Stockley's Drug Interactions

A source book of interactions, their mechanisms, clinical importance and management

Eighth edition

Edited by

Karen Baxter

BSc, MSc, MRPharmS

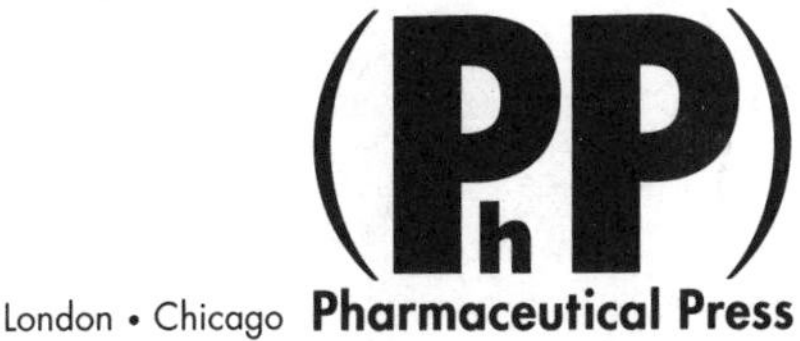

London • Chicago Pharmaceutical Press

Published by the Pharmaceutical Press
An imprint of RPS Publishing

1 Lambeth High Street, London SE1 7JN, UK
100 South Atkinson Road, Suite 200, Grayslake, IL 60030-7820, USA

First edition 1981
Second edition 1991
Third edition 1994
Fourth edition 1996
Fifth edition 1999
Sixth edition 2002
Seventh edition 2006
Eighth edition 2008

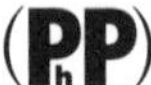 is a trade mark of RPS Publishing

RPS Publishing is the publishing organisation of the Royal Pharmaceutical Society of Great Britain

Printed in Great Britain by William Clowes Ltd, Beccles, Suffolk

ISBN 978 0 85369 754 1

A catalogue record for this book is available from the British Library

Stockley's Drug Interactions

Editor: Karen Baxter, BSc, MSc, MRPharmS

Editorial Staff: Mildred Davis, BA, BSc, PhD, MRPharmS
Samuel Driver, BSc
Chloë SAJ Hatwal, BSc, MRes
C Rhoda Lee, BPharm, PhD, MRPharmS
Alison Marshall, BPharm, DipClinPharm, PG CertClinEd, MRPharmS
Rosalind McLarney, BPharm, MSc, MRPharmS
Jennifer M Sharp, BPharm, DipClinPharm, MRPharmS
Elen R Shute, BA, MPhil

Digital Products Team: Julie McGlashan, BPharm, DipInfSc, MRPharmS
Elizabeth King, Dip BTEC PharmSci

Editorial Consultants: Ivan H Stockley, BPharm, PhD, FRPharmS, CBiol, MIBiol
Sean C Sweetman, BPharm, FRPharmS

Contents

Preface

The aim of *Stockley's Drug Interactions* is to inform busy doctors, pharmacists, surgeons, nurses and other healthcare professionals, of the facts about drug interactions, without their having to do the time-consuming literature searches and full assessment of the papers for themselves. These therefore are the practical questions which this book attempts to answer:

- Are the drugs and substances in question known to interact or is the interaction only theoretical and speculative?
- If they do interact, how serious is it?
- Has it been described many times or only once?
- Are all patients affected or only a few?
- Is it best to avoid these two substances altogether or can the interaction be accommodated in some way?
- And what alternative and safer drugs can be used instead?

To précis the mass of literature into a concise and easy-to-read form, the text has been organised into a series of individual monographs, all with a common format. If you need some insight into the general philosophy underlying the way all this information is handled in this publication, you should have a look at the section, 'Before using this book. . .'.

There have been several changes for the 8th edition. All of the existing monographs have, as with each edition, been reviewed, revalidated and updated, and many new ones have been added, making a total in excess of 3100 monographs. Many new monographs on herbal interactions have been added, although good quality human studies remain sparse. A new chapter has been added to cover the growing number of interactions about anorectics, and the chapter on sympathomimetics has been removed, with the information redistributed according to the therapeutic use of the drugs in question, to give a better indication of precisely which drugs from this disparate group are likely to interact. We have continued to add information provided by regulatory bodies outside of the UK, which further enhances the international flavour of the publication.

This edition has also seen the growth in our editorial team, with two practising clinical pharmacists recruited to help us ensure we maintain the practical nature of the information given. This has also allowed us to develop our product range, with the publication of the first *Stockley's Drug Interactions Pocket Companion*, which we have developed for delivery on PDA.

As always, the Editorial team have had assistance from many other people in developing this publication , and the Editor gratefully acknowledges the assistance and guidance that they have provided. The Martindale team continue to be a great source of advice and support, and particular thanks is due to the editor, Sean Sweetman. Thanks are also due to John Wilson and Tamsin Cousins, who handle the various aspects of producing our publications in print. We are also grateful for the support of both Paul Weller and Charles Fry. Ivan Stockley remains an important part of the publication, taking a keen interest in the development of new products, and as ever, we find his advice invaluable.

Stockley's Drug Interactions continues to be available on the Pharmaceutical Press platform, MedicinesComplete, as well as being available on other platforms, both in English and Spanish. With the further development of the integratable Alerts product and the new PDA, we remain indebted to Julie McGlashan, Michael Evans, Elizabeth King, and all those involved in the development of these products, for their advice and support. For more details about these digital products please visit:
www.pharmpress.com/Stockley

As ever, we have had feedback from pharmacists and doctors about the content of the publication, which is always valuable, especially in ensuring the publication meets the needs of the users. We are particularly grateful to those who have taken the time to answer our questions about specific aspects of practice. Anyone who wishes to contact the Stockley team can do so at the following address: stockley@rpsgb.org

London, September 2007

Abbreviations

ACE—angiotensin-converting enzyme
ADP—adenosine diphosphate
AIDS—acquired immunodeficiency syndrome
ALL—acute lymphoblastic leukaemia
ALT—alanine aminotransferase
am—*ante meridiem* (before noon)
AML—acute myeloid leukaemia
aPTT—activated partial thromboplastin time
AST—aspartate aminotransferase
AUC—area under the time–concentration curve
AUC_{0-12}—area under the time–concentration curve measured over 0 to 12 hours
AV—atrioventricular
BNF—British National Formulary
BP—blood pressure
BP—British Pharmacopoeia
BPC—British Pharmaceutical Codex
BPH—benign prostatic hyperplasia
bpm—beats per minute
BUN—blood urea nitrogen
CAPD—continuous ambulatory peritoneal dialysis
CDC—Centers for Disease Control (USA)
CNS—central nervous system
COPD—chronic obstructive pulmonary disease
CPR—cardiopulmonary resuscitation
CSF—cerebrospinal fluid
CSM—Committee on Safety of Medicines (UK) (now subsumed within the Commission on Human Medicines)
DNA—deoxyribonucleic acid
ECG—electrocardiogram
ECT—electroconvulsive therapy
ED_{50}—the dose at which 50% of subjects respond
EEG—electroencephalogram
e.g.—*exempli gratia* (for example)
EMEA—The European Agency for the Evaluation of Medicinal Products
FDA—Food and Drug Administration (USA)
FEF_{25-75}—maximum expiratory flow over the middle 50% of the vital capacity
FEV_1—forced expiratory volume in one second
FSH—follicle simulating hormone
ft—foot (feet)
FVC—forced vital capacity
GGT—gamma glutamyl transpeptidase
g—gram(s)
h—hour(s)
HAART—highly active antiretroviral therapy
HCV—hepatitis C virus
HIV—human immunodeficiency virus
HRT—hormone replacement therapy
ibid—*ibidem*, in the same place (journal or book)
i.e.—*id est* (that is)
INR—international normalised ratio
ITU—intensive therapy unit
IU—International Units
IUD—intra-uterine device
kg—kilogram(s)
l—litre
lbs—pound(s) avoirdupois
LDL—low-density lipoprotein
LFT—liver function test
LH—luteinising hormone
LMWH—low-molecular-weight heparin
MAC—minimum alveolar concentration
MAOI—monoamine oxidase inhibitor
MAOI-A—monoamine oxidase inhibitor, type A
MAOI-B—monoamine oxidase inhibitor, type B
MCA—Medicines Control Agency (UK) (now MHRA)
MHRA—Medicines and Healthcare products Regulatory Agency (UK)
MIC—minimum inhibitory concentration
mEq—milliequivalent(s)
mg—milligram(s)
mL—millilitre(s)
mmHg—millimetre(s) of mercury
mmol—millimole
mol—mole
MRSA—methicillin resistant *Staphylococcus aureus*
NICE—National Institue for Health and Clinical Excellence (UK) (formerly the National Institute for Clinical Excellence)
nM—nanomole
nmol—nanomole
NNRTI—non-nucleoside reverse transcriptase inhibitor
NRTI—nucleoside reverse transcriptase inhibitor
NSAID—non-steroidal anti-inflammatory drug
PABA—para-amino benzoic acid
PCP—pneumocystis pneumonia
pH—the negative logarithm of the hydrogen ion concentration
pm—*post meridiem* (after noon)
pO_2—plasma partial pressure (concentration) of oxygen
PPI—proton pump inhibitor
ppm—parts per million
PTT—partial thromboplastin time
PUD—peptic ulcer disease
RIMA—reversible inhibitor of monoamine oxidase type A
RNA—ribonucleic acid
sic—written exactly as it appears in the original
SNRI—serotonin and noradrenaline reuptake inhibitor
SSRI—selective serotonin reuptake inhibitor
STD—sexually transmitted disease
SVT—supraventricular tachycardia
TPN—total parenteral nutrition
TSH—thyroid-stimulating hormone
UK—United Kingdom
US and USA—United States of America
USP—The United States Pharmacopeia
UTI—urinary tract infection

Before using this book . . .

. . . you should read this short explanatory section so that you know how the drug interaction data have been set out here, and why – as well as the basic philosophy that has been followed in presenting it.

The monographs

This publication has over 3100 monographs with a common format, which are subdivided into sections like these:

- An abstract or summary for quick reading.
- **Clinical evidence**, detailing one, two or more illustrative examples of the interaction, followed by most or all of other supportive clinical evidence currently available.
- **Mechanism**, in brief.
- **Importance and management**, a short discussion designed to aid rapid clinical decision making. For example:
  - – Is the interaction established or not?
  - – What is its incidence?
  - – How important is it?
  - – How can it be managed?
  - – And what, if any, are the non-interacting alternatives?
- **References**, a list of all of the relevant references. The length of the references list gives a very fair indication of the extent of the documentation. A long list indicates a well documented interaction, whereas a short list indicates poor documentation.

Some of the monographs have been compressed into fewer subsections instead of the more usual five, simply where information is limited or where there is little need to be more expansive.

The monographs do not carry the drug interaction Hazard/Severity ratings as used in the electronic *Stockley Interactions Alerts* because of the difficulties of applying them to monographs that cover multiple pairs of drug–drug interactions, but what is written in each monograph should speak for itself.

Quality of information on interactions

The data on interactions are of widely varying quality and reliability. The best come from clinical studies carried out on large numbers of patients under scrupulously controlled conditions. The worst are anecdotal, uncontrolled, or based solely on *animal* studies. Sometimes they are no more than speculative and theoretical scaremongering guesswork, hallowed by repeated quotation until they become virtually set in stone.

The aim has been to filter out as much useless noise as possible, so wherever possible 'secondary' references are avoided, and 'primary' references which are available in good medical and scientific libraries are used instead – although sometimes unpublished, good quality, in-house reports on drug company files have been used where the drug company has kindly allowed access to the information. Product literature (the Summary of Product Characteristics in the UK and the Prescribing Information in the US) rather than the research reports that lie behind them are also cited because they are the only source of published information about new drugs.

The quality of drug company literature is very variable. Some of it is excellent, helpful and very reliable, but regrettably a growing proportion contains a welter of speculative and self-protective statements, probably driven more by the company's medico-legal policy than anything else, and the nervousness of drug regulatory authorities. It is almost unbelievable (but true all the same) that drug companies that are scrupulous in the way they do their research, come out with statements about possible interactions that are little more than guesswork.

When drawing your own conclusions

The human population is a total mixture, unlike selected batches of laboratory animals (same age, weight, sex, and strain etc.). For this reason human beings do not respond uniformly to one or more drugs. Our genetic make up, ethnic background, sex, renal and hepatic functions, diseases and nutritional states, ages and other factors (the route of administration, for example) all contribute towards the heterogeneity of our responses. This means that the outcome of giving one or more drugs to any individual for the first time is never totally predictable because it is a new and unique 'experiment'. Even so, some idea of the probable outcome of using a drug or a pair of drugs can be based on what has been seen in other patients: the more extensive the data, the firmer the predictions.

The most difficult decisions concern isolated cases of interaction, many of which only achieved prominence because they were serious. Do you ignore them as 'idiosyncratic' or do you, from that moment onwards, contraindicate the use of the two drugs totally?

There is no simple 'yes' or 'no' answer to these questions, but one simple rule-of-thumb is that isolated cases of interaction with old and very well-tried pairs of drugs are unlikely to be of general importance, whereas those with new drugs may possibly be the tip of an emerging iceberg and should therefore initially be taken much more seriously until more is known. The delicate balance between these two has then to be set against the actual severity of the reaction reported and weighed up against how essential it is to use the drug combination in question.

When deciding the possible first-time use of any two drugs in any particular patient, you need to put what is currently known about these drugs against the particular profile of your patient. Read the monograph. Consider the facts and conclusions, and then set the whole against the backdrop of your patients unique condition (age, disease, general condition, and so forth) so that what you eventually decide to do is well thought out and soundly based. We do not usually have the luxury of knowing absolutely all the facts, so that an initial conservative approach is often the safest.

I

General considerations and an outline survey of some basic interaction mechanisms

A. What is a drug interaction?

An interaction is said to occur when the effects of one drug are changed by the presence of another drug, herbal medicine, food, drink or by some environmental chemical agent. Much more colourful and informal definitions by patients are that it is "... when medicines fight each other...", or "... when medicines fizz together in the stomach ...", or "...what happens when one medicine falls out with another..."

The outcome can be harmful if the interaction causes an increase in the toxicity of the drug. For example, there is a considerable increase in risk of severe muscle damage if patients on statins start taking azole antifungals (see 'Statins + Azoles', p.1093). Patients taking monoamine oxidase inhibitor antidepressants (MAOIs) may experience an acute and potentially life-threatening hypertensive crisis if they eat tyramine-rich foods such as 'cheese', (p.1153).

A reduction in efficacy due to an interaction can sometimes be just as harmful as an increase: patients taking warfarin who are given rifampicin need more warfarin to maintain adequate and protective anticoagulation (see 'Coumarins + Antibacterials; Rifamycins', p.375), while patients taking 'tetracyclines', (p.347) or 'quinolones', (p.332) need to avoid antacids and milky foods (or separate their ingestion) because the effects of these antibacterials can be reduced or even abolished if admixture occurs in the gut.

These unwanted and unsought-for interactions are adverse and undesirable but there are other interactions that can be beneficial and valuable, such as the deliberate co-prescription of antihypertensive drugs and diuretics in order to achieve antihypertensive effects possibly not obtainable with either drug alone. The mechanisms of both types of interaction, whether adverse or beneficial, are often very similar, but the adverse interactions are the focus of this publication.

Definitions of a drug interaction are not rigidly adhered to in this publication because the subject inevitably overlaps into other areas of adverse reactions with drugs. So you will find in these pages some 'interactions' where one drug does not actually affect another at all, but the adverse outcome is the simple additive effects of two drugs with similar effects (for example the combined effects of two or more CNS depressants, or two drugs which affect the QT interval). Sometimes the term 'drug interaction' is used for the physico-chemical reactions that occur if drugs are mixed in intravenous fluids, causing precipitation or inactivation. The long-established and less ambiguous term is 'pharmaceutical incompatibilities'. Incompatibilities are not covered by this publication.

B. What is the incidence of drug interactions?

The more drugs a patient takes the greater the likelihood that an adverse reaction will occur. One hospital study found that the rate was 7% in those taking 6 to 10 drugs but 40% in those taking 16 to 20 drugs, which represents a disproportionate increase.[1] A possible explanation is that the drugs were interacting.

Some of the early studies on the frequency of interactions uncritically compared the drugs that had been prescribed with lists of possible drug interactions, without appreciating that many interactions may be clinically trivial or simply theoretical. As a result, an unrealistically high incidence was suggested. Most of the later studies have avoided this error by looking at only potentially clinically important interactions, and incidences of up to 8.8% have been reported.[2-4] Even so, not all of these studies took into account the distinction that must be made between the incidence of potential interactions and the incidence of those where clinical problems actually arise. The simple fact is that some patients experience quite serious reactions while taking interacting drugs, while others appear not to be affected at all.

A screening of 2 422 patients over a total of 25 005 days revealed that 113 (4.7%) were taking combinations of drugs that could interact, but evidence of interactions was observed in only seven patients, representing only 0.3%.[2] In another hospital study of 44 patients over a 5-day period taking 10 to 17 drugs, 77 potential drug interactions were identified, but only one probable and four possible adverse reactions (6.4%) were detected.[5] A further study among patients taking anticonvulsant drugs found that 6% of the cases of toxicity were due to drug interactions.[6] These figures are low compared with those of a hospital survey that monitored 927 patients who had received 1004 potentially interacting drug combinations. Changes in drug dosage were made in 44% of these cases.[7] A review of these and other studies found that the reported incidence rates ranged from 2.2 to 70.3%, and the percentage of patients actually experiencing problems was less than 11.1%. Another review found a 37% incidence of interactions among 639 elderly patients.[8] Yet another review of 236 geriatric patients found an 88% incidence of clinically significant interactions, and a 22% incidence of potentially serious and life-threatening interactions.[9] A 4.1% incidence of drug interactions on prescriptions presented to community pharmacists in the USA was found in a further survey,[10] whereas the incidence was only 2.9% in another American study,[11] and just 1.9% in a Swedish study.[12] An Australian study found that about 10% of hospital admissions were drug-related, of which 4.4% were due to drug interactions.[13] A very high incidence (47 to 50%) of potential drug interactions was found in a study carried out in an Emergency Department in the US.[14] One French study found that 16% of the prescriptions for a group of patients taking antihypertensive drugs were contraindicated or unsuitable,[15] whereas another study on a group of geriatrics found only a 1% incidence.[16] The incidence of problems would be expected to be higher in the elderly because ageing affects the functioning of the kidneys and liver.[17,18]

These discordant figures need to be put into the context of the under-reporting of adverse reactions of any kind by medical professionals, for reasons that may include pressure of work or the fear of litigation. Both doctors and patients may not recognise adverse reactions and interactions, and some patients simply stop taking their drugs without saying why. None of these studies give a clear answer to the question of how frequently drug interactions occur, but even if the incidence is as low as some of the studies suggest, it still represents a very considerable number of patients who appear to be at risk when one thinks of the large numbers of drugs prescribed and taken every day.

1. Smith JW, Seidl LG, Cluff LE. Studies on the epidemiology of adverse drug reactions. V. Clinical factors influencing susceptibility. *Ann Intern Med* (1969) 65, 629.
2. Puckett WH, Visconti JA. An epidemiological study of the clinical significance of drug-drug interaction in a private community hospital. *Am J Hosp Pharm* (1971) 28, 247.
3. Shinn AF, Shrewsbury RP, Anderson KW. Development of a computerized drug interaction database (Medicom) for use in a patient specific environment. *Drug Inf J* (1983) 17, 205.
4. Ishikura C, Ishizuka H. Evaluation of a computerized drug interaction checking system. *Int J Biomed Comput* (1983) 14, 311.
5. Schuster BG, Fleckenstein L, Wilson JP, Peck CC. Low incidence of adverse reactions due to drug-drug interaction in a potentially high risk population of medical inpatients. *Clin Res* (1982) 30, 258A.
6. Manon-Espaillat R, Burnstine TH, Remler B, Reed RC, Osorio I. Antiepileptic drug intoxication: factors and their significance. *Epilepsia* (1991) 32, 96–100.
7. Haumschild MJ, Ward ES, Bishop JM, Haumschild MS. Pharmacy-based computer system for monitoring and reporting drug interactions. *Am J Hosp Pharm* (1987) 44, 345.
8. Manchon ND, Bercoff E, Lamarchand P, Chassagne P, Senant J, Bourreille J. Fréquence et gravité des interaction médicamenteuses dans une population âgée: étude prospective concernant 639 malades. *Rev Med Interne* (1989) 10, 521–5.
9. Lipton HL, Bero LA, Bird JA, McPhee SJ. The impact of clinical pharmacists' consultations on physicians' geriatric drug prescribing. *Med Care* (1992) 30, 646–58.

10. Rupp MT, De Young M, Schondelmeyer SW. Prescribing problems and pharmacist interventions in community practice. *Med Care* (1992) 30, 926–40.
11. Rotman BL, Sullivan AN, McDonald T, DeSmedt P, Goodnature D, Higgins M, Suermond HJ, Young CY, Owens DK. A randomized evaluation of a computer-based physician's workstation; design considerations and baseline results. *Proc Annu Symp Comput Appl Med Care* (1995) 693–7.
12. Linnarsson R. Drug interactions in primary health care. A retrospective database study and its implications for the design of a computerized decision support system. *Scand J Prim Health Care* (1993) 11, 181–6.
13. Stanton LA, Peterson GM, Rumble RH, Cooper GM, Polack AE. Drug-related admissions to an Australian hospital. *J Clin Pharm Ther* (1994) 19, 341–7.
14. Goldberg RM, Mabee J, Chan L, Wong S. Drug-drug and drug-disease interactions in the ED; analysis of a high-risk population. *Am J Emerg Med* (1996) 14, 447–50.
15. Paille R, Pissochet P. L'ordonnance et les interactions medicamenteuses: etude prospective chez 896 patients traites pour hypertension arterielle en medicine generale. *Therapie* (1995) 50, 253–8.
16. Di Castri A, Jacquot JM, Hemmi P, Moati L, Rouy JM, Compan B, Nachar H, Bossy-Vassal A. Interactions medicamenteuses: etude de 409 ordannances etablies a l'issue d'une hospitalisation geriatrique. *Therapie* (1995) 50, 259–64.
17. Cadieux RJ. Drug interactions in the elderly. *Postgrad Med* (1989) 86, 179–86.
18. Tinawi M, Alguire P. The prevalence of drug interactions in hospitalized patients. *Clin Res* (1992) 40, 773A.

C. How seriously should interactions be regarded and handled?

It would be very easy to conclude after browsing through this publication that it is extremely risky to treat patients with more than one drug at a time, but this would be an over-reaction. The figures quoted in the previous section illustrate that many drugs known to interact in some patients, simply fail to do so in others. This partially explains why some quite important drug interactions remained virtually unnoticed for many years, a good example of this being the increase in serum digoxin levels seen with quinidine (see 'Digitalis glycosides + Quinidine', p.936).

Examples of this kind suggest that patients apparently tolerate adverse interactions remarkably well, and that many experienced physicians accommodate the effects (such as rises or falls in serum drug levels) without consciously recognising that what they are seeing is the result of an interaction.

One of the reasons it is often difficult to detect an interaction is that, as already mentioned, patient variability is considerable. We now know many of the predisposing and protective factors that determine whether or not an interaction occurs but in practice it is still very difficult to predict what will happen when an individual patient is given two potentially interacting drugs. An easy solution to this practical problem is to choose a non-interacting alternative, but if none is available, it is frequently possible to give interacting drugs together if appropriate precautions are taken. If the effects of the interaction are well-monitored they can often be allowed for, often simply by adjusting the dosages. Many interactions are dose-related so that if the dosage of the causative drug is reduced, the effects on the other drug will be reduced accordingly. Thus a non-prescription dosage of cimetidine may fail to inhibit the metabolism of phenytoin, whereas a larger dose may clearly increase phenytoin levels (see 'Phenytoin + H_2-receptor antagonists', p.559).

The dosage of the affected drug may also be critical. For example, isoniazid causes the levels of phenytoin to rise, particularly in those individuals who are slow acetylators of isoniazid, and levels may become toxic. If the serum phenytoin levels are monitored and its dosage reduced appropriately, the concentrations can be kept within the therapeutic range (see 'Phenytoin + Antimycobacterials', p.550). Some interactions can be accommodated by using another member of the same group of drugs. For example, the serum levels of doxycycline can become subtherapeutic if phenytoin, barbiturates or carbamazepine are given, but other 'tetracyclines' (p.346) do not seem to be affected. Erythromycin causes serum lovastatin levels to rise because it inhibits its metabolism, but does not affect pravastatin levels because these two statins are metabolised in different ways (see 'Statins', (p.1086)). It is therefore clearly important not to uncritically extrapolate the interactions seen with one drug to all members of the same group.

It is interesting to note in this context that a study in two hospitals in Maryland, USA, found that when interacting drugs were given with warfarin (but not theophylline) the length of hospital stay increased by a little over 3 days, with a rise in general costs because of the need to do more tests to get the balance right.[1] So it may be easier, quicker and cheaper to use a non-interacting alternative drug (always provided that its price is not markedly greater).

The variability in patient response has lead to some extreme responses among prescribers. Some clinicians have become over-anxious about interactions so that their patients are denied useful drugs that they might reasonably be given if appropriate precautions are taken. This attitude is exacerbated by some of the more alarmist lists and charts of interactions, which fail to make a distinction between interactions that are very well documented and well established, and those that have only been encountered in a single patient, and which in the final analysis are probably totally idiosyncratic. 'One swallow does not make a summer', nor does a serious reaction in a single patient mean that the drugs in question should never again be given to anyone else.

At the other extreme, there are some health professionals who, possibly because they have personally encountered few interactions, fail to consider drug interactions, so that some of their patients are potentially put at risk. An example of this is the fact that cisapride continued to be prescribed with known interacting drugs, even after the rare risk of fatal torsade de pointes arrhythmias, which can cause sudden death, was well established[2] (see 'Cisapride + Miscellaneous', p.963). The responsible position lies between these two extremes, because a very substantial number of interacting drugs can be given together safely, if the appropriate precautions are taken. There are relatively few pairs of drugs that should always be avoided.

Table 1.1 Some drug absorption interactions

Drug affected	*Interacting drugs*	*Effect of interaction*
Digoxin	Metoclopramide Propantheline	Reduced digoxin absorption Increased digoxin absorption (due to changes in gut motility)
Digoxin Levothyroxine Warfarin	Colestyramine	Reduced absorption due to binding/complexation with colestyramine
Ketoconazole	Antacids H_2-receptor antagonists Proton pump inhibitors	Reduced ketoconazole absorption due to reduced dissolution
Penicillamine	Antacids (containing Al^{3+} and/or Mg^{2+}), iron compounds, food	Formation of less soluble penicillamine chelates resulting in reduced absorption of penicillamine
Methotrexate	Neomycin	Neomycin-induced malabsorption state
Quinolones	Antacids (containing Al^{3+} and/or Mg^{2+}), milk, Zn^{2+}(?), Fe^{2+}	Formation of poorly absorbed complexes
Tetracyclines	Antacids (containing Al^{3+}, Ca^{2+}, Mg^{2+}, and/or Bi^{2+}), milk, Zn^{2+}, Fe^{2+}	Formation of poorly soluble chelates resulting in reduced antibacterial absorption (see Fig. 1.1, p.3)

1. Jankel CA, McMillan JA, Martin BC. Effect of drug interactions on outcomes of patient receiving warfarin or theophylline. *Am J Hosp Pharm* (1994) 51, 661–6.
2. Smalley W, Shatin D, Wysowski DK, Gurwitz J, Andrade SE, Goodman M, Chan KA, Platt R, Schech SD, Ray WA. Contraindicated use of cisapride: impact of food and drug administration regulatory action. *JAMA* (2000) 284, 3036–9.

D. Mechanisms of drug interaction

Some drugs interact together in totally unique ways, but as the many examples in this publication amply illustrate, there are certain mechanisms of interaction that are encountered time and time again. Some of these common mechanisms are discussed here in greater detail than space will allow in the individual monographs, so that only the briefest reference need be made there.

Mechanisms that are unusual or peculiar to particular pairs of drugs are detailed within the monographs. Very many drugs that interact do so, not by a single mechanism, but often by two or more mechanisms acting in concert, although for clarity most of the mechanisms are dealt with here as though they occur in isolation. For convenience, the mechanisms of interactions can be subdivided into those that involve the pharmacokinetics of a drug, and those that are pharmacodynamic.

1. Pharmacokinetic interactions

Pharmacokinetic interactions are those that can affect the processes by which drugs are absorbed, distributed, metabolised and excreted (the so-called ADME interactions).

1.1. Drug absorption interactions

Most drugs are given orally for absorption through the mucous membranes of the gastrointestinal tract, and the majority of interactions that go on within the gut result in reduced rather than increased absorption. A clear distinction must be made between those that decrease the *rate* of absorption and those that alter the *total amount* absorbed. For drugs that are given long-term, in multiple doses (e.g. the oral anticoagulants) the rate of absorption is usually unimportant, provided the total amount of drug absorbed is not markedly altered. On the other hand for drugs that are given as single doses, intended to be absorbed rapidly (e.g. hypnotics or analgesics), where a rapidly achieved high concentration is needed, a reduction in the rate of absorption may result in failure to achieve an adequate effect. 'Table 1.1', (p.2) lists some of the drug interactions that result from changes in absorption.

(a) Effects of changes in gastrointestinal pH

The passage of drugs through mucous membranes by simple passive diffusion depends upon the extent to which they exist in the non-ionised lipid-soluble form. Absorption is therefore governed by the pKa of the drug, its lipid-solubility, the pH of the contents of the gut and various other parameters relating to the pharmaceutical formulation of the drug. Thus the absorption of salicylic acid by the stomach is much greater at low pH than at high. On theoretical grounds it might be expected that alterations in gastric pH caused by drugs such as the H_2-receptor antagonists would have a marked effect on absorption, but in practice the outcome is often uncertain because a number of other mechanisms may also come into play, such as chelation, adsorption and changes in gut motility, which can considerably affect what actually happens. However, in some cases the effect can be significant. Rises in pH due to 'proton pump inhibitors', (p.218), 'H_2-receptor antagonists', (p.217) can markedly reduce the absorption of ketoconazole.

(b) Adsorption, chelation and other complexing mechanisms

Activated charcoal is intended to act as an adsorbing agent within the gut for the treatment of drug overdose or to remove other toxic materials, but inevitably it can affect the absorption of drugs given in therapeutic doses. Antacids can also adsorb a large number of drugs, but often other mechanisms of interaction are also involved. For example, the tetracycline antibacterials can chelate with a number of divalent and trivalent metallic ions, such as calcium, aluminium, bismuth and iron, to form complexes that are both poorly absorbed and have reduced antibacterial effects (see 'Figure 1.1', (below)).

These metallic ions are found in dairy products and antacids. Separating the dosages by 2 to 3 hours goes some way towards reducing the effects of this type of interaction. The marked reduction in the bioavailability of penicillamine caused by some antacids seems also to be due to chelation, although adsorption may have some part to play. Colestyramine, an anionic exchange resin intended to bind bile acids and cholesterol metabolites in the gut, binds to a considerable number of drugs (e.g. digoxin, warfarin, levothyroxine), thereby reducing their absorption. 'Table 1.1', (p.2) lists some drugs that chelate, complex or adsorb other drugs.

(c) Changes in gastrointestinal motility

Since most drugs are largely absorbed in the upper part of the small intestine, drugs that alter the rate at which the stomach empties can affect absorption. Propantheline, for example, delays gastric emptying and reduces 'paracetamol (acetaminophen)' absorption, (p.192), whereas 'metoclopramide', (p.191), has the opposite effect. However, the total amount of drug absorbed remains unaltered. Propantheline also increases the absorption of 'hydrochlorothiazide', (p.959). Drugs with antimuscarinic effects decrease the motility of the gut, thus the tricyclic antidepressants can increase the absorption of 'dicoumarol', (p.457), probably because they increase the time available for dissolution and absorption but in the case of 'levodopa', (p.690), they may reduce the absorption, possibly because the exposure time to intestinal mucosal metabolism is increased. The same reduced levodopa absorption has also been seen with 'homatropine', (p.682). These examples illustrate that what actually happens is sometimes very unpredictable because the final outcome may be the result of several different mechanisms.

(d) Induction or inhibition of drug transporter proteins

The oral bioavailability of some drugs is limited by the action of drug transporter proteins, which eject drugs that have diffused across the gut lining back into the gut. At present, the most well characterised drug transporter is 'P-glycoprotein', (p.8). Digoxin is a substrate of P-glycoprotein, and drugs that induce this protein, such as rifampicin, may reduce the bioavailability of 'digoxin', (p.938).

(e) Malabsorption caused by drugs

Neomycin causes a malabsorption syndrome, similar to that seen with non-tropical sprue. The effect is to impair the absorption of a number of drugs including 'digoxin', (p.906) and 'methotrexate', (p.642).

1.2. Drug distribution interactions

(a) Protein-binding interactions

Following absorption, drugs are rapidly distributed around the body by the circulation. Some drugs are totally dissolved in the plasma water, but many others are transported with some proportion of their molecules in solution and the rest bound to plasma proteins, particularly the albumins. The extent of this binding varies enormously but some drugs are extremely highly bound. For example, dicoumarol has only four out of every 1000 molecules remaining unbound at serum concentrations of 0.5 mg%. Drugs can also become bound to albumin in the interstitial fluid, and some, such as digoxin, can bind to the heart muscle tissue.

The binding of drugs to the plasma proteins is reversible, an equilibrium being established between those molecules that are bound and those that are not. Only the unbound molecules remain free and pharmacologically active, while those that are bound form a circulating but pharmacologically inactive reservoir which, in the case of drugs with a low-extraction ratio, is temporarily protected from metabolism and excretion. As the free molecules become metabolised, some of the bound molecules become unbound and pass into solution to exert their normal pharmacological actions, before they, in their turn are metabolised and excreted.

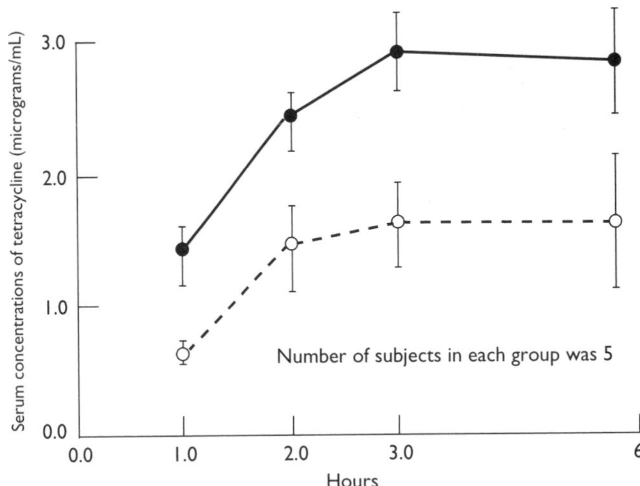

Fig. 1.1 A drug chelation interaction. Tetracycline forms a less-soluble chelate with iron if the two drugs are allowed to mix within the gut. This reduces the absorption and depresses the serum levels and the antibacterial effects (after Neuvonen PJ, *BMJ* (1970) 4, 532, with permission). The same interaction can occur with other ions such as Al^{3+}, Ca^{2+}, Mg^{2+}, Bi^{2+} and Zn^{2+}.

Depending on the concentrations and their relative affinities for the binding sites, one drug may successfully compete with another and displace it from the sites it is already occupying. The displaced (and now active) drug molecules pass into the plasma water where their concentration rises. So for example, a drug that reduces the binding from 99 to 95% would increase the unbound concentration of free and active drug from 1 to 5% (a fivefold increase). This displacement is only likely to raise the number of free and active molecules significantly if the majority of the drug is within the plasma rather than the tissues, so that only drugs with a low apparent volume of distribution (V_d) will be affected. Examples include the sulphonylureas, such as tolbutamide (96% bound, V_d 10 litres), oral anticoagulants, such as warfarin (99% bound, V_d 9 litres), and phenytoin (90% bound, V_d 35 litres). However, another important factor is clearance. Clinically important protein-binding interactions are unlikely if only a small proportion of the drug is eliminated during a single-passage through the eliminating organ (low-extraction ratio drugs), since any increase in free fraction will be effectively cleared. Most drugs that are extensively bound to plasma proteins and subject to displacement reactions (e.g. warfarin, sulphonylureas, phenytoin, methotrexate, and valproate) have low-extraction ratios, and drug exposure is therefore independent of protein-binding.

An example of displacement of this kind happens when patients stabilised on warfarin are given cloral hydrate because its major metabolite, trichloroacetic acid, is a highly bound compound that successfully displaces warfarin. This effect is only very short-lived because the now free and active warfarin molecules become exposed to metabolism as the blood flows through the liver, and the amount of drug rapidly falls. This transient increase in free warfarin levels is unlikely to change the anticoagulant effect of warfarin because the clotting factor complexes that are produced when warfarin is taken have a very long half-life, and thus take a long time to reach a new steady state. Normally no change in the warfarin dosage is needed (see 'Coumarins + Cloral and derivatives', p.396).

In vitro many commonly used drugs are capable of being displaced by others but in the body the effects seem almost always to be buffered so effectively that the outcome is not normally clinically important. It would therefore seem that the importance of this interaction mechanism has been grossly over-emphasised,[1-3] It is difficult to find an example of a clinically important interaction due to this mechanism alone. It has been suggested that this interaction mechanism is likely to be important only for drugs given intravenously that have a high-extraction ratio, a short pharmacokinetic-pharmacodynamic half-life and a narrow therapeutic index. Lidocaine has been given as an example of a drug fitting these criteria.[3] Some drug interactions that were originally assumed to be due to changes in protein binding have subsequently been shown to have other interaction mechanisms involved. For example, inhibition of metabolism has subsequently been shown to be important in the interactions between 'warfarin and phenylbutazone', (p.434), and 'tolbutamide and sulphonamide', (p.506).

However, knowledge of altered protein binding is important in therapeutic drug monitoring. Suppose for example a patient taking phenytoin was given a drug that displaced phenytoin from its binding sites. The amount of free phenytoin would rise but this would be quickly eliminated by metabolism and excretion thereby keeping the amount of free active phenytoin the same. However, the total amount of phenytoin would now be reduced. Therefore if phenytoin was monitored using an assay looking at total phenytoin levels it may appear that the phenytoin is subtherapeutic and that the dose may therefore need increasing. However, as the amount of free active phenytoin is unchanged this would not be necessary and may even be dangerous.

Basic drugs as well as acidic drugs can be highly protein bound, but clinically important displacement interactions do not seem to have been described. The reasons seem to be that the binding sites within the plasma are different from those occupied by acidic drugs (alpha-1-acid glycoprotein rather than albumin) and, in addition, basic drugs have a large V_d with only a small proportion of the total amount of drug being within the plasma.

(b) Induction or inhibition of drug transport proteins

It is increasingly being recognised that distribution of drugs into the brain, and some other organs such as the testes, is limited by the action of drug transporter proteins such as P-glycoprotein. These proteins actively transport drugs out of cells when they have passively diffused in. Drugs that are inhibitors of these transporters could therefore increase the uptake of drug substrates into the brain, which could either increase adverse CNS effects, or be beneficial. For more information see 'Drug transporter proteins', (p.8).

1. MacKichan JJ. Protein binding drug displacement interactions. Fact or fiction? *Clin Pharmacokinet* (1989) 16, 65–73.
2. Sansom LN, Evans AM. What is the true clinical significance of plasma protein binding displacement interactions? *Drug Safety* (1995) 12, 227–33.
3. Benet LZ, Hoener B-A. Changes in plasma protein binding have little clinical relevance. *Clin Pharmacol Ther* (2002) 71, 115–121.

Table 1.2 Drugs affecting or metabolised by the cytochrome P450 isoenzyme CYP1A2

Inhibitors	Cimetidine *Fluoroquinolones* Ciprofloxacin Enoxacin Grepafloxacin Fluvoxamine	Ipriflavone Mexiletine Rofecoxib Tacrine Ticlopidine Zileuton
Inducers	Barbiturates Phenytoin	Tobacco smoke
Substrates	Caffeine Clozapine Duloxetine Flecainide Olanzapine Rasagiline Ropinirole Tacrine Theophylline*	Tizanidine* *Tricyclic antidepressants* Amitriptyline Clomipramine Imipramine *Triptans* Frovatriptan Zolmitriptan R-Warfarin

*Considered the preferred *in vivo* substrates, see Bjornsson TD, Callaghan JT, Einolf HJ, *et al.* The conduct of *in vitro* and *in vivo* drug–drug interaction studies: a PhRMA perspective. *J Clin Pharmacol* (2003) 43, 443–69.

1.3. Drug metabolism (biotransformation) interactions

Although a few drugs are cleared from the body simply by being excreted unchanged in the urine, most are chemically altered within the body to less lipid-soluble compounds, which are more easily excreted by the kidneys. If this were not so, many drugs would persist in the body and continue to exert their effects for a long time. This chemical change is called 'metabolism', 'biotransformation', 'biochemical degradation' or sometimes 'detoxification'. Some drug metabolism goes on in the serum, the kidneys, the skin and the intestines, but the greatest proportion is carried out by enzymes that are found in the membranes of the endoplasmic reticulum of the liver cells. If liver is homogenised and then centrifuged, the reticulum breaks up into small sacs called microsomes which carry the enzymes, and it is for this reason that the metabolising enzymes of the liver are frequently referred to as the 'liver microsomal enzymes'.

We metabolise drugs by two major types of reaction. The first, so-called phase I reactions (involving oxidation, reduction or hydrolysis), turn drugs into more polar compounds, while phase II reactions involve coupling drugs with some other substance (e.g. glucuronic acid, known as glucuronidation) to make usually inactive compounds.

The majority of phase I oxidation reactions are carried out by the haem-containing enzyme cytochrome P450. Cytochrome P450 is not a single entity, but is in fact a very large family of related isoenzymes, about 30 of which have been found in human liver tissue. However, in practice, only a few specific subfamilies seem to be responsible for most (about 90%) of the metabolism of the commonly used drugs. The most important isoenzymes are: CYP1A2, CYP2C9, CYP2C19, CYP2D6, CYP2E1 and CYP3A4. Other enzymes involved in phase I metabolism include monoamine oxidases and epoxide hydrolases.

Less is known about the enzymes responsible for phase II conjugation reactions. However, UDP-glucuronyltransferases (UGT), methyltransferases, and N-acetyltransferases (NAT) are examples.

Although metabolism is very important in the body removing drugs, it is increasingly recognised that drugs can be adsorbed, distributed, or eliminated by transporters, the most well understood at present being 'P-glycoprotein', (p.8).

(a) Changes in first-pass metabolism

(i) Changes in blood flow through the liver

After absorption in the intestine, the portal circulation takes drugs directly to the liver before they are distributed by the blood flow around the rest of the body. A number of highly lipid-soluble drugs undergo substantial biotransformation during this first-pass through the gut wall and liver and there is some evidence that some drugs can have a marked effect on the extent of first pass metabolism by altering the blood flow through the liver. However, there are few clinically relevant examples of this, and many can be explained by other mechanisms, usually altered hepatic metabolism (see (ii) below). One possible example is the increase in rate of absorption of dofetilide with 'verapamil', (p.256), which has resulted in an increased incidence of torsade de pointes.

Another is the increase in bioavailability of high-extraction beta blockers with 'hydralazine', (p.847), possibly caused by altered hepatic blood flow, or altered metabolism.

(ii) Inhibition or induction of first-pass metabolism

The gut wall contains metabolising enzymes, principally the cytochrome P450 isoenzymes. In addition to the altered metabolism caused by changes in hepatic blood flow (see (i) above) there is evidence that some drugs can have a marked effect on the extent of first-pass metabolism by inhibiting or inducing the cytochrome P450 isoenzymes in the gut wall or in the liver. An example is the effect of grapefruit juice, which seems to inhibit the cytochrome P450 isoenzyme CYP3A4, mainly in the gut, and therefore reduces the metabolism of oral calcium-channel blockers. Although altering the amount of drug 'absorbed', these interactions are usually considered drug metabolism interactions. The effect of grapefruit on the metabolism of other drugs is discussed further under 'Drug-food interactions', (p.11).

(b) Enzyme induction

When barbiturates were widely used as hypnotics it was found necessary to keep increasing the dosage as time went by to achieve the same hypnotic effect, the reason being that the barbiturates increase the activity of the microsomal enzymes so that extent of metabolism and excretion increases. This phenomenon of enzyme stimulation or 'induction' not only accounts for the need for an increased barbiturate dose but if another drug that is metabolised by the same range of enzymes is also present, its enzymatic metabolism is similarly increased and larger doses are needed to maintain the same therapeutic effect. However, note that not all enzyme-inducing drugs induce their own metabolism (a process known as auto-induction). The metabolic pathway that is most commonly induced is phase I oxidation mediated by the cytochrome P450 isoenzymes. The main drugs responsible for induction of the most clinically important cytochrome P450 isoenzymes are listed in 'Table 1.2', (p.4), 'Table 1.3', (p.6), 'Table 1.4', (p.6). 'Figure 1.2', (see below) shows the reduction in trough ciclosporin levels when it is given with the enzyme inducer, St John's wort. 'St John's wort', (p.1037), induces the metabolism of ciclosporin by induction of CYP3A4 and possibly also P-glycoprotein. 'Figure 1.3', (see above) shows the effects of another enzyme inducer, rifampicin (rifampin) on the serum levels of 'ciclosporin', (p.1022), presumably via its effects on CYP3A4. Phase II glucuronidation can also be induced. An example is when rifampicin induces the glucuronidation of 'zidovudine', (p.792).

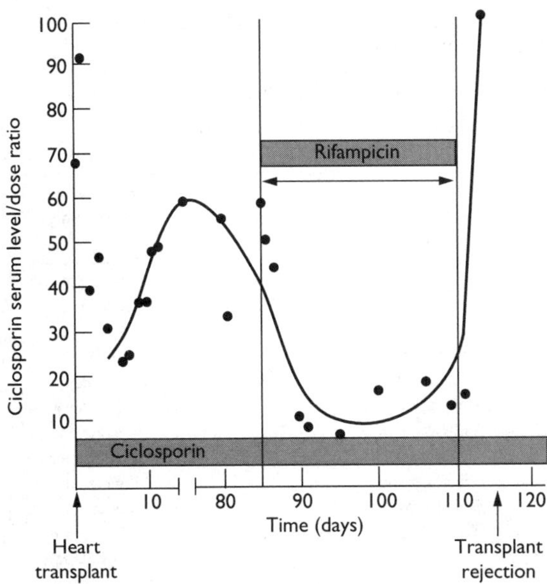

Fig. 1.3 An enzyme induction interaction. Rifampicin (600 mg daily plus isoniazid) increased the metabolism of ciclosporin in this patient, thereby reducing the trough serum levels. He subsequently died because his heart transplant was rejected (after *Transplant Proc*, 16, Van Buren D, Wideman CA, Ried M, Gibbons S, Van Buren CT, Jarowenko M, Flechner SM, Frazier OH, Cooley DA, Kahan BD. The antagonistic effect of rifampicin upon cyclosporine bioavailability. 1642–5, Copyright Elsevier (1984)).

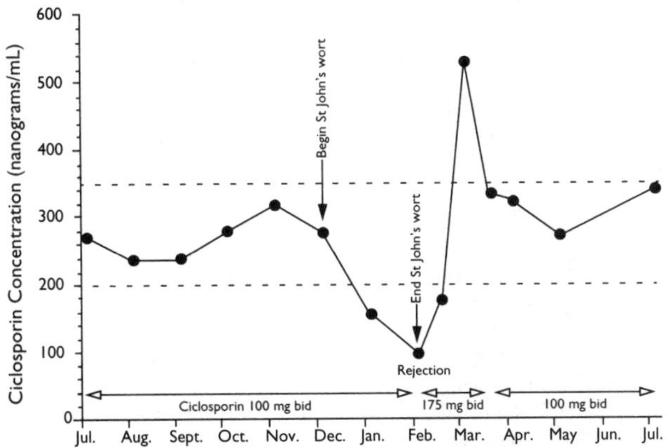

Fig. 1.2 An enzyme induction interaction. Chronology of ciclosporin trough concentrations (—●—) in a patient self-medicating with St John's wort. ---------- = desired ciclosporin therapeutic range (after Barone GW, Gurley BJ, Ketel BL, Lightfoot ML, Abul-Ezz SR. Drug interaction between St. John's Wort and Cyclosporine. *Ann Pharmacother* (2000) 34: 1013–16, with permission).

The extent of the enzyme induction depends on the drug and its dosage, but it may take days or even 2 to 3 weeks to develop fully, and may persist for a similar length of time when the enzyme inducer is stopped. This means that enzyme induction interactions are delayed in onset and slow to resolve. Enzyme induction is a common mechanism of interaction and is not confined to drugs; it is also caused by the chlorinated hydrocarbon insecticides such as dicophane and lindane, and smoking tobacco.

If one drug reduces the effects of another by enzyme induction, it may be possible to accommodate the interaction simply by raising the dosage of the drug affected, but this requires good monitoring, and there are obvious hazards if the inducing drug is eventually stopped without remembering to reduce the dosage again. The raised drug dosage may be an overdose when the drug metabolism has returned to normal.

(c) Enzyme inhibition

More common than enzyme induction is the inhibition of enzymes. This results in the reduced metabolism of an affected drug, so that it may begin to accumulate within the body, the effect usually being essentially the same as when the dosage is increased. Unlike enzyme induction, which may take several days or even weeks to develop fully, enzyme inhibition can occur within 2 to 3 days, resulting in the rapid development of toxicity. The metabolic pathway that is most commonly inhibited is phase I oxidation by the cytochrome P450 isoenzymes. The main drugs responsible for inhibition of the most clinically important cytochrome P450 isoenzymes are listed in 'Table 1.2', (p.4), 'Table 1.3', (p.6), 'Table 1.4', (p.6). For example a marked increase occurred in the plasma levels of a single dose of sildenafil after ritonavir had also been taken for 7 days, probably because ritonavir inhibits the metabolism of sildenafil by CYP3A4 (see 'Phosphodiesterase type-5 inhibitors + Protease inhibitors', p.1273).

An example of inhibition of phase I hydrolytic metabolism, is the inhibition of epoxide hydrolase by valpromide, which increases the levels of 'carbamazepine', (p.537). Phase II conjugative metabolism can also be inhibited. Examples are the inhibition of carbamazepine glucuronidation by

Table 1.3 Drugs affecting or metabolised by the CYP2 family of cytochrome P450 isoenzymes

Isoenzyme	*Inhibitors*	*Inducers*	*Substrates*
CYP2B6	Thiotepa	Phenobarbital Phenytoin	Cyclophosphamide Ifosfamide
CYP2C8	Gemfibrozil Rifampicin Trimethoprim		Pioglitazone Repaglinide Rosiglitazone
CYP2C9	Amiodarone *Azoles* Fluconazole Miconazole Voriconazole Fluvastatin *SSRIs* Fluoxetine Fluvoxamine Sulfinpyrazone Ticlopidine Zafirlukast	Aprepitant Rifampicin	Irbesartan Losartan Nateglinide *NSAIDs* Celecoxib Diclofenac Etoricoxib Valdecoxib Phenytoin *Statins* Fluvastatin Rosuvastatin *Sulphonylureas* Glibenclamide Gliclazide Glimepiride Glipizide Tolbutamide* S-Warfarin*
CYP2C19	Fluvoxamine Isoniazid *Proton pump inhibitors* Esomeprazole Omeprazole Ticlopidine Valdecoxib		Cilostazol Diazepam Escitalopram Moclobemide Omeprazole Phenytoin Proguanil
CYP2D6	Amiodarone Bupropion Cimetidine Dextropropoxyphene Diphenhydramine Duloxetine Propafenone Quinidine Ritonavir *SSRIs* Fluoxetine Paroxetine Sertraline Terbinafine Valdecoxib	Rifampicin	*Anticholinesterases, centrally-acting* Donepezil Galantamine *Antipsychotics* Clozapine Risperidone Thioridazine *Beta blockers* Carvedilol Metoprolol Propranolol Cyclobenzaprine Flecainide Mexiletine *Opioids* Codeine Dextromethorphan* Dihydrocodeine Hydrocodone Oxycodone Propafenone Tamoxifen Tolterodine *Tricyclics* Desipramine Imipramine Nortriptyline Trimipramine Venlafaxine
CYP2E1	Disulfiram	Alcohol Isoniazid	Chlorzoxazone* Paracetamol

*Considered the preferred *in vivo* substrates, see Bjornsson TD, Callaghan JT, Einolf HJ, *et al*. The conduct of *in vitro* and *in vivo* drug–drug interaction studies: a PhRMA perspective. *J Clin Pharmacol* (2003) 43, 443–69.

Table 1.4 Drugs affecting or metabolised by the cytochrome P450 isoenzyme CYP3A4

Inhibitors	Aprepitant *Azoles* Itraconazole Ketoconazole Voriconazole Cimetidine Delavirdine Diltiazem Grapefruit juice Imatinib	*Macrolides* Clarithromycin Erythromycin Troleandomycin Nefazodone Nicardipine Protease inhibitors *SSRIs* Fluoxetine Verapamil
Inducers	Aprepitant Bosentan Carbamazepine Dexamethasone Efavirenz Nevirapine	Phenobarbital (and probably other barbiturates) Phenytoin Rifabutin Rifampicin St John's wort (*Hypericum perforatum*)
Substrates	Amiodarone *Anticholinesterases, centrally-acting* Donepezil Galantamine *Antihistamines* Astemizole Terfenadine *Antineoplastics* Busulfan Cyclophosphamide Ifosfamide Irinotecan Taxanes Teniposide Vinblastine Vincristine Aprepitant *Azoles* Itraconazole Voriconazole *Benzodiazepines* Alprazolam Triazolam Midazolam* Bosentan Bromocriptine Buspirone* Cabergoline *Calcium-channel blockers* Diltiazem Felodipine* Lercanidipine Carbamazepine Ciclosporin Cilostazol Cisapride *Corticosteroids* Budesonide Dexamethasone Fluticasone Hydrocortisone Methylprednisolone Delavirdine Disopyramide Dutasteride Eletriptan Eplerenone Ergot derivatives	Imatinib Lidocaine, oral Maraviroc *Oestrogens* Combined hormonal contraceptives *Opioids* Alfentanil Buprenorphine Fentanyl Methadone Pimozide *Progestogens* Hormonal contraceptives Propafenone *Protease inhibitors* Amprenavir Atazanavir Darunavir Fosamprenavir Indinavir Nelfinavir Ritonavir Saquinavir Tipranavir Quetiapine Quinidine Reboxetine Rifabutin Sibutramine Sildenafil Sirolimus Solifenacin *Statins* Atorvastatin Lovastatin Simvastatin* Tacrolimus Tadalafil Tamoxifen Tolterodine Toremifene *Tricyclics* Amitriptyline Imipramine Vardenafil Zolpidem Zopiclone

*Considered the preferred *in vivo* substrates, see Bjornsson TD, Callaghan JT, Einolf HJ, *et al*. The conduct of *in vitro* and *in vivo* drug–drug interaction studies: a PhRMA perspective. *J Clin Pharmacol* (2003) 43, 443–69.

'sodium valproate', (p.537), and the inhibition of methyltransferase by aminosalicylates causing raised levels of 'azathioprine', (p.665).

The clinical significance of many enzyme inhibition interactions depends on the extent to which the serum levels of the drug rise. If the serum levels remain within the therapeutic range the interaction may not be clinically important.

(d) Genetic factors in drug metabolism

An increased understanding of genetics has shown that some of the cytochrome P450 isoenzymes are subject to 'genetic polymorphism', which simply means that some of the population have a variant of the isoenzyme with different (usually poor) activity. The best known example is CYP2D6, for which a small proportion of the population have the variant with low activity and are described as being poor or slow metabolisers (about 5 to 10% in white Caucasians, 0 to 2% in Asians and black people). Which group any particular individual falls into is genetically determined. The majority who possess the isoenzyme are called 'fast or extensive metabolisers'. It is possible to find out which group any particular individual falls into by looking at the way a single dose of a test or 'probe' drug is metabolised. This varying ability to metabolise certain drugs may explain why some patients develop toxicity when given an interacting drug while others remain symptom free. CYP2D6, CYP2C9 and CYP2C19 also show polymorphism, whereas CYP3A4 does not, although there is still some broad variation in the population without there being distinct groups. The effects of CYP2C19 polymorphism are discussed in more detail in 'Gastrointestinal drugs', (p.960). At present, genotyping of cytochrome P450 isoenzymes is primarily a research tool and is not used clinically. In the future, it may become standard clinical practice and may be used to individualise drug therapy.[1]

(e) Cytochrome P450 isoenzymes and predicting drug interactions

It is interesting to know which particular isoenzyme is responsible for the metabolism of drugs because by doing *in vitro* tests with human liver enzymes it is often possible to explain why and how some drugs interact. For example, ciclosporin is metabolised by CYP3A4, and we know that rifampicin (rifampin) is a potent inducer of this isoenzyme, whereas ketoconazole inhibits its activity, so that it comes as no surprise that rifampicin reduces the effects of ciclosporin and ketoconazole increases it.

What is very much more important than retrospectively finding out why two drugs interact, is the knowledge such *in vitro* tests can provide about forecasting which other drugs may possibly also interact. This may reduce the numbers of expensive clinical studies in subjects and patients and avoids waiting until significant drug interactions are observed in clinical use. A lot of effort is being put into this area of drug development.[2-6] However, at present such prediction is, like weather forecasting, still a somewhat hit-and-miss business because we do not know all of the factors that may modify or interfere with metabolism. It is far too simplistic to think that we have all the answers just because we know which liver isoenzymes are concerned with the metabolism of a particular drug, but it is a very good start.

'Table 1.2', (p.4), 'Table 1.3', (p.6), 'Table 1.4', (p.6) are lists of drugs that are inhibitors, inducers, or substrates of the clinically important cytochrome P450 isoenzymes, and each drug has a cross reference to a monograph describing a drug interaction thought to occur via that mechanism. If a new drug is shown to be an inducer, or an inhibitor, and/or a substrate of a given isoenzyme, these tables could be used to predict likely drug interactions. However, what may happen *in vitro* may not necessarily work in clinical practice because all of the many variables which can come into play are not known (such as how much of the enzyme is available, the concentration of the drug at the site of metabolism, and the affinity of the drug for the enzyme). Remember too that some drugs can be metabolised by more than one cytochrome P450 isoenzyme (meaning that this other isoenzyme may be able to 'pick up' more metabolism to compensate for the inhibited pathway); some drugs (and their metabolites) can both induce a particular isoenzyme and be metabolised by it; and some drugs (or their metabolites) can inhibit a particular isoenzyme but not be metabolised by it. With so many factors possibly impinging on the outcome of giving two or more drugs together, it is very easy to lose sight of one of the factors (or not even know about it) so that the sum of 2 plus 2 may not turn out to be the 4 that you have predicted.

For example, ritonavir and other protease inhibitors are well known potent inhibitors of CYP3A4, and in clinical use increase the levels of many drugs that are substrates of this isoenzyme. Methadone is a substrate of CYP3A4, and some *in vitro* data show that ritonavir (predictably) increased methadone levels. However, unexpectedly, in clinical use the protease inhibitors seem to decrease methadone levels, by a yet unknown mechanism (see, 'Opioids; Methadone + Protease inhibitors', p.182).

Another factor complicating the understanding of metabolic drug interactions is the finding that there is a large overlap between the inhibitors/inducers and substrates of P-glycoprotein (a 'drug transporter protein', (p.8)) and those of CYP3A4. Therefore, both mechanisms may be involved in many of the drug interactions previously thought to be due to effects on CYP3A4.

1. Phillips KA, Veenstra DL, Oren E, Lee JK, Sadee W. Potential role of pharmacogenomics in reducing adverse drug reactions: a systematic review. *JAMA* (2001) 286, 2270–79.
2. Bjornsson TD, Callaghan JT, Einolf HJ, Fischer V, Gan L, Grimm S, Kao J, King SP, Miwa G, Ni L, Kumar G, McLeod J, Obach RS, Roberts S, Roe A, Shah A, Snikeris F, Sullivan JT, Tweedie D, Vega JM, Walsh J, Wrighton SA. The conduct of in vitro and in vivo drug-drug interaction studies: a PhRMA perspective. *J Clin Pharmacol* (2003) 43, 443–69.
3. Bachmann KA, Ghosh R. The use of *in vitro* methods to predict *in vivo* pharmacokinetics and drug interactions. *Curr Drug Metab* (2001) 2, 299–314.
4. Yao C, Levy RH. Inhibition-based metabolic drug–drug interactions: predictions from *in vitro* data. *J Pharm Sci* (2002) 91, 1923–35.
5. Worboys PD, Carlile DJ. Implications and consequences of enzyme induction on preclinical and clinical drug development. *Xenobiotica* (2001) 31, 539–56.
6. Venkatakrishnan K, von Moltke LL, Obach RS, Greenblatt DJ. Drug metabolism and drug interactions: application and clinical value of *in vitro* models. *Curr Drug Metab* (2003) 4, 423–59.

1.4. Drug excretion interactions

With the exception of the inhalation anaesthetics, most drugs are excreted either in the bile or in the urine. Blood entering the kidneys along the renal arteries is, first of all, delivered to the glomeruli of the tubules where molecules small enough to pass through the pores of the glomerular membrane (e.g. water, salts, some drugs) are filtered through into the lumen of the tubules. Larger molecules, such as plasma proteins, and blood cells are retained within the blood. The blood flow then passes to the remaining parts of the kidney tubules where active energy-using transport systems are able to remove drugs and their metabolites from the blood and secrete them into the tubular filtrate. The renal tubular cells additionally possess active and passive transport systems for the reabsorption of drugs. Interference by drugs with renal tubular fluid pH, with active transport systems and with blood flow to the kidney can alter the excretion of other drugs.

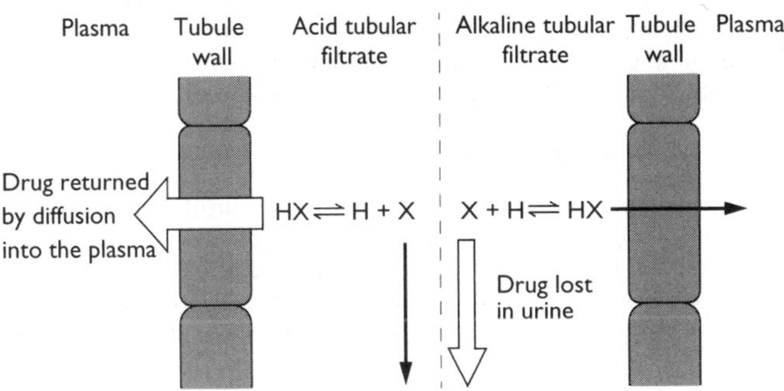

Fig. 1.4 An excretion interaction. If the tubular filtrate is acidified, most of the molecules of weakly acid drugs (HX) exist in an un-ionised lipid-soluble form and are able to return through the lipid membranes of the tubule cells by simple diffusion. Thus they are retained. In alkaline urine most of the drug molecules exist in an ionised non-lipid soluble form (X). In this form the molecules are unable to diffuse freely through these membranes and are therefore lost in the urine.

(a) Changes in urinary pH

As with drug absorption in the gut, passive reabsorption of drugs depends upon the extent to which the drug exists in the non-ionised lipid-soluble form, which in its turn depends on its pKa and the pH of the urine. Only the non-ionised form is lipid-soluble and able to diffuse back through the lipid membranes of the tubule cells. Thus at high pH values (alkaline), weakly acid drugs (pKa 3 to 7.5) largely exist as ionised lipid-insoluble molecules, which are unable to diffuse into the tubule cells and will therefore remain in the urine and be removed from the body. The converse will be true for weak bases with pKa values of 7.5 to 10.5. Thus pH changes that increase the amount in the ionised form (alkaline urine for acidic drugs, acid urine for basic drugs) increase the loss of the drug, whereas moving the pH in the opposite direction will increase their retention. 'Figure 1.4', (p.7) illustrates the situation with a weakly acidic drug. The clinical significance of this interaction mechanism is small, because although a very large number of drugs are either weak acids or bases, almost all are largely metabolised by the liver to inactive compounds and few are excreted in the urine unchanged. In practice therefore only a handful of drugs seem to be affected by changes in urinary pH (possible exceptions include changes in the excretion of 'quinidine', (p.277) or 'analgesic-dose aspirin', (p.135), due to alterations in urinary pH caused by antacids, and the increase in the clearance of 'methotrexate', (p.654), with urinary alkalinisers). In cases of overdose, deliberate manipulation of urinary pH has been used to increase the removal of drugs such as methotrexate and salicylates.

Table 1.5 Examples of interactions probably due to changes in renal transport

Drug affected	*Interacting drug*	*Result of interaction*
Cephalosporins Dapsone Methotrexate Penicillins Quinolones	Probenecid	Serum levels of drug affected raised; possibility of toxicity with some drugs
Methotrexate	Salicylates and some other NSAIDs	Methotrexate serum levels raised; serious methotrexate toxicity possible

(b) Changes in active renal tubular excretion

Drugs that use the same active transport systems in the renal tubules can compete with one another for excretion. For example, probenecid reduces the excretion of penicillin and other drugs. With the increasing understanding of drug transporter proteins in the kidneys, it is now known that probenecid inhibits the renal secretion of many other anionic drugs by organic anion transporters (OATs).[1] Probenecid possibly also inhibits some of the ABC transporters in the kidneys. The ABC transporter, P-glycoprotein, is also present in the kidneys, and drugs that alter this may alter renal drug elimination. See, 'Drug transporter proteins', (p.8), for further discussion. Some examples of drugs that possibly interact by alterations in renal transport are given in 'Table 1.5', (see above).

(c) Changes in renal blood flow

The flow of blood through the kidney is partially controlled by the production of renal vasodilatory prostaglandins. If the synthesis of these prostaglandins is inhibited the renal excretion of some drugs may be reduced. An interaction where this is the suggested mechanism is the rise in serum lithium seen with some NSAIDs, see 'Lithium + NSAIDs', p.1125.

(d) Biliary excretion and the entero-hepatic shunt

(i) Enterohepatic recirculation

A number of drugs are excreted in the bile, either unchanged or conjugated (e.g. as the glucuronide) to make them more water soluble. Some of the conjugates are metabolised to the parent compound by the gut flora and are then reabsorbed. This recycling process prolongs the stay of the drug within the body, but if the gut flora are diminished by the presence of an antibacterial, the drug is not recycled and is lost more quickly. This may possibly explain the rare failure of the oral contraceptives that can be brought about by the concurrent use of penicillins or tetracyclines, but see Mechanism in 'Hormonal contraceptives + Antibacterials; Penicillins', p.981. Antimicrobial-induced reductions in gut bacteria may reduce the activation of 'sulfasalazine', (p.973).

(ii) Drug transporters

Increasing research shows that numerous drug transporter proteins (both from the ABC family and SLC family, see 'Drug transporter proteins', (see below)) are involved in the hepatic extraction and secretion of drugs into the bile.[2] The relevance of many of these to drug interactions is still unclear, but the bile salt export pump (ABCB11) is known to be inhibited by a variety of drugs including ciclosporin, glibenclamide, and bosentan. Inhibition of this pump may increase the risk of cholestasis, and the manufacturer of bosentan says that they should be avoided in patients taking bosentan (see 'glibenclamide', (p.515) and 'ciclosporin', (p.1026)).

1. Lee W, Kim RB. Transporters and renal drug elimination. *Annu Rev Pharmacol Toxicol* (2004) 44, 137–66.
2. Faber KN, Müller M, Jansen PLM. Drug transport proteins in the liver. *Adv Drug Deliv Rev* (2003) 55, 107–24.

1.5. Drug transporter proteins

Drugs and endogenous substances are known to cross biological membranes, not just by passive diffusion, but by carrier-mediated processes, often known as transporters. Significant advances in the identification of various transporters have been made, although the contribution of many of these to drug interactions in particular, is still unclear.[1,2] The most well known is P-glycoprotein, which is a product of the MDR1 gene (ABCB1 gene) and a member of the ATP-binding cassette (ABC) family of efflux transporters.[1] Its involvement in drug interactions is discussed in (a) below.

Another ABC transporter is sister P-glycoprotein, otherwise called the bile salt export pump (BSEP or ABCB11).[1] It has been suggested that inhibition of this pump may increase the risk of cholestasis, see Drug transporters under 'Drug excretion interactions', (p.7).

Other transporters that are involved in some drug interactions are the organic anion transporters (OATs), organic anion-transporting polypeptides (OATPs) and organic cation transporters (OCTs), which are members of the solute carrier superfamily (SLC) of transporters.[1] The best known example of an OAT inhibitor is probenecid, which affects the renal excretion of a number of drugs, see Changes in active kidney tubule excretion under 'Drug excretion interactions', (p.7).

Table 1.6 Some possible inhibitors and inducers of P-glycoprotein shown to alter the levels of P-glycoprotein substrates in clinical studies[1]

Inhibitors		*Inducers*
Atorvastatin	Ketoconazole	Rifampicin
Clarithromycin	Propafenone	St John's wort (*Hypericum perforatum*)
Dipyridamole	Quinidine	
Erythromycin	Valspodar	
Itraconazole	Verapamil	

1. Mizuno N, Niwa T, Yotsumoto Y, Sugiyama Y. Impact of drug transporter studies on drug discovery and development. *Pharmacol Rev* (2003) 55, 425-61.

(a) P-glycoprotein interactions

More and more evidence is accumulating to show that some drug interactions occur because they interfere with the activity of P-glycoprotein. This is an efflux pump found in the membranes of certain cells, which can push metabolites and drugs out of the cells and have an impact on the extent of drug absorption (via the intestine), distribution (to the brain, testis, or placenta) and elimination (in the urine and bile). So, for example, the P-glycoprotein in the cells of the gut lining can eject some already-absorbed drug molecules back into the intestine resulting in a reduction in the total amount of drug absorbed. In this way P-glycoprotein acts as a barrier to absorption. The activity of P-glycoprotein in the endothelial cells of the blood-brain barrier can also eject certain drugs from the brain, limiting CNS penetration and effects.

The pumping actions of P-glycoprotein can be induced or inhibited by some drugs. So for example, the induction (or stimulation) of the activity of P-glycoprotein by rifampicin (rifampin) within the lining cells of the gut causes digoxin to be ejected into the gut more vigorously. This results in a fall in the plasma levels of digoxin (see 'Digitalis glycosides + Rifamycins', p.938). In contrast, verapamil appears to inhibit the activity of P-glycoprotein, and is well known to increase digoxin levels (see 'Digitalis glycosides + Calcium-channel blockers; Verapamil', p.916). Ketoconazole also has P-glycoprotein inhibitory effects, and has been shown to increase CSF levels of ritonavir, possibly by preventing the efflux of ritonavir from the CNS (see 'Protease inhibitors + Azoles; Ketoconazole', p.814). Thus the induction or inhibition of P-glycoprotein can have an impact on the pharmacokinetics of some drugs. Note that there is evidence that P-glycoprotein inhibition may have a greater impact on drug distribution (e.g. into the brain) than on drug absorption (e.g. plasma levels).[2]

There is an overlap between CYP3A4 and P-glycoprotein inhibitors, inducers and substrates. Therefore, both mechanisms may be involved in many of the drug interactions traditionally thought to be due to changes in CYP3A4. 'Table 1.6', (p.8) lists some possible P-glycoprotein inhibitors and inducers. Many drugs that are substrates for CYP3A4 (see 'Table 1.4', (p.6)) are also substrates for P-glycoprotein. Digoxin and talinolol are examples of the few drugs that are substrates for P-glycoprotein but not CYP3A4.

P-glycoprotein is also expressed in some cancer cells (where it was first identified). This has led to the development of specific P-glycoprotein inhibitors, such as valspodar, with the aim of improving the penetration of cytotoxic drugs into cancer cells.

1. Mizuno N, Niwa T, Yotsumoto Y, Sugiyama Y. Impact of drug transporter studies on drug discovery and development. *Pharmacol Rev* (2003) 55, 425–61.
2. Lin JH, Yamazaki M. Clinical relevance of P-glycoprotein in drug therapy. *Drug Metab Rev* (2003) 35, 417–54.

2. Pharmacodynamic interactions

Pharmacodynamic interactions are those where the effects of one drug are changed by the presence of another drug at its site of action. Sometimes the drugs directly compete for particular receptors (e.g. $beta_2$ agonists, such as salbutamol, and beta blockers, such as propranolol) but often the reaction is more indirect and involves interference with physiological mechanisms. These interactions are much less easy to classify neatly than those of a pharmacokinetic type.

2.1. Additive or synergistic interactions

If two drugs that have the same pharmacological effect are given together the effects can be additive. For example, alcohol depresses the CNS and, if taken in moderate amounts with normal therapeutic doses of any of a large number of drugs (e.g. anxiolytics, hypnotics, etc.), may cause excessive drowsiness. Strictly speaking (as pointed out earlier) these are not interactions within the definition given in 'What is a drug interaction?', (p.1). Nevertheless, it is convenient to consider them within the broad context of the clinical outcome of giving two drugs together.

Additive effects can occur with both the main effects of the drugs as well as their adverse effects, thus an additive 'interaction' can occur with antimuscarinic antiparkinson drugs (main effect) or butyrophenones (adverse effect) that can result in serious antimuscarinic toxicity (see 'Antipsychotics + Antimuscarinics', p.708).

Sometimes the additive effects are solely toxic (e.g. additive ototoxicity, nephrotoxicity, bone marrow depression, QT interval prolongation). Examples of these reactions are listed in 'Table 1.7', (see below). It is common to use the terms 'additive', 'summation', 'synergy' or 'potentiation' to describe what happens if two or more drugs behave like this. These words have precise pharmacological definitions but they are often used rather loosely as synonyms because in practice it is often very difficult to know the extent of the increased activity, that is to say whether the effects are greater or smaller than the sum of the individual effects.

The serotonin syndrome

In the 1950s a serious and life-threatening toxic reaction was reported in patients taking iproniazid (an MAOI) when they were given 'pethidine (meperidine)', (p.1140). The reasons were then not understood and even now we do not have the full picture. What happened is thought to have been due to over-stimulation of the 5-HT_{1A} and 5-HT_{2A} receptors and possibly other serotonin receptors in the central nervous system (in the brain stem and spinal cord in particular) due to the combined effects of these two drugs. It can occur exceptionally after taking only one drug, which causes over-stimulation of these 5-HT receptors, but much more usually it develops when two or more drugs (so-called serotonergic or serotomimetic drugs) act in concert. The characteristic symptoms (now known as the serotonin syndrome) fall into three main areas, namely altered mental status (agitation, confusion, mania), autonomic dysfunction (diaphoresis, diarrhoea, fever, shivering) and neuromuscular abnormalities (hyperreflexia, incoordination, myoclonus, tremor). These are the 'Sternbach diagnostic criteria' named after Dr Harvey Sternbach who drew up this list of clinical features and who suggested that at least three of them need to be seen before classifying this toxic reaction as the serotonin syndrome rather than the neuroleptic malignant syndrome.[1]

The syndrome can develop shortly after one serotonergic drug is added to another, or even if one is replaced by another without allowing a long enough washout period in between, and the problem usually resolves within about 24 hours if both drugs are withdrawn and supportive measures given. Non-specific serotonin antagonists (cyproheptadine, chlorpromazine, methysergide) have also been used for treatment. Most patients recover uneventfully, but there have been a few fatalities.

Table 1.7 Additive, synergistic or summation interactions

Drugs	*Result of interaction*
Antipsychotics + Antimuscarinics	Increased antimuscarinic effects; heat stroke in hot and humid conditions, adynamic ileus, toxic psychoses
Antihypertensives + Drugs that cause hypotension (e.g. Phenothiazines, Sildenafil)	Increased antihypertensive effects; orthostasis
Beta-agonist bronchodilators + Potassium-depleting drugs	Hypokalaemia
CNS depressants + CNS depressants Alcohol + Antihistamines Benzodiazepines + Anaesthetics, general Opioids + Benzodiazepines	Impaired psychomotor skills, reduced alertness, drowsiness, stupor, respiratory depression, coma, death
Drugs that prolong the QT interval + Other drugs that prolong the QT interval Amiodarone + Disopyramide	Additive prolongation of QT interval, increased risk of torsade de pointes
Methotrexate + Co-trimoxazole	Bone marrow megaloblastosis due to folic acid antagonism
Nephrotoxic drugs + Nephrotoxic drugs (e.g. Aminoglycosides, Ciclosporin, Cisplatin, Vancomycin)	Increased nephrotoxicity
Neuromuscular blockers + Drugs with neuromuscular blocking effects (e.g. Aminoglycosides)	Increased neuromuscular blockade; delayed recovery, prolonged apnoea
Potassium supplements + Potassium-sparing drugs (e.g. ACE inhibitors, Angiotensin II receptor antagonists, Potassium-sparing diuretics)	Hyperkalaemia

Following the first report of this syndrome, many other cases have been described involving 'tryptophan and MAOIs', (p.1151), the 'tricyclic antidepressants and MAOIs', (p.1149), and, more recently, the 'SSRIs', (p.1142) but other serotonergic drugs have also been involved and the list continues to grow.

It is still not at all clear why many patients can take two, or sometimes several serotonergic drugs together without problems, while a very small number develop this serious toxic reaction, but it certainly suggests that there are as yet other factors involved that have yet to be identified. The full story is likely to be much more complex than just the simple additive effects of two drugs.

1. Sternbach H. The serotonin syndrome. *Am J Psychiatry* (1991) 148, 705–13.

2.2. Antagonistic or opposing interactions

In contrast to additive interactions, there are some pairs of drugs with activities that are opposed to one another. For example the coumarins can prolong the blood clotting time by competitively inhibiting the effects of dietary vitamin K. If the intake of vitamin K is increased, the effects of the oral anticoagulant are opposed and the prothrombin time can return to normal, thereby cancelling out the therapeutic benefits of anticoagulant treatment (see 'Coumarins and related drugs + Vitamin K substances', p.458). Other examples of this type of interaction are listed in 'Table 1.8', (see below).

Table 1.8 Opposing or antagonistic interactions

Drug affected	*Interacting drugs*	*Results of interaction*
ACE inhibitors or Loop diuretics	NSAIDs	Antihypertensive effects opposed
Anticoagulants	Vitamin K	Anticoagulant effects opposed
Antidiabetics	Glucocorticoids	Blood glucose-lowering effects opposed
Antineoplastics	Megestrol	Antineoplastic effects possibly opposed
Levodopa	Antipsychotics (those with dopamine antagonist effects)	Antiparkinsonian effects opposed
Levodopa	Tacrine	Antiparkinsonian effects opposed

2.3. Drug or neurotransmitter uptake interactions

A number of drugs with actions that occur at adrenergic neurones can be prevented from reaching those sites of action by the presence of other drugs. The tricyclic antidepressants prevent the re-uptake of noradrenaline (norepinephrine) into peripheral adrenergic neurones. Thus patients taking tricyclics and given parenteral noradrenaline have a markedly increased response (hypertension, tachycardia); see 'Tricyclic antidepressants + Inotropes and Vasopressors', p.1237. Similarly, the uptake of guanethidine (and related drugs guanoclor, betanidine, debrisoquine, etc.) is blocked by 'chlorpromazine, haloperidol, tiotixene', (p.887), a number of 'amfetamine-like drugs', (p.886) and the 'tricyclic antidepressants', (p.888) so that the antihypertensive effect is prevented. The antihypertensive effects of clonidine are also prevented by the tricyclic antidepressants, one possible reason being that the uptake of clonidine within the CNS is blocked (see 'Clonidine + Tricyclic and related antidepressants', p.884). Some of these interactions at adrenergic neurones are illustrated in 'Figure 1.5', (see below).

E. Drug-herb interactions

The market for herbal medicines and supplements in the Western world has markedly increased in recent years, and, not surprisingly, reports of interactions with 'conventional' drugs have arisen. The most well known and documented example is the interaction of St John's wort (*Hypericum perforatum*) with a variety of drugs, see below. There have also been isolated reports of other herbal drug interactions, attributable to various mechanisms, including additive pharmacological effects.

Based on these reports, there are a growing number of reviews of herbal medicine interactions, which seek to predict likely interactions based on the, often hypothesised, actions of various herbs. Many of these predictions seem tenuous at best.

Rather than add to the volume of predicted interactions, at present, *Stockley's Drug Interactions* includes only those interactions for which there are published reports.

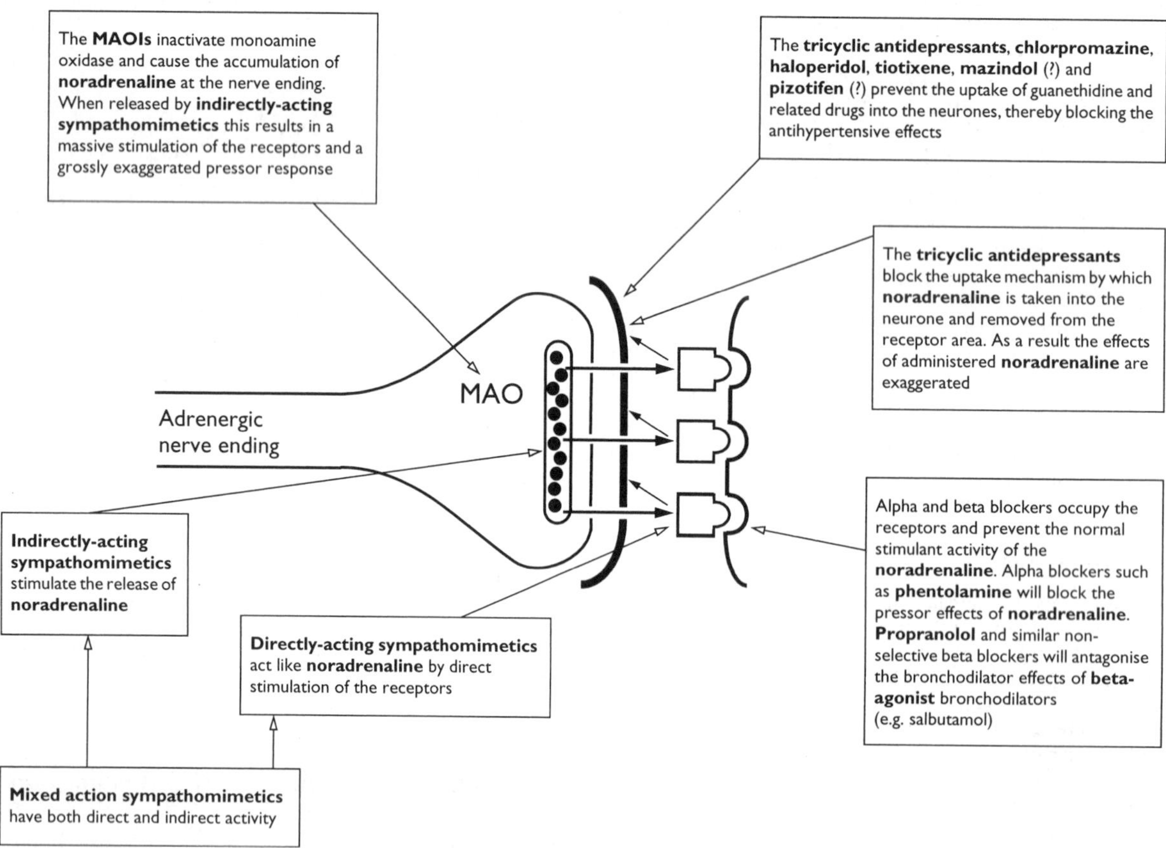

Fig. 1.5 Interactions at adrenergic neurones. A highly simplified composite diagram of an adrenergic neurone (molecules of noradrenaline (norepinephrine) indicated as (•) contained in a single vesicle at the nerve-ending) to illustrate in outline some of the different sites where drugs can interact. More details of these interactions are to be found in individual monographs.

To aid collection of data in this area, health professionals should routinely ask patients about their use of herbal medicines and supplements, and report any unexpected responses to treatment.

An additional problem in interpreting these interactions, is that the interacting constituent of the herb is usually not known and is therefore not standardised for. It could vary widely between different products, and batches of the same product.

St John's wort

An increasing number of reports have implicated St John's wort (*Hypericum perforatum*) in drug interactions. Evidence has shown that the herb can induce the cytochrome P450 isoenzyme CYP3A4, and can also induce 'P-glycoprotein', (p.8). Hence St John's wort decreases the levels of 'ciclosporin', (p.1037) and 'digoxin', (p.927), respectively. Other less certain evidence suggests that CYP2E1 and CYP1A2 may also be induced. St John's wort has serotonergic properties, and this has resulted in a pharmacodynamic interaction with the 'SSRIs', (p.1224), namely the development of the serotonin syndrome. St John's wort contains many possible constituents that could be responsible for its pharmacological effects. The major active constituents are currently considered to be hyperforin (a phloroglucinol) and hypericin (a naphthodianthrone). Hypericin is the only constituent that is standardised for, and then only in some St John's wort preparations.

General references

1. Miller LG. Herbal medicinals. Selected clinical considerations focusing on known or potential drug-herb interactions. *Arch Intern Med* (1998) 158, 2200–11.
2. Fugh-Berman A. Herb-drug interactions. *Lancet* (2000) 355, 134–8. Correction. ibid. 1020.
3. Wang Z, Gorski JC, Hamman MA, Huang S-M, Lesko LJ, Hall SD. The effects of St John's wort *(Hypericum perforatum)* on human cytochrome P450 activity. *Clin Pharmacol Ther* (2001) 70, 317–26.
4. Williamson EM. Drug interactions between herbal and prescription medicines. *Drug Safety* (2003) 26, 1075–92.
5. Henderson L, Yue QY, Bergquist C, Gerden B, Arlett P. St John's wort (*Hypericum perforatum*): drug interactions and clinical outcomes. *Br J Clin Pharmacol* (2002) 54, 349–56.
6. Gurley BJ, Gardner SF, Hubbard MA, Williams DK, Gentry WB, Cui Y, Ang CYW. Cytochrome P450 phenotypic ratios for predicting herb-drug interactions in humans. *Clin Pharmacol Ther* (2002) 72, 276–87.
7. Dresser GK, Schwarz UI, Wilkinson GR, Kim RB. Coordinate induction of both cytochrome P4503A and MDR1 by St John's wort in healthy subjects. *Clin Pharmacol Ther* (2003) 73, 41–50.

F. Drug-food interactions

It is well established that food can cause clinically important changes in drug absorption through effects on gastrointestinal motility or by drug binding, see 'Drug absorption interactions', (p.3). In addition, it is well known that tyramine (present in some foodstuffs) may reach toxic concentrations in patients taking 'MAOIs', (p.1153). With the growth in understanding of drug metabolism mechanisms, it has been increasingly recognised that some foods can alter drug metabolism. Currently, grapefruit juice causes the most clinically relevant of these interactions, see (b) below.

(a) Cruciferous vegetables and charcoal-broiled meats

Cruciferous vegetables, such as brussels sprouts, cabbage, and broccoli, contain substances that are inducers of the cytochrome P450 isoenzyme CYP1A2. Chemicals formed by 'burning' meats additionally have these properties. These foods do not appear to cause any clinically important drug interactions in their own right, but their consumption may add another variable to drug interaction studies, so complicating interpretation. In drug interaction studies where alteration of CYP1A2 is a predicted mechanism, it may be better for patients to avoid these foods during the study.

(b) Grapefruit juice

By chance, grapefruit juice was chosen to mask the taste of alcohol in a study of the effect of alcohol on felodipine, which led to the discovery that grapefruit juice itself markedly increased felodipine levels, see 'Calcium-channel blockers + Grapefruit juice', p.869. In general, grapefruit juice inhibits intestinal CYP3A4, and only slightly affects hepatic CYP3A4. This is demonstrated by the fact that intravenous preparations of drugs that are metabolised by CYP3A4 are not much affected, whereas oral preparations of the same drugs are. These interactions result in increased drug levels.

Some drugs that are not metabolised by CYP3A4 show decreased levels with grapefruit juice, such as 'fexofenadine', (p.588). The probable reason for this is that grapefruit juice is an inhibitor of some drug transporters (see 'Drug transporter proteins', (p.8)), and possibly affects organic anion-transporting polypeptides (OATPs), although inhibition of P-glycoprotein has also been suggested.

The active constituent of grapefruit juice is uncertain. Grapefruit contains naringin, which degrades during processing to naringenin, a substance known to inhibit CYP3A4. Because of this, it has been assumed that whole grapefruit will not interact, but that processed grapefruit juice will. However, subsequently some reports have implicated the whole fruit. Other possible active constituents in the whole fruit include bergamottin and dihydroxybergamottin.

General references

1. Ameer B, Wientraub RA. Drug interactions with grapefruit juice. *Clin Pharmacokinet* (1997) 33, 103–21.

G. Conclusions

It is now quite impossible to remember all the known clinically important interactions and how they occur, which is why this reference publication has been produced, but there are some broad general principles that need little memorising:

- Be on the alert with any drugs that have a narrow therapeutic window or where it is necessary to keep serum levels at or above a suitable level (e.g. anticoagulants, antidiabetic drugs, antiepileptics, antihypertensives, anti-infectives, antineoplastic cytotoxics, digitalis glycosides, immunosuppressants, etc.).
- Remember some of those drugs that are key enzyme inducers (e.g. phenytoin, barbiturates, rifampicin, etc) or enzyme inhibitors (e.g. azole antifungals, HIV-protease inhibitors, erythromycin, SSRIs).
- Think about the basic pharmacology of the drugs under consideration so that obvious problems (additive CNS depression for example) are not overlooked, and try to think what might happen if drugs that affect the same receptors are used together. And don't forget that many drugs affect more than one type of receptor.
- Keep in mind that the elderly are at risk because of reduced liver and renal function on which drug clearance depends.

2

ACE inhibitors and Angiotensin II receptor antagonists

ACE inhibitors (angiotensin-converting enzyme inhibitors) prevent the production of angiotensin II from angiotensin I. The angiotensin II receptor antagonists are more selective, and target the angiotensin II type I (AT_1) receptor, which is responsible for the pressor actions of angiotensin II.

Angiotensin II is involved in the renin-angiotensin-aldosterone system, which regulates blood pressure, sodium and water homoeostasis by the kidneys, and cardiovascular function. Angiotensin II stimulates the synthesis and secretion of aldosterone and raises blood pressure via a direct vasoconstrictor effect.

Angiotensin converting enzyme (ACE) is identical to bradykinase, so ACE inhibitors may additionally reduce the degradation of bradykinin and affect enzymes involved in the production of prostaglandins.

Many of the interactions of the ACE inhibitors and angiotensin II receptor antagonists involve drugs that affect blood pressure. Consequently in most cases the result is either an increase in the hypotensive effect (e.g. 'alcohol', (p.48)) or a decrease in the hypotensive effect (e.g. 'indometacin', (p.28)).

In addition, due to their effects on aldosterone, the ACE inhibitors and angiotensin II antagonists may increase potassium concentrations and can therefore have additive hyperkalaemic effects with other drugs that cause elevated potassium levels. Furthermore, drugs that affect renal function may potentiate the adverse effects of ACE inhibitors and angiotensin II antagonists on the kidneys.

Most ACE inhibitor and angiotensin II receptor antagonist interactions are pharmacodynamic, that is, interactions that result in an alteration in drug effects rather than drug disposition, so in most cases interactions of individual drugs will be applicable to the group. *In vitro* experiments suggest that the role of cytochrome P450 isoenzymes in the metabolism and interactions of the angiotensin II receptor antagonists (candesartan, eprosartan, irbesartan, losartan and valsartan) is small, although losartan, irbesartan, and to a minor extent, candesartan, are metabolised by CYP2C9. Only losartan and irbesartan were considered to have a theoretical potential for pharmacokinetic drug interactions involving the CYP2C9 enzyme.[1] See 'Angiotensin II receptor antagonists + Azoles', p.35. The ACE inhibitors do not appear to undergo interactions via cytochrome P450 isoenzymes.

'Table 2.1', (see below) lists the ACE inhibitors and the angiotensin II receptor antagonists. Although most of the interactions of the ACE inhibitors or angiotensin II receptor antagonists are covered in this section, if the ACE inhibitor or angiotensin II receptor antagonist is the affecting drug, the interaction is dealt with elsewhere.

1. Taavitsainen P, Kiukaanniemi K, Pelkonen O. In vitro inhibition screening of human hepatic P_{450} enzymes by five angiotensin-II receptor antagonists. *Eur J Clin Pharmacol* (2000) 56, 135–40.

Table 2.1 ACE inhibitors and Angiotensin II receptor antagonists

Group	*Drugs*
ACE inhibitors	Benazepril, Captopril, Cilazapril, Delapril, Enalapril, Fosinopril, Imidapril, Lisinopril, Moexipril, Perindopril, Quinapril, Ramipril, Spirapril, Temocapril, Trandolapril, Zofenopril
Angiotensin II receptor antagonists	Candesartan, Eprosartan, Irbesartan, Losartan, Olmesartan, Telmisartan, Valsartan

ACE inhibitors + Allopurinol

Three cases of Stevens-Johnson syndrome (one fatal) and two cases of hypersensitivity have been attributed to the use of captopril with allopurinol. Anaphylaxis and myocardial infarction occurred in one man taking enalapril when given allopurinol. The combination of ACE inhibitors and allopurinol may increase the risk of leucopenia and serious infection, especially in renal impairment.

Clinical evidence

An elderly man with hypertension, chronic renal failure, congestive heart failure and mild polyarthritis receiving multiple drug treatment, which included **captopril** 25 mg twice daily and diuretics, developed fatal Stevens-Johnson syndrome about 5 weeks after starting to take allopurinol 100 mg twice daily.[1] The authors of the report noted that the manufacturer of **captopril** was aware of two other patients who developed the syndrome 3 to 5 weeks after allopurinol was started.[1] Another report describes fever, arthralgia and myalgia in a diabetic man with chronic renal failure who was also given **captopril** and allopurinol. He improved when the **captopril** was withdrawn.[2] Exfoliatory facial dermatitis occurred in a patient with renal failure who was taking **captopril** and allopurinol.[3] A man taking **enalapril** had an acute anaphylactic reaction with severe coronary spasm, culminating in myocardial infarction, within 20 minutes of taking allopurinol 100 mg. He recovered and continued to take **enalapril** without allopurinol.[4]

The UK manufacturer of **captopril** also warns that neutropenia and agranulocytosis, resulting in serious infection, have occurred in patients taking **captopril** and other ACE inhibitors, and that concurrent treatment with allopurinol may be a complicating factor, especially in those with renal impairment.[5] However, the US manufacturer notes that, while renal impairment and a relatively high dose of **captopril** markedly increases the risk of neutropenia, no association between allopurinol and **captopril** and neutropenia has appeared in US reports.[6]

No significant pharmacokinetic changes were seen in 12 healthy subjects given allopurinol and **captopril** alone and in combination.[7]

Mechanism

Not understood. It is uncertain whether these are interactions because allopurinol alone can cause severe hypersensitivity reactions, particularly in the presence of renal failure and in conjunction with diuretic use. Captopril can also induce a hypersensitivity reaction.

Importance and management

These interactions are not clearly established, and the reaction appears to be rare and unpredictable. All that can be constructively said is that patients taking both drugs should be very closely monitored for any signs of hypersensitivity (e.g. skin reactions) or low white cell count (sore throat, fever), especially if they have renal impairment. The UK manufacturer of captopril recommends that differential white blood cell counts should be performed before adding allopurinol, then every 2 weeks during the first 3 months of treatment, and periodically thereafter.[5] Similar caution and advice is given by the UK manufacturers of several other ACE inhibitors. For other possible interactions with ACE inhibitors that might result in an increased risk of leucopenia see also 'ACE inhibitors + Azathioprine', p.18 and 'ACE inhibitors + Procainamide', p.33.

1. Pennell DJ, Nunan TO, O'Doherty MJ, Croft DN. Fatal Stevens-Johnson syndrome in a patient on captopril and allopurinol. *Lancet* (1984) i, 463.
2. Samanta A, Burden AC. Fever, myalgia, and arthralgia in a patient on captopril and allopurinol. *Lancet* (1984) i, 679.
3. Beeley L, Daly M, Stewart P. *Bulletin of the West Midlands Centre for Adverse Drug Reaction Reporting* (1987) 24, 9.
4. Ahmad S. Allopurinol and enalapril. Drug induced anaphylactic coronary spasm and acute myocardial infarction. *Chest* (1995) 108, 586.
5. Capoten (Captopril). E. R. Squibb & Sons Ltd. UK Summary of product characteristics, June 2005.
6. Capoten (Captopril). Par Pharmaceutical, Inc. US Prescribing information, June 2003.
7. Duchin KL, McKinstry DN, Cohen AI, Migdalof BH. Pharmacokinetics of captopril in healthy subjects and in patients with cardiovascular diseases. *Clin Pharmacokinet* (1988) 14, 241–59.

ACE inhibitors + Angiotensin II receptor antagonists

The combined use of ACE inhibitors and angiotensin II receptor antagonists increases the risk of hypotension, renal impairment and hyperkalaemia in patients with heart failure.

Clinical evidence, mechanism, importance and management

Both ACE inhibitors and angiotensin II receptor antagonists can have adverse renal effects and can cause hyperkalaemia. These effects might be expected to be additive when they are used together. In one randomised clinical study in patients with heart failure taking ACE inhibitors, the addition of **candesartan** resulted in higher rates of withdrawals than placebo for renal impairment (increase in creatinine 7.8% versus 4.1%) and hyperkalaemia (3.4% versus 0.7%).[1] In another double-blind study in patients with heart failure, the combination of **valsartan** and captopril resulted in a higher incidence of adverse events leading to a dose reduction or a discontinuation of study treatment than either drug alone. For hypotension, treatment was discontinued in 90 (1.9%) of patients in the combined group, 70 (1.4%) of patients in the valsartan group, and 41 (0.8%) of patients in the captopril group. For renal causes the corresponding figures were 61 (1.3%), 53 (1.1%) and 40 (0.8%) of patients, respectively, and for hyperkalaemia the figures were 12 (0.2%), 7 (0.1%) and 4 (0.1%) of patients, respectively.[2]

Monitor renal function and serum potassium carefully when combination therapy is used.

1. McMurray JJV, Östergren J, Swedberg K, Granger CB, Held P, Michelson EL, Olofsson B, Yusuf S, Pfeffer MA; CHARM Investigators and Committees. Effects of candesartan in patients with chronic heart failure and reduced left-ventricular systolic function taking angiotensin-converting-enzyme inhibitors: the CHARM-Added trial. *Lancet* (2003) 362, 767–71.
2. Pfeffer MA, McMurray JJV, Velazquez EJ, Rouleau J-L, Køber L, Maggioni AP, Solomon SD, Swedberg K, Van de Werf F, White H, Leimberger JD, Henis M, Edwards S, Zelenkofske S, Sellers MA, Califf RM; Valsartan in Acute Myocardial Infarction Trial Investigators. Valsartan, captopril, or both in myocardial infarction complicated by heart failure, left ventricular dysfunction, or both. *N Engl J Med* (2003) 349, 1893–1906.

ACE inhibitors + Antacids

An aluminium/magnesium hydroxide antacid reduced the bioavailability of captopril by 40%, but this did not seem to be clinically important. The bioavailability of fosinopril was reduced by about one-third by *Mylanta*. An antacid did not affect ramipril pharmacokinetics.

Clinical evidence

In 10 healthy subjects an antacid containing **aluminium/magnesium hydroxide** and **magnesium carbonate** reduced the AUC of a single 50-mg dose of **captopril** by about 40%, when compared with the fasting state. However, this did not alter the extent of the reduction in blood pressure.[1]

Another study found that ***Mylanta*** [**aluminium/magnesium hydroxide** and simeticone[2]] reduced the bioavailability of **fosinopril** 20 mg by about one-third.[3]

It is briefly noted in a review that antacid use did not affect the pharmacokinetics of ramiprilat, the active metabolite of **ramipril**.[4]

Mechanism

The mechanism of this interaction is uncertain, but is unlikely to be due to elevated gastric pH since cimetidine did not have a similar effect.[3]

Importance and management

Note that greater decreases in **captopril** bioavailability (caused by 'food', (p.26)) were found not to be clinically relevant, therefore, it is unlikely the change seen with antacids will be clinically important.

However, with **fosinopril**, the manufacturers[2,5] suggest separating administration of antacids by at least 2 hours.

The UK manufacturers of **quinapril**[6] and **trandolapril**[7] also warn that antacids may reduce the bioavailability of ACE inhibitors, quite possibly based on the way these named ACE inhibitors interact, but there seems to be no evidence of a clinically significant interaction in practice.

1. Mäntylä R, Männistö PT, Vuorela A, Sundberg S, Ottoila P. Impairment of captopril bioavailability by concomitant food and antacid intake. *Int J Clin Pharmacol Ther Toxicol* (1984) 22, 626–9.
2. Monopril (Fosinopril sodium). Bristol-Myers Squibb Company. US Prescribing information, July 2003.
3. Moore L, Kramer A, Swites B, Kramer P, Tu J. Effect of cimetidine and antacid on the kinetics of the active diacid of fosinopril in healthy subjects. *J Clin Pharmacol* (1988) 28, 946.
4. Todd PA, Benfield P. Ramipril. A review of its pharmacological properties and therapeutic efficacy in cardiovascular disorders. *Drugs* (1990) 39, 110–35.
5. Staril (Fosinopril sodium). E. R. Squibb & Sons Ltd. UK Summary of product characteristics, June 2005.
6. Accupro (Quinapril hydrochloride). Pfizer Ltd. UK Summary of product characteristics, March 2007.
7. Gopten (Trandolapril). Abbott Laboratories Ltd. UK Summary of product characteristics, May 2007.

ACE inhibitors + Antipsychotics

Marked postural hypotension occurred in a patient given chlorpromazine and captopril. The hypotensive adverse effects of antipsychotics such as the phenothiazines may be additive with the effects of ACE inhibitors.

Clinical evidence, mechanism, importance and management

A patient fainted and developed marked postural hypotension (standing blood pressure 66/48 mmHg) when given **captopril** 6.25 mg twice daily and **chlorpromazine** 200 mg three times daily. He had previously taken **chlorpromazine** with nadolol, prazosin and hydrochlorothiazide without any problems, although his blood pressure was poorly controlled on these drugs. Since the patient's blood pressure was quite elevated when taking **chlorpromazine** or **captopril** alone, there appeared to be a synergistic hypotensive effect between the two drugs.[1]

The manufacturers of several ACE inhibitors warn that ACE inhibitors may enhance the hypotensive effects of certain antipsychotics, and that postural hypotension may occur. Some of these warnings are based, not unreasonably, on the adverse reactions seen with other ACE inhibitors or antihypertensives, but not necessarily on direct observations.[2] If postural hypotension occurs warn patients to lay down and elevate their legs if they feel faint or dizzy, and, when recovered, to get up slowly. Dosage adjustments may be necessary to accommodate this interaction.

1. White WB. Hypotension with postural syncope secondary to the combination of chlorpromazine and captopril. *Arch Intern Med* (1986) 146, 1833–4.
2. Knoll Ltd. Personal communication,1993.

ACE inhibitors + Aprotinin

Aprotinin suppressed the hypotensive action of captopril and enalapril in *rats*.

Clinical evidence, mechanism, importance and management

A study in spontaneously hypertensive *rats* found that aprotinin suppressed the hypotensive responses of **captopril** and **enalapril**.[1] Aprotinin is a proteolytic enzyme inhibitor that has many actions including antagonism of the kallikrein-kinin system, which in turn affects bradykinins and renin. It would therefore be expected to have complex interactions with the ACE inhibitors,[2] which also affect these proteins. However, there does not appear to be any evidence to suggest that this theoretical interaction is of clinical relevance.

1. Sharma JN, Amrah SS, Noor AR. Suppression of hypotensive responses of captopril and enalapril by the kallikrein inhibitor aprotinin in spontaneously hypertensive rats. *Pharmacology* (1995) 50, 363–9.
2. Waxler B, Rabito SF. Aprotinin: a serine protease inhibitor with therapeutic actions: its interaction with ACE inhibitors. *Curr Pharm Des* (2003) 9, 777–87.

ACE inhibitors + Aspirin

The antihypertensive efficacy of captopril and enalapril may be reduced by high-dose aspirin in about 50% of patients. Low-dose aspirin (less than or equal to 100 mg daily) appears to have little effect. It is unclear whether aspirin attenuates the benefits of ACE inhibitors in heart failure. The likelihood of an interaction may depend on disease state and its severity.
Renal failure has been reported in a patient taking captopril and aspirin.

Clinical evidence

A. Effects on blood pressure

(a) Captopril

Aspirin 600 mg every 6 hours for 5 doses did not significantly alter the blood pressure response to a single 25 to 100-mg dose of captopril in 8 patients with essential hypertension. However, the prostaglandin response to captopril was blocked in 4 of the 8, and in these patients, the blood pressure response to captopril was blunted.[1] In another study, aspirin 75 mg daily did not alter the antihypertensive effects of captopril 25 mg twice daily in 15 patients with hypertension.[2]

(b) Enalapril

Two groups of 26 patients, one with mild to moderate hypertension taking enalapril 20 mg twice daily and the other with severe primary hypertension taking enalapril 20 mg twice daily (with nifedipine 30 mg and atenolol 50 mg daily), were given test doses of aspirin 100 and 300 mg daily for 5 days. The 100-mg dose of aspirin did not alter the efficacy of the antihypertensive drugs, but the 300-mg dose reduced the antihypertensive efficacy in about half the patients in both groups. In these patients, the antihypertensive effects were diminished by 63% in those with mild to moderate hypertension and by 91% in those with severe hypertension.[3] In contrast, another study in 7 patients with hypertension taking enalapril (mean daily dose 12.9 mg) found that aspirin 81 mg or 325 mg daily for 2 weeks did not have any significant effect on blood pressure.[4] A further study in 18 patients also found that aspirin 100 mg daily for 2 weeks did not alter the antihypertensive effect of enalapril 20 or 40 mg daily.[5]

(c) Unspecified ACE inhibitors

In a randomised study, the use of low-dose aspirin 100 mg daily for 3 months did not alter blood pressure control in patients taking calcium-channel blockers or ACE inhibitors, when compared with placebo.[6] Similarly, in a re-analysis of data from the Hypertension Optimal Treatment (HOT) study, long-term low-dose aspirin 75 mg daily did not interfere with the blood pressure-lowering effects of the antihypertensive drugs studied, when compared with placebo. Of 18 790 treated hypertensive patients, about 82% received a calcium-channel blocker, usually felodipine alone or in combination, and 41% received an ACE inhibitor, usually in combination with felodipine.[7]

B. Effects in coronary artery disease and heart failure

Various pharmacological studies have looked at the *short-term* effects of the combination of ACE inhibitors and aspirin on haemodynamic parameters. In one study in 40 patients with decompensated heart failure, aspirin 300 mg given on the first day and 100 mg daily thereafter antagonised the short-term haemodynamic effects of **captopril** 50 mg given every 8 hours for 4 days. The **captopril**-induced increase in cardiac index and the reduction in peripheral vascular resistance and pulmonary wedge pressure were all abolished.[8] In another study, in 15 patients with chronic heart failure receiving treatment with ACE inhibitors (mainly **enalapril** 10 mg twice daily), aspirin in doses as low as 75 mg impaired vasodilatation induced by arachidonic acid.[9] In yet another study, aspirin 325 mg daily worsened pulmonary diffusion capacity and made the ventilatory response to exercise less effective in patients taking **enalapril** 10 mg twice daily, but did not exert this effect in the absence of ACE inhibitors.[10] However, results from studies are inconsistent. In a review,[11] five of 7 studies reported aspirin did not alter the haemodynamic effects of ACE inhibitors whereas the remaining two did. In one of these studies showing an adverse interaction between aspirin and **enalapril**, **ticlopidine** did not interact with **enalapril**.[12]

A number of large clinical studies of ACE inhibitors, mostly post-myocardial infarction, have been re-examined to see if there was a difference in outcome between those receiving aspirin at baseline, and those not. The results are summarised in 'Table 2.2', (p.15). However, in addition to the problems of retrospective analysis of non-randomised parameters, the studies vary in the initiation and duration of aspirin and ACE inhibitor treatment and the length of follow-up, the degree of heart failure or ischaemia, the prognosis of the patients, and the final end point (whether compared with placebo or with the benefits of aspirin or ACE inhibitors). The conclusions are therefore conflicting, and, although two meta-analyses of

Table 2.2 Sub-group analyses of clinical studies assessing the interaction between aspirin and ACE inhibitors

Study and patients	*Aspirin dose*	*ACE inhibitor*	*Follow-up*	*Finding*	*Refs*
Evidence of an interaction					
SOLVD 6512 patients treated for heart failure or prevention of heart failure	Not reported	Enalapril	37 to 41 months	Combined treatment associated with reduced benefits compared with enalapril alone.	1
CONSENSUS II 6090 patients with acute MI	Not reported	Enalapril	6 months	Effect of enalapril less favourable in those taking aspirin at baseline.	2
GUSTO-I 31622 post-MI patients without heart failure	Not reported	Not reported	11 months (starting 30 days post MI)	Combined use associated with higher mortality than aspirin alone (mortality rates 3.3 vs 1.6%).	3
EPILOG 2619 patients undergoing coronary angioplasty	325 mg daily	Not reported	12 months	Combined use associated with higher mortality than aspirin alone (mortality rates 3.7 vs 1.2%).	3
AIRE 1986 patients after acute MI, with heart failure	Not reported	Ramipril 2.5 to 5 mg twice daily started 3 to 10 days after MI	15 months (average)	Trend towards greater benefit of ramipril in those not receiving aspirin.	4
No evidence of an interaction					
BIP Secondary prevention of MI in 1197 patients with coronary artery disease	250 mg daily	Captopril or enalapril	5 years (average)	Lower death rate in those on combined therapy than those on ACE inhibitor alone (19 vs 27%).	5
SAVE 2231 patients with left ventricular dysfunction after MI	Not reported	Captopril 75 to 150 mg daily	42 months (average)	Trend towards greater benefits of captopril when taken with aspirin.	6
HOPE Prevention of cardiovascular events in 9297 patients without left ventricular dysfunction or heart failure	Not reported	Ramipril 10 mg daily	About 4.5 years	Benefits of ramipril not affected by aspirin.	7
CATS Early treatment of acute MI in 298 patients	80 to 100 mg daily	Captopril	1 year	Benefits of captopril not affected by aspirin. Better prognosis in those on aspirin.	8
ISIS-4 Early treatment of acute MI in 58050 patients	Not reported	Captopril 100 mg daily	At 5 weeks and 1 year	Benefits of captopril not affected by aspirin.	9
Meta analysis of AIRE, SAVE, SOLVD and TRACE 12763 patients with left ventricular dysfunction or heart failure with or without MI	Not reported	Captopril, enalapril, ramipril, trandolapril	35 months (average)	Benefits of ACE inhibitors observed even if aspirin given.	10
Meta analysis of CCS-1, CONSENSUS II, GISSI-3, and ISIS-4 Early treatment of MI in 96712 patients	160 to 325 mg daily	Captopril, enalapril, lisinopril	30 days	ACE inhibitor reduced 30-day mortality from 15.1 to 13.8%. ACE inhibitor plus aspirin reduced 30-day mortality from 6.7 to 6.3%.	11
TRACE 1749 patients with left ventricular dysfunction after acute MI	Not reported	Trandolapril 1 to 4 mg daily	24 to 50 months	Trend towards greater benefit of trandolapril in those receiving aspirin (mortality of 45% with ACE inhibitor, and 34% with ACE inhibitor plus aspirin).	12
SMILE 1556 patients with acute MI	Not reported	Zofenopril 7.5 mg increasing to 30 mg twice daily for 6 weeks	At 6 weeks and 1 year	Benefits of zofenopril not significantly affected by aspirin.	13

Continued

Table 2.2 Sub-group analyses of clinical studies assessing the interaction between aspirin and ACE inhibitors (continued)

Study and patients	Aspirin dose	ACE inhibitor	Follow-up	Finding	Refs
Meta analysis of AIRE, HOPE, SAVE, SOLVD, and TRACE 22060 patients with either; left ventricular dysfunction or heart failure without MI, coronary artery disease without left ventricular dysfunction, or acute MI	Not reported	Captopril, enalapril, ramipril, trandolapril	More than 3 years	Benefits of ACE inhibitors observed even if aspirin given.	14

1. Al-Khadra AS, Salem DN, Rand WM, Udelson JE, Smith JJ, Konstam MA. Antiplatelet agents and survival: a cohort analysis from the Studies of Left Ventricular Dysfunction (SOLVD) trial. *J Am Coll Cardiol* (1998) 31, 419-25.
2. Nguyen KN, Aursnes I, Kjekshus J. Interaction between enalapril and aspirin on mortality after acute myocardial infarction: subgroup analysis of the Cooperative New Scandanavian Enalapril Survival Study II (CONSENSUS II). *Am J Cardiol* (1997) 79, 115-19.
3. Peterson JG, Topol EJ, Sapp SK, Young JB, Lincoff AM, Lauer MS. Evaluation of the effects of aspirin combined with angiotensin-converting enzyme inhibitors in patients with coronary artery disease. *Am J Med* (2000) 109, 371-7.
4. The Acute Infarction Ramipril Efficacy (AIRE) Study Investigators. Effect of ramipril on mortality and morbidity of survivors of acute myocardial infarction with clinical evidence of heart failure. *Lancet* (1993) 342, 821-8.
5. Leor J, Reicher-Reiss H, Goldbourt U, Boyko V, Gottlieb S, Battler A, Behar S. Aspirin and mortality in patients treated with angiotensin-converting enzyme inhibitors. A cohort study of 11,575 patients with coronary artery disease. *J Am Coll Cardiol* (1999) 33, 1920-5.
6. Pfeffer MA, Braunwald E, Moyé LA, Basta L, Brown EJ, Cuddy TE, Davis BR, Geltman EM, Goldman S, Flaker GC, Klein M, Lamas GA, Packer M, Rouleau J, Rouleau JL, Rutherford J, Wertheimer JH, Hawkins CM, on behalf of the SAVE Investigators. Effect of captopril on mortality and morbidity in patients with left ventricular dysfunction after myocardial infarction. Results of the survival and ventricular enlargement trial. *N Engl J Med* (1992) 327, 669-77.
7. The Heart Outcomes Prevention Evaluation Study Investigators. Effect of an angiotensin-converting-enzyme inhibitor, ramipril, on cardiovascular events in high-risk patients. *N Engl J Med* (2000) 342, 145-53.
8. Oosterga M, Anthonio RL, de Kam PJ, Kingma JH, Crijns HJ, van Gilst WH. Effects of aspirin on angiotensin-converting enzyme inhibition and left ventricular dilation one year after myocardial infarction. *Am J Cardiol* (1998) 81, 1178-81.
9. ISIS-4 (Fourth International Study of Infarct Survival) Collaborative Group. ISIS-4: a randomised factorial trial assessing early oral captopril, oral mononitrate, and intravenous magnesium sulphate in 58,050 patients with suspected acute myocardial infarction. *Lancet* (1995) 345; 669-85.
10. Flather MD, Yusuf S, Køber L, Pfeffer M, Hall A, Murray G, Trop-Pedersen C, Ball S, Pogue J, Moyé L, Braunwald E, for the ACE-inhibitor Myocardial Infarction Collaborative. Long-term ACE-inhibitor therapy in patients with heart failure or left-ventricular dysfunction: a systematic overview of data from individual patients. *Lancet* (2000) 335, 1575-81.
11. Latini R, Tognoni G, Maggioni AP, Baigent C, Braunwald E, Chen Z-M, Collins R, Flather M, Franzosi MG, Kjekshus J, Køber L, Liu L-S, Peto R, Pfeffer M, Pizzetti F, Santoro E, Sleight P, Swedberg K, Tavazzi L, Wang W, Yusuf S. Clinical effects of early angiotensin-converting enzyme inhibitor treatment for myocardial infarction are similar in the presence and absence of aspirin. *J Am Coll Cardiol* (2000) 35 1801-7.
12. Køber L, Torp-Pedersen C, Carlsen JE, Bagger H, Eliasen P, Lyngborg K, Videbæk J, Cole DS, Auclert L, Pauly NC, Aliot E, Persson S, Camm AJ, for the Trandolapril Cardiac Evaluation (TRACE) Study Group. A clinical trial of the angiotensin-converting-enzyme inhibitor trandolapril in patients with left ventricular dysfunction after myocardial infarction. *N Engl J Med* (1995) 333, 1670-6.
13. Ambrosioni E, Borghi C, Magnani B, for the Survival of Myocardial Infarction Long-Term Evaluation (SMILE) Study Investigators. The effect of the angiotensin-converting-enzyme inhibitor zofenopril on mortality and morbidity after anterior myocardial infarction. *N Engl J Med* (1995) 332, 80-5.
14. Teo KK, Yusuf S, Pfeffer M, Kober L, Hall A, Pogue J, Latini R, Collins R, for the ACE Inhibitors Collaborative Group. Effects of long-term treatment with angiotensin-converting-enzyme inhibitors in the presence or absence of aspirin: a systematic review. *Lancet* (2002) 360, 1037-43.

these studies found no interaction, an editorial[13] disputes the findings of one of these analyses.[14] In addition to these sub-group analyses, there have been a number of retrospective cohort studies. A retrospective study involving 576 patients with heart failure requiring hospitalisation, showed a trend towards an increased incidence of early readmissions (within 30 days after discharge) for heart failure among subjects treated with ACE inhibitors and aspirin, compared with those treated with ACE inhibitors without aspirin (16% versus 10%). In patients without coronary artery disease the increase in readmissions was statistically significant (23% versus 10%).[15] However, long-term survival in heart failure was not affected by the use of aspirin with ACE inhibitors. Furthermore, among patients with coronary artery disease there was a trend towards improvement in mortality in patients treated with the combination, compared with ACE inhibitor without aspirin (40% versus 56%).[16] Similarly, a lack of adverse interaction was found in a retrospective study involving 14 129 elderly patients who survived a hospitalisation for acute myocardial infarction. However, the added benefit of the combination over patients who received either aspirin or ACE inhibitors alone was not statistically significant.[17] Similarly, in another cohort of patients discharged after first hospitalisation for heart failure, there was no increase in mortality rates or readmission rates in those taking aspirin and ACE inhibitors.[18] In another retrospective analysis in patients with stable left ventricular systolic dysfunction, no decrease in survival was seen in patients receiving ACE inhibitors, when comparing those also receiving aspirin (mean dose 183 mg daily, 74% 200 mg or less) and those not.[19] Conversely, another study found that, compared to patients not taking aspirin, the use of high-dose aspirin (325 mg daily or more) with an ACE inhibitor was associated with a small but statistically significant 3% increase in the risk of death, whereas low-dose aspirin (160 mg daily or less) was not.[20]

C. Effects on renal function

Acute renal failure developed in a woman taking **captopril** when she started to take aspirin for arthritis. Renal function improved when both were stopped.[21] However, in a re-analysis of data from the Hypertension Optimal Treatment (HOT) study, long-term low-dose aspirin 75 mg daily had no effect on changes in serum creatinine, estimated creatinine clearance or the number of patients developing renal impairment, when compared with placebo. Of 18 790 treated hypertensive patients, 41% received an ACE inhibitor.[7]

D. Pharmacokinetic studies

A single-dose study in 12 healthy subjects found that the pharmacokinetics of **benazepril** 20 mg and aspirin 325 mg were not affected by concurrent use.[22]

Mechanism

Some, but not all the evidence suggests that prostaglandins may be involved in the hypotensive action of ACE inhibitors, and that aspirin, by inhibiting prostaglandin synthesis, may partially antagonise the effect of ACE inhibitors on blood pressure. This effect appears to depend on the dose of aspirin and may also be dependent on sodium status and plasma renin, and therefore it does not occur in all patients.

The beneficial effects of ACE inhibitors in heart failure and ischaemic heart disease are thought to be due, in part, to the inhibition of the breakdown of kinins, which are important regulators of prostaglandin and nitric oxide synthesis. Such inhibition promotes vasodilatation and afterload reduction. Aspirin may block these beneficial effects by inhibiting cyclo-oxygenase (COX) and thus prostaglandin synthesis, causing vasoconstriction, decreased cardiac output and worsening heart failure.[11,23]

Importance and management

Low-dose aspirin (less than or equal to 100 mg daily) does not alter the **antihypertensive efficacy** of captopril and enalapril. No special precautions would therefore seem to be required with ACE inhibitors and these low doses of aspirin. A high dose of aspirin (2.4 g daily) has been reported to interact in 50% of patients in a single study. Aspirin 300 mg daily has been reported to interact in about 50% of patients in another study, whereas 325 mg daily did not interact in further study. Thus, at present, it appears that if an ACE inhibitor is used with aspirin in doses higher than 300 mg daily, blood pressure should be monitored more closely, and the ACE inhibitor dosage raised if necessary. Intermittent use of aspirin should be considered as a possible cause of erratic control of blood pressure in patients on ACE inhibitors.

Both ACE inhibitors and aspirin are often taken by patients with **coronary artery disease**, and ACE inhibitors are used in **chronic heart failure**, which is often associated with coronary heart disease. The information about a possible interaction between ACE inhibitors and aspirin in heart failure is conflicting. This may be due to much of the clinical data being obtained from retrospective non-randomised analyses.[23] It may also be a factor of different disease states. For example, an interaction may be less likely to be experienced in patients with heart failure of ischaemic aetiology than those with non-ischaemic causes, because of the added benefits of aspirin in ischaemic heart disease.[24] The available data, and its implications, have been extensively reviewed and commented on.[11,13,23-32] Some commentators have advised that, if possible, aspirin should be avoided in patients requiring long-term treatment for heart failure, particularly if heart failure is severe.[13,27] Others suggest avoiding aspirin in heart failure unless there are clear indications, such as atherosclerosis.[11,23,28,29] The use of lower doses of aspirin (80 to 100 mg daily rather than greater than or equal to 325 mg daily) in those with heart failure taking ACE inhibitors has also been suggested.[24,25,28] US guidelines from 2005 on chronic heart failure[33] state that, "Many physicians believe the data justify prescribing aspirin and ACE inhibitors together when there is an indication for use of aspirin," while recognising that not all physicians agree. The guidelines say that further study is needed. European guidelines state that there is little evidence to support using ACE inhibitors and aspirin together in heart failure. The guidelines say aspirin can be used as prophylaxis after prior myocardial infarction, but that it should be avoided in patients with recurrent hospitalisation for worsening heart failure.[34] NICE guidelines in the UK make no comment about the combination of ACE inhibitors and aspirin. They say that all patients with heart failure due to left ventricular systolic dysfunction should be considered for treatment with an ACE inhibitor, and that aspirin (75 to 150 mg once daily) should be prescribed for patients with the combination of heart failure and atherosclerotic arterial disease (including coronary heart disease).[35] Data from ongoing randomised studies may provide further insight. Until these are available, combined low-dose aspirin and ACE inhibitors may continue to be used where there is a clear indication for both.

An increased risk of deterioration in **renal function** or **acute renal failure** appears to occur rarely with the combination of aspirin and ACE inhibitors. The routine monitoring of renal function, which is advised with ACE inhibitors, should be sufficient to detect any interaction.

1. Moore TJ, Crantz FR, Hollenberg NK, Koletsky RJ, Leboff MS, Swartz SL, Levine L, Podolsky S, Dluhy RG, Williams GH. Contribution of prostaglandins to the antihypertensive action of captopril in essential hypertension. *Hypertension* (1981) 3, 168–73.
2. Smith SR, Coffman TM, Svetkey LP. Effect of low-dose aspirin on thromboxane production and the antihypertensive effect of captopril. *J Am Soc Nephrol* (1993) 4, 1133–9.
3. Guazzi MD, Campodonico J, Celeste F, Guazzi M, Santambrogio G, Rossi M, Trabattoni D, Alimento M. Antihypertensive efficacy of angiotensin converting enzyme inhibition and aspirin counteraction. *Clin Pharmacol Ther* (1998) 63, 79–86.
4. Nawarskas JJ, Townsend RR, Cirigliano MD, Spinler SA. Effect of aspirin on blood pressure in hypertensive patients taking enalapril or losartan. *Am J Hypertens* (1999) 12, 784–9.
5. Polónia J, Boaventura I, Gama G, Camões I, Bernardo F, Andrade P, Nunes JP, Brandão F, Cerqueira-Gomes M. Influence of non-steroidal anti-inflammatory drugs on renal function and 24 h ambulatory blood pressure-reducing effects of enalapril and nifedipine gastrointestinal therapeutic system in hypertensive patients. *J Hypertens* (1995) 13, 925–31.
6. Avanzini F, Palumbo G, Alli C, Roncaglioni MC, Ronchi E, Cristofari M, Capra A, Rossi S, Nosotti L, Costantini C, Pietrofeso R. Collaborative Group of the Primary Prevention Project (PPP)–Hypertension study. Effects of low-dose aspirin on clinic and ambulatory blood pressure in treated hypertensive patients. *Am J Hypertens* (2000) 13, 611–16.
7. Zanchetti A, Hansson L, Leonetti G, Rahn K-H, Ruilope L, Warnold I, Wedel H. Low-dose aspirin does not interfere with the blood pressure-lowering effects of antihypertensive therapy. *J Hypertens* (2002) 20, 1015–22.
8. Viecili PR, Pamplona D, Park M, Silva SR, Ramires JAF, da Luz PL. Antagonism of the acute hemodynamic effects of captopril in decompensated congestive heart failure by aspirin administration. *Braz J Med Biol Res* (2003) 36, 771–80.
9. Davie AP, Love MP, McMurray JJV. Even low-dose aspirin inhibits arachidonic acid-induced vasodilation in heart failure. *Clin Pharmacol Ther* (2000) 67, 530–7.
10. Guazzi M, Pontone G, Agostoni P. Aspirin worsens exercise performance and pulmonary gas exchange in patients with heart failure who are taking angiotensin-converting enzyme inhibitors. *Am Heart J* (1999) 138, 254–60.
11. Mahé I, Meune C, Diemer M, Caulin C, Bergmann J-F. Interaction between aspirin and ACE inhibitors in patients with heart failure. *Drug Safety* (2001) 24, 167–82.
12. Spaulding C, Charbonnier B, Cohen-Solal A, Juillière Y, Kromer EP, Benhamda K, Cador R, Weber S. Acute hemodynamic interaction of aspirin and ticlopidine with enalapril. Results of a double-blind, randomized comparative trial. *Circulation* (1998) 98, 757–65.
13. Hall D. The aspirin—angiotensin-converting enzyme inhibitor tradeoff: to halve and halve not. *J Am Coll Cardiol* (2000) 35, 1808–12.
14. Latini R, Tognoni G, Maggioni AP, Baigent C, Braunwald E, Chen Z-M, Collins R, Flather M, Franzosi MG, Kjekshus J, Køber L, Liu L-S, Peto R, Pfeffer M, Pizzetti F, Santoro E, Sleight P, Swedberg K, Tavazzi L, Wang W, Yusuf S, on behalf of the Angiotensin-converting Enzyme Inhibitor Myocardial Infarction Collaborative Group. Clinical effects of early angiotensin-converting enzyme inhibitor treatment for acute myocardial infarction are similar in the presence and absence of aspirin. Systematic overview of individual data from 96,712 randomized patients. *J Am Coll Cardiol* (2000) 35 1801–7.
15. Harjai KJ, Nunez E, Turgut T, Newman J. Effect of combined aspirin and angiotensin-converting enzyme inhibitor therapy versus angiotensin-converting enzyme inhibitor therapy alone on readmission rates in heart failure. *Am J Cardiol* (2001) 87, 483–7.
16. Harjai KJ, Solis S, Prasad A, Loupe J. Use of aspirin in conjunction with angiotensin-converting enzyme inhibitors does not worsen long-term survival in heart failure. *Int J Cardiol* (2003) 88, 207–14.
17. Krumholz HM, Chen Y-T, Wang Y, Radford MJ. Aspirin and angiotensin-converting enzyme inhibitors among elderly survivors of hospitalization for an acute myocardial infarction. *Arch Intern Med* (2001) 161, 538–44.
18. McAlister FA, Ghali WA, Gong Y, Fang J, Armstrong PW, Tu JV. Aspirin use and outcomes in a community-based cohort of 7352 patients discharged after first hospitalization for heart failure. *Circulation* (2006) 113, 2572–8.
19. Auméqeat V, Lamblin N, de Groote P, Mc Fadden EP, Millaire A, Bauters C, Lablanche J-M. Aspirin does not adversely affect survival in patients with stable congestive heart failure treated with angiotensin-converting enzyme inhibitors. *Chest* (2003) 124, 1250–8.
20. Guazzi M, Brambilla R, Rèina G, Tumminello G, Guazzi MD. Aspirin-angiotensin-converting enzyme inhibitor coadministration and mortality in patients with heart failure: a dose-related adverse effect of aspirin. *Arch Intern Med* (2003) 163, 1574–9.
21. Seelig CB, Maloley PA, Campbell JR. Nephrotoxicity associated with concomitant ACE inhibitor and NSAID therapy. *South Med J* (1990) 83, 1144–8.
22. Sioufi A, Pommier F, Gauducheau N, Godbillon J, Choi L, John V. The absence of a pharmacokinetic interaction between aspirin and the angiotensin-converting enzyme inhibitor benazepril in healthy volunteers. *Biopharm Drug Dispos* (1994) 15, 451–61.
23. Massie BM, Teerlink JR. Interaction between aspirin and angiotensin-converting enzyme inhibitors: real or imagined. *Am J Med* (2000) 109, 431–3.
24. Nawarskas JJ, Spinler SA. Update on the interaction between aspirin and angiotensin-converting enzyme inhibitors. *Pharmacotherapy* (2000) 20, 698–710.
25. Stys T, Lawson WE, Smaldone GC, Stys A. Does aspirin attenuate the beneficial effects of angiotensin-converting enzyme inhibition in heart failure? *Arch Intern Med* (2000) 160, 1409–13.
26. Barbash IM, Goldbourt U, Gottlieb S, Behar S, Leor J. Possible interaction between aspirin and ACE inhibitors: update on unresolved controversy. *Congest Heart Fail* (2000) 6, 313–18.
27. Cleland JGF, John J, Houghton T. Does aspirin attenuate the effect of angiotensin-converting enzyme inhibitors in hypertension or heart failure? *Curr Opin Nephrol Hypertens* (2001) 10, 625–31.
28. Peterson JG, Lauer MS. Using aspirin and ACE inhibitors in combination: why the hullabaloo? *Cleve Clin J Med* (2001) 68, 569–74.
29. Olson KL. Combined aspirin/ACE inhibitor treatment for CHF. *Ann Pharmacother* (2001) 35, 1653–8.
30. Park MH. Should aspirin be used with angiotensin-converting enzyme inhibitors in patients with chronic heart failure? *Congest Heart Fail* (2003) 9, 206–11.
31. Konstam MA. Aspirin and heart failure: square evidence meets a round patient. *Congest Heart Fail* (2003) 9, 203–5.
32. Brunner-La Rocca HP. Interaction of angiotensin-converting enzyme inhibition and aspirin in congestive heart failure: long controversy finally resolved? *Chest* (2003) 124, 1192–4.
33. Hunt SA, Abraham WT, Chin MH, Feldman AM, Francis GS, Ganiats TG, Jessup M, Konstam MA, Mancini DM, Michl K, Oates JA, Rahko PS, Silver MA, Stevenson LW, Yancy CW, Antman EM, Smith SC Jr, Adams CD, Anderson JL, Faxon DP, Fuster V, Halperin JL, Hiratzka LF, Hunt SA, Jacobs AK, Nishimura R, Ornato JP, Page RL, Riegel B; American College of Cardiology; American Heart Association Task Force on Practice Guidelines; American College of Chest Physicians; International Society for Heart and Lung Transplantation; Heart Rhythm Society. ACC/AHA 2005 Guideline Update for the Diagnosis and Management of Chronic Heart Failure in the Adult: a report of the American College of Cardiology/American Heart Association Task Force on Practice Guidelines (Writing Committee to Update the 2001 Guidelines for the Evaluation and Management of Heart Failure): developed in collaboration with the American College of Chest Physicians and the International Society for Heart and Lung Transplantation: endorsed by the Heart Rhythm Society. *Circulation* (2005) 112, e154–235. Available at: http://circ.ahajournals.org/cgi/content/full/112/12/e154 (accessed 14/08/07).
34. Swedberg K, Cleland J, Dargie H, Drexler H, Follath F, Komajda M, Tavazzi L, Smiseth OA, Gavazzi A, Haverich A, Hoes A, Jaarsma T, Korewicki J, Lévy S, Linde C, Lopez-Sendon J-L, Nieminen MS, Piérard L, Remme WJ; The Task Force for the Diagnosis and Treatment of CHF of the European Society of Cardiology. Guidelines for the diagnosis and treatment of chronic heart failure: full text (update 2005): The Task Force for the Diagnosis and Treatment of Chronic Heart Failure of the European Society of Cardiology. *Eur Heart J* (2005) 26, 1115–40. Available at: http://www.escardio.org/NR/rdonlyres/8A2848B4-5DEB-41B9-9A0A-5B5A90494B64/0/CHFFullTexteh205FVFW170505.pdf (accessed 14/08/07).
35. National Institute for Clinical Excellence. Chronic heart failure: management of chronic heart failure in adults in primary and secondary care (issued July 2003). Available at http://www.nice.org.uk/pdf/CG5NICEguideline.pdf (accessed 14/08/07).

ACE inhibitors + Azathioprine

Anaemia has been seen in patients given azathioprine with enalapril or captopril. Leucopenia occasionally occurs when captopril is given with azathioprine.

Clinical evidence

(a) Anaemia

Nine out of 11 kidney transplant patients taking ACE inhibitors (**enalapril** or **captopril**) had a fall in their haematocrit from 34% to 27%, and a fall in their haemoglobin from 11.6 g/dL to 9.5 g/dL when ciclosporin was replaced by azathioprine. Two patients were switched back to ciclosporin, and had a prompt rise in their haematocrit. Another 10 patients taking both drugs similarly developed a degree of anaemia, when compared with 10 others not taking an ACE inhibitor (haematocrit of 33% compared with 41%, and a haemoglobin of 11.5 g/dL compared with 13.9 g/dL).[1] A later study by the same group of workers (again in patients taking **enalapril** or **captopril**) confirmed these findings: however, no pharmacokinetic interaction was found between **enalapril** and azathioprine.[2]

(b) Leucopenia

A patient whose white cell count fell sharply when taking both **captopril** 50 mg daily and azathioprine 150 mg daily, did not develop leucopenia when each drug was given separately.[3] Another patient who was given **captopril** (increased to 475 mg daily [sic] then reduced to 100 mg daily) immediately after discontinuing azathioprine, developed leucopenia. She was later successfully treated with **captopril** 4 to 6 mg daily [sic].[4] Other patients have similarly shown leucopenia when given both drugs;[5,6] in one case this did not recur when the patient was rechallenged with **captopril** alone (at a lower dose).[6]

Mechanism

The anaemia appears to be due to suppression of erythropoietin by the ACE inhibitors, and azathioprine may cause patients to be more susceptible to this effect.[2] The cause of the leucopenia is unknown. It may just be due to the additive effects of both drugs.

Importance and management

Anaemia caused by captopril and enalapril has been seen in kidney transplant patients and in dialysis patients (see 'ACE inhibitors and Angiotensin II receptor antagonists + Epoetin', p.25). The evidence that this effect can be potentiated by azathioprine is limited, but it would be prudent to monitor well if these drugs are used together.

The evidence that the concurrent use of ACE inhibitors and azathioprine increases the risk of leucopenia is also limited. However, the UK manufacturer of captopril recommends that captopril should be used with extreme caution in patients receiving **immunosuppressants**, especially if there is renal impairment. They advise that in such patients differential white blood cell counts should be performed before starting captopril, then every 2 weeks in the first 3 months of treatment, and periodically thereafter.[7] The UK manufacturers of a number of other ACE inhibitors also state in their prescribing information that the use of ACE inhibitors with **cytostatic** or **immunosuppressive drugs** may lead to an increased risk of leucopenia. For other potential interactions with ACE inhibitors that might lead to an increased risk of leucopenia, see also 'ACE inhibitors + Allopurinol', p.13, and 'ACE inhibitors + Procainamide', p.33.

1. Gossmann J, Kachel H-G, Schoeppe W, Scheuermann E-H. Anemia in renal transplant recipients caused by concomitant therapy with azathioprine and angiotensin-converting enzyme inhibitors. *Transplantation* (1993) 56, 585–9.
2. Gossmann J, Thürmann P, Bachmann T, Weller S, Kachel H-G, Schoeppe W, Scheuermann E-H. Mechanism of angiotensin converting enzyme inhibitor-related anemia in renal transplant recipients. *Kidney Int* (1996) 50, 973–8.
3. Kirchertz EJ, Gröne HJ, Rieger J, Hölscher M, Scheler F. Successful low dose captopril rechallenge following drug-induced leucopenia. *Lancet* (1981) i, 1363.
4. Case DB, Whitman HH, Laragh JH, Spiera H. Successful low dose captopril rechallenge following drug-induced leucopenia. *Lancet* (1981) i, 1362–3.
5. Elijovisch F, Krakoff LR. Captopril associated granulocytopenia in hypertension after renal transplantation. *Lancet* (1980), i, 927–8.
6. Edwards CRW, Drury P, Penketh A, Damluji SA. Successful reintroduction of captopril following neutropenia. *Lancet* (1981) i, 723.
7. Capoten (Captopril). E. R. Squibb & Sons Ltd. UK Summary of product characteristics, June 2005.

ACE inhibitors + Beta blockers

The combination of an ACE inhibitor with a beta blocker is in established clinical use. Enhanced blood pressure-lowering effects occur, as would be expected. Although not all combinations have been studied, no clinically significant pharmacokinetic interactions appear to occur between the ACE inhibitors and beta blockers.

Clinical evidence

(a) Atenolol

In a double-blind, crossover study in hypertensive subjects, the combination of atenolol 50 mg once daily and **enalapril** 20 mg once daily increased the hypotensive effect of either drug alone, but the effect was 30 to 50% less than additive.[1]

(b) Bisoprolol

In a single-dose, placebo-controlled, crossover study in 16 healthy men, bisoprolol 5 mg given with **imidapril** 10 mg did not significantly influence the pharmacokinetics of its active metabolite imidaprilat, and the pharmacodynamic effects, including blood pressure and heart rate reductions, were mainly additive.[2]

(c) Propranolol

Propranolol 80 mg three times daily did not affect the pharmacokinetics of a single 20-mg dose of **quinapril** in 10 healthy subjects.[3] The pharmacokinetics of **ramipril** 5 mg daily were unaffected by propranolol 40 mg twice daily.[4] Similarly, the manufacturer of **fosinopril** reports that the bioavailability of fosinoprilat, its active metabolite, was not altered by propranolol.[5,6] Another study found no significant pharmacokinetic interaction between **cilazapril** 2.5 mg daily and propranolol 120 mg daily in healthy subjects, but the reductions in blood pressure were about doubled and long-lasting in healthy subjects and in patients with hypertension.[7,8]

Mechanism, importance and management

Both ACE inhibitors and beta blockers lower blood pressure by different mechanisms, and therefore the enhanced blood pressure-lowering effects of the combination would be expected. No pharmacokinetic interactions have been demonstrated. The combination of an ACE inhibitor and a beta blocker is clinically useful in a number of cardiovascular disorders.

1. Wing LMH, Chalmers JP, West MJ, Russell AE, Morris MJ, Cain MD, Bune AJC, Southgate DO. Enalapril and atenolol in essential hypertension: attenuation of hypotensive effects in combination. *Clin Exp Hypertens* (1988) 10, 119–33.
2. Breithaupt-Grögler K, Ungethüm W, Meurer-Witt B, Belz GG. Pharmacokinetic and dynamic interactions of the angiotensin-converting enzyme inhibitor imidapril with hydrochlorothiazide, bisoprolol and nilvadipine. *Eur J Clin Pharmacol* (2001) 57, 275–84.
3. Horvath AM, Pilon D, Caillé G, Colburn WA, Ferry JJ, Frank GJ, Lacasse Y, Olson SC. Multiple-dose propranolol administration does not influence the single dose pharmacokinetics of quinapril and its active metabolite (quinaprilat). *Biopharm Drug Dispos* (1990) 11, 191–6.
4. van Griensven JMT, Seibert-Grafe M, Schoemaker HC, Frölich M, Cohen AF. The pharmacokinetic and pharmacodynamic interactions of ramipril with propranolol. *Eur J Clin Pharmacol* (1993) 45, 255–60.
5. Staril (Fosinopril sodium). E. R. Squibb & Sons Ltd. UK Summary of product characteristics, June 2005.
6. Monopril (Fosinopril sodium). Bristol-Myers Squibb Company. US Prescribing information, July 2003.
7. Belz GG, Essig J, Kleinbloesem CH, Hoogkamer JFW, Wiegand UW, Wellstein A. Interactions between cilazapril and propranolol in man; plasma drug concentrations, hormone and enzyme responses, haemodynamics, agonist dose-effect curves and baroreceptor reflex. *Br J Clin Pharmacol* (1988) 26, 547–56.
8. Belz GG, Essig J, Erb K, Breithaupt K, Hoogkamer JFW, Kneer J, Kleinbloesem CH. Pharmacokinetic and pharmacodynamic interactions between the ACE inhibitor cilazapril and β-adrenoceptor antagonist propranolol in healthy subjects and in hypertensive patients. *Br J Clin Pharmacol* (1989) 27, 317S–322S.

ACE inhibitors + Calcium-channel blockers

The combination of an ACE inhibitor and a dihydropyridine calcium-channel blocker is in established clinical use for hypertension, and, although only certain combinations have been studied, no clinically significant pharmacokinetic interactions appear to

occur between the dihydropyridine-type calcium-channel blockers and ACE inhibitors.

Clinical evidence

(a) Amlodipine

A study in 12 healthy subjects indicated that there was no pharmacokinetic interaction between single doses of amlodipine 5 mg and **benazepril** 10 mg.[1]

(b) Felodipine

No pharmacokinetic interaction occurred between single doses of felodipine 10 mg and **ramipril** 5 mg in healthy subjects. The blood pressure-lowering effect of the combination was greater, and **ramipril** attenuated the reflex tachycardia caused by felodipine.[2]

(c) Manidipine

In a single-dose crossover study in 18 healthy subjects, the concurrent use of manidipine 10 mg and **delapril** 30 mg did not significantly alter the pharmacokinetics of either drug or their main metabolites.[3]

(d) Nicardipine

In a study in 12 patients with hypertension taking **enalapril** 20 mg daily, the addition of nicardipine 30 mg three times daily for 2 weeks did not alter the pharmacokinetics of **enalapril**.[4] The manufacturer of **spirapril** briefly noted in a review that the concurrent use of spirapril and nicardipine increased **spirapril** plasma levels by about 25% and those of its active metabolite, spiraprilat, by about 45%. The bioavailability of nicardipine was reduced by 30%. It was assumed that the interaction took place at the absorption site. However, the changes were not considered clinically relevant.[5]

(e) Nifedipine

No evidence of either a pharmacokinetic or adverse pharmacodynamic interaction was seen in 12 healthy subjects given single doses of nifedipine retard 20 mg and **lisinopril** 20 mg; the effects on blood pressure were additive.[6] Similarly, there was no pharmacokinetic interaction between single doses of slow-release nifedipine 20 mg and **benazepril** 10 mg in healthy subjects; the effects on blood pressure were additive and the tachycardic effect of nifedipine was attenuated by benazepril.[7] The manufacturer of **fosinopril** notes that the bioavailability of fosinoprilat, the active metabolite, was not altered by nifedipine.[8,9] Similarly, the manufacturer of **moexipril** notes that no clinically important pharmacokinetic interaction occurred with nifedipine in healthy subjects.[10]

(f) Nilvadipine

In a single-dose, placebo-controlled, crossover study in 16 healthy subjects, no pharmacokinetic interaction occurred between nilvadipine 8 mg and **imidapril** 10 mg, and the pharmacodynamic effects, including the reduction in blood pressure and the decrease in total peripheral resistance, were mostly additive.[11]

Mechanism

No pharmacokinetic interactions are expected. Enhanced blood pressure-lowering effects occur, as would be expected.

Importance and management

No important pharmacokinetic interactions have been demonstrated. The combination of an ACE inhibitor and a dihydropyridine calcium-channel blocker is clinically useful in the treatment of hypertension. A number of products combining an ACE inhibitor with a calcium-channel blocker are available. It is generally advised that these combination products are only used in patients who have already been stabilised on the individual components in the same proportions.

1. Sun JX, Cipriano A, Chan K, John VA. Pharmacokinetic interaction study between benazepril and amlodipine in healthy subjects. *Eur J Clin Pharmacol* (1994) 47, 285–9.
2. Bainbridge AD, MacFadyen RJ, Lees KR, Reid JL. A study of the acute pharmacodynamic interaction of ramipril and felodipine in normotensive subjects. *Br J Clin Pharmacol* (1991) 31, 148–53.
3. Stockis A, Gengler C, Goethals F, Jeanbaptiste B, Lens S, Poli G, Acerbi D. Single oral dose pharmacokinetic interaction study of manidipine and delapril in healthy volunteers. *Arzneimittelforschung* (2003) 53, 627–34.
4. Donnelly R, Elliott HL, Reid JL. Nicardipine combined with enalapril in patients with essential hypertension. *Br J Clin Pharmacol* (1986) 22, 283S–287S.
5. Grass P, Gerbeau C, Kutz K. Spirapril: pharmacokinetic properties and drug interactions. *Blood Pressure* (1994) 3 (Suppl 2), 7–13.
6. Lees KR, Reid JL. Lisinopril and nifedipine: no acute interaction in normotensives. *Br J Clin Pharmacol* (1988) 25, 307–13.
7. Jakobsen J, Glaus L, Graf P, Degen P, Maurice NP, Bellet M, Ménard J. Unmasking of the hypotensive effect of nifedipine in normotensives by addition of the angiotensin converting enzyme inhibitor benazepril. *J Hypertens* (1992) 10, 1045–51.
8. Staril (Fosinopril sodium). E. R. Squibb & Sons Ltd. UK Summary of product characteristics, June 2005.
9. Monopril (Fosinopril sodium). Bristol-Myers Squibb Company. US Prescribing information, July 2003.
10. Perdix (Moexipril hydrochloride). Schwarz Pharma Ltd. UK Summary of product characteristics, July 2006.
11. Breithaupt-Grögler K, Ungethüm W, Meurer-Witt B, Belz GG. Pharmacokinetic and dynamic interactions of the angiotensin-converting enzyme inhibitor imidapril with hydrochlorothiazide, bisoprolol and nilvadipine. *Eur J Clin Pharmacol* (2001) 57, 275–84.

ACE inhibitors + Capsaicin

An isolated report describes a woman taking an ACE inhibitor who developed a cough each time she used a topical cream containing capsaicin.

Clinical evidence, mechanism, importance and management

A 53-year-old woman who had been taking an unnamed ACE inhibitor for several years, complained of cough each time she applied *Axsain*, a cream containing capsaicin 0.075%, to her lower extremities. Whether this reaction would have occurred without the ACE inhibitor was not determined,[1] but cough is a recognised adverse effect of ACE inhibitors and pre-treatment with an ACE inhibitor has been shown to enhance the cough caused by inhaled capsaicin.[1] This potential interaction is probably of little general clinical importance.

1. Hakas JF. Topical capsaicin induces cough in patient receiving ACE inhibitor. *Ann Allergy* (1990) 65, 322.

ACE inhibitors + Clonidine

Potentiation of the antihypertensive effect of clonidine by ACE inhibitors can be clinically useful.[1] However, limited evidence suggests that the effects of captopril may be delayed when patients are switched from clonidine.[2] Note that sudden withdrawal of clonidine may cause rebound hypertension.

1. Catapres Tablets (Clonidine hydrochloride). Boehringer Ingelheim Ltd. UK Summary of product characteristics, May 2006.
2. Gröne H-J, Kirchertz EJ, Rieger J. Mögliche Komplikationen und Probleme der Captopriltherapie bei Hypertonikern mit ausgeprägten Gefäßschäden. *Therapiewoche* (1981) 31, 5280–7.

ACE inhibitors + Colloids

Acute hypotension has been seen in a few patients taking enalapril when they were given a rapid infusion of albumin-containing stable plasma protein solution (SPPS). Another case occurred in an infant taking captopril when given albumin 4%. A few other cases have been described with gelatin-type colloids in patients taking ACE inhibitors (cilazapril, enalapril, lisinopril).

Clinical evidence

(a) Albumin

A woman taking **enalapril** 10 mg in the morning, underwent surgery for groin lymph node resection under spinal and general anaesthesia. When she was given a rapid infusion of 500 mL of the albumin solution, **stable plasma protein solution** (**SPPS**, *Commonwealth Serum Laboratories, Melbourne, Australia*), her pulse rose to 90 to 100 bpm and systolic blood pressure fell from 100 to 60 mmHg and a red flush was noted on all exposed skin. The blood pressure was controlled at 90 to 95 mmHg with metaraminol 4.5 mg, given over 10 minutes. When the **SPPS** was finished, the blood pressure and pulse rate spontaneously restabilised.[1] **SPPS** is a 5% plasma protein solution prepared by the cold ethanol fractionation process and pasteurisation from human plasma (volunteer donors). It contains sodium octanoate as a stabiliser.[1] Two very similar cases have been recorded in patients taking **enalapril** when given **SPPS**.[2,3] The manufacturer of **SPPS** notes that **captopril** has also been involved in this hypotensive interaction.[4]

A 20-month-old infant taking **captopril** was haemodynamically stable for 35 minutes after induction of anaesthesia while awaiting a donor kidney, but then developed hypotension after a bolus dose of 20 mL of albumin 4% (*Albumex*) was given. This was reversed with dopamine infusion.[5]

(b) Gelatin-based colloids

A report describes 3 cases of severe hypotension in patients taking ACE inhibitors (**lisinopril, enalapril**) while undergoing joint replacement surgery, and after they had been given a gelatin-based plasma expander (*Gelofusin*), which contains 4% succinylated gelatin in saline. The hypotension was resistant to ephedrine and methoxamine, and responded to adrenaline or dobutamine, which was required for 24 hours and 3 days in two cases. Anaphylactoid reactions were excluded as a cause of the hypotension.[6] In another similar case, a patient taking **cilazapril** developed hypotension refractory to sodium chloride 0.9% after induction of anaesthesia, and this worsened when a gelatin-type colloid (*Gelafundina*) was given.[7]

Mechanism

Not fully established, but it is believed that SPPS contains low levels of pre-kallikrein activator, which stimulates the production of bradykinin, which can cause vasodilatation and hypotension. Normally the bradykinin is destroyed by kininase II (ACE), but this is delayed by the ACE inhibitor so that the hypotensive effects are exaggerated and prolonged.[3,8] In the case with albumin 4%, a sample of the albumin used was analysed, and it was found to contain less prekallikrein activating factor than maximum permissible levels.[5] It was suggested that the infusion of gelatin-based colloids somehow resulted in raised plasma kinin levels associated with inhibition of ACE.[6]

Importance and management

The interaction with SPPS would appear to be established and of clinical importance, and would apply to all ACE inhibitors. The author of one report suggested that if rapid expansion of intravascular volume is needed in patients taking ACE inhibitors, an artificial colloid might be a safer choice than SPPS.[1] The manufacturer of SPPS also recommended using an alternative plasma volume expander, including other albumin solutions.[4] It should be noted that following these reports SPPS was withdrawn from the Australasian market.[9] However, note that a case has also occurred with albumin 4%, and cases have also been attributed to synthetic colloid solutions containing gelatin. It may be that this is just an unpredictable effect of colloids in patients taking ACE inhibitors. See also 'Anaesthetics, general + Antihypertensives', p.94, for discussion of the marked hypotension sometimes seen during induction of anaesthesia in patients taking ACE inhibitors.

1. McKenzie AJ. Possible interaction between SPPS and enalapril. *Anaesth Intensive Care* (1990) 18, 124–6.
2. Young K. Enalapril and SPPS. *Anaesth Intensive Care* (1990) 18, 583.
3. Young K. Hypotension from the interaction of ACE inhibitors with stable plasma protein solution. *Anaesthesia* (1993) 48, 356.
4. Schiff P. SPPS, hypotension and ACE inhibitors. *Med J Aust* (1992) 156, 363.
5. Fong SY, Hansen TG. Perioperative hypotension following plasma volume expansion with albumin in an angiotensin-converting enzyme inhibited infant. *Br J Anaesth* (2000) 84, 537–8.
6. Powell CG, Unsworth DJ, McVey FK. Severe hypotension associated with angiotensin-converting enzyme inhibition in anaesthesia. *Anaesth Intensive Care* (1998) 26, 107–9.
7. Barber L, Barrio J, de Rojas MD, Ibañez F, Añó C, Alepuz R, Montero R. Hipotensión refractaria y sostenida durante una anestesia general asociada al tratamiento crónico con inhibidores de la enzima conversiva de la angiotensina. Rev Esp Anestesiol Reanim. (2001) 48, 34–7.
8. Bönner G, Preis S, Schunk U, Toussaint C, Kaufmann W. Hemodynamic effects of bradykinin on systemic and pulmonary circulation in healthy and hypertensive humans. *J Cardiovasc Pharmacol* (1990) 15 (Suppl 6), S46–S56.
9. McKenzie AJ. ACE inhibitors, colloid infusions and anaesthesia. *Anaesth Intensive Care* (1998) 26, 330.

ACE inhibitors + Co-trimoxazole or Trimethoprim

Two reports describe serious hyperkalaemia, apparently caused by the use of trimethoprim with enalapril or quinapril in association with renal impairment.

Clinical evidence

A 40-year-old woman with a lung transplant (taking ciclosporin, azathioprine, prednisolone, **enalapril**, gentamicin inhalation, salbutamol and acetylcysteine) developed life-threatening hyperkalaemia of 6.8 mmol/L when she was treated with high-dose co-trimoxazole 120 mg/kg daily for suspected Pneumocystis pneumonia. The co-trimoxazole (sulfamethoxazole/trimethoprim) and **enalapril** were stopped and she was treated with sodium chloride 0.9%, mannitol and furosemide. After 12 hours her serum potassium had decreased to 4.6 mmol/L and she began to recover over a period of a week, but she then developed fatal septic shock with multi-organ failure.[1]

In another case, an elderly man treated with **quinapril** 20 mg daily for essential hypertension was found to have hyperkalaemia (serum potassium 7 to 7.4 mmol/L) and azotaemia after 20 days of treatment with co-trimoxazole for mild acute pyelonephritis. Co-trimoxazole and **quinapril** were stopped, and nifedipine was given to control blood pressure. After treatment with dextrose, insulin, sodium polystyrene sulfonate and calcium gluconate, the azotaemia and hyperkalaemia resolved over 36 hours.[2]

Mechanism

Hyperkalaemia has been reported in patients receiving co-trimoxazole alone.[3] This is attributed to the trimethoprim component, which can have a potassium-sparing effect on the distal part of the kidney tubules. ACE inhibitors reduce aldosterone synthesis, which results in reduced renal loss of potassium. The interaction is probably due to the additive effects of these two mechanisms, compounded by impaired renal function.[1,2]

Importance and management

Clinical examples of this interaction seem to be few, but the possibility of hyperkalaemia with either trimethoprim or ACE inhibitors alone, particularly with other factors such as renal impairment, is well documented. Thus it may be prudent to monitor potassium levels if this combination is used. It has been suggested that trimethoprim should probably be avoided in elderly patients with chronic renal impairment taking ACE inhibitors, and that patients with AIDS taking an ACE inhibitor for associated nephropathy should probably discontinue this treatment during treatment with high-dose co-trimoxazole.[2]

1. Bugge JF. Severe hyperkalaemia induced by trimethoprim in combination with an angiotensin-converting enzyme inhibitor in a patient with transplanted lungs. *J Intern Med* (1996) 240, 249–52.
2. Thomas RJ. Severe hyperkalemia with trimethoprim-quinapril. *Ann Pharmacother* (1996) 30, 413–14.
3. Alappan R, Perazella MA, Buller GK. Hyperkalemia in hospitalized patients treated with trimethoprim-sulfamethoxazole. *Ann Intern Med* (1996) 124, 316–20.

ACE inhibitors + Dialysis or Transfusion membranes

An anaphylactoid reaction can occur in patients taking ACE inhibitors within a few minutes of starting haemodialysis using high-flux polyacrylonitrile membranes ('AN 69'). Anaphylactoid reactions have also been reported in patients taking ACE inhibitors undergoing low-density lipoprotein apheresis. In addition, hypotensive reactions associated with blood transfusions through leucoreduction filters have occurred in patients taking ACE inhibitors.

Clinical evidence, mechanism, importance and management

(a) High-flux dialysis

In a retrospective study, 9 of 236 haemodialysis patients treated with **high-flux polyacrylonitrile membranes ('AN 69')** were found to have had anaphylactoid reactions (severe hypotension, flushing, swelling of face and/or tongue, and dyspnoea) within 5 minutes of starting haemodialysis. Treatment with an ACE inhibitor had been recently started in all 9 patients (7 **enalapril**, 1 **captopril**, 1 **lisinopril**). The anaphylactoid reactions disappeared in all 6 patients who discontinued the ACE inhibitor. Two other patients were given a filter rinsing procedure (the 'Bioprime' rinse method) and a new dialysis membrane, and in the final patient further anaphylactoid reactions were prevented by cellulose-triacetate haemofiltration while the ACE inhibitor was continued.[1] Similar reactions have been reported elsewhere and are thought to be bradykinin mediated.[2,3] The CSM in the UK has advised that the combination of ACE inhibitors and such membranes should be avoided, either by substituting an alternative membrane or an alternative antihypertensive drug.[4]

(b) Lipoprotein apheresis

Anaphylactoid reactions occurred in 2 patients taking ACE inhibitors during removal of low-density lipoproteins (LDL apheresis) with dextran sulfate adsorption.[5] Further reactions were reported in 6 patients taking either **captopril** or **enalapril** and dextran sulfate apheresis. When the interval between the last dose of the ACE inhibitor and the apheresis was prolonged to 12 to 30 hours no further adverse reactions occurred.[6] However, other workers found lengthening the interval to be ineffective in one patient.[7] The manufacturer of **enalapril** suggests temporarily withholding the ACE inhibitor before each apheresis,[8] but other manufacturers of ACE inhibitors recommend using a different class of antihypertensive drug[9,10] or changing the method of lipoprotein reduction.[9,11]

(c) Transfusion reactions

A report describes 8 patients receiving ACE inhibitors and blood transfusions through bedside **leucoreduction filters** who experienced severe hypotensive reactions. The reactions were attributed to bradykinin generation during blood filtration and prevention of bradykinin breakdown due to the ACE inhibitors. Six of the patients tolerated subsequent transfusions, but 3 had discontinued their medication the day before the planned transfusion and one received washed (plasma-depleted) components. One patient experienced a second reaction, but then received washed red cells and had no reaction.[12]

1. Verresen L, Waer M, Vanrenterghem Y, Michielsen P. Angiotensin-converting-enzyme inhibitors and anaphylactoid reactions to high-flux membrane dialysis. *Lancet* (1990) 336, 1360–2.
2. Tielemans C, Madhoun P, Lenaers M, Schandene L, Goldman M, Vanherweghem JL. Anaphylactoid reactions during hemodialysis on AN69 membranes in patients receiving ACE inhibitors. *Kidney Int* (1990) 38, 982–4.
3. Tielemans C, Vanherweghem JL, Blumberg A, Cuvelier R, de Fremont JF, Dehout F, Dupont P, Richard C, Stolear JC, Wens R. ACE inhibitors and anaphylactoid reactions to high-flux membrane dialysis. *Lancet* (1991) 337, 370–1.
4. Committee on Safety of Medicines. Anaphylactoid reactions to high-flux polyacrylonitrile membranes in combination with ACE inhibitors. *Current Problems* (1992) 33, 2.
5. Olbricht CJ, Schaumann D, Fischer D. Anaphylactoid reactions, LDL apheresis with dextran sulphate, and ACE inhibitors. *Lancet* (1992) 340, 908–9.
6. Keller C, Grützmacher P, Bahr F, Schwarzbeck A, Kroon AA, Kiral A. LDL-apheresis with dextran sulphate and anaphylactoid reactions to ACE inhibitors. *Lancet* (1993) 341, 60–1.
7. Davidson DC, Peart I, Turner S, Sangster M. Prevention with icatibant of anaphylactoid reactions to ACE inhibitor during LDL apheresis. *Lancet* (1994) 343, 1575.
8. Innovace (Enalapril). Merck Sharp & Dohme Ltd. UK Summary of product characteristics, October 2005.
9. Capoten (Captopril). E. R. Squibb & Sons Ltd. UK Summary of product characteristics, June 2005.
10. Perdix (Moexipril hydrochloride). Schwarz Pharma Ltd. UK Summary of product characteristics, July 2006.
11. Accupro (Quinapril hydrochloride). Pfizer Ltd. UK Summary of product characteristics, March 2007.
12. Quillen K. Hypotensive transfusion reactions in patients taking angiotensin-converting-enzyme inhibitors. *N Engl J Med* (2000) 343, 1422–3.

ACE inhibitors + Diuretics; Loop, Thiazide and related

The combination of captopril or other ACE inhibitors with loop or thiazide diuretics is normally safe and effective, but 'first dose hypotension' (dizziness, lightheadedness, fainting) can occur, particularly if the dose of diuretic is high, and often in association with various predisposing conditions. Renal impairment, and even acute renal failure, have been reported. Diuretic-induced hypokalaemia may still occur when ACE inhibitors are used with these potassium-depleting diuretics.

Clinical evidence

(a) First dose hypotensive reaction

The concurrent use of **captopril** or other ACE inhibitors and loop or thiazide diuretics is normally safe and effective, but some patients experience 'first dose hypotension' (i.e. dizziness, lightheadedness, fainting) after taking the first one or two doses of the ACE inhibitor. This appears to be associated with, and exaggerated by, certain conditions (such as heart failure, renovascular hypertension, haemodialysis, high levels of renin and angiotensin, low-sodium diet, dehydration, diarrhoea or vomiting) and/or hypovolaemia and sodium depletion caused by diuretics, particularly in high doses. A study describes one woman whose blood pressure of 290/150 mmHg failed to respond to a 10-mg intravenous dose of **furosemide**. After 30 minutes she was given **captopril** 50 mg orally and within 45 minutes her blood pressure fell to 135/60 mmHg, and she required an infusion of saline to maintain her blood pressure.[1] In another study, a man developed severe postural hypotension shortly after **furosemide** was added to **captopril** treatment.[2]

Starting with a low dose of the ACE inhibitor reduces the risk of first-dose hypotension. In a study in 8 patients with hypertension, treated with a diuretic (mainly **furosemide** or **hydrochlorothiazide**) for at least 4 weeks, **captopril** was started in small increasing doses from 6.25 mg. Symptomatic postural hypotension was seen in 2 of the 8 patients, but was only mild and transient.[3]

Hypotension is more common in patients with heart failure who are receiving large doses of diuretics. In a study in 124 patients with severe heart failure, all receiving **furosemide** (mean dose 170 mg daily; range 80 to 500 mg daily) and 90 also receiving the potassium-sparing diuretic spironolactone, the addition of **captopril** caused transient symptomatic hypotension in 44% of subjects. The **captopril** dose had to be reduced, and in 8 patients it was later discontinued. In addition, four patients developed symptomatic hypotension after 1 to 2 months of treatment, and **captopril** was also discontinued in these patients.[4]

There is some evidence that in patients with heart failure the incidence of marked orthostatic hypotension requiring treatment discontinuation in the first 36 hours was lower with **perindopril** 2 mg once daily than **captopril** 6.25 mg three times daily (6 of 357 cases versus 16 of 368 cases, respectively).[5]

(b) Hypokalaemia

In one study, the reduction in plasma potassium was greater with **hydrochlorothiazide** 25 mg daily than with **hydrochlorothiazide** combined with **cilazapril** 2.5 mg daily, showing that cilazapril reduced the potassium-depleting effect of **hydrochlorothiazide**.[6] In one analysis, 7 of 21 patients taking potassium-depleting diuretics given ACE inhibitors for heart failure developed hypokalaemia. This was corrected by potassium supplementation in 2 cases, an increase in the ACE inhibitor dose in 3 cases, and the use of a potassium-sparing diuretic in the remaining 2 cases.[7] In another report, a woman taking **furosemide** 80 to 120 mg daily remained hypokalaemic despite also taking **ramipril** 10 mg daily and spironolactone 50 to 200 mg daily.[8] However, note that the addition of 'spironolactone', (p.23) to ACE inhibitors and loop or thiazide diuretics has generally resulted in an increased incidence of hyperkalaemia.

(c) Hyponatraemia

An isolated report describes a patient who developed severe hyponatraemia 3 days after **bendroflumethiazide** 10 mg daily was added to treatment with **enalapril** 20 mg daily and atenolol 100 mg daily. However, on 2 other occasions she only developed mild hyponatraemia when given **bendroflumethiazide** alone.[9] An earlier study reported changes in sodium balance due to **captopril** in all 6 patients with renovascular hypertension and in 11 of 12 patients with essential hypertension; sodium loss occurred in 12 of the 18 patients.[1]

(d) Impairment of renal function

The risk of ACE inhibitor-induced renal impairment in patients with or without renovascular disease can be potentiated by diuretics.[10-13] In an analysis of 74 patients who had been treated with **captopril** or **lisinopril**, reversible acute renal failure was more common in those who were also treated with a diuretic (**furosemide** and/or **hydrochlorothiazide**) than those who were not (11 of 33 patients compared with 1 of 41 patients).[12] Similarly, in a prescription-event monitoring study, **enalapril** was associated with raised creatinine or urea in 75 patients and it was thought to have contributed to the deterioration in renal function and subsequent deaths in 10 of these patients. However, 9 of these 10 were also receiving loop or thiazide diuretics, sometimes in high doses.[14] Retrospective analysis of a controlled study in patients with hypertensive nephrosclerosis identified 8 of 34 patients who developed reversible renal impairment when treated with **enalapril** and various other antihypertensives including a diuretic (**furosemide** or **hydrochlorothiazide**). In contrast, 23 patients treated with placebo and various other antihypertensives did not develop renal impairment. Subsequently, **enalapril** was tolerated by 7 of the 8 patients without deterioration in renal function and 6 of these patients later received diuretics.[15] One patient was again treated with **enalapril** with recurrence of renal impairment, but discontinuation of the diuretics (**furosemide**, **hydrochlorothiazide**, and triamterene) led to an improvement in renal function despite the continuation of **enalapril**.[16]

Renal impairment in patients taking ACE inhibitors and diuretics has also been described in patients with heart failure. A patient with congestive heart failure and pre-existing moderate renal impairment developed acute non-oliguric renal failure while taking **enalapril** 20 mg daily and **furosemide** 60 to 80 mg daily, which resolved when the sodium balance was restored.[17] In a study involving 90 patients with severe congestive heart failure who were receiving **furosemide** and spironolactone, a decline in renal function occurred in 18 patients during the first month after initiation of **captopril** treatment; mean serum creatinine levels rose from 220 to 300 micromol/L. All the patients were receiving high daily doses of **furosemide** and all had renal impairment before receiving the first dose of **captopril**.[4]

Acute, fatal, renal failure developed in 2 patients with cardiac failure within 4 weeks of being treated with **enalapril** and **furosemide**, and in 2 similar patients renal impairment developed over a longer period.[18] Reversible renal failure developed in a patient with congestive heart failure when **captopril** and **metolazone** were given.[19]

(e) Pharmacokinetic and diuresis studies

1. Furosemide. A study in healthy subjects given single doses of **enalapril** and furosemide found no evidence of any pharmacokinetic interaction between these drugs.[20] Another study in hypertensive patients found that **captopril** did not affect the urinary excretion of furosemide, nor its subsequent diuretic effects.[21] However, a further study in healthy subjects showed that, although **captopril** did not alter urinary excretion of furosemide, it did reduce diuresis.[22] Yet another study in healthy subjects found that **captopril** reduced the urinary excretion of furosemide, and reduced the diuretic response during the first 20 minutes to approximately 50%, and the natriuretic response to almost 30%, whereas **enalapril** and **ramipril** did not significantly alter the diuretic effects of furosemide.[23] In one single-dose study in healthy subjects the concurrent use of **benazepril** and furosemide reduced the urinary excretion of furosemide by 10 to 20%, whereas **benazepril** pharmacokinetics were unaffected.[24] **Lisinopril** did not alter plasma levels or urinary excretion of furosemide in one study, nor did it alter urinary electrolyte excretion.[25] Similarly, furosemide did not affect the pharmacokinetics of **lisinopril** either in single-dose or multiple-dose regimens.[26]

2. Hydrochlorothiazide. In a single-dose, randomised, crossover study in 19 elderly patients the pharmacokinetics of **enalapril** 10 mg were unaffected by hydrochlorothiazide 25 mg. However, there was a significant reduction in renal clearance and a significant increase in the AUC of its metabolite, enalaprilat, resulting in higher serum levels of the active drug. This acute interaction was not thought to be clinically significant for long-term use.[27] No pharmacokinetic interaction occurred between **cilazapril** and hydrochlorothiazide in healthy subjects or patients with hypertension.[6] Similarly, no significant pharmacokinetic interaction occurred between **imidapril** and hydrochlorothiazide in healthy subjects[28] and neither **captopril** nor **ramipril** altered the diuresis induced by hydrochlorothiazide.[23] The manufacturer of **spirapril** briefly noted in a review that there was no clinically relevant pharmacokinetic interaction between **spirapril** and hydrochlorothiazide.[29] Furthermore no pharmacokinetic interaction was found when **spirapril** and hydrochlorothiazide were given together as a bi-layer tablet.[30] There was no clinically important pharmacokinetic interaction when **moexipril** was given with hydrochlorothiazide in a single-dose study in healthy subjects.[31]

Mechanism

The first dose hypotension interaction is not fully understood. One suggestion is that if considerable amounts of salt and water have already been lost as a result of using a diuretic, the resultant depletion in the fluid volume (hypovolaemia) transiently exaggerates the hypotensive effects of the ACE inhibitor.

The cases of hypokalaemia are simply a result of the potassium-depleting effects of the diuretics outweighing the potassium-conserving effects of the ACE inhibitor. The converse can also occur.

Thiazides can cause hyponatraemia, but this enhanced effect may have been due to an alteration in renal haemodynamics caused by the ACE inhibitor; sustained angiotensin-converting enzyme blockade can produce natriuresis.[1]

Marked decreases in blood pressure may affect renal function, and in addition, the renin-angiotensin system plays an important role in the maintenance of the glomerular filtration rate when renal artery pressure is diminished.[11] However, diuretic-induced sodium depletion may also be an important factor in the renal impairment sometimes observed with ACE inhibitors.

Importance and management

The **'first dose hypotension'** interaction between ACE inhibitors and diuretics is well established. The BNF in the UK notes that the risk is higher when the dose of diuretic is greater than furosemide 80 mg daily or equivalent,[32] and suggest that, in patients taking these doses of diuretics, consideration should be given to temporarily stopping the diuretic or reducing its dosage a few days before the ACE inhibitor is added. If this is not considered clinically appropriate, the first dose of the ACE inhibitor should be given under close supervision. In all patients taking diuretics, therapy with ACE inhibitors should be started with a very low dose, even in patients at low risk (e.g. those with uncomplicated essential hypertension on low-dose thiazides). To be on the safe side, all patients should be given a simple warning about what can happen and what to do when they first start concurrent use. The immediate problem (dizziness, lightheadedness, faintness), if it occurs, can usually be solved by the patient lying down. Taking the first dose of the ACE inhibitor just before bedtime is also preferable. Any marked hypotension is normally transient, but if problems persist it may be necessary temporarily to reduce the diuretic dosage. There is usually no need to avoid the combination just because an initially large hypotensive response has occurred.

A number of products combining an ACE inhibitor with a thiazide diuretic are available for the treatment of hypertension. These products should be used only in those patients who have been stabilised on the individual components in the same proportions.

The use of ACE inhibitors in patients taking potassium-depleting diuretics does not always prevent **hypokalaemia** developing. Serum potassium should be monitored.

There is only an isolated report of **hyponatraemia**, but be aware that ACE inhibitors may affect the natriuresis caused by diuretics.

The cases of **renal impairment** cited emphasise the need to monitor renal function in patients on ACE inhibitors and diuretics. If increases in blood urea and creatinine occur, a dosage reduction and/or discontinuation of the diuretic and/or ACE inhibitor may be required. In a statement, the American Heart Association comments that acute renal failure complicating ACE inhibitor therapy is almost always reversible and repletion of extracellular fluid volume and discontinuation of diuretic therapy is the most effective approach. In addition, withdrawal of interacting drugs, supportive management of fluid and electrolytes, and temporary dialysis, where indicated, are the mainstays of therapy.[13] Combined use of ACE inhibitors, diuretics and NSAIDs may be particularly associated with an increased risk of renal failure, see 'ACE inhibitors + NSAIDs', p.28.

The possibility of undiagnosed renal artery stenosis should also be considered.

None of the **pharmacokinetic** changes observed appear to be clinically significant.

1. Case DB, Atlas SA, Laragh JH, Sealey JE, Sullivan PA, McKinstry DN. Clinical experience with blockade of the renin-angiotensin-aldosterone system by an oral converting-enzyme inhibitor (SQ 14,225, captopril) in hypertensive patients. *Prog Cardiovasc Dis* (1978) 21, 195–206.
2. Ferguson RK, Vlasses PH, Koplin JR, Shirinian A, Burke JF, Alexander JC. Captopril in severe treatment-resistant hypertension. *Am Heart J* (1980) 99, 579–85.
3. Koffer H, Vlasses PH, Ferguson RK, Weis M, Adler AG. Captopril in diuretic-treated hypertensive patients. *JAMA* (1980) 244, 2532–5.
4. Dahlström U, Karlsson E. Captopril and spironolactone therapy for refractory congestive heart failure. *Am J Cardiol* (1993) 71, 29A–33A.
5. Haïat R, Piot O, Gallois H, Hanania G. Blood pressure response to the first 36 hours of heart failure therapy with perindopril versus captopril. French General Hospitals National College of Cardiologists. *J Cardiovasc Pharmacol* (1999) 33, 953–9.
6. Nilsen OG, Sellevold OFM, Romfo OS, Smedsrud A, Grynne B, Williams PEO, Kleinbloesem CH. Pharmacokinetics and effects on renal function following cilazapril and hydrochlorothiazide alone and in combination in healthy subjects and hypertensive patients. *Br J Clin Pharmacol* (1989) 27 (Suppl 2), 323S–328S.
7. D'Costa DF, Basu SK, Gunasekera NPR. ACE inhibitors and diuretics causing hypokalaemia. *Br J Clin Pract* (1990) 44, 26–7.
8. Jolobe OM. Severe hyperkalaemia induced by trimethoprim in combination with an angiotensin-converting enzyme inhibitor in a patient with transplanted lungs. *J Intern Med* (1997) 242, 88–9.
9. Collier JG, Webb DJ. Severe thiazide-induced hyponatraemia during treatment with enalapril. *Postgrad Med J* (1987) 63, 1105–6.
10. Watson ML, Bell GM, Muir AL, Buist TAS, Kellett RJ, Padfield PL. Captopril/diuretic combinations in severe renovascular disease: a cautionary note. *Lancet* (1983) ii, 404–5.
11. Hoefnagels WHL, Strijk SP, Thien T. Reversible renal failure following treatment with captopril and diuretics in patients with renovascular hypertension. *Neth J Med* (1984) 27, 269–74.
12. Mandal AK, Markert RJ, Saklayen MG, Mankus RA, Yokokawa K. Diuretics potentiate angiotensin converting enzyme inhibitor-induced acute renal failure. *Clin Nephrol* (1994) 42, 170–4.

13. Schoolwerth AC, Sica DA, Ballermann BJ, Wilcox CS. Renal considerations in angiotensin converting enzyme inhibitor therapy. A statement for healthcare professionals from the Council on the Kidney in Cardiovascular Disease and the Council for High Blood Pressure Research of the American Heart Association. *Circulation* (2001) 104, 1985–91.
14. Speirs CJ, Dollery CT, Inman WHW, Rawson NSB, Wilton LV. Postmarketing surveillance of enalapril. II: Investigation of the potential role of enalapril in deaths with renal failure. *BMJ* (1988) 297, 830–2.
15. Toto RD, Mitchell HC, Lee H-C, Milam C, Pettinger WA. Reversible renal insufficiency due to angiotensin converting enzyme inhibitors in hypertensive nephrosclerosis. *Ann Intern Med* (1991) 115, 513–19.
16. Lee H-C, Pettinger WA. Diuretics potentiate the angiotensin converting-enzyme inhibitor-associated acute renal dysfunction. *Clin Nephrol* (1992) 38, 236–7.
17. Funck-Brentano C, Chatellier G, Alexandre J-M. Reversible renal failure after combined treatment with enalapril and frusemide in a patient with congestive heart failure. *Br Heart J* (1986) 55, 596–8.
18. Stewart JT, Lovett D, Joy M. Reversible renal failure after combined treatment with enalapril and frusemide in a patient with congestive heart failure. *Br Heart J* (1986) 56, 489–90.
19. Hogg KJ, Hillis WS. Captopril/metolazone induced renal failure. *Lancet* (1986) 1, 501–2.
20. Van Hecken AM, Verbesselt R, Buntinx A, Cirillo VJ, De Schepper PJ. Absence of a pharmacokinetic interaction between enalapril and frusemide. *Br J Clin Pharmacol* (1987) 23, 84–7.
21. Fujimura A, Shimokawa Y, Ebihara A. Influence of captopril on urinary excretion of furosemide in hypertensive subjects. *J Clin Pharmacol* (1990) 30, 538–42.
22. Sommers De K, Meyer EC, Moncrieff J. Acute interaction of furosemide and captopril in healthy salt-replete man. *S Afr Tydskr Wet* (1991) 87, 375–7.
23. Toussaint C, Masselink A, Gentges A, Wambach G, Bönner G. Interference of different ACE-inhibitors with the diuretic action of furosemide and hydrochlorothiazide. *Klin Wochenschr* (1989) 67, 1138–46.
24. De Lepeleire I, Van Hecken A, Verbesselt R, Kaiser G, Barner A, Holmes I, De Schepper PJ. Interaction between furosemide and the converting enzyme inhibitor benazepril in healthy volunteers. *Eur J Clin Pharmacol* (1988) 34, 465–8.
25. Sudoh T, Fujimura A, Shiga T, Tateishi T, Sunaga K, Ohashi K, Ebihara A. Influence of lisinopril on urinary electrolytes excretion after furosemide in healthy subjects. *J Clin Pharmacol* (1993) 33, 640–3.
26. Beermann B. Pharmacokinetics of lisinopril. *Am J Med* (1988) 85 (Suppl 3B) 25–30.
27. Weisser K, Schloos J, Jakob S, Mühlberg W, Platt D, Mutschler E. The influence of hydrochlorothiazide on the pharmacokinetics of enalapril in elderly patients. *Eur J Clin Pharmacol* (1992) 43, 173–7.
28. Breithaupt-Grögler K, Ungethüm W, Meurer-Witt B, Belz GG. Pharmacokinetic and dynamic interactions of the angiotensin-converting enzyme inhibitor imidapril with hydrochlorothiazide, bisoprolol and nilvadipine. *Eur J Clin Pharmacol* (2001) 57, 275–84.
29. Grass P, Gerbeau C, Kutz K. Spirapril: pharmacokinetic properties and drug interactions. *Blood Pressure* (1994) 3 (Suppl 2), 7–13.
30. Schürer M, Erb K, Junge K, Schäfer HF, Schulz H-U, Amschler S, Krupp S, Hermann R. Drug interaction of spirapril hydrochloride monohydrate and hydrochlorothiazide. *Arzneimittelforschung* (2003) 53, 414–19.
31. Hutt V, Michaelis K, Verbesselt R, De Schepper PJ, Salomon P, Bonn R, Cawello W, Angehrn JC. Lack of a pharmacokinetic interaction between moexipril and hydrochlorothiazide. *Eur J Clin Pharmacol* (1996) 51, 339–44.
32. British National Formulary. 53rd ed. London: The British Medical Association and The Pharmaceutical Press; 2007. p. 98–100.

ACE inhibitors + Diuretics; Potassium-sparing

Combining ACE inhibitors with potassium-sparing diuretics (e.g. amiloride), including the aldosterone antagonists (eplerenone, spironolactone) can result in clinically relevant or severe hyperkalaemia, particularly if other important risk factors are present.

Clinical evidence

(a) Amiloride

The serum potassium levels of two patients taking furosemide and unnamed potassium-sparing diuretics and potassium supplements rose by 18% and 24%, respectively, when they were given **captopril** 37.5 to 75 mg daily. The rises occurred within one or two days. No clinical signs or symptoms of hyperkalaemia were seen, but one of the patients had an increase in serum potassium to above the upper limits of normal.[1] In a post-marketing survey, 2 patients who had **enalapril**-associated renal impairment and died were also receiving amiloride and furosemide; one was also taking potassium supplements.[2] Four diabetic patients, with some renal impairment, developed life-threatening hyperkalaemia with severe cardiac arrhythmias and deterioration of renal function, within 8 to 18 days of having an amiloride/hydrochlorothiazide diuretic added to their **enalapril** treatment. Two suffered cardiac arrest and both died. Potassium levels were between 9.4 and 11 mmol/L. A fifth diabetic patient with normal renal function developed hyperkalaemia soon after receiving amiloride/hydrochlorothiazide and **captopril** in combination.[3] A further case of hyperkalaemia and cardiac arrest was associated with **enalapril** and furosemide/amiloride.[4] In a brief report, the manufacturers of **enalapril** noted that, of 47 serious cases of hyperkalaemia, 25 patients were taking one or more (unnamed) potassium-sparing drugs.[5]

However, a retrospective comparison of 35 patients treated for congestive heart failure found no differences in the serum potassium levels of 16 patients taking furosemide, amiloride and **enalapril**, when compared with another group of 19 patients taking furosemide and amiloride alone. Patients were excluded from the comparison if they had significant renal impairment or were taking other drugs likely to affect serum potassium.[6]

(b) Eplerenone

In the large Eplerenone Post-Acute Myocardial Infarction Heart Failure Efficacy and Survival Study (EPHESUS)[7] the rate of serious hyperkalaemia (defined as serum potassium 6 mmol/L or greater) was 5.5% in patients randomised to eplerenone 25 mg to 50 mg daily (mean 43 mg daily[8]) compared with 3.9% in those receiving placebo: this represented a 1.4-fold increase. More eplerenone recipients required hospitalisation for serious hyperkalaemia than placebo recipients (12 versus 3). The risk of serious hyperkalaemia was increased in those with a baseline creatinine clearance of less than 50 mL/minute (10.1% in the eplerenone group and 5.9% in the placebo group). Eplerenone reduced the risk of serious hypokalaemia (defined as serum potassium 3.5 mmol/L or less) by 1.6-fold (8.4% versus 13.1%). About 86% of patients in this study were also receiving an ACE inhibitor or an angiotensin II receptor antagonist, and about 60% were receiving a (loop[8]) diuretic.[7] However, the US manufacturer states that the rate of maximum potassium levels greater than 5.5 mmol/L were similar in EPHESUS regardless of the use of ACE inhibitor or angiotensin II receptor antagonist.[8] Nevertheless, they mention another study in diabetics with microalbuminuria, where a higher dose of eplerenone 200 mg combined with **enalapril** 10 mg increased the frequency of hyperkalaemia (defined as serum potassium greater than 5.5 mmol/L) from 17% with enalapril alone to 38% with the combination: this represented a 2.2-fold increase.[8]

(c) Spironolactone

Twenty-five of 262 patients treated with ACE-inhibitors and spironolactone, and admitted to hospital for medical emergencies, were found to have serious hyperkalaemia (defined as serum potassium levels greater than 6 mmol/L: 11 patients had levels of at least 8 mmol/L). These 25 patients were elderly (mean age 74 years) and being treated for hypertension, heart failure, diabetic nephropathy, proteinuria, or nephrotic syndrome; 22 had associated renal impairment and 12 had signs of volume depletion. Combined treatment had been started an average of 25 weeks before the admission. The ACE inhibitors involved were **enalapril**, **captopril**, **lisinopril** or **perindopril**, and the average dose of spironolactone used was 57 mg daily; 10 patients were also receiving a loop or thiazide diuretic. Nineteen patients had ECG changes associated with hyperkalaemia; 2 of them died, another 2 required temporary pacing for third-degree heart block, and 2 others survived after sustained ventricular tachycardia and fibrillation. Of the 19 patients, 17 required at least one haemodialysis session and 12 were admitted to intensive care.[9] Other authors reported a higher 36% incidence of hyperkalaemia (serum potassium levels greater than 5 mmol/L) in 42 patients hospitalised for heart failure and prescribed spironolactone. It was suggested that this may be due to the excessively large doses of spironolactone prescribed,[10] although the specific doses were not mentioned.

Similar risk factors were found in an analysis of 44 patients with congestive heart failure who were taking spironolactone and ACE inhibitors or angiotensin II receptor antagonists, and were admitted for treatment of life-threatening hyperkalaemia. Their mean age was 76 years, the mean dose of spironolactone was 88 mg daily (range 25 to 200 mg daily) and 40 patients also received loop diuretics. In addition, 35 patients had type II diabetes. Haemodialysis was given to 37 patients, but in 6 patients renal function did not recover and 2 patients developed fatal complications.[11] A number of other cases of serious hyperkalaemia have been described in patients taking ACE inhibitors (**captopril**, **enalapril**, **lisinopril**), spironolactone, and loop (furosemide or bumetanide) or thiazide (hydroflumethiazide) diuretics.[2,12-16] Many of the patients were elderly and were receiving spironolactone 50 to 100 mg daily,[2,12,15] but one diabetic patient with moderate renal impairment was receiving just 25 mg of spironolactone daily.[14] In one report, the 4 cases had associated **enalapril**-induced deterioration in renal function and died.[2] Another patient died from complete heart block.[12]

One of the factors that affects the incidence of hyperkalaemia appears to be the dose of spironolactone. In a preliminary investigation for the Randomised Aldactone Evaluation Study (RALES), 214 patients with congestive heart failure taking an ACE inhibitor and a loop diuretic with or without digitalis, were randomised to receive placebo or various doses of spironolactone for 12 weeks. The incidence of hyperkalaemia (defined as serum potassium level of 5.5 mmol/L or greater) was 5% for the placebo group, whereas it was 5%, 13%, 20%, and 24% when spironolactone was given in single daily doses of 12.5, 25, 50, or 75 mg, respectively.[17] The main RALES study involving 1663 patients showed a 30% reduction in the risk of mortality in patients with severe heart failure when they were given spironolactone in addition to treatment including an ACE inhibitor, a loop diuretic and in most cases digoxin. During the first year of follow-up, the median creatinine concentration in the spironolactone group increased by about 4 to 9 micromol/L and the median potassium level increased by 0.03 mmol/L, but there was a low incidence of serious hyperkalaemia (2% in the spironolactone group compared with 1% in the placebo group). However, the dose of spironolactone was fairly low (mean dose 26 mg daily; range 25 mg every other day to 50 mg daily depending on serum potassium levels and response). In addition, patients with a serum creatinine of more than 221 micromol/L or a serum potassium of more than 5 mmol/L were excluded.[18] In a Canadian population-based time-series analysis, the increase in use of spironolactone for heart failure in patients taking ACE inhibitors after publication of the RALES study was found be associated with 50 additional hospitalisations for hyperkalaemia for every 1000 additional prescriptions for spironolactone, and there was a 6.7-fold increase in numbers of patients dying from hyperkalaemia. The authors say that spironolactone-related hyperkalaemia is a much greater problem in every day practice than in the setting of a clinical study, and give a number of reasons for this including, less frequent monitoring of potassium levels, presence of conditions predisposing to hyperkalaemia, failure to detect subsequent development of renal impairment, inappropriately high doses of spironolactone, increase in dietary potassium intake, and use of spironolactone in heart failure with causes not included in the RALES study.[19] In another study, use of spironolactone with ACE inhibitors in patients with class IV chronic heart failure was associated with a 14.6 odds ratio for developing hyperkalaemia when compared with ACE inhibitors alone. Predictors for hyperkalaemia included increases in creatinine following treatment, and diabetes.[20]

(d) Triamterene

A retrospective analysis found that **captopril**, given to 6 patients on *Dyazide* (hydrochlorothiazide/triamterene), had not increased the potassium levels.[21]

Mechanism

ACE inhibitors reduce the levels of aldosterone, which results in the retention of potassium. This would be expected to be additive with the potassium-retaining effects of amiloride and triamterene and aldosterone antagonists such as spironolactone and eplerenone, leading to hyperkalaemia, but usually only if other risk factors are present (see *Importance and management* below).

Importance and management

Hyperkalaemia with ACE inhibitors and potassium-sparing diuretics, and particularly the aldosterone antagonist spironolactone, is well documented and well established. If it occurs it can be serious and potentially life threatening. Its incidence depends on the presence of other risk factors, and clinically important hyperkalaemia usually only appears to develop if one or more of these are also present, particularly renal impairment. Other risk factors in patients with heart failure include advanced age[15] and diabetes[11,22] (hyperkalaemia has been found to be relatively common in both non-insulin-dependent and insulin-dependent diabetics).[23] In addition, doses of spironolactone greater than 25 mg daily increase the risk of hyperkalaemia.

Because ACE inhibitors have potassium-sparing effects, potassium-sparing diuretics such as amiloride and triamterene should normally not be given concurrently. If, however, the use of both drugs is thought to be appropriate the serum potassium levels should be closely monitored so that any problems can be quickly identified. Note that the concurrent use of a potassium-depleting diuretic (a 'loop or thiazide diuretic', (p.21)) with the potassium-sparing diuretic may not necessarily prevent the development of hyperkalaemia. The combination of an ACE inhibitor and spironolactone can be beneficial in some types of heart failure, but close monitoring of serum potassium and renal function is needed, especially with any changes in treatment or the patient's clinical condition. The combination should be avoided in patients with renal impairment with a glomerular filtration rate of less than 30 mL/min.[22] In addition, the dose of spironolactone should not exceed 25 mg daily.[22] Similarly, the UK manufacturer of eplerenone says that caution is required when it is given with ACE inhibitors, especially in renal impairment, and that potassium levels and renal function should be monitored.[24]

1. Burnakis TG, Mioduch HJ. Combined therapy with captopril and potassium supplementation. A potential for hyperkalemia. *Arch Intern Med* (1984) 144, 2371–2.
2. Speirs CJ, Dollery CT, Inman WHW, Rawson NSB, Wilton LV. Postmarketing surveillance of enalapril. II: Investigation of the potential role of enalapril in deaths with renal failure. *BMJ* (1988) 297, 830–2.
3. Chiu T-F, Bullard MJ, Chen J-C, Liaw S-J, Ng C-J. Rapid life-threatening hyperkalemia after addition of amiloride HCl/hydrochlorothiazide to angiotensin-converting enzyme inhibitor therapy. *Ann Emerg Med* (1997) 30, 612–15.
4. Johnston RT, de Bono DP, Nyman CR. Preventable sudden death in patients receiving angiotensin converting enzyme inhibitors and loop/potassium sparing diuretic combinations. *Int J Cardiol* (1992) 34, 213–15.
5. Brown C, Rush J. Risk factors for the development of hyperkalemia in patients treated with enalapril for heart failure. *Clin Pharmacol Ther* (1989) 45, 167.
6. Radley AS, Fitzpatrick RW. An evaluation of the potential interaction between enalapril and amiloride. *J Clin Pharm Ther* (1987) 12, 319–23.
7. Pitt B, Remme W, Zannad F, Neaton J, Martinez F, Roniker B, Bittman R, Hurley S, Kleiman J, Gatlin M; Eplerenone Post-Acute Myocardial Infarction Heart Failure Efficacy and Survival Study Investigators. Eplerenone, a selective aldosterone blocker, in patients with left ventricular dysfunction after myocardial infarction. *N Engl J Med* (2003) 348, 1309–21.
8. Inspra (Eplerenone). Pfizer Inc. US Prescribing information, May 2005.
9. Schepkens H, Vanholder R, Billiouw J-M, Lameire N. Life-threatening hyperkalemia during combined therapy with angiotensin-converting enzyme inhibitors and spironolactone: an analysis of 25 cases. *Am J Med* (2001) 110, 438–41.
10. Berry C, McMurray J. Life-threatening hyperkalemia during combined therapy with angiotensin-converting enzyme inhibitors and spironolactone. *Am J Med* (2001) 111, 587.
11. Wrenger E, Müller R, Moesenthin M, Welte T, Frölich JC, Neumann KH. Interaction of spironolactone with ACE inhibitors or angiotensin receptor blockers: analysis of 44 cases. *BMJ* (2003) 327, 147–9.
12. Lakhani M. Complete heart block induced by hyperkalaemia associated with treatment with a combination of captopril and spironolactone. *BMJ* (1986) 293, 271.
13. Lo TCN, Cryer RJ. Complete heart block induced by hyperkalaemia associated with treatment with a combination of captopril and spironolactone. *BMJ* (1986) 292, 1672.
14. Odawara M, Asano M, Yamashita K. Life-threatening hyperkalaemia caused by angiotensin-converting enzyme inhibitor and diuretics. *Diabet Med* (1997) 14, 169–70.
15. Vanpee D, Swine C. Elderly heart failure patients with drug-induced serious hyperkalemia. *Aging Clin Exp Res* (2000) 12, 315–19.
16. Dahlström U, Karlsson E. Captopril and spironolactone therapy for refractory congestive heart failure. *Am J Cardiol* (1993) 71, 29A–33A.
17. The RALES Investigators. Effectiveness of spironolactone added to an angiotensin-converting enzyme inhibitor and a loop diuretic for severe chronic congestive heart failure (The Randomized Aldactone Evaluation Study [RALES]). *Am J Cardiol* (1996) 78, 902–7.
18. Pitt B, Zannad F, Remme WJ, Cody R, Castaigne A, Perez A, Palensky J, Wittes J, for the Randomized Aldactone Evaluation Study Investigators. The effect of spironolactone on morbidity and mortality in patients with severe heart failure. *N Engl J Med* (1999) 341, 709–17.
19. Juurlink DN, Mamdani MM, Lee DS, Kopp A, Austin PC, Laupacis A, Redelmeier DA. Rates of hyperkalemia after publication of the Randomized Aldactone Evaluation Study. *N Engl J Med* (2004) 351, 543–51.
20. Cruz CS, Cruz ÁA, Marcílio de Souza CA. Hyperkalaemia in congestive heart failure patients using ACE inhibitors and spironolactone. *Nephrol Dial Transplant* (2003) 18, 1814–19.
21. Schuna AA, Schmidt GR, Pitterle ME. Serum potassium concentrations after initiation of captopril therapy. *Clin Pharm* (1986) 5, 920–3.
22. Palmer BF. Managing hyperkalemia caused by inhibitors of the renin-angiotensin-aldosterone system. *N Engl J Med* (2004) 351, 585–92.
23. Jarman PR, Keheley AM, Mather HM. Life-threatening hyperkalaemia caused by ACE inhibitor and diuretics. *Diabet Med* (1997) 14, 808.
24. Inspra (Eplerenone). Pfizer Ltd. UK Summary of product characteristics, May 2006.

ACE inhibitors + Dopamine agonists

A single report describes severe hypotension when a patient taking lisinopril was given pergolide. Dopamine agonists are well known to be associated with hypotensive reactions during the first few days of treatment.

Clinical evidence

A man successfully treated for hypertension with **lisinopril** 10 mg daily experienced a severe hypotensive reaction within four hours of taking a single 50-microgram dose of **pergolide** for periodic leg movements during sleep. He needed hospitalisation and treatment with intravenous fluids.[1]

Mechanism

All dopamine agonists can cause hypotensive reactions during the first few days of treatment. It is not clear whether this patient was extremely sensitive to the pergolide or whether what occurred was due to an interaction. However, it is not unreasonable to assume that the hypotensive effects of dopamine agonists and antihypertensives might be additive.

Importance and management

Postural hypotension on starting dopamine agonists is a well recognised adverse effect, but this appears to be the only report that this might be of more concern in patients taking antihypertensives. The manufacturers of pergolide recommend caution when it is given with antihypertensives because of the risk of postural and/or sustained hypotension. The authors of the case report suggest that in patients taking antihypertensives the initial dose of pergolide should be 25 micrograms.[1] It would seem prudent to exercise extra caution with the initial use of pergolide and other dopamine agonists in patients treated with antihypertensives.

1. Kando JC, Keck PE, Wood PA. Pergolide-induced hypotension. *Ann Pharmacother* (1990) 24, 543.

ACE inhibitors and Angiotensin II receptor antagonists + Epoetin

Epoetin may cause hypertension and thereby reduce the effects of antihypertensive drugs. An additive hyperkalaemic effect is theoretically possible with ACE inhibitors or angiotensin II receptor antagonists and epoetin. It is not entirely clear whether captopril, enalapril, fosinopril or other ACE inhibitors affect the efficacy of epoetin or not, but any interaction may take many months to develop.

Clinical evidence

(A) Antihypertensive effects

The most frequent adverse effect of epoetin is an increase in blood pressure, so it is important to control any existing hypertension before epoetin is started (the manufacturers contraindicate epoetin in uncontrolled hypertension). Blood pressure should be monitored before and during epoetin treatment, and if necessary antihypertensive drug treatment should be started or increased if the pressure rises.[1-3]

(B) Epoetin efficacy

(a) Decreased epoetin effects

In a retrospective analysis of 43 haemodialysis patients given epoetin regularly for about 10 months, the dose of epoetin was not significantly different between patients taking **captopril** (20 patients) and a control group (23 patients) who did not receive any ACE inhibitors (116.7 versus 98.3 units/kg per week, respectively). However, the haemoglobin and haematocrit values were significantly less at 6.2 mmol/L and 29.3%, respectively, in the **captopril** group than the values of 7.1 mmol/L and 33.3% in the control group.[4] Another retrospective study of 40 dialysis patients found that the 20 patients taking an ACE inhibitor (**captopril** 12.5 to 75 mg daily, **enalapril** 2.5 to 5 mg daily or **fosinopril** 10 to 20 mg daily) had some evidence of increased epoetin requirements after 1 year, when compared with the control group. However, this was not significant until 15 months when the cumulative epoetin dosage requirements were about doubled (12 092 versus 6 449 units/kg).[5] Similarly, a prospective study with a 12-month follow-up period found that 20 patients receiving **enalapril** 5 to 20 mg daily required significantly higher doses of epoetin compared with 20 patients receiving nifedipine or 20 patients receiving no antihypertensive therapy.[6] Higher epoetin requirements with ACE inhibitors were also reported in a small study in peritoneal dialysis patients.[7] Furthermore, another prospective study found that 15 patients in whom ACE inhibitors (**enalapril**, **captopril**, or **perindopril**) were withdrawn and replaced with amlodipine, felodipine or doxazosin, had an increase in their mean haematocrit level and a decrease in their mean epoetin dose requirement.[8]

(b) No interaction

A retrospective review of 14 haemodialysis patients receiving epoetin, compared the haematocrit and dosage of epoetin for 16 weeks before, and 16 weeks after, starting ACE inhibitors (8 taking **captopril**, mean dose 35 mg daily and 6 taking **enalapril**, mean dose 7.85 mg daily). This study failed to find any evidence of a clinically significant interaction when ACE inhibitors were added.[9] Another study involving 17 chronic haemodialysis patients found that ACE inhibitors (5 taking **captopril** and 12 taking **enalapril**) for 3 and 12 months did not increase the epoetin dose requirements or reduce the haematocrits.[10] However, given the results of the study[5] reported in *(a)* above, it is possible that these studies were not continued for long enough to detect an effect. Another study in 14 haemodialysis patients found no difference in epoetin requirements between patients receiving **losartan** 25 mg daily or placebo,[11] but again the **losartan** was only given for 3 months. A further study (length not specified) in 604 dialysis patients also found that the use of ACE inhibitors or angiotensin II receptor blockers was not associated with epoetin resistance.[12]

(c) ACE inhibitors compared with Angiotensin II receptor antagonists

In one retrospective analysis of dialysis patients, 18 of 24 receiving losartan had decreases in haemoglobin, and 14 of these were using epoetin. A three to fourfold increase in the epoetin dose was required in these patients to restore the haemoglobin levels.[13] This study suggests that angiotensin II receptor antagonists can behave similarly to ACE inhibitors. However, in a prospective study in 25 patients who had been undergoing haemodialysis for more than one year, 12 patients were given **temocapril** 2 mg daily and 13 patients received **losartan** 25 to 50 mg daily for 12 months. **Temocapril** significantly decreased haemoglobin levels from 9.8 to 9.1 g/dL at 3 months and reached a minimum of 9 g/dL at 6 months; haemoglobin levels recovered to 9.7 g/dL at the end of the study by increasing the dosage of epoetin. In contrast, no change was found in haemoglobin values in the patients receiving **losartan**. The dosage of epoetin was gradually increased from 76 to 121 units/kg per week in the **temocapril** group, but in the **losartan** group the epoetin dose was not significantly increased (94 versus 101 units/kg per week).[14] Similar results were found in a study with **captopril** and **losartan**.[15]

(C) Hyperkalaemia

The manufacturers of epoetin comment that increased potassium levels have been reported in a few patients with chronic renal failure receiving epoetin, and that serum potassium levels should be monitored regularly.[1-3] An additive hyperkalaemic effect is therefore theoretically possible with patients also receiving ACE inhibitors or angiotensin II receptor antagonists.

Mechanism

(A) Epoetin can cause hypertension, possibly associated with haemodynamic changes produced by the increase in haematocrit.[16]
(B) It has been argued that ACE inhibitors might possibly reduce the efficacy of epoetin in haemodialysis patients for several reasons. Firstly, because patients with chronic renal failure have a reduction in their haematocrit when given ACE inhibitors, secondly because ACE inhibitors reduce polycythaemia following renal transplantation, and thirdly because ACE inhibitors reduce the plasma levels of endogenous erythropoietin.[4,9,17] Many other factors have also been proposed.[18]
(C) Drugs that block angiotensin II cause reduced levels of aldosterone, which results in the retention of potassium. This would be expected to be additive with other drugs that cause hyperkalaemia.

Importance and management

Blood pressure should be routinely monitored in patients using epoetin, and this monitoring would seem sufficient to detect any interaction that affects the blood pressure-lowering effects of the ACE inhibitors. The dose of ACE inhibitor may need to be increased, but if blood pressure rises cannot be controlled, a transient interruption of epoetin therapy is recommended. Similarly, serum electrolytes, including potassium, should be routinely monitored in patients using epoetin. If potassium levels rise, consider ceasing epoetin until the level is corrected.[1,2]

The overall picture of the effect of ACE inhibitors on epoetin resistance is unclear, and it would seem that an interaction, if it happens, takes a long time to develop. There is even less evidence regarding any interaction with angiotensin II antagonists. As epoetin dosage is governed by response, no immediate intervention is generally necessary. More long-term study is needed.

1. NeoRecormon Solution (Epoetin beta). Roche Products Ltd. UK Summary of product characteristics, January 2007.
2. Eprex (Epoetin alfa). Janssen-Cilag Ltd. UK Summary of product characteristics, July 2006.
3. Epogen (Epoetin alfa). Amgen Inc. US Prescribing information, March 2007.
4. Walter J. Does captopril decrease the effect of human recombinant erythropoietin in haemodialysis patients? *Nephrol Dial Transplant* (1993) 8, 1428.
5. Heß E, Sperschneider H, Stein G. Do ACE inhibitors influence the dose of human recombinant erythropoietin in dialysis patients? *Nephrol Dial Transplant* (1996) 11, 749–51.
6. Albitar S, Genin R, Fen-Chong M, Serveaux M-O, Bourgeon B. High dose enalapril impairs the response to erythropoietin treatment in haemodialysis patients. *Nephrol Dial Transplant* (1998) 13, 1206–10.
7. Mora C, Navarro JF. Negative effect of angiotensin-converting enzyme inhibitors on erythropoietin response in CAPD patients. *Am J Nephrol* (2000) 20 248.
8. Ertürk Ş, Nergizoğlu G, Ateş K, Duman N, Erbay B, Karatan O, Ertuğ AE. The impact of withdrawing ACE inhibitors on erythropoietin responsiveness and left ventricular hypertrophy in haemodialysis patients. *Nephrol Dial Transplant* (1999) 14, 1912–16.
9. Conlon PJ, Albers F, Butterly D, Schwab SJ. ACE inhibitors do not affect erythropoietin efficacy in haemodialysis patients. *Nephrol Dial Transplant* (1994) 9, 1358.

10. Schwenk MH, Jumani AQ, Rosenberg CR, Kulogowski JE, Charytan C, Spinowitz BS. Potential angiotensin-converting enzyme inhibitor–epoetin alfa interaction in patients receiving chronic hemodialysis. *Pharmacotherapy* (1998) 18, 627–30.
11. Chew CG, Weise MD, Disney APS. The effect of angiotensin II receptor antagonist on the exogenous erythropoietin requirement of haemodialysis patients. *Nephrol Dial Transplant* (1999) 14, 2047–9.
12. Saudan P, Halabi G, Perneger T, Wasserfallen J-B, Wauters J-P, Martin P-Y. Use of ace inhibitors or angiotensin II receptors blockers is not associated with erythropoietin resistance in dialysis patients. *J Am Soc Nephrol* (2002) 13, 443A.
13. Schwarzbeck A, Wittenmeier KW, Hällfritzsch U. Anaemia in dialysis patients as a side-effect of sartanes. *Lancet* (1998) 352, 286.
14. Kato A, Takita T, Furuhashi M, Takahashi T, Maruyama Y, Hishida A. No effect of losartan on response to erythropoietin therapy in patients undergoing hemodialysis. *Nephron* (2000) 86, 538–9.
15. Schiffl H, Lang SM. Angiotensin-converting enzyme inhibitors but not angiotensin II AT 1 receptor antagonists affect erythropoiesis in patients with anemia of end-stage renal disease. *Nephron* (1999) 81, 106–8.
16. Sweetman SC, ed. Martindale: The complete drug reference. 35th ed. London: Pharmaceutical Press; 2007. p. 956.
17. Pratt MC, Lewis-Barned NJ, Walker RJ, Bailey RR, Shand BI, Livesey J. Effect of angiotensin converting enzyme inhibitors on erythropoietin concentrations in healthy volunteers. *Br J Clin Pharmacol* (1992) 34, 363–5.
18. Macdougall IC. ACE inhibitors and erythropoietin responsiveness. *Am J Kidney Dis* (2001) 38, 649–51.

ACE inhibitors + Food

Food has little or no effect on the absorption of cilazapril, enalapril, fosinopril, lisinopril, quinapril, ramipril, spirapril, and trandolapril. Although food may reduce the absorption of captopril, this does not appear to be clinically important. Food reduced the absorption of imidapril and moexipril, and reduced the conversion of perindopril to perindoprilat, but the clinical relevance of these effects has not been assessed.

Clinical evidence, mechanism, importance and management

(a) No interaction

Although food reduced the AUC of **captopril** 25 to 100 mg by up to 56%[1-4] this had no effect on the maximum decrease in blood pressure.[1,3,4] One study in 10 healthy subjects reported a one-hour delay in the maximum hypotensive effect.[1] Another study, in 10 hypertensive patients, found that the extent and duration of the antihypertensive efficacy of **captopril** 50 mg twice daily for one month was not affected by whether it was taken before or after food.[5] However, decreasing the dose of an ACE inhibitor might reduce the duration of the hypotensive effect and it has been suggested that these results should be confirmed with lower doses of **captopril**.[5]

Other single-dose studies have shown that food had no statistically significant effect on the pharmacokinetics of **lisinopril**,[6] or **enalapril**, and its active metabolite, enalaprilat.[7] Similarly, food had minimal effects on the pharmacokinetics of **cilazapril** (AUC decreased by only 14%).[8] Food caused small, but statistically significant increases in the time to reach maximum plasma levels of **quinapril** and its active metabolite. However, as the increase was less than 30 minutes this is not expected to alter the therapeutic effect.[9] Likewise, the manufacturers of **spirapril** briefly mention in a review that food delayed its absorption by 1 hour, it did not affect the bioavailability of **spirapril** or spiraprilat, its active metabolite.[10] Other manufacturers state that food had no effect on the absorption of **fosinopril**,[11,12] **ramipril**,[13,14] or **trandolapril**.[15,16]

(b) Possible interaction

In one study, food reduced the AUC of the active metabolite of **moexipril** (moexiprilat) by 40 to 50%.[17,18] Food did not reduce **moexipril**-induced ACE-inhibition and therefore the reduced bioavailability was not expected to be clinically relevant.[19] However, the US manufacturers suggest taking moexipril one hour before food.[18]

Although food did not significantly affect the pharmacokinetics of a single 4-mg dose of **perindopril**, the AUC of its active metabolite perindoprilat was reduced by 44%.[20] The blood pressure-lowering effects were not assessed, but it seems possible that they would not be affected (see captopril, above). Nevertheless, the UK manufacturer recommends that **perindopril** should be taken in the morning before a meal.[21]

The UK manufacturer of **imidapril** states that a fat-rich meal significantly reduces the absorption of **imidapril**, and recommends that the drug be taken at the same time each day, about 15 minutes before a meal.[22]

1. Mäntylä R, Männistö PT, Vuorela A, Sundberg S, Ottoila P. Impairment of captopril bioavailability by concomitant food and antacid intake. *Int J Clin Pharmacol Ther Toxicol* (1984) 22, 626–9.
2. Singhvi SM, McKinstry DN, Shaw JM, Willard DA, Migdalof BH. Effect of food on the bioavailability of captopril in healthy subjects. *J Clin Pharmacol* (1982) 22, 135–40.
3. Öhman KP, Kågedal B, Larsson R, Karlberg BE. Pharmacokinetics of captopril and its effects on blood pressure during acute and chronic administration and in relation to food intake. *J Cardiovasc Pharmacol* (1985) 7 (Suppl 1), S20–S24.
4. Müller H-M, Overlack A, Heck I, Kolloch R, Stumpe KO. The influence of food intake on pharmacodynamics and plasma concentration of captopril. *J Hypertens* (1985) 3 (Suppl 2), S135–S136.
5. Salvetti A, Pedrinelli R, Magagna A, Abdel-Haq B, Graziadei L, Taddei S, Stornello M. Influence of food on acute and chronic effects of captopril in essential hypertensive patients. *J Cardiovasc Pharmacol* (1985) 7 (Suppl 1), S25–S29.
6. Mojaverian P, Rocci ML, Vlasses PH, Hoholick C, Clementi RA, Ferguson RK. Effect of food on the bioavailability of lisinopril, a nonsulfhydryl angiotensin-converting enzyme inhibitor. *J Pharm Sci* (1986) 75, 395–7.
7. Swanson BN, Vlasses PH, Ferguson RK, Bergquist PA, Till AE, Irvin JD, Harris K. Influence of food on the bioavailability of enalapril. *J Pharm Sci* (1984) 73, 1655–7.
8. Massarella JW, DeFeo TM, Brown AN, Lin A, Wills RJ. The influence of food on the pharmacokinetics and ACE inhibition of cilazapril. *Br J Clin Pharmacol* (1989) 27, 205S–209S.
9. Ferry JJ, Horvath AM, Sedman AJ, Latts JR, Colburn WA. Influence of food on the pharmacokinetics of quinapril and its active diacid metabolite, CI-928. *J Clin Pharmacol* (1987) 27, 397–9.
10. Grass P, Gerbeau C, Kutz K. Spirapril: pharmacokinetic properties and drug interactions. *Blood Pressure* (1994) 3 (Suppl 2), 7–13.
11. Staril (Fosinopril sodium). E. R. Squibb & Sons Ltd. UK Summary of product characteristics, June 2005.
12. Monopril (Fosinopril sodium). Bristol-Myers Squibb Company. US Prescribing information, July 2003.
13. Tritace (Ramipril). Aventis Pharma Ltd. UK Summary of product characteristics, February 2004.
14. Altace Capsules (Ramipril). Monarch Pharmaceuticals, Inc. US Prescribing information, September 2005.
15. Gopten (Trandolapril). Abbott Laboratories Ltd. UK Summary of product characteristics, May 2007.
16. Mavik (Trandolapril). Abbott Laboratories. US Prescribing information, July 2003.
17. Perdix (Moexipril). Schwarz Pharma. Product Monograph, October 1995.
18. Univasc (Moexipril hydrochloride). Schwarz Pharma. US Prescribing information, May 2003.
19. Stimpel M, Cawello W. Pharmacokinetics and ACE-inhibition of the new ACE-inhibitor moexipril: is coadministration with food of clinical relevance? *Hypertension* (1995) 25, 1384.
20. Lecocq B, Funck-Brentano C, Lecocq V, Ferry A, Gardin M-E, Devissaguet M, Jaillon P. Influence of food on the pharmacokinetics of perindopril and the time course of angiotensin-converting enzyme inhibition in serum. *Clin Pharmacol Ther* (1990) 47, 397–402.
21. Coversyl (Perindopril). Servier Laboratories Ltd. UK Summary of product characteristics, November 2005.
22. Tanatril (Imidapril). Trinity Pharmaceuticals Ltd. UK Summary of product characteristics, May 2003.

ACE inhibitors + Garlic

In a single report, a patient taking lisinopril developed marked hypotension and became faint after taking garlic capsules.

Clinical evidence, mechanism, importance and management

A man whose blood pressure was 135/90 mmHg while taking **lisinopril** 15 mg daily began to take garlic 4 mg daily (*Boots odourless garlic oil capsules*). After 3 days he became faint on standing and was found to have a blood pressure of 90/60 mmHg. Stopping the garlic restored his blood pressure to 135/90 mmHg within a week. The garlic on its own did not lower his blood pressure. The reasons for this interaction are not known, although garlic has been reported to cause vasodilatation and blood pressure reduction.[1] This seems to be the first and only report of this reaction, so its general importance is small. There seems to be nothing documented about garlic and any of the other ACE inhibitors.

1. McCoubrie M. Doctors as patients: lisinopril and garlic. *Br J Gen Pract* (1996) 46, 107.

ACE inhibitors + Gold

Peripheral vasodilatation has occurred when some patients receiving gold were given ACE inhibitors.

Clinical evidence, mechanism, importance and management

A report describes 4 patients receiving long-term gold for rheumatoid arthritis who developed nitritoid reactions (adverse effects associated with **sodium aurothiomalate** treatment, consisting of facial flushing, nausea, dizziness, and occasionally, hypotension, as a result of peripheral vasodilatation). These reactions occurred soon after starting treatment with an ACE inhibitor (**captopril**, **enalapril**, or **lisinopril**). All the patients had been receiving a monthly injection of **sodium aurothiomalate** 50 mg for at least 2 years and none had ever had such a reaction before. The reactions were controlled by changing treatment to aurothioglucose (1 patient), discontinuing the ACE inhibitor (2), or reducing the dose of **sodium aurothiomalate** to 25 mg (1).[1] There appear to be few reports of this interaction, possibly because the nitritoid reaction is an established adverse effect of gold. However, a possible interaction should be borne in mind if a patient experiences these reactions and is also taking an ACE inhibitor.

1. Healey LA, Backes MB, Mason V. Nitritoid reactions and angiotensin-converting-enzyme inhibitors. *N Engl J Med* (1989) 321, 763.

ACE inhibitors + H_2-receptor antagonists

In general, no clinically significant interactions appear to occur between the H_2-receptor antagonists (including cimetidine) and the ACE inhibitors. However, note that cimetidine modestly reduces the bioavailability of temocapril.

Clinical evidence, mechanism, importance and management

Cimetidine did not appear to alter the pharmacokinetics or pharmacological effects of **captopril**[1] or **enalapril**,[2] or the pharmacokinetics of **fosinopril**[3] or **quinapril**[4] in studies in healthy subjects. The manufacturers of **cilazapril** say that no clinically significant interaction occurred with H_2-receptor antagonists (not specifically named)[5] and the manufacturers of **moexipril**,[6,7] **ramipril**,[8] and **trandolapril**[9] say that no important pharmacokinetic interaction occurred with **cimetidine**. The manufacturers of **spirapril** briefly note in a review that **cimetidine** did not alter the plasma concentrations of **spirapril** or its active metabolite spiraprilat.[10] None of these pairs of drugs appears to interact to a clinically relevant extent, and no special precautions appear to be necessary.

Preliminary findings suggest that **cimetidine** 400 mg twice daily had no effect on the metabolism of **temocapril** 20 mg daily in 18 healthy subjects, but the AUC was reduced by 26% on the fifth day of concurrent use.[11] The clinical relevance of this is uncertain, but changes of this magnitude with other ACE inhibitors have often not been clinically relevant.

1. Richer C, Bah M, Cadilhac M, Thuillez C, Giudicelli JF. Cimetidine does not alter free unchanged captopril pharmacokinetics and biological effects in healthy volunteer. *J Pharmacol* (1986) 17, 338–42.
2. Ishizaki T, Baba T, Murabayashi S, Kubota K, Hara K, Kurimoto F. Effect of cimetidine on the pharmacokinetics and pharmacodynamics of enalapril in normal volunteers. *J Cardiovasc Pharmacol* (1988) 12, 512–9.
3. Moore L, Kramer A, Swites B, Kramer P, Tu J. Effect of cimetidine and antacid on the kinetics of the active diacid of fosinopril in healthy subjects. *J Clin Pharmacol* (1988) 28, 946.
4. Ferry JJ, Cetnarowski AB, Sedman AJ, Thomas RW, Horvath AM. Multiple-dose cimetidine administration does not influence the single-dose pharmacokinetics of quinapril and its active metabolite (CI-928). *J Clin Pharmacol* (1988) 28, 48–51.
5. Vascace (Cilazapril monohydrate). Roche Products Ltd. UK Summary of product characteristics, September 2005.
6. Perdix (Moexipril hydrochloride). Schwarz Pharma Ltd. UK Summary of product characteristics, July 2006.
7. Univasc (Moexipril hydrochloride). Schwarz Pharma. US Prescribing information, May 2003.
8. Altace Capsules (Ramipril). Monarch Pharmaceuticals, Inc. US Prescribing information, September 2005.
9. Mavik (Trandolapril). Abbott Laboratories. US Prescribing information, July 2003.
10. Grass P, Gerbeau C, Kutz K. Spirapril: pharmacokinetic properties and drug interactions. *Blood Pressure* (1994) 3 (Suppl 2), 7–13.
11. Trenk D, Schaefer A, Eberle E, Jähnchen E. Effect of cimetidine on the pharmacokinetics of the ACE-inhibitor temocapril. *Eur J Clin Pharmacol* (1996) 50, 556.

ACE inhibitors and Angiotensin II receptor antagonists + Heparins

Heparin may increase the risk of hyperkalaemia with ACE inhibitors or angiotensin II receptor antagonists.

Clinical evidence, mechanism, importance and management

An extensive review of the literature found that heparin (both **unfractionated** and **low-molecular-weight heparins**) and **heparinoids** inhibit the secretion of aldosterone, which can cause hyperkalaemia.[1] The CSM in the UK suggests that plasma-potassium levels should be measured in all patients with risk factors (including those taking potassium-sparing drugs) before starting heparin, and monitored regularly thereafter, particularly if heparin is to be continued for more than 7 days.[2] Note that ACE inhibitors and angiotensin II receptor antagonists are potassium sparing, via their effects on aldosterone. Some workers[1] have suggested that the monitoring interval should probably be no greater than 4 days in patients at a relatively high risk of hyperkalaemia. Other risk factors include renal impairment, diabetes mellitus, pre-existing acidosis or raised plasma potassium.[2]

If hyperkalaemia occurs, the offending drugs should be stopped (although this may not be practical in the case of heparin). When the hyperkalaemia has been corrected (by whatever medical intervention is deemed appropriate) the drugs can cautiously be reintroduced.

1. Oster JR, Singer I, Fishman LM. Heparin-induced aldosterone suppression and hyperkalemia. *Am J Med* (1995) 98, 575–86.
2. Committee on Safety of Medicines/Medicines Control Agency. Suppression of aldosterone secretion by heparin. *Current Problems* (1999) 25, 6.

ACE inhibitors + Insect allergen extracts

There are a few case reports of severe anaphylactoid reactions in patients receiving ACE inhibitors during desensitisation with bee or wasp venom. Extra caution is required, and some suggest temporarily withholding the ACE inhibitor before each venom injection.

Clinical evidence

A report describes 2 cases of anaphylactoid reactions during **wasp venom immunotherapy** in patients taking **enalapril**. In one patient, generalised pruritus and severe hypotension occurred within a few minutes of the first **venom** injection. Desensitisation was achieved after the **enalapril** was stopped, and then the immunotherapy was maintained by discontinuing the **enalapril** 24 hours before the monthly **venom** injection. However, on one occasion, when the **enalapril** had not been stopped, the patient experienced a severe anaphylactoid reaction 30 minutes after the **venom** injection. In the other patient an anaphylactoid reaction occurred after the second dose of **venom**. The ACE inhibitor was replaced with nifedipine so that **venom immunotherapy** could be continued.[1]

In another report, a 43-year-old man who had been taking ACE inhibitors for 2 years (**lisinopril** 40 mg daily for the previous 5 months) had a hypotensive reaction to an insect sting. After skin testing, he received venom immunotherapy. About 4 months later, he had a severe anaphylactic reaction 5 minutes after being given a maintenance dose of **wasp venom** and **mixed vespid venom**. The ACE inhibitor was replaced with a calcium-channel blocker, and he subsequently tolerated full-strength venom immunotherapy injections.[2]

Mechanism

ACE inhibitors might potentiate the hypotension associated with anaphylactic reactions by inhibiting the breakdown of bradykinin and decreasing concentrations of the vasoconstrictor angiotensin II.[3] It has also been suggested that similar reactions may occur after an insect sting.[3] This is supported by a case report that describes a woman who had generalised angiooedema in response to bee stings on at least three occasions while taking captopril and then cilazapril, but experienced only localised swelling before and after treatment with an ACE inhibitor.[4]

Importance and management

On the basis of these few reports, it cannot be said with certainty that an interaction occurs; however, it is possible that ACE inhibitors could exacerbate the response to insect venom immunotherapy. Because of the potential severity of the reaction, extra caution should be taken in patients taking ACE inhibitors and undergoing desensitising treatment with **Hymenoptera** (bee or wasp) **venom**. Some authors[1-3] and manufacturers advise temporarily withholding the ACE inhibitor before each desensitisation (24 hours was sufficient in one case), while others suggest temporary substitution of a different antihypertensive e.g. a calcium-channel blocker. Note that some evidence suggests that anaphylactic shock in patients taking beta blockers may be resistant to treatment with adrenaline (epinephrine), see 'Beta blockers + Inotropes and Vasopressors', p.848. Therefore beta blockers are probably not a suitable alternative.

1. Tunon-de-Lara JM, Villanueva P, Marcos M, Taytard A. ACE inhibitors and anaphylactoid reactions during venom immunotherapy. *Lancet* (1992) 340, 908.
2. Ober AI, MacLean JA, Hannaway PJ. Life-threatening anaphylaxis to venom immunotherapy in a patient taking an angiotensin-converting enzyme inhibitor. *J Allergy Clin Immunol* (2003) 112, 1008–9.

3. Stumpf JL, Shehab N, Patel AC. Safety of angiotensin-converting enzyme inhibitors in patients with insect venom allergies. *Ann Pharmacother* (2006) 40, 699–703.
4. Black PN, Simpson IJ. Angio-oedema and ACE inhibitors. *Aust N Z J Med* (1995) 25, 746.

ACE inhibitors + Interleukin-3

Marked hypotension occurred when three patients taking ACE inhibitors were given interleukin-3.

Clinical evidence, mechanism, importance and management

Twenty-six patients with ovarian or small-cell undifferentiated cancers were treated with chemotherapy followed by recombinant human interleukin-3. Three of the 26 were taking ACE inhibitors (not named) and all three developed marked hypotension (WHO toxicity grade 2 or 3) within 1 to 4 hours of the first interleukin-3 injection. Their blood pressures returned to normal while continuing the interleukin-3 when the ACE inhibitors were stopped. When the interleukin-3 was stopped, they once again needed the ACE inhibitors to control their blood pressure. None of the other 23 patients had hypotension, except one who did so during a period of neutropenic fever.[1] The authors of the report suggest (and present some supporting evidence) that the drugs act synergistically to generate large amounts of nitric oxide in the blood vessel walls. This relaxes the smooth muscle in the blood vessel walls causing vasodilatation and consequent hypotension.[1] Information seems to be limited to this single report, but it would be prudent to monitor blood pressure even more closely in patients receiving interleukin-3 while taking ACE inhibitors.

1. Dercksen MW, Hoekman K, Visser JJ, ten Bokkel Huinink WW, Pinedo HM, Wagstaff J. Hypotension induced by interleukin-3 in patients on angiotensin-converting enzyme inhibitors. *Lancet* (1995) 345, 448.

ACE inhibitors + Iron compounds

Serious systemic reactions occurred when three patients taking enalapril were given infusions of ferric sodium gluconate; however, there was no increase in the incidence of such adverse reactions in patients taking ACE inhibitors in a very large clinical study. Oral ferrous sulfate may decrease the absorption of captopril, but this is probably of little clinical importance.

Clinical evidence

(a) Intravenous iron

A man with iron-deficiency anaemia taking furosemide and digoxin was given 125 mg of **ferric sodium gluconate** (*Ferlixit*[1]) intravenously in 100 mL of saline daily. Four days later, **enalapril** 5 mg daily was started. After the infusion of only a few drops of his next dose of **ferric sodium gluconate**, he developed diffuse erythema, abdominal cramps, hypotension, nausea and vomiting. He recovered after being given hydrocortisone 200 mg. Three days later, in the absence of the **enalapril**, he restarted the iron infusions for a further 10 days without problems, and was later treated uneventfully with the **enalapril**.[2] Two other patients taking **enalapril** reacted similarly when given intravenous infusions of **ferric sodium gluconate**. Neither was given any more intravenous iron and later had no problems while taking **enalapril** alone. During the same 13-month period in which these three cases occurred, 15 other patients, who were not taking ACE inhibitors, also received intravenous iron therapy with no adverse reactions.[2] In contrast, an interim report of a randomised, crossover study involving 1117 dialysis patients given a placebo or a single intravenous dose of 125 mg of **ferric sodium gluconate complex** (*Ferrlecit*) in sucrose, found no evidence of any significant difference in the incidence of immediate allergic reactions or other adverse reactions to the iron in the 308 patients also taking ACE inhibitors.[3] The findings of the full study, which included 707 patients taking ACE inhibitors, were the same.[4] Similarly, the longer-term follow-up of patients from this study who continued to receive intravenous **ferric sodium gluconate complex**, found that there was no difference in the incidence or severity of adverse events in the 372 patients taking ACE inhibitors, when compared with the 949 patients who were not.[5]

(b) Oral iron

A double-blind study in 7 healthy subjects, given single 300-mg doses of **ferrous sulfate** or placebo with **captopril** 25 mg, found that the AUC of unconjugated plasma **captopril** (the active form) was reduced by 37% although the maximum plasma levels were not substantially changed. The AUC of total plasma **captopril** was increased by 43%, although this was not statistically significant. There were no significant differences in blood pressure between treatment and placebo groups.[6]

Mechanism

(a) Uncertain. Intravenous iron may cause a variety of systemic reactions including fever, myalgia, arthralgia, hypotension, and nausea and vomiting, which are believed to be due to the release of various inflammatory mediators such as bradykinin, caused by iron-catalysed toxic free radicals. The authors of the report suggest that ACE inhibitors like enalapril decrease the breakdown of kinins so that the toxic effects of the iron become exaggerated.[2]
(b) Reduced levels of unconjugated captopril in the plasma are probably due to reduced absorption resulting from a chemical interaction between ferric ions and captopril in the gastrointestinal tract.[6]

Importance and management

(a) The interaction with intravenous iron is not firmly established because up to 25% of all patients given iron by this route develop a variety of systemic reactions, ranging from mild to serious anaphylactoid reactions. In addition, information from the large clinical study indicates that there is no increased risk in patients taking ACE inhibitors. This suggests that no extra precautions are required if intravenous iron is given to patients taking any ACE inhibitor.
(b) There is limited evidence that oral iron may reduce the absorption of captopril. The clinical relevance of this is unknown, but probably small. Information about the effect of oral iron on other ACE inhibitors is lacking.

1. Rolla G. Personal communication, 1994.
2. Rolla G, Bucca C, Brussino L. Systemic reactions to intravenous iron therapy in patients receiving angiotensin converting enzyme inhibitor. *J Allergy Clin Immunol* (1994) 93, 1074–5.
3. Warnock DG, Adkinson F, Coyne DW, Strobos J, Ferrlecit® Safety Study Group. ACE inhibitors and intravenous sodium ferric gluconate complex in sucrose (SFGC): lack of any significant interaction. *J Am Soc Nephrol* (2000) 11, 170A.
4. Michael B, Coyne DW, Fishbane S, Folkert V, Lynn R, Nissenson AR, Agarwal R, Eschbach JW, Fadem SZ, Trout JR, Strobos J, Warnock DG; Ferrlecit Publication Committee. Sodium ferric gluconate complex in hemodialysis patients: adverse reactions compared to placebo and iron dextran. *Kidney Int* (2002) 61, 1830–9.
5. Michael B, Coyne DW, Folkert VW, Dahl NV, Warnock DG; Ferrlecit Publication Committee. Sodium ferric gluconate complex in haemodialysis patients: a prospective evaluation of long-term safety. *Nephrol Dial Transplant* (2004) 19, 1576–80.
6. Schaefer JP, Tam Y, Hasinoff BB, Tawfik S, Peng Y, Reimche L, Campbell NRC. Ferrous sulphate interacts with captopril. *Br J Clin Pharmacol* (1998) 46, 377–81.

ACE inhibitors + Moracizine

Moracizine causes some moderate alterations in the pharmacokinetics of free captopril, but these are unlikely to be clinically important.

Clinical evidence, mechanism, importance and management

In a pharmacokinetic study, 19 healthy subjects were given moracizine 250 mg or **captopril** 50 mg, both every 8 hours, either alone or together, for 22 doses. When taken together the pharmacokinetics of the moracizine and total **captopril** remained unchanged, but the maximum blood levels of the free **captopril** and its AUC decreased by 32% and 14%, respectively. The half-life of the free **captopril** was reduced by 44%.[1] These modest changes are unlikely to be clinically relevant.

1. Pieniaszek HJ, Shum L, Widner P, Garner DM, Benedek IH. Pharmacokinetic interaction of moricizine and captopril in healthy volunteers. *J Clin Pharmacol* (1993) 33, 1005.

ACE inhibitors + NSAIDs

There is evidence that most NSAIDs can increase blood pressure in patients taking antihypertensives, including ACE inhibitors, although some studies have not found the increase to be clinically relevant. Some variation between drugs possibly occurs, with in-

dometacin appearing to have the most significant effect. The combination of an NSAID and an ACE inhibitor can increase the risk of renal impairment and hyperkalaemia.

Clinical evidence

(A) Effects on blood pressure

Various large epidemiological studies and meta-analyses of clinical studies have been conducted to assess the effect of NSAIDs on blood pressure in patients taking **antihypertensives**, and the findings of these are summarised in 'Table 23.2', (p.862). In these studies, NSAIDs were not always associated with an increase in blood pressure, and the maximum increase was 6.2 mmHg. The effect has been shown for both coxibs and non-selective NSAIDs. In two meta-analyses,[1,2] the effects were evaluated by NSAID. The confidence intervals for all the NSAIDs overlapped, showing that there was no statistically significant difference between them, with the exception of the comparison between **indometacin** and **sulindac** in one analysis.[2] Nevertheless, an attempt was made at ranking the NSAIDs based on the means. In one analysis,[1] the effect was said to be greatest for **piroxicam**, **indometacin**, and **ibuprofen**, intermediate for **naproxen**, and least for **sulindac** and **flurbiprofen**. In the other meta-analysis,[2] the effect was said to be greatest for **indometacin** and **naproxen**, intermediate for **piroxicam**, and least for **ibuprofen** and **sulindac**. An attempt was also made to evaluate the effect by **antihypertensive**.[1] The mean effect was greatest for beta blockers, intermediate for vasodilators (this group included ACE inhibitors and calcium-channel blockers), and least for diuretics. However, the differences between the groups were not significant.

The findings of individual studies that have studied the effects of specific NSAIDs on ACE inhibitors are outlined in the subsections below.

(a) Celecoxib

In a double-blind study in hypertensive patients taking **lisinopril** 10 to 40 mg daily, celecoxib did not have a clinically or statistically significant effect on blood pressure. The 24-hour blood pressure increased by 2.6/1.5 mmHg in 91 patients taking celecoxib 200 mg twice daily for 4 weeks compared with 1/0.3 mmHg in 87 patients taking placebo.[3] In another large study in 810 elderly patients with osteoarthritis and controlled hypertension given either celecoxib 200 mg or rofecoxib 25 mg daily for 6 weeks, approximately 40% of the patients randomised to the celecoxib group were receiving ACE inhibitors. Systolic blood pressure increased by a clinically significant amount (greater than 20 mmHg) in 11% of patients receiving celecoxib,[4] while in another study, only 4 of 87 (4.6%) of hypertensive patients taking ACE inhibitors had clinically significant increases in blood pressure after taking celecoxib 200 mg twice daily for 4 weeks.[5] A further study in 25 hypertensive patients with osteoarthritis taking **trandolapril** (with or without hydrochlorothiazide) found that the 24-hour blood pressure was not significantly increased by celecoxib 200 mg daily, but, at its peak activity, celecoxib increased blood pressure by about 5/4 mmHg.[6] In another randomised study, 16% of 138 patients given celecoxib 200 mg daily developed hypertension within 6 weeks (defined as a 24-hour systolic blood pressure greater than 135 mmHg). These patients had well-controlled hypertension at baseline; 83% were receiving an ACE inhibitor and 64% an additional antihypertensive.[7] The proportion of patients who developed hypertension was similar to that with naproxen (19%) and less than that with rofecoxib (30%).

(b) Ibuprofen

In 90 patients taking ACE inhibitors, giving ibuprofen for 4 weeks resulted in clinically significant increases in blood pressure in 15 of the patients. For the group as a whole, diastolic blood pressure was increased by 3.5 mmHg.[5] In one single-dose study, ibuprofen 800 mg or indometacin 50 mg abolished the hypotensive effect of **captopril** 50 mg in 8 healthy subjects when they took a high sodium diet, but not when they took a low sodium diet.[8] A case report describes attenuation of the antihypertensive effects of **captopril** by ibuprofen in an elderly woman.[9] However, two studies in African women found that ibuprofen 800 mg three times daily for one month did not alter the antihypertensive effect of either **fosinopril** 10 to 40 mg daily or **lisinopril** 10 to 40 mg daily (given with hydrochlorothiazide 25 mg daily).[10,11] It was thought that the diuretic might have enhanced salt depletion and renin stimulation making the antihypertensive action of the combination less prostaglandin dependent.[10]

(c) Indometacin

1. Captopril. In a randomised, double-blind study, 105 patients with hypertension were given captopril 25 to 50 mg twice daily for 6 weeks, which reduced their blood pressure by a mean of 8.6/5.6 mmHg. Indometacin 75 mg once daily was then added for one week, which caused a rise in blood pressure in the group as a whole of 4.6/2.7 mmHg (an attenuation of the effect of captopril of about 50%). Clear attenuation was seen in 67% of the patients, and occurred regardless of baseline blood pressure.[12] This same interaction has been described in numerous earlier studies, in both patients with hypertension and healthy subjects, given indometacin.[8,13-20] A man whose blood pressure was well controlled with captopril 75 mg daily had a rise in his blood pressure from 145/80 to 220/120 mmHg when he started using indometacin suppositories 200 mg daily.[21] In contrast, a randomised, placebo-controlled, crossover study in 11 patients found that indometacin 50 mg twice daily did not alter the antihypertensive efficacy of captopril 50 mg twice daily.[22]

2. Enalapril. In 9 patients with hypertension indometacin 50 mg twice daily for 1 week significantly reduced the antihypertensive effect of enalapril 20 to 40 mg once daily by about 18 to 22%.[23] In another study in 18 patients, indometacin 25 mg three times daily attenuated the antihypertensive effect of enalapril 20 to 40 mg daily. The reduction in hypotensive effect was about 42% when assessed by 24-hour ambulatory blood-pressure monitoring (9.4/4.1 mmHg increase in blood pressure with indometacin), and 12 to 23% when assessed by clinic blood pressure monitoring.[24] Similar results were found in other studies.[25-28] A further study in 10 normotensive subjects receiving a fixed sodium intake and enalapril 20 mg daily, with or without indometacin 50 mg twice daily for one week, found that indometacin reduced the natriuretic response to the ACE inhibitor.[29] A single case report describes a patient taking enalapril 10 mg daily whose hypertension was not controlled when indometacin 100 mg daily in divided doses was added.[30] However, other studies found indometacin did not significantly alter the blood pressure response to enalapril.[19,22,31]

3. Lisinopril. In a placebo-controlled, crossover study, indometacin 50 mg twice daily for 2 weeks produced mean blood pressure increases of 5.5/3.2 mmHg in 56 patients taking lisinopril 10 to 20 mg daily.[32] Similarly, results of an earlier study suggested that indometacin increased the blood pressure of 9 patients taking lisinopril.[26] In contrast in a placebo-controlled study in 16 patients, indometacin 50 mg twice daily for 4 weeks was found to have little effect on the antihypertensive efficacy of lisinopril 40 mg daily.[33]

4. Other ACE inhibitors. A placebo-controlled, randomised, crossover study in 16 hypertensive patients found that indometacin 50 mg twice daily reduced the blood pressure-lowering effects of **cilazapril** 2.5 mg daily. The reduction was greater when **cilazapril** was added to indometacin than when indometacin was added to **cilazapril** (approximately 60% versus 30% reduction in hypotensive effect measured 3 hours after the morning dose).[34] The antihypertensive effects of **perindopril** 4 to 8 mg daily were also found to be reduced by about 30% by indometacin 50 mg twice daily in 10 hypertensive patients.[35] A brief mention is made in a review that the pharmacodynamics of **ramipril** were unaffected by indometacin (dosage not stated) given to healthy subjects for 3 days.[36] Indometacin 25 mg three times daily did not alter the hypotensive effects of **trandolapril** 2 mg daily in 17 hypertensive patients.[37]

(d) Naproxen

In a randomised study, 19% of 130 patients given naproxen 500 mg twice daily developed hypertension within 6 weeks (defined as a 24-hour systolic blood pressure greater than 135 mmHg). These patients had well-controlled hypertension at baseline; 83% were receiving an ACE inhibitor and 66% an additional antihypertensive.[7] The proportion of patients who developed hypertension was similar to that with celecoxib (16%) and less than that with rofecoxib (30%).

(e) Rofecoxib

The manufacturer of rofecoxib noted that in patients with mild-to-moderate hypertension, rofecoxib 25 mg daily, taken with **benazepril** 10 to 40 mg daily, for four weeks, was associated with a small attenuation of the antihypertensive effect (average increase in mean arterial pressure of 2.8 mmHg).[38] Similarly, a case report describes a patient taking **lisinopril** 10 mg daily whose blood pressure rose from 127/78 to 143/89 mmHg when he was given rofecoxib 25 mg daily. His blood pressure was controlled by increasing the dose of **lisinopril** to 20 mg daily.[39]

In another study in 810 elderly patients with osteoarthritis and controlled hypertension given either celecoxib 200 mg or rofecoxib 25 mg daily for

6 weeks, approximately 29% of the patients randomised to the rofecoxib group were receiving ACE inhibitors. Systolic blood pressure increased by a clinically significant amount (greater than 20 mmHg) in 17% of the patients receiving rofecoxib.[4] In another similar randomised study, 30% of 138 patients given rofecoxib 25 mg daily developed hypertension within 6 weeks (defined as a 24-hour systolic blood pressure greater than 135 mmHg). These patients had well-controlled hypertension at baseline; 84% were receiving an ACE inhibitor and 62% an additional antihypertensive.[7] The proportion of patients who developed hypertension was greater than with celecoxib (16%) or naproxen (19%).

(f) Sulindac

In one study, sulindac 200 mg twice daily given to patients taking **captopril** 100 to 200 mg twice daily caused only a small rise in blood pressure (from 132/92 to 137/95 mmHg).[15] Sulindac 150 mg twice daily did not attenuate the blood pressure response to **captopril** when it was substituted for ibuprofen in an elderly woman.[9] Similarly, sulindac 200 mg twice daily did not blunt the antihypertensive effect of **enalapril** in 9 patients with hypertension.[31] Two studies in black women also found that sulindac 200 mg twice daily for one month did not alter the antihypertensive effect of **fosinopril** 10 to 40 mg daily or **lisinopril** 10 to 40 mg daily (given with hydrochlorothiazide 25 mg daily).[10,11]

(g) Other NSAIDs

A single 8-mg dose of **lornoxicam** was found to have no effect on the systolic blood pressure of 6 hypertensive patients taking **enalapril**, but a small rise in diastolic pressure (from 88.2 to 93.3 mmHg) occurred after 2 hours.[25] In 29 patients with hypertension **oxaprozin** 1.2 g daily for 3 weeks did not affect the pharmacodynamics of **enalapril** 10 to 40 mg daily.[40]

Twenty-five hypertensive patients with osteoarthritis taking **trandolapril** 2 to 4 mg daily (with or without hydrochlorothiazide) had an increase in blood pressure of about 3/4 mmHg when they were given **diclofenac** 75 mg twice daily.[6] However, **diclofenac** 75 mg twice daily for one month did not alter the antihypertensive effect of **lisinopril** 10 to 40 mg daily (given with hydrochlorothiazide).[11]

A study found that only 5 of 91 (5.5%) hypertensive patients stabilised on ACE inhibitors had clinically significant increases in blood pressure when they were given **nabumetone** 1 g twice daily for 4 weeks.[5] A study in 17 black women found that **nabumetone** 1 g twice daily for one month did not alter the antihypertensive effect of **fosinopril** 10 to 40 mg daily (given with hydrochlorothiazide).[10]

(B) Effects on renal function

In a retrospective analysis, 3 of 162 patients who had been taking ACE inhibitors and NSAIDs developed reversible renal failure, compared with none of 166 patients taking ACE inhibitors alone and none of 2116 patients taking NSAIDs alone. One patient was taking **naproxen** or **salsalate** and had a progressive decline in renal function over 19 months after **captopril** was started. Another man taking unnamed NSAIDs developed reversible renal failure 4 days after starting to take **captopril**.[41] In another similar analysis, in patients aged over 75 years, 2 out of 12 patients given an ACE inhibitor and an NSAID developed acute renal failure (1 died) and a further 4 showed deterioration in renal function. All of these 6 patients were also taking 'diuretics', (p.21), but of the 6 with unaffected renal function, only two were taking diuretics.[42] A randomised, crossover study in 17 black patients receiving **fosinopril** with hydrochlorothiazide and NSAIDs for a month, found that acute renal failure (a decrease in glomerular filtration rate of greater than or equal to 25%) occurred in 4 of the 17 patients when receiving **ibuprofen**, 1 of 17 receiving **sulindac** and 0 of 17 receiving **nabumetone**.[10] In a multivariate analysis, significant renal impairment was associated with use of two or more of ACE inhibitors or angiotensin II receptor antagonists with NSAIDs or diuretics.[43] In a case-control study, recently starting an NSAID was associated with a 2.2-fold increased risk of hospitalisation for renal impairment in patients taking ACE inhibitors.[44] In 2002, 28 of 129 reports to the Australian Adverse Drug Reactions Advisory Committee of acute renal failure were associated with the combined use of ACE inhibitors (or angiotensin II receptor antagonists), diuretics, and NSAIDs (including coxibs), and these cases had a fatality rate of 10%. In patients taking this triple combination, renal failure appeared to be precipitated by mild stress such as diarrhoea or dehydration. In other patients, the addition of a third drug (usually an NSAID) to a stable combination of the other two, resulted in acute renal failure.[45]

In contrast, another retrospective analysis found no evidence that the adverse effects of ACE inhibitors on renal function were greater in those taking NSAIDs.[46] A further study in 17 hypertensive patients with normal baseline renal function, found that **indometacin** 25 mg three times daily did not adversely affect renal function when it was given with **trandolapril** 2 mg daily for 3 weeks.[47]

(C) Hyperkalaemia

Hyperkalaemia, resulting in marked bradycardia, was attributed to the use of **loxoprofen** in an elderly woman taking **imidapril**.[48] A 77-year-old woman with mild hypertension and normal renal function taking **enalapril** 2.5 mg daily arrested and died 5 days after starting treatment with **rofecoxib** for leg pain. Her potassium was found to be 8.8 mmol/L. Infection and dehydration could have contributed to the hyperkalaemia in this patient.[49]

(D) Pharmacokinetic studies

The manufacturer of **spirapril** briefly noted in a review that there was no relevant pharmacokinetic interaction between **spirapril** and **diclofenac**.[50] **Oxaprozin** 1.2 g daily for 3 weeks did not affect the pharmacokinetics of **enalapril** 10 to 40 mg daily in 29 patients with hypertension.[40] A brief mention is made in a review that, in healthy subjects, the pharmacokinetics of **ramipril** were unaffected by **indometacin** [dosage not stated] given for 3 days.[36]

Mechanism

Some, but not all the evidence suggests that prostaglandins may be involved in the hypotensive action of ACE inhibitors, and that NSAIDs, by inhibiting prostaglandin synthesis, may partially antagonise the effect of ACE inhibitors. Another suggestion is that NSAIDs promote sodium retention and so blunt the blood pressure lowering effects of several classes of antihypertensive drugs, including ACE inhibitors. This interaction may be dependent on sodium status and on plasma renin, and so drugs that affect sodium status e.g. diuretics may possibly influence the effect. Therefore, the interaction does not occur in all patients. It may also depend on the NSAID, with indometacin being frequently implicated, and sulindac less so, as well as on the dosing frequency.[6]

Both NSAIDs and ACE inhibitors alone can cause renal impairment. In patients whose kidneys are underperfused, they may cause further deterioration in renal function when used together.[51] Impaired renal function is a risk factor for hyperkalaemia with ACE inhibitors.

Importance and management

The interaction between indometacin and ACE inhibitors is well established, with several studies showing that indometacin can reduce the **blood pressure-lowering** effect of a number of ACE inhibitors. The interaction may not occur in all patients. If indometacin is required in a patient taking any ACE inhibitor, it would be prudent to monitor blood pressure. In a few small comparative studies, indometacin has been shown to have less effect on the calcium-channel blockers amlodipine, felodipine, and nifedipine, than on enalapril.[24,27,28] See also, 'Calcium-channel blockers + Aspirin or NSAIDs', p.861. Therefore, a calcium-channel blocker may sometimes be an alternative to an ACE inhibitor in a patient requiring indometacin.

Limited information suggests that sulindac has little or no effect on ACE inhibitors, and may therefore be less likely to cause a problem, but further study is needed. The coxibs appear to have similar (celecoxib) or greater (rofecoxib) effects on ACE inhibitors than conventional NSAIDs (naproxen).

Although information about other NSAIDs is limited, the mechanism suggests that all of them are likely to interact similarly. Until more is known, it may be prudent to increase blood pressure monitoring when any NSAID is added or discontinued in a patient taking any ACE inhibitor, and intermittent use of NSAIDs should be considered as a possible cause of erratic control of blood pressure. In addition, sodium status and therefore diuretic use may affect any interaction. However, some consider that the clinical importance of an interaction between NSAIDs and antihypertensives is less than has previously been suggested.[52] While their findings do not rule out a 2/1 mmHg increase in blood pressure with NSAIDs in treated hypertensives, they suggest that if patients in primary care have inadequate control of blood pressure, other reasons may be more likely than any effect of concurrent NSAIDs.[52] Further study is needed. For the effects of NSAIDs on other antihypertensive drug classes see 'beta blockers', (p.835), 'calcium-channel blockers', (p.861) and 'thiazide diuretics', (p.956).

There is an increased risk of **deterioration in renal function** or acute renal failure with the combination of NSAIDs and ACE inhibitors, especially if poor renal perfusion is present. Renal function should be monitored periodically in patients taking ACE inhibitors with NSAIDs, particularly in volume depleted patients. In a statement, the American Heart Association comments that acute renal failure complicating ACE inhibitor therapy is almost always reversible and repletion of extracellular fluid volume and discontinuation of diuretic therapy is the best approach. In addition, withdrawal of interacting drugs, supportive management of fluid and electrolytes, and temporary dialysis, where indicated, are the mainstays of therapy.[53] The Australian Adverse Drug Reactions Advisory Committee consider that the triple combination of ACE inhibitors, 'diuretics', (p.21) and NSAIDs (including coxibs) should be avoided if possible, and that great care should be taken when giving ACE inhibitors and NSAIDs to patients with renal impairment.[45] Deterioration in renal function increases the risk of **hyperkalaemia**.

1. Johnson AG, Nguyen TV, Day RO. Do nonsteroidal anti-inflammatory drugs affect blood pressure? A meta-analysis. *Ann Intern Med* (1994) 121, 289–300.
2. Pope JE, Anderson JJ, Felson DT. A meta-analysis of the effects of nonsteroidal anti-inflammatory drugs on blood pressure. *Arch Intern Med* (1993) 153, 477–84.
3. White WB, Kent J, Taylor A, Verburg K, Lefkowith JB, Whelton A. Effects of celecoxib on ambulatory blood pressure in hypertensive patients on ACE inhibitors. *Hypertension* (2002) 39, 929–34.
4. Whelton A, Fort JG, Puma JA, Normandin D, Bello AE, Verburg KM, for the SUCCESS VI Study Group. Cyclooxygenase-2-specific inhibitors and cardiorenal function: a randomized, controlled trial of celecoxib and rofecoxib in older hypertensive osteoarthritis patients. *Am J Ther* (2001) 8, 85–95.
5. Palmer R, Weiss R, Zusman RM, Haig A, Flavin S, MacDonald B. Effects of nabumetone, celecoxib, and ibuprofen on blood pressure control in hypertensive patients on angiotensin converting enzyme inhibitors. *Am J Hypertens* (2003) 16, 135–9.
6. Izhar M, Alausa T, Folker A, Hung E, Bakris GL. Effects of COX inhibition on blood pressure and kidney function in ACE inhibitor-treated blacks and hispanics. *Hypertension* (2004) 43, 573–7.
7. Sowers JR, White WB, Pitt B, Whelton A, Simon LS, Winer N, Kivitz A, van Ingen H, Brabant T, Fort JG; Celecoxib Rofecoxib Efficacy and Safety in Comorbidities Evaluation Trial (CRESCENT) Investigators. *Arch Intern Med* (2005) 165, 161–8.
8. Goldstone R, Martin K, Zipser R, Horton R. Evidence for a dual action of converting enzyme inhibitor on blood pressure in normal man. *Prostaglandins* (1981) 22, 587–98.
9. Espino DV, Lancaster MC. Neutralization of the effects of captopril by the use of ibuprofen in an elderly woman. *J Am Board Fam Pract* (1992) 5, 319–21.
10. Thakur V, Cook ME, Wallin JD. Antihypertensive effect of the combination of fosinopril and HCTZ is resistant to interference by nonsteroidal antiinflammatory drugs. *Am J Hypertens* (1999) 12, 925–8.
11. Bhagat K. Effects of non-steroidal anti-inflammatory drugs on hypertension control using angiotensin converting enzyme inhibitors and thiazide diuretics. *East Afr Med J* (2001) 78, 507–9.
12. Conlin PR, Moore TJ, Swartz SL, Barr E, Gazdick L, Fletcher C, DeLucca P, Demopoulos L. Effect of indomethacin on blood pressure lowering by captopril and losartan in hypertensive patients. *Hypertension* (2000) 36, 461–5.
13. Moore TJ, Crantz FR, Hollenberg NK, Koletsky RJ, Leboff MS, Swartz SL, Levine L, Podolsky S, Dluhy RG, Williams GH. Contribution of prostaglandins to the antihypertensive action of captopril in essential hypertension. *Hypertension* (1981) 3, 168–73.
14. Swartz SL, Williams GH. Angiotensin-converting enzyme inhibition and prostaglandins. *Am J Cardiol* (1982) 49, 1405–9.
15. Salvetti A, Pedrinelli R, Magagna A, Ugenti P. Differential effects of selective and non-selective prostaglandin-synthesis inhibition on the pharmacological responses to captopril in patients with essential hypertension. *Clin Sci* (1982) 63, 261S–263S.
16. Silberbauer K, Stanek B, Templ H. Acute hypotensive effect of captopril in man modified by prostaglandin synthesis inhibition. *Br J Clin Pharmacol* (1982) 14, 87S–93S.
17. Witzgall H, Hirsch F, Scherer B, Weber PC. Acute haemodynamic and hormonal effects of captopril are diminished by indomethacin. *Clin Sci* (1982) 62, 611–15.
18. Ogihara T, Maruyama A, Hata T, Mikami H, Nakamaru M, Naka T, Ohde H, Kumahara Y. Hormonal responses to long-term converting enzyme inhibition in hypertensive patients. *Clin Pharmacol Ther* (1981) 30, 328–35.
19. Koopmans PP, Van Megen T, Thien T, Gribnau FWJ. The interaction between indomethacin and captopril or enalapril in healthy volunteers. *J Intern Med* (1989) 226, 139–42.
20. Fujita T, Yamashita N, Yamashita K. Effect of indomethacin on antihypertensive action of captopril in hypertensive patients. *Clin Exp Hypertens* (1981) 3, 939–52.
21. Robles Iniesta A, Navarro de León MC, Morales Serna JC. Bloqueo de la acción antihipertensiva del captoprilo por indometacina. *Med Clin (Barc)* (1991) 96, 438.
22. Gerber JG, Franca G, Byyny RL, LoVerde M, Nies AS. The hypotensive action of captopril and enalapril is not prostacyclin dependent. *Clin Pharmacol Ther* (1993) 54, 523–32.
23. Salvetti A, Abdel-Haq B, Magagna A, Pedrinelli R. Indomethacin reduces the antihypertensive action of enalapril. *Clin Exp Hypertens A* (1987) 9, 559–67.
24. Polónia J, Boaventura I, Gama G, Camões I, Bernardo F, Andrade P, Nunes JP, Brandão F, Cerqueira-Gomes M. Influence of non-steroidal anti-inflammatory drugs on renal function and 24 h ambulatory blood pressure-reducing effects of enalapril and nifedipine gastrointestinal therapeutic system in hypertensive patients. *J Hypertens* (1995) 13, 925–31.
25. Walden RJ, Owens CWI, Graham BR, Snape A, Nutt J, Prichard BNC. NSAIDs and the control of hypertension: a pilot study. *Br J Clin Pharmacol* (1992) 33, 241P.
26. Duffin D, Leahey W, Brennan G, Johnston GD. The effects of indomethacin on the antihypertensive responses to enalapril and lisinopril. *Br J Clin Pharmacol* (1992) 34, 456P.
27. Morgan T, Anderson A. Interaction of indomethacin with felodipine and enalapril. *J Hypertens* (1993) 11 (Suppl 5), S338–S339.
28. Morgan TO, Anderson A, Bertram D. Effect of indomethacin on blood pressure in elderly people with essential hypertension well controlled on amlodipine or enalapril. *Am J Hypertens* (2000), 13, 1161–7.
29. Fricker AF, Nussberger J, Meilenbrock S, Brunner HR, Burnier M. Effect of indomethacin on the renal response to angiotensin II receptor blockade in healthy subjects. *Kidney Int* (1998) 54, 2089–97.
30. Ahmad S. Indomethacin-enalapril interaction: an alert. *South Med J* (1991) 84, 411–2.
31. Oparil S, Horton R, Wilkins LH, Irvin J, Hammett DK. Antihypertensive effect of enalapril in essential hypertension: role of prostacyclin. *Am J Med Sci* (1987) 294, 395–402.
32. Fogari R, Zoppi A, Carretta R, Veglio F, Salvetti A: Italian Collaborative Study Group. Effect of indomethacin on the antihypertensive efficacy of valsartan and lisinopril: a multicentre study. *J Hypertens* (2002) 20: 1007–14.
33. Shaw W, Shapiro D, Antonello J, Cressman M, Vlasses P, Oparil S. Indomethacin does not blunt the antihypertensive effect of lisinopril. *Clin Pharmacol Ther* (1987) 41, 219.
34. Kirch W, Stroemer K, Hoogkamer JFW, Kleinbloesem CH. The influence of prostaglandin inhibition by indomethacin on blood pressure and renal function in hypertensive patients treated with cilazapril. *Br J Clin Pharmacol* (1989) 27, 297S–301S.
35. Abdel-Haq B, Magagna A, Favilla S, Salvetti A. Hemodynamic and humoral interactions between perindopril and indomethacin in essential hypertensive subjects. *J Cardiovasc Pharmacol* (1991) 18 (Suppl 7), S33–S36.
36. Quoted as data on file (Hoechst) by Todd PA, Benfield P. Ramipril. A review of its pharmacological properties and therapeutic efficacy in cardiovascular disorders. *Drugs* (1990) 39, 110–35.
37. Pritchard G, Lyons D, Webster J, Petrie JC, MacDonald TM. Indomethacin does not attenuate the hypotensive effect of trandolapril. *J Hum Hypertens* (1996) 10, 763–7.
38. Vioxx (Rofecoxib). Merck Sharp & Dohme Ltd. UK Summary of product characteristics, August 2003.
39. Brown CH. Effect of rofecoxib on the antihypertensive activity of lisinopril. *Ann Pharmacother* (2000) 34, 1486.
40. Noveck RJ, McMahon FG, Bocanegra T, Karem A, Sugimoto D, Smith M. Effects of oxaprozin on enalapril and enalaprilat pharmacokinetics, pharmacodynamics: blood pressure, heart rate, plasma renin activity, aldosterone and creatinine clearances, in hypertensive patients. *Clin Pharmacol Ther* (1997), 61, 208.
41. Seelig CB, Maloley PA, Campbell JR. Nephrotoxicity associated with concomitant ACE inhibitor and NSAID therapy. *South Med J* (1990) 83, 1144–8.
42. Adhiyaman V, Asghar M, Oke A, White AD, Shah IU. Nephrotoxicity in the elderly due to co-prescription of angiotensin converting enzyme inhibitors and nonsteroidal anti-inflammatory drugs. *J R Soc Med* (2001) 94, 512–14.
43. Loboz KK, Shenfield GM. Drug combinations and impaired renal function –the 'triple whammy'. *Br J Clin Pharmacol* (2005) 59, 239–43.
44. Bouvy ML, Heerdink ER, Hoes AW, Leufkens HGM. Effects of NSAIDs on the incidence of hospitalisations for renal dysfunction in users of ACE inhibitors. *Drug Safety* (2003) 26, 983–9.
45. ADRAC. ACE inhibitor, diuretic and NSAID: a dangerous combination. *Aust Adverse Drug React Bull* (2003) 22, 14–15. Available at: http://www.tga.gov.au/adr/aadrb/aadr0308.pdf (accessed 14/08/07).
46. Stürmer T, Erb A, Keller F, Günther K-P, Brenner H. Determinants of impaired renal function with use of nonsteroidal anti-inflammatory drugs: the importance of half-life and other medications. *Am J Med* (2001) 111, 521–7.
47. Pritchard G, Lyons D, Webster J, Petrie JC, MacDonald TM. Do trandolapril and indomethacin influence renal function and renal functional reserve in hypertensive patients? *Br J Clin Pharmacol* (1997) 44, 145–9.
48. Kurata C, Uehara A, Sugi T, Yamazaki K. Syncope caused by nonsteroidal anti-inflammatory drugs and angiotensin-converting enzyme inhibitors. *Jpn Circ J* (1999) 63, 1002–3.
49. Hay E, Derazon H, Bukish N, Katz L, Kruglyakov I, Armoni M. Fatal hyperkalaemia related to combined therapy with a COX-2 inhibitor, ACE inhibitor and potassium rich diet. *J Emerg Med* (2002) 22, 349–52.
50. Grass P, Gerbeau C, Kutz K. Spirapril: pharmacokinetic properties and drug interactions. *Blood Pressure* (1994) 3 (Suppl 2), 7–13.
51. Sturrock NDC, Struthers AD. Non-steroidal anti-inflammatory drugs and angiotensin converting enzyme inhibitors: a commonly prescribed combination with variable effects on renal function. *Br J Clin Pharmacol* (1993) 35, 343–8.
52. Sheridan R, Montgomery AA, Fahey T. NSAID use and BP in treated hypertensives: a retrospective controlled observational study. *J Hum Hypertens* (2005) 19, 445–50.
53. Schoolwerth AC, Sica DA, Ballermann BJ, Wilcox CS. Renal considerations in angiotensin converting enzyme inhibitor therapy. A statement for healthcare professionals from the Council on the Kidney in Cardiovascular Disease and the Council for High Blood Pressure Research of the American Heart Association. *Circulation* (2001) 104, 1985–91.

ACE inhibitors and other antihypertensives + Orlistat

In a handful of cases, patients taking enalapril and/or losartan and other antihypertensive drugs (amlodipine, atenolol, hydrochlorothiazide) had marked increases in blood pressure, hypertensive crises and, in one case, intracranial haemorrhage, within 7 to 60 days of starting orlistat.

Clinical evidence

The Argentinian System of Pharmacovigilance identified the following 3 cases of a possible interaction of orlistat with antihypertensives. An obese man whose hypertension was controlled at 120/80 mmHg with daily doses of **losartan** 100 mg, **atenolol** 100 mg, and **hydrochlorothiazide** 12.5 mg developed a hypertensive crisis (BP 260/140 mmHg) 7 days after starting to take orlistat 120 mg three times daily. The orlistat was stopped and the crisis was controlled. When later rechallenged with orlistat, his diastolic blood pressure rose to 100 to 110 mmHg after 5 days, but the systolic blood pressure increased only slightly. His blood pressure returned to baseline values 3 days after stopping the orlistat.[1] Two other patients reacted similarly. One whose blood pressure was controlled at 130/85 mmHg with **enalapril** 20 mg daily and **losartan** 50 mg daily developed an intracranial haemorrhage and hypertension (BP 160/100 mmHg) with occasional systolic peaks of around 200 mmHg one week after starting orlistat 120 mg three times daily. The other patient who was taking **enalapril** 20 mg daily and **amlodipine** 5 mg daily began to develop hypertensive peaks (BP 180/120 mmHg) 60 days after starting orlistat 120 mg twice daily. The hypertension responded to a change to **losartan** with **hydrochlorothiazide**, but 20 days later new hypertensive peaks developed (BP 180/110 to 120 mmHg). When the orlistat was withdrawn, the hypertension was controlled within 48 hours.[1]

The Uppsala Adverse Drug Reaction database has two reports of aggravated hypertension in women taking antihypertensives and orlistat.[1] Hypertension has also been reported in previously normotensive individuals taking orlistat, which, in one case, responded to stopping orlistat.[2,3]

However, the manufacturer has found no evidence of an association between orlistat and hypertension. In clinical studies, orlistat use was associated with a small reduction in blood pressure compared with placebo, which was as a result of weight reduction. Moreover, the incidence of hypertension of new onset and hypertensive crisis did not differ between orlistat and placebo (1.2% versus 1.3%, and 0% versus 0.1%, respectively).[4] In studies in healthy subjects, orlistat had no effect on steady-state **losartan** pharmacokinetics,[5] and no clinically significant effect on the pharmacokinetics of single-dose **captopril**, **atenolol**, **furosemide** or **nifedipine**.[6]

Mechanism

Not understood. Suggestions include a decrease in the absorption of the drugs due to accelerated gastrointestinal transit, increased defaecation, diarrhoea, or an increase in the amount of fat in the chyme.[1] An explanation for the difference between the clinical cases and pharmacokinetic studies may be that the latter tended to be single-dose studies and in healthy subjects only. Alternatively, these cases could just be idiosyncratic and not related to orlistat treatment.

Importance and management

The interactions between the antihypertensives and orlistat seem to be confined to the reports cited here, and their general significance is unclear. Given that the manufacturers report that specific drug interaction studies have not found any evidence of an interaction, the incidence seems likely to be small.

1. Valsecia ME, Malgor LA, Farias EF, Figueras A, Laporte J-R. Interaction between orlistat and antihypertensive drugs. *Ann Pharmacother* (2001) 35, 1495–6.
2. Persson M, Vitols S, Yue Q-Y. Orlistat associated with hypertension. *BMJ* (2000) 321, 87.
3. Persson M, Vitols S, Yue Q-Y. Orlistat associated with hypertension. Author's reply. *BMJ* (2001) 322, 111.
4. Huber MH. Orlistat associated with hypertension. Roche concludes that there is no evidence of a causal association. *BMJ* (2001) 322, 110.
5. Zhi J, Moore R, Kanitra L, Mulligan TE. Pharmacokinetic evaluation of the possible interaction between selected concomitant medications and orlistat at steady state in healthy subjects. *J Clin Pharmacol* (2002) 42, 1011–19.
6. Weber C, Tam YK, Schmidtke-Schrezenmeier G, Jonkmann JHG, van Brummelen P. Effect of the lipase inhibitor orlistat on the pharmacokinetics of four different antihypertensive drugs in healthy volunteers. *Eur J Clin Pharmacol* (1996) 51, 87–90.

ACE inhibitors + Potassium compounds

ACE inhibitors maintain serum potassium levels. Hyperkalaemia is therefore a possibility if potassium supplements or potassium-containing salt substitutes are given, particularly in those patients where other risk factors are present, such as decreased renal function.

Clinical evidence

(a) Potassium levels increased by concurrent use

1. Potassium supplements. The serum potassium levels of a patient taking a potassium supplement rose by 66% when **captopril** was added, with signs of a deterioration in renal function. Four others taking potassium supplements and furosemide (2 also taking unnamed potassium-sparing diuretics) had rises in their potassium levels of only 8 to 24% when given **captopril**. The rises occurred within 1 or 2 days. No clinical signs or symptoms of hyperkalaemia were seen, but 3 of the 5 patients had rises to above the upper limits of normal.[1] A post-marketing survey identified 10 patients in whom **enalapril** appeared to have been associated with renal impairment and death. Eight of them were also taking potassium supplements and/or potassium-sparing diuretics, and hyperkalaemia appeared to have been the immediate cause of death in two of them.[2] In a review of 47 patients treated with **enalapril** for heart failure, and who experienced serious hyperkalaemia, 8 had also received potassium supplements.[3]
In another survey of 53 patients taking ACE inhibitors who had hyperkalaemia in the absence of significant renal impairment, less than 5% were taking a potassium supplement, but 30% were using a potassium-containing **salt substitute** (see *2.* below).[4]

2. Dietary potassium. Two patients with renal impairment, one taking **lisinopril** and the other **enalapril**, developed marked hyperkalaemia shortly after starting to take *'Lo salt'* (a salt substitute containing 34.6 g potassium in every 100 g). One developed a life-threatening arrhythmia.[5] A similar report describes a man taking **captopril** who developed hyperkalaemia and collapsed 2 weeks after starting to use a **salt substitute** containing potassium.[6] In a further report, severe hyperkalaemia occurred in a patient on a very-low-calorie diet with a protein supplement who was taking **lisinopril** 10 mg daily. The protein supplement contained 48 mmol of potassium and salad topped with lemon juice and potassium chloride salt added at least another 72 mmol daily.[7] In 53 patients taking ACE inhibitors who had hyperkalaemia in the absence of significant renal impairment, 30% were using a **salt substitute**, and 72% were eating a moderate-to-high potassium diet, consisting of 2 or more servings of a potassium-rich food daily.[4] Hyperkalaemia and acute renal failure has also been reported in a diabetic patient taking **lisinopril** 20 mg twice daily following the use of a potassium-based water softener.[8]

(b) Potassium levels unaltered by concurrent use

A retrospective analysis of 14 patients without renal impairment taking potassium supplements and either furosemide or hydrochlorothiazide, found that the levels of serum potassium, during a 4-year period, had not significantly increased after the addition of **captopril**.[9] Another study in 6 healthy subjects found that intravenous potassium chloride caused virtually the same rise in serum potassium levels in those given **enalapril** as in those given a placebo.[10]

Mechanism

The potassium-retaining effects of ACE inhibitors (due to reduced aldosterone levels) are additive with an increased intake of potassium, particularly when there are other contributory factors such as poor renal function or diabetes.

Importance and management

The documentation of this interaction appears to be limited, but it is well established. In practice, a clinically relevant rise in potassium levels usually occurs only if other factors are also present, the most important of which is impaired renal function. In general, because ACE inhibitors have potassium-sparing effects, potassium supplements should not routinely be given concurrently. If a supplement is needed, serum potassium should be closely monitored. This is especially important where other possible contributory risk factors are known to be present.

Other sources of dietary potassium should also be borne in mind. Patients with heart disease and hypertension are often told to reduce their salt (sodium) intake. One way of doing this is to use potassium-containing salt substitutes. However, it appears that there is some risk associated with excess use of these substitutes, especially in patients taking ACE inhibitors.

1. Burnakis TG, Mioduch HJ. Combined therapy with captopril and potassium supplementation. A potential for hyperkalemia. *Arch Intern Med* (1984) 144, 2371–2.
2. Speirs CJ, Dollery CT, Inman WHW, Rawson NSB, Wilton LV. Postmarketing surveillance of enalapril. II: Investigation of the potential role of enalapril in deaths with renal failure. *BMJ* (1988) 297, 830–2.
3. Brown C, Rush J. Risk factors for the development of hyperkalemia in patients treated with enalapril for heart failure. *Clin Pharmacol Ther* (1989) 45, 167.
4. Good CB, McDermott L, McCloskey B. Diet and serum potassium in patients on ACE inhibitors. *JAMA* (1995) 274, 538.
5. Ray KK, Dorman S, Watson RDS. Severe hyperkalaemia due to the concomitant use of salt substitutes and ACE inhibitors in hypertension: a potentially life threatening interaction. *J Hum Hypertens* (1999) 13, 717–20.
6. Packer M, Lee WH. Provocation of hyper- and hypokalemic sudden death during treatment with and withdrawal of converting-enzyme inhibition in severe chronic congestive heart failure. *Am J Cardiol* (1986) 57, 347–8.
7. Stoltz ML, Andrews CE. Severe hyperkalemia during very-low-calorie diets and angiotensin converting enzyme use. *JAMA* (1990) 264, 2737–8.
8. Graves JW. Hyperkalemia due to a potassium-based water softener. *N Engl J Med* (1998) 339,1790–1.
9. Schuna AA, Schmidt GR, Pitterle ME. Serum potassium concentrations after initiation of captopril therapy. *Clin Pharm* (1986) 5, 920–3.
10. Scandling JD, Izzo JL, Pabico RC, McKenna BA, Radke KJ, Ornt DB. Potassium homeostasis during angiotensin-converting enzyme inhibition with enalapril. *J Clin Pharmacol* (1989) 29, 916–21.

ACE inhibitors + Probenecid

Probenecid decreases the renal clearance of captopril, but this is probably not clinically important. Probenecid decreases the renal clearance of enalapril, and raises its serum levels.

Clinical evidence, mechanism, importance and management

Steady-state levels of unchanged and total **captopril**, given by intravenous infusion, were slightly increased (14% and 36%, respectively) by the use of probenecid in 4 healthy subjects. Renal clearance of unchanged **captopril** decreased by 44%, but total clearance was reduced by only 19%.[1] These moderate changes are unlikely to be clinically important.

In 12 healthy subjects probenecid 1 g twice daily for 5 days increased the AUC of a single 20-mg oral dose of **enalapril** and its active metabolite, enalaprilat by about 50%. The renal clearance of **enalapril** decreased by 73%.[2] A moderate increase in the hypotensive effects might be expected, but there do not appear to be any reports of adverse effects.

1. Singhvi SM, Duchin KL, Willard DA, McKinstry DN, Migdalof BH. Renal handling of captopril: effect of probenecid. *Clin Pharmacol Ther* (1982) 32, 182–9.
2. Noormohamed FH, McNabb WR, Lant AF. Pharmacokinetic and pharmacodynamic actions of enalapril in humans: effect of probenecid pretreatment. *J Pharmacol Exp Ther* (1990) 253, 362–8.

ACE inhibitors + Procainamide

The combination of captopril or other ACE inhibitors and procainamide possibly increases the risk of leucopenia. No pharmacokinetic interaction occurs between captopril and procainamide.

Clinical evidence, mechanism, importance and management

In 12 healthy subjects the concurrent use of **captopril** 50 mg twice daily and procainamide 250 mg every 3 hours did not affect the pharmacokinetics of either drug.[1] The US manufacturer of **captopril** notes that in patients with heart failure who developed neutropenia, about 50% had a serum creatinine of 1.6 mg/dL or greater, and more than 75% were also receiving procainamide.[2] Similarly, the UK manufacturer of **captopril** notes that neutropenia or agranulocytosis and serious infection have occurred in patients taking **captopril**, and that concurrent treatment with procainamide may be a complicating factor. They recommend that the combination should be used with caution, especially in patients with impaired renal function. They suggest that differential white blood cell counts should be performed before concurrent use, then every 2 weeks in the first 3 months of treatment and periodically thereafter.[3] The UK manufacturers of a number of other ACE inhibitors suggest that concurrent use of ACE inhibitors and procainamide may lead to an increased risk of leucopenia. For reports of other possible interactions with ACE inhibitors that might result in an increased risk of leucopenia see also 'ACE inhibitors + Allopurinol', p.13 and 'ACE inhibitors + Azathioprine', p.18.

1. Levinson B, Sugerman AA, McKown J. Lack of kinetic interaction of captopril (CP) and procainamide (PA) in healthy subjects. *J Clin Pharmacol* (1985) 25, 460.
2. Capoten (Captopril). Par Pharmaceutical, Inc. US Prescribing information, June 2003.
3. Capoten (Captopril). E. R. Squibb & Sons Ltd. UK Summary of product characteristics, June 2005.

ACE inhibitors + Rifampicin (Rifampin)

An isolated report describes a rise in blood pressure in one hypertensive patient, which was attributed to an interaction between enalapril and rifampicin. Rifampicin may reduce the plasma levels of the active metabolites of imidapril and spirapril.

Clinical evidence

A man taking **enalapril** and a variety of other drugs (warfarin, acebutolol, bendroflumethiazide, dipyridamole, metoclopramide and *Gaviscon*) developed a fever. He was given streptomycin, oxytetracycline and rifampicin, because of a probable *Brucella abortus* infection, whereupon his blood pressure rose from 164/104 to 180/115 mmHg over the next 5 to 6 days. It was suspected that an interaction with the rifampicin was possibly responsible. Subsequent studies in the same patient showed that rifampicin, reduced the AUC_{0-7} of enalaprilat, the active metabolite of **enalapril**, by 31%, although the AUC of **enalapril** was unchanged.[1] There is also the hint of this interaction in another report, where **enalapril** failed to control blood pressure in a patient taking rifampicin.[2]

The manufacturer of **spirapril** briefly noted in a review that the use of rifampicin with **spirapril** modestly decreased plasma levels of **spirapril** and its active metabolite, spiraprilat.[3] The manufacturer of **imidapril** notes that rifampicin reduced plasma levels of imidaprilat, the active metabolite of **imidapril**.[4]

Mechanism

The mechanism of this interaction is not clear, because rifampicin is a potent liver enzyme inducer, which might have been expected to cause the production of more, rather than less, of the active metabolites of these ACE inhibitors. However, the authors of one of the reports postulated that the rifampicin might have increased the loss of the enalaprilat in the urine,[1] and others suggested that rifampicin stimulates the elimination of spiraprilat non-specifically.[3]

Importance and management

The general importance of these interactions is uncertain. The isolated reports with enalapril suggest minor clinical relevance. The manufacturers of spirapril did not consider the modest pharmacokinetic changes to be clinically relevant.[3] However, the manufacturers of imidapril state that rifampicin might reduce the antihypertensive efficacy of imidapril,[4] but this awaits clinical assessment.

1. Kandiah D, Penny WJ, Fraser AG, Lewis MJ. A possible drug interaction between rifampicin and enalapril. *Eur J Clin Pharmacol* (1988) 35, 431–2.
2. Tada Y, Tsuda Y, Otsuka T, Nagasawa K, Kimura H, Kusaba T, Sakata T. Case report: nifedipine-rifampicin interaction attenuates the effect on blood pressure in a patient with essential hypertension. *Am J Med Sci* (1992) 303, 25–7.
3. Grass P, Gerbeau C, Kutz K. Spirapril: pharmacokinetic properties and drug interactions. *Blood Pressure* (1994) 3 (Suppl 2), 7–13.
4. Tanatril (Imidapril). Trinity Pharmaceuticals Ltd. UK Summary of product characteristics, May 2003.

ACE inhibitors + Sevelamer

Sevelamer did not alter the pharmacokinetics of enalapril.

Clinical evidence, mechanism, importance and management

The concurrent use of a single 2.418-g dose of sevelamer hydrochloride (equivalent to 6 capsules) and did not alter the AUC of a single 20-mg dose of **enalapril** or its active metabolite, enalaprilat, in 28 healthy subjects.[1] Thus it appears that sevelamer does not bind to **enalapril** within the gut to reduce its absorption.

1. Burke SK, Amin NS, Incerti C, Plone MA, Lee JW. Sevelamer hydrochloride (Renagel®), a phosphate-binding polymer, does not alter the pharmacokinetics of two commonly used antihypertensives in healthy volunteers. *J Clin Pharmacol* (2001) 41, 199–205.

ACE inhibitors + Sibutramine

Sibutramine had only a minimal effect on blood pressure control with ACE inhibitors.

Clinical evidence, mechanism, importance and management

In a randomised, double-blind study over 52 weeks in 220 obese, hypertensive patients, whose hypertension was well controlled with an ACE inhibitor (**benazepril**, **enalapril** or **lisinopril**) with or without a thiazide diuretic, two-thirds of the patients were also given sibutramine and one-third were given placebo. Sibutramine 20 mg daily caused small increases in mean blood pressure compared with placebo (133.1/85.5 mmHg compared with 130.4/82.8 mmHg, at 52 weeks, respectively), but overall, hypertension remained well controlled.[1]

1. McMahon FG, Weinstein SP, Rowe E, Ernst KR, Johnson F, Fujioka K, and the Sibutramine in Hypertensives Clinical Study Group. Sibutramine is safe and effective for weight loss in obese patients whose hypertension is well controlled with angiotensin-converting enzyme inhibitors. *J Hum Hypertens* (2002) 16, 5–11.

Angiotensin II receptor antagonists + Antacids

Antacids slightly reduce irbesartan and olmesartan absorption, but this is not clinically relevant.

Clinical evidence, mechanism, importance and management

In a single-dose, crossover study in 18 healthy subjects, 10 mL of an antacid containing **aluminium/magnesium hydroxides** (*Unimaalox*) given with, or 2 hours before, a single 300-mg dose of **irbesartan** had little effect on irbesartan pharmacokinetics The only difference was that the AUC was reduced by 10% when the antacid was given 2 hours before irbesartan, when compared with irbesartan alone. However, this change is not considered to be clinically relevant.[1]

The steady-state AUC of **olmesartan** 20 mg daily was 12% lower when it was given 15 minutes after a daily dose of an **aluminium/magnesium hydroxide** antacid, when compared with **olmesartan** alone, but this was not considered to be clinically significant.[2]

1. Marino MR, Vachharajani NN. Drug interactions with irbesartan. *Clin Pharmacokinet* (2001) 40, 605–14.
2. Laeis P, Püchler K, Kirch W. The pharmacokinetic and metabolic profile of olmesartan medoxomil limits the risk of clinically relevant drug interaction. *J Hypertens* (2001) 19 (Suppl 1), S21–S32.

Angiotensin II receptor antagonists + Aspirin or NSAIDs

Indometacin may attenuate the antihypertensive effect of losartan, valsartan, or other angiotensin II receptor antagonists. However, low-dose aspirin does not appear to alter the antihypertensive effect of losartan. No clinically relevant *pharmacokinetic* interactions occur between telmisartan and ibuprofen or paracetamol (acetaminophen), or between valsartan and indometacin. The combination of an NSAID and angiotensin II receptor antagonist can increase the risk of renal impairment and hyperkalaemia.

Clinical evidence

(A) Effects on blood pressure

Various large epidemiological studies and meta-analyses of clinical studies have been conducted to assess the effect of NSAIDs on blood pressure in patients treated with **antihypertensives**, and the findings of these are summarised in 'Table 23.2', (p.862). In these studies, NSAIDs were not always associated with an increase in blood pressure, and the maximum increase was 6.2 mmHg.

(a) Aspirin

A double-blind, placebo-controlled study in 10 patients with hypertension taking **losartan** (mean daily dose 47.5 mg) found that neither aspirin 81 mg nor 325 mg daily for 2 weeks had any significant effect on blood pressure.[1]

(b) Indometacin

In a study in 111 patients with hypertension, **losartan** 50 mg once daily for 6 weeks reduced their blood pressure by a mean of 7.9/5.3 mmHg. Indometacin 75 mg once daily was then added for one week and this caused a rise in blood pressure in the group as a whole of 3.8/2.2 mmHg (reduction of about 45% in the effect of **losartan**). A rise in ambulatory diastolic blood pressure was seen in 69% of the **losartan**-treated patients during indometacin use.[2] In contrast, a much smaller study in 10 patients with essential hypertension taking **losartan** found that indometacin 50 mg twice daily for one week caused sodium and fluid retention, but did not significantly attenuate the antihypertensive effects of **losartan**.[3]

In a placebo-controlled, crossover study in 56 hypertensive patients whose blood pressure was adequately controlled by **valsartan** 80 to 160 mg daily, the addition of indometacin 50 mg twice daily for 2 weeks produced an increase in mean blood pressure of 2.1/1.9 mmHg.[4] A study in normotensive subjects given a fixed sodium intake and **valsartan** 80 mg daily, with or without indometacin 50 mg twice daily for one week, demonstrated that indometacin reduced the natriuretic response to the angiotensin receptor blockade.[5]

(B) Effects on renal function

In 2002, 28 of 129 reports to the Australian Adverse Drug Reactions Advisory Committee of acute renal failure were associated with the combined use of ACE inhibitors or angiotensin II receptor antagonists, diuretics, and NSAIDs (including coxibs), and these cases had a fatality rate of 10%. In patients taking this triple combination, renal failure appeared to be precipitated by mild stress such as diarrhoea or dehydration. In other patients, the addition of a third drug (usually an NSAID) to a stable combination of the other two, resulted in acute renal failure.[6] In a multivariate analysis, significant renal impairment was associated with the use of two or more of an ACE inhibitor or angiotensin II receptor antagonist, and NSAIDs or diuretics.[7]

(C) Pharmacokinetic studies

(a) Ibuprofen

In a crossover study in 12 healthy subjects, **telmisartan** 120 mg daily had no effect on the pharmacokinetics of ibuprofen 400 mg three times a day for 7 days. Similarly, the pharmacokinetics of **telmisartan** were unaffected by the concurrent use of ibuprofen, when compared with previous studies of **telmisartan** alone.[8]

(b) Indometacin

In 12 healthy subjects the pharmacokinetics of single oral doses of **valsartan** 160 mg or indometacin 100 mg were not significantly changed when the drugs were given together, although the pharmacokinetics of **valsartan** showed wide variations between subjects.[9]

(c) Paracetamol (Acetaminophen)

Telmisartan 120 mg had no effect on the pharmacokinetics of paracetamol 1 g in a single-dose study in 12 healthy subjects. The pharmacokinetics of **telmisartan** were also unaffected by paracetamol, when compared with previous studies of **telmisartan** alone.[8]

Mechanism

Some evidence suggests that prostaglandins may be partially involved in the hypotensive action of angiotensin II receptor antagonists, and that NSAIDs, by inhibiting prostaglandin synthesis, may antagonise their effects. However, a non-specific mechanism such as sodium retention may also be involved, as indometacin has been shown to reduce the hypotensive effect of other classes of antihypertensive drugs.[4,5] Both NSAIDs and angiotensin II receptor antagonists alone can cause renal impairment. In patients whose kidneys are underperfused, they may cause further deterioration in renal function when used together. Renal impairment increases the risk of hyperkalaemia.

Importance and management

As with other antihypertensives, the **antihypertensive effect** of angiotensin II receptor antagonists may be attenuated by NSAIDs such as indometacin. Patients taking losartan or valsartan or other angiotensin II receptor antagonists, who require indometacin and probably other NSAIDs, should be monitored for alterations in blood pressure control. See also 'ACE inhibitors + NSAIDs', p.28. Low-dose aspirin is unlikely to alter the blood pressure-lowering effect of angiotensin II receptor antagonists. However, for a discussion of the controversy as to whether low-dose aspirin might attenuate the benefits of ACE inhibitors in patients with heart failure, see 'ACE inhibitors + Aspirin', p.14.

Poor renal perfusion may increase the risk of **renal failure** if angiotensin II receptor antagonists are given with NSAIDs and so regular hydration of the patient and monitoring of renal function is recommended.[10] The Australian Adverse Drug Reactions Advisory Committee consider that the triple combination of angiotensin II receptor antagonists or ACE inhibitors with diuretics and NSAIDs (including coxibs) should be avoided if possible.[6] See also 'ACE inhibitors + NSAIDs', p.28.

1. Nawarskas JJ, Townsend RR, Cirigliano MD, Spinler SA. Effect of aspirin on blood pressure in hypertensive patients taking enalapril or losartan. *Am J Hypertens* (1999) 12, 784–9.
2. Conlin PR, Moore TJ, Swartz SL, Barr E, Gazdick L, Fletcher C, DeLucca P, Demopoulos L. Effect of indomethacin on blood pressure lowering by captopril and losartan in hypertensive patients. *Hypertension* (2000) 36, 461–5.
3. Olsen ME, Thomsen T, Hassager C, Ibsen H, Dige-Petersen H. Hemodynamic and renal effects of indomethacin in losartan-treated hypertensive individuals. *Am J Hypertens* (1999) 12, 209–16.
4. Fogari R, Zoppi A, Carretta R, Veglio F, Salvetti A: Italian Collaborative Study Group. Effect of indomethacin on the antihypertensive efficacy of valsartan and lisinopril: a multicentre study. *J Hypertens* (2002) 20: 1007–14.
5. Fricker AF, Nussberger J, Meilenbrock S, Brunner HR, Burnier M. Effect of indomethacin on the renal response to angiotensin II receptor blockade in healthy subjects. *Kidney Int* (1998) 54, 2089–97.

6. ADRAC. ACE inhibitor, diuretic and NSAID: a dangerous combination. *Aust Adverse Drug React Bull* (2003) 22, 14–15. Available at: http://www.tga.gov.au/adr/aadrb/aadr0308.pdf (accessed 14/08/07).
7. Loboz KK, Shenfield GM. Drug combinations and impaired renal function –the 'triple whammy'. *Br J Clin Pharmacol* (2005) 59, 239–43.
8. Stangier J, Su C-APF, Fraunhofer A, Tetzloff W. Pharmacokinetics of acetaminophen and ibuprofen when coadministered with telmisartan in healthy volunteers. *J Clin Pharmacol* (2000) 40, 1338–46.
9. Ciba. Data on file, Protocol 43.
10. Olmetec (Olmesartan medoxomil). Daiichi Sankyo UK Ltd. UK Summary of product characteristics, August 2006.

Angiotensin II receptor antagonists + Azoles

Fluconazole reduces the conversion of losartan to its active metabolite and decreases the metabolism of irbesartan, but the clinical relevance of these changes is uncertain. Fluconazole does not appear to influence the pharmacokinetics of eprosartan; candesartan and valsartan. Itraconazole does not significantly affect the pharmacokinetics or antihypertensive effects of losartan, and ketoconazole does not affect the pharmacokinetics of eprosartan or losartan.

Clinical evidence, mechanism, importance and management

(a) Fluconazole

In a study of 32 healthy subjects, half were given **losartan** 100 mg daily and half were given **eprosartan** 300 mg twice daily for 20 days. Fluconazole 200 mg daily was given to both groups on days 11 to 20. Fluconazole increased the AUC and maximum plasma levels of **losartan** by 69% and 31%, respectively, and reduced those of E-3174, the active metabolite of **losartan**, by 41% and 54%, respectively. However, fluconazole had no significant effect on the pharmacokinetics of **eprosartan**.[1] In a randomised, crossover study, 11 healthy subjects were given a single 50-mg dose of **losartan** after 4 days of fluconazole (400 mg on day 1 and 200 mg daily on days 2 to 4). The AUC of **losartan** was increased by 27% while its maximum plasma level was reduced by 23%. The AUC and the maximum plasma levels of E-3174 were reduced by 47% and 77%, respectively. However, no significant changes in the hypotensive effect of **losartan** were noted.[2] It is thought that fluconazole inhibits the conversion of **losartan** to its active metabolite mainly by inhibiting the cytochrome P450 isoenzyme CYP2C9,[1-4] although other isoenzymes may play a minor role. The lack of pharmacodynamic changes suggests that this pharmacokinetic interaction may not be clinically important, but the possibility of a decreased therapeutic effect should be kept in mind.[2]

A study in 15 healthy subjects given **irbesartan** 150 mg daily for 20 days found that the steady-state AUC and maximum blood levels were increased by about 55% and 18%, respectively, by fluconazole 200 mg daily on days 11 to 20. **Irbesartan** is primarily metabolised by CYP2C9,[4] and these increased levels probably occur as a result of CYP2C9 inhibition by fluconazole.[5] These modest increases were considered unlikely to be clinically relevant and a dosage reduction would not generally be required.[6] Other angiotensin II receptor antagonists would not be expected to interact, see the 'introduction', (p.12), to this section.

(b) Itraconazole

In 11 healthy subjects the pharmacokinetics and hypotensive effects of a single 50-mg dose of **losartan** and its active metabolite, E-3174, were not significantly affected by itraconazole 200 mg daily for 4 days.[2] Inhibition of the cytochrome P450 isoenzyme CYP3A4 alone (caused by itraconazole) does not appear to prevent the conversion of **losartan** to E-3174. No special precautions would appear to be needed if these drugs are used concurrently.

(c) Ketoconazole

A placebo-controlled, crossover study in 11 healthy subjects given a single 30-mg intravenous dose of **losartan**, found that ketoconazole 400 mg daily for 4 days did not affect the conversion of **losartan** to its active metabolite, E-3174, or the plasma clearance of **losartan**.[7] Inhibition of the cytochrome P450 isoenzyme CYP3A4 alone (caused by ketoconazole) does not appear to prevent the conversion of **losartan** to E-3174.

The plasma clearance of a 20-mg intravenous dose of E-3174 was also unaffected by pretreatment with ketoconazole.[7] Similar results were found in a study involving 27 healthy subjects. Ketoconazole 200 mg daily for 5 days was found to have no effect on the pharmacokinetics of **eprosartan** or **losartan** and its active metabolite.[8] No special precautions would appear to be needed if these drugs are used concurrently.

1. Kazierad DJ, Martin DE, Blum RA, Tenero DM, Ilson B, Boike SC, Etheredge R, Jorkasky DK. Effect of fluconazole on the pharmacokinetics of eprosartan and losartan in healthy male volunteers. *Clin Pharmacol Ther* (1997) 62, 417–25.
2. Kaukonen K-M, Olkkola KT, Neuvonen PJ. Fluconazole but not itraconazole decreases the metabolism of losartan to E-3174. *Eur J Clin Pharmacol* (1998) 53, 445–9.
3. Parnell K, Rodgers J, Graff D, Allen T, Hinderliter A, Patterson J, Pieper J. Inhibitory effect of fluconazole and erythromycin plus fluvastatin on losartan disposition in normal volunteers. *Clin Pharmacol Ther* (2000) 67, 121.
4. Taavitsainen P, Kiukaanniemi K, Pelkonen O. In vitro inhibition screening of human hepatic P_{450} enzymes by five angiotensin-II receptor antagonists. *Eur J Clin Pharmacol* (2000) 56, 135–40.
5. Kovacs SJ, Wilton JH, Blum RA. Steady state pharmacokinetics of irbesartan alone and in combination with fluconazole. *Clin Pharmacol Ther* (1999) 65, 132.
6. Marino MR, Vachharajani NN. Drug interactions with irbesartan. *Clin Pharmacokinet* (2001) 40, 605–14.
7. McCrea JB, Lo MW, Furtek CI, Ritter MA, Carides A, Waldman SA, Bjornsson TD, Goldberg MR. Ketoconazole does not effect the systemic conversion of losartan to E-3174. *Clin Pharmacol Ther* (1996) 59, 169.
8. Blum RA, Kazierad DJ, Tenero DM. A review of eprosartan pharmacokinetic and pharmacodynamic drug interaction studies. *Pharmacotherapy* (1999) 19, 79S–85S.

Angiotensin II receptor antagonists + Beta blockers

There appears to be no clinically significant pharmacokinetic interaction between atenolol and valsartan, and concurrent use enhances the hypotensive effects. The combination of angiotensin II receptor antagonists and beta blockers is in established clinical use.

Clinical evidence, mechanism, importance and management

In a single-dose, crossover study in 12 healthy subjects, the pharmacokinetics of **valsartan** 160 mg and **atenolol** 100 mg were not significantly altered by concurrent use. The combination had some additive effects on resting blood pressure.[1]

Although pharmacokinetic information is apparently limited to this drug pair, no significant adverse interaction would be expected between angiotensin II receptor antagonists and beta blockers, and the combination is clinically useful in a number of cardiovascular disorders.

1. Czendlik CH, Sioufi A, Preiswerk G, Howald H. Pharmacokinetic and pharmacodynamic interaction of single doses of valsartan and atenolol. *Eur J Clin Pharmacol* (1997) 52, 451–9.

Angiotensin II receptor antagonists + Calcium-channel blockers

No significant pharmacokinetic interactions occur between nifedipine and candesartan or irbesartan, or between amlodipine and telmisartan or valsartan. Calcium-channel blockers have been given safely with eprosartan or irbesartan.

Clinical evidence, mechanism, importance and management

(a) Amlodipine

In a study in 12 healthy subjects, **telmisartan** 120 mg daily had no clinically relevant effect on the pharmacokinetics of amlodipine 10 mg daily for 9 days, and there was no evidence of any marked effect of amlodipine on the pharmacokinetics of **telmisartan**. Although there were no serious adverse effects, mild to moderate adverse events (most commonly headache) occurred slightly more frequently with the combination, compared with amlodipine alone (19 events versus 12 events).[1]

In 12 healthy subjects the pharmacokinetics of single oral doses of **valsartan** 160 mg and amlodipine 5 mg were not significantly altered on concurrent use, although the pharmacokinetics of **valsartan** showed wide variations between subjects.[2]

No special precautions would therefore appear to be necessary if any of these drugs are given together, although be aware that an increase in adverse effects may occur.

(b) Nifedipine

In 12 healthy subjects nifedipine 30 mg daily did not significantly affect the pharmacokinetics of **candesartan** 16 mg daily.[3]

In vitro studies indicated that nifedipine inhibited the oxidation of **irbesartan**, which was mediated by the cytochrome P450 isoenzyme CYP2C9.[4] However, a randomised, crossover study in 11 healthy subjects given **irbesartan** 300 mg daily alone or with nifedipine 30 mg daily for 4 days, found that nifedipine did not alter the pharmacokinetics of **irbesartan**.[4] The manufacturer says that **irbesartan** has been safely given with antihypertensives such as long-acting calcium-channel blockers.[5] Similarly the manufacturer of **eprosartan** notes that it has been safely given with calcium-channel blockers (such as sustained-release nifedipine).[6]

1. Stangier J, Su C-APF. Pharmacokinetics of repeated oral doses of amlodipine and amlodipine plus telmisartan in healthy volunteers. *J Clin Pharmacol* (2000) 40, 1347–54.
2. Novartis Pharmaceuticals Ltd. Data on file, Protocol 37.
3. Jonkman JHG, van Lier JJ, van Heiningen PNM, Lins R, Sennewald R, Högemann A. Pharmacokinetic drug interaction studies with candesartan cilexetil. *J Hum Hypertens* (1997) 11 (Suppl 2), S31–S35.
4. Marino MR, Hammett JL, Ferreira I, Ford NF, Uderman HD. Effect of nifedipine on the steady-state pharmacokinetics and pharmacodynamics of irbesartan in healthy subjects. *J Cardiovasc Pharmacol Ther* (1998) 3, 111–17.
5. Aprovel (Irbesartan). Sanofi-Aventis. UK Summary of product characteristics, May 2006.
6. Teveten (Eprosartan mesilate). Solvay Healthcare Ltd. UK Summary of product characteristics, June 2006.

Angiotensin II receptor antagonists + Diuretics; Loop, Thiazide and related

Symptomatic hypotension may occur when an angiotensin II receptor antagonist is started in patients taking high-dose diuretics. Potassium levels may be either increased, decreased or not affected. No clinically relevant pharmacokinetic interactions appear to occur between candesartan, eprosartan, irbesartan, losartan, telmisartan or valsartan and hydrochlorothiazide, although the bioavailability of hydrochlorothiazide may be modestly reduced. Similarly, there is no clinically significant pharmacokinetic interaction between valsartan and furosemide.

Clinical evidence, mechanism, importance and management

(a) Hypotension

Angiotensin II receptor antagonists and thiazide or related diuretics have useful additive effects in the control of hypertension and are generally well tolerated. For example, in one double-blind, placebo-controlled study in 604 patients with hypertension, **losartan** 50 mg given with **hydrochlorothiazide** 12.5 mg once daily produced an additive reduction in trough sitting systolic and diastolic blood pressure, and the incidence of dizziness and headache was not significantly different from placebo.[1] However, symptomatic hypotension, especially after the first dose, may occur when angiotensin II receptor antagonists are started in patients with heart failure or those with hypertension who also have sodium and/or volume depletion, such as those taking **high-dose diuretics**. It is recommended that any volume and/or sodium depletion should be corrected before the angiotensin II receptor antagonist is given. In some situations it may be appropriate to reduce the dose of the diuretic and/or use a lower starting dose of the angiotensin II receptor antagonist.

A similar problem occurs with the ACE inhibitors, see 'ACE inhibitors + Diuretics; Loop, Thiazide and related', p.21.

(b) Pharmacokinetic studies

The changes in **furosemide** and **hydrochlorothiazide** pharmacokinetics appear to be of no practical importance, and the combination with an angiotensin II receptor antagonist can produce a significant and useful additional reduction in blood pressure. Details of these studies are given below.

1. Furosemide. In 12 healthy subjects the relative bioavailability of furosemide 40 mg was reduced by about 26% when it was given with **valsartan** 160 mg. However, this pharmacokinetic interaction had no influence on the diuretic effect of furosemide. Simultaneous use of **valsartan** and furosemide did not modify the pharmacokinetics of **valsartan**.[2]

2. Hydrochlorothiazide. In 18 healthy subjects the concurrent use of hydrochlorothiazide 25 mg daily and **candesartan** 12 mg daily for 7 days increased the AUC and maximum serum levels of **candesartan** by 18% and 23%, respectively, and reduced the AUC of hydrochlorothiazide by 14%, but these changes were not considered to be clinically relevant.[3] **Eprosartan** 800 mg also decreased the AUC of hydrochlorothiazide 25 mg by about 20% in 18 healthy subjects, but again this was not considered to be clinically important. In addition, hydrochlorothiazide had no effect on **eprosartan** pharmacokinetics.[4] Similarly, in a study of 12 patients with mild or moderate hypertension given **losartan** 50 mg alone or with hydrochlorothiazide 12.5 mg daily for 7 days, the AUC of hydrochlorothiazide was decreased by 17% during concurrent use (not clinically significant) while the pharmacokinetics of **losartan** were unchanged.[5] A single-dose study in 12 healthy subjects found that **valsartan** 160 mg reduced the systemic availability of hydrochlorothiazide 25 mg (AUC decreased by 31%), but the mean amount of hydrochlorothiazide excreted in the urine did not seem to change significantly. The pharmacokinetics of **valsartan** were not significantly affected by hydrochlorothiazide.[6]

In a randomised, crossover study in 13 healthy subjects, **telmisartan** 160 mg daily was given with hydrochlorothiazide 25 mg daily for 7 days. There was no difference in AUC and maximum plasma concentrations of either drug compared with when they were given alone.[7] Similarly, no pharmacokinetic interactions were found between **irbesartan** and hydrochlorothiazide.[8]

(c) Serum potassium levels

Angiotensin receptor II antagonists are potassium sparing, whereas loop and thiazide diuretics are potassium depleting. Giving an angiotensin receptor II antagonist with a diuretic could result in an increase, a decrease, or no change to the potassium levels, although logically adding an angiotensin II receptor antagonist to established treatment with a diuretic would seem more likely to raise potassium, and vice versa. Serum potassium should be routinely monitored when angiotensin II antagonists are used in patients with heart failure, renal impairment, or in the elderly.

1. MacKay JH, Arcuri KE, Goldberg AI, Snapinn SM, Sweet CS. Losartan and low-dose hydrochlorothiazide in patients with essential hypertension. A double-blind, placebo-controlled trial of concomitant administration compared with individual components. *Arch Intern Med* (1996) 156, 278–85.
2. Bindschedler M, Degen P, Flesch G, de Gasparo M, Preiswerk G. Pharmacokinetic and pharmacodynamic interaction of single oral doses of valsartan and furosemide. *Eur J Clin Pharmacol* (1997) 52, 371–8.
3. Jonkman JHG, van Lier JJ, van Heiningen PNM, Lins R, Sennewald R, Högemann A. Pharmacokinetic drug interaction studies with candesartan cilexetil. *J Hum Hypertens* (1997) 11 (Suppl 2), S31–S35.
4. Blum RA, Kazierad DJ, Tenero DM. A review of eprosartan pharmacokinetic and pharmacodynamic drug interaction studies. *Pharmacotherapy* (1999) 19, 79S–85S.
5. McCrea JB, Lo M-W, Tomasko L, Lin CC, Hsieh JY-K, Capra NL, Goldberg MR. Absence of a pharmacokinetic interaction between losartan and hydrochlorothiazide. *J Clin Pharmacol* (1995) 35, 1200–6.
6. Novartis Pharmaceuticals Ltd. Data on file, Protocol 07.
7. Yong C-L, Dias VC, Stangier J. Multiple-dose pharmacokinetics of telmisartan and of hydrochlorothiazide following concurrent administration in healthy subjects. *J Clin Pharmacol* (2000) 40, 1323–30.
8. Marino MR, Vachharajani NN. Drug interactions with irbesartan. *Clin Pharmacokinet* (2001) 40, 605–14.

Angiotensin II receptor antagonists + Diuretics; Potassium-sparing

There is an increased risk of hyperkalaemia if angiotensin II receptor antagonists are given with potassium-sparing diuretics (such as amiloride and the aldosterone antagonists, eplerenone and spironolactone), particularly if other risk factors are also present.

Clinical evidence

Life-threatening hyperkalaemia occurred in 6 patients with congestive heart failure who were taking **spironolactone** and an angiotensin II receptor antagonist (**candesartan**, **losartan** or **telmisartan**). Analysis of these patients, together with another 38 similar patients who had received ACE inhibitors, identified certain conditions that may lead to the development of severe hyperkalaemia in such patients. These were advanced age, dose of **spironolactone** greater than 25 mg, reduced renal function and type II diabetes.[1]

Mechanism

Angiotensin II receptor antagonists reduce the levels of aldosterone, which results in the retention of potassium. This would be expected to be additive with the potassium-retaining effects of amiloride, triamterene, spironolactone and eplerenone, leading to hyperkalaemia, but usually only if other risk factors are present.

Importance and management

Concurrent use of potassium-sparing diuretics (namely **amiloride**, **triamterene** and the aldosterone antagonists **eplerenone** and spironolactone) may increase serum potassium. There is a greater risk of hyperkalaemia if renal impairment and/or heart failure or diabetes are present. Because angiotensin II receptor antagonists have potassium-sparing effects, amiloride and triamterene should not normally be given concurrently. Aldosterone antagonists such as spironolactone may be useful in heart failure, but the combined use of angiotensin II receptor antagonists requires increased monitoring of serum potassium. Note that the combination should be avoided in patients with a glomerular filtration rate of less than 30 mL/minute.[2] In addition, the dose of spironolactone should not exceed 25 mg daily.[2] Similarly, the UK manufacturer of eplerenone says that caution is required when it is combined with angiotensin II receptor antagonists, especially in renal impairment, and that potassium levels and renal function should be monitored.[3]

Consider also 'ACE inhibitors + Diuretics; Potassium-sparing', p.23.

1. Wrenger E, Müller R, Moesenthin M, Welte T, Frölich JC, Neumann KH. Interaction of spironolactone with ACE inhibitors or angiotensin receptor blockers: analysis of 44 cases. *BMJ* (2003) 327, 147–9.
2. Palmer BF. Managing hyperkalemia caused by inhibitors of the renin-angiotensin-aldosterone system. *N Engl J Med* (2004) 351, 585–92
3. Inspra (Eplerenone). Pfizer Ltd. UK Summary of product characteristics, May 2006.

Angiotensin II receptor antagonists + Food

Food slightly increases the AUC of eprosartan and losartan, slightly reduces the AUC of telmisartan, and modestly reduces the AUC of valsartan. However, none of these changes is likely to be clinically important. Food has no effect on the AUC of candesartan, irbesartan or olmesartan.

Clinical evidence, mechanism, importance and management

(a) Candesartan

Food does not affect the bioavailability of candesartan,[1,2] and the manufacturer states that it may be given with or without food.

(b) Eprosartan

Food delays eprosartan absorption, and slightly increases its AUC and maximum serum concentrations by up to 25%. The UK manufacturer recommends that eprosartan is given with food,[3] but the US manufacturer suggests that the change in absorption is not clinically significant, and that eprosartan may be taken with or without food.[4]

(c) Irbesartan

In a study in 16 healthy men, a **high-fat breakfast** had no clinically relevant effects on the bioavailability of a single 300-mg dose of irbesartan,[5] therefore it may be taken with or without food.

(d) Losartan

In a crossover study in healthy subjects, the AUC and maximum levels of a single 100-mg dose of losartan, given 30 minutes before a **high-fat breakfast** was increased by 17% and 35%, respectively, when compared to the fasted state. Food caused a less than 10% decrease in AUC and maximum level of the losartan metabolite, E-3174.[6] These minor changes are unlikely to be clinically significant, and the manufacturer says that losartan may be given with or without food.[7,8]

(e) Olmesartan

Food does not affect the bioavailability of olmesartan,[9,10] and the manufacturer states that it may be given with or without food.

(f) Telmisartan

Food slightly reduces the AUC of telmisartan by about 6 to 20% depending on dose,[11,12] but this would not be expected to cause a reduction in therapeutic efficacy,[11] and telmisartan may be taken with or without food.[12]

(g) Valsartan

Food modestly decreased the AUC of valsartan by 40%,[13] but the manufacturer states that it may be taken with or without food.[13,14]

1. Amias (Candesartan cilexetil). Takeda UK Ltd. UK Summary of product characteristics, November 2006.
2. Atacand (Candesartan cilexetil). AstraZeneca. US Prescribing information, February 2007.
3. Teveten (Eprosartan mesilate). Solvay Healthcare Ltd. UK Summary of product characteristics, June 2006.
4. Teveten (Eprosartan mesylate). Kos Pharmaceuticals, Inc. US Prescribing information, September 2005.
5. Vachharajani NN, Shyu WC, Mantha S, Park J-S, Greene DS, Barbhaiya RH. Lack of effect of food on the oral bioavailability of irbesartan in healthy male volunteers. *J Clin Pharmacol* (1998) 38, 433–6.
6. Marier J-F, Guilbaud R, Kambhampati SRP, Mathew P, Moberly J, Lee J, Salazar DE. The effect of AST-120 on the single-dose pharmacokinetics of losartan and losartan acid (E-3174) in healthy subjects. *J Clin Pharmacol* (2006) 46, 310–20.
7. Cozaar (Losartan potassium). Merck Sharp & Dohme Ltd. UK Summary of product characteristics, December 2006.
8. Cozaar (Losartan potassium). Merck & Co., Inc. US Prescribing information, December 2005.
9. Benicar (Olmesartan medoxomil). Daiichi Sankyo, Inc. US Prescribing information, October 2006.
10. Olmetec (Olmesartan medoxomil). Daiichi Sankyo UK Ltd. UK Summary of product characteristics, August 2006.
11. Micardis (Telmisartan). Boehringer Ingelheim Pharmaceuticals Inc. US Prescribing information, May 2006.
12. Micardis (Telmisartan). Boehringer Ingelheim Ltd. UK Summary of product characteristics, March 2007.
13. Diovan (Valsartan). Novartis. US Prescribing information, June 2007.
14. Diovan (Valsartan). Novartis Pharmaceuticals UK Ltd. UK Summary of product characteristics, September 2006.

Angiotensin II receptor antagonists + H_2-receptor antagonists

Cimetidine may cause a small rise in plasma concentrations of valsartan, but this is unlikely to be clinically significant. Cimetidine did not significantly affect the pharmacokinetics and blood pressure-lowering effect of losartan, and ranitidine did not significantly alter the pharmacokinetics of eprosartan.

Clinical evidence, mechanism, importance and management

(a) Cimetidine

1. Losartan. In a randomised, crossover study in 8 healthy subjects when losartan 100 mg was given after cimetidine 400 mg four times daily for 6 days, the pharmacokinetics and pharmacodynamics of losartan and its active metabolite, E-3174, were not changed to a clinically relevant extent, although there was a minor increase of 18% in the AUC of losartan.[1] No special precautions are needed if these drugs are used concurrently.

2. Valsartan. In a single-dose, crossover study, cimetidine 800 mg, given one hour before valsartan 160 mg, increased the initial rate of absorption of valsartan (attributed to a raised gastric pH) resulting in a roughly 50% increase in its maximum plasma concentration. However, the AUC was only slightly increased and there were large inter-subject variations in the pharmacokinetics of valsartan.[2] The changes in valsartan pharmacokinetics seen with cimetidine are unlikely to be clinically relevant.

(b) Ranitidine

A single 400-mg dose of **eprosartan** was given to 17 healthy subjects, both alone and after ranitidine 150 mg twice daily for 3 days. The ranitidine caused some slight, but statistically insignificant, changes in the pharmacokinetics of the **eprosartan** (maximum plasma concentration and AUC reduced by about 7% and 11%, respectively).[3]

1. Goldberg MR, Lo M-W, Bradstreet TE, Ritter MA, Höglund P. Effects of cimetidine on pharmacokinetics and pharmacodynamics of losartan, an AT_1-selective non-peptide angiotensin II receptor antagonist. *Eur J Clin Pharmacol* (1995) 49, 115–19.

2. Schmidt EK, Antonin K-H, Flesch G, Racine-Poon A. An interaction study with cimetidine and the new angiotensin II antagonist valsartan. *Eur J Clin Pharmacol* (1998) 53, 451–8.
3. Tenero DM, Martin DE, Ilson BE, Boyle DA, Boike SC, Carr AM, Lundberg DE, Jorkasky DK. Effect of ranitidine on the pharmacokinetics of orally administered eprosartan, an angiotensin II antagonist, in healthy male volunteers. *Ann Pharmacother* (1998) 32, 304–8.

Angiotensin II receptor antagonists + Mannitol

A report describes mannitol-induced acute renal failure in a diabetic patient taking losartan.

Clinical evidence, mechanism, importance and management

A man with diabetic nephropathy taking **losartan** 25 mg twice daily for hypertension developed acute renal failure after being given a total of 420 g of intravenous mannitol over 4 days for haemorrhagic glaucoma. The patient recovered after the mannitol and **losartan** were discontinued, and after receiving haemodialysis.[1] It is not fully understood why this combination caused acute renal failure, but it may result in a marked decrease in glomerular filtration rate. Caution is recommended.[1] For comment on the potentiation of ACE inhibitor-induced renal damage by diuretics, see 'ACE inhibitors + Diuretics; Loop, Thiazide and related', p.21.

1. Matsumura M. Mannitol-induced toxicity in a diabetic patient receiving losartan. *Am J Med* (2001) 110, 331.

Angiotensin II receptor antagonists + Potassium compounds

There may be a risk of hyperkalaemia if angiotensin II receptor antagonists are given with potassium supplements or potassium-containing salt substitutes, particularly in those patients where other risk factors are present, such as decreased renal function, heart failure, or diabetes.

Clinical evidence, mechanism, importance and management

Angiotensin II receptor antagonists are potassium-sparing, via their effects on aldosterone, and their potential to cause clinically important hyperkalaemia is well established. The incidence of hyperkalaemia varies depending on the clinical indication and other disease conditions, being lowest in essential hypertension, and highest in heart failure, diabetes, and renal impairment. For example, the incidence of hyperkalaemia in clinical studies in patients with hypertension was 0.9% with **eprosartan**[1,2] and 1.5% with **losartan**;[3] in type II diabetic patients with nephropathy, the incidence was 9.9% with **losartan**[3] and 18.6% with **irbesartan**;[4] and in those with heart failure the incidence was 6.3% with **candesartan**.[5]

The concurrent use of potassium-containing supplements or **salt substitutes** and angiotensin II receptor antagonists is likely to further increase serum potassium. Therefore potassium supplements are generally unlikely to be needed in patients taking angiotensin II receptor antagonists, particularly if they have other risk factors for hyperkalaemia, and it may be prudent for such patients to be told to avoid using potassium-containing **salt substitutes**. If concurrent use is considered necessary, potassium levels should be closely monitored. For reports of hyperkalaemia associated with ACE inhibitors and *dietary* potassium, see 'ACE inhibitors + Potassium compounds', p.32.

1. Teveten (Eprosartan mesilate). Solvay Healthcare Ltd. UK Summary of product characteristics, June 2006.
2. Teveten (Eprosartan mesylate). Kos Pharmaceuticals, Inc. US Prescribing information, September 2005.
3. Cozaar (Losartan potassium). Merck Sharp & Dohme Ltd. UK Summary of product characteristics, December 2006.
4. Avapro (Irbesartan). Bristol-Myers Squibb. US Prescribing information, October 2005.
5. Atacand (Candesartan cilexetil). AstraZeneca. US Prescribing information, February 2007.

Angiotensin II receptor antagonists + Rifampicin (Rifampin)

Rifampicin increases the metabolism of losartan and its active metabolite, E-3174, which may result in reduced antihypertensive effects.

Clinical evidence, mechanism, importance and management

Ten healthy subjects were given **losartan** 50 mg daily for a week and then, after a 6-day washout period, **losartan** 50 mg daily with rifampicin 300 mg twice daily for a week. It was found that rifampicin reduced the AUC of **losartan** by 36%, reduced its half-life from 2 to 0.9 hours, and increased its clearance by 60%. The AUC of the active metabolite, E3174, was reduced by 41% and its half-life was reduced from 5.1 to 2.5 hours. Diastolic blood pressure was significantly reduced by **losartan** alone, but not by the combination.[1] The presumed reason for this interaction is that rifampicin (a recognised enzyme inducer) increases the metabolism of **losartan** to its active metabolite by the cytochrome P450 isoenzyme CYP2C9.

The clinical importance of this interaction still awaits assessment, but it would seem likely that the antihypertensive effects of **losartan** would be reduced by rifampicin. If both drugs are used, be alert for the need to increase the **losartan** dosage. More study is needed. There seems to be no information regarding other angiotensin II receptor antagonists, but note that **irbesartan**, and to a limited extent **candesartan**, are also metabolised by CYP2C9 (see the 'introduction', (p.12)).

1. Williamson KM, Patterson JH, McQueen RH, Adams KF, Pieper JA. Effects of erythromycin or rifampin on losartan pharmacokinetics in healthy volunteers. *Clin Pharmacol Ther* (1998) 63, 316–23.

Angiotensin II receptor antagonists; Losartan + AST-120

AST-120 does not appears to have an important effect on the pharmacokinetics of losartan.

Clinical evidence, mechanism, importance and management

When a single 100-mg dose of losartan was given 30 minutes before a high-fat breakfast, with AST-120 3 g three times daily for 48 hours started 30 minutes after the breakfast, the AUC of losartan was not significantly altered, although there was a minor 12.3% decrease in the maximum losartan level. Similarly, various other schedules (losartan with breakfast, then AST-120 started 30 minutes later, or AST-120 started 30 minutes after breakfast, then losartan given 30 minutes after that), did not significantly alter the AUC of losartan, when compared with losartan given 30 minutes before breakfast. However, there were minor to modest increases in the AUC of losartan (of up to 37%) when these schedules were compared with losartan given in the fasting state, which was attributed to the effect of food.[1]

AST-120 is a predominantly carbon-based oral absorbent, and might therefore interfere with absorption of other drugs.

Data from this pharmacokinetic study indicate that AST-120 has minimal effects on the pharmacokinetics of losartan. The authors suggest that giving AST-120 one hour after losartan may be preferred.[1]

1. Marier JF, Guilbaud R, Kambhampati SR, Mathew P, Moberly J, Lee J, Salazar DE. The effect of AST-120 on the single-dose pharmacokinetics of losartan and losartan acid (E-3174) in healthy subjects. *J Clin Pharmacol* (2006) 46, 310–20.

Angiotensin II receptor antagonists; Losartan + Erythromycin

The pharmacokinetics and blood pressure-lowering effect of losartan do not seem to be affected by erythromycin.

Clinical evidence, mechanism, importance and management

When 10 healthy subjects were given **losartan** 50 mg daily for a week and then, after a 6-day washout period, **losartan** 50 mg daily with erythromycin 500 mg four times daily for a week, it was found that erythromycin had no significant effect on the pharmacokinetics of **losartan** or its active metabolite, E-3174. In addition, erythromycin did not alter the blood pressure-lowering effect of **losartan**.[1] Inhibition of the cytochrome P450 isoenzyme CYP3A4 alone does not appear to prevent the conversion of **losartan** to E-3174. There would therefore appear to be no reason to take any special precautions if both drugs are used concurrently.

1. Williamson KM, Patterson JH, McQueen RH, Adams KF, Pieper JA. Effects of erythromycin or rifampin on losartan pharmacokinetics in healthy volunteers. *Clin Pharmacol Ther* (1998) 63, 316–23.

Angiotensin II receptor antagonists; Losartan + Grapefruit juice

Grapefruit juice has a minor effect on the pharmacokinetics of losartan and its active metabolite, E-3174, which is unlikely to be clinically relevant.

Clinical evidence, mechanism, importance and management

In a study in 9 healthy subjects, grapefruit juice approximately doubled the time for a single 50-mg dose of **losartan** to be detected in the serum (from 0.6 to 1.3 hours) and reduced the AUC of its active metabolite, E-3174, by 21%. **Losartan** is partly metabolised by the cytochrome P450 isoenzyme CYP3A4 and transported by P-glycoprotein, both of which can be affected by grapefruit juice. This may explain the minor changes seen.[1] However, this interaction is unlikely to be clinically relevant.

1. Zaidenstein R, Soback S, Gips M, Avni B, Dishi V, Weissgarten Y, Golik A, Scapa E. Effect of grapefruit juice on the pharmacokinetics of losartan and its active metabolite E3174 in healthy volunteers. *Ther Drug Monit* (2001) 23, 369–73.

Angiotensin II receptor antagonists; Losartan + Phenobarbital

Phenobarbital minimally alters the levels of losartan and its active metabolite.

Clinical evidence, mechanism, importance and management

In a placebo-controlled study 15 healthy subjects were given phenobarbital 100 mg daily for 16 days with a single 100-mg dose of **losartan**. Phenobarbital slightly reduced the AUC of **losartan** and its active metabolite, E-3174, by about 20%, but this was not considered to be clinically significant.[1]

1. Goldberg MR, Lo MW, Deutsch PJ, Wilson SE, McWilliams EJ, McCrea JB. Phenobarbital minimally alters plasma concentrations of losartan and its active metabolite E-3174. *Clin Pharmacol Ther* (1996) 59, 268–74.

Angiotensin II receptor antagonists; Losartan + Phenytoin

Phenytoin inhibited the metabolism of losartan to its active metabolite, E-3174, but the clinical relevance of the changes seen are unknown.

Clinical evidence, mechanism, importance and management

The concurrent use of phenytoin and losartan for 10 days reduced the AUC of the active metabolite of losartan, E-3174, by 63%, but did not significantly alter the AUC of losartan. The pharmacokinetics of phenytoin were not affected by losartan. In this crossover study in 16 healthy subjects, phenytoin was given at a dose of 4 mg/kg rounded to the nearest 100 mg, not to exceed 400 mg daily, and the dose was adjusted on the fourth day, if necessary, based on serum phenytoin levels. The losartan dose was 50 mg daily. Phenytoin did not alter the effect of losartan on blood pressure. The effect of phenytoin appeared to be CYP2C9 genotype-specific, with increases in losartan AUC seen in the 14 subjects who were extensive metabolisers of CYP2C9, and decreases in the 2 subjects who were poor metabolisers.[1]

Both phenytoin and losartan are substrates for the cytochrome P450 isoenzyme CYP2C9. It appears that phenytoin had an inhibitory effect on losartan metabolism. The conversion of losartan to E3174 represents about 5 to 15% of the clearance of an oral losartan dose,[1] but E3174 is much more active than losartan.

The clinical importance of this interaction still awaits assessment. Until more is known, if phenytoin is added to established losartan therapy, it may be prudent to initially monitor blood pressure more closely. More study is needed.

1. Fischer TL, Pieper JA, Graff DW, Rodgers JE, Fischer JD, Parnell KJ, Goldstein JA, Greenwood R, Patterson JH. Evaluation of potential losartan-phenytoin drug interactions in healthy volunteers. *Clin Pharmacol Ther* (2002) 72, 238–46.

3

Alcohol

For social and historical reasons alcohol is usually bought from a store or in a bar or restaurant, rather than from a pharmacy, because it is considered to be a drink and not a drug. However, pharmacologically it has much in common with medicinal drugs that depress the central nervous system. Objective tests show that as blood-alcohol levels rise, the ability to perform a number of skills gradually deteriorates as the brain becomes progressively disorganised. The myth that alcohol is a stimulant has arisen because at parties and social occasions it helps people to lose some of their inhibitions and it allows them to relax and unwind. Professor JH Gaddum put it amusingly and succinctly when, describing the early effects of moderate amounts of alcohol, he wrote that "logical thought is difficult but after dinner speeches easy." The expansiveness and loquaciousness that are socially acceptable can lead on, with increasing amounts of alcohol, to unrestrained behaviour in normally well-controlled individuals, through to drunkenness, unconsciousness, and finally death from respiratory failure. These effects are all a reflection of the progressive and deepening depression of the CNS.

'Table 3.1', (p.41) gives an indication in very broad terms of the reactions of men and women to different amounts and concentrations of alcohol.

On the whole women have a higher proportion of fat in which alcohol is not very soluble, their body fluids represent a smaller proportion of their total body mass, and their first-pass metabolism of alcohol is less than men because they have less alcohol dehydrogenase in their stomach walls. Consequently if a man and woman of the same weight matched each other, drink for drink, the woman would finish up with a blood alcohol level about 50% higher than the man. The values shown assume that the drinkers regularly drink, have had a meal and weigh between 9 and 11 stones (55 to 70 kg). Higher blood-alcohol levels would occur if alcohol was drunk on an empty stomach and lower values in much heavier individuals. The liver metabolises about one unit per hour so the values will fall with time.

Since alcohol impairs the skills needed to drive safely, almost all national and state authorities have imposed maximum legal blood alcohol limits (see 'Table 3.2', (p.41)). In a number of countries this has been set at 80 mg/100 mL (35 micrograms per 100 mL in the breath) but impairment is clearly detectable at lower concentrations, for which reason some countries have imposed much lower legal limits.

Alcohol can interact with many drugs both by pharmacokinetic and/or pharmacodynamic mechanisms. The quantity and frequency of alcohol consumption can affect the bioavailability of alcohol and other drugs. Several hepatic enzymes are important in the metabolism of alcohol; primarily alcohol dehydrogenases convert alcohol into acetaldehyde, but other enzymes, in particular the cytochrome P450 isoenzyme CYP2E1, are also involved, especially in moderate to heavy alcohol consumption. Enzyme induction of CYP2E1 (and possibly other isoenzymes) occurs after prolonged heavy alcohol intake, and this can result in an increased metabolic rate and lower blood levels of drugs metabolised via this system. Conversely, short term binge drinking is likely to cause inhibition of this enzyme group by direct competition for binding sites and therefore decrease the metabolism of other drugs.

Probably the most common drug interaction of all occurs if alcohol is drunk by those taking other drugs that have CNS depressant activity, the result being even further CNS depression. Blood-alcohol levels well within the legal driving limit may, in the presence of other CNS depressants, be equivalent to blood-alcohol levels at or above the legal limit in terms of worsened driving and other skills. This can occur with some antihistamines, antidepressants, anxiolytics, hypnotics, opioid analgesics, and others. This section contains a number of monographs that describe the results of formal studies of alcohol combined with a number of recognised CNS depressants, but there are still many other drugs that await study of this kind, and which undoubtedly represent a real hazard.

A less common interaction that can occur between alcohol and some drugs, chemical agents, and fungi, is the flushing (*Antabuse*) reaction. This is exploited in the case of disulfiram (*Antabuse*) as a drink deterrent (see 'Alcohol + Disulfiram', p.61), but it can occur unexpectedly with some other drugs, such as some antifungals and cephalosporins, chlorpropamide and metronidazole, and can be both unpleasant and possibly frightening, but it is not usually dangerous.

Table 3.1 Reactions to different concentrations of alcohol in the blood

Amounts of alcohol drunk				
Man 11 stones (70 kg)	**Woman 9 stones (55 kg)**	**Blood-alcohol levels mg% (mg per 100 mL)**	**Reactions to different % of alcohol in the blood**	
2 units	1 unit	25 to 30	Sense of well-being enhanced. Reaction times reduced	
4 units	2 units	50 to 60	Mild loss of inhibition, judgement impaired, increased risk of accidents at home, at work and on the road; no overt signs of drunkenness	
5 units	3 units	75 to 80	Physical co-ordination reduced, more marked loss of inhibition; noticeably under the influence; at the maximum legal limit for driving in some countries	
7 units	4 units	100 or more	Clumsiness, loss of physical control, tendency to extreme responses; definite intoxication	
10 units	6 units	150	Slurred speech, possible loss of memory the following day, probably drunk and disorderly	
24 units	14 units	360	Dead drunk, sleepiness, possible loss of consciousness	
33 units	20 units	500	Coma and possibly death	
1 unit	= half a pint (300 mL medium strength beer)	= glass of wine (100 mL)	= single sherry or martini (50 mL)	= single spirit (25 mL)
	alcohol 3 to 4%	alcohol 11%	alcohol 17 to 20%	alcohol 37 to 40%

After *Which?* October 1984, page 447 and others.

Table 3.2 Maximum legally allowable blood alcohol limits when driving in various countries

80 mg%	Belize, Canada,* Cape Verde, Central African Republic, Ghana, Guatemala, Ireland, Kenya, Luxembourg, Malaysia, Malta, Mexico, New Zealand,* Nicaragua, Niger, Paraguay, Seychelles, Singapore, Suriname, Switzerland, Uganda, United Kingdom, United States of America,* Uruguay, Zambia
70 mg%	Bolivia, Ecuador, Honduras
60 mg%	Brazil, Sri Lanka
52 mg%	Republic of Korea
50 mg%	Argentina, Australia,* Austria, Belarus, Benin, Bosnia & Herzegovina, Bulgaria, Cambodia, Croatia, Denmark, El Salvador, Finland, France, French Polynesia, Germany, Greece, Guinea-Bissau, Iceland, Israel, Italy, Kyrgyzstan, Mauritius, Micronesia (Federated States of), Namibia, Netherlands, Peru, Philippines, Portugal, Slovenia, South Africa, Spain, Thailand, The former Yugoslav Republic of Macedonia, Turkey, United Republic of Tanzania, Venezuela
49 mg%	Chile, Costa Rica, Latvia
40 mg%	Lithuania
35 mg%	Jamaica
33 mg%	Turkmenistan
30 mg%	Georgia, India, Japan, Republic of Moldova
20 mg%	Estonia, Mongolia, Norway, Poland, Sweden
10 mg%	Guyana, Palau
0 mg%	Armenia, Azerbaijan, Colombia, Czech Republic, Equatorial Guinea, Eritrea, Gambia, Guinea, Hungary, Islamic Republic of Iran, Jordan, Kazakhstan, Malawi, Nepal, Nigeria, Panama, Romania, Russian Federation, Slovakia
No legislation	China, Comoros, Congo (Brazzaville), Dominican Republic, Ethiopia, Lao People's Democratic Republic, Togo, Ukraine

Note: For easy comparison the legally allowable blood alcohol limits have all been expressed as mg%. Thus: blood alcohol levels of 80 mg% = 80 mg of alcohol in 100 mL blood = 0.8 g/L.

*Variations occur within these countries e.g. in Australia no alcohol is allowed for drivers of heavy, dangerous goods, public transport vehicles; learners and drivers under 25 years of age for first three years of driving.

Adapted from the WHO Global Status Report: Alcohol policy, Geneva, 2004.

Alcohol + Alpha blockers

The plasma levels of both indoramin and alcohol may be raised by concurrent use. The combination of alcohol and indoramin has been reported to increase drowsiness, which may possibly increase the risks when driving or using machinery. Prazosin appears to enhance the hypotensive effects of alcohol.

Clinical evidence

(a) Indoramin

When 10 healthy subjects were given a single 50-mg oral dose of indoramin together with alcohol 0.5 g/kg in 600 mL of alcohol-free lager, the AUC of indoramin was increased by 25% and the peak plasma levels were raised by 58%.[1,2] When the subjects were given a single 175-microgram/kg intravenous dose of indoramin together with the same oral dose of alcohol, a 26% rise in blood-alcohol levels occurred during the first 1.25 hours after dosing, but no change in indoramin pharmacokinetics were seen. The combination of alcohol and indoramin caused more sedation than either drug alone.[2]

(b) Prazosin

A study in 10 Japanese hypertensive patients found that alcohol 1 mL/kg decreased blood pressure for several hours. Treatment with prazosin 1 mg three times daily caused a significant reduction in blood pressure and enhanced alcohol-induced hypotension.[3] These effects may be restricted to Oriental/Asian patients because the alcohol flush syndrome, caused by accumulation of vasodilative acetaldehyde due to a genetic alteration in aldehyde dehydrogenase, is rare in whites and blacks.[3] The clinical significance is uncertain as the dose of prazosin in the study was relatively small and the dose of alcohol was relatively large, therefore these findings may not apply to more moderate drinking or higher doses of prazosin.

Mechanism

Uncertain. Increased absorption of indoramin from the gut or reduced liver metabolism may be responsible for the raised indoramin serum levels. The increase in sedation would appear to be due to the additive sedative effects of the two drugs.

Importance and management

Information is limited but the interaction between indoramin and alcohol appears to be established. The clinical importance of the raised levels of both drugs is uncertain. However since indoramin sometimes causes drowsiness when it is first given, there is the possibility that alertness will be reduced, which could increase the risks of driving or handling machinery. Patients should be warned. Prazosin appears to enhance the hypotensive effect of alcohol, see also, 'Alcohol + Antihypertensives', p.48.

1. Abrams SML, Pierce DM, Franklin RA, Johnston A, Marrott PK, Cory EP, Turner P. Effect of ethanol on indoramin pharmacokinetics. *Br J Clin Pharmacol* (1984) 18, 294P–295P.
2. Abrams SML, Pierce DM, Johnston A, Hedges A, Franklin RA, Turner P. Pharmacokinetic interaction between indoramin and ethanol. *Hum Toxicol* (1989) 8, 237–41.
3. Kawano Y, Abe H, Kojima S, Takishita S, Omae T. Interaction of alcohol and an α_1-blocker on ambulatory blood pressure in patients with essential hypertension. *Am J Hypertens* (2000) 13, 307–12.

Alcohol + Amfetamines

Dexamfetamine can reduce the deleterious effects of alcohol to some extent, but some impairment still occurs making it unsafe to drive. Another report suggests the combination of metamfetamine and alcohol produces an increase in perceived total intoxication, and may also increase cardiac adverse effects.

Clinical evidence

In 12 healthy subjects alcohol 0.85 g/kg (2 mL/kg of 100 proof vodka in orange juice) worsened the performance of a SEDI task (Simulator Evaluation of Drug Impairment).[1] This task is believed to parallel the skills needed to drive safely, and involves tests of attention, memory, recognition, decision making and reaction times. When the subjects were also given **dexamfetamine** 90 or 180 micrograms/kg, there was a dose-related improvement in the performance of the SEDI task, but the subjective assessment of intoxication was unchanged. Blood alcohol levels reached a maximum of about 100 mg% at approximately one hour. The bioavailability of the alcohol was slightly increased.[1]

Earlier reports using different testing methods found that in some tests **dexamfetamine** modified the effects of alcohol,[2,3] but the total picture was complex. Other reports found no antagonism.[4,5] Another study found that in stress situations, where relief of fatigue or boredom alone will not produce improved performance, **dexamfetamine** failed to improve attentive motor performance impaired by alcohol.[6] A later study found that, while the combination of alcohol and **metamfetamine** diminished the subjective feelings of alcohol intoxication, there was actually an increase in feelings of total intoxication.[7] The combination of alcohol and **metamfetamine** may increase cardiac toxicity.[7]

Mechanism

Not understood. Although alcohol is a CNS depressant and the amfetamines are CNS stimulants, there is no simple antagonism between the two.[3]

Importance and management

Clear-cut conclusions cannot be drawn from the evidence presented in the reported studies. There is some evidence that the effects of alcohol are modified or reduced, but driving skills appear to remain impaired to some extent. There is also evidence of an increased risk of adverse cardiac effects. The increase in perceived total intoxication noted in one report has been suggested as a possible reason for the popularity of the illicit use of the combination.[7] Consider also 'Alcohol + Ecstasy', p.62.

1. Perez-Reyes M, White WR, McDonald SA, Hicks RE. Interaction between ethanol and dextroamphetamine: effects on psychomotor performance. *Alcohol Clin Exp Res* (1992) 16, 75–81.
2. Kaplan HL, Forney RB, Richards AB, Hughes FW. Dextro-amphetamine, alcohol, and dextro-amphetamine-alcohol combination and mental performance. In Harger RN, ed. Alcohol and traffic safety. Bloomington, Indiana: Indiana Univ Press; 1966 p. 211–14.
3. Wilson L, Taylor JD, Nash CW, Cameron DF. The combined effects of ethanol and amphetamine sulfate on performance of human subjects. *Can Med Assoc J* (1966) 94, 478–84.
4. Hughes FW, Forney RB. Dextro-amphetamine, ethanol and dextro-amphetamine-ethanol combinations on performance of human subjects stressed with delayed auditory feedback (DAF). *Psychopharmacologia* (1964) 6, 234–8.
5. Newman HW, Newman EJ. Failure of dexedrine and caffeine as practical antagonists of the depressant effect of ethyl alcohol in man. *Q J Stud Alcohol* (1956) 17, 406–10.
6. Brown DJ, Hughes FW, Forney RB, Richards AB. Effect of d-amphetamine and alcohol on attentive motor performance in human subjects. In Harger RN, ed. Alcohol and traffic safety. Bloomington, Indiana: Indiana Univ Press; 1966 p. 215–19.
7. Mendelson J, Jones RT, Upton R, Jacob P. Methamphetamine and ethanol interactions in humans. *Clin Pharmacol Ther* (1995) 57, 559–68.

Alcohol + Aminosalicylic acid

Alcohol can abolish the lipid-lowering effects of aminosalicylic acid.

Clinical evidence, mechanism, importance and management

The effectiveness of PAS-C (purified aminosalicylic acid recrystallised in vitamin C) and diet on the treatment of hyperlipidaemia types IIa and IIb was studied in a group of 63 subjects. It was noted that when 3 of the subjects drank unstated amounts of alcohol (beer or cocktails), the effects of the PAS-C on lowering serum cholesterol, triglyceride and LDL-cholesterol levels were completely abolished.[1] The reasons are not understood.

There seems to be no evidence that alcohol affects the treatment of tuberculosis with aminosalicylic acid.

1. Kuo PT, Fan WC, Kostis JB, Hayase K. Combined para-aminosalicylic acid and dietary therapy in long-term control of hypercholesterolemia and hypertriglyceridemia (types II_a and II_b hyperlipoproteinemia). *Circulation* (1976) 53, 338–41.

Alcohol + Amisulpride

No pharmacokinetic interaction appears to occur between amisulpride and alcohol.

Clinical evidence, mechanism, importance and management

No significant pharmacokinetic interactions were seen in 18 healthy subjects given single 50- and 200-mg doses of amisulpride with alcohol 0.8 g/kg, nor were the detrimental effects of alcohol on performance increased by amisulpride.[1] Nevertheless, the manufacturer advises that the central effects of alcohol may be enhanced by amisulpride, and so they do not recommend the combination.[2]

1. Mattila MJ, Patat A, Seppälä T, Kalska H, Jalava M-L, Vanakoski J, Lavanant C. Single oral doses of amisulpride do not enhance the effects of alcohol on the performance and memory of healthy subjects. *Eur J Clin Pharmacol* (1996) 51, 161–6.
2. Solian (Amisulpride). Sanofi-Aventis. UK Summary of product characteristics, December 2004.

Alcohol + Antibacterials; Cephalosporins

Disulfiram-like reactions can occur in those who take cefamandole, cefmenoxime, cefoperazone, cefotetan, latamoxef (moxalactam) and possibly cefonicid, and drink alcohol. This is not a general reaction of the cephalosporins, but is confined to those with particular chemical structures.

Clinical evidence

A young man with cystic fibrosis was given **latamoxef** 2 g intravenously every 8 hours for pneumonia. After 3 days of treatment he drank, as was his custom, a can of **beer** with lunch. He rapidly became flushed with a florid macular eruption over his face and chest. This faded over the next 30 minutes but he complained of severe nausea and headache. Similarly, a patient taking **latamoxef** became flushed, diaphoretic and nauseated after drinking a cocktail of **vodka** and tomato juice.[1] This reaction has also been described in two subjects who drank alcohol while receiving **latamoxef**,[2] two of 10 subjects given **latamoxef** and alcohol,[3] and a patient taking **latamoxef** given theophylline elixir containing alcohol 20%.[4] It has also been seen in a patient taking **latamoxef** following the injection of alcohol into the para-aortic space for coeliac plexus block.[5] The symptoms experienced by these patients have included flushing of the face, arms and neck, shortness of breath, headache, tachycardia, dizziness, hyper- and hypotension, and nausea and vomiting.

Similar reactions have been described in patients or subjects receiving **cefamandole**,[6,7] **cefoperazone**,[8-15] **cefmenoxime**,[16] **cefonicid**[17] and **cefotetan**,[18] after drinking **wine**, **beer**, or other alcoholic drinks, or after the ingestion of an 8.5% alcoholic elixir.[16]

This disulfiram-like reaction is not a general reaction of all the cephalosporins. One study found no interaction in those taking **cefpirome** and alcohol,[19] and in another **ceftizoxime** was reported not to interact with alcohol.[20] No interaction was seen with **cefonicid** and alcohol in one placebo-controlled study,[21] however a case report describes a disulfiram-reaction in one patient taking the combination.[17]

Mechanism

These reactions appear to have the same pharmacological basis as the disulfiram/alcohol reaction (see 'Alcohol + Disulfiram', p.61). Three of these cephalosporins (latamoxef, cefamandole and cefoperazone) can raise blood acetaldehyde levels in *rats* when alcohol is given, but to a lesser extent than disulfiram.[2,11,22] It appears that any reaction normally only occurs with cephalosporins that possess a methyltetrazolethiol group in the 3-position on the cephalosporin molecule,[11,23] but it has also been seen with cefonicid, which possesses a methyl sulphonthiotetrazolic group instead.[17] Some amine-containing cephalosporins (**cefalexin, cefadroxil** and **cefradine**) have also been reported to interact with acetaldehyde *in vitro,* but the clinical significance of this is unknown.[24]

Importance and management

Established but unpredictable interactions of varying incidence. In studies, two out of 10 subjects given latamoxef and alcohol reacted,[3] five out of 8 taking cefotetan reacted,[18] and 8 out of 9 receiving cefoperazone reacted.[14,15] The reaction appears normally to be more embarrassing or unpleasant and frightening than serious, with the symptoms subsiding spontaneously after a few hours. There is evidence that the severity varies; in one study cefoperazone was said to be worse than latamoxef, which in turn was said to be worse than **cefmetazole**.[25] Treatment is not usually needed but there are two reports[4,6] of two elderly patients who needed treatment for hypotension, which was life-threatening in one case;[4] plasma expanders and dopamine have been used as treatment.[4,6]

Because the reaction is unpredictable, warn all patients taking these potentially interacting cephalosporins that it can occur during and up to 3 days after the course of treatment is over. Advise them to avoid alcohol. Those with renal or hepatic impairment in whom the drug clearance is prolonged should wait a week. It should not be forgotten that some foods and pharmaceuticals contain substantial amounts of alcohol, and a reaction with some topically applied products cannot be excluded (see 'Alcohol + Disulfiram', p.61).

A number of other cephalosporins are possible candidates for this reaction because they possess the methyltetrazolethiol group in the 3-position. These include, **ceforanide**, **cefotiam**, and **cefpiramide**,[11,23] but there do not appear to be any reports of an interaction between alcohol and these drugs.

1. Neu HC, Prince AS. Interaction between moxalactam and alcohol. *Lancet* (1980), i, 1422.
2. Buening MK, Wold JS, Israel KS, Kammer RB. Disulfiram-like reaction to β-lactams. *JAMA* (1981) 245, 2027–8.
3. Elenbaas RM, Ryan JL, Robinson WA, Singsank MJ, Harvey MJ, Klaasen CD. On the disulfiram-like activity of moxalactam. *Clin Pharmacol Ther* (1982) 32, 347–55.
4. Brown KR, Guglielmo BJ, Pons VG, Jacobs RA. Theophylline elixir, moxalactam, and a disulfiram-like reaction. *Ann Intern Med* (1982) 97, 621–2.
5. Umeda S, Arai T. Disulfiram-like reaction to moxalactam after celiac plexus alcohol block. *Anesth Analg* (1985) 64, 377.
6. Portier H, Chalopin JM, Freysz M, Tanter Y. Interaction between cephalosporins and alcohol. *Lancet* (1980), ii, 263.
7. Drummer S, Hauser WE, Remington JS. Antabuse-like effect of β-lactam antibiotics. *N Engl J Med* (1980) 303, 1417–18.
8. Foster TS, Raehl CL, Wilson HD. Disulfiram-like reaction associated with parenteral cephalosporin. *Am J Hosp Pharm* (1980) 37, 858–9.
9. Allaz A-F, Dayer P, Fabre J, Rudhardt M, Balant L. Pharmacocinétique d'une nouvelle céphalosporine, la céfopérazone. *Schweiz Med Wochenschr* (1979), 109, 1999–2005.
10. Kemmerich B, Lode H. Cefoperazone – another cephalosporin associated with a disulfiram type alcohol incompatibility. *Infection* (1981) 9, 110.
11. Uri JV, Parks DB. Disulfiram-like reaction to certain cephalosporins. *Ther Drug Monit* (1983) 5, 219–24.
12. Bailey RR, Peddie B, Blake E, Bishop V, Reddy J. Cefoperazone in the treatment of severe or complicated infections. *Drugs* (1981) 22 (Suppl 1), 76–86.
13. Ellis-Pegler RB, Lang SDR. Cefoperazone in Klebsiella meningitis: A case report. *Drugs* (1981) 22 (Suppl 1), 69–71.
14. Reeves DS, Davies AJ. Antabuse effect with cephalosporins. *Lancet* (1980) ii, 540.
15. McMahon FG. Disulfiram-like reaction to a cephalosporin. *JAMA* (1980), 243, 2397.
16. Kannangara DW, Gallagher K, Lefrock JL. Disulfiram-like reactions with newer cephalosporins: cefmenoxime. *Am J Med Sci* (1984) 287, 45–7.
17. Marcon G, Spolaor A, Scevola M, Zolli M, Carlassara GB. Effetto disulfiram-simile da cefonicid: prima segnalazione. *Recenti Prog Med* (1990) 81, 47–8.
18. Kline SS, Mauro VF, Forney RB, Freimer EH, Somani P. Cefotetan-induced disulfiram-type reactions and hypoprothrombinemia. *Antimicrob Agents Chemother* (1987) 31, 1328–31.
19. Lassman HB, Hubbard JW, Chen B-L, Puri SK. Lack of interaction between cefpirome and alcohol. *J Antimicrob Chemother* (1992) 29 (Suppl A), 47–50.
20. McMahon FG, Noveck RJ. Lack of disulfiram-like reactions with ceftizoxime. *J Antimicrob Chemother* (1982) 10 (Suppl C), 129–33.
21. McMahon FG, Ryan JR, Jain AK, LaCorte W, Ginzler F. Absence of disulfiram-type reactions to single and multiple doses of cefonicid: a placebo-controlled study. *J Antimicrob Chemother* (1987) 20, 913–8.
22. Yanagihara M, Okada K, Nozaki M, Tsurumi K, Fujimura H. Cephem antibiotics and alcohol metabolism. Disulfiram-like reaction resulting from intravenous administration of cephem antibiotics. *Folia Pharmacol Japon* (1982) 79, 551–60.
23. Norrby SR. Adverse reactions and interactions with newer cephalosporin and cephamycin antibiotics. *Med Toxicol* (1986) 1, 32–46.
24. Nuñez-Vergara LJ, Yudelevich J, Squella JA, Speisky H. Drug-acetaldehyde interactions during ethanol metabolism *in vitro*. *Alcohol Alcohol* (1991) 26, 139–46.
25. Nakamura K, Nakagawa A, Tanaka M, Masuda H, Hayashi Y, Saionji K. Effects of cephem antibiotics on ethanol metabolism. *Folia Pharmacol Japon* (1984) 83, 183–91.

Alcohol + Antibacterials; Ciprofloxacin

Ciprofloxacin does not significantly affect the pharmacokinetics of alcohol or the psychomotor performance observed with alcohol alone. There is an isolated report of a cutaneous reaction to ciprofloxacin, which may have been precipitated by alcohol ingestion.

Clinical evidence, mechanism, importance and management

A 3-day course of ciprofloxacin 500 mg twice daily had no significant effect on the pharmacokinetics of a single 30-g oral dose of alcohol (75 mL of vodka) in 12 healthy subjects, nor was the performance of a number of psychomotor tests affected.[1]

There is an isolated report of red blotches developing on the face and body of a tetraplegic patient receiving ciprofloxacin 250 mg twice daily, which developed within 10 minutes of drinking 2 cans of beer containing alcohol 4.7%. He did not feel unwell or drowsy and the blotches faded over a period of 30 minutes. Previous courses of ciprofloxacin had not produced any adverse effects and the same brand of alcohol caused no problems in the absence of ciprofloxacin.[2] The general clinical importance of this report is unknown, but it seems likely to be small.

1. Kamali F. No influence of ciprofloxacin on ethanol disposition: a pharmacokinetic-pharmacodynamic interaction study. *Eur J Clin Pharmacol* (1994) 47, 71–4.
2. Vaidyanathan S, Singh G, Sett P, Watt JWH, Soni BM, Oo T. Cutaneous adverse reaction to ciprofloxacin precipitated by ingestion of alcohol in a tetraplegic patient. *Spinal Cord* (1999) 37, 663–4. Correction. ibid. 807.

Alcohol + Antibacterials; Co-trimoxazole

A disulfiram-like reaction has been reported when two patients taking co-trimoxazole drank beer.

Clinical evidence, mechanism, importance and management

A 31-year-old man who had been taking prophylactic double-strength co-trimoxazole twice daily for 3 days experienced flushing, palpitations, dyspnoea, headache and nausea 10 to 20 minutes after drinking two 12-oz beers (about 340 mL each). Symptoms resolved gradually over 2 to 3 hours, but occurred again the next day when he drank 6 oz of beer. A similar experience occurred in another man taking double-strength co-trimoxazole after drinking three 12-oz beers. However, on the previous day, he had ingested 4 to 5 beers without a problem, even though he had taken co-trimoxazole.[1] The clinical and practical significance of these case reports is unknown as there do not appear to be any other reports of this interaction.

1. Heelon MW, White M. Disulfiram-cotrimoxazole reaction. *Pharmacotherapy* (1998) 18, 869–70.

Alcohol + Antibacterials; Erythromycin

Alcohol can cause a moderate reduction in the absorption of erythromycin ethylsuccinate. There is some evidence that intravenous erythromycin can raise blood-alcohol levels but the extent and the practical importance of this is unknown.

Clinical evidence, mechanism, importance and management

(a) Effects on alcohol

A study in 10 healthy subjects found that erythromycin base 500 mg three times daily did not alter the pharmacokinetics of oral alcohol 0.8 g/kg, and the subjects' perception of intoxication was unaltered.[1] In contrast, another study in 8 healthy subjects, primarily investigating the effects of intravenous erythromycin lactobionate 3 mg/kg on gastric emptying, found that when they were given a liquid meal of orange juice, alcohol 0.5 g/kg and lactulose 10 g immediately after a solid meal, the mean peak blood-alcohol levels were raised by about 40% and the AUC over the first hour was increased by 33%. After that the curve was virtually the same as that seen with a saline placebo. The authors suggest that the increased blood-alcohol levels are a result of erythromycin causing more rapid gastric emptying, so that the alcohol is exposed to metabolism by the gastric mucosa for a shorter time.[2]

What this means in terms of an increase in the effects of alcohol (e.g. on driving) is not known.

(b) Effects on erythromycin

When a single 500-mg dose of erythromycin ethylsuccinate was taken by 9 healthy subjects with two 150-mL alcoholic drinks (one immediately and the other 2.5 hours later) the erythromycin AUC was decreased by about 27% and its absorption was delayed. One subject had a 185% *increase* in absorption. The alcoholic drink was pisco sour, which contains lemon juice, sugar and pisco (a brandy-like liqueur). Blood alcohol levels achieved were about 50 mg%.[3]

The reason for the reduced absorption of erythromycin is not understood but it is suggested that the slight delay occurs because alcohol delays gastric emptying, so erythromycin reaches its absorption site in the duodenum a little later.[3] The extent to which this reduced absorption might affect the control of an infection is uncertain but it seems likely to be small.

1. Min DI, Noormohamed SE, Flanigan MJ. Effect of erythromycin on ethanol's pharmacokinetics and perception of intoxication. *Pharmacotherapy* (1995) 15, 164–9.
2. Edelbroek MAL, Horowitz M, Wishart JM, Akkermans LMA. Effects of erythromycin on gastric emptying, alcohol absorption and small intestinal transit in normal subjects. *J Nucl Med* (1993) 34, 582–8.
3. Morasso MI, Chávez J, Gai MN, Arancibia A. Influence of alcohol consumption on erythromycin ethylsuccinate kinetics. *Int J Clin Pharmacol Ther Toxicol* (1990) 28, 426–9.

Alcohol + Antibacterials; Metronidazole

A disulfiram-like reaction has occurred when some patients taking oral metronidazole have drunk alcohol. There is one report of its occurrence when metronidazole was applied as a vaginal insert, and another when metronidazole was given intravenously. Some clinical studies have not confirmed the interaction, and its existence is disputed in some reports. The interaction is alleged to occur with all other 5-nitroimidazoles (e.g. tinidazole).

Clinical evidence

A man who had been in a drunken stupor for 3 days was given two metronidazole tablets (a total of 500 mg) one hour apart by his wife in the belief that they might sober him up. Twenty minutes after the first tablet he was awake and complaining that he had been given disulfiram (which he had taken some months before). Immediately after the second tablet, he took another drink and developed a classic disulfiram-like reaction with flushing of the face and neck, nausea and epigastric discomfort.[1] Other individual cases have been reported,[2] including a reaction with a metronidazole vaginal insert.[3]

In a test of the value of metronidazole 250 mg twice daily as a possible drink-deterrent, all 10 alcoholic patients studied experienced some disulfiram-like reactions of varying intensity (facial flushing, headaches, sensation of heat, fall in blood pressure, vomiting) when given alcohol.[4] In another study in 60 alcoholic patients, given metronidazole 250 to 750 mg daily, most developed mild to moderate disulfiram-like reactions during an alcohol tolerance test.[5] A lower incidence of this reaction, between 2 and 24%, has been reported.[6-8]

Pharmaceutical preparations containing alcohol have also been implicated. A 2-year-old child became flushed and dyspnoeic when metronidazole was given with both *Stopayne* syrup and a phenobarbital syrup, both of which contained alcohol.[9] Another reaction has been seen in a patient receiving intravenous metronidazole and a trimethoprim-sulfamethoxazole (co-trimoxazole) preparation containing alcohol 10%.[10] A further patient who had just finished a 7-day course of metronidazole developed severe, prolonged nausea and vomiting postpartum: she had received a single 800-mg dose of prophylactic clindamycin intravenously before the birth and it was thought that the benzyl alcohol present in the clindamycin preparation could have caused the reaction. However, other factors such as intrathecal anaesthesia may have also contributed to the adverse effects.[11] For mention of other preparations containing alcohol, see 'Alcohol + Disulfiram', p.61.

An interaction has also been reported in association with metabolic acidosis in an intoxicated man 4 hours after he was given intravenous metronidazole as prophylaxis following injury.[12] A fatality occurred in a frail 31-year old woman, which was attributed to cardiac arrhythmia caused by acetaldehyde toxicity resulting from the alcohol/metronidazole interaction, linked to autonomic distress caused by a physical assault.[13] Alcohol is also said to taste unpleasant[1,4] or to be less pleasurable[8] while taking metronidazole. Some drug abusers apparently exploit the reaction for 'kicks'.[14]

In contrast, a study in 207 patients with inflammatory bowel disease assessed (using a phone survey) the presence of adverse reactions to alcohol in patients taking chronic metronidazole and/or mercaptopurine or neither drug; all of the patients consumed less than 4 alcoholic beverages per day. There was a trend towards more adverse effects in both the metronidazole and mercaptopurine study groups, but no statistically significant interaction between alcohol and metronidazole was found.[15] There are other reports, including two well-controlled studies, showing that metronidazole has no disulfiram-like effects.[16-18]

Mechanism

Not understood. In the disulfiram reaction, the accumulation of acetaldehyde appears to be responsible for most of the symptoms (see 'Alcohol + Disulfiram', p.61). Some workers have reported an increase in acetaldehyde levels due to the metronidazole/alcohol interaction,[13] but others have reported no effect[18] or a reduction in plasma acetaldehyde levels.[19] Furthermore, some studies with metronidazole indicate a lack of a disulfiram-like reaction,[16,17] and it has been suggested that if such a reaction does occur it may be by a mechanism other than the inhibition of hepatic acetaldehyde dehydrogenase.[18] It appears that metronidazole, like disulfiram, can inhibit other enzymes related to alcohol metabolism including xanthine oxidase and alcohol dehydrogenase.[20,21] Inhibition of xanthine oxidase may cause noradrenaline excess, and inhibition of alcohol dehydrogenase can lead to activation of microsomal enzyme oxidative pathways that generate ketones and lactate, which could produce acidosis.[12]

Importance and management

A reasonably well studied interaction, but it remains a controversial issue. The incidence is variously reported as between 0 and 100%, with more recent reports disputing its existence.[18,19] Nevertheless because of the uncertainty, all patients given metronidazole should be warned about what may happen if they drink alcohol. The manufacturer recommends avoidance of alcohol when metronidazole is taken, and for at least 48 hours after it has been stopped.[22] However, the authors of one report suggest a cautious trial of alcohol in patients that are starting and will be taking metronidazole on a chronic basis.[15]

The reaction, when it occurs, normally seems to be more unpleasant and possibly frightening than serious, and usually requires no treatment, although one report describes a serious reaction when intravenous metronidazole was given to an intoxicated man,[12] and one possible fatality has been reported.[13] The risk of a reaction with metronidazole used intravaginally seems to be small because the absorption is low (about 20% compared with about 100% orally), but evidently it can happen, even if only rarely.[3] Patients should be warned. It has been alleged that the disulfiram-like reaction with alcohol occurs with all of the related 5-nitroimidazoles,[23,24] but there do not appear to be any published reports of it occurring with **nimorazole**, **ornidazole**, **secnidazole** or **tinidazole**. The manufacturer of **tinidazole** notes that, as with related compounds, there is a possibility of a disulfiram-like reaction with alcoholic beverages, and recommends that alcohol should be avoided until 72 hours after discontinuing tinidazole.[25]

1. Taylor JAT. Metronidazole—a new agent for combined somatic and psychic therapy for alcoholism: a case study and preliminary report. *Bull Los Angel Neuro Soc* (1964) 29, 158–62.
2. Alexander I. 'Alcohol—Antabuse' syndrome in patients receiving metronidazole during gynaecological treatment. *Br J Clin Pract* (1985) 39, 292–3.
3. Plosker GL. Possible interaction between ethanol and vaginally administered metronidazole. *Clin Pharm* (1987) 6, 189 and 192–3.
4. Ban TA, Lehmann HE, Roy P. Rapport préliminaire sur l'effect thérapeutique du Flagyl dans l'alcoolisme. *Union Med Can* (1966) 95, 147–9.
5. Sansoy OM. Evaluation of metronidazole in the treatment of alcoholism. A comprehensive three-year study comprising 60 cases. *Rocky Mtn Med J* (1970) 67, 43–7.
6. de Mattos H. Relações entre o alcoolismo e aparelho digestivo. Experiência com metronidazol. *Hospital (Rio J)* (1968) 74, 1669–76.
7. Channabasavanna SM, Kaliaperumal VG, Mathew G, Itty A. Metronidazole in the treatment of alcoholism: a controlled trial. *Indian J Psychiatry* (1979) 21, 90–3.
8. Penick SB, Carrier RN, Sheldon JB. Metronidazole in the treatment of alcoholism. *Am J Psychiatry* (1969) 125, 1063–6.
9. Tunguy-Desmarais GP. Interaction between alcohol and metronidazole. *S Afr Med J* (1983) 63, 836.
10. Edwards DL, Fink PC, Van Dyke PO. Disulfiram-like reaction associated with intravenous trimethoprim–sulfamethoxazole and metronidazole. *Clin Pharm* (1986) 5, 999–1000.
11. Krulewitch CJ. An unexpected adverse drug effect. *J Midwifery Womens Health* (2003) 48, 67–8.
12. Harries DP, Teale KFH, Sunderland G. Metronidazole and alcohol: potential problems. *Scott Med J* (1990) 35, 179–180.
13. Cina SJ, Russell RA, Conradi SE. Sudden death due to metronidazole/ethanol interaction. *Am J Forensic Med Pathol* (1996) 17, 343–6.
14. Giannini AJ, DeFrance DT. Metronidazole and alcohol—potential for combinative abuse. *J Toxicol Clin Toxicol* (1983) 20, 509–15.
15. Ginzburg L, Present DH. Alcohol is well tolerated in IBD patients taking either metronidazole or 6-mercaptopurine. *Am J Gastroenterol* (2003) 98 (Suppl), S241.
16. Goodwin DW. Metronidazole in the treatment of alcoholism: a negative report. *Am J Psychiatry* (1967) 123, 1276–8.
17. Gelder MG, Edwards G. Metronidazole in the treatment of alcohol addiction: a controlled trial. *Br J Psychiatry* (1968) 114, 473–5.
18. Visapää J-P, Tillonen JS, Kaihovaara PS, Salaspuro MP. Lack of disulfiram-like reaction with metronidazole and ethanol. *Ann Pharmacother* (2002) 36, 971–4.
19. Williams CS, Woodcock KR. Do ethanol and metronidazole interact to produce a disulfiram-like reaction? *Ann Pharmacother* (2000) 34, 255–7.
20. Fried R, Fried LW. The effect of Flagyl on xanthine oxidase and alcohol dehydrogenase. *Biochem Pharmacol* (1966) 15, 1890–4.
21. Gupta NK, Woodley CL, Fried R. Effect of metronidazole on liver alcohol dehydrogenase. *Biochem Pharmacol* (1970) 19, 2805–8.
22. Flagyl Tablets (Metronidazole). Winthrop Pharmaceuticals UK Ltd. UK Summary of product characteristics, July 2005.
23. Ralph ED. Nitroimidazoles. In: Koren G, Prober CG, Gold R, eds. Antimicrobial therapy in infants and children. New York: Marcel Dekker; 1988 p. 729–45.
24. Andersson KE. Pharmacokinetics of nitroimidazoles. Spectrum of adverse reactions. *Scand J Infect Dis* (1981) 26 (Suppl), 60–7.
25. Fasigyn (Tinidazole). Pfizer Ltd. UK Summary of product characteristics, July 2005.

Alcohol + Antibacterials; Nitrofurantoin

There appears to be no good clinical evidence for an alleged interaction between alcohol and nitrofurantoin.

Clinical evidence, mechanism, importance and management

Despite claims in some books and reviews, an extensive literature search failed to find any experimental or clinical evidence for an alleged disulfiram-like reaction between alcohol and nitrofurantoin.[1] A study in healthy subjects failed to demonstrate any such interaction[2] and a survey of the reports in the manufacturer's database also failed to find good evidence for alcohol intolerance.[3] It is concluded that this 'interaction' is erroneous.[1]

1. Rowles B, Worthen DB. Clinical drug information: a case of misinformation. *N Engl J Med* (1982) 306, 113–4.
2. Miura K, Reckendorf HK. The nitrofurans. *Prog Med Chem* (1967) 5, 320–81.
3. D'Arcy PF. Nitrofurantoin. *Drug Intell Clin Pharm* (1985) 19, 540–7.

Alcohol + Antibacterials; Penicillins

No adverse interaction normally occurs between alcohol and phenoxymethylpenicillin or amoxicillin.

Clinical evidence, mechanism, importance and management

A long-standing and very common belief among members of the general public (presumably derived from advice given by doctors and pharmacists) is that alcohol should be strictly avoided while taking any antibacterial. It has been claimed that alcohol increases the degradation of penicillin in the gut and reduces the amount available for absorption.[1] However, one study showed that the pharmacokinetics of **phenoxymethylpenicillin (penicillin V)** were unaffected by alcoholic drinks,[2] and another study found that alcohol delayed the absorption of **amoxicillin** but did not affect the total amount absorbed.[3] An *in vitro* study did report that acetaldehyde, at concentrations occurring *in vivo* during alcohol metabolism, reacted with amine containing penicillins (**amoxicillin**, **ampicillin**, and **ciclacillin**), which theoretically could lead to decreased drug bioavailability and possibly adverse effects.[4] However, there seems to be no clinical evidence to support claims of an adverse interaction.

1. Kitto W. Antibiotics and ingestion of alcohol. *JAMA* (1965) 193, 411.
2. Lindberg RLP, Huupponen RK, Viljanen S and Pihlajamäki KK. Ethanol and the absorption of oral penicillin in man. *Int J Clin Pharmacol Ther Toxicol* (1987) 25, 536–8.
3. Morasso MI, Hip A, Márquez M, González C, Arancibia A. Amoxicillin kinetics and ethanol ingestion. *Int J Clin Pharmacol Ther Toxicol* (1988) 26, 428–31.
4. Nuñez-Vergara LJ, Yudelevich J, Squella JA, Speisky H. Drug-acetaldehyde interactions during ethanol metabolism *in vitro*. *Alcohol Alcohol* (1991) 26, 139–46.

Alcohol + Antibacterials; Tetracyclines

Doxycycline serum levels may fall below minimum therapeutic concentrations in alcoholic patients, but tetracycline is not affected. There is nothing to suggest that moderate amounts of alcohol have a clinically relevant effect on the serum levels of any tetracycline in non-alcoholic subjects.

Clinical evidence

(a) Alcoholic patients

A study into the effects of alcohol on **doxycycline** and **tetracycline** pharmacokinetics found that the half-life of **doxycycline** was 10.5 hours in 6 alcoholics (with normal liver function) compared with 14.7 hours in 6 healthy subjects. The serum **doxycycline** levels of 3 of the alcoholic patients fell below the generally accepted minimum inhibitory concentration at 24 hours. The half-life of **tetracycline** was the same in both groups. All of the subjects were given **doxycycline** 100 mg daily after a 200-mg loading dose, and **tetracycline** 500 mg twice daily after an initial 750-mg loading dose.[1]

(b) Non-alcoholic patients

Single 500-mg doses of **tetracycline** were given to 9 healthy subjects with water or alcohol 2.7 g/kg. The alcohol caused a 33% rise in the maximum serum levels of **tetracycline** from 9.3 to 12.4 micrograms/mL, and a 50%

rise in the AUC of **tetracycline**.[2] The clinical relevance of this rise is unknown.

Another study in healthy subjects found that cheap red wine, but not whisky (both 1 g/kg) delayed the absorption of **doxycycline**, probably because of the presence of acetic acid, which slows gastric emptying. However, the total absorption was not affected. The authors concluded that acute intake of alcoholic beverages has no clinically relevant effects on the pharmacokinetics of **doxycycline**.[3]

Mechanism

Heavy drinkers can metabolise some drugs much more quickly than non-drinkers due to the enzyme-inducing effects of alcohol.[4] The interaction with doxycycline would seem to be due to this effect, possibly allied with some reduction in absorption from the gut.

Importance and management

Information is limited, but the interaction between doxycycline and alcohol appears to be established and of clinical significance in alcoholics but not in non-alcoholic individuals. One possible solution to the problem of enzyme induction is to give alcoholic subjects double the dose of doxycycline.[5] Alternatively tetracycline may be a suitable non-interacting alternative. There is nothing to suggest that moderate or even occasional heavy drinking has a clinically relevant effect on any of the tetracyclines in non-alcoholic subjects.

1. Neuvonen PJ, Penttilä O, Roos M, Tirkkonen J. Effect of long-term alcohol consumption on the half-life of tetracycline and doxycycline in man. *Int J Clin Pharmacol Biopharm* (1976) 14, 303–7.
2. Seitz C, Garcia P, Arancibia A. Influence of ethanol ingestion on tetracycline kinetics. *Int J Clin Pharmacol Ther* (1995) 33, 462–4.
3. Mattila MJ, Laisi U, Linnoila M, Salonen R. Effect of alcoholic beverages on the pharmacokinetics of doxycycline in man. *Acta Pharmacol Toxicol (Copenh)* (1982) 50, 370–3.
4. Misra PS, Lefèvre A, Ishii H, Rubin E, Lieber CS. Increase of ethanol, meprobamate and pentobarbital metabolism after chronic ethanol administration in man and in rats. *Am J Med* (1971) 51, 346–51.
5. Neuvonen PJ, Penttilä O, Lehtovaara R and Aho K. Effect of antiepileptic drugs on the elimination of various tetracycline derivatives. *Eur J Clin Pharmacol* (1975) 9, 147–54.

Alcohol + Antiepileptics

Moderate social drinking does not appear to affect the serum levels of carbamazepine, ethosuximide or phenytoin. Some small changes are seen in the serum levels of phenobarbital and sodium valproate, but no changes in the control of epilepsy seem to occur. No pharmacokinetic interaction was detected between tiagabine and alcohol, and tiagabine did not alter the cognitive effect of alcohol. The adverse effects of both alcohol and antiepileptics, such as enhanced sedation, may be additive.

Clinical evidence, mechanism, importance and management

A study in 29 non-drinking epileptics found that when they drank 1 to 3 glasses of an alcoholic beverage (1 to 3 units) over a 2-hour period, twice a week for 16 weeks the serum levels of **carbamazepine**, **ethosuximide** and **phenytoin** were unchanged, when compared with those from a control group of 23 epileptics given drinks without alcohol. There was a marginal change in **phenobarbital** levels, and some increase in serum **valproate** levels. However, this effect is hard to interpret as **valproate** levels are known to fluctuate and are hard to reproduce. Other antiepileptics used were **clonazepam**, **primidone** and **sultiame**, but too few patients used these for a valid statistical analysis to be carried out. Maximum blood-alcohol levels ranged from 5 to 33 mg%. More important than any changes that occurred in serum antiepileptic levels, was the finding that this social drinking had no effect on the frequency of tonic-clonic convulsions, partial complex seizures, or on the epileptic activity as measured by EEGs.[1] Another study in healthy subjects excluded any pharmacodynamic or pharmacokinetic interaction between **tiagabine** and alcohol. In this study, **tiagabine** 4 mg three times daily did not alter the effect of a single dose of alcohol as assessed in a range of cognitive tests.[2]

For the effect of chronic heavy drinking on the pharmacokinetics of carbamazepine or phenytoin, see 'carbamazepine', (p.46) and 'phenytoin', (p.47).

There are very few studies, but there seem to be no reasons for epileptics to avoid alcohol in moderate social amounts (1 or 2 drinks per occasion; no more than 3 to 6 drinks per week).[3] However, patients who drink moderate to heavy amounts of alcohol (3 to 4 drinks or more) should be warned that they are at increased risk of seizures, with the greatest risk occurring 7 to 48 hours after the last drink.[3] The British Epilepsy Association comments that most people with epilepsy find they can have one or two units of alcohol, perhaps more, without increasing the chances of having a seizure, whereas other people find that even a small amount of alcohol triggers their seizures.[4] Patients who drink heavily may also get alcohol withdrawal seizures and binge drinking has been associated with seizures even in non-epileptic people. They also say that anyone taking antiepileptics is likely to be more sensitive to the effects of alcohol and can exaggerate the adverse effects of the antiepileptics.[4] Some antiepileptics such as **carbamazepine**, **clonazepam**, **'phenobarbital'**, (p.52), **primidone**, and **topiramate** have sedative effects, which may be additive with those of alcohol.

Individuals need to decide what level of alcohol intake is appropriate for them, and be aware that a change in medication, or an increase in dose of antiepileptic, may make them more susceptible to the effects of alcohol. Patients should also be made aware that drinking alcohol when taking antiepileptics may reduce their ability to perform certain skilled tasks, such as driving.

1. Höppener RJ, Kuyer A, van der Lugt PJM. Epilepsy and alcohol: the influence of social alcohol intake on seizures and treatment in epilepsy. *Epilepsia* (1983) 24, 459–71.
2. Kastberg H, Jansen JA, Cole G, Wesnes K. Tiagabine: absence of kinetic or dynamic interactions with ethanol. *Drug Metabol Drug Interact* (1998) 14, 259–73.
3. Gordon E, Devinsky O. Alcohol and marijuana: effects on epilepsy and use by patients with epilepsy. *Epilepsia* (2001) 42, 1266–72.
4. British Epilepsy Association. Epilepsy information: sports and leisure. Epilepsy, alcohol and recreational drugs. Epilepsy Action. Available at: http://www.epilepsy.org.uk/info/sportsandleisure/alcohol.html (accessed 24/8/07).

Alcohol + Antiepileptics; Carbamazepine

Moderate social drinking does not affect the serum levels of carbamazepine. Heavy drinking may possibly increase the metabolism of carbamazepine, and this may be further increased in alcoholics who abstain from drinking alcohol.

Clinical evidence, mechanism, importance and management

(a) Heavy drinking and alcohol withdrawal

A study in 7 alcoholics who consumed a mean dose of 750 mL of spirits (240 g of alcohol) daily found that the early (0 to 4 hours) bioavailability of a single 400-mg dose of carbamazepine was not affected by 9 days of controlled alcohol withdrawal. However, over the 4 to 12-hour period, carbamazepine levels were higher and those of its epoxy metabolite lower in alcoholics following alcohol exposure, when compared with abstinence. This effect was thought to be due to the acute inhibition of carbamazepine metabolism by alcohol and/or accelerated carbamazepine metabolism in the abstinence phase. The absorption rate of carbamazepine in alcoholics appeared to be slower compared with 8 healthy subjects, probably due to alcoholism-induced chronic gastrointestinal changes although this did not significantly affect the maximum serum levels of alcohol. However, adverse effects occurred in all of the healthy subjects but in none of the alcoholics, possibly indicating that long-term alcohol exposure may make the patient less sensitive to acute carbamazepine exposure.[1]

The long-term use of alcohol can cause induction of hepatic enzyme systems possibly resulting in increased metabolism and reduced plasma levels of carbamazepine. The risk of seizures may also increase on tapering or stopping alcohol because of an increase in metabolism and elimination caused by the relative lack of a competing substrate.[2]

(b) Moderate social drinking

Alcohol 25 g did not affect the bioavailability of carbamazepine in 8 healthy subjects.[1] A study in non-drinking epileptics (21 in the experimental alcohol group, 18 in the control group) found that the serum levels of carbamazepine were unchanged by moderate drinking (1 to 3 glasses of an alcoholic beverage, containing 9.85 g of alcohol, twice weekly), and there was no influence on tonic-clonic convulsions or partial complex seizures.[3]

For comment on moderate social drinking in epileptics and also the possible increased sedative effect of carbamazepine with alcohol, see 'Alcohol + Antiepileptics', above.

1. Sternebring B, Lidén A, Andersson K, Melander A. Carbamazepine kinetics and adverse effects during and after ethanol exposure in alcoholics and in healthy volunteers. *Eur J Clin Pharmacol* (1992) 43, 393–7.

2. Gordon E, Devinsky O. Alcohol and marijuana: effects on epilepsy and use by patients with epilepsy. *Epilepsia* (2001) 42, 1266–72.
3. Höppener RJ, Kuyer A, van der Lugt PJM. Epilepsy and alcohol: the influence of social alcohol intake on seizures and treatment in epilepsy. *Epilepsia* (1983) 24, 459–71.
10. Rubin E, Lieber CS. Hepatic microsomal enzymes in man and rat: induction and inhibition by ethanol. *Science* (1968) 162, 690–1.
11. Tanaka E. Toxicological interactions involving psychiatric drugs and alcohol: an update. *J Clin Pharm Ther* (2003) 28, 81–95.

Alcohol + Antiepileptics; Phenytoin

Acute alcohol intake may possibly increase serum phenytoin levels, but moderate social drinking appears to have little clinical effect. However, chronic heavy drinking reduces serum phenytoin levels so that above-average doses of phenytoin may be needed to maintain adequate levels.

Clinical evidence

(a) Acute alcohol ingestion

In a study designed to test the effects of acute alcohol intoxication in epileptics, 25 patients were given a 12 oz (about 340 mL) drink of alcohol 25%. Blood-alcohol levels ranged from 39 to 284 mg%. All patients had signs of alcohol intoxication without any effect on seizure frequency.[1] The metabolism of a single dose of phenytoin was not affected in one study in healthy subjects by the acute ingestion of alcohol.[2] However, the manufacturers say that acute alcoholic intake may increase phenytoin serum levels.[3,4]

(b) Heavy drinking

In a group of 15 drinkers (consuming a minimum of 200 g of ethanol daily for at least 3 months) phenytoin levels measured 24 hours after the last dose of phenytoin were approximately half those of 76 non-drinkers. The phenytoin half-life was reduced by 30%.[5]

Another study confirmed that alcoholics without liver disease have lower than usual plasma levels of phenytoin after taking standard doses while drinking.[6] Two reports describes a chronic alcoholic who was resistant to large doses of phenytoin,[7] and seizures, which developed in a man when an increase in his alcohol consumption appeared to cause a reduction in his serum phenytoin levels.[8]

(c) Moderate social drinking

A study in non-drinking epileptics (17 in the experimental group, 14 in the control group) found that the serum levels of phenytoin were unchanged by moderate drinking, and there was no influence on tonic-clonic convulsions or partial complex seizures. The experimental group drank 1 to 3 glasses of an alcoholic beverage (equivalent to a glass of beer containing 9.85 g of ethanol) over a 2-hour period, twice a week, for 16 weeks, and their maximum blood alcohol levels ranged from 5 to 33 mg%.[9]

Mechanism

Supported by *animal* data,[10] the evidence suggests that repeated exposure to large amounts of alcohol induces liver microsomal enzymes so that the rate of metabolism and clearance of phenytoin is increased. Conversely, acute alcohol intake may decrease hepatic metabolism.[11]

Importance and management

An established and clinically important interaction, although the documentation is limited. Heavy drinkers may need above-average doses of phenytoin to maintain adequate serum levels. However, be aware that patients with liver impairment usually need lower doses of phenytoin, so the picture may be more complicated. Moderate drinking appears to be safe in those taking phenytoin.[1,9] Consider also 'Alcohol + Antiepileptics', p.46.

1. Rodin EA, Frohman CE, Gottlieb JS. Effect of acute alcohol intoxication on epileptic patients. *Arch Neurol* (1961) 4, 115–18.
2. Schmidt D. Effect of ethanol intake on phenytoin metabolism in volunteers. *Experientia* (1975) 31, 1313–14.
3. Epanutin Capsules (Phenytoin sodium). Pfizer Ltd. UK Summary of product characteristics, February 2007.
4. Dilantin Kapseals (Phenytoin sodium). Pfizer Inc. US Prescribing information, September 2006.
5. Kater RMH, Roggin G, Tobon F, Zieve P, Iber FL. Increased rate of clearance of drugs from the circulation of alcoholics. *Am J Med Sci* (1969) 258, 35–9.
6. Sandor P, Sellers EM, Dumbrell M, Khouw V. Effect of short- and long-term alcohol use on phenytoin kinetics in chronic alcoholics. *Clin Pharmacol Ther* (1981) 30, 390–7.
7. Birkett DJ, Graham GG, Chinwah PM, Wade DN, Hickie JB. Multiple drug interactions with phenytoin. *Med J Aust* (1977) 2, 467–8.
8. Bellibas SE, Tuglular I. A case of phenytoin-alcohol interaction. *Therapie* (1995) 50, 487–8.
9. Höppener RJ, Kuyer A, van der Lugt PJM. Epilepsy and alcohol: the influence of social alcohol intake on seizures and treatment in epilepsy. *Epilepsia* (1983) 24, 459–71.

Alcohol + Antihistamines

Some antihistamines cause drowsiness, which can be increased by alcohol. The detrimental effects of alcohol on driving skills are considerably increased by the use of the older more sedative antihistamines and appear to be minimal or absent with the newer non-sedating antihistamines.

Clinical evidence

(a) Non-sedating antihistamines

A double-blind study found that **terfenadine** 60 to 240 mg alone did not affect psychomotor skills, nor did it affect the adverse effects of alcohol.[1] Another study had similar findings.[2] However, a later study found that **terfenadine** 240 mg slowed brake reaction times in the laboratory when given either alone or with alcohol.[3] **Acrivastine** 4 and 8 mg, given with and without alcohol, was found in a study to behave like **terfenadine** (which interacts minimally or not at all).[4] Other studies have shown that **astemizole** 10 to 30 mg daily,[5-7] **desloratadine**,[8] **ebastine** 20 mg,[9] **fexofenadine** 120 to 240 mg,[10,11] **levocabastine** 2 nasal puffs of 0.5 mg/mL,[12] **loratadine** 10 to 20 mg[2,13] and **mizolastine** 10 mg[14] do not interact with alcohol. **Cetirizine** 10 mg did not appear to interact with alcohol in two studies[14,15] but some slight additive effects were detected in other studies.[13,16] Similarly, a single oral dose of **rupatadine** 10 mg did not interact with alcohol, but a 20-mg dose given with alcohol produced more cognitive and psychomotor impairment than alcohol alone.[16]

(b) Sedating antihistamines

The effects of alcohol (blood levels about 50 mg%) and antihistamines, alone or together, on the performance of tests designed to assess mental and motor performance were examined in 16 subjects. **Clemizole** 40 mg or **tripelennamine** 50 mg alone did not significantly affect the performance under the stress of delayed auditory feedback, neither did they potentiate the effect of alcohol.[17] **Clemastine** in 3-mg doses had some additive detrimental effects with alcohol on co-ordination, whereas **clemastine** 1.5 mg and 1 mg did not.[18,19] A study in 5 subjects showed that the detrimental effects of 100 mL of whiskey on the performance of driving tests on a racing car simulator (blood alcohol estimated as less than 80 mg% were not increased by **cyclizine** 50 mg.[20] However 3 of the subjects experienced drowsiness after **cyclizine**, and other studies have shown that **cyclizine** alone causes drowsiness in the majority of subjects.[21] Significant impairment of psychomotor performance was seen in healthy subjects given **chlorphenamine** 12 mg with alcohol 0.5 g/kg.[5] A further study similarly found significant impairment in driving skills when chlorphenamine was given with alcohol, see (*c*) below. In 13 healthy subjects alcohol 0.75 g/kg given with **dexchlorpheniramine** 4 mg/70 kg significantly impaired the performance of a number of tests (standing steadiness, reaction time, manual dexterity, perception, etc.).[22] A study in 17 subjects found that **mebhydrolin** 0.71 mg/kg enhanced the alcohol-induced deficits in the performance of a number of tests on perceptual, cognitive and motor functions.[23] No interaction was detected in one study of the combined effects of **pheniramine aminosalicylate** 50 mg or **cyproheptadine hydrochloride** 4 mg and alcohol 0.95 mL/kg.[24] **Triprolidine** 10 mg alone can significantly affect driving performance,[2] and marked deterioration in driving skills has been demonstrated with 10 mL of *Actifed Syrup* (**triprolidine** with pseudoephedrine) alone and with a double whiskey.[25]

(c) Significantly-sedating antihistamines

Diphenhydramine in doses of 25 or 50 mg was shown to increase the detrimental effects of alcohol on the performance of choice reaction and co-ordination tests in subjects who had taken 0.5 g/kg of alcohol.[18] The interaction between **diphenhydramine** in doses of 50, 75 or 100 mg and alcohol in doses of 0.5 to 0.75 g/kg has been confirmed in other reports.[1,17,26-28] **Emedastine** in oral doses of 2 or 4 mg twice daily was found to be sedating and impair driving ability in 19 healthy subjects. The addition of alcohol increased this impairment.[29] A marked interaction can also occur with **hydroxyzine**[11,16] or **promethazine**.[30] A very marked deterioration in driving skills was clearly demonstrated in a test of car drivers given 20 mL of *Beechams Night Nurse* (**promethazine** with dextromethorphan), 10 mL of *Benylin* (**diphenhydramine** with dextromethorphan), or 30 mL of *Lemsip Night time flu medicine* (**chlorphenamine** with dextromethorphan). Very poor scores were seen when they were also given a double Scotch whiskey about 1.5 hours later.[25]

Mechanism

When an interaction occurs it appears to be due to the combined or additive central nervous depressant effects of both the alcohol and the antihistamine. The 'highly-sedating antihistamines' are highly lipophilic and readily cross the blood-brain barrier; consequently they have considerable sedative effects that may persist into the next day. The 'sedating antihistamines' do not cross the blood-brain barrier so readily, and are therefore less sedating. Most of the non-sedating antihistamines, such as fexofenadine, do not appear to cross the blood-brain barrier.[11] The authors of one study found that the sedating effects of cetirizine and emedastine were more marked in women than in men, and they noted that they had also previously seen this with acrivastine, clemastine and mizolastine.[29] The reason for this is not established although it has been suggested that a smaller volume of distribution in women may result in higher plasma antihistamine levels.

Importance and management

An adverse interaction between alcohol and the **highly-sedating antihistamines** (see 'Table 15.1', (p.582)) is well established and clinically important. Marked drowsiness can occur with these antihistamines taken alone, which makes driving or handling other potentially dangerous machinery much more hazardous. This can be further worsened by alcohol. Patients should be strongly warned. Remember that some of these antihistamines are present in non-prescription products licensed as antiemetics and sedatives, and as components of cough, cold and influenza remedies (e.g. some preparations of *Benylin*, *Lemsip* or *Night Nurse*). Emedastine may also cause marked sedation when used orally, but it is usually given as eye drops.

The situation with some of the **sedating antihistamines** is less clear cut, and tests with some of them failed to detect an interaction with normal doses and moderate amounts of alcohol; however, it has been clearly seen with *Actifed Syrup* (containing triprolidine). It would therefore be prudent to issue some cautionary warning, particularly if the patient is likely to drive.

The **non-sedating antihistamines** seem to cause little or no drowsiness in most patients and the risks if taken alone or with alcohol appear to be minimal or absent. However, the incidence of sedation varies with the non-sedating antihistamine (e.g. sedation appears to be lower with fexofenadine and loratadine than with acrivastine or cetirizine)[31] and with the individual (e.g. women may be more affected than men).[29] Therefore, patients should be advised to be alert to the possibility of drowsiness if they have not taken the drug before. Any drowsiness would be apparent after the first few doses. The patient information leaflets for acrivastine and cetirizine suggest avoidance of alcohol or excessive amounts of alcohol,[32-34] and caution is advised with **levocetirizine**.[35]

The possible interactions of alcohol with other antihistamines not cited here do not seem to have been formally studied, but increased drowsiness and increased driving risks would be expected with any that cause some sedation. Patients should be warned about drinking alcohol when taking sedative antihistamines. The risks with antihistamines given as eye drops or nasal spray (e.g. **azelastine, epinastine**) are probably minimal, but this needs confirmation.

1. Moser L, Hüther KJ, Koch-Weser J, Lundt PV. Effects of terfenadine and diphenhydramine alone or in combination with diazepam or alcohol on psychomotor performance and subjective feelings. *Eur J Clin Pharmacol* (1978) 14, 417–23.
2. O'Hanlon JF. Antihistamines and driving performance: The Netherlands. *J Respir Dis* (1988) (Suppl), S12–S17.
3. Bhatti JZ, Hindmarch I. The effects of terfenadine with and without alcohol on an aspect of car driving performance. *Clin Exp Allergy* (1989) 19, 609–11.
4. Cohen AF, Hamilton MJ, Peck AW. The effects of acrivastine (BW825C), diphenhydramine and terfenadine in combination with alcohol on human CNS performance. *Eur J Clin Pharmacol* (1987) 32, 279–88.
5. Hindmarch I, Bhatti JZ. Psychomotor effects of astemizole and chlorpheniramine, alone and in combination with alcohol. *Int Clin Psychopharmacol* (1987) 2, 117–19.
6. Bateman DN, Chapman PH, Rawlins MD. Lack of effect of astemizole on ethanol dynamics or kinetics. *Eur J Clin Pharmacol* (1983) 25, 567–8.
7. Moser L, Plum H, Bückmann M. Interaktionen eines neuen Antihistaminikums mit Diazepam und Alkohol. *Med Welt* (1984) 35, 296–9.
8. Rikken G, Scharf M, Danzig M, Staudinger H. Desloratadine and alcohol coadministration: no increase in impairment of performance over that induced by alcohol alone. Poster at EAACI (European Academy of Allergy and Clinical Immunology) Conference, Lisbon, Portugal. 2-4 July 2000.
9. Mattila MJ, Kuitunen T, Plétan Y. Lack of pharmacodynamic and pharmacokinetic interactions of the antihistamine ebastine with ethanol in healthy subjects. *Eur J Clin Pharmacol* (1992) 43, 179–84.
10. Vermeeren A, O'Hanlon JF. Fexofenadine's effects, alone and with alcohol, on actual driving and psychomotor performance. *J Allergy Clin Immunol* (1998) 101, 306–11.
11. Ridout F, Shamsi Z, Meadows R, Johnson S, Hindmarch I. A single-center, randomized, double-blind, placebo-controlled, crossover investigation of the effects of fexofenadine hydrochloride 180 mg alone and with alcohol, with hydroxyzine hydrochloride 50 mg as a positive internal control, on aspects of cognitive and psychomotor function related to driving a car. *Clin Ther* (2003) 25, 1518–38.
12. Nicholls A, Janssens M, James R. The effects of levocabastine and ethanol on psychomotor performance in healthy volunteers. *Allergy* (1993) 48 (Suppl 16), 34.
13. Ramaekers JG, Uiterwijk MMC, O'Hanlon JF. Effects of loratadine and cetirizine on actual driving and psychometric test performance, and EEG during driving. *Eur J Clin Pharmacol* (1992) 42, 363–9.
14. Patat A, Stubbs D, Dunmore C, Ulliac N, Sexton B, Zieleniuk I, Irving A, Jones W. Lack of interaction between two antihistamines, mizolastine and cetirizine, and ethanol in psychomotor and driving performance in healthy subjects. *Eur J Clin Pharmacol* (1995) 48, 143–50.
15. Doms M, Vanhulle G, Baelde Y, Coulie P, Dupont P, Rihoux J-P. Lack of potentiation by cetirizine of alcohol-induced psychomotor disturbances. *Eur J Clin Pharmacol* (1988) 34, 619–23.
16. Barbanoj MJ, García-Gea C, Antonijoan R, Izquierdo I, Donado E, Pérez I, Solans A, Jané F. Evaluation of the cognitive, psychomotor and pharmacokinetic profiles of rupatadine, hydroxyzine and cetirizine, in combination with alcohol, in healthy volunteers. *Hum Psychopharmacol* (2006) 21, 13–26.
17. Hughes FW, Forney RB. Comparative effect of three antihistaminics and ethanol on mental and motor performance. *Clin Pharmacol Ther* (1964) 5, 414–21.
18. Linnoila M. Effects of antihistamines, chlormezanone and alcohol on psychomotor skills related to driving. *Eur J Clin Pharmacol* (1973) 5, 247–54.
19. Franks HM, Hensley VR, Hensley WJ, Starmer GA, Teo RKC. The interaction between ethanol and antihistamines. 2. Clemastine. *Med J Aust* (1979) 1, 185–6.
20. Hughes DTD, Cramer F, Knight GJ. Use of a racing car simulator for medical research. The effects of marzine and alcohol on driving performance. *Med Sci Law* (1967) 7, 200–4.
21. Brand JJ, Colquhoun WP, Gould AH, Perry WLM. (–)-Hyoscine and cyclizine as motion sickness remedies. *Br J Pharmacol Chemother* (1967) 30, 463–9.
22. Franks HM, Hensley VR, Hensley WJ, Starmer GA, Teo RKC. The interaction between ethanol and antihistamines. 1: Dexchlorpheniramine. *Med J Aust* (1978) 1, 449–52.
23. Franks HM, Lawrie M, Schabinsky VV, Starmer GA, Teo RKC. Interaction between ethanol and antihistamines. 3. mebhydrolin. *Med J Aust* (1981) 2, 477–9.
24. Landauer AA, Milner G. Antihistamines, alone and together with alcohol, in relation to driving safety. *J Forensic Med* (1971) 18, 127–39.
25. Carter N. Cold cures drug alert. *Auto Express* (1992) November Issue 218, 15–16.
26. Baugh R, Calvert RT. The effect of diphenhydramine alone and in combination with ethanol on histamine skin response and mental performance. *Eur J Clin Pharmacol* (1977) 12, 201–4.
27. Burns M, Moskowitz H. Effects of diphenhydramine and alcohol on skills performance. *Eur J Clin Pharmacol* (1980) 17, 259–66.
28. Burns M. Alcohol and antihistamine in combination: effects on performance. *Alcohol Clin Exp Res* (1989) 13, 341.
29. Vermeeren A, Ramaekers JG, O'Hanlon JF. Effects of emedastine and cetirizine, alone and with alcohol, on actual driving of males and females. *J Psychopharmacol* (2002) 16, 57–64.
30. Hedges A, Hills M, Maclay WP, Newman-Taylor AJ, Turner P. Some central and peripheral effects of meclastine, a new antihistaminic drug, in man. *J Clin Pharmacol* (1971) 11, 112–19.
31. Mann RD, Pearce GL, Dunn N, Shakir S. Sedation with "non-sedating" antihistamines: four prescription-event monitoring studies in general practice. *BMJ* (2000) 320, 1184–6.
32. Semprex (Acrivastine). Glaxo Wellcome. UK Patient information leaflet, February 2002.
33. Cetirizine. Actavis UK Ltd. UK Patient information leaflet, January 2004.
34. Zirtek Allergy (Cetirizine). UCB Pharma Ltd. UK Patient information leaflet, December 2005.
35. Xyzal (Levocetirizine). UCB Pharma Ltd. Patient information leaflet, February 2006.

Alcohol + Antihypertensives

Chronic moderate to heavy drinking raises the blood pressure and reduces, to some extent, the effectiveness of antihypertensive drugs. A few patients may experience postural hypotension, dizziness and fainting shortly after having drank alcohol. Alpha blockers may enhance the hypotensive effect of alcohol in subjects susceptible to the alcohol flush syndrome.

Clinical evidence, mechanism, importance and management

(a) Hypertensive reaction

A study in 40 men with essential hypertension (taking **beta blockers, captopril, diuretics, methyldopa, prazosin** or **verapamil**) who were moderate to heavy drinkers, found that when they reduced their drinking over a 6-week period from an average of 450 mL of alcohol weekly (about 6 drinks daily) to 64 mL of alcohol weekly, their average blood pressure fell by 5/3 mmHg.[1] The reasons for this effect are uncertain.

The Atherosclerosis Risk in Communities (ARIC) study involving 8334 subjects who were free from hypertension at baseline and were assessed after 6 years, found that higher levels of consumption of alcoholic beverages (210 g or more of alcohol per week; approximately 3 drinks or more per day) were associated with a higher risk of hypertension. Low to moderate consumption of alcohol (up to 3 drinks/day) was associated with an increase in blood pressure in black, but not in white men.[2] A study in Japanese men found that the effect of alcohol intake on the risk of developing hypertension was dose-dependent, starting at low-to-moderate levels of alcohol (less than 23 g/day).[3]

These findings are consistent with those of other studies in hypertensive[4] and normotensive[5] subjects. It seems likely that this effect will occur with any antihypertensive. Patients with hypertension who are moderate to heavy drinkers should be encouraged to reduce their intake of alcohol. It may then become possible to reduce the dosage of the antihypertensive. It should be noted that epidemiological studies show that regular light to moderate alcohol consumption is associated with a *lower* risk of cardiovascular disease.[6]

(b) Hypotensive reaction

A few patients taking some antihypertensives feel dizzy or begin to 'black out' or faint if they stand up quickly or after exercise. This orthostatic and exertional hypotension may be exaggerated in some patients shortly after drinking alcohol, possibly because it can lower the cardiac output (noted in patients with various types of heart disease[7,8]). For other reports of postural hypotension with alcohol, see 'alpha blockers', (p.42), and 'calcium channel blockers', (p.57). Some manufacturers of antihypertensives e.g. **ACE inhibitors**[9,10] and **thiazide diuretics**[11] warn that acute alcohol intake may enhance the hypotensive effects, particularly at the start of treatment,[10] and this could apply to any antihypertensive. Patients just beginning antihypertensive treatment should be warned.

(c) CNS and other effects

For mention of the possibility of increased sedation with alcohol and clonidine or indoramin, see 'Clonidine and related drugs + CNS depressants', p.883 and 'Alcohol + Alpha blockers', p.42.

For the possible CNS effects of beta blockers and alcohol, see 'Alcohol + Beta blockers', p.55.

For mention of the disulfiram-like reaction when tolazoline is given with alcohol, see 'Alcohol + Tolazoline', p.79.

1. Puddey IB, Beilin LJ, Vandongen R. Regular alcohol use raises blood pressure in treated hypertensive subjects. A randomised controlled trial. *Lancet* (1987) i, 647–51.
2. Fuchs FD, Chambless LE, Whelton PK, Nieto FJ, Heiss G. Alcohol consumption and the incidence of hypertension. The Atherosclerosis Risk in Communities Study. *Hypertension* (2001) 37, 1242–50.
3. Nakanishi N, Yoshida H, Nakamura K, Suzuki K, Tatara K. Alcohol consumption and risk for hypertension in middle-aged Japanese men. *J Hypertens* (2001) 19, 851–5.
4. Potter JF, Beevers DG. Pressor effect of alcohol in hypertension. *Lancet* (1984) i, 119–22.
5. Puddey IB, Beilin LJ, Vandongen R, Rouse IL, Rogers P. Evidence for a direct effect of alcohol on blood pressure in normotensive men — a randomized controlled trial. *Hypertension* (1985) 7, 707–13.
6. Sesso HD. Alcohol and cardiovascular health: recent findings. *Am J Cardiovasc Drugs* (2001) 1, 167–72.
7. Gould L, Zahir M, DeMartino A, Gomprecht RF. Cardiac effects of a cocktail. *JAMA* (1971) 218, 1799–1802.
8. Conway N. Haemodynamic effects of ethyl alcohol in patients with coronary heart disease. *Br Heart J* (1968) 30, 638–44.
9. Innovace (Enalapril). Merck Sharp & Dohme Ltd. UK Summary of product characteristics, October 2005.
10. Capoten (Captopril). E. R. Squibb & Sons Ltd. UK Summary of product characteristics, June 2005.
11. Moduret (Amiloride/Hydrochlorothiazide). Bristol-Myers Squibb Pharmaceuticals Ltd. UK Summary of product characteristics, September 2006.

Alcohol + Antimuscarinics

Propantheline appears not to affect blood-alcohol levels, whereas atropine may cause a modest reduction. Marked impairment of attention can occur if alcohol is taken in the presence of atropine or glycopyrronium (glycopyrrolate), probably making driving more hazardous. No adverse interaction usually appears to occur with transdermal hyoscine and alcohol.

Clinical evidence, mechanism, importance and management

Oral **propantheline** (15 mg four times daily or 30 mg three times daily for 5 days, and 30 mg or 60 mg 2 hours before alcohol) did not affect blood-alcohol levels in 3 subjects.[1] A single 3-mg oral dose of **atropine** 2 hours before alcohol reduced the AUC of alcohol by a modest 20% in 3 subjects.[1] Another study in healthy subjects found that oral **atropine** 500 micrograms or **glycopyrronium** 1 mg given with alcohol 0.5 g/kg either did not affect or improved reaction times and co-ordination, there was a marked impairment of attention, which was large enough to make driving more hazardous.[2] Patients should be warned.

A double-blind crossover study in 12 healthy subjects found that a transdermal **hyoscine** preparation (*Scopoderm-TTS*) did not alter the effects of alcohol on the performance of several psychometric tests (Critical Flicker Fusion Frequency, Choice Reaction Tasks), nor was the clearance of alcohol or **hyoscine** changed. Blood-alcohol levels of up to 80 mg%, and 130 mg%, were studied.[3] Nevertheless, the manufacturer suggests caution in patients receiving drugs that act on the CNS, and advise that patients should not drink alcohol while using *Scopoderm-TTS*.[4] This is presumably because drowsiness and other CNS adverse effects have occasionally been reported with the transdermal preparation.[4,5] The manufacturers of travel tablets and injections containing **hyoscine hydrobromide** recommend avoidance of alcohol.[6,7] However, unlike **hyoscine** and **hyoscine hydrobromide**, the quaternary derivatives such as **hyoscine butylbromide** or **hyoscine methobromide** do not readily pass the blood-brain barrier,[8] and would be expected to be less likely to cause additive adverse effects with alcohol.

1. Gibbons DO, Lant AF. Effects of intravenous and oral propantheline and metoclopramide on ethanol absorption. *Clin Pharmacol Ther* (1975) 17, 578–84.
2. Linnoila M. Drug effects on psychomotor skills related to driving: interaction of atropine, glycopyrrhonium and alcohol. *Eur J Clin Pharmacol* (1973) 6, 107–12.
3. Gleiter CH, Antonin K-H, Schoenleber W, Bieck PR. Interaction of alcohol and transdermally administered scopolamine. *J Clin Pharmacol* (1988) 28, 1123–7.
4. Scopoderm TTS (Hyoscine). Novartis Consumer Health. UK Summary of product characteristics, March 2001.
5. Transderm Scop (Hyoscine). Novartis Consumer Health, Inc. US Prescribing information, March 2004.
6. Joy-Rides (Hyoscine hydrobromide). GlaxoSmithKline. UK Patient information leaflet, November 2002.
7. Hyoscine Injection (Hyoscine hydrobromide). UCB Pharma Ltd. UK Summary of product characteristics, June 2005.
8. Sweetman SC, ed. Martindale: The complete drug reference. 35th ed. London: Pharmaceutical Press; 2007 p. 1564.

Alcohol + Antimycobacterials

The hepatotoxicity of some antimycobacterials may possibly be increased by high alcohol consumption. Alcohol may increase the risk of epileptic episodes in patients taking cycloserine. A psychotoxic reaction in a patient taking ethionamide was attributed to concurrent heavy alcohol consumption. Isoniazid slightly increases the hazards of driving after drinking alcohol. Isoniazid-induced hepatitis may also possibly be increased by alcohol, and the effects of isoniazid are possibly reduced in some heavy drinkers. Acute alcohol intake does not appear to affect the pharmacokinetics of a single-dose of isoniazid.

Clinical evidence, mechanism, importance and management

(a) Combined antitubercular regimens

Hepatotoxicity can occur with several antituberculous drugs including **ethionamide, isoniazid, pyrazinamide** and **rifampicin** and high alcohol consumption/chronic alcoholism has been reported to increase the risk.[1,2] However, one study in patients with active tuberculosis taking **rifampicin** and **pyrazinamide**, found that of the 14 patients who developed hepatotoxicity, only 5 of these reported alcohol use (not quantified), and alcohol was not found to be associated with an increased risk of hepatotoxicity.[3] Similarly, another study found that alcohol consumption was not a risk factor for antimycobacterial-induced hepatotoxicity.[4]

(b) Cycloserine

A brief report describes an enhancement of the effects of alcohol in 2 patients taking cycloserine.[5] The clinical significance of this case report is unclear. However, the manufacturers of cycloserine state that it is 'incompatible' with alcohol because of an increased risk of epileptic episodes, and contraindicate its use in alcohol abuse.[6,7]

(c) Ethionamide

A psychotoxic reaction seen in a patient taking ethionamide was attributed to the concurrent heavy consumption of alcohol.[8] It is unclear whether this represents a clinically meaningful interaction but it appears to be the only case on record. However, the manufacturers advise avoidance of excessive alcohol ingestion.[9]

(d) Isoniazid

The effects of isoniazid 750 mg with alcohol 0.5 g/kg were examined in 100 subjects given various psychomotor tests, and in a further 50 drivers using a driving simulator. No major interaction was seen in the psychomotor tests, but the number of drivers who drove off the road on the simulator was increased.[10,11] There would therefore appear to be some extra risks for patients taking isoniazid who drink and drive, but the effect does not appear to be large. Patients should nevertheless be warned.

The incidence of severe progressive liver damage due to isoniazid is said to be higher in those who drink alcohol regularly.[12-14] The clinical effects of isoniazid are also said to be reduced by heavy drinking in some patients;[12] however, acute alcohol intake in 16 healthy subjects did not have any effect on the pharmacokinetics of a single 200-mg dose of isoniazid.[15] Alcohol is metabolised to acetaldehyde in the liver and isoniazid has been found to interact with acetaldehyde *in vitro*. The clinical significance of this is unknown, but if this binding occurs *in vivo,* it could lead to decreased bioavailability of isoniazid and possibly the acetaldehyde-modified drug formed could mediate some adverse effects.[16] The manufacturer advises care in giving isoniazid to patients with chronic alcoholism.[17]

1. Wada M. The adverse reactions of anti-tuberculosis drugs and its management. *Nippon Rinsho* (1998) 56, 3091–5.
2. Fernández-Villar A, Sopeña B, Fernández-Villar J, Vázquez-Gallardo R, Ulloa F, Leiro V, Mosteiro M, Piñeiro L. The influence of risk factors on the severity of anti-tuberculosis drug-induced hepatotoxicity. *Int J Tuberc Lung Dis* (2004) 8, 1499–1505.
3. Lee AM, Mennone JZ, Jones RC, Paul WS. Risk factors for hepatotoxicity associated with rifampin and pyrazinamide for the treatment of latent tuberculosis infection: experience from three public health tuberculosis clinics. *Int J Tuberc Lung Dis* (2002) 6, 995–1000.
4. Døssing M, Wilcke JTR, Askgaard DS, Nybo B. Liver injury during antituberculosis treatment: an 11-year study. *Tubercle Lung Dis* (1996) 77, 335–40.
5. Glaß F, Mallach HJ, Simsch A. Beobachtungen und Untersuchungen über die gemeinsame Wirkung von Alkohol und D-Cycloserin. *Arzneimittelforschung* (1965) 15, 684–8.
6. Cycloserine. King Pharmaceuticals Ltd. UK Summary of product characteristics, March 2007.
7. Seromycin (Cycloserine). Eli Lilly and Company. US Prescribing information, April 2005.
8. Lansdown FS, Beran M, Litwak T. Psychotoxic reaction during ethionamide therapy. *Am Rev Respir Dis* (1967) 95, 1053–5.
9. Trecator (Ethionamide). Wyeth Pharmaceuticals Inc. US Prescribing information, September 2006.
10. Linnoila M, Mattila MJ. Effects of isoniazid on psychomotor skills related to driving. *J Clin Pharmacol* (1973) 13, 343–50.
11. Linnoila M, Mattila MJ. Interaction of alcohol and drugs on psychomotor skills as demonstrated by a driving simulator. *Br J Pharmacol* (1973) 47, 671P–672P.
12. Anon. Interactions of drugs with alcohol. *Med Lett Drugs Ther* (1981) 23, 33–4.
13. Kopanoff DE, Snider DE, Caras GJ. Isoniazid-related hepatitis. *Am Rev Respir Dis* (1978) 117, 991–1001.
14. Wada M. The adverse reactions of anti-tuberculosis drugs and its management. *Nippon Rinsho* (1998) 56, 3091–5.
15. Dattani RG, Harry F, Hutchings AD, Routledge PA. The effects of acute ethanol intake on isoniazid pharmacokinetics. *Eur J Clin Pharmacol* (2004) 60, 679–82.
16. Nuñez-Vergara LJ, Yudelevich J, Squella JA, Speisky H. Drug-acetaldehyde interactions during ethanol metabolism *in vitro*. *Alcohol Alcohol* (1991) 26, 139–46.
17. Isoniazid. Celltech Manufacturing Services Ltd. UK Summary of product characteristics, November 2001.

Alcohol + Antipsychotics

The detrimental effects of alcohol on the skills related to driving are made worse by chlorpromazine, and, to a lesser extent, by flupentixol, sulpiride and thioridazine. Small or single-dose studies with haloperidol or tiapride suggest that any interaction would seem to be mild; nevertheless, all antipsychotic drugs which cause drowsiness have the potential to enhance the effects of alcohol. There is evidence that drinking can precipitate the emergence of extrapyramidal adverse effects in patients taking antipsychotics.

Clinical evidence

(a) Effect on driving and other skills

Twenty-one subjects showed a marked deterioration in the performance of a number of skills related to driving when given **chlorpromazine** 200 mg daily and alcohol (blood levels 42 mg%). Many complained of feeling sleepy, lethargic, dull, groggy, and poorly coordinated; and most considered themselves more unsafe to drive than with alcohol alone.[1] A later study confirmed these findings with **chlorpromazine** 1 mg/kg and blood-alcohol levels of 80 mg%.[2] Increased sedation was clearly seen in another study with alcohol and **chlorpromazine**,[3] and clear impairment of psychomotor skills related to driving have also been found.[4]

Single 500-microgram doses of **haloperidol** or **flupentixol** strongly impaired attention, but did not significantly interact with alcohol in one study.[5] However, a double-blind study in subjects given **flupentixol** 500 micrograms three times a day for 2 weeks found that, when combined with alcohol 0.5 g/kg, their performance of a number of tests (choice reaction, coordination, attention) was impaired to such an extent that driving or handling other potentially dangerous machinery could be hazardous.[6]

Sulpiride 50 mg three times daily for 2 weeks caused a mild decrease in psychomotor skills with alcohol in healthy subjects, but not as much as that seen with **chlorpromazine** and alcohol.[4,7] **Thioridazine** 25 mg caused some additive effects with alcohol, with a moderately deleterious effect on attention.[5] Another study found that **thioridazine** and alcohol affected skills related to driving, but not as much as the effects seen with **chlorpromazine**.[2] A further study found no difference between the effects of **thioridazine** and a placebo with alcohol.[4,8]

A study in 9 alcoholics given **tiapride** 400 to 600 mg daily showed that wakefulness was not impaired when alcohol 0.5 g/kg was given, and in fact appeared to be improved, but the effect on driving skills was not studied.[9]

(b) Precipitation of extrapyramidal adverse effects

A report describes 7 patients who developed acute extrapyramidal adverse effects (akathisia, dystonia) while taking **trifluoperazine**, **fluphenazine**, **perphenazine**, or **chlorpromazine** and drinking alcohol.[10] The author stated that these were examples of numerous such alcohol-induced toxicity reactions observed by him over an 18-year period involving phenothiazines and butyrophenones. Elsewhere he describes the emergence of drug-induced parkinsonism in a woman taking **perphenazine** and amitriptyline when she began to drink alcohol.[11] Eighteen cases of **haloperidol**-induced extrapyramidal reactions among young drug abusers, in most instances associated with the ingestion of alcohol, have also been described.[12] Similarly, a study involving 41 patients with schizophrenia found that those with a substance use disorder (alcohol or cannabis ± cocaine) displayed more extrapyramidal symptoms compared with non-abusing patients.[13]

(c) Toxicity

A study involving 332 fatal poisonings in Finland found that alcohol was present in 65% of cases involving **promazine**, and when alcohol was present, relatively small overdoses of **promazine** could result in fatal poisoning.[14] It appears that **promazine** and possibly **levomepromazine** may be more toxic when combined with alcohol.[15]

(d) Pharmacokinetic studies

A study in 12 patients receiving **chlorpromazine** 600 mg to 1.2 g daily long-term, found that **chlorpromazine** had no apparent effect on alcohol metabolism. However, about half of the patients had a statistically significant decrease (up to 33%) in urinary excretion of **chlorpromazine** and its metabolites during the 24-hour period following the consumption of 50 to 75 mL of alcohol.[16]

A study in 7 schizophrenics found that when they were given 40 g of alcohol to drink at about the same time as their regular injection of **fluphenazine decanoate** (25 to 125 mg every 2 weeks), their serum **fluphenazine** levels were reduced by 30% at 2 hours and by 16% at 12 hours.[17]

Mechanism

Uncertain. Additive CNS depressant effects are one explanation of this interaction. One suggestion to account for the emergence of the drug adverse effects is that alcohol lowers the threshold of resistance to the neurotoxicity of these drugs. Also alcohol may possibly impair the activity of tyrosine hydroxylase so that the dopamine/acetylcholine balance within the corpus striatum is upset.[11] In addition, chlorpromazine has been found to inhibit alcohol dehydrogenase, which may facilitate the formation of biogenic amines that have been implicated in extrapyramidal adverse effects.[18]

Pharmacokinetic interactions between acute and chronic alcohol ingestion, and single or multiple doses of antipsychotic drug are complex; acute alcohol intake can decrease metabolic clearance, whereas chronic intake can increase clearance.[19] Alcohol may also affect the peripheral circulation and membrane permeability, which might affect absorption from an injection site.[17]

Importance and management

The documentation is limited. The manufacturers of flupentixol[20] and haloperidol[21] warn that, in common with other antipsychotic drugs, the effects of alcohol maybe enhanced. Warn patients that if they drink alcohol while taking chlorpromazine, and to a lesser extent flupenthixol, sulpiride or thioridazine (probably other related drugs as well), they may become very drowsy, and should not drive or handle other potentially dangerous machinery. Some risk is possible with any antipsychotic that causes drowsiness, including those used as antiemetics, such as **prochlorperazine**.

The authors of the reports describing the emergence of serious adverse effects to antipsychotics in those who drink alcohol, consider that patients should routinely be advised to abstain from alcohol during antipsychotic treatment.

It has been suggested that a less dangerous alternative to promazine, and possibly levomepromazine, should be chosen when indications of alcohol abuse or suicide risk are present.[15]

The clinical importance of the pharmacokinetic studies is uncertain.

1. Zirkle GA, King PD, McAtee OB. Van Dyke R. Effects of chlorpromazine and alcohol on coordination and judgement. *JAMA* (1959) 171, 1496–9.
2. Milner G, Landauer AA. Alcohol, thioridazine and chlorpromazine effects on skills related to driving behaviour. *Br J Psychiatry* (1971) 118, 351–2.
3. Sutherland VC, Burbridge TN, Adams JE, Simon A. Cerebral metabolism in problem drinkers under the influence of alcohol and chlorpromazine hydrochloride. *J Appl Physiol* (1960) 15, 189–96.
4. Seppälä T, Saario I, Mattila MJ. Two weeks' treatment with chlorpromazine, thioridazine, sulpiride, or bromazepam: actions and interactions with alcohol on psychomotor skills related to driving. *Mod Probl Pharmacopsychiatry* (1976) 11, 85–90.
5. Linnoila M. Effects of diazepam, chlordiazepoxide, thioridazine, haloperidole, flupenthixole and alcohol on psychomotor skills related to driving. *Ann Med Exp Biol Fenn* (1973) 51, 125–32.
6. Linnoila M, Saario I, Olkoniemi J, Liljequist R, Himberg JJ, Mäki M. Effect of two weeks' treatment with chlordiazepoxide or flupenthixole, alone or in combination with alcohol, on psychomotor skills related to driving. *Arzneimittelforschung* (1975) 25, 1088–92.
7. Seppälä T. Effect of chlorpromazine or sulpiride and alcohol on psychomotor skills related to driving. *Arch Int Pharmacodyn Ther* (1976) 223, 311–23.
8. Saario I. Psychomotor skills during subacute treatment with thioridazine and bromazepam, and their combined effects with alcohol. *Ann Clin Res* (1976) 8, 117–23.
9. Vandel B, Bonin B, Vandel S, Blum D, Rey E, Volmat R. Étude de l'interaction entre le tiapride et l'alcool chez l'homme. *Sem Hop Paris* (1984) 60, 175–7.
10. Lutz EG. Neuroleptic-induced akathisia and dystonia triggered by alcohol. *JAMA* (1976) 236, 2422–3.
11. Lutz EG. Neuroleptic-induced parkinsonism facilitated by alcohol. *J Med Soc New Jers* (1978) 75, 473–4.
12. Kenyon-David D. Haloperidol intoxication. *N Z Med J* (1981) 93, 165.
13. Potvin S, Pampoulova T, Mancini-Marië A, Lipp O, Bouchard R-H, Stip E. Increased extrapyramidal symptoms in patients with schizophrenia and a comorbid substance use disorder. *J Neurol Neurosurg Psychiatry* (2006) 77, 796–8.
14. Koski A, Vuori E, Ojanperä I. Relation of postmortem blood alcohol and drug concentrations in fatal poisonings involving amitriptyline, propoxyphene and promazine. *Hum Exp Toxicol* (2005) 24, 389–96.
15. Koski A, Ojanperä I, Vuori E. Interaction of alcohol and drugs in fatal poisonings. *Hum Exp Toxicol* (2003) 22, 281–7.
16. Forrest F-M, Forrest I-S, Finkle B-S. Alcohol-chlorpromazine interaction in psychiatric patients. *Agressologie* (1972) 13, 67–74.
17. Soni SD, Bamrah JS, Krska J. Effects of alcohol on serum fluphenazine levels in stable chronic schizophrenics. *Hum Psychopharmacol* (1991) 6, 301–6.
18. Messiha FS. Cerebral and peripheral neurotoxicity of chlorpromazine and ethanol interaction: implications for alcohol and aldehyde dehydrogenase. *Neurotoxicology* (1991) 12, 559–70.
19. Tanaka E. Toxicological interactions involving psychiatric drugs and alcohol: an update. *J Clin Pharm Ther* (2003) 28, 81–95.
20. Depixol (Flupentixol). Lundbeck Ltd. UK Summary of product characteristics, September 2004.
21. Haldol (Haloperidol). Janssen-Cilag Ltd. UK Summary of product characteristics, June 2007.

Alcohol + Antiretrovirals

Heavy alcohol intake may affect the virological response to HAART. Theoretically, alcohol consumption may induce liver enzymes, which interfere with the metabolism of some antivirals such as the protease inhibitors. Alcohol reduces the metabolism of abacavir but this does not appear to be clinically significant.

Clinical evidence, mechanism, importance and management

(a) Alcohol and HAART regimens

A study of 94 HIV-positive patients receiving HAART, which included 2 '**nucleoside analogues**' plus either **indinavir**, **ritonavir**, **saquinavir**, **nelfinavir**, or **ritonavir/saquinavir**, found that the amount of alcohol consumed did not affect the antiviral response. However, the proportion of complete responders was slightly lower (57%) in heavy drinkers (more than 60 g of alcohol per day) compared with 68% in both non-drinkers and moderate drinkers (less than 60 g of alcohol per day), although this was not a significant finding. There was also a high prevalence of infection with hepatitis C virus, and liver decompensation occurred in 2 patients (both heavy drinkers).[1] Alcohol may affect thymus-induced immune repletion in HIV-positive patients and it has been reported that heavy alcohol users taking antiretrovirals are twice as likely not to achieve a positive virological response, compared with those who do not use alcohol.[2]

Alcohol consumption can induce the cytochrome P450 isoenzyme CYP3A4 and there is concern that HAART may not be as effective in some individuals who consume alcohol.[3] CYP3A4 is involved in the metabolism of the protease inhibitors **amprenavir**, **fosamprenavir**, **indinavir**, **lopinavir**, **nelfinavir**, **ritonavir**, and **saquinavir** and the NNRTIs **delavirdine**, **efavirenz**, and **nevirapine**, and therefore CYP3A4 induction may result in enhanced drug metabolism and reduced therapeutic levels.[4] Avoidance of alcohol has been suggested for HIV-positive patients receiving protease inhibitor therapy,[3,4] but at present there does not seem to be any clinical data to support this. Nevertheless, a reduction in alcohol consumption would seem sensible. More studies are needed. Note that some preparations of **ritonavir** contain alcohol, see 'Alcohol + Disulfiram', p.61.

(b) Effect of alcohol on abacavir

A study in 24 HIV-positive patients found that alcohol 0.7 g/kg increased the AUC of a single 600-mg dose of abacavir by 41%. The half-life of abacavir was increased by 26%, from 1.42 to 1.79 hours. The pharmacokinetics of alcohol were not affected by abacavir.[5] Alcohol may inhibit the formation of abacavir carboxylate resulting in a trend towards increased abacavir glucuronide formation and reduced abacavir metabolism. The increase in exposure to abacavir was not considered to be clinically significant, since it is within levels seen in other studies using higher doses, which demonstrated no additional safety concerns at doses of up to three times the recommended daily dose of abacavir.[5] No special precautions therefore appear to be necessary.

1. Fabris P, Tositti G, Manfrin V, Giordani MT, Vaglia A, Cattelan AM, Carlotto A. Does alcohol intake affect highly active antiretroviral therapy (HAART) response in HIV-positive patients? *J Acquir Immune Defic Syndr* (2000) 25, 92–3.
2. Miguez MJ, Burbano X, Morales G, Shor-Posner G. Alcohol use and HIV infection in the HAART era. *Am Clin Lab* (2001) 20, 20–3.
3. Flexner CW, Cargill VA, Sinclair J, Kresina TF, Cheever L. Alcohol use can result in enhanced drug metabolism in HIV pharmacotherapy. *AIDS Patient Care STDS* (2001) 15, 57–8.
4. Kresina TF, Flexner CW, Sinclair J, Correia MA, Stapleton JT, Adeniyi-Jones S, Cargill V, Cheever LW. Alcohol use and HIV pharmacotherapy. *AIDS Res Hum Retroviruses* (2002) 18, 757–70.
5. McDowell JA, Chittick GE, Stevens CP, Edwards KD, Stein DS. Pharmacokinetic interaction of abacavir (1592U89) and ethanol in human immunodeficiency virus-infected adults. *Antimicrob Agents Chemother* (2000) 44, 1686–90.

Alcohol + Aspirin

A small increase in the gastrointestinal blood loss caused by aspirin occurs in patients if they drink alcohol, but any increased damage to the lining of the stomach is small and appears usually to be of minimal importance in most healthy individuals. However, heavy drinkers who regularly take aspirin should be warned of the increased risk of gastric bleeding. Some limited information suggests that aspirin can raise or lower blood alcohol levels.

Clinical evidence

(a) Effect on blood loss

The mean daily blood loss from the gut of 13 healthy men was 0.4 mL while taking no medication, 3.2 mL while taking 2.1 g of soluble unbuffered aspirin (*Disprin*) and 5.3 mL while taking aspirin with 180 mL of Australian whiskey (alcohol 31.8%). In this study, alcohol alone did not cause gastrointestinal bleeding.[1] Similar results were reported in another study in healthy subjects.[2]

An epidemiological study of patients admitted to hospital with gastrointestinal haemorrhage showed a statistical association between bleeding and the ingestion of aspirin alone, and the combination with alcohol produced a significant synergistic effect.[3] A large case-controlled study found similar results: the overall relative risk of bleeding with regular use of aspirin at doses greater than 325 mg was 7 among drinkers and 5.1 among people who never drank alcohol. For those who drank less than 1 to 20 drinks a week there was no evidence of a trend of increasing or decreasing relative risk as levels of alcohol consumption increased, but among those who consumed 21 or more drinks a week there was a large association with upper gastrointestinal bleeding (crude estimated risk 27). For regular aspirin use at doses of 325 mg or less, the overall relative risk among all current drinkers was 2.8 and among people who never drank alcohol was 2.2.[4]

Endoscopic examination revealed that aspirin and alcohol have additive damaging effects on the gastric mucosa (not on the duodenum), but the extent is small.[5] However, a further case-control study found that large amounts of red wine (roughly over 500 mL of wine daily) increased the risk of upper gastrointestinal bleeding associated with low-dose aspirin, and small amounts of red wine (roughly less than 200 mL of wine daily) reduced this risk.[6] Another study using gastric mucosal potential difference as a measure of mucosal damage found that aspirin with alcohol caused additive damage to the mucosa.[7] In a review of the evidence, it was considered that while more study was needed, data available are highly suggestive that the gastrointestinal toxicity of alcohol and aspirin are combined in individuals who are heavy daily drinkers and heavy aspirin users.[8] Consider also 'Alcohol + NSAIDs', p.71.

No increased gastrointestinal bleeding occurred in 22 healthy subjects given three double gins or whiskies (equivalent to 142 mL of alcohol 40%) and 728 mg of buffered sodium acetylsalicylate (*Alka-Seltzer*).[9]

(b) Effect on blood alcohol levels

Five healthy subjects were given a standard breakfast with and without aspirin 1 g followed by alcohol 0.3 g/kg an hour later. The aspirin increased the peak blood alcohol levels by 39% and the AUC by 26%.[10] Similarly, in another study, 28 healthy subjects were given a midday meal (two sandwiches and a cup of tea or coffee), followed 90 minutes later by 600 mg of aspirin or a placebo, and then 30 minutes later by two standard drinks (35.5 mL of vodka 37.5% (21.6 g of alcohol) plus 60 mL of orange juice), which were drunk within a 15-minute period. The blood alcohol levels of the men were raised by 31% after one hour (from 24.29 to 31.85 mg%) and by 18% (from 20.82 to 24.57 mg%) after two hours. The blood alcohol levels of the women were raised by 32% (from 37.39 to 49.23 mg%) after one hour and by 21% (from 37.56 to 45.54 mg%) after two hours.[11]

However, a later study (effectively a repeat of a study[10] above) in 12 healthy subjects failed to find any effect on blood alcohol levels, but peak aspirin levels were reduced 25%.[12] A crossover study in 10 healthy male subjects found that after taking aspirin 75 mg daily for one week, their mean blood alcohol AUC following a 0.3 g/kg-dose was not significantly altered. However, individual *maximum* blood levels varied; one subject showed a rise, two were unchanged, and five were lowered: overall the reduction was 23%.[13]

Mechanism

(a) Effect on blood loss

Aspirin and alcohol can damage the mucosal lining of the stomach, one measure of the injury being a fall in the gastric potential difference. Once the protective mucosal barrier is breached, desquamation of the cells occurs and damage to the capillaries follows. Aspirin causes a marked prolongation in bleeding times, and this can be increased by alcohol.[14] The total picture is complex.

(b) Effect on blood alcohol levels

The increased blood alcohol levels in the presence of food and aspirin may possibly occur because the aspirin reduces the enzymic oxidation of the alcohol by alcohol dehydrogenase in the gastric mucosa, so that more remains available for absorption.[10] Any decreases with low-dose aspirin may possibly be due to delayed gastric emptying.[13]

Importance and management

The combined effect of aspirin and alcohol on the stomach wall is established. Aspirin 3 g daily for a period of 3 to 5 days induces an average blood loss of about 5 mL or so. Some increased loss undoubtedly occurs with alcohol, but it seems to be quite small and unlikely to be of much importance in most healthy individuals using moderate doses. In one study it was found that alcohol was a mild damaging agent or a mild potentiating agent for other damaging drugs.[5] On the other hand it should be remembered that chronic and/or gross overuse of salicylates and alcohol may result in gastric ulceration. People who consume at least 3 or more alcoholic drinks daily and who regularly take more than 325 mg of aspirin have been shown to have a high risk of bleeding.[15] The FDA in the US has ruled that non-prescription pain relievers and fever reducers, containing aspirin or salicylates, must carry a warning label advising people who consume 3 or more alcoholic drinks every day to consult their doctor before using these drugs, and that stomach bleeding may occur with these drugs.[16] However, the Australian Medicines Evaluation Committee has decided against such action as, for most people with mild to moderate alcohol intake, there is little risk especially if the aspirin is taken only as needed.[15]

Information about the increase in blood alcohol levels caused by aspirin after food is very limited and contradictory, and of uncertain practical importance. However, no practically relevant interaction has been seen with other drugs (such as the 'H_2-receptor antagonists', (p.64)), which have been extensively studied, and which appear to interact by the same mechanism. The pattern for these drugs is that the increases in blood alcohol levels are appreciable with small doses of alcohol, but usually they become proportionately too small to matter with larger doses of alcohol (i.e. those that give blood and breath levels at or around the legal driving limit in the UK).

1. Goulston K, Cooke AR. Alcohol, aspirin, and gastrointestinal bleeding. *BMJ* (1968) 4, 664–5.
2. DeSchepper PJ, Tjandramaga TB, De Roo M, Verhaest L, Daurio C, Steelman SL, Tempero KF. Gastrointestinal blood loss after diflunisal and after aspirin: effect of ethanol. *Clin Pharmacol Ther* (1978) 23, 669–76.
3. Needham CD, Kyle J, Jones PF, Johnston SJ, Kerridge DF. Aspirin and alcohol in gastrointestinal haemorrhage. *Gut* (1971) 12, 819–21.
4. Kaufman DW, Kelly JP, Wiholm B-E, Laszlo A, Sheehan JE, Koff RS, Shapiro S. The risk of acute major upper gastrointestinal bleeding among users of aspirin and ibuprofen at various levels of alcohol consumption. *Am J Gastroenterol* (1999) 94, 3189–96.
5. Lanza FL, Royer GL, Nelson RS, Rack MF, Seckman CC. Ethanol, aspirin, ibuprofen, and the gastroduodenal mucosa: an endoscopic assessment. *Am J Gastroenterol* (1985) 80, 767–9.
6. Lanas A, Serrano P, Bajador E, Fuentes J, Guardia J, Sainz R. Effect of red wine and low dose aspirin on the risk or upper gastrointestinal bleeding. A case-control study. *Gastroenterology* (2000) 118 (Suppl. 2) A251.
7. Murray HS, Strottman MP, Cooke AR. Effect of several drugs on gastric potential difference in man. *BMJ* (1974) 1, 19–21.
8. Pfau PR, Lichtenstein GR. NSAIDs and alcohol: never the twain shall mix? *Am J Gastroenterol* (1999) 94, 3098–3101.
9. Bouchier IAD, Williams HS. Determination of faecal blood-loss after combined alcohol and sodium acetylsalicylate intake. *Lancet* (1969) i, 178–80.
10. Roine R, Gentry T, Hernández-Munõz R, Baraona E, Lieber CS. Aspirin increases blood alcohol concentrations in humans after ingestion of ethanol. *JAMA* (1990) 264, 2406–8.
11. Sharma SC, Feeley J. The influence of aspirin and paracetamol on blood concentrations of alcohol in young adults. *Br J Clin Pharmacol* (1996) 41, 467P.
12. Melander O, Lidén A, Melander A. Pharmacokinetic interactions of alcohol and acetylsalicylic acid. *Eur J Clin Pharmacol* (1995) 48, 151–3.
13. Kechagias S, Jönsson K-Å, Norlander B, Carlsson B, Jones AW. Low-dose aspirin decreases blood alcohol concentrations by delaying gastric emptying. *Eur J Clin Pharmacol* (1997) 53, 241–6.
14. Rosove MH, Harwig SSL. Confirmation that ethanol potentiates aspirin-induced prolongation of the bleeding time. *Thromb Res* (1983) 31, 525–7.
15. Newgreen DB. Should consumers be warned about aspirin, alcohol and gastric bleeding? *Aust Prescriber* (2005) 28, 18–19.
16. Food and Drug Administration. FDA announces new alcohol warnings for pain relievers and fever reducers. HHS News. Available at: http://www.fda.gov/bbs/topics/NEWS/NEW00659.html (accessed 15/08/07).

Alcohol + Barbiturates

Alcohol and the barbiturates are CNS depressants, which together can have additive and possibly even synergistic effects. Activities requiring alertness and good co-ordination, such as driving a car or handling other potentially dangerous machinery, can be made more difficult and more hazardous. Alcohol may also continue to interact the next day if the barbiturate has hangover effects.

Clinical evidence

A study in healthy subjects of the effects of a single 0.5-g/kg dose of alcohol, taken in the morning after a dose of **amobarbital** 100 mg every night for 2 weeks, found that the performance of co-ordination skills was much more impaired than with either drug alone.[1]

This increased CNS depression due to the combined use of alcohol and barbiturates has been described in other clinical studies with **phenobarbital**.[2,3] However, a study in healthy subjects found that although **phenobarbital** 45 mg daily for one week and alcohol (35 to 45 mg%) affected some perceptual-motor tests when given separately, these effects were not always found when they were given together.[4] Nevertheless, high doses of **phenobarbital** can affect driving skills[5] and increased CNS depression has featured very many times in coroners' reports of fatal accidents and suicides involving barbiturates and alcohol.[6] A study of the fatalities due to this interaction indicated that with some barbiturates the CNS depressant effects are more than additive.[7] There is also some evidence that blood-alcohol levels may be reduced in the presence of a barbiturate.[8,9]

For the interaction between thiopental and alcohol, see 'Anaesthetics, general + Alcohol', p.92.

Mechanism

Both alcohol and the barbiturates are CNS depressants, and simple additive CNS depression provides part of the explanation. Acute alcohol ingestion may inhibit the liver enzymes concerned with the metabolism of barbiturates such as phenobarbital and **pentobarbital**, but chronic exposure to alcohol increases hepatic microsomal enzyme activity and may reduce sedation from barbiturates in patients without liver impairment.[10,11] Similarly, chronic exposure to a barbiturate such as phenobarbital may increase alcohol metabolism due to enzyme induction and consequently reduce blood-alcohol levels.[7]

Importance and management

Few formal studies in normal clinical situations have been made of the interactions between alcohol and the barbiturates, and most of these studies are old and involved barbiturates used as hypnotics. However, the effects (particularly those that result in fatalities) are very well established, serious, and of clinical importance. The most obvious hazards are increased drowsiness, lack of alertness and impaired co-ordination, which make the handling of potentially dangerous machinery (e.g. car driving), and even the performance of everyday tasks (e.g. walking downstairs) more difficult and dangerous. Only amobarbital and phenobarbital appear to have been specifically studied, but this interaction would be expected with all of the barbiturates. Some barbiturate hangover effects may be present the next morning and may therefore continue to interact significantly with alcohol. Patients should be warned.

For comments on the use of alcohol in epileptic patients taking antiepileptics including phenobarbital, see 'Alcohol + Antiepileptics', p.46.

1. Saario I, Linnoila M. Effect of subacute treatment with hypnotics, alone or in combination with alcohol, on psychomotor skills relating to driving. *Acta Pharmacol Toxicol (Copenh)* (1976) 38, 382–92.
2. Kielholz P, Goldberg L, Obersteg JI, Pöldinger W, Ramseyer A, Schmid P. Fahrversuche zur Frage der Beeinträchtigung der Verkehrstüchtigkeit durch Alkohol, Tranquilizer und Hypnotika. *Dtsch Med Wochenschr* (1969) 94, 301–6.
3. Morselli PL, Veneroni E, Zaccala M, Bizzi A. Further observations on the interaction between ethanol and psychotropic drugs. *Arzneimittelforschung* (1971) 21, 20–3.
4. Michiels W, Fryc O, Meyer JJ. Effet du tétrabamate, du phénobarbital et d'une faible quantité d'alcool sur quelques aspects perceptivo-moteurs en relation avec la conduite automobile. *Schweiz Med Wochenschr* (1978) 108, 640–6.
5. Cary PL, Johnson CA, Foltz RL, Pape BE. Driving under the influence of phenobarbital. *J Forensic Sci* (1983) 28, 502–4.
6. Gupta RC, Kofoed J. Toxicological statistics for barbiturates, other sedatives, and tranquillizers in Ontario: a 10-year survey. *Can Med Assoc J* (1966) 94, 863–5.
7. Stead AH, Moffat AC. Quantification of the interaction between barbiturates and alcohol and interpretation of fatal blood concentrations. *Hum Toxicol* (1983) 2, 5–14.
8. Mould GP, Curry SH, Binns TB. Interaction of glutethimide and phenobarbitone with ethanol in man. *J Pharm Pharmacol* (1972) 24, 894–9.
9. Mezey E, Robles EA. Effects of phenobarbital administration on rates of ethanol clearance and on ethanol-oxidizing enzymes in man. *Gastroenterology* (1974) 66, 248–53.
10. Rubin E, Gang H, Misra PS, Lieber CS. Inhibition of drug metabolism by acute ethanol intoxication. A hepatic microsomal mechanism. *Am J Med* (1970) 49, 801–6.
11. Weller RA, Preskorn SH. Psychotropic drugs and alcohol: pharmacokinetic and pharmacodynamic interactions. *Psychosomatics* (1984) 25, 301–3, 305–6, 309.

Alcohol + Benzodiazepines and related drugs

Benzodiazepine and related hypno-sedatives increase the CNS depressant effects of alcohol to some extent. The risks of car driving and handling other potentially dangerous machinery are increased. The risk is heightened because the patient may be unaware of being affected. Some benzodiazepines used at night for sedation are still present in appreciable amounts the next day and therefore may continue to interact. Alcohol may also increase the plasma levels of brotizolam, clobazam, diazepam, and possibly triazolam, whereas alprazolam may increase blood-alcohol levels. Alcohol has been reported to increase aggression or amnesia and/or reduce the anxiolytic effects of some benzodiazepines.

Clinical evidence

(a) Additive CNS depressant effects

It is very difficult to assess and compare the results of the very many studies of this interaction because of the differences between the tests, their duration, the dosages of the benzodiazepines and alcohol, whether given chronically or acutely, and a number of other variables. However, the overall picture seems to be that benzodiazepines and related drugs including **diazepam**,[1-12] **alprazolam**,[13-15] **bromazepam**,[16] **brotizolam**,[17] **chlordiazepoxide**,[12,18-22] **clobazam**,[23] **dipotassium clorazepate**,[24] **flunitrazepam**,[25,26] **flurazepam**,[27-31] **loprazolam**,[28,32] **lorazepam**,[10,33-36] **lormetazepam**,[37] **medazepam**,[38] **midazolam**,[39] **nitrazepam**,[3,40,41] **oxazepam**,[6] **temazepam**,[41-43] **triazolam**,[29,42,44-46] and **zopiclone**[46] enhance the effects of alcohol i.e. cause increased drowsiness, impaired performance and driving skills.

Patients taking benzodiazepines including **lorazepam**[34] or **triazolam**[44] may be unaware of the extent of the impairment that occurs. Furthermore, changes in CNS functioning may possibly occur in heavy social drinkers; a placebo-controlled study in 20-year-olds suggested that **lorazepam** 2 mg had more impairment on delayed auditory verbal memory performance in those who were heavy social drinkers (more than 20 drinks; 200 g of alcohol per week) than light social drinkers (20 g or less of alcohol per week).[47]

Some of the benzodiazepines and related drugs that are used primarily to aid sleep, such as **flunitrazepam**,[25,26] **flurazepam**,[27,28,30,31,48] **nitrazepam**,[3,40] and **temazepam**,[48,49] when taken the night before alcohol or in the evening with alcohol, can still interact with alcohol the next morning. However, **midazolam**,[39] **loprazolam**,[28] **lormetazepam**,[37] **triazolam**,[31,46] **zolpidem**,[50] and **zopiclone**[25,30,46] have been reported not to do so. The sedative effects of **midazolam** alone, and **midazolam** with fentanyl have been shown to have dissipated within 4 hours, and to not be affected by alcohol after this time.[51,52] However, some patients may metabolise **midazolam** more slowly and so an interaction could still be possible,[53] especially in older patients or those receiving additional drugs.[54]

Some contrasting effects have also been reported. One study suggested that alcohol might mitigate the effects of **loprazolam** on psychological performance.[32] Similarly, some antagonism has been reported between **chlordiazepoxide** and alcohol, but this is unlikely to be of practical importance.[18,19] The development of tolerance between benzodiazepines and alcohol with chronic use has also been suggested.[55,56]

(b) Increased aggression, anxiety, or amnesia

The anxiolytic effects of **lorazepam**[35] and possibly **chlordiazepoxide**[20] may be opposed by alcohol. **Alprazolam** and alcohol together may possibly increase behavioural aggression.[57] Similarly, **flunitrazepam** abuse can cause violent behaviour, impulsive decision-making and anterograde amnesia: a report looking at violent crimes committed by abusers of **flunitrazepam** found that alcohol was almost always also present.[58] Alcoholic drinks also enhance the effects of **flunitrazepam** when it is used as a 'date rape' drug.[59]

((c) Pharmacokinetic effects

Several studies have reported that alcohol increases plasma levels of **diazepam**[13,60] and that alcohol accelerates the absorption of **diazepam**,[5] but others have suggested that alcohol has no significant effect on diazepam pharmacokinetics.[9,11,61] Plasma levels of **brotizolam**[17] and **clobazam**[23] may be increased by alcohol. One study reported that the plasma levels of **triazolam** were increased by alcohol,[44] but other studies have found only a minimal pharmacokinetic interaction.[45,46] However, an *in vitro* study demonstrated that alcohol inhibited the metabolism of **triazolam** by the cytochrome P450 isoenzyme CYP3A.[62] Another *in vitro* study reported that the formation of **flunitrazepam** metabolites was weakly inhibited by alcohol,[63] but a pharmacokinetic study suggested that there was no interaction.[26] Alcohol appears to have minimal effects on the pharmacokinetics of **alprazolam**,[13] and **zopiclone**.[46,64]

The pharmacokinetics of alcohol do not appear to be affected to a clinically significant extent by **diazepam**,[11] **flunitrazepam**,[26] **zolpidem**,[50] or **zopiclone**[46] but **alprazolam**[13] may increase blood-alcohol levels.

Mechanism

The CNS depressant actions of the benzodiazepines and alcohol are mainly additive and it appears that different aspects of CNS processing may be involved.[41,65]

A pharmacokinetic interaction can sometimes occur, but the mechanisms seem to be quite complex. Acute alcohol intake increases the absorption and raises the serum levels of some benzodiazepines[23,60] and there may be direct competitive *inhibition* of metabolism.[66] It has been suggested that clearance of benzodiazepines via phase I metabolism, by *N*-demethylation and/or hydroxylation, tends to be more affected by alcohol intake than that of drugs such as lorazepam, oxazepam or lormetazepam that only undergo phase II conjugation. In addition, phase I metabolism is inhibited or decreases with increasing age and liver disease.[66] However, phase I metabolism is *increased* by chronic administration of substances that induce the cytochrome P450 isoenzyme system, such as alcohol,[66] and moderate alcohol consumption may cause intestinal CYP3A induction resulting in reduced bioavailability of some benzodiazepines, such as midazolam.[67]

Importance and management

Extensively studied, well established and clinically important interactions. The overall picture is that these drugs worsen the detrimental effects of alcohol.[68] Up to a 20 to 30% increase in the impairment of psychomotor function has been suggested.[44] The deterioration in skills will depend on the particular drug in question, its dosage and the amounts of alcohol taken. With modest amounts of alcohol the effects may be quite small in most patients (although a few may be more markedly affected[11]), but anyone taking any of these drugs should be warned that their usual response to alcohol may be greater than expected, and their ability to drive a car, or carry out any other tasks requiring alertness, may be impaired. They may be quite unaware of the deterioration or that the effects may still be present the following day. Benzodiazepines and alcohol are frequently found in the blood of car drivers involved in traffic accidents, which suggests that the risks are real.[56,68-71] Furthermore, alcohol may contribute to fatal poisonings and other deaths involving benzodiazepines, particularly diazepam[72-75] and temazepam.[76] Alcohol may contribute to drug-related accidents and deaths due to a disregard for safety;[71,77] and there is also an association between alcohol and benzodiazepines and violence-related accidents.[71]

1. Morselli PL, Veneroni E, Zaccala M, Bizzi A. Further observations on the interaction between ethanol and psychotropic drugs. *Arzneimittelforschung* (1971) 21, 20–3.
2. Linnoila M, Häkkinen S. Effects of diazepam and codeine, alone and in combination with alcohol, on simulated driving. *Clin Pharmacol Ther* (1974) 15, 368–73.
3. Linnoila M. Drug interaction on psychomotor skills related to driving: hypnotics and alcohol. *Ann Med Exp Biol Fenn* (1973) 51, 118–24.
4. Missen AW, Cleary W, Eng L, McMillan S. Diazepam, alcohol and drivers. *N Z Med J* (1978) 87, 275–7.
5. Laisi U, Linnoila M, Seppälä T, Himberg J-J, Mattila MJ. Pharmacokinetic and pharmacodynamic interactions of diazepam with different alcoholic beverages. *Eur J Clin Pharmacol* (1979) 16, 263–70.
6. Molander L, Duvhök C. Acute effects of oxazepam, diazepam and methylperone, alone and in combination with alcohol on sedation, coordination and mood. *Acta Pharmacol Toxicol (Copenh)* (1976) 38, 145–60.
7. Curry SH, Smith CM. Diazepam-ethanol interaction in humans: addition or potentiation? *Commun Psychopharmacol* (1979) 3, 101–13.
8. Smiley A, Moskowitz H. Effects of long-term administration of buspirone and diazepam on driver steering control. *Am J Med* (1986) 80 (Suppl 3B), 22–9.
9. Erwin CW, Linnoila M, Hartwell J, Erwin A, Guthrie S. Effects of buspirone and diazepam, alone and in combination with alcohol, on skilled performance and evoked potentials. *J Clin Psychopharmacol* (1986) 6, 199–209.
10. Aranko K, Seppälä T, Pellinen J, Mattila MJ. Interaction of diazepam or lorazepam with alcohol. Psychomotor effects and bioassayed serum levels after single and repeated doses. *Eur J Clin Pharmacol* (1985) 28, 559–65.
11. van Steveninck AL, Gieschke R, Schoemaker HC, Pieters MSM, Kroon JM, Breimer DD, Cohen AF. Pharmacodynamic interactions of diazepam and intravenous alcohol at pseudo steady state. *Psychopharmacology (Berl)* (1993) 110, 471–8.
12. Hughes FW, Forney RB, Richards AB. Comparative effect in human subjects of chlordiazepoxide, diazepam, and placebo on mental and physical performance. *Clin Pharmacol Ther* (1965) 6, 139–45.
13. Linnoila M, Stapleton JM, Lister R, Moss H, Lane E, Granger A, Eckardt MJ. Effects of single doses of alprazolam and diazepam, alone and in combination with ethanol, on psychomotor and cognitive performance and on autonomic nervous system reactivity in healthy volunteers. *Eur J Clin Pharmacol* (1990) 39, 21–8.
14. Rush CR, Griffiths RR. Acute participant-rated and behavioral effects of alprazolam and buspirone, alone and in combination with ethanol, in normal volunteers. *Exp Clin Psychopharmacol* (1997) 5, 28–38.
15. Bond AJ, Silveira JC, Lader MH. The effects of alprazolam alone and combined with alcohol on central integrative activity. *Eur J Clin Pharmacol* (1992) 42, 495–8.
16. Seppälä T, Saario I, Mattila MJ. Two weeks' treatment with chlorpromazine, thioridazine, sulpiride, or bromazepam: actions and interactions with alcohol on psychomotor skills relating to driving. *Mod Probl Pharmacopsychiatry* (1976) 11, 85–90.
17. Scavone JM, Greenblatt DJ, Harmatz JS, Shader RI. Kinetic and dynamic interaction of brotizolam and ethanol. *Br J Clin Pharmacol* (1986) 21, 197–204.
18. Dundee JW, Isaac M. Interaction of alcohol with sedatives and tranquillisers (a study of blood levels at loss of consciousness following rapid infusion). *Med Sci Law* (1970) 10, 220–4.
19. Linnoila M. Effects of diazepam, chlordiazepoxide, thioridazine, haloperidole, flupenthixole and alcohol on psychomotor skills related to driving. *Ann Med Exp Biol Fenn* (1973) 51, 125–32.
20. Linnoila M, Saario I, Olkoniemi J, Liljequist R, Himberg JJ, Mäki M. Effect of two weeks' treatment with chlordiazepoxide or flupenthixole, alone or in combination with alcohol, on psychomotor skills related to driving. *Arzneimittelforschung* (1975) 25, 1088–92.
21. Hoffer A. Lack of potentiation by chlordiazepoxide (Librium) of depression or excitation due to alcohol. *Can Med Assoc J* (1962) 87, 920–1.
22. Kielholz P, Goldberg L, Obersteg JI, Pöldinger W, Ramseyer A, Schmid P. Fahrversuche zur Frage der Beeinträchtigung der Verkehrstüchtigkeit durch Alkohol, Tranquilizer und Hypnotika. *Dtsch Med Wochenschr* (1969) 94, 301–6.
23. Taeuber K, Badian M, Brettel HF, Royen T, Rupp K, Sittig W, Uihlein M. Kinetic and dynamic interaction of clobazam and alcohol. *Br J Clin Pharmacol* (1979) 7, 91S-97S.
24. Staak M, Raff G, Nusser W. Pharmacopsychological investigations concerning the combined effects of dipotassium clorazepate and ethanol. *Int J Clin Pharmacol Biopharm* (1979) 17, 205–12.
25. Seppälä T, Nuotto E, Dreyfus JF. Drug–alcohol interactions on psychomotor skills: zopiclone and flunitrazepam. *Pharmacology* (1983) 27 (Suppl 2), 127–35.
26. Linnoila M, Erwin CW, Brendle A, Logue P. Effects of alcohol and flunitrazepam on mood and performance in healthy young men. *J Clin Pharmacol* (1981) 21, 430–5.
27. Saario I, Linnoila M. Effect of subacute treatment with hypnotics, alone or in combination with alcohol, on psychomotor skills related to driving. *Acta Pharmacol Toxicol (Copenh)* (1976) 38, 382–92.
28. Hindmarch I, Gudgeon AC. Loprazolam (HR158) and flurazepam with ethanol compared on tests of psychomotor ability. *Eur J Clin Pharmacol* (1982) 23, 509–12.
29. Hill SY, Goodwin DW, Reichman JB, Mendelson WB, Hopper S. A comparison of two benzodiazepine hypnotics administered with alcohol. *J Clin Psychiatry* (1982) 43, 408–10.
30. Mamelak M, Buck L, Csima A, Price V, Smiley A. Effects of flurazepam and zopiclone on the performance of chronic insomniac patients: a study of ethanol-drug interaction. *Sleep* (1987) 10 (Suppl 1), 79–87.
31. Mendelson WB, Goodwin DW, Hill SY, Reichman JD. The morning after: residual EEG effects of triazolam and flurazepam, alone and in combination with alcohol. *Curr Ther Res Clin Exp* (1976) 19, 155–63.
32. McManus IC, Ankier SI, Norfolk J, Phillips M, Priest RG. Effects on psychological performance of the benzodiazepine, loprazolam, alone and with alcohol. *Br J Clin Pharmacol* (1983) 16, 291–300.
33. Allen D, Baylav A, Lader M. A comparative study of the interaction of alcohol with alpidem, lorazepam and placebo in normal subjects. *Int Clin Psychopharmacol* (1988) 3, 327–41.
34. Seppälä T, Aranko K, Mattila MJ, Shrotriya RC. Effects of alcohol on buspirone and lorazepam actions. *Clin Pharmacol Ther* (1982) 32, 201–7.
35. Lister RG, File SE. Performance impairment and increased anxiety resulting from the combination of alcohol and lorazepam. *J Clin Psychopharmacol* (1983) 3, 66–71.
36. Soo-Ampon S, Wonqwitdecha N, Plasen S, Hindmarch I, Boyle J. Effects of word frequency on recall memory following lorazepam, alcohol, and lorazepam alcohol interaction in healthy volunteers. *Psychopharmacology (Berl)* (2004) 176, 420–5.
37. Willumeit H-P, Ott H, Neubert W, Hemmerling K-G, Schratzer M, Fichte K. Alcohol interaction of lormetazepam, mepindolol sulphate and diazepam measured by performance on the driving simulator. *Pharmacopsychiatry* (1984) 17, 36–43.
38. Landauer AA, Pocock DA, Prott FW. The effect of medazepam and alcohol on cognitive and motor skills used in car driving. *Psychopharmacologia* (1974) 37, 159–68.
39. Hindmarch I, Subhan Z. The effects of midazolam in conjunction with alcohol on sleep, psychomotor performance and car driving ability. *Int J Clin Pharmacol Res* (1983) 3, 323–9.
40. Saario I, Linnoila M, Mäki M. Interaction of drugs with alcohol on human psychomotor skills related to driving: effect of sleep deprivation or two weeks' treatment with hypnotics. *J Clin Pharmacol* (1975) 15, 52–9.
41. Taberner PV, Roberts CJC, Shrosbree E, Pycock CJ, English L. An investigation into the interaction between ethanol at low doses and the benzodiazepines nitrazepam and temazepam on psychomotor performance in normal subjects. *Psychopharmacology (Berl)* (1983) 81, 321–26.
42. Simpson CA, Rush CR. Acute performance-impairing and subject-rated effects of triazolam and temazepam, alone and in combination with ethanol, in humans. *J Psychopharmacol* (2002) 16, 23–34.
43. Lehmann W, Liljenberg B. Effect of temazepam and temazepam-ethanol on sleep. *Eur J Clin Pharmacol* (1981) 20, 201–5.
44. Dorian P, Sellers EM, Kaplan HL, Hamilton C, Greenblatt DJ, Abernethy D. Triazolam and ethanol interaction: kinetic and dynamic consequences. *Clin Pharmacol Ther* (1985) 37, 558–62.
45. Ochs HR, Greenblatt DJ, Arendt RM, Hübbel W, Shader RI. Pharmacokinetic noninteraction of triazolam and ethanol. *J Clin Psychopharmacol* (1984) 4,106–7.
46. Kuitunen T, Mattila MJ, Seppala T. Actions and interactions of hypnotics on human performance: single doses of zopiclone, triazolam and alcohol. *Int Clin Psychopharmacol* (1990) 5 (Suppl 2), 115–30.
47. Nichols JM, Martin F. The effect of lorazepam on long-term verbal recall in heavy and light social drinkers. *Alcohol* (1997) 14, 455–61.
48. Betts TA, Birtle J. Effect of two hypnotic drugs on actual driving performance next morning. *BMJ* (1982) 285, 852.
49. Hindmarch I. The effects of repeated doses of temazepam taken in conjunction with alcohol on aspects of psychomotor performance the morning following night time medication. *Arzneimittelforschung* (1978) 28, 2357–60.
50. Wilkinson CJ. The acute effects of zolpidem, administered alone and with alcohol, on cognitive and psychomotor function. *J Clin Psychiatry* (1995) 56, 309–18.
51. Lichtor JL, Zacny J, Korttila K, Apfelbaum JL, Lane BS, Rupani G, Thisted RA, Dohrn C. Alcohol after midazolam sedation: does it really matter? *Anesth Analg* (1991) 72, 661–6.
52. Lichtor JL, Zacny J, Apfelbaum JL, Lane BS, Rupani G, Thisted RA, Dohrn C, Korttila K. Alcohol after sedation with i.v. midazolam–fentanyl: effects on psychomotor functioning. *Br J Anaesth* (1991) 67, 579–84.
53. Dundee JW. Safety of alcohol after midazolam. *Anesth Analg* (1991) 73, 829.
54. Lichtor JL, Zacny J, Korttila K, Apfelbaum JL. Safety of alcohol after midazolam. Response. *Anesth Analg* (1991) 73, 829.
55. Palva ES, Linnoila M, Saario I, Mattila MJ. Acute and subacute effects of diazepam on psychomotor skills: interaction with alcohol. *Acta Pharmacol Toxicol (Copenh)* (1979) 45, 257–64.
56. Chan AWK. Effects of combined alcohol and benzodiazepine: a review. *Drug Alcohol Depend* (1984) 13, 315–41.
57. Bond AJ, Silveira JC. Behavioural aggression following the combination of alprazolam and alcohol. *J Psychopharmacol* (1990) 4, 315.
58. Dåderman AM, Fredriksson B, Kristiansson M, Nilsson L-H, Lidberg L. Violent behavior, impulsive decision-making, and anterograde amnesia while intoxicated with flunitrazepam and alcohol or other drugs: a case study in forensic psychiatric patients. *J Am Acad Psychiatry Law* (2002) 30, 238–51.
59. Schwartz RH, Milteer R, LeBeau MA. Drug-facilitated sexual assault ('date rape'). *South Med J* (2000) 93, 558–61.
60. MacLeod SM, Giles HG, Patzalek G, Thiessen JJ, Sellers EM. Diazepam actions and plasma concentrations following ethanol ingestion. *Eur J Clin Pharmacol* (1977) 11, 345–9.
61. Divoll M, Greenblatt DJ. Alcohol does not enhance diazepam absorption. *Pharmacology* (1981) 22, 263–8.
62. Patki KC, Greenblatt DJ, von Moltke LL. Ethanol inhibits in-vitro metabolism of nifedipine, triazolam and testosterone in human liver microsomes. *J Pharm Pharmacol* (2004) 56, 963–6.
63. Tanaka E, Nakamura T, Terada T, Shinozuka T, Honda K. Preliminary study of the *in vitro* interaction between alcohol, high-dose flunitrazepam and its three metabolites using human liver microsomes. *Basic Clin Pharmacol Toxicol* (2005) 96, 88–90.
64. Larivière L, Caillé G, Elie R. The effects of low and moderate doses of alcohol on the pharmacokinetic parameters of zopiclone. *Biopharm Drug Dispos* (1986) 7, 207–10.
65. Martin FH, Siddle DA. The interactive effects of alcohol and temazepam on P300 and reaction time. *Brain Cogn* (2003) 53, 58–65.
66. Tanaka E, Misawa S. Pharmacokinetic interactions between acute alcohol ingestion and single doses of benzodiazepines, and tricyclic and tetracyclic antidepressants–an update. *J Clin Pharm Ther* (1998) 23, 331–6.
67. Liangpunsakul S, Kolwankar D, Pinto A, Gorski JC, Hall SD, Chalasani N. Activity of CYP2E1 and CYP3A enzymes in adults with moderate alcohol consumption: a comparison with nonalcoholics. *Hepatology* (2005) 41, 1144–50.
68. Schuster R, Bodem M. Evaluation of ethanol-benzodiazepine-interactions using blood sampling protocol data. *Blutalkohol* (1997) 34, 54–65.
69. Staub C, Lacalle H, Fryc O. Présence de psychotropes dans le sang de conducteurs responsables d'accidents de la route ayant consommé en même temps de l'alcool. *Soz Praventivmed* (1994) 39, 143–9.
70. Longo MC, Hunter CE, Lokan RJ, White JM, White MA. The prevalence of alcohol, cannabinoids, benzodiazepines and stimulants amongst injured drivers and their role in driver culpability. Part II: The relationship between drug prevalence and drug concentration, and driver culpability. *Accid Anal Prev* (2000) 32, 623–32.

71. Kurzthaler I, Wambacher M, Golser K, Sperner G, Sperner-Unterweger B, Haidekker A, Pavlic M, Kemmler G, Fleischhacker WW. Alcohol and/or benzodiazepine use: different accidents – different impacts? *Hum Psychopharmacol* (2005) 20, 583–9.
72. Serfaty M, Masterton G. Fatal poisonings attributed to benzodiazepines in Britain during the 1980s. *Br J Psychiatry* (1993) 163, 386–93.
73. Kovac C. Airline passenger dies after being sedated by doctor. *BMJ* (1999) 318, 12.
74. Macdonald HA. Airline passenger dies after being sedated. Death may have been due to positional asphyxia. *BMJ* (1999) 318, 1491.
75. Samer Abdalla M. Airline passenger dies after being sedated. ...or to potentiating effects on diazepam. *BMJ* (1999) 318, 1491.
76. Koski A, Ojanperä I, Vuori E. Alcohol and benzodiazepines in fatal poisonings. *Alcohol Clin Exp Res* (2002) 26, 956–9.
77. Gable RS. Acute toxic effects of club drugs. *J Psychoactive Drugs* (2004) 36, 303–13.

Alcohol + Beta blockers

The haemodynamic and pharmacokinetic effects of atenolol and metoprolol in healthy subjects do not appear to be changed by alcohol. There is some evidence that alcohol modestly reduces the haemodynamic effects of propranolol, and some of the effects of sotalol may also be changed by alcohol. Some evidence suggests that the effects of alcohol and atenolol/chlortalidone or propranolol are additive on the performance of some psychomotor tests, but the importance of this is uncertain.

Clinical evidence, mechanism, importance and management

(a) CNS effects

In 12 healthy subjects the performance of a number of psychomotor tests was found to be impaired by alcohol 0.6 g/kg and by one tablet of *Tenoretic* (**atenolol** 100 mg with chlortalidone 25 mg). When alcohol and *Tenoretic* were taken together there was some evidence of additive effects but the practical importance of this is not clear.[1]

In 12 healthy subjects **propranolol** 40 mg every 6 hours had no effect on the alcohol-induced impairment of performance on a number of psychomotor tests given 50 mL/70 kg of alcohol, except that **propranolol** antagonised the effect of alcohol in one test (pursuit meter).[2] However, in another study, **propranolol** enhanced the effects of alcohol on some tests (inebriation and divided attention).[3]

The manufacturer of **oxprenolol** warns that the effects of alcohol and beta blockers on the CNS have been observed to be additive and it is possible that symptoms such as dizziness may be exaggerated if they are taken together.[4]

(b) Haemodynamic and pharmacokinetic effects

In 8 healthy subjects the pharmacokinetics of single 100-mg doses of **atenolol** or **metoprolol** were unaffected 6 hours after they had drunk the equivalent of 200 mL of absolute alcohol. No clinically significant changes in blood pressure or pulse rate were seen.[5] A study in 6 healthy subjects found that alcohol (sufficient to maintain blood-alcohol levels of 80 mg%) raised the mean AUC of a single 80-mg oral dose of **propranolol** by 17.4% in 5 subjects and decreased it by 37% in the other subject, but this was considered unlikely to be clinically important. No changes in heart rate or blood pressure were seen.[6] In contrast, a double-blind study in 14 healthy subjects found that alcohol (equivalent to 32 to 72 mL of absolute alcohol) increased the clearance of a single 80-mg dose of **propranolol** and diminished its ability to lower blood pressure. **Propranolol** was not able to abolish the alcohol-induced rise in heart rate.[7] Similarly, another study found that alcohol decreased the rate of absorption and increased the rate of elimination of **propranolol**, but the clinical significance of this small alteration was not assessed.[8]

A further study in 6 healthy subjects found that although the blood pressure lowering effects of **sotalol** 160 mg were increased by alcohol, **sotalol** did not cancel out the alcohol-induced rise in heart rate.[7]

It would seem prudent to be alert for changes in response to beta blockers that may be due to alcohol. See also, 'Alcohol + Antihypertensives', p.48.

1. Gerrard L, Wheeldon NM, McDevitt DG. Psychomotor effects of combined atenolol/chlorthalidone administration: interaction with alcohol. *Br J Clin Pharmacol* (1994) 37, 517P–518P.
2. Lindenschmidt R, Brown D, Cerimele B, Walle T, Forney RB. Combined effects of propranolol and ethanol on human psychomotor performance. *Toxicol Appl Pharmacol* (1983) 67, 117–21.
3. Alkana RL, Parker ES, Cohen HB, Birch H, Noble EP. Reversal of ethanol intoxication in humans: an assessment of the efficacy of propranolol. *Psychopharmacology (Berl)* (1976) 51, 29–37.
4. Trasicor (Oxprenolol). Amdipharm plc. UK Summary of product characteristics, September 2005.
5. Kirch W, Spahn H, Hutt HJ, Ohnhaus EE, Mutschler E. Interaction between alcohol and metoprolol or atenolol in social drinking. *Drugs* (1983) 25 (Suppl 2), 152.
6. Dorian P, Sellers EM, Carruthers G, Hamilton C, Fan T. Propranolol-ethanol pharmacokinetic interaction. *Clin Pharmacol Ther* (1982) 31, 219.
7. Sotaniemi EA, Anttila M, Rautio A, Stengård J, Saukko P, Järvensivu P. Propranolol and sotalol metabolism after a drinking party. *Clin Pharmacol Ther* (1981) 29, 705–10.
8. Grabowski BS, Cady WJ, Young WW, Emery JF. Effects of acute alcohol administration on propranolol absorption. *Int J Clin Pharmacol Ther Toxicol* (1980) 18, 317–19.

Alcohol + Bicalutamide, Flutamide or Nilutamide

Alcohol intolerance (facial flushing, malaise, hypotension) has been reported in patients receiving nilutamide but not bicalutamide or flutamide.

Clinical evidence, mechanism, importance and management

Several studies have described alcohol intolerance (facial flushes, malaise, hypotension) in patients taking nilutamide.[1-3] The incidence has been reported to be between 3% and 19%.[1-4] It is recommended that patients who experience this reaction should avoid drinking alcohol.[4]

Flutamide and bicalutamide have not been reported to produce these effects when patients drink alcohol,[3] so they may be considered as an alternative option to nilutamide.

1. Boccardo F, Decensi AU, Guarneri D, Martorana G, Fioretto L, Mini E, Macaluso MP, Giuliani L, Santi L, Periti P; the Italian Prostatic Cancer Project. Anandron (RU 23908) in metastatic prostate cancer: preliminary results of a multicentric Italian study. *Cancer Detect Prev* (1991), 15, 501–3.
2. Decensi AU, Boccardo F, Guarneri D, Positano N, Paoletti MC, Costantini M, Martorana G, Giuliani L; for the Italian Prostatic Cancer Project. Monotherapy with nilutamide, a pure nonsteroidal antiandrogen, in untreated patients with metastatic carcinoma of the prostate. *J Urol (Baltimore)* (1991) 146, 377–81.
3. McLeod DG. Tolerability of nonsteroidal antiandrogens in the treatment of advanced prostate cancer. *Oncologist* (1997) 2, 18–27.
4. Nilandron (Nilutamide). Sanofi-Aventis US LLC. US Prescribing information, June 2006.

Alcohol + Bromocriptine

There is some very limited evidence to suggest that the adverse effects of bromocriptine may possibly be increased by alcohol.

Clinical evidence, mechanism, importance and management

Intolerance to alcohol, which improved on continued treatment, has been briefly mentioned in a report about patients taking bromocriptine for acromegaly.[1] In another report two patients with high prolactin levels were said to have developed bromocriptine adverse effects, even in low doses, while continuing to drink. When they abstained, the frequency and the severity of the adverse effects fell, even with higher doses of bromocriptine.[2] This, it is suggested, may be due to some alcohol-induced increase in the sensitivity of dopamine receptors.[2] There would seem to be little reason, on the basis of this extremely sparse evidence, to tell all patients taking bromocriptine not to drink alcohol, but it would be reasonable to warn them to try avoiding alcohol if adverse effects develop.

1. Wass JAH, Thorner MO, Morris DV, Rees LH, Mason AS, Jones AE, Besser GM. Long-term treatment of acromegaly with bromocriptine. *BMJ* (1977) 1, 875–8.
2. Ayres J, Maisey MN. Alcohol increases bromocriptine's side effects. *N Engl J Med* (1980) 302, 806.

Alcohol + Bupropion

The concurrent use of bupropion and alcohol does not appear to affect the pharmacokinetics of either drug.

Clinical evidence, mechanism, importance and management

Single-dose studies in healthy subjects found that the pharmacokinetics of bupropion 100 mg were not affected by the concurrent use of alcohol, and bupropion did not affect blood-alcohol levels.[1,2] However, bupropion may reduce alcohol tolerance and there is an increased risk of seizures if alcohol is withdrawn abruptly, see 'Bupropion + Miscellaneous', p.1206.

1. Posner J, Bye A, Jeal S, Peck AW, Whiteman P. Alcohol and bupropion pharmacokinetics in healthy male volunteers. *Eur J Clin Pharmacol* (1984) 26, 627–30.
2. Hamilton MJ, Bush MS, Peck AW. The effect of bupropion, a new antidepressant drug, and alcohol and their interaction in man. *Eur J Clin Pharmacol* (1984) 27, 75–80.

Alcohol + Buspirone

Buspirone with alcohol may cause drowsiness and weakness, although it does not appear to impair the performance of a number of psychomotor tests.

Clinical evidence, mechanism, importance and management

A study in 12 healthy subjects showed that, in contrast to lorazepam, buspirone 10 or 20 mg did not appear to interact with alcohol (i.e. worsen the performance of certain psychomotor tests), but it did make the subjects feel drowsy and weak.[1,2] Similarly, another study in 13 healthy subjects found that combining buspirone (15 and 30 mg/70 kg) and alcohol caused sedation, but very little impairment of performance. In this study, the sedative effects were broadly similar to those seen with alprazolam plus alcohol, but alprazolam plus alcohol clearly impaired performance.[3] Similar findings were reported in another earlier comparison with diazepam.[4] A further study reported that single 5 to 15-mg doses of buspirone had a minimal effect on performance in both light and moderate female social drinkers.[5]

The UK manufacturer notes that there is no information on higher therapeutic doses of buspirone combined with alcohol, and they suggest that it would be prudent to avoid alcohol while taking buspirone.[6] They also caution patients of the potential hazards of driving or handling other potentially dangerous machinery until they are certain that buspirone does not adversely affect them.[6]

1. Mattila MJ, Aranko K, Seppala T. Acute effects of buspirone and alcohol on psychomotor skills. *J Clin Psychiatry* (1982) 43, 56–60.
2. Seppälä T, Aranko K, Mattila MJ, Shrotriya RC. Effects of alcohol on buspirone and lorazepam actions. *Clin Pharmacol Ther* (1982) 32, 201–7.
3. Rush CR, Griffiths RR. Acute participant-rated and behavioral effects of alprazolam and buspirone, alone and in combination with ethanol, in normal volunteers. *Exp Clin Psychopharmacol* (1997) 5, 28–38.
4. Erwin CW, Linnoila M, Hartwell J, Erwin A, Guthrie S. Effects of buspirone and diazepam, alone and in combination with alcohol, on skilled performance and evoked potentials. *J Clin Psychopharmacol* (1986) 6, 199–209.
5. Evans SM, Levin FR. The effects of alprazolam and buspirone in light and moderate female social drinkers. *Behav Pharmacol* (2002) 13, 427–39.
6. Buspar (Buspirone hydrochloride). Bristol-Myers Pharmaceuticals. UK Summary of product characteristics, March 2007.

Alcohol + Butyraldoxime

A disulfiram-like reaction can occur in those exposed to *N*-butyraldoxime if they drink alcohol.

Clinical evidence, mechanism, importance and management

Workers in a printing company complained of flushing of the face, neck and upper trunk, shortness of breath, tachycardia and drowsiness very shortly after drinking alcohol (1.5 oz (about 45 mL) of whiskey), and were found to have increased levels of acetaldehyde in their blood. The reason appeared to be that the printing ink they were using contained *N*-butyraldoxime, an antioxidant which, like disulfiram, can inhibit the metabolism of alcohol causing acetaldehyde to accumulate (see 'Alcohol + Disulfiram', p.61).[1] It is possible that it is a metabolite of *N*-butyraldoxime that causes this effect, rather than *N*-butyraldoxime itself.[2] This reaction would seem to be more unpleasant and socially disagreeable than serious. No treatment normally seems necessary.

1. Lewis W, Schwartz L. An occupational agent (N-butyraldoxime) causing reaction to alcohol. *Med Ann Dist Columbia* (1956) 25, 485–90.
2. DeMaster EG, Redfern B, Shirota FN, Crankshaw DL, Nagasawa HT. Metabolic activation of *n*-butyraldoxime by rat liver microsomal cytochrome P450. A requirement for the inhibition of aldehyde dehydrogenase. *Biochem Pharmacol* (1993) 46, 117–23.

Alcohol + Caffeine

Objective tests show that caffeine may counteract some of the effects of alcohol. However, it does not completely sober up those who have drunk too much, and may even make them more accident-prone.

Clinical evidence

A study in a large number of healthy subjects given a cup of **coffee** containing caffeine 300 mg/70 kg, either alone or immediately after drinking alcohol 0.75 g/kg, found that caffeine did not antagonise the deleterious effect of alcohol on the performance of psychomotor skill tests. Only reaction times were reversed.[1] Two other studies also found that caffeine did not antagonise the effects of alcohol in a variety of tests.[2,3] A further study in 8 subjects found that, contrary to expectations, caffeine increased the frequency of errors in the performance of a serial reaction time task,[4] and similarly, caffeine has been reported to increase the detrimental effects of alcohol.[5]

In contrast, more recent studies usually using caffeine in capsule form, have found that some of the performance-impairing effects of alcohol such as increased simple reaction time,[6,7] increased errors with four choice reaction time,[8] sedation,[9] and slowing of psychomotor speed[8] can be antagonised by caffeine given with the alcohol. However, caffeine does not appear to restore most subjective effects e.g. feeling of drunkenness.[6,9,10] One study found that the alcohol-caffeine combination typically altered the effects of caffeine alone rather than altering the effects of alcohol alone. For example the addition of alcohol reduced the jitteriness and alertness produced by caffeine, and although caffeine modestly antagonised alcohol impairment of driving, there was still a 9% increase in brake-response time, when compared with placebo.[10]

In a double-blind, placebo-controlled, crossover study in 8 healthy subjects, the AUC of a 400-mg caffeine capsule was 30% greater when it was taken with alcohol 0.8 g/kg than when taken alone. Blood-alcohol levels were not affected by caffeine use.[6] Similarly, other studies reported that alcohol increases serum-caffeine levels[2] and that blood-alcohol levels were not modified by caffeine.[1,2,7]

Mechanism

Not fully understood. Caffeine is a CNS stimulant, which seems to oppose some of the CNS depressant effects of alcohol. It appears that only those objective tests able to detect an enhancement due to a CNS stimulant show the clearest antagonistic effects.[6]

Alcohol appears to inhibit the hepatic metabolism of caffeine.[2]

Importance and management

It is not known why some studies report that caffeine antagonises some of the detrimental effects of alcohol and others report no interaction. However, the type of psychomotor tests, the amount of alcohol and caffeine consumed, and the timing and administration of the caffeine may affect the results.

Caffeine does appear to improve some of the detrimental effects of alcohol in some psychomotor tests, which is probably why there is a long-standing and time-hallowed belief in the value of strong black coffee to sober up those who have drunk too much. In addition, it is just possible that the time taken to drink the coffee gives the liver just a little more time to metabolise some of the alcohol. However, it seems that it is not effective in all aspects of alcohol impairment, particularly subjective effects. In addition, caffeine does not reduce blood-alcohol levels. **Coffee** and other sources of caffeine do not make it safe to drive or handle dangerous machinery, and it may even make drivers more accident-prone.

1. Franks HM, Hagedorn H, Hensley VR, Hensley WJ, Starmer GA. The effect of caffeine on human performance, alone and in combination with alcohol. *Psychopharmacologia* (1975) 45, 177–81.
2. Nuotto E, Mattila MJ, Seppälä T, Konno K. Coffee and caffeine and alcohol effects on psychomotor function. *Clin Pharmacol Ther* (1982) 31, 68–76.
3. Newman HW, Newman EJ. Failure of dexedrine and caffeine as practical antagonists of the depressant effect of ethyl alcohol in man. *Q J Stud Alcohol* (1956) 17, 406–10.
4. Lee DJ, Lowe G. Interaction of alcohol and caffeine in a perceptual-motor task. *IRCS Med Sci* (1980) 8, 420.
5. Oborne DJ, Rogers Y. Interactions of alcohol and caffeine on human reaction time. *Aviat Space Environ Med* (1983) 54, 528–34.
6. Azcona O, Barbanoj MJ, Torrent J, Jané F. Evaluation of the central effects of alcohol and caffeine interaction. *Br J Clin Pharmacol* (1995) 40, 393–400.
7. Marczinski CA, Fillmore MT. Dissociative antagonistic effects of caffeine on alcohol-induced impairment of behavioral control. *Exp Clin Psychopharmacol* (2003) 11, 228–36.

8. Mackay M, Tiplady B, Scholey AB. Interactions between alcohol and caffeine in relation to psychomotor speed and accuracy. *Hum Psychopharmacol* (2002) 17, 151–6.
9. Drake CL, Roehrs T, Turner L, Scofield HM, Roth T. Caffeine reversal of ethanol effects on the multiple sleep latency test, memory, and psychomotor performance. *Neuropsychopharmacology* (2003) 28, 371–8.
10. Liguori A, Robinson JH. Caffeine antagonism of alcohol-induced driving impairment. *Drug Alcohol Depend* (2001) 63, 123–9.

Alcohol + Calcium carbimide

Alcohol causes a disulfiram-like reaction in patients taking calcium carbimide. Calcium carbimide has been used as an alcohol deterrent.

Clinical evidence, mechanism, importance and management

Calcium carbimide interacts with alcohol in a similar way to disulfiram and by a similar mechanism[1] (see 'Alcohol + Disulfiram', p.61). Both of these drugs bind to aldehyde dehydrogenase, but calcium carbimide is said to have fewer adverse effects because it does not bind to dopamine beta hydroxylase.[2] However, marked cardiovascular effects and fatalities have occurred in those who drank alcohol while taking calcium carbimide.[3,4] Like disulfiram it is used to deter alcoholics from continuing to drink.[1,2]

1. Peachey JE, Brien JF, Roach CA, Loomis CW. A comparative review of the pharmacological and toxicological properties of disulfiram and calcium carbimide. *J Clin Psychopharmacol* (1981) 1, 21–6.
2. Monteiro MG. Pharmacological treatment of alcoholism. *Aust N Z J Med* (1992) 22, 220–3.
3. Kupari M, Hillbom M, Lindros K, Nieminen M. Possible cardiovascular hazards of the alcohol-calcium carbimide interaction. J Toxicol Clin Toxicol. (1982) 19, 79–86.
4. Brien JF, Peachey JE, Loomis CW. Calcium carbimide–ethanol interaction. *Clin Pharmacol Ther* (1980) 27, 426–33.

Alcohol + Calcium-channel blockers

Blood-alcohol levels can be raised and may remain elevated for a much longer period of time in patients taking verapamil. Alcohol may also increase the bioavailability of felodipine and nifedipine, but amlodipine appears not to interact. An increased incidence of postural hypotension has been reported in patients who took felodipine with alcohol

Clinical evidence

(a) Amlodipine

A study in 30 healthy subjects found that single and multiple doses of amlodipine 10 mg for 15 days (with or without lisinopril and simvastatin) had no effect on the pharmacokinetics of alcohol 0.8 g/kg nor on subjective psychological performance. Alcohol did not alter the pharmacokinetics of amlodipine.[1]

(b) Felodipine

A study in 8 healthy subjects given enough alcohol to maintain their blood levels at 80 to 120 mg% found that their felodipine levels (following a single 10-mg oral dose) were approximately doubled (AUC increased by 77%, maximum blood levels increased by 98%). Diuresis was approximately doubled and heart rates were increased.[2]

A double-blind, crossover study in 10 patients found that alcohol 0.75 g/kg in grapefruit juice enhanced the haemodynamic effects of a single 5-mg dose of felodipine. Four hours after dosing, felodipine with alcohol in grapefruit juice produced lower total peripheral resistance and diastolic blood pressure, and a higher heart rate, compared with felodipine with grapefruit juice alone. Furthermore, the greater blood pressure reduction caused symptoms in 50% of the patients; postural lightheadedness occurred in 5 patients given alcohol and felodipine, compared with 1 patient given felodipine without alcohol. However, felodipine plasma levels were higher than expected, although this may have largely been due to the 'grapefruit juice', (p.869), and the incidence of adverse effects for both groups was also higher.[3]

In a study, 8 non-smoking, healthy subjects were given a single 10-mg dose of an extended-release preparation of felodipine with 250 mL red wine on an empty stomach and 4 hours before a meal. Plasma felodipine levels were lower for the first 4 hours of the study than when taken with 250 mL water, but rose rapidly at 5 hours after dosing, resulting in a peak level that was higher than when taken with water.[4]

(c) Nifedipine

Alcohol (75 mL of alcohol 94% with 75 mL of orange juice) given to 10 healthy subjects increased the AUC of a single 20-mg dose of nifedipine by 54%, but no significant changes in heart rate or blood pressure were seen.[5] Another study, involving 226 patients receiving sustained-release nifedipine, found that reported alcohol use was associated with reduced nifedipine clearance (8.6 compared with 10.8 mL/minute per kg for alcohol use and no alcohol, respectively).[6] In another study no evidence was found that nifedipine 10 or 20 mg antagonised the effects of alcohol.[7]

(d) Verapamil

Ten healthy subjects given verapamil 80 mg three times daily for 6 days were given alcohol 0.8 g/kg on day 6. Peak blood-alcohol levels were found to be raised by 16.7% (from 106.45 to 124.24 mg%) and the $AUC_{0\text{-}12}$ was raised by almost 30%. The time that blood-alcohol levels exceeded 100 mg% was prolonged from 0.2 to 1.3 hours and the subjects said they felt more intoxicated.[8] In another study no evidence was found that verapamil 80 or 160 mg antagonised the effects of alcohol.[7]

Mechanism

Not understood. It seems possible that verapamil inhibits the metabolism of alcohol by the liver, thereby reducing its loss from the body. Alcohol also appears to inhibit the metabolism of nifedipine, and to increase the bioavailability of felodipine. Red wine may have caused "dose dumping" of felodipine from the extended-release preparation which altered its pharmacokinetic profile, but the reason why the felodipine levels remained low until after a meal is unclear.[4] An *in vitro* study demonstrated that alcohol inhibited the oxidative metabolism of nifedipine by the cytochrome P450 isoenzyme CYP3A.[9]

Importance and management

Information seems to be limited to these reports and they need confirmation. An alcohol concentration rise of almost 17% as caused by **verapamil** is quite small, but it could be enough to raise legal blood levels to illegal levels if driving. Moreover the intoxicant effects of alcohol may persist for a much longer period of time (five times longer in this instance).[8]

The bioavailability of **felodipine** and **nifedipine** appear to be increased by alcohol. The manufacturers of some calcium-channel blockers warn that inter-individual variations in the response to these drugs can occur and some patients ability to drive or operate machinery may be impaired, particularly at the start of treatment and in conjunction with alcohol.[10,11] Patients should therefore be advised about these effects. Note that long-term moderate to heavy drinking can impair the efficacy of antihypertensives. See also 'Alcohol + Antihypertensives', p.48.

1. Vincent J, Colangelo P, Baris B, Willavize S. Single and multiple doses of amlodipine do not alter the pharmacokinetics of alcohol in man. *Therapie* (1995) (Suppl) 50, 509.
2. Pentikainen PJ, Virolainen T, Tenhunen R, Aberg J. Acute alcohol intake increases the bioavailability of felodipine. *Clin Pharmacol Ther* (1994) 55, 148.
3. Bailey DG, Spence JD, Edgar B, Bayliff CD, Arnold JMO. Ethanol enhances the hemodynamic effects of felodipine. *Clin Invest Med* (1989) 12, 357–62.
4. Bailey DG, Dresser GK, Bend JR. Bergamottin, lime juice, and red wine as inhibitors of cytochrome P450 3A4 activity: Comparison with grapefruit juice. *Clin Pharmacol Ther* (2003) 73, 529–37.
5. Qureshi S, Laganière S, Caillé G, Gossard D, Lacasse Y, McGilveray I. Effect of an acute dose of alcohol on the pharmacokinetics of oral nifedipine in humans. *Pharm Res* (1992) 9, 683–6.
6. Krecic-Shepard ME, Park K, Barnas C, Slimko J, Kerwin DR, Schwartz JB. Race and sex influence clearance of nifedipine: results of a population study. *Clin Pharmacol Ther* (2000) 68, 130–42.
7. Perez-Reyes M, White WR, Hicks RE. Interaction between ethanol and calcium channel blockers in humans. *Alcohol Clin Exp Res* (1992) 16, 769–75.
8. Bauer LA, Schumock G, Horn J, Opheim K. Verapamil inhibits ethanol elimination and prolongs the perception of intoxication. *Clin Pharmacol Ther* (1992) 52, 6–10.
9. Patki KC, Greenblatt DJ, von Moltke LL. Ethanol inhibits in-vitro metabolism of nifedipine, triazolam and testosterone in human liver microsomes. *J Pharm Pharmacol* (2004) 56, 963–6.
10. Adalat Retard (Nifedipine). Bayer plc. UK Summary of product characteristics, September 2006.
11. Securon (Verapamil hydrochloride). Abbott Laboratories Ltd. UK Summary of product characteristics, August 2003.

Alcohol + Cannabis

The detrimental effects of drinking alcohol and smoking cannabis may be additive on some aspects of driving performance. However, there is some evidence that regular cannabis use *per se* does not potentiate the effects of alcohol. Smoking cannabis may alter the bioavailability of alcohol.

Clinical evidence and mechanism

(a) Enhanced CNS-depressant effects

Simultaneous use of alcohol and oral **Δ⁹-tetrahydrocannabinol** (THC, the major active ingredient of cannabis) reduced the performance of psychomotor tests, suggesting that those who use both drugs together should expect the deleterious effects to be additive.[1] In a further placebo-controlled study, subjects smoked cannabis containing 100 or 200 micrograms/kg of **Δ⁹-tetrahydrocannabinol** and drank alcohol (to achieve an initial blood level of 70 mg%, with further drinks taken to maintain levels at 40 mg%) 30 minutes before driving. They found that cannabis, even in low to moderate doses, negatively affected driving performance in real traffic situations. Further, the effect of combining moderate doses of both alcohol and cannabis resulted in dramatic performance impairment as great as that observed with blood-alcohol levels of 140 mg% alone.[2,3]

(b) Opposing or no additive CNS effects

One study in 14 regular cannabis users (long-term daily use) and 14 infrequent cannabis users found that regular use reduced the disruptive effects of alcohol on some psychomotor skills relevant to driving, whereas infrequent use did not have this effect. In this study, neither group had smoked any cannabis in the 12 hours before the alcohol test.[4] Another study found that moderate doses of alcohol and cannabis, consumed either alone or in combination, did not produce significant behavioural or subjective impairment the following day.[5]

A study in 12 healthy subjects who regularly used both cannabis and alcohol found that alcohol 0.5 g/kg significantly increased break latency without affecting body sway, whereas cannabis given as a cigarette containing **tetrahydrocannabinol** 3.33%, increased body sway but did not affect brake latency. There were no significant additive effects on brake latency, body sway, or mood when the two drugs were used together.[6] A population-based study of 2,777 drivers involved in fatal road crashes, who drank alcohol and/or used cannabis, found that although both cannabis and alcohol increased the risk of being responsible for a fatal crash, no statistically significant interaction was observed between the two drugs.[7]

(c) Pharmacokinetic studies

Fifteen healthy subjects given alcohol 0.7 g/kg developed peak plasma alcohol levels of 78.25 mg% at 50 minutes, but if they smoked a cannabis cigarette 30 minutes after the drink, their peak plasma alcohol levels were only 54.8 mg% and they occurred 55 minutes later. In addition, their subjective experience of the drugs decreased when used together.[8] However, another study found that smoking cannabis 10 minutes before alcohol consumption did not affect blood-alcohol levels.[5] A further study found that blood-alcohol levels were not affected by **Δ⁹-tetrahydrocannabinol** given orally one hour before alcohol.[1]

Importance and management

Several studies have found that cannabis and alcohol produce additive detrimental effects on driving performance, but other studies have failed to show any potentiation. This is probably due to the variety of simulated driving tests used and possibly the time lag between the administration of alcohol and cannabis; behavioural impairment after cannabis has been reported to peak within 30 minutes of smoking.[5] Nevertheless, both drugs have been shown to affect some aspects of driving performance and increase the risk of fatal car accidents. Concurrent use of cannabis and alcohol before driving should therefore be avoided.

1. Bird KD, Boleyn T, Chesher GB, Jackson DM, Starmer GA, Teo RKC. Intercannabinoid and cannabinoid-ethanol interactions and their effects on human performance. *Psychopharmacology (Berl)* (1980) 71, 181–8.
2. National Highway Traffic Safety Administration. Marijuana and alcohol combined severely impede driving performance. *Ann Emerg Med* (2000) 35, 398–9.
3. Jolly BT. Commentary: drugged driving—different spin on an old problem. *Ann Emerg Med* (2000) 35, 399–400.
4. Wright KA, Terry P. Modulation of the effects of alcohol on driving-related psychomotor skills by chronic exposure to cannabis. *Psychopharmacology (Berl)* (2002) 160, 213–19.
5. Chait LD, Perry JL. Acute and residual effects of alcohol and marijuana, alone and in combination, on mood and performance. *Psychopharmacology (Berl)* (1994) 115, 340–9.
6. Liguori A, Gatto CP, Jarrett DB. Separate and combined effects of marijuana and alcohol on mood, equilibrium and simulated driving. *Psychopharmacology (Berl)* (2002) 163, 399–405.
7. Laumon B, Gadeqbeku B, Martin J-L, Biecheler M-B; the SAM Group. Cannabis intoxication and fatal road crashes in France: population based case-control study. *BMJ* (2005) 331, 1371–6. Correction. ibid. (2006) 332, 1298.
8. Lukas SE, Benedikt R, Mendelson JH, Kouri E, Sholar M, Amass L. Marihuana attenuates the rise in plasma ethanol levels in human subjects. *Neuropsychopharmacology* (1992) 7, 77–81.

Alcohol + Carmofur

A disulfiram-like reaction occurred in a patient taking carmofur when he was given a coeliac plexus blockade with alcohol.

Clinical evidence, mechanism, importance and management

A man with pancreatic carcinoma taking carmofur 500 mg daily for 25 days experienced a disulfiram-like reaction (facial flushing, diaphoresis, hypotension with BP 60/30 mmHg, and tachycardia of 128 bpm) within 30 minutes of being given a coeliac plexus alcohol blockade for pain relief. Blood acetaldehyde levels were found to have risen sharply, supporting the belief that the underlying mechanism is similar to the disulfiram-alcohol interaction (see 'Alcohol + Disulfiram', p.61). It is suggested that alcohol blockade should be avoided for 7 days after treatment with carmofur.[1]

1. Noda J, Umeda S, Mori K, Fukunaga T, Mizoi Y. Disulfiram-like reaction associated with carmofur after celiac plexus alcohol block. *Anesthesiology* (1987) 67, 809–10.

Alcohol + Clomethiazole

Clomethiazole has been successfully used to treat alcohol withdrawal, but the long-term use of alcohol with clomethiazole can cause serious, even potentially fatal CNS depression, due to additive CNS depressant effects; fatal respiratory depression can occur even with short-term use in alcoholics with cirrhosis. The concurrent use of clomethiazole and alcohol may also affect driving skills. Clomethiazole bioavailability may be increased by alcohol.

Clinical evidence, mechanism, importance and management

(a) Enhanced adverse effects and bioavailability

The following is taken from an editorial in the British Medical Journal, which was entitled 'Chlormethiazole and alcohol: a lethal cocktail'.[1]

Clomethiazole is commonly used to treat withdrawal from alcohol because of its hypnotic, anxiolytic and anticonvulsant effects. It is very effective if a rapidly reducing dosage regimen is followed over six days, but if it is used long-term and drinking continues it carries several serious risks.

Alcoholics readily transfer dependency to clomethiazole and may visit several practitioners and hospitals to get their supplies. Tolerance develops so that very large amounts may need to be taken (up to 25 g daily). Often alcohol abuse continues and the combination of large amounts of alcohol and clomethiazole can result in coma and even fatal respiratory depression, due mainly to simple additive CNS depression.[1]

Other factors are that alcohol increases the bioavailability of clomethiazole (probably by impairing first pass metabolism),[2] and in the case of those with alcoholic cirrhosis, the systemic bioavailability may be increased tenfold because of venous shunting.[3] However, one study in 6 healthy subjects reported that intravenous alcohol 0.8 mL/kg given acutely had no effect on the disposition or elimination of clomethiazole. It was proposed that alcohol given orally might affect the absorption or rate of uptake of clomethiazole.[4]

Clomethiazole should not be given long-term for alcohol withdrawal states[1] or to those who continue to drink alcohol.[5] Use for more than 9 days is not recommended.[5,6] It has been said that if prescribers choose to manage detoxification at home, it should be done under very close supervision, issuing prescriptions for only one day's supply to ensure daily contact and to minimise the risk of abuse. And if the patient shows evidence of tolerance or clomethiazole dependency or of continuing to drink alcohol, the only safe policy is rapid admission for inpatient care.[1] The manufacturer warns that alcohol combined with clomethiazole particularly in alcoholics with cirrhosis can lead to fatal respiratory depression even with short-term use.[5]

(b) Effects on driving and related skills

There do not appear to be any studies on the combined effects of clomethiazole and alcohol on driving and related skills, but concurrent use would be expected to increase the risks.

There is a report of a man who had a blood-alcohol level of 23 mg% who was driving dangerously and caused a traffic accident. The clinical signs of impairment were far greater than expected and further analysis of the blood sample identified a high level of clomethiazole (5 mg/L). In 13 other impaired driving cases where clomethiazole was detected in blood samples, the concentrations ranged from 0.3 to 3.3 mg/L.[7] The manufacturer warns that clomethiazole may potentiate or be potentiated by CNS depressant drugs, including alcohol.[5]

1. McInnes GT. Chlormethiazole and alcohol: a lethal cocktail. *BMJ* (1987) 294, 592.
2. Neuvonen PJ, Pentikäinen PJ, Jostell KG, Syvälahti E. The pharmacokinetics of chlormethiazole in healthy subjects as affected by ethanol. *Clin Pharmacol Ther* (1981) 29, 268–9.
3. Pentikäinen PJ, Neuvonen PJ, Tarpila S, Syvälahti E. Effect of cirrhosis of the liver on the pharmacokinetics of chlormethiazole. *BMJ* (1978) 2, 861–3.
4. Bury RW, Desmond PV, Mashford ML, Westwood B, Shaw G, Breen KJ. The effect of ethanol administration on the disposition and elimination of chlormethiazole. *Eur J Clin Pharmacol* (1983) 24, 383–5.
5. Heminevrin Capsules (Clomethiazole). AstraZeneca UK Ltd. UK Summary of product characteristics, April 2007.
6. Morgan MY. The management of alcohol withdrawal using chlormethiazole. *Alcohol Alcohol* (1995) 30, 771–4.
7. Jones, AW. Driving under the influence of chlormethiazole. *Forensic Sci Int* (2005) 153, 213–17.

Alcohol + Cloral hydrate

Both alcohol and cloral hydrate are CNS depressants, and their effects may be at least additive, or possibly even synergistic. Some patients may experience a disulfiram-like flushing reaction if they drink alcohol after taking cloral hydrate for several days.

Clinical evidence

Studies in 5 healthy subjects given cloral hydrate 15 mg/kg and alcohol 0.5 g/kg found that both drugs given alone impaired their ability to carry out complex motor tasks. When taken together, the effects were additive, and possibly even more than additive. After taking cloral hydrate for 7 days, one of the subjects experienced a disulfiram-like reaction (bright red-purple flushing of the face, tachycardia, hypotension, anxiety and persistent headache) after drinking alcohol.[1,2]

The disulfiram-like reaction has been described in other reports.[3] Note that the earliest report was published more than a century ago in 1872 and described two patients taking cloral hydrate who experienced this reaction after drinking half a bottle of beer.[2]

Mechanism

Alcohol, cloral and trichloroethanol (to which cloral hydrate is metabolised) are all CNS depressants. During concurrent use, the metabolic pathways used for their elimination are mutually inhibited: blood-alcohol levels rise because the trichloroethanol competitively depresses the oxidation of alcohol to acetaldehyde, while trichloroethanol levels also rise because its production from cloral hydrate is increased and its further conversion and clearance as the glucuronide is inhibited. As a result the rises in the blood levels of alcohol and trichloroethanol are exaggerated, and their effects are accordingly greater.[1,2,4,5] In one subject, blood levels of acetaldehyde during the use of cloral hydrate with alcohol were only 50% of those after alcohol alone, so that the flushing reaction, despite its resemblance to the disulfiram reaction, may possibly have a partially different basis.[2]

Importance and management

A well-documented and established interaction, which has been comprehensively reviewed.[1,2] Only a few references are given here. Patients given cloral hydrate should be warned about the extensive CNS depression that can occur if they drink, and of the disulfiram-like reaction that may occur after taking cloral hydrate for a period of time. Its incidence is uncertain. The legendary Mickey Finn, which is concocted of cloral hydrate and alcohol, is reputed to be so potent that deep sleep can be induced in an unsuspecting victim within minutes of ingestion, but the evidence seems to be largely anecdotal. Very large doses of both drugs would be likely to cause serious and potentially life-threatening CNS depression.

It seems likely that **cloral betaine**, **triclofos** and other compounds closely related to cloral hydrate will interact with alcohol in a similar manner, but this requires confirmation.

1. Sellers EM, Lang M, Koch-Weser J, LeBlanc E, Kalant H. Interaction of chloral hydrate and ethanol in man. I. Metabolism. *Clin Pharmacol Ther* (1972) 13, 37–49.
2. Sellers EM, Carr G, Bernstein JG, Sellers S, Koch-Weser J. Interaction of chloral hydrate and ethanol in man. II. Hemodynamics and performance. *Clin Pharmacol Ther* (1972) 13, 50–8.
3. Bardoděj Z. Intolerance alkoholu po chloralhydrátu. *Cesk Farm* (1965) 14, 478–81.
4. Wong LK, Biemann K. A study of drug interaction by gas chromatography–mass spectrometry—synergism of chloral hydrate and ethanol. *Biochem Pharmacol* (1978) 27, 1019–22.
5. Weller RA, Preskorn SH. Psychotropic drugs and alcohol: pharmacokinetic and pharmacodynamic interactions. *Psychosomatics* (1984) 25, 301–3, 305–6, 309.

Alcohol + CNS depressants

The concurrent use of small or moderate amounts of alcohol and therapeutic doses of drugs that are CNS depressants can increase drowsiness and reduce alertness. These drugs include antidepressants, antiemetics, antiepileptics, antihistamines, antipsychotics, anxiolytics, barbiturates, hypnotics, opioid analgesics, skeletal muscle relaxants, and others. This increases the risk of accident when driving or handling other potentially dangerous machinery, and may make the performance of everyday tasks more difficult and hazardous.

Clinical evidence, mechanism, importance and management

Alcohol is a CNS depressant (see 'alcohol', (p.40)). With only small or moderate amounts of alcohol and with blood-alcohol levels well within legal driving limits, it may be quite unsafe to drive if another CNS depressant is being taken concurrently. The details of most of the drugs that have been tested are set out in the monographs in this section, but there are others that nobody seems to have tested formally. The summary above contains a list of some of those that commonly cause drowsiness. Quite apart from driving, almost everyone meets potentially dangerous situations every day at home, in the garden, in the street and at work. Crossing a busy street or even walking downstairs can become much more risky under the influence of CNS depressant drugs and alcohol. Elderly patients may be particularly susceptible.[1] A cause for concern is that patients may be partially or totally unaware of the extent of the deterioration in their skills: they should be warned.

1. Gerbino PP. Complications of alcohol use combined with drug therapy in the elderly. *J Am Geriatr Soc* (1982) 30 (11 Suppl), S88–S93.

Alcohol + Cocaine

Alcohol increases cocaine levels and the active metabolite cocaethylene. Subjective effects such as euphoria are enhanced and some of the CNS-depressant effects of alcohol, such as sedation, are attenuated by cocaine. The combination may be potentially more toxic, with increased cardiovascular effects particularly heart rate. The use of alcohol with cocaine may increase violent behaviour.

Clinical evidence

A study in 8 cocaine users found that intranasal cocaine 100 mg and alcohol 0.8 g/kg produced a greater euphoria and feeling of well-being than cocaine alone, and reduced alcohol sedation without altering the feeling of drunkenness. Compared with placebo, the peak heart-rate was increased by 17, 23, and 41 bpm, with alcohol, cocaine, or the combination, respectively. In addition, the combination resulted in higher plasma levels of cocaine and the appearance of cocaethylene, an active and potentially toxic metabolite produced by the interaction of the two drugs.[1] Another similar study with intranasal cocaine 1 mg/kg every 30 minutes for 4 doses and oral alcohol 1 g/kg reported very similar findings.[2] A further study found that intranasal cocaine 96 mg/70 kg improved behavioural performance, measured by the digit symbol substitution test (DSST), whereas alcohol 1 g/kg decreased DSST performance. The combination of alcohol 1 g/kg with intranasal cocaine 48 or 96 mg/70 kg reduced the DSST below that found with cocaine alone. The combination also additively increased heart rate and diastolic blood pressure. The blood-alcohol levels were not significantly affected by the concurrent use of intranasal cocaine.[3]

Mechanism

In the presence of alcohol, cocaine is metabolised in the liver to cocaethylene which appears to have the same stimulant effects as cocaine, but a longer half-life (2 hours compared with about 38 minutes for cocaine). *Animal* studies suggest that this metabolite is more toxic than cocaine.[4] In addition, chronic alcohol exposure may facilitate the metabolism of cocaine, promoting the formation of intermediate metabolites that may cause liver damage, potentiating the hepatotoxic properties of alcohol.[5]

Importance and management

It has been suggested that the enhanced psychological effects associated with alcohol and cocaine may lead to the use of larger amounts of the combination with an increased risk for toxic effects,[2] such as cardiotoxicity.[1] It has been reported that users of alcohol and cocaine who also have coronary artery disease have 21.5 times the risk for sudden death than users of cocaine alone.[4] The longer half-life of the metabolite cocaethylene explains why many people who experience cocaine-related heart attacks and strokes do so when the cocaine levels in their blood are low, as cocaethylene can remain active in the body for 7 hours after cocaine has disappeared.[4] Patients with coronary artery disease or alcoholics may be particularly vulnerable to the combined toxic effects of alcohol and cocaine.

1. Farré M, de la Torre R, González ML, Terán MT, Roset PN, Menoyo E, Camí J. Cocaine and alcohol interactions in humans: neuroendocrine effects and cocaethylene metabolism. *J Pharmacol Exp Ther* (1997) 283, 164–76.
2. McCance-Katz EF, Kosten TR, Jatlow P. Concurrent use of cocaine and alcohol is more potent and potentially more toxic than use of either alone--a multiple-dose study. *Biol Psychiatry* (1998) 44, 250–9.
3. Higgins ST, Rush CR, Bickel WK, Hughes JR, Lynn M, Capeless MA. Acute behavioral and cardiac effects of cocaine and alcohol combinations in humans. *Psychopharmacology (Berl)* (1993) 111, 285–94.
4. Randall T. Cocaine, alcohol mix in body to form even longer lasting, more lethal drug. *JAMA* (1992) 267, 1043–4.
5. Hoyumpa AM. Alcohol interactions with benzodiazepines and cocaine. *Adv Alcohol Subst Abuse* (1984) 3, 21–34.

Alcohol + Codergocrine mesilate (Ergoloid mesylates)

Codergocrine mesilate causes a very small reduction in blood-alcohol levels.

Clinical evidence, mechanism, importance and management

Thirteen subjects were given 0.5 g/kg of alcohol 25% in orange juice after breakfast, before and after taking 4.5 mg of codergocrine mesilate (ergoloid mesylates, *Hydergine*) every 8 hours for nine doses. The codergocrine caused a small reduction in blood-alcohol levels (maximum serum levels reduced from 59 mg% to 55.7 mg%), and the clearance was reduced by a modest 11%.[1] The reason is not understood. This interaction is almost certainly not of clinical importance.

1. Savage IT, James IM. The effect of Hydergine on ethanol pharmacokinetics in man. *J Pharm Pharmacol* (1993) 45 (Suppl 2), 1119.

Alcohol + Cyproterone acetate

Excessive alcohol consumption may reduce the antiandrogenic effect of cyproterone acetate in the treatment of hypersexuality, but the relevance of this in prostatic carcinoma is not known; there seems to be no evidence that normal social amounts of alcohol interact.

Clinical evidence, mechanism, importance and management

The UK manufacturer of cyproterone acetate says that alcohol appears to reduce its effects, and so it is of no value in chronic alcoholics.[1] This appears to be based solely on a simple and unelaborated statement in an abstract of studies[2] in 84 men whose hyper- or abnormal sexuality was treated with cyproterone acetate, which stated that "antiandrogens do not inhibit male sexual behaviour during alcohol excess."

The suggested reasons for this reaction are unknown, but it may possibly be due to several factors. These include enzyme induction by the alcohol, which could possibly increase the metabolism and clearance of cyproterone; increased sexual drive caused by alcohol, which might oppose the effects of cyproterone; and reduced compliance by alcoholic patients who forget to take their tablets while drinking to excess.[3]

It seems therefore that cyproterone may not be effective in alcoholic patients, but there is nothing to suggest that the effects of cyproterone are opposed by normal moderate social amounts of alcohol. The relevance of this in prostatic carcinoma is not known, nevertheless, it has been suggested that the use of alcohol during treatment with cyproterone acetate is not advisable.[4] It would seem prudent to limit alcohol intake in patients taking cyproterone.

1. Androcur (Cyproterone acetate). Schering Health Care Ltd. UK Summary of product characteristics, April 2004.
2. Laschet U, Laschet L. Three years clinical results with cyproterone-acetate in the inhibiting regulation of male sexuality. *Acta Endocrinol (Copenh)* (1969) 138 (Suppl), 103.
3. Schering Health Care Limited. Personal communication, January 1997.
4. Androcur (Cyproterone acetate). Bayer Inc. Canadian Prescribing information, March 2007.

Alcohol + Dimethylformamide

A disulfiram-like reaction can occur in workers exposed to dimethylformamide vapour if they drink alcohol; incidences of 20% and 70% have been reported. Alcohol may possibly enhance the toxic effects of dimethylformamide on liver function.

Clinical evidence

A 3-year study in a chemical plant where dimethylformamide (DMF) was used found that about 20% (19 out of 102 men) exposed to DMF vapour experienced flushing of the face, and often of the neck, arms, hands, and chest, after drinking alcohol. Sometimes dizziness, nausea and tightness of the chest also occurred. A single glass of beer was enough to induce a flush lasting 2 hours. The majority of the men experienced the reaction within 24 hours of exposure to DMF, but it could occur even after 4 days.[1] Three further cases of this interaction are described in other reports.[2,3]

One study in 126 factory workers exposed to DMF and 54 workers who had no contact with DMF indicated that DMF adversely affected liver function, and that concurrent alcohol had a synergistic effect (both drugs are hepatotoxic), although individual differences in tolerance to the interaction were observed. Flush symptoms after alcohol consumption were reported by 86 out of 126 (approximately 70%) of workers exposed to DMF, compared with 2 out of 54 (4%) of controls.[4]

Mechanism

Subjects exposed to DMF vapour develop substantial amounts of DMF and its metabolite (*N*-methylformamide) in their blood and urine.[1] This latter compound in particular has been shown in *rats* given alcohol to raise their blood acetaldehyde levels by a factor of five, so it would seem probable that the *N*-methylformamide is similarly responsible for this disulfiram-like reaction in man (see 'Alcohol + Disulfiram', p.61).[5]

Importance and management

An established interaction, with the incidence reported to be between about 20% and 70%.[1] Those who come into contact with DMF, even in very low concentrations, should be warned of this possible interaction with alcohol. It would appear to be more unpleasant than serious in most instances, and normally requires no treatment, however the hepatotoxic effects are clearly more of a concern.

1. Lyle WH, Spence TWM, McKinneley WM, Duckers K. Dimethylformamide and alcohol intolerance. *Br J Ind Med* (1979) 36, 63–6.
2. Chivers CP. Disulfiram effect from inhalation of dimethylformamide. *Lancet* (1978) i, 331.
3. Reinl W, Urban HJ. Erkrankungen durch dimethylformamid. *Int Arch Gewerbepathol Gewerbehyg* (1965) 21, 333–46.
4. Wrbitzky R. Liver function in workers exposed to *N,N*-dimethylformamide during the production of synthetic textiles. *Int Arch Occup Environ Health* (1999) 72, 19–25.
5. Hanasono GK, Fuller RW, Broddle WD, Gibson WR. Studies on the effects of *N,N'*-dimethylformamide on ethanol disposition and monoamine oxidase activity in rats. *Toxicol Appl Pharmacol* (1977) 39, 461–72.

Alcohol + Disopyramide

In healthy subjects, the renal clearance of disopyramide may be slightly increased by alcohol-induced diuresis.

Clinical evidence, mechanism, importance and management

A crossover study in 6 healthy subjects found that the half-life and total body clearance of disopyramide were not affected by alcohol, but the amount of the metabolite mono-*N*-dealkylated disopyramide excreted in the urine was reduced. Alcohol increased diuresis in 5 of the 6 subjects, and the renal clearance of disopyramide was increased by 19% in these subjects.[1] The overall clinical effect is likely to be minimal.

1. Olsen H, Bredesen JE, Lunde PKM. Effect of ethanol intake on disopyramide elimination by healthy volunteers. *Eur J Clin Pharmacol* (1983) 25, 103–5.

Alcohol + Disulfiram

The ingestion of alcohol while taking disulfiram will result in flushing and fullness of the face and neck, tachycardia, breathlessness, giddiness, hypotension, and nausea and vomiting. This is called the disulfiram or *Antabuse* reaction. It is used to deter alcoholic patients from drinking. A mild flushing reaction of the skin may possibly occur in particularly sensitive individuals if alcohol is applied to the skin or if the vapour is inhaled.

Clinical evidence

(a) Alcoholic drinks

One of the earliest descriptions of this toxic interaction was made in 1937 by Dr EE Williams[1] who noted it amongst workers in the rubber industry who were handling **tetramethylthiuram disulphide**:

"Even beer will cause a flushing of the face and hands, with rapid pulse, and some of the men describe palpitations and a terrible fullness of the face, eyes and head. After a glass of beer the blood pressure falls about 10 points, the pulse is slightly accelerated and the skin becomes flushed in the face and wrists. In 15 minutes the blood pressure falls another 10 points, the heart is more rapid, and the patient complains of fullness in the head."

The later observation[2] by Hald and his colleagues of the same reaction with the ethyl congener of **tetramethylthiuram disulphide**, disulfiram, led to its introduction as an alcoholic drink deterrent. Patients experience throbbing in head and neck, giddiness, sweating, nausea, vomiting, thirst, chest pain, difficulty in breathing, and headache. The severity of the reaction can depend upon the amount of alcohol ingested, but some individuals are extremely sensitive. Respiratory depression, cardiovascular collapse, cardiac arrhythmias, unconsciousness, and convulsions may occur. There have been fatalities.[3]

An unusual and isolated report describes painful, intermittent and transient myoclonic jerking of the arms and legs as the predominant manifestation of the disulfiram reaction in one patient.[4] Another unusual case has been reported in which a woman with a history of bipolar disorder and alcoholism, who was taking disulfiram, was admitted to hospital with a 3- to 4-day history of changes in her mental state, including difficulties with orientation, concentration and visual hallucinations. The confusional state was attributed to alcohol consumption while taking disulfiram, and the probability of this was supported by an earlier similar, though shorter, episode experienced by the patient.[5] Some alcoholics find that disulfiram potentiates the euphoric effects of low doses of alcohol, which alone would be relatively ineffective.[6]

(b) Products containing alcohol

A mild disulfiram reaction is said to occur in some patients who apply alcohol to the skin, but it is probably largely due to inhalation of the vapour.[7] It has been reported after using **after-shave lotion** (50% alcohol),[7] **tar gel** (33% alcohol)[8] and a **beer-containing shampoo** (3% alcohol).[9] A **contact lens wetting solution** (containing **polyvinyl alcohol**) used to irrigate the eye has also been implicated in a reaction,[10,11] although the probability of an interaction with this secondary alcohol has been disputed.[12] It has also been described in a patient who inhaled vapour from paint in a poorly ventilated area and from the inhalation of '**mineral spirits**'.[13] Furthermore, an unusual case describes a woman taking disulfiram who reported vaginal stinging and soreness during sexual intercourse, and similar discomfort to her husband's penis, which seemed to be related to the disulfiram dosage and how intoxicated her husband was.[14]

The UK manufacturer of the oral solution of **ritonavir** *(Norvir)* says that since it contains alcohol 43% v/v (which they say is about equivalent to 27 mL of wine per dose) the preparation should not be taken with disulfiram or other drugs such as **metronidazole** because a disulfiram-like reaction is possible.[15] However, in practice the risk is probably fairly small because the recommended dose of **ritonavir** in this form is only 7.5 mL. **Ritonavir** *(Norvir)* soft capsules also contain alcohol 12% w/w.[16] The oral concentrate of sertraline *(Zoloft oral concentrate)* is contraindicated with disulfiram due to the alcohol content (12%).[17]

Mechanism

Partially understood. Alcohol is normally rapidly metabolised within the liver, firstly by alcohol dehydrogenase to acetaldehyde, then by acetaldehyde dehydrogenase, and then by a series of biochemical steps to water and carbon dioxide. Disulfiram inhibits the enzyme acetaldehyde dehydrogenase so that the acetaldehyde accumulates.[3] The symptoms of the disulfiram-alcohol reaction are due partly to the high levels of acetaldehyde. However, not all of the symptoms can be reproduced by injecting acetaldehyde, so that some other biochemical mechanism(s) must also be involved. The conversion of dopamine to noradrenaline is also inhibited and the depletion of noradrenaline in the heart and blood vessels allows acetaldehyde to act directly on these tissues to cause flushing, tachycardia and hypotension.[18] Prostaglandin release may also be involved.[19] It has been suggested that the mild skin flush that can occur if alcohol is applied to the skin is not a true disulfiram reaction.[20]

However, some individuals appear to be more sensitive than others, which might be partially due to liver function and variations in the metabolism of disulfiram to its active metabolite by the cytochrome P450 isoenzymes.[21,22] Disulfiram is eliminated slowly from the body and ingestion of alcohol may produce unpleasant symptoms up to 14 days after taking the last dose of disulfiram.[23]

Importance and management

An extremely well-documented and important interaction exploited therapeutically to deter alcoholics from drinking alcohol. Initial treatment should be closely supervised because an extremely intense and potentially serious reaction occurs in a few individuals, even with quite small doses of alcohol. Apart from the usual warnings about drinking alcohol, patients should also be warned about the unwitting ingestion of alcohol in some pharmaceutical preparations.[24] The risk of a reaction is real. It has been seen following a single-dose of an alcohol-containing **cough mixture**,[25] whereas the ingestion of small amounts of **communion wine** and the absorption of alcohol from a **bronchial nebuliser spray** or **ear drops** did not result in any reaction in 3 individuals.[26] The severity of the reaction is reported to be proportional to the dosage of both disulfiram and alcohol.[23] Patients should also be warned about the exposure to alcohol from some foods, cosmetics, solvents etc. The manufacturers advise that certain foods (sauces and vinegars), liquid medicines, remedies (cough mixtures, tonics, back rubs), and toiletries (aftershave, perfumes and aerosol sprays) may contain sufficient alcohol to elicit a reaction.[18,23] Caution should also be exercised with low-alcohol and "non-alcohol" or "alcohol-free" beers and wines, which may provoke a reaction when consumed in sufficient quantities.[18]

Treatment

The disulfiram reaction can be treated, if necessary, with ascorbic acid. A dose of 1 g given orally is reported to be effective in mild cases (heart rate less than 100 bpm and general condition good). It works within 30 to 45 minutes. Moderately severe cases (heart rate 100 to 150 bpm, blood pressure 150/100 mmHg) can be treated with 1 g of intravenous ascorbic acid and this is effective within 2 to 5 minutes. Critically ill patients may need other standard supportive emergency measures.[27]

1. Williams EE. Effects of alcohol on workers with carbon disulfide. *JAMA* (1937) 109, 1472.
2. Hald J, Jacobsen E, Larsen V. The sensitizing effects of tetraethylthiuramdisulphide (Antabuse) to ethylalcohol. *Acta Pharmacol* (1948) 4, 285–96.
3. Kwentus J, Major LF. Disulfiram in the treatment of alcoholism: a review. *J Stud Alcohol* (1979) 40, 428–46.
4. Syed J, Moarefi G. An unusual presentation of a disulfiram-alcohol reaction. *Del Med J* (1995) 67, 183.
5. Park CW, Riggio S. Disulfiram-ethanol induced delirium. *Ann Pharmacother* (2001) 35, 32–5.
6. Brown ZW, Amit Z, Smith BR, Sutherland EA, Selvaggi N. Alcohol-induced euphoria enhanced by disulfiram and calcium carbimide. *Alcohol Clin Exp Res* (1983) 7, 276–8.
7. Mercurio F. Antabuse®-alcohol reaction following the use of after-shave lotion. *JAMA* (1952) 149, 82.
8. Ellis CN, Mitchell AJ, Beardsley GR. Tar gel interaction with disulfiram. *Arch Dermatol* (1979) 115, 1367–8.
9. Stoll D, King LE. Disulfiram-alcohol skin reaction to beer-containing shampoo. *JAMA* (1980) 244, 2045.
10. Newsom SR, Harper BS. Disulfiram-alcohol reaction caused by contact lens wetting solution. *Contact Intraocul Lens Med J* (1980) 6, 407–8.
11. Newsom SR. Letter to the editor. *Contact Intraocul Lens Med J* (1981) 7, 172.
12. Refojo MF. Letter to Editor. *Contact Intraocul Lens Med J* (1981) 7, 172.
13. Scott GE, Little FW. Disulfiram reaction to organic solvents other than ethanol. *N Engl J Med* (1985) 312, 790.
14. Chick JD. Disulfiram reaction during sexual intercourse. *Br J Psychiatry* (1988) 152, 438.

15. Norvir Oral Solution (Ritonavir). Abbott Laboratories Ltd. UK Summary of product characteristics, May 2007.
16. Norvir Soft Capsules (Ritonavir). Abbott Laboratories Ltd. UK Summary of product characteristics, May 2007.
17. Zoloft (Sertraline hydrochloride). Pfizer Inc. US Prescribing information, June 2007.
18. Antabuse (Disulfiram). Actavis UK Ltd. UK Summary of product characteristics, August 1999.
19. Truitt EB, Gaynor CR, Mehl DL. Aspirin attenuation of alcohol-induced flushing and intoxication in oriental and occidental subjects. *Alcohol Alcohol* (1987) 22 (Suppl 1), 595–9.
20. Haddock NF, Wilkin JK. Cutaneous reactions to lower aliphatic alcohols before and during disulfiram therapy. *Arch Dermatol* (1982) 118, 157–9.
21. Poikolainen K. The disulfiram-ethanol reaction (DER) experience. *Addiction* (2004) 99, 26.
22. Beyeler C, Fisch H-U, Preisig R. The disulfiram-alcohol reaction: factors determining and potential tests predicting severity. *Alcohol Clin Exp Res* (1985) 9, 118–24.
23. Antabuse (Disulfiram). Odyssey Pharmaceuticals, Inc. US Prescribing information, December 2003.
24. Parker WA. Alcohol-containing pharmaceuticals. *Am J Drug Alcohol Abuse* (1982–3) 9, 195–209.
25. Koff RS, Papadimas I, Honig EG. Alcohol in cough medicines: hazards to the disulfiram user. *JAMA* (1971) 215, 1988–9.
26. Rothstein E. Use of disulfiram (Antabuse) in alcoholism. *N Engl J Med* (1970) 283, 936.
27. McNichol RW, Sowell JM, Logsdon SA, Delgado MH, McNichol J. Disulfiram: a guide to clinical use in alcoholism treatment. *Am Fam Physician* (1991) 44, 481–4.

Alcohol + Ecstasy

Ecstasy may reduce subjective sedation associated with alcohol, without reversing the effects of alcohol on impulsivity or psychomotor skills. Alcohol may enhance the transient immune dysfunction associated with ecstasy. Alcohol may slightly increase the plasma levels of ecstasy, while alcohol levels may be slightly reduced by ecstasy.

Clinical evidence, mechanism, importance and management

Note that the chemical name of ecstasy is methylenedioxymethamphetamine (MDMA).

(a) Effect on behaviour or psychomotor skills

A study in 9 healthy subjects found that the combination of alcohol 0.8 g/kg and ecstasy 100 mg induced a longer lasting euphoria and sense of well-being than either ecstasy or alcohol alone. Ecstasy reversed the subjective feelings of sedation associated with alcohol, but did not reverse feelings of drunkenness, or the effects of alcohol on psychomotor performance.[1] Similarly, in a double-blind, placebo-controlled, crossover study in 18 recreational users of ecstasy, alcohol-induced impairment in response inhibition tasks was not affected by single 75- or 100-mg doses of ecstasy. This indicated that the CNS-stimulating effects of ecstasy do not overcome alcohol-induced impairment of impulse-control or risk-taking behaviour.[2] This may have implications for road safety, as subjects may consider they are driving better when actual performance is impaired by alcohol.[1] More study is needed. Consider also 'Alcohol + Amfetamines', p.42.

(b) Effect on immune system

A study in 6 healthy subjects found that a single dose of ecstasy produced a time-dependent immune dysfunction. Ecstasy impaired CD4 T-cell function, which is responsible for cellular immunity. Alcohol alone may produce a decrease in T-helper cells and in B lymphocytes, which are responsible for humoral immunity. Concurrent ecstasy and alcohol increased the suppressive effect of ecstasy on CD4 T-cells and increased natural killer cells. It was suggested that the transient defect in immunological homoeostasis could have clinical consequences such as increased susceptibility to infectious diseases.[3] More study is needed.

(c) Pharmacokinetic studies

A study in 9 healthy subjects found that alcohol 0.8 g/kg increased the maximum plasma levels of a single 100-mg dose of ecstasy by 13%, with no change in AUC. The AUC and maximum plasma levels of alcohol were reduced by 9% and 15%, respectively, after ecstasy use.[1] Another single-dose study in 18 recreational users of ecstasy found a similar decrease in mean blood-alcohol levels and a small increase in ecstasy levels when the two drugs were given together, but the results were not statistically significant.[2]

1. Hernández-López C, Farré M, Roset PN, Menoyo E, Pizarro N, Ortuño J, Torrens M, Camí J, de la Torre R. 3,4-Methylenedioxymethamphetamine (Ecstasy) and alcohol interactions in humans: psychomotor performance, subjective effects, and pharmacokinetics. *J Pharmacol Exp Ther* (2002) 300, 236–44.
2. Ramaekers JG, Kuypers KPC. Acute effects of 3,4-methylenedioxymethamphetamine (MDMA) on behavioral measures of impulsivity: alone and in combination with alcohol. *Neuropsychopharmacology* (2006) 31, 1048–55.
3. Pacifici R, Zuccaro P, Hernández López C, Pichini S, Di Carlo S, Farré M, Roset PN, Ortuño J, Segura J, de la Torre R. Acute effects of 3,4-methylenedioxymethamphetamine alone and in combination with ethanol on the immune system in humans. *J Pharmacol Exp Ther* (2001) 296, 207–15.

Alcohol + Edible fungi

A disulfiram-like reaction can occur if alcohol is taken after eating the smooth ink(y) cap fungus (*Coprinus atramentarius*) or certain other edible fungi.

Clinical evidence

A man who drank 3 pints of **beer** 2 hours after eating a meal of freshly picked and fried **ink(y) caps** (***Coprinus atramentarius***) developed facial flushing and a blotchy red rash over the upper half of his body. His face and hands swelled and he became breathless, sweated profusely, and vomited during the 3 hours when the reaction was most severe. On admission to hospital he was tachycardic and 12 hours later he was in atrial fibrillation, which lasted for 60 hours. The man's wife, who ate the same meal but without an alcoholic drink, did not show the reaction.[1]

This reaction has been described on many occasions in medical and pharmacological reports[2-7] and in books devoted to descriptions of edible and poisonous fungi. Only a few are listed here. Mild hypotension and ". . .alarming orthostatic features. . ." are said to be common symptoms[8] but the arrhythmia seen in the case cited here[1] appears to be rare. Recovery is usually spontaneous and uncomplicated. A similar reaction has been described after eating ***Boletus luridus***,[6,9] and other fungi including ***Coprinus micaceus***, ***Clitocybe claviceps*** and certain **morels**.[9,10] An African relative of ***Coprinus atramentarius***, ***Coprinus africanus***, which also causes this reaction, is called the **Ajeimutin** fungus by the Nigerian Yoruba people. The literal translation of this name is the 'eat-without-drinking-alcohol' mushroom.[11]

Mechanism

An early and attractive idea was that the reaction with *Coprinus atramentarius* was due to the presence of disulfiram (one group of workers actually claimed to have isolated it from the fungus[12]), but this was not confirmed by later work,[13,14] and it now appears that the active ingredient is coprine (*N*-5-(1-hydroxycyclopropyl)-glutamine).[15,16] This is metabolised in the body to 1-aminocyclopropanol, which appears, like disulfiram, to inhibit aldehyde dehydrogenase (see 'Alcohol + Disulfiram', p.61). The active ingredients in the other fungi are unknown.

Importance and management

An established and well-documented interaction. It is said to occur up to 24 hours after eating the fungus. The intensity depends upon the quantity of fungus and alcohol consumed, and the time interval between them.[1,4,17] Despite the widespread consumption of edible fungi and alcohol, reports of this reaction in the medical literature are few and far between, suggesting that even though it can be very unpleasant and frightening, the outcome is usually uncomplicated. Treatment appears normally not to be necessary.

The related fungus ***Coprinus comatus*** (the '**shaggy ink cap**' or '**Lawyers wig**') is said not to interact with alcohol,[8,18] nor is there anything to suggest that it ever occurs with the **common field mushroom** (***Agaricus campestris***) or the cultivated variety (***Agaricus bisporis***).[18]

1. Caley MJ, Clarke RA. Cardiac arrhythmia after mushroom ingestion. *BMJ* (1977) 2, 1633.
2. Reynolds WA, Lowe FH. Mushrooms and a toxic reaction to alcohol: report of four cases. *N Engl J Med* (1965) 272, 630–1.
3. Wildervanck LS. Alcohol en de kale inktzwam. *Ned Tijdschr Geneeskd* (1978) 122, 913–14.
4. Buck RW. Mushroom toxins—a brief review of the literature. *N Engl J Med* (1961) 265, 681–6.
5. Marty H. Von Pilzen und Schnäpsen. *Schweiz Med Wochenschr* (1998) 128, 598.
6. Flammer R. Brechdurchfälle als Leitsymptom – Pilze und Alkohol. Emesis and diarrhea – mushrooms and alcohol. *Schweiz Rundsch Med Prax* (1985) 74, 992–6.
7. Oteo Revuelta JA, Grandival García R, Olarte Arce A. Reaccíon disulfiram-like por ingesta de hongos [Disulfiram-like reaction caused by mushroom ingestion]. *Rev Clin Esp* (1989) 184, 394–5.
8. Broadhurst-Zingrich L. Ink caps and alcohol. *BMJ* (1978) 1, 511.
9. Budmiger H, Kocher F. Hexenröhrling (Boletus luridus) mit Alkohol: ein kasuistischer beitrag. *Schweiz Med Wochenschr* (1982) 112, 1179–81.
10. Cochran KW, Cochran MW. *Clitocybe clavipes:* antabuse-like reaction to alcohol. *Mycologia* (1978) 70, 1124–6.
11. Oso BA. Mushrooms and the Yoruba people of Nigeria. *Mycologia* (1975) 67, 311–19.

12. Simandl J, Franc J. Isolace tetraethylthiuramdisulfidu z hníku inko ustového (*Coprinus atramentarius*). *Chem Listy* (1956) 50, 1862–3.
13. Vanhaelen M, Vanhaelen-Fastré R, Hoyois J, Mardens Y. Reinvestigation of disulfiram-like biological activity of *Coprinus atramentarius* (Bull. *ex* Fr.) Fr. extracts. *J Pharm Sci* (1976) 65, 1774–6.
14. Wier JK, Tyler VE. An investigation of *Coprinus atramentarius* for the presence of disulfiram. *J Am Pharm Assoc* (1960) 49, 426–9.
15. Hatfield GM, Schaumberg JP. Isolation and structural studies of coprine, the disulfiram-like constituent of *Coprinus atramentarius*. *Lloydia* (1975) 38, 489–96.
16. Lindberg P, Bergman R, Wickberg B. Isolation and structure of coprine, the *in vivo* aldehyde dehydrogenase inhibitor in *Coprinus atramentarius*; syntheses of coprine and related cyclopropanone derivatives. *J Chem Soc* (1977) (6) 684–91.
17. Fujiyama Y, Naitoh M, Nakamura M, Minezaki K, Shigeta Y, Okubo M. [Mushroom poisoning whose symptoms were relevant to the amount of alcohol taken]. *Nippon Naika Gakkai Zasshi* (2002) 91, 2189–91.
18. Radford AP. Ink caps and mushrooms. *BMJ* (1978) 1, 112.

Alcohol + Fluvastatin

Alcohol does not significantly interact with fluvastatin.

Clinical evidence, mechanism, importance and management

Ten healthy subjects took a single 40-mg dose of fluvastatin and 70 g of alcohol diluted in lemonade. This acute ingestion of alcohol had no effect on the peak serum levels of fluvastatin or its AUC, but the half-life was reduced by almost one-third.[1] In a second related study, 20 patients with hypercholesterolaemia were given 40 mg of fluvastatin and 20 g of alcohol daily for 6 weeks. The AUC of fluvastatin was slightly increased and the half-life was increased by almost one-third, but the lipid profile with fluvastatin plus alcohol was little different from fluvastatin alone.[1,2] The conclusion was reached that although long-term moderate drinking has some small effect on the pharmacokinetics of fluvastatin, its safety and efficacy are unaltered.[1] There would seem to be no reason for patients taking fluvastatin to avoid alcohol.

1. Smit JWA, Wijnne HJA, Schobben F, Sitsen A, de Bruin TWA, Erkelens DW. Effects of alcohol consumption on pharmacokinetics, efficacy, and safety of fluvastatin. *Am J Cardiol* (1995) 76, 89A–96A.
2. Smit JW, Wijnne HJ, Schobben F, Sitsen A, De Bruin TW, Erkelens DW. Effects of alcohol and fluvastatin on lipid metabolism and hepatic function. *Ann Intern Med* (1995) 122, 678–80.

Alcohol + Food

Food and milk decrease the absorption of alcohol and meals increase the metabolism of alcohol. Foods rich in serotonin (e.g. bananas) taken with alcohol may produce adverse effects such as diarrhoea and headache. Previous alcohol consumption and the glycaemic load of a meal appear to interact to influence both mood and memory.

Clinical evidence, mechanism, importance and management

(a) Alcohol absorption and metabolism

In one study 10 subjects were given 25 mL of alcohol (equivalent to a double whiskey) after drinking a pint and a half of water or **milk** during the previous 90 minutes. Blood-alcohol levels at 90 minutes were reduced by about 40%, and at 120 minutes by about 25% by the presence of the **milk**. The intoxicant effects of the alcohol were also clearly reduced.[1] In a randomised, crossover study, 24 healthy subjects were given alcohol 0.3 g/kg either one hour before or after an **evening meal**. It was found that the maximum alcohol levels were increased by 87% from 21.3 to 39.9 mg%, and the AUC was increased by 63% when alcohol was given in the fasting rather than the fed state. However there was large inter and intra-individual variability in alcohol bioavailability.[2] Other studies have shown similar effects,[3-5] and shown that this is not limited to specific components of food,[4,5] as well as demonstrating that food reduces the feeling of intoxication and reduces the time required to eliminate alcohol from the body.[3]

After food, the rate of gastric emptying is slower, and hepatic blood flow and the activities of alcohol-metabolising enzymes are increased, which allows greater first-pass metabolism of alcohol. Thus, the effects of alcohol are greatest when taken on an empty stomach.

(b) Dietary serotonin

Serotonin (5-hydroxytryptamine, 5-HT) is excreted in the urine as 5-hydroxyindole-3-acetic acid (5-HIAA) and 5-hydroxytryptophol (5-HTOL) and the ratio of 5-HTOL to 5-HIAA is normally very low (less than 0.01). A study in 10 healthy subjects found that 4 hours after the ingestion of alcohol 0.5 g/kg the ratio was increased by about 70-fold. When the same amount of alcohol was given with 3 **bananas**, a food rich in 5-HT, the ratio was increased about 100-fold at 4 hours and was still significantly raised at 24 hours. Within 4 hours, 7 of the 10 subjects experienced adverse effects including diarrhoea, headache and fatigue. The symptoms were attributed to high levels of 5-HTOL, which is usually a minor metabolite of serotonin. Other foods rich in serotonin such as **pineapple**, **kiwi fruit** or **walnuts** may produce similar effects if taken with even moderate amounts of alcohol.[6]

(c) Glycaemic load

Breakfasts that release glucose at different speeds were found to interact with alcohol drunk the previous evening to influence cognition and mood. When less that 4.5 g of alcohol had been drunk, a breakfast high in rapidly available glucose was associated with better memory later in the morning. In contrast, when more than 4.5 g of alcohol had been drunk, a breakfast high in slowly available glucose resulted in better memory. After a high glycaemic-load lunch, the rapidly available glucose breakfast resulted in a more confused feeling than the slowly available glucose breakfast or fasting in those who had drunk more than 4.5 g of alcohol the previous evening.[7]

1. Miller DS, Stirling JL, Yudkin J. Effect of ingestion of milk on concentrations of blood alcohol. *Nature* (1966) 212, 1051.
2. Fraser AG, Rosalki SB, Gamble GD, Pounder RE. Inter-individual and intra-individual variability of ethanol concentration-time profiles: comparison of ethanol ingestion before or after an evening meal. *Br J Clin Pharmacol* (1995) 40, 387–92.
3. Jones AW, Jönsson KÅ. Food-induced lowering of blood-ethanol profiles and increased rate of elimination immediately after a meal. *J Forensic Sci* (1994) 39, 1084–93.
4. Jones AW, Jönsson KÅ, Kechagias S. Effect of high-fat, high-protein, and high-carbohydrate meals on the pharmacokinetics of a small dose of ethanol. *Br J Clin Pharmacol* (1997) 44, 521–6.
5. Ramchandani VA, Kwo PY, Li T-K. Effect of food and food composition on alcohol elimination rates in healthy men and women. *J Clin Pharmacol* (2001) 41, 1345–50.
6. Helander A, Some M. Dietary serotonin and alcohol combined may provoke adverse physiological symptoms due to 5-hydroxytryptophol. *Life Sci* (2000) 67, 799–806.
7. Benton D, Nabb S. Breakfasts that release glucose at different speeds interact with previous alcohol intake to influence cognition and mood before and after lunch. *Behav Neurosci* (2004) 118, 936–43.

Alcohol + Furazolidone

A disulfiram-like reaction may occur in patients taking furazolidone if they drink alcohol.

Clinical evidence

A patient taking furazolidone 200 mg four times daily complained of facial flushing, lachrymation, conjunctivitis, weakness, and light-headedness within 10 minutes of drinking beer. It occurred on several occasions and lasted 30 to 45 minutes.[1] A man prescribed furazolidone 100 mg four times daily and who had taken only three doses, developed intense facial flushing, wheezing and dyspnoea (lasting one hour), within one hour of drinking 2 oz (about 60 mL) of brandy. The same thing happened again the next day after drinking a *Martini* cocktail. No treatment was given.[2] A report originating from the manufacturers of furazolidone stated that by 1976, 43 cases of a disulfiram-like reaction had been reported, of which 14 were produced experimentally using above-normal doses of furazolidone.[3] A later study in 1986 described 9 out of 47 patients (19%) who complained of a disulfiram-like reaction after drinking alcohol while taking furazolidone 100 mg four times daily for 5 days.[4]

Mechanism

Uncertain. It seems possible that furazolidone acts like disulfiram by inhibiting the activity of acetaldehyde dehydrogenase (see 'Alcohol + Disulfiram', p.61).

Importance and management

An established and clinically important interaction of uncertain incidence. One report suggests that possibly about 1 in 5 may be affected.[4] Reactions of this kind appear to be more unpleasant and possibly frightening than serious, and normally need no treatment, however patients should be warned about what may happen if they drink alcohol.

1. Calesnick B. Antihypertensive action of the antimicrobial agent furazolidone. *Am J Med Sci* (1958) 236, 736–46.
2. Kolodny AL. Side-effects produced by alcohol in a patient receiving furazolidone. *Md State Med J* (1962) 11, 248.

3. Chamberlain RE. (Eaton Laboratories, Norwich Pharmacal Co.) Chemotherapeutic properties of prominent nitrofurans. *J Antimicrob Chemother* (1976) 2, 325–36.
4. DuPont HL, Ericsson CD, Reves RR, Galindo E. Antimicrobial therapy for travelers' diarrhea. *Rev Infect Dis* (1986) 8, (Suppl 2), S217–S222.

Alcohol + Glutethimide

The combination of glutethimide and alcohol results in greater impairment in some psychomotor tests, but improvement in others. Alcohol does not interact with glutethimide taken the previous night.

Clinical evidence, mechanism, importance and management

In a series of studies, blood-alcohol levels were raised a mean of 11% by glutethimide, while plasma and urinary glutethimide levels were reduced.[1] Neither glutethimide nor alcohol alone significantly impaired reaction times, but the combination did. However, in two other tests (tracking efficacy and finger tapping) impairment was greatest after glutethimide alone and reduced by the presence of alcohol.[1] In contrast, a later study found that glutethimide did not subjectively or objectively impair the performance of a number of psychomotor skill tests related to driving, and did not interact with alcohol given the morning after the glutethimide dose.[2] Both drugs are CNS depressants and their effects would be expected to be additive.

The information is limited and somewhat contradictory, nevertheless patients should be warned about the probable results of taking glutethimide and alcohol together. Driving, handling dangerous machinery, or undertaking any task needing alertness and full co-ordination, is likely to be made more difficult and hazardous. There is no evidence of a hangover effect, which could result in an interaction with alcohol the next day.[2]

1. Mould GP, Curry SH, Binns TB. Interactions of glutethimide and phenobarbitone with ethanol in man. *J Pharm Pharmacol* (1972) 24, 894–9.
2. Saario I, Linnoila M. Effect of subacute treatment with hypnotics, alone or in combination with alcohol, on psychomotor skills related to driving. *Acta Pharmacol Toxicol (Copenh)* (1976) 38, 382–92.

Alcohol + Glyceryl trinitrate (Nitroglycerin)

Patients who take glyceryl trinitrate while drinking may feel faint and dizzy.

Clinical evidence, mechanism, importance and management

The results of studies[1,2] on the combined haemodynamic effects of alcohol and glyceryl trinitrate give support to earlier claims that concurrent use increases the risk of exaggerated hypotension and fainting.[3,4] Their vasodilatory effects[5] would appear to be additive. The greatest effect was seen when the glyceryl trinitrate was taken one hour or more after starting to drink alcohol.[1] It is suggested that this increased susceptibility to postural hypotension should not be allowed to stop patients from using glyceryl trinitrate if they want to drink alcohol, but they should be warned about the possible effects and told what to do if they feel faint and dizzy (i.e. sit or lie down).[1]

1. Kupari M, Heikkilä J, Ylikahri R. Does alcohol intensify the hemodynamic effects of nitroglycerin? *Clin Cardiol* (1984) 7, 382–6.
2. Abrams J, Schroeder K, Raizada V, Gibbs D. Potentially adverse effects of sublingual nitroglycerin during consumption of alcohol. *J Am Coll Cardiol* (1990) 15, 226A.
3. Shafer N. Hypotension due to nitroglycerin combined with alcohol. *N Engl J Med* (1965) 273, 1169.
4. Opie. LH. Drugs and the heart. II. Nitrates. *Lancet* (1980) i, 750–3.
5. Allison RD, Kraner JC, Roth GM. Effects of alcohol and nitroglycerin on vascular responses in man. *Angiology* (1971) 22, 211–22.

Alcohol + Griseofulvin

An isolated case report describes a very severe disulfiram-like reaction when a man taking griseofulvin drank a can of beer. Another isolated report notes flushing and tachycardia. A few others have shown increased alcohol effects.

Clinical evidence

A man took griseofulvin 500 mg daily for about 2 weeks without problems. Subsequently he drank a can of beer, took his usual dose of griseofulvin about one hour later, and within 30 to 60 minutes developed a severe disulfiram-like reaction (flushing, severe nausea, vomiting, diarrhoea, hypotension and paraesthesias of all extremities). He was successfully treated with intravenous sodium chloride 0.9%, potassium, dopamine, and intramuscular promethazine.[1]

Another isolated case of flushing and tachycardia attributed to the concurrent use of alcohol and griseofulvin has also been described; rechallenge produced the same effects.[2]

It has been suggested that griseofulvin can increase the effects of alcohol, but the descriptions of this response are very brief. One of them describes[3] a man who had a decreased tolerance to alcohol and emotional instability manifested by crying and nervousness, which was said to be so severe that the drug was stopped. Another[4] states that this effect has been noted in a very small number of patients, but gives no further information.

Mechanism

Not understood. The reaction described above might possibly have the same pharmacological basis as the disulfiram/alcohol reaction (see 'Alcohol + Disulfiram', p.61).

Importance and management

The documentation is extremely sparse, which would seem to suggest that adverse interactions between alcohol and griseofulvin are uncommon. Concurrent use need not be avoided but it may be prudent to warn patients about the possible effects. The disulfiram-like reaction described was unusually severe. The manufacturer cautions that the effects of alcohol may be potentiated by griseofulvin, producing such adverse effects as tachycardia and flush.[5]

1. Fett DL, Vukov LF. An unusual case of severe griseofulvin-alcohol interaction. *Ann Emerg Med* (1994) 24, 95–7.
2. Robinson MM. Griseofulvin therapy of superficial mycoses. *Antibiot Annu* (1959–60) 7, 680–6.
3. Drowns BV, Fuhrman DL, Dennie CC. Use, abuse and limitations of griseofulvin. *Mo Med* (1960) 57, 1473–6.
4. Simon HJ, Randz LA. Untoward reactions to antimicrobial agents. *Annu Rev Med* (1961) 12, 111–34.
5. Gris-PEG (Griseofulvin). Pedinol Pharmacal Inc. US Prescribing information, 2005.

Alcohol + H_2-receptor antagonists

Although some studies have found that blood-alcohol levels can be raised to some extent in those taking some H_2-receptor antagonists and possibly remain elevated for longer than usual, others report that no significant interaction occurs. Drinking may worsen the gastrointestinal disease for which these H_2-receptor antagonists are being given. Hypoglycaemia associated with alcohol may be enhanced by H_2-receptor antagonists.

Clinical evidence

(a) Evidence of an interaction

A double-blind study in 6 healthy subjects found that **cimetidine** 300 mg four times daily for 7 days, increased the peak plasma levels of alcohol 0.8 g/kg by about 12% (from 146 to 163 mg%) and increased the AUC by about 7%. The subjects assessed themselves as being more intoxicated while taking **cimetidine** and alcohol than with alcohol alone.[1]

An essentially similar study[2,3] found that the blood-alcohol levels were raised by 17% (from 73 to 86 mg%) by **cimetidine** but not by **ranitidine**. However, another study found that **cimetidine** almost doubled peak blood-alcohol levels, whereas **ranitidine** raised the levels by about 50%.[4] A study in 6 healthy subjects also found that **cimetidine** 400 mg twice daily for one week approximately doubled the AUC following a single 0.15-g/kg oral dose of alcohol and raised peak alcohol levels by about 33%. No changes were seen when the alcohol was given intravenously.[5] A further study in healthy subjects given **cimetidine** or **ranitidine** for only 2 days found that peak plasma alcohol levels were raised by 17% and 28%, respectively, and the time that blood levels remained above the 80 mg% mark (the legal driving limit in some countries) was prolonged by about one-third.[6]

A study in subjects given 0.75 g/kg of alcohol found that single doses of **cimetidine** 800 mg, **nizatidine** 300 mg, or **ranitidine** 300 mg raised blood alcohol levels at 45 minutes by 26% (from 75.5 to 95.2 mg%), 17.5% (from 75.5 to 88.7 mg%) and 3.3% (75.5 to 78 mg%), respectively, and the AUCs at 120 minutes were increased by 25%, 20% and 9.8%, respectively. Each of the subjects said they felt more inebriated after taking **cimetidine** or **nizatidine**.[7] Another report briefly mentions that both **nizatidine** and **ranitidine** have similar effects on alcohol absorption to **cimetidine**.[8]

In subjects with substantial first-pass metabolism of alcohol, **cimetidine** increased the blood levels of repeated small drinks of alcohol to a greater degree than that which occurred after an equivalent single dose. The levels reached were associated with psychomotor impairment.[9] Similarly, **ranitidine** 150 mg twice daily for 7 days considerably increased blood-alcohol levels and the high levels persisted for longer in social drinkers (with substantial first-pass metabolism) receiving 4 drinks of 0.15 g/kg of alcohol at 45-minute intervals.[10]

In contrast, another study found that a combination of chlorphenamine (which blocks H_1-receptors) and **cimetidine** reduced the rate of absorption and peak blood alcohol levels, and suppressed alcohol-induced flushing.[11]

(b) Evidence of no interaction

The manufacturers of **cimetidine** have on file three unpublished studies that did not find any evidence to suggest that **cimetidine** or **ranitidine** significantly increased the blood levels of alcohol. One study was in 6 healthy subjects given single 400-mg doses of **cimetidine**, another in 6 healthy subjects given **cimetidine** 1 g daily for 14 days, and the last in 10 healthy subjects given either **cimetidine** 400 mg twice daily or **ranitidine** 150 mg twice daily.[12] A number of other studies have also found that no significant interaction occurs between **cimetidine**, **famotidine**, **nizatidine**, or **ranitidine**, and a number of different alcoholic drinks (low to high dose), either on an empty stomach or after eating.[13-26] Two other studies showing an interaction between other H_2-receptor antagonists and alcohol found that **famotidine** had no significant effect on blood-alcohol levels.[4,7]

(c) Hypoglycaemia

A study in 10 healthy subjects given alcohol 0.5 g/kg before and after **cimetidine** 400 mg twice daily, **ranitidine** 150 mg twice daily, or **famotidine** 40 mg once daily, all taken for 7 days, found that hypoglycaemia following alcohol ingestion was enhanced by all three H_2-receptor antagonists. The effect was especially marked with **famotidine**.[27]

Mechanism

It would appear that the interacting H_2-receptor antagonists inhibit the activity of alcohol dehydrogenase (ADH) in the gastric mucosa so that more alcohol passes unmetabolised into the circulation, thereby raising the levels.[28-32] Most of the studies assessing the interaction of H_2-receptor antagonists with larger quantities of alcohol have not found an interaction. The decrease in first pass metabolism with increasing amounts of alcohol could explain this, as it implies that a significant interaction with H_2-receptor antagonists would be more likely with smaller quantities of alcohol.[9,33] Other factors that affect the first pass metabolism of alcohol, such as fasting, chronic alcoholism and female gender may also affect the outcome. The increase in blood-alcohol levels with cimetidine or ranitidine and a low alcohol dose may also be explained by the effect of H_2-receptor antagonists or alcohol on gastric emptying times.[24,33] In one study the decrease in first-pass metabolism correlated with a ranitidine-induced increase in the rate of gastric emptying and an increase in blood-alcohol levels.[34] However, with small quantities of alcohol the magnitude of the effect on peak levels may be too small to increase effects on psychomotor performance,[33,35] although two studies suggested that an effect might occur.[9]

The hypoglycaemic effect is not considered to be due to effects on alcohol absorption but may be an effect of H_2-receptor antagonists on glucose metabolism.[27]

Importance and management

The contrasting and apparently contradictory results cited here clearly show that this interaction is by no means established. Extensive reviews of the data concluded that the interaction is, in general, clinically insignificant.[32,33,36-38] Under conditions mimicking social drinking there is some evidence that H_2-receptor antagonists may[10,27] or may not[26] increase blood-alcohol levels to those associated with impairment of psychomotor skills. However, as yet, there are insufficient grounds to justify any general warning regarding alcohol and H_2-receptor antagonists. However, note that many of the conditions for which H_2-receptor antagonists are used may be made worse by alcohol, so restriction of alcohol intake may be prudent.

1. Feely J, Wood AJJ. Effects of cimetidine on the elimination and actions of alcohol. *JAMA* (1982) 247, 2819–21.
2. Seitz HK, Bösche J, Czygan P, Veith S, Simon B, Kommerell B. Increased blood ethanol levels following cimetidine but not ranitidine. *Lancet* (1983) i, 760.
3. Seitz HK, Veith S, Czygan P, Bösche J, Simon B, Gugler R, Kommerell B. *In vivo* interactions between H_2-receptor antagonists and ethanol metabolism in man and in rats. *Hepatology* (1984) 4, 1231–4.
4. DiPadova C, Roine R, Frezza M, Gentry T, Baraona E, Lieber CS. Effects of ranitidine on blood alcohol levels after ethanol ingestion: comparison with other H_2-receptor antagonists. *JAMA* (1992) 267, 83–6.
5. Caballeria J, Baraona E, Rodamilans M, Lieber CS. Effects of cimetidine on gastric alcohol dehydrogenase activity and blood ethanol levels. *Gastroenterology* (1989) 96, 388–92.
6. Webster LK, Jones DB, Smallwood RA. Influence of cimetidine and ranitidine on ethanol pharmacokinetics. *Aust N Z J Med* (1985) 15, 359–60.
7. Guram M, Howden CW, Holt S. Further evidence for an interaction between alcohol and certain H_2-receptor antagonists. *Alcohol Clin Exp Res* (1991) 15, 1084–5.
8. Palmer RH. Cimetidine and alcohol absorption. *Gastroenterology* (1989) 97, 1066–8.
9. Gupta AM, Baraona E, Lieber CS. Significant increase of blood alcohol by cimetidine after repetitive drinking of small alcohol doses. *Alcohol Clin Exp Res* (1995) 19, 1083–7.
10. Arora S, Baraona E, Lieber CS. Alcohol levels are increased in social drinkers receiving ranitidine. *Am J Gastroenterol* (2000) 95, 208–13.
11. Tan OT, Stafford TJ, Sarkany I, Gaylarde PM, Tilsey C, Payne JP. Suppression of alcohol-induced flushing by a combination of H_1 and H_2 histamine antagonists. *Br J Dermatol* (1982) 107, 647–52.
12. Smith Kline and French. Personal communication, February 1989.
13. Dobrilla G, de Pretis G, Piazzi L, Chilovi F, Comberlato M, Valentini M, Pastorino A, Vallaperta P. Is ethanol metabolism affected by oral administration of cimetidine and ranitidine at therapeutic doses? *Hepatogastroenterology* (1984) 31, 35–7.
14. Johnson KI, Fenzl E, Hein B. Einfluß von Cimetidin auf den Abbau und die Wirkung des Alkohols. *Arzneimittelforschung* (1984) 34, 734–6.
15. Tanaka E, Nakamura K. Effects of H_2-receptor antagonists on ethanol metabolism in Japanese volunteers. *Br J Clin Pharmacol* (1988) 26, 96–9.
16. Holtmann G, Singer MV. Histamine H_2 receptor antagonists and blood alcohol levels. *Dig Dis Sci* (1988) 33, 767–8.
17. Holtmann G, Singer MV, Knop D, Becker S, Goebell H. Effect of histamine-H_2-receptor antagonists on blood alcohol levels. *Gastroenterology* (1988) 94, A190. (abs).
18. Fraser AG, Prewett EJ, Hudson M, Sawyerr AM, Rosalki SB, Pounder RE. The effect of ranitidine, cimetidine or famotidine on low-dose post-prandial alcohol absorption. *Aliment Pharmacol Ther* (1991) 5, 263–72.
19. Jönsson K-Å, Jones AW, Boström H, Andersson T. Lack of effect of omeprazole, cimetidine, and ranitidine on the pharmacokinetics of ethanol in fasting male volunteers. *Eur J Clin Pharmacol* (1992) 42, 209–12.
20. Fraser AG, Hudson M, Sawyerr AM, Smith M, Rosalki SB, Pounder RE. Ranitidine, cimetidine, famotidine have no effect on post-prandial absorption of ethanol 0.8 g/kg taken after an evening meal. *Aliment Pharmacol Ther* (1992) 6, 693–700.
21. Fraser AG, Prewett EJ, Hudson M, Sawyerr AM, Rosalki SB, Pounder RE. Ranitidine has no effect on post-prandial absorption of alcohol (0.6 g/kg) after an evening meal. *Eur J Gastroenterol Hepatol* (1992) 4, 43–7.
22. Kendall MJ, Spannuth F, Walt RP, Gibson GJ, Hale KA, Braithwaite R, Langman MJS. Lack of effect of H2-receptor antagonists on the pharmacokinetics of alcohol consumed after food at lunchtime. *Br J Clin Pharmacol* (1994) 37, 371–4.
23. Pipkin GA, Mills JG, Wood JR. Does ranitidine affect blood alcohol concentrations? *Pharmacotherapy* (1994) 14, 273–81.
24. Bye A, Lacey LF, Gupta S, Powell JR. Effect of ranitidine hydrochloride (150 mg twice daily) on the pharmacokinetics of increasing doses of ethanol (0.15, 0.3, 0.6 g kg^{-1}). *Br J Clin Pharmacol* (1996) 41, 129–33.
25. Hindmarch I, Gilburt S. The lack of CNS effects of nizatidine, with and without alcohol, on psychomotor ability and cognitive function. *Hum Psychopharmacol* (1990) 5, 25–32.
26. Brown ASJM, James OFW. Omeprazole, ranitidine and cimetidine have no effect on peak blood ethanol concentrations, first pass metabolism or area under the time–ethanol curve under 'real-life' drinking conditions. *Aliment Pharmacol Ther* (1998) 12, 141–5.
27. Czyżyk A, Lao B, Szutowski M, Szczepanik Z, Muszyński J. Enhancement of alcohol-induced hypoglycaemia by H_2-receptor antagonists. *Arzneimittelforschung* (1997) 47, 746–9.
28. Caballería J. Interactions between alcohol and gastric metabolizing enzymes: practical implications. *Clin Ther* (1991) 13, 511–20.
29. Fiatarone JR, Bennett MK, Kelly P, James OFW. Ranitidine but not gastritis or female sex reduces the first pass metabolism of ethanol. *Gut* (1991) 32, A594.
30. Caballería J, Baraona E, Deulofeu R, Hernández-Muñoz R, Rodés J, Lieber CS. Effects of H_2-receptor antagonists on gastric alcohol dehydrogenase activity. *Dig Dis Sci* (1991) 36, 1673–9.
31. Brown ASJM, Fiaterone JR, Day CP, Bennett MK, Kelly PJ, James OFW. Ranitidine increases the bioavailability of postprandial ethanol by the reduction of first pass metabolism. *Gut* (1995) 37, 413–17.
32. Gugler R. H_2-antagonists and alcohol: Do they interact? *Drug Safety* (1994) 10, 271–80.
33. Fraser AG. Is there an interaction between H_2-antagonists and alcohol? *Drug Metabol Drug Interact* (1998) 14, 123–145.
34. Amir I, Anwar N, Baraona E, Lieber CS. Ranitidine increases the bioavailability of imbibed alcohol by accelerating gastric emptying. *Life Sci* (1996) 58, 511–18.
35. Baraona E, Gentry RT, Lieber CS. Bioavailability of alcohol: role of gastric metabolism and its interaction with other drugs. *Dig Dis* (1994) 12, 351–57.
36. Levitt MD. Review article: lack of clinical significance of the interaction between H_2-receptor antagonists and ethanol. *Aliment Pharmacol Ther* (1993) 7, 131–8.
37. Monroe ML, Doering PL. Effect of common over-the-counter medications on blood alcohol levels. *Ann Pharmacother* (2001) 35, 918–24.
38. Weinberg DS, Burnham D, Berlin JA. Effect of histamine-2 receptor antagonists on blood alcohol levels: a meta-analysis. *J Gen Intern Med* (1998) 13, 594–9.

Alcohol + Herbal medicines; Ginseng

Ginseng increases the clearance of alcohol and lowers blood-alcohol levels.

Clinical evidence, mechanism, importance and management

Fourteen healthy subjects, each acting as their own control, were given alcohol (72 g/65 kg as a 25% solution) with and without a ginseng extract (3 g/65 kg) mixed in with it. They drank the alcohol or the alcohol/ginseng mixture over a 45-minute period in 7 portions, the first four at 5-minute intervals and the next three at 10-minute intervals. Measurements taken 40 minutes later showed that the presence of the ginseng lowered blood-alcohol levels by an average of 38.9%. The alcohol levels of 10 subjects were lowered by 32 to 51% by the ginseng, 3 showed reductions of 14 to 18% and one showed no changes at all.[1]

The reasons for this interaction are uncertain, but it is suggested that ginseng possibly increases the activity of the enzymes (alcohol and aldehyde dehydrogenase)[2] that are concerned with the metabolism of the alcohol, thereby increasing the clearance of the alcohol. What this means in practical terms is not clear but the authors of the report suggest the possibility of using ginseng to treat alcoholic patients and those with acute alcohol intoxication.[1] *Panax ginseng* has been shown to reduce voluntary alcohol intake in *animals.*[3]

1. Lee FC, Ko JH, Park KJ, Lee JS. Effect of *Panax ginseng* on blood alcohol clearance in man. *Clin Exp Pharmacol Physiol* (1987) 14, 543–6.
2. Choi CW, Lee SI, Huh K. Effect of ginseng on the hepatic alcohol metabolizing enzyme system activity in chronic alcohol-treated mice. *Korean J Pharmacol* (1984) 20, 13–21.
3. Carai MAM, Agabio R, Bombardelli E, Bourov I, Gessa GL, Lobina C, Morazzoni P, Pani M, Reali R, Vacca G, Colombo G. Potential use of medicinal plants in the treatment of alcoholism. *Fitoterapia* (2000) 71 (Suppl 1), S38–S42.

Alcohol + Herbal medicines; Kava

There is some evidence that kava may worsen the CNS depressant effects of alcohol.

Clinical evidence, mechanism, importance and management

Forty healthy subjects underwent a number of cognitive tests and visuomotor tests after taking alcohol alone, kava (Kava-Kava; the pepper plant *Piper methysticum*) alone, or both together. The subjects took 0.75 g/kg of alcohol (enough to give blood alcohol levels above 50 mg%) and the kava dose was 1 g/kg. The kava drink was made by mixing middle grade Fijian kava with water and straining it to produce about 350 mL of kava liquid. It was found that kava alone had no effect on the tests, but when given with alcohol it potentiated both the perceived and measured impairment that occurred with alcohol alone.[1] However, another study found that a kava extract (WS 1490) did not enhance the negative effects of alcohol on performance tests.[2]

No very strong conclusions can be drawn from the results of the studies, but it is possible that car driving and handling other machinery may be more hazardous if kava and alcohol are taken together. However, note that the use of kava-kava is restricted in the UK because of reports of idiosyncratic hepatotoxicity.[3]

1. Foo H, Lemon J. Acute effects of kava, alone or in combination with alcohol, on subjective measures of impairment and intoxication and on cognitive performance. *Drug Alcohol Rev* (1997) 16, 147–55.
2. Herberg K-W. Zum Einfluß von Kava-Spezialextrakt WS 1490 in Kombination mit Ethylalkohol auf sicherheitsrelevante Leistungsparameter. The influence of kava-special extract WS 1490 on safety-relevant performance alone and in combination with ethyl alcohol. *Blutalkohol* (1993) 30, 96–105.
3. Committee on Safety of Medicines/Medicines and Healthcare Regulatory Authority. Kava-kava and hepatotoxicity. *Current Problems* (2003) 29, 8.

Alcohol + Herbal medicines; Liv.52

***Liv.52*, an Ayurvedic herbal remedy, appears to reduce the hangover symptoms after drinking, reducing both urine and blood-alcohol and acetaldehyde levels at 12 hours. However it also raises the blood alcohol levels of moderate drinkers for the first few hours after drinking.**

Clinical evidence

Nine healthy subjects who normally drank socially (alcohol 40 to 100 g weekly) took six tablets of *Liv.52* two hours before drinking alcohol (four 60 mL doses of whiskey, equivalent to 90 g of alcohol). Their blood-alcohol levels at one hour were increased by 15% (from 75 to 86.2 mg%). After taking three tablets of *Liv.52* daily for two weeks, their 1-hour blood-alcohol levels were raised by 27% (from 75 to 95.3 mg%).[1] Acetaldehyde levels in the blood and urine were markedly lowered at 12 hours, and hangover symptoms seemed to be reduced.[1] In a similar study, the blood-alcohol levels of 9 moderate drinkers were raised over the first 2 hours by about 28 to 44% after taking three tablets of *Liv.52* twice daily for two weeks, and by 17 to 19% over the following 2 hours.[2] Only a minor increase in the blood-alcohol levels of 8 occasional drinkers occurred.[2]

Mechanism

Not understood. *Liv.52* contains the active principles from *Capparis spinosa*, *Cichorium intybus*, *Solanum nigrum*, *Cassia occidentalis*, *Terminalia arjuna*, *Achillea millefolium*, *Tamarix gallica* and *Phyllanthus amarus*.[1] These appear to increase the absorption of alcohol, or reduce its metabolism by the liver, thereby raising the blood-alcohol levels. It is suggested that the reduced hangover effects may possibly occur because it prevents the binding of acetaldehyde to cell proteins allowing a more rapid elimination.[1]

Importance and management

Direct pharmacokinetic evidence seems to be limited to these two studies.[1,2] *Liv.52* appears to reduce the hangover effects after drinking, but at the same time it can significantly increase the blood alcohol levels of moderate drinkers, for the first few hours after drinking. Increases of up to 30% may be enough to raise the blood alcohol from legal to illegal levels when driving. Moderate drinkers should be warned. Occasional drinkers appear to develop higher blood-alcohol levels than moderate drinkers but *Liv.52* does not seem to increase them significantly.[2]

1. Chauhan BL, Kulkarni RD. Alcohol hangover and Liv.52. *Eur J Clin Pharmacol* (1991) 40, 187–8.
2. Chauhan BL, Kulkarni RD. Effect of Liv.52, a herbal preparation, on absorption and metabolism of ethanol in humans. *Eur J Clin Pharmacol* (1991) 40, 189–91.

Alcohol + Hormonal contraceptives

The detrimental effects of alcohol may be reduced to some extent in women taking oral contraceptives, but alcohol clearance may also possibly be reduced. Alcohol does not affect the pharmacokinetics of ethinylestradiol.

Clinical evidence, mechanism, importance and management

(a) Effect of oral contraceptives on alcohol

A controlled study in 54 women found that those taking a combined oral contraceptive (30, 35, or 50 micrograms of **oestrogen**) unexpectedly tolerated the effects of alcohol better than those not taking oral contraceptives (as measured by a reaction-time test and a bead-threading test), but their blood-alcohol levels and its rate of alcohol clearance were unchanged.[1] For mention of a trend towards improved cognitive performance with small amounts of alcohol and oestrogen replacement therapy, see 'Alcohol + HRT', p.67.

The authors say that they do not recommend women taking oral contraceptives should attempt to drink more than usual, since even if alcohol is tolerated better, blood-alcohol levels are not reduced.[1] However, two other studies suggest that peak blood-alcohol levels may be reduced in those taking oral contraceptives, but alcohol clearance is also reduced and so alcohol may be present longer in women who are taking oral contraceptives.[2,3]

(b) Effect of alcohol on oral contraceptives

Alcohol ingestion did not have any significant effect on **ethinylestradiol** pharmacokinetics in 9 healthy women taking a combined oral contraceptive (ethinylestradiol/gestodene 30/75 micrograms). In this study, alcohol was given as a single dose of 0.4 g/kg (2 to 3 standard drinks) on day 14 then 0.4 g/kg twice daily for 7 days. The findings of this study contrast with those of the effect of alcohol on estradiol in postmenopausal women (see 'Alcohol + HRT', below). This may be because the ethinyl group in **ethinylestradiol** confers protection from the effects of alcohol.[4]

1. Hobbes J, Boutagy J, Shenfield GM. Interactions between ethanol and oral contraceptive steroids. *Clin Pharmacol Ther* (1985) 38, 371–80.
2. Jones MK, Jones BM. Ethanol metabolism in women taking oral contraceptives. *Alcohol Clin Exp Res* (1984) 8, 24–8.
3. Zeiner AR, Kegg PS. Menstrual cycle and oral contraceptive effects on alcohol pharmacokinetics in caucasian females. *Curr Alcohol* (1981) 8, 47–56.
4. Sarkola T, Ahola L, von der Pahlen B, Eriksson CJP. Lack of effect of alcohol on ethinylestradiol in premenopausal women. *Contraception* (2001) 63, 19–23.

Alcohol + HRT

Acute ingestion of alcohol markedly increases the levels of circulating estradiol in women using oral HRT; a smaller increase is seen with transdermal HRT. In addition, alcohol intake appears to increase the risk of breast cancer in women receiving HRT. Small amounts of alcohol may possibly improve some aspects of cognitive function in patients using HRT. Estradiol does not affect blood-alcohol levels.

Clinical evidence, mechanism, importance and management

(a) Hormone and blood-alcohol levels

Twelve healthy postmenopausal women receiving HRT (**estradiol** 1 mg daily and **medroxyprogesterone acetate** 10 mg daily for 10 out of each 25 days) were given an alcoholic drink (0.7 g/kg, a dose shown to achieve mean peak alcohol serum levels of about 97 mg% after about 1 hour) during the oestrogen-only phase of the HRT cycle. It was found that their peak **estradiol** levels rose threefold and were significantly above the baseline for 5 hours. No significant increases in the levels of circulating estrone (an oestrogen secreted by the ovaries) were seen, and blood-alcohol levels were not changed.[1] A similar, smaller 1.2-fold increase in peak **estradiol** levels was seen in another study when women using **transdermal estradiol** were given alcohol.[2]

The reasons for these changes are not understood. Alcohol can increase *endogenous* **estradiol** levels in postmenopausal women, although the findings are variable. Another possible explanation is altered clearance of **estradiol** in women who drink alcohol.[3] Note that alcohol does not affect ethinylestradiol levels, see 'Alcohol + Hormonal contraceptives', p.66.

(b) Risk of breast cancer

Since both alcohol and HRT are linked with a small increase in breast cancer risk, it has been postulated that the combination of HRT and alcohol could be additive.[4] A prospective study of 51 847 postmenopausal women confirmed an association with alcohol intake and breast cancer risk (for oestrogen receptor-positive (ER+) tumours, but not ER– tumours). Furthermore, among women who consumed alcohol, postmenopausal hormone use was associated with an increased risk for the development of ER+ tumours. For women with the highest alcohol intake (10 g (approximately 1 drink) or more daily) the relative risk of developing oestrogen receptor-positive/progesterone receptor-positive (ER+PR+) breast cancer was 1.2 and 1.8 for non-users and users of HRT, respectively, compared with non-drinkers who had never used postmenopausal hormones; the relative risk of developing ER+PR– tumours was even greater, being approximately 2.5 and 3.5, respectively.[5] Another study also reported a similar increased risk of developing ER+PR+ tumours with alcohol and oestrogen replacement therapy, but only a slight risk for ER+PR– tumours; the risk for ER–PR– breast cancer was, however, greatest.[6]

Regular consumption of alcohol as low as 1 to 2 drinks per day may possibly contribute to a modest increased risk,[3] and it has been suggested that women taking HRT should limit their alcohol intake;[4] about one drink or less per day has been proposed.[3] More study is needed to confirm the amount and frequency of alcohol consumption needed to have a deleterious effect both in women who use HRT and in non-users.

(c) Visuospatial performance

A study of 214 postmenopausal women suggested that small amounts of alcohol may enhance visuospatial processes (improved cognitive function measured by block design performance). HRT also appeared to be linked with better visuospatial performance, but only when the task was difficult. There was a trend (not statistically significant) towards improved performance with alcohol consumption (up to approximately half a standard drink per day) and oestrogen replacement therapy.[7] For mention of improved tolerance to alcohol in premenopausal women taking oestrogen, see 'Alcohol + Hormonal contraceptives', p.66.

1. Ginsburg ES, Mello NK, Mendelson JH, Barbieri RL, Teoh SK, Rothman M, Gao X, Sholar JW. Effects of alcohol ingestion on estrogens in postmenopausal women. *JAMA* (1996) 276, 1747–51.
2. Ginsburg ES, Walsh BW, Gao X, Gleason RE, Feltmate C, Barbieri RL. The effect of acute ethanol ingestion on estrogen levels in postmenopausal women using transdermal estradiol. *J Soc Gynecol Investig* (1995) 2, 26–9.
3. Singletary KW, Gapstur SM. Alcohol and breast cancer. Review of epidemiologic and experimental evidence and potential mechanisms. *JAMA* (2001) 286, 2143–51.
4. Gorins A. Responsabilité croisée des estrogènes et de l'alcool dans le cancer du sein. *Presse Med* (2000) 29, 670–2.
5. Suzuki R, Ye W, Rylander-Rudqvist T, Saji S, Colditz GA, Wolk A. Alcohol and postmenopausal breast cancer risk defined by estrogen and progesterone receptor status: a prospective cohort study. *J Natl Cancer Inst* (2005) 97, 1601–8.
6. Gapstur SM, Potter JD, Drinkard C, Folsom AR. Synergistic effect between alcohol and estrogen replacement therapy on risk of breast cancer differs by estrogen/progesterone receptor status in the Iowa Women's Health Study. *Cancer Epidemiol Biomarkers Prev* (1995) 4, 313–18.
7. Tivis LJ, Green MD, Nixon SJ, Tivis RD. Alcohol, estrogen replacement therapy, and visuospatial processes in postmenopausal women. *Alcohol Clin Exp Res* (2003) 27, 1055–63.

Alcohol + Interferons

A study found a reduced response to interferon in patients who drank alcohol.

Clinical evidence, mechanism, importance and management

In a study involving 245 patients, alcohol intake, and its effect on treatment were retrospectively evaluated between 1 and 3 years after diagnosis of hepatitis C virus-related chronic liver disease. Less than 50% of the patients who drank alcohol stopped after being diagnosed with liver disease, despite being advised to abstain from alcohol. Alcohol intake affected fibrosis, especially in women, and response to interferon therapy. Seventeen out of 65 patients (26.1%) who were treated with **interferon alfa** had a sustained response to therapy. However, the number of responders decreased as alcohol intake increased; there were more drinkers (63.1%) than abstainers (10.7%) among the 73.8% of patients who did not respond.[1] One manufacturer notes that hepatotoxicity has been reported with **interferon beta-1a** and the potential additive toxicity with hepatotoxic drugs such as alcohol has not been determined, and caution is warranted.[2]

There appears to be insufficient information to suggest that patients receiving interferons should avoid alcohol completely, however, alcohol intake, particularly heavy drinking, may increase the risk of hepatotoxicity with interferon.

1. Loguercio C, Di Pierro M, Di Marino MP, Federico A, Disalvo D, Crafa E, Tuccillo C, Baldi F, del Vecchio Blanco C. Drinking habits of subjects with hepatitis C virus-related chronic liver disease: prevalence and effect on clinical, virological and pathological aspects. *Alcohol Alcohol* (2000) 35, 296–301.
2. Avonex (Interferon beta-1a). Biogen Idec Ltd. UK Summary of product characteristics, February 2007.

Alcohol + Ivermectin

Alcohol may increase the bioavailability of ivermectin.

Clinical evidence, mechanism, importance and management

Anecdotal reports from Nigeria suggest that ivermectin is more potent when taken with palm wine, a local alcoholic drink, and a few cases of ataxia and postural hypotension occurring with ivermectin were considered to be due to an interaction with alcohol.[1] Ivermectin formulated as an alcoholic solution has been found to have about twice the systemic availability of tablets and capsules.[2] In another study, 20 healthy subjects were given ivermectin 150 micrograms/kg with either 750 mL of beer (alcohol 4.5%) or 750 mL of water. Plasma levels of ivermectin at 1 to 4 hours were increased by about 51% to 66%, respectively, when it was given with beer, when compared with water. No adverse effects were reported in either group.[1] The evidence suggest that concurrent use may be of benefit, if adverse effects such as postural hypotension are not troublesome; this may be more of a problem in those with pre-existing heart disease.

1. Shu EN, Onwujekwe EO, Okonkwo PO. Do alcoholic beverages enhance availability of ivermectin? *Eur J Clin Pharmacol* (2000) 56, 437–8.
2. Edwards G, Dingsdale A, Helsby N, Orme MLE, Breckenridge AM. The relative systemic bioavailability of ivermectin after administration as capsule, tablet, and oral solution. *Eur J Clin Pharmacol* (1988) 35, 681–4.

Alcohol + Ketoconazole

A few cases of disulfiram-like reactions have been reported in patients who drank alcohol while taking ketoconazole.

Clinical evidence, mechanism, importance and management

One patient (an alcoholic), out of group of 12 patients with Candida infections taking ketoconazole 200 mg daily, experienced a disulfiram-like reaction (nausea, vomiting, facial flushing) after drinking alcohol.[1] No further details are given, and the report does not say whether any of the others drank alcohol. A woman taking ketoconazole 200 mg daily developed a disulfiram-like reaction when she drank alcohol.[2] Another report describes a transient 'sunburn-like' rash or flush on the face, upper chest and back of a patient taking ketoconazole 200 mg daily when she drank modest quantities of wine or beer.[3] The reasons for the reactions are not known but it seems possible that ketoconazole may act like disulfiram and inhibit the activity of acetaldehyde dehydrogenase (see 'Alcohol + Disulfiram', p.61). The incidence of this reaction appears to be very low (these appear to be the only reports) and its importance is probably small. Reactions of this kind are usually more unpleasant than serious, with symptoms resolving within a few hours.[4] Nevertheless, the manufacturer advises avoidance of alcohol while taking ketoconazole.[5]

1. Fazio RA, Wickremesinghe PC, Arsura EL. Ketoconazole treatment of *Candida esophagitis*—a prospective study of 12 cases. *Am J Gastroenterol* (1983) 78, 261–4.
2. Meyboom RHB, Pater BW. Overgevoeligheid voor alcoholische dranken tijdens behandeling met ketoconazol. *Ned Tijdschr Geneeskd* (1989) 133, 1463–4.
3. Magnasco AJ, Magnasco LD. Interaction of ketoconazole and ethanol. *Clin Pharm* (1986) 5, 522–3.
4. Nizoral Tablets (Ketoconazole). Janssen-Cilag Ltd. UK Summary of product characteristics, October 2006.
5. Nizoral Tablets (Ketoconazole). Janssen-Cilag Ltd. UK Patient information leaflet, October 2006.

Alcohol + Lithium

Some limited evidence suggests that lithium carbonate combined with alcohol may make driving more hazardous.

Clinical evidence, mechanism, importance and management

In 9 out of 10 healthy subjects alcohol 0.5 g/kg raised the serum levels of a single 600-mg dose of lithium carbonate by 16%. Four subjects had at least a 25% increase in lithium levels. However these rises were not considered to be clinically important.[1] In contrast a study in 20 healthy subjects given lithium carbonate (to achieve lithium serum levels of 0.75 mmol/L) and alcohol 0.5 g/kg, and who were subjected to various psychomotor tests (choice reaction, coordination, attention) to assess any impairment of skills related to driving, indicated that lithium carbonate both alone and with alcohol may increase the risk of an accident. In this study, lithium did not affect blood-alcohol levels.[2] Information is very limited but patients should be warned about the possible increased risk of driving or other potentially hazardous activities when taking both drugs.

1. Anton RF, Paladino JA, Morton A, Thomas RW. Effect of acute alcohol consumption on lithium kinetics. *Clin Pharmacol Ther* (1985) 38, 52–5.
2. Linnoila M, Saario I, Maki M. Effect of treatment with diazepam or lithium and alcohol on psychomotor skills related to driving. *Eur J Clin Pharmacol* (1974) 7, 337–42.

Alcohol + Mefloquine

Mefloquine does not normally appear to interact with alcohol, although excessive alcohol may possibly contribute to its adverse effects on the liver. An isolated report describes two incidents of severe psychosis and depression in a man taking mefloquine who drank large quantities of alcohol.

Clinical evidence, mechanism, importance and management

Mefloquine 250 mg or placebo was given to two groups of 20 healthy subjects on three occasions, each time the day before they took enough alcohol to achieve blood levels of about 35 mg%. Mefloquine did not affect blood-alcohol levels, nor did it increase the effects of alcohol on two real-highway driving tests or on psychomotor tests done in the laboratory. In fact, the mefloquine group actually drove better than the placebo group.[1]

A 40-year old man with no previous psychiatric history taking mefloquine 250 mg weekly for malaria prophylaxis had no problems with the first 2 doses. However, on two separate occasions when taking the third and fourth doses he also drank about half a litre of whisky, whereupon he developed severe paranoid delusions, hallucinations and became suicidal. When he stopped drinking he had no further problems while taking subsequent doses of mefloquine. He was used to drinking large amounts of alcohol and had experienced no problems while previously taking proguanil and chloroquine.[2]

The broad picture is that mefloquine appears not to worsen the psychomotor effects of moderate amounts of alcohol. Just why an unusual toxic reaction developed in one individual is not known, although mefloquine alone can increase the risk of psychiatric events.[3,4] It has been postulated that many of the adverse effects of mefloquine are associated with liver damage, and concurrent insults to the liver, such as from alcohol and dehydration, may be related to the development of severe or prolonged adverse reactions to mefloquine. In a review of 516 published case reports of mefloquine adverse effects, 11 cited alcohol as a possible contributing factor.[4] It was suggested that travellers taking mefloquine should avoid alcohol particularly within 24 hours of their weekly mefloquine dose.[4] However, the manufacturers have not issued such a warning.[5,6] More study is needed.

1. Vuurman EFPM, Muntjewerff ND, Uiterwijk MMC, van Veggel LMA, Crevoisier C, Haglund L, Kinzig M, O'Hanlon JF. Effects of mefloquine alone and with alcohol on psychomotor and driving performance. *Eur J Clin Pharmacol* (1996) 50, 475–82.
2. Wittes RC, Saginur R. Adverse reaction to mefloquine associated with ethanol ingestion. *Can Med Assoc J* (1995) 152, 515–17.
3. van Riemsdijk MM, Sturkenboom MCJM, Pepplinkhuizen L, Stricker BHC. Mefloquine increases the risk of serious psychiatric events during travel abroad: a nationwide case-control study in the Netherlands. *J Clin Psychiatry* (2005) 66, 199–204.
4. Croft AM, Herxheimer A. Hypothesis: Adverse effects of the antimalaria drug, mefloquine: due to primary liver damage with secondary thyroid involvement? *BMC Public Health* (2002) 2:6.
5. Lariam (Mefloquine hydrochloride). Roche Products Ltd. UK Summary of product characteristics, September 2005.
6. Lariam (Mefloquine hydrochloride). Roche Pharmaceuticals. US Prescribing information, May 2004.

Alcohol + Meprobamate

The intoxicant effects of alcohol can be considerably increased by the presence of normal daily doses of meprobamate. Driving or handling other potentially dangerous machinery is made much more hazardous.

Clinical evidence

A study in 22 subjects, given meprobamate 400 mg four times daily for one week, showed that with blood-alcohol levels of 50 mg% their performance of a number of coordination and judgement tests was much more impaired than with either drug alone.[1] Four of the subjects were quite obviously drunk while taking both meprobamate and alcohol showed marked incoordination and social disinhibition. Two could not walk without assistance. The authors say this effect was much greater than anything seen with alcohol alone.

Other studies confirm this interaction, although the effects appeared to be less pronounced.[2-6]

Mechanism

Both meprobamate and alcohol are CNS depressants, which appear to have additive effects. There is also some evidence that alcohol may inhibit or increase meprobamate metabolism, depending on whether it is taken acutely or chronically, but the contribution of this to the enhanced CNS depression is uncertain.[7,8] Meprobamate does not appear to increase blood alcohol levels.[5]

Importance and management

A well-documented and potentially serious interaction. Normal daily dosages of meprobamate in association with relatively moderate blood-alcohol levels, well within the UK legal limit for driving, can result in obviously hazardous intoxication. Patients should be warned; the patient information leaflet for meprobamate says that alcohol should be avoided.[9]

1. Zirkle GA, McAtee OB, King PD, Van Dyke R. Meprobamate and small amounts of alcohol: effects on human ability, coordination, and judgement. *JAMA* (1960) 173, 1823–5.
2. Reisby N, Theilgaard A. The interaction of alcohol and meprobamate in man. *Acta Psychiatr Scand* (1969) 208 (Suppl), 5–204.
3. Forney RB, Hughes FW. Meprobamate, ethanol or meprobamate-ethanol combinations on performance of human subjects under delayed audiofeedback (DAF). *J Psychol* (1964) 57, 431–6.
4. Ashford JR, Cobby JM. Drug interactions. The effects of alcohol and meprobamate applied singly and jointly in human subjects. III. The concentrations of alcohol and meprobamate in the blood and their effects on performance; application of mathematical models. *J Stud Alcohol* (1975) (Suppl 7), 140–61.
5. Cobby JM, Ashford JR. Drug interactions. The effects of alcohol and meprobamate applied singly and jointly in human subjects. IV. The concentrations of alcohol and meprobamate in the blood. *J Stud Alcohol* (1975) (Suppl 7), 162–76.
6. Ashford JR, Carpenter JA. Drug interactions. The effect of alcohol and meprobamate applied singly and jointly in human subjects. V. Summary and conclusions. *J Stud Alcohol* (1975) (Suppl 7), 177–87.
7. Misra PS, Lefèvre A, Ishii H, Rubin E, Lieber CS. Increase of ethanol, meprobamate and pentobarbital metabolism after chronic ethanol administration in man and in rats. *Am J Med* (1971) 51, 346–51.
8. Rubin E, Gang H, Misra PS, Lieber CS. Inhibition of drug metabolism by acute ethanol intoxication: a hepatic microsomal mechanism. *Am J Med* (1970) 49, 801–6.
9. Meprobamate. Genus Pharmaceuticals. UK Patient information leaflet, September 2004.

Alcohol + Mercaptopurine

Alcohol has been tolerated in patients receiving mercaptopurine.

Clinical evidence, mechanism, importance and management

A study in 207 patients with inflammatory bowel disease assessed (using a phone survey) the presence of adverse reactions to alcohol in patients taking chronic mercaptopurine and/or metronidazole or neither drug. All of the patients consumed less than 4 alcoholic beverages per day. The proportion of patients experiencing any clinically significant adverse effects was: metronidazole group 16.3%, mercaptopurine group 14.5%, control group (not taking either drug) 8.97%. Although there was a trend towards more adverse effects in the drug study groups, this was not statistically significant. The authors suggest a cautious trial of alcohol is advisable in patients that are starting and will be taking either of the medications on a chronic basis.[1]

1. Ginzburg L, Present DH. Alcohol is well tolerated in IBD patients taking either metronidazole or 6-mercaptopurine. *Am J Gastroenterol* (2003) 98 (Suppl), S241.

Alcohol + Methaqualone

The CNS depressant effects of alcohol and its detrimental effects on the skills relating to driving or handling other potentially dangerous machinery are increased by the concurrent use of methaqualone with or without diphenhydramine.

Clinical evidence

(a) Methaqualone

A retrospective study of drivers arrested for driving under the influence of drugs and/or alcohol found that, generally speaking, those with blood methaqualone levels of 1 mg/L or less had no symptoms of sedation, whereas those with levels above 2 mg/L demonstrated staggering gait, drowsiness, incoherence and slurred speech. These effects were increased if the drivers had also been drinking alcohol. The authors state that the levels of methaqualone needed for driving skills to become impaired are considerably lowered by alcohol, but no precise measure of this is presented in the paper.[1]

(b) Methaqualone with diphenhydramine

A double-blind study in 12 healthy subjects given two *Mandrax* tablets (methaqualone 250 mg with diphenhydramine 25 mg) showed that the resulting sedation and reduction in cognitive skills were enhanced by alcohol 0.5 g/kg. Residual amounts of a single-dose of *Mandrax* continued to interact for as long as 72 hours. Methaqualone blood levels are also raised by regular moderate amounts of alcohol.[2] Enhanced effects were also seen in another study.[3]

Mechanism

Alcohol, methaqualone and 'diphenhydramine', (p.47), are all CNS depressants, the effects of which are additive. A hangover can occur because the elimination half-life of methaqualone is long (10 to 40 hours).

Importance and management

An established interaction of importance. Those taking either methaqualone or methaqualone with diphenhydramine should be warned that handling machinery, driving a car, or any other task requiring alertness and full coordination, will be made more difficult and hazardous if they drink alcohol. Levels of alcohol below the legal driving limit with normal amounts of methaqualone may cause considerable sedation. Patients should also be told that a significant interaction may possibly occur the following day, because it has a long half-life.

Note that methaqualone has been withdrawn from the market in many countries because of problems of abuse.

1. McCurdy HH, Solomons ET, Holbrook JM. Incidence of methaqualone in driving-under-the-influence (DUI) cases in the State of Georgia. *J Anal Toxicol* (1981) 5, 270–4.
2. Roden S, Harvey P, Mitchard M. The effect of ethanol on residual plasma methaqualone concentrations and behaviour in volunteers who have taken Mandrax. *Br J Clin Pharmacol* (1977) 4, 245–7.
3. Saario I, Linnoila M. Effect of subacute treatment with hypnotics, alone or in combination with alcohol, on psychomotor skills related to driving. *Acta Pharmacol Toxicol (Copenh)* (1976) 38, 382–92.

Alcohol + Methotrexate

There is some inconclusive evidence that the consumption of alcohol may increase the risk of methotrexate-induced hepatic cirrhosis and fibrosis.

Clinical evidence, mechanism, importance and management

It has been claimed that alcohol can increase the hepatotoxic effects of methotrexate.[1] Two reports of patients treated for psoriasis indicate that this may be so; in one, 3 out of 5 patients with methotrexate-induced cirrhosis were reported to have taken alcohol concurrently (2 patients greater than 85 g, one patient 25 to 85 g of alcohol per week),[2] and in the other, the subject was known to drink excessively.[3] The evidence is by no means conclusive and no direct causal relationship has been established. However, the manufacturers of methotrexate advise the avoidance of drugs, including alcohol, which have hepatotoxic potential,[4] and contraindicate its use in patients with alcoholism or alcoholic liver disease.[4,5]

1. Almeyda J, Barnardo D, Baker H. Drug reactions XV. Methotrexate, psoriasis and the liver. *Br J Dermatol* (1971) 85, 302–5.
2. Tobias H, Auerbach R. Hepatotoxicity of long-term methotrexate therapy for psoriasis. *Arch Intern Med* (1973) 132, 391–400.
3. Pai SH, Werthamer S, Zak FG. Severe liver damage caused by treatment of psoriasis with methotrexate. *N Y State J Med* (1973) 73, 2585–7.
4. Methotrexate sodium. Wyeth Pharmaceuticals. UK Summary of product characteristics, September 2006.
5. Rheumatrex (Methotrexate). Stada Pharmaceuticals, Inc. US Prescribing information, October 2003.

Alcohol + Methylphenidate

Alcohol may increase methylphenidate levels and exacerbate some of its CNS effects.

Clinical evidence, mechanism, importance and management

In 17 subjects who had taken methylphenidate orally or intranasally with alcohol on at least 10 separate occasions, the primary reason for concurrent use was given as an alteration in psychotropic effects with increased euphoria and energy and a diminished sense of drunkenness. In addition, a minority of subjects also reported occasionally experiencing unpleasant adverse effects such as increased nausea (3 subjects), insomnia (2), and 'jaw clenching' (1).[1] In a study in 20 subjects alcohol 0.6 g/kg was given either 30 minutes before or 30 minutes after a single 0.3-mg/kg dose of methylphenidate. Alcohol significantly increased the AUC and maximum serum levels of methylphenidate, regardless of the timing of administration, by about 25% and 40%, respectively.[2]

Methylphenidate has a short half-life mainly due to conversion to the inactive metabolite ritalinic acid, but co-administration of alcohol and methylphenidate has been reported to result in production of a minor metabolite, ethylphenidate, which has CNS activity.[3,4] However, a more recent study found that the ethylphenidate formed is predominantly of the inactive enantiomer, so is unlikely to contribute to the additive CNS effects of alcohol and methylphenidate.[2]

The manufacturer of methylphenidate advises that alcohol may exacerbate the CNS effects of methylphenidate and therefore recommends that alcohol should be avoided during treatment.[5] In addition, methylphenidate should be given cautiously to patients with a history of drug dependence or alcoholism because of its potential for abuse.[1,5,6]

1. Barrett SP, Pihl RO. Oral methylphenidate-alcohol co-abuse. *J Clin Psychopharmacol* (2002) 22, 633–4.
2. Patrick KS, Straughn AB, Minhinnett RR, Yeatts SD, Herrin AE, DeVane CL, Malcolm R, Janis GC, Markowitz JS. Influence of ethanol and gender on methylphenidate pharmacokinetics and pharmacodynamics. *Clin Pharmacol Ther* (2007) 81, 346–53.
3. Markowitz JS, DeVane CL, Boulton DW, Nahas Z, Risch SC, Diamond F, Patrick KS. Ethylphenidate formation in human subjects after the administration of a single dose of methylphenidate and ethanol. *Drug Metab Dispos* (2000) 28, 620–4.
4. Markowitz JS, Logan BK, Diamond F, Patrick KS. Detection of the novel metabolite ethylphenidate after methylphenidate overdose with alcohol coingestion. *J Clin Psychopharmacol* (1999) 19, 362–6.
5. Ritalin (Methylphenidate hydrochloride). Novartis Pharmaceuticals UK Ltd. UK Summary of product characteristics, June 2007.
6. Ritalin (Methylphenidate hydrochloride). Novartis Pharmaceuticals Corporation. US Prescribing information, April 2007.

Alcohol + Metoclopramide

There is some evidence that metoclopramide can increase the rate of absorption of alcohol, raise maximum blood-alcohol levels, and possibly increase alcohol-related sedation.

Clinical evidence, mechanism, importance and management

A study in 7 subjects found that 20 mg of intravenous metoclopramide increased the rate of alcohol absorption, and the peak blood levels were raised from 55 to 86 mg%. Similar results were seen in 2 healthy subjects given metoclopramide orally.[1] Another study in 7 healthy subjects found that 10 mg of intravenous metoclopramide accelerated the rate of absorption of alcohol 70 mg/kg given orally, and increased its peak levels, but not to a statistically significant extent. Blood alcohol levels remained below 12 mg%. More importantly the sedative effects of the alcohol were increased.[2] The reasons for this effect are not fully understood, but it appears to be related to an increase in gastric emptying. These two studies were done to find out more about intestinal absorption mechanisms rather than to identify daily practicalities, so the importance of the findings is uncertain. However, it seems possible that the effects of alcohol will be increased. Metoclopramide alone can sometimes cause drowsiness, and if affected, patients should not drive or operate machinery.

1. Gibbons DO, Lant AF. Effects of intravenous and oral propantheline and metoclopramide on ethanol absorption. *Clin Pharmacol Ther* (1975) 17, 578–84.
2. Bateman DN, Kahn C, Mashiter K, Davies DS. Pharmacokinetic and concentration-effect studies with intravenous metoclopramide. *Br J Clin Pharmacol* (1978) 6, 401–7.

Alcohol + Mirtazapine

The sedative effects of mirtazapine may be increased by alcohol.

Clinical evidence, mechanism, importance and management

In 6 healthy subjects alcohol (equivalent to 60 g) had a minimal effect on plasma levels of mirtazapine 15 mg.[1] However the sedation and CNS impairment seen with mirtazapine is additive with that produced by alcohol, and the manufacturers recommend avoiding concurrent use.[1,2] Mirtazapine does not affect the absorption of alcohol.[3]

1. Remeron (Mirtazapine). Organon USA Inc. US Prescribing information, June 2005.
2. Zispin (Mirtazapine). Organon Laboratories Ltd. UK Summary of product characteristics, September 2005.
3. Sitsen JMA, Zivkov M. Mirtazapine: clinical profile. *CNS Drugs* (1995) 4 (Suppl 1), 39–48.

Alcohol + Muscle relaxants

Three reported cases of overdosage with methocarbamol and alcohol resulted in death due to combined CNS depression. Concurrent use of small or moderate amounts of alcohol with muscle relaxants may increase drowsiness and reduce alertness.

Clinical evidence, mechanism, importance and management

(a) Baclofen

The manufacturer of baclofen warns that baclofen may enhance the sedative effect of alcohol.[1] However, tolerance to baclofen's sedative effect has been reported in alcohol-addicted patients after a period of abstinence, as well as after a relapse.[2]

(b) Dantrolene

The manufacturer of dantrolene advises caution if it is given with alcohol[3] and the patient information leaflet suggests that alcohol should be avoided because it may increase drowsiness.[4]

(c) Methocarbamol

Fatal cerebral anoxia produced by CNS respiratory depression occurred in a 31-year-old man after ingestion of significant amounts of methocarbamol and alcohol. Two other lethal overdoses have been reported with these 2 drugs. In all 3 cases the methocarbamol doses exceeded the recommended daily dosages, but were estimated to be less than the reported maximum tolerated single dose of 12 g. Acute alcohol intoxication combined with methocarbamol usage can lead to combined CNS depression, which may be sufficient to cause death.[5] The manufacturers of methocarbamol warn that it may potentiate the effects of alcohol[6,7] and the patient information leaflet suggests that patients taking methocarbamol should avoid alcohol.[8]

(d) Other muscle relaxants

For enhanced CNS effects with alcohol with other muscle relaxants, see 'benzodiazepines', (p.53), 'meprobamate', (p.68), and 'tizanidine', (p.1287).

1. Lioresal Tablets (Baclofen). Novartis Pharmaceuticals UK Ltd. UK Summary of product characteristics, February 2005.
2. Addolorato G, Leggio L, Abenavoli L, Caputo F, Gasbarrini G. Tolerance to baclofen's sedative effect in alcohol-addicted patients: no dissipation after a period of abstinence. *Psychopharmacology (Berl)* (2005) 178, 351–2.
3. Dantrium Capsules (Dantrolene sodium). Procter & Gamble Pharmaceuticals UK Ltd. UK Summary of product characteristics, October 2002.
4. Dantrium (Dantrolene sodium). Procter & Gamble Pharmaceuticals UK Ltd. UK Patient information leaflet, February 2003.
5. Ferslew KE, Hagardorn AN, McCormick WF. A fatal interaction of methocarbamol and ethanol in an accidental poisoning. *J Forensic Sci* (1990) 35, 477–82.
6. Robaxin (Methocarbamol). Shire Pharmaceuticals Ltd. UK Summary of product characteristics, October 2003.
7. Robaxin (Methocarbamol). Schwarz Pharma. US Prescribing information, September 2003.
8. Robaxin (Methocarbamol). Shire Pharmaceuticals Ltd. UK Patient information leaflet, May 2003.

Alcohol + Nefazodone

In one study nefazodone 400 mg was found not to increase the sedative-hypnotic effects of alcohol.[1]

1. Frewer LJ, Lader M. The effects of nefazodone, imipramine and placebo, alone and combined with alcohol, in normal subjects. *Int Clin Psychopharmacol* (1993) 8, 13–20.

Alcohol + Niclosamide

Alcohol may possibly increase the adverse effects of niclosamide.

Clinical evidence, mechanism, importance and management

The manufacturer of niclosamide advises avoiding alcohol while taking niclosamide. The reasoning behind this is that while niclosamide is virtually insoluble in water, it is slightly soluble in alcohol, which might possibly increase its absorption by the gut, resulting in an increase in its adverse effects. There are no formal reports of this but the manufacturer says that they have some anecdotal information that is consistent with this suggestion.[1]

1. Bayer. Personal communication, July 1992.

Alcohol + Nicotine

Nicotine (as a patch) may possibly enhance the effect of alcohol on heart rate and reduce the time to peak alcohol levels. The concur-

rent use of alcohol and a nicotine nasal spray did not affect the pharmacokinetics of either drug.

Clinical evidence, mechanism, importance and management

A placebo-controlled study in 12 otherwise healthy tobacco smokers found that alcohol-induced increases in heart rate were enhanced by pre-treatment with a 21-mg nicotine transdermal patch. The time to peak alcohol levels with a 0.4 g/kg dose of ethanol was faster with nicotine pretreatment (43 minutes compared with 52 minutes, respectively); however, this effect was not seen with a 0.7 g/kg dose of ethanol.[1] Another study in 12 otherwise healthy tobacco smokers found that although alcohol 0.4 or 0.8 g/kg (equivalent to approximately 2 or 4 drinks, respectively) influenced selected subjective responses and heart rate, pre-treatment with alcohol did not affect the subjects responses to low-dose nicotine 3 to 20 micrograms/kg given as a nasal spray (20 microgram/kg dose is equivalent to about one-half of a cigarette). Neither nicotine or alcohol influenced the blood levels of the other.[2]

1. Kouri EM, McCarthy EM, Faust AH, Lukas SE. Pretreatment with transdermal nicotine enhances some of ethanol's acute effects in men. *Drug Alcohol Depend* (2004) 75, 55–65.
2. Perkins KA, Fonte C, Blakesley-Ball R, Stolinski A, Wilson AS. The influence of alcohol pretreatment on the discriminative stimulus, subjective, and relative reinforcing effects of nicotine. *Behav Pharmacol* (2005) 16, 521–9.

Alcohol + Nicotinic acid (Niacin)

An isolated report describes delirium and metabolic acidosis when a patient taking nicotinic acid for hypercholesterolaemia drank about one litre of wine. The manufacturers warn that the concurrent use of nicotinic acid and alcohol may result in an increase in adverse effects such as flushing and pruritus, and possibly liver toxicity.

Clinical evidence, mechanism, importance and management

An isolated report describes delirium and metabolic acidosis after a patient taking nicotinic acid 3 g daily for hypercholesterolaemia drank about one litre of wine. Delirium had occurred on a previous similar occasion after he drank a large quantity of beer while taking nicotinic acid. It is suggested that the nicotinic acid may have caused liver impairment, which was exacerbated by the large amount of alcohol. The patient did have some elevations in liver enzymes.[1] Acidosis has been associated with alcohol intoxication[2] and there has been a report of lactic acidosis associated with high-dose (3 g daily) nicotinic acid treatment,[3] and therefore a combined effect would seem possible. However, no general conclusions can be drawn from this single case.

Hepatic toxicity can occur with nicotinic acid and the manufacturers advise caution in patients who consume substantial quantities of alcohol. They also suggest the avoidance of alcohol around the same time as ingestion of nicotinic acid as the adverse effects of flushing and pruritus may be increased.[4,5]

1. Schwab RA, Bachhuber BH. Delirium and lactic acidosis caused by ethanol and niacin coingestion. *Am J Emerg Med* (1991) 9, 363–5.
2. Zehtabchi S, Sinert R, Baron BJ, Paladino L, Yadav K. Does ethanol explain the acidosis commonly seen in ethanol-intoxicated patients? *Clin Toxicol* (2005) 43, 161–6.
3. Earthman TP, Odom L, Mullins CA. Lactic acidosis associated with high-dose niacin therapy. *South Med J* (1991) 84, 496–7.
4. Niaspan (Nicotinic acid). Merck Pharmaceuticals. UK Summary of product characteristics, January 2006.
5. Niaspan (Nicotinic acid). Kos Pharmaceuticals, Inc. US Prescribing information, April 2007.

Alcohol + Nitrous oxide

In a double-blind study in 11 healthy subjects there were several instances when alcohol 0.25 to 5 g/kg (equivalent to 1 to 3 drinks) enhanced the effects of nitrous oxide 30% in oxygen, inhaled for 35 minutes. Some effects were seen with the drug combination, which were not seen with either drug alone; these included subjective effects and delayed free recall.[1] For mention of the effect of alcohol following anaesthesia, see 'Anaesthetics, general + Alcohol', p.92.

1. Zacny JP, Camarillo VM, Sadeghi P, Black M. Effects of ethanol and nitrous oxide, alone and in combination, on mood, psychomotor performance and pain reports in healthy volunteers. *Drug Alcohol Depend* (1998) 52, 115–23.

Alcohol + NSAIDs

Alcohol may increase the risk of gastrointestinal haemorrhage associated with NSAIDs. The skills related to driving are impaired by indometacin and phenylbutazone and this is made worse if patients drink alcohol while taking phenylbutazone, but this does not appear to occur with indometacin. A few isolated reports attribute acute renal failure to the concurrent use of NSAIDs and acute excessive alcohol consumption.

Clinical evidence, mechanism, importance and management

(a) Gastrointestinal complications

In healthy subjects the concurrent use of alcohol with **ibuprofen** 2.4 g over 24 hours increased the damaging effect of **ibuprofen** on the stomach wall, although this did not reach statistical significance.[1] A case-control study involving 1224 patients admitted to hospital with upper gastrointestinal bleeding and 2945 controls found that alcohol consumption was associated with a threefold increase in the incidence of acute upper gastrointestinal haemorrhage from light drinking (less than one alcoholic drink per week) to heavy drinking (21 alcoholic drinks or more per week). There was some evidence to suggest that the risk of upper gastrointestinal bleeding was increased by the concurrent use of **ibuprofen**.[2] Another case-control study found that the use of prescription NSAIDs or non-prescription **naproxen** or **ibuprofen** in those with a history of alcohol abuse produced a risk ratio of adverse gastrointestinal effects that was greater than the expected additive risk. Both NSAID use and excessive alcohol consumption carry the risk of gastrointestinal adverse effects. This information suggests that NSAIDs should be used with caution in heavy drinkers.[3] The FDA in the US has ruled that non-prescription pain relievers and fever reducers containing **ibuprofen**, **ketoprofen**, or **naproxen** must carry a warning label advising people who consume 3 or more alcoholic drinks every day to consult their doctor before using these drugs, and that stomach bleeding may occur with these drugs.[4] Consider also 'Alcohol + Aspirin', p.51.

(b) Psychomotor skills and alcohol levels

A study in a large number of healthy subjects showed that the performance of various psychomotor skills related to driving (choice reaction, coordination, divided attention tests) were impaired by single doses of **indometacin** 50 mg or **phenylbutazone** 200 mg. Alcohol 0.5 g/kg made things worse in those taking **phenylbutazone**, but the performance of those taking **indometacin** was improved to some extent.[5] The reasons are not understood. The study showed that the subjects were subjectively unaware of the adverse effects of **phenylbutazone**. Information is very limited, but patients should be warned if they intend to drive. In two studies, **ibuprofen** 800 mg had no significant effect on blood-alcohol levels of healthy subjects.[6,7]

The pharmacokinetics of alcohol 1 g/kg and the results of performance tests were found to be similar in subjects given **dipyrone** 1 g or a placebo.[8] No special precautions seem to be necessary.

(c) Renal complications

After taking **ibuprofen** 400 mg the evening before, 400 mg the following morning, and then 375 mL of **rum** later in the day, followed by two further 400-mg tablets of **ibuprofen**, a normal healthy young woman with no history of renal disease developed acute renal failure.[9] Another similar case was reported in a 22-year-old woman who had taken **ibuprofen** 1.2 g the morning after binge drinking.[10] Both recovered.[9,10] A further case describes renal impairment in a young woman, which was associated with the use of **ketoprofen** 600 mg and binge drinking.[11] It is suggested that volume depletion caused by the alcohol (and compounded by vomiting) predisposed these patients to NSAID-induced renal toxicity.[10,11] The general importance of these isolated cases remains to be determined.

1. Lanza FL, Royer GL, Nelson RS, Rack MF, Seckman CC. Ethanol, aspirin, ibuprofen, and the gastroduodenal mucosa: an endoscopic assessment. *Am J Gastroenterol* (1985) 80, 767–9.
2. Kaufman DW, Kelly JP, Wiholm B-E, Laszlo A, Sheehan JE, Koff RS, Shapiro S. The risk of acute major upper gastrointestinal bleeding among users of aspirin and ibuprofen at various levels of alcohol consumption. *Am J Gastroenterol* (1999) 94, 3189–96.
3. Neutel CI, Appel WC. The effect of alcohol abuse on the risk of NSAID-related gastrointestinal events. *Ann Epidemiol* (2000) 10, 246–50.
4. Food and Drug Administration. FDA announces new alcohol warnings for pain relievers and fever reducers. HHS News. Available at: http://www.fda.gov/bbs/topics/NEWS/NEW00659.html (accessed 15/08/07).

5. Linnoila M, Seppälä T, Mattila MJ. Acute effect of antipyretic analgesics, alone or in combination with alcohol, on human psychomotor skills related to driving. *Br J Clin Pharmacol* (1974) 1, 477–84.
6. Barron SE, Perry JR, Ferslew KE. The effect of ibuprofen on ethanol concentration and elimination rate. *J Forensic Sci* (1992) 37, 432–5.
7. Melander O, Lidén A, Melander A. Pharmacokinetic interactions of alcohol and acetylsalicylic acid. *Eur J Clin Pharmacol* (1995) 48, 151–3.
8. Badian LM, Rosenkrantz B. Quoted as personal communication by Levy M, Zylber-Katz E, Rosenkranz B. Clinical pharmacokinetics of dipyrone and its metabolites. *Clin Pharmacokinet* (1995) 28, 216–34.
9. Elsasser GN, Lopez L, Evans E, Barone EJ. Reversible acute renal failure associated with ibuprofen ingestion and binge drinking. *J Fam Pract* (1988) 27, 221–2.
10. Johnson GR, Wen S-F. Syndrome of flank pain and acute renal failure after binge drinking and nonsteroidal anti-inflammatory drug ingestion. *J Am Soc Nephrol* (1995) 5, 1647–52.
11. Galzin M, Brunet P, Burtey S, Dussol B, Berland Y. Nécrose tubulaire après prise d'anti-inflammatoire non stéroïdien et intoxication éthylique aiguë. *Nephrologie* (1997) 18, 113–15.

Alcohol + Olanzapine

Postural hypotension and possibly drowsiness may be increased when alcohol is given with olanzapine.

Clinical evidence, mechanism, importance and management

The manufacturer says that patients taking olanzapine have shown an increased heart rate and accentuated postural hypotension when given a single-dose of alcohol.[1] In a study, 9 of 11 subjects experienced orthostatic hypotension when they drank alcohol one hour after taking olanzapine 10 mg.[2] No pharmacokinetic interaction has been seen.[1-3] In practical terms this means that patients should be warned of the risk of faintness and dizziness if they stand up quickly. The manufacturers also say that drowsiness is a common adverse effect of olanzapine, and they warn about taking other products that can cause CNS depression, including alcohol.[3,4] The US manufacturer[3] says that patients should not drink alcohol with olanzapine because of the potential drowsiness that would result.

1. Zyprexa (Olanzapine). Eli Lilly. Clinical and Laboratory Experience A Comprehensive Monograph, August 1996.
2. Callaghan JT, Bergstrom RF, Ptak LR, Beasley CM. Olanzapine. Pharmacokinetic and pharmacodynamic profile. *Clin Pharmacokinet* (1999) 37, 177–93.
3. Zyprexa (Olanzapine). Eli Lilly and Company. US Prescribing information, November 2006.
4. Zyprexa (Olanzapine). Eli Lilly and Company Ltd. UK Summary of product characteristics, September 2006.

Alcohol + Opioids

In general the opioid analgesics can enhance the CNS depressant effects of alcohol, which has been fatal in some cases: this appears to be a particular problem with dextropropoxyphene. Alcohol has been associated with rapid release of hydromorphone and morphine from extended-release preparations, which could result in potentially fatal doses. Acute administration of alcohol and methadone appears to increase the blood levels of methadone. The bioavailability of dextropropoxyphene is increased by alcohol.

Clinical evidence

(a) Buprenorphine

See under *methadone*, below.

(b) Codeine

Double-blind studies in a large number of professional army drivers found that 50 mg of codeine and alcohol 0.5 g/kg, both alone and together, impaired their ability to drive safely on a static driving simulator. The number of 'collisions', neglected instructions and the times they 'drove off the road' were increased.[1,2] Alcohol does not appear to affect the pharmacokinetics of codeine.[3] See also, *controlled-release opioids*, below.

(c) Dextropropoxyphene

In a study in 8 healthy subjects, alcohol alone (blood levels of 50 mg%) impaired the performance of various psychomotor tests (motor co-ordination, mental performance and stability of stance) more than dextropropoxyphene 65 mg alone. When given together there was some evidence that the effects were greater than with either drug alone, but in some instances the impairment was no greater than with just alcohol. The effect of alcohol clearly predominated.[4] In contrast, other studies have found that dextropropoxyphene does not enhance the psychomotor impairment seen with alcohol,[5,6] but the bioavailability of the dextropropoxyphene has been reported to be raised by 25 to 31% by alcohol.[6,7] A retrospective study involving 332 fatal poisonings in Finland found that alcohol was present in 73% of cases involving dextropropoxyphene and, when alcohol was present, relatively small overdoses of dextropropoxyphene could result in fatal poisoning.[8] Further reports describe alcohol reducing the lethal dose of dextropropoxyphene.[9-11]

(d) Hydromorphone

A young man died from the combined cardiovascular and respiratory depressant effects of hydromorphone and alcohol.[12] He fell asleep, the serious nature of which was not recognised by those around him. Post-mortem analysis revealed alcohol and hydromorphone concentrations of 90 mg% and 100 nanograms/mL, respectively, neither of which is particularly excessive. A study in 9 healthy subjects found that pre-treatment with hydromorphone 1 or 2 mg did not significantly affect the subject-rated effects of alcohol 0.5 or 1 g/kg. However, hydromorphone enhanced the sedative scores of alcohol on the adjective rating scale.[13] See also, *controlled-release opioids*, below.

(e) Methadone

A study in 21 opioid-dependent subjects who had been receiving maintenance methadone or buprenorphine for 3 months, and 21 matched non-drug-using controls, found that although alcohol (target blood-alcohol level around 50 mg%) resulted in decreased driving performance, there appeared to be no difference in simulated driving tests in the opioid-treated patients, when compared with controls. It was suggested that restrictions on opioids and driving are not necessary in stabilised patients receiving maintenance buprenorphine or methadone treatment, but little is known about the effects in the initial treatment period.[14] This study also found that blood-alcohol levels were lower in the opioid-treated patients when compared with the controls despite receiving the same amount of alcohol.

However, clinical anecdotal reports have indicated that co-ingestion of alcohol and methadone produces an additive and/or synergistic response,[15] which may result in serious respiratory depression and hypotension.[16]

(f) Controlled-release opioids

Pharmacokinetic data in healthy subjects has shown that consuming alcohol with a particular 24-hour extended-release formulation of **hydromorphone** *(Palladone XL Capsules; Purdue Pharma, USA)* could lead to rapid release (dose dumping) and absorption of a potentially fatal dose of hydromorphone.[17,18] Although no reports of serious problems had been received, the FDA in the US asked for the product to be withdrawn from the market.[19] Health Canada warned that this interaction might occur with other slow-release opioid painkillers.[20] However, the Canadian distributor of hydromorphone has commented that the controlled-release technology employed in *Palladone XL* is not the same as that of many other controlled-release opioid formulations. Dose-dumping with alcohol is said not to occur with:

- **morphine** sustained-release tablets: *MS Contin*,[21,22] *MST continus* suspension and tablets, *MXL* capsules,[22]
- **codeine** controlled-release tablets: *Codeine Contin*,[21,22]
- **dihydrocodeine** controlled-release tablets: *DHC Continus* tablets,[22]
- **hydromorphone** controlled-release capsules: *Hydromorph Contin*,[21] *Palladone SR*,[22]
- **oxycodone** controlled-release tablets: *OxyContin*,[21,22]
- or **tramadol** (once daily and twice daily formulations).[22]

In contrast, in laboratory studies, an extended-release capsule preparation of **morphine** *(Avinza; Ligand Pharmaceuticals, USA)* was found to release morphine earlier than expected when exposed to alcohol, and this effect increased dramatically with increasing alcohol concentration.[23,24] The product literature for *Avinza* now carries a warning to avoid alcohol, including medications containing alcohol, while taking this preparation.[24]

Although most opioid preparations do not appear to interact with alcohol in this way, co-ingestion of alcohol and opioid analgesics is never advisable because of the potential for an interaction between CNS depressant drugs, see above.

Mechanism

Both opioids and alcohol are CNS depressants, and there may be enhanced suppression of the medullary respiratory control centre.[9-11] Acute administration of alcohol appears to increase methadone effects due to inhibition of hepatic microsomal enzymes, but chronic alcoholism reduces the AUC and half-life of methadone because of induction of cytochrome P450 isoenzymes.[15]

Importance and management

The fatality and increased sedation emphasise the importance of warning patients about the potentially hazardous consequences of drinking while taking potent CNS depressants like the opioids. This seems to be a particular risk with dextropropoxyphene overdosage, and it has been suggested that a less dangerous alternative could be chosen when indications of alcohol abuse or suicide risk are present.[25] The US manufacturers recommend caution when prescribing dextropropoxyphene in patients who use alcohol in excess.[26] There is less information about therapeutic doses of dextropropoxyphene with moderate social drinking. In general it is suggested that alcohol intake should be avoided where possible, or limited in those taking opioids, but some manufacturers actually contraindicate alcohol. The objective evidence is that the interaction with moderate doses of alcohol and opioids is quite small (with the exception of the dose dumping effect). It would seem prudent to warn patients that opioids can cause drowsiness and this may be exaggerated to some extent by alcohol. They should be warned that driving or handling potentially hazardous machinery may be more risky, but total abstinence from alcohol does not seem to be necessary. Smaller doses, such as those available without a prescription, would be expected to have a smaller effect, but this does not appear to have been studied.

1. Linnoila M, Häkkinen S. Effects of diazepam and codeine, alone and in combination with alcohol, on simulated driving. *Clin Pharmacol Ther* (1974) 15, 368–73.
2. Linnoila M, Mattila MJ. Interaction of alcohol and drugs on psychomotor skills as demonstrated by a driving simulator. *Br J Pharmacol* (1973) 47, 671P–672P.
3. Bodd E, Beylich KM, Christophersen AS, Mørland J. Oral administration of codeine in the presence of ethanol: a pharmacokinetic study in man. *Pharmacol Toxicol* (1987) 61, 297–300.
4. Kiplinger GF, Sokol G, Rodda BE. Effects of combined alcohol and propoxyphene on human performance. *Arch Int Pharmacodyn Ther* (1974) 212, 175–80.
5. Edwards C, Gard PR, Handley SL, Hunter M, Whittington RM. Distalgesic and ethanol-impaired function. *Lancet* (1982) ii, 384.
6. Girre C, Hirschhorn M, Bertaux L, Palombo S, Dellatolas F, Ngo R, Moreno M, Fournier PE. Enhancement of propoxyphene bioavailability by ethanol: relation to psychomotor and cognitive function in healthy volunteers. *Eur J Clin Pharmacol* (1991) 41, 147–52.
7. Sellers EM, Hamilton CA, Kaplan HL, Degani NC, Foltz RL. Pharmacokinetic interaction of propoxyphene with ethanol. *Br J Clin Pharmacol* (1985) 19, 398–401.
8. Koski A, Vuori E, Ojanperä I. Relation of postmortem blood alcohol and drug concentrations in fatal poisonings involving amitriptyline, propoxyphene and promazine. *Hum Exp Toxicol* (2005) 24, 389–96.
9. Carson DJL, Carson ED. Fatal dextropropoxyphene poisoning in Northern Ireland: review of 30 cases. *Lancet* (1977) i, 894–7.
10. Whittington RM, Barclay AD. The epidemiology of dextropropoxyphene (Distalgesic) overdose fatalities in Birmingham and the West Midlands. *J Clin Hosp Pharm* (1981) 6, 251–7.
11. Williamson RV, Galloway JH, Yeo WW, Forrest ARW. Relationship between blood dextropropoxyphene and ethanol levels in fatal co-proxamol overdosage. *Br J Clin Pharmacol* (2000) 50, 388–9.
12. Levine B, Saady J, Fierro M, Valentour J. A hydromorphone and ethanol fatality. *J Forensic Sci* (1984) 29, 655–9.
13. Rush CR. Pretreatment with hydromorphone, a μ-opioid agonist, does not alter the acute behavioral and physiological effects of ethanol in humans. *Alcohol Clin Exp Res* (2001) 25, 9–17.
14. Lenné MG, Dietze P, Rumbold GR, Redman JR, Triggs TJ. The effects of the opioid pharmacotherapies methadone, LAAM and buprenorphine, alone and in combination with alcohol, on simulated driving. *Drug Alcohol Depend* (2003) 72, 271–8.
15. Schlatter J, Madras JL, Saulnier JL, Poujade F. Interactions médicamenteuses avec la méthadone. *Presse Med* (1999) 28, 1381–4.
16. Methadone Oral Solution. Rosemont Pharmaceuticals Ltd. UK Summary of product characteristics, January 2005.
17. Palladone (Hydromorphone hydrochloride). Purdue Pharma L.P. US Prescribing information, November 2004.
18. Murray S, Wooltorton E. Alcohol-associated rapid release of a long-acting opioid. *CMAJ* (2005) 173, 756.
19. FDA News. FDA asks Purdue Pharma to withdraw Palladone for safety reasons (issued 13th July 2005). Available at: http://www.fda.gov/bbs/topics/NEWS/2005/NEW01205.html (accessed 15/08/07).
20. Health Canada. Potentially fatal interaction between slow-release opioid painkillers and alcohol (issued 3rd August 2005). Available at: http://www.hc-sc.gc.ca/ahc-asc/media/advisories-avis/2005/2005_84_e.html (accessed 15/08/07).
21. Darke AC. Controlled-release opioids and alcohol. *CMAJ* (2006) 174, 352.
22. Mundi Pharma, Personal Communication, May 2007.
23. FDA Patient Safety News. Potentially hazardous interaction between Avinza and alcohol (issued March 2006). Available at: http://www.accessdata.fda.gov/scripts/cdrh/cfdocs/psn/printer.cfm?id=412 (accessed 15/08/07).
24. Avinza (Morphine sulfate extended-release capsules). King Pharmaceuticals Inc. US Prescribing information, October 2006.
25. Koski A, Ojanperä I, Vuori E. Interaction of alcohol and drugs in fatal poisonings. *Hum Exp Toxicol* (2003) 22, 281–7.
26. Darvon (Propoxyphene hydrochloride). AAI Pharma. US Prescribing information, February 2006.

Alcohol + Orlistat

A study in healthy subjects found that orlistat 120 mg three times daily for 6 days had no significant effect on the pharmacokinetics of alcohol.[1] There is nothing to suggest that alcohol should be avoided while taking orlistat.

1. Melia AT, Zhi J, Zelasko R, Hartmann D, Güzelhan C, Guerciolini R, Odink J. The interaction of the lipase inhibitor orlistat with ethanol in healthy volunteers. *Eur J Clin Pharmacol* (1998) 54, 773–7.

Alcohol + Paracetamol (Acetaminophen)

Many case reports describe severe liver damage, sometimes fatal, in some alcoholics and persistent heavy drinkers who take only moderate doses of paracetamol. However, other controlled studies have found no association between alcoholism and paracetamol-induced hepatotoxicity. There is controversy about the use of paracetamol in alcoholics. Some consider standard therapeutic doses can be used, whereas others recommend the dose of paracetamol should be reduced, or paracetamol avoided. Occasional and light to moderate drinkers do not seem to be at any extra risk. One study found that chronic alcohol intake, but not acute alcohol intake, enhanced paracetamol hepatotoxicity following overdose.

Clinical evidence

(a) Increased hepatotoxicity

Three chronic alcoholic patients developed severe liver damage after taking paracetamol. They had AST levels of about 7 000 to 10 000 units. Two of them had taken 10 g of paracetamol over 24 or 48 hours before admission (normal dosage is up to 4 g daily), and the third patient had taken about 50 g of paracetamol over 72 hours. One of them developed hepatic encephalopathy and died, and subsequent post-mortem revealed typical paracetamol toxicity. Two of them also developed renal failure.[1] A case of severe liver impairment has also been reported in a moderate social drinker who regularly drank 3 glasses of wine with dinner, but had stopped drinking alcohol whilst taking paracetamol for a viral infection.[2]

There are numerous other case reports of liver toxicity in alcoholics or chronic heavy alcohol users attributed to the concurrent use of alcohol and paracetamol. In the reports cited here, which include a total of about 30 patients, about one-third had been taking daily paracetamol doses of up to 4 g daily, and one-third had taken doses within the range 4 to 8 g daily.[3-19] Fasting possibly makes things worse.[20] A later survey reviewed a total of 94 cases from the literature, and described a further 67 patients who were regular users of alcohol, 64% of whom were alcoholics, who developed liver toxicity after taking paracetamol. In 60% of cases the paracetamol dose did not exceed 6 g daily and in 40% of cases the dose did not exceed 4 g daily. More than 90% of the patients developed AST levels ranging from 3 000 to 48 000 units.[21] A study of 209 consecutive cases of paracetamol overdose admitted to a liver unit in Denmark (57 identified as chronic alcohol intake and 45 as acute alcohol intake), found that chronic alcohol intake enhanced paracetamol hepatotoxicity. The relative risks for hepatic encephalopathy and death were 5.3 and 1.4, respectively, in the chronic alcohol intake group, compared with the non-chronic alcohol intake group, when adjusted for factors such as the total quantity of paracetamol ingested and the time to treatment with N-acetylcysteine. Acute alcohol intake did not affect the clinical course of paracetamol overdose.[22]

(b) No effect on hepatotoxicity

In a retrospective review of 553 cases of paracetamol-induced severe hepatotoxicity treated at a liver failure unit over a 7-year period, there was no association between the level of alcohol consumption and the severity of the hepatotoxicity (mean INR and serum creatinine levels in the first 7 days after overdose). Alcohol consumption was categorised into 4 groups ranging from non-drinkers to heavy drinkers (greater than 60 g of alcohol daily in men and 40 g daily in women).[23]

In a randomised, placebo-controlled study, there was no difference in measures of hepatotoxicity (mean AST levels, mean INR) between 102 alcoholic patients who received paracetamol 1 g four times daily for 2 days, and 99 alcoholic patients who received placebo. In this study, patients had entered an alcohol detoxification centre, and were given paracetamol immediately after stopping alcohol use[24] (the assumed time of greatest susceptibility, see Mechanism, below). A systematic review by the same research group concluded that the use of therapeutic doses of paracetamol in alcoholic patients is not associated with hepatic injury.[25]

(c) Effect on alcohol levels

Paracetamol 1 g was found to have no effect on the single-dose pharmacokinetics of alcohol in 12 healthy subjects.[26] Another study found that blood-alcohol levels were raised by 1 g of paracetamol but this was not statistically significant.[27]

Mechanism

Uncertain. The paracetamol-alcohol interaction is complex, because acute and chronic alcohol consumption can have opposite effects.[28,29] Paracetamol is usually predominantly metabolised by the liver to non-toxic sulfate and glucuronide conjugates. Persistent heavy drinking appears to stimulate a normally minor biochemical pathway involving the cytochrome P450 isoenzyme CYP2E1, and possibly CYP3A, which allows the production of unusually large amounts of highly hepatotoxic metabolites via oxidation.[20,29,30] Unless sufficient glutathione is present to detoxify these metabolites (alcoholics often have an inadequate intake of protein), they become covalently bound to liver macromolecules and damage results. Fasting may also make things worse by reducing the availability of glucose, and thus shifting paracetamol metabolism from glucuronidation towards microsomal oxidation.[20] However, most studies have failed to demonstrate an increase in hepatotoxic metabolites in alcoholics.[28,31] In fact alcoholics may possibly be most susceptible to toxicity during alcohol withdrawal because, while drinking, alcohol may possibly compete with the paracetamol for metabolism, and even inhibit it. Acute ingestion of alcohol by non-alcoholics may possibly protect them against damage because the damaging biochemical pathway is inhibited rather than stimulated. The relative timing of alcohol and paracetamol intake is therefore critical.[28]

Importance and management

The incidence of unexpected paracetamol toxicity in chronic alcoholics is uncertain, but possibly fairly small, bearing in mind the very wide-spread use of paracetamol and alcohol. Note that most of the evidence for an interaction comes from anecdotal case reports and case series, albeit in large numbers. However, the damage, when it occurs, can be serious and therefore some have advised that alcoholics and those who persistently drink heavily should avoid paracetamol or limit their intake considerably.[21] The normal daily recommended 'safe' maximum of 4 g is said to be too high in some alcoholics.[21] Because of this, the FDA in the US have required that all paracetamol-containing non-prescription products bear the warning that those consuming 3 or more alcoholic drinks every day should ask their doctor whether they should take paracetamol.[32] However, others consider that the evidence does not prove that there is an increase in paracetamol hepatotoxicity in alcoholics,[25,28] and is insufficient to support any change in paracetamol use or dose in alcoholics.[25,33] They note that the alternatives, aspirin and NSAIDs, are associated with a greater risk of gastrointestinal adverse effects in alcoholics,[25] see 'Alcohol + Aspirin', p.51 and 'Alcohol + NSAIDs', p.71. Further study is needed. The risk for non-alcoholics, moderate drinkers and those who very occasionally drink a lot appears to be low, although some chronic moderate social drinkers may be at risk, especially if alcohol intake is abruptly stopped.[34]

It is still prudent to consider patients who are alcoholics as being at high risk of hepatotoxicity after a paracetamol overdose, and to treat them with acetylcysteine.[28,30] Some workers have questioned the use of a lower plasma-paracetamol concentration threshold for the treatment of paracetamol poisoning in alcoholics,[31] but most advocate treatment at the lower threshold.[28,30] Possible malnutrition and fasting in these patients would further support the need for such treatment.[30]

1. McClain CJ, Kromhout JP, Peterson FJ, Holtzman JL. Potentiation of acetaminophen hepatotoxicity by alcohol. *JAMA* (1980) 244, 251–3.
2. Slattery JT, Nelson SD, Thummel KE. The complex interaction between ethanol and acetaminophen. *Clin Pharmacol Ther* (1996) 60, 241–6.
3. Emby DJ, Fraser BN. Hepatotoxicity of paracetamol enhanced by ingestion of alcohol. *S Afr Med J* (1977) 51, 208–9.
4. Goldfinger R, Ahmed KS, Pitchumoni CS, Weseley SA. Concomitant alcohol and drug abuse enhancing acetaminophen toxicity. *Am J Gastroenterol* (1978) 70, 385–8.
5. Barker JD, de Carle DJ, Anuras S. Chronic excessive acetaminophen use and liver damage. *Ann Intern Med* (1977) 87, 299–301.
6. O'Dell JR, Zetterman RK, Burnett DA. Centrilobular hepatic fibrosis following acetaminophen-induced hepatic necrosis in an alcoholic. *JAMA* (1986) 255, 2636–7.
7. McJunkin B, Barwick KW, Little WC, Winfield JB. Fatal massive hepatic necrosis following acetaminophen overdosage. *JAMA* (1976) 236, 1874–5.
8. LaBrecque DR, Mitros FA. Increased hepatotoxicity of acetaminophen in the alcoholic. *Gastroenterology* (1980) 78, 1310.
9. Johnson MW, Friedman PA, Mitch WE. Alcoholism, nonprescription drugs and hepatotoxicity. The risk from unknown acetaminophen ingestion. *Am J Gastroenterol* (1981) 76, 530–3.
10. Licht H, Seeff LB, Zimmerman HJ. Apparent potentiation of acetaminophen hepatotoxicity by alcohol. *Ann Intern Med* (1980) 92, 511.
11. Black M, Cornell JF, Rabin L, Shachter N. Late presentation of acetaminophen hepatotoxicity. *Dig Dis Sci* (1982) 27, 370–4.
12. Fleckenstein JL. *Nyquil* and acute hepatic necrosis. *N Engl J Med* (1985) 313, 48.
13. Gerber MA, Kaufmann H, Klion F, Alpert LI. Acetaminophen associated hepatic injury: report of two cases showing unusual portal tract reactions. *Hum Pathol* (1980) 11, 37–42.
14. Leist MH, Gluskin LE, Payne JA. Enhanced toxicity of acetaminophen in alcoholics: report of three cases. *J Clin Gastroenterol* (1985) 7, 55–9.
15. Himmelstein DU, Woolhandler SJ, Adler RD. Elevated SGOT/SGPT ratio in alcoholic patients with acetaminophen hepatotoxicity. *Am J Gastroenterol* (1984) 79, 718–20.
16. Levinson M. Ulcer, back pain and jaundice in an alcoholic. *Hosp Pract* (1983) 18, 48N, 48S.
17. Seeff LB, Cuccherini BA, Zimmerman HJ, Adler E, Benjamin SB. Acetaminophen hepatotoxicity in alcoholics. A therapeutic misadventure. *Ann Intern Med* (1986) 104, 399–404.
18. Florén C-H, Thesleff P, Nilsson Å. Severe liver damage caused by therapeutic doses of acetaminophen. *Acta Med Scand* (1987) 222, 285–8.
19. Edwards R, Oliphant J. Paracetamol toxicity in chronic alcohol abusers – a plea for greater consumer awareness. *N Z Med J* (1992) 105, 174–5.
20. Whitcomb DC, Block GD. Association of acetaminophen hepatotoxicity with fasting and ethanol use. *JAMA* (1994) 272, 1845–50.
21. Zimmerman HJ, Maddrey WC. Acetaminophen (paracetamol) hepatotoxicity with regular intake of alcohol: analysis of instances of therapeutic misadventure. *Hepatology* (1995) 22, 767–73.
22. Schiødt FV, Lee WM, Bondesen S, Ott P, Christensen E. Influence of acute and chronic alcohol intake on the clinical course and outcome in acetaminophen overdose. *Aliment Pharmacol Ther* (2002) 16, 707–15.
23. Makin A, Williams R. Paracetamol hepatotoxicity and alcohol consumption in deliberate and accidental overdose. *Q J Med* (2000) 93, 341–9.
24. Kuffner EK, Dart RC, Bogdan GM, Hill RE, Casper E, Darton L. Effect of maximal daily doses of acetaminophen on the liver of alcoholic patients: a randomized, double-blind, placebo-controlled trial. *Arch Intern Med* (2001) 161, 2247–52.
25. Dart RC, Kuffner EK, Rumack BH. Treatment of pain or fever with paracetamol (acetaminophen) in the alcoholic patient: a systematic review. *Am J Ther* (2000) 7, 123–4.
26. Melander O, Lidén A, Melander A. Pharmacokinetic interactions of alcohol and acetylsalicylic acid. *Eur J Clin Pharmacol* (1995) 48, 151–3.
27. Sharma SC, Feely J. The influence of aspirin and paracetamol on blood concentrations of alcohol in young adults. *Br J Clin Pharmacol* (1996) 41, 467P.
28. Prescott LF. Paracetamol, alcohol and the liver. *Br J Clin Pharmacol* (2000) 49, 291–301.
29. Tanaka E, Yamazaki K, Misawa S. Update: the clinical importance of acetaminophen hepatotoxicity in non-alcoholic and alcoholic subjects. *J Clin Pharm Ther* (2000) 25, 325–32.
30. Buckley NA, Srinivasan J. Should a lower treatment line be used when treating paracetamol poisoning in patients with chronic alcoholism? A case for. *Drug Safety* (2002) 25, 619–24.
31. Dargan PI, Jones AL. Should a lower treatment line be used when treating paracetamol poisoning in patients with chronic alcoholism? A case against. *Drug Safety* (2002) 25, 625–32.
32. Food and Drug Administration. FDA announces new alcohol warnings for pain relievers and fever reducers. HHS News. Available at: http://www.fda.gov/bbs/topics/NEWS/NEW00659.html (accessed 15/08/07).
33. Rumack BH. Acetaminophen hepatotoxicity: the first 35 years. *J Toxicol Clin Toxicol* (2002) 40, 3–20.
34. Draganov P, Durrence H, Cox C, Reuben A. Alcohol-acetaminophen syndrome. Even moderate social drinkers are at risk. *Postgrad Med* (2000) 107, 189–95.

Alcohol + Paraldehyde

Both alcohol and paraldehyde have CNS depressant effects, which can be additive. The use of paraldehyde in the treatment of acute alcohol intoxication has caused fatalities.

Clinical evidence, mechanism, importance and management

A report describes 9 patients who died suddenly and unexpectedly after treatment for acute alcohol intoxication with 30 to 90 mL of paraldehyde (the authors quote a normal dose range of 8 to 30 mL; fatal dose 120 mL or more, usually preceded by coma). None of the patients had hepatic impairment, although one did have some fatty changes.[1] Both drugs are CNS depressants and may therefore be expected to have additive effects at any dosage, although an *animal* study suggested that it might be less than additive,[2] and cross-tolerance may occur as paraldehyde is pharmacologically similar to alcohol.[3]

1. Kaye S, Haag HB. Study of death due to combined action of alcohol and paraldehyde in man. *Toxicol Appl Pharmacol* (1964) 6, 316–20.
2. Gessner PK, Shakarjian MP. Interactions of paraldehyde with ethanol and chloral hydrate. *J Pharmacol Exp Ther* (1985) 235, 32–6.
3. Weller RA, Preskorn SH. Psychotropic drugs and alcohol: pharmacokinetic and pharmacodynamic interactions. *Psychosomatics* (1984) 25, 301–3, 305–6, 309.

Alcohol + Phosphodiesterase type-5 inhibitors

Sildenafil, tadalafil and vardenafil do not usually alter the effects of alcohol on blood pressure, although postural hypotension has been seen in some subjects given tadalafil and alcohol, and headache and flushing has been reported in one patient taking sildena-

fil and alcohol. Alcohol does not affect the pharmacokinetics of tadalafil or vardenafil.

Clinical evidence, mechanism, importance and management

(a) Sildenafil

Sildenafil 50 mg did not potentiate the hypotensive effect of alcohol (mean maximum blood-alcohol levels of 80 mg%) in healthy subjects.[1,2] A study in 8 healthy subjects also found that sildenafil 100 mg did not affect the haemodynamic effects of red wine (e.g. heart rate, mean arterial pressure).[3] However, a case report describes potentiation of the adverse effects of sildenafil when alcohol was consumed within one hour of taking the drug. A 36-year-old hypertensive patient receiving regular treatment with a calcium-channel blocker (amlodipine) was additionally prescribed sildenafil 25 mg, which he used 3 times a week without any adverse effects. However, after having 2 drinks of whiskey (55.2 g of alcohol) he experienced severe headache and flushing about 15 minutes after taking sildenafil. The next day he took sildenafil 25 mg without any alcohol and no symptoms developed, but one week later, a challenge dose of sildenafil was given after a single 30-mL drink of whiskey and similar symptoms of severe headache and flushing occurred.[4] The UK patient information leaflet says that drinking alcohol can temporarily impair the ability to get an erection and advises patients not to drink large amounts of alcohol before taking sildenafil.[5]

(b) Tadalafil

Studies in subjects given alcohol 0.6 or 0.7 g/kg found that the effect of alcohol on blood pressure was unchanged by tadalafil 20 mg, although some subjects experienced dizziness and postural hypotension. In addition, the effects of alcohol on cognitive function were unchanged by tadalafil 10 mg.[6] The pharmacokinetics of tadalafil 10 or 20 mg and alcohol were also unaffected by concurrent use.[6,7] However, the manufacturers say that because both alcohol and tadalafil can cause peripheral vasodilation, additive blood pressure lowering effects are possible,[7,8] especially with substantial amounts of alcohol (5 units) and the US manufacturer states that this may result in postural hypotension, increased heart rate, dizziness and headache.[7] Alcohol may also affect the ability to have an erection.[8]

(c) Vardenafil

Alcohol (mean blood level of 73 mg%) did not affect the pharmacokinetics of vardenafil 20 mg.[9] The effects of alcohol on heart rate and blood pressure were also not affected by vardenafil.[9,10] There would therefore seem to be no need to avoid the combination. However, alcoholic drink can worsen erection difficulties.[11]

1. Viagra (Sildenafil citrate). Pfizer Ltd. UK Summary of product characteristics, June 2006.
2. Viagra (Sildenafil citrate). Pfizer Inc. US Prescribing information, October 2006.
3. Leslie SJ, Atkins G, Oliver JJ, Webb DJ. No adverse hemodynamic interaction between sildenafil and red wine. *Clin Pharmacol Ther* (2004) 76, 365–70.
4. Bhalla A. Is sildenafil safe with alcohol? *J Assoc Physicians India* (2003) 51, 1125–6.
5. Viagra (Sildenafil). Pfizer Ltd. UK Patient information leaflet, February 2007.
6. Cialis (Tadalafil). Eli Lilly and Company Ltd. UK Summary of product characteristics, July 2006.
7. Cialis (Tadalafil). Eli Lilly and Company Ltd. US Prescribing information, January 2007.
8. Cialis (Tadalafil). Eli Lilly and Company Ltd. UK Patient information leaflet, February 2007.
9. Levitra (Vardenafil hydrochloride trihydrate). Bayer plc. UK Summary of product characteristics, November 2006.
10. Levitra (Vardenafil hydrochloride). Bayer Pharmaceuticals Corporation. US Prescribing information, March 2007.
11. Levitra (Vardenafil). Bayer plc. UK Patient information leaflet, June 2006.

Alcohol + Procainamide

Alcohol may modestly increase the clearance of procainamide.

Clinical evidence, mechanism, importance and management

In 11 healthy subjects alcohol 0.73 g/kg, followed by alcohol 0.11 g/kg every hour increased the clearance and decreased the elimination half-life of a single 10-mg/kg oral dose of procainamide by 34% and 25%, respectively. This was due to increased acetylation of procainamide to its active metabolite *N*-acetylprocainamide.[1] The clinical relevance of these modest changes is probably small.

1. Olsen H, Mørland J. Ethanol-induced increase in procainamide acetylation in man. *Br J Clin Pharmacol* (1982) 13, 203–8.

Alcohol + Procarbazine

A flushing reaction has been seen in patients taking procarbazine who drank alcohol.

Clinical evidence

One report describes 5 patients taking procarbazine whose faces became very red and hot for a short time after drinking wine.[1] Another says that flushing occurred in 3 patients taking procarbazine after they drank beer.[2] Two out of 40 patients taking procarbazine in a third study complained of facial flushing after taking a small alcoholic drink, and one patient thought that the effects of alcohol were markedly increased.[3] Yet another study describes a 'flush syndrome' in 3 out of 50 patients who drank alcohol while taking procarbazine.[4]

Mechanism

Unknown, but it seems possible that in man, as in *rats*,[5] the procarbazine inhibits acetaldehyde dehydrogenase in the liver causing a disulfiram-like reaction (see 'Alcohol + Disulfiram', p.61).

Importance and management

An established interaction but of uncertain incidence. It seems to be more embarrassing, possibly frightening, than serious and if it occurs it is unlikely to require treatment, however patients should be warned. The manufacturers say it is best to avoid alcohol.[6] Procarbazine is also a weak MAOI and therefore interactions with certain foodstuffs, including alcoholic drinks, especially heavy red wines, although very rare, must be borne in mind (see 'Procarbazine + Sympathomimetics', p.657).

1. Mathé G, Berumen L, Schweisguth O, Brule G, Schneider M, Cattan A, Amiel JL, Schwarzenberg L. Methyl-hydrazine in the treatment of Hodgkin's disease and various forms of haematosarcoma and leukaemia. *Lancet* (1963) ii, 1077–80.
2. Dawson WB. Ibenzmethyzin in the management of late Hodgkin's disease. In 'Natulan, Ibenzmethyzin'. Report of the proceedings of a symposium, Downing College, Cambridge, June 1965. Jelliffe AM and Marks J (Eds). Bristol: John Wright; 1965. P. 31–4.
3. Todd IDH. Natulan in management of late Hodgkin's disease, other lymphoreticular neoplasms, and malignant melanoma. *BMJ* (1965) 1, 628–31.
4. Brulé G, Schlumberger JR, Griscelli C. *N*-isopropyl-α-(2-methylhydrazino)-*p*-toluamide, hydrochloride (NSC-77213) in treatment of solid tumors. *Cancer Chemother Rep* (1965) 44, 31–8.
5. Vasiliou V, Malamas M, Marselos M. The mechanism of alcohol intolerance produced by various therapeutic agents. *Acta Pharmacol Toxicol (Copenh)* (1986) 58, 305–10.
6. Matulane (Procarbazine hydrochloride). Sigma-tau Pharmaceuticals, Inc. US Prescribing Information, February 2004.

Alcohol + Proton pump inhibitors

Lansoprazole, omeprazole and pantoprazole do not interact with alcohol: other proton pump inhibitors therefore seem unlikely to interact.

Clinical evidence

(a) Lansoprazole

A study in 30 healthy subjects given 0.6 g/kg of alcohol before and after taking lansoprazole 30 mg daily for 3 days found that the pharmacokinetics of alcohol were not significantly changed, and blood-alcohol levels were not raised, by lansoprazole.[1]

(b) Omeprazole

A number of studies have shown that omeprazole does not affect blood alcohol levels.[2-6]

(c) Pantoprazole

Pantoprazole 40 mg daily or placebo were given to 16 healthy subjects for 7 days. On day 7 they were also given alcohol 0.5 g/kg in 200 mL of orange juice 2 hours after a standard breakfast. The maximum serum levels and the AUC of alcohol were not significantly changed by pantoprazole.[7]

Mechanism

The proton pump inhibitors do not affect alcohol dehydrogenase activity[3,8] (compare with the 'H_2-receptor antagonists', (p.64)), and would not be expected to alter the first-pass metabolism of alcohol.

Importance and management

The proton pump inhibitors do not appear to interact with alcohol, and no special precautions are necessary with concurrent use. But note that some of the conditions for which these drugs are used may be made worse by alcohol, so restriction of drinking of alcohol may be prudent.

1. Girre C, Coutelle C, David P, Fleury B, Thomas G, Palmobo S, Dally S, Couzigou P. Lack of effect of lansoprazole on the pharmacokinetics of ethanol in male volunteers. *Gastroenterology* (1994) 106, A504.
2. Guram M, Howden CW, Holt S. Further evidence for an interaction between alcohol and certain H_2-receptor antagonists. *Alcohol Clin Exp Res* (1991) 15, 1084–5.
3. Roine R, Hernández-Muñoz R, Baraona E, Greenstein R, Lieber CS. Effect of omeprazole on gastric first-pass metabolism of ethanol. *Dig Dis Sci* (1992) 37, 891–6.
4. Jönsson K-Å, Jones AW, Boström H, Andersson T. Lack of effect of omeprazole, cimetidine, and ranitidine on the pharmacokinetics of ethanol in fasting male volunteers. *Eur J Clin Pharmacol* (1992) 42, 209–212.
5. Minocha A, Rahal PS, Brier ME, Levinson SS. Omeprazole therapy does not affect pharmacokinetics of orally administered ethanol in healthy male subjects. *J Clin Gastroenterol* (1995) 21, 107–9.
6. Brown AS, James OF. Omeprazole, ranitidine, and cimetidine have no effect on peak blood ethanol concentrations, first pass metabolism or area under the time-ethanol curve under 'real-life' drinking conditions. *Aliment Pharmacol Ther* (1998) 12, 141–5.
7. Heinze H, Fischer R, Pfützer R, Teyssen S, Singer MV. Lack of interaction between pantoprazole and ethanol: a randomised, double-blind, placebo-controlled study in healthy volunteers. *Clin Drug Invest* (2001) 21, 345–51.
8. Battiston L, Tulissi P, Moretti M, Pozzato G. Lansoprazole and ethanol metabolism: comparison with omeprazole and cimetidine. *Pharmacol Toxicol* (1997) 81, 247–52.

Alcohol + Quetiapine

Postural hypotension and possibly drowsiness may be increased when alcohol is given with quetiapine. Quetiapine does not appear to affect the pharmacokinetics of alcohol.

Clinical evidence, mechanism, importance and management

A randomised, crossover study in 8 men with psychotic disorders found that quetiapine 250 mg three times daily did not affect the mean breath-alcohol concentration after they took 0.8 g/kg of alcohol in orange juice. Some statistically significant changes in the performance of psychomotor tests were seen, but these were considered to have little clinical relevance. However, the US manufacturers of quetiapine say that, in clinical studies, the motor and cognitive effects of alcohol were potentiated by quetiapine. Therefore the US manufacturers of quetiapine[1] advise avoiding alcohol, and the UK manufacturers[2] advise caution with the concurrent use of alcohol.[3] Note that drowsiness is the most common adverse effect of quetiapine, occurring in over 10% of patients.[1,2] Quetiapine may occasionally induce postural hypotension,[1,2] which could be exacerbated by alcohol administration.

1. Seroquel (Quetiapine fumarate). AstraZeneca. US Prescribing information, July 2007.
2. Seroquel (Quetiapine fumarate). AstraZeneca UK Ltd. UK Summary of product characteristics, November 2006.
3. Zeneca Pharma. Personal communication, October 1997.

Alcohol + Reboxetine

A study in 10 healthy subjects found that reboxetine does not affect cognitive or psychomotor function, and there is no interaction with alcohol.[1]

1. Kerr JS, Powell J, Hindmarch I. The effects of reboxetine and amitriptyline, with and without alcohol on cognitive function and psychomotor performance. *Br J Clin Pharmacol* (1996) 42, 239–41.

Alcohol + Retinoids

There is evidence that the consumption of alcohol may increase the serum levels of etretinate in patients taking acitretin. A single case report describes a marked reduction in the effects of isotretinoin following the acute intake of alcohol.

Clinical evidence, mechanism, importance and management

(a) Acitretin

A study in 10 patients with psoriasis taking acitretin found that the concurrent use of alcohol seemed to be associated with an increase in the formation of its metabolite etretinate, which has a much longer half-life than acitretin. The implications of this study are not known, but it is suggested that it may have some bearing on the length of the period after acitretin therapy during which women are advised not to conceive.[1]

(b) Isotretinoin

A former alcoholic, who no longer drank alcohol, was treated for acne conglobata, with some success, with isotretinoin 60 mg daily for 3 months. When for 2 weeks he briefly started to drink alcohol again as part of his job (he was a sherry taster) his skin lesions reappeared and the isotretinoin adverse effects (mucocutaneous dryness) vanished. When he stopped drinking alcohol his skin lesions became controlled again and the drug adverse effects re-emerged. The following year, while receiving another course of isotretinoin, the same thing happened when he started and stopped drinking alcohol. The reasons are not known, but one suggestion is that the alcohol briefly induced the liver microsomal enzymes responsible for the metabolism of isotretinoin, thereby reducing both its therapeutic and adverse effects.[2] The general importance of this apparent interaction is not known.

1. Larsen FG, Jakobsen P, Knudsen J, Weismann K, Kragballe K, Nielsen-Kudsk F. Conversion of acitretin to etretinate in psoriatic patients is influenced by ethanol. *J Invest Dermatol* (1993) 100, 623–7.
2. Soria C, Allegue F, Galiana J, Ledo A. Decreased isotretinoin efficacy during acute alcohol intake. *Dermatologica* (1991) 182, 203.

Alcohol + Salbutamol (Albuterol)

A patient with high blood-alcohol levels developed lactic acidosis after being exposed to smoke and receiving salbutamol.

Clinical evidence, mechanism, importance and management

An isolated report describes a 49-year-old male alcoholic who developed severe lactic acidosis after exposure to fire smoke and treatment of bronchospasm with salbutamol. The correction of lactic acidosis followed salbutamol withdrawal and a transitory increase in lactate after salbutamol re-introduction suggested hypersensitivity to salbutamol. However, the patient also had a very high plasma-alcohol level (240 mg%), and the metabolism of the alcohol was thought to have competed with the conversion of lactate to pyruvate resulting in reduced lactate clearance, thus potentiating the acidosis caused by the salbutamol.[1] The clinical significance of this report is unclear as beta agonist-induced exacerbation of lactic acidosis has been reported in asthmatics, both adults and children. The authors of the above report suggest close monitoring of lactate levels in alcoholic patients receiving beta-agonists.[1]

1. Taboulet P, Clemessy J-L, Fréminet A, Baud FJ. A case of life-threatening lactic acidosis after smoke inhalation – interference between ß-adrenergic agents and ethanol? *Intensive Care Med* (1995) 21, 1039–42.

Alcohol + Sibutramine

There does not seem to be a clinically relevant interaction between sibutramine and alcohol.

Clinical evidence, mechanism, importance and management

In a randomised study, 20 healthy subjects were given sibutramine 20 mg with 0.5 g/kg of alcohol diluted in ginger beer, or placebo. Sibutramine did not potentiate the cognitive or psychomotor effects of alcohol, and in one test, sibutramine slightly reduced the impairment caused by alcohol.[1]

However, the manufacturer notes that the consumption of alcohol is generally not compatible with recommended adjuvant dietary modification.[2]

1. Wesnes KA, Garratt C, Wickens M, Gudgeon A, Oliver S. Effects of sibutramine alone and with alcohol on cognitive function in healthy volunteers. *Br J Clin Pharmacol* (2000) 49, 110–17.
2. Reductil (Sibutramine hydrochloride monohydrate). Abbott Laboratories Ltd. UK Summary of product characteristics, November 2005.

Alcohol + SNRIs

No important psychomotor interaction normally appears to occur between duloxetine or venlafaxine and alcohol. However, the manufacturer warns that use of duloxetine with heavy alcohol intake may be associated with severe liver injury.

Clinical evidence, mechanism, importance and management

(a) Duloxetine

In a single-dose study in healthy subjects, duloxetine 60 mg, and alcohol given in a dose sufficient to produce blood levels of about 100 mg%, did not worsen the psychomotor impairment observed with alcohol alone.[1] Nevertheless, the UK manufacturer advises caution,[2] and the US manufacturer warns that duloxetine should ordinarily not be prescribed for patients with substantial alcohol use as severe liver injury may result.[3]

(b) Venlafaxine

Venlafaxine 50 mg every 8 hours was found to have some effect on psychomotor tests (digit symbol substitution, divided attention reaction times, profile of mood scales) in 15 healthy subjects, but these changes were small and not considered to be clinically significant. No pharmacodynamic or pharmacokinetic interactions occurred when alcohol 0.5 g/kg was also given.[4]

In therapeutic doses venlafaxine does not appear to interact significantly with alcohol, however, the manufacturers state that, as with all centrally-active drugs, patients should be advised to avoid alcohol whilst taking venlafaxine.[5,6] This is presumably because both drugs act on the CNS and also because alcohol is more likely to be abused by depressed patients.

1. Skinner MH, Weerakkody G. Duloxetine does not exacerbate the effects of alcohol on psychometric tests. *Clin Pharmacol Ther* (2002) 71, 53.
2. Cymbalta (Duloxetine hydrochloride). Eli Lilly and Company Ltd. UK Summary of product characteristics, November 2006.
3. Cymbalta (Duloxetine hydrochloride). Eli Lilly and Company. US Prescribing information, May 2007.
4. Troy SM, Turner MB, Unruh M, Parker VD, Chiang ST. Pharmacokinetic and pharmacodynamic evaluation of the potential drug interaction between venlafaxine and ethanol. *J Clin Pharmacol* (1997) 37, 1073–81.
5. Efexor (Venlafaxine hydrochloride). Wyeth Pharmaceuticals. UK Summary of product characteristics, May 2006.
6. Effexor (Venlafaxine hydrochloride). Wyeth Pharmaceuticals Inc. US Prescribing information, June 2007.

Alcohol + Sodium cromoglicate (Cromolyn sodium)

No adverse interaction occurs between sodium cromoglicate and alcohol.

Clinical evidence, mechanism, importance and management

A double-blind, crossover study in 17 healthy subjects found that the inhalation of 40 mg of sodium cromoglicate had little or no effect on the performance of a number of tests on human perceptual, cognitive, and motor skills, whether taken alone or with alcohol 0.75 g/kg. Nor did it affect blood-alcohol levels.[1] This is in line with the common experience of patients, and no special precautions seem to be necessary.

1. Crawford WA, Franks HM, Hensley VR, Hensley WJ, Starmer GA, Teo RKC. The effect of disodium cromoglycate on human performance, alone and in combination with ethanol. *Med J Aust* (1976) 1, 997–9.

Alcohol + SSRIs

Citalopram, escitalopram, fluoxetine, paroxetine and sertraline have no significant pharmacokinetic interaction with alcohol, but some modest increase in sedation may possibly occur with fluvoxamine and paroxetine.

Clinical evidence and mechanism

(a) Citalopram

The manufacturers of citalopram say that no pharmacodynamic interactions have been noted in clinical studies in which citalopram was given with alcohol.[1,2]

(b) Escitalopram

The manufacturers of escitalopram say that no pharmacokinetic or pharmacodynamic interactions are expected to occur with concurrent use of alcohol and escitalopram.[3]

(c) Fluoxetine

The concurrent use of fluoxetine 30 to 60 mg and alcohol (4 oz of whiskey) did not affect the pharmacokinetics of either drugs in healthy subjects, and fluoxetine did not alter the effect of alcohol on psychomotor activity (stability of stance, motor performance, manual co-ordination).[4] Similarly, blood-alcohol levels of 80 mg% impaired the performance of a number of psychomotor tests in 12 healthy subjects, but the addition of fluoxetine 40 mg daily taken for 6 days before the alcohol had little further effect.[5] Another study also found no change in the performance of a number of psychophysiological tests when fluoxetine was combined with alcohol.[6] No problems were found in a study of 20 alcohol-dependent patients taking fluoxetine 60 mg daily when they drank alcohol, or in approximately 31 patients taking fluoxetine 20 mg daily who drank unspecified small quantities of alcohol.[7]

(d) Fluvoxamine

One study found that fluvoxamine 150 mg daily with alcohol impaired alertness and attention more than alcohol alone,[8] whereas another study in subjects given 40 g of alcohol (blood-alcohol levels up to 70 mg%) found no evidence to suggest that the addition of fluvoxamine 50 mg twice daily worsened the performance of the psychomotor tests, and it even appeared to reverse some of the effects.[9] The pharmacokinetics of alcohol were hardly affected by fluvoxamine, but the steady state maximum plasma levels of the fluvoxamine were increased by 20%, although the fluvoxamine AUC was unchanged.[9] It was suggested that administration of alcohol may have promoted dissolution of fluvoxamine and increased the absorption rate without affecting bioavailability.[9] Another study also found that fluvoxamine does not appear to enhance the detrimental effects of alcohol on the performance of psychomotor tests.[10]

(e) Paroxetine

Studies have found that paroxetine alone caused little impairment of a series of psychomotor tests related to car driving, and with alcohol the effects were unchanged, except for a significant decrease in attentiveness and an increase in reaction time.[11,12] Another study suggested that the alcohol-induced sedation was antagonised by paroxetine.[13]

(f) Sertraline

Sertraline (in doses of up to 200 mg for 9 days) was found not to impair cognitive or psychomotor performance, and it also appeared not to increase the effects of alcohol.[14]

Importance and management

The results of the few studies reported above suggest that no pharmacokinetic or pharmacodynamic interactions occur with most SSRIs and alcohol, although modest effects were seen with fluvoxamine and possibly paroxetine. However, most manufacturers of SSRIs suggest that concurrent use with alcohol is not advisable. This is presumably because both drugs act on the CNS and also because of the risk of alcohol abuse in depressed patients.[15]

1. Cipramil (Citalopram hydrobromide). Lundbeck Ltd. UK Summary of product characteristics, January 2007.
2. Celexa (Citalopram hydrobromide). Forest Pharmaceuticals, Inc. US Prescribing information, May 2007.
3. Cipralex (Escitalopram oxalate). Lundbeck Ltd. UK Summary of product characteristics, December 2005.
4. Lemberger L, Rowe H, Bergstrom RF, Farid KZ, Enas GG. Effect of fluoxetine on psychomotor performance, physiologic response, and kinetics of ethanol. *Clin Pharmacol Ther* (1985) 37, 658–64.

5. Allen D, Lader M, Curran HV. A comparative study of the interactions of alcohol with amitriptyline, fluoxetine and placebo in normal subjects. *Prog Neuropsychopharmacol Biol Psychiatry* (1988) 12, 63–80.
6. Schaffler K. Study on performance and alcohol interaction with the antidepressant fluoxetine. *Int Clin Psychopharmacol* (1989) 4 (Suppl 1), 15–20.
7. Florkowski A, Gruszczyñski W. Alcohol problems and treating patients with fluoxetine. *Pol J Pharmacol* (1995) 47, 547.
8. Duphar Laboratories. Study of the effects of the antidepressant fluvoxamine on driving skills and its interaction with alcohol. Data on file, 1981.
9. van Harten J, Stevens LA, Raghoebar M, Holland RL, Wesnes K, Cournot A. Fluvoxamine does not interact with alcohol or potentiate alcohol-related impairment of cognitive function. *Clin Pharmacol Ther* (1992) 52, 427–35.
10. Linnoila M, Stapleton JM, George DT, Lane E, Eckardt MJ. Effects of fluvoxamine, alone and in combination with ethanol, on psychomotor and cognitive performance and on autonomic nervous system reactivity in healthy volunteers. *J Clin Psychopharmacol* (1993) 13, 175–80.
11. Cooper SM, Jackson D, Loudon JM, McClelland GR, Raptopoulos P. The psychomotor effects of paroxetine alone and in combination with haloperidol, amylobarbitone, oxazepam, or alcohol. *Acta Psychiatr Scand* (1989) 80 (Suppl 350), 53–55.
12. Hindmarch I, Harrison C. The effects of paroxetine and other antidepressants in combination with alcohol on psychomotor activity related to car driving. *Acta Psychiatr Scand* (1989) 80 (Suppl 350), 45.
13. Kerr JS, Fairweather DB, Mahendran R, Hindmarch I. The effects of paroxetine, alone and in combination with alcohol on psychomotor performance and cognitive function in the elderly. *Int Clin Psychopharmacol* (1992) 7, 101–8.
14. Warrington SJ. Clinical implications of the pharmacology of sertraline. *Int Clin Psychopharmacol* (1991) 6 (Suppl 2), 11–21.
15. Eli Lilly and Company Ltd. Personal communication, October 2006.

Alcohol + Sulfiram

Disulfiram-like reactions have been seen in at least three patients who drank alcohol after using a solution of sulfiram on the skin for the treatment of scabies.

Clinical evidence

A man who used undiluted *Tetmosol* (a solution of sulfiram) for 3 days on the skin all over his body developed a disulfiram-like reaction (flushing, sweating, skin swelling, severe tachycardia and nausea) on the third day, after drinking 3 double whiskies. The same thing happened on two subsequent evenings again after drinking 3 double whiskies.[1] Similar reactions have been described in 2 other patients who drank alcohol while using *Tetmosol* or *Ascabiol* (also containing sulfiram).[2,3]

Mechanism

Sulfiram (tetraethylthiuram *monosulphide*) is closely related to disulfiram (tetraethylthiuram *disulphide*) and can apparently undergo photochemical conversion to disulfiram when exposed to light. The longer it is stored, the higher the concentration.[4,5] The reaction with alcohol appears therefore to be largely due to the presence of disulfiram,[6] see 'Alcohol + Disulfiram', p.61.

Importance and management

An established interaction. The manufacturers of sulfiram preparations and others advise abstention from alcohol before, and for at least 48 hours after application, but this may not always be necessary. The writer of a letter,[7] commenting on one of the cases cited,[1] wrote that he had never encountered this reaction when using a diluted solution of *Tetmosol* on patients at the Dreadnought Seamen's Hospital in London who he described as "not necessarily abstemious". This would suggest that the reaction is normally uncommon and unlikely to occur if the solution is correctly diluted (usually with 2 to 3 parts of water), thereby reducing the amount absorbed through the skin. However, one unusually sensitive patient is said to have had a reaction (flushing, sweating, tachycardia) after using diluted *Tetmosol*, but without drinking alcohol. It was suggested that she reacted to the alcohol base of the formulation passing through her skin.[8]

1. Gold S. A skinful of alcohol. *Lancet* (1966) ii, 1417.
2. Dantas W. Monosulfiram como causa de síndrome do acetaldeído. *Arq Cat Med* (1980) 9, 29–30.
3. Blanc D, Deprez Ph. Unusual adverse reaction to an acaricide. *Lancet* (1990) 335, 1291–2.
4. Lipsky JJ, Mays DC, Naylor S. Monosulfiram, disulfiram, and light. *Lancet* (1994) 343, 304.
5. Mays DC, Nelson AN, Benson LM, Johnson KL, Naylor S, Lipsky JJ. Photolysis of monosulfiram: a mechanism for its disulfiram-like reaction. *Clin Pharmacol Ther* (1994) 55, 191.
6. Lipsky JJ, Nelson AN, Dockter EC. Inhibition of aldehyde dehydrogenase by sulfiram. *Clin Pharmacol Ther* (1992) 51, 184.
7. Erskine D. A skinful of alcohol. *Lancet* (1967) i, 54.
8. Burgess I. Adverse reactions to monosulfiram. *Lancet* (1990) 336, 873.

Alcohol + Sumatriptan

Alcohol does not alter the pharmacokinetics of sumatriptan.

Clinical evidence, mechanism, importance and management

A single 0.8-g/kg dose of alcohol was given to 16 healthy subjects, followed 30 minutes later by 200 mg of sumatriptan. No statistically significant changes were seen in the pharmacokinetics of sumatriptan.[1] There is nothing to suggest that alcohol should be avoided while taking sumatriptan.

1. Kempsford RD, Lacey LF, Thomas M, Fowler PA. The effect of alcohol on the pharmacokinetic profile of oral sumatriptan. *Fundam Clin Pharmacol* (1991) 5, 470.

Alcohol + Tacrolimus or Pimecrolimus

Alcohol may cause facial flushing or skin erythema in patients being treated with tacrolimus ointment; this reaction appears to be fairly common. Alcohol intolerance has been reported rarely with pimecrolimus cream.

Clinical evidence

Six patients reported facial flushing with small quantities of beer or wine during facial treatment with tacrolimus ointment. Re-exposure to tacrolimus 0.1% ointment, applied to the face twice daily for 4 days, followed by 100 mL of white wine on the fifth day, resulted in a facial flush reaction in all the patients, which occurred within 5 to 15 minutes of alcohol ingestion. The intensity of the erythema varied among the patients and was not confined to the treated areas, but started to fade after 30 minutes; a slight headache occurred in one patient. Forearm skin was also exposed to an epicutaneous patch containing 70 mg of tacrolimus 0.1% ointment, but these sites remained unchanged following alcohol exposure. After a tacrolimus washout period of at least 4 weeks, controlled exposure to alcohol in 2 patients was tolerated normally.[1] Another report describes one patient using tacrolimus ointment for mild eyelid eczema who experienced eyelid erythema, limited to the area the tacrolimus ointment was applied, after wine ingestion. Two other patients experienced an erythematous rash after alcohol when using topical tacrolimus; areas affected included the elbows, ears, eyes and face. The response to alcohol disappeared within 2 weeks of discontinuing tacrolimus ointment.[2]

Three patients experienced application site erythema following the consumption of alcohol after using topical tacrolimus or pimecrolimus for the treatment of facial dermatoses. Two of the patients then participated in a double-blind, controlled evaluation of the reaction. Both patients consumed alcohol (240 mL of red or white wine) without experiencing flushing, but following tacrolimus or pimecrolimus application, they experienced moderate or severe facial flushing (limited to the area of application) 5 to 10 minutes after alcohol consumption. The intensity of the erythema was sharply reduced after taking aspirin 325 mg twice daily for 3 days before alcohol consumption, but cetirizine 10 mg daily with cimetidine 400 mg twice daily for 3 days appeared to have little effect.[3]

There are other reports of this interaction between tacrolimus and alcohol.[3-7] The reaction is usually confined to the face and the intensity may be related to the amount of alcohol ingested.[4] In an open study of 316 patients, alcohol intolerance (facial flushing) was observed in 19% of the patients using tacrolimus 0.1% ointment[6] and in a controlled study, 6.9% of patients experienced the reaction with tacrolimus 0.1% ointment, and 3.4% of patients experienced the reaction with tacrolimus 0.03% ointment.[5]

Mechanism

The mechanism of this interaction is not understood. It has been proposed that tacrolimus may act on the same biochemical pathway as alcohol potentiating a capsaicin-mediated release of neuropeptides, which increase vasodilatory effects. Alternatively, cutaneous aldehyde dehydrogenase inhibition in areas where tacrolimus has been applied may increase cutaneous aldehyde levels that, through prostaglandins as mediators, could lead to vasodilation following alcohol consumption.[1,4]

Importance and management

The interaction between topical tacrolimus and alcohol is established and appears to occur in about 6 to 7% of patients treated with tacrolimus 0.1% ointment. Patients should be warned of the possibility of a flushing reaction with alcohol and that consumption of alcohol may need to be avoided if this occurs. Clinicians should be aware of the interaction and obtain a careful history, including alcohol use, in patients who present with new acute symptoms while using tacrolimus. It has been suggested that aspirin may possibly reduce the symptoms of this reaction,[3] but this needs further study. Alcohol intolerance with pimecrolimus has been reported,[3,8] but appears to be rare.[9]

1. Milingou M, Antille C, Sorg O, Saurat J-H, Lübbe J. Alcohol intolerance and facial flushing in patients treated with topical tacrolimus. *Arch Dermatol* (2004) 140, 1542–4.
2. Knight AK, Boxer M, Chandler MJ. Alcohol-induced rash caused by topical tacrolimus. *Ann Allergy Asthma Immunol* (2005) 95, 291–2.
3. Ehst BD, Warshaw EM. Alcohol-induced application site erythema after topical immunomodulator use and its inhibition by aspirin. *Arch Dermatol* (2004) 140, 1014–15.
4. Morales-Molina JA, Mateu-de Antonio J, Grau S, Ferrández O. Alcohol ingestion and topical tacrolimus: a disulfiram-like interaction? *Ann Pharmacother* (2005) 39, 772–3.
5. Soter NA, Fleischer AB, Webster GF Monroe E, Lawrence I; the Tacrolimus Ointment Study Group. Tacrolimus ointment for the treatment of atopic dermatitis in adult patients: part II, safety. *J Am Acad Dermatol* (2001) 44 (Suppl 1), S39–S46.
6. Reitamo S, Wollenberg A, Schöpf E, Perrot JL, Marks R, Ruzicka T, Christophers E, Kapp A, Lahfa M, Rubins A, Jablonska S, Rustin M.; the European Tacrolimus Ointment Study Group. Safety and efficacy of 1 year of tacrolimus ointment monotherapy in adults with atopic dermatitis. *Arch Dermatol* (2000) 136, 999–1006.
7. Lübbe J, Milingou M. Tacrolimus ointment, alcohol, and facial flushing. *N Engl J Med* (2004) 351, 2740.
8. Elidel (Pimecrolimus). Novartis Pharmaceuticals Corp. US Prescribing information, January 2006.
9. Elidel (Pimecrolimus). Novartis Pharmaceuticals UK Ltd. UK Summary of product characteristics, February 2007.

Alcohol + Tetracyclic antidepressants

Mianserin and maprotiline can cause drowsiness and impair the ability to drive or handle other dangerous machinery, particularly during the first few days of treatment. This impairment may be increased by alcohol. Pirlindole does not appear to interact with alcohol.

Clinical evidence

(a) Maprotiline

A double-blind, crossover study in 12 healthy subjects found that a single 75-mg oral dose of maprotiline subjectively caused drowsiness, which was increased by 1 g/kg of alcohol. The performance of a number of psychomotor tests was also worsened after the addition of alcohol.[1] However, in a later study the same group found that maprotiline 50 mg twice daily, for 15 days, did not increase the detrimental effects of alcohol.[2]

(b) Mianserin

A double-blind, crossover study in 13 healthy subjects given 10 to 30 mg of mianserin twice daily for 8 days, with and without alcohol 1 g/kg, found that their performance in a number of psychomotor tests (choice reaction, coordination, critical flicker frequency) were impaired both by mianserin alone and by concurrent use with alcohol. The subjects were aware of feeling drowsy, muzzy, and less able to carry out the tests.[3] These results confirm the findings of other studies.[4,5]

(c) Pirlindole

A study in healthy subjects given pirlindole 75 to 150 mg daily for 4 days indicated that it did not affect the performance of a number of psychomotor tests, both with and without 0.4 g/kg of alcohol.[6]

Mechanism

The CNS depressant effects of mianserin, and possibly maprotiline, appear to be additive with those of alcohol.

Importance and management

Drowsiness is a frequently reported adverse effect of mianserin, particularly during the first few days of treatment. Patients should be warned that driving or handling dangerous machinery will be made more hazardous if they drink. It would also be prudent to warn patients taking maprotiline of the possible increased risk if they drink.[2] Pirlindole appears not to interact.

1. Strömberg C, Seppälä T, Mattila MJ. Acute effects of maprotiline, doxepin and zimeldine with alcohol in healthy volunteers. *Arch Int Pharmacodyn Ther* (1988) 291, 217–228.
2. Strömberg C, Suokas A, Seppälä T. Interaction of alcohol with maprotiline or nomifensine: echocardiographic and psychometric effects. *Eur J Clin Pharmacol* (1988) 35, 593–99.
3. Seppälä T, Strömberg C, Bergman I. Effects of zimeldine, mianserin and amitriptyline on psychomotor skills and their interaction with ethanol: a placebo controlled cross-over study. *Eur J Clin Pharmacol* (1984) 27, 181–9.
4. Seppälä T. Psychomotor skills during acute and two-week treatment with mianserin (Org GB 94) and amitriptyline, and their combined effects with alcohol. *Ann Clin Res* (1977) 9, 66–72.
5. Strömberg C, Mattila MJ. Acute comparison of clovoxamine and mianserin, alone and in combination with ethanol, on human psychomotor performance. *Pharmacol Toxicol* (1987) 60, 374–9.
6. Ehlers T, Ritter M. Effects of the tetracyclic antidepressant pirlindole on sensorimotor performance and subjective condition in comparison to imipramine and during interaction of ethanol. *Neuropsychobiology* (1984) 12, 48–54.

Alcohol + Tianeptine

Alcohol reduced the absorption of tianeptine and lowered plasma levels by about 30%.

Clinical evidence, mechanism, importance and management

In 12 healthy subjects the absorption and peak plasma levels of a single 12.5-mg dose of tianeptine were reduced by about 30% by alcohol. The subjects were given vodka diluted in orange juice to give blood alcohol levels between 64 and 77 mg%. The plasma levels of the major metabolite of tianeptine were unchanged.[1] No behavioural studies were done so that the clinical significance of these studies is as yet uncertain.

1. Salvadori C, Ward C, Defrance R, Hopkins R. The pharmacokinetics of the antidepressant tianeptine and its main metabolite in healthy humans — influence of alcohol co-administration. *Fundam Clin Pharmacol* (1990) 4, 115–25.

Alcohol + Tolazoline

A disulfiram-like reaction may occur in patients taking tolazoline if they drink alcohol.

Clinical evidence, mechanism, importance and management

Seven healthy subjects were given tolazoline 25 mg daily for 4 days. Within 15 to 90 minutes of drinking 90 mL of port wine (alcohol 18.2%), 2 hours after the last dose of tolazoline, 6 experienced tingling over the head, and 4 developed warmth and fullness of the head.[1] The reasons are not understood, but this reaction is not unlike a mild disulfiram reaction, and may possibly have a similar mechanism (see 'Alcohol + Disulfiram', p.61). Patients given tolazoline should be warned about this reaction if they drink alcohol, and advised to limit their consumption. Reactions of this kind with drugs other than disulfiram are usually more unpleasant or frightening than serious, and treatment is rarely needed. In infants given tolazoline, it would seem sensible to avoid preparations containing alcohol, where possible.

1. Boyd EM. A search for drugs with disulfiram-like activity. *Q J Stud Alcohol* (1960) 21, 23–5.

Alcohol + Trazodone

Trazodone can make driving or handling other dangerous machinery more hazardous, particularly during the first few days of treatment, and further impairment may occur with alcohol.

Clinical evidence, mechanism, importance and management

A study in 6 healthy subjects comparing the effects of single-doses of amitriptyline 50 mg and trazodone 100 mg found that both drugs impaired the performance of a number of psychomotor tests, causing drowsiness and reducing 'clearheadedness' to approximately the same extent. Only manual dexterity was further impaired when the subjects taking trazodone were given sufficient alcohol to give blood levels of about 40 mg%.[1]

Another study similarly found that the impairment of psychomotor performance by trazodone was increased by alcohol.[2] This appears to be due to a simple additive depression of the CNS. This is an established interaction, and of practical importance. Patients should be warned that their ability to drive, handle dangerous machinery or to do other tasks needing complex psychomotor skills might be impaired by trazodone, and further worsened by alcohol.

1. Warrington SJ, Ankier SI, Turner P. Evaluation of possible interactions between ethanol and trazodone or amitriptyline. *Neuropsychobiology* (1986) 15 (Suppl 1), 31–7.
2. Tiller JWG. Antidepressants, alcohol and psychomotor performance. *Acta Psychiatr Scand* (1990) (Suppl 360), 13–17.

Alcohol + Trichloroethylene

A flushing skin reaction similar to a mild disulfiram reaction can occur in those who drink alcohol following exposure to trichloroethylene. Alcohol may also increase the risk of liver toxicity due to solvent exposure.

Clinical evidence

An engineer from a factory where trichloroethylene was being used as a degreasing agent, developed facial flushing, a sensation of increased pressure in the head, lachrymation, tachypnoea and blurred vision within 12 minutes of drinking 85 mL of bourbon whiskey. The reaction did not develop when he was no longer exposed to the trichloroethylene. Other workers in the same plant reported the same experience.[1] Vivid red blotches in a symmetrical pattern on the face, neck, shoulders and back were seen in other workers when they drank about 2 pints of beer[2] after having been exposed for a few hours each day for 3 weeks to increasing concentrations of trichloroethylene vapour (up to 200 ppm). Note that this was twice the maximum permissible level for trichloroethylene in air at that time.[3] This reaction has been described as the "degreasers' flush".[2]

A later study involving 188 workers occupationally exposed to trichloroethylene found a statistically significant synergistic toxic interaction between trichloroethylene and alcohol. There were 30 cases (15.9%) of degreasers' flush and 10 cases (5.3%) of clinical liver impairment.[4]

There is also some evidence that short-term exposure to the combination may possibly reduce mental capacity, although in this study the concentration of trichloroethylene was quite high (200 ppm).[5]

Another study investigated the metabolism of trichloroethylene in 5 healthy subjects who inhaled trichloroethylene 50 ppm for 6 hours per day for 5 days and then again 2 weeks later in the presence of alcohol. Inhalation of trichloroethylene with blood-alcohol concentrations of 0.6% resulted in increased blood and expired air concentrations of trichloroethylene 2 to 3 times greater than without alcohol.[6] A simulation study suggested that ingestion of moderate amounts of alcohol (0.23 to 0.92 g/kg) before the start of work or at lunchtime, but not at the end of work, could cause pronounced increases in blood-trichloroethylene concentrations and decreases in the urinary excretion rates of trichloroethylene metabolites. However, the effect of enzyme induction on trichloroethylene metabolism by consumption of alcohol the previous evening was negligible when exposure to trichloroethylene was below 100 ppm.[7]

Mechanism

Uncertain. One suggested mechanism is a disulfiram-like inhibition of acetaldehyde metabolism by trichloroethylene (see 'Alcohol + Disulfiram', p.61). Another suggested mechanism is inhibition of trichloroethylene metabolism in the presence of alcohol, resulting in increased plasma levels and possibly an accumulation of trichloroethylene in the CNS.[6]

Importance and management

The flushing reaction is an established interaction that has been reported to occur in about 16% of workers exposed to trichloroethylene when they drink alcohol. It would seem to be more unpleasant and socially disagreeable than serious, and normally requires no treatment. However, the hepatotoxicity of trichloroethylene and other organic solvents may be increased by alcohol. Several factors have been shown to affect the handling of solvents by the liver and the final toxicity. Increased body fat has been reported to increase the risk of solvent toxicity and heavy alcohol consumption may further increase the risk of liver toxicity.[8]

1. Pardys S, Brotman M. Trichloroethylene and alcohol: a straight flush. *JAMA* (1974) 229, 521–2.
2. Stewart RD, Hake CL, Peterson JE. "Degreasers' Flush": dermal response to trichloroethylene and ethanol. *Arch Environ Health* (1974) 29, 1–5.
3. Smith GF. Trichloroethylene: a review. *Br J Ind Med* (1966) 23, 249–62.
4. Barret L, Faure J, Guilland B, Chomat D, Didier B, Debru JL. Trichloroethylene occupational exposure: elements for better prevention. *Int Arch Occup Environ Health* (1984) 53, 283–9.
5. Windemuller FJB, Ettema JH. Effects of combined exposure to trichloroethylene and alcohol on mental capacity. *Int Arch Occup Environ Health* (1978) 41, 77–85.
6. Müller G, Spassowski M, Henschler D. Metabolism of trichloroethylene in man. III. Interaction of trichloroethylene and ethanol. *Arch Toxicol* (1975) 33, 173–89.
7. Sato A, Endoh K, Kaneko T, Johanson G. Effects of consumption of ethanol on the biological monitoring of exposure to organic solvent vapours: a simulation study with trichloroethylene. *Br J Ind Med* (1991) 48, 548–56.
8. Brautbar N, Williams J. Industrial solvents and liver toxicity: risk assessment, risk factors and mechanisms. *Int J Hyg Environ Health* (2002) 205, 479–91.

Alcohol + Tricyclic antidepressants

The ability to drive, to handle dangerous machinery or to do other tasks requiring complex psychomotor skills may be impaired by amitriptyline, and to a lesser extent by doxepin or imipramine, particularly during the first few days of treatment. This impairment can be increased by alcohol. Amoxapine, clomipramine, desipramine, and nortriptyline appear to interact with alcohol only minimally. Information about other tricyclics appears to be lacking, although most manufacturers of tricyclics warn that the effects of alcohol may be enhanced. There is also evidence that alcoholics (without liver disease) may need larger doses of desipramine and imipramine to control depression. However, the toxicity of some tricyclics may be increased by alcohol, and in alcoholics with liver disease.

Clinical evidence

(a) Amitriptyline

A single-dose, crossover study in 5 healthy subjects found that the plasma levels of amitriptyline 25 mg over an 8-hour period were markedly increased by alcohol (blood-alcohol concentration maintained at approximately 80 mg%). Compared with amitriptyline alone, the AUC_{0-8} increased by a mean of 44% following alcohol consumption, and was associated with decreased standing steadiness, recent memory and alertness.[1] Amitriptyline 800 micrograms/kg impaired the performance of three motor skills tests related to driving in 21 healthy subjects. When alcohol to produce blood levels of about 80 mg% was also given the performance was even further impaired.[2] Similar results have been very clearly demonstrated in considerable numbers of subjects using a variety of psychomotor skill tests,[1-6] the interaction being most marked during the first few days of treatment, but tending to wane as treatment continues.[5] Unexplained blackouts lasting a few hours have been described in 3 women after they drank only modest amounts of alcohol;[7] they had been taking amitriptyline or imipramine for a month. There is some limited evidence from *animal* studies that amitriptyline may possibly enhance the fatty changes induced in the liver by alcohol,[8] but this still needs confirmation from human studies.

A study involving 332 fatal poisonings in Finland found that alcohol was present in 67% of cases involving amitriptyline, and when alcohol was present, relatively small overdoses of amitriptyline could result in fatal poisoning.[9] It appears that amitriptyline may be more toxic when given with alcohol and it has been suggested that a less dangerous alternative could be chosen when indications of alcohol abuse or suicide risk are present.[10]

(b) Amoxapine

The interaction between amoxapine and alcohol is said to be slight,[11] but two patients have been described who experienced reversible extrapyramidal symptoms (parkinsonism, akathisia) while taking amoxapine, apparently caused by drinking alcohol.[12]

(c) Clomipramine

Studies in subjects with blood-alcohol levels of 40 to 60 mg% found that clomipramine had only slight or no effects on various choice reaction, coordination, memory and learning tests.[4,13,14] A case describes a fatal poisoning in a chronic alcoholic patient taking clomipramine for depression. The ultimate toxic effect was thought to be due to alcohol-induced decreased biotransformation of clomipramine, as post-mortem examination revealed toxic liver damage, and low levels of the metabolite were found in blood and hair samples.[15]

(d) Desipramine

Plasma desipramine levels were transiently, but non-significantly increased after healthy subjects drank alcohol, and breath-alcohol concentrations were not affected by the antidepressant. Further, skilled performance tests in subjects given desipramine 100 mg indicated that no significant interaction occurred with alcohol.[16] The half-life of oral desipramine was about 30% lower in recently detoxified alcoholics (without liver disease), when compared with healthy subjects, and the intrinsic clearance was 60% greater.[17]

(e) Doxepin

A double-blind, crossover study in 20 healthy subjects given various combinations of alcohol and either doxepin or a placebo found that with blood-alcohol levels of 40 to 50 mg% their choice reaction test times were prolonged and the number of mistakes increased. Coordination was obviously impaired after 7 days of treatment with doxepin, but not after 14 days.[4] In an earlier study doxepin appeared to cancel out the deleterious effects of alcohol on the performance of a simulated driving test.[18] It appears that doxepin may be more toxic when given with alcohol and it has been suggested that a less dangerous alternative could be chosen when indications of alcohol abuse or suicide risk are present.[10]

(f) Imipramine

Imipramine 150 mg daily has also been reported to enhance some of the hypno-sedative effects of alcohol,[19] and unexplained blackouts lasting a few hours have been described in 3 women after they drank only modest amounts of alcohol;[7] they had been taking amitriptyline or imipramine for only a month. The half-life of oral imipramine was about 45% lower in recently detoxified alcoholics (without liver disease) compared with healthy subjects, and the intrinsic clearance was 200% greater.[17]

(g) Nortriptyline

Studies in subjects with blood-alcohol levels of 40 to 60 mg% found that nortriptyline had only slight or no effects on various choice reaction, coordination, memory and learning tests,[4,13,20] although the acute use of alcohol with nortriptyline impaired learning in one study.[13]

Mechanism

Part of the explanation for the increased CNS depression is that both alcohol and some of the tricyclics, particularly amitriptyline, cause drowsiness and other CNS depressant effects, which can be additive with the effects of alcohol.[6] The sedative effects have been reported to be greatest with amitriptyline, then doxepin and imipramine, followed by nortriptyline, and least with amoxapine, clomipramine, desipramine, and **protriptyline**.[21-24] In addition acute alcohol intake causes marked increases (100 to 200%) in the plasma levels of amitriptyline, probably by inhibiting its first pass metabolism.[1,25] Alcohol-induced liver damage could also result in impaired amitriptyline metabolism.[23] The lower serum levels of imipramine and desipramine seen in abstinent alcoholics are attributable to induction of the cytochrome P450 isoenzymes by alcohol.[17]

Importance and management

The increased CNS depression resulting from the interaction between amitriptyline and alcohol is well documented and clinically important. The interaction between alcohol and doxepin or imipramine is less well documented and the information is conflicting. Amoxapine, clomipramine, desipramine, and nortriptyline appear to interact only minimally with alcohol. Direct information about other tricyclics seems to be lacking, but there appear to be no particular reasons for avoiding concurrent use, although tricyclics with greater sedation such as **trimipramine** are more likely to interact. During the first 1 to 2 weeks of treatment many tricyclics (without alcohol) may temporarily impair the skills related to driving.[11] Therefore it would seem prudent to warn any patient given a tricyclic that driving or handling dangerous machinery may be made more hazardous if they drink alcohol, particularly during the first few days of treatment, but the effects of the interaction diminish during continued treatment. Most manufacturers of tricyclic antidepressants warn that the effects of alcohol may be enhanced by tricyclics and several suggest avoidance of alcohol whilst taking tricyclic antidepressants.

Also be aware that alcoholic patients (without liver disease) may need higher doses of imipramine (possibly doubled) and desipramine to control depression, and if long-term abstinence is achieved the dosages may then eventually need to be reduced.

1. Dorian P, Sellers EM, Reed KL, Warsh JJ, Hamilton C, Kaplan HL, Fan T. Amitriptyline and ethanol: pharmacokinetic and pharmacodynamic interaction. *Eur J Clin Pharmacol* (1983) 25, 325–31.
2. Landauer AA, Milner G, Patman J. Alcohol and amitriptyline effects on skills related to driving behavior. *Science* (1969) 163, 1467–8.
3. Seppälä T. Psychomotor skills during acute and two-week treatment with mianserin (ORG GB 94) and amitriptyline, and their combined effects with alcohol. *Ann Clin Res* (1977) 9, 66–72.
4. Seppälä T, Linnoila M, Elonen E, Mattila MJ, Mäki M. Effect of tricyclic antidepressants and alcohol on psychomotor skills related to driving. *Clin Pharmacol Ther* (1975) 17, 515–22.
5. Seppälä T, Strömberg C, Bergman I. Effects of zimeldine, mianserin and amitriptyline on psychomotor skills and their interaction with ethanol: a placebo controlled cross-over study. *Eur J Clin Pharmacol* (1984) 27, 181–9.
6. Scott DB, Fagan D, Tiplady B. Effects of amitriptyline and zimelidine in combination with alcohol. *Psychopharmacology (Berl)* (1982) 76, 209–11.
7. Hudson CJ. Tricyclic antidepressants and alcoholic blackouts. *J Nerv Ment Dis* (1981) 169, 381–2.
8. Milner G, Kakulas BA. The potentiation by amitriptyline of liver changes induced by ethanol in mice. *Pathology* (1969) 1, 113–18.
9. Koski A, Vuori E, Ojanperä I. Relation of postmortem blood alcohol and drug concentrations in fatal poisonings involving amitriptyline, propoxyphene and promazine. *Hum Exp Toxicol* (2005) 24, 389–96.
10. Koski A, Ojanperä I, Vuori E. Interaction of alcohol and drugs in fatal poisonings. *Hum Exp Toxicol* (2003) 22, 281–7.
11. Wilson WH, Petrie WM, Ban TA, Barry DE. The effects of amoxapine and ethanol on psychomotor skills related to driving: a placebo and standard controlled study. *Prog Neuropsychopharmacol* (1981) 5, 263–70.
12. Shen WW. Alcohol, amoxapine, and akathisia. *Biol Psychiatry* (1984) 19, 929–30.
13. Liljequist R, Linnoila M, Mattila M. Effect of two weeks' treatment with chlorimipramine and nortriptyline, alone or in combination with alcohol, on learning and memory. *Psychopharmacologia* (1974) 39, 181–6.
14. Berlin I, Cournot A, Zimmer R, Pedarriosse A-M, Manfredi R, Molinier P, Puech AJ. Evaluation and comparison of the interaction between alcohol and moclobemide or clomipramine in healthy subjects. *Psychopharmacology (Berl)* (1990) 100, 40–5.
15. Kłys M, Ścisłowski M, Rojek S, Kołodziej J. A fatal clomipramine intoxication case of a chronic alcoholic patient: application of postmortem hair analysis method of clomipramine and ethyl glucuronide using LC/APCI/MS. *Leg Med* (2005) 7, 319–25.
16. Linnoila M, Johnson J, Dubyoski K, Buchsbaum MS, Schneinin M, Kilts C. Effects of antidepressants on skilled performance. *Br J Clin Pharmacol* (1984) 18, 109S–120S.
17. Ciraulo DA, Barnhill JG, Jaffe JJ. Clinical pharmacokinetics of imipramine and desipramine in alcoholics and normal volunteers. *Clin Pharmacol Ther* (1988) 43, 509–18.
18. Milner G, Landauer AA. The effects of doxepin, alone and together with alcohol, in relation to driving safety. *Med J Aust* (1973) 1, 837–41.
19. Frewer LJ, Lader M. The effects of nefazodone, imipramine and placebo, alone and combined with alcohol, in normal subjects. *Int Clin Psychopharmacol* (1993) 8, 13–20.
20. Hughes FW, Forney RB. Delayed audiofeedback (DAF) for induction of anxiety: effect of nortriptyline, ethanol, or nortriptyline-ethanol combinations on performance with DAF. *JAMA* (1963) 185, 556–8.
21. Marco LA, Randels RM. Drug interactions in alcoholic patients. *Hillside J Clin Psychiatry* (1981) 3, 27–44.
22. Linnoila M, Seppala T. Antidepressants and driving. *Accid Anal Prev* (1985) 17, 297–301.
23. Weathermon R, Crabb DW. Alcohol and medication interactions. *Alcohol Res Health* (1999) 23, 40–54.
24. Weller RA, Preskorn SH. Psychotropic drugs and alcohol: pharmacokinetic and pharmacodynamic interactions. *Psychosomatics* (1984) 25, 301–3, 305–6, 309.
25. Fraser AG. Pharmacokinetic interactions between alcohol and other drugs. *Clin Pharmacokinet* (1997) 33, 79–90.

Alcohol + Trinitrotoluene

Men exposed to trinitrotoluene (TNT) in a munitions factory were found to have a greater risk of TNT-induced liver damage if they had a long history of heavy alcohol drinking than if they were non-drinkers.[1]

1. Li J, Jiang Q-G, Zhong W-D. Persistent ethanol drinking increases liver injury induced by trinitrotoluene exposure: an in-plant case-control study. *Hum Exp Toxicol* (1991) 10, 405–9.

Alcohol + Vitamin A (Retinol)

Heavy consumption of alcohol may also increase betacarotene levels and affect vitamin A metabolism; there have been reports of possible increased toxicity.

Clinical evidence, mechanism, importance and management

A study involving 30 abstinent male alcoholics found that 5 of 15 given high-dose vitamin A (10 000 units daily by mouth) for 4 months developed liver abnormalities during treatment, compared with 1 of 15 patients given placebo. Two of the 6 patients admitted intermittent alcohol consumption. Five of these patients continued with vitamin A and the abnormal liver function tests resolved in 4 of these patients.[1]

The interaction between alcohol and vitamin A is complex. They have overlapping metabolic pathways; a similar 2-step process is involved in the metabolism of both alcohol and vitamin A, with alcohol dehydrogenases and acetaldehyde dehydrogenases being implicated in the conversion of vitamin A to retinoic acid.[2,3] Alcohol appears to act as a competitive inhibitor of vitamin A oxidation.[2,4] In addition, chronic alcohol intake can induce cytochrome P450 isoenzymes that appear to increase the breakdown of vitamin A (retinol and retinoic acid) into more polar metabolites in the liver, which can cause hepatocyte death. So chronic alcohol consumption may enhance the intrinsic hepatotoxicity of high-dose vitamin A. Alcohol has also been shown to alter retinoid homoeostasis by increasing vitamin A mobilisation from the liver to extrahepatic tissues, which could result in depletion of hepatic stores of vitamin A.[2,3]

It appears that consumption of substantial amounts of alcohol is associated with vitamin A deficiency partially due to poor nutrition and also the direct effects of alcohol on the metabolism of vitamin A. Vitamin A supplementation may therefore be indicated in heavy drinkers, but is complicated by the hepatotoxicity of large amounts of vitamin A, which may be potentiated by alcohol.[3] It would therefore seem reasonable to try to control drinking of alcohol when vitamin A supplementation is required. Patients who consume alcohol, particularly heavy drinkers or alcoholics, should be questioned about their use of vitamin supplements as some non-prescription vitamin A and D supplements contain substantial amounts of vitamin A.

1. Worner TM, Gordon GG, Leo MA, Lieber CS. Vitamin A treatment of sexual dysfunction in male alcoholics. *Am J Clin Nutr* (1988) 48, 1431–5.
2. Wang X-D. Alcohol, vitamin A, and cancer. *Alcohol* (2005) 35, 251–8.
3. Leo MA, Lieber CS. Alcohol, vitamin A, and ß-carotene: adverse interactions, including hepatotoxicity and carcinogenicity. *Am J Clin Nutr* (1999) 69, 1071–85.
4. Crabb DW, Pinairs J, Hasanadka R, Fang M, Leo MA, Lieber CS, Tsukamoto H, Motomura K, Miyahara T, Ohata M, Bosron W, Sanghani S, Kedishvili N, Shiraishi H, Yokoyama H, Miyagi M, Ishii H, Bergheim I, Menzl I, Parlesak A, Bode C. Alcohol and retinoids. *Alcohol Clin Exp Res* (2001) 25 (5 Suppl ISBRA), 207S–217S.

Alcohol + Xylene

Some individuals exposed to xylene vapour, who subsequently drink alcohol, may experience dizziness and nausea. A flushing skin reaction has also been seen.

Clinical evidence, mechanism, importance and management

Studies in subjects exposed to *m*-xylene vapour at concentrations of approximately 145 or 280 ppm for 4 hours who were then given 0.4 or 0.8 g/kg of alcohol found that about 10 to 20% experienced dizziness and nausea.[1,2] One subject exposed to 300 ppm of *m*-xylene vapour developed a conspicuous dermal flush on his face, neck, chest and back. He also showed some erythema with alcohol alone.[3] A study using a population-based pharmacokinetic and pharmacodynamic model predicted that the probability of experiencing CNS effects following exposure to xylene at the current UK occupational exposure standard (100 ppm time-weighted average over 8 hours) increased markedly and non-linearly with alcohol dose.[4]

The reasons for these reactions are not fully understood, but it is possible that xylene plasma levels are increased because alcohol impairs its metabolic clearance by the cytochrome P450 isoenzyme CYP2E1.[4] After alcohol intake, blood xylene levels have been reported to rise about 1.5- to 2-fold;[2] acetaldehyde levels may also be transiently increased.[2]

Alcoholic beverages are quite often consumed during lunchtime or after work, and since the excretion of xylene is delayed by its high solubility and storage in lipid-rich tissues, the simultaneous presence of xylene and alcohol in the body is probably not uncommon and could result in enhancement of the toxicity of xylene.[5]

1. Savolainen K, Riihimäki V, Vaheri E, Linnoila M. Effects of xylene and alcohol on vestibular and visual functions in man. *Scand J Work Environ Health* (1980) 6, 94–103.
2. Riihimäki V, Savolainen K, Pfäffli P, Pekari K, Sippel HW, Laine A. Metabolic interaction between m-xylene and ethanol. *Arch Toxicol* (1982) 49, 253–63.
3. Riihimäki V, Laine A, Savolainen K, Sippel H. Acute solvent-ethanol interactions with special reference to xylene. *Scand J Work Environ Health* (1982) 8, 77–9.
4. MacDonald AJ, Rostami-Hodjegan A, Tucker GT, Linkens DA. Analysis of solvent central nervous system toxicity and ethanol interactions using a human population physiologically based kinetic and dynamic model. *Regul Toxicol Pharmacol* (2002) 35, 165–76.
5. Lieber CS. Microsomal ethanol-oxidizing system. *Enzyme* (1987) 37, 45–56.

4

Alpha blockers

The selective and non-selective alpha blockers are categorised and listed in 'Table 4.1', (see below). The principal interactions of the alpha blockers are those relating to enhanced hypotensive effects. Early after the introduction of the selective alpha blockers it was discovered that, in some individuals, they can cause a rapid reduction in blood pressure on starting treatment (also called the 'first-dose effect' or 'first-dose hypotension'). The risk of this may be higher in patients already taking other antihypertensive drugs. The first-dose effect has been minimised by starting with a very low dose of the alpha blocker, and then escalating the dose slowly over a couple of weeks. A similar hypotensive effect can occur when the dose of the alpha blocker is increased, or if treatment is interrupted for a few days and then re-introduced. Some manufacturers recommend giving the first dose on retiring to bed, or if not, avoiding tasks that are potentially hazardous if syncope occurs (such as driving) for the first 12 hours. If symptoms such as dizziness, fatigue or sweating develop, patients should be warned to lie down, and to remain lying flat until they abate completely.

It is unclear whether there are any real differences between the alpha blockers in their propensity to cause this first-dose effect. With the exception of indoramin, postural hypotension, syncope, and dizziness are listed as adverse effects of the alpha blockers available in the UK and for most it is recommended that they should be started with a low dose and titrated as required. Tamsulosin is reported to have some selectivity for the alpha receptor 1A subtype, which are found mostly in the prostate, and therefore have less effect on blood pressure: an initial titration of the dose is therefore not considered to be necessary. Nevertheless, it would be prudent to exercise caution with all the drugs in this class.

Alpha blockers are also used to increase urinary flow-rate and improve obstructive symptoms in benign prostatic hyperplasia. In this setting, their effects on blood pressure are more of an adverse effect, and their additive hypotensive effect with other antihypertensives may not be beneficial.

Table 4.1 Alpha blockers

Drug	*Principal indications*
Selective alpha$_1$ blockers (Alpha blockers)	
Alfuzosin	BPH
Bunazosin	Hypertension
Doxazosin	BPH; Hypertension
Indoramin	BPH; Hypertension; Migraine
Prazosin	BPH; Heart failure; Hypertension; Raynaud's syndrome
Tamsulosin	BPH
Terazosin	BPH; Hypertension
Other drugs with alpha-blocking actions	
Moxisylate	Peripheral vascular disease; Erectile dysfunction
Phenoxybenzamine	Hypertensive episodes in phaeochromocytoma; Neurogenic bladder; Shock
Phentolamine	Erectile dysfunction; Hypertensive episodes in phaeochromocytoma
Urapidil	Hypertension

Alpha blockers + ACE inhibitors

Severe first-dose hypotension, and synergistic hypotensive effects that occurred when a patient taking enalapril was given bunazosin have been replicated in healthy subjects. The first-dose effect seen with other alpha blockers (particularly alfuzosin, prazosin and terazosin) is also likely to be potentiated by ACE inhibitors. In one small study tamsulosin did not have any clinically relevant effects on blood pressure that was already well controlled by enalapril.

Clinical evidence

After a patient taking **enalapril** developed severe first-dose hypotension after being given **bunazosin**, this interaction was further studied in 6 healthy subjects. When given **enalapril** 10 mg or **bunazosin** 2 mg, their mean blood pressure over 6 hours was reduced by 9.5/6.7 mmHg. When **bunazosin** was given one hour after **enalapril** the blood pressure fell by 27/28 mmHg, and still fell by 19/22 mmHg, even when the dose of **enalapril** was reduced to 2.5 mg.[1]

The manufacturers of **alfuzosin**[2] and **prazosin**[3] warn that patients receiving antihypertensive drugs (the manufacturers of **prazosin** specifically name the ACE inhibitors) are at particular risk of developing postural hypotension after the first dose of alpha blocker.

Retrospective analysis of a large multinational study in patients given **terazosin** 5 or 10 mg daily found that **terazosin** only affected the blood pressure of patients taking ACE inhibitors (**enalapril**, **lisinopril** or **perindopril**) if the blood pressure was uncontrolled. No change in blood pressure was seen in those with normal blood pressure (i.e. those without hypertension and those with hypertension controlled by ACE inhibitors). The most common adverse effect in the 10-week **terazosin** phase was dizziness, and the incidence of this appeared to be lower in those taking antihypertensives (13 to 16%) than those not (21 to 25%).[4] However, the manufacturer of **terazosin** notes that the incidence of dizziness in patients with BPH taking **terazosin** was higher when they were also receiving an ACE inhibitor.[5]

In a placebo-controlled study in 6 hypertensive men with blood pressure well controlled by **enalapril**, the addition of **tamsulosin** 400 micrograms daily for 7 days then 800 micrograms daily for a further 7 days had no clinically relevant effects on blood pressure (assessed after 6 and 14 days of **tamsulosin**). In addition, no first-dose hypotensive effect was seen on the day **tamsulosin** was started, or on the day the **tamsulosin** dose was increased.[6]

Mechanism

The first-dose effect of alpha blockers (see 'Alpha blockers', (p.83)) may be potentiated by ACE inhibitors. Tamsulosin possibly has less effect on blood pressure since it has some selectivity for alpha receptors in the prostate.

Importance and management

Direct information is limited. Acute hypotension (dizziness, fainting) sometimes occurs unpredictably with the first dose of some alpha blockers (particularly, alfuzosin, prazosin and terazosin; but see 'Alpha blockers', (p.83)), and this can be exaggerated if the patient takes or is already taking a beta blocker or a calcium-channel blocker (see 'Alpha blockers + Beta blockers', below, and 'Alpha blockers + Calcium-channel blockers', p.85). It would therefore seem prudent to apply the same precautions to ACE inhibitors, namely reducing the dose of the ACE inhibitor to a maintenance level if possible, then starting the alpha blocker at the lowest dose, with the first dose given at bedtime. Note that the acute hypotensive reaction appears to be short-lived. There is limited evidence that terazosin and tamsulosin may not cause an additional hypotensive effect in the longer term in patients with BPH who have hypertension already well-controlled with ACE inhibitors. Nevertheless, caution should be exercised in this situation, and a dose reduction of the ACE inhibitor may be required.

1. Baba T, Tomiyama T, Takebe K. Enhancement by an ACE inhibitor of first-dose hypotension caused by an alpha$_1$-blocker. *N Engl J Med* (1990) 322, 1237.
2. Xatral (Alfuzosin hydrochloride). Sanofi-Aventis. UK Summary of product characteristics, April 2005.
3. Hypovase (Prazosin hydrochloride). Pfizer Ltd. UK Summary of product characteristics, May 2007.
4. Kirby RS. Terazosin in benign prostatic hyperplasia: effects on blood pressure in normotensive and hypertensive men. *Br J Urol* (1998) 82, 373–9.
5. Hytrin (Terazosin). Abbott Laboratories Ltd. UK Summary of product characteristics, January 2006.
6. Lowe FC. Coadministration of tamsulosin and three antihypertensive agents in patients with benign prostatic hyperplasia: pharmacodynamic effect. *Clin Ther* (1997) 19, 730–42.

Alpha blockers + Beta blockers

The risk of first-dose hypotension with prazosin is higher if the patient is already taking a beta blocker. This is also likely to be true of other alpha blockers, particularly alfuzosin, bunazosin and terazosin. In a small study tamsulosin did not have any clinically relevant effects on blood pressure that was already well controlled by atenolol. Alpha blockers and beta blockers may be combined for additional lowering of blood pressure in patients with hypertension.

Clinical evidence

(a) Alfuzosin

No pharmacokinetic interaction occurred between alfuzosin 2.5 mg and atenolol 100 mg in a single-dose study in 8 healthy subjects.[1] The manufacturer notes that postural hypotension may occur in patients receiving antihypertensives when they start alfuzosin,[2,3] and note a study in which the combination of single doses of alfuzosin 2.5 mg and atenolol 100 mg caused significant reductions in mean heart rate and blood pressure. The AUCs of both drugs were raised up to about 20%.[3]

(b) Doxazosin

The manufacturer of doxazosin states that no adverse drug interaction has been observed between doxazosin and beta blockers,[4,5] although they do note that the most common adverse reactions associated with doxazosin are of a postural hypotension type.[4] They specifically note that doxazosin has been given with atenolol and propranolol without evidence of an adverse interaction.[5]

(c) Indoramin

The manufacturer of indoramin states that concurrent use with beta blockers may enhance their hypotensive action, and that titration of the dose of the beta blocker may be needed when initiating therapy.[6]

(d) Prazosin

A marked hypotensive reaction (dizziness, pallor, sweating) occurred in 3 out of 6 hypertensive patients taking alprenolol 400 mg twice daily when they were given the first 500-microgram dose of prazosin. All 6 patients had a greater reduction in blood pressure after the first prazosin dose than after 2 weeks of treatment with prazosin 500 microgram three times daily with no beta blocker (mean reduction 22/11 mmHg compared with 4/4 mmHg). A further 3 patients already taking prazosin 500 microgram three times daily had no unusual fall in blood pressure when they were given the first dose of alprenolol 200 mg.[7] Two studies have shown that the pharmacokinetics of prazosin are not affected by either alprenolol[7] or propranolol.[8]

The severity and the duration of the first-dose effect of prazosin was also found to be increased in healthy subjects given a single dose of propranolol.[9]

(e) Tamsulosin

In a placebo-controlled study in 8 hypertensive men with blood pressure well controlled by atenolol, the addition of tamsulosin 400 micrograms daily for 7 days, then 800 micrograms daily for a further 7 days, had no clinically relevant effect on blood pressure (assessed after 6 and 14 days of tamsulosin). No hypotension was seen with the first dose of tamsulosin or when the dose of tamsulosin was increased.[10]

(f) Terazosin

Retrospective analysis of a large multinational study in patients given terazosin 5 or 10 mg daily found that terazosin only affected the blood pressure of patients taking beta blockers (atenolol, labetalol, metoprolol, sotalol, and timolol) if the blood pressure was uncontrolled. No change in blood pressure was seen in those with normal blood pressure (i.e. those without hypertension and those with hypertension controlled by beta blockers). The most common adverse effect in the 10-week terazosin phase was dizziness, and the incidence of this appeared to be lower in those taking antihypertensives (13 to 16%) than those not (21 to 25%).[11]

In addition to these drugs the manufacturers of terazosin note that it has been taken by at least 50 patients with propranolol without evidence of an adverse interaction.[12]

Mechanism

The normal cardiovascular response (a compensatory increased heart output and rate) that should follow the first-dose hypotensive reaction to alpha blockers is apparently compromised by the presence of a beta blocker. The problem is usually only short-lasting because some physiological compensation occurs within hours or days, and this allows the blood pressure to be lowered without falling precipitously. Tamsulosin possibly has less effect on blood pressure since it has some selectivity for alpha receptors in the prostate (see 'Alpha blockers', (p.83)).

Importance and management

An established interaction. Some patients experience acute postural hypotension, tachycardia and palpitations when they begin to take prazosin or other alpha blockers (particularly alfuzosin, bunazosin and terazosin; but see also 'Alpha blockers', (p.83)). A few patients even collapse in a sudden faint within 30 to 90 minutes, and this can be exacerbated if they are already taking a beta blocker. It is recommended that those already taking a beta blocker should have their dose of beta blocker reduced to a maintenance dose and begin with a low-dose of these alpha blockers, with the first dose taken just before going to bed. They should also be warned about the possibility of postural hypotension and how to manage it (i.e. lay down, raise the legs and get up slowly). Similarly, when adding a beta blocker to an alpha blocker, it may be prudent to decrease the dose of the alpha blocker and re-titrate as necessary. There is limited evidence that terazosin and tamsulosin may not cause an additional hypotensive effect in the longer term in patients with BPH who have hypertension already well-controlled with beta blockers. Nevertheless, caution should be exercised in this situation, and a dose reduction of the beta blocker may be required.

1. Bianchetti G, Padovani P, Coupez JM, Guinebault P, Hermanns P, Coupez-Lopinot R, Guillet P, Thénot JP, Morselli PL. Pharmacokinetic interactions between hydrochlorothiazide, atenolol, and alfuzosin: a new antihypertensive drug. *Acta Pharmacol Toxicol (Copenh)* (1986) 59 (Suppl 5), 197.
2. Xatral (Alfuzosin hydrochloride). Sanofi-Aventis. UK Summary of product characteristics, April 2005.
3. Uroxatral (Alfuzosin hydrochloride extended-release tablets). Sanofi-Aventis US LLC. US Prescribing information, March 2007.
4. Cardura (Doxazosin mesilate). Pfizer Ltd. UK Summary of product characteristics, February 2007.
5. Cardura (Doxazosin mesylate). Pfizer Inc. US Prescribing information, April 2002.
6. Doralese Tiltab (Indoramin hydrochloride). GlaxoSmithKline UK. UK Summary of product characteristics, June 2007.
7. Seideman P, Grahnén A, Haglund K, Lindström B, von Bahr C. Prazosin first dose phenomenon during combined treatment with a β-adrenoceptor in hypertensive patients. *Br J Clin Pharmacol* (1982) 13, 865–70.
8. Rubin P, Jackson G, Blaschke T. Studies on the clinical pharmacology of prazosin. II: The influence of indomethacin and of propranolol on the action and the disposition of prazosin. *Br J Clin Pharmacol* (1980) 10, 33–9.
9. Elliott HL, McLean K, Sumner DJ, Meredith PA, Reid JL. Immediate cardiovascular responses to oral prazosin-effects of β-blockers. *Clin Pharmacol Ther* (1981) 29, 303–9.
10. Lowe FC. Coadministration of tamsulosin and three antihypertensive agents in patients with benign prostatic hyperplasia: pharmacodynamic effect. *Clin Ther* (1997) 19, 730–42.
11. Kirby RS. Terazosin in benign prostatic hyperplasia: effects on blood pressure in normotensive and hypertensive men. *Br J Urol* (1998) 82, 373–9.
12. Hytrin (Terazosin hydrochloride). Abbott Laboratories. US Prescribing information, February 2001.

Alpha blockers + Calcium-channel blockers

Blood pressure may fall sharply when calcium-channel blockers are first given to patients already taking alpha blockers (particularly prazosin and terazosin), and vice versa. In a small study, tamsulosin did not have any clinically relevant effects on blood pressure well controlled by nifedipine. Verapamil may increase the AUC of prazosin and terazosin. Alpha blockers and calcium-channel blockers may be combined for additional blood pressure lowering in patients with hypertension.

Clinical evidence

(a) Dihydropyridine calcium-channel blockers

1. Doxazosin. Although there was a tendency for first-dose hypotension no serious adverse events or postural symptoms were seen in 6 normotensive subjects given **nifedipine** 20 mg twice daily for 20 days, with doxazosin 2 mg once daily for the last 10 days. The same results were noted in 6 other normotensive subjects given the drugs in the opposite order. No pharmacokinetic interactions were found.[1] However, the US manufacturers note a study in which slight (less than 20%) alterations were found in the pharmacokinetics of **nifedipine** and doxazosin when they were given concurrently. As would be expected, blood pressures were lower when both drugs were given.[2]

2. Prazosin. In a placebo-controlled, crossover study 12 hypertensive subjects were given **nifedipine** 20 mg and prazosin 2 mg, separated by one hour. Concurrent use reduced blood pressure more than either drug alone, but when prazosin was given after **nifedipine** its effects were delayed.[3] Two patients with severe hypertension given prazosin 4 or 5 mg experienced a sharp fall in blood pressure shortly after being given **nifedipine** *sublingually*. One of them complained of dizziness and had a reduction in standing blood pressure from 232/124 to 88/48 mmHg about 20 minutes after taking **nifedipine** 10 mg. However, in a further 8 patients with hypertension taking prazosin, the reduction in blood pressure 20 minutes after the addition of *sublingual* nifedipine was smaller (mean reduction of 25/12 mmHg when lying and 24/17 mmHg when standing).[4] It is not clear what contribution prazosin had to the effect seen with *sublingual* **nifedipine**, since the experiment was not repeated using a prazosin placebo, but blood pressure in these patients had earlier remained unchanged 1 hour after taking prazosin alone. Note that *sublingual* **nifedipine** alone may cause a dangerous drop in blood pressure.

3. Tamsulosin. In a placebo-controlled study in 8 hypertensive men with blood pressure well controlled by **nifedipine**, the addition of tamsulosin 400 micrograms daily for 7 days then 800 micrograms daily for a further 7 days had no clinically relevant effect on blood pressure (assessed after 6 and 14 days of tamsulosin). In addition, no first-dose hypotension was seen on the first day of tamsulosin, or when the tamsulosin dose was increased.[5]

4. Terazosin. Retrospective analysis of a large multinational study in patients given terazosin 5 or 10 mg daily found that terazosin only affected the blood pressure of patients taking calcium-channel blockers (**amlodipine**, **felodipine**, **flunarizine**, **isradipine** and **nifedipine**) if the blood pressure was uncontrolled. No change in blood pressure was seen in those with normal blood pressure (i.e. those without hypertension and those with hypertension controlled by calcium-channel blockers). The most common adverse effect in the 10-week terazosin phase was dizziness, and the incidence of this appeared to be lower in those taking antihypertensives (13 to 16%) than those not taking antihypertensives (21 to 25%).[6]

(b) Diltiazem

The US manufacturers note that when diltiazem 240 mg daily was given with **alfuzosin** 2.5 mg three times daily the maximum serum levels and AUC of **alfuzosin** were raised by 50% and 30%, respectively, and the maximum serum levels and AUC of diltiazem were raised by 40%. However, no changes in blood pressure were seen.[7]

(c) Verapamil

1. Prazosin. A study in 8 normotensive subjects given a single 1-mg dose of prazosin found that the peak serum prazosin levels were raised by 85% (from 5.2 to 9.6 nanograms/mL) and the prazosin AUC was increased by 62% when it was given with a single 160-mg dose of verapamil. The standing blood pressure, which was unchanged after verapamil alone, fell from 114/82 to 99/81 mmHg with prazosin alone, and was further reduced to 89/68 mmHg when both drugs were given together.[8] A similar pharmacokinetic interaction was noted in another study in hypertensive patients.[9] In this study, the first 1-mg dose of prazosin alone caused a 23 mmHg fall in standing systolic blood pressure, and half the patients (3 of 6) experienced symptomatic postural hypotension. A similar fall in blood pressure occurred when the first 1-mg dose of prazosin was given to 6 patients who had been taking verapamil for 5 days, and 2 patients experienced symptomatic postural hypotension.[9]

2. Tamsulosin. A study into the safety of tamsulosin, with particular regard to the use of other medications, found that the concurrent use of verapamil increased the risk of adverse events related to tamsulosin treatment by threefold. The use of other calcium-channel blockers (not specified) did not appear to increase adverse effects, although there was a trend towards an increase.[10]

3. Terazosin. When verapamil 120 mg twice daily was added to terazosin 5 mg daily in 12 hypertensive patients, the peak plasma levels and the AUC of the terazosin were increased by about 25%. In contrast, in another 12 patients taking verapamil 120 mg twice daily, the addition of terazosin

(1 mg increased to 5 mg daily) had no effect on verapamil pharmacokinetics.[11] Both groups of patients had significant falls in standing blood pressure when they first started taking both drugs. Symptomatic orthostatic hypotension (which lessened within about 3 weeks) occurred in 4 patients when verapamil was first added to terazosin, and in 2 patients when terazosin was first added to verapamil.[11]

Mechanism

Not fully understood. It would seem that the vasodilatory effects of the alpha blockers and the calcium-channel blockers can be additive or synergistic, particularly after the first dose.[1,12] The fall in blood pressure seen with prazosin and verapamil may, in part, result from a pharmacokinetic interaction,[12] as does the interaction between alfuzosin and diltiazem. Tamsulosin possibly has less effect on blood pressure since it has some selectivity for alpha receptors in the prostate (see 'Alpha blockers', (p.83)).

Importance and management

The interaction between calcium-channel blockers and alpha blockers would appear to be established and of clinical importance, although the documentation is limited. Marked additive hypotensive effects can occur when concurrent use is first started, particularly with alfuzosin, bunazosin, prazosin and terazosin; but see also 'Alpha blockers', (p.83). It is recommended that patients already taking calcium-channel blockers should have their dose of calcium-channel blocker reduced and begin with a low-dose of alpha blocker, with the first dose taken just before going to bed. Caution should also be exercised when calcium-channel blockers are added to established treatment with an alpha blocker. Patients should be warned about the possibilities of exaggerated hypotension, and told what to do if they feel faint and dizzy. There is limited evidence that terazosin and tamsulosin may not cause an additional hypotensive effect in the longer term in patients with BPH who have hypertension already well-controlled with calcium-channel blockers. Nevertheless, caution should be exercised in this situation, and a dose reduction of the calcium-channel blocker may be required. It seems likely that any pharmacokinetic interaction will be accounted for by this dose titration.

1. Donnelly R, Elliott HL, Meredith PA, Howie CA, Reid JL. The pharmacodynamics and pharmacokinetics of the combination of nifedipine and doxazosin. *Eur J Clin Pharmacol* (1993) 44, 279–82.
2. Adalat CC (Nifedipine). Bayer HealthCare. US Prescribing information, August 2005.
3. Kiss I, Farsang C. Nifedipine-prazosin interaction in patients with essential hypertension. *Cardiovasc Drugs Ther* (1989) 3, 413–15.
4. Jee LD, Opie LH. Acute hypotensive response to nifedipine added to prazosin in treatment of hypertension. *BMJ* (1983) 287, 1514.
5. Starkey LP, Yasukawa K, Trenga C, Miyazawa Y, Ito Y. Study of possible pharmacodynamic interaction between tamsulosin and nifedipine in subjects with essential hypertension. *J Clin Pharmacol* (1994) 34, 1019.
6. Kirby RS. Terazosin in benign prostatic hyperplasia: effects on blood pressure in normotensive and hypertensive men. *Br J Urol* (1998) 82, 373–9.
7. Uroxatral (Alfuzosin hydrochloride extended-release tablets). Sanofi-Aventis US LLC. US Prescribing information, March 2007.
8. Pasanisi F, Elliott HL, Meredith PA, McSharry DR, Reid JL. Combined alpha adrenoceptor antagonism and calcium channel blockade in normal subjects. *Clin Pharmacol Ther* (1984) 36, 716–23.
9. Elliott HL, Meredith PA, Campbell L, Reid JL. The combination of prazosin and verapamil in the treatment of essential hypertension. *Clin Pharmacol Ther* (1988) 43, 554–60.
10. Michel MC, Bressel H-U, Goepel M, Rübben H. A 6-month large-scale study into the safety of tamsulosin. *Br J Clin Pharmacol* (2001) 51, 609–14.
11. Lenz ML, Pool JL, Laddu AR, Varghese A, Johnston W, Taylor AA. Combined terazosin and verapamil therapy in essential hypertension. Hemodynamic and pharmacodynamic interactions. *Am J Hypertens* (1995) 8, 133–45.
12. Meredith PA, Elliott HL. An additive or synergistic drug interaction: application of concentration-effect modeling. *Clin Pharmacol Ther* (1992) 51, 708–14.

Alpha blockers + Cimetidine

No important interaction occurs between cimetidine and either alfuzosin or doxazosin. Tamsulosin does not appear to have a clinically significant interaction with cimetidine, but caution is recommended with high tamsulosin doses.

Clinical evidence, mechanism, importance and management

In 10 healthy subjects cimetidine 1 g daily in divided doses for 20 days was found to have minimal effects on the pharmacokinetics of a single 5-mg dose of **alfuzosin**. The maximum serum levels and AUC of **alfuzosin** were increased by up to 24%, (not statistically significant) and the half-life was shortened by 14%. Cimetidine did not appear to increase the incidence of postural hypotension seen with **alfuzosin**.[1] These changes are not clinically relevant, and there would seem to be no reason for avoiding concurrent use.

The manufacturers of **doxazosin** note that in a placebo-controlled study in healthy subjects cimetidine 400 mg twice daily increased the AUC of a single 1-mg dose of **doxazosin** given on day 4 by 10%.[2,3] This seems unlikely to be of clinical significance, especially as this is within the expected intersubject variation of the **doxazosin** AUC.[3]

A study in 10 healthy subjects found that giving cimetidine 400 mg four times daily with a single 400-microgram dose of **tamsulosin** resulted in a 44% increase in the AUC of **tamsulosin** and a 26% reduction in **tamsulosin** clearance. Adverse events were not increased by concurrent use.[4] The UK manufacturer of **tamsulosin** considers that no dosage adjustment is necessary.[5] However, the US manufacturers advise caution, particularly with doses greater than 400 micrograms.[6] In practice this probably means being aware that any increase in the adverse effects of **tamsulosin** occur as a result of this interaction. If adverse effects do occur, consider changing to a non-interacting, alternative alpha blocker, such as alfuzosin. Other H_2-receptor antagonists would not be expected to interact, but there does not seem to be any evidence to support this suggestion.

1. Desager JP, Harvengt C, Bianchetti G, Rosenzweig P. The effect of cimetidine on the pharmacokinetics of single oral doses of alfuzosin. *Int J Clin Pharmacol Ther Toxicol* (1993) 31, 568–71.
2. Cardura (Doxazosin mesylate). Pfizer Inc. US Prescribing information, April 2002.
3. Cardura (Doxazosin mesilate). Pfizer Ltd. UK Summary of product characteristics, February 2007.
4. Miyazawa Y, Forrest A, Schentag JJ, Kamimura H, Swarz H, Ito Y. Effect of concomitant administration of cimetidine hydrochloride on the pharmacokinetic and safety profile of tamsulosin hydrochloride 0.4 mg in healthy subjects. *Curr Ther Res* (2002) 63, 15–26.
5. Flomaxtra XL (Tamsulosin hydrochloride). Astellas Pharma Ltd. UK Summary of product characteristics, October 2006.
6. Flomax (Tamsulosin hydrochloride). Boehringer Ingelheim Pharmaceuticals Inc. US Prescribing information, February 2007.

Alpha blockers + CYP3A4 inhibitors

Potent CYP3A4 inhibitors may increase the levels of alfuzosin.

Clinical evidence, mechanism, importance and management

The US manufacturers of alfuzosin XL briefly cite a study in which **ketoconazole** 400 mg increased the AUC and maximum levels of a 10-mg dose of alfuzosin by 3.2-fold and 2.3-fold, respectively. They therefore contraindicate the concurrent use of potent CYP3A4 inhibitors (they name **itraconazole**, **ketoconazole** and **ritonavir**).[1]

Based on the information available the contraindication with alfuzosin seems somewhat cautious, although the **protease inhibitors** may be expected to have a greater effect than **ketoconazole**. If any of the potent CYP3A4 inhibitors named is given with alfuzosin it would seem prudent to use the minimum dose of the alpha blocker and titrate the dose as necessary, monitoring for adverse effects, particularly first-dose hypotension when the dose is increased. Be aware that risks are likely to be greater in patients also taking other antihypertensives. There is no evidence to suggest that other alpha blockers interact similarly, and they may therefore be suitable alternatives in some patients.

1. Uroxatral (Alfuzosin hydrochloride extended-release tablets). Sanofi-Aventis US LLC. US Prescribing information, March 2007.

Alpha blockers + Diuretics

As would be expected, the use of an alpha blocker with a diuretic may result in an additive hypotensive effect, but aside from first-dose hypotension, this usually seems to be a beneficial interaction in patients with hypertension. The effects in patients with congestive heart failure may be more severe.

Clinical evidence, mechanism, importance and management

(a) Alfuzosin

No pharmacokinetic interaction occurred between alfuzosin 5 mg and **hydrochlorothiazide** 25 mg in a single-dose study in 8 healthy subjects.[1] The manufacturer notes that postural hypotension may occur in patients receiving antihypertensives when they start alfuzosin.[2]

(b) Doxazosin

The manufacturer of doxazosin notes that no adverse drug interaction has been seen between doxazosin and **thiazides**[3,4] or **furosemide**.[3] However, they point out that doxazosin doses of greater then 4 mg daily increase the likelihood of adverse effects such as postural hypotension and syncope.[4]

(c) Indoramin

The manufacturer of indoramin states that concurrent use with diuretics may enhance their hypotensive action, and that titration of the dose of the diuretic may be needed.[5]

(d) Prazosin

The acute first-dose hypotension that can occur with alpha blockers such as prazosin can be exacerbated by 'beta blockers', (p.84) and 'calcium-channel blockers', (p.85), but there seems to be no direct evidence that diuretics normally do the same. However, the manufacturer of prazosin suggests that it is particularly important that patients with congestive heart failure who have undergone vigorous diuretic treatment should be given the initial dose of prazosin at bedtime and started on the lowest dose (500 micrograms two to four times daily). The reason is that left ventricular filling pressure may decrease in these patients with a resultant fall in cardiac output and systemic blood pressure.[6] There seems to be no reason for avoiding concurrent use if these precautions are taken.

(e) Tamsulosin

The US manufacturer of tamsulosin[7] notes that when 10 healthy subjects taking tamsulosin 800 micrograms daily were given a single 20-mg intravenous dose of **furosemide** the AUC of tamsulosin was reduced by 12%. Both the UK and US manufacturers note that as levels remained within the normal range no change in dosage is necessary.[7,8]

(f) Terazosin

Retrospective analysis of a large multinational study in patients given terazosin 5 or 10 mg daily found that terazosin only affected the blood pressure of patients taking diuretics (**amiloride**, **bendroflumethiazide**, **chlortalidone**, **hydrochlorothiazide** and **spironolactone**) if the blood pressure was uncontrolled. No change in blood pressure was seen in those with normal blood pressure (i.e. those without hypertension and those with hypertension controlled by diuretics). The most common adverse effect in the 10-week terazosin phase was dizziness, and the incidence of this appeared to be lower in those taking antihypertensives (13 to 16%) than those not taking antihypertensives (21 to 25%).[9] However, the UK manufacturer of terazosin notes that the incidence of dizziness in patients with BPH taking terazosin was higher when they were also taking a diuretic.[10] Similarly, in clinical studies in patients with hypertension, a higher proportion experienced dizziness when they took terazosin with a diuretic, than when they took a placebo with a diuretic (20% versus 13%).[11] The manufacturer states that when terazosin is added to a diuretic, dose reduction and re-titration may be necessary.[10,12] In addition to these drugs the manufacturers of terazosin note that it has been given to at least 50 patients taking **methyclothiazide** without evidence of an adverse interaction.[12]

1. Bianchetti G, Padovani P, Coupez JM, Guinebault P, Hermanns P, Coupez-Lopinot R, Guillet P, Thénot JP, Morselli PL. Pharmacokinetic interactions between hydrochlorothiazide, atenolol, and alfuzosin: a new antihypertensive drug. *Acta Pharmacol Toxicol (Copenh)* (1986) 59 (Suppl 5), 197.
2. Xatral (Alfuzosin hydrochloride). Sanofi-Aventis. UK Summary of product characteristics, April 2005.
3. Cardura (Doxazosin mesilate). Pfizer Ltd. UK Summary of product characteristics, February 2007.
4. Cardura (Doxazosin mesylate). Pfizer Inc. US Prescribing information, April 2002.
5. Doralese Tiltab (Indoramin hydrochloride). GlaxoSmithKline UK. UK Summary of product characteristics, June 2007.
6. Hypovase (Prazosin hydrochloride). Pfizer Ltd. UK Summary of product characteristics, May 2007.
7. Flomax (Tamsulosin hydrochloride). Boehringer Ingelheim Pharmaceuticals Inc. US Prescribing information, February 2007.
8. Flomaxtra XL (Tamsulosin hydrochloride). Astellas Pharma Ltd. UK Summary of product characteristics, October 2006.
9. Kirby RS. Terazosin in benign prostatic hyperplasia: effects on blood pressure in normotensive and hypertensive men. *Br J Urol* (1998) 82, 373–9.
10. Hytrin (Terazosin). Abbott Laboratories Ltd. UK Summary of product characteristics, January 2006.
11. Rudd P. Cumulative experience with terazosin administered in combination with diuretics. *Am J Med* (1986) 80 (Suppl 5B), 49–54.
12. Hytrin (Terazosin hydrochloride). Abbott Laboratories. US Prescribing information, February 2001.

Alpha blockers + Dutasteride or Finasteride

No clinically important interaction has been found to occur between finasteride and doxazosin. In one study terazosin did not interact with finasteride, but in another there was a suggestion of modestly increased finasteride levels. No clinically significant interaction appears to occur between dutasteride and tamsulosin or terazosin.

Clinical evidence, mechanism, importance and management

(a) Dutasteride

A study in 24 subjects given dutasteride 500 micrograms daily for 14 days found that when **tamsulosin** 400 micrograms or **terazosin** (titrated to 10 mg) were also given once daily for 14 days, the pharmacokinetics of the alpha blockers remained unchanged.[1] Furthermore, a clinical study in 327 men demonstrated that the combination of **tamsulosin** and dutasteride was well-tolerated over a period of 6 months.[2]

(b) Finasteride

In a parallel study, 48 healthy subjects were divided into three groups. One group took **terazosin** 10 mg daily for 18 days, another took finasteride 5 mg daily for 18 days, and the third group took both drugs. The pharmacokinetics and pharmacodynamics of both drugs remained unchanged, and the serum levels of testosterone and dihydrotestosterone were also unaltered by concurrent use.[3] However, another study, comparing groups of healthy subjects taking finasteride and alpha blockers found that after 5 days of combined use the group taking finasteride and **terazosin** had an 11% lower maximum plasma level of finasteride and a 12% higher AUC, compared with the group taking finasteride alone (both differences were not statistically significant). Conversely, after 10 days of combined use, the maximum finasteride level was 16% higher and the AUC 31% higher, which was statistically significant. The levels of the group taking finasteride and **doxazosin** were not significantly different. The clinical significance of the possible modest increased finasteride levels with **terazosin** is not clear,[4] but is likely to be small.

1. GlaxoSmithKline. Personal Communication, August 2003.
2. Barkin J, Guimarães M, Jacobi G, Pushkar D, Taylor S, van Vierssen Trip OB on behalf of the SMART-1 investigator group. Alpha-blocker therapy can be withdrawn in the majority of men following initial combination therapy with the dual 5α-reductase inhibitor dutasteride. *Eur Urol* (2003) 44, 461–6.
3. Samara E, Hosmane B, Locke C, Eason C, Cavanaugh J, Granneman GR. Assessment of the pharmacokinetic-pharmacodynamic interaction between terazosin and finasteride. *J Clin Pharmacol* (1996) 36, 1169–78.
4. Vashi V, Chung M, Hilbert J, Lawrence V, Phillips K. Pharmacokinetic interaction between finasteride and terazosin, but not finasteride and doxazosin. *J Clin Pharmacol* (1998) 38, 1072–6.

Alpha blockers + Miscellaneous

The manufacturers of several of the alpha blockers provide lists of drugs that are not expected to interact. These are shown in 'Table 4.2', (p.88). In some cases these predictions are based on *in vitro* studies or from observation of clinical usage. Although this type of data can provide a guide, remember that it gives only the broadest indication of whether or not a drug interacts.

Alpha blockers + NSAIDs

Indometacin reduces the blood pressure-lowering effects of prazosin in some individuals. Other alpha blockers do not appear to interact with NSAIDs.

Clinical evidence

A study in 9 healthy subjects found that **indometacin** 50 mg twice daily for 3 days had no statistically significant effect on the hypotensive effect of a single 5-mg dose of **prazosin**. However, in 4 of the subjects it was noted that the maximum fall in the mean standing blood pressure due to the **prazosin** was 20 mmHg less when they were taking **indometacin**. Three of these 4 felt faint when given **prazosin** alone, but not while taking the **indometacin** as well.[1]

Table 4.2 Drugs that are not expected to interact with alpha blockers as listed by the manufacturers

	Doxazosin[1]	*Prazosin*[2]	*Tamsulosin*[3,4]	*Terazosin*[5]
Amitriptyline			No expected interaction (*in vitro* study)	
Amoxicillin	No expected interaction			
Antacids	No expected interaction			No expected interaction
Antidiabetic drugs	No expected interaction	No expected interaction with chlorpropamide, insulin, phenformin, tolazamide, or tolbutamide	No expected interaction with glibenclamide (*in vitro* study)	No expected interaction
Antigout drugs		No expected interaction with allopurinol, colchicine, or probenecid		No expected interaction with allopurinol
Anxiolytics and Hypnotics	No expected interaction with diazepam	No expected interaction with chlordiazepoxide or diazepam	No expected interaction with diazepam (*in vitro* study)	No expected interaction with diazepam
Chlorphenamine	No expected interaction			No expected interaction
Codeine	No expected interaction			No expected interaction
Cold and flu remedies	No expected interaction			No expected interaction with phenylephrine, phenylpropanolamine, or pseudoephedrine
Corticosteroids	No expected interaction			No expected interaction
Co-trimoxazole	No expected interaction			No expected interaction
Dextropropoxyphene (Propoxyphene)		No expected interaction		
Erythromycin	No expected interaction			No expected interaction
Phenobarbital		No expected interaction		
Paracetamol (Acetaminophen)	No expected interaction			No expected interaction
Procainamide		No expected interaction		
Quinidine		No expected interaction		
Salbutamol			No expected interaction (*in vitro* study)	
Simvastatin			No expected interaction (*in vitro* study)	

1. Cardura (Doxazosin mesylate). Pfizer Inc. US Prescribing information, April 2002.
2. Hypovase (Prazosin hydrochloride). Pfizer Ltd. UK Summary of product characteristics, May 2007.
3. Stronazon MR Capsules (Tamsulosin hydrochloride). Actavis UK Ltd. UK Summary of product characteristics, August 2006.
4. Omnic MR (Tamsulosin hydrochloride). Astellas Pharma Ltd. UK Summary of product characteristics, October 2006.
5. Hytrin (Terazosin hydrochloride). Abbott Laboratories. US Prescribing information, February 2001.

Mechanism

Not established. It seems probable that indometacin inhibits the production of hypotensive prostaglandins by the kidney.

Importance and management

Direct information seems to be limited to this study but what occurred is consistent with the way indometacin reduces the effects of many other different antihypertensives (e.g. see 'ACE inhibitors + NSAIDs', p.28, and 'Beta blockers + Aspirin or NSAIDs', p.835). It apparently does not affect every patient. If indometacin is added to established treatment with prazosin, be alert for a reduced antihypertensive response. It is not known exactly what happens in patients taking both drugs long-term, but note that with other interactions between antihypertensives and NSAIDs the effects seem to be modest. The manufacturers say that prazosin has been given with indometacin (and also **aspirin** and **phenylbutazone**) without any adverse interaction in clinical experience to date.[2] Other manufacturers also note that no adverse interaction has been seen between **doxazosin** and NSAIDs, or **terazosin** and **aspirin**, **ibuprofen**, or indometacin.[3,4]

1. Rubin P, Jackson G, Blaschke T. Studies on the clinical pharmacology of prazosin. II: The influence of indomethacin and of propranolol on the action and disposition of prazosin. *Br J Clin Pharmacol* (1980) 10, 33–9.
2. Hypovase (Prazosin hydrochloride). Pfizer Ltd. UK Summary of product characteristics, May 2007.
3. Cardura (Doxazosin mesylate). Pfizer Inc. US Prescribing information, April 2002.
4. Hytrin (Terazosin hydrochloride). Abbott Laboratories. US Prescribing information, February 2001.

Bunazosin + Rifampicin (Rifampin)

Rifampicin markedly reduces bunazosin serum levels.

Clinical evidence, mechanism, importance and management

In 15 healthy subjects a 7-day course of rifampicin 600 mg daily reduced the mean maximum serum levels of bunazosin 6 mg daily by 82% (from 11.6 to 2.1 nanograms/mL). The bunazosin AUC was reduced by more than sevenfold. The duration of the blood pressure-lowering effect of bunazosin was shortened, the heart rate increase was less pronounced, and some adverse effects of bunazosin treatment (fatigue, headache) disappeared.[1,2] The probable reason is that the rifampicin (a recognised, potent enzyme inducer) increases the metabolism of bunazosin by the liver so that its levels are reduced, and its effects therefore diminished.

The evidence seems to be limited to this study, but anticipate the need to raise the bunazosin dosage if rifampicin is added. Information about other alpha blockers does not seem to be available.

1. Al-Hamdan Y, Otto U, Kirch W. Interaction of rifampicin with bunazosin, an alpha$_1$-adrenoceptor antagonist. *J Clin Pharmacol* (1993) 33, 998.
2. Nokhodian A, Halabi A, Ebert U, Al-Hamdan Y, Kirch W. Interaction of rifampicin with bunazosin, an α_1-adrenoceptor antagonist, in healthy volunteers. *Drug Invest* (1993) 6, 362–4.

Indoramin + MAOIs

Based on early theoretical considerations, the manufacturers of indoramin contraindicate its use with MAOIs.

Clinical evidence, mechanism, importance and management

The concurrent use of MAOIs is contraindicated by the manufacturers of indoramin.[1] This was included in the datasheet at the time indoramin was first licensed, and was based on a theoretical suggestion that the effects of noradrenaline (norepinephrine) may be potentiated by indoramin,[2] leading to vasoconstriction with a possible increase in blood pressure. However, the pharmacology of these drugs suggests just the opposite, namely that hypotension is the more likely outcome. (Note that the hypertensive effects of noradrenaline (norepinephrine) may be treated with a non-selective alpha blocker such as phentolamine.) The manufacturers are not aware of any reported interactions between indoramin and MAOIs.[2] Note that the MAOIs are not contraindicated with any of the other alpha blockers.

1. Doralese Tiltab (Indoramin hydrochloride). GlaxoSmithKline UK. UK Summary of product characteristics, June 2007.
2. GlaxoSmithKline. Personal communication, August 2003.

5

Anaesthetics and Neuromuscular blockers

This section is concerned with the interactions where the effects of anaesthetics (both general and local) and neuromuscular blocking drugs are affected by the presence of other drugs. Where the anaesthetics or neuromuscular blocking drugs are responsible for an interaction they are dealt with under the heading of the drug affected.

Many patients undergoing anaesthesia may be taking long-term medication, which may affect their haemodynamic status during anaesthesia. This section is limited to drug interactions and therefore does not cover the many precautions relating to patients taking long-term medication and undergoing anaesthesia in general (for example, drugs affecting coagulation).

(a) General anaesthetics and neuromuscular blockers

In general anaesthesia a balanced approach is often used to meet the main goals of the anaesthetic procedure. These goals are unconsciousness/amnesia, analgesia, muscle relaxation, and maintenance of homoeostasis. Therefore general anaesthesia often involves the use of several drugs, including benzodiazepines, opioids, and anticholinesterases, as well as general anaesthetics (sometimes more than one) and neuromuscular blockers. The use of several different types of drugs in anaesthesia means that there is considerable potential for drug interactions to occur in the peri-operative period, but this section is limited to the effects of drugs on general anaesthetics and neuromuscular blockers. The interactions of drugs affecting these other drugs used in anaesthesia are covered in other sections ('anticholinesterases', (p.352), 'benzodiazepines', (p.706), and 'opioids', (p.133)).

There may be difficulty in establishing which of the drugs being used in a complex regimen are involved in a suspected interaction. It should also be borne in mind that disease processes and the procedure for which anaesthesia is used may also be factors to be taken into account when evaluating a possible interaction.

Some established interactions are advantageous and are employed clinically. For example, the hypnotic and anaesthetic effects of 'propofol and midazolam', (p.96), are found to be greater than the expected additive effects and this synergy allows for lower dosage regimens in practice. Similarly nitrous oxide reduces the required dose of inhalational general anaesthetics (see 'Anaesthetics, general + Anaesthetics, general', p.92). Anticholinesterases oppose the actions of competitive neuromuscular blockers, and are used to restore muscular activity after surgery (see 'Neuromuscular blockers + Anticholinesterases', p.114).

The general anaesthetics mentioned in this section are listed in 'Table 5.1', (p.91). Barbiturates used as anaesthetics (e.g. thiopental) are largely covered here, whereas those used predominantly for their antiepileptic or sedative properties (e.g. phenobarbital or secobarbital) are dealt with in the appropriate sections.

The competitive (non-depolarising) neuromuscular blockers and depolarising neuromuscular blockers mentioned in this section are listed in 'Table 5.2', (p.91). The modes of action of the two types of neuromuscular blocker are discussed in the monograph 'Neuromuscular blockers + Neuromuscular blockers', p.128. It should be noted that mivacurium (a competitive blocker) and suxamethonium (a depolarising blocker) are hydrolysed by cholinesterase, so share some interactions in common that are not relevant to other competitive neuromuscular blockers.

(b) Local anaesthetics

The local anaesthetics mentioned in this section are listed in 'Table 5.1', (p.91). The interactions discussed in this section mainly involve the interaction of drugs with local anaesthetics used for epidural or spinal anaesthesia. The interactions of lidocaine used as an antiarrhythmic is dealt with in 'Antiarrhythmics', (p.243).

Table 5.1 Anaesthetics

General anaesthetics			
Halogenated inhalational anaesthetics	**Miscellaneous inhalational anaesthetics**	**Barbiturate parenteral anaesthetics**	**Miscellaneous parenteral anaesthetics**
Chloroform	Anaesthetic ether	Methohexital	Alfadolone
Desflurane	Cyclopropane	Thiamylal	Alfaxolone
Enflurane	Nitrous oxide	Thiopental	Etomidate
Halothane	Xenon		Ketamine
Isoflurane			Propofol
Methoxyflurane			
Sevoflurane			
Trichloroethylene			
Local anaesthetics			
Amide-type	**Ester-type (ester of benzoic acid)**	**Ester-type (ester of para-aminobenzoic acid)**	
Articaine	Cocaine	Chloroprocaine	
Bupivacaine		Procaine	
Etidocaine		Propoxycaine	
Levobupivacaine		Tetracaine	
Lidocaine			
Mepivacaine			
Prilocaine			
Ropivacaine			

Table 5.2 Neuromuscular blockers

Competitive (Non-depolarising) blockers - Aminosteroid type	*Competitive (Non-depolarising) blockers - Benzylisoquinolinium type*	*Depolarising blockers*
Pancuronium	Alcuronium	Decamethonium
Pipecuronium	Atracurium	Suxamethonium (Succinylcholine)
Rapacuronium	Cisatracurium	
Rocuronium	Doxacurium	
Vecuronium	Gallamine	
	Metocurine	
	Mivacurium	
	Tubocurarine (d-Tubocurarine)	

Anaesthetics, general + Alcohol

Those who regularly drink alcohol may need more thiopental or propofol than those who do not. In theory, alcohol may increase the risk of renal damage with sevoflurane. It is also probably unsafe to drink for several hours following anaesthesia because of the combined central nervous depressant effects.

Clinical evidence, mechanism, importance and management

A study in 532 healthy patients, aged from 20 to over 80 years, found that those who normally drank alcohol (more than 40 g weekly, roughly 400 mL of wine) needed more **thiopental** to achieve anaesthesia than non-drinkers. After adjusting for differences in age and weight distribution, men and women who were heavy drinkers (more than 40 g alcohol daily) needed 33% and 44% more **thiopental**, respectively, for induction than non-drinkers.[1] Chronic alcohol intake is known to increase barbiturate metabolism by cytochrome P450 enzymes.[2]

Another study found that 26 chronic alcoholics (drinkers of about 40 g of alcohol daily, with no evidence of liver impairment) needed about one-third more **propofol** to induce anaesthesia than another 20 patients who only drank socially. However, there was great interindividual variation in the alcoholic group.[3]

When 12 healthy subjects were given 0.7 g/kg of alcohol 4 hours after receiving 5 mg/kg of **thiopental** 2.5%, body sway and lightheadedness were accentuated.[4] This suggests that an interaction may occur if an ambulatory patient drinks alcohol within 4 hours of receiving an induction dose of **thiopental**. Patients should be cautioned not to drink alcohol following anaesthesia and surgery.

The manufacturer of **sevoflurane** notes that its metabolism may be increased by known inducers of the cytochrome P450 isoenzyme CYP2E1 including alcohol.[5,6] This may increase the risk of kidney damage because of an increase in plasma fluoride, although no cases appear to have been reported.

1. Dundee JW, Milligan KR. Induction dose of thiopentone: the effect of alcohol intake. *Br J Clin Pharmacol* (1989) 27, 693P–694P.
2. Weathermon R, Crabb DW. Alcohol and medication interactions. *Alcohol Res Health* (1999) 23, 40–54.
3. Fassoulaki A, Farinotti R, Servin F, Desmonts JM. Chronic alcoholism increases the induction dose of propofol in humans. *Anesth Analg* (1993) 77, 553–6.
4. Lichtor JL, Zacny JP, Coalson DW, Flemming DC, Uitvlugt A, Apfelbaum JL, Lane BS, Thisted RA. The interaction between alcohol and the residual effects of thiopental anesthesia. *Anesthesiology* (1993) 79, 28–35.
5. Sevoflurane. Abbott Laboratories Ltd. UK Summary of product characteristics, June 2007.
6. Ultane (Sevoflurane). Abbott Laboratories. US Prescribing information, September 2006.

Anaesthetics, general + Anaesthetics, general

In general, the effects of the combined use of general anaesthetics are at least additive. The required dose of propofol will be lower if it is given with nitrous oxide, halothane or isoflurane. The anaesthetic effects of propofol and sevoflurane appear to be additive in ECT, and synergy has been reported between propofol and etomidate.

The dose requirement of inhalational anaesthetics and barbiturate anaesthetics is reduced by nitrous oxide, and the effect of ketamine may be prolonged by barbiturate anaesthetics.

An isolated report described myoclonic seizures in a man anaesthetised with *Alfathesin* (alfaxalone/alfadolone) when he was also given enflurane.

Clinical evidence, mechanism, importance and management

In general, the effects of the combined use of general anaesthetics are at least additive.

(a) Propofol

In a study in 20 healthy patients the concurrent use of either **halothane** or **isoflurane** increased the serum concentrations of propofol by about 20% during the maintenance of general anaesthesia.[1] The US manufacturer of propofol notes that **inhalational anaesthetics** (such as **halothane** or **isoflurane**) would be expected to increase the effects of propofol. The manufacturer also states that the dosage of propofol required may be reduced if it is given with supplemental **nitrous oxide**.[2]

Synergy has been reported between propofol and **etomidate** – patients given induction doses of either **etomidate** or propofol alone required about a 15% higher dose than those given half etomidate and half propofol in sequence.[3]

For reports of enhanced sedation when propofol is given with midazolam, **thiopental** or other anaesthetics, see 'Anaesthetics, general + Benzodiazepines', p.96.

In a study of the induction of anaesthesia in patients undergoing ECT, subjects were given one of three treatments: propofol 1.5 mg/kg intravenously, **sevoflurane** 5% in oxygen, or propofol followed by **sevoflurane** in oxygen. **Sevoflurane** alone was associated with greater increases in heart rate and blood pressure than the other regimens and seizure duration was greatest in patients receiving propofol alone. Recovery time was longest with the propofol/**sevoflurane** combination, possibly because the combination produced deeper anaesthesia than the individual drugs alone.[4] The manufacturer of **sevoflurane** notes that lower concentrations may be required following the use of an intravenous anaesthetic such as propofol.[5] Note that the UK manufacturers of propofol do not recommend its use in ECT.[6]

(b) Miscellaneous anaesthetics

Nitrous oxide usually reduces the MAC of **inhalational anaesthetics** in a simple additive manner; an inspired concentration of 60 to 70% nitrous oxide is commonly used with volatile anaesthetics.[7] Similarly, the concurrent use of **nitrous oxide** reduces the dose of intravenous **barbiturate anaesthetics**[8] and **sevoflurane**[9] required for anaesthesia.

The manufacturers of **ketamine** note that **barbiturates** may prolong the effects of **ketamine** and delay recovery.[10,11]

Myoclonic activity occurred in a healthy 23-year-old man after anaesthesia was induced with 2.5 mL of *Alfathesin* (**alfaxalone/alfadolone**) given intravenously over 2 minutes, and then maintained with 2% **enflurane** in oxygen. The myoclonic activity subsided after stopping the **enflurane**, and anaesthesia was maintained with **nitrous oxide/oxygen**. The myoclonus recurred when the **enflurane** was restarted, but it resolved when the **enflurane** was replaced with **halothane**.[12] Since both *Alfathesin* and **enflurane** can cause CNS excitation, it seems possible that these effects might have been additive, and it was suggested that concurrent use should be avoided, particularly in patients with known convulsive disorders.[12] However, note that *Alfathesin* has been withdrawn from general use.

1. Grundmann U, Ziehmer M, Kreienmeyer J, Larsen R, Altmayer P. Propofol and volatile anaesthetics. *Br J Anaesth* (1994) 72 (Suppl 1) 88.
2. Diprivan (Propofol). AstraZeneca. US Prescribing information, August 2005.
3. Drummond GB, Cairns DT. Do propofol and etomidate interact kinetically during induction of anaesthesia? *Br J Anaesth* (1994) 73, 272P.
4. Wajima Z, Shiga T, Yoshikawa T, Ogura A. Inoue T, Ogawa R. Propofol alone, sevoflurane alone, and combined propofol-sevoflurane anaesthesia in electroconvulsive therapy. *Anaesth Intensive Care* (2003) 31, 396–400.
5. Sevoflurane. Abbott Laboratories Ltd. UK Summary of product characteristics, June 2007.
6. Diprivan (Propofol). AstraZeneca UK Ltd. UK Summary of product characteristics, May 2007.
7. Dale O. Drug interactions in anaesthesia: focus on desflurane and sevoflurane. *Baillieres Clin Anaesthesiol* (1995) 9, 105–17.
8. Aitkenhead AR, ed. Textbook of anaesthesia. 4th ed. Edinburgh: Churchill Livingstone; 2001 P. 172–4
9. Ultane (Sevoflurane). Abbott Laboratories. US Prescribing information, September 2006.
10. Ketalar (Ketamine hydrochloride). Pfizer Ltd. UK Summary of product characteristics, January 2006.
11. Ketalar (Ketamine hydrochloride). Monarch Pharmaceuticals. US Prescribing information, April 2004.
12. Hudson R, Ethans CT. Alfathesin and enflurane: synergistic central nervous system excitation? *Can Anaesth Soc J* (1981) 28, 55–6.

Anaesthetics, general + Anaesthetics, local

An isolated report describes convulsions associated with the use of propofol with topical cocaine. Cocaine abuse may increase the risk of cardiovascular complications during inhalational anaesthesia. Abstinence from cocaine or the avoidance of anaesthetics with sympathomimetic properties has been suggested.

The dosage of propofol may need to be reduced after the use of bupivacaine or lidocaine (e.g. during regional anaesthetic techniques). Similarly, epidural lidocaine reduces sevoflurane requirements, and is likely to have the same effect on other inhalational anaesthetics.

Clinical evidence, mechanism, importance and management

(a) Cocaine

A patient with no history of epilepsy, undergoing septorhinoplasty for cosmetic reasons, was premedicated with papaveretum and hyoscine, and intubated after **propofol** and suxamethonium (succinylcholine) were given. Anaesthesia was maintained with **nitrous oxide/oxygen** and 2% **isoflurane**. During anaesthesia a paste containing 10% **cocaine** was applied to the nasal mucosa. During recovery the patient experienced a dystonic reaction, which developed into a generalised convulsion. The authors of the report suggest that a possible interaction between the **propofol** and **cocaine** might have been responsible, although they also suggest that the convulsions may have been an adverse effect of the propofol.[1]

Reviews of the anaesthetic implications of illicit drug use have stated that anaesthetists should be aware of the medical complications of cocaine abuse, such as myocardial ischaemia, hypertension and tachycardia due to sympathetic nervous system stimulation.[2,3] It was suggested that the concurrent use of **cocaine** and **inhalational anaesthetics**, such as **halothane**, that are known to significantly sensitise the myocardium to circulating catecholamines, should be avoided, and that other halogenated anaesthetics should be used with caution.[2,3] Theoretically, **isoflurane** would be a better choice of inhalational anaesthetic since it has less cardiovascular effects.[2] **Ketamine** should also be avoided because of its sympathomimetic effects. **Nitrous oxide**, **thiopental** and fentanyl were considered to be useful for general anaesthesia in patients who regularly abuse **cocaine**.[2,3] Although it has been suggested that anaesthesia is safe for patients with chronic cocaine abuse after abstinence for 24 hours, the occurrence of ventricular fibrillation in one such patient during anaesthesia with **thiopental** and **isoflurane**, led the authors of the case report to conclude that there should be a cocaine-free interval of at least one week before elective surgical procedures. They also suggest that if an emergency operation is required during acute **cocaine** intoxication, all sympathomimetic anaesthetic drugs should be avoided.[4]

(b) Lidocaine or Bupivacaine

A double-blind, randomised study of 17 patients requiring ventilatory support demonstrated that hourly laryngotracheal instillation of 5 mL of 1% lidocaine significantly reduced the dose of **propofol** required to maintain adequate sedation (overall reduction of 50%) when compared with prestudy values.[5]

In a placebo-controlled, double-blind study of 90 patients undergoing minor gynaecological surgery, intramuscular administration of 4% lidocaine (1 to 3 mg/kg) 10 minutes before induction of anaesthesia or 0.5% bupivacaine (500 to 1000 micrograms/kg) 30 minutes before induction of anaesthesia, significantly enhanced the hypnotic effect of intravenous **propofol** in a dose-dependent manner. Only the lowest doses of lidocaine and bupivacaine tested (500 and 250 micrograms/kg, respectively) lacked a significant effect on the hypnotic dose of **propofol**. The highest doses of lidocaine and bupivacaine (3 and 1 mg/kg, respectively) reduced the hypnotic requirements for **propofol** by about 34% and 40%, respectively. The dose of **propofol** should therefore be modified after the intramuscular use of lidocaine or bupivacaine.[6] The UK manufacturer of **propofol** also notes that required doses may be lower when general anaesthesia is used in association with regional anaesthetic techniques.[7] An *in vitro* study using liver microsomes found that **propofol** inhibited the metabolism of lidocaine by cytochrome P450 isoenzymes.[8] However, a further study by the same authors in 31 patients undergoing anaesthesia with either **propofol** or **sevoflurane**, and receiving epidural lidocaine, found that, compared with **sevoflurane** (which does not inhibit lidocaine metabolism), **propofol** similarly did not affect the metabolism of epidural lidocaine. The lack of interaction in the latter study could be due to the lower doses of **propofol** involved and because other isoenzymes or extrahepatic metabolism of lidocaine might possibly be involved.[9]

A randomised, double-blind, placebo-controlled study involving 44 patients found that lidocaine epidural anaesthesia (15 mL of 2% plain lidocaine) reduced the MAC of **sevoflurane** required for general anaesthesia by approximately 50% (from 1.18 to 0.52%). This implies that a lower dose of **inhalational anaesthetic** provides adequate anaesthesia during combined epidural-general anaesthesia than for general anaesthesia alone.[10]

(c) Adrenaline in local anaesthetics

Note that drugs such as adrenaline (epinephrine), which are used with local anaesthetics, may interact with inhalational anaesthetics such as halothane to increase the risk of arrhythmias, see 'Anaesthetics, general + Inotropes and Vasopressors', p.99.

1. Hendley BJ. Convulsions after cocaine and propofol. *Anaesthesia* (1990) 45, 788–9.
2. Voigt L. Anesthetic management of the cocaine abuse patient. *J Am Assoc Nurse Anesth* (1995) 63, 438–43.
3. Culver JL, Walker JR. Anesthetic implications of illicit drug use. *J Perianesth Nurs* (1999) 14, 82–90.
4. Vagts DA, Boklage C, Galli C. Intraoperatives Kammerflimmern bei einer Patientin mit chronischem Kokainmissbrauch – Eine Kasuistik. Intraoperative ventricular fibrillation in a patient with chronic cocaine abuse – a case report. *Anaesthesiol Reanim* (2004) 29, 19–24.
5. Mallick A, Smith SN, Bodenham AR. Local anaesthesia to the airway reduces sedation requirements in patients undergoing artificial ventilation. *Br J Anaesth* (1996) 77, 731–4.
6. Ben-Shlomo I, Tverskoy M, Fleyshman G, Cherniavsky G. Hypnotic effect of i.v. propofol is enhanced by i.m. administration of either lignocaine or bupivacaine. *Br J Anaesth* (1997) 78, 375–7.
7. Diprivan (Propofol). AstraZeneca UK Ltd. UK Summary of product characteristics, May 2007.
8. Inomata S, Nagashima A, Osaka Y, Kazama T, Tanaka E, Sato S, Toyooka H. Propofol inhibits lidocaine metabolism in human and rat liver microsomes. *J Anesth* (2003) 17, 246–50.
9. Nakayama S, Miyabe M, Kakiuchi Y, Inomata S, Osaka Y, Fukuda T, Kohda Y, Toyooka H. Propofol does not inhibit lidocaine metabolism during epidural anesthesia. *Anesth Analg* (2004) 99, 1131–5.
10. Hodgson PS, Liu SS, Gras TW. Does epidural anesthesia have general anesthetic effects? *Anesthesiology* (1999) 91, 1687–92.

Anaesthetics, general + Anthracyclines

Pretreatment with anthracyclines may result in prolongation of the QT interval during isoflurane anaesthesia.

Clinical evidence, mechanism, importance and management

A study in women with breast cancer found that the QTc interval was prolonged (to more than 440 milliseconds) during anaesthesia with **isoflurane** (end-tidal concentration 0.5 vol%) in more than 50% of the 20 patients who had received treatment (about 1 month before surgery) with fluorouracil and cyclophosphamide and either **doxorubicin** or **epirubicin**, compared with only 1 of 20 patients who had not previously received chemotherapy. However, QTc intervals of 600 milliseconds and above, which may be associated with serious arrhythmias, were not observed. Anthracyclines (such as **doxorubicin** and **epirubicin**) and **isoflurane** can prolong the QT interval. The patients had also received midazolam, which is reported to reduce QTc prolongation induced by other anaesthetics. It was noted that the use of higher **isoflurane** concentrations in patients given anthracyclines could result in greater QTc interval prolongation.[1] In patients treated with anthracyclines or other drugs that prolong the QT interval, it should also be borne in mind that several drugs used in anaesthesia may affect the QT interval. For example **thiopental** and **sufentanil** are also reported to prolong the QT interval, while **propofol** and **halothane** are said to shorten it.[1]

1. Owczuk R, Wujtewicz MA, Sawicka W, Wujtewicz M, Swierblewski M. Is prolongation of the QTc interval during isoflurane anaesthesia more prominent in women pretreated with anthracyclines for breast cancer? *Br J Anaesth* (2004) 92, 658–61.

Anaesthetics, general + Anticholinesterases

Inhalation anaesthetics may impair the efficacy of anticholinesterases in reversing neuromuscular blockade. Propofol does not affect the reversal of rocuronium block by neostigmine. Physostigmine pre-treatment increased propofol requirements by 20% in one study.

Clinical evidence, mechanism, importance and management

(a) Inhalational anaesthetics

Inhalational anaesthetics can impair **neostigmine** reversal of neuromuscular blockade. In one study, **neostigmine** took longer to reverse **pancuronium** blockade after anaesthesia with **enflurane** compared with fentanyl or **halothane**.[1] Another study demonstrated that the reversal of **vecuronium** block with **neostigmine** 40 micrograms/kg was more dependent on the concentration of **sevoflurane** than the degree of block present. At the lowest concentration of **sevoflurane** (0.2 MAC), adequate reversal was obtained in all patients within 15 minutes, but with increasing concentrations (up to 1.2 MAC) satisfactory restoration of neuromuscular function was not achieved within 15 minutes, probably because of a greater contribution of **sevoflurane** to the degree of block.[2] In another study, 120 patients were randomly allocated maintenance of anaesthesia with one of three drugs: **sevoflurane** or **isoflurane** (adjusted to 1.5 MAC), or intravenous **propofol** 6 to 12 mg/kg per hour. Neuromuscular block was induced with **rocuronium** and monitored using train-of-four stimulation (TOF) of the ulnar nerve. **Neostigmine** was given when the first response in TOF had recovered to 20 to 25%. At this point **isoflurane** or **sevoflurane** was stopped, or the **propofol** dose reduced, in half of the patients in each of the three groups. The times to recovery of the TOF ratio to 0.8 were 12 and 6.8 minutes in the **sevoflurane** continued and stopped groups respectively, 9 and 5.5 minutes in the **isoflurane** continued and stopped groups respectively, and 5.2 and 4.7 minutes in the **propofol** continued and reduced groups respectively. Only 9/20 and 15/20 patients in the **sevoflurane** and **isoflurane** continued groups, respectively, achieved a TOF ratio of 0.8 within 15 minutes. This showed that the reversal of **rocuronium** block by **neostigmine** is slowed by **sevoflurane** and to a lesser extent by **isoflurane**, but not significantly affected by **propofol**.[3]

Note that inhalation anaesthetics potentiate neuromuscular blockers, see 'Anaesthetics, general + Neuromuscular blockers', p.101.

(b) Intravenous anaesthetics

A study of 40 patients found that **physostigmine** pre-treatment (2 mg intravenously 5 minutes before induction) increased **propofol** requirements by 20%.[4] **Propofol** does not appear to delay the reversal of **rocuronium** block by **neostigmine**. See (a) above.

1. Delisle S, Bevan DR. Impaired neostigmine antagonism of pancuronium during enflurane anaesthesia in man. *Br J Anaesth* (1982) 54, 441–5.
2. Morita T, Kurosaki D, Tsukagoshi H, Shimada H, Sato H, Goto F. Factors affecting neostigmine reversal of vecuronium block during sevoflurane anaesthesia. *Anaesthesia* (1997) 52, 538–43.
3. Reid JE, Breslin DS, Mirakhur RK, Hayes AH. Neostigmine antagonism of rocuronium block during anesthesia with sevoflurane, isoflurane or propofol. *Can J Anaesth* (2001) 48, 351–5.
4. Fassoulaki A, Sarantopoulos C, Derveniotis C. Physostigmine increases the dose of propofol required to induce anaesthesia. *Can J Anaesth* (1997) 44, 1148–51.

Anaesthetics, general + Antiemetics

Metoclopramide pre-treatment reduces the dosage requirements of propofol and thiopental. Droperidol, but not ondansetron, reduces the dose requirements of thiopental.

Clinical evidence

(a) Metoclopramide or Droperidol

In a randomised, placebo-controlled, double-blind study of 60 surgical patients, half of whom were given metoclopramide 150 micrograms/kg 5 minutes before induction, it was found that the induction dose of **propofol** was reduced by 24% in the group given metoclopramide.[1] Similar results were seen in another study of 21 patients, in which metoclopramide 10 or 15 mg reduced the dose requirements of **propofol** by 24.5% and 41.2%, respectively.[2] In a randomised, double-blind, placebo-controlled study in 96 women patients, both metoclopramide and droperidol reduced the amount of **thiopental** needed to induce anaesthesia by about 45%.[3]

(b) Ondansetron

In a double-blind, placebo-controlled, randomised study of 168 female patients ondansetron 100 or 200 micrograms/kg given intravenously 5 minutes before **thiopental** induction did not influence the hypnotic requirements of the **thiopental**.[4]

Mechanism

The exact mechanism by which metoclopramide reduces propofol or thiopental dose requirements is unclear, but it appears to involve the blockade of dopamine (D_2) receptors.

Importance and management

Although the evidence is limited these interactions between metoclopramide and thiopental or propofol, and between droperidol and thiopental would appear to be established. Droperidol has not been studied with propofol, but, on the basis of other interactions it would be expected to behave like metoclopramide. When patients are pretreated with either metoclopramide or droperidol, be alert for the need to use less propofol and thiopental to induce anaesthesia. Ondansetron appears not to interact.

1. Page VJ, Chhipa JH. Metoclopramide reduces the induction dose of propofol. *Acta Anaesthesiol Scand* (1997) 41, 256–9.
2. Santiveri X, Castillo J, Buil JA, Escolano F, Castaño J. Efectos de la metoclopramida sobre las dosis hipnóticas de propofol. *Rev Esp Anestesiol Reanim* (1996) 43, 297–8.
3. Mehta D, Bradley EL, Kissin I. Metoclopramide decreases thiopental hypnotic requirements. *Anesth Analg* (1993) 77, 784–7.
4. Kostopanagiotou G, Pouriezis T, Theodoraki K, Kottis G, Andreadou I, Smyrniotis V, Papadimitriou L. Influence of ondansetron on thiopental hypnotic requirements. *J Clin Pharmacol* (1998) 38, 825–9.

Anaesthetics, general + Antihypertensives

The concurrent use of general anaesthetics and antihypertensives generally need not be avoided but it should be recognised that the normal homoeostatic responses of the cardiovascular system will be impaired. For example, marked hypotension has been seen in patients taking ACE inhibitors or angiotensin-II receptor antagonists during anaesthetic induction. Profound hypotension may occur in patients taking alfuzosin during general anaesthesia.

Clinical evidence, mechanism, importance and management

The antihypertensive drugs differ in the way they act, but they all interfere with the normal homoeostatic mechanisms that control blood pressure and, as a result, the reaction of the cardiovascular system during anaesthesia to fluid and blood losses, body positioning, etc. is impaired to some extent. For example, enhanced hypotension was seen in a study of the calcium-channel blocker **nimodipine** during general anaesthesia (see 'Anaesthetics, general + Calcium-channel blockers', p.98), and marked hypotension has also been seen with ACE inhibitors in this setting (see below). This instability of the cardiovascular system needs to be recognised and allowed for, but it is widely accepted that antihypertensive treatment should normally be continued.[1-5] In some cases there is a real risk in stopping, for example a hypertensive rebound can occur if **clonidine** or the beta blockers are suddenly withdrawn. See also 'Anaesthetics, general + Beta blockers', p.97.

(a) ACE inhibitors

Marked hypotension (systolic BP 75 mmHg), which did not respond to surgical stimulation, occurred in a 42-year-old man taking **enalapril** when he was anaesthetised with **propofol**. He responded slowly to the infusion of one litre of Hartmann's solution.[6] Severe and unexpected hypotension has been seen during anaesthetic induction in patients taking **captopril**.[7] In a randomised clinical study, the incidence of hypotension during anaesthetic induction was higher in patients who had taken **captopril** or **enalapril** on the day of surgery than in those who had stopped these drugs 12 or 24 hours prior to surgery.[8] In 18 patients induction of anaesthesia for coronary artery bypass surgery resulted in a significant reduction in blood pressure and heart rate, irrespective of whether or not they were taking ACE inhibitors. The patients taking ACE inhibitors showed a marked decrease in cardiac index but no changes in systemic vascular resistance compared with the patients not taking ACE inhibitors.[9] In another study in patients undergoing coronary artery bypass surgery, short-lasting hypotensive episodes (less than 60 seconds) occurred in 9 of 16 patients receiving **captopril, enalapril, perindopril** or **lisinopril**, compared with 2 of 16 who were not taking ACE inhibitors. The patients experiencing hypotension required additional intravenous fluids and vasoconstrictors to maintain haemodynamic stability.[10] Similar findings are reported in another study which included patients taking **captopril, enalapril, ramipril**, or **lisinopril**.[11] Another experimental study found that a single dose of **captopril** at induction of anaesthesia caused a small reduction in cerebral blood flow, when compared with control patients or patients given metoprolol.[12]

Particular care would seem to be needed with patients taking ACE inhibitors, but there is insufficient evidence to generally recommend discontinuing ACE inhibitors before surgery. It is noted that whether ACE inhibitors are discontinued or continued, haemodynamic instability may occur after induction of anaesthesia.[4] One report in patients undergoing cardiac surgery found that intravenous **enalaprilat** effectively reduced blood pressure and also exerted a beneficial effect on the endocrine regulators of macro- and microcirculation by blunting the increase in vasoconstrictors.[13]

One recommendation is that intravenous fluids should be given to all patients taking ACE inhibitors who are anaesthetised.[6] If hypotension occurs, blood pressure can be restored in most patients by giving sympathomimetics such as phenylephrine.[4] However, sympathomimetics may not be fully effective in treating hypotension due to ACE inhibitors and anaesthesia because ACE inhibitor administration may result in a decrease in the adrenergic vasoconstrictive response.[5,10] Terlipressin (a vasopressin analogue that has some effects as a vasopressin agonist) is reported to be an effective treatment for refractory hypotension during anaesthesia in patients taking ACE inhibitors.[4,14,15] One study found that severe hypotension during anaesthetic induction in patients chronically taking ACE inhibitors could be controlled with an intravenous injection of angiotensin II (*Hypertensine*).[16]

(b) Alpha blockers

The UK manufacturers of **alfuzosin** note that the use of general anaesthetics in patients taking **alfuzosin** could cause profound hypotension, and they recommend that **alfuzosin** should be withdrawn 24 hours before surgery.[17]

(c) Angiotensin II receptor antagonists

A study in 12 hypertensive patients taking angiotensin-II receptor antagonists found that hypotension occurred in all patients after induction of anaesthesia. This was more frequent than that found in matched groups of hypertensive patients receiving either beta blockers and/or calcium-channel blockers (27 out of 45) or ACE inhibitors (18 of 27). The magnitude of hypotension was also significantly greater in those treated with angiotensin II receptor antagonists and it was less responsive to ephedrine and phenylephrine.[14] Terlipressin has been found to be effective in patients with refractory hypotension taking angiotensin II receptor antagonists.[14,15]

1. Craig DB, Bose D. Drug interactions in anaesthesia: chronic antihypertensive therapy. *Can Anaesth Soc J* (1984) 31, 580–8.
2. Foëx P, Cutfield GR, Francis CM. Interactions of cardiovascular drugs with inhalational anaesthetics. *Anasth Intensivmed* (1982) 150, 109–28.
3. Anon. Drugs in the peri-operative period: 4 – Cardiovascular drugs. *Drug Ther Bull* (1999) 37, 89–92.
4. Colson P, Ryckwaert F, Coriat P. Renin angiotensin system antagonists and anesthesia. *Anesth Analg* (1999) 89, 1143–55.
5. Licker M, Neidhart P, Lustenberger S, Valloton MB, Kalonji T, Fathi M, Morel DR. Long-term angiotensin-converting enzyme inhibitor treatment attenuates adrenergic responsiveness without altering hemodynamic control in patients undergoing cardiac surgery. *Anesthesiology* (1996) 84, 789–800.
6. Littler C, McConachie I, Healy TEJ. Interaction between enalapril and propofol. *Anaesth Intensive Care* (1989) 17, 514–15.
7. McConachie I, Healy TEJ. ACE inhibitors and anaesthesia. *Postgrad Med J* (1989) 65, 273–4.
8. Coriat P, Richer C, Douraki T, Gomez C, Hendricks K, Giudicelli J-F, Viars P. Influence of chronic angiotensin-converting enzyme inhibition on anesthetic induction. *Anesthesiology* (1994) 81, 299–307.
9. Ryckwaert F, Colson P. Hemodynamic effects of anesthesia in patients with ischemic heart failure chronically treated with angiotensin-converting enzyme inhibitors. *Anesth Analg* (1997) 84, 945–9.
10. Licker M, Schweizer A, Höhn L, Farinelli C, Morel DR. Cardiovascular responses to anesthetic induction in patients chronically treated with angiotensin-converting enzyme inhibitors. *Can J Anaesth* (2000) 47, 433–40.
11. Colson P, Saussine M, Séguin JR, Cuchet D, Chaptal P-A, Roquefeuil B. Hemodynamic effects of anesthesia in patients chronically treated with angiotensin-converting enzyme inhibitors. *Anesth Analg* (1992) 74, 805–8.
12. Jensen K, Bunemann L, Riisager S, Thomsen LJ. Cerebral blood flow during anaesthesia: influence of pretreatment with metoprolol or captopril. *Br J Anaesth* (1989) 62, 321–3.
13. Boldt J, Schindler E, Härter K, Görlach G, Hempelmann G. Influence of intravenous administration of angiotensin-converting enzyme inhibitor enalaprilat on cardiovascular mediators in cardiac surgery patients. *Anesth Analg* (1995) 80, 480–5.
14. Brabant SM, Bertrand M, Eyraud D, Darmon P-L, Coriat P. The hemodynamic effects of anesthetic induction in vascular surgical patients chronically treated with angiotensin II receptor antagonists. *Anesth Analg* (1999) 88, 1388–92.
15. Eyruad D, Brabant S, Nathalie D, Fléron M-H, Gilles G, Bertrand M, Coriat P. Treatment of intraoperative refractory hypotension with terlipressin in patients chronically treated with an antagonist of the renin-angiotensin system. *Anesth Analg* (1999) 88, 980–4.
16. Eyraud D, Mouren S, Teugels K, Bertrand M, Coriat P. Treating anesthesia-induced hypotension by angiotensin II in patients chronically treated with angiotensin-converting enzyme inhibitors. *Anesth Analg* (1998) 86, 259–63.
17. Xatral (Alfuzosin hydrochloride). Sanofi-Aventis. UK Summary of product characteristics, April 2005.

Anaesthetics, general + Antipsychotics

An isolated report describes a grand mal seizure in a man taking chlorpromazine and flupentixol when he was anaesthetised with enflurane. The sedative properties of antipsychotics may be enhanced by thiopental. Lower etomidate doses are recommended in patients taking antipsychotics.

Clinical evidence, mechanism, importance and management

An isolated report[1] describes an unexpected grand mal seizure in a schizophrenic patient without a history of epilepsy when he was given **enflurane** anaesthesia. He was taking **chlorpromazine** 50 mg three times daily (irregularly) and **flupentixol** 40 mg intramuscularly every 2 weeks. The suggested reason is that the **enflurane** had a synergistic effect with the two antipsychotics, all of which are known to lower the seizure threshold. The general importance of this interaction is not known.

The manufacturer of thiopental notes that, as would be expected, the sedative properties of antipsychotics may be potentiated by **thiopental.**[2] The manufacturer of etomidate recommends that the dose of **etomidate** should be reduced in patients taking antipsychotics.[3] **Droperidol** reduces the dose requirements of **thiopental**, see 'Anaesthetics, general + Antiemetics', p.94.

1. Vohra SB. Convulsions after enflurane in a schizophrenic patient receiving neuroleptics. *Can J Anaesth* (1994) 41, 420–2.
2. Thiopental Injection. Link Pharmaceuticals Ltd. UK Summary of product characteristics, January 2003.
3. Hypnomidate (Etomidate). Janssen-Cilag Ltd. UK Summary of product characteristics, February 2004.

Anaesthetics, general + Aspirin or Probenecid

The anaesthetic dosage of thiopental is reduced, and its effects prolonged by pretreatment with aspirin or probenecid.

Clinical evidence

A study in patients about to undergo surgery found that pretreatment with aspirin 1 g (given as intravenous **lysine acetylsalicylate**) one minute before induction reduced the dosage of thiopental by 34%, from 5.3 to 3.5 mg/kg. Initially thiopental 2 mg/kg was given followed by increments of 25 mg until the eyelash reflex was abolished.[1] The same study[1] also found that oral probenecid 1 g given one hour before anaesthesia reduced the thiopental dosage by 23%, from 5.3 to 4.1 mg/kg.

A further double-blind study[2] in 86 women found that probenecid given 3 hours before surgery prolonged the duration of anaesthesia with thiopental:

- In patients premedicated with atropine 7.5 micrograms/kg, pethidine (meperidine) 1 mg/kg, and 500 mg of probenecid, the duration of anaesthesia with thiopental 7 mg/kg was prolonged by 65%,
- In patients premedicated with atropine 7.5 micrograms/kg, pethidine 1 mg/kg, and *1 g of probenecid*, the duration of anaesthesia with thiopental 7 mg/kg was prolonged by 46%,
- In patients premedicated with atropine 7.5 micrograms/kg (*no pethidine*) and 500 mg of probenecid, the duration of anaesthesia with thiopental 7 mg/kg was prolonged by 26%,
- In patients premedicated with atropine 7.5 micrograms/kg (*no pethidine*) and 500 mg of probenecid, and *no surgical stimulus* the duration of anaesthesia with *thiopental 4 mg/kg* was prolonged by 109%.

Mechanism

Not understood. It has been suggested that aspirin and probenecid increase the amount of free (and active) thiopental in the plasma since they compete for the binding sites on the plasma albumins.[1]

Importance and management

Information is limited but what is known shows that the effects of thiopental are increased by aspirin and probenecid. Be alert for the need to reduce the dosage. However, note also that regular aspirin use may increase the risk of bleeding during surgery, and it is often recommended that aspirin should not be taken in the week before surgery.[3]

1. Dundee JW, Halliday NJ, McMurray TJ. Aspirin and probenecid pretreatment influences the potency of thiopentone and the onset of action of midazolam. *Eur J Anaesthesiol* (1986) 3, 247–51.
2. Kaukinen S, Eerola M, Ylitalo P. Prolongation of thiopentone anaesthesia by probenecid. *Br J Anaesth* (1980) 52, 603–7.
3. Anon. Drugs in the peri-operative period: 4 – Cardiovascular drugs. *Drug Ther Bull* (1999) 37, 89–92.

Anaesthetics, general + Baclofen

Severe seizures occurred during induction of anaesthesia with propofol in a patient taking baclofen.

Clinical evidence, mechanism, importance and management

A 48-year-old man with syringomyelia taking baclofen for flexor spasms underwent surgery for the relief of obstructive hydrocephalus. His last dose of baclofen was 6 hours before induction of anaesthesia with pethidine (meperidine) 40 mg followed by **propofol**. After he had received about 60 mg of **propofol** he developed severe myoclonic seizures, which lasted about 3 minutes. The patient was given additional **propofol** 40 mg because he appeared to be awakening, and severe generalised seizures lasting 2 minutes occurred. He was then given vecuronium and anaesthesia was maintained with isoflurane and nitrous oxide/oxygen without further problem.[1]

Seizures have been reported in patients with and without epilepsy receiving **propofol**. They mainly occur at induction or emergence or are delayed after anaesthesia, suggesting changes in cerebral levels of **propofol** may be causal.[2] Baclofen can cause acute desensitisation of $GABA_B$ receptors producing persistent epileptiform discharges.[1] It was suggested that in this patient the seizures were mediated by both baclofen and **propofol**.[1] Opioid analgesics may induce seizures and opisthotonos has been reported in patients given opioids and **propofol** (see 'Anaesthetics, general + Opioids', p.103). However, generalised seizures attributed to pethidine are probably due to a metabolite. The time course therefore makes pethidine an unlikely cause of the seizure in this patient.[1]

1. Manikandan S, Sinha PK, Neema PK, Rathod RC. Severe seizures during propofol induction in a patient with syringomyelia receiving baclofen. *Anesth Analg* (2005) 100, 1468–9.
2. Walder B, Tramèr MR, Seeck M. Seizure-like phenomena and propofol. A systematic review. *Neurology* (2002) 58, 1327–32.

Anaesthetics, general + Benzodiazepines

Midazolam markedly potentiates the anaesthetic action of halothane. Similarly, the effects of propofol or thiopental are greater than would be expected by simple addition when midazolam is given concurrently, although the extent varies between the end-points measured (analgesic, motor, hypnotic). Quazepam reduces induction time for propofol anaesthesia and premedication with diazepam reduces the dose of ketamine required.

Clinical evidence

(a) Halothane

In a study in 50 women undergoing surgery **midazolam** markedly potentiated the anaesthetic action of halothane: a mean **midazolam** dose of 278 micrograms/kg reduced the halothane MAC by 51.3%.[1]

(b) Ketamine

A study in patients undergoing major abdominal surgery found that in 10 patients premedicated with rectal **diazepam** one hour before induction, the haemodynamic effects of ketamine (increases in heart rate and blood pressure) were significantly reduced, when compared with 31 controls. Also, a lower rate of ketamine infusion was required during the initial 30 minutes of anaesthesia, the half-life of ketamine was significantly increased and the plasma levels of the hydroxylated metabolites were reduced. These findings suggest that both pharmacodynamic and pharmacokinetic interactions exist between **diazepam** and ketamine. In the same study, 3 patients were given 20 mg of intravenous **clorazepate** about one hour before induction of anaesthesia, but this did not affect either the dose of ketamine required or its pharmacokinetics.[2]

(c) Propofol

Two studies found that if propofol and **midazolam** were given together, the hypnotic and anaesthetic effects were greater than would be expected by the simple additive effects of both drugs.[3,4] In one of these studies, the ED_{50} (the dose required for 50% of the patients to respond) for hypnosis was 44% less than that expected of the individual drugs and the addition of **midazolam** 130 micrograms/kg caused a 52% reduction in the ED_{50} of propofol required for anaesthesia.[3] A pharmacokinetic study found a very modest 20% increase in the levels of free **midazolam** in the plasma when it was given with propofol, but this was considered too small to explain the considerable synergism.[5] In a further double-blind, placebo-controlled study in 24 patients, premedication with intravenous **midazolam**, 50 micrograms/kg given 20 minutes before induction of anaesthesia, reduced the propofol dose requirements for multiple anaesthetic end-points, including hypnotic, motor, EEG and analgesia. However, the potentiating effect and the mechanism of the interaction appeared to vary with the anaesthetic end-point and the dose of propofol. Notably, the interaction was most marked for analgesia.[6] Another double-blind, placebo-controlled study in 60 children aged 1 to 3 years found that oral **midazolam** 500 micrograms/kg approximately 30 minutes before the induction of anaesthesia delayed early recovery from anaesthesia, which was induced with propofol and maintained with **sevoflurane** and **nitrous oxide/oxygen**. However, the time to hospital discharge was not prolonged.[7]

A further double-blind, placebo-controlled study in 24 patients found that propofol decreased the clearance of **midazolam** by 37% and increased its elimination half-life by 61%.[8]

A study in 33 patients found that **quazepam** 15 or 30 mg given the night before induction of anaesthesia with propofol and fentanyl reduced the induction time when compared with a third group of patients not given a hypnotic. **Quazepam** did not affect blood pressure or heart rate, but the 30 mg dose of **quazepam** did increase anterograde amnesia.[9]

(d) Thiopental

Thiopental has been shown to act synergistically with **midazolam** at induction of anaesthesia in two studies.[10,11] In one of these studies, **midazolam** reduced the dose of thiopental required to produce anaesthesia by 50%.[11] In a further double-blind, placebo-controlled study in 23 patients, premedication with intravenous **midazolam** 50 micrograms/kg, given 20 minutes before the induction of anaesthesia, reduced the thiopental dose requirements for multiple anaesthetic end-points, including hypnotic, motor, EEG and analgesia. Potentiation was greatest for the motor end-point (about 40%) and smallest for analgesia (18%).[12]

Mechanism

Propofol, barbiturates and halothane appear to interact with benzodiazepines through their effects on the gamma-aminobutyric acid (GABA) receptor.

Diazepam appears to undergo similar oxidative processes as ketamine and therefore competitively inhibits ketamine metabolism.[2] Clorazepate is only slowly decarboxylated and is therefore not affected.[2]

An *in vitro* study suggests that propofol may reduce the clearance of midazolam by inhibition of the cytochrome P450 isoenzyme CYP3A4.[8]

Importance and management

The interactions between propofol or thiopental and midazolam are well established. This synergy has been utilised for the induction of anaesthesia.[13] Midazolam also reduces the dose requirements of halothane. Other benzodiazepines may also potentiate the effects of general anaesthetics.

1. Inagaki Y, Sumikawa K, Yoshiya I. Anesthetic interaction between midazolam and halothane in humans. *Anesth Analg* (1993) 76, 613–17.
2. Idvall J, Aronsen KF, Stenberg P, Paalzow L. Pharmacodynamic and pharmacokinetic interactions between ketamine and diazepam. *Eur J Clin Pharmacol* (1983) 24, 337–43.
3. Short TG, Chui PT. Propofol and midazolam act synergistically in combination. *Br J Anaesth* (1991) 67, 539–45.
4. McClune S, McKay AC, Wright PMC, Patterson CC, Clarke RSJ. Synergistic interactions between midazolam and propofol. *Br J Anaesth* (1992) 69, 240–5.
5. Teh J, Short TG, Wong J, Tan P. Pharmacokinetic interactions between midazolam and propofol: an infusion study. *Br J Anaesth* (1994) 72, 62–5.
6. Wilder-Smith OHG, Ravussin PA, Decosterd LA, Despland PA, Bissonnette B. Midazolam premedication reduces propofol dose requirements for multiple anesthetic endpoints. *Can J Anesth* (2001) 48, 439–45.
7. Viitanen H, Annila P, Viitanen M, Yli-Hankala A. Midazolam premedication delays recovery from propofol-induced sevoflurane anesthesia in children 1-3 yr. *Can J Anesth* (1999) 46, 766–71.
8. Hamaoka N, Oda Y, Hase I, Mizutani K, Nakamoto T, Ishizaki T, Asada A. Propofol decreases the clearance of midazolam by inhibiting CYP3A4: in vivo and in vitro study. *Clin Pharmacol Ther* (1999) 66, 110–17.
9. Imamachi N, Saito Y, Sakura S, Doi K, Nomura T. Effects of quazepam given the night before surgery on amnesia and induction and recovery characteristics of propofol anesthesia. Annual Meeting of the American Society of Anesthesiologists, Orlando USA, 2002. Abstract A-444.
10. Tverskoy M, Fleyshman G, Bradley EL, Kissin I. Midazolam–thiopental anesthetic interaction in patients. *Anesth Analg* (1988) 67, 342–5.
11. Short TG, Galletly DC, Plummer JL. Hypnotic and anaesthetic action of thiopentone and midazolam alone and in combination. *Br J Anaesth* (1991) 66, 13–19.
12. Wilder-Smith OHG, Ravussin PA, Decosterd LA, Despland PA, Bissonnette B. Midazolam premedication and thiopental induction of anaesthesia: interactions at multiple end-points. *Br J Anaesth* (1999) 83, 590–5.
13. Orser BA, Miller DR. Propofol-benzodiazepine interactions: insights from a "bench to bedside" approach. *Can J Anesth* (2001) 48, 431–4.

Anaesthetics, general + Beta-agonist bronchodilators

Two patients developed arrhythmias when terbutaline was given to patients anaesthetised with halothane.

Clinical evidence, mechanism, importance and management

Two patients developed ventricular arrhythmias while anaesthetised with **halothane** and nitrous oxide/oxygen when given terbutaline 250 to 350 micrograms subcutaneously for wheezing. Both developed unifocal premature ventricular contractions followed by bigeminy, which responded to lidocaine.[1] **Halothane** was replaced by **enflurane** in one case, which allowed the surgery to be completed without further incident.[1]

Halothane is known to cause arrhythmias and it has been suggested that it may increase susceptibility to the adverse cardiac effect of beta-agonist bronchodilators,[2] which can cause arrhythmias. Note that beta agonists such as **terbutaline** are sympathomimetics (see 'Table 24.1', (p.879)), like adrenaline (epinephrine), which has also been shown to cause arrhythmias in the presence of **halothane** (see 'Anaesthetics, general + Inotropes and Vasopressors', p.99).

1. Thiagarajah S, Grynsztejn M, Lear E, Azar I. Ventricular arrhythmias after terbutaline administration to patients anesthetized with halothane. *Anesth Analg* (1986) 65, 417–8.
2. Combivent UDVs (Ipratropium bromide/Salbutamol sulfate). Boehringer Ingelheim Ltd. UK Summary of product characteristics, June 2006.

Anaesthetics, general + Beta blockers

Anaesthesia in the presence of beta blockers normally appears to be safer than withdrawal of the beta blocker before anaesthesia, provided certain inhalational anaesthetics are avoided (methoxyflurane, cyclopropane, ether, trichloroethylene) and atropine is used to prevent bradycardia. Bradycardia and marked hypotension occurred in a man using timolol eye drops when he was anaesthetised.

Acute peri-operative administration of beta blockers may reduce the dose of anaesthetic required for induction and may result in deeper anaesthesia.

Clinical evidence and mechanism

A. Cardiac depressant effects

It used to be thought that beta blockers should be withdrawn from patients before surgery because of the risk that their cardiac depressant effects would be additive with those of inhalational anaesthetics, resulting in a reduction in cardiac output and blood pressure, but it seems that any effect depends on the anaesthetic used.[1] It has been suggested that the ranking order of compatibility (from the least to the most compatible with beta blockers) is as follows: **methoxyflurane, ether, cyclopropane, trichloroethylene, enflurane, halothane, isoflurane.**[1]

(a) Cyclopropane, Ether, Methoxyflurane, and Trichloroethylene

A risk of cardiac depression certainly seems to exist with cyclopropane and ether because their depressant effects on the heart are normally counteracted by the release of catecholamines, which would be blocked by the presence of a beta blocker. There is also some evidence (clinical and/or *animal*) that unacceptable cardiac depression may occur with methoxyflurane and trichloroethylene when a beta blocker is present. This has been the subject of two reviews.[2,3] For these four inhalational anaesthetics it has been stated that an absolute indication for their use should exist before giving them in combination with a beta blocker.[1]

(b) Enflurane, Halothane, and Isoflurane

Although a marked reduction in cardiac performance has been described in a study in *dogs* given **propranolol** and enflurane (discussed in two reviews[2,3]) these drugs have been widely used without apparent difficulties.[1] Normally beta blockers and halothane or isoflurane appear to be safe. On the positive side there appear to be considerable benefits to be gained from the continued use of beta blockers during anaesthesia. Their sudden withdrawal from patients treated for angina or hypertension can result in the development of acute and life-threatening cardiovascular complications whether the patient is undergoing surgery or not.

In the peri-operative period patients benefit from beta blockade because it can minimise the effects of sympathetic overactivity of the cardiovascular system during anaesthesia and surgery (for example during endotracheal intubation, laryngoscopy, bronchoscopy and various surgical manoeuvres), which can cause cardiac arrhythmias and hypertension.

(c) Unnamed general anaesthetic

A 75-year-old man being treated with **timolol** eye drops for glaucoma developed bradycardia and severe hypotension when anaesthetised [drug not named], and responded poorly to intravenous atropine, dextrose-saline infusion and elevation of his feet.[4] It would seem that there was sufficient systemic absorption of the **timolol** for its effects to be additive with the anaesthetic and cause marked cardiodepression.

B. Reduction of anaesthetic requirements

Intra-operative intravenous **atenolol** given in 5-mg stepwise doses (median dose 20 mg; range 10 to 80 mg) was found to reduce the **isoflurane** requirement by about 40% without affecting the bispectral index (BIS; a predictor of the depth of anaesthesia). Patients also received on average 21% less fentanyl compared with control patients who were not given **atenolol**.[5]

Several studies have similarly found that the use of **esmolol** reduced the required dose of **isoflurane** or **propofol**, or resulted in a deeper anaesthesia (as measured by BIS), but only in the presence of an opioid.[6-10] As there appears to be no pharmacokinetic interaction between **esmolol** and **propofol**[6,8] it has been suggested that **esmolol** could be interacting with the opioid.[6,10]

However, in one study 60 patients were given one of three treatments before induction of anaesthesia with **propofol**: **esmolol** 1 mg/kg followed by an infusion of 250 micrograms/kg per minute; midazolam; or placebo (sodium chloride 0.9%). No opioids were given. **Esmolol** and midazolam reduced the required induction doses of **propofol** by 25% and 45%, respectively. **Esmolol** reduced the mean heart rate by 7.6 bpm compared with placebo in the pre-induction period, and the only adverse effect noted was a transient episode of bradycardia (44 bpm) in one patient receiving **esmolol**. **Esmolol** reduces cardiac output by reduction of heart rate and stroke volume and this possibly reduces the required induction dose of **propofol** by changing its distribution.[11]

Another study found that a single 80-mg dose of **esmolol** after induction of anaesthesia with **propofol** and either fentanyl or placebo did not affect the depth of anaesthesia (measured by BIS) in either group of patients, even though cardiovascular effects were seen (reduction in systolic arterial pressure and heart rate).[12]

Importance and management

A. The consensus of opinion is that beta blockers should not be withdrawn before anaesthesia and surgery[13,14] because of the advantages of maintaining beta-blockade, and because the risks accompanying withdrawal are considerable. But, if inhalational anaesthetics are used, it is important to select the safest anaesthetics (isoflurane, halothane), and avoid those that appear to be most risky (methoxyflurane, ether, cyclopropane, trichloroethylene: most of which are no longer regularly used), as well as ensuring that the patient is protected against bradycardia by atropine.

The authors of the report[4] concerning topically applied beta blockers suggest that if such patients are to be anaesthetised, low concentrations of timolol should be used (possibly withhold the drops pre-operatively), and that "induction agents should be used judiciously and beta-blocking antagonists kept readily available." It is easy to overlook the fact that systemic absorption from eye drops can be high enough to cause adverse interactions.

B. Several studies suggest that beta blockers, such as atenolol and esmolol, given before induction reduce the anaesthetic dose requirement and may potentiate hypnosis. However, there are concerns that reducing the dose of anaesthetic may increase the risk of intra-operative awareness and it has been suggested that the use of BIS to predict the depth of anaesthesia in the presence of beta blockers may not be valid.[15] There is a possibility that acute as well as chronic administration of beta blockers may prevent peri-operative cardiac complications,[12,14] but more study is needed on this.[14,15]

1. Lowenstein E. Beta-adrenergic blockers. In: Smith NT, Miller RD, Corbascio AN, eds. Drug Interactions in Anesthesia. Philadelphia: Lea and Febiger; 1981 p. 83–101.
2. Foëx P, Cutfield GR, Francis CM. Interactions of cardiovascular drugs with inhalational anaesthetics. *Anasth Intensivmed* (1982) 150, 109–28.
3. Foëx P, Francis CM, Cutfield GR. The interactions between β-blockers and anaesthetics. Experimental observations. *Acta Anaesthesiol Scand* (1982) (Suppl 76), 38–46.
4. Mostafa SM, Taylor M. Ocular timolol and induction agents during anaesthesia. *BMJ* (1985) 290, 1788.
5. Zaugg M, Tagliente T, Silverstein JH, Lucchinetti E. Atenolol may not modify anesthetic depth indicators in elderly patients – a second look at the data. *Can J Anaesth* (2003) 50, 638–42.
6. Johansen JW, Flaishon R. Sebel PS. Esmolol reduces anesthetic requirement for skin incision during propofol/nitrous oxide/morphine anesthesia. *Anesthesiology* (1997) 86, 364–71.
7. Johansen JW, Schneider G, Windsor AM, Sebel PS. Esmolol potentiates reduction of minimum alveolar isoflurane concentration by alfentanil. *Anesth Analg* (1998) 87, 671–6.
8. Johansen JW. Esmolol promotes electroencephalographic burst suppression during propofol/alfentanil anesthesia. *Anesth Analg* (2001) 93, 1526–31.
9. Menigaux C, Guignard B, Adam F, Sessler DI, Joly V, Chauvin M. Esmolol prevents movement and attenuates the BIS response to orotracheal intubation. *Br J Anaesth* (2002) 89, 857–62.

10. Orme R, Leslie K, Umranikar A, Ugoni A. Esmolol and anesthetic requirement for loss of responsiveness during propofol anesthesia. *Anesth Analg* (2002) 93, 112–16.
11. Wilson ES, McKinlay S, Crawford JM, Robb HM. The influence of esmolol on the dose of propofol required for induction of anaesthesia. *Anaesthesia* (2004) 59, 122–6.
12. Berkenstadt H, Loebstein R, Faibishenko I, Halkin H, Keidan I, Perel A. Effect of a single dose of esmolol on the bispectral index scale (BIS) during propofol/fentanyl anaesthesia. *Br J Anaesth* (2002) 89, 509–11.
13. Anon. Drugs in the peri-operative period: 4 – Cardiovascular drugs. *Drug Ther Bull* (1999) 37, 89–92.
14. Howell SJ, Sear JW, Foex P. Peri-operative β-blockade: a useful treatment that should be greeted with cautious enthusiasm. *Br J Anaesth* (2001) 86, 161–4.
15. Yang H, Fayad A. Are β-blockers anesthetics?/Les β-bloquants sont-ils des anesthésiques? *Can J Anaesth* (2003) 50, 627–30.

Anaesthetics, general + Calcium-channel blockers

Impaired myocardial conduction has been seen in two patients taking diltiazem after they were anaesthetised with enflurane, and prolonged anaesthesia has been seen with verapamil and etomidate, but it has been suggested that chronic administration of oral calcium-channel blockers up to the day of surgery is usually beneficial. Intravenous dihydropyridines have been used to control peri-operative hypertension, but the use of intravenous verapamil is not recommended in patients anaesthetised with either halothane or enflurane.

Clinical evidence, mechanism, importance and management

(a) Dihydropyridines

Enhanced hypotension was seen in a study in which patients were given intravenous **nimodipine** during general anaesthesia, which included either **halothane** or **isoflurane**.[1]

The presence of low concentrations of **isoflurane** (0.6%) or **sevoflurane** (0.9%) are reported not to have a marked effect on the pharmacological action of **nicardipine**.[2] In one study intravenous **nicardipine** 17 micrograms/kg was given to 30 neurosurgical patients anaesthetised with either **enflurane**, **isoflurane** or **sevoflurane**. Peak reductions in blood pressure occurred 3 minutes after **nicardipine** was given and were greatest in the group receiving **sevoflurane**. However, peak reductions in blood pressure persisted for longer (30 minutes), as did increases in heart rate, with **isoflurane**. However, clearance of **nicardipine** was most rapid in patients given **isoflurane** anaesthesia.[3]

Some caution is clearly appropriate, especially with intravenous calcium-channel blockers given during surgery, but general experience suggests that long-term treatment with *oral* dihydropyridine calcium-channel blockers need not be avoided in most patients undergoing anaesthesia, and may be continued until the day of surgery. Further, *intravenous* dihydropyridines have been reported to be safe and effective for the control of peri-operative hypertension.[4]

(b) Diltiazem or Verapamil

The author of a review about calcium-channel blockers and anaesthetics concludes that their concurrent use in patients with reasonable ventricular function is normally beneficial, except where there are other complicating factors. Thus he warns about possible decreases in ventricular function in patients undergoing open chest surgery given *intravenous* verapamil or diltiazem.[5] A report describes a patient taking diltiazem and atenolol who had impaired AV and sinus node function before anaesthesia, which worsened following the use of **enflurane**.[6] Another patient also taking diltiazem (and atenolol) had to be paced due to bradycardia of 35 bpm at induction, but despite this he developed severe sinus bradycardia, which progressed to asystole when **enflurane** was given.[6] The authors of this latter report suggest that **enflurane** and diltiazem can have additive depressant effects on myocardial conduction. Two cases of prolonged anaesthesia and Cheyne-Stokes respiration have been reported in patients who were undergoing cardioversion. Both received verapamil and were induced with **etomidate**.[7] The presence of low concentrations of **isoflurane** (0.6%) or **sevoflurane** (0.9%) are reported not to have a marked effect on the pharmacological action of diltiazem.[2]

The authors of a review concluded that *intravenous* verapamil or diltiazem are not recommended in patients anaesthetised with either **halothane** or **enflurane**, especially if the patients have cardiac failure or conduction disturbances.[8]

1. Müller H, Kafurke H, Marck P, Zierski J, Hempelmann G. Interactions between nimodipine and general anaesthesia – clinical investigations in 124 patients during neurosurgical operations. *Acta Neurochir (Wien)* (1988) 45 (Suppl), 29–35.
2. Fukusaki M, Tomiyasu S, Tsujita T, Ogata K, Goto Y. Interaction of cardiovascular effect of calcium channel blocking drugs and those of inhalation anesthetics in humans. *Masui* (1993) 42, 848–55.
3. Nishiyama T, Matsukawa T, Hanaoka K, Conway CM. Interactions between nicardipine and enflurane, isoflurane, and sevoflurane. *Can J Anaesth* (1997) 44, 1071–6.
4. Tobias JD. Nicardipine: applications in anesthesia practice. *J Clin Anesth* (1995) 7, 525–33.
5. Merin RG. Calcium channel blocking drugs and anesthetics: is the drug interaction beneficial or detrimental? *Anesthesiology* (1987) 66, 111–13.
6. Hantler CB, Wilton N, Learned DM, Hill AEG, Knight PR. Impaired myocardial conduction in patients receiving diltiazem therapy during enflurane anesthesia. *Anesthesiology* (1987) 67, 94–6.
7. Moore CA, Hamilton SF, Underhill AL, Fagraeus L. Potentiation of etomidate anesthesia by verapamil: a report of two cases. *Hosp Pharm* (1989) 24, 24–5.
8. Durand P-G, Lehot J-J, Foëx P. Calcium-channel blockers and anaesthesia. *Can J Anaesth* (1991) 38, 75–89.

Anaesthetics, general + Dexmedetomidine

Dexmedetomidine can reduce the dose requirements of thiopental, isoflurane, and other similar anaesthetics.

Clinical evidence, mechanism, importance and management

Dexmedetomidine reduced the **thiopental** dose requirement for EEG burst suppression by 30% in 7 patients, when compared with 7 control patients given placebo. In this study, dexmedetomidine was given for 35 minutes before anaesthesia and during anaesthesia at a dose of 100 nanograms/kg per minute for the first 10 minutes, 30 nanograms/kg per minute for the following 15 minutes, and 6 nanograms/kg per minute thereafter. There was no pharmacodynamic synergism, and pharmacokinetic analysis showed that dexmedetomidine significantly reduced the **thiopental** distribution, probably due to reduced cardiac output and decreased regional blood flow.[1]

A placebo-controlled study in women undergoing abdominal hysterectomy found that a dexmedetomidine infusion started 15 minutes before induction of anaesthesia caused a dose-dependent reduction in **isoflurane** MAC (by 35% and 47% with dexmedetomidine plasma levels maintained at 0.37 and 0.69 nanograms/mL, respectively).[2] In another study, dexmedetomidine reduced the ED_{50} dose requirement of **isoflurane** for anaesthesia (motor response) in 9 healthy subjects. Dexmedetomidine plasma levels of 0.35 and 0.75 nanograms/mL reduced the requirements for **isoflurane** by about 30% and 50%, respectively. Subjects who had received dexmedetomidine took longer to wake up.[3] Dexmedetomidine has sedative, analgesic and anxiolytic effects[4] and therefore, like other sedatives, may reduce the dose requirements of anaesthetics. However, it may also affect the distribution of **thiopental** and possibly other **intravenous anaesthetics**.

1. Bührer M, Mappes A, Lauber R, Stanski DR, Maitre PO. Dexmedetomidine decreases thiopental dose requirement and alters distribution pharmacokinetics. *Anesthesiology* (1994) 80, 1216–27.
2. Aantaa R, Jaakola M-L, Kallio A, Kanto J. Reduction of the minimum alveolar concentration of isoflurane by dexmedetomidine. *Anesthesiology* (1997) 86, 1055–60.
3. Khan ZP, Munday IT, Jones RM, Thornton C, Mant TG, Amin D. Effects of dexmedetomidine on isoflurane requirements in healthy volunteers. 1: Pharmacodynamic and pharmacokinetic interactions. *Br J Anaesth* (1999) 83, 372–80.
4. Bhana N, Goa KL, McClellan KJ. Dexmedetomidine. *Drugs* (2000) 59, 263–8.

Anaesthetics, general + Herbal medicines

***Animal* data suggest that valerian may prolong the effect of thiopental. It has been predicted that kava kava and St John's wort may also prolong the effects of anaesthetics. There is an isolated report of profound hypotension during anaesthesia following the long-term use of St John's wort, and a tentative report of increased bleeding attributed to the concurrent use of sevoflurane and aloe vera. The American Society of Anesthesiologists recommends that all herbal medicines should be stopped two weeks prior to elective surgery.**

Clinical evidence and mechanism

(a) Aloe vera

A case report describes a 35-year-old woman undergoing surgery for a hemangioma of the left thigh, who had twice the expected intra-operative blood loss. The patient had been taking 4 tablets of aloe vera for 2 weeks prior to surgery, and so the blood loss was attributed to an interaction between the herbal medicine and the **sevoflurane**, which was used to maintain anaesthesia.[1] **Sevoflurane** can inhibit platelet aggregation by inhibiting thromboxane A_2, and aloe vera affects prostaglandin synthesis, which may also impair platelet aggregation. However, it should be noted that the patient's aPTT and INR were not assessed pre-operatively and the authors do state that the vascularity and size of the haemangioma were the most important factors in the blood loss,[1] so an interaction is by no means proven.

(b) Kava kava

There is one case report of kava kava potentiating the effect of benzodiazepines (see 'Benzodiazepines + Kava', p.730), and it has been suggested that it could potentiate other CNS depressants including **barbiturates**[2,3] (e.g. **thiopental**), and may prolong or potentiate the effects of anaesthetics.[4-6] Kava may act via GABA receptors, and kavalactones (one group of active constituents) also have skeletal muscle relaxant and local anaesthetic properties.[2,3] Toxic doses can produce muscle weakness and paralysis.[2,3]

(c) St John's wort (Hypericum perforatum)

It has been suggested that St John's wort *(Hypericum perforatum)* may prolong anaesthesia,[4-7] but there are no reports of this. This appears to have been based on the possibility that St John's wort acts as an MAOI,[5,7,8] (although this has been disputed[9]) and the limited evidence that MAOIs may cause hepatic enzyme inhibition and potentiate the effects of barbiturates (see 'MAOIs + Barbiturates', p.1132). However, there is now increasing evidence that St John's wort induces hepatic enzymes, and might therefore increase the metabolism of barbiturates (see 'Antiepileptics + St John's wort *(Hypericum perforatum)*', p.523), which suggests that it could increase requirements for **thiopental** anaesthesia. The possible MAOI activity of St John's wort has led to the recommendation that the same considerations apply as for other MAOIs and general anaesthetics,[7,8] see 'Anaesthetics, general + MAOIs', p.100. A case report describes a healthy 23-year-old woman who had been taking St John's wort on a daily basis for 6 months, who developed severe hypotension (BP 60/20 mmHg) during general anaesthesia, which responded poorly to ephedrine and phenylephrine (BP increased to 70/40 mmHg). It was suggested that the St John's wort might have caused adrenergic desensitisation with decreased responsiveness to the vasopressors.[10]

(d) Valerian

An ethanol extract of valerian *(Valeriana officinalis)* was shown to modestly prolong **thiopental** anaesthesia in *mice*, possibly via its effects on the GABA-benzodiazepine receptor.[11]

Importance and management

Not established. The evidence presented suggests that some caution may be warranted in patients using valerian, kava kava, or St John's wort if they are given general anaesthetics. The situation with aloe vera is less clear. Many other herbs have the potential to cause problems in the care of patients undergoing surgery (other than via drug interactions with anaesthetics) and these have been reviewed.[5-7] Because of the limited information, the American Society of Anesthesiologists have recommended discontinuation of all herbal medicines 2 weeks before an elective anaesthetic[4,6] and if there is any doubt about the safety of a product, this may be a prudent precaution.[5]

1. Lee A, Chui PT, Aun CST, Gin T, Lau ASC. Possible interaction between sevoflurane and aloe vera. *Ann Pharmacother* (2004) 38, 1651–4.
2. Anon. Piper methysticum (kava kava). *Altern Med Rev* (1998) 3, 458–60.
3. Pepping J. Kava: *Piper methysticum. Am J Health-Syst Pharm* (1999) 56, 957–8 and 960.
4. Larkin, M. Surgery patients at risk for herb–anaesthesia interactions. *Lancet* (1999) 354, 1362.
5. Cheng B, Hung CT, Chiu W. Herbal medicine and anaesthesia. *Hong Kong Med J* (2002) 8, 123–30.
6. Leak JA. Perioperative considerations in the management of the patient taking herbal medicines. *Curr Opin Anaesthesiol* (2000) 13, 321–5.
7. Lyons TR. Herbal medicines and possible anesthesia interactions. *AANA J* (2002) 70, 47–51.
8. Klepser TB, Klepser ME. Unsafe and potentially safe herbal therapies. *Am J Health-Syst Pharm* (1999) 56, 125–38.
9. Miller LG. Herbal medicinals. Selected clinical considerations focusing on known or potential drug-herb interactions. *Arch Intern Med* (1998) 158, 2200–11.
10. Irefin S, Sprung J. A possible cause of cardiovascular collapse during anesthesia: long-term use of St John's wort. *J Clin Anesth* (2000) 12, 498–9.
11. Hiller K-O, Zetler G. Neuropharmacological studies on ethanol extracts of *Valeriana officinalis* L.; behavioural and anticonvulsant properties. *Phytother Res* (1996) 10,145–51.

Anaesthetics, general + Inotropes and Vasopressors

Patients anaesthetised with inhalational anaesthetics (particularly cyclopropane and halothane, and to a lesser extent desflurane, enflurane, ether, isoflurane, methoxyflurane, and sevoflurane) can develop cardiac arrhythmias if they are given adrenaline (epinephrine) or noradrenaline (norepinephrine), unless the dosages are very low. Children appear to be less susceptible to this interaction. The addition of adrenaline to intrathecal tetracaine enhances the sedative effects of propofol.

Clinical evidence, mechanism, importance and management

As early as 1895, it was noted that an adrenal extract could cause ventricular fibrillation in a *dog* anaesthetised with **chloroform**,[1] and it is now very well recognised that similar cardiac arrhythmias can be caused by **adrenaline** and **noradrenaline** in humans anaesthetised with **inhalational anaesthetics**. The mechanism appears to be a sensitisation of the myocardium to β-adrenergic stimulation, caused by the **inhalational anaesthetic**. The likelihood of arrhythmias is increased by hypoxia and marked hypercapnia. It has been reported that the highest incidence of complications has been in patients anaesthetised with **cyclopropane**, but that the incidence is also high with **trichloroethylene** and **halothane**.[2] A suggested listing of inhalational anaesthetics in order of decreasing sensitising effect on the myocardium is as follows:[3] **cyclopropane**, **halothane**, **enflurane/methoxyflurane**, **isoflurane**, **ether**. **Sevoflurane**[4] and **desflurane**[5] appear to behave like **isoflurane**.

It has been recommended that if **adrenaline** is used to reduce surgical bleeding in patients anaesthetised with **halothane/nitrous oxide/oxygen** the dosage should not exceed 10 mL of 1:100 000 in any given 10 minute period, nor 30 mL per hour (i.e. about a 100 microgram bolus or 1.5 micrograms/kg per 10 minutes for a 70 kg person), and adequate alveolar ventilation must be assured.[6] This dosage guide should also be safe for use with other inhalational anaesthetics since **halothane** is more arrhythmogenic than the others,[3] with the exception of **cyclopropane**, which is no longer widely used. However, some have suggested that concurrent **halothane** and **adrenaline** may have been a contributing factor in 3 deaths in patients undergoing tooth implant surgery.[7] Others consider that if **adrenaline** is used for haemostasis during surgery, **isoflurane** or **sevoflurane** carry less risk of cardiac arrhythmias than **halothane**.[8] Solutions containing 0.5% **lidocaine** with **adrenaline** 1:200 000 also appear to be safe because lidocaine may help to control the potential dysrhythmic effects. For example, a study in 19 adult patients anaesthetised with **halothane** found that the dose of **adrenaline** needed to cause three premature ventricular contractions in half the group was 2.11 micrograms/kg when it was given in saline, but 3.69 micrograms/kg when it was given in 0.5% **lidocaine**. Note that both these values were less than that in 16 patients anaesthetised with **isoflurane** (6.72 micrograms/kg), demonstrating that **isoflurane** was still safer.[9] It should be borne in mind that the arrhythmogenic effects of **adrenaline** are increased if sympathetic activity is increased, and in hyperthyroidism and hypercapnia.[3]

Children appear to be much less susceptible to these effects than adults. A retrospective study of 28 children found no evidence of arrhythmia during **halothane** anaesthesia with **adrenaline** doses of up to 8.8 micrograms/kg, and a subsequent study in 83 children (aged 3 months to 17 years) found that 10 micrograms/kg doses of **adrenaline** were safe.[10]

A study in 20 patients undergoing spinal anaesthesia with tetracaine found that **propofol** sedation (as measured by bispectral index monitoring (BIS)) was enhanced when **adrenaline** was added to the intrathecal tetracaine.[11] A study in *sheep* found that **adrenaline**, **noradrenaline** and **dopamine** decreased **propofol** concentrations during a continuous propofol infusion, with the result that **propofol** anaesthesia was reversed. This was thought to be due to increased first pass clearance of **propofol** secondary to increased cardiac output. It was concluded that this could be of clinical importance if **propofol** is used in hyperdynamic circulatory conditions induced by either catecholamine infusions or disease states such as sepsis.[12]

1. Oliver G, Schäfer EA. The physiological effects of extracts of the suprarenal capsules. J Physiol (1895) 18, 230–76.
2. Gibb D. Drug interactions in anaesthesia. *Clin Anaesthesiol* (1984) 2, 485–512.
3. Wong KC. Sympathomimetic drugs. In: Smith NT, Miller RD, Corbascio AN, eds. Drug Interactions in Anesthesia. Philadelphia: Lea and Febiger, 1981 p. 55–82.

4. Navarro R, Weiskopf RB, Moore MA, Lockhart S, Eger EI, Koblin D, Lu G, Wilson C. Humans anesthetized with sevoflurane or isoflurane have similar arrhythmic response to epinephrine. *Anesthesiology* (1994) 80, 545–9.
5. Moore MA, Weiskopf RB, Eger EI, Wilson C, Lu G. Arrhythmogenic doses of epinephrine are similar during desflurane or isoflurane anesthesia in humans. *Anesthesiology* (1993) 79, 943–7.
6. Katz RL, Matteo RS, Papper EM. The injection of epinephrine during general anesthesia with halogenated hydrocarbons and cyclopropane in man. 2. Halothane. *Anesthesiology* (1962) 23, 597–600.
7. Buzik SC. Fatal interaction? Halothane, epinephrine and tooth implant surgery. *Can Pharm J* (1990) 123, 68–9 and 81.
8. Ransom ES, Mueller RA. Safety considerations in the use of drug combinations during general anaesthesia. *Drug Safety* (1997) 16, 88–103.
9. Johnston RR, Eger EI, Wilson C. A comparative interaction of epinephrine with enflurane, isoflurane, and halothane in man. *Anesth Analg* (1976) 55, 709–12.
10. Karl HW, Swedlow DB, Lee KW, Downes JJ. Epinephrine–halothane interactions in children. *Anesthesiology* (1983) 58, 142–5.
11. Yotsui T, Kitamura A, Ogawa R. Addition of epinephrine to intrathecal tetracaine augments depression of the bispectral index during intraoperative propofol sedation. *J Anesth* (2004) 18, 147–50.
12. Myburgh JA, Upton RN, Grant C, Martinez A. Epinephrine, norepinephrine and dopamine infusions decrease propofol concentrations during continuous propofol infusion in an ovine model. *Intensive Care Med* (2001) 27, 276–82.

Anaesthetics, general + Isoniazid

Isoniazid may increase the metabolism of enflurane, isoflurane or sevoflurane and thereby increase plasma-fluoride concentrations. However, this does not seem to have resulted in clinically important renal impairment.

Clinical evidence, mechanism, importance and management

A 46-year-old woman underwent anaesthesia for renal transplantation 6 days after starting isoniazid 300 mg daily. Anaesthesia was induced with intravenous thiopental and maintained for 4 hours with 60% nitrous oxide, fentanyl and **isoflurane**. Serum fluoride ions increased from 4.3 micromol preoperatively to approximately 30 micromol between 2 and 8 hours after starting **isoflurane**. However, no impairment of renal function occurred. A second patient who was given 5 times the first patient's exposure to **isoflurane** and who had received isoniazid for 13 years showed no increase in serum fluoride concentrations over preoperative values, but did show an increase in trifluoroacetic acid levels.[1]

When **enflurane** was given to 20 patients who had been taking isoniazid 300 mg daily for between one week and one year, 9 had an increase in peak fluoride ion levels. These 9 patients had a fourfold higher fluoride level than 36 control subjects not taking isoniazid and the 11 other subjects taking isoniazid. By 48 hours after anaesthesia, there was no difference in fluoride levels. Despite the increase in fluoride levels, there was no change in renal function.[2]

Isoniazid may increase the metabolism of **enflurane**, **isoflurane** or **sevoflurane**[3,4] in some patients (probably related to isoniazid acetylator phenotype[2]) and so increase the release of fluoride ions that may cause nephrotoxicity. However, there do not appear to be any reports of a significant clinical effect on renal function.

1. Gauntlett IS, Koblin DD, Fahey MR, Konopka K, Gruenke LD, Waskell L, Eger EI. Metabolism of isoflurane in patients receiving isoniazid. *Anesth Analg* (1989) 69, 245–9.
2. Mazze RI, Woodruff RE, Heerdt ME. Isoniazid-induced enflurane defluorination in humans. *Anesthesiology* (1982) 57, 5–8.
3. Sevoflurane. Abbott Laboratories Ltd. UK Summary of product characteristics, June 2007.
4. Ultane (Sevoflurane). Abbott Laboratories. US Prescribing information, September 2006.

Anaesthetics, general + Levothyroxine

Marked hypertension and tachycardia occurred in two patients taking levothyroxine when they were given ketamine.

Clinical evidence, mechanism, importance and management

Two patients taking levothyroxine developed severe hypertension (240/140 and 210/130 mmHg, respectively) and tachycardia (190 and 150 bpm) when they were given **ketamine**. Both were effectively treated with 1 mg of intravenous propranolol.[1] It was not clear whether this was an interaction or simply a particularly exaggerated response to **ketamine**, but care is clearly needed if **ketamine** is given to patients taking thyroid replacement.

1. Kaplan JA, Cooperman LH. Alarming reactions to ketamine in patients taking thyroid medication — treatment with propranolol. *Anesthesiology* (1971) 35, 229–30.

Anaesthetics, general + MAOIs

It is generally recommended that MAOIs should be withdrawn at least 2 weeks before anaesthesia. Individual cases of both hypo- and hypertension have been seen and MAOIs can interact dangerously with other drugs sometimes used during surgery (particularly pethidine (meperidine) and ephedrine).

Clinical evidence

The absence of problems during emergency general anaesthesia in 2 patients taking MAOIs prompted further study in 6 others receiving long-term treatment with unnamed MAOIs. All 6 were premedicated with 10 to 15 mg of diazepam 2 hours before surgery, induced with **thiopental**, given suxamethonium (succinylcholine) before intubation, and maintained with **nitrous oxide/oxygen** with either **halothane** or **isoflurane**. Pancuronium was used for muscle relaxation, and morphine was given postoperatively. One patient experienced hypotension that responded to repeated 100-microgram intravenous doses of phenylephrine without hypertensive reactions. No other untoward events occurred either during or after the anaesthesia.[1]

No adverse reactions occurred in 27 other patients taking MAOIs (**tranylcypromine**, **phenelzine**, **isocarboxazid**, **pargyline**) when they were anaesthetised.[2] A retrospective review of 32 patients taking **isocarboxazid** 10 mg daily who underwent elective surgery (involving **thiopental** or **ketamine** for induction of anaesthesia and maintenance with an inhalation anaesthetic with or without a muscle relaxant or analgesic) found that 5 patients experienced intra-operative hypotension, another patient had hypertension, and bradycardia occurred in 4 patients. No postoperative complications were attributed to interaction between the MAOI and the drugs given peri-operatively.[3]

No problems were seen in *dogs* given **tranylcypromine**, anaesthetised with **enflurane** and fentanyl, and then given the vasopressors noradrenaline (norepinephrine) and ephedrine.[4] Two case reports describe the safe and uneventful use of **propofol** in a patient taking **phenelzine**[5] and another taking **tranylcypromine**.[6] The latter was also given alfentanil. No problems were seen in one patient taking **tranylcypromine** when **ketamine** was given,[7] and in another taking **selegiline** when fentanyl, **isoflurane** and midazolam were given.[8] No problems were seen in another patient taking **phenelzine** when anaesthetised firstly with **sevoflurane** in oxygen, followed by **isoflurane**, oxygen, air and an infusion of remifentanil.[9]

Unexplained hypertension has been described in a patient taking **tranylcypromine** when **etomidate** and atracurium were given.[10] Severe and prolonged cardiovascular collapse occurred in one patient in whom long-term **tranylcypromine** 10 mg four times daily therapy was discontinued 20 days before surgery. During surgery **etomidate** and suxamethonium were given for induction, and **isoflurane** and **nitrous oxide/oxygen** for maintenance, as well as epidural anaesthesia with bupivacaine, but without an opioid.[11] **Moclobemide** was stopped on the morning of surgery in a patient who was anaesthetised with **propofol** and later **isoflurane** in **nitrous oxide** and oxygen. Atracurium, morphine and droperidol were also used. No adverse reactions occurred.[12] Ketorolac, **propofol** and midazolam were used uneventfully in one patient taking **phenelzine**.[13]

There are a few anecdotal reports of MAOIs potentiating the effects of amobarbital, butobarbital and secobarbital–see 'MAOIs + Barbiturates', p.1132.

Mechanism, importance and management

There seems to be little documentary evidence that the withdrawal of MAOIs before giving an anaesthetic is normally necessary. Scrutiny of reports[14] alleging an adverse reaction usually shows that what happened could be attributed to an interaction between other drugs used during the surgery (e.g. either 'directly-acting sympathomimetics', (p.1146), 'indirectly-acting sympathomimetics', (p.1147), 'pethidine', (p.1140), or 'fentanyl', (p.1138)) rather than with the anaesthetics.

The authors of two of the reports cited here offer the opinion that 'general and regional anaesthesia may be provided safely without discontinuation of MAOI therapy, provided proper monitoring, adequate preparation, and prompt treatment of anticipated reactions are utilised'.[1,2] This implies that the possible interactions between the MAOI and other drugs are fully recognised, but be alert for the rare unpredictable response. The conclusion of another report was that patients on low-dose MAOIs could be safely anaesthetised.[3]

The BNF[15] states that 'in view of their hazardous interactions MAOIs should normally be stopped 2 weeks before surgery.' It has also been suggested that a longer period of time (more than 20 days) between discontinuing MAOIs and surgery may be required, not so much to recover MAO enzyme activity but to recover depressed adrenergic receptor function.[11] These warnings are probably more to avoid interactions with the anaesthetic adjuncts mentioned above, rather than the MAOIs themselves. Therefore in an emergency situation it would seem possible to anaesthetise a patient, but it must be remembered that the choice of anaesthetic adjuncts is likely to be restricted.

1. El-Ganzouri A, Ivankovich AD, Braverman B, Land PC. Should MAOI be discontinued preoperatively? *Anesthesiology* (1983) 59, A384.
2. El-Ganzouri AR, Ivankovich AD, Braverman B, McCarthy R. Monoamine oxidase inhibitors: should they be discontinued preoperatively? *Anesth Analg* (1985) 64, 592–6.
3. Ebrahim ZY, O'Hara J, Borden L, Tetzlaff J. Monoamine oxidase inhibitors and elective surgery. *Cleve Clin J Med* (1993) 60, 129–30.
4. Braverman B, Ivankovich AD, McCarthy R. The effects of fentanyl and vasopressors on anesthetized dogs receiving MAO inhibitors. *Anesth Analg* (1984) 63, 192.
5. Hodgson CA. Propofol and mono-amine oxidase inhibitors. *Anaesthesia* (1992) 47, 356.
6. Powell H. Use of alfentanil in a patient receiving monoamine oxidase inhibitor therapy. *Br J Anaesth* (1990) 64, 528–9.
7. Doyle DJ. Ketamine induction and monoamine oxidase inhibitors. *J Clin Anesth* (1990) 2, 324–5.
8. Noorily SH, Hantler CB, Sako EY. Monoamine oxidase inhibitors and cardiac anesthesia revisited. *South Med J* (1997) 90, 836–8.
9. Ure DS, Gillies MA, James KS. Safe use of remifentanil in a patient treated with the monoamine oxidase inhibitor phenelzine. *Br J Anaesth* (2000) 84, 414–16.
10. Sides CA. Hypertension during anaesthesia with monoamine oxidase inhibitors. *Anaesthesia* (1987) 42, 633–5.
11. Sprung J, Distel D, Grass J, Bloomfield EL, Lavery IC. Cardiovascular collapse during anesthesia in a patient with preoperatively discontinued chronic MAO inhibitor therapy. *J Clin Anesth* (1996) 8, 662–5.
12. McFarlane HJ. Anaesthesia and the new generation monoamine oxidase inhibitors. *Anaesthesia* (1994) 49, 597–9.
13. Fischer SP, Mantin R, Brock-Utne JG. Ketorolac and propofol anesthesia in a patient taking chronic monoamine oxidase inhibitors. *J Clin Anesth* (1996) 8, 245–7.
14. Stack CG, Rogers P, Linter SPK. Monoamine oxidase inhibitors and anaesthesia: a review. *Br J Anaesth* (1988) 60, 222–7.
15. British National Formulary. 53rd ed. London: The British Medical Association and The Pharmaceutical Press; 2007. p. 654.

Anaesthetics, general + Methylphenidate

A single report described difficulty in sedating a child taking methylphenidate, and a possible delayed interaction between ketamine and methylphenidate, which resulted in nausea, vomiting and dehydration. The use of methylphenidate after ketamine anaesthesia increased the incidence of vomiting, excessive talking, and limb movements in one study. Methylphenidate should probably be withheld before surgery using inhalational anaesthetics, because of the potential risk of hypertension and/or arrhythmias.

Clinical evidence, mechanism, importance and management

A 6-year-old boy weighing 22 kg, who was taking methylphenidate 5 mg twice daily for attention deficit disorder, was found to be difficult to sedate for an echocardiogram. Sedation was attempted with oral cloral hydrate 75 mg/kg without success. One week later he received midazolam 20 mg orally, but was only mildly sedated 20 minutes later and would not lie still. Despite an additional oral dose of midazolam 10 mg mixed with oral **ketamine** 60 mg the child was still alert and uncooperative 20 minutes later. He was finally given intravenous glycopyrronium (glycopyrrolate) 100 micrograms followed by intravenous midazolam 5 mg given over 5 minutes and was successfully sedated. He recovered from sedation uneventfully, but developed nausea, vomiting and lethargy after discharge from hospital, which responded to rehydration treatment.[1] In a double-blind study, methylphenidate was given as a single 20-mg intravenous dose to try to speed recovery at the end of **ketamine** anaesthesia for short urological procedures. However, methylphenidate did not improve recovery, and increased the incidence of vomiting, excessive talking, and limb movements.[2]

In the first case, the stimulant effect of the methylphenidate was thought to have antagonised the sedative effect of the midazolam and **ketamine**. The methylphenidate may also have delayed the absorption of the oral drugs. In addition, methylphenidate may inhibit liver microsomal enzymes and could therefore possibly delay elimination of both **ketamine** and midazolam so that hazardous plasma concentrations could develop.[1] However, the study did not find evidence of these effects.

These appear to be the only reports, so any effect is not established. Be aware that methylphenidate may possibly antagonise the effect of sedative drugs, and may also be associated with an increased incidence of vomiting. Note that methylphenidate is an indirectly-acting sympathomimetic, and as such might be expected to increase the risk of hypertension and arrhythmias if used with **inhalational anaesthetics** (consider 'Anaesthetics, general + Inotropes and Vasopressors', p.99). Because of this, the manufacturer of one brand of methylphenidate recommends that, if surgery with halogenated anaesthetics is planned, methylphenidate treatment should not be given on the day of surgery.[3] Taken together, these reports suggest this advice may be a prudent precaution for any form of sedation and/or general anaesthesia.

1. Ririe DG, Ririe KL, Sethna NF, Fox L. Unexpected interaction of methylphenidate (Ritalin®) with anaesthetic agents. *Paediatr Anaesth* (1997) 7, 69–72.
2. Attalah MM, Saied MMA, Yahya R, Ibrahiem EI. Ketamine anesthesia for short transurethral urologic procedures. *Middle East J Anesthesiol* (1993) 12, 123–33.
3. Concerta XL (Methylphenidate hydrochloride). Janssen-Cilag Ltd. UK Summary of product characteristics, June 2007.

Anaesthetics, general + Neuromuscular blockers

The inhalational anaesthetics increase the effects of the neuromuscular blockers to differing extents, but nitrous oxide appears not to interact significantly. Ketamine has been reported to potentiate the effects of atracurium. Propofol does not appear to interact with mivacurium or vecuronium. Xenon is reported not to interact with mivacurium or rocuronium, and has less effect than sevoflurane on vecuronium neuromuscular blockade. Bradycardia has been seen in patients given vecuronium with etomidate or thiopental. Propofol can cause serious bradycardia if it is given with suxamethonium (succinylcholine) without adequate antimuscarinic premedication, and asystole has been seen when fentanyl, propofol and suxamethonium were given sequentially.

Clinical evidence, mechanism, importance and management

A. Effects of anaesthetics on neuromuscular blockade

(a) Inhalational anaesthetics

The effects of neuromuscular blockers are increased by inhalational anaesthetics, the greater the dosage of the anaesthetic the greater the increase in blockade. In broad terms **desflurane**, **ether**, **enflurane**, **isoflurane**, **methoxyflurane** and **sevoflurane** have a greater effect than **halothane**, which is more potent than **cyclopropane**, whereas **nitrous oxide** appears not to interact significantly with competitive blockers.[1-7]

The mechanism is not fully understood but seems to be multifactorial. It has been suggested that the anaesthetic may:

- have an effect via the CNS (including depression of spinal motor neurones);
- have an effect on the neuromuscular junction (including a decrease in the release of acetylcholine and in the sensitivity of the motor end-plate to acetylcholine);
- affect the muscle tissue itself.[6,8]

It has also been suggested that for **mivacurium**, higher plasma levels, especially of the potent *trans-trans* isomer, occur in the presence of **isoflurane**, and these could contribute to the enhanced neuromuscular blockade observed.[9]

One study in children found that the potentiation of **vecuronium** was greater with **isoflurane** than with **enflurane**, and **halothane** had a lesser effect.[10]

The dosage of the neuromuscular blocker may need to be adjusted according to the anaesthetic in use. For example, the dosage of **atracurium** can be reduced by 25 to 30% if, instead of balanced anaesthesia (with **thiopental**, fentanyl and **nitrous oxide/oxygen**),[11] **enflurane** is used, and by up to 50% if **isoflurane** or **desflurane** are used.[4,12,13] Another study recommended reduced doses of neuromuscular blockers such as **atracurium** and **tubocurarine** in children undergoing anaesthesia with **enflurane** or **isoflurane**.[14] In one study, **enflurane** and **isoflurane** reduced the **vecuronium** infusion rate requirements by as much as 70%, when compared with fentanyl anaesthesia.[15] Another study demonstrated that although **halothane** and **isoflurane** could both increase the neuromuscular potency of **vecuronium**, only **isoflurane** prolonged the recovery from neuromuscular blockade.[16]

The duration of exposure to the anaesthetic and the duration of effect of the various neuromuscular blockers also appear to affect the degree of potentiation that occurs.[8,17] In a study in which the muscle relaxant was given about 5 minutes after the start of inhalational anaesthesia, **enflurane** prolonged the action of **atracurium**, **pipecuronium** and **pancuronium**, but did not significantly affect **vecuronium**. However, **halothane** did not significantly prolong the clinical duration of any of the neuromuscular blockers.[17] It was suggested that more prolonged exposure to the anaesthetic, allowing equilibration of the anaesthetic to the tissues, might result in more significant potentiation of the neuromuscular blockers. In addition, the duration of effect of the **vecuronium** may have been too short for interaction with a volatile anaesthetic that had not had time to equilibrate with the tissues.[17] The duration of exposure to **sevoflurane** also influences the dose-response of **vecuronium,** but it has been suggested that sevoflurane-induced potentiation of neuromuscular blockers might be more rapid than with other inhalational anaesthetics.[8] In one study when the volatile anaesthetics were given about 10 minutes before the neuromuscular blocker, **sevoflurane** was reported to increase and prolong the blockade of **rocuronium** more than **isoflurane** or **propofol**.[18] However, another study found that after a 40-minute equilibration period of the inhalation anaesthetic (steady-state conditions), there was no significant difference between **desflurane**, **isoflurane** and **sevoflurane** in relation to potency, infusion requirements or recovery characteristics of **rocuronium**; the potency of **rocuronium** was increased by 25 to 40% under inhalational anaesthesia compared with **propofol**.[19] Another study demonstrated considerable prolongation of neuromuscular blockade with **rapacuronium** in the presence of **sevoflurane**; the recovery times were approximately doubled compared with those given in the published literature using thiopental/opioid-nitrous oxide anaesthesia. This led to the study being prematurely terminated as spontaneous recovery of neuromuscular function was required after short surgical procedures.[20] Marked potentiation of neuromuscular block following the combination of **sevoflurane** and a small dose of **cisatracurium** 25 micrograms/kg has been reported in a myasthenic patient.[21]

Although it is generally assumed that **nitrous oxide** does not affect the potency of neuromuscular blockers, one study found that the administration of **nitrous oxide** increased **suxamethonium (succinylcholine)** neuromuscular blockade.[22]

Xenon is reported not to prolong the neuromuscular blocking effects of **rocuronium**.[23] It is also reported to have less effect on recovery from **vecuronium**-induced neuromuscular block than **sevoflurane**.[24] **Xenon** is also reported not to affect the onset time, duration and recovery from **mivacurium**.[25]

In two early studies, **halothane** was found to shorten the recovery from **pancuronium**[26] and **gallamine**.[27]

(b) Intravenous anaesthetics

Ketamine prolonged the duration of neuromuscular blockade induced by **atracurium**,[28] but did not influence **suxamethonium (succinylcholine)**-induced neuromuscular blockade.[29] However, the UK manufacturers of **suxamethonium** still warn of a possible interaction because they say that **ketamine** may reduce normal plasma cholinesterase activity.[30]

In *animals*, **ketamine** and **thiopental** potentiated the neuromuscular blocking effects of **rocuronium**, whereas **propofol** had no effect.[31]

The original formulation of **propofol** in *Cremophor* was found to increase the blockade due to **vecuronium**,[32] but the more recent formulation in soybean oil and egg phosphatide has been found in an extensive study not to interact with **vecuronium**.[33] Propofol also appears not to interact with **mivacurium**.[9]

B. Cardiac effects

Serious sinus bradycardia (heart rates of 30 to 40 bpm) developed rapidly in two young women when they were anaesthetised with a slow intravenous injection of **propofol** 2.5 mg/kg, followed by **suxamethonium (succinylcholine)** 1.5 mg/kg. This was controlled with 600 micrograms of intravenous atropine. Four other patients premedicated with 600 micrograms of intramuscular atropine given 45 minutes before induction of anaesthesia did not develop bradycardia.[34] It would appear that **propofol** lacks central vagolytic activity and can exaggerate the muscarinic effects of **suxamethonium**.[34] Another report describes a woman who became asystolic when given an anaesthetic induction sequence of fentanyl, **propofol** and **suxamethonium**.[35] Bradycardia and asystole has also been seen following the sequential administration of **propofol** and fentanyl in 2 patients.[36,37] All of these three drugs (fentanyl, **propofol**, **suxamethonium**) alone have been associated with bradycardia and their effects can apparently be additive.

Bradycardia and asystole occurred in another patient given **propofol**, fentanyl and **atracurium**.[38] The authors of one report suggest that atropine or glycopyrrolate pretreatment should attenuate or prevent such reactions.[35]

Bradycardia occurring during anaesthetic induction with **vecuronium** and **etomidate**, or to a lesser extent **thiopental**, has also been reported, particularly in patients also receiving fentanyl,[39] see also 'Neuromuscular blockers + Opioids', p.130.

C. Muscle effects

In children receiving **suxamethonium**, those who had anaesthesia induced and maintained with **halothane** had much higher levels of serum myoglobulin than those undergoing intravenous induction with **thiopental** followed by **halothane**. This suggests that prior use of **halothane** may have potentiated **suxamethonium**-induced muscle damage.[40]

1. Schuh FT. Differential increase in potency of neuromuscular blocking agents by enflurane and halothane. *Int J Clin Pharmacol Ther Toxicol* (1983) 21, 383–6.
2. Fogdall RP, Miller RD. Neuromuscular effects of enflurane, alone and combined with *d*-tubocurarine, pancuronium, and succinylcholine, in man. *Anesthesiology* (1975) 42, 173–8.
3. Miller RD, Way WL, Dolan WM, Stevens WC, Eger EI. Comparative neuromuscular effects of pancuronium, gallamine, and succinylcholine during Forane and halothane anesthesia in man. *Anesthesiology* (1971) 35, 509–14.
4. Lee C, Kwan WF, Chen B, Tsai SK, Gyermek L, Cheng M, Cantley E. Desflurane (I-653) potentiates atracurium in humans. *Anesthesiology* (1990) 73, A875.
5. Izawa H, Takeda J, Fukushima K. The interaction between sevoflurane and vecuronium and its reversibility by neostigmine in man. *Anesthesiology* (1992) 77, A960.
6. Østergaard D, Engbaek J, Viby-Mogensen J. Adverse reactions and interactions of the neuromuscular blocking drugs. *Med Toxicol Adverse Drug Exp* (1989) 4, 351–68.
7. Vanlinthout LEH, Booij LHDJ, van Egmond J, Robertson EN. Effect of isoflurane and sevoflurane on the magnitude and time course of neuromuscular block produced by vecuronium, pancuronium and atracurium. *Br J Anaesth* (1996) 76, 389–95.
8. Suzuki T, Iwasaki K, Fukano N, Hariya S, Saeki S, Ogawa S. Duration of exposure to sevoflurane affects dose–response relationship of vecuronium. *Br J Anaesth* (2000) 85, 732–4.
9. Ledowski T, Wulf H, Ahrens K, Weindlmayr-Goettel M, Kress H-G, Geldner G, Scholz J. Neuromuscular block and relative concentrations of mivacurium isomers under isoflurane versus propofol anaesthesia. *Eur J Anaesthesiol* (2003) 20, 821–5.
10. Lynas AGA, Fitzpatrick KTJ, Black GW, Mirakhur RK. Influence of volatile anaesthetics on the potency of vecuronium in children. *Br J Anaesth* (1988) 61, 506P.
11. Ramsey FM, White PA, Stullken EH, Allen LL, Roy RC. Enflurane potentiation of neuromuscular blockade by atracurium. *Anesthesiology* (1982) 57, A255.
12. Sokoll MD, Gergis SD, Mehta M, Ali NM, Lineberry C. Safety and efficacy of atracurium (BW33A) in surgical patients receiving balanced or isoflurane anesthesia. *Anesthesiology* (1983) 58, 450–5.
13. Smiley RM, Ornstein E, Mathews D, Matteo RS. A comparison of the effects of desflurane and isoflurane on the action of atracurium in man. *Anesthesiology* (1990) 73, A882.
14. Lynas AGA, Fitzpatrick KTJ, Black GW, Mirakhur RK, Clarke RSJ. Influence of volatile anaesthetics on the potency of tubocurarine and atracurium. *Br J Clin Pharmacol* (1988) 26, 617P–618P.
15. Cannon JE, Fahey MR, Castagnoli KP, Furuta T, Canfell PC, Sharma M, Miller RD. Continuous infusion of vecuronium: the effect of anesthetic agents. *Anesthesiology* (1987) 67, 503–6.
16. Pittet J-F, Melis A, Rouge J-C, Morel DR, Gemperle G, Tassonyi E. Effect of volatile anesthetics on vecuronium-induced neuromuscular blockade in children. *Anesth Analg* (1990) 70, 248–52.
17. Swen J, Rashkovsky OM, Ket JM, Koot HWJ, Hermans J, Agoston S. Interaction between nondepolarizing neuromuscular blocking agents and inhalational anesthetics. *Anesth Analg* (1989) 69, 752–5.
18. Lowry DW, Mirakhur RK, McCarthy GJ, Carroll MT, McCourt KC. Neuromuscular effects of rocuronium during sevoflurane, isoflurane, and intravenous anesthesia. *Anesth Analg* (1998) 87, 936–40.
19. Bock M, Klippel K, Nitsche B, Bach A, Martin E, Motsch J. Rocuronium potency and recovery characteristics during steady-state desflurane, sevoflurane, isoflurane or propofol anaesthesia. *Br J Anaesth* (2000) 84, 43–7.
20. Cara DM, Armory P, Mahajan RP. Prolonged duration of neuromuscular block with rapacuronium in the presence of sevoflurane. *Anesth Analg* (2000) 91, 1392–3.
21. Baraka AS, Taha SK, Kawkabani NI. Neuromuscular interaction of sevoflurane - cisatracurium in a myasthenic patient. *Can J Anesth* (2000) 47, 562–5.
22. Szalados JE, Donati F, Bevan DR. Nitrous oxide potentiates succinylcholine neuromuscular blockade in humans. *Anesth Analg* (1991) 72, 18–21.
23. Kunitz O, Baumert J-H, Hecker K, Beeker T, Coburn M, Zühlsdorff A, Rossaint R. Xenon does not prolong neuromuscular block of rocuronium. *Anesth Analg* (2004) 99, 1398–1401.
24. Nakata Y, Goto T, Morita S. Vecuronium-induced neuromuscular block during xenon or sevoflurane anaesthesia in humans. *Br J Anaesth* (1998) 80, 238–40.
25. Kunitz O, Baumert H-J, Hecker K, Coburn M, Beeker T, Zühlsdorff A, Fassl J, Rossaint R. Xenon does not modify mivacurium induced neuromuscular block. *Can J Anesth* (2005) 52, 940–3.
26. Barth L. Paradoxical interaction between halothane and pancuronium. *Anaesthesia* (1973) 28, 514–20.
27. Feldman SA, Andrew D. Paradoxical interaction between halothane and pancuronium. *Anaesthesia* (1974) 29, 100–2.
28. Toft P, Helbo-Hansen S. Interaction of ketamine with atracurium. *Br J Anaesth* (1989) 62, 319–20.
29. Helbo-Hansen HS, Toft P, Kirkegaard Neilsen H. Ketamine does not affect suxamethonium-induced neuromuscular blockade in man. *Eur J Anaesthesiol* (1989) 6, 419–23.
30. Anectine (Suxamethonium). GlaxoSmithKline. UK Summary of product characteristics, April 2003.
31. Muir AW, Anderson KA, Pow E. Interaction between rocuronium bromide and some drugs used during anaesthesia. *Eur J Anaesthesiol* (1994) 11 (Suppl 9), 93–8.
32. Robertson EN, Fragen RJ, Booij LHDJ, van Egmond J, Crul JF. Some effects of diisopropyl phenol (ICI 35 868) on the pharmacodynamics of atracurium and vecuronium in anaesthetized man. *Br J Anaesth* (1983) 55, 723–7.
33. McCarthy GJ, Mirakhur RK, Pandit SK. Lack of interaction between propofol and vecuronium. *Anesth Analg* (1992) 75, 536–8.

34. Baraka A. Severe bradycardia following propofol-suxamethonium sequence. *Br J Anaesth* (1988) 61, 482–3.
35. Egan TD, Brock-Utne JG. Asystole after anesthesia induction with a fentanyl, propofol, and succinylcholine sequence. *Anesth Analg* (1991) 73, 818–20.
36. Guise PA. Asystole following propofol and fentanyl in an anxious patient. *Anaesth Intensive Care* (1991) 19, 116–18.
37. Dorrington KL. Asystole with convulsion following a subanaesthetic dose of propofol plus fentanyl. *Anaesthesia* (1989) 44, 658–9.
38. Ricós P, Trillo L, Crespo MT, Guilera N, Puig MM. Bradicardia y asistolia asociadas a la administración simultánea de propofol y fentanilo en la inducción anestésica. *Rev Esp Anestesiol Reanim* (1994) 41, 194–5.
39. Inoue K, El-Banayosy A, Stolarski L, Reichelt W. Vecuronium induced bradycardia following induction of anaesthesia with etomidate or thiopentone, with or without fentanyl. *Br J Anaesth* (1988) 60, 10–17.
40. Laurence AS, Henderson P. Serum myoglobin after suxamethonium administration to children: effect of pretreatment before i.v. and inhalation induction. *Br J Anaesth* (1986) 58, 126P.

Anaesthetics, general + Opioids

The respiratory depressant effects of ketamine and morphine may be additive. The dose requirements of desflurane, etomidate, propofol and thiopental may be lower after opioid use. Opisthotonos or grand mal seizures have rarely been associated with the use of propofol with alfentanil and/or fentanyl. The effects of inhalational anaesthetics may be enhanced by opioid analgesics.

Clinical evidence, mechanism, importance and management

(a) Inhalational anaesthetics

Opioid analgesics have been reported to reduce the MAC values of inhalational anaesthetics. For example, **fentanyl** has been shown to lower the MAC value of **desflurane**, probably in a dose-dependent manner, and this has been the subject of a review.[1] The manufacturer notes that lower doses of **desflurane** are required in patients receiving opioids.[2] **Remifentanil** at a target-controlled plasma level of 1 nanogram/mL was found to decrease the MAC of **sevoflurane** with nitrous oxide by 60%, and **remifentanil** 3 nanograms/mL produced a further 30% decrease in the MAC of **sevoflurane**.[3] Another study found that **remifentanil** (dose-dependently) decreased the level of **sevoflurane** required to maintain anaesthesia.[4] However, 100 microgram/kg doses of **morphine** given during anaesthesia did not alter the awakening concentration of **sevoflurane**.[5]

(b) Etomidate

The manufacturer of etomidate recommends that the dose of etomidate should be reduced in patients who have already received opioids.[6]

(c) Ketamine

Ketamine is a respiratory depressant like **morphine**, but less potent, and its effects can be additive with morphine.[7] The manufacturer notes that prolonged recovery time may occur if opioids are used with ketamine.[8]

A study in 11 healthy subjects found that the combination of ketamine and **morphine** almost abolished windup-like pain (progressive increase in pain intensity on repeated stimulation) in a skin burn injury. This effect was not found with either drug alone. Further, ketamine alone, but not **morphine** reduced the area of secondary hyperalgesia of the local burn and increased the pain threshold, but the combination did not appear to enhance this effect. The reduction of wind-up pain may be due to ketamine-induced prevention of acute tolerance to **morphine**.[9]

Another study in healthy subjects using various experimental pain models found that ketamine *antagonised* the respiratory depressant effect of **remifentanil**. **Remifentanil** alone produced analgesic effects with all pain tests, but ketamine only enhanced the effect of **remifentanil** on intramuscular electrical stimulation. Acute **remifentanil**-induced hyperalgesia and tolerance were detected only by the pressure pain test and were not suppressed by ketamine. The combined effects of **remifentanil** and ketamine probably depend on the type of pain.[10]

(d) Propofol

A 71-year-old man undergoing a minor orthopaedic operation was given a 500-microgram intravenous injection of **alfentanil** followed by a slow injection of propofol 2.5 mg/kg. Approximately 15 seconds after the propofol, the patient developed strong bilateral fits and grimaces, which lasted for 10 seconds. Anaesthesia was maintained with nitrous oxide/oxygen and halothane and there were no other intra- or postoperative complications. The patient had no history of convulsions.[11] Propofol has also been associated with opisthotonos (a spasm where the head and heels bend backwards and the body arches forwards) in two patients given **fentanyl** with or without **alfentanil**.[12] There is a further report of opisthotonos during recovery from anaesthesia with **alfentanil**, propofol and nitrous oxide.[13] Seizures have been reported in patients with and without epilepsy receiving propofol. They mainly occur during induction and emergence or are delayed after anaesthesia, suggesting that they may be caused by changes in cerebral levels of propofol,[14] and postanaesthetic opisthotonos may be due to a propofol-induced tolerance to inhibitory transmitters (glycine and gamma-aminobutyric acid).[13] Any association with the opioid remains unknown, although it has been suggested that opioids may aggravate propofol-induced opisthotonos by antagonising the actions of glycine.[13]

Alfentanil has been found to reduce the amount of propofol needed for loss of eyelash reflex and loss of consciousness, as well as increasing the blood pressure fall produced by propofol.[15] Propofol inhibits both **alfentanil** and **sufentanil** metabolism causing an increase in plasma concentrations of these opioids, while **alfentanil** also increases propofol concentrations (reviewed by Vuyk[16] and also described in more recent reports[17-20]). Pretreatment with **fentanyl** may also decrease the propofol requirements for induction of anaesthesia,[16] and increase blood concentrations of propofol.[21] However, another study was unable to confirm an effect on blood propofol concentrations.[22] **Remifentanil** has been reported to reduce the dose of propofol needed for anaesthesia and also to reduce the recovery time.[23,24] Further, propofol and **remifentanil** caused dose-dependent respiratory-depression, which, during combined use, was synergistic.[25] One study using EEG-controlled dosing of propofol and **remifentanil** for anaesthesia found their pharmacodynamic effects were no more than additive.[26] Although **remifentanil** alone appears to be ineffective at countering the response to stimuli, a study in healthy subjects has found that **remifentanil** can significantly reduce the levels of propofol required to ablate response to shouting, shaking or laryngoscopy (synergistic effect), but the effects on EEG measures were additive.[27] In another study in healthy subjects, the synergy that occurred for both analgesic and hypnotic endpoints was found to be greatest at lower levels of the drugs which for each drug alone would not be producing maximal effects.[28] Another study found changes in BIS (Bispectral Index) that suggested that **remifentanil** may have some hypnotic properties or that it can potentiate the hypnotic effect of propofol.[29] It has been suggested that the increased hypnotic effects may be due to a dose-dependent decrease in cardiac output by **remifentanil**, resulting in an increase in arterial and brain propofol with increased anaesthetic effect.[30] One pharmacokinetic study found that the levels of **remifentanil** may be increased during concurrent propofol infusion,[31] while another study found that concurrent propofol reduced volume of distribution and distribution clearance of **remifentanil** by 41%. It was concluded that although propofol affects **remifentanil** bolus dose pharmacokinetics, maintenance infusion rates and recovery times would not be significantly affected.[32]

The manufacturer notes that the required induction dose of propofol may be reduced in patients who have received opioids, and that these drugs may increase the anaesthetic and sedative effects of propofol, and also cause greater reductions in blood pressure and cardiac output. They also state that the rate of propofol administration for maintenance of anaesthesia may be reduced in the presence of supplemental analgesics such as opioids.[33]

Two reviews have discussed the use of opioids and propofol in anaesthesia, their pharmacokinetic and pharmacodynamic interactions, and administration and monitoring techniques.[34,35]

(e) Thiopental

Opioid analgesics would be expected to potentiate the respiratory depressant effects of barbiturate anaesthetics. A study has found that the dose of thiopental required to induce anaesthesia was reduced by pretreatment with **fentanyl**.[36] The manufacturer recommends reduced doses of thiopental in patients premedicated with opioids.[37]

1. Dale O. Drug interactions in anaesthesia: focus on desflurane and sevoflurane. *Baillieres Clin Anaesthesiol* (1995) 9, 105–17.
2. Suprane (Desflurane). Baxter Healthcare Corporation. US Prescribing information, November 2005.
3. Albertin A, Casati A, Bergonzi P, Fano G, Torri G. Effects of two target-controlled concentrations (1 and 3 ng/ml) of remifentanil on MAC_{BAR} of sevoflurane. *Anesthesiology* (2004) 100, 255–9.
4. Coltura MJ-J, Van Belle K, Van Hemelrijck JH. Influence of remifentanil (Ultiva, Glaxo Wellcome) and nitrous oxide on sevoflurane (Sevorane, Abbott) requirement during surgery. 2001 Annual Meeting of the American Society of Anesthesiologists, New Orleans USA, 2002. Abstract A-462.
5. Katoh T, Suguro Y, Kimura T, Ikeda K. Morphine does not affect the awakening concentration of sevoflurane. *Can J Anaesth* (1993) 40, 825–8.
6. Hypnomidate (Etomidate). Janssen-Cilag Ltd. UK Summary of product characteristics, February 2004.

7. Bourke DL, Malit LA, Smith TC. Respiratory interactions of ketamine and morphine. *Anesthesiology* (1987) 66, 153–6.
8. Ketalar (Ketamine hydrochloride). Pfizer Ltd. UK Summary of product characteristics, January 2006.
9. Schulte H, Sollevi A, Segerdahl M. The synergistic effect of combined treatment with systemic ketamine and morphine on experimentally induced windup-like pain in humans. *Anesth Analg* (2004) 98, 1574–80.
10. Luginbühl M, Gerber A, Schnider TW, Petersen-Felix S, Arendt-Nielsen L, Curatolo M. Modulation of remifentanil-induced analgesia, hyperalgesia, and tolerance by small-dose ketamine in humans. *Anesth Analg* (2003) 96, 726–32.
11. Wittenstein U, Lyle DJR. Fits after alfentanil and propofol. *Anaesthesia* (1989) 44, 532–3.
12. Laycock GJA. Opisthotonos and propofol: a possible association. *Anaesthesia* (1988) 43, 257.
13. Ries CR, Scoates PJ, Puil E. Opisthotonos following propofol: a nonepileptic perspective and treatment strategy. *Can J Anaesth* (1994) 41, 414–19.
14. Walder B, Tramèr MR, Seeck M. Seizure-like phenomena and propofol. A systematic review. *Neurology* (2002) 58, 1327–32.
15. Vuyk J, Griever GER, Engbers FHM, Burm AGL, Bovill JG, Vletter AA. The interaction between propofol and alfentanil during induction of anesthesia. *Anesthesiology* (1994) 81, A400.
16. Vuyk J. Pharmacokinetic and pharmacodynamic interactions between opioids and propofol. *J Clin Anesth* (1997) 9, 23S–26S.
17. Ihmsen H, Albrecht S, Fechner J, Hering W, Schuttler J. The elimination of alfentanil is decreased by propofol. 2000 Annual Meeting of the American Society of Anesthesiologists, San Francisco USA, 2002. Abstract 531.
18. Mertens MJ, Vuyk J, Olofsen E, Bovill JG, Burm AGL. Propofol alters the pharmacokinetics of alfentanil in healthy male volunteers. *Anesthesiology* (2001) 94, 949–57.
19. Mertens MJ, Olofsen E, Burm AGL, Bovill JG, Vuyk J. Mixed-effects modeling of the influence of alfentanil on propofol pharmacokinetics. *Anesthesiology* (2004) 100, 795–805.
20. Schwilden H, Fechner J, Albrecht S, Hering W, Ihmsen H, Schüttler J. Testing and modelling the interaction of alfentanil and propofol on the EEG. *Eur J Anaesthesiol* (2003) 20, 363–72.
21. Cockshott ID, Briggs LP, Douglas EJ, White M. Pharmacokinetics of propofol in female patients. Studies using single bolus injections. *Br J Anaesth* (1987) 59, 1103–10.
22. Dixon J, Roberts FL, Tackley RM, Lewis GTR, Connell H, Prys-Roberts C. *Br J Anaesth* (1990) 64, 142–7.
23. O'Hare R, Reid J, Breslin D, Hayes A, Mirakhur RK. Propofol–remifentanil interaction: influence on recovery. *Br J Anaesth* (1999) 83, 180P.
24. Drover DR, Litalien C, Wellis V, Shafer SL, Hammer GB. Determination of the pharmacodynamic interaction of propofol and remifentanil during esophagogastroduodenoscopy in children. *Anesthesiology* (2004) 100, 1382–6.
25. Nieuwenhuijs, DJF, Olofsen E, Romberg RR, Sarton E, Ward D, Engbers F, Vuyk J, Mooren R, Teppema LJ, Dahan A. Response surface modeling of remifentanil-propofol interaction on cardiorespiratory control and bispectral index. *Anesthesiology* (2003) 98, 312–22.
26. Fechner J, Hering W, Ihmsen H, Palmaers T, Schüttler J, Albrecht S. Modelling the pharmacodynamic interaction between remifentanil and propofol by EEG-controlled dosing. *Eur J Anaesthesiol* (2003) 20, 373–9.
27. Bouillon TW, Bruhn J, Radulescu L, Andresen C, Shafer TJ, Cohane C, Shafer SL. Pharmacodynamic interaction between propofol and remifentanil regarding hypnosis, tolerance of laryngoscopy, bispectral index and electroencephalographic approximate entropy. *Anesthesiology* (2004) 100, 1353–72.
28. Kern SE, Xie G, White JL, Egan TD. Opioid-hypnotic synergy. *Anesthesiology* (2004) 100, 1373–81.
29. Koitabashi T, Johansen JW, Sebel PS. Remifentanil dose/electroencephalogram bispectral response during combined propofol/regional anesthesia. *Anesth Analg* (2002) 94, 1530–3.
30. Ludbrook GL, Upton RN. Pharmacokinetic drug interaction between propofol and remifentanil? *Anesth Analg* (2003) 97, 924–5.
31. Crankshaw DP, Chan C, Leslie K, Bjorksten AR. Remifentanil concentration during target-controlled infusion of propofol. *Anaesth Intensive Care* (2002) 30, 578–83.
32. Bouillon T, Bruhn J, Radu-Radulescu L, Bertaccini E, Park S, Shafer S. Non-steady state analysis of the pharmacokinetic interaction between propofol and remifentanil. *Anesthesiology* (2002) 97, 1350–62.
33. Diprivan (Propofol). AstraZeneca. US Prescribing information, August 2005.
34. Lichtenbelt B-J, Mertens M, Vuyk J. Strategies to optimise propofol-opioid anaesthesia. *Clin Pharmacokinet* (2004) 43, 577–93.
35. Vuyk J. Clinical interpretation of pharmacokinetic and pharmacodynamic propofol-opioid interactions. *Acta Anaesthesiol Belg* (2001) 52, 445–51.
36. Wang LP, Hermann C, Westrin P. Thiopentone requirements in adults after varying pre-induction doses of fentanyl. *Anaesthesia* (1996) 51, 831–5.
37. Thiopental Injection. Link Pharmaceuticals Ltd. UK Summary of product characteristics, January 2003.

Anaesthetics, general + Parecoxib

Limited evidence suggests parecoxib does not affect the pharmacokinetics or clinical effects of propofol. Parecoxib does not appear to interact with nitrous oxide and isoflurane.

Clinical evidence, mechanism, importance and management

A randomised, placebo-controlled, double-blind, crossover study in 12 healthy subjects found that pretreatment with 40 mg of intravenous parecoxib given one hour before a 2 mg/kg intravenous bolus of **propofol** did not significantly affect the pharmacokinetics of the **propofol**. Moreover, parecoxib did not alter the clinical effects of **propofol** (e.g. the time to loss of consciousness or the speed of awakening).[1] These limited data suggest that no special precautions should be required during concomitant use.

The UK manufacturer of parecoxib says that no formal interaction studies have been done with inhalational anaesthetics, but in surgical studies, where parecoxib was given preoperatively, there was no evidence of pharmacodynamic interactions in patients who had been given **nitrous oxide** and **isoflurane**.[2]

1. Ibrahim A, Park S, Feldman J, Karim A, Kharasch ED. Effects of parecoxib, a parenteral COX-2–specific inhibitor, on the pharmacokinetics and pharmacodynamics of propofol. *Anesthesiology* (2002) 96, 88–95.
2. Dynastat Injection (Parecoxib sodium). Pfizer Ltd. UK Summary of product characteristics, April 2007.

Anaesthetics, general + Phenylephrine, topical

Phenylephrine eye drops given to patients undergoing general anaesthesia caused marked cyanosis and bradycardia in a baby, and hypertension in a woman.

Clinical evidence, mechanism, importance and management

A 3-week-old baby anaesthetised with **halothane** and **nitrous oxide/oxygen** became cyanosed shortly after 2 drops of 10% phenylephrine solution were put into one eye. The heart rate decreased from 160 to 60 bpm, S-T segment and T wave changes were seen, and blood pressure measurements were unobtainable. The baby recovered uneventfully when anaesthesia was stopped and oxygen given. It was suggested that the phenylephrine caused severe peripheral vasoconstriction, cardiac failure and reflex bradycardia.[1] A 54-year-old woman anaesthetised with **isoflurane** developed hypertension (a rise from 125/70 to 200/90 mmHg) shortly after having two drops of 10% phenylephrine put into one eye. The hypertension responded to nasal glyceryl trinitrate (nitroglycerin) and increasing concentrations of isoflurane.[1] The authors of this report consider that general anaesthesia may have contributed to the systemic absorption of the phenylephrine. They suggest that phenylephrine should be given 30 to 60 minutes prior to anaesthesia, and not during anaesthesia. However, if it is necessary, use the lowest concentrations of phenylephrine (2.5%). They also point out that the following are effective mydriatics: single drop combinations of 0.5% cyclopentolate and 2.5% phenylephrine or 0.5% tropicamide and 2.5% phenylephrine.

Phenylephrine is a sympathomimetic, and as such may carry some risk of potentiating arrhythmias if it is used with inhalational anaesthetics such as halothane –see 'Anaesthetics, general + Inotropes and Vasopressors', p.99. However, it is considered that it is much less likely than adrenaline (epinephrine) to have this effect, since it has primarily alpha-agonist activity.[2]

1. Van der Spek AFL, Hantler CB. Phenylephrine eyedrops and anesthesia. *Anesthesiology* (1986) 64, 812–14.
2. Smith NT, Miller RD, Corbascio AN, eds. Sympathomimetic drugs, in Drug Interactions in Anesthesia. Philadelphia: Lea and Febiger; 1981 P. 55–82.

Anaesthetics, general + Phenytoin, Phenobarbital or Rifampicin (Rifampin)

Phenytoin toxicity occurred in a child following halothane anaesthesia. A near fatal hepatic reaction occurred in a woman given rifampicin (rifampin) after halothane anaesthesia, and hepatitis occurred in a patient taking phenobarbital who was given halothane anaesthesia. See also 'Anaesthetics, general + Isoniazid', p.100 and 'Anaesthetics, general; Methoxyflurane + Antibacterials or Barbiturates', p.107.

Clinical evidence

A 10-year-old girl receiving long-term treatment with phenytoin 300 mg daily was found to have phenytoin plasma levels of 25 micrograms/mL before surgery. Three days after anaesthesia with **halothane** her plasma phenytoin levels had risen to 41 micrograms/mL and she had marked signs of phenytoin toxicity.[1]

A woman taking promethazine and phenobarbital 60 mg three times daily died from **halothane** associated hepatitis within 6 days of being given **halothane** for the first time.[2] A nearly fatal shock-producing hepatic reaction occurred in a woman 4 days after having **halothane** anaesthesia immediately followed by a course of rifampicin 600 mg daily and isoniazid 300 mg daily.[3]

Mechanism

It seems possible that the general adverse hepatotoxic effects of halothane can slow the normal rate of phenytoin metabolism. One suggested explanation for the increased adverse effects on the liver is that, just as in *animals*, pre-treatment with phenobarbital and phenytoin increases the rate of drug metabolism and therefore the hepatotoxicity of halogenated hydrocarbons, including carbon tetrachloride and halothane.[4,5] As well as increased metabolism, the halothane-rifampicin interaction might also involve additive hepatotoxicity.

Importance and management

No firm conclusions can be drawn from these isolated cases, but they serve to emphasise the potential hepatotoxicity when halogenated anaesthetics are given to patients taking these drugs. It has been suggested that patients taking enzyme-inducing drugs such as phenobarbital and phenytoin may constitute a high-risk group for liver damage after halogenated anaesthetics.[6] Consider also 'Anaesthetics, general + Isoniazid', p.100 and 'Anaesthetics, general; Methoxyflurane + Antibacterials or Barbiturates', p.107.

1. Karlin JM, Kutt H. Acute diphenylhydantoin intoxication following halothane anesthesia. *J Pediatr* (1970) 76, 941–4.
2. Patial RK, Sarin R, Patial SB. Halothane associated hepatitis and phenobarbitone. *J Assoc Physicians India* (1989) 37, 480.
3. Most JA, Markle GB. A nearly fatal hepatotoxic reaction to rifampin after halothane anesthesia. *Am J Surg* (1974) 127, 593–5.
4. Garner RC, McLean AEM. Increased susceptibility to carbon tetrachloride poisoning in the rat after pretreatment with oral phenobarbitone. *Biochem Pharmacol* (1969) 18, 645–50.
5. Jenner MA, Plummer JL, Cousins MJ. Influence of isoniazid, phenobarbital, phenytoin, pregnenolone 16-α carbonitrile, and β-naphthoflavone on halothane metabolism and hepatotoxicity. *Drug Metab Dispos* (1990) 18, 819–22.
6. Sweetman SC, ed. Martindale: The complete drug reference. 35th ed. London: Pharmaceutical Press; 2007. p. 1608.

Anaesthetics, general + Sparteine sulfate

Patients given thiamylal sodium had a marked increase in cardiac arrhythmias when they were given intravenous sparteine sulfate, but those given thiopental or etomidate did not.

Clinical evidence, mechanism, importance and management

A group of 109 women undergoing dilatation and curettage were premedicated with atropine and fentanyl, and given either 2% **thiamylal sodium** (5 mg/kg), 0.2% **etomidate** (0.3 mg/kg) or 2.5% **thiopental** (4 mg/kg) to induce anaesthesia, which was maintained with **nitrous oxide/oxygen**. During the surgical procedure they were given a slow intravenous injection of sparteine sulfate 100 mg. Fourteen out of 45 patients given **thiamylal sodium** developed cardiac arrhythmias; 10 had bigeminy and 4 had frequent ventricular premature contractions. Only two patients given **etomidate** or **thiopental** developed any cardiac arrhythmias. It is not understood why sparteine should interact with **thiamylal sodium** in this way. Although the arrhythmias were effectively treated with lidocaine, the authors of this report suggest that the concurrent use of sparteine and thiamylal sodium should be avoided.[1]

1. Cheng C-R, Chen S-Y, Wu K-H, Wei T-T. Thiamylal sodium with sparteine sulfate inducing dysrhythmia in anesthetized patients. *Ma Zui Xue Za Zhi* (1989) 27, 297–8.

Anaesthetics, general + SSRIs

One patient had a seizure when she was given methohexital while taking paroxetine. Spontaneous movements have been seen in two patients taking fluoxetine when they were anaesthetised with propofol.

Clinical evidence, mechanism, importance and management

(a) Methohexital

A generalised tonic-clonic seizure occurred in a 42-year-old woman immediately after she was anaesthetised with 120 mg of intravenous methohexital for the last in a series of six electroconvulsive therapies. She had been receiving **paroxetine** 40 mg daily throughout the series.[1] The authors suggest that paroxetine should be given with caution to patients receiving ECT or methohexital anaesthesia.[1] Note that this appears to be an isolated report.

(b) Propofol

Two women in their mid-twenties, who had been taking **fluoxetine** 20 mg daily for 4 to 6 months, had pronounced involuntary upper limb movements lasting 20 to 30 seconds immediately after anaesthetic induction with 180 mg of propofol (2 to 2.5 mg/kg). The movements ceased spontaneously and the rest of the anaesthesia and surgery were uneventful. Neither had any history of epilepsy or movement disorders. It is not clear whether this was an interaction between propofol and **fluoxetine** or just a rare (but previously reported) reaction to propofol.[2]

1. Folkerts H. Spontaneous seizure after concurrent use of methohexital anesthesia for electroconvulsive therapy and paroxetine: a case report. *J Nerv Ment Dis* (1995) 183, 115–16.
2. Armstrong TSH, Martin PD. Propofol, fluoxetine and spontaneous movement. *Anaesthesia* (1997) 52, 809–10.

Anaesthetics, general + Sulfonamides

The anaesthetic effects of thiopental are increased but shortened by sulfafurazole. Phenobarbital appears not to affect the pharmacokinetics of sulfafurazole or sulfisomidine.

Clinical evidence

A study in 48 patients found that intravenous **sulfafurazole** 40 mg/kg reduced the required anaesthetic dosage of **thiopental** by 36%, but the duration of action was shortened.[1] This interaction has also been observed in *animal* experiments.[2] A study in children showed that **phenobarbital** did not affect the pharmacokinetics of **sulfafurazole** or **sulfisomidine**.[3]

Mechanism

It has been suggested that sulfafurazole successfully competes with thiopental for plasma protein binding sites,[4] the result being that more free and active barbiturate molecules remain in circulation to exert their anaesthetic effects and therefore smaller doses are required.

Importance and management

The evidence for an interaction between sulfafurazole and thiopental is limited, but it appears to be strong. Less thiopental than usual may be required to achieve adequate anaesthesia, but since the awakening time is shortened repeated doses may be needed. Phenobarbital does not appear to affect the pharmacokinetics of the sulfonamides.

1. Csögör SI, Kerek SF. Enhancement of thiopentone anaesthesia by sulphafurazole. *Br J Anaesth* (1970) 42, 988–90.
2. Csögör SI, Pálffy B, Feszt G, Papp J. Influence du sulfathiazol sur l'effet narcotique du thiopental et de l'hexobarbital. *Rev Roum Physiol* (1971) 8, 81–5.
3. Krauer B. Vergleichende Untersuchung der Eliminationskinetik zweier Sulfonamide bei Kindern mit und ohne Phenobarbitalmedikation. *Schweiz Med Wochenschr* (1971) 101, 668–71.
4. Csögör SI, Papp J. Competition between sulphonamides and thiopental for the binding sites of plasma proteins. *Arzneimittelforschung* (1970) 20, 1925–7.

Anaesthetics, general and/or Neuromuscular blockers + Theophylline

Cardiac arrhythmias can develop during the concurrent use of halothane and aminophylline but this seems less likely with isoflurane. One report attributes seizures to an interaction between ketamine and aminophylline. Supraventricular tachycardia occurred in a patient taking aminophylline when pancuronium was given. Isolated cases suggest that the effects of pancuronium, but not vecuronium, can be opposed by aminophylline.

Clinical evidence, mechanism, importance and management

(a) Development of arrhythmias

A number of reports describe arrhythmias apparently due to an interaction between **halothane** and theophylline or aminophylline. One describes intraoperative arrhythmias in three out of 45 adult asthmatics who had received preoperative theophylline or aminophylline then **halothane** anaesthesia.[1] Nine other patients developed heart rates exceeding 140 bpm when given aminophylline and **halothane**, whereas tachycardia did not occur in 22 other patients given only **halothane**.[1] There are other reports of individual adult and child patients who developed ventricular tachycardias attributed to this interaction.[2-5] One child had a cardiac arrest.[5] The same interaction has been reported in *animals*.[6,7] One suggested reason for the interaction with **halothane** is that theophylline causes the release of endogenous catecholamines (adrenaline (epinephrine), noradrenaline (norepinephrine)), which are known to sensitise the myocardium (see also 'Anaesthetics, general + Inotropes and Vasopressors', p.99). Another report describes supraventricular tachycardia in a patient taking aminophylline who was anaesthetised with **thiopental** and fentanyl, and then given **pancuronium**. Three minutes later his heart rate rose to 180 bpm and an ECG revealed supraventricular tachycardia.[8] The authors of this report attributed this reaction to an interaction between the **pancuronium** and the aminophylline, because previous surgery with these drugs in the absence of aminophylline had been without incident.[8]

The authors of one of the reports advise the avoidance of concurrent use i.e. to wait approximately 13 hours after the last dose of aminophylline before using **halothane**[2] but another[9] says that: "... my own experience with the liberal use of these drugs has convinced me of the efficacy and wide margin of safety associated with their use in combination." A possibly safer anaesthetic may be **isoflurane**, which in studies with *dogs* has been shown not to cause cardiac arrhythmias in the presence of aminophylline,[10] and is considered to be less arrhythmogenic than halothane.

(b) Development of seizures

Over a period of 9 years, tachycardia and extensor-type seizures were observed in 4 patients taking theophylline or aminophylline, who were initially anaesthetised with **ketamine**, and later with **halothane** or **enflurane**.[11] Based on subsequent study in *mice,* the authors attributed the seizures to an interaction between **ketamine** and theophylline or aminophylline, and they suggest that the combination should perhaps be avoided in some, or antiseizure premedication be given to patients at risk. However, these cases come from one isolated report. Note that, in *mice,* **ketamine** had no effect on aminophylline-induced seizures.[12]

(c) Altered neuromuscular blockade

Marked resistance to the effects of **pancuronium** (but not **vecuronium**) was seen in one patient receiving an aminophylline infusion.[13] Two other patients are reported to have shown a similar resistance but they had also been given hydrocortisone, which could have had a similar effect[14,15] (see also 'Neuromuscular blockers + Corticosteroids', p.121). These appear to be the only reports of such an interaction.

A study in *rabbits* showed that, at therapeutic concentrations of theophylline, the effects of **tubocurarine** were increased,[16] but there do not appear to have been any studies done in humans.

1. Barton MD. Anesthetic problems with aspirin-intolerant patients. *Anesth Analg* (1975) 54, 376–80.
2. Roizen MF, Stevens WC. Multiform ventricular tachycardia due to the interaction of aminophylline and halothane. *Anesth Analg* (1978) 57, 738–41.
3. Naito Y, Arai T, Miyake C. Severe arrhythmias due to the combined use of halothane and aminophylline in an asthmatic patient. *Jpn J Anesthesiol* (1986) 35, 1126–9.
4. Bedger RC, Chang J-L, Larson CE, Bleyaert AL. Increased myocardial irritability with halothane and aminophylline. *Anesth Prog* (1980) 27, 34–6.
5. Richards W, Thompson J, Lewis G, Levy DS, Church JA. Cardiac arrest associated with halothane anesthesia in a patient receiving theophylline. *Ann Allergy* (1988) 61, 83–4
6. Takaori M, Loehning RW. Ventricular arrhythmias induced by aminophylline during halothane anaesthesia in dogs. *Can Anaesth Soc J* (1967) 14, 79–86.
7. Stirt JA, Berger JM, Roe SD, Ricker SM, Sullivan SF. Halothane-induced cardiac arrhythmias following administration of aminophylline in experimental animals. *Anesth Analg* (1981) 60, 517–20.
8. Belani KG, Anderson WW, Buckley JJ. Adverse drug interaction involving pancuronium and aminophylline. *Anesth Analg* (1982) 61, 473–4.
9. Zimmerman BL. Arrhythmogenicity of theophylline and halothane used in combination. *Anesth Analg* (1979) 58, 259–60.
10. Stirt JA, Berger JM, Sullivan SF. Lack of arrhythmogenicity of isoflurane following administration of aminophylline in dogs. *Anesth Analg* (1983) 62, 568–71.
11. Hirshman CA, Krieger W, Littlejohn G, Lee R, Julien R. Ketamine-aminophylline-induced decrease in seizure threshold. *Anesthesiology* (1982) 56, 464–7.
12. Czuczwar SJ, Janusz W, Wamil A, Kleinrok Z. Inhibition of aminophylline-induced convulsions in mice by antiepileptic drugs and other agents. *Eur J Pharmacol* (1987) 144, 309–15.
13. Daller JA, Erstad B, Rosado L, Otto C, Putnam CW. Aminophylline antagonizes the neuromuscular blockade of pancuronium but not vecuronium. *Crit Care Med* (1991) 19, 983–5.
14. Doll DC, Rosenberg H. Antagonism of neuromuscular blockage by theophylline. *Anesth Analg* (1979) 58, 139–40.
15. Azar I, Kumar D, Betcher AM. Resistance to pancuronium in an asthmatic patient treated with aminophylline and steroids. *Can Anaesth Soc J* (1982) 29, 280–2.
16. Fuke N, Martyn J, Kim C, Basta S. Concentration-dependent interaction of theophylline with *d*-tubocurarine. *J Appl Physiol* (1987) 62, 1970–4.

Anaesthetics, general + Topiramate

A placebo-controlled study in healthy subjects found that pretreatment with topiramate 50 mg did not affect the reaction time after sub-anaesthetic doses of ketamine (slow intravenous injection of 120 micrograms/kg followed by 500 micrograms/kg over one hour).[1]

1. Micallef J, Gavaudan G, Burle B, Blin O, Hasbroucq T. A study of a topiramate pre-treatment on the effects induced by a subanaesthetic dose of ketamine on human reaction time. *Neurosci Lett* (2004) 369, 99–103.

Anaesthetics, general + Trichloroethane

Two patients with chronic cardiac toxicity after repeated exposure to trichloroethane had a deterioration in cardiac function following halothane anaesthesia.

Clinical evidence, mechanism, importance and management

Two patients who had been repeatedly exposed to trichloroethane (one during solvent abuse including *Tipp-Ex* typewriter correcting fluid thinner and the other due to industrial exposure including *Genklene* for degreasing steel) showed evidence of chronic cardiac toxicity. In both cases there was circumstantial evidence of cardiac deterioration after routine anaesthesia with **halothane**. Some **solvents** have a close chemical similarity to **inhalational anaesthetic** drugs, particularly the halogenated hydrocarbons, and these related compounds might have a toxic interaction.[1]

1. McLeod AA, Marjot R, Monaghan MJ, Hugh-Jones P, Jackson G. Chronic cardiac toxicity after inhalation of 1,1,1-trichloroethane. *BMJ* (1987) 294, 727–9.

Anaesthetics, general and/or Neuromuscular blockers + Tricyclic and related antidepressants

Tricyclic antidepressants may increase the risk of arrhythmias and hypotension during anaesthesia. Tachyarrhythmias have been seen in patients taking imipramine who were given halothane and pancuronium. Some very limited evidence suggests that amitriptyline may increase the likelihood of enflurane-induced seizure activity. A man taking maprotiline and lithium developed a tonic-clonic seizure when given propofol. Tricyclics may cause an increase in the duration of barbiturate anaesthesia and lower doses of barbiturates may be required.

Clinical evidence, mechanism, importance and management

(a) Development of arrhythmias

Two patients who were taking **nortriptyline** (one also taking fluphenazine) developed prolonged cardiac arrhythmias during general anaesthesia with **halothane**.[1] Two further patients taking **imipramine** developed marked tachyarrhythmias when anaesthetised with **halothane** and given **pancuronium**.[2] This adverse interaction was subsequently clearly demonstrated in *dogs*.[2] The authors concluded on the basis of their studies that:

- **pancuronium** should be given with caution to patients taking any **tricyclic antidepressant** if **halothane** is used;
- **gallamine** probably should be avoided but **tubocurarine** may be an acceptable alternative to **pancuronium**;
- **pancuronium** is probably safe in the presence of a tricyclic if **enflurane** is used.

However, this last conclusion does not agree with that reached by the authors of another report[3], who found that this combination increased the risk of seizures.

Some manufacturers[4] have recommended stopping tricyclics several days before elective surgery where possible. However, the BNF advises that tricyclic antidepressants need not be stopped, but there may be an increased risk of arrhythmias and hypotension (and dangerous interaction with vasopressor drugs–see 'Tricyclic antidepressants + Inotropes and Vasopressors', p.1237). Therefore, the anaesthetist should be informed if they are not stopped.[5]

(b) Development of seizures

1. Enflurane + Tricyclics. Two patients taking **amitriptyline** developed clonic movements of the leg, arm and hand during surgery while anaesthetised with enflurane and **nitrous oxide**. The movements stopped when the enflurane was replaced by **halothane**.[3] A possible reason is that **amitriptyline** can lower the seizure threshold at which enflurane-induced seizure activity occurs. It is suggested that it may be advisable to avoid enflurane in patients needing tricyclic antidepressants, particularly in those who have a history of seizures, or when hyperventilation or high concentrations of enflurane are likely to be used.[3]

2. Propofol + Maprotiline. A man with a bipolar disorder taking maprotiline 200 mg four times daily and lithium carbonate 300 mg daily, underwent anaesthesia during which he received fentanyl, **tubocurarine** and propofol 200 mg. Shortly after the injection of the propofol the patient complained of a burning sensation in his face. He then became rigid, his back and neck extended and his eyes turned upwards. After 15 seconds, rhythmic twitching developed in his eyes, arms and hands. This apparent seizure lasted about 1 minute until suxamethonium (succinylcholine) was given. The patient regained consciousness after several minutes and the surgery was cancelled.[6] It is not known whether the reaction was due to an interaction between propofol and the antidepressants, or due to just one of the drugs, because both propofol[7,8] and maprotiline[9] have been associated with seizures. However, the authors of this report suggest that it would now be prudent to avoid using propofol in patients taking drugs that significantly lower the convulsive threshold. More study of this possible interaction is needed.

(c) Increased duration of anaesthesia

A study in *dogs* found that **imipramine** caused about a 50% increase in the duration of **thiopental**-induced sleep.[10] In an early review of electroconvulsive therapy and anaesthetic considerations, it was noted that tricyclics interact with **barbiturates** resulting in an increased sleep time and duration of anaesthesia, and therefore it was suggested that lower doses of barbiturate anaesthetics such as **thiopental** should be employed during concurrent use.[11] However, in a later review, it was noted that no complications have been attributed to the use of ECT (which is often undertaken using methohexital or possibly propofol) in patients taking tricyclic antidepressants.[12] Apart from the study in *animals,*[10] there seems little published information to suggest that tricyclics interact significantly with barbiturate anaesthetics, but even if there is an interaction, as the dose of barbiturate should be carefully adjusted according to the patient's response any interaction will probably be accounted for by standard anaesthetic procedures. See also 'Tricyclic antidepressants + Barbiturates', p.1231.

1. Plowman PE, Thomas WJW. Tricyclic antidepressants and cardiac dysrhythmias during dental anaesthesia. *Anaesthesia* (1974) 29, 576–8.
2. Edwards RP, Miller RD, Roizen MF, Ham J, Way WL, Lake CR, Roderick L. Cardiac responses to imipramine and pancuronium during anesthesia with halothane or enflurane. *Anesthesiology* (1979) 50, 421–5.
3. Sprague DH, Wolf S. Enflurane seizures in patients taking amitriptyline. *Anesth Analg* (1982) 61, 67–8.
4. Amitriptyline Oral Solution. Rosemont Pharmaceuticals Ltd. UK Summary of product characteristics, March 2007.
5. British National Formulary. 53rd ed. London: The British Medical Association and The Pharmaceutical Press; 2007. p. 654.
6. Orser B, Oxorn D. Propofol, seizure and antidepressants. *Can J Anaesth* (1994) 41, 262.
7. Bevan JC. Propofol-related convulsions. *Can J Anaesth* (1993) 40, 805–9.
8. Committee on Safety of Medicines. Propofol – convulsions, anaphylaxis and delayed recovery from anaesthesia. *Current Problems* (1989) 26.
9. Jabbari B, Bryan GE, Marsh EE, Gunderson CH. Incidence of seizures with tricyclic and tetracyclic antidepressants. *Arch Neurol* (1985) 42, 480–1.
10. Dobkin AB. Potentiation of thiopental anesthesia by derivatives and analogues of phenothiazine. *Anesthesiology* (1960) 21, 292–6.
11. Gaines GY, Rees DI. Electroconvulsive therapy and anesthetic considerations. *Anesth Analg* (1986) 65, 1345–56.
12. Wagner KJ, Möllenberg O, Rentrop M, Werner C, Kochs EF. Guide to anaesthetic selection for electroconvulsive therapy. *CNS Drugs* (2005) 19, 745–58.

Anaesthetics, general; Methoxyflurane + Antibacterials or Barbiturates

The nephrotoxic effects of methoxyflurane appear to be increased by the use of tetracyclines, and possibly some aminoglycoside antibacterials and barbiturates.

Clinical evidence, mechanism, importance and management

Methoxyflurane has been withdrawn in many countries because it is nephrotoxic. This damage can be exacerbated by the concurrent use of other nephrotoxic drugs or possibly by the chronic use of hepatic enzyme-inducing drugs. Five out of 7 patients anaesthetised with methoxyflurane who had been given **tetracycline** before or after surgery showed rises in blood urea nitrogen, and three died. Post-mortem examination showed pathological changes (oxalosis) in the kidneys.[1] Another study identified renal tubular necrosis associated with calcium oxalate crystals in 6 patients who had been anaesthetised with methoxyflurane and given **tetracycline** (4 patients) and **penicillin** with **streptomycin** (2 patients).[2] Other reports support the finding of increased nephrotoxicity with **tetracycline** and methoxyflurane.[3-5] Another study suggested that **penicillin**, **streptomycin** and **chloramphenicol** appear not to increase the renal toxicity of methoxyflurane,[1] but **gentamicin** and **kanamycin** possibly do so.[6] There is also some evidence that **barbiturates** can exacerbate the renal toxicity because they enhance the metabolism of the methoxyflurane and increase the production of nephrotoxic metabolites.[7,8]

The risk of nephrotoxicity with methoxyflurane would therefore appear to be increased by some of these drugs and the concurrent use of **tetracycline** or **nephrotoxic antibiotics** should be avoided. Similarly, methoxyflurane should only be used with great caution, if at all, following the chronic use of hepatic enzyme-inducing drugs.

1. Kuzucu EY. Methoxyflurane, tetracycline, and renal failure. *JAMA* (1970) 211, 1162–4.
2. Dryden GE. Incidence of tubular degeneration with microlithiasis following methoxyflurane compared with other anesthetic agents. *Anesth Analg* (1974) 53, 383–5.
3. Albers DD, Leverett CL, Sandin JH. Renal failure following prostatovesiculectomy related to methoxyflurane anesthesia and tetracycline—complicated by Candida infection. *J Urol (Baltimore)* (1971) 106, 348–50.
4. Proctor EA, Barton FL. Polyuric acute renal failure after methoxyflurane and tetracycline. *BMJ* (1971) 4, 661–2.
5. Stoelting RK, Gibbs PS. Effect of tetracycline therapy on renal function after methoxyflurane anesthesia. *Anesth Analg* (1973) 52, 431–5.
6. Cousins MJ, Mazze RI. Tetracycline, methoxyflurane anaesthesia, and renal dysfunction. *Lancet* (1972) i, 751–2.
7. Churchill D, Yacoub JM, Siu KP, Symes A, Gault MH. Toxic nephropathy after low-dose methoxyflurane anesthesia: drug interaction with secobarbital? *Can Med Assoc J* (1976) 114, 326–33.
8. Cousins MJ, Mazze RI. Methoxyflurane nephrotoxicity: a study of dose response in man. *JAMA* (1973) 225, 1611–16.

Anaesthetics, local + Acetazolamide

The mean procaine half-life in 6 healthy subjects was increased by 66% (from 1.46 to 2.43 minutes) 2 hours after they were given acetazolamide 250 mg orally. This appears to be because the hydrolysis of the procaine is inhibited by the acetazolamide.[1] As the evidence of this interaction is limited to one report, its general significance is unclear.

1. Calvo R, Carlos R, Erill S. Effects of disease and acetazolamide on procaine hydrolysis by red blood cell enzymes. *Clin Pharmacol Ther* (1980) 27, 179–83.

Anaesthetics, local + Alcohol and/or Antirheumatics

Limited evidence suggests that the failure rate of spinal anaesthesia with bupivacaine may be markedly increased in patients who are receiving antirheumatic drugs and/or who drink alcohol.

Clinical evidence, mechanism, importance and management

The observation that regional anaesthetic failures seemed to be particularly high among patients undergoing orthopaedic surgery who were suffering from rheumatic joint diseases, prompted further study of a possible interaction. It was found that the failure rate of low-dose spinal anaesthesia with 0.5% **bupivacaine** (average volume of 2 mL) increased from 5% in the control group (no alcohol or long-term treatment) to 32% to 42% in those who had been taking antirheumatic drugs (**indometacin** or unspecified) for at least 6 months or who drank at least 80 g of ethanol daily, or both. The percentage of those patients who had a reduced response (i.e. an extended latency period and/or a reduced duration of action) also increased from 3% up to 39 to 42%.[1] The reasons are not understood. This appears to be the only report of such an effect.

1. Sprotte G, Weis KH. Drug interaction with local anaesthetics. *Br J Anaesth* (1982) 54, 242P–243P.

Anaesthetics, local + Anaesthetics, local

Mixtures of local anaesthetics are sometimes used to exploit the most useful characteristics of each drug. This normally seems to be safe although it is sometimes claimed that it increases the risk of toxicity. There is a case report of a man who developed toxicity when bupivacaine and mepivacaine were mixed together. Spinal bupivacaine followed by epidural ropivacaine may also interact to produce profound motor blockade. However, the effectiveness of bupivacaine in epidural anaesthesia may be reduced if it is preceded by chloroprocaine.

Clinical evidence and mechanism

(a) Evidence of no interaction

A study designed to assess the possibility of adverse interactions retrospectively studied the records of 10 538 patients over the period 1952 to 1970 who had been given **tetracaine** combined with **chloroprocaine**, **lidocaine**, **mepivacaine**, **prilocaine** or **propoxycaine** for caudal, epidural, or peripheral nerve block. The incidence of systemic toxic reactions was found to be no greater than when used singly and the conclusion was reached that combined use was advantageous and safe.[1] An *animal* study using combinations of **bupivacaine**, **lidocaine** and **chloroprocaine** also found no evidence that the toxicity was greater than if the anaesthetics were used singly.[2]

A study on the use of **chloroprocaine** 3%, **bupivacaine** 0.5% or a mixture of **chloroprocaine** 1.5% with **bupivacaine** 0.375% in obstetric epidural anaesthesia found that time to onset of analgesia, time to maximum analgesia, and effectiveness of analgesia were similar irrespective of the treatment regimen. **Bupivacaine** 0.5% alone had a longer duration of action than **chloroprocaine** or the mixture of anaesthetics.[3] Another study found that **lidocaine** did not affect the pharmacokinetics of **bupivacaine**.[4]

(b) Evidence of reduced analgesia

A study set up to examine the clinical impression that **bupivacaine** given epidurally did not relieve labour pain effectively if preceded by **chloroprocaine** confirmed that this was so. Using an initial 10-mL dose of 2% **chloroprocaine** followed by an 8-mL dose of 0.5% **bupivacaine**, given when pain recurred, the pain relief was less and the block took longer to occur, had a shorter duration of action and had to be augmented more frequently than if only **bupivacaine** was used.[5] This interaction could not be corrected by adjusting the pH of the local anaesthetics.[6]

(c) Evidence of enhanced effect/toxic interaction

There is a single case report of a patient given 0.75% **bupivacaine** and 2% **mepivacaine** who demonstrated lethargy, dysarthria and mild muscle tremor, which the authors of the report correlated with a marked increase in the percentage of unbound (active) **mepivacaine**. They attributed this to its displacement by the **bupivacaine** from protein binding sites.[7] **Bupivacaine** has also been shown *in vitro* to displace **lidocaine** from α_1-acid glycoprotein.[8] Two cases of prolonged, profound motor blockade, with patient-controlled epidural analgesia using 0.1% **ropivacaine** following spinal **bupivacaine** for caesarean section, have been reported. Including these two patients, a total of 11 out of 23 patients given regional anaesthesia with **bupivacaine** had clinical evidence of motor weakness 8 hours after starting **ropivacaine**.[9]

Importance and management

Well studied interactions. The overall picture is that combined use does not normally result in increased toxicity, although there may be some exceptions. For example, until more is known, caution should be exercised when giving epidural ropivacaine postoperatively to patients who have had bupivacaine spinal anaesthesia, as unexpected motor block may occur.[9] Reduced effectiveness might be seen if bupivacaine is preceded by chloroprocaine.

1. Moore DC, Bridenbaugh LD, Bridenbaugh PO, Thompson GE, Tucker GT. Does compounding of local anesthetic agents increase their toxicity in humans? *Anesth Analg* (1972) 51, 579–85.
2. de Jong RH, Bonin JD. Mixtures of local anesthetics are no more toxic than the parent drugs. *Anesthesiology* (1981) 54, 177–81.
3. Cohen SE, Thurlow A. Comparison of a chloroprocaine–bupivacaine mixture with chloroprocaine and bupivacaine used individually for obstetric epidural analgesia. *Anesthesiology* (1979) 51, 288–92.
4. Freysz M, Beal JL, D'Athis P, Mounie J, Wilkening M, Escousse A. Pharmacokinetics of bupivacaine after axillary brachial plexus block. *Int J Clin Pharmacol Ther Toxicol* (1987) 25, 392–5.
5. Hodgkinson R, Husain FJ, Bluhm C. Reduced effectiveness of bupivacaine 0.5% to relieve labor pain after prior injection of chloroprocaine 2%. *Anesthesiology* (1982) 57, A201.
6. Chen B-J, Kwan W-F. pH is not a determinant of 2-chloroprocaine-bupivacaine interaction: a clinical study. *Reg Anesth* (1990) 15 (Suppl 1), 25.
7. Hartrick CT, Raj PP, Dirkes WE, Denson DD. Compounding of bupivacaine and mepivacaine for regional anesthesia. A safe practice? *Reg Anesth* (1984) 9, 94–7.
8. Goolkasian DL, Slaughter RL, Edwards DJ, Lalka D. Displacement of lidocaine from serum α_1-acid glycoprotein binding sites by basic drugs. *Eur J Clin Pharmacol* (1983) 25, 413–17.
9. Buggy DJ, Allsager CM, Coley S. Profound motor blockade with epidural ropivacaine following spinal bupivacaine. *Anaesthesia* (1999) 54, 895–8.

Anaesthetics, local + Antihypertensives

Severe hypotension and bradycardia have been seen in patients taking captopril or verapamil when they were given epidural anaesthesia with bupivacaine. Acute hypotension also occurred in a man taking prazosin when he was given epidural anaesthesia with bupivacaine. Clonidine may increase the duration of caudal block with bupivacaine, although there are reports of reduced plasma levels of lidocaine with concurrent clonidine. Verapamil does not appear to interact with epidural lidocaine.

Clinical evidence

(a) ACE inhibitors

An 86-year-old man who had been receiving **captopril** 25 mg twice daily and bendroflumethiazide 25 mg daily [sic] for hypertension, underwent a transurethral resection of his prostate under spinal anaesthesia using 3 to 3.5 mL of 'heavy' **bupivacaine** 0.5%. At the end of surgery, he was returned to the supine position and suddenly developed a severe sinus bradycardia (35 bpm), his arterial blood pressure fell to 65/35 mmHg and he became unrousable. Treatment with head-down tilt, oxygen and 1.2 mg of atropine produced rapid improvement in cardiovascular and cerebral function. A further hypotensive episode (without bradycardia) occurred approximately one hour later, which responded rapidly to 4 mg of methoxamine.[1]

(b) Alpha blockers

A man taking **prazosin** (5 mg three times daily for hypertension) developed marked hypotension (BP 60/40 mmHg) within 3 to 5 minutes of receiving 100 mg of **bupivacaine** through an L3–4 lumbar epidural catheter.[2] He was unresponsive to intravenous phenylephrine (five 100-microgram boluses) but his blood pressure rose within 3 to 5 minutes of starting an infusion of adrenaline (epinephrine) 0.05 micrograms/kg per minute.

(c) Beta blockers

See 'Anaesthetics, local + Beta blockers', p.110.

(d) Calcium-channel blockers

Four patients taking long-term **verapamil** developed severe hypotension (systolic pressure as low as 60 mmHg) and bradycardia (48 bpm) 30 to 60 minutes after an epidural block with **bupivacaine** 0.5% and adrenaline (epinephrine). This was totally resistant to atropine and ephedrine, and responded only to calcium gluconate or chloride. No such interaction was seen in a similar group of patients when epidural **lidocaine** was used.[3]

Animal experiments have shown that the presence of **verapamil** increases the toxicity of **lidocaine**, and greatly increases the toxicity of **bupivacaine**, and that pretreatment with calcium chloride blocked this effect.[4] Another *animal* study found that **bupivacaine** had a more marked cardiodepressant effect than **lidocaine** when given with either **verapamil** or **diltiazem**.[5] One *animal* study found that **bupivacaine** accentuates the cardiovascular depressant effects of **verapamil**.[6] Other studies in *animals* have found that **diltiazem**,[7-9] **felodipine**,[10] **nifedipine**,[10,11] **nitren-**

dipine,[10] and **verapamil**[7,8,10] increase the toxicity of **bupivacaine**. However, another *animal* study indicated that pretreatment with **nimodipine** or **verapamil** reduced **bupivacaine** cardiotoxicity.[12]

(e) Clonidine

A study in 35 children undergoing ureteroneocystostomy found that the addition of clonidine 1 microgram/kg increased the duration of caudal block with **bupivacaine** 0.125% (with adrenaline (epinephrine) 1:400 000) and reduced the postoperative morphine requirements.[13] A study in *animals* found that clonidine increased the levels of **bupivacaine** and decreased its clearance.[14] However, another study in children found that oral clonidine premedication reduced the plasma levels of **lidocaine** by 25 to 50%.[15] Similar findings are reported in another study in which clonidine was given with epidural **lidocaine**.[16]

Mechanism

Spinal anaesthesia can produce bradycardia and a fall in cardiac output resulting in arterial hypotension, which may be magnified by the action of the antihypertensive drug, and by hypovolaemia. Other factors probably contributed to the development of this interaction in these particular patients.

The reported differences in effects of clonidine on levels of local anaesthetics are not fully understood. An *in vitro* study using liver microsomes found that clonidine at clinical levels is unlikely to affect the metabolism of lidocaine.[17] However, the haemodynamic effects of clonidine may lead to decreased hepatic blood flow and reduced metabolism.[17]

Importance and management

Direct information seems to be limited to the reports cited. Their general relevance is uncertain, but they serve to emphasise the importance of recognising that all antihypertensive drugs interfere in some way with the normal homoeostatic mechanisms that control blood pressure, so that the normal physiological response to hypotension during epidural anaesthesia may be impaired. In this context lidocaine would appear to be preferable to bupivacaine. Intravenous calcium effectively controls the hypotension and bradycardia produced by verapamil toxicity by reversing its calcium-channel blocking effects.[3,18]

Accidental intravenous administration of local anaesthetics during spinal anaesthesia may cause cardiovascular collapse and, on theoretical grounds, the serious cardiac depressant effects could be enhanced in patients taking antihypertensives, especially elderly patients with impaired cardiovascular function.[11] Particular care would seem to be important with any patient given epidural anaesthesia while taking antihypertensives.

1. Williams NE. Profound bradycardia and hypotension following spinal anaesthesia in a patient receiving an ACE inhibitor: an important 'drug' interaction? *Eur J Anaesthesiol* (1999) 16, 796–8.
2. Lydiatt CA, Fee MP, Hill GE. Severe hypotension during epidural anesthesia in a prazosin-treated patient. *Anesth Analg* (1993) 76, 1152–3.
3. Collier C. Verapamil and epidural bupivacaine. *Anaesth Intensive Care* (1984) 13, 101–8.
4. Tallman RD, Rosenblatt RM, Weaver JM, Wang Y. Verapamil increases the toxicity of local anesthetics. *J Clin Pharmacol* (1988) 28, 317–21.
5. Edouard AR, Berdeaux A, Ahmad R, Samii K. Cardiovascular interactions of local anesthetics and calcium entry blockers in conscious dogs. *Reg Anesth* (1991) 16, 95–100.
6. Edouard A, Froidevaux R, Berdeaux A, Ahmad R, Samii K, Noviant Y. Bupivacaine accentuates the cardiovascular depressant effects of verapamil in conscious dogs. *Eur J Anaesthesiol* (1987) 4, 249–59.
7. Bruguerolle B. Effects of calcium channel blockers on bupivacaine-induced toxicity. *Life Sci* (1993) 53, 349–53.
8. Jacob D, Grignon S, Attolini L, Gantenbein M, Bruguerolle B. Effects of calcium antagonists on binding of local anesthetics to plasma proteins and erythrocytes in mice. *Pharmacology* (1996) 53, 219–23.
9. Finegan BA, Whiting RW, Tam YK, Clanachan AS. Enhancement of bupivacaine toxicity by diltiazem in anaesthetised dogs. *Br J Anaesth* (1992) 69, 492–7.
10. Herzig S, Ruhnke L, Wulf H. Functional interaction between local anaesthetics and calcium antagonists in guineapig myocardium: 1. Cardiodepressant effects in isolated organs. *Br J Anaesth* (1994) 73, 357–63.
11. Howie MB, Mortimer W, Candler EM, McSweeney TD, Frolicher DA. Does nifedipine enhance the cardiovascular depressive effects of bupivacaine? *Reg Anesth* (1989) 14, 19–25.
12. Adsan H, Tulunay M, Onaran O. The effects of verapamil and nimodipine on bupivacaine-induced cardiotoxicity in rats: an *in vivo* and *in vitro* study. *Anesth Analg* (1998) 86, 818–24.
13. Tripi PA, Palmer JS, Thomas S, Elder JS. Clonidine increases duration of bupivacaine caudal analgesia for ureteroneocystostomy: a double-blind prospective trial. *J Urol (Baltimore)* (2005) 174, 1081–3.
14. Bruguerolle B, Attolini L, Lorec AM, Gantenbein M. Kinetics of bupivacaine after clonidine pretreatment in mice. *Can J Anaesth* (1995) 42, 434–7.
15. Inomata S, Tanaka E, Miyabe M, Kakiuchi Y, Nagashima A, Yamasaki Y, Nakayama S, Baba Y, Toyooka H, Okuyama K, Kohda Y. Plasma lidocaine concentrations during continuous thoracic epidural anesthesia after clonidine premedication in children. *Anesth Analg* (2001) 93, 1147–51.
16. Mazoit JX, Benhamou D, Veillette Y, Samii K. Clonidine and or adrenaline decrease lignocaine plasma peak concentration after epidural injection. *Br J Clin Pharmacol* (1996) 42, 242–5.
17. Inomata S, Nagashima A, Osaka Y, Tanaka E, Toyooka H. Effects of clonidine on lidocaine metabolism in human or rat liver microsomes. *J Anesth* (2003) 17, 281–3.
18. Coaldrake LA. Verapamil overdose. *Anaesth Intensive Care* (1984) 12, 174–5.

Anaesthetics, local + Azoles or Macrolides

Itraconazole may reduce the clearance of bupivacaine, and itraconazole, ketoconazole or clarithromycin may slightly decrease ropivacaine clearance, but the clinical importance of these interactions appears to be limited.

Clinical evidence, mechanism, importance and management

(a) Bupivacaine

In a double-blind, placebo-controlled, crossover study in 7 healthy subjects pretreatment with **itraconazole** 200 mg once daily for 4 days reduced the clearance of bupivacaine (0.3 mg/kg given intravenously over 60 minutes) by 20 to 25%. The increase in plasma concentrations of bupivacaine should be taken into account when **itraconazole** is used concurrently, although the interaction is probably of limited clinical significance.[1]

(b) Ropivacaine

Pretreatment with **itraconazole** 200 mg daily or **clarithromycin** 250 mg twice daily for 4 days did not significantly affect the pharmacokinetics of ropivacaine 600 microgram/kg given intravenously to 8 healthy subjects. However, there was considerable interindividual variation. A small but insignificant 20% increase in the AUC of ropivacaine occurred, and the peak plasma concentrations of the metabolite 2′,6′-pipecoloxylidide were significantly decreased by **clarithromycin** and **itraconazole**, by 44% and 74%, respectively. Both **itraconazole** and **clarithromycin** inhibit the formation of this metabolite by the cytochrome P450 isoenzyme CYP3A4.[2] Similar results were found with **ketoconazole** and ropivacaine.[3] Potent inhibitors of CYP3A4 appear to cause only a minor decrease in clearance of ropivacaine, which is unlikely to be of clinical relevance.[3] For a report of **erythromycin**, an inhibitor of CYP3A4 enhancing the effect of fluvoxamine, an inhibitor of CYP1A2, on the clearance of ropivacaine, see 'Anaesthetics, local + Fluvoxamine', p.110.

1. Palkama VJ, Neuvonen PJ, Olkkola KT. Effect of itraconazole on the pharmacokinetics of bupivacaine enantiomers in healthy volunteers. *Br J Anaesth* (1999) 83, 659–61.
2. Jokinen MK, Ahonen J, Neuvonen PJ, Olkkola KT. Effect of clarithromycin and itraconazole on the pharmacokinetics of ropivacaine. *Pharmacol Toxicol* (2001) 88, 187–91.
3. Arlander E, Ekström G, Alm C, Carrillo JA, Bielenstein M, Böttiger Y, Bertilsson L, Gustafsson LL. Metabolism of ropivacaine in humans is mediated by CYP1A2 and to a minor extent by CYP3A4: An interaction study with fluvoxamine and ketoconazole as in vivo inhibitors. *Clin Pharmacol Ther* (1998) 64, 484–91.

Anaesthetics, local + Benzodiazepines

Diazepam may increase the maximum plasma concentrations of bupivacaine, but its rate of elimination may also be increased. Midazolam has been reported to cause a modest decrease in lidocaine but not mepivacaine levels. Spinal anaesthesia with bupivacaine, lidocaine, or tetracaine may increase the sedative effects of midazolam. A case of possible lidocaine toxicity has been described when a woman taking sertraline was given flurazepam before intraoperative lidocaine.

Clinical evidence, mechanism, importance and management

(a) Effect of benzodiazepines on local anaesthetics

Twenty-one children aged 2 to 10 years were given single 1-mL/kg caudal injections of a mixture of 0.5% **lidocaine** and 0.125% **bupivacaine** for regional anaesthesia. Pretreatment with **diazepam** 10 mg rectally half-an-hour before the surgery had no significant effect on the plasma levels of **lidocaine**, but the AUC and maximum plasma **bupivacaine** levels were increased by 70 to 75%.[1] In another study, prior use of intravenous **diazepam** in adult patients slightly, but not significantly, increased the mean maximum plasma levels of epidural **bupivacaine** or **etidocaine**. However, the elimination half-lives of both anaesthetics were significantly decreased by about a half.[2]

A study in 20 children aged 2 to 7 years receiving caudal block with 1 mL/kg of a solution containing 0.5% **lidocaine** and 0.125% **bupi-**

vacaine, found that **midazolam** 400 micrograms/kg given rectally half-an-hour before surgery caused a slight but not significant reduction in the AUC and serum levels of **bupivacaine**, whereas the AUC of **lidocaine** was reduced by 24%.[3] In contrast, **midazolam** 400 micrograms/kg given rectally as a premedication was found to have no significant effect on plasma **mepivacaine** levels.[4]

There has been a single report of possible **lidocaine** toxicity following tumescent liposuction in a patient given perioperative sedation with **flurazepam** 30 mg orally. Ten hours after the completion of the procedure, in which a total of 58 mg/kg of lidocaine was used, the patient had nausea and vomiting, unsteady gate, mild confusion, and speech impairment. Her lidocaine level was 6.3 mg/L (levels greater than 6 mg/L were considered to be associated with an increased risk of toxicity). The patient was also on long-term treatment with sertraline. The authors suggested that sertraline and **flurazepam** may have had an additive effect on reducing the rate of **lidocaine** metabolism via inhibition of cytochrome P450 isoenzyme CYP3A4.[5]

The clinical importance of these interactions is uncertain, but anaesthetists should be aware that increased **bupivacaine** plasma levels have been seen with **diazepam**, and reduced **lidocaine** levels have been seen with **midazolam**. More study is needed.

(b) Effect of local anaesthetics on benzodiazepines

Twenty patients undergoing surgery were given repeated 1-mg intravenous doses of **midazolam** as induction anaesthesia every 30 seconds until they failed to respond to three repeated commands to squeeze the anaesthetist's hand. This was considered as the induction end-point 'titrated' dose. It was found that the 10 who had been given prior spinal anaesthesia with **tetracaine** 12 mg needed only half the dose of **midazolam** (7.6 mg) than the 10 other patients who had not received tetracaine (14.7 mg). The reasons are not known. The authors of this report simply advise care in this situation.[6] In another study in which patients were given intravenous **midazolam** following an intramuscular injection of either **bupivacaine**, **lidocaine** or saline, it was found that both anaesthetics enhanced the effect of **midazolam**. This effect was dose-dependent and it was concluded that the use of **lidocaine** or **bupivacaine** for regional blocks or local infiltration could alter the effect of **midazolam** from sedative to hypnotic.[7]

1. Giaufre E, Bruguerolle B, Morisson-Lacombe G, Rousset-Rouviere B. The influence of diazepam on the plasma concentrations of bupivacaine and lignocaine after caudal injection of a mixture of the local anaesthetics in children. *Br J Clin Pharmacol* (1988) 26, 116–18.
2. Giasi RM, D'Agostino E, Covino BG. Interaction of diazepam and epidurally administered local anesthetic agents. *Reg Anesth* (1980) 5, 8–11.
3. Giaufre E, Bruguerolle B, Morrison-Lacombe G, Rousset-Rouviere B. The influence of midazolam on the plasma concentrations of bupivacaine and lidocaine after caudal injection of a mixture of the local anesthetics in children. *Acta Anaesthesiol Scand* (1990) 34, 44–6.
4. Giaufre E, Bruguerolle B, Morisson-Lacombe G, Rousset-Rouviere B. Influence of midazolam on the plasma concentrations of mepivacaine after lumbar epidural injection in children. *Eur J Clin Pharmacol* (1990) 38, 91–2.
5. Klein JA, Kassarjdian N. Lidocaine toxicity with tumescent liposuction: a case report of probable drug interactions. *Dermatol Surg* (1997) 23, 1169–74.
6. Ben-David B, Vaida S, Gaitini L. The influence of high spinal anesthesia on sensitivity to midazolam sedation. *Anesth Analg* (1995) 81, 525–8.
7. Ben-Shlomo I, Tverskoy M, Fleyshman G, Melnick V, Katz Y. Intramuscular administration of lidocaine or bupivacaine alters the effect of midazolam from sedation to hypnosis in a dose-dependent manner. *J Basic Clin Physiol Pharmacol* (2003) 14, 257–63.

Anaesthetics, local + Beta blockers

Propranolol reduces the clearance of bupivacaine and so theoretically the toxicity of bupivacaine may be increased. There has been a single report of enhanced bupivacaine cardiotoxicity in a patient also receiving metoprolol and digoxin. The coronary vasoconstriction caused by cocaine is increased by propranolol. Beta blockers may interact with adrenaline (epinephrine)-containing local anaesthetics.

Clinical evidence, mechanism, importance and management

(a) Bupivacaine

1. Metoprolol. There is a case report of possible enhanced bupivacaine cardiotoxicity in a patient who was taking enalapril 5 mg daily, metoprolol 25 mg twice daily and digoxin 250 micrograms four times a day (serum digoxin level 1.1 nanograms/mL). Cardiac arrest occurred 15 minutes after the injection of 0.5% bupivacaine with adrenaline (epinephrine) for intercostal nerve block (total dose 100 mg). The cardiodepressant effects of metoprolol, digoxin and bupivacaine may have combined to produce toxicity at a dose of bupivacaine not usually considered toxic. The authors caution that patients taking digoxin with a calcium channel blocker and/or beta blocker should be considered at higher risk for bupivacaine cardiotoxicity.[1]

2. Propranolol. The clearance of bupivacaine was reduced by about 35% in 6 healthy subjects given bupivacaine 30 to 50 mg intravenously over 10 to 15 minutes after taking propranolol 40 mg every 6 hours for a day. The reason is thought to be that the propranolol inhibits the activity of the liver microsomal enzymes, thereby reducing the metabolism of the bupivacaine. Changes in blood flow to the liver are unlikely to affect bupivacaine metabolism substantially because it is relatively poorly extracted from the blood. The clinical importance of this interaction is uncertain, but it is suggested that an increase in local anaesthetic toxicity might occur and caution should be exercised if multiple doses of bupivacaine are given.[2]

(b) Cocaine

A study in 30 patients being evaluated for chest pain found that 2 mg/kg of a 10% intranasal solution of cocaine reduced coronary sinus flow by about 14% and coronary artery diameter by 6 to 9%. The coronary vascular resistance increased by 22%. The addition of propranolol 400 micrograms/minute by intracoronary infusion, (to a total of 2 mg) reduced coronary sinus flow by a further 15% and increased the coronary vascular resistance by 17%. The probable reason is that the cocaine stimulates the alpha-receptors of the coronary blood vessels causing vasoconstriction. When the beta-receptors are blocked by propranolol, the resultant unopposed alpha-adrenergic stimulation may lead to enhanced coronary vasoconstriction (see also 'Beta blockers + Inotropes and Vasopressors', p.848). The clinical importance of these findings is uncertain but the authors of the report suggest that beta blockers should be avoided in patients with myocardial ischaemia or infarction associated with the use of cocaine.[3]

(c) Local anaesthetics with vasoconstrictors

In a double-blind, randomised, placebo-controlled, crossover study in 10 healthy subjects, the upper lateral incisor teeth were anaesthetised using lidocaine with or without adrenaline (epinephrine). The mean duration of anaesthesia using 1 mL of 2% lidocaine containing 1:100 000 adrenaline was increased by 58% (17 minutes) for pulpal anaesthesia and 19% (16.5 minutes) for soft-tissue anaesthesia in subjects pretreated with **nadolol** 80 mg orally. Pretreatment with the beta blocker did not affect the duration of anaesthesia when lidocaine without adrenaline was used.[4] It is likely that the combined effects of adrenaline and **nadolol** caused increased local vasoconstriction, which resulted in the lidocaine persisting for longer. Therefore when a small amount of local anaesthetic with adrenaline is injected for dental procedures an increased duration of analgesia may result. Also note that a case report describes a transient hypertensive reaction in a patient taking **propranolol** when injections of 2% mepivacaine with 1:20 000 corbadrine were given for dental anaesthesia.[5] Larger doses of adrenaline have resulted in serious hypertension and bradycardia because of the interaction between non-selective beta blockers and adrenaline (see 'Beta blockers + Inotropes and Vasopressors', p.848). It has been suggested that, for dental procedures, the minimum amount of local anaesthetic containing the lowest concentration of adrenaline should be used. Alternatively, if excessive bleeding is unlikely, a local anaesthetic without adrenaline is preferred.[4]

Propranolol and some other beta blockers are known to reduce the metabolism of lidocaine—see 'Lidocaine + Beta blockers', p.263.

1. Roitman K, Sprung J, Wallace M, Matjasko J. Enhancement of bupivacaine cardiotoxicity with cardiac glycosides and β-adrenergic blockers: a case report. *Anesth Analg* (1993) 76, 658–61.
2. Bowdle TA, Freund PR, Slattery JT. Propranolol reduces bupivacaine clearance. *Anesthesiology* (1987) 66, 36–8.
3. Lange RA, Cigarroa RG, Flores ED, McBride W, Kim AS, Wells PJ, Bedotto JB, Danziger RS, Hillis LD. Potentiation of cocaine-induced coronary vasoconstriction by beta-adrenergic blockade. *Ann Intern Med* (1990) 112, 897–903.
4. Zhang C, Banting DW, Gelb AW, Hamilton JT. Effect of β-adrenoreceptor blockade with nadolol on the duration of local anesthesia. *J Am Dent Assoc* (1999) 130, 1773–80.
5. Mito RS, Yagiela JA. Hypertensive response to levonordefrin in a patient receiving propranolol: report of a case. *J Am Dent Assoc* (1988) 116, 55–7.

Anaesthetics, local + Fluvoxamine

Fluvoxamine inhibits the clearance of ropivacaine; therefore, prolonged administration of ropivacaine should be avoided in patients taking fluvoxamine.

Clinical evidence, mechanism, importance and management

Fluvoxamine decreased the mean total plasma clearance of **ropivacaine** by 68% from 354 to 112 mL/minute, and almost doubled the half-life of **ropivacaine** in a randomised, crossover study in 12 healthy subjects. Fluvoxamine was given at a dose of 25 mg twice daily for 2 days, and a single 40 mg intravenous dose of **ropivacaine** was given over 20 minutes one hour after the morning dose of fluvoxamine on the second day.[1]

Fluvoxamine is a potent inhibitor of the cytochrome P450 isoenzyme CYP1A2 and so reduces the metabolism of **ropivacaine** to its major metabolite 3-hydroxyropivacaine. In one study in healthy subjects the combination of fluvoxamine with **erythromycin**, an inhibitor of CYP3A4, which on its own has little effect on the pharmacokinetics of **ropivacaine**, was found to decrease the clearance of **ropivacaine** more than fluvoxamine alone.[2]

The UK manufacturer recommends that prolonged administration of **ropivacaine** should be avoided in patients concurrently treated with potent CYP1A2 inhibitors such as fluvoxamine.[3] Be aware that CYP3A4 inhibitors such as erythromycin in combination with CYP1A2 inhibitors may further reduce **ropivacaine** clearance.[2]

1. Arlander E, Ekström G, Alm C, Carrillo JA, Bielenstein M, Böttiger Y, Bertilsson L, Gustafsson LL. Metabolism of ropivacaine in humans is mediated by CYP1A2 and to a minor extent by CYP3A4: An interaction study with fluvoxamine and ketoconazole as in vivo inhibitors. *Clin Pharmacol Ther* (1998) 64, 484–91.
2. Jokinen MJ, Ahonen J, Neuvonen PJ, Olkkola KT. The effect of erythromycin, fluvoxamine, and their combination on the pharmacokinetics of ropivacaine. *Anesth Analg* (2000) 91, 1207–12.
3. Naropin (Ropivacaine). AstraZeneca UK Ltd. UK Summary of product characteristics, March 2007.

Anaesthetics, local + H_2-receptor antagonists

Some studies suggest that both cimetidine and ranitidine can raise plasma bupivacaine levels, whereas other evidence suggests that no significant interaction occurs. Ranitidine does not appear to significantly affect lidocaine. Some studies found that cimetidine does not affect lidocaine when used as an anaesthetic. Other studies found that cimetidine increased plasma lidocaine levels and that famotidine had less effect. See also 'Lidocaine + H_2-receptor antagonists', p.264 for interactions of lidocaine used as an antiarrhythmic.

Clinical evidence

(a) Cimetidine + Bupivacaine

Pretreatment with cimetidine 300 mg intramuscularly 1 to 4 hours before epidural anaesthesia with 0.5% bupivacaine (for caesarean section) had no effect on the pharmacokinetics of bupivacaine in 16 women or their foetuses when compared with 20 control women, although the maternal unbound bupivacaine plasma levels rose by 22%.[1] These findings were confirmed in two similar studies[2,3] in which women were pretreated with cimetidine before caesarean section, and a further study[4] in 7 healthy subjects (6 women and one man) given two oral doses of cimetidine 400 mg before intramuscular bupivacaine. However, the AUC of bupivacaine in 4 healthy male subjects was increased by 40% (when compared to placebo) by cimetidine 400 mg at 10 pm the previous evening and 8 am on the study day, followed by a 50-mg infusion of bupivacaine at 11 am.[5]

(b) Cimetidine + Lidocaine

In 5 women given epidural anaesthesia for caesarean section, the pharmacokinetics of 400 mg of lidocaine 2% (administered with adrenaline (epinephrine) 1:200 000) were unchanged by a single 400-mg oral dose of cimetidine given about 2 hours preoperatively.[6] Another very similar study in 9 women found no statistically significant rises in whole blood lidocaine levels (although they tended to be higher), in the presence of cimetidine 300 mg, given intramuscularly, at least an hour preoperatively.[7] However, in patients pretreated with cimetidine (200 mg orally on the night before surgery and 400 mg one hour before induction) peak plasma levels of epidural lidocaine 2% (with adrenaline 1:200 000) were 3.2 micrograms/mL. Lidocaine levels in patients who did not receive pretreatment with H_2-receptor antagonists were 2.3 micrograms/mL.[8]

(c) Famotidine + Lidocaine

In patients pretreated with famotidine (20 mg orally on the night before surgery plus 20 mg intramuscularly one hour before induction) peak plasma levels of epidural lidocaine 2% (with adrenaline 1:200 000) were 2.4 micrograms/mL. Lidocaine levels in patients who did not receive pretreatment with H_2-receptor antagonists were 2.3 micrograms/mL.[8] In another study the effects of famotidine on lidocaine were found to be less than those of cimetidine but greater than in patients not given an H_2-receptor antagonist.[9]

(d) Ranitidine + Bupivacaine

Pretreatment with oral ranitidine 150 mg 1.5 to 2 hours before bupivacaine for extradural anaesthesia for caesarean section, increased the maximum plasma levels of bupivacaine in 10 patients by about 36%, when compared with 10 patients given no pretreatment.[3] Another study found that two oral doses of ranitidine 150 mg caused a 25% increase in the mean AUC of bupivacaine, but this was not statistically significant.[5] No increased bupivacaine toxicity was described in any of these reports. However, two other studies in 36 and 28 women undergoing caesarean section found no measurable effect on the bupivacaine disposition when given ranitidine 150 mg the night before and on the morning of anaesthesia,[2] or ranitidine 50 mg intramuscularly 2 hours before anaesthesia, respectively.[10]

(e) Ranitidine + Lidocaine

In 7 women given epidural anaesthesia for caesarean section the pharmacokinetics of 400 mg of lidocaine 2%, (given with adrenaline (epinephrine) 1:200 000) were unchanged after a single 150-mg oral dose of ranitidine given about 2 hours preoperatively.[6] A similar study in 8 women also found no statistically significant rises in whole blood lidocaine levels in the presence of ranitidine 150 mg given orally at least 2 hours preoperatively.[7]

Mechanism

Not understood. It has been suggested that cimetidine reduces the hepatic metabolism of bupivacaine. Protein binding displacement has also been suggested.

Importance and management

A confusing situation. No clinically important interaction has been established, but be alert for any evidence of increased bupivacaine toxicity resulting from raised total plasma levels and rises in unbound bupivacaine levels during the concurrent use of cimetidine and possibly ranitidine. Cimetidine (but not ranitidine) has been shown to raise plasma lidocaine levels when lidocaine is used as an antiarrhythmic (see 'Lidocaine + H_2-receptor antagonists', p.264), but some of the studies cited above found cimetidine did not affect lidocaine levels when lidocaine is used as an anaesthetic. However, in the studies comparing the effects of cimetidine and famotidine, cimetidine was found to increase lidocaine levels and it was suggested that famotidine may be preferable to cimetidine as pretreatment before epidural lidocaine.[8,9]

1. Kuhnert BR, Zuspan KJ, Kuhnert PM, Syracuse CD, Brashear WT, Brown DE. Lack of influence of cimetidine on bupivacaine levels during parturition. *Anesth Analg* (1987) 66, 986–90.
2. O'Sullivan GM, Smith M, Morgan B, Brighouse D, Reynolds F. H_2 antagonists and bupivacaine clearance. *Anaesthesia* (1988) 43, 93–5.
3. Flynn RJ, Moore J, Collier PS, McClean E. Does pretreatment with cimetidine and ranitidine affect the disposition of bupivacaine? *Br J Anaesth* (1989) 62, 87–91.
4. Pihlajamäki KK, Lindberg RLP, Jantunen ME. Lack of effect of cimetidine on the pharmacokinetics of bupivacaine in healthy subjects. *Br J Clin Pharmacol* (1988) 26, 403–6.
5. Noble DW, Smith KJ, Dundas CR. Effects of H-2 antagonists on the elimination of bupivacaine. *Br J Anaesth* (1987) 59, 735–7.
6. Flynn RJ, Moore J, Collier PS, Howard PJ. Single dose oral H_2-antagonists do not affect plasma lidocaine levels in the parturient. *Acta Anaesthesiol Scand* (1989) 33, 593–6.
7. Dailey PA, Hughes SC, Rosen MA, Healey K, Cheek DBC, Shnider SM. Effect of cimetidine and ranitidine on lidocaine concentrations during epidural anesthesia for cesarean section. *Anesthesiology* (1988) 69, 1013–17.
8. Kishikawa K, Namiki A, Miyashita K, Saitoh K. Effects of famotidine and cimetidine on plasma levels of epidurally administered lignocaine. *Anaesthesia* (1990) 45, 719–21.
9. Sabatakaki A, Daifotis Z, Karayannacos P, Danou K, Kaniaris P. La famotidine ne modifie pas les taux plasmatiques de la lidocaïne pour rachianesthésie. Étude comparative de la famotidine et de la cimétidine. *Cah Anesthesiol* (1992) 40, 317–20.
10. Brashear WT, Zuspan KJ, Lazebnik N, Kuhnert BR, Mann LI. Effect of ranitidine on bupivacaine disposition. *Anesth Analg* (1991) 72, 369–76.

Anaesthetics, local + Ondansetron

In a placebo-controlled study oral ondansetron 4 mg was given to patients the evening before surgery, followed by intravenous ondansetron 4 mg given over 15 minutes before subarachnoid anaesthesia with lidocaine 5% in dextrose 8%. Ondansetron

significantly reduced the sensory block measured at 30 minutes. In this study 54 patients were enrolled, but not all patients were assessed for both motor and sensory block.[1]

1. Fassoulaki A, Melemeni A, Zotou M, Sarantopoulos C. Systemic ondansetron antagonizes the sensory block produced by intrathecal lidocaine. *Anesth Analg* (2005) 100, 1817–21.

Anaesthetics, local + Quinolones

Ciprofloxacin may decrease the clearance of ropivacaine and this could be significant in some patients. It is also likely that enoxacin will inhibit the metabolism of ropivacaine. Therefore prolonged administration of ropivacaine should be avoided in patients taking enoxacin.

Clinical evidence, mechanism, importance and management

A study in 9 healthy subjects found that **ciprofloxacin** 500 mg twice daily decreased the mean clearance of a single 0.6-mg/kg intravenous dose of **ropivacaine**, by 31%, but there was considerable inter-individual variation. **Ciprofloxacin** modestly decreases the clearance of **ropivacaine** by inhibiting the cytochrome P450 isoenzyme CYP1A2-mediated metabolism of **ropivacaine** to its major metabolite **3-hydroxyropivacaine**. For some patients concurrent use may cause toxicity.[1] On the basis of data with 'fluvoxamine', (p.110), the UK manufacturer of **ropivacaine** has recommended that prolonged administration of ropivacaine should be avoided in patients taking strong CYP1A2 inhibitors such as **enoxacin**.[2]

1. Jokinen MJ, Olkkola KT, Ahonen J, Neuvonen PJ. Effect of ciprofloxacin on the pharmacokinetics of ropivacaine. *Eur J Clin Pharmacol* (2003) 58, 653–7.
2. Naropin (Ropivacaine). AstraZeneca UK Ltd. UK Summary of product characteristics, March 2007.

Anaesthetics, local + Rifampicin (Rifampin) and/or Tobacco

Rifampicin increases the metabolism of ropivacaine, but this probably has little clinical relevance to its use as a local anaesthetic. Smoking appears to have only a minor effect on ropivacaine pharmacokinetics. Tobacco smoking may enhance cocaine-associated myocardial ischaemia.

Clinical evidence, mechanism, importance and management

(a) Cocaine

In a study involving 42 smokers (36 with proven coronary artery disease) the mean product of the heart rate and systolic arterial pressure increased by 11% after intranasal cocaine 2 mg/kg, by 12% after one cigarette and by 45% after both cocaine use and one cigarette. Compared with baseline measurements, the diameters of non-diseased coronary arterial segments decreased on average by 7% after cocaine use, 7% after smoking and 6% after cocaine and smoking. However, the diameters of diseased segments decreased by 9%, 5% and 19%, respectively.[1] Cigarette smoking increases myocardial oxygen demand and induces coronary-artery vasoconstriction through an alpha-adrenergic mechanism similar to cocaine and therefore tobacco smoking may enhance cocaine-associated myocardial ischaemia.[1,2]

(b) Ropivacaine

A study in 10 healthy non-smokers and 8 healthy smokers given ropivacaine 600 micrograms/kg by intravenous infusion over 30 minutes found that smoking increased the urinary excretion of the metabolite 3-hydroxyropivacaine and decreased the urinary excretion of 2′,6′-pipecoloxylidide by 62%, but did not significantly affect the ropivacaine AUC. However, pretreatment with rifampicin 600 mg daily for 5 days increased the clearance (by 93% and 46%) and decreased the AUC by 52% and 38% and half-life of ropivacaine in both non-smokers and smokers, respectively.[3] Ropivacaine undergoes oxidative hepatic metabolism mainly by the cytochrome P450 isoenzymes CYP1A2 and CYP3A4. Cigarette smoking may increase CYP1A2-mediated metabolism of ropivacaine, and the elimination of ropivacaine may be considerably accelerated by rifampicin, which is a potent cytochrome P450 enzyme inducer. However, in clinical use the local anaesthetic is given near the nerves to be desensitised and induction of isoenzymes is not likely to affect the local anaesthetic before it enters the systemic blood circulation.[3] This interaction is therefore of little clinical relevance.

Rifampicin may also increase the metabolism of lidocaine to a minor extent, see 'Lidocaine + Rifampicin (Rifampin)', p.267, and smoking may reduce the *oral* bioavailability of 'lidocaine', (p.267).

1. Moliterno DJ, Willard JE, Lange RA, Negus BH, Boehrer JD, Glamann DB, Landau C, Rossen JD, Winniford MD, Hillis LD. Coronary-artery vasoconstriction induced by cocaine, cigarette smoking, or both. *N Engl J Med* (1994) 330, 454–9.
2. Hollander JE. The management of cocaine-associated myocardial ischemia. *N Engl J Med* (1995) 333, 1267–72.
3. Jokinen MJ, Olkkola KT, Ahonen J, Neuvonen PJ. Effect of rifampin and tobacco smoking on the pharmacokinetics of ropivacaine. *Clin Pharmacol Ther* (2001) 70, 344–50.

Anaesthetics, local; Cocaine + Adrenaline (Epinephrine)

Arrhythmias occurred in 3 patients given a concentrated nasal paste containing cocaine and adrenaline (epinephrine).

Clinical evidence, mechanism, importance and management

Two children and one adult patient undergoing general anaesthesia[1] developed arrhythmias shortly after nasal application of a paste containing cocaine 25% and adrenaline (epinephrine) 0.18%. All 3 patients received doses of cocaine that exceeded the maximum dose (1.5 mg/kg) currently recommended in the BNF[2] for healthy adults.

Cocaine has sympathomimetic actions (tachycardia, peripheral vasoconstriction, and hypertension). Combined use with sympathomimetics such as adrenaline increases these effects, and the risk of life-threatening arrhythmias. This risk may be further increased if halothane anaesthesia is used (two of the above patients received halothane[1]). See also 'Anaesthetics, general + Anaesthetics, local', p.92 and 'Anaesthetics, general + Inotropes and Vasopressors', p.99.

The use of adrenaline with topical cocaine is controversial. Some consider that the addition of adrenaline is of doubtful value and that the combination should not be used, especially in the form of a concentrated paste.[1] However, others consider the combination to be safe and useful.[3] Whether or not adrenaline is combined with cocaine, the BNF considers that topical cocaine should be used only by those skilled in the precautions needed to minimise absorption and the consequent risk of arrhythmias.[2]

Note also that the use of local anaesthetics containing adrenaline should be avoided in patients who abuse cocaine, unless it is certain that they have not used cocaine for at least 24 hours.[4]

1. Nicholson KEA, Rogers JEG. Cocaine and adrenaline paste: a fatal combination? *BMJ* (1995) 311, 250–1.
2. British National Formulary. 53rd ed. London: The British Medical Association and The Pharmaceutical Press; 2007. p. 673.
3. De R, Uppal HS, Shehab ZP, Hilger AW, Wilson PS, Courteney-Harris R. Current practices of cocaine administration by UK otorhinolaryngologists. *J Laryngol Otol* (2003) 117, 109–12.
4. Goulet J-P, Pérusse R, Turcotte J-Y. Contraindications to vasoconstrictors in dentistry: part III. *Oral Surg Oral Med Oral Pathol* (1992) 74, 692–7.

Botulinum toxin + Miscellaneous

Theoretically, the neuromuscular blocking effects of botulinum toxin can be increased by other drugs with neuromuscular blocking effects, such as the aminoglycosides and muscle relaxants, but no such interactions have been reported.

Clinical evidence, mechanism, importance and management

A case report describes a 5-month-old baby boy who was admitted to hospital because of lethargy, poor feeding, constipation and muscle weakness (later identified as being due to a *Clostridium botulinum* infection). An hour after starting intravenous treatment with ampicillin and **gentamicin** 7.5 mg/kg daily in divided doses every 8 hours for presumed sepsis, he stopped breathing and died. The reason appeared to be the additive neuromuscular blocking effects of the systemic botulinum toxin produced by the *Clostridium botulinum* infection and the **gentamicin**.[1] *Animal* studies confirm that **gentamicin** and **tobramycin** potentiate the neuromuscular blocking effects of systemic botulinum toxin (used to mimic botulism),[1] and there is every reason to believe that any of the other drugs known to cause neuromuscular blockade (**aminoglycosides**, conventional **neuromuscular blockers**, etc.) will behave similarly. However, note that clinically, botulinum A toxin is injected for local effect in specific muscles, and is not used systemically; and so the situation is not analogous to that described in the case of the child with systemic botulism.

Up until 2002, the UK manufacturers of botulinum A toxin stated in their prescribing information that the **aminoglycosides** and **spectinomycin** were contraindicated. They also advised caution with **polymyxins, tetracyclines** and **lincomycin**, and a reduced starting dose with **muscle relaxants** with a long-lasting effect, or the use of an intermediate action drug such as vecuronium or atracurium.[2] Later prescribing information notes that these interactions are theoretical.[3] Similarly the UK manufacturer of botulinum B cautions use with aminoglycosides or other drugs that affect neuromuscular transmission.[4]

1. Santos JI, Swensen P, Glasgow LA. Potentiation of *Clostridium botulinum* toxin by aminoglycoside antibiotics: clinical and laboratory observations. *Pediatrics* (1981) 68, 50–4.
2. Botox (Botulinum A toxin). Allergan Ltd. UK Summary of product characteristics, December 2002.
3. Botox (Botulinum A toxin). Allergan Ltd. UK Summary of product characteristics, June 2007.
4. Neurobloc (Botulinum B toxin). Elan Pharma Ltd. UK Summary of product characteristics, July 2003.

Neuromuscular blockers + Aminoglycosides

The aminoglycoside antibacterials possess neuromuscular blocking activity. Appropriate measures should be taken to accommodate the increased neuromuscular blockade and the prolonged and potentially fatal respiratory depression that can occur if these antibacterials are used with conventional neuromuscular blocking drugs.

Clinical evidence

Two examples from many:

A 38-year-old patient anaesthetised with cyclopropane experienced severe respiratory depression after being given intraperitoneal **neomycin** 500 mg. She had also received **suxamethonium (succinylcholine)** and **tubocurarine**. This antibacterial-induced neuromuscular blockade was resistant to treatment with edrophonium.[1]

A 71-year-old woman received a standard bowel preparation consisting of oral erythromycin and **neomycin** (a total of 3 g). Surgery was postponed for one day and she received a second similar bowel preparation pre-operatively. Anaesthesia was induced with sufentanil and etomidate and maintained with isoflurane and sufentanil. **Rocuronium** (total dose of 60 mg over 2 hours) was used to facilitate tracheal intubation and maintain muscle relaxation. Despite clinical appearance of a reversal of the neuromuscular blockade by neostigmine 3.5 mg and glycopyrrolate 400 micrograms, the patient complained of dyspnoea and required reintubation twice. The effects of additional doses of neostigmine were inconsistent and the use edrophonium 50 mg or calcium chloride 500 mg intravenously did not result in an improvement.[2]

Many other reports confirm that some degree of respiratory depression or paralysis can occur if aminoglycosides are given to anaesthetised patients. When a conventional neuromuscular blocker is also used, the blockade is deepened and recovery prolonged. If the antibacterial is given towards the end of surgery the result can be that a patient who is recovering normally from neuromuscular blockade suddenly develops serious apnoea which can lead on to prolonged and in some cases fatal respiratory depression. A review of the literature[3] lists more than 100 cases over the period 1956 to 1970 involving:

- **tubocurarine** with **neomycin** or **streptomycin,**
- **gallamine** with **neomycin, kanamycin** or **streptomycin**,
- **suxamethonium** with **neomycin**, **kanamycin** or **streptomycin**.

The routes of antibacterial administration were oral, intraperitoneal, oesophageal, intraluminal, retroperitoneal, intramuscular, intrapleural, cystic, beneath skin flaps, extradural and intravenous. Later reports involve:

- **pancuronium**; with **amikacin,**[4] **gentamicin,**[5] **neomycin,**[6] or **streptomycin,**[7,8]
- **pipecuronium** with **netilmicin,**[9]
- **suxamethonium** with **dibekacin,**[10]
- **tubocurarine**; with **amikacin,**[11] **dibekacin,**[10,12] **framycetin** (eye irrigation),[13] **ribostamycin,**[10,12] or **tobramycin,**[14]
- **vecuronium**; with **amikacin/polymyxin,**[15] **gentamicin,**[16-18] **gentamicin/clindamycin,**[19] or **tobramycin.**[17,20]

Aminoglycosides and neuromuscular blockers that have been reported not to interact are:

- **tobramycin** with **alcuronium,**[21] **atracurium**[17] or **suxamethonium,**[10]
- **gentamicin** with **atracurium,**[17]
- **ribostamycin** with **suxamethonium.**[10]

Mechanism

The aminoglycosides appear to reduce or prevent the release of acetylcholine at neuromuscular junctions (related to an impairment of calcium influx) and they may also lower the sensitivity of the post-synaptic membrane, thereby reducing transmission. These effects would be additive with those of conventional neuromuscular blockers, which act at the post-synaptic membrane.

Importance and management

Extremely well documented, very long established, clinically important and potentially serious interactions. Ten out of the 111 cases in one review[3] were fatal, related directly or indirectly to aminoglycoside-induced respiratory depression. Concurrent use need not be avoided, but be alert for increased and prolonged neuromuscular blockade with every aminoglycoside and neuromuscular blocker although the potencies of the aminoglycosides differ to some extent. In *animal* studies at concentrations representing the maximum therapeutic levels, the neuromuscular blocking potency of various aminoglycosides was rated (from highest to lowest) neomycin, streptomycin, gentamicin, kanamycin.[22] The postoperative recovery period should also be closely monitored because of the risk of recurarisation if the aminoglycoside is given during surgery. High-risk patients appear to be those with renal disease and hypocalcaemia, who may have elevated serum antibacterial levels, and those with pre-existing muscular weakness. Treatment of the increased blockade with anticholinesterases and calcium has met with variable success because the response seems to be inconsistent.

1. LaPorte J, Mignault G, L'Allier R, Perron P. Un cas d'apnée à la néomycine. *Union Med Can* (1959) 88, 149–52.
2. Hasfurther DL, Bailey PL. Failure of neuromuscular blockade reversal after rocuronium in a patient who received oral neomycin. *Can J Anaesth* (1996) 43, 617–20.
3. Pittinger CB, Eryasa Y, Adamson R. Antibiotic-induced paralysis. *Anesth Analg* (1970) 49, 487–501.
4. Monsegur JC, Vidal MM, Beltrán J, Felipe MAN. Parálisis neuromuscular prolongada tras administración simultánea de amikacina y pancuronio. *Rev Esp Anestesiol Reanim* (1984) 31, 30–3.
5. Regan AG, Perumbetti PPV. Pancuronium and gentamicin interaction in patients with renal failure. *Anesth Analg* (1980) 59, 393.
6. Giala M, Sareyiannis C, Cortsaris N, Paradelis A, Lappas DG. Possible interaction of pancuronium and tubocurarine with oral neomycin. *Anaesthesia* (1982) 37, 776.
7. Giala MM, Paradelis AG. Two cases of prolonged respiratory depression due to interaction of pancuronium with colistin and streptomycin. *J Antimicrob Chemother* (1979) 5, 234–5.
8. Torresi S, Pasotti EM. Su un caso di curarizzazione prolungata da interazione tra pancuronio e streptomicina. *Minerva Anestesiol* (1984) 50, 143–5.
9. Stanley JC, Mirakhur RK, Clarke RSJ. Study of pipecuronium-antibiotic interaction. *Anesthesiology* (1990) 73, A898.
10. Arai T, Hashimoto Y, Shima T, Matsukawa S, Iwatsuki K. Neuromuscular blocking properties of tobramycin, dibekacin and ribostamycin in man. *Jpn J Antibiot* (1977) 30, 281–4.
11. Singh YN, Marshall IG, Harvey AL. Some effects of the aminoglycoside antibiotic amikacin on neuromuscular and autonomic transmission. *Br J Anaesth* (1978) 50, 109–17.
12. Hashimoto Y, Shima T, Matsukawa S, Iwatsuki K. Neuromuscular blocking properties of some antibiotics in man. *Tohoku J Exp Med* (1975) 117, 339–400.
13. Clark R. Prolonged curarization due to intraocular soframycin. *Anaesth Intensive Care* (1975) 3, 79–80.
14. Waterman PM, Smith RB. Tobramycin-curare interaction. *Anesth Analg* (1977) 56, 587–8.
15. Kronenfeld MA, Thomas SJ, Turndorf H. Recurrence of neuromuscular blockade after reversal of vecuronium in a patient receiving polymyxin/amikacin sternal irrigation. *Anesthesiology* (1986) 65, 93–4.
16. Harwood TN, Moorthy SS. Prolonged vecuronium-induced neuromuscular blockade in children. *Anesth Analg* (1989) 68, 534–6.
17. Dupuis JY, Martin R, Tétrault J-P. Atracurium and vecuronium interaction with gentamicin and tobramycin. *Can J Anaesth* (1989) 36, 407–11.
18. Dotan ZA, Hana R, Simon D, Geva D, Pfeffermann RA, Ezri T. The effect of vecuronium is enhanced by a large rather than a modest dose of gentamicin as compared with no preoperative gentamicin. *Anesth Analg* (2003) 96, 750–4.
19. Jedeikin R, Dolgunski E, Kaplan R, Hoffman S. Prolongation of neuromuscular blocking effect of vecuronium by antibiotics. *Anaesthesia* (1987) 42, 858–60.
20. Vanacker BF, Van de Walle J. The neuromuscular blocking action of vecuronium in normal patients and in patients with no renal function and interaction vecuronium-tobramycin in renal transplant patients. *Acta Anaesthesiol Belg* (1986) 37, 95–9.
21. Boliston TA, Ashman R. Tobramycin and neuromuscular blockade. *Anaesthesia* (1978) 33, 552.
22. Caputy AJ, Kim YI, Sanders DB. The neuromuscular blocking effects of therapeutic concentrations of various antibiotics on normal rat skeletal muscle: a quantitative comparison. *J Pharmacol Exp Ther* (1981) 217: 369–78.

Neuromuscular blockers + Anaesthetics, local

The neuromuscular blockade due to suxamethonium (succinylcholine) can be increased and prolonged by lidocaine, procaine and possibly procainamide. These local anaesthetics all have some neuromuscular blocking activity and may theoretically also enhance the block produced by competitive neuromuscular blockers. Increased toxicity occurred when mivacurium and prilocaine were given together for regional anaesthesia.

Clinical evidence

A patient anaesthetised with fluroxene and nitrous oxide demonstrated 100% blockade with **suxamethonium (succinylcholine)** and **tubocurarine**. About 50 minutes later when twitch height had fully returned and tidal volume was 400 mL, she was given **lidocaine** 50 mg intravenously for premature ventricular contractions. She immediately stopped breathing and the twitch disappeared. About 45 minutes later the tidal volume was 450 mL. Later it was found that the patient had a dibucaine number (a measure of cholinesterase activity) of 23%.[1]

A study in 10 patients has confirmed that **lidocaine** and **procaine** prolong the apnoea following the use of **suxamethonium** 700 micrograms/kg. A dose-relationship was established. The duration of apnoea was approximately doubled by 5 mg/kg of lidocaine or 2.2 mg/kg of procaine intravenously, and tripled by 16.6 mg/kg and 11.2 mg/kg, respectively, although the effects of procaine at higher doses were more marked.[2]

Procainamide has been reported to increase the effects of **suxamethonium** in *animals*,[3] increase muscle weakness in a myasthenic patient,[4] and reduce plasma cholinesterase activity in healthy subjects.[5] An *animal* study demonstrated potentiation of the neuromuscular blocking effect of **tubocurarine** by **lidocaine** alone and combined with antibiotics having neuromuscular blocking activity (**neomycin** or **polymyxin B**).[6]

In a study of 10 healthy subjects, prolonged muscle weakness and symptoms of local anaesthetic toxicity were experienced after deflation of the tourniquet when 40 mL of **prilocaine** 0.5% and **mivacurium** 600 micrograms were used together for intravenous regional anaesthesia of the forearm. Giving **prilocaine** or **mivacurium** alone did not produce these effects. The slow recovery suggested that **mivacurium** was not broken down in the ischaemic limb,[7] but inhibition of plasma cholinesterase by **prilocaine** would not fully explain the prolonged weakness once the cuff was deflated.[8]

Mechanism

Uncertain. Some local anaesthetics (ester-type[9]) such as procaine appear to inhibit plasma cholinesterase,[10] which might prolong the activity of suxamethonium. There may additionally be competition between suxamethonium and procaine for hydrolysis by plasma cholinesterase, which metabolises them both.[2,5] These effects are particularly important in patients with abnormal plasma cholinesterase.[11] Therapeutic procainamide plasma concentrations of 5 to 10 micrograms/mL have been found to inhibit cholinesterase activity by 19 to 32%.[5]

All local anaesthetics have some neuromuscular blocking activity and may enhance the block produced by competitive neuromuscular blockers if given in sufficient doses.[11,12] Procainamide also has acetylcholine receptor channel blocking activity.[12]

Importance and management

Information is limited but the interactions of suxamethonium with lidocaine, and suxamethonium with procaine appear to be established and of clinical importance. Be alert for signs of increased blockade and/or recurarisation with apnoea during the recovery period from suxamethonium.

Despite the potential for an interaction between suxamethonium and procainamide, no marked interaction has yet been reported. Nevertheless be aware that some increase in the neuromuscular blocking effects is possible.

Lidocaine, procaine and procainamide all have some neuromuscular blocking activity and may also enhance the block produced by competitive neuromuscular blockers if given in sufficient doses. However, again, there seems to be an absence of reports of this, probably because the amount of local anaesthetic absorbed into the circulation following a local block is usually modest.[12]

Animal studies indicate that low and otherwise safe doses of lidocaine given with other drugs having neuromuscular blocking activity (e.g. polymyxin B, aminoglycosides) may possibly be additive with conventional neuromuscular blockers and so some caution may be warranted.[6]

1. Miller RD. Neuromuscular blocking agents. In: Smith NT, Miller RD, Corbascio AN, eds. Drug Interactions in Anesthesia. Philadelphia: Lea and Febiger; 1981 p. 249–69.
2. Usubiaga JE, Wikinski JA, Morales RL, Usubiaga LEJ. Interaction of intravenously administered procaine, lidocaine and succinylcholine in anesthetized subjects. *Anesth Analg* (1967) 46, 39–45.
3. Cuthbert MF. The effect of quinidine and procainamide on the neuromuscular blocking action of suxamethonium. *Br J Anaesth* (1966) 38, 775–9.
4. Drachman DA, Skom JH. Procainamide—a hazard in myasthenia gravis. *Arch Neurol* (1965) 13, 316–20.
5. Kambam JR, Naukam RJ, Sastry BVR. The effect of procainamide on plasma cholinesterase activity. *Can J Anaesth* (1987) 34, 579–81.
6. Brueckner J, Thomas KC, Bikhazi GB, Foldes FF. Neuromuscular drug interactions of clinical importance. *Anesth Analg* (1980) 59, 533–4.
7. Torrance JM, Lewer BMF, Galletly DC. Low-dose mivacurium supplementation of prilocaine i.v. regional anaesthesia. *Br J Anaesth* (1997) 78, 222–3.
8. Torrance JM, Lewer BMF, Galletly DC. Interactions between mivacurium and prilocaine. *Br J Anaesth* (1997) 79, 262.
9. Sweetman SC, ed. Martindale: The complete drug reference. 35th ed. London: Pharmaceutical Press; 2007. p. 1751.
10. Reina RA, Cannavà N. Interazione di alcuni anestetici locali con la succinilcolina. *Acta Anaesthesiol Ital* (1972) 23, 1–10
11. Østergaard D, Engbaek J, Viby-Mogensen J. Adverse reactions and interactions of the neuromuscular blocking drugs. *Med Toxicol Adverse Drug Exp* (1989) 4, 351–68.
12. Feldman S, Karalliedde L. Drug interactions with neuromuscular blockers. *Drug Safety* (1996) 15, 261–73.

Neuromuscular blockers + Anticholinesterases

Anticholinesterases oppose the actions of competitive neuromuscular blockers (e.g. tubocurarine) and can therefore be used as an antidote to restore muscular activity following their use. Conversely, anticholinesterases increase and prolong the actions of the depolarising neuromuscular blockers (e.g. suxamethonium (succinylcholine)). Anticholinesterases used to treat Alzheimer's disease may also interact with neuromuscular blockers.

Clinical evidence, mechanism, importance and management

There are two main types of neuromuscular blockers: competitive (non-depolarising) and depolarising, see 'Table 5.2', (p.91).

(a) Competitive (non-depolarising) neuromuscular blockers

Competitive (non-depolarising) neuromuscular blockers (e.g. **tubocurarine**) compete with acetylcholine for receptors on the motor endplate. Anticholinesterases (e.g. **ambenonium**, **edrophonium**, **neostigmine**, **physostigmine**, **pyridostigmine**, etc.) can be used as an antidote to this kind of neuromuscular blockade, because they inhibit the enzymes that destroy acetylcholine so that the concentration of acetylcholine at the neuromuscular junction builds up. In this way the competition between the molecules of the blocker and the acetylcholine for occupancy of the receptors swings in favour of the acetylcholine so that transmission is restored. These drugs are used routinely following surgery to reactivate paralysed muscles. However, note that the **aminoglycosides** can act as neuromuscular blockers (see 'Neuromuscular blockers + Aminoglycosides', p.113) and therefore their use may unintentionally antagonise the effects of the anticholinesterases.

Some inhalational anaesthetics can impair the effect of anticholinesterases on neuromuscular blockers (see 'Anaesthetics, general + Anticholinesterases', p.93).

(b) Depolarising neuromuscular blockers

The depolarising blockers (such as **suxamethonium (succinylcholine)**) act like acetylcholine to depolarise the motor endplate, but unlike acetylcholine, they are not immediately removed by cholinesterase. The anticholinesterase drugs increase the concentration of acetylcholine at the neuromuscular junction, which enhances and prolongs this type of blockade, and therefore anticholinesterases cannot be used as an antidote for this kind of blocker. Care should be taken if an anticholinesterase has been given to antagonise a competitive neuromuscular block prior to the use of **suxamethonium**, as the duration of the **suxamethonium** block may be prolonged.[1]

(c) Tacrine and other centrally-acting anticholinesterases

Tacrine, like other anticholinesterases, has been used *intravenously* in anaesthetic practice to reverse the effects of competitive (non-depolarising) blockers such as **tubocurarine**[2] and to prolong the effects of depolarising blockers such as **suxamethonium**.[2-6] For example, one study found that only one-third of the normal dosage of **suxamethonium** was needed in the presence of 15 mg of intravenous tacrine.[7]

However, tacrine is now more commonly used *orally* for its central effects in the treatment of Alzheimer's disease. Therefore be alert for changes in the effects of both types of neuromuscular blocking drugs in patients in whom tacrine is being used. Other cholinesterase inhibitors (including **galantamine**, **rivastigmine** and possibly **donepezil**) will behave like tacrine. There is a report of such an interaction in a 72-year-old woman taking **donepezil** who had prolonged paralysis after induction of anaesthesia with propofol and **suxamethonium**. It is possible that levels of **donepezil** in this patient were high due to concurrent omeprazole and fluoxetine and this may have contributed to the prolonged action of **suxamethonium**.[8] Another report describes an 85-year-old woman taking **donepezil**, who developed prolonged neuromuscular blockade after the administration of **neostigmine** to reverse the effects of pancuronium (she had also received suxamethonium). This patient probably had atypical pseudocholinesterase activity, and the authors suggest the interaction may not be clinically relevant in patients with normal enzyme activity.[9]

(d) Organophosphorus compounds

Organophosphorus compounds are potent anticholinesterases, see 'Neuromuscular blockers + Organophosphorus compounds', p.130.

1. Fleming NW, Macres S, Antognini JF, Vengco J. Neuromuscular blocking action of suxamethonium after antagonism of vecuronium by edrophonium, pyridostigmine or neostigmine. *Br J Anaesth* (1996) 77, 492–5.
2. Hunter AR. Tetrahydroaminacrine in anaesthesia. *Br J Anaesth* (1965) 37, 505–13.
3. Oberoi GS, Yaubihi N. The use of tacrine (THA) and succinylcholine compared with alcuronium during laparoscopy. *P N G Med J* (1990) 33, 25–8.
4. Davies-Lepie SR. Tacrine may prolong the effect of succinylcholine. *Anesthesiology* (1994) 81, 524.
5. Norman J, Morgan M. The effect of tacrine on the neuromuscular block produced by suxamethonium in man. *Br J Anaesth* (1975) 47, 1027.
6. Lindsay PA, Lumley J. Suxamethonium apnoea masked by tetrahydroaminacrine. *Anaesthesia* (1978) 33, 620–2.
7. El-Kammah BM, El-Gafi SH, El-Sherbiny AM, Kader MMA. Biochemical and clinical study for the role of tacrine as succinylcholine extender. *J Egypt Med Assoc* (1975) 58, 559–67.
8. Crowe S, Collins L. Suxamethonium and donepezil: a cause of prolonged paralysis. *Anesthesiology* (2003) 98, 574–5.
9. Sprung J, Castellani WJ, Srinivasan V, Udayashankar S. The effects of donepezil and neostigmine in a patient with unusual pseudocholinesterase activity. *Anesth Analg* (1998) 87, 1203–5.

Neuromuscular blockers + Antiepileptics

The effects of many competitive neuromuscular blockers are reduced and shortened if carbamazepine or phenytoin are given for longer than one week, but they appear to be increased if phenytoin, and possibly carbamazepine, are given acutely (e.g. during surgery). Carbamazepine and phenytoin appear not to interact with mivacurium.

Clinical evidence

(a) Carbamazepine given long term: neuromuscular blocking effects reduced

The recovery from neuromuscular blockade with **pancuronium** in 18 patients undergoing craniotomy for tumours, seizure foci or cerebrovascular surgery was on average 65% shorter in those taking carbamazepine.[1] Another 9 patients taking carbamazepine for at least a week and undergoing surgery were given **doxacurium** took 66 minutes to reach 50% recovery compared with 161 minutes in the control group.[2] Similar findings were obtained in another study.[3] Further studies found that carbamazepine significantly shortened the recovery time from **vecuronium** blockade in adults[4] and in children.[5] Several reports and studies have demonstrated a shorter duration of action of **rocuronium** following long-term carbamazepine use,[6-9] although preliminary investigations found no effect.[10,11] A reduced duration of action has been reported with **rapacuronium** in a patient taking carbamazepine.[12] The effects of **pipecuronium** are also reduced by carbamazepine.[13,14] In one study it was found that the *onset* time for **pipecuronium** blockade was lengthened (although this was not statistically significant) in patients with therapeutic plasma concentrations of carbamazepine or phenytoin, but not in those with subtherapeutic levels. However, a shorter duration of action was seen regardless of anticonvulsant levels.[14] One study found that the recovery time from intravenous **atracurium** 500 micrograms/kg was significantly shorter in 14 patients taking long-term carbamazepine (5.93 minutes) when compared with 21 nonepileptic patients (8.02 minutes). This was assessed using the recovery index (time between 25% and 75% recovery of baseline electromyogram values).[15] However, other studies have reported no effect, see (e) below. Another study found that the recovery time from intravenous **cisatracurium** was shorter in patients taking carbamazepine or **phenytoin** than in patients not receiving these antiepileptics; the recovery index (times between 25% and 75% recovery) was 16.2 and 21.2 minutes, respectively. Clearance of **cisatracurium** was increased by about 25% in patients taking the antiepileptics. The steady-state plasma level of **cisatracurium** required to maintain 95% block was increased by 20% in the patients taking antiepileptics, indicating increased resistance to the action of **cisatracurium**.[16]

(b) Carbamazepine given short term: neuromuscular blocking effects increased

An *in vitro* study found that the acute neuromuscular effects of **carbamazepine** reduced the concentrations required for 50% paralysis with both a depolarising neuromuscular blocker (**suxamethonium (succinylcholine)**) and a competitive neuromuscular blocker (**atracurium**) by about 30%.[17]

(c) Phenytoin given long term: neuromuscular blocking effects reduced

In the preliminary report of a study, the reduction in the time to recover from 25 to 75% of the response to ulnar nerve stimulation, in patients who had received phenytoin for longer than one week was: **metocurine** 58%, **pancuronium** 40%, **tubocurarine** 24%, **atracurium** 8% (the last two were not statistically significant).[18] The **metocurine** results are published in full elsewhere.[19] In another study about 80% more **pancuronium** was needed by 9 patients taking long-term phenytoin (58 micrograms/kg per hour) than in 18 others not receiving phenytoin (32 micrograms/kg per hour).[20] Resistance to **pancuronium** and a shortening of the recovery period due to long-term phenytoin[3,21] or unspecified antiepileptics[22] has also been described in other reports. The recovery period from **doxacurium**,[2,3] **pipecuronium**,[13,14] **rapacuronium** (case report),[12] **rocuronium**[23,24] and **vecuronium**[5,25-28] is also reduced by phenytoin. In one study it was found that the *onset* time for **pipecuronium** blockade was lengthened (although this was not statistically significant) for patients with therapeutic plasma concentrations of phenytoin or carbamazepine, but not in those with subtherapeutic levels. However, a shorter duration of action occurred regardless of the anticonvulsant level.[14]

A reduced recovery time from **atracurium**-induced neuromuscular blockade was found in one study in patients taking long-term antiepileptics including phenytoin[15] but other studies have reported a minimal effect, see (e) below. For a report of reduced recovery time, increased clearance of **cisatracurium** and increased resistance to its actions in the presence of phenytoin, see (a) above.

(d) Phenytoin given short term: neuromuscular blocking effects increased

A retrospective review of 8 patients taking long-term phenytoin (greater than 2 weeks) and 3 others given phenytoin within 8 hours of surgery found that the average doses of **vecuronium** used from induction to extubation were 155 micrograms/kg per hour (long term) and 61.5 micrograms/kg per hour (acute).[29] Others have reported similar results.[26] Short-term phenytoin use may have been a contributing factor in the prolonged clearance of **vecuronium** in another patient.[30,31] Another study found that the sensitivity of patients to **vecuronium** was increased by phenytoin given intravenously during surgery,[32] and this has also been seen in *animal* studies using **tubocurarine** and phenytoin.[33] Similarly, a study of 20 patients undergoing craniotomy found that phenytoin (10 mg/kg over about 30 minutes) given during the operation augmented the neuromuscular block produced by **rocuronium**.[34]

(e) Antiepileptics given long term: neuromuscular blocking effects not significantly affected

Long-term (greater than 4 weeks) **carbamazepine** appears not to affect **mivacurium**-induced neuromuscular blockade.[35] Similarly, a study in 32 patients who had been taking **carbamazepine** alone or with **phenytoin** or **valproic acid** for greater than 2 weeks found no resistance to **mivacurium**,[36] although an earlier preliminary study by the same research group found a trend towards a shorter recovery from **mivacurium** in 13 patients taking unspecified antiepileptics (not statistically significant).[37] **Carbamazepine** has also been reported to have no effect on **atracurium**[4,38] and two studies suggest that **atracurium** is normally minimally affected by **phenytoin**.[25,39] However, one study[15] found that the recovery time from **atracurium** blockade was significantly reduced in patients on long-term anticonvulsant therapy, see (a) and (c) above.

Eight patients who had been taking **phenytoin** and/or **carbamazepine** for at least one month took longer to recover from **suxamethonium (succinylcholine)** blockade compared with 9 control patients; the time for return to baseline twitch height was 14.3 and 10 minutes, respectively. The slight prolongation of **suxamethonium** action was considered to have few clinical implications.[40]

Mechanism

Not fully understood, but it appears to be multifactorial. Acute administration of phenytoin or carbamazepine may result in neuromuscular block and potentiation of the action of competitive (non-depolarising) blockers.[17]

Long-term therapy with antiepileptics may produce subclinical neuromuscular blockade thought to be due to modest blockade of acetylcholine effects and a decrease in acetylcholine release; this antagonism may induce changes at the neuromuscular junction including increased number of acetylcholine receptors on the muscle membrane (up-regulation), with decreased sensitivity.[5,40,41] Other suggestions to account for the reduced response with chronic antiepileptics include: induction of liver enzyme activity (phenytoin and carbamazepine are both potent inducers of cytochrome P450 isoenzymes), which would increase the metabolism and clearance of the neuromuscular blocker; and changes in plasma protein binding.[5,40,41] It has been shown that carbamazepine doubles the clearance of vecuronium[5,42] and phenytoin possibly increases the plasma clearance of pancuronium[21] and rocuronium.[23]

Importance and management

Established and clinically important interactions. More is known about phenytoin and carbamazepine than other antiepileptics.

Anticipate the need to use more (possibly up to twice as much) doxacurium, metocurine, pancuronium, pipecuronium, rocuronium and vecuronium in patients who have taken these antiepileptics for more than a week,[26] and expect an accelerated recovery. The effects on tubocurarine and atracurium appear only to be small or moderate, whereas mivacurium appears not to interact.

Anticipate the need to use a smaller neuromuscular blocker dosage, or prepare for a longer recovery time if phenytoin and possibly carbamazepine are given acutely.

1. Roth S, Ebrahim ZY. Resistance to pancuronium in patients receiving carbamazepine. *Anesthesiology* (1987) 66, 691–3.
2. Ornstein E, Matteo RS, Weinstein JA, Halevy JD, Young WL, Abou-Donia MM. Accelerated recovery from doxacurium-induced neuromuscular blockade in patients receiving chronic anticonvulsant therapy. *J Clin Anesth* (1991) 3, 108–11.
3. Desai P, Hewitt PB, Jones RM. Influence of anticonvulsant therapy on doxacurium and pancuronium-induced paralysis. *Anesthesiology* (1989) 71, A784.
4. Ebrahim Z, Bulkley R, Roth S. Carbamazepine therapy and neuromuscular blockade with atracurium and vecuronium. *Anesth Analg* (1988) 67, S55.
5. Soriano SG, Sullivan LJ, Venkatakrishnan K, Greenblatt DJ, Martyn JAJ. Pharmacokinetics and pharmacodynamics of vecuronium in children receiving phenytoin or carbamazepine for chronic anticonvulsant therapy. *Br J Anaesth* (2001) 86, 223–9.
6. Baraka A, Idriss N. Resistance to rocuronium in an epileptic patient on long-term carbamazepine therapy. *Middle East J Anesthesiol* (1996) 13, 561–4.
7. Loan PB, Connolly FM, Mirakhur RK, Kumar N, Farling P. Neuromuscular effects of rocuronium in patients receiving beta-adrenoreceptor blocking, calcium entry blocking and anticonvulsant drugs. *Br J Anaesth* (1997) 78, 90–1.
8. Spacek A, Neiger FX, Krenn CG, Hoerauf K, Kress HG. Rocuronium-induced neuromuscular block is affected by chronic carbamazepine therapy. *Anesthesiology* (1999) 90, 109–12.
9. Soriano SG, Kaus SJ, Sullivan LJ, Martyn JAJ. Onset and duration of action of rocuronium in children receiving chronic anticonvulsant therapy. *Paediatr Anaesth* (2000) 10, 133–6.
10. Spacek A, Neiger FX, Katz RL, Watkins WD, Spiss CK. Chronic carbamazepine therapy does not affect neuromuscular blockade by rocuronium. *Anesth Analg* (1995) 80 (Suppl 2), S463.
11. Spacek A, Neiger FX, Krenn C-G, Spiss CK, Kress HG. Does chronic carbamazepine therapy influence neuromuscular blockade by rocuronium? *Anesthesiology* (1997) 87, A833.
12. Tobias JD, Johnson JO. Rapacuronium administration to patients receiving phenytoin or carbamazepine. *J Neurosurg Anesthesiol* (2001) 13, 240–2.
13. Jellish WS, Modica PA, Tempelhoff R. Accelerated recovery from pipecuronium in patients treated with chronic anticonvulsant therapy. *J Clin Anesth* (1993) 5, 105–8.
14. Hans P, Ledoux D, Bonhomme V, Brichant JF. Effect of plasma anticonvulsant level on pipecuronium-induced neuromuscular blockade: preliminary results. *J Neurosurg Anesthesiol* (1995) 7, 254–8.
15. Tempelhoff R, Modica PA, Jellish WS, Spitznagel EL. Resistance to atracurium-induced neuromuscular blockade in patients with intractable seizure disorders treated with anticonvulsants. *Anesth Analg* (1990) 71, 665–9.
16. Richard A, Girard F, Girard DC, Boudreault D, Chouinard P, Moumdjian R, Bouthilier A, Ruel M, Couture J, Varin F. Cisatracurium-induced neuromuscular blockade is affected by chronic phenytoin or carbamazepine treatment in neurosurgical patients. *Anesth Analg* (2005) 100, 538–44.
17. Nguyen A, Ramzan I. Acute in vitro neuromuscular effects of carbamazepine and carbamazepine-10,11-epoxide. *Anesth Analg* (1997) 84, 886–90.
18. Ornstein E, Matteo RS, Silverberg PA, Schwartz AE, Young WL, Diaz J. Chronic phenytoin therapy and nondepolarizing muscular blockade. *Anesthesiology* (1985) 63, A331.
19. Ornstein E, Matteo RS, Young WL, Diaz J. Resistance to metocurine-induced neuromuscular blockade in patients receiving phenytoin. *Anesthesiology* (1985) 63, 294–8.
20. Chen J, Kim YD, Dubois M, Kammerer W, Macnamara TE. The increased requirement of pancuronium in neurosurgical patients receiving Dilantin chronically. *Anesthesiology* (1983) 59, A288.
21. Liberman BA, Norman P, Hardy BG. Pancuronium-phenytoin interaction: a case of decreased duration of neuromuscular blockade. *Int J Clin Pharmacol Ther Toxicol* (1988) 26, 371–4.
22. Messick JM, Maass L, Faust RJ, Cucchiara RF. Duration of pancuronium neuromuscular blockade in patients taking anticonvulsant medication. *Anesth Analg* (1982) 61, 203–4.
23. Szenohradszky J, Caldwell JE, Sharma ML, Gruenke LD, Miller RD. Interaction of rocuronium (ORG 9426) and phenytoin in a patient undergoing cadaver renal transplantation: a possible pharmacokinetic mechanism? *Anesthesiology* (1994) 80, 1167–70.
24. Hernández-Palazón J, Tortosa JA, Martínez-Lage JF, Pérez-Ayala M. Rocuronium-induced neuromuscular blockade is affected by chronic phenytoin therapy. *J Neurosurg Anesthesiol* (2001) 13, 79–82.
25. Ornstein E, Matteo RS, Schwartz AE, Silverberg PA, Young WL, Diaz J. The effect of phenytoin on the magnitude and duration of neuromuscular block following atracurium or vecuronium. *Anesthesiology* (1987) 67, 191–6.
26. Platt PR, Thackray NM. Phenytoin-induced resistance to vecuronium. *Anaesth Intensive Care* (1993) 21, 185–91.
27. Caldwell JE, McCarthy GJ, Wright PMC, Szenohradszky J, Sharma ML, Gruenke LD, Miller RD. Influence of chronic phenytoin administration on the pharmacokinetics and pharmacodynamics of vecuronium. *Br J Anaesth* (1999) 83, 183P–184P.
28. Wright PMC, McCarthy G, Szenohradszky J, Sharma ML, Caldwell JE. Influence of chronic phenytoin administration on the pharmacokinetics and pharmacodynamics of vecuronium. *Anesthesiology* (2004) 100, 626–33.
29. Baumgardner JE, Bagshaw R. Acute versus chronic phenytoin therapy and neuromuscular blockade. *Anaesthesia* (1990) 45, 493–4.
30. Kainuma M, Miyake T, Kanno T. Extremely prolonged vecuronium clearance in a brain death case. *Anesthesiology* (2001) 95, 1023–4.
31. Gronert GA. Vecuronium sensitivity in part due to acute use of phenytoin. *Anesthesiology* (2002) 97, 1035.
32. Gray HSJ, Slater RM, Pollard BJ. The effect of acutely administered phenytoin on vecuronium-induced neuromuscular blockade. *Anaesthesia* (1989) 44, 379–81.
33. Gandhi IC, Jindal MN, Patel VK. Mechanism of neuromuscular blockade with some antiepileptic drugs. *Arzneimittelforschung* (1976) 26, 258–61.
34. Spacek A, Nickl S, Neiger FX, Nigrovic V, Ullrich O-W, Weindlmayr-Goettel M, Schwall B, Taeger K, Kress HG. Augmentation of the rocuronium-induced neuromuscular block by the acutely administered phenytoin. *Anesthesiology* (1999) 90, 1551–5.
35. Spacek A, Neiger FX, Spiss CK, Kress HG. Chronic carbamazepine therapy does not influence mivacurium-induced neuromuscular block. *Br J Anaesth* (1996) 77, 500–2.
36. Jellish WS, Thalji Z, Brundidge PK, Tempelhoff R. Recovery from mivacurium-induced neuromuscular blockade is not affected by anticonvulsant therapy. *J Neurosurg Anesthesiol* (1996) 8, 4–8.
37. Thalji Z, Jellish WS, Murdoch J, Tempelhoff R. The effect of chronic anticonvulsant therapy on recovery from mivacurium induced paralysis. *Anesthesiology* (1993) 79 (Suppl 3A), A965.
38. Spacek A, Neiger FX, Spiss CK, Kress HG. Atracurium-induced neuromuscular block is not affected by chronic anticonvulsant therapy with carbamazepine. *Acta Anaesthesiol Scand* (1997) 41, 1308–11.
39. deBros F, Okutani R, Lai A, Lawrence KW, Basta S. Phenytoin does not interfere with atracurium pharmacokinetics and pharmacodynamics. *Anesthesiology* (1987) 67, A607.
40. Melton AT, Antognini JF, Gronert GA. Prolonged duration of succinylcholine in patients receiving anticonvulsants: evidence for mild up-regulation of acetylcholine receptors? *Can J Anaesth* (1993) 40, 939–42.
41. Kim CS, Arnold FJ, Itani MS, Martyn JAJ. Decreased sensitivity to metocurine during long-term phenytoin therapy may be attributable to protein binding and acetylcholine receptor changes. *Anesthesiology* (1992) 77, 500–6.
42. Alloul K, Whalley DG, Shutway F, Ebrahim Z, Varin F. Pharmacokinetic origin of carbamazepine-induced resistance to vecuronium neuromuscular blockade in anesthetized patients. *Anesthesiology* (1996) 84, 330–9.

Neuromuscular blockers + Antineoplastics

The effects of suxamethonium (succinylcholine) can be increased and prolonged in patients receiving cyclophosphamide because their plasma cholinesterase levels are depressed. Respiratory insufficiency and prolonged apnoea have been reported. Irinotecan may prolong the neuromuscular blocking effects of suxamethonium and antagonise that of non-depolarising drugs. *Animal* data suggests that thiotepa may also enhance the effects of suxamethonium. An isolated report describes a marked increase in the neuromuscular blocking effects of pancuronium in a myasthenic patient who was given thiotepa, but normally it appears not to interact with competitive neuromuscular blockers.

Clinical evidence

(a) Cyclophosphamide

Respiratory insufficiency and prolonged apnoea occurred in a patient on two occasions while receiving cyclophosphamide and undergoing anaesthesia during which **suxamethonium (succinylcholine)** and **tubocurarine** were used. Plasma cholinesterase levels were found to be low. Anaesthesia without the **suxamethonium** was uneventful. Seven out of 8 patients subsequently examined also showed depressed plasma cholinesterase levels while taking cyclophosphamide.[1]

Respiratory depression and low plasma cholinesterase levels have been described in other reports in patients receiving cyclophosphamide.[2-4] Similarly, in the discussion of an *in vitro* study, the authors report preliminary results from a study in patients, showing a 35 to 70% reduction in cholinesterase activity for several days after cyclophosphamide use.[2] See also (d) below.

(b) Irinotecan

The manufacturer warns that irinotecan could possibly prolong the neuromuscular blocking effects of suxamethonium (succinylcholine) and antagonise the neuromuscular blockade of competitive (non-depolarising) drugs.[5] This is based on the fact that irinotecan has anticholinesterase activity[5,6] (see also 'Neuromuscular blockers + Anticholinesterases', p.114, for an explanation of this mechanism).

(c) Thiotepa

A myasthenic patient developed very prolonged respiratory depression very shortly after being given thiotepa intraperitoneally, following the use of **pancuronium**.[7] Thiotepa has also been shown to increase the duration of **suxamethonium (succinylcholine)** neuromuscular blockade in *dogs*.[8] However, an *in vitro* study showed that thiotepa was a poor inhibitor of plasma cholinesterase.[2] See also (d) below.

(d) Other antineoplastics

A patient with myasthenia gravis and thymoma experienced severe myasthenic crises during 2 cycles of treatment with **doxorubicin**, **cisplatin** and **etoposide**. He also received dexamethasone with the first but not the second cycle of treatment. It was suggested that at least one of the antineoplastics had a direct inhibitory effect on neuromuscular transmission leading to exacerbation of pre-existing myasthenia gravis.[9]

An *in vitro* study found that human motor endplate or red blood cell acetylcholinesterase was inhibited by alkylating antineoplastics, with **chlormethine** exerting the greatest effect, followed by **dacarbazine**, **nimustine**, **cyclophosphamide** and **ifosfamide**. **Chlormethine** and **cyclophosphamide** inhibited plasma pseudocholinesterase most strongly, followed by **thiotepa**, **nimustine**, **dacarbazine**, **ifosfamide**, and **carmustine**.[10]

Mechanism

Cyclophosphamide inhibits the activity of plasma cholinesterase,[4] and as a result the metabolism of the suxamethonium is reduced and its actions are enhanced and prolonged. Other alkylating agents are also reported to reduce plasma cholinesterase activity.[10]

Importance and management

The interaction between suxamethonium and cyclophosphamide is well documented and established. It is of clinical importance, but whether all patients are affected to the same extent is uncertain. The depression of the plasma cholinesterase levels may last several days, possibly weeks, so that ideally plasma cholinesterase levels should be checked before using suxamethonium. In patients taking cyclophosphamide it should certainly be used with caution, and the dosage should be reduced.[2] Some have suggested that concurrent use should be avoided.[1] Irinotecan may possibly enhance the effects of suxamethonium and antagonise the effects of non-depolarising drugs. *Animal* data suggest thiotepa may enhance the effects of suxamethonium and *in vitro* data suggest some other antineoplastics may also have an effect. The general silence in the literature would seem to indicate that no special precautions are normally necessary. However, patients with malignant tumours often have a reduced plasma cholinesterase activity, so care is warranted in these patients.[11]

1. Walker IR, Zapf PW, Mackay IR. Cyclophosphamide, cholinesterase and anaesthesia. *Aust N Z J Med* (1972) 3, 247–51.
2. Zsigmond EK, Robins G. The effect of a series of anti-cancer drugs on plasma cholinesterase activity. *Can Anaesth Soc J* (1972) 19, 75–82.
3. Mone JG, Mathie WE. Qualitative and quantitative defects of pseudocholinesterase activity. *Anaesthesia* (1967) 22, 55–68.
4. Wolff H. Die Hemmung der Serumcholinesterase durch Cyclophosphamid (Endoxan®). *Klin Wochenschr* (1965) 43, 819–21.
5. Campto (Irinotecan). Pfizer Ltd. UK Summary of product characteristics, January 2007.
6. Hyatt JL, Tsurkan L, Morton CL, Yoon KJP, Harel M, Brumshtein B, Silman I, Sussman JL, Wadkins RM, Potter PM. Inhibition of acetylcholinesterase by the anticancer prodrug CPT-11. *Chem Biol Interact* (2005) 157–8, 247–52.
7. Bennett EJ, Schmidt GB, Patel KP, Grundy EM. Muscle relaxants, myasthenia, and mustards? *Anesthesiology* (1977) 46, 220–1
8. Cremonesi E, Rodrigues I de J. Interação de agentes curarizantes com antineoplásico. *Rev Bras Anestesiol* (1982) 32, 313–15.
9. Ng CVT. Myasthenia gravis and a rare complication of chemotherapy. *Med J Aust* (2005) 182, 120.
10. Fujii M, Ohnoshi T, Namba T, Kimura I. Inhibitory effect of antineoplastic agents on human cholinesterases. *Gan To Kagaku Ryoho* (1982) 9, 831–5.
11. Viby Mogensen J. Cholinesterase and succinylcholine. *Dan Med Bull* (1983) 30, 129–50.

Neuromuscular blockers + Antipsychotics

An isolated report describes prolonged apnoea in a patient given promazine while recovering from neuromuscular blockade with suxamethonium (succinylcholine). Recovery from the neuromuscular blocking effects of suxamethonium is prolonged by fentanyl/droperidol.

Clinical evidence

(a) Suxamethonium (succinylcholine) + Fentanyl/droperidol

The observation that patients who had received *Innovar* (fentanyl/droperidol) before anaesthesia appeared to have prolonged suxamethonium effects, seen as apnoea, prompted further study of this possible interaction.[1] An average delay in recovery from neuromuscular blockade of 36% to 80% was seen in two studies.[1,2] Another study[3] showed that the droperidol component of *Innovar* was probably responsible for this interaction.

(b) Suxamethonium (succinylcholine) + Promazine

A woman recovering from surgery during which she had received suxamethonium, was given promazine 25 mg intravenously for sedation. Within 3 minutes she had become cyanotic and apnoeic, and required assisted respiration for 4 hours.[4]

Mechanism

Not understood. It has been suggested that promazine[4] and droperidol[3] depress plasma cholinesterase levels, which would reduce the metabolism of the suxamethonium and thereby prolong recovery. It has also been suggested that droperidol might act as a membrane stabiliser at neuromuscular junctions.[3]

Importance and management

Some caution would seem appropriate if promazine is given to any patient who has been given suxamethonium. There seems to be no information about other phenothiazines and other neuromuscular blockers.

Delayed recovery should be anticipated in patients given suxamethonium if droperidol is used. This is an established interaction.

1. Wehner RJ. A case study: the prolongation of Anectine® effect by Innovar®. *J Am Assoc Nurse Anesth* (1979) 47, 576–9.
2. Moore GB, Ciresi S, Kallar S. The effect of Innovar® versus droperidol or fentanyl on the duration of action of succinylcholine. *J Am Assoc Nurse Anesth* (1986) 54, 130–6.
3. Lewis RA. A consideration of prolonged succinylcholine paralysis with Innovar®: is the cause droperidol or fentanyl? *J Am Assoc Nurse Anesth* (1982) 50, 55–9.
4. Regan AG, Aldrete JA. Prolonged apnea after administration of promazine hydrochloride following succinylcholine infusion. *Anesth Analg* (1967) 46, 315–18.

Neuromuscular blockers + Aprotinin

Apnoea developed in a number of patients after they were given aprotinin while recovering from neuromuscular blockade with suxamethonium (succinylcholine) alone or with tubocurarine.

Clinical evidence

Three patients undergoing surgery who had received **suxamethonium (succinylcholine)**, alone or with **tubocurarine**, were given aprotinin intravenously in doses of 2500 to 12 000 KIU (kallikrein inactivator units) at the end of, or shortly after the operation, when spontaneous breathing had resumed. In each case respiration rapidly became inadequate and apnoea lasting periods of 7, 30 and 90 minutes occurred.[1] Seven other cases have been reported elsewhere.[2]

Mechanism

Not fully understood. Aprotinin is only a very weak inhibitor of serum cholinesterase (100 000 KIU caused a maximal 16% inhibition in man)[3] and on its own would have little effect on the metabolism of suxamethonium. However, it might tip the balance in those whose cholinesterase was already very depressed.

Importance and management

The incidence of this interaction is uncertain but probably low. Only a few cases have been reported. It seems probable that it only affects those whose plasma cholinesterase levels are already very low for other reasons. No difficulties should arise in those whose plasma cholinesterase levels are normal.

1. Chasapakis G, Dimas C. Possible interaction between muscle relaxants and the kallikrein-trypsin inactivator "Trasylol". *Br J Anaesth* (1966) 38, 838–9.
2. Marcello B, Porati U. Trasylol e blocco neuromuscolare. *Minerva Anestesiol* (1967) 33, 814–15.
3. Doenicke A, Gesing H, Krumey I, Schmidinger St. Influence of aprotinin (Trasylol) on the action of suxamethonium. *Br J Anaesth* (1970) 42, 948–60.

Neuromuscular blockers + Benzodiazepines

A few studies report that diazepam and other benzodiazepines increase the effects of neuromuscular blockers, but many others have not found an interaction. If an interaction does occur, the response is likely to be little different from the individual variations in response of patients to neuromuscular blockers.

Clinical evidence

(a) Increased blockade

A comparative study of 10 patients given **gallamine** and 4 others given **gallamine** with intravenous **diazepam** 150 to 200 micrograms/kg found that the **diazepam** prolonged the duration of activity of the blocker by a factor of three, and doubled the depression of the twitch response.[1] Persistent muscle weakness and respiratory depression was seen in 2 other patients given **tubocurarine** after premedication with **diazepam**.[2] A small reduction (approximately 10%) in neuromuscular blocker requirement has been described with **diazepam** and **tubocurarine**[3] or **suxamethonium (succinylcholine)**, but see also (b) below.[4]

Another study found that recovery to 25% and 75% of the twitch height after **vecuronium** was prolonged by about 25% by 15 mg of intravenous **midazolam**, when compared with control patients.[5] The same study found that **midazolam** prolonged the recovery from the effects of **atracurium** by about 20%. However, the increased recovery time due to **midazolam** was not statistically significant when compared with control patients, but was significantly longer when compared with patients receiving 20 mg of intravenous **diazepam**.[5] See also (b) below.

(b) Reduced blockade or no effect

The duration of paralysis due to **suxamethonium** was reduced in one study by 20% when **diazepam** (150 micrograms/kg) was also given and the recovery time was shortened.[1] **Diazepam** also slightly reduced the time to 25% and 75% recovery of twitch height in patients given **vecuronium** by about 15% (not statistically significant).[5] In *animals,* **diazepam** increased the mean dose of **rocuronium** required by 13%, but this was not statistically significant.[6]

In other studies **diazepam** was found to have no significant effect on the neuromuscular blockade due to **alcuronium**,[7] **atracurium**,[5] **gallamine**,[8] **pancuronium**,[7,9] **suxamethonium**[7,10] or **tubocurarine**.[7,8,10,11] **Lorazepam** and **lormetazepam** have been reported to have little or no effects on **atracurium** or **vecuronium**,[5] and **midazolam** has been reported to have no effect on **suxamethonium** or **pancuronium**.[12]

Mechanism

Not understood. One suggestion is that where some alteration in response is seen it may be a reflection of a central depressant action rather than a direct effect on the myoneural junction.[8] Another study instead suggests that a direct action on the muscle may be responsible.[13]

Importance and management

There is no obvious explanation for these discordant observations. What is known shows that the benzodiazepines may sometimes unpredictably alter the depth and prolong the recovery period from neuromuscular blockade, but the extent may not be very great and may possibly be little different from the individual variations in the response of patients to neuromuscular blockers.

Given that benzodiazepines are commonly given as pre-medication it seems likely that any significant interaction would have come to light by now.

1. Feldman SA, Crawley BE. Interaction of diazepam with the muscle-relaxant drugs. *BMJ* (1970) 2, 336–8.
2. Feldman SA, Crawley BE. Diazepam and muscle relaxants. *BMJ* (1970) 1, 691.
3. Stovner J, Endresen R. Intravenous anaesthesia with diazepam. *Acta Anaesthesiol Scand* (1966) 24 (Suppl), 223–7.
4. Jörgensen H. Premedicinering med diazepam, Valium®. Jämförelse med placebo i en dubbel-blind-undersökning. *Nord Med* (1964) 72, 1395–9.
5. Driessen JJ, Crul JF, Vree TB, van Egmond J, Booij LHDJ. Benzodiazepines and neuromuscular blocking drugs in patients. *Acta Anaesthesiol Scand* (1986) 30, 642–6.
6. Muir AW, Anderson KA, Pow E. Interaction between rocuronium bromide and some drugs used during anaesthesia. *Eur J Anaesthesiol* (1994) 11 (Suppl 9), 93–8.
7. Bradshaw EG, Maddison S. Effect of diazepam at the neuromuscular junction. A clinical study. *Br J Anaesth* (1979) 51, 955–60.
8. Dretchen K, Ghoneim MM, Long JP. The interaction of diazepam with myoneural blocking agents. *Anesthesiology* (1971) 34, 463–8.
9. Asbury AJ, Henderson PD, Brown BH, Turner DJ, Linkens DA. Effect of diazepam on pancuronium-induced neuromuscular blockade maintained by a feedback system. *Br J Anaesth* (1981) 53, 859–63.
10. Stovner J, Endresen R. Diazepam in intravenous anaesthesia. *Lancet* (1965) ii, 1298–9.
11. Hunter AR. Diazepam (Valium) as a muscle relaxant during general anaesthesia: a pilot study. *Br J Anaesth* (1967) 39, 633–7.
12. Tassonyi E. Effects of midazolam (Ro 21-3981) on neuromuscular block. *Pharmatherapeutica* (1984) 3, 678–81.
13. Ludin HP, Dubach K. Action of diazepam on muscular contraction in man. *Z Neurol* (1971) 199, 30–8.

Neuromuscular blockers + Beta-agonist bronchodilators

Bambuterol can prolong the recovery time from neuromuscular blockade with suxamethonium (succinylcholine) or mivacurium. A case report describes modestly enhanced neuromuscular blockade when pancuronium or vecuronium were given after intravenous salbutamol.

Clinical evidence

(a) Bambuterol

A double-blind study in 25 patients found that the recovery time from neuromuscular blockade with **suxamethonium (succinylcholine)** was prolonged by about 30% in those who had received 10 mg of bambuterol 10 to 16 hours before surgery, and by about 50% in those who had received 20 mg of bambuterol.[1]

This confirms two previous studies,[2,3] one of which found that 30 mg of bambuterol given about 10 hours before surgery approximately doubled the duration of **suxamethonium** blockade.[2] Furthermore, in 7 patients who were heterozygous for abnormal plasma cholinesterase, 20 mg of bambuterol taken 2 hours before surgery prolonged **suxamethonium** blockade two- to threefold, and in 4 patients a phase II block occurred.[4]

Similar results have been found in a study involving 27 patients given **mivacurium**. A marked decrease in plasma cholinesterase activity, leading to reduced clearance and prolonged elimination half-life of **mivacurium,** occurred when oral bambuterol 20 mg was given 2 hours before induction of anaesthesia. The duration of action of **mivacurium** was prolonged three- to fourfold compared with placebo.[5]

(b) Salbutamol

A case report describes a 28-year-old man undergoing elective surgery who was given three intravenous doses of salbutamol 125 micrograms over 3.5 hours for treatment and prophylaxis of bronchospasm. Muscle relaxation was maintained with **pancuronium** and then **vecuronium**. The neuromuscular blockade (measured by the force of contraction of the adductor pollicis in response to ulnar nerve stimulation) increased following salbutamol injection, from 45 to 66% during **pancuronium** blockade and from 66 to 86% following **vecuronium**. In addition, recovery of neuromuscular function with neostigmine appeared to be slower than expected.[6]

Mechanism

Bambuterol is an inactive prodrug which is slowly converted enzymatically in the body to its active form, terbutaline. The carbamate groups that are split off can selectively inhibit the plasma cholinesterase that is necessary for the metabolism of suxamethonium and mivacurium. As a result, the metabolism of these neuromuscular blockers is reduced and their effects are thereby prolonged. The effect appears to be related to the dose of the bambuterol and the time lag after administration; maximal depression of plasma cholinesterase activity appears to occur about 2 to 6 hours following oral administration, but is still markedly depressed after 10 hours.[2]

The effect of intravenous salbutamol was probably a direct effect at the neuromuscular junction.[6]

Importance and management

The interaction with bambuterol is an established interaction, which anaesthetists should be aware of. It may be more important where other factors reduce plasma cholinesterase activity or affect the extent of blockade in other ways (e.g. subjects heterozygous for abnormal plasma cholinesterase). This interaction only applies to beta agonists that are metabolised to carbamic acid (bambuterol appears to be the only one available).

The interaction between intravenous salbutamol and pancuronium or vecuronium appears to be limited to this single report and is probably of only minor clinical importance.

1. Staun P, Lennmarken C, Eriksson LI, Wirén J-E. The influence of 10 mg and 20 mg of bambuterol on the duration of succinylcholine-induced neuromuscular blockade. *Acta Anaesthesiol Scand* (1990) 34, 498–500.
2. Fisher DM, Caldwell JE, Sharma M, Wirén J-E. The influence of bambuterol (carbamylated terbutaline) on the duration of action of succinylcholine-induced paralysis in humans. *Anesthesiology* (1988) 69, 757–9.
3. Bang U, Viby-Mogensen J, Wirén JE, Skovgaard LT. The effect of bambuterol (carbamylated terbutaline) on plasma cholinesterase activity and suxamethonium-induced neuromuscular blockade in genotypically normal patients. *Acta Anaesthesiol Scand* (1990) 34, 596–9.
4. Bang U, Viby-Mogensen J, Wirén JE. The effect of bambuterol on plasma cholinesterase activity and suxamethonium-induced neuromuscular blockade in subjects heterozygous for abnormal plasma cholinesterase. *Acta Anaesthesiol Scand* (1990) 34, 600–4.
5. Østergaard D, Rasmussen SN, Viby-Mogensen J, Pedersen NA, Boysen R. The influence of drug-induced low plasma cholinesterase activity on the pharmacokinetics and pharmacodynamics of mivacurium. *Anesthesiology* (2000) 92, 1581–7.
6. Salib Y, Donati F. Potentiation of pancuronium and vecuronium neuromuscular blockade by intravenous salbutamol. *Can J Anaesth* (1993) 40, 50–3.

Neuromuscular blockers + Beta blockers

Increases or decreases (often only modest) in the extent of neuromuscular blockade have been seen in patients taking beta blockers. The bradycardia and hypotension sometimes caused by anaesthetics and beta blockers is not counteracted by atracurium.

Clinical evidence

(a) Reduced neuromuscular blockade

The effects of **suxamethonium** (**succinylcholine**) were slightly, but not significantly, reduced in 8 patients given a dose of **propranolol** of 1 mg/15 kg body weight intravenously 15 minutes pre-operatively. In another 8 patients, **propranolol**, given intravenously 20 to 40 minutes after the onset of action of **tubocurarine**, was also observed to shorten the recovery from **tubocurarine**.[1] Another study described a shortened recovery period from **tubocurarine** due to **oxprenolol** or **propranolol**, but **pindolol** only slightly affected a few subjects.[2]

(b) Increased neuromuscular blockade

Two patients with thyrotoxicosis showed prolonged neuromuscular blockade with **tubocurarine** after they had received **propranolol** 120 mg daily for 14 days prior to surgery.[3] In 8 patients, intravenous **esmolol** 300 to 500 micrograms/kg per minute reduced the increase in heart rate during intubation, and slightly but significantly prolonged the recovery from blockade with **suxamethonium** by approximately 3 minutes when compared with 8 patients given placebo.[4] See also (d) below.

(c) Bradycardia and hypotension

Eight out of 42 patients taking unnamed beta blockers given **atracurium** developed bradycardia (less than 50 bpm) and hypotension (systolic pressure less than 80 mmHg). Most of them had been premedicated with diazepam, induced with methohexital, and maintained with droperidol, fentanyl and nitrous oxide/oxygen. A further 24 showed bradycardia, associated with hypotension on 9 occasions. All responded promptly to 300 to 600 micrograms of intravenous atropine.[5]

Another patient using **timolol** 0.5% eye drops for glaucoma similarly developed bradycardia and hypotension when **atracurium** was given.[6] Bradycardia and hypotension have been seen in 2 other patients, one given **alcuronium** while using **timolol** eye drops for glaucoma, and the other given **atracurium** while taking **atenolol** for hypertension.[7]

For reports of bradycardia associated with **vecuronium** and opioids in patients also receiving beta blockers, see 'Neuromuscular blockers + Opioids', p.130.

(d) No interaction

A study of 16 patients who had been taking various beta blockers (**propranolol** 5, **atenolol** 5, **metoprolol** 2, **bisoprolol** 2, **oxprenolol** 1, **celiprolol** 1) for longer than one month found no difference in the onset and duration of action of **rocuronium**, when compared with a control group.[8] Similarly, intra-operative **esmolol** did not affect the onset and recovery time from **suxamethonium** (**succinylcholine**) blockade in patients with normal plasma cholinesterase (pseudocholinesterase) activity,[9] but see also (b) above.

Mechanism

The changes in the degree of blockade are not understood but the interaction appears to occur at the neuromuscular junction. It has been seen in *animal* studies.[10,11] The bradycardia and hypotension (c) were probably due to the combined depressant effects on the heart of the anaesthetics and the beta blocker not being offset by atracurium, which has little or no effect on the vagus nerve at doses within the recommended range. Note that neuromuscular blockers with vagolytic activity can cause tachycardia and hypotension.

Importance and management

Information is fairly sparse, but these interactions appear normally to be of relatively minor importance. Be aware that changes in neuromuscular blockade (increases or decreases) can occur if beta blockers are used, but they seem to be unpredictable, and then often only modest in extent. The possible combined cardiac depressant effects of beta blockade and anaesthesia are well known (see 'Anaesthetics, general + Beta blockers', p.97). These effects may not be prevented when a neuromuscular blocker is used that has little or no effect on the vagus (such as atracurium or vecuronium).

1. Varma YS, Sharma PL, Singh HW. Effect of propranolol hydrochloride on the neuromuscular blocking action of d-tubocurarine and succinylcholine in man. *Indian J Med Res* (1972) 60, 266–72.
2. Varma YS, Sharma PL, Singh HW. Comparative effect of propranolol, oxprenolol and pindolol on neuromuscular blocking action of d-tubocurarine in man. *Indian J Med Res* (1973) 61, 1382–6.
3. Rozen MS, Whan FM. Prolonged curarization associated with propranolol. *Med J Aust* (1972) 1, 467–8.
4. Murthy VS, Patel KD, Elangovan RG, Hwang T-F, Solochek SM, Steck JD, Laddu AR. Cardiovascular and neuromuscular effects of esmolol during induction of anesthesia. *J Clin Pharmacol* (1986) 26, 351–7.
5. Rowlands DE. Drug interaction? *Anaesthesia* (1984) 39, 1252.
6. Glynne GL. Drug interaction? *Anaesthesia* (1984) 39, 293.
7. Yate B, Mostafa SM. Drug interaction? *Anaesthesia* (1984) 39, 728–9.
8. Loan PB, Connolly FM, Mirakhur RK, Kumar N, Farling P. Neuromuscular effects of rocuronium in patients receiving beta-adrenoreceptor blocking, calcium entry blocking and anticonvulsant drugs. *Br J Anaesth* (1997) 78, 90–1.
9. McCammon RL, Hilgenberg JC, Sandage BW, Stoelting RK. The effect of esmolol on the onset and duration of succinylcholine-induced neuromuscular blockade. *Anesthesiology* (1985) 63, A317.
10. Usubiaga JE. Neuromuscular effects of beta-adrenergic blockers and their interaction with skeletal muscle relaxants. *Anesthesiology* (1968) 29, 484–92.
11. Harrah MD, Way WL, Katzung BG. The interaction of d-tubocurarine with antiarrhythmic drugs. *Anesthesiology* (1970) 33, 406–10.

Neuromuscular blockers + Bretylium

In theory there is the possibility of increased and prolonged neuromuscular blockade if bretylium is given with neuromuscular blockers.

Clinical evidence, mechanism, importance and management

Although case reports seem to be lacking, there is some evidence from *animal* studies that the effects of **tubocurarine** can be increased and prolonged by bretylium.[1] There is a theoretical possibility that if the bretylium were to be given during surgery to control arrhythmias, its effects (which are delayed) might be additive with the residual effects of the neuromuscular blocker during the recovery period, resulting in apnoea.

1. Welch GW, Waud BE. Effect of bretylium on neuromuscular transmission. *Anesth Analg* (1982) 61, 442–4.

Neuromuscular blockers + Calcium-channel blockers

Limited evidence indicates that intra-operative intravenous diltiazem, nicardipine, nifedipine and verapamil can increase the neuromuscular blocking effects of vecuronium and other competitive neuromuscular blockers. Intravenous nimodipine did not alter vecuronium effects in one study.

An isolated case report describes potentiation of tubocurarine and pancuronium by oral verapamil. However, long-term oral nifedipine did not alter vecuronium or atracurium effects, and long-term therapy with various calcium-channel blockers did not interact with rocuronium. Calcium-channel blockers do not increase the plasma potassium rise due to suxamethonium (succinylcholine).

Clinical evidence

(a) Competitive (non-depolarising) neuromuscular blockers + Intravenous calcium-channel blockers

A study in 24 surgical patients[1] anaesthetised with nitrous oxide and isoflurane found that **diltiazem** 5 or 10 microgram/kg per minute decreased the **vecuronium** requirements by up to 50%. Another study in 24 surgical patients found that **diltiazem** (5 mg bolus followed by a 4-microgram/kg per minute infusion) decreased **vecuronium** requirements by 45% when compared with a control group (no **diltiazem**), or those receiving **diltiazem** at half the infusion dose.[2] Reductions in the requirements for **vecuronium** were also noted in other surgical patients receiving intravenous **diltiazem** or **nicardipine**.[3] A study in patients given **vecuronium** 100 micrograms/kg for tracheal intubation found that **nicardipine** 10 micrograms/kg shortened the onset of blockade, making it the same as in other patients given a higher dose of **vecuronium** 150 micrograms/kg alone. Recovery times were unaffected by the **nicardipine**.[4] Yet another study showed that **nicardipine** reduced the requirements for **vecuronium** in a dose-dependent manner: nicardipine 1, 2 and 3 micrograms/kg per minute reduced the vecuronium dose requirement to 79%, 60% and 53% of control, respectively.[5] A study involving 44 patients anaesthetised with isoflurane in nitrous oxide/oxygen found that 1 mg of intravenous **nifedipine** prolonged the neuromuscular blockade due to **atracurium** from 29 to 40 minutes, and increased the neuromuscular blockade of **atracurium** or **vecuronium** from 75 to 90%.[6] In contrast, a study involving 20 patients found that an intravenous infusion of **nimodipine** had no significant effect on the time course of action of **vecuronium**.[7]

A 66-year-old woman with renal impairment, receiving 5 mg of intravenous **verapamil** three times a day for supraventricular tachycardia, underwent abdominal surgery during which she was initially anaesthetised with thiopental and then maintained on nitrous oxide/oxygen with fentanyl. **Vecuronium** was used as the muscle relaxant. The effects of the **vecuronium** were increased and prolonged, and at the end of surgery reversal of the blockade using neostigmine was difficult and extended.[8] Intravenous **verapamil** alone has caused respiratory failure in a patient with poor neuromuscular transmission (Duchenne's dystrophy).[9] Note that *in vitro* and *animal* studies have confirmed that the neuromuscular blocking effects of **tubocurarine**, **pancuronium**, **vecuronium**, **atracurium** and **suxamethonium (succinylcholine)** are increased by **diltiazem**, **verapamil** and **nifedipine**.[9-11]

(b) Competitive (non-depolarising) neuromuscular blockers + Oral calcium-channel blockers

A report describes increased neuromuscular blockade in a patient taking long-term **verapamil** 40 mg three times daily who was given **pancuronium** 2 mg and **tubocurarine** 5 mg. The neuromuscular blockade was difficult to reverse with neostigmine, but which responded well to edrophonium.[12] However, the authors of this report say that many patients taking long-term **verapamil** do not show a clinically significant increase in sensitivity to muscle relaxants.[12] This case also contrasts with another study in which 30 predominantly elderly patients taking chronic **nifedipine** (mean daily dose 33 mg) showed no changes in the time of onset to maximum block nor the duration of clinical relaxation in response to **atracurium** or **vecuronium**, when compared with 30 control patients.[13] Similarly, a study of 17 patients taking calcium-channel blockers (**nifedipine** 12, **diltiazem** 2, **nicardipine** 2, **amlodipine** 1) found no changes in the neuromuscular blocking effects of **rocuronium**.[14]

(c) Suxamethonium + Oral calcium-channel blockers

A comparative study in 21 patients taking calcium-channel blockers long term (**diltiazem**, **nifedipine**, **verapamil**) and 15 other patients not taking calcium-channel blockers found that, although suxamethonium (succinylcholine) caused a modest average peak rise of 0.5 mmol/L in plasma potassium levels, there were no differences between the two groups.[15] See also (a) above.

Mechanism

Not fully understood. Although one suggested explanation has been given: nerve impulses arriving at nerve endings release calcium ions, which in turn causes the release of acetylcholine. Calcium-channel blockers can reduce the concentration of calcium ions within the nerve so that less acetylcholine is released. This would be additive with the effects of a neuromuscular blocker.[11,12]

Importance and management

Direct information so far seems to be limited. Be alert for increased neuromuscular blockade in any patient given an intravenous calcium-channel blocker during surgery. However, this may not apply to nimodipine. From the limited evidence available it appears that increased blockade is not likely in patients taking long-term oral calcium-channel blockers, although one case has been reported with verapamil.

It would seem from the study quoted above[15] that patients taking chronic calcium-channel blocker treatment are at no greater risk of hyperkalaemia with suxamethonium than other patients.

1. Sumikawa K, Kawabata K, Aono Y, Kamibayashi T, Yoshiya I. Reduction in vecuronium infusion dose requirements by diltiazem in humans. *Anesthesiology* (1992) 77, A939.
2. Takasaki Y, Naruoka Y, Shimizu C, Ochi G, Nagaro T, Arai T. Diltiazem potentiates the neuromuscular blockade by vecuronium in humans. *Jpn J Anesthesiol* (1995) 44, 503–7.
3. Takiguchi M, Takaya T. Potentiation of neuromuscular blockade by calcium channel blockers. *Tokai J Exp Clin Med* (1994) 19, 131–7.
4. Yamada T, Takino Y. Can nicardipine potentiate vecuronium induced neuromuscular blockade? *Jpn J Anesthesiol* (1992) 41, 746–50.
5. Kawabata K, Sumikawa K, Kamibayashi T, Kita T, Takada K, Mashimo T, Yoshiya I. Decrease in vecuronium infusion dose requirements by nicardipine in humans. *Anesth Analg* (1994) 79, 1159–64.
6. Jelen-Esselborn S, Blobner M. Wirkungsverstärkung von nichtdepolarisierenden Muskelrelaxanzien durch Nifedipin i.v. in Inhalationsanaesthesie. *Anaesthesist* (1990) 39, 173–8.
7. Aysel İ, HepağuŞlar H, Balcioğlu T, Uyar M. The effects of nimodipine on vecuronium-induced neuromuscular blockade. *Eur J Anaesthesiol* (2000) 17, 383–9.
8. van Poorten JF, Dhasmana KM, Kuypers RSM, Erdmann W. Verapamil and reversal of vecuronium neuromuscular blockade. *Anesth Analg* (1984) 63, 155–7.
9. Durant NN, Nguyen N, Katz RL. Potentiation of neuromuscular blockade by verapamil. *Anesthesiology* (1984) 60, 298–303.
10. Bikhazi GB, Leung I, Foldes FF. Interaction of neuromuscular blocking agents with calcium channel blockers. *Anesthesiology* (1982) 57, A268.
11. Wali FA. Interactions of nifedipine and diltiazem with muscle relaxants and reversal of neuromuscular blockade with edrophonium and neostigmine. *J Pharmacol* (1986) 17, 244–53.
12. Jones RM, Cashman JN, Casson WR, Broadbent MP. Verapamil potentiation of neuromuscular blockade: failure of reversal with neostigmine but prompt reversal with edrophonium. *Anesth Analg* (1985) 64, 1021–5.
13. Bell PF, Mirakhur RK, Elliott P. Onset and duration of clinical relaxation of atracurium and vecuronium in patients on chronic nifedipine therapy. *Eur J Anaesthesiol* (1989) 6, 343–6.
14. Loan PB, Connolly FM, Mirakhur RK, Kumar N, Farling P. Neuromuscular effects of rocuronium in patients receiving beta-adrenoreceptor blocking, calcium entry blocking and anticonvulsant drugs. *Br J Anaesth* (1997) 78, 90–1.
15. Rooke GA, Freund PR, Tomlin J. Calcium channel blockers do not enhance increases in plasma potassium after succinylcholine in humans. *J Clin Anesth* (1994) 6, 114–18.

Neuromuscular blockers + Chloroquine or Quinine

A report describes respiratory insufficiency during the recovery period following surgery, which was attributed to the use of chloroquine diorotate. An isolated report describes recurarisation and dyspnoea in a patient given intravenous quinine after recovering from neuromuscular blockade with suxamethonium (succinylcholine) and pancuronium.

Clinical evidence, mechanism, importance and management

(a) Chloroquine

Studies were carried out on the possible neuromuscular blocking actions of chloroquine diorotate in *animals,* because it was noticed that when it was used in the peritoneal cavity to prevent adhesions following abdominal surgery in man, it caused respiratory insufficiency during the recovery period. These studies found that it had a non-depolarising blocking action at the neuromuscular junction, which was opposed by neostigmine.[1] It would seem therefore that during the recovery period the effects of the chloroquine can be additive with the residual effects of the conventional neuromuscular blocker used during the surgery.

Although this appears to be the only report of this interaction, it is consistent with the way chloroquine can unmask or aggravate myasthenia gravis, or oppose the effects of drugs used in its treatment. Be alert for this reaction if chloroquine is used.

(b) Quinine

A 47-year-old man with acute pancreatitis, taking quinine 600 mg three times daily, was given penicillin and gentamicin intravenously before undergoing surgery, during which **pancuronium** and **suxamethonium (succinylcholine)** were used uneventfully. After surgery the neuromuscular blockade was reversed with neostigmine and atropine, and the patient awoke and was breathing well. A 6-hour intravenous infusion of quinine 500 mg was started 90 minutes postoperatively. Within 10 minutes (after receiving about 15 mg of quinine) he became dyspnoeic, his breathing became totally ineffective and he needed re-intubation. Muscle flaccidity persisted for 3 hours.[2] The reason for this reaction is not fully understood. A possible explanation is that it may have been the additive neuromuscular blocking effects of the gentamicin (well recognised as having neuromuscular blocking activity; see 'Neuromuscular blockers + Aminoglycosides', p.113) and the quinine (an optical isomer of quinidine; see 'Neuromuscular blockers + Quinidine', p.131) and the residual effects of the **pancuronium** and **suxamethonium**.

There seem to be no other reports of problems in patients receiving neuromuscular blockers with quinine, but this isolated case serves to emphasise the importance of being alert for any signs of recurarisation in patients concurrently treated with one or more drugs possessing some neuromuscular blocking activity.

1. Jui-Yen T. Clinical and experimental studies on mechanism of neuromuscular blockade by chloroquine diorotate. *Jpn J Anesthesiol* (1971) 20, 491–503.
2. Sher MH, Mathews PA. Recurarization with quinine administration after reversal from anaesthesia. *Anaesth Intensive Care* (1983) 11, 241–3.

Neuromuscular blockers + Clonidine

There is limited evidence to suggest that clonidine modestly increases the duration of action of vecuronium.

Clinical evidence, mechanism, importance and management

In a study of 16 surgical patients, 8 took oral clonidine 4 to 5.5 micrograms/kg 90 minutes before their operation. Anaesthesia was induced by thiamylal, and maintained with nitrous oxide/isoflurane/oxygen supplemented by fentanyl. Clonidine increased the duration of neuromuscular blockade following the use of vecuronium by 26.4%, when compared with the patients not taking clonidine.[1]

The reasons are not understood. The clinical importance of this interaction would appear to be small.

1. Nakahara T, Akazawa T, Kinoshita Y, Nozaki J. The effect of clonidine on the duration of vecuronium-induced neuromuscular blockade in humans. *Jpn J Anesthesiol* (1995) 44, 1458–63.

Neuromuscular blockers + Corticosteroids

Two reports describe antagonism of the neuromuscular blocking effects of pancuronium by high-dose prednisone, or prednisolone and hydrocortisone. A third report in a patient with adrenocortical insufficiency describes reversal of the pancuronium block by hydrocortisone. Some evidence suggests the dosage of vecuronium may need to be almost doubled in those receiving intramuscular betamethasone. However, prolonged coadministration of high-dose corticosteroids and neuromuscular blockers may increase the risk of myopathy, resulting in prolonged paralysis following the discontinuation of the neuromuscular blocker.

Clinical evidence

(a) Neuromuscular blocking effects

A man undergoing surgery who was taking **prednisone** 250 mg daily by mouth, had good muscular relaxation in response to intravenous **pancuronium** 8 mg (100 micrograms/kg) early in the operation, but an hour later he began to show signs of inadequate relaxation, and continued to do so for the next 75 minutes despite being given four additional 2-mg doses of **pancuronium**.[1] Another patient taking large doses of **hydrocortisone**, **prednisolone** and aminophylline proved to be resistant to the effects of **pancuronium**.[2] A hypophysectomised man taking **cortisone** developed profound paralysis when given **pancuronium**, which was rapidly reversed with 100 mg of **hydrocortisone sodium succinate**.[3]

Inadequate neuromuscular blockade with **vecuronium** (presenting as unexpected movements) occurred in 2 patients during neurosurgery. They had both been given a preoperative course of **betamethasone** 4 mg four times daily to reduce raised intracranial pressure.[4] This prompted a retrospective search of the records of 50 other patients, which revealed that those given intramuscular **betamethasone** preoperatively had needed almost double the dose of **vecuronium** (134 compared with 76 micrograms/kg per hour).[4]

These reports contrast with another,[5] in which 25 patients who had no adrenocortical dysfunction or histories of corticosteroid therapy were given **pancuronium**, **metocurine**, **tubocurarine** or **vecuronium**. They showed no changes in their neuromuscular blockade when given a single intravenous dose of **dexamethasone** 400 micrograms/kg or **hydrocortisone** 10 mg/kg.

(b) Increased risk of myopathy

A report describes 3 patients in status asthmaticus who developed acute reversible myopathy after treatment with high-dose intravenous **methylprednisolone** 320 to 750 mg daily and steroidal neuromuscular blockers (**vecuronium** or **pancuronium**), used concurrently for at least 8 days.[6] A review of the literature from 1977 to 1995 found over 75 cases of prolonged weakness associated with combined use of neuromuscular blockers and **corticosteroids**.[7] This condition has been referred to as 'blocking agent–corticosteroid myopathy' (BACM). Prior to 1994, virtually all cases involved either **pancuronium** or **vecuronium**, leading some authors to suggest that **atracurium** might be safer as it does not have the steroidal structure of these neuromuscular blockers.[6] However, there have since been reports of prolonged paralysis associated with extended treatment with high-dose **corticosteroids** and **atracurium**[8,9] or **cisatracurium**.[10]

Mechanism

Not understood. For the partial reversal of neuromuscular blockade, one idea, based on *animal* studies, is that adrenocortical insufficiency causes a defect in neuromuscular transmission, which is reversed by the corticosteroids.[3] Another idea is that the effects seen are connected in some way with the steroid nucleus of the pancuronium and vecuronium, and are mediated presynaptically.[4,11]

The increased myopathy may be due to an additive effect as both neuromuscular blockers and corticosteroids can cause myopathy. Results of an *in vitro* study suggested that the combination of vecuronium and methylprednisolone might augment pharmacologic denervation, which may lead to myopathy and contribute to the prolonged weakness observed in some critically ill patients.[12]

Importance and management

The evidence for antagonism of neuromuscular blocking effects seems to be limited to the reports cited, and involve only pancuronium and vecuronium. Careful monitoring is clearly needed if either is used in patients who have been treated with corticosteroids, being alert for the need to increase the dosage of the neuromuscular blocker. Note that *animal* studies suggest that atracurium may also possibly be affected by betamethasone to the same extent as vecuronium.[11] However, also be aware that prolonged coadministration of competitive neuromuscular blockers and corticosteroids, particularly in patients in intensive care, may result in a marked prolongation of muscle weakness (several months' rehabilitation have been needed in some cases[6]). The complex state of the critically ill patient means that the effects of neuromuscular blockers may be unpredictable.

1. Laflin MJ. Interaction of pancuronium and corticosteroids. *Anesthesiology* (1977) 47, 471–2.
2. Azar I, Kumar D, Betcher AM. Resistance to pancuronium in an asthmatic patient treated with aminophylline and steroids. *Can Anaesth Soc J* (1982) 29, 280–2.
3. Meyers EF. Partial recovery from pancuronium neuromuscular blockade following hydrocortisone administration. *Anesthesiology* (1977) 46, 148–50.
4. Parr SM, Galletly DC, Robinson BJ. Betamethasone-induced resistance to vecuronium: a potential problem in neurosurgery? *Anaesth Intensive Care* (1991) 19, 103–5.
5. Schwartz AE, Matteo RS, Ornstein E, Silverberg PA. Acute steroid therapy does not alter nondepolarizing muscle relaxant effects in humans. *Anesthesiology* (1986) 65, 326–7.
6. Griffin D, Fairman N, Coursin D, Rawsthorne L, Grossman JE. Acute myopathy during treatment of status asthmaticus with corticosteroids and steroidal muscle relaxants. *Chest* (1992) 102, 510–14.

7. Fischer JR, Baer RK. Acute myopathy associated with combined use of corticosteroids and neuromuscular blocking agents. *Ann Pharmacother* (1996) 30, 1437–45.
8. Branney SW, Haenel JB, Moore FA, Tarbox BB, Schreiber RH, Moore EE. Prolonged paralysis with atracurium infusion: a case report. *Crit Care Med* (1994) 22, 1699–1701.
9. Meyer KC, Prielipp RC, Grossman JE, Coursin DB. Prolonged weakness after infusion of atracurium in two intensive care unit patients. *Anesth Analg* (1994) 78, 772–4.
10. Fodale V, Praticò C, Girlanda P, Baradello A, Lucanto T, Rodolico C, Nicolosi C, Rovere V, Santamaria LB, Dattola R. Acute motor axonal polyneuropathy after a cisatracurium infusion and concomitant corticosteroid therapy. *Br J Anaesth* (2004) 92, 289–93.
11. Robinson BJ, Lee E, Rees D, Purdie GL, Galletly DC. Betamethasone-induced resistance to neuromuscular blockade: a comparison of atracurium and vecuronium in vitro. *Anesth Analg* (1992) 74, 762–5.
12. Kindler CH, Verotta D, Gray AT, Gropper MA, Yost CS. Additive inhibition of nicotinic acetylcholine receptors by corticosteroids and the neuromuscular blocking drug vecuronium. *Anesthesiology* (2000) 92, 821–32.

Neuromuscular blockers + Danazol or Tamoxifen

Two isolated case reports describe prolonged atracurium effects, which were attributed to tamoxifen and danazol.

Clinical evidence, mechanism, importance and management

A case report describes a 67-year-old mastectomy patient taking methyldopa, hydrochlorothiazide, triamterene and long-term tamoxifen 10 mg twice daily who showed prolonged neuromuscular blockade after a single 500-microgram/kg dose of **atracurium**, which the authors suggest might be due to an interaction between **atracurium** and tamoxifen.[1] The authors also point out an earlier report[2] of prolonged **atracurium** blockade where the patient was taking danazol. These interactions are probably not of general importance.

1. Naguib M, Gyasi HK. Antiestrogenic drugs and atracurium – a possible interaction? *Can Anaesth Soc J* (1986) 33, 682–3.
2. Bizzarri-Schmid MD, Desai SP. Prolonged neuromuscular blockade with atracurium. *Can Anaesth Soc J* (1986) 33, 209–12.

Neuromuscular blockers + Dantrolene

One patient developed increased vecuronium effects when given dantrolene, whereas two others were unaffected.

Clinical evidence, mechanism, importance and management

A 60-year-old woman, given a total of 350 mg of dantrolene orally during the 28 hours before surgery to prevent malignant hyperthermia, developed increased neuromuscular blockade and a slow recovery rate when **vecuronium** was subsequently given.[1] This report contrasts with another describing two patients taking long-term dantrolene 20 to 50 mg daily who had no changes in **vecuronium**-induced neuromuscular blockade during or after surgery.[2] Dantrolene is a muscle relaxant that acts directly on the muscle by lowering intracellular calcium concentrations in skeletal muscle; it reduces the release of calcium from the sarcoplasmic reticulum. It may also possibly inhibit calcium-dependent pre-synaptic neurotransmitter release.[3] Be alert for any increased effects if both drugs are used. These case reports indicate that the effects could be dose-related, and so patients receiving higher doses of dantrolene may be at greater risk, although more study is needed to confirm this.

1. Driessen JJ, Wuis EW, Gielen MJM. Prolonged vecuronium neuromuscular blockade in a patient receiving orally administered dantrolene. *Anesthesiology* (1985) 62, 523–4.
2. Nakayama M, Iwasaki H, Fujita S, Narimatsu E, Namiki A. Neuromuscular effects of vecuronium in patients receiving long-term administration of dantrolene. *Jpn J Anesthesiol* (1993) 42, 1508–10.
3. Dantrium Capsules (Dantrolene sodium). Procter & Gamble Pharmaceuticals UK Ltd. UK Summary of product characteristics, October 2002.

Neuromuscular blockers + Dexmedetomidine

Dexmedetomidine caused a minor increase in plasma rocuronium levels.

Clinical evidence, mechanism, importance and management

A study in 10 healthy subjects under general anaesthesia with alfentanil, propofol and nitrous oxide/oxygen, found that an intravenous infusion of dexmedetomidine (950 to 990 nanograms/kg) increased plasma **rocuronium** levels by 7.6%, which was not clinically significant, and decreased the twitch tension from 51% to 44% after 45 minutes. Dexmedetomidine also decreased finger blood flow and increased systemic blood pressure. It was suggested these pharmacokinetic changes occurred due to peripheral vasoconstriction.[1] These effects are unlikely to be of clinical significance.

1. Talke PO, Caldwell JE, Richardson CA, Kirkegaard-Nielsen H, Stafford M. The effects of dexmedetomidine on neuromuscular blockade in human volunteers. *Anesth Analg* (1999) 88, 633–9.

Neuromuscular blockers + Dexpanthenol

An isolated report of an increase in the neuromuscular blocking effects of suxamethonium (succinylcholine) was attributed to the concurrent use of dexpanthenol in one patient, but a further study using pantothenic acid failed to confirm this interaction.

Clinical evidence, mechanism, importance and management

A study in 6 patients under general anaesthesia found that their response to **suxamethonium (succinylcholine)** was unaffected by the infusion of 500 mg of **pantothenic acid**.[1] This study was conducted in response to an earlier case report, which reported respiratory depression requiring re-intubation following the use of intramuscular **dexpanthenol** (which is converted to pantothenic acid in the body) shortly after stopping a **suxamethonium** infusion.[1]

Apart from the single unconfirmed report there seems to be little other reason for avoiding concurrent use or for taking particular precautions. However, the US manufacturer of **dexpanthenol** recommends that it should not be given within one hour of **suxamethonium**.[2]

1. Smith RM, Gottshall SC, Young JA. Succinylcholine-pantothenyl alcohol: a reappraisal. *Anesth Analg* (1969) 48, 205–208.
2. Dexpanthenol Injection. American Reagent, Inc. US Prescribing information, January 2003.

Neuromuscular blockers + Disopyramide

An isolated case report suggests that disopyramide may oppose the effects of neostigmine used to reverse neuromuscular blockade with vecuronium.

Clinical evidence, mechanism, importance and management

A case report[1] suggests that the normal antagonism by neostigmine of **vecuronium** neuromuscular blockade may be opposed by therapeutic serum levels of disopyramide (5 micrograms/mL). Disopyramide has also been shown to decrease the antagonism by neostigmine of the neuromuscular blockade of **tubocurarine** on the *rat* phrenic nerve-diaphragm preparation.[2] The general clinical importance of these observations is not known.

1. Baurain M, Barvais L, d'Hollander A, Hennart D. Impairment of the antagonism of vecuronium-induced paralysis and intra-operative disopyramide administration. *Anaesthesia* (1989) 44, 34–6.
2. Healy TEJ, O'Shea M, Massey J. Disopyramide and neuromuscular transmission. *Br J Anaesth* (1981) 53, 495–8.

Neuromuscular blockers + Ecothiopate iodide

The neuromuscular blocking effects of suxamethonium (succinylcholine) are markedly increased and prolonged in patients receiving ecothiopate iodide. The dosage of suxamethonium should be reduced appropriately.

Clinical evidence

In 1965 a study[1] showed that ecothiopate iodide eye drops could markedly lower pseudocholinesterase levels. It was noted that "... within a few days of commencing therapy, levels are reached at which protracted apnoea could occur, should these patients require general anaesthesia in which muscle relaxation is obtained with **succinylcholine**". Cases of apnoea due to this interaction were reported the following year,[2,3] and other cases have been subsequently reported.[4,5] In one case a woman given **suxamethonium (succinylcholine)** 200 mg showed apnoea for 5½ hours.[2] Other studies have confirmed that ecothiopate given orally[6] or as eye drops[7] markedly reduced the levels of plasma cholinesterase, and can prolong recovery after **suxamethonium**.[6] On discontinuing ecothiopate, it takes several weeks to 2 months for enzyme activity to return to normal.[7]

Mechanism

Suxamethonium is metabolised in the body by plasma cholinesterase. Ecothiopate iodide depresses the levels of this enzyme so that the metabolism of the suxamethonium is reduced and its effects are thereby enhanced and prolonged.[3,6] One study in 71 patients found that two drops of ecothiopate iodide 0.06% three times a week in each eye caused a twofold reduction in plasma cholinesterase (pseudocholinesterase) activity in about one-third of the patients, and a fourfold reduction in 1 in 7 patients.[8]

Importance and management

An established, adequately documented and clinically important interaction. The dosage of suxamethonium should be reduced appropriately because of the reduced plasma cholinesterase levels caused by ecothiopate. The study cited above[8] suggests that prolonged apnoea is likely in about 1 in 7 patients. One report describes the successful use of approximately one-fifth of the normal dosage of suxamethonium in a patient receiving 0.125% ecothiopate iodide solution, one drop twice a day in both eyes, and with a plasma cholinesterase activity 62% below normal. Recovery from the neuromuscular blockade was rapid and uneventful.[9] Another report describes the successful and uneventful use of atracurium in a patient receiving ecothiopate.[5] **Mivacurium** is also metabolised by plasma cholinesterase, and would be expected to interact with ecothiopate in the same way as suxamethonium.[10] Consider also 'Neuromuscular blockers + Anticholinesterases', p.114.

1. McGavi DDM. Depressed levels of serum-pseudocholinesterase with ecothiophate-iodide eyedrops. *Lancet* (1965) ii, 272–3.
2. Gesztes T. Prolonged apnoea after suxamethonium injection associated with eye drops containing an anticholinesterase agent. *Br J Anaesth* (1966) 38, 408–409.
3. Pantuck EJ. Ecothiopate iodide eye drops and prolonged response to suxamethonium. *Br J Anaesth* (1966) 38, 406–407.
4. Mone JG, Mathie WE. Qualitative and quantitative defects of pseudocholinesterase activity. *Anaesthesia* (1967) 22, 55–68.
5. Messer GJ, Stoudemire A, Knos G, Johnson GC. Electroconvulsive therapy and the chronic use of pseudocholinesterase-inhibitor (echothiophate iodide) eye drops for glaucoma. A case report. *Gen Hosp Psychiatry* (1992) 14, 56–60.
6. Cavallaro RJ, Krumperman LW, Kugler F. Effect of echothiophate therapy on the metabolism of succinylcholine in man. *Anesth Analg* (1968) 47, 570–4.
7. de Roetth A, Dettbarn W-D, Rosenberg P, Wilensky JG, Wong A. Effect of phospholine iodide on blood cholinesterase levels of normal and glaucoma subjects. *Am J Ophthalmol* (1965) 59, 586–92.
8. Eilderton TE, Farmati O, Zsigmond EK. Reduction in plasma cholinesterase levels after prolonged administration of echothiophate iodide eyedrops. *Can Anaesth Soc J* (1968) 15, 291–6.
9. Donati F, Bevan DR. Controlled succinylcholine infusion in a patient receiving echothiophate eye drops. *Can Anaesth Soc J* (1981) 28, 488–90.
10. Feldman S, Karalliedde L. Drug interactions with neuromuscular blockers. *Drug Safety* (1996) 15, 261–73.

Neuromuscular blockers + Ephedrine

A study in 80 patients found that premedication with ephedrine 10 mg reduced the onset time of rocuronium by roughly 30% but did not significantly affect that of atracurium.[1] The clinical significance of these effects is unclear.

1. Santiveri X, Mansilla R, Pardina B, Navarro J, Álvarez JC, Castillo J. La efedrina acorta el inicio de acción del rocuronio pero no del atracurio. *Rev Esp Anestesiol Reanim* (2003) 50, 176–81.

Neuromuscular blockers + Furosemide

The effects of the neuromuscular blockers have been both increased and decreased by furosemide.

Clinical evidence

(a) Increased neuromuscular blockade

Three patients receiving kidney transplants[1] developed increased neuromuscular blockade with **tubocurarine** (seen as a pronounced decrease in twitch tension) when given furosemide 40 or 80 mg and mannitol 12.5 g intravenously. One of them had the same reaction when later given only 40 mg of furosemide but no mannitol. The residual blockade was easily antagonised with pyridostigmine 14 mg or neostigmine 3 mg with atropine 1.2 mg.

(b) Decreased neuromuscular blockade

Ten neurosurgical patients given furosemide 1 mg/kg 10 minutes before induction of anaesthesia, took 14.7 minutes to recover from 95 to 50% blockade with **pancuronium** (as measured by a twitch response) compared with 21.8 minutes in 10 similar patients who had not received furosemide.[2]

Mechanism

Uncertain. *Animal* studies indicate that what happens probably depends on the dosage of furosemide: 0.1 to 10 micrograms/kg increased the blocking effects of tubocurarine and suxamethonium (succinylcholine) whereas 1 to 4 mg/kg opposed the blockade.[3] One suggestion is that low doses of furosemide may inhibit protein kinase causing a reduction in neuromuscular transmission, whereas higher doses cause inhibition of phosphodiesterase resulting in increased cyclic AMP activity and causing antagonism of neuromuscular blockade. It has also been suggested that large doses of loop diuretics may affect the renal excretion of neuromuscular blockers that are cleared by this route, resulting in more rapid recovery from the blockade.[3]

Importance and management

The documentation is very limited. Be on the alert for changes in the response to any blocker if furosemide is used.

1. Miller RD, Sohn YJ, Matteo RS. Enhancement of *d*-tubocurarine neuromuscular blockade by diuretics in man. *Anesthesiology* (1976) 45, 442–5.
2. Azar I, Cottrell J, Gupta B, Turndorf H. Furosemide facilitates recovery of evoked twitch response after pancuronium. *Anesth Analg* (1980) 59, 55–7.
3. Scappaticci KA, Ham JA, Sohn YJ, Miller RD, Dretchen KL. Effects of furosemide on the neuromuscular junction. *Anesthesiology* (1982) 57, 381–8.

Neuromuscular blockers + H_2-receptor antagonists

One report suggests that recovery from the neuromuscular blocking effects of suxamethonium (succinylcholine) is prolonged by cimetidine, but this may possibly have been due to the presence of metoclopramide. Four other reports say that no interaction occurs between suxamethonium and either cimetidine, famotidine or ranitidine. Cimetidine, but not ranitidine, has been reported to increase the effects of vecuronium. Cimetidine does not alter the effects of atracurium or rocuronium and ranitidine does not alter the effects of atracurium.

Clinical evidence

(a) Evidence of increased neuromuscular blockade

A study in 10 patients given **cimetidine** 300 mg orally at bedtime and another 300 mg 2 hours before anaesthesia, found that while the onset of action of **suxamethonium (succinylcholine)** 1.5 mg/kg intravenously was unchanged, when compared with 10 control patients, the time to recover 50% of the twitch height was prolonged 2 to 2.5-fold (from 8.6 to 20.3 minutes). One patient took 57 minutes to recover. His plasma cholinesterase levels were found to be normal.[1] It was later reported that some patients were also taking **metoclopramide**, which is known to interact in this way.[2] See also 'Neuromuscular blockers + Metoclopramide', p.127.

Another study[3] in 24 patients found that **cimetidine** 400 mg significantly prolonged the recovery (T1–25 period) from **vecuronium**, but few patients had any response to **cimetidine** 200 mg or **ranitidine** 100 mg. This slight prolongation of action of **vecuronium** due to **cimetidine** 400 mg was confirmed in another placebo-controlled study (mean time to return of T1 was 30 versus 22.5 minutes).[4] A study using a *rat* phrenic nerve diaphragm preparation found that **cimetidine** increased the neuromuscular blocking effects of **tubocurarine** and **pancuronium**, but there seem to be no reports confirming this in man.[5]

(b) Evidence of unchanged neuromuscular blockade

A study in 10 patients given 400 mg of **cimetidine** orally at bedtime and again 90 minutes before anaesthesia found no evidence of an effect on the neuromuscular blockade caused by **suxamethonium**, nor on its duration or recovery period, when compared with 10 control patients.[6] Another controlled study in patients given **cimetidine** 300 mg or **ranitidine** 150 mg, both the night before and 1 to 2 hours before surgery, found no evidence that the duration of action of **suxamethonium** or the activity of plasma cholinesterase were altered.[2] A study in 15 patients undergoing caesarean section also found no evidence that either **cimetidine** or **ranitidine** affected the neuromuscular blocking effects of **suxamethonium**.[7] A study in 70 patients[8] found no changes in the neuromuscular blocking effects of **suxamethonium** in those given **cimetidine** 400 mg, **ranitidine** 80 mg or **famotidine** 20 mg.

Cimetidine and **ranitidine** appear not to affect **atracurium**, **cimetidine** appears not to affect **rocuronium**,[9] and **ranitidine** appears not to affect **vecuronium**.[4] Another study found that premedication with **ranitidine** did not affect **vecuronium** blockade in postpartum patients, but that the neuromuscular blockade was prolonged in these patients compared with non-pregnant controls.[10]

Mechanism

Not understood. Studies with human plasma failed to find any evidence that cimetidine in therapeutic concentrations inhibits the metabolism of suxamethonium.[2,11] However, metoclopramide may do and therefore is possibly the drug responsible for any interaction seen. *In vitro* studies with very high cimetidine concentrations found inhibition of plasma cholinesterase (pseudocholinesterase) activity.[12] The cimetidine/vecuronium interaction is not understood, but it has been suggested that cimetidine may reduce the hepatic metabolism of vecuronium.[4]

Importance and management

Information seems to be limited to the reports cited. The most likely explanation for the discord between the cimetidine/suxamethonium results is that in the one study reporting increased suxamethonium effects[1] some of the patients were also given metoclopramide, which can inhibit plasma cholinesterase and prolong the effects of suxamethonium[2,8] (see also 'Neuromuscular blockers + Metoclopramide', p.127). In four other studies, cimetidine and other H_2-receptor antagonists did not alter suxamethonium effects. Therefore, it seems unlikely that an interaction exists. There is some evidence that cimetidine may slightly prolong the effects of vecuronium, but ranitidine appears not to interact. Atracurium and rocuronium appear not to be affected. Overall these possible interactions seem to be of little clinical significance.

1. Kambam JR, Dymond R, Krestow M. Effect of cimetidine on duration of action of succinylcholine. *Anesth Analg* (1987) 66, 191–2.
2. Woodworth GE, Sears DH, Grove TM, Ruff RH, Kosek PS, Katz RL. The effect of cimetidine and ranitidine on the duration of action of succinylcholine. *Anesth Analg* (1989) 68, 295–7.
3. Tryba M, Wruck G. Interaktionen von H_2-Antagonisten und nichtdepolarisierenden Muskelrelaxantien. *Anaesthesist* (1989) 38, 251–4.
4. McCarthy G, Mirakhur RK, Elliott P, Wright J. Effect of H_2-receptor antagonist pretreatment on vecuronium- and atracurium-induced neuromuscular block. *Br J Anaesth* (1991) 66, 713–15.
5. Galatulas I, Bossa R, Benvenuti C. Cimetidine increases the neuromuscular blocking activity of aminoglycoside antibiotics: antagonism by calcium. *Chem Indices Mec Proc Symp* (1981) 321–5.
6. Stirt JA, Sperry RJ, DiFazio CA. Cimetidine and succinylcholine: potential interaction and effect on neuromuscular blockade in man. *Anesthesiology* (1988) 69, 607–8.
7. Bogod DG, Oh TE. The effect of H_2 antagonists on duration of action of suxamethonium in the parturient. *Anaesthesia* (1989) 44, 591–3.
8. Turner DR, Kao YJ, Bivona C. Neuromuscular block by suxamethonium following treatment with histamine type 2 antagonists or metoclopramide. *Br J Anaesth* (1989) 63, 348–50.
9. Latorre F, de Almeida MCS, Stanek A, Weiler N, Kleemann PP. Beeinflussung der Pharmakodynamik von Rocuronium durch Cimetidin. *Anaesthesist* (1996) 45, 900–2.
10. Hawkins JL, Adenwala J, Camp C, Joyce TH. The effect of H_2-receptor antagonist premedication on the duration of vecuronium-induced neuromuscular blockade in postpartum patients. *Anesthesiology* (1989) 71, 175–7.
11. Cook DR, Stiller RL, Chakravorti S, Mannenhira T. Cimetidine does not inhibit plasma cholinesterase activity. *Anesth Analg* (1988) 67, 375–6.
12. Hansen WE, Bertl S. The inhibition of acetylcholinesterase and pseudocholinesterase by cimetidine. *Arzneimittelforschung* (1983) 33, 161–3.

Neuromuscular blockers + Immunosuppressants

There is limited evidence to suggest that the neuromuscular blocking effects of atracurium, pancuronium and vecuronium may be increased in some patients taking ciclosporin. There is also some evidence of reduced neuromuscular blockade with azathioprine and antilymphocyte immunoglobulins, but other evidence suggests that there is no clinically relevant interaction with azathioprine.

Clinical evidence

(a) Azathioprine or Antilymphocyte immunoglobulins

A retrospective study found that patients taking azathioprine or antilymphocyte immunoglobulins following organ transplantation needed an increased dosage of unspecified **muscle relaxants** to achieve satisfactory muscle relaxation.[1] A control group of 74 patients not receiving immunosuppression needed 0 to 10 mg of a **competitive (non-depolarising) muscle relaxant**; 13 patients taking azathioprine needed 12.5 to 25 mg; 11 patients receiving antilymphocyte immunoglobulins (antilymphocyte globulin) needed 10 to 20 mg and two patients taking azathioprine and guanethidine needed 55 and 90 mg.[1] However, a controlled study of 28 patients undergoing renal transplantation, who were receiving **atracurium, pancuronium** or **vecuronium** at a constant infusion rate, found that an injection of azathioprine 3 mg/kg given over 3 minutes caused a rapid, but only small and transient decrease of neuromuscular blockade. Ten minutes after the end of the azathioprine injection, a residual interaction was only detectable in those patients who had received **pancuronium**.[2]

(b) Ciclosporin

A retrospective study found that 4 of 36 patients receiving **atracurium** and 4 of 29 patients receiving **vecuronium** experienced prolonged neuromuscular blockade after anaesthesia for kidney transplantation. Respiratory failure occurred more often in patients who received intravenous ciclosporin during surgery.[3] Extended recovery times after **atracurium** and **vecuronium** are described in another report in renal transplant patients who had been taking oral ciclosporin.[4] Similarly, a prolonged duration of action of **vecuronium** was noted in 7 kidney transplant recipients, when compared with patients with normal renal function, and ciclosporin was considered to be a factor in this.[5] Two case reports describe prolonged neuromuscular blockade attributed to intravenous ciclosporin.

In the first report,[6] a woman with a 2-year renal transplant underwent surgery during which **pancuronium** 5.5 mg was used as the neuromuscular blocker. She was also given intravenous ciclosporin before and after surgery. The surgery lasted for 4 hours and no additional doses of **pancuronium** were given. Residual paralysis was inadequately reversed with neostigmine and atropine, and so edrophonium was given prior to extubation. However, she had to be re-intubated 20 minutes later because of increased respiratory distress.

In the second report,[7] a 15-year-old girl receiving intravenous ciclosporin with serum levels of 138 micrograms/L was anaesthetised using fentanyl, thiopental and **vecuronium** 100 micrograms/kg. Anaesthesia was maintained with nitrous oxide, oxygen and isoflurane. Attempts were later made to reverse the blockade with edrophonium, atropine and neostigmine but full neuromuscular function was not restored until 3 hours and 20 minutes after the **vecuronium** was given. Another report describes a prolongation of the effects of **vecuronium** in a renal-transplant recipient taking oral ciclosporin, azathioprine, and prednisolone.[8]

Mechanism

The reasons for the reduction in neuromuscular blockade with azathioprine and antilymphocyte immunoglobulins are not understood. It has been suggested that azathioprine may inhibit phosphodiesterase at the motor nerve terminal resulting in increased release of acetylcholine.[9]

The ciclosporin interaction may be partly due to the vehicle used in intravenous preparations. One idea is that *Cremophor*, a surfactant which has been used as a solvent for the ciclosporin, may increase the effective concentration of pancuronium at the neuromuscular junction.[6] Both compounds have been observed in *animal* studies to increase vecuronium blockade,[10] and *Cremophor* has also been seen to decrease the onset time of pancuronium blockade in patients given *Cremophor*-containing anaesthetics.[11] However, this is not the entire answer because the interaction has also been seen with oral ciclosporin, which does not contain *Cremophor*.[8]

Importance and management

Direct information seems to be limited to the reports cited, and the interactions are not established. Although retrospective data suggest that azathioprine and antilymphocyte immunoglobulins can cause a reduction in the effects of neuromuscular blockers, and in some cases the dosage may need to be increased two- to fourfold,[1] the only prospective study found that the interaction with azathioprine was not clinically significant.[2] The general importance of the ciclosporin interaction is also uncertain, but be alert for an increase in the effects of atracurium, pancuronium or vecuronium in any patient receiving ciclosporin. Not all patients appear to develop this interaction.[3] More study is needed.

1. Vetten KB. Immunosuppressive therapy and anaesthesia. *S Afr Med J* (1973) 47, 767–70.
2. Gramstad L. Atracurium, vecuronium and pancuronium in end-stage renal failure. Dose-response properties and interactions with azathioprine. *Br J Anaesth* (1987) 59, 995–1003.
3. Sidi A, Kaplan RF, Davis RF. Prolonged neuromuscular blockade and ventilatory failure after renal transplantation and cyclosporine. *Can J Anaesth* (1990) 37, 543–8.
4. Lepage JY, Malinowsky JM, de Dieuleveult C, Cozian A, Pinaud M, Souron R. Interaction cyclosporine atracurium et vecuronium. *Ann Fr Anesth Reanim* (1989) 8 (Suppl), R135.
5. Takita K, Goda Y, Kawahigashi H, Okuyama A, Kubota M, Kemmotsu O. Pharmacodynamics of vecuronium in the kidney transplant recipient and the patient with normal renal function. *Jpn J Anesthesiol* (1993) 42, 190–4.
6. Crosby E, Robblee JA. Cyclosporine-pancuronium interaction in a patient with a renal allograft. *Can J Anaesth* (1988) 35, 300–2.
7. Wood GG. Cyclosporine-vecuronium interaction. *Can J Anaesth* (1989) 36, 358.
8. Ganjoo P, Tewari P. Oral cyclosporine-vecuronium interaction. *Can J Anaesth* (1994) 41, 1017.
9. Viby-Mogensen J. Interaction of other drugs with muscle relaxants. *Semin Anesth* (1985) 4, 52–64.
10. Gramstad L, Gjerløw JA, Hysing ES, Rugstad HE. Interaction of cyclosporin and its solvent, cremophor, with atracurium and vecuronium: studies in the cat. *Br J Anaesth* (1986) 58, 1149–55.
11. Gramstad L, Lilleaasen P, Minsaas B. Onset time for alcuronium and pancuronium after cremophor-containing anaesthetics. *Acta Anaesthesiol Scand* (1981) 25, 484–6.

Neuromuscular blockers + Lansoprazole

There is some evidence that lansoprazole increases the duration of action of vecuronium.

Clinical evidence, mechanism, importance and management

In a study of 50 adult surgical patients, half of whom received lansoprazole 30 mg on the night before their operation, it was found that there was no significant difference between the time of onset of neuromuscular blockade by **vecuronium** in the two groups, but lansoprazole increased the duration of effect by about 34%.[1] This needs confirmation but be alert for this interaction in any patient treated with lansoprazole.

1. Ahmed SM, Panja C, Khan RM, Bano S. Lansoprazole potentiates vecuronium paralysis. *J Indian Med Assoc* (1997) 95, 422–3.

Neuromuscular blockers + Lithium

The concurrent use of neuromuscular blockers and lithium is normally safe and uneventful, but four patients taking lithium experienced prolonged blockade and respiratory difficulties after receiving standard doses of pancuronium and/or suxamethonium (succinylcholine).

Clinical evidence

A manic depressive woman taking lithium carbonate with a lithium level of 1.2 mmol/L, underwent surgery and was given thiopental, 310 mg of **suxamethonium** (**succinylcholine**) over a period of 2 hours, and 500 micrograms of **pancuronium**. Prolonged neuromuscular blockade with apnoea occurred.[1]

Three other patients taking lithium experienced enhanced neuromuscular blockade when given **pancuronium** alone,[2] with **suxamethonium**,[3] or both.[4] The authors of one of these reports[4] say that "...We have seen potentiation of the neuromuscular blockade produced by **succinylcholine** in several patients taking lithium carbonate..." but give no further details. In contrast, a retrospective analysis of data from 17 patients taking lithium carbonate, who received **suxamethonium** during a total of 78 ECT treatments, failed to reveal any instances of unusually prolonged recovery.[5] Interactions between lithium and pancuronium[1] or suxamethonium[6,7] have been demonstrated in *dogs,* and an interaction between lithium and **tubocurarine** has been demonstrated in *cats*,[8] but no clear interaction has been demonstrated with any other neuromuscular blocker.[7,9] A case of lithium toxicity has been described in a woman taking lithium who was given **suxamethonium**, but it is doubtful if it arose because of an interaction.[10]

Mechanism

Uncertain. One suggestion is that, when the interaction occurs, it may be due to changes in the electrolyte balance caused by the lithium, which results in changes in the release of acetylcholine at the neuromuscular junction.[8,11]

Importance and management

Information is limited. There are only four definite reports of this interaction in man, and good evidence that no adverse interaction normally occurs. Concurrent use need not be avoided but it would be prudent to be on the alert for this interaction in any patient taking lithium who is given any neuromuscular blocker.

1. Hill GE, Wong KC, Hodges MR. Potentiation of succinylcholine neuromuscular blockade by lithium carbonate. *Anesthesiology* (1976) 44, 439–42.
2. Borden H, Clarke MT, Katz H. The use of pancuronium bromide in patients receiving lithium carbonate. *Can Anaesth Soc J* (1974) 21, 79–82.
3. Rabolini V, Gatti G. Potenziamento del blocco neuro-muscolare di tipo depolarizzante da sali di litio (relazione su un caso). *Anest Rianim* (1988) 29, 157–9.
4. Rosner TM, Rosenberg M. Anesthetic problems in patients taking lithium. *J Oral Surg* (1981) 39, 282–5.
5. Martin BA, Kramer PM. Clinical significance of the interaction between lithium and a neuromuscular blocker. *Am J Psychiatry* (1982) 139, 1326–8.
6. Reimherr FW, Hodges MR, Hill GE, Wong KC. Prolongation of muscle relaxant effects by lithium carbonate. *Am J Psychiatry* (1977) 134, 205–6.
7. Hill GE, Wong KC, Hodges MR. Lithium carbonate and neuromuscular blocking agents. *Anesthesiology* (1977) 46, 122–6.
8. Basuray BN, Harris CA. Potentiation of d-tubocurarine (d-Tc) neuromuscular blockade in cats by lithium chloride. *Eur J Pharmacol* (1977) 45, 79–82.
9. Waud BE, Farrell L, Waud DR. Lithium and neuromuscular transmission. *Anesth Analg* (1982) 61, 399–402.
10. Jephcott G, Kerry RJ. Lithium: an anaesthetic risk. *Br J Anaesth* (1974) 46, 389–90.
11. Dehpour AR, Samadian T, Roushanzamir F. Interaction of aminoglycoside antibiotics and lithium at the neuromuscular junctions. *Drugs Exp Clin Res* (1992) 18, 383–7.

Neuromuscular blockers + Magnesium compounds

The effects of cisatracurium, mivacurium, pancuronium, rocuronium, tubocurarine, vecuronium, and probably other competitive neuromuscular blockers can be increased and prolonged by magnesium sulfate given parenterally. There is some evidence that magnesium may interact similarly with suxamethonium (succinylcholine), but also evidence from well-controlled trials that it does not.

Clinical evidence

(a) Competitive (non-depolarising) neuromuscular blockers

A pregnant 40-year-old with severe pre-eclampsia and receiving magnesium sulfate by infusion, underwent emergency caesarean section during which she was initially anaesthetised with thiopental, maintained with nitrous oxide/oxygen and enflurane, and given firstly suxamethonium and later **vecuronium** as muscle relaxants. At the end of surgery she rapidly recovered from the anaesthesia but the neuromuscular blockade was very prolonged (an eightfold increase in duration).[1] In a series of randomised studies involving 125 patients, pretreatment with intravenous magnesium sulfate 40 mg/kg reduced the dose requirement of **vecuronium** by 25%, approximately halved the time to the onset of action, and prolonged the duration of action from 25.2 to 43.3 minutes.[2] Another study found that pretreatment with 40 mg/kg of magnesium sulfate decreased the onset and prolonged the recovery time from **vecuronium** blockade, but magnesium sulfate 20 mg/kg had no effect.[3] Evidence of enhanced **vecuronium** neuromuscular blockade by magnesium sulfate is described in one other study,[4] and case report.[5] Another study in 20 patients found that recurarisation (sufficient to compromise respiration) occurred when magnesium sulfate 60 mg/kg was given in the postoperative period, shortly after recovery from neuromuscular block with **vecuronium**.[6] Neostigmine-induced recovery from **vecuronium** block was attenuated by about 30% in patients pretreated with magnesium sulfate in a randomised study. The authors demonstrated this was due to slower spontaneous recovery and not decreased response to neostigmine.[7]

In two patients who underwent cardiac surgery, neuromuscular block with either **pancuronium**, or **pancuronium** and **rocuronium** was prolonged by more than 10 hours. This was attributed to the effects of high doses of neuromuscular blockers potentiated by magnesium sulfate 2.5 g: moderate renal impairment may also have been a factor.[8] A fourfold increase in the duration of neuromuscular blockade of **rocuronium** 0.9 mg/kg was reported in a pregnant woman receiving magnesium sulfate.[9] A further randomised placebo-controlled study confirmed that pretreatment with magnesium sulfate 60 mg/kg increased the duration of neuromuscular block produced by **rocuronium** (time to initial recovery increased from 25.1 to 42.1 minutes), but the onset time was not affected.[10]

A patient given **cisatracurium** 14 mg during induction of anaesthesia, which was reversed postoperatively with 2 doses of neostigmine and glycopyrrolate, was then given intravenous magnesium sulfate 2 g over 5 minutes for atrial fibrillation, which had developed about 15 minutes after the end of surgery. Within a few minutes of receiving magnesium, recurarisation occurred and the patient required re-intubation and artificial ventilation for about 20 minutes.[11] A study in 20 patients undergoing elective cardiac surgery found that magnesium sulfate 70 mg/kg prior to induction followed by 30 mg/kg per hour prolonged the neuromuscular blockade induced with the first maintenance dose of **cisatracurium** by just over 30 minutes.[12]

The infusion rate of **mivacurium** required to obtain relaxation in women undergoing a caesarean section was about threefold lower in 12 women who had received magnesium sulfate for pre-eclampsia than in 12 women who had not.[13]

Prolonged neuromuscular block with **rapacuronium** has also been reported in a patient undergoing emergency caesarean section who received magnesium sulfate and clindamycin, although the clindamycin was thought to be mainly responsible (see also 'Neuromuscular blockers + Miscellaneous anti-infectives', p.127).[14]

Prolonged neuromuscular blockade has been described in three women with pre-eclampsia who were given magnesium sulfate and either **tubocurarine** alone or with **suxamethonium**.[15,16] Increased blockade by magnesium has been demonstrated with **tubocurarine** in *animals*.[15,17]

(b) Depolarising neuromuscular blockers

An early study in 59 women undergoing caesarean section found that those given magnesium sulfate for eclampsia and pre-eclampsia needed less **suxamethonium (succinylcholine)** than control patients (4.73 compared with 7.39 mg/kg per hour).[18] A 71-year-old woman given magnesium sulfate and lidocaine for ventricular tachycardia underwent emergency cardioversion and had a delayed onset and prolonged neuromuscular blockade when she was given **suxamethonium**.[19] Increased blockade by magnesium has been seen with **suxamethonium** in *animals*.[15,17]

However, a randomised study involving 20 patients found that pretreatment with a single 60-mg/kg bolus dose of magnesium sulfate did not significantly affect the onset or prolong the block produced by **suxamethonium**.[20] Similar results were found in a non-randomised study[4] and in a double-blind randomised study.[21] In randomised studies, the use of magnesium sulfate has also been reported to reduce **suxamethonium**-associated fasciculations[21] and reduce the increase in serum potassium levels produced by **suxamethonium**.[20]

Mechanism

Not fully understood. Magnesium sulfate has direct neuromuscular blocking activity by inhibiting the normal release of acetylcholine from nerve endings, reducing the sensitivity of the postsynaptic membrane and depressing the excitability of the muscle membranes. These effects are seen when serum magnesium levels rise above the normal range (hypermagnesaemia) and are possibly simply additive (or perhaps more than additive) with the effects of competitive neuromuscular blockers.

Importance and management

The interaction between competitive (non-depolarising) neuromuscular blockers and parenteral magnesium is established. Magnesium may decrease the time to onset (vecuronium but not rocuronium), prolong the duration of action and reduce the dose requirement of competitive neuromuscular blockers. Be alert for an increase in the effects of any competitive neuromuscular blocker if intravenous magnesium sulfate has been used, and anticipate the need to reduce the dose. Some have suggested that the decreased time to onset with vecuronium may be of use clinically to improve the intubating conditions for rapid sequence induction if suxamethonium is not suitable.[2] Intravenous calcium gluconate was used to assist recovery in one case of prolonged block.[15] Also be aware that recurarisation may occur when intravenous magnesium compounds are used in the postoperative period.[6,11] The authors of one report suggest that magnesium sulfate should be avoided for at least 30 minutes after reversal of residual neuromuscular block, to minimise the risk of recurarisation.[11] Hypermagnesaemia can occur in patients receiving magnesium in antacids, enemas or parenteral nutrition, especially if there is impaired renal function, but an interaction would not normally be expected, as oral magnesium compounds generally result in lower systemic levels than intravenous magnesium due to poor absorption.[22]

The interaction between magnesium and suxamethonium is not established. Although some *animal* and clinical evidence suggests potentiation of suxamethonium can occur, well-controlled studies have not confirmed this. Therefore some authors consider that magnesium sulfate does not significantly affect the clinical response to suxamethonium.[4,23]

1. Sinatra RS, Philip BK, Naulty JS, Ostheimer GW. Prolonged neuromuscular blockade with vecuronium in a patient treated with magnesium sulfate. *Anesth Analg* (1985) 64, 1220–2.
2. Fuchs-Buder T, Wilder-Smith OHG, Borgeat A, Tassonyi E. Interaction of magnesium sulphate with vecuronium-induced neuromuscular block. *Br J Anaesth* (1995) 74, 405–9.
3. Okuda T, Umeda T, Takemura M, Shiokawa Y, Koga Y. Pretreatment with magnesium sulphate enhances vecuronium-induced neuromuscular block. *Jpn J Anesthesiol* (1998) 47, 704–8.
4. Baraka A, Yazigi A. Neuromuscular interaction of magnesium with succinylcholine-vecuronium sequence in the eclamptic parturient. *Anesthesiology* (1987) 67, 806–8.
5. Hino H, Kaneko I, Miyazawa A, Aoki T, Ishizuka B, Kosugi K, Amemiya A. Prolonged neuromuscular blockade with vecuronium in patient with triple pregnancy treated with magnesium sulfate. *Jpn J Anesthesiol* (1997) 46, 266–70.
6. Fuchs-Buder T, Tassonyi E. Magnesium sulphate enhances residual neuromuscular block induced by vecuronium. *Br J Anaesth* (1996) 76, 565–6.
7. Fuchs-Buder T, Ziegenfuß T, Lysakowski K, Tassonyi E. Antagonism of vecuronium-induced neuromuscular block in patients pretreated with magnesium sulphate: dose-effect relationship of neostigmine. *Br J Anaesth* (1999) 82, 61–5.
8. Olivieri L, Plourde G. Prolonged (more than ten hours) neuromuscular blockade after cardiac surgery: report of two cases. *Can J Anesth* (2005) 52, 88–93.
9. Gaiser RR, Seem EH. Use of rocuronium in a pregnant patient with an open eye injury, receiving magnesium medication, for preterm labour. *Br J Anaesth* (1996) 77, 669–71.
10. Kussman B, Shorten G, Uppington J, Comunale ME. Administration of magnesium sulphate before rocuronium: effects on speed of onset and duration of neuromuscular block. *Br J Anaesth* (1997) 79, 122–4.
11. Fawcett WJ, Stone JP. Recurarization in the recovery room following the use of magnesium sulphate. *Br J Anaesth* (2003) 91, 435–8.
12. Pinard AM, Donati F, Martineau R, Denault AY, Taillefer J, Carrier M. Magnesium potentiates neuromuscular blockade with cisatracurium during cardiac surgery. *Can J Anesth* (2003) 50, 172–8.
13. Ahn EK, Bai SJ, Cho BJ, Shin Y-S. The infusion rate of mivacurium and its spontaneous neuromuscular recovery in magnesium-treated parturients. *Anesth Analg* (1998) 86, 523–6.
14. Sloan PA, Rasul M. Prolongation of rapacuronium neuromuscular blockade by clindamycin and magnesium. *Anesth Analg* (2002) 94, 123–4.
15. Ghoneim MM, Long JP. The interaction between magnesium and other neuromuscular blocking agents. *Anesthesiology* (1970) 32, 23–7.
16. de Silva AJC. Magnesium intoxication: an uncommon cause of prolonged curarization. *Br J Anaesth* (1973) 45, 1228–9.
17. Giesecke AH, Morris RE, Dalton MD, Stephen CR. Of magnesium, muscle relaxants, toxemic parturients, and cats. *Anesth Analg* (1968) 47, 689–95.
18. Morris R, Giesecke AH. Potentiation of muscle relaxants by magnesium sulfate therapy in toxemia of pregnancy. *South Med J* (1968) 61, 25–8.
19. Ip-Yam C, Allsop E. Abnormal response to suxamethonium in a patient receiving magnesium therapy. *Anaesthesia* (1994) 49, 355–6.
20. James MFM, Cork RC, Dennett JE. Succinylcholine pretreatment with magnesium sulfate. *Anesth Analg* (1986) 65, 373–6.
21. Stacey MRW, Barclay K, Asai T, Vaughan RS. Effects of magnesium sulphate on suxamethonium-induced complications during rapid-sequence induction of anaesthesia. *Anaesthesia* (1995) 50, 933–6.
22. Cammu G. Interactions of neuromuscular blocking drugs. *Acta Anaesthesiol Belg* (2001) 52, 357–63.
23. Guay J, Grenier Y, Varin F. Clinical pharmacokinetics of neuromuscular relaxants in pregnancy. *Clin Pharmacokinet* (1998) 34, 483–96.

Neuromuscular blockers + MAOIs

The effects of suxamethonium (succinylcholine) were enhanced in 3 patients taking phenelzine.

Clinical evidence, mechanism, importance and management

Two patients, one taking **phenelzine** and the other who had ceased to do so 6 days previously, developed apnoea following ECT during which **suxamethonium (succinylcholine)** was used. Both responded to injections of nikethamide and positive pressure ventilation with oxygen.[1] A later study observed the same response in another patient taking **phenelzine**.[2] This would appear to be explained by the finding that **phenelzine** caused a reduction in the levels of plasma cholinesterase (pseudocholinesterase) in 4 out of 10 patients studied. Since the metabolism of **suxamethonium** depends on this enzyme, reduced levels of the enzyme would result in a reduced rate of **suxamethonium** metabolism and in a prolongation of its effects. None of 12 other patients taking **tranylcypromine**, **isocarboxazid** or **mebanazine** had reduced plasma cholinesterase levels.[2]

It would clearly be prudent to be on the alert for this interaction in patients taking **phenelzine**. **Phenelzine** may be anticipated to react similarly with **mivacurium** as it is also metabolised by plasma cholinesterase.[3] On the basis of limited evidence this interaction seems less likely to occur with the other MAOIs cited.

1. Bleaden FA, Czekanska G. New drugs for depression. *BMJ* (1960) 1, 200.
2. Bodley PO, Halwax K, Potts L. Low serum pseudocholinesterase levels complicating treatment with phenelzine. *BMJ* (1969) 3, 510–12.
3. Feldman S, Karalliedde L. Drug interactions with neuromuscular blockers. *Drug Safety* (1996) 15, 261–73.

Neuromuscular blockers + Metoclopramide

The neuromuscular blocking effects of suxamethonium (succinylcholine) and mivacurium can be increased and prolonged in patients taking metoclopramide.

Clinical evidence

Metoclopramide 10 mg given intravenously 1 to 2 hours before induction of anaesthesia prolonged the time to 25% recovery after **suxamethonium** (**succinylcholine**) by 1.83 minutes (23%) in 19 patients, when compared with 21 control patients.[1,2] A larger 20-mg dose of metoclopramide prolonged the time to recovery by 56% in a further 10 patients.[1] In another study by the same research group, the recovery from neuromuscular blockade (time from 95% to 25% suppression of the activity of the adductor pollicis muscle) due to **suxamethonium** was prolonged by 67% in 11 patients who were given metoclopramide 10 mg intravenously during surgery, one minute before the **suxamethonium**.[3]

A randomised, placebo-controlled, double-blind study in 30 patients found that 150 micrograms/kg of intravenous metoclopramide given prior to anaesthetic induction about 10 minutes before **mivacurium** 150 micrograms/kg prolonged the duration of action of **mivacurium** by about 30%.[4] Another report found that infusion rates of **mivacurium** were reduced by up to about 80% in patients given metoclopramide 10 or 20 mg intravenously, 5 minutes before induction, and metoclopramide delayed complete recovery from neuromuscular block after **mivacurium** by 36% (10 mg dose) and 50% (20 mg dose).[5] Delays in recovery from **mivacurium** block of 78% after metoclopramide 20 mg were found in another study.[6]

Mechanism

Metoclopramide is postulated to reduce the activity of plasma cholinesterase, which is responsible for the metabolism of suxamethonium and mivacurium. One *in vitro* study found that a metoclopramide level of 800 nanograms/mL inhibited plasma cholinesterase activity by 50%. However, a 10-mg dose of metoclopramide in adult patients weighing 50 to 70 kg produces peak plasma levels five times less than this (140 nanograms/mL).[7] Further, in an *in vivo* study, metoclopramide had only minimal inhibitory effects on plasma cholinesterase, and there was no difference in plasma cholinesterase levels in patients who had received metoclopramide and those who had not.[4]

Importance and management

The interaction between metoclopramide and suxamethonium is an established but not extensively documented interaction of only moderate or minor clinical importance. However anaesthetists should be aware that some enhancement of blockade can occur. The interaction between metoclopramide and mivacurium has only more recently been demonstrated. Metoclopramide appears to allow a reduction in the infusion rate of mivacurium and it causes a significant delay in recovery from neuromuscular block. Care is recommended during combined use.[5] The authors of the suxamethonium reports also point out that plasma cholinesterase activity is reduced in pregnancy and so suxamethonium sensitivity is more likely in obstetric patients. Ester-type local anaesthetics also depend on plasma cholinesterase activity for metabolism[1,7] and their effects would therefore be expected to be additive with the effects of metoclopramide, see 'Neuromuscular blockers + Anaesthetics, local', p.114.

1. Kao YJ, Tellez J, Turner DR. Dose-dependent effect of metoclopramide on cholinesterases and suxamethonium metabolism. *Br J Anaesth* (1990) 65, 220–4.
2. Turner DR, Kao YJ, Bivona C. Neuromuscular block by suxamethonium following treatment with histamine type 2 antagonists or metoclopramide. *Br J Anaesth* (1989) 63, 348–50.
3. Kao YJ, Turner DR. Prolongation of succinylcholine block by metoclopramide. *Anesthesiology* (1989) 70, 905–8.
4. Skinner HJ, Girling KJ, Whitehurst A, Nathanson MH. Influence of metoclopramide on plasma cholinesterase and duration of action of mivacurium. *Br J Anaesth* (1999) 82, 542–5.
5. El Ayass N, Hendrickx P. Decreased mivacurium infusion rate and delayed neuromuscular recovery after metoclopramide: a randomized double blind placebo-controlled study. *Eur J Anaesthesiol* (2005) 22, 197–201.
6. Motamed C, Kirov K, Combes X, Dhonneur G, Duvaldestin P. Effect of metoclopramide on mivacurium-induced neuromuscular block. *Acta Anaesthesiol Scand* (2002) 46, 214–16.
7. Kambam JR, Parris WCV, Franks JJ, Sastry BVR, Naukam R, Smith BE. The inhibitory effect of metoclopramide on plasma cholinesterase activity. *Can J Anaesth* (1988) 35, 476–8.

Neuromuscular blockers + Miscellaneous anti-infectives

Colistin, colistimethate sodium, polymyxin B, clindamycin, lincomycin, some penicillins (apalcillin, azlocillin, mezlocillin, piperacillin) and vancomycin possess some neuromuscular blocking activity. Increased and prolonged neuromuscular blockade is possible if these antibacterials are used with neuromuscular blocking drugs. In theory amphotericin B might also interact, but the tetracyclines probably do not. No clinically significant interaction has been seen with cefoxitin, cefuroxime, chloramphenicol or metronidazole. See also 'Neuromuscular blockers + Aminoglycosides', p.113.

Clinical evidence

(a) Amphotericin B

Amphotericin B can induce hypokalaemia resulting in muscle weakness,[1] which might be expected to enhance the effects of neuromuscular blockers, but there appear to be no reports in the literature confirming that a clinically significant interaction actually occurs.

(b) Cephalosporins

No change in neuromuscular blockade was seen in patients given intravenous **cefuroxime** shortly before **pipecuronium**[2] or **rocuronium**[3] in a controlled study. Similarly, intravenous **cefoxitin** given before, during and after surgery was not associated with a clinically important prolongation of **vecuronium** blockade.[4]

(c) Chloramphenicol

No interaction was seen in myasthenic patients given chloramphenicol.[5]

(d) Clindamycin, Lincomycin

Enhanced blockade has been seen in patients given **pancuronium** and lincomycin, which was reversed by neostigmine.[6] Respiratory paralysis was seen 10 minutes after lincomycin 600 mg was given intramuscularly to a man recovering from neuromuscular blockade with **tubocurarine**[7] and this interaction was confirmed in another report.[8] Other case reports[9-11] and clinical studies[12] describe minor to marked increases in neuromuscular blockade in patients receiving **pancuronium**,[10] **pipecuronium**,[12] **rapacuronium**[11] or **suxamethonium** (**succinylcholine**)[9] when they were given **clindamycin**. One patient developed very prolonged blockade after being unintentionally given clindamycin 2.4 g instead of 600 mg shortly after recovery from **suxamethonium** and **tubocurarine**.[13] Prolongation of the neuromuscular blocking effects of **vecuronium** has also been reported in a patient who received both clindamycin and gentamicin.[14]

(e) Metronidazole

An increase in the neuromuscular blocking effects of **vecuronium** with metronidazole has been reported in *cats*,[15] but a later study in patients failed to find any evidence of an interaction,[16] and another study with **rocuronium** also found no evidence of an interaction with metronidazole.[3] Similarly, no interaction was seen with **rocuronium** and metronidazole/**cefuroxime**.[3] Another study found no significant interaction between **pipecuronium** and metronidazole.[2]

(f) Penicillins

A study in patients found that the neuromuscular blocking effects of **vecuronium** were prolonged by a number of penicillins: apalcillin 26%, **azlocillin** 55%, **mezlocillin** 38%, and **piperacillin** 46%.[17] Reinstitution of neuromuscular blockade and respiratory failure occurred in a patient given **piperacillin** 3 g by intravenous infusion postoperatively, following the reversal of **vecuronium** blockade.[18] However, a randomised, double-blind study involving 30 patients found that **piperacillin** or **cefoxitin**, given by intravenous infusion, pre- and intraoperatively, were not associated with clinically important prolongation of the neuromuscular block induced by **vecuronium**. Of 27 patients who could be evaluated, 22 showed a modest overall decrease in recovery time and 5 patients (2 patients after receiving **piperacillin** and 3 patients after **cefoxitin**) exhibited a slight prolongation in recovery time, but these patients all responded readily to neostigmine or other anticholinesterases and subsequent recurarisation did not occur.[4] No interaction was seen in a myasthenic patient given **ampicillin**.[19]

(g) Polymyxins

A literature review of interactions between antibiotics and neuromuscular blockers identified 17 cases over the period 1956 to 1970 period in which **colistin (polymyxin E)** or **colistimethate sodium**, with or without conventional neuromuscular blockers, were responsible for the development of increased blockade and respiratory muscle paralysis. Some of the patients had renal disease.[20] A later report describes prolonged respiratory depression in a patient receiving **pancuronium** and **colistin**.[21] Calcium gluconate was found to reverse the blockade.[21] A placebo-controlled study found that one million units of **colistin** also considerably prolonged the recovery time from **pipecuronium** blockade.[12] Six cases of enhanced neuromuscular blockade involving **polymyxin B** have also been reported.[20] An increase in the blockade due to **pancuronium** by **polymyxin B** and bacitracin wound irrigation is described in another report; pyridostigmine, neostigmine and edrophonium were ineffective antagonists of this block and only partial improvement occurred after calcium chloride was given.[22] Prolonged and fatal apnoea occurred in another patient given **suxamethonium** when his peritoneal cavity was instilled with a solution containing 100 mg of **polymyxin B** and 100 000 units of bacitracin.[23]

(h) Tetracyclines

Four cases of enhanced neuromuscular blockade with **rolitetracycline** or **oxytetracycline** in myasthenic patients have been reported[20] (2 cases originally reported elsewhere[19]) but there seem to be no reports of interactions in patients without myasthenia given neuromuscular blocking drugs.

(i) Vancomycin

A man recovering from neuromuscular blockade with **suxamethonium** (with some evidence of residual Phase II block) developed almost total muscle paralysis and apnoea when given an intravenous infusion of vancomycin. He recovered spontaneously when the vancomycin was stopped, but it took several hours.[24] The neuromuscular blockade due to **vecuronium** was increased in a patient when given an infusion of vancomycin (1 g in 250 mL of saline over 35 minutes).[25] Transient apnoea and apparent cardiac arrest have also been described in a patient following a 1-g intravenous injection of vancomycin given over 2 minutes.[26] However, in both of these cases[25,26] the vancomycin was given more rapidly than the current recommendations. It is now known that rapid infusion of vancomycin can provoke histamine release, which can result in apnoea, hypotension, anaphylaxis and muscular spasm, effects similar to those seen in these two patients.

Mechanism

Not fully understood but several sites of action at the neuromuscular junction (pre and/or post, effects on ion-channels or receptors) have been suggested.

The neuromuscular blocking properties of the polymyxins (polymyxin B, colistin, colistimethate sodium) involve a number of mechanisms, which may explain the difficulty in reversing the blockade.[27]

Importance and management

The interactions involving polymyxin B, colistin, colistimethate sodium, lincomycin, and clindamycin are established and clinically important. The incidence is uncertain. Concurrent use need not be avoided, but be alert for increased and prolonged neuromuscular blockade. The recovery period should be well monitored because of the risk of recurarisation. Check the outcome of using amphotericin. No interaction would be expected with the tetracyclines, cefuroxime, cefoxitin, metronidazole or metronidazole/cefuroxime, and probably with ampicillin and chloramphenicol, but some caution would seem appropriate with azlocillin, mezlocillin and piperacillin. The situation with vancomycin is less clear. The evidence does suggest a link between vancomycin and increased neuromuscular blockade following the use of suxamethonium, and possibly vecuronium. However, vancomycin is given routinely as antibiotic prophylaxis before surgical procedures. The sparsity of reports therefore suggests that in practice vancomycin rarely causes a clinically significant interaction with neuromuscular blockers.

1. Drutz DJ, Fan JH, Tai TY, Cheng JT, Hsieh WC. Hypokalemic rhabdomyolysis and myoglobinuria following amphotericin B therapy. *JAMA* (1970) 211, 824–6.
2. Stanley JC, Mirakhur RK, Clarke RSJ. Study of pipecuronium-antibiotic interaction. *Anesthesiology* (1990) 73, A898.
3. Cooper R, Maddineni VR, Mirakhur RK. Clinical study of interaction between rocuronium and some commonly used antimicrobial agents. *Eur J Anaesthesiol* (1993) 10, 331–5.
4. Condon RE, Munshi CA, Arfman RC. Interaction of vecuronium with piperacillin or cefoxitin evaluated in a prospective, randomized, double-blind clinical trial. *Am Surg* (1995) 61, 403–6.
5. Gibbels E. Weitere Beobachtungen zur Nebenwirkung intravenöser Reverin-Gaben bei Myasthenia gravis pseudoparalytica. *Dtsch Med Wochenschr* (1967) 92, 1153–4.
6. Booij LHDJ, Miller RD, Crul JF. Neostigmine and 4-aminopyridine antagonism of lincomycin-pancuronium neuromuscular blockade in man. *Anesth Analg* (1978) 57, 316–21.
7. Samuelson RJ, Giesecke AH, Kallus FT, Stanley VF. Lincomycin-curare interaction. *Anesth Analg* (1975) 54, 103–5.
8. Hashimoto Y, Iwatsuki N, Shima T, Iwatsuki K. Neuromuscular blocking properties of lincomycin and Kanendomycin® in man. *Jpn J Anesthesiol* (1971) 20, 407–11.
9. Avery D, Finn R. Succinylcholine-prolonged apnea associated with clindamycin and abnormal liver function tests. *Dis Nerv Syst* (1977) 38, 473–5.
10. Fogdall RP, Miller RD. Prolongation of a pancuronium-induced neuromuscular blockade by clindamycin. *Anesthesiology* (1974) 41, 407–8.
11. Sloan PA, Rasul M. Prolongation of rapacuronium neuromuscular blockade by clindamycin and magnesium. *Anesth Analg* (2002) 94, 123–4.
12. de Gouw NE, Crul JF, Vandermeersch E, Mulier JP, van Egmond J, Van Aken H. Interaction of antibiotics on pipecuronium-induced neuromuscular blockade. *J Clin Anesth* (1993) 5, 212–5.
13. Al Ahdal O, Bevan DR. Clindamycin-induced neuromuscular blockade. *Can J Anaesth* (1995) 42, 614–7.
14. Jedeikin R, Dolgunski E, Kaplan R, Hoffman S. Prolongation of neuromuscular blocking effect of vecuronium by antibiotics. *Anaesthesia* (1987) 42, 858–60.
15. McIndewar IC, Marshall RJ. Interactions between the neuromuscular blocking drug ORG NC 45 and some anaesthetic, analgesic and antimicrobial agents. *Br J Anaesth* (1981) 53, 785–92.
16. d'Hollander A, Agoston S, Capouet V, Barvais L, Bomblet JP, Esselen M. Failure of metronidazole to alter a vecuronium neuromuscular blockade in humans. *Anesthesiology* (1985) 63, 99–102.
17. Tryba M. Wirkungsverstärkung nicht-depolarisierender Muskelrelaxantien durch Acylaminopenicilline. Untersuchungen am Beispiel von Vecuronium. *Anaesthesist* (1985) 34, 651–55.
18. Mackie K, Pavlin EG. Recurrent paralysis following piperacillin administration. *Anesthesiology* (1990) 72, 561–3.
19. Wullen F, Kast G, Bruck A. Über Nebenwirkungen bei Tetracyclin-Verabreichung an Myastheniker. *Dtsch Med Wochenschr* (1967) 92, 667–9.
20. Pittinger CB, Eryasa Y, Adamson R. Antibiotic-induced paralysis. *Anesth Analg* (1970) 49, 487–501.
21. Giala MM, Paradelis AG. Two cases of prolonged respiratory depression due to interaction of pancuronium with colistin and streptomycin. *J Antimicrob Chemother* (1979) 5, 234–5.
22. Fogdall RP, Miller RD. Prolongation of a pancuronium-induced neuromuscular blockade by polymyxin B. *Anesthesiology* (1974) 40, 84–7.
23. Small GA. Respiratory paralysis after a large dose of intraperitoneal polymyxin B and bacitracin. *Anesth Analg* (1964) 43, 137–9.
24. Albrecht RF, Lanier WL. Potentiation of succinylcholine-induced phase II block by vancomycin. *Anesth Analg* (1993) 77, 1300–1302.
25. Huang KC, Heise A, Shrader AK, Tsueda K. Vancomycin enhances the neuromuscular blockade of vecuronium. *Anesth Analg* (1990) 71, 194–6.
26. Glicklich D, Figura I. Vancomycin and cardiac arrest. *Ann Intern Med* (1984) 101, 880–1.
27. Østergaard D, Engbaek J, Viby-Mogensen J. Adverse reactions and interactions of the neuromuscular blocking drugs. *Med Toxicol Adverse Drug Exp* (1989) 4, 351–68.

Neuromuscular blockers + Neuromuscular blockers

Combinations of competitive neuromuscular blockers may have additive or synergistic effects. However, the sequence of administration may also affect the interaction. Prior administration of a small dose of a competitive neuromuscular blocker (e.g. vecuronium) generally reduces the effects of a depolarising blocker (e.g. suxamethonium), but if the depolarising blocker is given during recovery from a competitive neuromuscular blocker, antagonism, enhancement or a combination of the two may occur. The effects of a competitive blocker may be increased if it is given after a depolarising blocker.

Clinical evidence, mechanism, importance and management

Neuromuscular blockers are of two types: **competitive (non-depolarising)** and **depolarising**:

The **competitive** or **non-depolarising** blockers (**atracurium** and others listed in 'Table 5.2', (p.91)) compete with acetylcholine for the receptors on the endplate of the neuromuscular junction. Thus the receptors fail to be stimulated and muscular paralysis results. Competitive neuromuscular blockers may be divided by chemical structure into the **aminosteroid** group (e.g. **pancuronium**) and the **benzylisoquinolinium** group (e.g. **atracurium**), see also 'Table 5.2', (p.91).

The **depolarising** blockers (**suxamethonium (succinylcholine)** and **decamethonium**) also occupy the receptors on the endplate but they act like acetylcholine to cause depolarisation. However, unlike acetylcholine, they are not immediately removed by cholinesterase so that the depolarisation persists and the muscle remains paralysed.

(a) Competitive neuromuscular blockers + Competitive neuromuscular blockers

Combinations of competitive (non-depolarising) neuromuscular blockers may have additive or synergistic effects. Structural differences between the interacting neuromuscular blockers may have an effect; it has been suggested that structurally similar neuromuscular blockers tend to produce an additive response, whereas structurally different blockers may be synergistic.[1,2] For example, additive effects have been found between the structurally similar combinations of:

- **atracurium** and **cisatracurium**[3] or **mivacurium**,[4]
- **pancuronium** and **vecuronium**,[5]
- **pipecuronium** and **vecuronium**,[6]
- **tubocurarine** and **metocurine**.[1]

Potentiation of neuromuscular blockade or synergy has been reported between the structurally different combinations of:

- **cisatracurium** and **rocuronium**[3,7,8] or **vecuronium**,[3]
- **metocurine** and **pancuronium**,[1]
- **mivacurium** and **pancuronium**[2,9] or **rocuronium**,[10]
- **tubocurarine** and **pancuronium**[1] or **vecuronium**.[11]

However, contrary to the prediction, synergism has been reported with the structurally similar combinations of:

- **cisatracurium** and **mivacurium**,[3]
- **tubocurarine** and **atracurium**.[11]

In addition to affecting response, the initial blocker may modify the duration of action of the supplemental blocker.[12,13] The blocking action of **pancuronium** was shortened when it was given during **vecuronium**-induced partial neuromuscular blockade.[13] Conversely, the duration of action of **mivacurium**[2,14] or **vecuronium**[13] was lengthened when they were given after **pancuronium**-induced neuromuscular block. Therefore, care should be taken if a small dose of a short-acting blocker is given near the end of an operation in which a longer-acting blocker has already been given.

(b) Competitive then depolarising neuromuscular blockers

The combination of a competitive and a depolarising neuromuscular blocker has an intrinsic antagonistic effect. This interaction has been used clinically to reduce muscle fasciculations caused by **suxamethonium**. A small dose of competitive neuromuscular blocker given shortly before the **suxamethonium** generally reduces effects and the duration of action of the suxamethonium.[15] However, following **pancuronium** pretreatment, the duration of **suxamethonium** blockade appears to be prolonged,[15] and this is probably due to the inhibition of cholinesterase by pancuronium.[16] Antagonism of **decamethonium** has also been seen when it was given after a small dose of **vecuronium**.[17]

If **suxamethonium** is given during the recovery from a paralysing dose of a competitive neuromuscular blocker, the resultant neuromuscular block is influenced by the depth of residual block and the dose of suxamethonium used.[18,19] In a study involving 38 patients recovering from **atracurium** 400 micrograms/kg, lower intravenous doses of **suxamethonium** 0.25 to 1 mg/kg mainly antagonised the partial block, whereas higher doses 1.5 to 3 mg/kg usually enhanced the blockade.[18] However, the degree of recovery from the underlying block also influences the effects of **suxamethonium**: early on when the residual block is still considerable, suxamethonium may appear to have no effect or produce a partial antagonism of the block, but later, a biphasic response may be seen (antagonism of the competitive block initially before superimposing a depolarising block); a combination of antagonism and enhancement may also occur in different muscle groups.[19] Partial antagonism of **vecuronium** block has been seen in 5 patients given **decamethonium** during the recovery from vecuronium block.[20] The neuromuscular blockade will also be affected by the competitive neuromuscular blocker used and whether or not an anticholinesterase has been given.[18,19] See also, 'Neuromuscular blockers + Anticholinesterases', p.114.

Suxamethonium and **decamethonium** would be expected to antagonise competitive neuromuscular blockers due to their opposite mechanisms of action (**suxamethonium** and **decamethonium** exert a receptor agonist-type activity whereas competitive blockers exhibit receptor antagonism). However, the depolarising blockers may also reverse a competitive block by enhancing the effect of acetylcholine postsynaptically.[20,21]

(c) Depolarising then competitive neuromuscular blockers

In general, when a competitive blocker is given following **suxamethonium**, the onset time may be reduced and the potency or duration of the block may be increased, although not always significantly. In a study involving 350 patients, prior administration of **suxamethonium** 1 mg/kg significantly accelerated the onset of neuromuscular blockade with **atracurium, pancuronium, pipecuronium** and **vecuronium**, when these were given after full recovery from the **suxamethonium** block. However, the duration of blockade was only significantly prolonged with **vecuronium**.[22] One study found potentiation of **vecuronium** when it was given up to 30 minutes after full recovery from a single intravenous dose of **suxamethonium** 1 mg/kg.[23] Another study found the effects of **vecuronium** or **pancuronium** were potentiated for at least 2 hours after full recovery from an intubating dose of **suxamethonium**.[24] Another study showed that the effect of prior administration of **suxamethonium** on **atracurium** neuromuscular block appears to depend on the level of recovery from **suxamethonium**. As with previous studies, the onset of **atracurium** blockade was shortened when given after full recovery from the **suxamethonium**. However, this effect was less apparent when the **atracurium** was given before full suxamethonium recovery.[25] Pretreatment with **suxamethonium** reduced the time to onset of **cisatracurium** block, but did not potentiate it or prolong recovery.[26] Pretreatment with **suxamethonium** decreased the onset time and increased the duration of action or **rocuronium**[27] although a study in *animals* suggested **rocuronium** is not affected by **suxamethonium**.[28]

Prior administration of **decamethonium** 100 micrograms/kg caused a sevenfold increase in sensitivity to **vecuronium** (reducing the ED_{50} from 24 to 3.5 micrograms/kg).[20]

It has been suggested that depolarising neuromuscular blockers such as **decamethonium** and **suxamethonium** may have a presynaptic action resulting in reduced acetylcholine output.[20] Although not always clinically significant, be aware that a reduction in the dose of competitive blocker may be necessary following the use of a depolarising neuromuscular blocker.

1. Lebowitz PW, Ramsey FM, Savarese JJ, Ali HH. Potentiation of neuromuscular blockade in man produced by combinations of pancuronium and metocurine or pancuronium and *d*-tubocurarine. *Anesth Analg* (1980) 59, 604–9.
2. Kim KS, Shim JC, Kim DW. Interactions between mivacurium and pancuronium. *Br J Anaesth* (1997) 79, 19–23.
3. Kim KS, Chun YS, Chon SU, Suh JK. Neuromuscular interaction between cisatracurium and mivacurium, atracurium, vecuronium or rocuronium administered in combination. *Anaesthesia* (1998) 53, 872–8.
4. Naguib M, Abdulatif M, Al-Ghamdi A, Selim M, Seraj M, El-Sanbary M, Magboul MA. Interactions between mivacurium and atracurium. *Br J Anaesth* (1994) 73, 484–9.
5. Ferres CJ, Mirakhur RK, Pandit SK, Clarke RSJ, Gibson FM. Dose-response studies with pancuronium, vecuronium and their combination. *Br J Clin Pharmacol* (1984) 18, 947–50.
6. Smith I, White PF. Pipecuronium-induced prolongation of vecuronium neuromuscular block. *Br J Anaesth* (1993) 70, 446–8.
7. Naguib M, Samarkandi AH, Ammar A, Elfaqih SR, Al-Zahrani S, Turkistani A. Comparative clinical pharmacology of rocuronium, cisatracurium, and their combination. *Anesthesiology* (1998) 89, 1116–24.
8. Breslin DS, Jiao K, Habib AS, Schultz J, Gan TJ. Pharmacodynamic interactions between cisatracurium and rocuronium. *Anesth Analg* (2004) 98, 107–10.
9. Motamed C, Menad R, Farinotti R, Kirov K, Combes X, Bouleau D, Feiss P, Duvaldestin P. Potentiation of mivacurium blockade by low dose of pancuronium. A pharmacokinetic study. *Anesthesiology* (2003) 98, 1057–62.
10. Naguib M. Neuromuscular effects of rocuronium bromide and mivacurium chloride administered alone and in combination. *Anesthesiology* (1994) 81, 388–95.
11. Middleton CM, Pollard BJ, Healy TEJ, Kay B. Use of atracurium or vecuronium to prolong the action of tubocurarine. *Br J Anaesth* (1989) 62, 659–63.
12. Okamoto T, Nakai T, Aoki T, Satoh T. Interaction between vecuronium and pancuronium. *Jpn J Anesthesiol* (1993) 42, 534–9.
13. Rashkovsky OM, Agoston S, Ket JM. Interaction between pancuronium bromide and vecuronium bromide. *Br J Anaesth* (1985) 57, 1063–6.
14. Erkola O, Rautoma P, Meretoja OA. Mivacurium when preceded by pancuronium becomes a long-acting muscle relaxant. *Anesthesiology* (1996) 84, 562–5.
15. Ferguson A, Bevan DR. Mixed neuromuscular block. The effect of precurarization. *Anaesthesia* (1981) 36, 661–6.
16. Stovner J, Oftedal N, Holmboe J. The inhibition of cholinesterases by pancuronium. *Br J Anaesth* (1975) 47, 949–54.
17. Campkin NTA, Hood JR, Feldman SA. Resistance to decamethonium neuromuscular block after prior administration of vecuronium. *Anesth Analg* (1993) 77, 78–80.

18. Scott RPF, Norman J. Effect of suxamethonium given during recovery from atracurium. *Br J Anaesth* (1988) 61, 292–6.
19. Black AMS. Effect of suxamethonium given during recovery from atracurium. *Br J Anaesth* (1989) 62, 348–9.
20. Feldman S, Fauvel N. Potentiation and antagonism of vecuronium by decamethonium. *Anesth Analg* (1993) 76, 631–4.
21. Braga MFM, Rowan EG, Harvey AL, Bowman WC. Interactions between suxamethonium and non-depolarizing neuromuscular blocking drugs. *Br J Anaesth* (1994) 72, 198–204.
22. Swen J, Koot HWJ, Bencini A, Ket JM, Hermans J, Agoston S. The interaction between suxamethonium and the succeeding non-depolarizing neuromuscular blocking agent. *Eur J Anaesthesiol* (1990) 7, 203–9.
23. d'Hollander AA, Agoston S, De Ville A, Cuvelier F. Clinical and pharmacological actions of a bolus injection of suxamethonium: two phenomena of distinct duration. *Br J Anaesth* (1983) 55, 131–4.
24. Ono K, Manabe N, Ohta Y, Morita K, Kosaka F. Influence of suxamethonium on the action of subsequently administered vecuronium or pancuronium. *Br J Anaesth* (1989) 62, 324–6.
25. Roed J, Larsen PB, Olsen JS, Engbæk J. The effect of succinylcholine on atracurium-induced neuromuscular block. *Acta Anaesthesiol Scand* (1997) 41, 1331–4.
26. Pavlin EG, Forrest AP, Howard M, Quessy S, McClung C. Prior administration of succinylcholine does not affect the duration of Nimbex (51W89) neuromuscular blockade. *Anesth Analg* (1995) 80, S374.
27. Robertson EN, Driessen JJ, Booij LHDJ. Suxamethonium administration prolongs the duration of action of subsequent rocuronium. *Eur J Anaesthesiol* (2004) 21, 734–7.
28. Muir AW, Anderson KA, Pow E. Interaction between rocuronium bromide and some drugs used during anaesthesia. *Eur J Anaesthesiol* (1994) 11 (Suppl 9), 93–8.

Neuromuscular blockers + Ondansetron

Ondansetron does not affect atracurium-induced neuromuscular blockade.

Clinical evidence, mechanism, importance and management

A double-blind placebo-controlled study of 30 patients undergoing elective surgery found that intravenous ondansetron 8 or 16 mg given over 5 minutes had no effect on subsequent neuromuscular blockade with **atracurium**.[1] No special precautions would therefore seem necessary. The authors suggest that no interaction is likely with other non-depolarising neuromuscular blockers, but this needs confirmation.

1. Lien CA, Gadalla F, Kudlak TT, Embree PB, Sharp GJ, Savarese JJ. The effect of ondansetron on atracurium-induced neuromuscular blockade. *J Clin Anesth* (1993) 5, 399–403.

Neuromuscular blockers + Opioids

A woman experienced hypertension and tachycardia when she was given pancuronium after induction of anaesthesia with morphine and nitrous oxide/oxygen. Bradycardia has been reported with vecuronium and alfentanil, fentanyl, or sufentanil, sometimes in patients receiving beta blockers and/or calcium channel blockers.

Clinical evidence, mechanism, importance and management

(a) Pancuronium

A woman about to receive a coronary by-pass graft was premedicated with **morphine** 10 mg and hyoscine 400 micrograms, intramuscularly, one hour before the induction of anaesthesia. **Morphine** 1 mg/kg was then slowly infused while the patient was ventilated with 50% nitrous oxide/oxygen. With the onset of neuromuscular relaxation with pancuronium 150 micrograms/kg, her blood pressure rose sharply from 120/60 to 200/110 mmHg and her pulse rate increased from 54 to 96 bpm, persisting for several minutes but restabilising when 1% halothane was added.[1] The suggested reason is that pancuronium can antagonise the vagal tone (heart slowing) induced by the **morphine**, thus allowing the blood pressure and heart rate to rise. The authors of the report point out the undesirability of this in those with coronary heart disease.

(b) Vecuronium

Two patients, one aged 72 and the other aged 84, undergoing elective carotid endarterectomy developed extreme bradycardia following induction with **alfentanil** and vecuronium; both were premedicated with **morphine**. The first was taking **propranolol** 20 mg 8-hourly and as the drugs were injected his heart rate fell from 50 to 35 bpm, and his blood pressure fell from 160/70 to 75/35 mmHg. He responded to atropine, ephedrine and phenylephrine. The other patient was taking nifedipine and quinidine. His heart rate fell from 89 to 43 bpm, and his blood pressure dropped from 210/80 to 120/45 mmHg. Both heart rate and blood pressures recovered following skin incision.[2]

Bradycardia in the presence of vecuronium has been seen during anaesthetic induction with other drugs including **fentanyl**,[3,4] and **sufentanil** (in 3 patients taking beta blockers with or without diltiazem).[5] The lack of vagolytic effects associated with vecuronium may mean that opioid-induced bradycardia is unopposed.[4,5] The beta blockers and diltiazem may also have played a part in the bradycardia seen in some of these patients[5] (see also 'Neuromuscular blockers + Beta blockers', p.119). Be alert for this effect if vecuronium is given with any of these drugs. Atropine 500 micrograms given intravenously at the time of induction may prevent the bradycardia.[4]

For reports of bradycardia occurring with **atracurium** or **suxamethonium** used with propofol and **fentanyl**, see 'Anaesthetics, general + Neuromuscular blockers', p.101.

1. Grossman E, Jacobi AM. Hemodynamic interaction between pancuronium and morphine. *Anesthesiology* (1974) 40, 299–301.
2. Lema G, Sacco C, Urzúa J. Bradycardia following induction with alfentanil and vecuronium. *J Cardiothorac Vasc Anesth* (1992) 6, 774–5.
3. Mirakhur RK, Ferres CJ, Clarke RSJ, Bali IM, Dundee JW. Clinical evaluation of Org NC 45. *Br J Anaesth* (1983) 55, 119–24.
4. Inoue K, El-Banayosy A, Stolarski L, Reichelt W. Vecuronium induced bradycardia following induction of anaesthesia with etomidate or thiopentone, with or without fentanyl. *Br J Anaesth* (1988) 60, 10–17.
5. Starr NJ, Sethna DH, Estafanous FG. Bradycardia and asystole following the rapid administration of sufentanil with vecuronium. *Anesthesiology* (1986) 64, 521–3.

Neuromuscular blockers + Organophosphorus compounds

Exposure to organophosphorus insecticides such as malathion and dimpylate (diazinon) can markedly prolong the neuromuscular blocking effects of suxamethonium (succinylcholine).

Clinical evidence

A man admitted to hospital for an appendectomy became apnoeic during the early part of the operation when given **suxamethonium (succinylcholine)** 100 mg to facilitate tracheal intubation, and remained so throughout the 40 minutes of surgery. Restoration of neuromuscular activity occurred about 180 minutes after he had received the **suxamethonium**. Later studies showed that he had an extremely low plasma cholinesterase activity (3 to 10%), even though he had a normal phenotype. It subsequently turned out that he had been working with **malathion** for 11 weeks without any protection.[1]

Another report describes a man whose recovery from neuromuscular blockade with **suxamethonium** was very prolonged. He had attempted suicide approximately 2 weeks earlier with **dimpylate (diazinon)**, a household insecticide. His pseudocholinesterase was found to be 2.5 units/L (normal values 7 to 19) and his dibucaine number (a measurement of cholinesterase activity) was too low to be measured.[2]

Other cases of prolonged **suxamethonium**-induced paralysis associated with organophosphate poisoning have been reported.[3-7] These cases have involved accidental ingestion of **chlorpyrifos**[3] or **dichlorvos**[7] in children, and one case resulted from subclinical exposure to **chlorpyrifos** and **propetamphos** following the treatment of carpets for pests.[4] Also, prolonged **suxamethonium**-induced paralysis has occurred following suicide attempts in adults with **chlorpyrifos**[6] or *Diazinon* **[dimpylate]**.[5] In one report ECT was performed 2 weeks after attempted suicide with **chlorpyrifos** and, despite low plasma cholinesterase levels, paralysis with **suxamethonium** was carried out successfully using one fifth of the normal dose.[6]

Mechanism

Malathion, dimpylate, and other organophosphorus insecticides inhibit the activity of plasma cholinesterase, thereby reducing the metabolism of the suxamethonium and prolonging its effects.

Importance and management

An established and well understood interaction. The organophosphorus pesticides are potent anticholinesterases used in agriculture and horticulture to control insects on crops, and in veterinary practice to control various ectoparasites. They are applied as sprays and dips. Anyone who is exposed to these toxic pesticides may therefore show changes in their responses to neuromuscular blockers. Widely used organophosphorus pesticides include **azamethiphos**, **bromophos**, **chlorpyrifos**, **clofenvinfos**,

coumafos, cythioate, dichlorvos, dimethoate, dimpylate, dioxation, ethion, famphur, fenitrothion, fenthion, heptenophos, iodofenphos, malathion, naled, parathion, phosmet, phoxim, pirimiphos-methyl, propetamphos, pyraclofos, temefos.[8] A number of the **nerve gases** (such as **sarin, soman, tabun** and **VX**) are also potent anticholinesterases. Consider also 'Neuromuscular blockers + Anticholinesterases', p.114

1. Guillermo FP, Pretel CMM, Royo FT, Macias MJP, Ossorio RA, Gomez JAA, Vidal CJ. Prolonged suxamethonium-induced neuromuscular blockade associated with organophosphate poisoning. *Br J Anaesth* (1988) 61, 233–6.
2. Ware MR, Frost ML, Berger JJ, Stewart RB, DeVane CL. Electroconvulsive therapy complicated by insecticide ingestion. *J Clin Psychopharmacol* (1990) 10, 72–3.
3. Selden BS, Curry SC. Prolonged succinylcholine-induced paralysis in organophosphate insecticide poisoning. *Ann Emerg Med* (1987) 16, 215–17.
4. Weeks DB, Ford D. Prolonged suxamethonium-induced neuromuscular block associated with organophosphate poisoning. *Br J Anaesth* (1989) 62, 237.
5. Jaksa RJ, Palahniuk RJ. Attempted organophosphate suicide: a unique cause of prolonged paralysis during electroconvulsive therapy. *Anesth Analg* (1995) 80, 832–3.
6. Dillard M, Webb J. Administration of succinylcholine for electroconvulsive therapy after organophosphate poisoning: a case study. *AANA J* (1999) 67, 513–17.
7. Sener EB, Ustun E, Kocamanoglu S, Tur A. Prolonged apnea following succinylcholine administration in undiagnosed acute organophosphate poisoning. *Acta Anaesthesiol Scand* (2002) 46, 1046–8.
8. Sweetman SC, ed. Martindale: The complete drug reference. 35th ed. London: Pharmaceutical Press; 2007. p. 1851.

Neuromuscular blockers + Quinidine

The effects of both depolarising neuromuscular blockers (e.g. suxamethonium (succinylcholine)) and competitive neuromuscular blockers (e.g. tubocurarine) can be increased by quinidine. Recurarisation and apnoea have been seen in patients when quinidine was given during the recovery period from neuromuscular blockade.

Clinical evidence

A patient given **metocurine** during surgery regained her motor functions and was able to talk coherently during the recovery period. However, within 15 minutes of additionally being given quinidine sulfate 200 mg by injection she developed muscular weakness and respiratory depression. She needed intubation and assisted respiration for a period of two and a half hours. Edrophonium and neostigmine were used to aid recovery.[1]

This interaction has also been described in case reports involving **tubocurarine**[2] and **suxamethonium (succinylcholine)**,[3,4] and has been confirmed in *animal* studies.[5-7]

Mechanism

Not fully understood, but it has been shown that quinidine can inhibit the enzyme (choline acetyltransferase), which is concerned with the synthesis of acetylcholine at nerve endings.[8] Neuromuscular transmission would be expected to be reduced if the synthesis of acetylcholine is reduced. Quinidine also inhibits the activity of plasma cholinesterase, which is concerned with the metabolism of suxamethonium.[4]

Importance and management

The interaction between quinidine and neuromuscular blockers is an established interaction of clinical importance, but the documentation is limited. The incidence is uncertain, but it was seen in one report cited to a greater or lesser extent in 5 of the 6 patients studied.[3] It has only been reported clinically with metocurine, tubocurarine and suxamethonium, but it occurs in *animals* with **gallamine**, and it seems possible that it could occur clinically with any depolarising or non-depolarising neuromuscular blocker. Be alert for increased neuromuscular blocking effects during and after surgery.

1. Schmidt JL, Vick NA, Sadove MS. The effect of quinidine on the action of muscle relaxants. *JAMA* (1963) 183, 669–71.
2. Way WL, Katzung BG, Larson CP. Recurarization with quinidine. *JAMA* (1967) 200, 163–4.
3. Grogono AW. Anaesthesia for atrial defibrillation: effect of quinidine on muscular relaxation. *Lancet* (1963) ii, 1039–40.
4. Kambam JR, Franks JJ, Naukam R, Sastry BVR. Effect of quinidine on plasma cholinesterase activity and succinylcholine neuromuscular blockade. *Anesthesiology* (1987) 67, 858–60.
5. Miller RD, Way WL, Katzung BG. The neuromuscular effects of quinidine. *Proc Soc Exp Biol Med* (1968) 129, 215–18.
6. Miller RD, Way WL, Katzung BG. The potentiation of neuromuscular blocking agents by quinidine. *Anesthesiology* (1967) 28, 1036–41.
7. Cuthbert MF. The effect of quinidine and procainamide on the neuromuscular blocking action of suxamethonium. *Br J Anaesth* (1966) 38, 775–9.
8. Kambam JR, Day P, Jansen VE, Sastry BVR. Quinidine inhibits choline acetyltransferase activity. *Anesthesiology* (1989) 71, A819.

Neuromuscular blockers + Testosterone

An isolated report describes marked resistance to the effects of suxamethonium (succinylcholine) and vecuronium, apparently due to the long-term use of testosterone. Another case reports resistance to vecuronium in a patient with elevated plasma testosterone levels.

Clinical evidence, mechanism, importance and management

A woman transsexual who had been receiving testosterone enantate 200 mg intramuscularly twice monthly for 10 years was resistant to 100 mg of intravenous **suxamethonium (succinylcholine)**, and needed 100 micrograms/kg of intravenous **vecuronium** for effective tracheal intubation before surgery. During the surgery it was found necessary to use a total of 22 mg of **vecuronium** over a 50-minute period to achieve acceptable relaxation of the abdominal muscles for a hysterectomy and salpingo-oophorectomy to be carried out.[1] Considerably higher than usual doses of **vecuronium** were required in a patient with testicular feminisation and elevated plasma testosterone levels.[2]

The reasons are not understood. However, it has been suggested that the close structural similarity between testosterone and **vecuronium**, with respect to their common steroidal core, might mean that they share similar metabolic pathways. Chronic elevation of circulating testosterone may up-regulate the hepatic metabolism of steroidal molecules in general, and so enhance the hepatic elimination of **vecuronium**.[2]

1. Reddy P, Guzman A, Robalino J, Shevde K. Resistance to muscle relaxants in a patient receiving prolonged testosterone therapy. *Anesthesiology* (1989) 70, 871–3.
2. Lee HT, Appel MI. Increased tolerance to vecuronium in a patient with testicular feminization. *J Clin Anesth* (1998) 10, 156–9.

Neuromuscular blockers + Tobacco

There is some evidence that smokers may need more vecuronium and possibly more rocuronium, but less atracurium to achieve the same effects as non-smokers. However, results are variable and another study found that rocuronium appeared to be unaffected by smoking.

Clinical evidence, mechanism, importance and management

Variable results have been reported on the effect of smoking on neuromuscular blockers. The amount of **atracurium** required was about 25% lower in smokers, when compared with non-smokers.[1] However, in another study, smokers required more **vecuronium** than non-smokers did (96.8 compared with 72.11 micrograms/kg per hour, respectively; a 34% increase).[2] Similarly another study involving patients undergoing minor surgery found that the 20 smokers required about 20% more **rocuronium** than the 20 non-smokers.[3] However, this study has been criticised for having too few patients, which meant that it was unable to properly detect a statistically significant difference between the smokers and non-smokers.[4] In yet another study, the onset and recovery times from the neuromuscular blocking effects of **rocuronium** 600 micrograms/kg were reported to be not significantly affected by smoking more than 10 cigarettes daily.[5]

Tobacco smoke contains many different compounds and has enzyme-inducing properties, which may affect the dose requirements of neuromuscular blockers. In addition, the time interval in refraining from smoking will affect plasma nicotine concentrations; small doses of nicotine may stimulate the neuromuscular junction, but larger doses may block transmission.[2] More studies are needed.

1. Kroeker KA, Beattie WS, Yang H. Neuromuscular blockade in the setting of chronic nicotine exposure. *Anesthesiology* (1994) 81, A1120.
2. Teiriä H, Rautoma P, Yli-Hankala A. Effect of smoking on dose requirements for vecuronium. *Br J Anaesth* (1996) 76, 154–5.
3. Rautoma P, Svartling N. Smoking increases the requirement for rocuronium. *Can J Anaesth* (1998) 45, 651–4.
4. Pühringer FK, Benzer A, Keller P, Luger TJ. Does smoking really increase the requirements for rocuronium? *Can J Anaesth* (1999) 46, 513.
5. Latorre F, de Almeida MCS, Stanek A, Kleemann PP. Die Wechselwirkung von Rocuronium und Rauchen. Der Einfluß des Rauchens auf die neuromuskuläre Übertragung nach Rocuronium. *Anaesthesist* (1997) 46, 493–5.

Neuromuscular blockers + Trimetaphan

Trimetaphan can increase the effects of suxamethonium (succinylcholine), which may result in prolonged apnoea. This may possibly occur with other neuromuscular blocking drugs, such as alcuronium.

Clinical evidence

A man undergoing neurosurgery was given **tubocurarine** and **suxamethonium (succinylcholine)**. Neuromuscular blockade was prolonged postoperatively, lasting about 2.5 hours, and was attributed to the concurrent use of trimetaphan 4.5 g, given over a 90-minute period. Later when he underwent further surgery using essentially the same anaesthetic techniques and drugs, but with a very much smaller dose of trimetaphan (35 mg over a 10-minute period), the recovery was normal.[1]

Nine out of 10 patients receiving ECT treatment and given **suxamethonium** showed an almost 90% prolongation in apnoea (from 142 to 265 seconds) when trimetaphan 10 to 20 mg was used instead of 1.2 mg of atropine.[2] Prolonged apnoea has been seen in another patient given **suxamethonium** and trimetaphan.[3] On the basis of an *in vitro* study it was calculated that a typical dose of trimetaphan would double the duration of paralysis due to **suxamethonium**.[4] Prolonged neuromuscular blockade was also seen in a man given **alcuronium** and trimetaphan.[5]

Mechanism

Not fully understood. Trimetaphan can inhibit plasma cholinesterase to some extent,[2,5] which would reduce the metabolism of the suxamethonium and thereby prolong its activity. Studies in *rats*[6,7] and case reports[8] also indicate that trimetaphan has direct neuromuscular blocking activity. Its effects are at least additive with the neuromuscular blocking effects of the **aminoglycosides**.[7]

Importance and management

Information is limited but the interaction appears to be established. If trimetaphan and suxamethonium are used concurrently, be alert for enhanced and prolonged neuromuscular blockade. This has also been seen with alcuronium, and trimetaphan may interact with other competitive neuromuscular blockers.[5] Respiratory arrest has been seen when large doses of trimetaphan were given in the absence of a neuromuscular blocker, so that caution is certainly needed.[8] *Animal* studies suggested that the blockade might not be reversed by neostigmine or calcium chloride,[7] but neostigmine and calcium gluconate were successfully used to reverse the effects of alcuronium and trimetaphan in one case.[5]

1. Wilson SL, Miller RN, Wright C, Hasse D. Prolonged neuromuscular blockade associated with trimethaphan: a case report. *Anesth Analg* (1976) 55, 353–6.
2. Tewfik GI. Trimetaphan. Its effect on the pseudo-cholinesterase level of man. *Anaesthesia* (1957) 12, 326–9.
3. Poulton TJ, James FM, Lockridge O. Prolonged apnea following trimethaphan and succinylcholine. *Anesthesiology* (1979) 50, 54–6.
4. Sklar GS, Lanks KW. Effects of trimethaphan and sodium nitroprusside on hydrolysis of succinylcholine *in vitro*. *Anesthesiology* (1977) 47, 31–3.
5. Nakamura K, Koide M, Imanaga T, Ogasawara H, Takahashi M, Yoshikawa M. Prolonged neuromuscular blockade following trimetaphan infusion. *Anaesthesia* (1980) 35, 1202–7.
6. Pearcy WC, Wittenstein ES. The interactions of trimetaphan (Arfonad), suxamethonium and cholinesterase inhibitor in the rat. *Br J Anaesth* (1960) 32, 156–9.
7. Paradelis AG, Crassaris LG, Karachalios DN, Triantaphyllidis CJ. Aminoglycoside antibiotics: interaction with trimethaphan at the neuromuscular junctions. *Drugs Exp Clin Res* (1987) 13, 233–6.
8. Dale RC, Schroeder ET. Respiratory paralysis during treatment of hypertension with trimethaphan camsylate. *Arch Intern Med* (1976) 136, 816–18.

Neuromuscular blockers + Ulinastatin

Ulinastatin delays the onset and hastens the recovery from vecuronium neuromuscular block.

Clinical evidence, mechanism, importance and management

A randomised, placebo-controlled study involving 60 patients found that a 5000 unit/kg intravenous bolus dose of ulinastatin given before induction of anaesthesia, and again 2 minutes before intravenous **vecuronium** 100 micrograms/kg, delayed the onset of neuromuscular blockade compared with placebo (250 compared with 214 seconds). The recovery from neuromuscular block (measured as return of post-tetanic count) was significantly shorter after ulinastatin than placebo (11 compared with 17.7 minutes). The effects of ulinastatin were thought to be due to an increase in the release of acetylcholine at the neuromuscular junction and enhanced **vecuronium** elimination due to increases in liver blood flow and urine volume.[1]

1. Saitoh Y, Fujii Y, Oshima T. The ulinastatin-induced effect on neuromuscular block caused by vecuronium. *Anesth Analg* (1999) 89, 1565–9.

6

Analgesics and NSAIDs

The drugs dealt with in this section include aspirin and other salicylates, NSAIDs, opioid analgesics, and the miscellaneous analgesics, such as nefopam and paracetamol. 'Table 6.1', (p.134) contains a listing, with a further classification of the NSAIDs.

Interactions

(a) Aspirin and NSAIDs

Aspirin and the NSAIDs generally undergo few clinically significant pharmacokinetic interactions. The majority are highly protein bound, and have the potential to interact with other drugs via this mechanism. However, with a few exceptions, most of these interactions are not clinically important (see 'Protein-binding interactions', (p.3)).

Of the newer NSAIDs, celecoxib is metabolised by the cytochrome P450 isoenzyme CYP2C9, and inhibits CYP2D6. Rofecoxib, now withdrawn, inhibits CYP1A2, see 'Tizanidine + CYP1A2 inhibitors', p.1286. Nevertheless, most of the important interactions with NSAIDs and aspirin are pharmacodynamic. Aspirin and all non-selective NSAIDs inhibit platelet aggregation, and so can increase the risk of bleeding and interact with other drugs that have this effect. NSAIDs that are highly selective for cyclo-oxygenase-2 (COX-2) do not inhibit platelet aggregation.

Aspirin and all NSAIDs (including COX-2 selective NSAIDs) affect the synthesis of renal prostaglandins, and so can cause salt and water retention. This can increase blood pressure and affect antihypertensive therapy.

Aspirin and non-selective NSAIDs inhibit the mechanisms that protect the gastrointestinal mucosa and so cause gastrointestinal toxicity. COX-2 selective NSAIDs (coxibs) are less likely to have this effect.

(b) Opioids

Morphine is metabolised by glucuronidation by UDP-glucuronyltransferases, mainly to one active and one inactive metabolite. The glucuronidation of morphine can be induced or inhibited by various drugs. Morphine is not significantly affected by the cytochrome P450 isoenzymes. The semi-synthetic morphine analogues, hydromorphone and oxymorphone, are metabolised similarly.

Codeine, dihydrocodeine, and hydrocodone are thought to be pro-drugs, and require metabolic activation, possibly by CYP2D6 or UGT enzymes. Inhibitors of these enzymes may therefore reduce their efficacy. Oxycodone is also metabolised by CYP2D6 and CYP3A4.

Pethidine is metabolised via several cytochrome P450 isoenzymes. If the metabolism of pethidine is increased it can lead to increased production of the toxic metabolite, norpethidine, and increased CNS adverse effects.

Methadone is principally metabolised by CYP3A4 and CYP2D6, although CYP2C8 may also play a role. Buprenorphine is metabolised by CYP3A4.

Alfentanil is extensively metabolised by CYP3A4, and has been used as a probe drug for assessing CYP3A4 activity. Fentanyl and sufentanil are also metabolised, but because they are high hepatic-extraction drugs (see 'Changes in first-pass metabolism', (p.4)) they are less affected by inhibitors or inducers of CYP3A4, although in some instances this may still lead to clinically significant effects.

(c) Paracetamol

Paracetamol is not absorbed from the stomach, and the rate of absorption is well correlated with the gastric emptying rate. Paracetamol has therefore been used as a marker drug in studies of gastric emptying. Paracetamol is primarily metabolised by the liver to a variety of metabolites, principally the glucuronide and sulfate conjugates. Hepatotoxicity of paracetamol is thought to be due to a minor metabolite, *N*-acetyl-p-benzoquinone imine (NAPQI), which is inactivated with glutathione and excreted as mercapturate and cysteine conjugates. When the liver stores of glutathione are depleted, and the rate of production of NAPQI exceeds the rate of production of glutathione, excess NAPQI attaches to liver proteins and causes liver damage. CYP2E1 may be involved in the formation of this hepatotoxic metabolite.

General references

1. Brouwers JRBJ, de Smet PAGM. Pharmacokinetic-pharmacodynamic drug interactions with nonsteroidal anti-inflammatory drugs. *Clin Pharmacokinet* (1994) 27, 462–5.
2. Rumack BH. Acetaminophen hepatotoxicity: the first 35 years. *J Toxicol Clin Toxicol* (2002) 40, 3–20.
3. Armstrong AC, Cozza KL. Pharmacokinetic drug interactions of morphine, codeine, and their derivatives: theory and clinical reality, Part I. *Psychosomatics* (2003) 44, 167–71.
4. Armstrong AC, Cozza KL. Pharmacokinetic drug interactions of morphine, codeine, and their derivatives: theory and clinical reality, Part II. *Psychosomatics* (2003) 44, 515–20.

Table 6.1 Analgesics and NSAIDs

Group	*Drugs*
Aspirin and oral salicylates	Aloxiprin, Aspirin, Benorilate, Choline salicylate, Diflunisal, Ethenzamide, Lysine aspirin, Magnesium salicylate, Salsalate, Sodium salicylate
NSAIDs	
Fenamates	Floctafenine, Flufenamic acid, Meclofenamic acid, Mefenamic acid, Tolfenamic acid
Indole- and indene-acetic acids	Acemetacin, Indometacin, Sulindac
Oxicams	Lornoxicam, Meloxicam, Piroxicam, Tenoxicam
Phenylacetic acid derivatives	Alclofenac, Diclofenac
Propionic acid derivatives	Dexketoprofen, Fenoprofen, Flurbiprofen, Ibuprofen, Ketoprofen, Naproxen, Oxaprozin, Tiaprofenic acid
Pyrazolone derivatives	Azapropazone, Feprazone, Kebuzone, Metamizole sodium (Dipyrone), Oxyphenbutazone, Phenylbutazone
Selective inhibitors of cyclo-oxygenase-2 (Coxibs)	Celecoxib, Etodolac, Etoricoxib, Meloxicam (see under *Oxicams*), Nimesulide, Parecoxib, Rofecoxib, Valdecoxib
Other	Benzydamine hydrochloride, Felbinac, Ketorolac, Nabumetone, Phenazone (Antipyrine), Tolmetin
Opioid and related analgesics	
Anaesthetic adjuncts	Alfentanil, Fentanyl, Remifentanil, Sufentanil
Mild to moderate pain	Codeine, Dextropropoxyphene (Propoxyphene), Dihydrocodeine
Moderate to severe pain:	
Partial agonists and agonists/antagonists	Buprenorphine (also used for opioid dependence), Butorphanol, Meptazinol, Nalbuphine, Pentazocine
Pure agonists	Dextromoramide, Diamorphine (Heroin), Dipipanone, Hydrocodone, Hydromorphone, Methadone (also used for opioid dependence), Morphine, Oxycodone, Oxymorphone, Papaveretum, Pethidine (Meperidine), Tramadol
Miscellaneous	Nefopam, Paracetamol (Acetaminophen)

Aspirin or other Salicylates + Antacids

The serum salicylate levels of patients taking large, anti-inflammatory doses of aspirin or other salicylates can be reduced to subtherapeutic levels by some antacids. The maximum plasma levels of aspirin may be increased by antacids, although the extent of absorption is unaltered.

Clinical evidence

A child with rheumatic fever taking aspirin 600 mg five times daily had a serum salicylate level of between 82 and 118 mg/L while taking 30 mL of *Maalox* (**aluminium/magnesium hydroxide** suspension). When the *Maalox* was withdrawn, the urinary pH fell from a range of 7 to 8 down to a range of 5 to 6.4, whereupon the serum salicylate level rose three- to fourfold to about 380 mg/L, which required a dosage reduction.[1] An associated study in 13 healthy subjects taking aspirin 4 g daily for a week found that **sodium bicarbonate** 4 g daily reduced serum salicylate levels by 44%, from 270 to 150 mg/L. This reflected a rise in the urinary pH from a range of 5.6 to 6.1 up to around 6.2 to 6.9.[1,2] Similar changes have been reported in other studies with: aspirin or **choline salicylate** and **aluminium/magnesium hydroxide**; aspirin and **magnesium trisilicate/aluminium hydroxide**; and aspirin or **sodium salicylate** and **sodium bicarbonate**.[3-7] There is some evidence to suggest that this effect does not occur at low serum salicylate levels,[4,5] or if the pH of the urine is unchanged by the antacid.[5]

A study in 10 healthy subjects found that the mean maximum plasma level of a single 650-mg dose of aspirin was about 70% higher when it was given 10 minutes after an antacid (**aluminium/magnesium hydroxide**), when compared with aspirin alone. However, there was no change in the time to reach the peak level or the AUC. There were also no significant changes in the pharmacokinetics of the metabolites, salicylic acid and salicyluric acid.[8]

Mechanism

Aspirin and other salicylates are acidic compounds that are excreted by the kidney tubules and are ionised in solution. In alkaline solution, much of the drug exists in the ionised form, which is not readily reabsorbed, and therefore is lost in the urine. If the urine is made more acidic (e.g. with ammonium chloride), much more of the drug exists in the un-ionised form, which is readily reabsorbed, so that less is lost in the urine and the drug is retained in the body.[6,7]

In vitro data show that magnesium oxide and aluminium hydroxide strongly adsorb aspirin and sodium salicylate.[9] However, in three of the studies above aluminium hydroxide-containing antacids had no effect on the extent of absorption of salicylate,[3,5,8] although the rate of absorption may be increased as a result of an increase in the solubility of salicylate in a less acidic gastric environment.[8]

Importance and management

A well established and clinically important interaction for those receiving long-term treatment with large doses of salicylates because the serum salicylate level may become subtherapeutic. This interaction can occur with both 'systemic' antacids (e.g. sodium bicarbonate) as well as some 'non-systemic' antacids (e.g. aluminium/magnesium hydroxide), but only appears to occur if there is an increase in the urinary pH. Care should be taken to monitor serum salicylate levels if any antacid is started or stopped in patients where the control of salicylate levels is critical.

No important adverse interaction would be expected in those taking occasional doses of aspirin for analgesia. Some aspirin formulations actually include antacids as buffering agents to increase absorption rates and raise peak serum levels,[10] which gives more rapid analgesia, and/or in an attempt to decrease gastric irritation. Note that antacids may also increase the rate of absorption of aspirin given as enteric-coated tablets.[11]

1. Levy G. Interaction of salicylates with antacids. In: Blondheim SH, Alkan WJ, Brunner D, eds. Frontiers of Internal Medicine. 12th Int Congr Intern Med, Tel Aviv, 1974. Basel: Karger; 1975 p. 404–8.
2. Levy G, Leonards JR. Urine pH and salicylate therapy. *JAMA* (1971) 217, 81.
3. Levy G, Lampman T, Kamath BL, Garrettson LK. Decreased serum salicylate concentration in children with rheumatic fever treated with antacid. *N Engl J Med* (1975) 293, 323–5.
4. Hansten PD, Hayton WL. Effect of antacid and ascorbic acid on serum salicylate concentration. *J Clin Pharmacol* (1980) 20, 326–31.
5. Shastri RA. Effect of antacids on salicylate kinetics. *Int J Clin Pharmacol Ther Toxicol* (1985) 23, 480–4.
6. Macpherson CR, Milne MD, Evans BM. The excretion of salicylate. *Br J Pharmacol* (1955) 10, 484–9.
7. Hoffman WS, Nobe C. The influence of urinary pH on the renal excretion of salicyl derivatives during aspirin therapy. *J Lab Clin Med* (1950) 35, 237–48.
8. Itthipanichpong C, Sirivongs P, Wittayalertpunya S, Chaiyos N. The effect of antacid on aspirin pharmacokinetics in healthy Thai volunteers. *Drug Metabol Drug Interact* (1992) 10, 213–28.
9. Naggar VF, Khalil SA, Daabis NA. The in-vitro adsorption of some antirheumatics on antacids. *Pharmazie* (1976) 31, 461–5.
10. Nayak RK, Smyth RD, Polk A, Herczeg T, Carter V, Visalli AJ, Reavey-Cantwell NH. Effect of antacids on aspirin dissolution and bioavailability. *J Pharmacokinet Biopharm* (1977) 5, 597–613.
11. Feldman S, Carlstedt BC. Effect of antacid on absorption of enteric-coated aspirin. *JAMA* (1974) 227, 660–1.

Aspirin + Bile-acid binding resins

Colestyramine and colestipol do not appear to have any clinically important effects on the absorption of aspirin.

Clinical evidence, mechanism, importance and management

(a) Colestipol

In 12 healthy subjects the extent of absorption of a single 650-mg dose of aspirin was unaffected by colestipol 10 g. However, the rate of aspirin absorption was increased by colestipol: at 60 minutes after the dose the plasma level was increased by about 40%.[1] No particular precautions seem to be necessary during concurrent use.

(b) Colestyramine

A study in 3 healthy subjects and 3 patients, and a later study in 7 healthy subjects, found that colestyramine 4 g delayed the absorption of a single 500-mg dose of aspirin (time to peak levels extended from 30 to 60 minutes) but the total amount absorbed was only reduced by 5 to 6%. Some of the subjects had slightly higher serum aspirin levels while taking colestyramine.[2] Similar results were reported in another study (a 31% lower plasma aspirin level at 60 minutes, but no difference in total absorption).[1] There would seem to be little reason for avoiding concurrent use unless rapid analgesia is needed.

1. Hunninghake DB, Pollack E. Effect of bile acid sequestering agents on the absorption of aspirin, tolbutamide, and warfarin. *Fedn Proc* (1977) 35, 996.
2. Hahn K-J, Eiden W, Schettle M, Hahn M, Walter E, Weber E. Effect of cholestyramine on the gastrointestinal absorption of phenprocoumon and acetylosalicylic acid in man. *Eur J Clin Pharmacol* (1972) 4, 142–5.

Aspirin or other Salicylates + Carbonic anhydrase inhibitors

A severe and even life-threatening toxic reaction can occur in patients taking high-dose salicylates if they are given carbonic anhydrase inhibitors (acetazolamide, diclofenamide).

Clinical evidence

An 8-year-old boy with chronic juvenile arthritis, taking prednisolone, indometacin and **aloxiprin**, was admitted to hospital with drowsiness, vomiting and hyperventilation (diagnosed as metabolic acidosis) within a month of the **aloxiprin** dosage being increased from 3 to 3.6 g daily and starting to take **diclofenamide** 25 mg three times daily for glaucoma.[1]

Other cases of toxicity (metabolic acidosis) have included a 22-year-old woman taking **salsalate** with **acetazolamide** 250 mg four times daily,[1] and 2 elderly women taking large doses of aspirin with **acetazolamide** or **diclofenamide**.[2] A 50-year-old woman taking **acetazolamide** for glaucoma was admitted to hospital with confusion and cerebellar ataxia, associated with hyperchloraemic acidosis, 14 days after starting to take aspirin for acute pericarditis.[3] A man taking **diclofenamide** developed salicylate poisoning within 10 days of starting to take aspirin 3.9 g daily.[4] Coma developed in an 85-year-old woman taking aspirin 3.9 g daily when her dosage of **acetazolamide** was increased from 500 mg to 1 g daily,[5,6] and toxicity was seen in a very elderly man given both drugs: levels of unbound **acetazolamide** were found to be unusually high.[6] An elderly man became confused, lethargic, incontinent and anorexic while taking **acetazolamide** and **salsalate**. He needed intravenous hydration.[7]

Mechanism

Not fully established. One idea is that these carbonic anhydrase inhibitors (acetazolamide, diclofenamide) affect the plasma pH, so that more of the salicylate exists in the un-ionised (lipid-soluble) form, which can enter the CNS and other tissues more easily, leading to salicylate toxicity.[2] However, carbonic anhydrase inhibitors also make the urine more alkaline, which increases the loss of salicylate[8] (see also 'Aspirin or other Salicylates + Antacids', p.135). *Animal* studies confirm that carbonic anhydrase inhibitors increase the lethal toxicity of aspirin.[4] An alternative suggestion is that because salicylate inhibits the plasma protein binding of acetazolamide and its excretion by the kidney, acetazolamide toxicity, which mimics salicylate toxicity, may occur.[6]

Importance and management

Although there are few clinical reports on record, the interaction between carbonic anhydrase inhibitors and salicylates is established, well confirmed by *animal* studies, and potentially serious. One study recommended that carbonic anhydrase inhibitors should probably be avoided in those receiving high-dose salicylate treatment.[6] If they are used, the patient should be well monitored for any evidence of toxicity (confusion, lethargy, hyperventilation, tinnitus) because the interaction may develop slowly and insidiously.[2] In this context NSAIDs may be a safer alternative. Naproxen proved to be a satisfactory substitute in one case.[1] The authors of one study suggest that **methazolamide** may possibly be a safer alternative to acetazolamide because it is minimally bound to plasma proteins. They also suggest paracetamol (acetaminophen) as an alternative to salicylate in patients taking acetazolamide.[6] The reports cited here concern carbonic anhydrase inhibitors given orally, not as eye drops. It is not known whether the latter interact similarly, but there appear to be no reports.

1. Cowan RA, Hartnell GG, Lowdell CP, McLean Baird I, Leak AM. Metabolic acidosis induced by carbonic anhydrase inhibitors and salicylates in patients with normal renal function. *BMJ* (1984) 289, 347–8.
2. Anderson CJ, Kaufman PL, Sturm RJ. Toxicity of combined therapy with carbonic anhydrase inhibitors and aspirin. *Am J Ophthalmol* (1978) 86, 516–19.
3. Hazouard E, Grimbert M, Jonville-Berra A-P, De Toffol M-C, Legras A. Salicylisme et glaucome: augmentation réciproque de la toxicité de l'acétazolamide et de l'acide acétyl salicylique. *J Fr Ophtalmol* (1999) 22, 73–5.
4. Hurwitz GA, Wingfield W, Cowart TD, Jollow DJ. Toxic interaction between salicylates and a carbonic anhydrase inhibitor: the role of cerebral edema. *Vet Hum Toxicol* (1980) 22 (Suppl), 42–4.
5. Chapron DJ, Brandt JL, Sweeny KR, Olesen-Zammett L. Interaction between acetazolamide and aspirin — a possible unrecognized cause of drug-induced coma. *J Am Geriatr Soc* (1984) 32, S18.
6. Sweeney KR, Chapron DJ, Brandt JL, Gomolin IH, Feig PU, Kramer PA. Toxic interaction between acetazolamide and salicylate: case reports and a pharmacokinetic explanation. *Clin Pharmacol Ther* (1986) 40, 518–24.
7. Rousseau P, Fuentevilla-Clifton A. Acetazolamide and salicylate interaction in the elderly: a case report. *J Am Geriatr Soc* (1993) 41, 868–9.
8. Macpherson CR, Milne MD, Evans BM. The excretion of salicylate. *Br J Pharmacol* (1955) 10, 484–9.

Aspirin or other Salicylates + Corticosteroids or Corticotropin

Serum salicylate levels are reduced by corticosteroids and therefore salicylate levels may rise, possibly to toxic concentrations, if the corticosteroid is withdrawn without first reducing the salicylate dosage. Concurrent use increases the risk of gastrointestinal bleeding and ulceration.

Clinical evidence

A 5-year-old boy taking long-term **prednisone** in doses of at least 20 mg daily, was given **choline salicylate** 3.6 g daily, and the **prednisone** was gradually tapered off to 3 mg daily over a 3-month period. Severe salicylate toxicity developed, and in a retrospective investigation of the cause, using frozen serum samples drawn for other purposes, it was found that the serum salicylate levels had risen from less than 100 mg/L up to 880 mg/L during the withdrawal of the **prednisone**.[1] Later studies in 3 other patients taking **choline salicylate** or aspirin and either **prednisone** or another unnamed corticosteroid, found about a threefold rise in salicylate levels during corticosteroid withdrawal.[1] **Hydrocortisone** was also found to increase the clearance of **sodium salicylate** in 4 other patients.[1]

A serum salicylate rise has been described in a patient taking **aloxiprin** when **prednisolone** was withdrawn.[2] Other studies in both adults and children show that **prednisone**, **methylprednisolone**, **betamethasone** and **corticotropin** reduce serum salicylate levels.[3-5] Two studies also found that intra-articular **dexamethasone**, **methylprednisolone**, and **triamcinolone** transiently reduced serum salicylate levels in patients given enteric-coated aspirin.[6,7] However one study in patients found that **prednisone** 12 to 60 mg daily had no effect on the clearance of single doses of **sodium salicylate**.[8]

Mechanism

Uncertain. One idea is that the presence of the corticosteroid increases the glomerular filtration rate, which increases salicylate clearance. When the corticosteroid is withdrawn, the clearance returns to normal and the salicylate accumulates. Another suggestion is that the corticosteroids increase the metabolism of the salicylate.[3]

Importance and management

Well established interactions.Patients should be monitored to ensure that salicylate levels remain adequate when corticosteroids are added[4] and do not become excessive if they are withdrawn. It should also be remembered that concurrent use may increase the incidence of gastrointestinal bleeding and ulceration. See also 'Corticosteroids + NSAIDs', p.1058.

1. Klinenberg JR, Miller F. Effect of corticosteroids on blood salicylate concentration. *JAMA* (1965) 194, 601–4.
2. Muirden KD, Barraclough DRE. Drug interactions in the management of rheumatoid arthritis. *Aust N Z J Med* (1976) 6 (Suppl 1), 14–17.
3. Graham GG, Champion GD, Day RO, Paull PD. Patterns of plasma concentrations and urinary excretion of salicylate in rheumatoid arthritis. *Clin Pharmacol Ther* (1977) 22, 410–20.
4. Bardare M, Cislaghi GU, Mandelli M, Sereni F. Value of monitoring plasma salicylate levels in treating juvenile rheumatoid arthritis. *Arch Dis Child* (1978) 53, 381–5.
5. Koren G, Roifman C, Gelfand E, Lavi S, Suria D, Stein L. Corticosteroids-salicylate interaction in a case of juvenile rheumatoid arthritis. *Ther Drug Monit* (1987) 9, 177–9.
6. Edelman J, Potter JM, Hackett LP. The effect of intra-articular steroids on plasma salicylate concentrations. *Br J Clin Pharmacol* (1986) 21, 301–7.
7. Baer PA, Shore A, Ikeman RL. Transient fall in serum salicylate levels following intraarticular injection of steroid in patients with rheumatoid arthritis. *Arthritis Rheum* (1987) 30, 345–7.
8. Day RO, Harris G, Brown M, Graham GG, Champion GD. Interaction of salicylate and corticosteroids in man. *Br J Clin Pharmacol* (1988) 26, 334–7.

Aspirin + Dapsone

Dapsone does not significantly affect the pharmacokinetics of aspirin.

Clinical evidence, mechanism, importance and management

A comparison of the pharmacokinetics of aspirin in 8 healthy subjects and 8 patients with uncomplicated lepromatous leprosy found that the pharmacokinetics of a single 600-mg dose of aspirin was not affected by either leprosy, or by treatment with dapsone 100 mg daily for 8 days.[1] No special precautions would seem likely to be needed on concurrent use.

1. Garg SK, Kumar B, Shukla VK, Bakaya V, Lal R, Kaur S. Pharmacokinetics of aspirin and chloramphenicol in normal and leprotic patients before and after dapsone therapy. *Int J Clin Pharmacol Ther Toxicol* (1988) 26, 204–5.

Aspirin + Food

Food delays the absorption of aspirin.

Clinical evidence, mechanism, importance and management

A study in 25 subjects given aspirin 650 mg in five different preparations showed that food roughly halved their serum salicylate levels (measured 10 and 20 minutes later), compared with those seen when the same dose of aspirin was taken while fasting.[1] Similar results were found in subjects given calcium aspirin 1.5 g.[2] In another study in 8 healthy subjects who were given effervescent aspirin 900 mg, serum salicylate levels at 15 minutes were roughly halved by food, but were more or less unchanged after one hour.[3]

A further study in 16 healthy subjects showed that the extent of absorption of a single 900-mg dose of soluble aspirin was not significantly affected by a high-fat meal. The rate of absorption was reduced by food and the maximum plasma level was reduced by 18%, which was not considered to be clinically significant. Furthermore, there was no statistically significant change in the time to maximum plasma levels (20 minutes fasted; 30 minutes fed).[4]

A possible reason for the reduced rate of absorption is that food delays gastric emptying. Thus if rapid analgesia is needed, aspirin should be taken without food, but if aspirin is needed long-term, giving it with food is thought to help to protect the gastric mucosa.

1. Wood JH. Effect of food on aspirin absorption. *Lancet* (1967) ii, 212.
2. Spiers ASD and Malone HF. Effect of food on aspirin absorption. *Lancet* (1967) i, 440.
3. Volans GN. Effects of food and exercise on the absorption of effervescent aspirin. *Br J Clin Pharmacol* (1974) 1, 137–41.
4. Stillings M, Havlik I, Chetty M, Clinton C, Schall R, Moodley I, Muir N, Little S. Comparison of the pharmacokinetic profiles of soluble aspirin and solid paracetamol tablets in fed and fasted volunteers. *Curr Med Res Opin* (2000) 16, 115–24.

Aspirin + Griseofulvin

An isolated report describes a marked fall in serum salicylate levels in a child given aspirin and griseofulvin.

Clinical evidence, mechanism, importance and management

An 8-year-old boy with rheumatic fever taking aspirin 110 mg/kg daily and furosemide, digoxin, captopril, potassium, aluminium/magnesium hydroxide and iron, had a very marked fall in his serum salicylate levels (from a range of 18.3 to 30.6 mg/dL to less than 0.2 mg/dL) within 2 days of starting griseofulvin 10 mg/kg daily. Two days after the griseofulvin was stopped, the salicylate levels were back to their former levels. The reasons for this effect are not known, but it was suggested that the salicylate absorption was impaired in some way.[1] This appears to be the first and only report of this interaction so that its general importance is uncertain.

1. Phillips KR, Wideman SD, Cochran EB, Becker JA. Griseofulvin significantly decreases serum salicylate concentrations. *Pediatr Infect Dis J* (1993) 12, 350–2.

Aspirin + Kaolin-pectin

Kaolin-pectin causes a small reduction in the absorption of aspirin, which is not clinically relevant.

Clinical evidence, mechanism, importance and management

In 10 healthy subjects the absorption of aspirin 975 mg was reduced by 5 to 10% by 30 or 60 mL of kaolin-pectin.[1] A likely explanation is that the aspirin becomes adsorbed by the kaolin so that the amount available for absorption through the gut wall is reduced. However, this small reduction in absorption is unlikely to be of clinical importance.

1. Juhl RP. Comparison of kaolin-pectin and activated charcoal for inhibition of aspirin absorption. *Am J Hosp Pharm* (1979) 36, 1097–8.

Aspirin + Laxatives

Sodium sulfate and castor oil used as laxatives can cause a modest, but probably clinically unimportant, reduction in aspirin absorption.

Clinical evidence, mechanism, importance and management

In an experimental study of the possible effects of laxatives on drug absorption, healthy subjects were given 10 to 20 g of oral **sodium sulfate** and 20 g of **castor oil** (doses sufficient to provoke diarrhoea). Absorption, measured by the amount of drug excreted in the urine, was decreased at 4 hours. The reduction was 21% for **castor oil** and aspirin, and 27% for **sodium sulfate** and aspirin. However, serum levels of aspirin were relatively unchanged. The overall picture was that while these laxatives can alter the pattern of absorption, they do not seriously impair the total amount of drug absorbed.[1]

1. Mattila MJ, Takki S, Jussila J. Effect of sodium sulphate and castor oil on drug absorption from the human intestine. *Ann Clin Res* (1974) 6, 19–24.

Aspirin + Levamisole

The salicylate levels of a patient taking aspirin rose when levamisole was given, but this effect was not confirmed in a subsequent controlled study.

Clinical evidence, mechanism, importance and management

A preliminary report of a patient who had an increase in salicylate levels when levamisole was given with aspirin[1] prompted a study in 9 healthy subjects of this possible interaction. Sustained-release aspirin 3.9 g daily in two divided doses was given over a period of 3 weeks, with levamisole 50 mg three times a day for a week, each subject acting as his own control. No significant changes in plasma salicylate levels were found.[2]

1. Laidlaw D'A. Rheumatoid arthritis improved by treatment with levamisole and L-histidine. *Med J Aust* (1976) 2, 382–5.
2. Rumble RH, Brooks PM, Roberts MS. Interaction between levamisole and aspirin in man. *Br J Clin Pharmacol* (1979) 7, 631–3.

Aspirin + Pentazocine

A man regularly taking large doses of aspirin developed renal papillary necrosis when he was given pentazocine.

Clinical evidence, mechanism, importance and management

An isolated report describes a man, regularly taking aspirin 1.8 to 2.4 g daily, who developed renal papillary necrosis within 6 months of also starting to take pentazocine 800 to 850 mg daily. He developed abdominal pain, nausea and vomiting, and passed tissue via his urethra. Before starting the pentazocine and after it was stopped, no necrosis was apparent. The postulated reason for this reaction is that a pentazocine-induced reduction in blood flow through the kidney potentiated the adverse effects of chronic aspirin use.[1] The general importance of this case is uncertain, but it emphasises the risks of long-term use (possibly abuse) of aspirin with pentazocine.

1. Muhalwas KK, Shah GM, Winer RL. Renal papillary necrosis caused by long-term ingestion of pentazocine and aspirin. *JAMA* (1981) 246, 867–8.

Aspirin + Phenylbutazone

Phenylbutazone reduces the uricosuric effects of high-dose aspirin. Concurrent use is likely to be associated with an increased risk of gastrointestinal damage.

Clinical evidence

The observation that several patients given aspirin and phenylbutazone developed elevated serum urate levels, prompted a study in 4 patients without gout. This found that aspirin 2 g daily had little effect on the excretion of uric acid in the urine, but marked uricosuria occurred with aspirin 5 g daily. When phenylbutazone 200, 400 and then 600 mg daily (over 3 days) was also given the uricosuria was abolished. Serum uric acid levels rose from an average of about 40 mg/L to 60 mg/L. The interaction was confirmed in a patient with tophaceous gout. The retention of uric acid also occurs if the phenylbutazone is given first.[1]

Mechanism

Not understood. Phenylbutazone is structurally related to sulfinpyrazone, which interacts similarly, see 'Aspirin or other Salicylates + Sulfinpyrazone', p.138.

Importance and management

An established but sparsely documented interaction. The potential problems arising from this interaction should be recognised in any patient given aspirin and phenylbutazone. The concurrent use of aspirin and NSAIDs increases the risk of gastrointestinal damage and is not recommended. Although there does not appear to be any specific evidence for phenylbutazone, it would be expected to interact in the same way as other NSAIDs, see 'NSAIDs + Aspirin; Anti-inflammatory dose', p.142.

1. Oyer JH, Wagner SL, Schmid FR. Suppression of salicylate-induced uricosuria by phenylbutazone. *Am J Med Sci* (1966) 225, 39–45.

Aspirin or other Salicylates + Probenecid

The uricosuric effects of high doses of aspirin or other salicylates and probenecid are not additive as might be expected but are mutually antagonistic. Low dose, enteric-coated aspirin appears not to interact with probenecid.

Clinical evidence

A study found that the average urinary uric acid excretion in 24 hours was 673 mg with a single 3-g daily dose of probenecid, 909 mg with a 6-g daily dose of **sodium salicylate**, but only 114 mg when both drugs were given.[1] Similar antagonism has been seen in other studies in patients given aspirin 2.6 to 5.2 g daily.[2-4] No antagonism is seen until serum salicylate levels of 50 to 100 mg/L are reached.[4] Therefore no interaction would be expected with low, antiplatelet dose aspirin. This was confirmed by a crossover study in 11 patients with gouty arthritis, regularly taking probenecid, which found that enteric-coated aspirin 325 mg daily, taken either with probenecid or 6 hours after probenecid, had no effect on serum urate levels or on the 24-hour urate excretion.[5]

Mechanism

Not understood. The interaction probably occurs at the site of renal tubular secretion, but it also seems that both drugs can occupy the same site on plasma albumins.

Importance and management

A well established and clinically important interaction. Regular dosing with substantial amounts of salicylates should be avoided if this antagonism is to be avoided, but small very occasional analgesic doses probably do not matter. Serum salicylate levels of 50 to 100 mg/L are necessary before this interaction occurs. Low-dose aspirin (325 mg or less daily) does not seem to interact.

1. Seegmiller JE, Grayzel AI. Use of the newer uricosuric agents in the management of gout. *JAMA* (1960) 173, 1076–80.
2. Pascale LR, Dubin A, Hoffman WS. Therapeutic value of probenecid (Benemid®) in gout. *JAMA* (1952) 149, 1188–94.
3. Gutman AB, Yü TF. Benemid (*p*-di-*n*-propylsulfamyl-benzoic acid) as uricosuric agent in chronic gouty arthritis. *Trans Assoc Am Physicians* (1951) 64, 279–88.
4. Pascale LR, Dubin A, Bronsky D, Hoffman WS. Inhibition of the uricosuric action of Benemid by salicylate. *J Lab Clin Med* (1955) 45, 771–7.
5. Harris M, Bryant LR, Danaher P, Alloway J. Effect of low dose daily aspirin on serum urate levels and urinary excretion in patients receiving probenecid for gouty arthritis. *J Rheumatol* (2000) 27, 2873–6.

Aspirin or other Salicylates + Sulfinpyrazone

The uricosuric effects of the salicylates and sulfinpyrazone are not additive, as might be expected, but are mutually antagonistic.

Clinical evidence

When **sodium salicylate** 6 g was given with sulfinpyrazone 600 mg daily to one patient the average urinary uric acid excretion in 24 hours was 30 mg, whereas when each drug was used alone in the same doses the average 24-hour urinary excretion was 281 mg for **sodium salicylate** and 527 mg for sulfinpyrazone.[1] A later study in 5 men with gout given a sulfinpyrazone infusion for about an hour (300 mg bolus followed by 10 mg/minute) found that the additional infusion of **sodium salicylate** (3 g bolus followed by 10 to 20 mg/minute) virtually abolished the uricosuria. When the drugs were given in the reverse order to 3 other patients the same result was seen.[2]

In another study, the uricosuria caused by sulfinpyrazone 400 mg daily was found to be completely abolished by aspirin 3.5 g.[3] The clearance of a single 400-mg dose of sulfinpyrazone was modestly increased by 12 to 27% in 5 healthy subjects given four doses of aspirin 325 mg over 24 hours.[4]

Mechanism

Not fully understood. Sulfinpyrazone competes successfully with salicylate for secretion by the kidney tubules so that salicylate excretion is reduced, but the salicylate blocks the inhibitory effect of sulfinpyrazone on the tubular reabsorption of uric acid causing the uric acid to accumulate within the body.[2]

Importance and management

An established and clinically important interaction. Concurrent use for uricosuria should be avoided. Doses of aspirin as low as 700 mg can cause an appreciable fall in uric acid excretion,[3] but the effects of an occasional small dose are probably of little practical importance.

1. Seegmiller JE, Grayzel AI. Use of the newer uricosuric agents in the management of gout. *JAMA* (1960) 173, 1076–80.
2. Yu TF, Dayton PG, Gutman AB. Mutual suppression of the uricosuric effects of sulfinpyrazone and salicylate: a study in interactions between drugs. *J Clin Invest* (1963) 42, 1330–9.
3. Kersley GD, Cook ER, Tovey DCJ. Value of uricosuric agents and in particular of G.28 315 in gout. *Ann Rheum Dis* (1958) 17, 326–33.
4. Buchanan MR, Endrenyi L, Giles AR, Rosenfeld J. The effect of aspirin on the pharmacokinetics of sulfinpyrazone in man. *Thromb Res* (1983) (Suppl 4), 145–52.

Nefopam + Miscellaneous

The manufacturer states that nefopam should not be given to patients taking non-selective MAOIs and caution should be used in those taking tricyclic antidepressants, antimuscarinics and sympathomimetics. The intensity and incidence of adverse effects are somewhat increased when nefopam is given with codeine, pentazocine or dextropropoxyphene (propoxyphene), and the CNS depressant effect of dihydrocodeine may have contributed to a fatal overdose with nefopam. However, a morphine-sparing effect has been reported. Nefopam may also have a synergistic analgesic effect with ketoprofen.

Clinical evidence, mechanism, importance and management

Detailed information about adverse interactions between nefopam and other drugs does not seem to be available.[1] The manufacturer advises caution if nefopam is given with a **tricyclic antidepressant** because they lower the convulsive threshold; convulsions have been seen in some patients taking nefopam. In addition, the antimuscarinic adverse effects of nefopam may be additive with those of **tricyclics** and other drugs with antimuscarinic effects.[1] For example, the CSM in the UK has a number of reports of urinary retention caused by nefopam[2], which would be expected to be worsened by drugs with antimuscarinic activity. Nefopam appears to have sympathomimetic activity and the manufacturer therefore says it should not be given with the **MAOIs**[1] (see 'MAOIs or RIMAs + Sympathomimetics; Indirectly-acting', p.1147).

A controlled study was conducted in 45 healthy subjects divided into nine groups of five, each given oral nefopam 60 mg three times daily for 3 days with either **aspirin** 650 mg, **diazepam** 5 mg, **phenobarbital** 60 mg, **dextropropoxyphene** (**propoxyphene**) 65 mg, **codeine** 60 mg, **pentazocine** 50 mg, **indometacin** 25 mg or **hydroxyzine** 50 mg (all three times daily). The only changes were a possible additive increase in the intensity and incidence of adverse effects with nefopam and **codeine**, **pentazocine** or **dextropropoxyphene**. There was no evidence that the bioavailability of nefopam was change by the other drugs.[3]

The incidence of sedation with nefopam is 20 to 30% which, depending on the circumstances, may present a problem if it is given with other **sedative drugs**.[4] A report describes a fatal overdose with nefopam, which was complicated by the CNS depressant effect of **dihydrocodeine**.[5]

In a study in *animals,* nefopam enhanced the analgesic potency of **morphine**,[6] but in a study in patients the effects were found to be less than additive.[7] However, another study in patients undergoing orthopaedic surgery found that the concurrent use of intravenous nefopam 20 mg every 4 hours with **morphine** given as patient-controlled analgesia (PCA) had a significant morphine-sparing effect, without major adverse effects. The amount of **morphine** used over 24 hours was 22% less for those receiving nefopam compared with placebo; the analgesic effect was particularly notable for patients with intense preoperative pain who required 35% less morphine with nefopam.[8] A study in 72 surgical patients found that the use of nefopam with **ketoprofen** had a synergistic analgesic effect.[9]

1. Acupan (Nefopam hydrochloride). 3M Health Care Ltd. UK Summary of product characteristics, November 2000.
2. Committee on Safety of Medicines (CSM). Nefopam hydrochloride (Acupan). Current Problems No 24, January 1989.
3. Lasseter KC, Cohen A, Back EL. Nefopam HCl interaction study with eight other drugs. *J Int Med Res* (1976) 4, 195–201.
4. Heel RC, Brogden RN, Pakes GE, Speight TM, Avery GS. Nefopam: a review of its pharmacological properties and therapeutic efficacy. *Drugs* (1980) 19, 249–67.
5. Urwin SC, Smith HS. Fatal nefopam overdose. *Br J Anaesth* (1999) 83, 501–2.
6. Girard P, Pansart Y, Gillardin JM. Nefopam potentiates morphine antinociception in allodynia and hyperalgesia in the rat. *Pharmacol Biochem Behav* (2004) 77, 695–703.
7. Beloeil H, Delage N, Nègre I, Mazoit J-X, Benhamou D. The median effective dose of nefopam and morphine administered intravenously for postoperative pain after minor surgery: a prospective randomized double-blinded isobolographic study of their analgesic action. *Anesth Analg* (2004) 98, 395–400.
8. Du Manoir B, Aubrun F, Langlois M, Le Guern ME, Alquier C, Chauvin M, Fletcher D. Randomized prospective study of the analgesic effect of nefopam after orthopaedic surgery. *Br J Anaesth* (2003) 91, 836–41.
9. Delage N, Maaliki H, Beloeil H, Benhamou D, Mazoit J-X. Median effective dose (ED_{50}) of nefopam and ketoprofen in postoperative patients: a study of interaction using sequential analysis and isobolographic analysis. *Anesthesiology* (2005) 102, 1211–16.

NSAIDs + Allopurinol

Allopurinol does not affect indometacin clearance or phenylbutazone levels.

Clinical evidence, mechanism, importance and management

Allopurinol 300 mg each morning was given to 8 patients for 5 days with **indometacin** 50 mg every 8 hours. The allopurinol had no significant effect on the AUC of **indometacin** and the amounts of **indometacin** excreted in the urine were not significantly altered.[1]

Allopurinol 100 mg three times daily for a month had no effect on the elimination of a 200-mg daily dose of **phenylbutazone** in 6 healthy subjects, and no effect on the steady-state plasma levels of **phenylbutazone** 200 or 300 mg daily in 3 patients.[2] In another study in 8 patients with acute gouty arthritis it was found that allopurinol 100 mg every 8 hours produced small but clinically unimportant effects on the half-life of **phenylbutazone** 6 mg/kg.[3]

There seems to be no reason for avoiding the concurrent use of these NSAIDs and allopurinol.

1. Pullar T, Myall O, Haigh JRM, Lowe JR, Dixon JS, Bird HA. The effect of allopurinol on the steady-state pharmacokinetics of indomethacin. *Br J Clin Pharmacol* (1988) 25, 755–7.
2. Rawlins MD, Smith SE. Influence of allopurinol on drug metabolism in man. *Br J Pharmacol* (1973) 48, 693–8.
3. Horwitz D, Thorgeirsson SS, Mitchell JR. The influence of allopurinol and size of dose on the metabolism of phenylbutazone in patients with gout. *Eur J Clin Pharmacol* (1977) 12, 133–6.

NSAIDs + Amoxicillin

A study in healthy subjects found that diclofenac increased the clearance of amoxicillin. An isolated report describes acute interstitial nephritis with nephrotic syndrome associated with the use of naproxen and amoxicillin.

Clinical evidence, mechanism, importance and management

(a) Diclofenac

In a study in 20 healthy subjects diclofenac 100 mg caused a slight reduction in the AUC and a slight increase in the mean renal clearance of a single 2-g dose of amoxicillin.[1] It should be noted that there was considerable individual variation and overlapping between the two groups, and the clinical significance of this finding is unclear.

An *animal* study found that diclofenac caused an 8.5-fold reduction in amoxicillin serum levels, when compared with amoxicillin alone. However, amoxicillin retained its efficacy despite lowered serum levels and it was suggested that diclofenac was unlikely to cause an increase in renal clearance of amoxicillin, nor an effect on its liver metabolism.[2] These studies therefore suggest that a clinically significant interaction would not be expected.

(b) Naproxen

A man without any previous renal problems developed acute interstitial nephritis with nephrotic syndrome after taking naproxen for 4 days (total 4 g) and amoxicillin for 10 days (total 24 g). He appeared to recover when the drugs were stopped, but 3 months later he developed renal failure and needed haemodialysis.[3] Acute interstitial nephritis is not only a rare syndrome (reported to be only 55 cases in the world literature in 1988)[3] but this is the first case involving both of these drugs. No special precautions would normally seem to be necessary.

1. de Cássia Bergamaschi C, Motta RHL, Franco GCN, Cogo K, Montan MF, Ambrosano GMB, Rosalen PL, de Sá Del Fiol F, Groppo FC. Effect of sodium diclofenac on the bioavailability of amoxicillin. *Int J Antimicrob Agents* (2006) 27, 417–22.
2. Groppo FC, Simões RP, Ramacciato JC, Rehder V, de Andrade ED, Mattos-Filho TR. Effect of sodium diclofenac on serum and tissue concentration of amoxicillin and on staphylococcal infection. *Biol Pharm Bull* (2004) 27, 52–5.
3. Nortier J, Depierreux M, Bourgeois V, Dupont P. Acute interstitial nephritis with nephrotic syndrome after intake of naproxen and amoxycillin. *Nephrol Dial Transplant* (1990) 5, 1055.

NSAIDs + Anabolic steroids

Serum oxyphenbutazone levels are raised about 40% by the use of methandienone (methandrostenolone). Phenylbutazone appears to be unaffected.

Clinical evidence

The serum levels of oxyphenbutazone 300 to 400 mg daily for 2 to 5 weeks were raised by 43% (range 5 to 100%) in 6 subjects given **methandienone**. Neither prednisone 5 mg nor dexamethasone 1.5 mg daily were found to affect oxyphenbutazone levels.[1]

Two other studies confirm this interaction with oxyphenbutazone.[2,3] One of them found no interaction with phenylbutazone.[2]

Mechanism

Uncertain. One idea is that the anabolic steroids alter the distribution of oxyphenbutazone between the tissues and plasma so that more remains in circulation. There may also possibly be some changes in metabolism.

Importance and management

The interaction is established but its importance is uncertain. There seem to be no reports of toxicity arising from concurrent use but the possibility should be borne in mind.

1. Weiner M, Siddiqui AA, Shahani RT, Dayton PG. Effect of steroids on disposition of oxyphenbutazone in man. *Proc Soc Exp Biol Med* (1967) 124, 1170–3.
2. Hvidberg E, Dayton PG, Read JM, Wilson CH. Studies of the interaction of phenylbutazone, oxyphenbutazone and methandrostenolone in man. *Proc Soc Exp Biol Med* (1968) 129, 438–43.
3. Weiner M, Siddiqui AA, Bostanci N, Dayton PG. Drug interactions.The effect of combined administration on the half-life of coumarin and pyrazolone drugs in man. *Fedn Proc* (1965) 24, 153.

NSAIDs; Azapropazone + Antacids or Laxatives

A study in 15 patients taking azapropazone 300 mg three times daily found that antacids (dihydroxyaluminium sodium carbonate, aluminium magnesium silicate), bisacodyl or anthraquinone laxatives only caused a minor (5 to 7%) reduction in azapropazone plasma levels.[1] No special precautions would seem to be needed if any of these drugs are given together with azapropazone. Consider also 'NSAIDs; Miscellaneous + Antacids', p.142.

1. Faust-Tinnefeldt G, Geissler HE, Mutschler E. Azapropazon-Plasmaspiegel unter Begleitmedikation mit einem Antacidum oder Laxans. *Arzneimittelforschung* (1977) 27, 2411–14.

NSAIDs; Coxibs + Antacids

The manufacturers say that antacids (unspecified) do not affect the pharmacokinetics of etoricoxib to a clinically relevant extent.[1] Aluminium/magnesium hydroxides had no clinically significant effect on the bioavailability of celecoxib,[2,3] or lumiracoxib.[4]

1. Arcoxia (Etoricoxib). Merck Sharp & Dohme Ltd. UK Summary of product characteristics, January 2007.
2. Celebrex (Celecoxib). Pharmacia Ltd. UK Summary of product characteristics, February 2007.

3. Celebrex (Celecoxib). Pfizer Inc. US Prescribing information, February 2007.
4. Scott G, Vinluan Reynolds C, Milosavljev S, Langholff W, Shenouda M, Rordorf C. Lack of effect of omeprazole or of an aluminium hydroxide/magnesium hydroxide antacid on the pharmacokinetics of lumiracoxib. *Clin Pharmacokinet* (2004) 43, 341–8.

NSAIDs; Diclofenac + Antacids

The absorption of diclofenac is not affected by aluminium hydroxide, magnesium hydroxide, or the combination.

Clinical evidence, mechanism, importance and management

About 10 mL of a 5.8% suspension of **aluminium hydroxide** had no effect on the bioavailability of a single 50-mg dose of diclofenac in 7 healthy subjects.[1] In another study, 10 mL of **magnesium hydroxide** suspension (850 mg) was found to have no significant effect on the rate or extent of absorption of a single 50-mg dose of diclofenac in 6 healthy, fasted subjects.[2] However, there was a tendency to an increased rate of absorption. *Aluco Gel* (**aluminium/magnesium hydroxide**) had no effect on the extent of absorption of enteric-coated diclofenac, but may have reduced the rate of absorption.[3] No particular precautions would seem to be needed if these antacids are given with diclofenac.

1. Schumacher A, Faust-Tinnefeldt G, Geissler HE, Gilfrich HJ, Mutschler E. Untersuchungen potentieller Interaktionen von Diclofenac-Natrium (Voltaren) mit einem Antazidum und mit Digitoxin. *Therapiewoche* (1983) 33, 2619–25.
2. Neuvonen PJ. The effect of magnesium hydroxide on the oral absorption of ibuprofen, ketoprofen and diclofenac. *Br J Clin Pharmacol* (1991) 31, 263–6.
3. Sioufi A, Stierlin H, Schweizer A, Botta L, Degen PH, Theobald W, Brechbühler S. Recent findings concerning clinically relevant pharmacokinetics of diclofenac sodium. In: Voltarol — New Findings, ed Kass E. Proc Int Symp Voltarol, Paris June 22nd, 1981. 15th Int Congress of Rheumatology. p 19–30.

NSAIDs; Diflunisal + Antacids

Antacids containing aluminium with or without magnesium can reduce the absorption of diflunisal by up to 40%, but no important interaction occurs if food is taken at the same time. Magnesium hydroxide can increase the rate of diflunisal absorption.

Clinical evidence

A study in 4 healthy, fasted subjects found that when a single 500-mg oral dose of diflunisal was given 2 hours before, together with, and 2 hours after three 15-mL doses of *Aludrox* (**aluminium hydroxide**), the diflunisal AUC was reduced by about 40%.[1] Another study found that the AUC of a single 500-mg dose of diflunisal was reduced by 13% when given with a single 30-mL dose of *Maalox* (**aluminium/magnesium hydroxide**), by 21% when given 1 hour after the antacid, and by 32% when the antacid was given four times daily.[2] However, in another study, **aluminium/magnesium hydroxide** had no effect on the AUC diflunisal when the diflunisal was given 30 minutes after food.[3] This study also found that the AUC of diflunisal was reduced by 26% by 15 mL of **aluminium hydroxide** gel in fasted subjects, but not when the diflunisal was given after food.[3] **Magnesium hydroxide** suspension markedly increased the rate of diflunisal absorption in fasted subjects. The plasma diflunisal level was increased by 130% at 30 minutes, and by 64% at one hour but the AUC was only increased by a modest 10%.[3]

Mechanism

Just how aluminium antacids reduce the absorption of diflunisal is not clear, but adsorption or formation of insoluble salts has been suggested. Food appears to diminish the effect of antacids on diflunisal absorption.[3] By raising the pH, magnesium hydroxide may promote the dissolution of diflunisal, so increasing its absorption.[3] Consider also 'NSAIDs; Fenamates + Antacids', below.

Importance and management

Aluminium-containing antacids appear to reduce the absorption of diflunisal in the fasted state, but not if taken with food. Since NSAIDs should be taken with or after food, it appears that this interaction has little clinical relevance. See also 'NSAIDs; Miscellaneous + Antacids', p.142. Magnesium hydroxide increases the absorption of diflunisal in the fasted state, which may improve the onset of analgesia. However, note that magnesium hydroxide increased the endoscopically-detected gastric toxicity of ibuprofen in one study, see 'NSAIDs; Ibuprofen and related drugs + Antacids', below.

1. Verbeeck R, Tjandramaga TB, Mullie A, Verbesselt R, De Schepper PJ. Effect of aluminium hydroxide on diflunisal absorption. *Br J Clin Pharmacol* (1979) 7, 519–22.
2. Holmes GI, Irvin JD, Schrogie JJ, Davies RO, Breault GO, Rogers JL, Huber PB, Zinny MA. Effects of Maalox on the bioavailability of diflunisal. *Clin Pharmacol Ther* (1979) 25, 229.
3. Tobert JA, DeSchepper P, Tjandramaga TB, Mullie A, Buntinx AP, Meisinger MAP, Huber PB, Hall TLP, Yeh KC. Effect of antacids on the bioavailability of diflunisal in the fasting and postprandial states. *Clin Pharmacol Ther* (1981) 30, 385–9.

NSAIDs; Fenamates + Antacids

The absorption of mefenamic acid and tolfenamic acid is markedly accelerated by magnesium hydroxide in fasted subjects. The rate of tolfenamic acid absorption is reduced by aluminium hydroxide alone or combined with magnesium hydroxide/magnesium carbonate, but is not affected by sodium bicarbonate.

Clinical evidence

Studies in 6 healthy, fasted subjects given a single dose of **mefenamic acid** 500 mg or **tolfenamic acid** 400 mg found that **magnesium hydroxide** accelerated the absorption of both drugs (the **mefenamic acid** AUC after 1 hour was increased threefold and the **tolfenamic acid** AUC was increased sevenfold) but the total bioavailability was only slightly increased. In contrast, **aluminium hydroxide**, alone and in combination with **magnesium hydroxide/magnesium carbonate** (*Medisan Forte*), markedly reduced the rate of absorption of **tolfenamic acid** without causing a marked change in the total amount absorbed. **Sodium bicarbonate** 1 g did not significantly alter the absorption of **tolfenamic acid**.[1]

Mechanism

Uncertain. It is suggested that magnesium hydroxide increases the solubility of acidic drugs such as the fenamates, possibly by forming a soluble salt and therefore enhancing their dissolution. In contrast, aluminium antacids may form insoluble salts of the drug. Note that food may reduce these effects, see 'NSAIDs; Diflunisal + Antacids', above.

Importance and management

Information is very limited but it would appear that if rapid analgesia is needed with either mefenamic acid or tolfenamic acid, magnesium hydroxide can be given concurrently but aluminium hydroxide should be avoided. However, note that this applies to the fasted state, whereas NSAIDs are usually taken with or after food. Also note that magnesium hydroxide increased the endoscopically-detected gastric toxicity of ibuprofen in one study, see 'NSAIDs; Ibuprofen and related drugs + Antacids', below. Aluminium hydroxide markedly reduces the speed of absorption. Sodium bicarbonate does not interact. Consider also 'NSAIDs; Miscellaneous + Antacids', p.142.

1. Neuvonen PJ, Kivistö KT. Effect of magnesium hydroxide on the absorption of tolfenamic and mefenamic acids. *Eur J Clin Pharmacol* (1988) 35, 495–501.

NSAIDs; Ibuprofen and related drugs + Antacids

Magnesium hydroxide increased the initial absorption of ibuprofen and flurbiprofen, but had no effect on ketoprofen. Unexpectedly, a pharmacodynamic study showed increased gastric erosions when ibuprofen was formulated with magnesium hydroxide.

A small reduction in ketoprofen absorption occurred with aluminium-magnesium hydroxide, but dexketoprofen, ibuprofen and flurbiprofen were not affected, and naproxen showed a slight increase in rate and extent of absorption. Aluminium phosphate had no effect on ketoprofen absorption.

Sodium bicarbonate increased the rate of naproxen absorption, and aluminium hydroxide and magnesium oxide decreased it.

Dimeticone did not affect ketoprofen bioavailability.

Clinical evidence

(a) Dexketoprofen

In 24 healthy subjects an **aluminium/magnesium hydroxide** antacid (*Maalox*) had no effect on the rate or extent of absorption of a single 25-mg dose of dexketoprofen, although the maximum level was slightly (13%) lower.[1]

(b) Flurbiprofen

Maalox (**aluminium/magnesium hydroxide**) 30 mL, taken 30 minutes before a single 100-mg dose of flurbiprofen, was found to affect neither the rate nor extent of flurbiprofen absorption in a group of young and old fasting healthy subjects. Similarly, the antacid had no effect on steady-state flurbiprofen pharmacokinetics when both drugs were given 90 minutes before food.[2] Another study found that **magnesium hydroxide** increased the AUC_{0-2} by 61%, but the AUC_{0-8} was not changed in fasted subjects, which demonstrated an increased rate of flurbiprofen absorption.[3]

(c) Ibuprofen

In 8 healthy, fasted subjects an antacid containing **aluminium/magnesium hydroxide**, given before, with, and after a single 400-mg dose of ibuprofen, did not alter the pharmacokinetics of ibuprofen.[4] In another study, the absorption of ibuprofen formulated with **aluminium** was delayed and reduced, when compared to that of ibuprofen without **aluminium**.[5] Another study in 6 healthy fasted subjects found that **magnesium hydroxide** 850 mg increased the AUC_{0-1} and the peak levels of a single 400-mg dose of ibuprofen by 65% and 31%, respectively. The time to the peak was shortened by about 30 minutes but the total bioavailability was unchanged.[6] In a pharmacodynamic study in healthy subjects, a 400-mg ibuprofen tablet buffered with 200 mg of **magnesium hydroxide**, given at a dose of two tablets three times daily for 5 days resulted in about a threefold increase in number of endoscopically-detected gastric erosions, when compared with the same dose of conventional ibuprofen tablets.[7]

A **sodium/potassium salt** (kanwa), often taken as an antacid in some West African countries, appeared to reduce the absorption of ibuprofen. The bioavailability of ibuprofen 400 mg given to 6 healthy subjects with a millet meal containing the salt extract (pH of 8.9) was reduced, compared with the millet meal alone (pH 5.3) or following overnight fasting (approximate AUCs 20, 120, 110 micrograms/mL per hour, respectively).[8]

(d) Ketoprofen

Five healthy, fasted subjects had a 22% reduction in the absorption of a 50-mg dose of ketoprofen (as measured by the amount excreted in the urine) when they were given a 1-g dose of **aluminium hydroxide**.[9] Conversely, **aluminium phosphate** 11 g (as a single then a daily dose) had no effect on the pharmacokinetics of ketoprofen 100 mg in 10 patients.[10] Another study in 12 healthy, fasted subjects showed that **dimeticone** did not significantly affect the bioavailability of a single 100-mg dose of ketoprofen.[11] In another study 10 mL of **magnesium hydroxide** suspension (equivalent to 850 mg) was found to have no significant effect on the rate or extent of absorption of ketoprofen 50 mg in fasted subjects, although the rate of ketoprofen absorption was already noted to be fast.[6]

(e) Naproxen

Sodium bicarbonate 700 mg or 1.4 g increased the rate of absorption of a single 300-mg dose of naproxen in 14 healthy fasted subjects, whereas **magnesium oxide** or **aluminium hydroxide** 700 mg had the opposite effect, and reduced the rate of absorption. **Magnesium carbonate** had little effect.[12] On the other hand when 15 or 60 mL of **aluminium/magnesium hydroxide** (*Maalox*) was given, the rate and extent of absorption of naproxen were slightly increased.[12]

Mechanism

Magnesium hydroxide appears to improve the rate of absorption of some acidic NSAIDs (which become more soluble as the pH rises) such as ibuprofen and flurbiprofen. Why this increased the gastric toxicity of ibuprofen in the one pharmacodynamic study is unclear.[7] Sodium bicarbonate appears to have a similar effect on rate of absorption. Aluminium antacids do not produce soluble salts with these NSAIDs, and may therefore reduce the rate/extent of absorption.

Importance and management

It would appear that the initial absorption of both ibuprofen and flurbiprofen is increased by magnesium hydroxide, but not if aluminium hydroxide is present as well. Thus if rapid analgesia is needed, an antacid containing magnesium hydroxide but without aluminium hydroxide could be used with these NSAIDs. However, the unexpected finding that magnesium hydroxide increased the endoscopically-detected gastric toxicity of ibuprofen[7] suggests that caution may be warranted, particularly on long-term use. Further study is needed.

Sodium bicarbonate and aluminium hydroxide appear to have a similar effect on naproxen, namely an increased and decreased effect, respectively, on the rate of absorption. However, note that these effects were seen in the fasted state, and may not apply when the NSAIDs are taken with or after food (as is recommended), as is the case with 'diflunisal', (p.140).

No particular precautions would seem to be needed if dimeticone, aluminium phosphate or magnesium hydroxide are given with ketoprofen, and it seems doubtful if the effects of ketoprofen will be reduced to any great extent by aluminium hydroxide.

1. McEwen J, De Luca M, Casini A, Gich I, Barbanoj MJ, Tost D, Artigas R, Mauleón D. The effect of food and an antacid on the bioavailability of dexketoprofen trometamol. *J Clin Pharmacol* (1998) 38 (Suppl), 41S–45S.
2. Caillé G, du Souich P, Vézina M, Pollock SR, Stalker DJ. Pharmacokinetic interaction between flurbiprofen and antacids in healthy volunteers. *Biopharm Drug Dispos* (1989) 10, 607–15.
3. Rao TRK, Ravisekhar K, Shobha JC, Sekhar EC, Naidu MUR, Krishna DR. Influence of magnesium hydroxide on the oral absorption of flurbiprofen. *Drug Invest* (1992) 4, 473–6.
4. Gontarz N, Small RE, Comstock TJ, Stalker DJ, Johnson SM, Willis HE. Effect of antacid suspension on the pharmacokinetics of ibuprofen. *Clin Pharm* (1987) 6, 413–16.
5. Laska EM, Sunshine A, Marrero I, Olson N, Siegel C, McCormick N. The correlation between blood levels of ibuprofen and clinical analgesic response. *Clin Pharmacol Ther* (1986) 40, 1–7.
6. Neuvonen PJ. The effect of magnesium hydroxide on the oral absorption of ibuprofen, ketoprofen and diclofenac. *Br J Clin Pharmacol* (1991) 31, 263–6.
7. Mäenpää J, Tarpila A, Jouhikainen T, Ikävalko H, Löyttyniemi E, Perttunen K, Neuvonen PJ, Tarpila S. Magnesium hydroxide in ibuprofen tablet reduces the gastric mucosal tolerability of ibuprofen. *J Clin Gastroenterol* (2004) 38, 41–5.
8. Yakasai IA. Effect of sodium/potassium salt (potash) on the bioavailability of ibuprofen in healthy human volunteers. *Eur J Drug Metab Pharmacokinet* (2003) 28, 93–9.
9. Ismail FA, Khalafallah N, Khalil SA. Adsorption of ketoprofen and bumadizone calcium on aluminium-containing antacids and its effect on ketoprofen bioavailability in man. *Int J Pharmaceutics* (1987) 34, 189–96.
10. Brazier JL, Tamisier JN, Ambert D, Bannier A. Bioavailability of ketoprofen in man with and without concomitant administration of aluminium phosphate. *Eur J Clin Pharmacol* (1981) 19, 305–7.
11. Presle N, Lapicque F, Gillet P, Herrmann M-A, Bannwarth B, Netter P. Effect of dimethicone (polysilane gel) on the stereoselective pharmacokinetics of ketoprofen. *Eur J Clin Pharmacol* (1998) 54, 351–4.
12. Segre EJ, Sevelius H, Varady J. Effects of antacids on naproxen absorption. *N Engl J Med* (1974) 291, 582–3.

NSAIDs; Indometacin or Sulindac + Antacids

Although a variety of different antacids have slightly altered the absorption of indometacin the changes are probably not clinically important. Aluminium/magnesium hydroxide had no effect on sulindac absorption.

Clinical evidence

In 12 healthy, fasted subjects the AUC of a single 50-mg dose of indometacin was reduced by 35% when formulated with 80% *Mergel* (an antacid formulation of **aluminium/magnesium hydroxide**, and **magnesium carbonate**) and by 18% when taken with 90% *Mergel*.[1]

In another single-dose study in 6 healthy, fasted subjects, **aluminium hydroxide** suspension 700 mg reduced the rate of indometacin absorption, and reduced the peak indometacin plasma levels. Conversely, **sodium bicarbonate** 1.4 g appeared to increase the rate of absorption, but this did not reach significance because of wide inter-individual variation.[2] In a further study 30 mL of **aluminium/magnesium hydroxide** caused only slight changes in the absorption of a 50-mg dose of indometacin in fasted subjects.[3]

The manufacturer of sulindac notes that an antacid (**aluminium/magnesium hydroxide** suspension) had no effect on the absorption of sulindac.[4]

Mechanism

Not known. Aluminium compounds might form insoluble salts with indometacin.[2] Food might reduce this effect, see 'NSAIDs; Diflunisal + Antacids', p.140.

Importance and management

Adequately but not extensively documented. Some small reduction in plasma indometacin levels is possible with some aluminium containing antacids. Despite this the manufacturers of indometacin recommend that it be taken with food, milk or an antacid to minimise gastrointestinal disturbances.[5] Sulindac absorption is not affected.

1. Galeazzi RL. The effect of an antacid on the bioavailability of indomethacin. *Eur J Clin Pharmacol* (1977) 12, 65–8.
2. Garnham JC, Kaspi T, Kaye CM and Oh VMS. The different effects of sodium bicarbonate and aluminium hydroxide on the absorption of indomethacin in man. *Postgrad Med J* (1977) 53, 126–9.
3. Emori HW, Paulus H, Bluestone R, Champion GD, Pearson C. Indomethacin serum concentrations in man. Effects of dosage, food and antacid. *Ann Rheum Dis* (1976) 35, 333–8.
4. Clinoril (Sulindac). Merck Sharp & Dohme Ltd. UK Summary of product characteristics, May 2007.
5. Pardelprin MR (Indometacin). Actavis UK Ltd. UK Summary of product characteristics, March 2007.

NSAIDs; Miscellaneous + Antacids

The rate and extent of absorption of ketorolac, metamizole and tolmetin was not significantly affected by aluminium/magnesium hydroxide. Nabumetone absorption was not affected by aluminium hydroxide, and an unspecified antacid did not affect etodolac absorption.

Clinical evidence

(a) Etodolac

A study in 18 healthy, fasted subjects found that when given a single 400-mg dose of etodolac with 30 mL of an unnamed antacid neither the rate nor the extent of etodolac absorption were altered.[1]

(b) Ketorolac

The AUC of oral ketorolac 10 mg was found to be reduced by 11% (not statistically significant) when taken with an unstated amount of **aluminium/magnesium hydroxide** suspension (*Maalox*) in 12 healthy fasted subjects. The rate of absorption was not affected.[2]

(c) Metamizole sodium (Dipyrone)

The concurrent use of 20 mL of *Maaloxan* (**aluminium/magnesium hydroxide** gel) was reported to have had no effect on the pharmacokinetics of the metabolites of metamizole sodium.[3]

(d) Nabumetone

The absorption of a single 1-g dose of nabumetone (as assessed by AUC and maximum plasma level) was not significantly altered by 160 mL of **aluminium hydroxide** suspension (*Aludrox*) in 15 healthy fasted subjects.[4]

(e) Tolmetin

A pharmacokinetic study in 24 healthy, fasted subjects showed that **aluminium/magnesium hydroxide** suspension (*Maalox*), given as a single 20-mL dose four times daily for 3 days, had no significant effect on the absorption of a single 400-mg dose of **tolmetin**.[5]

Mechanism

None.

Importance and management

Although information is limited, no particular precautions would seem to be needed if aluminium or aluminium/magnesium antacids are given with any of these antacids. Note that antacids have been frequently given with NSAIDs to reduce their gastric irritant effects. Consider also 'coxibs', (p.139), 'diclofenac', (p.140), 'diflunisal', (p.140), 'ibuprofen and related drugs', (p.140), 'indometacin', (p.141), 'fenamates', (p.140), and 'oxicams', (below) for information about the interaction of other NSAIDs with antacids.

1. Troy S, Sanda M, Dressler D, Chiang S, Latts J. The effect of food and antacid on etodolac bioavailability. *Clin Pharmacol Ther* (1990) 47, 192.
2. Mroszczak EJ, Jung D, Yee J, Bynum L, Sevelius H, Massey I. Ketorolac tromethamine pharmacokinetics and metabolism after intravenous, intramuscular, and oral administration in humans and animals. *Pharmacotherapy* (1990) 10 (Suppl 6), 33S–39S.
3. Scholz W, Rosenkrantz B. Clinical pharmacokinetics of dipyrone and its metabolites. *Clin Pharmacokinet* (1995) 28, 216–34.
4. von Schrader HW, Buscher G, Dierdorf D, Mügge H, Wolf D. Nabumetone — a novel anti-inflammatory drug: the influence of food, milk, antacids, and analgesics on bioavailability of single oral doses. *Int J Clin Pharmacol Ther Toxicol* (1983) 21, 311–21.
5. Ayres JW, Weidler DJ, MacKichan J, Sakmar E, Hallmark MR, Lemanowicz EF, Wagner JG. Pharmacokinetics of tolmetin with and without concomitant administration of antacid in man. *Eur J Clin Pharmacol* (1977) 12, 421–8.

NSAIDs; Oxicam derivatives + Antacids

The pharmacokinetics of lornoxicam, meloxicam, piroxicam and tenoxicam were not affected by aluminium/magnesium hydroxide antacids. Lornoxicam pharmacokinetics were also not altered by tripotassium dicitratobismuthate or aluminium hydroxide with calcium carbonate.

Clinical evidence, mechanism, importance and management

(a) Lornoxicam

Neither 10 mL of *Maalox* (**aluminium/magnesium hydroxide**) nor 10 g of *Solugastril* (**aluminium hydroxide** with **calcium carbonate**) had any effect on the pharmacokinetics of a 4-mg lornoxicam film-coated tablet in 18 healthy fasted subjects.[1] A later study similarly found no changes in the absorption or pharmacokinetics of a lornoxicam film-coated tablet given with **bismuth chelate (tripotassium dicitratobismuthate)** 120 mg twice daily.[2] There would seem to be no reason for avoiding concurrent use.

(b) Meloxicam

In an open, randomised, crossover study 9 healthy, fasted subjects were given meloxicam 30 mg alone or with *Maalox* suspension (**aluminium/magnesium hydroxide** 900/600 mg) four times daily for 4 days. *Maalox* had no significant effect on the pharmacokinetics of the meloxicam.[3] Therefore no adjustments of the dosage of meloxicam are needed if given with this type of antacid.

(c) Piroxicam

A multiple-dose study in 20 healthy subjects found that *Mylanta* (**aluminium/magnesium hydroxide**) and *Amphojel* (**aluminium hydroxide**) did not significantly affect the bioavailability of piroxicam 20 mg daily taken after food.[4] Concurrent use need not be avoided.

(d) Tenoxicam

The bioavailability of tenoxicam 20 mg was found to be unaffected in 12 healthy subjects by **aluminium hydroxide** (*Amphojel*) or **aluminium/magnesium hydroxide** (*Mylanta*) whether taken before, with, or after the tenoxicam, and in the fasted state or with food.[5] No special precautions seem necessary.

1. Dittrich P, Radhofer-Welte S, Magometschnigg D, Kukovetz WR, Mayerhofer S, Ferber HP. The effect of concomitantly administered antacids on the bioavailability of lornoxicam, a novel highly potent NSAID. *Drugs Exp Clin Res* (1990) 16, 57–62.
2. Ravic M, Johnston A, Turner P, Foley K, Rosenow D. Does bismuth chelate influence lornoxicam absorption? *Hum Exp Toxicol* (1992) 11, 59–60.
3. Busch U, Heinzel G, Narjes H, Nehmiz G. Interaction of meloxicam with cimetidine, Maalox or aspirin. *J Clin Pharmacol* (1996) 36, 79–84.
4. Hobbs DC, Twomey TM. Piroxicam pharmacokinetics in man: aspirin and antacid interaction studies. *J Clin Pharmacol* (1979) 19, 270–81.
5. Day RO, Lam S, Paull P, Wade D. Effect of food and various antacids on the absorption of tenoxicam. *Br J Clin Pharmacol* (1987) 24, 323–8.

NSAIDs + Aspirin; Anti-inflammatory dose

The combined use of aspirin and NSAIDs increases the risk of gastrointestinal damage. There is no clinical rationale for the combined use of anti-inflammatory/analgesic doses of aspirin and NSAIDs, and such use should be avoided. There are numerous early pharmacokinetic studies of aspirin and NSAIDs, many of which showed that aspirin reduced the levels of NSAIDs.

Clinical evidence

A. Gastrointestinal damage

In a case-control study of data from 1993 to 1998 in the UK General Practice Research Database the risk of upper gastrointestinal bleeding or perforation was increased by slightly more than an additive effect in patients taking both aspirin and NSAIDs (8.2-fold), when compared with aspirin alone (2.4-fold), or NSAIDs alone (3.6-fold). The specific NSAIDs were not mentioned.[1] Another study provided similar findings,[2] as have studies specifically looking at low-dose aspirin (325 mg or less daily), see 'NSAIDs + Aspirin; Antiplatelet dose', p.144. Analysis of Yellow Card reports to the CSM in the UK gastrointestinal perforation/obstruction, ulceration or bleeding with **diclofenac**, **naproxen**, and **ibuprofen** revealed that 28% of the patients were receiving concurrent aspirin (dose not stated).[3]

The one pharmacodynamic study below, that also measured gastrointestinal blood loss, found increased bleeding when anti-inflammatory doses of aspirin were given with **sodium meclofenamate**.[4]

A case report described acute ulcerative colitis in a woman taking **rofecoxib** 25 mg daily who also took aspirin.[5] See also *gastrointestinal effects*, in 'NSAIDs + Aspirin; Antiplatelet dose', p.144.

B. Pharmacokinetic and pharmacodynamic studies

Early studies evaluating non-aspirin NSAIDs in rheumatoid arthritis commonly permitted the concurrent use of aspirin, which was then in wide use for this condition. The unexpected finding that **indometacin** was no more effective than placebo in patients taking aspirin in one study led to a number of pharmacokinetic studies with this combination (see *Indometacin*, below), and subsequently other NSAID/aspirin combinations. These studies generally have little clinical relevance to current clinical practice where anti-inflammatory doses of aspirin should not be used in combination with NSAIDs because of the increased risk of gastrointestinal bleeding (see above) and lack of proven additional benefit. However, the pharmacokinetic studies are briefly summarised below.

(a) Diclofenac

Aspirin 900 mg reduced the AUC of diclofenac 50 mg by about one-third in a single-dose study.[6] In a clinical study, there was no significant difference in efficacy between diclofenac 50 mg three times daily alone or with aspirin 900 mg three times daily.[7]

(b) Fenamates

A study in 20 healthy subjects given aspirin 600 mg and **sodium meclofenamate** 100 mg both three times daily for 14 days found no significant reductions in plasma salicylate levels, but plasma **meclofenamate** levels were reduced to some extent. However, gastrointestinal blood loss was approximately doubled compared with either drug alone.[4]

(c) Ibuprofen and related drugs

Aspirin 1.3 to 3.6 g daily more than halved the serum levels of ibuprofen 800 mg to 2.4 g daily,[8,9] without affecting salicylate levels.[9] There was little additional clinical benefit from the combination.[9] Similarly, aspirin reduced the AUC of **flurbiprofen** by about two-thirds,[10] but without any clear changes in clinical effectiveness.[11] The pharmacokinetics of the aspirin were unchanged by **flurbiprofen**.[10] Aspirin 3.9 g daily also virtually halved the AUC of **fenoprofen** 2.4 g daily,[12] and reduced the AUC of **ketoprofen** 200 mg daily[13] by about one-third. The AUC of **naproxen** was only minimally reduced (by 10 to 15%).[14,15] **Choline magnesium trisalicylate** increased the clearance of **naproxen** by 56% and decreased its serum levels by 26% in one study.[16]

(d) Indometacin

The overall picture with aspirin and indometacin is confusing and contradictory. One early study found that indometacin had no additional benefit in patients already taking aspirin.[17] Consequently, a number of studies were conducted to see if there was a drug interaction. Some studies reported that aspirin reduced serum indometacin levels[12,18-20] or its efficacy,[21] or that the combination was no more effective than either drug alone.[22] Others report that no change in indometacin levels occurred.[23-25] Further studies using buffered aspirin claimed that it increased the rate of absorption of indometacin and was associated with an increase in adverse effects (tiredness, lack of coordination).[26,27] One study found that indometacin 50 mg given as suppositories at night was found to have a significant additive effect when given with slow-release aspirin 2 or 4.5 g daily, estimated by articular index and subjective ratings of pain and morning stiffness. However, the dose of aspirin (most often the 4.5 g dose) had to be reduced in 7 of the 24 treatment periods due to adverse effects.[28]

(e) Oxicams

Aspirin 3 g daily increased the maximum plasma levels of **meloxicam** 30 mg daily by 25% and its AUC by 10%.[29] Plasma levels of **piroxicam** 40 mg then 20 mg daily were not significantly affected by aspirin 3.9 g daily, and salicylate levels were unaffected by **piroxicam**.[30] Aspirin 2.6 to 3.9 g daily more than halved the serum levels of **tenoxicam** 20 mg daily.[31]

(f) Miscellaneous NSAIDs

Aspirin 600 mg four times daily caused a 15% reduction in the plasma levels of **diflunisal** 250 mg twice daily for 3 days.[32] Single-dose studies have shown that the absorption of **nabumetone** 1 g is not significantly altered by aspirin 1.5 g.[33] The plasma levels of **tolmetin** 1.2 g daily were slightly reduced by aspirin 3.9 g daily.[34]

Mechanism

The damaging effects of aspirin and NSAIDs on the gut appear to be additive. The mechanisms behind the pharmacokinetic changes have not been resolved. Changes in the rates of absorption and renal clearance and competition for plasma protein binding have been proposed.

Importance and management

The additive risk of gastrointestinal damage from combining aspirin and NSAIDs is established. Because of this, and the lack of clear benefit from the combination, the use of anti-inflammatory/analgesic doses of aspirin with NSAIDs should be avoided. For information on low-dose aspirin and NSAIDs see 'NSAIDs + Aspirin; Antiplatelet dose', p.144. Consider also 'NSAIDs + NSAIDs', p.151.

1. García Rodríguez LA, Hernández-Díaz S. The risk of upper gastrointestinal complications associated with nonsteroidal anti-inflammatory drugs, glucocorticoids, acetaminophen, and combinations of these agents. *Arthritis Res* (2001) 3, 98–101.
2. Mellemkjaer L, Blot WJ, Sørensen HT, Thomassen L, McLaughlin JK, Nielsen GL, Olsen JH. Upper gastrointestinal bleeding among users of NSAIDs: a population-based cohort study in Denmark. *Br J Clin Pharmacol* (2002) 53, 173–81.
3. Committee on Safety of Medicines/Medicines Control Agency. Non-steroidal anti-inflammatory drugs (NSAIDs) and gastrointestinal safety. *Current Problems* (2002) 28, 5.
4. Baragar FD, Smith TC. Drug interaction studies with sodium meclofenamate (Meclomen®). *Curr Ther Res* (1978) 23 (April Suppl), S51–S59.
5. Charachon A, Petit T, Lamarque D, Soulé J-C. Colite aiguë hémorragique chez une malade traitée par rofécoxib associé à une auto-médication par aspirine. *Gastroenterol Clin Biol* (2003) 27, 511–13.
6. Willis JV, Kendall MJ, Jack DB. A study of the effect of aspirin on the pharmacokinetics of oral and intravenous diclofenac sodium. *Eur J Clin Pharmacol* (1980) 18, 415–18.
7. Bird HA, Hill J, Leatham P, Wright V. A study to determine the clinical relevance of the pharmacokinetic interaction between aspirin and diclofenac. *Agents Actions* (1986) 18, 447–9.
8. Albert KS, Gernaat CM. Pharmacokinetics of ibuprofen. *Am J Med* (1984) 77(1A), 40–6.
9. Grennan DM, Ferry DG, Ashworth ME, Kenny RE, Mackinnon M. The aspirin-ibuprofen interaction in rheumatoid arthritis. *Br J Clin Pharmacol* (1979) 8, 497–503.
10. Kaiser DG, Brooks CD, Lomen PL. Pharmacokinetics of flurbiprofen. *Am J Med* (1986) 80 (Suppl 3A), 10–15.
11. Brooks PM, Khong TK. Flurbiprofen-aspirin interaction: a double-blind crossover study. *Curr Med Res Opin* (1977) 5, 53–7.
12. Rubin A, Rodda BE, Warrick P, Gruber CM, Ridolfo AS. Interactions of aspirin with nonsteroidal antiinflammatory drugs in man. *Arthritis Rheum* (1973) 16, 635–45.
13. Williams RL, Upton RA, Buskin JN, Jones RM. Ketoprofen-aspirin interactions. *Clin Pharmacol Ther* (1981) 30, 226–31.
14. Segre EJ, Chaplin M, Forchielli E, Runkel R, Sevelius H. Naproxen-aspirin interactions in man. *Clin Pharmacol Ther* (1974) 15, 374–9.
15. Segre E, Sevelius H, Chaplin M, Forchielli E, Runkel R, Rooks W. Interaction of naproxen and aspirin in the rat and in man. *Scand J Rheumatol* (1973) (Suppl 2), 37–42.
16. Furst DE, Sarkissian E, Blocka K, Cassell S, Dromgoole S, Harris ER, Hirschberg JM, Josephson N, Paulus HE. Serum concentrations of salicylate and naproxen during concurrent therapy in patients with rheumatoid arthritis. *Arthritis Rheum* (1987) 30, 1157–61.
17. The Cooperating Clinics Committee of the American Rheumatism Association. A three-month trial of indomethacin in rheumatoid arthritis, with special reference to analysis and inference. *Clin Pharmacol Ther* (1967) 8, 11–37.
18. Kaldestad E, Hansen T, Brath HK. Interaction of indomethacin and acetylsalicylic acid as shown by the serum concentrations of indomethacin and salicylate. *Eur J Clin Pharmacol* (1975) 9, 199–207.
19. Jeremy R, Towson J. Interaction between aspirin and indomethacin in the treatment of rheumatoid arthritis. *Med J Aust* (1970) 3, 127–9.
20. Kwan KC, Breault GO, Davis RL, Lei BW, Czerwinski AW, Besselaar GH, Duggan DE. Effects of concomitant aspirin administration on the pharmacokinetics of indomethacin in man. *J Pharmacokinet Biopharm* (1978) 6, 451–76.
21. Pawlotsky Y, Chales G, Grosbois B, Miane B, Bourel M. Comparative interaction of aspirin with indomethacin and sulindac in chronic rheumatic diseases. *Eur J Rheumatol Inflamm* (1978) 1, 18–20.
22. Brooks PM, Walker JJ, Bell MA, Buchanan WW, Rhymer AR. Indomethacin—aspirin interaction: a clinical appraisal. *BMJ* (1975) 3, 69–71.
23. Champion D, Mongan E, Paulus H, Sarkissian E, Okun R, Pearson C. Effect of concurrent aspirin (ASA) administration on serum concentrations of indomethacin (I). *Arthritis Rheum* (1971) 14, 375.
24. Lindquist B, Jensen KM, Johansson H, Hansen T. Effect of concurrent administration of aspirin and indomethacin on serum concentrations. *Clin Pharmacol Ther* (1974) 15, 247–52.
25. Barraclough DRE, Muirden KD, Laby B. Salicylate therapy and drug interaction in rheumatoid arthritis. *Aust N Z J Med* (1975) 5, 518–23.
26. Turner P,Garnham JC. Indomethacin-aspirin interaction. *BMJ* (1975) 2, 368.
27. Garnham JC, Raymond K, Shotton E, Turner P. The effect of buffered aspirin on plasma indomethacin. *Eur J Clin Pharmacol* (1975) 8, 107–13.
28. Alván G, Ekstrand R. Clinical effects of indomethacin and additive clinical effect of indomethacin during salicylate maintenance therapy. *Scand J Rheumatol* (1981) Suppl 39, 29–32.
29. Busch U, Heinzel G, Narjes H, Nehmiz G. Interaction of meloxicam with cimetidine, Maalox or aspirin. *J Clin Pharmacol* (1996) 36, 79–84.
30. Hobbs DC, Twomey TM. Piroxicam pharmacokinetics in man: aspirin and antacid interaction studies. *J Clin Pharmacol* (1979) 19, 270–81.

31. Day RO, Paull PD, Lam S, Swanson BR, Williams KM, Wade DN. The effect of concurrent aspirin upon plasma concentrations of tenoxicam. *Br J Clin Pharmacol* (1988) 26, 455–62.
32. Schulz P, Perrier CV, Ferber-Perret F, VandenHeuvel WJA, Steelman SL. Diflunisal, a new-acting analgesic and prostaglandin inhibitor: effect of concomitant acetylsalicylic acid therapy on ototoxicity and on disposition of both drugs. *J Int Med Res* (1979) 7, 61–8.
33. von Schrader HW, Buscher G, Dierdorf D, Mügge H, Wolf D. Nabumetone — a novel anti-inflammatory drug: the influence of food, milk, antacids, and analgesics on bioavailability of single oral doses. *Int J Clin Pharmacol Ther Toxicol* (1983) 21, 311–21.
34. Cressman WA, Wortham GF, Plostnieks J. Absorption and excretion of tolmetin in man. *Clin Pharmacol Ther* (1976) 19, 224–33.

NSAIDs + Aspirin; Antiplatelet dose

There is some evidence that non-selective NSAIDs such as ibuprofen antagonise the antiplatelet effects of low-dose aspirin, but that COX-2-selective NSAIDs (coxibs) do not. Some, but not other, epidemiological studies have shown that non-selective NSAIDs reduce the cardioprotective effects of low-dose aspirin. Furthermore, some NSAIDs (particularly coxibs) are associated with increased thrombotic risk. Combined use of NSAIDs and low-dose aspirin increases the risk of gastrointestinal bleeds. This seems to apply equally to coxibs.

Clinical evidence

(a) Cardioprotective effects

A number of pharmacodynamic studies have investigated whether or not NSAIDs affect the antiplatelet effects of aspirin. **Celecoxib** 200 mg twice daily,[1] **diclofenac** 75 mg twice daily,[2] **etoricoxib** 120 mg daily,[3] **lumiracoxib** 400 mg daily,[4] **meloxicam** 15 mg daily,[5] **naproxen** 500 mg twice daily,[6] **parecoxib** 40 mg twice daily,[7] and **rofecoxib** 25 mg daily[2] have all been shown not to alter the antiplatelet effects of aspirin in doses of 75 to 325 mg daily. The effects of **ibuprofen** are less clear, and may be related to the order of drug administration.

As a consequence of these pharmacodynamic studies, various cohort/case-control studies or sub-group analyses have been conducted to see if **ibuprofen** and/or other NSAIDs reduce the cardioprotective effect of low-dose aspirin in patients, see 'Table 6.2', (below). Because these studies are neither prospective nor randomised, their findings are suggestive only, nevertheless they provide some useful insight.

(b) Gastrointestinal effects

Low-dose aspirin alone (300 mg or less daily) was associated with an increased risk of hospitalisation for bleeding peptic ulcer in a case-control study. The odds ratios were 2.3 for aspirin 75 mg daily, 3.2 for aspirin

Table 6.2 Summary of studies on the effect of NSAIDs on the cardioprotective effect of antiplatelet dose aspirin

Study type	*Criteria*	*Outcome*	*Drugs (Number of patients)*	*Comments*	*Refs*
Studies showing a decrease in the cardioprotection of aspirin with NSAIDs					
Retrospective cohort	Discharge after CVD	Mortality	Aspirin alone (6285) Aspirin with Ibuprofen (187) Aspirin with Diclofenac (206) Aspirin with other NSAID (429)	Increased all-cause mortality and cardiovascular mortality in those taking aspirin with ibuprofen compared with the other groups.	1
Subgroup analysis of an RCT	Male physicians randomised to aspirin 325 mg on alternate days or placebo	First MI	Aspirin alone (5273) Aspirin with intermittent NSAID (5147) Aspirin with regular NSAID (598)	Use of NSAIDs for 60 days or more per year was associated with an increased risk of MI in those taking aspirin.	2
Case-control		First non-fatal MI	Aspirin alone (694) Aspirin with NSAIDs (170) NSAIDs alone (128)	Both aspirin alone, and NSAIDs alone were associated with a reduced risk of MI, but combined use was not.	3
Studies showing no effect of NSAIDs on the cardioprotection of aspirin					
Retrospective cohort	Discharge after MI	Death in first year	Aspirin alone (36211) NSAID alone (736) Aspirin with NSAID (2096) Neither (9541)	Risk of death reduced to a similar extent by aspirin, NSAIDs, and the combination.	4
Retrospective cohort	Discharge after MI and on aspirin	Death in first year	Aspirin alone (66739) Aspirin with Ibuprofen (844) Aspirin with other NSAID (2733)	Risk of death comparable between the 3 groups.	5
Retrospective cohort	General Practice Research Database	Acute MI or death from coronary heart disease	NSAID alone (417) NSAID with aspirin (163) Aspirin alone (1119) Non-NSAID users (1878)	Incidence of acute MI unaffected by NSAID alone. NSAID with aspirin similar to aspirin alone.	6
Studies showing an increase in the cardioprotection of aspirin with NSAIDs					
Retrospective cohort	Two consecutive prescriptions for aspirin or ibuprofen	Biochemical evidence of MI	Aspirin alone (10239) Aspirin with Ibuprofen (3859)	The aspirin alone group experienced 0.0044 MIs per patient month, compared with 0.0026 in the aspirin with ibuprofen group.	7

1. MacDonald TM, Wei L. Effect of ibuprofen on cardioprotective effect of aspirin. *Lancet* (2003) 361, 573-4.
2. Kurth T, Glynn RJ, Walker AM, Chan KA, Buring JE, Hennekens CH, Gaziano JM. Inhibition of clinical benefits of aspirin on first myocardial infarction by nonsteroidal antiinflammatory drugs. *Circulation* (2003) 108, 1191-5.
3. Kimmel SE, Berlin JA, Reilly M, Jaskowiak J, Kishel L, Chittams J, Strom BL. The effects of nonselective non-aspirin non-steroidal anti-inflammatory medications on the risk of nonfatal myocardial infarction and their interaction with aspirin. *J Am Coll Cardiol* (2004) 43, 985-90.
4. Ko D, Wang Y, Berger AK, Radford MJ, Krumholz HM. Nonsteroidal antiinflammatory drugs after acute myocardial infarction. *Am Heart J* (2002) 143, 475-81.
5. Curtis JP, Wang Y, Portnay EL, Masoudi FA, Havranek EP, Krumholz HM. Aspirin, ibuprofen, and mortality after myocardial infarction: retrospective cohort study. *BMJ* (2003) 327, 1322-3.
6. García Rodríguez LA, Varas-Lorenzo C, Maguire A, González-Pérez A. Nonsteroidal antiinflammatory drugs and the risk of myocardial infarction in the general population. *Circulation* (2004) 109, 3000-6.
7. Patel TN,Goldberg KC. Use of aspirin and ibuprofen compared with aspirin alone and the risk of myocardial infarction. *Arch Intern Med* (2004) 164, 852-6.

150 mg daily, and 3.9 for aspirin 300 mg daily. Use of NSAIDs combined with low-dose aspirin was associated with a greater risk of bleeding (odds ratio 7.7) than use of either NSAIDs alone (5.4) or low-dose aspirin alone (3.3).[8] Similar findings were reported in a cohort study (rate ratio for gastrointestinal bleed for low-dose aspirin 2.6, and for combined use with NSAIDs, 5.6).[9]

Patients taking low-dose aspirin (325 mg or less daily) with **celecoxib** had a higher frequency of gastrointestinal complications than those taking **celecoxib** alone. Moreover, there was no difference in frequency of gastrointestinal complications between those taking low-dose aspirin with **celecoxib** and those taking low-dose aspirin with **ibuprofen** or **diclofenac**. This was despite **celecoxib** alone being associated with a lower frequency of gastrointestinal adverse effects than **ibuprofen** or **diclofenac** alone.[10] Similar results were found with **rofecoxib** 25 mg daily, which increased the incidence of ulcers in patients taking enteric-coated aspirin 81 mg per day.[11]

Mechanism

Aspirin irreversibly blocks the production of thromboxane A2 by binding to cyclo-oxygenase (COX-1) in platelets, and so inhibits platelet aggregation. The beneficial cardiovascular effects are attributed to this effect. Other NSAIDs that are COX-1 inhibitors also have this effect, but it is more short-lived since they bind reversibly. These NSAIDs can therefore competitively inhibit the binding of aspirin to platelets (a fact that was shown *in vitro* as early as the 1980s[12]). When these NSAIDs are present in sufficient quantities when a daily low-dose of aspirin is given, they therefore reduce its antiplatelet effect. *In vitro* study confirms that COX-2 selective NSAIDs have less effect.[13]

It is well known that aspirin and NSAIDs have additive gastrointestinal adverse effects (see 'NSAIDs + Aspirin; Anti-inflammatory dose', p.142). This occurs even at the low doses of aspirin used for antiplatelet effects (doses as low as 75 mg daily).[8]

Importance and management

The evidence currently available on the antagonism of antiplatelet effects is insufficient to recommend that ibuprofen is not used with low-dose aspirin. Nevertheless, some have concluded that when patients taking low-dose aspirin for cardioprotection require long-term NSAIDs for inflammatory conditions, the use of diclofenac or naproxen would seem preferable to ibuprofen.[14] A coxib was also suggested as an alternative,[14] but the subsequent suggestion of an increased risk of serious cardiovascular effects with the coxibs (as a class[15]) probably precludes this. Recently the Commission on Human Medicines (CHM) in the UK has advised that there may be a small increased risk of thrombotic events with the non-selective NSAIDs, particularly when used at high doses and for long-term treatment.[16]

It is important to also consider the possible increased risk of gastrointestinal adverse effects from any combination. From a gastrointestinal perspective, the lowest dose of aspirin should be used (75 mg).[8] However, when combined with low-dose aspirin, the available evidence indicates that there is no gastrointestinal benefit to be obtained from using a coxib as opposed to diclofenac or ibuprofen.[10] Note that the CSM in the UK has advised that the combination of a non-aspirin NSAID and low-dose aspirin should be used only if absolutely necessary.[17,18] They state that patients taking long-term aspirin should be reminded to avoid NSAIDs, including those bought without prescription.[18] If concurrent use is necessary, where appropriate, the use of a proton pump inhibitor may be considered for prophylaxis of NSAID-induced gastrointestinal damage.

1. Wilner KD, Rushing M, Walden C, Adler R, Eskra J, Noveck R, Vargas R. Celecoxib does not affect the antiplatelet activity of aspirin in healthy volunteers. *J Clin Pharmacol* (2002) 42, 1027–30.
2. Catella-Lawson F, Reilly MP, Kapoor SC, Cucchiara AJ, De Marco S, Tournier B, Vyas SN, FitzGerald GA. Cyclooxygenase inhibitors and the antiplatelet effects of aspirin. *N Engl J Med* (2001) 345, 1809–17.
3. Arcoxia (Etoricoxib). Merck Sharp & Dohme Ltd. UK Summary of product characteristics, January 2007.
4. Jermany J, Branson J, Schmouder R, Guillaume M, Rordorf C. Lumiracoxib does not affect the ex vivo antiplatelet aggregation activity of low-dose aspirin in healthy subjects. *J Clin Pharmacol* (2005) 45, 1172–8.
5. Van Ryn J, Kink-Eiband M, Kuritsch I, Feifel U, Hanft G, Wallenstein G, Trummlitz G, Pairet M. Meloxicam does not affect the antiplatelet effect of aspirin in healthy male and female volunteers. *J Clin Pharmacol* (2004) 44, 777–84.
6. Capone ML, Sciulli MG, Tacconelli S, Grana M, Ricciotti E, Renda G, Di Gregorio P, Merciaro G, Patrignani P. Pharmacodynamic interaction of naproxen with low-dose aspirin in healthy subjects. *J Am Coll Cardiol* (2005) 45, 1295–1301.
7. Noveck RJ, Kuss ME, Qian J, North J, Hubbard RC. Parecoxib sodium, injectable COX-2 specific inhibitor, does not affect aspirin-mediated platelet function. *Reg Anesth Pain Med* (2001) 26 (Suppl), 19.
8. Weil J, Colin-Jones D, Langman M, Lawson D, Logan R, Murphy M, Rawlins M, Vessey M, Wainwright P. Prophylactic aspirin and risk of peptic ulcer bleeding. *BMJ* (1995) 310, 827–30.
9. Sorensen HT, Mellemkjaer L, Blot WJ, Nielsen GL, Steffensen FH, McLaughlin JK, Olsen JH. Risk of upper gastrointestinal bleeding associated with use of low-dose aspirin. *Am J Gastroenterol* (2000) 95, 2218–24.
10. Silverstein FE, Faich G, Goldstein JL, Simon LS, Pincus T, Whelton A, Makuch R, Eisen G, Agrawal NM, Stenson WF, Burr AM, Zhao WW, Kent JD, Lefkowith JB, Verburg KM, Geis GS. Gastrointestinal toxicity with celecoxib vs nonsteroidal anti-inflammatory drugs for osteoarthritis and rheumatoid arthritis: the CLASS study: a randomized controlled trial. *JAMA* (2000) 284, 1247–55.
11. Laine L, Maller ES, Yu C, Quan H, Simon T. Ulcer formation with low-dose enteric-coated aspirin and the effect of COX-2 selective inhibition: a double-blind trial. *Gastroenterology* (2004) 127, 395–402.
12. Parks WM, Hoak JC, Czervionke RL. Comparative effect of ibuprofen on endothelial and platelet prostaglandin synthesis. *J Pharmacol Exp Ther* (1981) 219, 415–19.
13. Ouellet M, Riendeau D, Percival MD. A high level of cyclooxygenase-2 inhibitor selectivity is associated with a reduced interference of platelet cyclooxygenase-1 inactivation by aspirin. *Proc Natl Acad Sci U S A* (2001) 98, 14583–8.
14. FitzGerald GA. Parsing an enigma: the pharmacodynamics of aspirin resistance. *Lancet* (2003) 361, 542–4.
15. FitzGerald GA. Coxibs and cardiovascular disease. *N Engl J Med* (2004) 351, 1709–11.
16. Commission on Human Medicines. NSAIDs letter to healthcare professionals: Safety of selective and non-selective NSAIDs. October 2006. Available at: http://www.mhra.gov.uk/home/idcplg?IdcService=SS_GET_PAGE&nodeId=227 (accessed 16/08/07).
17. Committee on Safety of Medicines/Medicines Control Agency. Non-steroidal anti-inflammatory drugs (NSAIDs) and gastrointestinal safety. *Current Problems* (2002) 28, 5.
18. Committee on Safety of Medicines/Medicines and Healthcare products Regulatory Agency. Reminder: Gastrointestinal toxicity of NSAIDs. *Current Problems* (2003) 29, 8–9.

NSAIDs + Azoles

Fluconazole markedly raises celecoxib levels, whereas ketoconazole has no effect on celecoxib levels. Fluconazole and ketoconazole moderately increase the levels of valdecoxib (the main metabolite of parecoxib). Ketoconazole moderately raises etoricoxib plasma levels, but this is unlikely to be of clinical relevance. Fluconazole has no clinically relevant effect on lumiracoxib pharmacokinetics.

Clinical evidence

(a) Celecoxib

The manufacturer notes that **fluconazole** 200 mg daily increased the AUC of a single 200-mg dose of celecoxib by 130% and increased the maximum level by 60%. Conversely, **ketoconazole** had no effect on the pharmacokinetics of celecoxib.[1]

(b) Etoricoxib

A single 60-mg dose of etoricoxib was given to healthy subjects on day 7 of an 11-day course of **ketoconazole** 400 mg daily. The AUC of etoricoxib was increased by 43% and the maximum plasma levels was increased by 29%.[2]

(c) Lumiracoxib

A placebo-controlled, crossover study in 13 healthy subjects[3] found that **fluconazole** 400 mg on day 1 and 200 mg on days 2 to 4 had no clinically relevant effect on the pharmacokinetics of a single 400-mg dose of lumiracoxib given on day 4.

(d) Parecoxib

The manufacturer of parecoxib reports a study in which **fluconazole** increased the plasma levels of valdecoxib (the main metabolite of parecoxib) by 19% and raised its AUC by 62%.[4] **Ketoconazole** had a similar, but more moderate effect on the levels of valdecoxib (maximum plasma levels increased by 24%, AUC increased by 38%).[4]

Mechanism

Fluconazole is a potent inhibitor of the cytochrome P450 isoenzyme CYP2C9 and ketoconazole inhibits CYP3A4. Celecoxib is extensively metabolised by CYP2C9, and therefore shows marked rises in plasma levels when given with fluconazole but not ketoconazole. Etoricoxib is partially metabolised by CYP3A4, therefore shows moderate rises in plasma levels with ketoconazole. Valdecoxib is metabolised by both CYP2C9 and CYP3A4, therefore was modestly affected by both fluconazole and ketoconazole. Parecoxib is a valdecoxib prodrug, and interacts similarly. From the study with lumiracoxib it appears that its pharmacokinetics are unlikely to be affected by inhibitors of CYP2C9, because, even though lumiracoxib is largely metabolised by CYP2C9, other pathways are also important (e.g. glucuronidation).[3]

Importance and management

These pharmacokinetic interactions are established, although their effect in clinical practice has not been assessed. The marked rise in celecoxib levels with fluconazole could be important, and the UK manufacturer recommends that the dose of celecoxib should be halved in patients receiving fluconazole,[1] whereas the US manufacturer suggests starting with the lowest recommended dose.[5] The rise in valdecoxib levels with fluconazole is less marked, nevertheless the manufacturer recommends that for parecoxib the dosage should be reduced (but they do not suggest by how much).[4] No dosage adjustments are thought to be necessary if etoricoxib or parecoxib are given with ketoconazole, and if lumiracoxib is given with fluconazole.

1. Celebrex (Celecoxib). Pharmacia Ltd. UK Summary of product characteristics, February 2007.
2. Agrawal NGB, Matthews CZ, Mazenko RS, Woolf EJ, Porras AG, Chen X, Miller JL, Michiels N, Wehling M, Schultz A, Gottlieb AB, Kraft WK, Greenberg HE, Waldman SA, Curtis SP, Gottesdiener KM. The effects of modifying in vivo cytochrome P450 3A (CYP3A) activity on etoricoxib pharmacokinetics and of etoricoxib administration on CYP3A activity. *J Clin Pharmacol* (2004) 44, 1125–31.
3. Scott G, Yih L, Yeh C-M, Milosavljev S, Laurent A, Rordorf C. Lumiracoxib: pharmacokinetic and pharmacodynamic profile when coadministered with fluconazole in healthy subjects. *J Clin Pharmacol* (2004) 44, 193–9.
4. Dynastat Injection (Parecoxib sodium). Pfizer Ltd. UK Summary of product characteristics, April 2007.
5. Celebrex (Celecoxib). Pfizer Inc. US Prescribing information, February 2007.

NSAIDs + Bile-acid binding resins

Simultaneous colestyramine markedly reduced the absorption of diclofenac and sulindac, modestly reduced the absorption of ibuprofen, but only delayed and did not reduce the extent of absorption of naproxen. Administration of colestyramine three or more hours after oral sulindac, piroxicam, or tenoxicam still markedly reduced their plasma levels. Markedly reduced NSAID levels have also been found when colestyramine is given after intravenous meloxicam or tenoxicam.

Simultaneous colestipol modestly reduced the oral absorption of diclofenac, but had no effect on ibuprofen absorption.

Clinical evidence

(a) Diclofenac

A single-dose, crossover study in 6 healthy, fasting subjects found that the simultaneous use of **colestyramine** 8 g markedly reduced the AUC of a single 100-mg oral dose of enteric-coated diclofenac by 62% and reduced its maximum plasma levels by 75%. **Colestipol** 10 g reduced the diclofenac AUC by 33% and its maximum plasma levels by 58%.[1]

(b) Ibuprofen and related drugs

A single-dose, crossover study in 6 healthy fasting subjects found that the simultaneous use of **colestyramine** 8 g modestly reduced the AUC of a single 400-mg oral dose of ibuprofen by 26% and reduced its maximum serum levels by 34%. The rate of absorption was also reduced. Conversely, **colestipol** 10 g had no significant effect on the pharmacokinetics of ibuprofen.[2]

The absorption of a single 250-mg dose of **naproxen** was delayed but not reduced in 8 healthy fasting subjects by the simultaneous use of **colestyramine** 4 g in 100 mL of orange juice. The amount absorbed after 2 hours was reduced from 96% to 51%, but was complete after 5 hours.[3]

(c) Oxicams

A study in 12 healthy subjects found that **colestyramine** 4 g taken 2 hours before a 30 mg *intravenous* dose of **meloxicam** increased its clearance by 49% and reduced its mean residence time in the body by 39%.[4]

Another study in 8 healthy subjects found that **colestyramine** increased the clearance of a single 20-mg oral dose of **piroxicam** and a single 20-mg *intravenous* dose of **tenoxicam** by 52% and 105%, respectively, and reduced their half-lives by 40% and 52%, respectively. In this study, **colestyramine** 4 g three times daily was started 2 hours before the intravenous **tenoxicam** and 3.5 hours after the oral **piroxicam**.[5] In another multiple-dose study **colestyramine**, given 4 hours after oral **piroxicam** or oral **tenoxicam**, gave similar results,[6] as did a study starting **colestyramine** 24 hours after the last dose of a 14-day course of **piroxicam** 20 mg daily [which has a long half-life].[7] The elimination half-life of both analgesics was roughly doubled by **colestyramine** 24 g daily.[6]

(d) Sulindac

In 6 healthy subjects **colestyramine** 4 g twice daily with meals was found to reduce the AUC of a simultaneous single 400-mg dose of sulindac by 78%: the AUC of its sulfide metabolite was reduced by 84%. Even when the sulindac was given 3 hours before the **colestyramine**, its AUC of colestyramine and its sulphide metabolite were reduced by 44% and 55%, respectively.[8]

Mechanism

The studies of simultaneous oral use suggest that the anion exchange resin colestyramine, and to a lesser extent colestipol, bind anionic NSAIDs (e.g. diclofenac) in the gut, so reducing their absorption. The studies showing reduced plasma levels when colestyramine was given after intravenous oxicams or separated by at least 3 hours from some oral NSAIDs, suggest that colestyramine can reduce the enterohepatic recirculation of these drugs.

Importance and management

Established interactions. Colestyramine markedly reduces the initial absorption of some NSAIDs (shown for diclofenac), and if these NSAIDs also undergo enterohepatic recirculation, their clearance will also be increased (shown for meloxicam, piroxicam, sulindac, and tenoxicam). This latter interaction cannot be avoided by separating the doses, and it may be best not to use colestyramine with these NSAIDs. Colestyramine can be used to speed the removal of piroxicam and tenoxicam following overdosage.[3] Diclofenac has been formulated with colestyramine in an attempt to reduce gastric mucosal damage by reducing direct mucosal contact: 140 mg of diclofenac-colestyramine is considered equivalent to 70 mg of diclofenac.[9]

The reduction in absorption of ibuprofen with colestyramine is probably not clinically important, and naproxen is not affected. Nevertheless, colestyramine delayed the absorption of both ibuprofen and naproxen, which may be relevant if they are being taken for the management of acute pain. Information on many other NSAIDs appears to be lacking. Animal studies suggest that **mefenamic acid**, **flufenamic acid** and **phenylbutazone** will also be affected by colestyramine.[10,11] Note that it is usually recommended that other drugs are given 1 hour before or 4 to 6 hours after colestyramine.

The reduction in diclofenac absorption with colestipol may be clinically relevant; if the combination is required monitor well. Note that it is usually recommended that other drugs are given 1 hour before or 4 hours after colestipol.

1. Al-Balla SR, El-Sayed YM, Al-Meshal MA, Gouda MW. The effects of cholestyramine and colestipol on the absorption of diclofenac in man. *Int J Clin Pharmacol Ther* (1994) 32, 441–5.
2. Al-Meshal MA, El-Sayed YM, Al-Balla SR, Gouda MW. The effect of colestipol and cholestyramine on ibuprofen bioavailability in man. *Biopharm Drug Dispos* (1994) 15, 463–71.
3. Calvo MV, Dominguez-Gil A. Interaction of naproxen with cholestyramine. *Biopharm Drug Dispos* (1984) 5, 33–42.
4. Busch U, Heinzel G, Narjes H. The effect of cholestyramine on the pharmacokinetics of meloxicam, a new non-steroidal anti-inflammatory drug (NSAID), in man. *Eur J Clin Pharmacol* (1995) 48, 269–72.
5. Guentert TW, Defoin R, Mosberg H. The influence of cholestyramine on the elimination of tenoxicam and piroxicam. *Eur J Clin Pharmacol* (1988) 34, 283–9.
6. Benveniste C, Striberni R, Dayer P. Indirect assessment of the enterohepatic recirculation of piroxicam and tenoxicam. *Eur J Clin Pharmacol* (1990) 38, 547–9.
7. Ferry DG, Gazeley LR, Busby WJ, Beasley DMG, Edwards IR, Campbell AJ, Enhanced elimination of piroxicam by administration of activated charcoal or cholestyramine. *Eur J Clin Pharmacol* (1990) 39, 599–601.
8. Malloy MJ, Ravis WR, Pennell AT, Hagan DR, Betagari S, Doshi DH. Influence of cholestyramine resin administration on single dose sulindac pharmacokinetics. *Int J Clin Pharmacol Ther* (1994) 32, 286–9.
9. Suárez-Otero R, Robles-San Román M, Jaimes-Hernández J, Oropeza-de la Madrid E, Medina-Peñaloza RM, Rosas-Ramos R, Castañeda-Hernández G. Efficacy and safety of diclofenac-cholestyramine and celecoxib in osteoarthritis. *Proc West Pharmacol Soc* (2002) 45, 26–8.
10. Rosenberg HA, Bates TR. Inhibitory effect of cholestyramine on the absorption of flufenamic and mefenamic acids in rats. *Proc Soc Exp Biol Med* (1974) 145, 93–8.
11. Gallo D G, Bailey K R, Sheffner A L. The interaction between cholestyramine and drugs. *Proc Soc Exp Biol Med* (1965) 120, 60–5.

NSAIDs or Aspirin + Caffeine

Caffeine modestly increases the bioavailability, rate of absorption and plasma levels of aspirin. Adding caffeine to diclofenac may improve its efficacy in the treatment of migraine.

Clinical evidence, mechanism, importance and management

Caffeine citrate 120 mg given to healthy subjects with a single 650-mg dose of aspirin increased the aspirin AUC by 36%, increased the maximum plasma levels by 15%, and increased the rate of absorption by 30%.[1] This confirms the results of previous studies.[2,3] These studies suggest that caffeine may modestly potentiate the efficacy of aspirin via a pharmacokinetic mechanism.

A meta analysis of randomised, controlled studies concluded that there was no therapeutic advantage of adding caffeine to analgesic doses of aspirin in patients experiencing postoperative pain.[4] In a placebo-controlled study in patients with migraine, there was a non significant trend towards improved analgesic effect in patients receiving diclofenac softgel 100 mg and caffeine 100 mg compared with diclofenac alone, although the sample size was too small to provide meaningful results.[5]

1. Thithapandha A. Effect of caffeine on the bioavailability and pharmacokinetics of aspirin. *J Med Assoc Thai* (1989) 72, 562–6.
2. Yoovathaworn KC, Sriwatanakul K, Thithapandha A. Influence of caffeine on aspirin pharmacokinetics. *Eur J Drug Metab Pharmacokinet* (1986) 11, 71–6.
3. Dahanukar SA, Pohujani S, Sheth UK. Bioavailability of aspirin and interacting influence of caffeine. *Indian J Med Res* (1978) 68, 844–8.
4. Zhang WY, Po ALW. Do codeine and caffeine enhance the analgesic effect of aspirin?--A systematic overview. *J Clin Pharm Ther* (1997) 22, 79–97.
5. Peroutka SJ, Lyon JA, Swarbrick J, Lipton RB, Kolodner K, Goldstein J. Efficacy of diclofenac sodium softgel 100 mg with or without caffeine 100 mg in migraine without aura: a randomized, double-blind, crossover study. *Headache* (2004) 44, 136–41.

NSAIDs + Food

In general, food has no clinically significant effect on the absorption of the NSAIDs; however, the delay in absorption that occurs may be important if NSAIDs are given in acute pain management.

Clinical evidence

(a) Coxibs

A study in 50 children showed that a single 250-mg/m^2 dose of **celecoxib,** given with high-fat food, increased the maximum plasma concentration by 82% and the AUC by 60%. When steady-state levels were achieved with **celecoxib** 250 mg/m^2 twice daily, food increased the maximum plasma concentration by 99% and the AUC by 75%.[1] The manufacturers of **celecoxib** note that a **high-fat meal** delayed absorption by about one to 2 hours[2,3] and the total absorption was increased by 10% to 20%.[3]

A **high-fat meal** reduced the maximum level of **etoricoxib** by 36% and delayed it by 2 hours, without affecting the extent of absorption.[4]

(b) Diclofenac

Thirteen healthy subjects were given a single 105-mg dose of diclofenac potassium suspension (*Flogan*) while fasting and after food. The pharmacokinetics of diclofenac were not changed to a clinically relevant extent by food, except that absorption was delayed (time to maximum level increased by about 30 minutes).[5] Similar findings (an increase in time to maximum level of 1.5 to 3 hours) were reported for single doses of enteric-coated diclofenac tablets.[6] However, there was no difference in steady state levels of diclofenac 50 mg twice daily when given before or after food.[6]

(c) Etodolac

When 18 healthy subjects were given etodolac 400 mg after a **high-fat meal**, peak serum levels were roughly halved, and delayed, from 1.4 to 3.8 hours, but the total amount absorbed was not markedly changed, when compared to the fasting state.[7]

(d) Ibuprofen and related drugs

1. Aceclofenac. The manufacturer states that the rate, but not the extent, of aceclofenac absorption was affected by food.[8]

2. Dexketoprofen. The absorption of a single 25-mg dose of dexketoprofen was delayed by food (maximum level reduced by 45% and time to maximum level delayed by about 1 hour), but the AUC was not affected.[9]

3. Flurbiprofen. Food slightly increased the maximum plasma level and AUC of sustained-release flurbiprofen (*Froben SR*) by 15% and 25%, respectively, but delayed the time to achieve the maximum level by about 5 hours.[10] In a study in 14 healthy subjects the pharmacokinetics of flurbiprofen were not affected by **cranberry juice**, **grape juice** or **tea**.[11]

4. Ibuprofen. Food had no effect on the pharmacokinetics of the *S*- and *R*-enantiomers of ibuprofen in one study.[12] However, in another study, food significantly delayed the absorption of both enantiomers of ibuprofen, and slightly increased the ratio of the *S*- to *R*-enantiomer.[13] A study considering the effect of food on ibuprofen pharmacokinetics also showed that the maximum level of a single 400-mg dose of a standard release ibuprofen tablet and two readily soluble preparations (ibuprofen lysinate and ibuprofen extrudate), was consistently lower and appeared later when the dose was given after a standardised breakfast; the extent of ibuprofen absorption was also reduced by food for all three formulations.[14] However, in a further study, food increased the maximum plasma level of sustained-release ibuprofen (*Brufen Retard*) by 42% without affecting the time to achieve the maximum level or the bioavailability.[10]

5. Ketoprofen. Food significantly decreased the rate and extent of absorption of ketoprofen in both single and multiple dose studies in healthy subjects. The AUC was decreased by about 40% and the time to maximum levels decreased by about 5 hours.[15] A further study found that the rate of absorption and the peak plasma levels of ketoprofen were reduced by food, although the AUC was unaltered.[16] In another study, the absorption of ketoprofen (200 mg daily, as a gastric-juice resistant, sustained-release formulation, given 4 hours before the first meal of the day) was about 15 to 24% greater when 16 healthy subjects were given a **low-calorie/low-fat diet** rather than a **high-calorie/high-fat diet.**[17] In a further study in 4 healthy subjects, which measured the urinary excretion of ketoprofen after a single 50-mg dose given with water, whole skimmed milk, or a traditional Egyptian breakfast, it was concluded that the rate and extent of absorption of ketoprofen had been reduced by the presence of food, and the extent of absorption was also reduced by **milk.**[18]

6. Naproxen. Food did not have any clinically relevant effect on the pharmacokinetics of sustained-release **naproxen** in two studies.[19,20] Taking a single 550-mg dose of **naproxen sodium** with **a meal** had no effect on its analgesic efficacy in postoperative pain, when compared with the fasted state.[21] However, the rate of absorption of a single 550-mg dose of *S*-naproxen betainate sodium salt monohydrate was found to be reduced by a high-fat meal, when compared with the fasting state.[22]

(e) Indometacin

Studies in patients and healthy subjects, given single or multiple oral doses of indometacin, found that food delayed and reduced peak serum indometacin levels, but fluctuations in levels were somewhat reduced.[23]

(f) Nabumetone

The absorption of a single 1-g dose of nabumetone was increased by food and **milk**, as shown by an increase of about 50% in the maximum levels and a 40% increase in the AUC_{0-24}. However, the AUC_{0-72} was not significantly increased.[24]

(g) Oxicams

Food caused some delay in the time to reach maximum levels of **piroxicam** in a single-dose study, but had no effect on total absorption.[25] In another study, the steady-state plasma levels of **piroxicam** 20 mg daily were unaffected by food.[26] The bioavailability of **tenoxicam** 20 mg was unaffected by food in 12 healthy subjects, although the time taken to reach peak serum levels was delayed by about 4 hours.[27] The rate (time to peak serum levels) and extent of absorption (AUC) of **meloxicam** 30 mg was not altered by food intake.[28]

(h) Sulindac

The manufacturer of sulindac notes that food delayed the time to achieve peak plasma levels of the active metabolite by 1 to 2 hours.[29]

Mechanism

Food delays gastric emptying, therefore frequently affects the rate, but not the extent, of absorption of the NSAIDs.

Importance and management

Food reduces the rate of absorption, but has little or no effect on the extent of absorption, of most of the NSAIDs studied. This was seen to vary with different formulations of NSAIDs; however, these changes in absorption will have no clinical relevance when these drugs are being used regularly to treat chronic pain and inflammation. If these drugs are being used for the treatment of acute pain, administration on an empty stomach would be preferable in terms of onset of effect, and is suggested by the manufacturers of dexketoprofen[30] and etoricoxib.[4] However, administration with or after food is a usual recommendation for NSAIDs in an attempt to minimise their gastrointestinal adverse effects.

Although food delayed the absorption of celecoxib, the UK manufacturer says that it can be taken with or without food.[2] However, high-fat food may increase the total absorption of celecoxib and the US manufacturer suggests that higher doses (400 mg twice daily) should be administered with food to improve absorption.[3]

1. Stempak D, Gammon J, Halton J, Champagne M, Koren G, Baruchel S. Modulation of celecoxib pharmacokinetics by food in pediatric patients. *Clin Pharmacol Ther* (2005) 77, 226–8.
2. Celebrex (Celecoxib). Pharmacia Ltd. UK Summary of product characteristics, February 2007.
3. Celebrex (Celecoxib). Pfizer Inc. US Prescribing information, February 2007.
4. Arcoxia (Etoricoxib). Merck Sharp & Dohme Ltd. UK Summary of product characteristics, January 2007.
5. Poli A, Moreno RA, Ribiero W, Dias HB, Moreno H, Muscara MN, De Nucci G. Influence of gastric acid secretion blockade and food intake on the bioavailability of a potassium diclofenac suspension in healthy male volunteers. *Int J Clin Pharmacol Ther* (1996) 34, 76–9.
6. Sioufi A, Stierlin H, Schweizer A, Botta L, Degen PH, Theobald W, Brechbühler S. Recent findings concerning clinically relevant pharmacokinetics of diclofenac sodium. In: Voltarol — New Findings, ed Kass E. Proc Int Symp Voltarol, Paris June 22nd, 1981. 15th Int Congress of Rheumatology. p 19–30.
7. Troy S, Sanda M, Dressler D, Chiang S, Latts J. The effect of food and antacid on etodolac bioavailability. *Clin Pharmacol Ther* (1990) 47, 192.
8. Preservex (Aceclofenac). UCB Pharma Ltd. UK Summary of product characteristics, May 2005.
9. McEwen J, De Luca M, Casini A, Gich I, Barbanoj MJ, Tost D, Artigas R, Mauleón D. The effect of food and an antacid on the bioavailability of dexketoprofen trometamol. *J Clin Pharmacol* (1998) 38 (Suppl), 41S–45S.
10. Pargal A, Kelkar MG, Nayak PJ. The effect of food on the bioavailability of ibuprofen and flurbiprofen from sustained release formulation. *Biopharm Drug Dispos* (1996) 17, 511–19.
11. Greenblatt DJ, von Moltke LL, Perloff ES, Luo Y, Harmatz JS, Zinny MA. Interaction of flurbiprofen with cranberry juice, grape juice, tea, and fluconazole: in vitro and clinical studies. *Clin Pharmacol Ther* (2006) 79, 125–33.
12. Levine MA, Walker SE, Paton TW. The effect of food or sucralfate on the bioavailability of S(+) and R(-) enantiomers of ibuprofen. *J Clin Pharmacol* (1992) 32, 1110–14.
13. Siemon D, de Vries JX, Stötzer F, Walter-Sack I, Dietl R. Fasting and postprandial disposition of R(-)- and S(+)-ibuprofen following oral administration of racemic drug in healthy individuals. *Eur J Med Res* (1997) 2, 215–19.
14. Klueglich M, Ring A, Scheuerer S, Trommeshauser D, Schuijt C, Liepold B, Berndl G. Ibuprofen extrudate, a novel, rapidly dissolving ibuprofen formulation: relative bioavailability compared to ibuprofen lysinate and regular ibuprofen, and food effect on all formulations. *J Clin Pharmacol* (2005) 45, 1055–61.
15. Caillé G, du Souich P, Besner JG, Gervais P, Vèzina M. Effects of food and sucralfate on the pharmacokinetics of naproxen and ketoprofen in humans. *Am J Med* (1989) 86 (Suppl 6A) 38–44. Correction. ibid. (1990) 89, 838.
16. Bannwarth B, Lapicque F, Netter P, Monot C, Tamisier JN, Thomas P, Royer RJ. The effect of food on the systemic availability of ketoprofen. *Eur J Clin Pharmacol* (1988) 33, 643–5.
17. Le Liboux A, Teule M, Frydman A, Oosterhuis B, Jonkman JHG. Effect of diet on the single- and multiple-dose pharmacokinetics of sustained-release ketoprofen. *Eur J Clin Pharmacol* (1994) 47, 361–6.
18. Eshra AG, Etman MA, Naggar VF. Effect of milk and food on the bioavailability of ketoprofen in man. *Int J Pharmaceutics* (1988) 44, 9–14.
19. Mroszczak E, Yee JP, Bynum L. Absorption of naproxen controlled-release tablets in fasting and postprandial volunteers. *J Clin Pharmacol* (1988) 28, 1128–31.
20. Palazzini E, Cristofori M, Babbini M. Bioavailability of a new controlled-release oral naproxen formulation given with and without food. *Int J Clin Pharmacol Res* (1992) 12, 179–84.
21. Forbes JA, Sandberg RÅ, Bood-Björklund L. The effect of food on bromfenac, naproxen sodium, and acetaminophen in postoperative pain after orthopedic surgery. *Pharmacotherapy* (1998) 18, 492–503.
22. Marzo A, Dal Bo L, Wool C, Cerutti R. Bioavailability, food effect and tolerability of S-naproxen betainate sodium salt monohydrate in steady state. *Arzneimittelforschung* (1998) 48, 935–40.
23. Emori HW, Paulus H, Bluestone R, Champion GD, Pearson C. Indomethacin serum concentrations in man. Effects of dosage, food, and antacid. *Ann Rheum Dis* (1976) 35, 333–8.
24. von Schrader HW, Buscher G, Dierdorf D, Mügge H, Wolf D. Nabumetone — a novel anti-inflammatory drug: the influence of food, milk, antacids, and analgesics on bioavailability of single oral doses. *Int J Clin Pharmacol Ther Toxicol* (1983) 21, 311–21.
25. Ishizaki T, Nomura T, Abe T. Pharmacokinetics of piroxicam, a new nonsteroidal anti-inflammatory agent, under fasting and postprandial states in man. *J Pharmacokinet Biopharm* (1979) 7, 369–81.
26. Tilstone WJ, Lawson DH, Omara F, Cunningham F. The steady-state pharmacokinetics of piroxicam: effect of food and iron. *Eur J Rheumatol Inflamm* (1981) 4, 309–13.
27. Day RO, Lam S, Paull P, Wade D. Effect of food and various antacids on the absorption of tenoxicam. *Br J Clin Pharmacol* (1987) 24, 323–8.
28. Busch U, Heinzel G, Narjes H. Effect of food on pharmacokinetics of meloxicam, a new non steroidal anti-inflammatory drug (NSAID). *Agents Actions* (1991) 32, 52–3.
29. Clinoril (Sulindac). Merck Sharp & Dohme Ltd. UK Summary of product characteristics, May 2007.
30. Keral (Dexketoprofen trometamol). A. Menarini Pharmaceuticals UK SRL. UK Summary of product characteristics, November 2004.

NSAIDs + *Ginkgo biloba*

An isolated case describes fatal intracerebral bleeding in a patient taking *Ginkgo biloba* with ibuprofen, and another case describes prolonged bleeding and subdural haematomas in another patients taking *Ginkgo biloba* with rofecoxib. Studies involving diclofenac and flurbiprofen showed that *Ginkgo biloba* had no effect on the pharmacokinetics of these drugs.

Clinical evidence

A case of fatal intracerebral bleeding has been reported in a 71-year-old patient taking a *Ginkgo biloba* supplement (*Gingium*) 4 weeks after he started to take **ibuprofen** 600 mg daily.[1] A 69-year-old man taking a *Ginkgo biloba* supplement and **rofecoxib** had a subdural haematoma after a head injury, then recurrent small spontaneous haematomas. He was subsequently found to have a prolonged bleeding time, which returned to normal one week after stopping the *Ginkgo biloba* supplement and **rofecoxib**, and remained normal after restarting low-dose **rofecoxib**.[2]

A placebo-controlled study in 11 healthy subjects who were given *Ginkgo biloba* leaf *(Ginkgold)* 120 mg twice daily for three doses, followed by a single 100-mg dose of **flurbiprofen**, found that the pharmacokinetics of flurbiprofen were unchanged.[3]

A study in 12 healthy subjects who were given **diclofenac** 50 mg twice daily for 14 days, with *Ginkgo biloba* extract *(Ginkgold)* 120 mg twice daily on days 8 to 15, found no alteration in the AUC or oral clearance of diclofenac.[4]

Mechanism

The reason for the bleeding is not known, but *Ginkgo biloba* extract contains ginkgolide B, which is a potent inhibitor of platelet-activating factor that is needed for arachidonate-independent platelet aggregation. On their own, *Ginkgo biloba* supplements have been associated with prolonged bleeding times,[5,6] left and bilateral subdural haematomas,[5,7] a right parietal haematoma,[8] post-laparoscopic cholecystectomy bleeding,[9] and subarachnoid haemorrhage.[6] Ibuprofen is an inhibitor of platelet aggregation, but selective inhibitors of COX-2 such as rofecoxib have no effect on platelets and would not be expected to potentiate any bleeding effect of *Ginkgo biloba*.

The pharmacokinetic study involving diclofenac was designed to identify whether *Ginkgo biloba* exerted an inhibitory effect on cytochrome P450 isoenzyme CYP2C9, which is involved in the metabolism of diclofenac. Although an indication that such an effect may occur was noted in studies *in vitro* using *S*-warfarin, the *in vivo* study did not confirm that this interaction would be seen clinically.[4]

Importance and management

The evidence from these reports is too slim to forbid patients to take NSAIDs and *Ginkgo biloba* concurrently, but some do recommend caution.[10] Medical professionals should be aware of the possibility of increased bleeding tendency with *Ginkgo biloba*, and report any suspected cases.[8] Consider also 'Antiplatelet drugs + Herbal medicines', p.699.

1. Meisel C, Johne A, Roots I. Fatal intracerebral mass bleeding associated with *Ginkgo biloba* and ibuprofen. *Atherosclerosis* (2003) 167, 367.
2. Hoffman T. Ginko, Vioxx and excessive bleeding – possible drug-herb interactions: case report. *Hawaii Med J* (2001) 60, 290.
3. Greenblatt DJ, von Moltke LL, Luo Y, Perloff ES, Horan KA, Bruce A, Reynolds RC, Harmatz JS, Avula B, Khan IA, Goldman P. Ginkgo biloba does not alter clearance of flurbiprofen, a cytochrome P450-2C9 substrate. *J Clin Pharmacol* (2006) 46, 214–21.
4. Mohutsky MA, Anderson GD, Miller JW, Elmer GW. *Ginkgo biloba:* evaluation of CYP2C9 drug interactions in vitro and in vivo. *Am J Ther* (2006) 13, 24–31.
5. Rowin J, Lewis SL. Spontaneous bilateral subdural hematomas associated with chronic *Ginkgo biloba* ingestion. *Neurology* (1996) 46, 1775–6.
6. Vale S. Subarachnoid haemorrhage associated with *Ginkgo biloba*. *Lancet* (1998) 352, 36.
7. Gilbert GJ. *Ginkgo biloba*. *Neurology* (1997) 48, 1137.
8. Benjamin J, Muir T, Briggs K, Pentland B. A case of cerebral haemorrhage – can *Ginkgo biloba* be implicated? *Postgrad Med J* (2001) 77, 112–13.
9. Fessenden JM, Wittenborn W, Clarke L. Gingko biloba: a case report of herbal medicine and bleeding postoperatively from a laparoscopic cholecystectomy. *Am Surg* (2001) 67, 33–5.
10. Griffiths J, Jordan S, Pilon S. Natural health products and adverse reactions. *Can Adverse React News* (2004) 14, 2–3.

NSAIDs or Aspirin + Gold

Gold appears to increase the risk of aspirin-induced liver damage. The use of gold with fenoprofen seems to be safer with regard to liver toxicity. An isolated report suggested that naproxen may have contributed to gold-induced pneumonitis.

Clinical evidence, mechanism, importance and management

A study in rheumatoid patients given aspirin 3.9 g or **fenoprofen** 2.4 g daily suggested that gold induction therapy (**sodium aurothiomalate**, by intramuscular injection, to a total dose of 985 mg over 6 months) increased aspirin-induced hepatotoxicity. Levels of AST, lactate dehydrogenase, and alkaline phosphatase were higher during aspirin than during

fenoprofen treatment. These indicators of liver impairment suggest that **fenoprofen** is safer than aspirin in this context. Combined treatment with gold and NSAIDs was more effective than the NSAIDs alone.[1]

A patient with rheumatoid arthritis taking gold (**sodium aurothiomalate**) developed pneumonitis soon after **naproxen** 500 mg twice daily was added. An *in vitro* study suggested the pneumonitis was due to hypersensitivity to gold. However, the patient's condition continued to deteriorate despite stopping the gold, then showed marked improvement when the **naproxen** was also stopped. The authors suggest that the **naproxen** may have altered the patient's immune system in some way to make them more sensitive to the gold.[2] This appears to be the only report of such an effect, and is therefore unlikely to be of general relevance.

1. Davis JD, Turner RA, Collins RL, Ruchte IR, Kaufmann JS. Fenoprofen, aspirin, and gold induction in rheumatoid arthritis. *Clin Pharmacol Ther* (1977) 21, 52–61.
2. McFadden RG, Fraher LJ, Thompson JM. Gold-naproxen pneumonitis: a toxic drug interaction? *Chest* (1989) 96, 216–18.

NSAIDs or Aspirin + H_2-receptor antagonists

The H_2-receptor antagonists have no effect or cause only modest and normally clinically unimportant changes in the serum levels of aspirin and the NSAIDs. More importantly H_2-receptor antagonists may protect the gastric mucosa from the irritant effects of the NSAIDs.

Clinical evidence

(a) Aspirin

Cimetidine 300 mg, given 1 hour before a single 1.2-g dose of aspirin caused only a modest increase in the serum salicylate levels of 3 out of 6 healthy subjects.[1] When 13 patients with rheumatoid arthritis taking enteric-coated aspirin were given **cimetidine** 300 mg four times daily for 7 days the total amount of aspirin absorbed was unaltered, but aspirin levels were slightly raised, from 161 to 180 micrograms/mL.[2] The pharmacokinetics of a single 1-g dose of aspirin were largely unchanged in 6 healthy subjects given **ranitidine** 150 mg twice daily for a week.[3] **Famotidine** has been found to cause some small changes in the pharmacokinetics of aspirin, but this is of doubtful clinical importance.[4]

(b) Azapropazone

A randomised pharmacokinetic study in 12 healthy subjects found that after taking **cimetidine** 300 mg every 6 hours for 6 days the AUC of a single 600-mg dose of azapropazone was increased by 25%, and the AUC of **cimetidine** was altered by less than 20%. No significant changes in laboratory values (blood counts, enzyme levels) were seen, and adverse effects were minor (headaches in 3 subjects).[5]

(c) Diclofenac

In 14 healthy subjects **famotidine** 40 mg raised the peak plasma levels of enteric-coated diclofenac 100 mg from 5.84 to 7.04 mg/L. Peak plasma diclofenac levels also occurred more rapidly (2 versus 2.75 hours). The extent of the absorption was unchanged.[6] Diclofenac did not affect the pharmacokinetics of **ranitidine** nor its ability to suppress gastric pH.[7] Another study also found that the pharmacokinetics of diclofenac were unaffected by **ranitidine**.[8]

(d) Dipyrone

In a study in 12 patients with confirmed duodenal ulcer, but no gastrointestinal bleeding, **cimetidine** 200 mg was given three times daily with another 400 mg at night for 20 days. A single 1.5-g or 750-mg dose of dipyrone was given on days 8 and 13 of cimetidine treatment. In the presence of **cimetidine**, the AUC of the active metabolite of dipyrone, 4-methyl-amino-antipyrine (4-MAA), was significantly increased, by 74%, with dipyrone doses of 1.5 g, but the renal clearance of 4-MAA remained unchanged.[9]

(e) Flurbiprofen

In 30 patients with rheumatoid arthritis **cimetidine** 300 mg three times daily for 2 weeks increased the maximum serum level of flurbiprofen 150 to 300 mg daily, but **ranitidine** 150 mg twice daily had no effect. The efficacy of the flurbiprofen (assessed by Ritchie score, 50 foot walking time, grip strength) was not altered.[10] Another study in healthy subjects found that **cimetidine** 300 mg four times daily slightly increased the serum levels of a single 200-mg dose of flurbiprofen, and raised the flurbiprofen AUC by 13%.[11] No statistically significant interaction occurred with **ranitidine** 150 mg twice daily.[11] Although the activity of flurbiprofen is thought to be related to the *S*-enantiomer, neither **cimetidine** nor **ranitidine** were shown to interact preferentially with one enantiomer over the other.[12]

(f) Ibuprofen

Cimetidine 400 mg three times daily raised the peak serum levels and AUC of a 600-mg dose of ibuprofen by 14% and 6%, respectively. No changes were seen with **ranitidine** 300 mg daily.[13] Another study found that the (AUC of *R*-ibuprofen and *S*-ibuprofen increased by 37% and 19%, respectively, but these were not statistically significant.[14] However, five other studies with ibuprofen found no interaction with **cimetidine** or **ranitidine**,[15-19] or **nizatidine**.[16] However, analysis of the results of one study showed that peak serum ibuprofen levels in black subjects (USA) were 54% higher and occurred sooner, whereas in white subjects (USA) they were 27% lower and delayed.[17,20]

(g) Indometacin

Cimetidine 1 g daily for 2 weeks was given to 10 patients with rheumatoid arthritis taking indometacin 100 to 200 mg daily for over a year. The plasma indometacin levels fell by an average of 18%, but there was no significant change in the clinical effectiveness of the anti-inflammatory treatment (as measured by articular index, pain, grip strength and erythrocyte sedimentation rate).[21] Another study found no changes in the pharmacokinetics of indometacin in healthy subjects given **ranitidine**.[22] No marked changes in the bioavailability of either **cimetidine** or **ranitidine** were seen when they were given with indometacin in a single-dose study in healthy subjects.[23]

(h) Ketoprofen

Cimetidine 600 mg twice daily was found not to affect the pharmacokinetics of enteric-coated ketoprofen 100 mg twice daily in 12 healthy subjects.[24]

(i) Lornoxicam

In 12 healthy subjects **cimetidine** 400 mg twice daily increased the maximum serum levels and AUC of lornoxicam 8 mg twice daily by 28% and 9%, respectively. **Ranitidine** 150 mg twice daily had no significant effect on lornoxicam pharmacokinetics in these same subjects, except that one subject had a very marked increase in serum lornoxicam levels while taking both drugs. He dropped out of the study after 6 days because of severe gastric irritation. It is not clear what part, if any, the **ranitidine** had to play in this effect.[25]

(j) Meloxicam

In an open, randomised, crossover study, a group of 9 healthy subjects was given meloxicam 30 mg either alone, or with **cimetidine** 200 mg four times daily for 5 days. **Cimetidine** had no significant effect on the pharmacokinetics of the meloxicam.[26]

(k) Naproxen

One study found no adverse interaction between naproxen and **cimetidine** and no alteration in the beneficial effects of **cimetidine** on gastric acid secretion,[27] but another study found that cimetidine caused a moderate 39 to 60% decrease in the naproxen half-life,[28,29] and a 20% reduction in the AUC of naproxen.[29] In one of these studies the half-life of naproxen was reduced by about 40% by **ranitidine** and 50% by **famotidine**.[29] A further study found that **nizatidine** does not affect the pharmacokinetics of naproxen.[30]

(l) Piroxicam

In 10 healthy subjects **cimetidine** 300 mg four times daily for 7 days slightly increased the half-life and the AUC of a single 20-mg dose of piroxicam by 8% and 16%, respectively.[31] Another study found that **cimetidine** caused a 15% rise in the AUC of piroxicam.[32] In 12 healthy subjects the half-life and AUC of a single-dose of piroxicam were increased by 41% and 31%, respectively, by **cimetidine** 200 mg three times daily, and the plasma levels were raised accordingly:[33] for example, at 4 hours they were raised by almost 25%.[33] **Ranitidine** was not found to affect the pharmacokinetics of piroxicam.[34] No clinically significant changes occurred in the steady-state serum levels of piroxicam in a further study when either **cimetidine** or **nizatidine** were given.[35]

(m) Tenoxicam

The pharmacokinetics of a single 20-mg oral dose of tenoxicam was unaltered in 6 healthy subjects after they took **cimetidine** 1 g daily for 7 days.[36]

Mechanism

Uncertain. Azapropazone, 4-MAA (the active metabolite of dipyrone), lornoxicam, and piroxicam serum levels are possibly increased because their metabolism via the cytochrome P450 system is reduced by the cimetidine.[5,9,25,33] There may also be some effects on renal excretion.[5]

Importance and management

Most of these interactions between the NSAIDs and cimetidine, famotidine, nizatidine or ranitidine appear to be of no particular clinical importance. The general relevance of the isolated case of increased lornoxicam levels and severe gastric irritation with ranitidine is uncertain, but probably small. The H_2-receptor antagonists as a group may protect the gastric mucosa from the irritant effects of the NSAIDs and concurrent use may therefore be advantageous.

1. Khoury W, Geraci K, Askari A, Johnson M. The effect of cimetidine on aspirin absorption. *Gastroenterology* (1979) 76, 1169.
2. Willoughby JS, Paton TW, Walker SE, Little AH. The effect of cimetidine on enteric-coated ASA disposition. *Clin Pharmacol Ther* (1983) 33, 268.
3. Corrocher R, Bambara LM, Caramaschi P, Testi R, Girelli M, Pellegatti M, Lomeo A. Effect of ranitidine on the absorption of aspirin. *Digestion* (1987) 37, 178–83.
4. Domecq C, Fuentes A, Hurtado C, Arancibia A. Effect of famotidine on the bioavailability of acetylsalicylic acid. *Med Sci Res* (1993) 21, 219–20.
5. Maggon KK, Lam GM. Azapropazone: 20 years of clinical use. Rainsford KD, ed. Kluwer Academic Pub; 1989 p. 136–45.
6. Suryakumar J, Chakrapani T, Krishna DR. Famotidine affects the pharmacokinetics of diclofenac sodium. *Drug Invest* (1992) 4, 66–8.
7. Blum RA, Alioth C, Chan KKH, Furst DE, Ziehmer BA, Schentag JJ. Diclofenac does not affect the pharmacodynamics of ranitidine. *Clin Pharmacol Ther* (1992) 51, 192.
8. Dammann HG, Simon-Schultz J, Steinhoff I, Damaschke A, Schmoldt A, Sallowsky E. Differential effects of misoprostol and ranitidine on the pharmacokinetics of diclofenac and gastrointestinal symptoms. *Br J Clin Pharmacol* (1993) 36, 345–9.
9. Bacracheva N, Tyutyulkova N, Drenska A, Gorantcheva J, Schinzel S, Scholl T, Stoinov A, Tchakarski I, Tentcheva J, Vlahov V. Effect of cimetidine on the pharmacokinetics of the metabolites of metamizol. *Int J Clin Pharmacol Ther* (1997) 35, 275–81.
10. Kreeft JH, Bellamy N, Freeman D. Do H_2-antagonists alter the kinetics and effects of chronically-administered flurbiprofen in rheumatoid arthritis? *Clin Invest Med* (1987) 10 (4 Suppl B), B58.
11. Sullivan KM, Small RE, Rock WL, Cox SR, Willis HE. Effects of cimetidine or ranitidine on the pharmacokinetics of flurbiprofen. *Clin Pharm* (1986) 5, 586–9.
12. Small RE, Cox SR, Adams WJ. Influence of H_2 receptor antagonists on the disposition of flurbiprofen enantiomers. *J Clin Pharmacol* (1990) 30, 660–4.
13. Ochs HR, Greenblatt DJ, Matlis R, Weinbrenner J. Interaction of ibuprofen with the H-2 receptor antagonists ranitidine and cimetidine. *Clin Pharmacol Ther* (1985) 38, 648–51.
14. Li G, Treiber G, Klotz U. The ibuprofen-cimetidine interaction. Stereochemical considerations. *Drug Invest* (1989) 1, 11–17.
15. Conrad KA, Mayersohn M, Bliss M. Cimetidine does not alter ibuprofen kinetics after a single dose. *Br J Clin Pharmacol* (1984) 18, 624–6.
16. Forsyth DR, Jayasinghe KSA, Roberts CJC. Do nizatidine and cimetidine interact with ibuprofen? *Eur J Clin Pharmacol* (1988) 35, 85–8.
17. Stephenson DW, Small RE, Wood JH, Willis HE, Johnson SM, Karnes HT, Rajasekharaiah K. Effect of ranitidine and cimetidine on ibuprofen pharmacokinetics. *Clin Pharm* (1988) 7, 317–21.
18. Evans AM, Nation RL, Sansom LN. Lack of effect of cimetidine on the pharmacokinetics of R(-)- and S(+)-ibuprofen. *Br J Clin Pharmacol* (1989) 28, 143–9.
19. Small RE, Wilmot-Pater MG, McGee BA, Willis HE. Effects of misoprostol or ranitidine on ibuprofen pharmacokinetics. *Clin Pharm* (1991) 10, 870–2.
20. Small RE, Wood JH. Influence of racial differences on effects of ranitidine and cimetidine on ibuprofen pharmacokinetics. *Clin Pharm* (1989) 8, 471–2.
21. Howes CA, Pullar T, Sourindhrin I, Mistra PC, Capel H, Lawson DH, Tilstone WJ. Reduced steady-state plasma concentrations of chlorpromazine and indomethacin in patients receiving cimetidine. *Eur J Clin Pharmacol* (1983) 24, 99–102.
22. Kendall MJ, Gibson R, Walt RP. Co-administration of misoprostol or ranitidine with indomethacin: effects on pharmacokinetics, abdominal symptoms and bowel habit. *Aliment Pharmacol Ther* (1992) 6, 437–46.
23. Delhotal-Landes B, Flouvat B, Liote F, Abel L, Meyer P, Vinceneux P, Carbon C. Pharmacokinetic interactions between NSAIDs (indomethacin or sulindac) and H_2-receptor antagonists (cimetidine or ranitidine) in human volunteers. *Clin Pharmacol Ther* (1988) 44, 442–52.
24. Verbeeck RK, Corman CL, Wallace SM, Herman RJ, Ross SG, Le Morvan P. Single and multiple dose pharmacokinetics of enteric coated ketoprofen: effect of cimetidine. *Eur J Clin Pharmacol* (1988) 35, 521–7.
25. Ravic M, Salas-Herrera I, Johnston A, Turner P, Foley K, Rosenow DE. A pharmacokinetic interaction between cimetidine or ranitidine and lornoxicam. *Postgrad Med J* (1993) 69, 865–66.
26. Busch U, Heinzel G, Narjes H, Nehmiz G. Interaction of meloxicam with cimetidine, Maalox or aspirin. *J Clin Pharmacol* (1996) 36, 79–84.
27. Holford NHG, Altman D, Riegelman S, Buskin JN, Upton RA. Pharmacokinetic and pharmacodynamic study of cimetidine administered with naproxen. *Clin Pharmacol Ther* (1981) 29, 251–2.
28. Vree TB, van den Biggelaar-Martea M, Verwey-van Wissen CPWGM, Vree ML, Guelen PJM. The pharmacokinetics of naproxen, its metabolite *O*-desmethylnaproxen, and their acyl glucuronides in humans. Effect of cimetidine. *Br J Clin Pharmacol* (1993) 35, 467–72.
29. Vree TB, van den Biggelaar-Martea M, Verwey-van Wissen CPWGM, Vree ML, Guelen PJM. The effects of cimetidine, ranitidine and famotidine on the single-dose pharmacokinetics of naproxen and its metabolites in humans. *Int J Clin Pharmacol Ther Toxicol* (1993) 31, 597–601.
30. Satterwhite JH, Bowsher RR, Callaghan JT, Cerimele BJ, Levine LR. Nizatidine: lack of drug interaction with naproxen. *Clin Res* (1992) 40, 706A.
31. Mailhot C, Dahl SL, Ward JR. The effect of cimetidine on serum concentrations of piroxicam. *Pharmacotherapy* (1986) 6, 112–17.
32. Freeman DJ, Danter WR, Carruthers SG. Pharmacokinetic interaction between cimetidine and piroxicam in normal subjects. *Clin Invest Med* (1988) 11, C19.
33. Said SA, Foda AM. Influence of cimetidine on the pharmacokinetics of piroxicam in rat and man. *Arzneimittelforschung* (1989) 39, 790–2.
34. Dixon JS, Lacey LF, Pickup ME, Langley SJ, Page MC. A lack of pharmacokinetic interaction between ranitidine and piroxicam. *Eur J Clin Pharmacol* (1990) 39, 583–6.
35. Milligan PA, McGill PE, Howden CW, Kelman AW, Whiting B. The consequences of H_2 receptor antagonist-piroxicam coadministration in patients with joint disorders. *Eur J Clin Pharmacol* (1993) 45, 507–12.
36. Day RO, Geisslinger G, Paull P, Williams KM. Neither cimetidine nor probenecid affect the pharmacokinetics of tenoxicam in normal volunteers. *Br J Clin Pharmacol* (1994) 37, 79–81.

NSAIDs or Aspirin + Hormonal contraceptives or HRT

Oral contraceptives increase diflunisal clearance in women, but only to the level normally seen in men. One study showed modestly reduced levels of ibuprofen with oral contraceptives, but another study did not. Oral contraceptives reduced the levels of aspirin, but not phenylbutazone. There are no clinically relevant changes in the pharmacokinetics of oxaprozin with conjugated oestrogens.

Clinical evidence, mechanism, importance and management

(a) Aspirin

The AUCs of single 300- and 600-mg doses of aspirin were lower in 10 women after they started to take a combined oral contraceptive (**ethinylestradiol/norethisterone** 30 micrograms/1 mg). After the oral contraceptive had been discontinued, the pharmacokinetics of aspirin returned to baseline values.[1]

(b) Coxibs

For a report of pulmonary embolism in a patient taking valdecoxib with a combined oral contraceptive, and for the effects of coxibs on contraceptive metabolism, see 'Hormonal contraceptives or HRT + Coxibs', p.994.

(c) Diflunisal

The clearance of a single 250-mg dose of diflunisal was 53% higher in 6 women taking oral contraceptives than in 6 control women, but was similar to the clearance in 6 men.[2] This difference is unlikely to be of clinical importance.

(d) Ibuprofen

In one study, the pharmacokinetics of *R*-ibuprofen did not differ between women taking combined oral contraceptives, control women, and control men.[3] However, in another study, the median AUC_{0-12} of *S*-ibuprofen lysinate was 29% lower in users of oral contraceptives, and pain-intensity was higher (possibly due to reduced pain tolerance).[4]

(e) Oxaprozin

There was no difference in the pharmacokinetics of a single 1.2-g dose of oxaprozin in 11 women taking **conjugated oestrogens** (*Premarin*) than in 11 control women, except that the time to peak concentration was shorter (4 versus 8.9 hours).[5] This difference is unlikely to be of clinical importance.

(f) Phenylbutazone

The pharmacokinetics of a single 400-mg dose of phenylbutazone did not change in 10 women after they started to take a combined oral contraceptive containing **ethinylestradiol/norethisterone** 30 micrograms/1 mg.[1]

1. Gupta KC, Joshi JV, Hazari K, Pohujani SM, Satoskar RS. Effect of low estrogen combination oral contraceptive on metabolism of aspirin and phenylbutazone. *Int J Clin Pharmacol Ther Toxicol* (1982) 20, 511–13.
2. Macdonald JI, Herman RJ, Verbeeck RK. Sex-difference and the effects of smoking and oral contraceptive steroids on the kinetics of diflunisal. *Eur J Clin Pharmacol* (1990) 38, 175–9.
3. Knights KM, McLean CF, Tonkin AL, Miners JO. Lack of effect of gender and oral contraceptive steroids on the pharmacokinetics of (R)-ibuprofen in humans. *Br J Clin Pharmacol* (1995) 40, 153–6.
4. Warnecke J, Pentz R, Siegers C-P. Effects of smoking and contraceptives on the pharmacokinetics and pharmacodynamics of S(+)-ibuprofen lysinate in humans. *Naunyn Schmiedebergs Arch Pharmacol* (1996) 354 (Suppl 1), R33.
5. Scavone JM, Ochs HR, Greenblatt DJ, Matlis R. Pharmacokinetics of oxaprozin in women receiving conjugated estrogen. *Eur J Clin Pharmacol* (1988) 35, 105–8.

NSAIDs or Salicylates + Mazindol

Mazindol does not appear to interact adversely with indometacin or salicylates.

Clinical evidence, mechanism, importance and management

In an 8-week, placebo-controlled, double-blind study, mazindol was given to 26 patients with obesity and arthritis, 15 of whom were taking **sali-**

cylates, 11 were taking **indometacin** and one was taking dextropropoxyphene (propoxyphene) with paracetamol (acetaminophen). Additional analgesic and anti-inflammatory drugs used were ibuprofen (4 patients), phenylbutazone (1), dextropropoxyphene (7) and paracetamol (3). No symptoms attributable to salicylism or **indometacin** toxicity (gastric intolerance, headache) were observed.[1]

1. Thorpe PC, Isaac PF, Rodgers J. A controlled trial of mazindol (Sanjorex, Teronac) in the management of obese rheumatic patients. *Curr Ther Res* (1975) 17, 149–55.

NSAIDs or Aspirin + Metoclopramide

Metoclopramide increases the rate of absorption of aspirin and tolfenamic acid. Conversely, metoclopramide reduces the bioavailability of ketoprofen.

Clinical evidence

(a) Aspirin

In one study, intramuscular metoclopramide given before oral effervescent aspirin increased the rate of aspirin absorption during a migraine attack to that seen when aspirin was given alone to subjects who were headache free.[1] Similarly, in another study, intramuscular or oral metoclopramide 10 mg increased the rate of absorption of aspirin in patients with migraine.[2] However, in healthy subjects metoclopramide did not alter the pharmacokinetics of aspirin.[3] In addition, in one clinical study there was no difference in analgesic efficacy between aspirin with metoclopramide (*Migravess*) and aspirin alone (*Alka-Seltzer*) for migraine attacks.[4]

(b) Ketoprofen

In a single-dose study in 4 healthy subjects, metoclopramide 10 mg reduced the AUC of a 50-mg capsule of ketoprofen by 28%. The maximum plasma levels of ketoprofen were almost halved and the time to reach this maximum was prolonged by 30%.[5]

(c) Tolfenamic acid

Rectal metoclopramide 20 mg, given to 8 healthy subjects 30 minutes before oral tolfenamic acid 300 mg, caused a threefold increase in the serum tolfenamic acid levels at 45 minutes. There was no change in the maximum level or the AUC.[6] In another study, rectal metoclopramide similarly enhanced the rate of oral absorption of tolfenamic acid when given during a migraine attack.[7]

Mechanism

Metoclopramide speeds up gastric emptying. The relatively poorly soluble ketoprofen spends less time in the stomach where it dissolves, and as a result less is available for absorption in the small intestine. Conversely, the absorption rate of tolfenamic acid is increased, without a change in the extent of absorption.

Importance and management

The clinical importance of the reduction in ketoprofen levels is unknown, but the authors of the study recommend that ketoprofen (and possibly other NSAIDs that are poorly soluble) should be taken 1 to 2 hours before metoclopramide. Conversely, for aspirin, tolfenamic acid, and other NSAIDs, metoclopramide can be used to increase the rate of absorption, and therefore possibly speed up the onset of analgesic effect in conditions such as migraine.

1. Volans GN. The effect of metoclopramide on the absorption of effervescent aspirin in migraine. *Br J Clin Pharmacol* (1975) 2, 57–63.
2. Ross-Lee LM, Eadie MJ, Heazlewood V, Bochner F, Tyrer JH. Aspirin pharmacokinetics in migraine: the effect of metoclopramide. *Eur J Clin Pharmacol* (1983) 24, 777–85.
3. Manniche PM, Dinneen LC, Langemark M. The pharmacokinetics of the individual constituents of an aspirin-metoclopramide combination ('Migravess'). *Curr Med Res Opin* (1984) 9, 153–6.
4. Tfelt-Hansen P, Olesen J. Effervescent metoclopramide and aspirin (Migravess) versus effervescent aspirin or placebo for migraine attacks: a double-blind study. *Cephalalgia* (1984) 4, 107–11.
5. Etman MA, Ismail FA, Nada AH. Effect of metoclopramide on ketoprofen pharmacokinetics in man. *Int J Pharmaceutics* (1992) 88, 433–5.
6. Tokola RA, Anttila V-J, Neuvonen PJ. The effect of metoclopramide on the absorption of tolfenamic acid. *Int J Clin Pharmacol Ther Toxicol* (1982) 20, 465–8.
7. Tokola RA, Neuvonen PJ. Effects of migraine attack and metoclopramide on the absorption of tolfenamic acid. *Br J Clin Pharmacol* (1984) 17, 67–75.

NSAIDs + NSAIDs

The concurrent use of two or more NSAIDs increases the risk of gastrointestinal damage. Diflunisal raises serum indometacin levels about twofold but does not affect naproxen levels. The concurrent use of indometacin and flurbiprofen does not appear to affect the pharmacokinetics of either drug. Floctafenine does not alter diclofenac levels. Indometacin caused renal impairment in a patient recovering from phenylbutazone-induced acute renal failure.

Clinical evidence

(a) Gastrointestinal effects

The risk of serious upper gastrointestinal bleeding was increased by the use of more than one NSAID in a meta-analysis of data from three case-controlled studies (odds ratio 4.9 with one NSAID and 10.7 with two).[1] Another study provided similar findings: the odds ratio was 7.1 with one NSAID and 12.3 with two or more NSAIDs.[2] Similar findings have been reported with aspirin and NSAIDs, see 'NSAIDs + Aspirin; Anti-inflammatory dose', p.142. Analysis of yellow card reports to the CSM in the UK, of gastrointestinal perforation, obstruction, ulceration or bleeding with **diclofenac**, **naproxen**, and **ibuprofen**, revealed that 6% of the patients were receiving another non-aspirin NSAID.[3]

One pharmacodynamic study in healthy subjects found that gastric instillation of a solution of **diflunisal** before an **indometacin** solution prevented the fall in transmucosal potential difference seen with **indometacin** alone. This was interpreted as evidence that **diflunisal** protects the human gastric mucosa against the damaging effects of **indometacin**.[4] However, the relevance of this test to the adverse effects of NSAIDs used clinically is unknown. Note that fatal gastrointestinal haemorrhage has been reported in a patient taking **diflunisal** and **indometacin**.[5]

(b) Pharmacokinetic studies

No clinically significant changes in the pharmacokinetics of either **indometacin** 75 mg daily or **flurbiprofen** 150 mg daily occurred when both drugs were given together.[6]

Diflunisal 250 mg twice daily had no effect on plasma levels or urinary excretion of **naproxen** 250 mg twice daily.[7]

A study in 16 healthy subjects showed that **diflunisal** 500 mg twice daily raised the steady-state plasma levels and the AUC of **indometacin** 50 mg twice daily about twofold. Combined use was associated with more gastrointestinal and CNS adverse effects, but there was no clear effect on blood loss in the faeces.[8] Another study produced similar findings.[9]

No change in free **diclofenac** levels was seen when 6 healthy subjects were given **floctafenine** 400 mg with **diclofenac** 75 mg daily for a week.[10]

(c) Renal effects

An isolated report describes deterioration in renal function in a patient during recovery from **phenylbutazone**-induced renal failure when **indometacin** 25 mg three times a day was given. The **indometacin** was discontinued with improvement of renal function.[11]

Mechanism

The damaging effects of the NSAIDs on the gut appear to be additive. Diflunisal may inhibit the glucuronidation of indometacin, or could compete for renal clearance of unmetabolised indometacin.[9] All NSAIDs have the propensity to cause renal impairment.

Importance and management

The gastrointestinal toxicity of the NSAIDs is well documented, and it appears that combined use increases this risk. The CSM in the UK state that not more than one NSAID should be used concurrently.[3,12] The marked rise in plasma levels of indometacin with diflunisal gives an additional reason why this combination in particular should not be used. Some NSAIDs cause more gastrointestinal toxicity than others, a suggested broad 'rank order' of seven NSAIDs is as follows. Highest risk (**azapropazone**); intermediate risk (diclofenac, indometacin, **ketoprofen** and naproxen, with **piroxicam** more risky); lowest risk (ibuprofen),[12] which has been borne out in another analysis.[3] The ranking was based on epidemiological studies and the yellow card database. **Ketorolac** may also be particularly associated with gastrointestinal bleeding, and concurrent use with other NSAIDs has been identified as a risk factor,[13] therefore the manufacturer consequently specifically contraindicates its use with other NSAIDs.[14]

1. Lewis SC, Langman MJS, Laporte J-R, Matthews JNS, Rawlins MD, Wiholm B-E. Dose-response relationships between individual nonaspirin nonsteroidal anti-inflammatory drugs (NANSAIDs) and serious upper gastrointestinal bleeding: a meta-analysis based on individual patient data. *Br J Clin Pharmacol* (2002) 54, 320–6.
2. Anon. Do not combine several NSAIDs. *Prescrire Int* (2003) 12, 20.
3. Committee on Safety of Medicines/Medicines Control Agency. Non-steroidal anti-inflammatory drugs (NSAIDs) and gastrointestinal safety. *Current Problems* (2002) 28, 5.
4. Cohen MM. Diflunisal protects human gastric mucosa against damage by indomethacin. *Dig Dis Sci* (1983) 28, 1070–77.
5. Edwards IR. Medicines Adverse Reactions Committee: eighteenth annual report, 1983. *N Z Med J* (1984) 97, 729–32.
6. Rudge SR, Lloyd-Jones JK, Hind ID. Interaction between flurbiprofen and indomethacin in rheumatoid arthritis. *Br J Clin Pharmacol* (1982) 13, 448–51.
7. Dresse A, Gerard MA, Quinaux N, Fischer P, Gerardy J. Effect of diflunisal on human plasma levels and on the urinary excretion of naproxen. *Arch Int Pharmacodyn Ther* (1978) 236, 276–84.
8. Van Hecken A, Verbesselt R, Tjandra-Maga TB, De Schepper PJ. Pharmacokinetic interaction between indomethacin and diflunisal. *Eur J Clin Pharmacol* (1989) 36, 507–12.
9. Eriksson L-O, Wåhlin-Boll E, Liedholm H, Seideman P, Melander A. Influence of chronic diflunisal treatment on the plasma levels, metabolism and excretion of indomethacin. *Eur J Clin Pharmacol* (1989) 37, 7–15.
10. Sioufi A, Stierlin H, Schweizer A, Botta L, Degen PH, Theobald W, Brechbühler S. Recent findings concerning clinically relevant pharmacokinetics of diclofenac sodium. In: Voltarol — New Findings, ed Kass E. Proc Int Symp Voltarol, Paris June 22nd, 1981. 15th Int Congress of Rheumatology. p 19–30.
11. Kimberly R, Brandstetter RD. Exacerbation of phenylbutazone-related renal failure by indomethacin. *Arch Intern Med* (1978) 138, 1711–12.
12. Committee on the Safety of Medicines/Medicines Control Agency. Relative safety of oral non-aspirin NSAIDs. *Current Problems* (1994) 20, 9–11.
13. Committee on Safety of Medicines/Medicines Control Agency. Ketorolac: new restrictions on dose and duration of treatment. *Current Problems* (1993) 19, 5–6.
14. Toradol (Ketorolac trometamol). Roche Products Ltd. UK Summary of product characteristics, May 2007.

NSAIDs or Aspirin + Paracetamol (Acetaminophen)

Paracetamol levels are increased by diflunisal. Aspirin, diclofenac, nabumetone and sulindac pharmacokinetics do not appear to be affected by paracetamol. There is no pharmacokinetic interaction between ibuprofen and paracetamol. Propacetamol, and possibly paracetamol, increase the antiplatelet effects of diclofenac, although the evidence is limited and the clinical relevance of this is uncertain.

One epidemiological study found that paracetamol alone, and particularly when combined with NSAIDs, was associated with an increased risk of gastrointestinal bleeding, but other studies have not found such an effect. Two isolated case reports describe renal toxicity in three patients taking ibuprofen or flurbiprofen in which paracetamol use was a theoretical contributing factor.

Clinical evidence, mechanism, importance and management

(a) Antiplatelet effects

In healthy subjects combining single doses of intravenous **propacetamol** 30 mg/kg and **diclofenac** 1.1 mg/kg augmented the platelet inhibitory effect of **diclofenac** by about one-third at 90 minutes post dose. At 5 minutes, the inhibitory effect of both **diclofenac** alone and the combination was 100%, and by 22 to 24 hours, neither **diclofenac** alone nor the combination had any inhibitory effect.[1] In a previous study, the authors had shown that **propacetamol** (which is hydrolysed to paracetamol) also inhibited platelet function, and they suggested that the effects of **diclofenac** and **propacetamol** were additive.[1] The clinical relevance of these findings is unclear, but the authors say it should be considered when assessing the risk of surgical bleeding.[1] Further study is needed.

An *in vitro* study suggested that high doses of paracetamol, and a combination of paracetamol and **diclofenac**, may cause platelet inhibition and may increase the risk of bleeding, particularly post-surgery.[2]

Intravenous **parecoxib** 40 mg was found not to alter the platelet function in 18 healthy subjects when given with intravenous paracetamol 1 g, when compared with paracetamol alone.[3]

(b) Gastrointestinal damage

In a case-control study of the UK General Practice Research Database from 1993 to 1998 the risk of upper gastrointestinal bleeding or perforation was slightly increased in those taking both aspirin and paracetamol (relative risk 3.3), when compared with aspirin alone (2.4), or paracetamol alone (2.4). Moreover, the risk was markedly increased in those taking NSAIDs and paracetamol (16.6), when compared with NSAIDs alone (3.6). The paracetamol doses used were at least 2 g daily. Paracetamol in doses of less than 2 g daily was not associated with an increased risk. Other drug doses and specific NSAIDs were not mentioned.[4] However, other epidemiological studies have not found any increased risk of upper gastrointestinal bleeding with paracetamol at any dose.[5] Paracetamol is usually considered not to increase the risk of upper gastrointestinal adverse effects, and the results of this case-control study are probably insufficient to change prescribing practice. Further studies are needed, controlled for the dose of the NSAID and indication for treatment.

(c) Pharmacokinetic studies

1. Aspirin. In a study in 6 healthy subjects, two doses of dextropropoxyphene with paracetamol 65 mg/650 mg, given one hour before and 3 hours after a single 1.2-g dose of soluble aspirin did not affect the plasma salicylate levels. A reduction in plasma salicylate levels was seen in one subject after a single 1.2-g dose of enteric-coated aspirin was taken with dextropropoxyphene and paracetamol, although the authors suggested that this was related to erratic absorption rather than a pharmacokinetic interaction.[6]

2. Diclofenac. Diclofenac 25 mg given with paracetamol 500 mg, both three times daily for 14 days, had no effect on the pharmacokinetics of diclofenac in 6 healthy subjects.[7]

3. Diflunisal. Diflunisal significantly raised serum paracetamol levels by 50% but the total bioavailability was unchanged in healthy subjects. Diflunisal levels were not affected.[8,9] This interaction has not been shown to be clinically important. Nevertheless, the manufacturer of diflunisal recommends that the combination should be used with caution, because of the association of high levels of paracetamol with hepatotoxicity.[9]

4. Ibuprofen. Ibuprofen 400 mg given with paracetamol 650 mg, both every 6 hours for 2 days, had no effect on the pharmacokinetics of either drug in a crossover study in 20 healthy subjects.[10]

5. Nabumetone. In a single-dose study, the absorption of nabumetone 1 g was not significantly altered by paracetamol 1.5 g.[11]

6. Sulindac. The manufacturer of sulindac notes that paracetamol had no effect on the plasma levels of sulindac or its sulfide metabolite.[12]

(d) Renal effects

Two children (aged 12 and 14 years) developed acute flank pain and reversible renal function impairment during the short-term use of **flurbiprofen** or **ibuprofen**. They had also taken paracetamol.[13] Similarly, a 14-month-old infant with febrile status epilepticus was treated with an alternating regimen of paracetamol and **ibuprofen**, and subsequently developed acute renal failure.[14] NSAIDs can cause renal toxicity, whereas paracetamol is less likely to cause renal toxicity, except perhaps in overdose.[15] The authors of the first case report proposed that tubular toxicity of NSAIDs and paracetamol are theoretically synergistic.[13] This is because NSAIDs inhibit the production of glutathione (needed to prevent the accumulation of toxic metabolites of paracetamol) and renal ischaemia (possibly induced by NSAIDs, or by dehydration) might lead to the accumulation of paracetamol in the renal medulla.[13]

A review concluded that the available evidence does not support an increased risk of renal toxicity with the use of combination products of aspirin and paracetamol when compared with either drug alone.[16] Paracetamol is often combined with NSAIDs in the management of chronic pain. In addition, paracetamol and **ibuprofen** are often used concurrently (as alternating doses) in the management of fever, particularly in children. This latter practice has become controversial. Opponents cite the lack of efficacy data to support combined use (rather than appropriate doses of single agents), and the theoretical increased risk of overdose and renal toxicity.[17,18] Others consider that, in the absence of true safety issues, professional judgement should be used for recommending combined treatment.[19] Further study is clearly needed.

1. Munsterhjelm E, Niemi TT, Syrjälä MT, Ylikorkala O, Rosenberg PH. Propacetamol augments inhibition of platelet function by diclofenac in volunteers. *Br J Anaesth* (2003) 91, 357–62.
2. Munsterhjelm E, Niemi TT, Ylikorkala O, Silvanto M, Rosenberg PH. Characterization of inhibition of platelet function by paracetamol and its interaction with diclofenac *in vitro*. *Acta Anaesthesiol Scand* (2005) 49, 840–6.
3. Munsterhjelm E, Niemi TT, Ylikorkala O, Neuvonen PJ, Rosenberg PH. Influence on platelet aggregation of i.v. parecoxib and acetaminophen in healthy volunteers. *Br J Anaesth* (2006) 97, 226–31.

4. García Rodríguez LA, Hernández-Díaz S. The risk of upper gastrointestinal complications associated with nonsteroidal anti-inflammatory drugs, glucocorticoids, acetaminophen, and combinations of these agents. *Arthritis Res* (2001) 3, 98–101.
5. Lewis SC, Langman MJS, Laporte J-R, Matthews JNS, Rawlins MD, Wiholm B-E. Dose-response relationships between individual nonaspirin nonsteroidal anti-inflammatory drugs (NANSAIDs) and serious upper gastrointestinal bleeding: a meta-analysis based on individual patient data. *Br J Clin Pharmacol* (2002) 54, 320–6.
6. Hemming JD, Bird HA, Pickup ME, Saunders A, Lowe JR, Dixon JS. Bioavailability of aspirin in the presence of dextropropoxyphene/paracetamol combination. *Pharmatherapeutica* (1981) 2, 543–6.
7. Sioufi A, Stierlin H, Schweizer A, Botta L, Degen PH, Theobald W, Brechbühler S. Recent findings concerning clinically relevant pharmacokinetics of diclofenac sodium. In: Voltarol — New Findings, ed Kass E. Proc Int Symp Voltarol, Paris June 22nd, 1981. 15th Int Congress of Rheumatology. p 19–30.
8. Merck Sharp & Dohme Ltd. Personal communication, 1988.
9. Dolobid (Diflunisal). Merck Sharp & Dohme Ltd. UK Summary of product characteristics, March 2000.
10. Wright CE, Antal EJ, Gillespie WR, Albert KS. Ibuprofen and acetaminophen kinetics when taken concurrently. *Clin Pharmacol Ther* (1983) 34, 707–10.
11. von Schrader HW, Buscher G, Dierdorf D, Mügge H, Wolf D. Nabumetone — a novel anti-inflammatory drug: the influence of food, milk, antacids, and analgesics on bioavailability of single oral doses. *Int J Clin Pharmacol Ther Toxicol* (1983) 21, 311–21.
12. Clinoril (Sulindac). Merck Sharp & Dohme Ltd. UK Summary of product characteristics, May 2007.
13. McIntire SC, Rubenstein RC, Gartner JC, Gilboa N, Elllis D. Acute flank pain and reversible renal dysfunction associated with nonsteroidal anti-inflammatory drug use. *Pediatrics* (1993) 92, 459–60.
14. Del Vecchio MT, Sundel ER. Alternating antipyretics: is this an alternative? *Pediatrics* (2001) 108, 1236–7.
15. Whelton A. Renal effects of over-the-counter analgesics. *J Clin Pharmacol* (1995) 35, 454–63.
16. Bach PH, Berndt WO, Delzell E, Dubach U, Finn WF, Fox JM, Hess R, Michielsen P, Sandler DP, Trump B, Williams G. A safety assessment of fixed dose combinations of acetaminophen and acetylsalicylic acid, coformulated with caffeine. *Ren Fail* (1998) 20, 749–62.
17. Carson SM. Alternating acetaminophen and ibuprofen in the febrile child: examination of the evidence regarding efficacy and safety. *Pediatr Nurs* (2003) 29, 379–82.
18. Anon. No evidence for practice of alternating doses of paracetamol and ibuprofen in children with fever. *Pharm J* (2004) 272, 4.
19. Conroy S, Tomlin S, Soor S. Unsubstantiated alarmist declarations need to be examined. *Pharm J* (2004) 272, 152.

NSAIDs + Pentoxifylline

A review of bleeding events associated with the use of postoperative ketorolac revealed that a small number of patients were also taking pentoxifylline.[1] The UK manufacturers therefore recommend that this drug combination should be avoided,[2] whereas the US manufacturers[3] make no mention of this tentative interaction. There seems to be no evidence regarding this interaction with other NSAIDs.

1. Syntex Pharmaceuticals Limited. Personal communication, January 1995.
2. Toradol (Ketorolac trometamol). Roche Products Ltd. UK Summary of product characteristics, May 2007.
3. Toradol (Ketorolac tromethamine). Roche Pharmaceuticals. US Prescribing information, September 2002.

NSAIDs + Pesticides

Chronic exposure to lindane and other chlorinated pesticides can slightly increase the rate of metabolism of phenazone (antipyrine) and phenylbutazone.

Clinical evidence, mechanism, importance and management

(a) Phenazone (Antipyrine)

A study in 26 men occupationally exposed to a mixture of insecticides, predominantly **DDT**, **chlordane** and **lindane**, found that the half-life of phenazone 10 or 15 mg/kg was reduced from 13.1 hours, in a group of 33 unexposed subjects, to 7.7 hours in the exposed group.[1] The significance of this is unclear as changes in working practices have reduced occupational exposure to such chemicals.

(b) Phenylbutazone

The plasma half-life of phenylbutazone in a group of men who regularly used **chlorinated insecticide** sprays (mainly **lindane**) as part of their work, was found to be 20% shorter (51 hours) than in a control group (64 hours), due, it is believed, to the enzyme-inducing effects of the **pesticides**.[2] This modest increase in rate of metabolism is of doubtful direct clinical importance, but it illustrates the changed metabolism that can occur in those exposed to environmental chemical agents.

1. Kolmodin B, Azarnoff DL, Sjöqvist F. Effect of environmental factors on drug metabolism: decreased plasma half-life of antipyrine in workers exposed to chlorinated hydrocarbon insecticides. *Clin Pharmacol Ther* (1969) 10, 638–42.
2. Kolmodin-Hedman B. Decreased plasma half-life of phenylbutazone in workers exposed to chlorinated pesticides. *Eur J Clin Pharmacol* (1973) 5, 195–8.

NSAIDs + Phenobarbital

Phenobarbital modestly decreases the AUC of fenoprofen and increases the clearance of phenylbutazone.

Clinical evidence, mechanism, importance and management

In 6 healthy subjects pretreatment with phenobarbital 15 or 60 mg every 6 hours for 10 days reduced the AUC of a single 200-mg dose of **fenoprofen** by 23% and 37%, respectively.[1]

In 5 healthy subjects the half-life of a single 6-mg/kg dose of **phenylbutazone** was reduced by 38% after pretreatment with phenobarbital 2 to 3 mg/kg daily for 3 weeks.[2] Other studies confirm that phenobarbital increases the clearance of **phenylbutazone**.[3,4]

The probable reason is that the phenobarbital increases the metabolism of these NSAIDs by the liver, thereby hastening their clearance. **Phenazone** is metabolised by mixed function oxidase enzymes in the liver, for which reason it is extensively used as a model drug for studying whether other drugs induce or inhibit liver enzymes. In one study phenobarbital caused about a 40% reduction thereby demonstrating that the liver enzymes were being stimulated to metabolise the phenazone more rapidly.[5]

The clinical importance of these interactions is uncertain (probably small) but be alert for any evidence of reduced NSAID effects if phenobarbital is added.

1. Helleberg L, Rubin A, Wolen RL, Rodda BE, Ridolfo AS, Gruber CM. A pharmacokinetic interaction in man between phenobarbitone and fenoprofen, a new anti-inflammatory agent. *Br J Clin Pharmacol* (1974) 1, 371–4.
2. Anderson KE, Peterson CM, Alvares AP, Kappas A. Oxidative drug metabolism and inducibility by phenobarbital in sickle cell anemia. *Clin Pharmacol Ther* (1977) 22, 580–7.
3. Levi AJ, Sherlock S, Walker D. Phenylbutazone and isoniazid metabolism in patients with liver disease in relation to previous drug therapy. *Lancet* (1968) i, 1275–9.
4. Whittaker JA, Price Evans DA. Genetic control of phenylbutazone metabolism in man. *BMJ* (1970) 4, 323–8.
5. Vesell ES, Page JG. Genetic control of the phenobarbital-induced shortening of plasma antipyrine half-lives in man. *J Clin Invest* (1969) 48, 2202–9.

NSAIDs + Probenecid

Probenecid reduces the clearance of dexketoprofen, diflunisal, indometacin (toxicity seen), ketoprofen, ketorolac, naproxen, sodium meclofenamate, tenoxicam and tiaprofenic acid and raises their levels. Ketorolac and probenecid are specifically contraindicated. The uricosuric effects of probenecid are not affected by indometacin but may be slightly reduced by sulindac.

Clinical evidence

(a) Diflunisal

In 8 healthy subjects probenecid 500 mg twice daily increased the steady-state plasma levels of diflunisal 250 mg twice daily by 65%, and reduced the clearances of the glucuronide metabolites.[1]

(b) Indometacin

A study in 28 patients with osteoarthritis, taking indometacin 50 to 150 mg daily orally or rectally, showed that probenecid 500 mg to 1 g daily roughly doubled their indometacin plasma levels and this paralleled the increased effectiveness (relief of morning stiffness, joint tenderness and raised grip strength indices). However, 4 patients developed indometacin toxicity.[2]

Other studies have also demonstrated the marked rise in plasma indometacin levels caused by probenecid.[3-5] Clear signs of indometacin toxicity (nausea, headache, tinnitus, confusion and a rise in blood urea) occurred when a woman with stable mild renal impairment was given probenecid.[6] The uricosuric effects of probenecid were not altered.[3]

(c) Ketoprofen and Dexketoprofen

In 6 healthy subjects probenecid 500 mg every 6 hours reduced the clearance of ketoprofen 50 mg every 6 hours by 67%.[7] The manufacturer of dexketoprofen notes that plasma levels may be increased by probenecid, and adjustment of the dose of dexketoprofen is required.[8]

(d) Ketorolac

Probenecid 500 mg four times daily for 4 days increased the total AUC of a single 10-mg dose of ketorolac in 8 subjects by more than threefold, increased its half-life from 6.6 to 15.1 hours, raised its maximum plasma levels by 24% and reduced its clearance by 67%.[9]

(e) Meclofenamate

Single-dose studies in 6 healthy subjects on the pharmacokinetics of sodium meclofenamate 100 mg found that pretreatment with probenecid (dosage unstated) increased its AUC and reduced its apparent plasma clearance by 60%, primarily due to a decrease in non-renal clearance.[10]

(f) Naproxen

Probenecid 500 mg twice daily increased the plasma levels of naproxen 250 mg twice daily by 50% in 12 healthy subjects.[11]

(g) Sulindac

The manufacturers of sulindac note that probenecid increased plasma levels of sulindac and its sulfone metabolite, but had little effect on the active sulfide metabolite. Sulindac produced a modest reduction in the uricosuric action of probenecid,[12,13] which is said not to be clinically significant in most circumstances.[13]

(h) Tenoxicam

Probenecid 1 g twice daily for 4 days increased the maximum serum levels of a single 20-mg oral dose of tenoxicam by 25%. None of the other pharmacokinetic parameters was significantly altered.[14]

(i) Tiaprofenic acid

Probenecid appeared to reduce the urinary excretion of tiaprofenic acid in one healthy subject. The maximum urinary excretion rate was reduced by 66% and delayed by 2 hours.[15]

Mechanism

Probenecid is a known substrate for renal glucuronidation, and possibly competitively inhibits the renal glucuronidation of these NSAIDs.[8,16]

Importance and management

The interaction between indometacin and probenecid is established and adequately documented. Concurrent use should be well monitored because, while clinical improvement can undoubtedly occur, some patients may develop indometacin toxicity (headache, dizziness, light-headedness, nausea, etc.). This is particularly likely in those with some renal impairment. Reduce the indometacin dosage as necessary. Information about other NSAIDs is limited, but these interactions also appear to be established. The clinical importance of most of them is uncertain, but probably small. Reports of adverse effects seem to be lacking, but it would still be prudent to be alert for any evidence of increased adverse effects. Reduce the NSAID dosage if necessary. The exception is ketorolac, which its manufacturers[17,18] contraindicate with probenecid because of the marked increases seen in its plasma levels.

1. Macdonald JI, Wallace SM, Herman RJ, Verbeeck RK. Effect of probenecid on the formation and elimination kinetics of the sulphate and glucuronide conjugates of diflunisal. *Eur J Clin Pharmacol* (1995) 47, 519–23.
2. Brooks PM, Bell MA, Sturrock RD, Famaey JP, Dick WC. The clinical significance of indomethacin-probenecid interaction. *Br J Clin Pharmacol* (1974) 1, 287–90.
3. Skeith MD, Simkin PA, Healey LA. The renal excretion of indomethacin and its inhibition by probenecid. *Clin Pharmacol Ther* (1968) 9, 89–93.
4. Emori W, Paulus HE, Bluestone R, Pearson CM. The pharmacokinetics of indomethacin in serum. *Clin Pharmacol Ther* (1973) 14, 134.
5. Baber N, Halliday L, Littler T, Orme ML'E, Sibeon R. Clinical studies of the interaction between indomethacin and probenecid. *Br J Clin Pharmacol* (1978) 5, 364P.
6. Sinclair H, Gibson T. Interaction between probenecid and indomethacin. *Br J Rheumatol* (1986) 25, 316–17.
7. Upton RA, Williams RL, Buskin JN, Jones RM. Effects of probenecid on ketoprofen kinetics. *Clin Pharmacol Ther* (1982) 31, 705–12.
8. Keral (Dexketoprofen trometamol). A. Menarini Pharmaceuticals UK SRL. UK Summary of product characteristics, November 2004.
9. Mroszczak EJ, Combs DL, Goldblum R, Yee J, McHugh D, Tsina I, Fratis T. The effect of probenecid on ketorolac pharmacokinetics after oral dosing of ketorolac tromethamine. *Clin Pharmacol Ther* (1992) 51, 154.
10. Waller ES. The effect of probenecid on the disposition of meclofenamate sodium. *Drug Intell Clin Pharm* (1983) 17, 453–4.
11. Runkel R, Mroszczak E, Chaplin M, Sevelius H, Segre E. Naproxen-probenecid interaction. *Clin Pharmacol Ther* (1978) 24, 706–13.
12. Clinoril (Sulindac). Merck Sharp & Dohme Ltd. UK Summary of product characteristics, May 2007.
13. Clinoril (Sulindac). Merck & Co Inc. US Prescribing information, February 2007.
14. Day RO, Geisslinger G, Paull P, Williams KM. Neither cimetidine nor probenecid affect the pharmacokinetics of tenoxicam in normal volunteers. *Br J Clin Pharmacol* (1994) 37, 79–81.
15. Jamali F, Russell AS, Lehmann C, Berry BW. Pharmacokinetics of tiaprofenic acid in healthy and arthritic subjects. *J Pharm Sci* (1985) 74, 953–6.
16. Vree TB, van den Biggelaar-Martea M, Verwey-van Wissen CPWGM, van Ewijk-Beneken Kolmer EWJ. Probenecid inhibits the glucuronidation of indomethacin and *O*-desmethylindomethacin in humans: a pilot experiment. *Pharm World Sci* (1994) 16, 22–6.
17. Toradol (Ketorolac trometamol). Roche Products Ltd. UK Summary of product characteristics, May 2007.
18. Toradol (Ketorolac tromethamine). Roche Pharmaceuticals. US Prescribing information, September 2002.

NSAIDs or Aspirin + Prostaglandins

Misoprostol increases the incidence of abdominal pain and diarrhoea when used with diclofenac or indometacin. Isolated cases of neurological adverse effects have been seen with naproxen or phenylbutazone given with misoprostol. However, no important pharmacokinetic interactions seem to occur between aspirin, diclofenac, ibuprofen or indometacin and misoprostol. NSAIDs are reported not to affect the abortive effects of intravaginal misoprostol.

Clinical evidence, mechanism, importance and management

(A) Oral misoprostol

(a) Gastrointestinal adverse effects

A higher incidence of abdominal pain, diarrhoea, nausea and dyspepsia occurred when **diclofenac** was combined with misoprostol.[1,2] Concurrent use of **indometacin** and misoprostol also resulted in an increase in frequency and severity of abdominal symptoms, frequency of bowel movements and a decrease in faecal consistency.[3] The most frequent adverse effect of misoprostol alone is diarrhoea, and this may limit the dose tolerated. When using misoprostol with NSAIDs, warn patients about the possibility of increased stomach pain and diarrhoea. Preparations combining **diclofenac** or **naproxen** with misoprostol are available.

(b) Neurological adverse effects

A man with rheumatoid arthritis taking long-term **naproxen** developed ataxic symptoms a few hours after starting to take misoprostol. He said he felt like a drunk person, staggering about and vomiting. He rapidly improved when he stopped the misoprostol but the adverse symptoms recurred on two further occasions when he restarted misoprostol.[4]

Adverse effects developed in 3 patients taking **phenylbutazone** 200 to 400 mg daily when they took misoprostol 400 to 800 micrograms daily.[5] One had headaches, dizziness and ambulatory instability that disappeared and then reappeared when the misoprostol was stopped and then restarted. No problems occurred when the **phenylbutazone** was replaced by **etodolac** 400 mg daily. The other 2 patients developed symptoms including headache, tingles, dizziness, hot flushes and transient diplopia.[5,6] No problems developed when one of them was given **naproxen** and misoprostol.[6] The reasons for this reaction are not understood but theoretically it could possibly be due to a potentiation of the adverse effects of **phenylbutazone**. The general relevance of these few reports is unclear, but bear them in mind should unexpected neurological effects occur.

(c) Pharmacokinetic studies

No clinically important pharmacokinetic interactions have been found to occur between **aspirin** 975 mg and misoprostol 200 micrograms,[7] or between **ibuprofen** and misoprostol.[8] One study found that misoprostol 800 micrograms daily decreased the AUC of a single 100-mg dose of **diclofenac** by a modest 20%.[2] However, other studies have found that misoprostol had no effect on steady-state **diclofenac** pharmacokinetics.[9] One study found that misoprostol 200 micrograms raised the steady-state levels of **indometacin** 50 mg three times daily by about 30%,[10] whereas another found that **misoprostol** 400 micrograms twice daily reduced the AUC of **indometacin** 50 mg twice daily by 13% after one dose and reduced the maximum steady-state plasma concentration by 24%.[3] These modest changes in serum **indometacin** levels are unlikely to be clinically important.

(B) Vaginal prostaglandins

NSAIDs and aspirin are frequently avoided before the use of **prostaglandins** for induction of uterine contractions, because of the theoretical concern that they may inhibit efficacy.[11] For example, the UK manufacturer of **dinoprostone** says that NSAIDs including aspirin should be stopped before giving intravaginal **dinoprostone** for induction of labour.[12] However, a study involving 416 women given intravaginal misoprostol to induce early abortion found that the concurrent use of oral NSAIDs did not interfere with the efficacy of misoprostol,[11] and the US manufacturer of **dinoprostone** does not list NSAIDs or aspirin as possible interacting drugs.[13] Further study is needed. Consider also 'Mifepristone + Aspirin or NSAIDs', p.1265.

1. Gagnier P. Review of the safety of diclofenac/misoprostol. *Drugs* (1993) 45 (Suppl 1), 31–5.
2. Dammann HG, Simon-Schultz J, Steinhoff I, Damaschke A, Schmoldt A, Sallowsky E. Differential effects of misoprostol and ranitidine on the pharmacokinetics of diclofenac and gastrointestinal symptoms. *Br J Clin Pharmacol* (1993) 36, 345–9.
3. Kendall MJ, Gibson R, Walt RP. Co-administration of misoprostol or ranitidine with indomethacin: effects on pharmacokinetics, abdominal symptoms and bowel habit. *Aliment Pharmacol Ther* (1992) 6, 437–46.
4. Huq M. Neurological adverse effects of naproxen and misoprostol combination. *Br J Gen Pract* (1990) 40, 432.
5. Jacquemier JM, Lassoued S, Laroche M, Mazières B. Neurosensory adverse effects after phenylbutazone and misoprostol combined treatment. *Lancet* (1989) 2, 1283.
6. Chassagne Ph, Humez C, Gourmelen O, Moore N, Le Loet X, Deshayes P. Neurosensory adverse effects after combined phenylbutazone and misoprostol. *Br J Rheumatol* (1991) 30, 392.
7. Karim A, Rozek LF, Leese PT. Absorption of misoprostol (Cytotec), an antiulcer prostaglandin, or aspirin is not affected when given concomitantly to healthy human subjects. *Gastroenterology* (1987) 92, 1742.
8. Small RE, Wilmot-Pater MG, McGee BA, Willis HE. Effects of misoprostol or ranitidine on ibuprofen pharmacokinetics. *Clin Pharm* (1991) 10, 870–2.
9. Karim A. Pharmacokinetics of diclofenac and misoprostol when administered alone or as a combination product. *Drugs* (1993) 45 (Suppl 1), 7–14.
10. Rainsford KD, James C, Hunt RH, Stetsko PI, Rischke JA, Karim A, Nicholson PA, Smith M, Hantsbarger G. Effects of misoprostol on the pharmacokinetics of indomethacin in human volunteers. *Clin Pharmacol Ther* (1992) 51, 415–21.
11. Creinin MD, Shulman T. Effect of nonsteroidal anti-inflammatory drugs on the action of misoprostol in a regimen for early abortion. *Contraception* (1997) 56, 165–8.
12. Propess (Dinoprostone). Ferring Pharmaceuticals Ltd. UK Summary of product characteristics, December 2005.
13. Prostin E2 (Dinoprostone). Pfizer Inc. US Prescribing information, April 2006.

NSAIDs or Aspirin + Proton pump inhibitors

The antiplatelet activity and the pharmacokinetics of aspirin do not appear to be affected by omeprazole. There was no clinically relevant pharmacokinetic interaction between omeprazole and diclofenac, enteric-coated ketoprofen, naproxen or piroxicam, or between pantoprazole and diclofenac or naproxen, or between esomeprazole and naproxen or rofecoxib.

Clinical evidence

(a) Aspirin

In a preliminary study in 11 healthy subjects, **omeprazole** 20 mg daily for 2 days reduced the serum levels of the salicylic acid metabolite of aspirin at 30 and 90 minutes after a single 650-mg dose of aspirin by 40% and 52%, respectively.[1] However, another study in 14 healthy subjects given **omeprazole** 20 mg daily for 4 days with a final dose one hour before a single 125-mg dose of aspirin found that **omeprazole** did not significantly affect the plasma levels of either aspirin or salicylic acid. **Omeprazole** also did not affect the antiplatelet effects of aspirin.[2] Similarly, **omeprazole** had no effect on the bioavailability of aspirin (uncoated or enteric-coated tablets) in another study, although it increased the rate of absorption of aspirin from enteric-coated tablets.[3]

(b) Diclofenac

A single 105-mg dose of diclofenac potassium suspension (*Flogan*) was given to 13 healthy subjects while fasting and after gastric acid secretion blockade with **omeprazole**. The pharmacokinetics of the diclofenac were not changed to a clinically relevant extent by **omeprazole**.[4] Similarly, **omeprazole** 20 mg daily given with diclofenac 50 mg twice daily for one week had no effect on the pharmacokinetics of either drug in 24 healthy subjects.[5]

In another study a single 40-mg oral dose of **pantoprazole** and diclofenac 100 mg (as enteric-coated *Voltarol*) were given to 24 healthy subjects together and separately. Neither drug affected the pharmacokinetics of the other.[6]

(c) Ketoprofen

There were no significant changes in the pharmacokinetics of enteric-coated ketoprofen, given with or without **omeprazole**, although a trend towards higher plasma concentrations with omeprazole was noted, indicating the possibility of increased drug release in the stomach in the presence of an elevated pH.[7]

(d) Naproxen

Naproxen 250 mg twice daily given to healthy subjects with **omeprazole** 20 mg daily,[5] **pantoprazole** 40 mg daily,[8] or **esomeprazole** 40 mg daily[9] for one week had no effect on the pharmacokinetics of either naproxen or the proton pump inhibitor.

(e) Phenazone (Antipyrine)

The pharmacokinetics of **pantoprazole** 40 mg orally daily for 8 days was not altered to a clinically relevant extent by a single 5-mg/kg oral dose of phenazone given on day 8 of the study. **Pantoprazole** did not affect the pharmacokinetics of phenazone.[10]

(f) Piroxicam

Omeprazole 20 mg daily given to 24 healthy subjects with piroxicam 10 mg daily for one week had no effect on the pharmacokinetics of either drug.[5]

(g) Rofecoxib

Esomeprazole 40 mg daily given to 30 healthy subjects with rofecoxib 12.5 mg daily for one week had no effect on the pharmacokinetics of either drug apart from a slight increase in the maximum level and AUC of rofecoxib, which was not thought to be clinically relevant.[9]

Mechanism

Data from *animal* studies suggest that the absorption and thus the effects of aspirin and NSAIDs can be reduced by omeprazole and H_2-receptor antagonists via a pH dependent mechanism.[11,12] However, note that clinical studies have not found H_2-receptor antagonists to have any important effect on the pharmacokinetics of aspirin or NSAIDs, see 'NSAIDs or Aspirin + H_2-receptor antagonists', p.149. It has been suggested that reducing gastric acidity with omeprazole results in the earlier disruption of enteric-coated tablets, and an increased absorption rate.[3]

Importance and management

The interaction between aspirin and omeprazole is not established. The balance of evidence suggests that omeprazole is unlikely to have an important effect on the pharmacokinetics and efficacy of aspirin. However, because of the uncertainty generated by the *animal* and preliminary clinical data,[1,11,12] it would be of benefit to confirm this in further studies.[2,13]

No clinically significant pharmacokinetic interactions have been identified between any of the other NSAIDs and PPIs cited here, and no special precautions are needed during concurrent use. For mention that valdecoxib raises plasma levels of omeprazole see 'NSAIDs; Parecoxib + Miscellaneous', p.160. Note that omeprazole and other proton pump inhibitors are widely used in the management of the gastrointestinal complications of aspirin and NSAIDs.

1. Anand BS, Sanduja SK, Lichtenberger LM. Effect of omeprazole on the bioavailability of aspirin: a randomized controlled study on healthy volunteers. *Gastroenterology* (1999) 116: A371.
2. Iñarrea P, Esteva F, Cornudella R, Lanas A. Omeprazole does not interfere with the antiplatelet effect of low-dose aspirin in man. *Scand J Gastroenterol* (2000) 35, 242–6.
3. Nefesoglu FZ, Ayanoglu-Dülger G, Ulusoy NB, Imeryüz N. Interaction of omeprazole with enteric-coated salicylate tablets. *Int J Clin Pharmacol Ther* (1998) 36, 549–53.
4. Poli A, Moreno RA, Ribeiro W, Dias HB, Moreno H, Muscara MN, De Nucci G. Influence of gastric acid secretion blockade and food intake on the bioavailability of a potassium diclofenac suspension in healthy male volunteers. *Int J Clin Pharmacol Ther* (1996) 34, 76–9.
5. Andersson T, Bredberg E, Lagerström P-O, Naesdal J, Wilson I. Lack of drug-drug interaction between three different non-steroidal anti-inflammatory drugs and omeprazole. *Eur J Clin Pharmacol* (1998) 54, 399–404.
6. Bliesath H, Huber R, Steinijans VW, Koch HJ, Wurst W, Mascher H. Lack of pharmacokinetic interaction between pantoprazole and diclofenac. *Int J Clin Pharmacol Ther* (1996) 34, 152–6.
7. Qureshi SA, Caillé G, Lacasse Y, McGilveray IJ. Pharmacokinetics of two enteric-coated ketoprofen products in humans with or without coadministration of omeprazole and comparison with dissolution findings. *Pharm Res* (1994) 11, 1669–72.
8. Schulz H-U, Hartmann M, Krupp S, Schuerer M, Huber R, Luehmann R, Bethke T, Wurst W. Pantoprazole lacks interaction with the NSAID naproxen. *Gastroenterology* (2000) 118 (Suppl 2), A1304.
9. Hassan-Alin M, Naesdal J, Nilsson-Pieschl C, Långström G, Andersson T. Lack of pharmacokinetic interaction between esomeprazole and the nonsteroidal anti-inflammatory drugs naproxen and rofecoxib in healthy subjects. *Clin Drug Invest* (2005) 25, 731–40.

10. De Mey C, Meineke I, Steinijans VW, Huber R, Hartmann M, Bliesath H, Wurst W. Pantoprazole lacks interaction with antipyrine in man, either by inhibition or induction. *Int J Clin Pharmacol Ther* (1994) 32, 98–106.
11. Lichtenberger LM, Ulloa C, Romero JJ, Vanous AL, Illich PA, Dial EJ. Nonsteroidal anti-inflammatory drug and phospholipid prodrugs: combination therapy with antisecretory agents in rats. *Gastroenterology* (1996) 111, 990–5.
12. Giraud M-N, Sanduja SK, Felder TB, Illich PA, Dial EJ, Lichtenberger LM. Effect of omeprazole on the bioavailability of unmodified and phospholipid-complexed aspirin in rats. *Aliment Pharmacol Ther* (1997) 11, 899–906.
13. Fernández-Fernández FJ. Might proton pump inhibitors prevent the antiplatelet effects of low- or very low-dose aspirin? *Arch Intern Med* (2002) 162, 2248.

NSAIDs + Rifampicin (Rifampin)

The plasma levels of celecoxib, diclofenac, and etoricoxib are reduced by rifampicin. Metamizole (dipyrone) increased the maximum level of rifampicin. Piroxicam appears unaffected by rifampicin.

Clinical evidence

(a) Celecoxib

In 12 healthy subjects pretreatment with rifampicin 600 mg daily for 5 days reduced the AUC of a single 200-mg dose of celecoxib by 64% and increased the clearance by 185%.[1] A preliminary report of another study found broadly similar results.[2]

(b) Diclofenac

A study in 6 healthy subjects found that after taking rifampicin 450 mg daily for 6 days, the maximum serum level of diclofenac, measured 8 hours after a single 100-mg dose of an enteric-coated tablet, was reduced by 43% and the AUC was reduced by 67%.[3]

(c) Etoricoxib

The AUC of a single 60-mg dose of etoricoxib has been found to be reduced by 65% when given on day 8 of a 12-day course of rifampicin 600 mg daily. The maximum plasma concentration of etoricoxib was reduced by 40%.[4]

(d) Metamizole sodium (Dipyrone)

A study in untreated patients with leprosy showed that the pharmacokinetics of a single 600-mg dose of rifampicin were not markedly changed by 1 g of metamizole sodium (dipyrone), but peak serum rifampicin levels occurred sooner (at 3 instead of 4 hours) and were about 50% higher.[5]

(e) Phenazone (Antipyrine)

Plasma concentrations following treatment with single 1.2-g oral doses of phenazone were lower after a 13-day course of rifampicin 600 mg daily. The mean AUC of phenazone was reduced by 59% and had not returned to the pre-rifampicin level 13 days after the final rifampicin dose.[6]

(f) Piroxicam

A study in 6 healthy subjects given a single 40-mg dose of piroxicam before and after a 7-day course of rifampicin 600 mg daily found that rifampicin did not significantly alter the pharmacokinetics of piroxicam.[7]

Mechanism

Rifampicin is a potent inducer of hepatic enzymes, and it is likely that it increased the metabolism of these NSAIDs.

Importance and management

Although information is limited, these pharmacokinetic interactions appear to be established. Their clinical relevance remains to be determined, but it seems likely that the efficacy of these NSAIDs will be reduced by rifampicin. Combined use should be well monitored, and the NSAID dosage increased if necessary. See also 'NSAIDs; Parecoxib + Miscellaneous', p.160. The clinical relevance of the increase in rifampicin maximum levels with metamizole is uncertain.

1. Jayasagar G, Krishna Kumar M, Chandrasekhar K, Madhusudan RY. Influence of rifampicin pretreatment on the pharmacokinetics of celecoxib in healthy male volunteers. *Drug Metabol Drug Interact* (2003) 19, 287–95.
2. Porras AG, Gertz B, Buschmeier A, Constanzer M, Gumbs C, Gottesdiener K, Waldman S, Gelmann A, Greenberg H, Schwartz J. The effects of metabolic induction by rifampin (Rf) on the elimination of celecoxib (CXB) and the effect of CXB on CYP2D6 metabolism. *Clin Pharmacol Ther* (2001) 69, P58.
3. Kumar JS, Mamidi NVSR, Chakrapani T, Krishna DR. Rifampicin pretreatment reduces bioavailability of diclofenac sodium. *Indian J Pharmacol* (1995) 27, 183–5.
4. Agrawal NGB, Matthews CZ, Mazenko RS, Woolf EJ, Porras AG, Chen X, Miller JL, Michiels N, Wehling M, Schultz A, Gottlieb AB, Kraft WK, Greenberg HE, Waldman SA, Curtis SP, Gottesdiener KM. The effects of modifying in vivo cytochrome P450 3A (CYP3A) activity on etoricoxib pharmacokinetics and of etoricoxib administration on CYP3A activity. *J Clin Pharmacol* (2004) 44, 1125–31.
5. Krishna DR, Appa Rao AVN, Ramanakar TV, Reddy KSC, Prabhakar MC. Pharmacokinetics of rifampin in the presence of dipyrone in leprosy patients. *Drug Dev Ind Pharm* (1984) 10, 101–110.
6. Bennett PN, John VA, Whitmarsh VB. Effect of rifampicin on metoprolol and antipyrine kinetics. *Br J Clin Pharmacol* (1982) 13, 387–91.
7. Patel RB, Shah GF, Jain SM. The effect of rifampicin on piroxicam kinetics. *Indian J Physiol Pharmacol* (1988) 32, 226–228.

NSAIDs or Aspirin + SSRIs

SSRIs may increase the risk of bleeding, including upper gastrointestinal bleeding, and the risk appears to be further increased by concurrent use of NSAIDs and/or aspirin (including low-dose aspirin).

Clinical evidence

A retrospective study of the UK general practice research database identified 1651 cases of upper gastrointestinal bleeding diagnosed between 1993 and 1997. Concurrent use of an SSRI significantly increased the risk of bleeding threefold when compared with 10,000 controls. In addition, the concurrent use of an SSRI with an NSAID greatly increased the risk of upper gastrointestinal bleeding (relative risk of bleeding compared with non-use of either drug: 15.6 for SSRIs with NSAIDs, 3.7 for NSAIDs alone, and 2.6 for SSRIs alone); the use of SSRIs with low-dose aspirin was associated with a relative risk of 7.2. Another study found a significant association between the degree of serotonin reuptake inhibition by antidepressants and risk of hospital admission for abnormal bleeding.[1] A retrospective cohort study in elderly patients taking antidepressants found a trend towards an increased risk of upper gastrointestinal bleeding for patients taking antidepressants with greater inhibition of serotonin reuptake. This association was statistically significant when controlled for previous upper gastrointestinal bleeding or age, and octogenarians, in particular, were at high risk.[2] Other studies or case reports have also found that SSRIs increase the risk of upper gastrointestinal bleeding,[3-6] and this effect is potentiated by the concurrent use of NSAIDs[3,4] or low-dose aspirin.[3]

In contrast, some workers have disagreed with these results and found no evidence to suggest that SSRIs are more likely to cause gastrointestinal bleeding than other drugs.[7] Another study reported both SSRIs and NSAIDs were associated with a twofold increase in risk of gastrointestinal bleeding, but that the risk of bleeding was not substantially increased when both drugs were taken together (odds ratio for NSAIDs was 2.19, SSRIs was 2.63 and combined use was 2.93).[8]

Mechanism

Serotonin is not synthesised by platelets but is taken up into platelets from the bloodstream. Serotonin released from platelets has an important role in regulating the haemostatic response to injury as it potentiates platelet aggregation. At therapeutic doses SSRIs can block this reuptake of serotonin by platelets leading to serotonin depletion, impairment of haemostatic function and so increase the risk of bleeding.[2,9-11]

Importance and management

Serotonin released by platelets plays an important role in haemostasis and there appears to be an association between the use of antidepressant drugs that interfere with serotonin reuptake and the occurrence of bleeding, including gastrointestinal bleeding. In addition, the concurrent use of an NSAID or aspirin (including low-dose aspirin) may potentiate the risk of bleeding. Therefore, the manufacturers of SSRIs advise caution in patients taking SSRIs with NSAIDs, aspirin or other drugs that affect coagulation or platelet function. Alternatives such as paracetamol (acetaminophen) or less gastrotoxic NSAIDs such as ibuprofen may be considered, but if the combination of an SSRI and NSAID cannot be avoided, prescribing of gastroprotective drugs such as proton pump inhibitors, H_2-receptor antagonists, or prostaglandin analogues should be considered, especially in elderly patients or those with a history of gastrointestinal bleeding. Patients, particularly those taking multiple drugs that may cause bleeding, should be advised to seek informed medical opinion before using non-prescription drugs such as ibuprofen on a regular basis.

1. Meijer WE, Heerdink ER, Nolen WA, Herings RM, Leufkens HG, Egberts AC. Association of risk of abnormal bleeding with degree of serotonin reuptake inhibition by antidepressants. *Arch Intern Med* (2004) 164, 2367–70.
2. Van Walraven C, Mamdani MM, Wells PS, Williams JI. Inhibition of serotonin reuptake by antidepressants and upper gastrointestinal bleeding in elderly patients: retrospective cohort study. *BMJ* (2001) 323, 655–8.
3. Dalton SO, Johansen C, Mellemkjær L, Nørgård B, Sørensen HT, Olsen JH. Use of selective serotonin reuptake inhibitors and risk of upper gastrointestinal tract bleeding. A population-based cohort study. *Arch Intern Med* (2003) 163, 59–64.
4. De Jong JCF, van den Berg PB, Tobi H, de Jong-van den Berg LTW. Combined use of SSRIs and NSAIDs increases the risk of gastrointestinal adverse effects. *Br J Clin Pharmacol* (2003) 55, 591–5.
5. Ceylan ME, Alpsan-Omay MH. Bleeding induced by SSRIs. *Eur Psychiatry* (2005) 20, 570–1.
6. Weinrieb RM, Auriacombe M, Lynch KG, Chang KM, Lewis JD. A critical review of selective serotonin reuptake inhibitor-associated bleeding: balancing the risk of treating hepatitis C-infected patients. *J Clin Psychiatry* (2003) 64, 1502–10.
7. Dunn NR, Pearce GL, Shakir SAW. Association between SSRIs and upper gastrointestinal bleeding. SSRIs are no more likely than other drugs to cause such bleeding. *BMJ* (2000) 320, 1405.
8. Tata LJ, Fortun PJ, Hubbard RB, Smeeth L, Hawkey CJ, Smith CJ, Whitaker HJ, Farrington CP, Card TR, West J. Does concurrent prescription of selective serotonin reuptake inhibitors and non-steroidal anti-inflammatory drugs substantially increase the risk of upper gastrointestinal bleeding? *Aliment Pharmacol Ther* (2005) 22, 175–81.
9. De Abajo FJ, Rodríguez LAG, Montero D. Association between selective serotonin reuptake inhibitors and upper gastrointestinal bleeding population based case-control study. *BMJ* (1999) 319, 1106–9.
10. Serebruany VL. Selective serotonin reuptake inhibitors and increased bleeding risk: are we missing something? *Am J Med* (2006) 119, 113–6.
11. Dalton SO, Sørensen HT, Johansen C. SSRIs and upper gastrointestinal bleeding. What is known and how should it influence prescribing? *CNS Drugs* (2006) 20, 143–51.

NSAIDs or Aspirin + Sucralfate

Sucralfate appears not to have a clinically important effect on the pharmacokinetics of aspirin, choline-magnesium trisalicylate, diclofenac, ibuprofen, indometacin, ketoprofen, naproxen or piroxicam.

Clinical evidence, mechanism, importance and management

Sucralfate 2 g was given to 18 healthy subjects 30 minutes before single-doses of **ketoprofen** 50 mg, **indometacin** 50 mg, or **naproxen** 500 mg. Some statistically significant changes were seen (modestly reduced maximum serum levels of **ketoprofen**, **indometacin**, and **naproxen**, reduced the rate of absorption of **naproxen** and **indometacin**, and increased the time to achieve maximal serum levels with **indometacin**) but no alterations in bioavailability occurred.[1] A delay, but no reduction in the total absorption of **naproxen** is described in two studies:[2,3] it is unlikely that its clinical efficacy will be reduced.[2] Sucralfate 1 g four times daily for 2 days was found not to decrease the rate of absorption of a single 400-mg dose of **ibuprofen**[4] or of a single 650-mg dose of **aspirin**.[5] Sucralfate 5 g in divided doses did not significantly alter the absorption of a single 600-mg dose of **ibuprofen**.[6] Similarly, another study also found that sucralfate had no important effect on the pharmacokinetics of **ibuprofen** enantiomers.[7] In one study, sucralfate 2 g was found not to affect significantly the pharmacokinetics of either **piroxicam** 20 mg or **diclofenac** 50 mg.[8] However, in another study, sucralfate 2 g twice daily modestly reduced the AUC_{0-8} and maximum serum levels of a single 105-mg dose of **diclofenac potassium** by 20% and 38%, respectively.[9] Sucralfate 1 g every 6 hours was found not to affect the pharmacokinetics of **choline-magnesium trisalicylate** 1.5 g every 12 hours.[10]

Single dose studies do not necessarily reliably predict what will happen when patients take drugs regularly, but most of the evidence available suggests that sucralfate is unlikely to have an adverse effect on treatment with these NSAIDs.

1. Caillé G, Du Souich P, Gervais P, Besner J-G. Single dose pharmacokinetics of ketoprofen, indomethacin, and naproxen taken alone or with sucralfate. *Biopharm Drug Dispos* (1987) 8, 173–83.
2. Caille G, du Souich P, Gervais P, Besner JG, Vezina M. Effects of concurrent sucralfate administration on pharmacokinetics of naproxen. *Am J Med* (1987) 83 (Suppl 3B), 67–73.
3. Lafontaine D, Mailhot C, Vermeulen M, Bissonnette B, Lambert C. Influence of chewable sucralfate or a standard meal on the bioavailability of naproxen. *Clin Pharm* (1990) 9, 773–7.
4. Anaya AL, Mayersohn M, Conrad KA, Dimmitt DC. The influence of sucralfate on ibuprofen absorption in healthy adult males. *Biopharm Drug Dispos* (1986) 7, 443–51.
5. Lau A, Chang C-W, Schlesinger PK. Evaluation of a potential drug interaction between sucralfate and aspirin. *Clin Pharmacol Ther* (1986) 39, 151–5.
6. Pugh MC, Small RE, Garnett WR, Townsend RJ, Willis HE. Effect of sucralfate on ibuprofen absorption in normal volunteers. *Clin Pharm* (1984) 3, 630–3.
7. Levine MAH, Walker SE, Paton TW. The effect of food or sucralfate on the bioavailability of S(+) and R(-) enantiomers of ibuprofen. *J Clin Pharmacol* (1992) 32, 1110–14.
8. Ungethüm W. Study on the interaction between sucralfate and diclofenac/piroxicam in healthy volunteers. *Arzneimittelforschung* (1991) 41, 797–800.
9. Pedrazzoli J, Pierossi M de A, Muscará MN, Dias HB, da Silva CMF, Mendes FD, de Nucci G. Short-term sucralfate administration alters potassium diclofenac absorption in healthy male volunteers. *Br J Clin Pharmacol* (1997) 43, 104–8.
10. Schneider DK, Gannon RH, Sweeney KR, DeFusco PA. Influence of sucralfate on trilisate bioavailability. *J Clin Pharmacol* (1991) 31, 377–9.

NSAIDs or Aspirin + *Tamarindus indica*

***Tamarindus indica* fruit extract markedly increases the absorption and plasma levels of aspirin and ibuprofen.**

Clinical evidence, mechanism, importance and management

(a) Aspirin

A study in 6 healthy subjects found that the bioavailability of a single 600-mg dose of aspirin was increased when it was taken with a millet meal containing *Tamarindus indica* fruit extract, compared with the millet meal alone or following overnight fasting. The aspirin AUC rose sixfold, the maximum plasma levels rose almost threefold (from about 10 micrograms/mL with the meal or fasting to about 29 micrograms/mL with the *Tamarindus indica* extract) and the half-life increased moderately (from about 1.04 to 1.5 hours).[1] The reasons are not known, nor has the clinical importance of these large increases been evaluated, but this interaction should be borne in mind if high (analgesic or anti-inflammatory) doses of aspirin are taken with this fruit extract. There would seem to be the possible risk of aspirin toxicity.

(b) Ibuprofen

A study in 6 healthy subjects found that the bioavailability of a single 400-mg dose of ibuprofen was increased when it was taken with a millet meal containing *Tamarindus indica* fruit extract compared with the millet meal alone, or following overnight fasting. The ibuprofen AUC rose approximately twofold and the maximum plasma levels rose from about 38 micrograms/mL to 45 micrograms/mL. There was also an increase in the plasma levels of the metabolites of ibuprofen. Ingestion of the meal containing *Tamarindus indica* was thought to favour the absorption of ibuprofen. This might result in an increased risk of toxicity.[2]

1. Mustapha A, Yakasai IA, Aguye IA. Effect of *Tamarindus indica* L. on the bioavailability of aspirin in healthy human volunteers. *Eur J Drug Metab Pharmacokinet* (1996) 21, 223–6.
2. Garba M, Yakasai IA, Bakare MT, Munir HY. Effect of *Tamarindus indica* L. on the bioavailability of ibuprofen in healthy human volunteers. *Eur J Drug Metab Pharmacokinet* (2003) 28, 179–84.

NSAIDs + Tobacco

The clearance of diflunisal, phenazone (antipyrine) and phenylbutazone is greater in smokers than in non-smokers.

Clinical evidence, mechanism, importance and management

(a) Diflunisal

The clearance of a single 250-mg dose of diflunisal was 35% higher in 6 women who smoked 10 to 20 cigarettes a day than in 6 non-smoking women.[1] This change does not appear to be large enough to be of clinical importance.

(b) Phenazone (Antipyrine)

The clearance of phenazone was increased by 63% and the half-life reduced from 13.2 to 8 hours when a single 1-g dose of phenazone was given intravenously to 10 healthy women who smoked cigarettes, when compared with a control group of 26 non-smoking women.[2] Similar results were reported in another study.[3] This is likely to be as a result of cigarette smoking causing induction of CYP1A2, the enzyme involved in the metabolism of phenazone.[2]

(c) Phenylbutazone

The half-life of a single 6-mg/kg dose of phenylbutazone was 37 hours in a group of smokers (10 or more cigarettes daily for 2 years) compared with 64 hours in a group of non-smokers. The metabolic clearance was roughly doubled.[4] The conclusion to be drawn is that those who smoke may possibly need larger or more frequent doses of phenylbutazone to achieve the same therapeutic response, but this needs confirmation.

1. Macdonald JI, Herman RJ, Verbeeck RK. Sex-difference and the effects of smoking and oral contraceptive steroids on the kinetics of diflunisal. *Eur J Clin Pharmacol* (1990) 38, 175–9.
2. Scavone JM, Greenblatt DJ, Abernethy DR, Luna BG, Harmatz JS, Shader RI Influence of oral contraceptive use and cigarette smoking, alone and together, on antipyrine pharmacokinetics. *J Clin Pharmacol* (1997) 37, 437–41.
3. Scavone JM, Greenblatt DJ, LeDuc BW, Blyden GT, Luna BG, Harmatz JS. Differential effect of cigarette smoking on antipyrine oxidation versus acetaminophen conjugation. *Pharmacology* (1990) 40, 77–84.
4. Garg SK, Kiran TNR. Effect of smoking on phenylbutazone disposition. *Int J Clin Pharmacol Ther Toxicol* (1982) 20, 289–90.

NSAIDs + Tricyclic antidepressants

The tricyclic antidepressants can delay the absorption of phenylbutazone and oxyphenbutazone from the gut, but their antirheumatic effects are probably not affected.

Clinical evidence, mechanism, importance and management

The absorption of a single 400-mg dose of phenylbutazone in 4 depressed women was considerably delayed (time to maximum level, 4 to 10 hours compared with 2 hours), but the total amount absorbed (measured by the urinary excretion of oxyphenbutazone) remained unchanged when they were pretreated with **desipramine** 75 mg daily for 7 days.[1] In another 5 depressed women the half-life of oxyphenbutazone was found to be unaltered by 75 mg of **desipramine** or **nortriptyline** daily.[2] *Animal* studies have confirmed that the absorption of phenylbutazone and oxyphenbutazone are delayed by the tricyclic antidepressants, probably because their antimuscarinic effects reduce the motility of the gut,[3,4] but there seems to be no direct clinical evidence that the antirheumatic effects of either drug are reduced by this interaction. No particular precautions appear to be needed.

1. Consolo S, Morselli PL, Zaccala M, Garattini S. Delayed absorption of phenylbutazone caused by desmethylimipramine in humans. *Eur J Pharmacol* (1970) 10, 239–42.
2. Hammer W, Mårtens S, Sjöqvist F. A comparative study of the metabolism of desmethylimipramine, nortriptyline, and oxyphenylbutazone in man. *Clin Pharmacol Ther* (1969) 10, 44–9.
3. Consolo S. An interaction between desipramine and phenylbutazone. *J Pharm Pharmacol* (1968) 20, 574–5.
4. Consolo S, Garattini S. Effect of desipramine on intestinal absorption of phenylbutazone and other drugs. *Eur J Pharmacol* (1969) 6, 322–6.

NSAIDs; Acemetacin + Miscellaneous

Acemetacin is a glycolic acid ester of indometacin, and its major metabolite is indometacin. Therefore the interactions of indometacin would be expected.

NSAIDs; Azapropazone + Chloroquine

The plasma levels of azapropazone are not significantly altered by chloroquine.

Clinical evidence, mechanism, importance and management

A study in 12 subjects given azapropazone 300 mg three times daily found that the plasma levels of azapropazone, measured at 4 hours, were not affected by chloroquine 250 mg daily for 7 days.[1] No special precautions would seem to be needed if these drugs are given together.

1. Faust-Tinnefeldt G, Geissler HE. Azapropazon und rheumatologische Basistherapie mit Chloroquin unter dem Aspekt der Arzneimittelinteraktion. *Arzneimittelforschung* (1977) 27, 2170–4.

NSAIDs; Celecoxib + Selenium

Selenium enriched baker's yeast does not appear to affect the pharmacokinetics of celecoxib.

Clinical evidence, mechanism, importance and management

In a study in 73 healthy subjects, celecoxib 400 mg was given daily for 2 weeks, then selenium enriched baker's yeast *(Saccharomyces cerevisiae)* 200 micrograms daily or matched placebo were added for 30 days. Following blood chemistry analysis (urea and electrolytes, full blood count etc), there were no clinically significant changes from baseline, nor were there any changes in celecoxib steady-state plasma levels.[1]

1. Frank DH, Roe DJ, Chow H-HS, Guillen JM, Choquette K, Gracie D, Francis J, Fish A, Alberts DS. Effects of a high-selenium yeast supplement on celecoxib plasma levels: a randomized phase II trial. *Cancer Epidemiol Biomarkers Prev* (2004) 13, 299–303.

NSAIDs; Diclofenac + Cephalosporins

Cefadroxil does not alter the pharmacokinetics of diclofenac. The biliary excretion of ceftriaxone is increased by diclofenac.

Clinical evidence, mechanism, importance and management

The pharmacokinetics of diclofenac 100 mg daily were unaffected by either **cefadroxil** 2 g daily (8 patients) or doxycycline 100 mg daily (7) for one week.[1] No special precautions are needed while taking either of these drugs and diclofenac.

A pharmacokinetic study in 8 patients who had undergone cholecystectomy and who had a T-drain in the common bile duct, found that diclofenac 50 mg every 12 hours increased the excretion of intravenous **ceftriaxone** 2 g in the bile by about fourfold and roughly halved the urinary excretion.[2] The clinical importance of this is uncertain, but probably small.

Animal studies have shown that diclofenac may alter the pharmacokinetics of some cephalosporins (the AUCs of **cefotiam** and **ceftriaxone** were increased by diclofenac, although the pharmacokinetics of **cefmenoxime** were not affected). The significance of these findings in humans is unknown and further studies are required before any valid conclusions can be drawn from this data.[3]

1. Schumacher A, Geissler HE, Mutschler E, Osterburg M. Untersuchungen potentieller Interaktionen von Diclofenac-Natrium (Voltaren) mit Antibiotika. *Z Rheumatol* (1983) 42, 25–7.
2. Merle-Melet M, Bresler L, Lokiec F, Dopff C, Boissel P, Dureux JB. Effects of diclofenac on ceftriaxone pharmacokinetics in humans. *Antimicrob Agents Chemother* (1992) 36, 2331–3.
3. Joly V, Pangon B, Brion N, Vallois J-M, Carbon C. Enhancement of the therapeutic effect of cephalosporins in experimental endocarditis by altering their pharmacokinetics with diclofenac. *J Pharmacol Exp Ther* (1988) 246, 695–700.

NSAIDs; Diclofenac topical + Miscellaneous

Topical diclofenac intended for use on the skin is very unlikely to interact adversely with any of the drugs known to interact with diclofenac given orally.

Clinical evidence, mechanism, importance and management

The manufacturer of *Pennsaid* (a topical solution containing diclofenac 16 mg/mL in dimethyl sulfoxide) says that when the maximum dosage of 1 mL is used on the skin, the maximum plasma levels of diclofenac achieved are less than 10 nanograms/mL.[1] This is 50 times lower than the maximum plasma levels achieved with oral diclofenac 25 mg. Despite these very low concentrations, the manufacturer lists all the interactions that have been observed after systemic administration of diclofenac sodium (**aspirin**, **digoxin**, **lithium**, **oral hypoglycaemic agents**, **diuretics**, **NSAIDs** including other **diclofenac** preparations, **methotrexate**, **ciclosporin**, **quinolones** and **antihypertensives**).[1] They note that the risk of these interactions in association with topical use is not known, but is probably low.[1] None of the drugs listed have yet been reported to interact with topical diclofenac.

The manufacturers of other topical preparations (*Solaraze* 3% w/w gel and *Voltarol* 1% w/w gel patch) state that interactions are not anticipated due to the low level of systemic absorption,[2,3] although one manufacturer still warns not to administer concurrently, by either the topical or systemic route, any medicinal product containing diclofenac or other NSAIDs.[3]

1. Pennsaid (Diclofenac sodium). Dimethaid International. UK Summary of product characteristics, February 2004.

2. Solaraze 3% Gel (Diclofenac sodium). Shire Pharmaceuticals Ltd. UK Summary of product characteristics, December 2006.
3. Voltarol Gel Patch (Diclofenac epolamine). Novartis Consumer Health. UK Summary of product characteristics, March 2004.

NSAIDs; Etoricoxib + Miscellaneous

The manufacturer of etoricoxib recommends care when using etoricoxib with drugs that are metabolised by human sulfotransferases (they name oral salbutamol and minoxidil). This is because etoricoxib is an inhibitor of human sulfotransferase activity, and may increase the levels of these drugs. The increase in ethinylestradiol levels with etoricoxib is thought to be via this mechanism,[1] see 'Hormonal contraceptives or HRT + Coxibs', p.994.

1. Arcoxia (Etoricoxib). Merck Sharp & Dohme Ltd. UK Summary of product characteristics, January 2007.

NSAIDs; Ibuprofen + Moclobemide

Moclobemide did not alter the pharmacokinetics of ibuprofen, or ibuprofen-induced faecal blood loss in one study. Ibuprofen does not affect the pharmacokinetics of moclobemide.

Clinical evidence, mechanism, importance and management

A study in 24 healthy subjects found that moclobemide 150 mg three times daily for 7 days had no effect on the steady-state pharmacokinetics of ibuprofen 600 mg three times daily, and the amount of ibuprofen-induced faecal blood loss was unaffected.[1] Ibuprofen did not affect the pharmacokinetics of moclobemide. No special precautions appear to be required during concurrent use.

1. Güntert TW, Schmitt M, Dingemanse J, Jonkman JHG. Influence of moclobemide on ibuprofen-induced faecal blood loss. *Psychopharmacology (Berl)* (1992) 106, S40–S42.

NSAIDs; Indometacin + Cocaine

An isolated report describes marked oedema, anuria and haematemesis in a premature child attributed to an interaction between cocaine and indometacin, which were taken by the mother before the birth.

Clinical evidence, mechanism, importance and management

A woman who was a cocaine abuser and who was in premature labour was unsuccessfully treated with terbutaline and magnesium sulfate. Indometacin proved to be more effective, but after being given 400 mg over 2 days she gave birth to a boy estimated at 34 to 35 weeks. Before birth the child was noted to be anuric and at birth showed marked oedema, and later haematemesis. The suggested reasons for this effect are that the anuria and oedema were due to renal vascular constriction of the foetus caused by the cocaine combined with an adverse effect of indometacin on ADH-mediated water reabsorption. Both drugs can cause gastrointestinal bleeding, which would account for the haematemesis. The authors of this report point out that one of the adverse effects of cocaine is premature labour, and that the likelihood is high that indometacin may be used to control it. They advise screening likely addicts in premature labour for evidence of cocaine usage before indometacin is given.[1]

1. Carlan SJ, Stromquist C, Angel JL, Harris M, O'Brien WF. Cocaine and indomethacin: fetal anuria, neonatal edema and gastrointestinal bleeding. *Obstet Gynecol* (1991) 78, 501–3.

NSAIDs; Indometacin + Vaccines

Some very limited evidence suggests that the response to immunisation with live vaccines may be more severe than usual in the presence of indometacin.

Clinical evidence, mechanism, importance and management

A man with ankylosing spondylitis taking indometacin 25 mg three times daily had a strong primary-type reaction 12 days after **smallpox vaccination**. He experienced 3 days of severe malaise, headache and nausea, as well as enlarged lymph nodes. The scab that formed was unusually large (3 cm in diameter) but he suffered no long term ill-effects.[1] The suggestion was that indometacin alters the response of the body to viral infections, whether originating from vaccines or not.[1] This suggestion is supported by the case of a child taking indometacin who developed haemorrhagic chickenpox during a ward outbreak of the disease.[2] These appear to be isolated reports, and of little general importance. Note that NSAIDs such as indometacin may mask some of the signs and symptoms of infection.

1. Maddocks AC. Indomethacin and vaccination. *Lancet* (1973) ii, 210–11.
2. Rodriguez RS, Barbabosa E. Hemorrhagic chickenpox after indomethacin. *N Engl J Med* (1971) 285, 690.

NSAIDs; Ketorolac + Vancomycin

An isolated report describes temporary acute renal failure and gastrointestinal bleeding following the use of ketorolac and vancomycin.

Clinical evidence, mechanism, importance and management

A previously healthy middle-aged man developed complete kidney shut down and subsequent gastrointestinal bleeding following uncomplicated surgery and treatment with ketorolac trometamol and vancomycin. The reason for the temporary kidney failure is not known, but the authors of the report suggest that the ketorolac inhibited the normal production of the vasodilatory renal prostaglandins so that renal blood flow was reduced. This would seem to have been additive with nephrotoxic effects of the vancomycin. Note that a vancomycin level taken on postoperative day 3 was found to be above the normal therapeutic range (although the timing of the sample was not stated).[1] Ketorolac alone can cause dose-related and transient renal impairment.[1] It has also been suggested that the trometamol component may be associated with hyperkalaemia.[2] The gastrointestinal bleeding appeared to be due to the direct irritant effects of the ketorolac, possibly made worse by the previous use of piroxicam[1] (see also 'NSAIDs + NSAIDs', p.151). The general importance of this interaction is uncertain, but it may be prudent to monitor renal function during concurrent use.

1. Murray RP, Watson RC. Acute renal failure and gastrointestinal bleed associated with postoperative Toradol and vancomycin. *Orthopedics* (1993) 16, 1361–3.
2. Waters JH. Ketorolac-induced hyperkalaemia. *Am J Kidney Dis* (1995) 26, 266.

NSAIDs; Naproxen + Diphenhydramine

There appears to be no significant pharmacokinetic interaction between diphenhydramine and naproxen.

Clinical evidence, mechanism, importance and management

Diphenhydramine hydrochloride 50 mg had no clinically significant effects on the pharmacokinetics of a single 220-mg dose of naproxen sodium in 27 healthy subjects. The pharmacokinetics of diphenhydramine were similarly unaffected by naproxen.[1] No special precautions appear to be necessary.

1. Toothaker RD, Barker SH, Gillen MV, Helsinger SA, Kindberg CG, Hunt TL, Powell JH. Absence of pharmacokinetic interaction between orally co-administered naproxen sodium and diphenhydramine hydrochloride. *Biopharm Drug Dispos* (2000) 21, 229–33.

NSAIDs; Naproxen + Sulglicotide

Sulglicotide does not affect the absorption of naproxen.

Clinical evidence, mechanism, importance and management

Sulglicotide 200 mg had no significant effects on the pharmacokinetics of a single 500-mg dose of naproxen in 12 healthy subjects.[1] Sulglicotide may therefore be used to protect the gastric mucosa from possible injury by naproxen without altering its absorption.

1. Berté F, Feletti F, De Bernardi di Valserra M, Nazzari M, Cenedese A, Cornelli U. Lack of influence of sulglycotide on naproxen bioavailability in healthy volunteers. *Int J Clin Pharmacol Ther Toxicol* (1988) 26, 125–8.

NSAIDs; Naproxen + Zileuton

There appears to be no clinically significant pharmacokinetic or pharmacodynamic interaction between naproxen and zileuton.

Clinical evidence, mechanism, importance and management

In a randomised, placebo-controlled study in 24 healthy subjects zileuton 800 mg every 12 hours was given with naproxen 500 mg every 12 hours for 5 days. No clinically significant change was found in the pharmacokinetics of either drug. Naproxen did not affect the inhibitory effect of zileuton on leukotriene B_4 levels and similarly zileuton did not affect the inhibitory effect of naproxen on thromboxane B_2. The inhibition of the 5-lipoxygenase pathway by zileuton did not appear to worsen the gastrointestinal effects associated with naproxen. No special precautions would seem necessary.[1]

1. Awni WM, Braeckman RA, Cavanaugh JH, Locke CS, Linnen PJ, Granneman GR, Dube LM. The pharmacokinetic and pharmacodynamic interactions between the 5-lipoxygenase inhibitor zileuton and the cyclo-oxygenase inhibitor naproxen in human volunteers. *Clin Pharmacokinet* (1995) 29 (Suppl 2) 112–24.

NSAIDs; Parecoxib + Miscellaneous

As parecoxib is rapidly metabolised to valdecoxib, the interactions are usually considered to be due to the effects of valdecoxib. The manufacturer of parecoxib cautions the concurrent use with carbamazepine, dexamethasone and rifampicin as their effects on parecoxib have not been studied. Valdecoxib increases the levels of dextromethorphan and omeprazole. Because of these interactions, caution is advised with drugs that are metabolised by the same isoenzymes, namely flecainide, metoprolol, propafenone, omeprazole, diazepam, imipramine and phenytoin. No interaction appears to occur between parecoxib and midazolam.

Clinical evidence, mechanism, importance and management

Parecoxib is a parenteral drug that is rapidly metabolised in the liver to the active COX-2 inhibitor valdecoxib. Valdecoxib is predominantly metabolised by the cytochrome P450 isoenzymes CYP3A4 and CYP2C9. The interactions therefore are usually considered to be due to the effects of valdecoxib.

The manufacturers have done several interaction studies to find out whether parecoxib or valdecoxib can inhibit or induce the cytochrome P450 isoenzymes CYP2C9, CYP2D6, CYP2C19, and CYP3A4 and thereby determine their potential to interact with drugs metabolised by these isoenzymes.

1. CYP2C19. The manufacturers say that the AUC of **omeprazole** 40 mg was increased by 46% by valdecoxib 40 mg twice daily for a week. This indicates that valdecoxib is an inhibitor of CYP2C19 and although the manufacturers consider it to be a weak inhibitor[1] they suggest that caution should be observed with drugs that have a narrow therapeutic margin and are known to be metabolised by CYP2C19. They list **diazepam, imipramine** and **phenytoin**.[2] The implication is that the serum levels of these drugs and their effects may possibly be increased by the use of parecoxib.

2. CYP2D6. The manufacturers say that treatment with 40 mg of valdecoxib twice daily for a week caused a threefold increase in the serum levels of **dextromethorphan**. This indicates that valdecoxib is an inhibitor of CYP2D6, and therefore the manufacturers[1] suggest that caution should be observed with drugs that have a narrow therapeutic margin and are known to be predominantly metabolised by CYP2D6. They list **flecainide, metoprolol** and **propafenone**.[2] The implication is that the serum levels of these drugs and their effects may possibly be increased by the use of parecoxib, but so far there appears to be no direct clinical reports of any problems with concurrent use.

3. CYP3A4. A study in 12 healthy adults found no significant changes in the pharmacokinetics of **midazolam** 70 micrograms/kg given an hour after a 40-mg dose of intravenous parecoxib.[3] This suggests that parecoxib and valdecoxib are unlikely to inhibit or induce the activity of CYP3A4. This means that parecoxib would not be expected to affect other drugs that are metabolised by CYP3A4.

4. Enzyme inducers. The effects of the enzyme inducers **carbamazepine, dexamethasone, phenytoin** and **rifampicin** have not been studied with parecoxib. Nevertheless, the manufacturer of parecoxib warns that they may increase the metabolism of valdecoxib.[2]

1. Pharmacia Ltd. Personal communication, May 2002.
2. Dynastat Injection (Parecoxib sodium). Pfizer Ltd. UK Summary of product characteristics, April 2007.
3. Ibrahim A, Karim A, Feldman J, Kharasch E. The influence of parecoxib, a parenteral cyclooxygenase-2 specific inhibitor, on the pharmacokinetics and clinical effects of midazolam. *Anesth Analg* (2002) 95, 667–73.

NSAIDs; Phenylbutazone + Methylphenidate

Methylphenidate significantly increased the serum levels of phenylbutazone 200 to 400 mg daily in 5 out of 6 patients, due, it is suggested, to inhibition of liver metabolising enzymes.[1] The clinical importance of this is uncertain, especially as the report does not indicate the magnitude of the interaction.

1. Sellers EM ed. Clinical Pharmacology of Psychoactive Drugs. Ontario: Addiction Research Foundation, 1973. p183–202.

NSAIDs; Sulindac + Dimethyl sulfoxide (DMSO)

Isolated case reports describe serious peripheral neuropathy, which occurred when DMSO was applied to the skin of two patients taking sulindac.

Clinical evidence, mechanism, importance and management

A man with a long history of degenerative arthritis took sulindac 400 mg daily uneventfully for 6 months until, without his doctor's knowledge, he began regularly to apply a topical preparation containing DMSO 90% to his upper and lower extremities. Soon afterwards he began to experience pain, weakness in all his extremities, and difficulty in standing or walking. He was found to have both segmental demyelination and axonal neuropathy. He made a partial recovery but was unable to walk without an artificial aid.[1]

A second case describes a 68-year-old man with a history of mild osteoarthritis of the knees who was taking sulindac 150 mg twice daily. He later started to apply aqueous solutions of DMSO to his lower extremities, whilst continuing to take sulindac. Within 3 months he reported difficulty in climbing stairs, and myalgia of the thighs and legs. Over the next 5 months he experienced a progressive loss of gait, wasting of thigh and leg muscles, and more intense myalgia, cramps and fasciculations. Nerve conduction studies revealed damage to the nerves. During the year after discontinuing the DMSO, and supplementing his diet with vitamins B_6 and B_{12}, the patient showed improvement in the myalgia and physical disabilities, and a return to normal muscle strength. He continued to take the sulindac at a dose of 200 mg twice daily.[2]

The reason for this reaction is not known, but studies in *rats* have shown that DMSO can inhibit a reductase enzyme by which sulindac is metabolised,[3] and it may be that the high concentrations of unmetabolised sulindac increased the neurotoxic activity of the DMSO. Although there are only these two cases on record, its seriousness suggests that patients should not use sulindac and DMSO-containing preparations concurrently.

1. Reinstein L, Mahon R, Russo GL. Peripheral neuropathy after concomitant dimethyl sulfoxide use and sulindac therapy. *Arch Phys Med Rehabil* (1982) 63, 581–4.
2. Swanson BN, Ferguson RK, Raskin NH, Wolf BA. Peripheral neuropathy after concomitant administration of dimethyl sulfoxide and sulindac. *Arthritis Rheum* (1983) 26, 791–3.
3. Swanson BN, Mojaverian P, Boppana VK, Dudash M. Dimethylsulfoxide (DMSO) interaction with sulindac (SO). *Pharmacologist* (1981) 23, 196.

Opioids + Amfetamines and related drugs

Dexamfetamine and methylphenidate increase the analgesic effects of morphine and other opioids and reduce their sedative and respiratory depressant effects.

Clinical evidence, mechanism, importance and management

Dexamfetamine increased the analgesic effect of **morphine** and reduced its respiratory depressant effects to some extent in studies during postoperative analgesia[1] and in healthy subjects.[2] **Methylphenidate** 15 mg daily similarly increased the analgesic effects of various opioids (**morphine**, **hydromorphone**, **levorphanol**, **oxycodone**) and reduced the sedative effects in patients with chronic pain due to advanced cancer.[3] Therefore, the analgesic dose of an opioid may be lower than expected in patients on these drugs.

1. Forrest WH, Brown BW, Brown CR, Defalque R, Gold M, Gordon HE, James KE, Katz J, Mahler DL, Schroff P, Teutsch G. Dextroamphetamine with morphine for the treatment of postoperative pain. *N Engl J Med* (1977) 296, 712–15.
2. Bourke DL, Allen PD, Rosenberg M, Mendes RW, Karabelas AN. Dextroamphetamine with morphine: respiratory effects. *J Clin Pharmacol* (1983) 23, 65–70.
3. Bruera E, Chadwick S, Brenneis C, Hanson J, MacDonald RN. Methylphenidate associated with narcotics for the treatment of cancer pain. *Cancer Treat Rep* (1987) 71, 67–70.

Opioids + Antiemetics

Metoclopramide increases the rate of absorption of oral morphine and increases its rate of onset and sedative effects. However, opioids may antagonise the effects of metoclopramide on gastric emptying. The use of droperidol with opioids can be beneficial, but an increase in sedation appears to occur.

Clinical evidence

(a) Alizapride

Intravenous alizapride 100 mg given to 60 women undergoing caesarean section under spinal anaesthesia, reduced **morphine**-induced pruritus, and the amount of sedation (8.3% both peri- and postoperatively) was less than with droperidol,[1] see below.

(b) Droperidol

1. Fentanyl. Epidural droperidol given with epidural fentanyl improved postsurgical analgesia following anorectal surgery and there was less nausea compared with fentanyl alone.[2]

2. Hydromorphone. Early respiratory depression has been reported when droperidol was given 10 minutes before epidural hydromorphone 1.25 mg; the patient became apnoeic 15 minutes after the epidural was given. Naloxone did not reverse the respiratory depression, but spontaneous ventilation resumed within 3 minutes of a 1-mg intravenous dose of physostigmine.[3]

3. Morphine. In a double-blind study in 179 patients following abdominal hysterectomy, droperidol 50 micrograms given with morphine 1 mg on demand via patient-controlled analgesia (PCA) provided a morphine-sparing effect and reduced the frequency of postoperative nausea and vomiting, when compared with morphine PCA alone.[4] However, in a study of 107 patients undergoing caesarean section, intravenous droperidol 2.5 mg given just after delivery, reduced the incidence and severity of epidural morphine-induced pruritus, but the incidence of nausea and vomiting was not affected. Furthermore, somnolence was greater in the droperidol-treated patients (17% versus 2% in the control group) but it was never incapacitating.[5] Similar sedative effects were seen with spinal morphine and intravenous droperidol in another study.[1]

(c) Metoclopramide

1. Butorphanol. The pharmacokinetics of a single 1-mg intranasal dose of butorphanol were unaffected by a single 10-mg oral dose of metoclopramide in 24 healthy women. The pharmacokinetics of metoclopramide were also not affected, except for a delay in the time to reach maximum plasma levels (increased from 1 to 2 hours), which was probably due to reduction of gastrointestinal motility by butorphanol.[6] Metoclopramide reduced the nausea associated with butorphanol, probably by antagonism of central and peripheral dopamine receptors.[7]

2. Morphine. A single 10-mg dose of oral metoclopramide, given to 10 patients before surgery, markedly increased the extent and speed of sedation due to a 20-mg oral dose of modified-release morphine (*MST Continus Tablets*) in the first 1.5 hours after the dose. The time to peak plasma levels of morphine was almost halved, but peak plasma morphine levels and the total absorption remained unaltered.[7] A study involving 40 patients found that intravenous metoclopramide 10 mg antagonised the reduction in gastric emptying caused by premedication with intramuscular morphine 10 mg given 20 minutes earlier. However, intramuscular metoclopramide given at the same time as the morphine had no effect on the reduced gastric emptying.[8]

Mechanism

Metoclopramide increases the rate of gastric emptying so that the rate of morphine absorption from the small intestine is increased. An alternative idea is that both drugs act additively on opiate receptors to increase sedation.[7] Droperidol may also enhance adverse effects such as sedation, and in some cases respiratory depression, possibly through opioid and other receptor sites in the CNS.[2] In one case the respiratory depression was not reversed by naloxone, suggesting that the droperidol was at least partially if not completely responsible.[3]

Importance and management

The effect of metoclopramide on oral morphine absorption is an established interaction that can be usefully exploited in anaesthetic practice, but the increased sedation may also represent a problem if the morphine is being given long-term. The morphine-sparing effect of droperidol is also a useful interaction, but the increased sedation and possible respiratory depression and hypotension should be borne in mind. One manufacturer of fentanyl specifically warns that concurrent use with droperidol can result in a higher incidence of hypotension.[9]

Morphine appears to antagonise the effects of metoclopramide on gastric emptying. As a reduction in gastric motility occurs with all opioids they would all be expected to interact with metoclopramide, and other motility stimulants such as **domperidone**. However, these drugs are commonly used together and the clinical significance of such effects is not clear.

Consider also 'Opioids + Antiemetics; Ondansetron', below.

1. Horta ML, Morejon LCL, da Cruz AW, dos Santos GR, Welling LC, Terhorst L, Costa RC, Alam RUZ. Study of the prophylactic effect of droperidol, alizapride, propofol and promethazine on spinal morphine-induced pruritus. *Br J Anaesth* (2006) 96, 796–800.
2. Kotake Y, Matsumoto M, Ai K, Morisaki H, Takeda J. Additional droperidol, not butorphanol, augments epidural fentanyl analgesia following anorectal surgery. *J Clin Anesth* (2000) 12, 9–13.
3. Cohen SE, Rothblatt AJ, Albright GA. Early respiratory depression with epidural narcotic and intravenous droperidol. *Anesthesiology* (1983) 59, 559–60.
4. Lo Y, Chia Y-Y, Liu K, Ko N-H. Morphine sparing with droperidol in patient-controlled analgesia. *J Clin Anesth* (2005) 17, 271–5.
5. Horta ML, Horta BL. Inhibition of epidural morphine-induced pruritus by intravenous droperidol. *Reg Anesth* (1993) 18, 118–20.
6. Vachharajani NN, Shyu WC, Barbhaiya RH. Pharmacokinetic interaction between butorphanol nasal spray and oral metoclopramide in healthy women. *J Clin Pharmacol* (1997) 37, 979–85.
7. Manara AR, Shelly MP, Quinn K, Park GR. The effect of metoclopramide on the absorption of oral controlled release morphine. *Br J Clin Pharmacol* (1988) 25, 518–21.
8. McNeill MJ, Ho ET, Kenny GNC. Effect of i.v. metoclopramide on gastric emptying after opioid premedication. *Br J Anaesth* (1990) 64, 450–2.
9. Sublimaze (Fentanyl citrate). Janssen-Cilag Ltd. UK Summary of product characteristics, January 2005.

Opioids + Antiemetics; Ondansetron

Ondansetron reduces the analgesic efficacy of tramadol and at least double the dose was required in one clinical study. This resulted in more vomiting despite the ondansetron. In contrast, in studies in healthy subjects, ondansetron had no effect on the analgesic effects of morphine and alfentanil.

Clinical evidence

(a) Alfentanil

In a study in healthy subjects single doses of intravenous ondansetron 8 or 16 mg were found to have no effect on the sedation or ventilatory depression due to alfentanil (a continuous infusion of 0.25 to 0.75 micrograms/kg following a 5 microgram/kg bolus dose) and had no effect on the rate of recovery.[1] Similarly, in another study, intravenous ondansetron 8 mg had no effect on the reaction of 8 healthy subjects to pressure, cold, or electrical stimulation, nor did it oppose the analgesic effect of intramuscular alfentanil 30 micrograms/kg.[2]

(b) Morphine

A double-blind, placebo-controlled study in 12 healthy subjects found that a single 16-mg intravenous dose of ondansetron given 30 minutes after a single 10-mg intravenous dose of morphine did not alter the pharmacokinetics of morphine or its metabolites, morphine-3- and morphine-6-glucuronides. The analgesic effect of morphine (as measured by a contact thermode system) was also unaffected by ondansetron.[3]

(c) Tramadol

Patients who were given a single 4-mg dose of ondansetron one minute before induction of anaesthesia required 26 to 35% more tramadol by patient controlled analgesia (PCA) from 1 to 4 hours postoperatively than those who received placebo.[4] Similarly, a 1-mg/hour ondansetron infusion increased the dose of postoperative tramadol used during PCA by two- to threefold in 30 patients, when compared with 29 patients who received placebo. Moreover, in this study the group receiving ondansetron actually experienced more vomiting, probably because they used more tramadol, which caused an emetic effect not well controlled by the ondansetron.[5]

Mechanism

On theoretical grounds ondansetron (a 5-HT_3-receptor antagonist) might be expected to decrease the effects of drugs that reduce pain transmission because serotonin (5-HT) is thought to affect pain responses via presynaptic 5-HT_3 receptors in the spinal dorsal horn. This has been demonstrated for tramadol, which is not a pure opioid and also acts by enhancing the effects of serotonin and noradrenaline (norepinephrine). However, ondansetron had no effect on alfentanil or morphine analgesia in healthy subjects.

Importance and management

The interaction between ondansetron and tramadol appears to be established and of clinical importance. Ondansetron may double the dose requirement of tramadol, and so result in increased emetic effects, consequently ondansetron does not appear to be the best antiemetic to use with tramadol.[3] Although not tested, other 5-HT_3-receptor antagonists would be expected to interact similarly. Ondansetron appears to have no effect on alfentanil or morphine.

1. Dershwitz M, Di Biase PM, Rosow CE, Wilson RS, Sanderson PE, Joslyn AF. Ondansetron does not affect alfentanil-induced ventilatory depression or sedation. *Anesthesiology* (1992) 77, 447–52.
2. Petersen-Felix S, Arendt-Nielsen L, Bak P, Bjerring P, Breivik H, Svensson P, Zbinden AM. Ondansetron does not inhibit the analgesic effect of alfentanil. *Br J Anaesth* (1994) 73, 326–30.
3. Crews KR, Murthy BP, Hussey EK, Passannante AN, Palmer JL, Maixner W, Brouwer KLR. Lack of effect of ondansetron on the pharmacokinetics and analgesic effects of morphine and metabolites after single-dose morphine administration in healthy volunteers. *Br J Clin Pharmacol* (2001) 51, 309–16.
4. De Witte JL, Schoenmaekers B, Sessler DI, Deloof T. The analgesic efficacy of tramadol is impaired by concurrent administration of ondansetron. *Anesth Analg* (2001) 92, 1319–21.
5. Arcioni R, della Rocca M, Romanò S, Romano R, Pietropaoli P, Gasparetto A. Ondansetron inhibits the analgesic effects of tramadol: a possible 5-HT_3 spinal receptor involvement in acute pain in humans. *Anesth Analg* (2002) 94, 1553–7.

Opioids + Antiepileptics; Enzyme-inducing

Patients taking enzyme-inducing antiepileptics appear to need more fentanyl than those not taking antiepileptics. Similarly, the efficacy of buprenorphine may be reduced by carbamazepine, phenobarbital and phenytoin. Carbamazepine appears to increase the production of a more potent metabolite of codeine, normorphine. The plasma levels of tramadol are reduced by carbamazepine, and the analgesic efficacy would be expected to be reduced. There is also an increased risk of seizures with tramadol. An isolated report describes pethidine toxicity in a man taking phenytoin. A pharmacokinetic study confirms that phenytoin increases the production of the toxic metabolite of pethidine.

Clinical evidence, mechanism, importance and management

(a) Buprenorphine

Although interaction studies have not been performed, the metabolism of buprenorphine is mediated by the cytochrome P450 isoenzyme CYP3A4 and therefore drugs that induce this enzyme such as **carbamazepine**, **phenobarbital** and **phenytoin** may induce the metabolism and increase clearance of buprenorphine.[1,2] The manufacturers of buprenorphine comment that inducers of CYP3A4 may reduce the efficacy of buprenorphine[1-3] and, if necessary, dose adjustments should be considered,[2] or the combination avoided.[1]

(b) Codeine

An experimental study in 7 epileptic patients to find out if **carbamazepine** induces the enzymes concerned with the metabolism of codeine found that it increased *N*-demethylation (to norcodeine and normorphine) by two- to threefold, but did not affect *O*-demethylation (to morphine). The patients were given a single 25-mg dose of codeine before and 3 weeks after starting to take **carbamazepine** 400 to 600 mg daily.[4] Similarly, an *in vitro* study found that **carbamazepine** and **phenytoin** did not alter the *O*-demethylation of codeine (methylmorphine) into morphine.[5]

Normorphine is an active metabolite, so that the authors of the first study suggest those taking both codeine and **carbamazepine** may possibly experience a stronger analgesic effect.[4] However, this needs further study. There would seem to be no reason for avoiding concurrent use.

(c) Dextropropoxyphene (Propoxyphene)

Dextropropoxyphene may increase the plasma levels of antiepileptics, particularly carbamazepine, see 'Carbamazepine or Oxcarbazepine + Dextropropoxyphene (Propoxyphene)', p.527.

(d) Fentanyl

Twenty-eight patients, undergoing craniotomy for seizure focus excision and receiving long-term treatment with antiepileptics in various combinations, needed 48 to 144% more fentanyl during anaesthesia than a control group of 22 patients who were not taking antiepileptics.[6] The fentanyl maintenance requirements in micrograms/kg per hour were:

- 2.7 in the control group,
- 4.0 in patients taking **carbamazepine**,
- 4.7 in patients taking **carbamazepine** and **phenytoin** or **valproate**,
- 6.3 in patients taking **carbamazepine**, **valproate** and either **phenytoin** or **primidone**.

Similar results were reported by the same authors in a study involving 61 patients.[7] The increased opioid requirement probably occurs because these antiepileptics are potent enzyme inducers (with the exception of **valproate**), which increase the metabolism of fentanyl by the liver, so that its levels are reduced.[6] Changes in the state of opiate receptors induced by chronic antiepileptic exposure may also be involved.[7] A marked increase in the fentanyl requirements should therefore be anticipated in any patient receiving long-term treatment with these interacting antiepileptics, but not **valproate**.

(e) Methadone

Methadone levels can be reduced by carbamazepine, phenobarbital or phenytoin. See 'Opioids; Methadone + Antiepileptics', p.163.

(f) Pethidine (Meperidine)

A 61-year-old man who was addicted to pethidine, taking 5 to 10 g weekly, developed repeated seizures and myoclonus when he also took **phenytoin**. The problem resolved when both drugs were stopped.[8]

It is known that **phenytoin** increases the metabolism of pethidine with increased production of norpethidine,[9,10] the metabolic product of pethidine that is believed to be responsible for its neurotoxicity (seizures, myoclonus, tremors etc). A study[11] in healthy subjects found that **phenytoin** 300 mg daily for 9 days decreased the elimination half-life of pethidine (100 mg orally and 50 mg intravenously) from 6.4 to 4.3 hours, and the systemic clearance increased by 27%. This seems to be the only report[8] of an adverse interaction between **phenytoin** and pethidine so its general importance is uncertain. Since the study cited[11] found that pethidine given orally produced more of the toxic metabolite (norpethidine) than when given intravenously, it may be preferable to give pethidine intravenously in patients taking **phenytoin**, or use an alternative opioid.

Consider also 'Opioids + Barbiturates', p.165.

(g) Tramadol

An unpublished study by the manufacturers found that the maximum plasma levels and the elimination half-life of a single 50-mg dose of tramadol were reduced by 50% by **carbamazepine** 400 mg twice daily for 9 days.[12] It is likely that **carbamazepine** increases the metabolism of tramadol. On the basis of this study the manufacturers say that the analgesic effectiveness of tramadol[13,14] and its duration of action would be expected to be reduced.[12,14] The US manufacturer recommends avoidance of concurrent use because of the increased metabolism and also the seizure risk associated with tramadol.[13] The UK manufacturer says that patients with a history of epilepsy or those susceptible to seizures should only be given tramadol if there are compelling reasons.[14] Monitor carefully if tramadol and antiepileptics, particularly **carbamazepine**, are required.

1. Temgesic Sublingual Tablets (Buprenorphine hydrochloride). Schering-Plough Ltd. UK Summary of product characteristics, April 2004.
2. Buprenorphine Hydrochloride Injection. Bedford Laboratories. US Prescribing information, August 2004.
3. Transtec Transdermal Patch (Buprenorphine). Napp Pharmaceuticals Ltd. UK Summary of product characteristics, May 2007.
4. Yue Q-Y, Tomson T, Säwe J. Carbamazepine and cigarette smoking induce differentially the metabolism of codeine in man. *Pharmacogenetics* (1994) 4, 193–8.
5. Dayer P, Desmeules J, Striberni R. In vitro forecasting of drugs that may interfere with codeine bioactivation. *Eur J Drug Metab Pharmacokinet* (1992) 17, 115–20.
6. Tempelhoff R, Modica P, Spitznagel E. Increased fentanyl requirement in patients receiving long-term anticonvulsant therapy. *Anesthesiology* (1988) 69, A594.
7. Tempelhoff R, Modica PA, Spitznagel EL. Anticonvulsant therapy increases fentanyl requirements during anaesthesia for craniotomy. *Can J Anaesth* (1990) 37, 327–32.
8. Hochman MS. Meperidine-associated myoclonus and seizures in long-term hemodialysis patients. *Ann Neurol* (1983) 14, 593.
9. Pethidine Injection (pethidine hydrochloride). Wockhardt UK Ltd. UK Summary of product characteristics, March 2005.
10. Demerol (Meperidine hydrochloride). Sanofi-Aventis US LLC. US Prescribing information, July 2007.
11. Pond SM, Kretschzmar KM. Effect of phenytoin on meperidine clearance and normeperidine formation. *Clin Pharmacol Ther* (1981) 30, 680–6.
12. GD Searle. Personal Communication, November 1994.
13. Ultram ER (Tramadol hydrochloride). Ortho-McNeil Pharmaceutical Inc. US Prescribing information, December 2006.
14. Zydol SR (Tramadol hydrochloride). Grünenthal Ltd. UK Summary of product characteristics, February 2005.

Opioids + Antiepileptics; Gabapentin

Gabapentin has been reported to enhance the analgesic effects of morphine and other opioids. Morphine can increase the bioavailability of gabapentin.

Clinical evidence, mechanism, importance and management

A single-dose, placebo-controlled study in 12 healthy subjects given controlled-release **morphine** 60 mg found that gabapentin 600 mg given after an interval of 2 hours had no effect on the pharmacokinetics of morphine, morphine-3- and morphine-6-glucuronides. In the presence of **morphine** the gabapentin AUC increased by 44% and its oral clearance and apparent renal clearance decreased by 23% and 16%, respectively. Analgesic effect was evaluated by changes in the area under the curve of pain tolerance. Gabapentin plus placebo had no significant analgesic effect, but a significant increase in the pain threshold and pain tolerance was found when gabapentin was given with morphine, when compared with placebo. The opioid adverse effects were similar in the gabapentin/morphine and gabapentin/placebo groups.[1] Other clinical studies have reported that gabapentin used in conjunction with opioids has an analgesic and opioid-sparing effect in acute postoperative pain management[2,3] and neuropathic pain.[4] The manufacturer of gabapentin warns that patients should be carefully observed for signs of CNS depression, such as somnolence, and the dose of gabapentin or **morphine** should be reduced appropriately.[5]

A study in *animals* reported a synergistic antinociceptive interaction between **tramadol** and gabapentin.[6]

1. Eckhardt K, Ammon S, Hofmann U, Riebe A, Gugeler N, Mikus G. Gabapentin enhances the analgesic effect of morphine in healthy volunteers. *Anesth Analg* (2000) 91, 185–91.
2. Ho K-Y, Gan TJ, Habib AS. Gabapentin and postoperative pain–a systematic review of randomised controlled trials. *Pain* (2006) 126, 91–101.
3. Turan A, White PF, Karamanlioğlu B, Memis D, Taşdoğan M, Pamukçu Z, Yavuz E. Gabapentin: an alternative to the cyclooxygenase-2 inhibitors for perioperative pain management. *Anesth Analg* (2006) 102, 175–81.
4. Vadalouca A, Siafaka I, Argyra E, Vrachnou E, Moka E. Therapeutic management of chronic neuropathic pain: an examination of pharmacologic treatment. *Ann N Y Acad Sci* (2006) 1088, 164–86.
5. Neurontin (Gabapentin). Pfizer Ltd. UK Summary of product characteristics, August 2006.
6. Granados-Soto V, Argüelles CF. Synergic antinociceptive interaction between tramadol and gabapentin after local, spinal and systemic administration. *Pharmacology* (2005) 74, 200–8.

Opioids; Methadone + Antiepileptics

Methadone levels can be reduced by carbamazepine, phenobarbital or phenytoin. Valproate appears not to interact. An isolated report describes lamotrigine-associated rash and blood dyscrasias, which may have been associated with methadone use.

Clinical evidence

(a) Enzyme-inducing antiepileptics

A study in 37 patients taking methadone maintenance found that those receiving enzyme-inducing drugs (10 patients: taking **carbamazepine**, **phenobarbital** or **phenytoin**) had low trough methadone levels of less than 100 nanograms/mL. One patient taking carbamazepine complained of daily withdrawal symptoms and had signs of opioid withdrawal.[1] Withdrawal symptoms have been seen in other patients taking **carbamazepine**,[2] **phenobarbital**,[3] and **phenytoin**.[1,2,4,5] Similarly methadone withdrawal symptoms developed in 5 patients within 3 to 4 days of starting to take **phenytoin** 300 to 500 mg daily. Methadone plasma levels were reduced about 60%. The symptoms disappeared within 2 to 3 days of stopping the **phenytoin** and the plasma methadone levels rapidly climbed to their former values.[6]

A further patient experienced methadone-induced respiratory depression after discontinuing **carbamazepine**.[7]

(b) Lamotrigine

Lamotrigine-associated rash and blood dyscrasias occurred in a 40-year-old opioid-dependent woman with hepatitis C. Lamotrigine was considered to be the causal factor as haematological values returned to normal 53 days after discontinuation. However, the woman was also receiving methadone maintenance treatment and it was thought that the methadone together with liver impairment might possibly have caused elevated levels of lamotrigine [not measured].[8]

(c) Valproate

Two patients who had methadone withdrawal symptoms while taking phenytoin 300 to 400 mg daily, and one of them later when taking carbamazepine 600 mg daily, became free from withdrawal symptoms when they were given valproate instead. It was also found possible to virtually halve their daily methadone dosage.[2]

Mechanism

Not fully established, but all of these antiepileptics (except lamotrigine and valproate) are recognised enzyme-inducers that can increase the metabolism of other drugs by the liver, thereby hastening their loss from the body. In one study it was found that phenytoin increased the urinary excretion of the main metabolite of methadone.[6]

Importance and management

Information is limited but the interaction between methadone and these enzyme-inducing antiepileptics appears to be established and of clinical importance. Anticipate the need to increase the methadone dosage in patients taking carbamazepine, phenytoin or phenobarbital. It may be necessary to give the methadone twice daily to prevent withdrawal symptoms appearing towards the end of the day. It seems probable that **primidone** will interact similarly because it is metabolised to phenobarbital. Also be aware of the need to reduce the methadone dose if any enzyme-inducing antiepileptic is stopped. Valproate appears not to interact.

It is unclear whether the methadone or the liver impairment contributed to the lamotrigine-associated rash and blood dyscrasias and therefore this isolated cases is of unknown significance.

1. Bell J, Seres V, Bowron P, Lewis J, Batey R. The use of serum methadone levels in patients receiving methadone maintenance. *Clin Pharmacol Ther* (1988) 43, 623–9.
2. Saxon AJ, Whittaker S, Hawker CS. Valproic acid, unlike other anticonvulsants, has no effect on methadone metabolism: two cases. *J Clin Psychiatry* (1989) 50, 228–9.
3. Liu S-J, Wang RIH. Case report of barbiturate-induced enhancement of methadone metabolism and withdrawal syndrome. *Am J Psychiatry* (1984) 141, 1287–8.
4. Finelli PF. Phenytoin and methadone tolerance. *N Engl J Med* (1976) 294, 227.
5. Knoll B, Haefeli WE, Ladewig D, Stohler R. Early recurrence of withdrawal symptoms under phenytoin and chronic alcohol use. *Pharmacopsychiatry* (1997) 30, 72–3.
6. Tong TG, Pond SM, Kreek MJ, Jaffery NF, Benowitz NL. Phenytoin-induced methadone withdrawal. *Ann Intern Med* (1981) 94, 349–51.
7. Benítez-Rosario MA, Salinas Martín A, Gómez-Ontañón E, Feria M. Methadone-induced respiratory depression after discontinuing carbamazepine administration. *J Pain Symptom Manage* (2006) 32, 99–100.
8. Alleyne S, Alao A, Batki SL. Lamotrigine-associated rash and blood dyscrasias in a methadone-treatment patient with hepatitis C. *Psychosomatics* (2006) 47, 257–8.

Opioids + Antihistamines

Increased respiratory depression has been seen with hydroxyzine and opioids in one study,[1] but not in two others.[2,3] The US manufacturers warn that hydroxyzine may enhance the effects of opio-

ids and particularly pethidine (meperidine).[4] A reduction in dosage may be necessary. All sedating antihistamines (see 'Table 15.1', (p.582)) would be expected to have additive CNS depressant effects with opioids. This may lead to increased sedation and respiratory depression, and therefore some caution is warranted when both drugs are given.

1. Reier CE, Johnstone RE. Respiratory depression: narcotic versus narcotic-tranquillizer combinations. *Anesth Analg* (1970) 49, 119–124.
2. Zsigmond EK, Flynn K, Shively JG. Effect of hydroxyzine and meperidine on arterial blood gases in healthy human volunteers. *J Clin Pharmacol* (1989) 29, 85–90.
3. Zsigmond EK, Flynn K, Shively JG. Effect of hydroxyzine and meperidine on arterial blood gases in patients with chronic obstructive pulmonary disease. *Int J Clin Pharmacol Ther Toxicol* (1993) 31, 124–9.
4. Hydroxyzine. Watson Laboratories, Inc. US Prescribing information, September 2004.

Opioids + Azoles

Several of the opioids (buprenorphine, hydromorphone, methadone) are metabolised by CYP3A, at least in part, and their metabolism is expected to be reduced by the azoles, which, to varying extents, inhibit CYP3A4. This has been seen when fluconazole and voriconazole are given with methadone, and when ketoconazole is given with buprenorphine. It has been suggested that ketoconazole inhibits the metabolism of morphine and oxycodone, but evidence for this is sparse.

Clinical evidence

(a) Buprenorphine

Ketoconazole increases the AUC of buprenorphine by 50% and increases its maximum level by 70% or more; levels of the metabolite norbuprenorphine are less affected.[1]

(b) Hydromorphone

An *in vitro* study found that **ketoconazole** reduced norhydromorphone formation by about 50%.[2]

(c) Methadone

1. Fluconazole. A randomised, double-blind, placebo-controlled study in 25 patients taking methadone found that fluconazole 200 mg daily for 2 weeks increased the steady-state serum methadone levels and AUC by about 30%, but no signs of methadone overdose were seen and no changes in the methadone dosage were needed.[3] However, a case report describes a man with advanced cancer who had received regular methadone 20 mg every 8 hours and one to three 5-mg rescue doses daily for 10 days, and who rapidly developed respiratory depression of 4 breaths per minute and became unresponsive 4 days after starting fluconazole 100 mg daily, initially orally, then intravenously. Within a few minutes of receiving naloxone he regained consciousness and his respiratory rate increased.[4]

2. Ketoconazole. An *in vitro* study suggests that clinically relevant concentrations of ketoconazole decreased the hepatic metabolism of methadone by about 50 to 70%.[5]

3. Voriconazole. In a double-blind, placebo-controlled study in 23 patients taking methadone, voriconazole 400 mg twice daily for one day then 200 mg twice daily for 4 days increased the AUC of *R*-methadone (active) by 47% and *S*-methadone (inactive) by 103%. Methadone appeared to have no effect on voriconazole pharmacokinetics when compared with a reference study in healthy subjects. There were no signs or symptoms of significant opioid withdrawal or overdose and the combination was generally well tolerated.[6]

(d) Morphine

In an *in-vitro* study **ketoconazole** inhibited morphine glucuronidation to morphine-3-glucuronide and morphine-6-glucuronide.[7] The clinical relevance of this is unknown.

(e) Oxycodone

The UK manufacturer of oxycodone suggests that inhibitors of CYP3A enzymes such as **ketoconazole** may inhibit the metabolism of oxycodone,[8] although oxycodone is also metabolised via CYP2D6.[8]

Mechanism

Since the metabolism of methadone is mainly mediated by the cytochrome P450 isoenzyme CYP3A4, methadone clearance can be decreased by drugs that inhibit CYP3A4 activity such as azole antifungals.[9] Buprenorphine is also metabolised by CYP3A4[10] and may therefore be similarly affected. Most azoles inhibit CYP3A4 to a greater or lesser extent.

Importance and management

It has been suggested that although a statistically significant pharmacokinetic interaction occurs between methadone and fluconazole, it is unlikely to be clinically important in patients taking methadone.[3] However, the case report introduces a note of caution. The authors of the second study suggest caution should be exercised if voriconazole is given with methadone and a dose reduction of methadone may be required.[6] Caution may also be warranted with ketoconazole. Further study is needed.

One manufacturer recommends that the dose of buprenorphine should be halved when starting treatment with ketoconazole, and then further titrated as clinically indicated.[1] Other manufacturers recommend close monitoring and possibly a dose reduction if buprenorphine is given with inhibitors of CYP3A4 including azole antifungals such as ketoconazole.[11] The clinical significance of the potential effects of azoles on other opioids, such as hydromorphone, morphine and oxycodone is unclear.

Consider also 'Opioids; Fentanyl and related drugs + Azoles', below.

1. Subutex (Buprenorphine hydrochloride). Schering-Plough Ltd. UK Summary of product characteristics, January 2006.
2. Benetton SA, Borges VM, Chang TKH, McErlane KM. Role of individual human cytochrome P450 enzymes in the *in vitro* metabolism of hydromorphone. *Xenobiotica* (2004) 34, 335–44.
3. Cobb MN, Desai J, Brown LS, Zannikos PN, Rainey PM. The effect of fluconazole on the clinical pharmacokinetics of methadone. *Clin Pharmacol Ther* (1998) 63, 655–62.
4. Tarumi Y, Pereira J, Watanabe S. Methadone and fluconazole: respiratory depression by drug interaction. *J Pain Symptom Manage* (2002) 23, 148–53.
5. Wang J-S, DeVane CL. Involvement of CYP3A4, CYP2C8, and CYP2D6 in the metabolism of (*R*)- and (*S*)-methadone in vitro. *Drug Metab Dispos* (2003) 31, 742–7.
6. Liu P, Foster G, Labadie R, Somoza E, Sharma A. Pharmacokinetic interaction between voriconazole and methadone at steady state in patients on methadone therapy. *Antimicrob Agents Chemother* (2007) 51, 110–18.
7. Takeda S, Kitajima Y, Ishii Y, Nishimura Y, Mackenzie PI, Oguri K, Yamada H. Inhibition of UDP-glucuronosyltransferase 2B7-catalyzed morphine glucuronidation by ketoconazole: dual mechanisms involving a novel noncompetitives mode. *Drug Metab Dispos* (2006) 34, 1277–82.
8. OxyNorm (Oxycodone hydrochloride). Napp Pharmaceuticals Ltd. UK Summary of product characteristics, March 2007.
9. Methadone Injection (Methadone hydrochloride). Rosemont Pharmaceuticals Ltd. UK Summary of product characteristics, January 2005.
10. Iribarne C, Picart D, Creano Y, Bail JP, Berthou F. Involvement of cytochrome P450 3A4 in N-dealkylation of buprenorphine in human liver microsomes. *Life Sci* (1997) 60, 1953–64.
11. Buprenorphine Hydrochloride Injection. Bedford Laboratories. US Prescribing information, August 2004.

Opioids; Fentanyl and related drugs + Azoles

Some patients may experience prolonged and increased alfentanil effects if they are given fluconazole or voriconazole. *In vitro* data suggest itraconazole and ketoconazole may interact similarly. Intravenous fentanyl does not appear to interact with itraconazole in healthy subjects, but one case of possible opioid toxicity from transdermal fentanyl has been reported.

Clinical evidence

(a) Alfentanil

A double-blind, randomised, crossover study in 9 healthy subjects given intravenous alfentanil 20 micrograms/kg after receiving **fluconazole** 400 mg, orally or by infusion, found that fluconazole reduced alfentanil clearance by about 60%. Both the alfentanil-induced ventilatory depression and its subjective effects were increased.[1]

A randomised, crossover study in 12 healthy subjects found that oral **voriconazole** (400 mg twice daily on the first day and 200 mg twice daily on the second day) caused an approximately fivefold increase in the mean AUC of alfentanil 20 micrograms/kg, given intravenously one hour after the last dose of the antifungal. The mean plasma clearance of alfentanil was decreased by 85% and its elimination half-life was prolonged from 1.5 to 6.6 hours. Nausea occurred in 5 subjects and vomiting in 4 subjects.[2]

(b) Fentanyl

In a crossover study in 10 healthy subjects the pharmacokinetics and pharmacodynamics of a single 3-micrograms/kg intravenous dose of fentanyl were not altered by **itraconazole** 200 mg once daily for 4 days.[3] However, the manufacturer says that increased fentanyl plasma concentrations have been observed in individual subjects taking itraconazole,[4] and a case report describes a man with cancer and severe oropharyngeal candidiasis receiving transdermal fentanyl 50 micrograms/hour who developed signs of opioid toxicity (agitated delirium, bilateral myoclonus of muscles in the hand) the day after starting oral **itraconazole** 200 mg twice daily.[5]

Mechanism

Fluconazole, itraconazole, and voriconazole inhibit the cytochrome P450 isoenzyme CYP3A4 in the liver, which is concerned with the metabolism of alfentanil and fentanyl. However, fentanyl has a high hepatic extraction, and so is more affected by changes in hepatic blood flow than changes in the isoenzymes responsible for its metabolism; it is therefore less affected by CYP3A inhibitors than alfentanil. **Sufentanil** also has a high hepatic extraction, see 'Opioids; Fentanyl and related drugs + Macrolides', p.174.

Importance and management

The interaction of alfentanil with fluconazole and voriconazole appears to be established and clinically important. *In vitro* data indicate that **ketoconazole** and itraconazole may interact in a similar way.[6-8] Alfentanil should be given with care to those who have recently received these drugs, and it may be necessary to use a lower alfentanil dose.[7] Be alert for evidence of prolonged alfentanil effects and respiratory depression.

Intravenous fentanyl was not affected by itraconazole in healthy subjects, but the single case report involving transdermal fentanyl introduces a note of caution, particularly in those with unstable advanced disease. Further study is needed. The manufacturers comment that concurrent use of potent CYP3A4 inhibitors including azole antifungals (e.g. fluconazole, itraconazole, ketoconazole) with oral[9] or transdermal[4,10] fentanyl may result in increased plasma concentrations of fentanyl. This may increase or prolong both the therapeutic effects and the adverse reactions, which may cause severe respiratory depression. Careful monitoring is required, with dosage adjustment if necessary.

1. Palkama VJ, Isohanni MH, Neuvonen PJ, Olkkola KT. The effect of intravenous and oral fluconazole on the pharmacokinetics and pharmacodynamics of intravenous alfentanil. *Anesth Analg* (1998) 87, 190–4.
2. Saari TI, Laine K, Leino K, Valtonen M, Neuvonen PJ, Olkkola KT. Voriconazole, but not terbinafine, markedly reduces alfentanil clearance and prolongs its half-life. *Clin Pharmacol Ther* (2006) 80, 502–8.
3. Palkama VJ, Neuvonen PJ, Olkkola KT. The CYP3A4 inhibitor itraconazole has no effect on the pharmacokinetics of i.v. fentanyl. *Br J Anaesth* (1998) 81, 598–600.
4. Matrifen (Fentanyl). Nycomed UK Ltd. UK Summary of product characteristics, June 2007.
5. Mercadante S, Villari P, Ferrera P. Itraconazole–fentanyl interaction in a cancer patient. *J Pain Symptom Manage* (2002) 24, 284–6.
6. Labroo RB, Thummel KE, Kunze KL, Podoll T, Trager WF, Kharasch ED. Catalytic role of cytochrome P4503A4 in multiple pathways of alfentanil metabolism. *Drug Metab Dispos* (1995) 23, 490–6.
7. Rapifen (Alfentanil hydrochloride). Janssen-Cilag Ltd. UK Summary of product characteristics, May 2007.
8. Klees TM, Sheffels P, Dale O, Kharasch ED. Metabolism of alfentanil by cytochrome P4503A (CYP3A) enzymes. *Drug Metab Dispos* (2005) 33, 303–11.
9. Actiq (Fentanyl citrate lozenge). Cephalon Ltd. UK Summary of product characteristics, October 2005.
10. Duragesic (Fentanyl transdermal system). Janssen Pharmaceutica Products, L.P. US Prescribing information, April 2007.

Opioids + Baclofen

The effects of fentanyl and morphine, but probably not pentazocine, may be increased by baclofen.

Clinical evidence, mechanism, importance and management

A study in three groups of 10 patients found that pretreatment with baclofen 0.6 mg/kg, either in four intramuscular doses for 5 days, or intravenously in 100 mL of glucose 5%, 45 minutes before surgery, prolonged the duration of **fentanyl** anaesthesia from 18 to 30 minutes. The baclofen reduced the amounts of **fentanyl** needed by 30 to 40%.[1]

In a placebo-controlled study in 69 patients undergoing surgery for the removal of third molar teeth, oral baclofen (5 mg three times daily for 3 days and then a 10-mg dose 6 hours before surgery and again immediately before surgery) enhanced postoperative analgesia due to intravenous **morphine** 6 mg. However, analgesia due to intravenous **pentazocine** 30 mg was not enhanced.[2]

These limited reports suggest that baclofen may potentiate the effects of **fentanyl** and **morphine**. The reasons for this effect are not understood, but it may be connected in some way with the action of baclofen on GABA receptors, since the spinal cord circuits that are important in opioid analgesia contain GABAergic receptors.[1,2] It appears that baclofen enhances the analgesic effect of **fentanyl** and **morphine**, which are pure opioid agonists that act primarily through μ-opioid receptors, whereas it does not affect pentazocine, a predominantly κ-opioid analgesic.[2]

The manufacturer of baclofen warns that increased sedation may occur if baclofen is taken with synthetic opioids and that the risk of respiratory depression is also increased. Careful monitoring of respiratory and cardiovascular functions is essential.[3]

1. Panerai AE, Massei R, De Silva E, Sacerdote P, Monza G, Mantegazza P. Baclofen prolongs the analgesic effect of fentanyl in man. *Br J Anaesth* (1985) 57, 954–5.
2. Gordon NC, Gear RW, Heller PH, Paul S, Miaskowski C, Levine JD. Enhancement of morphine analgesia by the $GABA_B$ agonist baclofen. *Neuroscience* (1995) 69, 345–9.
3. Lioresal Tablets (Baclofen). Novartis Pharmaceuticals UK Ltd. UK Summary of product characteristics, February 2005.

Opioids + Barbiturates

A single case report describes greatly increased sedation with severe CNS toxicity in a woman given pethidine after she took phenobarbital for two weeks. The analgesic effects of pethidine can be reduced by barbiturates. Secobarbital increases the respiratory depressant effects of morphine. Other barbiturates would also be expected to increase the CNS depressant effects of opioids.

Clinical evidence

(a) Codeine

A study found that codeine 60 mg increased the hypnotic actions of **secobarbital** 100 mg resulting in synergism in the sedative effects in pain-free patients.[1]

(b) Morphine

In 30 healthy subjects it was found that both intravenous **secobarbital** and intravenous **morphine** depressed respiration when given alone, and a much greater and more prolonged respiratory depression occurred when they were given together.[2] The combination should be used with caution.

A study in *animals* demonstrated that **pentobarbital** caused a synergistic enhancement of **morphine** analgesia and morphine significantly enhanced pentobarbital-induced anaesthesia.[3]

(c) Pethidine (Meperidine)

1. Increased pethidine toxicity. A woman whose pain had been satisfactorily controlled with pethidine without particular CNS depression, had prolonged sedation with severe CNS toxicity when she was given pethidine after taking **phenobarbital** 30 mg four times daily for 2 weeks.[4]

2. Pethidine effects reduced. Studies in women undergoing dilatation and curettage found that **thiopental** and **pentobarbital** increased their sensitivity to pain, and opposed the analgesic effects of pethidine.[5] This confirmed the findings of previous studies.[6] A marked anti-analgesic effect has been seen for up to 5 hours after high doses (6 to 10 mg/kg) of **thiopental**.[5] This anti-analgesic effect also occurred with **phenobarbital**.[5]

(d) Miscellaneous

Increased CNS depression may occur with opioids and other CNS depressants such as hypnotics and manufacturers of several opiates specifically mention that barbiturates can potentiate sedation, respiratory depression, and hypotension. A reduction in dosage may be required. One manufacturer of **methadone** contraindicates the use of the injection, but not the oral solution, with other CNS depressants including barbiturates;[7,8] however, other manufacturers warn of the potential for increased CNS depression, but do not contraindicate barbiturates.[9,10]

For comment on the effect of enzyme inducers such as phenobarbital on opioid metabolism, see 'Opioids + Antiepileptics; Enzyme-inducing', p.162 and 'Opioids; Methadone + Antiepileptics', p.163.

Mechanism

Studies suggest that phenobarbital stimulates the liver enzymes concerned with the metabolism (*N*-demethylation) of pethidine so that the production of its more toxic metabolite (norpethidine) is increased. The toxicity seen appears to be the combined effects of this compound and the directly sedative effects of the barbiturate.[4,11]

Importance and management

There is only one report of toxicity when phenobarbital was given with pethidine, but metabolic changes have been seen in other patients and subjects. The general clinical importance is uncertain but concurrent use should be undertaken with care. It has also been suggested that if the pethidine is continued but the barbiturate suddenly withdrawn, the toxic levels of norpethidine might lead to convulsions in the absence of an antiepileptic.[4] Be aware that the barbiturates may reduce analgesia. The metabolic product of pethidine is a less effective analgesic than the parent compound. Both the barbiturates and the opioids have CNS depressant effects, which would be expected to be additive. Therefore care is warranted on concurrent use.

1. Bellville JW, Forrest WH, Shroff P, Brown BW. The hypnotic effects of codeine and secobarbital and their interaction in man. *Clin Pharmacol Ther* (1971) 12, 607–12.
2. Zsigmond EK, Flynn K. Effect of secobarbital and morphine on arterial blood gases in healthy human volunteers. *J Clin Pharmacol* (1993) 33, 453–7.
3. Craft RM, Leitl MD. Potentiation of morphine antinociception by pentobarbital in female vs. male rats. *Pain* (2006) 121, 115–25.
4. Stambaugh JE, Wainer IW, Hemphill DM, Schwartz I. A potentially toxic drug interaction between pethidine (meperidine) and phenobarbitone. *Lancet* (1977) i, 398–9.
5. Dundee JW. Alterations in response to somatic pain associated with anaesthesia. II. The effect of thiopentone and pentobarbitone. *Br J Anaesth* (1960) 32, 407–14.
6. Clutton-Brock J. Some pain threshold studies with particular reference to thiopentone. *Anaesthesia* (1960) 15, 71–2.
7. Methadone Injection (Methadone hydrochloride). Rosemont Pharmaceuticals Ltd. UK Summary of product characteristics, January 2005.
8. Methadone Oral Solution (Methadone hydrochloride). Rosemont Pharmaceuticals Ltd. UK Summary of product characteristics, January 2005.
9. Methadone Injection (Methadone hydrochloride). Wockhardt UK Ltd. UK Summary of product characteristics, April 2000.
10. Methadone Hydrochloride Tablets for Oral Suspension. Mallinckrodt Inc. US Prescribing information, January 2005.
11. Stambaugh JE, Wainer IW, Schwartz I. The effect of phenobarbital on the metabolism of meperidine in normal volunteers. *J Clin Pharmacol* (1978) 18, 482–90.

Opioids + Benzodiazepines

In general the concurrent use of opioids and benzodiazepines results in both beneficial analgesic effects, and enhanced sedation and respiratory depression; however, in some cases benzodiazepines have antagonised the respiratory depressant effects of opioids, and, rarely, have antagonised their analgesic effects.

Clinical evidence, mechanism, importance and management

(a) Analgesia

In one study, low-dose **midazolam** (given to achieve levels of 50 nanograms/mL) reduced the dose of **morphine** required for postoperative analgesia in the first 12 hours.[1] However, in another study postoperative pain scores were higher in patients premedicated with oral **diazepam** 10 mg than with placebo, although **morphine** consumption did not differ.[2] Similarly, in another study, the benzodiazepine antagonist flumazenil enhanced **morphine** analgesia in patients who had been premedicated with **diazepam**.[3] It is suggested that benzodiazepines antagonise the analgesic effect of opioids via their effect on supraspinal GABA receptors. Why this has been shown in some studies, but not others, is unclear. Benzodiazepines and opioids are commonly used in surgical anaesthesia, and the relevance of these findings to clinical practice is uncertain.

(b) Overdose

Sudden deaths in patients who abuse opioids are frequently associated with ingestion of other CNS depressants, particularly **benzodiazepines**. Cases have been reported with **buprenorphine**,[4,5] **oxycodone**,[6] and **tramadol**[7] taken with various **benzodiazepines**. It has not been established exactly why this occurs, but both pharmacodynamic and pharmacokinetic mechanisms are possible. The deleterious interaction of benzodiazepines and opioids on respiration is possibly due to central effects and/or additive actions on the different neuromuscular components of respiration.[8] For **buprenorphine**, it is considered most likely that excessive CNS depression is solely due to combined pharmacological effects, and not to any pharmacokinetic interaction.[9-11] See also *Pharmacokinetics*, below.

(c) Pharmacokinetics

Intramuscular **pethidine** 100 mg and intramuscular **morphine** 10 mg delayed the absorption of oral **diazepam** 10 mg. **Diazepam** levels were found to be lower and peak levels were not reached in the 90-minute study period, when compared with the peak level at 60 minutes in the control group.[12] The underlying mechanism is that the opioid analgesics delay gastric emptying so that the rate of absorption of the **diazepam** is reduced. The maximal effect of **diazepam** would be expected to be delayed in patients receiving these opioids.

Another study in healthy subjects found that **dextropropoxyphene** 65 mg every 6 hours prolonged the **alprazolam** half-life from 11.6 to 18.3 hours, and decreased the clearance from 1.3 to 0.8 mL/minute per kg. The pharmacokinetics of single doses of **diazepam** and **lorazepam** were not significantly affected.[13] It would seem that **dextropropoxyphene** inhibits the metabolism (hydroxylation) of the **alprazolam** by the liver, thereby reducing its loss from the body, but has little or no effect on the *N*-demethylation or glucuronidation of the other two benzodiazepines. The clinical importance of this is uncertain, but the inference to be drawn is that the CNS depressant effects of **alprazolam** will be increased, over and above the simple additive CNS depressant effects likely when other benzodiazepines and **dextropropoxyphene** are taken together. More study is needed.

Extended-release **oxymorphone** did not affect the metabolism of **midazolam** in healthy subjects.[14] An *in vitro* study found that **buprenorphine** metabolism to norbuprenorphine was only weakly or negligibly inhibited by benzodiazepines, but **midazolam** had some modest effects and it was suggested that it may possibly cause some clinically relevant inhibition of buprenorphine metabolism.[15]

(d) Respiratory depression

A 14-year-old boy with staphylococcal pneumonia secondary to influenza developed adult respiratory distress syndrome. It was decided to suppress his voluntary breathing with opioids and use assisted ventilation and he was therefore given **phenoperidine** and **diazepam** for 11 days, and later **diamorphine** with **lorazepam**. Despite receiving **diamorphine** 19.2 mg in 24 hours his respiratory drive was not suppressed. On day 17, despite serum morphine and **lorazepam** levels of 320 and 5.3 micrograms/mL, respectively, he remained conscious and his pupils were not constricted.[16] Later *animal* studies confirmed that **lorazepam** opposed the respiratory depressant effects of morphine.[16]

In contrast, intravenous **diazepam** 150 micrograms/kg did not alter the respiratory depressant effect of intravenous **pethidine** 1.5 mg/kg in a study in healthy subjects[17] or in patients with chronic obstructive pulmonary disease.[18] Moreover, in the setting of overdose (see (b) above), benzodiazepines might increase the respiratory depressant effects of opioids.

(e) Sedation

The sedative effects of **midazolam** and **morphine** were additive in a study in patients given these drugs intravenously prior to surgery.[19] A prospective study of 80 patients undergoing elective endoscopy found that deep sedation occurred frequently (68% of patients) with **pethidine** and **midazolam** used with the intent of moderate sedation.[20] Another study found that single oral doses of **diazepam** 10 or 20 mg given to 8 **buprenorphine**-maintained patients increased subjective effects such as sedation and strength of drug effects, and also caused a deterioration in performance measures such as cancellation time, compared with placebo.[21]

1. Gilliland HE, Prasad BK, Mirakhur RK, Fee JPH. An investigation of the potential morphine sparing effect of midazolam. *Anaesthesia* (1996) 51, 808–11.
2. Caumo W, Hidalgo MPL, Schmidt AP, Iwamoto CW, Adamatti LC, Bergmann J, Ferreira MBC. Effect of pre-operative anxiolysis on postoperative pain response in patients undergoing total abdominal hysterectomy. *Anaesthesia* (2002) 57, 740–6.
3. Gear RW, Miaskowski C, Heller PH, Paul SM, Gordon NC, Levine JD. Benzodiazepine mediated antagonism of opioid analgesia. *Pain* (1997) 71, 25–9.
4. Reynaud M, Petit G, Potard D, Courty P. Six deaths linked to concomitant use of buprenorphine and benzodiazepines. *Addiction* (1998) 93, 1385–92.
5. Kintz P. A new series of 13 buprenorphine-related deaths. *Clin Biochem* (2002) 35, 513–16.
6. Burrows DL, Hagardorn AN, Harlan GC, Wallen EDB, Ferslew KE. A fatal drug interaction between oxycodone and clonazepam. *J Forensic Sci* (2003) 48, 683–6.
7. Clarot F, Goullé JP, Vaz E, Proust B. Fatal overdoses of tramadol: is benzodiazepine a risk factor of lethality? *Forensic Sci Int* (2003) 134, 57–61.
8. Megarbane B, Gueye P, Baud F. Interactions entre benzodiazépines et produits opioïdes. *Ann Med Interne (Paris)* (2003) 154 (Spec No 2) S64–S72.
9. Ibrahim RB, Wilson JG, Thorsby ME, Edwards DJ. Effect of buprenorphine on CYP3A activity in rat and human liver microsomes. *Life Sci* (2000) 66, 1293–8.

10. Kilicarslan T, Sellers EM. Lack of interaction of buprenorphine with flunitrazepam metabolism. *Am J Psychiatry* (2000) 157, 1164–6.
11. Elkader A, Sproule B. Buprenorphine: clinical pharmacokinetics in the treatment of opioid dependence. *Clin Pharmacokinet* (2005) 44, 661–80.
12. Gamble JAS, Gaston JH, Nair SG, Dundee JW. Some pharmacological factors influencing the absorption of diazepam following oral administration. *Br J Anaesth* (1976) 48, 1181–5.
13. Abernethy DR, Greenblatt DJ, Morse DS, Shader RI. Interaction of propoxyphene with diazepam, alprazolam and lorazepam. *Br J Clin Pharmacol* (1985) 19, 51–7.
14. Adams M, Pieniaszek HJ, Gammaitoni AR, Ahdieh H. Oxymorphone extended release does not affect CYP2C9 or CYP3A4 metabolic pathways. *J Clin Pharmacol* (2005) 45, 337–45.
15. Chang Y, Moody DE. Effect of benzodiazepines on the metabolism of buprenorphine in human liver microsomes. *Eur J Clin Pharmacol* (2005) 60, 875–81.
16. McDonald CF, Thomson SA, Scott NC, Scott W, Grant IWB, Crompton GK. Benzodiazepine-opiate antagonism — a problem in intensive-care therapy. *Intensive Care Med* (1986) 12, 39–42.
17. Zsigmond EK, Flynn K, Martinez OA. Diazepam and meperidine on arterial blood gases in healthy volunteers. *J Clin Pharmacol* (1974) 14, 377–81.
18. Zsigmond EK, Shively JG, Flynn K. Diazepam and meperidine on arterial blood gases in patients with chronic obstructive pulmonary disease. *J Clin Pharmacol* (1975) 15, 464–68.
19. Tverskoy M, Fleyshman G, Ezry J, Bradley EL, Kissin I. Midazolam-morphine sedative interaction in patients. *Anesth Analg* (1989) 68, 282–5.
20. Patel S, Vargo JJ, Khandwala F, Lopez R, Trolli P, Dumot JA, Conwell DL, Zuccaro G. Deep sedation occurs frequently during elective endoscopy with meperidine and midazolam. *Am J Gastroenterol* (2005) 100, 2689–95.
21. Lintzeris N, Mitchell TB, Bond A, Nestor L, Strang J. Interactions on mixing diazepam with methadone or buprenorphine in maintenance patients. *J Clin Psychopharmacol* (2006) 26, 274–83.

Opioids; Fentanyl and related drugs + Benzodiazepines

In general the combined use of benzodiazepines with alfentanil or fentanyl is synergistic but may also result in additive effects on respiratory depression and/or hypotension. A pharmacokinetic study found that fentanyl reduced the metabolism of midazolam. Retrospective evidence suggests that midazolam can increase the dose requirement of sufentanil, but midazolam did not alter the analgesic efficacy of fentanyl in healthy subjects.

Clinical evidence

(a) Anaesthetic induction

Combining **midazolam** and **alfentanil** or **fentanyl** for the induction of anaesthesia reduces the dose required of both the benzodiazepine and the opioid, when compared with either drug alone.[1-3] The interaction is synergistic.[2]

(b) Analgesic effects

An analysis of 43 patients who were mechanically ventilated following major trauma, and who were given infusions of **sufentanil** alone or **sufentanil** plus **midazolam**, found that **midazolam** appeared to reduce the efficacy of the **sufentanil**. The rate of **sufentanil** infusion in the group given both drugs (21 patients) was increased by more than 50%, when compared with the group given **sufentanil** alone (22 patients). It was found possible to reduce the **sufentanil** infusion in 8 of the patients given **sufentanil** alone, whereas this was possible in only one patient given both drugs.[4]

Conversely, in a study in healthy subjects, intravenous **midazolam** 500 micrograms to 2 mg per 70 kg did not affect the analgesia produced by intravenous **fentanyl** 100 micrograms per 70 kg in a cold pressor test.[5]

(c) Hypotension and respiratory depression

1. Neonates. Hypotension occurred in 6 neonates with respiratory distress who were given **midazolam** (a bolus of 200 micrograms/kg and/or an infusion of 60 micrograms/kg per hour) for sedation during the first 12 to 36 hours of life. Five of them were also given **fentanyl** either as an infusion (1 to 2 micrograms/kg per hour) or a bolus (1.5 to 2.5 micrograms/kg), or both. Blood pressures fell from an average of 55/40 mmHg to 36/24 mmHg in 5 of them, and from 42/28 to less than 20 mmHg in one.[6] Another report describes respiratory arrest in a child of 14 months who was given both drugs.[7]

2. Adults. **Midazolam** 50 micrograms/kg alone caused no episodes of apnoea or hypoxaemia in 12 healthy subjects, whereas **fentanyl** 2 micrograms/kg alone caused hypoxaemia in 6 subjects but no apnoea. When both drugs were given together 6 subjects had apnoea and 11 subjects had hypoxaemia.[8] Similarly, **fentanyl** with **diazepam** caused more respiratory depression in 12 healthy subjects than either drug alone.[9] Hypotension has also been seen in adult patients given **fentanyl** with **midazolam**[10] or **diazepam**.[11]

Acute hypotension occurred in a man receiving clonidine, captopril and furosemide who was premedicated with intramuscular **midazolam** 5 mg and anaesthetised with **sufentanil** 150 micrograms.[12] This is consistent with another report of sudden hypotension during anaesthetic induction in 4 patients given high-dose **sufentanil** who had been given **lorazepam** before induction.[13]

(d) Pharmacokinetics

A double-blind, placebo-controlled study in 30 patients undergoing orthopaedic surgery found that a single 200-microgram dose of **fentanyl** given one minute before intravenous **midazolam** 200 micrograms/kg decreased the systemic clearance of midazolam by 30%. The elimination half-life of midazolam was prolonged by approximately 50%.[14]

(e) Sedation

A study in patients undergoing an abdominal hysterectomy under **alfentanil** and **midazolam** anaesthesia found that although the pharmacokinetics of **midazolam** were unchanged, postoperative sedation was more pronounced, when compared with a group of patients that did not receive **alfentanil**.[15]

Mechanism

Uncertain. The additional use of other CNS depressants may produce additive respiratory depressant and sedative effects. Reduced metabolism of midazolam might also enhance its effects. Why midazolam appeared to increase the analgesic dose requirement for sufentanil is unknown. An *in vitro* study found that fentanyl competitively inhibited the metabolism of **midazolam** by the cytochrome P450 isoenzyme CYP3A4.[16]

Importance and management

Increased sedative and respiratory depressant effects are to be expected when benzodiazepines are used with opioids. The manufacturers of sufentanil[17] and alfentanil[18] suggest that clinically important hypotension may occur and this may be exacerbated by the use of benzodiazepines: it would seem prudent to be alert for this. The manufacturers of transdermal fentanyl also warn of the possibility of respiratory depression, hypotension, profound sedation and potentially coma with concurrent CNS depressants[19] including benzodiazepines.[20] When such combined therapy is contemplated, the dose of one or both drugs should be significantly reduced.[20]

What effect the use of midazolam has on the dose requirement of sufentanil and other opioids in the intensive care setting is unclear, although it would seem that hypotension is a risk.

1. Ben-Shlomo I, Abd-El-Khalim H, Ezry J, Zohar S, Tverskoy M. Midazolam acts synergistically with fentanyl for induction of anaesthesia. *Br J Anaesth* (1990) 64, 45–7.
2. Vinik HR, Bradley EL, Kissin I. Midazolam–alfentanil synergism for anesthetic induction in patients. *Anesth Analg* (1989) 69, 213–17.
3. Kissin I, Vinik HR, Castillo R, Bradley EL. Alfentanil potentiates midazolam-induced unconsciousness in subanalgesic doses. *Anesth Analg* (1990) 71, 65–9.
4. Luger TJ, Hill HF, Schlager A. Can midazolam diminish sufentanil analgesia in patients with major trauma? A retrospective study with 43 patients. *Drug Metabol Drug Interact* (1992) 10, 177–84.
5. Zacny JP, Coalson DW, Klafta JM, Klock PA, Alessi R, Rupani G, Young CJ, Patil PG, Apfelbaum JL. Midazolam does not influence intravenous fentanyl-induced analgesia in healthy volunteers. *Pharmacol Biochem Behav* (1996) 55, 275–80.
6. Burtin P, Daoud P, Jacqz-Aigrain E, Mussat E, Moriette G. Hypotension with midazolam and fentanyl in the newborn. *Lancet* (1991) 337, 1545–6.
7. Yaster M, Nichols DG, Deshpande JK, Wetzel RC. Midazolam-fentanyl intravenous sedation in children: case report of respiratory arrest. *Pediatrics* (1991) 86, 463–6.
8. Bailey PL, Moll JWB, Pace NL, East KA, Stanley TH. Respiratory effects of midazolam and fentanyl: potent interaction producing hypoxemia and apnea. *Anesthesiology* (1988) 69, 3A, A813.
9. Bailey PL, Andriano KP, Pace NL, Westenskow DR, Stanley TH. Small doses of fentanyl potentiate and prolong diazepam induced respiratory depression. *Anesth Analg* (1984) 63, 183.
10. Heikkïlä J, Jalonen J, Arola M, Kanto J, Laaksonen V. Midazolam as adjunct to high-dose fentanyl anaesthesia for coronary artery bypass grafting operation. *Acta Anaesthesiol Scand* (1984) 28, 683–89.
11. Tomicheck RC, Rosow CE, Philbin DM, Moss J, Teplick RS, Schneider RC. Diazepam-fentanyl interaction — hemodynamic and hormonal effects in coronary artery surgery. *Anesth Analg* (1983) 62, 881–4.
12. West JM, Estrada S, Heerdt M. Sudden hypotension associated with midazolam and sufentanil. *Anesth Analg* (1987) 66, 693–4.
13. Spiess BD, Sathoff RH, El-Ganzouri ARS, Ivankovich AD. High-dose sufentanil: four cases of sudden hypotension on induction. *Anesth Analg* (1986) 65, 703–5.
14. Hase I, Oda Y, Tanaka K, Mizutani K, Nakamoto T, Asada A. I.v. fentanyl decreases the clearance of midazolam. *Br J Anaesth* (1997) 79, 740 –3.
15. Persson MP, Nilsson A, Hartvig P. Relation of sedation and amnesia to plasma concentrations of midazolam in surgical patients. *Clin Pharmacol Ther* (1988) 43, 324–31.
16. Oda Y, Mizutani K, Hase I, Nakamoto T, Hamaoka N, Asada A. Fentanyl inhibits metabolism of midazolam: competitive inhibition of CYP3A4 *in vitro*. *Br J Anaesth* (1999) 82, 900–3.
17. Sufenta (Sufentanil citrate injection). Taylor Pharmaceuticals. US Prescribing information, April 2006.

18. Rapifen (Alfentanil hydrochloride). Janssen-Cilag Ltd. UK Summary of product characteristics, May 2007.
19. Durogesic DTrans (Fentanyl). Janssen-Cilag Ltd. UK Summary of product characteristics, July 2007.
20. Duragesic (Fentanyl transdermal system). Janssen Pharmaceutica Products, L.P. US Prescribing information, April 2007.

Opioids; Methadone + Benzodiazepines

Patients taking methadone who are given diazepam may experience increased drowsiness and possibly enhanced opioid effects. Temazepam may have contributed to the sudden death of a patient taking methadone.

Clinical evidence, mechanism, importance and management

A study in patients taking methadone noted that **diazepam** abuse was prevalent, and that many patients reported that **diazepam** boosted the effects of methadone.[1] The possible reasons for this have been studied. Four addicts, taking methadone for at least 6 months, were given **diazepam** 300 micrograms/kg for 9 days. The pharmacokinetics of methadone were unaltered and the opioid effects of the methadone remained unchanged, but all 4 subjects were sedated.[2] However, another study suggested that the opioid effects of methadone (subjective effects and pupil constriction) may be enhanced by **diazepam**. This was significant at higher doses (methadone at 150% of the maintenance dose with **diazepam** 40 mg).[3] Later analysis of blood samples from this study confirmed that there is no pharmacokinetic interaction between methadone and **diazepam**.[4] It has been suggested that the absence of increased opioid effects in the earlier study[2] may possibly be explained by the relatively low regular daily doses of diazepam they used, in contrast to the higher more intermittent doses used in the later study,[3] which is the pattern of dosage reportedly used by patients. A further study in patients taking methadone found that single oral doses of **diazepam** 10 or 20 mg, which are within the usual therapeutic range, increased subjective effects such as sedation, strength of drug effects and euphoria, and also caused a significant deterioration in performance measures such as reaction time, when compared with placebo.[5]

A 39-year-old man taking methadone 60 mg daily and **temazepam** 20 mg twice daily was found dead. Blood levels of methadone and **temazepam** were not particularly high, and revealed that amitriptyline had also been taken. The cause of death was considered to be accidental owing to methadone toxicity enhanced by **temazepam** and amitriptyline.[6] Another case is reported of ventricular arrhythmias associated with high-dose methadone given with CYP3A4 substrates including **midazolam**.[7]

Concurrent use involving low-to-moderate diazepam dosage need not be avoided, but patients given both drugs are likely to experience increased drowsiness and reduced psychomotor performance and should be warned against driving or operating machinery under these circumstances. With a high diazepam dose the possibility of opioid enhancement should be borne in mind. Bear in mind that concurrent use of benzodiazepines appears to be a risk factor in sudden death in patients taking methadone.

1. Stitzer ML, Griffiths RR, McLellan AT, Grabowski J, Hawthorne JW. Diazepam use among methadone maintenance patients: patterns and dosages. *Drug Alcohol Depend* (1981) 8, 189–9.
2. Pond SM, Tong TG, Benowitz NL, Jacob P, Rigod J. Lack of effect of diazepam on methadone metabolism in methadone-maintained addicts. *Clin Pharmacol Ther* (1982) 31, 139–43.
3. Preston KL, Griffiths RR, Stitzer ML, Bigelow GE, Liebson IA. Diazepam and methadone interactions in methadone maintenance. *Clin Pharmacol Ther* (1984) 36, 534–41.
4. Preston KL, Griffiths RR, Cone EJ, Darwin WD, Gorodetzky CW. Diazepam and methadone blood levels following concurrent administration of diazepam and methadone. *Drug Alcohol Depend* (1986) 18, 195–202.
5. Lintzeris N, Mitchell TB, Bond A, Nestor L, Strang J. Interactions on mixing diazepam with methadone or buprenorphine in maintenance patients. *J Clin Psychopharmacol* (2006) 26, 274–83.
6. Fahey T, Law F, Cottee H, Astley P. Sudden death in an adult taking methadone: lessons for general practice. *Br J Gen Pract* (2003) 53, 471–2.
7. Walker PW, Klein D, Kasza L. High dose methadone and ventricular arrhythmias: a report of three cases. *Pain* (2003) 103, 321–4.

Opioids + Calcium-channel blockers

Bradycardia and hypotension may be enhanced in patients taking opioids with calcium-channel blockers. The analgesic effects of morphine appear to be enhanced by some calcium-channel blockers. Diltiazem prolonged the effects of alfentanil in one study.

Clinical evidence, mechanism, importance and management

(a) Cardiovascular effects

The manufacturers of **remifentanil** and **sufentanil** caution that cardiovascular effects (bradycardia and hypotension) may be greater in patients also taking calcium-channel blockers.[1,2]

(b) Delayed recovery from anaesthesia

A 24% increase in the AUC of **alfentanil** and a 50% increase in its half-life were seen in 15 patients anaesthetised with midazolam and alfentanil (induced with 50 micrograms/kg, then maintained with 1 microgram/kg per minute) when they were given **diltiazem** 60 mg orally 2 hours before induction, then an infusion for 23 hours starting at induction. Tracheal extubation was performed on average 2.5 hours later in the patients receiving **diltiazem** than in a placebo group.[3] **Diltiazem** is an inhibitor of the cytochrome P450 isoenzyme CYP3A4, which is responsible for the metabolism of **alfentanil**.[3] Caution is required as there could be an increased risk of prolonged or delayed respiratory depression. The manufacturer says that the concurrent use of **diltiazem** and **alfentanil** requires special patient care and observation; it may be necessary to lower the dose of alfentanil.[4]

(c) Enhanced analgesia

A double-blind, placebo-controlled study in 26 patients undergoing surgery found that 2 doses of slow-release **nifedipine** 20 mg given on the day preceding surgery and a further dose given 60 to 90 minutes before surgery increased the analgesic effect of **morphine**.[5] A study in *animals* found that **verapamil** potentiated **morphine** analgesia.[6] A further study in *animals* found that **diltiazem**, **nimodipine** and **verapamil**, given before **morphine**, potentiated the analgesic effect of morphine and markedly increased morphine serum levels.[7]

1. Ultiva (Remifentanil hydrochloride). GlaxoSmithKline. UK Summary of product characteristics, May 2005.
2. Sufenta (Sufentanil citrate injection). Taylor Pharmaceuticals. US Prescribing information, April 2006.
3. Ahonen J, Olkkola KT, Salmenperä M, Hynynen M, Neuvonen PJ. Effect of diltiazem on midazolam and alfentanil disposition in patients undergoing coronary artery bypass grafting. *Anesthesiology* (1996) 85, 1246–52.
4. Rapifen (Alfentanil hydrochloride). Janssen-Cilag Ltd. UK Summary of product characteristics, May 2007.
5. Carta F, Bianchi M, Argenton S, Cervi D, Marolla G, Tamburini M, Breda M, Fantoni A, Panerai AE. Effect of nifedipine on morphine-induced analgesia. *Anesth Analg* (1990) 70, 493–8.
6. Shimizu N, Kishioka S, Maeda T, Fukazawa Y, Dake Y, Yamamoto C, Ozaki M, Yamamoto H. Involvement of peripheral mechanism in the verapamil-induced potentiation of morphine analgesia in mice. *J Pharmacol Sci* (2004) 95, 452–7.
7. Shimizu N, Kishioka S, Maeda T, Fukazawa Y, Yamamoto C, Ozaki M, Yamamoto H. Role of pharmacokinetic effects in the potentiation of morphine analgesia by L-type calcium channel blockers in mice. *J Pharmacol Sci* (2004) 94, 240–5.

Opioids + Cannabis

Low doses of cannabis enhanced the effect of morphine in three patients. *Animal* studies have shown that cannabinoids may enhance the potency of opioids.

Clinical evidence, mechanism, importance and management

A report of 3 patients with chronic pain (due to multiple sclerosis, HIV-related peripheral neuropathy, and lumbar spinal damage) found that small doses of smoked cannabis potentiated the antinociceptive effects of **morphine**. The patients were able to decrease the dose of opioid by 60 to 100%.[1] Studies in *animals* have shown that Δ^9-tetrahydrocannabinol, the major psychoactive constituent of cannabis, enhances the potency of opioids such as **morphine**, **codeine**, **hydromorphone**, **methadone**, **oxymorphone** and **pethidine (meperidine)**.[2-4] It has been suggested that low doses of Δ^9-tetrahydrocannabinol given with low doses of **morphine** may increase opioid potency without increasing adverse effects.[5] Cannabis use in **methadone**-maintained patients did not appear to affect treatment progress, although some psychological difficulties were slightly more prevalent.[6] However, other workers have suggested that heavy cannabis use is associated with poorer progress when methadone is given in the treatment of opioid addiction.[7]

1. Lynch ME, Clark AJ. Cannabis reduces opioid dose in the treatment of chronic non-cancer pain. *J Pain Symptom Manage* (2003) 25, 496–8. .
2. Smith FL, Cichewicz D, Martin ZL, Welch SP. The enhancement of morphine antinociception in mice by Δ^9-tetrahydrocannabinol. *Pharmacol Biochem Behav* (1998) 60, 559–66.
3. Cichewicz DL, Martin ZL, Smith FL, Welch SP. Enhancement of μ opioid antinociception by oral Δ^9-tetrahydrocannabinol: dose-response analysis and receptor identification. *J Pharmacol Exp Ther* (1999) 289, 859–67.

4. Cichewicz DL, McCarthy EA. Antinociceptive synergy between Δ^9-tetrahydrocannabinol and opioids after oral administration. *J Pharmacol Exp Ther* (2003) 304, 1010–15.
5. Cichewicz DL. Synergistic interactions between cannabinoid and opioid analgesics. *Life Sci* (2004) 74, 1317–24.
6. Epstein DH, Preston KL. Does cannabis use predict poor outcome for heroin-dependent patients on maintenance treatment? Past findings and more evidence against. *Addiction* (2003) 98, 269–79. Erratum. ibid., 538.
7. Nixon LN. Cannabis use and treatment outcome in methadone maintenance. *Addiction* (2003) 98, 1321–2.

Opioids + Carisoprodol

Carisoprodol may enhance the CNS depressant effects of opioids.

Clinical evidence, mechanism, importance and management

A 49-year-old woman who had been taking **oxycodone** *(OxyContin)* 40 mg twice daily for more than a year was given carisoprodol 350 mg (one tablet) four times daily because of muscle spasm and uncontrolled pain. After taking this regimen for a week without relief, she increased the dosage to 8 to 10 tablets daily. She was found unconscious, was responsive only to painful stimuli, and her respiration was also depressed. She rapidly returned to full alertness when she was given naloxone 2 mg intravenously, although she had not taken any extra **oxycodone** tablets. The adverse effects were thought to be due to additive CNS depressant effects of both **oxycodone** and carisoprodol.[1] In a retrospective review of deaths recorded in Jefferson County over a 12-year period, carisoprodol was present in the blood of 24 cases, but was never the sole drug detected; **dextropropoxyphene** (**propoxyphene**) was also present in 8 of the 24 cases. Respiratory depression was a major cause of death and as carisoprodol causes respiratory depression, it was considered to be probably responsible, in part, for those deaths.[2]

The manufacturer of carisoprodol reports that effects of overdosage can be additive with other CNS depressants and that concurrent use of other CNS depressants should be avoided. Dependence has occurred with carisoprodol.[3]

1. Reeves RR, Mack JE. Possible dangerous interaction of OxyContin and carisoprodol. *Am Fam Physician* (2003) 67, 941–2.
2. Davis GG, Alexander CB. A review of carisoprodol deaths in Jefferson County, Alabama. *South Med J* (1998) 91, 726–30.
3. Carisoma (Carisoprodol). Forest Laboratories UK Ltd. UK Summary of product characteristics, July 2006.

Opioids + Chlorobutanol

Chlorobutanol used as a preservative may possibly contribute to the QT prolongation seen with methadone. Higher maximum total bilirubin levels were observed among newborns exposed to morphine that contained chlorobutanol than those exposed to morphine without chlorobutanol. Somnolence in a patient on high-dose morphine may have been due to the effects of morphine and also to a high intake of chlorobutanol preservative.

Clinical evidence, mechanism, importance and management

(a) Methadone

A study in patients receiving intravenous methadone found an approximately linear relationship between the log-dose of methadone and QTc measurements. In addition, methadone and chlorobutanol (a preservative used in intravenous methadone preparations) were both found to block cardiac potassium ion channels *in vitro,* and chlorobutanol potentiated this effect with methadone.[1] High doses of methadone have been reported to cause torsades de pointes, but chlorobutanol used as a preservative in methadone injection may possibly contribute to the QT prolongation.[1]

(b) Morphine

A report describes a 19-year-old woman who required increasing doses of morphine to control pain, reaching a peak of 275 mg/hour, which was maintained for 4 days. After palliative radiotherapy the rate was reduced to 100 to 150 mg/hour, but only partial pain relief was achieved; however the patient was somnolent, which was attributed to an effect of the chlorobutol. At doses of morphine 275 mg/hour, chlorobutanol intake was 90 mg/hour, which is in excess of the dose used to aid sleep (150 mg); chlorobutol accumulation may also have occurred as it has a long half-life.[2] This appears to be an isolated report, the general importance of which is unknown.

1. Kornick CA, Kilborn MJ, Santiago-Palma J, Schulman G, Thaler HT, Keefe DL, Katchman AN, Pezzullo JC, Ebert SN, Woosley RL, Payne R, Manfredi PL. QTc interval prolongation associated with intravenous methadone. *Pain* (2003) 105, 499–506.
2. DeChristoforo R, Corden BJ, Hood JC, Narang PK, Magrath IT. High-dose morphine infusion complicated by chlorobutanol-induced somnolence. *Ann Intern Med* (1983) 98, 335–6.

Opioids + Cocaine

Cocaine-related torsade de pointes occurred in a patient taking methadone. Ventricular arrhythmias and increased cardiovascular effects have been reported when other patients taking methadone were given cocaine. The cardiovascular effects of cocaine and morphine appear to be similar to those seen with cocaine alone.

Clinical evidence, mechanism, importance and management

A 46-year-old woman who had been taking **methadone** 80 mg daily for over one year, started abusing cocaine by inhalation and injection and subsequently developed frequent self-limiting episodes of syncope. These syncopal events consistently occurred within an hour of cocaine use. She was admitted to hospital after collapsing and becoming comatose and was found to have torsade de pointes arrhythmia. She developed irreversible anoxic brain injury secondary to cardiac arrest. Although **methadone** can cause QT prolongation, the serum methadone level was well within the therapeutic range and it was felt that several factors might have contributed to the arrhythmias including cocaine abuse.[1] Another patient taking **methadone** was withdrawn from a study due to the occurrence of premature ventricular contractions for several minutes after a single 32-mg/70 kg intravenous dose of cocaine.[2] Furthermore increased cardiovascular effects (e.g. increased diastolic pressure and heart rate) have been reported when cocaine is given to patients taking **methadone**.[2] Both cocaine and **methadone** are considered to have effects on the QTc interval and both are potassium-channel blockers. The combination of these two drugs creates a potentially dangerous risk for torsade de pointes.[3]

In contrast, a study in 9 healthy subjects found that although the combination of **morphine** and cocaine produced significant cardiovascular and subjective effects, for the most part, the cardiovascular effects were similar to those produced by cocaine alone. Neither cocaine nor **morphine** altered the plasma levels of the other drug.[4]

1. Krantz MJ, Rowan SB, Mehler PS. Cocaine-related torsade de pointes in a methadone maintenance patient. *J Addict Dis* (2005) 24, 53–60.
2. Foltin RW, Christiansen I, Levin FR, Fischman MW. Effects of single and multiple intravenous cocaine injections in humans maintained on methadone. *J Pharmacol Exp Ther* (1995) 275, 38–47.
3. Krantz MJ, Baker WA, Schmittner J. Cocaine and methadone: parallel effects on the QTc interval. *Am J Cardiol* (2006) 98, 1121.
4. Foltin RW, Fischman MW. The cardiovascular and subjective effects of intravenous cocaine and morphine combinations in humans. *J Pharmacol Exp Ther* (1992) 261, 623–32.

Opioids + Food

Food can delay the absorption of dextropropoxyphene (propoxyphene), but the total amount absorbed may be slightly increased. Food increases the bioavailability of oral morphine solution and produces a sustained serum level, however, the absorption of some controlled-release preparations of morphine may be delayed by food. Food may also increase the bioavailability of oxycodone solution, but sustained-release preparations of oxycodone and tramadol and immediate-release hydromorphone appear not to be affected by food.

Clinical evidence, mechanism, importance and management

Studies in *animals* suggest that ingestion of **sucrose** for short duration may activate the endogenous opioid system and may modify **morphine** withdrawal.[1,2] Sucrose ingestion has also been shown to alleviate pain and distress in infants and adults.[1]

(a) Dextropropoxyphene (Propoxyphene)

A study in healthy subjects given a single 130-mg dose of dextropropoxyphene (as capsules) found that while fasting, peak plasma dextropropoxyphene levels were reached after about 2 hours. **High-fat** and **high-carbohydrate meals** delayed peak serum levels by about 1 hour, and **high protein** delayed the peak serum levels by about 2 hours. Both the **protein** and **carbohydrate meals** caused a small 25 to 30% increase in the total amount of dextropropoxyphene absorbed.[3] The delay in absorption probably occurs because food delays gastric emptying. Avoid food if rapid analgesic effects are needed.

(b) Hydromorphone

A crossover study in 24 healthy subjects found that food had no clinically relevant effect on the pharmacokinetics of a single 8-mg dose of immediate-release hydromorphone.[4]

(c) Morphine

Twelve patients with chronic pain were given oral morphine hydrochloride 50 mg in 200 mL of water either while fasting or after a **high-fat breakfast** (fried eggs and bacon, toast with butter, and milk). The maximum blood morphine levels and the time to achieve these levels were not significantly altered by the presence of the food, but the AUC was increased by 34% and blood morphine levels were maintained at higher levels over the period from 4 to 10 hours after the morphine had been given.[5] The reasons are not understood. The inference to be drawn is that pain relief is likely to be increased if the morphine solution is given with food. This appears to be an advantageous interaction. More confirmatory study is needed.

Some differences in pharmacokinetic parameters have also been reported between the fed and fasted states for controlled-release formulations, but these are not necessarily translated into measurable differences in the pharmacodynamic effects of pain relief and adverse effects.[6] One single-dose study found that the AUC, maximum plasma level, and time to maximum plasma level were increased by food, when compared with the fasting state for two modified-release morphine tablets available in the United Kingdom (*MST Continus*; *Oramorph SR*).[7] Whereas in another single-dose study, no difference in these pharmacokinetic parameters was found for *MS Contin (Purdue Frederick Company, USA)* between the fed and fasted states.[8] Yet another single-dose study reported that the rate of absorption of morphine from sustained-release morphine sulfate capsules (*Kapanol*; *Purdue Frederick Company USA*) was slower with food; there was a 28% increase in the absorption half-life and a 19% increase in the time to maximum plasma level, but the AUC and maximum plasma level were not significantly affected.[9] However, another study reported that sustained-release capsules (*Kapanol*) were bioequivalent under fed and fasting conditions, but the rate and extent of morphine absorption from modified-release capsules (*MXL*) was significantly reduced by food.[10]

Most of these studies used single doses in healthy subjects and food was given in the form of a **high-fat breakfast** and although it appears that there might be some delay in the absorption of some sustained-release preparations of morphine with food, the overall effect is unlikely to be clinically significant.

(d) Oxycodone

A study in 22 healthy subjects found that the bioavailability of oxycodone as an immediate-release solution was significantly altered by consumption of a **high-fat meal**; the AUC was increased by 20% and the maximum plasma level was decreased by 18%, when compared with the fasted state. However, there was no significant effect of food on the bioavailability of oxycodone given as a controlled-release tablet.[11]

(e) Tramadol

In an open, crossover study in 24 healthy subjects, tramadol sustained-release capsules were found to be bioequivalent with and without concurrent food intake (**high-fat breakfast**).[12]

1. Bhattacharjee M, Mathur R. Antinociceptive effect of sucrose ingestion in the human. *Indian J Physiol Pharmacol* (2005) 49, 383–94.
2. Jain R, Mukherjee K, Singh R. Influence of sweet tasting solutions on opioid withdrawal. *Brain Res Bull* (2004) 64, 319–22.
3. Musa MN, Lyons LL. Effect of food and liquid on the pharmacokinetics of propoxyphene. *Curr Ther Res* (1976) 19, 669–74.
4. Durnin C, Hind ID, Channon E, Yates DB, Cross M. Effect of food on the pharmacokinetics of oral immediate-release hydromorphone (Dilaudid® IR). *Proc West Pharmacol Soc* (2001) 44, 75–6.
5. Gourlay GK, Plummer JL, Cherry DA, Foate JA, Cousins MJ. Influence of a high-fat meal on the absorption of morphine from oral solutions. *Clin Pharmacol Ther* (1989) 46, 463–8.
6. Gourlay GK. Sustained relief of chronic pain. Pharmacokinetics of sustained release morphine. *Clin Pharmacokinet* (1998) 35, 173–90.
7. Drake J, Kirkpatrick CT, Aliyar CA, Crawford FE, Gibson P, Horth CE. Effect of food on the comparative pharmacokinetics of modified-release morphine tablet formulations: Oramorph SR and MST Continus. *Br J Clin Pharmacol* (1996) 41, 417–20.
8. Kaiko RF, Lazarus H, Cronin C, Grandy R, Thomas G, Goldenheim P. Controlled-release morphine bioavailability (MS Contin® tablets) in the presence and absence of food. *Hosp J* (1990) 6, 17–30.
9. Kaiko RF. The effect of food intake on the pharmacokinetics of sustained-release morphine sulfate capsules. *Clin Ther* (1997) 19, 296–303.
10. Broomhead A, West R, Eglinton L, Jones M, Bubner R, Sienko D, Knox K. Comparative single-dose pharmacokinetics of sustained-release and modified-release morphine sulfate capsules under fed and fasting conditions. *Clin Drug Invest* (1997) 13, 162–70.
11. Benziger DP, Kaiko RF, Miotto JB, Fitzmartin RD, Reder RF, Chasin M. Differential effects of food on the bioavailability of controlled-release oxycodone tablets and immediate-release oxycodone solution. *J Pharm Sci* (1996) 85, 407–10.
12. Raber M, Schulz H-U, Schürer M, Bias-Imhoff U, Momberger H. Pharmacokinetic properties of tramadol sustained release capsules. 2nd communication: investigation of relative bioavailability and food interaction. *Arzneimittelforschung* (1999) 49, 588–93.

Opioids + Glutethimide

A study in *animals* suggested that glutethimide might potentiate and prolong the analgesic effect of codeine by increasing plasma levels of morphine.[1] Glutethimide combined with codeine can produce a euphoric state and may be addictive; seizures and psychosis have been reported.[2]

1. Popa D, Loghin F, Imre S, Curea E. The study of codeine-glutetimide pharmacokinetic interaction in rats. *J Pharm Biomed Anal* (2003) 32, 867–77.
2. Shamoian CA. Codeine and glutethimide: euphoretic, addicting combination. *N Y State J Med* (1975) 75, 97–9.

Opioids + Grapefruit juice

Grapefruit juice has been associated with a modest increase in oral methadone bioavailability. Grapefruit juice does not appear to affect the bioavailability of intravenous alfentanil or transmucosal fentanyl to a clinically significant extent; the clearance of oral alfentanil may be reduced.

Clinical evidence, mechanism, importance and management

(a) Alfentanil

A study in 10 healthy subjects found that grapefruit juice had no effect on the bioavailability of intravenous alfentanil. However, the clearance of oral alfentanil was reduced by about 40% and the maximum plasma level and oral bioavailability were increased by approximately 40% and 60%, respectively. This was thought to be due to selective inhibition of intestinal CYP3A by grapefruit juice.[1] Therefore should alfentanil be given orally its effects would be expected to be increased and prolonged.

(b) Fentanyl

In a study in 12 healthy subjects, grapefruit juice had minimal effect on peak plasma levels or clinical effects of oral transmucosal fentanyl, despite a considerable proportion of the dose being swallowed and absorbed enterally.[2]

(c) Methadone

A study in 8 patients taking methadone found that 200 mL of grapefruit juice given 30 minutes before and also with their daily dose of methadone was associated with a modest increase in methadone bioavailability. The mean AUC and the maximum plasma levels increased by about 17%.[3] A study in healthy subjects found that grapefruit juice caused a similar modest increase in methadone bioavailability following oral methadone, but had no effect on intravenous methadone bioavailability.[4] The increase in methadone levels were not considered to be clinically significant in the patients studied.[3] On the basis of this evidence dosage adjustments of methadone seem unlikely to be necessary in the presence of grapefruit juice.

1. Kharasch ED, Walker A, Hoffer C, Sheffels P. Intravenous and oral alfentanil as in vivo probes for hepatic and first-pass cytochrome P450 3A activity: non-invasive assessment by use of pupillary miosis. *Clin Pharmacol Ther* (2004) 76, 452–66.
2. Kharasch ED, Whittington D, Hoffer C. Influence of hepatic and intestinal cytochrome P4503A activity on the acute disposition and effects of oral transmucosal fentanyl citrate. *Anesthesiology* (2004) 101, 729–37.

3. Benmebarek M, Devaud C, Gex-Fabry M, Powell Golay K, Brogli C, Baumann P, Gravier B, Eap CB. Effects of grapefruit juice on the pharmacokinetics of the enantiomers of methadone. *Clin Pharmacol Ther* (2004) 76, 55–63.
4. Kharasch ED, Hoffer C, Whittington D, Sheffels P. Role of hepatic and intestinal cytochrome P450 3A and 2B6 in the metabolism, disposition, and miotic effects of methadone. *Clin Pharmacol Ther* (2004) 76, 250–69.

Opioids + H_2-receptor antagonists

No clinically significant interaction appears to occur between cimetidine and butorphanol (intranasal), hydromorphone, morphine, pethidine or tramadol; between famotidine and hydromorphone; or between ranitidine and hydromorphone, morphine, or pethidine. However, isolated reports describe adverse reactions in patients taking methadone, morphine or mixed opium alkaloids with cimetidine, or morphine with ranitidine.

Clinical evidence

(a) Butorphanol

The pharmacokinetics of intranasal butorphanol 1 mg every 6 hours and oral **cimetidine** 300 mg every 6 hours for 4 days were not significantly altered by concurrent use in 16 healthy subjects, except for a moderate increase in the elimination half-life of **cimetidine**.[1]

(b) Hydromorphone

The US manufacturer of hydromorphone says that the concurrent use of H_2-receptor antagonists (**cimetidine**, **famotidine**, **ranitidine**) had no significant effect on hydromorphone steady-state pharmacokinetics.[2]

(c) Methadone

An *in vitro* study briefly mentions an elderly patient receiving methadone 25 mg daily who developed apnoea 2 days after starting **cimetidine** 1.2 g daily.[3] Another elderly patient taking methadone 5 mg every 8 hours by mouth and subcutaneous **morphine** 8 mg every 3 hours also developed apnoea (respiratory rate 2 breaths per minute) after receiving intravenous **cimetidine** 300 mg every 6 hours for 6 days. This was controlled with naloxone. The patient had previously shown no ill effects from the administration of morphine while taking **cimetidine** and methadone.[4]

(d) Morphine

1. Cimetidine. In a study in 7 healthy subjects cimetidine 300 mg four times daily for 4 days had no effect on the pharmacokinetics of a single 10-mg dose of intravenous morphine. The extent and duration of the morphine-induced pupillary miosis was also unchanged.[5] In other healthy subjects, cimetidine 600 mg, given one hour before a 10-mg dose of intramuscular morphine prolonged the respiratory depression due to morphine, but the extent was small and not considered to be clinically significant.[6] Another study in 118 patients undergoing major abdominal surgery found that there were no significant differences between the effects of preoperative or postoperative intravenous cimetidine 4 mg/kg or placebo on postoperative pain intensity, sedation score, cumulative morphine consumption, or the incidence of adverse effects.[7]

In contrast, an acutely ill patient with grand mal epilepsy, gastrointestinal bleeding and an intertrochanteric fracture who was undergoing haemodialysis three times a week, was taking cimetidine 300 mg three times daily. After being given the sixth dose of intramuscular morphine (15 mg every 4 hours) he became apnoeic (three breaths per minute), which was managed with naloxone. He remained confused and agitated for the next 80 hours with muscular twitching and further periods of apnoea controlled with naloxone. He had received nine 10-mg intramuscular doses of morphine on a previous occasion in the absence of cimetidine without problems. About a month later he experienced the same adverse reactions when given opium alkaloids while still taking cimetidine (see below).[8] Apnoea has also been reported in a patient receiving morphine, methadone and cimetidine, see (c) above.

2. Ranitidine. A man with terminal cancer receiving intravenous ranitidine 150 mg every 8 hours became confused, disorientated and agitated when given the ranitidine after an intravenous infusion of morphine 50 mg daily was started. When the ranitidine was stopped his mental state improved but worsened when he was given ranitidine again 8 hours and 16 hours later. He again improved when the ranitidine was stopped.[9]

Similarly, another report describes hallucinations in a patient receiving ranitidine and sustained-release morphine followed by rectal methadone, but the author discounted the possibility of an interaction.[10]

(e) Opium alkaloids, mixed

A patient taking **cimetidine** 150 mg twice daily developed apnoea, confusion, and muscle twitching after receiving 7 doses of intramuscular *Pantopon* (hydrochlorides of mixed opium alkaloids) postoperatively. He required 4 doses of naloxone over the next 24 hours.[8]

(f) Pethidine (Meperidine)

Cimetidine 600 mg twice daily for one week reduced the total body clearance of a single 70-mg intravenous dose of pethidine in 8 healthy subjects by a modest 22%.[11] In a similar study by the same research group, **ranitidine** 150 mg twice daily had no effect on pethidine pharmacokinetics.[12]

(g) Tramadol

In an unpublished study on file with the manufacturers, **cimetidine** increased the AUC of tramadol by 15% to 27% and decreased the total body clearance by 14% to 22% in healthy subjects.[13] The manufacturers say that these changes are not clinically significant.[14,15]

Mechanism

Cimetidine inhibits the activity of the liver enzymes concerned with the *N*-demethylation of methadone[3] and pethidine,[11,12] reducing their metabolism, so they accumulate in the body, thereby exaggerating their respiratory depressant effects. A reduction in liver function might possibly have contributed towards, or even been largely responsible for the cases with methadone, because both patients were elderly.

The isolated cases of possible interactions between morphine and H_2-receptor antagonists remain unexplained.[8,9] *In vitro* studies have shown that the conjugation of morphine is not affected by cimetidine or ranitidine,[16] although one study in 8 healthy subjects suggested that ranitidine might slightly increase the bioavailability of morphine.[17]

Importance and management

The virtual absence of a generally important interaction between morphine and cimetidine is adequately documented. Concurrent use normally causes only a slight and normally unimportant prolongation of the respiratory depression due to morphine, but it might possibly have some importance in patients with pre-existing respiratory disorders. One manufacturer warns that cimetidine may inhibit the metabolism of morphine[18] and another warns that, because of the isolated report (see (d) above), patients should be monitored for increased respiratory and CNS depression.[19] *In vitro* evidence suggests that ranitidine is unlikely to interact with morphine,[8] although one pharmacokinetic study indicated that ranitidine might cause a slight increase in morphine levels.[17]

Information about the interaction between pethidine and cimetidine is very limited, and its clinical importance is uncertain, but probably small given the minor changes in pharmacokinetics. However, some manufacturers warn that cimetidine may inhibit the metabolism of pethidine[20,21] and thus caution should be used with concurrent use.[21] Ranitidine has been shown not to affect the pharmacokinetics of pethidine.

It also seems doubtful if the interaction between methadone and cimetidine is of any general importance when the two isolated reports cited here are viewed against the background of the widespread use of both of these two drugs for a good number of years and the lack of other published adverse reports. However, some manufacturers warn that methadone clearance may be decreased when it is given with drugs that inhibit CYP3A4 activity including cimetidine.[22,23] There is no clinically important pharmacokinetic interaction between intranasal butorphanol and oral cimetidine, between hydromorphone and H_2-receptor antagonists, or between tramadol and cimetidine. Consider also 'Opioids; Fentanyl and related drugs + H_2-receptor antagonists', p.172.

1. Shyu WC, Barbhaiya RH. Lack of pharmacokinetic interaction between butorphanol nasal spray and cimetidine. *Br J Clin Pharmacol* (1996) 42, 513–17.
2. Palladone (Hydromorphone hydrochloride). Purdue Pharma L.P. US Prescribing information, November 2004.
3. Dawson GW, Vestal RE. Cimetidine inhibits the *in vitro* N-demethylation of methadone. *Res Commun Chem Pathol Pharmacol* (1984) 46, 301–4.
4. Sorkin EM, Ogawa GS. Cimetidine potentiation of narcotic action. *Drug Intell Clin Pharm* (1983) 17, 60–1.
5. Mojaverian P, Fedder IL, Vlasses PH, Rotmensch HH, Rocci ML, Swanson BN, Ferguson RK. Cimetidine does not alter morphine disposition in man. *Br J Clin Pharmacol* (1982) 14, 809–13.
6. Lam AM, Clement JL. Effect of cimetidine premedication on morphine-induced ventilatory depression. *Can Anaesth Soc J* (1984) 31, 36–43.
7. Chia Y-Y, Chiang H-L, Liu K, Ko N-H. Randomized, double-blind study comparing postoperative effects of treatment timing with histamine H_2-receptor antagonist cimetidine. *Acta Anaesthesiol Scand* (2005) 49, 865–9.
8. Fine A, Churchill DN. Potentially lethal interaction of cimetidine and morphine. *Can Med Assoc J* (1981) 124, 1434–6.

9. Martinez-Abad M, Delgado Gomis F, Ferrer JM, Morales-Olivas FJ. Ranitidine-induced confusion with concomitant morphine. *Drug Intell Clin Pharm* (1988) 22, 914–5.
10. Jellema JG. Hallucination during sustained-release morphine and methadone administration. *Lancet* (1987) ii, 392.
11. Guay DRP, Meatherall RC, Chalmers JL, Grahame GR. Cimetidine alters pethidine disposition in man. *Br J Clin Pharmacol* (1984) 18, 907–14.
12. Guay DRP, Meatherall RC, Chalmers JL, Grahame GR, Hudson RJ. Ranitidine does not alter pethidine disposition in man. *Br J Clin Pharmacol* (1985) 20, 55–9.
13. Data on file. Cited in: Raffa RB, Nayak RK, Liao S, Minn FL. The mechanism(s) of action and pharmacokinetics of tramadol hydrochloride. *Rev Contemp Pharmacother* (1995) 6, 485–97.
14. Zydol XL (Tramadol hydrochloride). Grünenthal Ltd. UK Summary of product characteristics, December 2005.
15. Ultram ER (Tramadol hydrochloride). Ortho-McNeil Pharmaceutical, Inc. US Prescribing information, December 2006.
16. Knodell RG, Holtzman JL, Crankshaw DL, Steele NM, Stanley LN. Drug metabolism by rat and human hepatic microsomes in response to interaction with H_2-receptor antagonists. *Gastroenterology* (1982) 82, 84–8.
17. Aasmundstad TA, Størset P. Influence of ranitidine on the morphine-3-glucuronide to morphine-6-glucuronide ratio after oral administration of morphine in humans. *Hum Exp Toxicol* (1998) 17, 347–52.
18. Morphgesic SR (Morphine sulfate). Amdipharm. UK Summary of product characteristics, January 2003.
19. Avinza (Morphine sulfate extended-release capsules). King Pharmaceuticals, Inc. US Prescribing information, October 2006.
20. Pethidine Injection (Pethidine hydrochloride). Wockhardt UK Ltd. UK Summary of product characteristics, March 2005.
21. Demerol (Meperidine hydrochloride). Sanofi-Aventis US LLC. US Prescribing information, July 2007.
22. Methadone Injection (Methadone hydrochloride). Rosemont Pharmaceuticals Ltd. UK Summary of product characteristics, January 2005.
23. Methadone Injection (Methadone hydrochloride). Wockhardt UK Ltd. UK Summary of product characteristics, April 2000.

Opioids; Fentanyl and related drugs + H_2-receptor antagonists

Cimetidine, but not ranitidine, increases the plasma levels of alfentanil. Some preliminary observations suggest that the effects of fentanyl may be increased by cimetidine.

Clinical evidence, mechanism, importance and management

(a) Alfentanil

In a pharmacokinetic study in 19 intensive care patients, intravenous **cimetidine** 1.2 g daily for 2 days was given with a single 125-microgram/kg intravenous dose of alfentanil. When compared with an oral aluminium/magnesium hydroxide antacid or intravenous **ranitidine** 300 mg daily the cimetidine increased the alfentanil half-life by 75 and 61%, respectively, and reduced the clearance by 64 and 54%, respectively. The alfentanil plasma levels were significantly raised by the **cimetidine**, probably because **cimetidine** inhibits the metabolism of the alfentanil.[1] Whether the alfentanil effects are increased to a clinically important extent awaits assessment. However, be alert for increased alfentanil effects because pharmacokinetic changes of this size are known to be clinically important in some patients (see 'macrolides', (p.174) and 'azoles', (p.164)). The manufacturer of alfentanil warns that alfentanil is metabolised mainly by CYP3A4, and therefore inhibitors of this enzyme, including **cimetidine**, could increase the risk of prolonged or delayed respiratory depression. The concurrent use of such drugs requires special patient care and observation; it may be necessary to lower the dose of alfentanil.[2,3]

Ranitidine does not appear to interact.[1]

(b) Fentanyl

The terminal half-life of fentanyl 100 micrograms/kg was reported to be more than doubled, from 155 to 340 minutes, by pretreatment with **cimetidine** (10 mg/kg the night before and 5 mg/kg 90 minutes before the fentanyl dose). This increase in half-life probably occurs because **cimetidine** inhibits the metabolism of fentanyl by the liver, thereby delaying its clearance from the body.[4] The clinical importance of this interaction has not been assessed, but if both drugs are used concurrently, be alert for increased and prolonged fentanyl effects.

1. Kienlen J, Levron J-C, Aubas S, Roustan J-P, du Cailar J. Pharmacokinetics of alfentanil in patients treated with either cimetidine or ranitidine. *Drug Invest* (1993) 6, 257–62.
2. Rapifen (Alfentanil hydrochloride). Janssen-Cilag Ltd. UK Summary of product characteristics, May 2007.
3. Alfenta Injection (Alfentanil hydrochloride). Taylor Pharmaceuticals. US Prescribing information, July 1998.
4. Unpublished data quoted by Maurer PM, Barkowski RR. Drug interactions of clinical significance with opioid analgesics. *Drug Safety* (1993) 8, 30–48.

Opioids + Haloperidol

A patient treated with long-term haloperidol and morphine experienced extrapyramidal symptoms when naloxone was given.

Clinical evidence, mechanism, importance and management

An 18-year-old woman with nasopharyngeal carcinoma who had been treated with long-term haloperidol and **morphine** developed profound extrapyramidal adverse effects during an attempt to reverse an intrathecal morphine overdose with naloxone. It was suggested that long-term morphine treatment might suppress haloperidol-induced extrapyramidal symptoms through its antimuscarinic and dopaminergic effects. Abrupt opioid withdrawal could be potentially hazardous in patients who are also taking haloperidol.[1]

1. Guo S-L, Lin C-J, Huang H-H, Chen L-K, Sun W-Z. Reversal of morphine with naloxone precipitates haloperidol-induced extrapyramidal side effects. *J Pain Symptom Manage* (2006) 31, 391–2.

Opioids + Herbal medicines

St John's wort reduces the plasma concentrations of methadone and withdrawal symptoms may occur. Some herbal teas may contain opioids.

Clinical evidence, mechanism, importance and management

Some herbal preparations may actually contain opioids; the **morphine** content of two herbal teas containing *Papaveris fructus* was found to be 10.4 micrograms/mL and 31.5 micrograms/mL, respectively. Furthermore, **morphine** was detected in the urine of 5 healthy subjects one hour after drinking 2 cups of either of the herbal teas and was maximal at 4 to 6 hours: positive urine samples were detected up to 6 to 9 hours after drinking the teas.[1] Therefore it may be expected that additive CNS depressant effects will occur if teas such as this are taken with other opioid preparations.

In contrast, a study in 4 patients taking **methadone** found that **St John's wort** *(Jarsin)* 900 mg daily for 14 to 47 days decreased methadone plasma concentration-to-dose ratios (indicating decreased methadone levels) by 19 to 60%. Two patients reported symptoms that suggested a withdrawal syndrome.[2] **St John's wort** *(Hypericum perforatum)* is metabolised in the liver and induces the cytochrome P450 enzyme CYP3A4 and P-glycoprotein, and so could affect plasma levels of drugs metabolised in this way including methadone[2] and other natural or some synthetic opioids.[3]

1. Van Thuyne W, Van Eenoo P, Delbeke FT. Urinary concentrations of morphine after the administration of herbal teas containing *Papaveris fructus* in relation to doping analysis. *J Chromatogr B Analyt Technol Biomed Life Sci* (2003) 785, 245–51.
2. Eic-Höchli D, Oppliger R, Powell Golay K, Baumann P, Eap CB. Methadone maintenance treatment and St John's wort. *Pharmacopsychiatry* (2003) 36, 35–7.
3. Kumar NB, Allen K, Bel H. Perioperative herbal supplement use in cancer patients: potential implications and recommendations for presurgical screening. *Cancer Control* (2005) 12, 149–57.

Opioids + Hormonal contraceptives

The clearance of morphine is roughly doubled by combined oral contraceptives. Combined oral contraceptives do not appear to alter the pharmacokinetics of pethidine. The manufacturer of buprenorphine predicts that gestodene may increase plasma levels of buprenorphine.

Clinical evidence, mechanism, importance and management

(a) Buprenorphine

Although no data from clinical studies are available, the manufacturer predicts that inhibitors of the cytochrome P450 isoenzyme CYP3A4 such as **gestodene** may increase exposure levels to buprenorphine and a dose reduction should be considered when initiating treatment.[1] Halving the starting dose of buprenorphine has been suggested for patients taking CYP3A4 inhibitors and receiving buprenorphine as a substitute for opioid dependence.[1] However, the same manufacturer suggests that, since the magnitude of an inhibitory effect is unknown, such drug combinations should be avoided when buprenorphine is used parenterally or sublingually as a strong analgesic.[2,3] Note that, there appear to be no cases or studies reporting interactions where **gestodene** is acting as a CYP3A4 inhibitor.

(b) Morphine

The clearance of intravenous morphine 1 mg and oral morphine 10 mg was increased by 75% and 120%, respectively, in 6 young women taking a combined oral contraceptive.[4] It is suggested that the oestrogen component of the contraceptive increases the activity of the liver enzyme (glucuronyl transferase) concerned with the metabolism of morphine, which results in an increased clearance. This implies that the dosage of morphine would need to be increased to achieve the same degree of analgesia. Whether this is so in practice requires confirmation.

(c) Pethidine (Meperidine)

One early study suggested that 4 of 5 women taking a combined oral contraceptive (**mestranol** with **noretynodrel** or **norethisterone**) excreted more unchanged pethidine in the urine than a control group of 4 women not taking contraceptives, who were found to excrete more of the demethylated metabolite.[5] However a later, well-controlled, comparative study in 24 healthy subjects (8 women taking a combined oral contraceptive containing **ethinylestradiol/norgestrel** 50/500 micrograms, and 8 women and 8 men not taking contraceptives) found no differences between the plasma levels or excretion patterns of pethidine between the three groups.[6] No special precautions appear to be needed if pethidine is given to women taking combined oral contraceptives.

1. Subutex (Buprenorphine hydrochloride). Schering-Plough Ltd. UK Summary of product characteristics, January 2006.
2. Temgesic Injection (Buprenorphine hydrochloride). Schering-Plough Ltd. UK Summary of product characteristics, April 2004.
3. Temgesic Sublingual Tablets (Buprenorphine hydrochloride). Schering-Plough Ltd. UK Summary of product characteristics, April 2004.
4. Watson KJR, Ghabrial H, Mashford ML, Harman PJ, Breen KJ, Desmond PV. The oral contraceptive pill increases morphine clearance but does not increase hepatic blood flow. *Gastroenterology* (1986) 90, 1779.
5. Crawford JS, Rudofsky S. Some alterations in the pattern of drug metabolism associated with pregnancy, oral contraceptives, and the newly-born. *Br J Anaesth* (1966) 38, 446–54.
6. Stambaugh JE, Wainer IW. Drug interactions I: meperidine and combination oral contraceptives. *J Clin Pharmacol* (1975) 15, 46–51.

Opioids + Interferons

Peginterferon alfa does not affect the pharmacokinetics of methadone, but an isolated report describes a patient who relapsed to heroin use following treatment with peginterferon. Methadone maintenance does not appear to affect the pharmacokinetics of peginterferon alfa or the virological response to interferons. Similarly, buprenorphine does not appear to influence the effect of interferon.

Clinical evidence, mechanism, importance and management

A study involving 22 patients with chronic hepatitis C who had been receiving **methadone** maintenance for a least 3 months found that subcutaneous **peginterferon alfa-2a** 180 micrograms once weekly for 4 weeks did not influence the pharmacokinetics of methadone to a clinically significant extent. The pharmacokinetics of **peginterferon alfa-2a** did not appear to be altered by **methadone** when compared with values from other patients.[1] However, a case report describes a patient who stopped taking **methadone** and then relapsed to heroin use approximately 5 months after completing treatment of chronic hepatitis C with **peginterferon** and ribavirin.[2] Although interferon does not appear to affect **methadone** levels pharmacokinetically, patients taking methadone may experience increased cravings while receiving antiviral therapy because the adverse effects may mimic opioid withdrawal symptoms. Craving may also be secondary to mood changes caused by antiviral therapy or be related to the use of needles used to deliver interferon.[2] It may, therefore, be necessary to increase the dose of **methadone** during interferon treatment.[2,3]

Although opioids may possibly facilitate the outbreak of infections through immunomodulating effects on the immune response against a virus, several studies suggest that the use of opioids (**buprenorphine**,[3] **methadone**[3,4]) has no effect on the outcome of treatment with interferons[4-6] (**peginterferon alfa-2b**[4,5]) in heroin addicts with chronic hepatitis C.[3-5]

1. Sulkowski M, Wright T, Rossi S, Arora S, Lamb M, Wang K, Gries J-M, Yalamanchili S. Peginterferon alfa-2a does not alter the pharmacokinetics of methadone in patients with chronic hepatitis C undergoing methadone maintenance therapy. *Clin Pharmacol Ther* (2005) 77, 214–24.
2. Matthews AM, Fireman M, Zucker B, Sobel M, Hauser P. Relapse to opioid use after treatment of chronic hepatitis C with pegylated interferon and ribavirin. *Am J Psychiatry* (2006) 163, 1342–7.
3. Verrando R, Robaeys G, Mathei C, Buntinx F. Methadone and buprenorphine maintenance therapies for patients with hepatitis C virus infected after intravenous drug use. *Acta Gastroenterol Belg* (2005) 68, 81–5.
4. Sergio N, Salvatore T, Gaetano B, Davide P, Claudio I, Massimo L, Barbara M, Giuseppe A, Stefano C, Danila C, Aikaterini T, Luca I, Daniela C, Luciano C. Immune response in addicts with chronic hepatitis C treated with interferon and ribavirine. *J Gastroenterol Hepatol* (2007) 22, 74–9.
5. Mauss S, Berger F, Goelz J, Jacob B, Schmutz G. A prospective controlled study of interferon-based therapy of chronic hepatitis C in patients on methadone maintenance. *Hepatology* (2004) 40, 120–4.
6. Van Thiel DH, Anantharaju A, Creech S. Response to treatment of hepatitis C in individuals with a recent history of intravenous drugs abuse. *Am J Gastroenterol* (2003) 98, 2281–8.

Opioids + Local anaesthetics

Chloroprocaine can reduce the efficacy of epidural morphine and fentanyl analgesia. Bupivacaine may enhance the local anaesthetic effect of fentanyl, but does not appear to affect respiration. Similarly, lidocaine does not appear to increase respiratory depressant effects of morphine. However, two cases of respiratory depression have been reported with lidocaine and opioids. Morphine given as an intravenous bolus does not alter lidocaine serum levels given as a continuous intravenous infusion.

Clinical evidence, mechanism, importance and management

(a) Bupivacaine

A study involving 40 elderly patients undergoing spinal anaesthesia found that bupivacaine 9 mg, with **fentanyl** 20 micrograms reduced the incidence of hypotension compared with bupivacaine 11 mg alone. Respiratory rates were not depressed in either group. The rate of failed spinal block and discomfort was similar in both groups. The addition of the fentanyl allowed a reduction in the minimum dose of bupivacaine to produce an adequate block, and consequently less hypotension.[1]

(b) Chloroprocaine

Two studies[2,3] have found that chloroprocaine decreases the duration of epidural **morphine** analgesia (16 hours for chloroprocaine compared with 24 hours for lidocaine[2]). Another study found that **morphine** requirements after caesarean section were much higher in women who had received chloroprocaine for epidural anaesthesia than in those receiving lidocaine.[4] The authors of one of the studies suggest that chloroprocaine should be avoided if epidural **morphine** is used.[2] Epidural **fentanyl** also appears to be antagonised by chloroprocaine.[5]

(c) Lidocaine

A double-blind study in 10 patients who were receiving continuous lidocaine infusions during suspected myocardial infarction found that a 10-mg intravenous **morphine sulfate** bolus did not significantly alter the steady-state serum levels of lidocaine.[6] In another study, giving lidocaine with extradural **morphine** did not increase the risk of respiratory depression associated with the morphine.[7] However, in one case, respiratory depression occurred within 5 minutes of giving intravenous lidocaine for an episode of ventricular tachycardia in a patient who had previously been given spinal **fentanyl** and **morphine**. Naloxone successfully reversed this.[8] Similarly, respiratory depression occurred in a 3-year-old boy given lidocaine with adrenaline (epinephrine) about 5 minutes after a submucosal injection of the narcotic **alphaprodine**. Again naloxone reversed the respiratory depression.[9]

1. Martyr JW, Stannard KJD, Gillespie G. Spinal-induced hypotension in elderly patients with hip fracture. A comparison of glucose-free bupivacaine with glucose-free bupivacaine and fentanyl. *Anaesth Intensive Care* (2005) 33, 64–8.
2. Eisenach JC, Schlairet TJ, Dobson CE, Hood DH. Effect of prior anesthetic solution on epidural morphine analgesia. *Anesth Analg* (1991) 73, 119–23.
3. Phan CQ, Azar I, Osborn IP, Lear E. The quality of epidural morphine analgesia following epidural anesthesia with chloroprocaine or chloroprocaine mixed with epinephrine for cesarean delivery. *Anesth Analg* (1988) 67, S171.
4. Karambelkar DJ, Ramanathan S. 2-Chloroprocaine antagonism of epidural morphine analgesia. *Acta Anaesthesiol Scand* (1997) 41, 774–8.

5. Coda B, Bausch S, Haas M, Chavkin C. The hypothesis that antagonism of fentanyl analgesia by 2-chloroprocaine is mediated by direct action on opioid receptors. *Reg Anesth* (1997) 22, 43–52.
6. Vacek JL, Wilson DB, Hurwitz A, Gollub SB, Dunn MI. The effect of morphine sulfate on serum lidocaine levels. *Clin Res* (1988) 36, 325A.
7. Saito Y, Sakura S, Kaneko M, Kosaka Y. Interaction of extradural morphine and lignocaine on ventilatory response. *Br J Anaesth* (1995) 75, 394–8.
8. Jensen E, Nader ND. Potentiation of narcosis after intravenous lidocaine in a patient given spinal opioids. *Anesth Analg* (1999) 89, 758–9.
9. Moore PA. Local anesthesia and narcotic drug interaction in pediatric dentistry. *Anesth Prog* (1988) 35, 17.

Opioids + Macrolides

An isolated report describes a marked increase in the effects of dextromoramide, resulting in coma, in a man treated with troleandomycin. Macrolides including troleandomycin and erythromycin are predicted to increase buprenorphine bioavailability. Similarly, the metabolism of hydromorphone is reduced by troleandomycin *in vitro*. Some manufacturers have suggested that the metabolism of methadone and oxycodone may be decreased by these macrolides, but there do not appear to be any clinical reports confirming this.

Clinical evidence, mechanism, importance and management

(a) Buprenorphine

Although no data from clinical studies are available, the manufacturers predict that inhibitors of the cytochrome P450 isoenzyme CYP3A4 such as macrolide antibacterials including **erythromycin**[1] and **troleandomycin**[2-4] may increase the levels of buprenorphine. Some manufacturers recommend close monitoring and possibly a dose reduction;[1] however, it has also been said that, since the magnitude of an inhibitory effect is unknown, such drug combinations should be avoided when buprenorphine is used parenterally or sublingually as an analgesic.[3,4] The manufacturers of buprenorphine for the treatment of opioid addiction suggest using half the dose if potent CYP3A4 inhibitors, such as some macrolides, are given.[2]

(b) Dextromoramide

A man taking dextromoramide developed signs of overdosage (a morphine-like coma, mydriasis and depressed respiration) 3 days after he started to take **troleandomycin** for a dental infection. He recovered when given naloxone. A possible explanation is that the **troleandomycin** reduced the metabolism of the dextromoramide, thereby increasing its serum levels and effects.[5] The general importance of this interaction is uncertain but concurrent use should be well monitored.

(c) Hydromorphone

An *in vitro* study found that the cytochrome P450 isoenzyme subfamily CYP3A, and to a lesser extent the isoenzyme CYP2C9, catalyse hydromorphone *N*-demethylation to norhydromorphone. **Troleandomycin** (an inhibitor of CYP3A) reduced norhydromorphone formation by about 45%.[6] The clinical relevance of this is unknown.

(d) Methadone

A randomised, crossover study in 12 healthy subjects found that **troleandomycin** did not significantly affect oral or intravenous methadone bioavailability. **Troleandomycin** caused only a small reduction in methadone *N*-demethylation after oral methadone, suggesting only a small role for CYP3A4 in human methadone metabolism.[7] However, one manufacturer of methadone warns that its clearance may be decreased if it is given with drugs that inhibit CYP3A4 activity, such as some macrolide antibacterials.[8]

(e) Oxycodone

The UK manufacturer of oxycodone suggests that inhibitors of CYP3A enzymes such as **erythromycin** may inhibit the metabolism of oxycodone,[9] although oxycodone is also metabolised via CYP2D6,[9] which would make a clinically significant interaction seem unlikely.

1. Buprenorphine Hydrochloride Injection. Bedford Laboratories. US Prescribing information, August 2004.
2. Subutex (Buprenorphine hydrochloride). Schering-Plough Ltd. UK Summary of product characteristics, January 2006.
3. Temgesic Injection (Buprenorphine hydrochloride). Schering-Plough Ltd. UK Summary of product characteristics, April 2004.
4. Temgesic Sublingual Tablets (Buprenorphine hydrochloride). Schering-Plough Ltd. UK Summary of product characteristics, April 2004.
5. Carry PV, Ducluzeau R, Jourdan C, Bourrat Ch, Vigneau C, Descotes J. De nouvelles interactions avec les macrolides? *Lyon Med* (1982) 248, 189–90.
6. Benetton SA, Borges VM, Chang TKH, McErlane KM. Role of individual human cytochrome P450 enzymes in the *in vitro* metabolism of hydromorphone. *Xenobiotica* (2004) 34, 335–44.
7. Kharasch ED, Hoffer C, Whittington D, Sheffels P. Role of hepatic and intestinal cytochrome P450 3A and 2B6 in the metabolism, disposition, and miotic effects of methadone. *Clin Pharmacol Ther* (2004) 76, 250–69.
8. Methadone Injection (Methadone hydrochloride). Rosemont Pharmaceuticals Ltd. UK Summary of product characteristics, January 2005.
9. OxyNorm (Oxycodone hydrochloride). Napp Pharmaceuticals Ltd. UK Summary of product characteristics, March 2007.

Opioids; Fentanyl and related drugs + Macrolides

Some patients may experience prolonged and increased alfentanil effects if they are given erythromycin or particularly troleandomycin. Troleandomycin also interacts with fentanyl but to a lesser extent. Erythromycin appears not to interact with sufentanil.

Clinical evidence

(a) Erythromycin

Erythromycin 500 mg twice daily for 7 days increased the mean half-life of **alfentanil** in 6 subjects from 84 to 131 minutes and decreased the clearance by 26%. The two most sensitive subjects had considerable changes with only one day of erythromycin treatment, and overall showed a marked change. The other 4 subjects had only small or moderate changes.[1]

A 32-year old man undergoing exploratory laparotomy was given erythromycin 1 g and neomycin 1 g, both three times daily, on the day before surgery. During the induction and maintenance of anaesthesia he received a total of 20.9 mg of **alfentanil**. An hour after recovery he was found to be unrousable and with a respiratory rate of only 5 breaths per minute. He was successfully treated with naloxone.[2] Another patient given **alfentanil** and erythromycin is said to have developed respiratory arrest during recovery.[3]

In contrast, in 6 healthy subjects erythromycin 500 mg twice daily for 7 days did not to affect the pharmacokinetics of intravenous **sufentanil** 3 micrograms/kg in the 9 hours following administration.[4] Two of the subjects were the same as those who had shown an alfentanil/erythromycin interaction cited above.

(b) Troleandomycin

A study in 9 healthy subjects given troleandomycin 500 mg orally found that the clearance of intravenous **alfentanil** 20 micrograms/kg was reduced by almost 70%, when compared with subjects given placebo.[5] Similar results were found in another study.[6] A further study found that oral troleandomycin (500 mg starting 105 minutes before alfentanil infusion then 250 mg every 6 hours for 3 doses) reduced the clearance of **alfentanil** by 88%.[7] This study found that troleandomycin only reduced intravenous **fentanyl** clearance by 39%. In another study in 12 healthy subjects, peak **fentanyl** concentrations and maximum miosis following oral transmucosal fentanyl 10 micrograms/kg were minimally affected by oral troleandomycin (500 mg given about 3 hours before and 9 hours after the opioid), but fentanyl metabolism, elimination and duration of effects were significantly affected (fentanyl AUC increased by 77%; norfentanyl AUC decreased by 36%; AUC_{0-10} of miosis increased 53%).[8]

Mechanism

Troleandomycin, and to a lesser extent erythromycin, inhibit the cytochrome P450 isoenzyme CYP3A4 in the liver, which is involved in the metabolism of alfentanil, fentanyl and sufentanil. In addition, troleandomycin has been reported to inhibit CYP3A5 as well as CYP3A4 and alfentanil appears to be metabolised by multiple CYP3A enzymes including CYP3A5.[9] Alfentanil is a low-extraction drug cleared mainly by hepatic metabolism,[6] whereas fentanyl and sufentanil are high extraction drugs (see 'Changes in first-pass metabolism', (p.4)) and are therefore less likely to be affected by changes in liver metabolism.[7,10] Alterations in intestinal or hepatic CYP3A activity also appear to have little influence on oral transmucosal fentanyl absorption and onset of effect, however, a significant proportion (approximately 75%) is swallowed and its systemic clearance may be decreased by CYP3A inhibitors.[8,11]

Importance and management

The interactions of alfentanil with erythromycin and troleandomycin appear to be established and clinically important. Alfentanil should be given in reduced amounts or avoided in those who have recently taken either of these drugs.[1] Be alert for evidence of prolonged alfentanil effects and respiratory depression. The interaction appears not to affect all patients given erythromycin. Alternatively, sufentanil in doses of 3 micrograms/kg or less may be used instead, but much larger doses of sufentanil should be given with caution.[4] Fentanyl is another alternative for use with erythromycin, but should probably be used with caution with troleandomycin. Caution is also advised if transmucosal fentanyl is given with CYP3A4 inhibitors including macrolide antibacterials (e.g. **clarithromycin**, erythromycin, troleandomycin) as there may be increased bioavailability of swallowed fentanyl resulting in increased or prolonged opioid effects:[11,12] the patient should be carefully monitored and dosage adjustments made if necessary.[12,13] Consider also 'Opioids + Macrolides', p.174.

1. Bartkowski RR, Goldberg ME, Larijani GE and Boerner T. Inhibition of alfentanil metabolism by erythromycin. *Clin Pharmacol Ther* (1989) 46, 99–102.
2. Bartkowski RR, McDonnell TE. Prolonged alfentanil effect following erythromycin administration. *Anesthesiology* (1990) 73, 566–8.
3. Yate PM, Thomas D, Short TSM, Sebel PS, Morton J. Comparison of infusions of alfentanil or pethidine for sedation of ventilated patients on ITU. *Br J Anaesth* (1986) 58, 1091–9.
4. Bartkowski RR, Goldberg ME, Huffnagle S, Epstein RH. Sufentanil disposition. Is it affected by erythromycin administration? *Anesthesiology* (1993) 78, 260–5.
5. Kharasch ED, Russell M, Mautz D, Thummel KE, Kunze KL, Bowdle A, Cox K. The role of cytochrome P450 3A4 in alfentanil clearance: implications for interindividual variability in disposition and perioperative drug interactions. *Anesthesiology* (1997) 87, 36–50.
6. Kharasch ED, Walker A, Hoffer C, Sheffels P. Intravenous and oral alfentanil as in vivo probes for hepatic and first-pass cytochrome P450 3A activity: non-invasive assessment by use of pupillary miosis. *Clin Pharmacol Ther* (2004) 76, 452–66.
7. Ibrahim AE, Feldman J, Karim A, Kharasch ED. Simultaneous assessment of drug interactions with low- and high-extraction opioids. Application to parecoxib effects on the pharmacokinetics and pharmacodynamics of fentanyl and alfentanil. *Anesthesiology* (2003) 98, 853–61.
8. Kharasch ED, Whittington D, Hoffer C. Influence of hepatic and intestinal cytochrome P4503A activity on the acute disposition and effects of oral transmucosal fentanyl citrate. *Anesthesiology* (2004) 101, 729–37.
9. Klees TM, Sheffels P, Dale O, Kharasch ED. Metabolism of alfentanil by cytochrome P4503A (CYP3A) enzymes. *Drug Metab Dispos* (2005) 33, 303–11.
10. Kharasch ED, Thummel KE. Human alfentanil metabolism by cytochrome P450 3A3/4. An explanation for the interindividual variability in alfentanil clearance? *Anesth Analg* (1993) 76, 1033–9.
11. Actiq (Fentanyl citrate lozenge). Cephalon Ltd. UK Summary of product characteristics, October 2005.
12. Duragesic (Fentanyl transdermal system). Janssen Pharmaceutica Products, L.P. US Prescribing information, April 2007.
13. Matrifen (Fentanyl). Nycomed UK Ltd. UK Summary of product characteristics, June 2007.

Opioids + Magnesium compounds

Magnesium compounds can potentiate opioid analgesia, although some studies have failed to find an effect. Magnesium sulfate may also reduce opioid requirements during anaesthesia.

Clinical evidence, mechanism, importance and management

Several clinical studies have found that magnesium enhances the analgesic effect of opioids, including intrathecal magnesium with intrathecal **fentanyl**,[1] and intravenous magnesium with intravenous **remifentanil**,[2] or intravenous **tramadol**.[3] However, one placebo-controlled study found that perioperative administration of intravenous magnesium sulfate did not decrease postoperative pain and patient-controlled **pethidine** (**meperidine**) consumption following caesarean delivery. Furthermore, intraoperative blood loss appeared to increase.[4] Another study found a similar lack of effect of intravenous magnesium on the amount of **morphine** used postoperatively.[5]

Magnesium sulfate infusion also decreased **sufentanil** requirements for sedation[6] and reduced the drug requirements of propofol, rocuronium and **fentanyl** during anaesthesia.[7] Intrathecal magnesium sulfate prolonged the period of spinal anaesthesia induced by bupivacaine and **fentanyl** without additional adverse effects, but the onset of anaesthesia was also significantly delayed.[8] Magnesium sulfate may also prolong the effects of the 'competitive neuromuscular blockers', (p.125).

Divalent cations appear to be involved in the pain pathway and magnesium sulfate can potentiate the opioid analgesic effect,[6] possibly by antagonism of *N*-methyl-D-aspartate receptor ion channels.[3,6] It has been suggested that as magnesium ions do not easily cross the blood brain barrier, the intrathecal use of magnesium may modulate pain relief via central effects, whereas the intravenous route mainly only affects peripheral mechanisms.[2]

1. Buvanendran A, McCarthy RJ, Kroin JS, Leong W, Perry P, Tuman KJ. Intrathecal magnesium prolongs fentanyl analgesia: a prospective, randomized, controlled trial. *Anesth Analg* (2002) 95, 661–6.
2. Steinlechner B, Dworschak M, Birkenberg B, Grubhofer G, Weigl M, Schiferer A, Lang T, Rajek A. Magnesium moderately decreases remifentanil dosage required for pain management after cardiac surgery. *Br J Anaesth* (2006) 96, 444–9.
3. Ünlügenç H, Gündüz M, Özalevli M, Akman H. A comparative study on the analgesic effect of tramadol, tramadol plus magnesium, and tramadol plus ketamine for postoperative pain management after major abdominal surgery. *Acta Anaesthesiol Scand* (2002) 46, 1025–30.
4. Paech MJ, Magann EF, Doherty DA, Verity LJ, Newnham JP. Does magnesium sulfate reduce the short- and long-term requirements for pain relief after caesarean delivery? A double-blind placebo-controlled trial. *Am J Obstet Gynecol* (2006) 194, 1596–1603.
5. Machowska B, Duda K. [Does intravenous administration of magnesium affect postoperative analgesia?]. *Folia Med Cracov* (2001) 42, 255–62.
6. Memiş D, Turan A, Karamanlioğlu B, Oğuzhan N, Pamukçu Z. Comparison of sufentanil with sufentanil plus magnesium sulphate for sedation in the intensive care unit using bispectral index. *Crit Care* (2003) 7, R123–R128.
7. Gupta K, Vohra V, Sood J. The role of magnesium as an adjuvant during general anaesthesia. *Anaesthesia* (2006) 61, 1058–63.
8. Özalevli M, Cetin TO, Unlugenc H, Guler T, Isik G. The effect of adding intrathecal magnesium sulphate to bupivacaine-fentanyl spinal anaesthesia. *Acta Anaesthesiol Scand* (2005) 49, 1514–19.

Opioids + NRTIs

Zidovudine had no effect on methadone levels in one study, but there is one report of a patient requiring a modest increase in methadone dose after starting zidovudine. Similarly case reports describe patients requiring a modest increase in methadone dose after starting abacavir. Methadone can increase zidovudine serum levels, and reduce levels of abacavir, stavudine, and didanosine from the tablet formulation, but not the enteric-coated capsule preparation. Tenofovir, and a single dose of zidovudine/lamivudine had no effect on methadone pharmacokinetics.

Clinical evidence

(a) Abacavir

Eleven patients given methadone with abacavir had a 23% increase in the rate of methadone clearance but no change in the half-life or renal clearance. In addition, there was a delay, and a 34% decrease in the peak concentration of abacavir, but no change in abacavir clearance or half-life.[1] Of 3 patients taking methadone who started taking abacavir, lamivudine and zidovudine, 2 required methadone dosage increases (31% and 46%, respectively). The abacavir was thought to be responsible for this effect.[2] A patient receiving methadone experienced torsades de pointes when receiving abacavir, lamivudine and zidovudine.[3]

(b) Didanosine

A study in 17 subjects taking methadone found that the AUC and maximum levels of didanosine tablets were 57% and 66% lower, respectively, when compared with 10 control subjects. Trough levels of methadone did not differ from historical controls, suggesting that didanosine had no effect on methadone pharmacokinetics.[4] A later study found that there was no reduction in the AUC of didanosine given as enteric-coated capsules.[5]

(c) Stavudine

A study in 17 subjects taking methadone found that the AUC and maximum levels of stavudine were 23% and 44% lower, respectively, when compared with 10 control subjects. Trough levels of methadone did not differ from historical controls suggesting that stavudine had no effect on methadone pharmacokinetics.[4]

(d) Tenofovir

In a study in 13 healthy subjects receiving methadone, tenofovir 300 mg daily for 2 weeks did not alter the pharmacokinetics of methadone, and no symptoms of opioid toxicity or opioid withdrawal were detected.[6]

(e) Zidovudine

1. Buprenorphine. In one study, there was no difference in the pharmacokinetics of oral zidovudine between patients receiving buprenorphine and control subjects.[7] Buprenorphine is not expected to cause zidovudine toxicity.

2. Methadone effects reduced or unaffected. A drug abuser with AIDS needed an increase in his levomethadone (*R*-methadone) dosage from 40 to 60 mg daily, within a month of starting to take zidovudine 1 g daily.[8]

In contrast, a study found no evidence of any change in the pharmacokinetics of methadone in HIV-positive patients taking methadone 14 days after they started zidovudine 200 mg every 4 hours. No methadone withdrawal symptoms occurred.[9] Another study in 16 patients taking methadone found that a single-dose of a fixed combination of zidovudine 300 mg with lamivudine 150 mg *(Combivir)* had no effect on the pharmacokinetics of methadone, and there was no evidence of withdrawal or toxicity.[10]

3. Zidovudine effects increased. In one study the mean AUC of zidovudine was increased by 43% by methadone, and in 4 of 9 patients it was doubled.[9] In another study, 8 HIV-positive patients starting methadone found a 29% increase in the AUC of oral zidovudine and a 41% increase in the AUC of intravenous zidovudine. Three of the 8 patients stopped zidovudine because of adverse effects or haematologic toxicity.[11] Decreased zidovudine clearance in patients taking methadone is described in another report.[12]

Mechanism

Uncertain. It appears that methadone reduces the bioavailability of didanosine, and to a lesser extent, stavudine, possibly because it delays gastric emptying. Thus, the enteric-coated didanosine preparation appears not to be affected.[4,5] Conversely, methadone apparently reduces the glucuronidation of the zidovudine by the liver, resulting in an increase in its serum levels.[13] Methadone may also reduce renal clearance of zidovudine.[11]

Importance and management

The increase in zidovudine levels with methadone is established, although the clinical relevance is uncertain. Be alert for any increase in zidovudine adverse effects. The balance of evidence suggests that zidovudine is unlikely to reduce methadone levels, and the one case reported remains unexplained, although note that some of the adverse effects of zidovudine may be mistaken for opioid withdrawal effects.

The reduction in didanosine levels with methadone may be clinically relevant, and the authors suggest increasing the dose of the tablet formulation. Monitor virological response. The enteric-coated didanosine preparation is not affected and it may therefore be worth considering using this preparation instead.

The reduction in stavudine levels and the changes in abacavir peak levels with methadone are probably not clinically relevant, but again, further data are required. The reports with abacavir suggest that it would be prudent to monitor methadone dose requirements when this drug is started. Tenofovir does not appear to affect methadone levels.

1. Sellers E, Lam R, McDowell J, Corrigan B, Hedayetullah N, Somer G, Kirby L, Kersey K, Yuen G. The pharmacokinetics of abacavir and methadone following coadministration: CNAA1012. *Intersci Conf Antimicrob Agents Chemother* (1999) 39, 663.
2. Pardo López MA, Cuadrado Pastor JM, Pérez Hervás MP, Fernández Villalba E. Síndrome de abstinencia a opiáceos tras la administración de zidovudina + lamivudina + abacavir en pacientes infectados por el virus de la inmunodeficiencia humana en tratamiento con metadona. *Rev Clin Esp* (2003) 203, 407–8.
3. Anon. Torsades de pointes with methadone. *Prescrire Int* (2005) 14, 61–2.
4. Rainey PM, Friedland G, McCance-Katz EF, Andrews L, Mitchell SM, Charles C, Jatlow P. Interaction of methadone with didanosine and stavudine. *J Acquir Immune Defic Syndr* (2000) 24, 241–8.
5. Friedland G, Rainey P, Jatlow P, Andrews L, Damle B, McCance-Katz E. Pharmacokinetics of didanosine from encapsulated enteric coated bead formulation vs chewable tablet formulation in patients on chronic methadone therapy. XIV International AIDS Conference, Barcelona, 2002. Abstract TuPeB4548.
6. Smith PF, Kearney BP, Liaw S, Cloen D, Bullock JM, Haas CE, Yale K, Booker BM, Berenson CS, Coakley DF, Flaherty JF. Effect of tenofovir disoproxil fumarate on the pharmacokinetics and pharmacodynamics of total, R-, and S-methdone. *Pharmacotherapy* (2004) 24, 970–77.
7. McCance-Katz EF, Rainey PM, Friedland G, Kosten TR, Jatlow P. Effect of opioid dependence pharmacotherapies on zidovudine disposition. *Am J Addict* (2001) 10, 296–307.
8. Brockmeyer NH, Mertins L, Goos M. Pharmacokinetic interaction of antimicrobial agents with levomethadon in drug-addicted AIDS patients. *Klin Wochenschr* (1991) 69, 16–18.
9. Schwartz EL, Brechbühl A-B, Kahl P, Miller MA, Selwyn PA, Friedland GH. Pharmacokinetic interactions of zidovudine and methadone in intravenous drug-using patients with HIV infection. *J Acquir Immune Defic Syndr* (1992) 5, 619–26.
10. Rainey PM, Friedland GH, Snidow JW, McCance-Katz EF, Mitchell SM, Andrews L, Lane B, Jatlow P. The pharmacokinetics of methadone following co-administration with a lamivudine/zidovudine combination tablet in opiate-dependent subjects. *Am J Addict* (2002) 11, 66–74.
11. McCance-Katz EF, Rainey PM, Jatlow P, Friedland G. Methadone effects on zidovudine disposition (AIDS clinical trials group 262). *J Acquir Immune Defic Syndr Hum Retrovirol* (1998) 18, 435–43.
12. Burger DM, Meenhorst PL, ten Napel CHH, Mulder JW, Neef C, Koks CHW, Bult A, Beijnen JH. Pharmacokinetic variability of zidovudine in HIV-infected individuals: subgroup analysis and drug interactions. *AIDS* (1994) 8, 1683–9.
13. Cretton-Scott E, de Sousa G, Nicolas F, Rahmani R, Sommadossi J-P. Methadone and its metabolite N-demethyl methadone, inhibit AZT glucuronidation in vitro. *Clin Pharmacol Ther* (1996) 59, 168.

Opioids; Methadone + NNRTIs

Methadone plasma levels can be markedly reduced by efavirenz or nevirapine and withdrawal symptoms have been seen. In contrast, delavirdine slightly increased methadone levels in one study.

Clinical evidence

(a) Delavirdine

The pharmacokinetics of delavirdine 600 mg twice daily did not differ between 16 HIV-negative subjects taking methadone and 15 healthy control subjects.[1] In another study methadone did not affect delavirdine pharmacokinetics. However, delavirdine decreased methadone clearance and increased its AUC by 19%.[2]

(b) Efavirenz

An HIV-positive woman who had been taking methadone for over a year began to complain of discomfort within 4 weeks of having nelfinavir replaced by efavirenz 600 mg daily, and by 8 weeks typical methadone withdrawal symptoms were occurring late in the afternoon. It was found that the levels of *R*-methadone (the active enantiomer) had fallen from 168 to 90 nanograms/mL, and those of the *S*-methadone from 100 to 28 nanograms/mL. The methadone dosage had to be increased from 100 mg to 180 mg daily before the symptoms disappeared.[3] A further case is reported in which a man taking methadone stopped taking efavirenz 600 mg daily because of the occurrence of withdrawal symptoms in spite of increased methadone dosage.[4] Another report describes a man who required a 133% increase in his methadone dose over 4 weeks after starting efavirenz, and mentions two other patients who complained of opioid withdrawal shortly after starting efavirenz. They also required methadone dose increases.[5]

In a pharmacokinetic study, 11 patients taking methadone 35 to 100 mg daily were given efavirenz with two nucleoside analogues. Nine of the patients developed methadone withdrawal symptoms and needed dose increases of 15 to 30 mg (mean 22%). A pharmacokinetic study of these patients found that 3 weeks after starting efavirenz their mean methadone AUCs were reduced by 57% and their maximum plasma levels by 48%.[6] Similar results were found in another study in 5 HIV-positive patients taking methadone: 4 patients experienced opioid withdrawal symptoms and a mean methadone dose increase of 52% was required.[7] In another retrospective study, 6 out of 7 patients needed methadone dosage increases of 8% to 200% within 2 weeks to 8 months of starting an efavirenz-based regimen.[8]

(c) Nevirapine

A retrospective review revealed 7 cases of patients taking methadone who developed withdrawal symptoms after starting regimens including nevirapine. The symptoms developed within 4 to 8 days, and methadone dose increases of 21% to 186% were required. Despite this, 3 patients did not respond. They elected to discontinue nevirapine, and in 2 of them somnolence developed within 2 weeks, so the methadone dosage was reduced. Methadone plasma levels were available in 2 patients, and these suggested that nevirapine decreased methadone levels by about 90%.[9] In a pilot study of a once daily nevirapine-containing regimen, 30% of patients required an increase in methadone dosage.[10] In another study 4 of 5 patients taking methadone developed withdrawal symptoms on starting nevirapine-containing regimens and 2 refused further nevirapine, despite increasing their methadone dose. Another 2 patients were successfully treated with increases in their methadone doses of 33% and 100%.[11] Three other similar cases have been reported.[4,12,13]

In a pharmacokinetic study, 8 patients taking methadone 30 to 120 mg daily had methadone levels measured before and 14 days after starting an antiretroviral regimen including nevirapine 200 mg daily. The methadone AUC decreased by 52%, and the maximum level by 36%. Six patients complained of symptoms of methadone withdrawal, and required a mean increase in methadone dose of 16%.[14]

Mechanism

Efavirenz and nevirapine induce the metabolism of methadone (possibly by the cytochrome P450 isoenzyme CYP3A4, or CYP2B6[15]), which results in reduced levels and effects. In contrast, delavirdine is an inhibitor of various cytochrome P450 isoenzymes, and might therefore be expected to inhibit the metabolism of methadone, although the effects appear small.

Importance and management

The interaction between methadone and efavirenz or nevirapine is established and of clinical importance. Some authors have found that the dosage increase required is much less than that predicted based on the reduction in methadone levels,[6,14] whereas others have questioned this.[5,16] It may be important not to confuse the adverse effects of the NNRTIs with withdrawal symptoms.[6] It has been suggested that patients taking methadone who are given these drugs should be screened for opioid withdrawal beginning on the fourth day of the new medication. If symptoms develop, the methadone dose should be increased by 10 mg every 2 to 3 days until symptoms abate.[17] However, others have suggested dose increments should be made at one-week intervals to avoid overdose, as methadone has a long half-life (reported to range form 13 to 47 hours).[18] Note that some patients may require an increase in methadone dose frequency to twice daily.[11] If efavirenz or nevirapine is stopped, the methadone dose should be gradually reduced to pretreatment levels over the course of 1 to 2 weeks.[17]

The US manufacturers of delavirdine[19] suggest that the methadone dose may need to be reduced; however, the effects in the study reported are small, and would not be expected to be of clinical significance.

1. Booker B, Smith P, Forrest A, DiFrancesco R, Morse G, Cottone P, Murphy M, McCance-Katz E. Lack of effect of methadone on the pharmacokinetics of delavirdine & N-delavirdine. *Intersci Conf Antimicrob Agents Chemother* (2001) 41, 14.
2. McCance-Katz EF, Rainey PM, Smith P, Morse GD, Friedland G, Boyarsky B, Gourevitch M, Jatlow P. Drug interactions between opioids and antiretroviral medications: interaction between methadone, LAAM, and delavirdine. *Am J Addict* (2006) 15, 23–34.
3. Marzolini C, Troillet N, Telenti A, Baumann P, Decosterd LA, Eap CB. Efavirenz decreases methadone blood concentrations. *AIDS* (2000) 14, 1291–2.
4. Pinzani V, Faucherre V, Peyriere H, Blayac J-P. Methadone withdrawal symptoms with nevirapine and efavirenz. *Ann Pharmacother* (2000) 34, 405–7.
5. Boffito M, Rossati A, Reynolds HE, Hoggard PG, Back DJ, di Perri G. Undefined duration of opiate withdrawal induced by efavirenz in drug users with HIV infection and undergoing chronic methadone treatment. *AIDS Res Hum Retroviruses* (2002) 18, 341–2.
6. Clarke SM, Mulcahy FM, Tjia J, Reynolds HE, Gibbons SE, Barry MG, Back DJ. The pharmacokinetics of methadone in HIV-positive patients receiving the non-nucleoside reverse transcriptase inhibitor efavirenz. *Br J Clin Pharmacol* (2001) 51, 213–7.
7. McCance-Katz EF, Gourevitch MN, Arnsten J, Sarlo J, Rainey P, Jatlow P. Modified directly observed therapy (MDOT) for injection drug users with HIV disease. *Am J Addict* (2002) 11, 271–8.
8. Tashima K, Bose T, Gormley J, Sousa H, Flanigan TP. The potential impact of efavirenz on methadone maintenance. Poster presented at 9th European Conference on Clinical Microbiology and Infectious Diseases, Berlin, March 23rd 1999 (Poster PO552).
9. Altice FL, Friedland GH, Cooney EL. Nevirapine induced opiate withdrawal among injection drug users with HIV infection receiving methadone. *AIDS* (1999) 13, 957–62.
10. Staszewski S, Haberl A, Gute P, Nisius G, Miller V, Carlebach A. Nevirapine/didanosine/lamivudine once daily in HIV-1-infected intravenous drug users. *Antivir Ther* (1998) 3 (Suppl 4), 55–6.
11. Otero M-J, Fuertes A, Sánchez R, Luna G. Nevirapine-induced withdrawal symptoms in HIV patients on methadone maintenance programme: an alert. *AIDS* (1999) 13, 1004–5.
12. Heelon MW, Meade LB. Methadone withdrawal when starting an antiretroviral regimen including nevirapine. *Pharmacotherapy* (1999) 19, 471–2.
13. de la Cruz Pellin M, Esteban J, Gimeno C, Mora E. Interacción entre metadona y antirretrovirales (estavudina, indinavir, ritonavir, nevirapina). *Med Clin (Barc)* (2003) 121, 439.
14. Clarke SM, Mulcahy FM, Tjia J, Reynolds HE, Gibbons SE, Barry MG, Back DJ. Pharmacokinetic interactions of nevirapine and methadone and guidelines for use of nevirapine to treat injection drug users. *Clin Infect Dis* (2001) 33, 1595–7.
15. Gerber JG, Rhodes RJ, Gal J. Stereoselective metabolism of methadone N-demethylation by cytochrome P4502B6 and 2C19. *Chirality* (2004) 16, 36–44.
16. Calvo R, Lukas JC, Rodriguez M, Carlos MA, Suarez E. Pharmacokinetics of methadone in HIV-positive patients receiving the non-nucleoside reverse transcriptase efavirenz. *Br J Clin Pharmacol* (2002) 53, 212–14.
17. Bruce RD, Altice FL, Gourevitch MN, Friedland GH. Pharmacokinetic drug interactions between opioid agonist therapy and antiretroviral medications: implications and management for clinical practice. *J Acquir Immune Defic Syndr* (2006) 41, 563–72.
18. Anon. Torsades de pointes with methadone. *Prescrire Int* (2005) 14, 61–2.
19. Rescriptor (Delavirdine mesylate). Pfizer Inc. US Prescribing information, June 2006.

Opioids; Buprenorphine + NNRTIs

Preliminary evidence suggests that buprenorphine does not affect the antiretroviral efficacy or pharmacokinetics of delavirdine and efavirenz. Delavirdine may increase buprenorphine plasma levels and efavirenz may decrease buprenorphine levels, but the clinical significance has not been fully investigated. Delavirdine given with buprenorphine/naloxone has been shown to slightly prolong the QT interval.

Clinical evidence

A study in 20 opioid-dependent subjects taking **buprenorphine** with naloxone found that **efavirenz** 600 mg daily for 15 days decreased the AUC of buprenorphine and its metabolite, norbuprenorphine, by approximately 50% and 71%, respectively. **Delavirdine** 600 mg twice daily for 7 days caused a greater than fourfold increase in the buprenorphine AUC, but norbuprenorphine AUC was decreased by about 60%.[1] In this study buprenorphine did not alter the pharmacokinetics of **delavirdine** or **efavirenz**.[1]

In a study in 50 opioid-dependent patients treated with sublingual buprenorphine/naloxone alone for at least 2 weeks and then additionally given an antiretroviral agent (**delavirdine**, **efavirenz**, **nelfinavir**, **lopinavir/ritonavir**, or **ritonavir**) for 5 to 15 days investigated the effect of these drugs on QT interval. Buprenorphine/naloxone alone did not significantly alter the QT interval; however, when delavirdine and efavirenz were given there was a statistically, but probably not clinically, significant increase in the QT interval. The greatest increase in QTc intervals were seen in patients taking **delavirdine** 600 mg twice daily.[2]

Mechanism

Buprenorphine is a substrate for the cytochrome P450 isoenzyme CYP3A4 and inducers of CYP3A enzymes such as **efavirenz** would be expected to increase buprenorphine clearance, whereas **delavirdine**, which is an inhibitor of CYP3A, would be expected to reduce the CYP3A-mediated metabolism of buprenorphine to norbuprenorphine.

Importance and management

Despite the magnitude of the changes in buprenorphine levels seen with efavirenz and delavirdine, clinically significant consequences of these interactions (opioid withdrawal symptoms, cognitive effects and adverse effects) were not observed and it was suggested that dosage adjustments were not likely to be necessary.[1] However, the study was in HIV-negative subjects and it has been suggested that the interaction may be of significance in HIV-positive individuals.[3] More clinical studies in HIV-positive patients are needed. Furthermore, the study showing QT-prolongation with these NNRTIs and buprenorphine suggest that some caution would be prudent.

The manufacturers predict that inhibitors of the cytochrome P450 isoenzyme CYP3A4 [such as delavirdine] may increase the exposure to buprenorphine.[4-7] One manufacturer recommends close monitoring and possibly a dose reduction;[7] halving the starting dose of buprenorphine has been suggested by another manufacturer for patients taking CYP3A4 inhibitors and receiving buprenorphine as a substitute for opioid dependence.[4] However, the same manufacturer suggests that, since the magnitude of an inhibitory effect is unknown, such drug combinations should be avoided when buprenorphine is used parenterally or sublingually as a strong analgesic.[5,6]

1. McCance-Katz EF, Moody DE, Morse GD, Friedland G, Pade P, Baker J, Alvanzo A, Smith P, Ogundele A, Jatlow P, Rainey PM. Interactions between buprenorphine and antiretrovirals. I: The nonnucleoside reverse-transcriptase inhibitors efavirenz and delavirdine. *Clin Infect Dis* (2006) 43 (Suppl 4), S224– S234.
2. Baker JR, Best AM, Pade PA, McCance-Katz EF. Effect of buprenorphine and antiretroviral agents on the QT interval in opioid-dependent patients. *Ann Pharmacother* (2006) 40, 392–6.
3. Bruce RD, McCance-Katz E, Kharasch ED, Moody DE, Morse GD. Pharmacokinetic interactions between buprenorphine and antiretroviral medications. *Clin Infect Dis* (2006) 43 (Suppl 4), S216–S223.
4. Subutex (Buprenorphine hydrochloride). Schering-Plough Ltd. UK Summary of product characteristics, January 2006.
5. Temgesic Injection (Buprenorphine hydrochloride). Schering-Plough Ltd. UK Summary of product characteristics, April 2004.
6. Temgesic Sublingual Tablets (Buprenorphine hydrochloride). Schering-Plough Ltd. UK Summary of product characteristics, April 2004.
7. Buprenorphine Hydrochloride Injection. Bedford Laboratories. US Prescribing information, August 2004.

Opioids + NSAIDs

Ketoprofen reduced morphine-associated respiratory depression, and did not alter morphine pharmacokinetics. Similarly, diclofenac did not alter morphine pharmacokinetics in one study. Improved pain relief and reduced adverse effects have been found when morphine was given with lornoxicam, ketoprofen, or ketorolac. However, in another, diclofenac slightly increased respiratory depression despite reducing morphine use, possibly because of persistent levels of an active metabolite of morphine. Diclofenac did not affect the pharmacokinetics or analgesic effects of codeine in healthy subjects. Intramuscular diclofenac did not affect the pharmacokinetics of methadone solution in cancer patients. Ibuprofen did not appear to interact

pharmacokinetically with oxycodone. No pharmacokinetic interaction occurred between meclofenamate and dextropropoxyphene, and dextropropoxyphene did not alter sulindac plasma levels. A single case report describes marked respiratory depression in a man given buprenorphine when ketorolac was added. An isolated report describes grand mal seizures in a patient given diclofenac and pentazocine. For mention of other NSAIDs see 'coxibs', (p.179).

Clinical evidence, mechanism, importance and management

NSAIDs are often administered with opioids because they usually reduce the opioid requirements and some of the opioid-induced adverse effects.[1]

Enhanced pain relief has been reported with various combinations including **dextromethorphan** with **ketorolac**[2] or **tenoxicam,**[3] **oxycodone** with **ibuprofen,**[4] and **tramadol** with **ketorolac**[5] without increased adverse effects. See also 'coxibs', (p.179). However, cases of respiratory depression have been reported, see *Morphine* below. Myoclonus has been reported with high does of morphine administered with NSAIDs, see 'Opioids; Morphine + Miscellaneous', p.190.

(a) Buprenorphine

A man underwent thoracotomy for carcinoma of the middle third of his oesophagus. An hour after transfer to the recovery ward he complained of severe pain at the operative site and was given epidural buprenorphine 150 micrograms (3 micrograms/kg), and 2 hours later intramuscular **ketorolac** 30 mg because of continued pain. During the next hour he became more drowsy, stopped obeying commands and his respiratory rate dropped to 6 breaths per minute. He recovered after 6 hours of mechanical ventilation. The authors of this report suggest that it may be necessary to use less buprenorphine in the presence of ketorolac to avoid the development of these respiratory depressant effects.[6] This appears to be the only report of this possible interaction.

As with other opioids, NSAIDs such as **etodolac** have been used with buprenorphine to reduce the postoperative pain score without increasing side effects.[7]

(b) Codeine

A single 50-mg dose of **diclofenac sodium** did not have an important effect on the pharmacokinetics of a single 100-mg dose of codeine phosphate in a placebo-controlled crossover study in 12 healthy subjects. There was no effect on the metabolic clearance of morphine, and only a slight (about 5% to 10%) increase in the levels of glucuronide metabolites. In addition, **diclofenac** did not alter the analgesic effects of codeine as assessed in a cold pressor test (a test in which opioids, but not NSAIDs, are effective).[8]

These findings are in contrast to an earlier *in vitro* study by the same research group, which found that **diclofenac** markedly inhibited the glucuronidation of codeine in human liver tissue.[9]

Although this interaction perhaps requires confirmation in a multiple-dose study in a clinical setting, the findings in healthy subjects suggest that no special precautions are required during the concurrent use of **diclofenac** and codeine.

Single oral-dose studies in 24 healthy subjects showed that the bioavailability of both codeine phosphate 25 mg and **ibuprofen** 200 mg were unaffected by concurrent use.[10]

(c) Dextropropoxyphene (Propoxyphene)

In healthy subjects dextropropoxyphene 260 mg daily and **sodium meclofenamate** 400 mg daily for a week was found to have no effect on the plasma levels of either drug.[11]

The manufacturer of **sulindac** notes that dextropropoxyphene had no effect on the plasma levels of **sulindac** or its sulfide metabolite.[12]

(d) Methadone

Intramuscular **diclofenac** 75 mg twice daily given for 5 days with oral methadone solution every 8 hours had no effect on the AUC or maximum plasma levels of methadone in 16 patients with cancer pain.[13] No special precautions would appear to be necessary during concurrent use.

(e) Morphine

An infusion of **ketoprofen** 1.5 mg/kg with morphine 100 micrograms/kg reduced the respiratory depression associated with morphine alone in 11 healthy subjects. There was no change in plasma morphine levels.[14] Another study in 6 patients found that intramuscular **diclofenac** 75 mg twice daily for 5 days did not affect the half-life and AUC of oral morphine solution.[15] Other studies have reported superior pain relief with morphine and NSAIDs e.g. **lornoxicam,**[2] **ketoprofen,**[16] and **ketorolac,**[17]with fewer adverse effects. See also 'coxibs', (p.179).

However, in contrast to these reports, a study in 7 patients on the first postoperative day after spinal surgery found that, although **diclofenac** 100 mg rectally reduced patient-controlled morphine consumption by 20%, respiratory rates were significantly lower after the **diclofenac**, and minimal at about 200 minutes. Levels of an active metabolite, morphine-6-glucuronide did not significantly decrease until 420 minutes.[18]

NSAIDs are frequently used with opioids because of their lack of respiratory depression and opioid-sparing effects. However, this study demonstrates that there may be a risk of respiratory depression and other adverse effects due to persistently high levels of morphine-6-glucuronide for a number of hours after receiving an NSAID. During this time period, patients should be more closely monitored.[18]

For mention of the suggestion that NSAIDs may increase the incidence of myoclonus with high-dose morphine, see 'Opioids; Morphine + Miscellaneous', p.190.

(f) Oxycodone

A study involving 23 healthy subjects found that the single-dose pharmacokinetics of **ibuprofen** 400 mg and oxycodone 5 mg were similar when given as monotherapy or in combination.[19]

(g) Pentazocine

A man with Buerger's disease had a grand mal seizure while watching television 2 hours after being given a single 50-mg suppository of **diclofenac**. He was also taking pentazocine 50 mg three times daily. He may possibly have had a previous seizure some months before after taking a single 100-mg slow-release **diclofenac** tablet.[8] The reasons for this reaction are not known, but on rare occasions **diclofenac** alone has been associated with seizures (incidence said to be 1 in 100 000) and seizures have also been seen with pentazocine alone. It is not clear what part the disease itself, or watching television, had in the development of this adverse reaction.[20]

No interaction between **diclofenac** and pentazocine is established, but be aware of this case if concurrent use is being considered, particularly in patients who are known to be seizure-prone.

1. Kehlet H. Postoperative opioid sparing to hasten recovery: what are the issues? *Anesthesiology* (2005) 102, 1083–5.
2. Lu C-H, Liu J-Y, Lee M-S, Borel CO, Yeh C-C, Wong C-S, Wu C-T. Preoperative cotreatment with dextromethorphan and ketorolac provides an enhancement of pain relief after laparoscopic-assisted vaginal hysterectomy. *Clin J Pain* (2006) 22, 799–804.
3. Yeh C-C, Wu C-T, Lee M-S, Yu J-C, Yang C-P, Lu C-H, Wong C-S. Analgesic effects of preincisional administration of dextromethorphan and tenoxicam following laparoscopic cholecystectomy. *Acta Anaesthesiol Scand* (2004) 48, 1049–53.
4. Oldfield V, Perry CM. Oxycodone/ibuprofen combination tablet: a review of its use in the management of acute pain. *Drugs* (2005) 65, 2337–54.
5. Lepri A, Sia S, Catinelli S, Casali R, Novelli G. Patient-controlled analgesia with tramadol *versus* tramadol plus ketorolac. *Minerva Anestesiol* (2006) 72, 59–67.
6. Jain PN, Shah SC. Respiratory depression following combination of epidural buprenorphine and intramuscular ketorolac. *Anaesthesia* (1993) 48, 898–9.
7. Koizuka S, Saito S, Obata H, Sasaki M, Nishikawa K, Takahashi K, Saito Y, Goto F. Oral etodolac, a COX-2 inhibitor, reduces postoperative pain immediately after fast-track cardiac surgery. *J Anesth* (2004) 18, 9–13.
8. Ammon S, Marx C, Behrens C, Hofmann U, Mürdter T, Griese E-U, Mikus G. Diclofenac does not interact with codeine metabolism in vivo: a study in healthy volunteers. *BMC Clin Pharmacol* (2002) 2, 2.
9. Ammon S, von Richter O, Hofmann U, Thon KP, Eichelbaum M, Mikus G. In vitro interaction of codeine and diclofenac. *Drug Metab Dispos* (2000) 28, 1149–52.
10. Laneury JP, Duchene P, Hirt P, Delarue A, Gleizes S, Houin G, Molinier P. Comparative bioavailability study of codeine and ibuprofen after administration of the two products alone or in association to 24 healthy volunteers. Eur J Drug Metab Pharmacokinet. (1998) 23, 185–9.
11. Baragar FD, Smith TC. Drug interaction studies with sodium meclofenamate (Meclomen®). *Curr Ther Res* (1978) 23 (April Suppl), S51–S59.
12. Clinoril (Sulindac). Merck Sharp & Dohme Ltd. UK Summary of product characteristics, May 2007.
13. Bianchi M, Clavenna A, Groff L, Zecca E, Ripamonti C. Diclofenac dose not modify methadone bioavailability in cancer patients. *J Pain Symptom Manage* (1999) 17, 227–9.
14. Moren J, Francois T, Blanloeil Y, Pinaud M. The effects of a nonsteroidal antiinflammatory drug (ketoprofen) on morphine respiratory depression: a double-blind, randomized study in volunteers. *Anesth Analg* (1997) 85, 400–5.
15. De Conno F, Ripamonti C, Bianchi M, Ventafridda V, Panerai AE. Diclofenac does not modify morphine bioavailability in cancer patients. *Pain* (1992) 48, 401–2.
16. Karaman S, Gunusen I, Uyar M, Firat V. The effect of pre-operative lornoxicam and ketoprofen application on the morphine consumption of post-operative patient-controlled analgesia. *J Int Med Res* (2006) 34, 168–75.
17. Safdar B, Dequtis LC, Landry K, Vedere SR, Moscovitz HC, D'Onofrio G. Intravenous morphine plus ketorolac is superior to either drug alone for treatment of acute renal colic. *Ann Emerg Med* (2006) 48, 173–81.

18. Tighe KE, Webb AM, Hobbs GJ. Persistently high plasma morphine-6-glucuronide levels despite decreased hourly patient-controlled analgesia morphine use after single-dose diclofenac: potential for opioid-related toxicity. *Anesth Analg* (1999) 88, 1137–42.

19. Kapil R, Nolting A, Roy P, Fiske W, Benedek I, Abramowitz W. Pharmacokinetic properties of combination oxycodone plus racemic ibuprofen: two randomized, open-label, crossover studies in healthy adult volunteers. *Clin Ther* (2004) 26, 2015–25.

20. Heim M, Nadvorna H, Azaria M. With comments by Straughan J and Hoehler HW. Grand mal seizures following treatment with diclofenac and pentazocine. *S Afr Med J* (1990) 78, 700–1.

Opioids + NSAIDs; Coxibs

Parecoxib had no effect on the pharmacokinetics of alfentanil or fentanyl, and celecoxib and rofecoxib appeared not to affect the pharmacokinetics of tramadol. Coxibs can reduce the perioperative opioid requirement, but adverse effects are not necessarily reduced.

Clinical evidence, mechanism, importance and management

(a) Pharmacokinetic studies

In a crossover study in 12 healthy subjects intravenous **parecoxib** 40 mg, given one hour before and 12 hours after an infusion of **alfentanil** 15 micrograms/kg or **fentanyl** 5 micrograms/kg, had no effect on the pharmacokinetics of these opioids.[1] Pupil diameter versus time curves were not affected by **parecoxib**. This interaction was investigated because both valdecoxib (the main metabolite of **parecoxib**) and **alfentanil** are substrates of the cytochrome P450 isoenzyme CYP3A4. The study suggests there should be no interaction during concurrent use. In a study in patients receiving stable doses of **celecoxib** or **rofecoxib**, the pharmacokinetics of **tramadol** (given with paracetamol) did not appear to be affected by the coxibs. **Tramadol** is metabolised by CYP2D6 and CYP3A4, but there appeared to be no difference in the clearance of tramadol given with **celecoxib** (potential to interact with CYP2D6 substrates and is itself metabolised in part by CYP3A4).[2]

(b) Pharmacodynamic studies

Many studies have reported reduced opioid requirements and reduced opioid-related adverse effects when coxibs including **celecoxib**,[3] **parecoxib**,[4] and **rofecoxib**[5] are given perioperatively or postoperatively with various opioids including **hydrocodone**[3] and **morphine**.[5] The timing of the coxib administration appears to affect the opioid-induced analgesia and post-infusion increases in sensitivity to pain. One study in healthy subjects found that pretreatment with **parecoxib** increased the analgesic effects of a **remifentanil** infusion and significantly diminished the increased sensitivity to pain after remifentanyl was withdrawn. Giving **parecoxib** at the start of the **remifentanil** infusion did not alter its analgesic effects.[6] In another study, patients given preoperative and postoperative rofecoxib, or placebo, found that rofecoxib reduced morphine requirements and pain scores. In another group of patients given placebo preoperatively and rofecoxib postoperatively, rofecoxib did not significantly affect morphine requirements or pain score at 24 hours after the operation compared to those given placebo pre-and postoperatively, but did show improvement at 48 hours and 72 hours after the operation. However, preoperative rofecoxib was considered to provide only moderate benefit and possibly offered little benefit over early postoperative administration.[5]

In a double-blind, placebo-controlled study in 72 patients undergoing laparoscopic cholecystectomy, oral **etoricoxib** 120 mg given 1.5 hours before surgery reduced the need for postoperative patient controlled analgesia (PCA) with **fentanyl**, but opioid-related adverse effects were not reduced.[7] Furthermore, the safety of short-term perioperative use of coxibs has been questioned, as some studies have reported more adverse effects (including myocardial infarction, cardiac arrest, stroke, and pulmonary embolism) with **parecoxib** or **valdecoxib** compared with placebo.[8]

1. Ibrahim AE, Feldman J, Karim A, Kharasch ED. Simultaneous assessment of drug interactions with low- and high-extraction opioids. Application to parecoxib effects on the pharmacokinetics and pharmacodynamics of fentanyl and alfentanil. *Anesthesiology* (2003) 98, 853–61.

2. Punwani NG. Tramadol pharmacokinetics and its possible interactions with cyclooxygenase 2-selective nonsteroidal anti-inflammatory drugs. *Clin Pharmacol Ther* (2004) 75, 363–5.

3. Ekman EF, Wahba M, Ancona F. Analgesic efficacy of perioperative celecoxib in ambulatory arthroscopic knee surgery: a double-blind, placebo-controlled study. *Arthroscopy* (2006) 22, 635–42.

4. Nussmeier NA, Whelton AA, Brown MT, Joshi GP, Langford RM, Singla NK, Boye ME, Verburg KM. Safety and efficacy of the cyclooxygenase-2 inhibitors parecoxib and valdecoxib after noncardiac surgery. *Anesthesiology* (2006) 104, 518–26.

5. Riest G, Peters J, Weiss M, Pospiech J, Hoffmann O, Neuhäuser M, Beiderlinden M, Eikermann M. Does perioperative administration of rofecoxib improve analgesia after spine, breast and orthopaedic surgery? *Eur J Anaesthesiol* (2006) 23, 219–26.

6. Tröster A, Sittl R, Singler B, Schmelz M, Schüttler J, Koppert W. Modulation of remifentanil-induced analgesia and postinfusion hyperalgesia by parecoxib in humans. *Anesthesiology* (2006) 105, 1016–23.

7. Puura A, Puolakka P, Rorarius M, Salmelin R, Lindgren L. Etoricoxib pre-medication for post-operative pain after laparoscopic cholecystectomy. *Acta Anaesthesiol Scand* (2006) 50, 688–93.

8. Babul N, Sloan P, Lipman AG. Postsurgical safety of opioid-sparing cyclooxygenase-2 inhibitors. *Anesthesiology* (2006) 104, 375.

Opioids + Opioids

The concurrent use of two opioid agonists may have enhanced effects, although acute opioid tolerance may also occur. Opioids with mixed agonist/antagonist properties (e.g. buprenorphine, butorphanol, nalbuphine, pentazocine) may precipitate opioid withdrawal symptoms in patients taking pure opioid agonists (e.g. fentanyl, methadone, morphine).

Clinical evidence, mechanism, importance and management

Many of the opioids used clinically act primarily at μ receptors including **morphine**, **codeine**, **fentanyl**, **methadone** and **diamorphine**, but they often have pharmacological differences, and patients tolerant to one opioid can frequently be switched to another opioid (opioid rotation) at doses lower than predicted by relative potencies.[1] Studies *in animals* have found synergistic or additive effects between μ-opioids.[1] The majority of studies in patients have reported enhanced analgesic effects with opioid combinations,[2,3] although combined opioids are not always beneficial;[4] in some cases adverse effects were increased and acute opioid tolerance has also occurred.[3] For example, a study in 69 patients who had undergone abdominal surgery and were receiving **morphine** found that the addition of a **tramadol** infusion was associated with improved patient-controlled analgesia and smaller **morphine** requirement with no increase in adverse effects.[2] However, another study found that the effects of this combination were less than additive.[5] Furthermore, the incidence of dry mouth occurred more frequently and it was concluded that the use of two μ-opioid agonists in combination might only increase the number of adverse effects.[5] Other studies have found that transdermal **fentanyl** reduced **morphine** requirements after hysterectomy[6,7] without affecting sedation scores.[6] However, the combination of **fentanyl** and **morphine** resulted in more pronounced respiratory depression than morphine alone.[6,7] In contrast, in a study of 49 patients undergoing major abdominal surgery, relatively large doses of intraoperative **remifentanil** (mean remifentanil infusion rate 300 nanograms/kg per minute) was reported to almost double **morphine** requirements in the first 24 hours postoperatively. The results suggested that **remifentanil** caused the development of acute opioid tolerance and excessive sensitivity to pain.[8] Therefore, although some opioid combinations are useful, clinical studies are needed to ascertain benefits and safety of specific combinations.[4]

Opioids with mixed agonist/antagonist properties (e.g. **buprenorphine**, **butorphanol**, **nalbuphine**, **pentazocine**) may precipitate opioid withdrawal symptoms in patients taking pure opioid agonists such as **fentanyl**, **methadone** and **morphine** (see 'Table 6.1', (p.134), for a classification). An example of this occurred in a 60-year-old woman who was taking slow-release **morphine** 90 mg twice daily for cancer pain and was additionally given **nalbuphine** 30 mg intravenously in an ambulance following a fractured femur. She became agitated and experienced involuntary movements, tachycardia, hypertension and sweating (typical of opioid withdrawal). Her management was further complicated by resistance to intravenous **morphine**, necessitating a femoral nerve block. The agitation, which lasted for about 4 hours after she was given the nalbuphine, was controlled with lorazepam.[9]

1. Bolan EA, Tallarida RJ, Pasternak GW. Synergy between μ opioid ligands: evidence for functional interactions among μ opioid receptor subtypes. *J Pharmacol Exp Ther* (2002) 303, 557–62.

2. Webb AR, Leong S, Myles PS, Burn SJ. The addition of a tramadol infusion to morphine patient-controlled analgesia after abdominal surgery: a double-blinded, placebo-controlled randomized trial. *Anesth Analg* (2002) 95, 1713–18.

3. Lötsch J, Skarke C, Tegeder I, Geisslinger G. Drug interactions with patient-controlled analgesia. *Clin Pharmacokinet* (2002) 41, 31–57.

4. Davis MP, LeGrand SB, Lagman R. Look before leaping: combined opioids may not be the rave. *Support Care Cancer* (2005) 13, 769–74.

5. Marcou TA, Marque S, Mazoit J-X, Benhamou D. The median effective dose of tramadol and morphine for postoperative patients: a study of interactions. *Anesth Analg* (2005) 100, 469–74.

6. Broome IJ, Wright BM, Bower S, Reilly CS. Postoperative analgesia with transdermal fentanyl following lower abdominal surgery. *Anaesthesia* (1995) 50, 300–3.

7. Sandler AN, Baxter AD, Katz J, Samson B, Friedlander M, Norman P, Koren G, Roger S, Hull K, Klein J. A double-blind, placebo-controlled trial of transdermal fentanyl after abdominal hysterectomy. Analgesic, respiratory, and pharmacokinetic effects. *Anesthesiology* (1994), 81, 1169–80.
8. Guignard B, Bossard AE, Coste C, Sessler DI, Lebrault C, Alfonsi P, Fletcher D, Chauvin M. Acute opioid tolerance: intraoperative remifentanil increases postoperative pain and morphine requirement. *Anesthesiology* (2000) 93, 409–17.
9. Smith J, Guly H. Nalbuphine and slow release morphine. *BMJ* (2004) 328, 1426.

Opioids + Phenothiazines

Chlorpromazine has been reported to increase the analgesic effect of pethidine, but increased respiratory depression, sedation, CNS toxicity and hypotension can also occur. Other phenothiazines such as levomepromazine, promethazine, prochlorperazine, propiomazine and thioridazine may also interact with pethidine to cause some of these effects. Additive CNS depressant effects would be expected when opioids are given with phenothiazines.

Clinical evidence

(a) Pethidine (Meperidine)

Chlorpromazine 25 mg/70 kg given alone had no consistent effect on respiratory function in 6 healthy subjects but the respiratory depression produced by pethidine 100 mg/70 kg was exacerbated when the two drugs were given together. One subject showed marked respiratory depression, beginning about 30 minutes after both drugs were given and lasting 2 hours.[1] No change in the pharmacokinetics of pethidine was found when **chlorpromazine** was given in a single-dose study in healthy subjects, but the excretion of the metabolites of pethidine was increased. The symptoms of light-headedness, dry mouth and lethargy were significantly increased and 4 subjects experienced such marked debilitation that they required assistance to continue the study. Systolic and diastolic blood pressures were also reduced.[2]

The respiratory depressant effects of pethidine can be increased by **promethazine** with pentobarbital,[3] **propiomazine**[4,5] and **levomepromazine**[6], but the effects of **prochlorperazine**[7] with pethidine on respiration were not statistically significant. A 12-year-old patient taking long-term **thioridazine** 50 mg twice daily, given premedication with pethidine, diphenhydramine and glycopyrrolate, was very lethargic after surgery and stopped breathing. He responded to naloxone.[8] For the effects of promethazine see below.

(b) Other opioids

There have been conflicting data as to whether or not phenothiazines potentiate narcotic analgesia,[9] and it has been suggested that some patients treated with an opioid and a phenothiazine are merely too sedated to report pain.[10] However, some studies have shown that **promethazine** reduces opioid requirements. The maintenance doses of a variety of opioid analgesics (**morphine**, **pethidine**, **oxymorphone**, **hydromorphone**, **fentanyl**, **pentazocine**) required during surgical anaesthesia were reduced by 28% to 46% when 132 patients were premedicated with intramuscular **promethazine**, 50 mg/70 kg, when compared with control patients. Similarly, on-demand **pentazocine** requirements post-caesarean section were reduced by 32% in women given **promethazine** as soon as the cord was clamped.[11] In a randomised, placebo-controlled study in 90 patients undergoing abdominal hysterectomy, the preoperative use of intravenous **promethazine** 100 micrograms/kg (given over 30 minutes, starting 30 minutes before induction), reduced the 24-hour postoperative **morphine** consumption by about 30%, when compared with placebo or postoperative **promethazine** use. Postoperative nausea and vomiting was reduced by both pre- and postoperative **promethazine** compared with placebo.[12]

Mechanism

There is evidence that chlorpromazine can increase the activity of the liver microsomal enzymes so that the metabolism of pethidine to norpethidine and norpethidinic acid are increased. These metabolites are toxic and probably account for the lethargy and hypotension seen in one study.[2] The effects of the phenothiazines on pethidine-induced respiratory depression may be related. Both the opioids and the phenothiazines are CNS depressants, and their effects may be additive.

Importance and management

The manufacturers of many opioids note that they can enhance the hypotensive, sedative, and respiratory depressant effects of phenothiazines. Patients should be monitored carefully, and dosage reductions made if necessary. One manufacturer of **methadone** contraindicates the use of the injection, but not the oral solution, with other CNS depressants including phenothiazines.[13,14] Although lower analgesic doses of pethidine have been used with chlorpromazine,[15] a marked increase in respiratory depression can occur in some susceptible individuals[1] and the authors of one study[2] suggested that the risks of using the combination of pethidine with chlorpromazine outweighed the advantages. Information about other adverse interactions with pethidine and phenothiazines seems to be very limited: the interaction with thioridazine seems to be the only one reported. Increased analgesia may occur but it may be accompanied by increased respiratory depression, which is undesirable in patients with existing respiratory insufficiency. The US manufacturer suggests that the dose of pethidine should be proportionally reduced (usually by 25 to 50%) when it is given with phenothiazines.[16]

For mention of myoclonus associated with high doses of morphine and chlorpromazine, see 'Opioids; Morphine + Miscellaneous', p.190.

1. Lambertsen CJ, Wendel H, Longenhagen JB. The separate and combined respiratory effects of chlorpromazine and meperidine in normal men controlled at 46 mmHg alveolar pCO_2. *J Pharmacol Exp Ther* (1961) 131, 381–93.
2. Stambaugh JE, Wainer IW. Drug interaction: meperidine and chlorpromazine, a toxic combination. *J Clin Pharmacol* (1981) 21, 140–6.
3. Pierce JA, Garofalvo ML. Preoperative medication and its effect on blood gases. *JAMA* (1965) 194, 487–90.
4. Hoffman JC, Smith TC. The respiratory effects of meperidine and propiomazine in man. *Anesthesiology* (1970) 32, 325–31.
5. Reier CE, Johnstone RE. Respiratory depression: narcotic versus narcotic-tranquillizer combinations. *Anesth Analg* (1970) 49, 119–124.
6. Zsigmond EK, Flynn K. The effect of methotrimeprazine on arterial blood gases in human volunteers. *J Clin Pharmacol* (1988) 28, 1033–7.
7. Steen SN, Yates M. The effects of benzquinamide and prochlorperazine, separately and combined, on the human respiratory center. *Anesthesiology* (1972) 36, 519–20.
8. Grothe DR, Ereshefsky L, Jann MW, Fidone GS. Clinical implications of the neuroleptic-opioid interaction. *Drug Intell Clin Pharm* (1986) 20, 75–7.
9. Warfield CA. Phenothiazines and analgesic potentiation. Reply. *Hosp Pract* (1984) 19, 24.
10. Creek K. Phenothiazines and analgesic potentiation. *Hosp Pract* (1984) 19, 22, 24.
11. Keèri-Szàntò M. The mode of action of promethazine in potentiating narcotic drugs. *Br J Anaesth* (1974) 46, 918–24.
12. Chia YY, Lo Y, Liu K, Tan PH, Chung NC, Ko NH. The effect of promethazine on postoperative pain: a comparison of preoperative, postoperative, and placebo administration in patients following total abdominal hysterectomy. *Acta Anaesthesiol Scand* (2004) 48, 625–30.
13. Methadone Injection (Methadone hydrochloride). Rosemont Pharmaceuticals Ltd. UK Summary of product characteristics, January 2005.
14. Methadone Oral Solution (Methadone hydrochloride). Rosemont Pharmaceuticals Ltd. UK Summary of product characteristics, January 2005.
15. Sadove MS, Levin MJ, Rose RF, Schwartz L, Witt FW. Chlorpromazine and narcotics in the management of pain of malignant lesions. *JAMA* (1954) 155, 626–8.
16. Demerol (Meperidine hydrochloride). Sanofi-Aventis US LLC. US Prescribing information, July 2007.

Opioids + Protease inhibitors

Ritonavir decreases pethidine (meperidine) and increases norpethidine levels, which may possibly increase toxicity on long-term use. Similarly, ritonavir and other protease inhibitors increase buprenorphine levels. Ritonavir may increase the metabolism of morphine, and decrease the metabolism of dextropropoxyphene (CYP3A4 substrate) and tramadol or other CYP2D6 substrates (such as codeine).

Clinical evidence

(a) Buprenorphine

One report describes 3 HIV-positive patients who experienced increased buprenorphine adverse effects (e.g. daytime sleepiness, dizziness, and reduced mental function) within about 2 days of starting to take **atazanavir** boosted by low-dose **ritonavir**. When the dose of buprenorphine was reduced there was a reduction in sedative symptoms within a week.[1]

In a study in opioid-dependent patients treated with sublingual buprenorphine and naloxone, patients were given an antiretroviral (**nelfinavir**, **lopinavir/ritonavir**, or **ritonavir**) for 5 to 15 days to investigate the effect of these drugs on the QT interval. Buprenorphine/naloxone alone did not significantly alter the QT interval, but when combined with an antiretroviral there was a statistically, but probably not clinically, significant increase in the QT interval. The greatest increase in QTc interval was seen in patients receiving buprenorphine/naloxone with **ritonavir** 100 mg twice daily (low booster dose).[2]

(b) Pethidine (Meperidine)

Ritonavir 500 mg twice daily for 10 days decreased the AUC of a single 50-mg dose of oral pethidine by 62% and increased the AUC of norpethidine by 47% in 8 healthy subjects.[3,4] Norpethidine is pharmacologically active, and is possibly less effective an analgesic than the parent compound, and more likely to cause CNS effects such as seizures.

Mechanism

In vitro and *in vivo* studies have demonstrated that ritonavir is a potent inhibitor of the cytochrome P450 isoenzyme CYP3A4 and to a lesser extent CYP2D6, and may also induce glucuronidation.[4] An *in vitro* study suggested that buprenorphine metabolism may be inhibited by **ritonavir** and to a lesser extent by **indinavir** and **saquinavir**,[5] which would be expected to lead to increased buprenorphine levels. Other opioids metabolised by CYP3A4 include **dextropropoxyphene** (propoxyphene), 'fentanyl and related drugs', (below), and 'methadone', (p.182). Substrates of CYP2D6 include **codeine**, **dihydrocodeine**, **oxycodone**, and **tramadol**. **Morphine** undergoes glucuronidation, and the morphine metabolite M6G [morphine-6 beta-glucuronide] is believed to contribute to the analgesic effects of morphine. Buprenorphine, and to some extent, **codeine** also undergo glucuronidation.[6]

Importance and management

Most of these interactions remain theoretical, but they are consistent with the way the protease inhibitors and the opioids interact with other drugs. The consequences of inhibition of CYP2D6 are most pronounced for **codeine**, and CYP2D6 inhibition will lead to decreased levels of the morphine metabolite of codeine and therefore, perhaps contrary to expectation, a reduced effect. The levels of other CYP2D6 substrates **dihydrocodeine**, **oxycodone**, and **tramadol** would be expected to be raised, and dose reductions may be necessary. This has been suggested for tramadol.[7] It would seem prudent to monitor for adverse effects such as sedation. However, note that *low-dose* ritonavir (i.e. the dose used as a pharmacokinetic enhancer with other protease inhibitors) has a less potent effect on CYP2D6 and dose reductions of drugs metabolised by CYP2D6 would not generally be required if this dose of ritonavir is given concurrently.[8]

Ritonavir is a potent inhibitor of CYP3A4 and therefore the UK manufacturer of ritonavir contraindicates its use with **dextropropoxyphene** as extremely raised dextropropoxyphene levels may occur, which would increase the risk of serious respiratory depression or other serious adverse events.[4] However, the US manufacturer only suggests that a dose decrease may be needed.[7]

The outcome of taking ritonavir with **morphine** is less clear, but it is expected that its levels will be decreased.[4,9] It would seem prudent to monitor closely to ensure morphine is effective in patients taking ritonavir. More study is needed.

It has been suggested that the starting dose of buprenorphine should be halved in patients taking CYP3A4 inhibitors, such as the protease inhibitors, when it is used for opioid dependence.[10] However, it has also been suggested that, since the magnitude of an inhibitory effect is unknown, such drug combinations should be avoided when buprenorphine is used parenterally or sublingually as a strong analgesic.[11,12]

The manufacturers of pethidine oral preparations and injection contraindicate or advise against its use with ritonavir because of the risk of norpethidine toxicity.[13,14] Long-term use of pethidine with other protease inhibitors e.g. tipranavir, which are given with low-dose ritonavir is also not recommended.[15,16]

1. Bruce RD, Altice FL. Three case reports of a clinical pharmacokinetic interaction with buprenorphine and atazanavir plus ritonavir. *AIDS* (2006) 20, 783–4.
2. Baker JR, Best AM, Pade PA, McCance-Katz EF. Effect of buprenorphine and antiretroviral agents on the QT interval in opioid-dependent patients. *Ann Pharmacother* (2006) 40, 392–6.
3. Piscitelli SC, Kress DR, Bertz RJ, Pau A, Davey R. The effect of ritonavir on the pharmacokinetics of meperidine and normeperidine. *Pharmacotherapy* (2000) 20, 549–53.
4. Norvir (Ritonavir). Abbott Laboratories Ltd. UK Summary of product characteristics, May 2007.
5. Iribarne C, Berthou F, Carlhant D, Dreano Y, Picart D, Lohezic F, Riche C. Inhibition of methadone and buprenorphine N-dealkylations by three HIV-1 protease inhibitors. *Drug Metab Dispos* (1998) 26, 257–60.
6. Lötsch J, Skarke C, Tegeder I, Geisslinger G. Drug interactions with patient-controlled analgesia. *Clin Pharmacokinet* (2002) 41, 31–57.
7. Norvir (Ritonavir). Abbott Laboratories. US Prescribing information, January 2006.
8. Aarnoutse RE, Kleinnijenhuis J, Koopmans PP, Touw DJ, Wieling J, Hekster YA, Burger DM. Effect of low-dose ritonavir (100 mg twice daily) on the activity of cytochrome P450 2D6 in healthy volunteers. *Clin Pharmacol Ther* (2005) 78, 664–74.
9. Abbott Laboratories Ltd (UK). Personal communication, March 1998.
10. Subutex (Buprenorphine hydrochloride). Schering-Plough Ltd. UK Summary of product characteristics, January 2006.
11. Temgesic Injection (Buprenorphine hydrochloride). Schering-Plough Ltd. UK Summary of product characteristics, April 2004.
12. Temgesic Sublingual Tablets (Buprenorphine hydrochloride). Schering-Plough Ltd. UK Summary of product characteristics, April 2004.
13. Pethidine Injection (Pethidine hydrochloride). Wockhardt UK Ltd. UK Summary of product characteristics, March 2005.
14. Demerol (Meperidine hydrochloride). Sanofi-Aventis US LLC. US Prescribing information, July 2007.
15. Aptivus (Tipranavir). Boehringer Ingelheim Ltd. UK Summary of product characteristics, March 2007.
16. Aptivus (Tipranavir). Boehringer Ingelheim. US Prescribing information, February 2007.

Opioids; Fentanyl and related drugs + Protease inhibitors

Ritonavir markedly increases the levels of fentanyl, and markedly increases alfentanil-induced miosis. Other protease inhibitors such as nelfinavir may have a similar effect. Care should also be taken if ritonavir is used with other protease inhibitors as a pharmacokinetic enhancer.

Clinical evidence

(a) Alfentanil

The miosis caused by oral and intravenous alfentanil was markedly increased by the short-term (1 to 3 days) and longer-term (14 days) use of **ritonavir** in healthy subjects.[1]

(b) Fentanyl

Ritonavir 200 mg increased to 300 mg three times daily for a total of 7 doses increased the AUC of a single 5-mg/kg intravenous dose of fentanyl by 83%, decreased its clearance by 67%, and increased the elimination half-life twofold in healthy subjects.[2]

Mechanism

Both fentanyl and alfentanil are metabolised by the cytochrome P450 isoenzyme CYP3A4. Ritonavir, and other protease inhibitors, are potent inhibitors of CYP3A4 and they therefore reduce the metabolism of these opioids, which results in increased levels and effects.

Importance and management

The evidence is limited, but is consistent with the way protease inhibitors and fentanyl or alfentanil interact with other drugs. The UK manufacturer of alfentanil warns that potent CYP3A4 inhibitors such as ritonavir could increase the risk of prolonged or delayed respiratory depression, and says the combination should be used with special care, and that a reduced dose of alfentanil may be necessary.[3] Similarly, caution is required in patients taking **ritonavir** given fentanyl by any route (oral, parenteral, or transdermal). In particular, the manufacturers suggest avoiding the combination of **ritonavir** and transdermal fentanyl, unless the patient is closely monitored.[4,5] Fentanyl dose reductions may be needed on long-term treatment to avoid fentanyl accumulation.[6] The US manufacturer also warns that other potent CYP3A4 inhibitors including **nelfinavir** may have a similar effect.[5] In addition, the manufacturers of saquinavir warn that, although specific studies have not been performed, the use of **saquinavir** or **saquinavir** with **ritonavir** may raise the levels of fentanyl and alfentanil and therefore these combinations should be given with caution.[7,8]

Consider also, 'Opioids + Protease inhibitors', p.180.

1. Kharasch ED, Hoffer C. Assessment of ritonavir effects on hepatic and first-pass CYP3A activity and methadone disposition using noninvasive pupillometry. *Clin Pharmacol Ther* (2004) 75, P96.
2. Olkkola KT, Palkama VJ, Neuvonen PJ. Ritonavir's role in reducing fentanyl clearance and prolonging its half-life. *Anesthesiology* (1999) 91, 681–5.
3. Rapifen (Alfentanil hydrochloride). Janssen-Cilag Ltd. UK Summary of product characteristics, May 2007.
4. Durogesic DTrans (Fentanyl). Janssen-Cilag Ltd. UK Summary of product characteristics, July 2007.
5. Duragesic (Fentanyl transdermal system). Janssen Pharmaceutica Products, L.P. US Prescribing information, April 2007.
6. Sublimaze (Fentanyl citrate). Janssen-Cilag Ltd. UK Summary of product characteristics, January 2005.
7. Invirase (Saquinavir mesylate). Roche Pharmaceuticals. US Prescribing information, July 2007.
8. Invirase Hard Capsules (Saquinavir mesilate). Roche Products Ltd. UK Summary of product characteristics, May 2007.

Opioids; Methadone + Protease inhibitors

Methadone serum levels can be reduced by amprenavir, nelfinavir, lopinavir/ritonavir, saquinavir/ritonavir, tipranavir/ritonavir, and possibly ritonavir. In addition, amprenavir levels may be reduced by methadone. No interaction appears to occur between methadone and indinavir, or possibly atazanavir or saquinavir, alone.

Clinical evidence

(a) Amprenavir

A study involving 16 opioid-dependent subjects found that amprenavir 1.2 g twice daily for 10 days decreased the AUCs for both *R*-methadone (active enantiomer) and *S*-methadone (inactive enantiomer) by 13% and 40%, respectively. No clinically significant changes were noted in opioid effects and there was no evidence of opioid withdrawal.[1] However, in another study methadone levels were reduced by 35% (range 28% to 87%) in 5 patients within 17 days of starting to take amprenavir 1.2 g twice daily and abacavir 600 mg twice daily. Two patients reported nausea before their daily methadone dose, which can be a sign of opiate withdrawal.[2] Note that 'abacavir', (p.175), may modestly reduce methadone levels, and could therefore have contributed to this effect.

The first study also found that amprenavir and methadone resulted in a 30% decrease in amprenavir AUC compared with non-matched historical controls.[1]

(b) Atazanavir

Atazanavir, given for 14 days, had little effect on the steady-state pharmacokinetics of methadone in 16 patients treated for opiate addiction, and symptoms of opiate withdrawal or excess were not detected.[3]

(c) Indinavir

A randomised, crossover study in 12 patients taking methadone found that the pharmacokinetics of methadone were unchanged by indinavir 800 mg every 8 hours for 8 days. A small decrease in indinavir peak levels and a small increase in trough levels were noted, when compared with historical controls.[4] Another study in 6 HIV-positive patients taking methadone and two nucleoside analogues similarly found that methadone serum levels remained unchanged when indinavir was added.[5,6]

There are also clinical reports about 2 patients whose methadone levels appeared to be unaltered while taking indinavir, but who later had reduced levels when treated with nelfinavir or ritonavir (see (e) and (g) below).[7,8] This would seem to confirm that indinavir does not have a clinically relevant effect on methadone levels.

(d) Lopinavir/ritonavir

A study in healthy subjects found that lopinavir/ritonavir 400 mg/100 mg twice daily for 10 days reduced the AUC of a single 5-mg dose of methadone by about 50%.[9] Similarly, in 15 healthy subjects taking methadone lopinavir/ritonavir 400 mg/100 mg twice daily for 7 days decreased the AUC of methadone by 26% and increased its clearance by 42%. Four of the subjects had clinically important increases in opioid-withdrawal scores, and were all found to have subtherapeutic trough methadone levels.[10] [Note that the same dose of ritonavir alone had no effect on methadone levels, see (f) below]. In another study in 8 HIV-positive patients taking methadone a lopinavir/ritonavir based antiretroviral regimen reduced the AUC of methadone by 36% after 14 days of treatment. However, none of these patients experienced methadone withdrawal during the study or during 6 weeks of follow-up.[11] In yet another study (that did not measure methadone levels), none of 18 patients experienced methadone withdrawal during the 28 days after starting lopinavir/ritonavir.[12]

In a further study, methadone appeared to have no effect on the pharmacokinetics of lopinavir or ritonavir (given as a combined preparation).[13]

(e) Nelfinavir

An HIV-positive man who had been taking methadone 100 mg daily for several years with indinavir 800 mg and zalcitabine 750 micrograms three times daily, developed opioid withdrawal symptoms within 6 weeks of starting to take stavudine and nelfinavir 750 mg three times daily. His methadone dosage was increased to 285 mg daily before therapeutic serum levels were achieved. When his antiretroviral treatment was withdrawn, his methadone dosage was successfully reduced to 125 mg daily.[8] Two other patients taking nucleoside analogues had a 40 to 50% fall in their serum methadone levels when nelfinavir was added.[5,6] Similarly, in another study, 4 of 6 patients developed symptoms of methadone withdrawal within 5 to 7 days of starting nelfinavir-based therapy. The mean AUC of methadone was reduced by 56% and the subjects required a mean increase in methadone dose of 15%.[14]

The manufacturers of nelfinavir say that in a pharmacokinetic study nelfinavir reduced the concentrations of methadone by 47%.[15,16] However, despite this reduction none of the subjects developed withdrawal symptoms, although due to the pharmacokinetic changes, it should be expected that some patients might experience withdrawal symptoms.[15] A retrospective study of HIV-positive patients taking methadone reported that 5 out of 30 patients (17%) required methadone adjustments (mean 26 mg). The use of nelfinavir with methadone was effective and well tolerated.[17]

A patient receiving methadone experienced torsades de pointes after starting treatment with nelfinavir.[18] Raised methadone levels are associated with QT-prolongation, and this case therefore suggests that nelfinavir raises methadone levels.

In a study looking at the levels of nelfinavir and its active metabolite M8, methadone had no significant effect on the AUC of nelfinavir, but the AUC_{0-12} of M8 was reduced by 48%.[19]

(f) Ritonavir

A patient taking lamivudine and zidovudine had a marked decrease in methadone serum levels when ritonavir was added.[5,6] Another patient receiving methadone experienced an opioid withdrawal syndrome when ritonavir was added to a similar antiretroviral regimen.[20]

Ritonavir (dose not stated) was given to 11 healthy subjects for 14 days, with a single 5-mg dose of methadone on day 11. Ritonavir reduced the maximum serum levels of methadone by 37.8% and the AUC by 36.3%.[21] However, in another study in 15 healthy subjects receiving methadone, ritonavir 100 mg twice daily for 7 days had no significant effect on methadone pharmacokinetics.[10]

In a further study, methadone apparently increased ritonavir exposure by 60%, when given alone, but had no effect on ritonavir pharmacokinetics when it was given with lopinavir.[13]

In healthy subjects the miosis caused by oral and intravenous methadone was increased by the acute use of ritonavir for 3 days but returned to below baseline after longer-term use for 14 days. It appeared that acute ritonavir inhibited, but chronic ritonavir mildly increased methadone elimination.[22]

(g) Ritonavir/saquinavir

An HIV-positive patient taking methadone 90 mg daily with indinavir, lamivudine and zidovudine, developed withdrawal symptoms and was hospitalised within a week of stopping these HIV drugs and starting ritonavir 400 mg, saquinavir 400 mg and stavudine 40 mg twice daily. The patient was eventually re-stabilised taking methadone 130 mg daily.[7]

A later study in 12 HIV-positive subjects taking methadone maintenance found that ritonavir/saquinavir 400 mg/400 mg twice daily decreased the *S*-methadone AUC by 40% and the *R*-methadone AUC by 32%. However, when these decreases were corrected for changes in protein binding, the free *R*-methadone AUC was decreased by only 19.6%, and the free *S*-methadone AUC by 24.6%. None of the subjects experienced methadone withdrawal or required a change in their methadone dosage.[23] Similarly, in another study ritonavir/saquinavir 100 mg/1600 mg daily for 14 days caused no clinically relevant changes in total or free levels of either enantiomer of methadone in 12 HIV-negative subjects taking methadone. None of the subjects experienced methadone withdrawal.[24]

(h) Saquinavir

A study in an HIV-positive patient taking methadone and two nucleoside analogues found that methadone serum levels remained unchanged when saquinavir was added.[5,6]

(i) Tipranavir/ritonavir

The manufacturers of tipranavir state that use of methadone with tipranavir boosted by low-dose ritonavir (200 mg) can result in a decrease in methadone levels of about 50%, which may require dose increase in some patients.[25,26]

Mechanism

Not known. The findings are the opposite of those originally predicted based on *in vitro* data showing *inhibition* of methadone metabolism (principally mediated by the cytochrome P450 isoenzyme CYP3A).[27] One study found a slight increase in methadone elimination,[22] but this was not mediated by CYP3A. It is possible that these protease inhibitors induce the activity of other isoenzymes or act via other mechanisms (e.g. glucuronyltransferases). The reduction in methadone levels has not always correlated with clinical effects, and it has been suggested that this may be because the pharmacokinetics of the enantiomers (one of which is inactive) are affected differently, and/or altered protein binding occurs.[19]

Importance and management

Information is limited but the interactions with amprenavir, nelfinavir, lopinavir/ritonavir, saquinavir/ritonavir, tipranavir/ritonavir and probably ritonavir would appear to be established. However the picture seems to be that not all patients experience withdrawal symptoms if given these drugs. Therefore, in methadone-maintained patients, care should be taken if any of these protease inhibitors is started or stopped. It has been suggested that patients taking methadone who are given a protease inhibitor should be screened for opioid withdrawal beginning on the fourth day of the new medication. If symptoms develop, the methadone dose should be increased by 10 mg every 2 to 3 days until symptoms abate.[28] However, others have suggested dose increments should be made at one-week intervals to avoid overdose, as methadone has a long half-life (reported to range form 13 to 47 hours).[18] If the protease inhibitor is stopped the methadone dose should be gradually reduced to pretreatment levels over the course of 1 to 2 weeks.[28]

Indinavir appears not to interact with methadone, and very limited evidence suggests that atazanavir and saquinavir alone do not interact either.

Note that amprenavir plasma levels may also be reduced by methadone. The US manufacturer says that amprenavir may be less effective if taken concurrently with narcotic analgesics and alternative antiretroviral therapy should be considered.[29]

1. Hendrix CW, Wakeford J, Wire MB, Lou Y, Bigelow GE, Martinez E, Christopher J, Fuchs EJ, Snidow JW. Pharmacokinetics and pharmacodynamics of methadone enantiomers after coadministration with amprenavir in opioid-dependent subjects. *Pharmacotherapy* (2004) 24, 1110–21.
2. Bart P-A, Rizzardi PG, Gallant S, Golay KP, Baumann P, Pantaleo G, Eap CB. Methadone blood concentrations are decreased by the administration of abacavir plus amprenavir. *Ther Drug Monit* (2001) 23, 553–5.
3. Friedland G, Andrews L, Schreibman T, Agarwala S, Daley L, Child M, Shi J, Wang Y, O'Mara E. Lack of an effect of atazanavir on steady-state pharmacokinetics of methadone in patients chronically treated for opiate addiction. *AIDS* (2005) 19, 1635–41.
4. Cantilena L, McCrea J, Blazes D, Winchell G, Carides A, Royce C, Deutsch P. Lack of a pharmacokinetic interaction between indinavir and methadone. *Clin Pharmacol Ther* (1999) 65, 135.
5. Touzeau D, Beauverie P, Bouchez J, Poisson N, Edel Y, Dessalles M-C, Lherm J, Furlan V, Lagarde B. Méthadone et nouveau anti-rétroviraux. Résultats du suivi thérapeutique. *Ann Med Interne (Paris)* (1999) 150, 355–6.
6. Beauverie P, Taburet A-M, Dessalles M-C, Furlan V, Touzeau D. Therapeutic drug monitoring of methadone in HIV-infected patients receiving protease inhibitors. *AIDS* (1998) 12, 2510–11.
7. Geletko SM, Erickson AD. Decreased methadone effect after ritonavir initiation. *Pharmacotherapy* (2000) 20, 93–4.
8. McCance-Katz EF, Farber S, Selwyn PA, O'Connor A. Decrease in methodone levels with nelfinavir mesylate. *Am J Psychiatry* (2000) 157, 481.
9. Bertz R, Hsu A, Lam W, Williams L, Renz C, Karol M, Dutta S, Carr R, Zhang Y, Wang Q, Schweitzer S, Foit C, Andre A, Bernstein B, Granneman GR, Sun E. Pharmacokinetic interactions between lopinavir/ritonavir (ABT-378r) and other non-HIV drugs [abstract P291]. *AIDS* (2000) 14 (Suppl 4), S100.
10. McCance-Katz EF, Rainey PM, Friedland G, Jatlow P. The protease inhibitor lopinavir-ritonavir may produce opiate withdrawal in methadone-maintained patients. *Clin Infect Dis* (2003) 37, 476–82.
11. Clarke S, Mulcahy F, Bergin C, Reynolds H, Boyle N, Barry M, Back DJ. Absence of opioid withdrawal symptoms in patients receiving methadone and the protease inhibitor lopinavir-ritonavir. *Clin Infect Dis* (2002) 34, 1143–5.
12. Stevens RC, Rapaport S, Maroldo-Connelly L, Patterson JB, Bertz R. Lack of methadone dose alterations or withdrawal symptoms during therapy with lopinavir/ritonavir. *J Acquir Immune Defic Syndr* (2003) 33, 650–1.
13. Smith P, McCance-Katz E, Sarlo J, Di Francesco R, Morse GD. Methadone increases ritonavir exposure when administered alone but not lopinavir/RTV combination. *Intersci Conf Antimicrob Agents Chemother* (2003) 43, 339.
14. Clarke S, Mulcahy F, Bergin C, Tjia J, Brown R, Barry M, Back DJ. The pharmacokinetic interaction between methadone and nelfinavir [abstract P276]. *AIDS* (2000) 14 (Suppl 4), S95.
15. Viracept (Nelfinavir mesilate). Roche Products Ltd. UK Summary of product characteristics, January 2007.
16. Viracept (Nelfinavir mesylate). Agouron Pharmaceuticals, Inc. US Prescribing information, January 2007.
17. Brown LS, Chu M, Aug C, Dabo S. The use of nelfinavir and two nucleosides concomitantly with methadone is effective and well-tolerated in HepC co-infected patients. *Intersci Conf Antimicrob Agents Chemother* (2001) 41, 311.
18. Anon. Torsades de pointes with methadone. *Prescrire Int* (2005) 14, 61–2.
19. McCance-Katz EF, Rainey PM, Smith P, Morse G, Friedland G, Gourevitch M, Jatlow P. Drug interactions between opioids and antiretroviral medications: interaction between methadone, LAAM, and nelfinavir. *Am J Addict* (2004) 13, 163 –80.
20. Jiménez-Lerma JM, Iraurgi I. Probable síndrome de abstinencia a opiáceos tras la administración de ritonavir en un paciente en tratamiento con metadona. *Rev Clin Esp* (1999) 199, 188–9.
21. Hsu A, Granneman GR, Carothers L, Dennis S, Chiu Y-L, Valdes J, Sun E. Ritonavir does not increase methadone exposure in healthy volunteers. 5th Conference on Retroviruses and Opportunistic Infection, Chicago, Feb 1–5, 1998, abstract 342.
22. Kharasch ED, Hoffer C. Assessment of ritonavir effects on hepatic and first-pass CYP3A activity and methadone disposition using noninvasive pupillometry. *Clin Pharmacol Ther* (2004) 75, P96.
23. Gerber JG, Rosenkranz S, Segal Y, Aberg J, D'Amico R, Mildvan D, Gulick R, Hughes V, Flexner C, Aweeka F, Hsu A, Gal J. Effect of ritonavir/saquinavir on stereoselective pharmacokinetics of methadone: Results of AIDS Clinical Trials Group (ACTG) 401. *J Acquir Immune Defic Syndr* (2001) 27, 153–60.
24. Shelton MJ, Cloen D, DiFrancesco R, Berenson CS, Esch A, de Caprariis PJ, Palic B, Schur JL, Buggé CJL, Ljungqvist A, Espinosa O, Hewitt RG. The effects of once-daily saquinavir/minidose ritonavir on the pharmacokinetics of methadone. *J Clin Pharmacol* (2004) 44, 293–304.
25. Aptivus (Tipranavir). Boehringer Ingelheim Ltd. UK Summary of product characteristics, March 2007.
26. Aptivus (Tipranavir). Boehringer Ingelheim. US Prescribing information, February 2007.
27. Iribarne C, Berthou F, Carlhant D, Dreano Y, Picart D, Lohezic F, Riche C. Inhibition of methadone and buprenorphine *N*-dealkylations by three HIV-1 protease inhibitors. *Drug Metab Dispos* (1998) 26, 257–60.
28. Bruce RD, Altice FL, Gourevitch MN, Friedland GH. Pharmacokinetic drug interactions between opioid agonist therapy and antiretroviral medications: implications and management for clinical practice. *J Acquir Immune Defic Syndr* (2006) 41, 563–72.
29. Agenerase (Amprenavir). GlaxoSmithKline. US Prescribing information, May 2005.

Opioids + Quinidine

Quinidine appears to increase the *oral* absorption and effects of fentanyl, methadone, and morphine, but does not significantly alter the opioid-induced miosis when these opioids are given *intravenously*. Care should be taken if high-dose methadone is used with quinidine as cardiac conduction might possibly be affected.

Clinical evidence, mechanism, importance and management

(a) Fentanyl

Quinidine sulfate 600 mg given one hour before an infusion of fentanyl 2.5 micrograms/kg did not alter the fentanyl-induced miosis in healthy subjects. However, the same dose of quinidine given before *oral* fentanyl 2.5 micrograms/kg (with ondansetron as an antiemetic) did increase fentanyl-induced miosis. This increase was considered proportionate to the increase in the AUC of fentanyl (160%). There was no change in the elimination half-life of fentanyl.[1] It was suggested that quinidine inhibits the intestinal P-glycoprotein and so allows an increase in oral fentanyl absorption, and a consequent increase in its effects. The effects on miosis indicate that quinidine did not alter brain access of fentanyl.[1]

The clinical importance of this finding to the use of *buccal* fentanyl citrate (of which a significant proportion is swallowed) remains to be determined, but be aware that effects may be increased.

(b) Hydromorphone

An *in vitro* study suggested that quinidine did not significantly affect the metabolism of hydromorphone to norhydromorphone. Hydromorphone appears to be mainly metabolised by CYP3A, and to a lesser extent CYP2C9, but the inhibition of CYP2D6 by quinidine does not appear to affect norhydromorphone formation.[2]

(c) Methadone

Quinidine sulfate 600 mg, given one hour before *intravenous* methadone hydrochloride 10 mg, did not alter methadone-induced miosis in healthy subjects. However, the same dose of quinidine given before *oral* methadone hydrochloride 10 mg (with ondansetron as an antiemetic) increased the peak methadone-induced miosis by 34% and increased the plasma levels of oral methadone in the absorption phase, but had no effect on the maximum plasma level or AUC of methadone.[3] Methadone is primarily metabolised by CYP3A and quinidine does not affect the hepatic metabolism of methadone. However, quinidine can inhibit P-glycoprotein and this may affect methadone intestinal transport and absorption.[3]

The absorption of oral methadone may possibly be affected by quinidine, but the clinical relevance is not known. However, note that both high doses of methadone and quinidine can affect the QT interval, see 'Drugs that prolong the QT interval + Other drugs that prolong the QT interval', p.257.

(d) Morphine

Quinidine sulfate 600 mg, given one hour before *intravenous* morphine sulfate 150 micrograms/kg, did not alter morphine-induced miosis in healthy subjects. However, the same dose of quinidine given before *oral* morphine sulfate 30 mg (with ondansetron as an antiemetic) increased morphine-induced miosis by 56%. This increase was considered proportionate to the increase in morphine AUC (60%) and maximum level (88%). There was no change in the elimination half-life of morphine.[4] Similarly, in another study in healthy subjects, quinidine 800 mg, given one hour before intravenous morphine 7.5 mg did not alter the respiratory depressant nor mitotic effects of morphine, and there was no change in plasma morphine or morphine glucuronide levels.[5]

It was suggested that quinidine inhibits P-glycoprotein and so allows an increase in oral morphine absorption.[4] In addition, the effects on miosis suggest that quinidine has no effect on the brain distribution of morphine.[4,5]

The clinical importance of these findings remains to be determined, but it appears that quinidine may increase the effects of oral morphine.

(e) Tramadol

A placebo-controlled study in 12 healthy subjects found that quinidine 50 mg had virtually no effect on the analgesic effects of tramadol 100 mg but it inhibited its effect on pupil size.[6] The manufacturers say that quinidine increases the tramadol AUC and maximum level by 25%, but this is within the normal pharmacokinetic variation seen with tramadol.[7] Tramadol is partially metabolised to the active metabolite *O*-desmethyltramadol (which affects opioid receptors), by the cytochrome P450 isoenzyme CYP2D6, and it is this enzyme that is inhibited by quinidine. Blockade of the production of this metabolite appears to have little effect on the analgesic effect of tramadol.[6] No special precautions seem to be needed.

1. Kharasch ED, Hoffer C, Altuntas TG, Whittington D. Quinidine as a probe for the role of P-glycoprotein in the intestinal absorption and clinical effects of fentanyl. *J Clin Pharmacol* (2004) 44, 224–33.
2. Benetton SA, Borges VM, Chang TKH, McErlane KM. Role of individual human cytochrome P450 enzymes in the *in vitro* metabolism of hydromorphone. *Xenobiotica* (2004) 34, 335–44.
3. Kharasch ED, Hoffer C, Whittington D. The effect of quinidine, used as a probe for the involvement of P-glycoprotein, on the intestinal absorption and pharmacodynamics of methadone. *Br J Clin Pharmacol* (2004) 57, 600–10.
4. Kharasch ED, Hoffer C, Whittington D, Sheffels. Role of P-glycoprotein in the intestinal absorption and clinical effects of morphine. *Clin Pharmacol Ther* (2003) 74, 543–54.
5. Skarke S, Jarrar M, Erb K, Schmidt H, Geisslinger G, Lotsch J. Respiratory and miotic effects of morphine in healthy volunteers when P-glycoprotein is blocked by quinidine. *Clin Pharmacol Ther* (2003) 74, 303–11.
6. Collart L, Luthy C, Dayer P. Multimodel analgesic effect of tramadol. *Clin Pharmacol Ther* (1993) 53, 223.
7. Zydol SR (Tramadol hydrochloride). Grünenthal Ltd. UK Summary of product characteristics, February 2005.

Opioids; Codeine and related drugs + Quinidine

The analgesic effects of codeine, and probably also hydrocodone, are reduced or abolished by quinidine. Quinidine alters the pharmacokinetics of dihydrocodeine and oxycodone, but this does not appear to alter their effects.

Clinical evidence

(a) Codeine

Codeine 100 mg was given to 16 extensive metabolisers of the cytochrome P450 isoenzyme CYP2D6 with and without a single 200-mg dose of quinidine. The quinidine reduced the peak morphine levels by about 80% (from a mean of 18 nanomol/L to less than 4 nanomol/L). Codeine given alone increased the pain threshold (pin-prick pain test using an argon laser) but no significant analgesic effects were detectable when quinidine was also present.[1] Another study found that the effects of codeine in extensive metabolisers of CYP2D6 who were given quinidine were virtually the same as codeine alone in poor metabolisers of CYP2D6.[2]

These studies confirm the preliminary findings of an earlier study using codeine 100 mg and quinidine 50 mg.[3] The quinidine reduced the peak morphine plasma levels by more than 90% (by 92% in 7 extensive metabolisers, and by 97% in one poor metaboliser) and similarly abolished the analgesic effects.[3]

(b) Dihydrocodeine

A study in which 4 extensive metabolisers of the cytochrome P450 isoenzyme CYP2D6 were given dihydrocodeine 40 or 60 mg found that when they were pretreated with quinidine 200 mg almost none of the morphinoid metabolites of dihydrocodeine normally present in the serum could be detected.[4] The same authors found essentially the same results in a later study in 10 extensive metabolisers of CYP2D6 given dihydrocodeine 60 mg and quinidine 50 mg.[5] However, a single-dose study involving 10 healthy subjects who were extensive metabolisers of CYP2D6 investigated the effect of quinidine on the visceral and somatic analgesic effects of dihydrocodeine and its metabolite, dihydromorphine. It was found that although quinidine reduced dihydromorphine plasma levels (by inhibition of CYP2D6 reducing the metabolism of dihydrocodeine to dihydromorphine), this did not result in diminished pain tolerance thresholds. This suggested that the metabolism of dihydrocodeine to dihydromorphine may not be clinically important for analgesia.[6] Further study is needed.

(c) Hydrocodone

In a comparative study, 5 extensive metabolisers and 6 poor metabolisers of the cytochrome P450 isoenzyme CYP2D6 were given hydrocodone, and another 4 extensive metabolisers of CYP2D6 were given hydrocodone after pre-treatment with quinidine. The metabolism of the hydrocodone to its active metabolite hydromorphone was found to be high in the extensive metabolisers who described 'good opiate effects' but poor in the poor metabolisers and the extensive metabolisers pre-treated with quinidine who described 'poor opiate effects'.[7] For the effect of quinidine on hydromorphone metabolism, see 'Opioids + Quinidine', p.183.

(d) Oxycodone

Quinidine, given as 200 mg 3 hours before and 100 mg 6 hours after a single 20-mg dose of oxycodone almost completely inhibited the formation of the metabolite, oxymorphone in 10 healthy extensive metabolisers of the cytochrome P450 isoenzyme CYP2D6. Despite this, the psychomotor and subjective effects of oxycodone were not altered (note that analgesia was not assessed). The AUC of the metabolite noroxycodone was increased about 85%, and the oxycodone AUC was slightly increased by 13%.[8] Similar results were found in the preliminary report of another study.[9]

Mechanism

The evidence available shows that the conversion of codeine, dihydrocodeine and hydrocodone to their active analgesic metabolites in the body (morphine, morphinoid metabolites and hydromorphone, respectively) probably depends upon the activity of the cytochrome P450 isoenzyme CYP2D6 in the liver. If this isoenzyme is inhibited by quinidine, these conversions largely fail to occur and the analgesic effects may be reduced or lost. This interaction is only likely to occur in extensive metabolisers, and not in poor metabolisers, who have minimal CYP2D6 activity and who therefore may only derive minimal benefit from analgesics such as codeine, whose principal pharmacological effect appears to depend on this metabolism.[2] However, one study in healthy subjects has suggested that the analgesic effect of dihydrocodeine does not necessarily depend on its systemic metabolism to dihydromorphine.[6] Similarly, although quinidine also blocks conversion of oxycodone to oxymorphone, it appears that this is not important for the pharmacodynamic effects of this drug.

Importance and management

The interaction between codeine and quinidine is well established and clinically important. Codeine will be virtually ineffective as an analgesic in extensive metabolisers of CYP2D6 (most patients) taking quinidine. An alternative analgesic should be used (possibly dihydrocodeine, see below, or tramadol, see 'Opioids + Quinidine', p.183). No interaction would be expected in poor metabolisers (about 7% of Caucasians), but codeine is probably unlikely to be effective in these patients in any case. Whether the antitussive effects of codeine are similarly affected is not established, but it seems likely. Note that this interaction has been used clinically in an attempt to treat codeine dependence.[10]

The interaction of hydrocodone is less well established, but the evidence suggests that the analgesic effect will similarly be reduced or lost if quinidine is given. Further study is needed.

The available evidence suggests that the efficacy of dihydrocodeine, hydromorphone, or oxycodone may not be significantly affected by quinidine, but this needs confirmation.

1. Sindrup SH, Arendt-Nielsen L, Brøsen K, Bjerring P, Angelo HR, Eriksen B, Gram LF. The effect of quinidine on the analgesic effect of codeine. *Eur J Clin Pharmacol* (1992) 42, 587–92.
2. Caraco Y, Sheller J, Wood AJ. Pharmacogenetic determination of the effects of codeine and prediction of drug interactions. *J Pharmacol Exp Ther* (1996) 278, 1165–74.
3. Desmeules J, Dayer P, Gascon M-P, Magistris M. Impact of genetic and environmental factors on codeine analgesia. *Clin Pharmacol Ther* (1989) 45, 122.
4. Hufschmid E, Theurillat R, Martin U, Thormann W. Exploration of the metabolism of dihydrocodeine via determination of its metabolites in human urine using micellar electrokinetic capillary chromatography. *J Chromatogr B Biomed Appl* (1995) 668, 159–70.
5. Hufschmid E, Theurillat R, Wilder-Smith CH, Thormann W. Characterization of the genetic polymorphism of dihydrocodeine O-demethylation in man via analysis of urinary dihydrocodeine and dihydromorphine by micellar electrokinetic capillary chromatography. *J Chromatogr B Biomed Appl* (1996) 678, 43–51.
6. Wilder-Smith CH, Hufschmid E, Thormann W. The visceral and somatic antinociceptive effects of dihydrocodeine and its metabolite, dihydromorphine. A cross-over study with extensive and quinidine-induced poor metabolizers. *Br J Clin Pharmacol* (1998) 45, 575–81.
7. Otton SV, Schadel M, Cheung SW, Kaplan, Busto UE, Sellers EM. CYP2D6 phenotype determines the metabolic conversion of hydrocodone to hydromorphone. *Clin Pharmacol Ther* (1993) 54, 463–72.
8. Heiskanen T, Olkkola KT, Kalso E. Effects of blocking CYP2D6 on the pharmacokinetics and pharmacodynamics of oxycodone. *Clin Pharmacol Ther* (1998) 64, 603–11.

9. Colucci R, Kaiko R, Grandy R. Effects of quinidine on the pharmacokinetics and pharmacodynamics of oxycodone. *Clin Pharmacol Ther* (1998) 63, 141.
10. Fernandes LC, Kilicarslan T, Kaplan HL, Tyndale RF, Sellers EM, Romach MK. Treatment of codeine dependence with inhibitors of cytochrome P450 2D6. *J Clin Psychopharmacol* (2002) 22, 326–9.

Opioids + Rifampicin (Rifampin)

Rifampicin markedly increases the metabolism of codeine and morphine, and reduces their effects. Rifampicin dramatically reduced the effects of oxycodone in one patient.

Clinical evidence, mechanism, importance and management

(a) Codeine

A study in 9 extensive metabolisers and 6 poor metabolisers of the cytochrome P450 isoenzyme CYP2D6 found that after taking rifampicin 600 mg daily for 3 weeks, the metabolism of a single 120-mg oral dose of codeine phosphate was markedly increased in both phenotypes. The AUC of codeine was decreased by 79.4% in extensive metabolisers and 83.5% in poor metabolisers and in both the *N*-demethylation and glucuronidation metabolic pathways were induced. However, the *O*-demethylation of codeine (mediated by CYP2D6) was induced only in extensive metabolisers, and in these subjects there was a 56% reduction in the AUC of morphine (the main active metabolite of codeine), and a 173% increase in the AUC normorphine (another active metabolite). Note that morphine and its metabolites were not detected in poor metabolisers, either before or after rifampicin was given because the pathway that leads to these metabolites is deficient or absent in these subjects. Rifampicin reduced the respiratory and psychomotor effects of the codeine in extensive metabolisers, but not in poor metabolisers. In contrast, rifampicin did not alter the pupillary effect of codeine in extensive metabolisers, but decreased it in poor metabolisers. The clinically more relevant question of whether, and to what extent, the analgesic effects of the codeine were reduced by this interaction was not addressed by this study.[1] However, some reduction in effect might be expected. Therefore, if these drugs are used concurrently, be alert for the need to raise the codeine dosage. More study is needed.

(b) Morphine

In a randomised study, 10 healthy subjects were given a single 10-mg oral dose of morphine sulfate with rifampicin 600 mg daily. It was found that the rifampicin increased the clearance of the morphine by 49% and its analgesic effects (using a modified cold pressor test) were abolished.[2] The mechanism of this interaction is uncertain since morphine is principally metabolised by glucuronidation (see 'opioids', (p.133)), but the findings of this study could not be attributed to rifampicin induction of glucuronosyltransferases (UGTs).[2] Be alert for the need to use an increased dosage of morphine in patients taking rifampicin. More study is needed.

(c) Oxycodone

A 60-year-old man who was taking rifampicin as well as oxycodone had 3 consecutive negative urine oxycodone screens in a 2-month period, which would normally suggest that he was not taking the oxycodone. However, oxycodone metabolites were found in his urine confirming compliance with his medication. An interaction between rifampicin and oxycodone was suspected and his oxycodone dose was increased to optimise his pain control.[3]

1. Caraco Y, Sheller J, Wood AJJ. Pharmacogenetic determinants of codeine induction by rifampin: the impact on codeine's respiratory, psychomotor and miotic effects. *J Pharmacol Exp Ther* (1997) 281, 330–6.
2. Fromm MF, Eckhardt K, Li S, Schänzle G, Hofmann U, Mikus G, Eichelbaum M. Loss of analgesic effect of morphine due to coadministration of rifampin. *Pain* (1997) 72, 261–7.
3. Lee HK, Lewis LD, Tsongalis GJ, McMullin M, Schur BC, Wong SH, Yeo KT. Negative urine opioid screening caused by rifampin-mediated induction of oxycodone hepatic metabolism. *Clin Chim Acta* (2006) 367, 196–200.

Opioids; Fentanyl and related drugs + Rifampicin (Rifampin)

The serum levels and effects of transdermal fentanyl were decreased when one patient took rifampicin. Studies in healthy subjects have shown that the bioavailability of transmucosal fentanyl is reduced, and the clearance of intravenous alfentanil is markedly increased, by rifampicin.

Clinical evidence, mechanism, importance and management

(a) Alfentanil

A study in 9 healthy subjects found that when they were given intravenous alfentanil 20 micrograms/kg after taking rifampicin 600 mg orally for 5 days, alfentanil clearance was increased almost threefold.[1] This increased clearance probably occurs because rifampicin increases the activity of the cytochrome P450 isoenzyme CYP3A4 in the liver, which is concerned with the metabolism of alfentanil (see 'opioids', (p.133)). This study was primarily designed to investigate the role of CYP3A4 in the metabolism of alfentanil, but it also provides good evidence that alfentanil is likely be much less effective in patients taking rifampicin. A much larger dose of alfentanil will almost certainly be needed.

(b) Fentanyl

A 61-year-old man with lung metastases was given transdermal fentanyl (1.67 mg patch every 3 days). Serum fentanyl levels were measured 48 and 72 hours after the first day of treatment were 0.9 and 0.77 nanograms/mL, respectively (within the reported minimal effective therapeutic range of 0.2 to 1.2 nanograms/mL). On day 5, due to insufficient pain control, the fentanyl patch was increased to 2.5 mg every 3 days. However, on day 7, oral rifampicin 300 mg daily, isoniazid and ethambutol were started for pulmonary tuberculosis. The following day severe pain developed and fentanyl serum levels 48 and 72 hours after treatment on day 8 were 0.53 and 0.21 nanograms/mL, respectively (i.e. in the presence of rifampicin a higher dose of fentanyl had led to lower levels). Even after the dose was titrated up to 7.5 mg every 3 days, the patient still complained of moderate pain and the fentanyl serum level 72 hours after treatment was only 0.69 nanograms/mL (i.e. less than the level achieved with the 1.67 mg dose).[2]

In a study in 12 healthy subjects, peak levels and maximum miosis after oral, transmucosal fentanyl 10 micrograms/kg were minimally affected by oral rifampicin 600 mg daily for 5 days, but the AUC of fentanyl was decreased by 63%; the AUC of its metabolite, norfentanyl, was increased by 73%, and the AUC_{0-10} of miosis was decreased by 54%.[3]

Fentanyl is metabolised by the cytochrome P450 isoenzyme CYP3A4 and rifampicin, a potent inducer of CYP3A4, appears to reduce its serum levels and pharmacological efficacy. Thus an increase in fentanyl dosage may be needed in patients taking rifampicin.[2]

Consider also 'Opioids + Rifampicin (Rifampin)', above.

1. Kharasch ED, Russell M, Mautz D, Thummel KE, Kunze KL, Bowdle TA, Cox K. The role of cytochrome P450 3A4 in alfentanil clearance: implications for interindividual variability in disposition and perioperative drug interactions. *Anesthesiology* (1997) 87, 36–50.
2. Takane H, Nosaka A, Wakushima H, Hosokawa K, Ieiri I. Rifampin reduces the analgesic effect of transdermal fentanyl. *Ann Pharmacother* (2005) 39, 2139–40.
3. Kharasch ED, Whittington D, Hoffer C. Influence of hepatic and intestinal cytochrome P4503A activity on the acute disposition and effects of oral transmucosal fentanyl citrate. *Anesthesiology* (2004) 101, 729–37.

Opioids; Methadone + Rifamycins

Serum methadone levels can be markedly reduced by rifampicin, and withdrawal symptoms have occurred in some patients. Rifabutin appears to interact similarly, but to a lesser extent.

Clinical evidence

(a) Rifabutin

A study in 24 HIV-positive patients taking methadone found that after taking rifabutin 300 mg daily for 13 days the pharmacokinetics of the methadone were minimally changed. However 75% of the patients reported at least one mild symptom of methadone withdrawal, but this was not enough for any of them to withdraw from the study. Only 3 of them asked for and received an increase in their methadone dosage. The authors offered the opinion that over-reporting of withdrawal symptoms was likely to be due to the warnings that the patients had received.[1]

(b) Rifampicin

The observation that former diamorphine (heroin) addicts taking methadone complained of withdrawal symptoms when given rifampicin, prompted a study[2] in 30 patients taking methadone. Withdrawal symptoms developed in 21 of the 30 within 1 to 33 days of starting rifampicin 600 to 900 mg daily and isoniazid daily. In 6 of the 7 most severely affected, the symptoms developed within a week, and their plasma methadone levels fell by 33 to 68%. Of 56 other patients taking methadone with other antitubercular treatment (which included isoniazid but not rifampicin), none developed withdrawal symptoms.[2-4]

Other cases of this interaction have been reported.[5-9] Some patients needed two to threefold increases in the methadone dosage while taking rifampicin to control the withdrawal symptoms.[6,7,9]

Mechanism

Rifampicin is a potent enzyme-inducer, which increases the activity of the intestinal and liver enzymes concerned with the metabolism of methadone, resulting in a marked decrease in its levels.[10] In 4 patients in the study cited, the urinary excretion of the major metabolite of methadone rose by 150%.[2] Rifabutin has only a small enzyme-inducing effect and therefore the effects are not as great.

Importance and management

The interaction between methadone and rifampicin is established, adequately documented and of clinical importance. The incidence is high. Two-thirds (21) of the narcotic-dependent patients in one study[2] developed this interaction, 14 of whom were able to continue treatment. Withdrawal symptoms may develop within 24 hours. The analgesic effects of methadone would also be expected to be reduced. Concurrent use need not be avoided, but the effects should be monitored and appropriate dosage increases (as much as two to threefold) made where necessary.

Rifabutin appears to interact to a very much lesser extent so that fewer, if any, patients are likely to need a methadone dosage increase.

1. Brown LS, Sawyer RC, Li R, Cobb MN, Colborn DC, Narang PK. Lack of a pharmacologic interaction between rifabutin and methadone in HIV-infected former injecting drug users. *Drug Alcohol Depend* (1996) 43, 71–7.
2. Kreek MJ, Garfield JW, Gutjahr CL, Giusti LM. Rifampin-induced methadone withdrawal. *N Engl J Med* (1976) 294, 1104–6.
3. Garfield JW, Kreek MJ, Giusti L. Rifampin-methadone relationship. 1. The clinical effects of rifampin-methadone interaction. *Am Rev Respir Dis* (1975) 111, 926.
4. Kreek MJ, Garfield JW, Gutjahr CL, Bowen D, Field F, Rothschild M. Rifampin-methadone relationship. 2. Rifampin effects on plasma concentration, metabolism, and excretion of methadone. *Am Rev Respir Dis* (1975) 111, 926–7.
5. Bending MR, Skacel PO. Rifampicin and methadone withdrawal. *Lancet* (1977) i, 1211.
6. Van Leeuwen DJ. Rifampicine leidt tot onthoudingsverschijnselen bij methadongebruikers. *Ned Tijdschr Geneeskd* (1986) 130, 548–50.
7. Brockmeyer NH, Mertins L, Goos M. Pharmacokinetic interaction of antimicrobial agents with levomethadon in drug-addicted AIDS patients. *Klin Wochenschr* (1991) 69, 16–18.
8. Holmes VF. Rifampin-induced methadone withdrawal in AIDS. *J Clin Psychopharmacol* (1990) 10, 443–4.
9. Raistrick D, Hay A, Wolff K. Methadone maintenance and tuberculosis treatment. *BMJ* (1996) 313, 925–6.
10. Kharasch ED, Hoffer C, Whittington D, Sheffels P. Role of hepatic and intestinal cytochrome P450 3A and 2B6 in the metabolism, disposition, and miotic effects of methadone. *Clin Pharmacol Ther* (2004) 76, 250–69.

Opioids + Tobacco

Smokers who discontinue smoking appear to require more opioid analgesics for postoperative pain control than non-smokers; this has been seen with both fentanyl and morphine patient controlled analgesia. Atmospheric pollution has a similar effect on pentazocine. Codeine metabolism was not affected to a clinically relevant extent by smoking in one study.

Clinical evidence

A retrospective study of coronary artery bypass graft patients found that 20 patients who had abruptly discontinued smoking prior to surgery required more postoperative opioid analgesics than 69 non-smokers. The opioid analgesics included **dextropropoxyphene (propoxyphene)**, **fentanyl**, **hydrocodone**, **oxycodone**, **morphine**, **nalbuphine** and **pethidine (meperidine)**, but the most commonly used postoperative opioid analgesic was **fentanyl** (used in approximately two-thirds of the patients) given by patient controlled analgesia (PCA). Smokers deprived of nicotine had an increase in opioid requirement (converted to morphine equivalents), during the first 48 hours after surgery, ranging from 29 to 33% (when normalised for body weight or body mass index).[1] Similarly, another retrospective study in 171 women found that average postoperative narcotic use (expressed as equivalent doses of morphine) was 10.9 mg/12 hours for patients who had never smoked, 13 mg/12 hours for former smokers, and 13.1 mg/12 hours for current smokers.[2]

(a) Codeine

The metabolism of a single 25-mg dose of codeine did not differ between 9 heavy smokers (greater than 20 cigarettes daily) and 9 non-smoking control subjects, except that smokers had a slightly higher rate of codeine glucuronidation.[3] This is unlikely to be clinically important. Another study found no clinically important differences in the systemic availability of single 60-mg oral or intramuscular doses of codeine between 10 smokers and 12 non-smokers. There was no significant difference in the plasma half-life of codeine or in the conversion of codeine to morphine, however, there was a slightly higher plasma clearance of codeine in smokers than in non-smokers.[4] No differences in the efficacy of codeine are expected between smokers and non-smokers.

(b) Dextropropoxyphene (Propoxyphene)

A study in 835 patients who were given dextropropoxyphene for mild or moderate pain or headache found that its efficacy as an analgesic was decreased by smoking. The drug was rated as ineffective in about 10% of 335 non-smokers, 15% of 347 patients who smoked up to 20 cigarettes daily, and 20% of 153 patients who smoked more than 20 cigarettes daily.[5]

(c) Morphine

A study in 7 women during acute post-caesarean recovery found that intravenous morphine use (as patient-controlled analgesia; PCA), was significantly higher in smokers compared with non-smokers: weight-adjusted morphine use was 1.8 mg/kg per 24 hours compared with 0.64 mg/kg per 24 hours, respectively). It was suggested that a history of nicotine use and/or short-term nicotine abstinence could modulate morphine use and analgesia during postoperative recovery.[6] Similarly, another retrospective study found increased morphine PCA requirements in smokers compared with non-smokers.[7]

(d) Pentazocine

A study in which pentazocine was used to supplement nitrous oxide relaxant anaesthesia found that patients who came from an urban environment needed about 50% more pentazocine than those who lived in the country (3.6 micrograms/kg per minute compared with 2.4 micrograms/kg per minute). Roughly the same difference was seen between those who smoked and those who did not (3.8 micrograms/kg per minute compared with 2.5 micrograms/kg per minute).[8] In another study it was found that pentazocine metabolism was 40% higher in smokers than in non-smokers.[9]

Mechanism

It is thought that tobacco smoke contains compounds that increase the activity of the liver enzymes concerned with the metabolism of dextropropoxyphene, pentazocine and other opioids, which increases their metabolism, decreases their levels and diminishes their effectiveness as analgesics.[2,5] However, former smokers have also been found to have increased opioid requirements and it has been suggested that smoking might have an effect on pain perception and/or opioid response, or that nicotine addiction and opioid requirements may be genetically linked.[2]

Importance and management

The interaction appears to be well established. Prescribers should be aware that smokers may require a greater amount of opioids postoperatively than non-smokers. In contrast, codeine metabolism does not appear to be affected to a clinically important extent by smoking.

1. Creekmore FM, Lugo RA, Weiland KJ. Postoperative opiate analgesia requirements of smokers and nonsmokers. *Ann Pharmacother* (2004) 38, 949–53.
2. Woodside JR. Female smokers have increased postoperative narcotic requirements. *J Addict Dis* (2000) 19, 1–10.
3. Yue Q-Y, Tomson T, Säwe J. Carbamazepine and cigarette smoking induce differentially the metabolism of codeine in man. *Pharmacogenetics* (1994) 4, 193–8.
4. Hull JH, Findlay JWA, Rogers JF, Welch RM, Butz RF, Bustrack JA. An evaluation of the effects of smoking on codeine pharmacokinetics and bioavailability in normal human volunteers. *Drug Intell Clin Pharm* (1982) 16, 849–54.
5. Boston Collaborative Drug Surveillance Program. Decreased clinical efficacy of propoxyphene in cigarette smokers. *Clin Pharmacol Ther* (1973) 14, 259–63.
6. Marco AP, Greenwald MK, Higgins MS. A preliminary study of 24-hour post-cesarean patient controlled analgesia: postoperative pain reports and morphine requests/utilization are greater in abstaining smokers than non-smokers. *Med Sci Monit* (2005) 11, CR255–CR261.
7. Glasson JC, Sawyer WT, Lindley CM, Ginsberg B. Patient-specific factors affecting patient-controlled analgesia dosing. *J Pain Palliat Care Pharmacother* (2002) 16, 5–21.
8. Keeri-Szanto M, Pomeroy JR. Atmospheric pollution and pentazocine metabolism. *Lancet* (1971) i, 947–9.
9. Vaughan DP, Beckett AH, Robbie DS. The influence of smoking on the intersubject variation in pentazocine elimination. *Br J Clin Pharmacol* (1976) 3, 279–83.

Opioids + Tricyclic and related antidepressants

In general, the concurrent use of most opioids and tricyclics is uneventful, although lethargy, sedation, and respiratory depression have been reported. Tramadol should be used with caution with tricyclic antidepressants because of the possible risk of seizures and the serotonin syndrome. Dextropropoxyphene may cause moderate rises in the serum levels of amitriptyline and nortriptyline, and methadone may moderately raise desipramine levels. The bioavailability and the degree of analgesia of oral morphine is increased by clomipramine, desipramine and possibly amitriptyline.

Clinical evidence

(a) Buprenorphine

A study in 12 healthy subjects found that both sublingual buprenorphine 400 micrograms and oral **amitriptyline** 50 mg impaired the performance of a number of psychomotor tests (digit symbol substitution, flicker fusion, Maddox wing, hand-to-eye coordination, reactive skills), and the subjects felt drowsy, feeble, mentally slow and muzzy. When **amitriptyline** 30 mg, increased to 75 mg daily was given for 4 days before a single dose of buprenorphine, the psychomotor effects were not significantly increased, but the respiratory depressant effects of the buprenorphine were enhanced.[1]

(b) Dextropropoxyphene (Propoxyphene)

An elderly man taking **doxepin** 150 mg daily developed lethargy and daytime sedation when he started to take dextropropoxyphene 65 mg every 6 hours. His plasma **doxepin** levels rose by almost 150% (from 20 to 48.5 nanograms/mL) and desmethyldoxepin levels were similarly increased (from 8.8 to 20.7 nanograms/mL).[2]

The **amitriptyline** concentration/dose ratio in 12 patients given **amitriptyline** and dextropropoxyphene was raised by about 20% (suggesting raised amitriptyline levels), when compared with other patients taking **amitriptyline** alone. Similarly, the plasma levels of the **amitriptyline** metabolite nortriptyline was raised by about 30% in 14 patients given dextropropoxyphene;[3] and in another study **nortriptyline** plasma levels were raised by 16% by dextropropoxyphene.[3]

Fifteen patients with rheumatoid arthritis given a single 25-mg dose of **amitriptyline** and dextropropoxyphene (up to 65 mg three times daily) experienced some drowsiness and mental slowness. They complained of being clumsier and had more pain, but these effects were said to be mild.[4]

(c) Methadone

The mean serum levels of **desipramine** 2.5 mg/kg daily were approximately doubled in 5 men who took methadone 500 micrograms/kg daily for 2 weeks. Previous observations in patients given both drugs had shown that **desipramine** levels were higher than expected and adverse effects developed at relatively low doses.[5] Further evidence of an increase in plasma **desipramine** levels due to methadone is described in another study.[6]

(d) Morphine

Clomipramine or **amitriptyline**, in doses of 20 or 50 mg daily, increased the AUC of oral morphine by 28 to 111% in 24 patients with cancer pain. The half-life of morphine was also prolonged.[7] A previous study[8] found that **desipramine**, but not **amitriptyline**, increased and prolonged morphine analgesia, and a later study by the same group confirmed the value of **desipramine**.[9]

(e) Oxycodone

Pretreatment with **amitriptyline** 10 mg increased to 50 mg daily for 4 days caused no major changes in the psychomotor effects of a single 280-microgram/kg oral dose of oxycodone in 9 healthy subjects.[10] Respiratory effects were not assessed.

(f) Pentazocine

Both pentazocine and **amitriptyline** given alone caused 11 healthy subjects to feel drowsy, muzzy and clumsy, and reduced the performance of a number of psychomotor tests. However, when the same subjects were given intramuscular pentazocine 30 mg after taking **amitriptyline** 50 mg daily for a week, the combination of drugs appeared not to impair driving or occupational skills more than either drug given alone.[11] Respiratory depression was increased more by the combination than either drug alone. **Amitriptyline** modestly decreased pentazocine plasma levels by about 20% at 1.5 and 3.5 hours.[11]

(g) Tramadol

The CSM in the UK has publicised 27 reports of convulsions and one of worsening epilepsy with tramadol, a reporting rate of 1 in 7000 patients. Some of the patients were given doses well in excess of those recommended, and 8 patients were also taking tricyclic antidepressants, which are known to reduce the convulsive threshold.[12] Similarly, the FDA in the US has received 124 reports of seizures associated with tramadol, 28 of which included the concurrent use of tricyclic antidepressants,[13] and the Australian Adverse Drug Reaction Advisory Committee (ADRAC) has received 26 cases of convulsions associated with tramadol, some of which included the concurrent use of tricyclic antidepressants.[14] ADRAC have also received reports of the serotonin syndrome, which were associated with the use of tramadol and tricyclic antidepressants.[14] Furthermore two case reports suggest that tramadol may have contributed to the development of the serotonin syndrome, one in a patient abusing tramadol, moclobemide and **clomipramine**,[15] and the other in a 79-year-old patient taking morphine *(MST)*, co-proxamol (dextropropoxyphene with paracetamol) and **amitriptyline**, after she started to take tramadol.[16,17] In both of these cases the patient died. For this reason tramadol should be used with caution with tricyclic antidepressants.

Similarly, seizures and the serotonin syndrome have been reported in a woman who took **mirtazapine** with tramadol, but this may have been due to over-use of the tramadol rather than an interaction.[18] Lethargy, confusion, hypotension, bronchospasm and hypoxia has also been seen following the use of tramadol and **mirtazapine**, which resolved within hours of both drugs being stopped.[19]

Mechanism

The CNS depressant effects of opioids and the tricyclic antidepressants are expected to be additive. The reasons for the increased morphine levels and analgesic effects that occur with some tricyclics are not understood. The increased analgesia may be due not only to the increased serum levels of morphine, but possibly also to some alteration in the way the morphine affects its receptors. Dextropropoxyphene probably inhibits liver metabolism of some tricyclic antidepressants[3] by inhibiting the activity of the cytochrome P450 isoenzyme CYP2D6, and as a result the serum levels of the tricyclic antidepressants rise. It is suggested that the methadone may possibly inhibit the hydroxylation of the desipramine, thereby raising its levels.[6]

Importance and management

The majority of the evidence, and general clinical experience suggests that, in most cases, the use of opioids with tricyclic antidepressants is uneventful. Furthermore, limited evidence suggests that concurrent use may be beneficial in pain management. However, the CNS depressant effects of both these classes of drugs should be considered when prescribing the combination, especially as there is some evidence to suggest that the respiratory depressant effects are increased: this may be clinically important in patients with a restricted respiratory capacity.[11] Certain opioids appear to have a greater propensity to interact. Both **tramadol** and the tricyclics can lower the seizure threshold and cause the serotonin syndrome. Therefore particular caution is warranted with this combination, especially in epileptic patients or those taking other drugs that affect serotonin. Mirtazapine appears to interact in the same way as the tricyclics. Be aware that as **dextropropoxyphene** and **methadone** may raise tricyclic levels: however, the general clinical significance of these interactions is uncertain but be alert for any evidence of increased CNS depression and increased tricyclic antidepressant adverse effects. In this context it is worth noting that one study reported that the incidence of hip fractures in the elderly was found to be increased by a factor of 1.6 in those taking dextropropoxyphene, and further increased to 2.6 when antidepressants, benzodiazepines or antipsychotics were added.[20]

For mention of the suggestion that antidepressants and antipsychotics may increase the incidence of myoclonus with high-dose morphine, see 'Opioids; Morphine + Miscellaneous', p.190.

1. Saarialho-Kere U, Mattila MJ, Paloheimo M, Seppälä T. Psychomotor, respiratory and neuroendocrinological effects of buprenorphine and amitriptyline in healthy volunteers. *Eur J Clin Pharmacol* (1987) 33, 139–46.
2. Abernethy DR, Greenblatt DJ, Steel K. Propoxyphene inhibition of doxepin and antipyrine metabolism. *Clin Pharmacol Ther* (1982) 31, 199.
3. Jerling M, Bertilsson L, Sjöqvist F. The use of therapeutic drug monitoring data to document kinetic drug interactions: an example with amitriptyline and nortriptyline. *Ther Drug Monit* (1994) 16, 1–12.
4. Saarialho-Kere U, Julkunen H, Mattila MJ, Seppälä T. Psychomotor performance of patients with rheumatoid arthritis: cross-over comparison of dextropropoxyphene, dextropropoxyphene plus amitriptyline, indomethacin and placebo. *Pharmacol Toxicol* (1988) 63, 286–92.
5. Maany I, Dhopesh V, Arndt IO, Burke W, Woody G, O'Brien CP. Increase in desipramine serum levels associated with methadone treatment. *Am J Psychiatry* (1989) 146, 1611–13.
6. Kosten TR, Gawin FH, Morgan C, Nelson JC, Jatlow P. Desipramine and its 2-hydroxy metabolite in patients taking or not taking methadone. *Am J Psychiatry* (1990) 147, 1379–80.
7. Ventafridda V, Ripamonti C, De Conno F, Bianchi M, Pazzuconi F, Panerai AE. Antidepressants increase bioavailability of morphine in cancer patients. *Lancet* (1987) i, 1204.
8. Levine JD, Gordon NC, Smith R, McBryde R. Desipramine enhances opiate postoperative analgesia. *Pain* (1986) 27, 45–9.
9. Gordon NC, Heller PH, Gear RW, Levine JD. Temporal factors in the enhancement of morphine analgesia by desipramine. *Pain* (1993) 53, 273–6.
10. Pöyhiä R, Kalso E, Seppälä T. Pharmacodynamic interactions of oxycodone and amitriptyline in healthy volunteers. *Curr Ther Res* (1992) 51, 739–49.
11. Saarialho-Kere U, Mattila MJ, Seppälä T. Parenteral pentazocine: effects on psychomotor skills and respiration, and interactions with amitriptyline. *Eur J Clin Pharmacol* (1988) 35, 483–9.
12. Committee on Safety of Medicines/Medicines Control Agency. In focus—tramadol. *Current Problems* (1996) 22, 11.
13. Kahn LH, Alderfer RJ, Graham DJ. Seizures reported with tramadol. *JAMA* (1997) 278, 1661.
14. Adverse Drug Reactions Advisory Committee (ADRAC). Tramadol – four years' experience. *Aust Adverse Drug React Bull* (2003) 22, 2.
15. Hernandez AF, Montero MN, Pla A, Villanueva E. Fatal moclobemide overdose or death caused by serotonin syndrome? *J Forensic Sci* (1995) 40, 128–30.
16. Kitson R, Carr B. Tramadol and severe serotonin syndrome. *Anaesthesia* (2005) 60, 934–5.
17. Gillman K. A response to 'Tramadol and severe serotonin syndrome'. *Anaesthesia* (2006) 61, 76. Author reply. Ibid., 76–77.
18. Freeman WD, Chabolla DR. 36-Year-old woman with loss of consciousness, fever, and tachycardia. *Mayo Clin Proc* (2005) 80, 667–70.
19. Gnanadesigan N, Espinoza RT, Smith R, Israel M, Reuben DB. Interaction of serotonergic antidepressants and opioid analgesics: is serotonin syndrome going undetected? *J Am Med Dir Assoc* (2005) 6, 265–9.
20. Shorr RI, Griffin MR, Daugherty JR, Ray WA. Opioid analgesics and the risk of hip fracture in the elderly: codeine and propoxyphene. *J Gerontol* (1992) 47, M111–M115.

Opioids + Urinary acidifiers or alkalinisers

Urinary methadone clearance is increased if the urine is made acid (e.g. by giving ammonium chloride) and reduced if it is made alkaline (e.g. by giving sodium bicarbonate). The urinary clearance of dextropropoxyphene (propoxyphene) and pethidine (meperidine) may also be increased by acidification of the urine.

Clinical evidence

(a) Dextropropoxyphene (Propoxyphene)

A study in 6 healthy subjects found that the cumulative 72-hour urinary excretion of unchanged dextropropoxyphene was increased sixfold by acidification of the urine with oral **ammonium chloride** and reduced by 95% by alkalinisation with **sodium bicarbonate**; the half-life of dextropropoxyphene was also shortened by ammonium chloride. The excretion of the active metabolite norpropoxyphene was much less dependent on urinary pH. However, the cumulative excretion of dextropropoxyphene and norpropoxyphene, even into acidic urine, accounted for less than 25% of the dose during 72 hours.[1]

(b) Methadone

A study in patients taking methadone found that the urinary clearance in those with urinary pHs of less than 6 was greater than those with higher urinary pHs.[2] When the urinary pH of one subject was lowered from 6.2 to 5.5, the loss of unchanged methadone in the urine was nearly doubled.[3]

A pharmacokinetic study in 5 healthy subjects given a 10-mg intramuscular dose of methadone found that the plasma half-life was 19.5 hours when the urine was made acidic (pH 5.2) with **ammonium chloride**, compared with 42.1 hours when the urine was made alkaline (pH 7.8) with **sodium bicarbonate**. The clearance of the methadone fell from 134 to 91.9 mL/minute when the urine was changed from acidic to alkaline.[4]

For isolated reports of respiratory depression when cimetidine or ranitidine were given with opioids, see 'H_2-receptor antagonists', (p.171).

(c) Pethidine (Meperidine)

A study in 6 healthy subjects given intravenous pethidine 21.75 mg found that urinary acidification with **ammonium chloride** increased the 48-hour urinary recovery of pethidine and norpethidine from about 7% and 12%, respectively, with no control of urinary pH, to about 20% and 24%, respectively. Urinary alkalinisation reduced the urinary recovery of pethidine and norpethidine to less than 1% and 7%, respectively. These pronounced effects had negligible effects on the blood concentration/time profiles.[5] A study in 10 healthy Chinese subjects given intravenous pethidine 150 micrograms/kg found large variations in the 48-hour urinary recovery of pethidine and norpethidine depending on urinary pH; mean urinary recovery values under acidic conditions were 24.3% and 33.0%, respectively, and under alkaline conditions were 0.4% and 3.8%, respectively. The bioavailability was slightly lower under acidic urinary conditions due to the greater renal clearance of the drug.[6]

Mechanism

Methadone is eliminated from the body both by liver metabolism and excretion of unchanged methadone in the urine. Above pH 6 the urinary excretion is less important, but with urinary pH below 6 the half-life becomes dependent on both excretion (30%) and metabolism (70%).[3,4,7] Methadone is a weak base (pKa 8.4) so that in acidic urine little of the drug is in the un-ionised form and little is reabsorbed by simple passive diffusion. On the other hand, in alkaline solution most of the drug is in the un-ionised form, which is readily reabsorbed by the kidney tubules, and little is lost in the urine.

Acidification of the urine may also increase the renal clearance of unchanged pethidine and norpethidine again probably due to reduced reabsorption in the renal tubule.[6] Dextropropoxyphene appears to be similarly affected.

Importance and management

The effect of urinary pH on the clearance of methadone is an established interaction, but of uncertain importance. Be alert for any evidence of reduced methadone effects in patients whose urine becomes acidic because they are taking large doses of ammonium chloride. Lowering the urinary pH to 5 with ammonium chloride to increase the clearance can also be used to treat toxicity. Theoretically, urinary alkalinisers such as sodium bicarbonate and **acetazolamide** may increase the effect of methadone.

Similarly, the urinary clearance of dextropropoxyphene and pethidine appear to be increased to some extent by acidification of the urine, although their bioavailabilities do not appear to be significantly affected and the clinical effect is probably small. However, be aware of the potential for increased urinary excretion.

1. Kärkkäinen S, Neuvonen PJ. Effect of oral charcoal and urine pH on dextropropoxyphene pharmacokinetics. *Int J Clin Pharmacol Ther Toxicol* (1985) 23, 219–25.
2. Bellward GD, Warren PM, Howald W, Axelson JE, Abbott FS. Methadone maintenance: effect of urinary pH on renal clearance in chronic high and low doses. *Clin Pharmacol Ther* (1977) 22, 92–9.
3. Inturrisi CE, Verebely K. Disposition of methadone in man after a single oral dose. *Clin Pharmacol Ther* (1972) 13, 923–30.
4. Nilsson M-I, Widerlöv E, Meresaar U, Änggård E. Effect of urinary pH on the disposition of methadone in man. *Eur J Clin Pharmacol* (1982) 22, 337–42.
5. Verbeeck RK, Branch RA, Wilkinson GR. Meperidine disposition in man: influence of urinary pH and route of administration. *Clin Pharmacol Ther* (1981) 30, 619–28.
6. Chan K, Tse J, Jennings F, Orme ML'E. Influence of urinary pH on pethidine kinetics in healthy volunteer subjects. 2. A study of ten Chinese subjects. *Methods Find Exp Clin Pharmacol* (1987) 9, 49–54.
7. Baselt RC, Casarett LJ. Urinary excretion of methadone in man. *Clin Pharmacol Ther* (1972) 13, 64–70.

Opioids; Alfentanil + Reserpine

An isolated report describes ventricular arrhythmias when a patient taking reserpine was given alfentanil during anaesthesia.

Clinical evidence, mechanism, importance and management

A hypertensive woman taking reserpine 250 micrograms daily was given intravenous alfentanil 800 micrograms over 5 minutes, before anaesthesia with thiopental and suxamethonium (succinylcholine). During surgery she was given nine 100-microgram doses of alfentanil and 70% N_2O/O_2. Bradycardia developed and frequent unifocal premature ventricular contractions occurred throughout the surgery, but they disappeared 3 to 4 hours afterwards. The arrhythmia was attributed to an interaction between reserpine and alfentanil, but just why this should occur is not understood.[1]

1. Jahr JS, Weber S. Ventricular dysrhythmias following an alfentanil anesthetic in a patient on reserpine for hypertension. *Acta Anaesthesiol Scand* (1991) 35, 788–9.

Opioids; Alfentanil + Terbinafine

Terbinafine 250 mg daily for 3 days had no statistically significant effect on alfentanil pharmacokinetics and no adverse effects were reported.[1]

1. Saari TI, Laine K, Leino K, Valtonen M, Neuvonen PJ, Olkkola KT. Voriconazole, but not terbinafine, markedly reduces alfentanil clearance and prolongs its half-life. *Clin Pharmacol Ther* (2006) 80, 502–8.

Opioids; Codeine + Kaolin

An isolated report describes patients suffering from chronic diarrhoea, who were stabilised taking codeine phosphate, but who experienced a relapse when the codeine was added to *Kaolin Mixture*. An *in vitro* study suggested the bioavailability of codeine may be reduced by adsorption onto kaolin.[1]

1. Yu SKS, Oppenheim RC, Stewart NF. Codeine phosphate adsorbed by kaolin. *Aust J Pharm* (1976) 57, 468.

Opioids; Codeine + Somatostatin analogues

Lanreotide and octreotide partially inhibit the metabolism of codeine, which may possibly reduce its analgesic effects.

Clinical evidence, mechanism, importance and management

A study in 6 patients with gastrointestinal carcinoid tumours found that **lanreotide** or **octreotide** 750 micrograms subcutaneously three times daily for 3 days decreased the partial metabolic clearance of **codeine** by *N*-demethylation (by the cytochrome P450 isoenzyme CYP3A) by an average of 44% and the *O*-demethylation (by CYP2D6) by 35%. However, the partial clearance by 6-glucuronidation and the total systemic clearance of **codeine** were not consistently changed. The effects of the somatostatins were thought to be mediated by a suppression of growth hormone secretion. The reduction in *O*-demethylation can reduce the active metabolite of codeine, morphine, which could reduce the analgesic effect of the drug.[1]

1. Rasmussen E, Eriksson B, Öberg K, Bondesson U, Rane A. Selective effects of somatostatin analogs on human drug-metabolizing enzymes. *Clin Pharmacol Ther* (1998) 64, 150–9.

Opioids; Dextropropoxyphene (Propoxyphene) + Orphenadrine

An alleged adverse interaction between dextropropoxyphene and orphenadrine, which is said to cause mental confusion, anxiety, and tremors, seems to be very rare, if indeed it ever occurs.

Clinical evidence, mechanism, importance and management

The manufacturers of orphenadrine used to state in their package insert that mental confusion, anxiety and tremors have been reported in patients receiving both orphenadrine and dextropropoxyphene. The manufacturers of dextropropoxyphene issued a similar warning. However, in correspondence with both manufacturers, two investigators[1] of this interaction were told that the basis of these statements consisted of 6 anecdotal reports from clinicians to one manufacturer and 7 to the other (some could represent the same cases). Of the 7 cases to one manufacturer, 4 occurred where patients had received twice the recommended dose of orphenadrine. In every case the adverse reactions seen were similar to those reported with either drug alone. A brief study in 5 patients given both drugs to investigate this alleged interaction failed to reveal an adverse interaction.[2] One case has been reported separately.[3]

The documentation is therefore sparse, and no case of interaction has been firmly established. The investigators calculated that the two drugs were probably being used together on 300 000 prescriptions a year, and that these few cases would be less than significant.[1] There seems therefore little reason for avoiding concurrent use.

1. Pearson RE, Salter FJ. Drug interaction? — Orphenadrine with propoxyphene. *N Engl J Med* (1970) 282, 1215.
2. Puckett WH, Visconti JA. Orphenadrine and propoxyphene (cont.). *N Engl J Med* (1970) 283, 544.
3. Renforth W. Orphenadrine and propoxyphene. *N Engl J Med* (1970) 283, 998.

Opioids; Diamorphine + Pyrithyldione

A single case report describes a fatality due to the combined CNS depressant effects of diamorphine and pyrithyldione.

Clinical evidence, mechanism, importance and management

A diamorphine (heroin) addict was found dead after taking pyrithyldione (a sedative and hypnotic) with diamorphine. His blood pyrithyldione and brain morphine levels were found to be 590 nanograms/mL and 0.06 nanograms/g respectively, suggesting that he had taken only a therapeutic dose of the pyrithyldione and a moderate dose of diamorphine. The presumed cause of death was the combined CNS depressant effects of both drugs. The authors of the report draw the conclusion that the pyrithyldione potentiated the effects of the diamorphine.[1]

1. Jorens PG, Coucke V, Selala MI, Schepens PJC. Fatal intoxication due to the combined use of heroin and pyrithyldione. *Hum Exp Toxicol* (1992) 11, 296–7.

Opioids; Levacetylmethadol + Miscellaneous

Levacetylmethadol has been withdrawn in Europe and the USA because of cases of life-threatening cardiac arrhythmias associated with QT prolongation.[1,2] Its use was contraindicated with MAOIs and drugs that prolong the QT interval.[3,4] In addition, the manufacturers warned about the possible effects of inducers or inhibitors of the cytochrome P450 isoenzyme CYP3A4, which may increase or reduce its activity, respectively;[3,5] the additive effects of alcohol or other CNS depressants; and the possible risk of oral contraceptive failure.[3] They also advised the avoidance of pethidine (meperidine), dextropropoxyphene (propoxyphene) or naloxone (except when used for overdosage).[3]

1. Important safety message: Orlaam (Levacetylmethadol) – CPMP opinion to suspend the marketing authorisation (MA), April 2001. Available at: http://www.mhra.gov.uk (accessed 16/08/07).
2. Product discontinuation notice. Orlaam. Letter from Roxane, August 2003. Available at: http://www.fda.gov/cder/drug/shortages/orlaam.htm (accessed 16/08/07).
3. OrLAAM (Levacetylmethadol). Britannia Pharmaceuticals UK. Product Information, January 2000.
4. Deamer RL, Wilson DR, Clark DS, Prichard JG. Torsades de pointes associated with high dose levomethadyl acetate (ORLAAM). *J Addict Dis* (2001) 20, 7–15.
5. Moody DE, Alburges ME, Parker RJ, Collins JM, Strong JM. The involvement of cytochrome P450 3A4 in the *N*-demethylation of l-α-acetylmethadol (LAAM), norLaam and methadone. *Drug Metab Dispos* (1997) 25, 1347–53.

Opioids; Methadone + Ciprofloxacin

An isolated case describes sedation, confusion and respiratory depression, which was attributed to the inhibition of methadone metabolism by ciprofloxacin.

Clinical evidence

A woman taking methadone 140 mg daily for 6 years to manage pain due to chronic intestinal pseudo-obstruction was admitted to hospital because of a urinary tract infection and given ciprofloxacin 750 mg twice daily. Two days later she became sedated and confused. Ciprofloxacin was replaced with co-trimoxazole and the patient recovered within 48 hours. She was treated with ciprofloxacin for recurrent urinary-tract infections a further three times and on each occasion the patient became sedated, with her normal alertness regained on discontinuing ciprofloxacin. On the last occasion, when the venlafaxine that she had also been taking was replaced by fluoxetine, she also developed respiratory depression, which was reversed with naloxone.[1]

Mechanism

The cytochrome P450 isoenzymes CYP1A2, CYP2D6 and CYP3A4 are involved in the metabolism of methadone. Ciprofloxacin is a potent inhibitor of CYP1A2 and possibly has some effect on CYP3A4. It is therefore probable that the confusion and sedation seen in the patient were due to the inhibition of methadone metabolism. The use of 'fluoxetine', (p.1221) and the fact that the patient was a smoker, may also have contributed.

Importance and management

This seems to be the only report of this interaction but it would appear to be of clinical importance. Care is needed if ciprofloxacin and methadone are given concurrently, especially if there are other factors such as smoking or the use of other enzyme inhibitors, which may also contribute to the interaction. Be alert for the need to change the methadone dosage. Consider also 'Quinolones + Opioids', p.338.

1. Herrlin K, Segerdahl M, Gustafsson LL, Kalso E. Methadone, ciprofloxacin, and adverse drug reactions. *Lancet* (2000) 356, 2069–70.

Opioids; Methadone + Disulfiram

No adverse interaction was seen when patients taking methadone were given disulfiram.

Clinical evidence, mechanism, importance and management

Seven opioid addicts, without chronic alcoholism or liver disease, and who were receiving methadone maintenance treatment (45 to 65 mg daily) had an increase in the urinary excretion of the major pyrrolidine metabolite of methadone (an indicator of increased *N*-demethylation) when given disulfiram 500 mg daily for 7 days. However, there was no effect on the degree of opioid intoxication, nor were withdrawal symptoms experienced.[1] No special precautions would seem to be necessary if both drugs are given.

1. Tong TG, Benowitz NL, Kreek MJ. Methadone-disulfiram interaction during methadone maintenance. *J Clin Pharmacol* (1980) 20, 506–13.

Opioids; Methadone + Fusidic acid

There is evidence that long-term fusidic acid may modestly reduce the effects of methadone.

Clinical evidence, mechanism, importance and management

A drug abuser with AIDS needed an increase in his levomethadone (*R*-methadone) dosage from 60 to 80 mg daily within 6 months of starting to take fusidic acid 1.5 g daily.[1] The patient showed evidence of liver enzyme induction (using antipyrine as a marker), from which it was concluded that fusidic acid increases the metabolism and loss of methadone from the body.[1] A subsequent study confirmed that fusidic acid 500 mg daily for 28 days increased antipyrine clearance in 10 patients taking levomethadone, and some of them developed clinical signs of underdosage. In contrast, fusidic acid 500 mg daily for 14 days had no effect in another 10 patients taking levomethadone.[2]

Information appears to be limited to these reports. Bear them in mind in the event of any unexpected reduction in efficacy of methadone in a patient taking long-term fusidic acid.

1. Brockmeyer NH, Mertins L, Goos M. Pharmacokinetic interaction of antimicrobial agents with levomethadon in drug-addicted AIDS patients. *Klin Wochenschr* (1991) 69, 16–18.
2. Reimann G, Barthel B, Rockstroh JK, Spatz D, Brockmeyer NH. Effect of fusidic acid on the hepatic cytochrome P450 enzyme system. *Int J Clin Pharmacol* (1999) 37, 562–6.

Opioids; Morphine + Miscellaneous

Some limited evidence suggests that antidepressants, antipsychotics, NSAIDs and thiethylperazine may increase the myoclonus caused by high doses of morphine.

Clinical evidence, mechanism, importance and management

In 19 patients with malignant disease taking high doses of morphine (daily doses of 500 mg or more orally or 250 mg or more parenterally), an analysis was made of the relationship between myoclonus and the use of supplemental drugs. In the 12 patients with myoclonus, 8 patients were taking antidepressants (**amitriptyline**, **doxepin**) or antipsychotics (**chlorpromazine**, **haloperidol**) compared with none of 6 patients without myoclonus. In addition, there was a higher use of NSAIDs (**indometacin**, **naproxen**, **piroxicam**, **aspirin**) and an antiemetic (**thiethylperazine**).[1] The reasons are not understood, and the findings of this paper have been questioned.[2]

Consider also 'Opioids + Phenothiazines', p.180, 'Opioids + NSAIDs', p.177, and 'Opioids + Tricyclic and related antidepressants', p.187.

1. Potter JM, Reid DB, Shaw RJ, Hackett P, Hickman PE. Myoclonus associated with treatment with high doses of morphine: the role of supplemental drugs. *BMJ* (1989) 299, 150–3.
2. Quinn N. Myoclonus associated with high doses of morphine. *BMJ* (1989) 299, 683–4.

Opioids; Pethidine (Meperidine) + Aciclovir

An isolated report describes pethidine toxicity associated with the use of high-dose aciclovir.

Clinical evidence, mechanism, importance and management

A man with Hodgkin's disease was treated with high-dose intravenous aciclovir for localised herpes zoster, and with intramuscular pethidine, oral methadone and carbidopa-levodopa. On the second day he experienced nausea, vomiting and confusion, and later dysarthria, lethargy and ataxia. Despite vigorous treatment he later died. It was concluded that some of the adverse effects were due to pethidine toxicity arising from norpethidine accumulation, associated with renal impairment caused by the aciclovir.[1] The US manufacturer of pethidine says that plasma concentrations of pethidine, and its metabolite norpethidine may be increased by aciclovir, thus caution should be used if both drugs are given.[2]

1. Johnson R, Douglas J, Corey L, Krasney H. Adverse effects with acyclovir and meperidine. *Ann Intern Med* (1985) 103, 962–3.
2. Demerol (Meperidine hydrochloride). Sanofi-Aventis US LLC. US Prescribing information, July 2007.

Opioids; Tramadol + Pseudoephedrine

An isolated report describes ischaemic colitis when a patient taking tramadol took a decongestant containing pseudoephedrine.

Clinical evidence, mechanism, importance and management

Acute, self-limiting ischaemic colitis occurred in a 46-year-old patient taking regular tramadol, celecoxib and diazepam for back pain, who had self-medicated with an oral decongestant containing pseudoephedrine. He had taken the maximum recommended dose of pseudoephedrine (240 mg daily) for 7 days. A similar, but milder abdominal discomfort had occurred 3 months earlier when he had used the same medication for one week. The colitis was thought to be due to the pseudoephedrine, but the concurrent use of the tramadol might possibly have contributed by increasing adrenergic vasoconstriction.[1] The general significance of this isolated case is unclear.

1. Traino AA, Buckley NA, Bassett ML. Probable ischemic colitis caused by pseudoephedrine with tramadol as a possible contributing factor. *Ann Pharmacother* (2004) 38, 2068–70.

Paracetamol (Acetaminophen) + Amantadine

Amantadine had no clinically significant effect on the pharmacokinetics of paracetamol.

Clinical evidence, mechanism, importance and management

A single 650-mg dose of paracetamol was given to 5 healthy subjects who had taken amantadine 200 mg daily for 42 days, and also after a single dose of amantadine. Although the apparent volume of distribution of paracetamol was very slightly larger following long-term amantadine use, no other pharmacokinetic parameters were altered. Therefore, from this limited information it appears that no change in paracetamol dose is necessary if these two drugs are given together.[1]

1. Aoki FY, Sitar DS. Effects of chronic amantadine hydrochloride ingestion on its and acetaminophen pharmacokinetics in young adults. *J Clin Pharmacol* (1992) 32, 24–7.

Paracetamol (Acetaminophen) + Antiemetics

Metoclopramide increases the rate of absorption of paracetamol and raises its maximum plasma levels. Similarly, domperidone may increase the rate of absorption of paracetamol.

Clinical evidence, mechanism, importance and management

Intravenous metoclopramide 10 mg increased the peak plasma levels of a single 1.5-g dose of paracetamol by 64% in 5 healthy subjects (slow absorbers of paracetamol), and increased its rate of absorption (peak levels reached in 48 minutes instead of 120 minutes), but the total amount absorbed remained virtually unaltered.[1] Oral metoclopramide also increases the rate of paracetamol absorption,[2] probably because the rate of gastric emptying is increased. Similarly, the speed of absorption of paracetamol may also be increased by domperidone.[3] This interaction is exploited in *Paramax* (a proprietary oral preparation containing both paracetamol and metoclopramide) to increase the effectiveness and onset of analgesia for the treatment of migraine. This is obviously an advantageous interaction in this situation.

1. Nimmo J, Heading RC, Tothill P, Prescott LF. Pharmacological modification of gastric emptying: effects of propantheline and metoclopramide on paracetamol absorption. *BMJ* (1973) 1, 587–9.
2. Crome P, Kimber GR, Wainscott G, Widdop B. The effect of the simultaneous administration of oral metoclopramide on the absorption of paracetamol in healthy volunteers. *Br J Clin Pharmacol* (1981) 11, 430P–431P.
3. Calpol Infant Suspension (Paracetamol). Pfizer Consumer Healthcare. UK Summary of product characteristics, December 2005.

Paracetamol (Acetaminophen) + Antiepileptics

The metabolism of paracetamol is increased in patients taking enzyme-inducing antiepileptics (carbamazepine, phenytoin, phenobarbital, primidone). Isolated reports describe unexpected hepatotoxicity in patients taking phenobarbital, phenytoin, or carbamazepine after taking paracetamol. Valproate does not appear to affect paracetamol metabolism.
Paracetamol modestly reduces the AUC of lamotrigine but appears not to affect phenytoin or carbamazepine.

Clinical evidence

(a) Enzyme-inducing antiepileptics

The AUC of oral paracetamol 1 g was found to be 40% lower (and when given intravenously, 31% lower) in 6 epileptic subjects than in 6 healthy subjects. Five of the epileptic patients were taking at least two of the following drugs: **carbamazepine**, **phenobarbital**, **primidone**, **phenytoin**, and one was taking **phenytoin** alone.[1] Similar findings (a 38% decrease in AUC) were reported in another study in 13 patients taking enzyme-inducing antiepileptics and 2 patients taking rifampicin. In these patients, the amount of glucuronide, but not sulfate, metabolites of paracetamol were higher than controls, but the potentially hepatotoxic metabolite (assessed by mercapturic acid and cysteine conjugates) was not raised.[2] Similar changes in paracetamol metabolites were reported in Chinese patients taking **phenytoin** alone. However, in those taking **carbamazepine** alone there was no change in the paracetamol metabolites, when compared with control subjects.[3] Other studies have also reported a greater rate of paracetamol glucuronidation and unchanged sulfation in patients taking **phenytoin** alone[4] and patients taking **phenytoin** and/or **carbamazepine**.[5] In contrast, this latter study also found an increase in clearance of the glutathione-derived conjugates (mercapturic and cysteine conjugates), which may indicate an increased risk of paracetamol hepatotoxicity.[5]

An epileptic woman taking **phenobarbital** 100 mg daily developed hepatitis after taking paracetamol 1 g daily for 3 months for headaches. Within 2 weeks of stopping the paracetamol her serum transaminase levels had fallen within the normal range, which implied drug-induced liver damage.[6] Another patient taking **phenobarbital** developed liver and kidney toxicity after taking only 9 g of paracetamol over 48 hours.[7] **Phenobarbital** also appeared to have increased the toxic effects of paracetamol in an adolescent who took an overdose of both drugs, which resulted in fatal hepatic encephalopathy.[8]

Other case reports describe unexpected paracetamol hepatotoxicity in three patients taking **phenytoin**,[9-11] three patients taking **carbamazepine**,[12-14] and a patient taking **phenytoin** and **primidone**.[15] Another analysis of patients with paracetamol-induced fulminant hepatic failure suggested that mortality was higher in the group of patients receiving antiepileptics (including **phenytoin**, **phenobarbital**, **carbamazepine**, **primidone** and **valproate** alone or in combination).[16]

The serum levels of **phenytoin** and **carbamazepine** in 10 epileptics were not significantly affected by paracetamol 1.5 g daily for 3 days.[17]

(b) Lamotrigine

A study in 8 healthy subjects found that paracetamol 2.7 g daily reduced the AUC of a 300-mg dose of lamotrigine by 20% and reduced its half-life by 15%.[18]

(c) Valproate

Valproate is extensively metabolised in man and a significant proportion of the metabolism occurs via glucuronide conjugation. A study designed to determine whether valproate affected the disposition of drugs that are largely dependent on conjugation found that it did not affect the pharmacokinetics of paracetamol in 3 epileptic patients.[19]

Mechanism

The increased paracetamol clearance is due to the well-recognised enzyme inducing effects of the antiepileptics, which increase its metabolism (glucuronidation and oxidation) and loss from the body. It has been suggested that this could result in an increase in the production of the hepatotoxic oxidative metabolite of paracetamol, *N*-acetyl-*p*-benzoquinone imine. If this toxic metabolite then exceeds the normal glutathione binding capacity, liver damage may occur (see 'paracetamol', (p.133)). The production of the toxic metabolite *in vitro* in animals and humans seems to depend on several isoenzymes, but the available evidence indicates that the cytochrome P450 isoenzyme CYP2E1 is the primary enzyme in humans.[20] Therefore, since these enzyme-inducing antiepileptics do not induce this isoenzyme, some consider the few possible cases described merely represent idiosyncratic effects.[20] However, others have suggested that, when several drugs, including phenobarbital or phenytoin are taken, inhibition of uridine diphosphate glucuronosyltransferase (UGT) enzymes by one of these drugs can lead to decreased glucuronidation and increased systemic exposure and toxicity of the paracetamol.[21]

Importance and management

Information is limited. The clinical importance of these interactions is not established and further study is needed. However, paracetamol is possibly a less effective analgesic in patients taking enzyme-inducing antiepileptics as plasma-paracetamol levels may be reduced. However, levels of the potentially hepatotoxic metabolites may be increased. Some believe that the evidence indicates that the risk of liver damage after paracetamol overdose is increased, and they suggest that patients taking enzyme-inducing antiepileptics should be treated with antidotes at lower plasma levels of paracetamol.[9,11,12,15] In addition, some suggest that therapeutic doses of paracetamol should be used with caution in patients receiving these drugs.[10,11,16] Conversely, others consider that therapeutic doses of paracetamol are not associated with an increased risk of toxicity when used with enzyme-inducers. Moreover, phenytoin, by increasing glucuronidation, may actually have some hepato-protective effects.[20,22] The differences stem from different understandings of which mechanism and isoenzyme(s) are important in the production of the hepatotoxic metabolite of paracetamol[10,20] (see Mechanism, above).

It is unlikely that the interaction between lamotrigine and paracetamol is of practical importance, but this needs confirmation.

1. Perucca E, Richens A. Paracetamol disposition in normal subjects and in patients treated with antiepileptic drugs. *Br J Clin Pharmacol* (1979) 7, 201–6.
2. Prescott LF, Critchley JAJH, Balali-Mood M, Pentland B. Effects of microsomal enzyme induction on paracetamol metabolism in man. *Br J Clin Pharmacol* (1981) 12, 149–53.
3. Tomlinson B, Young RP, Ng MCY, Anderson PJ, Kay R, Critchley JAJH. Selective liver enzyme induction by carbamazepine and phenytoin in Chinese epileptics. *Eur J Clin Pharmacol* (1996) 50, 411–15.

4. Bock KW, Wiltfang J, Blume R, Ullrich D, Bircher J. Paracetamol as a test drug to determine glucuronide formation in man. Effects of inducers and of smoking. *Eur J Clin Pharmacol* (1987) 31, 677–83.
5. Miners JO, Attwood J, Birkett DJ. Determinants of acetaminophen metabolism: effect of inducers and inhibitors of drug metabolism on acetaminophen's metabolic pathways. *Clin Pharmacol Ther* (1984) 35, 480–6.
6. Pirotte JH. Apparent potentiation by phenobarbital of hepatotoxicity from small doses of acetaminophen. *Ann Intern Med* (1984) 101, 403.
7. Marsepoil T, Mahassani B, Roudiak N, Sebbah JL, Caillard G. Potentialisation de la toxicité hépatique et rénale du paracétamol par le phénobarbital. *JEUR* (1989) 2, 118–20.
8. Wilson JT, Kasantikul V, Harbison R, Martin D. Death in an adolescent following an overdose of acetaminophen and phenobarbital. *Am J Dis Child* (1978) 132, 466–73.
9. McClements BM, Hyland M, Callender ME, Blair TL. Management of paracetamol poisoning complicated by enzyme induction due to alcohol or drugs. *Lancet* (1990) 335, 1526.
10. Brackett CC, Bloch JD. Phenytoin as a possible cause of acetaminophen hepatotoxicity: case report and review of the literature. *Pharmacotherapy* (2000) 20, 229–33.
11. Suchin SM, Wolf DC, Lee Y, Ramaswamy G, Sheiner PA, Facciuto M, Marvin MR, Kim-Schluger L, Lebovics E. Potentiation of acetaminophen hepatotoxicity by phenytoin, leading to liver transplantation. *Dig Dis Sci* (2005) 50, 1836–8.
12. Smith JAE, Hine ID, Beck P, Routledge PA. Paracetamol toxicity: is enzyme-induction important? *Hum Toxicol* (1986) 5, 383–5.
13. Young CR, Mazure CM. Fulminant hepatic failure from acetaminophen in an anorexic patient treated with carbamazepine. *J Clin Psychiatry* (1998) 59, 622.
14. Parikh S, Dillon LC, Scharf SL. Hepatotoxicity possibly due to paracetamol with carbamazepine. Intern Med J. (2004) 34, 441–2.
15. Minton NA, Henry JA, Frankel RJ. Fatal paracetamol poisoning in an epileptic. *Hum Toxicol* (1988) 7, 33–4.
16. Bray GP, Harrison PM, O'Grady JG, Tredger JM, Williams R. Long-term anticonvulsant therapy worsens outcome in paracetamol-induced fulminant hepatic failure. *Hum Exp Toxicol* (1992) 11, 265–70.
17. Neuvonen PJ, Lehtovaara R, Bardy A, Elomaa E. Antipyretic analgesics in patients on antiepileptic drug therapy. *Eur J Clin Pharmacol* (1979) 15, 263–8.
18. Depot M, Powell JR, Messenheimer JA, Cloutier G, Dalton MJ. Kinetic effects of multiple oral doses of acetaminophen on a single oral dose of lamotrigine. *Clin Pharmacol Ther* (1990) 48, 346–55.
19. Kapetanović IM, Kupferberg HJ, Theodore W, Porter RJ. Lack of effect of valproate on paracetamol (acetaminophen) disposition in epileptic patients. *Br J Clin Pharmacol* (1981) 11, 391–3.
20. Rumack BH. Acetaminophen hepatotoxicity: the first 35 years. *J Toxicol Clin Toxicol* (2002) 40, 3–20.
21. Kostrubsky SE, Sinclair JF, Strom SC, Wood S, Urda E, Stolz DB, Wen YH, Kulkarni S, Mutlib A. Phenobarbital and phenytoin increased acetaminophen hepatotoxicity due to inhibition of UDP-glucuronosyltransferases in cultured human hepatocytes. *Toxicol Sci* (2005) 87, 146–55.
22. Cook MD, Williams SR, Clark RF. Phenytoin-potentiated hepatotoxicity following acetaminophen overdose? A closer look. *Dig Dis Sci* (2007) 52, 208–9.

Paracetamol (Acetaminophen) + Antimuscarinics

Propantheline reduced the rate, but not the extent, of paracetamol absorption. This would be expected to reduce the rate of onset of analgesia. Other antimuscarinic drugs that delay gastric emptying would be expected to interact similarly. In one case, the diphenhydramine component of a paracetamol product delayed paracetamol absorption after an overdose, and complicated the evaluation of the risk of toxicity.

Clinical evidence, mechanism, importance and management

Propantheline 30 mg intravenously delayed the peak serum levels of paracetamol 1.5 g in 6 convalescent patients from about 1 hour to 3 hours. Peak levels were lowered by about one-third, but the total amount of paracetamol absorbed was unchanged.[1] This effect occurs because **propantheline** is an antimuscarinic drug that slows the rate at which the stomach empties, so that the rate of absorption in the gut is reduced. The practical consequence of this is likely to be that rapid pain relief with single doses of paracetamol may be delayed and reduced by antimuscarinics (see 'Table 18.1', (p.672), and 'Table 18.2', (p.674) for a list) but this needs clinical confirmation. If the paracetamol is being taken in repeated doses over extended periods this seems unlikely to be an important interaction because the total amount absorbed is unchanged.

One study in 10 healthy subjects reported that **diphenhydramine** 250 mg taken with paracetamol 5 g (simulated paracetamol overdose) had little effect on the absorption of paracetamol.[2] However, a case has been described where the **diphenhydramine** component of a paracetamol product (*Tylenol PM*) taken in overdose (paracetamol 7.5 g and **diphenhydramine** 375 mg) delayed the absorption of paracetamol, so that the peak serum-paracetamol level did not occur until 8 hours after ingestion (usual maximum is 2 hours).[3] In this situation there is a danger that early paracetamol levels could be incorrectly assessed. Therefore, when assessing paracetamol overdoses, it is important to consider whether any concurrent drugs could delay the absorption of paracetamol.

1. Nimmo J, Heading RC, Tothill P, Prescott LF. Pharmacological modification of gastric emptying: effects of propantheline and metoclopramide on paracetamol absorption. *BMJ* (1973) 1, 587–9.
2. Halcomb SE, Sivilotti ML, Goklaney A, Mullins ME. Pharmacokinetic effects of diphenhydramine or oxycodone in simulated acetaminophen overdose. *Acad Emerg Med* (2005) 12, 169–72.
3. Tsang WO, Nadroo AM. An unusual case of acetaminophen overdose. *Pediatr Emerg Care* (1999) 15, 344–6.

Paracetamol (Acetaminophen) + Caffeine

Caffeine has been variously reported to increase, decrease, and have no effect on the absorption of paracetamol.

Clinical evidence, mechanism, importance and management

Caffeine citrate 120 mg increased the AUC of a single 500-mg dose of paracetamol in 10 healthy subjects by 29%, increased the maximum plasma levels by 15% and decreased the total body clearance by 32%. The decrease in time to maximum level and increase in absorption rate did not reach statistical significance.[1] However, in another study, although caffeine slightly increased the rate of absorption of paracetamol, it had no effect on the extent of absorption.[2] Moreover, a third study states that caffeine decreased plasma paracetamol levels and AUC and increased paracetamol elimination in healthy men.[3] Caffeine is commonly included in paracetamol preparations as an analgesic adjuvant. Its potential benefit and the mechanisms behind its possible effects remain unclear.

1. Iqbal N, Ahmad B, Janbaz KH, Gilani A-UH, Niazi SK. The effect of caffeine on the pharmacokinetics of acetaminophen in man. *Biopharm Drug Dispos* (1995) 16, 481–7.
2. Tukker JJ, Sitsen JMA, Gusdorf CF. Bioavailability of paracetamol after oral administration to healthy volunteers. Influence of caffeine on rate and extent of absorption. *Pharm Weekbl (Sci)* (1986) 8, 239–43.
3. Raińska-Giezek T. Influence of caffeine on toxicity and pharmacokinetics of paracetamol [Article in Polish]. *Ann Acad Med Stetin* (1995) 41, 69–85.

Paracetamol (Acetaminophen) + Chloroquine

Although modest pharmacokinetic effects occur when paracetamol and chloroquine are given together this is not thought to be clinically significant.

Clinical evidence, mechanism, importance and management

In a single-dose study, intravenous chloroquine increased the peak plasma paracetamol levels and the AUC by 47% and 22%, respectively.[1] Another single-dose study in 8 healthy subjects found that paracetamol 500 mg increased the maximum plasma level and AUC of chloroquine 600 mg by 17% and 24%, respectively.[2] These changes were thought unlikely to be clinically significant in therapeutic doses.[1] A further study in 5 healthy subjects found that the pharmacokinetics of a single 300-mg dose of chloroquine were not affected by a single 1-g dose of paracetamol.[3] This evidence therefore suggests that no dosage adjustments would be expected to be necessary when paracetamol is given with chloroquine.

1. Adjepon-Yamoah KK, Woolhouse NM, Prescott LF. The effect of chloroquine on paracetamol disposition and kinetics. *Br J Clin Pharmacol* (1986) 21, 322–4.
2. Raina RK, Bano G, Amla V, Kapoor V, Gupta KL. The effect of aspirin, paracetamol and analgin on pharmacokinetics of chloroquine. *Indian J Physiol Pharmacol* (1993) 37, 229–31.
3. Essien EE, Ette EI, Brown-Awala EA. Evaluation of the effect of co-administered paracetamol on the gastro-intestinal absorption and disposition of chloroquine. *J Pharm Biomed Anal* (1988) 6, 521–6.

Paracetamol (Acetaminophen) + Colestyramine

The absorption of paracetamol may be reduced if colestyramine is given at the same time, but the reduction in absorption is small if colestyramine is given an hour later.

Clinical evidence

When 4 healthy subjects took colestyramine 12 g and paracetamol 2 g together, the absorption of the paracetamol was reduced by 60% (range 30 to 98%) at 2 hours, but the results were said not to be statistically significant. When the colestyramine was given 1 hour after the paracetamol, the absorption was reduced by only 16%.[1]

Mechanism

Colestyramine reduces absorption, presumably because it binds with the paracetamol in the gut. Separating the dosages minimises mixing in the gut.

Importance and management

Although information is limited, it suggests that colestyramine should not be given within 1 hour of paracetamol if maximal analgesia is to be achieved. It is normally recommended that other drugs are given 1 hour before or 4 to 6 hours after colestyramine.

1. Dordoni B, Willson RA, Thompson RPH, Williams R. Reduction of absorption of paracetamol by activated charcoal and cholestyramine: a possible therapeutic measure. *BMJ* (1973) 3, 86–7.

Paracetamol (Acetaminophen) + Disulfiram

Disulfiram had no important effect on the metabolism of paracetamol in one study, but decreased the production of the glutathione (hepatotoxic) metabolites in another.

Clinical evidence, mechanism, importance and management

After taking disulfiram 200 mg daily for 5 days, the clearance of a single 500-mg intravenous dose of paracetamol was slightly reduced (by about 10%) in 5 healthy subjects without liver disease and 5 others with alcoholic liver cirrhosis. The fractional clearance of paracetamol to its glucuronide, sulfate and glutathione metabolites was not altered.[1] In contrast, another study found that pretreatment of healthy subjects with a single 500-mg dose of disulfiram 10 hours before a single 500-mg oral dose of paracetamol reduced the recovery of glutathione metabolites (a measure of the production of the hepatotoxic metabolite, see 'paracetamol', (p.133)) by 69%.[2]

Disulfiram is an inhibitor of the cytochrome P450 isoenzyme CYP2E1, which is involved in the metabolism of paracetamol. Previously, the authors of the first study[1] had shown that in *rats,* high doses of disulfiram protected against the hepatotoxicity of paracetamol. Therefore, it was suggested that disulfiram might be useful in reducing the risks of paracetamol overdose. However, the authors of the first study concluded that disulfiram at doses used clinically is unlikely to have any beneficial (or adverse) effect on paracetamol metabolism.[1] In contrast, the authors of the second study consider that disulfiram may be useful in reducing the formation of the hepatotoxic metabolite of paracetamol in some situations.[2] Further study is needed.

1. Poulson HE, Ranek L, Jørgensen L. The influence of disulfiram on acetaminophen metabolism in man. *Xenobiotica* (1991) 21, 243–9.
2. Manyike PT, Kharasch ED, Kalhorn TF, Slattery JT. Contribution of CYP2E1 and CYP3A to acetaminophen reactive metabolite formation. *Clin Pharmacol Ther* (2000) 67, 275–82.

Paracetamol (Acetaminophen) + Erythromycin

Erythromycin accelerates gastric emptying and increases paracetamol absorption but this does not appear to result in a clinically significant interaction.

Clinical evidence, mechanism, importance and management

In a study in healthy subjects, intravenous erythromycin 0.75 to 3 mg/kg accelerated gastric emptying in a dose-dependent manner and increased paracetamol absorption.[1] However, another study found that erythromycin 200 mg intravenously, given to promote gastrointestinal motility, did not alter the pharmacokinetics of an extended-release oral dose of paracetamol.[2] A further study in 7 healthy subjects reported that the pharmacokinetics of a single 1-g oral dose of paracetamol were not significantly affected by pretreatment with oral erythromycin 250 mg four times daily for 7 days.[3] It was suggested that the concurrent use of erythromycin and paracetamol is unlikely to result in a clinically significant interaction.[3]

1. Boivin MA, Carey MC, Levy H. Erythromycin accelerates gastric emptying in a dose-response manner in healthy subjects. *Pharmacotherapy* (2003) 23, 5–8.
2. Amato CS, Wang RY, Wright RO, Linakis JG. Evaluation of promotility agents to limit the gut bioavailability of extended-release acetaminophen. *J Toxicol Clin Toxicol* (2004) 42, 73–7.
3. Ridtitid W, Wongnawa M, Mahathanatrakul W, Rukthai D, Sunbhanich M. Effect of erythromycin administration alone or coadministration with cimetidine on the pharmacokinetics of paracetamol in healthy volunteers. *Asia Pac J Pharmacol* (1998) 13, 19–23.

Paracetamol (Acetaminophen) + Food

Food slows the rate of absorption of paracetamol, but the overall bioavailability is not usually affected. However, in some individuals food may delay and reduce peak paracetamol-plasma levels. A high fat meal may slightly reduce the extent of paracetamol absorption and certain foods, such as cabbage and brussels sprouts, may affect the metabolism of paracetamol, but this is unlikely to be clinically significant.
Consider also the food preservative 'sodium nitrate', (p.198).

Clinical evidence, mechanism, importance and management

(a) Absorption of paracetamol (acetaminophen)

Several studies have demonstrated that food slows the rate of absorption of paracetamol, but the overall bioavailability is not affected[1-5] and some studies have also reported that food has no effect on the analgesic effect of paracetamol[6] or its onset.[7] The absorption of paracetamol is affected by the rate of gastric emptying and most foods delay gastric emptying. **Carbohydrate**,[2] **fat**,[2] **guar gum** and **pectin**,[5] **protein**,[1] and particularly **fibre**,[2,4] may delay the absorption of paracetamol. Furthermore, the rate and extent of absorption, and peak plasma levels of a single dose of paracetamol have been found to be impaired in vegetarians compared with non-vegetarians.[8] A **high fat** diet has also been reported to slightly reduce the extent of absorption.[2]

Although overall bioavailability is not usually affected by food, there may be a delay in reaching therapeutic plasma paracetamol levels, particularly following a single dose of paracetamol. A reduction in the maximum plasma paracetamol level has been reported when it is given after food, when compared with the fasted state;[3,9] in one study the maximum plasma paracetamol level in some individuals did not reach the level reported to be required for effective analgesia.[9] The dosage form will also affect the absorption; many of the studies have used conventional paracetamol tablets, but some formulations (for example paracetamol with sodium bicarbonate)[3,7] are more rapidly absorbed and, although food may reduce the rate of absorption,[3,4] one study found that there was no difference in the onset of analgesia between the fed and fasted states.[7] Another study found that diet composition did not affect the systemic availability of paracetamol in a liquid dosage form, whereas absorption of the tablet form was delayed by a **fibre**-enriched diet.[4]

The clinical importance of these findings is uncertain. It appears that rapid pain relief with single doses of paracetamol tablets may possibly be delayed and reduced by food in some individuals, but liquid or rapidly absorbed preparations are less likely to be affected. If paracetamol is being taken in repeated doses, the interaction with food is unlikely to be clinically important as the total amount absorbed is usually unchanged.

(b) Fasting and hepatotoxicity of paracetamol

A prospective study found that, of 49 patients with paracetamol hepatotoxicity, all had taken more that the recommended limit of 4 g of paracetamol daily. Paracetamol hepatotoxicity after a dose of 4 to 10 g daily was associated with fasting and less commonly with alcohol use, and it was suggested that paracetamol hepatotoxicity after an overdose appears to be enhanced by fasting in addition to alcohol ingestion.[10] The metabolism of a lower 2-g dose of paracetamol was not, however, affected by food restriction in obese patients.[11] Fasting may possibly contribute to paracetamol toxicity by shunting paracetamol detoxification from the conjugative to the potentially toxic oxidative pathways.[11] See also, 'Alcohol + Paracetamol (Acetaminophen)', p.73.

(c) Metabolism of paracetamol

In a crossover study in 10 healthy subjects, a 10-day balanced diet including **cabbage** 100 g and **brussels sprouts** 150 g at lunch and dinner was found to stimulate the metabolism of paracetamol, at least in part by enhanced glucuronidation. Compared with a control diet (which included instead, lettuce, cucumber, green beans and peas), **cabbage** and **brussels sprouts** induced a 16% decrease in the mean AUC of paracetamol, a 17% increase in the mean metabolic clearance rate, and an 8% increase in the mean 24-hour urinary recovery of the glucuronide metabolite.[12] Consumption of **watercress** caused a decrease in the levels of plasma and urinary oxidative metabolites of paracetamol, but the urinary excretion of paracetamol, or its glucuronide and sulfate were not significantly altered.[13] However, **charcoal-broiled beef** (which accelerates the oxidative metabolism of some drugs) did not affect paracetamol metabolism.[14] It seems unlikely that these foods would have a significant clinical effect, except perhaps **cabbage** and **brussels sprouts** if eaten to excess.

1. Robertson DRC, Higginson I, Macklin BS, Renwick AG, Waller DG, George CF. The influence of protein containing meals on the pharmacokinetics of levodopa in healthy volunteers. *Br J Clin Pharmacol* (1991) 31, 413–17.
2. Wessels JC, Koeleman HA, Boneschans B, Steyn HS. The influence of different types of breakfast on the absorption of paracetamol among members of an ethnic group. *Int J Clin Pharmacol Ther Toxicol* (1992) 30, 208–13.
3. Rostami-Hodjegan A, Shiran MR, Ayesh R, Grattan TJ, Burnett I, Darby-Dowman A, Tucker GT. A new rapidly absorbed paracetamol tablet containing sodium bicarbonate. I. A four-way crossover study to compare the concentration-time profile of paracetamol from the new paracetamol/sodium bicarbonate tablet and a conventional paracetamol tablet in fed and fasted volunteers. *Drug Dev Ind Pharm* (2002) 28, 523–31.
4. Walter-Sack IE, de Vries JX, Nickel B, Stenzhorn G, Weber E. The influence of different formula diets and different pharmaceutical formulations on the systemic availability of paracetamol, gallbladder size, and plasma glucose. *Int J Clin Pharmacol Ther Toxicol* (1989) 27, 544–50.
5. Holt S, Heading RC, Carter DC, Prescott LF, Tothill P. Effect of gel fibre on gastric emptying and absorption of glucose and paracetamol. *Lancet* (1979) 1, 636–9.
6. Forbes JA, Sandberg RA, Bood-Bjorklund L. The effect of food on bromfenac, naproxen sodium, and acetaminophen in postoperative pain after orthopedic surgery. *Pharmacotherapy* (1998) 18, 492–503.
7. Burnett I, Schachtel B, Sanner K, Bey M, Grattan T, Littlejohn S. Onset of analgesia of a paracetamol tablet containing sodium bicarbonate: a double-blind, placebo-controlled study in adult patients with acute sore throat. *Clin Ther* (2006) 28, 1273–8.
8. Prescott LF, Yoovathaworn K, Makarananda K, Saivises R, Sriwatanakul K. Impaired absorption of paracetamol in vegetarians. *Br J Clin Pharmacol* (1993) 36, 237–40.
9. Stillings M, Havlik I, Chetty M, Clinton C, Schall R, Moodley I, Muir N, Little S. Comparison of the pharmacokinetic profiles of soluble aspirin and solid paracetamol tablets in fed and fasted volunteers. *Curr Med Res Opin* (2000) 16, 115–24.
10. Whitcomb DC, Block GD. Association of acetaminophen hepatotoxicity with fasting and ethanol use. *JAMA* (1994) 272, 1845–50.
11. Schenker S, Speeg KV, Perez A, Finch J. The effects of food restriction in man on hepatic metabolism of acetaminophen. *Clin Nutr* (2001) 20, 145–50.
12. Pantuck EJ, Pantuck CB, Anderson KE, Wattenberg LW, Conney AH, Kappas A. Effect of brussels sprouts and cabbage on drug conjugation. *Clin Pharmacol Ther* (1984) 35, 161–9.
13. Chen L, Mohr SN, Yang CS. Decrease of plasma and urinary oxidative metabolites of acetaminophen after consumption of watercress by human volunteers. *Clin Pharmacol Ther* (1996) 60, 651–60.
14. Anderson KE, Schneider J, Pantuck EJ, Pantuck CB, Mudge GH, Welch RM, Conney AH, Kappas A. Acetaminophen metabolism in subjects fed charcoal-broiled beef. *Clin Pharmacol Ther* (1983) 34, 369–74.

Paracetamol (Acetaminophen) + H_2-receptor antagonists

Cimetidine, nizatidine, and ranitidine do not appear to alter the pharmacokinetics of paracetamol to a clinically relevant extent.

Clinical evidence

(a) Cimetidine

Cimetidine (given as a single 200-mg dose or as 1 g daily in divided doses for 7 days) had no statistically significant effect on the pharmacokinetics of a single 750-mg dose of paracetamol in 4 healthy subjects.[1] Similarly, in another study, a single 800-mg dose of cimetidine given one hour before paracetamol 1 g had no effect on paracetamol half-life or plasma clearance, and no effect on urinary excretion of its principal metabolites (glucuronide, sulfate, mercapturate) in 10 healthy subjects.[2] Furthermore, the pharmacokinetics of a single 1-g dose of paracetamol were not altered by 2 months of treatment with cimetidine 400 mg twice daily in 10 patients. The only difference in urinary metabolites was a modest 37% decrease in paracetamol mercapturate (indicating a reduction in the hepatotoxic metabolite).[2] Other studies have shown that cimetidine does not alter the clearance[3-5] or metabolic pathways of paracetamol.[3,5]

In contrast, one study reported that cimetidine 300 mg every 6 hours decreased the fractional clearance of the oxidised metabolites (mercapturate and cysteine conjugates) of paracetamol in healthy subjects.[6] Another study showed that a single 400-mg dose of cimetidine given one hour before paracetamol 1 g in fasting subjects delayed the absorption of paracetamol (for instance, there was a 37% reduction in peak salivary level and a 63% increase in time to peak level). This effect was not seen when the two drugs were given simultaneously.[7]

(b) Nizatidine

Nizatidine 300 mg given to 5 healthy subjects with paracetamol 1 g modestly increased the paracetamol AUC in the first 3 hours by 25%. Over this time period, there was also a nonsignificant 4% reduction in formation of paracetamol glucuronide, but this did reach statistical significance at 30 and 45 minutes. Nizatidine 150 mg had a similar, but smaller, effect.[8]

(c) Ranitidine

In one study, ranitidine 300 mg twice daily for 4 days had no effect on the clearance and half-life of single 1-g intravenous and oral doses of paracetamol in 8 healthy subjects. In addition, there was no difference in the urinary excretion of paracetamol metabolites. In this study, ranitidine was given one hour before paracetamol.[9,10] Another study reported similar findings when ranitidine 300 mg was given one hour before paracetamol 1 g. However, when the two drugs were given simultaneously, there was a change in paracetamol pharmacokinetics. The AUC_{0-3} of paracetamol was increased by 63%, and there was a 35% decrease in the AUC_{0-3} of paracetamol glucuronide, but no change occurred in sulfate levels.[11] An isolated case describes a man who noted his urine was dark 3 weeks after starting ranitidine 150 mg twice daily and paracetamol 1.3 to 2 g daily. He was found to have raised liver enzyme levels (alkaline phosphatase 708 units/L; AST 196 mIU/mL), which returned to normal on discontinuing ranitidine.[12]

Mechanism

Cimetidine may inhibit the oxidative metabolism of paracetamol by cytochrome P450 isoenzymes, resulting in a reduction in the hepatotoxic metabolite, see 'paracetamol', (p.133). It was suggested that cimetidine delayed paracetamol absorption by reducing gastric emptying.[7] Nizatidine may cause a minor inhibition of glucuronyltransferases.[8] Ranitidine may also inhibit paracetamol glucuronyltransferases when given simultaneously, but this was not seen when given one hour apart.

Importance and management

Any changes in the pharmacokinetics of paracetamol with these H_2-receptor antagonists appear to be clinically unimportant. Thus, no special precaution would seem to be necessary when paracetamol is used with cimetidine, nizatidine or ranitidine. The effect of cimetidine on the oxidative metabolism of paracetamol has been investigated as a means of reducing paracetamol hepatotoxicity. However, it appears that cimetidine is not effective for this purpose.[13]

1. Chen MM, Lee CS. Cimetidine-acetaminophen interaction in humans. *J Clin Pharmacol* (1985) 25, 227–9.
2. Vendemiale G, Altomare E, Trizio T, Leandro G, Manghisi OG, Albano O. Effect of acute and chronic cimetidine administration on acetaminophen metabolism in humans. *Am J Gastroenterol* (1987) 82, 1031–4.
3. Slattery JT, McRorie TI, Reynolds R, Kalhorn TF, Kharasch ED, Eddy AC. Lack of effect of cimetidine on acetaminophen disposition in humans. *Clin Pharmacol Ther* (1989) 46, 591–7.
4. Abernethy DR, Greenblatt DJ, Divoll M, Ameer B, Shader RI. Differential effect of cimetidine on drug oxidation (antipyrine and diazepam) *vs* conjugation (acetaminophen and lorazepam): prevention of acetaminophen toxicity by cimetidine. *J Pharmacol Exp Ther* (1983) 224, 508–13.
5. Miners JO, Attwood J, Birkett DJ. Determinants of acetaminophen metabolism: effect of inducers and inhibitors of drug metabolism on acetaminophen's metabolic pathways. *Clin Pharmacol Ther* (1984) 35, 480–6.
6. Mitchell MC, Schenker S, Speeg KV. Selective inhibition of acetaminophen oxidation and toxicity by cimetidine and other histamine H_2-receptor antagonists in vivo and in vitro in rat and in man. *J Clin Invest* (1984) 73, 383–91.
7. Garba M, Odunola MT, Ahmed BH. Effect of study protocol on the interactions between cimetidine and paracetamol in man. *Eur J Drug Metab Pharmacokinet* (1999) 24, 159–62.
8. Itoh H, Nagano T, Takeyama M. Effect of nizatidine on paracetamol and its metabolites in human plasma. *J Pharm Pharmacol* (2002) 54, 869–73.
9. Thomas M, Michael MF, Andrew P, Scully N. A study to investigate the effects of ranitidine on the metabolic disposition of paracetamol in man. *Br J Clin Pharmacol* (1988) 25, 671P.
10. Jack D, Thomas M, Skidmore IF. Ranitidine and paracetamol metabolism. *Lancet* (1985) ii, 1067.
11. Itoh H, Nagano T, Hayashi T, Takeyama M. Ranitidine increases bioavailability of acetaminophen by inhibiting the first-pass glucuronidation in man. *Pharm Pharmacol Commun* (2000) 6, 495–500.
12. Bredfeldt JE, von Huene C. Ranitidine, acetaminophen, and hepatotoxicity. *Ann Intern Med* (1984) 101, 719.
13. Kaufenberg AJ, Shepherd MF. Role of cimetidine in the treatment of acetaminophen poisoning. *Am J Health-Syst Pharm* (1998) 55, 1516–19.

Paracetamol (Acetaminophen) + Herbal medicines

Studies in healthy subjects found that garlic and hibiscus extracts did not affect the pharmacokinetics of single-dose paracetamol to a clinically relevant extent, although the clearance of paracetamol was increased by hibiscus extract. Similarly, single-dose studies in healthy subjects found that Kakkonto did not affect the pharmacokinetics of paracetamol, but *animal* studies found increased paracetamol levels.

Clinical evidence, mechanism, importance and management

(a) Garlic

A study in 16 healthy subjects found that the use of an aged garlic extract (approximately equivalent to 6 to 7 cloves of garlic daily) for 3 months had little effect on the metabolism of a single 1-g oral dose of paracetamol. There was a very slight increase in glucuronidation after the long-term use of garlic, and some evidence that sulfate conjugation was enhanced, but no effect on oxidative metabolism.[1] No clinically significant interaction would therefore be expected if paracetamol is taken with garlic.

(b) Hibiscus

A study in 6 healthy subjects found that **Zobo** drink (***Hibiscus sabdariffa*** water extract), given 78 minutes before a single 1-g dose of paracetamol did not affect the absorption or AUC of paracetamol, but the total body clearance increased by 12%.[2] This is not expected to be clinically significant.

(c) Kakkonto

A study in 6 healthy subjects found that 5 g of Kakkonto extract, a Chinese herbal medicine containing extracts of *Puerariae*, *Ephedrae*, *Zingiberis*, *Cinnamomi*, *Glycyrrhizae*, *Paeoniae* and *Zizphi* spp. had no effects on the pharmacokinetics of a single 12-mg/kg dose of paracetamol. A further study in 19 healthy subjects found that 1.25 g of Kakkonto had no effect on the pharmacokinetics of paracetamol 150 mg (from a preparation also containing salicylamide, caffeine and promethazine methylene disalicylate). Because in *animal* studies high doses of Kakkonto for 7 days were found to significantly increase serum levels of paracetamol, the authors concluded that further investigations were required to assess safety and efficacy of concurrent use.[3]

1. Gwilt PR, Lear CL, Tempero MA, Birt DD, Grandjean AC, Ruddon RW, Nagel DL. The effect of garlic extract on human metabolism of acetaminophen. *Cancer Epidemiol Biomarkers Prev* (1994) 3, 155–60.
2. Kolawole JA, Maduenyi A. Effect of Zobo drink (Hibiscus sabdariffa water extract) on the pharmacokinetics of acetaminophen in human volunteers. *Eur J Drug Metab Pharmacokinet* (2004) 29, 25–9.
3. Qi J, Toyoshima A, Honda Y, Mineshita S. Pharmacokinetic study on acetaminophen: interaction with a Chinese medicine. *J Med Dent Sci* (1997) 44, 31–5.

Paracetamol (Acetaminophen) + Hormonal contraceptives or HRT

Paracetamol clearance is increased in women taking oral contraceptives, although the clinical relevance of this is uncertain. Paracetamol also increases the absorption of ethinylestradiol from the gut by about 20%. HRT appears not to interact with paracetamol.

Clinical evidence

(a) Effect on paracetamol

In 7 healthy women taking combined oral contraceptives (containing **ethinylestradiol**), the plasma clearance of a single 1.5-g dose of paracetamol was 64% higher and the elimination half-life 30% lower, when compared with 7 healthy women not taking oral contraceptives. The fractional clearance by glucuronidation and of the cysteine conjugate increased, but that of sulfation and the mercapturic acid conjugate were unchanged.[1] Similarly, other studies have found higher paracetamol clearances of 30 to 49%, and corresponding lower paracetamol half-lives, in women taking oral contraceptives, when compared with control subjects.[2-4]

One study found that the pharmacokinetics of a single 650-mg intravenous dose of paracetamol did not differ between women who had taken **conjugated oestrogens** for at least 3 months and control subjects.[5]

(b) Effect on oral contraceptives

A single 1-g oral dose of paracetamol increased the AUC of **ethinylestradiol** by 22% in 6 healthy women, and decreased the AUC of ethinylestradiol sulfate by 41%. Plasma levels of **levonorgestrel** were not affected.[6]

Mechanism

The evidence suggests that oral contraceptives increase the metabolism (both oxidation and glucuronidation) of paracetamol by the liver so that it is cleared from the body more quickly.[3] The increased absorption of the ethinylestradiol probably occurs because the paracetamol reduces its metabolism by the gut wall during absorption.[6] It has been suggested that the differences between the effects of oral contraceptives and conjugated oestrogens on paracetamol may be attributable to the influence of progestogens on glucuronide and sulfate conjugation.[5] This needs confirmation.

Importance and management

The modest pharmacokinetic interaction between the oral contraceptives and paracetamol appears to be established, but its clinical importance has not been directly studied. The clinical importance of the modest increased ethinylestradiol absorption is also uncertain, but likely to be minor. HRT appears not to interact with paracetamol.

1. Mitchell MC, Hanew T, Meredith CG, Schenker S. Effects of oral contraceptive steroids on acetaminophen metabolism and elimination. *Clin Pharmacol Ther* (1983) 34, 48–53.
2. Abernethy DR, Divoll M, Ochs HR, Ameer B, Greenblatt DJ. Increased metabolic clearance of acetaminophen with oral contraceptive use. *Obstet Gynecol* (1982) 60, 338–41.
3. Miners JO, Attwood J, Birkett DJ. Influence of sex and oral contraceptive steroids on paracetamol metabolism. *Br J Clin Pharmacol* (1983) 16, 503–9.
4. Mucklow JC, Fraser HS, Bulpitt CJ, Kahn C, Mould G, Dollery CT. Environmental factors affecting paracetamol metabolism in London factory and office workers. *Br J Clin Pharmacol* (1980) 10, 67–74.
5. Scavone JM, Greenblatt DJ, Blyden GT, Luna BG, Harmatz JS. Acetaminophen pharmacokinetics in women receiving conjugated estrogen. *Eur J Clin Pharmacol* (1990) 38, 97–8.
6. Rogers SM, Back DJ, Stevenson PJ, Grimmer SFM, Orme ML'E. Paracetamol interaction with oral contraceptive steroids: increased plasma concentration of ethinyloestradiol. *Br J Clin Pharmacol* (1987) 23, 721–5.

Paracetamol (Acetaminophen) + 5-HT_3-receptor antagonists

A placebo-controlled, crossover study in 26 healthy subjects found that both intravenous granisetron 3 mg and tropisetron 5 mg blocked the analgesic effect of a single 1-g oral dose of paracetamol given 90 minutes later. The pharmacokinetics of paracetamol were unaffected by the two drugs. The interaction was thought to involve the serotonergic system,[1] see *Mechanism*, in 'Opioids + Antiemetics; Ondansetron', p.161.

1. Pickering G, Loriot M-A, Libert F, Eschalier A, Beaune P, Dubray C. Analgesic effect of acetaminophen in humans: first evidence of a central serotonergic mechanism. *Clin Pharmacol Ther* (2006) 79, 371–8.

Paracetamol (Acetaminophen) + Isoniazid

A number of reports suggest that the toxicity of paracetamol may be increased by isoniazid so that normal analgesic dosages (4 g daily) may not be safe in some individuals. Pharmacokinetic studies suggest that isoniazid usually inhibits the metabolism of paracetamol, but that metabolism to toxic metabolites may be induced shortly after stopping isoniazid, or late in the isoniazid dose-interval in fast acetylators of isoniazid.

Clinical evidence

A 21-year-old woman who had been taking isoniazid 300 mg for 6 months took 3.25 g of paracetamol for abdominal cramping. Within about 6 hours she developed marked evidence of liver damage (prolonged prothrombin time, elevated ammonia, transaminases, hyperbilirubinaemia).[1]

A young woman taking isoniazid who had taken up to 11.5 g of paracetamol in a suicide gesture, developed life-threatening hepatic and renal toxicity despite the fact that her serum paracetamol levels 13 hours later were only 15 micromol/L (toxicity normally associated with levels above 26 micromol/L).[2]

Three other similar cases were reported in patients taking isoniazid, rifampicin and pyrazinamide who had taken only 2 to 6 g of paracetamol daily.[3] Three other possible cases of this toxic interaction have been described.[4]

However, in a pharmacokinetic study in 10 healthy subjects of both slow and fast acetylator status, isoniazid 300 mg daily for 7 days modestly decreased the total clearance of a single 500-mg dose of paracetamol by 15%. Moreover, the clearance of paracetamol to oxidative metabolites was *decreased*.[5] Similarly, in a further study in 10 healthy slow acetylators of isoniazid, the formation of paracetamol thioether metabolites and oxidative metabolites was reduced by 63% and 49%, respectively, by isoniazid 300 mg daily. However, one day after stopping isoniazid, the formation of thioether metabolites was *increased* by 56%, and this returned to pretreatment values 3 days after the discontinuation of isoniazid.[6] In yet another study in 10 healthy subjects taking isoniazid prophylaxis, the formation clearance of paracetamol to *N*-acetyl-*p*-benzoquinone imine (NAPQI) was inhibited by 56% when the paracetamol was given simultaneously with the daily isoniazid dose, but when the paracetamol was taken 12 hours after the isoniazid, there was no difference in NAPQI formation clearance, compared with the control phase (1 to 2 weeks after isoniazid had been discontinued). However, when the results were analysed by acetylator status, it appeared that the NAPQI formation clearance was *increased* in fast acetylators taking paracetamol 12 hours after the isoniazid dose.[7]

Mechanism

Not established. A possible reason is that isoniazid induces the cytochrome P450 isoenzyme CYP2E1 by stabilisation.[8] This means that while the isoniazid is still present, the metabolism of substrates such as paracetamol is inhibited. However, when isoniazid levels drop sufficiently (as may be the case late in the dosing interval in fast acetylators), metabolism may be induced resulting in a greater proportion of the paracetamol being converted into toxic metabolites than would normally occur.[7]

Importance and management

Information is limited, but it would now seem prudent to consider warning patients taking isoniazid to limit their use of paracetamol because it seems that some individuals risk possible paracetamol-induced liver toxicity, even with normal recommended doses. Pharmacokinetic studies suggest that it is possible that the risk is greatest shortly after stopping isoniazid. The risk may also be higher if paracetamol is taken late in the isoniazid dosing interval, particularly in fast acetylators of isoniazid. More study is needed to clarify the situation.

1. Crippin JS. Acetaminophen hepatotoxicity: potentiation by isoniazid. *Am J Gastroenterol* (1993) 88, 590–2.
2. Murphy R, Swartz R, Watkins P B. Severe acetaminophen toxicity in a patient receiving isoniazid. *Ann Intern Med* (1990) 113, 799–800.
3. Nolan CM, Sandblom RE, Thummel KE, Slattery JT, Nelson SD. Hepatotoxicity associated with acetaminophen usage in patients receiving multiple drug therapy for tuberculosis. *Chest* (1994) 105, 408–11.
4. Moulding TS, Redeker AG, Kanel GC. Acetaminophen, isoniazid, and hepatic toxicity. *Ann Intern Med* (1991) 114, 431.
5. Epstein MM, Nelson SD, Slattery JT, Kalhorn TF, Wall RA, Wright JM. Inhibition of the metabolism of paracetamol by isoniazid. *Br J Clin Pharmacol* (1991) 31, 139–42.
6. Zand R, Nelson SD, Slattery JT, Thummel KE, Kalhorn TF, Adams SP, Wright JM. Inhibition and induction of cytochrome P4502E1-catalyzed oxidation by isoniazid in humans. *Clin Pharmacol Ther* (1993) 54, 142–9.
7. Chien JY, Peter RM, Nolan CM, Wartell C, Slattery JT, Nelson SD, Carithers RL, Thummel KE. Influence of polymorphic *N*-acetyltransferase phenotype on the inhibition and induction of acetaminophen bioactivation with long-term isoniazid. *Clin Pharmacol Ther* (1997) 61, 24–34.
8. Chien JY, Thummel KE, Slattery JT. Pharmacokinetic consequences of induction of CYP2E1 by ligand stabilization. *Drug Metab Dispos* (1997) 25, 1165–75.

Paracetamol (Acetaminophen) + Opioids

Diamorphine, morphine, oxycodone, pentazocine and pethidine delay gastric emptying so that the rate of absorption of paracetamol given orally is reduced. There is no pharmacokinetic interaction between codeine and paracetamol, but the combination may not always result in increased analgesia.

Clinical evidence

(a) Codeine

In 6 healthy subjects paracetamol 1 g every 8 hours for 7 doses had no effect on the pharmacokinetics of a single 30-mg oral dose of codeine, or its metabolites.[1] Similarly in other studies, codeine had no effect on the pharmacokinetics of paracetamol.[2,3] Paracetamol and codeine are often combined because the combination is more effective than either drug given alone. However, note that not all studies have found this. For example, in one clinical study of surgical removal of impacted third molar teeth, there was no difference in analgesic efficacy between patients given paracetamol alone (800 mg given 3, 6, and 9 hours after surgery, then 400 mg four times daily for 2 days) and those given the same dose of paracetamol with the addition of codeine phosphate 30 mg. Moreover, patients given codeine experienced more adverse effects (nausea, dizziness, drowsiness).[4]

(b) Diamorphine, Pethidine (Meperidine) and Pentazocine

In 8 healthy subjects the absorption of a single 20-mg/kg oral dose of paracetamol solution given 30 minutes after an intramuscular injection of either pethidine 150 mg or diamorphine 10 mg was markedly delayed and reduced. Peak plasma paracetamol levels were reduced by 31% and 74%, respectively, and delayed from 22 minutes to 114 minutes and 142 minutes, respectively.[5] This interaction was also observed, by the same study group, in women in labour who had been given paracetamol tablets after receiving pethidine, diamorphine or pentazocine.[6]

(c) Fentanyl

An *in vitro* study found that paracetamol inhibited the oxidation of fentanyl to norfentanyl, but the concentrations of paracetamol used were greater than those found therapeutically. A potential interaction was thought possible because fentanyl is metabolised by the cytochrome P450 isoenzyme CYP3A4 and paracetamol is also partially metabolised by the CYP3A family.[7]

(d) Morphine

A study in healthy subjects, who remained in the supine position, investigated the effect of morphine syrup (4 doses of 10 mg given every 4 hours) on the absorption of paracetamol. The time to the maximum plasma paracetamol level, for conventional tablets, was increased from 51 minutes to 160 minutes by morphine, whereas the time to the maximum plasma paracetamol level for dispersible tablets was only increased from 14 to 15 minutes.[8]

(e) Oxycodone

A crossover study in 10 healthy subjects investigated the effect of oxycodone 500 micrograms/kg on the absorption kinetics of a simulated paracetamol overdose (5 g). The maximum serum paracetamol level was reduced by 40%, the time to maximum level was increased by 68%, and the AUC_{0-8} was 27% lower, when compared with paracetamol alone.[9]

Mechanism, importance and management

The underlying mechanism of these interactions is that the opioid analgesics delay gastric emptying so that the rate of absorption of paracetamol is reduced, but the total amount absorbed is not affected. These were largely investigational studies in healthy subjects, where paracetamol was used as a measure of gastric emptying, and any clinical relevance has not been determined. Reducing the rate of paracetamol absorption would be expected to reduce the onset of analgesic effect, but this is probably not relevant in patients who are receiving regular doses of paracetamol. However, if speed of onset of action is important, one study[8] suggested that the use of dispersible paracetamol might help to reduce the delay in reaching therapeutic plasma levels.

In paracetamol overdose, it has been suggested that when an opioid is present there may be a potential role for the use of activated charcoal beyond the one-hour post ingestion, because of the delay in the absorption of paracetamol.[9] It is also worth noting that maximum plasma levels may be delayed when assessing treatment options.

1. Somogyi A, Bochner F, Chen ZR. Lack of effect of paracetamol on the pharmacokinetics and metabolism of codeine in man. *Eur J Clin Pharmacol* (1991) 41, 379–82.
2. Bajorek P, Widdop B, Volans G. Lack of inhibition of paracetamol absorption by codeine. *Br J Clin Pharmacol* (1978) 5, 346–8.
3. Sonne J, Poulsen HE, Loft S, Døssing M, Vollmer-Larsen A, Simonsen K, Thyssen H, Lundstrøm K. Therapeutic doses of codeine have no effect on acetaminophen clearance or metabolism. *Eur J Clin Pharmacol* (1988) 35, 109–11.
4. Skjelbred P, Løkken P. Codeine added to paracetamol induced adverse effects but did not increase analgesia. *Br J Clin Pharmacol* (1982) 14, 539–43.
5. Nimmo WS, Heading RC, Wilson J, Tothill P, Prescott LF. Inhibition of gastric emptying and drug absorption by narcotic analgesics. *Br J Clin Pharmacol* (1975) 2, 509–13.

6. Nimmo WS, Wilson J, Prescott LF. Narcotic analgesics and delayed gastric emptying during labour. *Lancet* (1975) i, 890–3.

7. Feierman DE. The effect of paracetamol (acetaminophen) on fentanyl metabolism *in vitro*. *Acta Anaesthesiol Scand* (2000) 44, 560–3.

8. Kennedy JM, Tyers NM, Davey AK. The influence of morphine on the absorption of paracetamol from various formulations in subjects in the supine position, as assessed by TDx measurement of salivary paracetamol concentrations. *J Pharm Pharmacol* (2003) 55, 1345–50.

9. Halcomb SE, Sivilotti ML, Goklaney A, Mullins ME. Pharmacokinetic effects of diphenhydramine or oxycodone in simulated acetaminophen overdose. *Acad Emerg Med* (2005) 12, 169–72.

Paracetamol (Acetaminophen) + Probenecid

Probenecid reduces the clearance of paracetamol.

Clinical evidence, mechanism, importance and management

A metabolic study in 10 healthy subjects found that the clearance of paracetamol 1.5 g was almost halved (from 6.23 to 3.42 mL/minute per kg) when it was taken 1 hour after a 1-g dose of probenecid. The amount of unchanged paracetamol in the urine stayed the same, but the glucuronide metabolite fell sharply.[1] Another study in 11 subjects also found that probenecid 500 mg every 6 hours almost halved (from 329 to 178 mL/minute) the clearance of a 650-mg intravenous dose of paracetamol. The urinary excretion of the glucuronide metabolite was decreased by 68% and the excretion of the sulfate metabolite increased by 49%.[2] These studies suggest that probenecid inhibits paracetamol glucuronidation, possibly by inhibiting glucuronyltransferase. See also 'paracetamol', (p.133). The practical consequences of this interaction are uncertain but there seem to be no adverse reports.

1. Kamali F. The effect of probenecid on paracetamol metabolism and pharmacokinetics. *Eur J Clin Pharmacol* (1993) 45, 551–3.

2. Abernethy DR, Greenblatt DJ, Ameer B, Shader RI. Probenecid impairment of acetaminophen and lorazepam clearance: direct inhibition of ether glucuronide formation. *J Pharmacol Exp Ther* (1985) 234, 345–9.

Paracetamol (Acetaminophen) + Propranolol

Propranolol may slightly increase the bioavailability of paracetamol, but this is unlikely to be clinically significant.

Clinical evidence, mechanism, importance and management

In a study in 10 healthy subjects, propranolol 80 mg twice daily for 4 days increased the half-life of a single 1.5-g dose of paracetamol by 25% and lowered its clearance by 14%. The partial clearance of paracetamol to its cysteine and mercapturate derivatives was decreased by 16% and 32%, respectively, and the clearance to the glucuronide conjugate was decreased by 27%, but the sulfate was not significantly affected.[1] Similarly, an earlier study found that propranolol 40 mg four times daily for one week increased the maximum plasma level of a single 1.5-g dose of paracetamol and reduced the time to peak plasma level. However, the increased rate of absorption of paracetamol was not thought to be clinically important.[2] In contrast, a study in 6 subjects found that a relatively small dose of propranolol (80 mg daily for 6 days) did not affect the pharmacokinetics of paracetamol.[3] Another study found that long-term propranolol use in patients with chronic liver disease did not influence the clearance of total or unconjugated paracetamol.[4]

The changes described here appear to be small, and therefore unlikely to be clinically significant. Note that, it has been postulated, based on studies in *animals,* that propranolol may have a protective effect on paracetamol hepatic toxicity by inhibiting the oxidative metabolism of paracetamol to toxic metabolites.[1,5]

1. Baraka OZ, Truman CA, Ford JM, Roberts CJC. The effect of propranolol on paracetamol metabolism in man. *Br J Clin Pharmacol* (1990) 29, 261–4.

2. Clark RA, Holdsworth CD, Rees MR, Howlett PJ. The effect on paracetamol absorption of stimulation and blockade of β-adrenoceptors. *Br J Clin Pharmacol* (1980) 10, 555–9.

3. Sanchez-Martinez V, Tucker GT, Jackson PR, Lennard MS, Bax NDS, Woods HF. Lack of effect of propranolol on the kinetics of paracetamol in man. *Br J Clin Pharmacol* (1985) 20, 548P.

4. Hayes PC, Bouchier IAD. Effect of acute and chronic propranolol administration on antipyrine and paracetamol clearance in patients with chronic liver disease. *Am J Gastroenterol* (1989) 84, 723–6.

5. Auty RM, Branch RA. Paracetamol toxicity and propranolol. *Lancet* (1973) 2, 1505.

Paracetamol (Acetaminophen) + Proton pump inhibitors

Lansoprazole modestly increased the rate, but not the extent, of absorption of paracetamol solution. Omeprazole does not appear to have any effect on the metabolism of phenacetin or paracetamol.

Clinical evidence

(a) Lansoprazole

In a study in 6 healthy subjects, lansoprazole 30 mg once daily for 3 days increased the peak level of paracetamol (given as a single 1-g dose in solution) by 43%, and decreased the time to peak paracetamol levels by half (from about 35 to 17.5 minutes). However, lansoprazole had no effect on the AUC and elimination half-life of paracetamol.[1]

(b) Omeprazole

Omeprazole 20 mg daily for 8 days had no effect on the pharmacokinetics of **phenacetin**, or paracetamol derived from **phenacetin**, in 10 healthy subjects, except that the peak plasma level of **phenacetin** was higher. There was no change in the metabolism (oxidative and conjugative) of phenacetin or derived paracetamol.[2] In another study, omeprazole 40 mg daily for 7 days had no effect on the formation of thioether metabolites of paracetamol in 5 rapid and 5 slow metabolisers of *S*-mephenytoin [a probe drug for CYP2C19 activity, see 'Genetic factors in drug metabolism', (p.4)].[3]

Mechanism

Lansoprazole may increase the absorption of paracetamol by indirectly increasing the rate of gastric emptying.[1] Phenacetin is metabolised to paracetamol by the cytochrome P450 isoenzyme CYP1A2, and it has been suggested that omeprazole can induce CYP1A2, and possibly increase the formation of hepatotoxic metabolites of paracetamol. However, the findings here suggest that omeprazole has no important effect on CYP1A2, or on phenacetin or paracetamol metabolism.

Importance and management

The findings from these studies suggest that neither lansoprazole nor omeprazole cause any clinically important changes in the pharmacokinetics of paracetamol. No special precautions appear to be needed on concurrent use.

1. Sanaka M, Kuyama Y, Mineshita S, Qi J, Hanada Y, Enatsu I, Tanaka H, Makino H, Yamanaka M. Pharmacokinetic interaction between acetaminophen and lansoprazole. *J Clin Gastroenterol* (1999) 29, 56–8.
2. Xiaodong S, Gatti G, Bartoli A, Cipolla G, Crema F, Perucca E. Omeprazole does not enhance the metabolism of phenacetin, a marker of CYP1A2 activity, in healthy volunteers. *Ther Drug Monit* (1994) 16, 248–50.
3. Sarich T, Kalhorn T, Magee S, Al-Sayegh F, Adams S, Slattery J, Goldstein J, Nelson S, Wright J. The effect of omeprazole pretreatment on acetaminophen metabolism in rapid and slow metabolizers of *S*-mephenytoin. *Clin Pharmacol Ther* (1997) 62, 21–8.

Paracetamol (Acetaminophen) + Rifampicin (Rifampin)

Rifampicin increases the metabolism of paracetamol. An isolated report describes hepatic failure, which may have been due to an interaction between paracetamol and rifampicin.

Clinical evidence, mechanism, importance and management

The metabolite to paracetamol ratio for glucuronides was twice as high in 10 patients treated with rifampicin 600 mg daily than in 14 healthy control subjects. In contrast the ratio for sulfates did not differ between the two groups.[1] In a crossover study in healthy subjects, rifampicin 600 mg daily for 1 week, given before paracetamol 500 mg, had no effect on the formation of *N*-acetyl-*p*-benzoquinone imine (NAPQI) or the recovery of thiol metabolites formed by conjugation of NAPQI with glutathione.[2] These studies suggest that rifampicin induces the glucuronidation of paracetamol, but that it does not increase the formation of hepatotoxic metabolites of 'paracetamol', (p.133).

However, a 32-year-old woman, who had taken paracetamol 2 to 4 g daily for several weeks, and who had not responded to doxycycline or clarithromycin for suspected cat scratch fever, became confused and agitated 2 days after starting to take rifampicin 600 mg twice daily. Her INR increased from 1.1 to 5.2 and her liver enzymes became raised. Rifampicin and paracetamol were stopped, and she was treated with vitamin K and acetylcysteine, and liver function returned to normal. Paracetamol hepatotoxicity, in doses not normally associated with such effects, occurred only after the addition of rifampicin. It was suggested that rifampicin, which alone may cause hepatitis, had in this case induced the metabolism of paracetamol to hepatotoxic metabolites.[3]

The clinical importance of the studies awaits further study, but they suggest that rifampicin may reduce the efficacy of paracetamol.

1. Bock KW, Wiltfang J, Blume R, Ullrich D, Bircher J. Paracetamol as a test drug to determine glucuronide formation in man. Effects of inducers and of smoking. *Eur J Clin Pharmacol* (1987) 31, 677–83.
2. Manyike PT, Kharasch ED, Kalhorn TF, Slattery JT. Contribution of CYP2E1 and CYP3A to acetaminophen reactive metabolite formation. *Clin Pharmacol Ther* (2000) 67, 275–82.
3. Stephenson I, Qualie M, Wiselka MJ. Hepatic failure and encephalopathy attributed to an interaction between acetaminophen and rifampicin. *Am J Gastroenterol* (2001) 96, 1310–1.

Paracetamol (Acetaminophen) + Sodium nitrate

An isolated report describes severe methaemoglobinaemia in a patient who had taken paracetamol after a meal consisting of 'yuke' (raw beef preserved with sodium nitrate). Both paracetamol and sodium nitrate may cause methaemoglobinaemia, so an interaction resulting in additive effects may have occurred, but a genetic cause was also considered to be a possibility.[1]

1. Kobayashi T, Kawabata M, Tanaka S, Maehara M, Mishima A, Murase T. Methemoglobinemia induced by combined use of sodium nitrate and acetoaminophen. *Intern Med* (2000) 39, 860.

Paracetamol (Acetaminophen) + Sucralfate

The bioavailability of paracetamol 1 g (using salivary paracetamol levels over 4 hours as a measure of paracetamol absorption) was found to be unchanged in 6 healthy subjects given sucralfate 1 g.[1]

1. Kamali F, Fry JR, Smart HL, Bell GD. A double-blind placebo-controlled study to examine effects of sucralfate on paracetamol absorption. *Br J Clin Pharmacol* (1985) 19, 113–14.

Paracetamol (Acetaminophen) + Sulfinpyrazone

Sulfinpyrazone modestly increases the clearance of paracetamol.

Clinical evidence, mechanism, importance and management

In 12 healthy subjects, sulfinpyrazone 200 mg given every 6 hours for one week, increased the clearance of a single 1-g dose of paracetamol by 23%. There was a 26% increase in metabolic clearance of the glucuronide conjugate, and a 43% increase in the glutathione-derived conjugates (indicating an increased production of the hepatotoxic metabolite), but no change in sulfation.[1] It has therefore been suggested that, in patients taking sulfinpyrazone, the risk of liver damage may be increased after paracetamol overdosage and perhaps during prolonged consumption,[1] (see also 'paracetamol', (p.133)) but there seem to be no adverse reports. The clinical importance of these findings awaits further study.

1. Miners JO, Attwood J, Birkett DJ. Determinants of acetaminophen metabolism: effect of inducers and inhibitors of drug metabolism on acetaminophen's metabolic pathways. *Clin Pharmacol Ther* (1984) 35, 480–6.

Paracetamol (Acetaminophen) + Tobacco

Heavy, but not moderate, smoking may increase the metabolism of paracetamol. The clearance of phenacetin is also increased in smokers. There is some evidence that smokers are at risk of a poorer outcome after paracetamol overdose.

Clinical evidence, mechanism, importance and management

There was no difference in the clearance of a single 1-g dose of paracetamol in 6 healthy smokers (more than 15 cigarettes per day) and 6 healthy non-smokers in one study, and no difference in the paracetamol metabolites.[1] Similarly, another study found no difference in the pharmacokinetics of a single 650-mg intravenous dose of paracetamol in 14 healthy smokers (range 8 to 35 cigarettes per day) and 15 non-smokers.[2] In contrast, in another study, the metabolite to paracetamol ratio for glucuronides was 83% higher in 9 heavy smokers (about 40 cigarettes daily), suggesting increased paracetamol metabolism, than in 14 healthy non-smokers. However, it was not higher in moderate smokers (about 10 cigarettes daily).[3]

A further study in 36 healthy Chinese subjects given a single 900-mg dose of phenacetin found that subjects who smoked cigarettes (7 to 40 daily; mean 20) had a 2.5-fold higher phenacetin apparent oral clearance, compared with non-smokers. Paracetamol plasma levels were also moderately lower in the smokers (phenacetin is metabolised to paracetamol). Cigarette smoke appears to induce the metabolism of phenacetin by the cytochrome P450 isoenzyme CYP1A2, and also appears to increase the metabolism of paracetamol either by stimulating a minor pathway involving CYP1A2 oxidation or by stimulating the conversion of phenacetin to compounds other than paracetamol.[4]

A retrospective study of patients treated for paracetamol poisoning found that there was a much higher proportion of smokers than in the general population (70% versus 31%). Moreover, smoking was independently associated with an increased risk of hepatic encephalopathy (odds ratio 2.68) and death (odds ratio 3.64) following paracetamol overdose.[5]

No interaction is established, but the above studies suggest that heavy smoking may increase the metabolism of paracetamol. The retrospective study also suggests that smoking is associated with a poorer outcome after paracetamol overdose. Further study is needed.

1. Miners JO, Attwood J, Birkett DJ. Determinants of acetaminophen metabolism: effect of inducers and inhibitors of drug metabolism on acetaminophen's metabolic pathways. *Clin Pharmacol Ther* (1984) 35, 480–6.
2. Scavone JM, Greenblatt DJ, LeDuc BW, Blyden GT, Luna BG, Harmatz JS. Differential effect of cigarette smoking on antipyrine oxidation versus acetaminophen conjugation. *Pharmacology* (1990) 40, 77–84.
3. Bock KW, Wiltfang J, Blume R, Ullrich D, Bircher J. Paracetamol as a test drug to determine glucuronide formation in man. Effects of inducers and of smoking. *Eur J Clin Pharmacol* (1987) 31, 677–83.
4. Dong SX , Ping ZZ, Xiao WZ, Shu CC, Bartoli A, Gatti G, D'Urso S, Perucca E. Effect of active and passive cigarette smoking on CYP1A2-mediated phenacetin disposition in Chinese subjects. *Ther Drug Monit* (1998) 20, 371–5.
5. Schmidt LE, Dalhoff K. The impact of current tobacco use on the outcome of paracetamol poisoning. *Aliment Pharmacol Ther* (2003) 18, 979–85.

7

Anorectics and Stimulants

This section covers the drugs used in the management of obesity (such as orlistat and sibutramine) as well as the older drugs, such as the amfetamines, which are now no longer widely indicated for this condition, and are now more generally considered as drugs of abuse. However, it should not be forgotten that the amfetamines (largely dexamfetamine) still have a limited therapeutic role in the management of narcolepsy. Ecstasy (MDMA, methylenedioxymethamfetamine), a drug of abuse that is structurally related to amfetamine, is also included in this section. The amfetamines are sympathomimetics, a diverse group, which have a number of interactions. The mechanism of action and classification of sympathomimetics is discussed in 'Cardiovascular drugs, miscellaneous', (p.878). Other stimulant drugs (such as atomoxetine; and methylphenidate, another sympathomimetic) have a role in attention deficit hyperactivity disorder (ADHD) and are also discussed in this section.

Amfetamines + Cocaine

An ischaemic stroke occurred in a patient who was abusing amfetamine and cocaine. *In vitro,* cocaine inhibits the demethylenation of ecstasy (MDMA, methylenedioxymethamfetamine), but the clinical significance of this is unknown.

Clinical evidence, mechanism, importance and management

A 16-year-old boy developed unsteadiness and double vision 5 minutes after intranasal inhalation of a small amount of amfetamine 'cut' with cocaine. Cranial MRI (magnetic resonance imaging) revealed a mesencephalic lesion that was seen to have decreased 12 days later, and he became symptom-free after 3 weeks. The ischaemic lesion was thought to be due to vasospasm caused by synergistic stimulation of the sympathetic nervous system: amfetamine causes the release of adrenaline (epinephrine) and noradrenaline (norepinephrine), while cocaine prevents their reuptake.[1]

An *in vitro* study showed that cocaine (a potent inhibitor of the cytochrome P450 isoenzyme CYP2D6) inhibited the CYP2D6-mediated demethylenation of **ecstasy** (MDMA, methylenedioxymethamfetamine). Therefore, theoretically, the use of cocaine would be expected to increase plasma and CNS concentrations of **ecstasy**,[2] but it is not known if this is significant in practice.

1. Strupp M, Hamann GF, Brandt T. Combined amphetamine and cocaine abuse caused mesencephalic ischemia in a 16-year-old boy – due to vasospasm? *Eur Neurol* (2000) 43, 181–2.
2. Ramamoorthy Y, Yu A, Suh N, Haining RL, Tyndale RF, Sellers EM. Reduced (±)-3,4-methylenedioxymethamphetamine ("Ecstasy") metabolism with cytochrome P450 2D6 inhibitors and pharmacogenetic variants *in vitro*. *Biochem Pharmacol* (2002) 63, 2111–19.

Amfetamines and related drugs + Lithium

The stimulant and/or cardiovascular effects of the amfetamines have been shown to be opposed by lithium in some, but not other studies.

Clinical evidence, mechanism, importance and management

Two depressed patients stopped abusing **metamfetamine** and cannabis, or **phenmetrazine** and 'other diet pills' because, while taking lithium carbonate, they were unable to get 'high'. Another patient complained that she felt no effects from amfetamines taken for weight reduction, including no decrease in appetite, until lithium carbonate was withdrawn.[1] A controlled study in 9 depressed patients confirmed that lithium carbonate taken for 10 days attenuated the subjective stimulant effects of **dexamfetamine** or L-**amfetamine**.[2] Another study found similar results with **dexamfetamine** in schizophrenic patients.[3] However, in a further study, only 4 of 8 subjects had an attenuation of the stimulant effects of **amfetamine**.[4] In this study, lithium attenuated the increase in systolic blood pressure caused by amfetamine (from an average increase of 31/15 mmHg down to 20/9 mmHg).[4] In contrast, in a controlled study in healthy subjects, there was no difference in subjective or cardiovascular effects of a single 20-mg dose of **dexamfetamine** between those receiving lithium 1.2 g daily for 7 days and those receiving placebo.[5] In yet another controlled study, in 9 subjects, the only significant effect of pretreatment with lithium 900 mg for 14 days was to attenuate the feeling of happiness after **dexamfetamine**.[6]

The reasons for these reactions, when they occur, are not known, but one suggestion is that amfetamines and lithium have mutually opposing pharmacological actions on noradrenaline (norepinephrine) release and uptake at adrenergic neurones.[1]

Information is contradictory, therefore an interaction is not established. Nevertheless, it may be prudent to be alert for evidence of reduced amfetamine effects in the presence of lithium.

1. Flemenbaum A. Does lithium block the effects of amphetamine? A report of three cases. *Am J Psychiatry* (1974) 131, 820–1.
2. van Kammen DP, Murphy D. Attenuation of the euphoriant and activating effects of *d*- and *l*-amphetamine by lithium carbonate treatment. *Psychopharmacologia* (1975) 44, 215–24.
3. van Kammen DP, Docherty JP, Marder SR, Rosenblatt JE, Bunney WE. Lithium attenuates the activation-euphoria but not the psychosis induced by *d*-amphetamine in schizophrenia. *Psychopharmacology (Berl)* (1985) 87, 111–15.
4. Angrist B, Gershon S. Variable attenuation of amphetamine effects by lithium. *Am J Psychiatry* (1979) 136, 806–10.
5. Silverstone PH, Pukhovsky A, Rotzinger S. Lithium does not attenuate the effects of D-amphetamine in healthy volunteers. *Psychiatry Res* (1998) 9, 219–26.
6. Willson MC, Bell EC, Dave S, Asghar SJ, McGrath BM, Silverstone PH. Valproate attenuates dextroamphetamine-induced subjective changes more than lithium. *Eur Neuropsychopharmacol* (2005) 15, 633–9.

Amfetamines and related drugs + Phenothiazines

The appetite suppressant and other effects of amfetamines, chlorphentermine and phenmetrazine are opposed by chlorpromazine. It seems possible that other phenothiazine will interact similarly. The antipsychotic effects of chlorpromazine can be opposed by dexamfetamine.

Clinical evidence

In a placebo-controlled study 10 obese schizophrenic patients who were taking drugs including **chlorpromazine**, **thioridazine**, imipramine and chlordiazepoxide did not respond to treatment with **dexamfetamine** for obesity. The expected sleep disturbance in response to **dexamfetamine** was also not seen.[1] In a double-blind, placebo-controlled study in 76 patients, **chlorpromazine** was found to diminish the weight-reducing effect of **phenmetrazine**,[2] and, in another study, patients taking **chlorpromazine** did not experience the expected weight loss when they were given **phenmetrazine** or **chlorphentermine**.[3] Similarly, antagonism of the effects of **amfetamines** by **chlorpromazine** has been described in other reports.[4,5]

A study in 462 patients taking **chlorpromazine** 200 to 600 mg daily indicated that the addition of **dexamfetamine** 10 to 60 mg daily had a detrimental effect on the control of their schizophrenic symptoms.[6]

This interaction has been deliberately exploited, with success, in the treatment of 22 children poisoned with various amfetamines or related compounds (**amfetamine**, **dexamfetamine**, **metamfetamine**, **phenmetrazine**).[4]

Mechanism

Not understood. It is known that chlorpromazine can inhibit adrenergic and dopaminergic activity, which could explain some part of the antagonism of the amfetamines, the euphoriant effects of which are said to be mediated by central dopamine receptors.

Importance and management

Established interactions. These reports suggest that it is not beneficial to attempt to treat patients taking chlorpromazine with amfetamines, such as dexamfetamine, or other central stimulants such as phenmetrazine. In one study, thioridazine also appeared to interact. However, it is not clear whether this interaction takes place with antipsychotics other than chlorpromazine, but it seems possible with the phenothiazines, especially if the suggested mechanism is correct. Note that central stimulants are no longer recommended for the treatment of obesity.

1. Modell W, Hussar AE. Failure of dextroamphetamine sulfate to influence eating and sleeping patterns in obese schizophrenic patients: clinical and pharmacological significance. *JAMA* (1965) 193, 275–8.
2. Reid AA. Pharmacological antagonism between chlorpromazine and phenmetrazine in mental hospital patients. *Med J Aust* (1964) 10, 187–8.
3. Sletten IW, Ognjanov V, Menendez S, Sundland D, El-Toumi A. Weight reduction with chlorphentermine and phenmetrazine in obese psychiatric patients during chlorpromazine therapy. *Curr Ther Res* (1967) 9, 570–5.
4. Espelin DE, Done AK. Amphetamine poisoning: effectiveness of chlorpromazine. *N Engl J Med* (1968) 278, 1361–65.
5. Jönsson L-E. Pharmacological blockade of amphetamine effects in amphetamine dependent subjects. *Eur J Clin Pharmacol* (1972) 4, 206–11.
6. Casey JF, Hollister LE, Klett CJ, Lasky JJ, Caffey EM. Combined drug therapy of chronic schizophrenics. Controlled evaluation of placebo, dextro-amphetamine, imipramine, isocarboxazid and trifluoperazine added to maintenance doses of chlorpromazine. *Am J Psychiatry* (1961) 117, 997–1003.

Amfetamines + Phenylpropanolamine

The effects of levamfetamine were attenuated in a hyperactive child by a nasal decongestant containing chlorphenamine and phenylpropanolamine.

Clinical evidence, mechanism, importance and management

The use of **levamfetamine succinate** 42 mg daily in was found to be ineffective a 12-year-old hyperactive boy on two occasions when he took ***Contac*** cold capsules and ***Allerest*** tablets for colds. Both of these proprietary nasal decongestants contain phenylpropanolamine and chlorphenamine.[1] The reason for this interaction is not understood and there is too little information to make any statement about the general importance of this reaction.

1. Huestis RD, Arnold LE. Possible antagonism of amphetamine by decongestant-antihistamine compounds. *J Pediatr* (1974) 85, 579.

Amfetamines and related drugs + Protease inhibitors

A man taking ritonavir suffered a fatal serotonergic reaction after taking ecstasy (MDMA, methylenedioxymethamfetamine). A similar fatal reaction occurred with metamfetamine and ritonavir.

Clinical evidence

(a) Ecstasy (MDMA, Methylenedioxymethamfetamine)

An HIV-positive man taking lamivudine and zidovudine was additionally given **ritonavir** 600 mg twice daily. About a fortnight later he went to a club and took ecstasy, in a dose estimated to be about 180 mg. He soon became unwell, and when seen by a nurse in the club was hypertonic, tachypnoeic (45 breaths per minute), tachycardic (more than 140 bpm), cyanosed and diaphoretic. He had a tonic-clonic seizure, his pulse rose to 200 bpm, he then vomited, had a cardiorespiratory arrest and died. A post mortem showed blood-alcohol concentrations of 24 mg% and an ecstasy level of 4.56 micrograms/mL, which was almost 10 times greater than might have been expected from the dose he had taken. The authors say that death was consistent with a severe serotonergic reaction.[1] Another report verifies that high ecstasy levels (4.05 micrograms/mL) result in these life-threatening symptoms.[2]

A patient with AIDS, taking **ritonavir** and **saquinavir**, experienced agitation that lasted for over a day, following a small dose of ecstasy. He then experienced a nearly fatal reaction to a small dose of **sodium oxybate (GHB, gamma-hydroxybutyrate, γ-hydroxybutyrate)**, becoming unresponsive within 20 minutes of ingestion of the drug and exhibiting a brief episode of repetitive clonic contractions.[3]

(b) Metamfetamine

A 49-year-old HIV-positive man taking protease inhibitors was found dead after injecting himself twice with metamfetamine as well as sniffing **amyl nitrate**. He had been taking an antiretroviral regimen of **ritonavir** 400 mg twice daily, soft gel **saquinavir** 400 mg twice daily and stavudine 40 mg twice daily for 4 months. Toxicology detected metamfetamine 500 nanograms/mL in the blood (considered to be in the fatal range, especially when used with other unnamed drugs). Cannabinoids and traces of diazepam and nordiazepam were also found in this patient.[4]

Mechanism

Ritonavir inhibits the cytochrome P450 isoenzyme CYP2D6, which is responsible for the demethylenation of ecstasy, so concurrent use leads to a sharp rise in ecstasy plasma levels. Poor liver function (due to alcoholism) may have been a contributory factor in one patient,[1] and further CYP inhibition by nitric oxide (the metabolite of amyl nitrate) may have contributed to another case.[4] An additional factor is that ecstasy may show non-linear pharmacokinetics.[5] Metamfetamine is also metabolised by CYP2D6 and its levels would therefore similarly be raised by ritonavir.

Importance and management

Although there are few reported cases, what happens is consistent with the known toxic effects and pharmacology of the drugs concerned. In addition, protease inhibitors may theoretically inhibit the metabolism of ecstasy via other isoenzymes (CYP3A4, CYP2B6), which could therefore also lead to increased levels.

It has been suggested that patients who are prescribed any protease inhibitor should be made aware of the potential risks of using any form of recreational drugs metabolised by CYP2D6.[4] In particular, some authors recommend that patients taking ritonavir should avoid using ecstasy, metamfetamine and other amfetamines.[6] Open discussions of illicit drug use would enable carers to warn patients that the use of these drugs may be even more dangerous while taking protease inhibitors. Appropriate precautions, apart from avoidance, include a reduction of the usual dose of ecstasy to about 25%, taking breaks from dancing, checking that a medical team are on site, maintaining adequate hydration by avoiding alcohol, and replenishing fluids regularly.[6]

1. Henry JA, Hill IR. Fatal interaction between ritonavir and MDMA. *Lancet* (1998) 352, 1751–2.
2. Roberts L, Wright H. Survival following intentional massive overdose of 'Ecstasy'. *J Accid Emerg Med* (1993) 11, 53–4.
3. Harrington RD, Woodward JA, Hooton TM, Horn JR. Life-threatening interactions between HIV-1 protease inhibitors and the illicit drugs MDMA and γ-hydroxybutyrate. *Arch Intern Med* (1999) 159, 2221–4.
4. Hales G, Roth N, Smith D. Possible fatal interaction between protease inhibitors and methamphetamine. *Antivir Ther* (2000) 5,19.
5. de la Torre, R, Ortuño J, Mas M, Farré M, Segura J. Fatal MDMA intoxication. *Lancet* (1999) 353, 593.
6. Antoniou T, Tseng AL. Interactions between recreational drugs and antiretroviral agents. *Ann Pharmacother* (2002) 36, 1598–1613.

Amfetamines and related drugs + SSRIs

The psychological effects of ecstasy (MDMA, methylenedioxymethamfetamine) may be reduced if citalopram has previously been given. It seems likely that other SSRIs will also reduce or block some of the effects of ecstasy, but increased serotonin effects may, in theory, also be possible. An isolated report describes a neurotoxic reaction in a man taking citalopram when he took unknown amounts of ecstasy. Fluoxetine and paroxetine may decrease the metabolism of ecstasy.

Clinical evidence

A double-blind, placebo-controlled psychometric study in 16 healthy subjects found that **ecstasy** (MDMA, methylenedioxymethamfetamine) 1.5 mg/kg produced an emotional state with heightened mood, increased self-confidence and extroversion, moderate derealisation and an intensification of sensory perception. Most of these effects were found to be markedly reduced by pretreatment with **citalopram** 40 mg by intravenous infusion, although their duration was prolonged by up to 2 hours.[1] Similarly a case report describes 2 patients taking **citalopram** 20 mg daily or **paroxetine** 20 mg daily who did not experience any effects from **ecstasy** after starting the SSRI. One patient continued to experience a 'high' from **amfetamines**.[2] However, an account of 4 **ecstasy** users who had taken **fluoxetine** 20 mg before taking **ecstasy** 100 to 250 mg, reported that they still experienced the subjective effects of euphoria, but one commented that the overall acute experience was "slightly calmer". Some of the adverse effects such as jaw clenching and insomnia were also attenuated and recovery was more rapid.[3]

When a man taking **citalopram** 60 mg daily additionally took unknown amounts of **ecstasy** he became aggressive, agitated, severely grandiose, restless and performed compulsive movements in a peculiar and joyless dance-like manner. He lacked normal movement control and said he could see little bugs. He was treated with haloperidol and chlordiazepoxide, and improved within 2 days of replacing the **citalopram** with promazine.[4]

In a placebo-controlled, randomised, crossover study, 7 healthy subjects were given **ecstasy** 100 mg on the last day of taking **paroxetine** 20 mg daily for 3 days. **Paroxetine** raised the maximum serum levels and AUC of **ecstasy** by 17% and 27%, respectively.[5]

Mechanism

Complex. It has been suggested that the psychological and neurotoxic effects of ecstasy may be caused by serotonin release in the brain.[3,6] This could potentially be blocked by serotonin reuptake inhibitors (such as citalopram) resulting in reduced ecstasy effects. However, ecstasy is also thought to inhibit serotonin reuptake,[6] so its use with the SSRIs could increase serotonin effects, which could result in neurotoxicity.[7] Furthermore, the SSRIs (to varying degrees) inhibit the cytochrome P450 isoenzyme CYP2D6, by which ecstasy is metabolised, so concurrent use could result in increased ecstasy levels.[5,8]

Importance and management

The study of ecstasy with citalopram was primarily undertaken to find out how ecstasy works, but on the basis of these results and *animal* studies it seems likely that patients already taking citalopram may not be able to get as 'high' on usual doses of ecstasy, and some adverse effects may also be reduced. Furthermore, if the proposed mechanism of interaction is correct, the same is also likely to be true if they are taking any other SSRI and some cases have been reported. However, be aware of possible pharmacokinetic interactions with some SSRIs that are potent CYP2D6 inhibitors (e.g. fluoxetine, paroxetine), which may increase ecstasy levels. There is also a risk of increased serotonergic activity and there have been a few reports of interactions involving other sympathomimetics and SSRIs or related drugs, see 'Phentermine + Fluoxetine', p.205.

The neurotoxic reaction cited seems to be an isolated case but it illustrates some of the risks attached to using 'recreational' drugs by patients already taking other medications, particularly antidepressant and psychotropic drugs that affect the same receptors in the CNS.

1. Liechti ME, Baumann C, Gamma A, Vollenweider FX. Acute psychological effects of 3,4-methylenedioxymethamphetamine (MDMA, "Ecstasy") are attenuated by the serotonin uptake inhibitor citalopram. *Neuropsychopharmacology* (2000) 22, 513–21.
2. Stein DJ, Rink J. Effects of "ecstasy" blocked by serotonin reuptake inhibitors. *J Clin Psychiatry* (1999) 60, 485.
3. McCann UD, Ricaurte GA. Reinforcing subjective effects of (±) 3,4-methylenedioxymethamphetamine ("Ecstasy") may be separable from its neurotoxic actions: clinical evidence. *J Clin Psychopharmacol* (1993) 13, 214–17.
4. Lauerma H, Wuorela M, Halme M. Interaction of serotonin reuptake inhibitor and 3,4-methylenedioxymethamphetamine? *Biol Psychiatry* (1998) 43, 929.
5. Segura M, Farré M, Pichini S, Peiró AM, Roset PN, Ramírez A, Ortuño J, Pacifici R, Zuccaro P, Segura J, de la Torre R. Contribution of cytochrome P450 2D6 to 3,4-methylenedioxymethamphetamine disposition in humans: use of paroxetine as a metabolic inhibitor probe. *Clin Pharmacokinet* (2005) 44, 649–60.
6. Lyles J, Cadet JL. Methylenedioxymethamphetamine (MDMA, Ecstasy) neurotoxicity: cellular and molecular mechanisms. *Brain Res Brain Res Rev* (2003) 42, 155–68.
7. Oesterheld JR, Armstrong SC, Cozza KL. Ecstasy: pharmacodynamic and pharmacokinetic interactions. *Psychosomatics* (2004) 45, 84–7.
8. Ramamoorthy Y, Yu A, Suh N, Haining RL, Tyndale RF, Sellers EM. Reduced (±)-3,4-methylenedioxymethamphetamine ("Ecstasy") metabolism with cytochrome P450 2D6 inhibitors and pharmacogenetic variants *in vitro*. *Biochem Pharmacol* (2002) 63, 2111–19.

Amfetamines + Urinary acidifiers or alkalinisers

The urinary excretion of amfetamines is increased by urinary acidifiers (ammonium chloride) and reduced by urinary alkalinisers (sodium bicarbonate).

Clinical evidence

A study in 6 healthy subjects given **dexamfetamine** 10 to 15 mg found that when the urine was made alkaline (pH of about 8) by giving **sodium bicarbonate**, only 3% of the original dose of amfetamine was excreted over a 16-hour period, compared with 55% when the urine was made acidic (pH of about 5) by taking **ammonium chloride**.[1] Similar results have been reported elsewhere for **amfetamine, dexamfetamine** and **metamfetamine**.[2-4] A further study found that the effects of **amfetamine** were increased and prolonged in subjects with alkaline urine.[5] Psychoses resulting from amfetamine retention in patients with **alkaline urine** has been described.[6]

Mechanism

Amfetamines are bases, which are excreted by the kidneys. If the urine is alkaline most of the drug exists in the unionised form, which is readily reabsorbed by the kidney tubules so that little is lost. In acid urine, little of the drug is in the unionised form so that little can be reabsorbed and much of it is lost. For more detail on this mechanism see 'Changes in urinary pH', (p.7).

Importance and management

A well established and well understood interaction but reports of problems in practice seem rare. The interaction has been exploited to increase the clearance of amfetamines in cases of overdose by acidifying the urine with ammonium chloride. Conversely it can represent an undesirable interaction if therapeutic doses of amfetamines are excreted too rapidly. Care is needed to ensure that amfetamine toxicity does not develop if the urine is made alkaline with sodium bicarbonate or another urinary alkaliniser, **acetazolamide**.

1. Beckett AH, Rowland M, Turner P. Influence of urinary pH on excretion of amphetamine. *Lancet* (1965) i, 303.
2. Rowland M, Beckett AH. The amphetamines: clinical and pharmacokinetic implications of recent studies of an assay procedure and urinary excretion in man. *Arzneimittelforschung* (1966) 16, 1369–73.
3. Beckett AH, Salmon JA, Mitchard M. The relation between blood levels and urinary excretion of amphetamine under controlled acidic and under fluctuating urinary pH values using [^{14}C]amphetamine. *J Pharm Pharmacol* (1969) 21, 251–8.
4. Davis JM, Kopin IJ, Lemberger L, Axelrod J. Effects of urinary pH on amphetamine metabolism. *Ann N Y Acad Sci* (1971) 179, 493–501.
5. Smart JV, Turner P. Influence of urinary pH on the degree and duration of action of amphetamine on the critical flicker fusion frequency in man. *Br J Pharmacol* (1966) 26, 468–72.
6. Änggård E, Jönsson L-E, Hogmark A-L, Gunne L-M. Amphetamine metabolism in amphetamine psychosis. *Clin Pharmacol Ther* (1973) 14, 870–80.

Atomoxetine + CYP2D6 inhibitors

Paroxetine markedly increases atomoxetine levels in extensive metabolisers of CYP2D6. Fluoxetine also raises atomoxetine levels. There is a possibility that this may increase adverse effects, and a slower titration of atomoxetine dose is suggested for patients taking paroxetine and other CYP2D6 inhibitors.

Clinical evidence

Paroxetine 20 mg daily for 17 days, with atomoxetine 20 mg twice daily on days 12 to 17, was given to 22 healthy subjects who were extensive metabolisers of the cytochrome P450 isoenzyme CYP2D6 (most common phenotype). **Paroxetine** increased the AUC of atomoxetine 6.5-fold, increased the maximum plasma level by 3.5-fold, and increased the elimination half-life by 2.5-fold, when compared with atomoxetine alone. No changes in paroxetine pharmacokinetics were seen.[1] The pharmacokinetics of atomoxetine with **paroxetine** in these subjects was similar to that previously seen with atomoxetine alone in poor metaboliser subjects.[1,2]

Following a small-scale study in which atomoxetine was given with **fluoxetine** without any adverse effects, 127 children with attention deficit hyperactivity disorder were randomised to receive **fluoxetine** 20 mg daily and 46 to placebo. After 3 weeks atomoxetine (starting at 0.5 mg/kg daily, increasing over 5 weeks to a maximum of 1.8 mg/kg daily) was also given to both groups. The **fluoxetine** group had 3.3-fold higher peak atomoxetine levels than the placebo group (1177 nanograms/mL compared with 351 nanograms/mL). However, despite a trend towards a greater incidence of decreased appetite with the combination (20% versus 6.8%), there was no significant difference in adverse events between the two groups.[3]

Mechanism

Atomoxetine is extensively metabolised by CYP2D6,[4] an isoenzyme that shows polymorphism, with up to 10% of the population lacking an active form (poor metabolisers). Paroxetine inhibits CYP2D6, and thereby increases atomoxetine levels in those with an extensive metaboliser phenotype. It would not be expected to have any effect in poor metabolisers. Fluoxetine can similarly inhibit CYP2D6.

Importance and management

An established pharmacokinetic interaction. Paroxetine effectively changes patients from an extensive metaboliser phenotype to a poor metaboliser phenotype, markedly raising atomoxetine levels. Although the clinical relevance has not been directly assessed, the manufacturer notes that some adverse effects of atomoxetine were up to twice as frequent in poor metaboliser patients in clinical studies.[2] Because of this, they suggest that patients already taking CYP2D6 inhibitors should undergo a slower titration of atomoxetine dose than usual,[5] with the dose only increased if symptoms fail to improve and if the initial dose is well tolerated.[2] This seems a sensible precaution. Note that in the fluoxetine study, which found that the concurrent use of atomoxetine was generally well-tolerated, dosage increases were made on a weekly basis, with a dose of 1.2 mg/kg daily achieved in 2 weeks.[3] The US manufacturers suggest a starting dose of atomoxetine 0.5 mg/kg daily and only increasing the dose to 1.2 mg/kg daily if symptoms fail to improve over 4 weeks and the initial dose is well tolerated.[2] The UK manufacturers say that the initial dose should be maintained for a minimum of 7 days before increasing it, if necessary, and that slower titration may be necessary in patients taking CYP2D6 inhibitors.[5]

It would also seem prudent to be alert to the possibility of an increase in adverse effects if CYP2D6 inhibitors are added to established atomoxetine treatment, and the US manufacturers specifically name fluoxetine, paroxetine and **quinidine**.[2] For a list of inhibitors of CYP2D6, see 'Table 1.3', (p.6).

Extra caution may be prudent with this combination in those with epilepsy, as both atomoxetine and SSRIs may lower the seizure threshold, and this risk appears to be increased by higher atomoxetine levels.[2]

1. Belle DJ, Ernest CS, Sauer J-M, Smith BP, Thomasson HR, Witcher JW. Effect of potent CYP2D6 inhibition by paroxetine on atomoxetine pharmacokinetics. *J Clin Pharmacol* (2002) 42, 1219–27.
2. Strattera (Atomoxetine hydrochloride). Eli Lilly and Company. US prescribing information, May 2007.
3. Kratochviol CJ, Newcorn JH, Arnold LE, Duesenberg D, Emslie GJ, Quintana H, Sarkis EH, Wagner KD, Gao H, Michelson D, Biederman J. Atomoxetine alone or combined with fluoxetine for treating ADHD with comorbid depressive or anxiety symptoms. *J Am Acad Child Adolesc Psychiatry* (2005) 44, 915–24.
4. Sauer J-M, Ponsler GD, Mattiuz EL, Long AJ, Witcher JW, Thomasson HR, Desante KA. Disposition and metabolic fate of atomoxetine hydrochloride: the role of CYP2D6 in human disposition and metabolism. *Drug Metab Dispos* (2003) 31, 98–107.
5. Strattera (Atomoxetine hydrochloride). Eli Lilly and Company Ltd. UK Summary of product characteristics, January 2007.

Atomoxetine + Miscellaneous

The manufacturer contraindicates the concurrent use of atomoxetine and MAOIs on theoretical grounds. Atomoxetine is predicted to have additive effects with pressor drugs and other sympathomimetics and has been seen to potentiate the increase in heart rate and blood pressure seen with intravenous salbutamol. However, no increase in cardiovascular effects was seen when atomoxetine was given with methylphenidate.

Atomoxetine did not alter desipramine pharmacokinetics and would therefore not be expected to affect other substrates of CYP2D6. Atomoxetine did not alter midazolam pharmacokinetics and would therefore not be expected to affect other substrates of CYP3A4. Antacids and omeprazole do not alter atomoxetine bioavailability.

Clinical evidence, mechanism, importance and management

Atomoxetine is a sympathomimetic that acts as a noradrenaline reuptake inhibitor. As such, it causes a modest increase in pulse and/or blood pressure in many patients.[1,2] It can also cause hypotension.[1,2]

(a) Antacids or Omeprazole

In a study in 20 extensive metabolisers of atomoxetine, **aluminium/magnesium hydroxide** (*Maalox*) and omeprazole did not affect the bioavailability of atomoxetine 40 mg.[3] No special precautions appear to be necessary on concurrent use.

(b) CYP2D6 substrates

Atomoxetine 40 or 60 mg twice daily for 13 days was given to 21 subjects who were extensive metabolisers of CYP2D6 (most common phenotype), with a single 50-mg dose of **desipramine** on day 4. Atomoxetine had no effect on **desipramine** pharmacokinetics.[4]

Desipramine is extensively metabolised by CYP2D6, and can be used as a probe drug for assessment of the effect of drugs on this isoenzyme in extensive metabolisers (see 'Genetic factors', (p.4)). It was concluded that atomoxetine, even at the maximum recommended dose, does not cause clinically relevant inhibition of CYP2D6 *in vivo*, and so will not affect the pharmacokinetics of other CYP2D6 substrates.[4] For a list of CYP2D6 substrates, see 'Table 1.3', (p.6).

(c) CYP3A4 substrates

Atomoxetine 60 mg twice daily for 12 days was given to 6 subjects who were poor metabolisers of CYP2D6, with a single 5-mg oral dose of **midazolam** on days 6 and 12. Atomoxetine increased the maximum level and AUC of midazolam by about 16%, which was not statistically or clinically significant.[4]

Midazolam is extensively metabolised by CYP3A4, and can be used as a probe drug for assessment of the effect of drugs on this isoenzyme. Poor metabolisers of CYP2D6 were chosen for this study, because they have much higher levels of atomoxetine than extensive metabolisers of CYP2D6. It was concluded that atomoxetine, even at the maximum recommended dose, does not cause clinically relevant inhibition of CYP3A4 *in vivo*, and so will not affect the pharmacokinetics of other CYP3A4 substrates.[4] For a list of CYP3A4 substrates, see 'Table 1.4', (p.6).

(d) MAOIs

The manufacturer contraindicates the concurrent use of atomoxetine with MAOIs, or within 2 weeks of stopping an MAOI,[1,2] because other drugs that affect brain monoamine levels have caused serious reactions (similar to the neuroleptic malignant syndrome) when taken with MAOIs.[2]

(e) Methylphenidate

A placebo-controlled, crossover study in 12 healthy subjects examined the effects of giving either atomoxetine 60 mg twice daily or and methylphenidate 60 mg daily for 5 days, with the other drug added for the final 2 days. No additional changes in blood pressure or heart rate were seen when the drugs were given together, and concurrent use did not increase the frequency of adverse effects.[5]

(f) Pressor drugs

The manufacturer recommends caution if atomoxetine is given concurrently with pressor drugs, because of the possible additive effects on blood pressure.[1,2]

(g) Salbutamol (Albuterol)

The manufacturer notes that atomoxetine 60 mg twice daily for 5 days potentiated the increase in heart rate and blood pressure caused by an infusion of salbutamol 600 micrograms over 2 hours.[2] Because of this, they recommend caution when atomoxetine is used in patients receiving intravenous or oral salbutamol or other $beta_2$ agonists[1,2] (for a list, see 'Table 33.1', (p.1159)). The UK manufacturer also extends this precaution to high-dose nebulised salbutamol.[1]

(h) Miscellaneous

The manufacturer recommends caution when atomoxetine is given concurrently with other drugs that affect noradrenaline, because of the potential for additive or synergistic pharmacological effects. Examples they name are antidepressants such as **imipramine**, **venlafaxine** and **mirtazapine**, and the decongestants **pseudoephedrine** or **phenylephrine**.[1] Until more is known, this would seem a sensible precaution.

1. Strattera (Atomoxetine hydrochloride). Eli Lilly and Company Ltd. UK Summary of product characteristics, January 2007.
2. Strattera (Atomoxetine hydrochloride). Eli Lilly and Company. US Prescribing information, April 2007.
3. DeSante KA, Long AJ, Smith PB, Thomasson HR, Sauer JM, Agbo F, Abeyratne A, Riggio AL, Sheets BA, Witcher JW. Atomoxetine absolute bioavailability and effects of food, Maalox or omeprazole on atomoxetine bioavailability. *AAPS PharmSci* (2001) 3(S1). Available at: http://www.aapspharmaceutica.com/search/abstract_view.asp?id=223&ct=01Abstracts (accessed 16/08/07).
4. Sauer J-M, Long AJ, Ring B, Gillespie JS, Sanburn NP, DeSante KA, Petullo D, Vanden-Branden MR, Jensen CB, Wrighton SA, Smith BP, Read HA, Witcher JW. Atomoxetine hydrochloride: clinical drug-drug interaction prediction and outcome. *J Pharmacol Exp Ther* (2004) 308, 410–18.
5. Kelly RP, Yeo KP, Teng C-H, Smith BP, Lowe S, Soon D, Read HA, Wise SD. Hemodynamic effects of acute administration of atomoxetine and methylphenidate. *J Clin Pharmacol* (2005) 45, 851–55.

Dexfenfluramine or Fenfluramine + Other anorectics

Fenfluramine and dexfenfluramine have generally been withdrawn worldwide because of the occurrence of serious and sometimes fatal valvular heart disease (aortic, mitral, tricuspid or mixed valve disease). Pulmonary hypertension has also sometimes been seen. These serious adverse effects occurred when these drugs were taken alone, and when combined with phentermine as *Fen-phen* and *Dexfen-phen*, but not with phentermine alone.[1-5]

There is also an isolated case of cardiomyopathy attributed to the use of fenfluramine with mazindol.[6] Before the withdrawal of the drug from the market, the manufacturer of fenfluramine recommended that concurrent use with other centrally acting anorectics should be avoided.[7]

1. Committee on Safety of Medicines/Medicines Control Agency. Fenfluramine and dexfenfluramine withdrawn. *Current Problems* (1997) 23, 12.
2. Food and Drugs Administration. FDA announces withdrawal fenfluramine and dexfenfluramine (Fen-Phen). September 15th, 1997.
3. Connolly HM, Crary JL, McGoon MD, Hensrud DD, Edwards BS, Edwards WD, Schaff HV. Valvular heart disease associated with fenfluramine-phentermine. *N Engl J Med* (1997) 337, 581–8.
4. Mark EJ, Patalas ED, Chang HT, Evans RJ, Kessler SC. Fatal pulmonary hypertension associated with short-term use of fenfluramine and phentermine. *N Engl J Med* (1997) 337, 602–6.
5. Graham DJ, Green L. Further cases of valvular heart disease associated with fenfluramine-phentermine. *N Engl J Med* (1997) 337, 635.

6. Gillis D, Wengrower D, Witztum E, Leitersdorf E. Fenfluramine and mazindol: acute reversible cardiomyopathy associated with their use. *Int J Psychiatry Med* (1985) 15, 197–200.
7. Ponderax Pacaps (Fenfluramine). Servier Laboratories Limited. ABPI Compendium of Datasheets and Summaries of Product Characteristics 1997–8, 1307.

Methylphenidate + Carbamazepine

Carbamazepine may reduce methylphenidate levels.

Clinical evidence, mechanism, importance and management

A 7-year-old boy with attention deficit disorder taking carbamazepine 1 g daily for grand mal epilepsy was referred because of unmanageable behaviour. He failed to respond to methylphenidate in doses of up to 30 mg every 4 hours, and his blood levels of both methylphenidate and its metabolites were undetectable. The authors of the report attributed this to an interaction with the carbamazepine.[1] Similarly, symptoms of attention deficit hyperactivity disorder worsened in a 13-year-old girl taking methylphenidate after she also took carbamazepine. Methylphenidate serum levels decreased markedly and the dose of methylphenidate had to be increased from 20 to 60 mg three times daily to regain a benefit similar to that achieved before the addition of carbamazepine.[2] However, another report describes 4 out of 7 children taking methylphenidate and carbamazepine in whom the combination was successful. Blood levels of methylphenidate were apparently not measured.[3] Despite the sparsity of the information, and the cases of apparently successful use, it would seem wise to consider carbamazepine as a possible cause if patients do not respond adequately to methylphenidate. If this occurs, consider increasing the methylphenidate dose.

1. Behar D, Schaller J, Spreat S. Extreme reduction of methylphenidate levels by carbamazepine. *J Am Acad Child Adolesc Psychiatry* (1998) 37, 1128–9.
2. Schaller JL, Behar D. Carbamazepine and methylphenidate in ADHD. *J Am Acad Child Adolesc Psychiatry* (1999) 38, 112–13.
3. Gross-Tsur V. Carbamazepine and methylphenidate. *J Am Acad Child Adolesc Psychiatry* (1999) 38, 637.

Methylphenidate + Clonidine

Much publicised fears about the serious consequences of using methylphenidate with clonidine appear to be unfounded. There is limited evidence to suggest that concurrent use can be both safe and effective.

Clinical evidence, mechanism, importance and management

There have been fears about serious adverse events when methylphenidate is taken with clonidine,[1] due to reports of 3 deaths in children taking both drugs. One child died from ventricular fibrillation due to cardiac abnormalities, one from cardiac arrest attributed to an overdose of fluoxetine, and the third death was unexplained. Studies of these 3 cases and one other failed to establish any link between the use of methylphenidate with clonidine and these deaths, the final broad conclusion being that the event was largely a media-inspired scare story built on inconclusive evidence.[2,3] A small scale pilot study in 24 patients suggested that the combination is both safe and effective for the treatment of attention deficit hyperactivity disorder,[4] and the manufacturers of one formulation of methylphenidate[1] said that, as of 2002, they were not aware of any reports describing adverse events when *Concerta XL* (methylphenidate) was used with clonidine.

1. Janssen-Cilag. Personal communication, April 2002.
2. Popper CW. Editorial commentary. Combining methylphenidate and clonidine: pharmacologic questions and news reports about sudden death. *J Child Adolesc Psychopharmacol* (1995) 5, 157–66.
3. Fenichel RR. Special communication. Combining methylphenidate and clonidine: the role of post-marketing surveillance. *J Child Adolesc Psychopharmacol* (1995) 5, 155–6.
4. Connor DF, Barkley RA, Davis HT. A pilot study of methylphenidate, clonidine, or the combination in ADHD comorbid with aggressive oppositional defiant or conduct disorder. *Clin Pediatr (Phila)* (2000) 39, 15–25.

Modafinil + Dexamfetamine

No pharmacokinetic interaction appears to occur between modafinil and dexamfetamine.

Clinical evidence, mechanism, importance and management

In a steady-state study, 23 healthy subjects were given modafinil 200 mg daily for 7 days, followed by 400 mg daily for 3 weeks. During the last week, 10 of the subjects were also given dexamfetamine 20 mg daily, 7 hours after their modafinil dose. Dexamfetamine caused no significant change in the pharmacokinetics of modafinil and the combination was well tolerated. In addition, the pharmacokinetics of dexamfetamine did not appear to be affected by modafinil, when compared with values reported in the literature.[1] Similar results were found in a single dose study.[2] No additional precautions appear to be necessary on concurrent use.

1. Hellriegel ET, Arora S, Nelson M, Robertson P. Steady-state pharmacokinetics and tolerability of modafinil administered alone or in combination with dextroamphetamine in healthy volunteers. *J Clin Pharmacol* (2002) 42, 448–58.
2. Wong YN, Wang L, Hartman L, Simcoe D, Chen Y, Laughton W, Eldon R, Markland C, Grebow P. Comparison of the single-dose pharmacokinetics and tolerability of modafinil and dextroamphetamine administered alone or in combination in healthy male volunteers. *J Clin Pharmacol* (1998) 38, 971–8.

Modafinil + Methylphenidate

No pharmacokinetic interaction appears to occur between modafinil and methylphenidate.

Clinical evidence, mechanism, importance and management

In a single-dose study in healthy subjects, modafinil 200 mg and methylphenidate 40 mg were given together without any clinically relevant changes in the pharmacokinetics of either drug.[1] In a steady-state study, 30 healthy subjects were given modafinil 200 mg daily for 7 days, followed by 400 mg daily for 3 weeks. During the last week, 16 of the subjects were also given methylphenidate 20 mg daily, taken 8 hours after their modafinil dose. Methylphenidate caused no significant change in the pharmacokinetics of modafinil. In addition, the pharmacokinetics of methylphenidate did not appear to be affected by modafinil, when compared with values reported in the literature.[2] No special precautions would appear to be necessary on concurrent use.

1. Wong YN, King SP, Laughton WB, McCormick GC, Grebow PE. Single-dose pharmacokinetics of modafinil and methylphenidate given alone or in combination in healthy male volunteers. *J Clin Pharmacol* (1998) 38, 276–82.
2. Hellriegel ET, Arora S, Nelson M, Robertson P. Steady-state pharmacokinetics and tolerability of modafinil given alone or in combination with methylphenidate in healthy volunteers. *J Clin Pharmacol* (2001) 41, 895–904.

Modafinil + Miscellaneous

The manufacturers caution if enzyme-inducing anticonvulsants, particularly phenytoin, are used with modafinil. There is speculation, based on *in vitro* studies, about some possible interactions with other drugs, such as warfarin. Modafinil is an inducer of CYP3A4 and therefore may be expected to interact with substrates of this isoenzyme.

Clinical evidence, mechanism, importance and management

(a) CYP3A4 inducers and inhibitors

Animal studies suggest that **phenobarbital** reduces the serum levels of modafinil; both drugs are inducers of the cytochrome P450 isoenzyme CYP3A4.[1] The manufacturers similarly suggest that this is a possibility.[2,3]

There is no clinical evidence of interactions with other potent enzyme inducers, but the manufacturers suggest that **carbamazepine**[2,3] and **rifampicin (rifampin)**[3] may reduce modafinil levels. Also, inhibitors of CYP3A4 (**itraconazole**, **ketoconazole** are specifically named) are predicted to possibly increase modafinil levels. However, clinically relevant interactions with either CYP3A4 inducers or inhibitors seem unlikely because CYP3A4 is not the only cytochrome P450 isoenzyme that is involved in the metabolism of modafinil.

(b) CYP3A4 substrates

Modafinil is an inducer of the cytochrome P450 isoenzyme CYP3A4. The manufacturers therefore predict that it may reduce the levels of drugs that are CYP3A4 substrates. They specifically name the protease inhibitors, **buspirone**, **calcium-channel blockers**, ciclosporin, **midazolam**, and the **statins** [note that only some statins, namely **atorvastatin**, **lovastatin** and

simvastatin, are CYP3A4 substrates], and triazolam.[2,3] Interactions have been seen with 'ciclosporin', (p.1039), and 'triazolam', (p.732).

(c) Phenytoin

Due to the enzyme inhibiting potential of modafinil, the manufacturers say that care should be taken if phenytoin is also given.[2] There is *in vitro* evidence to indicate that modafinil may possibly inhibit the metabolism of phenytoin by the cytochrome P450 isoenzymes CYP2C9 and CYP2C19, and so there is some reason for monitoring concurrent use for evidence of increased phenytoin effects and toxicity.[2,3]

(d) Warfarin

There is no clinical evidence of an interaction between warfarin and modafinil, but because warfarin is, in part, metabolised by the cytochrome P450 isoenzyme CYP2C9 (which is inhibited by modafinil) the manufacturers suggest that concurrent use should be monitored for the first 2 months of concurrent use.[2,3]

1. Moachon G, Kanmacher I, Clenet M, Matinier D. Pharmacokinetic profile of modafinil. *Drugs Today* (1996) 32 (Suppl 1), 23–33.
2. Provigil (Modafinil). Cephalon Ltd. UK Summary of product characteristics, July 2007.
3. Provigil (Modafinil), Cephalon, Inc. US Prescribing information, December 2004.

Orlistat + Sucrose polyesters

A single case report suggests that the concurrent use of orlistat and sucrose polyesters (*Olestra* – used in some foods as a fat substitute) can result in additive gastrointestinal adverse effects (soft, fatty/oily stools, increased flatus and abdominal pain). In the case in question, symptoms resolved when the patient stopped eating *Olestra*-containing food while continuing to take orlistat.[1]

1. Heck AM, Calis KA, McDuffie JR, Carobene SE, Yanovski JA. Additive gastrointestinal effects with concomitant use of olestra and orlistat. *Ann Pharmacother* (2002) 36, 1003–5.

Phenmetrazine + Barbiturates

The CNS adverse effects and the weight-reducing effects of phenmetrazine are reduced by amobarbital.

Clinical evidence, mechanism, importance and management

A comparative study in 50 overweight adults, of the effects of phenmetrazine 25 mg three times daily with or without amobarbital 30 mg three times daily, found that although the adverse CNS effects, particularly insomnia, headache and nervousness, were decreased by the presence of the barbiturate, the weight-reducing effects were also decreased (by 65%).[1]

1. Hadler AJ. Phenmetrazine vs. phenmetrazine with amobarbital for weight reduction: a double-blind study. *Curr Ther Res* (1969) 11, 750–4.

Phentermine + Fluoxetine

An isolated report describes phentermine toxicity, which occurred in a woman several days after she stopped taking fluoxetine.

Clinical evidence, mechanism, importance and management

A 22-year-old woman who had successfully and uneventfully taken fluoxetine 20 mg daily for 3 months, stopped the fluoxetine and then 8 days later took a single 30-mg tablet of phentermine. Within a few hours she experienced racing thoughts, stomach cramps, palpitations (pulse 84 bpm), tremors, dry eyes and diffuse hyper-reflexia. The problems had all resolved the following day after she took lorazepam 1.5 mg. The authors of this report suggested that the residual inhibitory effects of the fluoxetine on liver cytochrome P450 enzymes led to decreased phentermine metabolism, resulting in increased phentermine levels and sympathetic hyperstimulation. It is known that fluoxetine and its active metabolite are have a long half-life and can persist for weeks. The authors also alternatively wondered whether some of the symptoms might have fitted those of the serotonin syndrome.[1]

Although this is an isolated case and its general importance is unknown, the authors of the report draw attention to the possible risks of taking SSRIs and sympathomimetic drugs used for controlling diet.

A neurotoxic reaction has also been reported with ecstasy and citalopram, see 'Amfetamines and related drugs + SSRIs', p.201.

1. Bostwick JM, Brown TM. A toxic reaction from combining fluoxetine and phentermine. *J Clin Psychopharmacol* (1996) 16, 189–90.

Rimonabant + Miscellaneous

Ketoconazole doubled the AUC of rimonabant, and other potent CYP3A4 inhibitors are also expected to raise rimonabant levels. Potent CYP3A4 inducers are expected to lower rimonabant levels. Due to a lack of information the manufacturers suggest that rimonabant should not be taken with antidepressants. Rimonabant does not appear to affect the levels of oral contraceptives, digoxin, midazolam or warfarin, and alcohol, lorazepam, and orlistat do not appear to alter rimonabant levels.

Clinical evidence, mechanism, importance and management

(a) Antidepressants

Depressive disorders and mood alterations are common in patients taking rimonabant. The manufacturers say that as there is limited experience in using rimonabant with antidepressants, and concurrent use is not recommended.[1]

(b) CYP3A4 inducers and inhibitors

Rimonabant is partly metabolised by the cytochrome P450 isoenzyme CYP3A4. **Ketoconazole**, a potent CYP3A4 inhibitor, doubles the AUC of rimonabant. The manufacturers therefore expect that other potent CYP3A4 inhibitors (they name **clarithromycin**, **itraconazole**, **nefazodone**, **ritonavir**, and **telithromycin**) will also raise rimonabant levels, and they therefore advise caution on concurrent use.[1] They similarly suggest that potent CYP3A4 inducers (such as **carbamazepine**, **phenobarbital**, **phenytoin**, **rifampicin** (**rifampin**) and **St John's wort**) may lower rimonabant levels. If concurrent use is necessary monitor to ensure that rimonabant remains effective.[1] See 'Table 1.4', (p.6), for a list of clinically relevant CYP3A4 inducers and inhibitors.

(c) Miscellaneous

Digoxin, **midazolam**, and **warfarin** were given with rimonabant in clinical studies to assess the effect of rimonabant on P-glycoprotein, CYP3A4 and CYP2C9, respectively. As rimonabant did not interact with these drugs, the manufacturers say this confirms *in vitro* evidence that it has no effect on these isoenzymes or transporter, and would not be expected to interact with other substrates of P-glycoprotein, CYP3A4 and CYP2C9. The manufacturers also note that rimonabant had no effect on the pharmacokinetics of an oral contraceptive containing **ethinylestradiol** and **levonorgestrel**, and that **alcohol**, **lorazepam**, and **orlistat** did not affect the plasma levels of rimonabant.[1]

1. Acomplia (Rimonabant). Sanofi-Aventis. UK Summary of product characteristics, June 2006.

Sibutramine + Azoles

Ketoconazole modestly increases steady-state levels of sibutramine and its active metabolites. The UK manufacturers recommend caution when sibutramine is used with itraconazole or ketoconazole.

Clinical evidence, mechanism, importance and management

Twelve obese patients were given sibutramine hydrochloride monohydrate 20 mg daily for 14 days, with **ketoconazole** 200 mg twice daily for the last 7 days. **Ketoconazole** caused moderate increases in the serum levels of sibutramine and its two metabolites (AUC and maximum serum level increases of 58% and 36%, respectively, for metabolites M1, and 20% and 19%, respectively, for M2, probably through inhibition of the cytochrome P450 isoenzyme CYP3A4). Small increases in heart rates were seen (2.5 bpm at 4 hours and 1.4 bpm at 8 hours), while ECG parameters were unchanged.[1] Sibutramine alone can cause an increase in heart rate, and a rate increase of 10 bpm is an indication to withdraw the drug. Therefore, the manufacturers in the UK[2] suggest caution should be exercised when sibutramine is used with **ketoconazole**. They also suggest that due to its ability to inhibit CYP3A4 **itraconazole** should also be used with caution.

1. Hinson JL, Leone MB, Kisiki MJ, Moult JT, Trammel A and Faulkner RD. Steady-state interaction study of sibutramine (Meridia) and ketoconazole in uncomplicated obese subjects. *Pharm Res* (1996) 13 (9 Suppl), S116.
2. Reductil (Sibutramine hydrochloride monohydrate). Abbott Laboratories Ltd. UK Summary of product characteristics, November 2005.

Sibutramine + Macrolides

Although no interaction appears to occur between sibutramine and erythromycin, the UK manufacturers still caution the use of sibutramine with clarithromycin, erythromycin and troleandomycin.

Clinical evidence, mechanism, importance and management

Twelve obese patients were given sibutramine 20 mg daily for 14 days, with **erythromycin** 500 mg three times daily for the last 7 days. It was found that, apart from some slight and unimportant changes in the pharmacokinetics of the metabolites of sibutramine (probably caused by some inhibition of the cytochrome P450 isoenzyme CYP3A4), the pharmacokinetics of sibutramine were not significantly altered by **erythromycin**. No blood pressure changes were seen and only very small and clinically irrelevant increases in the QTc interval and heart rate occurred.[1] The extent of any interaction appears to be too small to matter,[1] and there would seem to be no reason for avoiding the concurrent use of these two drugs. Despite this the UK manufacturers still say that caution should be exercised, probably because sibutramine is principally metabolised by CYP3A4.[2] They also extrapolate their caution to the CYP3A4 inhibitors **clarithromycin** and **troleandomycin**.

1. Hinson JL, Leone MB, Leese PT, Moult JT, Carter FJ, Faulkner RD. Steady-state interaction study of sibutramine (Meridia) and erythromycin in uncomplicated obese subjects. *Pharm Res* (1996) 13 (9 Suppl), S116.
2. Reductil (Sibutramine hydrochloride monohydrate). Abbott Laboratories Ltd. UK Summary of product characteristics, November 2005.

Sibutramine + Miscellaneous

On theoretical grounds the manufacturers contraindicate the concurrent use of sibutramine with MAOIs, and they say that it should not be given with serotonergic drugs because of the risk of the serious serotonin syndrome. The manufacturers say that the use of sibutramine with other centrally acting appetite suppressants is contraindicated and they caution the use of cold and flu remedies. No clinically relevant interactions have been seen between sibutramine and cimetidine, and no interaction occurs with oral contraceptives.

Clinical evidence, mechanism, importance and management

(a) Cimetidine

When cimetidine 400 mg twice daily was given with sibutramine 15 mg once daily to 12 healthy subjects the maximum serum levels and AUCs of the combined sibutramine metabolites were increased by 3.4% and 7.3%, respectively.[1] These changes are too small to be of clinical significance, and there is no reason for avoiding the concurrent use of these two drugs.

(b) Centrally acting appetite suppressants, and drugs that raise blood pressure or heart rate

The UK manufacturers say that the concurrent use of sibutramine and other centrally acting appetite suppressants is contraindicated. No work appears to have been done to see what happens if sibutramine is given with **decongestants**, **cough**, **cold** and **allergy medications**, but the manufacturers advise caution because of the risk of raised blood pressure or heart rate. The manufacturers in the UK and US both list **ephedrine** and **pseudoephedrine**,[1,2] while in the UK **xylometazoline** is also specifically named.[2]

(c) CYP3A4 inducers

The UK manufacturers point out that **carbamazepine**, **dexamethasone**, **phenobarbital**, **phenytoin** and **rifampicin** are all inducers of CYP3A4, an isoenzyme involved in the metabolism of sibutramine.[2] These drugs might therefore increase the metabolism of sibutramine resulting in a fall in its serum levels. However, this has not been studied experimentally and, at the present time, the existence, the extent and the possible clinical relevance of any such interaction is unknown.

(d) MAOIs

There are no reports of adverse reactions between sibutramine and the MAOIs. However, sibutramine inhibits serotonin reuptake, and because the serious serotonin syndrome can occur when MAOIs and SSRIs are used together, the manufacturers warn that concurrent use of sibutramine and MAOIs is contraindicated. They say that 14 days should elapse between stopping either drug and starting the other.[1,2] The US manufacturers included **selegiline** in this warning.[1]

(e) Oral contraceptives

A crossover study in 12 subjects found that sibutramine 15 mg daily, given for 8 weeks, had no clinically significant effect on the inhibition of ovulation caused by an oral contraceptive, and it was concluded that there is no need to use alternative contraceptive methods while taking sibutramine.[1]

(f) Serotonergic drugs

Because sibutramine inhibits serotonin uptake, and because the serious serotonin syndrome has been seen when serotonergic drugs were taken with SSRIs, the manufacturers say that sibutramine should not be taken with any serotonergic drugs.[1,2] They name **dextromethorphan**, **dihydroergotamine**, **fentanyl**, **pentazocine**, **pethidine** (**meperidine**), SSRIs, **sumatriptan**, and **tryptophan**. Possible cases have been reported for sibutramine and 'SSRIs', (below).The US manufacturers also include **lithium** in their list.[1] Note that this list is not exhaustive (see MAOIs under (d) above) and a case of the serotonin syndrome has been seen when **venlafaxine** was given with sibutramine.[3]

The extent of the risk with these serotonergic drugs is not known, but because of the potential severity of the reaction this warning would seem to be a prudent precaution. For more information on the serotonin syndrome, see 'Additive or synergistic interactions', (p.9).

1. Meridia (Sibutramine hydrochloride monohydrate). Abbott Laboratories. US Prescribing information, December 2006.
2. Reductil (Sibutramine hydrochloride monohydrate). Abbott Laboratories Ltd. UK Summary of product characteristics, November 2005.
3. Trakas K, Shear NH. Serotonin syndrome risk with antiobesity drug. *Can J Clin Pharmacol* (2000) 7, 216.

Sibutramine + SSRIs

Two case reports suggest that the concurrent use of sertraline or citalopram with sibutramine may cause the serotonin syndrome.

Clinical evidence, mechanism, importance and management

A 43-year-old woman taking **citalopram** 40 mg daily was also given sibutramine hydrochloride monohydrate 10 mg daily. Within a few hours of taking the first dose of sibutramine she developed racing thoughts, hyperactivity, psychomotor agitation, shivering and diaphoresis, which continued for the 3 days that she continued to take sibutramine. The authors suggested that one of the reasons for the hypomania may have been the serotonin syndrome, which could have been caused by the use of two drugs with serotonergic action.[1] A letter briefly mentions another possible case of the serotonin syndrome, following the use of sibutramine and **sertraline**.[2] The manufacturers of sibutramine[3,4] say that concurrent use of any other drug that has serotonergic actions should be avoided where possible, or only undertaken with appropriate monitoring. For more information about the serotonin syndrome, see 'Additive or synergistic interactions', (p.9).

1. Benazzi F. Organic hypomania secondary to sibutramine-citalopram interaction. *J Clin Psychiatry* (2002) 63, 165.
2. Trakas K, Shear NH. Serotonin syndrome risk with antiobesity drug. *Can J Clin Pharmacol* (2000) 7, 216.
3. Meridia (Sibutramine hydrochloride monohydrate). Abbott Laboratories. US Prescribing information, December 2006.
4. Reductil (Sibutramine hydrochloride monohydrate). Abbott Laboratories Ltd. UK Summary of product characteristics, November 2005.

8

Anthelmintics, Antifungals and Antiprotozoals

'Table 8.1', (p.208) lists the drugs covered in this section by therapeutic group and drug class. If the anti-infective is the drug causing the interaction, the interaction is generally dealt with under the affected drug. Also note that drugs such as the 5-nitroimidazoles (e.g. metronidazole), which have actions against more than one type of organism (e.g. bacteria and protozoa) are covered under Antibacterials.

(a) Amphotericin B

Intravenous amphotericin B causes important pharmacodynamic interactions via additive nephrotoxicity and myelotoxicity, and may increase the cardiotoxicity of other drugs because of amphotericin-induced hypokalaemia. No important pharmacokinetic interactions are known. Lipid formulations such as liposomal amphotericin are less nephrotoxic than conventional amphotericin, and would therefore be expected to interact less frequently. Orally administered amphotericin is not absorbed systemically, and no interactions are known.

(b) Azole antifungals

The most important interactions affecting and caused by the azole antifungals are those resulting from inhibition and induction of cytochrome P450 isoenzymes.

Fluconazole is principally (80%) excreted unchanged in the urine, so is less affected by enzyme inducers and inhibitors than some other azoles. Fluconazole is a potent inhibitor of CYP2C9 and CYP2C19, and generally only inhibits CYP3A4 at high doses (greater than 200 mg daily). Interactions are less likely with single doses used for genital candidiasis than with longer term use.

Itraconazole is extensively metabolised by CYP3A4, and its metabolism may become saturated with multiple dosing. Itraconazole and its major metabolite, hydroxy-itraconazole are potent inhibitors of CYP3A4.

Ketoconazole is extensively metabolised, particularly by CYP3A4. It is also a potent inhibitor of CYP3A4.

Miconazole is a potent inhibitor of CYP2C9. Because this azole is generally used topically as pessaries, skin cream, or an oral gel, it is less likely to cause interactions, although it should be noted that interactions with 'warfarin', (p.388), have been reported, particularly for the oral gel.

Posaconazole is metabolised via UDP glucuronidation, and may also be a substrate for P-glycoprotein. Posaconazole is an inhibitor of CYP3A4.

Voriconazole is metabolised by CYP2C19, CYP2C9, and to a lesser extent by CYP3A4. Voriconazole is an inhibitor of CYP2C9, CYP2C19 and CYP3A4.

An number of other azole antifungals are only used topically in the form of skin creams or intravaginal preparations, and have not been associated with drug interactions, presumably since their systemic absorption is so low, see 'Azoles; Topical + Miscellaneous', p.222.

Fluconazole, ketoconazole and voriconazole have been associated with prolongation of the QT interval, although generally not to a clinically relevant extent. However, they may also raise the levels of other drugs that prolong the QT interval, and these combinations are often contraindicated, see 'Antihistamines + Azoles', p.584.

General references

1. Venkatakrishnan K, von Moltke LL, Greenblatt DJ. Effects of the antifungal agents on oxidative drug metabolism: clinical relevance. *Clin Pharmacokinet* (2000) 38, 111–80.

Table 8.1 Anthelmintics, antifungals and antimalarials and other antiprotozoals

Group	*Drugs*
Anthelmintics	
Benzimidazole derivatives	Albendazole, Flubendazole, Mebendazole, Tiabendazole (Thiabendazole)
Organophosphorous compounds	Metrifonate (Metriphonate)
Other	Diethylcarbamazine, Ivermectin, Levamisole, Niclosamide, Oxamniquine, Piperazine, Praziquantel, Pyrantel
Antifungals	
Allylamines	Naftifine, Terbinafine
Azoles:	
Imidazoles	Bifonazole,* Butoconazole,* Chlormidazole,* Clotrimazole,* Econazole,* Fenticonazole,* Isoconazole,* Ketoconazole, Miconazole, Oxiconazole,* Sertaconazole,* Sulconazole,* Tioconazole*
Triazoles	Fluconazole, Itraconazole, Posaconazole, Terconazole,* Voriconazole
Echinocandins	Anidulafungin, Caspofungin
Polyene antibiotics	Amphotericin B, Natamycin,* Nystatin*
Other	Amorolfine,* Butenafine,* Ciclopirox,* Flucytosine, Griseofulvin, Tolnaftate*
Antimalarials	
4-aminoquinolines	Amodiaquine, Chloroquine, Hydroxychloroquine
8-aminoquinolines	Primaquine
4-methanolquinolines	Mefloquine, Quinine
Other	Artemether, Artemotil, Artesunate, Atovaquone, Halofantrine, Lumefantrine, Proguanil, Pyrimethamine, Sulfadoxine
Antiprotozoals	
Antimony compounds	Sodium stibogluconate
Arsenicals	Melarsoprol
5-nitroimidazoles†	Metronidazole, Ornidazole, Tinidazole
Nitrofuran	Furazolidone, Nifurtimox
Other	Atovaquone, Diiodohydroxyquinoline, Diloxanide furoate, Eflornithine, Mepacrine, Pentamidine, Suramin

*Mainly used by topical application
†Covered under Antibacterials

Albendazole or Mebendazole + Antiepileptics

Phenytoin, carbamazepine and phenobarbital lower the plasma levels of albendazole and mebendazole, and they therefore might reduce their efficacy for systemic infections. Valproate does not lower plasma mebendazole levels.

Clinical evidence

(a) Albendazole

In one study, 32 patients with intraparenchymatous neurocysticercosis were given albendazole 7.5 mg/kg every 12 hours for 8 days. These patients were also taking either **phenytoin** 200 to 300 mg daily (9 patients), **carbamazepine** 600 to 1200 mg daily (9 patients), or **phenobarbital** 100 to 300 mg daily (5 patients) all for at least 3 months, and a control group consisting of 9 patients who did not receive any antiepileptics. The AUCs for (+)-albendazole sulfoxide were 66%, 49%, and 61% lower than the control group for the **phenytoin**, **carbamazepine**, and **phenobarbital** groups respectively. The maximum plasma levels of (+)-albendazole sulfoxide were 50 to 63% lower and the half lives about 3 to 4 hours shorter. The AUCs, peak plasma levels and half-life of (–)-albendazole sulfoxide (present in much lower levels than the (+)-isomer) were similarly reduced by the antiepileptics.[1]

(b) Mebendazole

A retrospective analysis found that patients with echinococcosis taking mebendazole and **phenytoin** or **carbamazepine** tended to have lower plasma mebendazole levels than patients not taking these antiepileptics.[2] **Valproic acid** tended to increase mebendazole levels, and some patients had a clinically important rise in mebendazole levels when they were switched from **phenytoin** or **carbamazepine** to **valproic acid**.[2]

Mechanism

Phenytoin, carbamazepine and phenobarbital appear to induce the oxidative metabolism of albendazole by the cytochrome P450 isoenzyme CYP3A to roughly the same extent, resulting in significantly reduced levels of albendazole sulfoxide. Phenytoin, and to a lesser extent carbamazepine, may also induce the metabolism of albendazole sulfone by CYP2C. Mebendazole is similarly affected.

Importance and management

These pharmacokinetic interactions are established, and are likely to be clinically important when these anthelmintics are used to treat systemic worm infections. For these infections it may be necessary to increase the albendazole or mebendazole dosage in patients taking phenytoin, carbamazepine or phenobarbital. Monitor the outcome of concurrent use. The interactions are of no importance when these anthelmintics are used for intestinal worm infections (where their action is a local effect on the worms in the gut), which is the most common use of mebendazole in particular.

1. Lanchote VL, Garcia FS, Dreossi SAC, Takayanagui OM. Pharmacokinetic interaction between albendazole sulfoxide enantiomers and antiepileptic drugs in patients with neurocysticercosis. *Ther Drug Monit* (2002) 24, 338–45.
2. Luder PJ, Siffert B, Witassek F, Meister F, Bircher J. Treatment of hydatid disease with high oral doses of mebendazole. Long-term follow-up of plasma mebendazole levels and drug interactions. *Eur J Clin Pharmacol* (1986) 31, 443–8.

Albendazole or Mebendazole + Cimetidine

Cimetidine raises serum mebendazole levels, and prolongs the half-life of albendazole sulfoxide. In some cases cimetidine appeared to increase the effectiveness of these anthelmintics against systemic infection.

Clinical evidence

(a) Albendazole

A study in 6 healthy subjects given albendazole 20 mg/kg and cimetidine 10 mg/kg twice daily found that cimetidine significantly inhibited the metabolism of albendazole sulfoxide as indicated by an increase in its elimination half-life from 7.4 to 19 hours. Cimetidine also reduced inter-individual variability in plasma albendazole levels.[1] Another study in patients with cystic echinococcosis given albendazole 20 mg/kg daily, for three 4-week courses separated by intervals of 10 days, found that levels of the active metabolite albendazole sulfoxide were higher in bile and hydatid cyst fluid in 7 patients who also received cimetidine 10 mg/kg daily. The therapeutic benefit of the combined treatment was reported to be greater than that with albendazole alone.[2]

(b) Mebendazole

A study in 8 patients (5 with peptic ulcers and 3 with hydatid cysts) taking mebendazole 1.5 g three times daily found that cimetidine 400 mg three times daily for 30 days raised the maximum plasma mebendazole levels by 48%. The previously unresponsive hepatic hydatid cysts resolved totally.[3] However, a previous study had found smaller increases in serum mebendazole levels with cimetidine 1 g daily in divided doses, which were considered too small to be clinically useful.[4]

Mechanism

It is suggested that the interaction is caused by the enzyme inhibitory actions of cimetidine, which result in a reduction in the metabolism of albendazole and mebendazole.[1,3] Cimetidine may also reduce albendazole absorption and minimise inter-patient variability by reducing gastric acidity,[1] but the reduction in absorption appears to be outweighed by the enzyme-inhibitory effects.

Importance and management

These pharmacokinetic interactions would appear to be established, but their clinical relevance is uncertain. Increased efficacy has been shown in some studies for systemic worm infections. There would seem to be no reason for avoiding concurrent use, but increased monitoring for efficacy and toxicity might be prudent.

1. Schipper HG, Koopmans RP, Nagy J, Butter JJ, Kager PA, Van Boxtel CJ. Effect of dose increase or cimetidine co-administration on albendazole bioavailability. *Am J Trop Med Hyg* (2000) 63, 270–3.
2. Wen H, Zhang HW, Muhmut M, Zou PF, New RRC, Craig PS. Initial observation on albendazole in combination with cimetidine for the treatment of human cystic echinococcosis. *Ann Trop Med Parasitol* (1994) 88, 49–52.
3. Bekhti A, Pirotte J. Cimetidine increases serum mebendazole concentrations. Implications for treatment of hepatic hydatid cysts. *Br J Clin Pharmacol* (1987) 24, 390–2.
4. Luder PJ, Siffert B, Witassek F, Meister F, Bircher J. Treatment of hydatid disease with high oral doses of mebendazole. Long-term follow-up of plasma mebendazole levels and drug interactions. *Eur J Clin Pharmacol* (1986) 31, 443–8.

Albendazole + Corticosteroids

Dexamethasone can raise levels of albendazole sulfoxide by 50%, which might increase its efficacy in systemic worm infections.

Clinical evidence

In one study albendazole 15 mg/kg daily in three divided doses was given to 8 patients with cysticercosis. The plasma levels of the active metabolite of albendazole (albendazole sulfoxide) were found to be increased by about 50% by the use of **dexamethasone** 8 mg every 8 hours.[1] Another study did not detect significantly increased maximum plasma levels of albendazole sulfoxide, when **dexamethasone** was given, but the AUC was increased twofold, and there was a decrease in its clearance.[2]

Mechanism

Uncertain. Dexamethasone is an inducer of the cytochrome P450 isoenzyme CYP3A4, and might therefore be expected to reduce levels of albendazole, so the finding is unexpected. Dexamethasone appears not to alter the rate of formation of albendazole sulfoxide, but decreases its elimination.[2]

Importance and management

Information about albendazole seems to be limited but the interaction would appear to be established. It would appear that albendazole can be given concurrently with dexamethasone without compromising treatment, and combined use may actually be beneficial.[3]

1. Jung H, Hurtado M, Tulio Medina M, Sanchez M, Sotelo J. Dexamethasone increases plasma levels of albendazole. *J Neurol* (1990) 237, 279–80.

2. Takayanagui OM, Lanchote VL, Marques MPC, Bonato PS. Therapy for neurocysticercosis: pharmacokinetic interaction of albendazole sulfoxide with dexamethasone. *Ther Drug Monit* (1997) 19, 51–5.
3. Sotelo J, Jung H. Pharmacokinetic optimisation of the treatment of neurocysticercosis. *Clin Pharmacokinet* (1998) 34, 503–15.

Albendazole + Diethylcarbamazine

There appears to be no pharmacokinetic interaction between albendazole and diethylcarbamazine.

Clinical evidence, mechanism, importance and management

There was no difference in the pharmacokinetics of single doses of diethylcarbamazine 6 mg/kg or albendazole 400 mg between groups of 14 amicrofilaraemic subjects given either drug alone and another group of 14 subjects given both drugs.[1] This study suggests there is no pharmacokinetic interaction between these two anthelmintic drugs, and the lack of adverse events[1] suggests that concurrent use is safe.

1. Shenoy RK, Suma TK, John A, Arun SR, Kumaraswami V, Fleckenstein LL, Na-Bangchang K. The pharmacokinetics, safety and tolerability of the co-administration of diethylcarbamazine and albendazole. *Ann Trop Med Parasitol* (2002) 96, 603–14.

Albendazole + Food

Giving albendazole with a fatty meal markedly increases the levels of its active metabolite. Albendazole should be taken with a meal.

Clinical evidence, mechanism, importance and management

A study in Sudanese men found that giving a single 400-mg dose of albendazole with a meal resulted in a 7.9-fold higher level of the active metabolite, albendazole sulfoxide, than when albendazole was given in the fasted state.[1] Similarly, a further study in healthy subjects found that when albendazole 10 mg/kg was given with a fatty meal, rather than with water, the peak plasma levels of the active metabolite were increased by more than sixfold and the half-life decreased from 8.8 to 8.2 hours.[2] Albendazole absorption is poor, and if it is being used for systemic infections, it is advisable to take it with a meal.

1. Homeida M, Leahy W, Copeland S, Ali MMM, Harron DWG. Pharmacokinetic interaction between praziquantel and albendazole in Sudanese men. *Ann Trop Med Parasitol* (1994) 88, 551–9.
2. Nagy J, Schipper HG, Koopmans RP, Butter JJ, Van Boxtel CJ, Kager PA. Effect of grapefruit juice or cimetidine coadministration on albendazole bioavailability. *Am J Trop Med Hyg* (2002) 66, 260–3.

Albendazole + Grapefruit juice

Grapefruit juice increases the plasma levels of albendazole.

Clinical evidence, mechanism, importance and management

Grapefruit juice increased albendazole sulfoxide levels by about threefold and shortened its half-life by 46%.[1] When albendazole was given with grapefruit juice and cimetidine the peak plasma level was reduced from 760 to 410 micrograms/L. However, the level achieved with cimetidine and grapefruit juice was still greater than that achieved when albendazole was given with water.

It was suggested that grapefruit juice inhibits the metabolism of albendazole by the cytochrome P450 isoenzyme CYP3A4 in the intestinal mucosa, and so albendazole levels are raised. The addition of cimetidine may decrease this effect by reducing albendazole absorption by affecting gastric pH.[1] (See also 'Albendazole or Mebendazole + Cimetidine', p.209.) The clinical relevance of the change with grapefruit juice is uncertain. For systemic infections, increased absorption might be beneficial, but the decrease in half-life might be detrimental.

1. Nagy J, Schipper HG, Koopmans RP, Butter JJ, Van Boxtel CJ, Kager PA. Effect of grapefruit juice or cimetidine coadministration on albendazole bioavailability. *Am J Trop Med Hyg* (2002) 66, 260–3.

Albendazole + Ivermectin

No pharmacokinetic interaction occurs between albendazole and ivermectin.

Clinical evidence, mechanism, importance and management

In a double-blind placebo-controlled study, 42 patients with onchocerciasis were given single doses of either ivermectin 200 micrograms/kg, albendazole 400 mg or both drugs together. There was no significant pharmacokinetic interaction, and although the combination seemed to offer no advantage over ivermectin alone for the treatment on onchocerciasis, the combination appeared safe. No dosage adjustments would be required during concurrent use.[1]

1. Awadzi K, Edwards G, Duke BOL, Opoku NO, Attah SK, Addy ET, Ardrey AE, Quarty BT. The co-administration of ivermectin and albendazole— safety, pharmacokinetics and efficacy against *Onchocerca volvulus*. *Ann Trop Med Parasitol* (2003) 97, 165–78.

Albendazole + Levamisole

Levamisole may markedly decrease the bioavailability of albendazole sulfoxide, but albendazole has no clinically significant effects on levamisole pharmacokinetics.

Clinical evidence, mechanism, importance and management

A study in 28 healthy subjects given levamisole 2.5 mg/kg alone or with albendazole 400 mg found that albendazole produced a modest reduction in the AUC of levamisole but no other pharmacokinetic parameters were affected. However, the AUC of albendazole sulfoxide (the active metabolite) was 75% lower when given with levamisole than historical values in subjects who had received levamisole alone.[1] An associated study in 44 patients found that levamisole with or without albendazole was not effective against *Onchocerca volvulus* infections. Both treatments caused a similar number of adverse effects.[1] The clinical relevance of these findings is unclear, but they suggest that caution is needed if both drugs are to be given for systemic worm infections.

1. Awadzi K, Edwards G, Opoku NO, Ardrey AE, Favager S, Addy ET, Attah SK, Yamuah LK, Quartey BT. The safety, tolerability and pharmacokinetics of levamisole alone, levamisole plus ivermectin, and levamisole plus albendazole, and their efficacy against *Onchocerca volvulus*. *Ann Trop Med Parasitol* (2004) 98, 595–614.

Albendazole + Praziquantel

Albendazole does not alter the bioavailability of praziquantel. Praziquantel markedly increases the bioavailability of albendazole sulfoxide in fasted subjects, but much less so when albendazole is given with a meal, as recommended. None of these changes appears to have adverse consequences.

Clinical evidence, mechanism, importance and management

(a) Effect on albendazole

In a study in Sudanese men, the AUC of albendazole sulfoxide (the active metabolite of albendazole), was increased 4.5-fold when a single 400-mg dose of albendazole was given with praziquantel 40 mg/kg to fasting subjects. However, this difference was much less marked (only a 1.5-fold increase) when the drugs were given with food.[1] The reasons for these changes and their practical consequences are not known, but the increases in albendazole sulfoxide levels seemed not to cause any problems.[1] If both drugs are given with food, as may be advisable (see 'Albendazole + Food', above), any interaction is modest. On the basis of these studies there do not seem to be any obvious reasons why the concurrent use of these two drugs should be avoided.

(b) Effect on praziquantel

In a study, 21 children treated for giardiasis were given a single 400-mg dose of albendazole either alone or with a single 20-mg/kg dose of praziquantel. It was found that the pharmacokinetics of albendazole were not significantly affected by praziquantel when the drugs were given with 200 mL of milk, one hour after breakfast. There were wide inter-individual variations in the plasma levels and AUC of the active metabolite, albendazole sulfoxide, but these were similar whether albendazole was given alone or with praziquantel.[2]

1. Homeida M, Leahy W, Copeland S, Ali MMM, Harron DWG. Pharmacokinetic interaction between praziquantel and albendazole in Sudanese men. *Ann Trop Med Parasitol* (1994) 88, 551–9.
2. Pengsaa K, Na-Bangchang K, Limkittikul K, Kabkaew K, Lapphra K, Sirivichayakul C, Wisetsing P, Pojjaroen-Anant C, Chanthavanich P, Subchareon A. Pharmacokinetic investigation of albendazole and praziquantel in Thai children infected with *Giardia intestinalis*. *Ann Trop Med Parasitol* (2004) 98, 349–57.

Amphotericin B + Antineoplastics

Use of conventional amphotericin B with nephrotoxic antineoplastics such as cisplatin and ifosfamide may increase the risk of renal impairment, and should generally be avoided. Liposomal amphotericin B may be an alternative, but renal function should still be closely monitored.

Clinical evidence, mechanism, importance and management

A multivariate analysis in patients receiving high-dose **cisplatin** with saline hydration and mannitol diuresis found that the concurrent use of amphotericin B was a predictor of renal failure.[1] Both cisplatin and amphotericin B are nephrotoxic, and their effects might be expected to be additive.

The manufacturer of conventional amphotericin B states that nephrotoxic antineoplastics should not be given concurrently except with great caution.[2] Of the antineoplastics, **cisplatin**, **ifosfamide** and **methotrexate** are well known for their nephrotoxicity. Amphotericin also reduces the renal clearance of 'methotrexate', (p.642).

Liposomal amphotericin B is licensed for use in the empirical treatment of presumed fungal infections in febrile neutropenic patients. It is therefore likely to be used in patients who have received antineoplastics and who may have antineoplastic-induced renal impairment. The manufacturer notes that it has been used successfully in a large number of patients with pre-existing renal impairment. Nevertheless, renal function should be closely monitored in these patients.[3]

1. Cooper BW, Creger RJ, Soegiarso W, Mackay WL, Lazarus HM. Renal dysfunction during high-dose cisplatin therapy and autologous hematopoietic stem cell transplantation: effect of aminoglycoside therapy. *Am J Med* (1993) 94, 497–504.
2. Fungizone Intravenous (Amphotericin B). E. R. Squibb & Sons Ltd. UK Summary of product characteristics, May 2006.
3. Ambisome (Liposomal Amphotericin B). Gilead Sciences International Ltd, UK Summary of product characteristics, August 2006.

Amphotericin B + Azoles

The effects of amphotericin B and azole antifungals would be expected to be antagonistic, and there is some clinical evidence to support this suggestion of reduced efficacy, and even increased adverse effects. However, other studies suggest that the combination of amphotericin B and fluconazole may be beneficial.

Clinical evidence

Studies in a few patients and *in vitro* experiments suggest that the antifungal effects of amphotericin B and **miconazole** used together may be antagonistic.[1,2] In another study, 4 out of 6 patients did not respond to amphotericin B treatment while also taking **ketoconazole**, whereas treatment was successful in 6 others, 5 of whom had stopped taking prophylactic **miconazole** or **ketoconazole**. The authors suggested that the numbers are too small to draw any definite conclusions, but antagonism is certainly a possibility.[3] A comparative study found that patients given **itraconazole** and amphotericin B had serum **itraconazole** levels of less than 1 microgram/mL, whereas those given **itraconazole** alone had serum **itraconazole** levels of 3.75 micrograms/mL, which suggests that amphotericin B may reduce **itraconazole** levels.[4] There are numerous *in vitro* and *animal* studies of the potential interaction of **azoles** with amphotericin B, which show conflicting results from antagonism to additive or synergistic effects, some of which have been the subject of a review.[5] In a recent large randomised study in 219 patients with candidaemia who were not neutropenic, high-dose **fluconazole** plus amphotericin B tended to be more effective than fluconazole plus placebo (69% versus 56% success rate). The combination was not antagonistic compared with fluconazole alone.[6] Similarly, in a randomised study in HIV-positive patients with cryptococcal meningitis, **fluconazole** plus amphotericin B was found to be more effective in reducing CSF fungal levels than amphotericin B alone. However, it was not as effective as amphotericin B plus flucytosine. All treatments were well tolerated.[7]

A retrospective study of **itraconazole** use found that 11 of 12 leukaemic patients given amphotericin B and **itraconazole** had raised liver enzymes. These abnormalities resolved in 7 patients when the amphotericin B was discontinued. **Itraconazole** alone, given to another 8 patients did not cause liver enzyme abnormalities, even though it was used in high doses.[8] Amphotericin B has only rarely been associated with adverse effects on the liver and increases in liver enzymes may occur in patients treated with itraconazole.

Mechanism

Uncertain. In theory, the combination of an antifungal that binds to ergosterol in fungal cell membranes (amphotericin B) with one that inhibits the synthesis of ergosterol (azoles) would be expected to exert antagonistic effects.[5,9,10] *In vitro* studies with *Candida albicans* found that azole exposure may allow the generation of cells that are unaffected by subsequent exposure to amphotericin B. The degree of resistance appears to depend on concentration and the azole involved, with itraconazole causing more resistance than fluconazole.[11] Resistance of *Candida* species. to amphotericin B appears to depend on the duration of pre-exposure to fluconazole and is also greater when amphotericin B is subsequently used in combination with fluconazole rather than alone.[10,12] Resistance may also depend on the organism involved and its sensitivity to azoles.[13,14]

Importance and management

Despite extensive *in vitro* and *animal* data, it is not entirely clear whether or not azoles inhibit the efficacy of amphotericin B.[9,15,16] The emergence of resistant strains of fungi and the fact that antifungal therapy for invasive fungal infections remains suboptimal, has meant that combinations of antifungals have continued to be tried. Critically ill patients are often given empirical treatment with amphotericin B, with a subsequent change to fluconazole if the organism is sensitive. The Infectious Disease Society of America advises that a combination of amphotericin B and fluconazole may be an option in selected patients.[17] However, combinations of azoles and amphotericin B should not be considered as routine practice, and until more is known it may be better to limit concurrent use to specific cases. The outcome of combined use should be well monitored for both a reduced antifungal response and an increase in adverse effects, such as a worsening of liver function tests.[8] Some recent reviews have usefully discussed the topic of antifungals combinations.[18-20]

1. Schacter LP, Owellen RJ, Rathbun HK, Buchanan B. Antagonism between miconazole and amphotericin B. *Lancet* (1976) ii, 318.
2. Cosgrove RF, Beezer AE, Miles RJ. In vitro studies of amphotericin B in combination with the imidazole antifungal compounds clotrimazole and miconazole. *J Infect Dis* (1978) 138, 681–5.
3. Meunier-Carpentier F, Cruciani M, Klastersky J. Oral prophylaxis with miconazole or ketoconazole of invasive fungal disease in neutropenic cancer patients. *Eur J Cancer Clin Oncol* (1983) 19, 43–8.
4. Pennick GJ, McGough DA, Barchiesi F, Rinaldi MG. Concomitant therapy with amphotericin B and itraconazole: Does this combination affect the serum concentration of itraconazole? *Intersci Conf Antimicrob Agents Chemother* (1994) 34, 39.
5. Sugar AM. Use of amphotericin B with azole antifungal drugs: what are we doing? *Antimicrob Agents Chemother* (1995) 39, 1907–12.
6. Rex JH, Pappas PG, Karchmer AW, Sobel J, Edwards JE, Hadley S, Brass C, Vazquez JA, Chapman SW, Horowitz HW, Zervos M, McKinsey D, Lee J, Babinchak T, Bradsher RW, Cleary JD, Cohen DM, Danziger L, Goldman M, Goodman J, Hilton E, Hyslop NE, Kett DH, Lutz J, Rubin RH, Scheld WM, Schuster M, Simmons B, Stein DK, Washburn RG, Mautner L, Chu TC, Panzer H, Rosenstein RB, Booth J; National Institute of Allergy and Infectious Diseases Mycoses Study Group. A randomized and blinded multicenter trial of high-dose fluconazole plus placebo versus fluconazole plus amphotericin B as therapy for candidemia and its consequences in nonneutropenic subjects. Clin Infect Dis. (2003) 36, 1221–8.
7. Brouwer AE, Rajanuwong A, Chierakul W, Griffen GE, Larsen RA, White NJ, Harrison TS. Combination antifungal therapies for HIV-associated cryptococcal meningitis: a randomised trial. *Lancet* (2004) 363, 1764–7.
8. Persat F, Schwartzbrod PE, Troncy J, Timour Q, Maul A, Piens MA, Picot S. Abnormalities in liver enzymes during simultaneous therapy with itraconazole and amphotericin B in leukaemic patients. *J Antimicrob Chemother* (2000) 45, 928–30.
9. Pahls S, Schaffner A. *Aspergillus fumigatus* pneumonia in neutropenic patients receiving fluconazole for infection due to *Candida* species: is amphotericin B combined with fluconazole the appropriate answer? *Clin Infect Dis* (1994) 18, 484–5.
10. Ernst EJ, Klepser ME, Pfaller MA. In vitro interaction of fluconazole and amphotericin B administered sequentially against *Candida albicans*: effect of concentration and exposure time. *Diagn Microbiol Infect Dis* (1998) 32, 205–10.
11. Vazquez JA, Arganoza MT, Vaishampayan JK, Akins RA. In vitro interaction between amphotericin B and azoles in Candida albicans. *Antimicrob Agents Chemother* (1996) 40, 2511–16.

12. Louie A, Kaw P, Banerjee P, Liu W, Chen G, Miller MH. Impact of order of initiation of fluconazole and amphotericin B in sequential or combination therapy on killing of Candida albicans in vitro and in rabbit model of endocarditis and pyelonephritis. *Antimicrob Agents Chemother* (2001) 45, 485–10.
13. Louie A, Banerjee P, Drusano GL, Shayegani M, Miller MH. Interaction between fluconazole and amphotericin B in mice with systemic infection due to fluconazole-susceptible or -resistant strains of Candida albicans. *Antimicrob Agents Chemother* (1999) 43, 2841–7.
14. LeMonte AM, Washum KE, Smedema ML, Schnizlein-Bick C, Kohler SM, Wheat LJ. Amphotericin B combined with itraconazole or fluconazole for treatment of histoplasmosis. *J Infect Dis* (2000) 182, 545–50.
15. Meis JF, Donnelly JP, Hoogkamp-Korstanje JA, De Pauw BE. Reply. *Clin Infect Dis* (1994) 18, 485–6.
16. Scheven M, Scheven M-L. Interaction between azoles and amphotericin B in the treatment of candidiasis. *Clin Infect Dis* (1995) 20, 1079.
17. Pappas PG, Rex JH, Sobel JD, Filler SG, Dismukes WE, Walsh TJ, Edwards JE. Infectious Disease Society of America: Guidelines for treatment of candidiasis. *Clin Infect Dis* (2004) 38:161–89
18. Baddley JW, Pappas PG. Antifungal combination therapy: clinical potential. *Drugs* (2005) 65, 1461–80.
19. Sobel JD. Combination therapy for invasive mycoses: evaluation of past clinical trial designs. *Clin Infect Dis* (2004) 39 (Suppl 4): S224–7.
20. Patterson TF. Advances and challenges in management of invasive mycoses. *Lancet* (2005) 366: 1013–25.

Amphotericin B + Corticosteroids

Both amphotericin B and corticosteroids can cause potassium loss and salt and water retention, which can have adverse effects on cardiac function.

Clinical evidence

Four patients treated with amphotericin B and **hydrocortisone** 25 to 40 mg daily developed cardiac enlargement and congestive heart failure. The cardiac size decreased and the heart failure disappeared within 2 weeks of stopping the **hydrocortisone**. The amphotericin B was continued successfully with the addition of potassium supplements.[1]

Mechanism

Amphotericin B causes potassium to be lost in the urine. Hydrocortisone can cause potassium to be lost, and salt and water to be retained, and occasional instances of hypernatraemia with amphotericin B have also been seen. Working in concert these could account for the hypokalaemic cardiopathy and the circulatory overload that was seen.

Importance and management

Information is limited but the interaction would seem to be established. Monitor electrolytes (especially potassium, which should be closely monitored in patients receiving amphotericin B in any case) and fluid balance if amphotericin B is given with corticosteroids. The elderly would seem to be particularly at risk. Note that hypokalaemia increases the risk of adverse interactions with 'digitalis glycosides', (p.923) and 'QT-interval prolonging drugs', (p.257). The manufacturer of conventional amphotericin B advises that corticosteroids should not be used concurrently unless necessary to control drug reactions.[2] However, in clinical practice, it is sometimes deemed necessary to use both drugs together. In this situation, close monitoring of the patient's fluid balance, potassium level and cardiovascular parameters is required.

1. Chung D-K, Koenig MG. Reversible cardiac enlargement during treatment with amphotericin B and hydrocortisone. Report of three cases. *Am Rev Respir Dis* (1971) 103, 831–41.
2. Fungizone Intravenous (Amphotericin B). E. R. Squibb & Sons Ltd. UK Summary of product characteristics, May 2006.

Amphotericin B + Diuretics

Amphotericin B commonly causes hypokalaemia. Loop diuretics or thiazides and related diuretics increase the risk of hypokalaemia when given with amphotericin.[1] In turn, this might increase the risk of interactions with 'digitalis glycosides', (p.923) and 'QT-interval prolonging drugs', (p.257). Conversely, potassium-sparing diuretics such as amiloride might reduce the incidence of hypokalaemia with amphotericin.[2]

1. Ambisome (Liposomal Amphotericin B). Gilead Sciences International Ltd. UK Summary of product characteristics, August 2006.
2. Wazny LD, Brophy DF. Amiloride for the prevention of amphotericin B–induced hypokalemia and hypomagnesemia. *Ann Pharmacother* (2000) 34, 94–7.

Amphotericin B + Low salt diet

The renal toxicity of amphotericin B can be associated with sodium depletion. When the sodium is replaced the renal function improves.[1,2]

1. Feeley J, Heidemann H, Gerkens J, Roberts LJ, Branch RA. Sodium depletion enhances nephrotoxicity of amphotericin B. *Lancet* (1981) i, 1422–3.
2. Heidemann HT, Gerkens JF, Spickard WA, Jackson EK, Branch RA. Amphotericin B nephrotoxicity in humans decreased by salt repletion. *Am J Med* (1983) 75, 476–81.

Amphotericin B + Pentamidine

There is some evidence to suggest that acute renal failure may develop in patients taking amphotericin B if they are also given parenteral pentamidine.

Clinical evidence, mechanism, importance and management

A retrospective study between 1985 and 1988 identified 101 patients with AIDS who had been given amphotericin B for various systemic mycoses. The patients were given amphotericin 0.6 to 0.8 mg/kg daily for 7 to 10 days, then a dose three times a week for about 9 weeks. Nine patients were concurrently treated for *Pneumocystis carinii* pneumonia, and of these the 4 who had been given pentamidine parenterally developed acute and rapid reversible renal failure. In all 4 cases, renal function returned to normal when the drugs were withdrawn. No renal failure was seen in 2 others given pentamidine by inhalation or 3 given intravenous co-trimoxazole.[1]

Both amphotericin B and pentamidine are known to be nephrotoxic and the renal impairment was attributed to additive effects of these drugs. The reason no toxicity occurred when the pentamidine was given by inhalation is probably because the serum levels achieved were low.

In general, conventional amphotericin B should not be used with other nephrotoxic drugs such as parenteral pentamidine. Renal function should be monitored closely with either drug (daily in the case of parenteral pentamidine), and it is essential that this recommendation is adhered to if both drugs are given. Anticipate the likelihood of renal failure and the need to withdraw the drugs.

1. Antoniskis D, Larsen RA. Acute, rapidly progressive renal failure with simultaneous use of amphotericin B and pentamidine. *Antimicrob Agents Chemother* (1990) 34, 470–2.

Amphotericin B; Oral + Miscellaneous

The manufacturer of amphotericin B[1] notes that its absorption from the gastrointestinal tract is negligible, and that no interactions have been noted with amphotericin B lozenges, or other oral formulations. For a theoretical interaction with sucralfate, see 'sucralfate', (below).

1. Fungilin Lozenge, Oral Suspension, Oral Tablets (Amphotericin B). E. R. Squibb & Sons Ltd. UK Summary of product characteristics, May 2006.

Amphotericin B; Oral + Sucralfate

An *in vitro* study with amphotericin B found that it became markedly and irreversibly bound to sucralfate at the pH values found in the gut. This suggests that efficacy for intestinal candidiasis or gut decontamination might be decreased, but no study appears to have been conducted to establish this.

Clinical evidence, mechanism, importance and management

To simulate what might happen in the gut, amphotericin B 25 mg/L was mixed with sucralfate 500 mg in 40 mL of water at pH 3.5 and allowed to stand for 90 minutes at 25°C. Analysis of the solution found that the amphotericin B concentration fell rapidly and progressively over 90 minutes to about 20%. When the pH of the mixture was then raised to about 6.5 to 7 for 90 minutes, there was no change in the concentration of amphotericin

B, suggesting that the interaction was irreversible.[1] The reason for this change is not known, but the suggestion is that sucralfate forms insoluble chelates with amphotericin B.[1]

It is not known how important this interaction is likely to be in practice, but the efficacy of amphotericin B for intestinal candidiasis or gut decontamination may be decreased. Separating the dosages might not be effective in some postoperative patients because their gastric function may not return to normal for up to 5 days, and some sucralfate might still be present when the next dose is given.[1] This study was conducted more than a decade ago, and nobody appears to have conducted a clinical study to establish its hypothesis. If both sucralfate and oral amphotericin are required, it would seem prudent to monitor concurrent use carefully, being alert for any evidence of reduced effects.

1. Feron B, Adair CG, Gorman SP, McClurg B. Interaction of sucralfate with antibiotics used for selective decontamination of the gastrointestinal tract. *Am J Hosp Pharm* (1993) 50, 2550–3.

Atovaquone + Co-trimoxazole

In one small study co-trimoxazole did not alter atovaquone levels, and atovaquone caused a minor decrease in co-trimoxazole levels, which was not considered clinically relevant.

Clinical evidence, mechanism, importance and management

As part of a larger study, 6 HIV-positive subjects received atovaquone 500 mg once daily, co-trimoxazole 960 mg (trimethoprim/sulfamethoxazole 160/800 mg) twice daily, or the combination, taken with food. There was no change in steady-state atovaquone levels but there was a minor 17% decrease in steady-state trimethoprim levels and a minor 8% decrease in sulfamethoxazole levels when both drugs were given together.[1]

This study shows there is no important pharmacokinetic interaction between atovaquone and co-trimoxazole. No dosage adjustments of either drug would be required on concurrent use.

1. Falloon J, Sargent S, Piscitelli SC, Bechtel C, LaFon SW, Sadler B, Walker RE, Kovacs JA, Polis MA, Davey RT, Lan HC, Masur H. Atovaquone suspension in HIV-infected volunteers: pharmacokinetics, pharmacodynamics, and TMP-SMX interaction study. *Pharmacotherapy* (1999) 19, 1050–6.

Atovaquone + Food

Taking atovaquone with fatty food markedly increases its AUC by two to threefold. Atovaquone/proguanil tablets should be taken with food or a milky drink, and atovaquone suspension should be taken with food, to maximise absorption and efficacy.

Clinical evidence

(a) Suspension

In a pharmacokinetic study in HIV-positive subjects designed to determine the dose of atovaquone suspension that would achieve specific steady-state plasma levels, administration with **high-fat** food increased the bioavailability of atovaquone by 1.4-fold when compared with the fasted state.[1] In another similar study, administration of atovaquone suspension with food (23 g of fat) increased average steady-state levels by 1.3-fold to 1.7-fold with different dosage regimens (using 500 mg to 1.5 g of atovaquone.[2]

In a single-dose study in healthy subjects, a **high-fat breakfast** (21 g of fat) increased the AUC of atovaquone by 2.4-fold, and an **enteral nutrition supplement** (*Sustacal Plus*, containing 28 g of fat) increased the AUC by 2.7-fold compared with the fasted state.[3]

(b) Tablets

In a crossover study in 18 healthy subjects after an overnight fast, administration of atovaquone 500 mg after a **high-fat standard breakfast** (23 g of fat) increased the AUC by 3.3-fold when compared with the fasted state.[4] In a further study of similar design, 2 slices of **toast** alone had no effect on atovaquone AUC, 2 slices of **toast with 23 g of butter** increased the AUC by threefold, and 2 slices of **toast with 56 g of butter** increased the AUC by 3.9-fold.[4]

Mechanism

Atovaquone is a highly lipophilic compound, which shows considerable inter-individual variability in absorption. Dietary fat increases the rate and extent of atovaquone absorption from both the suspension and the tablets, probably by increasing its solubility in the gut. The suspension has about a twofold higher oral bioavailability than the tablets when given with food or when fasting.

Importance and management

Established interactions of clinical importance. Atovaquone suspension used for the treatment or prevention of Pneumocystis pneumonia must be taken with food, since this is likely to increase the likelihood of successful treatment and survival.[5,6] Alternatively, an enteral nutritional supplement with a high-fat content appears to be suitable.[3] In the US, the manufacturer says that, for patients who have difficulty taking atovaquone suspension with food, parenteral therapy for Pneumocystis pneumonia should be considered.[6]

Similarly, atovaquone/proguanil tablets used for the treatment or prophylaxis of malaria should be taken with a milky drink or with food to maximise absorption.[7,8] Be aware that if patients are unable to tolerate food, the systemic exposure to atovaquone will be reduced.[7,8] In this situation, monitoring of parasitaemia to ensure efficacy would seem prudent.

1. Dixon R, Pozniak AL, Watt HM, Rolan P, Posner J. Single-dose and steady-state pharmacokinetics of a novel microfluidized suspension of atovaquone in human immunodeficiency virus-seropositive patients. *Antimicrob Agents Chemother* (1996) 40, 556–60.
2. Falloon J, Sargent S, Piscitelli SC, Bechtel C, LaFon SW, Sadler B, Walker RE, Kovacs JA, Polis MA, Davey RT, Lan HC, Masur H. Atovaquone suspension in HIV-infected volunteers: pharmacokinetics, pharmacodynamics, and TMP-SMX interaction study. *Pharmacotherapy* (1999) 19, 1050–6.
3. Freeman CD, Klutman NE, Lamp KC, Dall LH, Strayer AH. Relative bioavailability of atovaquone suspension when administered with an enteral nutrition supplement. *Ann Pharmacother* (1998) 32, 1004–7.
4. Rolan PE, Mercer AJ, Weatherley BC, Holdich T, Meire H, Peck RW, Ridout G, Posner J. Examination of some factors responsible for a food-induced increase in absorption of atovaquone. *Br J Clin Pharmacol* (1994) 37, 13–20.
5. Wellvone Oral Suspension (Atovaquone). GlaxoSmithKline UK. UK Summary of product characteristics, May 2006.
6. Mepron Suspension (Atovaquone). GlaxoSmithKline. US Prescribing information, November 2006.
7. Malarone (Atovaquone/Proguanil hydrochloride). GlaxoSmithKline UK. UK Summary of product characteristics, June 2007.
8. Malarone (Atovaquone/Proguanil hydrochloride). GlaxoSmithKline. US Prescribing information, November 2006.

Atovaquone + Miscellaneous

Preliminary evidence suggested that, of a number of drugs given with atovaquone in clinical trials, only metoclopramide caused any marked change (decreases) in the atovaquone serum levels. Until more is known, it may be prudent to monitor efficacy if metoclopramide is used with atovaquone.

Clinical evidence, mechanism, importance and management

An analysis of 191 patients with AIDS, given atovaquone as part of efficacy studies, found that when normalised for plasma albumin, bodyweight, and the absence of other drugs, the expected steady-state plasma levels of atovaquone were 14.8 micrograms/mL. Steady-state atovaquone plasma levels achieved in the presence of other drugs were examined in an attempt to identify possible interactions. **Fluconazole** and **prednisone** were associated with increases of 2.5 and 2.3 micrograms/mL, respectively, whereas **paracetamol (acetaminophen)**, **aciclovir**, **opioids**, **antidiarrhoeals**, **cephalosporins**, **benzodiazepines** and **laxatives** were associated with decreases of greater than 3.4 micrograms/mL. **Metoclopramide** was associated with a decrease of 7.2 micrograms/mL. **U plasma binders** [not defined], **erythromycin**, **clofazimine**, **antacids**, **clotrimazole**, **NSAIDs**, **ketoconazole**, **hydroxyzine**, **megestrol**, **antiemetics** (other than **metoclopramide**), **other systemic steroids**, and **H_2-receptor antagonists** were not associated with any change in steady-state atovaquone serum levels. **U plasma binders**, **erythromycin** and **clofazimine** were represented by fewer than 5 subjects.[1,2]

The kind of analysis described above[1,2] provides only the very broadest indication that interactions might or might not occur between atovaquone and these drugs, but it highlights the need to be vigilant if an apparently interacting drug is used concurrently. Only the changes caused by **metoclopramide** seem likely to have any potential clinical importance and the manufacturers recommend caution in its use with atovaquone/proguanil.[2,3] If an antiemetic is required in patients taking atovaquone/proguanil, they suggest that **metoclopramide** should be given only if other antiemetics are unavailable,[3] and that parasitaemia should be closely monitored.[4] In the UK, the manufacturers also say that **metoclopramide** should be given with caution to patients taking atovaquone suspension for Pneumocystis pneumonia, until the interaction has been further studied,[2] whereas the US manufacturers of atovaquone suspension do not mention **metoclopramide**.[5]

1. Sadler BM, Blum MR. Relationship between steady-state plasma concentrations of atovaquone (C_{ss}) and the use of various concomitant medications in AIDS patients with *Pneumocystis carinii* pneumonia. IXth Int Conf AIDS & IVth STD World Congr, Berlin, 1993. 504.
2. Wellvone Oral Suspension (Atovaquone). GlaxoSmithKline UK. UK Summary of product characteristics, May 2006.
3. Malarone (Atovaquone/Proguanil hydrochloride). GlaxoSmithKline. US Prescribing information, November 2006.
4. Malarone (Atovaquone/Proguanil hydrochloride). GlaxoSmithKline UK. UK Summary of product characteristics, June 2007.
5. Mepron Suspension (Atovaquone). GlaxoSmithKline. US Prescribing information, November 2006.

Atovaquone + Proguanil

There appears to be no clinically relevant pharmacokinetic interaction between atovaquone and proguanil.

Clinical evidence, mechanism, importance and management

Atovaquone did not affect the pharmacokinetics of proguanil in a comparative study of 4 patients taking proguanil 200 mg twice daily for 3 days and 12 patients taking proguanil 200 mg twice daily with atovaquone 500 mg twice daily for 3 days.[1] A similar lack of interaction was seen in 18 healthy subjects given proguanil 400 mg daily with atovaquone 1 g daily for 3 days.[2]

In contrast, in a longer study 13 healthy subjects were given a single 250/100-mg dose of atovaquone/proguanil, then after an interval of one week they were given daily doses for 13 days. There was no change in the AUC of atovaquone from single dose to steady state, indicating that accumulation did not occur. However, the AUC of proguanil was modestly increased at steady state, and the AUC of the active metabolite cycloguanil was modestly decreased, in the 9 subjects who were extensive metaboliser phenotypes for the cytochrome P450 isoenzyme CYP2C19 (see 'Genetic factors', (p.4)). It was suggested that atovaquone may have inhibited the production of cycloguanil by CYP3A4. However, since this study had no arm with each drug alone, it is impossible to determine whether these changes in pharmacokinetics were due to an interaction or not.[3]

A pharmacokinetic interaction is not established, and is anyway of little clinical relevance, since the efficacy of the combination product for malaria prophylaxis up to 12 weeks is established. The enhanced activity of the combination may, in part, be due to proguanil lowering the effective concentration at which atovaquone collapses the mitochondrial potential in malaria parasites.[4]

1. Edstein MD, Looareesuwan S, Viravan C, Kyle DE. Pharmacokinetics of proguanil in malaria patients treated with proguanil plus atovaquone. *Southeast Asian J Trop Med Public Health* (1996) 27, 216–20.
2. Gillotin C, Mamet JP, Veronese L. Lack of pharmacokinetic interaction between atovaquone and proguanil. *Eur J Clin Pharmacol* (1999) 55, 311–15.
3. Thapar MM, Ashton M, Lindegardh N, Bergqvist Y, Nivelius S, Johansson I, Bjorkman A. Time-dependent pharmacokinetics and drug metabolism of atovaquone plus proguanil (Malarone) when taken as chemoprophylaxis. *Eur J Clin Pharmacol* (2002) 58, 19–27.
4. Srivastava IK, Vaidya AB. A mechanism for the synergistic antimalarial action of atovaquone and proguanil. *Antimicrob Agents Chemother* (1999) 43, 1334–9.

Atovaquone + Rifamycins

Rifampicin reduces serum atovaquone levels by about 50% whereas atovaquone modestly raises serum rifampicin levels. The combination should be avoided because of the likelihood of sub-therapeutic atovaquone levels. Rifabutin caused a lesser 34% decrease in atovaquone levels, which the manufacturer considers may also reduce efficacy.

Clinical evidence

(a) Rifabutin

In 24 healthy subjects given atovaquone 750 mg twice daily and rifabutin 300 mg once daily for 14 days, there was a modest 34% decrease in the AUC of atovaquone and a small 19% decrease in the rifabutin levels.[1]

(a) Rifampicin (Rifampin)

A steady-state study in 13 HIV-positive subjects found that the use of atovaquone 750 mg twice daily with rifampicin 600 mg four times daily for 14 days resulted in a more than 50% reduction in the atovaquone AUC and serum levels, but a more than 30% rise in rifampicin AUC and serum levels.[2,3]

Mechanism

Uncertain. Atovaquone is predominantly excreted (greater than 90%) as unchanged drug in the faeces,[3,4] and would not therefore be expected to be affected by cytochrome P450 enzyme induction.

Importance and management

Information is limited but these pharmacokinetic interactions appear to be established. Their clinical importance is unknown, but it seems highly likely that the efficacy of atovaquone will be reduced in the presence of rifampicin. The combination should therefore be avoided.

The effect of rifabutin is less than rifampicin, and the authors of the above report suggested that no atovaquone dosage adjustment is needed.[1] However, in the UK, the manufacturer of atovaquone still considers that rifabutin use could result in subtherapeutic atovaquone levels in some patients, and they also advise against the concurrent use of this combination.[4]

1. Gillotin C, Grandpierre I, Sadler BM. Pharmacokinetic interaction between atovaquone (ATVQ) suspension and rifabutin (RFB). *Clin Pharmacol Ther* (1998) 63, 229.
2. Sadler BM, Caldwell P, Scott JD, Rogers M, Blum MR. Drug interaction between rifampin and atovaquone (Mepron®) in HIV+ asymptomatic volunteers. *Intersci Conf Antimicrob Agents Chemother* (1995) 35, 7.
3. Mepron Suspension (Atovaquone). GlaxoSmithKline. US Prescribing information, November 2006.
4. Wellvone Oral Suspension (Atovaquone). GlaxoSmithKline UK. UK Summary of product characteristics, May 2006.

Atovaquone + Tetracyclines

Tetracycline reduces the plasma levels of atovaquone by about 40%. The effect of doxycycline does not appear to have been studied.

Clinical evidence, mechanism, importance and management

The manufacturer of atovaquone/proguanil[1,2] notes that **tetracycline** may reduce plasma levels of atovaquone by about 40%.[1]

An *in vitro* study found that **doxycycline** potentiated the antimalarial activity of atovaquone,[3] but there appears to be no information on the effect of **doxycycline** on the absorption of atovaquone. A study looking at the population pharmacokinetics of atovaquone in 24 Thai patients found that neither the oral clearance nor the volume of distribution of atovaquone were significantly affected by the concurrent use of tetracycline.[4]

The manufacturers suggest that parasitaemia should be closely monitored in patients taking atovaquone/proguanil tablets with **tetracycline**.[1,2] In the UK, they also say that **tetracycline** should be given with caution to patients taking atovaquone suspension for Pneumocystis pneumonia, until the interaction has been further studied,[5] whereas the US manufacturers of atovaquone suspension do not mention **tetracycline**.[6]

1. Malarone (Atovaquone/Proguanil hydrochloride). GlaxoSmithKline. US Prescribing information, November 2006.
2. Malarone (Atovaquone/Proguanil hydrochloride). GlaxoSmithKline UK. UK Summary of product characteristics, June 2007.
3. Yeo AET, Edstein MD, Shanks GD, Rieckmann KH. Potentiation of the antimalarial activity of atovaquone by doxycycline against *Plasmodium falciparum* in vitro. *Parasitol Res* (1997) 83, 489–91.
4. Hussein Z, Eaves J, Hutchinson DB, Canfield CJ. Population pharmacokinetics of atovaquone in patients with acute malaria caused by *Plasmodium falciparum*. *Clin Pharmacol Ther* (1997) 61, 518–30.
5. Wellvone Oral Suspension (Atovaquone). GlaxoSmithKline UK. UK Summary of product characteristics, May 2006.
6. Mepron Suspension (Atovaquone). GlaxoSmithKline. US Prescribing information, November 2006.

Atovaquone/Proguanil + Artesunate

Artesunate does not appear to affect the pharmacokinetics of atovaquone/proguanil.

Clinical evidence, mechanism, importance and management

In a pharmacokinetic study, a single dose of atovaquone/proguanil 1 g/400 mg was given to 12 healthy subjects with and without artesunate 250 mg. No change was noted in the pharmacokinetics of either atovaquone or proguanil and no unexpected adverse events were seen.[1] Although artesunate does not therefore appear to interact pharmacokinetically with atovaquone/proguanil, this needs confirmation in a multiple-dose study. A study to investigate whether the addition of artesunate to atovaquone/proguanil increased the risk of cardiotoxicity found that the QT_c interval was not significantly different in those receiving all three drugs, when compared with those receiving atovaquone/proguanil alone.[2]

1. van Vugt M, Edstein MD, Proux S, Lay K, Ooh M, Looareesuwan S, White NJ, Nosten F. Absence of an interaction between artesunate and atovaquone – proguanil. *Eur J Clin Pharmacol* (1999) 55, 469–74.
2. Gupta RK, van Vugt M, Paiphun L, Slight T, Looareesuwan S, White NJ, Nosten F. Short Report: No evidence of cardiotoxicity of atovaquone-proguanil alone or in combination with artesunate. *Am J Trop Med Hyg* (2005) 73, 267–8.

Azoles + Antacids

The gastrointestinal absorption of ketoconazole is markedly reduced by antacids. Itraconazole may also be modestly affected. However, the absorption of fluconazole and posaconazole appears not be to significantly affected by antacids. Similarly, voriconazole is not expected to be affected.

Clinical evidence

(a) Fluconazole

Maalox forte (**aluminium/magnesium hydroxide**) 20 mL did not affect the absorption of a single 100-mg dose of fluconazole in 14 healthy subjects.[1]

(b) Itraconazole

For mention of a study in which some patients needed an increase in itraconazole dose when treated with ranitidine and an antacid [not named], see 'Azoles + H_2-receptor antagonists', p.217.

(c) Ketoconazole

A haemodialysis patient did not respond to treatment with ketoconazole 200 mg daily while taking cimetidine, **sodium bicarbonate** 2 g daily and **aluminium oxide** 2.5 g daily. Only when the ketoconazole dosage was increased to 200 mg four times daily did her serum levels rise. A later study in 3 healthy subjects found that when ketoconazole 200 mg was taken 2 hours after **cimetidine** 400 mg, the absorption was considerably reduced (AUC reduced by about 60%). When this was repeated with the addition of **sodium bicarbonate** 500 mg, the absorption was reduced by about 95%. In contrast, when this was again repeated, but with the ketoconazole in an acidic solution, the absorption was increased by about 50%.[2]

A study in 4 patients found that the concurrent use of *Maalox* reduced the absorption of ketoconazole but this was not statistically significant.[3] An anecdotal report suggested that giving ketoconazole 2 hours before a stomatitis cocktail containing *Maalox* seemed to prevent the cocktail reducing ketoconazole effectiveness.[4]

(d) Posaconazole

A study in 12 healthy subjects found that *Mylanta* (**aluminium/magnesium hydroxide**) 20 mL did not significantly affect the bioavailability of a single 200-mg dose of posaconazole, either when taken with food or when fasting.[5]

Mechanism

Ketoconazole is a poorly soluble base, which must be transformed by the acid in the stomach into the soluble hydrochloride salt. Agents that reduce gastric acidity, such as antacids, 'H_2-receptor antagonists', (p.217), and 'proton pump inhibitors', (p.218), raise the pH in the stomach so that the dissolution of the ketoconazole and its absorption are reduced. Conversely, anything that increases the gastric acidity (e.g. 'cola drinks', (p.215)) increases the dissolution and the absorption of ketoconazole. The absorption of itraconazole is also affected by changes in gastric pH, but fluconazole and posaconazole are minimally affected.

Importance and management

The interaction of antacids with **ketoconazole** is clinically important, but not extensively documented. Advise patients to take antacids not less than 2 to 3 hours before or after the ketoconazole so that absorption can take place with minimal changes in the pH of the gastric contents.[2] Monitor the effects to confirm that the ketoconazole is effective.

The situation with **itraconazole** is not entirely clear, but based on the data with 'H_2-receptor antagonists', (p.217), some reduction in its absorption might be expected with antacids, and it would therefore be prudent to separate administration.

Antacids do not significantly affect **posaconazole** or **fluconazole** levels, and, based on the data with 'H_2-receptor antagonists', (p.217), would not be expected to affect **voriconazole** levels.

1. Thorpe JE, Baker N, Bromet-Petit M. Effect of oral antacid administration on the pharmacokinetics of oral fluconazole. *Antimicrob Agents Chemother* (1990) 34, 2032–3.
2. Van der Meer JWM, Keuning JJ, Scheijgrond HW, Heykants J, Van Cutsem J, Brugmans J. The influence of gastric acidity on the bio-availability of ketoconazole. *J Antimicrob Chemother* (1980) 6, 552–4.
3. Brass C, Galgiani JN, Blaschke TF, Defelice R, O'Reilly RA, Stevens DA. Disposition of ketoconazole, an oral antifungal, in humans. *Antimicrob Agents Chemother* (1982) 21, 151–8.
4. Franklin MG. Nizoral and stomatitis cocktails may not mix. *Oncol Nurs Forum* (1991) 18, 1417.
5. Courtney R, Radwanski E, Lim J, Laughlin M. Pharmacokinetics of posaconazole coadministered with antacid in fasting or nonfasting healthy men. *Antimicrob Agents Chemother* (2004) 48, 804–8.

Azoles + Cola drinks

Some cola drinks can temporarily lower the stomach pH of patients with achlorhydria or hypochlorhydria due to disease or acid-suppressing drugs. This improves the bioavailability of itraconazole and ketoconazole.

Clinical evidence

Eight healthy subjects were given **itraconazole** 100 mg with either 325 mL of water or *Coca-Cola* (pH 2.5). Their peak serum **itraconazole** levels were more than doubled by the *Coca-Cola* and the **itraconazole** AUC was increased by 80%. Two of the subjects did not show this effect.[1]

Another study in 18 fasted AIDS patients who absorbed **itraconazole** poorly, found that the absorption was restored to that of fasted healthy subjects when the **itraconazole** was given with a cola drink.[2] A study in 30 healthy subjects compared the bioavailability of **itraconazole** alone or after ranitidine, both with and without a cola drink. Ranitidine reduced the absorption of **itraconazole** but this effect was countered by the cola drink.[3]

Yet another study used omeprazole to raise the pH and *Coca-Cola Classic* to lower it. Absorption was greatest when **ketoconazole** was given alone, and least when given with omeprazole. However, *Coca-Cola* increased the absorption of **ketoconazole** in the presence of omeprazole to 65% of that seen with **ketoconazole** alone.[4]

Mechanism

Itraconazole and ketoconazole are poorly soluble bases, which must be transformed by the acid in the stomach into a soluble hydrochloride salt. Therefore any condition that reduces gastric acidity (or any drug that raises stomach pH, see 'H_2-receptor antagonists', (p.217) and 'proton pump inhibitors', (p.218)) can reduce the dissolution and the absorption of these antifungals. Acidic drinks, which lower the pH, can increase the absorption.

Importance and management

The interactions of itraconazole and ketoconazole with cola drinks that lower the gastric pH are established. The interaction can be exploited to improve the absorption of these antifungals in patients with achlorhydria or hypochlorhydria, and those taking gastric acid suppressants (see 'H_2-receptor antagonists', (p.217) and 'proton pump inhibitors', (p.218)), and this is recommended by some manufacturers of ketoconazole[5] and itraconazole.[6,7] For a brief mention of the use of cola to increase itraconazole levels and thereby increase ciclosporin levels, see 'Ciclosporin + Azoles', p.1023. ***Coca-Cola Classic, Pepsi*** and ***Canada Dry Ginger Ale*** can be used because they can achieve stomach pH values of less than 3, but none of the other beverages examined in one study produced such a low pH. The authors suggest that these would be less effective, although they were not actually studied. They included ***Diet Coca-Cola, Diet Pepsi, Diet 7-Up, Diet Canada Dry Ginger Ale, Diet Canada Dry Orange juice, 7-Up*** and ***Canada Dry Orange juice***.[4] For mention that **glutamic acid** did not increase the absorption of itraconazole in fasted or fed subjects, or ketoconazole in subjects pre-treated with cimetidine, see 'Azoles + Food', below, and 'Azoles + H_2-receptor antagonists', p.217, respectively.

1. Jaruratanasirikul S, Kleepkaew A. Influence of an acidic beverage (Coca-Cola) on absorption of itraconazole. *Eur J Clin Pharmacol* (1997) 52, 235–7.
2. Hardin J, Lange D, Heykants J, Ding C, Van de Velde V, Slusser C, Klausner M. The effect of co-administration of a cola beverage on the bioavailability of itraconazole in AIDS patients. *Intersci Conf Antimicrob Agents Chemother* (1995) 35, 6.
3. Lange D, Pavao JH, Wu J, Klausner M. Effect of cola beverage on the bioavailability of itraconazole in the presence of H_2 blockers. *J Clin Pharmacol* (1997) 37, 535–40.
4. Chin TWF, Loeb M, Fong IW. Effects of an acidic beverage (Coca-Cola) on absorption of ketoconazole. *Antimicrob Agents Chemother* (1995) 39, 1671–5.
5. Nizoral Tablets (Ketoconazole). Janssen-Cilag Ltd. UK Summary of product characteristics, October 2006.
6. Sporanox Capsules (Itraconazole). Janssen-Cilag Ltd. UK Summary of product characteristics, March 2004.
7. Sporanox Capsules (Itraconazole). Janssen. US Prescribing information, June 2006.

Azoles + Food

Itraconazole capsules should be taken with or after food to improve absorption, whereas itraconazole solution should be taken at least one hour before food. Food increases the absorption of posaconazole suspension, and this should be taken with a meal or nutritional supplement. Some manufacturers advise taking ketoconazole with food, but two studies have shown little effect of food on absorption, and one actually showed a decrease. The bioavailability of voriconazole is modestly reduced by food, and the manufacturer recommends it be taken at least one hour before or after a meal. Food does not appear to affect the bioavailability of fluconazole capsules.

Clinical evidence

(a) Fluconazole

A study in 12 healthy subjects found that food had no therapeutically relevant effect on the pharmacokinetics of a single 100-mg dose of fluconazole in capsule form.[1]

(b) Itraconazole

A study in 24 patients with superficial dermatophyte, *Candida albicans* and pityriasis versicolor infections, given itraconazole 50 or 100 mg daily, found that taking the drug with or after breakfast produced higher serum levels and gave much better treatment results than taking it before breakfast.[2] A later study found that the relative bioavailability of itraconazole was 54% on an empty stomach, 86% after a light meal and 100% after a full meal.[1] Similar results were found in other studies.[3,4]

In contrast, studies with itraconazole oral solution give different results. A study in 30 healthy males given itraconazole solution 200 mg daily, either on an empty stomach or with a standard breakfast, found that the bioavailability was 29% higher when itraconazole was taken in the fasted state.[5]

In another study of 20 HIV positive patients, **glutamic acid** 1360 mg, given to acidify the stomach, either with or without food did not enhance itraconazole absorption.[3]

(c) Ketoconazole

One study found that the AUC and peak serum concentrations of a single 200-mg dose of ketoconazole tablets were *reduced* by about 40% (levels reduced from 4.1 to 2.3 micrograms/mL) when given to 10 healthy subjects after a standardised meal.[6]

In contrast, another study found that high carbohydrate and fat diets tended to reduce the rate, but not the overall amount of ketoconazole absorbed from tablets.[7] Similarly, a third study found that the absorption of single 200- or 800-mg doses of ketoconazole in 8 healthy subjects was not altered when they were taken after a standardised breakfast, although the peak serum levels were delayed. The absorption of single 400- and 600-mg doses were increased by about up to 50% with food, but this was not statistically significant.[8]

(d) Posaconazole

A study in 24 healthy subjects found that the maximum plasma levels and AUC of a single 400-mg dose of posaconazole oral suspension were increased 3.4- and 2.6-fold, respectively, when given with a **nutritional supplement** (*Boost Plus*) rather than in the fasting state.[9] In a further study in 20 healthy subjects, single 200-mg doses of posaconazole (as oral suspension) were given with either a high-fat meal, a non-fat breakfast or after a 10-hour fast. The AUC of the suspension was increased fourfold when given with a high-fat meal, and 2.7-fold when given with a non-fat breakfast when compared with fasting.[10]

(e) Voriconazole

In a study 12 healthy subjects were given voriconazole capsules 200 mg twice daily either with food or in the fasted state (2 hours before or after food). Food delayed the oral absorption of voriconazole by about one hour and reduced the AUC by 22%.[11]

Mechanism

Not understood.

Importance and management

Itraconazole absorption from the capsule formulation is best when it is taken with or after food, whereas absorption from the acidic liquid formulation appears to be better when it is taken at least one hour before food. Similarly, **posaconazole** absorption from the oral suspension is improved by food, and the manufacturer recommends that posaconazole should be taken with food.

A confusing and conflicting picture is presented by the studies with **ketoconazole**, two showing no significant change in absorption with food, and one showing a decrease. However, one manufacturer of ketoconazole says that the absorption of ketoconazole is maximal when it is taken during a meal, as it depends on stomach acidity, and it should therefore always be taken with meals.[12]

The manufacturers of **voriconazole** tablets and the US manufacturers of voriconazole suspension recommend that it should be taken at least 1 hour before or at least 1 hour after a meal. The UK manufacturers of voriconazole suspension suggest that it should be taken at least 1 hour before or at least *2* hours after a meal.[13,14]

There appears to be no relevant interaction between food and **fluconazole** capsules.

1. Zimmermann T, Yeates RA, Laufen H, Pfaff G, Wildfeuer A. Influence of concomitant food intake on the oral absorption of two triazole antifungal agents, itraconazole and fluconazole. *Eur J Clin Pharmacol* (1994) 46, 147–150.
2. Wishart JM. The influence of food on the pharmacokinetics of itraconazole in patients with superficial fungal infection. *J Am Acad Dermatol* (1987) 17, 220–3.
3. Carver P, Welage L, Kauffman C. The effect of food and gastric pH on the oral bioavailability of itraconazole in HIV+ patients. *Intersci Conf Antimicrob Agents Chemother* (1996) 36, 6.
4. Barone JA, Koh JG, Bierman RH, Colaizzi JL, Swanson KA, Gaffar MC, Moskovitz BL, Mechlinski W, Van De Velde V. Food interaction and steady-state pharmacokinetics of itraconazole capsules in healthy male volunteers. *Antimicrob Agents Chemother* (1993) 37, 778–84.
5. Barone JA, Moskovitz BL, Guarnieri J, Hassell AE, Colaizzi JL, Bierman RH, Jessen L. Food interaction and steady-state pharmacokinetics of itraconazole oral solution in healthy volunteers. *Pharmacotherapy* (1998) 18, 295–301.
6. Männistö PT, Mäntylä R, Nykänen S, Lamminsivu U, Ottoila P. Impairing effect of food on ketoconazole absorption. *Antimicrob Agents Chemother* (1982) 21, 730–33.
7. Lelawongs P, Barone JA, Colaizzi JL, Hsuan ATM, Mechlinski W, Legendre R, Guarnieri J. Effect of food and gastric acidity on absorption of orally administered ketoconazole. *Clin Pharm* (1988) 7, 228–35.
8. Daneshmend TK, Warnock DW, Ene MD, Johnson EM, Potten MR, Richardson MD, Williamson PJ. Influence of food on the pharmacokinetics of ketoconazole. *Antimicrob Agents Chemother* (1984) 25, 1–3.
9. Courtney R, Sansone A, Calzetta A, Martinho M, Laughlin. The effect of a nutritional supplement (Boost Plus) on the oral bioavailability of posaconazole. *Intersci Conf Antimicrob Agents Chemother* (2003) 43, 33.
10. Courtney R, Wexler D, Radwanski E, Lim J, Laughlin M. Effect of food on the relative bioavailability of two oral formulations of posaconazole in healthy adults. *Br J Clin Pharmacol* (2004) 57, 218–22.
11. Purkins L, Wood N, Kleinermans D, Greenhalgh K, Nichols D. Effect of food on the pharmacokinetics of multiple-dose oral voriconazole. *Br J Clin Pharmacol* (2003) 56 (Suppl 1) 17–23.
12. Nizoral Tablets (Ketoconazole). Janssen-Cilag Ltd. UK Summary of product characteristics, October 2006.
13. VFEND (Voriconazole). Pfizer Ltd. UK Summary of product characteristics, July 2007.
14. VFEND (Voriconazole). Pfizer Inc. US Prescribing information, November 2006.

Azoles + H_2-receptor antagonists

The gastrointestinal absorption of ketoconazole is markedly reduced by cimetidine and ranitidine. The absorption of itraconazole is reduced (possibly halved) by H_2-receptor antagonists, and, similarly, the absorption of posaconazole is reduced by about 40% by cimetidine. The absorption of fluconazole and voriconazole is not significantly affected by H_2-receptor antagonists.

Clinical evidence

(a) Fluconazole

The AUC_{0-48} of fluconazole 100 mg was reduced by only 13% when it was given to 6 healthy subjects with a single 400-mg dose of **cimetidine**.[1] Two other studies found that **cimetidine**[2] and **famotidine**[3] did not affect fluconazole absorption.

(b) Itraconazole

Twelve healthy subjects were given **cimetidine** 400 mg twice daily or **ranitidine** 150 mg twice daily for 3 days before and after a single 200-mg dose of itraconazole. The AUC and maximum serum levels of the itraconazole were reduced, but not significantly. The largest changes were 20% reductions in the AUC and maximum serum levels with **ranitidine**.[4] In contrast, another study in 30 healthy subjects found that **ranitidine** 150 mg twice daily for 3 days reduced the AUC of a single 200-mg dose of itraconazole by 44%, and reduced the maximum serum levels by 52%.[5] A study of the bioavailability of itraconazole in 12 lung transplant patients also given **ranitidine** 150 mg twice daily and an **antacid** four times daily found that the serum levels of itraconazole were highly variable. Half of the patients required the dose of itraconazole to be increased from 200 to 400 mg daily to achieve satisfactory serum levels.[6]

Famotidine 40 mg was found to reduce the serum levels of a 200-mg dose of itraconazole by about 50% in 12 healthy subjects.[3] **Famotidine** 20 mg twice daily was given with itraconazole 200 mg daily for 10 days to 16 patients undergoing chemotherapy for haematological malignancies. The minimum plasma levels of itraconazole were reduced by about 39%, and 8 patients did not achieve the levels considered necessary to protect neutropenic patients from fungal infections.[7]

A study in 8 healthy subjects found that itraconazole 200 mg twice daily for 3 days increased the AUC of intravenous **cimetidine** (loading dose 0.2 mg/kg followed by an infusion of 36 mg/hour for 4 hours) by 25%.[8]

(c) Ketoconazole

A haemodialysis patient did not respond to treatment with ketoconazole 200 mg daily while taking **cimetidine**, sodium bicarbonate 2 g daily and aluminium oxide 2.5 g daily. Only when the ketoconazole dosage was increased to 200 mg four times daily did her serum levels rise. A later study in 3 healthy subjects found that when ketoconazole 200 mg was taken 2 hours after **cimetidine** 400 mg, the absorption was considerably reduced (AUC reduced by about 60%). When this was repeated with the addition of sodium bicarbonate 500 mg, the absorption was reduced by about 95%. In contrast, when this was again repeated but with the ketoconazole in an acidic solution, the absorption was increased by about 50%.[9]

The AUC of a single 200-mg oral dose of ketoconazole was reduced by 91% in 12 fasting subjects who received **cimetidine** 300 mg two hours prior to ketoconazole, followed by sodium bicarbonate 2 g one hour prior to the ketoconazole. This effect was only slightly reversed by the use of **glutamic acid**.[10] Another study[2] in 24 healthy subjects found that intravenous **cimetidine** titrated to give a gastric pH of 6 or more reduced the absorption of ketoconazole by 95%. A study[11] in 6 healthy subjects found that **ranitidine** 150 mg given 2 hours before ketoconazole 400 mg reduced its AUC by about 95%.

(d) Posaconazole

A placebo-controlled study in 12 healthy subjects found that **cimetidine** 400 mg every 12 hours, given with posaconazole 200 mg once daily for 10 days, reduced the AUC and maximum plasma levels of posaconazole by about 40%.[12]

(e) Voriconazole

A study in 12 healthy subjects found that **cimetidine** 400 mg twice daily given with voriconazole 200 mg twice daily increased the maximum plasma levels and AUC of voriconazole by about 20%, but this is not considered sufficient to warrant a dosage adjustment.[13] **Ranitidine** 150 mg twice daily had no significant effect on the AUC and maximum plasma levels of voriconazole.[13]

Mechanism

Ketoconazole is a poorly soluble base, which must be transformed by the acid in the stomach into the soluble hydrochloride salt. Agents that reduce gastric acidity, such as H_2-receptor antagonists, 'proton pump inhibitors', (p.218) or 'antacids', (p.215), raise the pH in the stomach so that the dissolution of the ketoconazole and its absorption are reduced. Conversely, anything that increases the gastric acidity increases the dissolution and the absorption (e.g. 'cola drinks', (p.215)). The absorption of itraconazole is also affected by changes in gastric pH, but fluconazole is minimally affected. The manufacturer of posaconazole says that the reduced absorption is possibly secondary to a reduction in gastric acid.[14] The slight increase in cimetidine levels in the presence of itraconazole may be due to inhibition of P-glycoprotein mediated renal tubular secretion of cimetidine.[8]

Importance and management

The interactions with **ketoconazole** are clinically important but not extensively documented. Monitor the effects to confirm that the ketoconazole is effective. The situation with **itraconazole** is not entirely clear, but some reduction in its absorption apparently occurs and it would also therefore be prudent to confirm that it remains effective in the presence of H_2-receptor antagonists. It has been suggested[5] that the reduction in bioavailability due to H_2-receptor antagonists can be minimised by giving **itraconazole** and **ketoconazole** with an acidic drink such as 'cola', (p.215), and this is recommended by some manufacturers.[15-17]

The bioavailability of **posaconazole** also appears to be reduced by cimetidine. If this is due to the reduction in gastric acid, it could minimised by taking posaconazole with a cola drink, as for ketoconazole and itraconazole. However, the manufacturer currently recommends that the use of posaconazole with cimetidine or other H_2-receptor antagonists be avoided if possible, unless the benefit to the patient outweighs the risk.[14] Further study is needed.

Fluconazole only interacts to a small and clinically irrelevant extent with H_2-receptor antagonists and is therefore a possible alternative to ketoconazole and itraconazole. Similarly, no dosage adjustments are necessary if **voriconazole** is used with any of the H_2-receptor antagonists.[18]

1. Lazar JD, Wilner KD. Drug interactions with fluconazole. *Rev Infect Dis* (1990) 12 (Suppl 3), S327–S333.
2. Blum RA, D'Andrea DT, Florentino BM, Wilton JH, Hilligoss DM, Gardner MJ, Henry EB, Goldstein H, Schentag JJ. Increased gastric pH and the bioavailability of fluconazole and ketoconazole. *Ann Intern Med* (1991) 114, 755–7.
3. Lim SG, Sawyerr AM, Hudson M, Sercombe J, Pounder RE. Short report: The absorption of fluconazole and itraconazole under conditions of low intragastric acidity. *Aliment Pharmacol Ther* (1993) 7, 317–21.
4. Stein AG, Daneshmend TK, Warnock DW, Bhaskar N, Burke J, Hawkey CJ. The effects of H_2-receptor antagonists on the pharmacokinetics of itraconazole, a new oral antifungal. *Br J Clin Pharmacol* (1989) 27, 105P–106P.
5. Lange D, Pavao JH, Wu J, Klausner M. Effect of a cola beverage on the bioavailability of itraconazole in the presence of H_2 blockers. *J Clin Pharmacol* (1997) 37, 535–40.
6. PattersonTF, Peters J, Levine SM, Anzueto A, Bryan CL, Sako EY, LaWayne Miller O, Calhoon JH, Rinaldi MG. Systemic availability of itraconazole in lung transplantation. *Antimicrob Agents Chemother* (1996) 40, 2217–20.
7. Kanda Y, Kami M, Matsuyama T, Mitani K, Chiba S, Yazaki Y, Hirai H. Plasma concentration of itraconazole in patients receiving chemotherapy for hematological malignancies: the effect of famotidine on the absorption of itraconazole. *Hematol Oncol* (1998) 16, 33–7.
8. Karyekar CS, Eddington ND, Briglia A, Gubbins PO, Dowling TC. Renal interaction between itraconazole and cimetidine. *J Clin Pharmacol* (2004) 44, 919–27.
9. Van der Meer JWM, Keuning JJ, Scheijgrond HW, Heykants J, Van Cutsem J, Brugmans J. The influence of gastric acidity on the bio-availability of ketoconazole. *J Antimicrob Chemother* (1980) 6, 552–4.
10. Lelawongs P, Barone JA, Colaizzi JL, Hsuan ATM, Mechlinski W, Legendre R, Guarnieri J. Effect of food and gastric acidity on absorption of orally administered ketoconazole. *Clin Pharm* (1988) 7, 228–35.
11. Piscitelli SC, Goss TF, Wilton JH, D'Andrea DT, Goldstein H, Schentag JJ. Effects of ranitidine and sucralfate on ketoconazole bioavailability. *Antimicrob Agents Chemother* (1991) 35, 1765–71.
12. Courtney R, Wexler D, Statkevich P, Lim J, Batra V, Laughlin M. Effect of cimetidine on the pharmacokinetics of posaconazole in healthy volunteers. *Intersci Conf Antimicrob Agents Chemother* (2002) 42, 29.
13. Purkins L, Wood N, Kleinermans D, Nichols D. Histamine H_2-receptor antagonists have no clinically significant effect on the steady-state pharmacokinetics of voriconazole. *Br J Clin Pharmacol* (2003) 56, 51–5.
14. Noxafil (Posaconazole). Schering-Plough Ltd. UK Summary of product characteristics, October 2006.
15. Nizoral Tablets (Ketoconazole). Janssen-Cilag Ltd. UK Summary of product characteristics, October 2006.
16. Sporanox Capsules (Itraconazole). Janssen-Cilag Ltd. UK Summary of product characteristics, March 2004.
17. Sporanox Capsules (Itraconazole). Janssen. US Prescribing information, June 2006.
18. VFEND (Voriconazole). Pfizer Inc. US Prescribing information, November 2006.

Azoles + Proton pump inhibitors

The bioavailability of ketoconazole is reduced by both omeprazole and rabeprazole. Other proton pump inhibitors are expected to behave similarly. Omeprazole also markedly reduces the absorption of itraconazole capsules, but not the oral solution. Proton pump inhibitors are predicted to reduce the bioavailability of posaconazole. The bioavailabilities of fluconazole and voriconazole are not significantly affected by omeprazole. Esomeprazole levels may also be increased by voriconazole.Omeprazole levels are increased by ketoconazole, and markedly increased by fluconazole and voriconazole.

Clinical evidence

(a) Esomeprazole

Based on data for omeprazole (see below), and the known acid-lowering effect of esomeprazole,[1] the manufacturers predict that esomeprazole might reduce the absorption of **itraconazole** and **ketoconazole**, which depend on a low pH for optimal dissolution and absorption.[1] **Voriconazole** may more than double the levels of esomeprazole.[2]

(b) Omeprazole

1. Fluconazole. A study in 12 healthy subjects found that omeprazole 20 mg daily for 7 days did not affect the pharmacokinetics of a single 100-mg dose of fluconazole given after a standard breakfast.[3]
In another study in 18 healthy subjects, fluconazole 100 mg daily for 5 days markedly increased the peak plasma levels and AUC of a single 20-mg dose of omeprazole by 2.4- and 6.3-fold, respectively.[4]

2. Itraconazole. Itraconazole 200 mg [capsule] was given after a standard breakfast to 11 healthy subjects after 14 days pre-treatment with omeprazole 40 mg daily. The AUC and maximum serum level of itraconazole were both reduced by about 65%.[5] In contrast, another study in 15 healthy subjects found that omeprazole 40 mg daily did not significantly affect the pharmacokinetics of single 400-mg doses of itraconazole or its metabolite hydroxyitraconazole when given as an oral solution. However, there was a large interpatient variation in mean serum levels.[6] Another study similarly reported that omeprazole had little effect on the pharmacokinetics of itraconazole oral solution.[7]

3. Ketoconazole. A three-way crossover study in 9 healthy fasting subjects found that omeprazole 60 mg reduced the AUC of ketoconazole 200 mg by about 80%.[8]
Another study was carried out in 10 healthy subjects (both 'extensive' and 'poor' metabolisers) to find the extent to which cytochrome P450 isoenzyme CYP3A4 is involved in the metabolism (sulfoxidation) of omeprazole. This revealed that ketoconazole 100 to 200 mg, a known inhibitor of CYP3A4, reduced the formation of the omeprazole sulfone in both groups, and doubled the serum omeprazole levels in the poor metabolisers.[9]

4. Posaconazole. Based on the 40% reduction in posaconazole AUC when given with 'cimetidine', (p.217), the manufacturers consider that **proton pump inhibitors** might interact similarly.[10]

5. Voriconazole. A study in 18 healthy subjects found that omeprazole 40 mg daily for 7 days increased the maximum plasma levels and AUC of voriconazole by 15 and 41%, respectively. Food was prohibited within one hour before and after each dose.[11]
However, voriconazole 200 mg twice daily increased the maximum plasma levels and AUC of omeprazole 40 mg once daily by about twofold and fourfold respectively.[12]

(c) Rabeprazole

In a randomised placebo-controlled study 18 healthy subjects were given **ketoconazole** 400 mg before and after taking rabeprazole 20 mg daily or a placebo for 7 days. Significant decreases in the **ketoconazole** AUC and maximum serum levels were found,[13] representing about a 30% reduction in its bioavailability.[14] There was no evidence that **ketoconazole** affected rabeprazole metabolism.

Mechanism

Ketoconazole and itraconazole are poorly soluble bases, which must be transformed by the acid in the stomach into the soluble hydrochloride salt. Agents that reduce gastric secretions, such as proton pump inhibitors, 'H_2-receptor antagonists', (p.217), or 'antacids', (p.215), raise the pH in the stomach so that the dissolution and absorption of drugs such as itraconazole or ketoconazole are reduced. Conversely, anything that increases the gastric acidity increases their dissolution and absorption.[8]

Fluconazole and voriconazole almost certainly cause a rise in omeprazole and esomeprazole levels by inhibiting their metabolism by the cytochrome P450 isoenzymes CYP2C19 and CYP3A4. As esomeprazole is an inhibitor of and also a substrate for CYP2C19, it is likely to have the same effect as omeprazole.[1] Ketoconazole only inhibits CYP3A4 and therefore causes a less marked rise in omeprazole levels. Itraconazole would be expected to interact similarly to ketoconazole.

Importance and management

The interaction between **ketoconazole** and omeprazole appears to be established and of clinical importance. Direct evidence seems to be limited to this study, but other drugs that raise the gastric pH have a similar effect (see 'Azoles + Antacids', p.215 or 'H_2-receptor antagonists', p.217). Such a large reduction in the absorption of ketoconazole would be expected to result in the failure of treatment. Separating the dosages of the two drugs is unlikely to be the answer because the effect of omeprazole is so prolonged. An alternative would simply be to monitor for any inadequate response to ketoconazole if omeprazole or esomeprazole is also given and to raise the dosage if necessary. However, bear in mind that ketoconazole can double omeprazole levels, although the clinical relevance of this is uncertain. Giving ketoconazole with an acidic drink[8] such as 'cola', (p.215), appears to minimise the interaction, and is recommended by some manufacturers of ketoconazole for patients taking proton pump inhibitors.[15]

The interaction between ketoconazole and rabeprazole is also established, but the reduction in the bioavailability is only moderate (30%) and it may be possible to accommodate this by raising the antifungal dosage.

There seem to be no reports about ketoconazole and other proton pump inhibitors but they are also expected to interact to reduce the bioavailability of the ketoconazole, but the extent is not known.

The interaction between **itraconazole** and omeprazole also appears to be established, but it appears that this can be minimised by using an oral itraconazole solution. As with ketoconazole, giving itraconazole with an acidic drink such as 'cola', (p.215) would minimise the interaction, and is recommended by some manufacturers of itraconazole for patients taking proton pump inhibitors.[16,17] Monitor patients taking itraconazole if proton pump inhibitors are also given. The effect of itraconazole on omeprazole is unknown, but it might be expected to increase omeprazole levels similarly to ketoconazole.

The interaction between **voriconazole** and omeprazole is established but no adjustment to the dose of voriconazole is required.[12,18] The clinical importance of the marked rise in serum omeprazole levels caused by voriconazole is not established, but the manufacturers recommend that the omeprazole dose be halved,[12,18] although the US manufacturers restrict this to patients taking omeprazole 40 mg or more.[12] The increase in levels of esomeprazole by voriconazole does not routinely require a dose adjustment of esomeprazole However, patients taking esomeprazole in doses of more than 240 mg daily (e.g. for Zollinger-Ellison syndrome) may require a dose adjustment.[2]

Fluconazole is not affected by omeprazole, and is unlikely to be affected by other proton pump inhibitors. However, fluconazole markedly increases omeprazole levels. The clinical relevance of these changes is uncertain, but not likely to be important for single-dose fluconazole regimens. More study is needed to establish whether it is advisable to reduce the omeprazole dose in those given both drugs longer-term.

Because of the possibility that **posaconazole** levels might be reduced by proton pump inhibitors, the manufacturer currently recommends that concurrent use be avoided if possible.[10] Further study is needed.

1. Nexium Tablets (Esomeprazole magnesium trihydrate). AstraZeneca UK Ltd. UK Summary of product characteristics, May 2007.
2. Nexium (Esomeprazole magnesium). AstraZeneca. US Prescribing information, April 2007.
3. Zimmermann T, Yeates RA, Riedel K-D, Lach P, Laufen H. The influence of gastric pH on the pharmacokinetics of fluconazole: the effect of omeprazole. *Int J Clin Pharmacol Ther* (1994) 32, 491–6.
4. Kang BC, Yang CQ, Cho HK, Suh OK, Shin WG. Influence of fluconazole on the pharmacokinetics of omeprazole in healthy volunteers. *Biopharm Drug Dispos* (2002) 23, 77–81.
5. Jaruratanasirikul S, Sriwiriyajan S. Effect of omeprazole on the pharmacokinetics of itraconazole. *Eur J Clin Pharmacol* (1998) 54, 159–61.
6. Johnson MD, Hamilton CD, Drew RH, Sanders LL, Pennick GJ, Perfect JR. A randomized comparative study to determine the effect of omeprazole on the peak serum concentration of itraconazole oral solution. *J Antimicrob Chemother* (2003) 51, 453–7.
7. Levron JC, Chwetzoff E, Le Moing JP, Lappereau-Gallot A, Chrétien P. Lack of interaction of antacid drug omeprazole on the bioavailability of itraconazole oral solution. *Blood* (1998) 92 (Suppl 1, part 2), 54b.
8. Chin TWF, Loeb M, Fong IW. Effects of an acidic beverage (Coca-Cola) on absorption of ketoconazole. *Antimicrob Agents Chemother* (1995) 39, 1671–5.

9. Böttiger Y, Tybring G, Götharson E, Bertilsson L. Inhibition of the sulfoxidation of omeprazole by ketoconazole in poor and extensive metabolizers of S-mephenytoin. *Clin Pharmacol Ther* (1997) 62, 384–91.
10. Noxafil (Posaconazole). Schering-Plough Ltd. UK Summary of product characteristics, October 2006.
11. Wood N, Tan K, Purkins L, Layton G, Hamlin J, Kleinermans D, Nichols D. Effect of omeprazole on the steady-state pharmacokinetics of voriconazole. *Br J Clin Pharmacol* (2003) 56, 56–61.
12. VFEND (Voriconazole). Pfizer Inc. US Prescribing information, November 2006.
13. Humphries TJ, Nardi RV, Spera AC, Lazar JD, Laurent AL, Spanyers SA. Coadministration of rabeprazole sodium (E3810) and ketoconazole results in a predictable interaction with ketoconazole. *Gastroenterology* (1996) 110 (Suppl), A138.
14. Personal communication. Eisai Corporation of North America, October 1996.
15. Nizoral Tablets (Ketoconazole). Janssen-Cilag Ltd. UK Summary of product characteristics, October 2006.
16. Sporanox Capsules (Itraconazole). Janssen-Cilag Ltd. UK Summary of product characteristics, March 2004.
17. Sporanox Capsules (Itraconazole). Janssen. US Prescribing information, June 2006.
18. VFEND (Voriconazole). Pfizer Ltd. UK Summary of product characteristics, July 2007.

Azoles + Rifabutin

Rifabutin levels are increased by fluconazole, posaconazole, voriconazole, and possibly itraconazole. Patients taking this combination are at increased risk of rifabutin toxicity, specifically uveitis, and should be closely monitored. Rifabutin markedly reduces the plasma levels of itraconazole, posaconazole, and voriconazole. These azoles should be used cautiously with rifabutin, if at all. Rifabutin does not affect the metabolism of fluconazole.

Clinical evidence

(a) Fluconazole

Twelve HIV positive patients were given zidovudine 500 mg daily from day 1 to 44, fluconazole 200 mg daily from days 3 to 30 and rifabutin 300 mg daily from days 17 to 44. Rifabutin did not significantly affect the pharmacokinetics of fluconazole,[1] but fluconazole increased the AUC of rifabutin by 82%, and the AUC of the rifabutin metabolite LM565 was increased by 216%.[1] In another study in 10 patients with HIV infection, fluconazole 200 mg daily increased the AUC of rifabutin 300 mg daily by 76% and the maximum level by 91%. When the patients were also given clarithromycin 500 mg daily, the AUC of rifabutin was further increased to 152%.[2] There is some evidence that fluconazole increases the prophylactic efficacy of rifabutin against *M. avium* complex disease, although there was also an increase in incidence of leucopenia.[3] Uveitis developed in 6 HIV positive patients taking rifabutin 450 to 600 mg daily and fluconazole, 5 of whom were also taking clarithromycin,[4] which is also known to increase rifabutin levels, see 'Macrolides + Rifamycins', p.316. Uveitis has been attributed to the concurrent use of rifabutin and fluconazole in other reports.[5,6] Rifabutin does not appear to significantly affect the metabolism of fluconazole.[7,8]

(b) Itraconazole

1. Itraconazole serum levels reduced. In a three-period study, 6 HIV positive patients were given itraconazole 200 mg daily for 14 days, rifabutin 300 mg daily for 10 days, and then both drugs for 14 days. It was found that the rifabutin reduced the peak plasma levels of the itraconazole by 71% and reduced its AUC by 74%.[9]

2. Rifabutin serum levels raised. A 49-year-old HIV positive man taking rifabutin 300 mg daily was also given itraconazole 600 mg daily. Because of low plasma levels after 3 weeks the itraconazole dose was increased to 900 mg daily. A week later the patient developed anterior uveitis. It was found that the itraconazole trough serum levels were normal but rifabutin trough serum levels were raised to 153 nanograms/mL (expected to be less than 50 nanograms/mL after 24 hours). Rifabutin was stopped and the uveitis was treated. Symptoms resolved after 5 days.[10]

(c) Posaconazole

In a study in healthy subjects the concurrent use of posaconazole 200 mg once daily and rifabutin 300 mg once daily for 10 days increased the AUC of rifabutin by 72% and decreased the AUC of posaconazole by 51% when compared with either drug alone.[11]

(d) Voriconazole

Rifabutin 300 mg daily decreased the AUC and maximum plasma levels of voriconazole 200 mg twice daily by 79% and 67%, respectively. Increasing the dose of voriconazole to 350 mg twice daily in the presence of rifabutin gave an AUC of 68% of that achieved with voriconazole 200 mg twice daily alone while maximum plasma levels were more or less the same.[12,13] At a dose of 400 mg twice daily, voriconazole increased the maximum plasma level and AUC of rifabutin 300 mg twice daily by about threefold and fourfold, respectively.[12,13]

Mechanism

Rifabutin increases the metabolism of itraconazole, posaconazole and voriconazole, probably, at least in part, by inducing their metabolism by the cytochrome P450 CYP3A subfamily. Fluconazole is largely excreted unchanged in the urine and so it is not affected. The azoles apparently increase rifabutin levels by inhibiting its metabolism, probably by CYP3A4. Raised rifabutin levels can cause uveitis.

Importance and management

The interaction between rifabutin and **fluconazole** is established, the general picture being that concurrent use can be advantageous. However, because of the increased risk of uveitis, the UK Committee on Safety of Medicines says that full consideration should be given to reducing the dosage of rifabutin to 300 mg daily. The rifabutin should be stopped if uveitis develops and the patient referred to an ophthalmologist.[14] A later review suggests this 300 mg dose is associated with a reduced risk of uveitis and maintains efficacy.[15] The combination should be well monitored. Note that the effects of 'clarithromycin', (p.316), are additive with those of fluconazole.

Information on the interaction between **itraconazole** and rifabutin is very limited, but monitor for reduced antifungal activity, raising the itraconazole dosage as necessary, and watch for increased rifabutin levels and toxicity (in particular uveitis). More study is needed. Note that the manufacturers recommend that the combination should be avoided.[16,17]

The manufacturer of **ketoconazole** suggests that the levels of both drugs may be affected if rifabutin is also taken. They suggest that the rifabutin dose may need to be reduced.[18]

On the basis of the interaction between rifabutin and **posaconazole**, the manufacturer suggests that the combination be avoided unless the benefit to the patient outweighs the risk.[19] If the combination is used, monitor the efficacy of posaconazole and the toxicity of rifabutin, particularly full blood counts and uveitis.

The manufacturer in the US contraindicates the combination of **voriconazole** and rifabutin.[13] However, the UK manufacturer permits concurrent use if the benefits outweigh the risks.[12] If used together, it is recommended that the oral dose of voriconazole be increased from 200 mg twice daily to 350 mg twice daily (and from 100 to 200 mg twice daily in patients under 40 kg). The intravenous dose should also be increased from 4 to 5 mg/kg twice daily. Importantly, the manufacturer advises careful monitoring for rifabutin adverse effects (e.g. check full blood counts, monitor for uveitis).[12]

1. Trapnell CB, Narang PK, Li R, Lavelle JP. Increased plasma rifabutin levels with concomitant fluconazole therapy in HIV-infected patients. *Ann Intern Med* (1996) 124, 573–6.
2. Jordan MK, Polis MA, Kelly G, Narang PK, Masur H, Piscitelli SC. Effects of fluconazole and clarithromycin on rifabutin and 25-*O*-desacetylrifabutin pharmacokinetics. *Antimicrob Agents Chemother* (2000) 44, 2170–2.
3. Narang PK, Trapnell CB, Schoenfelder JR, Lavelle JP, Bianchine JR. Fluconazole and enhanced effect of rifabutin prophylaxis. *N Engl J Med* (1994) 330, 1316–17.
4. Becker K, Schimkat M, Jablonowski H, Häussinger D. Anterior uveitis associated with rifabutin medication in AIDS patients. *Infection* (1996) 24, 34–6.
5. Fuller JD, Stanfield LED, Craven DE. Rifabutin prophylaxis and uveitis. *N Engl J Med* (1994) 330, 1315–16.
6. Kelleher P, Helbert M, Sweeney J, Anderson J, Parkin J, Pinching A. Uveitis associated with rifabutin and macrolide therapy for *Mycobacterium avium intracellulare* infections in AIDS patients. *Genitourin Med* (1996) 72, 419–21.
7. Mycobutin (Rifabutin). Pfizer Inc. US Prescribing information, February 2006.
8. Mycobutin (Rifabutin). Pharmacia Ltd. UK Summary of product characteristics, October 2006.
9. Smith JA, Hardin TC, Patterson TF, Rinaldi MG, Graybill JR. Rifabutin (RIF) decreases itraconazole (ITRA) plasma levels in patients with HIV-infection. Am Soc Microbiol 2nd Nat Conf. Human retroviruses and related infections. Washington DC, Jan 29—Feb 2 1995, 77.
10. Lefort A, Launay O, Carbon C. Uveitis associated with rifabutin prophylaxis and itraconazole therapy. *Ann Intern Med* (1996) 125, 939–40.
11. Courtney RD, Statkevich P, Laughlin M, Radwanski E, Lim J, Clement RP, Batra VK. Potential for a drug interaction between posaconazole and rifabutin. *Intersci Conf Antimicrob Agents Chemother* (2001) 41, 4–5.
12. VFEND (Voriconazole). Pfizer Ltd. UK Summary of product characteristics, July 2007.
13. VFEND (Voriconazole). Pfizer Inc. US Prescribing information, November 2006.
14. Committee on Safety of Medicines/Medicines Control Agency. Stop Press: Rifabutin (Mycobutin) — uveitis. *Current Problems* (1994) 20, 4.
15. Committee on the Safety of Medicines/Medicines Control Agency. Revised indications and drug interactions of rifabutin. *Current Problems* (1997) 23, 14.
16. Sporanox Capsules (Itraconazole). Janssen-Cilag Ltd. UK Summary of product characteristics, March 2004.

17. Sporanox Capsules (Itraconazole). Janssen. US Prescribing information, June 2006.
18. Nizoral Tablets (Ketoconazole). Janssen-Cilag Ltd. UK Summary of product characteristics, October 2006.
19. Noxafil (Posaconazole). Schering-Plough Ltd. UK Summary of product characteristics, October 2006.

Azoles + Rifampicin (Rifampin) and/or Isoniazid

Although rifampicin causes only a modest increase in fluconazole clearance, the reduction in its effects may possibly be clinically important. Fluconazole does not appear to affect rifampicin pharmacokinetics. There is an isolated report of hypercalcaemia in a patient taking both fluconazole and rifampicin.
Rifampicin very markedly reduces serum itraconazole levels. This can reduce or abolish the antifungal effects of the itraconazole, possibly depending on the infection being treated.
The serum levels of ketoconazole can be reduced by 50 to 90% by rifampicin and/or isoniazid. Serum rifampicin levels can also be halved by ketoconazole, but are possibly unaffected if the drugs are given 12 hours apart.
Rifampicin markedly reduces voriconazole levels, and the combination should be avoided. Posaconazole is predicted to be similarly affected.

Clinical evidence

(a) Fluconazole

1. Fluconazole levels reduced. In a study in healthy subjects.rifampicin 600 mg daily for 19 days reduced the AUC of a single 200-mg dose of oral fluconazole by 23% and decreased the half-life by 19%.[1]
Similarly, a study in two groups of 12 patients with AIDS found that the AUC and peak plasma level of fluconazole 400 mg daily given for cryptococcal meningitis were reduced by 22% and 17% by rifampicin 600 mg daily when compared with the 12 patients not given rifampicin. The elimination rate constant of fluconazole was increased by 39% and the elimination half life was reduced by 28%. There were no significant changes in clinical outcome although the subsequent use of a lower prophylactic dose of fluconazole 200 mg with rifampicin was found to result in levels of fluconazole below the MIC of the infecting organism.[2] Also, 3 patients with AIDS being treated for cryptococcal meningitis with fluconazole 400 mg daily relapsed when rifampicin was added.[3] Another report briefly states that one of 5 patients taking fluconazole needed an increased dosage or a replacement antifungal when given rifampicin.[4]
In yet another study, the AUC of *intravenous* fluconazole was 52% lower in 2 patients also taking rifampicin than in 3 other patients not taking rifampicin.[5]

2. Rifampicin (Rifampin) levels unchanged. A study in 11 AIDS patients with cryptococcal meningitis found that fluconazole 200 mg twice daily for 14 days had no effect on the pharmacokinetics of rifampicin 300 mg daily.[6] Five AIDS patients with tuberculosis, taking rifampicin and fluconazole, had normal rifampicin levels compared with 14 similar patients taking rifampicin alone, but in both groups rifampicin levels were only about 28% of those predicted.[7]

3. Hypercalcaemia. There is an isolated report of severe hypercalcaemia attributed to the use of rifampicin and fluconazole in a patient with tuberculosis and pneumocystosis.[8] The clinical relevance of this case is uncertain.

(b) Itraconazole

A patient receiving antitubercular treatment including rifampicin 600 mg and isoniazid 300 mg daily was also given itraconazole 200 mg daily. After 2 weeks his serum itraconazole levels were negligible (0.011 mg/L). Even when the dosage was doubled the levels only reached a maximum of 0.056 mg/L. When the antitubercular drugs were stopped his serum itraconazole level was 3.23 mg/L with a 300 mg daily dose, and 2.35 to 2.6 mg/L with a 200 mg daily dose.[9]

A later study in 8 other patients confirmed that itraconazole levels were reduced by rifampicin but the clinical outcome depended on the mycosis being treated. Four out of 5 patients responded to treatment for a *Cryptococcus neoformans* infection, despite undetectable itraconazole levels, apparently because *in vitro* there is synergy between the two drugs. In contrast, 2 patients with coccidioidomycosis failed to respond, and 2 others with cryptococcosis suffered a relapse or persistence of seborrhoeic dermatitis (possibly due to *M. furfur*) while taking both drugs.[10] In a patient with AIDS the serum levels of itraconazole 400 to 600 mg daily in divided doses were undetectable in the presence of rifampicin, and took 3 to 5 days to recover after the rifampicin was stopped.[11] Undetectable itraconazole levels occurred in another patient given rifampicin who was treated for histoplasmosis.[12] In contrast, a study found that the AUC of a single 100-mg dose of itraconazole was reduced by 80% after 6 healthy subjects took rifampicin 600 mg daily for 3 days.[13] Very markedly reduced serum itraconazole levels (undetectable in some instances) have been seen in other healthy subjects and AIDS patients when given rifampicin.[14] Retrospective review of the medical records of 2 patients given itraconazole and rifampicin indicated that itraconazole was not effective until rifampicin was stopped, based on the finding of continued weight loss while on the combination, and a clear weight gain after rifampicin was stopped.[15]

(c) Ketoconazole

1. Ketoconazole levels. Rifampicin 600 mg daily reduced the AUC of ketoconazole 200 mg by 80% in a study in 6 healthy subjects.[16] Similarly, the serum levels of ketoconazole 200 mg daily were roughly halved by rifampicin 600 mg in one patient. After 5 months of concurrent use with rifampicin and **isoniazid** 300 mg daily, there was a ninefold decrease in peak serum levels and the AUC was reduced by nearly 90%.[17]
A study in a 3-year-old child who had responded poorly to treatment found that peak serum levels and AUC of ketoconazole were reduced by about 65 to 80% by rifampicin and/or **isoniazid**. The interaction also occurred when the dosages were separated by 12 hours. When all three drugs were given together the ketoconazole serum levels were undetectable.[18] Other reports confirm these reports of decreased ketoconazole levels with rifampicin.[19-23]

2. Rifampicin levels. The addition of ketoconazole 200 mg twice daily for one day then 200 mg once daily for 2 days to rifampicin 600 mg daily had little effect on the peak level and AUC of rifampicin in a study in 6 healthy subjects.[16] In contrast, the rifampicin serum levels of a child were roughly halved by ketoconazole, but when the rifampicin was given 12 hours after the ketoconazole, the serum levels of rifampicin were unaffected.[18] Other studies also show a reduction in rifampicin levels caused by ketoconazole,[21-23] one confirming that separation of the drugs by 12 hours minimised the interaction.[21]

(d) Voriconazole

The manufacturer[24] notes that rifampicin 600 mg once daily decreased the maximum plasma levels and AUC of voriconazole 200 mg twice daily by about 95%. Even doubling the dose of voriconazole did not give adequate exposure.[24] The concurrent use of voriconazole and rifampicin is therefore contraindicated.[24,25]

Mechanism

Rifampicin increases the metabolism of the azole antifungals by the liver. However, as fluconazole (unlike ketoconazole, itraconazole and voriconazole) is mainly excreted unchanged in the urine, changes to its metabolism would not be expected to have as marked an effect as on these other azoles.

The absorption of antitubercular drugs may be reduced in patients with AIDS and an increase in rifampicin levels may be due to increased absorption in the presence of fluconazole.[7] In contrast, it is suggested that ketoconazole impairs the absorption of rifampicin from the gut. Just how isoniazid interacts is uncertain.

Importance and management

The interaction between rifampicin and **fluconazole** appears to be established and of clinical importance. Although rifampicin has only a modest effect on fluconazole, the cases of relapse cited above[3] and the need for an increased dosage[4] indicate that this interaction can be clinically important. Monitor concurrent use and increase the fluconazole dosage if necessary. One study suggests a 30% increase in fluconazole dose may be considered for serious infections during concurrent rifampicin therapy. This may be especially important during prophylaxis of cryptococcal meningitis with lower doses of fluconazole, such as 200 mg daily.[2]

The interaction between **itraconazole** and rifampicin is established and clinically important. Monitor the effects of concurrent use, being alert for the need to increase the itraconazole dosage. The effect on serum itraconazole levels can be very marked indeed. The clinical importance of this interaction can apparently depend on the mycosis being treated. Note that the manufacturer considers that itraconazole should not be used with rifampicin, since its levels are so markedly reduced.[26,27]

The interactions between **ketoconazole** and rifampicin appear to be established and of clinical importance, but there is very much less information about the interaction with isoniazid. The effects on rifampicin can apparently be avoided by giving the ketoconazole at a different time (12 hours apart seems to be effective) but this does not solve the problem of the effects on ketoconazole. The dosage of at least one of the drugs will need to be increased to achieve both good antitubercular and antifungal responses. Concurrent use should be well monitored and dosage increases made if necessary. One manufacturer suggests that the combination should be avoided.[28]

The manufacturer predicts that **posaconazole** levels may be significantly lowered when used with rifampicin. They suggest that the combination be avoided unless the benefit to the patient outweighs the risk.[29]

Voriconazole levels are very markedly reduced by rifampicin and concurrent use is contraindicated.[24,25]

1. Apseloff G, Hilligoss M, Gardner MJ, Henry EB, Inskeep PB, Gerber N, Lazar JD. Induction of fluconazole metabolism by rifampin: *in vivo* study in humans. *J Clin Pharmacol* (1991) 31, 358–61.
2. Panomvana Na Ayudhya D, Thanompuangseree N, Tansuphaswadikul S. Effect of rifampicin on the pharmacokinetics of fluconazole in patients with AIDS. *Clin Pharmacokinet* (2004) 43, 725–32.
3. Coker RJ, Tomlinson DR, Parkin J, Harris JRW, Pinching AJ. Interaction between fluconazole and rifampicin. *BMJ* (1990) 301, 818.
4. Tett S, Carey D, Lee H-S. Drug interactions with fluconazole. *Med J Aust* (1992) 156, 365.
5. Nicolau DP, Crowe HM, Nightingale CH, Quintiliani R. Rifampin-fluconazole interaction in critically ill patients. *Ann Pharmacother* (1995) 29, 994–6.
6. Jaruratanasirikul S, Kleepaew A. Lack of effect of fluconazole on the pharmacokinetics of rifampicin in AIDS patients. *J Antimicrob Chemother* (1996) 38, 877–80.
7. Peloquin CA, Nitta AT, Burman WJ, Brudney KF, Miranda-Massari JR, McGuinness ME, Berning SE, Gerena GT. Low antituberculosis drug concentrations in patients with AIDS. *Ann Pharmacother* (1996) 30, 919–25.
8. Bani-Sadr F, Hoff J, Chiffoleau A, Allavena C, Raffi F. Hypercalcémie sévère chez une patiente traitée par fluconazole et rifampicine. *Presse Med* (1998) 27, 860.
9. Blomley M, Teare EL, de Belder A, Thway Y, Weston M. Itraconazole and anti-tuberculosis drugs. *Lancet* (1990) ii, 1255.
10. Tucker RM, Denning DW, Hanson LH, Rinaldi MG, Graybill JR, Sharkey PK, Pappagianis D, Stevens DA. Interaction of azoles with rifampin, phenytoin and carbamazepine: *in vitro* and clinical observations. *Clin Infect Dis* (1992) 14, 165–74.
11. Drayton J, Dickinson G, Rinaldi MG. Coadministration of rifampin and itraconazole leads to undetectable levels of serum itraconazole. *Clin Infect Dis* (1994) 18, 266.
12. Hecht FM, Wheat J, Korzun AH, Hafner R, Skahan KJ, Larsen R, Limjoco MT, Simpson M, Schneider D, Keefer MC, Clark R, Lai KK, Jacobsen JM, Squires K, Bartlett JA, Powderly W. Itraconazole maintenance treatment for histoplasmosis in AIDS: a prospective, multicenter trial. *J Acquir Immune Defic Syndr Hum Retrovirol* (1997) 16, 100–107.
13. Heykants J, Michiels M, Meuldermans W, Monbaliu J, Lavrijsen K, Van Peer A, Levron JC, Woestenborghs R, Cauwenbergh G. The pharmacokinetics of itraconazole in animals and man: an overview. In: Fromtling RA, ed. Recent Trends in the Discovery, Development and Evaluation of Antifungal Agents. SA: JR Prous Science Publishers, 1987 p 223–49.
14. Jaruratanasirikul S, Sriwiriyajan S. Effect of rifampicin on the pharmacokinetics of itraconazole in normal volunteers and AIDS patients. *Eur J Clin Pharmacol* (1998) 54, 155–8.
15. Todd JR, Arigala MR, Penn RL, King JW. Case report: possible clinically significant interaction of itraconazole plus rifampin. *AIDS Patient Care STDS* (2001) 15, 505–10.
16. Doble N, Shaw R, Rowland-Hill C, Lush M, Warnock DW, Keal EE. Pharmacokinetic study of the interaction between rifampicin and ketoconazole. *J Antimicrob Chemother* (1988) 21, 633–5.
17. Brass C, Galgiani JN, Blaschke TF, Defelice R, O'Reilly RA, Stevens DA. Disposition of ketoconazole, an oral antifungal, in humans. *Antimicrob Agents Chemother* (1982) 21, 151–8.
18. Engelhard D, Stutman HR,Marks MI. Interaction of ketoconazole with rifampin and isoniazid. *N Engl J Med* (1984) 311, 1681–3.
19. Drouhet E, Dupont B. Laboratory and clinical assessment of ketoconazole in deep-seated mycoses. *Am J Med* (1983) 74, 30–47.
20. Meunier F. Serum fungistatic and fungicidal activity in volunteers receiving antifungal agents. *Eur J Clin Microbiol* (1986) 5, 103–9.
21. Doble N, Hykin P, Shaw R, Keal EE. Pulmonary mycobacterium tuberculosis in acquired immune deficiency syndrome. *BMJ* (1985) 291, 849–50.
22. Abadie-Kemmerly S, Pankey GA, Dalvisio JR. Failure of ketoconazole treatment of *Blastomyces dermatidis* due to interaction of isoniazid and rifampin. *Ann Intern Med* (1988) 109, 844–5.
23. Pilheu JA, Galati MR, Yunis AS, De Salvo MC, Negroni R, Garcia Fernandez JC, Mingolla L, Rubio MC, Masana M, Acevedo C. Interaccion farmacocinetica entre ketoconazol, isoniacida y rifampicina. *Medicina (B Aires)* (1989) 49, 43–7.
24. VFEND (Voriconazole). Pfizer Inc. US Prescribing information, November 2006.
25. VFEND (Voriconazole). Pfizer Ltd. UK Summary of product characteristics, July 2007.
26. Sporanox Capsules (Itraconazole). Janssen-Cilag Ltd. UK Summary of product characteristics, March 2004.
27. Sporanox Capsules (Itraconazole). Janssen. US Prescribing information, June 2006.
28. Nizoral Tablets (Ketoconazole). Janssen. US Prescribing information, April 2001.
29. Noxafil (Posaconazole). Schering-Plough Ltd. UK Summary of product characteristics, October 2006.

Azoles + Sucralfate

The gastrointestinal absorption of ketoconazole is modestly reduced by sucralfate. The absorption of fluconazole appears not be to significantly affected by sucralfate.

Clinical evidence

(a) Fluconazole

Sucralfate 2 g was found to have no significant effect on the pharmacokinetics of a single 200-mg dose of fluconazole in 10 healthy subjects, confirming the results of an *in vitro* study.[1]

(b) Ketoconazole

A study[2] in 6 fasting healthy subjects found that sucralfate 1 g given 2 hours before ketoconazole 400 mg reduced its AUC by about 20%. Another study in fasting healthy subjects found that sucralfate 1 g given with glutamic acid hydrochloride reduced the AUC and maximum serum levels of a single 100-mg dose of ketoconazole by about 25%, but no significant changes were seen when the ketoconazole was given 2 hours after the sucralfate.[3]

Mechanism

There is *in vitro* evidence that an electrostatic interaction occurs between ketoconazole and sucralfate to form an ion pair that cannot pass through the gut wall.[4]

Importance and management

The interaction of sucralfate with ketoconazole is modest and of uncertain clinical importance. Any interaction may be minimised by taking sucralfate not less than 2 to 3 hours before or after the ketoconazole.

Fluconazole does not interact with sucralfate.

1. Carver PL, Hoeschele JD, Partipilo L, Kauffman CA, Mercer BT, Pecoraro VL. Fluconazole: a model compound for in vitro and in vivo interactions with sucralfate. *Pharmacotherapy* (1994) 14, 347.
2. Piscitelli SC, Goss TF, Wilton JH, D'Andrea DT, Goldstein H, Schentag JJ. Effects of ranitidine and sucralfate on ketoconazole bioavailability. *Antimicrob Agents Chemother* (1991) 35, 1765–71.
3. Carver PL, Berardi RR, Knapp MJ, Rider JM, Kauffman CA, Bradley SF, Atassi M. In vivo interaction of ketoconazole and sucralfate in healthy volunteers. *Antimicrob Agents Chemother* (1994) 38, 326–9.
4. Hoeschele JD, Roy AK, Pecoraro VL, Carver PL. In vitro analysis of the interaction between sucralfate and ketoconazole. *Antimicrob Agents Chemother* (1994) 38, 319–25.

Azoles; Fluconazole + Hydrochlorothiazide

Hydrochlorothiazide modestly increases the levels of fluconazole, but this is unlikely to be clinically relevant.

Clinical evidence, mechanism, importance and management

The manufacturer notes that, in 13 healthy subjects, hydrochlorothiazide 50 mg daily increased the AUC and plasma levels of fluconazole 100 mg daily for 10 days by about 40%.[1,2] They attribute these changes to a reduction in the renal clearance of fluconazole.[2] However they say it is unlikely that a change in the fluconazole dosage will be needed in patients taking diuretics, but that the interaction should be borne in mind.[1] Any interaction is almost certainly of no relevance in patients taking a single dose of fluconazole for genital candidiasis.

1. Diflucan (Fluconazole). Pfizer Ltd. UK Summary of product characteristics, April 2007.
2. Diflucan (Fluconazole). Pfizer Inc. US Prescribing information, August 2004.

Azoles; Itraconazole + Grapefruit and other fruit juices

Grapefruit juice impaired the absorption of itraconazole capsules in one study, but not in another. Grapefruit juice had no effect on the absorption of itraconazole oral solution. Orange juice impaired the absorption of itraconazole capsules in one study.

Clinical evidence

(a) Capsules

In one study, either 240 mL of double-strength **grapefruit juice** or water were given with, and 2 hours after a single 200-mg dose of itraconazole *(Sporanox capsules, Janssen)* to 11 healthy subjects immediately after a standard breakfast. **Grapefruit juice**, unexpectedly decreased the AUC of itraconazole on average by 43% (range 81% reduction to 105% increase), with a similar decrease in hydroxy-itraconazole levels.[1] However, another similar study found that **grapefruit juice** had no effect on the pharmacokinetics of itraconazole capsules *(Itrizole, Janssen)*. The only apparent differences in this study were that itraconazole was given at the lower dose of 100 mg, and that 350 mL of single-strength **grapefruit juice** was used.[2] Furthermore, in this study,[2] **orange juice** reduced the AUC of itraconazole by an average of 41%.

(b) Oral solution

A small 17% increase in the AUC of itraconazole was seen in 20 healthy subjects when given grapefruit juice. In this study, regular strength grapefruit juice 240 mL was given three times daily for 2 days, then together with itraconazole oral solution 200 mg on the morning of the third day in the fasted state, then again 2 hours later.[3]

Mechanism

As grapefruit juice is an inhibitor of intestinal cytochrome P450 isoenzyme CYP3A4, the major enzyme involved in itraconazole metabolism, it was predicted that it would enhance itraconazole absorption. Appearing to confirm this, a small increase in itraconazole levels was seen with itraconazole oral solution. However, with itraconazole capsules, one study showed decreased levels and one no change. The mechanism is not known, but grapefruit juice may impair the absorption of itraconazole capsules either by affecting P-glycoprotein or lowering the duodenal pH.[1]

Importance and management

The 40% reduction in itraconazole levels from itraconazole capsules seen with grapefruit juice would be anticipated to be clinically relevant in some situations, but it was seen in only one of two single-dose studies. Similarly, the reduction in levels with orange juice might be clinically relevant. However, at present, there is insufficient evidence to recommend avoiding concurrent use. Until more is known, in the event of unexpected inefficacy or low levels of itraconazole, bear the possibility in mind that grapefruit juice or orange juice may be a factor. Itraconazole oral solution, which is better absorbed than the capsules, did not appear to be affected by grapefruit juice.

1. Penzak SR, Gubbins PO, Gurley BJ, Wang P-L, Saccente M. Grapefruit juice decreases the systemic availability of itraconazole capsules in healthy volunteers. *Ther Drug Monit* (1999) 21, 304–309.
2. Kawakami M, Suzuki K, Ishizuka T, Hidaka T, Matsuki Y, Nakumara H. Effect of grapefruit juice on pharmacokinetics of itraconazole in healthy subjects. *Int J Clin Pharmacol Ther* (1998) 36, 306–308.
3. Gubbins PO, McConnell SA, Gurley BJ, Fincher TK, Franks AM, Williams DK, Penzak SR, Saccente M. Influence of grapefruit juice on the systemic availability of itraconazole oral solution in healthy adult volunteers. *Pharmacotherapy* (2004) 24, 460–7.

Azoles; Topical + Miscellaneous

Butoconazole, clotrimazole and fenticonazole are absorbed very poorly from the vagina so that the risk of an interaction with other drugs given systemically is small. Similarly, econazole, oxiconazole and sertaconazole are minimally absorbed through the skin, and would not be expected to cause drug interactions. However, note that there have been a few cases of miconazole cream or pessaries interacting with oral anticoagulants, see 'Coumarins and related drugs + Azoles; Miconazole', p.388.

Clinical evidence, mechanism, importance and management

(a) Intravaginal application

The manufacturer notes that 1.3% to 2.2% of the dose of intravaginal **butoconazole** cream 2% was absorbed in a study in three women.[1]

Early studies with intravaginal **clotrimazole** revealed that only a small fraction (3 to 10% of the dose) was absorbed systemically, and that this was rapidly metabolised.[2]

A study in 14 women (5 of them healthy, 4 with relapsing vulvovaginal candidiasis, and 5 with cervical carcinoma) found that the systemic absorption of **fenticonazole** nitrate from a single 1-g pessary was very small indeed. The amount absorbed, based on the amount recovered from the urine and faeces over 5 days, ranged from 0.58 to 1.81% of the original dose.[3]

The risk of a clinically relevant interaction with other drugs that may be present in the body would therefore seem to be very small with these antifungals used vaginally. However, for a few reports of raised INRs in women taking oral anticoagulants while using intravaginal miconazole, see 'Coumarins and related drugs + Azoles; Miconazole', p.388.

(b) Topical application to the skin

After topical application to the skin of normal subjects, systemic absorption was extremely low and less than 1% of the applied dose of **econazole** was recovered in the urine and faeces.[4] Systemically administered econazole does inhibit cytochrome P450 isoenzymes, but because of the low systemic availability after topical application, one manufacturer notes that clinically relevant interactions are rare.[5]

The manufacturer of **oxiconazole** notes that systemic absorption is low, and in healthy subjects less than 0.3% of the applied dose was recovered in the urine after topical application of the cream.[6]

Plasma levels of **sertaconazole** were below the limit of detection (2.5 nanograms/mL) when 5 patients with interdigital tinea pedis applied sertaconazole cream 2% every 2 hours for a total of 13 doses.[7]

Based on this information the risk of a clinically relevant drug interaction with systemically administered drugs and these topical azoles would seem to be very small. However, for a case report of raised INR in a man taking warfarin while using miconazole cream for a groin infection, see 'Coumarins and related drugs + Azoles; Miconazole', p.388.

1. Gynazole 1 (Butoconazole). Ther-Rx Corp. US Prescribing information, August 2003.
2. Ritter W. Pharmacokinetic fundamentals of vaginal treatment with clotrimazole. *Am J Obstet Gynecol* (1985) 152, 945–7.
3. Novelli A, Periti E, Massi GB, Mazzei T, Periti P. Systemic absorption of 3H-fenticonazole after vaginal administration of 1 gram in patients. *J Chemother* (1991) 3, 23–7.
4. Spectazole (Econazole). Ortho Pharmaceutical Corp. US Prescribing information, June 1996.
5. Pevaryl Topical Cream (Econazole). Janssen-Cilag Ltd. UK Summary of product characteristics, July 2004.
6. Oxistat (Oxiconazole). GlaxoSmithKline. US Prescribing information, March 2004.
7. Ertaczo (Sertaconazole). OrthoNeutrogena. US Prescribing information, November 2005.

Azoles; Voriconazole + St John's wort (*Hypericum perforatum*)

St John's wort, taken for two weeks, halved the levels of a single dose of voriconazole, which may be clinically relevant.

Clinical evidence, mechanism, importance and management

A single 400-mg dose of oral voriconazole was given alone and on the first and last day of St John's wort (*Jarsin, Lichtwer Pharma*) given at a dose of 300 mg three times daily for 15 days to 17 healthy subjects. One day of St John's wort had no effect on the voriconazole $AUC_{0-\infty}$, but slightly increased the maximum serum level and AUC_{0-10} by 22%. However, when voriconazole was given on day 15, the AUC of voriconazole was decreased by 59% and there was a 2.4-fold increase in oral clearance.[1]

These results suggest that the short-term effect of St John's wort is to slightly enhance the absorption of voriconazole, whereas the longer-term effect is to induce absorption-limiting transport proteins and intestinal metabolism via cytochrome P450 isoenzymes.[1]

The slight increase in voriconazole absorption with a single dose of St John's wort is not clinically relevant. However, the reduction in voriconazole levels after 15 days of St John's wort could impact on clinical efficacy. This suggests that patients requiring voriconazole should be asked about current or recent use of St John's wort, since this may indicate the need to use an increased voriconazole dose, at least initially. Patients taking voriconazole should be advised not to take St John's wort.

1. Rengelshausen J, Banfield M, Riedel KD, Burhenne J, Mikus G, et al. Opposite effects of short-term and long-term St John's wort on voriconazole pharmacokinetics. *Clin Pharmacol Ther* (2005) 78, 25–33.

Chloroquine or Hydroxychloroquine + Antacids or Kaolin

The absorption of chloroquine is moderately reduced by magnesium trisilicate and kaolin. Hydroxychloroquine is predicted to be similarly affected.

Clinical evidence

Six healthy subjects were given chloroquine phosphate 1 g (equivalent to 620 mg of chloroquine base) with either **magnesium trisilicate** 1 g or

kaolin 1 g after an overnight fast. The **magnesium trisilicate** reduced the AUC of the chloroquine by 18.2% and the **kaolin** reduced it by 28.6%.[1]

Related *in vitro* studies by the same authors using segments of *rat* intestine found that the absorption of chloroquine was decreased as follows: **magnesium trisilicate** 31.3%, **kaolin** 46.5%, **calcium carbonate** 52%, and **gerdiga** 36.1%. **Gerdiga** is a clay containing hydrated silicates with sodium and potassium carbonates and bicarbonates. It is used as an antacid and is similar to **attapulgite**.[2]

Mechanism

These antacid and antidiarrhoeal compounds adsorb chloroquine thereby reducing the amount available for absorption by the gut. Dissolution of chloroquine from tablets may also be delayed by adsorbent antacids.[3]

Importance and management

The modest pharmacokinetic interactions between chloroquine and magnesium trisilicate or kaolin are established, but their clinical importance does not seem to have been assessed. One way to minimise any interaction is to separate the dosages of the antimalarials and magnesium trisilicate or kaolin as much as possible (at least 2 to 3 hours) to reduce admixture in the gut. There do not appear to be any studies to see if other antacids behave similarly.

The manufacturer of **hydroxychloroquine** predicts that, as with chloroquine, antacids might decrease hydroxychloroquine absorption, and they recommend separating administration by 4 hours.[4]

1. McElnay JC, Mukhtar HA, D'Arcy PF, Temple DJ, Collier PS. The effect of magnesium trisilicate and kaolin on the *in vivo* absorption of chloroquine. *J Trop Med Hyg* (1982) 85, 159–63.
2. McElnay JC, Mukhtar HA, D'Arcy PF, Temple DJ. *In vitro* experiments on chloroquine and pyrimethamine absorption in the presence of antacid constituents of kaolin. *J Trop Med Hyg* (1982) 85, 153–8.
3. Iwuagwu MA, Aloko KS. Adsorption of paracetamol and chloroquine phosphate by some antacids. *J Pharm Pharmacol* (1992) 44, 655–8.
4. Plaquenil (Hydroxychloroquine sulfate). Sanofi-Aventis. UK Summary of product characteristics, March 2003.

Chloroquine + Colestyramine

Colestyramine can modestly reduce the absorption of chloroquine, but the clinical importance of this is uncertain.

Clinical evidence, mechanism, importance and management

Colestyramine 4 g reduced the absorption of chloroquine 10 mg/kg by about 30% in 5 children aged 6 to 13. Considerable inter-individual differences were seen.[1] This reduced absorption is consistent with the way colestyramine interacts with other drugs by binding to them in the gut. The clinical importance is uncertain but separating the dosages is effective in minimising this interaction with other drugs. It is generally advised that other drugs are given 1 hour before or 4 to 6 hours after colestyramine.

1. Gendrel D, Verdier F, Richard-Lenoble D, Nardou M. Interaction entre cholestyramine et chloroquine. *Arch Fr Pediatr* (1990) 47, 387–8.

Chloroquine or Hydroxychloroquine + H_2-receptor antagonists

Cimetidine reduces the metabolism and clearance of chloroquine, but the clinical importance of this is uncertain. Hydroxychloroquine is predicted to interact in the same way as chloroquine. Ranitidine appears not to interact with chloroquine.

Clinical evidence, mechanism, importance and management

Cimetidine 400 mg daily for 4 days approximately halved the clearance of a single 600-mg dose of chloroquine base in 10 healthy subjects. The elimination half-life was prolonged from 3.11 to 4.62 days.[1] It was suggested that these effects occurred because **cimetidine** inhibits the metabolism of chloroquine by the liver. The clinical importance of this interaction is uncertain, but it would seem prudent to be alert for any signs of chloroquine toxicity during concurrent use. A similar study by the same authors found that **ranitidine** does not interact with chloroquine.[2]

On the basis of these data for chloroquine and cimetidine, the manufacturer of **hydroxychloroquine** states that, even though specific reports have not appeared, **cimetidine** might inhibit **hydroxychloroquine** metabolism.[3]

1. Ette EI, Brown-Awala EA, Essien EE. Chloroquine elimination in humans: effect of low-dose cimetidine. *J Clin Pharmacol* (1987) 27, 813–16.
2. Ette EI, Brown-Awala EA, Essien EE. Effect of ranitidine on chloroquine disposition. *Drug Intell Clin Pharm* (1987) 21, 732–4.
3. Plaquenil (Hydroxychloroquine sulfate). Sanofi-Aventis. UK Summary of product characteristics, March 2003.

Chloroquine + Imipramine

No pharmacokinetic interaction was seen in 6 healthy subjects given single doses of chloroquine 300 mg and imipramine 50 mg.[1] See also 'Drugs that prolong the QT interval + Other drugs that prolong the QT interval', p.257.

1. Onyeji CO, Toriola TA, Ogunbona FA. Lack of pharmacokinetic interaction between chloroquine and imipramine. *Ther Drug Monit* (1993) 15, 43–6.

Chloroquine + Methylthioninium chloride (Methylene blue)

Methylthioninium chloride caused a small 20% reduction in exposure to chloroquine, which was not considered to be clinically relevant.

Clinical evidence, mechanism, importance and management

Methylthioninium chloride 130 mg twice daily given orally to 12 healthy subjects with a 3-day course of chloroquine tended to decrease the AUC of chloroquine (by 20%), without affecting renal clearance when compared with a control group of 12 patients receiving chloroquine alone. This small reduction would not be expected to be clinically relevant.[1]

1. Rengelshausen J, Burhenne J, Fröhlich M, Tayrouz Y, Kumar Singh S, Riedel K-D, Müller O, Hoppe-Tichy T, Haefeli WE, Mikus G, Walter-Sack I. Pharmacokinetic interaction of chloroquine and methylene blue combination against malaria. *Eur J Clin Pharmacol* (2004) 60, 709–15.

Chloroquine + Promethazine

Promethazine appears to increase the levels of intramuscular chloroquine and its metabolites.

Clinical evidence, mechanism, importance and management

A study in healthy subjects found that intramuscular promethazine hydrochloride 25 mg, given with intramuscular chloroquine phosphate 200 mg increased the AUC of chloroquine and its metabolites by 85%. This may be due to promethazine enhancing the absorption of chloroquine from the injection site or displacing it and its metabolites from binding sites in the blood. The initial rate of excretion of chloroquine and the total drug excreted within 3 hours was unaffected by promethazine.[1] The increased bioavailability of chloroquine may improve its therapeutic effects but could also increase toxicity. *In vitro* and *animal* studies suggest the combination may be effective in the treatment of uncomplicated chloroquine-resistant malaria.[2,3] More study is needed. For mention that chloroquine may increase chlorpromazine levels, see 'Phenothiazines + Antimalarials', p.759.

1. Ehiemua AO, Komolafe OO, Oyedeji GA, Olamijulo SK. Effect of promethazine on the metabolism of chloroquine. *Eur J Drug Metab Pharmacokinet* (1988) 13, 15–17.
2. Oduola OO, Happi TC, Gbotosho GO, Ogundahunsi OAT, Falade CO, Akinboye DO, Sowunmi A, Oduola AMJ. Plasmodium berghei: efficacy and safety of combinations of chloroquine and promethazine in chloroquine resistant infections in gravid mice. *Afr J Med Med Sci* (2004) 33, 77–81.
3. Oduola AMJ, Sowunmi A, Milhous WK, Brewer TG, Kyle DE, Gerena L, Rossan RN, Salako LA, Schuster BG. *In vitro* and *in vivo* reversal of chloroquine resistance in *Plasmodium falciparum* with promethazine. *Am J Trop Med Hyg* (1998) 58, 625–9.

Co-artemether + CYP2D6 substrates

The manufacturer of co-artemether[1] notes that *in vitro* data indicate that lumefantrine significantly inhibits CYP2D6. As a consequence, they contraindicate the use of co-artemether in patients taking any drug that is metabolised by CYP2D6, and they give flecainide, metoprolol, imipramine, amitriptyline, clomipramine as examples (for a list of CYP2D6 substrates, see 'Table 1.3', (p.6)). These contraindications seem unnecessarily restrictive, especially since none of the drugs they give as examples are contraindicated with other established inhibitors of CYP2D6. Until more is known, it would be prudent to closely monitor the effects of any CYP2D6 substrate in patients for whom co-artemether is considered the antimalarial drug of choice.

1. Riamet (Artemether/Lumefantrine). Novartis Pharmaceuticals UK Ltd. UK Summary of product characteristics, December 2006.

Co-artemether + CYP3A4 inhibitors

Ketoconazole doubles the AUC of artemether and lumefantrine, and other potent inhibitors of CYP3A4 are predicted to interact similarly. Although the clinical relevance of this is uncertain, the manufacturers of co-artemether currently advise against concurrent use.

Clinical evidence, mechanism, importance and management

In one study, 16 healthy subjects were given ketoconazole 400 mg on day one then 200 mg daily for 4 days increased the AUC of artemether 2.4-fold, its metabolite dihydroartemisinin 1.7-fold and lumefantrine 1.7-fold after a single dose of co-artemether 80/480 mg given with a high-fat breakfast.[1] The maximum levels of the drugs were increased to a similar extent. No changes in ECG parameters or increases in adverse events were noted.

It was suggested that ketoconazole probably increases the levels of artemether and lumefantrine via its effects on intestinal and/or hepatic cytochrome P450 isoenzyme CYP3A4.

A pharmacokinetic interaction with ketoconazole seems to be established, and would be predicted for other similar potent CYP3A4 inhibitors. However, the clinical relevance of a twofold increase in artemether and lumefantrine levels is unclear. The authors of this drug company-supported study suggest that this change is within the between subject variability in the pharmacokinetics of these drugs, and is therefore unlikely to be clinically relevant. They suggest that no dosage adjustment would appear necessary.[1] Nevertheless, the manufacturer of co-artemether contraindicates the use of co-artemether in patients who are taking any drug that inhibits CYP3A4, and they give **erythromycin**, **ketoconazole**, **itraconazole**, **cimetidine** and **protease inhibitors** as examples. They base this advice on the lack of clinical data and unknown effects on safety.[2] Given the data with ketoconazole, in the setting of acute *Plasmodium falciparum* malaria, when co-artemether is considered the appropriate treatment, this advice seems unnecessarily restrictive. If it is deemed necessary to use co-artemether in a patient on a CYP3A4 inhibitor, it may be prudent to closely monitor the ECG and potassium levels, since artemether may prolong the QT interval. Further study is needed.

1. Lefèvre G, Carpenter P, Souppart C, Schmidli H, McClean M, Stypinski D. Pharmacokinetics and electrocardiographic pharmacodynamics or artemether-lumefantrine (Riamet®) with concomitant administration of ketoconazole in healthy subjects. *Br J Clin Pharmacol* (2002) 54, 485–92.
2. Riamet (Artemether/Lumefantrine). Novartis Pharmaceuticals UK Ltd. UK Summary of product characteristics, December 2006.

Co-artemether + Food

High-fat food markedly increases the absorption of lumefantrine and moderately increases the absorption of artemether. As soon as patients can tolerate food they should be encouraged to take co-artemether with meals.

Clinical evidence, mechanism, importance and management

In a study in healthy Chinese subjects a single dose of artemether/lumefantrine 80/480 mg was taken after a high fat meal and in the fasted state. The relative bioavailabilities of artemether and its active metabolite dihydroartemisinin were increased by more than twofold, and the bioavailability of lumefantrine was increased 16-fold by the meal.[1] Based on these data, the manufacturer notes that if 100% absorption is assumed for lumefantrine taken with a high fat meal, then absorption in the fasted state is less than 10% of the dose.[2]

In a clinical trial in patients with malaria, intake of a light meal within one hour of lumefantrine increased the bioavailability by 48%, and intake of a normal meal increased absorption twofold, when compared with liquids alone. After 24 to 48 hours in this study, most patients were eating normally.[3] Artemether/lumefantrine should be taken with food. However, patients with acute uncomplicated malaria are unlikely to tolerate food. The manufacturer notes that patients should be encouraged to take artemether/lumefantrine with food as soon as this can be tolerated. They say that patients who remain averse to food during treatment should be closely monitored since they may be at greater risk of recrudescence (reappearance of the disease after a period of inactivity).[2]

1. Bindschedler M, et al. Comparative bioavailability of benflumetol after administration of single oral doses of co-artemether under fed and fasted conditions to healthy subjects. Cited in Lefèvre G, Thomsen MS. Clinical Pharmacokinetics of artemether and lumefantrine (Riamet®). *Clin Drug Invest* (1999) 18, 467–80.
2. Riamet (Artemether/Lumefantrine). Novartis Pharmaceuticals UK Ltd. UK Summary of product characteristics, December 2006.
3. Ezzet F, van Vugt M, Nosten F, Looareesuwan S, White NJ. Pharmacokinetics and pharmacodynamics of lumefantrine (Benflumetol) in acute falciparum malaria. *Antimicrob Agents Chemother* (2000) 44, 697–704.

Co-artemether + Grapefruit juice

Grapefruit juice doubles the AUC of artemether. Although the clinical relevance of this is uncertain, the manufacturers of co-artemether advise against concurrent use.

Clinical evidence, mechanism, importance and management

In a crossover study, healthy subjects were given a single 100-mg dose of artemether after breakfast with water, then after a 7-day washout period the study was repeated with 350 mL of double-strength grapefruit juice. Grapefruit juice increased the AUC of artemether by almost twofold, and the maximum level by more than twofold. The pharmacokinetics of the metabolite dihydroartemisinin were unaffected.[1] In a further multiple-dose study, artemether 100 mg was taken with water or 350 mL of double-strength grapefruit juice once daily for 5 days. Grapefruit juice increased the AUC and maximum level of artemether twofold on both day one and day 5, but the AUC of artemether was markedly lower on day 5, due to autoinduction of its metabolism.[2] This suggests that grapefruit juice might increase the levels of artemether via inhibition of intestinal CYP3A4, but that autoinduction does not affect this process.

The clinical relevance of a twofold increase in artemether levels is unclear. The authors suggest that the use of grapefruit juice might improve clinical efficacy in malaria, and might theoretically reduce the recrudescence (the reappearance of a disease after a period of inactivity) rate of artemether monotherapy.[2] However, artemether is used with lumefantrine to limit recrudescence. Further study is needed.

1. van Agtmael MA, Gupta V, van der Wosten TH, Rutten JP, van Boxtel CJ. Grapefruit juice increases the bioavailability of artemether. *Eur J Clin Pharmacol* (1999) 55, 405–10.
2. van Agtmael MA, Gupta V, van der Graaf CAA, van Boxtel CJ. The effect of grapefruit juice on the time-dependent decline of artemether plasma levels in healthy subjects. *Clin Pharmacol Ther* (1999) 66, 408–14.

Co-artemether + Mefloquine

The levels of lumefantrine were modestly reduced by mefloquine pretreatment, but the levels of artemether and of mefloquine were not affected. No adverse effects on the QT interval were seen. These data indicate that co-artemether may be used after mefloquine prophylaxis or treatment.

Clinical evidence, mechanism, importance and management

In a study, 6 doses of co-artemether 80/480 mg were given over 60 hours to 42 healthy subjects, starting 12 hours after a short course of mefloquine (3 doses totalling 1 g given over 12 hours). The pharmacokinetics of the mefloquine and the artemether were unaffected by sequential use, but the lumefantrine maximum plasma concentrations and AUC were reduced by 29 and 41% respectively. However, given that the plasma levels of lumefantrine are usually highly variable, these changes were not thought large enough to affect the efficacy of treatment.[1]

In another study, similar sequential use of these drugs did not affect the QT interval, and drug levels were also considered adequate for treatment.[2] The authors considered that adverse effects on the QT interval are unlikely to occur if co-artemether is used after mefloquine prophylaxis or treatment.

These data indicate that sequential use of mefloquine then co-artemether is unlikely to require any special precautions. The manufacturer of co-artemether notes that prolongation of the QT interval was seen in about 5% of patients in clinical trials (although they say this could be disease related). They state that, due to the limited data on safety and efficacy, co-artemether should not be given concurrently with any other antimalarial.[3] For mention of a study where artemether pretreatment modestly reduced mefloquine levels, see 'Mefloquine + Artemisinin derivatives', p.231.

1. Lefèvre G, Bindschedler M, Ezzet F, Schaeffer N, Meyer I, Thomsen MS. Pharmacokinetic interaction trial between co-artemether and mefloquine. *Eur J Pharm Sci* (2000) 10, 141–51.
2. Bindschedler M, Lefèvre G, Ezzet F, Schaeffer N, Meyer I, Thomsen MS. Cardiac effects of co-artemether (artemether/lumefantrine) and mefloquine given alone or in combination to healthy volunteers. *Eur J Clin Pharmacol* (2000) 56, 375–81.
3. Riamet (Artemether/Lumefantrine). Novartis Pharmaceuticals UK Ltd. UK Summary of product characteristics, December 2006.

Co-artemether + Quinine

No clinically significant pharmacokinetic interaction appears to occur between quinine and co-artemether. Quinine-induced QTc prolongation may be enhanced by artemether.

Clinical evidence, mechanism, importance and management

In a double-blind placebo-controlled study in healthy subjects, 6 doses of co-artemether 80/480 mg were given to 14 subjects, over a period of 60 hours, followed 2 hours after the last dose by intravenous quinine 10 mg/kg (to a maximum of 600 mg) over 2 hours. Another two groups, each containing 14 subjects, received quinine or co-artemether, with placebo. The pharmacokinetics of lumefantrine and quinine were unaffected by combined use but the AUC and plasma levels of artemether and its active metabolite dihydroartemisinin appeared to be lower when co-artemether was given with quinine. However, the levels prior to quinine use in this group were also lower and the reduction in the presence of quinine was not considered clinically significant. The transient prolongation of the QTc interval noted with quinine (average and peak increases of 3 and 6 milliseconds, respectively) was slightly greater when quinine was given after co-artemether (average and peak increases 7 and 15 milliseconds respectively).[1] Both quinine and artemether are known to prolong the QT interval. In general, it is advised that the concurrent use of drugs that prolong the QT interval should be avoided (see also 'Drugs that prolong the QT interval + Other drugs that prolong the QT interval', p.257). However, the authors of this study considered that the modest increased risk of QTc prolongation was outweighed by the potential benefit of the combined treatment in complicated or multidrug-resistant falciparum malaria.[1] If the combination is used, careful cardiac monitoring is recommended.

1. Lefèvre G, Carpenter P, Souppart C, Schmidli H, Martin JM, Lane A, Ward C, Amakye D. Interaction trial between artemether-lumefantrine (Riamet®) and quinine in healthy subjects. *J Clin Pharmacol* (2002) 42, 1147–58.

Diethylcarbamazine + Urinary acidifiers or alkalinisers

Urinary alkalinisers can reduce the loss of diethylcarbamazine in the urine, whereas urinary acidifiers can increase the loss. The clinical importance of this is unknown.

Clinical evidence

Two studies, one in healthy subjects[1] and the other in patients with onchocerciasis,[2] found that making the urine alkaline with **sodium bicarbonate** markedly increased the retention of the diethylcarbamazine. The urinary excretion of a 50-mg dose of diethylcarbamazine was 62.3% and its elimination half-life 4 hours when the urine was made acidic (pH less than 5.5) by giving ammonium chloride, compared with 5.1% and 9.6 hours respectively when the urine was made alkaline (pH more than 7.5) using sodium bicarbonate.[1]

Mechanism

In alkaline urine most of the diethylcarbamazine is non-ionised and is therefore easily reabsorbed in the kidney by simple diffusion through the lipid membrane. However, the conclusion was reached that in practice there is no advantage in making the urine alkaline in order to be able to use smaller doses of diethylcarbamazine because the severity of the adverse reactions (the Mazzotti reaction) is not reduced, and the microfilarial counts at the end of a month are not significantly different.[2]

Importance and management

The clinical importance of any unsought for changes in the urinary pH brought about by the use of other drugs during diethylcarbamazine treatment has not been assessed, but be aware that its pharmacokinetics and possibly the severity of its adverse effects can be changed.

1. Edwards G, Breckenridge AM, Adjepon-Yamoah KK, Orme M L'E, Ward SA. The effect of variations in urinary pH on the pharmacokinetics of diethylcarbamazine. *Br J Clin Pharmacol* (1981) 12, 807–12.
2. Awadzi K, Adjepon-Yamoah KK, Edwards G, Orme M L'E, Breckenridge AM, Gilles HM. The effect of moderate urine alkalinisation on low dose diethylcarbamazine therapy in patients with onchocerciasis. *Br J Clin Pharmacol* (1986) 21, 669–76.

Echinocandins + Amphotericin B

Limited evidence suggests that amphotericin B does not alter the pharmacokinetics of anidulafungin. The pharmacokinetics of caspofungin and amphotericin B are not altered by concurrent use.

Clinical evidence, mechanism, importance and management

(a) Anidulafungin

The manufacturer notes that population pharmacokinetic analysis showed no difference in the pharmacokinetics of anidulafungin in 27 patients who were also given liposomal amphotericin B when compared with data from patients receiving anidulafungin alone. This suggests that no dosage adjustment of anidulafungin is required if it is given with amphotericin B.[1]

(b) Caspofungin

The manufacturers of caspofungin say there were no pharmacokinetic interactions between caspofungin and amphotericin B in a study in healthy subjects.[2,3]

1. Eraxis (Anidulafungin). Pfizer Inc. US Prescribing information, May 2007.
2. Cancidas (Caspofungin acetate). Merck Sharp & Dohme Ltd. UK Summary of product characteristics, January 2007.
3. Cancidas (Caspofungin acetate). Merck & Co., Inc. US Prescribing information, February 2005.

Echinocandins + Azoles

No pharmacokinetic interaction appears to occur between anidulafungin and voriconazole or between caspofungin and itraconazole. No dosage adjustment of these drugs is necessary if they are used in combination.

Clinical evidence, mechanism, importance and management

(a) Anidulafungin

In a crossover study in 17 healthy subjects the steady state maximum level and AUC of both anidulafungin and **voriconazole** were not significantly altered by concurrent use, when compared with either drug given with placebo. Intravenous anidulafungin was given at a dose of 200 mg on the first day, then 100 mg daily for 3 days. **Voriconazole** was given orally, at a dose of 400 mg every 12 hours on the first day, then 200 mg every 12 hours for 3 days.[1] No dosage adjustment appears to be necessary with either drug when used together.

(b) Caspofungin

Caspofungin 70 mg on day 1 and 50 mg for the next 13 days did not alter the pharmacokinetics of **itraconazole** 200 mg daily.[2] The pharmacokinetics of caspofungin were also unaltered. No dosage adjustment of either drug appears to be necessary when they are used together.

1. Dowell JA, Schranz J, Baruch A, Foster G. Safety and pharmacokinetics of coadministered voriconazole and anidulafungin. *J Clin Pharmacol* (2005) 45, 1373–82.
2. Stone JA, McCrea JB, Wickersham PJ, Holland SD, Deutsch PJ, Bi S, Cicero T, Greenberg H, Waldman SA. A phase I study of caspofungin evaluating the potential for drug interactions with itraconazole, the effect of gender and the use of a loading dose regimen. *Intersci Conf Antimicrob Agents Chemother* (2000) 40, 26.

Echinocandins + Ciclosporin

Ciclosporin appears to modestly increase caspofungin levels, and concurrent use can apparently result in raised liver enzymes. Ciclosporin slightly raised anidulafungin levels in one study, without any serious adverse events.

Clinical evidence, mechanism, importance and management

(a) Anidulafungin

Intravenous anidulafungin 200 mg on day one, then 100 mg daily for 7 days was given to 12 healthy subjects with concurrent oral ciclosporin solution (*Neoral*) 1.25 mg/kg twice daily on the last 4 days. Ciclosporin caused a small 22% increase in the steady-state AUC of anidulafungin, which was not considered to be clinically relevant. No dose-limiting toxicities or serious adverse events were noted. One patient had a mild increase in liver enzymes on day 6 (after 2 days of concurrent use), and the study drugs were withdrawn at this point.[1]

Anidulafungin is not expected to alter ciclosporin levels based on an *in vitro* study where anidulafungin had no effect on the metabolism of ciclosporin.[1]

The manufacturer states that no dosage adjustment of either drug is needed on concurrent use.[2]

(b) Caspofungin

The manufacturers report that in two studies in healthy subjects, ciclosporin (a single 4-mg/kg dose, or two 3-mg/kg doses 12 hours apart) increased the AUC of caspofungin by 35%. Moreover, 5 of 12 subjects (43%) had increases in AST and ALT of up to threefold. The liver enzymes returned to normal on discontinuation of both drugs, and during concurrent use the levels of ciclosporin were not affected.[3-5] These findings led to the exclusion of patients receiving ciclosporin from phase II/III studies of caspofungin.[5] Note that elevated liver enzymes (typically mild and rarely leading to discontinuation) are a common adverse effect of caspofungin alone.[3] More recently, 3 studies have reported retrospective analyses of the clinical use of caspofungin in a total of 68 patients taking ciclosporin.[6-8] All three found no serious hepatic adverse events. Two reported no clinically significant elevations of liver enzymes,[6,8] but one found 2 of 40 patients had discontinued therapy because of abnormalities in hepatic enzymes, possibly related to caspofungin and/or ciclosporin.[7]

The manufacturers say that ciclosporin and caspofungin can be used together if the potential benefit outweighs the risk. If they are used together, close monitoring of liver enzymes is recommended.[3,4]

1. Dowell JA, Stogniew M, Krause D, Henkel T, Weston IE. Assessment of the safety and pharmacokinetics of anidulafungin when administered with cyclosporine. *J Clin Pharmacol* (2005) 45, 227–33.
2. Eraxis (Anidulafungin). Pfizer Inc. US Prescribing information, May 2007.
3. Cancidas (Caspofungin acetate). Merck Sharp & Dohme Ltd. UK Summary of product characteristics, January 2007.
4. Cancidas (Caspofungin acetate). Merck & Co., Inc. US Prescribing information, February 2005.
5. Sable CA, Nguyen B-YT, Chodakewitz JA, DiNubile MJ. Safety and tolerability of caspofungin acetate in the treatment of fungal infections. *Transpl Infect Dis* (2002) 4, 25–30.
6. Sanz-Rodriguez C, Lopez-Duarte M, Jurado M, Lopez J, Arranz R, Cisneros JM, Martino ML, Garcia-Sanchez PJ, Morales P, Olive T, Rovira M, Solano C. Safety of the concomitant use of caspofungin and cyclosporin A in patients with invasive fungal infections. *Bone Marrow Transplant* (2004) 34, 13–20.
7. Marr KA, Hachem R, Papanicolaou G, Somani J, Arduino JM, Lipka CJ, Ngai AL, Kartsonis N, Chodakewitz J, Sable C. Retrospective study of the hepatic safety profile of patients concomitantly treated with caspofungin and cyclosporin A. *Transpl Infect Dis* (2004) 6, 110–16.
8. Glasmacher A, Cornely OA, Orlopp K, Reuter S, Blaschke S, Eichel M, Silling G, Simons B, Egerer G, Siemann M, Florek M, Schnitzler R, Ebeling P, Ritter J, Reinel H, Schutt P, Fischer H, Hahn C, Just-Nuebling G. Caspofungin treatment in severely ill, immunocompromised patients: a case-documentation study of 118 patients. *J Antimicrob Chemother* (2006) 57, 127–34.

Echinocandins + Rifampicin (Rifampin) and other enzyme inducers

Rifampicin modestly reduces the trough levels of caspofungin after 2 weeks of concurrent use, but this is not thought to be due to increased metabolism. One case of caspofungin treatment failure has been reported in a patient taking rifampicin. Other enzyme inducers (carbamazepine, dexamethasone, efavirenz, nevirapine, and phenytoin) also appeared to reduce caspofungin levels. Rifampicin and other unnamed enzyme inducers did not appear to alter anidulafungin clearance.

Clinical evidence

(a) Anidulafungin

A population pharmacokinetic analysis of anidulafungin in patients with serious fungal infections found that the clearance of anidulafungin did not differ between 27 patients also taking **rifampicin** (**rifampin**) and 77 patients taking no known interacting drugs.[1] Similarly, anidulafungin clearance was not different in 40 patients given **inducers of cytochrome P450** (including **rifampicin**, but others not specifically named).[1] These findings suggest that no dosage adjustment of anidulafungin is needed in patients taking **rifampicin** or other **enzyme inducers**.[1,2]

(b) Caspofungin

A parallel-group study in healthy subjects looked at the effects of rifampicin on the pharmacokinetics of caspofungin. In the first group, **rifampicin** 600 mg daily was given with intravenous caspofungin 50 mg daily, started on the same day. It was found that the trough levels and AUC of caspofungin were increased by 170 and 61%, respectively, on day one. However, after 2 weeks the AUC had returned to normal, and, when compared to subjects not taking **rifampicin**, there was a trend to *lower* trough levels of caspofungin. In the second group of healthy subjects in this study, **rifampicin** 600 mg daily was given for 14 days alone and then for a further 14 days combined with caspofungin. In this study, no significant increase in the caspofungin AUC was seen on day one of concurrent use. On both day one and day 14, the trough levels of caspofungin were reduced by about 30%, without any change in the AUC, similar to the findings on day 14 in the first group. In this second group, caspofungin did not alter the pharmacokinetics of **rifampicin**.[3]

A case report describes a neutropenic patient with fungaemia who did not respond to intravenous caspofungin (70 mg on the first day then 50 mg daily) whilst taking **rifampicin** 600 mg daily. However, susceptibility testing showed that the isolate was not resistant to caspofungin and she was successfully treated with amphotericin B. Although this patient was treated with standard dose caspofungin, the authors note she weighed just 47 kg and showed not even an initial response. They suggest that caspofungin doses of more than 70 mg daily would have been required for efficacy in their patient.[4]

Mechanism

Caspofungin is a poor substrate for cytochrome P450 and is not a substrate for P-glycoprotein,[5] therefore these mechanisms are not thought to be involved in the interaction with rifampicin. It is possible that the modest effect of rifampicin on caspofungin is due to induction of tissue uptake transport proteins at steady-state.[3]

Importance and management

The manufacturers recommend that consideration should be given to increasing the dose of caspofungin from 50 to 70 mg daily in patients taking **rifampicin**.[5,6] This dose has been generally well tolerated in clinical studies.[3]. However, bear in mind the case report of possible caspofungin failure, even at this dose. The manufacturers also say that a population pharmacokinetic analysis suggested that the concurrent use of other metabolic inducers (**carbamazepine**, **dexamethasone**, **efavirenz**, **nevirapine** or **phenytoin**) may result in clinically meaningful reductions in caspofungin AUC.[5,6] They suggest considering increasing the dose of caspofungin from 50 to 70 mg daily if it is used with enzyme inducers such as these. Further study is needed.

1. Dowell J, Knebel W, Ludden T, Stogniew M, Krause D, Henkel T. Population pharmacokinetic analysis of anidulafungin, an echinocandin antifungal. *J Clin Pharmacol* (2004) 44, 590–8.
2. Eraxis (Anidulafungin). Pfizer Inc. US Prescribing information, May 2007.
3. Stone JA, Migoya EM, Hickey L, Winchell GA, Deutsch PJ, Ghosh K, Freeman A, Bi S, Desai R, Dilzer SC, Lasseter KC, Kraft WK, Greenberg H, Waldman SA. Potential for interactions between caspofungin and nelfinavir or rifampin. *Antimicrob Agents Chemother* (2004) 48, 4306–14.
4. Belmares J, Colaizzi L, Parada JP, Johnson S. Caspofungin treatment failure in a patient with invasive candidiasis and concomitant rifampicin treatment. *Int J Antimicrob Agents* (2005) 26, 264–5.
5. Cancidas (Caspofungin acetate). Merck Sharp & Dohme Ltd. UK Summary of product characteristics, January 2007.
6. Cancidas (Caspofungin acetate). Merck & Co., Inc. US Prescribing information, February 2005.

Echinocandins; Anidulafungin + Miscellaneous

A population pharmacokinetic analysis of anidulafungin in patients with serious fungal infections found that the clearance of anidulafungin did not differ between 140 patients taking drugs classified as cytochrome P450 isoenzyme inhibitors (none specifically named) and 77 patients who received no known interacting drugs.[1] For the lack of a pharmacokinetic interaction between anidulafungin and voriconazole, see 'Echinocandins + Azoles', p.225.

1. Dowell J, Knebel W, Ludden T, Stogniew M, Krause D, Henkel T. Population pharmacokinetic analysis of anidulafungin, an echinocandin antifungal. *J Clin Pharmacol* (2004) 44, 590–8.

Echinocandins; Caspofungin + Mycophenolate

The manufacturers of caspofungin say that the pharmacokinetics of caspofungin and mycophenolate are not altered by concurrent use.[1,2]

1. Cancidas (Caspofungin acetate). Merck Sharp & Dohme Ltd. UK Summary of product characteristics, January 2007.
2. Cancidas (Caspofungin acetate). Merck & Co., Inc. US Prescribing information, February 2005.

Echinocandins; Caspofungin + Nelfinavir

Nelfinavir does not have a clinically relevant effect on the pharmacokinetics of caspofungin.

Clinical evidence, mechanism, importance and management

In a parallel-group study healthy subjects were given nelfinavir 1250 mg every 12 hours, with intravenous caspofungin 50 mg daily, started on the same day. The AUC of caspofungin and the trough level were increased by 16 and 58%, respectively, on the first day when compared with subjects receiving caspofungin alone. However, after 2 weeks of combined use, there was no difference in the AUC or trough level of caspofungin.[1] The authors note that their previous population pharmacokinetic analysis had shown that nelfinavir might decrease the AUC and trough level of caspofungin, which in the light of the controlled study, they consider to be a spurious finding.

It appears that nelfinavir does not have a clinically significant effect on the pharmacokinetics of caspofungin, and no dosage adjustment of caspofungin is required on combined use.

1. Stone JA, Migoya EM, Hickey L, Winchell GA, Deutsch PJ, Ghosh K, Freeman A, Bi S, Desai R, Dilzer SC, Lasseter KC, Kraft WK, Greenberg H, Waldman SA. Potential for interactions between caspofungin and nelfinavir or rifampin. *Antimicrob Agents Chemother* (2004) 48, 4306–14.

Flucytosine + Amphotericin B

The combination of flucytosine with amphotericin B may be more effective than flucytosine alone for some fungal infections, but amphotericin B increases the toxicity of flucytosine. Close monitoring of flucytosine levels and renal function is required. Other drugs that impair glomerular filtration might also decrease flucytosine elimination and increase toxicity.

Clinical evidence, mechanism, importance and management

The combined use of flucytosine and **amphotericin B** is more effective than flucytosine alone in the treatment of cryptococcal meningitis, as demonstrated in an early study,[1] and is still the recommended treatment.[2,3] However, **amphotericin B** can cause deterioration in renal function, which reduces flucytosine elimination, and may result in raised flucytosine blood levels. In addition, amphotericin may increase the cellular uptake of flucytosine.[4] Whatever the exact mechanism, combined use increases flucytosine bone marrow toxicity. A study of 194 patients randomised to either a 4 or 6-week course of low-dose amphotericin B (initially 0.3 mg/kg daily) and maximal dose flucytosine (150 mg/kg daily, adjusted for renal function) found that severe adverse effects were common. These included azotaemia (51 patients), blood dyscrasias (52 patients), and hepatitis (13 patients).[5]

Flucytosine levels and renal function should be very closely monitored when the drugs are used concurrently. One manufacturer of flucytosine says that any drug that impairs glomerular filtration may prolong the half-life of flucytosine, which would increase the risk of toxicity.[6]

1. Bennett JE, Dismukes WE, Duma RJ, Medoff G, Sande MA, Gallis H, Leonard J, Fields BT, Bradshaw M, Haywood H, McGee ZA, Cate TR, Cobbs CG, Warner JF, Alling DW. A comparison of amphotericin B alone and combined with flucytosine in the treatment of cryptoccal meningitis. *N Engl J Med* (1979) 301, 126–31.
2. Working Party of the British Society for Antimicrobial Chemotherapy. Therapy of deep fungal infection in haematological malignancy. *J Antimicrob Chemother* (1997) 40, 779–88.
3. Saag MS, Graybill RJ, Larsen RA, Pappas PG, Perfect JR, Powderly WG, Sobel JD, Dismukes WE, for the Mycoses Study Group Cryptococcal Subproject. Practice guidelines for the management of cryptococcal disease. *Clin Infect Dis* (2000) 30, 710–18.
4. Fungizone Intravenous (Amphotericin B). E. R. Squibb & Sons Ltd. UK Summary of product characteristics, May 2006.
5. Stamm AM, Diasio RB, Dismukes WE, Shadomy S, Cloud GA, Bowles CA, Karam GH, Espinel-Ingroff A and members of the National Institute of Allergy and Infectious Diseases Mycoses Study group. Toxicity of amphotericin B plus flucytosine in 194 patients with cryptococcal meningitis. *Am J Med* (1987) 83, 236–42.
6. Ancobon Capsules (Flucytosine). ICN Pharmaceuticals Inc. US Prescribing information, March 2003.

Flucytosine + Antacids

Aluminium/magnesium hydroxide delays the absorption of flucytosine from the gut, but the total amount absorbed remains unaffected.[1] No special precautions appear to be needed if this antacid is given with oral flucytosine.

1. Cutler RE, Blair AD, Kelly MR. Flucytosine kinetics in subjects with normal and impaired renal function. *Clin Pharmacol Ther* (1978) 24, 333–42.

Flucytosine + Cytarabine

Some very limited evidence suggests that cytarabine may oppose the antifungal effects of flucytosine, or reduce flucytosine levels. Theoretically, their bone marrow suppressant effects might be additive.

Clinical evidence, mechanism, importance and management

A man with Hodgkin's disease treated for cryptococcal meningitis with flucytosine 100 mg/kg daily had reduced flucytosine serum and CSF levels, from a range of 30 to 40 mg/L down to undetectable levels, when given cytarabine intravenously. When the cytarabine was replaced by procarbazine, the flucytosine levels returned to their former values. *In vitro* tests found that cytarabine 1 mg/L completely abolished the activity of up to 50 mg/L of flucytosine against the patient's strain of *Cryptococcus*, whereas procarbazine did not.[1] In another study in a patient with acute myeloid leukaemia, the predose flucytosine level fell from 65 to 42 mg/L and the post-dose flucytosine level fell from and 80 to 53 mg/L when cytarabine and daunorubicin were given. However, these levels were still within the therapeutic range. The drop in levels was attributed to an improvement in renal function rather than antagonism between the two drugs.[2] In an *in vitro* study the antifungal effects of flucytosine against 14 out of 16 wild isolates of *Cryptococcus* were not changed in the presence of cytarabine. In the remaining two isolates, an increase in effect was seen in one and a decrease was seen the other.[2]

The evidence for any interaction is therefore very limited indeed and its general clinical importance remains uncertain. The manufacturers of flucytosine advise that strict monitoring of flucytosine levels is required if both drugs are given.[3] Of equal concern is the fact that both drugs are bone marrow suppressants, and this effect might be additive.

1. Holt RJ. Clinical problems with 5-fluorocytosine. *Mykosen* (1978) 21, 363–9.
2. Wingfield HJ. Absence of fungistatic antagonism between flucytosine and cytarabine *in vitro* and *in vivo*. *J Antimicrob Chemother* (1987) 20, 523–7.
3. Ancotil Solution for Infusion (Flucytosine). Valeant Pharmaceuticals Ltd. UK Summary of product characteristics, November 2004.

Furazolidone + Omeprazole

Omeprazole modestly reduces the serum levels of furazolidone. Note that the two drugs have been successfully combined in *H. pylori* eradication regimens.

Clinical evidence, mechanism, importance and management

A study in 18 healthy subjects found that omeprazole 20 mg twice daily for 5 days reduced the peak serum level of a single 200-mg dose of furazolidone by about 30%. The clinical relevance of this modest change is uncertain. Omeprazole may alter the bioavailability of furazolidone by reducing its dissolution or increasing its degradation before it reaches the intestine and/or inducing its first-pass metabolism.[1] Note that there are now a large number of clinical trials describing the successful combination of furazolidone with omeprazole in regimens to eradicate *H. pylori*. However, there is some evidence that success rates are unacceptable if low-dose furazolidone (100 mg twice daily) rather than standard dose (200 mg twice daily) is used.[2] It is possible that a pharmacokinetic interaction could play a part in this finding.

1. Calafatti SA, Ortiz RAM, Deguer M, Martinez M, Pedrazzoli J. Effect of acid secretion blockade by omeprazole on the relative bioavailability of orally administered furazolidone in healthy volunteers. *Br J Clin Pharmacol* (2001) 52, 205–9.
2. Fakheri H, Merat S, Hosseini C, Malekzadeh R. Low-dose furazolidone in triple and quadruple regimens for Helicobacter pylori eradication. *Aliment Pharmacol Ther* (2004) 19, 89–93.

Furazolidone + Sympathomimetics

After 5 to 10 days of use furazolidone has MAO-inhibitory activity about equivalent to that of the non-selective MAOIs. The concurrent use of furazolidone with indirectly-acting sympathomimetic amines (amfetamines, phenylpropanolamine, ephedrine, etc.) or with tyramine-rich foods and drinks may be expected to result in a potentially serious rise in blood pressure. However, direct evidence of accidental adverse reactions of this kind does not seem to have been reported. The pressor effects of noradrenaline (norepinephrine) are unchanged by furazolidone.

Clinical evidence

After 6 days of treatment with furazolidone 400 mg daily, the pressor responses to **tyramine** or **dexamfetamine** in 4 hypertensive patients had increased two to threefold, and after 13 days by about tenfold. These responses were about the same as those found in 2 other patients taking the MAOI **pargyline**.[1] The MAO-inhibitory activity of furazolidone was confirmed by measurements taken on jejunal specimens. The pressor effects of **noradrenaline (norepinephrine)** were unchanged by furazolidone.[1]

Mechanism

The MAO-inhibitory activity of furazolidone is not immediate and may in fact be due to a metabolite of furazolidone.[2] It develops gradually so that after 5 to 10 days of use, indirectly-acting sympathomimetics will interact with furazolidone in the same way as they do in the presence of other non-selective MAOIs.[3,4] More details of the mechanisms of this interaction are to be found elsewhere. See 'MAOIs or RIMAs + Tyramine-rich foods', p.1153 and 'MAOIs or RIMAs + Sympathomimetics; Indirectly-acting', p.1147.

Importance and management

The MAO-inhibitory activity of furazolidone after 5 to 10 days of use is established, but reports of hypertensive crises either with sympathomimetics or **tyramine-containing foods** or drinks appear to be lacking. This may be, in part, a reflection of the fact that furazolidone may be given for just 2 to 5 days. Notwithstanding, it would seem prudent to warn patients given furazolidone not to take any of the drugs, foods or drinks that are prohibited with non-selective MAOIs. See the appropriate monographs on MAOIs for more detailed lists of these 'drugs', (p.1130), 'foods', (p.1153), and 'drinks', (p.1151). No adverse interaction would be expected with 'directly-acting sympathomimetics', (p.1146), such as noradrenaline (norepinephrine).

1. Pettinger WA, Oates JA. Supersensitivity to tyramine during monoamine oxidase inhibition in man. Mechanism at the level of the adrenergic neurone. *Clin Pharmacol Ther* (1968) 9, 341–4.
2. Stern IJ, Hollifield RD, Wilk S, Buzard JA. The anti-monoamine oxidase effects of furazolidone. *J Pharmacol Exp Ther* (1967) 156, 492–9.
3. Pettinger WA, Soyangco FG, Oates JA. Monoamine-oxidase inhibition by furazolidone in man. *Clin Res* (1966) 14, 258.
4. Pettinger WA, Soyangco FG, Oates JA. Inhibition of monoamine oxidase in man by furazolidone. *Clin Pharmacol Ther* (1968) 9, 442–7.

Griseofulvin + Food

The rate and probably extent of griseofulvin absorption is markedly increased if it is taken with a high-fat meal.

Clinical evidence, mechanism, importance and management

A study in 5 healthy subjects found that the absorption of micronised griseofulvin 125 mg (*Fulcin*) was enhanced if it was given with a fatty meal rather than in the fasting state, as assessed by a 37% increase in urinary excretion.[1] Other studies similarly found that the absorption of griseofulvin at 4 and 8 hours was about doubled when it was taken with a high-fat meal.[2,3] A further study in 12 healthy subjects found that the higher the fat content of the meal the higher the bioavailability of griseofulvin (70% increase in bioavailability with a low-fat meal and 120% increase with a high-fat meal, when compared with fasting state absorption).[4] However, another study found that although food increased the rate of absorption of micronised and PEG-ultramicronised griseofulvin, the extent of absorption was not changed.[5] Another report suggested that giving griseofulvin with food tended to reduce the differences in the bioavailability of griseofulvin from micronised and ultramicronised tablets.[6] Enhanced absorption was also found with a formulation of griseofulvin in a **corn oil** emulsion, when compared with tablets or an aqueous suspension.[7]

This interaction is established and of clinical importance. Some manufacturers advise that griseofulvin should be given after meals, otherwise absorption is likely to be inadequate.[8]

1. Khalafalla N, Elgholmy ZA, Khalil SA. Influence of a high fat diet on GI absorption of griseofulvin tablets in man. *Pharmazie* (1981) 36, 692–3.
2. Crounse RG. Human pharmacology of griseofulvin: the effect of fat intake on gastrointestinal absorption. *J Invest Dermatol* (1961) 37, 529–33.
3. Crounse RG. Effective use of griseofulvin. *Arch Dermatol* (1963) 87, 176–8.
4. Ogunbona FA, Smith IF, Olawoye OS. Fat contents of meals and bioavailability of griseofulvin in man. *J Pharm Pharmacol* (1985) 37, 283–4.
5. Aoyagi N, Ogata H, Kaniwa N, Ejima A. Effect of food on the bioavailability of griseofulvin from microsize and PEG ultramicrosize (GRIS-PEG) plain tablets. *J Pharmacobiodyn* (1982) 4, 120–4.
6. Bijanzadeh M, Mahmoudian M, Salehian P, Khazainia T, Eshghi L, Khosravy A. The bioavailability of griseofulvin from microsized and ultramicrosized tablets in nonfasting volunteers. *Indian J Physiol Pharmacol* (1990) 34, 157–61.
7. Bates TR, Sequeria JA. Bioavailability of micronized griseofulvin from corn oil-in-water emulsion, aqueous suspension, and commercial tablet dosage forms in humans. *J Pharm Sci* (1975) 64, 793–7.
8. Grisovin (Griseofulvin). GlaxoSmithKline UK. UK Summary of product characteristics, July 2004.

Griseofulvin + Phenobarbital

The antifungal effects of griseofulvin can be reduced or even abolished by phenobarbital.

Clinical evidence

Two epileptic children taking phenobarbital 40 mg daily did not respond to long-term treatment for tinea capitis with griseofulvin 125 mg three times daily until the barbiturate was withdrawn.[1]

Five other patients (3 also taking phenytoin) similarly did not respond to griseofulvin while taking phenobarbital.[2-4] Two studies, in a total of 14 healthy subjects, found that phenobarbital 30 mg three times daily reduced the serum levels of oral griseofulvin by about one-third,[5] and the absorption was reduced from 58.1% without phenobarbital to 40.6% in the presence of phenobarbital.[6]

Mechanism

Not fully understood. Initially it was thought that the phenobarbital increased the metabolism and clearance of the griseofulvin,[7] but it has also been suggested that it reduces the absorption of griseofulvin from the gut.[6] One idea is that the phenobarbital increases peristalsis reducing the opportunity for absorption.[6] Another suggestion is that phenobarbital forms a complex with griseofulvin, which makes an already poorly soluble drug even less soluble, and therefore less readily absorbed.[8] A further suggestion is that phenobarbital may reduce the level of intestinal bile salts, which in turn may reduce the solubility and absorption of griseofulvin.[9]

Importance and management

An established interaction of clinical importance, although the evidence seems to be limited to the reports cited. If phenobarbital must be given, it has been suggested that the griseofulvin should be given in divided doses three times a day to give it a better chance of being absorbed.[6] However, divided doses were used in one of the reports describing an interaction.[1] The effect of increasing the dosage of griseofulvin appears not to have been studied. An alternative, where possible, is to use a non-interacting anticonvulsant such as sodium valproate. This proved to be successful in one of the cases cited.[1]

1. Beurey J, Weber M, Vignaud J-M. Traitement des teignes microsporiques. Interférence métabolique entre phénobarbital et griséofulvine. *Ann Dermatol Venereol* (1982) 109, 567–70.
2. Lorenc E. A new factor in griseofulvin treatment failures. *Mo Med* (1967) 64, 32–3.
3. Stepanova ZV, Sheklakova AA. Liuminal kak prichina neudachi griseoful'vinoterapii bol'no-go mikrospoviei. *Vestn Dermatol Venerol* (1975) 12, 63–5.
4. Hay RJ, Clayton YM, Moore MK, Midgely G. An evaluation of itraconazole in the management of onychomycosis. *Br J Dermatol* (1988) 119, 359–66.
5. Busfield D, Child KJ, Atkinson RM, Tomich EG. An effect of phenobarbitone on blood-levels of griseofulvin in man. *Lancet* (1963) ii, 1042–3.
6. Riegelman S, Rowland M, Epstein WL. Griseofulvin-phenobarbital interaction in man. *JAMA* (1970) 213, 426–31.
7. Busfield D, Child KJ, Tomich EG. An effect of phenobarbitone on griseofulvin metabolism in the rat. *Br J Pharmacol* (1964) 22, 137–42.
8. Abougela IKA, Bigford DJ, McCorquodale I, Grant DJW. Complex formation and other physico-chemical interactions between griseofulvin and phenobarbitone. *J Pharm Pharmacol* (1976) 28, 44P.
9. Jamali F, Axelson JE. Griseofulvin–phenobarbital interaction: a formulation-dependent phenomenon. *J Pharm Sci* (1978) 67, 466–70.

Halofantrine + Antacids

Magnesium carbonate halves the maximum plasma levels of halofantrine, which may be clinically relevant. Aluminium hydroxide and magnesium trisilicate seem less likely to interact.

Clinical evidence

Magnesium carbonate 1 g reduced the maximum plasma levels of halofantrine 500 mg by almost 50% in a single-dose study in healthy subjects. The AUC was also reduced by 28%, but this was not statistically significant. The active metabolite of halofantrine, which is equally potent, was similarly affected.[1]

Mechanism

Magnesium carbonate might decrease the absorption of halofantrine. *In vitro* study showed that the halofantrine absorptive capacity of various antacids was highest for magnesium carbonate, intermediate for **aluminium hydroxide**, and least for **magnesium trisilicate**.[1]

Importance and management

The pharmacokinetic interaction between halofantrine and magnesium carbonate appears to be established. Its clinical importance does not seem to have been assessed, but the authors note that the clinical efficacy of halofantrine is related to peak levels, and therefore they consider that magnesium carbonate might affect antimalarial efficacy.[1] One way to minimise the interaction is to separate the dosages of halofantrine and magnesium carbonate as much as possible (at least 2 to 3 hours) to reduce admixture in the gut. There do not appear to be any studies to see if other antacids behave similarly, but the *in vitro* data with aluminium hydroxide and magnesium trisilicate (see Mechanism, above) suggest they are less likely to interact.[1]

1. Aideloje SO, Onyeji CO, Ugwu NC. Altered pharmacokinetics of halofantrine by an antacid, magnesium carbonate. *Eur J Pharm Biopharm* (1998) 46, 299–303.

Halofantrine + Miscellaneous

Halofantrine prolongs the QT interval and therefore should not be used with other drugs that can prolong the QT interval because of the increased risk of cardiac arrhythmias. The concurrent and sequential use of halofantrine and mefloquine markedly increased the risk of clinically important increases in the QT interval.
Pyrimethamine/sulfadoxine and tetracycline have been shown to increase halofantrine levels, and may therefore increase its toxicity. Diltiazem, erythromycin, ketoconazole, mefloquine, quinine, and quinidine might also increase the toxicity of halofantrine because they have been shown to inhibit its metabolism *in vitro*. The manufacturer has therefore recommended caution with the concurrent use of potent CYP3A4 inhibitors. Fatty food markedly increases halofantrine levels, consequently it is recommended that halofantrine is taken on an empty stomach. Grapefruit juice has a similar effect. Note that halofantrine is no longer widely marketed.

Clinical evidence, mechanism, importance and management

(a) CYP3A4 inhibitors

A study in *animals* found that **ketoconazole** roughly doubled the AUC of halofantrine and inhibited its metabolism to the equipotent metabolite, desbutylhalofantrine.[1] In *in vitro* studies, **ketoconazole** markedly inhibited the metabolism of halofantrine by CYP3A4.[2,3] It has been suggested that the rise in halofantrine levels could reasonably be expected to increase toxicity.[2,3] Other CYP3A4 inhibitors, **diltiazem** and **erythromycin**, also inhibited the metabolism of halofantrine *in vitro*, and might therefore do so clinically.[3] The manufacturer recommended caution with the concurrent use of potent CYP3A4 inhibitors.[4] Further study is needed of these potential pharmacokinetic interactions. **Mefloquine**, **quinine** and **quinidine** may also inhibit the metabolism of halofantrine by CYP3A4, see (b) below.

(b) Drugs that prolong the QT interval

Halofantrine, in therapeutic doses, can prolong the QT interval in the majority of patients, causing ventricular arrhythmias in a very small number. The effect is increased if halofantrine is taken with **fatty foods** because of the marked increase in absorption, see (d) below. By 1993, worldwide, 14 cases of cardiac arrhythmias associated with halofantrine had been reported, and 8 patients were known to have died. In order to reduce the likelihood of arrhythmias, in 1994 the UK Committee on Safety of Medicines advised that halofantrine should not be taken with **meals**, or with certain other drugs that may induce arrhythmias. They list **chloroquine**, **mefloquine**, **quinine**, **tricyclic antidepressants**, **antipsychotics**, **certain antiarrhythmics**, **terfenadine** and **astemizole**, as well as drugs causing electrolyte disturbances.[5] Although not listed, it would seem prudent to avoid other drugs that prolong the QT interval. For a list, see 'Table 9.2', (p.257)'.

In addition to possible additive QT-prolonging effects, **quinidine** and **quinine** have been shown *in vitro* to inhibit the metabolism of halofantrine by CYP3A4, and so may increase halofantrine levels, which could reasonably be expected to increase toxicity.[2,3] *Animal* studies found that although **mefloquine** alone did not significantly alter the QTc interval, it enhanced the effects of halofantrine by increasing blood levels.[6] Similarly, a study in patients with malaria found that the risk of clinically relevant QT prolongation was increased twofold when halofantrine was used after **mefloquine** failure (7 of 10 patients) when compared with use as primary treatment (18 of 51 patients). However, the authors note that their population had longer baseline QT intervals than the average population, which may have made them more susceptible to the effects of halofantrine[7] The manufacturers of **mefloquine**[8,9] and halofantrine,[4] therefore contraindicated concurrent use, and the use of halofantrine after **mefloquine**.

(c) Food

A study in 6 healthy subjects found that the maximum plasma levels and AUC of a single 250-mg dose of halofantrine were increased by about 6.6-fold and 2.9-fold, respectively, when given with a **fatty meal** rather than in a fasting state. The AUC of the metabolite desbutylhalofantrine was also increased.[10] *Animal* data suggest that **fats** may reduce the presystemic metabolism of halofantrine.[1] As this is likely to increase the risk of halofantrine-induced arrhythmias, halofantrine should not be taken with **meals**, but should be taken on an empty stomach.

(d) Grapefruit juice or Orange juice

A crossover study in 12 healthy subjects given halofantrine 500 mg with 250 mL of either water, orange juice or grapefruit juice (standard strength), found that grapefruit juice increased the AUC and peak plasma levels of halofantrine by 2.8-fold and 3.2-fold, respectively. The QTc interval increased by 17 milliseconds with halofantrine, and by 31 milliseconds when grapefruit juice was also given. Orange juice did not affect the pharmacokinetics or pharmacodynamics of halofantrine.[11] These data suggest that grapefruit juice should be avoided by patients taking halofantrine due to the increased risk of arrhythmias.[11]

(e) Pyrimethamine/Sulfadoxine (Fansidar)

In a preliminary study in healthy subjects, **pyrimethamine/sulfadoxine** (*Fansidar*) raised the AUC_{0-6} and peak plasma levels of halofantrine by about 1.6-fold, without changing the overall AUC. This might lead to an increased incidence of arrhythmias,[12] see also (b) above.

(f) Tetracyclines

A study in 8 healthy subjects found that tetracycline 500 mg twice daily for 7 days increased the maximum plasma levels, AUC and elimination half-life of a single 500-mg dose of halofantrine by 146%, 99%, and 73%, respectively. Increases in the major metabolite of halofantrine also occurred in the presence of tetracycline.[13] As both halofantrine and tetracycline are excreted into the bile, competition for this elimination route may result in increased plasma levels. There may be an increased risk of halofantrine toxicity if it is used with higher doses of tetracycline.[13] In contrast, *in vitro* studies found that **doxycycline** does not inhibit the metabolism of halofantrine.[2]

1. Khoo S-M, Porter CJH, Edwards GA, Charman WN. Metabolism of halofantrine to its equipotent metabolite, desbutylhalofantrine, is decreased when orally administered with ketoconazole. *J Pharm Sci* (1998) 87, 1538–41.
2. Baune B, Furlan V, Taburet AM, Farinotti R. Effect of selected antimalarial drugs and inhibitors of cytochrome P-450 3A4 on halofantrine metabolism by human liver microsomes. *Drug Metab Dispos* (1999) 27, 565–8.
3. Baune B, Flinois JP, Furlan V, Gimenez F, Taburet AM, Becquemont L, Farinotti R. Halofantrine metabolism in microsomes in man: major role of CYP 3A4 and CYP 3A5. *J Pharm Pharmacol* (1999) 51, 419–26.
4. Halfan (Halofantrine). SmithKline Beecham Pharmaceuticals. US Prescribing information, October 2001.
5. Committee on Safety of Medicines/Medicines Control Agency. Cardiac arrhythmias with halofantrine (Halfan). *Current Problems* (1994) 20, 6.
6. Lightbown ID, Lambert JP, Edwards G, Coker SJ. Potentiation of halofantrine-induced QTc prolongation by mefloquine: correlation with blood concentrations of halofantrine. *Br J Pharmacol* (2001) 132, 197–204.
7. Nosten F, ter Kuile FO, Luxemburger C, Woodrow C, Kyle DE, Chongsuphajaisiddhi T, White NJ. Cardiac effects of antimalarial treatment with halofantrine. *Lancet* (1993) 341, 1054–6.
8. Lariam (Mefloquine hydrochloride). Roche Products Ltd. UK Summary of product characteristics, September 2005.
9. Lariam (Mefloquine hydrochloride). Roche Pharmaceuticals. US Prescribing information, May 2004.
10. Milton K, Edwards G, Ward SA, Orme ML'E, Breckenridge AM. Pharmacokinetics of halofantrine in man: effects of food and dose size. *Br J Clin Pharmacol* (1989) 28, 71–7.
11. Charbit B, Becquemont L, Lepère B, Peytavin G, Funck-Brentano C. Pharmacokinetic and pharmacodynamic interaction between grapefruit juice and halofantrine. *Clin Pharmacol Ther* (2002) 72, 514–23.
12. Hombhanje FW. Effect of a single dose of Fansidar™ on the pharmacokinetics of halofantrine in healthy volunteers: a preliminary report. *Br J Clin Pharmacol* (2000) 49, 283–4.
13. Bassi PU, Onyeji CO, Ukponmwan OE. Effects of tetracycline on the pharmacokinetics of halofantrine in healthy volunteers. *Br J Clin Pharmacol* (2004) 58, 52–5.

Hydroxychloroquine + Rifampicin (Rifampin)

A woman with discoid lupus, controlled by hydroxychloroquine, rapidly relapsed when rifampicin was started. Disease control was regained when the hydroxychloroquine dosage was doubled.

Clinical evidence, mechanism, importance and management

A woman with discoid lupus, which was controlled by hydroxychloroquine 200 mg daily, was also given rifampicin, isoniazid and pyrazinamide for tuberculosis. Within 1 to 2 weeks the discoid lupus flared-up again but it rapidly responded when the hydroxychloroquine dosage was doubled. The reason for this reaction is not known for certain but the authors of the report suggest that the rifampicin (a recognised and potent cytochrome P450 enzyme inducer) increased the metabolism and clearance of the hydroxychloroquine so that it was no longer effective.[1] It is already known that discoid lupus flare-ups can occur within 2 weeks of stopping hydroxychloroquine,[2] which gives support to this suggested mechanism. Neither isoniazid nor pyrazinamide is likely to have been responsible for what happened.

This seems to be the first and only report of this interaction, but what happened is consistent with the way rifampicin interacts with many other drugs. If rifampicin is added to hydroxychloroquine, the outcome should be well monitored. Be alert for the need to increase the hydroxychloroquine dosage.

1. Harvey CJ, Bateman NT, Lloyd ME, Hughes GRV. Influence of rifampicin on hydroxychloroquine. *Clin Exp Rheumatol* (1995) 13, 536.
2. The Canadian Hydroxychloroquine Study Group. A randomized study of the effect of withdrawing hydroxychloroquine sulfate in systemic lupus erythematosus. *N Engl J Med* (1991) 324, 150–4.

Hydroxyquinoline (Oxyquinoline) + Zinc oxide

The presence of zinc oxide inhibits the therapeutic effects of hydroxyquinoline in ointments.

Clinical evidence

The observation that a patient had an allergic reaction to hydroxyquinoline in ointments with a paraffin base, but not a zinc oxide base, prompted further study of a possible incompatibility. The subsequent study in 13 patients confirmed that zinc oxide reduces the eczematogenic (allergic) properties of the hydroxyquinoline. However, it also inhibits its antibacterial and antimycotic effects, and appears to stimulate the growth of *Candida albicans*.[1]

Mechanism

It seems almost certain that the zinc ions form chelates with hydroxyquinoline, which have little or no antibacterial properties.[1,2]

Importance and management

The documentation is limited but the reaction appears to be established. There is no point in using zinc oxide to reduce the allergic properties of hydroxyquinoline if, at the same time, the therapeutic effects disappear.

1. Fischer T. On 8-hydroxyquinoline-zinc oxide incompatibility. *Dermatologica* (1974) 149, 129–35.
2. Albert A, Rubbo SD, Goldacre RJ, Balfour BG. The influence of chemical constitution on antibacterial activity. Part III: A study of 8-hydroxyquinoline (oxine) and related compounds. *Br J Exp Pathol* (1947) 28, 69–87.

Ivermectin + Food

The manufacturer notes that the bioavailability of ivermectin 30 mg was increased by about 2.5-fold when it was taken after a high-fat meal (48.6 g of fat) when compared with the fasted state.[1] They recommend that ivermectin is taken on a empty stomach with water.[1]

1. Stromectol (Ivermectin). Merck & Co., Inc. US Prescribing information, March 2007.

Ivermectin + Levamisole

Levamisole may markedly increase the bioavailability of ivermectin. Ivermectin does not alter the pharmacokinetics of levamisole.

Clinical evidence, mechanism, importance and management

A study in 28 healthy subjects given levamisole 2.5 mg/kg, alone or with ivermectin 200 micrograms/kg, found that ivermectin had no effect on the AUC or maximum level of levamisole. However, the AUC of ivermectin was twofold higher when given with levamisole compared with historical values in subjects who had received ivermectin alone.[1] An associated study in 44 patients with *Onchocerca volvulus* infections found that levamisole given with ivermectin was neither macrofilaricidal nor more effective against microfilariae and adult worms than ivermectin alone. In addition, patients taking both drugs had a higher incidence of pruritus, arthralgia and fever than those on ivermectin alone.[1] Caution is recommended on concurrent use.

1. Awadzi K, Edwards G, Opoku NO, Ardrey AE, Favager S, Addy ET, Attah SK, Yamuah LK, Quartey BT. The safety, tolerability and pharmacokinetics of levamisole alone, levamisole plus ivermectin, and levamisole plus albendazole, and their efficacy against *Onchocerca volvulus*. *Ann Trop Med Parasitol* (2004) 98, 595–614.

Ivermectin + Orange juice

Orange juice modestly reduces the bioavailability of ivermectin.

Clinical evidence, mechanism, importance and management

A study in 16 healthy subjects found that the AUC and peak plasma levels of a single 150-micrograms/kg dose of ivermectin were reduced by 36% and 39%, respectively, when the ivermectin was given with orange juice (750 mL over 4 hours) rather than with water. The mechanism for the reduced bioavailability is not known but it does not seem related to P-glycoprotein activity.[1] The clinical relevance of these changes is uncertain.

1. Vanapalli SR, Chen Y, Ellingrod VL, Kitzman D, Lee Y, Hohl RJ, Fleckenstein L. Orange juice decreases the oral bioavailability of ivermectin in healthy volunteers. *Clin Pharmacol Ther* (2003) 73, P94.

Levamisole + Miscellaneous

There is some evidence that levamisole, taken with fluorouracil, can increase the effects of phenytoin, and that a disulfiram-like reaction can occur if patients taking levamisole drink alcohol.

Clinical evidence, mechanism, importance and management

The product information for levamisole states that levamisole, taken with fluorouracil, may increase in the plasma levels of **phenytoin**. Note that fluorouracil alone increases phenytoin levels, see 'Antiepileptics + Antineoplastics; Cytotoxic', p.518.

The information also notes that a disulfiram-like reaction has been reported with levamisole and **alcohol**.[1] The general importance of this interaction is uncertain, but bear it in mind when prescribing levamisole.

1. Ergamisol (Levamisole). Janssen Pharmaceutica Inc. US Prescribing information, August 1999.

Mefloquine + Ampicillin

Although ampicillin modestly increases the plasma levels of mefloquine and reduces its half-life, these effects are probably not clinically relevant.

Clinical evidence, mechanism, importance and management

In a study, 8 healthy subjects were given ampicillin 250 mg four times daily for 5 days, with a single 750-mg dose of mefloquine on day 2. The maximum plasma level and 5-day AUC of mefloquine were increased by 34% and 49%, respectively, although the $AUC_{0-\infty}$ was not significantly increased. The half-life and volume of distribution of mefloquine were reduced from 17.7 to 15.3 days and by 27%, respectively, by the ampicillin. No increase in adverse events was seen. The effects may be due to an increase in mefloquine bioavailability and a reduction in its enterohepatic recycling.[1] The clinical relevance of these changes is uncertain, but the authors consider that the changes in elimination are unlikely to be clinically significant, since these occur after the resolution of infection.[1]

1. Karbwang J, Na Bangchang K, Back DJ, Bunnag D. Effect of ampicillin on mefloquine pharmacokinetics in Thai males. *Eur J Clin Pharmacol* (1991) 40, 631–3.

Mefloquine + Artemisinin derivatives

Artemether pretreatment appears to modestly reduce mefloquine levels, whereas artemisinin and dihydroartemisinin do not affect the pharmacokinetics of mefloquine. If mefloquine is given shortly after artesunate its levels are lowered, but giving mefloquine two days in to artesunate treatment appears to raise mefloquine levels. The combined use of mefloquine with artemisinin derivatives might improve antimalarial activity. See also 'Co-artemether + Mefloquine', p.224

Clinical evidence, mechanism, importance and management

(a) Artemether

In a study in patients with acute uncomplicated falciparum malaria 15 patients were given a single 300-mg dose of artemether, with a single 750-mg dose of mefloquine 24 hours later. The AUC of mefloquine in these patients was found to be 27% lower than the AUC of 7 patients receiving mefloquine alone. However, the addition of artemether improved the rate of parasite clearance, and cure rates were similar between the groups.[1] For discussion of a study that found mefloquine pharmacokinetics did not appear to be altered when artemether/lumefantrine was given 12 hours after mefloquine treatment, see 'Co-artemether + Mefloquine', p.224. Note that co-artemether (artemether with lumefantrine) is one of the recommended treatment options in the WHO guidelines for the treatment of uncomplicated falciparum malaria.[2]

(b) Artemisinin or Dihydroartemisinin

In a single-dose three-way crossover study, 10 healthy subjects were given either mefloquine 750 mg, dihydroartemisinin 300 mg or both drugs together. The pharmacokinetics of the drugs were unchanged on concurrent use, except for the rate of absorption of mefloquine, which was increased. Also the activity of these drugs against *Plasmodium falciparum* was synergistic, rather than additive.[3] Another study in patients with falciparum malaria found no significant pharmacokinetic interaction between artemisinin and mefloquine. In this study, patients received mefloquine 750 mg alone or artemisinin 500 mg daily for 3 days with a single 750-mg dose of mefloquine either on day 1 or day 4. There was no difference in overall efficacy between treatments, although those treated with artemisinin together with mefloquine on the first day of treatment had the fastest parasite clearance rates.[4]

(c) Artesunate

A study in 20 patients with acute uncomplicated falciparum malaria given mefloquine (750 mg followed after 6 hours by 500 mg) found that the levels of mefloquine were reduced by 27% and its clearance rate was increased 2.6-fold when the doses of mefloquine were given 6 and 12 hours after artesunate 200 mg. However, the patients who received the combination had shorter fever clearance and parasite clearance times than those given mefloquine alone, but the cure rate was lower for combined treatment than for mefloquine alone (66% versus 75%). To prevent the pharmacokinetic interaction resulting in a reduction in its efficacy, mefloquine should be given when artesunate and its metabolites have cleared the circulation (the authors suggest possibly 24 hours after a dose).[5] This suggestion is supported by a study looking at the efficacy of mefloquine with artesunate. This study found that the AUC of mefloquine was about 30% higher in 22 children given mefloquine on day 2 of artesunate treatment, when compared with 24 children given mefloquine on day 0 (before artesunate was started). Both groups were given mefloquine without food.[6]

The combined use of artesunate and mefloquine is one of the recommended treatment options in the WHO guidelines for the treatment of uncomplicated falciparum malaria, and for uncomplicated vivax malaria in selected areas.[2] They say that mefloquine is usually given on day 2 of combined treatment.

1. Na-Bangchang K, Karbwang J, Molunto P, Banmairuroi V, Thanavibul A. Pharmacokinetics of mefloquine, when given alone and in combination with artemether, in patients with uncomplicated falciparum malaria. *Fundam Clin Pharmacol* (1995) 9, 576–82.

2. World Health Organisation. Guidelines for the treatment of malaria 2006. Available at: http://www.who.int/malaria/docs/TreatmentGuidelines2006.pdf (accessed 16/08/07).
3. Na-Bangchang K, Tippawangkosol P, Thanavibul A, Ubalee R, Karbwang J. Pharmacokinetic and pharmacodynamic interactions of mefloquine and dihydroartemisinin. *Int J Clin Pharmacol Res* (1999) 19, 9–17.
4. Svensson USH, Alin MH, Karlsson MO, Bergqvist Y, Ashton M. Population pharmacokinetic and pharmacodynamic modelling of artemisinin and mefloquine enantiomers in patients with falciparum malaria. *Eur J Clin Pharmacol* (2002) 58, 339–51.
5. Karbwang J, Na Bangchang K, Thanavibul A, Back DJ, Bunnag D, Harinasuta T. Pharmacokinetics of mefloquine alone or in combination with artesunate. *Bull WHO* (1994) 72, 83–7.
6. Price R, Simpson JA, Teja-Isavatharm P, Than MM, Luxemburger C, Heppner DG, Chongsuphajaisiddhi T, Nosten F, White NJ. Pharmacokinetics of mefloquine combined with artesunate in children with acute falciparum malaria. *Antimicrob Agents Chemother* (1999) 43, 341–6.

Mefloquine + Cardioactive drugs

An isolated report describes cardiopulmonary arrest in a patient taking mefloquine with propranolol. The WHO have issued a warning about the concurrent use of mefloquine with antiarrhythmics, beta blockers, calcium-channel blockers, antihistamines, phenothiazines, and some related antimalarials. For mention that halofantrine should not be used with or after mefloquine, because of a clinically significant lengthening of the QT interval, see 'Halofantrine + Miscellaneous', p.229.

Clinical evidence, mechanism, importance and management

The WHO[1] warn that the use of mefloquine with **antiarrhythmics, beta blockers, calcium-channel blockers, antihistamines** and **phenothiazines** may contribute to the prolongation of the QTc interval, but do not specifically contraindicate the use of mefloquine with these drugs.[1] Note that, of the classes mentioned, class Ic and class III antiarrhythmics, sotalol, astemizole and terfenadine are most frequently associated with QT-prolongation, and these drugs are therefore likely to present the greatest risk. It is also suggested that mefloquine and related drugs (e.g. **quinine** or **quinidine**) should only be given together under close medical supervision because of possible additive cardiotoxicity.[1] The manufacturers of mefloquine also give these warnings, pointing out that the interactions are theoretical, and that clinically significant QTc prolongation has not been found with mefloquine alone.[2,3] Apart from '**quinine**', (p.233) where two studies found minor QTc prolongation, no formal studies on the possible adverse effects of combining any of the above drugs with mefloquine seem to have been done. It remains to be confirmed whether the effects of mefloquine and these other drugs on cardiac function are normally additive, and whether the outcome is clinically important. However, until more is known it would seem prudent to err on the side of caution and to follow this cautionary advice. Drugs that prolong the QT interval are listed in 'Table 9.2', (p.257). There is also a theoretical interaction with QT-prolonging 'quinolones' (p.233). For mention that halofantrine should not be used with or after mefloquine, because of a clinically significant lengthening of the QT interval, which may be due to a pharmacokinetic interaction, see 'Halofantrine + Miscellaneous', p.229. One 1990 review[4] and the US prescribing information[3] briefly mention a single case of cardiopulmonary arrest (with full recovery[3]) when a patient taking **propranolol** was given a single dose[4] of mefloquine. It has been suggested that the concurrent use of beta blockers and mefloquine may lead to bradycardia, which is an uncommon adverse effect of mefloquine,[2,3] and a known effect of the beta blockers. However, there do not appear to be any reports of an adverse interaction in the literature.

1. WHO. International travel and health; Malaria. Geneva: WHO, 2007. Available at: http://www.who.int/ith/en (accessed 16/08/07).
2. Lariam (Mefloquine hydrochloride). Roche Products Ltd. UK Summary of product characteristics, September 2005.
3. Lariam (Mefloquine hydrochloride). Roche Pharmaceuticals. US Prescribing information, May 2004.
4. Anon. Mefloquine for malaria. *Med Lett Drugs Ther* (1990) 31, 13–14.

Mefloquine + Cimetidine

Mefloquine levels may be modestly increased and/or its elimination modestly reduced by cimetidine. The clinical importance of this is uncertain.

Clinical evidence, mechanism, importance and management

A single 500-mg dose of mefloquine was given to 10 healthy subjects before and after they took cimetidine 400 mg twice daily for 28 days. The cimetidine had no effect on the AUC or serum levels of mefloquine, but its half-life increased by 50% (from 9.6 to 14.4 days) and the oral clearance decreased by almost 40%.[1] In another study mefloquine was given to 6 healthy subjects and 6 patients with peptic ulcers, before and after cimetidine 400 mg twice daily for 3 days. In contrast to the first study, cimetidine increased the maximum plasma levels of mefloquine by about 42% and 20% and increased the AUC by about 37% and 32% in the healthy subjects and patients, respectively. The elimination half-life was increased, but not to a significant extent.[2]

The findings of the first study suggest that cimetidine (a recognised enzyme inhibitor) reduces the metabolism of the mefloquine by the liver.[1] However, the second study suggests that cimetidine may increase the rate of mefloquine absorption without significantly inhibiting its elimination.[2]

These two studies produced different findings, and an interaction is not therefore established. Nevertheless, the changes seen in both studies were modest, and unlikely to be clinically relevant in most patients taking lower doses of chloroquine for malaria prophylaxis. With higher doses of mefloquine used to treat malaria, to be on the safe side, prescribers should be alert for any evidence of increased mefloquine adverse effects (dizziness, nausea, vomiting, abdominal pain) and psychiatric or neurological reactions during concurrent use. Note that the UK Committee on Safety of Medicines say that any patient given mefloquine [for malaria prophylaxis] should be informed about its adverse effects, and advised that, if these occur, they should seek medical advice on alternative antimalarials before the next dose is due.[3]

1. Sunbhanichi M, Ridtitid W, Wongnawa M, Akesiripong S, Chamnongchob P. Effect of cimetidine on an oral single-dose mefloquine pharmacokinetics in humans. *Asia Pac J Pharmacol* (1997) 12, 51–5.
2. Kolawole JA, Mustapha A, Abudu-Aguye I, Ochekpe N. Mefloquine pharmacokinetics in healthy subjects and in peptic ulcer patients after cimetidine administration. *Eur J Drug Metab Pharmacokinet* (2000) 25, 165–70.
3. Committee on Safety of Medicines/Medicines Control Agency. Mefloquine (Lariam) and neuropsychiatric reactions. *Current Problems* (1996) 22, 6.

Mefloquine + Ketoconazole

Ketoconazole increased the AUC of mefloquine by 79%. The clinical relevance of this is uncertain, but an increase in adverse events is possible.

Clinical evidence, mechanism, importance and management

In a study in healthy subjects a single 500-mg dose of mefloquine, given on day 5 of a 10-day course of ketoconazole 400 mg daily, increased the mefloquine AUC by 79%, the maximum level by 64% and the half-life by 34%, when compared to mefloquine alone. A 28% decrease in the AUC of the carboxylic metabolite was also seen. No significant adverse effects were reported.[1] It is probable that ketoconazole inhibits the metabolism of mefloquine by cytochrome P450 isoenzyme CYP3A4. Although the clinical relevance of this increase in mefloquine levels is not known, it seems possible that it could increase the risk of adverse effects in some patients. Until more is known, it may be prudent to be cautious in the use of mefloquine in patients taking ketoconazole.

1. Ridtitid W, Wongnawa M, Mahatthanatrakul W, Raungsri N, Sunbhanich M. Ketoconazole increases plasma concentrations of antimalarial mefloquine in healthy human volunteers. *J Clin Pharm Ther* (2005) 30, 285–90.

Mefloquine + Metoclopramide

Although metoclopramide increases the rate of absorption of a single-dose of mefloquine and increases mefloquine peak levels, its gastrointestinal adverse effects are possibly reduced.

Clinical evidence, mechanism, importance and management

When 7 healthy subjects took a 10-mg dose of metoclopramide 15 minutes before a single 750-mg dose of mefloquine, the absorption half-life of the mefloquine was reduced from 3.2 to 2.4 hours and the peak blood levels were raised by 31%. However, although the rate of absorption was increased, the total amount absorbed was unchanged. A possible reason for these changes is that metoclopramide increases gastric emptying causing mefloquine to reach the small intestine more quickly, which would increase the rate of absorption. Despite these changes, the toxicity of mefloquine (dizziness, nausea, vomiting, abdominal pain) was noted to be reduced.[1] The modest increase in peak levels is probably not clinically relevant, especially with prophylactic mefloquine doses. More study is needed.

1. Na Bangchang K, Karbwang J, Bunnag D, Harinasuta T, Back DJ. The effect of metoclopramide on mefloquine pharmacokinetics. *Br J Clin Pharmacol* (1991) 32, 640–1.

Mefloquine + Primaquine

Although one study suggested that primaquine can increase both the peak serum levels and adverse effects of mefloquine, other studies have generally found no important interaction. Primaquine may be used after mefloquine to effect a radical cure of *P. vivax* malaria without any special precautions.

Clinical evidence

A preliminary report of a randomised crossover study in 14 healthy subjects given mefloquine 1 g found that the addition of primaquine 15 or 30 mg raised the peak serum levels of mefloquine by 48% and 29%, respectively. Those taking the larger dose of primaquine had a transient increase in peak primaquine serum levels, and its conversion to its inactive carboxyl metabolite was also increased. Significant CNS symptoms were also experienced by those taking the larger dose of primaquine.[1]

However, these results contrast with another single dose study in 8 healthy subjects, who were given mefloquine 750 mg with primaquine 45 mg. No increased adverse effects attributable to concurrent use were seen, and mefloquine pharmacokinetics (including the peak level) were not altered by primaquine.[2] Similarly, in a study in patients with malaria, there was no change in mefloquine pharmacokinetics when it was given with primaquine.[3] In another group in this study, the only difference in mefloquine pharmacokinetics was an 11% shorter terminal elimination half-life in those taking primaquine with mefloquine and sulfadoxine/pyrimethamine, when compared with those taking mefloquine with sulfadoxine/pyrimethamine.[3] Similarly, in another study in children given mefloquine with sulfadoxine/pyrimethamine, the addition of primaquine had no effect on the pharmacokinetics of mefloquine, and there was no serious adverse effects.[4]

The pharmacokinetics of a single 45-mg dose of primaquine were not altered by a single 10-mg/kg oral dose of mefloquine in healthy subjects.[5]

Mechanism

In vitro studies suggest that primaquine is a potent inhibitor of mefloquine metabolism.[6]

Importance and management

The bulk of the evidence suggests there is no important alteration in the pharmacokinetics or effect of mefloquine when it is given with primaquine. After treatment of vivax malaria, primaquine is used to eradicate hepatic parasites, so producing a radical cure, and the manufacturer of mefloquine specifically advises this.[7,8]

1. Macleod CM, Trenholme GM, Nora MV, Bartley EA, Frischer H. Interaction of primaquine with mefloquine in healthy males. *Intersci Conf Antimicrob Agents Chemother* (1990) 30, 213.
2. Karbwang J, Na Bangchang K, Thanavibul A, Back DJ, Bunnag D. Pharmacokinetics of mefloquine in the presence of primaquine. *Eur J Clin Pharmacol* (1992) 42, 559–60.
3. Karbwang J, Back DJ, Bunnag D, Breckenridge AM. Pharmacokinetics of mefloquine in combination with sulfadoxine-pyrimethamine and primaquine in male Thai patients with falciparum malaria. *Bull WHO* (1990) 68, 633–8.
4. Singhasivanon V, Chongsuphajaisiddhi T, Sabchareon A, Attanath P, Webster HK, Edstein MD, Lika ID. Pharmacokinetic study of mefloquine in Thai children aged 5–12 years suffering from uncomplicated falciparum malaria treated with MSP or MSP plus primaquine. *Eur J Drug Metab Pharmacokinet* (1994) 19, 27–32.
5. Edwards G, McGrath CS, Ward SA, Supanaranond W, Pukrittayakamee S, Davis TM, White NJ. Interactions among primaquine, malaria infection and other antimalarials in Thai subjects. *Br J Clin Pharmacol* (1993) 35, 193–8.
6. Na Bangchang K, Karbwang J, Back DJ. Mefloquine metabolism by human liver microsomes. Effect of other antimalarial drugs. *Biochem Pharmacol* (1992) 43, 1957–61.
7. Lariam (Mefloquine hydrochloride). Roche Products Ltd. UK Summary of product characteristics, September 2005.
8. Lariam (Mefloquine hydrochloride). Roche Pharmaceuticals. US Prescribing information, May 2004.

Mefloquine + Quinine and related drugs

Mefloquine serum levels may possibly be increased by quinine. In theory there is an increased risk of convulsions if mefloquine is given with quinine or chloroquine.

Clinical evidence, mechanism, importance and management

Mefloquine 750 mg was given to 7 healthy subjects either alone, or followed 24 hours later by quinine 600 mg. The combination did not affect the pharmacokinetics of either drug, but the number of adverse effects and the period of prolongation of the QT interval was greater with the combination, although no symptomatic cardiotoxicity was seen.[1] This absence of a change in pharmacokinetics is contrary to earlier *in vitro* data and unpublished clinical observations,[2] which suggested that quinine may inhibit the metabolism of mefloquine, thereby raising its serum levels. Another study in 13 patients with uncomplicated falciparum malaria given quinine dihydrochloride 10 mg/kg as a one-hour infusion and simultaneous oral mefloquine 15 mg/kg found no evidence of a pharmacokinetic interaction, but postural hypotension was common. The QTc interval was prolonged by 12%, although a clinically significant cardiovascular interaction was not reported.[3]

The manufacturers of mefloquine say that it should not be given with quinine or related compounds (e.g. **quinidine**, **chloroquine**) since this could increase the risk of ECG abnormalities and convulsions. They suggest that patients initially given intravenous quinine for 2 to 3 days should delay mefloquine until at least 12 hours after the last dosing of quinine to minimise interactions leading to adverse events.[4,5] However, there seem to be no documented adverse reports of this interaction leading to convulsions. Consider also 'Mefloquine + Cardioactive drugs' p.232, for further discussion of the potential for cardiotoxicity with these drugs.

1. Na-Bangchang K, Tan-Ariya P, Thanavibul A, Reingchainam S, Shrestha SB, Karbwang J. Pharmacokinetic and pharmacodynamic interactions of mefloquine and quinine. *Int J Clin Pharmacol Res* (1999) 19, 73–82.
2. Na Bangchang K, Karbwang J, Back DJ. Mefloquine metabolism by human liver microsomes. Effect of other antimalarial drugs. *Biochem Pharmacol* (1992) 43, 1957–61.
3. Supanaranond W, Suputtamongkol Y, Davis TME, Pukrittayakamee S, Teja-Isavadharm P, Webster HK, White NJ. Lack of a significant adverse cardiovascular effect of combined quinine and mefloquine therapy for uncomplicated malaria. *Trans R Soc Trop Med Hyg* (1997) 91, 694–6.
4. Lariam (Mefloquine hydrochloride). Roche Products Ltd. UK Summary of product characteristics, September 2005.
5. Lariam (Mefloquine hydrochloride). Roche Pharmaceuticals. US Prescribing information, May 2004.

Mefloquine + Quinolones

Three non-epileptic patients had convulsions when they were treated for fever with mefloquine and a quinolone. Also, some quinolones, such as moxifloxacin, prolong the QT interval and concurrent use with mefloquine might theoretically result in additive effects.

Clinical evidence, mechanism, importance and management

(a) Convulsions

A large scale survey in India of the adverse effects of mefloquine identified 3 cases of convulsions out of a total of 150 patients also taking **ciprofloxacin**, **ofloxacin** or **sparfloxacin**. All 3 patients were not epileptic, and had no family history of epilepsy. All were being treated for fever, which was due to *Plasmodium vivax* in one case, *P. falciparum* in the second, and was not established in the third. None of the patients had severe or complicated malaria. The **ofloxacin** was given 2 days before the mefloquine, and the other two quinolones were given together with the mefloquine.[1] The reason for the seizures is not known, but seizures are among the recognised adverse effects of both mefloquine and these quinolones. These adverse, apparently additive, effects are rare, but prescribers should be aware of the potential increased risk of convulsions when prescribing these drugs together.

(b) Prolongation of the QT interval

Gatifloxacin, **moxifloxacin**, and **sparfloxacin** may cause clinically relevant prolongation of the QT interval. Although mefloquine alone has not been shown to cause a clinically relevant lengthening of the QT interval, caution has still been recommended when it is combined with some other drugs that prolong the QT interval, see 'Mefloquine + Cardioactive drugs', p.232, and it may be prudent to extend this caution to these quinolones. The manufacturers of **moxifloxacin** note that an additive effect on QT prolongation between **moxifloxacin** and antimalarials cannot be excluded, and therefore contraindicates concurrent use, although they specifically mention only halofantrine.[2]

1. Mangalvedhekar SS, Gogtay NJ, Wagh VR, Waran MS, Mane D, Kshirsager NA. Convulsions in non-epileptics due to mefloquine-fluoroquinolone co-administration. *Natl Med J India* (2000) 13, 47.
2. Avelox (Moxifloxacin). Bayer plc. UK Summary of product characteristics, July 2006.

Mefloquine + Rifampicin (Rifampin)

Rifampicin significantly reduces the plasma concentrations of mefloquine. Until more is known, it may be prudent to avoid the combination.

Clinical evidence, mechanism, importance and management

Rifampicin 600 mg daily was given to 7 healthy subjects for 7 days with a single 500-mg dose of mefloquine on day 7. The maximum plasma level of mefloquine decreased by 19% and the AUC decreased by 68%. Rifampicin, a potent enzyme-inducer, increases the metabolism of mefloquine by the cytochrome P450 isoenzyme CYP3A4 in the liver and gut wall. The clinical relevance of this reduction in mefloquine levels uncertain, but the authors suggest that simultaneous use of rifampicin and mefloquine should be avoided to prevent treatment failure and the risk of *Plasmodium falciparum* resistance to mefloquine.[1] Until more is known, this would seem a sensible precaution.

1. Ridtitid W, Wongnawa M, Mahatthanatrakul W, Chaipol P, Sunbhanich M. Effect of rifampicin on plasma concentrations of mefloquine in healthy volunteers. *J Pharm Pharmacol* (2000) 52, 1265–9.

Mefloquine + Sulfadoxine/Pyrimethamine

Sulfadoxine/pyrimethamine caused a modest increase in exposure to mefloquine in healthy subjects, but not in a study in patients. Any changes seem unlikely to be clinically relevant.

Clinical evidence, mechanism, importance and management

In healthy subjects, a comparison of the pharmacokinetic parameters of a single 750-mg dose of mefloquine given alone or in combination with sulfadoxine/pyrimethamine found that the only difference was a 33% increase in mean residence time and 27% increase in the half-life of mefloquine.[1] However, in a further study in patients with malaria, there was no difference in any pharmacokinetic parameter of mefloquine 750 mg between 15 patients taking mefloquine alone and 16 taking mefloquine with sulfadoxine/pyrimethamine.[2] In both of these studies there was considerable inter-individual variability in the pharmacokinetics of mefloquine.[1,2] In another study in healthy subjects, the mefloquine AUC was increased by a non-significant 13% when mefloquine was given as a combination tablet containing mefloquine, sulfadoxine and pyrimethamine when compared with mefloquine given alone.[3]

These studies suggest that, at the most, a small increase in exposure to mefloquine may occur when it is given with sulfadoxine/pyrimethamine. It would seem that this is unlikely to be clinically relevant, especially in view of the inter-individual variability in mefloquine pharmacokinetics. No special precautions appear to be needed.

1. Karbwang J, Bunnag D, Breckenridge AM, Back DJ. The pharmacokinetics of mefloquine when given alone or in combination with sulphadoxine and pyrimethamine in Thai male and female subjects. *Eur J Clin Pharmacol* (1987) 32, 173–7.
2. Karbwang J, Back DJ, Bunnag D, Breckenridge AM. Pharmacokinetics of mefloquine in combination with sulfadoxine-pyrimethamine and primaquine in male Thai patients with falciparum malaria. *Bull WHO* (1990) 68, 633–8.
3. Schwartz DE, Weidekamm E, Ranalder UB, Dubach UC, Forgo I, Weber B. Absence of pharmacokinetic interaction between Fansidar and mefloquine. *Trans R Soc Trop Med Hyg* (1986) 80, 1001–2.

Mefloquine + Tetracycline

Mefloquine serum levels are modestly increased by tetracycline.

Clinical evidence, mechanism, importance and management

The maximum serum levels of a single 750-mg dose of mefloquine were increased by 38% (from 1.16 to 1.6 mg/mL) in 20 healthy Thai men who took tetracycline 250 mg four times daily for a week. The AUC was increased by 30% and the half-life reduced from 19.3 to 14.4 days, without any evidence of an increase in adverse effects. The suggested reason for the increased mefloquine levels is that its enterohepatic recycling is reduced because of competition with tetracycline for biliary excretion.[1] The authors of the report conclude that concurrent use may be valuable for treating multi-drug resistant falciparum malaria because higher mefloquine levels are associated with a more effective response. However, more study is needed to confirm these findings. There seems to be no reason for avoiding concurrent use.

1. Karbwang J, Na Bangchang K, Back DJ, Bunnag D, Rooney W. Effect of tetracycline on mefloquine pharmacokinetics in Thai males. *Eur J Clin Pharmacol* (1992) 43, 567–9.

Mefloquine + Typhoid vaccine; Oral

Some sources suggest that mefloquine should not be given at the same time as oral attenuated live typhoid vaccine, whereas others suggest that concurrent administration is acceptable. Note that this advice does not apply to the capsular polysaccharide typhoid vaccine for injection.

Clinical evidence

An *in vitro* study found that mefloquine killed a significant amount of *S.typhi* (Ty21a vaccine strain), which suggested that concurrent administration could possibly reduce the efficacy of the vaccine.[1] A study in healthy subjects investigated the use of mefloquine with a combination of cholera and oral typhoid vaccine (Ty21a vaccine strain). Cholera and typhoid vaccines had previously been shown not to affect each other, and the addition of mefloquine did not significantly reduce the serum antibody response to these vaccines. The authors therefore concluded that mefloquine could be given at the same time as oral typhoid vaccine without reducing its efficacy.[2]

Mechanism

Oral typhoid vaccine requires active replication of the attenuated *Salmonella typhi* strain in the ileum for the development of immunity. Mefloquine is thought to have some antibacterial effect, which may diminish the amount of *S. typhi* present, and therefore reduce the immune response produced by the vaccine.[2,3]

Importance and Management

As mefloquine is rapidly absorbed it has been suggested that by 8 hours after a dose, the levels of mefloquine will be insufficient to inhibit live oral typhoid vaccine.[4] Based on the results of the above study the US manufacturers note that mefloquine can be given at the same time as oral typhoid vaccine.[2,5] The UK manufacturers of the oral typhoid vaccine recommend separating the dose of oral typhoid vaccine and mefloquine by at least 12 hours.[6] However, the manufacturers of mefloquine say that immunisation with vaccines such as oral typhoid should be completed at least 3 days before the first dose of mefloquine.[7,8] The UK Department of Health say that mefloquine can be given 12 hours before or after vaccination with oral typhoid vaccine.[9] It would therefore seem acceptable to separate administration by 12 hours. Note that this advice does not apply to the capsular polysaccharide typhoid vaccine for injection.

1. Horowitz H, Carbonaro CA. Inhibition of *Salmonella typhi* oral vaccine strain Ty21a, by mefloquine and chloroquine. *J Infect Dis* (1992) 166, 1462–4.

2. Kollaritsch H, Que JU, Kunz C, Wiedermann G, Herzog C, Cryz SJ. Safety and immunogenicity of live oral cholera and typhoid vaccines administered alone or in combination with antimalarial drugs, oral polio vaccine, or yellow fever vaccine. *J Infect Dis* (1997) 175, 871–5.
3. Brachman PS, Metchock B, Kozarsky PE. Effects of antimalarial chemoprophylactic agents on the viability of the Ty21a typhoid vaccine strain. *Clin Infect Dis* (1992) 15, 1057–8.
4. Cryz SJ. Post-marketing experience with live oral Ty21a vaccine. *Lancet* (1993) 341, 49–50.
5. Vivotif (Typhoid Vaccine Live Oral Ty21a). US Prescribing information. February 2004.
6. Vivotif (Live attenuated *S. Typhi* Ty21a). Masta Ltd. UK Summary of product characteristics. March 2005.
7. Lariam (Mefloquine hydrochloride). Roche Products Ltd. UK Summary of product characteristics, September 2005.
8. Lariam (Mefloquine hydrochloride). Roche Pharmaceuticals. US Prescribing information, May 2004.
9. Department of Health. Immunisation Against Infectious Disease 2006: "The Green Book". Available at: http://www.dh.gov.uk/en/Policyandguidance/Healthandsocialcaretopics/Greenbook/ DH_4097254 (accessed 16/08/07).

Metrifonate + Antacids or H_2-receptor antagonists

The pharmacokinetics of a single dose of metrifonate were not altered by an antacid containing aluminium/magnesium hydroxide, nor by pretreatment with cimetidine or ranitidine.

Clinical evidence, mechanism, importance and management

(a) Antacids

The AUC and maximum level of metrifonate and its pharmacologically active metabolite were not altered by concurrent use of an **aluminium/magnesium hydroxide**-containing antacid in a single-dose study in healthy subjects.[1]

(b) H_2-receptor antagonists

The AUC and maximum level of metrifonate and its pharmacologically active metabolite were not altered by pretreatment with either **cimetidine** or **ranitidine** in a study in healthy subjects.[1] Based on these results it seems unlikely that other H_2-receptor antagonists will interact with metrifonate.

1. Heinig R, Boettcher M, Herman-Gnjidic Z, Pierce CH. Effects of magnesium/aluminium hydroxide-containing antacid, cimetidine or ranitidine on the pharmacokinetics of metrifonate and its metabolite DDVP. *Clin Drug Invest* (1999) 17, 67–77.

Piperazine + Chlorpromazine

An isolated case of convulsions in a child was attributed to the use of piperazine followed by chlorpromazine.

Clinical evidence, mechanism, importance and management

A child given piperazine for pin worms developed convulsions when treated with chlorpromazine several days later.[1] In a subsequent *animal* study using chlorpromazine 4.5 or 10 mg/kg, many of the *animals* died from respiratory arrest after severe clonic convulsions.[1] However, a later study did not confirm these findings[2] and it is by no means certain whether the adverse reaction in the child was due to an interaction or not. Given that both drugs may cause convulsions, there is probably enough evidence to warrant caution if they are used concurrently.

1. Boulos BM, Davis LE. Hazard of simultaneous administration of phenothiazine and piperazine. *N Engl J Med* (1969) 280, 1245–6.
2. Armbrecht BH. Reaction between piperazine and chlorpromazine. *N Engl J Med* (1970) 282, 1490–1.

Praziquantel + Antiepileptics

Phenytoin, phenobarbital and carbamazepine markedly reduce the serum levels of praziquantel, but whether this results in neurocysticercosis treatment failures is unclear. A case report suggests that the addition of 'cimetidine', (p.236) may control this interaction.

Clinical evidence

(a) Carbamazepine, Phenobarbital or Phenytoin

A comparative study of patients, taking long-term phenytoin or carbamazepine, and healthy subjects (10 in each group), both given a single 25-mg/kg oral dose of praziquantel, found that **phenytoin** and **carbamazepine** reduced the AUC of praziquantel by about 74% and 90%, respectively, and reduced the maximum serum levels by 76% and 92%, respectively, when compared with the controls.[1] Another study also reported low praziquantel levels (maximum levels of 42 to 540 nanograms/mL with undetectable trough levels) in 4 patients taking **phenytoin** and 8 patients taking **phenobarbital**. However, in this study praziquantel 45 mg/kg daily in 3 divided doses for 15 days was very effective for neurocysticercosis, with all patients showing a marked improvement.[2]

(b) Phenytoin/Phenobarbital and Cimetidine

A patient with neurocysticercosis taking phenytoin and phenobarbital for a seizure disorder had no response to praziquantel (four courses in doses of up to 50 mg/kg daily). Praziquantel 50 mg/kg daily and dexamethasone 12 mg daily were started and, after one week, cimetidine 400 mg four times daily was added. The patient's serum praziquantel levels more than doubled with the addition of cimetidine (maximum serum levels raised from 350 to 826 nanograms/mL) and the AUC rose about fourfold, and became similar to that found in control subjects taking praziquantel alone. The patient showed marginal improvement, and continued to slowly improve over the following 4 months.[3]

Mechanism

Not established, but the probable reason is that these anticonvulsants and 'dexamethasone', (p.236) have enzyme-inducing effects and can therefore increase the metabolism of praziquantel. 'Cimetidine', (p.236) (an enzyme inhibitor) appears to oppose this effect. However, the fact that praziquantel was still effective in one study suggests that metabolites of praziquantel might be active.[2]

Importance and management

Direct information appears to be limited to the reports cited, but the pharmacokinetic interactions appear to be established. However, the clinical relevance of the interaction is uncertain. When treating systemic worm infections such as neurocysticercosis some authors advise increasing the praziquantel dosage from 25 to 50 mg/kg if potent enzyme inducers such as carbamazepine or phenytoin are being used, in order to reduce the risk of treatment failure.[1] A 45 mg/kg daily dose was effective in one study in 11 patients taking antiepileptics, despite low praziquantel levels,[2] but a 50 mg/kg daily dose was not effective in another case.[3] Note that the manufacturer recommends giving praziquantel 50 mg/kg daily in 3 divided doses for neurocysticercosis, and they suggest that the use of drugs to prevent or alleviate convulsions should be decided on a case to case basis.[4] Adding cimetidine may reduce the effect of enzyme-inducing anticonvulsants. However, the authors of the case above[3] were not sure whether the improvement they saw was in fact due to the cimetidine or simply part of the natural history of the disease. It is clear that 'cimetidine', (p.236), alone can markedly increase praziquantel levels. The interaction with anticonvulsants is of no importance when praziquantel is used for intestinal worm infections (where its action is a local effect on the worms in the gut).

1. Bittencourt PRM, Gracia CM, Martins R, Fernandes AG, Diekmann HW, Jung W. Phenytoin and carbamazepine decrease oral bioavailability of praziquantel. *Neurology* (1992) 42, 492–6.
2. Na-Bangchang K, Vanijanonta S, Karbwang J. Plasma concentrations of praziquantel during the therapy of neurocysticerosis with praziquantel, in the presence of antiepileptics and dexamethasone. *Southeast Asian J Trop Med Public Health* (1995) 26, 120–3.
3. Dachman WD, Adubofour KO, Bikin DS, Johnson CH, Mullin PD, Winograd M. Cimetidine-induced rise in praziquantel levels in a patient with neurocysticercosis being treated with anticonvulsants. *J Infect Dis* (1994) 169, 689–91.
4. Cysticide (Praziquantel). Merck. UK package insert, January 2000.

Praziquantel + Chloroquine

Chloroquine reduces the bioavailability of praziquantel, which would be expected to reduce its efficacy in systemic worm infections such as schistosomiasis.

Clinical evidence, mechanism, importance and management

A single 40-mg/kg oral dose of praziquantel was given to 8 healthy subjects alone, and 2 hours after chloroquine 600 mg. The chloroquine reduced the praziquantel AUC by 65% and the maximum serum levels by 59%. The reasons for this effect are not understood. There were large individual variations in levels, and one subject was not affected. The effect of this interaction could be that some patients will not achieve high enough serum praziquantel levels to treat systemic worm infections such as schistosomiasis. After taking the chloroquine, the praziquantel serum levels of 4 out of the 8 subjects (50%) did not reach the threshold of 0.3 micrograms/mL for about 6 hours (which is required to effectively kill schistosomes), compared with only 2 of 8 (25%) during the control period. The authors conclude that an increased dosage of praziquantel should be considered if chloroquine is given (they do not suggest how much), particularly in anyone who does not respond to initial treatment with praziquantel.[1] More study of this interaction is needed.

The interaction is of no importance when praziquantel is used for intestinal worm infections (where its action is a local effect on the worms in the gut).

1. Masimirembwa CM, Naik YS, Hasler JA. The effect of chloroquine on the pharmacokinetics and metabolism of praziquantel in rats and in humans. *Biopharm Drug Dispos* (1994) 15, 33–43.

Praziquantel + Cimetidine

Cimetidine can double the serum levels of praziquantel, and may improve its efficacy in neurocysticercosis.

Clinical evidence

In a randomised crossover study 8 healthy subjects were given three 25-mg/kg oral doses of praziquantel at 2-hourly intervals with cimetidine 400 mg given 1 hour before each dose of praziquantel. Cimetidine was found to have roughly doubled the praziquantel serum levels and AUC.[1,2] A further study in patients with neurocysticercosis found that this short regimen of praziquantel with cimetidine (which increased plasma levels of praziquantel by about threefold), had similar efficacy to the traditional regimen of 50 mg/kg daily in divided doses for 15 days.[3] Of 6 patients receiving praziquantel with cimetidine, the clinical cure rate was 83% compared with only 50% in 6 patients receiving praziquantel while fasting.[3]

Mechanism

Cimetidine probably inhibits the metabolism of praziquantel.

Importance and management

Direct information appears to be limited to the reports cited, but the interaction appears to be established. It is clear that cimetidine can markedly increase praziquantel levels, and the authors say that concurrent use can reduce treatment for neurocysticercosis from 2 weeks to 1 day.[1,3] Cimetidine has been tried to reverse the effects of 'antiepileptics', (p.235) and 'corticosteroids', (below) on praziquantel.

1. Jung H, Medina R, Castro N, Corona T, Sotelo J. Pharmacokinetic study of praziquantel administered alone and in combination with cimetidine in a single-day therapeutic regimen. *Antimicrob Agents Chemother* (1997) 41, 1256–9.
2. Castro N, Gonzàlez-Esquivel D, Medina R, Sotelo J, Jung H. The influence of cimetidine on plasma levels of praziquantel after a single day therapeutic regimen. *Proc West Pharmacol Soc* (1997) 40, 33–4.
3. Castro N, González-Esquivel DF, López M, Jung H. Análisis comparativo de la influencia de los alimentos y la cimetidina en los niveles plasmáticos de prazicuantel. *Rev Invest Clin* (2003) 55, 655–61.

Praziquantel + Corticosteroids

The continuous use of dexamethasone can halve serum praziquantel levels. Two case reports suggest that this may reduce its efficacy in systemic worm infections, whereas another study suggests that efficacy is not affected.

Clinical evidence

Eight patients with parenchymal brain cysticercosis taking praziquantel 50 mg/kg (in three divided doses, taken every 8 hours) had a 50% reduction in steady-state serum levels, from 3.13 to 1.55 micrograms/mL, when given **dexamethasone** 8 mg every 8 hours.[1] Another patient with recurrent neurocysticercosis, who did not respond to praziquantel 50 mg/kg daily, was successfully treated with high-dose praziquantel 100 mg/kg daily, dexamethasone 12 mg daily and cimetidine 800 mg daily. As dexamethasone was thought to reduce the plasma levels of praziquantel, cimetidine was added to try to reverse this effect, as it has been reported to increase the bioavailability of praziquantel.[2] However, some patients have responded well to praziquantel, despite low serum levels.[3]

Mechanism

Uncertain. Dexamethasone is an inducer of the cytochrome P450 isoenzyme CYP3A4, and might therefore be expected to reduce levels of praziquantel. 'Cimetidine', (above) may reverse this effect.

Importance and management

Information seems to be limited but the pharmacokinetic interaction would appear to be established. Just how much it affects the outcome of treatment for systemic worm infections such as cysticercosis is unknown because the optimum praziquantel levels are still uncertain, and it is possible that the metabolites of praziquantel might be active.[3] The authors of one report suggest that dexamethasone should not be given continuously with praziquantel but only used transiently to resolve inflammatory reactions to praziquantel treatment.[1] Alternatively, limited information suggests the addition of cimetidine may allow dexamethasone to be used.[2]

Intravenous **methylprednisolone** has also been used for acute corticosteroid therapy with praziquantel, and oral **prednisone** has been used long-term to prevent further tissue damage associated with inflammation[4,5] but the effect of these corticosteroids on the plasma levels of praziquantel do not appear to have been studied.

The interaction with dexamethasone is of no importance when praziquantel is used for intestinal worm infections (where its action is a local effect on the worms in the gut).

1. Vazquez ML, Jung H, Sotelo J. Plasma levels of praziquantel decrease when dexamethasone is given simultaneously. *Neurology* (1987) 37, 1561–2.
2. Yee T, Barakos JA, Knight RT. High-dose praziquantel with cimetidine for refractory neurocysticercosis: a case report with clinical and MRI follow-up. *West J Med* (1999) 170, 112–15.
3. Na-Bangchang K, Vanijanonta S, Karbwang J. Plasma concentrations of praziquantel during the therapy of neurocysticerosis with praziquantel, in the presence of antiepileptics and dexamethasone. *Southeast Asian J Trop Med Public Health* (1995) 26, 120–3.
4. Sotelo J, Jung H. Pharmacokinetic optimisation of the treatment of neurocysticercosis. *Clin Pharmacokinet* (1998) 34, 503–15.
5. Silva LCS, Maciel PE, Ribas JGR, Souza-Pereira SR, Antunes CM, Lambertucci JR. Treatment of schistosomal myeloradiculopathy with praziquantel and corticosteroids and evaluation by magnetic resonance imaging: a longitudinal study. *Clin Infect Dis* (2004) 39, 1618–24.

Praziquantel + Food

Food increases the bioavailability of praziquantel.

Clinical evidence, mechanism, importance and management

The maximum plasma levels and AUC of a single 1.8-g dose of praziquantel were increased by 243% and 180% when it was given following a **high-fat** diet and by 515% and 271% after a **high-carbohydrate** diet, respectively.[1] In another study in healthy Sudanese men, when praziquantel was given with food the AUC was 2.6-fold higher than when it was given in the fasted state.[2]

A further study in patients with neurocysticercosis found that treatment with a short regimen of praziquantel 25 mg/kg every 2 hours for 3 doses with a **high-carbohydrate** diet, which increased plasma levels of praziquantel, provided an adequate clinical alternative to the traditional regimen of 50 mg/kg daily in divided doses for 15 days.[3] In 6 patients who took praziquantel with food, the clinical cure rate was 83%, compared with only 50% in 6 patients who took praziquantel while fasting.[3]

On the basis of the above studies, if praziquantel is used for systemic worm infections, administration with **food** is advisable, and this is recommended by the manufacturers.[4,5]

1. Castro N, Medina R, Sotelo J, Jung H. Bioavailability of praziquantel increases with concomitant administration of food. *Antimicrob Agents Chemother* (2000) 44, 2903–4.
2. Homeida M, Leahy W, Copeland S, Ali MM, Harron DWG. Pharmacokinetic interaction between praziquantel and albendazole in Sudanese men. *Ann Trop Med Parasitol* (1994) 88, 551–9.
3. Castro N, González-Esquivel DF, López M, Jung H. Análisis comparativo de la influencia de los alimentos y la cimetidina en los niveles plasmáticos de prazicuantel. *Rev Invest Clin* (2003) 55, 655–61.
4. Biltricide (Praziquantel). Bayer Healthcare. US Prescribing information, October 2004.
5. Cysticide (Praziquantel). Merck. UK package insert, January 2000.

Praziquantel + Grapefruit juice

Grapefruit juice increases the AUC of praziquantel.

Clinical evidence, mechanism, importance and management

In a study in healthy subjects the maximum plasma level of a single 1.8-g dose of praziquantel was increased by about 63% and the AUC by 90% when given with 250 mL of **grapefruit juice** rather than with water.[1] The authors suggested that grapefruit juice probably increased the absorption of praziquantel. The clinical effect of this interaction has not been assessed, but it may lead to improved efficacy. When compared with other studies, the authors noted that the effect of grapefruit juice was comparable to that of 'cimetidine', (p.236) and less than that of 'food', (p.236).

1. Castro N, Jung H, Medina R, González-Esquivel D, Lopez M, Sotelo J. Interaction between grapefruit juice and praziquantel in humans. *Antimicrob Agents Chemother* (2002) 46, 1614–16.

Praziquantel + Rifampicin (Rifampin)

The plasma levels of praziquantel were markedly reduced by rifampicin pretreatment, to undetectable levels in over half of the subjects in one study. It is predicted that rifampicin will reduce the efficacy of praziquantel.

Clinical evidence, mechanism, importance and management

Pretreatment with rifampicin 600 mg once daily for 5 days markedly reduced the AUC and maximum level of a single 40-mg/kg dose of praziquantel in 10 subjects. Seven of the subjects had undetectable praziquantel levels (less than 12.5 nanograms/mL), and the other 3 had an 85% reduction in the AUC of praziquantel. The same subjects were then given three doses of praziquantel 25 mg/kg at intervals of 8 hours, alone, and after pretreatment with rifampicin. In this multiple-dose study, 5 of the 10 subjects had undetectable praziquantel levels, and the remainder had an 80% reduction in AUC.[1] It was suggested that rifampicin induced the metabolism of praziquantel via cytochrome P450 isoenzyme CYP3A4. Although efficacy has not been assessed, the authors concluded that the levels of praziquantel after rifampicin pretreatment were less than those considered necessary for anthelmintic activity. They therefore recommend that the combination should be avoided,[1] a stance which is also taken by one of the manufacturers of praziquantel.[2]

1. Ridtitid W, Wongnawa M, Mahatthanatrakul W, Punyo J, Sunbhanich M. Rifampin markedly decreases plasma concentrations of praziquantel in healthy volunteers. *Clin Pharmacol Ther* (2002) 72, 505–13.

2. Biltricide (Praziquantel). Bayer Healthcare. US Prescribing information, October 2004.

Primaquine + Mepacrine (Quinacrine)

Theoretically, mepacrine would be expected to elevate the serum levels of primaquine, because it increased levels of a formerly used drug pamaquine, but there do not seem to be any reports confirming or disproving this.

Clinical evidence, mechanism, importance and management

Patients given pamaquine (a formerly used antimalarial that was a predecessor of primaquine, and almost identical in structure), had grossly elevated pamaquine serum levels when they were also given mepacrine.[1,2] The reason is unknown. On theoretical grounds primaquine might be expected to interact with mepacrine similarly, but there seem to be no reports confirming that a clinically important interaction actually takes place.

1. Zubrod CG, Kennedy TJ, Shannon JA. Studies on the chemotherapy of the human malarias. VIII. The physiological disposition of pamaquine. *J Clin Invest* (1948) 27 (Suppl), 114–120.

2. Earle DP, Bigelow FS, Zubrod CG, Kane CA. Studies on the chemotherapy of the human malarias. IX. Effect of pamaquine on the blood cells of man. *J Clin Invest* (1948) 27, (Suppl), 121–9.

Primaquine + Quinine

Quinine does not appear to affect the pharmacokinetics of primaquine.

Clinical evidence, mechanism, importance and management

Quinine 10 mg/kg three times daily had no effect on the pharmacokinetics of a single 45-mg dose of primaquine in 7 subjects, except for a 50% increase in the AUC of the carboxyprimaquine metabolite. The combination was effective for the treatment of malaria with no complications and no adverse effects reported.[1]

Usually quinine is used only for the treatment of falciparum malaria, and primaquine is used only to eliminate the liver stages of vivax and ovale malarias, and therefore the drugs are generally unlikely to be taken together. However, quinine may be used when the infective species is unknown or the infection mixed, when subsequent primaquine may then be required. The limited data from the above study suggest that no special precautions would be required.

1. Edwards G, McGrath CS, Ward SA, Supanaranond W, Pukrittayakamee S, Davis TM, White NJ. Interactions among primaquine, malaria infection and other antimalarials in Thai subjects. *Br J Clin Pharmacol* (1993) 35, 193–8.

Proguanil + Antacids

The absorption of proguanil is markedly reduced by magnesium trisilicate, and therefore the efficacy of proguanil may be reduced.

Clinical evidence

Magnesium trisilicate reduced the AUC of a 200-mg dose of proguanil by about 65% in 8 healthy subjects, as assessed by salivary proguanil levels.[1]

Mechanism

In vitro tests showed that magnesium trisilicate adsorbed proguanil. Two other antacids, **aluminium hydroxide** and light **magnesium carbonate**, had lesser effects.[1]

Importance and management

The interaction between proguanil and magnesium trisilicate appears to be established, but its clinical importance does not seem to have been assessed. Given the extent of reduction in levels, the antimalarial effects of proguanil might be expected to be reduced. One way to minimise the interaction is to separate the dosage of proguanil and magnesium trisilicate as much as possible (2 to 3 hours) to reduce admixture in the gut. There do not appear to be any studies to see if other antacids behave similarly. The manufacturers of proguanil recommend taking proguanil and antacids at least 2 to 3 hours apart.[2]

1. Onyeji CO, Babalola CP. The effect of magnesium trisilicate on proguanil absorption. *Int J Pharmaceutics* (1993) 100, 249–52.
2. Paludrine (Proguanil hydrochloride). AstraZeneca UK Ltd. UK Summary of product characteristics, April 2005.

Proguanil + Chloroquine

Chloroquine appears to increase the incidence of mouth ulcers by 1.5-fold in those taking prophylactic proguanil.

Clinical evidence, mechanism, importance and management

Following the observation that mouth ulcers appeared to be common in those taking prophylactic antimalarials, an extensive study was undertaken in 628 servicemen in Belize. Of those taking proguanil 200 mg daily, 24% developed mouth ulcers, and in those also taking chloroquine base 150 to 300 mg weekly, 37% developed mouth ulcers. The incidence of diarrhoea was also increased from 63% among those who did not develop ulcers to 83% in those that did develop ulcers (any treatment). The reasons are not understood. The authors of the study suggested that these two drugs should not be given together unnecessarily for prophylaxis against *Plasmodium falciparum*.[1] Nevertheless, chloroquine plus proguanil is an established prophylactic regimen that is commonly recommended in regions where there is some chloroquine resistance.

1. Drysdale SF, Phillips-Howard PA, Behrens RH. Proguanil, chloroquine, and mouth ulcers. *Lancet* (1990) 1, 164.

Proguanil + Cimetidine or Omeprazole

There is some evidence that omeprazole and cimetidine can moderately reduce the production of the active metabolite of proguanil, but also some evidence to suggest that this may not be clinically relevant.

Clinical evidence

(a) Cimetidine

In one study, 4 patients with peptic ulcer disease and 6 healthy subjects were given a single 200-mg dose of proguanil on the last day of a 3-day course of cimetidine 400 mg twice daily. In both groups the half-life and AUC of proguanil were significantly increased, but only the healthy subjects had an increase in the maximum serum concentration of 89%. In both groups these pharmacokinetic changes resulted in lower levels of the active metabolite, cycloguanil.[1] This decrease in cycloguanil supported the findings of an earlier study, which had found a 30% decrease in the urinary recovery of cycloguanil when proguanil and cimetidine were given together.[2]

(b) Omeprazole

In a steady-state study in 12 healthy subjects taking proguanil 200 mg daily it was found that omeprazole 20 mg daily roughly halved the AUC of the active metabolite of proguanil, cycloguanil.[3] However, an earlier study found that omeprazole 20 mg had no effect on the urinary recovery of cycloguanil (or proguanil) following a single 200-mg dose of proguanil.[2]

Mechanism

Cimetidine and omeprazole increase the gastric pH, which may lead to an increase in the absorption of proguanil. Cimetidine[1,2] and omeprazole[3] are also thought to inhibit the metabolism of proguanil, due to their inhibitory effects on cytochrome P450 isoenzyme CYP2C19.

Importance and management

The differences between the healthy subjects and patients with peptic ulcer disease seen in one study may have been because the disease itself alters the effects of the cimetidine in some way.[1] Patients with peptic ulcer disease are also likely to have an increased gastric pH, which will lead to altered proguanil absorption. The clinical relevance of all these findings is still unclear, although the implication is that decreased cycloguanil levels may lead to inadequate malaria prophylaxis. However, a subsequent clinical study reported that subjects who were poor metabolisers of proguanil (who had relatively low cycloguanil levels) did not have an increased risk of failure of proguanil prophylaxis.[4] Similarly, treatment of malaria with proguanil was as effective in 62 patients with CYP2C19 poor metaboliser genotype as in 33 patients with extensive metaboliser genotype, independent of cycloguanil levels.[5] This suggests that any interaction with omeprazole or cimetidine via this mechanism would be unlikely to be clinically relevant.

1. Kolawole JA, Mustapha A, Abdul-Aguye I, Ochekpe N, Taylor RB. Effects of cimetidine on the pharmacokinetics of proguanil in healthy subjects and in peptic ulcer patients. *J Pharm Biomed Anal* (1999) 20, 737–43.
2. Somogyi AA, Reinhard HA, Bochner F. Effects of omeprazole and cimetidine on the urinary metabolic ratio of proguanil in healthy volunteers. *Eur J Clin Pharmacol* (1996) 50, 417–19.
3. Funck-Bretano C, Becquemont L, Lenevu A, Roux A, Jaillon P, Beaune P. Inhibition by omeprazole of proguanil metabolism: mechanism of the interaction *in vitro* and prediction of *in vivo* results from the *in vitro* experiments. *J Pharmacol Exp Ther* (1997) 280, 730–8.
4. Mberu EK, Wansor T, Sato H, Nishikawa Y, Watkins WM. Japanese poor metabolizers of proguanil do not have an increased risk of malaria chemoprophylaxis breakthrough. Trans R Soc Trop Med Hyg. 1995 Nov-Dec;89(6):658–9.
5. Kaneko A, Bergqvist Y, Takechi M, Kalkoa M, Kaneko O, Kobayakawa T, Ishizaki T, Bjorkman A. Intrinsic efficacy of proguanil against falciparum and vivax malaria independent of the metabolite cycloguanil. *J Infect Dis* (1999) 179; 974–9.

Proguanil + Fluvoxamine

The conversion of proguanil to its active metabolite is markedly inhibited by fluvoxamine in those who are CYP2C19 extensive metabolisers. However, there is some evidence this may not be of any clinical relevance.

Clinical evidence

Twelve healthy subjects, 6 of whom were of CYP2C19 extensive metaboliser genotype and 6 of whom were CYP2C19 poor metabolisers, were given proguanil 200 mg daily for 8 days. This was followed by fluvoxamine 100 mg for 8 days, with a single 200-mg dose of proguanil on day 6. In the group of extensive metabolisers it was found that fluvoxamine reduced the total clearance of proguanil by about 40%. The partial clearance of proguanil via its two metabolites was reduced, by 85% for cycloguanil, and by 89% for 4-chlorophenylbiguanide. The concentrations of these two metabolites in the plasma were hardly detectable while fluvoxamine was being taken. No pharmacokinetic interaction occurred in the poor metabolisers.[1]

Mechanism

Proguanil, which is thought to be a prodrug, is metabolised to its active metabolite, cycloguanil by the cytochrome P450 isoenzyme CYP2C19. This isoenzyme is inhibited by fluvoxamine and so proguanil does not become activated.[2] Note that subjects with decreased CYP2C19 activity show slower metabolism of proguanil to cycloguanil,[3] but they may still respond to proguanil.[4]

Importance and management

Information appears to be limited to the studies cited, the purpose of which was to confirm that fluvoxamine is an inhibitor of CYP2C19. However, they also demonstrate that proguanil, which is a prodrug, will not be effectively converted into its active form in patients who are extensive metabolisers if fluvoxamine is also being taken, making them effectively poor metabolisers. There are as yet no reports of treatment failures due to this interaction, but if the activity of proguanil is virtually abolished by fluvoxamine, as the authors suggest,[2] then proguanil would also be expected to be ineffective in the proportion of the population that are poor metabolisers. However, a subsequent clinical study reported that subjects who were poor metabolisers of proguanil did not have an increased risk of failure of proguanil prophylaxis.[5] Similarly, treatment of malaria with proguanil was as effective in 62 patients with CYP2C19 poor metaboliser genotype as in 33 patients with extensive metaboliser genotype, independent of cycloguanil levels.[4] This suggests any interaction with fluvoxamine, or other CYP2C19 inhibitors, may not be clinically relevant.

1. Jeppesen U, Rasmussen BB, Brøsen K. Fluvoxamine inhibits the CYP2C19-catalyzed bioactivation of chloroguanide. *Clin Pharmacol Ther* (1997) 62, 279–86.
2. Rasmussen BB, Nielsen TL, Brøsen K. Fluvoxamine inhibits the CYP2C19-catalysed metabolism of proguanil in vitro. *Eur J Clin Pharmacol* (1998) 54, 735–40.
3. Herrlin K, Massele AY, Rimoy G, Alm C, Rais M, Ericsson Ö, Bertilsson L, Gustafsson LL. Slow chloroguanide metabolism in Tanzanians compared with white subjects and Asian subjects confirms a decreased CYP2C19 activity in relation to genotype. *Clin Pharmacol Ther* (2000) 68, 189–98.
4. Kaneko A, Bergqvist Y, Takechi M, Kalkoa M, Kaneko O, Kobayakawa T, Ishizaki T, Bjorkman A. Intrinsic efficacy of proguanil against falciparum and vivax malaria independent of the metabolite cycloguanil. *J Infect Dis* (1999) 179; 974–9.
5. Mberu EK, Wansor T, Sato H, Nishikawa Y, Watkins WM. Japanese poor metabolizers of proguanil do not have an increased risk of malaria chemoprophylaxis breakthrough. *Trans R Soc Trop Med Hyg* (1995) 89, 658–9.

Pyrantel + Piperazine

Piperazine opposes the anthelmintic actions of pyrantel.

Clinical evidence, mechanism, importance and management

Pyrantel acts as an anthelmintic because it depolarises the neuromuscular junctions of some intestinal nematodes causing the worms to contract. This paralyses the worms so that they are dislodged by peristalsis and expelled in the faeces. Piperazine also paralyses nematodes but it does so by causing hyperpolarisation of the neuromuscular junctions. These two pharmacological actions oppose one another, as was shown in two *in vitro* pharmacological studies. Strips of whole *Ascaris lumbricoides,* which contracted when exposed to pyrantel failed to do so when also exposed to piperazine.[1] Parallel electrophysiological studies using *Ascaris* cells confirmed that the depolarisation due to pyrantel (which causes the paralysis) was opposed by piperazine.[1]

In practical terms this means that piperazine does not add to the anthelmintic effect of pyrantel on *Ascaris* as might be expected, but opposes it. For this reason it is usually recommended that concurrent use should be avoided, but direct clinical evidence confirming that combined use is ineffective seems to be lacking. It seems reasonable to extrapolate the results of these studies on *Ascaris lumbricoides* (roundworm) to the other gastrointestinal parasites for which pyrantel is used, i.e. *Enterobius vermicularis* (threadworm or pinworm), *Ancylostoma duodenale*, *Necator americanus* (hookworm) and *Trichostrongylus* spp. However, no one seems to have studied this.

1. Aubry ML, Cowell P, Davey MJ, Shevde S. Aspects of the pharmacology of a new anthelmintic: pyrantel. *Br J Pharmacol* (1970) 38, 332–44.

Pyrimethamine + Artemether

Artemether raises pyrimethamine plasma levels, but this does not appear to cause an increase in adverse effects.

Clinical evidence, mechanism, importance and management

In a three-way single-dose crossover study, 8 healthy subjects were given either artemether 300 mg, pyrimethamine 100 mg, or both drugs together. Although there was large inter-individual variation in the pharmacokinetics of pyrimethamine, its maximum plasma levels were raised by 44%. As there was no corresponding increase in adverse effects the authors suggest that the interaction may be of benefit.[1] More study is warranted to confirm this result.

1. Tan-ariya P, Na-Bangchang K, Ubalee R, Thanavibul A, Thipawangkosol P, Karbwang J. Pharmacokinetic interaction or artemether and pyrimethamine in healthy male Thais. *Southeast Asian J Trop Med Public Health* (1998) 29, 18–23.

Pyrimethamine + Co-trimoxazole or Sulfonamides

Serious pancytopenia and megaloblastic anaemia have occasionally occurred in patients given pyrimethamine and either co-trimoxazole or other sulfonamides.

Clinical evidence

A woman taking pyrimethamine 50 mg weekly as malaria prophylaxis, developed petechial haemorrhages and widespread bruising within 10 days of starting to take co-trimoxazole (trimethoprim 320 mg with sulfamethoxazole 800 mg) daily for a urinary-tract infection. She was found to have gross megaloblastic changes and pancytopenia in addition to being obviously pale and ill. After withdrawal of the two drugs she responded rapidly to hydroxocobalamin and folic acid, and the pyrimethamine was changed to chloroquine for malaria prophylaxis.[1]

Similar cases have been described in other patients taking pyrimethamine with co-trimoxazole,[2-4] **sulfafurazole (sulfisoxazole)**,[5] or other sulfonamides.[6]

Mechanism

Uncertain, but a reasonable surmise can be made. Pyrimethamine and **trimethoprim** are both **folate antagonists** and both selectively inhibit the actions of the enzyme dihydrofolate reductase, which is concerned with the eventual synthesis of the nucleic acids needed for the production of new cells. The sulfonamides inhibit another part of the same synthetic chain. The adverse reactions seen would seem to reflect a gross reduction of the normal folate metabolism caused by the combined actions of both drugs. Megaloblastic anaemia and pancytopenia are among the adverse reactions of pyrimethamine and, more rarely, of co-trimoxazole taken alone.

Importance and management

Information seems to be limited to the reports cited, but the interaction appears to be established. Its incidence is unknown. Pyrimethamine is usually given with a sulfonamide for toxoplasmosis and malaria. Caution should be used in prescribing these combinations, especially in the presence of other drugs, such as folate antagonists, or disease states that may predispose to folate deficiency. Note that the manufacturer of sulfadoxine/pyrimethamine (*Fansidar*), which is indicated for the prophylaxis and treatment of malaria, recommends that concomitant treatment with folate antagonists such as other sulfonamides, trimethoprim, co-trimoxazole and some antiepileptics should be avoided.[7,8] When high-dose pyrimethamine is used for the treatment of toxoplasmosis, the manufacturer recommends that all patients should receive a folate supplement, preferably calcium folinate, to reduce the risk of bone marrow depression.[9,10]

1. Fleming AF, Warrell DA, Dickmeiss H. Co-trimoxazole and the blood. *Lancet* (1974) ii, 284–5.
2. Ansdell VE, Wright SG, Hutchinson DBA. Megaloblastic anaemia associated with combined pyrimethamine and co-trimoxazole administration. *Lancet* (1976) ii, 1257.
3. Malfatti S, Piccini A. Anemia megaloblastica pancitopenica in corso di trattamento con pirimetamina, trimethoprim e sulfametossazolo. *Haematologica* (1976) 61, 349–57.
4. Borgstein A, Tozer RA. Infectious mononucleosis and megaloblastic anaemia associated with Daraprim and Bactrim. *Cent Afr J Med* (1974) 20, 185.
5. Waxman S, Herbert V. Mechanism of pyrimethamine-induced megaloblastosis in human bone marrow. *N Engl J Med* (1969) 280, 1316–19.
6. Weißbach G. Auswirkungen kombinierter Behandlung der kindlichen Toxoplasmose mit Pyrimethamin (Daraprim) und Sulfonamiden auf Blut und Knochenmark. *Z Arztl Fortbild (Berl)* (1965) 59, 10–22.
7. Fansidar (Sulfadoxine/Pyrimethamine). Roche Products Ltd. UK Summary of product characteristics, September 2005.
8. Fansidar (Sulfadoxine/Pyrimethamine). Roche Pharmaceuticals. US Prescribing information, August 2004.
9. Daraprim (Pyrimethamine). GlaxoSmithKline UK. UK Summary of product characteristics, December 2005.
10. Daraprim (Pyrimethamine). GlaxoSmithKline. US Prescribing information, March 2003.

Pyrimethamine ± Sulfadoxine + Zidovudine

Pyrimethamine does not appear to alter zidovudine pharmacokinetics, and zidovudine does not appear to alter the prophylactic efficacy of sulfadoxine/pyrimethamine for toxoplasmosis. The combination of pyrimethamine and zidovudine may increase the risk of myelosuppression.

Clinical evidence, mechanism, importance and management

The addition of pyrimethamine (200 mg loading dose then 50 mg daily) and folinic acid 10 mg daily to zidovudine had no effect on zidovudine pharmacokinetics, based on data from 10 HIV positive patients for whom zidovudine pharmacokinetics were available before and after starting pyrimethamine. Of 26 patients receiving the combination, 5 developed leucopenia and one discontinued treatment because of anaemia.[1]

A study in patients with AIDS found that zidovudine 250 mg four times daily did not adversely affect the prevention of toxoplasma encephalitis with pyrimethamine/sulfadoxine (*Fansidar*), one tablet twice weekly for up to 8 months.[2] *In vitro* and animal data have shown that the combination of zidovudine and pyrimethamine caused synergistic decreases in lymphocyte and neutrophil numbers.[3]

The manufacturers of pyrimethamine note that the concurrent use of zidovudine may increase the risk of bone marrow depression.[4,5] They say that if signs of folate deficiency develop, then pyrimethamine should be discontinued and folinic acid given. Note that the prophylactic use of a folate supplement, preferably folinic acid, is recommended for all patients with toxoplasmosis taking high-dose pyrimethamine, to reduce the risk of bone marrow suppression.[4,5] See also 'NRTIs; Zidovudine + Myelosuppressive drugs', p.809

1. Jacobson JM, Davidian M, Rainey PM, Hafner R, Raasch RH, Luft BJ. Pyrimethamine pharmacokinetics in human immunodeficiency virus-positive patients seropositive for *Toxoplasma gondii*. *Antimicrob Agents Chemother* (1996) 40, 1360–5.
2. Eljaschewitsch J, Schürmann D, Pohle HD, Ruf B. Zidovudine does not antagonize Fansidar in preventing toxoplasma encephalitis in HIV infected patients. 7th International Conference on AIDS; Science Challenging AIDS, Florence, Italy, 1991. Abstract W.B.2334.
3. Freund YR, Dabbs J, Creek MR, Phillips SJ, Tyson CA, MacGregor JT. Synergistic bone marrow toxicity of pyrimethamine and zidovudine in murine *in vivo* and *in vitro* models: mechanism of toxicity. *Toxicol Appl Pharmacol* (2002) 181, 16–26.
4. Daraprim (Pyrimethamine). GlaxoSmithKline UK. UK Summary of product characteristics, December 2005.
5. Daraprim (Pyrimethamine). GlaxoSmithKline. US Prescribing information, March 2003.

Quinine + Colestyramine

Colestyramine does not appear to alter the pharmacokinetics of quinine.

Clinical evidence, mechanism, importance and management

Colestyramine 8 g did not alter the pharmacokinetics of quinine 600 mg, given concurrently to 8 healthy subjects. The authors warn that this lack of interaction may have been because only single doses were used, and suggest continuing to separate the administration of the two drugs until a lack of interaction is demonstrated in a multiple dose study.[1] It is usually recommended that other drugs are taken 1 hour before or 4 to 6 hours after colestyramine.

1. Ridtitid W, Wongnawa M, Kleekaew A, Mahatthanatrakul W, Sunbhanich M. Cholestyramine does not significantly decrease the bioavailability of quinine in healthy volunteers. *Asia Pac J Pharmacol* (1998) 13, 123–7.

Quinine + Fluvoxamine

Fluvoxamine had no effect on the pharmacokinetics of quinine.

Clinical evidence, mechanism, importance and management

In a study in healthy subjects, fluvoxamine 25 mg was given both 12-hours and 1-hour before a single 500-mg dose of quinine hydrochloride, followed by a further 4 doses of fluvoxamine, given every 12 hours.[1] Fluvoxamine had no effect on the apparent oral clearance of quinine and caused a minor 6% increase in the AUC of 3-hydroxyquinine, with no effect on the AUC of various other metabolites.[1,2]

Fluvoxamine is a known inhibitor of the cytochrome P450 isoenzyme CYP2C19, and it appears that this has little effect on the pharmacokinetics of quinine and therefore no dose adjustments would be necessary on concurrent use.

1. Mirghani RA, Helllgren U, Westerberg PA, Ericsson O, Bertilsson L, Gustafsson LL. The roles of cytochrome P450 3A4 and 1A2 in the 3-hydroxylation of quinine in vivo. *Clin Pharmacol Ther* (1999) 66, 454–60.
2. Mirghani RA, Hellgren U, Bertilsson L, Gustafsson LL, Ericsson Ö. Metabolism and elimination of quinine in healthy volunteers. *Eur J Clin Pharmacol* (2003) 59, 423–7.

Quinine + Grapefruit juice

Grapefruit juice had no effect on the pharmacokinetics of quinine.

Clinical evidence, mechanism, importance and management

In a study in 10 healthy subjects 200 mL full-strength grapefruit juice, half-strength grapefruit juice, or orange juice was given twice daily for 11 doses with a single 600-mg dose of quinine sulfate, given on day 6 with the last dose of grapefruit juice. There were no significant differences in the pharmacokinetics of quinine between the three treatments, although the maximum level of the 3-hydroxymetabolite was slightly reduced (by 19%) with full-strength grapefruit juice compared with orange juice or half-strength grapefruit juice.[1]

Grapefruit juice is a known inhibitor of intestinal cytochrome P450 isoenzyme CYP3A4, and it appears that this has little effect on the pharmacokinetics of quinine, which has a high oral bioavailability and is metabolised in the liver.

Grapefruit juice does not alter the pharmacokinetics of quinine, suggesting that patients requiring quinine may safely drink grapefruit juice if they wish.[1]

1. Ho PC, Chalcroft SC, Coville PF, Wanwimolruk S. Grapefruit juice has no effect on quinine pharmacokinetics. *Eur J Clin Pharmacol* (1999) 55, 393–8.

Quinine + H_2-receptor antagonists

Quinine clearance is reduced by cimetidine, but not ranitidine.

Clinical evidence, mechanism, importance and management

In a study in 6 healthy subjects **cimetidine** 200 mg three times daily and 400 mg at night for one week reduced the clearance of quinine by 27%, increased the half-life by 49% (from 7.6 to 11.3 hours), and increased the AUC by 42%. Peak levels were unchanged. No interaction was seen when **cimetidine** was replaced by **ranitidine** 150 mg twice daily.[1] The probable reason for this effect is that **cimetidine** (a recognised enzyme inhibitor) reduces the metabolism of the quinine by the liver, whereas **ranitidine** does not. It therefore seems likely that other H_2-receptor antagonists will not interact, although this needs confirmation. The clinical importance of this is uncertain, but prescribers should be alert for any evidence of quinine toxicity if cimetidine is also given.

1. Wanwimolruk S, Sunbhanich M, Pongmarutai M and Patamasucon P. Effects of cimetidine and ranitidine on the pharmacokinetics of quinine. *Br J Clin Pharmacol* (1986) 22, 346–50.

Quinine + Isoniazid

A study in 9 healthy subjects found that the clearance of a single 600-mg dose of quinine sulfate was not significantly affected by pretreatment with isoniazid 300 mg daily for a week.[1]

1. Wanwimolruk S, Kang W, Coville PF, Viriyayudhakorn S, Thitiarchakul S. Marked enhancement by rifampicin and lack of effect of isoniazid on the elimination of quinine in man. *Br J Clin Pharmacol* (1995) 40, 87–91.

Quinine + Ketoconazole

Ketoconazole modestly decreases the clearance of quinine, but this is probably not clinically relevant.

Clinical evidence, mechanism, importance and management

In a study in healthy subjects ketoconazole 100 mg twice daily was given for 3 days with a single 500-mg dose of quinine hydrochloride one hour after the second dose of ketoconazole. Ketoconazole decreased the apparent oral clearance of quinine by 31% and decreased the AUC of 3-hydroxyquinine by 30%,[1] with increases in the AUC of various other metabolites.[2]

It is likely that ketoconazole inhibits the metabolism of quinine to its major metabolite 3-hydroxyquinine via the cytochrome P450 isoenzyme CYP3A4. This pharmacokinetic interaction would appear to be established, but of unknown clinical relevance. The modest increase in quinine levels seen is probably unlikely to be of much significance.

1. Mirghani RA, Helllgren U, Westerberg PA, Ericsson O, Bertilsson L, Gustafsson LL. The roles of cytochrome P450 3A4 and 1A2 in the 3-hydroxylation of quinine in vivo. *Clin Pharmacol Ther* (1999) 66, 454–60.
2. Mirghani RA, Hellgren U, Bertilsson L, Gustafsson LL, Ericsson Ö. Metabolism and elimination of quinine in healthy volunteers. *Eur J Clin Pharmacol* (2003) 59, 423–7.

Quinine + Miscellaneous

Urinary alkalinisers can increase the retention of quinine in man, and antacids can reduce the absorption of quinine in *animals*. None of these interactions appears to be of general clinical importance.

Clinical evidence, mechanism, importance and management

(a) Antacids

Aluminium/magnesium hydroxide gel reduces the absorption of quinine from the gut of *rats* and reduces quinine blood levels by 50 to 70%.[1] This appears to occur because **aluminium hydroxide** slows gastric emptying, which reduces absorption, and also because **magnesium hydroxide** forms an insoluble precipitate with quinine. However, there seem to be no clinical reports of a reduction in the therapeutic effectiveness of quinine due to the concurrent use of antacids.

(b) Urinary alkalinisers and acidifiers

The excretion of unchanged quinine is virtually halved (from 17.4 to 8.9%) if the urine is alkalinised. This is because in alkaline urine more of the quinine exists in the non-ionised (lipid soluble) form, which is more easily reabsorbed by the kidney tubules.[2] However, there seem to be no reports of adverse effects arising from changes in excretion due to this interaction, and no special precautions seem to be necessary.

1. Hurwitz A. The effects of antacids on gastrointestinal drug absorption. II. Effect of sulfadiazine and quinine. *J Pharmacol Exp Ther* (1971) 179, 485–9.

2. Haag HB, Larson PS, Schwartz JJ. The effect of urinary pH on the elimination of quinine in man. *J Pharmacol Exp Ther* (1943) 79, 136–9.

Quinine + Rifampicin (Rifampin)

Rifampicin induces the metabolism of quinine, which may result in subtherapeutic quinine levels.

Clinical evidence, mechanism, importance and management

A study in 9 healthy subjects found that the clearance of a single 600-mg dose of quinine sulfate was increased more than sixfold by pretreatment with rifampicin 600 mg daily for 2 weeks. The elimination half-life of quinine was decreased from about 11 hours to 5.5 hours.[1]

A report describes a patient with myotonia, controlled with quinine, whose symptoms worsened within 3 weeks of starting to take rifampicin for the treatment of tuberculosis. Peak quinine levels were found to be low, but rose again when the rifampicin was stopped. Control of the myotonia was regained 6 weeks later.[2]

The effect of adding rifampicin to quinine was investigated in patients with uncomplicated falciparum malaria. They were taking quinine sulfate 10 mg/kg three times daily either alone (30 patients) or with rifampicin 15 mg/kg daily (29 patients) for 7 days. Peak plasma levels of quinine during monotherapy were attained within 2 days of treatment and remained within the therapeutic range for the 7-day treatment period. Levels of the main metabolite of quinine, 3-hydroxyquinine, followed a similar pattern. In patients taking quinine with rifampicin, quinine was more extensively metabolised and, after the second day of treatment, quinine levels were sharply reduced to below therapeutic levels. Acute malaria reduces the metabolic clearance of quinine (by a reduction in hepatic mixed function oxidase activity, mainly by the cytochrome P450 isoenzyme CYP3A4) and recovery is associated with a sharp decline in quinine levels. Rifampicin induces the cytochrome P450 isoenzymes and this probably more than countered their inhibition during acute malaria and resulted in increased metabolism of quinine. Although patients who received rifampicin with quinine had shorter parasite clearance times than those who received quinine alone, suggesting rifampicin may enhance the antimalarial activity of quinine, recrudescence rates were 5 times, higher suggesting increased resistance. [Note, recrudescence is the reappearance of the disease after a period of inactivity.] The authors suggest that rifampicin should not be given with quinine for the treatment of malaria. Patients receiving rifampicin who also require quinine for malaria may need increased doses of quinine.[3]

1. Wanwimolruk S, Kang W, Coville PF, Viriyayudhakorn S, Thitiarchakul S. Marked enhancement by rifampicin and lack of effect of isoniazid on the elimination of quinine in man. *Br J Clin Pharmacol* (1995) 40, 87–91.

2. Osborn JE, Pettit MJ, Graham P. Interaction between rifampicin and quinine: case report. *Pharm J* (1989) 243, 704.

3. Pukrittayakamee S, Prakongpan S, Wanwimolruk S, Clemens R, Looareesuwan S, White NJ. Adverse effect of rifampin on quinine efficacy in uncomplicated falciparum malaria. *Antimicrob Agents Chemother* (2003) 47, 1509–13.

Quinine + Tetracyclines

Doxycycline does not appear to alter the pharmacokinetics of quinine. Tetracycline increases quinine levels and has been found to improve efficacy.

Clinical evidence, mechanism, importance and management

(a) Doxycycline

In a study in 13 patients with acute falciparum malaria, the addition of intravenous **doxycycline** to treatment with intravenous quinine did not affect quinine pharmacokinetics, when compared with 13 patients taking quinine alone.[1] In contrast, *in vitro*, **doxycycline** appears to be a potent inhibitor of quinine metabolism.[2] However, given the above evidence from their use in patients, no special precautions would seem to be necessary on concurrent use.

(b) Tetracycline

A study in patients with acute falciparum malaria found that quinine levels were about doubled in those taking quinine 600 mg every 8 hours with **tetracycline** 250 mg every 6 hours, when compared with those taking quinine alone. Quinine levels were above the MIC for malaria with the combination but not for quinine alone. Two of 8 patients treated with quinine alone had malaria recrudescence (the reappearance of the disease after a period of inactivity) compared with none of 8 patients receiving the combination.[3] *In vitro* **tetracycline** is also a potent inhibitor of quinine metabolism.[2] The authors considered that this pharmacokinetic interaction might be part of the explanation why the combination has been found to be more effective.[3]

1. Couet W, Laroche R, Floch JJ, Istin B, Fourtillan JB, Sauniere JF. Pharmacokinetics of quinine and doxycycline in patients with acute falciparum malaria: a study in Africa. *Ther Drug Monit* (1991) 13, 496–501.

2. Zhao X-J, Ishizaki T. A further interaction study of quinine with clinically important drugs by human liver microsomes: determinations of inhibition constant (K_i) and type of inhibition. *Eur J Drug Metab Pharmacokinet* (1999) 24, 272–8.

3. Karbwang J, Molunto P, Bunnag D, Harinasuta T. Plasma quinine levels in patients with falciparum malaria given alone or in combination with tetracycline with or without primaquine. *Southeast Asian J Trop Med Public Health* (1991) 22, 72–6.

Quinine + Tobacco

Smokers cleared quinine from the body much more quickly than non-smokers in a single-dose study in healthy subjects. However, quinine metabolism is reduced in patients with falciparum malaria, which may negate this effect. Quinine pharmacokinetics and efficacy were unchanged by smoking in one study.

Clinical evidence

A comparative study in 10 smokers (averaging 17 cigarettes daily) and 10 non-smokers found that the AUC of a single 600-mg dose of quinine sulphate was reduced by 44%, the clearance was increased by 77% and the half-life was shortened (from 12 to 7.5 hours), when compared with the non-smokers.[1] In contrast, in a study in patients with uncomplicated falciparum malaria taking quinine sulfate 10 mg/kg three times daily for 7 days, there was no significant difference in fever clearance time, parasite clearance time, and cure rate between 10 regular smokers and 12 non-smokers. In addition pharmacokinetic parameters did not differ significantly between the smokers and non-smokers.[2]

Mechanism

Tobacco smoke contains polycyclic aromatic compounds and other substances, which are potent inducers of the liver enzymes that metabolise quinine. It is not yet clear which cytochrome P450 isoenzymes are affected. Smoking induces CYP1A, but the formation of the major metabolite of quinine, 3-hydroxyquinine, is catalysed by CYP3A, which suggests that other metabolic pathways of quinine are affected by smoking.[3]

Importance and management

Information seems to be limited but the pharmacokinetic interaction would appear to be established in healthy subjects. However, the clinical study in patients with falciparum malaria suggests that any pharmacokinetic differences are more limited probably due to the additional effect the disease has on quinine metabolism, and that smoking status does not appear to affect the clinical outcome of quinine treatment for malaria. The systemic clearance of quinine in acute falciparum malaria may be reduced by up to two-thirds, when compared to healthy subjects as malaria reduces hepatic microsomal enzyme activity. The authors say that this reduction in the clearance of quinine outweighs the possible effects of smoking-induced clearance.[2]

1. Wanwimolruk S, Wong SM, Coville PF, Viriyayudhakorn S, Thitiarchakul S. Cigarette smoking enhances the elimination of quinine. *Br J Clin Pharmacol* (1993) 36, 610–14.

2. Pukrittayakamee S, Pitisuttithum P, Zhang H, Jantra A, Wanwimolruk S, White NJ. Effects of cigarette smoking on quinine pharmacokinetics in malaria. *Eur J Clin Pharmacol* (2002) 58, 315–19.
3. Wanwimolruk S, Wong S-M, Zhang H, Coville PF, Walker RJ. Metabolism of quinine in man: identification of a major metabolite, and effects of smoking and rifampicin pretreatment. *J Pharm Pharmacol* (1995) 47, 957–63.

Terbinafine + H_2-receptor antagonists

Cimetidine modestly increases the AUC of terbinafine. However, no clinically relevant interactions appear to have been reported between terbinafine and cimetidine or ranitidine.

Clinical evidence, mechanism, importance and management

In a study in 12 healthy subjects **cimetidine** 400 mg twice daily for 5 days increased the AUC of a single 250-mg dose of terbinafine by 34% and reduced its clearance by 30%.[1] The likely reason is that **cimetidine** (a known enzyme inhibitor) reduces the metabolism of terbinafine by the liver. However, it seems that this modest increase in the serum levels of terbinafine is of little or no clinical relevance, because in a large scale post-marketing survey of patients taking terbinafine no interactions were reported in patients also taking **cimetidine** or **ranitidine** [number unknown].[2] Nevertheless, the manufacturer of terbinafine recommends that the dosage of terbinafine may need adjusting (presumably reduced) if cimetidine is given.[3]

1. Jensen JC. Pharmacokinetics of Lamisil® in humans. *J Dermatol Treat* (1990) 1 (Suppl 2), 15–18.
2. Hall M, Monka C, Krupp P, O'Sullivan D. Safety of oral terbinafine. Results of a postmarketing surveillance study in 25 884 patients. *Arch Dermatol* (1997) 133, 1213–19.
3. Lamisil Tablets (Terbinafine hydrochloride). Novartis Pharmaceuticals UK Ltd. UK Summary of product characteristics, February 2007.

Terbinafine + Rifampicin (Rifampin)

The serum levels of terbinafine are reduced by rifampicin.

Clinical evidence, mechanism, importance and management

In 12 subjects, rifampicin 600 mg daily for 6 days halved the AUC of terbinafine and roughly doubled its clearance.[1] Rifampicin is a potent enzyme inducer, which increases the metabolism of many drugs. Be alert, therefore, for the need to increase the dosage of terbinafine if rifampicin is given.

1. Jensen JC. Pharmacokinetics of Lamisil® in humans. *J Dermatol Treat* (1990) 1 (Suppl 2), 15–18.

9

Antiarrhythmics

This section is mainly concerned with the class I antiarrhythmics, which also possess some local anaesthetic properties, and with class III antiarrhythmics. Antiarrhythmics that fall into other classes are dealt with under 'beta blockers', (p.833), 'digitalis glycosides', (p.903), and 'calcium-channel blockers', (p.860). Some antiarrhythmics that do not fit into the Vaughan Williams classification (see 'Table 9.1', (below)) are also included in this section (e.g. adenosine). Interactions in which the antiarrhythmic drug is the affecting substance, rather than the drug whose activity is altered, are dealt with elsewhere.

Predicting interactions between two antiarrhythmics

It is difficult to know exactly what is likely to happen if two antiarrhythmics are used together. The hope is always that a combination will work better than just one drug, and many drug trials have confirmed that hope, but sometimes the combinations are unsafe. Predicting unsafe combinations is difficult, but there are some very broad general rules that can be applied if the general pharmacology of the drugs is understood.

If drugs with similar effects are used together, whether they act on the myocardium itself or on the conducting tissues, the total effect is likely to be increased (additive). The classification of the antiarrhythmics in 'Table 9.1', (see below) helps to predict what is likely to happen, but remember that the classification is not rigid so drugs in one class can share some characteristics with others. The following sections deal with some examples.

(a) Combinations of antiarrhythmics from the same class

The drugs in class Ia can prolong the QT interval so combining drugs from this class would be expected to show an increased effect on the QT interval. This prolongation carries the risk of causing torsade de pointes arrhythmias (see the monograph, 'Drugs that prolong the QT interval + Other drugs that prolong the QT interval', p.257). It would also be expected that the negative inotropic effects of quinidine would be additive with procainamide or any of the other drugs within class Ia. For safety therefore it is sometimes considered best to avoid drugs that fall into the same subclass or only to use them together with caution.

(b) Combinations of antiarrhythmics from different classes

Class III antiarrhythmics such as amiodarone can also prolong the QT interval, so they would also be expected to interact with drugs in other classes that do the same, namely class Ia drugs (see 'Drugs that prolong the QT interval + Other drugs that prolong the QT interval', p.257). Verapamil comes into class IV and has negative inotropic effects, so it can interact with other drugs with similar effects, such as the beta blockers, which fall into class III. For safety you should always look at the whole drug profile and take care with any two drugs, from any class, that share a common pharmacological action.

Table 9.1 Antiarrhythmics (modified Vaughan Williams classification)

Class I: Membrane stabilising drugs
(a) Ajmaline, Cibenzoline (Cifenline),* Disopyramide, Procainamide, Quinidine
(b) Aprindine, Lidocaine, Mexiletine, Tocainide
(c) Flecainide, Propafenone
Class I, but not easily fitting the above subgroups – Moracizine
Class II: Beta blocker activity
Atenolol, Bretylium,† Propranolol
Class III: Inhibitors of depolarisation
Amiodarone, Azimilide, Bretylium,† Cibenzoline (Cifenline),* Dofetilide, Dronedarone, Ibutilide, Sotalol
Class IV: Calcium-channel blocker activity
Cibenzoline (Cifenline),* Diltiazem, Verapamil
Drugs not fitting into this classification
Adenosine

*Cibenzoline has class Ia, and also some class III and IV activity

†Bretylium has class II and III activity

Adenosine + Dipyridamole

Dipyridamole reduces the bolus dose of adenosine necessary to convert supraventricular tachycardia to sinus rhythm by about fourfold. Profound bradycardia occurred in one patient taking dipyridamole when an adenosine infusion was given for myocardial stress testing.

Clinical evidence

(a) Adenosine bolus for supraventricular tachycardia

Adenosine by rapid intravenous bolus (10 to 200 micrograms/kg in stepwise doses) was found to restore sinus rhythm in 10 of 14 episodes of tachycardia in 7 patients with supraventricular tachycardia (SVT). The mean dose was 8.8 mg compared with only 1 mg in two patients also taking oral dipyridamole.[1] Another study in 6 patients found that dipyridamole (560 microgram/kg intravenous bolus, followed by a continuous infusion of 5 micrograms/kg/minute) reduced the minimum effective bolus dose of intravenous adenosine required to stop the SVT from 68 to 17 micrograms/kg in 5 patients. In the other patient, dipyridamole alone stopped the SVT.[2]

Other studies in healthy subjects have clearly shown that dipyridamole reduces the dose of adenosine required to produce an equivalent cardiovascular effect by fourfold[3] or six- to sixteenfold.[4] A brief report describes a woman with paroxysmal SVT who lost ventricular activity for 18 seconds when given adenosine 6 mg intravenously. She was also taking dipyridamole [dose unstated], which was considered to have contributed to the loss of ventricular function.[5] Another report describes 3 of 4 patients who had heart block of 3, 9 and 21-second duration respectively when given adenosine 3 to 6 mg by central venous bolus. The patient with the most profound heart block was also being treated with dipyridamole, which was thought to have contributed to the reaction.[6]

(b) Adenosine infusion for myocardial stress testing

A 79-year-old woman taking a combination of low-dose aspirin and extended-release dipyridamole *(Aggrenox)* became profoundly bradycardic (36 bpm), dizzy and almost fainted 2 minutes after the start of an adenosine infusion for radionuclide myocardial imaging. Adenosine was stopped, and she recovered within 2 minutes. The last dose of *Aggrenox* had been taken 12 hours previously.[7] However, note that bradycardia is a known adverse effect of adenosine.[8,9]

Mechanism

Not fully understood. Part of the explanation is that dipyridamole increases plasma levels of endogenous adenosine by inhibiting its uptake into cells.[2,4,10]

Importance and management

An established interaction.

(a) Patients will need much less adenosine to treat arrhythmias while taking dipyridamole. It has been suggested that the initial dose of adenosine should be reduced by twofold[5] or fourfold.[2] The UK manufacturers actually advise the avoidance of adenosine in patients taking dipyridamole. If it must be used for supraventricular tachycardia in a patient taking dipyridamole, they recommend that the adenosine dose should be reduced about fourfold.[8]

(b) The UK manufacturers advise the avoidance of adenosine in patients taking dipyridamole. If adenosine is considered necessary for myocardial imaging in a patient taking dipyridamole, they suggest that the dipyridamole should be stopped 24 hours before, or the dose of adenosine should be greatly reduced.[9] This may be insufficient for extended-release dipyridamole preparations: the authors of the above report recommend several days.[7] Xanthines, such as intravenous aminophylline, have been used to terminate persistent adverse effects of adenosine infusion given for myocardial imaging.[9] Consider also 'Adenosine + Xanthines', below.

1. Watt AH, Bernard MS, Webster J, Passani SL, Stephens MR, Routledge PA. Intravenous adenosine in the treatment of supraventricular tachycardia: a dose-ranging study and interaction with dipyridamole. *Br J Clin Pharmacol* (1986) 21, 227–30.
2. Lerman BB, Wesley RC, Belardinelli L. Electrophysiologic effects of dipyridamole on atrioventricular nodal conduction and supraventricular tachycardia. Role of endogenous adenosine. *Circulation* (1989) 80, 1536–43.
3. Biaggioni I, Onrot J, Hollister AS, Robertson D. Cardiovascular effects of adenosine infusion in man and their modulation by dipyridamole. *Life Sci* (1986) 39, 2229–36.
4. Conradson T-BG, Dixon CMS, Clarke B, Barnes PJ. Cardiovascular effects of infused adenosine in man: potentiation by dipyridamole. *Acta Physiol Scand* (1987) 129, 387–91.
5. Mader TJ. Adenosine: adverse interactions. *Ann Emerg Med* (1992) 21, 453.
6. McCollam PL, Uber WE, Van Bakel AB. Adenosine-related ventricular asystole. *Ann Intern Med* (1993) 118, 315–16.
7. Littmann L, Anderson JD, Monroe MH. Adenosine and Aggrenox: a hazardous combination. *Ann Intern Med* (2002) 137, W1.
8. Adenocor (Adenosine). Sanofi-Aventis. UK Summary of product characteristics, January 2005.
9. Adenoscan (Adenosine). Sanofi-Aventis. UK Summary of product characteristics, September 2005.
10. German DC, Kredich NM, Bjornsson TD. Oral dipyridamole increases plasma adenosine levels in human beings. *Clin Pharmacol Ther* (1989) 45, 80–4.

Adenosine + Nicotine

Nicotine appears to enhance the effects of adenosine, but the clinical relevance of this is unclear.

Clinical evidence, mechanism, importance and management

Nicotine chewing gum 2 mg (approximately equal to one cigarette) increased the circulatory effects of a 70 microgram/kg/minute infusion of adenosine in 10 healthy subjects. The increase in heart rate due to nicotine (5.5 bpm) was further increased to 14.9 bpm by the adenosine, and the diastolic blood pressure rise due to nicotine (7 mmHg) was reduced to 1.1 mmHg.[1] In another study, **nicotine chewing gum** 2 mg increased chest pain and the duration of AV block when it was given to 7 healthy subjects with intravenous bolus doses of adenosine.[2] What this means in practical terms is uncertain, but be aware that the effects of adenosine may be modified to some extent by nicotine-containing products (**tobacco smoking, nicotine gum**, etc).

1. Smits P, Eijsbouts A, Thien T. Nicotine enhances the circulatory effects of adenosine in human beings. *Clin Pharmacol Ther* (1989) 46, 272–8.
2. Sylvén C, Beerman B, Kaijser L, Jonzon B. Nicotine enhances angina pectoris-like chest pain and atrioventricular blockade provoked by intravenous bolus of adenosine in healthy volunteers. *J Cardiovasc Pharmacol* (1990) 16, 962–5.

Adenosine + Xanthines

Caffeine and theophylline can inhibit the effects of adenosine infusions used in conjunction with radionuclide myocardial imaging. Xanthines should be withheld 12 to 24 hours prior to the procedure or they will interfere with test results. Aminophylline has been used to terminate persistent adverse effects of adenosine infusions. Adenosine may still be effective for terminating supraventricular tachycardia in patients taking xanthines.

Clinical evidence

(a) Adenosine bolus for supraventricular tachycardia

It is usually considered that an adenosine bolus for the termination of paroxysmal supraventricular tachycardia will be ineffective in patients taking xanthines. However, one case describes a man taking **theophylline** (serum level 8 nanograms/mL) in whom adenosine 9 mg terminated supraventricular tachycardia. Two previous adenosine doses, one of 3 mg and one of 6 mg had not been effective.[1] Another report found that high adenosine doses, of 400 to 800 micrograms/kg (usual dose 50 to 200 micrograms/kg), were required to revert supraventricular tachycardia in a preterm infant receiving **theophylline**.[2]

(b) Adenosine infusion

Experimental studies in healthy subjects, on the way xanthine drugs possibly interact with adenosine, have shown that **caffeine** and **theophylline** (but not **enprofylline**) reduced the increased heart rate and the changes in blood pressure caused by infusions of adenosine,[3-6] and attenuated adenosine-induced vasodilatation.[7,8] **Theophylline** also attenuated adenosine-induced respiratory effects and chest pain.[5,6] Similarly, an adenosine infusion antagonised the haemodynamic effects of a single dose of **theophylline** in healthy subjects, but did not reduce the metabolic effects (reductions in plasma potassium and magnesium).[5]

Mechanism

Caffeine and theophylline have an antagonistic effect on adenosine receptors.[9] They appear to have opposite effects on the circulatory system: caffeine and theophylline cause vasoconstriction whereas adenosine infusions generally cause vasodilatation.[3] Consequently their concurrent use is likely to result in an interaction.

Importance and management

(a) Adenosine bolus injection for the termination of paroxysmal supraventricular tachycardia may still be effective in patients on xanthines. The usual dose schedule should be followed. However, note that adenosine has induced bronchospasm. The US manufacturers[10,11] state that adenosine preparations, whether used for supraventricular tachycardia or myocardial imaging, should be avoided in patients with bronchoconstriction or bronchospasm (e.g. asthma), and used cautiously in those with obstructive pulmonary disease not associated with bronchospasm (e.g. emphysema, bronchitis). The UK manufacturers similarly recommend that the product used for supraventricular tachycardia[12] should be avoided in asthma, and warn that adenosine may precipitate or aggravate bronchospasm. They also contraindicate the use of adenosine for diagnostic imaging[13] in both asthma and other obstructive pulmonary disease associated with bronchospasm. Whether an adenosine bolus can stop theophylline-induced supraventricular tachycardia appears not to have been studied.

(b) The manufacturers of adenosine state that theophylline, aminophylline and other xanthines should be avoided for 24 hours before using an adenosine infusion for radionuclide myocardial imaging, and that xanthine-containing drinks (tea, coffee, chocolate, cola drinks etc.) should be avoided for at least 12 hours before imaging.[13] In a recent study in 70 patients, measurable caffeine serum levels were found in 74% of patients after 12 hours of self-reported abstention from caffeine-containing products. Patients with caffeine serum levels of at least 2.9 mg/L had significantly fewer stress symptoms (chest tightness, chest pain, headache, dyspnoea, nausea, dizziness) than those with lower serum levels. The authors suggest that a 12-hour abstention from caffeine-containing products may be insufficient, and could result in false-negative results.[14] Xanthines, such as intravenous aminophylline, have been used to terminate persistent adverse effects of adenosine infusion given for myocardial imaging.[13]

1. Giagounidis AAN, Schäfer S, Klein RM, Aul C, Strauer BE. Adenosine is worth trying in patients with paroxysmal supraventricular tachycardia on chronic theophylline medication. *Eur J Med Res* (1998) 3, 380–2.
2. Berul CI. Higher adenosine dosage required for supraventricular tachycardia in infants treated with theophylline. *Clin Pediatr (Phila)* (1993) 32, 167–8.
3. Smits P, Schouten J, Thien T. Cardiovascular effects of two xanthines and the relation to adenosine antagonism. *Clin Pharmacol Ther* (1989) 45, 593–9.
4. Smits P, Boekema P, De Abreu R, Thien T, van 't Laar A. Evidence for an antagonism between caffeine and adenosine in the human cardiovascular system. *J Cardiovasc Pharmacol* (1987) 10, 136–43.
5. Minton NA, Henry JA. Pharmacodynamic interactions between infused adenosine and oral theophylline. *Hum Exp Toxicol* (1991) 10, 411–18.
6. Maxwell DL, Fuller RW, Conradson T-B, Dixon CMS, Aber V, Hughes JMB, Barnes PJ. Contrasting effects of two xanthines, theophylline and enprofylline, on the cardio-respiratory stimulation of infused adenosine in man. *Acta Physiol Scand* (1987) 131, 459–65.
7. Taddei S, Pedrinelli R, Salvetti A. Theophylline is an antagonist of adenosine in human forearm arterioles. *Am J Hypertens* (1991) 4, 256–9.
8. Smits P, Lenders JWM, Thien T. Caffeine and theophylline attenuate adenosine-induced vasodilation in humans. *Clin Pharmacol Ther* (1990) 48, 410–18.
9. Fredholm BB. On the mechanism of action of theophylline and caffeine. *Acta Med Scand* (1985) 217, 149–53.
10. Adenocard (Adenosine). Astellas Pharma Inc. US Prescribing information, July 2005.
11. Adenoscan (Adenosine). Astellas Pharma Inc. US Prescribing information, July 2005.
12. Adenocor (Adenosine). Sanofi-Aventis. UK Summary of product characteristics, January 2005.
13. Adenoscan (Adenosine). Sanofi-Aventis. UK Summary of product characteristics, September 2005.
14. Majd-Ardekani J, Clowes P, Menash-Bonsu V, Nunan TO. Time for abstention from caffeine before an adenosine myocardial perfusion scan. *Nucl Med Commun* (2000) 21, 361–4.

Ajmaline + Miscellaneous

An isolated report describes cardiac failure in a patient given ajmaline with lidocaine. Quinidine causes a very considerable increase in the plasma levels of ajmaline, and phenobarbital appears to cause a marked reduction.

Clinical evidence, mechanism, importance and management

A woman had a marked aggravation of her existing cardiac failure when she was given ajmaline orally and **lidocaine** intravenously for repeated ventricular tachycardias.[1]

A study[2] in 4 healthy subjects found that if a single 200-mg oral dose of **quinidine** was given with a single 50-mg oral dose of ajmaline, the AUC of ajmaline was increased 10- to 30-fold and the maximum plasma concentrations increased from 18 to 141 nanograms/mL. Another single-dose study in 5 healthy subjects found that the metabolism of ajmaline was inhibited by **quinidine**, possibly because the **quinidine** becomes competitively bound to the enzymes that metabolise ajmaline.[3]

The clearance of intravenous ajmaline was almost twice as high in 3 patients also taking **phenobarbital** when compared with 5 patients who were not taking **phenobarbital**. Therefore the clinical effects of ajmaline would be expected to be markedly diminished in those taking **phenobarbital**.[4]

The clinical importance of all of these interactions is uncertain but concurrent use should be well monitored.

1. Bleifeld W. Side effects of antiarrhythmics. *Naunyn Schmiedebergs Arch Pharmacol* (1971) 269, 282–97.
2. Hori R, Okumura K, Inui K-I, Yasuhara M, Yamada K, Sakurai T, Kawai C. Quinidine-induced rise in ajmaline plasma concentration. *J Pharm Pharmacol* (1984) 36, 202–4.
3. Köppel C, Tenczer J, Arndt I. Metabolic disposition of ajmaline. *Eur J Drug Metab Pharmacokinet* (1989) 14, 309–16.
4. Köppel C, Wagemann A, Martens F. Pharmacokinetics and antiarrhythmic efficacy of intravenous ajmaline in ventricular arrhythmia of acute onset. *Eur J Drug Metab Pharmacokinet* (1989) 14, 161–7.

Amiodarone + Anaesthesia

There is some evidence that the presence of amiodarone possibly increases the risk of complications (atropine-resistant bradycardia, hypotension, decreased cardiac output) during general anaesthesia. All cases were with fentanyl-based anaesthesia, but some other studies have shown no problems with fentanyl-based anaesthesia.

Clinical evidence

(a) Evidence for complications

Several case reports[1-4] and two studies[5,6] suggest that severe intra-operative complications (atropine-resistant bradycardia, myocardial depression, hypotension) may occur in patients receiving amiodarone. One of the studies, a comparative retrospective review of patients (16 receiving amiodarone 300 to 800 mg daily and 30 controls) having operations under anaesthesia (mainly open-heart surgery), showed that the incidence of slow nodal rhythm, complete heart block or pacemaker dependency rose from 17% in controls to 66% in amiodarone-treated patients. Intra-aortic balloon pump augmentation (reflecting poor cardiac output) was 50% in the amiodarone group compared with 7% in the control group, and a state of low systemic vascular resistance with normal to high cardiac output occurred in 13% of the amiodarone-treated patients, but none of the controls. Overall there were 3 fatalities; all of these patients had received amiodarone and had been on cardiopulmonary bypass during surgery. **Fentanyl** was used for all of the patients, often combined with **diazepam**, and sometimes also **isoflurane**, **enflurane** or **halothane**.[5]

Another study of 37 patients receiving amiodarone (mean dose about 250 mg daily) found no problems in 8 undergoing non-cardiac surgery. Of the 29 undergoing cardiac surgery, 52% had postoperative arrhythmias and 24% required a pacemaker, which was not considered exceptional for the type of surgery. However, one patient having coronary artery bypass surgery had fatal vasoplegia (a hypotensive syndrome), which was considered to be amiodarone-related. This occurred shortly after he was taken off of cardiopulmonary bypass. Anaesthesia in all patients was **fentanyl**-based.[6] It was suggested in one case report that serious hypotension in two patients on amiodarone undergoing surgery may have been further compounded by **ACE inhibitor** therapy.[3] For the interactions of ACE inhibitors and anaesthetics see 'Anaesthetics, general + Antihypertensives', p.94.

(b) Evidence for no complications

The preliminary report of one study in 21 patients taking amiodarone (mean dose 538 mg daily) and undergoing defibrillator implantation suggested that haemodynamic changes during surgery were not significantly different from those in matched controls not taking amiodarone.[7] Similarly, another study found no difference in haemodynamic status or pacemaker dependency between patients on short-term amiodarone 600 mg daily for 1 week then 400 mg daily for 2 weeks prior to surgery and a control group during valve replacement surgery with **thiopental-fentanyl** anaesthesia.[8] In a double-blind trial, there was no significant difference in haemodynamic instability during **fentanyl-isoflurane** anaesthesia between patients randomised to receive short-term amiodarone (3.4 g over 5 days or 2.2 g over 24 hours) or placebo before cardiac surgery. In this study, haemodynamic instability was assessed by fluid balance, use of dopamine or other vasopressors, and use of a phosphodiesterase inhibitor or intra-aortic balloon pump.[9] A case report describes the successful use of epidural anaesthesia with **fentanyl** then **chloroprocaine** during labour and caesarean section in a woman who had been taking amiodarone long-term for arrhythmia control. The only haemodynamic change of possible note was that the patient had a drop in systemic vascular resistance from high to almost normal levels shortly after receiving **fentanyl** during the first stage of labour, and again when **fentanyl** was given for postoperative pain relief.[10]

Mechanism

In vitro and *in vivo* studies in *animals* suggest that amiodarone has additive cardiodepressant and vasodilator effects with volatile anaesthetics such as halothane, enflurane and isoflurane.[2,11] The manufacturer notes that fentanyl is a substrate for the cytochrome P450 isoenzyme CYP3A4, and that amiodarone might inhibit CYP3A4, thereby increasing the toxicity of fentanyl.[12]

Importance and management

The assessment of this interaction is complicated by the problem of conducting studies in anaesthesia, most being retrospective and using matched controls. The only randomised study used short-term amiodarone to assess its safety in the prevention of post-operative atrial fibrillation, and its findings may not be relevant to patients taking long-term amiodarone.[9] It appears that potentially severe complications may occur in some patients taking amiodarone undergoing general anaesthesia, including bradycardia unresponsive to atropine, hypotension, conduction disturbances, and decreased cardiac output. Anaesthetists should take particular care in patients taking amiodarone who undergo surgery on cardiopulmonary bypass.[13] Amiodarone persists in the body for many weeks, which usually means it cannot be withdrawn before surgery, especially if there are risks in delaying surgery,[6] or the amiodarone is being used for serious arrhythmias.[13] A possible pharmacokinetic interaction exists between fentanyl and amiodarone, which could contribute to the interactions seen, and further study is needed on this.

1. Gallagher JD, Lieberman RW, Meranze J, Spielman SR, Ellison N. Amiodarone-induced complications during coronary artery surgery. *Anesthesiology* (1981) 55, 186–8.
2. MacKinnon G, Landymore R, Marble A. Should oral amiodarone be used for sustained ventricular tachycardia in patients requiring open-heart surgery? *Can J Surg* (1983) 26, 355–7.
3. Mackay JH, Walker IA, Bethune DW. Amiodarone and anaesthesia: concurrent therapy with ACE inhibitors—an additional cause for concern? *Can J Anaesth* (1991) 38, 687.
4. Navalgund AA, Alifimoff JK, Jakymec AJ, Bleyaert AL. Amiodarone-induced sinus arrest successfully treated with ephedrine and isoproterenol. *Anesth Analg* (1986) 65, 414–16.
5. Liberman BA, Teasdale SJ. Anaesthesia and amiodarone. *Can Anaesth Soc J* (1985) 32, 629–38.
6. Van Dyck M, Baele P, Rennotte MT, Matta A, Dion R, Kestens-Servaye Y. Should amiodarone be discontinued before cardiac surgery? *Acta Anaesthesiol Belg* (1988) 39, 3–10.
7. Elliott PL, Schauble JF, Rogers MC, Reid PR. Risk of decompensation during anesthesia in presence of amiodarone. *Circulation* (1983) 68 (Suppl 3), 280.
8. Chassard D, George M, Guiraud M, Lehot JJ, Bastien O, Hercule C, Villard J, Estanove S. Relationship between preoperative amiodarone treatment and complications observed during anaesthesia for valvular cardiac surgery. *Can J Anaesth* (1990) 37, 251–4.
9. White CM, Dunn A, Tsikouris J, Waberski W, Felton K, Freeman-Bosco L, Giri S, Kluger J. An assessment of the safety of short-term amiodarone therapy in cardiac surgical patients with fentanyl-isoflurane anesthesia. *Anesth Analg* (1999) 89, 585–9.
10. Koblin DD, Romanoff ME, Martin DE, Hensley FA, Larach DR, Stauffer RA, Luck JC. Anesthetic management of the parturient receiving amiodarone. *Anesthesiology* (1987) 66, 551–3.
11. Rooney RT, Marijic J, Stommel KA, Bosnjak ZJ, Aggarwai A, Kampine JP, Stowe DF. Additive cardiac depression by volatile anesthetics in isolated hearts after chronic amiodarone treatment. *Anesth Analg* (1995) 80, 917–24.
12. Cordarone X (Amiodarone hydrochloride). Sanofi-Aventis. UK Summary of product characteristics, April 2006.
13. Teasdale S, Downar E. Amiodarone and anaesthesia. *Can J Anaesth* (1990) 37, 151–5.

Amiodarone + Antihistamines

A case of torsade de pointes occurred in an elderly woman taking amiodarone when she was also given loratadine, an antihistamine generally viewed as unlikely to have clinically relevant effects on the QT-interval. Combined effects on the QT interval would be expected if amiodarone was given with terfenadine or astemizole, and possibly also mizolastine.

Clinical evidence, mechanism, importance and management

A 73-year-old woman taking amiodarone for atrial fibrillation was given **loratadine** and developed syncope and multiple episodes of torsade de pointes arrhythmia.[1]

Amiodarone alone is known to cause QT prolongation and torsade de pointes arrhythmia, but **loratadine** is not usually considered to have a clinically relevant effect on the QT interval, see 'Table 15.2', (p.583). Amiodarone may have inhibited the metabolism of loratadine by the cytochrome P450 isoenzyme CYP3A4.

The general clinical relevance of this one case is uncertain, but the authors consider that the QT interval should be monitored if **loratadine** is given with other drugs that may potentially prolong the QT interval. Note that it is recommended that antihistamines with known potential for QT prolongation such as **terfenadine** and **astemizole** (see 'Table 15.2', (p.583)) should not be used with amiodarone, and although there appear to be no cases of clinically relevant QT-prolongation with **mizolastine**, the manufacturers contraindicate concurrent amiodarone.[2,3]

1. Atar S, Freedberg NA, Antonelli D, Rosenfeld T. Torsade de pointes and QT prolongation due to a combination of loratadine and amiodarone. *Pacing Clin Electrophysiol* (2003) 26, 785–6.
2. Mizollen (Mizolastine). Schwarz Pharma Ltd. UK Summary of product characteristics, May 2006.
3. Cordarone X (Amiodarone hydrochloride). Sanofi-Aventis. UK Summary of product characteristics, April 2006.

Amiodarone + Beta blockers

Hypotension, bradycardia, ventricular fibrillation and asystole have been seen in a few patients given amiodarone with propranolol, metoprolol or sotalol (for sotalol, see also 'Drugs that prolong the QT interval + Other drugs that prolong the QT interval', p.257). However, analysis of clinical trials suggests that the combination can be beneficial. Amiodarone may inhibit the metabolism of beta blockers metabolised by CYP2D6, such as metoprolol, which might be a factor in the interaction.

Clinical evidence

(a) Case reports of problems

A 64-year-old woman was treated for hypertrophic cardiomyopathy with amiodarone 1.2 g daily and **atenolol** 50 mg daily. Five days later the **atenolol** was replaced by **metoprolol** 100 mg daily. Within 3 hours she complained of dizziness, weakness and blurred vision. On examination she was found to be pale and sweating with a pulse rate of 20 bpm. Her systolic blood pressure was 60 mmHg. Atropine 2 mg did not produce chronotropic or haemodynamic improvement. She responded to isoprenaline (isoproterenol).[1] Severe hypotension has been reported in another patient taking **sotalol** when intravenous amiodarone (total dose 250 mg) was given.[2] Another report describes cardiac arrest in one patient on amiodarone, and severe bradycardia and ventricular fibrillation (requiring defibrillation) in another, within 1.5 and 2 hours of starting to take **propranolol**.[3]

(b) Clinical studies showing benefits

In contrast to the above case reports, an analysis of data from two large clinical studies of the use of amiodarone for post-myocardial infarction arrhythmias found that the combination of **beta blockers** [unnamed] and amiodarone was beneficial (reduced cardiac deaths, arrhythmic deaths and resuscitated cardiac arrest) compared with either drug alone, or neither drug. Discontinuation of amiodarone because of excessive bradycardia was no more frequent when beta blockers were also given, although more patients taking amiodarone discontinued beta blockers than those taking placebo.[4] Similarly, in the analysis of another study in ischaemic heart failure, the benefits of **carvedilol** were still apparent in those patients already receiving amiodarone, and the combination was not associated with a greater incidence of adverse effects (worsened heart failure, hypotension/dizziness, bradycardia/atrioventricular block) than either drug alone.[5]

(c) Pharmacokinetics

In one study, 10 elderly patients (9 with symptomatic atrial fibrillation and one with an implanted defibrillator and frequent ventricular tachycardia) taking **metoprolol** (mean daily dose 119 mg) were also given amiodarone 1.2 g daily for 6 days. The **metoprolol** AUC and plasma levels were increased by about 80% and 75%, respectively, by the amiodarone, the extent varying by CYP2D6 genotype.[6] None of the patients included in the study were poor metabolisers.

Mechanism

Not understood. The clinical picture is that of excessive beta-blockade, and additive pharmacodynamic effects are possible. In addition, amiodarone increases the levels of metoprolol via inhibition of the cytochrome P450 isoenzyme CYP2D6, and this may be significant in fast metabolisers.[6] See 'Genetic factors', (p.4), for more information about fast metabolisers. Other beta blockers that are also substrates of CYP2D6, and which could therefore be similarly affected, include carvedilol and propranolol.

Importance and management

The isolated reports of adverse reactions cited here (they seem to be the only ones so far documented) emphasise the need for caution when amiodarone is used with beta blockers. The manufacturers of amiodarone recommend that the combination should not be used[7] or used with caution[8] because potentiation of negative chronotropic properties and conduction-slowing effects may occur. However, the concurrent use of beta blockers and amiodarone is not uncommon and may be therapeutically useful. The authors of one of the analyses suggest that post-myocardial infarction, if possible, beta blockers should be continued in patients for whom amiodarone is indicated.[4] A pharmacokinetic interaction between amiodarone and beta blockers that are substrates of CYP2D6, such as metoprolol, also appears to be established. Although this interaction with other inhibitors of CYP2D6 is generally not thought to be clinically relevant (e.g. see 'Beta blockers + SSRIs', p.855), it is possible that this pharmacokinetic interaction plays some part in the adverse reactions sometimes seen, or even in the clinical benefits.[6] See also 'Drugs that prolong the QT interval + Other drugs that prolong the QT interval', p.257, which deals with the possible risks of using amiodarone with sotalol.

1. Leor J, Levartowsky D, Sharon C, Farfel Z. Amiodarone and β-adrenergic blockers: an interaction with metoprolol but not with atenolol. *Am Heart J* (1988) 116, 206–7.
2. Warren R, Vohra J, Hunt D, Hamer A. Serious interactions of sotalol with amiodarone and flecainide. *Med J Aust* (1990) 152, 277.
3. Derrida JP, Ollagnier J, Benaim R, Haiat R, Chiche P. Amiodarone et propranolol; une association dangereuse? *Nouv Presse Med* (1979) 8, 1429.
4. Boutitie F, Boissel J-P, Connolly SJ, Camm AJ, Cairns JA, Julian DG, Gent M, Janse MJ, Dorian P, Frangin G. Amiodarone interaction with β-blockers: analysis of the merged EMIAT (European Myocardial Infarct Amiodarone Trial) and CAMIAT (Canadian Amiodarone Myocardial Infarction Trial) databases. *Circulation* (1999) 99, 2268–75.
5. Krum H, Shusterman N, MacMahon S, Sharpe N. Efficacy and safety of carvedilol in patients with chronic heart failure receiving concomitant amiodarone therapy. *J Card Fail* (1998) 4, 281–8.
6. Werner D, Wuttke H, Fromm MF, Schaefer S, Eschenhagen T, Brune K, Daniel WG, Werner U. Effect of amiodarone on the plasma levels of metoprolol. *Am J Cardiol* (2004) 94, 1319–21.
7. Cordarone X (Amiodarone hydrochloride). Sanofi-Aventis. UK Summary of product characteristics, April 2006.
8. Cordarone (Amiodarone hydrochloride). Wyeth Pharmaceuticals. US Prescribing information, May 2007.

Amiodarone + Calcium-channel blockers

Increased cardiac depressant effects would be expected if amiodarone is used with diltiazem or verapamil. One case of sinus arrest and serious hypotension occurred in a woman taking diltiazem when she was given amiodarone.

Clinical evidence, mechanism, importance and management

A woman with compensated congestive heart failure, paroxysmal atrial fibrillation and ventricular arrhythmias was treated with furosemide and **diltiazem** 90 mg every 6 hours. Four days after amiodarone, 600 mg every 12 hours was added, she developed sinus arrest and a life-threatening low cardiac output state (systolic blood pressure 80 mmHg) with oliguria. **Diltiazem** and amiodarone were stopped and she was treated with pressor drugs and ventricular pacing. She had previously had no problems when taking **diltiazem** or **verapamil** alone, and later she took amiodarone 400 mg daily alone without incident. This reaction is thought to be caused by the additive effects of both drugs on myocardial contractility, and on sinus and atrioventricular nodal function.[1] Before this isolated case report was published, another author predicted this interaction with **diltiazem** or **verapamil** on theoretical grounds, and warned of the risks if dysfunction of the sinus node (bradycardia or sick sinus syndrome) is suspected, or if partial AV block exists.[2] The manufacturers state that amiodarone should not be used,[3] or used with caution,[4] with certain calcium-channel blockers (**diltiazem**, **verapamil**) because potentiation of negative chronotropic properties and conduction-slowing effects may occur. Note that **diltiazem** has been used for rate control in patients developing postoperative atrial fibrillation despite the use of prophylactic amiodarone.[5] There do not appear to be any reports of adverse effects attributed to the use of amiodarone with the dihydropyridine class of calcium-channel blockers (e.g. **nifedipine**), which typically have little or no negative inotropic activity at usual doses.

1. Lee TH, Friedman PL, Goldman L, Stone PH, Antman EM. Sinus arrest and hypotension with combined amiodarone-diltiazem therapy. *Am Heart J* (1985) 109, 163–4.
2. Marcus FI. Drug interactions with amiodarone. *Am Heart J* (1983) 106, 924–30.
3. Cordarone X (Amiodarone hydrochloride). Sanofi-Aventis. UK Summary of product characteristics, April 2006.
4. Cordarone (Amiodarone hydrochloride). Wyeth Pharmaceuticals. US Prescribing information, May 2007.
5. Kim MH, Rachwal W, McHale C, Bruckman D, Decena BF, Russman P, Morady F, Eagle KA. Effect of amiodarone ± diltiazem ± beta blocker on frequency of atrial fibrillation, length of hospitalization, and hospital costs after coronary artery bypass grafting. *Am J Cardiol* (2002) 89, 1126–28.

Amiodarone + Cimetidine

Cimetidine possibly causes a modest rise in the serum levels of amiodarone in some patients.

Clinical evidence, mechanism, importance and management

The preliminary report of one study in 12 patients notes that the mean serum levels of amiodarone 200 mg twice daily rose by an average of 38%, from 1.4 to 1.93 micrograms/mL, when cimetidine 1.2 g daily was given for a week. The desethyl-amiodarone levels rose by 54%. However, these increases were not statistically significant, and only 8 of the 12 patients had any rise.[1] It is possible that cimetidine may inhibit the metabolism of amiodarone. Information seems to be limited to this study but this interaction may be clinically important in some patients. Monitor the effects when cimetidine is started, being alert for amiodarone adverse effects. Remember that amiodarone has a very long half-life of 25 to 100 days, so that the results of the one-week study cited here may possibly not adequately reflect the magnitude of this interaction. There does not appear to have been anything further published on this.

1. Hogan C, Landau S, Tepper D, Somberg J. Cimetidine-amiodarone interaction. *J Clin Pharmacol* (1988) 28, 909.

Amiodarone + Colestyramine

Colestyramine appears to reduce the serum levels of amiodarone.

Clinical evidence

When 4 doses of colestyramine 4 g were given to 11 patients at 1-hour intervals starting 1.5 hours after a single 400-mg dose of amiodarone, the serum amiodarone levels 7.5 hours later were reduced by about 50%.[1] In a further study, the amiodarone half-life was shorter in 3 patients given colestyramine 4 g daily after discontinuing long-term amiodarone (23.5, 29 and 32 days, respectively) compared with that in 8 patients discontinuing amiodarone and not given colestyramine (35 to 58 days).[1]

Mechanism

This interaction probably occurs because colestyramine binds with amiodarone in the gut, thereby reducing its absorption. It may also affect the enterohepatic recirculation of amiodarone.[1] This is consistent with the way colestyramine interacts with other drugs.

Importance and management

Information is very limited but a reduced response to amiodarone may be expected. Separating the dosages to avoid admixture in the gut would reduce or prevent any effects on absorption from the gut, but not the effects due to reduced enterohepatic recirculation. Monitor concurrent use closely and consider an alternative to colestyramine, or raise the amiodarone dosage if necessary.

1. Nitsch J, Luderitz B. Beschleunigte elimination von Amiodaron durch Colestyramin. *Dtsch Med Wochenschr* (1986) 111, 1241–44.

Amiodarone + Disopyramide

The risk of QT interval prolongation and torsade de pointes is increased if amiodarone is given with disopyramide.

Clinical evidence

A brief report describes 2 patients who developed torsade de pointes when they were given amiodarone with disopyramide. Their QT intervals became markedly prolonged to somewhere between 500 and 600 milliseconds.[1] In another study, 2 patients who had been taking disopyramide 300 mg daily for a number of months developed prolonged QT intervals from 450 to 640 milliseconds and from 390 to 680 milliseconds respectively, and developed torsade de pointes 2 and 5 days respectively, after starting amiodarone 800 mg daily.[2] However, one early report also described the successful and apparently safe use of amiodarone 100 to 600 mg daily with disopyramide 300 to 500 mg daily,[3] although the results on long-term follow-up were not reported in all cases.

Mechanism

Amiodarone is a class III antiarrhythmic and can prolong the QT interval. Disopyramide is a class Ia antiarrhythmic and also prolongs the QT interval. Their additive effects can result in the development of torsade de pointes arrhythmias.

Importance and management

An established and potentially serious interaction. In general, class Ia antiarrhythmics such as disopyramide (see 'Table 9.2', (p.257)) should be avoided or used with great caution with amiodarone because of their additive effects in delaying conduction. The manufacturers of amiodarone contraindicate[4] or urge caution[5] if it is used with class Ia antiarrhythmics. If amiodarone is started in a patient taking disopyramide, they suggest the dose of disopyramide should be reduced by 30 to 50% several days after the addition of amiodarone, and that the continued need for disopyramide should be monitored, and withdrawal attempted. If disopyramide is added to amiodarone, the initial dose of disopyramide should be about half of the usual recommended dose.[5] See also 'Drugs that prolong the QT interval + Other drugs that prolong the QT interval', p.257, and for the interactions of other class Ia antiarrhythmics see 'Procainamide + Amiodarone', p.271, and 'Quinidine + Amiodarone', p.276.

1. Tartini R, Kappenberger L, Steinbrunn W. Gefährliche Interaktionen zwischen Amiodaron und Antiarrhythmika der Klass I. *Schweiz Med Wochenschr* (1982) 112, 1585–87.
2. Keren A, Tzivoni D, Gavish D, Levi J, Gottlieb S, Benhorin J, Stern S. Etiology, warning signs and therapy of torsade de pointes. A study of 10 patients. *Circulation* (1981) 64, 1167–74.
3. James MA, Papouchado M, Vann Jonec J. Combined therapy with disopyramide and amiodarone: a report of 11 cases. *Int J Cardiol* (1986) 13, 248–52.
4. Cordarone X (Amiodarone hydrochloride). Sanofi-Aventis. UK Summary of product characteristics, April 2006.
5. Cordarone (Amiodarone hydrochloride). Wyeth Pharmaceuticals. US Prescribing information, May 2007.

Amiodarone + Grapefruit juice

Grapefruit juice inhibited the metabolism of oral amiodarone, and *decreased* its effects on the PR and QTc interval.

Clinical evidence, mechanism, importance and management

A single 17-mg/kg oral dose of amiodarone was given to 11 healthy subjects on two occasions, once with water and once with grapefruit juice (300 mL taken three times on the same day). Grapefruit juice completely inhibited the metabolism of amiodarone to its major metabolite *N*-desethylamiodarone (N-DEA) and increased the amiodarone AUC by 50% and the peak serum level by 84%. The effect of amiodarone on the PR and QTc intervals was *decreased*.[1] It is likely that grapefruit juice inhibits the cytochrome P450 isoenzyme CYP3A4 in the intestinal mucosa, thus inhibiting the formation of N-DEA from oral, but probably not intravenous, amiodarone.

This interaction appears to be established, but its clinical consequences remain to be determined. N-DEA is known to be active, so this could possibly result in decreased activity.[1] In addition, high amiodarone concentrations may increase toxicity.[1] Conversely, a reduction in QT prolongation is potentially beneficial.[1] Further study is needed. However, the US manufacturer recommends that grapefruit juice should not be taken during treatment with oral amiodarone.[2]

1. Libersa CC, Brique SA, Motte KB, Caron JF, Guédon-Moreau LM, Humbert L, Vincent A, Devos P, Lhermitte MA. Dramatic inhibition of amiodarone metabolism induced by grapefruit juice. *Br J Clin Pharmacol* (2000) 49, 373–8.
2. Cordarone (Amiodarone hydrochloride). Wyeth Pharmaceuticals. US Prescribing information, May 2007.

Amiodarone + Lithium

Hypothyroidism developed very rapidly in two patients taking amiodarone when lithium was added.

Clinical evidence, mechanism, importance and management

A patient who had taken amiodarone 400 mg daily for more than a year developed acute manic depression. He was started on 600 mg of lithium daily [salt unknown], but within 2 weeks he developed clinical signs of hypothyroidism, which were confirmed by clinical tests. He made a complete recovery within 3 weeks of stopping amiodarone while continuing lithium.[1] Similarly, another patient rapidly developed hypothyroidism, when taking amiodarone with lithium [dose and salt unknown]. It resolved when the amiodarone was stopped.[1] Both lithium and amiodarone on their own can cause hypothyroidism, (note that amiodarone can also cause hyperthyroidism). In these two cases the effects appear to have been additive, and very rapid.

These two cases appear to be the first and only reports of this interaction. Its general importance is therefore still uncertain. Note that lithium has been tried for the treatment of amiodarone-induced hyperthyroidism,[2] and regular monitoring of thyroid status is recommended throughout amiodarone treatment.[3,4] It would therefore seem prudent to be extra vigilant for any signs of hypothyroidism (lethargy, weakness, depression, weight gain, hoarseness) in any patient given both drugs.

Lithium therapy has rarely been associated with cardiac QT prolongation, and consequently the UK manufacturer of amiodarone contraindicates combined use.[3] However, note that QT-prolongation associated with lithium is usually as a result of lithium toxicity. See also 'Drugs that prolong the QT interval + Other drugs that prolong the QT interval', p.257.

1. Ahmad S. Sudden hypothyroidism and amiodarone-lithium combination: an interaction. *Cardiovasc Drugs Ther* (1995) 9, 827–8.
2. Dickstein G, Shechner C, Adawi F, Kaplan J, Baron E, Ish-Shalom S. Lithium treatment in amiodarone-induced thyrotoxicosis. *Am J Med* (1997) 102, 454–8.
3. Cordarone X (Amiodarone hydrochloride). Sanofi-Aventis. UK Summary of product characteristics, April 2006.
4. Cordarone (Amiodarone hydrochloride). Wyeth Pharmaceuticals. US Prescribing information, May 2007.

Amiodarone + Macrolides

Torsade de pointes occurred in a man taking amiodarone when he was also given intravenous erythromycin. QT prolongation occurred in another patient when azithromycin was added to established amiodarone therapy.

Clinical evidence

A 76-year-old man taking amiodarone 200 mg daily had a prolonged QT interval and a syncopal episode with torsade de pointes 24 hours after starting a course of intravenous **erythromycin lactobionate**. This occurred on rechallenge.[1] Marked QT prolongation and increased QT dispersion occurred when **azithromycin** was started in a patient on long-term amiodarone therapy, and resolved when it was stopped.[2]

Mechanism

Amiodarone alone can prolong the QT interval and increase the risk of torsade de pointes. Of the macrolides, *intravenous* erythromycin is known to prolong the QT interval, and there is also some evidence that clarithromycin may prolong the QT interval.[3] Amiodarone and these macrolides may therefore have additive effects on the QT interval.

Importance and management

In general the concurrent use of two or more drugs that prolong the QT interval should be avoided, because this increases the risk of torsade de pointes arrhythmias (see also 'Drugs that prolong the QT interval + Other drugs that prolong the QT interval', p.257). For this reason, the UK manufacturer of amiodarone contraindicates the concurrent use of *intravenous* erythromycin,[4] The authors of the above report suggest that the combination of azithromycin and amiodarone should be used with caution,[2] and this should probably also apply to **clarithromycin** until more is known. The US manufacturer recommends that a careful risk assessment should be done if amiodarone is to be given with a macrolide.[5]

1. Nattel S, Ranger S, Talajic M, Lemery R, Roy D. Erythromycin-induced long QT syndrome: concordance with quinidine and underlying cellular electrophysiologic mechanism. *Am J Med* (1990) 89, 235–8.
2. Samarendra P, Kumari S, Evans SJ, Sacchi TJ, Navarro V. QT prolongation associated with azithromycin/amiodarone combination. *Pacing Clin Electrophysiol* (2001) 24, 1572–4.
3. Lee KL, Man-Hong J, Tang SC, Tai Y-T. QT-prolongation and torsades de pointes associated with clarithromycin. *Am J Med* (1998) 104, 395–6.
4. Cordarone X (Amiodarone hydrochloride). Sanofi-Aventis. UK Summary of product characteristics, April 2006.
5. Cordarone (Amiodarone hydrochloride). Wyeth Pharmaceuticals. US Prescribing information, May 2007.

Amiodarone + Orlistat

Orlistat modestly reduces the absorption of amiodarone, but this is unlikely to be clinically important.

Clinical evidence, mechanism, importance and management

A randomised placebo-controlled study in 16 healthy subjects found that orlistat 120 mg three times daily reduced the AUC and peak serum level of a single 1.2-g dose of amiodarone by 23% and 27%, respectively. Levels of its active metabolite, desethylamiodarone, were similarly reduced. The half-life and time to maximum serum level were not significantly altered. It was suggested that orlistat, which inhibits dietary fat absorption, may also reduce the absorption of amiodarone, which is a lipophilic drug.[1]

Although the clinical effect of this modest reduction in amiodarone levels is not known, it is almost certainly unlikely to be clinically relevant.

1. Zhi J, Moore R, Kanitra L, Mulligan TE. Effects of orlistat, a lipase inhibitor, on the pharmacokinetics of three highly lipophilic drugs (amiodarone, fluoxetine, and simvastatin) in healthy volunteers. *J Clin Pharmacol* (2003) 43, 428–35.

Amiodarone + Oxygen

High-dose oxygen may increase the risks of amiodarone-induced postoperative adult respiratory distress syndrome.

Clinical evidence, mechanism, importance and management

A retrospective review of 20 patients who underwent cardiac surgery found that pulmonary complications were more common in those receiving amiodarone (73% versus 25%). Moreover, the incidence of pulmonary complications in patients taking amiodarone was higher in those exposed to 100% oxygen (6 of 7) than those not (2 of 4).[1]

Four other patients taking amiodarone (without preoperative amiodarone pulmonary toxicity), developed postoperative toxicity, and 2 patients died). The common intraoperative factor in the 4 patients was exposure to high inspired oxygen concentrations.[2] A further two reports describe 3 patients taking amiodarone who developed acute onset unilateral adult respiratory syndrome after receiving 100% oxygen ventilation of one lung during surgery. These reports also suggest that high-dose oxygen may be a risk factor in patients receiving amiodarone.[3,4]

Life-threatening pulmonary complications occurred in 4 patients with diagnosed amiodarone pulmonary toxicity who subsequently underwent cardiothoracic surgery: 2 patients died. These 4 patients were compared with 13 other patients taking amiodarone (only one of whom had preoperative amiodarone pulmonary toxicity) who were undergoing similar surgery and who did not develop pulmonary complications. The comparison indicated that *preoperative* amiodarone pulmonary toxicity appears to be a risk factor in the development of pulmonary complications, but other additional factors could include pump-oxygenator time and oxygen toxicity.[5]

Increased pulmonary toxicity (pulmonary oedema) with the combination of amiodarone and 100% oxygen has been confirmed in *mice*.[6]

The UK manufacturer of amiodarone suggests caution in patients receiving high-dose oxygen therapy.[7] Others have suggested that the concentration of oxygen should be maintained at the lowest possible level consistent with adequate oxygenation.[1,3,4,6]

1. Duke PK, Ramsay MAE, Herndon JC, Swygert TH, Cook AO. Acute oxygen induced amiodarone pulmonary toxicity after general anaesthesia. *Anesthesiology* (1991) 75, A228.
2. Kay GN, Epstein AE, Kirklin JK, Diethelm AG, Graybar G, Plumb VJ. Fatal postoperative amiodarone pulmonary toxicity. *Am J Cardiol* (1988) 62, 490–2.
3. Herndon JC, Cook AO, Ramsay AE, Swygert TH, Capehart J. Postoperative unilateral pulmonary edema: possible amiodarone pulmonary toxicity. *Anesthesiology* (1992) 76, 308–12.
4. Saussine M, Colson P, Alauzen M, Mary H. Postoperative acute respiratory distress syndrome. A complication of amiodarone associated with 100 percent oxygen ventilation. *Chest* (1992) 102, 980–1.
5. Nalos PC, Kass RM, Gang ES, Fishbein MC, Mandel WJ, Peter T. Life-threatening postoperative pulmonary complications in patients with previous amiodarone pulmonary toxicity undergoing cardiothoracic operations. *J Thorac Cardiovasc Surg* (1987) 93, 904–12.
6. Donica SK, Paulsen AW, Simpson BR, Ramsay MAE, Saunders CT, Swygert TH, Tappe J. Danger of amiodarone therapy and elevated inspired oxygen concentrations in mice. *Am J Cardiol* (1996) 77, 109–10.
7. Cordarone X (Amiodarone hydrochloride). Sanofi-Aventis. UK Summary of product characteristics, April 2006.

Amiodarone + Protease inhibitors

A case report describes increased amiodarone levels in a patient given indinavir. Other protease inhibitors are predicted to act similarly.

Clinical evidence

A patient taking amiodarone 200 mg daily was also given zidovudine, lamivudine, and **indinavir** for 4 weeks, as post HIV-exposure prophylaxis after a needlestick injury. Amiodarone serum levels increased, from 0.9 mg/L before antiretroviral prophylaxis, to 1.3 mg/L during therapy, and gradually decreased to 0.8 mg/L during the 77 days after stopping prophylaxis. Although the reference range for amiodarone levels is not established, these levels were not outside those usually considered to achieve good antiarrhythmic control.[1]

Mechanism

Protease inhibitors such as indinavir are inhibitors of cytochrome P450 enzymes and pharmacokinetic interactions are therefore possible. It was considered that the increase in serum amiodarone in this case was due to decreased metabolism of amiodarone, although no decrease in the serum levels of desethylamiodarone were observed.[1]

Importance and management

Although in the case cited the interaction was not clinically relevant, the authors considered that it could be in patients with higher initial amiodarone levels. They recommend monitoring amiodarone therapy if indinavir is also given.[1] In general the UK manufacturers of protease inhibitors suggest that they may increase amiodarone levels, and contraindicate concurrent use. The exception is **atazanavir**,[2] where caution is recommended. Similarly the US manufacturers of the protease inhibitors generally contraindicate concurrent use. The exceptions are **amprenavir**,[3] **atazanavir**,[4] **fosamprenavir**[5] and **lopinavir**,[6] where the manufacturers recommend increased monitoring, including taking amiodarone levels, where possible.

1. Lohman JJHM, Reichert LJM, Degen LPM. Antiretroviral therapy increases serum concentrations of amiodarone. *Ann Pharmacother* (1999) 33, 645–6.
2. Reyataz (Atazanavir sulfate). Bristol-Myers Squibb Pharmaceuticals Ltd. UK Summary of product characteristics, April 2007.
3. Agenerase (Amprenavir). GlaxoSmithKline. US Prescribing information, May 2005.
4. Reyataz (Atazanavir sulfate). Bristol-Myers Squibb Company. US Prescribing information, March 2007.
5. Lexiva (Fosamprenavir calcium). GlaxoSmithKline. US Prescribing information, June 2007.
6. Kaletra (Lopinavir/ritonavir). Abbott Laboratories. US Prescribing information, January 2007.

Amiodarone + Quinolones

Torsade de pointes has been reported in two patients taking amiodarone and levofloxacin. Post-marketing surveillance identified two cases with amiodarone and sparfloxacin. An increased risk of this arrhythmia would also be expected if amiodarone is used with gatifloxacin or moxifloxacin.

Clinical evidence, mechanism, importance and management

Torsade de pointes arrhythmia occurred in a patient taking **levofloxacin** and amiodarone.[1] The same authors subsequently encountered a second case of this reaction.[2] The FDA Adverse Events Reporting System database up to May 2001 was reviewed for cases of torsade de pointes associated with quinolones. Four cases [possibly including the two mentioned above] were noted in patients taking amiodarone and a quinolone (unspecified, but **ciprofloxacin**, **gatifloxacin**, **levofloxacin**, **moxifloxacin**, and **ofloxacin** were assessed). In total, 37 cases of torsade de pointes were identified, and 19 occurred in patients also taking other drugs known to prolong the QT interval.[3]

During post-marketing surveillance of **sparfloxacin** in France over a period of 8 months (about 750 000 patients) serious adverse cardiovascular effects were reported in 7 patients. All 7 patients had underlying risk factors including 3 patients who were also receiving amiodarone. Of these, 2 patients had documented QT prolongation and ventricular tachycardia.[4]

Amiodarone can prolong the QT interval and increase the risk of torsade de pointes. Of the quinolones used clinically, **gatifloxacin**, **moxifloxacin**, and **sparfloxacin** are known to prolong the QT interval (see 'Table 9.2', (p.257)). There is also evidence that **levofloxacin** may prolong the QT interval.[2,3]

In general the concurrent use of two or more drugs that prolong the QT interval should be avoided, because this increases the risk of torsade de pointes arrhythmias (see also 'Drugs that prolong the QT interval + Other drugs that prolong the QT interval', p.257). The above quinolones should probably be avoided in patients on amiodarone. **Ciprofloxacin** appears to have less effect on the QT interval.[3]

1. Iannini PB, Kramer H, Circiumaru I, Byazrova E, Doddamani S. QTc prolongation associated with levofloxacin. *Intersci Conf Antimicrob Agents Chemother* (2000) 40, 477.
2. Iannini P. Quinolone-induced QT interval prolongation: a not-so-unexpected class effect. *J Antimicrob Chemother* (2001) 47, 893–4.
3. Frothingham R. Rates of torsades de pointes associated with ciprofloxacin, ofloxacin, levofloxacin, gatifloxacin, and moxifloxacin. *Pharmacotherapy* (2001) 21, 1468–72.
4. Jaillon P, Morganroth J, Brumpt I, Talbot G, and the Sparfloxacin Safety Group. Overview of electrocardiographic and cardiovascular safety data for sparfloxacin. *J Antimicrob Chemother* (1996) 37 (Suppl A), 161–7.

Amiodarone + Rifampicin (Rifampin)

An isolated case report suggests that rifampicin may decrease the serum levels of amiodarone and its metabolite *N*-desethylamiodarone.

Clinical evidence, mechanism, importance and management

A woman with congenital heart disease and atrial and ventricular arrhythmias managed by an implanted cardioverter defibrillator, epicardial pacing and amiodarone 400 mg daily, experienced deterioration in the control of her condition. She developed palpitations and experienced a shock from the defibrillator. Her amiodarone serum levels were 40% lower than 2 months previously, and her *N*-desethylamiodarone levels were undetectable. It was noted that 5 weeks earlier rifampicin 600 mg daily had been started to treat an infection of the pacing system. The amiodarone dose was doubled, but the palpitations continued. Amiodarone and *N*-desethylamiodarone levels increased after rifampicin was discontinued.[1] Rifampicin is a potent enzyme inducer and it may have increased the metabolism and clearance of amiodarone. This case suggests that combined use of amiodarone and rifampicin should be well monitored.

1. Zarembski DG, Fischer SA, Santucci PA, Porter MT, Costanzo MR, Trohman RG. Impact of rifampin on serum amiodarone concentrations in a patient with congenital heart disease. *Pharmacotherapy* (1999) 19, 249–51.

Amiodarone + Sertraline

In an isolated report, a slight to moderate rise in plasma amiodarone levels was attributed to the concurrent use of sertraline.

Clinical evidence, mechanism, importance and management

A depressed patient taking amiodarone 200 mg twice daily had his treatment with carbamazepine 200 mg twice daily and sertraline 100 mg daily stopped, just before ECT treatment. After 4 days it was noted that his plasma amiodarone levels had fallen by nearly 20%. The authors of the report drew the conclusion that while taking all three drugs, the amiodarone levels had become slightly raised due to the enzyme inhibitory effects of the sertraline, despite the potential enzyme-inducing activity of the carbamazepine.[1] The patient had no changes in his cardiac status while amiodarone levels were reduced, suggesting that this interaction (if such it is) is of limited clinical importance.[1]

1. DeVane CL, Gill HS, Markowitz JS, Carson WH. Awareness of potential drug interactions may aid avoidance. *Ther Drug Monit* (1997) 19, 366–7.

Amiodarone + Trazodone

An isolated report describes the development of torsade de pointes when a woman taking amiodarone was also given trazodone.

Clinical evidence, mechanism, importance and management

A 74-year-old woman with a pacemaker, taking nifedipine, furosemide, aspirin and amiodarone 200 mg daily, began to have dizzy spells but no loss of consciousness soon after starting trazodone (initially 50 mg and eventually 150 mg daily by the end of 2 weeks). Both the amiodarone and trazodone were stopped when she was hospitalised. She had prolonged QT, QTc and JTc intervals on the ECG and recurrent episodes of torsade de pointes arrhythmia, which were controlled by increasing the ventricular pacing rate. The QTc and other ECG intervals shortened and she was later discharged on amiodarone without the trazodone, with an ECG similar to that seen 4 months before hospitalisation.[1] No general conclusions can be drawn from this apparent interaction, but prescribers should be aware of this case. The manufacturer notes that trazodone does have the potential to be arrhythmogenic.[2] See also, 'Drugs that prolong the QT interval + Other drugs that prolong the QT interval', p.257.

1. Mazur A, Strasberg B, Kusniec J, Sclarovsky S. QT prolongation and polymorphous ventricular tachycardia associated with trasodone-amiodarone combination. *Int J Cardiol* (1995) 52, 27–9.
2. Molipaxin (Trazodone hydrochloride). Sanofi-Aventis. UK Summary of product characteristics, July 2005.

Aprindine + Amiodarone

Serum aprindine levels can be increased by amiodarone. Toxicity may occur unless the dosage is reduced.

Clinical evidence, mechanism, importance and management

The serum aprindine levels of two patients rose, accompanied by signs of toxicity (nausea, ataxia, etc.), when they were also given amiodarone. One of them, taking aprindine 100 mg daily, had a progressive rise in trough serum levels from 2.3 to 3.5 mg/L over a 5-week period, when given 1.2 g and later 600 mg of amiodarone daily. Even when the aprindine dosage was reduced, serum levels remained higher than before amiodarone was started.[1] The authors say that those given both drugs generally need less aprindine than those on aprindine alone. This interaction has been briefly reported elsewhere.[2] Its mechanism is not understood. Monitor the effects of concurrent use and reduce the dosage of aprindine as necessary.

1. Southworth W, Friday KJ, Ruffy R. Possible amiodarone-aprindine interaction. *Am Heart J* (1982) 104, 323.
2. Zhang Z, Wang G, Wang H, Zhang J. Effect of amiodarone on the plasma concentration of aprindine [Abstract 115: 197745u in Chemical Abstracts (1991) 115, 22]. *Zhongguo Yao Xue Za Zhi* (1991) 26, 156–9.

Azimilide + Miscellaneous

There was no important pharmacokinetic interaction between azimilide and digoxin, and digoxin did not appreciably alter azimilide-induced QTc prolongation. Ketoconazole did not alter the pharmacokinetics of azimilide to a clinically relevant extent, and therefore other CYP3A4 inhibitors are also unlikely to affect azimilide pharmacokinetics. Azimilide did not alter the pharmacokinetics of omeprazole to a clinically relevant extent, and is therefore unlikely to interact with other substrates of CYP2C19.

***In vitro* studies suggest pharmacokinetic interactions between azimilide and drugs metabolised by CYP1A2, CYP2C9 and CYP2D6 are also unlikely. Azimilide was found to maintain its class III antiarrhythmic effect in the presence of isoprenaline.**

Clinical evidence, mechanism, importance and management

(a) Digoxin

A study in 18 healthy subjects found that, except for an increase in renal clearance of 36%, azimilide pharmacokinetics were not affected by digoxin. The pharmacokinetics of digoxin were unaffected by azimilide except for a 21% increase in maximum serum levels and a 10% increase in the AUC. In this study, azimilide dihydrochloride 175 mg was given orally once daily for 4 days then 100 mg on day 5 and digoxin was given as a loading dose of 750 micrograms on day one then as 250 micrograms daily for 4 days. Drugs were given alone, and then combined. Azimilide alone increased the QTc, whereas digoxin did not. The combination showed that digoxin caused about a 2 to 4% decrease in QTc when compared with azimilide alone. Neither the pharmacokinetic changes nor the effect of digoxin on the azimilide-induced QTc prolongation are likely to be clinically important.[1]

(b) Isoprenaline (Isoproterenol)

In a study, patients with cardiovascular disorders were given isoprenaline infusion titrated from 0.5 micrograms/minute up to a maximum of 4 micrograms/minute until the heart rate reached 125% of baseline (up to a maximum 120 bpm). Patients were then given azimilide infusion as a loading dose of 4.5 mg/kg over 15 minutes followed by a continuous infusion of 0.625 mg/kg per hour plus either a second dose of isoprenaline at the same final dose as the first then a saline infusion or *vice versa*. In the presence of isoprenaline, azimilide prolonged the action potential duration at 90% repolarisation by a mean of 8.7 milliseconds (isoprenaline alone shortened action potential duration by 2.6 milliseconds). Isoprenaline alone shortened the right ventricular effective period by 13.6 seconds, but in the presence of azimilide this period was essentially unaffected. Azimilide maintained its class III antiarrhythmic effect in the presence of isoprenaline and at increased heart rate.[2]

(c) Ketoconazole and other CYP3A4 inhibitors

In a randomised placebo-controlled study in 21 healthy subjects, ketoconazole 200 mg daily slightly increased the AUC and maximum blood levels of a single 125-mg dose of azimilide dihydrochloride given on day 8 by 16% and 12%, respectively. Azimilide half-life was prolonged by 13% and clearance was decreased by 14%. Azimilide is partly metabolised by the cytochrome P450 isoenzyme CYP3A4, which is inhibited by ketoconazole. The minor changes in azimilide pharmacokinetics with ketoconazole are not considered to be clinically important, and clinically significant pharmacokinetic interactions with other inhibitors of CYP3A4 are not expected.[3]

(d) Omeprazole

A randomised placebo-controlled study in 40 healthy subjects (extensive metabolisers of the cytochrome P450 isoenzyme CYP2C19) given azimilide dihydrochloride 125 mg every 12 hours for 3 days, then daily for 5 days found that the AUC of a single 20-mg dose of omeprazole given on day 8 was reduced by 12%. There were no significant changes in the pharmacokinetics of 5-hydroxyomeprazole. There was no change in the metabolite-to-parent AUC suggesting that azimilide had no effect on the CYP2C19-mediated metabolism of omeprazole.[4] The change in omeprazole AUC described would not be clinically significant.

The authors note that *in vitro* studies suggested that of the cytochrome P450 isoenzymes, azimilide had the lowest inhibitory concentration against CYP2C19. On this basis they suggest that azimilide is also unlikely to interact with drugs metabolised by CYP1A2, CYP2C9, CYP2D6 and CYP3A4.[4]

1. Toothaker RD, Corey AE, Valentine SN, Agnew JR, Parekh N, Moehrke W, Thompson GA, Powell JH. Influence of coadministration on the pharmacokinetics of azimilide dihydrochloride and digoxin. *J Clin Pharmacol* (2005) 45, 773–80.
2. Dorian P, Dunnmon P, Elstun L, Newman D. The effect of isoproterenol on the class III effect of azimilide in humans. *J Cardiovasc Pharmacol Ther* (2002) 7, 211–17.
3. El Mouelhi M, Worley DJ, Kuzmak B, Destefano AJ, Thompson GA. Influence of ketoconazole on azimilide pharmacokinetics in healthy subjects. *Br J Clin Pharmacol* (2004) 58, 641–7.
4. El Mouelhi M, Worley DJ, Kuzmak B, Destefano AJ, Thompson GA. Influence of azimilide on CYP2C19-mediated metabolism. *J Clin Pharmacol* (2004) 44, 373–8.

Bretylium + Sympathomimetics

The pressor effects of adrenaline (epinephrine) and noradrenaline (norepinephrine) are increased in the presence of bretylium. Amfetamine and protriptyline antagonise the blood pressure lowering effect of bretylium.

Clinical evidence

(a) Adrenaline (epinephrine) or Noradrenaline (norepinephrine)

A dose of bretylium sufficient to produce postural hypotension enhanced the pressor effect of noradrenaline in 4 healthy subjects. A similar effect was found with adrenaline.[1]

(b) Amfetamine

When 7 patients with hypertension, taking bretylium 600 mg to 4 g daily were given a single 25-mg dose of amphetamine, 6 patients had a rise in blood pressure.[2]

(c) Protriptyline

An experimental study found that protriptyline can return the blood pressure to normal in patients taking bretylium, without reducing its antiarrhythmic efficacy.[3]

Mechanism

Animal studies have shown that bretylium reduces blood pressure via its blocking effects on adrenergic neurones similar to guanethidine.[4,5] Bretylium therefore enhances the effects of directly-acting sympathomimetics such as noradrenaline, and is antagonised by drugs with indirect sympathomimetic activity such as the amfetamines and tricyclic antidepressants.

Importance and management

Although documentation is limited, based on the known pharmacology of bretylium, these interactions would appear to be established. The use of bretylium is now limited to the short-term control of ventricular arrhythmias. In this situation, if directly-acting sympathomimetics such as noradrenaline are required to reverse bretylium-induced hypotension, this should be undertaken with caution since their effects may be enhanced.

Bretylium is no longer used for the treatment of hypertension, therefore the interactions with amfetamines and tricyclics described above are unlikely to be of much clinical relevance.

1. Laurence DR, Nagle RE. The interaction of bretylium with pressor agents. *Lancet* (1961) i, 593–4.
2. Wilson R, Long C. Action of bretylium antagonised by amphetamine. *Lancet* (1960) ii, 262.
3. Woosley RL, Reele SB, Roden DM, Nies AS, Oates JA. Pharmacological reversal of hypotensive effect complicating antiarrhythmic therapy with bretylium. *Clin Pharmacol Ther* (1982) 32, 313–21.
4. Day MD. Effect of sympathomimetic amines on the blocking action of guanethidine, bretylium and xylocholine. *Br J Pharmacol* (1962) 18, 421–39.
5. Boura ALA, Green AF. Comparison of bretylium and guanethidine: tolerance and effects on adrenergic nerve function and responses to sympathomimetic amines. *Br J Pharmacol* (1962) 19, 13–41.

Cibenzoline (Cifenline) + H_2-receptor antagonists

Cimetidine increases the plasma levels of cibenzoline, but ranitidine does not interact.

Clinical evidence, mechanism, importance and management

Cimetidine 1.2 g daily raised the maximum plasma levels of a single 160-mg dose of cibenzoline in 12 healthy subjects by 27%, increased the AUC by 44%, and prolonged its half-life by 30%. **Ranitidine** 300 mg daily had no effect.[1] The probable reason is that **cimetidine**, an enzyme inhibitor, reduces the metabolism of the cibenzoline by the liver, whereas **ranitidine**, which has little enzyme inhibiting effects, does not. The clinical importance of this interaction is not known but be alert for increased cibenzoline effects.

1. Massarella JW, Defeo TM, Liguori J, Passe S, Aogaichi K. The effects of cimetidine and ranitidine on the pharmacokinetics of cifenline. *Br J Clin Pharmacol* (1991) 31, 481–3.

Disopyramide + Antacids

There is some inconclusive evidence that aluminium phosphate may possibly cause a small reduction in the absorption of disopyramide.

Clinical evidence, mechanism, importance and management

A single 11-g dose of an **aluminium phosphate** antacid had no statistically significant effect on the pharmacokinetics of a single 200-mg oral dose of disopyramide in 10 patients. However the antacid appeared to reduce the absorption of disopyramide to some extent in individual subjects.[1] The clinical importance of this interaction is uncertain, but probably small.

1. Albin H, Vincon G, Bertolaso D, Dangoumau J. Influence du phosphate d'aluminium sur la biodisponibilité de la procaïnamide et du disopyramide. *Therapie* (1981) 36, 541–6.

Disopyramide + Beta blockers

Severe bradycardia has been described after the use of disopyramide with beta blockers including practolol (3 cases, 1 fatal) pindolol (1 case, fatal) and metoprolol (1 case). Another patient given disopyramide and intravenous sotalol developed asystole (see also 'Drugs that prolong the QT interval + Other drugs that prolong the QT interval', p.257). Atenolol modestly decreased disopyramide clearance in one study. Oral propranolol and disopyramide have been combined without any increase in negative inotropic effects or pharmacokinetic changes in healthy subjects.

Clinical evidence

Two patients with supraventricular tachycardia (180 bpm) were treated, firstly with intravenous **practolol** (20 and 10 mg respectively) and shortly afterwards with disopyramide (150 and 80 mg respectively). The first patient rapidly developed sinus bradycardia of 25 bpm, lost consciousness and became profoundly hypotensive. He did not respond to 600 micrograms of atropine, but later his heart rate increased to 60 bpm while a temporary pacemaker was being inserted.[1] He was successfully treated with disopyramide 150 mg alone for a later episode of tachycardia. The second patient also developed severe bradycardia and asystole, despite the use of atropine. He was resuscitated with adrenaline (epinephrine) but later died.[1]

Severe bradycardia has been reported in another patient, similarly treated with intravenous **practolol** and then disopyramide.[2] Another patient developed severe bradycardia and died when treated for supraventricular tachycardia with **pindolol** 5 mg and disopyramide 250 mg (both orally).[3] Another patient taking oral disopyramide 250 mg twice daily developed asystole when given a total of 60 mg of intravenous **sotalol**.[4]

A patient with hypertrophic obstructive cardiomyopathy and paroxysmal atrial fibrillation taking disopyramide 450 mg daily developed hypotension, bradycardia and cardiac conduction disturbances 5 days after starting **metoprolol** 50 mg daily.[5]

Atenolol 100 mg daily has been shown to increase the serum disopyramide steady-state levels from 3.46 to 4.25 micrograms/mL and reduce the clearance of disopyramide by 16% in healthy subjects and patients with ischaemic heart disease.[6] None of the subjects developed any adverse reactions or symptoms of heart failure, apart from one of the subjects who had transient first degree heart block.[6]

In contrast, studies in healthy subjects have shown that the negative inotropic effect was no greater when oral **propranolol** and disopyramide were used concurrently,[7] nor were the pharmacokinetics of either drug affected.[8]

Mechanism

Not understood. Both disopyramide and the beta blockers can depress the contractility and conductivity of the heart muscle.

Importance and management

The general clinical importance of this interaction is uncertain. A clear risk seemed to exist in patients who were treated with disopyramide and practolol. Considerable caution should be exercised in patients treated with disopyramide and intravenous sotalol. More study is needed to find out what contributes to the development of this potentially serious interaction. The US manufacturers of disopyramide suggest that the combination of disopyramide and beta blockers should generally be avoided, except in the case of life-threatening arrhythmias unresponsive to a single drug.[9]

The UK manufacturer of sotalol also warns that both sotalol and disopyramide can prolong the QT interval, which may increase the risk of torsade de pointes arrhythmia if both are used together.[10] The US manufacturer recommends that this combination should be avoided.[11] See also 'Drugs that prolong the QT interval + Other drugs that prolong the QT interval', p.257.

1. Cumming AD, Robertson C. Interaction between disopyramide and practolol. *BMJ* (1979) 2, 1264.
2. Gelipter D, Hazell M. Interaction between disopyramide and practolol. *BMJ* (1980) 1, 52.
3. Pedersen C, Josephsen P, Lindvig K. Interaktion mellem disopyramid og pindolol efter oral indgift. *Ugeskr Laeger* (1983) 145, 3266.
4. Bystedt T, Vitols S. Sotalol-disopyramid ledde till asystoli. *Lakartidningen* (1994) 91, 2241.
5. Pernat A, Pohar B, Horvat M. Heart conduction disturbances and cardiovascular collapse after disopyramide and low-dose metoprolol in a patient with hypertrophic obstructive cardiomyopathy. *J Electrocardiol* (1997) 30, 341–4.
6. Bonde J, Bødtker S, Angelo HR, Svendsen TL, Kampmann JP. Atenolol inhibits the elimination of disopyramide. *Eur J Clin Pharmacol* (1986) 28, 41–3.
7. Cathcart-Rake WF, Coker JE, Atkins FL, Huffman DH, Hassanein KM, Shen DD, Azarnoff DL. The effect of concurrent oral administration of propranolol and disopyramide on cardiac function in healthy men. *Circulation* (1980) 61, 938–45.
8. Karim A, Nissen C, Azarnoff DL. Clinical pharmacokinetics of disopyramide. *J Pharmacokinet Biopharm* (1982) 10, 465–94.
9. Norpace (Disopyramide). Pharmacia. US Prescribing information, September 2001.
10. Beta-Cardone (Sotalol). Celltech Pharmaceuticals Ltd. UK Summary of product characteristics, June 2005.
11. Betapace (Sotalol). Berlex Laboratories. US Prescribing information, January 2004.

Disopyramide + H_2-receptor antagonists

A single-dose study has shown that cimetidine can slightly increase the serum levels of oral disopyramide. Cimetidine did not affect the pharmacokinetics of intravenous disopyramide. Ranitidine appears not to interact with disopyramide.

Clinical evidence, mechanism, importance and management

Oral cimetidine 400 mg twice daily for 14 days did not alter the pharmacokinetics of a single 150-mg intravenous dose of disopyramide in 7 healthy subjects.[1] Another study in 6 healthy subjects found that a single 400-mg dose of **cimetidine** increased the AUC of a single 300-mg oral dose of disopyramide by 8.5% and increased the maximum serum levels by 18.5%, but did not significantly affect the metabolism of disopyramide. **Ranitidine** 150 mg was found not to interact significantly.[2] The reasons are not known, but the authors of the report suggest that **cimetidine** may have increased disopyramide absorption.[2] **Cimetidine** is only a weak inhibitor of disopyramide metabolism *in vitro*.[3] The changes described are unlikely to be clinically important, but this should probably be confirmed in a more clinically realistic situation, using multiple oral doses of both drugs.

1. Bonde J, Pedersen LE, Nygaard E, Ramsing T, Angelo HR, Kampmann JP. Stereoselective pharmacokinetics of disopyramide and interaction with cimetidine. *Br J Clin Pharmacol* (1991) 31, 708–10.
2. Jou M-J, Huang S-C, Kiang F-M, Lai M-Y, Chao P-DL. Comparison of the effects of cimetidine and ranitidine on the pharmacokinetics of disopyramide in man. *J Pharm Pharmacol* (1997) 49, 1072–5.
3. Echuzen H, Kawasaki H, Chiba K, Tani M. Ishizaki T. A potent inhibitory effect of erythromycin and other macrolide antibiotics on the mono-N-dealkylation metabolism of disopyramide with human liver microsomes. *J Pharmacol Exp Ther* (1993) 264, 1425–31.

Disopyramide + Macrolides

The serum disopyramide levels of two patients rose when they were given erythromycin, and QT prolongation and cardiac arrhythmias developed. Another patient given both drugs developed heart block. One patient developed ventricular fibrillation and two patients developed torsade de pointes when given clarithromycin with disopyramide. Two other patients developed severe hypoglycaemia. Ventricular fibrillation occurred in a patient given azithromycin with disopyramide. See also 'Drugs that prolong the QT interval + Other drugs that prolong the QT interval', p.257.

Clinical evidence

(a) Azithromycin

A patient taking disopyramide 150 mg three times daily developed ventricular tachycardia requiring cardioversion 11 days after starting azithromycin 250 mg daily.[1] Her disopyramide level was found to have risen from 2.6 to 11.1 micrograms/mL.

(b) Clarithromycin

A 74-year-old woman who had been taking disopyramide 200 mg twice daily for 7 years collapsed with ventricular fibrillation 6 days after starting to take omeprazole 40 mg, metronidazole 800 mg and clarithromycin 500 mg daily. After successful resuscitation, her QTc interval, which had never previously been above 440 milliseconds, was found to have risen to 625 milliseconds. Her disopyramide plasma level was also elevated (4.6 micrograms/mL) and the half-life was markedly prolonged (40 hours). The QTc interval normalised as her plasma disopyramide levels fell.[2] A 76-year old woman taking disopyramide developed torsades de pointes when given clarithromycin 200 mg twice daily. Hypokalaemia (potassium 2.8 mmol/L) probably contributed to this case.[3]

An episode of torsade de pointes occurred in another elderly woman taking disopyramide 5 days after starting clarithromycin 250 mg twice daily.[4]

A haemodialysis patient, receiving disopyramide 50 mg daily because of paroxysmal atrial fibrillation, was hospitalised with hypoglycaemic coma after also taking clarithromycin 600 mg daily. Serum disopyramide levels increased from 1.5 to 8 micrograms/mL during treatment with clarithromycin. QT and QTc intervals were prolonged, but torsade de pointes did not occur.[5] Hypoglycaemic coma has also been reported in another patient taking disopyramide with clarithromycin.[6]

(c) Erythromycin

A woman with ventricular ectopy taking disopyramide (300 mg alternating with 150 mg every 6 hours) developed new arrhythmias (ventricular asystoles and later torsade de pointes) within 36 hours of starting erythromycin lactobionate 1 g intravenously every 6 hours, and cefamandole. Her QTc interval had increased from 390 to 600 milliseconds and her serum disopyramide level was found to be 16 micromol/L. The problem resolved when the disopyramide was stopped and bretylium given, but it returned when the disopyramide was restarted. It resolved again when the erythromycin was stopped.[7] Another patient with ventricular tachycardia, well controlled over 5 years with disopyramide 200 mg four times daily, developed polymorphic ventricular tachycardia within a few days of starting erythromycin 500 mg four times daily. His QTc interval had increased from 430 to 630 milliseconds and serum disopyramide levels were found to be elevated at 30 micromol/L. The problem resolved when both drugs were withdrawn and antiarrhythmics given.[7] Heart block is said to have developed in another patient treated with both drugs.[8]

Mechanism

Not fully established. An *in vitro* study using human liver microsomes indicated that erythromycin inhibits the metabolism (mono-*N*-dealkylation) of disopyramide which, *in vivo*, would be expected to reduce its loss from the body and increase its serum levels.[9] Clarithromycin and azithromycin probably do the same. The increased serum levels of disopyramide can result in adverse effects such as QT prolongation and torsade de pointes, and may result in enhanced insulin secretion and hypoglycaemia.[5,6] Both intravenous erythromycin[10] and clarithromycin[11] alone have been associated with prolongation of the QT interval and torsade de pointes. Therefore, disopyramide and macrolides may have additive effects on the QT interval in addition to the pharmacokinetic interaction.

Importance and management

An established interaction, although it is probably rare. Even so the effects of concurrent use should be well monitored if azithromycin, clarithromycin or erythromycin is added to disopyramide, being alert for the development of raised plasma disopyramide levels and prolongation of the QT interval. The manufacturer of disopyramide recommends[12] avoiding the combination of disopyramide and macrolides that inhibit the cytochrome P450 isoenzyme CYP3A, and this would certainly be prudent in situations where close monitoring is not possible. Although direct clinical information is lacking, *in vitro* studies with human liver microsomes[9] indicate that **josamycin** is likely to interact similarly, and **telithromycin** (an erythromycin derivative) might also be expected to interact in the same way. See also 'Drugs that prolong the QT interval + Other drugs that prolong the QT interval', p.257.

1. Granowitz EV, Tabor KJ, Kirchhoffer JB. Potentially fatal interaction between azithromycin and disopyramide. *Pacing Clin Electrophysiol* (2000) 23, 1433–5.
2. Paar D, Terjung B, Sauerbruch T. Life-threatening interaction between clarithromycin and disopyramide. *Lancet* (1997) 349, 326–7.
3. Hayashi Y, Ikeda U, Hashimoto T, Watanabe T, Mitsuhashi T, Shimada K. Torsade de pointes ventricular tachycardia induced by clarithromycin and disopyramide in the presence of hypokalaemia. *Pacing Clin Electrophysiol* (1999) 22, 672–4.
4. Choudhury L, Grais IM, Passman RS. Torsade de pointes due to drug interaction between disopyramide and clarithromycin. *Heart Dis* (1999) 1, 206–7.
5. Iida H, Morita T, Suzuki E, Iwasawa K, Toyo-oka T, Nakajima T. Hypoglycemia induced by interaction between clarithromycin and disopyramide. *Jpn Heart J* (1999) 40, 91–6.
6. Morlet-Barla N, Narbonne H, Vialettes B. Hypoglycémie grave et récidivante secondaire á l'interaction disopyramide-clarithromicine. *Presse Med* (2000) 29, 1351.
7. Ragosta M, Weihl AC, Rosenfeld LE. Potentially fatal interaction between erythromycin and disopyramide. *Am J Med* (1989) 86, 465–6.
8. Beeley L, Cunningham H, Carmichael A, Brennan A. *Bulletin of the West Midlands Centre for Adverse Drug Reaction Reporting* (1992) 35, 13.
9. Echizen H, Kawasaki H, Chiba K, Tani M. Ishizaki T. A potent inhibitory effect of erythromycin and other macrolide antibiotics on the mono-N-dealkylation metabolism of disopyramide with human liver microsomes. *J Pharmacol Exp Ther* (1993) 264, 1425–31.
10. Gitler B, Berger LS, Buffa SD. Torsades de pointes induced by erythromycin. *Chest* (1994) 105, 368–72.
11. Lee KL, Jim M-H, Tang SC, Tai Y-T. QT-prolongation and torsades de pointes associated with clarithromycin. *Am J Med* (1998) 104, 395–6.
12. Rythmodan Capsules (Disopyramide). Sanofi-Aventis. UK Summary of product characteristics, November 2005.

Disopyramide + Phenobarbital

Serum disopyramide levels are reduced by phenobarbital.

Clinical evidence

After taking phenobarbital 100 mg daily for 21 days, the half-life and AUC of a single 200-mg dose of disopyramide were reduced by about 35%. The apparent metabolic clearance more than doubled, and the fraction recovered in the urine as metabolite increased. Sixteen healthy subjects took part in the study and no significant differences were seen between those who smoked and those who did not.[1]

Mechanism

It seems probable that phenobarbital (a known enzyme inducer) increases the metabolism of disopyramide by the liver, and thereby increases its loss from the body.

Importance and management

This interaction appears to be established, but its clinical importance is uncertain. The extent to which it would reduce the control of arrhythmias by disopyramide is unknown, but monitor the effects and the serum levels of disopyramide if phenobarbital is added or withdrawn. The manufacturer of disopyramide[2] recommends avoiding using it in combination with inducers of the cytochrome P450 isoenzyme CYP3A, such as phenobarbital. Other barbiturates would be expected to interact similarly.

1. Kapil RP, Axelson JE, Mansfield IL, Edwards DJ, McErlane B, Mason MA, Lalka D, Kerr CR. Disopyramide pharmacokinetics and metabolism: effect of inducers. *Br J Clin Pharmacol* (1987) 24, 781–91.
2. Rythmodan Capsules (Disopyramide). Sanofi-Aventis. UK Summary of product characteristics, November 2005.

Disopyramide + Phenytoin

Serum disopyramide levels are reduced by phenytoin and may fall below therapeutic levels. Loss of arrhythmic control may occur.

Clinical evidence

Eight patients with ventricular tachycardia treated with disopyramide 600 mg to 2 g daily had a 54% fall in their serum disopyramide levels (from a mean of 3.99 to 1.82 micrograms/mL) when they were also given phenytoin 200 to 600 mg daily for a week. Two of the patients who responded to disopyramide and underwent Holter monitoring showed a 53- and 2000-fold increase in ventricular premature beat frequency as a result of this interaction.[1]

In other reports, 3 patients who had low levels of disopyramide and high levels of its metabolite were noted to be taking phenytoin,[2] and one patient receiving both drugs required an unusually high dose of disopyramide.[3] A marked fall in serum disopyramide levels (75% in one case) was seen in 2 patients who took phenytoin 300 to 400 mg daily for up to 2 weeks.[4] Pharmacokinetic studies[3,5] in a total of 12 healthy subjects confirm this interaction. In addition, one healthy epileptic taking phenytoin had a disopyramide AUC and elimination half-life that were 50% lower than those in control subjects.[5]

Mechanism

Phenytoin, which is a known enzyme-inducer, increases the metabolism of the disopyramide by the liver. Although, the major metabolite (*N*-dealkyldisopyramide) also possesses antiarrhythmic activity the net effect is a reduction in arrhythmic control.[1]

Importance and management

An established interaction of clinical importance. Some loss of arrhythmic control can occur during concurrent use. Disopyramide adverse effects (because of the potential for high metabolite levels) and the antiarrhythmic response should be well monitored. An increase in the dosage of disopyramide may be necessary. The interaction appears to resolve fully within 2 weeks of withdrawing the phenytoin. Note that the manufacturer of disopyramide[6] recommends avoiding using it in combination with inducers of the cytochrome P450 isoenzyme CYP3A, such as phenytoin.

1. Matos JA, Fisher JD, Kim SG. Disopyramide-phenytoin interaction. *Clin Res* (1981) 29, 655A.
2. Aitio M-L, Vuorenmaa T. Enhanced metabolism and diminished efficacy of disopyramide by enzyme induction? *Br J Clin Pharmacol* (1980) 9, 149–152.
3. Nightingale J, Nappi JM. Effect of phenytoin on serum disopyramide concentrations. *Clin Pharm* (1987) 6, 46–50.
4. Kessler JM, Keys PW, Stafford RW. Disopyramide and phenytoin interaction. *Clin Pharm* (1982) 1, 263–4.
5. Aitio M-L, Mansury L, Tala E, Haataja M, Aitio A. The effect of enzyme induction on the metabolism of disopyramide in man. *Br J Clin Pharmacol* (1981) 11, 279–85.
6. Rythmodan Capsules (Disopyramide). Sanofi-Aventis. UK Summary of product characteristics, November 2005.

Disopyramide + Quinidine

Disopyramide serum levels may be slightly raised by quinidine. Both drugs prolong the QT interval, and this effect may be additive on combined use.

Clinical evidence, mechanism, importance and management

After taking quinidine 200 mg four times daily, the peak serum levels of disopyramide, given as a single 150-mg dose to 16 healthy subjects, were raised by 20% from 2.68 to 3.23 micrograms/mL, and by 14% when given long-term, as 150 mg four times a day. Serum quinidine levels were decreased by 26%. However, there was no change in the half-life of either drug. Both quinidine and disopyramide caused a slight lengthening of the QTc interval, and when quinidine was added to disopyramide therapy additional lengthening of the QT interval occurred. The frequency of adverse effects such as dry mouth, blurred vision, urinary retention and nausea were also somewhat increased.[1] The mechanism of the effect on serum levels is not understood. The antimuscarinic adverse effects of disopyramide may be increased. Disopyramide and quinidine are both class Ia antiarrhythmics that prolong the QT interval, and, in general, such combinations should be avoided (see also 'Drugs that prolong the QT interval + Other drugs that prolong the QT interval', p.257).

1. Baker BJ, Gammill J, Massengill J, Schubert E, Karin A, Doherty JE. Concurrent use of quinidine and disopyramide: evaluation of serum concentrations and electrocardiographic effects. *Am Heart J* (1983) 105, 12–15.

Disopyramide + Rifampicin (Rifampin)

The plasma levels of disopyramide can be reduced by rifampicin.

Clinical evidence

After taking rifampicin for 14 days the plasma levels of disopyramide were approximately halved in 11 patients with tuberculosis who had taken a single 200- or 300-mg dose of disopyramide.[1] The disopyramide AUC was reduced by about two-thirds and the half-life was reduced from 5.9 to 3.25 hours by rifampicin. A woman who had been receiving rifampicin for 2 weeks started taking disopyramide 100 mg every 8 hours but only achieved subtherapeutic levels of 0.9 micromol/L. The dosage of disopyramide was increased to 300 mg every 8 hours, and the rifampicin was discontinued. Three days after discontinuing rifampicin the disopyramide level was 3.6 micromol/L and after 5 days it was 8.1 micromol/L. The patient was eventually maintained on disopyramide 250 mg every 8 hours.[2]

Mechanism

The most probable explanation is that rifampicin (a well-known enzyme inducer) increases the metabolism of the disopyramide by the liver so that it is cleared from the body much more quickly.

Importance and management

Information seems to be limited to these studies, but they indicate that the dosage of disopyramide will need to be increased in most patients taking rifampicin.

1. Aitio M-L, Mansury L, Tala E, Haataja M, Aitio A. The effect of enzyme induction on the metabolism of disopyramide in man. *Br J Clin Pharmacol* (1981) 11, 279–85.
2. Staum JM. Enzyme induction: rifampin-disopyramide interaction. *DICP Ann Pharmacother* (1990) 24, 701–3.

Disopyramide + Verapamil

Profound hypotension and collapse has occurred in a small number of patients taking verapamil who were also given disopyramide.

Clinical evidence, mechanism, importance and management

A group of clinicians who had used single 400-mg oral doses of disopyramide successfully and with few adverse effects for reverting acute supraventricular arrhythmias, reported 5 cases of profound hypotension and collapse. Three of the patients developed severe epigastric pain. All 5 had previous myocardial disease and/or were taking myocardial depressants, either beta blockers or verapamil in small quantities [not specified].[1]

On the basis of this report, and on reports of studies in *animals*,[2] and from the known risks associated with the concurrent use of beta blockers (see 'Disopyramide + Beta blockers', p.252), the UK manufacturer warns about combining disopyramide and other drugs [such as verapamil] that may have additive negative inotropic effects.[3] However, they do point out that in some specific circumstances combinations of antiarrhythmic drugs (they specifically name digoxin, beta blockers and verapamil for the control of atrial fibrillation) may be beneficial.[3] They note that severe hypotension caused by disopyramide has usually been associated with cardiomyopathy or uncompensated congestive heart failure.[3] However, the US manufacturer advises that until more data is available, disopyramide should not be given within 48 hours before or 24 hours after verapamil.[4]

1. Manolas EG, Hunt D, Dowling JT, Luxton M, Vohra J. Collapse after oral administration of disopyramide. *Med J Aust* (1979) 1, 20.
2. Lee JT, Davy J-M, Kates RE. Evaluation of combined administration of verapamil and disopyramide in dogs. *J Cardiovasc Pharmacol* (1985) 7, 501–7.
3. Rythmodan Capsules (Disopyramide). Sanofi-Aventis. UK Summary of product characteristics, November 2005.
4. Norpace (Disopyramide). Pharmacia. US Prescribing information, September 2001.

Dofetilide + Antacids

Antacids (aluminium/magnesium hydroxide) appear not to interact with dofetilide.

Clinical evidence, mechanism, importance and management

A study in 12 healthy subjects found that pretreatment with **aluminium/magnesium hydroxide** *(Maalox)* 30 mL (10, 2 and 0.5 hours before dofetilide) did not affect the pharmacokinetics of a single 500-microgram dose of dofetilide, nor the dofetilide-induced change in QTc interval.[1] No special precautions appear to be necessary.

1. Vincent J, Gardner MJ, Baris B, Willavize SA. Concurrent administration of omeprazole and antacid does not alter the pharmacokinetics and pharmacodynamic of dofetilide in healthy subjects. *Clin Pharmacol Ther* (1996) 59, 182.

Dofetilide + Diuretics

Hydrochlorothiazide and hydrochlorothiazide/triamterene modestly increased dofetilide plasma levels, and caused a marked increase in the QT interval.

Clinical evidence

The manufacturer notes that the concurrent use of dofetilide 500 micrograms twice daily with **hydrochlorothiazide** 50 mg daily for 7 days increased the dofetilide AUC by 14% and increased the QTc interval by 47.6 milliseconds.[1] Similar results were seen with the same dose of dofetilide combined with **hydrochlorothiazide/triamterene** 50/100 mg daily (18% increase in AUC, and 38.1 millisecond increase in QTc).[1]

Mechanism

Triamterene might be expected to increase dofetilide plasma levels by competing for its renal tubular secretion (see 'Dofetilide + Miscellaneous', p.255), but the effect of its combination with hydrochlorothiazide was no greater than with hydrochlorothiazide alone. Why hydrochlorothiazide should increase dofetilide levels is unclear. An increase in dofetilide levels would be expected to increase the QT interval, but the increase seen here was much greater than expected by the change in plasma levels. The manufacturer suggests that a reduction in serum potassium could have contributed to the extent of QT prolongation.[1] This makes sense for hydrochlorothiazide (a potassium-depleting diuretic), but the combination with triamterene (a potassium-sparing diuretic) might therefore have been expected to have less effect on the QT interval.

Importance and management

On the basis of the above findings, the manufacturer contraindicates the use of dofetilide with **hydrochlorothiazide** alone or in combination with **triamterene**.[2] Given the increase in QT interval, a risk factor for torsade de pointes arrhythmia, this appears a prudent precaution. Further study is needed. Any diuretic that depletes serum potassium (such as the **loop diuretics**) might be expected to increase the risk of QT prolongation and torsade de pointes with dofetilide, and serum potassium should be monitored.[2]

1. Pfizer Global Pharmaceuticals. Personal Communication, June 2004.
2. Tikosyn (Dofetilide). Pfizer Labs. US Prescribing information, March 2004.

Dofetilide + H_2-receptor antagonists

Cimetidine markedly increases plasma dofetilide levels, and hence increases dofetilide-induced QT prolongation and the risk of torsade de pointes arrhythmias. Its combined use with dofetilide should be avoided. Dofetilide appears not to interact with ranitidine.

Clinical evidence

A placebo-controlled study in 24 healthy subjects indicated that **cimetidine** 400 mg twice daily given with dofetilide 500 micrograms twice daily for 7 days significantly decreased the renal clearance of dofetilide by 44%, increased its AUC by 58%, and increased its peak blood levels by 50%, without significantly altering the QTc interval.[1] In a further study it was found that **cimetidine** 100 mg twice daily (non-prescription dose) or 400 mg twice daily (a common prescription dose) for 4 days reduced the renal clearance of a single 500-microgram dose of dofetilide by 13 and 33%, respectively. In addition, the respective **cimetidine** doses increased the QTc interval by 22 and 33%. Conversely, **ranitidine** 150 mg twice daily did not significantly affect the pharmacokinetics or pharmacodynamics of dofetilide.[2]

Mechanism

At least 50% of a dofetilide dose is eliminated unchanged in the urine by an active renal tubular secretion mechanism.[3,4] Drugs that inhibit this mechanism, such as cimetidine, increase dofetilide plasma levels.[2,3] There is a linear relationship between plasma dofetilide concentrations and prolongation of the QT interval, which increases the risk of torsade de pointes arrhythmias.[3]

Importance and management

An established interaction. Because of the likely increased risk of torsade de pointes, the manufacturer contraindicates the use of cimetidine in patients on dofetilide. This would seem to be a prudent precaution. This applies equally to cimetidine at over-the-counter doses, and patients on dofetilide should be warned to avoid this. No special precautions appear to be necessary with ranitidine. Note that 'omeprazole', (p.256) and 'antacids', (p.254) also appear not to interact with dofetilide.

1. Vincent J, Gardner MJ, Apseloff G, Baris B, Willavize S, Friedman HL. Cimetidine inhibits renal elimination of dofetilide without altering QTc activity on multiple dosing in healthy subjects. *Clin Pharmacol Ther* (1998) 63, 210.
2. Abel S, Nichols DJ, Brearly CJ, Eve MD. Effect of cimetidine and ranitidine on pharmacokinetics and pharmacodynamics of a single dose of dofetilide. *Br J Clin Pharmacol* (2000) 49, 64–71.
3. Tikosyn (Dofetilide). Pfizer Labs. US Prescribing information, March 2004.
4. Rasmussen HS, Allen MJ, Blackburn KJ, Butrous GS, Dalrymple HW. Dofetilide, a novel class III antiarrhythmic agent. *J Cardiovasc Pharmacol* (1992) 20 (Suppl 2), S96–S105.

Dofetilide + Ketoconazole

Ketoconazole markedly increases the plasma levels of dofetilide. This is likely to be associated with an increased risk of dofetilide-induced QT prolongation and torsade de pointes arrhythmias.

Clinical evidence

The manufacturer of dofetilide notes that ketoconazole 400 mg daily, given with dofetilide 500 micrograms twice daily for 7 days, increased the dofetilide peak levels by 53% in men and 97% in women, and the AUC by 41% in men and 69% in women.[1] Ketoconazole decreased the renal clearance of dofetilide by 31.3% and the non-renal clearance by 40.3%, resulting in a reduction in total clearance of 34.7%.[2]

Mechanism

Ketoconazole may inhibit the active renal tubular secretion mechanism by which dofetilide is eliminated, so reducing its loss from the body (see also 'Dofetilide + H_2-receptor antagonists', above).[1,2] Ketoconazole also inhibits the metabolism of dofetilide[2] by the cytochrome P450 isoenzyme CYP3A4. Both of these mechanisms contribute to the increase in dofetilide plasma levels. There is a linear relationship between plasma dofetilide concentrations and prolongation of the QT interval, which increases the risk for torsade de pointes.[1]

Importance and management

An established interaction. Because of the likely increased risk of torsade de pointes, the manufacturer contraindicates the use of ketoconazole in patients on dofetilide. This would seem to be a prudent precaution.

1. Tikosyn (Dofetilide). Pfizer Labs. US Prescribing information, March 2004.
2. Tikosyn (Dofetilide). Pfizer US Pharmaceuticals. Product monograph, March 2002. Available at http://www.tikosyn.com/pdf/prodmonograph.pdf (accessed 17/08/07).

Dofetilide + Miscellaneous

The manufacturer of dofetilide cautions about the use of various drugs that may have the potential to increase dofetilide plasma levels, so increasing the risk of QT prolongation and arrhythmias. Use with other drugs that prolong the QT interval should be avoided.

Clinical evidence, mechanism, importance and management

(a) Inhibitors/substrates for renal secretion

At least 50% of a dofetilide dose is eliminated unchanged in the urine by an active renal tubular secretion mechanism.[1,2] Some drugs that inhibit this mechanism have been shown to increase dofetilide plasma levels (e.g. see 'Dofetilide + H_2-receptor antagonists', above). The manufacturer contraindicates their concurrent use since there is a linear relationship between plasma dofetilide concentrations and prolongation of the QT interval, which is a risk factor for torsade de pointes arrhythmias.[1] The manufacturer also contraindicates the use of other drugs that inhibit the renal mechanism by which dofetilide is eliminated, such as **prochlorperazine** and **megestrol**,[1] although these have not been directly studied. Furthermore, the manufacturer suggests[1] that there is a potential for dofetilide plasma levels to be increased by other drugs undergoing active renal secretion (e.g. **amiloride, metformin** and **triamterene**), but this needs confirmation in direct studies (see also 'Dofetilide + Diuretics', p.255). Until then, these drugs should be used cautiously with dofetilide.

(b) Inhibitors of hepatic metabolism

Dofetilide is partially metabolised by the liver, primarily by the cytochrome P450 isoenzyme CYP3A4.[3] The manufacturer suggests[1] that there is a potential for dofetilide plasma levels to be increased by inhibitors of CYP3A4, and this has been shown for 'ketoconazole', (p.255). They recommend caution with other CYP3A4 inhibitors.

(c) Other drugs that prolong the QT interval

Dofetilide is a class III antiarrhythmic that prolongs the QT interval and can cause torsade de pointes arrhythmia. In general, use of two or more drugs that prolong the QT interval should be avoided. See also 'Drugs that prolong the QT interval + Other drugs that prolong the QT interval', p.257.

1. Tikosyn (Dofetilide). Pfizer Labs. US prescribing information, March 2004.
2. Rasmussen HS, Allen MJ, Blackburn KJ, Butrous GS, Dalrymple HW. Dofetilide, a novel class III antiarrhythmic agent. *J Cardiovasc Pharmacol* (1992) 20 (Suppl 2), S96–S105.
3. Walker DK, Alabaster CT, Congrave GS, Hargreaves MB, Hyland R, Jones BC, Reed LJ, Smith DA. Significance of metabolism in the disposition and action of the antidysrhythmic drug, dofetilide. *In vitro* studies and correlation with *in vivo* data. *Drug Metab Dispos* (1996) 24, 447–55.

Dofetilide + Omeprazole

Omeprazole appears not to interact with dofetilide.

Clinical evidence, mechanism, importance and management

A study in 12 healthy subjects found that pretreatment with omeprazole 40 mg (10 or 2 hours before dofetilide) did not affect the pharmacokinetics of a single 500-microgram dose of dofetilide nor the dofetilide-induced change in QTc interval.[1] No special precautions appear to be necessary.

1. Vincent J, Gardner MJ, Baris B, Willavize SA. Concurrent administration of omeprazole and antacid does not alter the pharmacokinetics and pharmacodynamic of dofetilide in healthy subjects. *Clin Pharmacol Ther* (1996) 59, 182.

Dofetilide + Phenytoin

There does not appear to be any interaction between dofetilide and phenytoin.

Clinical evidence, mechanism, importance and management

In one study, 24 healthy subjects were stabilised on phenytoin to achieve steady-state plasma levels of 8 to 20 micrograms/mL and then either dofetilide 500 micrograms twice daily or placebo was given. No changes in phenytoin pharmacokinetics or cardiac effects were seen.[1] Another study by the same researchers in 24 subjects given dofetilide 500 micrograms every 12 hours found that phenytoin 300 mg daily did not have a clinically important effect on either the pharmacokinetics of the dofetilide or on its cardiovascular pharmacodynamics (QTc, PR, QRS, RR intervals).[2] These findings confirm those of an *in vitro* study[3] showing that dofetilide did not inhibit the cytochrome P450 isoenzyme CYP2C9, thus suggesting that dofetilide is unlikely to affect the metabolism of phenytoin.

1. Vincent J, Gardner M, Scavone J, Ashton H, Willavize S, Friedman HL. The effect of dofetilide on the steady-state PK and cardiac effects of phenytoin in healthy subjects. *Clin Pharmacol Ther* (1997) 61, 233.
2. Gardner MJ, Ashton HM, Willavize SA, Friedman HL, Vincent J. The effects of phenytoin on the steady-state PK and PD of dofetilide in healthy subjects. *Clin Pharmacol Ther* (1997) 61, 205.
3. Walker DK, Alabaster CT, Congrave GS, Hargreaves MB, Hyland R, Jones BC, Reed LJ, Smith DA. Significance of metabolism in the disposition and action of the antidysrhythmic drug, dofetilide. *In vitro* studies and correlation with *in vivo* data. *Drug Metab Dispos* (1996) 24, 447–55.

Dofetilide + Theophylline

There does not appear to be any interaction between theophylline and dofetilide.

Clinical evidence, mechanism, importance and management

Studies in healthy subjects found that the concurrent use of theophylline 450 mg every 12 hours and dofetilide 500 micrograms every 12 hours did not alter the steady-state pharmacokinetics of either drug.[1,2] In addition, the increase in the QTc interval was no greater with the combination than with dofetilide alone.[1] No special precautions appear to be necessary.

1. Gardner MJ, Ashton HM, Willavize SA, Vincent J. The effects of concomitant dofetilide therapy on the pharmacokinetics and pharmacodynamics of theophylline. *Clin Pharmacol Ther* (1996) 59, 181.
2. Gardner MJ, Ashton HM, Willavize SA, Vincent J. The effects of orally administered theophylline on the pharmacokinetics and pharmacodynamics of dofetilide. *Clin Pharmacol Ther* (1996) 59, 182.

Dofetilide + Trimethoprim

Trimethoprim markedly increases the plasma levels of dofetilide. This is likely to be associated with an increased risk of dofetilide-induced QT prolongation and torsade de pointes.

Clinical evidence, mechanism, importance and management

The manufacturer of dofetilide notes that trimethoprim 160 mg (in combination with **sulfamethoxazole** 800 mg) twice daily given with dofetilide 500 micrograms twice daily for 4 days increased dofetilide peak levels by 93% and AUC by 103%.[1] Trimethoprim inhibits the active renal tubular secretion mechanism by which dofetilide is eliminated, so reducing its loss from the body (see also 'Dofetilide + H_2-receptor antagonists', p.255). There is a linear relationship between plasma dofetilide concentrations and prolongation of the QT interval, which increases the risk of torsade de pointes arrhythmia.[1] For this reason, the manufacturer contraindicates the use of trimethoprim in patients on dofetilide. This would seem to be a prudent precaution.

1. Tikosyn (Dofetilide). Pfizer Labs. US Prescribing information, March 2004.

Dofetilide + Verapamil

Verapamil transiently increases dofetilide plasma levels and QTc prolongation, and has been associated with an increased risk of torsade de pointes arrhythmia. Its use with dofetilide is contraindicated.

Clinical evidence

A study in 12 healthy subjects found that verapamil 80 mg three times daily given with dofetilide 500 micrograms twice daily for 3 days caused a 42% increase in the peak plasma levels of dofetilide from 2.4 to 3.43 nanograms/mL. There was a 26% increase in the AUC_{0-4}, which was associated with a transient simultaneous increase in QTc of 20 milliseconds for dofetilide alone and 26 milliseconds for the combination. However, the AUC_{0-8} was not significantly different.[1] The manufacturer notes that an analysis of clinical trial data for dofetilide revealed a higher occurrence of torsade de pointes when verapamil was used with dofetilide.[2]

Mechanism

Verapamil is postulated to interact with dofetilide by increasing its rate of absorption by increasing hepatic blood flow.[1] There is a linear relationship between plasma dofetilide concentrations and prolongation of the QT interval, which is a risk factor for torsade de pointes.[2]

Importance and management

The use of verapamil with dofetilide appears to be associated with a transient increase in dofetilide plasma concentrations, and an increased risk of torsade de pointes. For this reason, the combination is contraindicated.

1. Johnson BF, Cheng SL, Venitz J. Transient kinetic and dynamic interactions between verapamil and dofetilide, a class III antiarrhythmic. *J Clin Pharmacol* (2001) 41, 1248–56.
2. Tikosyn (Dofetilide). Pfizer Labs. US Prescribing information, March 2004.

Table 9.2 Drugs causing QT prolongation and torsade de pointes

High risk	*Some risk*
Amisulpride	Clarithromycin (increase in QTc interval less than 5 milliseconds; rare case reports of torsade de pointes)
Antiarrhythmics, class Ia (ajmaline, cibenzoline, disopyramide, hydroquinidine, procainamide, quinidine)	Chlorpromazine (rare case reports of torsade de pointes)
Antiarrhythmics, class III (amiodarone, azimilide, cibenzoline, dofetilide,† ibutilide,† sotalol†)	Erythromycin oral (see also high risk)
Arsenic trioxide (40% of patients had a QTc interval greater than 500 milliseconds)	Gatifloxacin (increase in QTc interval less than 10 milliseconds)
Artemisinin derivatives (artemisinin, artemether/lumefantrine - 5% of patients had an asymptomatic prolongation of QTc intervals by greater than 30 milliseconds, with an actual QTc of greater than 450 milliseconds in males and greater than 470 milliseconds in females)	Levofloxacin (rare case reports of torsade de pointes)
Astemizole† (if metabolism inhibited)	Lithium (greater risk if levels raised)
Cisapride† (if metabolism inhibited)	Methadone (in doses greater than 100 mg)
Droperidol†	Moxifloxacin (increase in QTc interval less than 10 milliseconds)
Erythromycin intravenous (see also some risk)	Pentamidine intravenous (case reports of torsade de pointes)
Halofantrine†	Quinine (greater risk with higher doses and intravenous use)
Haloperidol (also increased in high doses and with intravenous use)	Spiramycin
Ketanserin (30% of patients had an increase of greater than 30 milliseconds in a clinical trial)	Tricyclics (prolongation of QTc interval greater than 10 milliseconds, most notable risk occurs with clomipramine, risk with other tricyclics largely seems to be in overdose)
Mesoridazine†	
Pimozide†	
Ranolazine (dose-related QTc interval prolonged by up to 15 milliseconds, or more if metabolism inhibited)	
Sertindole†	
Sparfloxacin (10 millisecond increase in clinical trials)	
Terfenadine† (if metabolism inhibited)	
Thioridazine†	

†indicates drug suspended/restricted in some countries because of this effect
This list is not exhaustive

Drugs that prolong the QT interval + Drugs that lower potassium levels

The combined use of drugs that can cause hypokalaemia (e.g. amphotericin B, corticosteroids, thiazide and loop diuretics, and stimulant laxatives) and drugs that prolong the QT interval (e.g. class Ia and class III antiarrhythmics; see 'Table 9.2', (above)) should be well monitored because hypokalaemia increases the risk of torsade de pointes arrhythmias. There appear to be only a few reports of this interaction, for example, see 'Beta blockers + Potassium-depleting drugs', p.852.

Drugs that prolong the QT interval + Other drugs that prolong the QT interval

The consensus of opinion is that the concurrent use of drugs that have a high risk of prolonging the QTc interval should be avoided because of the risk of additive effects, leading to the possible development of serious and potentially life-threatening torsade de pointes cardiac arrhythmia. With drugs that have some risk of prolonging the QTc interval, some caution is appropriate, particularly in patients with other risk factors for QTc prolongation.

Clinical evidence, mechanism, importance and management

If the QT interval on the ECG becomes excessively prolonged, ventricular arrhythmias can develop, in particular a type of polymorphic tachycardia known as 'torsade de pointes'. On the ECG this arrhythmia can appear as an intermittent series of rapid spikes during which the heart fails to pump effectively, the blood pressure falls and the patient will feel dizzy and may possibly lose consciousness. Usually the condition is self-limiting but it may progress and degenerate into ventricular fibrillation, which can cause sudden death.

There are a number of reasons why QT interval prolongation can occur. These include:

- increasing age
- female sex
- congenital long QT syndrome
- cardiac disease
- thyroid disease
- some metabolic disturbances (hypocalcaemia, hypokalaemia, hypomagnesaemia)

Another important cause is the use of various QT-prolonging drugs including some antiarrhythmics, antipsychotics, antihistamines, antimalarials and others.[1,2] These drugs all appear to cause this effect by blocking the rapid component of the delayed rectifier (repolarisation) potassium channel.

At what degree of prolongation of corrected QT (QTc) interval torsade de pointes arrhythmia is likely to develop is uncertain. However a QTc interval exceeding 500 milliseconds is generally considered of particular concern, but this is not an exact figure. In addition, there is uncertainty about what constitutes an important change in QTc interval from baseline, although, in general, increases of 30 to 60 milliseconds should raise concern, and increases of over 60 milliseconds raise clear concerns about the potential for arrhythmias. Because of these uncertainties, many drug manufacturers and regulatory agencies contraindicated the concurrent use of drugs known to prolong the QT interval, and a 'blanket' warning was often issued because the QT prolonging effects of the drugs are expected to be additive. Regulatory guidance for the assessment of risk of a non-antiarrhythmic drug states that drugs causing an increase in mean QT/QTc interval of around 5 milliseconds or less do not appear to cause torsade de pointes. Data on drugs causing mean increases of around 5 and less than 20 are inconclusive, and some drugs causing this have been associated with proarrhythmic risk. Drugs with an increase of more than 20 milliseconds have a substantially increased likelihood of being proarrhythmic.[3,4] The extent of the drug-induced prolongation usually depends on the dosage of the drug and the particular drugs in question.

'Table 9.2', (p.257) is a list of drugs that are known to prolong the QT interval and cause torsade de pointes. Note that this list is not exhaustive of all the drugs that have ever been reported to be associated with QT interval prolongation and torsade de pointes. For some of the drugs listed, QT prolongation is a fairly frequent effect when the drug is used alone, and it is well accepted that use of these drugs requires careful monitoring (e.g. a number of the antiarrhythmics). For other drugs, QT prolongation is rare, but because of the relatively benign indications for these drugs, the risk-benefit ratio is considered poor, and use of these drugs has been severely restricted or discontinued (e.g. astemizole, terfenadine, cisapride). For others there is less clear evidence of the risk of QT prolongation (e.g. clarithromycin, chlorpromazine). Specific reports of additive QT prolonging effects with or without torsade de pointes are covered in individual monographs.

Drugs that do not themselves prolong the QT interval, but potentiate the effect of drugs that do (e.g. by pharmacokinetic mechanisms, lowering serum potassium, or by causing bradycardia) are not included in 'Table 9.2', (p.257). The interactions of these drugs (e.g. azole antifungals with cisapride, astemizole, or terfenadine, and potassium-depleting diuretics with sotalol) are dealt with in individual monographs. However, note that some drugs, for example the macrolide antibacterials, may cause QT prolongation by dual mechanisms—they appear to have both the intrinsic ability to prolong the QT interval, and they may inhibit the metabolism of drugs that prolong the QT interval.[5]

General references discussing the problems of QT-prolongation are given below.[6-14]

1. Zeltzer D, Justo D, Halkin A, Prokhorov V, Heller K, Viskin S. Torsade de pointes due to noncardiac drugs. Most patients have easily identifiable risk factors. *Medicine* (2003) 82, 282–90.
2. Benoit SR, Mendelsohn AB, Nourjah P, Staffa JA, Graham DJ. Risk factors for prolonged QTc among US adults: Third National Health and Nutrition Survey. *Eur J Cardiovasc Prev Rehabil* (2005) 12, 363–8.
3. European Medicines Agency. Note for guidance on the clinical evaluation of QT/QTc interval prolongation and proarrhythmic potential for non-antiarrhythmic drugs. November 2005. Available at: http://www.emea.eu.int/pdfs/human/ich/000204en.pdf (accessed 17/08/07).
4. US Food and Drug Administration. Guidance for Industry: E14 Clinical evaluation of QT/QTc interval prolongation and proarrhythmic potential for non-antiarrhythmic drugs. October 2005. Available at: http://www.fda.gov/cder/guidance/6922fnl.pdf (accessed 17/08/07).
5. Shaffer D, Singer S, Korvick J, Honig P. Concomitant risk factors in reports of torsades de pointes associated with macrolide use: review of the United States Food and Drug Administration Adverse Event Reporting System. *Clin Infect Dis* (2002) 35, 197–200.
6. Committee on Safety of Medicines/Medicines Control Agency. Drug-induced prolongation of the QT interval. *Current Problems* (1996) 22, 2.
7. Thomas SHL. Drugs, QT interval abnormalities and ventricular arrhythmias. *Adverse Drug React Toxicol Rev* (1994) 13, 77–102.
8. De Ponti F, Poluzzi E, Montanaro N. QT-interval prolongation by non-cardiac drugs: lessons to be learned from recent experience. *Eur J Clin Pharmacol* (2000) 56, 1–18.
9. Haverkamp W, Breithardt G, Camm AJ, Janse MJ, Rosen MR, Antzelevitch C, Escande D, Franz M, Malik M, Moss A, Shah R. The potential for QT prolongation and pro-arrhythmia by non-anti-arrhythmic drugs: clinical and regulatory implications. Report on a policy conference of the European Society of Cardiology. *Cardiovasc Res* (2000) 47, 219–33.
10. Bednar MM, Harrigan EP, Anziano RJ, Camm AJ, Ruskin JN. The QT interval. *Prog Cardiovasc Dis* (2001) 43 (Suppl 1): 1–45.
11. Kao LW, Furbee RB. Drug-induced Q–T prolongation. *Med Clin North Am* (2005) 89, 1125–44.
12. Glassman AH, Bigger JT. Antipsychotic drugs: prolonged QTc interval, torsade de pointes, and sudden death. *Am J Psychiatry* (2001) 158, 1774–82.
13. Stöllberger C, Huber JO, Finsterer J. Antipsychotic drugs and QT prolongation. *Int Clin Psychopharmacol* (2005) 20, 243–51.
14. Committee on Safety of Medicines/Medicines Control Agency. Risk of QT interval prolongation with methadone. *Current Problems* (2006) 31, 6.

Flecainide + Amiodarone

Serum flecainide levels are increased by amiodarone. The flecainide dosage should be reduced by between one-third and one-half. An isolated report describes a patient on amiodarone who developed torsade de pointes when given flecainide.

Clinical evidence

Amiodarone 1.2 g daily for 10 to 14 days then 600 mg daily was given to 7 patients taking oral flecainide 200 to 500 mg daily. The trough plasma levels of flecainide were increased by about 50%, and the flecainide dosage was reduced by one-third (averaging a reduction from 325 to 225 mg daily) to keep the flecainide levels constant. Observations in two patients suggest that the interaction begins soon after the amiodarone is added, and it takes 2 weeks or more to develop fully.[1]

Other authors have reported this interaction, and suggest reducing the flecainide dosage by between one-third to one-half when amiodarone is added.[2-5] Another study found that amiodarone raised steady-state flecainide plasma levels by 37% in extensive metabolisers, and 55% in poor metabolisers of dextromethorphan (a probe drug for CYP2D6 activity).[6] In a later report of this study the authors concluded that these differences were not clinically important, and that CYP2D6 phenotype does not affect the extent of the flecainide-amiodarone interaction.[7] An isolated report describes torsade de pointes in a patient on amiodarone when given flecainide.[8]

Mechanism

Amiodarone inhibits the cytochrome P450 isoenzyme CYP2D6, so that the flecainide is metabolised by the liver more slowly. Amiodarone also inhibits CYP2D6-independent mechanisms of flecainide elimination.[7]

Importance and management

An established interaction, but the documentation is limited. Reduce the flecainide dosage by one-third to one-half if amiodarone is added.[1-5,7] The manufacturers of flecainide recommend a 50% reduction in dose if amiodarone is given, and advise that adverse effects and plasma flecainide levels should be monitored.[9,10] There seems to be no need to treat extensive metabolisers differently from poor metabolisers.[7] Remember that the interaction may take 2 weeks or more to develop fully, and also that amiodarone is cleared from the body exceptionally slowly so that this interaction may persist for some weeks after it has been withdrawn.

1. Shea P, Lal R, Kim SS, Schechtman K, Ruffy R. Flecainide and amiodarone interaction. *J Am Coll Cardiol* (1986) 7, 1127–30.
2. Leclercq JF, Coumel P. La flécaïnide: un nouvel antiarythmique. *Arch Mal Coeur* (1983) 76, 1218–29.
3. Fontaine G, Frank R, Tonet JL. Association amiodarone-flécaïnide dans le traitement des troubles du rythme ventriculaires graves. *Arch Mal Coeur* (1984) 77, 1421.
4. Leclercq JF, Coumel P. Association amiodarone-flécaïnide dans le traitement des troubles du rythme ventriculaires graves. Résponse. *Arch Mal Coeur* (1984) 77, 1421–2.
5. Leclercq JF, Denjoy I, Mentré F, Coumel P. Flecainide acetate dose-concentration relationship in cardiac arrhythmias: influence of heart failure and amiodarone. *Cardiovasc Drugs Ther* (1990) 4, 1161–65.
6. Funck-Brentano C, Kroemer HK, Becquemont L, Bühl K, Eichelbaum M, Jaillon P. The interaction between amiodarone and flecainide is genetically determined. *Circulation* (1992) 86, (Suppl I), I–720.
7. Funck-Brentano C, Becquemont L, Kroemer HK, Bühl K, Knebel NG, Eichelbaum M, Jaillon P. Variable disposition kinetics and electrocardiographic effects of flecainide during repeated dosing in humans: contribution of genetic factors, dose-dependent clearance, and interaction with amiodarone. *Clin Pharmacol Ther* (1994) 55, 256–69.
8. Andrivet P, Beaslay V, Canh VD. Torsades de pointe with flecainide-amiodarone therapy. *Intensive Care Med* (1990) 16, 342–3.
9. Tambocor (Flecainide acetate). 3M Health Care Ltd. UK Summary of product characteristics, May 2006.
10. Tambocor (Flecainide). 3M Pharmaceuticals. US Prescribing information, June 1998.

Flecainide + Antacids or Food

The absorption of flecainide is not significantly altered if it is taken with food or an aluminium hydroxide antacid in adults, but it may possibly be reduced by milk in infants.

Clinical evidence, mechanism, importance and management

Neither food nor three 15-mL doses of *Aldrox* (280 mg of **aluminium hydroxide** per 5 mL) had any significant effect on the rate or extent of absorption of a single 200-mg dose of flecainide in healthy adult subjects.[1] No special precautions seem necessary if they are taken together.

A premature baby being treated for refractory atrio-ventricular tachycardia with high doses of flecainide (40 mg/kg daily or 25 mg every 6 hours) developed flecainide toxicity (seen as ventricular tachycardia) when his **milk feed** was replaced by **dextrose 5%**. His serum flecainide levels approximately doubled, the conclusion being that the **milk** had reduced the absorption.[2] **Milk**-fed infants on high doses of flecainide may therefore possibly need a reduced dosage if **milk** is reduced or stopped. Monitor the effects.

1. Tjandra-Maga TB, Verbesselt R, Van Hecken A, Mullie A, De Schepper PJ. Flecainide: single and multiple oral dose kinetics, absolute bioavailability and effect of food and antacid in man. *Br J Clin Pharmacol* (1986) 22, 309–16.
2. Russell GAB, Martin RP. Flecainide toxicity. *Arch Dis Child* (1989) 64, 860–2.

Flecainide + Antiepileptics

Limited data suggests that phenytoin or phenobarbital may modestly increase flecainide clearance, but this may not be clinically important.

Clinical evidence, mechanism, importance and management

Preliminary findings of a controlled study in 6 epileptic patients taking **phenytoin** or **phenobarbital** showed that the pharmacokinetics of a single 2-mg/kg intravenous dose of flecainide were not statistically different from those in a group of 7 healthy subjects. A 25 to 30% shorter flecainide half-life and urine clearance of unchanged drug was noted.[1] The authors say that this change may not require any adjustment in the flecainide dosage.

1. Pentikäinen PJ, Halinen MO, Hiepakorpi S, Chang SF, Conard GJ, McQuinn RL. Pharmacokinetics of flecainide in patients receiving enzyme inducers. *Acta Pharmacol Toxicol (Copenh)* (1986) 59 (Suppl 5), 91.

Flecainide + Benziodarone

A single case report describes ECG changes in a patient taking flecainide with benziodarone.

Clinical evidence, mechanism, importance and management

A 71-year-old woman who had undergone kidney transplantation 7 years earlier and who was taking amlodipine, losartan, furosemide, chlortalidone, calcitriol, aspirin, prednisone, ciclosporin, cyclophosphamide and insulin was also treated with flecainide, which controlled her paroxysmal atrial fibrillation. Atorvastatin was then restarted for hypercholesterolaemia and benziodarone 100 mg daily (because of intolerance to allopurinol) was added to treat hyperuricaemia. Three days later she presented with asthenia and poor overall condition and later an ECG showed QRS prolongation of 169 milliseconds (21% increase) caused by complete right bundle branch block with a previous anterior hemiblock, QTc interval prolongation of 482 milliseconds (22% increase) and PR interval prolongation of 203 milliseconds (18% increase). Creatinine levels were about 127 micromol/L, creatine phosphokinase 354 units/L and urea 155 mg/dL. Atorvastatin was stopped because of mild rhabdomyolysis. Flecainide and benziodarone were discontinued because an interaction was also suspected and symptoms resolved within 48 hours, with the ECG then showing values close to baseline. Flecainide was restarted and the dose gradually increased to 100 mg daily.[1]

It was suggested that benziodarone may inhibit the cytochrome P450 isoenzyme CYP2D6 which is concerned with the metabolism of flecainide.[1] Note that benziodarone is chemically related to amiodarone, which has a similar effect, see 'Flecainide + Amiodarone', p.258. Mild renal insufficiency in the patient may also have contributed to reduced flecainide elimination. More study is needed.

1. Gormaz CL, Page JCG, Fuentes FL. Pharmacological interaction between flecainide and benziodarone. *Rev Esp Cardiol* (2003) 56, 631–2.

Flecainide + Cimetidine

Cimetidine can increase flecainide plasma levels.

Clinical evidence

After taking cimetidine 1 g daily for a week, the AUC of a single 200-mg dose of flecainide was increased by 28% in 8 healthy subjects. The fraction of flecainide excreted unchanged in the urine was increased by 20%, but the total renal clearance was not altered.[1] In another study in 11 patients, cimetidine 1 g daily for 5 days almost doubled the plasma levels of flecainide 200 mg daily measured 2 hours after the morning dose.[2]

Mechanism

Uncertain, but it is thought that the cimetidine reduces the hepatic metabolism of flecainide.[1,2]

Importance and management

An established but not extensively documented interaction. The clinical importance appears not to have been assessed, but be alert for the need to reduce the flecainide dosage if cimetidine is added. Caution is recommended in patients with impaired renal function, as the interaction is likely to be enhanced.[1]

1. Tjandra-Maga TB, Van Hecken A, Van Melle P, Verbesselt R, De Schepper PJ. Altered pharmacokinetics of oral flecainide by cimetidine. *Br J Clin Pharmacol* (1986) 22, 108–110.
2. Nitsch J, Köhler U, Neyses L, Lüderitz B. Flecainid-Plasmakonzentraionen bei Hemmung des hepatischen Metabolismus durch Cimetidin. *Klin Wochenschr* (1987) 65 (Suppl IX), 250.

Flecainide + Colestyramine

An isolated report describes reduced plasma flecainide levels in a patient given colestyramine. However, studies in other subjects have not found an interaction.

Clinical evidence, mechanism, importance and management

A patient taking flecainide 100 mg twice daily had unusually low trough plasma levels (100 nanograms/mL) while taking colestyramine 4 g three times daily. When he stopped taking the colestyramine his plasma flecainide levels rose. However, a later study in 3 healthy subjects given flecainide 100 mg once daily and colestyramine 4 g three times daily, found little or no evidence of an interaction (steady-state flecainide levels of 63.1 and 59.1 nanograms/mL without and with colestyramine respectively). *In vitro* studies also did not find any binding between flecainide and colestyramine that might result in reduced absorption from the gut.[1] The authors however postulate that the citric acid contained in the colestyramine formulation might have altered the urinary pH, which could have increased the renal clearance of the flecainide.[1]

Information seems to be limited to this preliminary report. Its general importance seems to be minor, nevertheless the outcome of concurrent use should be monitored so that any unusual cases can be identified.

1. Stein H, Hoppe U. Is there an interaction between flecainide and cholestyramine? *Naunyn Schmiedebergs Arch Pharmacol* (1989) 339 (Suppl), R114.

Flecainide + Quinidine or Quinine

Quinidine and quinine cause a modest reduction in the clearance of flecainide.

Clinical evidence, mechanism, importance and management

(a) Quinidine

A single 50-mg oral dose of quinidine given to 6 healthy subjects the night before a single 150-mg intravenous dose of flecainide decreased the flecainide clearance by 23%. The flecainide half-life was increased by 22%

and its AUC by 28%.[1] In another study, 5 patients who were 'extensive metabolisers', (p.4), of the cytochrome P450 isoenzyme CYP2D6 and taking long-term flecainide were given quinidine 50 mg every 6 hours for 5 days. The plasma levels and clearance of S-(+)-flecainide were unchanged, but plasma levels of R-(−)-flecainide increased by about 15% and its clearance reduced by 15%. The effects of the flecainide were slightly but not significantly increased.[2] Quinidine inhibits CYP2D6, which is concerned with the metabolism of flecainide. The clinical importance of this interaction is uncertain, but it is probably minor.

(b) Quinine

Three 500-mg doses of quinine given to 10 healthy subjects over 24 hours increased the AUC of a single 150-mg intravenous infusion of flecainide (given over 30 minutes) by 21% and reduced the systemic clearance by 16.5%. Renal clearance remained unchanged. The increases in the PR and QRS intervals caused by flecainide were slightly, but not significantly, increased by quinine.[3] The evidence suggests that quinine reduces the metabolism of flecainide.[3] The clinical importance of this interaction is uncertain but a slight increase in the serum levels of flecainide would be expected, accompanied by some, probably minor, changes in its effects.

1. Munafo A, Buclin T, Tuto D, Biollaz J. The effect of a low dose of quinidine on the disposition of flecainide in healthy volunteers. *Eur J Clin Pharmacol* (1992) 43, 441–3.
2. Birgersdotter UM, Wong W, Turgeon J, Roden DM. Stereoselective genetically-determined interaction between chronic flecainide and quinidine in patients with arrhythmias. *Br J Clin Pharmacol* (1992) 33, 275–80.
3. Munafo A, Reymond-Michel G, Biollaz J. Altered flecainide disposition in healthy volunteers taking quinine. *Eur J Clin Pharmacol* (1990) 38, 269–73.

Flecainide + SSRIs

Paroxetine is an inhibitor of CYP2D6 and may, therefore, increase the plasma levels of flecainide, which is metabolised via this isoenzyme. The manufacturers suggest that escitalopram may have similar effects.

Clinical evidence, mechanism, importance and management

(a) Escitalopram

Although studies *in vitro* did not reveal an inhibitory effect of escitalopram on CYP2D6, limited *in vivo* data with 'desipramine', (p.1241) and 'metoprolol', (p.855) suggest a modest inhibitory effect.[1] The UK manufacturer recommends caution if escitalopram is given with drugs that are mainly metabolised by this enzyme, and that have a narrow therapeutic index. They specifically name flecainide.[1]

(b) Paroxetine

The manufacturer[2] states that paroxetine is an inhibitor of CYP2D6 and it may increase the plasma levels of drugs that are metabolised via this enzyme, such as flecainide. Several similarly metabolised drugs have been shown to interact (e.g. 'metoprolol', (p.855), and 'propafenone', (p.275)).

1. Cipralex (Escitalopram oxalate). Lundbeck Ltd. UK Summary of product characteristics, December 2005.
2. Seroxat (Paroxetine hydrochloride hemihydrate). GlaxoSmithKline UK. UK Summary of product characteristics, April 2007.

Flecainide + Tobacco

Tobacco smokers need larger doses of flecainide than non-smokers to achieve the same therapeutic effects.

Clinical evidence

Prompted by the chance observation that smokers appeared to have a reduced pharmacodynamic response to flecainide than non-smokers, a meta-analysis[1] was undertaken of the findings of 7 premarketing pharmacokinetic studies and 5 multicentre efficacy trials in which flecainide had been studied and in which the smoking habits of the subjects/patients had been also been recorded. In the pharmacokinetic studies, the clearance of flecainide was found to be about 50% higher in smokers than in non-smokers. In the efficacy studies, average clinically effective flecainide doses were found to be 338 mg daily for smokers and 288 mg daily for non-smokers, while trough plasma concentrations of flecainide were 1.74 and 2.18 nanograms/mL per mg dose for the smokers and non-smokers, respectively. This confirmed that smokers needed higher doses of flecainide to achieve the same steady-state serum levels.[1]

Mechanism

The probable reason for this interaction is that some components of the tobacco smoke stimulate the cytochrome P450 enzymes in the liver concerned with the *O*-dealkylation of flecainide, so that it is cleared from the body more quickly.[1]

Importance and management

An established interaction. Smokers seem likely to need higher doses of flecainide than non-smokers, but the way in which this interaction was identified suggests that in practice no specific action needs to be taken to accommodate it.

1. Holtzman JL, Weeks CE, Kvam DC, Berry DA, Mottonen L, Ekholm BP, Chang SF, Conard GJ. Identification of drug interactions by meta-analysis of premarketing trials: the effect of smoking on the pharmacokinetic and dosage requirements for flecainide acetate. *Clin Pharmacol Ther* (1989) 46, 1–8.

Flecainide + Urinary acidifiers or alkalinisers

The excretion of flecainide is increased if the urine is made acidic (e.g. with ammonium chloride) and reduced if the urine is made alkaline (e.g. with sodium bicarbonate). The clinical importance of these changes is not known.

Clinical evidence

Six healthy subjects were given single 300-mg oral doses of flecainide on two occasions. On the first occasion flecainide was taken after **ammonium chloride** 1 g orally every 3 hours, and 2 g at bedtime, for a total of 21 hours to make the urine acidic (pH range 4.4 to 5.4). On the second occasion flecainide was taken after **sodium bicarbonate** 4 g every 4 hours for a total of 21 hours (including night periods) to make the urine alkaline (pH range 7.4 to 8.3). Over the next 32 hours, 44.7% of unchanged flecainide appeared in the acidic urine, but only 7.4% in alkaline urine.[1] This compares with 25% found by other researchers when urinary pH was not controlled.[1] A later similar study from the same research group broadly confirmed these findings; the elimination half-life of the flecainide was 10.7 hours in acidic urine and 17.6 hours in alkaline urine.[2] Another study also confirmed the effect of urinary pH on the excretion of flecainide, and found that the fluid load and the urinary flow rate had little effect on flecainide excretion.[3]

Mechanism

In alkaline urine at pH 8, much of the flecainide exists in the kidney tubules in the non-ionised form (non-ionised fraction 0.04), which is therefore more readily reabsorbed. In acidic urine at pH 5 more exists in the ionised form (non-ionised fraction 0.0001), which is less readily reabsorbed and is therefore lost in the urine.[3]

Importance and management

Established interactions, but their clinical importance is still uncertain. The effects of these changes on the subsequent control of arrhythmias by flecainide in patients seem not to have been studied, but the outcome should be well monitored if patients are given drugs that alter urinary pH to a significant extent (such as ammonium chloride, sodium bicarbonate). Large doses of some **antacids** may possibly do the same, but nobody seems to have studied this.

1. Muhiddin KA, Johnston A, Turner P. The influence of urinary pH on flecainide excretion and its serum pharmacokinetics. *Br J Clin Pharmacol* (1984) 17, 447–51.
2. Johnston A, Warrington S, Turner P. Flecainide pharmacokinetics in healthy volunteers: the influence of urinary pH. *Br J Clin Pharmacol* (1985) 20, 333–8.
3. Hertrampf R, Gundert-Remy U, Beckmann J, Hoppe U, Elsäßer W, Stein H. Elimination of flecainide as a function of urinary flow rate and pH. *Eur J Clin Pharmacol* (1991) 41, 61–3.

Flecainide + Verapamil

Although flecainide and verapamil have been used together successfully, serious and potentially life-threatening cardiogenic shock and asystole have been seen in a few patients, because the cardiac depressant effects of the two drugs can be additive.

Clinical evidence

A man with triple coronary vessel disease and taking flecainide 200 mg daily for recurrent ventricular tachycardia, developed severe cardiogenic shock within 2 days of increasing the flecainide dosage to 300 mg daily and one day of starting verapamil 80 mg daily. His blood pressure fell to 60/40 mmHg and he had an idioventricular rhythm of 88 bpm.[1] Another patient with atrial flutter and fibrillation was given digitalis and verapamil 120 mg three times daily. He was also given flecainide 150 mg daily for 10 days, but 3 days after the dosage was raised to 200 mg daily he fainted, and later developed severe bradycardia (15 bpm) and asystoles of up to 14 seconds. He later died.[1]

Another report describes atrioventricular block in a patient with a pacemaker when treated with digoxin, flecainide and verapamil.[2]

Two earlier studies in patients[3] and healthy subjects[4] had found that the pharmacokinetics of flecainide and verapamil were only minimally affected by concurrent use, but the PR interval was increased by both drugs and additive depressant effects were seen on heart contractility and AV conduction. No serious adverse responses occurred.

Mechanism

Flecainide and verapamil have little or no effects on the pharmacokinetics of each other,[3,4] but they can apparently have additive depressant effects on the heart (negative inotropic and chronotropic) in both patients and healthy subjects.[1,3,4] Verapamil alone[5,6] and flecainide alone[7,8] have been responsible for asystole and cardiogenic shock in a few patients. In the cases cited above[1-3] the cardiac depressant effects were particularly serious because the patients already had compromised cardiac function.

Importance and management

An established interaction, but the incidence of serious adverse effects is probably not great. The additive cardiac depressant effects are probably of little importance in many patients, but may represent 'the last straw' in a few who have seriously compromised cardiac function. The authors of one of the reports cited[1] advise careful monitoring if both drugs are used and emphasise the potential hazards of combining **class Ic antiarrhythmics** and verapamil.

1. Buss J, Lasserre JJ, Heene DL. Asystole and cardiogenic shock due to combined treatment with verapamil and flecainide. *Lancet* (1992) 340, 546.
2. Tworek DA, Nazari J, Ezri M, Bauman JL. Interference by antiarrhythmic agents with function of electrical cardiac devices. *Clin Pharm* (1992) 11, 48–56.
3. Landau S, Hogan C, Butler B, Somberg J. The combined administration of verapamil and flecainide. *J Clin Pharmacol* (1988) 28, 909.
4. Holtzman JL, Finley D, Mottonen L, Berry DA, Ekholm BP, Kvam DC, McQuinn RL, Miller AM. The pharmacodynamic and pharmacokinetic interaction between single doses of flecainide acetate and verapamil: effects on cardiac function and drug clearance. *Clin Pharmacol Ther* (1989) 46, 26–32.
5. Perrot B, Danchin N, De La Chaise AT. Verapamil: a cause of sudden death in a patient with hypertrophic cardiomyopathy. *Br Heart J* (1984) 51, 532–4.
6. Cohen IL, Fein A, Nabi A. Reversal of cardiogenic shock and asystole in a septic patient with hypertrophic cardiomyopathy on verapamil. *Crit Care Med* (1990) 18, 775–6.
7. Forbes WP, Hee TT, Mohiuddin SM, Hillman DE. Flecainide-induced cardiogenic shock. *Chest* (1988) 94, 1121.
8. Echt DS, Liebson PR, Mitchell LB, Peters RW, Obias-Manno D, Barker AH, Arensberg D, Baker A, Friedman L, Greene HL, Huther ML, Richardson DW, CAST investigators. Mortality and morbidity in patients receiving encainide, flecainide or placebo. *N Engl J Med* (1991) 324, 781–8.

Ibutilide + Amiodarone

The concurrent use of ibutilide and amiodarone would be expected to further prolong the QT interval and increase the risk of torsade de pointes, but, despite this, one report describes their successful use for cardioversion.

Clinical evidence, mechanism, importance and management

When intravenous ibutilide 2 mg was used for cardioversion of atrial fibrillation or flutter in 70 patients taking long-term amiodarone the QT interval was further prolonged (from 371 to 479 milliseconds). However, only one patient had an episode of non-sustained torsade de pointes. Ibutilide was effective within 30 minutes of infusion in 39% of patients with atrial flutter, and 54% of patients with fibrillation.[1] Both amiodarone and ibutilide are class III antiarrhythmics and prolong the QT interval, with the consequent risk of torsade de pointes. The manufacturer recommends that they should not be used concurrently.[2] However, the authors of the above report suggest that ibutilide may be useful for cardioversion in those already taking amiodarone. Combined use should be very well monitored.

1. Glatter K, Yang Y, Chatterjee K, Modin G, Cheng J, Kayser S, Scheinman MM. Chemical cardioversion of atrial fibrillation or flutter with ibutilide in patients receiving amiodarone therapy. *Circulation* (2001) 103, 253–7.
2. Corvert (Ibutilide fumarate). Pharmacia & Upjohn. US Prescribing information. July 2002.

Ibutilide + Calcium-channel blockers

Calcium-channel blockers (predominantly non-dihydropyridine type) have not altered the safety or efficacy of ibutilide in clinical trials.

Clinical evidence, mechanism, importance and management

Retrospective analysis of three clinical trials showed that calcium-channel blockers did not alter the ECG effects (QT prolongation) or the efficacy of ibutilide. In these three studies, 68 of the 130 patients treated with ibutilide were also taking calcium-channel blockers. The report did not specify which calcium-channel blockers were used, except to say that only 12 of the 68 (19%) were taking a dihydropyridine-type.[1]

In vitro studies have shown that **nifedipine** (a dihydropyridine) attenuated the effects of ibutilide.[2] The findings of the above report[1] suggest that this may not be clinically important. However, since so few patients were taking a dihydropyridine, an effect specific to dihydropyridines cannot be excluded. Further study is needed.

1. Wood MA, Gilligan DM, Brown-Mahoney C, Nematzadeh F, Stambler BS, Ellenbogen KA. Clinical and electrophysiologic effects of calcium channel blockers in patients receiving ibutilide. *Am Heart J* (2002) 143, 176–80.
2. Lee KS, Lee EW. Ionic mechanism of ibutilide in human atrium: evidence for a drug-induced Na^+ current through a nifedipine inhibited inward channel. *J Pharmacol Exp Ther* (1998) 286, 9–22.

Ibutilide + Class Ic antiarrhythmics

Some evidence suggests that patients taking ibutilide have a less marked increase in QT interval, without a change in efficacy, when they are also given propafenone or flecainide.

Clinical evidence, mechanism, importance and management

The increase in QTc interval after intravenous ibutilide 2 mg was less in patients treated with **propafenone** (5 patients) or **flecainide** (1 patient) than in 85 other patients who had taken ibutilide alone (34 versus 65 milliseconds). The effect appeared to be dose-related, with higher propafenone doses causing the largest attenuation in the ibutilide-induced QT prolongation. The efficacy of ibutilide was unaltered.[1] In a further study, 71 patients with atrial fibrillation or atrial flutter receiving either propafenone 300 to 900 mg daily or flecainide 100 to 300 mg daily underwent cardioversion with a single intravenous dose of ibutilide 1 mg over 10 minutes, followed if necessary by a further dose after an interval of 10 minutes. Torsade de pointes occurred in one patient with profound sinus node suppression after cardioversion, but the mean ibutilide-induced QTc interval was attenuated (20 ± 54 milliseconds compared to reported range of 47 to 90 milliseconds) without a decrease in efficacy. However, the authors note that the risk of sustained torsade de pointes in this study appears to be similar to that seen in other studies of ibutilide.[2]

Ibutilide, a class III antiarrhythmic, is known to increase the QT interval, so increasing the risk of torsade de pointes arrhythmia. Class Ic antiarrhythmics such as **propafenone** and **flecainide** generally shorten the QT interval. It is possible that class Ic antiarrhythmics may usefully attenuate the risk of torsade de pointes with ibutilide,[1] and ibutilide may be useful in restoring sinus rhythm in patients taking class Ic antiarrhythmics,[2] but further study is needed.

1. Reiffel JA, Blitzer M. The actions of ibutilide and class Ic drugs on the slow sodium channel: new insights regarding individual pharmacologic effects elucidated through combination therapies. *J Cardiovasc Pharmacol Ther* (2000) 5, 177–81.
2. Hongo RH, Themistoclakis S, Raviele A, Bonso A, Rossillo A, Glatter A, Yang Y, Scheinman MM. Use of ibutilide in cardioversion of patients with atrial fibrillation or atrial flutter treated with Class IC agents. *J Am Coll Cardiol* (2004) 44, 864–8.

Ibutilide + Miscellaneous

Ibutilide can prolong the QT interval, therefore caution has been advised about the concurrent use of other drugs that can do the same. Ibutilide is reported not to interact with beta blockers or digoxin.

Clinical evidence, mechanism, importance and management

No specific drug interaction studies appear to have been undertaken with ibutilide, which is a class III antiarrhythmic, but because it can prolong the QT interval it has been recommended that other drugs that can do the same should be administered with caution, because of the potential additive effects.[1] The manufacturer of ibutilide specifically recommends that **class Ia** and other **class III antiarrhythmics** should not be given within 4 hours of an ibutilide infusion, and that ibutilide should not be given within five half-lives of these antiarrhythmics (but see also, 'Ibutilide + Amiodarone', p.261).[2] The concern is that a prolongation of the QT interval is associated with an increased risk of torsade de pointes arrhythmia, which is potentially life-threatening. See also 'Drugs that prolong the QT interval + Other drugs that prolong the QT interval', p.257.

The concurrent use of **beta blockers** and **digoxin** during clinical trials is reported not to affect the safety or efficacy of ibutilide.[1,2] Ibutilide is said not to affect the cytochrome P450 isoenzymes CYP3A4 or CYP2D6 and so metabolic interactions with drugs affected by these enzymes would not be expected.[1] Study is needed to confirm all of these predictions and findings.

1. Cropp JS, Antal EG, Talbert RL. Ibutilide: a new Class III antiarrhythmic agent. *Pharmacotherapy* (1997) 17, 1–9.
2. Corvert (Ibutilide fumarate). Pharmacia & Upjohn. US Prescribing information. July 2002.

Lidocaine + Amiodarone

One man receiving intravenous lidocaine had a seizure about two days after starting treatment with amiodarone, and another man with sick sinus syndrome taking amiodarone had a sinoatrial arrest during placement of a pacemaker under local anaesthesia with lidocaine. There is conflicting evidence as to whether or not amiodarone affects the pharmacokinetics of intravenous lidocaine.

Clinical evidence

(a) Effects on lidocaine levels, seizure

An elderly man taking digoxin, enalapril, amitriptyline and temazepam was treated for monomorphic ventricular tachycardia, firstly with procainamide, later replaced by a 2-mg/minute infusion of lidocaine, to which oral amiodarone 600 mg twice daily was added. After 12 hours his lidocaine level was 5.4 mg/L (therapeutic levels 1.5 to 5 mg/L), but 53 hours later he developed a seizure and his lidocaine level was found to have risen to 12.6 mg/L. A tomography brain scan showed no abnormalities that could have caused the seizure and it was therefore attributed to the toxic lidocaine levels.[1]

Six patients with symptomatic cardiac arrhythmias took part in a two-phase study. Initially, lidocaine 1 mg/kg was given intravenously over 2 minutes. In phase I, loading doses of amiodarone 500 mg daily for 6 days were given, followed by the same lidocaine dose. After 19 to 21 days, when the total cumulative amiodarone dose was 13 g, the same lidocaine dose was given again (phase II). The lidocaine AUC increased by about 20% and the systemic clearance decreased by about 20%. The elimination half-life and distribution volume at steady-state were unchanged. The pharmacokinetic parameters of lidocaine in phase II were the same as those in phase I, indicating that the interaction occurs early in the loading phase of amiodarone use.[2] This is in contrast to an earlier study, in which the pharmacokinetics of a bolus dose of lidocaine 1 mg/kg over 2 minutes were not altered in 10 patients who had taken amiodarone 200 to 400 mg daily (following an loading dose of 800 or 1200 mg) for 4 to 5 weeks.[3]

(b) Sinoatrial arrest

An elderly man with long standing brady-tachycardia was successfully treated for atrial flutter firstly with a temporary pacemaker (later withdrawn) and 600 mg amiodarone daily. Ten days later, and 25 minutes after a permanent pacemaker was inserted under local anaesthesia with 15 mL of 2% lidocaine, severe sinus bradycardia and long sinoatrial arrest developed. He was effectively treated with atropine plus isoprenaline, and cardiac massage.[4]

Mechanism

An *in vitro* study has demonstrated that amiodarone may inhibit lidocaine metabolism competitively and *vice versa*. The interaction *in vivo* may be due to inhibition of the cytochrome P450 isoenzyme CYP3A4 by amiodarone and/or its main metabolite desethylamiodarone.[3] CYP3A4 is partially involved in the metabolism of lidocaine.

The authors of the report describing the sinoatrial arrest suggest a synergistic depression by both drugs of the sinus node.

Importance and management

Evidence of a pharmacokinetic interaction between lidocaine and amiodarone is conflicting. However, the two reports of adverse interactions and the study in patients with arrhythmias illustrate the importance of good monitoring if both drugs are used.

1. Siegmund JB, Wilson JH, Imhoff TE. Amiodarone interaction with lidocaine. *J Cardiovasc Pharmacol* (1993) 21, 513–15.
2. Ha HR, Candinas R, Steiger B, Meyer UA, Follath F. Interactions between amiodarone and lidocaine. *J Cardiovasc Pharmacol* (1996) 28, 533–9.
3. Nattel S, Talajic M, Beaudoin D, Matthews C, Roy D. Absence of pharmacokinetic interaction between amiodarone and lidocaine. *Am J Cardiol* (1994) 73, 92–4.
4. Keidar S, Grenadier E, Palant A. Sinoatrial arrest due to lidocaine injection in sick sinus syndrome during amiodarone administration. *Am Heart J* (1982) 104, 1384–5.

Lidocaine + Barbiturates

Plasma lidocaine levels following slow intravenous injection may be modestly lower in patients who are taking barbiturates.

Clinical evidence

A single 2-mg/kg dose of lidocaine was given by slow intravenous injection (rate about 100 mg over 15 minutes) to 7 epileptic patients, firstly while taking their usual antiepileptic drugs and sedatives (including phenytoin, barbiturates, phenothiazines, benzodiazepines) and secondly after taking only **phenobarbital** 300 mg daily for 4 weeks. The same lidocaine dose was also given to 6 control subjects who had not received any drugs. When compared with the levels in the 6 control subjects, plasma lidocaine levels were somewhat lower when the patients took their standard antiepileptic treatment (18 and 29% lower at 30 and 60 minutes, respectively). When plasma lidocaine levels achieved during the **phenobarbital** phase were compared with those achieved during the standard antiepileptic treatment they were found to be 10 to 25% higher, suggesting that the effect of combined treatment caused a greater reduction in lidocaine levels than **phenobarbital**.[1]

Mechanism

Not fully understood. One suggestion is that the barbiturates increase the activity of the liver microsomal enzymes, thereby increasing the rate of metabolism of the lidocaine.[1]

Importance and management

Direct information is very limited. It may be necessary to increase the dosage of lidocaine to achieve the desired therapeutic response in patients on phenobarbital or other barbiturates.

1. Heinonen J, Takki S, Jarho L. Plasma lidocaine levels in patients treated with potential inducers of microsomal enzymes. *Acta Anaesthesiol Scand* (1970) 14, 89–95.

Lidocaine + Beta blockers

The plasma levels of lidocaine after intravenous, and possibly oral, use can be increased by propranolol. Isolated cases of toxicity attributed to this interaction have been reported. Nadolol and penbutolol possibly interact similarly, but there is uncertainty about metoprolol. Atenolol and pindolol appear not to interact.

Clinical evidence

(a) Atenolol

A study with oral atenolol 50 mg daily found that it did not affect the clearance of lidocaine after oral or intravenous use.[1]

(b) Metoprolol

In 6 healthy subjects, metoprolol 100 mg twice daily for 2 days did not affect the pharmacokinetics of a single intravenous dose of lidocaine.[2] Similarly, another study in 7 healthy subjects failed to find any changes in the pharmacokinetics of a single oral or intravenous dose of lidocaine after treatment with metoprolol 100 mg every 12 hours for a week.[1] In contrast, another study found that the clearance of a single intravenous dose of lidocaine was reduced by 31% by pretreatment with metoprolol 50 mg every 6 hours for a day.[3]

(c) Nadolol

A study in 6 healthy subjects receiving 30-hour infusions of lidocaine at a rate of 2 mg/minute found that pretreatment with nadolol 160 mg daily for 3 days raised the steady-state plasma lidocaine levels by 28% (from 2.1 to 2.7 micrograms/mL) and reduced the plasma clearance by 17%.[4]

(d) Penbutolol

In 7 healthy subjects, penbutolol 60 mg daily significantly increased the volume of distribution of a single 100-mg intravenous dose of lidocaine, thus prolonging its elimination half-life. However, the reduction in clearance of lidocaine did not reach significance.[5]

(e) Pindolol

A study with intravenous pindolol 23 micrograms/kg found that it did not affect the clearance of intravenous lidocaine.[6]

(f) Propranolol

A study in 6 healthy subjects receiving 30-hour infusions of lidocaine at a rate of 2 mg/minute found that pretreatment with propranolol 80 mg every 8 hours for 3 days raised the steady-state plasma lidocaine levels by 19% (from 2.1 to 2.5 micrograms/mL) and reduced the plasma clearance by 16%.[4] Other similar studies have found a 22.5 to 30% increase in steady-state serum lidocaine levels and a 14.7 to 46% fall in plasma clearance due to the concurrent use of propranolol.[3,6,7] Two cases of lidocaine toxicity attributed to a lidocaine-propranolol interaction were revealed by a search[8] of the FDA adverse drug reaction file in 1981. A further case of lidocaine toxicity (seizures) has been described in a man on propranolol after accidental *oral* ingestion of lidocaine for oesophageal anaesthesia. High serum levels of lidocaine were detected.[9]

(g) Unnamed beta blockers

A matched study in 51 cardiac patients taking a variety of beta blockers (including **propranolol**, **metoprolol**, **timolol**, **pindolol**) found no significant differences in either total or free concentrations of lidocaine during a lidocaine infusion, but there was a trend towards an increase in the adverse effects of lidocaine (bradycardias) with concurrent beta blocker treatment.[10]

Mechanism

Not fully agreed. There is some debate about whether the increased serum lidocaine levels largely occur because of the decreased cardiac output caused by the beta blockers, which decreases the flow of blood through the liver thereby reducing the metabolism of the lidocaine,[4] or because of direct liver enzyme inhibition.[11] There may also be a pharmacodynamic interaction, with an increased risk of myocardial depression.[10]

Importance and management

The lidocaine/propranolol interaction is established and of clinical importance. Monitor the effects of concurrent use and reduce the intravenous lidocaine dosage if necessary to avoid toxicity. The situation with other beta blockers is less clear. Nadolol appears to interact like propranolol, but it is uncertain whether metoprolol interacts or not. Atenolol and pindolol are reported not to interact pharmacokinetically. It has been suggested that a higher intravenous loading dose (but not a higher maintenance dose) of lidocaine may be needed if penbutolol is used.[5] The suggestion has been made that a significant pharmacokinetic interaction is only likely to occur with non-selective beta blockers without intrinsic sympathomimetic activity[11] e.g. nadolol or propranolol. Aside from the pharmacokinetic interactions, a pharmacodynamic interaction is possible, and so it would be prudent to monitor the effects of concurrent use with any beta blocker.

Note that local anaesthetic preparations of lidocaine often contain adrenaline (epinephrine), which may interact with beta blockers, see 'Beta blockers + Inotropes and Vasopressors', p.848.

1. Miners JO, Wing LMH, Lillywhite KJ, Smith KJ. Failure of 'therapeutic' doses of β-adrenoceptor antagonists to alter the disposition of tolbutamide and lignocaine. *Br J Clin Pharmacol* (1984) 18, 853–60.
2. Jordö L, Johnsson G, Lundborg P, Regårdh C-G. Pharmacokinetics of lidocaine in healthy individuals pretreated with multiple dose of metoprolol. *Int J Clin Pharmacol Ther Toxicol* (1984) 22, 312–15.
3. Conrad KA, Byers JM, Finley PR, Burnham L. Lidocaine elimination: effects of metoprolol and of propranolol. *Clin Pharmacol Ther* (1983) 33, 133–8.
4. Schneck DW, Luderer JR, Davis D, Vary J. Effects of nadolol and propranolol on plasma lidocaine clearance. *Clin Pharmacol Ther* (1984) 36, 584–7.
5. Ochs HR, Skanderra D, Abernethy DR, Greenblatt DJ. Effect of penbutolol on lidocaine kinetics. *Arzneimittelforschung* (1983) 33, 1680–1.
6. Svendsen TL, Tangø M, Waldorff S, Steiness E, Trap-Jensen J. Effects of propranolol and pindolol on plasma lignocaine clearance in man. *Br J Clin Pharmacol* (1982) 13, 223S–226S.
7. Ochs HR, Carstens G, Greenblatt DJ. Reduction in lidocaine clearance during continuous infusion and by co administration of propranolol. *N Engl J Med* (1980) 303, 373–7.
8. Graham CF, Turner WM, Jones JK. Lidocaine-propranolol interactions. *N Engl J Med* (1981) 304, 1301.
9. Parish RC, Moore RT, Gotz VP. Seizures following oral lidocaine for esophageal anesthesia. *Drug Intell Clin Pharm* (1985) 19, 199–201.
10. Wyse DG, Kellen J, Tam Y, Rademaker AW. Increased efficacy and toxicity of lidocaine in patients on beta-blockers. *Int J Cardiol* (1988) 21, 59–70.
11. Bax NDS, Tucker GT, Lennard MS, Woods HF. The impairment of lignocaine clearance by propranolol—major contribution from enzyme inhibition. *Br J Clin Pharmacol* (1985) 19, 597–603.

Lidocaine + Cocaine

Limited evidence suggests intravenous lidocaine use in patients with cocaine-associated myocardial infarction is not associated with significant toxicity.

Clinical evidence, mechanism, importance and management

A retrospective study, covering a 6-year period in 29 hospitals, identified 29 patients (27 available for review) who received lidocaine for prophylaxis or treatment of cocaine-associated myocardial infarction. No patient exhibited bradycardia, sustained ventricular tachycardia or ventricular fibrillation, and no patients died.[1]

Both lidocaine and cocaine exhibit class I antiarrhythmic effects and are proconvulsants. Lidocaine may potentiate the cardiac and CNS adverse effects of cocaine. Therefore the use of lidocaine for cocaine-associated myocardial infarction is controversial. The lack of adverse effects in this study may have been due to delays of more than 5 hours between last exposure to cocaine and lidocaine therapy. These authors[1] and others[2,3] consider that the cautious use of lidocaine does not appear to be contraindicated in patients with cocaine-associated myocardial infarction who require antiarrhythmic therapy. However, extra care should be taken in patients who receive lidocaine shortly after cocaine.[1]

1. Shih RD, Hollander JE, Burstein JL, Nelson LS, Hoffman RS, Quick AM. Clinical safety of lidocaine in patients with cocaine-associated myocardial infarction. *Ann Emerg Med* (1995) 26, 702–6.
2. Derlet RW. More on lidocaine use in cocaine toxicity. *J Emerg Nurs* (1998) 24, 303.
3. Friedman MB. Is lidocaine contraindicated with cocaine? *J Emerg Nurs* (1997) 23, 520.

Lidocaine + Dextromethorphan

Intravenous lidocaine does not inhibit the activity of CYP2D6, as assessed by its lack of effect on dextromethorphan pharmacokinetics, and is therefore unlikely to interact with drugs that are metabolised by this isoenzyme.

Clinical evidence, mechanism, importance and management

Although *in vitro* data suggested that lidocaine inhibited oxidative metabolism reactions mediated by the cytochrome P450 isoenzyme CYP2D6, a later *in vivo* study in 16 patients found that, while being given an infusion of lidocaine (serum level range 3.2 to 55.9 micromol/L), the metabolism of a single 30-mg dose of dextromethorphan remained unchanged. All of the patients were of the extensive metaboliser phenotype. Since dextromethorphan is a well-established marker of CYP2D6 activity, it was concluded that lidocaine is unlikely to interact with drugs that are extensively metabolised by this isoenzyme.[1]

1. Bartoli A, Gatt G, Chimienti M, Corbellini D, Perrucca E. Does lidocaine affect oxidative dextromethorphan metabolism *in vivo*? *G Ital Chim Clin* (1993/4) 18, 125–9.

Lidocaine + Disopyramide

***In vitro* studies show that disopyramide can increase the levels of unbound lidocaine, but it is not known whether their combined effects have a clinically important cardiac depressant effect in practice.**

Clinical evidence, mechanism, importance and management

An *in vitro* study using serum taken from 9 patients receiving intravenous lidocaine for severe ventricular arrhythmias showed that there was an average 20% increase in its free (unbound) fraction when disopyramide in a concentration of 14.7 micromol/L was added.[1] This appears to occur because disopyramide can displace lidocaine from its binding sites on plasma proteins (alpha-1-acid glycoprotein).

The importance of this possible displacement interaction in clinical practice is uncertain. The suggestion made by the authors[1] is that, although lidocaine has only a minor cardiac depressant effect, a transient 20% increase in levels of free and active lidocaine plus the negative inotropic effects of the disopyramide might possibly be hazardous in patients with reduced cardiac function.

1. Bonde J, Jensen NM, Burgaard P, Angelo HR, Graudal N, Kampmann JP, Pedersen LE. Displacement of lidocaine from human plasma proteins by disopyramide. *Pharmacol Toxicol* (1987) 60, 151–5.

Lidocaine + Erythromycin

Erythromycin may markedly increase plasma levels of oral lidocaine, but causes only a minor increase after intravenous lidocaine.

Clinical evidence

In a randomised double-blind crossover study 9 healthy subjects were given erythromycin 500 mg three times daily or placebo daily for 4 days. Erythromycin increased the AUC and peak plasma levels of a single 1-mg/kg *oral* dose of lidocaine by 50 and 40% respectively. Erythromycin also markedly increased the AUC of the metabolite of lidocaine, monoethylglycinexylidide (MEGX) by 60%.[1]

In a similar study,[2] erythromycin had no effect on the AUC or peak plasma level of a single 1.5-mg/kg intravenous dose of lidocaine, but still increased the AUC of MEGX by 70%. In yet another study, erythromycin ethylsuccinate 600 mg three times daily for 5 doses had a minor effect on the pharmacokinetics of a single 1-mg/kg intravenous dose of lidocaine (an 18% decrease in clearance), and caused a 33% increase in the AUC of MEGX. There was no difference in the results from the 10 healthy subjects and the 20 patients with biopsy proven cirrhosis.[3] In another study, 9 healthy subjects were given fluvoxamine 100 mg daily alone or with erythromycin 500 mg three times daily for 5 days before the administration of a single intravenous dose of lidocaine 1.5 mg/kg on day 6. The clearance of lidocaine was reduced 41% by fluvoxamine and 53% by concurrent fluvoxamine and erythromycin.[4]

Mechanism

Erythromycin is an inhibitor of the cytochrome P450 isoenzyme CYP3A4, the isoenzyme partially involved in the metabolism of lidocaine. Erythromycin appears to markedly reduce the first-pass metabolism of oral lidocaine so that its plasma levels rise.[1] The increase in MEGX could be due to either an increase in the production of this metabolite, or the inhibition of its further metabolism. Fluvoxamine, is an inhibitor of CYP1A2 which is also involved in lidocaine metabolism. Lidocaine clearance is reduced by fluvoxamine and further decreased by concurrent erythromycin.

Importance and management

Information seems limited, and since lidocaine is not usually given orally the practical importance is minor. However, lidocaine is used for oro-pharyngeal topical anaesthesia, and there have been cases of toxicity after accidental ingestion. Thus, in a patient on erythromycin, the toxicity of *oral* lidocaine may be markedly increased. Further study is required to assess the significance of the increase in MEGX during prolonged intravenous lidocaine infusions.

1. Isohanni MH, Neuvonen PJ, Olkkola KT. Effect of erythromycin and itraconazole on the pharmacokinetics of oral lignocaine. *Pharmacol Toxicol* (1999) 84, 143–6.
2. Isohanni MH, Neuvonen PJ, Palkama VJ, Olkkola KT. Effect of erythromycin and itraconazole on the pharmacokinetics of intravenous lignocaine. *Eur J Clin Pharmacol* (1998) 54, 561–5.
3. Orlando R, Piccoli P, De Martin S, Padrini R, Palatini P. Effect of the CYP3A4 inhibitor erythromycin on the pharmacokinetics of lignocaine and its pharmacologically active metabolites in subjects with normal and impaired liver function. *Br J Clin Pharmacol* (2003) 55, 86–93.
4. Olkkola KT, Isohanni MH, Hamunen K, Neuvonen PJ. The effect of erythromycin and fluvoxamine on the pharmacokinetics of intravenous lidocaine. *Anesth Analg* (2005) 100, 1352–6.

Lidocaine + Fluvoxamine

Fluvoxamine reduces the clearance of intravenous lidocaine.

Clinical evidence, mechanism, importance and management

In a study, 9 healthy subjects were given fluvoxamine 100 mg daily alone or with erythromycin 500 mg three times daily for 5 days before the administration of a single intravenous dose of lidocaine 1.5 mg/kg on day 6. The clearance of lidocaine was reduced 41% by fluvoxamine and 53% by concurrent fluvoxamine and erythromycin.[1]

The study found lidocaine clearance was reduced by fluvoxamine and further decreased by concurrent erythromycin. The cytochrome P450 isoenzymes CYP1A2 and CYP3A4 are involved in lidocaine metabolism. An *in vitro* study found that fluvoxamine (a CYP1A2 inhibitor) was a more potent inhibitor of lidocaine metabolism than erythromycin (a CYP3A4 inhibitor).[2] See also 'Lidocaine + Erythromycin', above and 'Anaesthetics, local + Fluvoxamine', p.110.

1. Olkkola KT, Isohanni MH, Hamunen K, Neuvonen PJ. The effect of erythromycin and fluvoxamine on the pharmacokinetics of intravenous lidocaine. *Anesth Analg* (2005) 100, 1352–6.
2. Wang JS, Backman JT, Wen X, Taavitsainen P, Neuvonen PJ, Kivisto KT. Fluvoxamine is a more potent inhibitor of lidocaine metabolism than ketoconazole and erythromycin in vitro. *Pharmacol Toxicol* (1999) 85, 201–5.

Lidocaine + H_2-receptor antagonists

Cimetidine modestly reduces the clearance of intravenous and possibly oral lidocaine, and raises its serum levels in some patients. Lidocaine toxicity may occur if the dosage is not reduced. Ranitidine appears to interact minimally. **See also 'Anaesthetics, local + H_2-receptor antagonists', p.111.**

Clinical evidence

(a) Cimetidine in cardiac patients

In one study, 15 patients were given a 1-mg/kg intravenous loading dose of lidocaine followed by a continuous infusion of 2 or 3 mg/minute over 26 hours. At 6 hours the patients were started on cimetidine (initial dose 300 mg intravenously, then 300 mg every 6 hours by mouth). After 26 hours (20 hours after cimetidine was started) the serum levels of lidocaine were 30% higher (5.6 micrograms/mL) than in a control group of 6 patients (4.3 micrograms/mL). The most substantial rise in levels occurred in the first 6 hours after cimetidine was started. Six patients developed toxic serum levels (over 5 micrograms/mL) and two (with levels of 10 and 11 micrograms/mL) experienced lethargy and confusion attributed to lidocaine toxicity, which disappeared when the lidocaine was stopped.[1]

A study in patients with suspected myocardial infarction given two 300-mg oral doses of cimetidine 4 hours apart, starting 11 to 20 hours after a 2 mg/minute infusion of lidocaine began, showed that total lidocaine serum levels had risen by 28%, and unbound levels by 18%, 24 hours after the initial cimetidine dose. In three of these patients whose diagnosis of myocardial infarction was subsequently confirmed, rises in total and unbound lidocaine serum levels of 24% and 9% occurred by 24 hours.[2] In contrast, a study in 6 patients with suspected myocardial infarction given lidocaine infusions, followed later by a cimetidine infusion, failed to find a significant increase in the plasma accumulation of lidocaine.[3]

An 89-year-old man with congestive heart failure taking oral cimetidine had two seizures 10 to 15 minutes after accidental *oral* ingestion of lidocaine solution for oesophageal anaesthesia. He had a high serum lidocaine level of 7.8 micrograms/mL.[4]

(b) Cimetidine in healthy subjects

In a study in 6 healthy subjects cimetidine 300 mg every 6 hours for one day raised the peak serum levels of intravenous lidocaine by 50%. Systemic clearance fell by about 25% (from 766 to 576 mL/minute) and 5 of the 6 experienced toxicity (light-headedness, paraesthesia).[5] Similarly, in another study, oral cimetidine 300 mg four times daily caused a 30% fall in the clearance of intravenous lidocaine.[6] In contrast, in other studies, oral cimetidine 300 mg four times daily caused only 18% and 15% falls in the clearance of intravenous lidocaine under both single-dose and steady-state conditions, which did not reach statistical significance.[7,8] In one study, the effect of intravenous cimetidine 300 mg four times daily was less than that of the oral cimetidine.[8]

Cimetidine pretreatment increased the *oral* bioavailability of lidocaine by 35% in healthy subjects, and reduced the apparent oral clearance by 42%.[9] Another study showed that 2 days of cimetidine pretreatment increased the AUC of lidocaine by 52% after aerosol application of lidocaine 120 mg (12 sprays of *Xylocaine* 10%) to the oropharynx.[10]

(c) Ranitidine in healthy subjects

A study in 10 healthy subjects given 150 mg ranitidine twice daily for 5 days found that it increased the systemic clearance of lidocaine by 9%, but did not alter the oral clearance.[11] In two other studies, ranitidine 150 mg twice daily for 1 to 2 days did not change the clearance of intravenous lidocaine.[7,12]

Mechanism

Not established. It seems possible that the metabolism of lidocaine is reduced both by a fall in blood flow to the liver and by direct inhibition of the activity of the liver microsomal enzymes. As a result its clearance is reduced and its serum levels rise.

Importance and management

The lidocaine/cimetidine interaction is well studied but controversial. It is confused by the differences between the studies (healthy subjects, patients with different diseases, different modes of drug administration, etc). A fall in the clearance of lidocaine (15% or more) and a resultant rise in the serum levels should be looked for if cimetidine is used, but a clinically significant alteration may not occur in every patient. It may possibly be of less importance in patients following a myocardial infarction because of the increased amounts of alpha-1-acid glycoprotein, which alters the levels of bound and free lidocaine.[2] Monitor all patients closely for evidence of toxicity and, where possible, check serum lidocaine levels regularly. A reduced infusion rate may be needed. Ranitidine would appear to be a suitable alternative to cimetidine. See also 'Anaesthetics, local + H_2-receptor antagonists', p.111.

1. Knapp AB, Maguire W, Keren G, Karmen A, Levitt B, Miura DS, Somberg JC. The cimetidine-lidocaine interaction. *Ann Intern Med* (1983) 98, 174–7.
2. Berk SI, Gal P, Bauman JL, Douglas JB, McCue JD, Powell JR. The effect of oral cimetidine on total and unbound serum lidocaine concentrations in patients with suspected myocardial infarction. *Int J Cardiol* (1987) 14, 91–4.
3. Patterson JH, Foster J, Powell JR, Cross R, Wargin W, Clark JL. Influence of a continuous cimetidine infusion on lidocaine plasma concentrations in patients. *J Clin Pharmacol* (1985) 25, 607–9.
4. Parish RC, Moore RT, Gotz VP. Seizures following oral lidocaine for esophageal anesthesia. *Drug Intell Clin Pharm* (1985) 19, 199–201.
5. Feely J, Wilkinson GR, McAllister CB, Wood AJJ. Increased toxicity and reduced clearance of lidocaine by cimetidine. *Ann Intern Med* (1982) 96, 592–4.
6. Bauer LA, Edwards WAD, Randolph FP, Blouin RA. Cimetidine-induced decrease in lidocaine metabolism. *Am Heart J* (1984) 108, 413–15.
7. Jackson JE, Bentley JB, Glass SJ, Fukui T, Gandolfi AJ, Plachetka JR. Effects of histamine-2 receptor blockade on lidocaine kinetics. *Clin Pharmacol Ther* (1985) 37, 544–8.
8. Powell JR, Foster J, Patterson JH, Cross R, Wargin W. Effect of duration of lidocaine infusion and route of cimetidine administration on lidocaine pharmacokinetics. *Clin Pharm* (1986) 5, 993–8.
9. Wing LMH, Miners JO, Birkett DJ, Foenander T, Lillywhite K, Wanwimolruk S. Lidocaine disposition—sex differences and effects of cimetidine. *Clin Pharmacol Ther* (1984) 35, 695–701.
10. Parish RC, Gotz VP, Lopez LM, Mehta JL, Curry SH. Serum lidocaine concentrations following application to the oropharynx: effects of cimetidine. *Ther Drug Monit* (1987) 9, 292–7.
11. Robson RA, Wing LMH, Miners JO, Lillywhite KJ, Birkett DJ. The effect of ranitidine on the disposition of lignocaine. *Br J Clin Pharmacol* (1985) 20, 170–3.
12. Feely J, Guy E. Lack of effect of ranitidine on the disposition of lignocaine. *Br J Clin Pharmacol* (1983) 15, 378–9.

Lidocaine + Itraconazole

Itraconazole may markedly increase the plasma levels of lidocaine after oral administration, but not after intravenous administration or inhalation via a nebuliser.

Clinical evidence

Nine healthy subjects were given either itraconazole 200 mg once daily or placebo for 4 days, in a randomised double-blind crossover study. Itraconazole increased the AUC and peak plasma levels of a single 1-mg/kg oral dose of lidocaine by 75 and 55% respectively. Itraconazole did not affect the concentration of the lidocaine metabolite, monoethylglycinexylidide (MEGX).[1] In similar studies, itraconazole had no effect on the AUC and peak plasma levels of lidocaine or MEGX after 1.5-mg/kg intravenous[2] or nebulised[3] doses of lidocaine.

Mechanism

Itraconazole is an inhibitor of the cytochrome P450 isoenzyme CYP3A4, which is partially involved in the metabolism of lidocaine. Itraconazole appears to markedly reduce the first-pass metabolism of orally administered lidocaine so that its plasma levels rise.[1]

Importance and management

Information seems to be limited, and since lidocaine is not usually given orally the practical importance is minor. However, lidocaine is used for oro-pharyngeal topical anaesthesia, and there have been cases of toxicity after accidental ingestion. There is also a possibility of accidental oral ingestion during inhalation of lidocaine. In patients on itraconazole, the toxicity of oral lidocaine may be markedly increased.

1. Isohanni MH, Neuvonen PJ, Olkkola KT. Effect of erythromycin and itraconazole on the pharmacokinetics of oral lignocaine. *Pharmacol Toxicol* (1999) 84, 143–6.
2. Isohanni MH, Neuvonen PJ, Palkama VJ, Olkkola KT. Effect of erythromycin and itraconazole on the pharmacokinetics of intravenous lignocaine. *Eur J Clin Pharmacol* (1998) 54, 561–5.
3. Isohanni MH, Neuvonen PJ, Olkkola KT. Effect of itraconazole on the pharmacokinetics of inhaled lidocaine. *Basic Clin Pharmacol Toxicol* (2004) 95, 120–3.

Lidocaine + Mexiletine

Mexiletine may increase the toxicity of lidocaine.

Clinical evidence, mechanism, importance and management

A patient with cardiomyopathy taking mexiletine 300 mg twice daily developed lidocaine CNS toxicity within one hour of receiving a total of 600 mg of oral lidocaine for oesophageal burning. Her lidocaine concentration was raised at 26.9 micrograms/mL.[1] Similarly, involuntary motion and muscular stiffness occurred in a man treated with oral mexiletine and an intravenous infusion of lidocaine for one day.[2] Studies in *animals* have shown that the concurrent use of mexiletine and intravenous lidocaine resulted in a decrease in the total clearance of lidocaine and an increase in plasma levels. It appeared that this was due to mexiletine displacing the tissue binding of lidocaine and reducing its distribution.[3] Mexiletine is an oral lidocaine analogue, so it is perhaps not surprising the two drugs may interact. The combination should be used with caution, especially during the initial stages of treatment. Where possible, lidocaine levels should be closely monitored.

1. Geraets DR, Scott SD, Ballew KA. Toxicity potential of oral lidocaine in a patient receiving mexiletine. *Ann Pharmacother* (1992) 26, 1380–1.
2. Christie JM, Valdes C, Markowsky SJ. Neurotoxicity of lidocaine combined with mexiletine. *Anesth Analg* (1993) 77, 1291–4.
3. Maeda Y, Funakoshi S, Nakamura M, Fukuzawa M, Kugaya Y, Yamasaki M, Tsukiai S, Murakami T, Takano M. Possible mechanism for pharmacokinetic interaction between lidocaine and mexiletine. *Clin Pharmacol Ther* (2002) 71, 389–97.

Lidocaine + Omeprazole

Omeprazole does not appear to alter the pharmacokinetics of intravenous lidocaine.

Clinical evidence, mechanism, importance and management

Omeprazole 40 mg daily for one week did not affect the AUC or half-life of lidocaine or its metabolite methylglycinexylidine when a single 1-mg/kg intravenous dose of lidocaine was given to 10 healthy subjects.[1] This study suggests that no special precautions are required during concurrent use.

1. Noble DW, Bannister J, Lamont M, Andersson T, Scott DB. The effect of oral omeprazole on the disposition of lignocaine. *Anaesthesia* (1994) 49, 497–500.

Lidocaine + Phenytoin

The incidence of central toxic adverse effects may be increased following the concurrent intravenous infusion of lidocaine and phenytoin. Sinoatrial arrest has been reported in one patient. In patients taking phenytoin, serum lidocaine levels may be slightly reduced when given intravenously, but markedly reduced if given orally.

Clinical evidence

(a) Cardiac depression and increased adverse effects

A study in 5 patients with suspected myocardial infarction, given lidocaine 0.5 to 3 mg/minute intravenously for at least 24 hours, followed by additional intravenous injections or infusions of phenytoin, found that plasma levels of both drugs remained unchanged but the incidence of adverse effects (vertigo, nausea, nystagmus, diplopia, impaired hearing) were unusually high.[1]

Sinoatrial arrest occurred in a man with heart block following a suspected myocardial infarction, after he received intravenous lidocaine 1 mg/kg over 1 minute, followed 3 minutes later by phenytoin 250 mg given over 5 minutes. The patient lost consciousness and his blood pressure could not be measured, but he responded to a 200-microgram dose of isoprenaline (isoproterenol).[2]

(b) Serum lidocaine levels

In the study described above,[1] intravenous phenytoin had no effect on plasma lidocaine levels during continuous infusion. However, in another study, lidocaine 2 mg/kg was given intravenously to 7 epileptic patients taking their usual anticonvulsants (including phenytoin, barbiturates, phenothiazines, benzodiazepines), and to 6 control subjects. Plasma lidocaine levels were 27 and 43% lower in the epileptic patients at 30 and 60 minutes, respectively.[3] Another study found that the clearance of intravenous lidocaine was slightly greater in patients taking anticonvulsants than in healthy subjects (850 compared with 770 mL/minute) but this difference was not statistically significant.[4] Other studies in epileptic patients and healthy subjects have shown that phenytoin halves the bioavailability of *oral* lidocaine.[4,5]

Mechanism

Phenytoin and lidocaine appear to have additive cardiac depressant actions.

The reduced lidocaine serum levels are possibly due to liver enzyme induction; when lidocaine is given orally the marked reduction in levels results from the stimulation of hepatic first-pass metabolism by phenytoin.[4,5] In addition, patients taking antiepileptics including phenytoin had higher plasma concentrations of alpha-1-acid glycoprotein, which may result in a lower free fraction of lidocaine in the plasma.[6]

Importance and management

Information is limited and the importance of this interaction is not well established. The case of sinoatrial arrest emphasises the need to exercise caution when giving two drugs that have cardiac depressant actions.

The reduction in serum lidocaine levels after intravenous use in patients taking antiepileptics, including phenytoin, is small and appears not to be of any clinical significance. Since lidocaine is not usually given orally, the practical importance of the marked reduction in bioavailability would also seem to be small.

1. Karlsson E, Collste P, Rawlins MD. Plasma levels of lidocaine during combined treatment with phenytoin and procainamide. *Eur J Clin Pharmacol* (1974) 7, 455–9.
2. Wood RA. Sinoatrial arrest: an interaction between phenytoin and lignocaine. *BMJ* (1971) i, 645.
3. Heinonen J, Takki S, Jarho L. Plasma lidocaine levels in patients treated with potential inducers of microsomal enzymes. *Acta Anaesthesiol Scand* (1970) 14, 89–95.
4. Perucca E, Richens A. Reduction of oral bioavailability of lignocaine by induction of first pass metabolism in epileptic patients. *Br J Clin Pharmacol* (1979) 8, 21–31.
5. Perucca E, Hedges A, Makki KA, Richens A. A comparative study of antipyrine and lignocaine disposition in normal subjects and in patients treated with enzyme-inducing drugs. *Br J Clin Pharmacol* (1980) 10, 491–7.
6. Routledge PA, Stargel WW, Finn AL, Barchowsky A, Shand DG. Lignocaine disposition in blood in epilepsy. *Br J Clin Pharmacol* (1981) 12, 663–6.

Lidocaine + Procainamide

An isolated case of delirium has been described in a patient given intravenous lidocaine with procainamide.

Clinical evidence, mechanism, importance and management

A man with paroxysmal tachycardia, treated with oral procainamide 1 g every 5 hours and increasing doses of lidocaine by intravenous infusion (550 mg within 3.5 hours), became restless, noisy and delirious when given a further 250 mg intravenous dose of procainamide.[1] The symptoms disappeared within 20 minutes of discontinuing the lidocaine. The reason is not understood but the symptoms suggest that the neurotoxic effects of the two drugs might be additive. Other studies in patients have shown that lidocaine plasma levels are unaffected by intravenous or oral procainamide.[2]

1. Ilyas M, Owens D, Kvasnicka G. Delirium induced by a combination of anti-arrhythmic drugs. *Lancet* (1969) ii, 1368–9.
2. Karlsson E, Collste P, Rawlins MD. Plasma levels of lidocaine during combined treatment with phenytoin and procainamide. *Eur J Clin Pharmacol* (1974) 7, 455–9.

Lidocaine + Propafenone

Propafenone has minimal effects on the pharmacokinetics of intravenous lidocaine, but the severity and duration of the CNS adverse effects of lidocaine are increased.

Clinical evidence, mechanism, importance and management

Twelve healthy subjects, who had been taking 225 mg propafenone every 8 hours for 4 days, were given a continuous infusion of lidocaine 2 mg/kg/hour for 22 hours. Propafenone increased the AUC of lidocaine by 7% and reduced the clearance by 7%. One poor metaboliser of propafenone had an increase in lidocaine clearance. Increases in the PR and QRS intervals of 10 to 20% were also seen. Combined use increased the severity and duration of adverse effects (lightheadedness, dizziness, paraesthesia, lethargy, somnolence). One subject withdrew from the study as a result.[1] In another study, the combined infusion of lidocaine (100 mg bolus then a 2 mg/minute infusion) and propafenone (1 or 2 mg/kg) produced a minor additional negative inotropic effect (which was not statistically significant) and reversed the prolongation in atrial and ventricular refractoriness produced by propafenone alone.[2]

There would therefore appear to be no marked or important pharmacokinetic interaction between these two drugs, but the increased CNS adverse effects may be poorly tolerated by some individuals, and cardiac depressant effects may be additive.

1. Ujhelyi MR, O'Rangers EA, Fan C, Kluger J, Pharand C, Chow MSS. The pharmacokinetic and pharmacodynamic interaction between propafenone and lidocaine. *Clin Pharmacol Ther* (1993) 53, 38–48.
2. Feld GK, Nademanee K, Singh BN, Kirsten E. Hemodynamic and electrophysiologic effects of combined infusion of lidocaine and propafenone in humans. *J Clin Pharmacol* (1987) 27, 52–9.

Lidocaine + Rifampicin (Rifampin)

Rifampicin may reduce the serum levels of lidocaine given intravenously.

Clinical evidence, mechanism, importance and management

Rifampicin 600 mg daily for 6 days increased the clearance of a 50-mg intravenous dose of lidocaine by 15% in 10 healthy subjects. In addition, plasma concentrations of the lidocaine metabolite monoethylglycinexylidide (MEGX) increased by 34%, although this did not reach statistical significance.[1] Using cultured human hepatocytes it was found that rifampicin increases the metabolism of lidocaine, probably because it induces the cytochrome P450 isoenzyme CYP3A4, which is partially concerned with the metabolism of lidocaine to MEGX.[2] These modest changes in lidocaine pharmacokinetics are unlikely to be of much importance, particularly as the intravenous lidocaine dose is usually titrated to effect.

1. Reichel C, Skodra T, Nacke A, Spengler U, Sauerbruch T. The lignocaine metabolite (MEGX) liver function test and P-450 induction in humans. *Br J Clin Pharmacol* (1998) 46, 535–9.
2. Li AP, Rasmussen A, Xu L, Kaminski DL. Rifampicin induction of lidocaine metabolism in cultured human hepatocytes. *J Pharmacol Exp Ther* (1995) 274, 673–7.

Lidocaine + Tobacco

Tobacco smoking reduces the bioavailability of oral but not intravenous lidocaine.

Clinical evidence, mechanism, importance and management

A study in healthy subjects found that the bioavailability of oral lidocaine was markedly lower in smokers (mean AUCs of 15.2 and 47.9 micrograms/mL per minute in 4 smokers and 5 non-smokers respectively), but when the lidocaine was given intravenously only moderate differences were seen.[1] The reason for the differences is probably due to liver enzyme induction caused by components of tobacco smoke. With oral lidocaine this could result in increased first-pass hepatic clearance. In the case of intravenous lidocaine, first-pass clearance is bypassed, and the enzyme induction was opposed by a smoking-related decrease in hepatic flow. In practical terms this interaction is unlikely to be of much importance since lidocaine is not usually given orally.

1. Huet P-M, Lelorier J. Effects of smoking and chronic hepatitis B on lidocaine and indocyanine green kinetics. *Clin Pharmacol Ther* (1980) 28, 208–15.

Lidocaine + Tocainide

A report describes a tonic-clonic seizure in a man during the period when his treatment was being changed from intravenous lidocaine to oral tocainide.

Clinical evidence, mechanism, importance and management

An elderly man taking furosemide and co-trimoxazole experienced a tonic-clonic seizure while his treatment with intravenous lidocaine was being changed to oral tocainide, although the serum levels of both antiarrhythmics remained within their therapeutic ranges. The patient became progressively agitated and disorientated about 8 hours after starting oral tocainide 600 mg every 6 hours while still receiving lidocaine 2 mg/minute intravenously. About 1 hour later he had a seizure. The patient subsequently tolerated each drug separately, at concentrations similar to those that preceded the seizure, without problems.[1] A study in *animals*[2] showed that tocainide reduces the lidocaine serum levels at which seizures occur by about 45%. Tocainide is no longer widely available, but the manufacturer previously noted that concurrent use of lidocaine and tocainide may cause an increased incidence of adverse effects, including CNS adverse reactions such as seizure, since the two drugs have similar pharmacodynamic effects.[3] Great care must therefore be exercised if tocainide is given during lidocaine use.

1. Forrence E, Covinsky JO, Mullen C. A seizure induced by concurrent lidocaine-tocainide therapy — Is it just a case of additive toxicity? *Drug Intell Clin Pharm* (1986) 20, 56–9.
2. Schuster MR, Paris PM, Kaplan RM, Stewart RD. Effect on the seizure threshold in dogs of tocainide/lidocaine administration. *Ann Emerg Med* (1987) 16, 749–51.
3. Tonocard (Tocainide). AstraZeneca. US Prescribing information, September 2000.

Mexiletine + Amiodarone

Amiodarone does not affect the clearance of mexiletine. The concurrent use of mexiletine and amiodarone can be clinically useful.

Clinical evidence, mechanism, importance and management

The clearance of mexiletine in 10 patients did not differ before and after 1, 3 and 5 months concurrent use of amiodarone. In addition, the clearance of mexiletine did not differ between these patients and 155 other patients not taking amiodarone.[1]

Torsade de pointes has been described in a patient taking amiodarone and mexiletine (a class Ib antiarrhythmic).[2] The manufacturers of mexiletine say that this seems to be an isolated case.[3]

Class Ib antiarrhythmics are usually associated with shortening of the QT interval, and could therefore be expected to reduce the QT prolongation and risk of torsade de pointes seen with amiodarone alone (for examples of this effect of mexiletine see also 'Mexiletine + Beta blockers', p.268 and 'Mexiletine + Quinidine', p.269. However, note that the UK manufacturer of mexiletine[4] says that it may exacerbate arrhythmias [as all antiarrhythmics may], but also that it may be used concurrently with amiodarone. The two drugs have been used together successfully.[5,6]

1. Yonezawa E, Matsumoto K, Ueno K, Tachibana M, Hashimoto H, Komamura K, Kamakura S, Miyatake K, Tanaka K. Lack of interaction between amiodarone and mexiletine in cardiac arrhythmia patients. *J Clin Pharmacol* (2002) 42, 342–6.
2. Tartini R, Kappenberger L, Steinbrunn W. Gefährliche Interaktionen zwischen Amiodaron und Antiarrhythmika der Klasse I. *Schweiz Med Wochenschr* (1982) 112, 1585–7.
3. Boehringer Ingelheim. Personal Communication, July 1995.
4. Mexitil (Mexiletine). Boehringer Ingelheim Ltd. UK Summary of product characteristics, May 2003.
5. Waleffe A, Mary-Rabine L, Legrand V, Demoulin JC, Kulbertus HE. Combined mexiletine and amiodarone treatment of refractory recurrent ventricular tachycardia. *Am Heart J* (1980) 100, 788–93.
6. Hoffmann A, Follath F, Burckhardt D. Safe treatment of resistant ventricular arrhythmias with a combination of amiodarone and quinidine or mexiletine. *Lancet* (1983) i, 704–5.

Mexiletine + Antacids, Atropine or Metoclopramide

The rate of absorption of mexiletine is slowed by the antacid almasilate and atropine and hastened by metoclopramide, but the extent of the absorption is unaltered.

Clinical evidence, mechanism, importance and management

The antacid almasilate (*Gelusil*), given one hour before a single 400-mg dose of mexiletine, resulted in a slight delay in absorption (time to maximum concentration prolonged from 1.7 to 2.9 hours), but had no effect on the extent of absorption in healthy subjects.[1]

A study in 8 healthy subjects found that a single 600-microgram dose of intravenous atropine reduced the rate of absorption of a single 400-mg oral dose of mexiletine, but the mexiletine AUC remained unaffected. Intravenous metoclopramide 10 mg hastened the absorption of mexiletine but similarly did not affect the AUC. Metoclopramide tended to reverse the effect of diamorphine on plasma mexiletine levels in one clinical trial[2] (see also 'Mexiletine + Opioids', p.268).

Since the achievement of steady-state mexiletine levels depends on the extent of absorption, not on its rate, it seems very unlikely that these drugs will affect the antiarrhythmic effects of mexiletine during chronic dosing.[3] However, these drugs may cause variations in the antiarrhythmic effects of initial oral mexiletine doses, which may be a problem if rapid control of the arrhythmia is essential. In general, no special precautions would appear necessary.

1. Herzog P, Holtermüller KH, Kasper W, Meinertz T, Trenk D, Jähnchen E. Absorption of mexiletine after treatment with gastric antacids. *Br J Clin Pharmacol* (1982) 14, 746–7.
2. Smyllie HC, Doar JW, Head CD, Leggett RJ. A trial of intravenous and oral mexiletine in acute myocardial infarction. *Eur J Clin Pharmacol* (1984) 26, 537–42.
3. Wing LMH, Meffin PJ, Grygiel JJ, Smith KJ, Birkett DJ. The effect of metoclopramide and atropine on the absorption of orally administered mexiletine. *Br J Clin Pharmacol* (1980) 9, 505–9.

Mexiletine + Beta blockers

The concurrent use of mexiletine and beta blockers can be clinically useful. Mexiletine may reduce the QT prolonging effects of sotalol.

Clinical evidence, mechanism, importance and management

A study in 4 patients found that a combination of mexiletine and **propranolol** 240 mg daily was more effective in blocking ventricular premature depolarisation (VPD) and ventricular tachycardia than mexiletine alone, and did not increase adverse effects. Plasma mexiletine concentrations were not changed significantly by **propranolol**.[1] Similar efficacy was reported for **metoprolol** with mexiletine.[2] Success in decreasing VPDs was noted in 30% of 44 patients taking mexiletine plus a beta blocker [unspecified] compared with only 14% of 185 subjects taking mexiletine alone.[3] The UK manufacturer of mexiletine states that it may be used concurrently with beta blockers.[4]

A study in *animals* showed that mexiletine reduced the QT prolonging effect of **sotalol** and reduced the risk of torsade de pointes.[5]

1. Leahey EB, Heissenbuttel RH, Giardina E-GV, Bigger JT. Combined mexiletine and propranolol treatment of refractory ventricular tachycardia. *BMJ* (1980) 281, 357–8.
2. Ravid S, Lampert S, Graboys TB. Effect of the combination of low-dose mexiletine and metoprolol on ventricular arrhythmia. *Clin Cardiol* (1991) 14, 951–5.
3. Bigger JT. The interaction of mexiletine with other cardiovascular drugs. *Am Heart J* (1984) 107, 1079–85.
4. Mexitil (Mexiletine). Boehringer Ingelheim Ltd. UK Summary of product characteristics, May 2003.
5. Chézalveil-Guilbert F, Davy J-M, Poirier J-M, Weissenburger J. Mexiletine antagonizes effects of sotalol on QT interval duration and its proarrhythmic effects in a canine model of torsade de pointes. *J Am Coll Cardiol* (1995) 26, 787–92.

Mexiletine + Ciprofloxacin

Ciprofloxacin slightly reduces the clearance of mexiletine, but this is unlikely to be clinically relevant.

Clinical evidence, mechanism, importance and management

A study in healthy subjects found that the oral clearance of mexiletine was reduced by about 8 to 20% when a single dose was given on day 3 of a 5-day course of ciprofloxacin 750 mg twice daily. This was due to a decrease in the metabolic clearance of mexiletine, presumed to occur as a result of ciprofloxacin-induced inhibition of the cytochrome P450 isoenzyme CYP1A2, which is involved in the metabolism of mexiletine.[1] It is unlikely that changes of this magnitude would be clinically relevant.

1. Labbé L, Robitaille NM, Lefez C, Potvin D, Gilbert M, O'Hara G, Turgeon J. Effects of ciprofloxacin on the stereoselective disposition of mexiletine in man. *Ther Drug Monit* (2004) 26, 492–8.

Mexiletine + Fluconazole

Fluconazole does not affect the pharmacokinetics of mexiletine.

Clinical evidence, mechanism, importance and management

Six healthy subjects were given a single 200-mg dose of mexiletine before and after taking fluconazole 200 mg daily for 7 days. Two of the subjects were given fluconazole 400 mg daily for a further 7 days. No significant changes in the pharmacokinetics of mexiletine were seen.[1] The clinical outcome of concurrent use in patients was not studied, but there appear to be no adverse reports in the literature. No special precautions appear to be necessary if these drugs are used concurrently.

1. Ueno K, Yamaguchi R, Tanaka K, Sakaguchi M, Morishima Y, Yamauchi K, Iwai A. Lack of a kinetic interaction between fluconazole and mexiletine. *Eur J Clin Pharmacol* (1996) 50, 129–31.

Mexiletine + H_2-receptor antagonists

The pharmacokinetics of mexiletine were not altered by cimetidine or ranitidine. Cimetidine can reduce the gastric adverse effects of mexiletine.

Clinical evidence, mechanism, importance and management

The peak and trough plasma mexiletine levels of 11 patients were unaltered when they were given **cimetidine** 300 mg four times daily for a week, and the frequency and severity of the ventricular arrhythmias for which they were being treated remained unchanged. Moreover the gastric adverse effects of mexiletine were reduced in half of the patients.[1] This study in patients confirms the findings of two other studies using **cimetidine** or **ranitidine** in healthy subjects.[2,3] There would seem to be no problems associated with giving these drugs concurrently, and some advantages.

1. Klein AL, Sami MH. Usefulness and safety of cimetidine in patients receiving mexiletine for ventricular arrhythmia. *Am Heart J* (1985) 109, 1281–6.
2. Klein A, Sami M, Selinger K. Mexiletine kinetics in healthy subjects taking cimetidine. *Clin Pharmacol Ther* (1985) 37, 669–73.
3. Brockmeyer NH, Breithaupt H, Ferdinand W, von Hattingberg M, Ohnhaus EE. Kinetics of oral and intravenous mexiletine: lack of effect of cimetidine and ranitidine. *Eur J Clin Pharmacol* (1989) 36, 375–8.

Mexiletine + Omeprazole

Omeprazole does not appear to affect the pharmacokinetics of mexiletine.

Clinical evidence, mechanism, importance and management

A crossover study in 9 healthy Japanese men found that when they were given mexiletine 200 mg after taking omeprazole 40 mg daily for 8 days, the mexiletine serum concentrations and its AUCs remained unchanged. It was concluded that omeprazole does not affect the metabolism of mexiletine,[1] and no special precautions would seem to be needed if these drugs are used concurrently.

1. Kusumoto M, Ueno K, Tanaka K, Takeda K, Mashimo K, Kameda T, Fujimura Y, Shibakawa M. Lack of pharmacokinetic interaction between mexiletine and omeprazole. *Ann Pharmacother* (1998) 32, 182–4.

Mexiletine + Opioids

The absorption of mexiletine is reduced following myocardial infarction, and very markedly reduced and delayed if diamorphine or morphine is used concurrently. A higher loading dose may be needed if oral mexiletine is required during the first few hours following a myocardial infarction.

Clinical evidence

A pharmacokinetic study showed that the mean plasma levels of mexiletine (400 mg orally followed by 200 mg 2 hours later) in the first 3 hours were more than 50% lower in 6 patients who had suffered a myocardial infarction and who had been given **diamorphine** 5 to 10 mg or **morphine** 10 to 15 mg than in 4 patients who had not been given opioids. In addition, the AUC_{0-8} was 38.6% lower in those who had received opioids.[1]

In a further study about the prophylactic use of mexiletine, the same authors found that plasma mexiletine levels 3 hours after the first oral dose were 31% lower in 10 patients who had received opioids than in 6 patients who had not. These patients were from a subset who were subsequently shown not to have had a myocardial infarction.[1] In another similar trial of mexiletine in acute myocardial infarction, use of **diamorphine** was associated with low plasma mexiletine levels at 3 hours, and possible reduced efficacy of mexiletine. In this study, pretreatment with intravenous metoclopramide tended to reduce the effect of **diamorphine** on mexiletine absorption,[2] although this was not noted in the other report.[1]

Mechanism

The reduced absorption of mexiletine would seem to result from inhibition of gastric emptying by the opioids. Other mechanisms probably contribute to the delayed clearance of mexiletine.

Importance and management

An established interaction although information is limited. The delay and reduction in the absorption would seem to limit the value of oral mexiletine during the first few hours after a myocardial infarction, particularly if opioid analgesics are used. The manufacturer suggests that a higher loading dose of oral mexiletine may be preferable in this situation. Alternatively, an intravenous dose of mexiletine may be given. In addition, they note that it may be necessary to titrate the dose against therapeutic effects and adverse effects.[3]

1. Pottage A, Campbell RWF, Achuff SC, Murray A, Julian DC, Prescott LF. The absorption of oral mexiletine in coronary care patients. *Eur J Clin Pharmacol* (1978) 13, 393–9.
2. Smyllie HC, Doar JW, Head CD, Leggett RJ. A trial of intravenous and oral mexiletine in acute myocardial infarction. *Eur J Clin Pharmacol* (1984) 26, 537–42.
3. Mexitil (Mexiletine). Boehringer Ingelheim Ltd. UK Summary of product characteristics, May 2003.

Mexiletine + Phenytoin

Plasma mexiletine levels are reduced by phenytoin. An increase in the dosage may be necessary.

Clinical evidence

The observation that 3 patients had unusually low plasma mexiletine levels while taking phenytoin prompted a pharmacokinetic study in 6 healthy subjects. After taking phenytoin 300 mg daily for a week, the mean AUC and half-life of a single 400-mg dose of mexiletine were reduced by an average of about 50% (half-life reduced from 17.2 to 8.4 hours).[1]

Mechanism

The most likely explanation is that phenytoin increases the metabolism of mexiletine by the cytochrome P450 isoenzyme CYP1A2.

Importance and management

Information seems to be limited to this report[1] but the interaction appears to be established. It seems likely that the fall in mexiletine levels will be clinically important in some individuals. Monitor for mexiletine efficacy, and where possible levels. Raise the dosage if necessary.

1. Begg EJ, Chinwah PM, Webb C, Day RO, Wade DN. Enhanced metabolism of mexiletine after phenytoin administration. *Br J Clin Pharmacol* (1982) 14, 219–23.

Mexiletine + Propafenone

Propafenone raises mexiletine serum levels in extensive metabolisers of the cytochrome P450 isoenzyme CYP2D6.

Clinical evidence, mechanism, importance and management

In one study in healthy subjects, propafenone reduced mexiletine clearance and increased plasma mexiletine concentrations in those subjects with extensive cytochrome P450 isoenzyme CYP2D6 activity, but had no effect in those of the poor metaboliser phenotype. The pharmacokinetics of mexiletine in extensive metabolisers after propafenone treatment became the same as those in poor metabolisers.[1] Mexiletine did not affect propafenone pharmacokinetics.[1] In this study, overall changes in ECG parameters were minor during the concurrent use of mexiletine and propafenone.[1] Propafenone is an inhibitor of CYP2D6, and inhibits the metabolism of mexiletine by this pathway.[1] Although the use of the combination was not associated with significant ECG changes, the potentiation of drug effects could predispose to proarrhythmias in patients with ischaemic heart disease. The authors suggest that slow dose titration of the combination may decrease the risk of adverse effects.[1] The UK manufacturer[2] notes that it may be necessary to reduce the dose of mexiletine when it is given with drugs causing inhibition of hepatic enzymes, especially CYP1A2 and CYP2D6.

1. Labbé L, O'Hara G, Lefebvre M, Lessard É, Gilbert M, Adedoyin A, Champagne J, Hamelin B, Turgeon J. Pharmacokinetic and pharmacodynamic interaction between mexiletine and propafenone in human beings. *Clin Pharmacol Ther* (2000) 68, 44–57.
2. Mexitil (Mexiletine). Boehringer Ingelheim Ltd. UK Summary of product characteristics, May 2003.

Mexiletine + Quinidine

The concurrent use of mexiletine and quinidine can be clinically useful. Mexiletine appears to limit the quinidine-induced increase in QT interval. Quinidine raises mexiletine serum levels in extensive metabolisers of cytochrome P450 isoenzyme CYP2D6.

Clinical evidence, mechanism, importance and management

Mexiletine and quinidine given concurrently were reported to be more effective than either drug alone, and the incidence of adverse effects was reduced. Mexiletine limited the quinidine-induced increase in QT interval.[1] A study in *animals* concluded that the benefit of combined use may be due to prolonged refractoriness and conduction time in the peri-infarct zone.[2] Two studies[3,4] in healthy subjects have shown that quinidine reduces the metabolism and excretion of mexiletine in extensive metabolisers of the cytochrome P450 isoenzyme CYP2D6 (total clearance reduced by 24%[4]), but not poor metabolisers. Quinidine is an inhibitor of CYP2D6, and inhibits the metabolism of mexiletine by this pathway. Thus, a pharmacokinetic mechanism may also contribute to the increased efficacy of the combination.[4] The UK manufacturer of mexiletine states that it may be used concurrently with quinidine.[5] They also note that it may be necessary to reduce the dose of mexiletine when used concurrently with drugs causing inhibition of hepatic enzymes, particularly the cytochrome P450 isoenzymes CYP1A2 and CYP2D6.[5]

1. Duff HJ, Roden D, Primm RK, Oates JA, Woosley RL. Mexiletine in the treatment of resistant ventricular arrhythmias: enhancement of efficacy and reduction of dose-related side effects by combination with quinidine. *Circulation* (1983) 67, 1124–8.
2. Duff HJ, Rahmberg M, Sheldon RS. Role of quinidine in the mexiletine-quinidine interaction: electrophysiologic correlates of enhanced antiarrhythmic efficacy. *J Cardiovasc Pharmacol* (1990) 16, 685–92.
3. Broly F, Vandamme N, Caron J, Libersa C, Lhermitte M. Single-dose quinidine treatment inhibits mexiletine oxidation in extensive metabolizers of debrisoquine. *Life Sci* (1991) 48, PL-123–128.
4. Turgeon J, Fiset C, Giguère R, Gilbert M, Moerike K, Rouleau JR, Kroemer HK, Eichelbaum M, Grech-Bélanger O, Bélanger PM. Influence of debrisoquine phenotype and of quinidine on mexiletine disposition in man. *J Pharmacol Exp Ther* (1991) 259, 789–98.
5. Mexitil (Mexiletine). Boehringer Ingelheim Ltd. UK Summary of product characteristics, May 2003.

Mexiletine + Rifampicin (Rifampin)

The clearance of mexiletine is increased by rifampicin. An increase in the dosage of mexiletine may be necessary.

Clinical evidence, mechanism, importance and management

After taking rifampicin 600 mg daily for 10 days, the half-life of a single 400-mg dose of mexiletine was reduced by 40% (from 8.5 to 5 hours) and the AUC fell by 39% in 8 healthy subjects.[1] The probable reason is that the rifampicin (a known, potent enzyme-inducer) increases the metabolism and clearance of mexiletine. It seems likely that the mexiletine dosage will need to be increased during concurrent use. Monitor concurrent use well.

1. Pentikäinen PJ, Koivula IH, Hiltunen HA. Effect of rifampicin treatment on the kinetics of mexiletine. *Eur J Clin Pharmacol* (1982) 23, 261–6.

Mexiletine + SSRIs

Fluvoxamine markedly increases the AUC of mexiletine by inhibiting CYP1A2. Fluoxetine and paroxetine might also be expected to interact, albeit by inhibiting CYP2D6, but sertraline is possibly unlikely to interact.

Clinical evidence, mechanism, importance and management

Fluvoxamine 50 mg twice daily for 7 days increased the AUC of a single 200-mg dose of mexiletine by 55%, and decreased the clearance by 37% in 6 healthy subjects.[1] It is likely that **fluvoxamine** decreases the metabolism of mexiletine by inhibiting the cytochrome P450 isoenzyme CYP1A2, which is partially responsible for the metabolism of mexiletine.[1] The large changes in mexiletine AUC suggest that concurrent therapy should be well monitored.

Mexiletine is also metabolised by CYP2D6 (e.g. see 'Mexiletine + Propafenone', p.269). In an *in vitro* study using human liver microsomes, **paroxetine**, **fluoxetine**, and **sertraline** extensively inhibited the metabolism of mexiletine. Using a model to predict *in vivo* interactions, it was suggested that both **fluoxetine** and **paroxetine** may interact with mexiletine to a clinically relevant extent, whereas **sertraline** is less likely to interact.[2]

The UK manufacturer notes that it may be necessary to reduce the dose of mexiletine when used concurrently with drugs causing inhibition of hepatic enzymes, in particular the cytochrome P450 isoenzymes CYP1A2 and CYP2D6,[3] which is consistent with the proposed mechanism of the interaction.

1. Kusumoto M, Ueno K, Oda A, Takeda K, Mashimo K, Takaya K, Fujimura Y, Nishihori T, Tanaka K. Effect of fluvoxamine on the pharmacokinetics of mexiletine in healthy Japanese men. *Clin Pharmacol Ther* (2001) 69, 104–7.
2. Hara Y, Nakajima M, Miyamoto K-I, Yokoi T. Inhibitory effects of psychotropic drugs on mexiletine metabolism in human liver microsomes: prediction of *in vivo* drug interactions. *Xenobiotica* (2005) 35, 549–60.
3. Mexitil (Mexiletine). Boehringer Ingelheim Ltd. UK Summary of product characteristics, May 2003.

Mexiletine + Urinary acidifiers or alkalinisers

Large changes in urinary pH caused by acidifying or alkalinising drugs can have a marked effect on the plasma levels of mexiletine in some patients.

Clinical evidence

In 4 healthy subjects, a single 200-mg intravenous dose of mexiletine was given, once when the urine was acidic (pH 5) after administration of **ammonium chloride**, and once when the urine was alkaline (pH 8) after administration of **sodium bicarbonate**. The plasma elimination half-life was significantly shorter when the urine was acidic (2.8 hours) compared with when it was alkaline (8.6 hours). In addition, the percentage of mexiletine excreted unchanged in the urine was 57.5% when acidic and just 0.6% when alkaline.[1] Similar results were found in another study.[2] A further study in patients with uncontrolled urine pH (range 5.04 to 7.86) given mexiletine orally for 5 days found that the plasma concentration of mexiletine correlated with urine pH. In addition, it was predicted that a normal variation in pH could cause more than a 50% variation in plasma mexiletine levels.[3] A later comprehensive pharmacokinetic study in 5 healthy subjects confirmed that renal clearance of mexiletine was 4 mL/minute in alkaline urine (pH 8) compared with 168 mL/minute in acidic urine (pH 5.2). In two subjects, this resulted in an increase in plasma concentrations of 61% and 96%, but in the other three the increase was less than 20%. Non-renal clearance (metabolic clearance) increased in the three subjects with little change in plasma concentrations, but was unaffected in the two with marked changes.[4]

Mechanism

Mexiletine is a basic drug, and undergoes greater reabsorption by the kidneys when in the non-ionised form in alkaline urine. Mexiletine is also extensively cleared from the body by liver metabolism and only about 10% is excreted unchanged in the urine at physiological pH, although this is variable. Any changes in the renal clearance of mexiletine that occur as a result of urinary pH changes might therefore be expected to be compensated by an increase in metabolic clearance, but this does not seem to occur in all patients.[4]

Importance and management

Although changes in urinary pH can affect the amount of mexiletine lost in the urine, the effect of diet or the concurrent use of alkalinisers (sodium bicarbonate, **acetazolamide**) or acidifiers (ammonium chloride etc.) on the plasma concentrations of mexiletine does not appear to be predictable. There appear to be no reports of adverse interactions but concurrent use should be monitored. The UK manufacturer of mexiletine recommends that the concomitant use of drugs that markedly acidify or alkalinise the urine should be avoided.[5]

1. Kiddie MA, Kaye CM, Turner P, Shaw TRD. The influence of urinary pH on the elimination of mexiletine. *Br J Clin Pharmacol* (1974) 1, 229–32.
2. Beckett AH, Chidomere EC. The distribution, metabolism and excretion of mexiletine in man. *Postgrad Med J* (1977) 53 (Suppl 1), 60–6.
3. Johnston A, Burgess CD, Warrington SJ, Wadsworth J, Hamer NAJ. The effect of spontaneous changes in urinary pH on mexiletine plasma concentrations and excretion during chronic administration to healthy volunteers. *Br J Clin Pharmacol* (1979) 8, 349–52.
4. Mitchell BG, Clements JA, Pottage A, Prescott LF. Mexiletine disposition: individual variation in response to urine acidification and alkalinisation. *Br J Clin Pharmacol* (1983) 16, 281–4.
5. Mexitil (Mexiletine). Boehringer Ingelheim Ltd. UK Summary of product characteristics, May 2003.

Moracizine + Cimetidine

Cimetidine increases the plasma levels of moracizine but the clinical importance of this is uncertain.

Clinical evidence, mechanism, importance and management

In a study in 8 healthy subjects cimetidine 300 mg four times daily for 7 days, halved the clearance of a single 500-mg dose of moracizine and increased both its half-life and AUC by 39%. It is believed that this is because the cimetidine reduces moracizine metabolism by the liver.[1] Despite the increase in plasma moracizine levels, the PR and QRS intervals were not further prolonged. One possible explanation (so it is postulated) is that some of the metabolites of moracizine, whose production is inhibited by cimetidine, could also be pharmacologically active. Concurrent use should be well monitored, but measuring plasma moracizine levels may be of limited value because of the potential effects of the moracizine metabolites.

1. Biollaz J, Shaheen O, Wood AJJ. Cimetidine inhibition of ethmozine metabolism. *Clin Pharmacol Ther* (1985) 37, 665–8.

Moracizine + Diltiazem

A pharmacokinetic interaction occurs between moracizine and diltiazem resulting in increased systemic availability of moracizine and decreased systemic availability of diltiazem.

Clinical evidence, mechanism, importance and management

After 16 healthy subjects took both diltiazem 60 mg and moracizine 250 mg every 8 hours for 7 days, the maximum plasma concentration of moracizine was increased by 89%, the AUC was increased by 121%, and clearance was decreased by 54%. In contrast, the maximum plasma concentration and AUC of diltiazem decreased by 36% and clearance was increased by 52%. The AUCs for the diltiazem metabolites were not significantly affected. No clinically significant changes in ECG parameters were seen. However, the frequency of adverse events (e.g. headache, dizziness, paraesthesia) was greater on concurrent use (76%) than with either drug alone (54 and 45% for moracizine and diltiazem respectively).[1] Diltiazem probably inhibits the hepatic metabolism of moracizine while moracizine increases that of diltiazem. The clinical significance of this interaction is not known. However, particular caution is advised if diltiazem and moracizine are given concurrently, in light of the increase in adverse events. Dose adjustments may also be required to obtain optimum therapeutic responses.[1]

1. Shum L, Pieniaszek HJ, Robinson CA, Davidson AF, Widner PJ, Benedek IH, Flamenbaum W. Pharmacokinetic interactions of moricizine and diltiazem in healthy volunteers. *J Clin Pharmacol* (1996) 36, 1161–8.

Moracizine + Propranolol

Moracizine appears not to interact adversely with propranolol.

Clinical evidence, mechanism, importance and management

The efficacy and tolerability of the combination of propranolol and moracizine was compared with either drug alone in patients with ventricular arrhythmias in controlled trials. The combination was well tolerated, with no evidence of any adverse interactions, nor any beneficial interactions.

However, the dose of propranolol used was fairly low at 120 mg daily.[1,2] Further study is needed.

1. Pratt CM, Butman SM, Young JB, Knoll M, English LD. Antiarrhythmic efficacy of Ethmozine® (moricizine HCl) compared with disopyramide and propranolol. *Am J Cardiol* (1987) 60, 52F–58F.
2. Butman SM, Knoll ML, Gardin JM. Comparison of ethmozine to propranolol and the combination for ventricular arrhythmias. *Am J Cardiol* (1987) 60, 603–7.

Pirmenol + Cimetidine

Cimetidine 300 mg four times daily for 8 days had no significant effect on the pharmacokinetics of single 150-mg oral doses of pirmenol in 8 healthy subjects.[1] No clinically important interaction would therefore be expected in patients given both drugs.

1. Stringer KA, Lebsack ME, Cetnarowski-Cropp AB, Goldfarb AL, Radulovic LL, Bockbrader HN, Chang T, Sedman AJ. Effect of cimetidine administration on the pharmacokinetics of pirmenol. *J Clin Pharmacol* (1992) 32, 91–4.

Pirmenol + Rifampicin (Rifampin)

Rifampicin markedly increases the loss of pirmenol from the body. A reduction in its antiarrhythmic effects is likely to occur.

Clinical evidence, mechanism, importance and management

Treatment with rifampicin 600 mg daily for 14 days markedly affected the pharmacokinetics of a single 150-mg dose of pirmenol in 12 healthy subjects.[1] The apparent plasma clearance increased sevenfold and the AUC decreased by 83%.[1] The probable reason is that rifampicin increases the hepatic metabolism of pirmenol. Monitor well and anticipate the need to increase the dosage of pirmenol if rifampicin is used concurrently.

1. Stringer KA, Cetnarowski AB, Goldfarb AB, Lebsack ME, Chang TS, Sedman AJ. Enhanced pirmenol elimination by rifampin. *J Clin Pharmacol* (1988) 28, 1094–7.

Procainamide + Amiodarone

When procainamide and amiodarone are used together the QT interval prolonging effects are increased, therefore the combination should generally be avoided. Serum procainamide levels are increased by about 60% and *N*-acetylprocainamide levels by about 30% by amiodarone. If the combination is used, the dosage of procainamide will need to be reduced to avoid toxicity.

Clinical evidence

Twelve patients were stabilised on procainamide (2 to 6 g daily, or about 900 mg every 6 hours). When amiodarone (600 mg loading dose every 12 hours for 5 to 7 days, then 600 mg daily) was also given their mean serum procainamide levels rose by 57% (from 6.8 to 10.6 micrograms/mL) and their serum levels of the metabolite *N*-acetylprocainamide (NAPA) rose by 32% (from 6.9 to 9.1 micrograms/mL). Procainamide levels increased by more than 3 micrograms/mL in 6 patients. The increases usually occurred within 24 hours, but in other patients they occurred as late as 4 or 5 days. Toxicity was seen in 2 patients. Despite lowering the procainamide dosages by 20%, serum procainamide levels were still higher (at 7.7 micrograms/mL) than before the amiodarone was started.[1]

In another study, intravenous procainamide was given once before (at a mean dose of 13 mg/kg), and once during (at a 30% reduced dose: mean 9.2 mg/kg) the use of amiodarone 1.6 g daily for 7 to 14 days. Amiodarone decreased the clearance of procainamide by 23% and increased its elimination half-life by 38%. Both drugs prolonged the QRS and QTc intervals, and the extent of prolongation was significantly greater with the combination than either drug alone.[2]

Mechanism

The mechanism behind the pharmacokinetic interaction is not understood. The QT prolonging effects of the two drugs would be expected to be additive.

Importance and management

Information appears to be limited to these studies, but the interaction would seem to be established and clinically important. The use of amiodarone with procainamide further prolongs the QTc interval, which can increase the risk of torsade de pointes. Therefore, the combination should generally be avoided. The UK manufacturers of amiodarone contraindicate its use with class Ia antiarrhythmics such as procainamide,[3] whereas the US manufacturers of amiodarone recommend that such combined therapy should be reserved for life-threatening ventricular arrhythmias incompletely responsive to either drug alone and recommend that the procainamide dosage should be reduced by one-third.[4] See also 'Drugs that prolong the QT interval + Other drugs that prolong the QT interval', p.257. This is similar to the recommendation made by the authors of the pharmacokinetic studies, who suggest that the dosage of procainamide may need to be reduced by 20 to 50%. They also suggest that serum levels should be monitored and patients observed for adverse effects.[1,2] Remember that the interaction can develop within 24 hours.

1. Saal AK, Werner JA, Greene HL, Sears GK, Graham EL. Effect of amiodarone on serum quinidine and procainamide levels. *Am J Cardiol* (1984) 53, 1264–7.
2. Windle J, Prystowsky EN, Miles WM, Heger JJ. Pharmacokinetic and electrophysiologic interactions of amiodarone and procainamide. *Clin Pharmacol Ther* (1987) 41, 603–10.
3. Cordarone X (Amiodarone hydrochloride). Sanofi-Aventis. UK Summary of product characteristics, April 2006.
4. Cordarone (Amiodarone hydrochloride). Wyeth Pharmaceuticals. US Prescribing information, May 2007.

Procainamide + Antacids or Antidiarrhoeals

There is some inconclusive evidence that aluminium phosphate may possibly cause a small reduction in the absorption of procainamide. Kaolin-pectin appears to reduce the bioavailability of procainamide.

Clinical evidence, mechanism, importance and management

A single 11-g dose of an **aluminium phosphate** antacid modestly reduced the AUC of a single 750-mg oral dose of procainamide by 14.6%.[1] The clinical importance of this interaction is uncertain, but probably small.

Kaolin-pectin was found to reduce the peak saliva concentrations and AUC of a single 250-mg dose of procainamide by about 30% in 4 healthy subjects. **Kaolin-pectin** and a variety of antacids (***Pepto-bismol***, ***Simeco***, and **magnesium trisilicate**) absorbed procainamide *in vitro*.[2] The clinical importance of this is also uncertain.

1. Albin H, Vincon G, Bertolaso D, Dangoumau J. Influence du phosphate d'aluminium sur la biodisponibilité de la procaïnamide et du disopyramide. *Therapie* (1981) 36, 541–6.
2. Al-Shora HI, Moustafa MA, Niazy EM, Gaber M, Gouda MW. Interactions of procainamide, verapamil, guanethidine and hydralazine with adsorbent antacids and antidiarrhoeal mixtures. *Int J Pharmaceutics* (1988) 47, 209–13.

Procainamide + Beta blockers

The pharmacokinetics of procainamide are little changed by either propranolol or metoprolol. Both sotalol and procainamide have QT-interval prolonging effects, which may be additive if they are used together.

Clinical evidence, mechanism, importance and management

Preliminary results of a study in 6 healthy subjects found that long-term treatment with **propranolol** [period and dosage not stated] increased the procainamide half-life from 1.71 to 2.66 hours and reduced the plasma clearance by 16%.[1] However, a later study in 8 healthy subjects found that the pharmacokinetics of a single 500-mg dose of procainamide were only slightly altered by **propranolol** 80 mg three times daily or **metoprolol** 100 mg twice daily. The procainamide half-life of 1.9 hours increased to 2.2 hours with **propranolol**, and to 2.3 hours with **metoprolol**, but no significant changes in total clearance occurred. No changes in the AUC of the metabolite *N*-acetylprocainamide were seen.[2] It seems unlikely that a clinically important adverse interaction normally occurs between these drugs.

A clinical study describes the successful use of procainamide with **sotalol**.[3] However, both **sotalol** and procainamide can prolong the QT interval, and there may be an increased risk of torsade de pointes arrhythmias if they are used together. See also 'Drugs that prolong the QT interval + Other drugs that prolong the QT interval', p.257.

1. Weidler DJ, Garg DC, Jallad NS, McFarland MA. The effect of long-term propranolol administration on the pharmacokinetics of procainamide in humans. *Clin Pharmacol Ther* (1981) 29, 289.
2. Ochs HR, Carstens G, Roberts G-M, Greenblatt DJ. Metoprolol or propranolol does not alter the kinetics of procainamide. *J Cardiovasc Pharmacol* (1983) 5, 392–5.
3. Dorian P, Newman D, Berman N, Hardy J, Mitchell J. Sotalol and type IA drugs in combination prevent recurrence of sustained ventricular tachycardia. *J Am Coll Cardiol* (1993) 22, 106–13.

Procainamide + H_2-receptor antagonists

Serum procainamide levels can be increased by cimetidine and toxicity may develop, particularly in those who have a reduced renal clearance, such as the elderly. Ranitidine and famotidine appear to interact only minimally or not at all.

Clinical evidence

(a) Cimetidine

In one study, 36 elderly patients (65 to 90 years old) taking sustained-release oral procainamide every 6 hours had rises in mean steady-state serum levels of procainamide and its metabolite *N*-acetylprocainamide of 55 and 36% respectively, after taking cimetidine 300 mg every 6 hours for 3 days. This was tolerated in 24 patients without adverse effects (serum procainamide and *N*-acetylprocainamide less than 12 mg/L and less than 15 mg/L respectively) but the other 12 had some adverse effects (nausea, weakness, malaise PR interval increases of less than 20%), which was dealt with by stopping one or both drugs.[1] Another report describes an elderly man who developed procainamide toxicity when given cimetidine 1.2 g daily. His procainamide dosage was roughly halved (from 937.5 to 500 mg every 6 hours) to bring his serum procainamide and *N*-acetylprocainamide levels into the accepted therapeutic range.[2]

Four studies in healthy subjects have found that cimetidine increased the procainamide AUC by 24 to 43%, and decreased the renal clearance by 31 to 40%,[3-6] these changes occurring even with single doses of cimetidine.[5] A steady-state procainamide serum level increase of 43% has been seen when cimetidine 1.2 g daily was also given.[6]

(b) Famotidine

Famotidine 40 mg daily for 5 days did not affect the pharmacokinetics or pharmacodynamics of a single 5-mg/kg intravenous dose of procainamide in 8 healthy subjects.[7]

(c) Ranitidine

One study[8] found that ranitidine 150 mg twice daily for one day reduced the absorption of procainamide from the gut by 10% and reduced its renal excretion by 19%, increasing the procainamide and *N*-acetylprocainamide AUC by about 14%. However, no change in the steady-state pharmacokinetics of procainamide was found with ranitidine 150 mg twice daily in another study, except that ranitidine delayed the time to maximum plasma concentration (from 1.4 to 2.7 hours).[6] In a further study, ranitidine 150 mg twice daily for 4 days caused no significant changes in the mean pharmacokinetics of oral procainamide 1 g in 13 healthy subjects. However, it appeared that subjects had either a modest 20% increase or decrease in procainamide clearance, with the direction of change related to their baseline procainamide clearance: the higher the baseline clearance the greater the decrease caused by ranitidine.[9]

Mechanism

Procainamide levels in the body are increased because cimetidine reduces its renal excretion by about one-third or more, but the precise mechanism is uncertain. One suggestion is that it interferes with the active secretion of procainamide by the kidney tubules.[3,4]

Importance and management

The interaction between procainamide and cimetidine is established. Concurrent use should be undertaken with care because the safety margin of procainamide is low. Reduce the procainamide dosage as necessary. This is particularly important in the elderly because they have a reduced ability to clear both drugs. Ranitidine and famotidine appear not to interact to a clinically important extent, but it should be appreciated that what is known is based on studies in healthy subjects rather than patients.

1. Bauer LA, Black D, Gensler A. Procainamide-cimetidine drug interaction in elderly male patients. *J Am Geriatr Soc* (1990) 38, 467–9.
2. Higbee MD, Wood JS, Mead RA. Case report. Procainamide-cimetidine interaction. A potential toxic interaction in the elderly. *J Am Geriatr Soc* (1984) 32, 162–4.
3. Somogyi A, McLean A, Heinzow B. Cimetidine-procainamide pharmacokinetic interaction in man: evidence of competition for tubular secretion of basic drugs. *Eur J Clin Pharmacol* (1983) 25, 339–45.
4. Christian CD, Meredith CG, Speeg KV. Cimetidine inhibits renal procainamide clearance. *Clin Pharmacol Ther* (1984) 36, 221–7.
5. Lai MY, Jiang FM, Chung CH, Chen HC, Chao PDL. Dose dependent effect of cimetidine on procainamide disposition in man. *Int J Clin Pharmacol Ther Toxicol* (1988) 26, 118–21.
6. Rodvold KA, Paloucek FP, Jung D, Gallastegui J. Interaction of steady-state procainamide with H_2-receptor antagonists cimetidine and ranitidine. *Ther Drug Monit* (1987) 9, 378–83.
7. Klotz U, Arvela P, Rosenkranz B. Famotidine, a new H_2-receptor antagonist, does not affect hepatic elimination of diazepam or tubular secretion of procainamide. *Eur J Clin Pharmacol* (1985) 28, 671–5.
8. Somogyi A, Bochner F. Dose and concentration dependent effect of ranitidine on procainamide disposition and renal clearance in man. *Br J Clin Pharmacol* (1984) 18, 175–81.
9. Rocci ML, Kosoglou T, Ferguson RK, Vlasses PH. Ranitidine-induced changes in the renal and hepatic clearances of procainamide are correlated. *J Pharmacol Exp Ther* (1989) 248, 923–8.

Procainamide + Para-aminobenzoic acid (PABA)

A single case report found that para-aminobenzoic acid (PABA) increased the serum levels of procainamide and reduced the serum levels of the procainamide metabolite *N*-acetylprocainamide. In contrast, a later pharmacokinetic study in healthy subjects found that PABA had no effect on serum procainamide levels, and increased serum *N*-acetylprocainamide levels.

Clinical evidence, mechanism, importance and management

A 61-year-old man who had sustained ventricular tachycardia, which did not respond adequately to oral procainamide, was found to be a fast acetylator of procainamide, which resulted in particularly high serum levels of the procainamide metabolite (*N*-acetylprocainamide) when compared with the procainamide levels. When he was also given para-aminobenzoic acid (PABA) 1.5 g every 6 hours for 30 hours, to suppress the production of this metabolite, the serum level of procainamide increased, that of *N*-acetylprocainamide decreased, and control of his arrhythmia improved.[1] However, a later study in 10 healthy subjects, who were also fast acetylators, found that PABA did not significantly affect the pharmacokinetics of procainamide. In addition, although PABA inhibited the production of *N*-acetylprocainamide, it also inhibited renal excretion, so that the AUC and elimination half-life were increased. This suggests that PABA may in fact not be useful for increasing the efficacy and safety of procainamide.[2]

These contradictory findings are difficult to explain, but neither report suggests that concurrent use need be avoided.

1. Nylen ES, Cohen AI, Wish MH, Lima JL, Finkelstein JD. Reduced acetylation of procainamide by para-aminobenzoic acid. *J Am Coll Cardiol* (1986) 7, 185–7.
2. Tisdale JE, Rudis MI, Padhi ID, Svensson CK, Webb CR, Borzak S, Ware JA, Krepostman A, Zarowitz BJ. Inhibition of N-acetylation of procainamide by para-aminobenzoic acid in humans. *J Clin Pharmacol* (1995) 35, 902–10.

Procainamide + Probenecid

The pharmacokinetics of a single 750-mg intravenous dose of procainamide and its effects on the QT interval were not altered by the prior administration of probenecid 2 g in 6 healthy subjects.[1] No special precautions appear to be necessary.

1. Lam YWF, Boyd RA, Chin SK, Chang D, Giacomini KM. Effect of probenecid on the pharmacokinetics and pharmacodynamics of procainamide. *J Clin Pharmacol* (1991) 31, 429–32.

Procainamide + Quinidine

A single case report describes a marked increase in the plasma procainamide levels of a patient when he was also given quinidine. The combination prolongs the QT interval, and should generally be avoided because of the increased risk of torsade de pointes.

Clinical evidence

A man with sustained ventricular tachycardia taking high-dose intravenous procainamide 2 g every 8 hours had a 70% increase in his steady-state plasma procainamide levels, from 9.1 to 15.4 nanograms/mL, when he also took quinidine gluconate 324 mg every 8 hours. The procainamide half-life increased from 3.7 to 7.2 hours and its clearance fell from 27 to 16 L/hour. His QTc interval increased from 648 to 678 milliseconds.[1] In another study in patients with ventricular arrhythmias, quinidine was combined with procainamide. The doses were adjusted based in part on the QT interval. The QTc interval was longer with the combination (499 milliseconds) than each drug alone (quinidine 470 milliseconds, procainamide 460 milliseconds) despite using reduced doses in the combination (mean quinidine dose reduced by 28%; mean procainamide dose reduced by 32%).[2]

Mechanism

It has been suggested that the quinidine interferes with one or more of the renal pathways by which procainamide is cleared from the body.[1]

Importance and management

Information on the possible pharmacokinetic interaction seems to be limited to this report. Both quinidine and procainamide are class Ia antiarrhythmics and prolong the QT interval, an effect that is increased with the combination. Such combinations should generally be avoided because of the increased risk of torsade de pointes. See also 'Drugs that prolong the QT interval + Other drugs that prolong the QT interval', p.257.

1. Hughes B, Dyer JE, Schwartz AB. Increased procainamide plasma concentrations caused by quinidine: a new drug interaction. *Am Heart J* (1987) 114, 908–9.
2. Kim SG, Seiden SW, Matos JA, Waspe LE, Fisher JD. Combination of procainamide and quinidine for better tolerance and additive effects for ventricular arrhythmias. *Am J Cardiol* (1985) 56, 84–8.

Procainamide + Quinolones

Ofloxacin and levofloxacin cause moderate increases in the serum levels of procainamide, whereas ciprofloxacin has a lesser effect. However, the ECG appears to be unaltered in studies in healthy subjects given these quinolones with procainamide. An increased risk of torsade de pointes would be expected if procainamide is used with gatifloxacin, moxifloxacin, or sparfloxacin, and possibly levofloxacin.

Clinical evidence

Nine healthy subjects were given a single 1-g oral dose of procainamide alone, then again with the fifth dose of **ofloxacin** (400 mg given twice daily for five doses). **Ofloxacin** increased the AUC of procainamide by 27%, increased the maximum plasma levels by 21% (from 4.8 to 5.8 micrograms/L) and reduced the total clearance by 22%, whereas the pharmacokinetics of the active metabolite of procainamide (*N*-acetylprocainamide) were not significantly altered.[1] In another study 10 healthy subjects were given **levofloxacin** 500 mg once daily or **ciprofloxacin** 500 mg twice daily and a single 15-mg/kg intravenous dose of procainamide on day 5. **Levofloxacin** increased the AUC of procainamide by 21% and prolonged the half-life by about 19% (from 2.7 to 3.2 hours). The clearance of procainamide was reduced by 17% (range 4 to 46%) with renal clearance reduced by 26% (range 11 to 58%) by **levofloxacin**. The pharmacokinetics of *N*-acetylprocainamide were similarly affected. **Ciprofloxacin** caused only minor changes in procainamide and *N*-acetylprocainamide pharmacokinetics, although the renal clearance of procainamide was reduced by 15% (range 3 to 26%).[2]

Despite the pharmacokinetic changes, no ECG changes were detected. However, these studies[1,2] involved only single doses of procainamide with average maximum serum levels (about 4 to 6 micrograms/mL) in the lower end of the therapeutic range for procainamide, although in one study individual levels of up to 8.5 micrograms/mL were found.[1]

One case of torsade de pointes was noted in a patient taking procainamide with a quinolone [unspecified] in an analysis of cases of torsade de pointes associated with quinolones on the FDA Adverse Events Reporting System database up to May 2001. The quinolones included were **ciprofloxacin, ofloxacin, levofloxacin, gatifloxacin**, and **moxifloxacin**, and in total there were 37 cases identified, of which 19 occurred in patients also taking other drugs known to prolong the QT interval.[3]

Mechanism

The probable reason for the interaction is that levofloxacin, ofloxacin and to a lesser extent ciprofloxacin, inhibit the secretion of unchanged procainamide by the kidney tubules via renal drug transporters. Levofloxacin also appears to inhibit the secretion of *N*-acetylprocainamide.

Importance and management

These results suggest that ofloxacin and levofloxacin interact to a modest extent and ciprofloxacin to a lesser extent with procainamide. The large interpatient variation found in these studies suggests it is possible that many patients will not experience a clinically significant interaction. However, in slow acetylators, in whom renal clearance contributes to a larger fraction of total clearance, and those on higher doses of procainamide (serum levels greater than 10 micrograms/mL), the use of quinolones could result in pharmacodynamic changes. Therefore, it would be prudent to monitor the outcome if procainamide and ofloxacin or ciprofloxacin are given together in patients. Monitoring has been recommended if procainamide is given with levofloxacin.[2] However, as there is also evidence that levofloxacin may prolong the QT interval (see 'Amiodarone + Quinolones', p.249) it may be best to avoid concurrent use of this quinolone and procainamide.

Of the quinolones used clinically, gatifloxacin, moxifloxacin, and **sparfloxacin** are known to prolong the QT interval (see 'Table 9.2', (p.257)) and would be expected to increase the risk of torsade de pointes arrhythmias when used with procainamide. These quinolones should probably be avoided in patients on procainamide (see also 'Drugs that prolong the QT interval + Other drugs that prolong the QT interval', p.257).

1. Martin DE, Shen J, Griener J, Raasch R, Patterson JH, Cascio W. Effects of ofloxacin on the pharmacokinetics and pharmacodynamics of procainamide. *J Clin Pharmacol* (1996) 36, 85–91.
2. Bauer LA, Black DJ, Lill JS, Garrison J, Raisys VA, Hooton TM. Levofloxacin and ciprofloxacin decrease procainamide and *N*-acetylprocainamide renal clearances. *Antimicrob Agents Chemother* (2005) 49, 1649–51.
3. Frothingham R. Rates of torsades de pointes associated with ciprofloxacin, ofloxacin, levofloxacin, gatifloxacin, and moxifloxacin. *Pharmacotherapy* (2001) 21, 1468–72.

Procainamide + Sucralfate

Sucralfate does not appear to affect the absorption of procainamide.

Clinical evidence, mechanism, importance and management

In 4 healthy subjects sucralfate 1 g taken 30 minutes before a single 250-mg dose of procainamide reduced the mean maximum salivary level of procainamide by 5.3%, but did not significantly affect either the AUC or the rate of absorption.[1] These results suggest that a clinically significant interaction is unlikely.

1. Turkistani AAA, Gaber M, Al-Meshal MA, Al-Shora HI, Gouda MW. Effect of sucralfate on procainamide absorption. *Int J Pharmaceutics* (1990) 59, R1–R3.

Procainamide + Trimethoprim

Trimethoprim causes a marked increase in the plasma levels of procainamide and its active metabolite, *N*-acetylprocainamide, which increases the risk of toxicity.

Clinical evidence

Eight healthy subjects were given procainamide 500 mg every 6 hours for 3 days. The concurrent use of trimethoprim 200 mg daily increased the AUC_{0-12} of procainamide and its active metabolite, *N*-acetylprocainamide (NAPA), by 63% and 51%, respectively. The renal clearance of procainamide and NAPA decreased by 47% and 13%, respectively. The QTc prolonging effects of procainamide were increased to a significant, but slight, extent by trimethoprim.[1] Another study found that trimethoprim 200 mg daily reduced the renal clearance of a single 1-g dose of procainamide by 45% and of NAPA by 26%. The QTc interval was increased from 400 to 430 milliseconds.[2]

Mechanism

Trimethoprim decreases the renal clearance of both procainamide and its active metabolite by competing for active tubular secretion. It may also cause a small increase in the conversion of procainamide to *N*-acetylprocainamide.[1]

Importance and management

An established interaction but its documentation is limited. The need to reduce the procainamide dosage should be anticipated if trimethoprim is given to patients already controlled on procainamide. In practice the effects may be greater than the studies cited suggest because the elderly lose procainamide through the kidneys more slowly than young healthy subjects. Remember too that the daily dosage of trimethoprim in **co-trimoxazole** (trimethoprim 160 mg with sulfamethoxazole 800 mg) may equal or exceed the dosages used in the studies cited.

1. Kosoglou T, Rocci ML, Vlasses PH. Trimethoprim alters the disposition of procainamide and N-acetylprocainamide. *Clin Pharmacol Ther* (1988) 44, 467–77.
2. Vlasses PH, Kosoglou T, Chase SL, Greenspon AJ, Lottes S, Andress E, Ferguson RK, Rocci ML. Trimethoprim inhibition of the renal clearance of procainamide and N-acetylprocainamide. *Arch Intern Med* (1989) 149, 1350–3.

Propafenone + Barbiturates

Phenobarbital increases the metabolism of propafenone and reduces its serum levels.

Clinical evidence, mechanism, importance and management

In a preliminary report of a study in 7 non-smoking subjects who were fast metabolisers of propafenone, **phenobarbital** 100 mg daily for 3 weeks reduced the levels of a single 300-mg dose of propafenone by 26 to 87% and the AUC by 10 to 89%. The intrinsic clearance increased by 11 to 84%. The results in a further 4 heavy smokers were similar.[1] These changes probably occur because **phenobarbital** (a potent stimulator of liver enzymes) increases the metabolism of the propafenone. The clinical importance of this awaits assessment, but check that propafenone remains effective if **phenobarbital** is added, and that toxicity does not occur if it is stopped. If the suggested mechanism is correct, other barbiturates would be expected to interact similarly.

1. Chan GL-Y, Axelson JE, Kerr CR. The effect of phenobarbital on the pharmacokinetics of propafenone in man. *Pharm Res* (1988) 5, S153.

Propafenone + Cimetidine

Cimetidine appears to interact minimally with propafenone.

Clinical evidence, mechanism, importance and management

A study in 12 healthy subjects (10 extensive metabolisers and 2 poor metabolisers of propafenone) given propafenone 225 mg every 8 hours found that the concurrent use of cimetidine 400 mg every 8 hours caused some changes in the pharmacokinetics and pharmacodynamics of the propafenone, with wide intersubject variability. Raised mean peak and steady-state plasma levels were seen (24 and 22%, respectively), but these did not reach statistical significance. A slight increase in the QRS duration also occurred.[1] However, none of the changes were considered clinically important.

1. Pritchett ELC, Smith WM, Kirsten EB. Pharmacokinetic and pharmacodynamic interactions of propafenone and cimetidine. *J Clin Pharmacol* (1988) 28, 619–24.

Propafenone + Erythromycin

Limited evidence suggests that erythromycin may inhibit the metabolism of propafenone.

Clinical evidence, mechanism, importance and management

The preliminary results of a study in 12 healthy subjects given a single 300-mg dose of propafenone with or without erythromycin 250 mg showed that the increase in propafenone AUC with erythromycin was greater in those with lower cytochrome P450 isoenzyme CYP2D6 activity. It was suggested[1] that low CYP2D6 activity shifts propafenone metabolism to the CYP3A4/1A2-mediated *N*-depropylpropafenone pathway increasing the interaction with erythromycin, which is an inhibitor of CYP3A4. This appears to be the only documentation of a possible interaction with erythromycin and its clinical significance is not certain. More study is needed.

1. Munoz CE, Ito S, Bend JR, Tesoro A, Freeman D, Spence JD, Bailey DG. Propafenone interaction with CYP3A4 inhibitors in man. *Clin Pharmacol Ther* (1997) 61, 154.

Propafenone + Grapefruit juice

Limited evidence suggests that grapefruit juice may inhibit the metabolism of propafenone.

Clinical evidence, mechanism, importance and management

Preliminary results of a study in 12 healthy subjects given a single 300-mg dose of propafenone with or without 250 mL of grapefruit juice showed that the increase in propafenone AUC with grapefruit juice was greater in those with lower cytochrome P450 isoenzyme CYP2D6 activity. It was suggested[1] that in the presence of low CYP2D6 activity a greater proportion of propafenone is eliminated by metabolism by CYP3A4 and CYP1A2 and the effect of grapefruit juice is increased since it is an inhibitor of CYP3A4. The clinical significance of this finding is not certain. Further study is needed.

1. Munoz CE, Ito S, Bend JR, Tesoro A, Freeman D, Spence JD, Bailey DG. Propafenone interaction with CYP3A4 inhibitors in man. *Clin Pharmacol Ther* (1997) 61, 154.

Propafenone + Ketoconazole

An isolated case report describes a man taking propafenone who had a seizure two days after taking a dose of ketoconazole. Limited evidence suggests ketoconazole may inhibit the metabolism of propafenone.

Clinical evidence

A man who had been taking captopril and hydrochlorothiazide for 6 years and propafenone 300 mg daily for 4 years, without problems, and without any history of convulsive episodes, experienced a tonic-clonic seizure while watching television. It was later found that he had started to take two capsules of ketoconazole daily 2 days previously for the treatment of a candidal infection.[1] The preliminary results of another study in 12 healthy subjects given a single 300-mg dose of propafenone with or without ketoconazole 200 mg found that the increase in propafenone AUC with ketoconazole was greater in those with lower cytochrome P450 isoenzyme CYP2D6 activity.[2]

Mechanism

The authors of the case report postulate that the ketoconazole may have inhibited the metabolism of the propafenone so that this patient, in effect, may have developed an overdose.[1] However, convulsions with propafenone, even in overdose, are extremely rare.[3] Ketoconazole is an inhibitor of the cytochrome P450 isoenzyme CYP3A4, by which propafenone is metabolised to *N*-depropylpropafenone. Propafenone is also extensively metabolised by CYP2D6 to 5-hydroxypropafenone but it was suggested that if CYP2D6 activity is low, propafenone metabolism may be shifted to the CYP3A4 pathway increasing the possibility of an interaction with ketoconazole.[2] The manufacturer states that drugs that inhibit CYP2D6 and CYP3A4, such as ketoconazole, might lead to increased levels of propafenone.[4]

Importance and management

The general importance of this interaction is uncertain. As of 2006, there had been no other cases reported to the manufacturer of propafenone.[4] As available data suggest that an interaction can occur, it would seem prudent to keep this interaction in mind during concurrent use. There seems to be nothing documented about the effects of other azole antifungals.

1. Duvelleroy Hommet C, Jonville-Bera AP, Autret A, Saudeau D, Autret E, Fauchier JP. Une crise convulsive chez un patient traité par propafénone et kétoconazole. *Therapie* (1995) 50, 164–5.
2. Munoz CE, Ito S, Bend JR, Tesoro A, Freeman D, Spence JD, Bailey DG. Propafenone interaction with CYP3A4 inhibitors in man. *Clin Pharmacol Ther* (1997) 61, 154.
3. Arythmol (Propafenone hydrochloride). Abbott Laboratories Ltd. UK Summary of product characteristics, December 2001.
4. Abbott Laboratories. Personal communication, April 2006.

Propafenone + Quinidine

Quinidine doubles the plasma levels of propafenone and halves the levels of its active metabolite in CYP2D6 extensive metabolisers. This interaction has been utilised clinically.

Clinical evidence

Nine patients taking propafenone for frequent isolated ventricular ectopic beats, firstly had their dosage reduced to 150 mg every 8 hours and then 4 days later the steady-state pharmacokinetics of propafenone were determined at this new dose. Quinidine was then added at a dose of 50 mg every 8 hours, and after a further 4 days the steady-state plasma propafenone levels in 7 CYP2D6 extensive metabolisers had more than doubled from 408 to 1100 nanograms/mL, and 5-hydroxypropafenone concentrations had approximately halved, but the ECG intervals and arrhythmia frequency were unaltered. The steady-state plasma propafenone levels remained unchanged in the other 2 patients with low levels of CYP2D6 ('poor' metabolisers).[1] Consider 'Genetic factors', (p.4), for more information on metaboliser status. The same research group conducted a similar study in healthy subjects, which confirmed that quinidine increased the plasma levels of propafenone in 'extensive' but not 'poor' metabolisers. In addition, it was found that quinidine increased the extent of the beta-blockade caused by the propafenone in 'extensive' metabolisers to approach that seen in 'poor' metabolisers.[2] Another study has shown that the inhibition of propafenone metabolism by low-dose quinidine also occurs in Chinese as well as Caucasian patients.[3] [CYP2D6 shows pronounced interethnic differences in expression.] A further study showed that combining low-dose quinidine (150 mg daily) with standard dose propafenone in patients with atrial fibrillation resulted in a similar control of the arrhythmia as increasing the propafenone dose, but caused less gastrointestinal adverse effects.[4]

Mechanism

Quinidine inhibits the CYP2D6-dependent 5-hydroxylation of propafenone by the liver in those who are 'extensive' metabolisers so that it is cleared more slowly. Its plasma levels are doubled as a result, but the overall antiarrhythmic effects remain effectively unchanged, possibly because the production of its active antiarrhythmic metabolite (5-hydroxypropafenone) is simultaneously halved.[1] Quinidine increases the beta-blocking effects of propafenone in extensive metabolisers because only the parent drug, and not the metabolites, has beta-blocking activity.[2]

Importance and management

Quinidine appears to raise propafenone levels, and may also affect the beta-blocking properties of propafenone in some patients. In one study the concurrent use of propafenone and quinidine was said to have an effect similar to increasing the propafenone dose.[4] The importance of CYP2D6 metaboliser status is unclear, and more study is needed to clarify this.

1. Funck-Brentano C, Kroemer HK, Pavlou H, Woosley RL, Roden DM. Genetically-determined interaction between propafenone and low dose quinidine: role of active metabolites in modulating net drug effect. *Br J Clin Pharmacol* (1989) 27, 435–44.
2. Mörike K, Roden D. Quinidine-enhanced β-blockade during treatment with propafenone in extensive metabolizer human subjects. *Clin Pharmacol Ther* (1994) 55, 28–34.
3. Fan C, Tang M, Lau C-P, Chow M. The effect of quinidine on propafenone metabolism in Chinese patients. *Clin Invest Med* (1998) (Suppl) S12.
4. Lau C-P, Chow MSS, Tse H-F, Tang M-O, Fan C. Control of paroxysmal atrial fibrillation recurrence using combined administration of propafenone and quinidine. *Am J Cardiol* (2000) 86, 1327–32.

Propafenone + Rifampicin (Rifampin)

Propafenone serum levels and therapeutic effects can be markedly reduced by rifampicin.

Clinical evidence

A man with ventricular arrhythmias successfully treated with propafenone had a marked fall in his plasma propafenone level from 993 to 176 nanograms/mL within 12 days of starting to take rifampicin 450 mg twice daily. Levels of the two active metabolites of propafenone, 5-hydroxypropafenone and *N*-depropylpropafenone, changed from 195 to 64 nanograms/mL and from 110 to 192 nanograms/mL, respectively. His arrhythmias returned, but 2 weeks after stopping the rifampicin his arrhythmias had disappeared and the propafenone and its 5-hydroxy and *N*-depropyl metabolites had returned to acceptable levels (1411, 78 and 158 nanograms/mL respectively).[1] In a study in young healthy subjects, rifampicin 600 mg daily for 9 days reduced the bioavailability of a single 300-mg oral dose of propafenone from 30 to 10% in CYP2D6 extensive metabolisers, and from 81 to 48% in those with low levels of CYP2D6 ('poor' metabolisers). Consider 'Genetic factors', (p.4), for more information on metaboliser status. QRS prolongation decreased during enzyme induction. In contrast, in this study, rifampicin had no substantial effect on the pharmacokinetics of propafenone given intravenously.[2] Similar findings were reported in a further study by the same research group in healthy elderly subjects.[3]

Mechanism

Rifampicin induces the CYP3A4/1A2-mediated metabolism and phase II glucuronidation of propafenone. The effect of rifampicin on gastrointestinal clearance of propafenone was greater than that of its hepatic clearance. Rifampicin had no effect on CYP2D6-mediated metabolism of propafenone (the usual main metabolic route in 'extensive' metabolisers).[2,3]

Importance and management

An established and clinically relevant metabolic drug interaction. The dosage of oral propafenone will need increasing during concurrent use of rifampicin.[3] Alternatively, if possible, the authors of the case report[1] advise the use of another antibacterial, where possible, because of the probable difficulty in adjusting the propafenone dosage.

1. Castel JM, Cappiello E, Leopaldi D, Latini R. Rifampicin lowers plasma concentrations of propafenone and its antiarrhythmic effect. *Br J Clin Pharmacol* (1990) 30, 155–6.
2. Dilger K, Greiner B, Fromm MF, Hofmann U, Kroemer HK, Eichelbaum M. Consequences of rifampicin treatment on propafenone disposition in extensive and poor metabolizers of CYP2D6. *Pharmacogenetics* (1999) 9, 551–9.
3. Dilger K, Hofmann U, Klotz U. Enzyme induction in the elderly: Effect of rifampin on the pharmacokinetics and pharmacodynamics of propafenone. *Clin Pharmacol Ther* (2000) 67, 512–20.

Propafenone + SSRIs

Fluoxetine markedly inhibits the metabolism of propafenone by 5-hydroxylation, and paroxetine would be expected to behave similarly, but the clinical consequences of this are unknown. Fluvoxamine would be expected to inhibit the metabolism of propafenone by *N*-dealkylation. Sertraline, citalopram (and probably escitalopram) would not be expected to interact to a significant extent.

Clinical evidence, mechanism, importance and management

In a study in healthy subjects **fluoxetine** 20 mg daily for 10 days decreased the oral clearance of a single 400-mg dose of propafenone by 34% for both the *R*- and *S*-enantiomers. The peak plasma levels increased by 39% for *S*-propafenone and by 71% for *R*-propafenone. However, there were no differences in the changes to the PR and QRS intervals.[1] **Fluoxetine** is an inhibitor of the cytochrome P450 isoenzyme CYP2D6, which is responsible for the metabolism of propafenone to its primary active metabolite 5-hydroxypropafenone (for more detail see mechanism under 'Propafenone + Quinidine', above). *In vitro* data have shown that, of the SSRIs, **fluoxetine** is the most potent inhibitor of propafenone 5-hydroxylation, and that **paroxetine** would also be expected to interact.[2] As with 'quinidine', (p.275), inhibition of 5-hydroxylation would be expected to increase the beta-blocking effects of propafenone.[2] Until more is known, it would be prudent to use caution when giving **fluoxetine** or **paroxetine** with propafenone. **Sertraline** and **citalopram** did not interact *in vitro*.[2] Similarly, **escitalopram** would not be expected to interact significantly because evidence with other drugs ('desipramine', (p.1241) and 'metoprolol', (p.855)) suggest that **escitalopram** has only a modest inhibitory effect on CYP2D6. However, the manufacturers[3] still warn about a possible interaction with propafenone.

Although **fluvoxamine** had no effect on propafenone 5-hydroxylation *in vitro*,[2] it did inhibit propafenone *N*-dealkylation[2] via its inhibitory effects on the cytochrome P450 isoenzyme CYP1A2. This isoenzyme has only a minor role in the metabolism of propafenone, but it may assume greater importance in those who have low levels of CYP2D6 ('poor' metabolisers).[2] Further study is needed.

1. Cai WM, Chen B, Zhou Y, Zhang YD. Fluoxetine impairs the CYP2D6-mediated metabolism of propafenone enantiomers in healthy Chinese volunteers. *Clin Pharmacol Ther* (1999) 66, 516–21.
2. Hemeryck A, De Vriendt C, Belpaire FM. Effect of selective serotonin reuptake inhibitors on the oxidative metabolism of propafenone: *in vitro* studies using human liver microsomes. *J Clin Psychopharmacol* (2000) 20, 428–34.
3. Cipralex (Escitalopram oxalate). Lundbeck Ltd. UK Summary of product characteristics, December 2005.

Quinidine + Amiloride

A single study has shown that the antiarrhythmic activity of quinidine can be opposed by amiloride.

Clinical evidence

A study in 10 patients with inducible sustained ventricular tachycardia was carried out to see whether a beneficial interaction occurred between quinidine and amiloride. Patients were given oral quinidine until their trough serum levels reached 10 micromol/L, or the maximum well-tolerated dose was reached. After electrophysiological studies, oral amiloride was added at a dosage of 5 mg twice daily, increased up to 10 mg twice daily (if serum potassium levels remained normal) for 3 days. The electrophysiological studies were then repeated. Unexpectedly, 7 of the 10 patients demonstrated adverse responses while taking both drugs. Three developed sustained ventricular tachycardia and 3 others had somatic adverse effects (hypotension, nausea, diarrhoea), which prevented further studies being carried out. One patient had 12 episodes of sustained ventricular tachycardia while taking both drugs. Amiloride had no effect on quinidine levels.[1]

Mechanism

Not understood. The combination of quinidine and amiloride increased the QRS interval, but did not prolong the QT interval more than quinidine alone.

Importance and management

So far the evidence seems to be limited to this single study but it suggests that amiloride can oppose the antiarrhythmic activity of quinidine. The full clinical implications of this interaction are not yet known, but it would now clearly be prudent to consider monitoring to confirm that the quinidine continues to be effective if amiloride is present.

1. Wang L, Sheldon RS, Mitchell B, Wyse DG, Gillis AM, Chiamvimonvat N, Duff HJ. Amiloride-quinidine interaction: adverse outcomes. *Clin Pharmacol Ther* (1994) 56, 659–67.

Quinidine + Amiodarone

The QT interval prolonging effects of quinidine and amiodarone are increased when they are used together, and torsade de pointes has occurred. Therefore the combination should generally be avoided. However, if the combination is used, note that amiodarone increases quinidine levels and dosage reductions are likely to be needed.

Clinical evidence

Eleven patients were stabilised on quinidine (daily doses of 1.2 to 4.2 g). When they were also given amiodarone (600 mg every 12 hours for 5 to 7 days, then 600 mg daily) their mean serum quinidine levels rose by an average of 32%, from 4.4 to 5.8 micrograms/mL and 3 of them had a substantial increase of 2 micrograms/mL. Signs of toxicity (diarrhoea, nausea, vomiting, hypotension) were seen in some, and the quinidine dosage was reduced in 9 of the patients by an average of 37%. Despite the dose reduction, the quinidine serum levels were still higher at 5.2 micrograms/mL than before the amiodarone was started.[1]

A test in a healthy subject showed that 3 days after amiodarone 600 mg was added to quinidine 1.2 g daily, the serum quinidine levels doubled and the relative QT interval was prolonged from 1 (no drugs) to 1.2 (quinidine alone) to 1.4 (quinidine plus amiodarone).[2] This report also described two patients with minor cardiac arrhythmias who developed QT prolongation and torsade de pointes when given both drugs.[2] A Russian study of the use of the combination in atrial fibrillation reported that one of 52 patients had a 50% increase in the QT interval resulting in torsade de pointes and subsequently ventricular fibrillation, which required repeated defibrillation over 6 hours.[3] A 76-year-old man taking quinidine and amiodarone had a number of episodes of loss of consciousness, and subsequently QT prolongation and torsade de pointes, which stopped when the quinidine was discontinued.[4]

Mechanism

The mechanism behind the pharmacokinetic interaction is not understood. The QT prolonging effects of the two drugs would be expected to be additive.

Importance and management

An established and clinically important pharmacokinetic and pharmacodynamic interaction. The use of amiodarone with quinidine further prolongs the QT interval and increases the risk of torsade de pointes. Therefore, the combination should generally be avoided. The UK manufacturer of amiodarone contraindicates its use with class Ia antiarrhythmics such as quinidine.[5] See also 'Drugs that prolong the QT interval + Other drugs that prolong the QT interval', p.257. The pharmacokinetic component appears to occur in most patients, and to develop rapidly. The US manufacturer[6] of amiodarone considers such combination therapy should be reserved for life-threatening ventricular arrhythmias incompletely responsive to either drug alone and recommend that the dose of quinidine should be reduced by one-third. Others suggest that if the two drugs are considered essential, the dosage of quinidine should be reduced by about 30 to 50% and the serum levels should be monitored.[1] The ECG should also be monitored for evidence of changes in the QT interval when combined therapy is started or stopped.[7] Successful and uneventful concurrent use has been described in a report of 4 patients taking quinidine [dose not stated] and amiodarone 200 mg five times weekly.[8] Another describes the successful use of a short course of quinidine to convert chronic atrial fibrillation to sinus rhythm in 9 of 15 patients on long-term amiodarone therapy. Patients were hospitalised and continuously monitored. No proarrhythmias occurred and the QT interval remained within acceptable limits.[9]

1. Saal AK, Werner JA, Greene HL, Sears GK, Graham EL. Effect of amiodarone on serum quinidine and procainamide levels. *Am J Cardiol* (1984) 53, 1265–7.
2. Tartini R, Kappenberger L, Steinbrunn W, Meyer UA. Dangerous interaction between amiodarone and quinidine. *Lancet* (1982) i, 1327–9.
3. Lipnitsky TN, Dorogan AV, Randin AG, Kotsuta GI. Clinical efficacy and potential hazards from combined cordarone-and-chinidine treatment in patients with atrial fibrillation (in Russian). *Klin Med (Mosk)* (1992) 70, 31–4.
4. Nattel S, Ranger S, Talajic M, Lemery R, Roy D. Erythromycin-induced long QT syndrome: concordance with quinidine and underlying cellular electrophysiologic mechanism. *Am J Med* (1990) 89, 235–8.
5. Cordarone X (Amiodarone hydrochloride). Sanofi-Aventis. UK Summary of product characteristics, April 2006.
6. Cordarone (Amiodarone hydrochloride). Wyeth Pharmaceuticals. US Prescribing information, May 2007.
7. Kinidin Durules (Quinidine). AstraZeneca UK Ltd. UK Summary of product characteristics, June 2002.
8. Hoffmann A, Follath F, Burckhardt D. Safe treatment of resistant ventricular arrhythmias with a combination of amiodarone and quinidine or mexiletine. *Lancet* (1983) i, 704–5.
9. Kerin NZ, Ansari-Leesar M, Faitel K, Narala C, Frumin H, Cohen A. The effectiveness and safety of the simultaneous administration of quinidine and amiodarone in the conversion of chronic atrial fibrillation. *Am Heart J* (1993) 125, 1017–21.

Quinidine + Antacids or Urinary alkalinisers

Large rises in urinary pH due to the concurrent use of some antacids, diuretics or alkaline salts can cause quinidine retention, which could lead to quinidine toxicity, but there seems to be only one case on record of an adverse interaction (with an aluminium/magnesium hydroxide antacid). Aluminium hydroxide alone appears not to interact.

Clinical evidence

The renal clearance of oral quinidine in 4 subjects taking 200 mg every 6 hours was reduced by an average of 50% (from 53 to 26 mL/minute) when their urine was made alkaline (i.e. changed from pH 6 to 7, up to pH 7 to 8) with **sodium bicarbonate** and **acetazolamide** 500 mg twice daily. Below pH 6 their urinary quinidine level averaged 115 mg/L, whereas when urinary pH values rose above 7.5 the average quinidine level fell to 13 mg/L. The quinidine urinary excretion rate decreased from 103 to 31 micrograms/minute. In 6 other subjects the rise in serum quinidine levels was reflected in a prolongation of the QT interval. Raising the urinary pH from about 6 to 7.5 in one individual increased serum quinidine levels from about 1.6 to 2.6 micrograms/mL.[1]

A patient on quinidine who took eight *Mylanta* tablets daily (**aluminium hydroxide** gel 200 mg, **magnesium hydroxide** 200 mg and simeticone 20 mg) for a week and a little over 1 litre of fruit juice (orange and grapefruit) each day developed a threefold increase in serum quinidine levels (from 8 to 25 mg/L) and toxicity. However, note that the 'grapefruit juice', (p.280) may have contributed. In 6 healthy subjects, this dose of *Mylanta* for 3 days produced consistently alkaline urine in 4 subjects, and in 5 subjects when combined with fruit juice.[2]

In 4 healthy subjects, 30 mL of **aluminium hydroxide** gel *(Amphogel)* given with, and one hour after, a single 200-mg dose of quinidine sulphate had no effect on serum quinidine levels, AUC or excretion (urine pH ranged from 5 to 6.2).[3] Two similar single-dose studies in healthy subjects found that the absorption and elimination of 400 mg of quinidine sulphate[4] or 648 mg of quinidine gluconate[5] was unaffected by 30 mL **aluminium hydroxide** gel, although the change in quinidine AUC did vary from a decrease of 18% to an increase of 35% in one study.[5] Urinary pH was unaffected in both studies.[4,5]

Mechanism

Quinidine is excreted unchanged in the urine. In acid urine much of the quinidine excreted by the kidney tubules is in the ionised (lipid-insoluble) form, which is unable to diffuse freely back into the cells and so is lost in the urine. In alkaline urine more of the quinidine is in the non-ionised (lipid-soluble) form, which freely diffuses back into the cells and is retained. In this way the pH of the urine determines how much quinidine is lost or retained and thereby governs the serum levels. *In vitro* data suggest that changes in pH and adsorption effects within the gut due to antacids could also affect the absorption of quinidine.[6,7]

Importance and management

An established interaction, but with the exception of the one isolated case cited,[2] there seem to be no reports of problems in patients given quinidine and antacids or urinary alkalinisers. However, in this case quinidine was given with grapefruit juice, which may potentially have had an effect of its own, see 'Quinidine + Grapefruit juice', p.280. Nevertheless you should monitor the effects if drugs that can markedly change urinary pH are started or stopped. Reduce the quinidine dosage as necessary.

It is difficult to predict which antacids, if any, are likely to increase the serum levels of quinidine. As noted above, aluminium hydroxide gel and magnesium hydroxide (*Mylanta*) alkalinises urine and can interact. Similarly, magnesium and aluminium hydroxide (*Maalox*) can raise the urinary pH by about 0.9 and could possibly interact.[8] Magnesium hydroxide (*Milk of magnesia*) and **calcium carbonate-glycine** (*Titralac*) in normal doses raise the urinary pH by about 0.5, so that a smaller effect is likely.[8] Aluminium hydroxide gel (*Amphogel*) and **dihydroxyaluminium glycinate** (*Robalate*) are reported to have no effect on urinary pH,[8] and the studies above confirm aluminium hydroxide gel does not generally interact.

1. Gerhardt RE, Knouss RF, Thyrum PT, Luchi RJ, Morris JJ. Quinidine excretion in aciduria and alkaluria. *Ann Intern Med* (1969) 71, 927–33.
2. Zinn MB. Quinidine intoxication from alkali ingestion. *Tex Med* (1970) 66, 64–6.
3. Romankiewicz JA, Reidenberg M, Drayer D, Franklin JE. The noninterference of aluminium hydroxide gel with quinidine sulfate absorption: an approach to control quinidine-induced diarrhea. *Am Heart J* (1978) 96, 518–20.
4. Ace LN, Jaffe JM, Kunka RL. Effect of food and antacid on quinidine bioavailability. *Biopharm Drug Dispos* (1983) 4, 183–90.
5. Mauro VF, Mauro LS, Fraker TD, Temesy-Armos PN, Somani P. Effect of aluminium hydroxide gel on quinidine gluconate absorption. *Ann Pharmacother* (1990) 24, 252–4.
6. Remon JP, Van Severen R, Braeckman P. Interaction entre antiarythmiques, antiacides et antidiarrhéiques. III. Influence d'antacides et d'antidiarrhéiques sur la réabsorption in vitro de sels de quinidine. *Pharm Acta Helv* (1979) 54, 19–22.
7. Moustafa MA, Al-Shora HI, Gaber M, Gouda MW. Decreased bioavailability of quinidine sulphate due to interactions with adsorbent antacids and antidiarrhoeal mixtures. *Int J Pharmaceutics* (1987) 34, 207–11.
8. Gibaldi M, Grundhofer B, Levy G. Effect of antacids on pH of urine. *Clin Pharmacol Ther* (1974) 16, 520–5.

Quinidine + Antiepileptics

Serum quinidine levels can be reduced by phenytoin, phenobarbital or primidone. Loss of arrhythmia control is possible if the quinidine dosage is not increased.

Clinical evidence

A man taking long-term **primidone** 500 mg daily was given quinidine 300 mg every 4 hours, but only attained a plasma quinidine level of 0.8 micrograms/mL with an estimated half-life of 5 hours. When **primidone** was discontinued, his quinidine level rose to 2.4 micrograms/mL and the half-life was 12 hours. **Phenobarbital** 90 mg daily was then started, and the quinidine level fell to 1.6 micrograms/mL with a half-life of 7.6 hours. In another case, a woman required doses of quinidine sulfate of up to 800 mg every 4 hours to achieve therapeutic levels while taking **phenytoin**. When the **phenytoin** was stopped, quinidine toxicity occurred, and the dose was eventually halved. Further study was then made in 4 healthy subjects. After 4 weeks of treatment with either **phenytoin** (in dosages adjusted to give levels of 10 to 20 micrograms/mL) or **phenobarbital**, the elimination half-life of a single 300-mg dose of quinidine sulphate was reduced by about 50% and the total AUC was reduced by about 60%.[1]

Similar results were found with **phenytoin** in another study in 3 healthy subjects.[2] Other cases have also been reported with **phenytoin, primidone, pentobarbital** and **phenobarbital**.[3-6] In one case, quinidine levels fell by 44% when **phenytoin** was given with quinidine to a patient with recurrent ventricular tachycardia.[3] In another report quinidine levels increased from a mean of 0.8 to 2.2 micrograms/mL 15 days after **pentobarbital** was discontinued.[4] Interestingly, in this case the patient was also on **digoxin**, and stopping phenobarbital precipitated **digoxin** toxicity by causing an increase in quinidine levels.

A 3-year-old child taking both **phenobarbital** and **phenytoin** required quinidine 300 mg every 4 hours to achieve therapeutic serum quinidine levels, and had an estimated quinidine half-life of only 1.4 hours.[5] Difficulty in achieving adequate serum quinidine levels was also reported in a woman taking **phenytoin** and **primidone**. Her quinidine half-life was 2.7 hours, about half that usually seen in adults.[6]

Quinidine 200 mg had no effect on the metabolism (4-hydroxylation) of **mephenytoin** 100 mg in 10 healthy subjects.[7]

Mechanism

The evidence suggests that phenytoin, primidone or phenobarbital (all known enzyme-inducers) increase the hepatic metabolism of quinidine and thereby reduce its levels.[2]

Importance and management

Established interactions of clinical importance although the documentation is limited. The concurrent use of phenytoin, primidone, phenobarbital or any other barbiturate need not be avoided, but be alert for the need to increase the quinidine dosage. If the anticonvulsants are withdrawn the quinidine dosage may need to be reduced to avoid quinidine toxicity. Where possible, quinidine serum levels should be monitored.

1. Data JL, Wilkinson GR, Nies AS. Interaction of quinidine with anticonvulsant drugs. *N Engl J Med* (1976) 294, 699–702.
2. Russo ME, Russo J, Smith RA, Pershing LK. The effect of phenytoin on quinidine pharmacokinetics. *Drug Intell Clin Pharm* (1982) 16, 480.
3. Urbano AM. Phenytoin-quinidine interaction in a patient with recurrent ventricular tachyarrhythmias. *N Engl J Med* (1983) 308, 225.
4. Chapron DJ, Mumford D, Pitegoff GI. Apparent quinidine-induced digoxin toxicity after withdrawal of pentobarbital. A case of sequential drug interactions. *Arch Intern Med* (1979) 139, 363–5.

5. Rodgers GC, Blackman MS. Quinidine interaction with anticonvulsants. *Drug Intell Clin Pharm* (1983) 17, 819–20.
6. Kroboth FJ, Kroboth PD, Logan T. Phenytoin-theophylline-quinidine interaction. *N Engl J Med* (1983) 308, 725.
7. Schellens JHM, Ghabrial H, van der Wart HHF, Bakker EN, Wilkinson GR, Breimer DD. Differential effects of quinidine on the disposition of nifedipine, sparteine and mephenytoin in humans. *Clin Pharmacol Ther* (1991) 50, 520–8.

Quinidine + Aspirin

A patient and two healthy subjects given quinidine and aspirin had a two- to threefold increase in bleeding times. The patient developed petechiae and gastrointestinal bleeding.

Clinical evidence, mechanism, importance and management

A patient with a prolonged history of paroxysmal atrial tachycardia was given quinidine 800 mg daily and aspirin 325 mg twice daily. After a week he developed generalised petechiae and blood in his faeces. His prothrombin and partial prothrombin times were normal but the template bleeding time was more than 35 minutes (normal 2 to 10 minutes). Further study in two healthy subjects showed that quinidine 975 mg daily given alone for 5 days and aspirin 650 mg three times a day given alone for 5 days prolonged bleeding times by 125% and 163% respectively; given together for 5 days the bleeding times were prolonged by 288%.[1] The underlying mechanism is not totally understood but it is believed to be the outcome of the additive effects of two drugs, both of which can reduce platelet aggregation,[1] although with quinidine this antiplatelet effect usually only occurs as the result of a hypersensitivity reaction.

This seems to be the only study of this adverse interaction, and its general importance is uncertain. It may be prudent to monitor concurrent use to check that bleeding does not occur.

1. Lawson D, Mehta J, Mehta P, Lipman BC, Imperi GA. Cumulative effects of quinidine and aspirin on bleeding time and platelet α_2-adrenoceptors: potential mechanism of bleeding diathesis in patients receiving this combination. *J Lab Clin Med* (1986) 108, 581–6.

Quinidine + Calcium-channel blockers

A few patients have shown increased serum quinidine levels when stopping nifedipine, but in others no interaction has occurred and one study even suggests that quinidine serum levels may be slightly raised by nifedipine. Nifedipine levels may be modestly raised by quinidine. Verapamil reduces the clearance of quinidine and in one patient the serum quinidine levels doubled and quinidine toxicity developed. Acute hypotension has also been seen in three patients taking quinidine when they were given verapamil intravenously. Felodipine and nisoldipine appear not to interact, and the situation with diltiazem is unclear.

Clinical evidence

(a) Diltiazem

A study in 10 healthy subjects given quinidine 600 mg twice daily and diltiazem 120 mg daily for 7 days found that the pharmacokinetics of neither drug was affected by the presence of the other.[1] These findings contrast with another crossover study in 12 healthy subjects in which a single 60-mg dose of diltiazem was given before and after quinidine 100 mg twice daily for 5 doses, and a single 200-mg dose of quinidine was given before and after diltiazem 90 mg twice daily for 5 doses. The pharmacokinetics of diltiazem were unaffected by quinidine, but the AUC of quinidine was increased by 51% by diltiazem.[2] When quinidine was given after diltiazem pretreatment, there were significant increases in QTc and PR intervals, and a significant decrease in heart rate and diastolic blood pressure. Pretreatment with quinidine did not significantly alter the effects of diltiazem.[2]

(b) Felodipine

Felodipine 10 mg daily for 3 days was found to have no clinically significant effect on the pharmacokinetics or haemodynamic and ECG effects of a single 400-mg dose of quinidine in 12 healthy subjects. Felodipine did cause a modest 22% decrease in the AUC of the quinidine metabolite 3-hydroxyquinidine.[3]

(c) Nifedipine

1. Quinidine serum levels. The quinidine serum levels of 2 patients taking quinidine sulfate 300 or 400 mg every 6 hours and nifedipine 10 or 20 mg every 6 or 8 hours doubled (from a range of 2 to 2.5 up to 4.6 micrograms/mL and from 1.6 to 1.8 up to 3.5 micrograms/mL respectively) when the nifedipine was withdrawn. The increased serum quinidine levels were reflected in a prolongation of the QTc interval. However, in the first patient there had been no change in quinidine levels when nifedipine was initially added to his existing quinidine therapy. Further, 4 other patients did not develop this interaction.[4] Two other reports[5,6] describe a similar response: the quinidine serum level doubled in one patient when the nifedipine was stopped,[5] and in the other it was found difficult to achieve adequate serum quinidine levels when nifedipine was added, even when the quinidine dosage was increased threefold. When the nifedipine was withdrawn, the quinidine levels rose once again.[6] A study in 12 patients found no significant change in serum quinidine levels in the group as a whole when given nifedipine, but one patient had a 41% decrease in quinidine levels.[7] Two other studies in healthy subjects found that the quinidine AUC was unchanged by nifedipine.[3,8]
A further study in 12 healthy subjects found that the AUC of a single 200-mg oral dose of quinidine sulphate was increased by 16% by nifedipine 20 mg. The quinidine clearance was reduced by 14% and the maximum serum level was raised by almost 20%. These modest changes were not considered clinically relevant.[9]

2. Nifedipine serum levels. In a study in 10 healthy subjects quinidine sulfate 200 mg every 8 hours increased the AUC of nifedipine by 37%, and heart rates were significantly increased. Quinidine levels were unchanged.[8] Another study found that quinidine had a modest inhibitory effect on the metabolism of nifedipine (half-life prolonged by 40%).[10] A further study in 12 healthy subjects found that the AUC of a single 20-mg dose of nifedipine was increased 16% by quinidine 200 mg and its clearance was reduced by 17%, but these modest changes were not considered clinically relevant.[9]

(d) Nisoldipine

An open crossover study in 20 healthy subjects found that nisoldipine 20 mg had no effect on the bioavailability of quinidine gluconate 648 mg.[11]

(e) Verapamil

After taking verapamil 80 mg three times daily for 3 days, the clearance of a single 400-mg dose of quinidine sulphate in 6 healthy subjects was decreased by 32% and the half-life was increased by 35% from 6.87 to 9.29 hours.[12]

A patient given quinidine gluconate 648 mg every 6 hours had an increase in serum quinidine levels from 2.6 to 5.7 micrograms/mL when given verapamil 80 mg every 8 hours for a week. He became dizzy and had blurred vision and was found to have atrioventricular block (heart rate 38 bpm) and a systolic blood pressure of 50 mmHg. In a subsequent study in this patient it was found that the verapamil halved the quinidine clearance and almost doubled the serum half-life.[13]

Three other patients given quinidine orally developed marked hypotension when given intravenous verapamil 2.5 or 5 mg (blood pressure fall from 130/70 to 80/50 mmHg, systolic pressure fall from 140 to 85 mmHg and a mean arterial pressure fall from 100 to 60 mmHg, in the 3 patients respectively). In two of the patients, after quinidine was discontinued, the same dose of verapamil did not cause a drop in blood pressure.[14]

Mechanism

Suggestions for how nifedipine could alter quinidine levels include changes in cardiovascular haemodynamics,[4] and effects on metabolism.[7] Quinidine probably inhibits the metabolism of nifedipine by competing for metabolism by the cytochrome P450 isoenzyme CYP3A4.[10] The interaction with verapamil is probably due to an inhibitory effect of verapamil on the metabolism of quinidine (inhibition of cytochrome P450 isoenzyme CYP3A).[12,15] The marked hypotension observed may be related to the antagonistic effects of the two drugs on catecholamine-induced alpha-receptor induced vasoconstriction.[14]

Importance and management

The results of studies of the interaction between quinidine and nifedipine are inconsistent and contradictory, so that the outcome of concurrent use is uncertain. Monitor the response, being alert for the need to modify the dosage. More study of this interaction is needed. Quinidine appears to increase nifedipine levels, but the importance of this is uncertain.

What is known about the interaction between quinidine and verapamil suggests that a reduction in the dosage of the quinidine may be needed to avoid toxicity. If the verapamil is given intravenously, use with caution and be alert for evidence of acute hypotension. Monitor the effects of concurrent use closely. There is actually a fixed dose preparation containing verapamil and quinidine *(Cordichin)* available in Germany, which is used for the management of atrial fibrillation. No interaction apparently occurs between quinidine and felodipine or nisoldipine. The situation with diltiazem is as yet uncertain but be alert for the need to reduce the quinidine dosage.

1. Matera MG, De Santis D, Vacca C, Fici F, Romano AR, Marrazzo R, Marmo E. Quinidine-diltiazem: pharmacokinetic interaction in humans. *Curr Ther Res* (1986) 40, 653–6.
2. Laganière S, Davies RF, Carignan G, Foris K, Goernert L, Carrier K, Pereira C, McGilveray I. Pharmacokinetic and pharmacodynamic interactions between diltiazem and quinidine. *Clin Pharmacol Ther* (1996) 60, 255–64.
3. Bailey DG, Freeman DJ, Melendez LJ, Kreeft JH, Edgar B, Carruthers SG. Quinidine interaction with nifedipine and felodipine: pharmacokinetic and pharmacodynamic evaluation. *Clin Pharmacol Ther* (1993) 53, 354–9.
4. Farringer JA, Green JA, O'Rourke RA, Linn WA, Clementi WA. Nifedipine-induced alterations in serum quinidine concentrations. *Am Heart J* (1984) 108, 1570–2.
5. Van Lith RM, Appleby DH. Quinidine-nifedipine interaction. *Drug Intell Clin Pharm* (1985) 19, 829–31.
6. Green JA, Clementi WA, Porter C, Stigelman W. Nifedipine-quinidine interaction. *Clin Pharm* (1983) 2, 461–5.
7. Munger MA, Jarvis RC, Nair R, Kasmer RJ, Nara AR, Urbancic A, Green JA. Elucidation of the nifedipine-quinidine interaction. *Clin Pharmacol Ther* (1989) 45, 411–16.
8. Bowles SK, Reeves RA, Cardozo L, Edwards DJ. Evaluation of the pharmacokinetic and pharmacodynamic interaction between quinidine and nifedipine. *J Clin Pharmacol* (1993) 33, 727–31.
9. Hippius M, Henschel L, Sigusch H, Tepper J, Brendel E. Hoffmann A. Pharmacokinetic interactions of nifedipine and quinidine. *Pharmazie* (1995) 50 613–16.
10. Schellens JHM, Ghabrial H, van der Wart HHF, Bakker EN, Wilkinson GR, Breimer DD. Differential effects of quinidine on the disposition of nifedipine, sparteine and mephenytoin in humans. *Clin Pharmacol Ther* (1991) 50, 520–8.
11. Schall R, Müller FO, Groenewoud G, Hundt HKL, Luus HG, Van Dyk M, Van Schalkwyk AMC. Investigation of a possible pharmacokinetic interaction between nisoldipine and quinidine in healthy volunteers. *Drug Invest* (1994) 8, 162–170.
12. Edwards DJ, Lavoie R, Beckman H, Blevins R, Rubenfire M. The effect of coadministration of verapamil on the pharmacokinetics and metabolism of quinidine. *Clin Pharmacol Ther* (1987) 41, 68–73.
13. Trohman RG, Estes DM, Castellanos A, Palomo AR, Myerburg RJ, Kessler KM. Increased quinidine plasma concentrations during administration of verapamil; a new quinidine-verapamil interaction. *Am J Cardiol* (1986) 57, 706–7.
14. Maisel AS, Motulsky HJ, Insel PA. Hypotension after quinidine plus verapamil. Possible additive competition at alpha-adrenergic receptors. *N Engl J Med* (1985) 312, 167–70.
15. Kroemer HK, Gautier J-C, Beaune P, Henderson C, Wolf CR, Eichelbaum M. Identification of P450 enzymes involved in metabolism of verapamil in humans. *Naunyn Schmiedebergs Arch Pharmacol* (1993) 348, 332–7.

Quinidine + Colesevelam

A single 4.5-g dose of colesevelam had no significant effect on the pharmacokinetics of a single 324-mg dose of quinidine in 25 healthy subjects.[1] This suggests that colesevelam does not reduce the absorption of quinidine. No special precautions appear to be needed during concurrent use.

1. Donovan JM, Stypinski D, Stiles MR, Olson TA, Burke SK. Drug interactions with colesevelam hydrochloride, a novel, potent lipid-lowering agent. *Cardiovasc Drugs Ther* (2000) 14, 681–90.

Quinidine + Co-phenotrope (Atropine/Diphenoxylate)

Co-phenotrope slightly reduced the rate, but not the extent, of absorption of a single dose of quinidine.

Clinical evidence, mechanism, importance and management

In one study, 8 healthy subjects were given a single 300-mg dose of quinidine sulfate alone and after taking two tablets of co-phenotrope (atropine sulfate 25 micrograms, diphenoxylate 2.5 mg; *Lomotil*) at midnight on the evening before and another two tablets the next morning an hour before the quinidine.[1] It was found that the maximum plasma quinidine levels were reduced by 21% from 2.1 to 1.65 micrograms/mL by the co-phenotrope, the time to maximum level was prolonged from 0.89 to 1.21 hours, and there was a slight increase in elimination half-life from 5.7 to 6.8 hours. While these results were statistically significant, the changes were relatively small and it seems doubtful if they are clinically relevant, particularly as the extent of absorption was unchanged. However it needs to be emphasised that because the quinidine formulation used was an immediate-release preparation, these results may not necessarily apply to sustained-release preparations, and also may not apply if multiple doses of quinidine are used.

1. Ponzillo JJ, Scavone JM, Paone RP, Lewis GP, Rayment CM, Fitzsimmons WE. Effect of diphenoxylate with atropine sulfate on the bioavailability of quinidine sulfate in healthy subjects. *Clin Pharm* (1988) 7, 139–42.

Quinidine + Diazepam

A single dose study suggests that diazepam does not affect the pharmacokinetics of quinidine.

Clinical evidence, mechanism, importance and management

A comparative study in 8 healthy subjects found that the pharmacokinetics of a single 250-mg dose of quinidine sulfate was unaltered by a single 10-mg dose of diazepam.[1] This suggests that no interaction between these drugs is likely but it needs confirmation by further studies using multiple doses of both drugs.

1. Rao BR, Rambhau D. Absence of a pharmacokinetic interaction between quinidine and diazepam. *Drug Metabol Drug Interact* (1995) 12, 45–51.

Quinidine + Diclofenac

Diclofenac inhibits the metabolism (*N*-oxidation) of quinidine but does not affect other pharmacokinetic parameters. *In vitro* and *animal* data suggest that quinidine may increase the metabolism of diclofenac.

Clinical evidence, mechanism, importance and management

In an open study, 6 healthy subjects were given a single 200-mg dose of quinidine sulfate before and on day 5 of a 6-day course of diclofenac 100 mg daily. Diclofenac reduced the *N*-oxidation of quinidine by 33%, but no other pharmacokinetic changes were found.[1] Diclofenac is a substrate for, and therefore a possible competitive inhibitor of the cytochrome P450 isoenzyme CYP2C9. These results suggest that CYP2C9 does not appear to have a major role in quinidine metabolism,[1] and so clinically relevant changes in quinidine pharmacokinetics with diclofenac would seem unlikely.

A study in *monkeys* found that plasma levels of diclofenac were approximately halved when diclofenac was given with quinidine (both by portal vein infusion).[2] *In vitro* study[3] has shown that quinidine stimulates the metabolism of diclofenac to its 5-hydroxylated derivative, via its effects on CYP3A4. Further study is required to assess the clinical relevance of these findings.

1. Damkier P, Hansen LL, Brøsen K. Effect of diclofenac, disulfiram, itraconazole, grapefruit juice and erythromycin on the pharmacokinetics of quinidine. *Br J Clin Pharmacol* (1999) 48, 829–38.
2. Tang W, Stearns RA, Kwei GY, Iliff SA, Miller RR, Egan MA, Yu NX, Dean DC, Kumar S, Shou M, Lin JH, Baillie TA. Interaction of diclofenac and quinidine in monkeys: stimulation of diclofenac metabolism. *J Pharmacol Exp Ther* (1999) 291, 1068–74.
3. Ngui JS, Tang W, Stearns RA, Shou M, Miller RR, Zhang Y, Lin JH, Baillie TA. Cytochrome P450 3A4-mediated interaction of diclofenac and quinidine. *Drug Metab Dispos* (2000) 28, 1043–50.

Quinidine + Disulfiram

Disulfiram does not affect the pharmacokinetics of quinidine.

Clinical evidence, mechanism, importance and management

In an open study, 6 healthy subjects were given a single 200-mg dose of quinidine sulfate before and on day 5 of a 6-day course of disulfiram 200 mg daily. There were no changes in quinidine pharmacokinetics during disulfiram administration.[1] Disulfiram is thought to be an inhibitor of the cytochrome P450 isoenzyme CYP2E1, but this isoenzyme does not appear to have a major role in quinidine metabolism.[1] Clinically relevant pharmacokinetic interactions between quinidine and disulfiram therefore seem unlikely. Concurrent use need not be avoided.

1. Damkier P, Hansen LL, Brøsen K. Effect of diclofenac, disulfiram, itraconazole, grapefruit juice and erythromycin on the pharmacokinetics of quinidine. *Br J Clin Pharmacol* (1999) 48, 829–38.

Quinidine + Erythromycin

Erythromycin can increase quinidine levels and cause a small further increase in the QTc interval. An isolated report describes a moderate rise in serum quinidine levels in an elderly man attributed to the concurrent use of intravenous erythromycin, which was possibly a factor in an episode of torsade de pointes. Another isolated report describes the development of torsade de pointes arrhythmia in a very elderly man when he was given quinidine and erythromycin orally. See also 'Drugs that prolong the QT interval + Other drugs that prolong the QT interval', p.257.

Clinical evidence

A 74-year-old man with a history of cardiac disease (coronary artery bypass graft surgery, ventricular tachycardia) treated with quinidine sulfate 200 mg every 6 hours and several other drugs (mexiletine, hydralazine, dipyridamole, aspirin and paracetamol (acetaminophen)), was hospitalised with suspected implantable cardioverter defibrillator infection. Within 2 days of starting to take erythromycin lactobionate 500 mg every 6 hours and ceftriaxone 1 g daily, both given intravenously, his trough serum quinidine levels had risen by about one-third from about 2.8 to 4.2 mg/L. On day 7 metronidazole 500 mg every 8 hours was added and the erythromycin dosage was doubled, and the patient experienced an episode of torsade de pointes. By day 12 his serum quinidine levels had further risen to 5.8 mg/L, whereupon the quinidine dosage was reduced by 25%. Because an interaction between quinidine and erythromycin had by then been suspected, the antibacterials were replaced by doxycycline and ciprofloxacin. By day 21 the quinidine serum levels had fallen to their former levels. The patient had a prolonged QTc interval of 504 milliseconds on admission, and this did not change.[1]

A 95-year-old man developed QT interval prolongation, torsade de pointes arrhythmia and subsequent cardiac arrest when given quinidine and erythromycin, both orally.[2]

Preliminary results of a randomised, placebo-controlled crossover study in 12 subjects found that when a single 400-mg dose of quinidine was given after oral erythromycin 500 mg three times daily or a placebo for 5 days, the total QTc AUC was significantly prolonged by about 6% during the erythromycin phase.[3] In a parallel study by the same group, peak levels of quinidine were increased by 39%, from 587 to 816 nanograms/mL, and the AUC by 62%, by day 5 of the erythromycin phase. Peak levels of the main metabolite of quinidine, 3-hydroxyquinidine, were significantly reduced.[4] Another study in 6 healthy subjects found that oral erythromycin 250 mg four times daily for 6 days reduced the total clearance of a single 200-mg dose of quinidine sulfate by 34% and increased its maximum serum concentration by 39%.[5]

Mechanism

Not fully understood, but erythromycin inhibits the metabolism of quinidine,[4] possibly by inhibition of the cytochrome P450 isoenzyme CYP3A4,[5] thereby reducing its clearance from the body and increasing its effects. There are also a number of cases on record of prolongation of the QT interval and torsade de pointes associated with the use of intravenous erythromycin alone.[6] Therefore, quinidine and erythromycin may have additive effects on the QT interval in addition to the pharmacokinetic interaction.

Importance and management

Information about this interaction appears to be limited to these reports, but it would appear to be established. If erythromycin is essential in a patient taking quinidine, the effects of concurrent use should be well monitored, being alert for the development of raised plasma quinidine levels and prolongation of the QT interval (see also 'Drugs that prolong the QT interval + Other drugs that prolong the QT interval', p.257).

1. Spinler SA, Cheng JWM, Kindwall KE, Charland SL. Possible inhibition of hepatic metabolism of quinidine by erythromycin. *Clin Pharmacol Ther* (1995) 57, 89–94.
2. Lin JC, Quasny HA. QT prolongation and development of torsades de pointes with the concomitant administration of oral erythromycin base and quinidine. *Pharmacotherapy* (1997) 17, 626–30.
3. Stanford RH, Geraets DR, Lee H-C, Min DI. Effect of oral erythromycin on quinidine pharmacodynamics in healthy volunteers. *Pharmacotherapy* (1997) 17, 1111.
4. Stanford RH, Park JM, Geraets Dr, Min DI, Lee H-C. Effect of oral erythromycin on quinidine pharmacokinetics in healthy volunteers. *Pharmacotherapy* (1998) 18, 426–7.
5. Damkier P, Hansen LL, Brøsen K. Effect of diclofenac, disulfiram, itraconazole, grapefruit juice and erythromycin on the pharmacokinetics of quinidine. *Br J Clin Pharmacol* (1999) 48, 829–38.
6. Gitler B, Berger LS, Buffa SD. Torsades de pointes induced by erythromycin. *Chest* (1994) 105, 368–72.

Quinidine + Fluvoxamine

Fluvoxamine appears to inhibit the metabolism and clearance of quinidine.

Clinical evidence, mechanism, importance and management

Six healthy subjects were given a single 250-mg dose of quinidine sulfate before and on day 5 of a 6-day course of fluvoxamine 100 mg daily.[1] The total apparent oral clearance of quinidine was reduced by 29%, and *N*-oxidation and 3-hydroxylation were reduced by 33 and 44% respectively. Renal clearance and the elimination half-life were unchanged. It was concluded that fluvoxamine inhibited the metabolism of quinidine by the cytochrome P450 isoenzyme CYP3A4, although a role for CYP1A2 and CYP2C19 was not excluded. The clinical relevance of these findings is unclear. However, it would seem prudent to monitor the concurrent use of quinidine with fluvoxamine. More study is needed to assess the effect of multiple dosing and to establish the clinical significance of this interaction.

1. Damkier P, Hansen LL, Brøsen K. Effect of fluvoxamine on the pharmacokinetics of quinidine. *Eur J Clin Pharmacol* (1999) 55, 451–6.

Quinidine + Grapefruit juice

Grapefruit juice delays the absorption of quinidine and reduces its metabolism to some extent, but no clinically relevant adverse interaction seems to occur.

Clinical evidence, mechanism, importance and management

In one study, 12 healthy subjects were given quinidine sulfate 400 mg orally on two occasions, once with 240 mL of water and once with grapefruit juice. The pharmacokinetics of the quinidine were unchanged, except that its absorption was delayed (the time to reach maximum plasma concentrations was doubled from 1.6 to 3.3 hours), for reasons that are not understood. The AUC of its metabolite (3-hydroxyquinidine) was decreased by one-third, suggesting that the grapefruit juice inhibits the metabolism of the quinidine.[1] No important changes in the QTc interval were seen.[1] Similarly, another study in 6 healthy subjects found the total clearance of a single 200-mg dose of quinidine sulfate was reduced by 15% by 250 mL of grapefruit juice, with no change in maximum level. There was a small reduction in metabolite formation suggesting only minor inhibition of metabolism.[2] Grapefruit is known to inhibit the cytochrome P450 isoenzyme CYP3A4, which is involved with the metabolism of quinidine, so it seems likely that any interaction would occur via this pathway.[1,2] These studies suggest that it is not necessary for patients on quinidine to avoid grapefruit juice. Nevertheless, grapefruit juice may have contributed to raised quinidine levels and toxicity in a woman who took an antacid and one litre of fruit juice daily for a week, see 'Quinidine + Antacids or Urinary alkalinisers', p.277.

1. Min DI, Ku Y-M, Geraets DR, Lee H-C. Effect of grapefruit juice on the pharmacokinetics and pharmacodynamics of quinidine in healthy volunteers. *J Clin Pharmacol* (1996) 36, 469–76.
2. Damkier P, Hansen LL, Brøsen K. Effect of diclofenac, disulfiram, itraconazole, grapefruit juice and erythromycin on the pharmacokinetics of quinidine. *Br J Clin Pharmacol* (1999) 48, 829–38.

Quinidine + H_2-receptor antagonists

Quinidine serum levels can rise and toxicity may develop in some patients when they take cimetidine. An isolated case of ventricular bigeminy (a form of arrhythmia) occurred in a patient taking quinidine and ranitidine.

Clinical evidence

Cimetidine 300 mg four times daily for 7 days prolonged the elimination half-life of a single 400-mg dose of quinidine sulfate by 55%, from 5.8 to 9 hours, and decreased its clearance by 37% in 6 healthy subjects. Peak plasma levels were raised by 21%. These changes were reflected in ECG changes, with 51% and 28% increases in the mean areas under the QT and QTc time curves, respectively, but these were not considered to be statistically significant.[1]

A later study in healthy subjects, prompted by the observation of two patients who developed toxic quinidine levels when given **cimetidine**, found essentially the same effects. The AUC and half-life of quinidine were increased by 14.5 and 22.6% respectively, and the clearance was decreased by 25% by **cimetidine** 300 mg four times daily.[2] A further study in 4 healthy subjects found that **cimetidine** 300 mg four times daily for 5 days prolonged the elimination half-life of quinidine by 54% and decreased its total clearance by 36%.[3,4] **Cimetidine** prolonged the QT interval by 30% more than the effect of quinidine alone.[4] A case report describes marked increases in both quinidine and digitoxin concentrations in a woman also given **cimetidine**.[5] Similarly, quinidine levels increased by up to 50%, without causing any adverse effects, when a man taking quinidine was given **cimetidine**.[6]

Ventricular bigeminy (a form of arrhythmia) occurred when a man taking quinidine was given **ranitidine**. His serum quinidine levels remained unchanged.[7]

Mechanism

It was originally suggested that the cimetidine inhibits the metabolism of the quinidine by the liver so that it is cleared more slowly.[2] However, further data suggest that cimetidine successfully competes with quinidine for its excretion by the kidneys.[8]

Importance and management

The interaction between quinidine and cimetidine is established and of clinical importance. The incidence is unknown. Be alert for changes in the response to quinidine if cimetidine is started or stopped. Ideally the quinidine serum levels should be monitored and the dosage reduced as necessary. Reductions of 25% (oral) and 35% (intravenous) have been suggested.[3] Those at greatest risk are likely to be patients with impaired renal function, patients with impaired liver function, the elderly, and those with serum quinidine levels already at the top end of the therapeutic range.[2] The situation with ranitidine is uncertain.

1. Hardy BG, Zador IT, Golden L, Lalka D, Schentag JJ. Effect of cimetidine on the pharmacokinetics and pharmacodynamics of quinidine. *Am J Cardiol* (1983) 52, 172–5.
2. Kolb KW, Garnett WR, Small RE, Vetrovec GW, Kline BJ, Fox T. Effect of cimetidine on quinidine clearance. *Ther Drug Monit* (1984) 6, 306–12.
3. MacKichan JJ, Boudoulas H, Schaal SF. Effect of cimetidine on quinidine bioavailability. *Biopharm Drug Dispos* (1989) 10, 121–5.
4. Boudoulas H, MacKichan JJ, Schaal SF. Effect of cimetidine on the pharmacodynamics of quinidine. *Med Sci Res* (1988) 16, 713–14.
5. Polish LB, Branch RA, Fitzgerald GA. Digitoxin-quinidine interaction: potentiation during administration of cimetidine. *South Med J* (1981) 74, 633–4.
6. Farringer JA, McWay-Hess K, Clementi WA. Cimetidine–quinidine interaction. *Clin Pharm* (1984) 3, 81–3.
7. Iliopoulou A, Kontogiannis D, Tsoutsos D, Moulopoulos S. Quinidine-ranitidine adverse reaction. *Eur Heart J* (1986) 7, 360.
8. Hardy BG, Schentag JJ. Lack of effect of cimetidine on the metabolism of quinidine: effect on renal clearance. *Int J Clin Pharmacol Ther Toxicol* (1988) 26, 388–91.

Quinidine + Itraconazole

Itraconazole increases the plasma levels of quinidine.

Clinical evidence

In a double-blind, randomised, two-phase crossover study, 9 healthy subjects were given a single 100-mg dose of quinidine sulfate on the final day of a 4-day course of either itraconazole 200 mg daily or placebo. The itraconazole caused a 1.6-fold increase in the peak plasma quinidine levels, a 2.4-fold increase in its AUC, a 1.6-fold increase in its elimination half-life and a 50% decrease in its renal clearance.[1] Similarly, another study in 6 healthy subjects found that itraconazole 100 mg daily for 6 days reduced the total clearance of a single 200-mg dose of quinidine sulfate by 61%, increased its elimination half-life by 35%, and decreased its renal clearance by 60%.[2]

Mechanism

The most likely explanation is that itraconazole not only inhibits the metabolism of quinidine by the cytochrome P450 isoenzyme CYP3A4 in the gut wall and liver, but possibly also inhibits the active secretion of quinidine by the kidney tubules.[1,2]

Importance and management

Direct information appears to be limited to these studies, but the evidence suggests that this interaction is clinically important. What happens is consistent with the way that itraconazole interacts with other drugs. If larger doses of itraconazole were to be used and for longer periods, it seems likely that the effects would be even greater. The concurrent use of these drugs should therefore be well monitored and the dosage of quinidine reduced accordingly. More study is needed. Consider also 'Quinidine + Ketoconazole', below.

1. Kaukonen K-M, Olkkola KT, Neuvonen PJ. Itraconazole increases plasma concentrations of quinidine. *Clin Pharmacol Ther* (1997) 62, 510–17.
2. Damkier P, Hansen LL, Brøsen K. Effect of diclofenac, disulfiram, itraconazole, grapefruit juice and erythromycin on the pharmacokinetics of quinidine. *Br J Clin Pharmacol* (1999) 48, 829–38.

Quinidine + Kaolin-pectin

There is some evidence that kaolin-pectin can reduce the absorption of quinidine and lower its serum levels.

Clinical evidence, mechanism, importance and management

When 4 patients were given 30 mL of kaolin-pectin (*Kaopectate*), after a single 100-mg oral dose of quinidine, the maximal salivary quinidine concentration was reduced by 54% and the AUC by 58%, without any effect on absorption rate.[1] There is a correlation between salivary and serum concentrations after a single (but not repeated) doses of quinidine.[2] This is consistent with *in vitro* data showing quinidine is adsorbed onto kaolin,[3] pectin,[3] and kaolin-pectin.[1] Documentation appears to be limited to these two studies, but be alert for the need to increase the quinidine dosage if kaolin-pectin is used concurrently.

1. Moustafa MA, Al-Shora HI, Gaber M, Gouda MW. Decreased bioavailability of quinidine sulphate due to interactions with adsorbent antacids and antidiarrhoeal mixtures. *Int J Pharmaceutics* (1987) 34, 207–11.
2. Narang PK, Carliner NH, Fisher ML, Crouthamel WG. Quinidine saliva concentrations: absence of correlation with serum concentrations at steady state. *Clin Pharmacol Ther* (1983) 34, 695–702.
3. Bucci AJ, Myre SA, Tan HSI, Shenouda LS. In vitro interaction of quinidine with kaolin and pectin. *J Pharm Sci* (1981) 70, 999–1002.

Quinidine + Ketoconazole

An isolated report describes a temporary marked increase in plasma quinidine levels in man when he was also given ketoconazole.

Clinical evidence, mechanism, importance and management

An elderly man with chronic atrial fibrillation, treated with quinidine sulfate 300 mg four times daily, was also given ketoconazole 200 mg daily, for candidal oesophagitis after antineoplastic therapy. Within 7 days his plasma quinidine levels had risen from a range of 1.4 to 2.7 mg/L up to 6.9 mg/L (normal range 2 to 5 mg/L) but he showed no evidence of toxicity. The elimination half-life of quinidine was found to be 25 hours (normal values in healthy subjects 6 to 7 hours). The quinidine dosage was reduced to 200 mg twice daily, but it needed to be increased to the former dose by the end of a month, even though ketoconazole was continued at the same dosage. The reasons for this reaction are not understood, but may be that the ketoconazole initially inhibits the metabolism of quinidine, causing the plasma levels to rise, and then later induces the metabolism of quinidine, causing the levels to fall.[1] This is an isolated case so that its general importance is uncertain. See also 'Quinidine + Itraconazole', p.281.

1. McNulty RM, Lazor JA, Sketch M. Transient increase in plasma quinidine concentrations during ketoconazole-quinidine therapy. *Clin Pharm* (1989) 8, 222–5.

Quinidine + Laxatives

Quinidine plasma levels can be reduced by the anthraquinone laxative senna.

Clinical evidence, mechanism, importance and management

A study in 7 patients with cardiac arrhythmias taking quinidine bisulfate 500 mg every 12 hours found that the anthraquinone laxative **senna** (***Liquedepur***) reduced plasma quinidine levels, measured 12 hours after the last dose of quinidine, by about 25%.[1] This might be of clinical importance in patients whose plasma levels are barely adequate to control their arrhythmia.

1. Guckenbiehl W, Gilfrich HJ, Just H. Einfluß von Laxantien und Metoclopramid auf die Chindin-Plasmakonzentration während Langzeittherapie bei Patienten mit Herzrhythmusstörugen. *Med Welt* (1976) 27, 1273–6.

Quinidine + Lidocaine

A single case report describes a man taking quinidine who had sinoatrial arrest when he was given intravenous lidocaine.

Clinical evidence, mechanism, importance and management

A man with Parkinson's disease was given quinidine 300 mg every 6 hours for the control of ventricular ectopic beats. After receiving two doses he was given lidocaine as well, initially as a bolus of 80 mg, followed by an infusion of 4 mg/minute because persistent premature ventricular beats developed. Within 2.5 hours the patient complained of dizziness and weakness, and was found to have sinus bradycardia, sinoatrial arrest and atrioventricular escape rhythm. Normal sinus rhythm resumed when the lidocaine was stopped. Whether quinidine was a contributing factor in this reaction is uncertain.[1] However, this case emphasises the need to exercise caution when giving two drugs that have cardiac depressant actions.

1. Jeresaty RM, Kahn AH, Landry AB. Sinoatrial arrest due to lidocaine in a patient receiving quinidine. *Chest* (1972) 61, 683–5.

Quinidine + Metoclopramide

Metoclopramide slightly reduced the absorption of quinidine from a sustained-release formulation in one study, but modestly increased quinidine levels in another.

Clinical evidence

A study of this interaction was prompted by the case of a patient who was taking sustained-release quinidine (*Quinidex*) and whose arrhythmia became uncontrolled when metoclopramide was added. In a crossover study, 9 healthy subjects were given either metoclopramide 10 mg every 6 hours for 24 hours before, and 48 hours after, a single 600- or 900-mg oral dose of quinidine sulfate or quinidine alone. It was found that metoclopramide caused a mean 10% decrease in the AUC of quinidine, although two subjects had decreases of 22.5 and 28.1%, respectively. The elimination rate constant was unaffected.[1] Another study in patients taking a sustained-release formulation of quinidine bisulfate 500 mg every 12 hours found that metoclopramide 10 mg three times daily increased the mean plasma levels measured 3.5 hours after the last dose of quinidine by almost 20%, from 1.6 to 1.9 micrograms/mL, and at 12 hours by about 16%, from 2.4 to 2.8 micrograms/mL.[2]

Mechanism

Not understood. Metoclopramide alters both the gastric emptying time and gastrointestinal motility, which can affect quinidine absorption.

Importance and management

Direct information seems to be limited to these studies using different quinidine preparations. The outcome of concurrent use is uncertain, but generally seems small.

1. Yuen GJ, Hansten PD, Collins J. Effect of metoclopramide on the absorption of an oral sustained-release quinidine product. *Clin Pharm* (1987) 6, 722–5.
2. Guckenbiehl W, Gilfrich HJ, Just H. Einfluß von Laxantien und Metoclopramid auf die Chindin-Plasmakonzentration während Langzeittherapie bei Patienten mit Herzrhythmusstörugen. *Med Welt* (1976) 27, 1273–6.

Quinidine + Omeprazole

Omeprazole does not appear to alter the pharmacokinetics or QT-interval prolonging effects of quinidine.

Clinical evidence, mechanism, importance and management

Omeprazole 40 mg daily for one week had no effect on the pharmacokinetics of a single 400-mg dose of quinidine sulfate in 8 healthy subjects. In addition, the corrected QT interval was not significantly changed.[1] There would not appear to be the need for any special precautions during concurrent use.

1. Ching MS, Elliott SL, Stead CK, Murdoch RT, Devenish-Meares S, Morgan DJ, Smallwood RA. Quinidine single dose pharmacokinetics and pharmacodynamics are unaltered by omeprazole. *Aliment Pharmacol Ther* (1991) 5, 523–31.

Quinidine + Quinolones

Ciprofloxacin normally appears not to interact with quinidine to a clinically relevant extent. An increased risk of torsade de pointes might be expected if quinidine is used with gatifloxacin, moxifloxacin, or sparfloxacin, and possibly levofloxacin.

Clinical evidence, mechanism, importance and management

The pharmacokinetics of a single 400-mg oral dose of quinidine sulfate and QRS and QTc prolongation were not significantly changed in 7 healthy subjects after they took **ciprofloxacin** 750 mg daily for 6 days. The decrease in clearance ranged from a decrease of 10% to an increase of 20%, with a mean 1% increase, which is unlikely to be clinically relevant.[1] However an isolated case report describes a woman who started taking quinidine gluconate 324 mg every 8 hours while she was taking **ciprofloxacin** and metronidazole. Her first trough serum quinidine levels was raised a little above normal at 6.3 micrograms/mL compared with the normal range of 2 to 5 micrograms/mL, without evidence of toxicity. Quinidine therapy was continued unchanged, and her next trough serum quinidine level was only 2.3 micrograms/mL, 3 days after finishing the course of antibacterials. This was tentatively attributed to the possible enzyme inhibitory effects of **ciprofloxacin** and metronidazole. This case is far from clear and so no firm conclusions can be reached.[2] There would seem to be little reason for avoiding concurrent use.

Some quinolones can prolong the QT interval, and would be expected to increase the risk of torsade de pointes arrhythmias when used with quinidine. Of the quinolones used clinically, **gatifloxacin**, **moxifloxacin**, and **sparfloxacin** are known to prolong the QT interval (see 'Table 9.2', (p.257)). There is also evidence that **levofloxacin** may prolong the QT interval (see 'Amiodarone + Quinolones', p.249). These quinolones should probably be avoided in patients taking quinidine (see also 'Drugs that prolong the QT interval + Other drugs that prolong the QT interval', p.257).

1. Bleske BE, Carver PL, Annesley TM, Bleske JRM, Morady F. The effect of ciprofloxacin on the pharmacokinetic and ECG parameters of quinidine. *J Clin Pharmacol* (1990) 30, 911–15.
2. Cooke CE, Sklar GE, Nappi JM. Possible pharmacokinetic interaction with quinidine: ciprofloxacin or metronidazole? *Ann Pharmacother* (1996) 30, 364–6.

Quinidine + Rifamycins

The serum levels and therapeutic effects of quinidine can be markedly reduced by rifampicin.

Clinical evidence

It was noted that the control of ventricular arrhythmia deteriorated in a patient taking quinidine sulfate 800 mg daily within a week of starting to take **rifampicin** 600 mg daily. His serum quinidine level fell from 4 to 0.5 micrograms/mL, and remained low despite doubling the quinidine dose to 1.6 g daily. The **rifampicin** was discontinued, and quinidine levels gradually increased over a week. Some signs of quinidine toxicity then occurred, and the quinidine dose was reduced back to 800 mg daily.[1] Further study in 4 healthy subjects found that treatment with **rifampicin** 600 mg daily for 7 days reduced the mean half-life of a single 6-mg/kg oral dose of quinidine sulfate by about 62% (from 6.1 to 2.3 hours) and the AUC by 83%.[2] Similar findings were reported in 4 other subjects receiving the same dose of quinidine intravenously.[2]

Another case report describes a patient taking **rifampicin** who did not achieve adequate serum quinidine levels despite large daily doses of up to 3.2 g of quinidine. When the **rifampicin** was stopped, ultimately, a reduced quinidine dosage of 1.8 g daily achieved a serum level of 2 micrograms/mL, reflecting a 44% decrease in dose and a 43% increase in level.[3] In a further case, a 'double interaction' was seen when a patient taking quinidine and digoxin was given **rifampicin**: the quinidine levels fell, resulting in a fall in digoxin levels.[4]

Mechanism

Rifampicin is a potent enzyme-inducer, which markedly increases the metabolism of the quinidine by 3-hydroxylation and N-oxidation, thereby reducing its levels and effects.[5] It has been suggested that two of the quinidine metabolites (3-hydroxyquinidine and 2-oxoquinidinone) may be active, which might, to some extent, offset the effects of this interaction.[4]

Importance and management

An established and clinically important interaction, although documentation is limited. The dosage of quinidine will need to be increased if rifampicin is given concurrently. Monitor the serum levels. Doubling the dose may not be sufficient.[2,4] An equivalent dosage reduction will be needed if the rifampicin is stopped. There does not seem to be any information regarding the other rifamycins, **rifabutin** (a weak enzyme inducer) and **rifapentine** (a moderate enzyme inducer). However, the manufacturers and the CSM in the UK warn that **rifabutin** may possibly reduce the effects of a number of drugs, including quinidine.[6,7]

1. Ahmad D, Mathur P, Ahuja S, Henderson R, Carruthers G. Rifampicin-quinidine interaction. *Br J Dis Chest* (1979) 73, 409–11.
2. Twum-Barima Y, Carruthers SG. Quinidine-rifampin interaction. *N Engl J Med* (1981) 304, 1466–9.
3. Schwartz A, Brown JR. Quinidine-rifampin interaction. *Am Heart J* (1984) 107, 789–90.
4. Bussey HI, Merritt GJ, Hill EG. The influence of rifampin on quinidine and digoxin. *Arch Intern Med* (1984) 144, 1021–3.
5. Damkier P, Hansen LL, Brøsen K. Rifampicin treatment greatly increases the apparent oral clearance of quinidine. *Pharmacol Toxicol* (1999) 85, 257–62.
6. Mycobutin (Rifabutin). Pharmacia Ltd. UK Summary of product characteristics, October 2006.
7. Committee on the Safety of Medicines/Medicines Control Agency. Revised indication and drug interactions of rifabutin. *Current Problems* (1997) 23, 14.

Quinidine + Sucralfate

An isolated report describes a marked reduction in serum quinidine levels, which was attributed to the concurrent use of sucralfate.

Clinical evidence, mechanism, importance and management

An elderly woman was found to have subtherapeutic levels of warfarin, digoxin and sustained-release quinidine (serum quinidine level 0.31 micromol/L), even though they were given 2 hours apart from sucralfate. On hospitalisation, a variety of other medications were then started for chest pain (glyceryl trinitrate, diltiazem, pethidine, promethazine), and on day 4 the sucralfate was stopped. On day 5, her serum quinidine level was 5.55 micromol/L.[1] The patient denied noncompliance, and the suggestion was that sucralfate can bind with quinidine within the gut and reduce its absorption. However, a study in *dogs* found sucralfate did not alter quinidine bioavailability.[2] This isolated case report is of doubtful general importance.

1. Rey AM, Gums JG. Altered absorption of digoxin, sustained-release quinidine, and warfarin with sucralfate administration. *DICP Ann Pharmacother* (1991) 25, 745–6.
2. Lacz JP, Groschang AG, Geising DH, Browne RK. The effect of sucralfate on drug absorption in dogs. *Gastroenterology* (1982) 82, 1108.

Tocainide + Antacids or Urinary alkalinisers

Raising the pH of the urine (e.g. with some antacids, diuretics or alkaline salts) can modestly reduce the loss of tocainide from the body.

Clinical evidence

Preliminary findings of a study found that when 5 healthy subjects took 30 mL of an unnamed antacid four times a day for 48 hours before and 58 hours after a single 600-mg dose of tocainide, the urinary pH rose from 5.9 to 6.9, the total clearance of tocainide fell by 28%, the peak serum levels fell by 19% from 4.2 to 3.4 micrograms/mL, the AUC rose by 33% and the half-life was prolonged from 13.2 to 15.4 hours.[1]

Mechanism

Tocainide is a weak base so that its loss in the urine will be affected by the pH of the urine. Alkalinisation of the urine increases the number of non-ionised molecules available for passive reabsorption, thereby reducing the urinary loss and raising the serum levels.

Importance and management

An established interaction of uncertain but probably limited clinical importance. There seem to be no reports of adverse reactions in patients as a result of this interaction, but be alert for any evidence of increased tocainide effects if other drugs are given that can raise the urinary pH significantly (e.g. **sodium bicarbonate** and **acetazolamide**). Reduce the tocainide dosage if necessary. Of the antacids,[2] **aluminium/magnesium hydroxide** (*Maalox*) can raise urinary pH by about 0.9 whereas **magnesium hydroxide** (*Milk of magnesia*) and **calcium carbonate-glycine** (*Titralac*) in normal doses raise the pH by about 0.5. **Aluminium hydroxide** (*Amphogel*) and **dihydroxyaluminium glycinate** (*Robalate*) are reported to have no effect on urinary pH.[2]

1. Meneilly GP, Scavone JM, Meneilly GS, Wei JY. Tocainide: pharmacokinetic alterations during antacid-induced urinary alkalinization. *Clin Pharmacol Ther* (1987) 41, 178.
2. Gibaldi M, Grundhofer B, Levy G. Effect of antacids on pH of urine. *Clin Pharmacol Ther* (1974) 16, 520–5.

Tocainide + H_2-receptor antagonists

There is some evidence that cimetidine can reduce the bioavailability and serum levels of tocainide, but ranitidine appears not to interact.

Clinical evidence, mechanism, importance and management

In a preliminary report of a study, 4 days of treatment with **cimetidine** [dose not stated] in 11 healthy subjects had a small effect on the pharmacokinetics of tocainide 500 mg given intravenously over 15 minutes, which was not considered clinically important.[1] In another study, **cimetidine** 300 mg four times daily for 2 days reduced the AUC of a single 400-mg oral dose of tocainide in 7 healthy subjects by about one-third. The peak serum levels were also reduced, from 2.81 to 1.7 micrograms/mL, but no changes in the half-life or renal clearance occurred.[2] The reasons for this, and its clinical importance are uncertain, but be alert for evidence of a reduced response to tocainide in the presence of **cimetidine**. **Ranitidine** 150 mg twice daily has been found not to interact.[2]

1. Price BA, Holmes GI, Antonello J, Yeh KC, Demetriades J, Irvin JD, McMahon FG. Intravenous tocainide (T) maintains safe therapeutic levels when administered concomitantly with cimetidine (C). *Clin Pharmacol Ther* (1987), 41, 237.

2. North DS, Mattern AL, Kapil RP, Lalonde RL. The effect of histamine-2 receptor antagonists on tocainide pharmacokinetics. *J Clin Pharmacol* (1988) 28, 640–3.

Tocainide + Phenobarbital

Phenobarbital does not appear to alter the pharmacokinetics of tocainide.

Clinical evidence, mechanism, importance and management

Phenobarbital 100 mg daily for 15 days did not alter the AUC of a single 600-mg dose of tocainide in 6 healthy subjects. In addition, the percentage of the dose excreted unchanged in the urine and as the glucuronide metabolite did not differ.[1] Phenobarbital at this dosage does not appear to alter the metabolism of tocainide. No special precautions appear to be necessary.

1. Elvin AT, Lalka D, Stoeckel K, du Souich P, Axelson JE, Golden LH, McLean AJ. Tocainide kinetics and metabolism: effects of phenobarbital and substrates of glucuronyl transferase. *Clin Pharmacol Ther* (1980) 28, 652–8.

Tocainide + Rifampicin (Rifampin)

The loss of tocainide from the body is increased by rifampicin.

Clinical evidence, mechanism, importance and management

The AUC of a single 600-mg oral dose of tocainide was reduced by almost 30% and the half-life was also reduced by about 30%, from 13.2 to 9.4 hours, in 8 healthy subjects given rifampicin 300 mg twice daily for 5 days.[1]

This response is consistent with the well-recognised enzyme inducing effects of rifampicin. Information is limited to this single dose study, but the interaction would seem to be established and may be of clinical importance. Monitor any patients given rifampicin for evidence of reduced tocainide serum levels and reduced effects. Increase the dosage as necessary. Reduce the tocainide dosage if the rifampicin is withdrawn. More study is needed.

1. Rice TL, Patterson JH, Celestin C, Foster JR, Powell JR. Influence of rifampin on tocainide pharmacokinetics in humans. *Clin Pharm* (1989) 8, 200–205.

10

Antibacterials

This section deals with interactions where the effects of the antibacterial are altered. In many cases the antibacterial drugs interact by affecting other drugs, and these interactions are dealt with elsewhere in this publication. Some of the macrolides and the quinolones are potent enzyme inhibitors; the macrolides exert their effects on the cytochrome P450 isoenzyme CYP3A4, whereas many quinolones inhibit CYP1A2. Rifampicin (rifampin) is a potent non-specific enzyme inducer and therefore lowers the levels of many drugs.

Many of the interactions covered in this section concern absorption interactions, such as the ability of the tetracyclines and quinolones to chelate with divalent cations. More information on the mechanism of these interactions can be found in 'Drug absorption interactions', (p.3).

Many monographs concern the use of multiple antibacterials. One of the great difficulties with these interactions is the often poor correlation between *in vitro* and *in vivo* studies, so that it is difficult to get a thoroughly reliable indication of how antibacterial drugs will behave together in clinical practice. Two antibacterials may actually be less effective than one on its own, because, in theory, the effects of a bactericidal drug, which requires actively dividing cells for it to be effective, may be reduced by a bacteriostatic drug. However, in practice this seems to be less important than might be supposed and there are relatively few well-authenticated clinical examples.

The antibacterials covered in this section are listed in 'Table 10.1', (see below).

Table 10.1 Antibacterials

Group	*Drugs*
Aminoglycosides	Amikacin, Astromicin, Dibekacin, Dihydrostreptomycin, Framycetin, Gentamicin, Isepamicin, Kanamycin, Micronomicin, Neomycin, Netilmicin, Paromomycin, Sisomicin, Streptomycin, Tobramycin
Antimycobacterials and related drugs	Aminosalicylic acid (PAS), Capreomycin, Clofazimine, Cycloserine, Dapsone, Ethambutol, Ethionamide, Isoniazid, Methaniazide, Protionamide, Pyrazinamide, Rifabutin, Rifampicin (Rifampin), Rifamycin, Rifapentine, Rifaximin
Carbapenems	Biapenem, Ertapenem, Faropenem, Imipenem, Meropenem, Panipenem
Cephalosporins	Cefaclor, Cefadroxil, Cefalexin, Cefaloglycin, Cefaloridine, Cefalotin, Cefamandole, Cefapirin, Cefatrizine, Cefazolin, Cefbuperazone, Cefcapene, Cefdinir, Cefditoren, Cefepime, Cefetamet, Cefixime, Cefmenoxime, Cefmetazole, Cefminox, Cefodizime, Cefonicid, Cefoperazone, Ceforanide, Cefotaxime, Cefotetan, Cefotiam, Cefoxitin, Cefpiramide, Cefpirome, Cefpodoxime, Cefprozil, Cefradine, Cefsulodin, Ceftazidime, Cefteram, Ceftezole, Ceftibuten, Ceftizoxime, Ceftriaxone, Cefuroxime, Flomoxef, Latamoxef
Macrolides	Azithromycin, Clarithromycin, Dirithromycin, Erythromycin, Flurithromycin, Josamycin, Midecamycin, Rokitomycin, Roxithromycin, Spiramycin, Telithromycin, Troleandomycin
Penicillins	Amoxicillin, Ampicillin, Azidocillin, Azlocillin, Bacampicillin, Benzylpenicillin (Penicillin G), Carbenicillin, Carindacillin, Ciclacillin, Clometocillin, Cloxacillin, Dicloxacillin, Flucloxacillin, Mecillinam, Meticillin, Mezlocillin, Nafcillin, Oxacillin, Phenethicillin, Phenoxymethylpenicillin (Penicillin V), Piperacillin, Pivampicillin, Pivmecillinam, Procaine benzylpenicillin (Procaine penicillin), Propicillin, Sulbenicillin, Temocillin, Ticarcillin
Polypeptides	Bacitracin, Colistimethate sodium, Colistin, Polymyxin B, Teicoplanin, Vancomycin
Quinolones	Cinoxacin, Ciprofloxacin, Enoxacin, Fleroxacin, Flumequine, Gatifloxacin, Gemifloxacin, Grepafloxacin, Levofloxacin, Lomefloxacin, Moxifloxacin, Nadifloxacin, Nalidixic acid, Norfloxacin, Ofloxacin, Oxolinic Acid, Pazufloxacin, Pefloxacin, Pipemidic Acid, Rosoxacin, Rufloxacin, Sparfloxacin, Temafloxacin, Tosufloxacin, Trovafloxacin
Sulfonamides	Co-trimoxazole, Phthalylsulfathiazole, Sulfadiazine, Sulfadimidine (Sulfamethazine), Sulfafurazole (Sulfisoxazole), Sulfaguanidine, Sulfamerazine, Sulfamethizole, Sulfamethoxazole, Sulfametopyrazine, Sulfametrole
Tetracyclines	Chlortetracyline, Demeclocycline, Doxycycline, Lymecycline, Methacycline, Minocycline, Oxytetracycline, Rolitetracycline, Tetracycline, Tigecycline
Miscellaneous	Aztreonam, Carumonam, Chloramphenicol, Cilastatin, Clindamycin, Daptomycin, Fosfomycin, Fusidic acid, Lincomycin, Linezolid, Loracarbef, Methenamine, Metronidazole, Mupirocin, Nitrofurantoin, Novobiocin, Pristinamycin, Quinupristin/Dalfopristin, Spectinomycin, Trimethoprim, Vancomycin

Aminoglycosides + Amphotericin B

One study suggested that amphotericin B decreased the clearance of amikacin and gentamicin. The concurrent use of aminoglycosides and amphotericin B can result in nephrotoxicity.

Clinical evidence, mechanism, importance and management

A study found that **amikacin** or **gentamicin** clearance was impaired in 12 of 17 children given amphotericin B. Serum creatinine increased by 50% or more in 3 of them, but there was no significant increase in creatinine levels in 7 others. As a result, the aminoglycoside dose was decreased or the dose interval lengthened in 7 children.[1]

The renal function of 4 patients receiving moderate doses of **gentamicin** deteriorated when they were given amphotericin B. Both drugs are known to be nephrotoxic and it is suggested, on the basis of what was seen, that combined use may have had additive nephrotoxic effects.[2] A further retrospective analysis found that the use of **amikacin** tended to increase amphotericin B-related nephrotoxicity.[3]

A study assessing the risk factors for nephrotoxicity with aminoglycosides (**tobramycin** and **gentamicin**) enrolled 1489 patients, 157 of whom developed clinical nephrotoxicity. Of these patients 118 had no immediately identifiable cause (such as acute renal failure) and further evaluation of other risk factors found that the concurrent use of amphotericin B significantly increased the risk of nephrotoxicity.[4]

The nephrotoxicity of various combinations of antibiotics was assessed in 171 cancer patients (139 treated with a combination of aminoglycoside with penicillin or cephalosporin; 32 treated with amphotericin B or vancomycin with other antibacterials). The highest nephrotoxicity (based on changes in urea and electrolytes) was found in patients treated with amphotericin B with an aminoglycoside and a cephalosporin.[5]

Two other studies did not find aminoglycosides increased the risk of amphotericin B-associated toxicity (defined as a 100% or greater increase in serum creatinine),[6,7] although in one of the studies[7] the frequency of concurrent aminoglycoside use may have been too low to identify any evidence of increased nephrotoxic risk.

As aminoglycosides are generally considered to be nephrotoxic, avoidance of use with other nephrotoxic drugs (such as amphotericin B) is generally recommended. However, concurrent use may be essential. Renal function and drug levels should be routinely monitored during aminoglycoside therapy, and it may be prudent to increase the frequency of such monitoring in the presence of amphotericin B. Lipid formulations of amphotericin B are less nephrotoxic than the conventional formulation.[8] One manufacturer notes there was significantly less nephrotoxicity in patients receiving concurrent aminoglycosides and liposomal amphotericin B (*Ambisome*) compared to aminoglycosides and conventional amphotericin B.[9]

1. Goren MP, Viar MJ, Shenep JL, Wright RK, Baker DK, Kalwinsky DK. Monitoring serum aminoglycoside concentrations in children with amphotericin B nephrotoxicity. *Pediatr Infect Dis J* (1988) 7, 698–703.
2. Churchill DN, Seely J. Nephrotoxicity associated with combined gentamicin-amphotericin B therapy. *Nephron* (1977) 19, 176–181.
3. Harbath S, Pestotnik SL, Lloyd JF, Burke JP, Samore MH. The epidemiology of nephrotoxicity associated with conventional amphotericin B therapy. *Am J Med* (2001) 111, 528–34.
4. Bertino JS, Booker LA, Franck PA, Jenkins PL, Franck KR, Nafziger AN. Incidence of and significant risk factors for aminoglycoside-associated nephrotoxicity in patients dosed by using individualized pharmacokinetic monitoring. *J Infect Dis* (1993) 167, 173–9.
5. Krčméry V, Fuchsberger P, Gočár M, Šalát T, Bodnárová J, Sobota R, Koza I, Švec J. Nephrotoxicity of aminoglycosides, polypeptides and cephalosporins in cancer patients. *Chemotherapy* (1991) 37, 287–91.
6. Fisher MA, Talbot GH, Maislin G, McKeon BP, Tynan KP, Strom BL. Risk factors for amphotericin B-associated nephrotoxicity. *Am J Med* (1989) 87, 547–52.
7. Zager RA, O'Quigley J, Zager BK, Alpers CE, Shulman HM, Gamelin LM, Stewart P, Thomas ED. Acute renal failure following bone marrow transplantation: a retrospective study of 272 patients. *Am J Kidney Dis* (1989) 13, 210–16.
8. Dupont B. Overview of the lipid formulations of amphotericin B. *J Antimicrob Chemother* (2002) 49, (Suppl S1) 31–6.
9. Ambisome (Liposomal Amphotericin B). Gilead Sciences International Ltd. UK Summary of product characteristics, August 2006.

Aminoglycosides + Cephalosporins

The nephrotoxic effects of gentamicin and tobramycin can be increased by cefalotin. This may also occur with other aminoglycosides and cephalosporins.

Clinical evidence

(a) Gentamicin and Cefaloridine

Acute renal failure has been reported in a patient given gentamicin and cefaloridine.[1] One study reported an increase in the incidence of nephrotoxicity when cefaloridine was given with gentamicin (or other unnamed aminoglycosides), although other factors such as excessive dosage or pre-existing renal impairment were also associated with the increase in cephalosporin nephrotoxicity in most cases.[2]

(b) Gentamicin or Tobramycin and Cefalotin

A randomised, double-blind study[3] in patients with sepsis showed the following incidence of definite nephrotoxicity;

- **gentamicin** with **cefalotin** 30.4% (7 of 23 patients),
- **tobramycin** with **cefalotin** 20.8% (5 of 24),
- **gentamicin** with **methicillin** 10% (2 of 20),
- **tobramycin** with **methicillin** 4.3% (1 of 23).

A very considerable number of studies and case reports confirm an increase in the incidence of nephrotoxicity when **gentamicin**[2,4-14] or **tobramycin**[15,16] are used with **cefalotin**. However, some other studies have found no increase in nephrotoxicity with the combination.[17-20]

(c) Aminoglycosides and other Cephalosporins

The nephrotoxicity of various combinations of antibiotics was assessed in 171 cancer patients. In those receiving an aminoglycoside with a third generation cephalosporin, the most nephrotoxic combinations were found to be **gentamicin** with **cefotaxime** (although another study did not find this combination to be nephrotoxic[21]) and **amikacin** with **ceftriaxone**, where 5 of 20 and 5 of 13 patients, respectively, had increased serum creatinine. The following combinations were found to be safer: **amikacin** with **cefoxitin** or **ceftazidime**, **gentamicin** with **cefoxitin**, and **netilmicin** with **cefotaxime**.[22]

Another study assessing the risk factors for nephrotoxicity with aminoglycosides (**tobramycin** and **gentamicin**) enrolled 1489 patients, 157 of whom developed clinical nephrotoxicity. Of these patients 118 had no immediately identifiable cause (such as acute renal failure) and further evaluation of other risk factors found that the concurrent use of cephalosporins (including **cefazolin**, **cefotaxime**, **cefoxitin**, **cefamandole**, **cefuroxime**, **ceftriaxone**, and **ceftazidime**) significantly increased the risk of nephrotoxicity.[23]

Hypokalaemia has also been described in patients taking cytotoxic drugs for leukaemia when they were given **gentamicin** and **cefalexin**.[24]

A study in healthy subjects found that **ceftazidime** may increase the levels of **amikacin**.[25]

Some studies have reported no adverse interactions between;

- **amikacin** and **cefepime**[26]
- **gentamicin** and **cefuroxime**,[27] or **cefazolin**,[20]
- **tobramycin** and **cefuroxime**,[28] **cefotaxime**,[29] **ceftazidime**[30] or **cefazolin**[20]

Mechanism

Uncertain. The nephrotoxic effects of gentamicin and tobramycin are well documented, and some (mostly older) cephalosporins are known to be nephrotoxic, especially in high dose. However, it appears that doses that are well tolerated separately can be nephrotoxic when given together.[11]

Importance and management

The interaction between gentamicin and cefalotin is very well documented and potentially serious, but there is less information about tobramycin with cefalotin. The risk of nephrotoxicity is probably greatest if high doses of antibacterial are used in those with some existing renal impairment. One study suggests that short courses of treatment are sometimes justified,[12] but renal function should be very closely monitored and dosages kept to a minimum. The combination of gentamicin or tobramycin and cefalotin is probably best avoided in high-risk patients wherever possible.

Whether other aminoglycosides or cephalosporins interact similarly is uncertain, but the possibility should be borne in mind. Risk factors for this interaction are said to include raised aminoglycoside trough levels, decreased albumin, male gender, advanced age, increased length of treatment, liver disease or ascites, and some other diseases, including leukaemia,[23,31] although their significance in practice has been questioned.[23]

1. Zazgornik J, Schmidt P, Lugscheider R, Kopsa H. Akutes Nierenversagen bei kombinierter Cephaloridin-Gentamycin-Therapie. *Wien Klin Wochenschr* (1973) 85, 839–41.
2. Foord RD. Cephaloridine, cephalothin and the kidney. *J Antimicrob Chemother* (1975) 1(suppl) 119–33.
3. Wade JC, Smith CR, Petty BG, Lipsky JJ, Conrad G, Ellner J, Lietman PS. Cephalothin plus an aminoglycoside is more nephrotoxic than methicillin plus an aminoglycoside. *Lancet* (1978) ii, 604–6.
4. Opitz A, Herrmann I, von Harrath D, Schaefer K. Akute niereninsuffizienz nach Gentamycin-Cephalosporin-Kombinationstherapie. *Med Welt* (1971) 22, 434–8.
5. Plager JE. Association of renal injury with combined cephalothin-gentamicin therapy among patients severely ill with malignant disease. *Cancer* (1976) 37, 1937–43.
6. The EORTC International Antimicrobial Therapy Project Group. Three antibiotic regimens in the treatment of infection in febrile granulocytopenic patients with cancer. *J Infect Dis* (1978) 137, 14–29.
7. Kleinknecht D, Ganeval D, Droz D. Acute renal failure after high doses of gentamicin and cephalothin. *Lancet* (1973) i, 1129.
8. Bobrow SN, Jaffe E, Young RC. Anuria and acute tubular necrosis associated with gentamicin and cephalothin. *JAMA* (1972) 222, 1546–7.
9. Fillastre JP, Laumonier R, Humbert G, Dubois D, Metayer J, Delpech A, Leroy J, Robert M. Acute renal failure associated with combined gentamicin and cephalothin therapy. *BMJ* (1973) 2, 396–7.
10. Cabanillas F, Burgos RC, Rodríguez RC, Baldizón C. Nephrotoxicity of combined cephalothin-gentamicin regimen. *Arch Intern Med* (1975) 135, 850–52.
11. Tvedegaard E. Interaction between gentamicin and cephalothin as cause of acute renal failure. *Lancet* (1976) ii, 581.
12. Hansen MM, Kaaber K. Nephrotoxicity in combined cephalothin and gentamicin therapy. *Acta Med Scand* (1977) 201, 463–7.
13. Schwartz JH, Schein P. Fanconi syndrome associated with cephalothin and gentamicin therapy. *Cancer* (1978) 41, 769–72.
14. Bailey RR. Renal failure in combined gentamicin and cephalothin therapy. *BMJ* (1973) 2, 776–7.
15. Tobias JS, Whitehouse JM, Wrigley PFM. Severe renal dysfunction after tobramycin/cephalothin therapy. *Lancet* (1976) i, 425.
16. Klastersky J, Hensgens C, Debusscher L. Empiric therapy for cancer patients: comparative study of ticarcillin-tobramycin, ticarcillin-cephalothin, and cephalothin-tobramycin. *Antimicrob Agents Chemother* (1975) 7, 640–45.
17. Fanning WL, Gump D, Jick H. Gentamicin- and cephalothin-associated rises in blood urea nitrogen. *Antimicrob Agents Chemother* (1976) 10, 80–82.
18. Stille W, Arndt I. Argumente gegen eine Nephrotoxizität von cephalothin und gentamycin. *Med Welt* (1972) 23, 1603–5.
19. Wellwood JM, Simpson PM, Tighe JR, Thompson AE. Evidence of gentamicin nephrotoxicity in patients with renal allografts. *BMJ* (1975) 3, 278–81.
20. Schentag JJ, Cerra FB, Plaut ME. Clinical and pharmacokinetic characteristics of aminoglycoside nephrotoxicity in 201 critically ill patients. *Antimicrob Agents Chemother* (1982) 21, 721–6.
21. Bethke RO, v. Gablenz E, Malerczyk V, Seidel G. Nierenverträglichkeit der kombinierten Behandlung mit Cefotaxim und Gentamicin. *Dtsch Med Wochenschr* (1981) 106, 334–6.
22. Krčméry V, Fuchsberger P, Gočár M, Šalát T, Bodnárová J, Sobota R, Koza I, Švec J. Nephrotoxicity of aminoglycosides, polypeptides and cephalosporins in cancer patients. *Chemotherapy* (1991) 37, 287–91.
23. Bertino JS, Booker LA, Franck PA, Jenkins PL, Franck KR, Nafziger AN. Incidence of and significant risk factors for aminoglycoside-associated nephrotoxicity in patients dosed by using individualized pharmacokinetic monitoring. *J Infect Dis* (1993) 167, 173–9.
24. Young GP, Sullivan J, Hurley A. Hypokalæmia due to gentamicin/cephalexin in leukaemia. *Lancet* (1973) ii, 855.
25. Adamis G, Papaioannou MG, Giamarellos-Bourboulis EJ, Gargalianos P, Kosmidis J, Giamarellou H. Pharmacokinetic interactions of ceftazidime, imipenem and aztreonam with amikacin in healthy volunteers. *Int J Antimicrob Agents* (2004) 23, 144–9.
26. Barbhaiya RH, Knupp CA, Pfeffer M, Pittman KA. Lack of pharmacokinetic interaction between cefepime and amikacin in humans. *Antimicrob Agents Chemother* (1992) 36, 1382–6.
27. Cockram CS, Richards P, Bax RP. The safety of cefuroxime and gentamicin in patients with reduced renal function. *Curr Med Res Opin* (1980) 6, 398–403.
28. Trollfors B, Alestig K, Rödjer S, Sandberg T, Westin J. Renal function in patients treated with tobramycin-cefuroxime or tobramycin-penicillin G. *J Antimicrob Chemother* (1983) 12, 641–5.
29. Kuhlmann J, Seidel G, Richter E, Grötsch H. Tobramycin nephrotoxicity: failure of cefotaxime to potentiate injury in patient. *Naunyn Schmiedebergs Arch Pharmacol* (1981) 316 (Suppl), R80.
30. Aronoff GR, Brier RA, Sloan RS, Brier ME. Interactions of ceftazidime and tobramycin in patients with normal and impaired renal function. *Antimicrob Agents Chemother* (1990) 34, 1139–42.
31. Streetman DS, Nafziger AN, Destache CJ, Bertino JS. Individualized pharmacokinetic monitoring results in less aminoglycoside-associated nephrotoxicity and fewer associated costs. *Pharmacotherapy* (2001) 21, 443–51.

Aminoglycosides + Clindamycin

Three cases of acute renal failure have been tentatively attributed to the use of gentamicin with clindamycin, and another report identified the combination as a risk factor for nephrotoxicity. However, other reports note no increased nephrotoxicity when gentamicin or tobramycin was given with clindamycin.

Clinical evidence, mechanism, importance and management

Acute renal failure has been reported in 3 patients with normal renal function when they were given **gentamicin** 3.9 to 4.9 mg/kg daily and clindamycin 0.9 to 1.8 mg/kg daily for 13 to 18 days. They recovered within 3 to 5 days of discontinuing the antibacterials[1] but in one patient acute renal failure only developed after the clindamycin was stopped. The reasons for the renal failure are not known, but given the long courses of **gentamicin** involved, the possibility that renal impairment occurred as an adverse effect of the aminoglycoside alone cannot be excluded. However, one report identified concurrent clindamycin as one of several factors that increased the risk of aminoglycoside-associated nephrotoxicity.[2]

Clindamycin with an aminoglycoside seems to be a fairly common antibacterial combination, especially following abdominal trauma. A study assessing the risk factors for nephrotoxicity with aminoglycosides (**tobramycin** and **gentamicin**) enrolled 1489 patients, 157 of whom developed clinical nephrotoxicity. Of these patients 118 had no immediately identifiable cause (such as acute renal failure) and further evaluation of other risk factors found that the concurrent use of clindamycin was not significantly associated with increased risk of nephrotoxicity.[3] This suggests that treatment with the combination is without nephrotoxic risk above and beyond that seen with an aminoglycoside alone. A short report has also indicated that the combination of **tobramycin** and clindamycin is not nephrotoxic.[4]

As renal function should be routinely monitored during the use of aminoglycosides, no additional precautions should be necessary if clindamycin is also given.

1. Butkus DE, de Torrente A, Terman DS. Renal failure following gentamicin in combination with clindamycin. Gentamicin nephrotoxicity. *Nephron* (1976) 17, 307–13.
2. Streetman DS, Nafziger AN, Destache CJ, Bertino JS. Individualized pharmacokinetic monitoring results in less aminoglycoside-associated nephrotoxicity and fewer associated costs. *Pharmacotherapy* (2001) 21, 443–51.
3. Bertino JS, Booker LA, Franck PA, Jenkins PL, Franck KR, Nafziger AN. Incidence of and significant risk factors for aminoglycoside-associated nephrotoxicity in patients dosed by using individualized pharmacokinetic monitoring. *J Infect Dis* (1993) 167, 173–9.
4. Gillett P, Wise R, Melikian V, Falk R. Tobramycin/cephalothin nephrotoxicity. *Lancet* (1976) i, 547.

Aminoglycosides + Loop diuretics

The concurrent use of aminoglycosides and etacrynic acid should be avoided because their damaging actions on the ear can be additive. Even sequential use may not be safe. Bumetanide and piretanide have been shown to interact similarly in *animals*. Although some patients have developed nephrotoxicity and/or ototoxicity while taking furosemide and an aminoglycoside, it has not been established that this was as a result of an interaction.

Clinical evidence

(a) Bumetanide

There seem to be no clinical reports of an interaction between aminoglycosides and bumetanide, but ototoxicity has been described in *animals* given **kanamycin** and bumetanide.[1,2]

(b) Etacrynic acid

Four patients with renal impairment became permanently deaf after they were given intramuscular **kanamycin** 1 to 1.5 g and intravenous etacrynic acid 50 to 150 mg. One patient also received **streptomycin**, and another also received oral **neomycin**. Deafness took between 30 minutes and almost 2 weeks to develop. In some cases deafness developed despite the doses being given on separate days, and in all cases it appeared irreversible.[3] A patient receiving **gentamicin** rapidly developed deafness when furosemide was replaced by intravenous etacrynic acid.[4]

There are other reports describing temporary, partial or total permanent deafness as a result of giving intravenous etacrynic acid with **gentamicin**,[5] intramuscular **kanamycin**,[5-7] oral **neomycin**,[8] or **streptomycin**.[6,9] This interaction has been extensively demonstrated in *animals*.

(c) Furosemide

An analysis of three, controlled, randomised, studies found that furosemide did not increase either aminoglycoside-induced nephrotoxicity, or ototoxicity (the aminoglycosides used were **amikacin**, **gentamicin**, and **tobramycin**). Nephrotoxicity developed in 20% (10 of 50 patients) given furosemide and 17% (38 of 222) not given furosemide. Auditory toxicity developed in 22% (5 of 23) given furosemide and 24% (28 of 119) not given furosemide.[4]

A study assessing the risk factors for nephrotoxicity with aminoglycosides (**tobramycin** and **gentamicin**) enrolled 1489 patients, 157 of whom developed clinical nephrotoxicity. Of these patients 118 had no immediately identifiable cause (such as acute renal failure) and further evaluation of other risk factors found that the concurrent use of furosemide significantly increased the risk of nephrotoxicity.[10] A clinical study evaluating a possible interaction found that furosemide increased aminoglycoside-induced renal damage,[11] whereas two other clinical studies found no interaction.[12,13] There are clinical reports claiming that concurrent use results in ototoxicity, but usually only small numbers of patients were involved and control groups were not included.[14-18] A retrospective study of neonates suggested the possibility of increased ototoxicity but no firm conclusions could be drawn.[19] Studies in patients and healthy subjects have shown that furosemide reduces the renal clearance of **gentamicin**[20,21] and can cause a rise in both serum **gentamicin**[21] and **tobramycin** levels.[22] Ototoxicity has been described in *animals* given **kanamycin** and furosemide.[1,2]

(d) Piretanide

There seem to be no clinical reports of an interaction between aminoglycosides and piretanide, but ototoxicity has been described in *animals* given **kanamycin** and piretanide.[23]

Mechanism

Aminoglycosides or etacrynic acid alone can damage the ear and cause deafness, the site of action of the aminoglycosides being the hair cell and that of etacrynic acid the stria vascularis. Other loop diuretics can similarly damage hearing.

Animal studies have shown that intramuscular neomycin can cause a fivefold increase in the concentration of etacrynate in cochlear tissues, and it is possible that the aminoglycoside has some effect on the tissues, which allows the etacrynic acid to penetrate more easily.[24] Similar results have been found with gentamicin.[25]

Importance and management

The interaction between etacrynic acid and aminoglycoside is well established and well documented. The concurrent or sequential use of etacrynic acid with parenteral aminoglycosides should be avoided because permanent deafness may result. Patients with renal impairment seem to be particularly at risk, most likely because the drugs are less rapidly cleared. Most of the reports describe deafness after intravenous use, but it has also been seen when etacrynic acid is given orally alone.[9] If it is deemed absolutely necessary to use etacrynic acid and intravenous aminoglycosides, minimal doses should be used and the effects on hearing should be monitored continuously. Not every aminoglycoside has been implicated, but their ototoxicity is clearly established and they may be expected to interact in a similar way. For this reason the same precautions should be used.

Although there is ample evidence of an adverse interaction between furosemide and aminoglycosides in *animals*,[2,26] the weight of clinical evidence suggests that furosemide does not normally increase either the nephrotoxicity or ototoxicity of the aminoglycosides. Nevertheless as there is still some uncertainty about the safety of concurrent use it would be prudent to monitor for any evidence of changes in aminoglycoside serum levels, and renal or hearing impairment. The authors of the major study cited[4] suggest that an interaction may possibly exist if high dose infusions of furosemide are used. The same precautions would seem to be appropriate with bumetanide and piretanide. Note that it is generally advised that aminoglycosides should not be used with other drugs that may cause ototoxicity or nephrotoxicity, such as etacrynic acid and furosemide.

1. Ohtani I, Ohtsuki K, Omata T, Ouchi J, Saito T. Interaction of bumetanide and kanamycin. *ORL J Otorhinolaryngol Relat Spec* (1978) 40, 216–25.
2. Brummett RE, Bendrick T, Himes D. Comparative ototoxicity of bumetanide and furosemide when used in combination with kanamycin. *J Clin Pharmacol* (1981) 21, 628–36.
3. Johnson AH, Hamilton CH. Kanamycin ototoxicity — possible potentiation by other drugs. *South Med J* (1970) 63, 511–13.
4. Smith CR, Lietman PS. Effect of furosemide on aminoglycoside-induced nephrotoxicity and auditory toxicity in humans. *Antimicrob Agents Chemother* (1983) 23, 133–7.
5. Meriwether WD, Mangi RJ, Serpick AA. Deafness following standard intravenous dose of ethacrynic acid. *JAMA* (1971) 216, 795–8.
6. Mathog RH, Klein WJ. Ototoxicity of ethacrynic acid and aminoglycoside antibiotics in uremia. *N Engl J Med* (1969) 280, 1223–4.
7. Ng PSY, Conley CE, Ing TS. Deafness after ethacrynic acid. *Lancet* (1969) i, 673–4.
8. Matz GJ, Beal DD, Krames L. Ototoxicity of ethacrynic acid. Demonstrated in a human temporal bone. *Arch Otolaryngol* (1969) 90, 152–5.
9. Schneider WJ, Becker EL. Acute transient hearing loss after ethacrynic acid therapy. *Arch Intern Med* (1966) 117, 715–17.
10. Bertino JS, Booker LA, Franck PA, Jenkins PL, Franck KR, Nafziger AN. Incidence of and significant risk factors for aminoglycoside-associated nephrotoxicity in patients dosed by using individualized pharmacokinetic monitoring. *J Infect Dis* (1993) 167, 173–9.
11. Prince RA, Ling MH, Hepler CD, Rainville EC, Kealey GP, Donta ST, LeFrock JL, Kowalsky SF. Factors associated with creatinine clearance changes following gentamicin therapy. *Am J Hosp Pharm* (1980) 37, 1489–95.
12. Bygbjerg IC, Møller R. Gentamicin-induced nephropathy. *Scand J Infect Dis* (1976) 8, 203–8.
13. Smith CR, Maxwell RR, Edwards CQ, Rogers JF, Lietman PS. Nephrotoxicity induced by gentamicin and amikacin. *Johns Hopkins Med J* (1978) 142, 85–90.
14. Gallagher KL, Jones JK. Furosemide-induced ototoxicity. *Ann Intern Med* (1979) 91, 744–5.
15. Noël P, Levy V-G. Toxicité rénale de l'association gentamicine-furosémide. Une observation. *Nouv Presse Med* (1978) 7, 351–3.
16. Brown CB, Ogg CS, Cameron JS, Bewick M. High dose frusemide in acute reversible intrinsic renal failure. A preliminary communication. *Scott Med J* (1974) 19, 35–9.
17. Thomsen J, Bech P, Szpirt W. Otological symptoms in chronic renal failure. The possible role of aminoglycoside-furosemide interaction. *Arch Otorhinolaryngol* (1976) 214, 71–9.
18. Bates DE, Beaumont SJ, Baylis BW. Ototoxicity induced by gentamicin and furosemide. *Ann Pharmacother* (2002) 36, 446–51.
19. Salamy A, Eldredge L, Tooley WH. Neonatal status and hearing loss in high-risk infants. *J Pediatr* (1989) 114, 847–52.
20. Lawson DH, Tilstone WJ, Semple PF. Furosemide interactions: studies in normal volunteers. *Clin Res* (1976) 24, 3.
21. Lawson DH, Tilstone WJ, Gray JMB, Srivastava PK. Effect of furosemide on the pharmacokinetics of gentamicin in patients. *J Clin Pharmacol* (1982) 22, 254–8.
22. Kaka JS, Lyman C, Kilarski DJ. Tobramycin-furosemide interaction. *Drug Intell Clin Pharm* (1984) 18, 235–8.
23. Brummett RE. Ototoxicity resulting from the combined administration of potent diuretics and other agents. *Scand Audiol* (1981) (Suppl 14), 215–24.
24. Orsulakova A, Schacht J. A biochemical mechanism of the ototoxic interaction between neomycin and ethacrynic acid. *Acta Otolaryngol* (1982) 93, 43–8.
25. Tran Ba Huy P, Meulemans A, Manuel C, Sterkers O, Wassef M. Critical appraisal of the experimental studies on the ototoxic interaction between ethacrynic acid and aminoglycoside antibiotics. A pharmacokinetical standpoint. *Scand Audiol* (1981) (Suppl 14), 225–32.
26. Ohtani I, Ohtsuki K, Omata T, Ouchi J, Saito T. Potentiation and its mechanism of cochlear damage resulting from furosemide and aminoglycoside antibiotics. *ORL J Otorhinolaryngol Relat Spec* (1978) 40, 53–63.

Aminoglycosides + Magnesium compounds

A neonate with elevated serum magnesium levels had a respiratory arrest when given gentamicin.

Clinical evidence

An infant born to a woman whose pre-eclampsia had been treated with magnesium sulfate was found to have muscle weakness and a serum magnesium concentration of 1.77 mmol/L. The neonate was given ampicillin 100 mg/kg intravenously and **gentamicin** 2.5 mg/kg intramuscularly every 12 hours, starting 12 hours after birth. Soon after the second dose of **gentamicin** she stopped breathing and needed intubation. The **gentamicin** was stopped and the child improved.[1] *Animal* studies confirmed this interaction.[1]

Mechanism

Magnesium ions and the aminoglycosides have neuromuscular blocking activity, which can be additive (see also 'Neuromuscular blockers + Magnesium compounds', p.125 and 'Neuromuscular blockers + Aminoglycosides', p.113). In the case cited here it seems that it was enough to block the actions of the respiratory muscles.

Importance and management

Direct information about this interaction is very limited, but it is well supported by the recognised pharmacological actions of magnesium and the aminoglycosides, and their interactions with conventional neuromuscular blockers. The aminoglycosides as a group should be avoided in hypermagnesaemic infants needing antibacterial treatment. If this is not possible, the effects on respiration should be closely monitored.

1. L'Hommedieu CS, Nicholas D, Armes DA, Jones P, Nelson T, Pickering LK. Potentiation of magnesium sulfate-induced neuromuscular weakness by gentamicin, tobramycin and amikacin. *J Pediatr* (1983) 102, 629–31.

Aminoglycosides + Miconazole

A report describes a reduction in serum tobramycin levels, which was attributed to the use of miconazole.

Clinical evidence, mechanism, importance and management

Intravenous miconazole significantly lowered the peak serum **tobramycin** levels from 9.1 to 6.7 micrograms/mL in 9 patients undergoing bone marrow transplantation. Six of them needed **tobramycin** dosage adjustments.[1] Miconazole was stopped in 4 patients, and **tobramycin** pharmacokinetic parameters returned to normal 4 to 8 days later. The reasons for this interaction are not understood. Although the use of **tobramycin** should be well monitored it would be prudent to increase the frequency in patients also given systemic miconazole (note that miconazole oral gel can have significant systemic absorption). There does not appear to be any information about other aminoglycosides and azole antifungals.

1. Hatfield SM, Crane LR, Duman K, Karanes C, Kiel RJ. Miconazole-induced alteration in tobramycin pharmacokinetics. *Clin Pharm* (1986) 5, 415–19.

Aminoglycosides + NSAIDs

There are conflicting reports as to whether or not serum gentamicin and amikacin levels are raised by indometacin or ibuprofen in premature infants.

Clinical evidence

(a) Amikacin

A study in 10 preterm infants with gestational ages ranging from 25 to 34 weeks, who were given amikacin, found that the use of **indometacin** 200 micrograms/kg every 8 hours, for up to 3 doses, caused a rise in the serum levels of amikacin. Trough and peak levels of amikacin were raised by 28% and 17%, respectively.[1]

In another study, preterm infants were given amikacin 20 mg/kg every 36 hours (gestational age less than 30 weeks) or every 24 hours (gestational age 30 to 31 weeks) with either **ibuprofen lysine** 10 mg/kg within 6 hours of birth, then a further 5 mg/kg dose 24 and 48 hours later, or placebo. The half-life of amikacin was increased from 12.4 to 16.4 hours and its clearance was reduced by 40% in infants who also received intravenous **ibuprofen lysine**.[2] Reductions in amikacin clearance, independent of gestational age were found by the same authors in another study in which preterm infants with gestational ages of between 24 and 34 weeks were given amikacin and **ibuprofen**.[3]

In contrast, another study in preterm infants given amikacin found no changes in its pharmacokinetics when **ibuprofen** or **indometacin** were given.[4]

(b) Gentamicin

A study in 10 preterm infants with gestational ages ranging from 25 to 34 weeks, who were given gentamicin, found that the use of **indometacin** 200 micrograms/kg every 8 hours, for up to 3 doses, caused a rise in the serum levels of gentamicin. Trough and peak levels of gentamicin were raised by 48% and 33%, respectively.[1] A later study[5] confirmed that **indometacin** (200 micrograms/kg given intravenously at 0 hours, then 100 micrograms/kg given at 12 and then 36 hours) decreased the clearance of 3-mg/kg daily doses of gentamicin by 23% in preterm infants weighing less than 1250 g.

In contrast, 8 out of 13 infants had no increase in their serum gentamicin levels when they were given **indometacin** 200 to 250 micrograms/kg every 12 hours for 3 doses. Of the remaining 5, slight to moderate rises occurred in 4, and a substantial rise occurred in just one.[6] In another study no significant changes in serum gentamicin levels were seen in 31 preterm newborns given parenteral **indometacin** 200 micrograms/kg every 12 hours for 3 doses.[7]

Mechanism

Aminoglycosides are excreted by renal filtration, which can be inhibited by indometacin or ibuprofen. This may result in the retention of the aminoglycoside.

Importance and management

Information seems to be limited to these conflicting studies, although supporting evidence for indometacin comes from the fact that it also causes the retention of digoxin in premature infants. The authors of one of the studies[6] suggest that the different results may be because aminoglycoside serum levels were lower in their study before the indometacin was given, and also because they measured the new steady-state levels after 40 to 60 hours instead of 24 hours. Whatever the explanation, concurrent use should be very closely monitored because toxicity is associated with raised aminoglycoside serum levels. It has been suggested that the aminoglycoside dosage should be reduced before giving indometacin and the serum levels and renal function well monitored during concurrent use.[1] It has also been suggested that the dose interval of amikacin should be increased by at least 6 to 8 hours if ibuprofen lysine is also given during the first days of life.[2] Other aminoglycosides possibly behave similarly. This interaction does not seem to have been studied in adults.

1. Zarfin Y, Koren G, Maresky D, Perlman M, MacLeod S. Possible indomethacin-aminoglycoside interaction in preterm infants. *J Pediatr* (1985) 106, 511–13.
2. Allegaert K, Cossey V, Langhendries JP, Naulaers G, Vanhole C, Devlieger H, Van Overmeire B. Effects of co-administration of ibuprofen-lysine on the pharmacokinetics of amikacin in preterm infants during the first days of life. *Biol Neonate* (2004) 86, 207–11.
3. Allegaert K, Cossey V, Debeer A, Langhendries JP, Van Overmeire B, de Hoon J, Devlieger H. The impact of ibuprofen on renal clearance in preterm infants is independent of the gestational age. *Pediatr Nephrol* (2005) 20, 740–3.
4. Cuesta Grueso C, Gimeno Navarro A, Marqués Miñana MR, Peris Ribera JE, Morcillo Sopena F, Poveda Andrés JL. Efecto de la administración concomitante de indometacina o ibuprofeno en la farmacocinética de amikacina en neonatos prematuros. *Farm Hosp* (2006) 30, 149–53.
5. Dean RP, Domanico RS, Covert RF. Prophylactic indomethacin alters gentamicin pharmacokinetics in preterm infants <1250 grams. *Pediatr Res* (1994) 35, 83A.
6. Jerome M, Davis JC. The effects of indomethacin on gentamicin serum levels. *Proc West Pharmacol Soc* (1987) 30, 85–7.
7. Grylack LJ, Scanlon JW. Interaction of indomethacin (I) and gentamicin (G) in preterm newborns. *Pediatr Res* (1988) 23, 409A.

Aminoglycosides + Penicillins or Carbapenems

The use of piperacillin is reported to be a risk factor for aminoglycoside-associated nephrotoxicity. A reduction in serum aminoglycoside levels can occur if aminoglycosides and penicillins are given together to patients with severe renal impairment. No pharmacokinetic interaction of importance appears to occur with intravenous aminoglycoside and penicillins in those with normal renal function or between aminoglycosides and carbapenems. The serum levels of oral phenoxymethylpenicillin can be halved by oral neomycin.

Clinical evidence

A. Intravenous or intramuscular aminoglycosides

(a) With carbapenems

The suspicion that low **tobramycin** levels in one patient might have been due to an interaction with **imipenem/cilastatin** was not confirmed in a later *in vitro* study.[1] It has also been suggested that the nephrotoxic effects of **imipenem** and the **aminoglycosides** might possibly be additive but this awaits confirmation.[2] A study in healthy subjects given single intravenous doses of **imipenem** and **amikacin** found there was a transient increase in **imipenem** levels but no effects on other pharmacokinetic parameters of either drug.[3] In a study in 12 healthy subjects the concurrent use of **tobramycin** and **biapenem** did not alter the pharmacokinetics of either drug.[4] No inactivation occurred in an *in vitro* assessment of these two drugs in urine.[5]

(b) With penicillins in patients with renal impairment

A study in 6 patients with renal failure requiring dialysis, who were receiving intravenous **carbenicillin** 8 to 15 g daily in 3 to 6 divided doses, found that in the presence of the penicillin serum **gentamicin** levels did not exceed 4 micrograms/mL. When the **carbenicillin** was stopped, serum **gentamicin** levels rose.[6]

Other reports similarly describe unusually low **gentamicin** levels in patients with impaired renal function, given **carbenicillin**,[7-10] **piperacillin**,[11] or **ticarcillin**.[8,10,12] The half-life of **gentamicin** has been reported to be reduced by **carbenicillin** or **piperacillin** by about one-half or one-third.[8,11,13] Similarly, unusually low **tobramycin** levels have been reported in patients with impaired renal function, who were given **carbenicillin**,[6] **piperacillin**[14] or **ticarcillin**.[12]

In 3 patients receiving long-term haemodialysis **piperacillin** doubled the clearance of **tobramycin** 2 mg/kg, and reduced its half-life from 73 to 22 hours.[15] A patient showed a reduction in the half-life of **tobramycin** from an expected 70 hours to 10.5 hours after being given **piperacillin**.[16] In contrast one study found that **piperacillin** or **piperacillin/tazobactam** did not change the pharmacokinetics of **tobramycin** in subjects with renal impairment.[17]

Piperacillin 4 g every 12 hours did not affect the pharmacokinetics of **netilmicin** 2 mg/kg in 3 patients receiving long-term haemodialysis.[15]

(c) With penicillins in patients with normal renal function

A patient with normal renal function was given **gentamicin** 80 mg intravenously, with and without **carbenicillin** 4 g. The serum **gentamicin** concentration profiles in both cases were very similar.[7]

No interaction was seen in 10 patients given **tobramycin** with **piperacillin**,[18] or in another 10 healthy subjects given once daily **gentamicin** with **piperacillin/tazobactam**.[19] Only minimal pharmacokinetic changes were seen in 9 healthy subjects given **tobramycin** with **piperacillin/tazobactam**,[20] and 18 cystic fibrosis patients (adults and children) given **tobramycin** with **ticarcillin**.[21]

However, a study assessing the risk factors for nephrotoxicity with aminoglycosides (**tobramycin** and **gentamicin**) enrolled 1489 patients,

157 of whom developed clinical nephrotoxicity. Of these patients 118 had no immediately identifiable cause (such as acute renal failure) and further evaluation of other risk factors found that the concurrent use of **piperacillin**, but not **ticarcillin** or **carbenicillin** significantly increased the risk of nephrotoxicity.[22]

B. Oral aminoglycosides

The serum concentrations of a 250-mg oral dose of **phenoxymethylpenicillin** were reduced by more than 50% in 5 healthy subjects after they took **neomycin** 3 g four times daily for 7 days. Normal penicillin pharmacokinetics were not seen until 6 days after the **neomycin** was withdrawn.[23]

Mechanism

The nephrotoxic effects of gentamicin and tobramycin are well documented. The reason why piperacillin but not carbenicillin or ticarcillin should increase the risk of nephrotoxicity is not clear. One suggestion is that sodium loading may protect the kidney from tobramycin toxicity and piperacillin has only 40% as much sodium as ticarcillin.[22]

In vitro, the amino groups on the aminoglycosides and the beta-lactam ring on the penicillins interact chemically to form biologically inactive amides.[24] It has been suggested that this reaction may also occur in the plasma, causing a drop in the levels of active antibacterial.[13] The interaction occurs in those with poor renal function as the drugs persist in the plasma for longer, allowing a greater time for inactivation. This therefore means the drug is lost more rapidly than has been accounted for by the renal function, and consequently lower than expected levels of the antibacterial result. However, the lack of interaction found in one study led to the conclusion that reported interactions in renal impairment may be due to *in vitro* inactivation after sample collection.[17]

In the case of phenoxymethylpenicillin, the levels are probably lowered because oral neomycin can cause a reversible malabsorption syndrome (histologically similar to nontropical sprue).

Importance and management

The concurrent use of piperacillin and aminoglycosides is reported to be a risk factor for nephrotoxicity.[22,25] The nephrotoxic effects of gentamicin and tobramycin are well documented. Risk factors for nephrotoxicity include raised aminoglycoside trough levels, decreased albumin, male gender, advanced age, increased length of treatment, liver disease or ascites, and some other diseases, including leukaemia,[22,25] although their significance in practice has been questioned.[22] Renal function and antibacterial serum levels should be monitored if piperacillin is given with an aminoglycoside.

Other reports suggest that a pharmacokinetic interaction between parenteral aminoglycosides and piperacillin or other penicillins, resulting in reduced levels of aminoglycoside, seems to occur in patients with renal impairment.

In those cases where concurrent use is thought necessary, it has been recommended that the serum levels of both antibacterials closely monitored.[6] However, note that antibacterial inactivation can continue in the assay sample, and one author[26] suggests that rapid assay is necessary, while others[17] note the importance of protecting samples against further inactivation.

There would seem to be no reason for avoiding concurrent use in patients with normal renal function because no significant *in vivo* inactivation appears to occur. Moreover there is good clinical evidence that concurrent use is valuable, especially in the treatment of Pseudomonas infections.[7,27]

Evidence for the oral neomycin/penicillin interaction seems limited to this one report and its clinical significance is unclear. It seems possible that oral **kanamycin** and **paromomycin** might interact similarly, but this needs confirmation.

1. Ariano RE, Kassum DA, Meatherall RC, Patrick WD. Lack of in vitro inactivation of tobramycin by imipenem/cilastatin. *Ann Pharmacother* (1992) 26, 1075–7.
2. Albrecht LM, Rybak MJ. Combination imipenem-aminoglycoside therapy. *Drug Intell Clin Pharm* (1986) 20, 506.
3. Adamis G, Papaionnou MG, Giamarellos-Bourboulis EJ, Gargalianos P, Kosmidis J, Giamarellou H. Pharmacokinetic interactions of ceftazidime, imipenem and aztreonam with amikacin in healthy volunteers. *Int J Antimicrob Agents* (2004) 23, 144–9.
4. Muralidharan G, Buice R, Depuis E, Carver A, Friederici D, Kinchelow T, Kinzig M, Kuye O, Sorgel F, Yacobi A, Mayer P. Pharmacokinetics of biapenem with and without tobramycin in healthy volunteers. *Pharm Res* (1993) 10 (10 Suppl), S-396.
5. Muralidharan G, Carver A, Mayer P. Lack of in vitro inactivation of tobramycin by biapenem in human urine. *Pharm Res* (1994) 11 (10 Suppl), S-398.
6. Weibert R, Keane W, Shapiro F. Carbenicillin inactivation of aminoglycosides in patients with severe renal failure. *Trans Am Soc Artif Intern Organs* (1976) 22, 439–43.
7. Eykyn S, Phillips I, Ridley M. Gentamicin plus carbenicillin. *Lancet* (1971) i, 545–6.
8. Davies M, Morgan JR, Anand C. Interactions of carbenicillin and ticarcillin with gentamicin. *Antimicrob Agents Chemother* (1975) 7, 431–4.
9. Weibert RT, Keane WF. Carbenicillin-gentamicin interaction in acute renal failure. *Am J Hosp Pharm* (1977) 34, 1137–9.
10. Kradjan WA, Burger R. In vivo inactivation of gentamicin by carbenicillin and ticarcillin. *Arch Intern Med* (1980) 140, 1668–70.
11. Thompson MIB, Russo ME, Saxon BJ, Atkin-Thor E, Matsen JM. Gentamicin inactivation by piperacillin or carbenicillin in patients with end-stage renal disease. *Antimicrob Agents Chemother* (1982) 21, 268–73.
12. Chow MSS, Quintiliani R, Nightingale CH. In vivo inactivation of tobramycin by ticarcillin. A case report. *JAMA* (1982) 247, 658–9.
13. Riff LJ, Jackson GG. Laboratory and clinical conditions for gentamicin inactivation by carbenicillin. *Arch Intern Med* (1972) 130, 887–91.
14. Uber WE, Brundage RC, White RL, Brundage DM, Bromley HR. In vivo inactivation of tobramycin by piperacillin. *Ann Pharmacother* (1991) 25, 357–9.
15. Matzke GR, Halstenson CE, Heim KL, Abraham PA, Keane WF. Netilmicin disposition is not altered by concomitant piperacillin administration. *Clin Pharmacol Ther* (1985) 41, 210.
16. Uber WE, Brundage RC, White RL, Brundage DM, Bromley HR. In vivo inactivation of tobramycin by piperacillin. *DICP Ann Pharmacother* (1991) 25, 357–9.
17. Dowell JA, Korth-Bradley J, Milisci M, Tantillo K, Amorusi P, Tse S. Evaluating possible pharmacokinetic interactions between tobramycin, piperacillin, and a combination of piperacillin and tazobactam in patients with various degrees of renal impairment. *J Clin Pharmacol* (2001) 41, 979–86.
18. Lau A, Lee M, Flascha S, Prasad R, Sharifi R. Effect of piperacillin on tobramycin pharmacokinetics in patients with normal renal function. *Antimicrob Agents Chemother* (1983) 24, 533–7.
19. Hitt CM, Patel KB, Nicolau DP, Zhu Z, Nightingale CH. Influence of piperacillin-tazobactam on pharmacokinetics of gentamicin given once daily. *Am J Health-Syst Pharm* (1997) 54, 2704–8.
20. Lathia C, Sia L, Lanc R, Greene D, Kuye O, Batra V, Yacobi A, Faulkner R. Pharmacokinetics of piperacillin/tazobactam IV with and without tobramycin IV in healthy adult male volunteers. *Pharm Res* (1991) 8, (10 Suppl), S-303.
21. Roberts GW, Nation RL, Jarvinen AO, Martin AJ. An *in vivo* assessment of the tobramycin/ticarcillin interaction in cystic fibrosis patients. *Br J Clin Pharmacol* (1993) 36, 372–5.
22. Bertino JS, Booker LA, Franck PA, Jenkins PL, Franck KR, Nafziger AN. Incidence of and significant risk factors for aminoglycoside-associated nephrotoxicity in patients dosed by using individualized pharmacokinetic monitoring. *J Infect Dis* (1993) 167, 173–9.
23. Cheng SH, White A. Effect of orally administered neomycin on the absorption of penicillin V. *N Engl J Med* (1962) 267, 1296–7.
24. Perényi T, Graber H, Arr M. Über die Wechselwirkung der Penizilline und Aminoglykosid-Antibiotika. *Int J Clin Pharmacol Ther Toxicol* (1974) 10, 50–5.
25. Streetman DS, Nafziger AN, Destache CJ, Bertino JS. Individualized pharmacokinetic monitoring results in less aminoglycoside-associated nephrotoxicity and fewer associated costs. *Pharmacotherapy* (2001) 21, 443–51.
26. Russo ME. Penicillin-aminoglycoside inactivation: another possible mechanism of interaction. *Am J Hosp Pharm* (1980) 37, 702–4.
27. Kluge RM, Standiford HC, Tatem B, Young VM, Schimpff SC, Greene WH, Calia FM, Hornick RB. The carbenicillin-gentamicin combination against *Pseudomonas aeruginosa*. Correlation of effect with gentamicin sensitivity. *Ann Intern Med* (1974) 81, 584–7.

Aminoglycosides + Polygeline (*Haemaccel*)

The incidence of acute renal failure appears to be increased in cardiac surgical patients given polygeline (*Haemaccel*) with gentamicin.

Clinical evidence

The observation of a differing incidence of acute renal failure in patients undergoing coronary artery bypass surgery in two similar units, prompted a retrospective review of patient records. This showed that the only management differences were related to antibacterial prophylaxis and the bypass prime content (i.e. the solution used to prime the cardiopulmonary bypass circuit).

Acute renal failure was defined as a more than 50% rise in serum creatinine on the first postoperative day in those patients whose creatinine was also greater than 120 micromol/L.

Four groups of patients were identified, and the incidence of renal failure was as follows:

A (polygeline plus **gentamicin** and flucloxacillin) 31% (28 of 91 patients);

B (polygeline plus cefalotin) 12% (9 of 72 patients);

C (crystalloid plus **gentamicin** and flucloxacillin) 7% (4 of 57 patients);

D (crystalloid plus cefalotin) 2% (1 of 47 patients).

Polygeline (*Haemaccel*) 1 litre, which is a urea linked gelatin colloid with a calcium concentration of 6.25 micromol/L, was used for groups A and B, with crystalloid - Hartmann's solution or Ringer's injection (calcium concentration 2 mmol/L) to make up the rest of the prime volume of 2 litres. Groups C and D received only crystalloid (no polygeline) in the prime. Albumin 100 mL was used in groups B and D.[1] However, the study has been criticised because other drugs affecting renal function (such as ACE inhibitors, cimetidine, NSAIDs or clonidine) which may have been taken by the patients were not considered.[2] This criticism has been refuted because of the large sample size involved.[3]

Mechanism

Not fully understood. It is thought that the relatively high calcium content of the polygeline may have potentiated gentamicin-associated nephrotoxicity. Hypercalcaemia has been shown in *animals* to increase aminoglycoside-induced nephrotoxicity.[4]

Importance and management

Information appears to be limited to this clinical study and *animal* studies, but the evidence available suggests that a clinically important adverse interaction occurs between these drugs. The incidence of acute renal failure in cardiac surgery patients is normally about 3 to 5%[5] which is low compared with the 31% shown by those given polygeline and gentamicin. The authors of the study advise avoidance of these two drugs. More study is needed.

1. Schneider M, Valentine S, Clarke GM, Newman MAJ, Peakcock J. Acute renal failure in cardiac surgical patients potentiated by gentamicin and calcium. *Anaesth Intensive Care* (1996) 24, 647–50.
2. Bolsin S, Jones S. Acute renal failure potentiated by gentamicin and calcium. *Anaesth Intensive Care* (1997) 25, 431–2.
3. Schneider M, Clarke GM, Valentine SJ, Peakcock J. Acute renal failure potentiated by gentamicin and calcium; reply. *Anaesth Intensive Care* (1997) 25, 432.
4. Elliott WC, Patchin DS, Jones DB. Effect of parathyroid hormone activity on gentamicin nephrotoxicity. *J Lab Clin Med* (1987) 109, 48–54.
5. Hilberman M, Myers BD, Carrie BJ, Derby G, Jamison RL, Stinson EB. Acute renal failure following cardiac surgery. *J Thorac Cardiovasc Surg* (1979) 77, 880–8.

Aminoglycosides + Vancomycin

The nephrotoxicity of the aminoglycosides appears to be potentiated by vancomycin.

Clinical evidence, mechanism, importance and management

A retrospective review of 105 patients who had received an aminoglycoside with vancomycin for at least 5 days found that nephrotoxicity occurred in 27% of the patients. Of these, 6 had no other identifiable cause for nephrotoxicity.[1] A study assessing the risks factors for nephrotoxicity with aminoglycosides (**tobramycin** and **gentamicin**) enrolled 1489 patients, 157 of whom developed clinical nephrotoxicity. Of these patients 118 had no immediately identifiable cause (such as acute renal failure) and further evaluation of other risk factors found that the concurrent use of vancomycin significantly increased the risk of nephrotoxicity.[2]

A number of other studies,[3-9] including those where patients have had individualised pharmacokinetic monitoring,[3] and those using both once daily and multiple daily dosing,[4] have all found that vancomycin independently increases the risk of nephrotoxicity in patients receiving aminoglycosides. In one meta-analysis of 8 studies, the incidence of nephrotoxicity with the combination was 4.3% greater than with aminoglycosides alone and 13.3% greater than with vancomycin alone.[8]

Risk factors are said to include vancomycin peak and trough levels,[1,6] aminoglycoside trough levels,[1,3,6] decreased albumin concentrations,[2] male gender,[1-3] advanced age,[1-3] increased length of treatment,[1-3] liver disease or ascites,[1,2] as well as a large number of other disease states (such as leukaemia,[2] peritonitis[1] or neutropenia),[1] although their significance in practice has been questioned.[2]

Concurrent use of these antibacterials is therapeutically useful, but the risk of increased nephrotoxicity should be borne in mind. Therapeutic drug monitoring and regular assessment of renal function is warranted, as is recommended with the use of either drug alone.

1. Pauly DJ, Musa DM, Lestico MR, Lindstrom MJ, Hetsko CM. Risk of nephrotoxicity with combination vancomycin-aminoglycoside antibiotic therapy. *Pharmacotherapy* (1990) 10, 378–82.
2. Bertino JS, Booker LA, Franck PA, Jenkins PL, Franck KR, Nafziger AN. Incidence of and significant risk factors for aminoglycoside-associated nephrotoxicity in patients dosed by using individualized pharmacokinetic monitoring. *J Infect Dis* (1993) 167, 173–9.
3. Streetman DS, Nafziger AN, Destache CJ, Bertino JS. Individualized pharmacokinetic monitoring results in less aminoglycoside-associated nephrotoxicity and fewer associated costs. *Pharmacotherapy* (2001) 21, 443–51.
4. Rybak MJ, Abate BJ, Kang SL, Ruffing MJ, Lerner SA, Drusano GL. Prospective evaluation on the effect of an aminoglycoside dosing regimen on rates of observed nephrotoxicity and ototoxicity. *Antimicrob Agents Chemother* (1999) 43, 1549–55.
5. Farber BF, Moellering RC. Retrospective study of the toxicity of preparations of vancomycin from 1974 to 1981. *Antimicrob Agents Chemother* (1983) 23, 138–41.
6. Cimino MA, Rotstein C, Slaughter RL, Emrich LJ. Relationship of serum antibiotic concentrations to nephrotoxicity in cancer patients receiving concurrent aminoglycoside and vancomycin therapy. *Am J Med* (1987) 83, 1091–7.
7. Rybak MJ, Frankowski JJ, Edwards DJ, Albrecht LM. Alanine aminopeptidase and β_2-microglobulin excretion in patients receiving vancomycin and gentamicin. *Antimicrob Agents Chemother* (1987) 31, 1461–4.
8. Goetz MB, Sayers J. Nephrotoxicity of vancomycin and aminoglycoside therapy separately and in combination. *J Antimicrob Chemother* (1993) 32, 325–34.
9. Rybak MJ, Albrecht LM, Boike SC, Chandrasekar PH. Nephrotoxicity of vancomycin, alone and with an aminoglycoside. *J Antimicrob Chemother* (1990) 25, 679–87.

Aminoglycosides + Verapamil

Verapamil appears to protect the kidney from damage caused by gentamicin.

Clinical evidence, mechanism, importance and management

In a comparative study, 9 healthy subjects were given **gentamicin** alone (2 mg/kg loading dose, followed by doses every 8 hours to achieve a peak concentration of 5.5 mg/L and a trough concentration of 0.5 mg/L), and 6 other subjects were given the same dosage of **gentamicin** with sustained-release verapamil 180 mg twice daily. The **gentamicin** AUCs of the two groups were virtually the same but the 24-hour urinary excretion of alanine aminopeptidase (AAP) was modestly reduced, by 18%, in the group given verapamil. The reduction in AAP excretion was particularly marked during the first 6 days.[1] The significance of urinary AAP is that this enzyme is found primarily in the brush border membranes of the proximal renal tubules, and its excretion is an early and sensitive marker of renal damage. Thus it seems that verapamil may modestly protect the kidneys from damage by **gentamicin**, but using a drug as potentially toxic as verapamil to provide this protection, when the risks of renal toxicity can be minimised by carefully controlling the **gentamicin** dosage, is unwarranted. Information about other aminoglycosides and other calcium-channel blockers seems to be lacking.

1. Kazierad DJ, Wojcik GJ, Nix DE, Goldfarb AL, Schentag JJ. The effect of verapamil on the nephrotoxic potential of gentamicin as measured by urinary enzyme excretion in healthy volunteers. *J Clin Pharmacol* (1995) 35, 196–201.

Aminoglycosides; Tobramycin + Sucralfate

An *in vitro* study with tobramycin found that it became markedly and irreversibly bound to sucralfate at the pH values found in the gut. This suggests that the efficacy of tobramycin in gut decontamination might be decreased.

Clinical evidence, mechanism, importance and management

To simulate what might happen in the gut, tobramycin 50 mg/mL was mixed with sucralfate 500 mg in 40 mL of water at pH 3.5 and allowed to stand for 90 minutes at 25°C. Analysis of the solution showed that the tobramycin concentration fell rapidly and progressively over 90 minutes to about 1%. When the pH of the mixture was then raised to 6.5 to 7 for 90 minutes, there was no change in the concentration of tobramycin, suggesting that the interaction was irreversible.[1] The reason for this change is not known, but the suggestion is that sucralfate forms insoluble chelates with tobramycin.[1]

It is not known how important this interaction is likely to be in practice, but the efficacy of tobramycin in gut decontamination may be decreased. Separating the dosages might not be effective in some postoperative patients because their gastric function may not return to normal for up to 5 days, and some sucralfate might still be present when the next dose is given.[1] More study is needed to find out whether this interaction is clinically important, but in the meanwhile it would seem prudent to monitor concurrent use carefully, being alert for any evidence of reduced effects.

1. Feron B, Adair CG, Gorman SP, McClurg B. Interaction of sucralfate with antibiotics used for selective decontamination of the gastrointestinal tract. *Am J Hosp Pharm* (1993) 50, 2550–3.

Aminosalicylic acid + Diphenhydramine

Diphenhydramine can cause a small reduction in the absorption of aminosalicylic acid from the gut.

Clinical evidence, mechanism, importance and management

A study in 9 healthy subjects[1] showed that diphenhydramine 50 mg given intramuscularly 10 minutes before a 2-g oral dose of aminosalicylic acid, reduced the mean peak serum aminosalicylic acid levels by about 15%.

This effect may occur because diphenhydramine reduces peristalsis in the gut, which in some way reduces aminosalicylic acid absorption. The extent to which diphenhydramine or any other anticholinergic drug diminishes the therapeutic response to long-term treatment with aminosalicylic acid is uncertain, but it is probably small.

1. Lavigne J-G, Marchand C. Inhibition of the gastrointestinal absorption of p-aminosalicylate (PAS) in rats and humans by diphenhydramine. *Clin Pharmacol Ther* (1973) 14, 404–12.

Aminosalicylic acid + Probenecid

The plasma levels of aminosalicylic acid can be raised up to fourfold by probenecid.

Clinical evidence, mechanism, importance and management

In a study in 7 patients, probenecid 500 mg every 6 hours increased the plasma levels of aminosalicylic acid 4 g by as much as fourfold.[1] Similar results are described in another report.[2]

The reasons for this effect are uncertain but it seems probable that probenecid successfully competes with aminosalicylic acid for active excretion by the kidney tubules, which results in the increased aminosalicylic acid levels.

The documentation of this interaction is limited but it appears to be established. Such large increases in plasma aminosalicylic acid levels would be expected to lead to toxicity. It also seems possible that the dosage of aminosalicylic acid could be reduced without losing the required therapeutic response. This needs confirmation. Monitoring aminosalicylic acid levels, where possible, would probably be useful. Concurrent use should be undertaken with caution.

1. Boger WP, Pitts FW. Influence of *p*-(Di-n-propylsulfamyl)-benzoic acid, 'Benemid' on para-aminosalicylic acid (PAS) plasma concentrations. *Am Rev Tuberc* (1950) 61, 862–7.
2. Carr DT, Karlson AG, Bridge EV. Concentration of PAS and tuberculostatic potency of serum after administration of PAS with and without Benemid. *Proc Staff Meet Mayo Clin* (1952) 27, 209–15.

Antibacterials + Immunoglobulins

One *animal* study found that for severe infections antibacterials were less effective in the presence of high-dose immunoglobulin, but this was not seen in less severe infections. The clinical relevance of this is uncertain.

Clinical evidence, mechanism, importance and management

A study in an *animal* model of severe group B streptococcal infection found the following mortalities:, 51% with **benzylpenicillin** 200 mg/kg alone, 88% with immunoglobulin and benzylpenicillin, and 100% with immunoglobulin 2 g/kg alone. A smaller dose of immunoglobulin 0.5 g/kg was not associated with an increase in mortality.[1] Roughly similar results were found when the penicillin was replaced by **ceftriaxone**.[1] In another study using a 1000-fold smaller inoculum of group B streptococci, there was no difference in mortality between **benzylpenicillin** 200 mg/kg daily alone and **benzylpenicillin** with immunoglobulin 0.25 to 2 g/kg, and there was some evidence of a lower incidence of bacteraemia with the combination.[1,2]

Immunoglobulins are used with antibacterials in the successful prevention of infections in clinical practice, and no special precautions appear to be needed in this situation. However, their clinical use for treating established infection is unclear, and the above findings suggest some caution is warranted.

1. Kim KS. High-dose intravenous immune globulin impairs antibacterial activity of antibiotics. *J Allergy Clin Immunol* (1989) 84, 579–88.
2. Kim KS. Efficacy of human immunoglobulin and penicillin G in treatment of experimental group B streptococcal infection. *Pediatr Res* (1987) 21, 289–92.

Aztreonam + Other antibacterials

There appear to be no clinically significant pharmacokinetic interactions between aztreonam and amikacin, cefradine, clindamycin, gentamicin, metronidazole or nafcillin.

Clinical evidence, mechanism, importance and management

A study in healthy subjects given a single 1-g intravenous dose of aztreonam found that maximum levels were reduced by 12.6% and 9.8% when it was given with **gentamicin** 80 mg and **metronidazole** 500 mg, respectively. Serum bound aztreonam fell by 5% when it was given with **nafcillin** 500 mg and increased by 5.1% when given with **cefradine** 1 g. When aztreonam 1 g and **clindamycin** 600 mg were given together, their renal excretion increased by 5.2% and 10.9%, respectively. None of these changes was statistically significant.[1] Another study in healthy subjects found that the AUC of a 1-g intravenous dose of aztreonam was reduced by 22% by amikacin 500 mg, and the AUC of amikacin was increased by 27% by aztreonam.[2]

1. Creasey WA, Adamovics J, Dhruv R, Platt TB, Sugerman AA. Pharmacokinetic interaction of aztreonam with other antibiotics. *J Clin Pharmacol* (1984) 24, 174–80.
2. Adamis G, Papaioannou MG, Giamarellos-Bourboulis EJ, Gargalianos P, Kosmidis J, Giamarellou H. Pharmacokinetic interactions of ceftazidime, imipenem and aztreonam with amikacin in healthy volunteers. *Int J Antimicrob Agents* (2004) 23, 144–9.

Carbapenems + Probenecid

Probenecid increases the serum levels of meropenem, but does not appear to interact with ertapenem to a clinically relevant extent.

Clinical evidence, mechanism, importance and management

(a) Ertapenem

The use of probenecid with ertapenem is reported to decrease the renal clearance of unbound ertapenem by about 50%, probably because probenecid inhibits the renal tubular secretion of ertapenem. Probenecid slightly increased the elimination half-life and AUC of ertapenem and therefore concurrent use is considered unlikely to increase the effects of ertapenem.[1]

(b) Meropenem

In 6 healthy subjects probenecid (1 g given orally 2 hours before meropenem and 500 mg given orally 1.5 hours after meropenem) increased the AUC of meropenem 500 mg by 43%.[2] Another study in 6 healthy subjects found that probenecid (1.5 g in divided doses the day before and 500 mg one hour before meropenem) increased the AUC of meropenem 1 g by up to 55% and increased its half-life by 33% (from 0.98 to 1.3 hours).[3] In both studies the serum levels of meropenem were modestly increased. This is possibly because meropenem and probenecid compete for active kidney tubular secretion.[4,5] The manufacturers say that because the potency and duration of meropenem are adequate without probenecid, they do not recommend concurrent use.[4,5]

1. Nix DE, Majumdar AK, DiNubile MJ. Pharmacokinetics and pharmacodynamics of ertapenem: an overview for clinicians. *J Antimicrob Chemother* (2004) 53 (Suppl S2), ii23–ii28.
2. Ishida Y, Matsumoto F, Sakai O, Yoshida M, Shiba K. The pharmacokinetic study of meropenem: effect of probenecid and hemodialysis. *J Chemother* (1993) 5 (Suppl 1), 124–6.
3. Bax RP, Bastain W, Featherstone A, Wilkinson DM, Hutchison M, Haworth SJ. The pharmacokinetics of meropenem in volunteers. *J Antimicrob Chemother* (1989) 24 (Suppl A), 311–20.
4. Meronem (Meropenem). AstraZeneca UK Ltd. UK Summary of product characteristics, January 2004.
5. Merrem (Meropenem). AstraZeneca. US Prescribing information, February 2007.

Cephalosporins + Antacids

No clinically significant interactions appear to occur between an aluminium/magnesium hydroxide antacid and cefaclor AF, cefalexin, cefetamet pivoxil, cefixime or cefprozil; between *Alka-Seltzer* and cefixime; or between ceftibuten and *Mylanta*. In contrast, antacids reduce the bioavailability of cefpodoxime proxetil.

Clinical evidence, mechanism, importance and management

(a) Cefaclor

A study with cefaclor AF (a formulation with a slow rate of release) found that an **aluminium/magnesium hydroxide** antacid (*Maalox*) given one hour after the cefaclor AF to fed subjects reduced the AUC by 18%.[1] This reduction is small and unlikely to be clinically important.

(b) Cefalexin

An **aluminium/magnesium hydroxide** antacid (*Maalox*) given as 8 doses of 10 mL on day one and 2 doses on day 2, had only small and therapeutically unimportant effects on the pharmacokinetics of cefalexin 1 g.[2]

(c) Cefetamet pivoxil

Cefetamet pivoxil 1 g was given to 18 healthy subjects after breakfast with or without 80 mL of an **aluminium/magnesium hydroxide** antacid (*Maalox 70*) given the evening before, 2 hours before, and after breakfast. The pharmacokinetics of the cefetamet were unaffected by the antacid.[3]

(d) Cefixime

An **aluminium/magnesium hydroxide** antacid (*Maalox*) and ***Alka-Seltzer*** (aspirin, calcium phosphate, citric acid and **sodium bicarbonate**) do not significantly affect the absorption of cefixime,[4,5]

(e) Cefpodoxime proxetil

A study in 10 healthy subjects found that 10 mL of an **aluminium/magnesium hydroxide** antacid (*Maalox*) reduced the bioavailability of cefpodoxime proxetil by about 40%. This was considered to be due to reduced dissolution at increased gastric pH values.[6] These results confirm the findings of a previous study with **sodium bicarbonate** and **aluminium hydroxide**.[7] It has been recommended that cefpodoxime is given at least 2 hours after antacids.[6]

(f) Cefprozil

An **aluminium/magnesium hydroxide** antacid (*Maalox*) does not affect the bioavailability of cefprozil.[8]

(g) Ceftibuten

In 18 healthy subjects, 60 mL of an antacid containing **aluminium/magnesium hydroxide** plus **simeticone** (*Mylanta II*) was found not to affect the pharmacokinetics of ceftibuten 400 mg.[9]

1. Satterwhite JH, Cerimele BJ, Coleman DL, Hatcher BL, Kisicki J, DeSante KA. Pharmacokinetics of cefaclor AF: effects of age, antacids and H_2-receptor antagonists. *Postgrad Med J* (1992) 68 (Suppl 3), S3–S9.
2. Deppermann K-M, Lode H, Höffken G, Tschink G, Kalz C, Koeppe P. Influence of ranitidine, pirenzepine, and aluminum magnesium hydroxide on the bioavailability of various antibiotics, including amoxicillin, cephalexin, doxycycline and amoxicillin-clavulanic acid. *Antimicrob Agents Chemother* (1989) 33, 1901–1907.
3. Blouin RA, Kneer J, Ambros RJ, Stoeckel K. Influence of antacid and ranitidine on the pharmacokinetics of oral cefetamet pivoxil. *Antimicrob Agents Chemother* (1990) 34, 1744–8.
4. Petitjean O, Brion N, Tod M, Montagne A, Nicolas P. Étude de l'interaction pharmacocinétique entre le céfixime et deux antiacides. Résultats préliminaires. *Presse Med* (1989) 18, 1596–8.
5. Healy DP, Sahai JV, Sterling LP, Racht EM. Influence of an antacid containing aluminum and magnesium on the pharmacokinetics of cefixime. *Antimicrob Agents Chemother* (1989) 33, 1994–7.
6. Saathoff N, Lode H, Neider K, Depperman KM, Borner K, Koeppe P. Pharmacokinetics of cefpodoxime proxetil and interactions with an antacid and an H_2 receptor antagonist. *Antimicrob Agents Chemother* (1992) 36, 796–800.
7. Hughes GS, Heald DL, Barker KB, Patel RK, Spillers CR, Watts KC, Batts DH, Euler AR. The effects of gastric pH and food on the pharmacokinetics of a new oral cephalosporin, cefpodoxime proxetil. *Clin Pharmacol Ther* (1989) 46, 674–85.
8. Shyu WC, Wilber RB, Pittman KA, Barbhaiya RH. Effect of antacid on the bioavailability of cefprozil. *Antimicrob Agents Chemother* (1992) 36, 962–5.
9. Radwanski E, Nomeir A, Cutler D, Affrime M, Lin C-C. Pharmacokinetic drug interaction study: administration of ceftibuten concurrently with the antacid Mylanta double-strength liquid or with ranitidine. *Am J Ther* (1998) 5, 67–72.

Cephalosporins + Calcium-channel blockers

Nifedipine increases the serum levels of cefixime but this is unlikely to be clinically important. Neither nifedipine nor diltiazem affect the pharmacokinetics of cefpodoxime proxetil.

Clinical evidence, mechanism, importance and management

In 8 healthy subjects the AUC and peak serum levels of a single 200-mg dose of **cefixime** were increased by about 70% and 50%, respectively, when **cefixime** was taken 30 minutes after a 20-mg dose of **nifedipine**. The rate of absorption was also increased. One suggested reason for this interaction is that the **nifedipine** increases the absorption of the **cefixime** by affecting the carrier system across the epithelial wall of the gut.[1] It seems doubtful if this increased **cefixime** bioavailability is clinically important (the combination was well-tolerated) and no particular precautions would seem to be necessary on concurrent use.

The pharmacokinetics of a single 200-mg dose of **cefpodoxime proxetil** were found to be unchanged by single doses of either **diltiazem** 60 mg or **nifedipine** 20 mg in 12 healthy subjects.[2] No special precautions would seem necessary during concurrent use.

Information about other cephalosporins and calcium-channel blockers seems to be lacking, but there seems to be no particular reason to suspect an interaction.

1. Duverne C, Bouten A, Deslandes A, Westphal J-F, Trouvin J-H, Farinotti R, Carbon C. Modification of cefixime bioavailability by nifedipine in humans: involvement of the dipeptide carrier system. *Antimicrob Agents Chemother* (1992) 36, 2462–7.
2. Deslandes A, Camus F, Lacroix C, Carbon C, Farinotti R. Effects of nifedipine and diltiazem on pharmacokinetics of cefpodoxime following its oral administration. *Antimicrob Agents Chemother* (1996) 40, 2879–81.

Cephalosporins + Colestyramine

Colestyramine binds with cefadroxil and cefalexin in the gut, which delays their absorption. The importance of this is probably small.

Clinical evidence

The peak serum levels of a 500-mg oral dose of **cefadroxil** were reduced and delayed in 4 subjects when it was taken with 10 g of colestyramine, but the total amount absorbed was not affected.[1] Similar results were found in a study involving **cefalexin** and colestyramine.[2]

Mechanism

Colestyramine is an ion-exchange resin, which binds with these two cephalosporins in the gut. This prevents the early and rapid absorption of the antibacterial, but as the colestyramine/cephalosporin complex passes along the gastrointestinal tract, the antibacterial is progressively released and eventually virtually all of it becomes available for absorption.[1]

Importance and management

Direct information seems to be limited to the studies cited. The clinical significance is uncertain, but as the total amount of antibacterial absorbed is not reduced this interaction is probably of little importance. This needs confirmation. Information about other cephalosporins seems to be lacking.

1. Marino EL, Vicente MT and Dominguez-Gil A. Influence of cholestyramine on the pharmacokinetic parameters of cefadroxil after simultaneous administration. *Int J Pharmaceutics* (1983) 16, 23–30.
2. Parsons RL, Paddock GM. Absorption of two antibacterial drugs, cephalexin and co-trimoxazole, in malabsorption syndromes. *J Antimicrob Chemother* (1975) 1 (Suppl), 59–67.

Cephalosporins + Food

The bioavailabilities of cefadroxil, cefalexin, cefixime, cefprozil, and cefradine are not affected by food. Cefaclor may be given without regard to food but absorption of an extended-release preparation may be increased by food. The bioavailabilities of cefetamet pivoxil and cefuroxime axetil may be increased by administration with food.

Clinical evidence, mechanism, importance and management

(a) Cefaclor

A study in 18 healthy subjects given a single 250-mg capsule of cefaclor after an overnight fast or within 30 minutes of different meals found the bioavailability was not significantly affected by food. The rate of absorption and maximum plasma levels were decreased: a low-fat vegetarian diet produced the smallest decrease in maximum plasma levels (26%) and a high-fat non-vegetarian diet produced the largest decrease (47%) compared with levels achieved after an overnight fast. None of the diets significantly affected the $AUC_{0-\infty}$ of cefaclor. Therapeutic efficacy (measured by time levels were above MIC_{50}) was not significantly altered.[1] In a further study, healthy subjects were given a single 500-mg dose of cefaclor as an extended-release tablet. The rate of absorption was decreased by food but compared to the fasting state, the maximum levels were increased; by 52% for rice-based diets, by 33% for low-fat-vegetarian food, by 29% for high-fat non-vegetarian food, by 12.5% for high-fat-vegetarian food, and by 7% for low-fat non-vegetarian food. Compared with the fasting state, all the diets increased the time above MIC_{90}, with a significant increase of almost 42% with low-fat vegetarian (wheat-based) food.[2] The manufacturers of immediate-release cefaclor capsules state that total absorption is the same whether the drug is given with or without food,[3] but for the extended-release preparation since absorption is enhanced by administration with food, the manufacturers recommend that this preparation should be taken with meals.[4]

(b) Cefadroxil

The manufacturers of cefadroxil state that the bioavailability of cefadroxil is unaffected by food so it may be taken either with meals or on an empty stomach.[5]

(c) Cefalexin

The manufacturers of cefalexin state that it is acid stable and may be given without regard to meals.[6]

(d) Cefetamet pivoxil

A study found that the bioavailability of cefetamet pivoxil was up to 25% higher when it was given 10 minutes after a standard breakfast rather than in the fasting state.[7,8] However, in another study, healthy subjects were given oral cefetamet pivoxil hydrochloride 1 g (equivalent to 693 mg of cefetamet free acid) either: 1 hour before food with 200 mL of water; with a standard breakfast and a cup of tea or coffee; or 1 hour after breakfast with 200 mL of water. The cefetamet maximum plasma levels were 5.5, 5.47. and 6.57 micrograms/mL, respectively, and the AUCs were 38, 35.7, and 42.8 micrograms.hour/mL, respectively, suggesting that bioavailability of cefetamet pivoxil is lowest when taken with food. The time to reach maximum plasma levels was increased from 3.3 hours when given before food to 4.3 hours when given with food, and 4.1 hours when given one hour after food.[9] It was thought possible that the amount of fluid taken with cefetamet may have affected absorption, but a study in which cefetamet 1 g was given under fasting conditions with either 250 or 450 mL of water found that increasing fluid intake did not affect absorption. Further, the absorption when taken with food, with or without 200 mL of water was similar. It was recommended that cefetamet pivoxil should be taken within an hour of a meal to improve absorption. The delay in absorption was not considered to be of significance, especially during multiple dose therapy.[9]

(e) Cefixime

A study in healthy subjects given a single 400-mg dose of cefixime, either in the fasting state or immediately after a standard breakfast found that the time to peak serum levels was increased from about 3.8 to 4.8 hours when cefixime was given with food, probably because of delayed gastric emptying. Serum levels, AUC and 24 hour urinary recovery were similar for fasted and fed states.[10] Cefixime may be given without regard to meals.[10,11]

(f) Cefpodoxime proxetil

In a study in healthy subjects, cefpodoxime proxetil 400 mg tablets were given with 180 mL of water after an overnight fast, or either 1 hour before, with, or 2 hours after the start of a high-fat meal. Dosing 1 hour before the meal was similar to dosing in the fasting state. However, when cefpodoxime was taken with, or 2 hours after the meal its peak plasma levels were increased by about 45% and 46%, respectively, when compared with the peak levels achieved in the fasting state. The AUC was also increased, by 40%. The rate of cefpodoxime absorption was not greatly affected by food.[12] Studies with a 200-mg dose of cefpodoxime have also found that food increases the extent, but not the rate, of cefpodoxime absorption.[13] However, the extent of the food effect appears to be greater with the 400 mg dose. This is possibly because the bioavailability of the 400-mg tablets is less than that of the 200-mg tablets, so food may have a greater effect on the higher strength preparation.[12] In another study by the same authors the AUC and urinary excretion of cefpodoxime proxetil 200 mg given as a suspension were higher (11% and 14%, respectively) when taken with a high-fat meal rather than in the fasting state. Maximum plasma levels were not affected by a high-fat meal but the time to achieve maximum levels was prolonged.[14]

The manufacturers state that the bioavailability of cefpodoxime proxetil 100 mg tablets and suspension is increased by food.[15,16] The studies[12-14] suggest the increased bioavailability of the tablets, but possibly not that of the suspension, when given with food may be clinically significant.

(g) Cefprozil

A study in healthy subjects found that, although food caused slight changes in the rate of absorption of a 1-g dose of cefprozil its pharmacokinetics (including total absorption) were not significantly affected.[17]

(h) Cefradine

A study in healthy subjects given cefradine 500 mg in the fasting state or immediately after a meal found the time to peak levels was increased from 0.8 hours to 2 hours by food. Peak serum levels of cefradine were reduced by 45% when it was given after food. However, the half-life and AUC were not affected.[18] The manufacturers state that cefradine may be given without regard to meals.[19]

(i) Cefuroxime axetil

A study in healthy subjects given cefuroxime axetil 500 mg intravenously or oral doses of 125 mg to 1 g with or without food found that 36% and 52% of a 500-mg oral dose was absorbed in the fasting and fed states respectively.[20] In another study in healthy subjects, a single 1-g dose of cefuroxime axetil was given 2 hours before or 35 minutes after a standard cooked breakfast. The bioavailability of cefuroxime was markedly enhanced by food.[21] The manufacturer notes that optimum absorption of cefuroxime axetil occurs when it is given after a meal.[22] This is probably because of delayed gastric emptying and transit which allowed more complete dissolution and absorption.[21]

1. Karim S, Ahmed T, Monif T, Saha N, Sharma PL. The effect of four different types of food on the bioavailability of cefaclor. *Eur J Drug Metab Pharmacokinet* (2003), 28, 185–90.
2. Khan BAH, Ahmed T, Karim S, Monif T, Saha N. Comparative effect of different types of food on the bioavailability of cefaclor extended release tablet. *Eur J Drug Metab Pharmacokinet* (2004) 29, 125–32.
3. Distaclor (Cefaclor monohydrate). Flynn Pharma Ltd. UK Summary of product characteristics, November 2005.
4. Distaclor MR (Cefaclor monohydrate). Flynn Pharma Ltd. UK Summary of product characteristics, December 2006.
5. Baxan (Cefadroxil monohydrate) Bristol-Myers Pharmaceuticals, UK Summary of product characteristics, July 2005.
6. Keflex (Cefalexin monohydrate). Flynn Pharma Ltd. UK Summary of product characteristics, September 2005.
7. Blouin RA, Kneer J, Stoeckel K. Pharmacokinetics of intravenous cefetamet (Ro 15-8074) and oral cefetamet pivoxil (R0-8075) in young and elderly subjects. *Antimicrob Agents Chemother* (1989) 33, 291–6.
8. Koup JR, Dubach UC, Brandt R, Wyss R, Stoeckel K. Pharmacokinetics of cefetamet (Ro 15-8074) and cefetamet pivoxil (Ro 15-8075) after intravenous and oral doses in humans. *Antimicrob Agents Chemother* (1988) 32, 573–9.
9. Tam YK, Kneer J, Dubach UC, Stoeckel K. Effects of timing of food and fluid volume on cefetamet pivoxil absorption in healthy normal volunteers. *Antimicrob Agents Chemother* (1990) 34, 1556–9.
10. Faulkner RD, Bohaychuk W, Haynes JD, Desjardins RE, Yacobi A, Silber BM. The pharmacokinetics of cefixime in the fasted and fed state. *Eur J Clin Pharmacol* (1988) 34, 525–8.
11. Suprax Tablets (Cefixime). Sanofi-Aventis. UK Summary of product characteristics, May 2006.
12. Borin MT, Driver MR, Forbes KK. Effect of timing of food on absorption of cefpodoxime proxetil. *J Clin Pharmacol* (1995) 35, 505–9.
13. Hughes GS, Heald DL, Barker KB, Patel RK, Spillers CR, Watts KC, Batts DH, Euler AR. The effects of gastric pH and food on the pharmacokinetics of a new oral cephalosporin, cefpodoxime proxetil. *Clin Pharmacol Ther* (1989) 46, 674–85.
14. Borin MT, Forbes KK. Effect of food on absorption of cefpodoxime proxetil oral suspension in adults. *Antimicrob Agents Chemother* (1995) 39, 273–5.
15. Orelox Tablets (Cefpodoxime proxetil). Sanofi-Aventis. UK Summary of product characteristics, April 2006.
16. Orelox Suspension (Cefpodoxime proxetil). Sanofi-Aventis. UK Summary of product characteristics, April 2006.
17. Shukla UA, Pittman KA, Barbhaiya RH. Pharmacokinetic interactions of cefprozil with food, propantheline, metoclopramide, and probenecid in healthy volunteers. *J Clin Pharmacol* (1992) 32, 725–31.
18. Mischler TW, Sugerman AA, Willard DA, Brannick LJ, Neiss ES. Influence of probenecid and food on the bioavailability of cephradine in normal male subjects. *J Clin Pharmacol* (1974) 14, 604–11.
19. Velosef (Cefradine). ER Squibb & Sons Ltd. UK Summary of product characteristics, June 2005.
20. Finn A, Straughn A, Meyer M, Chubb J. Effect of dose and food on the bioavailability of cefuroxime axetil. *Biopharm Drug Dispos* (1987) 8, 519–26.
21. Sommers DK, Van Wyk M, Moncrieff J, Schoeman HS. Influence of food and reduced gastric acidity on the bioavailability of bacampicillin and cefuroxime axetil. *Br J Clin Pharmacol* (1984) 18, 535–9.
22. Zinnat Tablets (Cefuroxime axetil). GlaxoSmithKline UK. UK Summary of product characteristics, January 2007.

Cephalosporins + Furosemide

The nephrotoxic effects of cefaloridine and possibly cefalotin or cefacetrile appear to be increased by furosemide. Cefradine brain levels are reduced by furosemide. No important interactions appear to occur between furosemide and cefoxitin, ceftazidime, ceftriaxone, or cefuroxime.

Clinical evidence

(a) Nephrotoxicity

Nine out of 36 patients who developed acute renal failure while taking **cefaloridine** had also been taking a diuretic: furosemide was used in 7 cases. Other factors such as patient age and drug dosage may also have been involved. The authors of this report related their observations to previous *animal* studies, which showed that potent diuretics such as furosemide and etacrynic acid enhanced the incidence and extent of tubular necrosis.[1] Several other reports describe nephrotoxicity in patients given both **cefalori-**

dine and furosemide.[2-4] There is a possibility that this effect also occurs with **cefalotin** and **cefacetrile** because *animal* studies found an increase in nephrotoxicity,[5,6] and there is a single report describing nephrotoxicity in one patient taking **cefalotin** with furosemide.[2] **Cefoxitin** seems to be relatively free of nephrotoxicity alone or with furosemide.[7]

(b) Changes in serum levels and clearance

A clinical study[8] found that furosemide 80 mg increased the serum half-life of **cefaloridine** by 25%, and in another study **cefaloridine** clearance was reduced by furosemide.[9] A further study found that brain concentrations of **cefradine** are markedly reduced by furosemide.[10] In a study in 6 healthy subjects, furosemide 40 mg, given 1 hour before a 1-g intramuscular dose of **ceftazidime**, raised the serum **ceftazidime** levels by about 20 to 40% over 8 hours and increased the AUC by 28%. Furosemide given 3 hours before **ceftazidime** had much smaller effects.[11] The serum half-lives of intravenous **cefoxitin** and **cefuroxime** were not affected by oral furosemide.[12] **Ceftriaxone** does not appear to interfere with the diuretic effects of furosemide.[13]

Mechanism

Cefaloridine is nephrotoxic, but why this should be increased by furosemide is not understood. It may possibly be related to a reduction in its clearance.[9]

Importance and management

The interaction between cefaloridine and furosemide is not well-established, but there is enough evidence to suggest that concurrent use should be undertaken with care. Age and/or renal impairment may possibly be predisposing factors. Renal function should be checked frequently if both drugs are given. A pharmacokinetic study suggests that the development of this adverse interaction may possibly depend on the time relationship of drug use, and it has been recommended that furosemide should be avoided for 3 or 4 hours before the cefaloridine.[14]

Although the manufacturers of ceftazidime issue a caution about the use of high doses of cephalosporins with other nephrotoxic drugs, they say that clinical experience has not shown this to be a problem with ceftazidime at the recommended doses.[15] The rest of the information about other cephalosporins and furosemide is fairly sparse. Most appear not to interact adversely, with a few possible exceptions, namely cefalotin (nephrotoxicity in a single case[2] and *animal* studies[5]) and cefacetrile (nephrotoxicity in *animal* studies[6]). Care is clearly prudent with these two cephalosporins.

1. Dodds MG, Foord RD. Enhancement by potent diuretics of renal tubular necrosis induced by cephaloridine. *Br J Pharmacol* (1970) 4, 227–36.
2. Simpson IJ. Nephrotoxicity and acute renal failure associated with cephalothin and cephaloridine. *N Z Med J* (1971) 74, 312–15.
3. Kleinknecht D, Jungers P, Fillastre J-P. Nephrotoxicity of cephaloridine. *Ann Intern Med* (1974) 80, 421–2.
4. Lawson DH, Macadam RF, Singh H, Gavras H, Linton AL. The nephrotoxicity of cephaloridine. *Postgrad Med J* (1970) 46 (Suppl), 36–9.
5. Lawson DH, Macadam RF, Singh H, Gavras H, Hartz S, Turnbull D, Linton AL. Effect of furosemide on antibiotic-induced renal damage in rats. *J Infect Dis* (1972) 126, 593–600.
6. Luscombe DK, Nichols PJ. Possible interaction between cephacetrile and frusemide in rabbits and rats. *J Antimicrob Chemother* (1975) 1, 67–77.
7. Trollfors B, Norrby R, Kristianson K, Nilsson NJ. Effects on renal function of treatment with cefoxitin alone or in combination with furosemide. *Scand J Infect Dis* (1978) (Suppl), 13, 73–7.
8. Norrby R, Stenqvist K, Elgefors B. Interaction between cephaloridine and furosemide in man. *Scand J Infect Dis* (1976) 8, 209–212.
9. Tilstone WJ, Semple PF, Lawson DH, Boyle JA. Effects of furosemide on glomerular filtration rate and clearance of practolol, digoxin, cephaloridine and gentamicin. *Clin Pharmacol Ther* (1977) 22, 389–94.
10. Adam D, Jacoby W, Raff WK. Beeinflussung der Antibiotika-Konzentration im Gewebe durch ein Saluretikum. *Klin Wochenschr* (1978) 56, 247–51.
11. Chrysos G, Gargalianos P, Lelekis M, Stefanou J, Kosmidis J. Pharmacokinetic interactions of ceftazidime and frusemide. *J Chemother* (1995) 7 (Suppl 4), 107–10.
12. Trollfors B, Norrby R. Effect of frusemide on the elimination of cefuroxime and cefoxitin. *J Antimicrob Chemother* (1989) 6, 405–7.
13. Korn A, Eichler HG, Gasic S. A drug interaction study of ceftriaxone and frusemide in healthy volunteers. *Int J Clin Pharmacol Ther Toxicol* (1986) 24, 262–4.
14. Kosmidis J, Polyzos A, Daikos GK. Pharmacokinetic interactions between cephalosporins and furosemide are influenced by administration time relationships. 11th International Congress of Chemotherapy, 1980. 673–5.
15. Fortum Injection (Ceftazidime pentahydrate). GlaxoSmithKline UK. UK Summary of product characteristics, May 2007.

Cephalosporins + H_2-receptor antagonists

Ranitidine and famotidine reduce the bioavailability of cefpodoxime proxetil. Ranitidine with sodium bicarbonate reduces the bioavailability of cefuroxime axetil, but not to an important extent if cefuroxime is taken with food. No clinically significant pharmacokinetic interactions appear to occur between cefaclor AF and cimetidine, or between cefetamet pivoxil, cefalexin or ceftibuten and ranitidine.

Clinical evidence

(a) Cefaclor

A study using cefaclor AF (a formulation with a slow rate of release) found that **cimetidine** 800 mg taken the previous night reduced its maximum plasma concentration by 12%.[1]

(b) Cefalexin

Ranitidine 150 mg for 3 doses had only small and therapeutically unimportant effects on the pharmacokinetics of cefalexin 1 g.[2] In another study in healthy subjects **ranitidine** 150 mg for 3 doses prolonged the time to attain peak serum levels of a single 500-mg dose of cefalexin from 1.19 to 1.48 hours. Other pharmacokinetic parameters were not significantly affected. Similar results were found when **omeprazole** was given instead of ranitidine.[3]

(c) Cefetamet pivoxil

Ranitidine 150 mg twice daily for 4 days did not affect the pharmacokinetics of cefetamet pivoxil 1 g given to 18 healthy subjects after breakfast.[4]

(d) Cefpodoxime proxetil

A study in 10 healthy fasted subjects showed that **famotidine** 40 mg reduced the bioavailability of cefpodoxime proxetil by about 40%.[5] This confirms the findings of a previous study with **ranitidine**.[6]

(e) Ceftibuten

Ranitidine 150 mg every 12 hours for 3 days raised the maximum plasma levels and AUC of ceftibuten by 23% and 16%, respectively, in 18 healthy subjects. However these values lie within the normal ranges seen in healthy subjects and no dosage adjustment is therefore thought to be needed.[7]

(f) Cefuroxime axetil

Ranitidine 300 mg with sodium bicarbonate 4 g reduced the AUC of cefuroxime axetil 1 g by 43% when the combination was given to fasted subjects. However, when cefuroxime was given after food, its bioavailability was higher, and minimally affected by **ranitidine** plus sodium bicarbonate (10% reduction in AUC).[8]

Mechanism

The reduction in the bioavailability of some of the cephalosporins is thought to be due to reduced dissolution at increased gastric pH values.[5]

Importance and management

In most cases the interactions between the cephalosporins and H_2-receptor antagonists are not clinically significant. The clinical importance of the interaction with cefpodoxime has not been studied, but the manufacturer recommends that cefpodoxime is given at least 2 hours before H_2-receptor antagonists.[9] As it is thought that a change in gastric pH is responsible for this interaction it would seem likely that **proton pump inhibitors** will interact similarly.

As long as cefuroxime is taken with food (as is recommended[10]), any interaction is minimal. The bioavailability of cefetamet pivoxil,[4] and cefpodoxime proxetil,[5,6] are also enhanced by food so it is probable that interaction with drugs which raise gastric pH may be similarly minimised.

1. Satterwhite JH, Cerimele BJ, Coleman DL, Hatcher BL, Kisicki J, DeSante KA. Pharmacokinetics of cefaclor AF: effects of age, antacids and H_2-receptor antagonists. *Postgrad Med J* (1992) 68 (Suppl 3), S3–S9.
2. Deppermann K-M, Lode H, Höffken G, Tschink G, Kalz C, Koeppe P. Influence of ranitidine, pirenzepine, and aluminum magnesium hydroxide on the bioavailability of various antibiotics, including amoxicillin, cephalexin, doxycycline and amoxicillin-clavulanic acid. *Antimicrob Agents Chemother* (1989) 33, 1901–1907.
3. Madaras-Kelly K, Michas P, George M, May MP, Adejare A. A randomized crossover study investigating the influence of ranitidine or omeprazole on the pharmacokinetics of cephalexin monohydrate. *J Clin Pharmacol* (2004) 44, 1391–7.
4. Blouin RA, Kneer J, Ambros RJ, Stoeckel K. Influence of antacid and ranitidine on the pharmacokinetics of oral cefetamet pivoxil. *Antimicrob Agents Chemother* (1990) 34, 1744–8.
5. Saathoff N, Lode H, Neider K, Depperman KM, Borner K, Koeppe P. Pharmacokinetics of cefpodoxime proxetil and interactions with an antacid and an H_2 receptor antagonist. *Antimicrob Agents Chemother* (1992) 36, 796–800.

6. Hughes GS, Heald DL, Barker KB, Patel RK, Spillers CR, Watts KC, Batts DH, Euler AR. The effects of gastric pH and food on the pharmacokinetics of a new oral cephalosporin, cefpodoxime proxetil. *Clin Pharmacol Ther* (1989) 46, 674–85.
7. Radwanski E, Nomeir A, Cutler D, Affrime M, Lin C-C. Pharmacokinetic drug interaction study: administration of ceftibuten concurrently with the antacid Mylanta double-strength liquid or with ranitidine. *Am J Ther* (1998) 5, 67–72.
8. Sommers De K, Van Wyk M, Moncrieff J, Schoeman HS. Influence of food and reduced gastric acidity on the bioavailability of bacampicillin and cefuroxime axetil. *Br J Clin Pharmacol* (1984) 18, 535–9.
9. Orelox Tablets (Cefpodoxime proxetil). Sanofi-Aventis. UK Summary of product characteristics, April 2006.
10. Zinnat Tablets (Cefuroxime axetil). GlaxoSmithKline UK. UK Summary of product characteristics, January 2007.

Cephalosporins + Probenecid

The serum levels of many cephalosporins are raised by probenecid. Possible exceptions include ceforanide, ceftazidime, ceftriaxone and latamoxef. The rise in serum levels may possibly increase the risk of nephrotoxicity with some cephalosporins such as cefaloridine and cefalotin.

Clinical evidence

Ten healthy subjects given a single 500-mg oral dose of **cefradine** or **cefaclor** developed markedly raised serum antibacterial concentrations when they were also given probenecid (500-mg doses taken 25, 13 and 2 hours before the antibacterial). Peak serum levels of the antibacterial were very roughly doubled.[1] Similar results were obtained in another study in healthy subjects given **cefradine** by mouth or intramuscularly.[2]

Although some cephalosporins don not appear to interact, in general, most have their clearance reduced, their serum levels raised and sometimes their half-lives prolonged by probenecid, see 'Table 10.2', (p.297).

Mechanism

Probenecid inhibits the excretion of most cephalosporins by the kidney tubules by successfully competing for the excretory mechanisms. A fuller explanation of this mechanism is set out in 'Drug excretion interactions', (p.7). Thus the cephalosporin is retained in the body and its serum levels rise. The extent of the rise cannot always be fully accounted for by this mechanism alone and it is suggested that some change in tissue distribution may sometimes have a part to play.[1]

Importance and management

An extremely well-documented interaction. The serum levels of many (but not all) cephalosporins will be higher if probenecid is given, but no special precautions are normally needed. The interaction has been used clinically. Elevated serum levels of some cephalosporins, in particular cefaloridine and cefalotin, might possibly increase the risk of nephrotoxicity.

1. Welling PG, Dean S, Selen A, Kendall MJ, Wise R. Probenecid: an unexplained effect on cephalosporin pharmacology. *Br J Clin Pharmacol* (1979) 8, 491–5.
2. Mischler TW, Sugerman AA, Willard DA, Brannick LJ, Neiss ES. Influence of probenecid and food on the bioavailability of cephradine in normal male subjects. *J Clin Pharmacol* (1974) 14, 604–11.

Cephalosporins; Cefalexin + Pirenzepine

Pirenzepine (50 mg for 4 doses) had only small and therapeutically unimportant effects on the pharmacokinetics of a 1-g dose of cefalexin.[1]

1. Deppermann K-M, Lode H, Höffken G, Tschink G, Kalz C, Koeppe P. Influence of ranitidine, pirenzepine, and aluminum magnesium hydroxide on the bioavailability of various antibiotics, including amoxicillin, cephalexin, doxycycline and amoxicillin-clavulanic acid. *Antimicrob Agents Chemother* (1989) 33, 1901–1907.

Cephalosporins; Cefalotin + Colistin

Renal failure has been attributed to the concurrent use of cefalotin and colistin.

Clinical evidence, mechanism, importance and management

Four patients developed acute renal failure, which appeared to be reversible, during treatment with colistin. Three were given cefalotin concurrently and the fourth had previously been taking this antibacterial.[1] An increase in renal toxicity associated with concurrent use has been described in another report.[2] The reason for this reaction is not known. What is known suggests that renal function should be closely monitored if these drugs are given concurrently or sequentially.

1. Adler S, Segal DP. Nonoliguric renal failure secondary to sodium colistimethate: a report of four cases. *Am J Med Sci* (1971) 262, 109–14.
2. Koch-Weser J, Sidel VW, Federman EB, Kanarek P, Finer DC, Eaton AE. Adverse effects of sodium colistimethate. Manifestations and specific reaction rates during 317 courses of therapy. *Ann Intern Med* (1970) 72, 857–68.

Cephalosporins; Cefdinir + Iron compounds

Ferrous sulfate markedly reduces the absorption of cefdinir.

Clinical evidence

When 6 healthy subjects were given **ferrous sulfate** (1050 mg of *Fero-Gradumet*, sustained release, equivalent to 210 mg of elemental iron) with cefdinir 200 mg the AUC of the cefdinir was reduced by 93%. When the **ferrous sulfate** was taken 3 hours after the cefdinir, the absorption of the cefdinir remained unchanged for 3 hours and then rapidly fell, the total AUC over 12 hours being reduced by 36%.[1]

Mechanism

It is believed that the ferrous sulfate chelates with the cefdinir in the gut to produce a poorly absorbed complex.

Importance and management

An established interaction of clinical importance. Avoid ferrous sulfate and other iron compounds while taking cefdinir. It is not yet known how far apart these drugs must be separated to avoid this interaction, but 3 hours improves the situation considerably even if it does not totally solve it. There is no information to suggest that other cephalosporins interact in this way.

1. Ueno K, Tanaka K, Tsujimura K, Morishima Y, Iwashige H, Yamazaki K, Nakata I. Impairment of cefdinir absorption by iron ion. *Clin Pharmacol Ther* (1993) 54, 473–5.

Cephalosporins; Cefotaxime + Penicillins

Azlocillin and mezlocillin may reduce the clearance of cefotaxime in subjects with normal or impaired renal function.

Clinical evidence, mechanism, importance and management

A patient with renal failure developed encephalopathy with focal motor status and generalised convulsions when given cefotaxime 2 g every 8 hours and **azlocillin** 5 g every 8 hours (high-dose).[1] In a study in subjects with either normal or impaired renal function, the clearance of a single dose of cefotaxime was reduced by 40 to 50% regardless of renal function.[2]

When intravenous cefotaxime 30 mg/kg and **mezlocillin** 50 mg/kg were given together over 30 minutes in 8 healthy subjects, the pharmacokinetics of the **mezlocillin** were unchanged but the clearance of the cefotaxime was reduced by about 40%. However, in a series of 5 patients with end-stage renal disease no significant decrease in cefotaxime clearance was seen when **mezlocillin** was given.[3]

Doses of cefotaxime may need to be reduced in the presence of either **azlocillin** or **mezlocillin**. One report suggests a dosage reduction of cefotaxime is advisable if the glomerular filtration rate is 20 to 40 mL/minute and **azlocillin** is also given.[2]

1. Wroe SJ, Ellershaw JE, Whittaker JA, Richens A. Focal motor status epilepticus following treatment with azlocillin and cefotaxime. *Med Toxicol* (1987) 2, 233–4.
2. Kampf D, Borner K, Möller M, Kessel M. Kinetic interactions between azlocillin, cefotaxime, and cefotaxime metabolites in normal and impaired renal function. *Clin Pharmacol Ther* (1984) 35, 214–20.
3. Rodondi LC, Flaherty JF, Schoenfeld P, Barriere SL, Gambertoglio JG. Influence of coadministration on the pharmacokinetics of mezlocillin and cefotaxime in healthy volunteers and in patients with renal failure. *Clin Pharmacol Ther* (1989) 45, 527–34.

Table 10.2 Effect of probenecid on the pharmacokinetics of the cephalosporins

Drug	*Route*	*Effect of probenecid*	*Refs*
Cefacetrile	Intramuscular	Mean serum half-life increased from 52 to 90 minutes	1
Cefaclor	Oral	Serum level approximately doubled; renal excretion inhibited; renal excretion after 4 hours reduced by 61%	2,3
Cefadroxil	Oral	Probenecid 500 mg every 8 hours for 5 doses increased the half-life of cefadroxil from 1.13 to 1.63 hours and reduced its renal excretion by 58%; probenecid slightly increased and prolonged cefadroxil serum levels	4
Cefalexin	Oral	Reduced clearance	5
Cefaloglycin	Oral	Increased peak serum levels and duration of antibacterial activity	6
Cefaloridine	Intramuscular/Intravenous	Plasma levels increased by 20%. Clearance reduced by 24% (intravenous); increased serum levels; prolonged antibacterial activity (intramuscular)	7,8
Cefalotin	Intravenous	Plasma levels increased by 70%. Clearance reduced by 59%	7
Cefamandole	Intramuscular	Peak serum levels almost doubled; half-life prolonged from 1.1 to 2 hours	9
Cefazedone	Intravenous	AUC increased more than threefold; elimination half-life increased from 1.58 to 4.44 hours; total clearance reduced by 68%	10
Cefazolin	Intramuscular/Intravenous	At 6 hours serum levels of intramuscular dose doubled; after intravenous dose elimination half-life increased from 1.6 to 2.7 hour and mean serum level after 24 hours was increased from 1.1 to 2 mg/L; therapeutic levels at steady-state maintained by once daily rather than three times daily dose regimen	11-13
Cefditoren	Oral	Increased plasma half-life; decreased excretion and renal clearance	14
Cefmenoxime	Intravenous	Renal clearance of cefmenoxime reduced from 159 to 66 mL/minute; AUC almost doubled	15
Cefmetazole	Intravenous	Mean AUC increased by about 58%; clearance reduced by about 36%; half-life increased from 1.5 to 2.27 hours	16
Cefonicid	Intramuscular	Probenecid 1 g increased the maximum levels of cefonicid 500 mg by 52%, increased the AUC twofold, increased the half-life from 3.5 to 7.5 hours, reduced elimination rates and decreased renal clearance	17
Ceforanide	Intramuscular	No significant effect	18
Cefotaxime	Intramuscular/Intravenous	Oral probenecid 500 mg every 6 hours for 24 hours before, and 1 g 30 minutes before, intravenous cefotaxime 1 g reduced renal clearance by about half and almost doubled its AUC. Delayed excretion and increased plasma levels due to effects on renal tubular transfer. Clearance of cefotaxime and also its metabolites decreased by probenecid	19-21
Cefoxitin	Intramuscular/Intravenous	Serum half-life increased from 39 to 129 minutes and clearance halved (intravenous); greater increase in AUC when probenecid given 1 hour before rather than with cefoxitin (intravenous); increasing dose of probenecid from 1 to 2 g increased AUC of cefoxitin (intramuscular)	21-23
Cefprozil	Oral	Significant increase in half-life and maximum levels, AUC approximately doubled, and clearance decreased by about 60%	24
Cefradine	Oral/Intramuscular	Serum levels approximately doubled. Delay to time of peak from 1 to 2 hours (oral) and 1 to 1.5 hours (intramuscular); half-lives prolonged	2,25
Ceftazidime	Intravenous	Probenecid 500 mg every 6 hours for 24 hours before and 1 g immediately before a single intravenous dose of ceftazidime 1 g did not significantly affect ceftazidime clearance. Pharmacokinetics of single 50-mg/kg dose of ceftazidime in patients with cystic fibrosis not affected by pre-treatment with probenecid 2 g	19,26
Ceftizoxime	Intramuscular/Intravenous	AUC increased by 49% (both routes); half-life increased from 1.7 to 2.3 hours (intravenous) and 1.9 to 2.8 hours (intramuscular)	27
Ceftriaxone	Intravenous	No significant effect	28
Cefuroxime	Intravenous	AUC increased by 44 to 50%; half-life prolonged by 63%; clearance decreased by 29%	29
Latamoxef	Intravenous	Probenecid 500 mg every 6 hours for 24 hours before and 1 g immediately before a single 1-g intravenous dose of latamoxef did not significantly affect latamoxef clearance	19

1. Wise R, Reeves DS. Pharmacological studies on cephacetrile in human volunteers. *Curr Med Res Opin* (1974) 2, 249–55.
2. Welling PG, Dean S, Selen A, Kendall MJ, Wise R. Probenecid: an unexplained effect on cephalosporin pharmacology. *Br J Clin Pharmacol* (1979) 8, 491–5.

Continued

Table 10.2 Effect of probenecid on the pharmacokinetics of the cephalosporins (continued)

3. Santoro J, Agarwal BN, Martinelli R, Wenger N, Levison ME. Pharmacology of cefaclor in normal volunteers and patients with renal failure. *Antimicrob Agents Chemother* (1978) 13, 951–4.
4. Mariño EL, Dominguez-Gil A. The pharmacokinetics of cefadroxil associated with probenecid. *Int J Clin Pharmacol Ther Toxicol* (1981) 19, 506–8.
5. Taylor WA, Holloway WJ. Cephalexin in the treatment of gonorrhea. *Int J Clin Pharmacol Ther Toxicol* (1972) 6, 7–9.
6. Applestein JM, Crosby EB, Johnson WD, Kaye D. In-vitro antimicrobial activity and human pharmacology of cephaloglycin. *Appl Microbiol* (1968) 16, 1006–10.
7. Tuano SB, Brodie JL, Kirby WMM. Cephaloridine versus cephalothin: relation of the kidney to blood level differences after parenteral administration. *Antimicrob Agents Chemother* (1966) 6, 101–6.
8. Kaplan KS, Reisberg BE, Weinstein L. Cephaloridine: antimicrobial activity and pharmacologic behaviour. *Am J Med Sci* (1967) 253, 667–74.
9. Griffith RS, Black HR, Brier GL, Wolny JD. Effect of probenecid on the blood levels and urinary excretion of cefamandole. *Antimicrob Agents Chemother* (1977) 11, 809–12.
10. Ungethüm W, Pabst J, Dingeldein E, Leopold G. Clinical pharmacology phase I of cefazedone, a new cephalosporin, in healthy volunteers; III. Investigations of the mechanism of renal elimination. *Arzneimittelforschung* (1979) 29, 443–8.
11. Duncan WC. Treatment of gonorrhea with cefazolin plus probenecid. *J Infect Dis* (1974) 130, 398–401.
12. Brown G, Zemcov SJV, Clarke AM. Effect of probenecid on cefazolin serum concentrations. *J Antimicrob Chemother* (1993) 31, 1009–1011.
13. Spina SP, Dillon EC. Effect of chronic probenecid therapy on cefazolin serum concentrations. *Ann Pharmacother* (2003) 37, 621–4.
14. Mayer M, Mulford D, Witt G. Effect of probenecid on the pharmacokinetics of cefditoren. 41st Annual Meeting of the Interscience Conference on Antimicrobial Agents and Chemotherapy, Chicago, Illinois. (2001) 41, Abstract 23.
15. Sennello LT, Quinn D, Rollins DE, Tolman KG, Sonders RC. Effect of probenecid on the pharmacokinetics of cefmenoxime. *Antimicrob Agents Chemother* (1983) 23, 803–7.
16. Ko H, Cathcart KS, Griffith DL, Peters GR, Adams WJ. Pharmacokinetics of intravenously administered cefmetazole and cefoxitin and effects of probenecid on cefmetazole elimination. *Antimicrob Agents Chemother* (1989) 33, 356–61.
17. Pitkin D, Dubb J, Actor P, Alexander F, Ehrlich S, Familiar R, Stote R. Kinetics and renal handling of cefonicid. *Clin Pharmacol Ther* (1981) 30, 587–93.
18. Jovanovich JF, Saravolatz LD, Burch K, Pohlod DJ. Failure of probenecid to alter the pharmacokinetics of ceforanide. *Antimicrob Agents Chemother* (1981) 20, 530–2.
19. Lüthy R, Blaser J, Bonetti A, Simmen H, Wise R, Siegenthaler W. Comparative multiple-dose pharmacokinetics of cefotaxime, moxalactam, and ceftazidime. *Antimicrob Agents Chemother* (1981) 20, 567–75.
20. Ings RMJ, Reeves DS, White LO, Bax RP, Bywater MJ, Holt HA. The human pharmacokinetics of cefotaxime and its metabolites and the role of renal tubular secretion on their elimination. *J Pharmacokinet Biopharm* (1985) 13, 121–42.
21. Bint AJ, Reeves DS, Holt HA. Effect of probenecid on serum cefoxitin concentrations. *J Antimicrob Chemother* (1977) 3, 627–8.
22. Reeves DS, Bullock DW, Bywater MJ, Holt HA, White LO, Thornhill DP. The effect of probenecid on the pharmacokinetics and distribution of cefoxitin in healthy volunteers. *Br J Clin Pharmacol* (1981) 11, 353–9.
23. Vlasses PH, Holbrook AM, Schrogie JJ, Rogers JD, Ferguson RK, Abrams WB. Effect of orally administered probenecid on the pharmacokinetics of cefoxitin. *Antimicrob Agents Chemother* (1980) 17, 847–55.
24. Shukla UA, Pittman KA, Barbhaiya RH. Pharmacokinetic interactions of cefprozil with food, propantheline, metoclopramide, and probenecid in healthy volunteers. *J Clin Pharmacol* (1992) 32, 725–31.
25. Mischler TW, Sugerman AA, Willard DA, Brannick LJ, Neiss ES. Influence of probenecid and food on the bioavailability of cephradine in normal male subjects. *J Clin Pharmacol* (1974) 14, 604–11.
26. Kercsmar CM, Stern RC, Reed MD, Myers CM, Murdell D, Blumer JL. Ceftazidime in cystic fibrosis: pharmacokinetics and therapeutic response. *J Antimicrob Chemother* (1983) 12 (Suppl. A) 289–95.
27. LeBel M, Paone RP, Lewis GP. Effect of probenecid on the pharmacokinetics of ceftizoxime. *J Antimicrob Chemother* (1983) 12, 147–55.
28. Stoeckel K, Trueb V, Dubach UC, McNamara PJ. Effect of probenecid on the elimination and protein binding of ceftriaxone. *Eur J Clin Pharmacol* (1988) 34, 151–6.
29. Garton AM, Rennie RP, Gilpin J, Marrelli M, Shafran SD. Comparison of dose doubling with probenecid for sustaining serum cefuroxime levels. *J Antimicrob Chemother* (1997) 40, 903–6.

Cephalosporins; Cefotaxime + Phenobarbital

A 30-month study noted a very marked increase in drug-induced reactions in children in intensive care who were given high-dose phenobarbital and beta-lactam antibacterials (mainly cefotaxime). Twenty-four out of 49 children developed drug-induced reactions, which were mainly exanthematous skin reactions.[1] The reasons are not known. It would seem prudent to consider this interaction in patients who develop skin reactions while taking both drugs.

1. Harder S, Schneider W, Bae ZU, Bock U, Zielen S. Unerwünschte Arzneimittelreaktionen bei gleichzeitiger Gabe von hochdosiertem Phenobarbital und Betalaktam-Antibiotika. *Klin Padiatr* (1990) 202, 404–7.

Cephalosporins; Cefpodoxime + Acetylcysteine

The pharmacokinetics of oral cefpodoxime proxetil are minimally affected by acetylcysteine and the interaction is unlikely to be of clinical importance.[1]

1. Kees F, Wellenhofer M, Bröhl K, Grobecker H. Bioavailability of cefpodoxime proxetil with co-administered acetylcysteine. *Arzneimittelforschung* (1996) 46, 435–8.

Cephalosporins; Cefprozil + Metoclopramide or Propantheline

The pharmacokinetics of cefprozil are minimally affected by propantheline and metoclopramide, and an interaction of clinical importance is unlikely.[1]

1. Shukla UA, Pittman KA, Barbhaiya RH. Pharmacokinetic interactions of cefprozil with food, propantheline, metoclopramide, and probenecid in healthy volunteers. *J Clin Pharmacol* (1992) 32, 725–31.

Cephalosporins; Ceftazidime + Indometacin

The clearance of ceftazidime is significantly reduced by indometacin in neonates, and dosage adjustments are likely to be necessary.

Clinical evidence, mechanism, importance and management

A study found the prenatal use of indometacin reduced the clearance of ceftazidime 25 mg/kg by 17.5% in 12 premature neonates (born at about 29 weeks) who were 10 days old. Further, in similar neonates who had not received indometacin, the clearance of ceftazidime increased over the first 10 days of life, but this was not seen when indometacin had been given.[1] A further study by the same authors intended to establish an appropriate dose of ceftazidime for premature neonates. This study found that in 25 subjects who had received indometacin prenatally, the clearance of ceftazidime was reduced by 31% and therefore the authors suggest that additional dose reductions are required. However, note that the effect of indometacin was cancelled out in neonates who had also received betamethasone prenatally.[2] *Animal* studies have shown that indometacin reduces ceftazidime excretion by decreasing its glomerular filtered load.[3] Dosage of ceftazidime in preterm infants in the first week of life should be based on gestational age and glomerular filtration rate. Additional dosage adjustments are recommended in preterm infants who are also given indometacin.[1,2]

1. van den Anker JN, Hop WCJ, Schoemaker RC, Van der Heijden BJ, Neijens HJ, De Groot R. Ceftazidime pharmacokinetics in preterm infants: effect of postnatal age and postnatal exposure to indomethacin. *Br J Clin Pharmacol* (1995) 40, 439–43.
2. van den Anker JN, Schoemaker RC, Hop WCJ, van der Heijden BJ, Weber A, Sauer PJJ, Neijens HJ, de Groot R. Ceftazidime pharmacokinetics in preterm infants: effects of renal function and gestational age. *Clin Pharmacol Ther* (1995) 58, 650–9,
3. Carbon C, Dromer F, Brion N, Cremieux A-C, Contrepois A. Renal disposition of ceftazidime illustrated by interferences by probenecid, furosemide and indomethacin in rabbits. *Antimicrob Agents Chemother* (1984) 26, 373–7.

Chloramphenicol + Cimetidine

Isolated reports describe fatal aplastic anaemia in two patients given intravenous chloramphenicol and cimetidine.

Clinical evidence, mechanism, importance and management

Pancytopenia and aplastic anaemia developed in a man taking cimetidine 1.2 g daily, within 18 days of being given intravenous chloramphenicol 1 g every 6 hours. It proved to be fatal.[1] Another patient, similarly treated, developed fatal aplastic anaemia after 19 days.[2] A drug interaction with cimetidine was suspected because the onset of pancytopenia was more rapid than in previous cases where chloramphenicol alone induced aplastic anaemia. This effect may occur because the bone marrow depressant effects of the two drugs are additive. There are at least 8 other cases of aplastic anaemia following the use of parenteral chloramphenicol in the absence of cimetidine.[2] The general importance of these observations is uncertain, but the authors of one of the reports suggest that these drugs should be used together with caution.

1. Farber BF, Brody JP. Rapid development of aplastic anemia after intravenous chloramphenicol and cimetidine therapy. *South Med J* (1981) 74, 1257–8.
2. West BC, DeVault GA, Clement JC, Williams DM. Aplastic anemia associated with parenteral chloramphenicol: review of 10 cases, including the second case of possible increased risk with cimetidine. *Rev Infect Dis* (1988) 10, 1048–51.

Chloramphenicol + Dapsone

Dapsone does not significantly affect the pharmacokinetics of oral chloramphenicol.

Clinical evidence, mechanism, importance and management

A comparison of the pharmacokinetics of oral chloramphenicol in 8 healthy subjects and 8 patients with uncomplicated lepromatous leprosy found that the half-life of a single 500-mg dose of chloramphenicol was prolonged from 4.3 to 6.4 hours in patients with leprosy, possibly due to changes in liver function. The elimination half-life of chloramphenicol was further increased, to about 8 hours, when the subjects were also given dapsone 100 mg daily for 8 days. However, this latter increase was not statistically significant. Although there was no clinically significant interaction between dapsone and chloramphenicol, the disposition of chloramphenicol may be altered in leprosy.[1]

1. Garg SK, Kumar B, Shukla VK, Bakaya V, Lal R, Kaur S. Pharmacokinetics of aspirin and chloramphenicol in normal and leprotic patients before and after dapsone therapy. *Int J Clin Pharmacol* (1988) 26, 204–5.

Chloramphenicol + Other antibacterials

An old report suggests that the use of chloramphenicol may antagonise the effects of ampicillin in bacterial meningitis. In contrast, no antagonism and even additive antibacterial effects have been described in other infections. Chloramphenicol levels have been markedly lowered by rifampicin (rifampin) in 4 children.

Clinical evidence

(a) Antibacterial antagonism

A study in 264 patients (adults, and children over two months old) with acute bacterial meningitis showed that when they were given **ampicillin** 150 mg/kg daily alone, the case-fatality ratio was 4.3% compared with 10.5% in comparable subjects given a combination of **ampicillin**, chloramphenicol 100 mg/kg daily up to 4 g and **streptomycin** 40 mg/kg daily up to 2 g. The neurological sequelae (hemiparesis, deafness, cranial nerve palsies) were also markedly increased by the combined use of these drugs.[1] Antibacterial antagonism was clearly seen in a 10-week-old infant with *Salmonella enteritidis* meningitis, who was treated with chloramphenicol and **ceftazidime**.[2]

However, in contrast a report claims that antibacterial antagonism was not seen in 65 of 66 patients given chloramphenicol and **benzylpenicillin** for bronchitis or bronchopneumonia.[3] **Ampicillin** with chloramphenicol is more effective than chloramphenicol alone in the treatment of typhoid,[4] and in a study of 700 patients, **procaine benzylpenicillin** with chloramphenicol was shown to be more effective than chloramphenicol alone in the treatment of gonorrhoea (failure rates of 1.8% compared with 8.5%).[5]

(b) Pharmacokinetic interactions

In a study in premature and full-term neonates, infants and small children, it was found that the presence of **penicillin** markedly raised chloramphenicol levels.[6]

Two children, aged 2 and 5 years, with *Haemophilus influenzae* meningitis, were given chloramphenicol 100 mg/kg per day in four divided doses by infusion over 30 minutes. Within 3 days of starting **rifampicin (rifampin)** 20 mg/kg per day their peak serum chloramphenicol levels were reduced by 86 and 64%, respectively, and only returned to the therapeutic range when the chloramphenicol dosage was increased to 125 mg/kg per day.[7]

Two other children, of 5 and 18 months, with *Haemophilus influenzae* infections, are also reported to have shown reductions of 75% and 94%, respectively, in serum chloramphenicol levels when given **rifampicin** 20 mg/kg daily for 4 days. These reductions occurred despite 20 to 25% increases in the chloramphenicol dosage.[8]

Mechanism

By no means fully understood. Chloramphenicol inhibits bacterial protein synthesis and can change an actively growing bacterial colony into a static one. Thus the effects of a bactericide, such as penicillin, which interferes with cell wall synthesis, are blunted, and the death of the organism occurs more slowly. This would seem to explain the antagonism seen with some organisms.

It is thought that rifampicin, a potent enzyme inducer, markedly increases the metabolism of the chloramphenicol by the liver, thereby lowering its serum levels.[7,8]

Importance and management

Proven cases of antibacterial antagonism of chloramphenicol in patients seem to be few in number, and there is insufficient evidence to impose a general prohibition, because, depending on the organism, penicillins and chloramphenicol have been used together with clear advantage.

So far only four cases of an interaction between rifampicin and chloramphenicol appear to have been reported. However, the evidence is of good quality and in line with the way rifampicin interacts with other drugs, so this interaction should be taken seriously. There is a risk that serum chloramphenicol levels will become subtherapeutic. The authors of the second report point out that raising the chloramphenicol dosage may possibly expose the patient to a greater risk of bone marrow aplasia. They suggest delaying rifampicin prophylaxis in patients with invasive *Haemophilus influenzae* infections until the end of chloramphenicol treatment.

1. Mathies AW, Leedom JM, Ivler D, Wehrle PF, Portnoy B. Antibiotic antagonism in bacterial meningitis. *Antimicrob Agents Chemother* (1967) 7, 218–24.
2. French GL, Ling TKW, Davies DP, Leung DTY. Antagonism of ceftazidime by chloramphenicol in vitro and in vivo during treatment of gram negative meningitis. *BMJ* (1985) 291, 636–7.
3. Ardalan P. Zur Frage des Antagonismus von Penicillin und Chloramphenicolus klinischer Sicht. *Prax Pneumol* (1969) 23, 772–6.
4. De Ritis R, Giammanco G, Manzillo G. Chloramphenicol combined with ampicillin in treatment of typhoid. *BMJ* (1972) 4, 17–18.
5. Gjessing HC, Ödegaard K. Oral chloramphenicol alone and with intramuscular procaine penicillin in the treatment of gonorrhoea. *Br J Vener Dis* (1967) 43, 133–6.

6. Windorfer A, Pringsheim W. Studies on the concentrations of chloramphenicol in the serum and cerebrospinal fluid of neonates, infants and small children. *Eur J Pediatr* (1977) 124, 129–38.

7. Prober CG. Effect of rifampin on chloramphenicol levels. *N Engl J Med* (1985) 312, 788–9.

8. Kelly HW, Couch RC, Davis RL, Cushing AH, Knott R. Interaction of chloramphenicol and rifampin. *J Pediatr* (1988) 112, 817–20.

Chloramphenicol + Paracetamol (Acetaminophen)

Although there is limited evidence to suggest that paracetamol may affect chloramphenicol pharmacokinetics its validity has been criticised. Evidence of a clinically relevant interaction appears to be lacking.

Clinical evidence, mechanism, importance and management

Three studies report alterations in the pharmacokinetics of chloramphenicol by paracetamol. The first was conducted in 6 adults in intensive care after an observation that the half-life of chloramphenicol was prolonged by paracetamol in children with kwashiorkor. The addition of 100 mg of intravenous paracetamol increased the half-life of chloramphenicol in the adults from 3.25 to 15 hours.[1] However, this study has been criticised because of potential errors in the method used to calculate the half-life,[2] the unusual doses and routes of administration used,[2,3] and because the pharmacokinetics of the chloramphenicol with and without paracetamol were calculated at different times after the administration of chloramphenicol.[4] It has also been pointed out that malnutrition (e.g. kwashiorkor) can increase the elimination rate and AUC of chloramphenicol independently of paracetamol.[2]

The second study demonstrated a different interaction, in that the clearance of chloramphenicol was *increased* and the half-life *reduced*.[5] This study has also been criticised as it does not account for the fact that chloramphenicol clearance increases over the duration of a treatment course, which suggests that the changes seen in the pharmacokinetics of chloramphenicol may be independent of the paracetamol.[6] The authors later admit this as a possibility.[7] The third study found no differences in the pharmacokinetics of chloramphenicol after the first dose, but at steady state, the AUC and peak serum levels of chloramphenicol were lower in children who also received paracetamol.[8]

Three other studies have failed to confirm the existence of a pharmacokinetic interaction between chloramphenicol and paracetamol.[2-4]

The clinical significance of these reports is unclear, and clinical evidence of toxicity or treatment failure of chloramphenicol appears to be lacking. It would seem prudent to remain aware of the potential for interaction, especially in malnourished patients, but routine monitoring would appear unnecessary without further evidence.

1. Buchanan N, Moodley GP. Interaction between chloramphenicol and paracetamol. *BMJ* (1979) 2, 307–308.

2. Kearns GL, Bocchini JA, Brown RD, Cotter DL, Wilson JT. Absence of a pharmacokinetic interaction between chloramphenicol and acetaminophen in children. *J Pediatr* (1985) 107, 134–9.

3. Rajpurohit R, Krishnaswamy K. Lack of effect of paracetamol on the pharmacokinetics of chloramphenicol in adult human subjects. *Indian J Pharm* (1984) 16, 124–8.

4. Stein CM, Thornhill DP, Neill P, Nyazema NZ. Lack of effect of paracetamol on the pharmacokinetics of chloramphenicol. *Br J Clin Pharmacol* (1989) 27, 262–4.

5. Spika JS, Davis DJ, Martin SR, Beharry K, Rex J, Aranda JV. Interaction between chloramphenicol and acetaminophen. *Arch Dis Child* (1986) 61, 1121–4.

6. Choonara IA. Interaction between chloramphenicol and acetaminophen. *Arch Dis Child* (1987) 62, 319.

7. Spika JS, Aranda JV. Interaction between chloramphenicol and acetaminophen. *Arch Dis Child* (1987) 62, 1087–8.

8. Bravo ME, Horwitz I, Contreras C, Olea I, Arancibia A. Influencia del paracetamol en la farmacocinética del cloramfenicol en pacientes con fiebre tifoidea. *Rev Chil Pediatr* (1987) 58, 117–20.

Chloramphenicol + Phenobarbital

Studies in children show that phenobarbital can markedly reduce serum chloramphenicol levels. There is a single report, in one adult, of markedly increased serum phenobarbital levels caused by chloramphenicol.

Clinical evidence

(a) Effects on chloramphenicol

A study in a group of infants and children (aged 1 month to 12 years) given chloramphenicol 25 mg/kg every 6 hours found that 6 of them, also taking phenobarbital, had reduced serum chloramphenicol levels, when compared with 17 controls. The peak levels were lowered by 34%, from 25.3 to 16.6 micrograms/mL, and the trough levels were lowered by 44%, from 13.4 to 7.5 micrograms/mL.[1] Two children aged 3 and 7 months were treated for *H. influenzae* meningitis with chloramphenicol 100 mg/kg daily, initially intravenously, and later orally. The chloramphenicol levels halved over the first 2 days of treatment, while the children were receiving phenobarbital 10 mg/kg/day to prevent convulsions. One child had serum chloramphenicol levels of only 5 micrograms/mL even though the initial doses used were expected to give levels of 15 to 25 micrograms/mL.[2]

Another study confirmed that this interaction occurred in 20 neonates, but no statistically significant effect was found in 40 infants.[3] Decreased chloramphenicol levels have been described in a single case report of a child who was also being treated with phenytoin and phenobarbital. The serum chloramphenicol levels were 35.1 micrograms/mL prior to the antiepileptics, 19.1 micrograms/mL after 2 days of phenytoin and 13.2 micrograms/mL a month after the addition of phenobarbital.[4] For more information on the interaction of chloramphenicol with phenytoin see 'Phenytoin + Chloramphenicol', p.555.

(b) Effects on phenobarbital

A man admitted to hospital on numerous occasions for pulmonary complications associated with cystic fibrosis, had average serum phenobarbital levels of 33 micrograms/mL while taking phenobarbital 200 mg daily and oral chloramphenicol 600 mg every 6 hours. One week after the antibacterial was withdrawn, his serum phenobarbital levels were 24 micrograms/mL even though the phenobarbital dosage was increased from 200 to 300 mg daily.[5]

Mechanism

Phenobarbital is a potent liver enzyme inducer, which can increase the metabolism and clearance of chloramphenicol (clearly demonstrated in *rats*[6]), so that its serum levels fall and its effects are reduced. Chloramphenicol inhibits the metabolism of the phenobarbital (also demonstrated in *animals*[7]) so that the effects of the barbiturate are increased.

Importance and management

This interaction appears to be established. The documentation is limited but what happened is consistent with the recognised enzyme-inducing actions of phenobarbital and the inhibitory actions of chloramphenicol. Concurrent use should be well monitored to ensure that chloramphenicol serum levels are adequate, and that phenobarbital levels do not become too high. Make appropriate dosage adjustments as necessary.

1. Krasinski K, Kusmiesz H, Nelson JD. Pharmacologic interactions among chloramphenicol, phenytoin and phenobarbital. *Pediatr Infect Dis* (1982) 1, 232–5.

2. Bloxham RA, Durbin GM, Johnson T, Winterborn MH. Chloramphenicol and phenobarbitone—a drug interaction. *Arch Dis Child* (1979) 54, 76–7.

3. Windorfer A, Pringsheim W. Studies on the concentrations of chloramphenicol in the serum and cerebrospinal fluid of neonates, infants, and small children. *Eur J Pediatr* (1977) 124, 129–38.

4. Powell DA, Nahata MC, Durrell DC, Glazer JP, Hilty MD. Interactions among chloramphenicol, phenytoin, and phenobarbital in a pediatric patient. *J Pediatr* (1981) 98, 1001–1003.

5. Koup JR, Gibaldi M, McNamara P, Hilligoss DM, Colburn WA, Bruck E. Interaction of chloramphenicol with phenytoin and phenobarbital. Case report. *Clin Pharmacol Ther* (1978) 24, 571–5.

6. Bella DD, Ferrari V, Marca G,Bonanomi L. Chloramphenicol metabolism in the phenobarbital-induced rat. Comparison with thiamphenicol. *Biochem Pharmacol* (1968) 17, 2381–90.

7. Adams HR. Prolonged barbiturate anesthesia by chloramphenicol in laboratory animals. *J Am Vet Med Assoc* (1970) 157, 1908–13.

Clindamycin or Lincomycin + Food or Drinks

The serum levels of lincomycin are markedly reduced (by up to two-thirds) if taken in the presence of food, but clindamycin is not significantly affected. Cyclamate sweeteners can also reduce the absorption of lincomycin.

Clinical evidence

In a study in 10 healthy subjects the mean peak serum levels of a single 500-mg oral dose of lincomycin were about 3 micrograms/mL when taken 4 hours before **breakfast**, 2 micrograms/mL when taken 1 hour before breakfast, and less than 1 microgram/mL when taken after breakfast. The mean total amounts of lincomycin recovered from the urine were 40.4, 23.8, and 8.9 mg, respectively.[1]

Reduced serum lincomycin levels due to the presence of **food** have been described in other reports,[2,3] but the absorption of clindamycin is not affected.[3,4]

Sodium cyclamate, an artificial sweetener found in diet foods, drinks and some pharmaceuticals, can also markedly reduce the absorption of lincomycin. The AUC of lincomycin 500 mg was reduced by about 75% by 1 Molar equivalent of **sodium cyclamate** (said to be an amount equal to only part of a bottle of diet drink, but exact quantity not stated).[5]

Mechanism

Not understood.

Importance and management

The food interaction with lincomycin is well established and of clinical importance. Lincomycin should not be taken with food or within several hours of eating a meal if adequate serum levels are to be achieved. An alternative is clindamycin, a synthetic derivative of lincomycin, which has the same antibacterial spectrum but is not affected by food.

1. McCall CE, Steigbigel NH, Finland M. Lincomycin: activity *in vitro* and absorption and excretion in normal young men. *Am J Med Sci* (1967) 254, 144–55.
2. Kaplan K, Chew WH, Weinstein L. Microbiological, pharmacological and clinical studies of lincomycin. *Am J Med Sci* (1965) 250, 137–46.
3. McGehee RF, Smith CB, Wilcox C, Finland M. Comparative studies of antibacterial activity in vitro and absorption and excretion of lincomycin and clinimycin. *Am J Med Sci* (1968) 256, 279–92.
4. Wagner JG, Novak E, Patel NC, Chidester CG, Lummis WL. Absorption, excretion and half-life of clinimycin in normal adult males. *Am J Med Sci* (1968) 256, 25–37.
5. Wagner JG. Aspects of pharmacokinetics and biopharmaceutics in relation to drug activity. *Am J Pharm Sci Support Public Health* (1969) 141, 5–20.

Clindamycin or Lincomycin + Kaolin

Kaolin-pectin can markedly reduce the absorption of lincomycin. This can be avoided by giving the lincomycin two hours after the kaolin. The rate but not the extent of clindamycin absorption is altered by kaolin-pectin. However, note that diarrhoea is often an indication that these antibacterials should be withdrawn.

Clinical evidence

About 85 mL of *Kaopectate* (kaolin-pectin) reduced the absorption of lincomycin 500 mg by about 90% in 8 healthy subjects. Giving the *Kaopectate* 2 hours before the antibacterial had little or no effect on its absorption, whereas when *Kaopectate* was given 2 hours after lincomycin, the absorption was reduced by about 50%. The absorption rate of clindamycin is markedly prolonged by kaolin, but the extent of its absorption remains unaffected.[1]

Mechanism

It seems probable that the lincomycin becomes adsorbed onto the kaolin, thereby reducing its bioavailability. The kaolin also coats the lining of the gut and acts as a physical barrier to absorption.[2]

Importance and management

Information seems to be limited to this study, but the interaction between lincomycin and kaolin appears to be established and of clinical importance. For good absorption and a good antibacterial response separate their administration as much as possible, ideally giving the kaolin at least 2 hours before the antibacterial. Clindamycin appears to be a suitable alternative to lincomycin.

However, note that marked diarrhoea is an indication that lincomycin or clindamycin should be stopped immediately. This is because it may be a sign of pseudomembranous colitis, which can be fatal.

1. Albert KS, DeSante KA, Welch RD, DiSanto AR. Pharmacokinetic evaluation of a drug interaction between kaolin-pectin and clindamycin. *J Pharm Sci* (1978) 67, 1579–82.
2. Wagner JG. Design and data analysis of biopharmaceutical studies in man. *Can J Pharm Sci*

Colistin + Sucralfate

An *in vitro* study with colistin sulfate found that it became markedly and irreversibly bound to sucralfate at the pH values found in the gut. This suggests that its efficacy for gut decontamination or gastrointestinal infections might be decreased by sucralfate.

Clinical evidence, mechanism, importance and management

To simulate what might happen in the gut, colistin sulfate 50 mg/L was mixed with sucralfate 500 mg in 40 mL of water at pH 3.5 and allowed to stand for 90 minutes at 25°C. Analysis of the solution showed that the colistin concentration fell rapidly and progressively over 90 minutes to about 40%. When the pH of the mixture was then raised to 6.5 to 7 for 90 minutes, there was no change in the concentration of colistin, suggesting that the interaction was irreversible.[1] The reason for this change is not known, but the suggestion is that sucralfate forms insoluble chelates with colistin.[1]

It is not known how important this interaction is likely to be in practice, but the efficacy of colistin in gut decontamination and gut infections may be decreased. Separating the dosages might not be effective in some post-operative patients because their gastric function may not return to normal for up to 5 days, and some sucralfate might still be present when the next dose is given.[1] More study is needed to find out whether this interaction is clinically important, but in the meanwhile it would seem prudent to monitor concurrent use carefully, being alert for any evidence of reduced effects.

1. Feron B, Adair CG, Gorman SP, McClurg B. Interaction of sucralfate with antibiotics used for selective decontamination of the gastrointestinal tract. *Am J Hosp Pharm* (1993) 50, 2550–3.

Co-trimoxazole + Azithromycin

Azithromycin does not alter the pharmacokinetics of co-trimoxazole.

Clinical evidence, mechanism, importance and management

A study in 12 healthy subjects given **co-trimoxazole** (trimethoprim and sulfamethoxazole) 960 mg daily for 7 days found that a single 1.2-g dose of azithromycin given on day 7 did not alter the pharmacokinetics of either trimethoprim or sulfamethoxazole to a clinically relevant extent.[1]

1. Amsden GW, Foulds G, Thakker K. Pharmacokinetic study of azithromycin with fluconazole and cotrimoxazole (trimethoprim-sulfamethoxazole) in healthy volunteers. *Clin Drug Invest* (2000) 20, 135–42.

Co-trimoxazole + Cimetidine

Cimetidine has no significant effect on the pharmacokinetics of co-trimoxazole.

Clinical evidence, mechanism, importance and management

In a placebo-controlled study, 6 healthy subjects were given cimetidine 400 mg every 6 hours for 6 days, with a single 960-mg dose of co-trimoxazole (trimethoprim with sulfamethoxazole) on day 6. Although trimethoprim levels were consistently slightly higher in the presence of cimetidine, they were not significantly different. Cimetidine had no effect on the pharmacokinetics sulfamethoxazole.[1]

1. Rogers HJ, James CA, Morrison PJ, Bradbrook ID. Effect of cimetidine on oral absorption of ampicillin and co-trimoxazole. *J Antimicrob Chemother* (1980) 6, 297–300.

Co-trimoxazole + Kaolin-pectin

Kaolin-pectin can cause a small but probably clinically unimportant reduction in serum trimethoprim levels, and has no effect on sulfamethoxazole pharmacokinetics.

Clinical evidence, mechanism, importance and management

Co-trimoxazole suspension (trimethoprim 160 mg with sulfamethoxazole 800 mg) was given to 8 healthy subjects, with and without 20 mL of kaolin-pectin suspension. The kaolin-pectin reduced the AUC and the maximum serum levels of the trimethoprim by about 12% and 20%, respectively. Changes in the sulfamethoxazole pharmacokinetics were not significant.[1] The probable reason for this reduction in AUC is that trimethoprim is adsorbed onto the kaolin-pectin, which reduces the amount available for absorption. However, the reductions are small and unlikely to be clinically relevant.

1. Gupta KC, Desai NK, Satoskar RS, Gupta C, Goswami SN. Effect of pectin and kaolin on bioavailability of co-trimoxazole suspension. *Int J Clin Pharmacol Ther Toxicol* (1987) 25, 320–1.

Co-trimoxazole + Prilocaine/Lidocaine cream

Methaemoglobinaemia developed in a baby treated with co-trimoxazole when *Emla* (prilocaine/lidocaine) cream was applied to his skin.

Clinical evidence, mechanism, importance and management

A 12-week-old child, given co-trimoxazole for 2 months for pyelitis, was treated with 5 g of *Emla* cream (prilocaine 25 mg and lidocaine 25 mg per gram) applied to the back of his hands and the cubital regions. Unfortunately his operation was delayed, and 5 hours later, just before the operation began, his skin was noted to be pale and his lips had a brownish cyanotic colour. This was found to be due to the presence of 28% methaemoglobin (reference range: less than 3%).[1] The authors of the report suggest that the prilocaine together with the sulfamethoxazole (both known to be able to cause methaemoglobin formation) suppressed the activity of two enzymes (NADH-dehydrogenase and NADP-diaphorase), which normally keep blood levels of methaemoglobin to a minimum.[1] A study in 20 children[2] confirmed that *Emla* cream can increase methaemoglobin levels, although levels *decreased* in 6 of them. However, the maximum increase was 1.2% (from 0.7 to 1.9%), and the highest value was 2%, which was still within the reference range. Another study showed similar small increases in methaemoglobin levels, and found that these remained elevated after 24 hours. The authors concluded that daily application may lead to accumulation, and a greater risk of toxicity.[3]

The case report appears to be unusual, but it has been suggested that there may be a special risk of methaemoglobinaemia with *Emla* in children with pre-existing anaemia, reduced renal excretion of the metabolites of prilocaine, or the concurrent use of sulfonamides.[3] It would seem prudent to keep *Emla* contact time to a minimum in these patients.

1. Jakobson B, Nilsson A. Methemoglobinemia associated with a prilocaine-lidocaine cream and trimethoprim-sulphamethoxazole. A case report. *Acta Anaesthesiol Scand* (1985) 29, 453–55.
2. Engberg G, Danielson K, Henneberg S, Nilsson A. Plasma concentrations of prilocaine and lidocaine and methaemoglobin formation in infants after epicutaneous application of a 5% lidocaine-prilocaine cream (Emla). *Acta Anaesthesiol Scand* (1987) 31, 624–8.
3. Frayling IM, Addison GM, Chattergee K, Meakin G. Methaemoglobinaemia in children treated with prilocaine-lignocaine cream. *BMJ* (1990) 301, 153–4.

Co-trimoxazole or Trimethoprim + Rifamycins

The pharmacokinetics of trimethoprim are not significantly affected by rifabutin, and probably not by rifampicin (rifampin). Rifabutin does not affect the pharmacokinetics of sulfamethoxazole, but significantly increases exposure to its hydroxylamine metabolite and as a result may increase adverse reactions to sulfamethoxazole in HIV-positive patients.
A significant reduction in co-trimoxazole levels and a decrease in prophylactic efficacy has been seen in HIV-positive patients taking rifampicin. Limited evidence suggests that co-trimoxazole can increase rifampicin serum levels. Trimethoprim does not affect the pharmacokinetics of rifampicin.

Clinical evidence, mechanism, importance and management

(a) Rifabutin

Twelve HIV-positive patients taking co-trimoxazole (sulfamethoxazole and trimethoprim; strength not stated) twice daily for 7 days were also given rifabutin 300 mg daily for a further 14 days. The sulfamethoxazole component remained unaffected by rifabutin but the trimethoprim AUC was decreased by 22%. This small reduction is not expected to be clinically significant.[1] However, another study in HIV-positive patients given co-trimoxazole (sulfamethoxazole 800 mg with trimethoprim 160 mg daily) found that although rifabutin 300 mg daily had minimal effects on the disposition of sulfamethoxazole and its acetylated metabolite, it significantly increased the AUC, urinary recovery and formation clearance of its hydroxylamine metabolite by about 50%. As the hydroxylamine metabolite may be one of the factors associated with adverse reactions to sulfamethoxazole in HIV-positive patients, concurrent rifabutin may increase the rate of adverse reactions.[2]

(b) Rifampicin (Rifampin)

No significant pharmacokinetic interaction seems to occur when healthy subjects are given trimethoprim 240 mg daily with rifampicin 900 mg daily (both in divided doses). After 4 to 5 days, less trimethoprim is recovered in the urine, as more is metabolised prior to excretion due to the enzyme-inducing effects of rifampicin, but this does not appear to be of clinical importance.[3,4] Another study also notes that no clinically significant pharmacokinetic interaction occurs between trimethoprim and rifampicin.[5]

However, a case-control study of the efficacy of co-trimoxazole in preventing toxoplasmosis in HIV-positive patients found a link between rifampicin use and co-trimoxazole failure,[6] which prompted the authors to conduct a pharmacokinetic study. When rifampicin 600 mg daily was given to 10 HIV-positive patients with co-trimoxazole 960 mg daily, it was found that the AUCs of trimethoprim and sulfamethoxazole were reduced by 56% and 28%, respectively. These changes are sufficient to reduce the efficacy of co-trimoxazole treatment.[7] It would therefore seem prudent to consider this interaction when giving rifampicin to HIV-positive patients taking co-trimoxazole prophylaxis.

In one study 15 patients with tuberculosis, who had taken rifampicin 450 mg daily for at least 15 days, were given co-trimoxazole (trimethoprim 320 mg and sulfamethoxazole 800 mg 12-hourly) for 5 to 10 days. Rifampicin levels were measured at 5 time points over 6 hours before and during co-trimoxazole treatment. At 4 and 6 hours, rifampicin levels were significantly higher (27% and 56%, respectively) during co-trimoxazole treatment, but peak levels were only increased by about 18%. Concurrent use did not result in any increase in adverse effects over the study period.[8]

1. Lee BL, Lampiris H, Colborn DC, Lewis RC, Narang PK, Sullam P. The effect of rifabutin (RBT) on the pharmacokinetics (PK) of trimethoprim-sulfamethoxazole (TMP-SMX) in HIV-infected patients. *Intersci Conf Antimicrob Agents Chemother* (1995) 35, 7.
2. Winter HR, Trapnell CB, Slattery JT, Jacobson M, Greenspan DL, Hooton TM, Unadkat JD. The effect of clarithromycin, fluconazole, and rifabutin on sulfamethoxazole hydroxylamine formation in individuals with human immunodeficiency virus infection (AACTG 283). *Clin Pharmacol Ther* (2004) 76, 313–22.
3. Buniva G, Palminteri R, Berti M. Kinetics of a rifampicin-trimethoprim combination. *Int J Clin Pharmacol Biopharm* (1979) 17, 256–9.
4. Emmerson AM, Grüneberg RN, Johnson ES. The pharmacokinetics in man of a combination of rifampicin and trimethoprim. *J Antimicrob Chemother* (1978) 4, 523–31.
5. Acocella G, Scotti R. Kinetic studies on the combination rifampicin-trimethoprim in man. *J Antimicrob Chemother* (1976) 2, 271–77.
6. Ribera E, Fernandez-Sola A, Juste C, Rovira A, Romero FJ, Armandas-Gil L, Ruiz I, Ocaña I, Pahissa A. Comparison of high and low doses of trimethoprim-sulfamethoxazole for primary prevention of toxoplasmic encephalitis in human immunodeficiency virus-infected patients. *Clin Infect Dis* (1999) 29, 1461–6.
7. Ribera E, Pou L, Fernandez-Sola A, Campos F, Lopez RM, Ocaña I, Ruiz I, Pahissa A. Rifampin reduces concentrations of trimethoprim and sulfamethoxazole in serum in human immunodeficiency virus infected patients. *Antimicrob Agents Chemother* (2001) 45, 3238–41.
8. Bhatia RS, Uppal R, Malhi R, Behera D, Jindal SK. Drug interaction between rifampicin and co-trimoxazole in patients with tuberculosis. *Hum Exp Toxicol* (1991) 10, 419–21.

Co-trimoxazole + Salbutamol (Albuterol)

Salbutamol reduces the rate but increases the extent of sulfamethoxazole absorption.

Clinical evidence, mechanism, importance and management

In 6 healthy subjects, oral salbutamol 4 mg four times daily for 2 weeks had no effect on the pharmacokinetics of a single 400-mg oral dose of sulfamethoxazole (in co-trimoxazole), although the absorption rate constant was reduced by about 40% and the extent of absorption over 72 hours was increased by 22.6%.[1] A possible reason for these effects is that salbutamol stimulates the beta receptors in the gut, causing relaxation, which allows an increased contact time, and therefore increased absorption of sulfamethoxazole.[1] The clinical significance of this interaction is unknown, but it seems unlikely to be of importance. No interaction would be expected with inhaled salbutamol.

1. Adebayo GI, Ogundipe TO. Effects of salbutamol on the absorption and disposition of sulphamethoxazole in adult volunteers. *Eur J Drug Metab Pharmacokinet* (1989) 14, 57–60.

Cycloserine + Ethionamide

Neurotoxic adverse effects may be potentiated by the concurrent use of cycloserine and ethionamide.

Clinical evidence, mechanism, importance and management

Three cases of encephalopathy have been reported in patients taking antitubercular regimens which included ethionamide (and in 2 cases, isoniazid): in one case symptoms occurred during treatment with ethionamide and cycloserine. All 3 patients recovered after withdrawal of either ethionamide (and isoniazid) or cycloserine, and treatment with nicotinamide and other vitamin B compounds.[1] The manufacturers note that the concurrent use of ethionamide can potentiate the neurotoxic adverse effects of cycloserine.[2,3] The US manufacturer of ethionamide notes that convulsions have been reported in patients also taking cycloserine and they recommend special care when the treatment regimen includes both drugs.[4]

1. Swash M, Roberts AH, Murnaghan DJ. Reversible pellagra-like encephalopathy with ethionamide and cycloserine. *Tubercle* (1972) 53, 132–6.
2. Cycloserine. King Pharmaceuticals Ltd. UK Summary of product characteristics, March 2007.
3. Seromycin (Cycloserine). Eli Lilly and Company. US Prescribing information, April 2005.
4. Trecator (Ethionamide). Wyeth Pharmaceuticals Inc. US Prescribing information, September 2006.

Cycloserine + Food or Antacids

Orange juice and an antacid (*Mylanta*) do not affect the pharmacokinetics of cycloserine, but a high-fat meal delays its absorption.

Clinical evidence, mechanism, importance and management

(a) Antacids

A study in 12 healthy subjects found that the bioavailability of a single 500-mg dose of cycloserine was not affected by 15 mL of ***Mylanta*** (**aluminium hydroxide** 400 mg, **magnesium hydroxide** 400 mg, **simeticone** 40 mg per 5 mL). ***Mylanta*** was given 9 hours before the cycloserine, at the same time as the cycloserine, immediately after meals, and at bedtime on the dosing day and following day.[1]

(b) Food

A study in 12 healthy subjects found that the bioavailability of a single 500-mg dose of cycloserine was not significantly affected by 240 mL of **orange juice**.[1] When cycloserine 500 mg was given 15 minutes after the start of a **high-fat meal**, which was completed within 30 minutes, the AUC was not affected, but the maximum serum levels were reduced by about 16% and the time to maximum levels was increased from 0.75 to 3.5 hours. It is possible that patients with relatively low plasma levels or patients receiving once rather than a twice daily dosage that the delay in absorption could result in increased periods of subinhibitory levels.[1] However, there is no evidence to suggest that this is clinically significant.

1. Zhu M, Nix DE, Adam RD, Childs JM, Peloquin CA. Pharmacokinetics of cycloserine under fasting conditions and with high-fat meal, orange juice, and antacids. *Pharmacotherapy* (2001) 21, 891–7.

Cycloserine + Isoniazid

The adverse CNS effects of cycloserine are increased by isoniazid.

Clinical evidence, mechanism, importance and management

A report describes both an increase and a decrease in serum cycloserine levels in some subjects, which were apparently caused by isoniazid; however, the mean level of cycloserine was not significantly changed. Only one out of 11 patients taking cycloserine alone developed adverse effects (drowsiness, dizziness, unstable gait), but when isoniazid was added, 9 of the 11 developed these effects.[1] The manufacturers recommend monitoring for these adverse effects and adjusting the doses as necessary to manage them.[2,3]

1. Mattila MJ, Nieminen E, Tiitinen H. Serum levels, urinary excretion, and side-effects of cycloserine in the presence of isoniazid and p-aminosalicylic acid. *Scand J Respir Dis* (1969) 50, 291–300.
2. Cycloserine. King Pharmaceuticals Ltd. UK Summary of product characteristics, March 2007.
3. Seromycin (Cycloserine). Eli Lilly and Company. US Prescribing information, April 2005.

Dapsone + Antacids

The absorption of dapsone is unaltered by an antacid containing aluminium/magnesium hydroxide and/or simeticone.

Clinical evidence, mechanism, importance and management

A study to see whether changes in gastric pH might affect the absorption of dapsone found that when a single 100-mg dose of dapsone was taken with the second of 11 doses of *Mylanta II* (**hydrated aluminium hydroxide**, **magnesium hydroxide** and **simeticone**), given every hour, the absorption of the dapsone remained unchanged. The mean gastric pH rose from 2.3 before using the antacid, to 4.5 or higher while taking dapsone and the antacid.[1] In another study, 8 subjects were given a single 100-mg dose of dapsone as a liquid oral preparation followed immediately by 12.5 mL of *Maalox TC* (**aluminium/magnesium hydroxide**). Peak plasma levels of dapsone were increased by about 11% and the time to peak levels was reduced from 1.9 to 1.3 hours. However, the dapsone AUC and elimination rate were not affected.[2] No special precautions would therefore seem to be needed if *Mylanta, Maalox TC* or any other similar antacid is used with dapsone. See also 'NRTIs + Dapsone', p.796, for a discussion of the effects of the buffer in didanosine tablets.

1. Breen GA, Brocavich JM, Etzel JV, Shah V, Schaefer P, Forlenza S. Evaluation of effects of altered gastric pH on absorption of dapsone in healthy volunteers. *Antimicrob Agents Chemother* (1994) 38, 2227–9.
2. Mirochnick M, Breña A, McNamara ER, Clarke D, Pelton S. Effect of antacid on dapsone absorption. *Pediatr AIDS HIV Infect* (1993) 4, 13–16.

Dapsone + Clarithromycin

Clarithromycin does not alter the metabolism of dapsone.

Clinical evidence, mechanism, importance and management

A study in 12 healthy subjects given single 100-mg doses of dapsone before and after taking clarithromycin 1 g twice daily for 10 days, found that the clearance of dapsone was unchanged. Of equal importance was finding that the AUC of the *N*-hydroxylation metabolite of dapsone, which appears to be responsible for the haematological toxicity (methaemoglobinaemia), was also unchanged.[1]

In another study, 11 HIV-positive patients were given dapsone 100 mg daily then clarithromycin 500 mg twice daily for 2 weeks. Clarithromycin had no effect on dapsone clearance or the production of the hydroxylamine metabolite of dapsone.[2]

These results suggest that the cytochrome P450 isoenzyme CYP3A4, which is inhibited by clarithromycin, is not involved in dapsone metabolism.[2]

Clarithromycin would not be expected to alter the toxicity of dapsone, and no special precautions are required during concurrent use.

1. Occhipinti DJ, Choi A, Deyo K, Danziger LH, Fischer JH. Influence of rifampin and clarithromycin on dapsone (D) disposition and methemoglobin concentrations. *Clin Pharmacol Ther* (1995) 57, 163.
2. Winter HR, Trapnell CB, Slattery JT, Jacobson M, Greenspan DL, Hooton TM, Unadkat JD. The effect of clarithromycin, fluconazole, and rifabutin on dapsone hydroxylamine formation in individuals with human immunodeficiency virus infection (AACTG 283). *Clin Pharmacol Ther* (2004) 76, 579–87.

Dapsone + Clofazimine

Dapsone can reduce the anti-inflammatory effects of clofazimine. Clofazimine does not affect the pharmacokinetics of dapsone.

Clinical evidence, mechanism, importance and management

Fourteen out of 16 patients with severe recurrent erythema nodosum leprosum (ENL) failed to respond adequately when given dapsone and clofazimine and needed additional treatment with corticosteroids. When the dapsone was stopped the patients responded to clofazimine alone, and in some instances the ENL was controlled by smaller doses.[1] Further evidence of this interaction comes from a laboratory study, which suggests that the actions of clofazimine may be related to its ability to inhibit neutrophil migration (resulting in decreased numbers of neutrophils in areas of inflammation), whereas dapsone can have the opposite effect.[1] Although the information is very limited, it would seem prudent to avoid the concurrent use of dapsone and clofazimine in the treatment of ENL. The authors of this report[1] are at great pains to emphasise that what they describe only relates to the effects of dapsone on the anti-inflammatory effects of clofazimine, and not to the beneficial effects of combined use when treating drug-resistant *Mycobacterium leprae*.

A study in patients taking clofazimine and dapsone[2] and 4 other studies in patients also taking isoniazid or rifampicin suggest that clofazimine does not affect the pharmacokinetics of dapsone.[3-6] However, one earlier study[7] found that clofazimine transiently increased the renal excretion of dapsone in 9 of 17 patients with leprosy who had recently discontinued dapsone.

1. Imkamp FMJH, Anderson R, Gatner EMS. Possible incompatibility of dapsone with clofazimine in the treatment of patients with erythema nodosum leprosum. *Lepr Rev* (1982) 53, 148–9.
2. George J, Balakrishnan S, Bhatia VN. Drug interaction during multidrug regimens for treatment of leprosy. *Indian J Med Res* (1988) 87, 151–6.
3. Venkatesan K, Mathur A, Girdhar BK, Bharadwaj VP. The effect of clofazimine on the pharmacokinetics of rifampicin and dapsone in leprosy. *J Antimicrob Chemother* (1986) 18, 715–18.
4. Pieters FAJM, Woonink F, Zuidema J. Influence of once-monthly rifampicin and daily clofazimine on the pharmacokinetics of dapsone in leprosy patients in Nigeria. *Eur J Clin Pharmacol* (1988) 34, 73–6.
5. Venkatesan K, Bharadwaj VP, Ramu R, Desikan KV. Study on drug interactions. *Lepr India* (1980) 52, 229–35.
6. Balakrishnan S, Seshadri PS. Drug interactions— the influence of rifampicin and clofazimine on the urinary excretion of DDS. *Lepr India* (1981) 53, 17–22.
7. Grabosz JAJ, Wheate HW. Effect of clofazimine on the urinary excretion of DDS (Dapsone). *Int J Lepr* (1975) 43, 61–2.

Dapsone + Drugs that affect gastric pH

Cimetidine raises serum dapsone levels, and may reduce methaemoglobinaemia due to dapsone. Cimetidine, ranitidine and omeprazole do not appear to affect the outcome of dapsone prophylaxis against Pneumocystis pneumonia. The absorption of dapsone does not appear to be altered by nizatidine-induced increases in gastric pH.

Clinical evidence, mechanism, importance and management

The AUC of a single 100-mg dose of dapsone was increased by 40% in 7 healthy subjects after they took **cimetidine** 400 mg three times daily for 3 days.[1] The probable reason is that the **cimetidine** (a known enzyme inhibitor) inhibits the metabolism of the dapsone by the liver. Although this might be expected to increase the risk of haematological adverse effects of dapsone by raising its serum levels, **cimetidine** also apparently markedly reduces the production of the hydroxylamine metabolite of dapsone (the AUC fell by more than half). Dapsone hydroxylamine appears to be responsible for the methaemoglobinaemia and haemolysis that may occur with dapsone treatment.[1] These findings were later confirmed in 6 patients taking long-term dapsone 75 to 350 mg daily who were given **cimetidine** 1.2 g daily for 2 weeks. Steady-state serum dapsone levels rose by about 47%, accompanied by a fall in serum methaemoglobin levels from 7.1 to 5.2% (reference range less than 2%), in the first week.[2] Similar findings were reported in a further 3-month study in 8 patients.[3] However, a sustained decrease in methaemoglobin was not seen, with levels returning to baseline at week 12, despite the continued use of **cimetidine**.[3] Another report on a small number of patients, comparing those treated with **cimetidine**, **ranitidine** or **omeprazole** with those not taking acid suppression, found no difference in the outcome of dapsone prophylaxis for Pneumocystis pneumonia in HIV-positive patients.[4] A study in healthy subjects found that the increase in pH produced by **nizatidine** did not result in any clinically significant changes in the rate or extent of dapsone absorption.[5] It would therefore seem that no additional precautions are needed if H_2-receptor antagonists or proton pump inhibitors are given to patients taking dapsone. Consider also 'Dapsone + Antacids', p.303.

1. Coleman MD, Scott AK, Breckenridge AM, Park BK. The use of cimetidine as a selective inhibitor of dapsone *N*-hydroxylation in man. *Br J Clin Pharmacol* (1990) 30, 761–7.
2. Coleman MD, Rhodes LE, Scott AK, Verbov JL, Friedmann PS, Breckenridge AM, Park BK. The use of cimetidine to reduce dapsone-dependent methaemoglobinaemia in dermatitis herpetiformis patients. *Br J Clin Pharmacol* (1992) 34, 244–9.
3. Rhodes LE, Tingle MD, Park BK, Chu P, Verbov JL, Friedmann PS. Cimetidine improves the therapeutic/toxic ratio of dapsone in patients on chronic dapsone therapy. *Br J Dermatol* (1995) 132, 257–62.
4. Huengsberg M, Castelino S, Sherrard J, O'Farrell N, Bingham J. Does drug interaction cause failure of PCP prophylaxis with dapsone? *Lancet* (1993) 341, 48.
5. Itokazu GA, Fischer JH, Manitpisitkul P, Hariharan R, Danziger LH. Lack of effect of nizatidine-induced elevation of gastric pH on the oral bioavailability of dapsone in healthy volunteers. *Pharmacotherapy* (2002) 22, 1420–5.

Dapsone + Fluconazole

Fluconazole decreases the production of the toxic metabolite of dapsone, and might therefore reduce the incidence of adverse reactions to dapsone.

Clinical evidence, mechanism, importance and management

Twelve HIV-positive patients were given dapsone 100 mg daily for 2 weeks and then in random order either fluconazole 200 mg daily, rifabutin 300 mg daily or fluconazole with rifabutin, each for 2 weeks. Dapsone pharmacokinetics were unaffected by fluconazole. However, fluconazole inhibited the production of the *N*-hydroxylamine metabolite of dapsone (AUC, urinary recovery, and formation clearance reduced by about 50%).[1]

Hydroxylamine is assumed to be responsible for the haematological toxicity of dapsone (methaemoglobinaemia). The findings of this study suggest that the production of this metabolite is mediated via the cytochrome P450 isoenzyme CYP2C9, which fluconazole inhibits.

On the basis of these results, fluconazole would not be expected to alter the efficacy of dapsone, but might reduce its toxicity. Further study is needed to assess this potential.

1. Winter HR, Trapnell CB, Slattery JT, Jacobson M, Greenspan DL, Hooton TM, Unadkat JD. The effect of clarithromycin, fluconazole, and rifabutin on dapsone hydroxylamine formation in individuals with human immunodeficiency virus infection (AACTG 283). *Clin Pharmacol Ther* (2004) 76, 579–87.

Dapsone + Probenecid

The serum levels of dapsone can be markedly raised by probenecid.

Clinical evidence

Twelve patients with quiescent tuberculoid leprosy were given dapsone 300 mg with probenecid 500 mg, and 5 hours later another 300-mg dose of dapsone. At 4 hours, the dapsone serum levels were raised about 50%. The urinary excretion of dapsone and its metabolites were reduced.[1]

Mechanism

Not fully examined. It seems probable that the probenecid inhibits the renal excretion of dapsone by the kidney.

Importance and management

The documentation is very limited. It is likely that the probenecid will raise the serum levels of dapsone given long-term. The importance of this is uncertain, but the extent of the rise and the evidence that the haematological toxicity of dapsone may be related to dapsone levels[2] suggests that it may well have some clinical importance. It would therefore seem prudent to monitor for dapsone adverse effects if probenecid is also given.

1. Goodwin CS, Sparell G. Inhibition of dapsone excretion by probenecid. *Lancet* (1969) ii, 884–5.
2. Ellard GA, Gammon PT, Savin JA, Tan RS-H. Dapsone acetylation in dermatitis herpetiformis. *Br J Dermatol* (1974) 90, 441–4.

Dapsone + Proguanil

No pharmacokinetic interaction appears to occur between dapsone and proguanil, and they have been successfully used together for malaria prophylaxis.

Clinical evidence, mechanism, importance and management

A study in 6 healthy subjects found that proguanil 200 mg daily had no effect on the pharmacokinetics of dapsone 10 mg daily, nor on its principal metabolite, monoacetyldapsone. However, the authors of this report are extremely cautious because, despite this lack of a pharmacokinetic interaction at these dosages, they say that increased dapsone toxicity cannot be ruled out.[1] Dapsone 25 mg was successfully used with proguanil 200 mg daily for malarial prophylaxis in the Vietnam war,[2] and the same regimen, but with the dapsone dosage every third day was successful as prophylaxis against proguanil-resistant falciparum malaria in Papua New Guinea.[1] Moreover, a different dosage (dapsone 4 or 12.5 mg with proguanil 200 mg daily), was well tolerated over a period of 80 days when used as malaria prophylaxis in Thailand.[3]

1. Edstein MD, Rieckmann KH. Lack of effect of proguanil on the pharmacokinetics of dapsone in healthy volunteers. *Chemotherapy* (1993) 39, 235–41.
2. Black RH. Malaria in the Australian army in South Vietnam. Successful use of a proguanil-dapsone combination for chemoprophylaxis of chloroquine-resistant falciparum malaria. *Med J Aust* (1973) 1, 1265–70.
3. Shanks GD, Edstein MD, Suriyamongkol V, Timsaad S, Webster HK. Malaria prophylaxis using proguanil/dapsone combinations on the Thai-Cambodian border. *Am J Trop Med Hyg* (1992) 46, 643–8.

Dapsone + Pyrimethamine

Pyrimethamine does not significantly affect the pharmacokinetics of dapsone.

Clinical evidence, mechanism, importance and management

A study in 7 healthy subjects given single doses of dapsone 100 mg, pyrimethamine 25 mg or both drugs together found that the peak plasma levels of dapsone fell by 17% and the half-life was unchanged, but the apparent volume of distribution was significantly increased from 1.53 to 1.93 L/kg. The pharmacokinetics of pyrimethamine were not affected by dapsone.[1] In another study HIV-positive patients were given dapsone 200 mg weekly (the maximum tolerated dose) either alone or with pyrimethamine 25 mg weekly. In contrast to the earlier study, there was a *decrease* in volume of distribution of dapsone when it was given with pyrimethamine, although dapsone levels were not significantly altered.[2] Furthermore, the tolerability of one-weekly dapsone plus pyrimethamine was found to be similar to that of once-weekly dapsone alone.[2]

1. Ahmad RA, Rogers HJ. Pharmacokinetics and protein binding interactions of dapsone and pyrimethamine. *Br J Clin Pharmacol* (1980) 10, 519–24.
2. Falloon J, Lavelle J, Ogata-Arakaki D, Byrne A, Graziani A, Morgan A, Amantea MA, Ownby K, Polis M, Davey RT, Kovacs JA, Lane HC, Masur H, MacGregor RR. Pharmacokinetics and safety of weekly dapsone and dapsone plus pyrimethamine for prevention of pneumocystis pneumonia. *Antimicrob Agents Chemother* (1994) 38, 1580–7.

Dapsone + Rifamycins

Rifampicin increases the urinary excretion of dapsone, lowers its serum levels and increases the risk of toxicity (methaemoglobinaemia). Similarly, rifabutin increases the clearance of dapsone, and may also increase its toxicity.

Clinical evidence

(a) Rifabutin

Twelve HIV-positive patients were given dapsone 100 mg daily for 2 weeks and then, in random order, either rifabutin 300 mg daily, fluconazole 200 mg daily, or fluconazole with rifabutin, each for 2 weeks. Rifabutin alone increased the clearance of dapsone by 67%. When combined with fluconazole, rifabutin increased the clearance of dapsone by 38%, which shows that fluconazole partially attenuated the enzyme-inducing effects of rifabutin. Rifabutin increased the formation clearance of dapsone by 92%, which was again attenuated by fluconazole. Rifabutin did not affect the AUC of the hydroxylamine metabolite of dapsone, which is thought to be associated with dapsone toxicity.[1]

(b) Rifampicin (Rifampin)

A study in 7 patients with leprosy given single doses of dapsone 100 mg and rifampicin 600 mg, alone or together, found that while the pharmacokinetics of rifampicin were not significantly changed, the half-life of the dapsone was roughly halved and the AUC was reduced by about 20%.[2] Other studies in patients given both drugs for several days, similarly found reduced dapsone serum levels and an increased urinary excretion.[3-7] Another study in 12 healthy subjects given a single 100-mg dose of dapsone before and after taking rifampicin 600 mg daily for 10 days, found that the clearance of the dapsone was considerably increased (from 2.01 to 7.17 litres/hour). Of equal importance was finding that the production of the hydroxylamine metabolite of dapsone, which appears to be responsible for the haematological toxicity (methaemoglobinaemia), was markedly increased. The 24-hour AUC of methaemoglobin was increased by more than 60%,[8] suggesting that this interaction increases dapsone toxicity.

Mechanism

Rifampicin and rifabutin increase the metabolism and clearance of dapsone. Rifampicin also increases the blood levels of the toxic hydroxylamine metabolite of dapsone. Similarly, rifabutin increased the formation of this metabolite, although increases in the AUC were not seen.

Importance and management

The interaction between dapsone and rifampicin is established but of uncertain clinical importance. Concurrent use should be well monitored to confirm that treatment is effective. It may be necessary to raise the dosage of dapsone. It has been pointed out that there is the risk of treatment failures for Pneumocystis pneumonia as well as for leprosy.[9] Also be alert for any evidence of methaemoglobinaemia.

Although there is less information, rifabutin appears to interact similarly to rifampicin. When dapsone is given with rifabutin, the dosage of dapsone may need to be increased, but this may increase exposure to the potentially toxic hydroxylamine metabolite.[1]

1. Winter HR, Trapnell CB, Slattery JT, Jacobson M, Greenspan DL, Hooton TM, Unadkat JD. The effect of clarithromycin, fluconazole, and rifabutin on dapsone hydroxylamine formation in individuals with human immunodeficiency virus infection (AACTG 283). *Clin Pharmacol Ther* (2004) 76, 579–87.
2. Krishna DR, Appa Rao AVN, Ramanakar TV, Prabhakar MC. Pharmacokinetic interaction between dapsone and rifampicin in leprosy patients. *Drug Dev Ind Pharm* (1986) 12, 443–59.
3. Balakrishnan S, Seshadri PS. Drug interactions – the influence of rifampicin and clofazimine on the urinary excretion of DDS. *Lepr India* (1981) 53, 17–22.
4. Peters JH, Murray JF, Gordon GR, Gelber RH, Laing ABG, Waters MFR. Effect of rifampin on the disposition of dapsone in Malaysian leprosy patients. *Fedn Proc* (1977) 36, 996.
5. George J, Balakrishnan S, Bhatia VN. Drug interaction during multidrug regimens for treatment of leprosy. *Indian J Med Res* (1988) 87, 151–6.
6. Pieters FAJM, Woonink F, Zuidema J. Influence of once-monthly rifampicin and daily clofazimine on the pharmacokinetics of dapsone in leprosy patients in Nigeria. *Eur J Clin Pharmacol* (1988) 34, 73–6.
7. Venkatesan K, Bharadwaj VP, Ramu G, Desikan KV. Study on drug interactions. *Lepr India* (1980) 52, 229–35.
8. Occhipinti DJ, Choi A, Deyo K, Danziger LH, Fischer JH. Influence of rifampin and clarithromycin on dapsone (D) disposition and methemoglobin concentrations. *Clin Pharmacol Ther* (1995) 57, 163.
9. Jorde UP, Horowitz HW, Wormser GP. Significance of drug interactions with rifampin in *Pneumocystis carinii* pneumonia prophylaxis. *Arch Intern Med* (1992) 152, 2348.

Dapsone + Trimethoprim

The serum levels of both drugs are possibly raised by concurrent use. Both increased efficacy and dapsone toxicity have been seen.

Clinical evidence

Eighteen patients with AIDS, treated for Pneumocystis pneumonia and taking dapsone 100 mg daily, were compared with 30 other patients taking dapsone with trimethoprim 20 mg/kg daily. The trimethoprim raised dapsone levels by 40%, from 1.5 to 2.1 micrograms/mL, at 7 days (steady-state). Dapsone toxicity (methaemoglobinaemia) was also increased.[1] Trimethoprim plasma levels were 48.4% higher in the 30 patients also taking dapsone when compared with another group of 30 patients given co-trimoxazole (trimethoprim with sulfamethoxazole), but the incidence of toxicity was higher in the co-trimoxazole group.[1] However, a later study by the same authors in 8 asymptomatic HIV-positive patients given dapsone 100 mg daily and trimethoprim 200 mg every 12 hours found that the steady-state pharmacokinetics of each drug was unaffected by the other, although the single dose pharmacokinetics showed higher serum levels than at steady state for both drugs.[2]

Mechanism

Not understood. Dapsone and trimethoprim appear to have mutually inhibitory effects on clearance.

Importance and management

Information is limited. The difference between the results of the two studies may be because the first was in AIDS patients with Pneumocystis pneumonia and the second was in asymptomatic HIV-positive patients whose drug metabolism may possibly be different. Concurrent use appears to be an effective form of treatment, but be alert for evidence of increased dapsone toxicity (methaemoglobinaemia).

1. Lee BL, Medina I, Benowitz NL, Jacob P, Wofsy CB, Mills J. Dapsone, trimethoprim, and sulfamethoxazole plasma levels during treatment of pneumocystis pneumonia in patients with acquired immunodeficiency syndrome (AIDS). *Ann Intern Med* (1989) 110, 606–11.
2. Lee BL, Safrin S, Makrides V, Gambertoglio JG. Zidovudine, trimethoprim, and dapsone pharmacokinetic interactions in patients with human immunodeficiency virus infection. *Antimicrob Agents Chemother* (1996) 40, 1231–6.

Dapsone + Ursodeoxycholic acid (Ursodiol)

A single case suggests that the effectiveness of dapsone in the treatment of dermatitis herpetiformis may be reduced by ursodeoxycholic acid.

Clinical evidence, mechanism, importance and management

A 61-year-old man taking dapsone 50 mg daily for dermatitis herpetiformis started taking ursodeoxycholic acid 450 mg twice daily for cholecystitis. Two weeks later the dermatitis herpetiformis worsened and the dose of dapsone was increased to 150 mg daily. However, his condition did not improve, so ursodeoxycholic acid was stopped and, as his condition improved, the dapsone dose was reduced to 100 mg, and then 50 mg daily. Two months later ursodeoxycholic acid was restarted and there was again an exacerbation of the dermatitis herpetiformis.[1] The general importance of this isolated report is unknown, but consider the possibility of reduced dapsone effects if ursodeoxycholic acid is also given.

1. Stroubou E, Dawn G, Forsyth A. Ursodeoxycholic acid causing exacerbation of dermatitis herpetiformis. *J Am Acad Dermatol* (2001) 45, 319–20.

Daptomycin + Miscellaneous

The use of statins and probably fibrates should be suspended during daptomycin use because of the possible increased risk of muscle toxicity. Daptomycin does not appear to interact with warfarin, but its use may result in falsely elevated prothrombin times. NSAIDs may reduce daptomycin excretion and concurrent use may increase the risks of renal impairment.

Clinical evidence, mechanism, importance and management

(a) Drugs causing myopathy

The US manufacturers describe a study in 20 healthy subjects taking **simvastatin** 40 mg daily, in which the addition of daptomycin 4 mg/kg per day for 14 days did not result in an increase in adverse effects, when compared to subjects given placebo. In contrast, in a phase III study of patients with bacteraemia, 5 out of 22 patients who were currently, or had recently, been taking a **statin** developed raised creatinine phosphokinase levels.[1] Furthermore, a case report describes a patient who was given daptomycin 6.5 mg/kg daily, who developed muscle pain and a raised creatinine phosphokinase (20 771 units/L). He had been taking **simvastatin**, but this had been discontinued when the daptomycin was started.[2] It is difficult to know whether this was a result of an interaction as another case of rhabdomyolysis (creatinine phosphokinase 21 243 units/L) was attributed to daptomycin alone: the patient was taking no other drugs known to cause myopathy (fibrates and statins specifically mentioned).[3] A review of patients with Gram-positive complicated skin and skin structure infections found that musculoskeletal pain or myalgia occurred in up to 0.4% of patients. In patients with similar infections treated with daptomycin the incidence of myopathy was slightly higher, at 0.2 to 0.9%,[4] suggesting that daptomycin increases the risk of muscle toxicity.

The manufacturers note that experience of the concurrent use of daptomycin with statins is limited, and therefore the use of a statin should be suspended if daptomycin is given,[1,5] unless the benefits of concurrent use outweigh the risks, in which case the patient's creatine kinase should be monitored more frequently than weekly.[5] See also 'muscle toxicity', (p.1086), for further guidance on monitoring for statin-associated myopathy, and risk factors for muscle toxicity. The UK manufacturers give the same guidance for **fibrates** and **ciclosporin**, both of which have been associated with myopathy.[1]

(b) NSAIDs

The UK manufacturers note that NSAIDs (including coxibs) may reduce the renal excretion of daptomycin and have additive detrimental effects on renal function if used with daptomycin.[5] They advise caution on concurrent use, which in practice probably means keeping a close eye on renal function and monitoring for possible daptomycin adverse effects.

(c) Warfarin

The US manufacturers describe a study in 16 healthy subjects in which daptomycin 6 mg/kg per day for 5 days did not affect either the pharmacokinetics or the INR in response to a single 25-mg dose of warfarin. The pharmacokinetics of daptomycin were also unchanged.[1] However, as experience is limited the manufacturers advise monitoring the INR for the first few days of concurrent use. Note that daptomycin causes a concentration-dependent false prolongation of prothrombin time.[1,5] This only appears to occur with recombinant thromboplastin reagents. Blood for INR testing should therefore be drawn during the daptomycin trough (i.e. immediately before the next dose). If a raised INR is found it is recommended that the INR should be re-tested, and alternative methods of monitoring should be considered.[1]

(d) Miscellaneous

The US manufacturers[1] briefly mention small studies in which daptomycin was given with **aztreonam** or **tobramycin** without any significant change in the pharmacokinetics of either drug. They also mention a study in which **probenecid** did not alter the pharmacokinetics of daptomycin.

1. Cubicin (Daptomycin). Cubist Pharmaceuticals, Inc. US Prescribing information, March 2007.
2. Echevarria K, Datta P, Cadena J, Lewis JS. Severe myopathy and possible hepatotoxicity related to daptomycin. *J Antimicrob Chemother* (2005) 55, 599–600.
3. Kazory A, Dibadj, K, Weiner ID. Rhabdomyolysis and acute renal failure in a patient treated with daptomycin. *J Antimicrob Chemother* (2006) 57, 578–9.
4. Fenton C, Keating GM, Curran MP. Daptomycin. *Drugs* (2004) 64, 445–55.
5. Cubicin (Daptomycin). Novartis Pharmaceuticals UK Ltd. UK Summary of product characteristics, July 2006.

Ethambutol + Antacids

Aluminium hydroxide and aluminium/magnesium hydroxide can cause a small but probably clinically unimportant reduction in the absorption of ethambutol in some patients.

Clinical evidence, mechanism, importance and management

A study in 13 patients with tuberculosis, given a single 50-mg/kg dose of ethambutol, found that when they were also given three 1.5-g doses of **aluminium hydroxide gel** (at the same time and 15 and 30 minutes later) their peak serum ethambutol levels were delayed and reduced. The average urinary excretion of ethambutol over a 10-hour period was reduced by about 15%, but there were marked variations between individual patients. Some showed no interaction, and others showed increased absorption.[1] No interaction was seen in 6 healthy subjects similarly treated.[1] A further study in 14 healthy subjects found that 30 mL of an **aluminium/magnesium hydroxide** antacid decreased the AUC and maximum serum levels of a 25-mg/kg dose of ethambutol by 10% and 29%, respectively.[2]

Just why this interaction occurs is not understood, but **aluminium hydroxide** can affect gastric emptying. The reduction in absorption is generally small and variable, and it seems doubtful if it will have a significant effect on the treatment of tuberculosis. However, the authors of the second study suggest avoiding giving antacid at the same time as ethambutol,[2] and the US manufacturer states that **aluminium hydroxide**-containing antacids should not be taken until 4 hours after a dose of ethambutol.[3]

1. Mattila MJ, Linnoila M, Seppälä T, Koskinen R. Effect of aluminium hydroxide and glycopyrrhonium on the absorption of ethambutol and alcohol in man. *Br J Clin Pharmacol* (1978) 5, 161–6.
2. Peloquin CA, Bulpitt AE, Jaresko GS, Jelliffe RW, Childs JM, Nix DE. Pharmacokinetics of ethambutol under fasting conditions, with food, and with antacids. *Antimicrob Agents Chemother* (1999) 43, 568–72.
3. Myambutol (Ethambutol). Dura Pharmaceuticals. US Prescribing information, November 2003.

Ethambutol + Food

The pharmacokinetics of ethambutol given with a high-fat breakfast were only slightly different to its pharmacokinetics when it is given in the fasting state.[1] Therefore ethambutol may be given without regard to meals.

1. Peloquin CA, Bulpitt AE, Jaresko GS, Jelliffe RW, Childs JM, Nix DE. Pharmacokinetics of ethambutol under fasting conditions, with food, and with antacids. *Antimicrob Agents Chemother* (1999) 43, 568–72.

Ethambutol + Rifabutin

Rifabutin does not appear to affect the pharmacokinetics of ethambutol.

Clinical evidence, mechanism, importance and management

Ten healthy subjects were given a single 1.2-g dose of ethambutol before and after taking rifabutin 300 mg daily for a week. No clinically relevant changes in the pharmacokinetics of ethambutol were seen.[1] Although 5 of the subjects experienced moderate to severe chills, and one had transient thrombocytopenia these reactions are unlikely to have been due to an interaction. No special precautions would appear to be necessary during concurrent use.

1. Breda M, Benedetti MS, Bani M, Pellizzoni C, Poggesi I, Brianceschi G, Rocchetti M, Dolfi L, Sassella D, Rimoldi R. Effect of rifabutin on ethambutol pharmacokinetics in healthy volunteers. *Pharmacol Res* (1999) 40, 351–6.

Ethionamide + Isoniazid

Isoniazid may contribute to acute psychotic reactions associated with ethionamide, but evidence for this is limited.

Clinical evidence, mechanism, importance and management

Acute psychotic reactions occurring during treatment with either isoniazid or ethionamide are reported to be uncommon.[1] Acute mania occurred in a patient treated with streptomycin, isoniazid and prednisolone for 4 months, and ethionamide and pyrazinamide for 27 days. It was thought that ethionamide was probably responsible for the psychotic reaction but that isoniazid and prednisolone may have potentiated the reaction.[2] In another patient, ethionamide was considered to be responsible for psychological changes, which resolved when the drug was stopped. However, the contribution of alcohol and other concurrent drugs such as isoniazid was not ruled out.[3] One study in patients found that ethionamide 750 mg increased serum levels of a single 10-mg/kg dose of isoniazid at 4 hours but not at 1 or 10 hours, but this was not considered to be of therapeutic significance[4] and the toxic symptoms reported with the combination[5,6] were considered not to be due to increased isoniazid levels.[4]

A clinically significant interaction therefore seems unlikely, but as both drugs can, rarely, cause psychotic reactions these tentative reports cannot entirely be dismissed.

1. Sharma GS, Gupta PK, Jain NK, Shanker A, Nanawati V. Toxic psychosis to isoniazid and ethionamide in a patient with pulmonary tuberculosis. *Tubercle* (1979) 60, 171–2.
2. Narang RK. Acute psychotic reaction probably caused by ethionamide. *Tubercle* (1972) 137–8.
3. Lansdown FS, Beran M, Litwak T. Psychotoxic reaction during ethionamide therapy. *Am Rev Respir Dis* (1967) 95,1053–5.
4. Tiitinen H. Isoniazid and ethionamide serum levels and inactivation in Finnish subjects. *Scand J Respir Dis* (1969) 50, 110–24.
5. Brouet G, Marche J, Rist N, Chevallier J, LeMeur G. Observations on the antituberculous effectiveness of alpha-ethyl-thioisonicotinamide in tuberculosis in humans. *Am Rev Tuberc* (1959) 79, 6–18.
6. Trendelenburg F. Antibakterielle chemotherapie der tuberkulose. *Fortschr Arzneimittelforsch* (1964) 7, 193–303.

Ethionamide + Miscellaneous

A study in 12 healthy subjects found that the bioavailability of a single 500-mg dose of ethionamide was not significantly affected by food, orange juice or antacids, when compared with ethionamide bioavailability under fasting conditions. It was suggested that ethionamide may be given with food if tolerance is a problem.[1]

1. Auclair B, Nix DE, Adam RD, James GT, Peloquin CA. Pharmacokinetics of ethionamide administered under fasting conditions or with orange juice, food, or antacids. *Antimicrob Agents Chemother* (2001) 45, 810–4.

Fosfomycin + Cimetidine

In a study in 9 healthy subjects the pharmacokinetics of a 50-mg dose of fosfomycin were not significantly altered by two 400 mg doses of cimetidine, given both the night before and 30 minutes before the fosfomycin.[1]

1. Bergan T, Mastropaolo G, Di Mario F, Naccarato R. Pharmacokinetics of fosfomycin and influence of cimetidine and metoclopramide on the bioavailability of fosfomycin trometamol. New Trends in Urinary Tract Infections (eds Neu and Williams) Int Symp Rome 1987, pp 157–66. Published in 1988.

Fosfomycin + Metoclopramide

Metoclopramide reduces fosfomycin bioavailability but the evidence suggests that this probably does not alter its efficacy in urinary tract infections.

Clinical evidence, mechanism, importance and management

Metoclopramide 20 mg given to 9 healthy subjects 30 minutes before fosfomycin 50 mg/kg reduced the peak serum levels of fosfomycin by 42% and reduced the AUC by 27%. These changes appear to occur because metoclopramide speeds the transit through the gut, so that less time is available for good absorption. However, despite these reductions, the urinary concentrations of fosfomycin remained above the minimum levels required for common urinary pathogens for at least 36 hours after the dose.[1] This suggests that the interaction is unlikely to be clinically important.

1. Bergan T, Mastropaolo G, Di Mario F, Naccarato R. Pharmacokinetics of fosfomycin and influence of cimetidine and metoclopramide on the bioavailability of fosfomycin trometamol. New Trends in Urinary Tract Infections (eds Neu and Williams) Int Symp Rome 1987, pp 157–66. Published in 1988.

Isoniazid + Aminosalicylic acid

Isoniazid serum levels are raised by aminosalicylic acid.

Clinical evidence, mechanism, importance and management

A study found that aminosalicylic acid significantly increased the plasma levels of isoniazid at 4 and 6 hours after administration by 32% and 114%, respectively in fast acetylators of isoniazid, and by 21% and 39%, respectively in slow acetylators. The half-life of isoniazid was increased from 1.32 to 2.89 hours in fast acetylators and from 3.05 to 4.27 hours in slow acetylators (see 'Genetic factors', (p.4), for more information about acetylator status). The effects were probably due to the inhibition of isoniazid metabolism by aminosalicylic acid.[1] There seem to be no reports of isoniazid toxicity arising from this interaction, but the manufacturers of isoniazid warn that adverse effects are more likely in the presence of aminosalicylic acid.[2]

1. Hanngren Å, Borgå O, Sjöqvist F. Inactivation of isoniazid (INH) in Swedish tuberculous patients before and during treatment with para-aminosalicylic acid (PAS). *Scand J Respir Dis* (1970) 51, 61–9.
2. Isoniazid. Celltech Manufacturing Services Ltd. UK Summary of product characteristics, November 2001.

Isoniazid + Antacids

The absorption of isoniazid from the gut is modestly reduced by aluminium hydroxide, less so by magaldrate, and not by affected by aluminium/magnesium hydroxide tablets or didanosine chewable tablets.

Clinical evidence

Aluminium hydroxide (***Amphojel***) 45 mL was given to 10 patients with tuberculosis at 6, 7 and 8 am, followed immediately by isoniazid and any other medication they were receiving. The plasma isoniazid levels at 1 hour were decreased, and peak plasma concentrations occurring between 1 and 2 hours after ingestion were reduced by about 25%, when adjusted for different dosages.[1] The effect of **magaldrate (hydrated magnesium aluminate)** was less,[1] and in another well-controlled study **aluminium/magnesium hydroxide** *(Mylanta)* had no effect.[2]

Didanosine chewable tablets contain antacids (**aluminium/magnesium hydroxide**) in the formulation, but it has been shown that they do not affect the bioavailability of isoniazid.[3]

Mechanism

Aluminium hydroxide delays gastric emptying,[4,5] causing retention of the isoniazid in the stomach. Since isoniazid is largely absorbed from the intestine, this explains the slight decrease in plasma isoniazid concentrations. Aluminium hydroxide also appears to inhibit the absorption of isoniazid.

Importance and management

Information on this interaction is limited, and it is not established. The clinical importance of the modest reductions in isoniazid levels with aluminium hydroxide in one study is uncertain, but likely to be small. However, aluminium/magnesium hydroxide did not interact, and neither did didanosine chewable tablets.

1. Hurwitz A, Schlozman DL. Effects of antacids on gastrointestinal absorption of isoniazid in rat and man. *Am Rev Respir Dis* (1974) 109, 41–7.
2. Peloquin CA, Namdar S, Dodge AA, Nix DE. Pharmacokinetics of isoniazid under fasting conditions, with food, and with antacids. *Int J Tuberc Lung Dis* (1999) 3, 703–710.
3. Gallicano K, Sahai J, Zaror-Behrens G, Pakuts A. Effect of antacids in didanosine tablet on bioavailability of isoniazid. *Antimicrob Agents Chemother* (1994) 38, 894–7.
4. Vats TS, Hurwitz A, Robinson RG, Herrin W. Effects of antacids on gastric emptying in children. *Pediatr Res* (1973) 7, 340.
5. Hava M, Hurwitz A. The relaxing effect of aluminium and lanthanum on rat and human gastric smooth muscle in vitro. *Eur J Pharmacol* (1973) 22, 156–61.

Isoniazid + Ciprofloxacin

Ciprofloxacin may cause a modest increase in the bioavailability of isoniazid.

Clinical evidence, mechanism, importance and management

In a single-dose study ciprofloxacin 500 mg was found to increase the absorption of isoniazid 300 mg by about 15%. The time to reach maximum plasma levels was increased from 3 hours to 4 hours. The rate of elimination and plasma half-life of isoniazid were not significantly affected. The effects on isoniazid absorption may be due to inhibition of gastric motility and emptying by ciprofloxacin.[1] However, these effects are modest and unlikely to be clinically significant.

1. Ofoefule SI, Obodo CE, Orisakwe OE, Ilondu NA, Afonne OJ, Maduka SO, Anusiem CA, Agbasi PU. Some plasma pharmacokinetic parameters of isoniazid in the presence of a fluoroquinolone antibacterial agent. *Am J Ther* (2001) 8, 243–6.

Isoniazid + Disulfiram

In most patients, the concurrent use of isoniazid and disulfiram is uneventful, but difficulties in co-ordination, with changes in mental status, behaviour, and drowsiness have been reported in a small number of patients.

Clinical evidence

Seven patients with tuberculosis who had been taking isoniazid for at least 30 days, without problems, experienced adverse reactions within 2 to 8 days of starting to take disulfiram 500 mg daily. Among the symptoms were dizziness, disorientation, a staggering gait, insomnia, irritability and querulous behaviour, listlessness, and lethargy. One patient became hypomanic. Most of them were also taking chlordiazepoxide, and other drugs included aminosalicylic acid, streptomycin and phenobarbital. The adverse reactions decreased or disappeared when the disulfiram was either reduced to 250 or 125 mg daily, or withdrawn. These 7 patients represented less than one-third of those who received both drugs.[1] As disulfiram is known to inhibit the metabolism of chlordiazepoxide,[2] another 4 patients were given only isoniazid and disulfiram. Although their reaction was not as severe, all 4 developed drowsiness and depression.[1]

In contrast, another report describes the concurrent use of both drugs, without problems, in 200 patients.[3] A retrospective study in patients treated with isoniazid-containing regimens for tuberculosis found no difference in rates of toxicity in 13 patients taking disulfiram, when compared to a large group of patients not taking disulfiram. However, the small number of patients taking disulfiram in this study limits the strength of the negative finding.[4] Another patient taking disulfiram with isoniazid and rifampicin (rifampin) also did not experience any problems.[5]

Mechanism

Not understood. One idea is that some kind of synergy occurs between the two drugs because both can produce similar adverse effects if given in high doses. The authors of one report[1] speculate that isoniazid and disulfiram together inhibit two of three biochemical pathways concerned with the metabolism of dopamine. This leaves a third pathway open, catalysed by COMT (catechol-*O*-methyl transferase), which produces a number of methylated products of dopamine. These methylated products may possibly have been responsible for the mental and physical reactions seen.

Importance and management

Information about this interaction appears to be limited to the reports cited. Its incidence is uncertain but apparently quite small. Two-thirds of the patients in one study, and at least 200 other patients showed no interaction. It would therefore seem that concurrent use need not be avoided, but the response should be monitored. If marked changes in mental status occur, or there is unsteady gait, the manufacturers recommend that the disulfiram should be withdrawn.[6]

1. Whittington HG, Grey L. Possible interaction between disulfiram and isoniazid. *Am J Psychiatry* (1969) 125, 1725–9.
2. Antabuse (Disulfiram). Actavis UK Ltd. UK Summary of product characteristics, August 1999.
3. McNichol RW, Ewing JA, Faiman MD, eds. Disulfiram (Antabuse), a unique medical aid to sobriety: history, pharmacology, research, clinical use. Springfield Ill: Thomas; 1987 p. 47–90.
4. Burman WJ, Terra M, Breese P, Cohn D, Reves R. Lack of toxicity from concomitant directly observed disulfiram and isoniazid-containing therapy for active tuberculosis. *Int J Tuberc Lung Dis* (2002) 6, 839–42.
5. Rothstein E. Rifampin with disulfiram. *JAMA* (1972) 219, 1216.
6. Antabuse (Disulfiram). Odyssey Pharmaceuticals, Inc. US Prescribing information, December 2003.

Isoniazid + Ethambutol

Ethambutol does not appear to affect serum isoniazid levels. However, it seems that the optic neuropathy caused by ethambutol may be increased by isoniazid.

Clinical evidence, mechanism, importance and management

The mean serum levels of a 300-mg dose of isoniazid were not significantly changed in 10 patients with tuberculosis when they were given a single 20-mg/kg dose of ethambutol.[1] The possible effects of concurrent use over a period of time were not studied. However, there is some evidence that the optic neuropathy caused by ethambutol may be increased by isoniazid, and any effects resolve more slowly after the use of isoniazid.[2-5] One group of authors recommends that both ethambutol and isoniazid should be stopped immediately if severe optic neuritis occurs. They further recommend that isoniazid should be stopped if less severe optic neuritis does not improve within 6 weeks after stopping ethambutol.[6]

1. Singhal KC, Varshney DP, Rathi R, Kishore K, Varshney SC. Serum concentration of isoniazid administered with and without ethambutol in pulmonary tuberculosis patients. *Indian J Med Res* (1986) 83, 360–2.
2. Renard G, Morax PV. Nevrite optique au cours des traitements antituberculeux. *Ann Ocul (Paris)* (1977) 210, 53–61.
3. Karmon G, Savir H, Zevin D, Levi J. Bilateral optic neuropathy due to combined ethambutol and isoniazid treatment. *Ann Ophthalmol* (1979) 11, 1013–17.
4. Garret CR. Optic neuritis in a patient on ethambutol and isoniazid evaluated by visual evoked potentials: Case report. *Mil Med* (1985) 150, 43–6.
5. Jimenez-Lucho VE, del Busto R, Odel J. Isoniazid and ethambutol as a cause of optic neuropathy. *Eur J Respir Dis* (1987) 71, 42–5.
6. Sivakumaran P, Harrison AC, Marschner J, Martin P. Ocular toxicity from ethambutol: a review of four cases and recommended precautions. *N Z Med J* (1998) 111, 428–30.

Isoniazid + Fluconazole

A double-blind, crossover study in 16 healthy subjects (8 'fast' and 8 'slow' acetylators of isoniazid) found that fluconazole 400 mg daily for a week had no clinically significant effect on the pharmacokinetics of isoniazid.[1] No special precautions would appear necessary during concurrent use.

1. Buss DC, Routledge PA, Hutchings A, Brammer KW, Thorpe JE. The effect of fluconazole on the acetylation of isoniazid. *Hum Exp Toxicol* (1991) 10, 85–6.

Isoniazid + Food

The absorption of isoniazid is reduced by food. See also 'Isoniazid + Food; Cheese or Fish', below, for toxic reactions between isoniazid and specific foods.

Clinical evidence

In 9 healthy subjects the mean peak serum levels of isoniazid 10 mg/kg were delayed, and reduced by 79%,when isoniazid was given with **breakfast** rather than when fasting. The AUC was reduced by 43%.[1] In another study in 14 healthy subjects given isoniazid with a **full fat breakfast**, the maximum serum levels of isoniazid were decreased by 51%, the absorption was delayed, and the AUC was decreased by 12%.[2] Similar results have been found in another study.[3]

Mechanism

Uncertain. Food delays gastric emptying so that absorption further along the gut is also delayed, but the reduction in absorption is not understood.

Importance and management

Information is limited but the interaction seems to be established. For maximum absorption isoniazid should be taken without food, hence the manufacturer's guidance to take it at least 30 minutes before or 2 hours after food.[4]

1. Melander A, Danielson K, Hanson A, Jansson L, Rerup C, Scherstén B, Thulin T, Wåhlin E. Reduction of isoniazid bioavailability in normal men by concomitant intake of food. *Acta Med Scand* (1976) 200, 93–7.
2. Peloquin CA, Namdar S, Dodge AA, Nix DE. Pharmacokinetics of isoniazid under fasting conditions, with food, and with antacids. *Int J Tuberc Lung Dis* (1999) 3, 703–710.
3. Männisto P, Mäntylä R, Klinge R, Nykänen S, Koponen A, Lamminsivu U. Influence of various diets on the bioavailability of isoniazid. *J Antimicrob Chemother* (1982) 10, 427–34.
4. Isoniazid. Celltech Manufacturing Services Ltd. UK Summary of product characteristics, November 2001.

Isoniazid + Food; Cheese or Fish

Patients taking isoniazid who eat some foods, particularly fish from the scombroid family (tuna, mackerel, salmon) that are not fresh, may experience an exaggerated histamine poisoning reaction. Cheese has also been implicated in this reaction, but the adverse effects may be due to the weak MAOI effects of isoniazid rather than histamine poisoning.

Clinical evidence

Three months after starting to take isoniazid 300 mg daily, a woman experienced a series of unpleasant reactions 10 to 30 minutes after eating cheese. These reactions included chills, headache (sometimes severe), itching of the face and scalp, slight diarrhoea, flushing of the face (and on one occasion the whole body), variable and mild tachycardia, and a bursting sensation in the head. Blood pressure measurements showed only a modest rise (from her normal level of 95/65 to 110/80 mmHg). No physical or biochemical abnormalities were found.[1]

Headache, dizziness, blurred vision, tachycardia, flushing and itching of the skin, redness of the eyes, burning sensation of the body, difficulty in breathing, abdominal colic, diarrhoea, vomiting, sweating and wheezing have all been described after other patients taking isoniazid ate cheese.[2-6] Certain tropical fish, including **tuna (skipjack** or **bonito** — ***Katsuwanus pelamis***),[7-11] ***Sardinella (Amblygaster) sirm***,[12] ***Rastrigella kanagurta***,[13] **saury** (**skipper** or **bill-fish**)[14] and others[15] are also implicated. There are a few hundred cases of this reaction on record.

Mechanism

The reaction appears to be an exaggeration of the histamine poisoning that can occur after eating some foods, such as members of the scombroid family of fish (tuna, mackerel, salmon, etc), if they are not fresh and adequately refrigerated. These fish (and some cheeses) have a high histidine content and under poor storage circumstances the histine is decarboxylated by bacteria to produce unusually large amounts of histamine. Normally this is inactivated by histaminase in the body, but isoniazid is a potent inhibitor of this enzyme, which means that the histamine is absorbed largely unchanged and histamine poisoning develops.[16] Histamine survives all but very prolonged cooking. Tuna fish can contain 180 to 500 mg histamine per 100 g, other types of fish may contain as little as 0.5 to 7.5 mg.[10]

Alternatively, it has been suggested that the cases of reactions to cheese are caused by tyramine content and the weak MAOI properties of isoniazid. See 'MAOIs or RIMAs + Tyramine-rich foods', p.1153 for more details of the mechanism of this interaction.

Importance and management

An established interaction of clinical importance. With the exception of one patient who appeared to have had a cerebrovascular accident,[9] the reactions experienced by the others were unpleasant and alarming but usually not serious or life-threatening. They required little or no treatment, although 'scombroid poisoning' in the absence of isoniazid is sometimes more serious. Two reports say that treatment with antihistamines can be effective.[10,15] Isoniazid has been in use since 1956 and there is little need to now introduce any general dietary restrictions, but if any of these reactions is experienced, examine the patient's diet and advise the avoidance of any probable offending foodstuffs. Very mature cheese and fish of the scombroid family (tuna, mackerel, salmon and other varieties of dark meat fish) that are not fresh are to be treated with suspicion, but the likely histamine or tyramine content of food cannot be assessed without undertaking a detailed analysis. See 'Table 32.2', (p.1152) and 'Table 32.3', (p.1154) for a list of tyramine rich foods and drinks.

1. Smith CK, Durack DT. Isoniazid and reaction to cheese. *Ann Intern Med* (1978) 88, 520–1.
2. Uragoda CG, Lodha SC. Histamine intoxication in a tuberculous patient after ingestion of cheese. *Tubercle* (1979) 60, 59–61.
3. Lejonc JL, Gusmini D, Brochard P. Isoniazid and reaction to cheese. *Ann Intern Med* (1979) 91, 793.
4. Hauser MJ, Baier H. Interactions of isoniazid with foods. *Drug Intell Clin Pharm* (1982) 16, 617–18.
5. Toutoungi M, Carroll R, Dick P. Isoniazide (INH) and tyramine-rich food. *Chest* (1986) 89 (Suppl 6), 540S.
6. Carvalho ACC, Manfrin M, Gore RP, Capone S, Scalvini A, Armellini A, Giovine T, Carosi G, Matteelli A. Reaction to cheese during TB treatment. *Thorax* (2004) 59, 635.
7. Uragoda CG, Kottegoda SR. Adverse reactions to isoniazid on ingestion of fish with a high histamine content. *Tubercle* (1977) 58, 83–9.
8. Uragoda CG. Histamine poisoning in tuberculous patients after ingestion of tuna fish. *Am Rev Respir Dis* (1980) 121, 157–9.
9. Senanayake N, Vyravanathan S, Kanagasuriyam S. Cerebrovascular accident after a 'skipjack' reaction in a patient taking isoniazid. *BMJ* (1978) 2, 1127–8.
10. Senanayake N, Vyravanathan S. Histamine reactions due to ingestion of tuna fish (*Thunnus argentivittatus*) in patients on antituberculosis therapy. *Toxicon* (1981) 19, 184–5.
11. Morinaga S, Kawasaki A, Hirata H, Suzuki S, Mizushima Y. Histamine poisoning after ingestion of spoiled raw tuna in a patient taking isoniazid. *Intern Med* (1997) 36, 198–200.
12. Uragoda CG. Histamine poisoning in tuberculous patients on ingestion of tropical fish. *J Trop Med Hyg* (1978) 81, 243–5.
13. Uragoda CG. Histamine intoxication with isoniazid and a species of fish. *Ceylon Med J* (1978) 23, 109–10.
14. Miki M, Ishikawa T, Okayama H. An outbreak of histamine poisoning after ingestion of the ground saury paste in eight patients taking isoniazid in a tuberculous ward. *Intern Med* (2005) 44, 1133–6.
15. Diao Y *et al*. Histamine like reaction in tuberculosis patients taking fishes containing much of histamine under treatment with isoniazid in 277 cases. *Zhonghua Jie He He Hu Xi Xi Ji Bing Za Zhi* (1986) 9, 267–9, 317–18.
16. O'Sullivan TL. Drug-food interaction with isoniazid resembling anaphylaxis. *Ann Pharmacother* (1997) 31, 928–9.

Isoniazid + H_2-receptor antagonists

Pharmacokinetic evidence suggests that neither cimetidine nor ranitidine interact with isoniazid.

Clinical evidence, mechanism, importance and management

In 13 healthy subjects **cimetidine** 400 mg or **ranitidine** 300 mg, three times a day, for 3 days had no effect on the pharmacokinetics of a single 10-mg/kg dose of isoniazid. Neither the absorption nor the metabolism of isoniazid were changed.[1] No special precautions would appear to be necessary on concurrent use. Although data about other H_2-receptor antagonists appears to be lacking, based on this study, they would not be expected to interact with isoniazid.

1. Paulsen O, Höglund P, Nilsson L-G, Gredeby H. No interaction between H_2 blockers and isoniazid. *Eur J Respir Dis* (1986) 68, 286–90.

Isoniazid + Laxatives

Sodium sulfate and castor oil used as laxatives can cause a modest but probably clinically unimportant reduction in isoniazid absorption.

Clinical evidence, mechanism, importance and management

In an experimental study of the possible effects of laxatives on isoniazid absorption, healthy subjects were given 10 to 20 g of oral **sodium sulfate** or 20 g of **castor oil** (doses sufficient to provoke diarrhoea). Absorption, measured by the amount of isoniazid excreted in the urine, was decreased by 50% with **castor oil** and by 41% with **sodium sulfate** at 4 hours. However, serum levels of isoniazid were relatively unchanged. The overall picture was that while these laxatives can alter the pattern of absorption, they do not seriously impair the total amount of drug absorbed.[1]

1. Mattila MJ, Takki S, Jussila J. Effect of sodium sulphate and castor oil on drug absorption from the human intestine. *Ann Clin Res* (1974) 6, 19–24.

Isoniazid + Pethidine (Meperidine)

An isolated case report describes hypotension and lethargy in a patient after he took isoniazid with pethidine.

Clinical evidence, mechanism, importance and management

A patient became lethargic and his blood pressure fell from 124/68 to 84/50 mmHg within 20 minutes of being given pethidine 75 mg intramuscularly. An hour before, he had been given isoniazid. There was no evidence of fever or cardiac arrhythmias, and his serum electrolytes, glucose levels and blood gases were normal. His blood pressure returned to normal over the next 3 hours. He had previously had both pethidine and isoniazid separately without incident. He was subsequently uneventfully given intravenous morphine sulfate, 4 mg every 2 to 4 hours.[1] The authors of the report attribute this reaction to the MAO-inhibitory properties of the isoniazid and equate it with the severe and potentially fatal 'MAOI-pethidine interaction', (p.1140), but in reality this reaction was mild and lacked many of the characteristics of the more serious reaction. Moreover, isoniazid possesses only mild MAO-inhibitory properties and does not normally interact to the same extent as the potent antidepressant and antihypertensive MAOIs.

There is too little evidence to advise against concurrent use, but bear this interaction in mind in the case of an unexpected response to treatment.

1. Gannon R, Pearsall W, Rowley R. Isoniazid, meperidine, and hypotension. *Ann Intern Med* (1983) 99, 415.

Isoniazid + Prednisolone

Prednisolone can lower plasma isoniazid levels, but this may not be clinically important.

Clinical evidence, mechanism, importance and management

Isoniazid 10 mg/kg daily was given to 26 patients with tuberculosis. The 13 slow acetylators of isoniazid had a 23% fall in plasma isoniazid levels when they were given **prednisolone** 20 mg, while the 13 fast acetylators showed a 38% fall over 8.5 hours (see 'Genetic factors', (p.4), for an explanation of acetylator status). The reasons for these changes are not understood but changes in the metabolism, and/or the excretion of the isoniazid by the kidney, are possibilities. Despite these changes the response to treatment was excellent.[1] In another group of 49 patients, both slow and fast acetylators of isoniazid, rifampicin 12 mg/kg largely counteracted the isoniazid-lowering effects of **prednisolone**.[1]

None of these interactions were of clinical importance, but the authors point out that if the dosage of isoniazid had been lower, its effects might have been reduced. Be aware of the possibility of a reduced response during concurrent use, and raise the isoniazid dosage if necessary. There seems to be no information about other corticosteroids.

1. Sarma GR, Kailasam S, Nair NGK, Narayana ASL, Tripathy SP. Effect of prednisolone and rifampin on isoniazid metabolism in slow and rapid inactivators of isoniazid. *Antimicrob Agents Chemother* (1980) 18, 661–6.

Isoniazid + Propranolol

Propranolol causes a small reduction in the clearance of isoniazid, which seems unlikely to be of much practical importance.

Clinical evidence, mechanism, importance and management

The clearance of a single 600-mg intravenous dose of isoniazid was reduced by 21%, from 16.4 to 13 L/hour, in 6 healthy subjects after they took propranolol 40 mg three times daily for 3 days.[1] It is suggested that propranolol reduces the clearance of isoniazid by inhibiting its metabolism (acetylation) by the liver.[1] However, as the increase in isoniazid levels is likely to be only modest this interaction is probably of little clinical importance.

1. Santoso B. Impairment of isoniazid clearance by propranolol. *Int J Clin Pharmacol Ther Toxicol* (1985) 23, 134–6.

Isoniazid + Pyrimethamine

A study in 19 patients with tuberculosis found that pyrazinamide did not affect serum levels of isoniazid.[1]

1. Levy D, Duysak S, Zylberberg B, Haapanen J, Russell WF, Middlebrook G. Effect of pyrazinamide on antimicrobially active serum isoniazid. *Dis Chest* (1960) 38, 148–51.

Isoniazid + Rifamycins

The concurrent use of a rifamycin and isoniazid is common and therapeutically valuable, but there is evidence that the incidence of hepatotoxicity may be increased, particularly in slow acetylators of isoniazid. One study suggests the bioavailability of rifampicin may be reduced by isoniazid but other studies found no pharmacokinetic interaction. Rifabutin and rifampicin do not alter the pharmacokinetics of isoniazid.

Clinical evidence, mechanism, importance and management

(a) Rifabutin

Rifabutin 300 mg, given daily for 7 days to 6 healthy subjects, had no significant effect on the pharmacokinetics of a single 300-mg dose of isoniazid or its metabolite acetylisoniazid.[1] Two of the 6 subjects were rapid acetylators of isoniazid (see 'Genetic factors', (p.4), for more information about acetylator status).

Although both drugs have been effectively used together in the treatment of tuberculosis, it is not clear whether concurrent use increases the incidence of hepatotoxicity, as occurs with isoniazid and rifampicin (see below). However, as regular monitoring of liver function is required for both isoniazid and rifabutin, no additional monitoring seems necessary on concurrent use. The manufacturer of rifabutin notes that haematological reactions of rifabutin could be increased by isoniazid, but, again, as regular monitoring of white blood cell and platelet counts is advised,[2] no additional monitoring seems necessary.

(b) Rifampicin (Rifampin)

Most studies have shown that the serum levels and half-lives of both drugs are not significantly affected by concurrent use,[3-6] even in those with hepatic impairment.[6] There was also no difference[4] between rapid and slow acetylators of isoniazid, (see 'Genetic factors', (p.4), for more information about acetylator status). One single-dose study in healthy subjects found that isoniazid 12 mg/kg reduced the AUC of rifampicin 10 mg/kg by about 25%.[7] There is some evidence that the incidence and severity of hepatotoxicity rises if both drugs are given together.[8] Reports from India suggest that the incidence can be as high as 8 to 10%, while much lower figures of

2 to 3% are reported in the US.[9] There is certainly one case report that appears to prove that hepatotoxicity can arise rapidly from the use of both drugs. The patient tolerated both drugs individually, but hepatotoxicity reappeared on concurrent use.[10] Increased isoniazid hepatotoxicity caused by rifampicin has been demonstrated *in vitro*.[11]

The reasons for the hepatotoxicity are not fully understood but rifampicin or isoniazid alone can cause liver damage by their own toxic action. One suggestion is that the rifampicin alters the metabolism of isoniazid, resulting in the formation of hydrazine, which has proven to be hepatotoxic.[9,10,12] Higher plasma levels of hydrazine are said to occur in slow acetylators of isoniazid,[9] but one study failed to confirm that this is so.[13] There has certainly been at least one fatality caused by this combination.[14] The manufacturers of rifampicin advise that caution is particularly needed in patients with impaired liver function, the elderly, malnourished patients, and children under two years of age. After baseline LFTs, further tests are only needed if fever, vomiting, or jaundice occur, or if the patient deteriorates.[15] However, the manufacturers of isoniazid suggest that liver function tests should be reviewed regularly in patients on combined treatment.[16]

1. Breda M, Painezzola E, Benedetti MS, Efthymiopoulos C, Carpentieri M, Sassella D, Rimoldi R. A study of the effects of rifabutin on isoniazid pharmacokinetics and metabolism in healthy volunteers. *Drug Metabol Drug Interact* (1993) 10, 323–40.
2. Mycobutin (Rifabutin). Pharmacia Ltd. UK Summary of product characteristics, October 2006.
3. Boman G. Serum concentration and half-life of rifampicin after simultaneous oral administration of aminosalicylic acid or isoniazid. *Eur J Clin Pharmacol* (1974) 7, 217–25.
4. Sarma GR, Kailasam S, Nair NGK, Narayana ASL, Tripathy SP. Effect of prednisolone and rifampin on isoniazid metabolism in slow and rapid inactivators of isoniazid. *Antimicrob Agents Chemother* (1980) 18, 661–6.
5. Venho VMK, Koskinen R. The effect of pyrazinamide, rifampicin and cycloserine on the blood levels and urinary excretion of isoniazid. *Ann Clin Res* (1971) 3, 277–80.
6. Acocella G, Bonollo L, Garimoldi M, Mainardi M, Tenconi LT. Kinetics of rifampicin and isoniazid administered alone and in combination to normal subjects and patients with liver disease. *Gut* (1972) 13, 47–53.
7. Immanuel C, Gurumurthy P, Ramachandran G, Venkatesan P, Chandrasekaran V, Prabhakar R. Bioavailability of rifampicin following concomitant administration of ethambutol or isoniazid or pyrazinamide or a combination of the three drugs. *Indian J Med Res* (2003) 118, 109–14.
8. Steele MA, Burk RF, DesPrez RM. Toxic hepatitis with isoniazid and rifampin. A meta-analysis. *Chest* (1991) 99, 465–71.
9. Gangadharam PRJ. Isoniazid, rifampin and hepatotoxicity. *Am Rev Respir Dis* (1986) 133, 963–5.
10. Askgaard DS, Wilcke T, Døssing M. Hepatotoxicity caused by the combined action of isoniazid and rifampicin. *Thorax* (1995) 50, 213–14.
11. Nicod L, Viollon C, Regnier A, Jacqueson A, Richert L. Rifampicin and isoniazid increase acetaminophen and isoniazid cytotoxicity in human HepG2 hepatoma cells. *Hum Exp Toxicol* (1997) 16(1), 28–34.
12. Pessayre D, Bentata M, Degott C, Nouel O, Miguet J-P, Rueff B, Benhamou J-P. Isoniazid-rifampin fulminant hepatitis. A possible consequence of the enhancement of isoniazid hepatotoxicity by enzyme induction. *Gastroenterology* (1977) 72, 284–9.
13. Jenner PJ, Ellard GA. Isoniazid-related hepatotoxicity: a study of the effect of rifampicin administration on the metabolism of acetylisoniazid in man. *Tubercle* (1989) 70, 93–101.
14. Lenders JWM, Bartelink AKM, van Herwaarden CLA, van Haelst UJGM, van Tongeren JHM. Dodelijke levercelnecrose na kort durende toediening van isoniazide en rifampicine aan een patiënt die reeds werd behandeld met anti-epileptica. *Ned Tijdschr Geneeskd* (1983) 127, 420–3.
15. Rifadin (Rifampicin), Sanofi-Aventis. UK Summary of product characteristics, March 2006.
16. Isoniazid. Celltech Manufacturing Services Ltd. UK Summary of product characteristics, November 2001.

Isoniazid + SSRIs and related antidepressants

A few reports suggest that no important interaction occurs between isoniazid and the SSRIs or nefazodone. However, adverse reactions have been seen during concurrent use and one report found an increased discontinuation rate in patients taking an SSRI with isoniazid.

Clinical evidence

Two HIV-positive patients taking **fluoxetine** 20 mg daily were also given isoniazid. One of them tolerated the use of both drugs, but the other developed vomiting and diarrhoea, and after 10 days the **fluoxetine** was stopped.[1]

A woman who had been hospitalised for serious depression was given **nefazodone** 300 mg daily. A few days later she began to take isoniazid 300 mg daily, and was later discharged on an increased **nefazodone** dose of 400 mg daily. She was reported to have had no problems while taking both drugs over a 5 month period.[2]

A woman with tuberculosis taking isoniazid 300 mg daily presented with depression and was given **sertraline** 50 mg daily, later raised to 150 mg daily, without problems. She responded well and was reported to have taken both drugs together for 8 months without problems.[2]

A retrospective review of HIV-positive patients who were taking either an SSRI, isoniazid, or both, found that the rate of discontinuation of the SSRI was higher in those also taking isoniazid (7 of 10 patients) than in the group of patients taking an SSRI alone (2 of 14). It is unclear why this rate was increased; little mention is made of the influence of other drugs or medical conditions.[3]

Mechanism, importance and management

Direct information about the concurrent use of isoniazid and SSRIs seems to be limited, but the case reports cited here[1,2,4] would suggest that the combination of isoniazid and these SSRIs is normally without problems. However, also be aware that one report suggests the possibility of an increase in adverse effects with the combination of SSRIs and isoniazid.[3]

In theory isoniazid could interact with the SSRIs[4] because it has some weak MAO inhibitory activity. However, isoniazid rarely interacts like the MAOIs. This is because isoniazid seems to lack activity on mitochondrial MAO even though it has activity on plasma MAO. Therefore no adverse MAOI/SSRI interaction would usually be expected.

1. Judd FK, Mijch AM, Cockram A, Norman TR. Isoniazid and antidepressants: is there cause for concern? *Int Clin Psychopharmacol* (1994) 9, 123–5.
2. Malek-Ahmadi P, Chavez M, Contreras SA. Coadministration of isoniazid and antidepressant drugs. *J Clin Psychiatry* (1996) 57, 550.
3. Doyle ME, Hicks D, Aronson NE. Selective serotonin reuptake inhibitors and isoniazid: evidence of a potential adverse interaction. *Mil Med* (2001) 166, 1054–6.
4. Evans ME, Kortas KJ. Potential interaction between isoniazid and selective serotonin-reuptake inhibitors. *Am J Health-Syst Pharm* (1995) 52, 2135–6.

Linezolid + Antacids

A study in healthy subjects found that *Maalox 70mVal* suspension 10 mL (aluminium/magnesium hydroxide) did not affect the pharmacokinetics of a single 600-mg dose of linezolid.[1]

1. Grunder G, Zysset-Aschmann Y, Vollenweider F, Maier T, Krähenbühl S, Drewe J. Lack of pharmacokinetic interaction between linezolid and antacid in healthy volunteers. *Antimicrob Agents Chemother* (2006) 50, 68–72.

Linezolid + Antidepressants

The serotonin syndrome has been reported in patients taking linezolid with an SSRI or venlafaxine. The serotonin syndrome is also predicted to occur if linezolid is given with tricyclic antidepressants.

Clinical evidence

(a) SSRIs

In an analysis of phase III studies, changes in vital signs did not differ between patients given linezolid and comparator drugs (i.e. antibiotics) when either were used with drugs known to interact with MAOIs, including unnamed SSRIs.[1,2] One patient taking **fluoxetine** had a transient episode of asymptomatic hypertension after one dose of linezolid, but since this patient had no other symptoms of serotonin syndrome, it was not considered an interaction.[2] However, a 4-year-old girl given **fluoxetine** 5 mg daily developed symptoms of the serotonin syndrome 2 days after starting linezolid 140 mg every 12 hours, and after a procedure for which she was given fentanyl 200 micrograms. Fentanyl may have been a contributing factor.[3] Another case report describes an 85-year-old woman taking **citalopram** who developed tremor, confusion, dysarthria, hyperreflexia, agitation, and restlessness after linezolid was started. **Citalopram** was stopped and the symptoms resolved over 72 hours.[4] There are several other case reports of this interaction between linezolid and SSRIs[5-8] including **citalopram**,[5,6] **sertraline**[6,7] and **paroxetine**.[8,9]

(b) Tricyclics

In an analysis of phase III studies, changes in vital signs did not differ between patients given linezolid and comparator drugs (i.e. antibiotics) when either were used with drugs known to interact with MAOIs, including unnamed cyclic antidepressants.[1,2] A case report describes the serotonin syndrome in an elderly patient treated with linezolid 600 mg every 12 hours, 21 days after amitriptyline 10 mg daily, paroxetine 20 mg daily and alprazolam 500 micrograms daily were started.[9]

(c) Other antidepressants

1. Mirtazapine. A patient taking linezolid 600 mg twice daily developed delirium, confusion and visual hallucinations 2 weeks after starting to take mirtazapine 15 or 30 mg daily and gabapentin 300 mg at night. Gabapentin was stopped and the delirium resolved. About 4 weeks later the delirium recurred and then resolved when the patient discontinued mirtazapine. Mirtazapine was restarted without recurrence of delirium. The patient subsequently took mirtazapine 15 mg daily with linezolid 600 mg twice daily without adverse effects.[10]

2. Venlafaxine. An 85-year-old man taking venlafaxine 150 mg daily was prescribed ciprofloxacin, rifampicin and linezolid 600 mg twice daily for a hip prosthesis infection. After 20 days he was found to be confused and disorientated, and 4 days later he was also drowsy, and suffering myoclonic jerks. Linezolid and venlafaxine were stopped and the symptoms resolved over 2 days.[11] However, another case report describes a 7-year-old boy treated with venlafaxine and methylphenidate who was prescribed linezolid for osteomyelitis. He was given all three drugs (doses not stated) for several days without any alterations in vital signs or evidence of the serotonin syndrome.[12]

Mechanism

Not fully understood. Linezolid has weak MAOI effects, and the serotonin syndrome is known to occur when MAOIs are given with 'SSRIs', (p.1142), 'tricyclics', (p.1149) and 'venlafaxine', (p.1156). In the case of the patient taking linezolid with amitriptyline and paroxetine, it is possible that an interaction between amitriptyline and paroxetine contributed to the development of the serotonin syndrome. Consider also 'Tricyclic and related antidepressants + SSRIs', p.1241.

Importance and management

Information on the reaction between linezolid and the SSRIs, tricyclics, mirtazapine or venlafaxine appears to be limited, but what is known suggests that the interaction is probably rare. The manufacturers of linezolid say that patients taking SSRIs and tricyclic antidepressants should have their blood pressure monitored and be closely observed if given linezolid. They say that if this is not possible, concurrent use should be avoided.[13] If linezolid is used with a drug with serotonergic actions it would seem prudent to monitor for symptoms of the serotonin syndrome, which may take several weeks to manifest. See 'The serotonin syndrome', (p.9), for further details.

1. Hartman CS, Leach TS, Todd WM, Hafkin B. Lack of drug-interaction with combination of linezolid and monoamine oxidase inhibitor-interacting medications. *Pharmacotherapy* (2000) 20, 1230.
2. Rubinstein E, Isturiz R, Standiford HC, Smith LG, Oliphant TH, Cammarata S, Hafkin B, Le V, Remington J. Worldwide assessment of linezolid's clinical safety and tolerability: comparator-controlled phase III studies. *Antimicrob Agents Chemother* (2003) 47, 1824–31.
3. Thomas CR, Rosenberg M, Blythe V, Meyer WJ. Serotonin syndrome and linezolid. *J Am Acad Child Adolesc Psychiatry* (2004) 43, 790.
4. Tahir N. Serotonin syndrome as a consequence of drug-resistant infections: an interaction between linezolid and citalopram. *J Am Med Dir Assoc* (2004) 5, 111–13.
5. Bernard L, Stern R, Lew D, Hoffmeyer P. Serotonin syndrome after concomitant treatment with linezolid and citalopram. *Clin Infect Dis* (2003) 36, 1197.
6. Hachem RY, Hicks K, Huen A, Raad I. Myelosuppression and serotonin syndrome associated with concurrent use of linezolid and selective serotonin reuptake inhibitors in bone marrow transplant recipients. *Clin Infect Dis* (2003) 37, 37: e8–e11.
7. Lavery S, Ravi H, McDaniel WW, Pushkin YR. Linezolid and serotonin syndrome. *Psychosomatics* (2001) 42, 432–4.
8. Willis CL, Goetz MB. Serotonin syndrome and linezolid. *Clin Infect Dis* (2002) 34, 1651–2.
9. Morales-Molina JA, Mateu-de Antonio J, Grau Cerrato S, Marín-Casino M. Probable síndrome serotoninérgico por interacción entre amitriptilina, paroxetina y linezolid. *Farm Hosp* (2005) 29, 1–2.
10. Aga VM, Barklage NE, Jefferson JW. Linezolid, a monoamine oxidase inhibiting antibiotic, and antidepressants. *J Clin Psychiatry* (2003) 64, 609–11.
11. Jones SL, Athan E, O'Brien D. Serotonin syndrome due to co-administration of linezolid and venlafaxine. *J Antimicrob Chemother* (2004) 54, 289–90.
12. Hammerness P, Parada H, Abrams A. Linezolid: MAOI activity and potential drug interactions. *Psychosomatics* (2002) 43, 248–9.
13. Zyvox (Linezolid). Pharmacia Ltd. UK Summary of product characteristics, July 2007.

Linezolid + Aztreonam

The pharmacokinetics of intravenous aztreonam 1 g and intravenous linezolid 375 mg were not affected when they were given together in a single-dose study in healthy subjects. Therefore dose alterations are unlikely to be needed during concurrent use.[1]

1. Sisson TL, Jungbluth GL, Hopkins NK. A pharmacokinetic evaluation of concomitant administration of linezolid and aztreonam. *J Clin Pharmacol* (1999) 39, 1277–82.

Linezolid + Dextromethorphan

There is no important pharmacokinetic interaction between linezolid and dextromethorphan, but one case of concurrent use resulted in the serotonin syndrome.

Clinical evidence, mechanism, importance and management

In a study in 14 healthy subjects, two 20-mg doses of dextromethorphan given 4 hours apart, before and during the use of linezolid 600 mg every 12 hours, had no effect on linezolid pharmacokinetics. The AUC and maximum level of the dextromethorphan metabolite, dextrorphan was decreased by 30%, but this was not considered sufficient to warrant any dosing alterations. There was no evidence of the serotonin syndrome, as measured by changes in body temperature, alertness and mental performance.[1] However, the manufacturers describe one case where the concurrent use of linezolid and dextromethorphan resulted in the serotonin syndrome.[2] Linezolid has mild reversible MAOI activity, and the serotonin syndrome has been described when dextromethorphan was taken by patients also taking antidepressant MAOIs, see 'MAOIs or RIMAs + Dextromethorphan', p.1134. If the concurrent use of linezolid and dextromethorphan is considered necessary, it would seem prudent to monitor for symptoms of 'the serotonin syndrome', (p.9).

1. Hendershot PE, Antal EJ, Welshman IR, Batts DH, Hopkins NK. Linezolid: pharmacokinetic and pharmacodynamic evaluation of coadministration with pseudoephedrine HCl, phenylpropanolamine HCl, and dextromethorphan HBr. *J Clin Pharmacol* (2001) 41, 563–72.
2. Zyvox (Linezolid). Pharmacia Ltd. UK Summary of product characteristics, July 2007.

Linezolid + Food

Linezolid modestly increases the blood pressure response to oral tyramine, and as a consequence patients receiving linezolid should not consume excessive amounts of tyramine-rich foods and drinks. The bioavailability of linezolid is not affected by enteral feeds or food.

Clinical evidence, mechanism, importance and management

(a) Enteral feeds

In a study a single 600-mg dose of linezolid was given as a suspension via a nasogastric tube or gastric tube to 9 patients receiving enteral feeds. The rate and extent of linezolid absorption was not significantly different to that found in another 6 patients not receiving enteral feeds. No dose adjustments are therefore thought to be required if linezolid is given with enteral feeds.[1]

(b) Food

A study in healthy subjects found that the plasma levels following a single 375-mg oral dose of linezolid as a tablet were 23% higher when given to fasted subjects than when it was taken immediately after a high-fat meal. However, the AUCs were not significantly different, indicating that the extent of absorption was not affected by food.[2] Another study in healthy subjects found that food delayed the rate but not the extent of absorption and distribution of linezolid into tissues.[3]

(c) Tyramine-rich food

In a pharmacodynamic study in healthy subjects, the dose of oral tyramine required to raise the systolic blood pressure by 30 mmHg was decreased by a factor of about 3.5 (from a range of 300 to 600 mg without linezolid to 100 to 200 mg with linezolid) when the subjects were pretreated with linezolid 625 mg twice daily for 4 to 7 days. This increase in the pressor response to tyramine was similar to that seen with moclobemide 150 mg three times daily.[4] Further, another placebo-controlled study in healthy subjects found that single doses of linezolid 600 mg and moclobemide 300 mg also caused similar increases in the pressor response to intravenous tyramine as measured by amount of tyramine required to raise the systolic blood pressure by 30 mmHg.[5]

Linezolid is a weak, non-selective inhibitor of MAO. As a consequence, it can inhibit the breakdown of the tyramine by MAO in the gut, and can also potentiate the effect of tyramine at nerve endings, therefore causing an increase in blood pressure (see Mechanism, under 'MAOIs or RIMAs + Tyramine-rich foods', p.1153). However, the extent of this rise was similar to that for moclobemide, which is much less than that seen with classical MAOIs.

The manufacturers of linezolid recommend that patients should avoid large amounts of tyramine-rich foods and drinks[6,7] and should not consume more than 100 mg of tyramine per meal.[7] For a list of the possible tyramine-content of various foods and drinks, see 'Table 32.2', (p.1152), 'Table 32.3', (p.1154) and 'Table 32.4', (p.1155). This is in line with the dietary restrictions recommended for RIMAs rather than the more stringent dietary recommendations required in patients taking non-selective MAOIs.

1. Nguyen M, Beringer P, Wong-Beringer A, Louie S, Gill M, Gurevitch A. Effect of continuous enteral feedings (TF) on oral bioavailability (F) of linezolid (LZD) in hospitalized patients. Abstracts of the 43rd Annual Interscience Conference on Antimicrobial Agents and Chemotherapy, Chicago, Il, 2003, 43, 36.
2. Welshman IR, Sisson TA, Jungbluth GL, Stalker D, Hopkins NK. Linezolid absolute bioavailability and the effect of food on oral bioavailability. *Biopharm Drug Dispos* (2001) 22, 91–7.
3. Islinger F, Dehghanyar P, Sauermann R, Burger C, Kloft C, Muller M, Joukhader C. The effect of food on plasma and tissue concentrations of linezolid after multiple doses. *Int J Antimicrob Agents* (2006) 27, 108–12.
4. Antal EJ, Hendershot PE, Batts DH, Sheu W-P, Hopkins NK, Donaldson KM. Linezolid, a novel oxazolidinone antibiotic: assessment of monoamine oxidase inhibition using pressor response to oral tyramine. *J Clin Pharmacol* (2001) 41, 552–62.
5. Cantarini MV, Painter CJ, Gilmore EM, Bolger C, Watkins CL, Hughes AM. Effect of oral linezolid on the pressor response to intravenous tyramine. *Br J Clin Pharmacol* (2004) 58, 470–5.
6. Zyvox (Linezolid). Pharmacia Ltd. UK Summary of product characteristics, July 2007.
7. Zyvox (Linezolid). Pharmacia & Upjohn. US Prescribing information, March 2007.

Linezolid + Other drugs with MAOI activity

The manufacturer of linezolid contraindicates its use with the MAOIs, including the selective MAO-B inhibitor selegiline and the RIMA moclobemide.

Clinical evidence, mechanism, importance and management

The UK manufacturer contraindicates the concurrent use of linezolid with or within 2 weeks of taking any other drug that inhibits MAO-A or MAO-B.[1] They specifically name the non-selective MAOIs **isocarboxazid** and **phenelzine**, the RIMA, **moclobemide**, and the MAO-B inhibitor, **selegiline**. Linezolid has reversible non-selective MAO-inhibitory activity, and this warning is based on the sometimes serious reactions that have occurred when non-selective MAOIs are given sequentially (see 'MAOIs + MAOIs or RIMAs', p.1137) or MAOIs are given with MAO-B inhibitors, see 'MAO-B inhibitors + MAOIs or RIMAs', p.692.

1. Zyvox (Linezolid). Pharmacia Ltd. UK Summary of product characteristics, July 2007.

Linezolid + Pethidine (Meperidine)

The UK manufacturer of linezolid[1] (a drug with weak, reversible, non-selective MAOI activity) contraindicates its use with pethidine, unless facilities are available for close observation and monitoring of blood pressure, because of the possibility of serious reactions, as have occurred with classical MAOIs and pethidine, see 'MAOIs or RIMAs + Opioids; Pethidine (Meperidine)', p.1140.

1. Zyvox (Linezolid). Pharmacia Ltd. UK Summary of product characteristics, July 2007.

Linezolid + Rifampicin (Rifampin)

Serum levels of intravenous linezolid are reduced by intravenous rifampicin.

Clinical evidence, mechanism, importance and management

A 31-year-old woman was given intravenous rifampicin 300 mg every 8 hours and linezolid 600 mg every 12 hours for an MRSA infection. During rifampicin treatment her linezolid peak and trough levels were 7.29 and 2.04 micrograms/mL, respectively. However, when the rifampicin was stopped the linezolid peak and trough levels were higher, at 12.46 and 5.03 micrograms/mL, respectively.[1]

In an earlier study, healthy subjects were given a single 600-mg dose of intravenous linezolid either alone or with a single 600-mg dose of intravenous rifampicin. This study also found that rifampicin reduced the serum levels of linezolid by 10%, 20% and 35% at 6, 9 and 12 hours, respectively.

Linezolid is not metabolised by the cytochrome P450 enzyme system so the reduction in levels is unlikely to be due to increased metabolism associated with rifampicin enzyme induction. The reduction in linezolid serum levels may be attributable to the induction of P-glycoprotein by rifampicin, resulting in increased excretion of linezolid.[1,2]

The clinical significance of this interaction is unclear and the concurrent use of rifampicin and linezolid is not established. The available evidence suggests that, where possible, linezolid levels should be monitored if both drugs are given. If this is not possible it would seem prudent to monitor concurrent use closely to ensure that the antibacterial treatment is effective.

1. Gebhart BC, Barker BC, Markewitz BA. Decreased serum linezolid levels in a critically ill patient receiving concomitant linezolid and rifampin. *Pharmacotherapy* (2007) 27, 476–9.
2. Egle H, Trittler R, Kümmerer K, Lemmen SW. Linezolid and rifampicin: drug interaction contrary to expectations? *Clin Pharmacol Ther* (2005) 77,451–3.

Linezolid + Sympathomimetics

Because of its weak MAO-inhibitory properties, the manufacturers of linezolid contraindicate its use with sympathomimetics (such as adrenergic bronchodilators, phenylpropanolamine, pseudoephedrine, adrenaline (epinephrine), noradrenaline (norepinephrine), dopamine and dobutamine) unless facilities for close observation and blood pressure monitoring are available. In one study the use of linezolid with phenylpropanolamine or pseudoephedrine resulted in additive hypertensive effects.

Clinical evidence

In a placebo-controlled study, 14 healthy patients were given two 60-mg doses of **pseudoephedrine** or two 25-mg doses of **phenylpropanolamine** 4 hours apart, with and without linezolid. The mean maximum blood pressure rise was 11 mmHg with placebo, 15 mmHg with linezolid, 18 mmHg with **pseudoephedrine** and 14 mmHg with **phenylpropanolamine**. When the subjects were given linezolid with **pseudoephedrine** the rise was 32 mmHg, which was similar to the 38 mmHg rise seen with linezolid plus **phenylpropanolamine**. However, these rises were transient, resolving in about 2 hours. No effects were seen on linezolid pharmacokinetics.[1]

Mechanism

Linezolid acts as a weak MAO-inhibitor, which allows the accumulation of some noradrenaline at adrenergic nerve endings associated with arterial blood vessels. Pseudoephedrine and phenylpropanolamine, both indirectly-acting sympathomimetics, can release these above-normal amounts of noradrenaline resulting in blood vessel constriction and a rise in blood pressure.

Importance and management

The manufacturers contraindicate the use of sympathomimetics (including adrenergic bronchodilators, pseudoephedrine, phenylpropanolamine, adrenaline (epinephrine), noradrenaline (norepinephrine), dopamine, dobutamine) with linezolid unless there are facilities available for close observation of the patient and monitoring of blood pressure.[2] Some indirectly-acting sympathomimetics occur in cough and cold remedies, which can be bought without prescription. To keep in line with the manufacturers recommendations, patients should be told to avoid these preparations. However, it should be said that the evidence available indicates that blood pressure rises are unlikely to be of the proportions seen with the antidepressant MAOIs, which result in hypertensive crises. Consider also 'MAOIs or RIMAs + Sympathomimetics; Indirectly-acting', p.1147.

1. Hendershot PE, Antal EJ, Welshman IR, Batts DH, Hopkins NK. Linezolid: pharmacokinetic and pharmacodynamic evaluation of coadministration with pseudoephedrine HCl, phenylpropanolamine HCl, and dextromethorphan HBr. *J Clin Pharmacol* (2001) 41, 563–72.
2. Zyvox (Linezolid). Pharmacia Ltd. UK Summary of product characteristics, July 2007.

Linezolid + Vitamins

The pharmacokinetics of linezolid are not affected by either vitamin C or vitamin E.

Clinical evidence, mechanism, importance and management

Healthy subjects were given vitamin C 1 g daily or vitamin E 800 units daily for 8 days with a single 600-mg dose of linezolid on the sixth day. As *in vitro* studies have indicated that endogenous reactive oxygen species (ROS) may affect linezolid clearance, it was considered possible that antioxidant supplements may affect the balance of ROS and linezolid clearance. However, the study found that antioxidants (vitamins C and E) given in doses far higher than the recommended daily intake did not affect linezolid pharmacokinetics. Therefore no dosage adjustments are considered necessary during concurrent use.[1]

1. Gordi T, Tan LH, Hong C, Hopkins NJ, Francom SF, Slatter JG, Antal EJ. The pharmacokinetics of linezolid are not affected by concomitant intake of the antioxidant vitamins C and E. *J Clin Pharmacol* (2003) 43, 1161–7.

Loracarbef + Acetylcysteine

A study in healthy subjects found that acetylcysteine 200 mg had no effect on the absorption of loracarbef 400 mg.[1]

1. Roller S, Lode H, Stelzer I, Deppermann KM, Boeckh M, Koeppe P. Pharmacokinetics of loracarbef and interaction with acetylcysteine. *Eur J Clin Microbiol Infect Dis* (1992) 11, 851–5.

Loracarbef + Food

Food reduces the maximum plasma levels of loracarbef, but does not alter its bioavailability.

Clinical evidence, mechanism, importance and management

Loracarbef 400 mg was given to 12 healthy subjects either in a fasting state or following a standard breakfast. Food slowed the rate of absorption, but not the total bioavailability of loracarbef.[1] In another study food was found to decrease the maximum plasma levels of a single 200-mg dose of loracarbef and increase the time to achieve maximum levels but the AUC of loracarbef was not significantly affected by food.[2] Loracarbef should be taken 1 hour before or 2 hours after food.[3]

1. Roller S, Lode H, Stelzer I, Deppermann KM, Boeckh M, Koeppe P. Pharmacokinetics of loracarbef and interaction with acetylcysteine. *Eur J Clin Microbiol Infect Dis* (1992) 11, 851–5.
2. DeSante KA, Zeckel ML. Pharmacokinetic profile of loracarbef. *Am J Med* (1992) 92 (Suppl 6A), 16S–19S.
3. Lorabid (Loracarbef). Monarch Pharmaceuticals, Inc. US Prescribing information, September 2002.

Loracarbef + Probenecid

Probenecid increases the half-life of loracarbef by about 50% but the clinical importance of this is unknown.[1]

1. Force RW, Nahata MC. Loracarbef: a new orally administered carbacephem antibiotic. *Ann Pharmacother* (1993) 27, 321–9.

Macrolides + Antacids

Aluminium/magnesium hydroxide antacids may reduce the peak levels of azithromycin. *Mylanta* can prolong the absorption of erythromycin, but this is unlikely to be clinically important. Aluminium/magnesium hydroxide antacids do not appear to significantly alter the pharmacokinetics of clarithromycin, roxithromycin or telithromycin.

Clinical evidence, mechanism, importance and management

In 10 healthy subjects the peak serum levels, but not the total absorption, of **azithromycin** was reduced by 30 mL *Maalox* (**aluminium/magnesium hydroxide**).[1] It is suggested therefore that **azithromycin** should not be given at the same time as antacids, but should be taken at least 1 hour before or 2 hours after.[2,3]

In 8 healthy subjects *Mylanta* (**aluminium/magnesium hydroxide, dimeticone**) 30 mL had no significant effect on the AUC, peak serum concentration, or time to peak serum concentration of **erythromycin stearate** 500 mg, but the mean elimination rate constant was more than doubled. It was suggested that the effect on elimination may be due to a possible prolonging of absorption, although the reason for this effect is unclear.[4] However, an *in vitro* study has suggested that the release and absorption of **erythromycin stearate** may be slowed in the presence of some antacids, including **aluminium** and **magnesium hydroxides**, **aluminium** and **magnesium trisilicates**, and **simeticone** because of adsorption of **erythromycin** by the antacids.[5] The clinical relevance of this is uncertain, but likely to be small.

Aluminium/magnesium hydroxide antacids are reported not to affect the pharmacokinetics of **clarithromycin**,[6] **roxithromycin**,[7] or **telithromycin**.[8,9]

1. Foulds G, Hilligoss DM, Henry EB, Gerber N. The effects of an antacid or cimetidine on the serum concentrations of azithromycin. *J Clin Pharmacol* (1991) 31, 164–7.
2. Hopkins S. Clinical toleration and safety of azithromycin. *Am J Med* (1991) 91 (Suppl 3A), 40S–45S.
3. Zithromax (Azithromycin). Pfizer Ltd. UK Summary of product characteristics, July 2006.
4. Yamreudeewong W, Scavone JM, Paone RP, Lewis GP. Effect of antacid coadministration on the bioavailability of erythromycin stearate. *Clin Pharm* (1989) 8, 352–4.
5. Arayne MS, Sultana N. Erythromycin-antacid interaction. *Pharmazie* (1993) 48, 599–602.
6. Zündorf H, Wischmann L, Fassenbender M, Lode H, Borner K, Koeppe P. Pharmacokinetics of clarithromycin and possible interaction with H_2 blockers and antacids. *Intersci Conf Antimicrob Agents Chemother* (1991) 31, 185.
7. Boeckh M, Lode H, Höffken G, Daeschlein S, Koeppe P. Pharmacokinetics of roxithromycin and influence of H_2-blockers and antacids on gastrointestinal absorption. *Eur J Clin Microbiol Infect Dis* (1992) 11, 465–8.
8. Ketek (Telithromycin). Sanofi-Aventis US LLC. US Prescribing information, February 2007.
9. Ketek (Telithromycin). Sanofi-Aventis. UK Summary of product characteristics, May 2007.

Macrolides + Azoles

Moderate pharmacokinetic interactions appear to occur between several of the azoles and macrolides but many of these are unlikely to be of clinical significance. However, clarithromycin may almost double itraconazole levels, and ketoconazole may almost double telithromycin levels.

Clinical evidence, mechanism, importance and management

(a) Azithromycin

Single doses of **fluconazole** 800 mg and azithromycin 1200 mg were given to 18 healthy subjects alone and together without any significant change in the pharmacokinetics of either drug.[1]

In healthy subjects, azithromycin 500 mg once daily for 3 days had no significant effect on the AUC and maximum plasma levels of **voriconazole** 200 mg twice daily.[2]

(b) Clarithromycin

Twenty healthy subjects were given clarithromycin 500 mg twice daily for 8 days. **Fluconazole** 400 mg daily was added on day 5, followed by 200 mg daily on days 6 to 8. The **fluconazole** increased the minimum plasma levels of the clarithromycin by 33% and the AUC_{0-12} by 18%.[3] These relatively small changes in the pharmacokinetics of clarithromycin are almost certainly of little or no clinical importance.

A study in 8 AIDS patients taking **itraconazole** 200 mg daily found that when clarithromycin 500 mg twice daily was also given, for 14 days, the maximum serum levels and the AUC of the **itraconazole** were increased by 90% and 92%, respectively.[4] Both clarithromycin and **itraconazole** are known to be metabolised by the hepatic cytochrome P450 isoenzyme CYP3A4 and it is therefore probable that competition for metabolism leads to a reduction in the clearance of **itraconazole**. This report does not comment on the outcome of this almost twofold increase in **itraconazole** levels, but it would seem prudent to be alert for the need to reduce its dosage. More study is needed.

(c) Erythromycin

The manufacturer notes that peak plasma levels and AUC of a single 200-mg dose of **itraconazole** were increased by 44% and 36%, respectively, by a single 1-g dose of erythromycin ethyl succinate.[5] However, no dosage adjustments are recommended.

In healthy subjects, erythromycin 1 g twice daily for 7 days had no significant effect on the AUC and maximum plasma levels of **voriconazole** 200 mg twice daily.[2]

(d) Telithromycin

In a study in which healthy subjects were given either telithromycin 800 mg, **ketoconazole** 800 mg or both drugs once daily, it was found that the AUC and peak plasma levels of telithromycin were increased by 94.5% and 51.3%, respectively. It may be prudent to monitor for telithromycin adverse effects on concurrent use. In a further related study healthy subjects were given **itraconazole** 200 mg daily instead of ketoconazole. **Itraconazole** was found to increase the AUC and peak plasma levels of telithromycin by 53.8% and 21.7%, respectively. No serious adverse effects were reported in either study and telithromycin did not increase the QTc intervals observed with either **ketoconazole** or **itraconazole** alone.[6] Another study[7] by the same authors, in subjects aged 60 years or older and with a creatinine clearance of 30 mL/minute or more, found that, when **ketoconazole** was given, levels of telithromycin were increased but only slightly higher than those found in younger healthy subjects[6] in the earlier study.

1. Amsden GW, Foulds G, Thakker K. Pharmacokinetic study of azithromycin with fluconazole and cotrimoxazole (trimethoprim-sulfamethoxazole) in healthy volunteers. *Clin Drug Invest* (2000) 20, 135–42.
2. Purkins L, Wood N, Ghahramani P, Kleinermans D, Layton G, Nichols. No clinically significant effect of erythromycin or azithromycin on the pharmacokinetics of voriconazole in healthy male volunteers. *Br J Clin Pharmacol* (2003) 56, 30–6.
3. Gustavson LE, Shi H, Palmer RN, Siepman NC, Craft JC. Drug interaction between clarithromycin and fluconazole in healthy subjects. *Clin Pharmacol Ther* (1996) 59, 185.
4. Hardin TC, Summers KS, Rinaldi MG, Sharkey PK. Evaluation of the pharmacokinetic interaction between itraconazole and clarithromycin following chronic oral dosing in HIV-infected patients. *Pharmacotherapy* (1997) 17, 195.
5. Sporanox Capsules (Itraconazole). Janssen. US Prescribing information, June 2006.
6. Shi J, Montay G, Leroy B, Bhargava V. Effects of ketoconazole and itraconazole on the pharmacokinetics of telithromycin, a new ketolide antibiotic. *Intersci Conf Antimicrob Agents Chemother* (2002) 42, 28.
7. Shi J, Chapel S, Montay G, Hardy P, Barrett JS, Sica D, Swan SK, Noveck R, Leroy B, Bhargava VO. Effect of ketoconazole on the pharmacokinetics and safety of telithromycin and clarithromycin in older subjects with renal impairment. *Int J Clin Pharmacol Ther* (2005) 43, 123–33.

Macrolides + Grapefruit juice

Grapefruit juice modestly increases the bioavailability of erythromycin, but does not affect the bioavailability of clarithromycin or telithromycin.

Clinical evidence

(a) Clarithromycin

In a study 12 healthy subjects were given a single 500-mg dose of clarithromycin and 240 mL of either water or freshly squeezed white grapefruit juice with and 2 hours after clarithromycin. Grapefruit juice increased the time to peak levels of both clarithromycin and its metabolite 14-hydroxy-clarithromycin from about 82 to 148 minutes and 84.5 to 172 minutes, respectively, but it did not affect the extent of clarithromycin absorption and had no significant effects on any other pharmacokinetic parameters.[1]

(b) Erythromycin

A study in 6 healthy subjects given a single 400-mg dose of erythromycin with either water or grapefruit juice found that grapefruit juice increased the AUC and maximum plasma level of erythromycin by about 49% and 52%, respectively. The time to achieve maximum levels and the half-life of erythromycin were not affected.[2]

(c) Telithromycin

A study in 16 healthy subjects given telithromycin 800 mg daily found that grapefruit juice did not affect telithromycin pharmacokinetics.[3]

Mechanism

Some components of grapefruit juice, possibly flavonoids such as naringenin, or a psoralen, dihydroxybergamottin, may inhibit the activity of the cytochrome P450 isoenzyme CYP3A4 in the gut.[1] The levels of drugs metabolised by CYP3A4, such as the macrolides, may therefore be raised by grapefruit juice. Erythromycin levels, but not those of clarithromycin or telithromycin appear to be affected by grapefruit juice. It has been suggested that a drug with low or variable bioavailability may be more likely to have its levels increased by grapefruit juice and it has been suggested that this may partly explain why the pharmacokinetics of clarithromycin (bioavailability of about 55%) and telithromycin (bioavailability of about 60%) are not significantly affected.[1]

Importance and management

Information is very limited but is would appear that there is unlikely to be a clinically significant interaction between grapefruit juice and either clarithromycin or telithromycin. The increased bioavailability of erythromycin was found in a single-dose study and it has been suggested that more prolonged administration of erythromycin with grapefruit juice could increase levels further and potentially increase the risk of adverse effects.[4] More study is needed.

1. Cheng KL, Nafziger AN, Peloquin CA, Amsden GW. Effect of grapefruit juice on clarithromycin pharmacokinetics. *Antimicrob Agents Chemother* (1998) 42, 927–9.
2. Kanazawa S, Ohkubo T, Sugawara K. The effects of grapefruit juice on the pharmacokinetics of erythromycin. *Eur J Clin Pharmacol* (2001) 56, 799–803.
3. Shi J, Montay G, Leroy B, Bhargava VO. Effects of itraconazole or grapefruit juice on the pharmacokinetics of telithromycin. *Pharmacotherapy* (2005) 25, 42–51.
4. Amory JK, Amory DW. Oral erythromycin and the risk of sudden death. *N Engl J Med* (2005) 352, 302–3.

Macrolides + H_2-receptor antagonists

Cimetidine doubled the serum levels of erythromycin in one single-dose study, and a single case report describes reversible deafness, which was attributed to this interaction. No clinically significant interaction appears to occur when cimetidine is given with azithromycin or clarithromycin, or when ranitidine is given with clarithromycin, roxithromycin, or telithromycin.

Clinical evidence

(a) Cimetidine

A 64-year-old woman was admitted to hospital with cough, dyspnoea and pleuritic pain and was found to have an atypical pneumonia and renal impairment. All her antihypertensive treatment (methyldopa, propranolol, co-amilofruse) was stopped, due to hypotension, and her treatment for duodenal ulcer was changed from ranitidine 150 mg twice daily to cimetidine 400 mg at night. She was then started on amoxicillin 500 mg three times daily and **erythromycin** stearate 1 g four times daily. Two days later she complained of 'fuzzy hearing' and audiometry showed a bilateral hearing loss. The **erythromycin** was stopped and her hearing returned to normal after 5 days.[1] This prompted a study of this possible interaction in 8 healthy subjects, which found that cimetidine 400 mg twice daily increased the AUC of a single 250-mg dose of **erythromycin** by 73%. Maximum serum **erythromycin** levels were doubled.[1]

The pharmacokinetics of **azithromycin** were not affected by a single 800-mg dose of cimetidine in one study,[2] and although cimetidine prolongs the absorption of **clarithromycin**, this is unlikely to be of clinical significance.[3]

(b) Ranitidine

The pharmacokinetics of **clarithromycin**,[4] **roxithromycin**[5] and **telithromycin**[6,7] are reported to be unaffected by ranitidine.

Mechanism

Cimetidine is known to inhibit the *N*-demethylation of erythromycin so that it is metabolised and cleared from the body more slowly and its serum levels rise. Deafness is known to be one of the adverse effects of erythromycin,[1] which usually occurs with high-doses or intravenous therapy, and was probably exacerbated by renal impairment[4] in the patient described above.

Importance and management

Clinical information about an interaction between cimetidine and erythromycin seems to be limited to this case and the associated single-dose study. The manufacturers[8] say that reversible hearing loss has been reported with erythromycin alone, usually in high doses (greater than 4 g daily[9]), usually when given by the intravenous route,[9] and in patients with renal impairment.[8] Most UK manufacturers do not include this interaction in their product information, and evidence for an interaction seems limited.

If deafness were to occur, the management would seem to be similar (withdraw the erythromycin) regardless of whether or not cimetidine was present, so no additional precautions seem necessary.

There is evidence that azithromycin and clarithromycin do not interact, and ranitidine does not interact with clarithromycin, roxithromycin or telithromycin. No interaction would be expected between the macrolides and other non-enzyme inducing H_2-receptor antagonists.

1. Mogford N, Pallett A, George C. Erythromycin deafness and cimetidine treatment. *BMJ* (1994) 309, 1620.
2. Foulds G, Hilligoss DM, Henry EB, Gerber N. The effects of an antacid or cimetidine on the serum concentrations of azithromycin. *J Clin Pharmacol* (1991) 31, 164–7.
3. Amsden GW, Cheng KL, Peloquin CA, Nafziger AN. Oral cimetidine prolongs clarithromycin absorption. *Antimicrob Agents Chemother* (1998) 42, 1578–80.
4. Zündorf H, Wischmann L, Fassenbender M, Lode H, Borner K, Koeppe P. Pharmacokinetics of clarithromycin and possible interaction with H_2 blockers and antacids. *Intersci Conf Antimicrob Agents Chemother* (1991) 31, 185.
5. Boeckh M, Lode H, Höffken G, Daeschlein S, Koeppe P. Pharmacokinetics of roxithromycin and influence of H_2-blockers and antacids on gastrointestinal absorption. *Eur J Clin Microbiol Infect Dis* (1992) 11, 465–8.
6. Ketek (Telithromycin). Sanofi-Aventis US LLC. US Prescribing information, May 2007.
7. Ketek (Telithromycin). Sanofi-Aventis. UK Summary of product characteristics, May 2007.
8. PCE (Erythromycin particles in tablets). Abbott Laboratories. US Prescribing information, September 2006.
9. Erymax Capsules (Erythromycin). Cephalon Ltd. UK Summary of product characteristics, December 2006.

Macrolides + Penicillins

Some *in vitro* evidence suggests that antagonism may occur between erythromycin (a bacteriostatic drug) and penicillins (bactericidal drugs) when they are used against staphylococci[1] and *Streptococcus pneumoniae*.[2] However, another study has suggested that this *in vitro* antagonism against *S. pneumoniae* between 'penicillin' and erythromycin is minimal and dependent on the interpretative criteria applied.[3] Clinical evidence for this interaction is apparently lacking, and the combination is generally used successfully for pneumonia.[4] In the UK, the combination of amoxicillin and erythromycin or another macrolide (e.g. azithromycin or clarithromycin) has been recommended by the British Thoracic Society (BTS) for adult patients with non-severe community-acquired pneumonia who require hospital admission.[5] More recently the BTS has recommended an intravenous combination of a beta-lactamase stable antibacterial such as co-amoxiclav (amoxicillin with clavulanic acid) with a macrolide (erythromycin or clarithromycin) for severe community-acquired pneumonia in hospitalised patients.[6]

1. Manten A. Synergism and antagonism between antibiotic mixtures containing erythromycin. *Antibiot Chemother* (1954) 4, 1228–33.
2. Johansen HK, Jensen TG, Dessau RB, Lundgren B, Frimodt-Møller N. Antagonism between penicillin and erythromycin against Streptococcus pneumoniae in vitro and in vivo. *J Antimicrob Chemother* (2000) 46, 973–80.
3. Deshpande LM, Jones RN. Antagonism between penicillin and erythromycin against Streptococcus pneumoniae: Does it exist? *Diagn Microbiol Infect Dis* (2003) 46, 223–5.
4. Feldman C. Clinical relevance of antimicrobial resistance in the management of pneumococcal community-acquired pneumonia. *J Lab Clin Med* (2004) 143, 269–83.
5. British Thoracic Society. BTS Guidelines for the management of community acquired pneumonia in adults. *Thorax* (2001) 56 (suppl IV) iv1–iv64.
6. British Thoracic Society. BTS Guidelines for the management of community acquired pneumonia in adults – 2004 update. Available at http://www.brit-thoracic.org.uk/c2/uploads/MACAPrevisedApr04.pdf (accessed 17/08/07).

Macrolides + Rifamycins

Rifabutin and azithromycin seem not to affect the serum levels of each other, but a very high incidence of neutropenia was seen in one study of the combination. Both rifabutin and rifampicin markedly reduce the serum levels of clarithromycin. Clarithromycin increases the serum levels of rifabutin and the combination is associated with an increased risk of uveitis and neutropenia. Rifampicin (rifampin) greatly reduces telithromycin levels and concurrent use is not recommended.

Clinical evidence

(a) Rifabutin

1. Neutropenia. A study in 12 healthy subjects was designed to investigate the safety and possible interactions between rifabutin 300 mg daily, and **azithromycin** 250 mg daily or **clarithromycin** 500 mg twice daily, for a course of 14 days. The subjects were matched against 18 healthy controls who received either of the macrolides or rifabutin alone. The study had to be abandoned after 10 days because 14 patients developed neutropenia; 2 taking rifabutin alone, and all 12 of those taking rifabutin with a macrolide. Eight subjects developed a fever, 5 required colony simulating factors, and 3 required hospitalisation.[1]

2. Pharmacokinetics. In a study[2] investigating a possible regimen for the prophylaxis of *Mycobacterium avium* complex (MAC) disease, 12 HIV-positive patients were treated with **clarithromycin** 500 mg daily, to which rifabutin 300 mg daily was added on day 15. By day 42 the **clarithromycin** AUC had fallen by 44%, and levels of the metabolite, 14-hydroxyclarithromycin, had risen by 57%. A related study[2] in 14 patients given **clarithromycin** 500 mg every 12 hours and rifabutin 300 mg daily found that after 28 days the AUC of the rifabutin had increased by 99%, and the AUC of the active metabolite, 25-*O*-desacetyl-rifabutin, had increased by 375%. Another group of patients with lung disease due to MAC were treated with **clarithromycin** 500 mg twice daily. When rifabutin 600 mg was added the **clarithromycin** levels fell by 63% (from 5.4 to 2 micrograms/mL).[3] Limited information from a randomised study in healthy subjects found similar results.[1,4] Fluconazole appears to further increase the effects of clarithromycin on rifabutin.[4] One study suggests that there is no pharmacokinetic interaction between **azithromycin** and rifabutin.[1]

3. Uveitis or arthralgias. Uveitis, and in some cases pseudojaundice, aphthous stomatitis and an arthralgia syndrome have been described in patients treated with both **clarithromycin** 1 to 2 g daily and rifabutin 300 to 600 mg daily.[5-8] The presence of fluconazole does not appear to affect the development of uveitis in patients taking clarithromycin with rifabutin,[6,7,9] but it has been suggested that this was because only small doses (50 mg) were used.[7]

Reports suggest that uveitis develops between 27 to 370 days after taking the combination.[6,7] The reaction appears to be dose-dependent. In patients taking rifabutin 600 mg with clarithromycin the incidence of uveitis was 14% in patients weighing more than 65 kg, 45% in those weighing between 55 and 65 kg and 64% in those weighing less than 55 kg. The risk of developing uveitis was reduced from a mean of 43% to 13% when the dose of rifabutin was reduced to 300 mg daily.[9]

Uveitis did not develop in 8 patients taking rifabutin and **azithromycin** 500 mg daily,[7] although cases of uveitis have been reported in patients taking rifabutin, fluconazole, and **azithromycin** 1.2 g weekly but they have been attributed to an interaction between rifabutin and fluconazole.[10] See 'Azoles + Rifabutin', p.219.

(b) Rifampicin (Rifampin)

Patients with lung disease due to MAC were treated with **clarithromycin** 500 mg twice daily. When rifampicin 600 mg daily was added, the mean serum levels of **clarithromycin** fell by almost 90% (from 5.4 to 0.7 micrograms/mL).[3] Similar results are reported in another study.[11]

The manufacturer notes that rifampicin reduces the AUC and maximum serum levels of **telithromycin** by 86% and 79%, respectively.[12]

Two cases of cholestatic jaundice have been reported in patients taking rifampicin with **troleandomycin**.[13,14]

Mechanism

Both rifabutin and rifampicin are known enzyme inducers, which can increase the metabolism of other drugs by the liver, thereby reducing their serum levels. Rifampicin is recognised as being the more potent inducer. Rifabutin is also a substrate for cytochrome P450 isoenzyme CYP3A4. Both clarithromycin and fluconazole are inhibitors of CYP3A4 and it is probable that clarithromycin and fluconazole exert additive effects resulting in greater inhibition of rifabutin metabolism than occurs with either drug alone.[4]

The reason for the uveitis is not known, but based on *animal* studies it has been suggested that it is associated with effective treatment of MAC and is due to release of a mycobacterial protein, rather than a toxic effect of the drugs.[15] It has been suggested that lower body weight and concurrent clarithromycin may result in toxic rifabutin serum levels, although concurrent fluconazole which increases levels does not appear to be a factor.[9] The hepatotoxicity seen with rifampicin and troleandomycin is probably due to additive effects as both drugs are known to be hepatotoxic.

Importance and management

(a) Rifabutin and Rifampicin: Pharmacokinetics

Direct information appears to be limited to the reports cited but the interactions would appear to be established. What is not entirely clear is whether these interactions result in treatment failures because of the potentially subtherapeutic clarithromycin serum levels. Because of the lack of information, be alert for evidence of reduced efficacy if clarithromycin and rifampicin are used.

Although rifabutin can lower clarithromycin levels, the efficacy of this combination for MAC infection is established, although not without risk, see *Uveitis*, below. Clarithromycin raises rifabutin levels and therefore increases the risks of adverse effects. Concurrent use may therefore be desirable, but monitoring for adverse effects is necessary.

Due to a pharmacokinetic interaction the UK manufacturers recommend that telithromycin should not be given during and for 2 weeks after the use of rifampicin.[12]

(b) Rifabutin: Neutropenia

Information regarding neutropenia with macrolides and rifamycins is very limited but what is known suggests that white cell counts should be monitored closely if rifabutin is given with azithromycin or clarithromycin. Rifabutin is known to cause polyarthritis on rare occasions, but in conjunction with clarithromycin it appears to happen at much lower doses.[8] Careful monitoring is necessary.

(c) Rifabutin: Uveitis

The CSM in the UK has warned about the need to be aware of the increased risk of uveitis with clarithromycin and rifabutin[16] and of the raised rifabutin levels. If uveitis occurs the CSM recommends that rifabutin should be stopped and the patient should be referred to an ophthalmologist.[16] Because of the increased risk of uveitis they also say that consideration should be given to reducing the dosage of rifabutin to 300 mg daily in the presence of macrolides.[16] Later review and a case-control study suggest that this dose is associated with a reduced risk of uveitis and maintains efficacy.[9,17]

1. Apseloff G, Foulds G, LaBoy-Goral L, Willavize S, Vincent J. Comparison of azithromycin and clarithromycin in their interactions with rifabutin in healthy volunteers. *J Clin Pharmacol* (1998) 38, 830–5.
2. Hafner R, Bethel J, Power M, Landry B, Banach M, Mole L, Standiford HC, Follansbee S, Kumar P, Raasch R, Cohn D, Mushatt D, Drusano G. Tolerance and pharmacokinetic interactions of rifabutin and clarithromycin in human immunodeficiency virus-infected volunteers. *Antimicrob Agents Chemother* (1998) 42, 631–9.
3. Wallace RJ, Brown BA, Griffith DE, Girard W, Tanaka K. Reduced serum levels of clarithromycin in patients treated with multidrug regimens including rifampin or rifabutin for *Mycobacterium avium-M. intracellulare* infection. *J Infect Dis* (1995) 171, 747–50.
4. Jordan MK, Polis MA, Kelly G, Narang PK, Masur H, Piscitelli SC. Effects of fluconazole and clarithromycin on rifabutin and 25-O-desacetylrifabutin pharmacokinetics. *Antimicrob Agents Chemother* (2000) 44, 2170–2.
5. Shafran SD, Deschênes J, Miller M, Phillips P, Toma E. Uveitis and pseudojaundice during a regimen of clarithromycin, rifabutin, and ethambutol. *N Engl J Med* (1994) 330, 438–9.
6. Becker K, Schimkat M, Jablonowski H, Häussinger D. Anterior uveitis associated with rifabutin medication in AIDS patients. *Infection* (1996) 24, 34–6.
7. Kelleher P, Helbert M, Sweeney J, Anderson J, Parkin J, Pinching A. Uveitis associated with rifabutin and macrolide therapy for *Mycobacterium avium intracellulare* infections in AIDS patients. *Genitourin Med* (1996) 72, 419–21.
8. Le Gars L, Collon T, Picard O, Kaplan G, Berenbaum F. Polyarthralgia-arthritis syndrome induced by low doses of rifabutin. *J Rheumatol* (1999) 26, 1201–2.
9. Shafran SD, Singer J, Zarowny DP, Deschênes J, Phillips P, Turgeon F, Aoki FY, Toma E, Miller M, Duperval R, Lemieux C, Schlech WF, for the Canadian HIV Trials Network Protocol 010 Study Group. Determinants of rifabutin-associated uveitis in patients treated with rifabutin, clarithromycin, and ethambutol for *Mycobacterium avium* complex bacteremia: a multivariate analysis. *J Infect Dis* (1998) 177, 252–5.
10. Havlir D, Torriani F, Dubé M. Uveitis associated with rifabutin prophylaxis. *Ann Intern Med* (1994) 121, 510–12.
11. Yamamoto F, Harada S, Mitsuyama T, Harada Y, Kitahara Y, Yoshida M, Nakanishi Y. Concentration of clarithromycin and 14-R-hydroxyclarithromycin in plasma of patients with *Mycobacterium avium* complex infection, before and after the addition of rifampicin. *Jpn J Antibiot* (2004) 57, 124–33.
12. Ketek (Telithromycin). Sanofi-Aventis. UK Summary of product characteristics, May 2007.
13. Piette F, Peyrard P. Ictère bénin médicamenteux lors d'un traitement associant rifampicine-triacétyloléandomycine. *Nouv Presse Med* (1979) 8, 368–9.
14. Givaudan JF, Gamby T, Privat Y. Ictère cholestatique après association rifampicine-troléandomycine: une nouvelle observation. *Nouv Presse Med* (1979) 8, 2357.
15. Opremcak EM, Cynamon M. Uveitogenic activity of rifabutin and clarithromycin in the *Mycobacterium avium*-infected beige mice. Am Soc Microbiol 2nd Nat Conf. Human retroviruses and related infections. Washington DC, Jan 29—Feb 2 1995, 74.
16. Committee on the Safety of Medicines. Rifabutin (Mycobutin) – uveitis. *Current Problems* (1994) 20, 4.
17. Committee on Safety of Medicines/Medicines Control Agency. Revised indications and drug interactions of rifabutin. *Current Problems* (1997) 23, 14.

Macrolides; Azithromycin + Ceftriaxone

A study in healthy subjects found that there did not appear to be a pharmacokinetic interaction between steady-state intravenous azithromycin and ceftriaxone and the combination was well-tolerated.[1]

1. Chiu LM, Menhinick AM, Johnson PW, Amsden GW. Pharmacokinetics of intravenous azithromycin and ceftriaxone when administered alone and concurrently to healthy volunteers. *J Antimicrob Chemother* (2002) 50, 1075–9.

Macrolides; Azithromycin + Chloroquine

A study in which healthy subjects were given azithromycin 1 g daily for 3 days either alone or with chloroquine base 600 mg daily on days 1 and 2, and 300 mg on day 3, found no pharmacokinetic interaction.[1]

1. Cook JA, Randinitis EJ, Bramson CR, Wesche DL. Lack of a pharmacokinetic interaction between azithromycin and chloroquine. *Am J Trop Med Hyg* (2006) 74, 407–12.

Macrolides; Azithromycin + Food

Food appears to halve azithromycin absorption from the capsule formulation, but does not alter the AUC of tablets or suspension.

Clinical evidence, mechanism, importance and management

A review by the manufacturers briefly mentions that food reduced the absorption of azithromycin by about half.[1] It is suggested therefore that azithromycin *capsules* should not be given at the same time as food, but should be taken at least 1 hour before or 2 hours after a meal.[1,2] However, the US prescribing information states that a high-fat meal increased the maximum levels of azithromycin *tablets* by 23%, and had no effect on the AUC.[3] Similarly, food increased the maximum levels of azithromycin *suspension* by 56%, without altering the AUC.[3] Azithromycin suspension[2,3] and tablets[3] may therefore be taken without regard to food.

1. Hopkins S. Clinical toleration and safety of azithromycin. *Am J Med* (1991) 91 (Suppl 3A), 40S–45S.
2. Zithromax (Azithromycin). Pfizer Ltd. UK Summary of product characteristics, July 2006.
3. Zithromax (Azithromycin). Pfizer Inc. US Prescribing information, March 2007.

Macrolides; Clarithromycin + Disulfiram

Fatal toxic epidermal necrolysis and fulminant hepatitis occurred in a patient taking disulfiram and clarithromycin.

Clinical evidence, mechanism, importance and management

A 47-year-old man who had taken disulfiram 250 mg daily for about a month, with clarithromycin 500 mg twice daily and paracetamol 500 mg three times daily for one week ,developed fatal toxic epidermal necrolysis and fulminant hepatitis. He had not drunk alcohol for several weeks and although he was taking paracetamol, the dose was below the toxic range and therefore an interaction between disulfiram and clarithromycin was considered probable.[1]

Disulfiram alone may cause hepatic toxicity, possibly as the result of hypersensitivity or toxic metabolites. It was suggested that inhibition of cytochrome P450 isoenzyme CYP3A4 by clarithromycin could have resulted in the accumulation of toxic metabolites of disulfiram. Hepatocellular damage is uncommon in patients receiving clarithromycin alone, but may occur in patients with underlying disease. Both clarithromycin and disulfiram alone may cause adverse skin reactions, but neither has been reported to cause toxic epidermal necrolysis. The reason why this should occur with concurrent use is not understood.[1] Information seems to be limited to this single report, so no general conclusions can be drawn.

1. Masiá M, Guliérrez F, Jimeno A, Navarro A, Borrás J, Matarredona J, Martín-Hidalgo A. Fulminant hepatitis and fatal toxic epidermal necrolysis (Lyell disease) coincident with clarithromycin administration in an alcoholic patient receiving disulfiram therapy. *Arch Intern Med* (2002) 162, 474–6.

Macrolides; Erythromycin + Carbimazole

An isolated case describes torsade de pointes in an elderly patient taking carbimazole and oral erythromycin.

Clinical evidence

A 75-year-old woman with known mild mitral stenosis taking digoxin, furosemide, warfarin and carbimazole was given oral erythromycin 250 mg four times daily for a urinary tract infection. Three days later she experienced presyncopal episodes, and 4 days later she was admitted to hospital with syncope and self-terminating episodes of torsade de pointes. She completed the 7-day course of erythromycin on the day before admission. Five days after admission, when the QT interval was back to normal, she was inadvertently rechallenged with erythromycin, given as prophylaxis before permanent pacemaker insertion. After two doses of erythromycin 500 mg given at an interval of 6 hours, she developed torsade de pointes associated with a prolonged QT interval (QTc 612 milliseconds). The QT interval returned to normal 4 days after erythromycin was discontinued.[1]

Mechanism

Intravenous erythromycin may cause QT prolongation and torsade de pointes. It is rare with oral erythromycin. Carbimazole is rapidly metabolised to thiamazole which is the active form of the drug. Thiamazole inhibits cytochrome P450 isoenzymes including CYP3A4 and it may therefore have inhibited the metabolism of erythromycin resulting in higher than normal levels. In addition, hypothyroidism can cause torsade de pointes, and therefore mild hypothyroidism induced by carbimazole could have contributed.[1] Furthermore, bradycardia (heart rate less than 60 bpm) may also have contributed.

Importance and management

It was suggested that the combination of oral erythromycin and carbimazole could lead to torsade de pointes in susceptible individuals. In this case, female sex, presence of valvular heart disease, bradycardia, hypokalaemia, and hypothyroidism may all have been contributory factors.[1] See also, 'Drugs that prolong the QT interval + Other drugs that prolong the QT interval', p.257.

1. Koh TW. Risk of torsades de pointes from oral erythromycin with concomitant carbimazole (methimazole) administration. *PACE* (2001) 24, 1575–6.

Macrolides; Erythromycin + Sucralfate

Sucralfate does not appear to affect the pharmacokinetics of erythromycin.

Clinical evidence, mechanism, importance and management

The pharmacokinetics (elimination rate constant, half-life, AUC) of a single 400-mg dose of erythromycin ethylsuccinate were not significantly altered by a single 1-g dose of sucralfate in 6 healthy subjects. It was concluded that the therapeutic effects of erythromycin are unlikely to be affected by concurrent use.[1]

1. Miller LG, Prichard JG, White CA, Vytla B, Feldman S, Bowman RC. Effect of concurrent sucralfate administration on the absorption of erythromycin. *J Clin Pharmacol* (1990) 30, 39–44.

Macrolides; Erythromycin + Urinary acidifiers or alkalinisers

In the treatment of urinary tract infections, the antibacterial activity of erythromycin is maximal in alkaline urine and minimal in acidic urine.

Clinical evidence

Urine taken from 7 subjects receiving erythromycin 1 g every 8 hours, was tested against 5 genera of Gram-negative bacilli (*Escherichia coli, Klebsiella pneumoniae, P. mirabilis, Ps. aeruginosa* and *Serratia* sp.) both before and after treatment with **acetazolamide** or **sodium bicarbonate**, given to alkalinise the urine. A direct correlation was found between the activity of the antibacterial and the pH of the urine. In general, acidic urine had little or no antibacterial activity, whereas alkalinised urine had activity.[1]

Clinical studies have confirmed the increased antibacterial effectiveness of erythromycin in the treatment of bacteriuria when the urine is made alkaline.[2,3]

Mechanism

The pH of the urine does not apparently affect the way the kidney handles the antibacterial (most of it is excreted actively rather than passively) but it does have a direct influence on the way the antibacterial affects the micro-organisms. Mechanisms suggested include effects on bacterial cell receptors, the induction of active transport mechanisms on bacterial cell walls, and changes in ionisation of the antibacterial, which enables it to enter the bacterial cell more effectively.

Importance and management

An established interaction, which can be exploited. Should erythromycin be used to treat urinary tract infections its efficacy can be maximised by making the urine alkaline (for example with acetazolamide or sodium bicarbonate). Treatment with urinary acidifiers will minimise the activity of the erythromycin for urinary tract infections and should be avoided. There is no evidence that the efficacy of erythromycin in other infections is affected by urinary acidifiers or alkalinisers.

1. Sabath LD, Gerstein DA, Loder PB, Finland M. Excretion of erythromycin and its enhanced activity in urine against gram-negative bacilli with alkalinization. *J Lab Clin Med* (1968) 72, 916–23.
2. Zinner SH, Sabath LD, Casey JI, Finland M. Erythromycin and alkalinisation of the urine in the treatment of urinary-tract infections due to gram-negative bacilli. *Lancet* (1971) i, 1267–8.
3. Zinner SH, Sabath LD, Casey JI, Finland M. Erythromycin plus alkalinization in treatment of urinary infections. *Antimicrob Agents Chemother* (1969) 9, 413–16.

Methenamine + Urinary acidifiers or alkalinisers

Urinary alkalinisers (e.g. potassium or sodium citrate) and those antacids that can raise the urinary pH above 5.5 should not be used during treatment with methenamine because they inhibit its activation.

Clinical evidence, mechanism, importance and management

Methenamine and methenamine mandelate are only effective as urinary antiseptics if the pH is about 5.5 or lower, when formaldehyde is released. This is normally achieved by giving urinary acidifiers such as ammonium chloride, ascorbic acid,[1,2] or sodium acid phosphate. In the case of methenamine hippurate, the acidification of the urine is achieved by the presence of hippuric acid. The concurrent use of substances that raise the urinary pH such as **acetazolamide**, **sodium bicarbonate**, **potassium** or **sodium citrate** is clearly contraindicated. **Potassium citrate mixture BPC** has been shown to raise the pH by more than 1 at normal therapeutic doses, thereby making the urine sufficiently alkaline to interfere with the activation of methenamine to formaldehyde.[3] Some **antacids** (containing magnesium, aluminium or calcium as well as sodium bicarbonate mentioned above) can also cause a significant rise in the pH of the urine.[4]

1. Strom JG, Jun HW. Effect of urine pH and ascorbic acid on the rate of conversion of methenamine to formaldehyde. *Biopharm Drug Dispos* (1993) 14, 61–9.
2. Nahata MC, Cummins BA, McLeod DC, Schondelmeyer SW, Butler R. Effect of urinary acidifiers on formaldehyde concentration and efficacy with methenamine therapy. *Eur J Clin Pharmacol* (1982) 22, 281–4.
3. Lipton JH. Incompatibility between sulfamethizole and methenamine mandelate. *N Engl J Med* (1963) 268, 92.
4. Blondheim SH, Alkan WJ, Brunner D, eds. Frontiers of Internal Medicine. 1974. Basel: Karger; 1975 p. 404–8.

Metronidazole + Antacids, Colestyramine or Kaolin-pectin

The absorption of metronidazole is unaffected by kaolin-pectin, but it is slightly reduced by an aluminium hydroxide antacid and colestyramine, although not to a clinically relevant extent.

Clinical evidence, mechanism, importance and management

The bioavailability of a single 500-mg dose of metronidazole in 5 healthy subjects was not significantly changed by 30 mL of a kaolin-pectin antidiarrhoeal mixture. However, a 14.5% reduction in metronidazole bioavailability occurred with 30 mL of an **aluminium hydroxide/simeticone** suspension, and a 21.3% reduction occurred with a single 4-g dose of colestyramine.[1] The clinical importance of these reductions is probably small, and no special precautions seem necessary.

1. Molokhia AM, Al-Rahman S. Effect of concomitant oral administration of some adsorbing drugs on the bioavailability of metronidazole. *Drug Dev Ind Pharm* (1987) 13, 1229–37.

Metronidazole + Barbiturates

Phenobarbital markedly increases the metabolism of metronidazole and treatment failure has been reported in both adults and children.

Clinical evidence

A woman with vaginal trichomoniasis was given metronidazole on several occasions over the course of a year, but the infection flared up again as soon as it was stopped. When it was realised that she was also taking **phenobarbital** 100 mg daily, the metronidazole dosage was doubled to 500 mg three times daily, and she was cured after a 7-day course.[1] A pharmacokinetic study found that the clearance of metronidazole was increased (half-life 3.5 hours compared with the normal half-life of 8 to 9 hours).[1]

A retrospective study in children who had not responded to metronidazole for giardiasis or amoebiasis found that 80% of them had been taking long-term **phenobarbital**. In a prospective study in 36 children the normal recommended metronidazole dosage had to be increased approximately threefold to 60 mg/kg to achieve a cure. The half-life of metronidazole in 15 other children taking **phenobarbital** was found to be 3.5 hours compared with the normal half-life of 8 to 9 hours.[2]

Other studies in patients with Crohn's disease and healthy subjects have shown that **phenobarbital** reduces the AUC of metronidazole by about one-third,[3] and increases the clearance of metronidazole 1.5-fold.[4]

Mechanism

Phenobarbital is a known, potent liver enzyme inducer, which increases the metabolism and clearance of metronidazole from the body.

Importance and management

An established and clinically important interaction. Monitor the effects of concurrent use and anticipate the need to increase the metronidazole dosage two to threefold if phenobarbital is given. All of the barbiturates are potent liver enzyme inducers and would therefore be expected to interact similarly.

1. Mead PB, Gibson M, Schentag JJ, Ziemniak JA. Possible alteration of metronidazole metabolism by phenobarbital. *N Engl J Med* (1982) 306, 1490.
2. Gupte S. Phenobarbital and metabolism of metronidazole. *N Engl J Med* (1983) 308, 529.
3. Eradiri O, Jamali F, Thomson ABR. Interaction of metronidazole with phenobarbital, cimetidine, prednisone, and sulfasalazine in Crohn's disease. *Biopharm Drug Dispos* (1988) 9, 219–27.
4. Loft S, Sonne J, Poulsen HE, Petersen KT, Jørgensen BG, Døssing M. Inhibition and induction of metronidazole and antipyrine metabolism. *Eur J Clin Pharmacol* (1987) 32, 35–41.

Metronidazole + Chloroquine

An isolated report describes acute dystonia in one patient, which was attributed to an interaction between metronidazole and chloroquine.

Clinical evidence, mechanism, importance and management

A patient was given a 7-day course of metronidazole and ampicillin, following a laparoscopic investigation. She developed acute dystonic reactions (facial grimacing, coarse tremors, and an inability to maintain posture) on day 6, within 10 minutes of being given chloroquine phosphate (equivalent to 200 mg of base) and intramuscular promethazine 25 mg. The dystonic symptoms started to subside within 15 minutes of being given diazepam 5 mg intravenously, and had completely resolved within 2 hours.[1]

The authors of the report attribute the dystonia to an interaction between metronidazole and chloroquine as she had taken both drugs alone without adverse effect. However, they do not fully assess the possible contribution of **promethazine**, which is known to cause dystonias. It is therefore possible that the reaction seen was an adverse effect of the **promethazine**, or perhaps even an interaction between **promethazine** and chloroquine. No general recommendations can therefore be made from this single report.

1. Achumba JI, Ette EI, Thomas WOA, Essien EE. Chloroquine-induced acute dystonic reactions in the presence of metronidazole. *Drug Intell Clin Pharm* (1988) 22, 308–10.

Metronidazole or Tinidazole + Cimetidine

Cimetidine reduces the metabolism of tinidazole, and possibly also metronidazole, but this is probably not clinically important.

Clinical evidence

(a) Metronidazole

The half-life of a 400-mg intravenous dose of metronidazole was increased from 6.2 to 7.9 hours in 6 healthy subjects after they took cimetidine 400 mg twice daily for 6 days. The total plasma clearance was reduced by almost 30%.[1] However, in another study in 6 patients with Crohn's disease, cimetidine 600 mg twice daily for 7 days was found not to affect either the AUC or the half-life of metronidazole,[2] and no evidence of an interaction was found in a further study in 6 healthy subjects.[3]

(b) Tinidazole

In a study in 6 healthy subjects cimetidine 400 mg twice daily for 7 days raised the peak serum levels of a single 600-mg dose of tinidazole by 21%, increased the 24-hour AUC by 40% and increased the half-life by 47%, from 7.66 to 11.23 hours.[4]

Mechanism

Cimetidine is a well known enzyme inhibitor, which probably inhibits the metabolism of the metronidazole and tinidazole by the liver.

Importance and management

The modest changes in the pharmacokinetics of tinidazole with cimetidine seem unlikely to be clinically significant, but bear them in mind in the case of an unexpected response to treatment. The interaction between metronidazole and cimetidine is not established, but any changes in metronidazole pharmacokinetics seem to be modest and unlikely to be important.

1. Gugler R, Jensen JC. Interaction between cimetidine and metronidazole. *N Engl J Med* (1983) 309, 1518–19.
2. Eradiri O, Jamali F, Thomson ABR. Interaction of metronidazole with phenobarbital, cimetidine, prednisone, and sulfasalazine in Crohn's disease. *Biopharm Drug Dispos* (1988) 9, 219–27.
3. Loft S, Døssing M, Sonne J, Dalhof K, Bjerrum K, Poulsen HE. Lack of effect of cimetidine on the pharmacokinetics and metabolism of a single oral dose of metronidazole. *Eur J Clin Pharmacol* (1988) 35, 65–8.
4. Patel RB, Shah GF, Raval JD, Gandhi TP, Gilbert RN. The effect of cimetidine and rifampicin on tinidazole kinetics in healthy human volunteers. *Indian Drugs* (1986) 23, 338–41.

Metronidazole + Diosmin

Diosmin reduces the metabolism of metronidazole to some extent, but the clinical importance of this is probably small.

Clinical evidence, mechanism, importance and management

A single 800-mg dose of metronidazole was given to 12 healthy subjects following 9 days of treatment with diosmin 500 mg daily. The metronidazole AUC and maximum plasma concentrations were raised by 27% and 25%, respectively.[1] This interaction is thought to occur because of an inhibitory effect of diosmin on metronidazole metabolism by hepatic enzymes, and inhibition of P-glycoprotein. The increase in metronidazole levels is similar to that seen with other drugs (e.g. 'cimetidine' (above)) that are not considered to be clinically significant. Therefore no clinically significant interaction is likely to occur if metronidazole is given with diosmin.

1. Rajnarayana K, Reddy MS, Krishna DR. Diosmin pretreatment affects bioavailability of metronidazole. *Eur J Clin Pharmacol* (2003) 58, 803–807.

Metronidazole + Disulfiram

Acute psychoses and confusion can be caused by the concurrent use of metronidazole and disulfiram.

Clinical evidence, mechanism, importance and management

In a double-blind study in 58 hospitalised chronic alcoholics taking disulfiram, 29 patients were also given metronidazole 750 mg daily for a month, then 250 mg daily thereafter. Six of the 29 subjects in the group receiving metronidazole developed acute psychoses or confusion. Five of the 6 had paranoid delusions and in 3 visual and auditory hallucinations were also seen. The symptoms persisted for 2 to 3 days after the drugs were withdrawn, but disappeared at the end of a fortnight and did not reappear when disulfiram alone was restarted.[1] Similar reactions have been described in two other reports.[2,3]

The reason for this interaction is not understood, but it appears to be established. Concurrent use should be avoided or very well monitored.

1. Rothstein E, Clancy DD. Toxicity of disulfiram combined with metronidazole. *N Engl J Med* (1969) 280, 1006–7.
2. Goodhue WW. Disulfiram-metronidazole (well-identified) toxicity. *N Engl J Med* (1969) 280, 1482–3.
3. Scher JM. Psychotic reaction to disulfiram. *JAMA* (1967) 201,1051.

Metronidazole + Mebendazole

A case-control study identified the concurrent use of metronidazole and mebendazole as a risk factor in an outbreak of Stevens-Johnson syndrome/toxic epidermal necrolysis.

Clinical evidence, mechanism, importance and management

A case control study was conducted in an attempt to identify risk factors associated with an outbreak of Stevens-Johnson syndrome/toxic epidermal necrolysis that occurred amongst Filipino workers in Taiwan. The risk of developing this serious condition was significantly higher in workers who had taken both metronidazole and mebendazole sometime in the preceding 6 weeks (odds ratio of 9.5). In addition, there was an increase in risk with higher doses of metronidazole.[1]

The information is limited to this report, which does not establish an interaction. However, Stevens-Johnson syndrome/toxic epidermal necrolysis is a serious condition, and therefore, the manufacturer of mebendazole states that the concurrent use of mebendazole and metronidazole should be avoided.[2] Caution would certainly seem appropriate if both drugs are considered essential.

1. Chen K-T, Twu S-J, Chang H-J, Lin R-S. Outbreak of Stevens-Johnson syndrome/toxic epidermal necrolysis associated with mebendazole and metronidazole use among Filipino laborers in Taiwan. *Am J Public Health* (2003) 93, 489–92.
2. Vermox (Mebendazole). Janssen-Cilag Ltd. UK Summary of product characteristics, June 2005.

Metronidazole + Prednisone

Prednisone modestly decreases the AUC of metronidazole.

Clinical evidence, mechanism, importance and management

In 6 patients with Crohn's disease the AUC of metronidazole 250 mg twice daily was reduced by 31% by prednisone 10 mg twice daily for 6 days, probably because prednisone induces the metabolism of metronidazole by liver enzymes.[1]

Information appears to be limited to this report and the interaction is probably of only limited clinical importance. Information about other corticosteroids is lacking.

1. Eradiri O, Jamali F, Thomson ABR. Interaction of metronidazole with phenobarbital, cimetidine, prednisone, and sulfasalazine in Crohn's disease. *Biopharm Drug Dispos* (1988) 9, 219–27.

Metronidazole or Tinidazole + Rifampicin (Rifampin)

Rifampicin modestly increases the clearance of metronidazole and tinidazole but the clinical importance of this is uncertain.

Clinical evidence

(a) Metronidazole

Intravenous metronidazole 500 mg or 1 g was given to 10 healthy subjects before and after taking rifampicin 450 mg daily for 7 days. Rifampicin reduced the AUC of metronidazole by 33% and increased its clearance by 44%. Results were the same with both metronidazole doses.[1]

(b) Tinidazole

After 6 healthy subjects took rifampicin 600 mg daily for 7 days the peak serum levels of a single 600-mg dose of tinidazole were reduced by 22%, the AUC_{0-24} was reduced by 30% and the half-life was reduced by 27% (from 7.66 to 5.6 hours).[2]

Mechanism

This interaction almost certainly occurs because rifampicin (a well-recognised and potent enzyme inducer) increases the metabolism of metronidazole and tinidazole by the liver.

Importance and management

The clinical significance of these interactions appear not to have been studied. A 30% reduction in metronidazole levels would not be expected to be of much clinical significance and there do not appear to be any reports of an interaction in practice. Rifampicin is known to act synergistically with metronidazole,[3] so it may be that any reduction in levels is offset by enhanced antimicrobial activity. Tinidazole acts very much like metronidazole, and therefore a clinically significant interaction between rifampicin and either of these drugs seems unlikely.

1. Djojosaputro M, Mustofa SS, Donatus IA, Santoso B. The effects of doses and pre-treatment with rifampicin on the elimination kinetics of metronidazole. *Eur J Pharmacol* (1990) 183, 1870–1.
2. Patel RB, Shah GF, Raval JD, Gandhi TP, Gilbert RN. The effect of cimetidine and rifampicin on tinidazole kinetics in healthy human volunteers. *Indian Drugs* (1986) 23, 338–41.
3. Metronidazole Tablets. Dumex-Alpharma A/S. UK Summary of product characteristics, October 2005.

Metronidazole + Silymarin

Silymarin (the active constituent of milk thistle) modestly reduces metronidazole levels, but the clinical significance of this is unclear.

Clinical evidence, mechanism, importance and management

Silymarin 140 mg daily was given to 12 healthy subjects for 9 days, with metronidazole 400 mg three times daily on days 7 to 10. Silymarin reduced the AUC of metronidazole and hydroxymetronidazole (a major active metabolite) by 28% and the maximum serum levels by 29% and 20%, respectively. The authors suggest that silymarin causes these pharmacokinetic changes by inducing P-glycoprotein and the cytochrome P450 isoenzyme CYP3A4, which are involved in the transport and metabolism of metronidazole.[1] The clinical significance of this interaction is unclear, but a 28% reduction in the AUC of metronidazole would not be expected to be of much clinical significance.

1. Rajnarayana K, Reddy MS, Vidyasagar J, Krishna DR. Study on the influence of silymarin pretreatment on metabolism and disposition of metronidazole. *Arzneimittelforschung* (2004) 54, 109–113.

Metronidazole + Sucralfate

Sucralfate does not alter the pharmacokinetics of metronidazole.

Clinical evidence, mechanism, importance and management

Because oral triple therapy to eradicate *H. pylori* using sucralfate instead of bismuth has yielded inconsistent results, a 5-day study was undertaken in 14 healthy subjects to investigate whether sucralfate interacts with metronidazole. It was found that sucralfate 2 g twice daily had no effect on the pharmacokinetics of a single 400-mg dose of metronidazole.[1] Sucralfate would therefore not be expected to alter the effects of metronidazole.

1. Amaral Moraes ME, De Almeida Pierossi M, Moraes MO, Bezerra FF, Ferreira De Silva CM, Dias HB, Muscará MN, De Nucci G, Pedrazzoli J. Short-term sucralfate administration does not alter the absorption of metronidazole in healthy male volunteers. *Int J Clin Pharmacol Ther* (1996) 34, 433–7.

Nitrofurantoin + Antacids

Magnesium trisilicate reduces the absorption of nitrofurantoin, but the clinical significance of this is unknown. Aluminium hydroxide is reported not to interact with nitrofurantoin. Whether other antacids interact adversely is uncertain.

Clinical evidence

Magnesium trisilicate 5 g in 150 mL of water reduced the absorption of a single 100-g oral dose of nitrofurantoin in 6 healthy subjects by more than 50%. The time during which the concentration of nitrofurantoin in the urine was at, or above 32 micrograms/mL (a level stated to be the minimum inhibitory concentration) was also reduced.[1] The amounts of nitrofurantoin adsorbed by other antacids in *in vitro* tests were as follows: **magnesium trisilicate** and **charcoal** 99%, **bismuth subcarbonate** and **talc** 50 to 53%, **kaolin** 31%, **magnesium oxide** 27%, **aluminium hydroxide** 2.5% and **calcium carbonate** 0%.[1]

A crossover study in 6 healthy subjects confirmed that **aluminium hydroxide gel** does not affect the absorption of nitrofurantoin from the gut (as measured by its excretion into the urine).[2] Another study in 10 healthy subjects found that an antacid containing **aluminium hydroxide, magnesium carbonate** and **magnesium hydroxide** reduced the absorption of nitrofurantoin by 22%.[3]

Mechanism

Antacids can, to a greater or lesser extent, adsorb nitrofurantoin onto their surfaces, as a result less is available for absorption by the gut and for excretion into the urine.

Importance and management

Information appears to be limited to these reports. There seems to be nothing in the literature confirming that a clinically important interaction occurs between nitrofurantoin and antacids. One reviewer offers the opinion that common antacid preparations are unlikely to interact with nitrofurantoin.[4]

It is not yet known whether magnesium trisilicate significantly reduces the antibacterial effectiveness of nitrofurantoin but the response should be monitored. While it is known that the antibacterial action of nitrofurantoin is increased by drugs that acidify the urine (so that reduced actions would be expected if the urine were made more alkaline by antacids) this again does not seem to have been confirmed. The results of the *in vitro* studies suggest that the possible effects of the other antacids are quite small, and aluminium hydroxide is reported not to interact.

1. Naggar VF, Khalil SA. Effect of magnesium trisilicate on nitrofurantoin absorption. *Clin Pharmacol Ther* (1979) 25, 857–63.
2. Jaffe JM, Hamilton B, Jeffers S. Nitrofurantoin-antacid interaction. *Drug Intell Clin Pharm* (1976) 10, 419–20.
3. Männistö P. The effect of crystal size, gastric content and emptying rate on the absorption of nitrofurantoin in healthy human volunteers. *Int J Clin Pharmacol Biopharm* (1978) 16, 223–8.
4. D'Arcy PF. Nitrofurantoin. *Drug Intell Clin Pharm* (1985) 19, 540–7.

Nitrofurantoin + Antigout drugs

On theoretical grounds the efficacy and toxicity of nitrofurantoin may possibly be increased by probenecid and sulfinpyrazone.

Clinical evidence, mechanism, importance and management

A study of the way the kidneys handle nitrofurantoin found that intravenous **sulfinpyrazone** 2.5 mg/kg reduced the secretion of nitrofurantoin by the kidney tubules by about 50%.[1] This reduction would be expected to reduce its urinary antibacterial efficacy, and the higher serum levels might lead to increased systemic toxicity, but there do not seem to be any reports suggesting that this represents a real problem in practice. The same situation would also seem likely with **probenecid**, but there do not appear to be any reports confirming this interaction.

The clinical importance of both of these interactions is therefore uncertain, but it would seem prudent to be alert for any evidence of reduced antibacterial efficacy and increased systemic toxicity if either sulfinpyrazone or probenecid is used with nitrofurantoin.

1. Schirmeister J, Stefani F, Willmann H, Hallauer W. Renal handling of nitrofurantoin in man. *Antimicrob Agents Chemother* (1965) 5, 223–6.

Nitrofurantoin + Antimuscarinics or Diphenoxylate

Diphenoxylate and anticholinergic drugs such as propantheline can double the absorption of nitrofurantoin in some patients, but the clinical importance of this is uncertain.

Clinical evidence, mechanism, importance and management

In 6 healthy subjects **propantheline** 30 mg given 45 minutes before nitrofurantoin approximately doubled the absorption of nitrofurantoin 100 mg (as measured by the urinary excretion).[1] In another study, **diphenoxylate** 200 mg daily for 3 days nearly doubled nitrofurantoin absorption in 2 out of 6 men.[2] **Atropine** 500 micrograms given subcutaneously 30 minutes before a single 100-mg dose of nitrofurantoin had little effect on the bioavailability of nitrofurantoin, but the absorption and excretion into the urine was delayed.[3]

It was suggested that the reduced gut motility caused by these drugs allows the nitrofurantoin to dissolve more completely so that it is absorbed by the gut more easily. Whether this is of any clinical importance is uncertain but it could possibly increase the incidence of dose-related adverse reactions. So far there appear to be no reports of any problems arising from concurrent use.

1. Jaffe JM. Effect of propantheline on nitrofurantoin absorption. *J Pharm Sci* (1975) 64, 1729–30.
2. Callahan M, Bullock FJ, Braun J, Yesair DW. Pharmacodynamics of drug interactions with diphenoxylate (Lomotil®). *Fedn Proc* (1974) 33, 513.
3. Männistö P. The effect of crystal size, gastric content and emptying rate on the absorption of nitrofurantoin in healthy human volunteers. *Int J Clin Pharmacol Biopharm* (1978) 16, 223–8.

Nitrofurantoin + Azoles

In an isolated case hepatic and pulmonary toxicity occurred when nitrofurantoin was given with fluconazole, but not with itraconazole.

Clinical evidence, mechanism, importance and management

A 73-year-old man who had taken nitrofurantoin 50 mg daily for 5 years was given **fluconazole** 150 mg weekly for onychomycosis. At the start of treatment with **fluconazole** his hepatic enzyme levels were slightly raised, and 3 weeks later they were increased more than twofold. Two months after starting **fluconazole** the patient's hepatic enzyme levels had increased fivefold and he had fatigue, dyspnoea on exertion, pleuritic pain, burning tracheal pain, and a cough. Bilateral pulmonary disease was confirmed by chest X-rays, and pulmonary function tests suggested nitrofurantoin toxicity. Both **fluconazole** and nitrofurantoin were discontinued, and hepatic and lung function gradually improved.[1]

Either **fluconazole** or nitrofurantoin could have caused the liver toxicity. However, it was considered that both the lung and liver toxicity may have been due to an interaction between nitrofurantoin and **fluconazole**, possibly due to increased nitrofurantoin concentrations resulting from competition with **fluconazole** for renal tubular secretion.

Some 2 years earlier the patient had received pulse **itraconazole** (less than 1% excreted in the urine as active drug) with nitrofurantoin without raised liver enzymes or any other adverse effects.[1]

Information appears to be limited to this report, but bear it in mind in the event of increased nitrofurantoin adverse effects. More study is needed.

1. Linnebur SA, Parnes BL. Pulmonary and hepatic toxicity due to nitrofurantoin and fluconazole treatment. *Ann Pharmacother* (2004) 38, 612–16.

Nitrofurantoin + Metoclopramide

Metoclopramide reduces the absorption of nitrofurantoin.

Clinical evidence, mechanism, importance and management

In 10 healthy subjects the urinary excretion of a 100-mg dose of nitrofurantoin was approximately halved by pretreatment with a 10-mg intramuscular dose of metoclopramide and a 10 mg oral dose of metoclopramide given 30 minutes before the nitrofurantoin.[1]

It is thought that metoclopramide increases the gastric emptying rate, thus decreasing nitrofurantoin absorption. The practical importance of this is uncertain because there seem to be no reports of an interaction in practice.

1. Männistö P. The effect of crystal size, gastric content and emptying rate on the absorption of nitrofurantoin in healthy human volunteers. *Int J Clin Pharmacol Biopharm* (1978) 16, 223–8.

Nitroxoline + Antacids

The antibacterial effects of nitroxoline have been found to be reduced *in vitro* by magnesium and calcium ions because they form chelates with the nitroxoline.[1] In the absence of any direct clinical information it would seem prudent to monitor concurrent use for any evidence that its antibacterial effects are reduced.

1. Pelletier C, Prognon P, Bourlioux P. Roles of divalent cations and pH in mechanism of action of nitroxoline against *Escherichia coli* strains. *Antimicrob Agents Chemother* (1995) 707–13.

Novobiocin + Rifampicin (Rifampin)

Rifampicin reduces the half-life of novobiocin but this is unlikely to be clinically significant.

Clinical evidence, mechanism, importance and management

When 10 healthy subjects were given novobiocin 1 g daily for 13 days with rifampicin 600 mg daily, the novobiocin half-life was reduced from 5.85 to 2.66 hours and the AUC was reduced by almost 50%. There were no significant changes to the half-life or AUC of rifampicin. The serum novobiocin and rifampicin levels were not significantly altered and the trough serum levels of both antibacterials when given alone or concurrently remained in excess of the MIC for 90% of the strains of MRSA tested.[1] No special precautions would therefore seem to be necessary during concurrent use.

1. Drusano GL, Townsend RJ, Walsh TJ, Forrest A, Antal EJ, Standiford HC. Steady-state serum pharmacokinetics of novobiocin and rifampin alone and in combination. *Antimicrob Agents Chemother* (1986) 30, 42–5.

Penicillins + Acacia or Guar gum

The absorption of amoxicillin may be significantly reduced when given with or 2 hours after acacia. Guar gum causes a small reduction in the absorption of phenoxymethylpenicillin (penicillin V).

Clinical evidence, mechanism, importance and management

(a) Acacia

In healthy subjects the maximum serum levels and AUC of a single 500-mg dose of **amoxicillin** were reduced by 73% and 79%, respectively, when given with acacia (gum arabic: amount not stated) and by 56% and 49%, respectively, when given 2 hours after ingestion of acacia. The pharmacokinetics of **amoxicillin** were not significantly affected when it was given 4 hours after acacia. Acacia is used in pharmaceutical preparations as a suspending, demulcent and emulsifying agent. Concurrent administration with **amoxicillin** could result in subtherapeutic levels of the antibacterial, but whether or not this would occur with the amount of acacia in a dose of a preparation containing it as an excipient is not known. In some countries acacia is given to patients with chronic renal failure. The authors suggest that if **amoxicillin** is used to treat urinary-tract infections in patients also treated with acacia, it should be given 4 hours before or after the acacia.[1]

(b) Guar gum

Guar gum 5 g (*Guarem*, 95% guar gum) reduced the absorption of a single 1980-mg dose of **phenoxymethylpenicillin** (penicillin V) in 10 healthy subjects. Peak serum penicillin levels were reduced by 25% and the AUC_{0-6} was reduced by 28%.[2] The reasons are not understood.

The clinical significance of this interaction is uncertain, but the reduction in serum levels is only small. It would clearly only be important if the reduced amount of penicillin absorbed was inadequate to control infection The effect of guar gum on other penicillins seems not to have been studied.

1. Eltayeb IB, Awad AI, Elderbi MA, Shadad SA. Effect of gum arabic on the absorption of a single oral dose of amoxicillin in healthy Sudanese volunteers. *J Antimicrob Chemother* (2004) 54, 577–8.
2. Huupponen R, Seppälä P, Iisalo E. Effect of guar gum, a fibre preparation, on digoxin and penicillin absorption in man. *Eur J Clin Pharmacol* (1984) 26, 279–81.

Penicillins + Allopurinol

The incidence of skin rashes in patients taking either ampicillin or amoxicillin is increased by allopurinol.

Clinical evidence

A retrospective search through the records of 1324 patients, 67 of whom were taking allopurinol and **ampicillin**, found that 15 of them (22%) developed a skin rash compared with 94 (7.5%) of the patients not taking allopurinol.[1] The types of rash were not defined. Another study found that 35 out of 252 patients (13.9%) taking allopurinol and **ampicillin** developed a rash, compared with 251 out of 4434 (5.9%) taking **ampicillin** alone.[2] A parallel study revealed that 8 out of 36 patients (22%) taking **amoxicillin** and allopurinol developed a rash, whereas only 52 out of 887 (5.9%) did so when taking **amoxicillin** alone.[2]

A case report describes a patient who developed erythema multiforme shortly after starting **amoxicillin** and allopurinol and who was found to have both allopurinol hypersensitivity and type IV amoxicillin hypersensitivity.[3]

In contrast, one study did not find that the incidence of penicillin-related rashes was increased by allopurinol, and the authors suggested that this contrasting finding may be because exposure to penicillins was shorter in their study.[4]

Mechanism

Not understood. One suggestion is that the hyperuricaemia was responsible.[1] Another is that hyperuricaemic individuals may possibly have an altered immunological reactivity.[5]

Importance and management

An established interaction of limited importance. There would seem to be no strong reason for avoiding concurrent use, but prescribers should recognise that the development of a rash is by no means unusual. Whether this also occurs with penicillins other than ampicillin or amoxicillin is uncertain, and does not seem to have been reported.

1. Boston Collaborative Drug Surveillance Programme. Excess of ampicillin rashes associated with allopurinol or hyperuricemia. *N Engl J Med* (1972) 286, 505–7.
2. Jick H, Porter JB. Potentiation of ampicillin skin reactions by allopurinol or hyperuricemia. *J Clin Pharmacol* (1981) 21, 456–8.
3. Pérez A, Cabrerizo S, de Barrio M, Díaz MP, Herrero T, Tornero P, Baeza ML. Erythema-multiforme-like eruption from amoxicillin and allopurinol. *Contact Dermatitis* (2001) 44, 113–14.
4. Sonntag MR, Zoppi M, Fritschy D, Maibach R, Stocker F, Sollberger J, Buchli W, Hess T, Hoigné R. Exantheme unter haufig angewandten Antibiotika und antibakteriellen Chemotherepeutika (Penicilline, speziell Aminopenicilline, Cephalosporine und Cotrimoxazol) sowie Allopurinol. *Schweiz Med Wochenschr* (1986) 116, 142–5.
5. Fessel WJ. Immunologic reactivity in hyperuricemia. *N Engl J Med* (1972) 286, 1218.

Penicillins + Antacids

Aluminium/magnesium hydroxide and aluminium hydroxide do not significantly affect the bioavailability of amoxicillin or amoxicillin with clavulanic acid (co-amoxiclav). Antacids may reduce the absorption of the hydrochloride salt of pivampicillin.

Clinical evidence, mechanism, importance and management

(a) Amoxicillin or Co-amoxiclav

The pharmacokinetics of amoxicillin 1 g, and both amoxicillin and clavulanic acid (given as co-amoxiclav 625 mg), were not significantly altered by 10 doses of **aluminium/magnesium hydroxide** (*Maalox*) 10 mL, with the last dose given 30 minutes before amoxicillin.[1] Another study found that four 40-mg doses of **aluminium hydroxide** (*Aludrox*) given at 20 minute intervals had no effect on the pharmacokinetics of either amoxicillin or clavulanic acid (given as co-amoxiclav 750 mg with the second dose of antacid).[2]

There would seem to be no reason for avoiding the concurrent use of antacids and amoxicillin or co-amoxiclav.

(b) Pivampicillin

The UK manufacturers[3] used to recommend that, because antacids may decrease pivampicillin absorption, concurrent use should be avoided. This warning relates to a hydrochloride salt formulation, which needs acidic conditions for optimal absorption, whereas the basic salt formulation should not be affected by any pH change.[4]

1. Deppermann K-M, Lode H, Höffken G, Tschink G, Kalz C, Koeppe P. Influence of ranitidine, pirenzepine, and aluminium magnesium hydroxide on the bioavailability of various antibacterials, including amoxicillin, cephalexin, doxycycline, and amoxicillin-clavulanic acid. *Antimicrob Agents Chemother* (1989) 33, 1901–7.
2. Staniforth DH, Clarke HL, Horton R, Jackson D, Lau D. Augmentin bioavailability following cimetidine, aluminum hydroxide and milk. *Int J Clin Pharmacol Ther Toxicol* (1985) 23, 145–7.
3. Pondocillin (Pivampicillin). Leo Laboratories Ltd. ABPI Compendium of Datasheets and Summaries of Product Characteristics, 1998–99, 625–6.
4. Leo Laboratories Limited. Personal communication, March 1995.

Penicillins + Catha (Khat)

Chewing khat reduces the absorption of ampicillin and, to a lesser extent, amoxicillin, but the effects are minimal 2 hours after khat chewing stops.

Clinical evidence, mechanism, importance and management

A study in 8 healthy Yemeni male subjects found that chewing khat reduced the absorption of oral **ampicillin** from the gut.[1] When **ampicillin** 500 mg was taken with 250 mL water 2 hours before or just before khat chewing started, or midway through a 4 hour chewing session, the amounts of unchanged **ampicillin** in the urine fell by 46%, 41% and 49%, respectively. Even when **ampicillin** was taken 2 hours after a chewing session had stopped, the amount of drug excreted unchanged in the urine fell by 12%. A parallel series of studies with **amoxicillin** 500 mg found much smaller reductions. The equivalent reductions were 14%, 9%, 22% and 13%. A similar study found that chewing khat resulted in variable reduction in the bioavailability of **amoxicillin** 500 mg, which was maximal (22%) when it was given midway during the 4-hour chewing period.[2]

The reasons for this interaction are not known, but the authors of the reports suggest that tannins from the khat might form insoluble and non-absorbable complexes with these penicillins, and possibly also directly reduce the way the gut absorbs them.[1]

Khat (the leaves and stem tips of *Catha edulis*) is chewed in some African and Arabian countries for its stimulatory properties. The authors of one of the studies concluded that both **ampicillin** and **amoxicillin** should be taken 2 hours after khat chewing to ensure that maximum absorption occurs.[1]

1. Attef OA, Ali A-AA, Ali HM. Effect of Khat chewing on the bioavailability of ampicillin and amoxycillin. *J Antimicrob Chemother* (1997) 39, 523–5.
2. Abdel Ghani YM, Etman MA, Nada AH. Effect of khat chewing on the absorption of orally administered amoxycillin. *Acta Pharm* (1999) 49, 43–50.

Penicillins + Chloroquine

Chloroquine reduces the absorption of ampicillin, but bacampicillin is unaffected.

Clinical evidence

Chloroquine 1 g reduced the absorption (as measured by excretion in the urine) of a single 1-g dose of oral **ampicillin** by about one-third (from 29 to 19%) in 7 healthy subjects.[1] Another study by the same author demonstrated that the absorption of **ampicillin** from **bacampicillin** tablets was unaffected by chloroquine.[2]

Mechanism

A possible reason for the reduction in absorption is that the chloroquine irritates the gut so that the ampicillin is moved through more quickly, thereby reducing the time for absorption.

Importance and management

Information appears to be limited to the studies cited, which used large doses of chloroquine (1 g) when compared with those usually used for malarial prophylaxis (300 mg base weekly) or for rheumatic diseases (150 mg daily). The reduction in the ampicillin absorption is also only moderate. The general clinical importance of this interaction is therefore uncertain. However, one report suggests separating the dosing by not less than 2 hours.[1] An alternative would be to use bacampicillin (an ampicillin pro-drug), which does not appear to interact with chloroquine.[2] More study is needed to confirm and evaluate the importance of this interaction.

1. Ali HM. Reduced ampicillin bioavailability following oral coadministration with chloroquine. *J Antimicrob Chemother* (1985) 15, 781–4.
2. Ali HM. The effect of Sudanese food and chloroquine on the bioavailability of ampicillin from bacampicillin tablets. *Int J Pharmaceutics* (1981) 9, 185–90.

Penicillins + Food

The absorption of many penicillins is not significantly affected by food. The exceptions are ampicillin (food may reduce its levels by up to 50%), cloxacillin, and possibly pivampicillin and phenoxymethylpenicillin.

Clinical evidence, mechanism, importance and management

(a) Dietary fibre

The AUC of a single 500-mg oral dose of **amoxicillin** was found to be 12.17 micrograms/mL per hour in 10 healthy subjects on a low fibre diet (7.8 g of insoluble fibre daily) but only 9.65 micrograms/mL per hour when they ate a high fibre diet (36.2 g of insoluble fibre daily); a difference of about 20%. Peak serum levels were the same and occurred at 3 hours.[1] The clinical relevance of these changes is likely to be minimal.

(b) Enteral and parenteral feeds

A single 250-mg intravenous dose of **ampicillin** was given to 7 healthy subjects 2 hours into a 12-hour infusion of parenteral nutrition or 4 hours after an enteral meal. The parenteral nutrition was of two types, one with and one without amino acids, calcium and phosphorus, both without lipids, and of similar calorific content and volume to the enteral feed. None of the three regimens altered the pharmacokinetics of intravenous **ampicillin**.[2] Note that the **ampicillin** was given in a separate limb to the parenteral nutrition.

(c) Food

1. Amoxicillin and co-amoxiclav. Food eaten immediately before amoxicillin reduced its serum levels by about 50% and reduced urinary excretion, when compared with the fasted state.[3] However, in another study, a standard breakfast had no effect on the AUC of a single 500-mg dose of amoxicillin in 16 healthy subjects.[4] Similarly, a crossover study in 18 healthy subjects given co-amoxiclav (amoxicillin 500 mg with **clavulanic acid** 250 mg), either 2 hours before or with a fried breakfast, found that the breakfast had no significant effect on the pharmacokinetics of amoxicillin or **clavulanic acid**. Moreover, a further study in 43 healthy subjects found that taking co-amoxiclav with food tended to minimise the incidence (but not the severity) of gastrointestinal adverse effects (watery stools, nausea and vomiting).[5] It would therefore be beneficial to take co-amoxiclav with a meal.

2. Ampicillin. Food eaten immediately before a single 500-mg dose of ampicillin reduced its serum levels by about 50% and reduced urinary excretion.[3] A standard breakfast reduced the AUC of a single 500-mg dose of ampicillin by 31% in 16 healthy subjects.[4] Another study found ampicillin absorption was delayed and the total absorption reduced when it was taken with food. Urinary excretion of ampicillin was about 30% of a dose when given on an empty stomach and about 20% when given with food.[6] It is recommended that ampicillin is taken one hour before food or on an empty stomach to optimise absorption.

3. Bacampicillin. The AUC of ampicillin was assessed when 6 healthy subjects took a 1.6-g dose of bacampicillin either 35 minutes after breakfast or 2 hours before breakfast. The AUC was 26% lower with the post-breakfast dose, but this difference was not statistically significant.[7] On the basis of other work that also suggests that no important interaction occurs with food,[8,9] the manufacturers say that bacampicillin can be given without regard to time of food intake.

4. Flucloxacillin. A study in children given flucloxacillin 12.5 mg/kg as either tablets or mixture found that while the absorption depended on both the formulation and age of the child, there was no difference in levels achieved when given to a subject when fasting or with a breakfast.[10] However, it is recommended that flucloxacillin is taken one hour before food or on an empty stomach to optimise absorption. The presence of food is reported to reduce the rate and extent of absorption of the related drug **cloxacillin,**[11] and therefore it may be prudent to follow the advice given for flucloxacillin.

5. Pivampicillin. A study in healthy subjects found the absorption of pivampicillin was delayed when it was given with food, but the amount absorbed was not affected. The urinary excretion of ampicillin following pivampicillin was about 60% of the dose when taken with or without food.[6] However, another study in which pivampicillin 350 mg was given in the fasting state or with a standardised cooked breakfast found that food both delayed and reduced the absorption of pivampicillin by almost 50%.[12]

6. Pivmecillinam. The manufacturers of pivmecillinam note that its absorption is practically unaffected when the tablets are taken with food.[13]

(d) Milk

The peak levels and the AUCs of oral **phenoxymethylpenicillin** and *oral* **benzylpenicillin** were reduced by 40 to 60% in infants and children when they were given with milk.[14] It is recommended that **phenoxymethylpenicillin** is taken one hour before food or on an empty stomach to optimise absorption.

Co-amoxiclav (**amoxicillin** 500 mg with **clavulanic acid** 250 mg) was given to 16 healthy subjects at the same time as the second of four 200-mL glasses of milk (taken at 20 minute intervals). Although the bioavailability of the **amoxicillin** and **clavulanic acid** tended to be decreased, and the time to peak levels delayed, the changes did not reach statistical significance.[15] No special precautions would seem to be necessary.

1. Lutz M, Espinoza J, Arancibia A, Araya M, Pacheco I, Brunser O. Effect of structured dietary fiber on bioavailability of amoxicillin. *Clin Pharmacol Ther* (1987) 42, 220–4.
2. Koo WWK, Ke J, Tam YK, Finegan BA, Marriage B. Pharmacokinetics of ampicillin during parenteral nutrition. *J Parenter Enteral Nutr* (1990) 14, 279–82.
3. Welling PG, Huang H, Koch PA, Craig WA, Madsen PO. Bioavailability of ampicillin and amoxicillin in fasted and nonfasted subjects. *J Pharm Sci* (1977) 66, 549–52.
4. Eshelman FN, Spyker DA. Pharmacokinetics of amoxicillin and ampicillin: crossover study of the effect of food. *Antimicrob Agents Chemother* (1978) 14, 539–43.
5. Staniforth DH, Lillystone RJ, Jackson D. Effect of food on the bioavailability and tolerance of clavulanic acid/amoxycillin combination. *J Antimicrob Chemother* (1982) 10, 131–9.
6. Neuvonen PJ, Elonen E, Pentikainen PJ. Comparative effect of food on absorption of ampicillin and pivampicillin. *J Int Med Res* (1977) 5, 71–6.
7. Sommers DK, van Wyk M, Moncrieff J, Schoeman HS. Influence of food and reduced gastric acidity on the bioavailability of bacampicillin and cefuroxime axetil. *Br J Clin Pharmacol* (1984) 18, 535–9.
8. Magni L, Sjöberg B, Sjövall J, Wessman J. Clinical pharmacological studies with bacampicillin. *Chemotherapy* (1976) 5, 109–114.
9. Ali HM. The effect of Sudanese food and chloroquine on the bioavailability of ampicillin from bacampicillin tablets. *Int J Pharmaceutics* (1981) 9, 185–90.
10. Bergdahl S, Eriksson M, Finkel Y, Lännergren K. Oral absorption of flucloxacillin in infants and young children. *Acta Pharmacol Toxicol (Copenh)* (1986) 58, 255–8.
11. Babalola CP, Iwheye GB, Olaniyi AA. Effect of proguanil interaction on bioavailability of cloxacillin. *J Clin Pharm Ther* (2002) 27, 461–4.
12. Fernandez CA, Menezes JP, Ximenes J. The effect of food on the absorption of pivampicillin and a comparison with the absorption of ampicillin potassium. *J Int Med Res* (1973) 1, 530–3.
13. Selexid (Pivmecillinam hydrochloride). Leo Laboratories Ltd. UK Summary of product characteristics, August 1999.
14. McCracken GH, Ginsburg CM, Clahsen JC, Thomas ML. Pharmacologic evaluation of orally administered antibiotics in infants and children: effect of feeding on bioavailability. *Pediatrics* (1978) 62, 738–43.
15. Staniforth DH, Clarke HL, Horton R, Jackson D, Lau D. Augmentin bioavailability following cimetidine, aluminium hydroxide and milk. *Int J Clin Pharmacol Ther Toxicol* (1985) 23, 154–7.

Penicillins + H_2-receptor antagonists

Cimetidine does not adversely affect the bioavailability of ampicillin or co-amoxiclav, but the bioavailability of oral benzylpenicillin may be increased in some subjects. Ranitidine does not affect the pharmacokinetics of amoxicillin, but may possibly reduce the bioavailability of bacampicillin.

Clinical evidence, mechanism, importance and management

(a) Amoxicillin and Co-amoxiclav

Cimetidine 200 mg, given three times daily the day before and with a single 200-mg dose of co-amoxiclav (amoxicillin with clavulanic acid), had no significant effect on the bioavailability of amoxicillin or clavulanic acid.[1] Another study found that **ranitidine** (300 mg given the day before and 150 mg given with the antibacterial) had no effect on the pharmacokinetics of a single 1-g dose of amoxicillin.[2]

(b) Ampicillin

The pharmacokinetics of ampicillin were unchanged in a placebo controlled study in which 6 healthy subjects were given **cimetidine** 400 mg every 6 hours for 6 days, with a single 500-mg dose of ampicillin on day 6.[3]

(c) Bacampicillin

One small study suggested that when bacampicillin was given with **ranitidine** 300 mg and **sodium bicarbonate** 4 g, the AUC was reduced by 78% when the drugs were given with breakfast and by 55% when the drugs were given without food.[4] However, these results have been criticised because the study only included 6 subjects and because of differences in methodology between compared groups.[5] The findings remain unconfirmed, and their clinical significance is uncertain.

(d) Benzylpenicillin

A study using a 600-mg *oral* dose of benzylpenicillin found that **cimetidine** raised the benzylpenicillin serum levels by about 3-fold in one subject, but did not significantly affect benzylpenicillin levels in another 4 subjects.[5] The clinical significance of these findings is unclear, especially as benzylpenicillin is more usually given parenterally.

1. Staniforth DH, Clarke HL, Horton R, Jackson D, Lau D. Augmentin bioavailability following cimetidine, aluminum hydroxide and milk. *Int J Clin Pharmacol Ther Toxicol* (1985) 23, 145–7.
2. Deppermann K-M, Lode H, Höffken G, Tschink G, Kalz C, Koeppe P. Influence of ranitidine, pirenzepine, and aluminium magnesium hydroxide on the bioavailability of various antibiotics, including amoxicillin, cephalexin, doxycycline, and amoxicillin-clavulanic acid. *Antimicrob Agents Chemother* (1989) 33, 1901–7.
3. Rogers HJ, James CA, Morrison PJ and Bradbrook ID. Effect of cimetidine on oral absorption of ampicillin and cotrimoxazole. *J Antimicrob Chemother* (1980) 6, 297–300.
4. Sommers DK, van Wyk M, Moncrieff J, Schoeman HS. Influence of food and reduced gastric acidity on the bioavailability of bacampicillin and cefuroxime axetil. *Br J Clin Pharmacol* (1984) 18, 535–9.
5. Fairfax AJ, Adam J and Pagan FS. Effect of cimetidine on absorption of oral benzylpenicillin. *BMJ* (1977) 2, 820.

Penicillins + Miscellaneous

Aspirin, indometacin, phenylbutazone, sulfaphenazole and sulfinpyrazone prolong the half-life of benzylpenicillin whereas chlorothiazide, sulfamethizole and sulfamethoxypyridazine do not. Some sulfonamides reduce oxacillin blood levels. Pirenzepine does not affect the pharmacokinetics of amoxicillin.

Clinical evidence, mechanism, importance and management

Studies in patients given different drugs for 5 to 7 days showed the following increases in the half-life of **benzylpenicillin**: **aspirin** 63%, **indometacin** 22%, **phenylbutazone** 139%, **sulfaphenazole** 44% and **sulfinpyrazone** 65%. It seems likely that competition between these drugs and **benzylpenicillin** for excretion by the kidney tubules caused these increases. Changes in the half-life with **chlorothiazide**, **sulfamethizole** and **sulfamethoxypyridazine** were not significant.[1]

In healthy subjects, **sulfamethoxypyridazine** 3 g given 8 hours before a 1-g dose of oral **oxacillin** reduced the 6-hour urinary recovery by 55%. **Sulfaethidole** 3.9 g given 3 hours before the **oxacillin** reduced the 6-hour urinary recovery by 42%.[2]

Pirenzepine 50 mg given three times daily on the day before and with a single 1-g dose of **amoxicillin** had no significant effect on the pharmacokinetics of the antibacterial.[3]

None of the interactions listed appears to be adverse, and no particular precautions would seem necessary during concurrent use of these drugs and the penicillins. The importance of the interaction between **oxacillin** and the sulfonamides is uncertain, but it can easily be avoided by choosing alternative drugs.

1. Kampmann J, Hansen JM, Siersboek-Nielsen K, Laursen H. Effect of some drugs on penicillin half-life in blood. *Clin Pharmacol Ther* (1972) 13, 516–19.
2. Kunin CM. Clinical pharmacology of the new penicillins. II. Effect of drugs which interfere with binding to serum proteins. *Clin Pharmacol Ther* (1966) 7, 180–88.
3. Deppermann K-M, Lode H, Höffken G, Tschink G, Kalz C, Koeppe P. Influence of ranitidine, pirenzepine, and aluminium magnesium hydroxide on the bioavailability of various antibiotics, including amoxicillin, cephalexin, doxycycline, and amoxicillin-clavulanic acid. *Antimicrob Agents Chemother* (1989) 33, 1901–7.

Penicillins + Nifedipine

Nifedipine increases the absorption of amoxicillin from the gut but this is unlikely to be clinically important. Nafcillin increases the clearance of nifedipine, but the clinical significance of this is unclear.

Clinical evidence, mechanism, importance and management

(a) Amoxicillin

In 8 healthy subjects when amoxicillin 1 g was given 30 minutes after a 20-mg nifedipine capsule, the peak serum amoxicillin levels were raised by 33%, the bioavailability was raised by 21% and the absorption rate was raised by 70%.[1] The authors speculate that the uptake of amoxicillin through the gut wall is increased by nifedipine in some way.[1] There would seem to be no good reason for avoiding concurrent use as overall the bioavailability was not significantly altered.

(b) Nafcillin

In a randomised, placebo-controlled study, 9 healthy subjects were given a single 10-mg nifedipine capsule after a 5-day course of nafcillin 500 mg four times daily. The nifedipine AUC was decreased by 63% and the clearance was increased by 145%, but the effect of these changes on nifedipine pharmacodynamics was not assessed. It was suggested that nafcillin is an inducer of cytochrome P450 isoenzymes, and increased the metabolism of nifedipine.[2] The clinical significance of these changes is unclear.

1. Westphal J-F, Trouvin J-H, Deslandes A, Carbon C. Nifedipine enhances amoxicillin absorption kinetics and bioavailability in humans. *J Pharmacol Exp Ther* (1990) 255, 312–17.
2. Lang CC, Jamal SK, Mohamed Z, Mustafa MR, Mustafa AM, Lee TC. Evidence of an interaction between nifedipine and nafcillin in humans. *Br J Clin Pharmacol* (2003) 55, 588–90.

Penicillins + Probenecid

Probenecid reduces the excretion of the penicillins.

Clinical evidence

(a) Amoxicillin

In 10 healthy subjects a single 3-g dose of amoxicillin was given with or without probenecid 1 g. Two hours after administration, the serum levels of amoxicillin taken with probenecid were 55% higher than those with amoxicillin alone, and they remained higher for up to 18 hours.[1] Similar results were found in another study.[2] Amoxicillin 3 g twice daily plus placebo, amoxicillin 1 g twice daily plus probenecid 1 g twice daily, and amoxicillin 1 g twice daily plus probenecid 500 mg four times daily were given to 6 patients to treat bronchiectasis. The maximum serum concentration and half-life of both high- and low-dose amoxicillin were similar, but in the regimens containing probenecid the clearance of amoxicillin was reduced by two-thirds, when compared with amoxicillin given alone.[3]

(b) Benzylpenicillin

Four healthy subjects were given infusions of benzylpenicillin at three different rates, either alone or with probenecid given as a separate infusion, at rates to provide low and high plasma levels. An infusion rate of probenecid 83 mg/hour, corresponding to a daily dose of 2 g was found to produce about 90% inhibition of the tubular excretion of benzylpenicillin (at plasma levels of 25 mg/L). Doses of probenecid above 2 g daily did not have a significantly greater effect.[4]

(c) Mezlocillin

A study in healthy subjects found that probenecid 1 g, given one hour before an intramuscular injection of mezlocillin, increased the peak serum levels and AUC of mezlocillin by 65% and decreased the total clearance, renal clearance and apparent volume of distribution by 38%, 52%, and 35%, respectively.[5]

(d) Nafcillin

A study in 5 healthy subjects given 500 mg of intravenous nafcillin sodium with probenecid, 1 g given orally the previous night and 1 g given 2 hours prior to the antibacterial, showed that the urinary recovery of nafcillin was reduced from 30% to 17%, and its AUC was approximately doubled.[6]

(e) Piperacillin/Tazobactam

In 10 healthy subjects probenecid 1 g given 1 hour before a single infusion of piperacillin 3 g/tazobactam 375 mg caused a decrease of about 25% in the clearance of both components. The half-life of tazobactam was increased by 72%.[7] A study in 8 healthy subjects found that oral probenecid 1 g, given one hour before an intramuscular injection of piperacillin 1 g, increased both the peak plasma level and terminal half-life of piperacillin by 30% and the AUC by 60%. The apparent volume of distribution of piperacillin was reduced by 20% and renal clearance was reduced by 40%.[8]

(f) Pivampicillin

In a crossover study healthy subjects were given either pivampicillin 350 mg every 8 hours or a tablet of MK-356 (approximately, pivampicillin 350 mg with probenecid 200 mg). Peak ampicillin levels of 4 to 5 micrograms/mL were found about 1 hour after administration of the first and last dose of both treatments suggesting that probenecid did not affect the ampicillin elimination. Administration of MK-356 (pivampicillin 700 mg with probenecid 400 mg) twice daily indicated that peak serum levels of ampicillin were increased and elimination rate slowed following successive doses.[9]

(g) Procaine benzylpenicillin

A study in patients given intramuscular procaine benzylpenicillin 2.4 or 4.8 million units with or without probenecid 2 g found the peak serum levels were higher in patients given probenecid, but because of wide interpatient variation, possibly associated with differences in the release of penicillin from the injection sites, the exact potentiating effect of probenecid could not be determined.[10] However, another study in men and women given procaine benzylpenicillin 2.4 million units and 4.8 million units, respectively (for uncomplicated gonorrhoea), found treatment failure after 1 week in 15.4% of men and 10.4% of women. Failure rates were reduced to 1.8% and 3.7%, respectively, when oral probenecid 1 g was given with the penicillin.[11]

(h) Ticarcillin

Probenecid, either 500 mg twice daily, 1 g daily, or 2 g daily was added to ticarcillin 3 g every 4 hours, which was being given to treat infections in adult cystic fibrosis patients. In all cases the clearance of ticarcillin was reduced: by about 27% with the 500-mg dose regimen, by about 32% with the 1-g dose regimen and by about 43% with the 2-g dose regimen.[12]

Mechanism

In each case the penicillin competes with the probenecid for excretion by the kidney tubules, although with nafcillin, non-renal clearance may also play a part.

Importance and management

In the case of amoxicillin, benzylpenicillin, nafcillin and ticarcillin the effects are of clinical significance. In the case of the ticarcillin study the authors suggest that a 12-hourly dosing regimen could be used if probenecid is given concurrently, which has implications for home treatment. With piperacillin/tazobactam the changes were not thought to provide any benefit in terms of dose reduction or alteration of the dosage interval. Note that this is generally considered to be a beneficial interaction, but bear in mind that, in some cases, such as in renal impairment, the increase in penicillin levels may be undesirably large.

1. Shanson DC, McNabb R, Hajipieris P. The effect of probenecid on serum amoxycillin concentrations up to 18 hours after a single 3 g oral dose of amoxycillin: possible implications for preventing endocarditis. *J Antimicrob Chemother* (1984) 13, 629–32.
2. Barbhaiya R, Thin RN, Turner P, Wadsworth J. Clinical pharmacological studies of amoxycillin: effect of probenecid. *Br J Vener Dis* (1979) 55, 211–13.
3. Allen MB, Fitzpatrick RW, Barratt A, Cole RB. The use of probenecid to increase the serum amoxycillin levels in patients with bronchiectasis. *Respir Med* (1990) 84, 143–6.
4. Overbosch D, Van Gulpen C, Hermans J, Mattie H. The effect of probenecid on the renal tubular excretion of benzylpenicillin. *Br J Clin Pharmacol* (1988) 25, 51–8.
5. Verbist L, Tjandramaga TB, Verbesselt R, De Schepper PJ. Pharmacocinétique de la mezlocilline. Comparaison avec l'ampicilline et influence du probénécide. *Nouv Presse Med* (1982) 11, 347–52.
6. Waller ES, Sharanevych MA, Yakatan GJ. The effect of probenecid on nafcillin disposition. *J Clin Pharmacol* (1982) 22, 482–9.
7. Ganes D, Batra V, Faulkner R, Greene D, Haynes J, Kuye O, Ruffner A, Shin K, Tonelli A, Yacobi A. Effect of probenecid on the pharmacokinetics of piperacillin and tazobactam in healthy volunteers. *Pharm Res* (1991) 8 (10 Suppl), S-299.
8. Tjandramaga TB, Mullie A, Verbesselt R, De Schepper PJ, Verbist L. Piperacillin: human pharmacokinetics after intravenous and intramuscular administration. *Antimicrob Agents Chemother* (1978) 14, 829–37.
9. Kampffmeyer HG, Hartmann I, Metz H, Breault GO, Skeggs HR, Till AE, Weidner L. Serum concentrations of ampicillin and probenecid and ampicillin excretion after repeated oral administration of a pivampicillin-probenecid salt (MK-356). *Eur J Clin Pharmacol* (1975) 9, 125–9.
10. Cornelius CE, Schroeter AL, Lester A, Martin JE. Variations in serum concentrations of penicillin after injections of aqueous procaine penicillin G with and without oral probenecid. *Br J Vener Dis* (1971) 47, 359–63.
11. Holmes KK, Karney WW, Harnisch JP, Wiesner PJ, Turck M, Pedersen AHB. Single-dose aqueous procaine penicillin G therapy for gonorrhea: use of probenecid and cause of treatment failure. *J Infect Dis* (1973) 127, 455–60.
12. Corvaia L, Li SC, Ioannides-Demos LL, Bowes G, Spicer WJ, Spelman DW, Tong N, McLean AJ. A prospective study of the effects of oral probenecid on the pharmacokinetics of intravenous ticarcillin in patients with cystic fibrosis. *J Antimicrob Chemother* (1992) 30, 875–8.

Penicillins + Tetracyclines

Data from the 1950s suggested that the tetracyclines can reduce the effectiveness of penicillins in the treatment of pneumococcal meningitis and probably scarlet fever. It is uncertain whether a similar interaction occurs with other infections. This interaction may possibly be important only with those infections where a rapid kill is essential.

Clinical evidence

When **chlortetracycline** originally became available it was tested as a potential treatment for meningitis. In patients with pneumococcal meningitis it was shown that **benzylpenicillin** one million units, intramuscularly every 2 hours was more effective than the same regimen of penicillin with **chlortetracycline** 500 mg intravenously every 6 hours. Out of 43 patients given penicillin alone, 70% recovered, compared with only 20% in another group of 14 essentially similar patients who had received both antibacterials.[1]

Another report about the treatment of pneumococcal meningitis with intramuscular or intravenous **penicillin** and intravenous tetracyclines (**chlortetracycline, oxytetracycline, tetracycline**) confirmed that the mortality was much lower in those given only penicillin, rather than the combination of penicillin and a tetracycline.[2] In the treatment of scarlet fever (Group A beta-haemolytic streptococci), no difference was seen in the initial response to treatment with penicillin (oral **procaine benzylpenicillin**) and **chlortetracycline** or the penicillin alone, but spontaneous re-infection occurred more frequently in those who had received both antibacterials.[3]

Mechanism

The generally accepted explanation is that bactericides such as the penicillins, which inhibit bacterial cell wall synthesis, require cells to be actively growing and dividing to be maximally effective, a situation that will not occur in the presence of bacteriostatic antibacterials, such as the tetracyclines.

Importance and management

Documentation is limited, but this is an apparently important interaction when treating pneumococcal meningitis and probably scarlet fever as well. However, the use of these antibacterials for such severe infections has largely been superseded. It has not been shown to occur when treating pneumococcal pneumonia.[4] It has been suggested that antagonism, if it occurs, may only be significant when it is essential to kill bacteria rapidly,[4] i.e. in serious infections such as meningitis. Any penicillin and any tetracycline would be expected to behave in this way.

Note that, the macrolides, which are also bacteriostatic would be expected to attenuate the action of penicillins, but this does not seem to occur in practice. See 'Macrolides + Penicillins', p.316.

1. Lepper MH, Dowling HF. Treatment of pneumococcic meningitis with penicillin compared with penicillin plus aureomycin: studies including observations on an apparent antagonism between penicillin and aureomycin. *Arch Intern Med* (1951) 88, 489–94.
2. Olsson RA, Kirby JC, Romansky MJ. Pneumococcal meningitis in the adult. Clinical, therapeutic and prognostic aspects in forty-three patients. *Ann Intern Med* (1961) 55, 545–9.
3. Strom J. The question of antagonism between penicillin and chlortetracycline, illustrated by therapeutical experiments in Scarlatina. *Antibiotic Med* (1955) 1,6–12.
4. Ahern JJ, Kirby WMM. Lack of interference of aureomycin with penicillin in treatment of pneumococcic pneumonia. *Arch Intern Med* (1953) 91, 197–203.

Penicillins; Amoxicillin + Amiloride

Amiloride can cause a small but probably clinically unimportant reduction in the absorption of amoxicillin.

Clinical evidence, mechanism, importance and management

When 8 healthy subjects were given amiloride 10 mg followed 2 hours later by a single 1-g oral dose of amoxicillin, the bioavailability and maximum serum levels of amoxicillin were reduced by 27% and 25%, respectively, and the time to reach maximum levels was delayed from 1 hour to 1.56 hours. When amoxicillin was given intravenously its bioavailability was unchanged by amiloride.[1] It is thought that the absorption of beta lactams like amoxicillin depends on a dipeptide carrier system in the cells lining the intestine (brush border membrane). This system depends on the existence of a pH gradient between the outside and inside of the cells, which is maintained by a Na-H exchanger. As this exchanger is inhibited by amiloride the reduced absorption would seem to be explained.

This reported reduction in the absorption of the amoxicillin is only small and unlikely to have very much clinical relevance. There seems to be no information about other penicillins.

1. Westphal JF, Jehl F, Brogard JM, Carbon C. Amoxicillin intestinal absorption reduction by amiloride: possible role of the Na(+)-H(+) exchanger. *Clin Pharmacol Ther* (1995) 57, 257–64.

Penicillins; Cloxacillin + Proguanil

Proguanil may reduce the bioavailability of cloxacillin.

Clinical evidence, mechanism, importance and management

A pharmacokinetic study in healthy subjects given cloxacillin 500 mg with or without proguanil 200 mg found the total amount of cloxacillin excreted in the urine in 12 hours was reduced by up to 48% by proguanil. The time to maximum excretion and the half-life were increased by 23% and 34%, respectively. The reasons why cloxacillin absorption is reduced by proguanil are not known, but it has been suggested that it may be due to adsorption of cloxacillin on to proguanil in the gut, formation of a drug-complex, increased gastric motility or increased beta-lactam ring hydrolysis leading to reduced cloxacillin bioavailability.[1] The clinical implications of the interaction are unknown.

1. Babalola CP, Iwheye GB, Olaniyi AA. Effect of proguanil interaction on bioavailability of cloxacillin. *J Clin Pharm Ther* (2002) 27, 461–4.

Penicillins; Dicloxacillin + Rifampicin

Rifampicin increases the oral clearance of dicloxacillin and reduces its plasma levels.

Clinical evidence, mechanism, importance and management

A study in 18 healthy subjects found that rifampicin 600 mg daily for 10 days decreased the maximum plasma level of a single 1-g dose of dicloxacillin by 27% and increased the mean oral clearance by 26%. The mean absorption time increased from 0.71 to 1.34 hours. Rifampicin increased the formation clearance, maximum level and AUC of the 5-hydroxymetabolite of dicloxacillin by 135%, 119%, and 59%, respectively. Dicloxacillin is a substrate of P-glycoprotein and it was suggested that the effects of rifampicin on dicloxacillin were due to induction of both intestinal P-glycoprotein and dicloxacillin metabolism.[1]

1. Putnam WS, Woo JM, Huang Y, Benet LZ. Effect of the *MDR1* C3435T variant and P-glycoprotein induction on dicloxacillin pharmacokinetics. *J Clin Pharmacol* (2005) 45, 411–21.

Penicillins; Piperacillin/tazobactam + Vancomycin

Vancomycin does not interact to a clinically relevant extent with piperacillin/tazobactam.

Clinical evidence, mechanism, importance and management

A randomised, crossover study in 9 healthy subjects found that infusions of vancomycin 500 mg and piperacillin 3 g with tazobactam 375 mg had little or no effect on the pharmacokinetics of any of the antibacterials, except that the piperacillin AUC was slightly raised, by about 7%. It was concluded that no dosage adjustments are needed if these drugs are given together.[1]

1. Vechlekar D, Sia L, Lanc R, Kuye O, Yacobi A, Faulkner R. Pharmacokinetics of piperacillin/tazobactam (Pip/Taz) IV with and without vancomycin IV in healthy adult male volunteers. *Pharm Res* (1992) 9 (10 Suppl), S-322.

Penicillins; Pivampicillin or Pivmecillinam + Valproate

An isolated report describes hyperammonaemic encephalopathy in an elderly patient during treatment with valproate and pivmecillinam. The manufacturers of both pivmecillinam and pivampicillin advise the avoidance of concurrent valproate because of the increased risk of carnitine deficiency.

Clinical evidence, mechanism, importance and management

There is a report of hyperammonaemic encephalopathy which developed in a 72-year-old woman taking valproate monotherapy for partial epilepsy after she started treatment with pivmecillinam 600 mg daily. She recovered after discontinuation of valproate and use of cefuroxime instead of pivmecillinam.[1] Valproate may reduce serum carnitine,[1] for reasons that are not well understood.[2] Valproate-induced hyperammonaemic encephalopathy may be due to reduced carnitine levels.[1]

Pivmecillinam and pivampicillin are hydrolysed to release mecillinam or ampicillin respectively, pivalic acid and formaldehyde. One of the potential problems of these drugs is that the pivalic acid can react with carnitine to form pivaloyl-carnitine, which is excreted in the urine, and so the body can become depleted of carnitine. Carnitine deficiency also manifests as muscle weakness and cardiomyopathy.

The risks of carnitine deficiency due to pivmecillinam or pivampicillin seem to be small in healthy adults, but the manufacturers of pivmecillinam and pivampicillin issue a warning about long-term or frequently repeated treatment.[3,4]

The authors of the report advise caution if pivmecillinam is added to treatment with valproate.[1] Although this appears to be the only report of an adverse effect due to the combined effects of pivmecillinam and valproate on carnitine levels, the manufacturers advise the avoidance of both pivampicillin or pivmecillinam with valproic acid or valproate or other medication liberating pivalic acid.[3,4]

1. Lokrantz C-M, Eriksson B, Rosén I, Asztely F. Hyperammonemic encephalopathy induced by a combination of valproate and pivmecillinam. *Acta Neurol Scand* (2004) 109, 297–301.
2. Melegh B, Kerner J, Jaszai V, Bieber LL. Differential excretion of xenobiotic acyl-esters of carnitine due to administration of pivampicillin and valproate. *Biochem Med Metab Biol* (1990) 43, 30–8.
3. Selexid (Pivmecillinam hydrochloride). Leo Laboratories Ltd. UK Summary of product characteristics, August 1999.
4. Pondocillin (Pivampicillin). Leo Laboratories Ltd. ABPI Compendium of Datasheets and Summaries of Product Characteristics, 1998–99, 625–6.

Protionamide + Other antimycobacterials

Protionamide appears to be very hepatotoxic and this is possibly increased by the concurrent use of rifampicin or rifandin. Protionamide does not affect the pharmacokinetics of either dapsone or rifampicin.

Clinical evidence

In a study of 39 patients with leprosy, 39% became jaundiced after treatment for 24 to 120 days with **dapsone** 100 mg daily, protionamide 300 mg daily and **rifandin** [isopiperazinylrifamycin SV] 300 to 600 mg monthly. Laboratory evidence of liver damage occurred in a total of 56% of patients and despite the withdrawal of the drugs from all the patients, 2 of them died.[1] All the patients except two had taken **dapsone** before, alone, for 3 to 227 months without reported problems.[1] In another group of leprosy patients, 22% (11 of 50) had liver damage after treatment with **dapsone** 100 mg and protionamide 300 mg given daily, and **rifampicin** 900 mg, protionamide 500 mg and **clofazimine** 300 mg given monthly over a period of 30 to 50 days. One patient died.[1] Most of the patients recovered within 30 to 60 days after withdrawing the treatment.

Jaundice, liver damage and deaths have occurred in other leprosy patients given **rifampicin** and protionamide or **ethionamide**.[2-4] Protionamide does not affect the pharmacokinetics of either **dapsone** or **rifampicin**.[5]

Mechanism

Although not certain, it seems probable that the liver damage was primarily caused by the protionamide, and possibly exacerbated by the rifampicin or the rifandin.

Importance and management

This serious and potentially life-threatening hepatotoxic reaction to protionamide is established, but the part played by the other drugs, particularly the rifampicin, is uncertain. Strictly speaking this may not be an interaction. If protionamide is given the liver function should be very closely monitored in order to detect toxicity as soon as possible.

1. Baohong J, Jiakun C, Chenmin W, Guang X. Hepatotoxicity of combined therapy with rifampicin and daily prothionamide for leprosy. *Lepr Rev* (1984) 55, 283–9.
2. Lesobre R, Ruffino J, Teyssier L, Achard F, Brefort G. Les ictères au cours du traitement par la rifampicine. *Rev Tuberc Pneumol (Paris)* (1969) 33, 393–403.
3. Report of the Third Meeting of the Scientific Working Group on Chemotherapy of Leprosy (THELEP) of the UNDP/World Bank/WHO Special Programme for Research and Training in Tropical Diseases. *Int J Lepr* (1981) 49, 431–6.
4. Cartel J-L, Millan J, Guelpa-Lauras C-C, Grosset JH. Hepatitis in leprosy patients treated by a daily combination of dapsone, rifampin, and a thioamide. *Int J Lepr* (1983) 51, 461–5.
5. Mathur A, Venkatesan K, Girdhar BK, Bharadwaj VP, Girdhar A, Bagga AK. A study of drug interactions in leprosy — 1. Effect of simultaneous administration of prothionamide on metabolic disposition of rifampicin and dapsone. *Lepr Rev* (1986) 57, 33–7.

Pyrazinamide + Antacids

In 14 healthy subjects 30 mL of *Mylanta* (aluminium/magnesium hydroxide) given 9 hours before, with, and after a single 30-mg/kg dose of pyrazinamide decreased the time to peak absorption by 17%, but had no effect on other pharmacokinetic parameters.[1] This change is not clinically important.

1. Peloquin CA, Bulpitt AE, Jaresko GS, Jelliffe RW, James GT, Nix DE. Pharmacokinetics of pyrazinamide under fasting conditions, with food, and with antacids. *Pharmacotherapy* (1998) 18, 1205–11.

Pyrazinamide + Antigout drugs

Pyrazinamide commonly causes hyperuricaemia and may therefore reduce the uricosuric effect of benzbromarone and probenecid. Allopurinol is unlikely to be effective against pyrazinamide-induced hyperuricaemia, and may exacerbate the situation, whereas benzbromarone may have modest efficacy in reducing hyperuricaemia caused by pyrazinamide.

Clinical evidence, mechanism, importance and management

The manufacturers of pyrazinamide warn that hyperuricaemia is a contraindication for its use, and that if hyperuricaemia accompanied by acute gouty arthritis occurs during treatment, the pyrazinamide should be stopped and not restarted. They also say that pyrazinamide should not be given unless regular uric acid determinations can be made.[1]

(a) Allopurinol

It is thought that pyrazinamide is hydrolysed in the body to pyrazinoic acid, which appears to be responsible for the hyperuricaemic effect of pyrazinamide. Pyrazinoic acid is oxidised by the enzyme xanthine oxidase to 5-hydroxypyrazoic acid.[2] Since allopurinol is an inhibitor of xanthine oxidase, its presence increases pyrazinoic acid concentrations[3] thereby probably worsening the pyrazinamide-induced hyperuricaemia.[4] Allopurinol would therefore appear to be unsuitable for treating pyrazinamide-induced hyperuricaemia.

(b) Benzbromarone

A single dose of pyrazinamide completely abolished the uricosuric effect of a single 160-mg dose of benzbromarone in 5 subjects with hyperuricaemia and gout.[5] Other authors also briefly mention the same finding.[6] However in another study, when benzbromarone 50 mg daily for 8 to 10 days was given to 10 patients taking pyrazinamide 35 mg/kg daily for tuberculosis, uric acid levels were reduced by an average of 24.3%, and returned to normal in four of them.[7] It is unclear from these studies whether or not pyrazinamide abolishes the uricosuric effects of benzbromarone. However, pyrazinamide commonly causes hyperuricaemia, and would be expected to antagonise the effects of uricosuric drugs such as benzbromarone. Benzbromarone may have modest efficacy in reducing hyperuricaemia caused by pyrazinamide, but further study is necessary. However, see above, for advice relating to hyperuricaemia caused by pyrazinamide.

(c) Probenecid

The interactions of probenecid and pyrazinamide and their effects on the excretion of uric acid are complex and intertwined. Probenecid increases the secretion of uric acid into the urine, apparently by inhibiting its reabsorption from the kidney tubules.[8] Pyrazinamide on the other hand decreases the secretion of uric acid into the urine by one-third to one-half,[9] resulting in a rise in the serum levels of urate in the blood, thereby causing hyperuricaemia.[9,10] The result of using probenecid and pyrazinamide together is not however merely the simple sum of these two effects. This is because pyrazinamide additionally decreases the metabolism of the probenecid and prolongs its uricosuric effects, and the effect of pyrazinamide is reduced. Also, probenecid inhibits the secretion of pyrazinamide, increasing its effects.[11]

The likely overall effect is that if probenecid were to be used to treat the hyperuricaemia caused by pyrazinamide, the normal uricosuric effects of probenecid would be diminished, and larger doses would be required. However, see above, for advice relating to hyperuricaemia caused by pyrazinamide.

1. Zinamide (Pyrazinamide). Merck Sharp & Dohme. UK Summary of product characteristics, January 1998.
2. Weiner IM, Tinker JP. Pharmacology of pyrazinamide: metabolic and renal function studies related to the mechanism of drug-induced urate retention. *J Pharmacol Exp Ther* (1972) 180, 411–34.
3. Lacroix C, Guyonnaud C, Chaou M, Duwoos H, Lafont O. Interaction between allopurinol and pyrazinamide. *Eur Respir J* (1988) 807–11.
4. Urban T, Maquarre E, Housset C, Chouaid C, Devin E, Lebeau B. Hypersensibilité à l'allopurinol. Une cause possible d'hépatite et d'éruption cutanéo-muqueuse chez un patient sous antituberculeux. *Rev Mal Respir* (1995) 12, 314–16.
5. Sinclair DS, Fox IH. The pharmacology of hypouricemic effect of benzbromarone. *J Rheumatol* (1975) 2, 437–45.
6. Sorensen LB, Levinson DJ. Clinical evaluation of benzbromarone. *Arthritis Rheum* (1976) 19, 183–90.
7. Kropp R. Zur urikosurischen Wirkung von Benzbromaronum an Modell der pyrizinamidbedingten Hyperurikämie. *Med Klin* (1970) 65, 1448–50.
8. Meisel AD, Diamond HS. Mechanism of probenecid-induced uricosuria: inhibition of reabsorption of secreted urate. *Arthritis Rheum* (1977) 20, 128.
9. Cullen JH, LeVine M, Fiore JM. Studies of hyperuricemia produced by pyrazinamide. *Am J Med* (1957) 23, 587–95.
10. Shapiro M, Hyde L. Hyperuricemia due to pyrazinamide. *Am J Med* (1957) 23, 596–9.
11. Yü T-F, Perel J, Berger L, Roboz J, Israili ZH, Dayton PG. The effect of the interaction of pyrazinamide and probenecid on urinary uric acid excretion in man. *Am J Med* (1977) 63, 723–8.

Pyrazinamide + Food

A single 30-mg/kg dose of pyrazinamide taken with a high-fat breakfast approximately doubled the time to peak absorption in 14 subjects but had no effect on other pharmacokinetic parameters.[1] It would therefore seem that pyrazinamide may be taken without regard to meals.

1. Peloquin CA, Bulpitt AE, Jaresko GS, Jelliffe RW, James GT, Nix DE. Pharmacokinetics of pyrazinamide under fasting conditions, with food, and with antacids. *Pharmacotherapy* (1998) 18, 1205–11.

Quinolones + Antacids or Calcium compounds

The serum levels of many of the quinolone antibacterials can be reduced by aluminium and magnesium antacids. Calcium compounds interact to a lesser extent, and bismuth compounds only minimally. Separating administration by 2 to 6 hours where significant interactions occur reduces admixture in the gut and can minimise the effects.

Clinical evidence

There is a wealth of information about the interaction between quinolones and antacids and for simplicity this is summarised in 'Table 10.3', (p.329). This table shows what happens to the maximum serum levels (C_{max}) and the relative bioavailabilities (%) when the quinolones listed have been given at the same time as antacids, and when separated by time intervals (e.g. –2 h; two hours before the antacid).

Mechanism

It is believed that certain of the quinolone functional groups (3-carboxyl and 4-oxo) form insoluble chelates with aluminium and magnesium ions within the gut, which reduces their absorption.[1-3] The stability of the chelate formed seems to be an important factor in determining the degree of interaction.[3] It has been suggested from *animal* studies that adsorption of quinolones by aluminium hydroxide re-precipitated in the small intestine may be a factor in the reduced bioavailability of quinolones.[4] See also 'Quinolones + Iron or Zinc compounds', p.336.

Importance and management

The interaction between quinolones and antacids are generally well documented, well established and, depending on the particular quinolone and antacid concerned, of clinical importance. The risk is that the serum levels of the antibacterial may fall below minimally inhibitory concentrations (i.e. become subtherapeutic, particularly against organisms such as staphylococci and *Ps. aeruginosa*[5]), resulting in treatment failures.[6] The overall picture is that the aluminium/magnesium antacids interact to a greater extent than the calcium compounds, and bismuth compounds hardly at all.

(a) Aluminium/magnesium antacids

'Table 10.3', (p.329) shows that the aluminium/magnesium antacids can greatly reduce the bioavailabilities of the quinolones. Separating their administration to reduce the admixture of the two drugs in the gut minimises the interaction, a very broad rule-of-thumb being that the quinolones should be taken at least 2 hours before and not less than 4 to 6 hours after the antacid.[1,7-12] The only obvious exception is **fleroxacin**, which appears to interact minimally.

(b) Bismuth compounds

As can be seen from 'Table 10.3', (p.329), bismuth compounds have little or no effect on the bioavailability of **ciprofloxacin**. Information about other quinolones appears to be lacking. However, using **ciprofloxacin** as a guide it would seem that any interaction is likely only to be of minimal clinical importance, and no action appears to be necessary.

(c) Calcium compounds

Information about the interactions with calcium carbonate is more limited than with the aluminium/magnesium antacids, but 'Table 10.3', (p.329) shows that the bioavailabilities of **ciprofloxacin** and **norfloxacin**, and to a lesser extent **gemifloxacin**, can be reduced. These reductions are less than those seen with the aluminium/magnesium antacids, but using **ciprofloxacin** as a guide a very broad rule-of-thumb would be to separate the drug administration by about 2 hours to minimise this interaction.[13,14] This is clearly not necessary with **levofloxacin**,[15] **lomefloxacin**,[16] **moxifloxacin**[17] or **ofloxacin**,[18] nor probably with some of the other qui-

Table 10.3 The effect of antacids on the pharmacokinetics of quinolone antibacterials

Quinolone (mg:time)*	*Antacid or other coadministered drug*	*Maximum level (micrograms/mL)* alone	with	*Relative bioavailability (%)*†	*Refs*
Ciprofloxacin					
250	$Mg(OH)_2 + Al(OH)_3$	3.69	less than 1.25	NR	1
500	$Mg(OH)_2 + Al(OH)_3$	2.6	0.88	NR	2
500: +24 h	$Mg(OH)_2 + Al(OH)_3$	1.7	0.1	NR	3
500: +24 h	$Mg(OH)_2 + Al(OH)_3$	1.9	0.13	9.5	4
750: –2 h	$Mg(OH)_2 + Al(OH)_3$	3.01	3.96	107	5
+0.08 h		3.42	0.68	15.1	
+2 h		3.42	0.88	23.2	
+4 h		3.01	2.62	70	
+6 h		2.63	2.64	108.5	
750:+0.08 h	$Al(OH)_3$	3.2	0.6	15.4	6
750	$Al(OH)_3$	2.3	0.8	NR	7
200	$Al(OH)_3$	1.3	0.2	12	8
250	$CaCO_3$	3.69	3.42 (ns)	NR	1
500	$CaCO_3$	1.53	1.37 (ns)	94 (ns)	9
500	$CaCO_3$	2.9	1.8	58.8	10
750:+0.08 h	$CaCO_3$	3.2	1.7	64.5	6
500:+2 h	$CaCO_3$	1.25	1.44	102.4	11
500	Mg citrate	2.4	0.6	21	12
500	Bismuth salicylate (subsalicylate)	3.8	2.9	83.8	13
750	Bismuth salicylate (subsalicylate)	2.95	2.57	87	14
500	Tripotassium dicitratobismuthate			100	12
400	Polycarbophil calcium	2.66	0.95	48	15
Enoxacin					
200	$Al(OH)_3$	2.26	0.46	15.4	16
400:+0.5 h	$Mg(OH)_2 + Al(OH)_3$	3.17	0.95	26.8	17
+2 h		3.17	1.95	52.3	
+8 h		3.17	2.88	82.7	
200	$Al(OH)_3$	2.3	0.5	15.8	8
Fleroxacin					
200	$Al(OH)_3$	2.4	1.8	82.8	8
Gatifloxacin					
200	$Al(OH)_3$	1.71	0.75	45.9	18
400	$Mg(OH)_2 + Al(OH)_3$	3.8	1.2	35.6	19
400:–2 h		3.8	2.1	57.9	
+2 h		3.4	3.3	82.5	
+4 h		3.4	3.5 (ns)	100 (ns)	
Gemifloxacin					
320:+3 h	$Mg(OH)_2 + Al(OH)_3$	0.91	0.75	85.9	20
–0.17 h		0.91	0.13	16.8	
–2 h		0.91	0.99	101.2	
320	$CaCO_3$	1.13	0.9	77	21
320:–2 h		1.13	1.13	93	
+2 h		1.11	1.01	90	
Grepafloxacin					
200	$Al(OH)_3$	NR	NR	60	22
Levofloxacin					
100	$Al(OH)_3$	1.82	0.64	56.3	23, 24
100	$Al(OH)_3$	1.8	0.6	54.8	8
100	MgO	1.82	1.13	78.2	23, 24
100	$CaCO_3$	1.45	1.12	96.7	23, 24
Lomefloxacin					
200	$Mg(OH)_2 + Al(OH)_3$	1.91	1.03	59.2	25
200	$Al(OH)_3$	2.2	1.0	65.2	8

Continued

Table 10.3 The effect of antacids on the pharmacokinetics of quinolone antibacterials (continued)

Quinolone	*Antacid or other*	*Maximum level (micrograms/mL)*		*Relative*	*Refs*
(mg:time)*	*coadministered drug*	*alone*	*with*	*bioavailability (%)†*	
NR:+2 h	$Mg(OH)_2$ + $Al(OH)_3$	2.85	2.67 (ns)	88.2	26
−2 h		2.85	2.16	80.4	
−4 h		2.85	2.67 (ns)	90.1	
400	$Mg(OH)_2$ + $Al(OH)_3$	3.25	1.31	52.1	27
400:+12 h		3.25	3.66 (ns)		
−4 h		3.25	3.69 (ns)		
400	$CaCO_3$	4.72	4.08	97.9 (ns)	28
Moxifloxacin					
400	$Mg(OH)_2$ + $Al(OH)_3$	2.57	1	74	29
400	Calcium lactate gluconate + $CaCO_3$	2.71	2.29	97.6	30
Norfloxacin					
200	$Al(OH)_3$	1.45	less than 0.01	2.7	16
400:+0.08 h	$Mg(OH)_2$ + $Al(OH)_3$	1.64	0.08	9 (based on urinary recovery)	31
−2 h		1.64	1.25	81.3	
200	$Al(OH)_3$	1.5	less than 0.1	3	8
400	$Al(OH)_3$	1.51	1.09	71.2 (from saliva)	32
400	Mg trisilicate	1.51	0.43	19.3 (from saliva)	32
400	$CaCO_3$	1.64	0.56	37.5	31
400	$CaCO_3$	1.51	1.08	52.8 (from saliva)	32
400	Bismuth salicylate (subsalicylate)			89.7 (ns)	33
400	Sodium bicarbonate	1.4	1.47	104.9 (ns)	32
Ofloxacin					
200	$Al(OH)_3$	3.23	1.31	52.1	16
200	$Al(PO)_4$			93.1 (ns)	34
200	MgO + $Al(OH)_3$	1.97	1.1	62	35
200:+24 h	$Mg(OH)_2$ + $Al(OH)_3$	2.6	0.7	30.8	4
400:+2 h	$Mg(OH)_2$ + $Al(OH)_3$	3.7	2.6	79.2	36
−2 h		3.7	3.8 (ns)	101.9 (ns)	
+24 h		3.7	3.5 (ns)	95.3 (ns)	
600	$Mg(OH)_2$ + $Al(OH)_3$	8.11	6.13	NR	37
200	$Al(OH)_3$	3.2	1.3	52.1	8
400:+2 h	$CaCO_3$	3.2	3.3 (ns)	103.6 (ns)	36
−2 h		3.2	3.3 (ns)	97.9 (ns)	
+24 h		3.2	3.5 (ns)	95.9 (ns)	
Pefloxacin					
400	$Mg(OH)_2$ + $Al(OH)_3$	5.14	1.95	44.2	38
400	$Mg(OH)_2$ + $Al(OH)_3$	3.95	1.25	NR	39
400	$Mg(OH)_2$ + $Al(OH)_3$	5.1	2	45.7	40
Rufloxacin					
400:+0.08 h	$Mg(OH)_2$ + $Al(OH)_3$	3.74	2.12	59.7	41
−4 h		3.74	3.97 (ns)	84.7	
Sparfloxacin					
400:−2 h	$Mg(OH)_2$ + $Al(OH)_3$	1.09	0.94	82.8	42
+2 h		1.09	0.77	77.2	
−4 h		1.09	1.17	93.4	
200	$Al(OH)_3$	1.09	1.17	94.7	8, 43
Tosufloxacin					
150	$Al(OH)_3$	0.3	0.1	29.2	8
Trovafloxacin					
300:−2 h	$Mg(OH)_2$ + $Al(OH)_3$	2.8	2.5	71.7	44
+0.5 h		2.8	1.1	33.7	

*Time interval between intake of quinolone and the other drug: - and + indicate that the quinolone was administered before and after, respectively, intake of the other drug.
†Calculated from AUC data.
NR = not reported; h = hour; ns = not significant.

Continued

Table 10.3 The effect of antacids on the pharmacokinetics of quinolone antibacterials (continued)

1. Fleming LW, Moreland TA, Stewart WK, Scott AC. Ciprofloxacin and antacids. *Lancet* (1986) ii, 294.
2. Preheim LC, Cuevas TA, Roccaforte JS, Mellencamp MA, Bittner MJ. Ciprofloxacin and antacids. *Lancet* (1986) ii, 48.
3. Höffken G, Borner K, Glatzel PD, Koeppe P, Lode H. Reduced enteral absorption of ciprofloxacin in the presence of antacids. *Eur J Clin Microbiol* (1985) 4, 345.
4. Höffken G, Lode H, Wiley R, Glatzel TD, Sievers D, Olschewski T, Borner K, Koeppe T. Pharmacokinetics and bioavailability of ciprofloxacin and ofloxacin: effect of food and antacid intake. *Rev Infect Dis* (1988) 10 (Suppl 1), S138–S139.
5. Nix DE, Watson WA, Lener ME, Frost RW, Krol G, Goldstein H, Lettieri J, Schentag JJ. Effects of aluminum and magnesium antacids and ranitidine on the absorption of ciprofloxacin. *Clin Pharmacol Ther* (1989) 46, 700–705.
6. Frost RW, Lasseter KC, Noe AJ, Shamblen EC, Lettieri JT. Effects of aluminum hydroxide and calcium carbonate antacids on the bioavailability of ciprofloxacin. *Antimicrob Agents Chemother* (1992) 36, 830–2.
7. Golper TA, Hartstein AI, Morthland VH, Christensen JM. Effects of antacids and dialysate dwell times on multiple-dose pharmacokinetics of oral ciprofloxacin in patients on continuous ambulatory peritoneal dialysis. *Antimicrob Agents Chemother* (1987) 31, 1787–90.
8. Shiba K, Sakamoto M, Nakazawa Y, Sakai O. Effect of antacid on absorption and excretion of new quinolones. *Drugs* (1995) 49 (Suppl 2), 360–1.
9. Lomaestro BM, Bailie GR. Effect of multiple staggered doses of calcium on the bioavailability of ciprofloxacin. *Ann Pharmacother* (1993) 27, 1325–8.
10. Sahai J, Healey DP, Stotka J, Polk RE. The influence of chronic administration of calcium carbonate on the bioavailability of oral ciprofloxacin. *Br J Clin Pharmacol* (1993) 35, 302–4.
11. Lomaestro BM, Bailie GR. Effect of staggered dose of calcium on the bioavailability of ciprofloxacin. *Antimicrob Agents Chemother* (1991) 35, 1004–1007.
12. Brouwers JRBJ, van der Kam HJ, Sijtsma J, Proost JH. Important reduction of ciprofloxacin absorption by sucralfate and magnesium citrate solution. *Drug Invest* (1990) 2, 197–9.
13. Sahai J, Oliveras L, Garber G. Effect of bismuth subsalicylate (Peptobismol. PB) on ciprofloxacin (C) absorption: a preliminary investigation. 17th Int Congr Chemother, June 1991, Berlin, Abstract 414.
14. Rambout L, Sahai J, Gallicano K, Oliveras L, Garber G. Effect of bismuth subsalicylate on ciprofloxacin bioavailability. *Antimicrob Agents Chemother* (1994) 38, 2187–90.
15. Kato R, Ueno K, Imano H, Kawai M, Kuwahara , Tsuchishita Y, Yonezawa E, Tanaka K. Impairment of ciprofloxacin absorption by calcium polycarbophil. *J Clin Pharmacol* (2002) 42, 806–11.
16. Shiba K, Saito A, Miyahara T, Tachizawa H, Fujimoto T. Effect of aluminium hydroxide, an antacid, on the pharmacokinetics of new quinolones in humans. Proc 15th Int Congr Chemother, Istanbul 1987, 168–9.
17. Grasela TH, Schentag JJ, Sedman AJ, Wilton JH, Thomas DJ, Schultz RW, Lebsack ME, Kinkel AW. Inhibition of enoxacin absorption by antacids or ranitidine. *Antimicrob Agents Chemother* (1989) 33, 615–17.
18. Shiba K, Kusajima H, Momo K. The effects of aluminium hydroxide, cimetidine, ferrous sulfate, green tea and milk on pharmacokinetics of gatifloxacin in healthy humans. *J Antimicrob Chemother* (1999) 44 (Suppl A), 141.
19. Lober S, Ziege S, Rau M, Schreiber G, Mignot A, Koeppe P, Lode H. Pharmacokinetics of gatifloxacin and interaction with an antacid containing aluminum and magnesium. *Antimicrob Agents Chemother* (1999) 43, 1067–71.
20. Allen A, Vousden M, Porter A, Lewis A. Effect of Maalox® on the bioavailability of oral gemifloxacin in healthy volunteers. *Chemotherapy* (1999) 45, 504–11.
21. Pletz MW, Petzold P, Allen A, Burkhardt O, Lode H. Effect of calcium carbonate on bioavailability of orally administered gemifloxacin. *Antimicrob Agents Chemother* (2003) 47, 2158–60.
22. Koneru B, Bramer S, Bricmont P, Maroli A, Shiba K. Effect of food, gastric pH and co-administration of antacid, cimetidine and probenecid on the oral pharmacokinetics of the broad spectrum antimicrobial agent grepafloxacin. *Pharm Res* (1996) 13 (9 Suppl), S414.
23. Shiba K, Sakai O, Shimada J, Okazaki O, Aoki H, Hakusui H. Effects of antacids, ferrous sulfate, and ranitidine on absorption of DR-3355 in humans. *Antimicrob Agents Chemother* (1992) 36, 2270–4.
24. Shiba K , Okazaki O, Aoki H, Shimada J, Sakai O. Influence of antacids and ranitidine on the absorption of levofloxacin in men. *Drugs* (1993) 45 (Suppl 3) 299–300.
25. Shimada J, Shiba K, Oguma T, Miwa H, Yoshimura Y, Nishikawa T, Okabayashi Y, Kitagawa T, Yamamoto S. Effect of antacid on absorption of the quinolone lomefloxacin. *Antimicrob Agents Chemother* (1992) 36, 1219–24.
26. Forster T, Blouin R. The effect of antacid timing on lomefloxacin bioavailability. Intersci Conf Antimicrob Agents Chemother (1989) 29, 318.
27. Kunka RL, Wong YY, Lyon JL. Effect of antacid on the pharmacokinetics of lemofloxacin. *Pharm Res* (1988) 5 (Suppl), S–165.
28. Lehto P, Kivistö KT. Different effects of products containing metal ions on the absorption of lomefloxacin. *Clin Pharmacol Ther* (1994) 56, 477–82.
29. Stass H, Böttcher M-F, Ochmann K. Evaluation of the influence of antacids and H2 antagonists on the absorption of moxifloxacin after oral administration of a 400-mg dose to healthy volunteers. *Clin Pharmacokinet* (2001) 40 (Suppl 1), 39–48.
30. Stass H, Wandel C, Delesen H, Möller J-G. Effect of calcium supplements on the oral bioavailability of moxifloxacin in healthy male volunteers. *Clin Pharmacokinet* (2001) 40 (Suppl 1), 27–32.
31. Nix DE, Wilton JH, Ronald B, Distlerath L, Williams VC, Norman A. Inhibition of norfloxacin absorption by antacids. *Antimicrob Agents Chemother* (1990) 34, 432–5.
32. Okhamafe AO, Akerele JO, Chukuka CS. Pharmacokinetic interactions of norfloxacin with some metallic medicinal agents. *Int J Pharmaceutics* (1991) 68, 11–18.
33. Campbell NRC, Kara M, Hasinoff BB, Haddara WM, McKay DW. Norfloxacin interaction with antacids and minerals. *Br J Clin Pharmacol* (1992) 33, 115–16.
34. Martínez Carbaga M, Sánchez Navarro A, Colino Gandarillas CI, Domínguez-Gil A. Effects of two cations on gastrointestinal absorption of ofloxacin. *Antimicrob Agents Chemother* (1991) 35, 2102–5.
35. Shiba K, Yoshida M, Kachi M, Shimada J, Saito A, Sakai N. Effects of peptic ulcer-healing drugs on the pharmacokinetics of new quinolone (OFLX). 17th Int Congr Chemother, June 1991, Berlin, Abstract 415.
36. Flor S, Guay DRP, Opsahl JA, Tack K, Matzke GR. Effects of magnesium-aluminum hydroxide and calcium carbonate antacids on bioavailability of ofloxacin. *Antimicrob Agents Chemother* (1990) 34, 2436–8.
37. Maesen FPV, Davies BI, Geraedts WH, Sumajow CA. Ofloxacin and antacids. *J Antimicrob Chemother* (1987) 19, 848–50.
38. Metz R, Jaehde U, Sörgel F, Wiesemann H, Gottschalk B, Stephan U, Schunack W. Pharmacokinetic interactions and non-interactions of pefloxacin. Proc 15th Int Congr Chemother, Istanbul, 1987, 997–9.
39. Vinceneux P, Weber P, Gaudin H, Boussougant Y. Diminution de l'absorption de la péfloxacine par les pansements gastriques. *Presse Med* (1986) 15, 1826.
40. Jaehde U, Sörgel F, Stephan U, Schunack W. Effect of an antacid containing magnesium and aluminum on absorption, metabolism and mechanism of renal elimination of pefloxacin in humans. *Antimicrob Agents Chemother* (1994) 38, 1129–33.
41. Lazzaroni M, Imbimbo BP, Bargiggia S, Sangaletti O, Dal Bo L, Broccali G, Bianchi Porro G. Effects of magnesium-aluminum hydroxide antacid on absorption of rufloxacin. *Antimicrob Agents Chemother* (1993) 37, 2212–16.
42. Johnson RD, Dorr MB, Talbot GH, Caille G. Effect of Maalox on the oral absorption of sparfloxacin. *Clin Ther* (1998) 20, 1149–58.
43. Shimada J, Saito A, Shiba K, Hojo T, Kaji M, Hori S, Yoshida M, Sakai O. Pharmacokinetics and clinical studies on sparfloxacin. *Chemotherapy (Tokyo)* (1991) 39 (Suppl 4), 234–44.
44. Teng R, Dogolo LC, Willavize SA, Freidman HL, Vincent J. Effect of Maalox and omeprazole on the bioavailability of trovafloxacin. *J Antimicrob Chemother* (1997) 39 (Suppl B), 93–7.

nolones that have yet to be studied, but in the absence of direct information a 2-hour separation errs on the side of caution.

(d) Sodium antacids

Sodium bicarbonate does not interact significantly with **norfloxacin**[19] but information about other quinolones appears to be lacking. However, bear in mind that in the case of **ciprofloxacin** an excessive rise in urinary pH (which can be caused by antacids like sodium bicarbonate) may possibly result in urinary crystalluria and kidney damage.[20]

Possible alternatives to the antacids, which do not appear to interact with the quinolones, include the 'H_2-receptor antagonists', (p.335) and 'omeprazole', (p.338).

1. Nix DE, Watson WA, Lener ME, Frost RW, Krol G, Goldstein H, Lettieri J, Schentag JJ. Effects of aluminum and magnesium antacids and ranitidine on the absorption of ciprofloxacin. *Clin Pharmacol Ther* (1989) 46, 700–705.
2. Shimada J, Shiba K, Oguma T, Miwa H, Yoshimura Y, Nishikawa T, Okabayashi Y, Kitagawa T, Yamamoto S. Effect of antacid on absorption of the quinolone lomefloxacin. *Antimicrob Agents Chemother* (1992) 36, 1219–24.
3. Mizuki Y, Fujiwara I, Yamaguchi T. Pharmacokinetic interactions related to the chemical structures of fluoroquinolones. *J Antimicrob Chemother* (1996) 37 (Suppl), A41–A55.
4. Tanaka M, Kurata T, Fujisawa C, Ohshima Y, Aoki H, Okazaki O, Hakusui H. Mechanistic study of inhibition of levofloxacin absorption by aluminium hydroxide. *Antimicrob Agents Chemother* (1993) 37, 2173–8.
5. Preheim LC, Cuevas TA, Roccaforte JS, Mellencamp MA, Bittner MJ. Ciprofloxacin and antacids. *Lancet* (1986) ii, 48.
6. Noyes M, Polk RE. Norfloxacin and absorption of magnesium-aluminium. *Ann Intern Med* (1988) 109, 168–9.
7. Grasela TH, Schentag JJ, Sedman AJ, Wilton JH, Thomas DJ, Schultz RW, Lebsack ME, Kinkel AW. Inhibition of enoxacin absorption by antacids or ranitidine. *Antimicrob Agents Chemother* (1989) 33, 615–17.
8. Nix DE, Wilton JH, Ronald B, Distlerath L, Williams VC, Norman A. Inhibition of norfloxacin absorption by antacids. *Antimicrob Agents Chemother* (1990) 34, 432–5.
9. Forster T, Blouin R. The effect of antacid timing on lomefloxacin bioavailability. *Intersci Conf Antimicrob Agents Chemother* (1989) 29, 318.
10. Johnson RD, Dorr MB, Talbot GH, Caille G. Effect of Maalox on the oral absorption of sparfloxacin. *Clin Ther* (1998) 20, 1149–58.
11. Lober S, Ziege S, Rau M, Schreiber G, Mignot A, Koeppe P, Lode H. Pharmacokinetics of gatifloxacin and interaction with an antacid containing aluminum and magnesium. *Antimicrob Agents Chemother* (1999) 43, 1067–71.
12. Misiak P, Toothaker R, Lebsack M, Sedman A, Colburn W. The effect of dosing-time intervals on the potential pharmacokinetic interaction between oral enoxacin and oral antacid. *Intersci Conf Antimicrob Agents Chemother* (1988) 28, 367.
13. Lomaestro BM, Bailie GR. Effect of staggered dose of calcium on the bioavailability of ciprofloxacin. *Antimicrob Agents Chemother* (1991) 35, 1004–1007.
14. Lomaestro BM, Bailie GR. Effect of multiple staggered doses of calcium on the bioavailability of ciprofloxacin. *Ann Pharmacother* (1993) 27, 1325–8.
15. Shiba K, Sakai O, Shimada J, Okazaki O, Aoki H, Hakusui H. Effects of antacids, ferrous sulfate, and ranitidine on absorption of DR-3355 in humans. *Antimicrob Agents Chemother* (1992) 36, 2270–4.
16. Lehto P, Kivistö KT. Different effects of products containing metal ions on the absorption of lomefloxacin. *Clin Pharmacol Ther* (1994) 56, 477–82.
17. Stass H, Kubitza D. Profile of moxifloxacin drug interactions. *Clin Infect Dis* (2001) 32, (Suppl 1), S47–S50.
18. Sánchez Navarro A, Martínez Cabarga M, Dominguez-Gil Hurlé A. Comparative study of the influence of Ca^{2+} on absorption parameters of ciprofloxacin and ofloxacin. *J Antimicrob Chemother* (1994) 34, 119–25.
19. Okhamafe AO, Akerele JO, Chukuka CS. Pharmacokinetic interactions of norfloxacin with some metallic medicinal agents. *Int J Pharmaceutics* (1991) 68, 11–18.
20. Ciproxin Tablets (Ciprofloxacin hydrochloride). Bayer plc. UK Summary of product characteristics, January 2006.

Quinolones + Antineoplastics

The absorption of ciprofloxacin and ofloxacin can be reduced by some cytotoxic antineoplastics but this seems unlikely to be clinically significant.

Clinical evidence

(a) Ciprofloxacin

Six patients with newly diagnosed haematological malignancies (5 with acute myeloid leukaemia and one with non-Hodgkin's lymphoma) were given ciprofloxacin 500 mg twice daily to control possible neutropenic infections. It was found that, after 13 days of chemotherapy, their mean maximum serum ciprofloxacin levels had fallen by 46%, from 3.7 to 2 mg/L and the AUC_{0-4} was reduced by 47%. There were large individual differences between the patients. The antineoplastics used were **cyclophosphamide**, **cytarabine**, **daunorubicin**, **doxorubicin**, **mitoxantrone** and **vincristine**.[1] Methotrexate toxicity has occurred in 2 patients during treatment with ciprofloxacin, see 'Methotrexate + Antibacterials; Ciprofloxacin', p.643.

(b) Ofloxacin

Ten patients with non-Hodgkin's lymphoma, hairy cell leukaemia or acute myeloid leukaemia were given ofloxacin 400 mg at breakfast time for antibacterial prophylaxis during neutropenia. Blood samples were taken 3 days before chemotherapy began and then at 2 to 3, 5 to 7, and 8 to 10 days. The maximum serum ofloxacin levels were reduced by 18% two to three days after the chemotherapy but none of the other pharmacokinetic measurements were changed by the antineoplastic treatment. The serum levels had returned to normal by days 5 to 7. At all times serum levels exceeded the expected MICs of the gram-negative potential pathogens. The antineoplastics used were **cyclophosphamide**, **cytarabine**, **doxorubicin**, **etoposide**, **ifosfamide** (with mesna), **vincristine**.[2]

Mechanism

Uncertain. The interaction seems to result from a reduction in the absorption of the quinolones by the small intestine, possibly related to the damaging effect cytotoxic antineoplastics have on the rapidly dividing cells of the intestinal mucosa.

Importance and management

Direct information is limited, but these reports are consistent with the way cytotoxic antineoplastics can reduce the absorption of some other drugs. The authors of both reports suggest that these changes are probably clinically unimportant, because the serum levels of achieved are likely to be sufficient to treat most infections. If the suggested mechanism of interaction is correct, no interaction should occur if quinolones are given parenterally. Nothing appears to be documented about any of the other quinolones.

1. Johnson EJ, MacGowan AP, Potter MN, Stockley RJ, White LO, Slade RR, Reeves DS. Reduced absorption of oral ciprofloxacin after chemotherapy for haematological malignancy. *J Antimicrob Chemother* (1990) 25, 837–42.
2. Brown NM, White LO, Blundell EL, Chown SR, Slade RR, MacGowan AP, Reeves DS. Absorption of oral ofloxacin after cytotoxic chemotherapy for haematological malignancy. *J Antimicrob Chemother* (1993) 32, 117–22.

Quinolones + Chinese herbal medicines

Sho-saiko-to, Rikkunshi-to and Sairei-to do not interact with ofloxacin, and Hotyu-ekki-to, Rikkunshi-to and Juzen-taiho-to do not interact with levofloxacin.

Clinical evidence, mechanism, importance and management

The bioavailability and urinary recovery of a single 200-mg oral dose of **ofloxacin** were not significantly altered in 7 healthy subjects by three Chinese herbal medicines (**Sho-saiko-to**, **Rikkunshi-to** or **Sairei-to**).[1] The bioavailability and renal excretion of a single 200-mg oral dose of **levofloxacin** was not affected in 8 healthy subjects given single 2.5-g doses of **Hotyu-ekki-to**, **Rikkunshi-to** or **Juzen-taiho-to**.[2] There would therefore seem to be no reason for avoiding concurrent use. Information about other quinolones is lacking. The ingredients of these herbal medicines are detailed in 'Table 10.4', (p.333).

1. Hasegawa T, Yamaki K, Nadai M, Muraoka I, Wang L, Takagi K, Nabeshima T. Lack of effect of Chinese medicines on bioavailability of ofloxacin in healthy volunteers. *Int J Clin Pharmacol Ther* (1994) 32, 57–61.
2. Hasegawa T, Yamaki K-I, Muraoka I, Nadai M, Takagi K, Nabeshima T. Effects of traditional Chinese medicines on pharmacokinetics of levofloxacin. *Antimicrob Agents Chemother* (1995) 39, 2135–7.

Quinolones + Dairy products

Dairy products reduce the bioavailability of ciprofloxacin and norfloxacin, and to a minor extent, gatifloxacin, but not enoxacin, lomefloxacin, moxifloxacin, ofloxacin and probably not fleroxacin.

Clinical evidence

(a) Ciprofloxacin

A study in 7 healthy subjects given a single 500-mg dose of ciprofloxacin found that 300 mL of **milk** or **yoghurt** reduced the peak plasma levels by 36% and 47%, respectively, and the AUC by 33% and 36%, respectively.[1] In another study 300 mL of **milk** reduced the AUC of ciprofloxacin 500 mg by about 30%.[2]

Table 10.4 Herbs contained in some Chinese herbal remedies[1,2]

Herb (plant part)	*Amounts of herbs in the medicines (mg/2.5 g)*				
	Hotyu-ekki-to	**Rikkunshi-to**	**Juzen-taiho-to**	**Sho-saiko-to**	**Sairei-to**
Atractylodis lanceae (rhizome)	278	248	175		125
Ginseng (root)	278	248	175	188	125
Glycyrrhizae (root)	104	662	688	125	83
Aurantii nobilis (pericarp)	139	124			
Zizyphi (fruit)	139	124		188	125
Zingiberis (rhizome)	635	631		63	42
Astragali (root)	278		175		
Angelicae (root)	208		175		
Bupleuri (root)	139			438	292
Cimicifugae (rhizome)	669				
Hoelen		248	175		125
Pinelliae (tuber)		248		313	208
Cinnamomi (cortex)			175		83
Rehmanniae (root)			175		
Paeoniae (root)			175		
Cnidii (rhizome)			175		
Scutellariae (root)				188	125
Alismatis (rhizome)					208
Polyporus					125

1. Hasegawa T, Yamaki K, Nadai M, Muraoka I, Wang L, Takagi K, Nabeshima T. Lack of effect of Chinese medicines on bioavailability of ofloxacin in healthy volunteers. *Int J Clin Pharmacol Ther* (1994) 32, 57-61.
2. Hasegawa T, Yamaki K-I, Muraoka I, Nadai M, Takagi K, Nabeshima T. Effects of traditional Chinese medicines on pharmacokinetics of levofloxacin. *Antimicrob Agents Chemother* (1995) 39, 2135-7.

(b) Enoxacin

A study found that **milk** and a standard breakfast had no effect on enoxacin absorption.[3]

(c) Fleroxacin

In a study, a **fat and liquid calcium meal** had no clinically significant effect on the pharmacokinetics of fleroxacin.[4] In another study, **milk** had no effect on fleroxacin pharmacokinetics.[2]

(d) Gatifloxacin

In one study 200 mL of **milk** reduced the AUC of gatifloxacin 200 mg by about 15%.[5]

(e) Lomefloxacin

Milk had no effect on the pharmacokinetics of lomefloxacin.[6]

(f) Moxifloxacin

A study found that the rate of absorption of a single 400-mg dose of moxifloxacin was slightly delayed by 250 g of **yoghurt**. The maximum plasma level of moxifloxacin was reduced by about 15%, but the bioavailability was unaffected.[7]

(g) Norfloxacin

A study found that 300 mL of **milk** or **yoghurt** reduced the absorption and the peak plasma levels of a single 200-mg dose of norfloxacin by roughly 50%.[8]

(h) Ofloxacin

A study in 21 healthy subjects found that 8 oz (about 250 mL) of **milk** had no clinically significant effects on the absorption of 300 mg of ofloxacin.[9] Another study confirmed the lack of a significant interaction between ofloxacin and both **milk** and **yoghurt**.[10]

Mechanism

The proposed reason for these changes is that the calcium in milk and yoghurt or other dairy products combines with the ciprofloxacin and norfloxacin to produce insoluble chelates. Compare also 'Quinolones + Antacids or Calcium compounds', p.328.

Importance and management

The effect of these changes to ciprofloxacin and norfloxacin pharmacokinetics on the control of infection is uncertain but until the situation is clear patients should be advised not to take these dairy products within 1 to 2 hours of either ciprofloxacin or norfloxacin to prevent admixture in the gut. The slight reduction in gatifloxacin levels is probably not clinically relevant.

The quinolones that do not interact significantly would appear to be enoxacin, lomefloxacin, moxifloxacin, ofloxacin and probably fleroxacin. They may provide a useful alternative to the interacting quinolones.

1. Neuvonen PJ, Kivistö KT, Lehto P. Interference of dairy products with the absorption of ciprofloxacin. *Clin Pharmacol Ther* (1991) 50, 498–502.
2. Hoogkamer JFW, Kleinbloesem CH. The effect of milk consumption on the pharmacokinetics of fleroxacin and ciprofloxacin in healthy volunteers. *Drugs* (1995) 49 (Suppl 2), 346–8.
3. Lehto P, Kivistö KT. Effects of milk and food on the absorption of enoxacin. *Br J Clin Pharmacol* (1995) 39, 194–6.
4. Bertino JS, Nafziger AN, Wong M, Stragand L, Puleo C. Effects of a fat- and calcium-rich breakfast on pharmacokinetics of fleroxacin administered in single and multiple doses. *Antimicrob Agents Chemother* (1994) 38, 499–503.
5. Shiba K, Kusajima H, Momo K. The effects of aluminium hydroxide, cimetidine, ferrous sulfate, green tea and milk on pharmacokinetics of gatifloxacin in healthy humans. *J Antimicrob Chemother* (1999) 44 (Suppl A), 141.
6. Lehto PL, Kivistö KT. Different effects of products containing metal ions on the absorption of lomefloxacin. *Clin Pharmacol Ther* (1994) 56, 477–82.
7. Stass H, Kubitza D. The effects of dairy products on the oral bioavailability of moxifloxacin, a novel 8-methoxyfluoroquinolone, in healthy volunteers. *Clin Pharmacokinet* (2001) 40 (Suppl 1) 33–8.
8. Kivistö KT, Ojala-Karlsson P, Neuvonen PJ. Inhibition of norfloxacin absorption by dairy products. *Antimicrob Agents Chemother* (1992) 36, 489–91.

9. Dudley MN, Marchbanks CR, Flor SC, Beals B. The effect of food or milk on the absorption kinetics of ofloxacin. *Eur J Clin Pharmacol* (1991) 41, 569–71.
10. Neuvonen PJ, Kivistö KT. Milk and yoghurt do not impair the absorption of ofloxacin. *Br J Clin Pharmacol* (1992) 33, 346–8.

Quinolones + Didanosine

An extremely marked reduction in the serum levels of ciprofloxacin occurs if it is given at the same time as didanosine tablets, because of an interaction with the antacid buffers in the didanosine formulation. Taking the ciprofloxacin 2 hours before or 6 hours after didanosine tablets minimises this interaction. Other quinolones are expected to interact similarly. Didanosine enteric-coated capsules do not interact with ciprofloxacin.

Clinical evidence

When 12 healthy subjects were given **ciprofloxacin** 750 mg with two didanosine placebo tablets (i.e. all of the antacid additives but no didanosine), the **ciprofloxacin** AUC and maximum serum levels were reduced by 98% and 93%, respectively.[1] The antacids in this formulation were dihydroxyaluminium sodium carbonate and magnesium hydroxide.

Other studies have looked at whether separating the administration times affects this interaction. When 16 HIV-positive patients were given **ciprofloxacin** 1.5 g daily 2 hours before didanosine tablets, the **ciprofloxacin** AUC was reduced by only 26%.[2] Another study in just one subject found that when **ciprofloxacin** 500 mg was given 2 hours after taking two didanosine placebo tablets the **ciprofloxacin** serum levels were reduced below minimal inhibitory concentrations, but giving the **ciprofloxacin** 2 hours before the didanosine placebo tablets resulted in normal blood levels.[3]

The enteric-coated capsule formulation of didanosine (which does not contain antacids) does not interact with **ciprofloxacin.**[4]

Mechanism

Didanosine is extremely acid labile at pH values below 3, so one of the formulations contains buffering agents (dihydroxyaluminium sodium carbonate and magnesium hydroxide) to keep the pH as high as possible to minimise the acid-induced hydrolysis. Ciprofloxacin forms insoluble non-absorbable chelates with these metallic ions in the buffer so that its bioavailability is markedly reduced. See also 'Quinolones + Antacids or Calcium compounds', p.328.

Importance and management

Direct information is limited to these reports but the interaction between buffered didanosine and ciprofloxacin appears to be clinically important. Such drastic reductions in serum ciprofloxacin levels mean that minimal inhibitory concentrations are unlikely to be achieved. Ciprofloxacin should be given at least 2 hours before or 6 hours after didanosine tablets (see 'Quinolones + Antacids or Calcium compounds', p.328). Other quinolone antibacterials that interact with antacids are also expected to interact with didanosine tablets, but so far reports are lacking. Didanosine enteric-coated capsules do not interact.

1. Sahai J, Gallicano K, Oliveras L, Khaliq S, Hawley-Foss N, Garber G. Cations in the didanosine tablet reduce ciprofloxacin bioavailability. *Clin Pharmacol Ther* (1993) 53, 292–7.
2. Knupp CA, Barbhaiya RH. A multiple-dose pharmacokinetic interaction study between didanosine (Videx®) and ciprofloxacin (Cipro®) in male subjects seropositive for HIV but asymptomatic. *Biopharm Drug Dispos* (1997) 18, 65–77.
3. Sahai J. Avoiding the ciprofloxacin-didanosine interaction. *Ann Intern Med* (1995) 123, 394–5.
4. Damle BD, Mummaneni V, Kaul S, Knupp C. Lack of effect of simultaneously administered didanosine encapsulated enteric bead formulation (Videx EC) on oral absorption of indinavir, ketoconazole, or ciprofloxacin. *Antimicrob Agents Chemother* (2002) 46, 385–91.

Quinolones + Enteral feeds or Food

The absorption of ciprofloxacin can be reduced by enteral feeds such as *Ensure, Jevity, Osmolite, Pulmocare* and *Sustacal*. An *in vitro* study found a significant reduction in the concentration of ciprofloxacin, levofloxacin and ofloxacin with *Ensure* but other studies suggest the interaction with moxifloxacin or ofloxacin is much smaller than that with ciprofloxacin and probably of little clinical importance.

Apart from 'dairy products' (p.332), most foods delay but do not reduce the absorption of ciprofloxacin, enoxacin, gemifloxacin, lomefloxacin, ofloxacin or sparfloxacin. A high-fat/high-calcium breakfast did not reduce ciprofloxacin levels. Calcium-fortified orange juice significantly reduces the absorption of ciprofloxacin, but not gatifloxacin or levofloxacin.

Clinical evidence

A. Enteral feeds

(a) Ciprofloxacin

The oral bioavailability of ciprofloxacin 750 mg was reduced by 28% and the mean maximum serum ciprofloxacin levels were reduced by 48% when it was given to 13 fasted subjects with ***Ensure***. In this study the subjects were given 120 mL of the study liquid (***Ensure*** or water) and this was repeated at 30-minute intervals for 5 doses. The ciprofloxacin was crushed and mixed with the second dose of the study liquid and the cup rinsed with another 60 mL of the study liquid.[1]

Other enteral feeds given orally (***Osmolite***, ***Pulmocare***, and ***Resource***) similarly reduced the bioavailability and maximum serum levels of ciprofloxacin by about one-quarter to one-third in two other studies.[2,3] One comparative study found that ***Ensure*** reduced the AUC of ciprofloxacin by 40.2% in men but by only 14.5% in women.[4]

Ciprofloxacin bioavailability was reduced by 53% and 67% by ***Jevity*** or ***Sustacal***, respectively, when given via gastrostomy or jejunostomy tubes in a study of 26 hospitalised patients. Despite this, the serum levels achieved with gastrostomy tubes were roughly equivalent to those seen in subjects taking tablets orally.[5] In another study in patients given ***Jevity*** or ***Osmolite***, the 4 patients with a nasoduodenal tube achieved a ciprofloxacin AUC that was about double that seen in the 3 patients with a nasogastric tube or a gastrostomy.[6] In contrast, in another study in healthy subjects, there was no difference in the bioavailability of ciprofloxacin when it was given alone or when it was given with ***Osmolite*** via a nasogastric tube.[7]

The bioavailability of ciprofloxacin 750 mg every 12 hours in 5 patients with severe gram-negative intra-abdominal infections was reduced by 47% when it was added to enteral feeding with ***Nutrison*** or ***Nutrison E+*** and given via nasogastric or nasoduodenal tubes. The serum levels were similar to those found in another 7 patients given ciprofloxacin with these enteral feeds and also to those found when the 5 original patients were given intravenous ciprofloxacin 400 mg every 12 hours.[8] In another study in 12 intensive care patients the AUC of ciprofloxacin 400 mg given by intravenous infusion was similar to that found after a dose of 750 mg given via nasogastric tube during enteral feeding with ***Normo-Réal fibres***.[9]

An *in vitro* study found an 83% decrease in the concentration of ciprofloxacin when a 500-mg ciprofloxacin tablet was crushed and mixed with ***Ensure***. Mixing with solutions of calcium chloride and/or magnesium chloride did not significantly reduce ciprofloxacin concentrations.[10]

(b) Levofloxacin

An *in vitro* study found a 61% decrease in the concentration of levofloxacin when a 500-mg levofloxacin tablet was crushed and mixed with ***Ensure***. Mixing with solutions of calcium chloride and/or magnesium chloride did not significantly reduce levofloxacin concentrations.[10]

(c) Moxifloxacin

Compared to oral administration of an uncrushed tablet with water, the oral bioavailability of a single 400-mg dose of moxifloxacin was slightly decreased (by 9%) when given to 12 healthy subjects as a suspension of a crushed tablet via a nasogastric tube with either water or ***Isosource Energy***. Maximum plasma levels were decreased by 5% and 12% after nasogastric administration with water and ***Isosource Energy***, respectively.[11]

(d) Ofloxacin

The oral bioavailability of **ofloxacin** 400 mg was reduced by 10% when given to 13 healthy subjects with ***Ensure***. The mean maximum serum **ofloxacin** levels were reduced by 36%. The same procedure as described in (a) was followed.[1] Only small reductions in the AUCs of **ofloxacin** were seen in another study (10.5% in men, 13.2% in women) with ***Ensure***.[4]

However, an *in vitro* study found a 46% decrease in the concentration of ofloxacin when a 300-mg tablet of ofloxacin was crushed and mixed with ***Ensure***. Mixing with solutions of calcium chloride and/or magnesium chloride did not significantly reduce ofloxacin concentrations.[10]

B. Food

Food delayed the absorption of **ciprofloxacin** and **ofloxacin** in 10 subjects, but their bioavailabilities remained unchanged.[12] A study in 12 healthy subjects found that standard or high-fat breakfasts did not affect the absorption of **ciprofloxacin**.[13] Another study in healthy subjects found that a standard breakfast reduced the bioavailability of a single 300-mg dose of **ofloxacin** by about 18%, but this was not considered clinically significant.[14] Other studies suggest that food delays the absorption of **ofloxacin**[15] and **lomefloxacin**[16] but the bioavailability is unchanged. Food also has no effect on the absorption of **enoxacin**, but high carbohydrate meals delayed the peak serum levels by almost an hour.[17] The pharmacokinetics of **gemifloxacin** 320 mg or 640 mg[18] or **sparfloxacin** 200 mg[19] were not significantly affected when they were given to healthy subjects with high fat or standard meals, although the absorption of **sparfloxacin** was slightly delayed.

C. Calcium-fortified foods

Calcium-fortified orange juice decreased the AUC of **ciprofloxacin** by 38% and the maximum plasma level by 41%, when compared to water.[20] However, in another study, a high-fat/high-calcium breakfast did not affect the absorption of **ciprofloxacin**.[13]

The AUC of **gatifloxacin** was reduced by only 12% by calcium-fortified orange juice.[21] Similarly, in two studies, orange juice, calcium-fortified orange juice,[22] or a breakfast of calcium-fortified orange juice and cereal with or without milk[23] were found to decrease the bioavailability of **levofloxacin**. However, the **levofloxacin** AUC was decreased by less than 16%, an amount that rarely proves to be clinically significant.

Mechanism

Not fully understood. The quinolone antibacterials can form insoluble chelates with divalent ions, which reduces their absorption from the gut. Enteral feeds such as those used above contain at least two divalent ions, calcium and magnesium. However, an *in vitro* study found no evidence of chelate formation with fluoroquinolones and calcium or magnesium, and therefore suggested that either other divalent cations may be involved, or that the quinolones may be adsorbed onto other metal ions, proteins or fat in the enteral feed.[10]

It has also been suggested that alteration in pH as well as the presence of cations are required to form chelates with ciprofloxacin and while this helps explain the lack of effect of high calcium in a high fat breakfast,[13] it does not explain the significant effect with enteral feeds or calcium-fortified orange juice. The differences seen in men and women are possibly due to a slower gastric emptying rate in men, which increases the exposure of the quinolone to the enteral feed.[4]

Importance and management

The interaction between ciprofloxacin and enteral feeds is established. No treatment failures have been reported but it may be clinically important. For example, if patients receiving enteral feeds were to be switched from parenteral to oral ciprofloxacin, there could be a significant reduction in serum ciprofloxacin levels. The authors of one study recommend that in patients with severe infections, such a switch from parenteral to nasogastric administration of ciprofloxacin should be restricted to those whose plasma ciprofloxacin levels can be routinely monitored. However, some have found the reduced levels with enteral feeding still provide adequate antibacterial levels,[8,24] but be alert for any evidence that ciprofloxacin is less effective and raise the dosage as necessary. Use of enteral feeds with lower concentrations of divalent ions or even stopping tube feeding for a short period of time have been suggested as methods to try to improve ciprofloxacin absorption.[24] The authors of one study suggest that *Ensure* should be given at least 2 hours before or after fluoroquinolones.[10]

The interaction between ofloxacin or moxifloxacin and enteral feeds is much smaller and probably not clinically important but this needs confirmation. There are no specific reports about other quinolones but be alert for this interaction with any of them.

Apart from 'dairy products' (p.332), quinolones can be given with food without any decrease in levels. However, calcium-fortified foods may cause significant interactions with ciprofloxacin.

1. Mueller BA, Brierton DG, Abel SR, Bowman L. Effect of enteral feeding with *Ensure* on oral bioavailabilities of ofloxacin and ciprofloxacin. *Antimicrob Agents Chemother* (1994) 38, 2101–5.
2. Noer BL, Angaran DM. The effect of enteral feedings on ciprofloxacin pharmacokinetics. *Pharmacotherapy* (1990) 10, 254.
3. Piccolo ML, Toossi Z, Goldman M. Effect of coadministration of a nutritional supplement on ciprofloxacin absorption. *Am J Hosp Pharm* (1994) 51, 2697–9.
4. Sowinski KM, Abel SR, Clark WR, Mueller BA. Effect of gender on relative oral bioavailability of ciprofloxacin and ofloxacin when administered with an enteral feeding product. *Pharmacotherapy* (1997) 17, 1112.
5. Healy DP, Brodbeck MC, Clendening CE. Ciprofloxacin absorption is impaired in patients given enteral feedings orally and via gastrostomy and jejunostomy tubes. *Antimicrob Agents Chemother* (1996) 40, 6–10.
6. Yuk JH, Nightingale CH, Quintiliani R, Yeston NS, Orlando R, Dobkin ED, Kambe JC, Sweeney KR, Buonpane EA. Absorption of ciprofloxacin administered through a nasogastric tube or a nasoduodenal tube in volunteers and patients receiving enteral nutrition. *Diagn Microbiol Infect Dis* (1990) 13, 99–102.
7. Yuk JH, Nightingale CH, Sweeney KR, Quintiliani R, Lettieri JT, Frost RW. Relative bioavailability in healthy volunteers of ciprofloxacin administered through a nasogastric tube with and without enteral feeding. *Antimicrob Agents Chemother* (1989) 33, 1118–20.
8. de Marie S, VandenBergh MFQ, Buijk SLCE, Bruining HA, van Vliet A, Kluytmans JAJW, Mouton JW. Bioavailability of ciprofloxacin after multiple enteral and intravenous doses in ICU patients with severe gram-negative intra-abdominal infections. *Intensive Care Med* (1998) 24, 343–6.
9. Mimoz O, Binter V, Jacolot A, Edouard A, Tod M, Petitjean O, Samii K. Pharmacokinetics and absolute bioavailability of ciprofloxacin administered through a nasogastric tube with continuous enteral feeding to critically ill patients. *Intensive Care Med* (1998) 24, 1047–51.
10. Wright DH, Pietz SL, Konstantinides FN, Rotschafer JC. Decreased *in vitro* fluoroquinolone concentrations after admixture with an enteral feeding formulation. *J Parenter Enteral Nutr* (2000) 24, 42–8.
11. Burkhardt O, Stass H, Thuss U, Borner K, Welte T. Effects of enteral feeding on the oral bioavailability of moxifloxacin in healthy volunteers. *Clin Pharmacokinet* (2005) 44, 969–76.
12. Höffken G, Lode H, Wiley R, Glatzel TD, Sievers D, Olschewski T, Borner K, Koeppe T. Pharmacokinetics and bioavailability of ciprofloxacin and ofloxacin: effect of food and antacid intake. *Rev Infect Dis* (1988) 10 (Suppl 1), S138–S139.
13. Frost RW, Carlson JD, Dietz AJ, Heyd A, Lettieri JT. Ciprofloxacin pharmacokinetics after a standard or high-fat/high-calcium breakfast. *J Clin Pharmacol* (1989) 29, 953–5.
14. Verho M, Malerczyk V, Dagrosa E, Korn A. The effect of food on the pharmacokinetics of ofloxacin. *Curr Med Res Opin* (1986) 10, 166–71.
15. Dudley MN, Marchbanks CR, Flor SC, Beals B. The effect of food or milk on the absorption kinetics of ofloxacin. *Eur J Clin Pharmacol* (1991) 41, 569–71.
16. Hooper WD, Dickinson RG, Eadie MJ. Effect of food on absorption of lomefloxacin. *Antimicrob Agents Chemother* (1990) 34, 1797–9.
17. Somogyi AA, Bochner F, Keal JA, Rolan PE, Smith M. Effect of food on enoxacin absorption. *Antimicrob Agents Chemother* (1987) 31, 638–9.
18. Allen A, Bygate E, Clark D, Lewis A, Pay V. The effect of food on the bioavailability of oral gemifloxacin in healthy volunteers. *Int J Antimicrob Agents* (2000) 16, 45–50.
19. Johnson RD, Dorr MB, Hunt TL, Jensen BK, Talbot GH. Effects of food on the pharmacokinetics of sparfloxacin. *Clin Ther* (1999) 21, 982–91.
20. Neuhofel AL, Wilton JH, Victory JM, Hejmanowski LG, Amsden GW. Lack of bioequivalence of ciprofloxacin when administered with calcium-fortified orange juice: a new twist on an old interaction. *J Clin Pharmacol* (2002) 42, 461–6.
21. Wallace AW, Victory JM, Amsden GW. Lack of bioequivalence of gatifloxacin when coadministered with calcium-fortified orange juice in healthy volunteers. *J Clin Pharmacol* (2003) 43, 92–6.
22. Wallace AW, Victory JM, Amsden GW. Lack of bioequivalence when levofloxacin and calcium-fortified orange juice are coadministered to healthy volunteers. *J Clin Pharmacol* (2003) 43, 539–44.
23. Amsden GW, Whitaker A-M. Johnson PW. Lack of bioequivalence of levofloxacin when coadministered with a mineral-fortified breakfast of juice and cereal. *J Clin Pharmacol* (2003) 43, 990–95.
24. Cohn SM, Sawyer MD, Burns GA, Tolomeo C, Milner KA. Enteric absorption of ciprofloxacin during tube feeding in the critically ill. *J Antimicrob Chemother* (1996) 38, 871–6.

Quinolones + H_2-receptor antagonists

Cimetidine can increase the serum levels of some quinolones (intravenous enoxacin or fleroxacin and oral clinafloxacin or pefloxacin). Famotidine can reduce the serum levels of norfloxacin, and ranitidine can reduce the absorption of enoxacin. None of these interactions appear to be clinically important.

Clinical evidence and mechanism

(a) Ciprofloxacin

Neither **cimetidine**[1,2] nor **ranitidine**[3,4] appear to have a clinically important effect on the pharmacokinetics of ciprofloxacin.

(b) Clinafloxacin

Cimetidine 300 mg four times daily for 4 days increased the maximum serum levels of clinafloxacin by 15% and increased its AUC by 44%.[5]

(c) Enoxacin

The plasma levels of a 400-mg intravenous dose of enoxacin were higher when **cimetidine** 300 mg four times daily was given concurrently. Renal clearance and systemic clearance were reduced by 26% and 20%, respectively, and the elimination half-life was increased by 30%.[6]

In one study **ranitidine** 150 mg twice daily did not affect the pharmacokinetics of a single 400-mg intravenous dose of enoxacin.[6] However, in another, **ranitidine** 50 mg given intravenously 2 hours before a single 400-mg oral dose of enoxacin reduced the absorption by 26 to 40%,[7,8] which seemed to be related to changes in gastric pH caused by the **ranitidine**.[8]

(d) Fleroxacin

Cimetidine decreased the total clearance of fleroxacin by about 25%, without much effect on renal clearance, and increased its elimination half-life by 32%.[9]

(e) Gatifloxacin

Cimetidine does not alter the pharmacokinetics of gatifloxacin.[10]

(f) Grepafloxacin

Cimetidine does not alter the pharmacokinetics of grepafloxacin.[11] Similarly, intravenous **famotidine** in a dose of up to 40 mg had no effect on the pharmacokinetics of a 400-mg dose of grepafloxacin.[12]

(g) Levofloxacin

Cimetidine reduced the clearance of levofloxacin by about 25% and increased its AUC by almost 30%,[13] whereas **ranitidine** did not affect the pharmacokinetics of levofloxacin.[14]

(h) Lomefloxacin

Ranitidine does not affect the pharmacokinetics of lomefloxacin.[15,16]

(i) Moxifloxacin

Ranitidine does not affect the pharmacokinetics of moxifloxacin.[17]

(j) Norfloxacin

Famotidine given 8 hours before norfloxacin significantly reduced its maximum serum concentrations in 6 healthy subjects, but the AUC and urinary recovery rate were unchanged.[18]

(k) Ofloxacin

Cimetidine does not alter the pharmacokinetics of ofloxacin.[19]

(l) Pefloxacin

Cimetidine increased the AUC of intravenous pefloxacin by about 40%. It increased the half-life from 10.3 to 15.3 hours and the clearance was reduced by almost by 30%.[20]

(m) Sparfloxacin

Cimetidine does not alter the pharmacokinetics of sparfloxacin.[21]

(n) Trovafloxacin

Cimetidine does not alter the pharmacokinetics of trovafloxacin.[22]

Importance and management

Although the pharmacokinetic changes seen in some of these studies are moderate, none has been shown to affect the outcome of treatment and they are probably only of minor clinical relevance.

1. Ludwig E, Graber H, Székely É, Csiba A. Metabolic interactions of ciprofloxacin. *Diagn Microbiol Infect Dis* (1990) 13, 135–41.
2. Prince RA, Liou W-S, Kasik JE. Effect of cimetidine on ciprofloxacin pharmacokinetics. *Pharmacotherapy* (1990) 10, 233.
3. Höffken G, Lode H, Wiley R, Glatzel TD, Sievers D, Olschewski T, Borner K, Koeppe T. Pharmacokinetics and bioavailability of ciprofloxacin and ofloxacin: effect of food and antacid intake. *Rev Infect Dis* (1988) 10 (Suppl 1), S138–9
4. Nix DE, Watson WA, Lener ME, Frost RW, Krol G, Goldstein H, Letterei J, Schentag JJ. Effects of aluminum and magnesium antacids and ranitidine on the absorption of ciprofloxacin. *Clin Pharmacol Ther* (1989) 46, 700–5.
5. Randinitis EJ, Koup JR, Bron NJ, Hounslow NJ, Rausch G, Abel R, Vassos AB, Sedman AJ. Drug interaction studies with clinafloxacin and probenecid, cimetidine, phenytoin and warfarin. *Drugs* (1999) 58 (Suppl 2), 254–5.
6. Misiak PM, Eldon MA, Toothaker RD, Sedman AJ. Effects of oral cimetidine or ranitidine on the pharmacokinetics of intravenous enoxacin. *J Clin Pharmacol* (1993) 33, 53–6.
7. Grasela TH, Schentag JJ, Sedman AJ, Wilton JH, Thomas DJ, Schultz RW, Lebsack ME, Kinkel AW. Inhibition of enoxacin absorption by antacids or ranitidine. *Antimicrob Agents Chemother* (1989) 33, 615–17.
8. Lebsack ME, Nix D, Ryerson B, Toothaker RD, Welage L, Norman AM, Schentag JJ, Sedman AJ. Effect of gastric acidity on enoxacin absorption. *Clin Pharmacol Ther* (1992) 52, 252–6.
9. Portmann R. Influence of cimetidine on fleroxacin pharmacokinetics. *Drugs* (1993) 45 (Suppl 3), 471.
10. Shiba K, Kusajima H, Momo K. The effects of aluminium hydroxide, cimetidine, ferrous sulfate, green tea and milk on pharmacokinetics of gatifloxacin in healthy humans. *J Antimicrob Chemother* (1999) 44 (Suppl A), 141.
11. Koneru B, Bramer S, Bricmont P, Maroli A, Shiba K. Effect of food, gastric pH and co-administration of antacid, cimetidine and probenecid on the oral pharmacokinetics of the broad spectrum antimicrobial agent grepafloxacin. *Pharm Res* (1996) 13 (9 Suppl), S414.
12. Efthymiopoulos C, Bramer SL, Maroli A. Effect of food and gastric pH on the bioavailability of grepafloxacin. *Clin Pharmacokinet* (1997) 33 (Suppl 1), 18–24.
13. Gaitonde MD, Mendes P, House ESA, Lehr KH. The effects of cimetidine and probenecid on the pharmacokinetics of levofloxacin (LFLX). *Intersci Conf Antimicrob Agents Chemother* (1995) 35, 8.
14. Shiba K, Sakai O, Shimada J, Okazaki O, Aoki H, Hakusui H. Effects of antacids, ferrous sulphate, and ranitidine on absorption of DR-3355 in humans. *Antimicrob Agents Chemother* (1992) 36, 2270–4.
15. Nix D, Schentag J. Lomefloxacin (L) absorption kinetics when administered with ranitidine (R) and sucralfate (S). *Intersci Conf Antimicrob Agents Chemother* (1989) 29, 317.
16. Sudoh T, Fujimura A, Harada K, Sunaga K, Ohmori M, Sakamoto K. Effect of ranitidine on renal clearance of lomefloxacin. *Eur J Clin Pharmacol* (1996) 51, 95–8.
17. Stass H, Böttcher M-F, Ochmann K. Evaluation of the influence of antacids and H_2 antagonists on the absorption of moxifloxacin after oral administration of a 400-mg dose to healthy volunteers. *Clin Pharmacokinet* (2001) 40 (Suppl 1), 39–48.
18. Shimada J, Hori S. Effect of antiulcer drugs on gastrointestinal absorption of norfloxacin. *Chemotherapy (Tokyo)* (1992) 40, 1141–7.
19. Shiba K, Yoshida M, Kachi M, Shimada J, Saito A, Sakai N. Effects of peptic ulcer-healing drugs on the pharmacokinetics of new quinolone (OFLX). 17th International Congress on Chemotherapy, Berlin, June 1991. Abstract 415.
20. Sörgel F, Mahr G, Koch HU, Stephan U, Wiesemann HG, Malter U. Effects of cimetidine on the pharmacokinetics of pefloxacin in healthy volunteers. *Rev Infect Dis* (1988) 10 (Suppl 1), S137.
21. Gries JM, Honorato J, Taburet AM, Alvarez MP, Sadaba B, Azanza JR, Singlas E. Cimetidine does not alter sparfloxacin pharmacokinetics. *Int J Clin Pharmacol Ther* (1995) 33, 585–7.
22. Purkins L, Oliver SD, Willavize SA. An open, controlled, crossover study on the effects of cimetidine on the steady-state pharmacokinetics of trovafloxacin. *Eur J Clin Microbiol Infect Dis* (1998) 17, 431–3.

Quinolones + Iron or Zinc compounds

Ferrous fumarate, gluconate, sulfate and other iron compounds can reduce the absorption of ciprofloxacin, gatifloxacin, levofloxacin, moxifloxacin, norfloxacin, ofloxacin and sparfloxacin from the gut. Serum levels of the antibacterial may become subtherapeutic as a result. Limited evidence suggests that fleroxacin is not affected and lomefloxacin is only minimally affected. Gemifloxacin does not appear to interact when given 2 hours before or 3 hours after ferrous sulfate. No interaction appears to occur with iron-ovotransferrin. Zinc appears to interact like iron.

Clinical evidence

(a) Ciprofloxacin

The absorption of ciprofloxacin is markedly reduced by iron and zinc compounds. Several studies have clearly demonstrated reductions in the AUC and maximum serum levels of 30 to 90% with **ferrous fumarate**,[1] **ferrous gluconate**,[2] **ferrous sulfate**,[2-5] **iron-glycine sulfate**,[6] ***Centrum Forte***[2] (a multi-mineral preparation containing iron, magnesium, zinc, calcium, copper and manganese) and with ***Stresstabs 600-with-zinc***[4] (a multivitamin-with-zinc preparation). However **iron-ovotransferrin** has been found to have no significant effect on the absorption of ciprofloxacin.[7]

(b) Fleroxacin

A study in 12 subjects found that **ferrous sulfate** (equivalent to 100 mg of elemental iron) had no significant effect on the pharmacokinetics of fleroxacin.[8]

(c) Gatifloxacin

A study in 6 healthy subjects found that **ferrous sulfate** 160 mg given with gatifloxacin 200 mg decreased the maximum serum levels and AUC of gatifloxacin by 49% and 29%, respectively.[9]

(d) Gemifloxacin

Gemifloxacin 320 mg was given either 3 hours before or 2 hours after **ferrous sulfate** 325 mg in a study in 27 healthy subjects. The pharmacokinetics of gemifloxacin were not significantly altered in either case.[10]

(e) Levofloxacin

Ferrous sulfate has been found to reduce the bioavailability of levofloxacin by 79%.[11]

(f) Lomefloxacin

When lomefloxacin 400 mg was given with **ferrous sulfate** (equivalent to 100 mg of elemental iron), the lomefloxacin maximum serum levels were reduced by about 28% and the AUC by about 14%.[12]

(g) Moxifloxacin

In 12 healthy subjects **ferrous sulfate** (equivalent to 100 mg of elemental iron) reduced the AUC and maximum plasma levels of a single 400-mg dose of moxifloxacin by 39% and 59%, respectively. The rate of absorption was reduced (time to maximum plasma level increased from a mean of 1 hour to 2.79 hours).[13]

(h) Norfloxacin

In 8 healthy subjects **ferrous sulfate** reduced the AUC and maximum serum levels of a single 400-mg dose of norfloxacin by 73% and 75%, respectively.[5] **Ferrous sulfate** caused a 51% reduction in the norfloxacin AUC in another study,[14,15] and a 97% reduction in bioavailability in a further single dose study.[16] The same authors also found that both **ferrous**

sulfate and **zinc sulfate** reduced the urinary recovery of norfloxacin by 55% and 56%, respectively.[17]

(i) Ofloxacin

In 8 healthy subjects **ferrous sulfate** (equivalent to 100 mg of elemental iron) reduced the AUC and maximum serum levels of a single 400-mg dose of ofloxacin by 25% and 36%, respectively.[5] In 9 healthy subjects **ferrous sulfate** 1050 mg decreased the absorption of ofloxacin 200 mg by 11%.[18] In 12 healthy subjects elemental iron 200 mg (in the form of an **iron-glycine-sulfate** complex) reduced the bioavailability of ofloxacin 400 mg by 36%.[6]

(j) Sparfloxacin

In a single dose study in 6 subjects, 525 mg of **ferrous sulfate** (equivalent to 170 mg of elemental iron) reduced the AUC of sparfloxacin 200 mg by 27%.[14,15]

Mechanism

It is believed that the quinolones form a complex with iron and zinc (by chelation between the metal ion and the 4-oxo and adjacent carboxyl groups), which is less easily absorbed by the gut. However, a study in *rats* using oral iron and intravenous ciprofloxacin suggested that the interaction may not be entirely confined to the gut.[19] This needs further study. Iron-ovotransferrin differs from other iron preparations in being able to combine directly with the transferrin receptors of intestinal cells, and appears to release little iron into the gut to interact with the quinolones.

Importance and management

The interactions between the quinolones and iron compounds are established and would appear to be of clinical importance because the serum antibacterial levels can become subtherapeutic. In descending order the extent of the interaction appears to be: norfloxacin, levofloxacin, ciprofloxacin, moxifloxacin, gatifloxacin, ofloxacin/sparfloxacin, then least affected, lomefloxacin.

None of these quinolones should be taken at the same time as any iron preparation that contains substantial amounts of iron (e.g. ferrous sulfate, ferrous gluconate, ferrous fumarate, iron-glycine sulfate). Since the quinolones are rapidly absorbed, taking them 2 hours before the iron should minimise the risk of admixture in the gut and largely avoid this interaction. Information about other quinolones seems to be lacking but the same precautions should be taken with all of them except fleroxacin, which appears not to interact, and lomefloxacin, which seems to interact only minimally.

Iron-ovotransferrin does not interact with ciprofloxacin and is not expected to interact with any of the quinolones (see 'Mechanism') but this awaits confirmation.

There seems to be very little data about the interactions between zinc compounds and quinolones, but zinc appears to interact like iron and therefore the same precautions suggested for iron should be followed.

1. Brouwers JRBJ, Van der Kam HJ, Sijtsma J, Proost JH. Decreased ciprofloxacin absorption with concomitant administration of ferrous fumarate. *Pharm Weekbl (Sci)* (1990) 12, 182–3.
2. Kara M, Hasinoff BB, McKay DW, Campbell NRC. Clinical and chemical interactions between iron preparations and ciprofloxacin. *Br J Clin Pharmacol* (1991) 31, 257–61.
3. Le Pennec MP, Kitzis MD, Terdjman M, Foubard S, Garbarz E, Hanania G. Possible interaction of ciprofloxacin with ferrous sulphate. *J Antimicrob Chemother* (1990) 25, 184–5.
4. Polk RE, Healy DP, Sahai J, Drwal L, Racht E. Effect of ferrous sulfate and multivitamins with zinc on absorption of ciprofloxacin in normal volunteers. *Antimicrob Agents Chemother* (1989) 33, 1841–4.
5. Lehto P, Kivistö KT, Neuvonen PJ. The effect of ferrous sulphate on the absorption of norfloxacin, ciprofloxacin and ofloxacin. *Br J Clin Pharmacol* (1994) 37, 82–5.
6. Lode H, Stuhlert P, Deppermann KH, Mainz D, Borner K, Kotvas K, Koeppe P. Pharmacokinetic interactions between oral ciprofloxacin (CIP)/ofloxacin (OFL) and ferro-salts. *Intersci Conf Antimicrob Agents Chemother* (1989) 29,136.
7. Pazzucconi F, Barbi S, Baldassarre D, Colombo N, Dorigotti F, Sirtori CR. Iron-ovotransferrin preparation does not interfere with ciprofloxacin absorption. *Clin Pharmacol Ther* (1996) 59, 418–22.
8. Sörgel F, Naber KG, Kinzig M, Frank A, Birner B. Effect of ferrous sulfate on fleroxacin analyzed by the confidence interval (CI) approach. *Pharm Res* (1995) 12 (9 Suppl), S-422.
9. Shiba K, Kusajima H, Momo K. The effects of aluminium hydroxide, cimetidine, ferrous sulfate, green tea and milk on pharmacokinetics of gatifloxacin in healthy humans. *J Antimicrob Chemother* (1999) 44 (Suppl A), 141.
10. Allen A, Bygate E, Faessel H, Isaac L, Lewis A. The effect of ferrous sulphate and sucralfate on the bioavailability of oral gemifloxacin in healthy volunteers. *Int J Antimicrob Agents* (2000) 15, 283–9.
11. Shiba K, Okazaki O, Aoki H, Sakai O, Shimada J. Inhibition of DR-3355 absorption by metal ions. *Intersci Conf Antimicrob Agents Chemother* (1991) 31, 198.
12. Lehto P, Kivistö KT. Different effects of products containing metal ions on the absorption of lomefloxacin. *Clin Pharmacol Ther* (1994) 56, 477–82.
13. Stass H, Kubitza D. Effects of iron supplements on the oral bioavailability of moxifloxacin, a novel 8-methoxyfluoroquinolone, in humans. *Clin Pharmacokinet* (2001) 40 (Suppl 1), 57–62.
14. Kanemitsu K, Hori S, Yanagawa A, Shimada J. Effect of ferrous sulfate on the pharmacokinetics of sparfloxacin. *Chemotherapy* (1994) 42, 6–13.
15. Kanemitsu K, Hori S, Yanagawa A, Shimada J. Effect of ferrous sulfate on the absorption of sparfloxacin in healthy volunteers and rats. *Drugs* (1995) 49 (Suppl 2), 352–6.
16. Okhamafe AO, Akerele JO, Chukuka CS. Pharmacokinetic interactions of norfloxacin with some metallic medicinal agents. *Int J Pharmaceutics* (1991) 68, 11–18.
17. Campbell NRC, Kara M, Hasinoff BB, Haddara WM, McKay DW. Norfloxacin interaction with antacids and minerals. *Br J Clin Pharmacol* (1992) 33, 115–16.
18. Martínez Cabarga M, Sánchez Navarro A, Colino Gandarillas CI, Domínguez-Gil A. Effects of two cations on gastrointestinal absorption of ofloxacin. *Antimicrob Agents Chemother* (1991) 35, 2102–5.
19. Wong PY, Zhu M, Li RC. Pharmacokinetic and pharmacodynamic interactions between intravenous ciprofloxacin and oral ferrous sulfate. *J Chemother* (2000) 12, 286–93.

Quinolones + NSAIDs

A number of cases of convulsions have been seen in Japanese patients given fenbufen with enoxacin, and there is also one possible case involving ofloxacin. Use of these particular drugs together should be avoided. Normally no interaction seems to occur with most quinolones and NSAIDs, except where there is a predisposition to convulsive episodes. Isolated cases of convulsions, other neurological toxicity or skin eruptions have been seen when ciprofloxacin was given with indometacin, mefenamic acid or naproxen. These appear to be very rare events.

Clinical evidence

(a) Ciprofloxacin

As of 1995 the manufacturer of ciprofloxacin had, on record, two confirmed spontaneous reports of convulsions in patients taking ciprofloxacin and an NSAID; one with **mefenamic acid** and the other with **naproxen**.[1] These appear to be the only medically validated reports of ciprofloxacin/NSAID reactions by 1995.[1]

A woman taking **chloroquine** 250 mg and **naproxen** 1 g daily developed dizziness, anxiety and tremors within a week of starting ciprofloxacin 1 g daily. The symptoms largely resolved when the **chloroquine** was stopped; it was not known if she also stopped the naproxen. Two months after **chloroquine** was discontinued, and while she was still taking ciprofloxacin, **indometacin** was started. This time she developed pain in her feet and became extremely tired. The pain partially subsided and the fatigue vanished when the ciprofloxacin was stopped. Later she was found to have some axonal demyelination, compatible with drug-induced polyneuropathy.[2]

A study in 8 healthy subjects found that the pharmacokinetics of ciprofloxacin were unaffected by treatment with **fenbufen** for 3 days.[3] Another study found that combined single doses of ciprofloxacin and **fenbufen** in 12 healthy subjects produced no evidence, using EEG recordings, of increased CNS excitatory effects.[4]

(b) Enoxacin

A total of 17 Japanese patients have been identified, with apparently no previous history of seizures, who in the 1986 to 1987 period developed convulsions when given **fenbufen** 400 mg to 1.2 g daily with enoxacin 200 to 800 mg.[5] Two case reports of this interaction have been published.[6,7] An 87-year-old Japanese woman taking enoxacin 200 mg also had convulsions after receiving a single 50-mg intravenous dose of **flurbiprofen**.[8]

(c) Levofloxacin

A study in 24 healthy subjects found plasma levels of single 125-mg and 500-mg doses of levofloxacin were increased by about 13%, 6.5 hours after they were given **fenbufen** 600 mg. No changes in CNS activity were found.[9]

(d) Ofloxacin

One patient taking **fenbufen** 800 mg had involuntary movements of the neck and upper extremities after taking ofloxacin 600 mg.[5] The pharmacokinetics of ofloxacin 200 mg twice daily were unchanged by **ketoprofen** 100 mg daily for 3 days in 10 healthy subjects.[10] The incidence of psychotic adverse effects (euphoria, hysteria, psychosis) in 151 patients on ofloxacin were not increased by the concurrent use of NSAIDs (**aspirin, diclofenac, indometacin, dipyrone**).[11]

(e) Pefloxacin

The pharmacokinetics of pefloxacin 400 mg twice daily were not affected by **ketoprofen** 100 mg daily for 3 days in 10 healthy subjects.[10]

(f) Sparfloxacin

A 62-year-old woman developed drug eruptions (erythematous papules), which were attributed to sparfloxacin hypersensitivity induced by **mefenamic acid**.[12]

Mechanism

Not fully understood. Convulsions have occurred in a few patients taking quinolones alone, some of whom were epileptics and some of whom were not (see 'Antiepileptics + Quinolones', p.522). Experiments in *mice* have shown that quinolones competitively inhibit the binding of gamma-amino butyric acid (GABA) to its receptors.[13] GABA is an inhibitory transmitter in the CNS, which is believed to be involved in the control of convulsive activity. Enoxacin and fenbufen are known to affect the GABA receptor site in the hippocampus and frontal cortex of *mice*, which is associated with convulsive activity.[14] It could be that, if and when an interaction occurs, the NSAID simply lowers the amount of quinolone needed to precipitate convulsions in already susceptible individuals.

Importance and management

The interaction between enoxacin and fenbufen is established, but it seems to be uncommon. Nevertheless, it would seem prudent to avoid fenbufen with enoxacin. There are very many alternatives.

Reports of adverse interactions between other quinolones and NSAIDs are extremely rare. The general warning about convulsions with quinolones and NSAIDs issued by the CSM in the UK[15] seems to be an extrapolation from the interaction between enoxacin and fenbufen, and from some *animal* experiments. In addition to the data cited above, an epidemiological study of 856 users of quinolones (ciprofloxacin, enoxacin, nalidixic acid) and a range of NSAIDs found no cases of convulsions.[16] The overall picture would therefore seem to be that although a potential for interaction exists, the risk is very small indeed and normally there would seem to be little reason for most patients taking quinolones to avoid NSAIDs. Epileptic patients are a possible exception (see 'Antiepileptics + Quinolones', p.522) and it would seem prudent to avoid quinolones and NSAIDs wherever possible in these patients.

1. Bomford J. Ciprofloxacin. *Pharm J* (1995) 255, 674.
2. Rollof J, Vinge E. Neurological adverse effects during concomitant treatment with ciprofloxacin, NSAIDS, and chloroquine: possible drug interaction. *Ann Pharmacother* (1993) 27, 1058–9.
3. Kamali F. Lack of a pharmacokinetic interaction between ciprofloxacin and fenbufen. *J Clin Pharm Ther* (1994) 19, 257–9.
4. Kamali F, Ashton CH, Marsh VR, Cox J. Is there a pharmacodynamic interaction between ciprofloxacin and fenbufen? *Br J Clin Pharmacol* (1997) 43, 545P–546P.
5. Lederle. Data on file. Personal Communication, December 1995.
6. Takeo G, Shibuya N, Motomura M, Kanazawa H, Shishido H. A new DNA gyrase inhibitor induces convulsions: a case report and animal experiments. *Chemotherapy (Tokyo)* (1989) 37, 1154–9.
7. Morita H, Maemura K, Sakai Y, Kaneda Y. A case with convulsion, loss of consciousness and subsequent acute renal failure caused by enoxacin and fenbufen. *Nippon Naika Gakkai Zasshi* (1988) 77, 744–5.
8. Mizuno J, Takumi Z, Kaneko A, Tsutsui T, Tsutsui T, Zushi N, Machida K. Convulsion following the combination of single preoperative oral administration of enoxacine and single postoperative intravenous administration of flurbiprofen axetil. *Jpn J Anesthesiol* (2001) 50, 425–8.
9. Hoechst Marion Roussel Ltd. Data on file. Personal communication, January 1999.
10. Fillastre JP, Leroy A, Borsa-Lebas F, Etienne I, Gy C, Humbert G. Effects of ketoprofen (NSAID) on the pharmacokinetics of pefloxacin and ofloxacin in healthy volunteers. *Drugs Exp Clin Res* (1992) 18, 487–92.
11. Jüngst G, Weidmann E, Breitstadt A, Huppertz E. Does ofloxacin interact with NSAIDs to cause psychotic side effects? 17th International Congress on Chemotherapy, Berlin, June 23–8, 1991. Abstract 412.
12. Oiso N, Taniguchi S, Goto Y, Hisa T, Mizuno N, Mochida K, Hamada T, Yorifuji T. A case of drug eruption due to sparfloxacin (SPFX) and mefenamic acid. *Skin Res* (1995) 37, 321–7.
13. Hori S, Shimada J, Saito A, Matsuda M, Miyahara T. Comparison of the inhibitory effects of new quinolones on γ-aminobutyric acid receptor binding in the presence of antiinflammatory drugs. *Rev Infect Dis* (1989) 11 (Suppl 5), S1397–S1398.
14. Motomura M, Kataoka Y, Takeo G, Shibayama K, Ohishi K, Nakamura T, Niwa M, Tsujihata M, Nagataki S. Hippocampus and frontal cortex are the potential mediatory sites for convulsions induced by new quinolones and non-steroidal anti-inflammatory drugs. *Int J Clin Pharmacol Ther Toxicol* (1991) 29, 223–7.
15. Committee on Safety of Medicines. Convulsions due to quinolone antimicrobial agents. *Current Problems* (1991) 32, 2.
16. Mannino S, Garcia-Rodriguez LA, Jick SS. NSAIDs, quinolones and convulsions: an epidemiological approach. *Post Marketing Surveillance* (1992) 6, 119–28.

Quinolones + Omeprazole

Omeprazole has no clinically important effect on the pharmacokinetics of ciprofloxacin, gemifloxacin, lomefloxacin, ofloxacin or trovafloxacin.

Clinical evidence, mechanism, importance and management

A single-dose study found that omeprazole 20 or 80 mg had no significant effect on the pharmacokinetics of single doses of **ofloxacin** 400 mg, **ciprofloxacin** 500 mg or **lomefloxacin** 250 or 400 mg.[1] Another study in 27 subjects found that omeprazole 40 mg daily for 3 days did not affect the pharmacokinetics of a single 1-g dose of an extended-release formulation of **ciprofloxacin** (*Depomed*).[2] Omeprazole 40 mg caused an 18% reduction in the AUC of a single 300-mg dose of **trovafloxacin** and a 32% reduction in the maximum serum levels, but this was considered not to be of clinical significance.[3] A double-blind, randomised, crossover study in 12 healthy subjects found that the maximum serum levels and the AUC of a single 320-mg dose of **gemifloxacin** were increased by 11% and 10%, respectively, after taking omeprazole 40 mg daily for 4 days. The confidence intervals indicated that the respective increases were unlikely to exceed 36% and 43%, and it was concluded that these two drugs could be given together without any need for dosage adjustments.[4]

1. Stuht H, Lode H, Koeppe P, Rost KL, Schaberg T. Interaction study of lomefloxacin and ciprofloxacin with omeprazole and comparative pharmacokinetics. *Antimicrob Agents Chemother* (1995) 39, 1045–9.
2. Washington C, Hou E, Hughes N, Berner B. Effect of omeprazole on bioavailability of an oral extended-release formulation of ciprofloxacin. *Am J Health-Syst Pharm* (2006) 63, 653–6.
3. Teng R, Dogolo LC, Willavize SA, Friedman HL, Vincent J. Effect of Maalox and omeprazole on the bioavailability of trovafloxacin. *J Antimicrob Chemother* (1997) 39 (Suppl B), 93–7.
4. Allen A, Vousden M, Lewis A. Effect of omeprazole on the pharmacokinetics of oral gemifloxacin in healthy volunteers. *Chemotherapy* (1999) 45, 496–503.

Quinolones + Opioids

Morphine modestly reduces the AUC of trovafloxacin, but this is not considered to be clinically significant. Trovafloxacin did not alter the effects or pharmacokinetics of morphine. Oxycodone does not appear to significantly affect the pharmacokinetics of either levofloxacin or gatifloxacin. It has been suggested that opiates decrease oral ciprofloxacin levels, but good evidence for this appears to be lacking.

Clinical evidence, mechanism, importance and management

(a) Ciprofloxacin

In one non-randomised study[1] the levels of oral ciprofloxacin were only 1.3 mg/L in the presence of intramuscular **papaveretum**, compared to 3.22 mg/L in a control group not receiving **papaveretum**. The authors say that this means the peak ciprofloxacin levels in the **papaveretum** group would not reach the MIC of a number of gut pathogens. They name *Bacteroides fragilis* (but it should be noted that the levels of the control group also did not reach the MIC of this organism), and *Enterococcus faecalis*, many strains of which are only moderately susceptible to ciprofloxacin anyway. Further, the **papaveretum** group in this study had only 4 patients, and, as the authors note, the control group was not matched.[1] Based on this rather slim evidence, the manufacturers of ciprofloxacin state that the use of ciprofloxacin tablets is not recommended with opiate premedicants due to the risks of inadequate ciprofloxacin levels.[2,3] This advice is also given by the manufacturers of **morphine** sulfate,[4] and was added at the request of the UK Medicines and Healthcare Regulatory Agency.[5]

(b) Gatifloxacin

In 12 healthy subjects, the pharmacokinetics of gatifloxacin 400 mg were not significantly altered by **oxycodone** 5 mg every 4 hours.[6]

(c) Levofloxacin

In 8 healthy subjects, the pharmacokinetics of oral levofloxacin 500 mg were not significantly altered by **oxycodone** 5 mg every 4 hours.[7]

(d) Trovafloxacin

An intravenous infusion of **morphine** 150 micrograms/kg given with oral trovafloxacin 200 mg to 18 healthy subjects caused a 36% reduction in the trovafloxacin AUC and a 46% reduction in the maximum serum levels. These levels were considered sufficient for prophylaxis of infection, and remained above the MICs of the most likely organisms to cause post-surgical infections. The bioavailability and effects of **morphine** were not significantly changed by trovafloxacin.[8]

1. Morran C, McArdle C, Petitt L, Sleigh D, Gemmell C, Hichens M, Felmingham D, Tillotson G. Brief report: pharmacokinetics of orally administered ciprofloxacin in abdominal surgery. *Am J Med* (1989) 87, (Suppl 5A), 86S–88S.

2. Ciproxin Tablets (Ciprofloxacin hydrochloride). Bayer plc. UK Summary of product characteristics, January 2006.
3. Bayer Health Care. Personal Communication, September 2003.
4. Morphine sulfate Injection. UCB Pharma Ltd. UK Summary of product characteristics, June 2005.
5. Celltech Pharmaceutical Ltd. Personal Communication, August 2003.
6. Grant EM, Nicolau DP, Nightingale C, Quintiliani R. Minimal interaction between gatifloxacin and oxycodone. *J Clin Pharmacol* (2002) 42, 928–32.
7. Grant EM, Zhong MK, Fitzgerald JF, Nicolau DP, Nightingale C, Quintiliani R. Lack of interaction between levofloxacin and oxycodone: pharmacokinetics and drug disposition. *J Clin Pharmacol* (2001) 41, 206–9.
8. Vincent J, Hunt T, Teng R, Robarge L, Willavize SA, Friedman HL. The pharmacokinetic effects of coadministration of morphine and trovafloxacin in healthy subjects. *Am J Surg* (1998) 176 (Suppl 6A), 32S–38S.

Quinolones + Other antibacterials

There appear to be few documented cases of clinically relevant interactions between the quinolones and other antibacterials. However, note that clindamycin may antagonise the effects of ciprofloxacin on *S. aureus*. Further, *in vitro* studies have demonstrated antagonistic antibacterial effects when nitrofurantoin and nalidixic acid are used together, and other quinolones are also said to antagonise the effects of nitrofurantoin.

Clinical evidence, mechanism, importance and management

(a) Aminoglycosides

A study found that a single 100-mg intravenous dose of **tobramycin** had no effect on the pharmacokinetics of **pefloxacin**, and **pefloxacin** did not affect the pharmacokinetics of **tobramycin**.[1] Similarly no pharmacokinetic interaction was found between **pefloxacin** and **amikacin**.[2]

(b) Cephalosporins

A study found that a single 2-g intravenous dose of **ceftazidime** had no effect on the pharmacokinetics of **pefloxacin**, and **pefloxacin** did not affect the pharmacokinetics of **ceftazidime**.[1]

In a study of 11 healthy subjects, the pharmacokinetics of **cefotaxime** and **ofloxacin** were similar, whether given alone or in combination, and the antimicrobial effect of the combination was additive for *S. aureus*, *S. pneumoniae*, *E. cloacae* and *K. pneumoniae*, but not for *Ps. aeruginosa*.[3]

(c) Clindamycin

One study found that the pharmacokinetics of intravenous **ciprofloxacin** 200 mg were not affected by intravenous clindamycin 600 mg and there is evidence that combined use may possibly enhance the antibacterial activity, particularly against *S. aureus* and *S. pneumoniae*.[4] However, another study found that the serum bactericidal activity of **ciprofloxacin** against *S. aureus* was completely antagonised by clindamycin, if the strains were susceptible to the latter.[5]

(d) Macrolides

A study designed to assess the potential interaction between **trovafloxacin** and **azithromycin** found no significant alteration in the pharmacokinetics of either drug.[6]

(e) Metronidazole

A study found that a single 400-mg oral dose of metronidazole had no effect on the pharmacokinetics of **pefloxacin**, and similarly **pefloxacin** did not affect the pharmacokinetics of metronidazole.[1] In another study no interaction was found between **ciprofloxacin** or **ofloxacin** (both 200 mg intravenously) and metronidazole 500 mg intravenously,[7] and metronidazole with **ciprofloxacin** orally.[8]

A further study, investigating the use of metronidazole 500 mg intravenously and **ciprofloxacin** 200 mg intravenously, also did not find any significant pharmacokinetic changes, although metronidazole reduced the **ciprofloxacin** volume of distribution by 20%.[4] This is not expected to be clinically significant.

(f) Nitrofurantoin

The antibacterial activity of **nalidixic acid** can be attenuated by sub-inhibitory concentrations of nitrofurantoin. In 44 out of 53 strains of *Escherichia coli*, *Salmonella* and *Proteus*, antagonism was shown.[9] Another study confirmed these findings.[10] Whether this similarly occurs if both antibacterials are given to patients is uncertain, but the advice that concurrent use should be avoided when treating urinary tract infections seems sound.[9] Active division of bacteria is required for the bactericidal activity of quinolones such as nalidixic acid, and the presence of a bacteriostatic drug such as nitrofurantoin may inhibit its action.[11] Other quinolone antibacterials (not named) and nitrofurantoin have been found to be antagonistic *in vitro* and although the clinical significance of this is unknown.[12,13]

(g) Penicillins

A single-dose study in 6 healthy subjects found that intravenous **azlocillin** 60 mg/kg reduced the clearance of intravenous **ciprofloxacin** 4 mg/kg by 35%. The pharmacokinetics of **azlocillin** were not affected.[14]

Another study found that when a single 4-g intravenous dose of **piperacillin** was given with **pefloxacin** 400 mg the pharmacokinetics of both drugs were unchanged.[1]

The absorption of **ofloxacin** 400 mg was not altered by **amoxicillin** 3 g in 6 healthy subjects.[15]

In another study in 12 healthy subjects, the serum bacterial activity of **ciprofloxacin** plus **piperacillin** against a variety of organisms was found to be additive, rather than antagonistic or synergistic despite the fact that the clearance of **ciprofloxacin** was reduced by 24%.[16]

(h) Rifampicin (Rifampin)

A single-dose study in 5 healthy subjects found that **ciprofloxacin** 500 mg decreased the peak serum levels of rifampicin 600 mg by 12%, and prolonged its half-life from 3.5 to 3.8 hours.[17] In a further study, **ciprofloxacin** did not affect the percentage of rifampicin recovered in the urine, but it did increase its initial rate of excretion.[18] **Ciprofloxacin** 750 mg and rifampicin 300 mg, both given every 12 hours for 2 weeks, did not significantly affect the pharmacokinetics of either drug in 12 elderly patients (aged 67 to 95).[19] This is confirmed by other pharmacokinetic studies, one of which also reported that combined use provided excellent serum bactericidal activity against *S. aureus* strains, although activity was modestly lower than rifampicin alone.[5,20,21]

A study in 8 healthy subjects found that rifampicin 900 mg daily for 10 days decreased the half-life and AUC_{0-12} of **pefloxacin** 400 mg twice daily by about 30%, due to a 35% increase in total plasma clearance.[22] Despite these changes the serum **pefloxacin** levels still remained well above the minimal inhibitory concentrations (0.5 mg/L) for 90% of strains of methicillin-sensitive *S. aureus* and *S. epidermis*.[22] A single-dose study in 5 healthy subjects found that **pefloxacin** 500 mg increased the AUC of a single 600-mg dose of rifampicin by about twofold.[23] In a further study the urinary recovery of rifampicin was increased from 15.6% of the dose to 20.1% by **pefloxacin**.[24]

Another study in 13 healthy subjects found that rifampicin 600 mg daily for a week increased the clearance of **fleroxacin** 400 mg daily by 15%. However, the **fleroxacin** levels remained above the MIC_{90} of methicillin-sensitive strains of *S. aureus* and *S. epidermis* for at least 24 hours.[25] No special precautions would seem necessary if rifampicin is given with any of these quinolones.

1. Metz R, Jaehde U, Wiesemann H, Gottschalk B, Stephan U, Schunack W. Pharmacokinetic interactions and non-interactions of pefloxacin. Proc 15th Int Congr Chemother, Istanbul, 1987, 997–9.
2. Sultan E, Richard C, Pezzano M, Auzepy P, Singlas E. Pharmacokinetics of pefloxacin and amikacin administered simultaneously to intensive care patients. *Eur J Clin Pharmacol* (1988) 34, 637–43.
3. Nix DE, Wilton JH, Hyatt J, Thomas J, Strenkoski-Nix LC, Forrest A, Schentag JJ. Pharmacodynamic modeling of the in vivo interaction between cefotaxime and ofloxacin by using serum ultrafiltrate inhibitory titers. *Antimicrob Agents Chemother* (1997) 41, 1108–14.
4. Deppermann K-M, Boeckh M, Grineisen S, Shokry F, Borner K, Koeppe P, Krasemann C, Wagner J, Lode H. Brief report: combination effects of ciprofloxacin, clindamycin, and metronidazole intravenously in volunteers. *Am J Med* (1989) 87 (Suppl 5A), 46S–48S.
5. Weinstein MP, Deeter RG, Swanson KA, Gross JS. Crossover assessment of serum bactericidal activity and pharmacokinetics of ciprofloxacin alone and in combination in healthy elderly volunteers. *Antimicrob Agents Chemother* (1991) 35, 2352–8.
6. Foulds G, Cohen MJ, Geffken A, Willavize S, Hunt T. Coadministration of azithromycin 1-g packet does not affect the bioavailability of trovafloxacin. *Intersci Conf Antimicrob Agents Chemother* (1998) 38, 31.
7. Boeckh M, Grineisen S, Shokry F, Koeppe P, Borner K, Krasemann C, Lode H. Pharmacokinetics and serum bactericidal activity (SBA) of ciprofloxacin (CIP) and ofloxacin (OFL) alone and in combination with metronidazole (METRO) or clindamycin (CLINDA). *Intersci Conf Antimicrob Agents Chemother* (1988) 28, 246.
8. Ludwig E, Graber H, Székely É, Csiba A. Metabolic interactions of ciprofloxacin. *Diagn Microbiol Infect Dis* (1990) 13, 135–41.
9. Stille W, Ostner KH. Antagonismus Nitrofurantoin-Nalidixinsaure. *Klin Wochenschr* (1966) 44, 155–6.
10. Piguet D. L'action inhibitrice de la nitrofurantoïne sur le pouvoir bactériostatique *in vitro* de l'acide nalidixique. *Ann Inst Pasteur (Paris)* (1969) 116, 43–8.
11. NegGram (Nalidixic acid) Sanofi-Synthelabo Inc. US Prescribing information, June 2004.
12. Macrobid (Nitrofurantoin monohydrate/macrocrystals). Proctor & Gamble Pharmaceuticals, US Prescribing information, December 2006.
13. Macrodantin (Nitrofurantoin macrocrystals) Proctor & Gamble Pharmaceuticals, US Prescribing information, December 2006.
14. Barriere SL, Catlin DH, Orlando PL, Noe A, Frost RW. Alteration in the pharmacokinetic disposition of ciprofloxacin by simultaneous administration of azlocillin. *Antimicrob Agents Chemother* (1990) 34, 823–6.
15. Paintaud G, Alván G, Hellgren U, Nilsson-Ehle I. Lack of effect of amoxycillin on the absorption of ofloxacin. *Eur J Clin Pharmacol* (1993) 44, 207–9.

16. Strenkoski-Nix LC, Forrest A, Schentag JJ, Nix DE. Pharmacodynamic interactions of ciprofloxacin, piperacillin, and piperacillin/tazobactam in healthy volunteers. *J Clin Pharmacol* (1998) 38, 1063–71.
17. Orisakwe OE, Agbasi PU, Afonne OJ, Ofoefule SI, Obi E, Orish CN. Rifampicin pharmacokinetics with and without ciprofloxacin. *Am J Ther* (2001) 8, 151–3.
18. Orisakwe OE, Afonne OJ, Agbasi PU, Ofoefule SI. Urinary excretion of rifampicin in the presence of ciprofloxacin. *Am J Ther* (2004) 11, 171–4.
19. Chandler MHH, Toler SM, Rapp RP, Muder RR, Korvick JA. Multiple-dose pharmacokinetics of concurrent oral ciprofloxacin and rifampin therapy in elderly patients. *Antimicrob Agents Chemother* (1990) 34, 442–7.
20. Polk RE. Drug-drug interactions with ciprofloxacin and other fluoroquinolones. *Am J Med* (1989) 87 (Suppl 5A), 76S–81S.
21. Jhaj R, Roy A, Uppal R, Behera D. Influence of ciprofloxacin on pharmacokinetics of rifampin. *Curr Ther Res* (1997) 58, 260–5.
22. Humbert G, Brumpt I, Montay G, Le Liboux A, Frydman A, Borsa-Lebas F, Moore N. Influence of rifampin on the pharmacokinetics of pefloxacin. *Clin Pharmacol Ther* (1991) 50, 682–7.
23. Orisakwe OE, Akunyili DN, Agbasi PU, Ezejiofor NA. Some plasma and saliva pharmacokinetic parameters of rifampicin in the presence of pefloxacin. *Am J Ther* (2004) 11, 283–7.
24. Orisakwe OE, Agbasi PU, Ofoefule SI, Ilondu NA, Afonne OJ, Anusiem CA, Ilo CE, Maduka SO. Effect of pefloxacin on the urinary excretion of rifampicin. *Am J Ther* (2004) 11, 13–16.
25. Schrenzel J, Dayer P, Leemann T, Weidekamm E, Portmann R, Lew DP. Influence of rifampin on fleroxacin pharmacokinetics. *Antimicrob Agents Chemother* (1993) 37, 2132–8.

Quinolones + Pirenzepine

Four doses of pirenzepine 50 mg delayed the absorption of ciprofloxacin and ofloxacin in 10 healthy subjects, but their bioavailabilities remained unchanged.[1] The delayed absorption is unlikely to be of clinical significance.

1. Höffken G, Lode H, Wiley R, Glatzel TD, Sievers D, Olschewski T, Borner K, Koeppe T. Pharmacokinetics and bioavailability of ciprofloxacin and ofloxacin: effect of food and antacid intake. *Rev Infect Dis* (1988) 10 (Suppl 1), S138–S139.

Quinolones + Probenecid

Probenecid increases the serum levels and/or decreases the urinary excretion of cinoxacin, ciprofloxacin, clinafloxacin, enoxacin, fleroxacin, levofloxacin, nalidixic acid and norfloxacin. The clinical importance of these changes is uncertain, but is seems likely they will only be important in the presence of other drugs that also affect renal excretion. Grepafloxacin, moxifloxacin, sparfloxacin, and probably ofloxacin, appear not to interact with probenecid.

Clinical evidence

(a) Cinoxacin

A study in 6 healthy subjects found that probenecid 500 mg three times daily roughly doubled the serum levels of a 3-hour intravenous infusion of cinoxacin. The renal clearance of cinoxacin was also reduced from 68 to 46% during and for the 4 hours after the infusion.[1]

(b) Ciprofloxacin

In one study, probenecid 1 g, given 30 minutes before ciprofloxacin 500 mg, was found to reduce the renal clearance of ciprofloxacin by up to 50%. Other pharmacokinetic parameters (maximum serum levels, AUC) were unchanged and no accumulation of ciprofloxacin appeared to occur, probably due to an increase in extra-renal elimination.[2]

Another study found that the renal clearance of ciprofloxacin was reduced by 64% by probenecid. However, in contrast to the other study cited, the AUC of ciprofloxacin was increased by 74% and the AUC of its 2-aminoethylamino metabolite was increased by 234%. As a consequence, levels of ciprofloxacin in tears, sweat and saliva were also increased, but probenecid had no direct effect on ciprofloxacin distribution into these fluids.[3]

(c) Clinafloxacin

Probenecid 1 g, given 1 hour before a single 400-mg dose of clinafloxacin, reduced the total and renal clearance of clinafloxacin by 24% and 36%, respectively, raised the AUC by 32% and increased the elimination half-life from 6.3 to 7 hours.[4]

(d) Enoxacin

In one subject, the renal clearance of enoxacin 600 mg was approximately halved, and the half-life increased from 3.5 to 4.5 hours by a single 2.5-g dose of probenecid.[5]

(e) Fleroxacin

A study in 6 healthy subjects given a single 200-mg dose of fleroxacin, followed by 500 mg of probenecid 0.5, 12, 24 and 36 hours later, found that the fleroxacin AUC was increased by 37%, and the fleroxacin urinary excretion was decreased by 22%.[6] Another study found that probenecid increased the AUC of fleroxacin 400 mg by 26% (not statistically significant), and had no effect on fleroxacin urinary excretion.[7]

(f) Grepafloxacin

A study in 32 healthy subjects found that probenecid had no effect on the pharmacokinetics of a single 200-mg dose of grepafloxacin.[8] In another 6 healthy subjects probenecid similarly had no significant effect on grepafloxacin pharmacokinetics.[9]

(g) Levofloxacin

A study in 12 healthy subjects found that although probenecid reduced the renal clearance of a single 500-mg oral dose of levofloxacin by about one-third and increased its AUC and half-life by similar amounts, the 72-hour urinary levofloxacin excretion was unaltered.[10]

(h) Moxifloxacin

A study in 12 healthy subjects found that probenecid had no clinically significant effects on the pharmacokinetics of a single 400-mg dose of moxifloxacin.[11]

(i) Nalidixic acid

Two volunteers, acting as their own controls, took nalidixic acid 500 mg with and without probenecid 500 mg. The peak serum levels of nalidixic acid were unaffected at 2 hours, but at 8 hours the levels were increased threefold by the probenecid.[12]

Another study in 5 women with urinary tract infections treated with nalidixic acid showed that probenecid increased the maximum serum nalidixic acid levels and AUC by 43% and 74%, respectively.[13]

(j) Norfloxacin

The mean 12-hour urinary recovery of norfloxacin 200 mg was reduced by about half in 5 subjects when they were given probenecid 1 g. Norfloxacin serum concentrations were unaffected.[14]

(k) Ofloxacin

A study in 8 healthy subjects found that probenecid 500 mg increased the AUC of a single 200-mg dose of ofloxacin by 16% and decreased the total body clearance by 14%. Other pharmacokinetic parameters were not significantly affected.[15]

(l) Sparfloxacin

Probenecid 1.5 g did not significantly affect the clearance, the AUC or the half-life of sparfloxacin 200 mg in 6 healthy subjects.[16]

Mechanism

The likely explanation for this interaction is that probenecid successfully competes with some quinolones for tubular excretion, so that their renal elimination is reduced. Some quinolones are more dependent on glomerular filtration (e.g. grepafloxacin)[9] than tubular excretion for elimination, and thus are unaffected by competition for tubular excretion.[7]

Importance and management

Established interactions, but their clinical importance seems not to have been assessed. There appears to be no reason for avoiding concurrent use.

The increased levels and decreased renal excretion of clinafloxacin caused by probenecid are not considered large enough to warrant dosage adjustment,[4] and most of the changes seen with the other quinolones were of a similar magnitude. However, caution has been advised in the presence of other drugs that may also compete for renal excretion (such as some penicillins or cephalosporins).[3,4] Grepafloxacin, moxifloxacin, sparfloxacin, and probably ofloxacin, appear not to interact.

1. Rodriguez N, Madsen PO, Welling PG. Influence of probenecid on serum levels and urinary excretion of cinoxacin. *Antimicrob Agents Chemother* (1979) 15, 465–69.
2. Wingender W, Beerman D, Förster D, Graefe K-H, Kuhlmann J. Interactions of ciprofloxacin with food intake and drugs. *Curr Clin Pract Ser* (1986) 34, 136–40.
3. Jaehde U, Sörgel F, Reiter A, Sigl G, Naber KG, Schunack W. Effect of probenecid on the distribution and elimination of ciprofloxacin in humans. *Clin Pharmacol Ther* (1995) 58, 532–41.
4. Randinitis EJ, Koup JR, Bron NJ, Hounslow NJ, Rausch G, Abel R, Vassos AB, Sedman AJ. Drug interaction studies with clinafloxacin and probenecid, cimetidine, phenytoin and warfarin. *Drugs* (1999) 58 (Suppl 2), 254–5.

5. Wijnands WJA, Vree TB, Baars AM, van Herwaarden CLA. Pharmacokinetics of enoxacin and its penetration into bronchial secretions and lung tissue. *J Antimicrob Chemother* (1988) 21 (Suppl B), 67–77.
6. Shiba K, Saito A, Shimada J, Hori S, Kaji M, Miyahara T, Kusajima H, Kaneko S, Saito S, Uchida H. Interactions of fleroxacin with dried aluminium hydroxide gel and probenecid. *Rev Infect Dis* (1989) 11 (Suppl 5), S1097–S1098.
7. Weidekamm E, Portmann R, Suter K, Partos C, Dell D, Lücker PW. Single- and multiple dose pharmacokinetics of fleroxacin, a trifluorinated quinolone, in humans. *Antimicrob Agents Chemother* (1987) 31, 1909–14.
8. Koneru B, Bramer S, Bricmont P, Maroli A, Shiba K. Effect of food, gastric pH and co-administration of antacid, cimetidine and probenecid on the oral pharmacokinetics of the broad spectrum antimicrobial agent grepafloxacin. *Pharm Res* (1996) 13 (9 Suppl), S414.
9. Shiba K, Yoshida M, Hori S, Shimada J, Saito A, Sakai O. Pharmacokinetic interaction of OPC-17116 with probenecid in healthy volunteers. *Intersci Conf Antimicrob Agents Chemother* (1991) 31, 346.
10. Gaitonde MD, Mendes P, House ESA, Lehr KH. The effects of cimetidine and probenecid on the pharmacokinetics of levofloxacin (LVFX). *Intersci Conf Antimicrob Agents Chemother* (1995) 35, 8.
11. Stass H, Sachse R. Effect of probenecid on the kinetics of a single oral 400-mg dose of moxifloxacin in healthy male volunteers. *Clin Pharmacokinet* (2001) 40 (Suppl 1), 71–76.
12. Dash H, Mills J. Severe metabolic acidosis associated with nalidixic acid overdose. *Ann Intern Med* (1976) 84, 570–1.
13. Ferry N, Cuisinaud G, Pozet N, Zech PY, Sassard J. Influence du probénécide sur la pharmacocinétique de l'acide nalidixique. *Therapie* (1982) 37, 645–9.
14. Shimada J, Yamaji T, Ueda Y, Uchida H, Kusajima H, Irikura T. Mechanism of renal excretion of AM-715, a new quinolonecarboxylic acid derivative, in rabbits, dogs, and humans. *Antimicrob Agents Chemother* (1983) 23, 1–7.
15. Nataraj B, Rao Mamidi NVS, Krishna DR. Probenecid affects the pharmacokinetics of ofloxacin in healthy volunteers. *Clin Drug Invest* (1998) 16, 259–62.
16. Shimada J, Saito A, Shiba K, Hojo T, Kaji M, Hori S, Yoshida M, Sakai O. Pharmacokinetics and clinical studies of sparfloxacin. *Chemotherapy (Tokyo)* (1991) 39 (Suppl 4), 234–44.

Quinolones + Sucralfate

Sucralfate causes a marked reduction in the absorption of ciprofloxacin, enoxacin, gemifloxacin, lomefloxacin, moxifloxacin, ofloxacin, norfloxacin and sparfloxacin, but only a modest reduction in fleroxacin levels.

Clinical evidence

(a) Ciprofloxacin

In a study in 8 healthy subjects sucralfate 1 g four times daily reduced the AUC and maximum serum concentration of ciprofloxacin 500 mg by 88% and 90%, respectively.[1]

A patient given sucralfate 1 g four times daily had serum ciprofloxacin levels which were 85 to 90% lower than 5 other patients who were not taking sucralfate.[2] A single dose study found a 96% reduction in the AUC of ciprofloxacin following a 2-g dose of sucralfate.[3] A study in 12 healthy subjects found that a 1-g dose of sucralfate given 6 and 2 hours before a single 750-mg dose of ciprofloxacin, reduced the ciprofloxacin AUC by about 30%. Three of the subjects showed little or no changes in AUC but a decrease of more than 50% was seen in 4 others.[4] A related study in 12 healthy subjects found that the bioavailability of ciprofloxacin 750 mg was reduced by 7%, 20%, and 95%, respectively, when sucralfate was given 6 hours before, 2 hours before, or at the same time as, the ciprofloxacin.[5] Oral sucralfate does not alter the effects of ciprofloxacin on aerobic bacteria in the gut.[6]

(b) Enoxacin

In 8 healthy subjects the bioavailability of enoxacin 400 mg was reduced by 54% and 88%, respectively, when sucralfate 1 g was given 2 hours before or with the enoxacin. When sucralfate was given 2 hours after the enoxacin the bioavailability was not affected.[7]

(c) Fleroxacin

The bioavailability of fleroxacin 400 mg was reduced by 24% in 20 healthy subjects taking sucralfate 1 g every 6 hours.[8]

(d) Gemifloxacin

In a study in 27 healthy subjects gemifloxacin 320 mg was given either 3 hours before or 2 hours after sucralfate 2 g. The pharmacokinetics of gemifloxacin were not significantly altered when sucralfate was given after the gemifloxacin, probably due to its rapid absorption. However, when sucralfate was given 3 hours before gemifloxacin, the AUC and maximum plasma levels were decreased by 53% and 69%, respectively.[9]

(e) Levofloxacin

The pharmacokinetics of levofloxacin are unaffected by sucralfate taken 2 hours after the quinolone.[10]

(f) Lomefloxacin

A study in 12 subjects found that when lomefloxacin 400 mg was given 2 hours after sucralfate 1 g the lomefloxacin AUC and maximum serum concentration was reduced by about 25% and 30%, respectively.[11] Another study in 8 healthy subjects found that when lomefloxacin 400 mg was given with sucralfate 1 g, the lomefloxacin AUC was reduced by 51%.[12]

(g) Moxifloxacin

In 12 healthy subjects a total of five doses of sucralfate 1 g, given at the same time as a single 400-mg dose of moxifloxacin and then 5, 10, 15, and 24 hours after the dose, reduced the AUC and maximum serum concentration of moxifloxacin by 40% and 29%, respectively.[13]

(h) Norfloxacin

A study in 8 healthy subjects found that sucralfate 1 g four times daily reduced the AUC of a single 400-mg dose of norfloxacin by 98%, when taken with the sucralfate, and by 42% when taken 2 hours after the sucralfate.[14] Another study found a reduction of 91% in the AUC of norfloxacin 400 mg when it was taken with sucralfate 1 g, but no reduction when it was taken 2 hours before sucralfate.[15]

(i) Ofloxacin

A single dose study found that sucralfate (dose not stated) reduced the maximum serum levels and AUC of a single 200-mg dose of ofloxacin by about two-thirds.[16] Another study found a reduction of 61% when ofloxacin 400 mg was taken with sucralfate 1 g, but no reduction when the ofloxacin was taken 2 hours before sucralfate.[15] Food reduced the extent of the interaction but it was still marked.[17]

(j) Sparfloxacin

In a study in 15 healthy subjects sucralfate 1 g four times daily reduced the maximum serum levels, the AUC and the relative bioavailability of sparfloxacin 400 mg daily by 39%, 47%, and 44%, respectively.[18] In a study assessing staggered dosing of sucralfate 1.5 g on the pharmacokinetics of sparfloxacin 300 mg, the AUC was unaffected when sucralfate was given 4 hours after the quinolone, but was decreased by 34% when given 2 hours before, and 51% when given at the same time as sucralfate.[19]

Mechanism

The aluminium hydroxide component of sucralfate (about 200 mg in each gram) forms an insoluble chelate between the cation and the 4-keto and 3-carboxyl groups of the quinolone, which reduces its absorption. See 'Quinolones + Antacids or Calcium compounds', p.328 for more on this mechanism.

Importance and management

Established and clinically important interactions. Because it seems probable that serum ciprofloxacin, enoxacin, gemifloxacin, levofloxacin, lomefloxacin, moxifloxacin, ofloxacin, norfloxacin and sparfloxacin levels will be reduced to subtherapeutic concentrations if given with the sucralfate, separate the dosages as much as possible (by 2 hours or more), giving the quinolone first. The study with moxifloxacin suggested that sucralfate should not be given for 2 hours before or 4 hours after the quinolone, but more study is needed to confirm both these findings and the effectiveness of separating the dosages. The interaction with fleroxacin is only modest (bioavailability reduced by 24%) and probably not clinically important, but some separation of the dosages may reduce the interaction further. This needs confirmation. **Pefloxacin** interacts with antacids containing aluminium hydroxide (see 'Quinolones + Antacids or Calcium compounds', p.328) and is therefore likely to interact with sucralfate. The 'H_2-receptor antagonists', (p.335) and 'omeprazole', (p.338) do not interact with the quinolones and may therefore be alternatives to sucralfate in many situations.

1. Garrelts JC, Godley PJ, Peterie JD, Gerlach EH, Yakshe CC. Sucralfate significantly reduces ciprofloxacin concentrations in serum. *Antimicrob Agents Chemother* (1990) 34, 931–3.
2. Yuk JH, Nightingale CN, Quintiliani R. Ciprofloxacin levels when receiving sucralfate. *JAMA* (1989) 262, 901.
3. Brouwers JRBJ, Van Der Kam HJ, Sijtsma J, Proost JH. Important reduction of ciprofloxacin absorption by sucralfate and magnesium citrate solution. *Drug Invest* (1990) 2, 197–9.
4. Nix DE, Watson WA, Handy L, Frost RW, Rescott DL, Goldstein HR. The effect of sucralfate pretreatment on the pharmacokinetics of ciprofloxacin. *Pharmacotherapy* (1989) 9, 377–80.
5. Van Slooten AD, Nix DE, Wilton JH, Love JH, Spivey JM, Goldstein HR. Combined use of ciprofloxacin and sucralfate. *DICP Ann Pharmacother* (1991) 25, 578–82.
6. Krueger WA, Ruckdeschel G, Unertl K. Influence of intravenously administered ciprofloxacin on aerobic intestinal microflora and fecal drug levels when administered simultaneously with sucralfate. *Antimicrob Agents Chemother* (1997) 41, 1725–30.

7. Ryerson B, Toothaker R, Schleyer I, Sedman A, Colburn W. Effect of sucralfate on enoxacin pharmacokinetics. *Intersci Conf Antimicrob Agents Chemother* (1989) 29, 136.
8. Lubowski TJ, Nightingale CH, Sweeney K, Quintiliani R. Effect of sucralfate on pharmacokinetics of fleroxacin in healthy volunteers. *Antimicrob Agents Chemother* (1992) 36, 2758–60.
9. Allen A, Bygate E, Faessel H, Isaac L, Lewis A. The effect of ferrous sulphate and sucralfate on the bioavailability of oral gemifloxacin in healthy volunteers. *Int J Antimicrob Agents* (2000) 15, 283–9.
10. Lee L-J, Hafkin B, Lee I-D, Hoh J, Dix R. Effect of food and sucralfate on a single oral dose of 500 milligrams of levofloxacin in healthy subjects. *Antimicrob Agents Chemother* (1997) 41, 2196–2200.
11. Nix D, Schentag J. Lomefloxacin (L) absorption kinetics when administered with ranitidine (R) and sucralfate (S). *Intersci Conf Antimicrob Agents Chemother* (1989) 29, 317.
12. Lehto P, Kivistö KT. Different effects of products containing metal ions on the absorption of lomefloxacin. *Clin Pharmacol Ther* (1994) 56, 477–82.
13. Stass H, Schühly U, Möller J-G, Delesen H. Effects of sucralfate on the oral bioavailability of moxifloxacin, a novel 8-methoxyfluoroquinolone, in healthy volunteers. *Clin Pharmacokinet* (2001) 40 (Suppl 1), 49–55.
14. Parpia SH, Nix DE, Hejmanowski LG, Goldstein HR, Witton JH, Schentag JJ. Sucralfate reduces the gastrointestinal absorption of norfloxacin. *Antimicrob Agents Chemother* (1989) 33, 99–102.
15. Lehto P, Kvistö KT. Effect of sucralfate on absorption of norfloxacin and ofloxacin. *Antimicrob Agents Chemother* (1994) 38, 248–51.
16. Shiba K, Yoshida M, Kachi M, Shimada J, Saito A, Sakai N. Effects of peptic ulcer-healing drugs on the pharmacokinetics of new quinolone (OFLX). 17th Int Congr Chemother, June 1991, Berlin, Abstract 415.
17. Kawakami J, Matsuse T, Kotaki H, Seino T, Fukuchi Y, Orimo H, Sawada Y, Iga T. The effect of food on the interaction of ofloxacin with sucralfate in healthy volunteers. *Eur J Clin Pharmacol* (1994) 47, 67–9.
18. Zix JA, Geerdes-Fenge HF, Rau M, Vöckler J, Borner K, Koeppe P, Lode H. Pharmacokinetics of sparfloxacin and interaction with cisapride and sucralfate. *Antimicrob Agents Chemother* (1997) 41, 1668–1672.
19. Kamberi M, Nakashima H, Ogawa K, Oda N, Nakano S. The effect of staggered dosing of sucralfate on oral bioavailability of sparfloxacin. *Br J Clin Pharmacol* (2000) 49, 98–103.

Quinolones; Ciprofloxacin + Pancreatic enzymes

The pharmacokinetics of ciprofloxacin are not affected by pancreatic enzyme supplements.

Clinical evidence, mechanism, importance and management

Six patients with cystic fibrosis, chronically infected with *Ps. aeruginosa* and treated with a range of drugs including ceftazidime, tobramycin, ticarcillin and salbutamol, demonstrated no significant changes in the pharmacokinetics of a single 250-mg dose of ciprofloxacin when it was given with standard doses of pancreatic enzymes (seven *Pancrease* capsules).[1] Another study in 12 patients with cystic fibrosis found that administration of pancreatic enzyme supplements 30 minutes before a single 750-mg dose of ciprofloxacin did not alter the pharmacokinetics of ciprofloxacin.[2] No special precautions would seem to be necessary during concurrent use.

1. Mack G, Cooper PJ, Buchanan N. Effects of enzyme supplementation on oral absorption of ciprofloxacin in patients with cystic fibrosis. *Antimicrob Agents Chemother* (1991) 35, 1484–5.
2. Reed MD, Stern RC, Myers CM, Yamashita TS, Blumer JL. Lack of unique pharmacokinetic characteristics in patients with cystic fibrosis. *J Clin Pharmacol* (1988) 28, 691–9.

Quinolones; Ciprofloxacin + Phenazopyridine

Phenazopyridine appears to increase the bioavailability of ciprofloxacin.

Clinical evidence, mechanism, importance and management

A study in 23 healthy subjects given a single 500-mg dose of ciprofloxacin either alone or with phenazopyridine 200 mg found that phenazopyridine increased the AUC and mean residence time of ciprofloxacin by about 30%. The time to achieve maximum plasma levels was increased from 1 to 1.5 hours.[1] If anything, this seems likely to be a beneficial, rather than adverse, interaction.

1. Marcelín-Jiménez G, Ángeles AP, Martínez-Rossier L, Fernández A. Ciprofloxacin bioavailability is enhanced by oral co-administration with phenazopyridine: a pharmacokinetic study in a Mexican population. *Clin Drug Invest* (2006) 26, 323–8.

Quinolones; Ciprofloxacin + Sevelamer

Sevelamer reduced the bioavailability of ciprofloxacin by 48% in one study.

Clinical evidence, mechanism, importance and management

In a crossover study in 15 healthy subjects the AUC of ciprofloxacin was reduced by 39% and the relative oral bioavailability was reduced by 48% when a single 750-mg dose of ciprofloxacin was taken with sevelamer 2.8 g The reduction was variable.[1] The mechanism of the interaction is unknown. Based on the results of this study, sevelamer should not be given at the same time as ciprofloxacin because the efficacy of ciprofloxacin might be reduced in some patients. Further study is needed to establish whether or not the interaction could be avoided by separation of the doses.

1. Kays MB, Overholser BR, Mueller BA, Moe SM, Sowinski KM. Effects of sevelamer hydrochloride and calcium acetate on the oral bioavailability of ciprofloxacin. *Am J Kidney Dis* (2003) 42, 1253–9.

Quinolones; Ciprofloxacin + Ursodeoxycholic acid (Ursodiol)

An isolated report describes a reduction in serum ciprofloxacin levels in a patient taking ursodeoxycholic acid.

Clinical evidence, mechanism, importance and management

A man with metastatic colon cancer had unusually low serum levels of ciprofloxacin following oral dosing; his only other medication was ursodeoxycholic acid 300 mg twice daily for gallstones. Despite the low antibacterial serum levels the bacteraemia cleared. Several months later when he was readmitted to hospital, both drugs were again given, initially staggered, and then later together. When taken together the AUC of the ciprofloxacin was reduced by 50% by ursodeoxycholic acid.[1] The reason for this interaction is not understood.

This seems to be the first and only report of an interaction between a quinolone and ursodeoxycholic acid and its importance is uncertain. More study is needed to establish this interaction, its importance, and its mechanism.

1. Belliveau PP, Nightingale CH, Quintiliani R, Maderazo EG. Reduction in serum concentrations of ciprofloxacin after administration of ursodiol to a patient with hepatobiliary disease. *Clin Infect Dis* (1994) 19, 354–5.

Quinolones; Levofloxacin + Antiretrovirals

There appears to be no clinically important pharmacokinetic interaction between levofloxacin and efavirenz or nelfinavir.

Clinical evidence, mechanism, importance and management

A study in HIV-positive patients who were taking antiretroviral therapy consisting of zidovudine and lamivudine with either **efavirenz** or **nelfinavir**, found that levofloxacin 500 mg daily for 4 days did not affect the steady-state pharmacokinetics of either **efavirenz** 600 mg daily or **nelfinavir** 750 mg three times daily. The pharmacokinetics of levofloxacin during concurrent treatment with **efavirenz** or **nelfinavir** were unaffected, except for the time to maximum levels, which was increased from 0.9 to 1.7 hours in control subjects, to 3.3 hours with **efavirenz**. This may have occurred as a result of delayed gastric emptying caused by the **efavirenz**. A clinically important interaction between levofloxacin and either **efavirenz** or **nelfinavir** is unlikely.[1]

1. Villani P, Viale P, Signorini L, Cadeo B, Marchetti F, Villani A, Fiocchi C, Regazzi MB, Carosi G. Pharmacokinetic evaluation of oral levofloxacin in human immunodeficiency virus-infected subjects receiving concomitant antiretroviral therapy. *Antimicrob Agents Chemother* (2001) 45, 2160–2.

Quinolones; Lomefloxacin + Furosemide

Furosemide causes a small, almost certainly unimportant, rise in the serum levels of lomefloxacin. The pharmacokinetics and diuretic effects of the furosemide are not changed.

Clinical evidence, mechanism, importance and management

A study in 8 healthy subjects found that when a single 200-mg dose of lomefloxacin was taken with furosemide 40 mg, the AUC of lomefloxacin was increased by 12%. The maximum serum levels and the half-life were also increased, but not to a statistically significant extent.[1] The suggested reason for the interaction is that there is some competition between the two drugs for excretion by the kidney tubules. No significant changes were seen in the pharmacokinetics of the furosemide nor in its diuretic effects.[1] The small rise in the serum levels of lomefloxacin is almost certainly too small to be important and there would seem to be no reason for avoiding concurrent use. Information about other quinolone antibacterials appears to be lacking.

1. Sudoh T, Fujimura A, Shiga T, Sasaki M, Harada K, Tateishi T, Ohashi K, Ebihara A. Renal clearance of lomefloxacin is decreased by furosemide. *Eur J Clin Pharmacol* (1994) 46, 267–9.

Quinolones; Moxifloxacin + Itraconazole

A study in healthy subjects found that itraconazole 200 mg daily for 9 days did not affect the pharmacokinetics of a single 200-mg dose of moxifloxacin given on day 7. No clinically relevant changes were found in the pharmacokinetics of itraconazole.[1] No special precautions would seem to be necessary during concurrent use.

1. Stass H, Nagelschmitz J, Moeller J-G, Delesen . Pharmacokinetics of moxifloxacin are not influenced by a 7-day pre-treatment with 200 mg oral itraconazole given once a day in healthy subjects. *Int J Clin Pharmacol Ther* (2004) 42, 23–9.

Quinolones; Ofloxacin + Cetraxate

A single-dose study found that cetraxate (dose not stated) did not affect the pharmacokinetics of a single 200-mg dose of ofloxacin.[1] No special precautions would seem to be necessary on concurrent use.

1. Shiba K, Yoshida M, Kachi M, Shimada J, Saito A, Sakai N. Effects of peptic ulcer-healing drugs on the pharmacokinetics of new quinolone (OFLX). 17th Int Congr Chemother, June 1991, Berlin, Abstract 415.

Quinupristin/Dalfopristin + Miscellaneous

***In vitro* studies have found that quinupristin/dalfopristin inhibits the CYP3A4-mediated metabolism of docetaxel, tamoxifen and terfenadine and is predicted to inhibit the metabolism of other drugs by this enzyme system.**

Clinical evidence, mechanism, importance and management

In vitro studies found quinupristin/dalfopristin inhibited the cytochrome P450 isoenzyme CYP3A4-mediated metabolism of **docetaxel**, **tamoxifen**, and **terfenadine**.[1] Quinupristin/dalfopristin is predicted to raise the levels of other drugs including antiarrhythmics (**disopyramide**, **lidocaine**, **quinidine**), antiretrovirals (such as **delavirdine**, **indinavir**, **nevirapine**, **ritonavir**), **astemizole**, **carbamazepine**, **cisapride**, **methylprednisolone**, **paclitaxel**, **statins** (but see 'Lipid regulating drugs', (p.1086)), and **vinca alkaloids**.[1] More study is needed.

1. Rubinstein E, Prokocimer P, Talbot GH. Safety and tolerability of quinupristin/dalfopristin: administration guidelines. *J Antimicrob Chemother* (1999) 44 (Topic A) 37–46.

Rifampicin (Rifampin) + Aminosalicylic acid

The serum levels of rifampicin are approximately halved if aminosalicylic acid granules containing bentonite are given.

Clinical evidence

In 30 patients with tuberculosis the serum levels of rifampicin 10 mg/kg were reduced by more than 50%, from 6.06 to 2.91 micrograms/mL, at 2 hours by aminosalicylate.[1,2] Later studies in 6 healthy subjects showed that this interaction was not due to the aminosalicylic acid itself but to the **bentonite**, which was the main excipient of the granules.[3] The rifampicin AUC was statistically unchanged in the presence of sodium aminosalicylate tablets (no **bentonite**), whereas it was reduced by more than 37% in the presence of **bentonite** from aminosalicylate granules.[3]

Other studies confirm this marked reduction in serum rifampicin levels in the presence of **bentonite** in aminosalicylic acid granules.[4]

Mechanism

The bentonite excipient in the aminosalicylic acid granules adsorbs the rifampicin onto its surface so that much less is available for absorption, which results in reduced serum levels.[3] Bentonite is a naturally occurring mineral (montmorillonite) consisting largely of hydrate aluminium silicate, and is similar to kaolin.

Importance and management

A well documented and clinically important interaction. Separating the administration of the two drugs by 8 to 12 hours to prevent their mixing in the gut has been suggested as an effective way to prevent this interaction.[1] An alternative is to give aminosalicylic acid preparations that do not contain bentonite.

1. Boman G, Hanngren Å, Malmborg A-S, Borgå O, Sjöqvist F. Drug Interaction: decreased serum concentrations of rifampicin when given with P.A.S. *Lancet* (1971) i, 800.
2. Boman G, Borgå O, Hanngren Å, Malmborg A-S and Sjöqvist F. Pharmacokinetic interactions between the tuberculostatics rifampicin, para-aminosalicylic acid and isoniazid. *Acta Pharmacol Toxicol (Copenh)* (1970) 28 (Suppl 1), 15.
3. Boman G, Lundgren P, Stjernström G. Mechanism of the inhibitory effect of PAS granules on the absorption of rifampicin: adsorption of rifampicin by an excipient, bentonite. *Eur J Clin Pharmacol* (1975) 8, 293–9.
4. Boman G. Serum concentration and half-life of rifampicin after simultaneous oral administration of aminosalicylic acid or isoniazid. *Eur J Clin Pharmacol* (1974) 7, 217–25.

Rifampicin (Rifampin) + Antacids

The absorption of rifampicin can be reduced up to about one-third by antacids, but the clinical importance of this is uncertain.

Clinical evidence

When 5 healthy subjects took a single 600-mg dose of rifampicin with various antacids the absorption of rifampicin was reduced. The antacids caused a fall in the urinary excretion of rifampicin as follows: 15 or 30 mL of **aluminium hydroxide gel** 29 to 31%; 2 or 4 g of **magnesium trisilicate** 31 to 36%; and 2 g of **sodium bicarbonate** 21%.[1]

Three groups of 15 patients with tuberculosis were given a single oral dose of rifampicin 10 to 12 mg/kg, isoniazid 300 mg and ethambutol 20 mg/kg either alone or with about 20 mL of antacid. A 'significant number' of patients had peak rifampicin concentrations below 6.5 micrograms/mL (serum level quoted as necessary to achieve adequate lung concentrations) in the group receiving *Aludrox* (**aluminium hydroxide**), but no significant effect was noted in the group receiving *Gelusil* (**aluminium hydroxide** plus **magnesium trisilicate**).[2] However, in a further study in 14 healthy subjects, 30 mL of *Mylanta* (**aluminium/magnesium hydroxide**) given 9 hours before, with and after rifampicin had no effect on rifampicin pharmacokinetics.[3]

Mechanism

It has been suggested that the rise in stomach pH caused by these antacids reduces the dissolution of the rifampicin and thereby inhibits its absorption. In addition, aluminium ions may form less soluble chelates with rifampicin, and magnesium trisilicate can adsorb rifampicin, both of which would also be expected to reduce bioavailability.[1]

Importance and management

Direct information seems to be limited to these reports. The effects of 20 to 35% reductions in rifampicin absorption do not appear to have been assessed, but if antacids are given it would be prudent to be alert for any evidence that treatment is less effective than expected. The US manufacturers of rifampicin advise giving rifampicin 1 hour before antacids.[4]

1. Khalil SAH, El-Khordagui LK, El-Gholmy ZA. Effect of antacids on oral absorption of rifampicin. *Int J Pharmaceutics* (1984) 20, 99–106.
2. Gupta PR, Mehta YR, Gupta ML, Sharma TN, Jain D, Gupta RB. Rifampicin-aluminium antacid interaction. *J Assoc Physicians India* (1988) 36, 363–4.
3. Peloquin CA, Namdar R, Singleton MD, Nix DE. Pharmacokinetics of rifampin under fasting conditions, with food, and with antacids. *Chest* (1999) 115, 12–18.
4. Rifadin (Rifampicin). Sanofi-Aventis US LLC. US Prescribing information, March 2007.

Rifampicin (Rifampin) + Clofazimine

There is no pharmacokinetic interaction between rifampicin and clofazimine.

Clinical evidence, mechanism, importance and management

Clofazimine 100 mg daily, given to 15 patients with leprosy taking rifampicin 600 mg daily and dapsone 100 mg daily, had no effect on the pharmacokinetics of rifampicin.[1] A single-dose study similarly found that the bioavailability of clofazimine remained unaltered when rifampicin was given, although a reduction in the rate of absorption was seen.[2] No special precautions would seem to be necessary on concurrent use.

1. Venkatesan K, Mathur A, Girdhar BK, Bharadwaj VP. The effect of clofazimine on the pharmacokinetics of rifampicin and dapsone in leprosy. *J Antimicrob Chemother* (1986) 18, 715–18.
2. Mehta J, Gandhi IS, Sane SB, Wamburkar MN. Effect of clofazimine and dapsone on rifampicin (Lositril) pharmacokinetics in multibacillary and paucibacillary leprosy cases. *Indian J Lepr* (1985) 57, 297–310.

Rifampicin (Rifampin) + Food

Food delays and reduces the absorption of rifampicin from the gut.

Clinical evidence

The absorption of a single 10-mg/kg dose of rifampicin was reduced when it was given to 6 healthy subjects with a **standard Indian breakfast** (125 g wheat, 10 g visible fat, 350 g vegetables). The AUC after 8 hours was reduced by 26% and the peak plasma levels were prolonged (from 11.84 micrograms/mL at 2 hours to 8.35 micrograms/mL at 4 hours) and reduced by about 30%.[1] In another study, a **high-fat breakfast** reduced the maximum serum level of rifampicin 600 mg by 36% and delayed the absorption, but the AUC was not significantly altered.[2]

Mechanism

Not understood.

Importance and management

An established interaction. Rifampicin should be taken on an empty stomach (at least 30 minutes before a meal, or 2 hours after a meal) to ensure rapid and complete absorption.

1. Polasa K, Krishnaswamy K. Effect of food on bioavailability of rifampicin. *J Clin Pharmacol* (1983) 23, 433–7.
2. Peloquin CA, Namdar R, Singleton MD, Nix DE. Pharmacokinetics of rifampin under fasting conditions, with food, and with antacids. *Chest* (1999) 155, 12–18.

Rifampicin (Rifampin) + H_2-receptor antagonists

No clinically significant interaction appears to occur between rifampicin and cimetidine or ranitidine.

Clinical evidence, mechanism, importance and management

(a) Cimetidine

In a study, 12 patients given daily doses of rifampicin 8 mg/kg, isoniazid 8 mg/kg and ethambutol 25 mg/kg, and 13 untreated control subjects were given intravenous cimetidine 300 mg. In the patients receiving antimycobacterials, the non-renal clearance of cimetidine was increased by 52% but the total clearance and volume of distribution were unchanged. The reduction in renal clearance in the patients may have been associated with age-related impairment of renal function, but it was suggested that the increased non-renal clearance may have been due to enzyme induction of cimetidine metabolism.[1] As total clearance was unchanged this interaction seems unlikely to be clinically significant.

(b) Ranitidine

In a controlled study, 112 patients with pulmonary tuberculosis were treated in 2 groups, one with a daily regimen of rifampicin 10 mg/kg, isoniazid 300 mg and ethambutol 20 mg/kg and ranitidine 150 mg twice daily, and the other with the same antimycobacterials but without ranitidine. The pharmacokinetics of rifampicin (as measured by the total and unchanged urinary excretion) were not affected by ranitidine. No changes occurred in the incidence of adverse hepatic reactions, while gastrointestinal reactions were reduced.[2] There would seem to be no reason for avoiding the use of ranitidine, or any other H_2-receptor antagonists, in patients taking rifampicin.

1. Keller E, Schollmeyer P, Brandenstein U, Hoppe-Seyler G. Increased nonrenal clearance of cimetidine during antituberculous therapy. *Int J Clin Pharmacol Ther Toxicol* (1984) 22, 307–11.
2. Purohit SD, Johri SC, Gupta PR, Mehta YR, Bhatnagar M. Ranitidine-rifampicin interaction. *J Assoc Physicians India* (1992) 40, 308–10.

Rifampicin (Rifampin) + Phenobarbital

Phenobarbital possibly modestly increases the clearance of rifampicin. The effect of rifampicin on phenobarbital levels is unknown, but note that rifampicin markedly increased the clearance of another barbiturate hexobarbital, used as a marker of drug metabolism.

Clinical evidence

In one study, the serum levels of rifampicin were reduced by 20 to 40% in 12 of 15 patients taking phenobarbital 100 mg daily.[1] In another study, although phenobarbital 100 mg daily for 7 days reduced the mean half-life of a single 600-mg dose of rifampicin by 15%, this was not statistically significant. However, in a further 5 patients with cirrhosis of the liver, phenobarbital did reduce the half-life of rifampicin by a mean of 2.2 hours.[2]

The effect of rifampicin on phenobarbital levels does not appear to have been studied, but rifampicin markedly increased the clearance of another barbiturate **hexobarbital**, used as a marker of drug metabolism.[3-6]

Mechanism

Both rifampicin and phenobarbital are potent liver enzyme inducers. The outcome of their effects when combined is not clear.

Importance and management

The documentation for this interaction is very limited, and the outcome of concurrent use is unclear. Concurrent use need not be avoided, but be alert for a reduced response to both drugs.

1. de Rautlin de la Roy Y, Beauchant G, Breuil K, Patte F. Diminution du taux sérique de rifampicine par le phénobarbital. *Presse Med* (1971) 79, 350.
2. Acocella G, Bonollo L, Mainardi M, Margaroli P, Nicolis FB. Kinetic studies on rifampicin. III. Effect of phenobarbital on the half-life of the antibiotic. *Tijdschr Gastroenterol* (1974) 17, 151–8.
3. Breimer DD, Zilly W, Richter E. Influence of rifampicin on drug metabolism: differences between hexobarbital and antipyrine. *Clin Pharmacol Ther* (1977) 21, 470–81.
4. Zilly W, Breimer DD, Richter E. Induction of drug metabolism in man after rifampicin treatment measured by increased hexobarbital and tolbutamide clearance. *Eur J Clin Pharmacol* (1975) 9, 219–27.
5. Zilly W, Breimer DD, Richter E. Stimulation of drug metabolism by rifampicin in patients with cirrhosis or cholestasis measured by increased hexobarbital and tolbutamide clearance. *Eur J Clin Pharmacol* (1977) 11, 287–93.
6. Smith DA, Chandler MHH, Shedlofsky SI, Wedlund PJ, Blouin RA. Age-dependent stereoselective increase in the oral clearance of hexobarbitone isomers caused by rifampicin. *Br J Clin Pharmacol* (1991) 32, 735–9.

Rifampicin (Rifampin) + Probenecid

Probenecid increased rifampicin levels in one study, but not in another.

Clinical evidence, mechanism, importance and management

A study in 6 healthy subjects given probenecid 2 g before and after a single 300-mg dose of rifampicin found that probenecid increased the mean peak serum rifampicin levels by 86%. At 4, 6, and 9 hours after the dose the increases were 118%, 90%, and 102%, respectively.[1] However, subsequent studies in patients taking either rifampicin 600 mg daily, or rifampicin 300 mg daily 30 minutes after a 2-g dose of probenecid found that the probenecid group achieved serum rifampicin levels that were only about half those achieved by those taking rifampicin 600 mg alone, suggesting that no interaction occurred.[2] The reasons for these discordant results are not understood, although it has been suggested that erratic rifampicin absorption may have played a part.[2] The interaction is not proven, but it seems possible that some patients will experience a rise in rifampicin levels. Consider this interaction as a possible cause if rifampicin adverse effects are troublesome.

1. Kenwright S, Levi AJ. Impairment of hepatic uptake of rifamycin antibiotics by probenecid, and its therapeutic implications. *Lancet* (1973) ii, 1401–5.
2. Fallon RJ, Lees AW, Allan GW, Smith J, Tyrrell WF. Probenecid and rifampicin serum levels. *Lancet* (1975) ii, 792–4.

Sodium fusidate + Colestyramine

***In vitro* studies have shown that colestyramine can bind with sodium fusidate in the gut, thereby reducing its activity,[1] and *in vivo animal* studies have shown peak fusidate levels are decreased by 33 to 77% by colestyramine,[2] but whether this also occurs clinically has not been confirmed. It is generally recommended that other drugs are given 1 hour before or 4 to 6 hours after colestyramine.**

1. Johns WH, Bates TR. Drug-cholestyramine interactions. I: Physicochemical factors affecting *in vitro* binding of sodium fusidate to cholestyramine. *J Pharm Sci* (1972) 61, 730–5.
2. Johns WH, Bates TR. Drug-cholestyramine interactions. II: Influence of cholestyramine on GI absorption of sodium fusidate. *J Pharm Sci* (1972) 61, 735–9.

Sulfonamides + Local anaesthetics

Para-aminobenzoic acid (PABA), derived from certain local anaesthetics, can reduce the effects of the sulfonamides and allow the development of local and even generalised infections. However, it should be noted that the limited evidence for this interaction is from the 1940s.

Clinical evidence

Four patients taking sulfonamides developed local infections in areas where **procaine** had been injected before diagnostic taps for meningitis, or draining procedures in empyema. Extensive cellulitis of the lumbar region occurred in one case, and abscesses appeared at the puncture sites in another. However, it should be noted that lumbar punctures were being done at least daily and up to four times a day in the 3 patients with meningitis.[1]

An *in vitro* study demonstrated that the amount of **procaine** in the pleural fluid after anaesthesia for thoracentesis was sufficient to inhibit the antibacterial activity of 0.005% **sulfapyridine** against type III pneumococci.[2] Another *in vitro* study found that some local anaesthetics derived from PABA inhibited the bacteriostatic activity of **sulfapyridine** and **sulfathiazole** but some other local anaesthetics not derived from PABA did not affect the antibacterial activity of these sulfonamides.[3] Other studies in *animals* confirm that both *in vitro*[4-6] and *in vivo*[7] antagonism can occur between sulfonamides and local anaesthetics that are hydrolysed to **PABA**.

Mechanism

The ester type of local anaesthetic is hydrolysed within the body to produce PABA. Sulfonamides work by inhibiting bacterial DNA synthesis by competitively inhibiting folate production. The PABA competes with the sulfonamides, so higher PABA concentrations effectively dilute the effects of the sulfonamides.

Importance and management

Clinical examples of this interaction seem to be few and of poor quality (note that the patients were given repeated lumbar punctures, up to four times daily in some instances). It should also be noted that the supporting evidence (human, *animal* and *in vitro* studies) dates back to the mid-1940s with nothing more recent apparently on record. Local anaesthetics of the ester type that are hydrolysed to PABA (e.g. tetracaine, procaine, benzocaine) present the greatest risk of a reaction, whereas those of the amide type (bupivacaine, cinchocaine, lidocaine, mepivacaine and prilocaine) would not be expected to interact adversely. The evidence seems to be too slim to preclude concurrent use of these drugs, but it is perhaps worth considering this interaction if high or repeated doses of the local anaesthetic are used. However, note that high doses or prolonged use of these ester-type anaesthetics are best avoided given their toxicity when used in this manner.

1. Peterson OL, Finland M. Sulfonamide inhibiting action of procaine. *Am J Med Sci* (1944) 207, 166–75.
2. Boroff DA, Cooper A, Bullowa JGM. Inhibition of sulfapyridine by procaine in chest fluids after procaine anesthesia. *Proc Soc Exp Biol Med* (1941) 47,182–3.
3. Keltch AK, Baker LA, Krahl ME, Clowes GHA. Anti-sulfapyridine and anti-sulfathiazole effect of local anaesthetics derived from p-aminobenzoic acid. *Proc Soc Exp Biol Med* (1941) 47, 533–8.
4. Casten D, Fried JJ, Hallman FA. Inhibitory effect of procaine on the bacteriostatic activity of sulfathiazole. *Surg Gynecol Obstet* (1943) 76, 726–8.
5. Powell HM, Krahl ME, Clowes GHA. Inhibition of chemotherapeutic action of sulfapyridine by local anesthetics. *J Indiana State Med Assoc* (1942) 35, 62–3.
6. Walker BS, Derow MA. The antagonism of local anesthetics against the sulfonamides. *Am J Med Sci* (1945) 210, 585–8.
7. Pfeiffer CC, Grant CW. The procaine-sulfonamide antagonism: an evaluation of local anesthetics for use with sulfonamide therapy. *Anesthesiology* (1944) 5, 605–14.

Sulfonamides; Sulfafurazole (Sulfisoxazole) + Laxatives

Sodium sulfate and castor oil used as laxatives can cause a modest but probably clinically unimportant reduction in sulfafurazole absorption.

Clinical evidence, mechanism, importance and management

In an experimental study of the possible effects of laxatives on the absorption of sulfafurazole, healthy subjects were given 10 to 20 g of oral **sodium sulfate** or 20 g of **castor oil** (doses sufficient to provoke diarrhoea). Absorption, measured by the amount of sulfafurazole excreted in the urine, was decreased by 50% with **castor oil**, and by 33% with **sodium sulfate** at 4 hours. However, serum levels of the drugs were relatively unchanged. The overall picture was that while these laxatives can alter the pattern of absorption, they do not seriously impair the total amount of drug absorbed.[1]

1. Mattila MJ, Takki S, Jussila J. Effect of sodium sulphate and castor oil on drug absorption from the human intestine. *Ann Clin Res* (1974) 6, 19–24.

Tetracyclines + Antacids

The serum levels and therefore the therapeutic effectiveness of the tetracyclines can be markedly reduced or even abolished by antacids containing aluminium, bismuth, calcium or magnesium. Other antacids, such as sodium bicarbonate, may also reduce the bioavailability of some tetracyclines. Even intravenous doxycycline levels can be reduced by antacids.

Clinical evidence

(a) Aluminium-containing antacids

A study in 5 patients and 6 healthy subjects found that within 48 hours of starting to take about 10 mL of aluminium hydroxide gel (*Amphogel*) every 6 hours with **chlortetracycline** 500 mg the serum levels of the antibacterial were reduced by 80 to 90%. One patient had a recurrence of her urinary tract infection, which only subsided when the antacid was withdrawn, and one patient maintained **chlortetracycline** levels despite antacid treatment.[1] Similar results were obtained in other studies.[2,3]

Further studies have shown similar interactions with other tetracyclines:

- 30 mL of aluminium hydroxide reduced **oxytetracycline** serum levels by more than 50%,[3]
- 20 mL of aluminium hydroxide caused a 75% reduction in **demeclocycline** serum levels,[4]
- 15 mL of aluminium hydroxide caused a 100% reduction in serum **doxycycline** levels,[5,6]
- 30 mL of aluminium/**magnesium** hydroxide (*Maalox*) caused a 90% reduction in **tetracycline** serum levels.[7]

Intravenous doxycycline also appears to be affected. The mean serum levels of an intravenous dose of **doxycycline** were found to be reduced by

36% when 30 mL of aluminium hydroxide was taken four times daily, for 2 days before and after the antibacterial.[8]

(b) Bismuth-containing antacids

Bismuth subsalicylate reduces the absorption of **tetracycline** by 34%[9] and reduces the maximum serum levels of **doxycycline** by 50%.[10] It has been suggested the excipient *Veegum* (**magnesium** aluminium silicate) in some bismuth subsalicylate formulations enhances this effect.[11] Bismuth carbonate similarly interacts with the tetracyclines *in vitro*.[12]

(c) Calcium-containing antacids

There seem to be no direct clinical studies with calcium-containing antacids, but a clinically important interaction seems almost a certainty, based on *in vitro* studies with calcium carbonate,[12] calcium in milk, (see 'Tetracyclines + Food or Drinks', p.347), dicalcium phosphate,[13] and calcium as an excipient in tetracycline capsules.[14]

(d) Magnesium-containing antacids

Magnesium sulfate certainly interacts with **tetracycline**, but in the only clinical study available[15] the amount of magnesium was much higher than would normally be found in the usual dose of antacid.

(e) Sodium-containing antacids

Sodium bicarbonate 2 g reduced the absorption of a 250-mg capsule of **tetracycline** by 50% in 8 subjects. If however **tetracycline** was dissolved before administration, the absorption was unaffected by the sodium bicarbonate.[16] Another study stated that sodium bicarbonate 2 g had an insignificant effect on **tetracycline** absorption.[7]

Mechanism

The tetracyclines bind with aluminium, bismuth, calcium, magnesium and other metallic ions to form compounds (chelates), which are much less soluble and therefore much less readily absorbed by the gut.[17] Because doxycycline undergoes enterohepatic recirculation, even intravenous doxycycline is affected, although less so than oral. It has also been suggested that the antacids reduce gastric acidity and thereby decrease the absorption of tetracyclines,[16] but studies demonstrating the lack of a significant interaction with 'H_2-receptor antagonists', (p.348) suggest that this is not the case. The reduced absorption with bismuth compounds may be because they adsorb tetracyclines.[9] The interaction of some tetracycline preparations with sodium bicarbonate is unexplained.

Importance and management

Extremely well-documented, and well-established interactions. Their clinical importance depends on how much the serum tetracycline levels are lowered, but with normal antacid dosages the reductions cited above (50 to 100%) are large enough to mean that many organisms will not be exposed to minimum inhibitory concentrations (MIC) of antibacterial. As a general rule none of the aluminium, bismuth, calcium or magnesium-containing antacids should be given at the same time as the tetracycline antibacterials. If they must be used, separate the dosages by 2 to 3 hours or more to prevent their admixture in the gut. This also applies to **quinapril** formulations containing substantial quantities of magnesium (such as *Accupro*), although the interaction is less pronounced (see 'Tetracyclines + Quinapril', p.349), and is also predicted to occur with **didanosine** tablets formulated with antacids,[18] but not with the enteric-coated capsule formulation (which contains no antacids).[19]

Patients should be warned about taking any antacids and indigestion preparations. Instead of using antacids to minimise the gastric irritant effects of the tetracyclines it is usually recommended that tetracyclines are taken after food, however it is not entirely clear how much this affects their absorption (see 'Tetracyclines + Food or Drinks', p.347). H_2-receptor antagonists may be suitable non-interacting alternatives to antacids in some situations, see 'Tetracyclines + H_2-receptor antagonists', p.348.

1. Waisbren BA, Hueckel JS. Reduced absorption of aureomycin caused by aluminum hydroxide gel (*Amphojel*). *Proc Soc Exp Biol Med* (1950) 73, 73–4.
2. Seed JC, Wilson CE. The effect of aluminum hydroxide on serum aureomycin concentrations after simultaneous oral administration. *Bull Johns Hopkins Hosp* (1950) 86, 415–8.
3. Michel JC, Sayer RJ, Kirby WMM. Effect of food and antacids on blood levels of aureomycin and terramycin. *J Lab Clin Med* (1950) 36, 632–4.
4. Scheiner J, Altemeier WA. Experimental study of factors inhibiting absorption and effective therapeutic levels of declomycin. *Surg Gynecol Obstet* (1962) 114, 9–14.
5. Rosenblatt JE, Barrett JE, Brodie JL, Kirby WMM. Comparison of in vitro activity and clinical pharmacology of doxycycline with other tetracyclines. *Antimicrob Agents Chemother* (1966) 6, 134–41.
6. Deppermann K-M, Lode H, Höffken G, Tschink G, Kalz C, Koeppe P. Influence of ranitidine, pirenzepine, and aluminum magnesium hydroxide on the bioavailability of various antibiotics, including amoxicillin, cephalexin, doxycycline, and amoxicillin-clavulanic acid. *Antimicrob Agents Chemother* (1989) 33, 1901–7.
7. Garty M, Hurwitz A. Effect of cimetidine and antacids on gastrointestinal absorption of tetracycline. *Clin Pharmacol Ther* (1980) 28, 203–7.
8. Nguyen VX, Nix DE, Gillikin S, Schentag JJ. Effect of oral antacid administration on the pharmacokinetics of intravenous doxycycline. *Antimicrob Agents Chemother* (1989) 33, 434–6.
9. Albert KS, Welch RD, De Sante KA, Disanto AR. Decreased tetracycline bioavailability caused by a bismuth subsalicylate antidiarrheal mixture. *J Pharm Sci* (1979) 68, 586–8.
10. Ericsson CD, Feldman S, Pickering LK, Cleary TG. Influence of subsalicylate bismuth on absorption of doxycycline. *JAMA* (1982) 247, 2266–7.
11. Healy DP, Dansereau RJ, Dunn AB, Clendening CE, Mounts AW, Deepe GS. Reduced tetracycline bioavailability caused by magnesium aluminum silicate in liquid formulations of bismuth subsalicylate. *Ann Pharmacother* (1997) 31, 1460–4.
12. Christensen EKJ, Kerckhoffs HPM, Huizinga T. De invloed van antacida op de afgifte in vitro van tetracycline hydrochloride. *Pharm Weekbl* (1967) 102, 463–73.
13. Boger WP, Gavin JJ. An evaluation of tetracycline preparations. *N Engl J Med* (1959) 261, 827–32.
14. Sweeney WM, Hardy SM, Dornbush AC, Ruegsegger JM. Absorption of tetracycline in human beings as affected by certain excipients. *Antibiotic Med Clin Ther* (1957) 4, 642–56.
15. Harcourt RS, Hamburger M. The effect of magnesium sulfate in lowering tetracycline blood levels. *J Lab Clin Med* (1957) 50, 464–8.
16. Barr WH, Adir J, Garrettson L. Decrease of tetracycline absorption in man by sodium bicarbonate. *Clin Pharmacol Ther* (1971) 12, 779–84.
17. Albert A, Rees CW. Avidity of the tetracyclines for the cations of metals. *Nature* (1956) 177, 433–4.
18. Videx Tablets (Didanosine). Bristol-Myers Squibb Pharmaceuticals Ltd. UK Summary of product characteristics, December 2006.
19. Videx EC (Didanosine). Bristol-Myers Squibb Pharmaceuticals Ltd. UK Summary of product characteristics, December 2006.

Tetracyclines + Antiepileptics

The serum levels of doxycycline are reduced and may fall below the accepted minimum inhibitory concentration in patients receiving long-term treatment with barbiturates, phenytoin or carbamazepine. Other tetracyclines do not appear to be affected.

Clinical evidence

A study in 14 patients taking **phenytoin** 200 to 500 mg daily, **carbamazepine** 300 mg to 1 g daily, or both, found that the half-life of **doxycycline** was approximately halved from 15.1 hours in patients not taking antiepileptics, to 7.2 hours in patients taking **phenytoin**, 8.4 hours in patients taking **carbamazepine**, and 7.4 hours in patients taking both drugs.[1]

Similar results were found in 16 other patients taking various combinations of **phenytoin**, **carbamazepine**, **primidone** or **phenobarbital**. The serum **doxycycline** levels of almost all of them fell below 0.5 micrograms/mL during the 12 to 24 hour period following their last dose of **doxycycline** 100 mg. **Tetracycline**, **methacycline**, **oxytetracycline**, **demeclocycline** and **chlortetracycline** levels were not significantly affected by these antiepileptics.[2] Other studies confirm this interaction between some **barbiturates (amobarbital**, **pentobarbital**, **phenobarbital)** and **doxycycline**.[3,4]

Mechanism

Uncertain. These antiepileptics and barbiturates are known enzyme inducers and it seems probable that they increase the metabolism of the doxycycline by the liver, thereby increasing its clearance from the body.

Importance and management

The interactions between doxycycline and the enzyme-inducing antiepileptics are established, but the clinical significance of the reduction in levels does not seem to have been studied. Serum doxycycline levels below 0.5 micrograms/mL are less than the minimum inhibitory concentration (MIC) quoted by the authors, so that it seems likely that the antibacterial will be less effective. To accommodate this potential problem it has been suggested that the doxycycline dosage could be doubled.[2] Alternatively any of the tetracyclines that are reported not to be affected by these antiepileptics (tetracycline, methacycline, oxytetracycline, demeclocycline and chlortetracycline) may provide a suitable alternative.[2]

1. Penttilä O, Neuvonen PJ, Aho K, Lehtovaara R. Interaction between doxycycline and some antiepileptic drugs. *BMJ* (1974) 2, 470–2.
2. Neuvonen PJ, Penttilä O, Lehtovaara R, Aho K. Effect of antiepileptic drugs on the elimination of various tetracycline derivatives. *Eur J Clin Pharmacol* (1975) 9, 147–54.
3. Neuvonen PJ, Penttilä O. Interaction between doxycycline and barbiturates. *BMJ* (1974) 1, 535–6.
4. Alestig K. Studies on the intestinal excretion of doxycycline. *Scand J Infect Dis* (1974) 6, 265–71.

Tetracyclines + Colestipol

Colestipol can reduce the absorption of tetracycline by about a half. Information about other tetracyclines is lacking but it seems likely that they will interact similarly.

Clinical evidence

Colestipol 30 g taken either in 180 mL of water or orange juice reduced the absorption of a single 500-mg dose of oral **tetracycline** in 9 healthy subjects by 54 to 56%, as measured by recovery in the urine.[1]

Mechanism

Colestipol binds to bile acids in the gut and can also bind with some drugs, thereby reducing their availability for absorption. An *in vitro* study found a 30% binding with tetracycline.[2] The presence of citrate ions in the orange juice, which can also bind to colestipol, appears not to have a marked effect on the binding of the tetracycline.

Importance and management

An established interaction. Direct information seems to be limited to the report cited, but it is consistent with the way colestipol interacts with other drugs. In practice up to 30 g of colestipol is given daily in single or two divided doses, and tetracycline 250 to 500-mg is given every 6 hours. As other drugs need to be given 1 hour before or 4 hours after colestipol it may be difficult to avoid some mixing in the gut. It seems very probable that a clinically important interaction will occur, but by how much the efficacy of tetracycline is affected seems not to have been determined. Tell patients to separate the dosages as much as possible. Monitor the outcome well. Information about other tetracyclines is lacking but it also seems likely that they will interact similarly, but those that can be given less often may prove easier to administer, although note that doxycycline undergoes enterohepatic recirculation and therefore separating dosages may not be completely effective..

1. Friedman H, Greenblatt DJ, LeDuc BW. Impaired absorption of tetracycline by colestipol is not reversed by orange juice. *J Clin Pharmacol* (1989) 29, 748–51.
2. Ko H, Royer ME. *In vitro* binding of drugs to colestipol hydrochloride. *J Pharm Sci* (1974) 63, 1914–20.

Tetracyclines + Diuretics

It has been recommended by some that the concurrent use of tetracyclines and diuretics should be avoided because of their association with rises in blood urea nitrogen levels.

Clinical evidence, mechanism, importance and management

A retrospective study of patient records as part of the Boston Collaborative Drug Surveillance Program showed that an association existed between tetracycline use with diuretics (not named) and rises in blood urea nitrogen (BUN) levels.[1] Both diuretics and tetracyclines are known to cause rises in BUN levels.[2] It was suggested that tetracyclines should be avoided in patients taking diuretics when alternative antibacterials could be substituted.[1] However, the results of this study have been much criticised as the authors could not exclude physician bias,[1,2] they did not define what was meant by 'clinically significant rise in BUN',[2] they did not state whether or not this rise affected patient outcomes,[2] they did not measure creatinine levels[3] and they did not specify which diuretics were involved.[2] The patients most affected also had the highest levels of BUN before starting tetracyclines. Tetracyclines alone are known to cause rises in BUN, especially where a degree of renal impairment exists, although it has been suggested that **doxycycline** is less prone to this effect.[4] It would seem that tetracyclines and diuretics may be used together safely, although it would be wise to give thought to the patient's renal function.

1. Boston Collaborative Drug Surveillance Program. Tetracycline and drug-attributed rises in blood urea nitrogen. *JAMA* (1972) 220, 377–9.
2. Tannenberg AM. Tetracyclines and rises in urea nitrogen. *JAMA* (1972) 221, 713.
3. Dijkhuis HJPM, van Meurs AJ. Tetracycline and BUN level. *JAMA* (1973) 223, 441.
4. Alexander MR. Tetracyclines and rises in urea nitrogen. *JAMA* (1972) 221, 713–14.

Tetracyclines + Food or Drinks

The calcium in food can complex with tetracycline to reduce its absorption. This is particularly notable with dairy products, which can reduce the absorption of the tetracyclines by up to 80%, thereby reducing or even abolishing their therapeutic effects. Doxycycline and minocycline are less affected by dairy products (25 to 30% reduction). Orange juice and coffee do not interact with tetracycline.

Clinical evidence, mechanism, importance and management

(a) Dairy products

1. Demeclocycline. The serum levels of a 300-mg dose of demeclocycline were 70 to 80% lower in 4 subjects given dairy products, when compared with those who took it with a meal containing no dairy products. The dairy products used were either 8 oz (about 250 mL) of **fresh pasteurized milk**, 8 oz of **buttermilk** or 4 oz of **cottage cheese**.[1]

2. Doxycycline. The plasma doxycycline levels were reduced by 20%, from 1.79 to 1.45 micrograms/mL, 2 hours after a single 100-mg oral dose was taken with 240 mL of **milk**.[2] Another study in 9 healthy subjects found a 30% reduction in the absorption, and a 24% reduction in the peak serum levels of doxycycline 200 mg when it was taken with 300 mL of **fresh milk**.[3] However, two other studies suggest that the absorption of 200 mg of doxycycline is unaffected by milk,[4,5] although in one the half-life was almost halved and the clearance increased.[5]

3. Methacycline. In one study 300 mL of **milk** reduced the absorption of methacycline 300 mg by about 63%.[4]

4. Minocycline. About 180 mL (6 oz) of **homogenised milk** reduced the absorption of minocycline 100 mg by 27% in one study.[6]

5. Oxytetracycline. In one study 300 mL of **milk** reduced the absorption of oxytetracycline 500 mg by about 64%.[4]

6. Tetracycline. About 180 mL (6 oz) of **homogenised milk** reduced the absorption of tetracycline hydrochloride 250 mg by 65% in one study.[6] In another study the absorption of tetracycline 500 mg was reduced by about 50% by 300 mL of **milk**.[4]

(b) Other calcium-containing foods or drinks

A study in 9 healthy subjects found that 200 mL of **orange juice** or **coffee** (milk content, if any, unstated) did not significantly affect the bioavailability of a single 250-mg dose of **tetracycline**. This is despite the fact that **orange juice** contains 35 to 70 mg calcium per 100 mL.[7]

Tetracycline 250 mg was given to 9 healthy subjects with 200 mL of water on an empty stomach. The **tetracycline** bioavailability was compared with its administration after a **standard meal** (two slices of bread, ham, tomato, and water, containing 145 mg calcium) and a **Mexican meal** (two tortillas, beans, two eggs, tomato and water, containing 235 mg calcium). The cumulative amounts of **tetracycline** excreted in the urine at 72 hours were about 151 mg (fasting), 90 mg (**standard meal**) and 68 mg (**Mexican meal**).[8] The absorption of a 300-mg dose of **demeclocycline** was not affected when it was given with a meal not containing dairy products,[1] and **doxycycline** seems to be minimally affected by food not containing dairy products.[2]

Mechanism

The tetracyclines have a strong affinity for the calcium ions that are found in abundance in dairy products and some foodstuffs. The tetracycline/calcium chelates formed are much less readily absorbed from the gastrointestinal tract and as a result the serum tetracycline levels achieved are much lower. Some tetracyclines have a lesser tendency to form chelates, which explains why their serum levels are reduced to a smaller extent.[9]

Orange juice appears not to interact, despite its calcium content, because at the relevant pH values in the gut, the calcium is bound to components within the orange juice (citric, tartaric and ascorbic acids) and is not free to combine with the tetracycline.[7]

Importance and management

Well documented and very well established interactions of clinical importance. Reductions in serum tetracycline levels of 50 to 80% caused by calcium-rich foods are sufficiently large to reduce or even abolish their antibacterial effects. For this reason tetracyclines should not be taken with milk or dairy products such as yoghurt or cheese. Separate the ingestion of these foods and tetracycline as much as possible. In the case of iron, which interacts by the same mechanism, 2 to 3 hours is enough. Doxycycline[3,10] and minocycline[6] are not affected as much by dairy products (reductions of about 25 to 30%) and in this respect have some advantages over other tetracyclines.

It is usual to recommend that tetracyclines are taken 1 hour before or 2 hours after food (which would be expected to contain at least some calcium), to minimise admixture in the gut and thereby reduce the effects of the interaction. The separation is something of a compromise, because food can help to minimise the gastric irritant effects of the tetracyclines.

1. Scheiner J, Altemeier WA. Experimental study of factors inhibiting absorption and effective therapeutic levels of declomycin. *Surg Gynecol Obstet* (1962) 114, 9–14.
2. Rosenblatt JE, Barrett JE, Brodie JL, Kirby WMM. Comparison of in vitro activity and clinical pharmacology of doxycycline with other tetracyclines. *Antimicrob Agents Chemother* (1966) 6, 134–41.
3. Meyer FP, Specht H, Quednow B, Walther H. Influence of milk on bioavailability of doxycycline — new aspects. *Infection* (1989) 17, 245–6.
4. Mattila MJ, Neuvonen PJ, Gothoni G, Hackman CR. Interference of iron preparations and milk with the absorption of tetracyclines. *Int Congr Ser* (1972) 254, 128–33.
5. Saux M-C, Mosser J, Pontagnier H, Leng B. Pharmacokinetic study of doxycycline polyphosphate after simultaneous ingestion of milk. *Eur J Drug Metab Pharmacokinet* (1983) 8, 43–9.
6. Leyden JJ. Absorption of minocycline hydrochloride and tetracycline hydrochloride. Effect of food, milk, and iron. *J Am Acad Dermatol* (1985) 12, 308–12.
7. Jung H, Rivera O, Reguero MT, Rodríguez JM, Moreno-Esparza R. Influence of liquids (coffee and orange juice) on the bioavailability of tetracycline. *Biopharm Drug Dispos* (1990) 11, 729–34.
8. Cook HJ, Mundo CR, Fonseca L, Gasque L, Moreno-Esparza R. Influence of the diet on bioavailability of tetracycline. *Biopharm Drug Dispos* (1993) 14, 549–53.
9. Albert A, Rees CW. Avidity of the tetracyclines for the cations of metals. *Nature* (1956) 177, 433–4.
10. Siewert M, Blume H, Stenzhorn G, Kieferndorf U, Lenhard G. Zur Qualitätsbeurteilung von doxycyclinhaltigen ertigarzneimitteln. 3. Mitteilung: Vergleichende Bioverfügbarkeitsstudie unter Berücksichtigung einer Einnahme mit Milch. *Pharm Ztg* (1990) 3, 96–102.

Tetracyclines + H_2-receptor antagonists

Cimetidine reduces the absorption of tetracycline but does not appear to affect its serum levels. Ranitidine seems not to affect the bioavailability of doxycycline. Information about other tetracyclines and H_2-receptor antagonists is lacking, but there would seem to be no reason to suspect that they will interact.

Clinical evidence, mechanism, importance and management

A study in 5 subjects found that **cimetidine** 200 mg three times daily and 400 mg at bedtime for 3 days reduced the absorption of a single 500-mg dose of a **tetracycline** capsule by about 30%, but had no effect when the **tetracycline** was given as a solution.[1] However, when **tetracycline** as either a tablet or a suspension was given to 6 subjects with **cimetidine** 1.6 g daily for 6 days, no changes in the plasma levels of **tetracycline** were seen.[2] Similar results were found in another study.[3]

In 10 healthy subjects, the bioavailability of **doxycycline** 200 mg was not altered by three 150-mg doses of **ranitidine**.[4]

No special precautions would seem necessary with either combination. Information about other tetracyclines seems to be lacking, but there would seem to be no reason to suspect that they will interact.

1. Cole JJ, Charles BG, Ravenscroft PJ. Interaction of cimetidine with tetracycline absorption. *Lancet* (1980) ii, 536.
2. Fisher P, House F, Inns P, Morrison PJ, Rogers HJ, Bradbrook ID. Effect of cimetidine on the absorption of orally administered tetracycline. *Br J Clin Pharmacol* (1980) 9, 153–8.
3. Garty M, Hurwitz A. Effect of cimetidine and antacids on gastrointestinal absorption of tetracycline. *Clin Pharmacol Ther* (1980) 28, 203–7.
4. Deppermann K-M, Lode H, Höffken G, Tschink G, Kalz C, Koeppe P. Influence of ranitidine, pirenzepine, and aluminum magnesium hydroxide on the bioavailability of various antibiotics, including amoxicillin, cephalexin, doxycycline, and amoxicillin-clavulanic acid. *Antimicrob Agents Chemother* (1989) 33, 1901–7.

Tetracyclines + Iron compounds

The absorption of both the tetracyclines and iron compounds is markedly reduced by concurrent use, leading to reduced serum levels of the tetracyclines. Their therapeutic effectiveness may be reduced or even abolished.

Clinical evidence

(a) Effect on tetracyclines

An investigation in 10 healthy subjects given single oral doses of tetracyclines showed that **ferrous sulfate** 200 mg decreased the serum antibacterial levels as follows: **doxycycline** 200 mg, 80 to 90%; **methacycline** 300 mg, 80 to 85%; **oxytetracycline** 500 mg, 50 to 60% and **tetracycline** 500 mg, 40 to 50%.[1] Another study in 2 groups of 8 healthy subjects found that **ferrous sulfate** 300 mg reduced the absorption of **tetracycline** and **minocycline** by 81% and 77%, respectively.[2]

Other studies found that in some instances iron caused the tetracycline serum levels to fall below minimum bacterial inhibitory concentrations.[3,4] If the iron was given 3 hours before or 2 hours after most tetracyclines the serum levels were not significantly reduced.[3-5] However, even when the iron was given up to 11 hours after **doxycycline**, serum concentrations were still lowered by 20 to 45%.[5] In contrast to this, another study found that four doses of **ferrous sulfate** (each equivalent to 80 mg of elemental iron) starting 11.5 hours after doxycycline did not affect the absorption of a 200-mg dose of **doxycycline**, and only reduced the AUC of a 100-mg dose of **doxycycline** by 17%.[6]

(b) Effect on iron

When **ferrous sulfate** 250 mg (equivalent to 50 mg of elemental iron) was given with **tetracycline** 500 mg, the absorption of iron was reduced by up to 78% in healthy subjects, and up to 65% in those with depleted iron stores.[7,8]

Mechanism

The tetracyclines have a strong affinity for iron and form poorly soluble tetracycline-iron chelates, which are much less readily absorbed by the gut, and as a result the serum tetracycline levels achieved are much lower.[9,10] There is also less free iron available for absorption. Separating the administration of the two prevents their admixture.[3,4] However, doxycycline undergoes enterohepatic recycling, which could affect any attempt to keep the iron and antibacterial apart, although the significance of the enterohepatic recycling has been said to be minimal.[6] Even when given intravenously the half-life of doxycycline is reduced.[5] The different extent to which iron compounds interact with the tetracyclines appears to be a reflection of their ability to liberate ferrous and ferric ions, which are free to combine with the tetracycline.[11]

Importance and management

The interactions between the tetracyclines and iron compounds are well-documented, well-established, and of clinical importance. The 30 to 90% reductions in serum tetracycline levels that are caused by iron are so large that tetracycline levels may fall below the MIC.[4] However, the extent of the reductions depends on a number of factors.

- *the particular tetracycline used:* tetracycline and oxytetracycline in the study cited above were the least affected.[1]
- *the time-interval between the administration of the two drugs:* giving the iron 3 hours before or 2 to 3 hours after the antibacterial is satisfactory with tetracycline itself,[3] but one study found that even 11 hours was inadequate for doxycycline.
- *the particular iron preparation used:* with tetracycline the reduction in serum levels with ferrous sulfate was 80 to 90%, with **ferrous fumarate, succinate** and **gluconate**, 70 to 80%; with **ferrous tartrate**, 50%; and with **ferrous sodium edetate**, 30%. This was with doses containing equivalent amounts of elemental iron.[11]

The interaction can therefore be accommodated by separating the dosages as much as possible. It would also seem logical to choose one of the iron preparations causing minimal interference, but it seems unlikely that there will be a clinically significant difference between those that are commonly available (i.e. sulfate, fumarate and gluconate).

Only tetracycline, oxytetracycline, methacycline, minocycline and doxycycline have been shown to interact with iron, but it seems reasonable to expect that the other tetracyclines will behave in a similar way.

1. Neuvonen PJ, Gothoni G, Hackman R, Björksten K. Interference of iron with the absorption of tetracyclines in man. *BMJ* (1970) 4, 532–4.
2. Leyden JJ. Absorption of minocycline hydrochloride and tetracycline hydrochloride. Effect of food, milk, and iron. *J Am Acad Dermatol* (1985) 12, 308–12.
3. Mattila MJ, Neuvonen PJ, Gothoni G, Hackman CR. Interference of iron preparations and milk with the absorption of tetracyclines. *Int Congr Ser* (1972) 254, 128–33.
4. Gothoni G, Neuvonen PJ, Mattila M, Hackman R. Iron-tetracycline interaction: effect of time interval between the drugs. *Acta Med Scand* (1972) 191, 409–11.

5. Neuvonen PJ, Penttilä O. Effect of oral ferrous sulphate on the half-life of doxycycline in man. *Eur J Clin Pharmacol* (1974) 7, 361–3.
6. Venho VMK, Salonen RO, Mattila MJ. Modification of the pharmacokinetics of doxycycline in man by ferrous sulphate or charcoal. *Eur J Clin Pharmacol* (1978) 14, 277–80.
7. Heinrich HC, Oppitz KH, Gabbe EE. Hemmung der Eisenabsorption beim Menschen durch Tetracyclin. *Klin Wochenschr* (1974) 52, 493–8.
8. Heinrich HC, Oppitz KH. Tetracycline inhibits iron absorption in man. *Naturwissenschaften* (1973) 60, 524–5.
9. Albert A, Rees CW. Avidity of the tetracyclines for the cations of metals. *Nature* (1956) 177, 433–4.
10. Albert A, Rees C. Incompatibility of aluminium hydroxide and certain antibiotics. *BMJ* (1955) 2, 1027–8.
11. Neuvonen PJ, Turakka H. Inhibitory effect of various iron salts on the absorption of tetracycline in man. *Eur J Clin Pharmacol* (1974) 7, 357–60.

Tetracyclines + Kaolin-pectin

Kaolin-pectin reduces the absorption of tetracycline by about 50%.

Clinical evidence, mechanism, importance and management

Healthy subjects were given **tetracycline** 250 mg as a solution or as a capsule, with and without 30 mL of kaolin-pectin (*Kaopectate*). The absorption of both formulations was reduced by about 50% by the kaolin-pectin. Even when the kaolin-pectin was given 2 hours before or after the **tetracycline**, the drug absorption was still reduced by about 20%.[1] The likely reason for this interaction is that **tetracycline** becomes adsorbed onto the kaolin-pectin so that less is available for absorption.

If these two drugs are given together, consider separating the dosages by at least 2 hours to minimise admixture in the gut. It may even then be necessary to increase the **tetracycline** dosage. Information about other tetracyclines is lacking, but be aware that they may interact similarly.

1. Gouda MW. Effect of an antidiarrhoeal mixture on the bioavailability of tetracycline. *Int J Pharmaceutics* (1993) 89, 75–7.

Tetracyclines + Metoclopramide

Metoclopramide 20 mg was found to double the rate of absorption and slightly reduce the maximum serum levels of a single 500-mg dose of tetracycline in 4 patients.[1] This appears to be of little clinical importance.

1. Nimmo J. The influence of metoclopramide on drug absorption. *Postgrad Med J* (1973) 49 (July Suppl), 25–8.

Tetracyclines + Quinapril

The absorption of oral tetracycline is reduced by the magnesium carbonate excipient in some quinapril formulations.

Clinical evidence

Quinapril, formulated as *Accupro* also contains **magnesium carbonate** (250 mg in a 40 mg quinapril capsule, 47 mg in a 5 mg capsule). A pharmacokinetic study in 12 healthy subjects investigating the potential interaction between the **magnesium carbonate** in these capsules and **tetracycline** found that single doses of both of these formulations of quinapril markedly reduced the **tetracycline** absorption. The 5 mg and 40 mg quinapril capsules reduced the **tetracycline** AUC by 28% and 37%, respectively, and the maximum serum levels were reduced by 25% and 34%, respectively.[1]

Mechanism

The reason for these reductions in tetracycline levels is that the magnesium carbonate and the tetracycline form a less soluble chelate in the gut which is less well absorbed (see 'Tetracyclines + Antacids', p.345).

Importance and management

An established interaction but the extent of the reduction is only moderate and its clinical importance is uncertain. However, the authors of the study recommend that the concurrent use of this formulation of quinapril and tetracycline should be avoided.[1] This is repeated by the manufacturers.[2] Other tetracyclines would be expected to behave similarly. One possible way to accommodate this interaction (as with the antacid interaction) is to separate the dosages as much as possible (by about 2 to 3 hours) to minimise admixture in the gut.

1. Parke Davis Ltd. Effect of magnesium-containing quinapril tablets on the single-dose pharmacokinetics of tetracycline in healthy volunteers, protocol 906–237. Data on file, Report RR 764–00872.
2. Accupro (Quinapril hydrochloride). Pfizer Ltd. UK Summary of product characteristics, March 2007.

Tetracyclines + Sucralfate

On theoretical grounds the absorption of tetracycline may possibly be reduced by sucralfate, but clinical confirmation of this appears to be lacking.

Clinical evidence, mechanism, importance and management

The manufacturers of sucralfate, point out that it may reduce the bioavailability of **tetracycline**, probably because the two become bound together in the gut, thereby reducing absorption. It is suggested that they should be given 2 hours apart to minimise their admixture in the gut.[1] There do not appear to be any clinical reports in the literature confirming this potential interaction so it has yet to be shown to be clinically relevant.

However, the *in vitro* formation of a **tetracycline**-sucralfate acid complex has been investigated in *animal* studies and indicates that the interaction may be clinically useful for *Helicobacter pylori* eradication because of direct delivery of **tetracycline** to the gastric mucosa for extended periods of time.[2-4]

1. Antepsin (Sucralfate). Chugai Pharma UK Ltd. UK Summary of product characteristics, November 2006.
2. Higo S, Ori K, Takeuchi H, Yamamoto H, Hino T, Kawashima Y. A novel evaluation method of gastric mucoadhesive property *in vitro* and the mucoadhesive mechanism of tetracycline-sucralfate acidic complex for eradication of *Helicobacter pylori*. *Pharm Res* (2004) 21, 413–9.
3. Higo S, Takeuchi H, Yamamoto H, Hino T, Kawashima Y. The acidic complexation of tetracycline with sucralfate for its mucoadhesive preparation. *Drug Dev Ind Pharm* (2004) 30, 715–24.
4. Yokel RA, Dickey KM, Goldberg AH. Selective adherence of a sucralfate-tetracycline complex to gastric ulcers: implications for the treatment of *Helicobacter pylori*. *Biopharm Drug Dispos* (1995) 16, 475–9.

Tetracyclines + Thiomersal

Patients being treated with tetracyclines who use contact lens solutions containing thiomersal may experience an inflammatory ocular reaction.

Clinical evidence, mechanism, importance and management

The observation that 2 patients had ocular reactions (red eye, irritation, blepharitis) when they used a 0.004% thiomersal-containing contact lens solution while taking a tetracycline, prompted further study of this interaction. A questionnaire revealed another 9 similar cases that suddenly began shortly after patients who had used thiomersal containing solutions for 6 months without problem started to take a tetracycline. In each case the reaction cleared when the thiomersal or the tetracycline was stopped. The same reaction was also clearly demonstrated in *rabbits*.[1] The reasons are not understood. It would seem prudent to avoid the concurrent use of these compounds.

1. Crook TG, Freeman JJ. Reactions induced by the concurrent use of thimerosal and tetracycline. *Am J Optom Physiol Opt* (1983) 60, 759–61.

Tetracyclines + Zinc compounds

The absorption of tetracycline can be reduced by as much as 50% by zinc sulphate. Separating their administration as much as possible minimises the effects of this interaction. Doxycycline interacts minimally with zinc.

Clinical evidence

When **tetracycline** 500 mg was given to 7 subjects either alone or with zinc sulfate 200 mg (equivalent to 45 mg of elemental zinc) the **tetracycline** serum concentrations and AUC were reduced by about 30 to 40%.[1]

This study was repeated with **doxycycline** 200 mg and zinc, but **doxycycline** absorption was not affected.[1] A reduction in **tetracycline** absorption of more than 50% has been seen in other studies when zinc was given concurrently.[2,3]

Tetracycline appears to cause minimal reductions in zinc concentrations.[2]

Mechanism

Zinc (like iron, calcium, magnesium and aluminium) forms a relatively stable and poorly absorbed chelate with tetracycline in the gut, which results in a reduction in the amount of antibacterial available for absorption.[4,5]

Importance and management

An established and moderately well documented interaction of clinical importance. Separate the administration of tetracycline and zinc compounds as much as possible to minimise admixture in the gut. In the case of 'iron', (p.348), which interacts by the same mechanism, 2 to 3 hours is usually enough. Alternatively it would seem that doxycycline is less affected, so it may be a useful alternative.[1] Other tetracyclines would be expected to interact like tetracycline itself, but this needs confirmation. The small reduction in serum zinc concentrations is likely to be of little practical importance.[2]

1. Penttilä O, Hurme H, Neuvonen PJ. Effect of zinc sulphate on the absorption of tetracycline and doxycycline in man. *Eur J Clin Pharmacol* (1975) 9, 131–4.
2. Andersson K-E, Bratt L, Dencker H, Kamme C, Lanner E. Inhibition of tetracycline absorption by zinc. *Eur J Clin Pharmacol* (1976) 10, 59–62.
3. Mapp RK, McCarthy TJ. The effect of zinc sulphate and of bicitropeptide on tetracycline absorption. *S Afr Med J* (1976) 50, 1829–30.
4. Albert A, Rees CW. Avidity of the tetracyclines for the cations of metals. *Nature* (1956) 177, 433–4.
5. Doluisio JT, Martin AN. Metal complexation of the tetracycline hydrochlorides. *J Med Chem* (1963) 16, 16.

Tetracyclines; Doxycycline + Dimeticone

A study in 8 healthy subjects found that dimeticone 2.25 g did not alter the bioavailability of a single 200-mg dose of doxycycline.[1]

1. Bistue C, Perez P, Becquart D, Vinçon G, Albin H. Effet du diméticone sur la biodisponibilité de la doxycycline. *Therapie* (1987) 42, 13–16.

Tetracyclines; Doxycycline + Rifampicin (Rifampin)

Rifampicin may cause a marked reduction in doxycycline levels, which has led to treatment failures in some cases.

Clinical evidence

Rifampicin 10 mg/kg daily caused a considerable reduction in the serum levels of doxycycline 200 mg daily in 7 patients. The reduction was very marked in 4 patients but not significant in the other 3 patients. The AUC of doxycycline was reduced by 54%, its clearance was approximately doubled, and its half-life was reduced from about 14 hours to 9 hours.[1,2]

Five patients with brucellosis taking doxycycline 200 mg daily had a reduction in the doxycycline half-life from 14.52 to 7.99 hours when they took rifampicin 200 mg daily.[3] Another study of 20 patients treated for brucellosis found that the mean AUC of doxycycline was nearly 60% lower in the presence of rifampicin as opposed to streptomycin. There were no treatment failures in the patients taking doxycycline and streptomycin, but 2 treatment failures occurred in the 10 patients taking doxycycline and rifampicin.[4]

A meta-analysis of 6 studies involving 544 patients with brucellosis found a significantly higher numbers of relapses and lower numbers of initial cures if doxycycline was given with rifampicin rather than streptomycin.[5]

Mechanism

Not established, but it seems almost certain that the rifampicin (a known potent enzyme inducer) increases the metabolism of the doxycycline thereby reducing its levels.

Importance and management

The interaction between doxycycline and rifampicin is established and of clinical importance. Monitor the effects of concurrent use and increase the doxycycline dosage as necessary. No clinically important adverse interaction appears to occur between doxycycline and streptomycin.

1. Garraffo R, Dellamonica P, Fournier JP, Lapalus P, Bernard E, Beziau H, Chichmanian RM. Effet de la rifampicine sur la pharmacocinétique de la doxycycline. *Pathol Biol (Paris)* (1987) 35, 746–9.
2. Garraffo R, Dellamonica P, Fournier JP, Lapalus P, Bernard E. The effect of rifampicin on the pharmacokinetics of doxycycline. *Infection* (1988) 16, 297–8.
3. Bessard G, Stahl JP, Dubois F, Gaillat J, Micoud M. Modification de la pharmacocinetique de la doxycycline par l'administration de rifampicine chez l'homme. *Med Mal Infect* (1983) 13, 138–41.
4. Colmenero JD, Fernández-Gallardo LC, Agúndez JAG, Sedeño J, Benítez J, Valverde E. Possible implications of doxycycline-rifampin interaction for the treatment of brucellosis. *Antimicrob Agents Chemother* (1994) 38, 2798–2802.
5. Solera J, Martínez-Alfaro E, Sáez L. Metaanálisis sobre la eficacia de la combinación de rifampicina y doxiciclina en el tratamiento de la brucelosis humana. *Med Clin (Barc)* (1994) 102, 731–8.

Tetracyclines; Minocycline + Ethinylestradiol

There is some evidence that ethinylestradiol may accentuate the facial pigmentation that can be caused by minocycline.

Clinical evidence

Two teenage sisters with severe acne vulgaris, taking minocycline 50 mg four times daily for 14 days then 50 mg twice daily thereafter, developed dark-brown pigmentation in their acne scars when they took *Dianette* (cyproterone acetate and ethinylestradiol) for about 15 months.[1] The type of pigmentation was not identified because they both declined to have a biopsy, but in other cases it has been found to consist of haemosiderin, iron, melanin and a metabolic degradation product of minocycline.[1] Two other reports describe facial pigmentation in patients taking minocycline, two of whom were taking oral contraceptives containing ethinylestradiol.[2,3] Other young women who have developed minocycline pigmentation may also have been taking **oral contraceptives** because they fall into the right age-group, but this is not specifically stated in any of the reports.

Mechanism

Not understood. It seems possible that the facial pigmentation (melasma, chloasma) that can occur with oral contraceptives may have been additive with the effects of the minocycline.[1]

Importance and management

Evidence is very limited but it has been suggested that all patients given long-term minocycline treatment should be well screened for the development of pigmentation, particularly if they are taking other drugs such as the oral contraceptives that are known to induce hyperpigmentation.[1] Remember also that very rarely contraceptive failure has been associated with the use of minocycline and other tetracyclines, see 'Hormonal contraceptives + Antibacterials; Tetracyclines', p.983.

1. Eedy DJ, Burrows D. Minocycline-induced pigmentation occurring in two sisters. *Clin Exp Dermatol* (1991) 16, 55–7.
2. Ridgeway HA, Sonnex TS, Kennedy CTC, Millard PR, Henderson WJ, Gold SC. Hyperpigmentation associated with oral minocycline. *Br J Dermatol* (1982) 107, 95–102.
3. Prigent F, Cavelier-Balloy B, Tollenaere C, Civatte J. Pigmentation cutanée induite par la minocycline: deux cas. *Ann Dermatol Venereol* (1986) 113, 227–33.

Tetracyclines; Minocycline + Phenothiazines

An isolated report describes black galactorrhoea, which was attributed to an interaction between minocycline and perphenazine.

Clinical evidence, mechanism, importance and management

A woman taking minocycline 100 mg twice daily for 4 years to control pustulocystic acne, and also taking **perphenazine**, amitriptyline and diphenhydramine, developed irregular darkly pigmented macules in the areas of acne scarring and later began to produce droplets of darkly coloured milk. The milk was found to contain macrophages filled with positive iron-staining particles, assumed to be haemosiderin. The situation resolved when the drugs were withdrawn: the galactorrhoea within a week and the skin staining over 6 months.[1] Galactorrhoea is a known adverse effect of the phenothiazines and is due to an elevation of serum prolactin levels caused by the blockade of dopamine receptors in the hypothalamus. The dark colour appeared to be an adverse effect of the **minocycline**, which can cause haemosiderin to be deposited in cells, and in this instance to be scavenged by the macrophages that were then secreted in the milk. The general significance of this isolated case is unknown, but it seems likely to be small.

1. Basler RSW, Lynch PJ. Black galactorrhea as a consequence of minocycline and phenothiazine therapy. *Arch Dermatol* (1985) 121, 417–18.

Trimethoprim + Food or Guar gum

Guar gum and food can modestly reduce the absorption of trimethoprim suspension.

Clinical evidence, mechanism, importance and management

In a study over a 24-hour period, 12 healthy subjects were given a single 3-mg/kg oral dose of a trimethoprim suspension with food, with or without guar gum. The mean peak serum levels were reduced by food and by food given with 5 g of guar gum by 21% and 15%, respectively. Food, both with guar gum and alone, reduced the AUC of trimethoprim by about 22%.[1] The greatest individual reductions in peak serum levels and AUC were 44% and 36%, respectively with food, and 48% and 38%, respectively, with food and guar gum.[1] The reasons are not understood but it may be due to adsorption of the trimethoprim onto the food and guar gum.

The clinical importance of this interaction is uncertain but a marked reduction in absorption can occur in some individuals. However, trimethoprim is generally taken without regard to food, so this interaction would not appear to be significant in most patients.

1. Hoppu K, Tuomisto J, Koskimies O and Simell O. Food and guar decrease absorption of trimethoprim. *Eur J Clin Pharmacol* (1987) 32, 427–9.

Vancomycin + Colestyramine

Colestyramine may bind with vancomycin in the gut.

Clinical evidence, mechanism, importance and management

Colestyramine binds with vancomycin within the gut, thereby reducing its biological activity (about tenfold according to *in vitro* studies). The combination of vancomycin and colestyramine used to be used in antibacterial-associated colitis (now no longer recommended) and to overcome this interaction it was suggested that a vancomycin dosage of 2 g daily should be used, and that administration of the vancomycin and colestyramine should be separated as much as possible to minimise their admixture in the gut.[1] It is usually recommended that other drugs should be taken 1 hour before or 4 to 6 hours after colestyramine.

1. Taylor NS, Bartlett JG. Binding of *Clostridium difficile* cytotoxin and vancomycin by anion-exchange resins. *J Infect Dis* (1980) 141, 92–7.

Vancomycin + Dobutamine, Dopamine and Furosemide

There is some evidence to suggest that dobutamine, dopamine and furosemide can markedly reduce vancomycin serum levels following cardiac surgery.

Clinical evidence, mechanism, importance and management

A retrospective evaluation of the records of 18 critically ill patients in intensive care units following cardiac surgery, suggested that drugs with important haemodynamic effects (dopamine, dobutamine, furosemide) may lower the serum levels of vancomycin. It was noted that withdrawal of the interacting drugs was followed by an increase of in the minimum steady-state serum levels of vancomycin, from 8.79 mg/L to 13.3 mg/L, despite no major changes in body weight or estimated renal clearance. This resulted in a mean dose reduction of 4.26 mg/kg per day.

It is suggested that this interaction occurs because these drugs increase cardiac output, which increases the renal clearance of vancomycin, and therefore reduces its serum levels.[1] The clinical implication is that in this particular situation creatinine clearance is a less good predictor of vancomycin clearance and consequently dose. Good therapeutic drug monitoring is needed to ensure that serum vancomycin levels are optimal. More confirmatory study is needed.

1. Pea F, Porreca L, Baraldo M, Furlanut M. High vancomycin dosage regimens required by intensive care unit patients cotreated with drugs to improve haemodynamics following cardiac surgical procedures. *J Antimicrob Chemother* (2000) 45, 329–35.

Vancomycin + Indometacin

Indometacin reduces the renal clearance of vancomycin in premature neonates. This interaction does not appear to have been studied in adults.

Clinical evidence, mechanism, importance and management

In 6 premature neonates with patent ductus arteriosus given indometacin, the half-life of vancomycin 15 to 20 mg/kg given intravenously over 1 hour was found to be 24.6 hours, compared with only 7 hours in 5 other premature neonates without patent ductus arteriosus who were not given indometacin.[1] The reason for this effect is uncertain but it seems possible that the indometacin reduces the renal clearance of vancomycin. The authors of this report suggest that the usual vancomycin maintenance dosage should be halved if indometacin is also being used. If vancomycin therapeutic drug monitoring is possible it would be advisable to take levels and adjust the vancomycin dose accordingly. It is not known whether indometacin has the same effect on vancomycin in adults.

1. Spivey JM, Gal P. Vancomycin pharmacokinetics in neonates. *Am J Dis Child* (1986) 140, 859.

Vancomycin + Nephrotoxic or Ototoxic drugs

The risk of nephrotoxicity and ototoxicity with vancomycin may possibly be increased if it is given with other drugs with similar toxic effects.

Clinical evidence, mechanism, importance and management

Vancomycin is both potentially nephrotoxic and ototoxic, and its manufacturers therefore suggest that it should be used with particular care, or avoided in patients with renal impairment or deafness.[1] They also advise the avoidance of other drugs that have nephrotoxic potential, because the effects could be additive. They list **amphotericin B**, **aminoglycosides**, **bacitracin**, **colistin**, **polymyxin B**, **viomycin** and **cisplatin**. They also list **etacrynic acid** and **furosemide** as potentially aggravating ototoxicity.

The monograph 'Aminoglycosides + Vancomycin', p.291 outlines some of the evidence that additive nephrotoxicity can occur with the **aminoglycosides**, but there seems to be no direct evidence about the other drugs. Even so, the general warning issued by the manufacturers to monitor carefully is a reasonable precaution.

1. Vancomycin hydrochloride. Mayne Pharma plc. UK Summary of product characteristics, December 2003.

Vancomycin + Theophylline

Theophylline appears not to interact with vancomycin in premature infants.

Clinical evidence, mechanism, importance and management

Five premature infants (mean gestational age of 25 weeks and weighing 1.1 kg) were given theophylline (serum levels of 6.6 mg/L) for apnoea of prematurity. It was found that the pharmacokinetics of vancomycin 20 mg/kg given every 12 to 18 hours for suspected sepsis were unchanged by the presence of the theophylline, when compared with previously published data on the pharmacokinetics of vancomycin in neonates.[1] There seems to be no other clinical reports about vancomycin with theophylline, and nothing to suggest that vancomycin has any effect on the serum levels of theophylline.

1. Ilagan NB, MacDonald JL, Liang K-C, Womack SJ. Vancomycin pharmacokinetics in low birth weight preterm neonates on therapeutic doses of theophylline. *Pediatr Res* (1996) 39, 74A.

11

Anticholinesterases

The anticholinesterase drugs (or cholinesterase inhibitors) can be classified as **centrally-acting**, **reversible** inhibitors such as donepezil (used in the treatment of Alzheimer's disease), **reversible** inhibitors with **poor CNS penetration**, such as neostigmine (used in the treatment of myasthenia gravis), or **irreversible** inhibitors, such as ecothiopate and metrifonate. The centrally-acting anticholinesterases and the reversible anticholinesterases form the basis of this section, and these are listed in 'Table 11.1', (see below). Interactions where the anticholinesterases are affecting other drugs are covered elsewhere in the publication.

Due to their differing pharmacokinetic characteristics, the centrally-acting anticholinesterases have slightly different interaction profiles, although they share a number of common pharmacodynamic interactions. Tacrine[1] is metabolised by the cytochrome P450 isoenzyme CYP1A2, and so interacts with 'fluvoxamine', (p.356), a potent inhibitor of this isoenzyme, whereas there is no evidence to suggest the other centrally acting anticholinesterases do. On the other hand, donepezil[1] and galantamine[1] are metabolised by the cytochrome P450 isoenzymes CYP3A4 and CYP2D6, and so they may interact with 'ketoconazole', (p.353) and 'quinidine', (p.356), respectively, whereas tacrine would not be expected to do so. Rivastigmine,[1] which is metabolised by conjugation, seems relatively free of *pharmacokinetic* interactions. Consideration of concurrent drug use would therefore seem to be an important factor in the choice of centrally-acting anticholinesterase.

Note that, organophosphorus compounds such as insecticides are also anticholinesterases.

1. Jann MW, Shirley KL, Small GW. Clinical pharmacokinetics and pharmacodynamics of cholinesterase inhibitors. *Clin Pharmacokinet* (2002) 719–39.

Table 11.1 Anticholinesterase drugs; reversible

Centrally-acting inhibitors used principally for Alzheimer's disease	*Inhibitors with poor CNS penetration used principally for myasthenia gravis*
Donepezil	Ambenonium
Galantamine	Distigmine
Rivastigmine	Edrophonium (mainly used diagnostically)
Tacrine	Neostigmine
	Physostigmine
	Pyridostigmine (also used for glaucoma)

Anticholinesterases; Centrally acting + Antipsychotics

No pharmacokinetic interaction appears to occur between risperidone and donepezil or galantamine, but extrapyramidal symptoms occurred in one patient given donepezil with risperidone. The pharmacokinetics of thioridazine are not affected by donepezil. Two isolated reports describe severe parkinsonism when haloperidol was given with tacrine.

Clinical evidence, mechanism, importance and management

(a) Donepezil

1. Risperidone. In a randomised, crossover study 24 healthy subjects were given risperidone 500 micrograms twice daily with donepezil 5 mg daily. Although donepezil caused slight changes in the levels of risperidone and 9-hydroxyrisperidone they did not exceed the limits for bioequivalence. Concurrent use did not increase adverse effects.[1] In one study 16 schizophrenic patients taking risperidone were given donepezil 5 mg daily for 7 days without any alteration in their risperidone and 9-hydroxyrisperidone levels. The pharmacokinetics of donepezil were similar in the risperidone-treated patients and healthy controls taking donepezil alone.[2] However, a case report describes the emergence of parkinsonian symptoms in an 80-year-old woman after she was given donepezil 5 mg daily, with risperidone 1 mg daily added 12 days later. Risperidone was discontinued and she recovered without treatment.[3] This appears to be an isolated report and its general significance is therefore unknown.

2. Thioridazine. In a crossover study 11 healthy subjects were given donepezil 5 mg daily for 16 days, with a single 50-mg dose of thioridazine on the final day. Although donepezil did not affect the pharmacokinetics of thioridazine or its effects on the QT interval, thioridazine, either alone or in combination with donepezil, was poorly tolerated and resulted in postural hypotension and increases in heart rate.[4] It would therefore seem prudent to use an alternative antipsychotic wherever possible.

(b) Galantamine

In a randomised, crossover study 16 patients over 60-years-old were given a 14-day dose escalation of galantamine, after which they were given galantamine 12 mg twice daily with risperidone 500 micrograms twice daily, both for 13 doses. Although galantamine caused slight changes in the levels of risperidone and 9-hydroxyrisperidone, their combined level (the active moiety) was unchanged. The combination was well-tolerated so no additional precautions would seem to be necessary on concurrent use.[5]

(c) Tacrine

An isolated report describes an 87-year-old man with dementia, who started taking haloperidol 5 mg daily for symptoms of agitation and paranoia. Doses of greater than 5 mg were noted to cause extrapyramidal symptoms. After 10 days, tacrine 10 mg four times daily was added. Within 72 hours he developed severe parkinsonian symptoms, which resolved within 8 hours of stopping both drugs.[6] Another isolated report describes a woman taking haloperidol 10 mg daily who similarly developed a disabling parkinsonian syndrome within one week of starting tacrine 10 mg four times daily.[7] One possible reason is that the haloperidol blocked the dopamine receptors in striatum, thereby increasing striatal acetylcholine activity, which was further increased by the tacrine.[1] It is not clear whether patients given other dopamine receptor blocking drugs and tacrine would similarly show this reaction.

1. Zhao Q, Xie C, Pesco-Koplowitz L, Jia X, Parier J-L. Pharmacokinetic and safety assessments of concurrent administration of risperidone and donepezil. *J Clin Pharmacol* (2003) 43, 180–6.
2. Reyes JF, Preskorn SH, Khan A, Kumar D, Cullen EI, Perdomo CA, Pratt RD. Concurrent administration of donepezil HCl and risperidone in patients with schizophrenia: assessment of pharmacokinetic changes and safety following multiple oral doses. *Br J Clin Pharmacol* (2004) 58, 50–7.
3. Liu H-C, Lin S-K, Sung S-M. Extrapyramidal side-effect due to drug combination of risperidone and donepezil. *Psychiatry Clin Neurosci* (2002) 54, 479.
4. Ravic M, Warrington S, Boyce M, Dunn K, Johnston A. Repeated dosing with donepezil does not affect the safety, tolerability or pharmacokinetics of single-dose thioridazine in young volunteers. *Br J Clin Pharmacol* (2004) 58 (Suppl 1), 34–40.
5. Huang F, Lasseter KC, Janssens L, Verhaeghe T, Lau H, Zhao Q. Pharmacokinetic and safety assessments of galantamine and risperidone after the two drugs are administered alone and together. *J Clin Pharmacol* (2002) 42, 1341–51.
6. McSwain ML, Forman LM. Severe parkinsonian symptom development on combination treatment with tacrine and haloperidol. *J Clin Psychopharmacol* (1995) 15, 284.
7. Maany I. Adverse interaction of tacrine and haloperidol. *Am J Psychiatry* (1996) 153, 1504.

Anticholinesterases; Centrally acting + CYP3A4 inducers and inhibitors

Ketoconazole modestly increases the levels of donepezil. Even though this was not considered to be clinically significant, the manufacturers suggest that potent inhibitors of CYP3A4 will raise donepezil levels and inducers of CYP3A4 will lower donepezil levels. Galantamine levels are also increased by ketoconazole.

Clinical evidence, mechanism, importance and management

(a) Donepezil

Donepezil 5 mg daily was given to 18 healthy subjects with **ketoconazole** 200 mg daily, which is a specific and potent inhibitor of the cytochrome P450 isoenzyme CYP3A4. After one week of concurrent use, the maximum serum levels and AUC of donepezil were increased by less than 30%. Donepezil had no effect on the pharmacokinetics of **ketoconazole**.[1] None of the increases in donepezil levels were considered to be clinically relevant, and the authors suggest that no dose modifications will be required with **ketoconazole** or other CYP3A4 inhibitors.[1] Despite this, the UK manufacturer recommends that donepezil should be used with CYP3A4 inhibitors with care, and they specifically name **itraconazole** and **erythromycin**. Furthermore, both the US and UK manufacturers suggest that CYP3A4 inducers (they name **carbamazepine**, **dexamethasone**, **phenobarbital**, **phenytoin** and **rifampicin**) may lower donepezil levels.[2,3] Be aware that a reduction in donepezil levels is possible with these drugs, but that a clinically significant interaction seems unlikely.

(b) Galantamine

The manufacturers note that **ketoconazole** increased the bioavailability of galantamine by 30%, probably as a result of CYP3A4 inhibition. They therefore predict that **ketoconazole** (and other potent CYP3A4 inhibitors such as **ritonavir**) may increase the incidence of nausea and vomiting with galantamine, and suggest that, based on tolerability, a decrease in the maintenance dose be considered.[4,5] Whether this is in fact necessary in practice remains to be established. **Erythromycin**, a moderate CYP3A4 inhibitor, only increased galantamine bioavailability by about 10%,[4,5] and so a clinically significant interaction would not be expected.

1. Tiseo PJ, Perdomo CA, Friedhoff LT. Concurrent administration of donepezil HCl and ketoconazole: assessment of pharmacokinetic changes following single and multiple doses. *Br J Clin Pharmacol* (1998) 46 (Suppl 1), 30–34.
2. Aricept (Donepezil hydrochloride). Eisai Ltd. UK Summary of product characteristics, January 2007.
3. Aricept (Donepezil hydrochloride). Eisai Inc. US Prescribing information, October 2006.
4. Reminyl (Galantamine hydrobromide). Shire Pharmaceuticals Ltd. UK Summary of product characteristics, July 2005.
5. Razadyne (Galantamine hydrobromide). Ortho-McNeil Neurologics, Inc. US Prescribing information, August 2006.

Anticholinesterases; Centrally acting + Diazepam

Diazepam does not appear to affect the pharmacokinetics of tacrine or rivastigmine.

Clinical evidence, mechanism, importance and management

In a small study a single 2-mg dose of diazepam did not affect the pharmacokinetics of **tacrine** 20 mg every 6 hours, when compared with subjects not taking diazepam.[1] Similarly the manufacturers of **rivastigmine** say that no pharmacokinetic interaction has been seen with diazepam in healthy subjects.[2,3] No special precautions would seem necessary if diazepam is given with **tacrine** or **rivastigmine**.

1. deVries TM, Siedlik P, Smithers JA, Brown RR, Reece PA, Posvar EL, Sedman AJ, Koup JR, Forgue ST. Effect of multiple-dose tacrine administration on single-dose pharmacokinetics of digoxin, diazepam, and theophylline. *Pharm Res* (1993) 10 (10 Suppl), S-333.
2. Exelon (Rivastigmine hydrogen tartrate). Novartis Pharmaceuticals UK Ltd. UK Summary of product characteristics, October 2006.
3. Exelon (Rivastigmine tartrate). Novartis Pharmaceuticals Corp. US Prescribing information, June 2006.

Anticholinesterases; Centrally acting + H_2-receptor antagonists

Cimetidine possibly increases the effects of tacrine. Cimetidine does not appear to significantly affect the pharmacokinetics of donepezil or galantamine, and ranitidine does not affect the bioavailability of galantamine.

Clinical evidence, mechanism, importance and management

(a) Donepezil

In one study, donepezil 5 mg daily was given to 18 healthy subjects with **cimetidine** 800 mg daily. It was found that after one week of concurrent use the maximum serum levels and AUC of donepezil were increased by 13% and 10%, respectively. Donepezil had no effect on the pharmacokinetics of **cimetidine**.[1] None of the increases in donepezil levels were considered to be clinically relevant.[1]

(b) Galantamine

The US manufacturer notes that when a single 40-mg dose of galantamine was given on day 2 of a 3-day course of **cimetidine** 800 mg daily the bioavailability of galantamine was increased by 16%, which would not be expected to be clinically significant. **Ranitidine** 300 mg daily had no effect on galantamine bioavailability.[2] No interaction would therefore be expected with any H_2-receptor antagonist.

(c) Tacrine

Cimetidine 300 mg four times daily for 2 days decreased the clearance of a single 40-mg dose of tacrine by 30%, and increased the AUC and maximum level by about 35% in 11 healthy subjects.[3] The manufacturers of tacrine also say that **cimetidine** increases the AUC and the maximum plasma level of tacrine by 64% and 54%, respectively.[4] The reason is not known, but it seems probable that **cimetidine** (a well-recognised liver enzyme inhibitor) reduces the metabolism of tacrine by the cytochrome P450 isoenzyme CYP1A2 (see also 'fluvoxamine', (p.356)).[3] An increase in the effects and possibly adverse effects of tacrine (nausea, vomiting, diarrhoea) seems possible. One patient in the study mentioned[3] had to be withdrawn due to nausea and vomiting, but none of the other 11 subjects particularly suffered from adverse effects. More study is needed to find out whether this interaction is generally clinically important. If the suggested mechanism of interaction is correct, the other H_2-receptor antagonists would not be expected to interact. Tacrine also increases the secretion of gastric acid but it is not clear whether this would oppose the actions of the H_2-receptor antagonists.

1. Tiseo PJ, Perdomo CA, Friedhoff LT. Concurrent administration of donepezil HCl and cimetidine: assessment of pharmacokinetic changes following single and multiple doses. *Br J Clin Pharmacol* (1998) 46 (Suppl 1), 25–29.
2. Razadyne (Galantamine hydrobromide). Ortho-McNeil Neurologics, Inc. US Prescribing information, August 2006.
3. Forgue ST, Reece PA, Sedman AJ, deVries TM. Inhibition of tacrine oral clearance by cimetidine. *Clin Pharmacol Ther* (1996) 59, 444–9.
4. Cognex (Tacrine hydrochloride). First Horizon Pharmaceutical™ Corp. US Prescribing information, January 2002.

Anticholinesterases; Centrally acting + HRT

A small study suggests that HRT treatment can almost double the serum levels of tacrine. Limited evidence suggests that oestrogens do not affect rivastigmine pharmacokinetics.

Clinical evidence, mechanism, importance and management

Following the observation that HRT appeared to increase the response of postmenopausal Alzheimer's patients to **tacrine**, a randomised, crossover, placebo-controlled study was undertaken in 10 healthy women who were given HRT (**estradiol** 2 mg with **levonorgestrel** 250 micrograms daily) with a single 40-mg dose of tacrine on day 10. The HRT increased the mean tacrine AUC by 60%, increased the mean peak serum level of tacrine by 46% and reduced the tacrine clearance by 31%. The AUC of one individual was increased threefold. These pharmacokinetic changes are thought to occur because HRT reduces the metabolism of the tacrine to its main metabolite (1-hydroxytacrine) by the cytochrome P450 isoenzyme CYP1A2.[1] The importance of this interaction is still uncertain, but increased tacrine levels would be expected to increase its adverse effects. Be alert therefore for the need to use a smaller tacrine dose in patients given HRT. More study of this interaction is needed.

In contrast, analysis of population data from 70 subjects found that oestrogens did not affect **rivastigmine** pharmacokinetics.[2]

1. Laine K, Palovaara S, Tapanainen P, Manninen P. Plasma tacrine concentrations are significantly increased by concomitant hormone replacement therapy. *Clin Pharmacol Ther* (1999) 66, 602–8.
2. Exelon (Rivastigmine tartrate). Novartis Pharmaceuticals Corp. US Prescribing information, June 2006.

Anticholinesterases; Centrally acting + Memantine

Memantine does not appear to attenuate the anticholinesterase effects of donepezil, galantamine, or tacrine, nor affect the pharmacokinetics of galantamine or donepezil.

Clinical evidence, mechanism, importance and management

(a) Donepezil

An *in vitro* study in *rats* suggested that memantine does not attenuate the anticholinesterase effects of donepezil at therapeutic concentrations.[1] In a later study 19 healthy subjects were given memantine 10 mg before and on the last day of taking donepezil (5 mg daily for 7 days then 10 mg daily for 22 days). The pharmacokinetics of both drugs were not significantly affected by concurrent use, and the effects of donepezil on anticholinesterase were also unaffected.[2] Furthermore, an efficacy and safety study of one year's duration has reported that the combination is well tolerated and beneficial.[3]

(b) Galantamine

An *in vitro* study in *rats* suggested that memantine does not attenuate the anticholinesterase effects of galantamine at therapeutic concentrations.[1] A study in 15 healthy subjects found that the concurrent use of extended-release galantamine 16 mg daily with memantine 10 mg twice daily for 12 days did not affect the pharmacokinetics of galantamine and generally did not increase the incidence of adverse effects, although dizziness may have been more common.[4]

Furthermore, a review of efficacy studies suggested that the effects of galantamine on anticholinesterase are unaffected, that the combination is safe and generally well tolerated.[5]

(c) Tacrine

An *in vitro* study in *rats* suggested that memantine does not attenuate the anticholinesterase effects of tacrine at therapeutic concentrations.[1]

1. Wenk GL, Quack G, Moebius H-J, Danysz W. No interaction of memantine with anticholinesterase inhibitors approved for clinical use. *Life Sci* (2000) 66, 1079–83.
2. Periclou AP, Ventura D, Sherman T, Rao N, Abramowitz WT. Lack of pharmacokinetic or pharmacodynamic interaction between memantine and donepezil. *Ann Pharmacother* (2004) 38, 1389–94.
3. Tariot PN, Farlow MR, Grossberg GT, Graham SM, McDonald S, Gergel I, for the Memantine Study Group. Memantine treatment in patients with moderate to severe Alzheimer Disease already receiving donepezil: a randomized controlled trial. *JAMA* (2004) 291, 317–24.
4. Yao C, Raoufinia A, Gold M, Nye JS, Ramael S, Padmanabhan M, Walschap Y, Verhaeghe T, Zhao Q. Steady-state pharmacokinetics of galantamine are not affected by addition of memantine in healthy subjects. *J Clin Pharmacol* (2005) 45, 519–28.
5. Grossberg GT, Edwards KR, Zhao Q. Rationale for combination therapy with galantamine and memantine in Alzheimer's disease. *J Clin Pharmacol* (2006) 46, 17S–26S.

Anticholinesterases + Miscellaneous

A number of drugs can affect myasthenia gravis, often by increasing muscular weakness. This is, strictly speaking, a drug-disease interaction, but such effects may be expected to oppose the actions of the drugs used to treat myasthenia gravis. A number of drugs (e.g. chlorpromazine, methocarbamol, and propafenone) are clearly contraindicated in patients with myasthenia, and, as this is not strictly a drug interaction, they

Table 11.2 Case reports of drugs aggravating or unmasking myasthenia gravis

Drug	*Effect seen*	*Refs*
Acetazolamide 500 mg intravenously	Aggravation of muscular weakness in patients with myasthenia gravis taking unnamed anticholinesterases.	1
Ampicillin up to 1.5 g daily	Aggravation of myasthenic symptoms in 2 patients taking pyridostigmine.	2
Aspirin	Mild aggravation of myasthenic symptoms in a patient taking neostigmine.	3
Beta blockers	See Beta blockers + Anticholinesterases, p. 834.	
Chloroquine	Persisting myasthenic symptoms, including muscular weakness, attributed to prior chloroquine use. Development of myasthenic symptoms in 3 patients, one who took chloroquine in overdose.	4-7
Ciprofloxacin	Aggravation of myasthenic symptoms in a patient taking pyridostigmine, and unmasking of myasthenia in one patient.	8, 9
Dipyridamole* 75 mg three times daily	Aggravation of myasthenic symptoms in a patient taking distigmine.	10
Erythromycin 500 mg intravenously	Precipitation of a myasthenic crisis in an undiagnosed 15-year-old girl.	11
Imipenem/cilastatin 500 mg four times daily	Aggravation of myasthenic symptoms in a patient taking pyridostigmine.	12
Ketoprofen 50 mg daily	Aggravation of myasthenic symptoms in a patient taking neostigmine.	3
Lithium carbonate 600 mg daily	Unmasking of myasthenia in one patient.	13
Norfloxacin*	Aggravation of myasthenic symptoms in a patient taking pyridostigmine.	14
Penicillamine	Aggravation of myasthenic symptoms in numerous patients taking anticholinesterases. Amitriptyline and imipramine also implicated in 2 cases.	15-18
Phenytoin 100 mg three times daily	Aggravation of myasthenic symptoms in an untreated patient.	19
Procainamide* 250 mg	Serious aggravation of myasthenic symptoms in a patient taking pyridostigmine. Two other less severe cases also reported.	20, 21
Quinidine* up to 970 mg daily	Mild aggravation of myasthenic symptoms in one patient taking pyridostigmine and another taking neostigmine. Development of myasthenic symptoms in 2 undiagnosed patients.	21-23

*Drugs that should be used with caution in myasthenia gravis.

1. Carmignani M, Scoppetta C, Ranelletti OF, Tonali P. Adverse interaction between acetazolamide and anticholinesterase drugs at the normal and myasthenic neuromuscular junction level. *Int J Clin Pharmacol Ther Toxicol* (1984) 22, 140–4.
2. Argov Z, Brenner T, Abramsky O. Ampicillin may aggravate clinical and experimental myasthenia gravis. *Arch Neurol* (1986) 43, 255–6.
3. McDowell IFW, McConnell JB. Cholinergic crisis in myasthenia gravis precipitated by ketoprofen. *BMJ* (1985) 291, 1094.
4. De Bleecker J, De Reuck J, Quatacker J, Meire F. Persisting chloroquine-induced myasthenia? *Acta Clin Belg* (1991) 46, 401–6.
5. Robberecht W, Bednarik J, Bourgeois P, van Hees J, Carton H. Myasthenic syndrome caused by direct effect of chloroquine on neuromuscular junction. *Arch Neurol* (1989) 46, 464–8.
6. Sghirlanzoni A, Mantegazza R, Mora M, Pareyson D, Cornelio F. Chloroquine myopathy and myasthenia-like syndrome. *Muscle Nerve* (1988) 11, 114–19.
7. Pichon P, Soichot P, Loche D, Chapelon M. Syndrome myasthenique induit par une intoxication a la choroquine: une forme clinique inhabituelle confirmee par une atteinte oculaire. *Bull Soc Ophtalmol Fr* (1984) 84, 219–22.
8. Moore B, Safani M, Keesey J. Possible exacerbation of myasthenia gravis by ciprofloxacin. *Lancet* (1988) 1, 882.
9. Mumford CJ, Ginsberg L. Ciprofloxacin and myasthenia gravis. *BMJ* (1990) 301, 818.
10. Haddad M, Zelikovski A, Reiss R. Dipyridamole counteracting distigmine in a myasthenic patient. *IRCS Med Sci* (1986) 14, 297.
11. Absher JR, Bale JF. Aggravation of myasthenia gravis by erythromycin. *J Pediatr* (1991) 119, 155–6.
12. O'Riordan J, Javed M, Doherty C, Hutchinson M. Worsening of myasthenia gravis on treatment with imipenem/cilastatin. *J Neurol Neurosurg Psychiatry* (1994) 57, 383.
13. Neil JF, Himmelhoch JM, Licata SM. Emergence of myasthenia gravis during treatment with lithium carbonate. *Arch Gen Psychiatry* (1976) 33, 1090–2.
14. Rauser EH, Ariano RE, Anderson BA. Exacerbation of myasthenia gravis by norfloxacin. *DICP Ann Pharmacother* (1990) 24, 207–8.
15. Vincent A, Newsom-Davis J, Martin V. Anti-acetylcholine receptor antibodies in D-penicillamine-associated myasthenia gravis. *Lancet* (1978) i, 1254.
16. Masters CL, Dawkins RL, Zilko PJ, Simpson JA, Leedman RJ, Lindstrom J. Penicillamine-associated myasthenia gravis, antiacetylcholine receptor and antistriational antibodies. *Am J Med* (1977) 63, 689–94.
17. Ferro J, Susano R, Gómez C, de Quirós FB. Miastenia inducida por penicilamina: ¿existe interacción con los antidepresivos tricíclicos? *Rev Clin Esp* (1993) 192, 358–9.
18. Russell AS, Linstrom JM. Penicillamine-induced myasthenia gravis associated with antibodies to acetylcholine receptor. *Neurology* (1978) 28, 847–9.
19. Brumlik J, Jacobs RS. Myasthenia gravis associated with diphenylhydantoin therapy for epilepsy. *Can J Neurol Sci* (1974) 1, 127–9.
20. Drachman DA, Skom JH. Procainamide - a hazard in myasthenia gravis. *Arch Neurol* (1965) 13, 316–20.
21. Kornfeld P, Horowitz SH, Genkins G, Papatestas AE. Myasthenia gravis unmasked by antiarrhythmic agents. *Mt Sinai J Med* (1976) 43, 10–14.
22. Stoffer SS, Chandler JH. Quinidine-induced exacerbation of myasthenia gravis in patient with Graves' disease. *Arch Intern Med* (1980) 140, 283–4.
23. Weisman SJ. Masked myasthenia gravis. *JAMA* (1949) 141, 917–18.

are not dealt with here. A number of case reports (see 'Table 11.2', (above)) describe the worsening or unmasking of myasthenia gravis with a range of different drugs. The evidence for many of these interactions is very sparse indeed, and in some instances they are simply rare and isolated cases. It would therefore be wrong to exaggerate their importance, but it would nevertheless be prudent to be alert for any evidence of worsening myasthenia if any of the drugs listed are added to established treatment.

Anticholinesterases + Other drugs that affect acetylcholine

The effects of centrally-acting anticholinesterases (e.g. donepezil) are expected to be additive with those of other anticholinesterases (e.g. neostigmine) and cholinergics (e.g. pilocarpine). The effects of centrally-acting anticholinesterases and drugs with antimuscarinic effects are expected to be antagonistic.

Clinical evidence, mechanism, importance and management

Anticholinesterases raise acetylcholine levels: some are more selective for raising acetylcholine levels in the brain (e.g. **donepezil**), whereas others (e.g. **neostigmine**) have a more generalised effect. Therefore if both drugs are given together their effects may be expected to be additive. Similarly, additive effects may be expected if anticholinesterases are given with cholinergic drugs, such as **bethanechol**, **carbachol**, and **pilocarpine**, which mimic the effects of acetylcholine,[1-6] and depolarising neuromuscular blockers, which act like acetylcholine to cause depolarisation (see 'Neuromuscular blockers + Anticholinesterases', p.114, for reports of this interaction).

In contrast, drugs with **antimuscarinic** (anticholinergic) effects (see 'Table 18.2', (p.674)), which block the actions of acetylcholine, would be expected to oppose the actions of the anticholinesterases.

A number of case reports describe an interaction between centrally-acting anticholinesterases and other antimuscarinics. Two patients taking **donepezil** and one taking **rivastigmine** were given **tolterodine** (an antimuscarinic). One patient (taking **donepezil**) developed confusion, while the other two developed delusional states. This is the opposite effect to the predicted interaction (where the anticholinesterase inhibitor may be expected to oppose the antimuscarinic effects of **tolterodine**). The authors suggest that the combination causes 'cholinergic neurogenic hypersensitivity' similar to that seen as a withdrawal reaction to anticholinesterases.[7] In contrast, a case report describes the successful use of **tolterodine** 6 mg daily in a patient taking **donepezil** 10 mg daily. The authors of this report suggest that, despite the predictions of an interaction, a trial of an **antimuscarinic** for urinary incontinence may be worthwhile in patients taking centrally-acting anticholinesterases.[8]

All of these interactions, additive or antagonistic, are in theory possible, but whether most of them are of real practical importance awaits confirmation. It would certainly be prudent to monitor the concurrent use of any of these potentially interacting groups of drugs.

1. Aricept (Donepezil hydrochloride). Eisai Ltd. UK Summary of product characteristics, January 2007.
2. Reminyl (Galantamine hydrobromide). Shire Pharmaceuticals Ltd. UK Summary of product characteristics, July 2005.
3. Exelon (Rivastigmine hydrogen tartrate). Novartis Pharmaceuticals UK Ltd. UK Summary of product characteristics, October 2006.
4. Cognex (Tacrine hydrochloride). First Horizon Pharmaceutical™ Corp. US Prescribing information, January 2002.
5. Exelon (Rivastigmine tartrate). Novartis Pharmaceuticals Corp. US Prescribing information, June 2006.
6. Razadyne (Galantamine hydrobromide). Ortho-McNeil Neurologics, Inc. US Prescribing information, August 2006.
7. Edwards KR, O'Connor JT. Risk of delirium with concomitant use of tolterodine and acetylcholinesterase inhibitors. *J Am Geriatr Soc* (2002) 50, 1165–6.
8. Siegler EL, Reidenberg M. Treatment of urinary incontinence with anticholinergics in patients taking cholinesterase inhibitors for dementia. *Clin Pharmacol Ther* (2004) 75, 484–8.

Anticholinesterases; Centrally acting + Quinidine

Quinidine does not affect the metabolism of tacrine, but is predicted to inhibit the metabolism of donepezil and galantamine.

Clinical evidence, mechanism, importance and management

(a) Donepezil

In vitro study has shown that quinidine inhibits donepezil metabolism, and, as no clinical information is available, the manufacturer suggests care with the combination,[1] as an increase in donepezil levels and adverse effects is theoretically possible.

(b) Galantamine

Quinidine, like paroxetine, is an inhibitor of the cytochrome P450 isoenzyme CYP2D6, an enzyme involved in the metabolism of galantamine. 'Paroxetine', (below) has been shown to increase galantamine levels and therefore quinidine is predicted to do the same. Consequently the manufacturers of galantamine suggest that concurrent treatment with quinidine may result in increased adverse effects (mainly nausea and vomiting), and, if this occurs, a reduction in the maintenance dose of galantamine should be considered.[2]

(c) Tacrine

Quinidine 83 mg every 8 hours did not affect the clearance of a single 40-mg dose of tacrine in 11 healthy subjects.[3] Since quinidine inhibits the cytochrome P450 isoenzyme CYP2D6 in the liver, it may be concluded that CYP2D6 does not have an important role to play in the metabolism of tacrine and therefore that other drugs that inhibit this enzyme are unlikely to interact with tacrine by this means.

1. Aricept (Donepezil hydrochloride). Eisai Ltd. UK Summary of product characteristics, January 2007.
2. Reminyl (Galantamine hydrobromide). Shire Pharmaceuticals Ltd. UK Summary of product characteristics, July 2005.
3. deVries TM, O'Connor-Semmes RL, Guttendorf RJ, Reece PA, Posvar EL, Sedman AJ, Koup JR, Forgue ST. Effect of cimetidine and low-dose quinidine on tacrine pharmacokinetics in humans. *Pharm Res* (1993) 10 (10 Suppl), S-337.

Anticholinesterases; Centrally acting + SSRIs

Fluvoxamine markedly increases the levels of tacrine, and increases its cholinergic adverse effects, whereas fluoxetine, paroxetine, and sertraline are not expected to interact. Paroxetine and fluoxetine may increase donepezil and galantamine levels. Sertraline does not appear to have a pharmacokinetic interaction with donepezil, and concurrent use seems generally well tolerated; however, one report describes hepatotoxicity, possibly as a result of their concurrent use. Rivastigmine and fluoxetine appear not to interact.

Clinical evidence, mechanism, importance and management

(a) Donepezil

Two case reports suggest that donepezil and **paroxetine** may interact, in one case with an increase in gastrointestinal adverse effects, and the other with increased CNS effects. These adverse effects were thought to occur because **paroxetine** may inhibit donepezil metabolism by the cytochrome P450 isoenzyme CYP2D6.[1] The manufacturer logically predicts that **fluoxetine** could also inhibit the metabolism of donepezil, and until more information is available, they suggest caution with concurrent use of donepezil and CYP2D6 inhibitors.[2]

In a crossover study 16 healthy subjects were given **sertraline** (50 mg daily increasing after 5 days to 100 mg daily) with donepezil 5 mg daily for 15 days. The pharmacokinetics of both drugs were not significantly altered by concurrent use, and, although there was some indication that digestive adverse effects may have been increased, overall adverse effects were not changed.[3] Another study has similarly found that the concurrent use of donepezil and **sertraline** is well tolerated.[4] A case report describes an 83-year-old woman taking **sertraline** 200 mg daily, who developed drug-induced cholestatic jaundice within 10 days of starting donepezil 5 mg daily. The authors suggest that although this reaction could have been in response to either drug, it may also have been precipitated by their concurrent use. The general significance of this report is unclear.[5]

(b) Galantamine

The manufacturers[6,7] note that interaction studies have shown that **paroxetine** 20 mg daily for 16 days increased the bioavailability of galantamine by about 40%, by inhibiting galantamine metabolism by the cytochrome P450 isoenzyme CYP2D6. They therefore warn about the increased risk of galantamine adverse effects (in particular nausea and vomiting) if **paroxetine** is added. If such adverse effects develop or worsen, the manufacturers suggest a reduction in the galantamine dosage.[6] They also predict that other SSRIs that are potent inhibitors of CYP2D6 may interact similarly, and they list **fluoxetine** and **fluvoxamine**,[6] although it should be noted that **fluvoxamine** is only a weak inhibitor of CYP2D6. Thus far there appear to be no reports of adverse reactions with any of these drugs.

(c) Rivastigmine

The manufacturers of rivastigmine report that in studies in healthy subjects no pharmacokinetic interactions were seen between rivastigmine and **fluoxetine**.[8,9] No special precautions appear necessary.

(d) Tacrine

Fluvoxamine is an inhibitor of cytochrome P450 isoenzyme CYP1A2, the main isoenzyme involved in the metabolism of tacrine. *In vitro* study showed that **fluvoxamine** is a potent inhibitor of tacrine metabolism, and it was therefore predicted that **fluvoxamine** may dramatically increase tacrine plasma levels in patients.[10] This prediction was confirmed in a placebo-controlled study in 13 healthy subjects who had an eightfold increase in the mean AUC of a single 40-mg dose of tacrine after taking **fluvoxamine** 100 mg for 6 days. A very large increase in the AUC of the hydroxylated metabolites of tacrine, and an eightfold fall in the clearance of tacrine was also seen. No subjects had any adverse effects when they took tacrine after placebo, but 5 had adverse effects (nausea, vomiting, sweating, and diarrhoea) when they took tacrine after **fluvoxamine**.[11] Another pilot study in one individual found that the total clearance of tacrine was reduced about tenfold and its half-life increased tenfold by **fluvoxamine** 100 mg daily.[12] A further study by the same authors found that the clearance of tacrine was reduced by about 85% in 18 healthy subjects taking **fluvoxamine** 50 or 100 mg.[13] It is likely that standard tacrine doses will be poorly tolerated in the presence of **fluvoxamine** because of cholinergic adverse effects, and a decrease in tacrine dose is probably necessary.[13] Alternatively, other SSRIs such as **fluoxetine**, **paroxetine**, or **sertraline** may be suitable alternatives, since these are unlikely to inhibit tacrine metabolism (they are only weak inhibitors of CYP1A2).

1. Carrier L. Donepezil and paroxetine: possible drug interaction. *J Am Geriatr Soc* (1999) 47, 1037.
2. Aricept (Donepezil hydrochloride). Eisai Ltd. UK Summary of product characteristics, January 2007.
3. Nagy CF, Kumar D, Perdomo CA, Wason S, Cullen EI, Pratt RD. Concurrent administration of donepezil HCl and sertraline HCl in healthy volunteers: assessment of pharmacokinetic changes and safety following single and multiple oral doses. *Br J Clin Pharmacol* (2004) 58, 25–33.
4. Finkel SI, Mintzer JE, Dysken M, Krishnan KR, Burt T, McRae T. A randomized, placebo-controlled study of the efficacy and safety of sertraline in the treatment of the behavioral manifestations of Alzheimer's disease in outpatients treated with donepezil. *Int J Geriatr Psychiatry* (2004) 19, 9–18.
5. Verrico MM, Nace DA, Towers AL. Fulminant chemical hepatitis possibly associated with donepezil and sertraline therapy. *J Am Geriatr Soc* (2000) 48, 1659–63.
6. Reminyl (Galantamine hydrobromide). Shire Pharmaceuticals Ltd. UK Summary of product characteristics, July 2005.
7. Razadyne (Galantamine hydrobromide). Ortho-McNeil Neurologics, Inc. US Prescribing information, August 2006.
8. Exelon (Rivastigmine hydrogen tartrate). Novartis Pharmaceuticals UK Ltd. UK Summary of product characteristics, October 2006.
9. Exelon (Rivastigmine tartrate). Novartis Pharmaceuticals Corp. US Prescribing information, June 2006.
10. Becquemont L, Le Bot MA, Riche C, Beaune P. Influence of fluvoxamine on tacrine metabolism in vitro: potential implication for the hepatotoxicity in vivo. *Fundam Clin Pharmacol* (1996) 10, 156–7.
11. Becquemont L, Ragueneau I, Le Bot MA, Riche C, Funck-Brentano C, Jaillon P. Influence of the CYP1A2 inhibitor fluvoxamine on tacrine pharmacokinetics in humans. *Clin Pharmacol Ther* (1997) 61, 619–27.
12. Larsen JT, Hansen LL, Brøsen K. Tacrine-fluvoxamine interaction study in healthy volunteers. *Eur J Clin Pharmacol* (1997) 52 (Suppl), A136.
13. Larsen JT, Hansen LL, Spigset O, Brøsen K. Fluvoxamine is a potent inhibitor of tacrine metabolism in vivo. *Eur J Clin Pharmacol* (1999) 55, 375–82.

Anticholinesterases; Centrally acting + Tobacco

Smoking tobacco reduces the serum levels of tacrine and increases the clearance of rivastigmine.

Clinical evidence, mechanism, importance and management

A comparative study in 7 tobacco smokers and 4 non-smokers found that the AUC of a single 40-mg dose of **tacrine** in the smokers was about 10% of that in the non-smokers. The elimination half-life in the smokers was also reduced, to about two-thirds of that in non-smokers. The increase in **tacrine** metabolism in smokers is thought to occur because some of the components of tobacco smoke increase the activity of the cytochrome P450 isoenzyme CYP1A2 in the liver, by which **tacrine** is metabolised.[1] In practical terms this means that smokers are likely to need larger doses of **tacrine** than non-smokers, although this needs confirmation in multiple dose studies. Other centrally acting anticholinesterases (**donepezil**, **galantamine**, **rivastigmine**) would not be expected to interact in this way, as they are not metabolised by CYP1A2. However, the US manufacturers[2] note that nicotine use increases **rivastigmine** clearance by 23%, and so other mechanisms may have a part to play. One observational study has suggested that patients with Alzheimer's disease who are smokers are more likely to improve if they are given centrally-acting anticholinesterases than non-smokers.[3] Whether this counteracts the effects of any pharmacokinetic interaction is unclear.

1. Welty D, Pool W, Woolf T, Posvar E, Sedman A. The effect of smoking on the pharmacokinetics and metabolism of Cognex® in healthy volunteers. *Pharm Res* (1993) 10 (10 Suppl), S-334.
2. Exelon (Rivastigmine tartrate). Novartis Pharmaceuticals Corp. US Prescribing information, June 2006.
3. Connelly PJ, Prentice NP. Current smoking and response to cholinesterase inhibitor therapy in Alzheimer's disease. *Dementia Geriatr Cogn Disord* (2005) 19, 11–14.

Donepezil + *Ginkgo biloba*

***Ginkgo biloba* does not appear to affect the pharmacokinetics or pharmacodynamics of donepezil.**

Clinical evidence, mechanism, importance and management

In a pharmacokinetic study 14 elderly patients with Alzheimer's disease were given donepezil 5 mg daily for at least 20 weeks, after which *Ginkgo biloba* extract 90 mg daily was also given for a further 30 days. Concurrent use did not affect the pharmacokinetics or cholinesterase activity of donepezil, and cognitive function appeared to be unchanged.[1] Therefore, over the course of 30 days, concurrent use appears neither beneficial nor detrimental.

1. Yasui-Furukori N, Furukori H, Kaneda A, Kaneko S, Tateishi T. The effects of *Ginkgo biloba* extracts on the pharmacokinetics and pharmacodynamics of donepezil. *J Clin Pharmacol* (2004) 44, 538–42.

Tacrine + Ibuprofen

An isolated report describes a woman taking tacrine who became delirious when she also started to take ibuprofen.

Clinical evidence, mechanism, importance and management

A 71-year-old diabetic woman with probable Alzheimer's disease developed delirium while taking tacrine 40 mg four times daily. The symptoms included delusions, hallucinations, and fluctuating awareness. She was also bradycardic, diaphoretic and dizzy.[1] She was eventually stabilised with tacrine 20 mg four times daily, and continued this for 8 months without problems, but became delirious again 2 weeks after starting to take ibuprofen 600 mg daily. The delirium resolved when both drugs were withdrawn. The reasons for this reaction are unknown. This is the first and only report of this apparent interaction and its general importance is probably small, especially as the patient had previously experienced delirium with tacrine alone.

1. Hooten WM, Pearlson G. Delirium caused by tacrine and ibuprofen interaction. *Am J Psychiatry* (1996) 153, 842.

Tacrine + Quinolones

Enoxacin possibly increases the effects of tacrine.

Clinical evidence, mechanism, importance and management

In vitro studies with human and *rat* liver microsomes found that enoxacin, a specific inhibitor of the cytochrome P450 isoenzyme CYP1A2, significantly inhibited all known routes by which tacrine is metabolised.[1] A reasonable conclusion to be drawn from this is that the effects of tacrine (both beneficial and adverse) would be increased by enoxacin, but this interaction does not appear to have been studied in patients or healthy subjects. The same study also suggested that enoxacin possibly inhibits the production of the hepatotoxic metabolites of tacrine.[1]

Other quinolones vary in the extent to which they inhibit CYP1A2 (see 'Theophylline + Quinolones', p.1192), so that any interaction with other quinolones would be expected to reflect this variation.

1. Madden S, Woolf TF, Pool WF, Park BK. An investigation into the formation of stable, protein-reactive and cytotoxic metabolites from tacrine *in vitro*. Studies with human and rat liver microsomes. *Biochem Pharmacol* (1993) 46, 13–20.

12

Anticoagulants

The blood clotting process

When blood is lost or clotting is initiated in some other way, a complex cascade of biochemical reactions is set in motion, which ends in the formation of a network or clot of insoluble protein threads enmeshing the blood cells. These threads are produced by the polymerisation of the molecules of fibrinogen (a soluble protein present in the plasma) into threads of insoluble fibrin. The penultimate step in the chain of reactions requires the presence of an enzyme, thrombin, which is produced from its precursor prothrombin, already present in the plasma. This is initiated by factor III (tissue thromboplastin), and subsequently involves various factors including activated factor VII, IX, X, XI and XII, and is inhibited by antithrombin III. Platelets are also involved in the coagulation process. Fibrinolysis is the mechanism of dissolution of fibrin clots, which can be promoted with thrombolytics. For further information on platelet aggregation and clot dissolution, see 'Antiplatelet drugs and thrombolytics', (p.697).

Mode of action of the anticoagulants

Anticoagulants may be divided into direct anticoagulants, which have an immediate effect, and the indirect anticoagulants, which inhibit the formation of coagulation factors, so have a delayed effect as they do not inactivate coagulation factors already formed. See 'Table 12.1', (p.359), for a list.

(a) Direct anticoagulants

The direct anticoagulants include **heparin**, which principally enhances the effect of antithrombin III, thereby inhibiting the effect of thrombin (factor IIa) and activated factor X (factor Xa). **Low-molecular-weight heparins** are salts of fragments of heparin and act similarly, except that they have a greater effect on factor Xa than factor IIa. They have a longer duration of action than heparin and usually require less monitoring. The **heparinoids** (such as **danaparoid**) are similar. A more recent introduction is the synthetic polysaccharide **fondaparinux**, which is an inhibitor of factor Xa. The other group of direct anticoagulants are the **thrombin inhibitors**, which bind to the active thrombin site. These include recombinant forms or synthetic analogues of **hirudin** such as bivalirudin and lepirudin. Megalatran and its oral prodrug **ximelagatran** act similarly, but have been withdrawn because of liver toxicity.

(b) Indirect anticoagulants

The indirect anticoagulants inhibit the vitamin K-dependent synthesis of factors VII, IX, X and II (prothrombin) in the liver, and may also be referred to as **vitamin K antagonists**. The most commonly used are the **coumarins**, principally warfarin, but also acenocoumarol and phenprocoumon. The **indanediones** such as phenindione are now less frequently used. The indirect anticoagulants have the advantage over currently available direct anticoagulants in that they are orally active. They are often therefore referred to as **oral anticoagulants**, but this term may become misleading with the development of direct-acting oral anticoagulants, such as ximelegatran, which have different monitoring requirements and interactions.

Coagulation tests

During anticoagulant therapy the aim is to give protection against intravascular clotting, without running the risk of bleeding. To achieve this, doses of heparin and oral anticoagulants should be individually titrated until the desired response is attained. With the coumarin and indanedione oral anticoagulants, this procedure normally takes several days because they do not act directly on the blood clotting factors already in circulation, but on the rate of synthesis of new factors by the liver. The successful titration is determined by one of a number of different but closely related laboratory tests, see 'Table 12.2', (p.360) and below. Note that routine monitoring of anticoagulant effect is not required for low-molecular weight heparins or heparinoids, except in patients at increased risk of bleeding, such as those with renal impairment or who are overweight. Also, note that these tests cannot be used to monitor the anticoagulant effect of fondaparinux or the direct thrombin inhibitors, and these require no routine monitoring.

(a) Prothrombin time

The prothrombin time test (PT, Pro-Time, tissue factor induced coagulation time) is the most common method employed in clinical situations. It measures the time taken for a fibrin clot to form in a citrated plasma sample containing calcium ions and tissue thromboplastin. The PT is usually reported as the International Normalised Ratio (INR).

1. International normalised ratio (INR). The INR was adopted by the WHO in 1982 to standardise (using the International Sensitivity Index) oral anticoagulant therapy to take into account the sensitivities of the different thromboplastins used in laboratories across the world. The formula for calculating the INR is as follows:

$$\text{INR} = (\text{patient's prothrombin time in seconds/mean normal prothrombin time in seconds})^{\text{ISI}}$$

The PT values obtained from the patient's sample are compared to a control, and this gives the INR. The higher the INR, the higher the PT value so if the patient's ratio is 2, this means the PT (and therefore clotting) is twice as long as the normal plasma. The British Corrected Ratio is essentially the same, but was calculated to a standard British thromboplastin.

2. Quick Value. The Quick Value is expressed as a percentage; the lower the value, the longer the blood takes to coagulate. Therefore as the Quick Value increases, the corresponding INR value gets smaller and vice versa.

(b) Activated partial thromboplastin time

The activated partial thromboplastin time (aPTT) is the second most common method for monitoring anticoagulant therapy, measuring all the clotting factors in the intrinsic pathway as opposed to the PT test, which measures the extrinsic pathway.

(c) Other methods of assessing clotting

Other tests used, which in some instances offer more sensitivity to specific aspects of therapy, include the prothrombin-proconvertin ratio (PP), the thrombotest, the thrombin clotting time test (TCT, activated clotting time, activated coagulation time), the platelet count and the bleeding time test. The use of the most appropriate test will depend on the situation and the desired result.

Anticoagulant interactions

Stable oral anticoagulant therapy is difficult to achieve even during close monitoring. For example, in one controlled study in patients with atrial fibrillation, only 61% of INR values were within the target range of 2 to 3, despite monitoring the INR monthly and adjusting the warfarin dose appropriately.[1] A large number of factors can influence levels of coagulation, including diet, disease (fever, diarrhoea, heart failure, thyroid dysfunction), and the use of other drugs. It must therefore be remembered that it is particularly difficult to ascribe a change in INR specifically to a drug interaction in a single case report, and single case reports or a few isolated reports for widely used drugs do not prove that an interaction occurs. Nevertheless, either the addition or the withdrawal of drugs may upset the

Table 12.1 Anticoagulants

Direct anticoagulants	*Indirect anticoagulants*
Fondaparinux sodium	**Coumarins**
Heparin	Acenocoumarol
Heparin calcium	Dicoumarol
Heparin sodium	Ethyl biscoumacetate
Heparinoids	Phenprocoumon
Danaparoid	Warfarin
Dermatan sulfate	**Indanediones**
Pentosan polysulfate	Fluindione
Suleparoid	Phenindione
Sulodexide	
Low-molecular-weight heparins	
Bemiparin	
Certoparin	
Dalteparin	
Enoxaparin	
Nadroparin	
Parnoparin	
Reviparin	
Tinzaparin	
Thrombin inhibitors	
Argotroban	
Bivalirudin	
Desirudin	
Hirudin	
Lepirudin	
Melagatran	
Ximelagatran	

balance in a patient already well stabilised on an anticoagulant. Some drugs are well known to increase the activity of the anticoagulants and can cause bleeding if the dosage of the anticoagulant is not reduced appropriately. Others reduce the activity and return the prothrombin time to normal. Both situations are serious and may be fatal, although excessive hypoprothrombinaemia manifests itself more obviously and immediately as bleeding and is usually regarded as the more serious. The interaction mechanism may be pharmacodynamic or pharmacokinetic: pharmacokinetic mechanisms are particularly well established and important for coumarin anticoagulants.

(a) Metabolism of the coumarins

The coumarins, warfarin, phenprocoumon and acenocoumarol, are racemic mixtures of *S*- and *R*-enantiomers. The *S*-enantiomers of these coumarins have several times more anticoagulant activity than the *R*-enantiomers. Reports suggest for example, that *S*-warfarin is three to five times more potent a vitamin K antagonist than *R*-warfarin. The *S*-enantiomer of warfarin is metabolised primarily by the cytochrome P450 isoenzyme CYP2C9, and to a much lesser extent, by CYP3A4. The metabolism of *R*-warfarin is more complex, but this enantiomer is primarily metabolised by CYP1A2, CYP3A4, and CYP2C19. *S*-warfarin is eliminated in the bile and *R*-warfarin is excreted in the urine as inactive metabolites. There is much more known about the metabolism of warfarin compared with other anticoagulants, but it is established that *S*-phenprocoumon and *S*-acenocoumarol are also substrates for CYP2C9 and that they differ from warfarin in their hepatic metabolism, and stereospecific potency.[2]

It makes sense to assume therefore, that an inhibitor of CYP2C9 (e.g. 'fluconazole', (p.387)) is likely to increase the concentration of the coumarin and enhance the anticoagulant effect. Drugs that induce CYP2C9 (e.g. 'rifampicin', (p.375)) reduce plasma levels of the coumarins by increasing the clearance.

'Genetic differences', (p.4), in the genes for these cytochrome P450 isoenzymes may have an important influence on drug metabolism of the coumarins. For example, different versions of the gene encoding CYP2C9 exist and the enzymatic activity of the most clinically important CYP2C9 variants, CYP2C9*2 and CYP2C9*3, is significantly reduced. Studies have suggested an association between patients possessing one or more of these variants and a low-dose requirement of warfarin. Similar observations have been seen with the CYP2C9*3 variant and acenocoumarol.

While the metabolism of the coumarins, especially warfarin, are well known, the numerous interaction pathways and the variability in patient responses, makes the clinical consequences difficult to predict.

(b) Other mechanisms for anticoagulant interactions

Some drugs, such as 'colestyramine', (p.393), may also prevent the absorption of the coumarins and reduce their bioavailability. See also 'Drug absorption interactions', (p.3). Additive anticoagulant effects can occur if anticoagulants are given with other drugs that also impair coagulation by other mechanisms such as 'antiplatelets', (p.700). Coumarins and indanediones act as vitamin K antagonists, and so dietary intake of 'vitamin K', (p.409) can also 'reduce or abolish', (p.9) their effects. 'Protein-binding displacement', (p.3) is another possible drug interaction mechanism but this usually plays a minor role compared with other mechanisms.[3]

Bleeding and its treatment

When prothrombin times become excessive, bleeding can occur. In order of decreasing frequency the bleeding shows itself as ecchymoses, blood in the urine, uterine bleeding, black faeces, bruising, nose-bleeding, haematoma, gum bleeding, coughing and vomiting blood.

Vitamin K is an antagonist of the coumarin and indanedione oral anticoagulants. The British Society for Haematology has given advice on the appropriate course of action if bleeding occurs in patients taking warfarin, and this is readily available in summarised form in the British National Formulary.

If the effects of heparin are excessive it is usually sufficient just to stop the heparin, but protamine sulfate is a specific antidote if a rapid effect is required. Protamine sulfate only partially reverses the effect of low molecular weight heparins.

There is currently no known specific antidote for fondaparinux, or for the direct thrombin inhibitors.

1. Stroke Prevention in Atrial Fibrillation Investigators. Adjusted-dose warfarin versus low-intensity, fixed dose warfarin plus aspirin for high-risk patients with atrial fibrillation: Stroke Prevention in Atrial Fibrillation III randomised clinical trial. *Lancet* (1996) 348, 633–8.
2. Ufer M. Comparative pharmacokinetics of vitamin-K antagonists. Warfarin, phenprocoumon and acenocoumarol. *Clin Pharmacokinet* (2005) 44, 1227–46.
3. Sands CD, Chan ES, Welty TE. Revisiting the significance of warfarin protein-binding displacement interactions. *Ann Pharmacother* (2002) 36, 1642–4.

Table 12.2 Coagulation tests

Test	*Normal range*	*Therapeutic/diagnostic range*
Activated partial thromboplastin time	20 to 39 seconds after reagents added	1.5 to 2.5 x control
Bleeding time	1 to 9 minutes depending on method used	Critical value greater than 15 minutes
International normalised ratio	0.9 to 1.2	2 to 4 depending on indication for anticoagulation
Plasma thrombin time test	10 to 15 seconds	Greater than 15 seconds
Prothrombin-proconvertin ratio	70 to 130%	10 to 30%
Prothrombin time	10 to 15 seconds	1 to 2 x control
Quick value	70 to 130%	10 to 20%
Thrombin clotting time	70 to 120 seconds	150 to 600 seconds depending on indication for anticoagulation
Thrombotest	100%	10 to 20%

Coumarins + ACE inhibitors

There is a single, isolated and unexplained case of melaena attributed to an interaction between acenocoumarol and fosinopril. No other ACE inhibitor studied has so far been shown to interact to a clinically relevant extent with the coumarins.

Clinical evidence

(a) Benazepril

Benazepril 20 mg daily for 7 days did not affect the steady-state plasma levels of either **warfarin** or **acenocoumarol** in healthy subjects. The anticoagulant activity of **acenocoumarol** was not altered. The effects of **warfarin** were slightly reduced, as demonstrated by a mean reduction in PT of about 4%, but this is not enough to be clinically important.[1]

(b) Cilazapril

Cilazapril 2.5 mg daily for 3 weeks had no effect on the thrombotest times or coagulation factors II, VII and X in 26 patients taking long-term **acenocoumarol** or **phenprocoumon**.[2]

(c) Enalapril

Enalapril 20 mg for 5 days did not affect the anticoagulant effects of **warfarin** 2.5 to 7.5 mg daily, according to a brief summary of unpublished data cited in a review.[3]

(d) Fosinopril

A 74-year-old patient stabilised on **acenocoumarol, enalapril**, piretanide, and digoxin had the piretanide and **enalapril** switched to furosemide and fosinopril. Eleven days later, he presented with dark faeces (melaena) and had a low haemoglobin. Fosinopril and acenocoumarol were stopped, and then **enalapril** and acenocoumarol were restarted. On gastrointestinal endoscopy, no explanation for the melaena was found, and his haemoglobin level had returned to normal 15 days later. This case was attributed to possible potentiation of the effect of acenocoumarol by fosinopril,[4] but as the drugs were not taken alone, the interaction is not proven.

(e) Moexipril

In 10 healthy subjects, the pharmacokinetics and pharmacodynamics of a single 50-mg dose of **warfarin** were not altered when it was given with the first dose of moexipril 15 mg daily for 6 days.[5]

(f) Ramipril

In 8 healthy subjects, ramipril 5 mg daily for 7 days had no effect on the steady-state pharmacokinetics or anticoagulant effects of **phenprocoumon**.[6] Similarly, ramipril 5 mg daily for 3 weeks did not alter the anticoagulant effects of **acenocoumarol** or **phenprocoumon** in patients stabilised on these anticoagulants, when compared with placebo.[7]

(g) Temocapril

In 24 healthy subjects, temocapril 20 mg daily for 2 weeks had no effect on the steady-state pharmacokinetics or pharmacodynamics of **warfarin**.[8] The absence of an interaction between **warfarin** and temocapril was also shown in another study.[9]

(h) Trandolapril

In a study in 19 healthy subjects,[10] **trandolapril** 2 mg daily for 13 days did not affect the pharmacodynamics of a single 25-mg dose of **warfarin** given on day 8.

Mechanism, importance and management

No important pharmacokinetic or pharmacodynamic interaction has been demonstrated for any ACE inhibitor and coumarin anticoagulant. Contrasting with all this evidence, there is a single, unexplained and isolated case of melaena attributed to an interaction between acenocoumarol and fosinopril. There seems to be no other evidence that fosinopril normally interacts with the oral anticoagulants and so this interaction is unlikely to be of general significance.

No special precautions would therefore seem necessary if any of these coumarin anticoagulants and ACE inhibitors are used concurrently.

1. Van Hecken A, De Lepeleire I, Verbesselt R, Arnout J, Angehrn J, Youngberg C, De Schepper PJ. Effect of benazepril, a converting enzyme inhibitor, on plasma levels and activity of acenocoumarol and warfarin. *Int J Clin Pharmacol Res* (1988) 8, 315–19.
2. Boeijinga JK, Breimer DD, Kraay CJ, Kleinbloesem CH. Absence of interaction between the ACE inhibitor cilazapril and coumarin derivatives in elderly patients on long term oral anticoagulants. *Br J Clin Pharmacol* (1992) 33, 553P.
3. Gomez HJ, Cirillo VJ, Irvin JD. Enalapril: a review of human pharmacology. *Drugs* (1985) 30 (Suppl 1), 13–24.
4. de Tomás ME, Sáez L, Beltrán S, Gato A. Probable interacción farmacológica entre fosinopril y acenocumarol. *Med Clin (Barc)* (1997) 108, 757.
5. Van Hecken A, Verbesselt R, Depré M, Tjandramaga TB, Angehrn J, Cawello W, De Schepper PJ. Moexipril does not alter the pharmacokinetics of pharmacodynamics of warfarin. *Eur J Clin Pharmacol* (1993) 45, 291–3.
6. Verho M, Malerczyk V, Grötsch H, Zenbil I. Absence of interaction between ramipril, a new ACE-inhibitor, and phenprocoumon, an anticoagulant agent. *Pharmatherapeutica* (1989) 5, 392–9.
7. Boeijinga JK, Matroos AW, van Maarschalkerweerd MW, Jeletich-Bastiaanse A, Breimer DD. No interaction shown between ramipril and coumarine derivatives. *Curr Ther Res* (1988) 44, 902–8.
8. Siepmann M, Kirch W, Kleinbloesem CH. Non-interaction of temocapril, an ACE-inhibitor, with warfarin. *Clin Pharmacol Ther* (1996) 59, 214.
9. Lankhaar G, Eckenberger P, Ouwerkerk MJA, Dingemanse J. Pharmacokinetic-pharmacodynamic investigation of a possible interaction between steady-state temocapril and warfarin in healthy subjects. *Clin Drug Invest* (1999) 17, 399–405.
10. Meyer BH, Muller FO, Badenhorst PN, Luus HG, De La Rey N. Multiple doses of trandolapril do not affect warfarin pharmacodynamics. *S Afr Med J* (1995) 85, 768–70.

Coumarins + Alcohol

A number of early studies showed that the effects of the coumarin oral anticoagulants are unlikely to be changed in those with normal liver function who drink small or moderate amounts of alcoholic beverages such as wine or spirits. An increase in bleeding time may occur in patients with liver disease who drink to excess.

Clinical evidence

(a) Patients and subjects free from liver disease

The daily consumption of 1 pint (about 560 mL) of Californian white table wine for a 3-week period at meal times by 8 healthy subjects anticoagulated with **warfarin**, was found to have no significant effects on either the serum **warfarin** levels or the anticoagulant response.[1]

Other studies in both patients[2,3] and healthy subjects[4,5] taking either **warfarin**[2,3,5] or **phenprocoumon**[4] have very clearly confirmed the absence of an interaction with wine[3,5] gin,[4] or 40% alcohol.[2] In one of these studies the subjects were given almost 600 mL of a table wine (12% alcohol) or 300 mL of a fortified wine (20% alcohol) without adverse effects on coagulation.[5]

In contrast to the above studies, a 58-year-old man stabilised on **warfarin** experienced a sharp rise in his INR to 8 when he started to drink half a can of light beer (5.35 g alcohol) every other day. In the previous 5 months he had an INR in the range of 1.9 to 2.5 with a stable warfarin dose, and no other explanation for the change in INR was found. He stopped taking the alcohol, and was eventually restabilised on the original dose of warfarin.[6]

(b) Chronic alcoholics or those with liver disease

In one study, 15 alcoholics who had been drinking heavily (250 g ethanol or more daily) for at least 3 months and 11 control subjects (minimal social drinkers or non-drinkers) were given a single 40-mg dose of **warfarin**. The half-life of **warfarin** was lower in the alcoholics (26.5 versus 41.1 hours), but a comparison of the prothrombin times with those of healthy subjects found no differences.[7]

One patient with liver cirrhosis had marked fluctuations in prothrombin times and **warfarin** levels associated with weekend binge drinking of vodka.[2] Another patient with abnormal liver function had a fall in plasma **warfarin** levels and effect when he stopped drinking 50 mL of whiskey daily. When rechallenged with alcohol, warfarin levels and effect rose, and he had a nosebleed.[8] In contrast, a large retrospective cohort study did not find a significantly increased risk of serious bleeding in 140 patients with a history of alcoholic binge drinking who were taking **warfarin**. The relative risk was 1.3 (0.8 to 1.9) compared with patients who had no record of alcohol abuse.[9]

Mechanism

It seems probable that, as in *rats*,[10] continuous heavy drinking stimulates the hepatic enzymes concerned with the metabolism of warfarin, leading to its more rapid elimination.[7,11] As a result the half-life shortens. The fluctuations in prothrombin times in those with liver impairment[2,8] may possibly occur because sudden large amounts of alcohol exacerbate the general dysfunction of the liver and this affects the way it metabolises warfarin. Alcohol may also change the ability of the liver to synthesise clotting factors.[12] Constituents of beer other than alcohol may affect warfarin metabolism.[6]

Importance and management

The absence of an interaction between warfarin or phenprocoumon and alcohol in those free from liver disease is well documented and well established. It appears to be quite safe for patients taking oral anticoagulants to drink small or moderate amounts of wine or spirits. Even much less conservative amounts (up to 8 oz/250 mL of spirits[4] or a pint of wine[1]) do not create problems with the anticoagulant control, so that there appears to be a good margin of safety even for the less than abstemious. Only warfarin and phenprocoumon have been investigated but other coumarin anticoagulants would be expected to behave similarly. The single case of increased INR in a patient who started to drink beer is unexplained. Further study specifically with beer is needed to throw light on this possible interaction.

On the other hand, those who drink heavily may possibly need above-average doses of the anticoagulant, while limited evidence suggests that those with liver damage who binge drink may experience marked fluctuations in their prothrombin times. It might be prudent to avoid anticoagulation in this type of patient unless they can abstain from drinking. Nevertheless, although one cohort study in patients taking warfarin found a slight trend towards serious bleeding events in patients with a history of binge drinking, this was not significant, and other risk factors were more important (highly variable prothrombin time ratio, or prothrombin time ratio greater than 2).[9]

1. O'Reilly RA. Lack of effect of mealtime wine on the hypoprothrombinemia of oral anticoagulants. *Am J Med Sci* (1979) 277, 189–94.
2. Udall JA. Drug interference with warfarin therapy. *Clin Med* (1970) 77, 20–25.
3. Karlson B, Leijd B, Hellström A. On the influence of vitamin K-rich vegetables and wine on the effectiveness of warfarin treatment. *Acta Med Scand* (1986) 220, 347–50.
4. Waris E. Effect of ethyl alcohol on some coagulation factors in man during anticoagulant therapy. *Ann Med Exp Biol Fenn* (1963) 41, 45–53.
5. O'Reilly RA. Lack of effect of fortified wine ingested during fasting and anticoagulant therapy. *Arch Intern Med* (1981) 141, 458–9.
6. Havrda DE, Mai T, Chonlahan J. Enhanced antithrombotic effect of warfarin associated with low-dose alcohol consumption. *Pharmacotherapy* (2005) 25, 303–7.
7. Kater RMH, Roggin G, Tobon F, Zieve P, Iber FL. Increased rate of clearance of drugs from the circulation of alcoholics. *Am J Med Sci* (1969) 258, 35–9.
8. Breckenridge A, Orme M. Clinical implications of enzyme induction. *Ann N Y Acad Sci* (1971) 179, 421–31.
9. Fihn SD, McDonell M, Martin D, Henikoff J, Vermes D, Kent D, White RH, for the Warfarin Optimized Oupatient Follow-up Study Group. Risk factors for complications of chronic anticoagulation: a multicenter study. *Ann Intern Med* (1993) 118, 511–20.
10. Rubin E, Hutterer F, Lieber CS. Ethanol increases hepatic smooth endoplasmic reticulum and drug-metabolizing enzymes. *Science* (1968) 159, 1469–70.
11. Kater RMH, Carruli N, Iber FL. Differences in the rate of ethanol metabolism in recently drinking alcoholic and nondrinking subjects. *Am J Clin Nutr* (1969) 22, 1608–17.
12. Riedler G. Einfluß des Alkohols auf die Antikoagulantientherapie. *Thromb Diath Haemorrh* (1966) 16, 613–35.

Coumarins + Aliskiren

Aliskiren did not alter the pharmacodynamics or pharmacokinetics of a single dose of warfarin.

Clinical evidence, mechanism, importance and management

In a placebo-controlled, crossover study in 15 healthy subjects, aliskiren 150 mg daily for 11 days did not alter the pharmacodynamics of a single dose of **warfarin** given on day 8. In addition, there was no change in the AUC or half-life of *R*- and *S*-warfarin.[1]

This study suggests that no **warfarin** dose adjustments would be expected to be needed if aliskiren is used in patients taking **warfarin**.

1. Dieterle W, Corynen S, Mann J. Effect of the oral renin inhibitor aliskiren on the pharmacokinetics and pharmacodynamics of a single dose of warfarin in healthy subjects. *Br J Clin Pharmacol* (2004) 58, 433–6.

Coumarins + Allopurinol

A number of studies and case reports suggest that allopurinol does not alter the pharmacokinetics or pharmacodynamics of warfarin. Nevertheless, a few case reports suggest that allopurinol might have increased the effect of warfarin. Two cases have also been reported with phenprocoumon. Allopurinol increased the half-life of dicoumarol in some healthy subjects, but there do not appear to be any reports of a clinically significant interaction.

Clinical evidence

(a) Dicoumarol

In 6 healthy subjects, allopurinol 2.5 mg/kg twice daily for 14 days increased the mean half-life of a single 4-mg/kg dose of dicoumarol from 51 to 153 hours, with large inter-individual variation.[1] In another similar study, only 1 of 3 healthy subjects showed an increase in dicoumarol half-life (from 13 to 17 hours) when they were also given allopurinol.[2]

(b) Phenprocoumon

Two patients stabilised for a few weeks taking phenprocoumon developed prolonged bleeding times, with haematuria in one of them, within 4 to 5 weeks of starting to take allopurinol 300 mg daily.[3]

(c) Warfarin

In a study in 8 healthy subjects, the half-life of a single 25-mg dose of warfarin was not altered by pretreatment with allopurinol 100 mg twice daily for 10 days.[2] Similarly, in 6 subjects, the elimination of a single 50-mg dose of warfarin was not altered by 2 or 4 weeks treatment with allopurinol 100 mg three times daily, although one subject had a 30% reduction in the elimination of warfarin after 4 weeks.[4] No change was seen in the prothrombin ratios of 2 patients taking warfarin who took allopurinol 100 mg three times daily for 3 weeks.[4] In contrast, one patient stabilised on warfarin had a 42% increase in his prothrombin ratio after taking allopurinol 100 mg daily for 2 days.[5]

In a retrospective study[6] of the adverse effects of allopurinol in 1835 patients, 3 patients were identified who had developed excessive anticoagulation while taking warfarin and allopurinol. One of them developed extensive intrapulmonary haemorrhage and had a prothrombin time of 71 seconds. An increase in prothrombin time was seen in an 82-year-old woman stabilised on warfarin when given both allopurinol 300 mg daily and 'indometacin', (p.432), but the precise role of allopurinol in this case is unclear.[7]

Mechanism

It has been suggested that, as in *rats*, allopurinol inhibits the metabolism of the anticoagulants by the liver, thereby prolonging their effects and half-lives.[1,2,5] There is a wide individual variability in the effects of allopurinol on drug metabolism,[4] so that only a few individuals are affected.

Importance and management

Documentation is poor, and a pharmacokinetic interaction is not established. There appear to be few case reports of any important interaction. Nevertheless, consider increased monitoring of the anticoagulant effect in any patient taking a coumarin with allopurinol.

1. Vesell ES, Passananti GT, Greene FE. Impairment of drug metabolism in man by allopurinol and nortriptyline. *N Engl J Med* (1970) 283, 1484–8.
2. Pond SM, Graham GG, Wade DN, Sudlow G. The effects of allopurinol and clofibrate on the elimination of coumarin anticoagulants in man. *Aust N Z J Med* (1975) 5, 324–8.
3. Jähnchen E, Meinertz T, Gilfrich HJ. Interaction of allopurinol with phenprocoumon in man. *Klin Wochenschr* (1977) 55, 759–61.
4. Rawlins MD, Smith SE. Influence of allopurinol on drug metabolism in man. *Br J Pharmacol* (1973) 48, 693–8.
5. Barry M, Feeley J. Allopurinol influences aminophenazone elimination. *Clin Pharmacokinet* (1990) 19, 167–9.
6. McInnes GT, Lawson DH, Jick H. Acute adverse reactions attributed to allopurinol in hospitalised patients. *Ann Rheum Dis* (1981) 40, 245–9.
7. Self TH, Evans WE, Ferguson T. Drug enhancement of warfarin activity. *Lancet* (1975) ii, 557–8.

Coumarins + Alpha blockers

Studies suggest that tamsulosin does not alter the pharmacokinetics or anticoagulant effect of acenocoumarol, and alfuzosin does not interact with warfarin. Doxazosin is said not to interact with anticoagulants.

Clinical evidence, mechanism, importance and management

In a double-blind, placebo-controlled, crossover study in 12 healthy subjects, **tamsulosin** 400 micrograms daily for 9 days had no effect on the pharmacokinetics or anticoagulant effects of a single 10-mg dose of **acenocoumarol** given on day five.[1]

The UK manufacturers of alfuzosin report that no pharmacodynamic or pharmacokinetic interaction was observed in healthy subjects given **alfuzosin** with **warfarin**,[2] and the US manufacturers report that in 6 healthy subjects **alfuzosin** 5 mg twice daily for 6 days did not affect the pharmacological response to a single 25-mg dose of **warfarin**.[3]

One UK manufacturer of **doxazosin** says that no adverse drug interaction has been observed with **anticoagulants** (unspecified).[4]

No coumarin dose adjustment would therefore be expected to be needed with concurrent use of these alpha blockers.

1. Rolan P, Terpstra IJ, Clarke C, Mullins F, Visser JN. A placebo-controlled pharmacodynamic and pharmacokinetic interaction study between tamsulosin and acenocoumarol. *Br J Clin Pharmacol* (2003) 55, 314–16.
2. Xatral (Alfuzosin hydrochloride). Sanofi-Aventis. UK Summary of product characteristics, April 2005.
3. Uroxatral (Alfuzosin hydrochloride extended-release tablets). Sanofi-Aventis US LLC. US Prescribing information, March 2007
4. Cardura (Doxazosin mesilate). Pfizer Ltd. UK Summary of product characteristics, February 2007.

Coumarins and related drugs + Amiodarone

The anticoagulant effects of warfarin, phenprocoumon and acenocoumarol are increased by amiodarone and bleeding may occur. The interaction may be maximal in 2 to 7 weeks, and may persist long after the amiodarone has been withdrawn.

Clinical evidence

A. Inhibition of coumarin metabolism

(a) Warfarin

In the one of the first reports of an interaction between amiodarone and warfarin, 5 out of 9 patients who were stabilised on warfarin showed signs of bleeding (4 had microscopic haematuria and one had diffuse ecchymoses) within 3 to 4 weeks of starting to take amiodarone (dosage not stated). All 9 had increases in their prothrombin times averaging 21 seconds. It was necessary to decrease the warfarin dosage by an average of a third (range 16 to 45%) to return their prothrombin times to the therapeutic range. The effects of amiodarone persisted for 6 to 16 weeks in 4 of the patients from whom it was withdrawn.[1]

Since then numerous other case reports have described a prolongation in prothrombin times and/or bleeding in patients taking **warfarin** and also given amiodarone (maintenance doses of 100 to 800 mg daily, sometimes with initial higher loading doses).[2-11] One patient died of haemorrhage.[6] Warfarin dose reductions varied between about 25 to 60%,[4,6,8,11] with only a few patients not needing a reduction.[4] In one retrospective study, the required dose of warfarin was related to the amiodarone maintenance dose, leading to the recommendation that the warfarin dose should be reduced by 40% for a daily maintenance dose of amiodarone of 400 mg, by 35% for 300 mg, by 30% for 200 mg and by 25% for 100 mg.[11]

A few pharmacokinetic studies have shown that amiodarone decreased the clearance of warfarin by 44 to 55% in patients receiving the drugs clinically[7,12] and by 20 to 37% in healthy subjects given a single dose of warfarin after taking amiodarone for 3 to 4 days.[13,14] In the two studies in healthy subjects, amiodarone caused a similar decrease in the clearance of both *R*- and *S*-warfarin.[13,14] However, a recent study in patients concluded that amiodarone had a much greater effect on *S*-warfarin than on *R*-warfarin.[15]

(b) Other coumarins

A number of retrospective studies[16-19] have shown that patients stabilised on **acenocoumarol** require a dose reduction when they are given amiodarone, the combined range in these studies being 4 to 69%. In a prospective study, 10 patients stabilised on **acenocoumarol** were given amiodarone 600 mg daily for a week, then 400 mg daily. Eight of the 10 had a decrease in prothrombin time after a mean of 4 days of amiodarone. Six patients required a decrease in **acenocoumarol** dose of 60% while taking amiodarone 600 mg daily, but by the third week of taking amiodarone 400 mg daily the effects had diminished, and only a 33% reduction in dose was necessary.[20] A couple of case reports of the interaction have also been published.[21,22] Amiodarone similarly interacts with **phenprocoumon**, with one case series in 7 patients reporting that a 9 to 59% phenprocoumon dose reduction was required within 1 to 3 weeks of starting amiodarone.[23] Conversely, an early study in 12 patients stabilised on **phenprocoumon** and given amiodarone 400 mg to 1 g daily failed to identify an interaction.[24]

B. Thyrotoxicosis (Hyperthyroidism)

The INR of a patient stabilised on **warfarin** and amiodarone was noted to increase from about 2 to 5.5 after he developed amiodarone-induced thyrotoxicosis.[25] Another 3 well-described cases of this potential interaction have been reported.[26]

Mechanism

Amiodarone inhibits the metabolism of warfarin, probably because it, and/or its metabolite desethylamiodarone,[27] inhibit the cytochrome P450 isoenzyme CYP2C9, CYP3A4 and CYP1A2 (see 'metabolism of the coumarins', (p.358)).

Thyrotoxicosis, which can be caused by amiodarone, potentiates the effect of warfarin, see 'Coumarins and related drugs + Thyroid and Antithyroid compounds', p.455. As a result less warfarin would be required to prolong the prothrombin time.[25,26]

Importance and management

The potentiating effect of amiodarone on coumarin anticoagulants is a well documented, established and clinically important interaction. It appears to occur in most patients.[1,4,8] It would seem prudent to adjust the doses of the coumarin anticoagulants based on INR measurements. Some recommend the dosage of warfarin should initially be reduced by 25%[8] or 50%[4] when amiodarone is added to established anticoagulant treatment, with increased INR monitoring until a new steady-state is achieved. The potentiation of coumarins starts within a few days and is usually maximal by 2 to 7 weeks.[8,11,15] The final reduction in warfarin dose required may depend on the amiodarone maintenance dose: average warfarin dose reductions of 25% have been required for amiodarone 100 mg daily, 30 to 35% for amiodarone 200 mg daily, 35% for amiodarone 300 mg daily, 40 to 50% for amiodarone 400 mg daily, and 65% for amiodarone 600 mg daily.[7,11] These suggested reductions are broad generalisations and individual patients may need more or less.[19,28] If established amiodarone therapy is withdrawn in a patient taking warfarin, it is likely that the dose of warfarin will need increasing gradually over the first few months after amiodarone is stopped. This is because amiodarone has such a long half-life. If warfarin is required in a patient on established amiodarone therapy, a lower initial dose of warfarin should be used.

Similar advice applies to acenocoumarol and phenprocoumon, and probably also other coumarins. Some recommend an initial reduction in acenocoumarol dose of 50% when amiodarone is added,[16] whereas others recommend that the INR should be closely monitored, and the dose of acenocoumarol only reduced in response to an increase in INR.[28]

In patients stabilised on warfarin and amiodarone, the possibility of amiodarone-induced thyrotoxicosis should be considered if an abrupt increase in INR occurs.[25,26]

Some sources appear to suggest that the **indanediones** may interact similarly, but this appears to be an extrapolation from the known interaction with warfarin. There seems no clinical evidence available to support this prediction.

1. Martinowitz U, Rabinovici J, Goldfarb D, Many A, Bank H. Interaction between warfarin sodium and amiodarone. *N Engl J Med* (1981) 304, 671–2.
2. Rees A, Dalal JJ, Reid PG, Henderson AH, Lewis MJ. Dangers of amiodarone and anticoagulant treatment. *BMJ* (1981) 282, 1756–7.
3. Serlin MJ, Sibeon RG, Green GJ. Dangers of amiodarone and anticoagulant treatment. *BMJ* (1981) 283, 58.
4. Hamer A, Peter T, Mandel WJ, Scheinman MM, Weiss D. The potentiation of warfarin anticoagulation by amiodarone. *Circulation* (1982) 65, 1025–29.
5. McGovern B, Garan H, Kelly E, Ruskin JN. Adverse reactions during treatment with amiodarone hydrochloride. *BMJ* (1983) 287, 175–80.
6. Raeder EA, Podrid PJ, Lown B. Side effects and complications of amiodarone therapy. *Am Heart J* (1985) 109, 975–83.
7. Almog S, Shafran N, Halkin H, Weiss P, Farfel Z, Martinowitz U, Bank H. Mechanism of warfarin potentiation by amiodarone: dose- and concentration-dependent inhibition of warfarin elimination. *Eur J Clin Pharmacol* (1985) 28, 257–61.
8. Kerin NZ, Blevins RD, Goldman L, Faitel K, Rubenfire M. The incidence, magnitude, and time course of the amiodarone-warfarin interaction. *Arch Intern Med* (1988) 148, 1779–81.
9. Cheung B, Lam FM, Kumana CR. Insidiously evolving, occult drug interaction involving warfarin and amiodarone. *BMJ* (1996) 312, 107–8.
10. Chan TYK. Drug interactions as a cause of over-anticoagulation and bleedings in Chinese patients receiving warfarin. *Int J Clin Pharmacol Ther* (1998) 36, 403–5.
11. Sanoski CA, Bauman JL. Clinical observations with the amiodarone/warfarin interaction: dosing relationships with long-term therapy. *Chest* (2002) 121, 19–23.
12. Watt AH, Stephens MR, Buss DC, Routledge PA. Amiodarone reduces plasma warfarin clearance in man. *Br J Clin Pharmacol* (1985) 20, 707–9.
13. Heimark LD, Wienkers L, Kunze K, Gibaldi M, Eddy AC, Trager WF, O'Reilly RA, Goulart DA. The mechanism of the interaction between amiodarone and warfarin in humans. *Clin Pharmacol Ther* (1992) 51, 398–407.
14. O'Reilly RA, Trager WF, Rettie AE, Goulart DA. Interaction of amiodarone with racemic warfarin and its separate enantiomorphs in humans. *Clin Pharmacol Ther* (1987) 42, 290–4.
15. Matsumoto K, Ueno K, Nakabayashi T, Komamura K, Kamakura S, Miyatake K. Amiodarone interaction time differences with warfarin and digoxin. *J Pharm Technol* (2003) 19, 83–90.

16. Caraco Y, Chajek-Shaul T. The incidence and clinical significance of amiodarone and acenocoumarol interaction. *Thromb Haemost* (1989) 62, 906–8.
17. Arboix M, Frati ME, Laporte J-R. The potentiation of acenocoumarol anticoagulant effect by amiodarone. *Br J Clin Pharmacol* (1984) 18, 355–60.
18. Pini M, Manotti C, Quintavalla R. Interaction between amiodarone and acenocoumarin. *Thromb Haemost* (1985) 54, 549.
19. Fondevila C, Meschengieser S, Lazzari MA. Amiodarone potentiates acenocoumarin. *Thromb Res* (1988) 53, 203–8.
20. Richard C, Riou B, Berdeaux A, Forunier C, Khayat D, Rimailho A, Giudicelli JF, Auzépy P. Prospective study of the potentiation of acenocoumarol by amiodarone. *Eur J Clin Pharmacol* (1985) 28, 625–9.
21. El Allaf D, Sprynger M, Carlier J. Potentiation of the action of oral anticoagulants by amiodarone. *Acta Clin Belg* (1984) 39, 306–8.
22. Bharat V, Mohanty B. Bleeding complication during coumarin therapy due to amiodarone and azithromycin. *J Assoc Physicians India* (2000) 48, 746–7.
23. Broekmans AW, Meyboom RHB. Bijwerkingen van geneesmiddelen. Potentiëring van het cumarine-effect door amiodaron (Cordarone). *Ned Tijdschr Geneeskd* (1982) 126, 1415–17.
24. Verstraete M, Vermylen J, Claeys H. Dissimilar effect of two anti-anginal drugs belonging to the benzofuran group on the action of coumarin derivatives. *Arch Int Pharmacodyn Ther* (1968) 176, 33–41.
25. Woeber KA, Warner I. Potentiation of warfarin sodium by amiodarone-induced thyrotoxicosis. *West J Med* (1999) 170, 49–51.
26. Kurnik D, Loebstein R, Farfel Z, Ezra D, Halkin H, Olchovsky D. Complex drug-drug-disease interactions between amiodarone, warfarin, and the thyroid gland. *Medicine* (2004) 83, 107–13.
27. Naganuma M, Shiga T, Nishikata K, Tsuchiya T, Kasaniki H, Fujii E. Role of desethylamiodarone in the anticoagulant effect of concurrent amiodarone and warfarin therapy. *J Cardiovasc Pharmacol Ther* (2001) 6, 363–7.
28. Fondevila C, Meschengieser S, Lazzari M. Amiodarone-acenocoumarin interaction. *Thromb Haemost* (1991) 65, 328.

Coumarins and related drugs + Anabolic steroids and Androgens

Increased anticoagulant effects and bleeding has been seen in patients taking a coumarin anticoagulant or the indanedione, phenindione and an anabolic steroid or testosterone.

Clinical evidence

(a) Anabolic steroids

Six patients stabilised on **warfarin** or **phenindione** were given **oxymetholone** 15 mg daily. One patient developed extensive subcutaneous bleeding and another had haematuria. After 15 to 30 days all 6 patients had thrombotests of less than 5%, which returned to the therapeutic range within a few days of **oxymetholone** being withdrawn.[1] Other similar cases have been reported with **oxymetholone** and **warfarin**,[2-4] or **acenocoumarol**.[5] In 3 of the reports[1,3,4] the interaction was severe enough to discontinue the **oxymetholone**. In one patient[2] the **warfarin** dose was reduced by 59%, and in another[5] the **acenocoumarol** dose was reduced by 66 to 75%.

Similarly increased anticoagulant effects and bleeding have been described in studies and case reports involving:

- **dicoumarol** with **norethandrolone**,[6]
- **dicoumarol** with **stanozolol**,[7]
- **phenindione** with **methandienone**,[8]
- **phenindione** with **ethylestrenol**,[9]
- **warfarin** with **methandienone**[2,8,10,11] (62% to 73% decrease in dose required in 3 cases[2] and 38% in 7 others[8])
- **warfarin** with **stanozolol**[12-15] (40% and 64% decrease in dose required in 2 patients and about a 70% increase required after stopping stanozolol[12]).

In a pharmacokinetic study in 15 healthy subjects, the manufacturer noted that the concurrent use of **warfarin** and **oxandrolone** 5 or 10 mg twice daily increased the *S*-warfarin AUC by 2.65-fold and doubled its half-life, and had similar effects on *R*-warfarin.[16] Microscopic haematuria occurred in 9 subjects and gingival bleeding in one. A 5.5-fold decrease in warfarin dose (about 80 to 85%) was necessary to maintain a target INR of 1.5.

(b) Androgens

A 58-year-old man receiving **methyltestosterone** replacement therapy 37.5 mg daily required a maintenance dose of **phenprocoumon** of just 0.94 mg daily: control subjects required 2.62 mg daily.[17]

One report notes that 3 patients receiving **warfarin** and *Sustanon* (containing four combined esters of **testosterone**) had no changes in their anticoagulant requirements,[4] whereas another report describes a woman who showed a 78% and a 65% increase in prothrombin times on two occasions when using a 2% **testosterone propionate** vaginal ointment twice daily. She needed a 25% reduction in **warfarin** dosage.[18]

Mechanism

Not understood. One study showed that norethandrolone did not alter the metabolism of dicoumarol, and did not alter the plasma levels of vitamin-K dependent clotting factors.[6] However, a more recent study of oxandrolone and warfarin shows a pharmacokinetic basis for this interaction.[16]

Importance and management

Well documented, well established and clinically important interactions that develop rapidly, possibly within 2 to 3 days. Most, if not all, patients are affected.[1,6] If concurrent use cannot be avoided, the dosage of the anticoagulant should be appropriately reduced. In a few cases, where patients have been able to be stabilised on the combination, up to 75% reductions in anticoagulant dose have been required, and the study[16] with oxandrolone suggests an 85% reduction in dose of warfarin might be necessary. After withdrawal of the interacting drug the anticoagulant dosage will need to be increased.

It seems probable that all the coumarin and indanedione anticoagulants will interact with any 17-alkyl substituted anabolic steroid. The situation with testosterone and other non 17-alkylated steroids is not clear as there are only case reports, which are conflicting. Until more is known it would seem prudent to increase the frequency of INR monitoring if these drugs are given with coumarins or indanediones.

1. Longridge RGM, Gillam PMS, Barton GMG. Decreased anticoagulant tolerance with oxymetholone. *Lancet* (1971) ii, 90.
2. Murakami M, Odake K, Matsuda T, Onchi K, Umeda T, Nishino T. Effects of anabolic steroids on anticoagulant requirements. *Jpn Circ J* (1965) 29, 243–50.
3. Robinson BHB, Hawkins JB, Ellis JE, Moore-Robinson M. Decreased anticoagulant tolerance with oxymetholone. *Lancet* (1971) i, 1356.
4. Edwards MS, Curtis JR. Decreased anticoagulant tolerance with oxymetholone. *Lancet* (1971) ii, 221.
5. de Oya JC, del Río A, Noya M, Villeneuva A. Decreased anticoagulant tolerance with oxymetholone in paroxysmal nocturnal hæmoglobinuria. *Lancet* (1971) ii, 259.
6. Schrogie JJ, Solomon HM. The anticoagulant response to bishydroxycoumarin. II. The effect of d-thyroxine, clofibrate, and norethandrolone. *Clin Pharmacol Ther* (1967) 8, 70–7.
7. Howard CW, Hanson SG, Wahed MA. Anabolic steroids and anticoagulants. *BMJ* (1977) 1, 1659–60.
8. Pyörälä K, Kekki M. Decreased anticoagulant tolerance during methandrostenolone therapy. *Scand J Clin Lab Invest* (1963) 15, 367–74.
9. Vere DW, Fearnley GR. Suspected interaction between phenindione and ethylœstrenol. *Lancet* (1968) ii, 281.
10. Dresdale FC, Hayes JC. Potential dangers in the combined use of methandrostenolone and sodium warfarin. *J Med Soc New Jers* (1967) 64, 609–12.
11. McLaughlin GE, McCarty DJ, Segal BL. Hemarthrosis complicating anticoagulant therapy. Report of three cases. *JAMA* (1966) 196, 1020–1.
12. Acomb C, Shaw PW. A significant interaction between warfarin and stanozolol. *Pharm J* (1985) 234, 73–4.
13. Cleverly CR. Personal communication, March 1987.
14. Shaw PW, Smith AM. Possible interaction of warfarin and stanozolol. *Clin Pharm* (1987) 6, 500–2.
15. Elwin C-E, Törngren M. Samtidigt intag av warfarin och stanozolol orsak till blödningar hos patienten. *Lakartidningen* (1988) 85, 3290.
16. Oxandrin (Oxandrolone). Savient Pharmaceuticals Inc. US Prescribing information, February 2006.
17. Husted S, Andreasen F, Foged L. Increased sensitivity to phenprocoumon during methyltestosterone therapy. *Eur J Clin Pharmacol* (1976) 10, 209–16.
18. Lorentz SM, Weibert RT. Potentiation of warfarin anticoagulation by topical testosterone ointment. *Clin Pharm* (1985) 4, 332–4.

Coumarins + Angiotensin II receptor antagonists

None of the angiotensin II receptor antagonists appear to interact to a clinically relevant extent with warfarin..

Clinical evidence

(a) Candesartan

In healthy subjects stabilised on individualised doses of **warfarin**, candesartan cilexetil 16 mg daily for 10 days reduced the trough serum levels of **warfarin** by 7%, but this had no effect on prothrombin times.[1]

(b) Eprosartan

No clinically relevant changes in anticoagulation occurred in 18 healthy subjects stabilised on **warfarin** with INRs between 1.3 and 1.6 when they were given eprosartan 300 mg twice daily for 7 days.[2]

(c) Irbesartan

Warfarin 2.5 to 10 mg daily was given to 16 healthy subjects for 2 weeks, with irbesartan 300 mg or a placebo daily for a further week. There was no evidence that irbesartan affected the pharmacokinetics or pharmacodynamics of warfarin.[3]

(d) Losartan

In a placebo-controlled, randomised, crossover study, 10 healthy subjects were given losartan 100 mg daily for 13 days with a single 30-mg dose of **warfarin** on day 7. The pharmacokinetics of **warfarin** (both *R*- and *S*-enantiomers) and its anticoagulant effects were not altered. Losartan, given alone for a week, also had no effect on prothrombin times.[4]

(e) Telmisartan

Telmisartan 120 mg daily for 10 days was given to 12 healthy subjects stabilised on **warfarin**, with INRs of between 1.2 and 1.8. A small 11% decrease in the mean trough plasma **warfarin** concentration occurred, but the anticoagulation effect remained unchanged.[5]

(f) Valsartan

In 12 healthy subjects, **warfarin** (10 mg daily for 3 days) and valsartan (160 mg daily for 3 days) were each given alone then valsartan 160 mg daily was given for 7 days with warfarin 10 mg daily for the first 3 of these. Warfarin had no effect on the pharmacokinetics of valsartan. Valsartan caused a small increase in prothrombin time of about 12%, which was not considered clinically important. Warfarin pharmacokinetics were not assessed.[6,7]

Mechanism

The angiotensin II antagonists, and warfarin, are substrates for the cytochrome P450 isoenzyme CYP2C9. It was therefore possible that they might affect warfarin metabolism. However, this does not appear to happen.

Importance and management

The available pharmacokinetic and pharmacodynamic studies showing that the angiotensin II receptor antagonists (candesartan, eprosartan, irbesartan, losartan, telmisartan, valsartan) do not interact with warfarin, and the lack of any published evidence to the contrary, suggest that no warfarin dose adjustments should be needed if these drugs are used.

1. Jonkman JHG, van Lier JJ, van Heiningen PNM, Lins R, Sennewald R, Högemann A. Pharmacokinetic drug interaction studies with candesartan cilexetil. *J Hum Hypertens* (1997) 11 (Suppl 2), S31–S35.
2. Kazierad DJ, Martin DE, Ilson B, Boike S, Zariffa N, Forrest A, Jorkasky DK. Eprosartan does not affect the pharmacodynamics of warfarin. *J Clin Pharmacol* (1998) 38, 649–53.
3. Mangold B, Gielsdorf W, Marino MR. Irbesartan does not affect the steady-state pharmacodynamics and pharmacokinetics of warfarin. *Eur J Clin Pharmacol* (1999) 55, 593–8.
4. Kong A-N T, Tomasko P, Waldman SA, Osborne B, Deutsch PJ, Goldberg MR, Bjornsson TD. Losartan does not affect the pharmacokinetics and pharmacodynamics of warfarin. *J Clin Pharmacol* (1995) 35, 1008–15.
5. Stangier J, Su C-APF, Hendriks MGC, van Lier JJ, Sollie FAE, Oosterhuis B, Jonkman JHG. Steady-state pharmacodynamics and pharmacokinetics of warfarin in the presence and absence of telmisartan in healthy male volunteers. *J Clin Pharmacol* (2000) 40, 1331–7.
6. Novartis Pharmaceuticals Ltd. Data on file, Protocol 40.
7. Knight H, Flesch G, Prasad P, Lloyd P, Douglas J. Lack of pharmacokinetic and pharmacodynamic interaction between valsartan and warfarin. *J Hypertens* (2000) 18 (Suppl 4), S89.

Coumarins + Antacids

There is some evidence that the absorption of dicoumarol may be increased by magnesium hydroxide, but there is no direct evidence that this is clinically important. Aluminium hydroxide does not interact with either warfarin or dicoumarol, and magnesium hydroxide does not interact with warfarin.

Clinical evidence

(a) Dicoumarol

Magnesium hydroxide (*Milk of Magnesia*) 15 mL taken with and 3 hours after a single dose of dicoumarol was found to raise the peak plasma levels and AUC of dicoumarol by 75% and 50%, respectively, in 6 healthy subjects. Conversely, **aluminium hydroxide** (*Amphogel)* 30 mL did not alter dicoumarol levels.[1]

(b) Warfarin

Aluminium/magnesium hydroxide (*Maalox*) 30 mL given with and for four 2-hourly doses after warfarin had no effect on the plasma warfarin levels or on the anticoagulant response in 6 subjects.[2] Similarly, neither **aluminium hydroxide** (*Amphogel*) 30 mL nor **magnesium hydroxide** (*Milk of Magnesia*) 15 mL taken with and 3 hours after a single 75-mg dose of warfarin had any effect on warfarin peak levels or AUC.[1]

Mechanism

It is suggested that dicoumarol forms a more readily absorbed chelate with magnesium so that its effects are increased.[1,3] An *in vitro* study suggested that the absorption of warfarin may be decreased by **magnesium trisilicate**,[4] where as another *in vitro* study found no effect.[5]

Importance and management

No special precautions need be taken if aluminium or magnesium hydroxide antacids are given to patients taking warfarin, or if aluminium hydroxide is given to those taking dicoumarol. Choosing these antacids avoids the possibility of an adverse interaction. Despite the evidence of increased absorption of dicoumarol with magnesium hydroxide, there seems to be no direct clinical evidence of any important adverse interaction for this combination, or indeed between any coumarin and an antacid.

1. Ambre JJ, Fischer LJ. Effect of coadministration of aluminum and magnesium hydroxides on absorption of anticoagulants in man. *Clin Pharmacol Ther* (1973) 14, 231–7.
2. Robinson DS, Benjamin DM, McCormack JJ. Interaction of warfarin and nonsystemic gastrointestinal drugs. *Clin Pharmacol Ther* (1971) 12, 491–5.
3. Akers MJ, Lach JL, Fischer LJ. Alterations in the absorption of dicoumarol by various excipient materials. *J Pharm Sci* (1973) 62, 391–5.
4. McElnay JC, Harron DWG, D'Arcy PF, Collier PS. Interaction of warfarin with antacid constituents. *BMJ* (1978) 2, 1166.
5. Khalil SA, Naggar VF, Zaghloul IA, Ismail AA. In vitro anticoagulant–antacid interactions. *Int J Pharmaceutics* (1984) 19, 307–21.

Coumarins + Antibacterials

Altered (usually enhanced) coumarin response has been reported with virtually every class of antibacterial. While some such as sulfamethoxazole, clearly have a pharmacokinetic interaction, for others there is no clear explanation for why an interaction might be expected. Theoretical mechanisms include reduced intestinal bacterial production of vitamin K_2 substances, or reduced enterohepatic recycling. Possible confounding mechanisms include a reduction in dietary vitamin K_1 intake because of illness, or the effect of fever or infection on coagulation or drug metabolism.

Clinical evidence and mechanism

Various studies have implicated antibacterials in general as being a risk factor for overanticoagulation. For example, in a large prospective cohort study, INR levels of greater than 7 were recorded in 31 patients. When compared with 100 patients with stable INRs, these 31 patients were more likely to have been treated with an antibacterial (not specified) in the previous 4 weeks (odds ratio 6.2), and more likely to have an intercurrent illness (odds ratio 4.48).[1] Various mechanisms may be responsible for these findings, and these are discussed below.

(a) Confounding effects relating to the infection

1. Dietary factors. Patients taking coumarins and related drugs are advised to maintain a constant dietary intake of 'vitamin K_1', (p.409), since sustained changes in intake of vitamin K_1-rich foods, such as green leafy vegetables, causes clinically relevant changes in anticoagulation. It is therefore possible that patients who stop eating for a more than a day or so could develop over-anticoagulation. The same could happen with a reduced appetite leading to a sustained reduction in intake of vitamin K_1-rich foods.

2. Fever. Fever might possibly be a confounding factor in reports of antibacterial warfarin interactions, because it might increase the catabolism of vitamin K-dependent coagulation factors by producing a hypermetabolic state. However, in one cohort study, there was no difference in the frequency of fever between patients who developed over-anticoagulation (INR greater than 6) while taking antibacterials and those who did not develop over-anticoagulation while taking antibacterials.[2]

3. Reduced metabolism. There is some evidence from *animal* studies that infection can down regulate cytochrome P450 isoenzymes, which might result in reduced drug metabolism.[3] Whether the metabolism of warfarin is different during an acute infection does not appear to have been studied.

(b) Effects relating to the antibacterial

1. Direct anticoagulant effects. Cephalosporins and related beta lactams with an *N*-methylthiotetrazole or similar side-chain can occasionally cause enough hypoprothrombinaemia for bleeding to occur when they are used alone, and this effect might therefore be additive with coumarins, although there is not that much evidence to support this, see 'Coumarins + Antibacterials; Cephalosporins and related beta lactams', p.367.

2. Intestinal production of vitamin K_2 substances by bacteria. The activity of intestinal microflora produces menaquinones (vitamin K_2 substances). Suppression of the microflora might therefore result in reduced vitamin K_2, and hence reduced synthesis of vitamin-K dependent clotting factors. There is some evidence from studies in healthy subjects receiving vitamin-K_1 restricted diets and taking warfarin that giving menaquinones (an extract of bacterially synthesised material) decreases the response to warfarin.[4] In addition, 'Natto', (p.408), which is a rich source of bacterially-derived menaquinones markedly inhibits the effect of warfarin. It is therefore possible that antibacterials that decimate gut microflora might increase the effect of warfarin by reducing vitamin K_2 levels. However, this effect might be important only if vitamin-K_1 intake from dietary sources is also reduced.

3. Protein-binding displacement. Many drugs can displace warfarin from protein-binding sites leading to an increase in unbound (active) concentrations. However, any effect is transient, as the unbound warfarin is quickly metabolised. The exception to this is if the metabolism of warfarin is markedly inhibited at the same time. The only drug that is known to interact via both these mechanisms is 'phenylbutazone', (p.434). Consider also 'Protein-binding interactions', (p.3). Altered protein binding has not clearly been shown to be an important mechanism in any interaction between warfarin and an antibacterial, but it is often suggested as one.

4. Reduced or increased metabolism. Sulfamethoxazole clearly inhibits the metabolism of warfarin by the cytochrome P450 isoenzyme CYP2C9, so enhancing its effect. Some macrolides such as erythromycin inhibit CYP3A4, and therefore have a minor inhibitory effect on warfarin, which would, on its own, be unlikely to be of any clinical relevance. Conversely, 'rifamycins', (p.375) are well established inducers of drug metabolism, and clearly reduce the effect of warfarin. Most other antibacterial classes have no effect on warfarin pharmacokinetics.

Importance and management

All these factors in their own right might affect the intensity of anticoagulation. Therefore, a few case reports of an enhanced response to warfarin on starting a specific antibacterial does not necessarily imply that the antibacterial has a direct interaction with warfarin. Conversely, demonstration of a lack of a specific interaction between an antibacterial and warfarin does not mean that a patient prescribed that drug for an infection will not have a change in coagulation status. Therefore, if a patient is unwell enough to require an antibacterial, it may be prudent to increase monitoring of coagulation status even if no interaction is expected. Monitor within 3 days of starting the antibacterial. The expectation of an interaction should not exclude the use of an antibacterial if it is considered clinically appropriate.

1. Panneerselvam S, Baglin C, Lefort W, Baglin T. Analysis of risk factors for over-anticoagulation in patient receiving long-term warfarin. *Br J Haematol* (1998) 103, 422–4.
2. Visser LE, Penning-van Beest FJA, Kasbergen AAH, De Smet PAGM, Vulto AG, Hofman A, Stricker BHC. Overanticoagulation associated with combined use of antibacterial drugs and acenocoumarol or phenprocoumon anticoagulants. *Thromb Haemost* (2002) 88, 705–10.
3. Eschenauer G, Collins CD, Regal RE. Azithromycin-warfarin interaction: are we fishing with a red herring? *Pharmacotherapy* (2005) 25, 630–1.
4. Conly JM, Stein K, Worobetz L, Rutledge-Harding S. The contribution of vitamin K2 (menaquinones) produced by the intestinal microflora to human nutritional requirements for vitamin K. *Am J Gastroenterol* (1994) 89, 915–23.

Coumarins and related drugs + Antibacterials; Aminoglycosides

Limited data suggest that no clinically significant interaction occurs between dicoumarol or warfarin and oral neomycin or paromomycin in most patients. However, individual patients have shown some alteration in anticoagulant effect (usually increases) when given oral neomycin and parenteral streptomycin.

Clinical evidence

Six out of 10 patients taking **warfarin** who were given oral **neomycin** (2 g daily[1] or 4 g daily[2]) over a 3-week period had a gradual increase in their prothrombin times averaging 5.6 seconds.[1,2]

In patients taking an unnamed anticoagulant, 2 of 5 given oral **neomycin** with bacitracin had a fall in their prothrombin-proconvertin concentration from a range of 10 to 30% to less than 6%. Similarly, one of 3 patients given parenteral **streptomycin** 500 mg twice daily, and 2 patients given parenteral **streptomycin** 500 mg twice daily with 1 million units of penicillin daily had a fall in their prothrombin-proconvertin concentration from a range of 10 to 30% down to 6 to 9%.[3] This suggests an *increase* in anticoagulant effect. Five of 7 patients taking unnamed anticoagulants had no change in their mean daily dose of anticoagulant when given oral **neomycin** 1 to 2 g daily for 18 weeks. Of the remaining two, one required an increase of about 100%, and one required a small 27% decrease.[4] The concurrent use of oral **paromomycin** 2 g daily with **dicoumarol** or **warfarin** did not alter anticoagulant requirements in 2 subjects.[5]

Mechanism

Not understood. One idea is that these antibacterials increase the anticoagulant effects by diminishing the bacterial population in the gut, thereby reducing their production of vitamin K_2 substances, see 'Coumarins + Antibacterials', p.365. Another suggestion is that these antibacterials decrease the vitamin K_1 absorption as part of a general antibacterial-induced malabsorption syndrome.[6]

Importance and management

A sparsely documented interaction but common experience seems to confirm that normally no interaction of any significance occurs. Concurrent use need not be avoided. Occasionally vitamin K deficiency and/or spontaneous bleeding is seen after the prolonged use of broad-spectrum antibacterials combined with a totally inadequate diet, starvation or some other condition in which the intake of vitamin K is very limited.[7,8] Under these circumstances the effects of the oral anticoagulants (coumarins and **indanediones**) would be expected to be significantly increased and appropriate precautions should be taken. There is nothing to suggest that an adverse interaction occurs between the oral anticoagulants and other parenteral aminoglycosides.

1. Udall JA. Drug interference with warfarin therapy. *Clin Med* (1970) 77, 20–25.
2. Udall JA. Human sources and absorption of vitamin K in relation to anticoagulation stability. *JAMA* (1965) 194, 107–9.
3. Magid E. Tolerance to anticoagulants during antibiotic therapy. *Scand J Clin Lab Invest* (1962) 14, 565–6.
4. Schade RWB, van't Laar A, Majoor CLH, Jansen AP. A comparative study of the effects of cholestyramine and neomycin in the treatment of type II hyperlipoproteinaemia. *Acta Med Scand* (1976) 199, 175–80.
5. Messinger WJ, Samet CM. The effect of a bowel sterilizing antibiotic on blood coagulation mechanisms. The anti-cholesterol effect of paromomycin. *Angiology* (1965) 16, 29–36.
6. Faloon WW, Paes IC, Woolfolk D, Nankin H, Wallace K, Haro EN. Effect of neomycin and kanamycin upon intestinal absorption. *Ann N Y Acad Sci* (1966) 132, 879–87.
7. Haden HT. Vitamin K deficiency associated with prolonged antibiotic administration. *Arch Intern Med* (1957) 100, 986–8.
8. Frick PG, Riedler G, Brögli H. Dose response and minimal daily requirement for vitamin K in man. *J Appl Physiol* (1967) 23, 387–9.

Coumarins + Antibacterials; Aminosalicylic acid and/or Isoniazid

A report attributes bleeding in a patient taking warfarin to the concurrent use of isoniazid. Another report describes a markedly increased anticoagulant response in a patient taking warfarin when the dose was doubled and aminosalicylic acid and isoniazid were started. In one study, isoniazid inhibited warfarin metabolism *in vitro*.

Clinical evidence

A man who had recently started to take **warfarin** 10 mg daily and isoniazid 300 mg daily began to bleed (haematuria, bleeding gums) within 10 days of accidentally doubling his dosage of isoniazid. His prothrombin time had increased from about 26 to 53 seconds.[1]

Another patient taking digoxin, potassium chloride, docusate, diazepam and **warfarin** 2.5 mg daily, was also given aminosalicylic acid 12 g, isoniazid 300 mg and pyridoxine 100 mg daily, and at the same time the warfarin dose was doubled to 5 mg daily. His prothrombin time increased from 18 to 130 seconds over 20 days but no signs of haemorrhage were seen.[2]

Mechanism

Not understood. It seems possible that isoniazid may inhibit the metabolism of the coumarin anticoagulants, since *in vitro* study in human liver microsomes has shown it inhibits *S*-warfarin 7-hydroxylation by the cytochrome P450 isoenzyme CYP2C9,[3] but this needs confirmation *in vivo*. Isoniazid increased the anticoagulant effects of dicoumarol in *dogs*[4] but not of warfarin in *rabbits*.[5] Two patients taking isoniazid, aminosalicylic acid and streptomycin (but not taking anticoagulants) developed haemorrhage attributed to the anticoagulant effects of isoniazid.[6]

Importance and management

These two isolated cases of possible interactions are far from conclusive, and the interactions of warfarin with isoniazid and aminosalicylic acid are not established. Nevertheless, given that the *in vitro* data suggest that isoniazid might inhibit warfarin metabolism, some caution might be appropriate. Further study is needed.

1. Rosenthal AR, Self TH, Baker ED, Linden RA. Interaction of isoniazid and warfarin. *JAMA* (1977) 238, 2177.
2. Self TH. Interaction of warfarin and aminosalicylic acid. *JAMA* (1973) 223, 1285.
3. Nishimura Y, Kurata N, Sakurai E, Yasuhara H. Inhibitory effect of antituberculosis drugs on human cytochrome P450-mediated activities. *J Pharmacol Sci* (2004) 96, 293–300.
4. Eade NR, McLeod PJ, MacLeod SM. Potentiation of bishydroxycoumarin in dogs by isoniazid and p-aminosalicylic acid. *Am Rev Respir Dis* (1971) 103, 792–9.
5. Kiblawi SS, Jay SJ, Bang NU, Rowe HM. Influence of isoniazid on the anticoagulant effect of warfarin. *Clin Ther* (1979) 2, 235–9.
6. Castell FA. Accion anticoagulante de la isoniazida. *Enferm Torax* (1969) 18, 153–62.

Coumarins + Antibacterials; Cephalosporins and related beta lactams

Cephalosporins and related beta lactams with an *N*-methylthiotetrazole or similar side-chain can occasionally cause enough hypoprothrombinaemia for bleeding to occur when they are used alone. These effects could therefore be additive with those of the coumarins, and this appears to have been shown in a study with cefamandole or cefazolin and warfarin. Similarly, a few cases of over-anticoagulation have been reported with cefonicid and cefotiam in patients taking acenocoumarol or warfarin. Although not having an *N*-methylthiotetrazole side-chain, the manufacturers of cefixime and cefaclor have on record a few cases of over-anticoagulation. Cephalosporins and related beta lactams that have caused increases in prothrombin times when used alone, and might therefore be predicted to interact, include aztreonam, cefalotin, cefoperazone, ceftriaxone, and latamoxef. Other cephalosporins with a related side-chain include cefmenoxime, cefmetazole, cefminox, ceforanide, cefotetan and cefpiramide.

Clinical evidence

(a) Cephalosporins with N-methylthiotetrazole or similar side-chains

1. Cefamandole or cefazolin. Two patients who had received prophylactic cefamandole before cardiac valve replacement developed unusually high prothrombin times, with bleeding in one case, within 48 hours of an initial dose of **warfarin** 10 mg. Because of this, the records of a total of 60 other patients who had undergoing heart valve replacement surgery were reviewed. They had been given antibacterials prophylactically before the chest incision was made, and every 6 hours thereafter for about 72 hours. The 44 patients given cefamandole 2 g showed a much greater anticoagulant response than the 16 patients given vancomycin 500 mg. Fourteen of the cefamandole group had a prothrombin time greater than 32 seconds after the initial warfarin dose, compared with only one of the vancomycin group.[1] In a later randomised study by the same workers, the prothrombin times as a percentage of activity after 3 days of concurrent use with **warfarin** were as follows: cefamandole 29%, cefazolin 38%, and vancomycin 51%, suggesting that cefamandole had a much greater effect on anticoagulant response than vancomycin.[2]

2. Cefonicid. In a study in 9 patients stabilised on **warfarin**, there was no change in prothrombin times when they were given intravenous cefonicid 2 g daily for 7 days.[3] In contrast, a later study identified 9 patients taking **acenocoumarol** who had increased INRs within 3 to 8 days of being given cefonicid. They needed a reduction in the anticoagulant dosage of about one-third to one-half.[4] Another patient stabilised on **acenocoumarol**, with a prothrombin index of 28% bled 2 days after starting cefonicid 1 g daily and had a prothrombin index of less than 5%.[5]

3. Cefotiam. Severe haemorrhage has been reported in 3 patients taking **acenocoumarol** with cefotiam. One developed an abdominal haematoma and an INR of 10.4 within 2 days. Another had gastrointestinal bleeding and melaena after one day of concurrent use. The third died from intracranial haemorrhage on the day she started cefotiam.[6]

(b) Cephalosporins without N-methylthiotetrazole or similar side-chains

1. Cefaclor. Over the period 1979 to 1997, there had been 3 cases of raised INRs with or without clinical bleeding in patients taking **acenocoumarol**, **warfarin** or an unknown anticoagulant and cefaclor reported to the CSM in the UK.[7] No cases seem to have been published.

2. Cefixime. Cefixime has also been implicated in a handful of cases of bleeding and/or increased INRs in patients taking **warfarin** or **phenindione**, but the evidence is inconclusive.[8] No cases seem to have been published.

(c) Unnamed cephalosporins

None of 36 patients taking warfarin and prescribed an oral cephalosporin (not named) experienced a change in their INR in a prospective study of the effect of antibacterials on anticoagulation.[9]

Mechanism

Cephalosporins with an *N*-methylthiotetrazole side-chain can, like the oral anticoagulants, act as vitamin K antagonists to reduce the production of some blood clotting factors. They can therefore cause bleeding on their own. For example, serious bleeding following the use of **cefamandole** (in the absence of an anticoagulant) has been described in 3 out of 37 patients in one report,[10] and a further report highlights a further 16 cases.[11] Other similar cephalosporins and related beta lactams that have been reported to cause hypoprothrombinaemia when used alone include cefoperazone,[12-16] cefotetan,[17] ceftriaxone,[18] cefalotin,[19] cefazolin,[20-22] and latamoxef.[23,24] The incidence is very variable: in some instances only isolated cases have been reported whereas a 15% bleeding rate was found in one study[24] with latamoxef alone, 22% in another[23], but only 8% with cefoxitin alone.[23] These cephalosporins might therefore worsen the risk of bleeding by simple addition if given with coumarin or **indanedione** anticoagulants. In addition, some of them may also inhibit platelet function.[25] Ceftriaxone seems to act similarly although it has an *N*-methylthio*triazine* ring instead, as does cefazolin, which has an *N*-methylthiadiazolethiol side-chain. **Aztreonam** can also increase the prothrombin time.[26-29] See also 'antibacterials', (p.365).

Importance and management

Most cephalosporins and related beta lactams do not normally cause bleeding so would not be expected to have an additive interaction with the oral anticoagulants. In contrast, cephalosporins with the *N*-methylthiotetrazole side-chain appear to increase the risk of bleeding, and might therefore interact. Both **cefamandole** and to a lesser extent **cefazolin** have been shown to increase the response to warfarin, and cases of over-anticoagulation have been reported for **cefonicid** and **cefotiam**. All other cephalosporins and related beta-lactams with the *N*-methylthiotetrazole or similar side-chain might be expected to behave similarly, but have not so far been reported to do so. These include **cefalotin**, **cefmenoxime**, **cefmetazole**, **cefminox**, **cefoperazone**, **ceforanide**, **cefotetan**, **cefpiramide**, **ceftriaxone**, and **latamoxef**. **Aztreonam** has also been predicted to interact similarly, although, again there are no reports. Although not having an *N*-methylthiotetrazole side-chain, the manufacturers of **cefixime** and **cefaclor** have on record a few cases of over-anticoagulation.

Patients most at risk seem to be those whose intake of vitamin K is restricted (poor diet, malabsorption syndromes, etc.) and those with renal failure. The use of an anticoagulant represents just another factor that may precipitate bleeding.

A possible solution to the problem is to use a non-interacting cephalosporin. Alternatively you should monitor the outcome closely, particularly in the early stages of treatment, adjusting the anticoagulant dosage if necessary. Excessive hypoprothrombinaemia can be controlled with vitamin K.

1. Angaran DM, Dias VC, Arom KV, Northrup WF, Kersten TE, Lindsay WG, Nicoloff DM. The influence of prophylactic antibiotics on the warfarin anticoagulation response in the postoperative prosthetic cardiac valve patient. *Ann Surg* (1984) 199, 107–111.

2. Angaran DM, Dias VC, Arom KV, Northrup WF, Kersten TG, Lindsay WG, Nicoloff DM. The comparative influence of prophylactic antibiotics on the prothrombin response to warfarin in the postoperative prosthetic cardiac valve patient. *Ann Surg* (1987) 206, 155–61.
3. Angaran DM, Tschida VH, Copa AK. Effect of cefonicid (CN) on prothrombin time (PT) in outpatients (OP) receiving warfarin (W) therapy. *Pharmacotherapy* (1988) 8, 120.
4. Puente Garcia M, Bécares Martínez FJ, Merlo Arroyo J, García Sánchez G, García Díaz B, Cervero Jiménez M. Potenciación del efecto anticoagulante del acenocoumarol por cefonicid. *Rev Clin Esp* (1999) 199, 620–1.
5. Riancho JA, Olmos JM, Sedano C. Life-threatening bleeding in a patient being treated with cefonicid. *Ann Intern Med* (1995) 123, 472–3.
6. Gras-Champel V, Sauvé L, Perault MC, Laine P, Gouello JP, Decocq G, Masson H, Touzard M, Andréjak M. Association cefotiam et acenocoumarol: a propos de 3 cas d'hémorragies. *Therapie* (1998) 53, 191.
7. Eli Lilly and Company Limited. Personal communication, December 1997.
8. Lederle Laboratories. Personal communication, December 1995.
9. Pharmacy Anticoagulant Clinic Study Group. A multicentre survey of antibiotics on the INR of anticoagulated patients. *Pharm J* (1996) 257 (Pharmacy Practice Suppl), R30.
10. Hooper CA, Haney BB, Stone HH. Gastrointestinal bleeding due to vitamin K deficiency in patients on parenteral cefamandole. *Lancet* (1980) i, 39–40.
11. Rymer W, Greenlaw CW. Hypoprothrombinemia associated with cefamandole. *Drug Intell Clin Pharm* (1980) 14, 780–3.
12. Meisel S. Hypoprothrombinemia due to cefoperazone. *Drug Intell Clin Pharm* (1984) 18, 316.
13. Cristiano P. Hypoprothrombinemia associated with cefoperazone treatment. *Drug Intell Clin Pharm* (1984) 18, 314–16.
14. Osborne JC. Hypoprothrombinemia and bleeding due to cefoperazone. *Ann Intern Med* (1985) 102, 721–2.
15. Freedy HR, Cetnarowski AB, Lumish RM, Schafer FJ. Cefoperazone-induced coagulopathy. *Drug Intell Clin Pharm* (1986) 20, 281–3.
16. Andrassy K, Koderisch J, Fritz S, Bechtold H, Sonntag H. Alteration of hemostasis associated with cefoperazone treatment. *Infection* (1986) 14, 27–31.
17. Conjura A, Bell W, Lipsky JJ. Cefotetan and hypoprothrombinemia. *Ann Intern Med* (1988) 108, 643.
18. Haubenstock A, Schmidt P, Zazgornik J, Balcke P, Kopsa H. Hypoprothrombinaemic bleeding associated with ceftriaxone. *Lancet* (1983) i, 1215–16.
19. Natelson EA, Brown CH, Bradshaw MW, Alfrey CP, Williams TW. Influence of cephalosporin antibiotics on blood coagulation and platelet function. *Antimicrob Agents Chemother* (1976) 9, 91–3.
20. Lerner PI, Lubin A. Coagulopathy with cefazolin in uremia. *N Engl J Med* (1974) 290, 1324.
21. Khaleeli M, Giorgio AJ. Defective platelet function after cephalosporin administration. *Blood* (1976) 48, 971.
22. Dupuis LL, Paton TW, Suttie JW, Thiessen JJ, Rachlis A. Cefazolin-induced coagulopathy. *Clin Pharmacol Ther* (1984) 35, 237.
23. Brown RB, Klar J, Lemeshow S, Teres D, Pastides H, Sands M. Enhanced bleeding with cefoxitin or moxalactam. Statistical analysis within a defined population of 1493 patients. *Arch Intern Med* (1986) 146, 2159–64.
24. Morris DL, Fabricius PJ, Ambrose NS, Scammell B, Burdon DW, Keighley MRB. A high incidence of bleeding is observed in a trial to determine whether addition of metronidazole is neeeded with latamoxef for prophylaxis in colorectal surgery. *J Hosp Infect* (1984) 5, 398–408.
25. Bang NU, Tessler SS, Heidenreich RO, Marks CA, Mattler LE. Effects of moxalactam on blood coagulation and platelet function. *Rev Infect Dis* (1982) 4 (Suppl), S546–S554.
26. Bodey G, Reuben A, Elting L, Kantarjian H, Keating M, Hagemeister F, Koller C, Velasquez W, Papadopoulos N. Comparison of two schedules of cefoperazone plus aztreonam in the treatment of neutropenic patients with fever. *Eur J Clin Microbiol Infect Dis* (1991) 10, 551–8.
27. Rusconi F, Assael BM, Boccazzi A, Colombo R, Crossignani RM, Garlaschi L, Rancilio L. Aztreonam in the treatment of severe urinary tract infections in pediatric patients. *Antimicrob Agents Chemother* (1986) 30, 310–14.
28. Giamarellou H, Galanakis N, Dendrinos CH, Kanellakopoulou K, Petrikkos G, Koratzanis G, Daikos GK. Clinical experience with aztreonam in a variety of gram-negative infections. *Chemioterapia* (1985) 4 (Suppl 1), 75–80.
29. Giamerellou H, Koratzanis G, Kanellakopoulou K, Galanakis N, Papoulias G, El Messidi M, Daikos G. Aztreonam versus cefamandole in the treatment of urinary tract infections. *Chemioterapia* (1984) 3, 127–31.

Coumarins + Antibacterials; Chloramphenicol

There is some limited evidence to suggest that the anticoagulant effects of acenocoumarol and dicoumarol can be increased by oral chloramphenicol. An isolated report attributes a marked INR rise in a patient taking warfarin to the use of chloramphenicol eye drops.

Clinical evidence

A study in 4 patients showed that the half-life of **dicoumarol** was increased on average from 8 to 25 hours when they were given oral chloramphenicol 2 g daily for 5 to 8 days.[1]

Three out of 9 patients taking an unnamed anticoagulant had a fall in their prothrombin-proconvertin values from a range of 10 to 30% down to less than 6% (suggesting an increased anticoagulant effect) when given oral chloramphenicol 1 to 2 g daily for 4 to 6 days. One patient had a smaller reduction.[2] In early clinical experience with **acenocoumarol**, one of 3 patients taking chloramphenicol had greater sensitivity to the anticoagulant.[3]

An isolated report describes an 83-year-old woman stabilised on **warfarin** who showed a rise in her INR to about 8.9 from her normal range of 1.9 to 2.8 within 2 weeks of starting to use eye drops containing chloramphenicol 5 mg/mL, dexamethasone sodium phosphate 1 mg/mL and tetrahydrozoline hydrochloride 0.25 mg/mL. She used one drop in each eye four times daily.[4] Hypoprothrombinaemia and bleeding have also been described in patients given intramuscular,[5] intravenous,[5] or oral[6] chloramphenicol in the absence of an anticoagulant.

Mechanism

Uncertain. One suggestion is that the chloramphenicol inhibits the liver enzymes concerned with the metabolism of the anticoagulants so that their effects are prolonged and increased.[4] *In vitro* work with human liver microsomes showed that chloramphenicol did not inhibit the hydroxylation of *S*-warfarin, but it did inhibit *R*-warfarin metabolism, probably via CYP3A4.[7] Another suggestion is that the antibacterial diminishes the gut bacteria thereby decreasing a source of vitamin K, but it is doubtful if these bacteria are normally an important source of the vitamin except in exceptional cases where dietary levels are very inadequate.[8] A third suggestion is that chloramphenicol blocks production of prothrombin by the liver.[5] See also 'antibacterials', (p.365)

Importance and management

The documentation for the interaction between anticoagulants and oral chloramphenicol is very sparse and poor (the best being the pharmacokinetic report about dicoumarol) so that this interaction is by no means adequately established. There would therefore appear to be little reason for avoiding concurrent use, but it would seem prudent to monitor prothrombin times if oral chloramphenicol is started in patients taking a coumarin, being alert for the need to reduce the anticoagulant dosage.

The report about an apparent interaction between warfarin and topical chloramphenicol is very surprising because the amount of chloramphenicol absorbed from eye drops is relatively small and because, despite the very widespread use of warfarin and chloramphenicol for very many years, this report appears to be the only one. This suggests that any such interaction is very unlikely indeed, however the ultracautious may wish to monitor the outcome if topical chloramphenicol is used.

1. Christensen LK, Skovsted L. Inhibition of drug metabolism by chloramphenicol. *Lancet* (1969) ii, 1397–9.
2. Magid E. Tolerance to anticoagulants during antibiotic therapy. *Scand J Clin Lab Invest* (1962) 14, 565–6.
3. Johnson R, David A, Chartier Y. Clinical experience with G-23350 (Sintrom). *Can Med Assoc J* (1957) 77, 756–61.
4. Leone R, Ghiotto E, Conforti A, Velo G. Potential interaction between warfarin and ocular chloramphenicol. *Ann Pharmacother* (1999) 33, 114.
5. Klippel AP, Pitsinger B. Hypoprothrombinemia secondary to antibiotic therapy and manifested by massive gastrointestinal hemorrhage. *Arch Surg* (1968) 96, 266–8.
6. Matsaniotis N, Messaritakis J, Vlachou C. Hypoprothrombinaemic bleeding in infants associated with diarrhoea and antibiotics. *Arch Dis Child* (1970) 45, 586–7.
7. Park J-Y, Kim K-A, Kim S-L. Chloramphenicol is a potent inhibitor of cytochrome P450 isoforms CYP2C19 and CYP3A4 in human liver microsomes. *Antimicrob Agents Chemother* (2003) 47, 3464–9.
8. Udall JA. Human sources and absorption of vitamin K in relation to anticoagulation stability. *JAMA* (1965), 194, 107–9.

Coumarins + Antibacterials; Clindamycin

An isolated report describes bleeding and a markedly increased INR in a woman stabilised on warfarin, which was tentatively attributed to an interaction with clindamycin. Another report found no cases of a serious increase in INR in patients taking acenocoumarol or phenprocoumon with clindamycin.

Clinical evidence, mechanism, importance and management

A 47-year-old woman with multiple medical problems stabilised on **warfarin** (and also taking azathioprine, captopril, furosemide, insulin, captopril, prednisone, levothyroxine, valproic acid and zolpidem) had all her teeth removed under general anaesthetic. Sixteen days later she needed a dental abscess drained and was given oral clindamycin 300 mg four times daily with ibuprofen 600 mg for any discomfort. On day 17 she needed a suture to stop some bleeding and her INR was found to be 3.5. By day 20 she had developed more severe oral bleeding, which needed emergency room treatment. Her INR was found to have risen to 13 and her haematocrit decreased to 18%. She was treated successfully with a blood transfusion and vitamin K.[1]

This appears to be an isolated case, from which no general conclusions should be drawn (see also 'antibacterials', (p.365)) because the whole picture is so uncertain. Note that in a cohort study, none of 37 patients stabilised on **acenocoumarol** or **phenprocoumon** developed over-anticoagulation (an INR greater than 6) when they were given clindamycin.[2]

1. Aldous JA, Olson CJ. Managing patients on warfarin therapy: a case report. *Spec Care Dentist* (2001) 21, 109–112.
2. Visser LE, Penning-van Beest FJA, Kasbergen AAH, De Smet PAGM, Vulto AG, Hofman A, Stricker BHC. Overanticoagulation associated with combined use of antibacterial drugs and acenocoumarol or phenprocoumon anticoagulants. *Thromb Haemost* (2002) 88, 705–10.

Coumarins + Antibacterials; Linezolid

Linezolid had only minor effects on the pharmacokinetics and anticoagulant activity of single-dose warfarin, which were not considered to be clinically significant.

Clinical evidence, mechanism, importance and management

Linezolid 600 mg twice daily was given to 13 healthy subjects for 5 days followed by a single 25-mg dose of **warfarin**. The pharmacokinetics of warfarin with linezolid were within 20% of those seen with warfarin alone, and the INR was minimally affected (about a 10% increase in maximal INR).[1] These effects were not considered to be clinically relevant. See also 'antibacterials', (p.365).

1. Azie NE, Stalker DJ, Jungbluth GL, Sisson T, Adams G. Effect of linezolid on CYP2C9 using racemic warfarin (W) as a probe. *Clin Pharmacol Ther* (2001) 69, 21.

Coumarins + Antibacterials; Macrolides

Most studies suggest that macrolides do not significantly alter the pharmacokinetics or anticoagulant effects of warfarin. There is less information about other anticoagulants but studies similarly suggest that acenocoumarol and phenprocoumon do not usually interact with the macrolides; however one study has suggested that clarithromycin increases the risk of bleeding in patients taking these coumarins. Furthermore, a number of case reports describe bleeding in patients taking coumarins and macrolides.

Clinical evidence

(a) Azithromycin

There are no studies of the effect of azithromycin on the pharmacokinetics of coumarins. One pharmacodynamic study and two case series suggest no interaction occurs with warfarin. However, at least 7 published case reports suggest an interaction might occur. These are discussed below.

The manufacturer notes that a 5-day course of azithromycin (500 mg on day one then 250 mg daily for 4 days) did not affect the prothrombin time response to a single 15-mg dose of warfarin in healthy subjects.[1,2] A retrospective study of 26 patients stabilised on warfarin found no evidence that treatment with azithromycin had any effect on their INRs. The patients had stable INRs for a least 2 consecutive records before receiving azithromycin, and an INR taken within 14 days (9 patients) or 30 days (17 patients) of starting the azithromycin.[3] The same finding was reported in another similar smaller study in 17 patients.[4] A major disadvantage of these 2 retrospective studies is the small numbers of patients who had an INR value within 7 days of starting azithromycin.

In contrast, there are now a number of published case reports suggesting that azithromycin might potentiate the activity of warfarin.[5-11] In one of these cases, a 57-year-old woman stabilised on warfarin with an INR ranging from 1.75 to 3.03 in the previous 3 months was prescribed a 5-day course of azithromycin (500 mg on day one, then 250 mg daily for 4 days) for a possible upper respiratory tract infection. Two days after completing the azithromycin, a routine INR was found to be 8.32. She had no signs or symptoms of bleeding. During the infection she had a fever on the second day, and she reduced her 'smoking', (p.456) from 1 pack of cigarettes daily to 1 pack over 3 days.[9] In other cases, a rise in INR of 1.4-fold to sixfold occurred within 1 to 7 days of starting azithromycin.[5-8,10,11] Three patients had bleeding complications,[6,7,10] and 4 required vitamin K administration.[6-8,10] Most of these patients had possible confounding factors such as recent increases in warfarin dose,[7,8] other concurrent antibacterials,[8,11] fever and decreased appetite,[5,10] or complex disease states and heart failure.[6-8,10]

The manufacturers[12] say that as of December 1998, they had received 47 reports (40 in the US, 7 elsewhere in the world, including 2 in the UK) of possible interactions between azithromycin and warfarin. A 2004 report from the Australian Adverse Drug Reactions Advisory Committee said they had received 3 reports of interactions between warfarin and azithromycin,[13] which presumably includes the 2 published cases.[8]

(b) Clarithromycin

There are no studies of the effect of clarithromycin on the pharmacokinetics or anticoagulant activity of coumarins. However, there are at least 13 cases of increased INRs in published reports, and one cohort study suggesting that the use of clarithromycin is associated with an increased risk of bleeding in patients taking coumarins. These are discussed below.

1. Acenocoumarol. The INR of a 75-year-old woman stabilised on acenocoumarol rose from 2.1 to 9 within a week of starting to take clarithromycin 250 mg twice daily.[14] Five patients stabilised on acenocoumarol had a mean increase in their INRs from about 2.5 to 5.5 when they took clarithromycin.[15] The largest increase was from 1.95 to 7.01. In one cohort study in patients taking acenocoumarol or phenprocoumon, clarithromycin significantly increased the risk of overanticoagulation (INR greater than 6: relative risk of 11.7 range 3.6 to 37.8). The risk was highest during the first 3 days of combined use.[16]

2. Phenprocoumon. A 70-year-old woman stabilised on phenprocoumon developed a marked increase in prothrombin time from a range of 140 to 180 seconds up to 304 seconds, but no bleeding, within 4 days of starting to take clarithromycin 500 mg daily. The phenprocoumon was stopped and phytomenadione given. When the antibacterial was withdrawn she was restabilised on the original dosage of phenprocoumon.[17] For discussion of a cohort study in patients stabilised on phenprocoumon or acenocoumarol, which showed an increased risk of over-anticoagulation with clarithromycin, see *Acenocoumarol*, above.

3. Warfarin. In 1992 the CSM in the UK notified prescribers in the UK of a case of a woman taking warfarin for mitral valve disease who suffered a fatal cerebrovascular bleed 3 days after starting to take clarithromycin.[18] Her INR was above 10. A further patient stabilised on warfarin had a suprachoroidal haemorrhage 7 days after starting clarithromycin 250 mg twice daily, with permanent vision loss. Her INR was 8.2. She had a normal INR (2.3) three days prior to starting clarithromycin, and also 3 days after starting the course (2.9).[19]
Other patients taking warfarin have been found to have INRs of 5.6 five days after starting clarithromycin,[20] of 90.3 five days after completing a 10-day course of clarithromycin,[20] of 17 five days after finishing a 14-day course of clarithromycin,[21] and of 7.3 within 12 days of starting clarithromycin.[22] None of these patients had bleeding complications. In a brief report in 2004, the Adverse Drug Reactions Advisory Committee of Australia state that they had received 6 reports of interactions between clarithromycin and warfarin (median INR of 7.6), two of which were symptomatic.[13]

(c) Dirithromycin

In a study in 15 healthy subjects the pharmacokinetics and pharmacodynamics of a single 0.5-mg/kg dose of warfarin were not altered when it was given on day 10 of a 14-day course of dirithromycin 500 mg daily.[23]

(d) Erythromycin

Erythromycin caused a minor inhibition of warfarin metabolism in three pharmacokinetic studies, and there are at least 11 published cases of interactions with coumarins, and 19 cases mentioned in a report from the Adverse Drug Reactions Advisory Committee of Australia. These are discussed below.

1. Acenocoumarol. Haematuria occurred in a patient stabilised on acenocoumarol on the last day of a 14-day course of erythromycin.[24] Another patient stabilised on acenocoumarol with an INR in the range of 3 to 4.5 was found to have an INR of 15 a week after starting to take erythromycin ethylsuccinate 1.5 g daily but no bleeding was seen.[25] Conversely, in one cohort study in patients taking acenocoumarol or phenprocoumon, no cases of over-anticoagulation (INR greater than 6) occurred in patients treated with erythromycin (78 patients received this antibacterial).[16] Note that this study did show an increase for *clarithromycin*, see above.

2. Warfarin. A study in 12 healthy subjects found that the clearance of a single 1-mg/kg dose of warfarin was reduced by an average of 14% (range 0 to about 30%) when taken on day 5 of an 8-day course of erythromycin 250 mg every 6 hours. This change was greatest in those subjects with relatively slow warfarin clearance rates.[26] In another similar study, warfarin 0.5 mg/kg, given on day 10 of a 14-day course of erythromycin 250 mg four times daily increased the AUC of *S*-warfarin by 11.2% and of *R*-warfarin by 11.9%. The INR increased by 10.2%.[23] Similar effects were seen in another study in 8 patients stabilised on warfarin and who did not have infections. In these patients, erythromycin 333 mg three times daily for 7 days caused a mean 9.9% increase in the prothrombin time ratio, which was maximal by day 2 to 5. There was also a mean 9.4% increase in total plasma warfarin level, which was similar for the *S*- and *R* -enantiomers, and was maximal by day 7. No patient had a prothrombin time ratio above the therapeutic range and none required a reduction in warfarin dose.[27]

In contrast to the modest effects in the above studies, various case reports have demonstrated a marked increase in INR. For example, an elderly woman taking warfarin developed haematuria and bruising within a week of starting to take erythromycin stearate 500 mg four times daily for a chest infection. Her prothrombin time had risen to 64 seconds (prothrombin time ratio about 5.5). Within the previous month she had started taking digoxin and quinidine, and had her warfarin dose increased because of a decrease in prothrombin time.[28] At least 8 other cases of bleeding and/or an increase in prothrombin time or INR have been described in patients taking warfarin with erythromycin (as the base, ethylsuccinate, stearate, or lactobionate).[29-35] In addition, in a brief report in 2004, the Adverse Drug Reactions Advisory Committee of Australia stated that they had received 19 reports of interactions between erythromycin and warfarin (median INR of 9.7), only 4 of which were symptomatic.[13]

There is also a case report of sulfonamide-induced bullous haemorrhagic eruption in a patient taking warfarin, 'co-trimoxazole', (p.376) and erythromycin, in which the authors considered an interaction between warfarin and erythromycin may have contributed to the haemorrhagic component.[36]

(e) Midecamycin diacetate

The pharmacokinetics of a single 8-mg oral dose of acenocoumarol were not significantly changed when it was taken on day 4 of a 9-day course of midecamycin diacetate 800 mg twice daily.[37]

(f) Roxithromycin

Roxithromycin did not alter the pharmacokinetics or effect of warfarin in one study. However, there are at least 2 published cases of interactions with coumarins, and one report reviewing 16 cases. These are discussed below.

1. Acenocoumarol. A 79-year-old man stabilised on acenocoumarol developed an abdominal wall haematoma 2 days after starting to take roxithromycin 150 mg twice daily for a lung infection.[38] Six days later, on admission to hospital, his INR was found to be 5.9. Conversely, in one cohort study in patients taking acenocoumarol or phenprocoumon, no cases of over-anticoagulation (INR greater than 6) occurred in patients treated with roxithromycin (only 14 patients received this antibacterial).[16] Note that this study did show an increase for *clarithromycin*, see above.

2. Phenprocoumon. A 75-year-old man taking phenprocoumon developed a marked increase in prothrombin time but no bleeding when he was given roxithromycin 300 mg daily for 5 days. The phenprocoumon was stopped and phytomenadione given. When the antibacterial was withdrawn he was restabilised on the original dosage of phenprocoumon.[17] For mention of a cohort study in patients stabilised on phenprocoumon or acenocoumarol showing no increased risk of overanticoagulation with roxithromycin, see *Acenocoumarol*, above.

3. Warfarin. In a study in which warfarin was given at a daily dose sufficient to maintain the thrombotest percentages at 10 to 20%, there was no difference in warfarin dose or AUC between 10 subjects given roxithromycin 150 mg twice daily for 2 weeks and 11 subjects given placebo. The dose of warfarin and the AUC of warfarin increased by about 10% in both the roxithromycin group and the placebo group, which was taken as indicating that steady state had not been achieved. Serum roxithromycin levels were unchanged by warfarin.[39] In contrast, during the 1992 to 1995 period The Centre for Adverse Reactions Monitoring of New Zealand received 7 reports of a possible interaction with roxithromycin resulting in increased warfarin effects, and, during the same period, the Adverse Drug Reactions Advisory Committee of Australia received 9 similar reports. Review of the 16 cases showed that 7 patients had clinical symptoms of over-anticoagulation, and the other 9 were asymptomatic and detected by routine testing.[40] In a 2004 update from ADRAC, it was noted that they now had on record 56 cases of an interaction between roxithromycin and warfarin, with 27 cases being symptomatic. The median INR was 8.8, and the median time to onset was 6 days. One fatality occurred in a 79-year-old woman who started taking warfarin and roxithromycin at the same time. By day 8, she had an INR of 11.6, and subsequently died from widespread bleeding.[13]

(g) Telithromycin

In a placebo-controlled, crossover study in healthy subjects, telithromycin 800 mg once daily for 7 days did not alter the pharmacodynamics of a single-dose of warfarin 25 mg given on day 4. There was a small 20% increase in the AUC of *R*-warfarin, and a 5% increase in the AUC of *S*-warfarin,[41] effects which the manufacturer does not consider to be clinically relevant.[42,43] Conversely, a 73-year-old man taking warfarin for a metallic valve replacement started taking telithromycin 800 mg daily for 5 days for a cough. On the last day of treatment he developed haemoptysis and was found to have an INR of 11. His INR 10 days before telithromycin was started was 3.1. The telithromycin was stopped and he was subsequently restabilised on warfarin.[44] Moreover, Health Canada reported that from May 2003 to September 2004 they had received 7 reports of suspected coagulation disorder interactions with telithromycin, 6 with warfarin and one with an unspecified oral anticoagulant. The INR was increased in 6 of the reports and decreased in the seventh.[45]

(h) Unspecified macrolides

The INR increased by an estimated 0.319 in 35 patients taking warfarin when prescribed an oral macrolide (not named) in a prospective study of the effect of antibacterials on anticoagulation.[46]

Mechanism

Erythromycin is a known inhibitor of the cytochrome P450 isoenzyme CYP3A4. However, this isoenzyme has only a minor role in the 'metabolism of warfarin', (p.358), specifically the less active *R*-isomer of warfarin. Consequently, only minor increases in the levels of warfarin have been seen in pharmacokinetic studies, which would generally not be expected to be clinically relevant. However, it is possible that even these small changes might be important in a very few patients, particularly those with a low prothrombin complex activity.[26] Other macrolides (azithromycin, clarithromycin, dirithromycin, roxithromycin) have less effect on CYP3A4 than erythromycin, and consequently would be expected to have even less effect on the pharmacokinetics of warfarin or acenocoumarol, which is borne out in the few studies available. Nevertheless, cases of interactions have been reported for nearly all these macrolides. Moreover, one cohort study found that clarithromycin increased the risk of an interaction and erythromycin did not. It is possible that there is some other, as yet unidentified, mechanism involved. Alternatively, it is equally possible that the relatively few cases just represent idiosyncratic effects attributable to other factors, and not to any interaction (see also 'Coumarins + Antibacterials', p.365).

Importance and management

The minor pharmacokinetic interaction with erythromycin and warfarin is established, but would not generally be expected to be clinically relevant. This is borne out by the relatively few published reports of an interaction (11 published case reports worldwide and 19 cases reported to the Adverse Drug Reactions Advisory Committee of Australia). Other macrolides would be even less likely to inhibit the metabolism of warfarin or acenocoumarol than erythromycin, and this is borne out by studies with dirithromycin, midecamycin and roxithromycin. Nevertheless, cases of important interactions have been reported for most of the other macrolides (azithromycin, clarithromycin, roxithromycin, and telithromycin). Moreover, one cohort study found an increased risk of over-anticoagulation with clarithromycin but not with erythromycin. Taken together, the available evidence suggests that because very occasionally and unpredictably the effects of warfarin and acenocoumarol or phenprocoumon appear to markedly increased by macrolides, it would be prudent to increase monitoring in all patients when they are first given any macrolide antibacterial. There is some evidence that this may be particularly important in those who clear warfarin and other anticoagulants slowly and who therefore only need low doses. The elderly in particular would seem to fall into this higher risk category. With azithromycin, bear in mind that, because of azithromycin's long half-life, the interaction may possibly not become apparent until a couple of days after a short course (i.e. 5 days) of azithromycin has been stopped.

1. Hopkins S. Clinical toleration and safety of azithromycin. *Am J Med* (1991) 91 (Suppl 3A), 40S–45S.

2. Zithromax (Azithromycin). Pfizer Ltd. UK Summary of product characteristics, July 2006.
3. Beckey NP, Parra D, Colon A. Retrospective evaluation of a potential interaction between azithromycin and warfarin in patients stabilized on warfarin. *Pharmacotherapy* (2000) 20, 1055–9.
4. McCall KL, Anderson HG, Jones AD. Determination of the lack of a drug interaction between azithromycin and warfarin. *Pharmacotherapy* (2004) 24, 188–94.
5. Lane G. Increased hypoprothrombinemic effect of warfarin possibly induced by azithromycin. *Ann Pharmacother* (1996) 30, 884–5.
6. Woldtveldt BR, Cahoon CL, Bradley LA, Miller SJ. Possible increased anticoagulation effect of warfarin induced by azithromycin. *Ann Pharmacother* (1998) 32, 269–70.
7. Foster DR, Milan NL. Potential interaction between azithromycin and warfarin. *Pharmacotherapy* (1999) 19, 902–8.
8. Wiese MD, Cosh DG. Raised INR with concurrent warfarin and azithromycin. *Aust J Hosp Pharm* (1999) 29, 159–161.
9. Shrader SP, Fermo JD, Dzikowski AL. Azithromycin and warfarin interaction. *Pharmacotherapy* (2004) 24, 945–9.
10. Williams D, Ponte CD. Warfarin associated hypoprothrombinemia: an unusual presentation. *Am J Health-Syst Pharm* (2003) 60, 274–8.
11. Rao KB, Pallaki M, Tolbert SR, Hornick TR. Enhanced hypoprothrombinemia with warfarin due to azithromycin. *Ann Pharmacother* (2004) 38, 982–5.
12. Pfizer Limited. Personal Communication, December 1998.
13. ADRAC. Macrolides and warfarin interaction. *Aust Adverse Drug React Bull* (2004) 23; 7.
14. Grau E, Real E, Pastor E. Interaction between clarithromycin and oral anticoagulants. *Ann Pharmacother* (1996) 30, 1495–6.
15. Sánchez B, Muruzábal MJ, Peralta G, Santiago G, Castilla A, Aguilera JP, Arjona R. Clarithromycin-oral anticoagulants interaction. Report of five cases. *Clin Drug Invest* (1997) 13, 220–2.
16. Visser LE, Penning-van Beest FJA, Kasbergen AAH, De Smet PAGM, Vulto AG, Hofman A, Stricker BHC. Overanticoagulation associated with combined use of antibacterial drugs and acenocoumarol or phenprocoumon anticoagulants. *Thromb Haemost* (2002) 88, 705–10.
17. Meyboom RHB, Heere FJ, Egberts ACG, Lastdrager CJ. Vermoedelijke potentiëring van fenprocoumon door claritromycine en roxitromycine. *Ned Tijdschr Geneeskd* (1996) 140, 375–7.
18. Committee on Safety of Medicines. Reminders: interaction between macrolide antibiotics and warfarin. *Current Problems* (1992) 35, 4.
19. Dandekar SS, Laidlaw DAH. Suprachoroidal haemorrhage after addition of clarithromycin. *J R Soc Med* (2001) 94, 583–4.
20. Oberg KC. Delayed elevation of international normalized ratio with concurrent clarithromycin and warfarin therapy. *Pharmacotherapy* (1998) 18, 386–91.
21. Recker MW, Kier KL. Potential interaction between clarithromycin and warfarin. *Ann Pharmacother* (1997) 31, 996–8.
22. Gooderham MJ, Bolli P, Fernandez PG. Concomitant digoxin toxicity and warfarin interaction in a patient receiving clarithromycin. *Ann Pharmacother* (1999) 33, 796–9.
23. Ellsworth A, Horn JR, Wilkinson W, Black DJ, Church L, Sides GD, Harris J, Cullen PD. An evaluation of the effect of dirithromycin (D) and erythromycin (E) on the pharmacokinetics and pharmacodynamics of warfarin (W). *Intersci Conf Antimicrob Agents Chemother* (1995) 35, 9.
24. Grau E, Fontcuberta J, Félez J. Erythromycin-oral anticoagulants interaction. *Arch Intern Med* (1986) 146, 1639.
25. Grau E, Real E, Pastor E. Macrolides and oral anticoagulants: a dangerous association. *Acta Haematol (Basel)* (1999) 102, 113–14.
26. Bachmann K, Schwartz JI, Forney R, Frogameni A, Jauregui LE. The effect of erythromycin on the disposition kinetics of warfarin. *Pharmacology* (1984) 28, 171–6.
27. Weibert RT, Lorentz SM, Townsend RJ, Cook CE, Klauber MR, Jagger PI. Effect of erythromycin in patients receiving long-term warfarin therapy. *Clin Pharm* (1989) 8, 210–14.
28. Bartle WR. Possible warfarin-erythromycin interaction. *Arch Intern Med* (1980) 140, 985–7.
29. Husserl FE. Erythromycin-warfarin interaction. *Arch Intern Med* (1983) 143, 1831, 1836
30. Sato RI, Gray DR, Brown SE. Warfarin interaction with erythromycin. *Arch Intern Med* (1984) 144, 2413–14.
31. Friedman HS, Bonventre MV. Erythromycin-induced digoxin toxicity. *Chest* (1982) 82, 202.
32. Hassell D, Utt JK. Suspected interaction: warfarin and erythromycin. *South Med J* (1985) 78, 1015–16.
33. Bussey HI, Knodel LC, Boyle DA. Warfarin-erythromycin interaction. *Arch Intern Med* (1985) 145, 1736–7.
34. O'Donnell D. Antibiotic-induced potentiation of oral anticoagulant agents. *Med J Aust* (1989) 150, 163–4.
35. Schwartz J, Bachmann K, Perigo E. Interaction between warfarin and erythromycin. *South Med J* (1983) 76, 91–3.
36. Wolf R, Elman M, Brenner S. Sulfonamide-induced bullous hemorrhagic eruption in a patient with low prothrombin time. *Isr J Med Sci* (1992), 28, 882–4.
37. Couet W, Istin B, Decourt JP, Ingrand I, Girault J, Fourtillan JB. Lack of effect of ponsinomycin on the pharmacokinetics of nicoumalone enantiomers. *Br J Clin Pharmacol* (1990) 30, 616–20.
38. Chassany O, Logeart I, Choulika S, Caulin C. Hématome pariétal abdominal lors d'un traitement associant acénocoumarol et roxithromycine. *Presse Med* (1998) 27, 1103.
39. Paulsen O, Nilsson L-G, Saint-Salvi B, Manuel C, Lunell E. No effect of roxithromycin on pharmacokinetic or pharmacodynamic properties of warfarin and its enantiomers. *Pharmacol Toxicol* (1988) 63, 215–20.
40. Ghose K, Ashton J, Rohan A. Possible interaction of roxithromycin with warfarin; updated review of ADR reports. *Clin Drug Invest* (1995) 10, 302–9.
41. Scholtz HE, Pretorius SG, Wessels DH, Mogilmicka EM, Van Niekerk N, Sultan E. HMR 3647, a new ketolide antimicrobial does not affect the pharmacodynamics or pharmacokinetics of warfarin in healthy adult males. Abstracts of the IDSA 37th Annual Meeting p. 976.
42. Ketek (Telithromycin). Sanofi-Aventis. UK Summary of product characteristics, May 2007.
43. Ketek (Telithromycin). Sanofi-Aventis US LLC. US Prescribing information, February 2007.
44. Kolilekas L, Anagnostopoulos GK, Lampaditis I, Eleftheriadis I. Potential interaction between telithromycin and warfarin. *Ann Pharmacother* (2004) 38, 1424–7.
45. Health Canada. Telithromycin (Ketek) and warfarin: suspected interaction. *Can Adverse React News* (2005) 15, 1.
46. Pharmacy Anticoagulant Clinic Study Group. A multicentre survey of antibiotics on the INR of anticoagulated patients. *Pharm J* (1996) 257 (Pharmacy Practice Suppl), R30.

Coumarins + Antibacterials; Metronidazole or Nimorazole

One early study found that metronidazole increased the half-life of a single dose of warfarin by one-third and increased its effects, and another cohort study showed that the combination caused a marked increase in INR, without bleeding. Case reports support these findings. There is a single case of a markedly increased INR and bleeding in a man taking phenprocoumon was given nimorazole.

Clinical evidence

(a) Metronidazole

Metronidazole 250 mg three times daily for a week increased the half-life of a single 1.5-mg/kg dose of **warfarin** by about one-third (from 35 to 46 hours) in 8 healthy subjects, and increased the prothrombin time from a mean of 100 to 142 seconds. When the warfarin enantiomers were given separately, the anticoagulant effects of ***S*-warfarin** were virtually doubled and the half-life increased by 60%, but the response to ***R*-warfarin** was only affected in one subject.[1] In a retrospective cohort study, 32 patients taking **warfarin** had an INR reading before and during concurrent metronidazole use. In these patients, the mean INR increased from 2.2 to a maximum of 4.3 by day 8 of concurrent use. Fourteen of the 32 had an INR above 4, but no bleeding events were recorded.[2]

Bleeding has been seen in 2 patients taking **warfarin** and metronidazole.[3,4] One of them had severe pain in one leg, ecchymoses, and haemorrhage of both legs, and an increase in her prothrombin time from 17 to 19 seconds to 147 seconds within 17 days of starting the metronidazole.[3] A further report describes 3 elderly patients taking warfarin, who developed raised INRs after being given intravenous metronidazole.[5] In the first patient the INR on admission was 4.6, and so warfarin was stopped. The next day metronidazole was given for about 24 hours, and on day 4 the INR had reached 10.3. In the second patient the INR on admission was 4.9 and so the warfarin was stopped. Later that day metronidazole was started, and the INR was reduced to 1.7 with fresh frozen plasma. Nevertheless by day 5 the INR had reached 6 (metronidazole had been stopped on day 2). In the third patient the INR on admission was 4 and so the warfarin was stopped. Later that day metronidazole was given, and the INR was reduced to 2.1 with fresh frozen plasma. Nevertheless by day 5 (while still receiving metronidazole) the INR had reached 10.

(b) Nimorazole

A 66-year-old man who had been taking **phenprocoumon** for 15 years with an INR around 2.5 was diagnosed with carcinoma of the glottis.[6] He received radiotherapy 6 times a week with nimorazole 2.5 g given 1.5 hours prior to the radiotherapy as a radiosensitiser. At the 16th dose, he had haemoptysis, on the 17th dose continuous haematuria, and then on the 22nd dose his INR was found to be 7.5. Fluconazole had been started 4 days previously. When the patient had recovered and restarted phenprocoumon, he was rechallenged with nimorazole prior to his last 5 days of radiotherapy, with an INR increase from 3.7 to 5.3.

Mechanism

In the early study, it was suggested that metronidazole probably inhibits the activity of the enzymes responsible for the metabolism (ring oxidation) of the more potent isomer *S*-warfarin, but not *R*-warfarin.[1] Reduction of protein binding coupled with reduced metabolism was suggested by other authors.[5] Nimorazole may act similarly, although there are other likely contributing factors in the case with this drug including concomitant 'fluconazole', (p.387), and reduced 'vitamin-K intake', (p.409). See also, 'antibacterials', (p.365).

Importance and management

The interaction between metronidazole and warfarin appears to be established and clinically important, although the documentation is limited. Monitor the INR when both drugs are used and adjust the warfarin dose accordingly. Nothing seems to be documented about other anticoagulants but it would be prudent to expect other coumarins to behave similarly. The single case with nimorazole suggests that caution may also be warranted with this drug.

1. O'Reilly RA. The stereoselective interaction of warfarin and metronidazole in man. *N Engl J Med* (1976) 295, 354–7.
2. Laine K, Forsström J, Grönroos P, Irjala K, Kailajärvi M, Scheinin M.. Frequency and clinical outcome of potentially harmful drug metabolic interactions in patients hospitalized on internal and pulmonary medicine wards: focus on warfarin and cisapride. *Ther Drug Monit* (2000) 22, 503–9.
3. Kazmier FJ. A significant interaction between metronidazole and warfarin. *Mayo Clin Proc* (1976) 51, 782–4.

4. Dean RP, Talbert RL. Bleeding associated with concurrent warfarin and metronidazole therapy. *Drug Intell Clin Pharm* (1980) 14, 864–6.
5. Tonna AP, Scott D, Keeling D, Tonna I. Metronidazole causes an unexpected rise in INR in anticoagulated patients even after warfarin has been stopped. *Hosp Pharm* (2007) 14, 65–7.
6. Bjarnason NH, Specht L, Dalhoff K. Nimorazole may increase the effect of phenprocoumon. *Radiother Oncol* (2005) 74, 345.

Coumarins + Antibacterials; Penicillins

Isolated cases of increased prothrombin times and/or bleeding have been seen in patients given amoxicillin (with or without clavulanic acid) intravenous benzylpenicillin, pheneticillin or talampicillin. An increased risk of over-anticoagulation was seen with amoxicillin with or without clavulanic acid in cohort studies, but not flucloxacillin. There is also some evidence that phenoxymethylpenicillin (penicillin V) does not interact.

In contrast, several cases of markedly reduced warfarin effects (warfarin resistance) have been seen with intravenous nafcillin, with a 75% reduction in warfarin half-life documented in one case. Similarly, other studies and cases suggest that dicloxacillin may cause a modest reduction in warfarin effects in many patients, and that some may experience greater reductions, with thrombosis being reported in one case.

Clinical evidence

(a) Amoxicillin ± clavulanic acid

An 81-year-old woman taking **acenocoumarol** 3 mg daily (INR 2.5 to 4) developed bruising and an increased INR of 7.1 within a week of starting amoxicillin 500 mg every 8 hours.[1] Another patient stabilised on **warfarin** (INR 2 to 3) had a normal INR (2.55) 4 days after completion of a 7-day course of co-amoxiclav (amoxicillin with clavulanic acid), but about 2.5 weeks after the course a routine INR was 6.2. A further 3 days later it was 8.7 and microscopic haematuria was detected.[2] In one case control study, use of co-amoxiclav was found to be associated with an increased risk of an INR of greater than 6 (odds ratio 4.1; range 0.9 to 19.2) in patients stabilised on either **acenocoumarol** or **phenprocoumon**. Amoxicillin alone was associated with a smaller increased risk (odds ratio 1.7; range 0.6 to 4.7).[3] Conversely, in a population-based cohort study in similar patients conducted by the same research group, the risk of over-anticoagulation (INR greater than or equal to 6) was greater for amoxicillin alone than amoxicillin plus an enzyme inhibitor. The relative risk for amoxicillin alone was 10.5 (range 5.1 to 21.7) and for amoxicillin plus an enzyme inhibitor was 5.1 (range 1.9 to 13.9).[4] The increased risk was observed in the early stages of concurrent use but was greater after 4 or more days of treatment.[4]

In contrast to these reports of increased anticoagulation, a very brief report states that in an audit of an anticoagulant clinic, 5 patients who had taken amoxicillin had an unspecified decrease in prothrombin time.[5]

(b) Ampicillin

A bulletin briefly mentions a case of an increased prothrombin time in a patient taking **warfarin** with ampicillin and **flucloxacillin**.[6]

(c) Benzylpenicillin

One patient stabilised on **warfarin** (prothrombin time 20 seconds) was found to have an increased prothrombin time of 32 seconds 8 days after starting intravenous benzylpenicillin 24 million units daily for subacute bacterial endocarditis. The benzylpenicillin was continued, and the warfarin dose reduced for 18 days. However, the prothrombin time dropped below the therapeutic range, and the warfarin dose was increased back to the original dose, still with continuation of the benzylpenicillin for a further 3 weeks.[7]

(d) Dicloxacillin

In a controlled study in 7 patients stabilised on **warfarin** and without infections, dicloxacillin 500 mg four times daily for 7 days reduced the mean prothrombin time by 1.9 seconds. One patient had a 5.6 second reduction.[8] This study was conducted because the authors had noted a case of a patient receiving **warfarin** who had a decrease in prothrombin time when dicloxacillin was started.[8] Another patient stabilised on **warfarin** had a 17% fall in prothrombin times within 4 to 5 days of starting dicloxacillin 500 mg four times daily, with a documented 20 to 25% reduction in both *S*- and *R*-warfarin levels.[9] In a retrospective review, 7 other patients similarly treated were also identified as having a 17% reduction in prothrombin times.[9] In yet another case, a patient who had previously required **warfarin** 10 mg daily subsequently needed an increased dosage of 15 mg daily while taking dicloxacillin 4 g daily long-term.[10] However, another case report suggested a greater effect of dicloxacillin—a patient taking 500 mg every 6 hours required an increase in **warfarin** dose from a range of 35 to 40 mg weekly up to 50 to 60 mg weekly, with INRs still being subtherapeutic (about 1.5).[11] Moreover, when a woman taking **warfarin** was given dicloxacillin 500 mg four times daily she developed a heart valve thrombosis, suggesting inadequate anticoagulation. Her INR was 1.4, and an increased **warfarin** dose was required for 3 weeks after she stopped dicloxacillin.[12]

(e) Flucloxacillin

In one cohort study in patients taking **acenocoumarol** or **phenprocoumon**, no cases of over-anticoagulation (INR greater than 6) occurred in patients taking flucloxacillin (25 patients received this antibacterial).[4] Note that this study did show an increase for *amoxicillin*, see above. A bulletin briefly mentions a case of an increased prothrombin time in a patient taking **warfarin** with **ampicillin** and flucloxacillin.[6]

(f) Nafcillin

The prothrombin time of a 29-year-old patient stabilised on **warfarin** fell from a range of 20 to 25 seconds down to 16 seconds five days after intravenous nafcillin 2 g every 4 hours was started for endocarditis.[13] Over the next 2 weeks the prothrombin time ranged between 14 and 17 seconds despite an eventual doubling of the warfarin dose, and heparin was substituted. In this patient the half-life of a single 30-mg dose of warfarin was 11 hours when nafcillin was taken, 17 hours 4 days after stopping nafcillin, and 44 hours eight months after the nafcillin was discontinued. At least 10 other cases of this warfarin resistance have been reported with high-dose nafcillin.[10,14-18]

(g) Pheneticillin

In one cohort study in patients taking **acenocoumarol** or **phenprocoumon**, one case of over-anticoagulation (INR greater than 6) occurred in a group of 219 patients treated with pheneticillin, giving a calculated relative risk of 0.9.[4]

(h) Phenoxymethylpenicillin (Penicillin V)

When 10 patients taking an unnamed anticoagulant were given intravenous phenoxymethylpenicillin calcium 300 000 units four times daily for 4 days, none had a change in their prothrombin-proconvertin value.[19] For mention that, in another study no patients taking penicillins including phenoxymethylpenicillin had an increase in INR see (j) below.

(i) Talampicillin

A bulletin briefly mentions a case of bleeding (haematuria, epistaxis) and an increase in the prothrombin ratio in a patient taking **warfarin** and talampicillin.[20]

(j) Unspecified penicillins

In one analysis of patients taking **warfarin** with antibacterials, there was no association between use of penicillins (**phenoxymethylpenicillin (penicillin V)** and **broad-spectrum penicillins**) and an increase in INR. The estimated change in INR was 0.117 in 109 patients given the combination.[21]

Mechanism

Not understood. The interaction between nafcillin and warfarin is possibly due to increases in the metabolism of warfarin by the liver. Dicloxacillin also possibly reduces serum warfarin levels.[9] Other penicillins (ampicillin,[22] benzylpenicillin,[22,23] carbenicillin,[24-29] methicillin,[22] ticarcillin[30]) have caused increased bleeding times when given alone, principally due to platelet inhibition,[22-24] which might be additive with the effects of oral anticoagulants. Broad-spectrum antibacterials may decrease the gut flora and thereby possibly decrease production of vitamin K. Other factors relating to the disease may be important, see 'Coumarins + Antibacterials' p.365.

Importance and management

The reduced effect of warfarin with **dicloxacillin** and **nafcillin** appears to be established. If these penicillins are used, increase monitoring of the INR and anticipate the need to increase the warfarin dose. Some patients taking nafcillin have been warfarin resistant, and needed heparin treatment.

Documented reports of interactions between oral anticoagulants and other penicillins are relatively rare, bearing in mind how frequently these drugs are used, so that the broad picture is that no clinically relevant interaction normally occurs with most other penicillins. This lack of interaction was supported by one clinical study.[21] However, in one case-control study, amoxicillin/clavulanic acid (co-amoxiclav) increased the risk of bleeding, and the authors recommended avoiding this combination,[3] although a later cohort study by the same authors just recommended increased monitoring with amoxicillin or co-amoxiclav.[4] Even though the general picture is of no interaction, there are a number of reports of adverse interactions between coumarins and penicillins. Although there appear to be no reports of an interaction, if the mechanism of the interaction is correct, the **indanediones** are also likely to be affected. However, these interactions may be due to a number of different factors, and these are discussed in detail in the monograph 'Coumarins + Antibacterials', p.365. Therefore concurrent use should be monitored so that the very occasional and unpredictable cases (increases or decreases in the anticoagulant effects) can be identified and handled accordingly.

1. Soto J, Sacristan JA, Alsar MJ, Fernandez-Viadero C, Verduga R. Probable acenocoumarol-amoxycillin interaction. *Acta Haematol (Basel)* (1993) 90, 195–7.
2. Davydov L, Yermolnik M, Cuni LJ. Warfarin and amoxicillin/clavulanate drug interaction. *Ann Pharmacother* (2003) 37, 367–70.
3. Penning-van Beest FJA, van Meegen E, Rosendaal FR, Stricker BH. Drug interactions as a cause of overanticoagulation on phenprocoumon or acenocoumarol predominantly concern antibacterial drugs. *Clin Pharmacol Ther* (2001) 69, 451–57.
4. Visser LE, Penning-van Beest FJA, Kasbergen AAH, De Smet PAGM, Vulto AG, Hofman A, Stricker BHC. Overanticoagulation associated with combined use of antibacterial drugs and acenocoumarol or phenprocoumon anticoagulants. *Thromb Haemost* (2002) 88, 705–10.
5. Radley AS, Hall J. Interactions. *Pharm J* (1992) 249, 81.
6. Beeley L, Stewart P. *Bulletin of the West Midlands Centre for Adverse Drug Reaction Reporting* (1987) 25, 21.
7. Brown MA, Korchinski ED, Miller DR. Interaction of penicillin-G and warfarin? *Can J Hosp Pharm* (1979) 32, 18–19.
8. Krstenansky PM, Jones WN, Garewal HS. Effect of dicloxacillin sodium on the hypoprothrombinemic response to warfarin sodium. *Clin Pharm* (1987) 6, 804–6.
9. Mailloux AT, Gidal BE, Sorkness CA. Potential interaction between warfarin and dicloxacillin. *Ann Pharmacother* (1996) 30, 1402–7.
10. Taylor AT, Pritchard DC, Goldstein AO, Fletcher JL. Continuation of warfarin-nafcillin interaction during dicloxacillin therapy. *J Fam Pract* (1994) 39, 182–5.
11. Lacey CS. Interaction of dicloxacillin with warfarin. *Ann Pharmacother* (2004) 38, 898.
12. Halvorsen S, Husebye T, Arnesen H. Prosthetic heart valve thrombosis during dicloxacillin therapy. *Scand Cardiovasc J* (1999) 33, 366–8.
13. Qureshi GD, Reinders TP, Somori GJ, Evans HJ. Warfarin resistance with nafcillin therapy. *Ann Intern Med* (1984) 100, 527–9.
14. Fraser GL, Miller M, Kane K. Warfarin resistance associated with nafcillin therapy. *Am J Med* (1989) 87, 237–8.
15. Davis RL, Berman W, Wernly JA, Kelly HW. Warfarin-nafcillin interaction. *J Pediatr* (1991) 118, 300–3.
16. Shovick VA, Rihn TL. Decreased hypoprothrombinemic response to warfarin secondary to the warfarin-nafcillin interaction. *DICP Ann Pharmacother* (1991) 25, 598–9.
17. Heilker GM, Fowler JW, Self TH. Possible nafcillin-warfarin interaction. *Arch Intern Med* (1994) 154, 822–4.
18. Baciewicz AM, Heugel AM, Rose PG. Probable nafcillin-warfarin interaction. *J Pharm Technol* (1999) 15, 5–7.
19. Magid E. Tolerance to anticoagulants during antibiotic therapy. *Scand J Clin Lab Invest* (1962) 14, 565–6.
20. Beeley L, Daly M. *Bulletin of the West Midlands Centre for Adverse Drug Reaction Reporting* (1986) 23, 13.
21. Pharmacy Anticoagulant Clinic Study Group. A multicentre survey of antibiotics on the INR of anticoagulated patients. *Pharm J* (1996) 257 (Pharmacy Practice Suppl), R30.
22. Brown CH, Bradshaw MW, Natelson EA, Alfrey CP, Williams TW. Defective platelet function following the administration of penicillin compounds. *Blood* (1976) 47, 949–56.
23. Roberts PL. High-dose penicillin and bleeding. *Ann Intern Med* (1974) 81, 267–8.
24. Brown CH, Natelson EA, Bradshaw MW, Williams TW, Alfrey CP. The hemostatic defect produced by carbenicillin. *N Engl J Med* (1974) 291, 265–70.
25. McClure PD, Casserly JG, Monsier C, Crozier D. Carbenicillin-induced bleeding disorder. *Lancet* (1970) ii, 1307–8.
26. Waisbren BA, Evani SV, Ziebert AP. Carbenicillin and bleeding. *JAMA* (1971) 217, 1243.
27. Yudis M, Mahood WH, Maxwell R. Bleeding problems with carbenicillin. *Lancet* (1972) ii, 599.
28. Lurie A, Ogilvie M, Townsend R, Gold C, Meyers AM, Goldberg B. Carbenicillin-induced coagulopathy. *Lancet* (1970) i, 1114–15.
29. Andrassy K, Ritz E, Weisschedel E. Bleeding after carbenicillin administration. *N Engl J Med* (1975) 292, 109.
30. Brown CH, Natelson EA, Bradshaw MW, Alfrey CP, Williams TW. Study of the effects of ticarcillin on blood coagulation and platelet function. *Antimicrob Agents Chemother* (1975) 7, 652–7.

Coumarins + Antibacterials; Quinolones

Most studies show that the quinolones have, at most, a small, clinically insignificant effect on the pharmacokinetics and pharmacodynamics of warfarin. Despite this, increased effects and even bleeding have been seen quite unpredictably in isolated cases in patients taking warfarin with ciprofloxacin, gatifloxacin, levofloxacin, moxifloxacin, nalidixic acid, norfloxacin or ofloxacin; or while taking acenocoumarol when given nalidixic acid, norfloxacin or pefloxacin, or phenprocoumon with norfloxacin. Furthermore, two studies suggest that there may be an increased risk of over-anticoagulation in patients taking acenocoumarol or phenprocoumon with norfloxacin, and warfarin with gatifloxacin.

Clinical evidence

(a) Ciprofloxacin

In a randomised, placebo-controlled study in 32 patients stabilised on **warfarin** and without infections, ciprofloxacin 750 mg twice daily for 12 days had no clinically relevant effect on measures of anticoagulation. There was a mean increase in prothrombin time ratio of just 3% (range 0 to 6%), with a 10 to 13% decrease in the levels of clotting factors II and VII. In this study, ciprofloxacin had no effect on *S*-warfarin levels, but did slightly increase *R*-warfarin levels by 14.7%.[1] Similarly, no clinically relevant effects on **warfarin** anticoagulation were seen in two other studies in a total of 16 patients without infections given ciprofloxacin 500 mg twice daily for 7 or 10 days.[2,3] In a population-based cohort study,[4] there were no cases of over-anticoagulation (INR greater than 6) in patients taking **acenocoumarol** or **phenprocoumon** with ciprofloxacin (just 19 received ciprofloxacin). Note that this study did find an increased risk for *norfloxacin*, see below.

In contrast, there are reports where ciprofloxacin has apparently been responsible for moderate to markedly increased prothrombin times and/or bleeding in patients taking **warfarin.** The FDA in the US has a total of 64 such cases over the 10 year period 1987 to 1997 on its Spontaneous Reporting System database. Those cases where details were available, plus an additional 2 cases, showed that the median prothrombin time was 38 seconds, the INR 10, and the median time to detection after starting ciprofloxacin was 5.5 days. Hospitalisation was reported in 15 cases, bleeding in 25 cases and death in one case.[5] There are a number of other individual published case reports from the USA describing moderate to marked increases in prothrombin times and/or bleeding in a total of 8 patients stabilised on **warfarin**, which was associated with taking ciprofloxacin.[6-12] For the period December 1989 to January 2004, Health Canada had received 10 reports of suspected coagulation disorders associated with ciprofloxacin and **warfarin**, 7 of which were considered serious, and in one case, fatal.[13] Similarly, in February 2006, the Australia Adverse Drug Reactions Advisory Committee stated they had received 9 reports of a suspected interaction between **warfarin** and ciprofloxacin.[14]

(b) Clinafloxacin

Clinafloxacin 200 mg twice daily for 14 days had no effect on the steady-state levels of *S*-warfarin in healthy subjects, but the levels of the less active enantiomer *R*-warfarin were increased by 32% and the mean INR was increased by 13%.[15]

(c) Enoxacin

When a single 25-mg dose of **warfarin** was given to 6 healthy subjects on day 8 of a 14-day course of enoxacin 400 mg twice daily, the pharmacokinetics of *S*-warfarin were not altered, but the clearance of *R*-warfarin was decreased by 32% and its elimination half-life was prolonged from 36.8 to 52.2 hours. The overall anticoagulant response to the **warfarin** was unaltered.[16] Another report about one patient taking **warfarin** also suggested that the use of enoxacin does not alter the prothrombin time ratio.[17]

(d) Fleroxacin

The pharmacokinetics of *R*- and *S*-warfarin, the prothrombin time and factor VII clotting time were unaffected when 12 healthy subjects were given a single 25-mg dose of **warfarin** on day 4 of a 9-day course of fleroxacin 400 mg daily.[18]

(e) Gatifloxacin

The manufacturer notes that gatifloxacin 400 mg daily for 11 days had no effect on the pharmacokinetics of a single 25-mg dose of **warfarin**, nor was the prothrombin time altered.[19] In contrast, in a review of 94 patients taking **warfarin** and given antibacterials for community-acquired pneumonia, 22 of the 40 patients treated with gatifloxacin (55%) had INRs greater than 3 during or within 48 hours after stopping gatifloxacin therapy, compared with 20 of 54 patients treated with ceftriaxone and/or azithromycin (37%). In the gatifloxacin group, 38% needed a **warfarin** dose adjustment, compared with 18% of patients taking other antibacterials. There was no difference in infection severity between the two groups.[20] For the period February 2001 to January 2004, Health Canada had received 13 reports of suspected coagulation disorders associated with gatifloxacin and **warfarin**, all of which were considered serious, and 2 of which were fatal.[13]

(f) Gemifloxacin

A double-blind, randomised, placebo-controlled study found that healthy subjects taking fixed doses of **warfarin** and with INRs in the range of 1.3 to 1.8 had no INR changes when they were given gemifloxacin 320 mg daily for 7 days.[21]

(g) Levofloxacin

Levofloxacin 500 mg twice daily for 9 days had no effect on the pharmacokinetics or pharmacodynamics of *R*- and *S*-warfarin in 15 healthy subjects given a single 30-mg dose of **warfarin** on day 4.[22] In a prospective study 18 patients stabilised on **warfarin** were given a course of levofloxacin. There was no difference in the mean INR obtained before levofloxacin and the first INR taken a median of 5 days after levofloxacin was started (2.61 versus 2.74). However, 4 patients had an increase in INR (to a range of 3.89 to 4.2) and 3 had a decrease in INR (to a range of 1.39 to 1.84) outside of the therapeutic range (2 to 3), and required **warfarin** dosage adjustments. Only 7 patients had INRs that were therapeutic (range 2 to 3) throughout the study (before, during, and after levofloxacin) and did not require adjustment in **warfarin** dose.[23] Similar findings were reported in a retrospective analysis of 22 patients taking **warfarin** with levofloxacin.[24]

However, two elderly patients taking **warfarin** were found to have increased INRs (of 5.7 and 7.9) on routine testing shortly after stopping levofloxacin 500 mg daily.[25] Six other cases of modest to markedly increased INRs have been reported in patients stabilised on **warfarin** who were given courses of levofloxacin 500 mg daily for 5 to 10 days;[26,27] epistaxis occurred in one patient.[27] Moreover, for the period November 1997 to January 2004, Health Canada had received 16 reports of suspected coagulation disorders associated with levofloxacin and **warfarin**, 14 of which were considered serious, and one of which was fatal.[13]

(h) Moxifloxacin

The pharmacokinetics of *R*- and *S*-warfarin were not altered when a single 25-mg dose of **warfarin** was given on day 5 of an 8-day course of moxifloxacin 400 mg once daily in healthy subjects. The prothrombin time increased by 3% (0 to 6%), which is not clinically relevant.[28]

In contrast, one report describes 2 patients stabilised on **warfarin** who had marked rises in their INRs (to 6.2 and 7.3), and another patient recently started on **warfarin** who had a more modest rise (to 4.2) within 1 to 5 days of starting moxifloxacin.[29] All these patients had recently been receiving other antibacterials, which complicates interpretation. For the period October 2000 to January 2004, Health Canada had received 12 reports of suspected coagulation disorders associated with moxifloxacin and **warfarin**, 11 of which were considered serious.[13] Similarly, in February 2006, the Australia Adverse Drug Reactions Advisory Committee stated they had received one report of a suspected interaction between **warfarin** and moxifloxacin. In this patient the INR rose from around 2 to greater than 10, four days after starting moxifloxacin.[14]

(i) Nalidixic acid

A patient stabilised on **warfarin** (prothrombin ratio 2), developed a purpuric rash and bruising within 6 days of starting nalidixic acid 500 mg four times daily. Her prothrombin ratio had risen to 3.46.[30] Another patient, previously well controlled on **warfarin**, developed a prothrombin time of 60 seconds 10 days after starting nalidixic acid 1 g three times daily.[31] The INR of an 84-year-old woman taking **warfarin** rose from 1.9 to 9.6 when nalidixic acid was added.[32] Similarly, a patient taking **acenocoumarol** developed hypoprothrombinaemia after receiving nalidixic acid 1 g daily.[33]

(j) Norfloxacin

In 10 healthy subjects norfloxacin 400 mg twice daily for 9 days was found not to alter either the pharmacokinetics or anticoagulant effects of a single 30-mg dose of **warfarin** given on day 4.[34]

In contrast, a 91-year-old woman taking **warfarin** and digoxin developed a brain haemorrhage within 11 days of starting to take norfloxacin (precise dose not stated). Her prothrombin times had risen from 21.6 to 36.5 seconds. At this time, the manufacturers of norfloxacin were said to have 6 other reports of an interaction between warfarin and norfloxacin on file.[35] In a population-based cohort study, patients taking **acenocoumarol** or **phenprocoumon** were found to have an increased risk of overanticoagulation (INR greater than or equal to 6) during norfloxacin treatment (relative risk 9.8). The risk was greatest during the first 3 days of treatment.[4] Furthermore, for the period December 1986 to January 2004, Health Canada had received 6 reports of suspected coagulation disorders associated with norfloxacin and **warfarin**, 4 of which were considered serious.[13] Similarly, in February 2006, the Australia Adverse Drug Reactions Advisory Committee stated they had received 11 reports of a suspected interaction between **warfarin** and norfloxacin.[14]

(k) Ofloxacin

Ofloxacin 200 mg daily for 7 days did not significantly affect the prothrombin times of 7 healthy subjects stabilised on **phenprocoumon**.[36] In a population-based cohort study,[4] there were no cases of over-anticoagulation (INR greater than 6) in patients taking **acenocoumarol** or **phenprocoumon** with ofloxacin (33 received ofloxacin. Note that this study did find an increased risk for *norfloxacin*, see (j) above. Furthermore, for the period December 1990 to January 2004, Health Canada had not received any reports of suspected coagulation disorders associated with ofloxacin and **warfarin**.[13]

In contrast, a woman who had recently started to take **warfarin** 5 mg daily, had a marked increase in her INR (from 2.5 to 4.4) within 2 days of starting to take ofloxacin 200 mg three times daily.[37] Two days later her INR had risen to 5.8. Another patient stabilised on **warfarin** developed gross haematuria and a prothrombin time of 78 seconds 5 days after starting to take ofloxacin 400 mg twice daily.[38]

(l) Pefloxacin

A patient had a marked increase in the effects of **acenocoumarol** (Quick time reduced from 26% to less than 5%) within 5 days of starting to take pefloxacin 800 mg daily and rifampicin 1.2 g daily.[39] Rifampicin is an enzyme inducer, which normally causes a reduction in the effects of the 'anticoagulants', (p.375), so the findings in this case are surprising.

(m) Trovafloxacin

Healthy subjects stabilised on **warfarin** with INRs in the range of 1.3 to 1.7 were additionally given trovafloxacin 200 mg daily for 7 days. No changes in the pharmacokinetics of either *S*- or *R*-warfarin occurred and no significant changes in mean INRs were seen.[40]

Mechanism

Uncertain. It is not clear what other factors might have been responsible in those cases where the effects of the anticoagulants were increased. Factors relating to acute infection rather than the antibacterial used to treat it may be responsible for increased INRs, see also 'Coumarins + Antibacterials', p.365. However, one study that controlled for severity of infection indicated this is not the case and that an interaction between the quinolone and anticoagulant probably occurs.[20] *In vitro* experiments[41,42] have shown that nalidixic acid can displace warfarin from its binding sites on human plasma albumin, but this mechanism on its own is almost certainly not the full explanation. In a single-dose study enoxacin was shown to inhibit the metabolism of the less potent *R*-warfarin isomer, without affecting the anticoagulant response.[16] This effect may become important if accumulation of the *R*-warfarin isomer (which is cleared slowly) occurred during prolonged dosing.[3] Other quinolones may have a similar effects. It has also been suggested that fluoroquinolones may suppress vitamin K-producing gut bacteria with resultant potentiation of anticoagulant effects,[37] see also 'Coumarins + Antibacterials', p.365.

Importance and management

The minor pharmacokinetic interaction between ciprofloxacin and warfarin in patients taking warfarin would appear to be established, but unlikely to be clinically relevant. Similarly no other quinolone has been shown to have a clinically significant interaction with warfarin. Despite this, there are isolated published case reports of marked over-anticoagulation with many of the quinolones, and other known unpublished cases reported to regulatory authorities. Given the widespread use of warfarin and quinolones, these interactions would appear to be rare.

The overall picture is that no adverse interaction normally occurs between these quinolones and coumarin anticoagulants, but rarely and unpredictably increased anticoagulant effects and even bleeding can occur with some of them. There is no need to avoid using any of the quinolones with oral anticoagulants but it would be prudent to monitor the effects when any quinolone antibacterial is first added to treatment with any coumarin so that any problems can be quickly identified.

1. Israel DS, Stotka J, Rock W, Sintek CD, Kamada AK, Klein C, Swaim WR, Pluhar RE, Toscano JP, Lettieri JT, Heller AH, Polk RE. Effect of ciprofloxacin on the pharmacokinetics and pharmacodynamics of warfarin. *Clin Infect Dis* (1996) 22, 251–6.

2. Rindone JP, Keuey CL, Jones WN, Garewal HS. Hypoprothrombinemic effect of warfarin not influenced by ciprofloxacin. *Clin Pharm* (1991) 10, 136–8. Erratum *ibid*, 429 [name].
3. Bianco TM, Bussey HI, Farnett LE, Linn WD, Roush MK, Wong YWJ. Potential warfarin-ciprofloxacin interaction in patients receiving long-term anticoagulation. *Pharmacotherapy* (1992) 12, 435–9.
4. Visser LE, Penning-van Beest FJA, Kasbergen AAH, De Smet PAGM, Vulto AG, Hofman A, Stricker BHC. Overanticoagulation associated with combined use of antibacterial drugs and acenocoumarol or phenprocoumon anticoagulants. *Thromb Haemost* (2002) 88, 705–10.
5. Ellis RJ, Mayo MS, Bodensteiner DM. Ciprofloxacin-warfarin coagulopathy: a case series. *Am J Hematol* (2000) 63, 28–31.
6. Mott FE, Murphy S, Hunt V. Ciprofloxacin and warfarin. *Ann Intern Med* (1989) 111, 542–3.
7. Linville D, Emory C, Graves L. Ciprofloxacin and warfarin interaction. *Am J Med* (1991) 90, 765.
8. Kamada AK. Possible interaction between ciprofloxacin and warfarin. *DICP Ann Pharmacother* (1990) 24, 27–8.
9. Johnson KC, Joe RH, Self TH. Drug interaction. *J Fam Pract* (1991) 33, 338.
10. Renzi R, Finkbeiner S. Ciprofloxacin interaction with warfarin: a potentially dangerous side-effect. *Am J Emerg Med* (1991) 9, 551–2.
11. Dugoni-Kramer BM. Ciprofloxacin-warfarin interaction. *DICP Ann Pharmacother* (1991) 25, 1397.
12. Jolson HM, Tanner A, Green L, Grasela TH. Adverse reaction reporting of interaction between warfarin and fluoroquinolones. *Arch Intern Med* (1991) 151, 1003–4.
13. Health Canada. Fluoroquinolones and warfarin: suspected interaction. *Can Adverse React News* (2004) 14, 1–2.
14. ADRAC. Fluoroquinolone antibiotics: interactions with warfarin. *Aust Adverse Drug React Bull* (2006) 25; 2.
15. Randinitis EJ, Koup JR, Bron NJ, Hounslow NJ, Rausch G, Abel R, Vassos AB, Sedman AJ. Drug interaction studies with clinafloxacin and probenecid, cimetidine, phenytoin and warfarin. *Drugs* (1999) 58 (Suppl 2), 254–5.
16. Toon S, Hopkins KJ, Garstang FM, Aarons L, Sedman A, Rowland M. Enoxacin-warfarin interaction: pharmacokinetic and stereochemical aspects. *Clin Pharmacol Ther* (1987) 42, 33–41.
17. McLeod AD, Burgess C. Drug interaction between warfarin and enoxacin. *N Z Med J* (1988) 101, 216.
18. Holazo AA, Soni PP, Kachevsky V, Min BH, Townsend L, Patel IH. Fleroxacin-warfarin interaction in humans. *Intersci Conf Antimicrob Agents Chemother* (1990) 30, 253.
19. Tequin (Gatifloxacin). Bristol-Myers Squibb Company. US Prescribing information, January 2006.
20. Artymowicz RJ, Cino BJ, Rossi JG, Walker JL, Moore S. Possible interaction between gatifloxacin and warfarin. *Am J Health-Syst Pharm* (2002) 59 1205–6.
21. Davy M, Bird N, Rost KL, Fuder H. Lack of effect of gemifloxacin on the steady-state pharmacodynamics of warfarin in healthy volunteers. *Chemotherapy* (1999) 45, 491–5.
22. Liao S, Palmer M, Fowler C, Nayak RK. Absence of an effect of levofloxacin on warfarin pharmacokinetics and anticoagulation in male volunteers. *J Clin Pharmacol* (1996) 36, 1072–7.
23. Yamreudeewong W, Lower DL, Kilpatrick DM, Enlow AM, Burrows MM, Greenwood MC. Effect of levofloxacin coadministration on the international normalized ratios during warfarin therapy. *Pharmacotherapy* (2003) 23, 333–8.
24. McCall KL, Scott JC, Anderson HG. Retrospective evaluation of a possible interaction between warfarin and levofloxacin. *Pharmacotherapy* (2005) 25, 67–73.
25. Ravnan SL, Locke C. Levofloxacin and warfarin interaction. *Pharmacotherapy* (2001) 21, 884–5.
26. Gheno G, Cinetto L. Levofloxacin-warfarin interaction. *Eur J Clin Pharmacol* (2001) 57, 427.
27. Jones CB, Fugate SE. Levofloxacin and warfarin interaction. *Ann Pharmacother* (2002) 36, 1554–7.
28. Müller FO, Hundt HKL, Muir AR, Potgieter MA, Terblanché J, Toerien CJ, Stass H. Study to investigate the influence of 400 mg BAY 12-8039 (M) given once daily to healthy volunteers on PK and PD of warfarin (W). *Intersci Conf Antimicrob Agents Chemother* (1998) 18, A-13.
29. Arnold LM, Nissen LR, Ng TMH. Moxifloxacin and warfarin: additional evidence for a clinically relevant interaction. *Pharmacotherapy* (2005) 25, 904–7.
30. Hoffbrand BI. Interaction of nalidixic acid and warfarin. *BMJ* (1974) 2, 666.
31. Leor J, Levartowsky D, Sharon C. Interaction between nalidixic acid and warfarin. *Ann Intern Med* (1987) 107, 601.
32. Gulløv AL, Koefoed BG, Petersen P. Interaktion mellem warfarin og nalidixinsyre. *Ugeskr Laeger* (1996) 158, 5174–5.
33. Potasman I, Bassan H. Nicoumalone and nalidixic acid interaction. *Ann Intern Med* (1980) 92, 571.
34. Rocci ML, Vlasses PH, Distlerath LM, Gregg MH, Wheeler SC, Zing W, Bjornsson TD. Norfloxacin does not alter warfarin's disposition or anticoagulant effect. *J Clin Pharmacol* (1990) 30, 728–32.
35. Linville T, Matanin D. Norfloxacin and warfarin. *Ann Intern Med* (1989) 110, 751–2.
36. Verho M, Malerczyk V, Rosenkranz B, Grötsch H. Absence of interaction between ofloxacin and phenprocoumon. *Curr Med Res Opin* (1987) 10, 474–9.
37. Leor J, Matetzki S. Ofloxacin and warfarin. *Ann Intern Med* (1988) 109, 761.
38. Baciewicz AM, Ashar BH, Locke TW. Interaction of ofloxacin and warfarin. *Ann Intern Med* (1993) 119, 1223.
39. Pertek JP, Helmer J, Vivin P, Kipper R. Potentialisation d'une antivitamine K par l'association péfloxacine-rifampicine. *Ann Fr Anesth Reanim* (1986) 5, 320–1.
40. Teng R, Apseloffl G, Vincent J, Pelletier SM, Willavize SA, Friedman JL. Effect of trovafloxacin (CP-99,219) on the pharmacokinetics and pharmacodynamics of warfarin in healthy male subjects. *Intersci Conf Antimicrob Agents Chemother* (1996) 36, A2.
41. Sellers EM, Koch-Weser J. Kinetics and clinical importance of displacement of warfarin from albumin by acidic drugs. *Ann N Y Acad Sci* (1971) 179, 213–25.
42. Sellers EM, Koch-Weser J. Displacement of warfarin from human albumin by diazoxide and ethacrynic, mefenamic, and nalidixic acids. *Clin Pharmacol Ther* (1970) 11, 524–9.

Coumarins + Antibacterials; Rifamycins

The anticoagulant effects of warfarin are markedly reduced by rifampicin (rifampin), with two to fivefold increases in dose needed to maintain efficacy in a number of case reports. Acenocoumarol and phenprocoumon are similarly affected.

Clinical evidence

(a) Acenocoumarol

The dosage of acenocoumarol needed to be markedly increased to maintain the Quick value within the therapeutic range in 18 patients stabilised on acenocoumarol who were given rifampicin 450 mg twice daily for 7 days. The effect was apparent 5 to 8 days after starting the rifampicin, and had not reached a maximum at 14 days, at which point a mean 76% increase in the acenocoumarol dosage was needed.[1] In another study the Quick time of a single dose of acenocoumarol, measured 35 hours after the dose, was reduced by 44% when rifampicin 10 mg/kg daily was given for 2 weeks.[2]

(b) Phenprocoumon

In a study in healthy subjects, rifampicin 600 mg daily for 14 days increased the clearance of a single dose of phenprocoumon by 2.2-fold.[3] Similarly, two patients stabilised on phenprocoumon required the dose to be doubled while taking rifampicin 600 mg daily (plus isoniazid with or without ethambutol). In one case, the patient developed severe gross haematuria 3 months after rifampicin had been discontinued because the phenprocoumon dose had not been reduced.[4]

(c) Warfarin

In one controlled study in 8 healthy subjects, rifampicin 600 mg daily for 21 days reduced the steady-state plasma warfarin levels by 85% (range 64% to 100%). In addition, rifampicin abolished the anticoagulant effect of warfarin (the prothrombin time averaged 27% of normal during warfarin alone, and 85% of normal when rifampicin was taken).[5] Similar findings were seen in 2 other single-dose warfarin studies.[6,7] One of these measured the isomers of warfarin separately and found that rifampicin increased the clearance of *R*-warfarin threefold and *S*-warfarin twofold.[7] This interaction has also been described in a number of case reports.[8-14] In these reports the dosage of warfarin was doubled[8,10] or even tripled[10] to accommodate this interaction, and reduced by an equivalent amount over two[9] to three weeks[12] following withdrawal of the rifampicin. In one more-recent well-described case, a threefold increase in warfarin dose from 5 to 15 mg daily over 4 months failed to achieve a therapeutic INR during long-term rifampicin therapy, and eventually a fivefold increase in dose (25 mg daily) attained an INR of 1.7 and 1.9. A gradual 70% dose reduction over 4 to 5 weeks was required when the rifampicin was discontinued.[14]

Mechanism

Rifampicin is a potent liver enzyme inducer, which increases the metabolism and clearance of the anticoagulants from the body, thereby reducing their effects.[7] Other mechanisms may also be involved.[12] See also 'antibacterials', (p.365).

Importance and management

The interaction between rifampicin and the coumarins is very well documented, clinically important, and occurs in most patients. A marked reduction in the anticoagulant effects may be expected within a week of starting the rifampicin, and persisting for about 2 to 5 weeks after the rifampicin has been withdrawn. With warfarin there is evidence that the dosage may need to be markedly increased (two to fivefold) over a number of weeks to accommodate this interaction, and reduced slowly by an equivalent amount following withdrawal of the rifampicin. Warfarin dose titrations should be carried out with close monitoring. There does not seem to be any information regarding the other rifamycins, **rifabutin** (a weak enzyme inducer) and **rifapentine** (a moderate enzyme inducer). However, the manufacturers and the CSM in the UK warn that rifabutin may possibly reduce the effects of a number of drugs, including oral anticoagulants.[15,16]

1. Michot F, Bürgi M, Büttner J. Rimactan (Rifampizin) und Antikoagulantientherapie. *Schweiz Med Wochenschr* (1970) 100, 583–4.
2. Sennwald G. Etude de l'influence de la rifampicine sur l'effet anticoagulant de l'acénocoumarol. *Rev Med Suisse Romande* (1974) 94, 945–54.
3. Ohnhaus EE, Kampschulte J, Mönig H. Effect of propranolol and rifampicin on liver blood flow and phenprocoumon elimination. *Acta Pharmacol Toxicol (Copenh)* (1986) 59 (Suppl 4), 92.
4. Boekhout-Mussert RJ, Bieger R, van Brummelen A, Lemkes HHPJ. Inhibition by rifampin of the anticoagulant effect of phenprocoumon. *JAMA* (1974) 229, 1903–4.
5. O'Reilly RA. Interaction of chronic daily warfarin therapy and rifampin. *Ann Intern Med* (1975) 83, 506–8.
6. O'Reilly RA. Interaction of sodium warfarin and rifampin. Studies in man. *Ann Intern Med* (1974) 81, 337–40.

7. Heimark LD, Gibaldi M, Trager WF, O'Reilly RA, Goulart DA. The mechanism of the warfarin-rifampicin drug interaction in humans. *Clin Pharmacol Ther* (1987) 42, 388–94.
8. Romankiewicz JA, Ehrman M. Rifampin and warfarin: a drug interaction. *Ann Intern Med* (1975) 82, 224–5.
9. Self TH, Mann RB. Interaction of rifampicin and warfarin. *Chest* (1975) 67, 490–1.
10. Fox P. Warfarin-rifampicin interaction. *Med J Aust* (1982) 1, 60.
11. Beeley L, Daly M, Stewart P. *Bulletin of the West Midlands Centre for Adverse Drug Reaction Reporting* (1987) 24, 23.
12. Almog S, Martinowitz U, Halkin H, Bank HZ, Farfel Z. Complex interaction of rifampin and warfarin. *South Med J* (1988) 81, 1304–6.
13. Casner PR. Inability to attain oral anticoagulation: warfarin-rifampin interaction revisited. *South Med J* (1996) 89, 1200–3.
14. Lee CR, Thrasher KA. Difficulties in anticoagulation management during coadministration of warfarin and rifampin. *Pharmacotherapy* (2001) 21, 1240–6.
15. Mycobutin (Rifabutin). Pharmacia Ltd. UK Summary of product characteristics, October 2006.
16. Committee on the Safety of Medicines/Medicines Control Agency. Revised indication and drug interactions of rifabutin. *Current Problems* (1997) 23, 14.

Coumarins and related drugs + Antibacterials; Sulfonamides and/or Trimethoprim

Co-trimoxazole modestly inhibits the metabolism of *S*-warfarin, and a number of case reports show that the anticoagulant effects of the coumarins warfarin, acenocoumarol, and phenprocoumon are increased by co-trimoxazole. Case reports suggest that sulfafurazole, sulfadoxine, and sulfamethizole may have similar effects. Two cohort studies have suggested that trimethoprim alone is associated with an increased risk of overanticoagulation, but this was less than that for co-trimoxazole in one of these studies. Anecdotal evidence suggests that the indanedione phenindione might not interact with co-trimoxazole, but in one study sulfaphenazole increased the effect of phenindione.

Clinical evidence

(a) Co-trimoxazole (Sulfamethoxazole with trimethoprim)

1. Coumarins. Six out of 20 patients taking **warfarin** had an increase in their prothrombin ratios (to about 4 to 6) within 2 to 6 days of starting to take co-trimoxazole 960 mg twice daily.[1] One patient had a gastrointestinal haemorrhage and needed to be given vitamin K. The **warfarin** was temporarily withdrawn from 5 patients and the dosage was reduced in one patient to control excessive hypoprothrombinaemia.[1]

Similarly, an increase in the effects of **warfarin**, with or without bleeding complications, in patients given co-trimoxazole has been described in a number of other case reports.[2-14] In one study in healthy subjects, co-trimoxazole 480 mg four times daily for 8 days increased the prothrombin time after a single dose of warfarin by 1.5-fold, but no change in the half-life of **warfarin** was seen.[15] However, a later similar study by the same research group, in which warfarin was given as its separate isomers, co-trimoxazole increased the AUC of *S*-warfarin by 22% and caused a 5% decrease in AUC of *R*-warfarin.[16]

In a population based cohort study[17] in patients taking **acenocoumarol** or **phenprocoumon**, co-trimoxazole was associated with an increased risk of over-anticoagulation (INR greater than or equal to 6); the adjusted relative risk of over-anticoagulation was noted to be 20.1 (range 10.7 to 37.9). The risk was increased in the first 3 days of use (RR 16.6), but was greatest after 4 days of concurrent use (RR 23.2).

2. Indanediones. In one anecdotal report, the author noted that in several years experience of the use of **phenindione** in an anticoagulant clinic serving 1000 patients, he had not come across a clinically important case of anticoagulant potentiation with co-trimoxazole.[18] Nothing else seems to have been published on the combination, but note that another sulphonamide, sulfaphenazole, potentiated the effect of phenindione, see (d) below.

(b) Sulfadoxine

A 19-year-old with a valve replacement and taking **warfarin** presented with melaena and coughing up blood about a week after self-medicating with *Fansidar* (sulfadoxine/pyrimethamine). He had not had his anticoagulant control monitored.[19]

(c) Sulfafurazole (Sulfisoxazole)

A man taking digitalis, diuretics, antacids and **warfarin** was later given sulfafurazole 500 mg every 6 hours. After 9 days, his prothrombin time had risen from 20 to 28 seconds, and after 14 days he bled (haematuria, haemoptysis, gum bleeding). His prothrombin time had risen to 60 seconds.[20]

Another patient who had recently started taking **warfarin** developed haematuria and had a prolonged prothrombin time 7 days after also starting sulfafurazole.[21]

(d) Sulfamethizole

The half-life of **warfarin** was increased by over 40% (from 65 to 93 hours) in 2 patients taking sulfamethizole 1 g four times daily for a week.[22]

(e) Sulfaphenazole

Sixteen patients given single oral doses of **phenindione** and sulfaphenazole 500 mg had prothrombin time increases after 24 hours of 16.8 seconds, compared with 10.3 seconds in 12 other patients who took **phenindione** alone.[23]

(f) Trimethoprim

Trimethoprim combined with sulfamethoxazole (co-trimoxazole) is known to interact with coumarins, see (a) above. However, there appear to be no controlled studies of the effect of trimethoprim alone on these drugs, and no case reports of any interaction. In one cohort study, 12 patients taking **warfarin** had a small INR increase of about 0.36 when given trimethoprim, but this was not statistically significant.[24] In another cohort study in patients taking **acenocoumarol** or **phenprocoumon**, the use of trimethoprim was associated with an increased risk of over-anticoagulation (INR greater than or equal to 6). The adjusted relative risk of over-anticoagulation was noted to be 5.6 (range 1.3 to 23.1), and the greatest risk was in the first 3 days of concurrent use. The risk from trimethoprim alone in this study was less than that for co-trimoxazole.[17]

Mechanism

Not fully understood. Sulfamethoxazole is a known inhibitor of the cytochrome P450 isoenzyme CYP2C9, by which *S*-warfarin in predominantly metabolised. The finding that co-trimoxazole caused a modest 22% increase in *S*-warfarin levels supports this mechanism.[16,25] Acenocoumarol and phenprocoumon are also metabolised by CYP2C9 and might be expected to be similarly affected. Plasma protein binding displacement has been suggested as a mechanism,[26,27] but on its own it does not provide an adequate explanation because the interaction is sustained.[17,25] Sulfonamides can drastically reduce the intestinal bacterial synthesis of vitamin K, but this is not normally an essential source of the vitamin unless dietary sources are exceptionally low,[25,28] see also 'Coumarins + Antibacterials', p.365.

Importance and management

The interaction between co-trimoxazole and coumarin anticoagulants is well documented and well established. The incidence appears to be high. If bleeding is to be avoided the INR should be well monitored and the warfarin, acenocoumarol, or phenprocoumon dosage should be reduced. Anecdotal evidence suggests that co-trimoxazole may not interact with the indanedione phenindione, but note that sulfaphenazole did, so some caution is still appropriate.

The other interactions are poorly documented. However, it would seem prudent to follow the precautions suggested for co-trimoxazole if any sulfonamide is given with a coumarin or indanedione.

The relative silence in the literature for trimethoprim alone would suggest that, in practice, any interaction, if it occurs, is of only minor importance, and the anticoagulant dosage probably needs little or no adjustment, but note that 2 cohort studies have shown some increased risk when trimethoprim was given with warfarin, acenocoumarol or phenprocoumon so an interaction cannot entirely be dismissed.

1. Hassall C, Feetam CL, Leach RH, Meynell MJ. Potentiation of warfarin by co-trimoxazole. *Lancet* (1975) ii, 1155–6.
2. Barnett DB, Hancock BW. Anticoagulant resistance: an unusual case. *BMJ* (1975) 1, 608–9.
3. Tilstone WJ, Gray JMB, Nimmo-Smith RH, Lawson DH. Interaction between warfarin and sulphamethoxazole. *Postgrad Med J* (1977) 53, 388–90.
4. Errick JK, Keys PW. Co-trimoxazole and warfarin: case report of an interaction. *Am J Hosp Pharm* (1979) 35, 1399–1401.
5. Greenlaw CW. Drug interaction between co-trimoxazole and warfarin. *Am J Hosp Pharm* (1979) 36, 1155.
6. Keys PW. Drug interaction between co-trimoxazole and warfarin. *Am J Hosp Pharm* (1979) 36, 1155–6.
7. Kaufman JM, Fauver HE. Potentiation of warfarin by trimethoprim-sulfamethoxazole. *Urology* (1980) 16, 601–3.
8. Beeley L, Ballantine N, Beadle F. *Bulletin of the West Midlands Centre for Adverse Drug Reaction Reporting* (1983) 16, 7.
9. McQueen EG. New Zealand Committee on Adverse Drug Reactions. 17th Annual Report 1982. *N Z Med J* (1983) 96, 95–9.
10. O'Donnell D. Antibiotic-induced potentiation of oral anticoagulant agents. *Med J Aust* (1989) 150, 163–4.

11. Wolf R, Elman M, Brenner S. Sulfonamide-induced bullous hemorrhagic eruption in a patient with low prothrombin time. *Isr J Med Sci* (1992) 28, 882–4.
12. Erichsen C, Sndenaa K, Sreide JA, Andersen E, Tysvær A. Spontaneous liver hematomas induced by anti-coagulation therapy. A case report and review of the literature. *Hepatogastroenterology* (1993) 40, 402–6.
13. Cook DE, Ponte CD. Suspected trimethoprim/sulfamethoxazole-induced hypoprothrombinemia. *J Fam Pract* (1994) 39, 589–91.
14. Chafin CC, Ritter BA, James A, Self TH. Hospital admission due to warfarin potentiation by TMP-SMX. *Nurse Pract* (2000) 25, 73–75.
15. O'Reilly RA, Motley CH. Racemic warfarin and trimethoprim-sulfamethoxazole interaction in humans. *Ann Intern Med* (1979) 91, 34–6.
16. O'Reilly RA. Stereoselective interaction of trimethoprim-sulfamethoxazole with the separated enantiomorphs of racemic warfarin in man. *N Engl J Med* (1980) 302, 33–5.
17. Visser LE, Penning-van Beest FJA, Kasbergen AAH, De Smet PAGM, Vulto AG, Hofman A, Stricker BHC. Overanticoagulation associated with combined use of antibacterial drugs and acenocoumarol or phenprocoumon anticoagulants. *Thromb Haemost* (2002) 88, 705–10.
18. De Swiet J. Potentiation of warfarin by co-trimoxazole. *BMJ* (1975) 3, 491.
19. Obasohan AO, Ukoh V, Ajuyah CO. Prosthetic valve dysfunction in a Nigerian. *Trop Geogr Med* (1993) 45, 183–5.
20. Self TH, Evans W, Ferguson T. Interaction of sulfisoxazole and warfarin. *Circulation* (1975) 52, 528.
21. Sioris LJ, Weibert RT, Pentel PR. Potentiation of warfarin anticoagulation by sulfisoxazole. *Arch Intern Med* (1980) 140, 546–7.
22. Lumholtz B, Siersbaek-Nielsen K, Skovsted L, Kampmann J, Hansen JM. Sulphamethizole-induced inhibition of diphenylhydantoin, tolbutamide and warfarin metabolism. *Clin Pharmacol Ther* (1975) 17, 731.
23. Varma DR, Gupta RK, Gupta S, Sharma KK. Prothrombin response to phenindione during hypoalbuminaemia. *Br J Clin Pharmacol* (1975) 2, 467–8.
24. Pharmacy Anticoagulant Clinic Study Group. A multicentre survey of antibiotics on the INR of anticoagulated patients. *Pharm J* (1996) 257 (Pharmacy Practice Suppl), R30.
25. Fredricks DA. Comment: TMP/SMX—warfarin interaction. *DICP Ann Pharmacother* (1989) 23, 619–20.
26. Seiler K, Duckert F. Properties of 3-(1-phenyl-propyl)-4-oxycoumarin (Marcoumar®) in the plasma when tested in normal cases and under the influence of drugs. *Thromb Diath Haemorrh* (1968) 19, 389–96.
27. Solomon HM, Schrogie JJ. The effect of various drugs on the binding of warfarin-^{14}C to human albumin. *Biochem Pharmacol* (1967) 16, 1219–26.
28. Udall JA. Human sources and absorption of vitamin K in relation to anticoagulation stability. *JAMA* (1965) 194, 107–9.

Coumarins + Antibacterials; Teicoplanin or Vancomycin

An isolated case report describes a marked reduction in the effects of warfarin, which was attributed to teicoplanin, but which could be equally be explained by rifampicin treatment. One study found that vancomycin possibly causes a small increase in the effects of warfarin, and a cohort study suggested that vancomycin increased risk of over-anticoagulation with acenocoumarol or phenprocoumon.

Clinical evidence, mechanism, importance and management

(a) Teicoplanin

A 60-year-old woman taking digoxin, furosemide and **warfarin** (INR 3.5 to 5) developed a fever after mitral valve replacement surgery and was given rifampicin 450 mg twice daily and teicoplanin 400 mg twice daily. Within 3 days her INR began to fall and by day 6 the anticoagulant effect was completely lost. Despite progressive **warfarin** increases to 10, 15, and then 20 mg daily, her INR stayed between 1.2 and 1.6, even when the rifampicin was stopped, and remained low for a further 20 days, at which point the teicoplanin was also stopped.[1]

Some of this resistance to **warfarin** was undoubtedly due to the rifampicin (a known and potent inducer of **warfarin** metabolism) but as the INRs remained depressed for a further 20 days after rifampicin was withdrawn the authors suggested that the teicoplanin had its own part to play. However, rifampicin has been shown is several cases to decrease the effects of warfarin for 3 or more weeks after its withdrawal (see 'Coumarins + Antibacterials; Rifamycins' p.375), so an interaction with teicoplanin would seem doubtful.

(b) Vancomycin

In a retrospective review of 60 patients undergoing heart valve replacement surgery and receiving prophylactic antibacterials, 44 patients given cefamandole had a much greater anticoagulant response to their first dose of **warfarin** than 16 patients given **vancomycin**.[2] In a later prospective study by the same workers, in patients taking warfarin with an antibacterial, after 3 days the prothrombin times as a percentage of activity were as follows: cefamandole 29%, cefazolin 38%, and **vancomycin** 51%, suggesting that 'cefamandole', (p.367) had a much greater effect on anticoagulant response than **vancomycin**.[3]

In a cohort study, the use of **vancomycin** was associated with an increased risk of over-anticoagulation (an INR greater than 6) in patients stabilised on **acenocoumarol** or **phenprocoumon**. The relative risk was 13.6; however, the confidence interval was very large (1.7 to 107), so it is not possible to draw any firm conclusions from this.[4] Consider also 'Coumarins + Antibacterials', p.365.

1. Agosta FG, Liberato NL, Chiofalo F. Warfarin resistance induced by teicoplanin. *Haematologica* (1997) 82, 637–40.
2. Angaran DM, Dias VC, Arom KV, Northrup WF, Kersten TE, Lindsay WG, Nicoloff DM. The influence of prophylactic antibiotics on the warfarin anticoagulation response in the postoperative prosthetic cardiac valve patient. *Ann Surg* (1984) 199, 107–111.
3. Angaran DM, Dias VC, Arom KV, Northrup WF, Kersten TG, Lindsay WG, Nicoloff DM. The comparative influence of prophylactic antibiotics on the prothrombin response to warfarin in the postoperative prosthetic cardiac valve patient. *Ann Surg* (1987) 206, 155–61.
4. Visser LE, Penning-van Beest FJA, Kasbergen AAH, De Smet PAGM, Vulto AG, Hofman A, Stricker BHC. Overanticoagulation associated with combined use of antibacterial drugs and acenocoumarol or phenprocoumon anticoagulants. *Thromb Haemost* (2002) 88, 705–10.

Coumarins and related drugs + Antibacterials; Tetracyclines

Isolated cases suggest that doxycycline and tetracycline can increase the effects of coumarins. Similarly, some small studies (none controlled) suggest that chlortetracycline (alone or with oxytetracycline), doxycycline, or the tetracyclines as a class may increase the risks of over-anticoagulation, but there appear to be no studies of the effect of tetracyclines on the pharmacokinetics of coumarins. However, the related antibacterial, tigecycline, increased the AUC of warfarin, and has been shown to increase the prothrombin time when given alone.

Clinical evidence

There are no controlled studies of the effect of any tetracycline on the pharmacokinetics or pharmacodynamics of warfarin or other coumarins, although there are data for tigecycline, a new glycylcycline antibacterial structurally related to tetracyclines.

(a) Chlortetracycline

Six out of 9 patients taking an unnamed anticoagulant had a fall in their prothrombin-proconvertin concentration from a range of 10 to 30% to less than 6% when given chlortetracycline 250 mg four times a day for 4 days. Although the anticoagulant effects were increased, there was no evidence of bleeding.[1] In one early study of **dicoumarol** and **ethyl biscoumacetate**, the authors briefly comment that 4 cases of combined use with chlortetracycline plus oxytetracycline increased the prothrombin response.[2]

(b) Doxycycline

A woman stabilised on **warfarin** developed menorrhagia after taking doxycycline 100 mg twice daily for 10 days, and her prothrombin time ratio had increased from about 2 to 4.4.[3] Two other patients stabilised on **acenocoumarol** or **warfarin** developed markedly increased prothrombin ratios (3.82 and 4.09, respectively) with bruising, haematomas and bleeding when they took doxycycline.[4] Another patient with multiple medical problems, taking **warfarin** and a range of drugs (alendronate, atorvastatin, salbutamol, diltiazem, fluticasone) developed peritoneal bleeding and an INR of 7.2 (previously 2.6) 6 days after starting doxycycline 100 mg twice daily.[5]

In a population-based cohort study in patients taking **acenocoumarol** or **phenprocoumon**, doxycycline was found to increase the risk of over-anticoagulation (INR greater than or equal to 6) with an adjusted relative risk of 4.3 (range 1.8 to 10.4). The risks were greatest after 4 or more days of concurrent use.[6]

(c) Oxytetracycline

In one early study of **dicoumarol** and **ethyl biscoumacetate**, the authors briefly comment that 4 cases of combined use with chlortetracycline plus **oxytetracycline** increased the prothrombin response.[2].

(d) Tetracycline

In one analysis of haemorrhagic events in patients taking **dicoumarol** and antibacterials, 1 patient out of 20 who received tetracycline had a bleeding event.[7] A patient stabilised on **warfarin** had a marked increase in INR (from about 2 to 7.7) 6 weeks after starting to take tetracycline 250 mg four times daily. Warfarin was withheld for a few days, then restarted at a 40% lower dose. The INR decreased over the following months, broadly in parallel with decreases in the tetracycline dosage.[8] A patient taking **warfarin** bled (right temporal lobe haematoma) and had an extended prothrombin time a week after starting to take tetracycline and nystatin.[9] Another patient taking **warfarin** also bled (epistaxis, haematemesis, melaena) 3 weeks after starting to take tetracycline and nystatin.[9]

(e) Tigecycline

The manufacturer notes that, in healthy subjects, intravenous tigecycline 100 mg then 50 mg every 12 hours decreased the clearance of *R*-warfarin by 40% and *S*-warfarin by 23% after a single 25-mg dose of **warfarin**. The AUC was increased by 68% and 29%, respectively. However, the INR was not affected.[10,11]

(f) Unnamed tetracyclines

In a prospective study of the effect of antibacterials on anticoagulation, there was an estimated 0.53 increase in the INR in 9 patients taking warfarin and a tetracycline (unnamed) The effect with tetracyclines was greater than the effect of other antibacterials studied (penicillins, cephalosporins, macrolides).[12]

Mechanism

Not understood. Tetracyclines in the absence of anticoagulants can reduce prothrombin activity,[13] and both hypoprothrombinaemia and bleeding have been described.[14,15] It seems possible that very occasionally the anticoagulant and the tetracycline have additive hypoprothrombinaemic effects. Tigecycline alone has commonly caused prolonged prothrombin time (incidence 1 to 10%) or uncommonly caused an increased INR (incidence 0.1 to 1%) in clinical studies.[10] It is also possible that antibacterials can diminish the intestinal flora of the gut thereby depleting the body of vitamin K_2, although this might be clinically important only where normal dietary intake of vitamin K_1 is extremely low, see 'Coumarins + Antibacterials', p.365. There appear to be no data on the effect of tetracyclines on the pharmacokinetics of coumarins. Although tigecycline decreased the clearance of warfarin, the mechanism for this is unclear.[10,11]

Importance and management

A relatively sparsely documented interaction, bearing in mind that the tetracyclines have been in very widespread use for many years. It can therefore reasonably be concluded that normally any changes are of little clinical relevance. As a few patients have unpredictably shown increased anticoagulant effects and even bleeding, bear this interaction in mind when a tetracycline is first added to established anticoagulant treatment with a coumarin. Because tigecycline decreased the clearance of warfarin, and because it could cause an increase in INR, it is recommended that the INR be closely monitored in patients taking warfarin when given tigecycline.[10,11] There appears to be no information about the indanediones, but if the mechanism suggested is correct they may also interact like the coumarins.

1. Magid E. Tolerance to anticoagulants during antibiotic therapy. *Scand J Clin Lab Invest* (1962) 14, 565–6.
2. Scarrone LA, Beck DF, Wright IS. A comparative evaluation of Tromexan and dicumarol in the treatment of thromboembolic conditions — based on experience with 514 patients. *Circulation* (1952) 6, 489–514.
3. Westfall LK, Mintzer DL, Wiser TH. Potentiation of warfarin by tetracycline. *Am J Hosp Pharm* (1980) 37, 1620, 1625.
4. Caraco Y, Rubinow A. Enhanced anticoagulant effect of coumarin derivatives induced by doxycycline coadministration. *Ann Pharmacother* (1992) 26, 1084–6.
5. Baciewicz AM, Bal BS. Bleeding associated with doxycycline and warfarin treatment. *Arch Intern Med* (2001) 161, 1231.
6. Visser LE, Penning-van Beest FJA, Kasbergen AAH, De Smet PAGM, Vulto AG, Hofman A, Stricker BHC. Overanticoagulation associated with combined use of antibacterial drugs and acenocoumarol or phenprocoumon anticoagulants. *Thromb Haemost* (2002) 88, 705–10.
7. Chiavazza F, Merialdi A. Sulle interferenze fra dicumarolo e antibiotici. *Minerva Ginecol* (1973) 25, 630–1.
8. Danos EA. Apparent potentiation of warfarin activity by tetracycline. *Clin Pharm* (1992) 11, 806–8.
9. O'Donnell D. Antibiotic-induced potentiation of oral anticoagulant agents. *Med J Aust* (1989) 150, 163–4.
10. Tygacil (Tigecycline). Wyeth Pharmaceuticals. UK Summary of product characteristics, April 2006.
11. Tygacil (Tigecycline). Wyeth Pharmaceuticals Inc. US Prescribing information, May 2007.
12. Pharmacy Anticoagulant Clinic Study Group. A multicentre survey of antibiotics on the INR of anticoagulated patients. *Pharm J* (1996) 257 (Pharmacy Practice Suppl), R30.
13. Searcy RL, Simms NM, Foreman JA, Bergquist LM. Evaluation of the blood-clotting mechanism in tetracycline-treated patients. *Antimicrob Agents Chemother* (1964) 4, 179–83.
14. Rios JF. Hemorrhagic diathesis induced by antimicrobials. *JAMA* (1968) 205, 142.
15. Klippel AP, Pitsinger B. Hypoprothrombinemia secondary to antibiotic therapy and manifested by massive gastrointestinal hemorrhage. *Arch Surg* (1968) 96, 266–8.

Coumarins + Anticholinesterases; Centrally acting

Donepezil, galantamine, rivastigmine and tacrine do not appear to alter the pharmacokinetics or effects of warfarin.

Clinical evidence, mechanism, importance and management

(a) Donepezil

In an open-label, crossover study, 12 healthy men were given donepezil 10 mg daily for 19 days with a single 25-mg dose of **warfarin** on day 14. The pharmacokinetics of *R*- and *S*-warfarin and the prothrombin times were unchanged by the presence of the donepezil, and vital signs, ECG and laboratory tests were unaltered.[1]

(b) Galantamine

The manufacturers of galantamine[2,3] say that galantamine 12 mg twice had no effect on the pharmacokinetics of *R*- and *S*-warfarin after a single 25-mg dose of **warfarin**. In addition, galantamine did not alter the prothrombin time.[3]

(c) Rivastigmine

The manufacturers of rivastigmine[4,5] say that no pharmacokinetic interaction has been noted between rivastigmine and **warfarin** in healthy subjects. In addition, rivastigmine did not affect the increase in prothrombin time seen with warfarin.

(d) Tacrine

A study in 10 patients stabilised on **warfarin** found that the addition of tacrine 20 mg four times daily for 5 days had no significant effect on prothrombin times.[6]

1. Tiseo PJ, Foley K, Friedhoff LT. The effect of multiple doses of donepezil hydrochloride on the pharmacokinetic and pharmacodynamic profile of warfarin. *Br J Clin Pharmacol* (1998) 46 (Suppl 1), 45–50.
2. Reminyl (Galantamine hydrobromide). Shire Pharmaceuticals Ltd. UK Summary of product characteristics, July 2005.
3. Razadyne (Galantamine hydrobromide). Ortho-McNeil Neurologics, Inc. US Prescribing information, August 2006.
4. Exelon (Rivastigmine hydrogen tartrate). Novartis Pharmaceuticals UK Ltd. UK Summary of product characteristics, October 2006.
5. Exelon (Rivastigmine tartrate). Novartis Pharmaceuticals Corp. US Prescribing information, June 2006.
6. Reece PA, Garnett WR, Rock WL, Taylor JR, Underwood B, Sedman AJ, Rajagopalan R. Lack of effect of tacrine administration on the anticoagulant activity of warfarin. *J Clin Pharmacol* (1995) 35, 526–8.

Coumarins + Antidiabetics; Alpha-glucosidase inhibitors

Acarbose, miglitol and voglibose did not appear to alter the pharmacokinetics or effects of warfarin. However, there are a few cases of reduced or increased INRs in patients given warfarin and acarbose.

Clinical evidence, mechanism, importance and management

(a) Acarbose

There are 3 isolated case reports of apparent interactions between **warfarin** and acarbose. A 66-year-old man taking fosinopril, hydrochlorothiazide, diphenhydramine, insulin, glipizide and **warfarin** started taking acarbose to improve the control of his diabetes. Four days before starting acarbose his INR was 3.09, but after 2 weeks (25 mg acarbose daily for week 1 and then 50 mg daily for week 2) his INR had *risen* to 4.85. The **warfarin** was temporarily stopped, then it was reintroduced at a lower dosage, and finally the acarbose was withdrawn, resulting in an INR of 2.84. No bleeding was seen.[1] In contrast, the manufacturer has on record 2 other cases of patients taking **warfarin** whose INRs were *reduced* when acarbose was added. One of them stopped taking the acarbose, whereupon her INR returned to its previous value. The other patient needed an increased **warfarin** dosage.[2]

The picture presented by these cases is that usually no interaction occurs, but in isolated cases some changes in **warfarin** requirements occur. Bear this potential interaction in mind if anticoagulant control alters in a patient taking acarbose.

(b) Miglitol

In a double-blind, randomised, placebo-controlled study, 24 healthy subjects were given miglitol 100 mg three times daily for 7 days, with a single 25-mg oral dose of **warfarin** on day 4. Neither the pharmacokinetics nor the pharmacodynamics of *R*- or *S*-warfarin was affected by the miglitol.[3] No special precautions would therefore appear to be needed if these two drugs are used concurrently.

(c) Voglibose

Twelve healthy male subjects were given individually adjusted doses of **warfarin** to give Quick values of 30 to 40%, and then from day 11 to 15 they were also given voglibose 5 mg three times daily. It was found that the voglibose had no effect on the pharmacokinetics of the **warfarin** nor on its anticoagulant effects.[4] No special precautions would therefore appear to be needed if these two drugs are used concurrently.

1. Morreale AP, Janetzky K. Probable interaction of warfarin and acarbose. *Am J Health-Syst Pharm* (1997) 54, 1551–2.
2. Bayer. Personal communication, December 1997.
3. Schall R, Müller FO, Hundt HKL, Duursema L, Groenewoud G, Middle MV. Study of the effect of miglitol on the pharmacokinetics and pharmacodynamics of warfarin in healthy males. *Arzneimittelforschung* (1996) 46, 41–6.
4. Fuder H, Kleist P, Birkel M, Ehrlich A, Emeklibas S, Maslak W, Stridde E, Wetzelsberger N, Wieckhorst G, Lücker PW. The α-glucosidase inhibitor voglibose (AO-128) does not change pharmacodynamics or pharmacokinetics of warfarin. *Eur J Clin Pharmacol* (1997) 53, 153–7.

Coumarins + Antidiabetics; Biguanides

One patient had a marked increase in the effects of phenprocoumon when she stopped taking metformin for a short period, and there is some evidence that metformin increases the metabolism of phenprocoumon.
One patient taking warfarin developed haematuria with a therapeutic prothrombin time three months after starting phenformin. Another patient developed metformin-induced lactic acidosis after warfarin-induced bleeding caused renal obstruction. However, these interactions are isolated and seem unlikely to be of general importance.

Clinical evidence

(a) Phenprocoumon

The Quick value of a 58-year old woman stabilised on **metformin** 1.7 g twice daily and phenprocoumon 3 to 4.5 mg daily fell from a range of 20 to 30% down to 0% when she stopped taking the **metformin** while on holiday. Despite the increased anticoagulant effect no signs of bleeding were observed, and she was eventually restabilised on the original doses of both drugs.[1] This case prompted a further observational study in 13 patients with type 2 diabetes. It was found that the 7 patients taking **metformin** 1.1 to 3 g daily were less well anticoagulated than those taking only 400 mg to 1 g of **metformin**, even though the mean phenprocoumon dosage was slightly higher in those taking the higher **metformin** dose (2.57 mg daily versus 2.27 mg daily).[1] In another study, the half-life of phenprocoumon was reduced by about one-third (from 123 to 85 hours) by **metformin** 1.7 g daily.[1]

(b) Warfarin

An elderly woman taking warfarin 5 mg daily and **metformin** 1 g twice daily developed fatigue, epistaxis, haematuria and gingival bleeding, with an INR of 16.9, which was treated with vitamin K. The following morning, she was given **metformin**, then she was found to have a retroperitoneal haematoma and bilateral perinephric blood with obstruction of both renal collecting systems. Over the next 8 hours, she developed progressive metabolic acidosis and suffered a cardiopulmonary arrest. Her **metformin** level was 7.3 micrograms/mL (therapeutic range 1 to 2 micrograms/mL). It was suggested that **metformin** accumulation occurred because of renal insufficiency caused by the site of renal bleeding secondary to the excessive effects of warfarin. This then resulted in metabolic acidosis.[2]

Haematuria occurred in a patient taking warfarin 3 months after **phenformin** was started. Her prothrombin values were normal.[3] **Phenformin** may have increased fibrinolysis to the point where it was additive with the effects of the warfarin.

Mechanism

Metformin possibly reduces the effects of phenprocoumon by altering blood flow to the liver and interfering with enterohepatic circulation.

Importance and management

The information about a biguanide interaction with warfarin appears to be limited to these isolated reports, neither of which definitively suggest that the biguanide altered anticoagulant effects. In general no interaction would be expected between metformin or phenformin and warfarin.

There is some evidence that a small increase in the dosage of phenprocoumon may be necessary if metformin is given but it seems likely that this can be managed with routine anticoagulant monitoring .

1. Ohnhaus EE, Berger W, Duckert F, Oesch F. The influence of dimethylbiguanide on phenprocoumon elimination and its mode of action. *Klin Wochenschr* (1983) 61, 851–8.
2. Schier JG, Hoffman RS, Nelson LS. Metformin-induced acidosis due to a warfarin adverse drug event. *Ann Pharmacother* (2003) 37, 1145.
3. Hamblin TJ. Interaction between warfarin and phenformin. *Lancet* (1971) ii, 1323.

Coumarins + Antidiabetics; Nateglinide or Repaglinide

Nateglinide and repaglinide do not appear to interact with warfarin, and nateglinide does not interact with acenocoumarol

Clinical evidence, mechanism, importance and management

(a) Nateglinide

In a randomised, double-blind study, 11 healthy subjects were given nateglinide 120 mg three times daily for 5 days, with a single 10-mg dose of **acenocoumarol** on day 3. Nateglinide had no effect on the tolerability, pharmacokinetics or anticoagulant activity of **acenocoumarol**.[1]

In another study,12 healthy subjects were given nateglinide 120 mg three times daily for 4 days with a single 30-mg dose of **warfarin** on day 2. No pharmacokinetic or pharmacodynamic interaction was noted.[2] No dosage adjustments would therefore be expected to be necessary if nateglinide is taken with either acenocoumarol or warfarin.

(b) Repaglinide

In a double-blind, placebo-controlled study in 28 healthy subjects who were stabilised on **warfarin**, repaglinide did not alter the anticoagulant effects of **warfarin** or the steady-state warfarin pharmacokinetics.[3] Therefore, no **warfarin** dosage adjustment would be anticipated on concurrent use.

1. Sunkara G, Bigler H, Wang Y, Smith H, Prasad P, McLeod J, Ligueros-Saylan M. The effect of nateglinide on the pharmacokinetics and pharmacodynamics of acenocoumarol. *Curr Med Res Opin* (2004) 20, 41–8.
2. Anderson DM, Shelley S, Crick N, Buraglio M. No effect of the novel antidiabetic agent nateglinide on the pharmacokinetics and anticoagulant properties of warfarin in healthy volunteers. *J Clin Pharmacol* (2002) 42, 1358–65.
3. Rosenberg M, Strange P, Cohen A. Assessment of pharmacokinetic (PK) and pharmacodynamic (PD) interaction between warfarin and repaglinide. *Diabetes* (1999) 48 (Suppl 1), A356.

Coumarins + Antidiabetics; Pioglitazone or Rosiglitazone

Pioglitazone does not appear to alter the pharmacokinetics or anticoagulant effect of warfarin or phenprocoumon. Rosiglitazone did not affect the pharmacokinetics of warfarin.

Clinical evidence

(a) Pioglitazone

Pioglitazone 45 mg daily for 7 days did not alter the steady-state pharmacokinetics of *R*- or *S*-warfarin and there was no significant change in prothrombin time.[1,2] Similar results were noted with **phenprocoumon**.[2] Pioglitazone had no effect on prothrombin time when it was given to patients stabilised on **warfarin**.[1]

(b) Rosiglitazone

Rosiglitazone has been found to have no clinically relevant effect on the steady-state pharmacokinetics of **warfarin**.[3]

Mechanism

In vitro, troglitazone (the first thiazolidinedione, which has now been withdrawn) significantly inhibited the cytochrome P450 isoenzyme CYP2C9-dependent 7-hydroxylation of *S*-warfarin; however, pioglitazone and rosiglitazone only slightly inhibited this activity.[4]

Importance and management

Controlled studies have shown no interaction between pioglitazone and warfarin or phenprocoumon, or between rosiglitazone and warfarin. This suggests that coumarin dose adjustments are unlikely to be needed when these antidiabetics are used.

1. Actos (Pioglitazone hydrochloride). Takeda Pharmaceutical Company Ltd. US Prescribing information, February 2007.
2. Kortboyer JM, Eckland DJA. Pioglitazone has low potential for drug interactions. *Diabetologia* (1999) 42 (Suppl 1), A228.
3. Avandia (Rosiglitazone maleate). GlaxoSmithKline. US Prescribing information, June 2007.
4. Yamazaki H, Suzuki M, Tane K, Shimada N, Nakajima M, Yokoi T. *In vitro* inhibitory effects of troglitazone and its metabolites on drug oxidation activities of human cytochrome P450 enzymes: comparison with pioglitazone and rosiglitazone. *Xenobiotica* (2000) 30, 61–70.

Coumarins and related drugs + Antidiabetics; Sulfonylureas

Dicoumarol inhibits the metabolism of tolbutamide and increases its effects; cases of hypoglycaemic coma have been reported. Chlorpropamide may be affected similarly. Although isolated cases of interactions (raised prothrombin times, bleeding or hypoglycaemia) have been seen in patients taking sulfonylureas and coumarins, in general, no important interaction appears to occur. There also appears to be no interaction between phenindione and tolbutamide.

Clinical evidence

A. Coumarins

(a) Chlorpropamide

1. Acenocoumarol. A woman with normal renal function had an increase in the half-life of chlorpropamide to 88 hours (normally about 36 hours) when she took acenocoumarol.[1]

2. Dicoumarol. A 67-year-old non-diabetic man taking chlorpropamide for Parkinson's disease developed severe hypoglycaemia about 3 months after starting dicoumarol. He had high chlorpropamide levels with a half-life of 80 to 90 hours. Dicoumarol was withdrawn, and 3 weeks later his chlorpropamide half-life was 30 hours.[2] This observation prompted further study in 3 other patients and 2 non-diabetics. Dicoumarol doubled the serum chlorpropamide levels within 3 to 4 days and also more than doubled the half-life.[2]

(b) Glibenclamide (Glyburide)

1. Phenprocoumon. The pharmacokinetics of glibenclamide remained unchanged by phenprocoumon.[3] Similarly, the plasma levels and half-life of single doses of phenprocoumon did not differ between patients with type 2 diabetes managed by diet alone (12 patients) and those taking glibenclamide (9 patients).[4]

2. Warfarin. There do not appear to be any controlled studies on the effect of glibenclamide on the pharmacokinetics of coumarins, although recent *in vitro* data suggest that an effect is possible because glibenclamide inhibited *S*-warfarin hydroxylation (a 7 to 37% *in vivo* inhibition was predicted).[5] Moreover, isolated reports describe increased warfarin effects (INR increased from 2.3 to 6.6 with haematomas in one instance[6]) in 2 patients given glibenclamide.[6,7]

(c) Glibornuride

Phenprocoumon, given to 3 subjects for 4 days, slightly increased the half-life of a single 25-mg dose of glibornuride by 29%.[8] The plasma levels and half-life of a single dose of **phenprocoumon** did not differ between patients with type 2 diabetes managed by diet alone (12 patients) and those taking glibornuride (12 patients).[4]

(d) Glimepiride

In healthy subjects, glimepiride 4 mg daily caused only minor, clinically unimportant changes in the prothrombin times (about 10% decrease in mean maximum prothrombin time) in response to single 25-mg doses of **warfarin**. In addition, glimepiride had no effect on the pharmacokinetics of *R*- and *S*-warfarin.[9]

(e) Tolbutamide

1. Dicoumarol. Dicoumarol has been shown to increase the serum levels of tolbutamide, prolong its half-life (more than threefold), and reduce blood-glucose levels in both diabetics[10] and healthy subjects.[10-12] This may become excessive in a few patients and hypoglycaemic coma has been described in 3 diabetics,[10,13,14] and one non-diabetic.[15]
Two patients taking dicoumarol had marked increases in prothrombin times (a rise from 33 to 60 seconds) within 2 days of starting to take tolbutamide, but no bleeding occurred. However, no increases were seen in 3 other patients taking dicoumarol when they started tolbutamide.[16] Conversely, the half-life of dicoumarol was approximately halved in 2 out of 4 healthy subjects given tolbutamide, but the hypoprothrombinaemic effects were unchanged.[12] However, in a retrospective study there was no difference in the initial or average dose of dicoumarol between 15 patients taking tolbutamide and 24 control subjects taking insulin.[17]

2. Phenprocoumon. Phenprocoumon did not alter the half-life of tolbutamide in 3 patients.[18]
The plasma levels and half-life of single doses of phenprocoumon did not differ between patients with type 2 diabetes managed by diet alone (12 patients) and those taking tolbutamide (10 patients).[4]

3. Warfarin. In a retrospective study, there was no difference in the initial or average dose of warfarin between 42 patients taking tolbutamide and 54 control subjects taking insulin.[17] However, a bulletin mentions an isolated report of an increased INR in a patient taking warfarin and tolbutamide.[19]

B. Indanediones

In one early study, phenindione given 6 days did not affect the half-life of **tolbutamide** in 2 healthy subjects. Similarly, the average plasma levels of **tolbutamide** in 3 patients taking phenindione were not different from 4 patients not taking phenindione.[10]

Mechanism

Dicoumarol appears to increase the effects of tolbutamide by inhibiting its metabolism by the liver.[10,11] This may also be true for chlorpropamide.[2] The increase in the anticoagulant effects of dicoumarol by tolbutamide may, in part, be due to a plasma protein binding interaction. In the case of phenprocoumon there seem to be several different mutually opposing processes going on, which cancel each other out.[12] There is no clear explanation for most of these interactions.

Importance and management

Information is patchy and very incomplete. The effect of dicoumarol on tolbutamide has been most thoroughly investigated, and the interaction is clinically important. Increased blood-glucose lowering effects may be expected if dicoumarol is given to patients taking tolbutamide, and there is a risk of hypoglycaemic coma. Whether tolbutamide alters the anticoagulant response to dicoumarol is unclear. Avoid concurrent use unless the outcome can be well monitored and dosage adjustments made. The same precautions should be taken with dicoumarol and chlorpropamide, but information is limited to one study.

Information on other interactions is limited to isolated cases, and these are therefore of doubtful general significance.

1. Petitpierrre B, Perrin L, Rudhardt M, Herrera A, Fabre J. Behaviour of chlorpropamide in renal insufficiency and under the effect of associated drug therapy. *Int J Clin Pharmacol* (1972) 6, 120–4.
2. Kristensen M, Hansen JM. Accumulation of chlorpropamide caused by dicoumarol. *Acta Med Scand* (1968) 183, 83–6.
3. Schulz E, Schmidt FH. Über den Einfluß von Sulphaphenazol, Phenylbutazon und Phenprocumarol auf die Elimination von Glibenclamid beim Menschen. *Verh Dtsch Ges Inn Med* (1970) 76, 435–8.
4. Heine P, Kewitz H, Wiegboldt K-A. The influence of hypoglycaemic sulphonylureas on elimination and efficacy of phenprocoumon following a single oral dose in diabetic patients. *Eur J Clin Pharmacol* (1976) 10, 31–6.
5. Kim K-A, Park J-Y. Inhibitory effect of glyburide on human cytochrome P450 isoforms in human liver microsomes. *Drug Metab Dispos* (2003) 3, 1090–2.
6. Jassal SV. Drug points. *BMJ* (1991) 303, 789.
7. Beeley L, Stewart P, Hickey FM. *Bulletin of the West Midlands Centre for Adverse Drug Reaction Reporting* (1988) 26, 27.
8. Eckhardt W, Rudolph R, Sauer H, Schubert WR, Undeutsch D. Zur pharmakologischen Interferenz von Glibornurid mit Sulfaphenazol, Phenylbutazon und phenprocoumon beim Menschen. *Arzneimittelforschung* (1972) 22, 2212–19.
9. Schaaf LJ, Sisson TA, Dietz AJ, Viveash DM, Oliver LK, Knuth DW, Carel BJ. Influence of multiple dose glimepiride on the pharmacokinetics and pharmacodynamics of racemic warfarin in healthy volunteers. *Pharm Res* (1994) 11 (10 Suppl), S-359.
10. Kristensen M, Hansen JM. Potentiation of the tolbutamide effect by dicoumarol. *Diabetes* (1967) 16, 211–14.

11. Solomon HM, Schrogie JJ. Effect of phenyramidol and bishydroxycoumarin on the metabolism of tolbutamide in human subjects. *Metabolism* (1967) 16, 1029–33.
12. Jähnchen E, Meinertz T, Gilfrich H-J, Groth U. Pharmacokinetic analysis of the interaction between dicoumarol and tolbutamide in man. *Eur J Clin Pharmacol* (1976) 10, 349–56.
13. Spurny OM, Wolf JW, Devins GS. Protracted tolbutamide-induced hypoglycemia. *Arch Intern Med* (1965) 115, 53–6.
14. Fontana G, Addarii F, Peta G. Su di un caso di coma ipoglicemico in corso di terapia con tolbutamide e dicumarolici. *G Clin Med* (1968) 49, 849–58.
15. Schwartz JF. Tolbutamide-induced hypoglycemia in Parkinson's disease. A case report. *JAMA* (1961) 176, 106–9.
16. Chaplin H, Cassell M. Studies on the possible relationship of tolbutamide to dicumarol in anticoagulant therapy. *Am J Med Sci* (1958) 235, 706–15.
17. Poucher RL, Vecchio TJ. Absence of tolbutamide effect on anticoagulant therapy. *JAMA* (1966) 197, 1069–70.
18. Skovsted L, Kristensen M, Hansen M, Siersbæk-Nielsen K. The effect of different oral anticoagulants on diphenylhydantoin (DPH) and tolbutamide metabolism. *Acta Med Scand* (1976) 199, 513–15.
19. Beeley L, Magee P, Hickey FN. *Bulletin of the West Midlands Centre for Adverse Drug Reaction Reporting* (1990) 30, 32.

Coumarins + Antihistamines

Findings from a retrospective review suggest that the anticoagulant effects of acenocoumarol may be reduced by loratadine, ebastine, or cetirizine. Conversely, an isolated report describes bleeding and a markedly raised INR in an elderly man taking acenocoumarol and cetirizine.

Clinical evidence, mechanism, importance and management

A retrospective review of patients taking **acenocoumarol** with **loratadine**, **ebastine**, or **cetirizine** found that INRs were decreased during concurrent use, but no thromboembolic event was noted. The authors consider that temporary increases in the anticoagulant dosage might be required.[1]

In contrast, there is a case report of an 88-year-old man taking **acenocoumarol** for a deep vein thrombosis who developed acute and severe epistaxis after a fall, and within 3 days of starting to take **cetirizine** 10 mg daily for allergic rhinitis.[2] His INR was found to have risen from 1.5 to 14. The **cetirizine** concentration may have been particularly high because of some renal impairment and because cetirizine may have displaced **acenocoumarol** from its plasma protein binding sites, although this mechanism on its own is now largely discredited as an explanation for interactions between anticoagulants and highly bound drugs.

Information is limited, and given the widespread use of these drugs any consistent clinically significant interaction might have been expected to have come to light by now. No specific precautions seem necessary if these drugs are given in combination, but bear the interaction in mind in the case of an unexpected response to treatment.

1. García Callejo FJ, Velert Vila MM, Marco Sanz M, Fernández Julián EN. Empleo simultáneo de antihistamínicos H_1 y anticoagulantes orales. *Acta Otorrinolaringol Esp* (2001) 52, 442–5.
2. Berod T, Mathiot I. Probable interaction between cetirizine and acenocoumarol. *Ann Pharmacother* (1997) 31, 122.

Coumarins + Antineoplastics; Fluorouracil and related prodrugs

Capecitabine markedly increases warfarin levels and increases its anticoagulant effects. A number of case reports describe over-anticoagulation in patients taking warfarin with capecitabine. Similarly, case reports describe overanticoagulation in patients taking warfarin and fluorouracil, ftorafur or tegafur.

Clinical evidence

(a) Capecitabine

In an open study, 4 patients with breast or colorectal cancer received a single 20-mg dose of **warfarin** 8 days before starting oral capecitabine (3 cycles of capecitabine 1250 mg/m^2 twice daily for 14 days, then 7 days rest), then again on day 12 of the third cycle of capecitabine. Capecitabine increased the AUC of *S*-warfarin was increased by 57%, and its elimination half-life by 51%, without any significant changes to *R*-warfarin. The maximum INR was increased by 1.9-fold and the AUC of the INR increased 2.8-fold. Three of the patients required vitamin K administration. Because of the clear, statistically significant findings in these 4 patients, the study was terminated early.[1]

Various cases of this interaction have been reported.[2-6] In one of these reports, 2 patients starting **warfarin** developed gastrointestinal bleeding with an INR of greater than 10, after 2 cycles of capecitabine.[2] In another case, a patient who had been taking long-term **warfarin** required a gradual 85% reduction in warfarin dose to 0.78 mg daily over 3 cycles of capecitabine and **irinotecan**, and required an increase to 4 mg daily over the 3 weeks after stopping chemotherapy.[4] Another patient required a 50% reduction in **warfarin** dose while taking capecitabine.

The manufacturers of **capecitabine** also report that this interaction has occurred with the coumarins including **phenprocoumon**.[7,8]

(a) Fluorouracil and fluorouracil-based regimens

In an early clinical study, 25 patients with colon cancer were given bolus fluorouracil 15 to 20 mg/kg weekly plus **warfarin** daily, titrated to maintain the prothrombin time in the 20 to 30% range, and modified weekly as necessary. Three patients developed blood loss from the gut, which was controlled by giving a transfusion and stopping the **warfarin**. This study did not report the required dose of warfarin, or how often it needed adjusting in these patients.[9]

Various case reports have described clinically important over-anticoagulation with concurrent use of dose adjusted **warfarin** (for treatment of deep vein thrombosis, or in patients with prosthetic heart valves) and fluorouracil, either alone,[10,11] with folinic acid (leucovorin),[12-15] or levamisole.[13,16,17] In one well-described case, an elderly man taking **warfarin** long-term was found to have an INR of almost 40 (usual INR 3) four weeks after he started taking fluorouracil (450 mg/m^2 daily for 5 days then once weekly) and **levamisole** (50 mg every 8 hours for 3 days every other week). He required a two-thirds reduction in **warfarin** dose. Later, when the chemotherapy was withheld for 5 weeks his INR became subtherapeutic, and then increased again when the chemotherapy was re-started.[16] In another retrospective case series, 4 patients taking **warfarin** long-term (target INR 2 to 3) required an 18 to 74% reduction in **warfarin** dose during treatment with fluorouracil and **folinic acid** or **levamisole**. The maximum INR in 3 of these patients was 3.66 to 8.15, and the other patient had a maximum INR of 23.7 and a retroperitoneal bleed.[13]

Other cases of overanticoagulation have been reported with **warfarin** and fluorouracil-based regimens including **CMF** (**cyclophosphamide**, **methotrexate** and fluorouracil),[13,18,19] CMF plus **vincristine** and prednisone,[20] fluorouracil, **cisplatin** and **etoposide**,[21] and fluorouracil, **cisplatin** and **mitomycin**.[11]

A case has also been reported with the use of fixed dose **warfarin** (1 mg daily) for prophylaxis of venous catheter-associated thrombosis in a patient receiving fluorouracil with **vinblastine**.[22] Similarly, in a large retrospective analysis of fixed dose **warfarin**, 31 of 95 patients given regimens based on continuous infusions of **fluorouracil** had INR elevations above 1.5, and, of these, 18 had an INR of 3 to 4.9 and seven had an INR of more than 5. Epistaxis and haematuria occurred in 8 of the patients. The regimens used were fluorouracil plus **folinic acid**; folinic acid, fluorouracil plus **oxaliplatin** (FOLFOX), and folinic acid, fluorouracil plus **irinotecan** (FOLFIRI).[23] In a further analysis of the use of fixed dose **warfarin** with the FOLFOX regimen, 25 of 50 patients had an INR greater than 1.5 (range 1.55 to 9.4). Two of these developed haematuria, and one had a nosebleed.[24]

(c) Ftorafur

Increased INRs and bleeding (haemoptysis) were seen in a patient taking **warfarin** when *Orzel* (**uracil/ftorafur** in a 4:1 molar ratio) was given, and a 63% reduction in the warfarin dose was needed.[25]

(d) Tegafur

The manufacturers of *Uftoral* (**tegafur**/**uracil**) say that marked elevations in prothrombin times and INRs have been reported in patients taking **warfarin** when *Uftoral* was added.[26]

Mechanism

Uncertain. However, in a pharmacokinetic study in *rats,* fluorouracil significantly reduced the total clearance of *S*-warfarin by inhibiting its metabolism.[27] Data from the clinical study with the fluorouracil prodrug, capecitabine, suggests this interacts similarly.[1]

Importance and management

Fairly well-documented and established interactions of clinical importance. Prothrombin times should be regularly monitored in patients taking warfarin and other **coumarins** and requiring fluorouracil, capecitabine or other fluorouracil pro-drugs, anticipating the need to reduce the warfarin dose. Note that, from a disease perspective, when treating venous thromboembolic disease in patients with cancer, warfarin is generally inferior (higher risk of major bleeds and recurrent thrombosis) to low-molecular-weight heparins.[28]

1. Camidge R, Reigner B, Cassidy J, Grange S, Abt M, Weidekamm, Jodrell D. Significant effect of capecitabine on the pharmacokinetics and pharmacodynamics of warfarin in patients with cancer. *J Clin Oncol* (2005) 23, 4719–25.
2. Copur MS, Ledakis P, Bolton M, Morse AK, Werner T, Norvell M, Muhvic J, Chu E. An adverse interaction between warfarin and capecitabine: a case report and review of the literature. *Clin Colorectal Cancer* (2001) 3, 182–4.
3. Buyck HCE, Buckley N, Leslie MD, Plowman PN. Capecitabine-induced potentiation of warfarin. *Clin Oncol* (2003) 15, 297.
4. Janney LM, Waterbury NV. Capecitabine–warfarin interaction. *Ann Pharmacother* (2005) 39, 1546–51.
5. Issacs K, Haim N. Adverse interaction between capecitabine and warfarin resulting in altered coagulation parameters and bleeding: case report and review of the literature. *J Chemother* (2005) 17, 339–42.
6. Yildirim Y, Ozyilkan O, Akcali Z, Basturk B. Drug interaction between capecitabine and warfarin: a case report and review of the literature. *Int J Clin Pharmacol Ther* (2006) 44, 80–2.
7. Xeloda (Capecitabine). Roche Products Ltd. UK Summary of product characteristics, March 2007.
8. Xeloda (Capecitabine). Roche Pharmaceuticals. US Prescribing information, April 2006.
9. Chlebowski RT, Gota CH, Chann KK, Weiner JM, Block JB, Batemen JR. Clinical and pharmacokinetic effects of combined warfarin and 5-fluorouracil in advanced colon cancer. *Cancer Res* (1982) 42, 4827–30.
10. Wajima T, Mukhopadhyay P. Possible interactions between warfarin and 5-fluorouracil. *Am J Hematol* (1992) 40, 238.
11. Morita N, Kashihara K, Tagashira H, Otsuka H, Yoneda K, Murase T, Tsujikawa T, Furutani S, Furutani K, Minato M, Nishitani H. Two cases of retroperitoneal hematoma caused by combination of anticoagulant therapy and 5-fluorouracil. *J Med Invest* (2005) 52, 114–17.
12. Brown MC. Multisite mucous membrane bleeding due to a possible interaction between warfarin and 5-fluorouracil. *Pharmacotherapy* (1997) 17, 631–3.
13. Kolesar JM, Johnson CL, Freeberg BL, Berlin JD, Schiller JH. Warfarin-5-FU interaction – a consecutive case series. *Pharmacotherapy* (1999) 19, 1445–9.
14. Carabino J, Wang F. International normalized ratio fluctuation with warfarin-fluorouracil therapy. *Am J Health-Syst Pharm* (2002), 59, 875.
15. Davis DA, Fugate SE. Increasing warfarin dosage reductions associated with concurrent warfarin and repeated cycles of 5-fluorouracil therapy. *Pharmacotherapy* (2005) 25, 442–7.
16. Scarfe MA, Israel MK. Possible drug interaction between warfarin and combination of levamisole and fluorouracil. *Ann Pharmacother* (1994) 28, 464–7.
17. Wehbe TW, Warth JA. A case of bleeding requiring hospitalisation that was likely caused by an interaction between warfarin and levamisole. *Clin Pharmacol Ther* (1996) 59, 360–2. Erratum *ibid.* 60, 137.
18. Seifter EJ, Brooks BJ, Urba WJ. Possible interactions between warfarin and antineoplastic drugs. *Cancer Treat Rep* (1985) 69, 244–5.
19. Malacarne P, Maestri A. Possible interactions between antiblastic agents and warfarin inducing prothrombin time abnormalities. *Recenti Prog Med* (1996) 87, 135.
20. Booth BW, Weiss RB. Venous thrombosis during adjuvant chemotherapy. *N Engl J Med* (1981) 305, 170.
21. Aki Z, Kotiloğlu G, Özyilkan Ö. A patient with a prolonged prothrombin time due to an adverse interaction between 5-fluorouracil and warfarin. *Am J Gastroenterol* (2000) 95, 1093–4.
22. Brown MC. An adverse interaction between warfarin and 5-fluorouracil; a case report and review of the literature. *Chemotherapy* (1999) 45, 392–5.
23. Masci G, Magagnoli M, Zucali PA, Castagna L, Carnaghi C, Sarina B, Pedicini V, Fallini M, Santoro A. Minidose warfarin prophylaxis for catheter-associated thrombosis in cancer patients: can it be safely associated with fluorouracil-based chemotherapy? *J Clin Oncol* (2003) 21, 736–9.
24. Magagnoli M, Masci G, Carnagi C, Zucali PA, Castagna L, Morenghi E, Santoro A. Minidose warfarin is associated with a high incidence of international normalized ratio elevation during chemotherapy with FOLFOX regimen. *Ann Oncol* (2003) 14, 959–60.
25. Karwal MW, Schlueter AJ, Arnold MM, Davis RT. Presumed drug interaction between Orzel® and warfarin. *Blood* (1999) 94 (10 Suppl 1, part 2), 106b.
26. Uftoral (Tegafur/uracil). Merck Pharmaceuticals. UK Summary of product characteristics, November 2006.
27. Zhou Q, Chan E. Effect of 5-fluorouracil on the anticoagulant activity and the pharmacokinetics of warfarin enantiomers in rats. *Eur J Pharm Sci* (2002) 17, 73–80.
28. Baglin TP, Keeling DM, Watson HG, for the British Committee for Standards in Haematology. Guidelines on oral anticoagulation (warfarin): third edition – 2005 update. *Br J Haematol* (2006) 132, 277–85.

Coumarins + Antineoplastics; Miscellaneous

A number of case reports describe an increase in the effects of warfarin, accompanied by bleeding in some cases, caused by antineoplastic regimens containing carboplatin, chlormethine, cyclophosphamide, doxorubicin, etoposide, gefitinib, gemcitabine, ifosfamide with mesna, methotrexate, procarbazine, trastuzumab, vincristine or vindesine. A decrease in the effects of warfarin has been seen with azathioprine, cyclophosphamide, mercaptopurine and mitotane, a decrease in the effects of acenocoumarol has been seen with mercaptopurine, and a decrease in the effects of phenprocoumon have been seen with azathioprine.

Clinical evidence

(a) Azathioprine

A survey of 103 patients with antiphospholipid syndrome found that azathioprine appeared to increase **warfarin** requirements.[1] A woman who was resistant to **warfarin**, needing 14 to 17 mg daily while taking azathioprine, began to bleed (epistaxes, haematemesis) when the azathioprine was stopped. She was restabilised on **warfarin** 5 mg daily.[2] Reduced **warfarin** effects were seen in 2 other patients taking azathioprine,[3,4] one of whom had a marked fall in serum **warfarin** levels during azathioprine treatment.[4] Two women with systemic lupus erythematosus taking **phenprocoumon**[5] and a third taking **warfarin**[6] had marked falls in their INRs during treatment with azathioprine, and another woman needed an almost fourfold increase in the dose of **warfarin** when she was given azathioprine.[7]

(b) Carboplatin

The INR of a man taking **warfarin** increased from a baseline range of 1.15 to 2.11 up to 12.6 within 16 days of a first course of chemotherapy with carboplatin and **etoposide**.[8]

(c) Cyclophosphamide

A woman taking **warfarin** had a marked rise in her prothrombin time when her treatment with cyclophosphamide was withdrawn.[9]

(d) Etoposide

The INR of a man taking **warfarin** increased from a baseline range of 1.15 to 2.11 up to 12.6 within 16 days of a first course of chemotherapy with **carboplatin** and etoposide.[8] Another elderly man taking **warfarin** had a marked increase in prothrombin times (prolongation of 8 to 15 seconds) on two occasions when he took etoposide 500 mg and **vindesine** 5 mg.[10]

(e) Gefitinib

A woman stabilised on **warfarin** required a gradual decrease in the dose from 4 mg to 2.5 mg daily after starting gefitinib 250 mg/m^2 daily for lung cancer. In contrast, a second patient did not have an increase in warfarin effect while taking gefitinib.[11]

(f) Gemcitabine

A 63-year-old man needed a reduction in his weekly **warfarin** dosage from 59.23 mg to 50.75 mg in order to keep his INR at about 2.5 during 2 cycles of gemcitabine. When the gemcitabine was stopped his **warfarin** dosage had to be increased again.[12] The manufacturers have information on 4 cases of suspected interactions between gemcitabine and **warfarin**, and one with **phenprocoumon** (reported by December 2000).[13] Based on 724 reports of the concurrent use of gemcitabine and **anticoagulants**,[13] they suggest that the incidence of the suspected interaction is 0.8%.

(g) Ifosfamide

Three patients taking **warfarin** had a marked and very rapid increase in their INRs when they took ifosfamide with **mesna**.[14]

(h) Mercaptopurine

A man well stabilised on **warfarin** had a marked reduction in his anticoagulant response on two occasions while taking mercaptopurine, but no changes occurred when he took **busulfan**, **cyclophosphamide**, **cytarabine**, **hydroxycarbamide**, **mitobronitol**, **demecolcine** or **melphalan**.[15] A woman needed a marked increase in her dosage of **acenocoumarol**, from 21 to 70 mg weekly, when she was given mercaptopurine 100 mg daily.[16] Another patient required about a 25% increase in **warfarin** dose while taking mercaptopurine 100 mg daily.[17]

(i) Mitotane

The anticoagulant effects of **warfarin** were progressively reduced in a woman taking mitotane.[18] Later this effect began to reverse.

(j) ProMace-Mopp

The prothrombin times of an elderly man given **warfarin** increased by 50 to 100% in the middle of three cycles of treatment with ProMace-Mopp (**cyclophosphamide**, **doxorubicin**, **etoposide**, **chlormethine**, **vincristine**, **procarbazine**, **methotrexate** and prednisone), and he developed a subconjunctival haemorrhage during the first cycle.[19]

(k) Trastuzumab

Two women stabilised on **warfarin** developed nosebleeds after 10 and 8 weekly doses of trastuzumab, respectively, and were found to have INRs of 6 and 5.8, respectively.[20] However, the manufacturer notes that in an analysis of clinical study data the rate of bleeding events was similar for patients receiving or not receiving trastuzumab, with or without anticoagulants.[21]

Mechanism

Not well understood. Mercaptopurine possibly increases the synthesis or activation of prothrombin.[22] Azathioprine is metabolised to mercaptopurine, and would therefore be expected to interact similarly.

Importance and management

The absence of problems in early small studies using warfarin as an adjunct to chemotherapy,[23,24] and the small number of reports describing difficulties, suggest that many of these interactions may be uncommon events. The concurrent use of these drugs need not be avoided but there is clearly a need to be aware that any antineoplastic regimen might increase the response to anticoagulants. It would also be prudent to note that mercaptopurine and azathioprine may decrease the anticoagulant response. The anticoagulant dosages may need adjustment. Note that, from a disease perspective, when treating venous thromboembolic disease in patients with cancer, warfarin is generally inferior (higher risk of major bleeds and recurrent thrombosis) to low-molecular-weight heparins.[25]

1. Khamashta MA, Cuadrado MJ, Mujic F, Taub N, Hunt BJ, Hughes GRV. Effect of azathioprine on the anticoagulant activity of warfarin in patients with the antiphospholipid syndrome. *Lupus* (1998) 7 (Suppl 2), S227.
2. Singleton JD, Conyers L. Warfarin and azathioprine: an important drug interaction. *Am J Med* (1992) 92, 217.
3. Rivier G, Khamashta MA, Hughes GRV. Warfarin and azathioprine: a drug interaction does exist. *Am J Med* (1993) 95, 342.
4. Rotenberg M, Levy Y, Shoenfeld Y, Almog S, Ezra D. Effect of azathioprine on the anticoagulant activity of warfarin. *Ann Pharmacother* (2000) 34, 120–2.
5. Jeppesen U, Rasmussen JM, Brøsen K. Clinically important interaction between azathioprine (Imurel) and phenprocoumon (Marcoumar). *Eur J Clin Pharmacol* (1997) 52, 503–4.
6. Walker J, Mendelson H, McClure A Smith MD. Warfarin and azathioprine: clinically significant drug interaction. *J Rheumatol* (2002) 29, 398–9.
7. Havrda DE, Rathbun S, Scheid D. A case report of warfarin resistance due to azathioprine and review of the literature. *Pharmacotherapy* (2001) 21, 355–7.
8. Le AT, Hasson NK, Lum BL. Enhancement of warfarin response in a patient receiving etoposide and carboplatin chemotherapy. *Ann Pharmacother* (1997) 31, 1006–8.
9. Tashima CK. Cyclophosphamide effect on coumarin anticoagulation. *South Med J* (1979) 72, 633–4.
10. Ward K, Bitran JD. Warfarin, etoposide, and vindesine interactions. *Cancer Treat Rep* (1984) 68, 817–18.
11. Onoda S, Mitsufuji H, Yanase N, Ryuge S, Kato E, Wada M, Ishii K, Hagiri S, Yamamoto M, Yokoba M, Yanaihara T, Kuboto M, Takada N, Katagiri M, Abe T, Tanaka M, Kobayashi H, Masuda N. Drug interaction between gefitinib and warfarin. *Jpn J Clin Oncol* (2005) 35, 478–82.
12. Kinikar SA, Kolesar JM. Identification of a gemcitabine-warfarin interaction. *Pharmacotherapy* (1999) 19, 1331–3.
13. Kilgour-Christie J, Czarnecki A. Gemcitabine and the interaction with anticoagulants. *Lancet Oncol* (2002) 3, 460.
14. Hall G, Lind MJ, Huang M, Moore A, Gane A, Roberts JT, Cantwell BMJ. Intravenous infusions of ifosfamide/mesna and perturbation of warfarin anticoagulant control. *Postgrad Med J* (1990) 66, 860–1.
15. Spiers ASD, Mibashan RS. Increased warfarin requirement during mercaptopurine therapy: a new drug interaction. *Lancet* (1974) ii, 221–2.
16. Fernádez MA, Regadera A, Aznar J. Acenocoumarol and 6-mercaptopurine: an important drug interaction. *Haematologica* (1999) 84, 664–5.
17. Martin LA, Mehta SD. Diminished anticoagulant effects of warfarin with concomitant mercaptopurine therapy. *Pharmacotherapy* (2003) 23, 260–4.
18. Cuddy PG, Loftus LS. Influence of mitotane on the hypoprothrombinemic effect of warfarin. *South Med J* (1986) 79, 387–8.
19. Seifter EJ, Brooks BJ, Urba WJ. Possible interactions between warfarin and antineoplastic drugs. *Cancer Treat Rep* (1985) 69, 244–5.
20. Nissenblatt MJ, Karp GI. Bleeding risk with trastuzumab (Herceptin) treatment. *JAMA* (1999) 282, 2299–2300.
21. Stewart SJ. Bleeding risk with trastuzumab (Herceptin) treatment. In reply. *JAMA* (1999) 282, 2300–1.
22. Martini A, Jähnchen E. Studies in rats on the mechanisms by which 6-mercaptopurine inhibits the anticoagulant effect of warfarin. *J Pharmacol Exp Ther* (1977) 201, 547–53.
23. Zacharski LR, Henderson WG, Rickles FR, Forman WB, Cornell CJ, Forcier RJ, Edwards RL, Headley E, Kim S-H, O'Donnell JR, O'Dell R, Tornyos K, Kwaan HC. Effect of warfarin anticoagulation on survival in carcinoma of the lung, colon, head and neck, and prostate. *Cancer* (1984) 53, 2046–52.
24. Zacharski LR, Henderson WG, Rickles FR, Forman WB, Cornell CJ, Forcier RJ, Edwards R, Headley E, Kim S-H, O'Donnell JR, O'Dell R, Tornyos K, Kwaan HC. Effect of warfarin on survival in small cell carcinoma of the lung. *JAMA* (1981) 245, 831–5.
25. Baglin TP, Keeling DM, Watson HG, for the British Committee for Standards in Haematology. Guidelines on oral anticoagulation (warfarin): third edition – 2005 update. *Br J Haematol* (2006) 132, 277–85.

Coumarins and related drugs + Antiplatelet drugs; Cilostazol

Cilostazol does not appear to have a clinically relevant effect on the pharmacokinetics or pharmacodynamics of warfarin. Nevertheless, as with other antiplatelet drugs, concurrent use might increase the bleeding risk.

Clinical evidence, mechanism, importance and management

In a randomised, double-blind, two-way crossover study in 15 healthy subjects, cilostazol 100 mg twice daily for 13 days did not alter the pharmacokinetics of a single 25-mg dose of warfarin given on day 7. Also, prothrombin times, aPTT time and Ivy bleeding time were unaffected.[1]

This suggests that no interaction is likely during concurrent use. Nevertheless, because cilostazol is an antiplatelet drug, the manufacturer advises caution with the concurrent use of anticoagulants, with more frequent monitoring to reduce the possibility of bleeding.[2]

1. Millakaarjun S, Bramer SL. Effect of cilostazol on the pharmacokinetics and pharmacodynamics of warfarin. *Clin Pharmacokinet* (1999) 37 (Suppl 2), 79–86.
2. Pletal (Cilostazol). Otsuka Pharmaceuticals (UK) Ltd. UK Summary of product characteristics, May 2006.

Coumarins and related drugs + Antiplatelet drugs; Clopidogrel

Clopidogrel does not appear to have a clinically relevant effect on the pharmacokinetics or pharmacodynamics of warfarin. Nevertheless, concurrent use might increase the bleeding risk.

Clinical evidence, mechanism, importance and management

In a randomised, double-blind, placebo-controlled study involving 43 patients who had been taking **warfarin** for at least 2 months, the addition of clopidogrel 75 mg daily for 8 days had no effect on plasma **warfarin** levels or INRs. No bleeding occurred with clopidogrel and no serious adverse events were reported.[1]

Nevertheless, as with other antiplatelet drugs, combined use might increase the risk or intensity of bleeding. Therefore, in the UK, the manufacturers of clopidogrel state that the concurrent use of **warfarin** is not recommended,[2] whereas the US manufacturers recommend caution.[3] This caution would be prudent with clopidogrel and any coumarin or **indanedione**.

1. Lidell C, Svedberg L-E, Lindell P, Bandh S, Job B, Wallentin L. Clopidogrel and warfarin: absence of interaction in patients receiving long-term anticoagulant therapy for non-valvular atrial fibrillation. *Thromb Haemost* (2003) 89, 842–6.
2. Plavix (Clopidogrel hydrogen sulfate). Bristol-Myers Squibb Pharmaceuticals Ltd. UK Summary of product characteristics, June 2007.
3. Plavix (Clopidogrel bisulfate). Sanofi-Aventis/Bristol Myers Squibb Company. US Prescribing information, February 2007.

Coumarins and related drugs + Antiplatelet drugs; Dipyridamole

The combination of dipyridamole and coumarin anticoagulants does not alter the prothrombin time, but might cause an increased risk of serious bleeding when compared with anticoagulants alone. There is some evidence that the risk of bleeding may be lower, without a reduction in efficacy, if the INR is maintained within a lower range.

Clinical evidence

(a) Prosthetic heart valves

In a short-term study in 6 patients stabilised on **warfarin**, the addition of dipyridamole 75 mg three times daily did not alter prothrombin time ratios measured 8 times over 17 days.[1]

A meta-analysis of 6 randomised, controlled studies of the combined use of an oral anticoagulant and dipyridamole compared with an oral anticoagulant alone, found no increased risk of *any* bleeding events when dipyridamole was given (odds ratio 1.001).[2] In contrast, in a later meta-analysis of the same studies, the risk of *major* bleeding with the addition of dipyridamole was increased (odds ratio 2.22). In addition to the difference in classification of bleeding events, the authors of the second analysis stated that they had used published data from two studies, which showed a slightly higher bleeding risk, whereas the earlier meta-analysis had used unpublished data from these studies, showing a lower bleeding risk.[3]

In one randomised study, the risk of excessive bleeding was 4% in patients taking **warfarin** and dipyridamole 400 mg daily, compared with 14% in patients taking **warfarin** and aspirin 500 mg daily. When compared with a non-randomised control group taking warfarin alone, the risk of excessive bleeding was not increased by dipyridamole (4% combined therapy versus 5% **warfarin** alone).[4]

In another randomised study, the risk of bleeding was lower (1% versus 3.7%) in patients receiving dipyridamole 225 mg daily with **phenindione** at a target INR range of 2 to 2.5 than in patients receiving **phenindione** alone with a target INR of 2.5 to 3.5, and the combination was more effective.[5] Similarly, the risk of bleeding was lower with a lower target INR of 2 to 3 than with a target INR of 3 to 4.5 (3.9% versus 20.8%) in patients taking **acenocoumarol**, aspirin 330 mg twice daily and dipyridamole 75 mg twice daily.[6]

(b) Other conditions

Thirty patients with glomerulonephritis stabilised on either **warfarin** (28 patients) or **phenindione** (2 patients) with a prothrombin activity of between 20 to 30% of control had no significant changes in prothrombin times when they were given dipyridamole in doses increased from 100 mg daily up to a maximum of 400 mg daily over about a month. Twelve to 19 days after starting dipyridamole, 3 patients with normal renal function developed mild bleeding (epistaxis, bruising, haematuria), which resolved when either drug was withdrawn or the dosage reduced.[7]

Mechanism

Dipyridamole reduces platelet adhesiveness or aggregation, which prolongs bleeding time. This may increase the risk or severity of bleeding if overanticoagulation occurs.

Importance and management

The combination of dipyridamole with coumarin anticoagulants is in established clinical use for the prophylaxis of thromboembolism associated with prosthetic heart valves. There is clearly some uncertainty regarding the increased risk of bleeding with the combination, with one analysis showing no increased risk,[2] and a second showing about a doubling of risk of serious bleeding.[3] The authors of the second analysis consider that their results represent a more conservative estimate of bleeding risk.[3] There is some evidence that maintaining anticoagulant control at the lower end of the therapeutic range minimises possible bleeding complications and it would therefore seem prudent to consider this wherever possible.

1. Donaldson DR, Sreeharan N, Crow MJ, Rajah SM. Assessment of the interaction of warfarin with aspirin and dipyridamole. *Thromb Haemost* (1982) 47, 77.
2. Pouleur H, Buyse M. Effects of dipyridamole in combination with anticoagulant therapy on survival and thromboembolic events in patients with prosthetic heart valves. A meta-analysis of the randomized trials. *J Thorac Cardiovasc Surg* (1995) 110, 463—72.
3. Little SH, Massel DR. Antiplatelet and anticoagulation for patients with prosthetic heart valves. Available in The Cochrane Database of Systematic Reviews; Issue 4. Chichester: John Wiley; 2003 (accessed 20070606).
4. Chesebro JH, Fuster V, Elveback LR, McGoon DC, Pluth JR, Puga FJ, Wallace RB, Danielson GK, Orszulak TA, Piehler JM, Schaff HV. Trial of combined warfarin plus dipyridamole or aspirin therapy in prosthetic heart valve replacement: danger of aspirin compared with dipyridamole. *Am J Cardiol* (1983) 51, 1537–41.
5. Hassouna A, Allam H, Awad A, Hassaballah F. Standard versus low-level anticoagulation combined to low-dose dipyridamole after mitral valve replacement. *Cardiovasc Surg* (2000) 8, 491–8.
6. Altman R, Rouvier J, Gurfinkel E, D'Ortencio O, Manzanel R, de La Fuente L, Favaloro RG. Comparison of two levels of anticoagulant therapy in patients with substitute heart valves. *J Thorac Cardiovasc Surg* (1991) 101, 427–31.
7. Kalowski S, Kincaid-Smith P. Interaction of dipyridamole with anticoagulants in the treatment of glomerulonephritis. *Med J Aust* (1973) 2, 164–6.

Coumarins and related drugs + Antiplatelet drugs; Ditazole

Ditazole does not alter the anticoagulant effects of acenocoumarol. Nevertheless, as with other antiplatelet drugs, concurrent use might increase bleeding risk.

Clinical evidence, mechanism, importance and management

Fifty patients with artificial heart valves taking **acenocoumarol** had no changes in their prothrombin times while taking ditazole 800 mg daily.[1] Nevertheless, as with other antiplatelet drugs, combined use with oral anticoagulants might increase the risk or intensity of bleeding. Some caution is therefore appropriate on concurrent use.

1. Jacovella G, Milazzotto F. Ricerca di interazioni fra ditazolo e anticoagulanti in portatori di protesi valvolari intracardiache. *Clin Ter* (1977) 80, 425–31.

Coumarins + Antiplatelet drugs; Picotamide

Picotamide did not alter the anticoagulant effects of warfarin. Nevertheless, as with other antiplatelet drugs, concurrent use might increase bleeding risk.

Clinical evidence, mechanism, importance and management

Picotamide 300 mg three times daily for 10 days did not alter the anticoagulant effects of established **warfarin** therapy in 10 patients with aortic or mitral valve prostheses.[1] No **warfarin** dose adjustments would therefore be expected to be needed on concurrent use. Nevertheless, as with other antiplatelet drugs, combined use with oral anticoagulants might increase the risk or intensity of bleeding. Some caution is therefore appropriate on concurrent use.

1. Parise P, Gresele P, Viola E, Ruina A, Migliacci R, Nenci GG. La picotamide non interferisce con l'attività anticoagulante del warfarin in pazienti portatori di protesi valvolari cardiache. *Clin Ter* (1990) 135, 479–82.

Coumarins + Antiplatelet drugs; Ticlopidine

In a retrospective analysis, the anticoagulant effects of acenocoumarol were modestly reduced by ticlopidine in 80% of patients, whereas, in a small prospective study, the anticoagulant effects of warfarin were unchanged by ticlopidine. As with other antiplatelet drugs, combined use might possibly increase bleeding risk. Cholestatic hepatitis has been reported in some patients given warfarin and ticlopidine.

Clinical evidence

(a) Acenocoumarol

A retrospective study of 36 patients with heart valve prostheses found that when they took ticlopidine 250 mg daily, 29 of them needed a mean 13% increase in acenocoumarol dosage from 15.5 to 17.5 mg weekly, accompanied by a small INR rise from 3.05 to 3.13. One patient needed a dosage increase from 14 to 22 mg weekly. INR changes were detectable with a week of starting the ticlopidine.[1]

(b) Warfarin

Ticlopidine 250 mg twice daily for 2 weeks given to 9 men taking warfarin long-term increased the mean *R*-warfarin levels by 25.7% but did not change *S*-warfarin levels or their INRs.[2] *R*-warfarin is the much less active of the two enantiomers.

In a Japanese study, 4 out of 132 patients (3%) given both warfarin and ticlopidine after cardiovascular surgery developed cholestatic hepatitis.[3]

Mechanism

It seems possible that ticlopidine inhibits the metabolism of *R*-warfarin, but the interaction with acenocoumarol is not understood. Ticlopidine alone can cause raised liver enzymes and cholestatic hepatitis,[4] and whether these cases represent an interaction is unclear.

Importance and management

Information seems to be limited to the reports cited. A small to moderate increase in the acenocoumarol dosage may be needed if ticlopidine is added, but none seems to be necessary with warfarin. However, as with other antiplatelet drugs, an increased risk of bleeding (a combination of anticoagulant and platelet anti-aggregant activity) might be anticipated on concurrent use. The manufacturer states that the long-term safety of concurrent use of ticlopidine with oral anticoagulants has not been established, and they recommend that if a patient is switched from an anticoagulant to ticlopidine, the anticoagulant should be discontinued prior to ticlopidine administration.[4] Whether the incidence of cholestatic hepatitis is higher with the combination of warfarin and ticlopidine than with ticlopidine alone is unclear.

1. Salar A, Domenech P, Martínez F. Ticlopidine antagonizes acenocoumarol treatment. *Thromb Haemost* (1997) 77, 223–4.
2. Gidal BE, Sorkness CA, McGill KA, Larson R, Levine RR. Evaluation of a potential enantioselective interaction between ticlopidine and warfarin in chronically anticoagulated patients. *Ther Drug Monit* (1995) 27, 33–8.

3. Takase K, Fujioka H, Ogasawara M, Aonuma H, Tameda Y, Nakano T, Kosaka Y. Drug-induced hepatitis during combination therapy of warfarin potassium and ticlopidine hydrochloride. *Mie Med J* (1990) 40, 27–32.
4. Ticlid (Ticlopidine hydrochloride). Roche Pharmaceuticals. US Prescribing information, March 2001.

Coumarins + Aprepitant

Aprepitant modestly reduces warfarin levels and slightly decreases the INR in healthy subjects. It is expected to interact similarly with acenocoumarol.

Clinical evidence, mechanism, importance and management

In a double-blind study, healthy subjects were stabilised on **warfarin** and then given either aprepitant (125 mg on day one, then 80 mg daily on days 2 and 3) or placebo. On day 3, there was no change in **warfarin** levels. However, by day 8 (5 days after stopping aprepitant) there was a 34% decrease in trough *S*-warfarin levels, and a 14% decrease in INR in the aprepitant group.[1]

Aprepitant is an inducer of the cytochrome P450 isoenzyme CYP2C9, by which *S*-warfarin is metabolised. The manufacturer recommends that, in patients taking **warfarin**, the INR should be monitored closely for 2 weeks, particularly at 7 to 10 days,[2] after each 3-day course of aprepitant,[2,3] and this seems a prudent precaution. They similarly recommend caution with **acenocoumarol**, which is also metabolised by CYP2C9.[3]

1. Depré M, Van Hecken A, Oeyen M, De Lepeleire I, Laethem T, Rothenberg P, Petty KJ, Majumdar A, Crumley T, Panebianco D, Bergman A, de Hoon JN. Effect of aprepitant on the pharmacokinetics and pharmacodynamics of warfarin. *Eur J Clin Pharmacol* (2005) 61, 341–6.
2. Emend (Aprepitant). Merck & Co., Inc. US Prescribing information, June 2006.
3. Emend (Aprepitant). Merck Sharp & Dohme Ltd. UK Summary of product characteristics, February 2007.

Coumarins + Aromatase inhibitors

The anticoagulant effects of warfarin and acenocoumarol can be markedly reduced by aminoglutethimide. The extent of the reduction appears to be related to the aminoglutethimide dosage. However, in controlled studies, anastrozole and letrozole did not interact with warfarin.

Clinical evidence

(a) Aminoglutethimide

In a study in 9 patients being treated for breast cancer, a low-dose aminoglutethimide regimen (125 mg twice daily) increased the clearance of a single-dose of *R*- or *S*-warfarin by 41.2% with marked variability between individuals (range 15 to 103%). A high-dose regimen (250 mg four times daily) increased the clearance by 90.8%. The effects of the interaction had developed fully by 14 days. Both enantiomers of **warfarin** were equally affected.[1]

One 79-year-old woman taking aminoglutethimide 250 mg four times daily showed resistance to **warfarin** requiring a dose of 17.5 to 20 mg daily. Two weeks after the aminoglutethimide was stopped, the required dose of warfarin gradually declined, eventually reaching a level of 3.75 and 5 mg on alternate days (about a fourfold reduction).[2] Another patient stabilised on warfarin gradually needed about a threefold increase in the **warfarin** dosage after starting aminoglutethimide 250 mg four times a day.[2] The increased requirement persisted for 2 weeks after the aminoglutethimide was stopped, and then declined. A study briefly mentions a patient who required greatly increased doses of **warfarin** after starting aminoglutethimide.[3] Three patients taking **acenocoumarol** needed a doubled dosage to maintain adequate anticoagulation when they took aminoglutethimide 250 mg four times daily for 3 to 4 weeks.[4]

(b) Anastrozole

A randomised, double-blind, placebo-controlled, crossover study[5] in 16 healthy men found that anastrozole (7 mg loading dose followed by 1 mg daily for a further 10 days) had no effect on the pharmacokinetics or pharmacodynamics of a single dose of **warfarin** given on day 3.

(c) Letrozole

The manufacturers report that letrozole had no clinically relevant effect on the pharmacokinetics of **warfarin**.[6,7]

Mechanism

Uncertain. The most likely explanation is that aminoglutethimide, like glutethimide, stimulates the activity of the liver enzymes concerned with the metabolism of the anticoagulants, thereby reducing their levels and efficacy. Alternatively, it has been suggested that aminoglutethimide may affect blood steroid levels, which in turn might affect coagulation.[2]

Importance and management

An established and clinically important interaction. Monitor the effects of adding aminoglutethimide to patients already taking warfarin or acenocoumarol and increase the anticoagulant dosage as necessary. Up to four times the dosage may be needed. The extent of the effects would appear to be related to the dosage of aminoglutethimide used. Monitor the INR and reduce the anticoagulant dosage accordingly if aminoglutethimide is withdrawn. Information about other coumarins is lacking but it would be prudent to apply the same precautions with any of them.

Conversely, controlled studies have shown no interaction between anastrozole or letrozole and warfarin. This suggests that coumarin dose adjustments are unlikely to be needed when these aromatase inhibitors are used.

1. Lønning PE, Ueland PM, Kvinnsland S. The influence of a graded dose schedule of aminoglutethimide on the disposition of the optical enantiomers of warfarin in patients with breast cancer. *Cancer Chemother Pharmacol* (1986) 17, 177–81.
2. Lønning PE, Kvinnsland S, Jahren G. Aminoglutethimide and warfarin. A new important drug interaction. *Cancer Chemother Pharmacol* (1984) 12, 10–12.
3. Murray RML, Pitt P, Jerums G. Medical adrenalectomy with aminoglutethimide in the management of advanced breast cancer. *Med J Aust* (1981) 1, 179–81.
4. Bruning PF, Bonfrèr JGM. Aminoglutethimide and oral anticoagulant therapy. *Lancet* (1983) ii, 582.
5. Yates RA, Wong J, Seiberling M, Merz M, März W, Nauck M. The effect of anastrozole on the single-dose pharmacokinetics and anticoagulant activity of warfarin in healthy volunteers. *Br J Clin Pharmacol* (2001) 51, 429–35.
6. Femara (Letrozole). Novartis Pharmaceuticals UK Ltd. UK Summary of product characteristics, May 2007.
7. Femara (Letrozole). Novartis Pharmaceuticals. US Prescribing information, December 2006.

Coumarins and related drugs + Aspirin

Low-dose aspirin (75 to 325 mg daily) increases the risk of bleeding when given with warfarin by about 1.5 to 2.5-fold, although, in most studies the absolute risks have been small. The overall benefits of concurrent use outweigh the risks in certain patient groups; however, for some warfarin indications, there is not enough data to assess this. In addition to increased bleeding, high doses of aspirin (4 g daily or more) can increase prothrombin times. Therefore, aspirin is not considered a suitable analgesic or anti-inflammatory drug for those taking oral anticoagulants.

Clinical evidence

A. Analgesic-dose aspirin

In a pharmacological study in patients stabilised on **acenocoumarol**, aspirin 2.4 g daily for one week increased faecal blood loss from an average of 1.1 mL to 4.7 mL. While taking aspirin, 11 of 17 patients required a 29% reduction in their **acenocoumarol** dose from a mean of 3.1 mg to 2.2 mg. One patient required a slight increase of 0.5 mg, and the remaining 5 required a dose reduction of less than 0.5 mg.[1]

In another study in healthy subjects, aspirin 1.95 g daily for 11 days had no effect on the prothrombin time response to a single dose of **warfarin** given on day 4. When 11 healthy subjects were stabilised on **dicoumarol** or **warfarin** and given aspirin 1.95 g daily, 7 had no significant change in prothrombin time activity, and 4 had a slight reduction (of 5 to 10% points). Of the 2 subjects showing signs of bleeding, neither had a reduction in prothrombin time activity. A further 4 subjects stabilised on **warfarin** received a higher dose of aspirin (3.9 g daily), and all 4 had a reduction in prothrombin time activity of 6 to 12% points and signs of bleeding occurred. Bleeding time was significantly prolonged by the combination of aspirin 1.95 g daily and **warfarin** than by **warfarin** alone (10.3 minutes versus 4 minutes).[2] In 2 further studies in healthy subjects, aspirin 6 g daily moderately prolonged prothrombin times,[3,4] and in one study this effect tended to be reversed by vitamin K.[3]

In contrast, in another study in 10 patients, adding aspirin 3 g daily to **warfarin** for 2 weeks had no effect on prothrombin times (20.9 versus 21.2 seconds).[5]

B. Antiplatelet-dose aspirin

In a study in healthy subjects, low-dose aspirin 75 mg daily doubled the normal blood loss from the gastric mucosa. However, concurrent **warfarin** (dose individualised to achieve an INR of 1.4 to 1.6) did not increase the gastric mucosal bleeding any further.[6]

(a) Atrial fibrillation

In a large study in patients with atrial fibrillation, the cumulative incidence of bleeding events after 3 years was no different in those receiving fixed low-dose **warfarin** 1.25 mg daily plus aspirin 300 mg daily (24.4%) than with fixed low-dose **warfarin** alone (24.7%) or aspirin 300 mg daily alone (30%).[7] This study also contained an adjusted-dose **warfarin**-only group, which proved more effective than the other group, so the study was terminated early. Other studies have found similar results.[8]

In another study, the combination of adjusted dose **fluindione** (INR 2 to 2.6) plus aspirin 100 mg daily was associated with a much higher incidence of haemorrhagic complications than **fluindione** alone (13.1% versus 1.2%). The overall balance of benefit to risk could not be assessed because of the low incidence of the primary endpoint (ischaemic events).[9]

(b) Coronary stents

In a retrospective analysis, a 20% incidence of severe upper gastrointestinal bleeding was seen in 138 coronary stent patients given heparin post-procedure, then **warfarin** with aspirin 325 mg daily. Ten of the patients needed a blood transfusion.[10] In another analysis of patients who had been taking **warfarin** long-term and who underwent stent implantation and were then discharged taking aspirin, clopidogrel and **warfarin**, the incidence of major bleeding was 6.6% and of minor bleeding was 14.9% This compared with 0% and 3.8% for major and minor bleeding, respectively, in patients not given aspirin with clopidogrel post-procedure (no **warfarin**).[11] Another study reported an incidence of 9.2% of bleeding in patients who had undergone stent placement and received **warfarin**, aspirin and clopidogrel.[12]

(c) Myocardial infarction

1. Primary prevention. In a large primary prevention study in men at high risk of ischaemic heart disease, the incidence of haematuria was twofold higher in those receiving both low-dose aspirin 75 mg daily and low-intensity **warfarin** (INR 1.5) than in those receiving low-dose aspirin alone, or low-intensity **warfarin** alone. Similarly, the incidence of minor episodes of bleeding (nose bleeds, bruising, rectal bleeding, pink/red urine) was 1.27-fold higher in those receiving the combination than in those receiving low-dose aspirin alone, or low-intensity **warfarin** alone (49% versus 38% and 39%, respectively), although the difference was not statistically significant. There was no difference in incidence of major and intermediate episodes of bleeding.[13]

2. Secondary prevention. In a meta-analysis of randomised, controlled studies[14] in patients following myocardial infarction or acute coronary syndrome, intensive **warfarin** (INR greater than 2) plus aspirin 80 to 325 mg daily was associated with 2.5-fold increased risk of major bleeding, when compared with aspirin alone, although the actual incidence was low (1.5% versus 0.6%). This analysis excluded studies of coronary stenting, see (b) above. In another similar meta-analysis, combined use of aspirin and **warfarin** (INR 2 to 3) was associated with a 2.3 odds ratio of a major bleed, when compared with aspirin alone.[15] The number needed to treat to cause one major bleed was 100. This compared with a number needed to treat to avoid one major adverse event (death, myocardial infarction or stroke) of 33.

Similarly, in an observational cohort study of elderly survivors of acute myocardial infarction, the rate of bleeding was higher in patients receiving **warfarin** with aspirin (0.08 per patient year), or the triple drug combination of **warfarin** and aspirin with either clopidogrel or ticlopidine (0.09 per patient-year), than in patients receiving aspirin alone (0.03 per patient-year).[16]

Using lower intensity **warfarin** with the low-dose aspirin was still associated with more major bleeding than aspirin alone (1.77 in one study, although this is less than higher intensity warfarin; 2.3 as mentioned above). Nevertheless, low-intensity **warfarin** with low-dose aspirin does not appear to be any more effective than aspirin alone.[15,17]

(d) Peripheral arterial disease

In a meta-analysis of studies of patients with peripheral arterial disease, combined use of **oral anticoagulants** together with aspirin increased the risk of major bleeding about twofold when compared with aspirin alone, and appeared to be associated with increased mortality.[18]

(e) Prosthetic heart valves

In one randomised study in patients with artificial heart valves, the risk of bleeding episodes requiring blood transfusion or hospitalisation was much higher among those taking aspirin 500 mg daily and **warfarin** (14%), compared with those taking **warfarin** and dipyridamole 400 mg daily (4%), and compared with a non-randomised control group taking **warfarin** alone (5%). Bleeding was mainly gastrointestinal or cerebral. All of those with intracerebral bleeding died.[19]

A further study found that aspirin 1 g daily combined with **unnamed anticoagulants** was associated with a threefold higher incidence of bleeding episodes than those taking anticoagulants alone (13.9 versus 4.7 per 100 patients per year).[20,21] However, in another study there was no difference in haemorrhagic risk between patients receiving aspirin 500 mg daily and **acenocoumarol** or **acenocoumarol** alone.[22]

More recent studies have used lower doses of aspirin. In one study in patients stabilised on **warfarin** with a target INR range of 3.0 to 4.5, the addition of aspirin 100 mg daily increased the risk of any bleeding by 55%, when compared with placebo (35% versus 22% per year), mainly due to an increase in minor haematuria, nosebleeds and bruising. However, the risk was more than offset by the overall reduction in mortality.[23]

The preliminary report of a meta-analysis of these four studies, concluded that the combined use of oral anticoagulants and aspirin (100 mg to 1 g daily) significantly reduced mortality and embolic complications in patients with prosthetic heart valves, with an estimated increased odds ratio of major bleeds of 1.7 and of total bleeds of 1.98. Nevertheless the overall picture was that the benefits possibly outweighed the problems.[24] In a more recent meta-analysis,[25] which excluded one non-randomised study,[19] but included 2 other randomised controlled studies, the risk of major bleeding for the combination of **warfarin** and aspirin was 1.53. For the two low-dose aspirin (100 mg daily) trials, there did not appear to be an excess risk of major bleeding.[25] Another analysis of these studies provided essentially the same risk of increased major bleeding with the combination.[26]

Mechanism

Aspirin has a direct irritant effect on the stomach lining and can cause gastrointestinal bleeding, even in doses as low as 75 mg daily.[27] It also decreases platelet aggregation and prolongs bleeding times. In addition, large doses of aspirin (4 g daily or more) alone are known to have a direct hypoprothrombinaemic effect, which is reversible by vitamin K.[3,4] The effects of the aspirin can be additive with the effects of the anticoagulant.

Importance and management

The interaction of aspirin and warfarin at high doses is not well documented, but is clinically important. It is usual to avoid normal analgesic and anti-inflammatory doses of aspirin while taking any coumarin anticoagulant, although only dicoumarol, acenocoumarol and warfarin appear to have been investigated. Patients should be told that many non-prescription analgesic, antipyretic, cold and influenza preparations may contain substantial amounts of aspirin. Warn them that it may be listed as acetylsalicylic acid. Paracetamol is a safer analgesic substitute (but not entirely without problems, see 'Coumarins + Paracetamol (Acetaminophen)', p.438).

The effect of low-dose aspirin (used for its antiplatelet effects) combined with warfarin has been far more extensively studied. Overall, the evidence shows that the combination is still associated with an increased risk of bleeding over either drug alone, and this is in the region of 1.5 to 2.5-fold. Nevertheless, the absolute risk is small. A twofold increased risk of haematuria and a slight increased risk of minor bleeding of 1.27 was still seen in the study using the lowest dose of warfarin (INR 1.5) combined with just 75 mg of aspirin a day.[13] In certain patient groups the benefits of combined use have been clearly shown to outweigh this increased risk of bleeding, such as patients with prosthetic heart valves at high risk of thromboembolism. However, in many of the common indications for warfarin such as atrial fibrillation, there is insufficient evidence to answer the question of whether the combination should be used.[26]

1. Watson RM, Pierson RN. Effect of anticoagulant therapy upon aspirin-induced gastrointestinal bleeding. *Circulation* (1961) 24, 613–16.
2. O'Reilly RA, Sahud MA, Aggeler PM. Impact of aspirin and chlorthalidone on the pharmacodynamics of oral anticoagulant drugs in man. *Ann N Y Acad Sci* (1971) 179, 173–86.
3. Shapiro S. Studies on prothrombin. VI. The effect of synthetic vitamin K on the prothrombinopenia induced by salicylate in man. *JAMA* (1944) 125, 546–8.
4. Quick AJ, Clesceri L. Influence of acetylsalicylic acid and salicylamide on the coagulation of blood. *J Pharmacol Exp Ther* (1960) 128, 95–8.
5. Udall JA. Drug interference with warfarin therapy. *Clin Med* (1970) 77, 20–5.
6. Prichard PJ, Kitchingman GK, Walt RP, Daneshmend TK, Hawkey CJ. Human gastric mucosal bleeding induced by low dose aspirin, but not warfarin. *BMJ* (1989) 298, 493–6.
7. Gulløv AL, Koefoed BG, Petersen P, Pedersen TS, Andersen ED, Godtfredsen J, Boysen G. Fixed minidose warfarin and aspirin alone and in combination vs adjusted-dose warfarin for stroke prevention in atrial fibrillation. Second Copenhagen atrial fibrillation, aspirin, and anticoagulant study. *Arch Intern Med* (1998) 158, 1513–21.
8. Stroke Prevention in Atrial Fibrillation Investigators. Adjusted-dose warfarin versus low-intensity, fixed-dose warfarin plus aspirin for high-risk patients with atrial fibrillation: Stroke Prevention in Atrial Fibrillation III randomised clinical trial. *Lancet* (1996) 348, 633–38.
9. Lechat P, Lardoux H, Mallet A, Sanchez P, Derumeaux G, Lecompte T, Maillard L, Mas JL, Mentre F, Pousset F, Lacomblez L, Pisica G, Solbes-Latourette S, Raynaud P, Chaumet-Riffaud P for the FFAACS Investigators. Anticoagulant (fluindione)-aspirin combination in patients with high-risk atrial fibrillation. A randomized trial. *Cerebrovasc Dis* (2001) 12, 245–52.
10. Younossi ZM, Strum WB, Cloutier D, Teirstein PS, Schatz RA. Upper GI bleeding in post-coronary stent patients following aspirin and anticoagulant treatment. *Gastroenterology* (1995) 108 (4 Suppl), A265.
11. Khurram Z, Chou E, Minutello R, Bergman G, Parikh M, Naidu S, Wong SC, Hong MK. Combination therapy with aspirin, clopidogrel and warfarin following coronary stenting is associated with a significant risk of bleeding. *J Invasive Cardiol* (2006) 18, 162–4.
12. Orford JL, Fasseas P, Melby S, Burger K, Steinhubl SR, Holmes DR, Berger PB. Safety and efficacy of aspirin, clopidogrel, and warfarin after coronary stent placement in patients with an indication for anticoagulation. *Am Heart J* (2004) 147, 463–7.
13. The Medical Research Council's General Practice Research Framework. Thrombosis prevention trial: randomised trial of low-intensity oral anticoagulation with warfarin and low-dose aspirin in the primary prevention of ischaemic heart disease in men at increased risk. *Lancet* (1998) 351, 233–41.
14. Rothberg MB, Celestin C, Fiore LD, Lawler E, Cook JR. Warfarin plus aspirin after myocardial infarction or the acute coronary syndrome: meta-analysis with estimates of risk and benefit. *Ann Intern Med* (2005) 143, 241–50.
15. Andreotti F, Testa L, Biondi-Zoccai GG, Crea F. Aspirin plus warfarin compared to aspirin alone after acute coronary syndromes: an updated and comprehensive meta-analysis of 25,307 patients. *Eur Heart J* (2006) 27, 519–26.
16. Buresly K, Eisenberg MJ, Zhang X, Pilote L. Bleeding complications associated with combinations of aspirin, thienopyridine derivatives, and warfarin in elderly patients following acute myocardial infarction. *Arch Intern Med* (2005) 165, 784–9.
17. Fiore LD, Ezekowitz MD, Brophy MT, Lu D, Sacco J, Peduzzi P. Department of Veterans Affairs Cooperative Studies Program clinical trial comparing combined warfarin and aspirin with aspirin alone in survivors of acute myocardial infarction: primary results of the CHAMP study. *Circulation* (2002) 105, 557–63.
18. WAVE investigators. The effects of oral anticoagulants in patients with peripheral arterial disease: rationale, design, and baseline characteristics of the Warfarin and Antiplatelet Vascular Evaluation (WAVE) trial, including a meta-analysis of trials. *Am Heart J* (2006) 151, 1–9.
19. Chesebro JH, Fuster V, Elveback LR, McGoon DC, Pluth JR, Puga FJ, Wallace RB, Danielson GK, Orszulak TA, Piehler JM, Schaff HV. Trial of combined warfarin plus dipyridamole or aspirin therapy in prosthetic heart valve replacement: danger of aspirin compared with dipyridamole. *Am J Cardiol* (1983) 51, 1537–41.
20. Dale J, Myhre E, Storstein O, Stormorken H, Efskind L. Prevention of arterial thromboembolism with acetylsalicylic acid. A controlled clinical study in patients with aortic ball valves. *Am Heart J* (1977) 94, 101–111.
21. Dale J, Myhre E, Loew D. Bleeding during acetylsalicylic acid and anticoagulant therapy in patients with reduced platelet reactivity after aortic valve replacement. *Am Heart J* (1980) 99, 746–52.
22. Altman R, Boullon F, Rouvier J, Rada R, de la Fuente L, Favaloro R. Aspirin and prophylaxis of thromboembolic complications in patients with substitute heart valves. *J Thorac Cardiovasc Surg* (1976) 72, 127–9.
23. Turpie AGG, Gent M, Laupacis A, Latour Y, Gunstensen J, Basile F, Klimek M, Hirsh J. A comparison of aspirin with placebo in patients treated with warfarin after heart-valve replacement. *N Engl J Med* (1993) 329, 524–9.
24. Fiore L, Brophy M, Deykin D, Cappelleri J, Lau J. The efficacy and safety of the addition of aspirin in patients treated with oral anticoagulants after heart valve replacement: a meta-analysis. *Blood* (1993) 82 (10 Suppl 1), 409a.
25. Little SH, Massel DR. Antiplatelet and anticoagulation for patients with prosthetic heart valves. Available in The Cochrane Database of Systematic Reviews; Issue 4. Chichester: John Wiley; 2006 (accessed 20070606).
26. Larson RJ, Fischer ES. Should aspirin be continued in patients started on warfarin? A systematic review and meta-analysis. *J Gen Intern Med* (2004) 19, 879–86.
27. Weil J, Colin-Jones D, Langman M, Lawson D, Logan R, Murphy M, Rawlins M, Vessey M, Wainwright P. Prophylactic aspirin and risk of peptic ulcer bleeding. *BMJ* (1995) 310: 827–30.

Coumarins + Azoles; Fluconazole

Fluconazole causes a dose-related inhibition of the metabolism of warfarin, and increases its anticoagulant effect. Cases of minor to major bleeding have been reported. There is one case report with acenocoumarol and fluconazole.

Clinical evidence

(a) Acenocoumarol

A patient stabilised on acenocoumarol suffered an intracranial haemorrhage (prothrombin time 170 seconds) 5 days after starting to take fluconazole 200 mg daily for the management of relapsed prosthetic valve candidal endocarditis.[1]

(b) Warfarin

1. Multiple-dose fluconazole. In a well-designed study in healthy subjects, fluconazole was given at three dose levels (100 mg, 200 mg and 400 mg daily) for 14 days with a single dose of warfarin given both before fluconazole and on day 7, at each fluconazole dose level. In this study, fluconazole markedly potentiated the anticoagulant effect of warfarin in a dose-related manner. The duration of anticoagulant effect was 4 to 7 days for the single dose of warfarin alone, 5 to 9 days with fluconazole 100 mg daily, 6 to 11 days with fluconazole 200 mg daily, and 8 to 15 days with fluconazole 400 mg daily. Fluconazole increased the levels of both *R*- and *S*-warfarin. The AUC of *R*-warfarin was increased 1.28-, 1.63-, and 1.7-fold with the 3 doses of fluconazole, respectively, and that of *S*-warfarin by 1.35-, 1.86-, and 2-fold, respectively.[2] Two other studies in healthy subjects have shown broadly similar results.[3-5]

The clinical importance of this interaction was shown in an earlier study, which found that when fluconazole 100 mg daily was given to 7 patients stabilised on warfarin, the prothrombin time increased from 15.8 seconds on day one, to 18.9 seconds on day 5, and 21.9 seconds on day 8. The fluconazole was stopped early in 3 of the patients due to high prothrombin times, but none exceeded an increase of 9.7 seconds, and no bleeding occurred.[6]

At least 7 reports have described increased prothrombin times or INRs in patients stabilised on warfarin who took fluconazole in doses of 50 to 400 mg daily.[7-14] Several patients had haemorrhagic effects (gastrointestinal bleeding, melaena, ocular haemorrhage, spinal epidural haematoma).[7,10,12-14]

2. Single-dose fluconazole. Six women on stable doses of warfarin with an INR between 2 and 3 were given a single 150-mg dose of fluconazole, and their prothrombin time measured on day 2, 5 and 8. The prothrombin time increased by 11% at day 2, and 34% on day 5, with a 2% increase on day 8, although none of these differences was statistically significant. However, three of the women had an increase in the INR to above 4 or had bleeding.[15]

Mechanism

In vitro studies using human liver microsomes clearly demonstrate that fluconazole inhibits the cytochrome P450 isoenzyme CYP2C9-mediated 7-hydroxylation of S-warfarin and the CYP3A4-mediated metabolism of *R*-warfarin, and possibly other isoenzymes involved in the metabolism of warfarin.[16] *In vivo,* this results in the accumulation of warfarin and in an increase in its effects, possibly leading to bleeding.[5]

Importance and management

An established and clinically important interaction. If fluconazole is added to treatment with warfarin or acenocoumarol the prothrombin times should be very well monitored and the anticoagulant dosage reduced as necessary. On the basis of pharmacokinetic studies it has been predicted that the warfarin dosage may need to be reduced by about 20% when using fluconazole 50 mg daily, ranging to a reduction of about 70% when using fluconazole 600 mg daily. These larger reductions should be gradual over 5 days or so.[17] However, remember that individual variations between patients can be considerable. Most of the available data relate to multiple-dose fluconazole, with just one small study with a single-dose of fluconazole 150 mg. Although the effect in this study was not as great as that for multiple-dose fluconazole, it suggests that careful monitoring of prothrombin times is still required.[15]

Of the other azole antifungals, 'ketoconazole', (p.388) and 'itraconazole', (p.388), appear less likely to interact.

1. Isalska BJ, Stanbridge TN. Fluconazole in the treatment of candidal prosthetic valve endocarditis. *BMJ* (1988) 297, 178–9.
2. Neal JM, Kunze KL, Levy RH, O'Reilly RA, Trager WF. K_iIV, an in vivo parameter for predicting the magnitude of a drug interaction arising from competitive enzyme inhibition. *Drug Metab Dispos* (2003) 31, 1043–8.
3. Lazar JD, Wilner KD. Drug interactions with fluconazole. *Rev Infect Dis* (1990) 12 (Suppl 3), S327–S333.
4. Rieth H, Sauerbrey N. Interaktionsstudien mit Fluconazol, einem neuen Triazolantimykotikum. *Wien Med Wochenschr* (1989) 139, 370–4.
5. Black DJ, Kunze KL, Wienkers LC, Gidal BE, Seaton TL, McDonnell ND, Evans JS, Bauwens JE, Trager WF. Warfarin-fluconazole II. A metabolically based drug interaction: *in vivo* studies. *Drug Metab Dispos* (1996) 24, 422–8.
6. Crussell-Porter LL, Rindone JP, Ford MA, Jaskar DW. Low-dose fluconazole therapy potentiates the hypoprothrombinemic response of warfarin sodium. *Arch Intern Med* (1993) 153, 102–4.
7. Seaton TL, Celum CL, Black DJ. Possible potentiation of warfarin by fluconazole. *DICP Ann Pharmacother* (1990) 24, 1177–8.

8. Tett S, Carey D, Lee H-S. Drug interactions with fluconazole. *Med J Aust* (1992) 156, 365.
9. Beeley L, Cunningham H, Brennan A. *Bulletin of the West Midlands Centre for Adverse Drug Reaction Reporting* (1993) 36, 17.
10. Kerr HD. Case report: potentiation of warfarin by fluconazole. *Am J Med Sci* (1993) 305, 164–5.
11. Gericke KR. Possible interaction between warfarin and fluconazole. *Pharmacotherapy* (1993) 13, 508–9.
12. Baciewicz AM, Menke JJ, Bokar JA, Baud EB. Fluconazole-warfarin interaction. *Ann Pharmacother* (1994) 28, 1111.
13. Mootha VV, Schluter ML, Das A. Intraocular hemorrhages due to warfarin-fluconazole drug interaction in a patient with presumed *Candida* endophthalmitis. *Arch Ophthalmol* (2002) 120, 94–5.
14. Allison EJ, McKinney TJ, Langenberg JN. Spinal epidural haematoma as a result of warfarin/fluconazole drug interaction. *Eur J Emerg Med* (2002) 9, 175–7.
15. Turrentine MA. Single dose fluconazole for vulvovaginal candidiasis; impact on prothrombin time in women taking warfarin. *Obstet Gynecol* (2006) 107, 310–3.
16. Kunze KL, Wienkers LC, Thummel KE, Trager WF. Warfarin-fluconazole I. Inhibition of the human cytochrome P450-dependent metablism of warfarin by fluconazole: *in vitro* studies. *Drug Metab Dispos* (1996) 24, 414–21.
17. Kunze KL, Trager WF. Warfarin-fluconazole III. A rational approach to management of a metabolically based drug interaction. *Drug Metab Dispos* (1996) 24, 429–35.

Coumarins + Azoles; Itraconazole

An isolated report describes a very marked increase in the anticoagulant effects of warfarin, accompanied by bruising and bleeding, in a patient given itraconazole. Limited evidence suggests that itraconazole may increase the risk of over-anticoagulation with acenocoumarol or phenprocoumon.

Clinical evidence

A woman stabilised on **warfarin** 5 mg daily and also taking ipratropium bromide, salbutamol, budesonide, quinine sulfate and omeprazole, was given itraconazole 200 mg twice daily for oral candidiasis caused by the inhaled steroid. Within 4 days she developed generalised bleeding and recurrent nosebleeds. Her INR had risen to more than 8. The **warfarin** and itraconazole were stopped, but next day she had to be admitted to hospital for intractable bleeding and increased bruising, for which she was treated with fresh frozen plasma. Two days later when the bleeding had stopped, and her INR had returned to 2.4, she was restarted on **warfarin** and later restabilised on her original dosage.[1]

In one cohort study in patients taking **acenocoumarol** or **phenprocoumon**, itraconazole significantly increased the risk of over-anticoagulation (INR greater than 6: relative risk of 13.9, range 1.7 to 115). However, the authors say this figure should be interpreted cautiously since it was based on just one case.[2]

Mechanism

Itraconazole is a known potent inhibitor of the cytochrome P450 isoenzyme CYP3A4, but this isoenzyme is involved only in the metabolism of the less potent *R*-warfarin, and therefore inhibition would not be expected to have a marked effect on 'warfarin metabolism', (p.358). However, there appear to be no pharmacological studies to confirm this. 'Omeprazole' (p.444) may also have had some minor part to play in the case described.[1]

Importance and management

A minor to modest pharmacokinetic interaction would be predicted, but as yet there appear to be no studies to confirm this. The case report and cohort study suggest that this interaction might be clinically important in some individuals. Therefore, it would be prudent to increase monitoring of anticoagulant control when any patient on a coumarin anticoagulant is given itraconazole. Further study is needed.

1. Yeh J, Soo S-C, Summerton C, Richardson C. Potentiation of action of warfarin by itraconazole. *BMJ* (1990) 301, 669.
2. Visser LE, Penning-van Beest FJA, Kasbergen AAH, De Smet PAGM, Vulto AG, Hofman A, Stricker BHC. Overanticoagulation associated with combined use of antifungal agents and coumarin anticoagulants. *Clin Pharmacol Ther* (2002) 71, 496–502.

Coumarins + Azoles; Ketoconazole

In two healthy subjects the anticoagulant effect of warfarin was unchanged when they were given ketoconazole. However, there are three isolated cases of an increase in the anticoagulant effects of warfarin in patients also taking ketoconazole. Some evidence suggests that topical ketoconazole does not interact with acenocoumarol or phenprocoumon.

Clinical evidence

Two healthy subjects had no changes in their anticoagulant response to **warfarin** when they were given ketoconazole 200 mg daily over a 3-week period.[1,2]

However, an elderly woman, stabilised on **warfarin** for 3 years, complained of spontaneous bruising 3 weeks after starting a course of ketoconazole 200 mg twice daily. Her British Comparative Ratio was found to have risen from 1.9 to 5.4. Her liver function was normal. She was restabilised on her previous **warfarin** dosage 3 weeks after the ketoconazole was withdrawn.[3] In 1984, the CSM in the UK had one report of an 84-year-old man taking **warfarin** whose British Comparative Ratio rose to 4.8 when he was given ketoconazole, and fell to 1.4 when it was withdrawn.[3] In 1986, the manufacturers of ketoconazole had one other report of an elderly man taking **warfarin** whose prothrombin time rose from a range of 34 to 39 seconds to over 60 seconds when he was given ketoconazole 400 mg daily.[4] In one cohort study in patients taking **acenocoumarol** or **phenprocoumon**, *topical* ketoconazole did not significantly increase the relative risk of over-anticoagulation (INR greater than 6; relative risk 1.1, range 0.3 to 4.3). However, this figure should be interpreted cautiously since it was based on just two patients.[5]

Mechanism

In *rats*,[6] ketoconazole potentiated the anticoagulant effect of acenocoumarol, but at much higher doses than 'miconazole', (p.388). It is now known that ketoconazole is an inhibitor of the cytochrome P450 isoenzyme CYP3A4, but this isoenzyme has only a minor role in the 'metabolism of warfarin' (p.358), specifically the less active *R*-isomer.

Importance and management

Information about this interaction seems to be limited to the reports cited. Its general importance and incidence is therefore uncertain, but it is probably quite small. However, it would seem prudent to monitor the anticoagulant response of any patient given both drugs, particularly the elderly, to ensure that excessive anticoagulation does not occur.

1. Brass C, Galgiani JN, Blaschke TF, Defelice R, O'Reilly RA, Stevens DA. Disposition of ketoconazole, an oral antifungal, in humans. *Antimicrob Agents Chemother* (1982) 21, 151–8.
2. Stevens DA, Stiller RL, Williams PL, Sugar AM. Experience with ketoconazole in three major manifestations of progressive coccidioidomycosis. *Am J Med* (1983) 74, 58–63.
3. Smith AG. Potentiation of oral anticoagulants by ketoconazole. *BMJ* (1984) 288, 188–9.
4. Janssen Pharmaceutical Limited. Personal communication, April 1986.
5. Visser LE, Penning-van Beest FJA, Kasbergen AAH, De Smet PAGM, Vulto AG, Hofman A, Stricker BHC. Overanticoagulation associated with combined use of antifungal agents and coumarin anticoagulants. *Clin Pharmacol Ther* (2002) 71, 496–502.
6. Niemegeers CJE, Levron JC, Awouters F, Janssen PAJ. Inhibition and induction of microsomal enzymes in the rat. A comparative study of four antimycotics: miconazole, econazole, clotrimazole and ketoconazole. *Arch Int Pharmacodyn Ther* (1981) 251, 26–38.

Coumarins and related drugs + Azoles; Miconazole

The anticoagulant effects of acenocoumarol, and warfarin can be markedly increased if miconazole is given orally as an oral (buccal) gel, and bleeding can occur. Oral miconazole has also been reported to interact with ethyl biscoumacetate, fluindione, phenindione and tioclomarol in a few reports. The interaction has also rarely been seen in some women using intravaginal miconazole, and in those using a miconazole cream on skin. In one cohort study, use of oral miconazole markedly increased the risk of over-anticoagulation with acenocoumarol and phenprocoumon, whereas intravaginal miconazole caused a non-statistically significant minor increase, and cutaneous miconazole barely increased the risk.

Clinical evidence

(a) Oral gel

In one early report, a patient with a prosthetic heart valve and stabilised on **warfarin** developed blood blisters and bruised easily 12 days after starting miconazole gel 250 g four times a day for a presumed fungal mouth infection. Her prothrombin time ratio had risen from less than 3 to about 16. She was subsequently restabilised in the absence of miconazole on her former dose of **warfarin**.[1]

Numerous other cases of this interaction with **warfarin** have been reported, and, where stated, often involved the use of 5 mL (125 mg) of the gel four times daily for oral candidiasis.[2-10] One case of an increase in INR to 11.4 with frank haematuria and spontaneous bruising was reported in a women who had used 30 g of non-prescription miconazole (*Daktarin*) over 8 days (estimated daily dose of 75 mg).[7] In 1996, the New Zealand Centre for Adverse Reactions Monitoring reported 5 patients taking **warfarin** whose INRs rose from normal values to between 7.5 and 18 within 7 to 15 days of starting to use miconazole oral gel.[5] In 2002, the Australian Adverse Drug Reactions Advisory Committee (ADRAC) stated that they had received 18 reports of this interaction. In the 17 cases for which it was documented, the INR was above 7.5. Eight of the cases had bleeding complications, 9 required vitamin K, and 5 fresh frozen plasma.[11]

A few similar cases have also been reported for **acenocoumarol**[12-14] or **fluindione**[15] with miconazole oral gel. In addition, in one cohort study in patients taking **acenocoumarol** or **phenprocoumon**, use of oral miconazole (form and doses not stated) markedly increased the risk of over-anticoagulation (INR greater than 6: adjusted relative risk 36.6; range 12.4 to 108). When analysed separately, the adjusted relative risk was higher for **acenocoumarol** than **phenprocoumon** (35.1 versus 16.5).[16]

(b) Tablets

In a study in 6 healthy subjects, miconazole 125 mg daily for 18 days (in the form of *tablets*) caused a very marked fivefold increase in prothrombin time response to a single dose of **warfarin** given on day 3. In addition, there was a threefold increase in the AUC of warfarin, with *S*-warfarin most affected (fourfold), and *R*-warfarin increased 1.7-fold.[17] In one early case report with warfarin, one patient with a prosthetic heart valve and stabilised on **warfarin** was found to have a prothrombin time ratio of 23.4 within 10 days of starting miconazole tablets 250 mg four times a day for a suspected fungal diarrhoea. He developed two haematomas soon after both drugs were withdrawn, and was subsequently restabilised, in the absence of miconazole, on his former dose of **warfarin**.[1]

The Centres de Pharmacovigilance Hospitalière in Bordeaux have on record 5 cases where miconazole (oral doses of 500 mg daily, where stated; form not mentioned) was responsible for a marked increase in prothrombin times and/or bleeding (haematomas, haematuria, gastrointestinal bleeding) in patients taking **acenocoumarol** (2 cases), **ethyl biscoumacetate** (1 case), **tioclomarol** (1 case) and **phenindione** (1 case).[18] Other cases and reports of this interaction involving **acenocoumarol** have been described elsewhere.[19-21]

(c) Skin creams

An 80-year-old man stabilised on **warfarin** with an INR of 2.2 to 3.1 was found to have an INR of 21.4 at a routine check 2 weeks after starting to use miconazole cream for a fungal infection in his groin. He showed no evidence of bruising or bleeding.[22] In 2001, Health Canada reported that they had on record a case of an 80-year-old man taking **warfarin** and using topical miconazole who had a cerebral vascular accident, although this case was complicated by multiple medical conditions and medications.[23] In 2002, the Australian Adverse Drug Reactions Advisory Committee stated that they had received one report of an interaction involving topical miconazole cream.[11]

In one cohort study in patients taking **acenocoumarol** or **phenprocoumon**, use of topical miconazole was associated with a small increased risk of over-anticoagulation (INR greater than 6: adjusted relative risk 1.4) but this was not statistically significant. Note that this was markedly less than the increased risk seen with oral miconazole (relative risk 36.6).[16]

(d) Vaginal dose forms

In 1999, the Netherlands Pharmacovigilance Foundation LAREB reported 2 elderly women patients taking **acenocoumarol** whose INRs rose sharply and rapidly when they were given a 3-day course of 400-mg miconazole pessaries.[24] Another report describes the development of bruising and an INR of about 9.78 in a 55-year-old woman taking **warfarin** on the third day of using 200-mg miconazole pessaries. For a subsequent course of intravaginal miconazole 100 mg daily for 7 days, the dose of warfarin was decreased by 28%, and her INR was 3.27.[25] Yet another report describes haemorrhage of the kidney in a 52-year old woman taking **warfarin** after she used vaginal miconazole for 12 days.[23] In one cohort study in patients taking **acenocoumarol** or **phenprocoumon**, use of vaginal miconazole was associated with a small increased risk of over-anticoagulation (INR greater than 6: adjusted relative risk 4.3) but this was not statistically significant. Note that this was markedly less than the increased risk seen with oral miconazole (relative risk 36.6).[16]

Mechanism

There is evidence that miconazole is a very potent inhibitor of the metabolism of *S*-warfarin by the cytochrome P450 isoenzyme CYP2C9, and that it also inhibits the metabolism of *R*-warfarin to a lesser extent.[17] Even low oral doses of miconazole (125 mg daily) markedly inhibit warfarin metabolism, so it is not surprising that prescription doses of miconazole oral gel (480 to 960 mg daily) interact, since this is swallowed after retaining in the mouth. Very unusually, absorption of miconazole from the vagina (see also comments below) and even exceptionally through the skin, can result in increased anticoagulant effects.

Importance and management

The interaction of miconazole oral gel and miconazole tablets with and coumarin anticoagulants is a very well established and potentially serious interaction. Most of the reports are about warfarin or acenocoumarol, but many other oral anticoagulants have been implicated. In some cases the bleeding has taken 7 to 15 days to develop,[1,3,18] whereas others have bled within only 3 days.[20,25] Raised INRs have been seen even sooner. Usual prescription doses of miconazole oral gel [5 to 10 mL (120 to 240 mg) four times daily] should therefore not be given to patients taking any oral anticoagulant unless the prothrombin times can be closely monitored and suitable dosage reductions made. Given the very large increased relative risk of over-anticoagulation seen in one cohort study, the authors suggest that the concurrent use of oral miconazole and coumarins should be discouraged.[16] The interaction has been seen with a lower oral dose of about 75 mg daily (one 30 g tube given over 8 days), which is not surprising in the context of the pharmacokinetic study, and suggests that patients taking oral anticoagulants should also avoid using non-prescription miconazole. Nevertheless, the UK patient information leaflet for non-prescription *Daktarin* oral gel contains no specific cautions regarding anticoagulants.[26] Nystatin and amphotericin are possible alternative antifungals to miconazole for mouth infections.

An interaction with **intravaginal miconazole** would not normally be expected because its systemic absorption is usually very low (less than 2%) in healthy women of child-bearing age.[27] However, the reports cited above show that significant absorption could apparently occur in a few patients with particular conditions (possibly in postmenopausal women with inflamed vaginal tissue), which allows an interaction to occur. Appropriate monitoring is therefore needed even with this route of administration in potentially at-risk women.

Topical (cutaneous) miconazole would also not be expected to interact, but the few reports cited shows that some caution might be warranted.

1. Watson PG, Lochan RG, Redding VJ. Drug interaction with coumarin derivative anticoagulants. *BMJ* (1982) 285, 1044–5
2. Colquhoun MC, Daly M, Stewart P, Beeley L. Interaction between warfarin and miconazole oral gel. *Lancet* (1987) i, 695–6.
3. Bailey GM, Magee P, Hickey FM, Beeley L. Miconazole and warfarin interaction. *Pharm J* (1989) 242, 183.
4. Shenfield GM, Page M. Potentiation of warfarin action by miconazole oral gel. *Aust N Z J Med* (1991) 21, 928.
5. Pillans P, Woods DJ. Interaction between miconazole oral gel (Daktarin) and warfarin. *N Z Med J* (1996) 109, 346.
6. Ariyaratnam S, Thakker NS, Sloan P, Thornhill MH. Potentiation of warfarin anticoagulant activity by miconazole oral gel. *BMJ* (1997) 314, 349.
7. Evans J, Orme DS, Sedgwick ML, Youngs GR. Treating oral candidiasis: potentially fatal. *Br Dent J* (1997) 182, 452.
8. Marco M, Guy AJ. Retroperitoneal haematoma and small bowel intramural haematoma caused by warfarin and miconazole interaction. *Int J Oral Maxillofac Surg* (1997) 27, 485.
9. Pemberton MN, Sloan P, Ariyaratnam S, Thakker NS, Thornhill MH. Derangement of warfarin anticoagulation by miconazole oral gel. *Br Dent J* (1998) 184, 68–9.
10. Øgard CG, Vestergaad H. Interaktion mellem warfarin og oral miconazol-gel. *Ugeskr Laeger* (2000) 162, 5511.
11. ADRAC. Miconazole oral gel elevates INR –a reminder. *Aust Adverse Drug React Bull* (2002) 21; 14–15.
12. Marotel C, Cerisay D, Vasseur P, Rouvier B, Chabanne JP. Potentialisation des effets de l'acénocoumarol par le gel buccal de miconazole. *Presse Med* (1986) 15, 1684–5.
13. Ducroix JP, Smail A, Sevenet F, Andrejak M, Baillet J. Hématome oesophagien secondaire à une potentialisation des effets de l'acénocoumarol par le gel buccal de miconazole. *Rev Med Interne* (1989) 10, 557–9.
14. Ortín M, Olalla JI, Muruzábal MJ, Peralta FG, Gutiérrez MA. Miconazole oral gel enhances acenocoumarol anticoagulant activity: a report of three cases. *Ann Pharmacother* (1999) 33, 175–77.
15. Ponge T, Rapp MJ, Fruneau P, Ponge A, Wassen-Hove L, Larousse C, Cottin S. Interaction médicamenteuse impliquant le miconazole en gel et la fluindione. *Therapie* (1987) 42, 412–13.

16. Visser LE, Penning-van Beest FJA, Kasbergen AAH, De Smet PAGM, Vulto AG, Hofman A, Stricker BHC. Overanticoagulation associated with combined use of antifungal agents and coumarin anticoagulants. *Clin Pharmacol Ther* (2002) 71, 496–502.
17. O'Reilly RA, Goulart DA, Kunze KL, Neal J, Gibaldi M, Eddy AC, Trager WF. Mechanisms of the stereoselective interaction between miconazole and racemic warfarin in human subjects. *Clin Pharmacol Ther* (1992) 51, 656–67.
18. Loupi E, Descotes J, Lery N, Evreux J C. Interactions médicamenteuses et miconazole. *Therapie* (1982) 37, 437–41
19. Anon. New possibilities in the treatment of systemic mycoses. Reports on the experimental and clinical evaluation of miconazole. Round table discussion and Chairman's summing up. *Proc R Soc Med* (1977), 70 (Suppl l), 51–4.
20. Ponge T, Barrier J, Spreux A, Guillou B, Larousse C, Grolleau JY. Potentialisation des effets de l'acénocoumarol par le miconazole. *Therapie* (1982) 37, 221–2.
21. Goenen M, Reynaert M, Jaumin P, Chalant CH, Tremouroux J. A case of candida albicans endocarditis three years after an aortic valve replacement. *J Cardiovasc Surg* (1977) 18, 391–6.
22. Devaraj A, O'Beirne JPO, Veasey R, Dunk AA. Interaction between warfarin and topical miconazole cream. *BMJ* (2002) 325, 77.
23. Anon. Miconazole-warfarin interaction: increased INR. *Can Med Assoc J* (2001) 165, 81.
24. Lansdorp D, Bressers HPHM, Dekens-Konter JAM, Meyboom RHB. Potentiation of acenocoumarol during vaginal administration of miconazole. *Br J Clin Pharmacol* (1999) 47, 225–6.
25. Thirion DJ, Zanetti LAF. Potentiation of warfarin's hypoprothrombinemic effect with miconazole vaginal suppositories. *Pharmacotherapy* (2000) 20, 98–9.
26. Daktarin Oral Gel (Miconazole). Janssen-Cilag Ltd. UK Patient information leaflet, December 2003.
27. Daneshmend TK. Systemic absorption of miconazole from the vagina. *J Antimicrob Chemother* (1986) 18, 507–11.

Coumarins + Azoles; Voriconazole

In one pharmacodynamic study, voriconazole approximately doubled the prothrombin time in response to warfarin.

Clinical evidence, mechanism, importance and management

When a single 30-mg dose of **warfarin** was given to 16 healthy subjects on day 7 of a 12-day course of voriconazole 300 mg twice daily, the maximal increase in prothrombin time was about doubled.[1] These increases in prothrombin time were still present 6 days after the **warfarin** dose, at which point the prothrombin time had returned to baseline with **warfarin** alone. Two subjects were withdrawn from the study because of an increased prothrombin time.[1]

Voriconazole is a known inhibitor of the cytochrome P450 isoenzymes CYP2C9 and CYP3A4, by which the coumarins (**phenprocoumon**, **acenocoumarol** and **warfarin**) are metabolised.[2,3] The manufacturers advise close monitoring of the prothrombin time in any patient on a coumarin anticoagulant who is given voriconazole. Dose adjustments of the coumarin should be made accordingly.[2,3]

1. Purkins L, Wood N, Kleinermans D, Nichols D. Voriconazole potentiates warfarin-induced prothrombin time prolongation. *Br J Clin Pharmacol* (2003) 56 (Suppl 1), 24–9.
2. VFEND (Voriconazole). Pfizer Ltd. UK Summary of product characteristics, July 2007.
3. VFEND (Voriconazole). Pfizer Ltd. US Prescribing information, November 2006.

Coumarins + Barbiturates

The effects of the coumarins are substantially reduced by the barbiturates. Primidone is metabolised to phenobarbital and is expected to interact similarly.

Clinical evidence

(a) Phenobarbital

A study in 16 patients stabilised on **warfarin** found that when they were also given phenobarbital 2 mg/kg their average daily **warfarin** requirements rose over a 4-week period by 25% (from 5.7 to 7.1 mg daily).[1] In another study, phenobarbital 100 mg at night for 4 weeks reduced the mean prothrombin time by 13% in patients stabilised on **warfarin**.[2] Other studies have shown that phenobarbital causes a 29% or 46% reduction in the half-life of **warfarin**,[3,4] and that the reduction was similar for both *R*- and *S*-warfarin.[5] A retrospective analysis in patients taking **warfarin** revealed that use of phenobarbital was associated with more erratic anticoagulation control, and that discontinuation of phenobarbital in a patient taking **warfarin** resulted in severe hypoprothrombinaemia and haematuria 2 weeks later.[6] In contrast, there is one isolated report of a woman stabilised on **warfarin** who developed haematuria three days after starting to take phenobarbital 60 mg four times daily.[7]

A reduced anticoagulant response has also been described in studies with **dicoumarol**,[8-10] and 2 cases have been reported with **ethyl biscoumacetate**.[11]

(b) Other barbiturates

An investigation in 12 patients taking either **warfarin** or **phenprocoumon** found that **secbutabarbital sodium**, 15 mg four times daily for the first week and 30 mg four times daily for the next two weeks, increased their anticoagulant requirements by 35 to 60%, reaching a maximum after 4 to 5 weeks.[12]

This interaction has also been described in pharmacological studies between:

- **acenocoumarol** and **pentobarbital**,[13] or **heptabarb**;[14]
- **dicoumarol** and **aprobarbitone**,[15] **heptabarb**,[14,16] or **vinbarbital**;[15]
- **ethyl biscoumacetate** and **heptabarb**;[14]
- **warfarin** and **amobarbital**,[17-19] **heptabarb**,[20] **secobarbital**,[2,17-19,21-23] or **secbutobarbital**.[12]

Cases have been described in patients taking **ethyl biscoumacetate** who were treated with **amobarbital**, **heptabarb**, or **secobarbital**.[11] Cases have also been described of apparent resistance to coumarins in patients taking barbiturates,[15,24] and of bleeding in patients who were stabilised on a coumarin and a barbiturate when they stopped taking the barbiturate.[15,24,25]

Mechanism

Pharmacokinetic studies in man and *animals*[3,4,18-20,22] clearly show that the barbiturates are potent liver enzyme inducers, which increase the metabolism and clearance of the coumarin anticoagulants from the body. The effect is similar for both *R*- and *S*-warfarin.[5,23] Barbiturates may also reduce the absorption of dicoumarol from the gut.[16]

Importance and management

The interactions between the anticoagulants and barbiturates are clinically important and very well documented. The reduced anticoagulant effects expose the patient to the risk of thrombus formation if the dosage is not increased appropriately. A very large number of anticoagulant/barbiturate pairs have been found to interact and the others may be expected to behave similarly. The reduction in the anticoagulant effects begins within a week, sometimes within 2 to 4 days, reaching a maximum after about 3 weeks, and it may still be evident up to 6 weeks after stopping the barbiturate.[12] Patients' responses can vary considerably. Stable anticoagulant control can be re-established[26] in the presence of the barbiturate by increasing the anticoagulant dosage by about 30 to 60%.[1,6,10,12] Care must be taken not to withdraw the barbiturate without also reducing the anticoagulant dosage, otherwise over-anticoagulation will occur. Alternative non-interacting drugs that are now considered more appropriate sedatives than the barbiturates include the 'benzodiazepines', (p.391).

Primidone is metabolised in the body to phenobarbital and is therefore expected to interact like phenobarbital, although there seem to be no reports of interactions with anticoagulants. Notwithstanding it would be prudent to be alert for reduced anticoagulant effects if primidone is given concurrently.

1. Robinson DS, MacDonald MG. The effect of phenobarbital administration on the control of coagulation achieved during warfarin therapy in man. *J Pharmacol Exp Ther* (1966) 153, 250–3.
2. Udall JA. Clinical implications of warfarin interactions with five sedatives. *Am J Cardiol* (1975) 35, 67–71.
3. Corn M. Effect of phenobarbital and glutethimide on biological half-life of warfarin. *Thromb Diath Haemorrh* (1966) 16, 606–12.
4. MacDonald MG, Robinson DS, Sylwester D, Jaffe JJ. The effects of phenobarbital, chloral betaine, and glutethimide administration on warfarin plasma levels and hypoprothrombinemic responses in man. *Clin Pharmacol Ther* (1969) 10, 80–4.
5. Orme M, Breckenridge A. Enantiomers of warfarin and phenobarbital. *N Engl J Med* (1976) 295, 1482.
6. MacDonald MG, Robinson DS. Clinical observations of possible barbiturate interference with anticoagulation. *JAMA* (1968) 204, 97–100.
7. Taylor PJ. Hemorrhage while on anticoagulant therapy precipitated by drug interaction. *Ariz Med* (1967) 24, 697–9.
8. Corn M, Rockett JF. Inhibition of bishydroxycoumarin activity by phenobarbital. *Med Ann Dist Columbia* (1965) 34, 578–9, 588.
9. Cucinell SA, Conney AH, Sansur M, Burns JJ. Drug interactions in man. I. Lowering effect of phenobarbital on plasma levels of bishydroxycoumarin (Dicumarol) and diphenylhydantoin (Dilantin). *Clin Pharmacol Ther* (1965) 6, 420–9.
10. Goss JE, Dickhaus DW. Increased bishydroxycoumarin requirements in patients receiving phenobarbital. *N Engl J Med* (1965) 273, 1094–5.
11. Avellaneda M. Interferencia de los barbituricos en la accion del Tromexan. *Medicina (B Aires)* (1955) 15, 109–15.
12. Antlitz AM, Tolentino M, Kosai MF. Effect of butabarbital on orally administered anticoagulants. *Curr Ther Res* (1968) 10, 70–3.
13. Kroon C, de Boer A, Hoogkamer JFW, Schoemaker HC, vd Meer FJM, Edelbroek PM, Cohen AF. Detection of drug interactions with single dose acenocoumarol: new screening method? *Int J Clin Pharmacol Ther Toxicol* (1990) 28, 355–60.
14. Dayton PG, Tarcan Y, Chenkin T, Weiner M. The influence of barbiturates on coumarin plasma levels and prothrombin response. *J Clin Invest* (1961) 40, 1797–1802.

15. Johansson S-A. Apparent resistance to oral anticoagulant therapy and influence of hypnotics on some coagulation factors. *Acta Med Scand* (1968) 184, 297–300.
16. Aggeler PM, O'Reilly RA. Effect of heptabarbital on the response to bishydroxycoumarin in man. *J Lab Clin Med* (1969) 74, 229–38.
17. Breckenridge A, Orme M. Clinical implications of enzyme induction. *Ann N Y Acad Sci* (1971) 179, 421–31.
18. Robinson DS, Sylwester D. Interaction of commonly prescribed drugs and warfarin. *Ann Intern Med* (1970) 72, 853–6.
19. Whitfield JB, Moss DW, Neale G, Orme M, Breckenridge A. Changes in plasma γ-glutamyl transpeptidase activity associated with alterations in drug metabolism in man. *BMJ* (1973) 1, 316–18.
20. Levy G, O'Reilly RA, Aggeler PM, Keech GM. Pharmacokinetic analysis of the effect of barbiturate on the anticoagulant action of warfarin in man. *Clin Pharmacol Ther* (1970) 11, 372–7.
21. Feuer DJ, Wilson WR, Ambre JJ. Duration of effect of secobarbital on the anticoagulant effect and metabolism of warfarin. *Pharmacologist* (1974) 16, 195.
22. Breckenridge A, Orme ML'E, Davies L, Thorgeirsson SS, Davies DS. Dose-dependent enzyme induction. *Clin Pharmacol Ther* (1973) 14, 514–20.
23. O'Reilly RA, Trager WF, Motley CH, Howald W. Interaction of secobarbital with warfarin pseudoracemates. *Clin Pharmacol Ther* (1980) 28, 187–95.
24. Reverchon F, Sapir M. Constatation clinique d'un antagonisme entre barbituriques et anticoagulants. *Presse Med* (1961) 69, 1570–1.
25. Macgregor AG, Petrie JC and Wood RA. Therapeutic conferences. Drug interaction. *BMJ* (1971) 1, 389–91.
26. Williams JRB, Griffin JP, Parkins A. Effect of concomitantly administered drugs on the control of long term anticoagulant therapy. *Q J Med* (1976) 45, 63–73.

Coumarins + Benfluorex

Benfluorex does not alter the anticoagulant effects of phenprocoumon.

Clinical evidence, mechanism, importance and management

No significant changes occurred in the prothrombin times of 22 patients stabilised on **phenprocoumon** when they were given benfluorex 150 mg three times daily for 9 weeks, when compared with equivalent periods before and after taking benfluorex.[1]

1. De Witte P, Brems HM. Co-administration of benfluorex with oral anticoagulant therapy. *Curr Med Res Opin* (1980) 6, 478–80.

Coumarins and related drugs + Benzbromarone or Benziodarone

The anticoagulant effects of warfarin are increased by benzbromarone and bleeding has been seen. Similarly, the anticoagulant effects of acenocoumarol, ethyl biscoumacetate, diphenadione and warfarin are increased by benziodarone.
Clorindione, dicoumarol and phenindione were not affected by benziodarone in one study. Phenprocoumon was not affected in one study, but was in another.

Clinical evidence

(a) Benzbromarone

The observation that 2 patients bled (haematuria, gastrointestinal bleeding) when given **warfarin** and benzbromarone, prompted a more detailed study in 7 other patients who were stabilised on both drugs. The thrombotest values of these 7 averaged 24.7% while taking both **warfarin** and benzbromarone (average dosage 57.1 mg daily), but when the benzbromarone was stopped for a week they rose to 47.3%. On restarting the benzbromarone the thrombotest values decreased to 30.3% (indicating an enhanced anticoagulant effect). The Factor II activity paralleled the thrombotest values. The total plasma **warfarin** levels were reduced during the period that benzbromarone was stopped.[1] Another later study found that the **warfarin** requirements of 13 patients given benzbromarone 50 mg daily were 36% lower than in 18 other patients given **warfarin** alone (3.9 versus 2.5 mg daily). The oral clearance of *S*-warfarin was 54% lower in the benzbromarone recipients, but the clearance of *R*-warfarin did not differ between the groups.[2] These two studies confirm observations in other patients with prosthetic valve replacements who showed haemorrhagic tendencies when given both drugs.[1]

Early information about benzbromarone noted that no increase in the anticoagulant effects of the coumarins **acenocoumarol** and **ethyl biscoumacetate** or the indanedione **phenindione** had been seen in a few patients also given benzbromarone.[3]

(b) Benziodarone

Benziodarone 200 mg three times daily for 2 days then 100 mg three times daily thereafter was given to 90 patients taking various anticoagulants. To maintain constant prothrombin-proconvertin percentages the coumarin anticoagulant dosages were reduced as follows: **ethyl biscoumacetate** 17% (9 patients), **acenocoumarol** 25% (7) and **warfarin** 46% (15). No changes in dose were needed in patients taking **dicoumarol** (9) or **phenprocoumon** (8). For the indanedione anticoagulants, a dose reduction of 42% was required in 8 patients taking **diphenadione**, but no changes were needed in those taking **clorindione** (5 patients) or **phenindione** (10 patients).[4] A parallel study in healthy subjects also found that benziodarone 300 mg or 600 mg daily increased the effects of a single dose of **warfarin**.[4]

In another study, benziodarone 300 to 600 mg daily increased the anticoagulant effects of **phenprocoumon** in just 9 out of 29 patients.[5] Plasma levels of **ethyl biscoumacetate** after a single intravenous dose were increased by pre-treatment with benziodarone 600 mg daily for 6 days.[5]

Mechanism

Benzbromarone selectively inhibits the metabolism of *S*-warfarin by the cytochrome P450 isoenzyme CYP2C9 so that its effects are increased. The metabolism of the *R*-warfarin remains unchanged.[2] Acenocoumarol and phenprocoumon are also known to be metabolised by CYP2C9, and would therefore be expected to interact similarly. Benziodarone is another benzofuran derivative with a similar structure to benzbromarone, and therefore probably interacts via a similar mechanism.

Importance and management

The interaction between warfarin and benzbromarone or benziodarone is established and clinically important. If benzbromarone is added to warfarin monitor prothrombin times and be alert for the need to reduce the dosage by about one-third to prevent over-anticoagulation. Information about other coumarins is limited, but what is known about the mechanism of action suggests that acenocoumarol and phenprocoumon would also be predicted to interact, and this has been shown for benziodarone and acenocoumarol or phenprocoumon, in a few patients. The limited evidence suggesting an interaction with some indanediones also suggests that some caution is appropriate with these drugs as well.

1. Shimodaira H, Takahashi K, Kano K, Matsumoto Y, Uchida Y, Kudo T. Enhancement of anticoagulant action by warfarin-benzbromarone interaction. *J Clin Pharmacol* (1996) 36, 168–74.
2. Takahashi H, Sato T, Shimoyama Y, Shioda N, Shimizu T, Kubo S, Tamura N, Tainaka H, Yasumori T, Echizen H. Potentiation of anticoagulant effect of warfarin caused by enantioselective metabolic inhibition by the uricosuric agent benzbromarone. *Clin Pharmacol Ther* (1999) 66, 569–81.
3. Masbernard A. Quoted as personal communication (1977) by Heel RC, Brogden RN, Speight TM, Avery GS. Benzbromarone: a review of its pharmacological properties and therapeutic use in gout and hyperuricaemia. *Drugs* (1977) 14, 349–66.
4. Pyörälä K, Ikkala E, Siltanen P. Benziodarone (Amplivix®) and anticoagulant therapy. *Acta Med Scand* (1963) 173, 385–9.
5. Verstraete M, Vermylen J, Claeys H. Dissimilar effect of two anti-anginal drugs belonging to the benzofuran group on the action of coumarin derivatives. *Arch Int Pharmacodyn Ther* (1968) 176, 33–41.

Coumarins + Benzodiazepines and related drugs

The anticoagulant effects of warfarin are not affected by chlordiazepoxide, diazepam, flurazepam, or nitrazepam, or the related hypnotics, eszopiclone, zaleplon, or zolpidem. The effects of phenprocoumon are not affected by nitrazepam or oxazepam, and those of ethyl biscoumacetate are not affected by chlordiazepoxide. An interaction between any oral anticoagulant and a benzodiazepine is unlikely, but there are three unexplained and unconfirmed cases of increased or decreased anticoagulant responses, which were attributed to an interaction.

Clinical evidence

A. Benzodiazepines

(a) Chlordiazepoxide

In a placebo-controlled study in 7 patients stabilised on **warfarin**, chlordiazepoxide 10 mg three times daily for 2 weeks had no effect on anticoagulant control.[1] Other studies in healthy subjects[2,3] and patients[4] have similarly shown that chlordiazepoxide does not alter the anticoagulant effect or the half-life of **warfarin**. Similarly, chlordiazepoxide 10 mg three times daily for 10 days had no effect on the half-life of a single intravenous dose of **ethyl biscoumacetate** in healthy subjects.[5] However, one patient stabilised on warfarin had a small 18% fall in mean plasma **warfarin** levels with a corresponding change in the anticoagulant response when given chlordiazepoxide 15 mg daily.[6]

(b) Diazepam

In 4 patients stabilised on **warfarin**, diazepam 5 mg three times daily for 30 days had no effect on anticoagulant control (thrombotest). In one of the patients, the half-life of **warfarin** was measured, and this was not changed by diazepam.[4] Similarly, diazepam 5 mg daily did not alter the anticoagulant response or the half-life of a single dose of **warfarin** in healthy subjects.[3]

However, there are two discordant reports. A patient stabilised on **dicoumarol** developed multiple ecchymoses and a prothrombin time of 53 seconds within 2 weeks of starting to take **diazepam** 5 mg four times daily.[7] The New Zealand Committee on Adverse Drug Reactions has received one report of an increased anticoagulant effect in a patient taking **warfarin** with **diazepam**.[8] It is by no means certain that these responses were due to an interaction.

(c) Flurazepam

In healthy subjects, flurazepam 30 mg at bedtime for 28 days had no effect on the half-life of a single dose of **warfarin** given on day 14 and 28, but there was a slight statistically significant reduction in prothrombin time. In a further placebo-controlled study in 12 patients stabilised on **warfarin**, flurazepam 30 mg at night for 28 days had no effect on prothrombin time or plasma warfarin concentrations.[9]

(d) Nitrazepam

In 2 reports by the same researchers, nitrazepam 10 mg at night for 30 days had no effect on steady-state warfarin levels or anticoagulant control in a few patients stabilised on **warfarin**.[4,6] In a placebo-controlled study in 22 patients stabilised on **phenprocoumon**, nitrazepam 5 mg at night for 2 weeks had no effect on thrombotest times.[10]

(e) Oxazepam

Oxazepam 10 mg in the morning and 10 to 20 mg in the evening for 3 weeks had no effect on anticoagulant response in 21 patients stabilised on **phenprocoumon**.[11]

B. Non-benzodiazepine hypnotics

(a) Eszopiclone

In a study in healthy subjects, eszopiclone 3 mg daily for 5 days had no effect on the AUC of *S*- or *R*-warfarin after a single 25-mg dose of **warfarin** and there was no change in the INR.[12]

(b) Zaleplon

In a study in healthy subjects, zaleplon 20 mg daily for 12 days had no effect on the AUC of *S*- or *R*-warfarin after a single 25-mg dose of **warfarin**. There was a minor 17% increase in the maximum serum levels of *S*-warfarin. However, zaleplon did not alter the prothrombin time response to **warfarin**.[13,14]

(c) Zolpidem

The prothrombin times of 8 healthy subjects given **warfarin** were unaffected by zolpidem 20 mg daily for 4 days.[15]

Mechanism

The three discordant reports are not understood. Enzyme induction is a possible explanation in one case with chlordiazepoxide,[6] because increases in the urinary excretion of 6-beta-hydroxycortisol (a marker of enzyme induction) have been described during chlordiazepoxide use.[4,6]

Importance and management

The weight of evidence and common experience shows that the benzodiazepines do not interact with the anticoagulants. Not all of the anticoagulant and benzodiazepines have been examined, but none of the possible pairs would be expected to interact. Similarly, based on pharmacodynamic studies, no interaction would be anticipated with the newer non-benzodiazepine hypnotics eszopiclone, zaleplon or zolpidem.

1. Lackner H, Hunt VE. The effect of Librium on hemostasis. *Am J Med Sci* (1968) 256, 368–72.
2. Robinson DS, Sylwester D. Interaction of commonly prescribed drugs and warfarin. *Ann Intern Med* (1970) 72, 853–6.
3. Solomon HM, Barakat MJ, Ashley CJ. Mechanisms of drug interaction. *JAMA* (1971) 216, 1997–9.
4. Orme M, Breckenridge A, Brooks RV. Interactions of benzodiazepines with warfarin. *BMJ* (1972) 3, 611–14.
5. van Dam FE, Gribnau-Overkamp MJH. The effect of some sedatives (phenobarbital, glutethimide, chlordiazepoxide, chloral hydrate) on the rate of disappearance of ethyl biscoumacetate from the plasma. *Folia Med Neerl* (1967) 10, 141–5.
6. Breckenridge A, Orme M. Clinical implications of enzyme induction. *Ann N Y Acad Sci* (1971) 179, 421–31.
7. Taylor PJ. Hemorrhage while on anticoagulant therapy precipitated by drug interaction. *Ariz Med* (1967) 24, 697–9.
8. McQueen EG. New Zealand Committee on Adverse Drug Reactions: Ninth Annual Report 1974. *N Z Med J* (1974) 80, 305–11.
9. Robinson DS, Amidon EL. Interaction of benzodiazepines with warfarin in man. In: Garattini S, Mussini E, Randall LO, eds. The Benzodiazepines. New York: Raven Press, 1973. p. 641–6.
10. Bieger R, De Jonge H, Loeliger EA. Influence of nitrazepam on oral anticoagulation with phenprocoumon. *Clin Pharmacol Ther* (1972) 13, 361–5.
11. Schneider J, Kamm G. Beeinflußt Oxazepam (Adumbran®) die Antikoagulanzientherapie mit Phenprocoumon? *Med Klin* (1978) 73, 153–6.
12. Maier G, Roach J, Rubens R. Evaluation of pharmacokinetic and pharmacodynamic interactions between eszopiclone and warfarin. *Sleep* (2004) 27 (Suppl), A56.
13. Darwish M. Overview of drug interaction studies with zaleplon. Poster presented at 13th Annual Meeting of Associated Professional Sleep Studies (APSS), Orlando, Florida, June 23rd, 1999.
14. Darwish M. Analysis of potential drug interactions with zaleplon. *J Am Geriatr Soc* (1999) 47, S62.
15. Sauvanet JP, Langer SZ, Morselli PL, eds. Imidazopyridines in Sleep Disorders. New York: Raven Press; 1988 p. 165–73.

Coumarins and related drugs + Beta blockers

The effects of the coumarins are not normally altered by any beta blocker. However, propranolol has caused small increases in warfarin levels in a couple of studies, and one or two isolated cases of increased warfarin and phenindione effects have been reported.

Clinical evidence

(a) Acenocoumarol

In a study in 4 patients stabilised on acenocoumarol there was no difference in anticoagulation tests when **atenolol** 100 mg daily, **metoprolol** 100 mg twice daily, or placebo, was given for 3 weeks.[1]

(b) Phenindione

In one early clinical study, haemorrhagic tendencies without any changes in Quick value or any other impairment of coagulation were described in three patients stabilised on phenindione within 6 weeks of starting **propranolol**.[2]

(c) Phenprocoumon

In healthy subjects, a single dose of **atenolol** 100 mg or **metoprolol** 100 mg did not affect the AUC of a single dose of **phenprocoumon**, although **phenprocoumon** levels were slightly higher at 4 and 6 hours after the **metoprolol** dose. Nevertheless, neither beta blocker altered the prothrombin time response.[3]

In healthy subjects, **carvedilol** 25 mg daily for 7 days had no effect on the pharmacokinetics of a single 15-mg dose of phenprocoumon given on day 5 phenprocoumon.[4]

In 12 patients stabilised on phenprocoumon, there was no difference in Quick time between those randomised to receive **pindolol** 5 mg three times daily for 6 weeks and those who received placebo.[5]

(d) Warfarin

In 6 patients stabilised on warfarin, **acebutolol** 300 mg three times daily for 3 days had no effect on prothrombin time response.[6] Similarly, in one patient taking warfarin, neither **atenolol** 100 mg daily nor metoprolol 100 mg twice daily for 3 weeks had any effect on prothrombin time.[1] Similarly, in studies in healthy subjects the following beta blockers had no clinically relevant effects on the pharmacokinetics and/or anticoagulant response to warfarin; **atenolol** 100 mg daily,[7] **betaxolol** 20 mg daily,[8] **bisoprolol** 10 mg daily,[9] **esmolol**,[10] or **metoprolol** 100 mg twice daily.[7]

In contrast, the minimum steady state plasma **warfarin** levels of 6 healthy subjects rose by 15% when they took **propranolol** 80 mg twice daily in one study.[11] Similarly, in another study in 6 healthy subjects given **propranolol** 80 mg twice daily for 7 days with a single dose of warfarin on day 4, the AUC of warfarin was increased by 16.3% and the in maximum serum level was increased by 23%, but there was no change in the prothrombin time.[7] A patient stabilised on **warfarin** had a rise in his British Corrected Ratio from a low of 1.3 up to 2.5 while taking **propranolol** 80 mg twice daily.[12]

Mechanism

None known.

Importance and management

Overall, the findings of these pharmacological studies in patients and healthy subjects confirm the general clinical experience that the effects of the coumarin anticoagulants are not normally altered by the beta blockers. No special precautions are needed on concurrent use. The only uncertainty is with propranolol, which has shown a small rise in warfarin levels in two studies, and for which there are a couple of reports of possible increased anticoagulant responses of warfarin and phenindione. Even so, a clinically significant interaction would seem to be extremely rare.

1. Mantero F, Procidano M, Vicariotto MA , Girolami A. Effect of atenolol and metoprolol on the anticoagulant activity of acenocoumarin. *Br J Clin Pharmacol* (1984) 17 (Suppl), 94S–96S.
2. Neilson GH, Seldon WA. Propranolol in angina pectoris. *Med J Aust* (1969) 1, 856–57.
3. Spahn H, Kirch W, Mutschler E, Ohnhaus EE, Kitteringham NR, Lögering HJ, Paar D. Pharmacokinetic and pharmacodynamic interactions between phenprocoumon and atenolol or metoprolol. *Br J Clin Pharmacol* (1984) 17, 97S–102S.
4. Harder S, Brei R, Caspary S, Merz PG. Lack of a pharmacokinetic interaction between carvedilol and digitoxin or phenprocoumon. *Eur J Clin Pharmacol* (1993) 44, 583–6.
5. Vinazzer H. Effect of the beta-receptor blocking agent Visken® on the action of coumarin. *Int J Clin Pharmacol* (1975) 12, 458–60.
6. Ryan JR. Clinical pharmacology of acebutolol. *Am Heart J* (1985) 109, 1131–6.
7. Bax NDS, Lennard MS, Tucker GT, Woods HF, Porter NR, Malia RG, Preston FE. The effect of β-adrenoceptor antagonists on the pharmacokinetics and pharmacodynamics of warfarin after a single dose. *Br J Clin Pharmacol* (1984) 17, 553–7.
8. Thiercelin JF, Warrington SJ, Thenot JP, Orofiamma B. Lack of interaction of betaxolol on warfarin induced hypocoagulability. In: Aiache JM, Hirtz J, eds. Proc 2nd Eur Cong Biopharm Pharmacokinet Vol III: Clinical Pharmacokinetics. Paris: Imprimerie de l'Université de Clermont Ferrand; 1984. pp 73–80.
9. Warrington SJ, Johnston A, Lewis Y, Murphy M. Bisoprolol: studies of potential interactions with theophylline and warfarin in healthy volunteers. *J Cardiovasc Pharmacol* (1990) 16 (Suppl 5), S164–S168.
10. Lowenthal DT, Porter RS, Saris SD, Bies CM, Slegowski MB, Staudacher A. Clinical pharmacology, pharmacodynamics and interactions with esmolol. *Am J Cardiol* (1985) 56, 14F–17F.
11. Scott AK, Park BK, Breckenridge AM. Interaction between warfarin and propranolol. *Br J Clin Pharmacol* (1984) 17, 559–64.
12. Bax NDS, Lennard MS, Al-Asady S, Deacon CS, Tucker GT, Woods HF. Inhibition of drug metabolism by β-adrenoceptor antagonists. *Drugs* (1983) 25 (Suppl 2), 121–6.

Coumarins + Bicalutamide, Flutamide or Nilutamide

The manufacturer has on record a few cases of flutamide possibly increasing the anticoagulant effects of warfarin. *In vitro,* bicalutamide displaced warfarin from its protein binding sites. The clinical relevance of this, if any, has not been assessed. *In vitro,* nilutamide inhibited P450 isoenzymes, and might therefore interact with coumarins, although there does not appear to be any further information on this.

Clinical evidence, mechanism, importance and management

(a) Bicalutamide

The manufacturers say[1,2] that *in vitro* studies show that bicalutamide can displace **warfarin** from its protein binding sites. They therefore recommended close monitoring of the prothrombin time. It used to be thought that the displacement of **warfarin** from its protein binding sites by other drugs normally resulted in clinically important interactions, but that is now known to rarely be true (see 'Protein-binding interactions', (p.3)). In 1995, the manufacturers said that they did not know of any reports of an interaction between **warfarin** and bicalutamide, apart from an isolated case of a raised INR in one patient taking **warfarin** with bicalutamide 150 mg, but no causal link with bicalutamide was established.[3] In a clinical study of bicalutamide and finasteride, it was briefly stated that one patient developed a prolonged prothrombin time while also taking warfarin.[4] To date, there appear to be no published cases of an interaction. There would therefore seem little reason to believe that bicalutamide interacts with **warfarin**, but until more is known it would seem prudent to remain aware of the possibility if it is started in any patient taking **warfarin**.

(b) Flutamide

In 1990, the manufacturer had on record, 5 cases of patients with prostatic cancer receiving **warfarin** whose prothrombin times had increased when they were given flutamide. For example, one patient needed reductions in his **warfarin** dosage from 35 to 22.5 mg weekly over a 2-month period. Another had a prothrombin time rise from 15 to 37 seconds within 4 days of starting flutamide 750 mg daily.[5] There appears to be no published information about this interaction, but the manufacturer recommends that prothrombin times are monitored if flutamide is given to patients taking **warfarin**, reducing the dosage when necessary.[6]

(c) Nilutamide

The manufacturer notes that, *in vitro,* nilutamide has been shown to inhibit cytochrome P450 isoenzymes (specific isoenzymes not stated). Because of this, they suggest that nilutamide might increase the toxicity of drugs with a low therapeutic margin such as the vitamin K antagonists (i.e. **coumarins** and **indanediones**). They therefore recommend that the prothrombin time be carefully monitored when nilutamide is given with these drugs, and their dosages reduced if necessary.[7] There does not appear to be any further information about this potential interaction.

1. Casodex (Bicalutamide). AstraZeneca UK Ltd. UK Summary of product characteristics, February 2007.
2. Casodex (Bicalutamide). AstraZeneca. US Prescribing information, March 2006.
3. Zeneca. Personal Communication, October 1995.
4. Tay M-H, Kaufman DS, Regan MM, Leibowitz SB, George DJ, Febbo PG, Manola J, Smith MR, Kaplan ID, Kantoff PW, Oh WK. Finasteride and bicalutamide as primary hormonal therapy in patients with advanced adenocarcinoma of the prostate. *Ann Oncol* (2004) 15, 974–8.
5. Schering-Plough Ltd. Personal communication, March 1990.
6. Drogenil (Flutamide). Schering-Plough Ltd. UK Summary of product characteristics. March 2005.
7. Nilandron (Nilutamide). Sanofi-Aventis US LLC. US Prescribing information, June 2006.

Coumarins + Bile-acid binding resins

The anticoagulant effects of phenprocoumon and warfarin can be reduced by colestyramine, especially if the coumarin is given at the same time. An isolated report describes unexpected sensitivity to warfarin in a patient taking colestyramine, which was attributed to a possible reduction in vitamin K absorption with colestyramine. Colestipol did not alter the absorption or effect of phenprocoumon or warfarin and colesevelam did not alter the pharmacokinetics of warfarin.

Clinical evidence

(a) Colesevelam

Colesevelam 4.5 g had no effect on the pharmacokinetics of **warfarin** 10 mg in a single-dose study in 24 healthy subjects.[1]

(b) Colestipol

In a placebo-controlled, single-dose study in 4 healthy subjects, **phenprocoumon** plasma levels and the prothrombin response were unaffected by colestipol 8 g given at the same time as **phenprocoumon** 12 mg.[2] Similarly, in an study quoted in a review,[3] the concurrent use of colestipol 10 g did not cause any changes in the absorption of a single 10-mg dose of **warfarin** in healthy subjects.

(c) Colestyramine

1. Phenprocoumon. It was noted that establishing effective anticoagulation was difficult in patients taking phenprocoumon with colestyramine, in spite of doubling the dose of phenprocoumon. This prompted a study in healthy subjects in which it was found that concurrent single doses of phenprocoumon and colestyramine markedly reduced phenprocoumon plasma levels and effect.[4] In another study using *intravenous* phenprocoumon, colestyramine reduced the effect of the anticoagulant by this route, presumably by reducing enterohepatic recycling.[5] This fact has been used clinically to enhance the elimination of phenprocoumon after phenprocoumon overdose. In one case, the half-life of phenprocoumon was measured as 6.8 days without colestyramine, and 3.5 days with colestyramine 4 g three times daily.[6]

A patient stabilised on phenprocoumon developed a fatal valve thrombosis after starting colestyramine, despite separation of doses in accordance with the manufacturer's instructions.[7]

2. Warfarin. Ten subjects were treated for one-week periods with warfarin alone then warfarin with colestyramine 8 g given three times daily, with the warfarin taken 30 minutes after colestyramine for one week, then 6 hours after colestyramine for one week. When warfarin was taken 30 minutes after colestyramine, peak warfarin levels were reduced by 52% and the prolongation in prothrombin times was reduced by 27%, compared with warfarin alone. However, when warfarin was taken 6 hours after colestyramine, peak warfarin levels were reduced by only 16%, and the prolongation in prothrombin times was the same as with warfarin alone.[8]

Comparable results were found in another similar study; simultaneous administration of warfarin and colestyramine reduced the prothrombin time response by 21%, and separation by 3 hours still caused an 11% reduction in the prothrombin time response.[9] Another study using *intravenous* warfarin has shown that colestyramine also reduces the effect of warfarin by this route, presumably by reducing enterohepatic recycling.[10]

Another report describes a patient taking colestyramine 4 g three times daily who was successfully stabilised on warfarin with alternating doses of 5 mg and 7.5 mg daily. The warfarin was given at 8 am, then the colestyramine at 12 noon with lunch, with dinner, and with an evening snack.[11]

In contrast, an isolated report describes a 77-year-old patient taking multiple medications including colestyramine who was found to have a very high prothrombin time of 78.9 seconds and microscopic haematuria 6 weeks after starting warfarin 5 mg daily. Four days after starting the warfarin her prothrombin time was 17.1 seconds, and it had not been checked again.[12] However, as it is not certain that this patient was properly stabilised on warfarin this may simply have been an effect of the warfarin alone.

Mechanism

Colestyramine binds to coumarin anticoagulants in the gut, thereby preventing their absorption.[4,9,13,14] Data with intravenous warfarin and phenprocoumon show that they undergo enterohepatic recycling, and that colestyramine can reduce this as well.[5,10] Long-term use of colestyramine also reduces the absorption of fat-soluble vitamins such as vitamin K so that it can have some direct hypoprothrombinaemic effects of its own.[15,16] This may to some extent offset the full effects of its interaction with anticoagulants. Colestipol on the other hand appears not to bind to any great extent at the pH values in the gut.[2] The paradoxical increase in the effects of warfarin in the isolated case cited above was attributed to the effect of colestyramine on vitamin K.[12]

Importance and management

The interaction of colestyramine with phenprocoumon and warfarin is established, and can be clinically important. If concurrent use is thought necessary, prothrombin times should be monitored and the dosage of the anticoagulant increased appropriately. Giving the colestyramine 4 to 6 hours after the anticoagulant has been shown to minimise the effects of this interaction,[8,11] and it is a standard recommendation that other drugs should be given 1 hour before or 4 to 6 hours after colestyramine. However, despite adequate separation of doses, one patient taking phenprocoumon developed fatal valve thrombosis when given colestyramine, leading the authors to suggest that colestyramine should not be used in patients taking oral anticoagulants.[7] Information about other anticoagulants is lacking but as colestyramine interacts with dicoumarol and ethyl biscoumacetate in *animals*[14] it would be prudent to expect all coumarins to interact similarly. Bear in mind that long-term colestyramine can reduce vitamin K absorption and can cause hypoprothrombinaemia. This might result in an increased effect of warfarin, as has been suggested in one unconfirmed case report but there seems to be no other evidence to suggest that this is clinically relevant.

No special precautions appear necessary if warfarin or phenprocoumon and colestipol or colesevelam are given concurrently.

1. Donovan JM, Stypinski D, Stiles MR, Olson TA, Burke SK. Drug interactions with colesevelam hydrochloride, a novel, potent lipid-lowering agent. *Cardiovasc Drugs Ther* (2000) 14, 681–90.
2. Harvengt C, Desager JP. Effects of colestipol, a new bile acid sequestrant, on the absorption of phenprocoumon in man. *Eur J Clin Pharmacol* (1973) 6, 19–21.
3. Heel RC, Brogden RN, Pakes GE, Speight TM, Avery GS. Colestipol: a review of its pharmacological properties and therapeutic effects in patients with hypercholesterolaemia. *Drugs* (1980) 19, 161–80.
4. Hahn KJ, Eiden W, Schettle M, Hahn M, Walter E, Weber E. Effect of cholestyramine on the gastrointestinal absorption of phenprocoumon and acetylosalicylic acid in man. *Eur J Clin Pharmacol* (1972) 4, 142–5.
5. Meinertz T, Gilfrich H-J, Groth U, Jonen HG, Jähnchen E. Interruption of the enterohepatic circulation of phenprocoumon by cholestyramine. *Clin Pharmacol Ther* (1977) 21, 731–5.
6. Meinertz T, Gilfrich H-J, Bork R, Jähnchen E. Treatment of phenprocoumon intoxication with cholestyramine. *BMJ* (1977) 2, 439.
7. Balmelli N, Domine F, Pfisterer M, Krähenbühl S, Marsch S. Fatal drug interaction between colestyramine and phenprocoumon. *Eur J Intern Med* (2002) 13, 210–11.
8. Kuentzel WP, Brunk SF. Cholestyramine-warfarin interaction in man. *Clin Res* (1970) 18, 594.
9. Robinson DS, Benjamin DM, McCormack JJ. Interaction of warfarin and nonsystemic gastrointestinal drugs. *Clin Pharmacol Ther* (1971) 12, 491–5.
10. Jähnchen E, Meinertz T, Gilfrich H-J, Kersting F, Groth U. Enhanced elimination of warfarin during treatment with cholestyramine. *Br J Clin Pharmacol* (1978) 5, 437–40.
11. Cali TJ. Combined therapy with cholestyramine and warfarin. *Am J Pharm Sci Support Public Health* (1975) 147, 166–9.
12. Lawlor DP, Hyers TM. Extreme prolongation of the prothrombin time in a patient receiving warfarin and cholestyramine. *Cardiovasc Rev Rep* (1993) April, 72–4.
13. Gallo DG, Bailey KR, Sheffner AL. The interaction between cholestyramine and drugs. *Proc Soc Exp Biol Med* (1965) 120, 60–5.
14. Tembo AV, Bates TR. Impairment by cholestyramine of dicumarol and tromexan absorption in rats: a potential drug interaction. *J Pharmacol Exp Ther* (1974) 191, 53–9.
15. Casdorph HR. Safe uses of cholestyramine. *Ann Intern Med* (1970) 72, 759.
16. Gross L, Brotman M. Hypoprothrombinemia and hemorrhage associated with cholestyramine therapy. *Ann Intern Med* (1970) 72, 95–6.

Coumarins + Bosentan

Bosentan modestly enhanced the metabolism of warfarin and reduced its anticoagulant effects in one study and in one case a patient needed a 64% increase in her warfarin dose after taking bosentan.

Clinical evidence

In a double-blind, randomised, placebo-controlled, crossover study, 12 healthy subjects were given bosentan 500 mg twice daily or placebo for 10 days, with a single 26-mg dose of **warfarin** on day 6. Bosentan reduced the AUC of *R*-warfarin by 38% and of *S*-warfarin by 29%. A significant decrease in the anticoagulant effects of **warfarin** was also noted, with a 23% reduction in prothrombin time occurring with bosentan.[1]

One case highlights the clinical significance of this interaction. A 35-year-old woman taking **warfarin** with a stable INR of 2 to 3 over three months started taking bosentan 62.5 mg twice daily. After 10 days her INR was 1.7, and remained at this level over the next 4 weeks, despite an increase in her weekly **warfarin** dose from 27.5 to 40 mg. The bosentan dose was then increased to the maintenance dose of 125 mg twice daily, and two further weekly increases in **warfarin** dose were made. The INR was then high (3.2 to 4.1) for 3 weeks, before she was finally stabilised on **warfarin** 45 mg each week.[2]

However, the manufacturer of bosentan notes that, in clinical experience, the use of bosentan with **warfarin** did not result in clinically relevant changes in the INR or **warfarin** dose. There was no difference in the frequency of **warfarin** dose changes (due to INR changes or adverse effects) between bosentan or placebo recipients.[3]

Mechanism

It has been suggested that bosentan induces both cytochrome P450 isoenzymes CYP3A4 and CYP2C9, which are involved in the metabolism of *R*-warfarin and *S*-warfarin, respectively.[1]

Importance and management

Both the reports suggest that a clinically significant interaction between warfarin and bosentan is possible, although exactly how frequently this may occur is unclear, since it was not detected in clinical studies. However, the INR should be closely monitored in any patient taking warfarin during the period that bosentan is started or stopped, or if the dose is altered.[3]

1. Weber C, Banken L, Birnboeck H, Schulz R. Effect of the endothelin-receptor antagonist bosentan on the pharmacokinetics and pharmacodynamics of warfarin. *J Clin Pharmacol* (1999) 39, 847–54.
2. Murphey LM, Hood EH. Bosentan and warfarin interaction. *Ann Pharmacother* (2003) 37, 1028–31.
3. Tracleer (Bosentan monohydrate). Actelion Pharmaceuticals UK. UK Summary of product characteristics, October 2006.

Coumarins + Broxuridine

A case report describes an increase in the effects of warfarin in a patient taking broxuridine.

Clinical evidence, mechanism, importance and management

A man taking **warfarin** and with grade III anaplastic astrocytoma was given intravenous broxuridine as a radiosensitiser. His prothrombin times were unaffected by the first course of broxuridine 1.4 g daily for 4 days, but became more prolonged with successive courses, and after the fourth course his prothrombin time reached about 45 seconds. This which was managed with 10 mg of vitamin K. Warfarin was stopped after a significant increase also took place with a fifth cycle of broxuridine 990 mg daily.[1] The clinical relevance of this single case is uncertain.

1. Oster SE, Lawrence HJ. Potentiation of anticoagulant effect of coumadin by 5-bromo-2′-deoxyuridine (BUDR). *Cancer Chemother Pharmacol* (1988) 22, 181.

Coumarins + Bucolome

Bucolome increases the anticoagulant effects of warfarin by inhibiting its metabolism.

Clinical evidence

A study in Japanese patients stabilised on **warfarin** found that the addition of bucolome 300 mg daily increased the INR of 21 patients 1.5-fold despite a 58% reduction in the **warfarin** dose, when compared with another group of 34 patients taking **warfarin** and not receiving bucolome.[1] In another 7-day study, 25 Japanese patients with heart disease on **warfarin** and bucolome 300 mg daily were compared with another control group of 30 patients taking **warfarin** alone. It was found that bucolome had no effect on the serum levels of *R*-warfarin but both the serum levels of *S*-warfarin and the prothrombin times rose. These changes were complete within 7 days.[2] In one analysis, the daily dose of **warfarin** was found to be about 40% lower in 78 patients taking bucolome, when compared with 99 patients not taking bucolome, although the thrombotest values were lower in those also taking bucolome (suggesting greater anticoagulation). Bucolome appeared to reduce the between patient variation in intrinsic hepatic clearance of warfarin.[3]

A patient who had been taking **warfarin** with bucolome for 18 days developed gross haematuria. He was found to have an intraluminal ureteral haematoma and an excessively prolonged prothrombin time, and was treated with intravenous vitamin K.[4]

Mechanism

In vitro studies show that the bucolome can inhibit the metabolism of the more potent enantiomer *S*-warfarin by the cytochrome P450 isoenzyme CYP2C9, thereby reducing its clearance and increasing its effects.[1]

Importance and management

Information appears to be limited to the reports cited here but the interaction would seem to be established and clinically important. Monitor the INR closely. A reduced warfarin dosage (the study cited above suggests a 30 to 60% reduction)[2] is likely to be needed if both drugs are used concurrently to avoid excessive anticoagulation and possible bleeding. Note that bucolome is sometimes used with warfarin to enhance its therapeutic effect.[3] Based on the mechanism of action, **acenocoumarol** and **phenprocoumon** would be anticipated to be similarly affected.

1. Takahashi H, Kashima T, Kimura S, Murata N, Takaba T, Iwade K, Abe T, Tainaka H, Yasumori T, Echizen H. Pharmacokinetic interaction between warfarin and a uricosuric agent, bucolome: application of in vitro approaches to predicting in vivo reduction of (S)-warfarin clearance. *Drug Metab Dispos* (1999) 27, 1179–86.
2. Matsumoto K, Ishida S, Ueno K, Hashimoto H, Takada M, Tanaka K, Kamakura S, Miyatake K, Shibakawa M. The stereoselective effects of bucolome on the pharmacokinetics and pharmacodynamics of racemic warfarin. *J Clin Pharmacol* (2001) 41, 459–64.
3. Osawa M, Hada N, Matsumoto K, Hasegawa T, Kobayashi D, Morimoto Y, Yamaguchi M, Kanamoto I, Nakagawa T, Sugibayashi K. Usefulness of coadministration of bucolome in warfarin therapy: pharmacokinetic and pharmacodynamic analysis using outpatient prescriptions. *Int J Pharm* (2005) 293, 43–9.
4. Murosaki N, Senoh H, Takemoto M. Intraluminal ureteral hematoma complicating anticoagulant therapy [In Japanese]. *Nippon Hinyokika Gakkai Zasshi* (2005) 96, 564–7.

Coumarins + Calcium-channel blockers

In pharmacological studies neither amlodipine nor felodipine affected the anticoagulant effects of warfarin. Similarly, although diltiazem may cause a minor decrease in warfarin metabolism, this did not alter the anticoagulant effect in two studies.

Clinical evidence

(a) Dihydropyridine calcium-channel blockers

The manufacturers say that **amlodipine** did not significantly alter the effect of **warfarin** on prothrombin times in healthy subjects.[1,2]

In healthy subjects given **warfarin** until at steady state, **felodipine** 10 mg daily for 14 days did not alter the dose of warfarin required to maintain a stable INR, or the pharmacokinetics of *S*- or *R*-warfarin.[3] Because **felodipine** does not interact with **warfarin** it has been used as a control drug in retrospective cohort studies assessing **warfarin** drug interactions.[4,5]

(b) Diltiazem

In a study, 11 healthy men were given racemic **warfarin**, and 8 were given *R*-warfarin, both as a single 1.5-mg/kg intravenous dose. Another 10 subjects were given *S*-warfarin as a single 0.75-mg/kg intravenous dose. After taking diltiazem 120 mg three times a day (for 4 days before and 9 days after the dose of **warfarin**) the clearance of *R*-warfarin was decreased by about 20% but the more potent *S*-warfarin remained unaffected. The total anticoagulant response remained unchanged.[6] Similarly, in another study in 20 healthy subjects, diltiazem 30 mg three times daily for one week caused no clinically relevant changes in the anticoagulant effects of a single dose of **warfarin**. There was a small 13% decrease in **warfarin** clearance and an 8% increase in AUC when given with diltiazem, which were not statistically significant.[7]

Mechanism

Diltiazem is a known inhibitor of the cytochrome P450 isoenzyme CYP3A4. However, this isoenzyme has only a minor role in the 'metabolism of warfarin', (p.358), specifically in the metabolism of the less active *R*-isomer of warfarin. Consequently, only minor increases in the levels of warfarin have been seen in pharmacokinetic studies, which would generally not be expected to be clinically relevant. **Verapamil** is also an inhibitor of CYP3A4, but the dihydropyridine calcium-channel blockers are not.

Importance and management

No special precautions would seem to be necessary during the concurrent use of warfarin and dihydropyridine calcium-channel blockers. Although the minor pharmacokinetic interaction between diltiazem and warfarin would appear to be established, in the studies cited this did not change anticoagulant control, and is therefore unlikely to be of clinical importance. **Verapamil** would be expected to cause a similar pharmacokinetic interaction, although no data appear to be available on this.

The absence of adverse reports about these very widely used drugs suggests that concurrent use is normally uneventful.

1. Istin (Amlodipine besilate). Pfizer Ltd. UK Summary of product characteristics, July 2007.
2. Norvasc (Amlodipine besylate). Pfizer Labs. US Prescribing information, September 2005.
3. Grind M, Murphy M, Warrington S, Åberg J. Method for studying drug-warfarin interactions. *Clin Pharmacol Ther* (1993) 54, 381–7.
4. McCall KL, Anderson HG, Jones AD. Determination of the lack of a drug interaction between azithromycin and warfarin. *Pharmacotherapy* (2004) 24, 188–94.
5. McCall KL, Scott JC, Anderson HG. Retrospective evaluation of a possible interaction between warfarin and levofloxacin. *Pharmacotherapy* (2005) 25, 67–73.
6. Abernethy DR, Kaminsky LS, Dickinson TH. Selective inhibition of warfarin metabolism by diltiazem in humans. *J Pharmacol Exp Ther* (1991) 257, 411–15.
7. Stoysich AM, Lucas BD, Mohiuddin SM, Hilleman DE. Further elucidation of pharmacokinetic interaction between diltiazem and warfarin. *Int J Clin Pharmacol Ther* (1996) 34, 56–60.

Coumarins + Carbamazepine or Oxcarbazepine

The anticoagulant effects of warfarin can be markedly reduced by carbamazepine, and two case reports suggest phenprocoumon is similarly affected. Oxcarbazepine appears not to interact significantly with warfarin.

Clinical evidence

(a) Carbamazepine

1. Phenprocoumon. A man in his mid-twenties developed multiple thrombotic episodes due to hereditary resistance to activated protein C. Because of cerebral embolic strokes he developed epileptic seizures and was given carbamazepine 400 mg daily, followed 6 days later by phenprocoumon. It was found that relatively large doses of phenprocoumon (8 mg daily) had to be given without achieving adequate anticoagulation (Quick value 50 to 60%; target 10 to 20%) until the carbamazepine was withdrawn, whereupon the phenprocoumon dosage could be reduced to 1.5 mg daily with a Quick value of 30 to 40%.[1] Similarly, another patient stabilised on phenprocoumon was found to have a markedly reduced anticoagulant effect (a dramatic increase in his Quick value) 21 days after he started taking carbamazepine 400 mg daily. The values returned to normal when the carbamazepine was stopped.[2]

2. Warfarin. In one study, 2 patients taking warfarin with carbamazepine (200 mg daily for the first week, 400 mg daily for the second and 600 mg for the third) had a fall of about 50% in serum warfarin levels, and sharp rises in their prothrombin-proconvertin percentages.[3] The half-life of a single intravenous dose of warfarin in three other patients fell by about 11%, 53%, and 60%, respectively, when they were similarly treated.[3] In another analysis, warfarin dose requirements were 2.3-fold higher in 5 patients stabilised on warfarin and carbamazepine than in 54 patients not taking any interacting drugs (median 9 mg daily versus 3.86 mg daily). These 5 patients had higher clearances of both *R*- and *S*-warfarin, and had about 11-fold higher plasma levels of the 10-hydroxymetabolite of warfarin.[4] This interaction has been described in 5 case reports.[5-9] One of them describes a patient stabilised on warfarin and carbamazepine who developed widespread dermal ecchymoses and a prothrombin time of 70 seconds, one week after stopping the carbamazepine. She was restabilised on approximately half the dose of warfarin in the absence of the carbamazepine.[9]

(b) Oxcarbazepine

In a study in 7 healthy subjects given warfarin until steady-state, oxcarbazepine 450 mg twice daily for one week slightly increased the mean Quick values from 36.6% to only 38.1%, which was not statistically significant.[10]

Mechanism

Carbamazepine is a known enzyme inducer, and increases the metabolism of warfarin. Phenprocoumon would be similarly affected. Oxcarbazepine on the other hand has relatively little enzyme-inducing activity.

Importance and management

The interaction between warfarin and carbamazepine is moderately well documented, established and clinically important. The incidence is uncertain, but monitor the anticoagulant response if carbamazepine is added to established treatment with warfarin and anticipate the need to double the dosage. Oxcarbazepine appears to be a relatively non-interacting alternative.

Information about an interaction between phenprocoumon and carbamazepine seems to be limited to the two reports cited. Nevertheless it would be prudent to monitor concurrent use in any patient, being alert for the need to increase the phenprocoumon dosage. The same precautions would seem sensible with any other coumarin but information appears to be lacking.

1. Böttcher T, Buchmann J, Zettl U-K, Benecke R. Carbamazepine-phenprocoumon interaction. *Eur Neurol* (1997) 38, 132–3.
2. Schlienger R, Kurmann M, Drewe J, Müller-Spahn F, Seifritz E. Inhibition of phenprocoumon anticoagulation by carbamazepine. *Eur Neuropsychopharmacol* (2000) 10, 219–21.
3. Hansen JM, Siersbæk-Nielsen K, Skovsted L. Carbamazepine-induced acceleration of diphenylhydantoin and warfarin metabolism in man. *Clin Pharmacol Ther* (1971) 12, 539–43.
4. Herman D, Locatelli I, Grabnar I, Peternel P, Stegnar M, Lainščak M, Mrhar A, Breskvar K, Dolžan V. The influence of co-treatment with carbamazepine, amiodarone and statins on warfarin metabolism and maintenance dose. *Eur J Clin Pharmacol* (2006) 62, 291–6.
5. Ross JRY, Beeley L. Interaction between carbamazepine and warfarin. *BMJ* (1980) 1, 1415–16.
6. Kendall AG, Boivin M. Warfarin-carbamazepine interaction. *Ann Intern Med* (1981) 94, 280.
7. Massey EW. Effect of carbamazepine on Coumadin metabolism. *Ann Neurol* (1983) 13, 691–2.
8. Beeley L, Stewart P, Hickey FM. *Bulletin of the West Midlands Centre for Adverse Drug Reaction Reporting* (1988) 26, 18.
9. Denbow CE, Fraser HS. Clinically significant hemorrhage due to warfarin-carbamazepine interaction. *South Med J* (1990) 83, 981.
10. Krämer G, Tettenborn B, Klosterkov Jensen P, Menge GP, Stoll KD. Oxcarbazepine does not affect the anticoagulant activity of warfarin. *Epilepsia* (1992) 33, 1145–8.

Coumarins + Carbon tetrachloride

A single case report describes an increase in the anticoagulant effects of dicoumarol in a patient who accidentally drank some cleaning liquid containing carbon tetrachloride.

Clinical evidence, mechanism, importance and management

A patient, well stabilised on **dicoumarol**, accidentally drank a small amount of cleaning liquid later estimated to contain just 0.1 mL of carbon tetrachloride. The next day his prothrombin time had risen to 41 seconds. This value was about the same after another day even though the **dicoumarol** had been withdrawn, and marked hypoprothrombinaemia persisted for another 5 days.[1]

The probable reason for this reaction is that carbon tetrachloride is very toxic to the liver, the changed anticoagulant response being a manifestation of this. Carbon tetrachloride, once used as an anthelmintic in man, is no longer used in human medicine, but is still employed as an industrial solvent and degreasing agent. On theoretical grounds it would seem possible for anticoagulated patients exposed to substantial amounts of the vapour to experience this interaction, but this has not been reported.

1. Luton EF. Carbon tetrachloride exposure during anticoagulant therapy. Dangerous enhancement of hypoprothrombinemic effect. *JAMA* (1965) 194, 1386–7.

Coumarins + Chlorpromazine

Chlorpromazine does not interact significantly with acenocoumarol.

Clinical evidence, mechanism, importance and management

Although in one early report, chlorpromazine 40 to 100 mg daily was said to have "slightly sensitised" 2 out of 8 patients to the effects of **acenocoumarol**[1] and in another was reported to increase its anticoagulant effects in *animals*,[2] there appears to be nothing else published to suggest that an interaction occurs. *In vitro* study in human liver microsomes[3] found that chlorpromazine did not inhibit CYP2C9, the cytochrome P450 isoenzyme predominantly involved in the 'metabolism of **warfarin**', (p.358) and other coumarins. No coumarin dose adjustments would therefore be anticipated to be needed on concurrent use.

1. Johnson R, David A, Chartier Y. Clinical experience with G-23350 (Sintrom). *Can Med Assoc J* (1957) 77, 756–61.
2. Weiner M. Effect of centrally active drugs on the action of coumarin anticoagulants. *Nature* (1966) 212, 1599–1600.
3. Shin J-G, Soukhova N, Flockhart DA. Effect of antipsychotic drugs on human liver cytochrome P-450 (CYP) isoforms in vitro: preferential inhibition of CYP2D6. *Drug Metab Dispos* (1999) 27, 1078–84.

Coumarins + Cloral and derivatives

The anticoagulant effects of warfarin are increased in the first few days of cloral hydrate use, but this is normally of little or no clinical importance. Cloral betaine and triclofos may be expected to behave similarly.

Clinical evidence

In a retrospective study in patients just starting **warfarin**, the same loading doses of **warfarin** were given to 32 patients taking **cloral hydrate** daily and 67 patient who did not receive cloral hydrate. The **warfarin** requirements of the **cloral** group during the first 4 days fell by about one-third, but rose again to control requirements by the fifth day.[1]

In a study in 8 subjects, the concurrent use of **warfarin** (loading dose 25 mg then 5 mg daily for 5 days) and **cloral hydrate** 1 g each night resulted in potentiation of the effect of **warfarin**, when compared with placebo (increase in prothrombin time of about 3 to 4 seconds). However, in a longer term study, the addition of **cloral hydrate** 500 mg at night for 4 weeks to subjects stabilised on **warfarin** did not alter the average prothrombin time before, during, and after the **cloral** treatment (18.9, 19.3, and 19.2 seconds, respectively).[2,3]

Similar results have been described in other studies in patients taking **warfarin** and **cloral hydrate**[4-8] or **triclofos**.[9] **Cloral betaine** appears to behave similarly.[10] An isolated and by no means fully explained case of fatal hypoprothrombinaemia occurred in a patient taking **dicoumarol** who was given **cloral hydrate** for 10 days, later replaced by secobarbital.[11] Another patient taking **dicoumarol** had a reduction in prothrombin times when given **cloral hydrate**.[11]

Mechanism

Cloral hydrate is mainly metabolised to trichloroacetic acid, which then successfully competes with warfarin for its binding sites on plasma proteins.[6] As a result, free and active molecules of warfarin are displaced into the plasma water and the effects of the warfarin are increased. But this is only short-lived because the warfarin molecules become exposed to metabolism by the liver, so the warfarin level is reduced.

Importance and management

The interaction between warfarin and cloral hydrate is well documented and well understood, but normally of little or no clinical importance. There is very good evidence that concurrent use need not be avoided.[1-8] However, it may be prudent to keep an eye on the anticoagulant response during the first 4 to 5 days, just to make sure it does not become excessive. It is not certain whether other anticoagulants behave in the same way because the evidence is sparse, indirect and inconclusive,[11,12] but what is known suggests that the coumarins probably do. Triclofos and cloral betaine appear to behave like cloral hydrate. Dichloralphenazone on the other hand interacts quite differently (see 'Coumarins + Dichloralphenazone', p.399).

1. Boston Collaborative Drug Surveillance Program. Interaction between chloral hydrate and warfarin. *N Engl J Med* (1972) 286, 53–5.
2. Udall JA. Warfarin-chloral hydrate interaction. Pharmacological activity and significance. *Ann Intern Med* (1974) 81, 341–4.
3. Udall JA. Warfarin interactions with chloral hydrate and glutethimide. *Curr Ther Res* (1975) 17, 67–74.
4. Griner PF, Raisz LG, Rickles FR, Wiesner PJ, Odoroff CL. Chloral hydrate and warfarin interaction: clinical significance? *Ann Intern Med* (1971) 74, 540–3.
5. Udall JA. Clinical implications of warfarin interactions with five sedatives. *Am J Cardiol* (1975) 35, 67–71.
6. Sellers EM, Koch-Weser J. Kinetics and clinical importance of displacement of warfarin from albumin by acidic drugs. *Ann N Y Acad Sci* (1971) 179, 213–25.
7. Breckenridge A, Orme ML'E, Thorgeirsson S, Davies DS, Brooks RV. Drug interactions with warfarin: studies with dichloralphenazone, chloral hydrate and phenazone (antipyrine). *Clin Sci* (1971) 40, 351–64.
8. Breckenridge A, Orme M. Clinical implications of enzyme induction. *Ann N Y Acad Sci* (1971) 179, 421–31.
9. Sellers EM, Lang M, Koch-Weser J, Colman RW. Enhancement of warfarin-induced hypoprothrombinemia by triclofos. *Clin Pharmacol Ther* (1972) 13, 911–15.
10. MacDonald MG, Robinson DS, Sylwester D, Jaffe JJ. The effects of phenobarbital, chloral betaine, and glutethimide administration on warfarin plasma levels and hypoprothrombinemic responses in man. *Clin Pharmacol Ther* (1969) 10, 80–4.
11. Cucinell SA, Odessky L, Weiss M, Dayton PG. The effect of chloral hydrate on bishydroxycoumarin metabolism. A fatal outcome. *JAMA* (1966) 197, 144–6.
12. van Dam FE, Gribnau-Overkamp MJH. The effect of some sedatives (phenobarbital, glutethimide, chlordiazepoxide, chloral hydrate) on the rate of disappearance of ethyl biscoumacetate from the plasma. *Folia Med Neerl* (1967) 10, 141–5.

Coumarins and related drugs + Colchicine

One report describes five cases of a possible marked increase in the effect of fluindione when colchicine was given for acute gout.

Clinical evidence, mechanism, importance and management

The national pharmacovigilance system in France have reported 5 cases where colchicine appeared to increase the anticoagulant effect of **fluindione**. All 5 patients were stabilised on **fluindione** and were given short-term colchicine 1 to 6 mg daily for an acute attack of gout. All 5 patients had markedly raised INRs (6.5 to in excess of 18), but only one had clinical bleeding (haemorrhoidal bleeding).[1] The authors consider that colchicine may have been a factor in a case of raised INR with **warfarin**, which was attributed to the 'SSRI', (p.448), fluvoxamine.

The mechanism of this interaction is unknown, although the authors rule out protein binding or P-glycoprotein alterations. They suggest that it may occur because colchicine decreases expression of various cytochrome P450 isoenzymes, so decreasing the metabolism of **fluindione**.[1]

This appears to be the only report of an interaction of anticoagulants with colchicine. Bear it in mind in the event of an unexpected response to treatment. Further study is needed.

1. Gras-Champel V, Ohlmann P, Polard E, Wiesel M-L, Imbs J-L, Andréjak M. Can colchicine potentiate the anticoagulant effect of fluindione? *Eur J Clin Pharmacol* (2005) 61, 555–6.

Coumarins + COMT inhibitors

Entacapone caused a slight increase in INR in subjects given warfarin, and slightly increased *R*-warfarin levels. These effects are unlikely to be generally clinically relevant, but some caution may be prudent. Tolcapone is not expected to interact with *S*-warfarin.

Clinical evidence

In a double-blind, crossover study in 12 healthy subjects given individualised **warfarin** doses to achieve an INR of between 1.4 and 1.8, **entacapone** 200 mg four times daily slightly increased the INR by 13%. The AUC of *R*-warfarin was increased by 18%, with no change in the AUC of *S*-warfarin.[1]

Mechanism

Not known. Based on *in vitro* data, both entacapone and **tolcapone** were thought to potentially interfere with the metabolism of drugs by the cytochrome P450 isoenzyme CYP2C9, such as *S*-warfarin.[2-4] However, the above study shows that entacapone does not alter *S*-warfarin pharmacokinetics, and tolcapone is also thought not expected to interact by this mechanism because it does not interact with 'tolbutamide', (p.516), another CYP2C9 substrate.

Importance and management

The minor pharmacokinetic interaction between entacapone and warfarin would appear to be established, but its clinical relevance is uncertain. Changes of this magnitude would not generally be expected to be clinically relevant, and there do not appear to be any published case reports of problems. Nevertheless, it is possible that some patients might show a greater effect, and the manufacturer in the UK recommends that the INR be monitored when entacapone is started in patients taking warfarin.[2]

Similarly, although the manufacturers do not predict a pharmacokinetic interaction between **tolcapone** and warfarin, they still recommend monitoring because of the limited clinical information on the combination.[3,4]

1. Dingemanse J, Meyerhoff C, Schadrack J. Effect of the catechol-*O*-methyltransferase inhibitor entacapone on the steady-state pharmacokinetics and pharmacodynamics of warfarin. *Br J Clin Pharmacol* (2002) 53, 485–91.
2. Comtess (Entacapone). Orion Pharma (UK) Ltd. UK Summary of product characteristics, February 2007.
3. Tasmar (Tolcapone). Valeant Pharmaceuticals Ltd. UK Summary of product characteristics, August 2006.
4. Tasmar (Tolcapone). Valeant Pharmaceuticals International. US Prescribing information, December 2006.

Coumarins and related drugs + Corticosteroids or Corticotropin

In two early studies, small increases or decreases in anticoagulation were reported when dicoumarol or phenindione were used with low-to-moderate doses of corticotropin or prednisone. In the most recent analysis, use of unspecified corticosteroids appeared to be associated with a slightly higher incidence of INRs over the target range in children taking warfarin. In one study, very marked prothrombin time increases were seen in patients taking fluindione or acenocoumarol when given high-dose intravenous methylprednisolone, and two cases of this interaction have been reported with warfarin.

Clinical evidence

(a) Corticotropin

Ten out of 14 patients receiving long-term treatment with either **dicoumarol** or **phenindione** had a small but definite increase in their anticoagulant responses when they were given intramuscular or intravenous corticotropin for 4 to 9 days.[1] A patient stable on **ethyl biscoumacetate** developed frank melaena and microscopic haematuria within 3 days of starting treatment with intravenous corticotropin 10 mg twice daily.[2]

In contrast, a decrease in the anticoagulant effects of **ethyl biscoumacetate** was described in one patient given corticotropin and one patient given **cortisone**.[3]

(b) Methylprednisolone

A sharp increase in the INR of a patient with APS (antiphospholipid syndrome) occurred after **methylprednisolone** was added to treatment with an unnamed oral anticoagulant.[4,5] This prompted a controlled study in 10 patients stabilised on anticoagulants (8 taking **fluindione** and 2 taking **acenocoumarol**) and 5 patients not taking an anticoagulant. It was found that pulse high-dose intravenous **methylprednisolone** (500 mg or 1 g) increased the mean INR of those taking an anticoagulant from a baseline of 2.75 to 8.04, but had no effect on the prothrombin time in those taking **methylprednisolone** alone.[4,5] Two patients stabilised on **warfarin** are also reported to have shown significant prolongations in their prothrombin times when given high-dose **methylprednisolone** (960 mg or 1 g, followed by **dexamethasone** 60 mg three times daily for 3 days in one case) for the treatment of multiple sclerosis.[6]

(c) Prednisone

A study in 24 patients anticoagulated for several days with **dicoumarol** found that 2 hours after receiving prednisone 10 mg their silicone coagulation time had decreased from 28 to 24 minutes, and 2 hours later was down to 22 minutes.[7]

(d) Unspecified corticosteroids

In an analysis of a cohort of children receiving **warfarin**, there was no difference in dose of **warfarin** required to achieve and maintain the target INR between **warfarin** courses if corticosteroids were given (38 courses) and courses where corticosteroids were not given (314). However, courses with corticosteroids were associated with a higher percentage of INR measurements greater than the target (21% versus 14%).[8]

Mechanism

Not understood. Corticotropin, cortisone and prednisone can increase the coagulability of the blood in the absence of anticoagulants.[9,10] It has been suggested that methylprednisolone may inhibit the metabolism of anticoagulants.[5]

Importance and management

The interaction of low to moderate doses of corticosteroids with coumarins is by no means established, and is very poorly documented. Most of the few reports are from the 1950s and 60s, with very little appearing to have been published since then, suggesting that any effects are generally not clinically relevant. In an analysis from the 1990s, the use of corticosteroids appeared to be associated with a slightly higher incidence of INRs over the target range in children. The most constructive thing that can be said is that if either corticotropin (corticotrophin, ACTH) or any corticosteroid is given to patients taking anticoagulants, be aware that an interaction might very rarely occur. Also note that corticosteroids are associated with a weak increase in peptic ulceration and gastrointestinal bleeding, and the risk of this could theoretically be increased if over-anticoagulation occurs.

The situation with high dose methylprednisolone is clearly different. Although the evidence is limited, marked INR increases have been reported and INRs should be closely monitored (daily has been recommended[5]) if this or other high-dose corticosteroids are added to established treatment with any coumarin or indanedione oral anticoagulant. More study is needed.

1. Hellem AJ, Solem JH. The influence of ACTH on prothrombin-proconvertin values in blood during treatment with dicumarol and phenylindanedione. *Acta Med Scand* (1954) 150, 389–93.
2. van Cauwenberge H, Jacques LB. Haemorrhagic effect of ACTH with anticoagulants. *Can Med Assoc J* (1958) 79, 536–40.
3. Chatterjea JB, Salomon L. Antagonistic effects of A.C.T.H. and cortisone on the anticoagulant activity of ethyl biscoumacetate. *BMJ* (1954) 2, 790–2.
4. Costedoat-Chalumeau N, Amoura Z, Wechsler B, Ankri A, Piette J-C. Implications of interaction between vitamin K antagonists and high-dose intravenous methylprednisolone in the APS. *J Autoimmun* (2000) 15, A22.
5. Costedoat-Chalumeau N, Amoura Z, Aymard G, Sevin O, Wechsler B, Cacoub P, Huong Du, Le Th, Diquet B, Ankri A, Piette J-C. Potentiation of vitamin K antagonists by high-dose intravenous methylprednisolone. *Ann Intern Med* (2000) 132, 631–5.
6. Kaufman M. Treatment of multiple sclerosis with high-dose corticosteroids may prolong the prothrombin time to dangerous levels in patients taking warfarin. *Multiple Sclerosis* (1997) 3, 248–9.
7. Menczel J, Dreyfuss F. Effect of prednisone on blood coagulation time in patients on dicumarol therapy. *J Lab Clin Med* (1960) 56, 14–20.
8. Streif W, Marzinotto AV, Massicotte P, Chan AKC, Julian JA, Mitchell L. Analysis of warfarin therapy in pediatric patients: a prospective cohort study of 319 patients. *Blood* (1999) 94, 3007–14.
9. Cosgriff SW, Diefenbach AF, Vogt W. Hypercoagulability of the blood associated with ACTH and cortisone therapy. *Am J Med* (1950) 9, 752–6.
10. Ozsoylu S, Strauss HS, Diamond LK. Effects of corticosteroids on coagulation of the blood. *Nature* (1962) 195, 1214–15.

Coumarins + Cranberry juice

A number of case reports suggest that cranberry juice can increase the INR of patients taking warfarin, and one patient has died as a result of this interaction. Limited evidence suggests that the use of cranberry juice in patients taking warfarin can result in unstable INRs, or, in one isolated case, a *reduced* INR.

Clinical evidence

In September 2003, the CSM in the UK noted that they had received 5 reports suggesting an interaction between **warfarin** and cranberry juice (*Vaccinium macrocarpon*) since 1999.[1] The most serious case involved a man taking **warfarin** whose INR markedly increased (INR greater than 50) 6 weeks after starting to drink cranberry juice. He died from gastrointestinal and pericardial haemorrhages.[1] Further details of this case included that he had recently been treated with cefalexin (not known to interact, although consider 'antibacterials', (p.365)) for a chest infection, and had been eating virtually nothing,[2] a fact that would have contributed to increased anticoagulation. Less marked INR increases (not specified) were seen in two other patients, one of whom was restabilised on a lower **warfarin** dosage, while the other regained normal INR values after cranberry juice was stopped.[1] A further patient had unstable INRs, while the final patient had a decrease in INR.[1]

In a further case,[3] a patient stabilised on **warfarin** was found to have INRs of 10 to 12 in the days prior to a surgical procedure, although he had no previous record of an INR greater than 4. Vitamin K was given, and heparin was substituted for warfarin. When **warfarin** was restarted postoperatively, the INR quickly rose to 8 and then to 11 with haematuria, and postoperative bleeding. The patient was drinking almost 2 litres of cranberry juice daily, because of recurrent urinary tract infections, and was advised to stop drinking this. After three days the INR had stabilised at 3.

In October 2004, the MHRA/CSM in the UK noted that they had now received 12 reports of a suspected interaction.[4] These included 5 additional cases of bleeding episodes and two additional cases of unstable INRs in patients drinking cranberry juice while taking warfarin.

In the US major bleeding and a high INR have been reported, which occurred shortly after cranberry juice was started.[5]

Mechanism

Not known. It was suggested that one or more of the constituents of cranberry juice might have inhibited the metabolism of warfarin by the cytochrome isoenzyme CYP2C9, thereby reducing its clearance from the body and increasing its effects.[1] However, doubt has been cast on this mechanism, since cranberry juice had no effect on flurbiprofen pharmacokinetics, a drug used as a surrogate index of CYP2C9 activity, and had only weak CYP2C9-inhibitory activity *in vitro*.[6] Alternatively, the salicylate constituent of cranberry juice might cause hypoprothrombinaemia,[7] similarly to high-dose 'aspirin', (p.385).

Importance and management

The incidence and general clinical importance of this interaction is unknown, but the current recommendation of the CSM/MHRA in the UK is that patients taking warfarin should avoid drinking cranberry juice unless the health benefits are considered to outweigh any risks. They recommend increased INR monitoring for any patient taking warfarin and a regular intake of cranberry juice.[4] They also advise similar precautions with other cranberry products (such as capsules or concentrates).[4] Further study is needed.

1. Committee on Safety of Medicines/Medicines and Healthcare products Regulatory Agency. Possible interaction between warfarin and cranberry juice. *Current Problems* (2003) 29, 8.
2. Suvarna R, Pirmohamed M, Henderson L. Possible interaction between warfarin and cranberry juice. *BMJ* (2003) 327, 1454.
3. Grant P. Warfarin and cranberry juice: an interaction? *J Heart Valve Dis* (2004) 13, 25–6.
4. Committee on Safety of Medicines/Medicines and Healthcare products Regulatory Agency. Interaction between warfarin and cranberry juice: new advice. *Current Problems* (2004) 30, 10.
5. Rindone JP, Murphy TW. Warfarin-cranberry juice interaction resulting in profound hypoprothrombinemia and bleeding. *Am J Ther* (2006) 13, 283–4.
6. Greenblatt DJ, von Moltke LL, Perloff ES, Luo Y, Harmatz JS, Zinny MA. Interaction of flurbiprofen with cranberry juice, grape juice, tea, and fluconazole: in vitro and clinical studies. *Clin Pharmacol Ther* (2006) 79, 125–33.
7. Isele H. Tödliche Blutung unter Warfarin plus Preiselbeersaft. Liegt's an der Salizylsäure? *MMW Fortschr Med* (2004) 146, 13.

Coumarins + Danazol or Gestrinone

Increased anticoagulant effects and bleeding have been seen in a few patients taking warfarin with danazol. A case describes similar effects in a patient taking warfarin and gestrinone.

Clinical evidence

(a) Danazol

A 40-year-old woman stabilised on **warfarin** 6 mg daily with a prothrombin ratio of 2.3 presented after vomiting blood. She was found to have a prothrombin ratio of 14, and required fresh frozen plasma and 2 litres of blood. Three weeks previously she had been prescribed danazol 200 mg twice daily.[1] Four other similar cases of this interaction with danazol have been reported.[2-4] In two of the cases the patients were subsequently stabilised on **warfarin** and danazol, but with 50 to 70% lower **warfarin** doses.[3,4]

(b) Gestrinone

A bulletin includes a brief mention of an increased INR with vaginal bleeding and multiple bruising in a woman taking **warfarin** and gestrinone.[5]

Mechanism

The reason for this interaction is unknown, but both danazol and gestrinone have androgenic properties, and 'anabolic steroids,' (p.364), are known to increase the effects of warfarin.

Importance and management

Although data are limited, the interaction with danazol would appear to be established, and close monitoring of the INR is advisable if danazol is added to established coumarin anticoagulant therapy. Some suggest that the initial dosage of anticoagulant should be halved when danazol is started.[2] However, others note that this may not be appropriate in patients at high thrombogenic risk, such as those with mechanical valves. In these patients, they recommend a cautious reduction in dose with weekly monitoring of the INR until it becomes stable (several weeks).[4] Gestrinone might be expected to interact similarly, and some caution is therefore appropriate.

1. Goulbourne IA, Macleod DAD. An interaction between danazol and warfarin. Case report. *Br J Obstet Gynaecol* (1981) 88, 950–1.
2. Small M, Peterkin M, Lowe GDO, McCune G, Thomson JA. Danazol and oral anticoagulants. *Scott Med J* (1982) 27, 331–2.
3. Meeks ML, Mahaffey KW, Katz MD. Danazol increases the anticoagulant effect of warfarin. *Ann Pharmacother* (1992) 26, 641–2.
4. Booth CD. A drug interaction between danazol and warfarin. *Pharm J* (1993) 250, 439.
5. Beeley L, Cunningham H, Carmichael A, Brennan A. *Bulletin of the West Midlands Centre for Adverse Drug Reaction Reporting* (1992) 35, 18.

Coumarins + Darifenacin or Solifenacin

Solifenacin did not alter the pharmacokinetics or effect of warfarin. Similarly, darifenacin did not alter the prothrombin time in response to warfarin.

Clinical evidence, mechanism, importance and management

(a) Darifenacin

The manufacturer notes that steady state darifenacin 30 mg daily did not alter the prothrombin time after a single 30-mg dose of **warfarin**.[1] No **warfarin** dose adjustment would be expected to be needed on concurrent use.

(b) Solifenacin

In a placebo-controlled, crossover study in healthy subjects, solifenacin 10 mg daily for 10 days had no effect on the pharmacokinetics of *S*- or *R*-warfarin after a single 25-mg dose of **warfarin** was given on day 10. In addition, solifenacin did not alter the prothrombin time.[2]

This study suggests that no pharmacokinetic or pharmacodynamic interaction occurs, and that no **warfarin** dose adjustment would be expected to be needed on concurrent use.

1. Enablex (Darifenacin hydrobromide). Novartis. US Prescribing information, February 2007.
2. Smulders RA, Kuipers ME, Krauwinkel WJJ. Multiple doses of the antimuscarinic agent solifenacin do not affect the pharmacodynamics or pharmacokinetics of warfarin or the steady-state pharmacokinetics of digoxin in healthy subjects. *Br J Clin Pharmacol* (2006) 62, 210–17.

Coumarins + Dichloralphenazone

The anticoagulant effects of warfarin are reduced by dichloralphenazone.

Clinical evidence

Five patients stabilised taking **warfarin** long-term and given dichloralphenazone 1.3 g each night for 30 days had a reduction of about 50% (range 20.2 to 68.5%) in plasma **warfarin** levels and a fall in the anticoagulant response during the last 14 days of concurrent use. Another patient given dichloralphenazone 1.3 g nightly for one month had a 70% fall in plasma **warfarin** levels and a thrombotest percentage rise from 9 to 55% (indicating a reduced anticoagulant effect). These values returned to normal when the hypnotic was withdrawn.[1,2]

Mechanism

The 'phenazone', (p.434) component of dichloralphenazone is a potent liver enzyme inducer, which increases the metabolism and clearance of the warfarin, thereby reducing its effects.[1,2] The effects of the 'cloral hydrate', (p.396) component appear to be minimal.

Importance and management

Information is limited, but the interaction between warfarin and dichloralphenazone appears to be an established and clinically important interaction, probably affecting most patients. The dosage of warfarin will need to be increased to accommodate this interaction. If the effect of warfarin has been reduced by using dichloralphenazone, it may take up to a month for it to restabilise. There does not appear to be any information about other anticoagulants, but other coumarins would be expected to be similarly affected. The 'benzodiazepines', (p.391) would now be preferred hypnotics, and do not interact.

1. Breckenridge A, Orme ML'E, Thorgeirsson S, Davies DS, Brooks RV. Drug interaction with warfarin: studies with dichloralphenazone, chloral hydrate and phenazone (antipyrine). *Clin Sci* (1971) 40, 351–64.
2. Breckenridge A, Orme M. Clinical implications of enzyme induction. *Ann N Y Acad Sci* (1971) 179, 421–31.

Anticoagulants + Dietary supplements; Ascorbic acid (Vitamin C)

Although two isolated cases have been reported in which the effects of warfarin were reduced by ascorbic acid, four subsequent prospective studies have not found any interaction.

Clinical evidence

In a woman recently stabilised on **warfarin** 7.5 mg daily, who began to simultaneously take ascorbic acid (dose not stated) with her warfarin, the prothrombin time fell steadily from 23 seconds, to 19, 17, and then 14 seconds, with no response to an increase in the dosage of **warfarin** to 10, 15, and finally 20 mg daily. The prothrombin time returned to 28 seconds within 2 days of stopping the ascorbic acid.[1] Another woman recently stabilised on warfarin 5 mg daily had a recurrence of acute thrombophlebitis with a prothrombin time of 12 seconds. She was unusually resistant to the actions of **warfarin** and required 25 mg daily before a significant increase in prothrombin times was achieved. On questioning, she had been taking massive amounts of ascorbic acid (about 16 g daily) for several weeks. She was eventually stabilised on warfarin 10 mg daily.[2]

In contrast, in prospective studies no changes in the effects of **warfarin** were seen:

- in 5 patients given ascorbic acid 1 g daily for a fortnight,[3]
- in 11 patients (some taking **dicoumarol**) given ascorbic acid 4 g daily for 2 weeks,[4]
- in 14 patients given ascorbic acid 3 g then 5 g daily for one week or 5 patients given 10 g daily for one week:[5] a mean fall of 17.5% in total plasma **warfarin** concentrations was seen at all doses.
- in a 10-week study, where the proportion of patients requiring a change in **warfarin** dose did not differ between 84 patients given ascorbic acid (dose unstated) and 96 control patients (31 versus 18 patients required a dose reduction, and 7 versus 13 required a dose increase, respectively).[6]

Mechanism

Not understood. One *animal* study has demonstrated this interaction[7] and others have not,[8,9] but none of them has provided any definite clues about why it ever occurs. One suggestion is that high doses of ascorbic acid can cause diarrhoea, which might prevent adequate absorption of the anticoagulant.

Importance and management

Four clinical studies in patients stabilised on warfarin have failed to confirm that ascorbic acid alters the anticoagulant effect of warfarin, even using very large doses of ascorbic acid (up to 10 g daily), even though there are two isolated reports of reduced warfarin efficacy. All these data are from the 1970s, and nothing further seems to have been published. Coumarin dose adjustments are therefore unlikely to be needed when ascorbic acid is also used.

1. Rosenthal G. Interaction of ascorbic acid and warfarin. *JAMA* (1971) 215, 1671.
2. Smith EC, Skalski RJ, Johnson GC, Rossi GV. Interaction of ascorbic acid and warfarin. *JAMA* (1972) 221, 1166.
3. Hume R, Johnstone JMS, Weyers E. Interaction of ascorbic acid and warfarin. *JAMA* (1972) 219, 1479.
4. Blakely JA. Interaction of warfarin and ascorbic acid. 1st Florence Conference on Haemostasis and Thrombosis, May 1977. Abstracts p 99.
5. Feetam CL, Leach RH, Meynell MJ. Lack of a clinically important interaction between warfarin and ascorbic acid. *Toxicol Appl Pharmacol* (1975) 31, 544–7.
6. Dedichen J. The effect of ascorbic acid given to patients on chronic anticoagulant therapy. *Boll Soc Ital Cardiol* (1973) 18, 690–2.
7. Sigell LT, Flessa HC. Drug interactions with anticoagulants. *JAMA* (1970) 214, 2035–8.
8. Weintraub M, Griner PF. Warfarin and ascorbic acid: lack of evidence for a drug interaction. *Toxicol Appl Pharmacol* (1974) 28, 53–6.
9. Deckert FW. Ascorbic acid and warfarin. *JAMA* (1973) 223, 440.

Coumarins + Dietary supplements; Fish oils

The use of warfarin with fish oils did not alter the INR in two studies, nor the incidence of bleeding episodes in another. However, in one study, fish oil significantly prolonged bleeding time, and there is one report of an increased in INR in a patient taking warfarin who doubled her fish oil dose.

Clinical evidence

In one early study, 40 patients took 4 g of a fish oil preparation daily for 4 weeks: 18 of these patients were taking **warfarin**. In the group as a whole (40 patients), the bleeding time was significantly prolonged from 240 to 270 seconds. In the subset of patients taking **warfarin** who had stable anticoagulant control in the preceding 3 months (15 patients), the thrombotest was shortened from 114 to 90 seconds, although no changes in warfarin dosage were made. One patient taking warfarin had a minor nosebleed.[1] In a large randomised study of the effect of fish oils or placebo, taken with either aspirin or **warfarin** over 9 months, there was no difference in the frequency of bleeding episodes between 132 patients taking **warfarin** and fish oil and 154 taking **warfarin** alone (17 versus 14, respectively).[2]

One case of a possible interaction with a rise in INR has been reported. A woman had INRs in the range of 2 to 3 for five months while taking **warfarin** 1.5 mg and 1 mg on alternate days. During this time, she starting taking 1 g of a fish oil preparation daily with no change in her INR. Her **warfarin** was then increased to 1.5 mg daily, with stable INRs for about 5 months. A routine INR was then found to be 4.3 (raised from 2.8 one month earlier). One week previously, she had started to take double the dose of fish oil (to 2 g daily). The dose of **warfarin** was reduced to 1.5 mg and 1 mg on alternate days, and she was asked to reduce the fish oil back to 1 g daily. Eight days later her INR was 1.6, and the **warfarin** was increased back to 1.5 mg daily.[3]

Mechanism

Fish oils contain omega-3 fatty acids particularly **eicosapentaenoic acid** and **docosahexaenoic acid**. These are considered to have some antithrombotic activity, and may prolong the bleeding time.

Importance and management

This interaction is not established. One large study found no increase in bleeding episodes in over 150 patients taking warfarin and fish oils, suggesting that most patients do not show any interaction. However, based on the possible moderate increase in bleeding times with high-dose fish oils, the manufacturers of one product, *Omacor* (omega-3-acid ethyl esters), say that patients receiving anticoagulants should be monitored, and the dose of anticoagulant adjusted as necessary.[4]

1. Smith P, Arnesen H, Opstad T, Dahl KH, Eritsland J. Influence of highly concentrated N-3 fatty acids on serum lipids and hemostatic variables in survivors of myocardial infarction receiving either oral anticoagulants or matching placebo. *Thromb Res* (1989) 53, 467–74.
2. Eritsland J, Arnesen H, Seljeflot I, Kierulf P. Long-term effects of *n*-3 polyunsaturated fatty acids on haemostatic variables and bleeding episodes in patients with coronary artery disease. *Blood Coagul Fibrinolysis* (1995) 6, 17–22.
3. Buckley MS, Goff AD, Knapp WE. Fish oil interaction with warfarin. *Ann Pharmacother* (2004) 38, 50–3.
4. Omacor (Omega-3-acid ethyl esters). Solvay Healthcare Ltd. UK Summary of product characteristics, January 2006.

Coumarins + Dietary supplements; Glucosamine ± Chondroitin

A few reports suggest that glucosamine with or without chondroitin may increase the INR in patients taking warfarin. In contrast, one case of a decreased INR has been reported when glucosamine was given with acenocoumarol.

Clinical evidence, mechanism, importance and management

A 69-year-old man stabilised on **warfarin** 47.5 mg weekly had an increase in his INR from 2.58 to 4.52 four weeks after starting to take 6 capsules of *Cosamin DS* (glucosamine hydrochloride 500 mg, sodium chondroitin sulfate 400 mg, manganese ascorbate per capsule) daily. His **warfarin** dose was reduced to 40 mg weekly, and his INR returned to the target range of 2 to 3 (INR 2.15) with continued *Cosamin DS* therapy.[1] A comment on this report noted that this is twice the usual dose of glucosamine.[2] The Canadian Adverse Drug Reaction Monitoring Program briefly reported that an increase in INR had been noted when glucosamine was given to patients on **warfarin**, and that INR values decreased when glucosamine was stopped.[3] Moreover, in 2006 the CHM in the UK reported that they had received 7 reports of an increase in INR in patients taking **warfarin** after they started taking glucosamine supplements.[4]

In contrast, a 71-year-old man stabilised on **acenocoumarol** 15 mg weekly had a *decrease* in his INR to 1.6 after taking glucosamine sulfate (*Xicil*) 1.5 g daily for 10 days. The glucosamine was stopped and the INR reached 2.1. When the glucosamine was restarted, with an increase in **acenocoumarol** dose to 17 mg weekly, the INR only reached 1.9. The glucosamine was eventually stopped.[5]

There do not appear to have been any controlled studies of the effects of glucosamine supplements on the pharmacodynamics or pharmacokinetics of oral anticoagulants. The cases described suggest it would be prudent to monitor the INR more closely if glucosamine is started. If a patient shows an unexpected change in INR, bear in mind the possibility of self-medication with supplements such as glucosamine. Note that the CHM in the UK recommend that patients taking **warfarin** do not take glucosamine.[4]

1. Rozenfeld V, Crain JL, Callahan AK. Possible augmentation of warfarin effect by glucosamine–chondroitin. *Am J Health-Syst Pharm* (2004) 61, 306–7.
2. Scott GN. Interaction of warfarin with glucosamine—chondroitin. *Am J Health-Syst Pharm* (2004) 61, 1186.
3. Canadian Adverse Drug Reaction Monitoring Program. Communiqué. Warfarin and glucosamine: interaction. *Can Adverse Drug React News* (2001) 11 (Apr), 8.
4. Commission on Human Medicines/Medicines and Healthcare Products Regulatory Agency. Glucosamine adverse reactions and interactions. *Current Problems* (2006) 31, 8.
5. Garrote García M, Iglesias Piñeiro MJ, Martín Álvarez R, Pérez González J. Interacción farmacológica del sulfato de glucosamina con acenocumarol. *Aten Primaria* (2004) 33, 162–4.

Coumarins + Dietary supplements; Levocarnitine

Two isolated reports describe a marked increase in the anticoagulant effects of acenocoumarol in patients taking levocarnitine (L-carnitine), one of which was associated with melaena.

Clinical evidence, mechanism, importance and management

A woman who had taken **acenocoumarol** for 17 years because of aortic and mitral prosthetic valves, was admitted to hospital with melaena within 5 days of starting to take levocarnitine (L-carnitine) 1 g daily, which she was prescribed for congestive heart failure. Her INR had risen from 2.1 to 7.

Endoscopy and colonoscopy revealed diffuse bleeding from superficial erosions in the gut. She was discharged 10 days later with the same dose of **acenocoumarol** and an INR of 2.1 without the carnitine.[1] A similar case has been described in a man stabilised on **acenocoumarol** (INR 1.99 to 2.94) who had a rise in INR to 4.65 despite a dose correction. The increases in INR occurred when he was using levocarnitine 1 g daily for 10 weeks in the form of a drink (*Maximize*) promoted for bodybuilding and fitness training. When this product was discontinued, the INR returned to the therapeutic range.[2]

The reason for this apparent interaction is not known. These seem to the only recorded cases of an interaction between an oral anticoagulant and levocarnitine, but it may be prudent to bear this interaction in mind if levocarnitine is taken with acenocoumarol, or possibly any coumarin, being alert for an increased response.

1. Martinez E, Domingo P, Roca-Cusachs A. Potentiation of acenocoumarol action by L-carnitine. *J Intern Med* (1993) 233, 94.
2. Bachmann HU, Hoffmann A. Interaction of food supplement L-carnitine with oral anticoagulant acenocoumarol. *Swiss Med Wkly* (2004) 134: 385.

Coumarins + Dietary supplements; Ubidecarenone (Coenzyme Q10)

Ubidecarenone did not alter the INR or required warfarin dose in a controlled study in patients stabilised on warfarin. However, two reports describe reduced anticoagulant effects of warfarin in four patients taking ubidecarenone. A transient increase in INR has been reported in one patient taking ubidecarenone and warfarin.

Clinical evidence

In a randomised, double-blind, crossover study in 21 patients stabilised on **warfarin**, ubidecarenone 100 mg daily (*Bio-Quinone*) for 4 weeks did not alter the INR or the required dose of **warfarin**, when compared with placebo.[1] Similarly, 2 patients taking ubidecarenone to treat alopecia caused by **warfarin** treatment did not have any notable changes in INR, except that one had a transient INR *increase* when ubidecarenone was started.[2]

In contrast, another report describes 3 patients taking **warfarin** who had a drop in INR while taking ubidecarenone. In two of these INR reductions from about 2.5 to 1.4 occurred when they took ubidecarenone 30 mg daily for 2 weeks. The INRs rapidly returned to normal when the ubidecarenone was stopped.[3] In another case, a patient appeared to have a reduced response to **warfarin** while taking ubidecarenone, and responded normally when it was stopped.[4]

Mechanism

The reasons for these INR changes are not known but it may be that ubidecarenone has some vitamin K-like activity. In a study in *rats,* ubidecarenone reduced the anticoagulant effect of warfarin and increased the clearance of both enantiomers of warfarin.[5]

Importance and management

The well-controlled study suggests that ubidecarenone does not interact with warfarin, and that no warfarin dose adjustment would be expected to be necessary in patients who take this substance. However, the finding in 2 reports of a decrease in warfarin effect introduces a note of caution. The authors of the controlled study do recommend close monitoring of the INR if a patient decides to use ubidecarenone, because the underlying health problem resulting in them choosing to take this substance may alter their response to warfarin.[1]

1. Engelsen J, Nielsen JD, Winther K. Effect of coenzyme Q_{10} and ginkgo biloba on warfarin dosage in stable, long-term warfarin treated outpatients. A randomised, double blind, placebo-crossover trial. *Thromb Haemost* (2002) 87, 1075–6.
2. Nagao T, Ibayashi S, Fujii K, Sugimori H, Sadoshima S, Fujishima M. Treatment of warfarin-induced hair loss with ubidecarenone. *Lancet* (1995) 346, 1104–5.
3. Spigset O. Reduced effect of warfarin caused by ubidecarenone. *Lancet* (1994) 344, 1372–3.
4. Landbo C, Almdal TP. Interaction mellem warfarin og coenzym Q10. *Ugeskr Laeger* (1998) 160, 3226–7.
5. Zhou S, Chan E. Effect of ubidecarenone on warfarin anticoagulation and pharmacokinetics of warfarin enantiomers in rats. *Drug Metabol Drug Interact* (2001) 18, 99–122.

Coumarins + Dietary supplements; Vitamin E substances

In two studies in patients the anticoagulant effects of warfarin were unchanged by small to large doses of vitamin E, although there is an isolated case of bleeding attributed to concurrent use. In three healthy subjects, the effects of dicoumarol were slightly increased by vitamin E.

Clinical evidence

(a) Dicoumarol

A study in 3 healthy subjects found that 42 units of vitamin E daily for a month increased the response to a single dose of dicoumarol after 36 hours (decrease in prothrombin activity from 52 to 33%).[1]

(b) Warfarin

In a double-blind, placebo-controlled study in 25 patients stabilised on warfarin, moderate to large daily doses of vitamin E (800 or 1200 units) for a month caused no clinically relevant changes in prothrombin times and INRs.[2] Similarly, in another study in 12 patients taking warfarin, the anticoagulant effects of warfarin were unchanged by smaller daily doses of 100 or 400 units of vitamin E given for 4 weeks.[3]

However, in one case, a patient taking warfarin (and multiple other drugs) developed ecchymoses and haematuria, which was attributed to him taking 1200 units of vitamin E daily over a 2-month period. His prothrombin time was found to be 36 seconds. A later study in this patient showed that 800 units of vitamin E daily for 6 weeks reduced his blood clotting factor levels, increased the prothrombin time from about 21 to 29 seconds, and caused ecchymoses.[4]

Mechanism

Not understood. The suggested explanation is that vitamin E interferes with the activity of vitamin K in producing the blood clotting factors,[4,5] and increases in the dietary requirements of vitamin K.[6,7]

Importance and management

Information is limited but the evidence suggests that most patients taking warfarin are unlikely to have problems if given even quite large daily doses (up to 1200 units) of vitamin E. Nevertheless the isolated case cited here shows that occasionally and unpredictably the warfarin effects can be changed. It has been recommended that prothrombin times should be monitored when vitamin E is first given (within 1 to 2 weeks has been recommended).[2] The same precautions could be applied to dicoumarol as well. However, as only one case of bleeding has been reported this does seem somewhat over-cautious. Information about other oral anticoagulants is lacking.

1. Schrogie JJ. Coagulopathy and fat-soluble vitamins. *JAMA* (1975) 232, 19.
2. Kim JM, White RH. Effect of vitamin E on the anticoagulant response to warfarin. *Am J Cardiol* (1996) 77, 545–6.
3. Corrigan JJ, Ulfers LL. Effect of vitamin E on prothrombin levels in warfarin-induced vitamin K deficiency. *Am J Clin Nutr* (1981) 34, 1701–5.
4. Corrigan JJ, Marcus FI. Coagulopathy associated with vitamin E ingestion. *JAMA* (1974) 230, 1300–1.
5. Booth SL, Golly I, Sacheck JM, Roubenoff R, Dallal GE, Hamada K, Blumberg JB. Effect of vitamin E supplementation on vitamin K status in adults with normal coagulation status. *Am J Clin Nutr* (2004) 80, 143–8.
6. Anon. Vitamin K, vitamin E and the coumarin drugs. *Nutr Rev* (1982) 40, 180–2.
7. Anon. Megavitamin E supplementation and vitamin K-dependent carboxylation. *Nutr Rev* (1983) 41, 268–70.

Coumarins + Dietary supplements; Vitamin K_1–containing

In patients with normal vitamin K status, multivitamin supplements containing 10 to 50 micrograms of vitamin K_1 (phytomenadione) will generally have no clinically important effect on the INR or anticoagulant requirements. Vitamin K doses of 150 micrograms daily are likely to require a dose adjustment in a proportion of patients. However, in patients with poor vitamin K status, even low vitamin K doses of 25 micrograms daily may have an important effect.

Clinical evidence

In a controlled study in healthy subjects stabilised on individual doses of **acenocoumarol**, the dose of vitamin K_1 tablets required to cause a statistically significant reduction in INR was 150 micrograms daily (INR 1.59 versus 2.04). Each dose of vitamin K_1 was taken daily for a week, and in successive weeks the dose was increased in increments of 50 micrograms from 50 to 300 micrograms daily, then 500 micrograms daily for the final week. The authors noted that their usual clinical criteria requiring an adjustment in **acenocoumarol** dose would have been met in 3 of the 12 subjects at a dose of vitamin K_1 of 150 micrograms daily.[1] However, in another study in 9 patients stabilised on **warfarin** with low vitamin K levels the median INR dropped by 0.51 requiring a **warfarin** dose increase of 5.3% after they took just one multivitamin tablet containing vitamin K_1 25 micrograms daily for 4 weeks. Conversely, in a control group with normal plasma vitamin K levels, the same multivitamin did not change the INR or warfarin requirement.[2] In another study in patients taking **phenprocoumon**, supplementation with vitamin K_1 50 micrograms daily for 3 weeks had little effect on the INR, and required just a 3% increase in **phenprocoumon** dose. A higher dose of vitamin K_1 of 100 micrograms daily resulted in a mean dose increase of 9%. On stopping the supplements, a mean 7% decrease in dose was needed. However, there was wide variation between patients.[3]

A patient who required **warfarin** 15 to 17.5 mg daily to maintain an INR of about 3 was found to be taking vitamin K (dose not stated) as part of a vitamin supplement. When he stopped taking the vitamin K, his **warfarin** dose requirement decreased to 10.5 to 12.5 mg daily.[4] In another report, a woman required an increase in her **warfarin** dose from 45 mg to 60 mg weekly when she started taking a daily multivitamin containing vitamin K_1 25 micrograms (*Centrum Plus*). Two weeks after stopping the multivitamin, she had haematuria and flank pain and was found to have a haematoma of the kidney and an INR of 13.2. A second patient had an acute occlusion of an aorto-bifemoral graft, requiring emergency surgery, 4 weeks after starting *Centrum Plus*. His INR had fallen from a mean of 2.48 to 1.1. A third patient had a fall in INR from a mean of 2.54 to 1.65 after taking *Centrum Plus* for 2 weeks. It was postulated that all three patients had low levels of vitamin K.[5]

Mechanism

Vitamin K_1 reduces the effect of vitamin K-antagonists (coumarins and **indanediones**). The dose of vitamin K_1 at which this becomes clinically important appears to depend on the vitamin K status of the individual.

Importance and management

The data from the controlled studies suggest that taking multivitamin supplements containing 10 to 50 micrograms of vitamin K_1 is probably acceptable in most patients taking anticoagulants, and is likely to require no change or only small changes to the anticoagulant dose. However, in patients with poor vitamin K status, even these low levels of vitamin K may be sufficient to antagonise the effect of their therapy. Note that a review of selected US supplements found that they contained 10 to 80 micrograms of vitamin K_1. Therefore, patients should be advised to *not* take a multivitamin preparation containing vitamin K_1 (phytomenadione) without increased monitoring when starting or stopping treatment. Because of this, and because of the increasing recognition of the importance of vitamin K in bone health, some consider that patients taking anticoagulants should be advised to consume sufficient vitamin K to meet the recommended adequate intakes,[6] see also 'Coumarins and related drugs + Foods; Vitamin K_1-rich', p.409. Others have even suggested that a low and steady vitamin K supplement may reduce the risk of excessive anticoagulation without altering efficacy.[7]

1. Schurgers LJ, Shearer MJ, Hamulyák K, Stöcklin E, Vermeer C. Effect of vitamin K intake on the stability of oral anticoagulant treatment: dose-response relationships in healthy subjects. *Blood* (2004) 104, 2682–9.
2. Kurnik D, Loebstein R, Rabinovitz H, Austerweil N, Halkin H, Almog S. Over-the-counter vitamin K_1-containing multivitamin supplements disrupt warfarin anticoagulation in vitamin K_1-depleted patients. A prospective, controlled trial. *Thromb Haemost* (2004) 92, 1018–24.
3. Rombouts EK, Rosendaal FR, van der Meer FJM. The effect of vitamin K supplementation on anticoagulant treatment. *J Thromb Haemost* (2006) 4, 691–2.
4. Eliason BC, Larson W. Acetaminophen and risk factors for excess anticoagulation with warfarin. *JAMA* (1998) 280, 696–7.
5. Kurnik D, Lubetsky A, Almog S, Halkin H. Multivitamin supplements may affect warfarin anticoagulation in susceptible patients. *Ann Pharmacother* (2003) 37, 1603–6.
6. Johnson MA. Influence of vitamin K on anticoagulant therapy depends on vitamin K status and the source and chemical forms of vitamin K. Nutr Rev 2003; 63, 91–7
7. Oldenburg J. Vitamin K intake and stability of oral anticoagulant treatment. *Thromb Haemost* (2005) 93, 799–800.

Coumarins + Disopyramide

In two small uncontrolled studies, the anticoagulant effects of warfarin were slightly reduced by disopyramide. In contrast, there is an isolated report of a patient who needed his warfarin dose to be doubled after *stopping* disopyramide.

Clinical evidence

In a preliminary report of a study in 10 patients with recent atrial fibrillation taking **warfarin** and with a British Corrected Ratio of 2 to 3, disopyramide (dose not stated) increased the clearance of **warfarin** by 21%.[1] Similarly, another study found that 2 out of 3 patients needed a slight **warfarin** dosage increase of about 10% after cardioversion and after starting disopyramide 200 mg three times daily for atrial fibrillation.[2]

In contrast, another report describes a patient who, following a myocardial infarction, was given **warfarin** 3 mg daily and disopyramide 100 mg every 6 hours with digoxin, furosemide and potassium supplements. When the disopyramide was withdrawn his **warfarin** requirements doubled over a 9-day period.[3,4]

Mechanism

Unknown. One idea is that when the disopyramide controls fibrillation, changes occur in cardiac output and in the flow of blood through the liver, which might have an effect on the synthesis of the blood clotting factors.[2,5] But the discordant response in the isolated case remains unexplained.

Importance and management

Very poorly documented and not established. Limited data suggest only a minor interaction occurs (a slight reduction in anticoagulant effect), but an isolated case suggests a greater and opposite effect. Bear the possibility of an interaction in mind in the case of an unexpected response to warfarin in a patient starting or stopping disopyramide.

1. Woo KS, Chan K, Pun CO. The mechanisms of warfarin-disopyramide interaction. *Circulation* (1987) 76 (Suppl 4), IV-520.
2. Sylvén C, Anderson P. Evidence that disopyramide does not interact with warfarin. *BMJ* (1983) 286, 1181.
3. Haworth E, Burroughs AK. Disopyramide and warfarin interaction. *BMJ* (1977) 2, 866–7.
4. Marshall J. Personal communication, 1987.
5. Ryll C, Davis LJ. Warfarin-disopyramide interaction? *Drug Intell Clin Pharm* (1979) 13, 260.

Coumarins + Disulfiram

The anticoagulant effects of warfarin were increased by disulfiram in two studies, and two cases showing this effect have also been reported.

Clinical evidence

In one study in 7 healthy subjects, **warfarin** (adjusted to maintain a prothrombin activity of 40%) was given alone for 21 days, then given with disulfiram 500 mg daily for 21 days. The plasma **warfarin** levels of 5 of the 7 subjects rose by an average of 20% and their prothrombin activity fell from about 34% to 24% of normal (suggesting an increased anticoagulant effect); one of the subjects had little change, and the other had the opposite effect.[1] Other experiments with single doses of **warfarin** confirm these results.[1] However, a further study found that, although disulfiram potentiated the effect of *S*-warfarin, it did not change the plasma levels of either *R*- or *S*-warfarin.[2]

An alcoholic patient stabilised on **warfarin** had an increase in his prothrombin time associated with gross haematuria when disulfiram 250 mg daily was given. Two subsequent attempts to introduce disulfiram 250 mg on alternate days also had a similar effect. He was eventually stabilised on a 43% lower daily dose of warfarin and disulfiram 250 mg daily.[3] Another case of increased prothrombin time and the need for a reduced warfarin dose has been reported.[4]

Mechanism

Not fully understood. The suggestion[1] that disulfiram inhibits the liver enzymes concerned with the metabolism of warfarin has not been confirmed by later studies.[2] It has instead been suggested[2] that disulfiram may chelate with the metal ions necessary for the production of active thrombin from prothrombin, thereby augmenting the actions of warfarin.

Importance and management

An interaction appears to be established, although direct information about patients is very limited. What is known suggests that most individuals will demonstrate this interaction. If concurrent use is thought appropriate, the effects of warfarin should be monitored and suitable dosage adjustments made when adding or withdrawing disulfiram. Care should be taken when starting warfarin in patients already taking disulfiram, and consideration should be given to using a smaller loading dose.

1. O'Reilly RA. Interaction of sodium warfarin and disulfiram (Antabuse®) in man. *Ann Intern Med* (1973) 78, 73–6.
2. O'Reilly RA. Dynamic interaction between disulfiram and separated enantiomorphs of racemic warfarin. *Clin Pharmacol Ther* (1981) 29, 332–6.
3. Rothstein E. Warfarin effect enhanced by disulfiram. *JAMA* (1968) 206, 1574–5.
4. Rothstein E. Warfarin effect enhanced by disulfiram (Antabuse). *JAMA* (1972) 221, 1052–3.

Coumarins + Diuretics

The loop diuretics, bumetanide, furosemide and torasemide, the potassium-sparing diuretic spironolactone, and the thiazides chlortalidone and chlorothiazide, have all been shown either not to interact or to cause only a small reduction in the effects of the coumarin anticoagulants of minimal or no clinical importance. The lack of reports of clinically relevant interactions suggests that, in general, diuretics do not interact with anticoagulants. The possible exception is etacrynic acid, which on rare occasions has caused a marked increase in the effects of warfarin.

Clinical evidence

A. Loop diuretics

(a) Bumetanide

In 10 healthy subjects, bumetanide 1 mg daily for 14 days did not alter the anticoagulant effect of a single-dose of **warfarin** given on day 8, and did not alter serum **warfarin** levels.[1] This confirms findings of a previous study in 5 healthy subjects given single-dose **warfarin** after bumetanide 2 mg daily for 5 days.[2]

(b) Etacrynic acid

A case report describes a marked increase in the anticoagulant effects of **warfarin** in a woman with hypoalbuminaemia on two occasions when she was given etacrynic acid 150 mg to 300 mg daily.[3] In a preliminary report of a cohort study, it was stated that a therapeutically significant interaction between **warfarin** and etacrynic acid was documented, but no details are given.[4]

(c) Furosemide

In 6 healthy subjects, plasma levels, half-lives and prothrombin times were not altered when a single 50-mg dose of **warfarin** was given after furosemide 80 mg daily for 5 days.[2] However, a 28% decrease in the INR of one patient taking **warfarin** was seen when furosemide was taken on a regular basis. This was attributed to volume depletion caused by the diuretic, although interpretation of this case is complicated by the patient's admission of previous non-compliance and abuse of alcohol and cocaine.[5] In a pharmacokinetic study in 17 healthy subjects, furosemide 40 mg twice daily had no effect on the pharmacokinetics of a single 0.22-mg/kg dose of **phenprocoumon**.[6] In another study in 22 patients with congestive heart failure stabilised on **phenprocoumon**, furosemide 40 mg daily for 8 days did not alter the anticoagulant effects or required dose of **phenprocoumon**.[7]

(d) Tienilic acid (Ticrynafen)

In 6 healthy subjects, tienilic acid 250 mg daily for about 14 days caused a mean 265% increase in the anticoagulant effect of a single dose of **warfarin** given on day 4. Analysis showed the interaction was stereoselective, with the AUC of *S*-warfarin increased by 192%, with the AUC for *R*-warfarin increased by only 8%.[8] Two patients taking **ethyl biscoumacetate** began to bleed spontaneously (haematuria, ecchymoses of the legs and gastrointestinal bleeding) when they started to take tienilic acid 250 mg daily. The thrombotest percentage of one of them was found to have fallen by 10%.[9] Increased anticoagulant effects and/or bleeding, which began within a few days, have been described in a number of other case reports in patients given tienilic acid while taking **ethyl biscoumacetate**,[10,11] **acenocoumarol**[12] or **warfarin**.[10,13]

(e) Torasemide

In a study in 24 patients with congestive heart failure stabilised on **phenprocoumon**, torasemide 20 mg daily for 8 days did not alter the anticoagulant effects or required dose of **phenprocoumon**.[7]

B. Potassium-sparing diuretics

(a) Spironolactone

In a study in 9 healthy subjects, spironolactone 50 mg four times daily for about 16 days reduced the prothrombin time response to a single dose of warfarin given on day 8 by 24%, when compared with **warfarin** alone. Plasma **warfarin** levels remained unchanged.[14]

C. Thiazides

(a) Chlortalidone

Six healthy subjects given a single 1.5-mg/kg dose of **warfarin** showed reduced hypoprothrombinaemia (prothrombin activity reduced from 77 to 58 units) when they were also given chlortalidone 100 mg daily for 7 days with the **warfarin** given on the first day, although the plasma **warfarin** levels remained unaltered.[15] Similarly, reduced anticoagulant effects have been described when chlortalidone was given with **phenprocoumon**, but no significant effects were seen when chlortalidone was given with **acenocoumarol**.[16]

(b) Chlorothiazide

A study in 8 healthy subjects given single 40 to 60-mg doses of **warfarin** before and after chlorothiazide 1 g daily for 21 days found that the mean half-life of the anticoagulant was increased from 39 to 44 hours, but the prothrombin time was only decreased by 0.3 seconds.[17]

Mechanism

It has been suggested that the diuresis induced by chlortalidone, furosemide and spironolactone reduces plasma water, which leads to a concentration of the blood clotting factors.[5,14,15] Etacrynic acid can displace warfarin from its plasma protein binding sites,[18] and it was originally thought that other diuretics also interacted by drug displacement.[9,19,20] Only 3% of total plasma warfarin is in the free active form, thus a small displacement could result in marked enhancement of activity,[3] but it is almost certain that this, on its own, does not explain the interaction described.[4] Tienilic acid (ticrynafen), which is structurally related to etacrynic acid, reduces the metabolism of *S*-warfarin (but not *R*-warfarin) thereby prolonging its stay in the body and increasing its effects.[8] It is possible that etacrynic acid interacts via a similar mechanism.

Importance and management

The documentation relating to diuretics in general (other than tienilic acid) is limited and seems to be confined to the reports cited here, most of which are single-dose pharmacological studies. The evidence suggests that these diuretics either do not interact at all with the coumarin anticoagulants, or only to an extent which is of little clinical relevance. This seems to be supported by the lack of case reports of problems with these combinations, and is in general agreement with common experience. No special precautions normally seem to be necessary, except possibly with etacrynic acid where it might be prudent to monitor the outcome particularly in those with hypoalbuminaemia or renal impairment.

The interaction between the coumarins and tienilic acid is established and of clinical importance, but the incidence is uncertain. Concurrent use should be avoided. If that is not possible, prothrombin times should be closely monitored and the anticoagulant dosage reduced as necessary. Tienilic acid has been withdrawn in many countries because of its hepatotoxicity.

1. Nipper H, Kirby S, Iber FL. The effect of bumetanide on the serum disappearance of warfarin sodium. *J Clin Pharmacol* (1981) 21, 654–6.
2. Nilsson CM, Horton ES, Robinson DS. The effect of furosemide and bumetanide on warfarin metabolism and anticoagulant response. *J Clin Pharmacol* (1978) 18, 91–4.
3. Petrick RJ, Kronacher N, Alcena V. Interaction between warfarin and ethacrynic acid. *JAMA* (1975) 231, 843–4.
4. Koch-Weser J. Hemorrhagic reactions and drug interactions in 500 warfarin-treated patients. *Clin Pharmacol Ther* (1973) 14, 139.
5. Laizure SC, Madlock L, Cyr M, Self T. Decreased hypoprothrombinemic effect of warfarin associated with furosemide. *Ther Drug Monit* (1997) 19, 361–3.
6. Mönig H, Böhm M, Ohnhaus EE, Kirch W. The effects of frusemide and probenecid on the pharmacokinetics of phenprocoumon. *Eur J Clin Pharmacol* (1990) 39, 261–5.

7. Piesche L, Bölke T. Comparative clinical trial investigating possible interactions of torasemide (20 mg o.d.) or furosemide (40 mg o.d.) with phenprocoumon in patients with congestive heart failure. *Int Congr Ser* (1993) 1023, 267–70.
8. O'Reilly RA. Ticrynafen-racemic warfarin interaction: hepatotoxic or stereoselective? *Clin Pharmacol Ther* (1982) 32, 356–61.
9. Detilleux M, Caquet R, Laroche C. Potentialisation de l'effet des anticoagulants coumariniques par un nouveau diurétique, l'acide tiénilique. *Nouv Presse Med* (1976) 5, 2395.
10. Prandota J, Pankow-Prandota L. Klinicznie znamienna interakcja nowego leku moczopednego kwasu tienylowego z lekami przeciwzakrzepowymi pochodnymi kumaryny. *Przegl Lek* (1982) 39, 385–8.
11. Portier H, Destaing F, Chauve L. Potentialisation de l'effet des anticoagulants coumariniques par l'acide tiénilique: une nouvelle observation. *Nouv Presse Med* (1977) 6, 468.
12. Grand A, Drouin B, Arche G-J. Potentialisation de l'action anticoagulante des anti-vitamines K par l'acide tiénilique. *Nouv Presse Med* (1977) 6, 2691.
13. McLain DA, Garriga FJ, Kantor OS. Adverse reactions associated with ticrynafen use. *JAMA* (1980) 243, 763–4.
14. O'Reilly RA. Spironolactone and warfarin interaction. *Clin Pharmacol Ther* (1980) 27, 198–201.
15. O'Reilly RA, Sahud MA, Aggeler PM. Impact of aspirin and chlorthalidone on the pharmacodynamics of oral anticoagulant drugs in man. *Ann N Y Acad Sci* (1971) 179, 173–86.
16. Vinazzer H. Die Beeinflussung der Antikoagulantientherapie durch ein Diuretikum. *Wien Z Inn Med* (1963) 44, 323–7.
17. Robinson DS, Sylwester D. Interaction of commonly prescribed drugs and warfarin. *Ann Intern Med* (1970) 72, 853–6.
18. Sellers EM, Koch-Weser J. Kinetics and clinical importance of displacement of warfarin from albumin by acidic drugs. *Ann N Y Acad Sci* (1971) 179, 213–25.
19. Slattery JT, Levy G. Ticrynafen effect on warfarin protein binding in human serum. *J Pharm Sci* (1979) 68, 393.
20. Prandota J, Albengres E, Tillement JP. Effect of tienilic acid (Diflurex) on the binding of warfarin ^{14}C to human plasma proteins. *Int J Clin Pharmacol Ther Toxicol* (1980) 18, 158–62.

Coumarins + Dofetilide

Dofetilide did not alter the anticoagulant effect of warfarin in one study.

Clinical evidence, mechanism, importance and management

In a placebo-controlled study in 14 healthy subjects dofetilide 750 micrograms twice daily for 8 days had no effect on the prothrombin time in response to a single 40-mg dose of **warfarin** given on day 5.[1] No dose adjustment of **warfarin** would be anticipated to be needed on concurrent use.

1. Nichols DJ, Dalrymple I, Newgreen MW, Kleinermans D. The effect of dofetilide on pharmacodynamics of warfarin and pharmacokinetics of digoxin. *Eur Heart J* (1999) 20 (Abstr Suppl), 586.

Coumarins + Etanercept

Etanercept did not alter the pharmacodynamics or pharmacokinetics of a single dose of warfarin.

Clinical evidence, mechanism, importance and management

In a study in 12 healthy subjects, subcutaneous etanercept 25 mg twice weekly for 7 doses did not alter the pharmacodynamics (INR) of a single dose of **warfarin** given with the last dose of etanercept. In addition, there was no change in the AUC of *R*- and *S*-warfarin.[1]

This study suggests that no **warfarin** dose adjustments would be expected to be needed if etanercept is used in patients taking **warfarin**.

1. Zhou H, Patat A, Parks V, Buckwalter M, Metzger D, Korth-Bradley J. Absence of a pharmacokinetic interaction between etanercept and warfarin. *J Clin Pharmacol* (2004) 44, 543–50.

Coumarins + Ethchlorvynol

The anticoagulant effects of dicoumarol and warfarin are reduced by ethchlorvynol.

Clinical evidence

Six patients who had recently started taking **dicoumarol** had a rise in their Quick index from 38 to 55% (suggesting a reduction in anticoagulant effect) while taking ethchlorvynol 1 g daily over an 18-day period. Another patient stabilised on **dicoumarol** became over-anticoagulated and developed haematuria on two occasions when ethchlorvynol was withdrawn for periods of 6 days and 4 days.[1] A marked reduction in the anticoagulant effects of **warfarin** occurred in another patient given ethchlorvynol.[2]

Mechanism

Uncertain. The idea that ethchlorvynol increases the metabolism of the anticoagulants by the liver has not been confirmed by studies in *dogs* and *rats*.[3]

Importance and management

Information is very sparse and limited to dicoumarol and warfarin, but the interaction seems to be established. Be alert for other coumarins to behave similarly. Anticipate the need to alter the anticoagulant dosage if ethchlorvynol is started or stopped. The benzodiazepines may be a useful non-interacting alternative to ethchlorvynol, see 'Coumarins + Benzodiazepines and related drugs', p.391.

1. Johansson S-A. Apparent resistance to oral anticoagulant therapy and influence of hypnotics on some coagulation factors. *Acta Med Scand* (1968) 184, 297–300.
2. Cullen SI and Catalano PM. Griseofulvin-warfarin antagonism. *JAMA* (1967) 199, 582–3.
3. Martin YC. The effect of ethchlorvynol on the drug-metabolizing enzymes of rats and dogs. *Biochem Pharmacol* (1967) 16, 2041–4.

Coumarins and related drugs + Ezetimibe

No clinically significant interaction occurred between ezetimibe and warfarin in one study. However, raised INRs have been seen in patients taking warfarin after they were also given ezetimibe.

Clinical evidence, mechanism, importance and management

In a two-way, crossover study, 12 healthy subjects were given ezetimibe 10 mg or placebo daily for 11 days, with a single 25-mg dose of **warfarin** on day 7. The pharmacokinetics and pharmacodynamics (prothrombin time) of **warfarin** were not significantly altered by ezetimibe. In addition, the pharmacokinetics of ezetimibe were similar to those previously seen with the drug alone.[1] However, the manufacturers of ezetimibe state that raised INRs have been seen in patients taking **warfarin** after they were also given ezetimibe. They therefore advise that the INR should be monitored if ezetimibe is given with any coumarin or **fluindione**,[2] (this is probably a prudent precaution for any **indanedione**).

1. Bauer KS, Kosoglou T, Statkevich P, Calzetta A, Maxwell SE, Patrick JE, Batra V. Ezetimibe does not affect the pharmacokinetics or pharmacodynamics of warfarin. *Clin Pharmacol Ther* (2001) 69, P5.
2. Ezetrol (Ezetimibe). MSD-SP Ltd. UK Summary of product characteristics, December 2006.

Coumarins + Felbamate

An isolated case report describes a marked increase in the effects of warfarin, which were attributed to felbamate.

Clinical evidence, mechanism, importance and management

A 62-year-old man with a seizure disorder who was receiving **warfarin** had his antiepileptic treatment with carbamazepine, phenobarbital and sodium valproate discontinued and replaced by felbamate 2.4 g daily and later 3.2 g daily. Within 14 days his INR had risen from a normal range of 2.5 to 3.5 up to 7.8. After stopping and later restarting the **warfarin** his INR rose within about another 14 days to 18.2. He was eventually restabilised on about half his former **warfarin** dosage. The authors of the report suggest that the withdrawal of the carbamazepine and phenobarbital was an unlikely reason for this reaction because no increases in **warfarin** dosage had been needed when they were started.[1] Suspicion therefore falls on the felbamate, but it is clearly difficult to be sure that the withdrawal of the enzyme-inducing antiepileptics did not have some part to play. A letter commenting on this report favours the idea that what occurred was in fact due to the withdrawal of the 'carbamazepine', (p.395) and 'phenobarbital', (p.390).[2]

The general importance of this interaction (if such it is) is uncertain, and this appears to be the only case. Bear it in mind in the event of an unexpected response to **warfarin**.

1. Tisdel KA, Israel DS, Kolb KW. Warfarin-felbamate interaction: first report. *Ann Pharmacother* (1994) 28, 805.
2. Glue P, Banfield CR, Colucci RD, Perhach JL. Comment: warfarin-felbamate interaction. *Ann Pharmacother* (1994) 28, 1412–13.

Coumarins and related drugs + Fibrates

Clofibrate increases the effects of coumarin and indanedione anticoagulants. This has been fatal in some cases. Other fibrates appear to interact similarly, although data in many cases is limited to case reports.

Clinical evidence

(a) Bezafibrate

In a study in patients with hyperlipidaemia and stabilised on **phenprocoumon**, it was necessary to reduce the anticoagulant dosage by about 20% when bezafibrate 450 mg daily was given for 4 weeks to 10 patients, and by 33% when bezafibrate 600 mg daily was given to 5 patients.[1] In another study in 22 patients taking bezafibrate 400 mg daily the dosage of **acenocoumarol** had to be reduced by 20% to maintain a constant INR.[2]

A patient (with hypoalbuminaemia due to nephrotic syndrome and chronic renal failure) stabilised on **acenocoumarol** developed severe haematemesis with an INR of 25.9, two weeks after starting to take bezafibrate 800 mg daily.[3] A woman stabilised on **warfarin** and bezafibrate 400 mg daily had an increase in her INR to 5.29 after being given an incorrect double dose of bezafibrate for a few days, and a man had a reduced response to **warfarin** (INR 1.5) when he stopped taking bezafibrate for a week.[4]

(b) Ciprofibrate

In a randomised, placebo-controlled, crossover study, 12 young healthy men were given a single 25-mg dose of **warfarin** on day 21 of a 26-day course of ciprofibrate 100 mg daily. The ciprofibrate increased the anticoagulant response to warfarin by 50% and caused a 28% decrease in the apparent intrinsic clearance of *S*-warfarin, which is the more active enantiomer.[5]

(c) Clofibrate

1. Coumarins. In a study including 11 patients stabilised on **warfarin**, clofibrate/androsterone (*Atromid*), given for 5 to 7 months, reduced the weekly **warfarin** dose requirement in all patients by a mean of 32%, with variability between patients.[6,7] This interaction has been confirmed in a number of other similar studies in patients stabilised on **warfarin** and given clofibrate,[8,9] or clofibrate with androsterone,[10] with only 2 of 10 patients affected in one study[8] but all 13 patients affected in another study.[10] One fatal case of haemorrhage has been reported in a man stabilised on **warfarin** who was given clofibrate 500 mg four times daily for a week.[11] The interaction has been studied in 4 healthy subjects given the enantiomers of **warfarin** separately. In this study, clofibrate increased the effect of *S*-warfarin without altering its clearance, whereas there was no alteration of the effect of *R*-warfarin and an increase in clearance.[12] In another study in 10 healthy subjects, clofibrate 500 mg four times daily for 18 days increased the anticoagulant effect of a single dose of **dicoumarol** given on day 14 without altering the half-life or plasma **dicoumarol** levels.[13]

2. Indanediones. Ten out of 15 patients stabilised on **phenindione** needed a 33% reduction in **phenindione** dose and 5 of them bled (haematuria or haematoma) when they were given clofibrate, or clofibrate with androsterone (*Atromid*).[7] In another series, of 13 patients stabilised on **phenindione** and given clofibrate/androsterone (*Atromid*) there were 5 cases of haemorrhagic episodes, two of which were not associated with a prolonged prothrombin time, and one of which was fatal.[14,15] In yet another study, clofibrate/androsterone appeared to be less effective in reducing serum cholesterol in the patients taking **phenindione** than in 12 other patients taking clofibrate alone.[16]

(d) Fenofibrate

In an early clinical study of fenofibrate, 2 patients stabilised on **acenocoumarol** needed a 30% reduction in their dosage to maintain the same prothrombin time when they were given long-term fenofibrate 200 mg in the morning and 100 mg in the evening.[17] In other similar studies, reductions in the dose of unnamed **coumarins** of 12% (range 0 to 21%)[18] or about one-third[19] were needed when fenofibrate was given. One patient developed haematuria.[20]

A number of case reports of this interaction have subsequently been published, as follows:

- A patient taking **warfarin** had a rise in his INR to 8.5 (from a previous range of 2 to 2.5) within a week of starting to take fenofibrate 200 mg daily. His INR later restabilised when the **warfarin** dosage was reduced by 27%.
- A patient taking **warfarin** had a marked INR rise from a range of 2.8 to 3.5 up to 5.6 within 10 days of starting to take fenofibrate (dosage not stated).[21]
- A patient taking **warfarin** bled, and was found to have an INR of 18 when his gemfibrozil was replaced by fenofibrate.[22]
- In 2 cases 30 to 40% reductions in the **warfarin** dose were required when fenofibrate was given.[23]

(e) Gemfibrozil

In a randomised, placebo-controlled, crossover study, gemfibrozil 600 mg twice daily for 8 days did not alter the anticoagulant effect of a single dose of **warfarin** given on day 3. In addition, gemfibrozil unexpectedly slightly decreased the AUC of both *R*- and *S*-warfarin (by 6% and 11%, respectively).[24] In contrast, a brief report describes bleeding ('menstrual cycle prolonged and lots of blood clots') and much higher prothrombin times (values not given) two weeks after a woman stabilised on **warfarin** started to take gemfibrozil 1.2 g daily in divided doses. Halving the **warfarin** dosage resolved the problem.[25] Another patient stabilised on **warfarin** developed severe hypoprothrombinaemia (INR 43) and bleeding (melaena, bruising) 4 weeks after starting to take gemfibrozil 1.2 g daily.[26]

Mechanism

Uncertain. Clofibrate can displace warfarin from its plasma protein binding sites,[5,27-29] but this does not adequately explain the interaction. Another suggestion is that the fibrates have an additive pharmacodynamic effect.[1,12] Altered metabolism may also account for the interaction with ciprofibrate, since this decreased the clearance of *S*-warfarin.[5] However, this did not occur with clofibrate[12,13] or gemfibrozil.[24]

Importance and management

The interactions of clofibrate with dicoumarol, warfarin and phenindione are established, clinically important and potentially serious. Severe bleeding (fatal in some instances) has been seen. The incidence of the interaction is reported to be between 20 and 100%, but it would be prudent to assume that all patients will be affected. Dosage reductions of one-third to one-half may be needed to avoid the risk of bleeding. Monitor the INR and adjust the dose accordingly. Information about other coumarins and indanediones is lacking but it would be prudent to assume that they will interact with clofibrate in a similar way.

Information about other fibrates is much less conclusive, and limited to case reports in many instances. Nevertheless, overall the evidence suggests that it would be prudent to monitor the INR in any patient taking a coumarin or indanedione with a fibrate.

1. Zimmermann R, Ehlers W, Walter E, Hoffrichter A, Lang PD, Andrassy K, Schlierf G. The effect of bezafibrate on the fibrinolytic enzyme system and the drug interaction with racemic phenprocoumon. *Atherosclerosis* (1978) 29, 477–85.
2. Manotti C, Quintavalla R, Pini M, Tomasini G, Vargiu G, Dettori AG. Interazione farmacologica tra bezafibrato in formulazione retard ed acenocumarolo. Studio clinico. *G Arterioscler* (1991) 16, 49–52.
3. Blum A, Seligmann H, Livneh A, Ezra D. Severe gastrointestinal bleeding induced by a probable hydroxycoumarin-bezafibrate interaction. *Isr J Med Sci* (1992) 28, 47–9.
4. Beringer TRO. Warfarin potentiation with bezafibrate. *Postgrad Med J* (1997) 73, 657–8.
5. Sanofi Withrop Ltd. Personal communication, December 1997.
6. Roberts SD, Pantridge JF. Effect of Atromid on requirements of warfarin. *J Atheroscler Res* (1963) 3, 655–7.
7. Oliver MF, Roberts SD, Hayes D, Pantridge JF, Suzman MM, Bersohn I. Effect of Atromid and ethyl chlorophenoxyisobutyrate on anticoagulant requirements. *Lancet* (1963) i, 143–4.
8. Udall JA. Drug interference with warfarin therapy. *Clin Med* (1970) 77, 20–5.
9. Eastham RD. Warfarin dosage, clofibrate, and age of patient. *BMJ* (1973) ii, 554.
10. Counihan TB, Keelan P. Atromid in high cholesterol states. *J Atheroscler Res* (1963) 3, 580–3.
11. Solomon RB, Rosner F. Massive hemorrhage and death during treatment with clofibrate and warfarin. *N Y State J Med* (1973) 73, 2002.
12. Bjornsson TD, Meffin PJ, Blaschke TF. Interaction of clofibrate with the optical enantiomorphs of warfarin. *Pharmacologist* (1976) 18, 207.
13. Schrogie JJ, Solomon HM. The anticoagulant response to bishydroxycoumarin. II. The effect of d-thyroxine, clofibrate, and norethandrolone. *Clin Pharmacol Ther* (1967) 8, 70–7.
14. Rogen AS, Ferguson JC. Clinical observations on patients treated with Atromid and anticoagulants. *J Atheroscler Res* (1963) 3, 671–6.
15. Rogen AS, Ferguson JC. Effect of Atromid on anticoagulant requirements. *Lancet* (1963) i, 272.

16. Williams GEO, Meynell MJ, Gaddie R. Atromid and anticoagulant therapy. *J Atheroscler Res* (1963) 3, 658–70.
17. Harvengt C, Heller F, Desager JP. Hypolipidemic and hypouricemic action of fenofibrate in various types of hyperlipoproteinemias. *Artery* (1980) 7, 73–82.
18. Stähelin HB, Seiler W, Pult N. Erfahrungen mit dem Lipidsenker Procetofen (Lipanthyl®). *Schweiz Rundsch Med Prax* (1979) 68, 24–8.
19. Raynaud P. Un nouvel hypolipidemiant: le procetofene. *Rev Med Tours* (1977) 11, 325–30.
20. Lauwers PL. Effect of procetofene on blood lipids of subjects with essential hyperlipidaemia. *Curr Ther Res* (1979) 26, 30–8.
21. Ascah KJ, Rock GA, Wells PS. Interaction between fenofibrate and warfarin. *Ann Pharmacother* (1998) 32, 765–8.
22. Aldridge MA, Ito MK. Fenofibrate and warfarin interaction. *Pharmacotherapy* (2001) 21, 886–9.
23. Kim KY, Mancano MA. Fenofibrate potentiates warfarin effects. *Ann Pharmacother* (2003) 37, 212–15.
24. Lilja JJ, Backman JT, Neuvonen PJ. Effect of gemfibrozil on the pharmacokinetics and pharmacodynamics of racemic warfarin in healthy subjects. *Br J Clin Pharmacol* (2004) 59, 433–9.
25. Ahmad S. Gemfibrozil interaction with warfarin sodium (Coumadin). *Chest* (1990) 98, 1041–2.
26. Rindone JP, Keng HC. Gemfibrozil-warfarin interaction resulting in profound hypoprothrombinemia. *Chest* (1998) 114, 641–2.
27. Solomon HM, Schrogie JJ, Williams D. The displacement of phenylbutazone-C^{14} and warfarin-C^{14} from human albumin by various drugs and fatty acids. *Biochem Pharmacol* (1968) 17, 143–51.
28. Solomon HM, Schrogie JJ. The effect of various drugs on the binding of warfarin-^{14}C to human albumin. *Biochem Pharmacol* (1967) 16, 1219–26.
29. Bjornsson TD, Meffin PJ, Swezey S, Blaschke TF. Clofibrate displaces warfarin from plasma proteins in man: an example of a pure displacement interaction. *J Pharmacol Exp Ther* (1979) 210, 316–21.

Coumarins + Flupirtine

In one study, flupirtine did not interact with phenprocoumon.

Clinical evidence, mechanism, importance and management

Twelve healthy subjects had no significant changes in their plasma levels of **phenprocoumon** 1.5 mg daily when they were given flupirtine 100 mg three times daily for 14 days. The prothrombin times were also not significantly changed.[1] There would therefore seem to be no reason for taking special precautions if these drugs are given concurrently.

1. Harder S, Thürmann P, Hermann R, Weller S, Mayer M. Effects of flupirtine coadministration on phenprocoumon plasma concentrations and prothrombin time. *Int J Clin Pharmacol Ther* (1994) 32, 577–581.

Coumarins + Fondaparinux

Warfarin did not alter the pharmacokinetics of fondaparinux, and fondaparinux did not alter the effect of warfarin on prothrombin time.

Clinical evidence, mechanism, importance and management

Subcutaneous fondaparinux 4 mg was given daily for 5 days to 12 healthy subjects, with warfarin 15 mg given on day 4 and 10 mg on day 5 in a placebo controlled study. Warfarin had no effect on fondaparinux pharmacokinetics. In addition, the effect of warfarin on prothrombin time was not altered by fondaparinux. The authors concluded that the prothrombin time (INR) can still be used to monitor the effect of oral anticoagulants during the switch from fondaparinux to oral anticoagulants.[1]

1. Faaij RA, Burggraaf J, Schoemaker RC, van Amsterdam RGM, Cohen AF. Absence of an interaction between the synthetic pentasaccharide fondaparinux and oral warfarin. *Br J Clin Pharmacol* (2002) 54, 304–8.

Coumarins + Food

The rate of absorption of dicoumarol can be increased by food. Two reports describe antagonism of the effects of warfarin by ice-cream, and another report attributes an increase in prothrombin time to the use of aspartame. However, the most common food-warfarin interaction is that due to foods containing vitamin K.

Clinical evidence

(a) Dicoumarol

A study in 10 healthy subjects showed that the peak serum concentrations of a single 250-mg dose of dicoumarol, were increased on average by 85% by food. Two subjects showed increases of 242% and 206%, respectively.[1]

(b) Warfarin

A very brief report states that a patient taking warfarin had a raised prothrombin time, possibly due to the use of **aspartame**.[2]

A woman taking warfarin 22.5 mg daily did not have the expected prolongation of her prothrombin times. It was then discovered that she took the warfarin in the evening and she always ate **ice cream** before going to bed. When the warfarin was taken in the mornings, the prothrombin times increased.[3] Another patient's warfarin requirements almost doubled when she started to eat very large quantities of **ice cream** (1 litre each evening). The effect was not seen when she ate normal amounts of **ice cream**. She took the warfarin at 6 pm and the **ice cream** at about 10 pm.[4]

Mechanism

Not understood. One suggestion for the interaction between food and dicoumarol[1] is that food may cause prolonged retention of dicoumarol in the upper part of the gut, leading to increased tablet dissolution and increased absorption.

Importance and management

None of these interactions is very well documented, and their clinical relevance is unclear. Note that vitamin K in food commonly interacts with warfarin, and these interactions are discussed in 'Coumarins and related drugs + Foods; Vitamin K_1-rich', p.409. See also 'cranberry juice', (p.398), 'enteral and parenteral nutrition', (below), 'grapefruit juice', (p.411), 'mango', (p.408) and 'soya bean products', (p.408).

1. Melander A, Wåhlin E. Enhancement of dicoumarol bioavailability by concomitant food intake. *Eur J Clin Pharmacol* (1978) 14, 441–4.
2. Beeley L, Beadle F, Lawrence R. *Bulletin of the West Midlands Centre for Adverse Drug Reaction Reporting* (1984) 19, 9.
3. Simon LS, Likes KE. Hypoprothrombinemic response due to ice cream. *Drug Intell Clin Pharm* (1978) 12, 121–2.
4. Blackshaw CA, Watson VA. Interaction between warfarin and ice cream. *Pharm J* (1990) 244, 318.

Coumarins and related drugs + Foods; Enteral and parenteral nutrition

A number of early case reports described warfarin resistance in patients taking enteral feeds that contained high levels of added vitamin K_1. These products were then reformulated to contain lower amounts of vitamin K_1, commonly now about 4 to 10 micrograms per 100 mL; however, some cases of interactions have still been reported, and one study in children reported that those receiving enteral nutrition (mostly vitamin K enriched formula) required 2.4-fold higher maintenance warfarin doses. Lipid emulsions containing soya oil might contain sufficient natural vitamin K_1 to alter warfarin requirements. Parenteral multivitamin preparations may also contain vitamin K_1.

Clinical evidence

A. Enteral feeds

Case reports from the early 1980s described patients stabilised on **warfarin** who had reversal of the anticoagulant effect when they started taking the liquid dietary supplements ***Ensure***,[1,2] or ***Osmolite***.[3] Other patients who were resistant to **warfarin** were found to be taking ***Ensure***[4] or ***Ensure Plus***[5,6]. At this time, these products contained high levels of vitamin K_1 (240 to 380 micrograms per 240 or 250 mL, an amount equivalent to approximately 1 mg of vitamin K_1 for every 1000 calories). Two of the patients were successfully anticoagulated with **warfarin** when their enteral nutrition was switched to ***Compleat B*** (vitamin K_1 16.6 micrograms/250 mL)[6] or ***Meritene*** (trace of vitamin K_1).[4]

In response to these reports, ***Ensure***, ***Ensure-Plus***, and ***Osmolite*** were reformulated to reduce the vitamin K_1 content to 50 micrograms in 240 mL (140 micrograms per 1000 calories).[4] However, further case reports for ***Ensure Plus***[7] and ***Osmolite***[8] suggested that this lower level of vitamin K may still be sufficient to cause an interaction. The vitamin K_1 content of these products was reduced further to 36 to 37 micrograms per 1000 calories,[9] but even then one further case of increased **warfarin** requirement was reported with ***Ensure***.[10] In another case, a patient taking

Osmolite and intermittent ***Ensure Plus*** (total mean vitamin K_1 dose 81 micrograms daily) only achieved satisfactory anticoagulation with **warfarin** when the ***Osmolite*** was stopped, which reduced the vitamin K_1 intake to 36 micrograms daily.[11] Another patient given ***Osmolite*** (vitamin K_1 68.4 micrograms daily), only achieved satisfactory anticoagulation with **warfarin** when the dose was given separately from the ***Osmolite***.[12]

In another case, ***Isocal*** 3550 mL daily (equivalent to 460 micrograms of vitamin K_1) caused an increase in **warfarin** requirement from 8 mg daily to 13 mg daily.[13] A further patient had a decrease in anticoagulant response requiring an increase in **warfarin** dose when she started a weight-reducing diet consisting solely of ***Nutrilite 330*** (vitamin K content unknown).[14]

Another patient required twice the dose of **acenocoumarol** during a period of enteral feeding (vitamin K_1 200 micrograms daily).[15]

In a prospective cohort study in 319 children, the use of enteral nutrition (mostly **vitamin K supplemented formula**, and some **vitamin K supplemented tube feeds**) was associated with a higher dose of **warfarin** to achieve a target INR (0.28 versus 0.16 mg/kg) and similarly a higher dose of **warfarin** was needed to maintain the INR (0.26 versus 0.11 mg/kg).[16]

B. Parenteral nutrition

(a) Intravenous lipids

Warfarin resistance was seen a in patient who was given a constant intravenous infusion of **soya oil emulsion** (***Intralipid***). In this case intravenous **warfarin** up to 15 mg daily only slightly prolonged the prothrombin time.[17] In another patient, an emulsified infusion of **propofol** containing 10% **soya oil** antagonised the effect of **warfarin**; anticoagulation was not achieved until the **propofol** was discontinued despite an increase in the **warfarin** dose to 30 mg daily. The dose of propofol given was estimated to provide about 154 to 231 micrograms of vitamin K_1 daily. The same effect was later see when the patient was given parenteral nutrition supplemented with 20% ***Liposyn II***, which also contains **soya oil**, and was estimated to provide 53 micrograms vitamin K_1 daily.[18]

(b) Multivitamins

The FDA in the US now require that multivitamin products for inclusion in total parenteral nutrition contain 150 micrograms of vitamin K_1. The aim of this is to provide a daily physiological amount of the vitamin, rather than the previous practice of giving a large single weekly dose. Previously, patients taking anticoagulants were not given this single large weekly dose, therefore it is anticipated that with the new multivitamin preparation, **warfarin** doses for anticoagulation may be higher than previously needed. What effect this level of vitamin K_1 will have on the fixed dose **warfarin** used for prophylaxis of catheter-associated thrombosis is not known.[19]

In the UK, ***Vitlipid N*** contains vitamin K_1 (phytomenadione) 15 micrograms/mL for adults and 20 micrograms/mL for children under 11 years.

Mechanism

The coumarin and **indanedione** anticoagulants are vitamin K antagonists, and consequently giving 'vitamin K_1', (p.458) reduces their effects. The dose at which this might become clinically important is not firmly established, but in one controlled study 150 micrograms of vitamin K_1 daily produced a clinically relevant effect in 25% of subjects (see 'Dietary supplements; Vitamin K_1-containing, (p.401)). There is also some evidence that a physicochemical interaction (possibly binding to protein) may occur between warfarin and enteral foods in the gut.[12,20]

Lipid emulsions given as part of parenteral nutrition often contain soya oil, which has a moderate level of vitamin K (see 'Table 12.3', (below)). These preparations may also have direct coagulation effects.[18] Parenteral nutrition may also be supplemented with vitamin K.

Importance and management

Established interactions of clinical importance. Be aware that enteral feeds might contain sufficient vitamin K to alter coagulation status, so starting or stopping these feeds might affect dose requirements of vitamin K antagonists such as warfarin. It is also possible that there is a local interaction in the gut, as in one case separating the administration of the warfarin and an enteral feed by 3 hours or more was effective.[12] Patients should be advised not to add or substitute dietary supplements such as *Ensure* without increased monitoring of their coagulation status.

Table 12.3 Foods with a moderate to high content of Vitamin K_1 (phytomenadione)

Foods	*Vitamin K_1 content (micrograms/100 g)*
Vegetables	
Asparagus	51 to 80
Beet greens	484
Broccoli	101 to 156
Brussels sprouts	122 to 289
Cabbage	50 to 98
Collards (non-heading cabbage)	440 to 623
Endive	231
Kale	817 to 882
Lettuce (iceberg to green leaf)	24 to 174
Parsley (fresh or dried)	360 to 1640
Spinach	270 to 575
Spring onions	207
Turnip greens	367 to 519
Fats and oils	
Soya oil	25 to 145
Rapeseed oil	112 to 150
Olive oil	30 to 60
Margarines	40 to 110
Fruit and nuts	
Avocado	14 to 20
Cashew nuts	19 to 64
Kiwi fruit	25 to 40
Pine nuts	33 to 74
Prunes, dried	1.4 to 68

Data from:

1. Booth SL, Sadowski JA, Pennington JAT. Phylloquinone (vitamin K1) content of foods in the U.S. Food and Drug Administration's Total Diet Study. *J Agric Food Chem* (1995) 43, 1574–9.
2. Piironen V, Koivu T, Tammisalo O, Mattila P. Determination of phylloquinone in oils, margarines and butter by high-performance liquid chromatography with electrochemical detection. *Food Chem* (1997) 59, 473–80.
3. Koivu TJ, Pirronen VI, Henttonen SK, Mattila PH. Determination of phylloquinone in vegetables, fruits and berries by high-performance liquid chromatography with electrochemical detection. *J Agric Food Chem* (1997) 45, 4644–49.
4. Bolton-Smith C, Price RJG, Fenton ST, Harrington DJ, Shearer MJ. Compliation of a provisional UK database for the phylloquinone (vitamin K1) content of foods. *Br J Nutr* (2000) 83, 389–99.
5. USDA National Nutrient Database for Standard Reference, Release 17. Vitamin K (phylloquinone) (μg) Content of selected foods per common measure. Available at: http://www.nal.usda.gov/fnic/foodcomp/Data/SR17/wtrank/sr17a430.pdf (accessed 29/11/06).
6. Dismore ML, Haytowitz DB, Gebhardt SE, Peterson JW, Booth SL. Vitamin K content of nuts and fruits in the US diet. *J Am Diet Assoc* (2003) 103, 1650–2.
7. Schurgers LJ, Vermeer C. Determination of phylloquinone and menaquinones in food. Effect of food matrix on circulating vitamin K concentrations. *Haemostasis* (2000) 30, 298–307.

Fat emulsions used for parenteral use containing soya oil may themselves contain sufficient vitamin K_1 for daily needs. Parenteral multivitamin preparations may also contain important levels of vitamin K_1. It would be advisable to keep the vitamin K_1 intake constant in any patient requiring long-term supplemental or total parenteral nutrition and warfarin. If the amount of lipid and/or multivitamins is altered, anticipate a change in warfarin requirement.

Although there is only a single case, bear in mind that propofol may interact because it is formulated with soya oil, which contains vitamin K_1.

1. O'Reilly RA, Rytand DA. 'Resistance' to warfarin due to unrecognized vitamin K supplementation. *N Engl J Med* (1980) 303, 160–1.
2. Westfall LK. An unrecognized cause of warfarin resistance. *Drug Intell Clin Pharm* (1981) 15, 131.
3. Lader EW, Yang L, Clarke A. Warfarin dosage and vitamin K in Osmolite. *Ann Intern Med* (1980) 93, 373–4.
4. Lee M, Schwartz RN, Sharifi R. Warfarin resistance and vitamin K. *Ann Intern Med* (1981) 94, 140–1.
5. Michaelson R, Kempin SJ, Navia B, Gold JWM. Inhibition of the hypoprothrombinemic effect of warfarin (Coumadin®) by Ensure-Plus, a dietary supplement. *Clin Bull* (1980) 10, 171–2.
6. Zallman JA, Lee DP, Jeffrey PL. Liquid nutrition as a cause of warfarin resistance. *Am J Hosp Pharm* (1981) 38, 1174.
7. Griffith LD, Olvey SE, Triplett WC, Stotter Cuddy ML. Increasing prothrombin times in a warfarin-treated patient upon withdrawal of Ensure Plus. *Crit Care Med* (1982) 10, 799–800.
8. Parr MD, Record KE, Griffith GL, Zeok JV, Todd EP. Effect of enteral nutrition on warfarin therapy. *Clin Pharm* (1982) 1, 274–6.
9. Kutsop JJ. Update on vitamin K_1 content of enteral products. *Am J Hosp Pharm* (1984) 41, 1762.
10. Howard PA, Hannaman KN. Warfarin resistance linked to enteral nutrition products. *J Am Diet Assoc* (1985) 85, 713–15.
11. Martin JE, Lutomski DM. Warfarin resistance and enteral feedings. *J Parenter Enteral Nutr* (1989) 13, 206–8.
12. Petretich DA. Reversal of Osmolite-warfarin interaction by changing warfarin administration time. *Clin Pharm* (1990) 9, 93.
13. Watson AJM, Pegg M, Green JRB. Enteral feeds may antagonise warfarin. *BMJ* (1984) 288, 557.
14. Oren B, Shvartzman P. Unsuspected source of vitamin K in patients treated with anticoagulants: a case report. *Fam Pract* (1989) 6, 151–2.
15. Van Iersel MB, Blenke AAM, Kremer HPH, Hekster YA. Een patiënt met verminderde gevoeligheid voor acenocoumarol tijdens gebruik van sondevoeding. *Ned Tijdschr Geneeskd* (2004) 148, 1155–6.
16. Streif W, Marzinotto AV, Massicotte P, Chan AKC, Julian JA, Mitchell L. Analysis of warfarin therapy in pediatric patients: a prospective cohort study of 319 patients. *Blood* (1999) 94, 3007–14.
17. Lutomski DM, Palascak JE, Bower RH. Warfarin resistance associated with intravenous lipid administration. *J Parenter Enteral Nutr* (1987) 11, 316–18.
18. MacLaren R, Wachsman BA, Swift DK, Kuhl DA. Warfarin resistance associated with intravenous lipid administration: discussion of propofol and review of the literature. *Pharmacotherapy* (1997) 17, 1331–7.
19. Helphingstine CJ, Bistrian BR. New Food and Drug Administration requirements for inclusion of vitamin K in adult parenteral multivitamins. *J Parenter Enteral Nutr* (2003) 27, 220–4.
20. Penrod LE, Allen JB, Cabacungan LR. Warfarin resistance and enteral feedings: 2 case reports and a supporting in vitro study. *Arch Phys Med Rehabil* (2001) 82, 1270–3.

Coumarins + Foods; Mango fruit (*Mangifera indica*)

A daily intake of 1 to 6 mangoes was considered the reason for a moderate increase in the anticoagulant effects of warfarin in one report. None of the patients in whom this interaction was seen showed any evidence of bleeding.

Clinical evidence, mechanism, importance and management

In 13 patients taking **warfarin**, eating mango fruit (*Mangifera indica*) appeared to increase their INRs by an average of 38% (from 2.79 to 3.85), but no bleeding occurred. No other explanation for the increased INRs could be identified. The patients were reported to have eaten 1 to 6 mangoes daily for 2 days to 1 month before attending the anticoagulant clinic. When mango was identified as a possible cause for their increased INRs, the patients were told to stop eating mango, whereupon their mean INR fell within 2 weeks, by almost 18%. When 2 of the patients whose mean INRs had originally risen by 13% were later rechallenged with mango (rather less than before), their mean INR rose by 9%.[1]

The reason for this apparent interaction is not known but the authors of the report speculate about the possible role of vitamin A (reported to be 8061 units in an average sized mango of 130 g, without seed). In practical terms this increase in INR would not seem to represent a serious problem, although note that one patient's INR rose to 5.1 (a 54% increase).

There appear to be no other reports in the literature of an interaction between mango and **warfarin**, nor of interactions between mango and any other oral anticoagulant. More study of this interaction is needed, but at the present time there is insufficient reason to suggest that patients taking **warfarin** should avoid mango fruit.

1. Monterrey-Rodríguez J, Feliú JF, Rivera-Miranda GC. Interaction between warfarin and mango fruit. *Ann Pharmacother* (2002) 36, 940–1.

Coumarins + Foods; Soya bean products

Natto, a Japanese food made from fermented soya bean, can markedly reduce the effects of warfarin and acenocoumarol, because of the high levels of vitamin K_2 substance produced in the fermentation process. In one study, soya bean protein also modestly reduced the effects of warfarin, and a similar case has been reported with soy milk.

Clinical evidence

(a) Fermented soya bean products (natto)

In a controlled study in 12 healthy subjects stabilised on **acenocoumarol**, a single meal containing 100 g of natto decreased the mean INR from 2.1 to 1.5 after 24 hours, and the INR had still not returned to the original level after 7 days (INR 1.75 one week later). The effect was considered clinically important in 6 of the 12 subjects.[1] Similarly, in an earlier retrospective study of 10 patients taking **warfarin**, eating natto caused the thrombotest values to rise from a range of 12 to 29% up to a range of 33 to 100%. The extent of the rise appeared to be related to the amount of natto eaten. The thrombotest values fell again when the natto was stopped. A healthy subject taking **warfarin**, with a thrombotest value of 40%, ate 100 g of natto. Five hours later the thrombotest value was unchanged, but 24 hours later it was 86%, and after 48 hours it was 90% (suggesting that the anticoagulant effect was decreased).[2]

(b) Soya milk

In a 70-year-old man stabilised on **warfarin** 3 mg daily, consumption of soya milk 480 mL daily (240 mL of both *Sun Soy* and *8th Continent* mixed together) decreased the INR from 2.5 to 1.6 after about 4 weeks.[3] One week after stopping the soya milk, his INR was 1.9, and 4 weeks after it was 2.5.

(c) Soya oil

Soya oil is an important source of dietary vitamin K, see 'Table 12.3', (p.407). For two cases of 'warfarin resistance' with intravenous soya oil emulsions, see 'Coumarins and related drugs + Foods; Enteral and parenteral nutrition', p.406.

(d) Soya protein

In a study in 10 patients with hypercholesterolaemia who were stabilised on **warfarin**, substitution of all animal protein for textured **soya protein** for 4 weeks caused a marked reduction (Quick value approximately doubled) in the anticoagulant effects of warfarin by the second week.[4]

Mechanism

Soya beans are a moderate source of vitamin K_1 (19 micrograms per 100 g),[5] and soya oil and products derived from it are an important dietary source of vitamin K (see 'Table 12.3', (p.407)). However, the soy milk brand taken in the case report did not contain vitamin K,[3] and another reference source lists soya milk as containing just 7.5 micrograms vitamin K per 250 mL,[5] which would not be expected to cause an interaction. Why this product decreased the effect of warfarin is therefore open to speculation. The vitamin K content of textured soya protein is unknown. Note that **soy sauce** made from soy and wheat is reported to contain no vitamin K, and soft **tofu** made from the curds by coagulating soy milk contains only low levels (2 micrograms per 100 g).[5]

In contrast, *fermented* soya bean products such as natto contain very high levels of a particular vitamin K_2 substance (MK-7)[6], because of the fermentation process with *Bacillus natto*. In addition, the bacteria might continue to act in the gut to increase the synthesis and subsequent absorption of vitamin K_2.[2] Although the role of vitamin K_2 in anticoagulation is less well established than vitamin K_1, it appears that this also opposes the actions of coumarins and indanediones, which are vitamin K antagonists.

Importance and management

The interaction with fermented soya bean products is established, marked, and is likely to be clinically relevant in all patients. Patients taking coumarin and probably **indanedione** anticoagulants should probably be advised to avoid natto, unless they want to consume a regular constant amount.

Although information is limited, it appears that soya protein might also modestly reduce the effect of warfarin. In particular, complete substitution of animal protein for soya protein appears to reduce the effect of warfarin. A single report suggests that soy milk may also interact. 'Soya oil', (p.406) has been reported to interact in a couple of cases. On the basis of known vitamin K-content, **whole soya beans** could potentially reduce the effect of warfarin, whereas **soy sauce** should not.[5]

1. Schurgers LJ, Shearer MJ, Hamulyák K, Stöcklin E, Vermeer C. Effect of vitamin K intake on the stability of oral anticoagulant treatment: dose-response relationships in healthy subjects. *Blood* (2004) 104, 2682–9.
2. Kudo T. Warfarin antagonism of natto and increase in serum vitamin K by intake of natto. *Artery* (1990) 17, 189–201.
3. Cambria-Kiely JA. Effect of soy milk on warfarin efficacy. *Ann Pharmacother* (2002) 36, 1893–6.
4. Gaddi A, Sangiorgi Z, Ciarrocchi A, Braiato A, Descovich GC. Hypocholesterolemic soy protein diet and resistance to warfarin therapy. *Curr Ther Res* (1989) 45, 1006–10.
5. USDA National Nutrient Database for Standard Reference, Release 17. Vitamin K (phylloquinone) (µg) Content of selected foods per common measure. Available at: http://www.nal.usda.gov/fnic/foodcomp/Data/SR17/wtrank/sr17a430.pdf (accessed 17/08/07)
6. Schurgers LJ, Vermeer C. Determination of phylloquinone and menaquinones in food. Effect of food matrix on circulating vitamin K concentrations. *Haemostasis* (2000) 30, 298–307.

Coumarins and related drugs + Foods; Vitamin K_1-rich

Unintentional and unwanted antagonism of warfarin has occurred in patients who ate exceptionally large amounts of some green vegetables, which can contain significant amounts of vitamin K_1. Isolated cases have also been reported with avocado, green tea, liver, and seaweed sushi. Patients should be advised to maintain a constant dietary intake of vitamin K_1. Foods containing significant amounts of vitamin K_2 substances such as fermented soya beans might also interact.

Clinical evidence and mechanism

The coumarin and indanedione oral anticoagulants are vitamin K antagonists, which inhibit the enzyme vitamin K epoxide reductase so reducing the synthesis of vitamin K-dependent blood clotting factors by the liver. If the intake of dietary vitamin K_1 increases, the synthesis of the blood clotting factors begins to return to normal. As a result the prothrombin time also begins to fall to its normal value. Naturally occurring vitamin K_1 (phytomenadione) is found only in plants.

A. Individual foods

(a) Avocado

Two women taking **warfarin** had a reduction in their INRs (from 2.5 to 1.7 and from 2.7 to 1.6, respectively) when they started to eat avocado 100 g daily, or 200 g of avocado on two consecutive days. Their INRs climbed again when the avocado was stopped.[1] Avocado contains a small to moderate amount of vitamin K_1, see 'Table 12.3', (p.407), so might occasionally reduce the efficacy of **warfarin** if eaten in these quantities.

(b) Green tea

A patient taking **warfarin** had a reduction in his INR from a range of 3.2 to 3.79 down to 1.37, which was attributed to the ingestion of very large quantities of green tea (about 2 to 4 litres each day for a week). This interaction was attributed to the vitamin-K content of the tea.[2] However, although dried tea, including green tea, is very high in vitamin-K_1, the brewed liquid made from the tea contains negligible amounts of vitamin K_1,[1,3] and is therefore not considered to contribute any vitamin K_1 to the diet.[3] The reason for this interaction is therefore unclear, unless the patient was eating some of the brewed tea leaves. A pharmacokinetic interaction also appears unlikely, because, although black tea inhibited CYP2C9 *in vitro*, brewed tea had no effect on the CYP2C9 substrate flurbiprofen in healthy subjects.[4] For discussion of a case where a patient had an increase in INR after stopping taking a herbal preparation of which green tea leaves were one of 25 ingredients, see 'Coumarins + Herbal medicines; Vitamin K_1–rich', p.418.

(c) Green vegetables

In a formal study in patients stabilised on **warfarin**, one day of a high intake of vitamin K_1-rich vegetables (**brussels sprouts** 400 g, **broccoli** 400 g, **lettuce** 750 g, or **spinach** 300 g, estimated to contain 1 mg of vitamin K_1 daily) decreased anticoagulant effects: the thrombotest values rose above the normal range of 10 to 25% in 2 of 5 patients in 2 to 3 days. Two days of a high intake of the same vegetable caused values above the therapeutic range in 3 of 7 patients, and 7 days intake did the same in 9 of 13 patients.[5] In another similar study, intake of **spinach** 250 g or **broccoli** 250 g daily for 7 days increased the mean thrombotest values to above the therapeutic limit of 15%, and the effect was similar to that of a supplement containing phytomenadione 250 micrograms daily. A reduction in the anticoagulant effect of **warfarin** was also seen in one healthy subject given about 450 g **spinach** daily.[6,7] In a pharmacokinetic study in healthy subjects, a daily intake of 400 g of **brussels sprouts** for 2 weeks slightly decreased the AUC of **warfarin** by 16% and increased its metabolic clearance by 27%.[8] This is probably because **brussels sprouts** induce the cytochrome P450 isoenzyme CYP1A2, which has a role in the 'metabolism of warfarin', (p.358).

A few cases of this interaction (often described as warfarin resistance) have been reported in patients taking **dicoumarol**,[9] or **warfarin**[10-13] when consuming diets containing large amounts of green vegetables (about 300 to 700 g daily),[11,12] such as **spinach**,[9,14] **broccoli**,[11,12] or a weight-loss diet consisting of **lettuce**, **turnip greens**, and **broccoli**.[13] The dietary vitamin K was estimated to be 1277 micrograms daily in one case,[10] and 6000 micrograms daily in another.[13] In two cases, patients suffered a serious thromboembolic event.[12,13] For discussion of a case where a patient had an increase in INR after stopping a herbal preparation, of which **spinach**, **broccoli** and **cabbage** were 3 of 25 ingredients, see 'Coumarins + Herbal medicines; Vitamin K_1–rich', p.418.

Conversely, a single intake of **spinach** 250 g or **broccoli** 250 g had no effect on thrombotest values over 7 days.[14] Similarly, in another study in healthy subjects stabilised on **acenocoumarol**, a single meal containing either **spinach** 400 g or **broccoli** 400 g with corn oil caused just 0.27 and 0.41 reductions in mean INR, an effect that was not considered clinically relevant. These reductions were equivalent to that seen with about 200 micrograms of vitamin K_1.[15]

(d) Liver

A patient taking **acenocoumarol** had a soft tissue bleed, and was found to have a very low thrombotest value of about 3%. She had always consumed about 142 g daily of green vegetables, but about 4 months previously had been advised to stop eating liver (750 g weekly) as part of a low-fat diet.[16] In another case, a man taking **warfarin** 5 mg daily had diffuse bruising and an INR of 5.6 two weeks after he was advised to stop eating pork **liver**[12] (1 kg per week). He was eventually restabilised on just 1.5 mg of warfarin daily. Early studies showed that liver contained high levels of vitamin K, but more recent studies using more specific detection techniques have shown that liver generally contains very low levels of vitamin K_1 (4 and 7 micrograms in 100 g).[17] However, liver may contain vitamin K_2 substances in sufficient levels to be of possible nutritional relevance.[17,18] The precise role of vitamin K_2 substances in anticoagulation control is less clear, but 'Natto', (p.408), which is a rich source of these, clearly reduces the effects of coumarins.

(e) Seaweed and Japanese food

A patient taking **warfarin** had, on two occasions, reduced INRs of 1.6 and 1.8 (usual range 2 to 3) within 24 hours of eating sushi with **seaweed** (***asakusa-nori***). It was estimated that she had consumed only about 45 micrograms of **phytomenadione**, but because her vitamin K stores may have been low, this amount could have accounted for a large percentage of her vitamin K intake or stores.[19] In an early report, a Japanese man recently stabilised on **warfarin** developed bleeding episodes on two occasions shortly after resuming his usual diet of Japanese food (specific foods not mentioned). However, ingestion of 3 similar Japanese meals in a 24-hour period had no effect on the prothrombin time in 6 Caucasian patients taking **warfarin**.[20]

B. Overall dietary vitamin K intake

(a) Relationship between dietary vitamin K and INR with anticoagulants

There is evidence that the average dietary vitamin K_1 intake is correlated with the efficacy of **warfarin**. In one study, patients consuming a diet containing more than 250 micrograms daily of vitamin K_1 had a lower INR five days after starting **warfarin** than patients consuming less dietary vitamin K_1 (median INR 1.9 versus 3). Also, the high-vitamin K_1 group needed a higher maintenance **warfarin** dose (5.7 mg/day versus 3.5 mg/day).[21] In another study, multiple regression analysis indicated that, in patients taking warfarin, the INR was altered by 1, by a weekly change in the intake of vitamin K of 714 micrograms.[22] Similarly, for each increase in daily dietary vitamin K_1 intake of 100 micrograms, the INR decreased by just 0.2 in another study.[23]

In a randomised, crossover study in patients taking **warfarin** or **phenprocoumon**, increasing the dietary intake of vitamin K_1 by 500% relative to the baseline value (from 118 to 591 micrograms daily) for 4 days only modestly decreased the INR from 3.1 to 2.8 on day 4. Decreasing the dietary intake of vitamin K_1 by 80% (from 118 to 26 micrograms daily) for 4 days increased the INR from just 2.6 to 3.3 on day 7.[24]

(b) Stability of anticoagulant control and dietary vitamin K

There is some evidence that patients with a very low dietary vitamin K_1 intake are more sensitive to alterations in vitamin K_1 intake, and have less stable anticoagulant control. For example, in one study, patients with unstable control of anticoagulation were found to have a much lower dietary intake of vitamin K_1, when compared with another group of patients with stable anticoagulant control (29 micrograms daily versus 76 micrograms daily).[25] In another study in 10 patients with poorly controlled anticoagulation taking **acenocoumarol**, and receiving a diet with a low, controlled vitamin K_1 content of 20 to 40 micrograms daily increased the percentage of INR values within the therapeutic range, when compared with a control group of 10 patients not subjected to any dietary restrictions.[26]

Importance and management

A very well established, well documented and clinically important drug-food interaction, expected to occur with every coumarin or indanedione anticoagulant because they have a common mode of action. The evidence suggests that, in patients with normal vitamin K_1 status, in general, clinically relevant changes in coagulation status require large continued changes in intake of vitamin K_1 from foods. However, there is some evidence to suggest that patients with low dietary vitamin K_1 intake may be sensitive to smaller changes in dietary vitamin K_1. This suggests that patients taking anticoagulants should be advised to eat a normal balanced diet, maintaining a relatively consistent amount of vitamin-K_1 rich foods. They should be told to avoid making major changes to their diet, including starting a weight-loss diet, without increased monitoring of their INR. It is estimated that a normal Western diet contains 300 to 500 micrograms of vitamin K_1 daily. The minimum daily requirement is about 1 micrograms/kg and, in the US, an adequate intake has been determined to be 120 micrograms for adult men and 90 micrograms daily for adult women. 'Table 12.3', (p.407), gives the vitamin K_1 content of some vitamin-K_1 rich foods; however, it is important to note that these are not the bioavailable contents, which may be much lower for green vegetables, particularly if they are eaten in the absence of fat.[18,27] Nevertheless, green leafy vegetables usually contribute 40 to 50% of the total intake, followed by certain vegetable oils and margarines made from these oils.[28] Also, processed foods can have moderate to high vitamin K_1 levels if they contain fats with high vitamin K_1 levels. Note that some foods that have a low vitamin K_1 content can contribute significantly to total intake because of how often they are eaten. Cooking and freezing do not alter the vitamin K_1 content, but vitamin K_1 in oils is degraded by exposure to light.[29] In the US, a chart has been devised to help patients and researchers determine the daily intake of vitamin K_1.[30]

For the effect of multivitamins containing vitamin K_1, see 'Coumarins + Dietary supplements; Vitamin K_1–containing', p.401, and for the effect of supplements in enteral and parenteral feeds, see 'Coumarins and related drugs + Foods; Enteral and parenteral nutrition', p.406.

There is growing evidence that vitamin K_2 substances (menaquinones) may also be important, and in one analysis rich dietary sources of these included goose liver paste, hard and soft cheeses, egg yolk,[18] and 'natto', (p.408), the effect of which is already established.

1. Blickstein D, Shaklai M, Inbal A. Warfarin antagonism by avocado. *Lancet* (1991) 337, 914–15.
2. Taylor JR, Wilt VM. Probable antagonism of warfarin by green tea. *Ann Pharmacother* (1999) 33, 426–8.
3. Booth SL, Madabushi HT, Davidson KW, Sadowski JA. Tea and coffee brews are not dietary sources of vitamin K-1 (phylloquinone). *J Am Diet Assoc* (1995) 95, 82–3.
4. Greenblatt DJ, von Moltke LL, Perloff ES, Luo Y, Harmatz JS, Zinny MA. Interaction of flurbiprofen with cranberry juice, grape juice, tea, and fluconazole: in vitro and clinical studies. *Clin Pharmacol Ther* (2006) 79, 125–33.
5. Pedersen FM, Hamberg O, Hess K, Ovesen L. The effect of dietary vitamin K on warfarin-induced anticoagulation. *J Intern Med* (1991) 229, 517–20.
6. Udall JA, Krock LB. A modified method of anticoagulant therapy. *Curr Ther Res* (1968) 10, 207–11.
7. Udall JA. Human sources and absorption of vitamin K in relation to anticoagulation stability. *JAMA* (1965) 194, 127–9.
8. Ovesen L, Lyduch S, Idorn ML. The effect of a diet rich in brussel sprouts on warfarin pharmacokinetics. *Eur J Clin Pharmacol* (1988) 33, 521–3.
9. Anon. Leafy vegetables in diet alter prothrombin time in patients taking anticoagulant drugs. *JAMA* (1964) 187, 27.
10. Qureshi GD, Reinders P, Swint JJ, Slate MB. Acquired warfarin resistance and weight-reducing diet. *Arch Intern Med* (1981) 141, 507–9.
11. Kempin SJ. Warfarin resistance caused by broccoli. *N Engl J Med* (1983) 308, 1229–30.
12. Chow WH, Chow TC, Tse TM, Tai YT, Lee WT. Anticoagulation instability with life-threatening complication after dietary modification. *Postgrad Med J* (1990) 66, 855–7.
13. Walker FB. Myocardial infarction after diet-induced warfarin resistance. *Arch Intern Med* (1984) 144, 2089–90.
14. Karlson B, Leijd B, Hellström A. On the influence of vitamin K-rich vegetables and wine on the effectiveness of warfarin treatment. *Acta Med Scand* (1986) 220, 347–50.
15. Schurgers LJ, Shearer MJ, HamulyáK K, Stöcklin E, Vermeer C. Effect of vitamin K intake on the stability of oral anticoagulant treatment: dose-response relationships in healthy subjects. *Blood* (2004) 104, 2682–9.
16. Kalra PA, Cooklin M, Wood G, O'Shea GM, Holmes AM. Dietary modification as a cause of anticoagulation instability. *Lancet* (1988) ii, 803.
17. Shearer MJ, Bach A, Kohlmeier M. Chemistry, nutritional sources, tissue distribution and metabolism of vitamin K with special reference to bone health. *J Nutr* (1996) 126, 1181S–1186S.
18. Schurgers LJ, Vermeer C. Determination of phylloquinone and menaquinones in food. Effect of food matrix on circulating vitamin K concentrations. *Haemostasis* (2000) 30, 298–307.
19. Bartle WR, Madorin P, Ferland G. Seaweed, vitamin K, and warfarin. *Am J Health-Syst Pharm* (2001) 58, 2300.
20. Flannery EP, MacDonald BS, O'Leary DS, McGinty JM. Japanese-restaurant syndrome. *N Engl J Med* (1971) 285, 414.
21. Lubetsky A, Dekel-Stern E, Chetrit A, Lubin F, Halkin H. Vitamin K intake and sensitivity to warfarin in patients consuming regular diets. *Thromb Haemost* (1999) 81, 396–9.
22. Couris R, Tataronis G, McCloskey W, Oertel L, Dallal G, Dwyer J, Blumberg JB. Dietary vitamin K variability affects International normalized ratio (INR) coagulation indices. *Int J Vitam Nutr Res* (2006) 76, 65–74.
23. Khan T, Wynne H, Wood P, Torrance A, Hankey C, Avery P, Kesteven P, Kamali F. Dietary vitamin K influences intra-individual variability in anticoagulant response to warfarin. *Br J Haematol* (2004) 124, 348–54.
24. Franco V, Polanczyk CA, Clausell N, Rohde LE. Role of dietary vitamin K intake in chronic oral anticoagulation: prospective evidence from observational and randomized protocols. *Am J Med* (2004) 116, 651–6.
25. Sconce E, Khan T, Mason J, Noble F, Wynne H, Kamali F. Patients with unstable control have a poorer dietary intake of vitamin K compared to patients with stable control of anticoagulation. *Thromb Haemost* (2005) 93, 872–5.
26. Sorano GG, Biondi G, Conti M, Mameli G, Licheri D, Marongiu F. Controlled vitamin K content diet for improving the management of poorly controlled anticoagulated patients: a clinical practice proposal. *Haemostasis* (1993) 23, 77–82.
27. Gijsbers BLMG, Jie K-SG, Vermeer C. Effect of food composition on vitamin K absorption in human volunteers. *Br J Nutr* (1996) 76, 223–9.
28. Booth SL, Suttie JW. Dietary intake and adequacy of vitamin K. *J Nutr* (1998) 128, 785–8.
29. Booth SL, Centurelli MA. Vitamin K: a practical guide to the dietary management of patients on warfarin. *Nutr Rev* (1999) 57, 288–96.
30. Couris RR, Tataronis GR, Booth SL, Dallal GE, Blumberg JB, Dwyer JT. Development of a self-assessment instrument to determine daily intake and variability of dietary vitamin K. *J Am Coll Nutr* (2000) 19, 801–6.

Coumarins + Glucagon

In one early analysis, the anticoagulant effects of warfarin were markedly increased by very large doses of glucagon (total dose exceeding 50 mg over 2 days), but not by doses of less than 30 mg over 1 to 2 days. Doses of glucagon this high are unlikely to be encountered in clinical use.

Clinical evidence

In an analysis of 24 patients taking **warfarin** who were given glucagon for inadequate cardiac contractility, no potentiation of the action of **warfarin** was noted in 11 patients given a total of less than 30 mg of glucagon over 1 to 2 days. However, 8 out of 9 patients had a marked increase in anticoagulant effects (prothrombin times of 30 to 50 seconds or more) when they were given higher doses of glucagon (62 to 362 mg over 3 to 8 days). Three of them bled. The interaction was not able to be assessed in 4 patients.[1]

Mechanism

Unknown. Changes in the production of blood clotting factors and an increase in the affinity of warfarin for its site of action have been proposed.[1] A study in *guinea pigs* using acenocoumarol suggested that changes in warfarin metabolism or its absorption from the gut are *not* responsible.[2]

Importance and management

Direct information is limited to the report cited,[1] which relates to doses far in excess of those used clinically for hypoglycaemia (1 mg) or in the management of beta blocker overdose (2 to 10 mg then 50 micrograms/kg per hour). As such, its findings are probably of no general relevance. Its authors recommend that if glucagon 25 mg per day or more is given for two or more days, the dosage of warfarin should be reduced in anticipation of the interaction, and prothrombin times closely monitored.[1]

1. Koch-Weser J. Potentiation by glucagon of the hypoprothrombinemic action of warfarin. *Ann Intern Med* (1970) 72, 331–5.
2. Weiner M, Moses D. The effect of glucagon and insulin on the prothrombin response to coumarin anticoagulants. *Proc Soc Exp Biol Med* (1968) 127, 761–3.

Coumarins + Glutethimide

The anticoagulant effects of warfarin and ethyl biscoumacetate can be decreased by glutethimide.

Clinical evidence

Ten subjects stabilised on **warfarin**, with average prothrombin times of 18.8 seconds, had a mean reduction of 2.7 seconds in their prothrombin times after they took glutethimide 500 mg at bedtime for 4 weeks.[1,2] Other studies have shown that up to 1 g of glutethimide daily for 1 to 3 weeks reduced the half-life of single-dose **warfarin** by between one-third to one-half.[3,4] Conversely, an unexplained report describes a paradoxical increase in prothrombin times and severe bruising in a patient stabilised on **warfarin** who took 3.5 g of glutethimide over a 5-day period.[5]

Glutethimide 500 or 750 mg daily for 10 days has been shown to reduce the half-life of single-dose **ethyl biscoumacetate** by about one-third,[6,7] whereas in contrast, an early study in 25 patients taking **ethyl biscoumacetate** found no evidence of an interaction.[8]

Mechanism

Glutethimide is a liver enzyme inducer, which increases the metabolism and clearance of the anticoagulants from the body, thereby reducing their effects.[1-4,6,7] There is no obvious explanation for the reports finding no interaction or increased effects.

Importance and management

The interaction of glutethimide with warfarin is established, while the interaction with ethyl biscoumacetate is uncertain. Information about both interactions is limited and there seems to be nothing documented about any other anticoagulant. However, it would be prudent to monitor the effect of adding glutethimide to patients taking any coumarin anticoagulant, being alert for the need to increase the anticoagulant dosage. Other interactions due to enzyme induction can take several weeks to develop fully and persist after withdrawal, so good monitoring and dosage adjustment should continue until anticoagulant stability has been achieved. The benzodiazepines may be a useful non-interacting alternative, see 'Coumarins + Benzodiazepines and related drugs', p.391.

1. Udall JA. Clinical implications of warfarin interactions with five sedatives. *Am J Cardiol* (1975) 35, 67–71.
2. Udall JA. Warfarin interactions with chloral hydrate and glutethimide. *Curr Ther Res* (1975) 17, 67–74.
3. Corn M. Effect of phenobarbital and glutethimide on biological half-life of warfarin. *Thromb Diath Haemorrh* (1966) 16, 606–12.
4. MacDonald MG, Robinson DS, Sylwester D, Jaffe JJ. The effects of phenobarbital, chloral betaine, and glutethimide administration on warfarin plasma levels and hypoprothrombinemic responses in man. *Clin Pharmacol Ther* (1969) 10, 80–4.
5. Taylor PJ. Hemorrhage while on anticoagulant therapy precipitated by drug interaction. *Ariz Med* (1967) 24, 697–9.
6. van Dam FE, Gribnau-Overkamp MJH. The effect of some sedatives (phenobarbital, glutethimide, chlordiazepoxide, chloral hydrate) on the rate of disappearance of ethyl biscoumacetate from the plasma. *Folia Med Neerl* (1967) 10, 141–5.
7. van Dam FE, Overkamp M, Haanen C. The interaction of drugs. *Lancet* (1966) ii, 1027.
8. Grilli H. Gluthetimida y tiempo de protrombina. Su aplicación en la terapéutica anticoagulante. *Prensa Med Argent* (1959) 46, 2867–9.

Coumarins + Grapefruit juice

Preliminary evidence from one study suggests that grapefruit juice might cause a modest rise in the INR of a few patients taking warfarin, and one case report describes a marked rise in INR, which was attributed to grapefruit juice. However, other studies have suggested that grapefruit juice does not interact with warfarin or acenocoumarol.

Clinical evidence

(a) Acenocoumarol

In the preliminary report of a single-dose, placebo-controlled study in 12 healthy subjects, 150 mL of grapefruit juice did not alter the maximum INR of a 10-mg dose of acenocoumarol, and the AUCs of *S*- and *R*-acenocoumarol were not altered.[1,2]

(b) Warfarin

In a study in 9 patients stabilised on warfarin, consumption of grapefruit juice 240 mL three times daily for one week had no effect on the INR or prothrombin times.[3] Similarly, in the preliminary report of a two-way crossover study in 24 patients stabilised on warfarin, the frequency of the **warfarin** dosage adjustments needed by the group as a whole, when taking 250 mL grapefruit juice daily for 4 weeks was the same as when taking a placebo (orange juice). However, 4 individuals had a clinically significant, progressive and sustained 12 to 25% decrease in the warfarin dose to INR ratio when taking grapefruit juice, but not orange juice.[4] A 64-year-old man stabilised on warfarin was found to have an INR of 6.29 on routine testing 10 days after starting to drink about 1.5 litres of grapefruit juice daily. However, when the author took warfarin to achieve an INR of 2 to 3 and then drank 1.5 litres of grapefruit juice daily there was no clinically relevant change in his INR.[5]

Mechanism

The patients who showed some evidence of an interaction between grapefruit juice and warfarin may possibly have had an increased susceptibility to the inhibitory effects of grapefruit juice on the activity of the cytochrome P450 isoenzyme CYP3A4 in the gut.[4]

Importance and management

Information is limited. One study with warfarin suggests that some patients might require a slight reduction in dose if they regularly consume grapefruit juice, but further study is needed. Current evidence suggests that routine testing should be sufficient to detect any interaction.

1. van Rooij J, van der Meer FJM, Schoemaker HC, Cohen AF. Comparison of the effect of grapefruit juice and cimetidine on pharmacokinetics and anticoagulant effect of a single dose of acenocoumarol. *Br J Clin Pharmacol* (1993) 35, 548P.
2. van der Meer FJM. Personal communication, April 1994.
3. Sullivan DM, Ford MA, Boyden TW. Grapefruit juice and the response to warfarin. *Am J Health-Syst Pharm* (1998) 55, 1581–3.
4. Dresser GK, Munoz C, Cruikshank M, Kovacs M, Spence JD. Grapefruit juice-warfarin interaction in anticoagulated patients. *Clin Pharmacol Ther* (1999) 65, 193.
5. Bartle WR. Grapefruit juice might still be factor in warfarin response. *Am J Health-Syst Pharm* (1999) 56, 676.

Coumarins + Griseofulvin

The anticoagulant effects of warfarin might be reduced by griseofulvin in some patients.

Clinical evidence

The anticoagulant effects of **warfarin** were modestly and markedly reduced, respectively, in 2 patients stabilised on **warfarin** when they were given griseofulvin 1 g daily in divided doses. Griseofulvin 1 g daily had no effect on the prothrombin time in one healthy subject given warfarin, whereas 2 g daily caused a marked reduction in the prothrombin time. Another healthy subject showed no interaction, even when the griseofulvin dosage was raised to 4 g daily for 2 weeks.[1]

In another study there was no change in the mean prothrombin time in 10 patients stabilised on **warfarin** when they were given griseofulvin 1 g daily in divided doses for 2 weeks. Four of the patients had an equivocal average reduction in prothrombin time of 4.2 seconds.[2] One case report describes decreased anticoagulant effects in a man stabilised on **warfarin** when he took griseofulvin 250 mg twice daily, which took 12 weeks to develop fully.[3] He eventually needed a 41% increase in his daily dose of **warfarin**. Another report very briefly mentions a case of a coagulation defect in a patient taking **warfarin** and griseofulvin.[4]

Mechanism

Not understood. It has been suggested that the griseofulvin acts as a liver enzyme inducer, which increases the metabolism of the warfarin, thereby reducing its effects.[1,3]

Importance and management

This interaction is poorly documented and not well established. It possibly affects some patients. Because of the uncertainty, the prothrombin times of all patients taking warfarin who are given griseofulvin should be monitored, and suitable warfarin dosage increases made as necessary.

1. Cullen SI, Catalano PM. Griseofulvin-warfarin antagonism. *JAMA* (1967) 199, 582–3.
2. Udall JA. Drug interference with warfarin therapy. *Clin Med* (1970) 77, 20–5.
3. Okino K, Weibert RT. Warfarin-griseofulvin interaction. *Drug Intell Clin Pharm* (1986) 20, 291–3.
4. McQueen EG. New Zealand Committee on Adverse Drug Reactions: 14th Annual Report 1979. *N Z Med J* (1980) 91, 226–9.

Coumarins and related drugs + H_2-receptor antagonists

The anticoagulant effects of warfarin can be increased by cimetidine. The effect is generally minor to modest, although severe bleeding has been reported in a few cases. Acenocoumarol seems to interact similarly, but phenprocoumon appears not to be affected. In one patient the effects of phenindione were modestly increased by cimetidine. Famotidine, nizatidine, ranitidine and roxatidine normally do not appear to interact, although isolated cases of bleeding have been reported.

Clinical evidence

(a) Cimetidine

A brief report in 1978, published as a letter by the manufacturers of cimetidine, stated that preliminary details of a study in healthy subjects indicated that cimetidine 1 g daily could cause a prothrombin time rise of about 20% in patients stabilised on **warfarin**. At that time, they were aware of 17 cases worldwide, most of moderate rises in prothrombin times.[1]

A number of studies[2,3] and case reports[4-8] have confirmed this interaction with **warfarin**. In the studies, plasma **warfarin** levels were reported to rise by 25% and 80%, and prothrombin times were increased by 18% and 20% by cimetidine 1.2 g daily. In the case reports, severe bleeding (haematuria, internal haemorrhages) and very prolonged prothrombin times have been seen in few patients given cimetidine 900 mg or 1.2 g daily.[4,6-8] In one study, 7 out of 14 patients stabilised on **warfarin** had a greater than 30 second increase in their prothrombin time, whereas the other 7 had no prolongation or only a minor prolongation in their prothrombin time when they were given cimetidine 1.2 g daily for 10 days.[9] In another study in 27 patients, although the AUC of **warfarin** was increased by 21 to 39% and its clearance fell by 22 to 28%, prothrombin times only increased by 2 to 2.6 seconds by cimetidine 800 mg or 1.2 g daily.[10] A pharmacokinetic study in 6 healthy subjects found that cimetidine did not affect *S*-warfarin but increased the trough plasma levels of *R*-warfarin by 28%, with minimal effect on prothrombin times.[11] Other pharmacokinetic studies have confirmed that the interaction affects only *R*-warfarin.[12-15] In one analysis of combined use of **warfarin** and H_2-receptor antagonists in inpatients, there was no difference in the intensity of prothrombin time monitoring, and no difference in bleeding rates between 35 patients receiving cimetidine, 38 patients receiving ranitidine, or 36 patients receiving famotidine. Two patients in the cimetidine group had a bleed after they had taken both drugs for one or two days but neither had abnormally high prothrombin times.[16]

In 3 studies, the AUC of single-dose **acenocoumarol** was increased by cimetidine, and the prothrombin time prolonged,[17-19] with the effect greatest for *R*-acenocoumarol.[19] However, another study found no interaction.[20] Data from one patient taking **acenocoumarol** and one taking **phenindione** showed that cimetidine increased their anticoagulant effects.[2] In one study in patients stabilised on **phenprocoumon**, cimetidine 400 mg twice daily did not alter the pharmacokinetics of **phenprocoumon** nor its anticoagulant effect.[21]

(b) Famotidine

In a study in 8 healthy subjects taking doses of **warfarin** titrated to prolong the prothrombin time by 2 to 5 seconds (mean dose 4 mg daily), treatment with famotidine 40 mg daily for 7 days did not affect prothrombin times, thrombotest coagulation times or steady-state plasma **warfarin** levels.[22] No changes in prothrombin times were seen in 3 patients stabilised on **acenocoumarol** or **fluindione** when they were given famotidine.[23] However, in another report 2 patients taking **warfarin** are said to have had prolonged prothrombin times and bled when they took famotidine.[24]

(c) Nizatidine

Nizatidine 300 mg daily for 2 weeks had no significant effect on the prothrombin times, kaolin-cephalin clotting times, the activity of factors II, VII, XI and X, or on steady-state serum **warfarin** levels in 7 healthy subjects taking warfarin.[25] A lack of a pharmacokinetic interaction was also reported in the preliminary results of another study.[26] An isolated case of gastrointestinal bleeding, associated with markedly prolonged prothrombin times, occurred after a 78-year-old took six doses of nizatidine 300 mg.[24]

(d) Ranitidine

Ranitidine 200 mg twice daily for 2 weeks had no effect on **warfarin** concentrations or prothrombin times in 5 healthy subjects.[27] In another study in 11 healthy subjects, ranitidine 150 mg twice daily for 3 days had no effect on the pharmacodynamics or pharmacokinetics of a single dose of **warfarin**.[3] The same finding was reported in another similar study.[15] In contrast, in a fourth study in 5 subjects, ranitidine 150 mg twice daily for a week reduced the clearance of a single dose of **warfarin** by almost 30%, but the half-life was not significantly changed and prothrombin times were not measured.[28] Ranitidine 750 mg daily given to 2 subjects reduced the **warfarin** clearance by more than 50%.[28] In an isolated case, a patient stabilised on ranitidine 150 mg twice daily and **warfarin** vomited blood one week after her ranitidine dose was doubled to 300 mg twice daily. Her prothrombin time had risen from 17.6 to 36.7 seconds. She was subsequently restabilised on ranitidine 150 mg twice daily and the original dose of warfarin with a prothrombin time between 19 and 20 seconds.[29]

In one study in 10 patients stabilised on **phenprocoumon**, ranitidine 150 mg twice daily for 14 days had no effect on anticoagulation or on phenprocoumon plasma levels.[30]

(e) Roxatidine

Roxatidine 150 mg daily for 4 days had no effect on the steady-state pharmacokinetics of **warfarin** or the prothrombin ratio in 12 healthy subjects.[31]

Mechanism

Cimetidine binds with the cytochrome P450 isoenzymes and inhibits oxidative metabolism in the liver. Although cimetidine is considered to be a general inhibitor, it exhibits a degree of specificity for certain isoenzymes such as CYP1A2 and CYP2C19. These isoenzymes are principally involved in the metabolism of *R*-warfarin and not *S*-warfarin (see 'metabolism of the coumarins', (p.358), for more detail). Thus, the interaction between warfarin and cimetidine has been found to be stereoselective (i.e. cimetidine interacts with the *R*-isomer but not with the *S*-isomer).[11-14] Because *R*-warfarin is the less active isomer, and the pharmacokinetic interaction is not marked, the interaction is generally modest.

Cimetidine also appears to interact with acenocoumarol, but not phenprocoumon. The other H_2-receptor antagonists normally do not act as enzyme inhibitors.

Importance and management

The interaction between warfarin and cimetidine is well documented, well established and potentially clinically important. Its effects are generally modest, but rarely, patients have shown a marked interaction. Because of this unpredictability, and to avoid bleeding, the response should be monitored well in every patient when cimetidine is first added, being alert for the need to reduce the warfarin dosage. The onset of the interaction appears rapid; effects have been seen within days,[4,7] and even as early as 24 hours.[9] The effect of low non-prescription doses of cimetidine on warfarin do not appear to have been studied. Acenocoumarol is reported to interact similarly, and there is one case of phenindione being affected. Expect other coumarins and indanediones to behave in the same way, with the possible exception of phenprocoumon, which was not affected in one study.

Famotidine, nizatidine, ranitidine and roxatidine normally appear not to interact with oral anticoagulants although note that, in rare cases, increases in prothrombin times and bleeding have been seen.

1. Flind AC. Cimetidine and oral anticoagulants. *Lancet* (1978) ii, 1054.
2. Serlin MJ, Sibeon RG, Mossman S, Breckenridge AM, Williams JRB, Atwood JL, Willoughby JMT. Cimetidine: interaction with oral anticoagulants in man. *Lancet* (1979) ii, 317–19.

3. O'Reilly RA. Comparative interaction of cimetidine and ranitidine with racemic warfarin in man. *Arch Intern Med* (1984) 144, 989–91.
4. Silver BA, Bell WR. Cimetidine potentiation of the hypoprothrombinemic effect of warfarin. *Ann Intern Med* (1979) 90, 348–9.
5. Hetzel D, Birkett D, Miners J. Cimetidine interaction with warfarin. *Lancet* (1979) ii, 639.
6. Wallin BA, Jacknowitz A, Raich PC. Cimetidine and effect of warfarin. *Ann Intern Med* (1979) 90, 993.
7. Kerley B, Ali M. Cimetidine potentiation of warfarin action. *Can Med Assoc J* (1982) 126, 116.
8. Devanesen S. Prolongation of prothrombin time with cimetidine. *Med J Aust* (1981) 1, 537.
9. Bell WR, Anderson KC, Noe DA, Silver BA. Reduction in the plasma clearance rate of warfarin induced by cimetidine. *Arch Intern Med* (1986) 146, 2325–8.
10. Sax MJ, Randolph WC, Peace KE, Chretien S, Frank WO, Braverman AJ, Gray DR, McCree LC, Wyle F, Jackson BJ, Beg MA, Young MD. Effect of two cimetidine regimens on prothrombin time and warfarin pharmacokinetics during long-term warfarin therapy. *Clin Pharm* (1987) 6, 492–5.
11. Niopas I, Toon S, Aarons L, Rowland M. The effect of cimetidine on the steady-state pharmacokinetics and pharmacodynamics of warfarin in humans. *Eur J Clin Pharmacol* (1999) 55, 399–404.
12. Choonara IA, Cholerton S, Haynes BP, Breckenridge AM, Park BK. Stereoselective interaction between the R enantiomer of warfarin and cimetidine. *Br J Clin Pharmacol* (1986) 21, 271–77.
13. Toon S, Hopkins KJ, Garstang FM, Diquet B, Gill TS, Rowland M. The warfarin-cimetidine interaction: stereochemical considerations. *Br J Clin Pharmacol* (1986) 21, 245–6.
14. Niopas I, Toon S, Rowland M. Further insight into the stereoselective interaction between warfarin and cimetidine in man. *Br J Clin Pharmacol* (1991) 32, 508–11.
15. Toon S, Hopkins KJ, Garstang FM, Rowland M. Comparative effects of ranitidine and cimetidine on the pharmacokinetics and pharmacodynamics of warfarin in man. *Eur J Clin Pharmacol* (1987) 32, 165–72.
16. Greaney JJ, Souney PF, Scavone JM. A review of monitoring intensity and bleeding complications in hospitalized patients receiving concurrent warfarin and histamine$_2$ antagonist therapy. *J Pharmacoepidemiol* (1994) 3, 27–45.
17. van Rooij J, van der Meer FJM, Schoemaker HC, Cohen AF. Comparison of the effect of grapefruit juice and cimetidine on pharmacokinetics and anticoagulant effect of a single dose of acenocoumarol. *Br J Clin Pharmacol* (1993) 35, 548P.
18. Kroon C, de Boer A, Hoogkamer JFW, Schoemaker HC, vd Meer FJM, Edelbroek PM, Cohen AF. Detection of drug interactions with single dose acenocoumarol: new screening method? *Int J Clin Pharmacol Ther Toxicol* (1990) 28, 355–60.
19. Gill TA, Hopkins KJ, Bottomley J, Gupta SK, Rowland M. Cimetidine-nicoumalone interaction in man: stereochemical considerations. *Br J Clin Pharmacol* (1989) 27, 469–74.
20. Thijssen HHW, Janssen GMJ, Baars LGM. Lack of effect of cimetidine on pharmacodynamics and kinetics of single oral doses of R- and S-acenocoumarol. *Eur J Clin Pharmacol* (1986) 30, 619–23.
21. Harenberg J, Staiger C, de Vries JX, Walter E, Weber E, Zimmermann R. Cimetidine does not increase the anticoagulant effect of phenprocoumon. *Br J Clin Pharmacol* (1982) 14, 292–3.
22. De Lepeleire I, van Hecken A, Verbesselt R, Tjandra-Maga TB, Buntinx A, Distlerath L, De Schepper PJ. Lack of interaction between famotidine and warfarin. *Int J Clin Pharmacol Res* (1990) 10, 167–71.
23. Chichmanian RM, Mignot G, Spreux A, Jean-Girard C, Hofliger P. Tolérance de la famotidine. Étude du réseau médecins sentinelles en pharmacovigilance. *Therapie* (1992) 47, 239–43.
24. Shinn AF. Unrecognized drug interactions with famotidine and nizatidine. *Arch Intern Med* (1991) 151, 814.
25. Cournot A, Berlin I, Sallord JC, Singlas E. Lack of interaction between nizatidine and warfarin during chronic administration. *J Clin Pharmacol* (1988) 28, 1120–2.
26. Callaghan JT, Nyhart EH. Drug interactions between H_2-blockers and theophylline (T) or warfarin (W). *Pharmacologist* (1988) 30, A14.
27. Serlin MJ, Sibeon RG, Breckenridge AM. Lack of effect of ranitidine on warfarin action. *Br J Clin Pharmacol* (1981) 12, 791–4.
28. Desmond PV, Mashford ML, Harman PJ, Morphett BJ, Breen KJ, Wang YM. Decreased oral warfarin clearance after ranitidine and cimetidine. *Clin Pharmacol Ther* (1984) 35, 338–41.
29. Baciewicz AM, Morgan PJ. Ranitidine-warfarin interaction. *Ann Intern Med* (1990) 112, 76–7.
30. Harenberg J, Zimmermann R, Kommerell B, Weber E. Interaktion von Ranitidin mit oralen Antikoagulantien. *Dtsch Med Wochenschr* (1983) 108, 1536.
31. Bender W, Brockmeier D. Pharmacokinetic characteristics of roxatadine. *J Clin Gastroenterol* (1989) 11 (Suppl 1), S6–S19.

Coumarins + Heparin

Heparin may prolong the prothrombin time, therefore a sufficient time interval should be allowed after the last heparin dose in a patient taking a coumarin to obtain a valid prothrombin time.

Clinical evidence, mechanism, importance and management

Heparin may prolong the one-stage prothrombin time.[1] The US manufacturer notes that, if a valid prothrombin time is to be obtained in a patient starting **warfarin** or other coumarins, a period of a least 5 hours after the last intravenous heparin dose or 24 hours after the last subcutaneous dose should be left before measuring the prothrombin time.[2] Note that it is usual clinical practice to start heparin and a coumarin anticoagulant at the same time. Further, it is clear that the concurrent use of warfarin and heparin will have an at least additive anticoagulant effect.

1. Lutomski DM, Djuric PE, Draeger RW. Warfarin therapy: the effect of heparin on prothrombin times. *Arch Intern Med* (1987) 147, 432–3.
2. Heparin Sodium Injection. Pharmacia & Upjohn. US Prescribing information, December 2000.

Coumarins and related drugs + Heparinoids

Some of the normal tests of anticoagulation (prothrombin time, thrombotest) are unreliable for a few hours after giving intravenous danaparoid to patients taking coumarins.
Oral pentosan polysulfate sodium did not alter the pharmacokinetics or pharmacodynamics of warfarin in healthy subjects, but note that this heparinoid is associated with rectal bleeding.
An isolated case report describes bleeding in a patient taking acenocoumarol after a heparinoid-impregnated bandage was applied.
In general, the use of heparinoids with coumarins or indanediones would be expected to increase the risk of bleeding.

Clinical evidence, mechanism, importance and management

(a) Intravenous danaparoid

A study in 6 healthy subjects given **acenocoumarol** (steady-state thrombotest values of 10 to 15%), found that a single intravenous bolus injection of 3250 anti-Xa units of danaparoid prolonged the prothrombin time and thrombotest for up to 1 hour and 5 hours, respectively, which was more than would have been expected by the simple addition of the effects of both drugs. However, no significant differences were seen in bleeding time, and danaparoid did not alter **acenocoumarol** pharmacokinetics.[1] The authors concluded that when monitoring the anticoagulant effects of **acenocoumarol**, the prothrombin time and the thrombotest may therefore be unreliable for at least one hour and five hours, respectively, after intravenous danaparoid has been given. This advice would apply equally to other coumarins and other drugs monitored using these tests, such as the indanediones.

(b) Oral pentosan polysulfate sodium

In a placebo-controlled, crossover study in 24 healthy subjects stabilised on **warfarin**, pentosan polysulfate sodium 100 mg every 8 hours for 7 days did not alter the anticoagulant effect of **warfarin** or the pharmacokinetics of *R*- or *S*-warfarin.[2] The authors consider it appears that, unlike intravenous administration, oral pentosan polysulfate sodium has no anticoagulant activity. However, the manufacturer notes that rectal haemorrhage was reported as an adverse effect in 6.3% of patients receiving pentosan polysulfate sodium at a dose of 300 mg daily.[3]

On the basis of the pharmacological study, the authors considered that it seems unnecessary to make changes in the warfarin dose or the oral pentosan polysulfate sodium dose when the two drugs are used together. However, they do recommend careful monitoring on starting concurrent therapy.[2] Logic would suggest that, if bleeding occurs, this could be more severe in anticoagulated patients. The patient information provided by the manufacturer states that concurrent use of pentosan polysulfate and warfarin should be avoided until they have spoken with their doctor.[3]

(c) Topical heparinoid

A man who was well stabilised on **acenocoumarol** and also taking metoprolol, dipyridamole and isosorbide dinitrate began to bleed within about 3 days of starting to use a medicated bandage on an inflamed lesion on his hand, probably caused by a mosquito bite. His prothrombin percentage was found to have fallen to less than 10%. The bandage was impregnated with a semi-synthetic heparinoid compound based on **xylane acid polysulfate** [possibly pentosan polysulfate].[4] It would appear that enough of the heparinoid had been absorbed through his skin to increase his anticoagulation to the point where he began to bleed. This case is unusual but it illustrates the need to keep a close watch on patients who are given several drugs that can potentially cause bleeding.

1. Stiekema JCJ, de Boer A, Danhof M, Kroon C, Broekmans AW, van Dinther TG, Voerman J, Breimer DD. Interaction of the combined medication with the new low-molecular-weight heparinoid Lomoparan® (Org 10172) and acenocoumarol. *Haemostasis* (1990) 20,136–46.
2. Modi NB, Kell S, Simon M, Vargas R. Pharmacokinetics and pharmacodynamics of warfarin when coadministered with pentosan polysulfate sodium. *J Clin Pharmacol* (2005) 45, 919–26.
3. Elmiron (Pentosan polysulfate sodium). Ortho-McNeil Pharmaceutical, Inc. US Prescribing information, September 2006.
4. Potel G, Maulaz B, Pabœuf C, Touze MD, Baron D. Potentialisation de l'acénocoumarol après application cutanée d'un héparinoïde semi-synthétique. *Therapie* (1989) 44, 67–8.

Coumarins + Herbal medicines

Many of the interactions of herbal medicines (health foods, dietary supplements) with warfarin in the published literature are solely hypothetical based on the postulated pharmacological effects of known chemical constituents of the plants. These mechanisms are discussed further below. Where specific clinical data on a herbal medicine interaction with warfarin are available, this is covered in a separate monograph.

All patients should be encouraged to report their use of herbal medicines and food supplements and cases of uneventful concurrent use should be published as well as cases of possible interactions to increase the clinical information available.

Clinical evidence and mechanism

(a) Antiplatelet effects

Antiplatelet doses of 'aspirin', (p.385), do not alter the anticoagulant efficacy of warfarin (INR); however, these doses of aspirin by themselves increase the risk of gastrointestinal bleeding, and the risk of this is higher in patients taking warfarin. On this basis, many herbs with antiplatelet activity *in vitro* are postulated to interact with warfarin, including 'ginger', (p.416) and 'garlic', (p.415). To establish the increased risk with antiplatelet doses of aspirin with warfarin, very large studies were needed because the absolute risks are small (about 1 in 100 in one study). Studies of this size are very unlikely to be conducted with herbals. One way might be to compare the *in vivo* antiplatelet activity of the herbal product with that of aspirin 75 mg, and then to extrapolate to the likely increased risk of bleeding.

(b) Coumarin constituents

There is a misconception that if a plant contains natural coumarins it will have anticoagulant properties. More than 3400 coumarins occur naturally throughout at least 160 plant families. Of these, just 13 have been tested for antithrombotic or anticoagulant activity, and only about half (7) were found to be active.[1] There are no established interactions between warfarin and herbal medicines that have been attributed to the coumarin content of the herb. Even in the classic case of hemorrhagic death of livestock that led to the discovery of dicoumarol, it was the action of the mould on the coumarin in the sweet clover ('melilot', (p.417)) that led to the production of the anticoagulant, so consumption of a spoiled product would seem to be necessary for this interaction to occur. This suggests that the occurrence of coumarins in dietary supplements or herbal medicines should not trigger immediate concern.[1]

(c) Hepatic cytochrome P450 metabolism

St John's wort is the most well established example of a herb that can induce the metabolism of drugs, principally by the cytochrome P450 isoenzyme CYP3A4. This herb appears to have a modest effect on 'warfarin', (p.418), which might be clinically important. 'Danshen', (p.415) might interact by increasing the bioavailability of warfarin. No other herbs appear to have an established effect on the metabolism of warfarin.

(d) Vitamin K content

Vitamin K is found in highest levels in 'green leafy vegetables', (p.409), which, if ingested in sufficient quantities, can markedly reduce the effects of warfarin and related drugs. It would therefore not be surprising if many herbal medicines derived from dark green leaves contain vitamin K. However, whether enough of these herbs could be taken to cause an interaction seems less likely than with foods. Nevertheless, two case reports of altered coagulation status attributed to the vitamin K content of herbal preparations have been reported, see 'vitamin K', (p.418).

Importance and management

There are many reviews of the effect of various herbal medicines on warfarin. Most of these include interactions based on theoretical data, based on the knowledge that a plant has been shown to contain antiplatelet substances or coumarins. The problem with these lists is that a suggested interaction might never be clinically relevant if, for example, the coumarins present are found not to be anticoagulants, or the substances are found in such small quantities and the herb cannot be ingested in sufficient amounts to cause an interaction. With natural substances, there is also the problem of chemical variations between batches of product if they are not standardised. Moreover, even isolated reports of an interaction between a herbal medicine and warfarin cannot definitively establish that such an interaction exists (see also 'anticoagulant interactions', (p.358)).

Because of the potential for interactions, some consider that patients taking warfarin would be well advised to avoid all herbal medications. However, this approach may not be practical: there are many papers showing that patients taking warfarin do use a number of herbal medicines and dietary supplements (19.2% in a UK survey;[2] 26% in a Hong Kong survey[3]). If patients have been told to avoid all herbal products, they may be less likely to admit to their use, and become less cautious in the future if they discover that the use of one product is uneventful. It may be better to advise patients to discuss the use of any products they wish to try, and to increase monitoring if this is thought advisable. Cases of uneventful use should be reported, as they are as useful as possible cases of adverse use.

1. Booth NL, Nikolic D, van Breemen RB, Geller SE, Banuvar S, Shulman LP, Farnsworth NR. Confusion regarding anticoagulant coumarins in dietary supplements. *Clin Pharmacol Ther* (2004) 76, 511–16.
2. Simth L, Ernst E, Ewings P, Myers P, Smith C. Co-ingestion of herbal medicines and warfarin. *Br J Gen Pract* (2004) 54, 439–41.
3. Wong RSM, Cheng G, Chan TYK. Use of herbal medicines by patients receiving warfarin. *Drug Safety* (2003) 26, 585–8.

Coumarins + Herbal medicines; Boldo or Fenugreek

A report describes a woman taking warfarin whose INR rose modestly when she began to take boldo and fenugreek.

Clinical evidence, mechanism, importance and management

A woman taking **warfarin** for atrial fibrillation whose INR was normally within the range 2 to 3 had a modest rise in her INR to 3.4, apparently due to the use of 10 drops of boldo after meals and one capsule of fenugreek before meals. A week after stopping these two herbal medicines her INR had fallen to 2.6. When she restarted them, her INR rose to 3.1 after a week, and to 3.4 after 2 weeks. Her INR was later restabilised in her normal range in the presence of these two medicines by reducing the **warfarin** dosage by 15%.[1] The mechanism of this apparent interaction remains unknown, and it is not known whether both herbs or just one was responsible for what happened. Boldo comes from *Peumus boldus,* and might have antiplatelet activity, and fenugreek comes from *Trigonella foenum-graecum*, which might contain coumarins (but see 'Coumarins + Herbal medicines', above).

This patient had no undesirable reactions (e.g. bruising or bleeding), but this case serves to draw attention to the possibility of an interaction in other patients taking anticoagulants if these herbal medicines are also taken.

1. Lambert JP, Cormier A. Potential interaction between warfarin and boldo-fenugreek. *Pharmacotherapy* (2001) 21, 509–12.

Coumarins + Herbal medicines; Chamomile

A single case report describes a woman stabilised on warfarin who developed a marked increase in her INR with bleeding complications five days after she started using two chamomile products.

Clinical evidence

A 70-year-old woman stabilised on **warfarin** with an INR of 3.6 started drinking 4 to 5 cups of chamomile tea daily for chest congestion, and using a chamomile-based skin lotion 4 to 5 times daily for foot oedema. About 5 days later she developed ecchymoses and was found to have an INR of 7.9, a retroperitoneal haematoma and other internal haemorrhages.[1]

Mechanism

Both species of chamomile used medicinally (*Matricaria recutita* also known as *Matricaria chamomilla* or *Chamomilla recutita* and *Anthemis nobilis* also known as *Chamaemelum nobile*) are known to contain coumarins, but natural coumarins are not always anticoagulants, see 'Coumarins + Herbal medicines', above. There appear to be no reports of chamomile alone causing bleeding.

Importance and management

This appears to be the first report of an interaction between warfarin and chamomile, and it may be that it was due to excessive use of two chamomile-based products. It serves to draw attention to the possibility of an interaction in other patients taking anticoagulants if chamomile is used concurrently. Further study is needed. However, note that there appear to be no reports of chamomile alone causing anticoagulation, which might suggest that the risk of an additive effect is small.

1. Segal R, Pilote L. Warfarin interaction with *Matricaria chamomilla. Can Med Assoc J* (2006) 174, 1281–2.

Coumarins + Herbal medicines; *Curbicin*

The INR of one patient taking warfarin modestly increased after he took *Curbicin* (saw palmetto, cucurbita, and vitamin E). This product has also been associated with an increased INR in a patient not taking anticoagulants.

Clinical evidence, mechanism, importance and management

A 61-year-old man taking **warfarin** and simvastatin, with a stable INR of around 2.4, had an increase in his INR to 3.4 within 6 days of starting to take 5 tablets of *Curbicin* daily. Within a week of stopping the *Curbicin*, his INR had fallen to its previous value. Another elderly man who was not taking any anticoagulants and was taking 3 tablets of *Curbicin* daily was found to have an INR of 2.1 (normal 0.9 to 1.2). His INR improved (1.3 to 1.4) when he was given vitamin K, but did not normalise until a week after stopping the *Curbicin*. *Curbicin* is a herbal remedy used for micturition problems, and contains extracts from the fruit of *Serenoa repens* (**saw palmetto**) and the seed of ***Cucurbita pepo***.[1]

The authors of this report suggest that what happened was possibly due to the presence of vitamin E in the *Curbicin* preparation (each tablet contains 10 mg), but 'vitamin E', (p.401) does not normally affect INRs. The clinical significance of this interaction is unknown, but bear it in mind in the case of an unexpected response to treatment.

1. Yue, Q-Y, Jansson K. Herbal drug Curbicin and anticoagulant effect with and without warfarin: possibly related to the vitamin E component. *J Am Geriatr Soc* (2001) 49, 838.

Coumarins and related drugs + Herbal medicines; Danshen (*Salvia miltiorrhiza*)

Two case reports and some *animal* data indicate that *Danshen*, a Chinese herbal remedy, can increase the effects of warfarin, resulting in bleeding.

Clinical evidence

A woman who had undergone venous mitral valve valvuloplasty and who was taking furosemide, digoxin and **warfarin**, began to take *Danshen* (the root of *Salvia miltiorrhiza*) every other day for intermittent influenza-like symptoms. After about a month she was hospitalised with malaise, breathlessness and fever and was found to be both very anaemic and over-anticoagulated (prothrombin time greater than 60 seconds, INR greater than 5.62). The anaemia was attributed to occult gastrointestinal bleeding and the over-anticoagulation to an interaction with the *Danshen*. She was later restabilised on the **warfarin** in the absence of the *Danshen* with an INR of 2.5, and within 4 months her haemoglobin levels were normal.[1]

Another report describes a man taking **warfarin**, digoxin, captopril and furosemide with an INR of about 3, who developed chest pain and breathlessness about 2 weeks after starting to take *Danshen*. He was found to have a massive pleural effusion, which was later drained of blood, and an INR of more than 8.4. He was later discharged on his usual dose of **warfarin** with an INR stable at 3, in the absence of the *Danshen*.[2]

Mechanism

Not fully understood. Studies in *rats* show that *Danshen* can increase the bioavailability of both *R*- and *S*-warfarin thereby increasing its effects.[3]

It may affect haemostasis by inhibiting platelet aggregation and by interfering with extrinsic coagulation, and it also has antithrombin III-like activity and can promote fibrinolytic activity. The additive effects of these activities might be expected to result in bleeding complications.

Importance and management

Clinical information appears to be limited to these two case reports and one other, which also involved 'methyl salicylate', (p.457), which is also known to increase the effects of warfarin. This interaction is therefore not very well established but there is enough evidence to suggest that normally patients on warfarin should avoid *Danshen* (although with very careful monitoring and warfarin dosage adjustments safe concurrent use might be possible). More study is needed. Information about other oral anticoagulants is lacking but, given the proposed mechanism of interaction, it would seem sensible to take the same precautions if using any indanedione or coumarin.

1. Yu CM, Chan JCN, Sanderson JE. Chinese herbs and warfarin potentiation by 'Danshen'. *J Intern Med* (1997) 241, 337–9.
2. Izzat MB, Yim APC, El-Zufari MH. A taste of Chinese medicine. *Ann Thorac Surg* (1998) 66, 941–2.
3. Lo ACT, Chan K, Yeung JHK, Woo KS. The effects of Danshen (*Salvia miltiorrhiza*) on pharmacokinetics and dynamics of warfarin in rats. *Eur J Drug Metab Pharmacokinet* (1992) 17, 257–62.

Coumarins + Herbal medicines; Dong quai (*Angelica sinensis*)

Two case reports describe a very marked increase in the anticoagulant effects of warfarin when dong quai was given.

Clinical evidence, mechanism, importance and management

A 46-year-old African-American woman with atrial fibrillation taking **warfarin** had a greater than twofold increase in her prothrombin time and INR after taking dong quai for 4 weeks. The prothrombin time and INR were back to normal 4 weeks after stopping the dong quai.[1] Another woman who had been taking **warfarin** for 10 years developed widespread bruising and an INR of 10, a month after starting to take dong quai.[2]

The reasons are not understood but dong quai is known to consist of natural coumarin derivatives, which may possibly have anticoagulant properties and inhibit platelet aggregation, but note that not all natural coumarins are anticoagulants, see 'Coumarins + Herbal medicines', p.414.

These seem to be only reports of this apparent interaction, but patients taking **warfarin** should be warned of the potential risks of also taking dong quai. For safety dong quai should be avoided unless the effects on anticoagulation can be monitored. More study is needed.

1. Page RL, Lawrence JD. Potentiation of warfarin by dong quai. *Pharmacotherapy* (1999) 19, 870–6.
2. Ellis GR, Stephens MR. Untitled report. *BMJ* (1999) 319, 650.

Coumarins + Herbal medicines; Garlic

An isolated report described increases in the anticoagulant effects of warfarin in two patients taking garlic supplements. Garlic supplements alone have also rarely been associated with bleeding. However, in one study, aged garlic extract did not increase the INR or risk of bleeding in patients taking warfarin.

Clinical evidence

The INR of a patient stabilised on **warfarin** more than doubled and haematuria occurred 8 weeks after the patient started to take three *Höfels garlic pearles* daily. The situation resolved when the garlic was stopped. The INR rose on a later occasion while the patient was taking two *Kwai* garlic tablets daily. The INR of another patient was also more than doubled by six *Kwai* garlic tablets daily.[1,2]

In contrast, in a placebo-controlled study in 48 patients stabilised on **warfarin**, there was no change in INR or evidence of increased bleeding in those receiving 5 mL of aged garlic extract twice daily.[3] Similarly, in a preliminary report of the use of alternative and complementary medicines in 156 patients taking **warfarin**, there was no apparent increased risk or bleeding or raised INRs in 57 patients taking potentially interacting complementary medicines (garlic in 10%), compared with 84 who did not.[4]

Mechanism

Garlic has been associated with decreased platelet aggregation, which has on at least two documented occasions led to spontaneous bleeding in the absence of an anticoagulant.[5,6] These effects might therefore increase the risk of bleeding with anticoagulants, see also 'Coumarins + Herbal medicines', p.414.

Importance and management

Information about an adverse interaction between warfarin and garlic seems to be limited to these two cases from one author. Bearing in mind the wide-spread use of garlic and garlic products, and the limited information from the review,[4] and study with aged garlic extract,[3] it seems most unlikely that garlic usually has any generally important interaction with anticoagulants. Nevertheless, bear the possibility in mind in the event of an unexpected response to treatment.

1. Sunter W. Warfarin and garlic. *Pharm J* (1991) 246, 722.
2. Sunter W. Personal communication, July 1991.
3. Macan H, Uykimpang R, Alconcel M, Takasu J, Razon R, Amagase H, Niihara Y. Aged garlic extract may be safe for patients on warfarin therapy. *J Nutr* (2006) 136 (3 Suppl), 793S–795S.
4. Shalansky S, Neall E, Lo M, Abd-Elmessih E, Vickars L, Lynd L. The impact of complementary and alternative medicine use on warfarin-related adverse outcomes. *Pharmacotherapy* (2002) 22, 1345.
5. German K, Kumar U, Blackford HN. Garlic and the risk of TURP bleeding. *Br J Urol* (1995) 76, 518.
6. Rose KD, Croissant PD, Parliament CF, Levin MP. Spontaneous spinal epidural hematoma with associated platelet dysfunction from excessive garlic ingestion: a case report. *Neurosurgery* (1990) 26, 880–2.

Coumarins + Herbal medicines; Ginger

Evidence from pharmacological studies suggests that ginger does not increase the anticoagulant effect of warfarin, neither does it alter coagulation or platelet aggregation on its own. However, two case reports describe markedly raised INRs with phenprocoumon and warfarin, which were associated with eating dried ginger and drinking ginger tea.

Clinical evidence, mechanism, importance and management

In a randomised, crossover study in 12 healthy subjects, 3 ginger capsules three times daily for 2 weeks did not affect either the pharmacokinetics or pharmacodynamics (INR) of a single 25-mg dose of **warfarin** taken on day 7. The brand of ginger used was *Blackmores Travel Calm Ginger,* each capsule containing an extract equivalent to 400 mg of ginger rhizome powder. Moreover, ginger alone did not affect the INR or platelet aggregation.[1]

However, a case report describes a rise in INR to greater than 10, with epistaxis, in a woman stabilised on **phenprocoumon** several weeks after she started to eat ginger regularly in the form of pieces of dried ginger and tea from ginger powder. She was eventually restabilised on the original dose of **phenprocoumon**, and was advised to stop taking ginger.[2] Another very similar case has been described in a woman taking **warfarin**.[3]

These appear to be the only reports of ginger as a probable cause of over-anticoagulation, despite the fact that prior to these Ginger (*Zingiber officinale*) has been sometimes listed as a herb that interacts with **warfarin**.[4,5] on the basis that *in vitro* it inhibits platelet aggregation. However, this antiplatelet effect has not been demonstrated in clinical studies (which have been the subject of a review[6]), see also 'Coumarins + Herbal medicines', p.414.

Evidence from pharmacological studies suggests that ginger does not increase the anticoagulant effect of **warfarin**, neither does it alter coagulation or platelet aggregation on its own. However, two case reports describe markedly raised INRs with **phenprocoumon** and **warfarin**, which were associated with ginger root and ginger tea. Bear the possibility in mind in the event of an unexpected response to treatment.

1. Jiang X, Williams KM, Liauw WS, Ammit AJ, Roufogalis BD, Duke CC, Day RO, McLachlan AJ. Effect of ginkgo and ginger on the pharmacokinetics and pharmacodynamics of warfarin in healthy subjects. *Br J Clin Pharmacol* (2005) 59, 425–32.
2. Krüth P, Brosi E, Fux R, Mörike K, Gleiter CH. Ginger-associated overanticoagulation by phenprocoumon. *Ann Pharmacother* (2004) 38, 257–60.
3. Lesho EP, Saullo L, Udvari-Nagy S. A 76-year-old woman with erratic anticoagulation. *Cleve Clin J Med* (2004) 71, 651–6 .
4. Argento A, Tiraferri E, Marzaloni M. Anticoagulanti orali e piante medicinali. Una interazione emergente. *Ann Ital Med Int* (2000) 15, 139–43
5. Braun L. Herb-drug interaction guide. *Aust Fam Physician* (2001) 30, 473–6.
6. Vaes LPJ, Chyka PA. Interactions of warfarin with garlic, ginger, ginkgo, or ginseng: nature of the evidence. *Ann Pharmacother* (2000) 34, 1478–82.

Coumarins + Herbal medicines; *Ginkgo biloba*

Evidence from pharmacological studies in patients and healthy subjects suggests that *Ginkgo biloba* extracts do not interact with warfarin. However, an isolated report describes intracerebral haemorrhage associated with the use of *Ginkgo biloba* and warfarin, and there are a few reports of bleeding associated with the use of ginkgo alone.

Clinical evidence

In a randomised, crossover study in 21 patients stabilised on **warfarin**, *Ginkgo biloba* extract 100 mg daily (*Bio-Biloba*) for 4 weeks did not alter the INR or the required dose of **warfarin**, when compared with placebo.[1] Similarly, in another study in healthy subjects,[2] *Tavonin* (containing standardised dry extract EGb 761 of *Ginkgo biloba* equivalent to 2 g of leaf) 2 tablets three times daily for 2 weeks did not affect either the pharmacokinetics or pharmacodynamics (INR) of a single dose of **warfarin** given on day 7. Moreover, a retrospective review of 21 clinical cases involving the concurrent use of ginkgo and **warfarin** also found no evidence of altered INRs.[3]

Conversely, a report describes an intracerebral haemorrhage in an elderly woman within 2 months of starting *Ginkgo biloba.* Her prothrombin time was found to be 16.9 and her partial thromboplastin time was 35.5 seconds. She had been taking **warfarin** uneventfully for 5 years.[4] The author of the report speculated that *Ginkgo biloba* may have contributed towards the haemorrhage.

Mechanism

Uncertain. Isolated cases of bleeding have been reported with ginkgo alone (which have been the subject of a review[5]). In pharmacological studies, *Ginkgo biloba* extract alone did not alter coagulation parameters or platelet aggregation.[2,3] However, in *animal* studies it was found that the AUC of warfarin was decreased by 23.4% during EGb 761 administration, and the prothrombin time was also reduced by EGb 761, which would suggest that ginkgo should *reduce* the effects of warfarin.[3] In healthy subjects, *Gingko biloba* extract had no effect on diclofenac or tolbutamide, which were used as marker substrates for the cytochrome P50 isoenzyme CYP2C9, suggesting that it will not alter the metabolism of *S*-warfarin.[6]

Importance and management

There is good evidence from pharmacological studies in patients and healthy subjects that *Ginkgo biloba* extract would not be expected to interact with warfarin. However, there is one case report of over-anticoagulation, and a few reports of bleeding with ginkgo alone. This is insufficient evidence to justify telling patients taking warfarin to avoid *Ginkgo biloba,* but they should be told to monitor for early signs of bruising or bleeding and seek informed professional advice if any bleeding problems arise.

1. Engelsen J, Nielsen JD, Winther K. Effect of coenzyme Q_{10} and ginkgo biloba on warfarin dosage in stable, long-term warfarin treated outpatients. A randomised, double blind, placebo-crossover trial. *Thromb Haemost* (2002) 87, 1075–6.
2. Jiang X, Williams KM, Liauw WS, Ammit AJ, Roufogalis BD, Duke CC, Day RO, McLachlan AJ. Effect of ginkgo and ginger on the pharmacokinetics and pharmacodynamics of warfarin in healthy subjects. *Br J Clin Pharmacol* (2005) 59, 425–32.
3. Lai C-F, Chang C-C, Fu C-H, Chen C-M. Evaluation of the interaction between warfarin and ginkgo biloba extract. *Pharmacotherapy* (2002) 22, 1326.
4. Matthews MK. Association of *Ginkgo biloba* with intracerebral hemorrhage. *Neurology* (1998) 50, 1933.
5. Vaes LPJ, Chyka PA. Interactions of warfarin with garlic, ginger, ginkgo, or ginseng: nature of the evidence. *Ann Pharmacother* (2000) 34, 1478–82.
6. Mohutsky MA, Anderson GA, Miller JW, Elmer GW. *Ginkgo biloba:* evaluation of CYP2C9 drug interactions in vitro and in vivo. *Am J Ther* (2006) 13, 24–31.

Coumarins + Herbal medicines; Ginseng

One pharmacological study found that American ginseng (*Panax quinquefolius*) modestly decreased the effect of warfarin, whereas another study found that *Panax ginseng* did not alter the effect of warfarin. Two case reports describe decreased warfarin effects, one with thrombosis, attributed to the use of ginseng (probably *Panax ginseng*).

Clinical evidence

In a placebo-controlled study, 20 healthy subjects were given **warfarin** 5 mg daily for 3 days alone then again on days 15 to 17 of a 3-week course of American ginseng 1 g twice daily. In the 12 subjects given ginseng, the peak INR was modesty reduced by 0.16, compared with a non-significant reduction of 0.02 in the 8 subjects given placebo. There was also a modest reduction in the AUC of **warfarin**. In this study, American ginseng (*Panax quinquefolius*) root was ground and capsulated.[1]

Evidence from two earlier case reports supports a reduction in warfarin effect. A man taking **warfarin** long-term, and also diltiazem, glyceryl trinitrate and salsalate, had a fall in his INR from 3.1 to 1.5 within 2 weeks of starting to take ginseng capsules (*Ginsana*) three times daily. This preparation contains 100 mg of standardised concentrated ginseng [probably *Panax ginseng*] in each capsule. Within 2 weeks of stopping the ginseng his INR had risen again to 3.3.[2] Another patient taking **warfarin** was found to have thrombosis of a prosthetic aortic valve, with a subtherapeutic INR of 1.4. Three months prior to this episode his INR had become persistently subtherapeutic, requiring a progressive increment in his **warfarin** dose. It was suggested that this might have been because he had begun using a ginseng product (not identified).[3] In contrast, in a randomised, crossover study in 12 healthy subjects, ginseng capsules 1 g three times daily for 2 weeks did not affect either the pharmacokinetics or pharmacodynamics (INR) of a single 25-mg dose of **warfarin** taken on day 7. The brand of ginseng used was *Golden Glow,* each capsule containing an extract equivalent to 0.5 g of *Panax ginseng* root.[4]

Mechanism

Ginseng can come from the root of *Panax ginseng* (known in the US as Asian ginseng) or *Panax quinquefolius* (American ginseng), which differ in the concentrations and specific ginsenosides.[5] The study showing a reduction in effect of warfarin used American ginseng, and the study showing no effect used *Panax ginseng*. A study in *rats* also failed to find any evidence of an interaction between warfarin and an extract from *Panax ginseng*.[6] Nevertheless, the two case reports of reduced warfarin effect are probably *Panax ginseng.*

In contrast there have been handful of reports of spontaneous bleeding in patients using ginseng preparations (unspecified) in the absence of an anticoagulant,[7,8] and, *in vitro*, *Panax ginseng* has been found to contain antiplatelet components.[9] See also 'Coumarins + Herbal medicines', p.414.

Importance and management

The available evidence suggests that ginseng might *decrease* the effect of warfarin. It is possible that the effect is greater with, or specific to, American ginseng (*Panax quinquefolius*), since this interacted in one study whereas *Panax ginseng* did not. Although the ginseng dose was higher in the *Panax ginseng* study, the treatment duration was not as long, which may have obscured an effect. Moreover, the two case reports of decreased warfarin effects attributed to the use of ginseng were probably *Panax ginseng.*

Until further information becomes available it would seem prudent to be alert for decreased effects of coumarins in patients using ginseng, particularly American ginseng. However, the possibility of an increased risk of bleeding due to the antiplatelet component of Panax ginseng cannot entirely be ruled out, but see also 'Coumarins + Herbal medicines', p.414.

1. Yuan C-S, Wei G, Dey L, Karrison T, Nahlik L, Maleckar S, Kasza K, Ang-Lee M, Moss J. Brief communication: American ginseng reduces warfarin's effect in healthy patients. *Ann Intern Med* (2004) 141, 23–27.
2. Janetzky K, Morreale AP. Probable interaction between warfarin and ginseng. *Am J Health-Syst Pharm* (1997) 54, 692–3.
3. Rosado MF. Thrombosis of a prosthetic aortic valve disclosing a hazardous interaction between warfarin and a commercial ginseng product. *Cardiology* (2003) 99, 111.
4. Jiang X, Williams KM, Liauw WS, Ammit AJ, Roufogalis BD, Duke CC, Day RO, McLachlan AJ. Effect of St John's wort and ginseng on the pharmacokinetics and pharmacodynamics of warfarin in healthy subjects. *Br J Clin Pharmacol* (2004) 57, 592–99.
5. Plotnikoff GA, McKenna D, Watanabe K, Blumenthal M. *Ann Intern Med* (2004) 141, 893–4.
6. Zhu M, Chan KW, Ng LS, Chang Q, Chang S, Li RC. Possible influences of ginseng on the pharmacokinetics and pharmacodynamics of warfarin in rats. *J Pharm Pharmacol* (1999) 51, 175–80.
7. Hopkins MP, Androff L, Benninghoff AS. Ginseng face cream and unexplained vaginal bleeding. *Am J Obstet Gynecol* (1988) 159, 1121–2.
8. Greenspan EM. Ginseng and vaginal bleeding. *JAMA* (1983) 249, 2018.
9. Kuo S-C, Teng C-M, Leed J-C, Ko F-N, Chen S-C, Wu T-S. Antiplatelet components in Panax ginseng. *Planta Med* (1990) 56, 164–7.

Coumarins + Herbal medicines; *Lycium barbarum*

There is an isolated report of a modest increase in the anticoagulant effects of warfarin in a patient taking a herbal tea made from *Lycium barbarum* L.

Clinical evidence, mechanism, importance and management

A 61-year-old Chinese woman stabilised on **warfarin** (INRs normally 2 to 3) had an unexpected rise in her INR to 4.1, which was identified during a routine monthly check. No bleeding was seen. She was also taking atenolol, benazepril, digoxin and fluvastatin. It was found that 4 days before visiting the clinic she had started to take one glass (about 170 mL) 3 or 4 times daily of a Chinese herbal tea made from the fruits of *Lycium barbarum* L (also known as Chinese wolfberry, gou qi zi, Fructus Lycii Chinensis, or *Lycium chinense*) to treat blurred vision caused by a sore eye. When the herbal treatment was stopped, her INRs rapidly returned to normal. Later *in vitro* studies showed that an infusion of *Lycium barbarum* L caused some inhibition of the cytochrome P450 isoenzyme CYP2C9, which is involved in the metabolism of warfarin, but this was apparently too weak to explain why this interaction occurred.[1] So far this is an isolated case but it draws attention to the possibility of problems with this herbal remedy in other patients.

1. Lam AY, Elmer GW, Mohutsky M. Possible interaction between warfarin and *Lycium barbarum. Ann Pharmacother* (2001) 35, 1199–1201.

Coumarins + Herbal medicines; Melilot

Increased anticoagulation was seen in a patient taking acenocoumarol after using a melilot-containing topical cream.

Clinical evidence

A 66-year-old taking **acenocoumarol**, levothyroxine and prazepam had an increase in her INR after massaging a proprietary topical cream (*Cyclo 3)* containing melilot (*Melilotus officinalis;* **sweet clover**) and butcher's broom (*Ruscus aculeatus*) on her legs three times daily. On the first occasion her INR rose from about 2 to 5.8 after 7 days of use, and on a later occasion it rose to 4.6 after 10 days of use.[1]

Mechanism

Melilot (sweet clover) is known to contain natural coumarins, which can be turned into dicoumarol by moulds, see 'Coumarins + Herbal medicines', p.414. In another report, a woman with unexplained abnormal menstrual bleeding was found to have a prothrombin time of 53 seconds, and laboratory tests showed that her blood clotting factors were abnormally low. When given parenteral vitamin K her prothrombin time rapidly returned to normal (suggesting that she was taking a vitamin K antagonist of some kind). She strongly denied taking any anticoagulant drugs, but it was eventually discovered that she had been drinking large quantities of a herbal tea containing among other ingredients **tonka beans**, **melilot** and **sweet woodruff**, all of which might contain natural coumarins, but see 'Coumarins + Herbal medicines', p.414.[2]

Importance and management

This case is isolated, but it shows that herbal preparations of this kind might affect anticoagulation. Absorption through the skin appears to be enough to upset the anticoagulant control.

1. Chiffoleau A, Huguenin H, Veyrac G, Argaiz V, Dupe D, Kayser M, Bourin M, Jolliet P. Interaction entre mélilot et acénocoumarol ? (mélilot-*ruscus aculeatus*). *Therapie* (2001) 56, 321–7.
2. Hogan RP. Hemorrhagic diathesis caused by drinking an herbal tea. *JAMA* (1983) 249, 2679–80.

Coumarins + Herbal medicines; Quilinggao

A single case report describes a man who had a marked increase in his INR with bleeding complications, nine days after he switched the brand of quilinggao he was using.

Clinical evidence

A 61-year-old man stabilised on **warfarin** with an INR in the range of 1.6 to 2.8 was found to have an INR greater than 6 and skin bruising, and complained of gum bleeding and epistaxis in the previous 3 days. For the past 3 years he had taken quilinggao, apparently without problems. However, 9 days previously he had started taking a different brand of quilinggao. He was eventually stabilised on the previous dose of **warfarin** with an INR of 2.5, but after discharge started taking a third brand of quilinggao, and 3 days later had an INR of 5.2.[1]

Mechanism

Quilinggao is a Chinese herbal product made from a mixture of herbs. The first brand did not contain any herbs suspected to have anticoagulant effects except one with possible antiplatelet activity, but the second brand contained Chinese peony (*Paeoniae rubra*), *Poncirus trifoliata* and a couple of other herbs known to contain substances with anticoagulant or antiplatelet effects *in vitro*, but see also 'Coumarins + Herbal medicines', p.414.

Importance and management

This appears to be the only case of a possible interaction, and as such the interaction is not established. Quilinggao did not affect anticoagulant control in this patient for a number of years, and then did after switching brands. Bear the possibility of an interaction in mind.

1. Wong ALN, Chan TYK. Interaction between warfarin and the herbal product *quilinggao*. *Ann Pharmacother* (2003) 37, 836–8.

Coumarins + Herbal medicines; St John's wort (*Hypericum perforatum*)

St John's wort can cause a moderate reduction in the anticoagulant effects of phenprocoumon and warfarin.

Clinical evidence

(a) Phenprocoumon

In a randomised, placebo-controlled crossover study in 10 healthy men,[1] St John's wort extract (*LI 160, Lichtwer Pharma*) 900 mg daily for 11 days reduced the AUC of a single 12-mg dose of phenprocoumon by a modest 17.4%. There is also a case report of a 75-year-old woman taking phenprocoumon who had a reduced anticoagulant response (a rise in the Quick value) 2 months after starting to take St John's wort.[2]

(b) Warfarin

In a randomised, crossover study in 12 healthy subjects, one tablet of St John's wort three times daily for 3 weeks modestly decreased the AUC of both *R*- and *S*-warfarin by about 25% after a single 25-mg dose of warfarin taken on day 14. In this study, the brand of St John's wort used was *Bioglan* tablets, each tablet containing an extract equivalent to 1 g of *Hypericum perforatum* flowering herb top containing 825 micrograms of hypericin and 12.5 mg of hyperforin.[3]

The Swedish Medical Products Agency received 7 case reports over the 1998 to 1999 period of patients stabilised on warfarin who showed decreased INRs when St John's wort was added. Their INRs fell from the normal therapeutic range of about 2 to 4 to about 1.5. Two patients needed warfarin dosage increases of 6.6% and 15% when St John's wort was added. The INRs of 4 of the patients returned to their former values when the St John's wort was stopped.[4]

Mechanism

Uncertain, but it is suggested that the St John's wort increases the metabolism and clearance of the anticoagulants[1,3,4] possibly by induction of cytochrome P450 isoenzymes. It affected both *R*- and *S*-warfarin.[3] Oral bioavailability was not altered.[3]

Importance and management

Information seems to be limited to these reports, but a modest pharmacokinetic interaction is established, which might be clinically important. It would be prudent to monitor the INRs of patients taking phenprocoumon, warfarin or any other coumarin if they start taking St John's wort, being alert for the need to slightly raise the anticoagulant dosage. However, note that the advice of the CSM in the UK is that St John's wort should not be used with warfarin. They note that the degree of induction of warfarin metabolism is likely to vary because levels of active ingredients may vary between St John's wort preparations. If a patient is already taking the combination, they advise checking the INR, stopping the St John's wort and then monitoring the INR closely and adjusting the anticoagulant dosage as necessary.[5]

1. Maurer A, Johne A, Bauer S, Brockmöller J, Donath F, Roots I, Langheinrich M, Hübner W-D. Interaction of St John's wort extract with phenprocoumon. *Eur J Clin Pharmacol* (1999) 55, A22.
2. Bon S, Hartmann, Kuhn M. Johanniskraut: Ein Enzyminduktor? *Schweiz Apothekerzeitung* (1999) 16, 535–6.
3. Jiang X, Williams KM, Liauw WS, Ammit AJ, Roufogalis BD, Duke CC, Day RO, McLachlan AJ. Effect of St John's wort and ginseng on the pharmacokinetics and pharmacodynamics of warfarin in healthy subjects. *Br J Clin Pharmacol* (2004) 57, 592–9.
4. Yue Q-Y, Bergquist C, Gerdén B. Safety of St John's wort *(Hypericum perforatum)*. *Lancet* (2000) 355, 576–7.
5. Committee on Safety of Medicines. Message from Professor A Breckenridge, Chairman, Committee on Safety of Medicines, and Fact Sheet for Health Care Professionals, February 2000. Available at http://www.mhra.gov.uk/home/idcplg?IdcService=SS_GET_PAGE&useSecondary=true&ssDocName=CON2015756&ssTargetNodeId=221 (accessed 17/08/07).

Coumarins + Herbal medicines; Vitamin K_1–rich

A man had a rise in his INR after stopping taking a herbal nutritional supplement *(Nature's Life Greens)*, which contained a number of plants known to be high in vitamin K_1. Another patient had a decrease in INR after starting to drink a plant extract juice (called *Noni Juice*).

Clinical evidence, mechanism, importance and management

(a) Nature's Life Greens

A 72-year-old man stabilised on **warfarin** was found to have an INR of 4.43 at a routine clinic visit, which was increased from 3.07 six weeks previously. The patient had stopped taking a herbal product *Nature's Life Greens* that month because he did not have enough money to buy it. He had been taking it for the past 7 years as a vitamin supplement because he had previously been instructed to limit his intake of green leafy vegetables. He was eventually restabilised on **warfarin** and the same nutritional product.

The product label listed 25 vegetables without stating the amounts or concentrations,[1] but at least 5 of the listed ingredients are known to contain high levels of vitamin K_1 including **parsley, green tea leaves, spinach, broccoli**, and **cabbage** (see also 'foods; vitamin K–rich', (p.409)). It is therefore likely it contained sufficient vitamin to antagonise the effect of the **warfarin** so that when it was stopped the warfarin requirements fell, and without an appropriate adjustment in dose, this resulted in an increased INR.

This case reinforces the view that all patients taking **warfarin** should seek advice when they want to stop or start any herbal medicine or nutritional supplement.

(b) Plant extracts juices

A 41-year-old woman stabilised on **warfarin** was found to have an INR of 1.6 at a routine clinic visit. The only possible cause identified was that the patient had begun to drink one to two small glasses daily of *Noni Juice 4 Everything.* This was identified as a brown liquid that contains extracts and derivates from more than 115 components. The authors noted that many of the listed plants contained vitamin K and that vitamin K was listed as a separate component, indicating that the juice might be fortified with vitamin K. The patient was given heparin and then discharged on her previous dose of **warfarin**, and advised to stop taking this brand of juice.[2]

This case reinforces the view that all patients taking **warfarin** should seek advice when they want to stop or start any herbal medicine or nutritional supplement.

1. Bransgrove LL. Interaction between warfarin and a vitamin K-containing nutritional supplement: a case report. *J Herb Pharmacother* (2001) 1, 85–89.
2. Carr ME, Klotz J, Bergeron M. Coumadin resistance and the vitamin supplement "Noni". *Am J Hematol* (2004) 77, 103–4.

Coumarins + Herbicides

An isolated report describes a marked increase in the anticoagulant effects of acenocoumarol, with bleeding, caused by use of a herbicide containing thiocarbamates.

Clinical evidence, mechanism, importance and management

A 55-year-old patient with mitral and aortic prostheses, stabilised on **acenocoumarol** 2 mg daily and with an INR of 3.6 to 4.2 was hospitalised because of severe and uncontrollable gum bleeding. He responded when given a transfusion of fresh plasma. The cause of the marked increase in the anticoagulant effects of the **acenocoumarol** was eventually identified as almost certainly being due to the use of a herbicide (*SATURN-S*) containing **thiobencarb** and **molinate** (two thiocarbamates), which the patient was using to spray his rice crop. The **thiobencarb** can be absorbed through the skin and the **molinate** by inhalation. Just how these two compounds interact with **acenocoumarol** is not known but the authors of the report suggest that these herbicides may possibly have inhibited the metabolism of the anticoagulant, thereby increasing its effects. The patient was later restabilised on his former dose of **acenocoumarol**.[1]

This seems to be the first and only report of this interaction but it highlights one of the possible risks of using chemical sprays that have never been formally tested for their potential to interact with drugs. See also 'Coumarins + Insecticides', p.421.

1. Fernández MA, Aznar J. Potenciación del efecto anticoagulante del acenocumarol por un herbicida. *Rev Iberoamer Tromb Hemostasia* (1988) 1, 40–1.

Coumarins + Hormonal contraceptives

One small study found that the acenocoumarol dose requirements were about 20% lower during the use of a combined hormonal contraceptive. An isolated report describes a marked INR increase in the INR of a woman taking warfarin when she was given emergency contraception with levonorgestrel. In contrast, in small single-dose studies in healthy subjects, the anticoagulant effects of dicoumarol and phenprocoumon were slightly decreased by oral contraceptives.

Note that, in general, the indications for the use of oral anticoagulants are contraindications to the use of combined oral contraceptives.

Clinical evidence

(a) Acenocoumarol

The anticoagulant requirements of 12 patients taking acenocoumarol were about 20% lower while they were taking a combined hormonal contraceptive (average 19 months) than when they were not taking the contraceptive (average 12 months). Even then, they were anticoagulated to a higher degree while taking the contraceptive (prothrombin ratio of 1.67 compared with 1.5) than with the anticoagulant alone. The contraceptives used were *Neogynona*, *Microgynon*, *Eugynon* (**ethinylestradiol** with **levonorgestrel**) or *Topasel* (intramuscular **estradiol enantate** with **algestone**).[1]

(b) Dicoumarol

A study in 4 healthy subjects given single 150- or 200-mg doses of dicoumarol on day 17 of a 20-day course of *Enovid* (**noretynodrel** and **mestranol**) found that the anticoagulant effects were decreased in 3 of the 4 subjects, although the dicoumarol half-life remained unaltered.[2]

(c) Phenprocoumon

In a controlled study in 14 healthy women, the clearance of a single 0.22-mg/kg dose of phenprocoumon was increased by 20% in the 7 subjects taking combined oral contraceptives, compared with that in the 7 not taking oral contraceptives.[3]

(d) Warfarin

A 39-year-old woman with familial type 1 antithrombin deficiency and a history of extensive deep vein thrombosis and pulmonary embolism, taking warfarin, was given **levonorgestrel** for emergency contraception. Within 3 days her INR had risen from 2.1 to 8.1. No bleeding occurred. Her INR returned to normal after stopping the warfarin for 2 days.[4]

Mechanism

Not understood. The oral contraceptives are well known to be associated with a small increased risk of venous thromboembolism in otherwise healthy women, and are therefore contraindicated in women who have had thrombosis. They can apparently increase the metabolism (glucuronidation) of phenprocoumon.[3] The authors of the report about levonorgestrel suggest that it might have displaced the warfarin from its binding sites thereby increasing its activity,[4] although this mechanism is now generally discounted.

Importance and management

Direct information seems to be limited to these reports. Oral contraceptives are normally contraindicated in those with thromboembolic disorders but if they must be used, be alert for any changes in the anticoagulant response if an oral contraceptive is started or stopped. The report about the apparent interaction between warfarin and postcoital levonorgestrel seems to be isolated and therefore its general importance is unknown.

1. de Teresa E, Vera A, Ortigosa J, Alonso Pulpon L, Puente Arus A, de Artaza M. Interaction between anticoagulants and contraceptives: an unsuspected finding. *BMJ* (1979) 2, 1260–1.
2. Schrogie JJ, Solomon HM, Zieve PD. Effect of oral contraceptives on vitamin K-dependent clotting activity. *Clin Pharmacol Ther* (1967) 8, 670–5.
3. Mönig H, Baese C, Heidemann HT, Ohnhaus EE, Schulte HM. Effect of oral contraceptive steroids on the pharmacokinetics of phenprocoumon. *Br J Clin Pharmacol* (1990) 30, 115–18.
4. Ellison J, Thomson AJ, Greer IA, Walker ID. Apparent interaction between warfarin and levonorgestrel used for emergency contraception. *BMJ* (2000) 321, 1382.

Coumarins and related drugs + HRT or Tibolone

A retrospective analysis of women starting HRT found that only three needed warfarin dose increases, of about 10 to 30%. A case report describes a woman who needed 75% more acenocoumarol when her HRT treatment with oral conjugated oestrogens was changed to transdermal estradiol.

Four women taking warfarin and one taking phenindione who started taking tibolone had modest to marked increases in INR and required 12% to 56% reductions in anticoagulant dose.

Note that, because of the increased risk of developing venous thromboembolism with HRT, the use of HRT in women already on anticoagulant therapy requires careful consideration of the risks and benefits. Whether tibolone is associated with the same risk is unknown, therefore similar caution would seem prudent.

Clinical evidence

(a) Oestrogens for menopausal HRT

In a retrospective analysis, 18 women were identified who had started HRT while taking **warfarin** (n=16) or **phenindione** (n=2). A wide variety of HRT preparations were being used, including topical and oral preparations, oestrogens with or without progestogens, and progestogens alone. Half of the women taking **warfarin** had no change in their warfarin dose requirement after starting HRT. Five required a less than 10% increase or decrease in average **warfarin** dose, and 3 required a 12.8%, 22%, and 28% increase in average **warfarin** dose, the latter two of these being the only 2 women taking oestrogen-only oral HRT. Of the 2 women taking **phenindione**, one needed no change in dose, and the other a 4.6% increase in dose.[1]

In one case, a postmenopausal 53-year-old woman needed an increase in her daily dose of **acenocoumarol** from 2 to 3.5 mg when her **HRT** was changed from **oral conjugated oestrogens** 0.625 mg daily to **transdermal estradiol** 50 micrograms daily. When the oral **HRT** was restarted, her **acenocoumarol** requirements returned to their former levels.[2]

(b) Tibolone

In a retrospective analysis, five women were identified who had started tibolone while taking **warfarin** or **phenindione**, and one who discontinued tibolone while taking **warfarin**. All of the 5 patients had an increase in INR to a range of 4.6 to 9.5 after starting tibolone, and required reductions

Table 12.4 Summary of the evidence for and against an interaction between influenza vaccine and coumarins

Study type (year)	*Group*	*Coumarin*	*Influenza vaccine*	*Route*	*Notes*	*Refs*
Studies showing no interaction						
Prospective (1983)	33 patients and 15 controls	Warfarin	Not stated	Not stated	No evidence of an interaction (one vaccinated patient had haematuria 27 days later, and one control patient had epistaxis)	1
Prospective series (1984)	21 patients	Stable warfarin	Trivalent type A and B, Wyeth	Not stated	No change in average prothrombin time at 0, 3, 7, 10 and 14 days after vaccination	2
Randomised, placebo-controlled (1984)	25 patients vaccinated and 25 placebo	Stable warfarin	Trivalent type A and B (*Fluvirin*)	Deep subcutaneous	No change in mean ratio of prothrombin times at 0, 2, 7 and 21 days after vaccination	3
Prospective (1984)	4 healthy subjects	Low-dose warfarin	*Influvac*	Intramuscular	No change in average prothrombin time at 7, 11, 14, 16, 21 and 28 days after vaccination, and no change in warfarin levels	4
Prospective series (1985)	7 patients	Stable warfarin	Trivalent type A and B, Wyeth	Not stated	No change in prothrombin time at 4, 6, 10, 14 and 21 days after vaccination	5
Prospective series (1986)	26 patients	Stable warfarin	Trivalent (subvirion) type A and B (*Fluogen*)	Intramuscular	No change in mean INR at day 14 after vaccination	6
Prospective series (1986)	7 patients and 9 controls	Stable warfarin	Trivalent type A and B, Wyeth	Not stated	No change in prothrombin time at 1, 3 and 5 weeks after vaccination, or compared with controls	7
Prospective series (1990)	9 patients	Stable warfarin	Trivalent, split virion, A and B (*MFV-Ject*)	Not stated	No significant change in INR at 3, 6, 8, 10, 13, 22 and 30 days after vaccination (mean decrease of 4.8%)	8
Prospective series (1993)	43 patients	Stable acenocoumarol	Trivalent type A and B	Subcutaneous	No change in mean INR at 7, 15 and 30 days after vaccination. INR values increased in 3 patients and decreased in 6 patients requiring modification in acenocoumarol dose	9
Prospective series (1995)	41 patients	Stable warfarin	Not stated	Intramuscular	No significant change in prothrombin time at 3, 7 and 14 days after vaccination, and no local complications	10
Studies showing an increase in effect						
Prospective series (1984)	8 patients	Stable warfarin	Trivalent type A and B	Not stated	All patients had an increase in prothrombin time to at least the upper limit of their range for the previous year (40% from baseline)*	11
Prospective series (1986)	10 patients	Stable warfarin	Trivalent (subvirion) type A and B (*Fluogen*)	Intramuscular	Slight maximal 7.6% increase in mean INR at day 14 after vaccination	6
Case-control (2003)	90 patients and 45 controls	Stable warfarin (98%) Acenocoumarol (2%)	*Inflexel V, Isiflu V, Fluad*, or *Agrippal*	Intramuscular	49 out of 90 patients had a clear increase in INR from a mean of 2.64 to 3.85, and 2 of these had bleeding episodes. In the remaining patients and controls there was no change in INR	12
Studies showing a decrease in effect						
Prospective series (1988)	24 patients	Stable warfarin	Trivalent type A and B	Not stated	A slight 8.3% decrease in prothrombin time occurred in the first 2 weeks after vaccination.	13
Prospective series (2002)	73 patients and 72 controls	Stable warfarin	Not stated	Subcutaneous	Overall, there was no change in anticoagulation, but the 34 vaccinated patients aged 70 or more had a slight reduction in INR in month after vaccination (mean 2.8 versus 2.99)	14

*Other researchers[5] state that their analysis of these data failed to show a statistical difference after vaccination.

1. Patriarca PA, Kendal AP, Stricof RL, Weber JA, Meissner MK, Dateno B. Influenza vaccination and warfarin or theophylline toxicity in nursing-home residents. *N Engl J Med* (1983) 308, 1601–2.
2. Lipsky BA, Pecoraro RE, Roben NJ, de Blaquiere P, Delaney CJ. Influenza vaccination and warfarin anticoagulation. *Ann Intern Med* (1984) 100, 835–7.
3. Farrow PR, Nicholson KG. Lack of effect of influenza and pneumococcal vaccines on anticoagulation by warfarin. *J Infect* (1984) 9, 157–60.
4. Scott AK, Cannon J, Breckenridge AM. Lack of effect of influenza vaccination on warfarin in healthy volunteers. *Br J Clin Pharmacol* (1984) 19, 144P–145P.
5. Gomolin IH, Chapron DJ, Luhan PA. Lack of effect of influenza vaccine on theophylline levels and warfarin anticoagulation in the elderly. *J Am Geriatr Soc* (1985) 33, 269–72.
6. Weibert RT, Lorentz SM, Norcross WA, Klauber MR, Jagger PI. Effect of influenza vaccine in patients receiving long-term warfarin therapy. *Clin Pharm* (1986) 5, 499–503.
7. Gomolin IH. Lack of effect of influenza vaccine on warfarin anticoagulation in the elderly. *Can Med Assoc J* (1986) 135, 39–41.
8. Arnold WSG, Mehta MK, Roberts JS. Influenza vaccine and anticoagulation control in patients receiving warfarin. *Br J Clin Pract* (1990) 44, 136–9.

Continued

Table 12.4 Summary of the evidence for and against an interaction between influenza vaccine and coumarins (continued)

9. Souto JC, Oliver A, Montserrat I, Mateo J, Sureda A, Fontcuberta J. Lack of effect of influenza vaccine on anticoagulation by acenocoumarol. *Ann Pharmacother* (1993) 27, 365–8.
10. Raj G, Kumar R, McKinney WP. Safety of intramuscular influenza immunization among patients receiving long-term warfarin anticoagulation therapy. *Arch Intern Med* (1995) 155, 1529–31.
11. Kramer P, Tsuru M, Cook CE, McClain CJ, Holtzman JL. Effect of influenza vaccine on warfarin anticoagulation. *Clin Pharmacol Ther* (1984) 35, 416–18.
12. Paliani U, Filippucci E, Gresele P. Significant potentiation of anticoagulation by flu-vaccine during the season 2001-2002. *Haematologica* (2003) 88, 599–600.
13. Bussey HI, Saklad JJ. Effect of influenza vaccine on chronic warfarin therapy. *Drug Intell Clin Pharm* (1988) 22, 198–201.
14. Poli D, Chiarugi L, Capanni M, Antonucci E, Abbate R, Gensini GF, Prisco D. Need of more frequent international normalized ratio monitoring in elderly patients on long-term anticoagulant therapy after influenza vaccination. *Blood Coag Fibrinol* (2002) 13, 297–300.

in their anticoagulant dose (range of 12% to 53% reductions in **warfarin** dose, and 56% for **phenindione**). The woman who discontinued tibolone required an increase in her **warfarin** dose from 6 to 7.5 mg daily.[1]

Mechanism

Not understood. Menopausal HRT alone is now known to be associated with a small increased risk of venous thromboembolism. Tibolone alone increases fibrinolytic activity without altering prothrombin time,[3] and might therefore be expected to increase the risk of bleeding with anticoagulants. However, this would not result in raised INRs, and it was suggested that the effect on the INR might be because of the androgenic effect of tibolone causing a reduction in factor VIIa.[1]

Importance and management

Published information on concurrent use of warfarin and HRT or tibolone appears to be very limited. The retrospective study suggests that usually HRT causes no or only minor changes in warfarin requirements, whereas tibolone causes more marked increases in INR and reduced warfarin requirements of up to about 50%.[1] Because of this, increased monitoring of the INR on starting tibolone in patients stabilised on warfarin, other coumarins, or indanediones is required.

Note that, because of the increased risk of developing venous thromboembolism with HRT, the use of HRT in women already taking an anticoagulant requires careful consideration of the risks and benefits. Whether tibolone is associated with the same risk is unknown,[4] therefore similar caution would seem prudent.

1. McLintock LA, Dykes A, Tait RC, Walker ID. Interaction between hormone replacement therapy preparations and oral anticoagulant therapy. *Br J Obstet Gynaecol* (2003) 110, 777–9.
2. Cotton F, Sorlin P, Corvilain B, Fockedey J-M, Capel P. Interference with oral anticoagulant treatment by oestrogen - influence of oestrogen administration route. *Thromb Haemost* (1999) 81, 471–2.
3. Cortes-Prieto J. Coagulation and fibrinolysis in post-menopausal women treated with Org OD 14. *Maturitas* (1987) Suppl 1, 67–72.
4. Livial (Tibolone). Organon Laboratories Ltd. UK Summary of product characteristics, May 2006.

Coumarins and related drugs + Influenza vaccines

The concurrent use of warfarin and influenza vaccine is usually safe and uneventful, but there are reports of bleeding in a handful of patients (life threatening in one case) attributed to an interaction. Acenocoumarol also does not normally interact.

Clinical evidence

(a) Effect on anticoagulant control

About 15 studies of the effect of influenza vaccine on the anticoagulant effect of coumarins have been published, and these are summarised in 'Table 12.4', (p.420). Most of these are non-controlled studies in small to moderate numbers of patients, and the majority were unable to demonstrate a significant change in prothrombin time or INR in patients taking coumarins, including the only randomised placebo-controlled study. Some studies found a slight change in anticoagulant effect (both slight increases and slight reductions), but they are probably of limited clinical relevance. However, in one larger case-control study, a clear increase in INR from 2.64 to 3.85 was seen in about half of the 90 patients, and 2 of these had bleeding episodes. The reasons for the clear difference between this study and the many others are not known.

There are also various brief case reports of a possible interaction. In one review paper, there is a very brief report of a patient receiving **warfarin** who had serious bleeding, which was almost fatal, after receiving a 'flu shot'. No further details are given.[1] An elderly man receiving **warfarin** developed bleeding (haematemesis and melaena) within 10 days of being given an influenza vaccination. His prothrombin time was found to be 36 seconds.[2] Another patient taking **warfarin** had raised INRs in two successive years when an influenza vaccination was given.[3]

(b) Route of injection of vaccine

In a randomised study in 26 patients stabilised on **warfarin**, there was no difference in injection site adverse events between intramuscular or subcutaneous injection of a standard trivalent influenza vaccine, and no patient had bruising or swelling. In addition, both routes of administration produced similar levels of antibody titres.[4] In another study that specifically assessed the local reactions to intramuscular influenza vaccination, there were no detectable local complications after intramuscular injection, including no change in arm circumference.[5]

Mechanism

Not understood. In a placebo-controlled study in healthy subjects, influenza vaccine did not alter the half-life of either *R*- or *S*-warfarin.[2] It has therefore been suggested that when an interaction occurs the synthesis of the blood clotting factors is altered.[2]

Importance and management

A well-investigated interaction, but with some contradictory data. The weight of evidence shows that influenza vaccination in those taking warfarin is normally safe and uneventful, nevertheless it would be prudent to be on the alert because very occasionally and unpredictably bleeding may occur. Acenocoumarol appears not to be affected.

Limited evidence suggests that intramuscular administration is not associated with increased local complications, but also that subcutaneous administration is effective. Because of the theoretical risk of local muscle haematoma, it may be preferable to give influenza vaccines by deep subcutaneous injection in patients taking coumarins and related anticoagulants.

1. Sumner HW, Holtzman JL, McClain CJ. Drug-induced liver disease. *Geriatrics* (1981) 36, 83–96.
2. Kramer P, Tsuru M, Cook CE, McClain CJ, Holtzman JL. Effect of influenza vaccine on warfarin anticoagulation. *Clin Pharmacol Ther* (1984) 35, 416–18.
3. Beeley L, Cunningham H, Carmichael A, Brennan A. *Bulletin of the West Midlands Centre for Adverse Drug Reaction Reporting* (1991), 33, 19.
4. Delafuente JC, Davis JA, Meuleman JR, Jones RA. Influenza vaccination and warfarin anticoagulation: a comparison of subcutaneous and intramuscular routes of administration in elderly men. *Pharmacotherapy* (1998) 18, 631–6.
5. Raj G, Kumar R, McKinney WP. Safety of intramuscular influenza immunization among patients receiving long-term warfarin anticoagulation therapy. *Arch Intern Med* (1995) 155, 1529–31.

Coumarins + Insecticides

A patient showed a marked increase in his response to acenocoumarol when exposed to insecticides containing ivermectin and methidathion. Another patient was resistant to the effects of warfarin after very heavy exposure to a toxaphene and lindane-containing insecticide.

Clinical evidence

(a) Acenocoumarol

A farmer in Spain, normally well stabilised on acenocoumarol and amiodarone, had marked rises in his INR, from 3.5 up to 7.9, requiring a reduction in his anticoagulant dosage (from 12 to 8 mg weekly), which occurred during the summer months. No bleeding occurred. It was then discovered that he was using insecticides containing **ivermectin** and an organophosphate **methidathion** on his trees without any protective clothing.[1]

(b) Warfarin

A rancher in the USA, who was taking warfarin, had a very marked reduction in his anticoagulant response after dusting his sheep with an insecticide containing 5% **toxaphene (camphechlor)** and 1% **lindane (gamma-benzene hexachloride)**. Over a 2-year period he had periods of considerable warfarin resistance, which were linked to the use of this insecticide. Normally warfarin 7.5 mg daily maintained his prothrombin time in the therapeutic range, but after exposure to the insecticide even 15 mg daily failed to have any effect at all.[2] The dusting was done by putting the insecticide in a sack and hitting the sheep with it in an enclosed barn.[2]

Mechanism

The interaction between acenocoumarol and ivermectin with methidathion is not understood. When used on its own, ivermectin used for onchocerciasis normally has no effect on prothrombin times,[3,4] but two unexplained cases of prolonged prothrombin times associated with the development of haematomas have been reported.[5] Methidathion is an organophosphate. Lindane and other chlorinated hydrocarbon insecticides are known liver enzyme inducers,[6] which increase the metabolism and clearance of the warfarin, thereby reducing or even abolishing its effects.

Importance and management

Information about these interactions appears to be limited to these isolated case reports. Neither interaction is well established and neither would appear to be of general clinical importance. The chlorinated hydrocarbon insecticides have been withdrawn from general use in most countries so that the possibility of an interaction with any anticoagulant is now very small. No other cases of an interaction between an anticoagulant and ivermectin, whether used as an insecticide or for the treatment of onchocerciasis, appear to have been reported.

As a general rule, farm workers and others should use proper protection (gloves, masks, protective clothing) if they are exposed to substantial amounts of any insecticide, because these can be both directly toxic and can also apparently interact with some prescribed drugs, including the anticoagulants, even if only very rarely.

1. Fernandéz MA, Ballasteros S, Aznar J. Oral anticoagulants and insecticides. *Thromb Haemost* (1998) 80, 724.
2. Jeffery WH, Ahlin TA, Goren C, Hardy WR. Loss of warfarin effect after occupational insecticide exposure. *JAMA* (1976) 236, 2881–2.
3. Richards FO, McNeeley MB, Bryan RT, Eberhard ML, McNeeley DF, Lammie PJ, Spencer HC. Ivermectin and prothrombin time. *Lancet* (1989) i, 1139–40.
4. Pacque MC, Munoz B, White AT, Williams PN, Greene BM, Taylor HR. Ivermectin and prothrombin time. *Lancet* (1989) i, 1140.
5. Homeida MMA, Bagi IA, Ghalib HW, El Sheikh H, Ismail A, Yousif MA, Sulieman S, Ali HM, Bennett JL, Williams J. Prolongation of prothrombin time with ivermectin. *Lancet* (1988) i, 1346–7.
6. Kolmodin B, Azarnoff DL, Sjöqvist F. Effect of environmental factors on drug metabolism: Decreased plasma half-life of antipyrine in workers exposed to chlorinated hydrocarbon insecticides. *Clin Pharmacol Ther* (1969) 10, 638–42.

Coumarins + Interferons

Isolated case reports indicate that the effects of acenocoumarol and warfarin may be increased by interferons.

Clinical evidence

A woman stabilised on long-term **warfarin** 2.5 to 3.5 mg daily had a prothrombin time rise from 16.7 to 20.4 seconds after receiving 6 million units of **interferon-alfa** daily for 10 days, then three times a week. Her serum **warfarin** levels rose from about 0.8 to 5.2 micrograms/mL. She responded to a reduction in the **warfarin** dosage to 2 mg daily. The authors of the report also say that they have seen 4 other patients taking **warfarin** who needed a dosage reduction when given interferon, two of them while taking **interferon beta** and the other two while taking **interferon alfa-2b**.[1] A woman taking **acenocoumarol** 1 and 2 mg on alternate days had gingival bleeding and a thrombotest change from 35% to 19% (indicating an increased anticoagulant effect) within 6 weeks of starting treatment with 3 million units of **interferon-alpha 2b** three times weekly. Her thrombotest percentages stabilised between 25 and 40% when the **acenocoumarol** dosage was reduced to 1 mg daily. A later reduction in the interferon dosage caused a decrease in the anticoagulant effects of acenocoumarol.[2]

Mechanism

Not understood. The authors of both reports suggest that interferon reduces the metabolism of the anticoagulants by the liver, thereby reducing their clearance and increasing their effects.[1,2]

Importance and management

These reports seem to be the only ones to describe this interaction so the interaction is not yet established. However it would seem prudent to monitor the effects if interferon is given to patients taking coumarins, reducing the dosage if necessary. For a case of decreased warfarin effects in a patient given interferon alfa-2b and ribavirin, see 'Coumarins + Ribavirin', p.447.

1. Adachi Y, Yokoyama Y, Nanno T, Yamamoto T. Potentation of warfarin by interferon. *BMJ* (1995) 311, 292.
2. Serratrice J, Durand J-M, Morange S. Interferon-alpha 2b interaction with acenocoumarol. *Am J Hematol* (1998) 57, 89–92.

Coumarins + Ispaghula (Psyllium)

Ispaghula (psyllium) did not affect either the absorption or the anticoagulant effects of warfarin in one study. A cohort study also found no evidence of an interaction in patients taking acenocoumarol or phenprocoumon.

Clinical evidence, mechanism, importance and management

In a study in 6 healthy subjects, ispaghula (given as a 14-g dose of colloid (*Metamucil*) in a small amount of water with a single 40-mg dose of **warfarin**, and three further doses of ispaghula every 2 hours thereafter) did not affect either the absorption or the anticoagulant effects of the **warfarin**.[1] Similarly, in a population-based cohort study in patients taking **acenocoumarol** or **phenprocoumon**, there was no increased risk of over-anticoagulation (INR greater than 6) associated with the use of ispaghula (psyllium seeds), although the number of people treated was small.[2] No alteration of the anticoagulant response would therefore be expected on concurrent use.

1. Robinson DS, Benjamin DM, McCormack JJ. Interaction of warfarin and nonsystemic gastrointestinal drugs. *Clin Pharmacol Ther* (1971) 12, 491–5.
2. Visser LE, Penning-van Beest FJA, Wilson JHP, Vulto AG, Kasbergen AAH, De Smet PAGM, Hofman A, Stricker BHC. Overanticoagulation associated with combined use of lactulose and acenocoumarol or phenprocoumon. *Br J Clin Pharmacol* (2003) 57, 522–4.

Coumarins + Lanthanum

Lanthanum did not alter the pharmacokinetics of a single dose of warfarin.

Clinical evidence, mechanism, importance and management

In a pharmacokinetic study in healthy subjects, lanthanum (3 doses of 1 g the day before **warfarin**, then 1 g thirty minutes before **warfarin**) had no effect on the pharmacokinetics of a single dose of **warfarin**.[1]

Lanthanum is a phosphate-binding drug, and does not appear to alter **warfarin** absorption. This suggests that no **warfarin** dose adjustments are expected to be needed on concurrent use. However, note that the pharmacodynamics of **warfarin** (e.g. the effects on INR) were not assessed in this study.

1. Fiddler G. Fosrenol (lanthanum carbonate) does not affect the pharmacokinetics of concomitant treatment with warfarin. *J Am Soc Nephrol* (2002) 13, 749A–750A.

Coumarins + Lasofoxifene

In a study, lasofoxifene caused a minor 16% decrease in prothrombin time without changing warfarin pharmacokinetics.

Clinical evidence, mechanism, importance and management

In 12 healthy postmenopausal women, lasofoxifene 4 mg on day one then 500 micrograms daily for 13 days had no effect on the pharmacokinetics of *R*- or *S*-warfarin when a single 20-mg dose of **warfarin** was given on day 8. Conversely, the maximum prothrombin time was decreased by 16%, with a similar decrease in maximum INR from 1.9 to 1.6.[1]

Because this slight decrease in **warfarin** effects has been seen with 'raloxifene', (p.446), the authors suggested that it might be because oestrogenic compounds increase plasma concentrations of vitamin K-dependent clotting factors.[1]

The authors suggest that the small decrease in **warfarin** effect with lasofoxifene may not be clinically relevant. Nevertheless, they say that until more data are available on longer-term concurrent use, it is recommended that prothrombin times should be monitored when starting or stopping lasofoxifene.[1] This seems a sensible precaution.

1. Quellet D, Bramson C, Carvajal-Gonzalez S, Roman D, Randinitis E, Remmers A, Gardner MJ. Effects of lasofoxifene on the pharmacokinetics and pharmacodynamics of single-dose warfarin. *Br J Clin Pharmacol* (2006) 61, 741–5.

Coumarins + Laxatives

In one cohort study, the long-term use of lactulose appeared to be associated with an increased risk of overanticoagulation. Limited evidence suggested no interaction occurred with liquid paraffin or colocynth.

Clinical evidence

In a population-based cohort study in patients taking **acenocoumarol** or **phenprocoumon**, lactulose significantly increased the risk of over-anticoagulation (INR greater than 6) (relative risk of 3.4, range 2.2 to 5.3). When analysed by duration of use, less than 27 days use of **lactulose** actually decreased the risk of over-anticoagulation, whereas longer use was associated with an increased risk. In this study, neither **liquid paraffin** nor **colocynth** preparations were associated with an increased risk of over-anticoagulation, but numbers of patients treated with these drugs was small.[1]

Mechanism

In theory, drugs that shorten gastrointestinal transit time such as laxatives and liquid paraffin (mineral oil) might be expected to decrease the absorption of both vitamin K and the oral anticoagulants. Decreasing the absorption of vitamin K would be expected to increase the effect of oral anticoagulants, which could be offset by the decrease in absorption of oral anticoagulants. In the case of short-term lactulose use, it was suggested that decreasing the colonic pH might have increased the absorption of vitamin K, thereby reducing the effect of the anticoagulant. On longer term use, it was postulated that lactulose might reduce faecal flora that produce vitamin K, so increasing the risk of over-anticoagulation.[1] Liquid paraffin might also be expected to impair the absorption of vitamin K.

Importance and management

The cohort study cited appears to be the first and only evidence of a possible interaction with laxatives, and it suggests that long-term use of lactulose may increase the effect of coumarins. This finding requires confirmation in a controlled pharmacological study. Until further data are available, it may be prudent to consider the possibility of an interaction in anybody taking lactulose long-term. Limited evidence suggested no interaction occurred with liquid paraffin or colocynth. Clinical evidence for an interaction with other laxatives is lacking, despite the theoretical considerations.

1. Visser LE, Penning-van Beest FJA, Wilson JHP, Vulto AG, Kasbergen AAH, De Smet PAGM, Hofman A, Stricker BHC. Overanticoagulation associated with combined use of lactulose and acenocoumarol or phenprocoumon. *Br J Clin Pharmacol* (2003) 57, 522–4.

Coumarins + Leflunomide

There are a few reports of increased INRs, some with bleeding complications, in patients taking warfarin with leflunomide.

Clinical evidence, mechanism, importance and management

A short report describes a patient taking **warfarin** whose INR rose from 2.5 to over 6, resulting in a hospital admission, shortly after she started taking leflunomide (3 days of 100 mg daily).[1]

Another report describes a patient taking **warfarin** who developed haematuria after taking leflunomide 100 mg daily for 2 days. His INR was found to have risen from 3.4 to over 11, and **warfarin** was discontinued. The haematuria spontaneously resolved, but as the INR remained elevated for the next 2 days he was given 1 mg of vitamin K, which brought his INR down to 1.9. He was later stabilised on **warfarin** 1 mg daily with a leflunomide maintenance dose of 20 mg daily.[2] The authors of this report stated that at that time (2002) the CSM in the UK had received over 300 reports of leflunomide raising the INRs of patients taking **warfarin**;[2] however, this was an error, and it should have read that of 300 reports of raised INRs with **warfarin** and another drug, *four* reports related to leflunomide.[3] An additional case describes a patient who required a 22% decrease in her weekly **warfarin** dose after starting leflunomide.[4]

The manufacturers of leflunomide note that *in vitro,* the active metabolite of leflunomide inhibits the cytochrome P450 isoenzyme CYP2C9. They therefore advise caution if leflunomide is given with drugs metabolised by CYP2C9, of which they give **warfarin** and **phenprocoumon** as examples.[5] On the basis of the cases seen, it would seem prudent to monitor the INR of any patient taking a coumarin anticoagulant who is started on leflunomide.

1. Mason JP. Warfarin and leflunomide. *Pharm J* (2000) 265, 267.
2. Lim V, Pande I. Leflunomide can potentiate the anticoagulant effect of warfarin. *BMJ* (2002) 325, 1333. Erratum *ibid.* (2003) 326, 432.
3. Anonymous. Corrections and clarifications: drug points. *BMJ* (2003) 326, 432.
4. Chonlahan J, Halloran MA, Hammonds A. Leflunomide and warfarin interaction: case report and review of the literature. *Pharmacotherapy* (2006) 26, 868–71.
5. Arava (Leflunomide). Sanofi-Aventis. UK Summary of product characteristics, January 2006.

Coumarins + Leukotriene antagonists

Zafirlukast increases the anticoagulant effects of warfarin and bleeding has been seen. Pranlukast is predicted to interact similarly. In contrast, montelukast did not alter the pharmacokinetics or anticoagulant effects of single-dose warfarin.

Clinical evidence

(a) Montelukast

In a double-blind, placebo-controlled, randomised study, 12 healthy subjects were given oral montelukast 10 mg daily for 12 days and a single 30-mg dose of **warfarin** on day 7. It was found that the pharmacokinetics of the **warfarin** were virtually unchanged by the montelukast, and prothrombin times and INRs were not significantly altered.[1]

(b) Zafirlukast

In a placebo-controlled study, 16 healthy subjects taking zafirlukast 80 mg twice daily for 10 days were given a single 25-mg dose of **warfarin** on day 5. The mean AUC of *S*-warfarin was increased by 63% and the half-life by 36%, but the pharmacokinetics of *R*-warfarin were not significantly changed. The mean prothrombin time increased by 35%.[2]

An 85-year-old woman taking **warfarin**, salbutamol (albuterol), diltiazem, digoxin, furosemide and potassium was admitted to hospital with various cardiac-related problems and bleeding (epistaxis, melaena, multiple bruising), which was attributed to the use of zafirlukast 20 mg twice daily. Her INR had risen from 1.1 (measured 6 months previously) to 4.5. The report does not say how long she had been taking the both drugs together.[3]

Mechanism

The reason for the interaction is thought to be that the zafirlukast inhibits the cytochrome P450 isoenzyme CYP2C9, which metabolises *S*-warfarin.[2,4] *In vitro* studies suggest that **pranlukast** has a similar effect.[5]

Importance and management

Information appears to be limited to these reports but the interaction with zafirlukast would seem to be established. If zafirlukast is given to patients stabilised on warfarin, monitor prothrombin times well and be alert for the need to reduce the warfarin dosage to avoid over-anticoagulation. Other coumarins might be expected to be affected similarly. Pranlukast is also predicted to interact, as it is also an inhibitor of CYP2C9. In contrast, montelukast does not appear to interact with warfarin, and no warfarin dose adjustments are predicted to be needed on concurrent use.

1. Van Hecken A, Depre M, Verbesselt R, Wynants K, De Lepeleire I, Arnoudt J, Wong PH, Freeman A, Holland S, Gertz B, De Schepper PJ. Effect of montelukast on the pharmacokinetics and pharmacodynamics of warfarin in healthy subjects. *J Clin Pharmacol* (1999) 39, 495–500.
2. Suttle AB, Vargo DL, Wilkinson LA, Birmingham BK, Lasseter K. Effect of zafirlukast on the pharmacokinetics of R- and S-warfarin in healthy men. *Clin Pharmacol Ther* (1997) 61, 186.
3. Morkunas A, Graeme K. Zafirlukast-warfarin drug interaction with gastrointestinal bleeding. *J Toxicol Clin Toxicol* (1997) 35, 501.
4. Accolate (Zafirlukast). AstraZeneca UK Ltd. UK Summary of product characteristics, December 2004.
5. Liu KH, Lee YM, Shon JH, Kim MJ, Lee SS, Yoon YR, Cha IJ, Shin JG. Potential of pranlukast and zafirlukast in the inhibition of human liver cytochrome P450 enzymes. *Xenobiotica* (2004) 34, 429–38.

Coumarins + Levetiracetam

In a controlled study, levetiracetam did not alter the pharmacokinetics or pharmacodynamics of warfarin.

Clinical evidence, mechanism, importance and management

In a randomised, double-blind, placebo-controlled study in 42 healthy subjects stabilised on **warfarin,** levetiracetam 1 g twice daily for 7 days had no significant effect on the pharmacokinetics of *R*- or *S*-warfarin and the INRs were not significantly altered.[1] No **warfarin** dose adjustments would therefore be expected to be needed on concurrent use.

1. Ragueneau-Majlessi I, Levy RH, Meyerhoff C. Lack of effect of repeated administration of levetiracetam on the pharmacodynamic and pharmacokinetic profiles of warfarin. *Epilepsy Res* (2001) 47, 55–63.

Coumarins + MAOIs or RIMAs

Although some *animal* data show that the non-selective MAOIs increase the effects of some oral anticoagulants, there appears to be no clinical evidence of an interaction. Moclobemide did not interact with phenprocoumon in a pharmacological study.

Clinical evidence, mechanism, importance and management

A number of studies in *animals*[1-4] have shown that some of the non-selective MAOIs can increase the effects of some oral anticoagulants. However, there appear to be no clinical studies or case reports of this interaction, and therefore no special precautions seem to be necessary. A study in healthy subjects found that **moclobemide** 200 mg three times daily for 7 days did not alter the anticoagulant effects of steady-state **phenprocoumon.**[5]

1. Fumarola D, De Rinaldis P. Ricerche sperimentali sugli inibitori della mono-aminossidasi. Influenza della nialamide sulla attività degli anticoagulanti indiretti. *Haematologica* (1964) 49, 1248–66.
2. Reber K, Studer A. Beeinflussung der Wirkung einiger indirekter Antikoagulantien durch Monoaminoxydase-Hemmer. *Thromb Diath Haemorrh* (1965) 14, 83–7.
3. de Nicola P, Fumarola D, de Rinaldis P. Beeinflussung der gerinnungshemmenden Wirkung der indirekten Antikoagulantien durch die MAO-Inhibitoren. *Thromb Diath Haemorrh* (1964) 12 (Suppl), 125–7.
4. Hrdina P, Rusnáková M, Kovalčík V. Changes of hypoprothrombinaemic activity of indirect anticoagulants after MAO inhibitors and reserpine. *Biochem Pharmacol* (1953) 12 (Suppl), 241.
5. Amrein R, Güntert TW, Dingemanse J, Lorscheid T, Stabl M, Schmid-Burgk W. Interactions of moclobemide with concomitantly administered medication: evidence from pharmacological and clinical studies. *Psychopharmacology (Berl)* (1992) 106, S24–S31.

Coumarins + Medroxyprogesterone acetate or Megestrol

High-dose medroxyprogesterone acetate and megestrol prolonged the half-life of single-dose warfarin in one small study in patients with advanced breast cancer. There is also a case of increased bleeding times when megestrol was given with unnamed anticoagulants.

Clinical evidence, mechanism, importance and management

In a study in patients with advanced breast cancer, a single 0.3-mg/kg doses of **warfarin** were given to 2 patients before and after oral medroxyprogesterone acetate 500 mg twice daily for 5 weeks and to 2 patients before and after megestrol 160 mg daily for 5 weeks. The half-life of **warfarin** was increased by 71% and the clearance decreased by 35%.[1] A bulletin includes a brief mention of increased bleeding times in a patient taking unnamed anticoagulants and given **megestrol** (dose not stated).[2]

Although the evidence is limited, what is known suggests that it would be prudent to monitor prothrombin times in patients taking **warfarin** who are high-dose medroxyprogesterone acetate or megestrol, being alert for any increased warfarin effects.

1. Lundgren S, Kvinnsland S, Utaaker E, Bakke O, Ueland PM. Effect of oral high-dose progestins on the disposition of antipyrine, digitoxin, and warfarin in patients with advanced breast cancer. *Cancer Chemother Pharmacol* (1986) 18, 270–5.
2. Beeley L, Stewart P, Hickey FM. *Bulletin of the West Midlands Centre for Adverse Drug Reaction Reporting* (1988) 27, 24.

Coumarins + Mefloquine

The effects of warfarin and an unnamed coumarin were increased in two patients who took mefloquine.

Clinical evidence, mechanism, importance and management

A 66-year-old man taking **warfarin** and various other drugs presented to an emergency department unwell with a distended abdomen while travelling in Kenya. His prothrombin time was grossly prolonged and the distension was found to be due to bleeding. One week before travel he had started mefloquine 250 mg weekly without a check of his prothrombin time. He was given subcutaneous enoxaparin instead of **warfarin** while continuing the mefloquine. Another patient taking a coumarin and oral antidiabetics presented with hypoglycaemia and a large haematoma of the right leg after taking 3 doses of mefloquine 250 mg weekly. His INR was 6.4.[1]

The author considered that mefloquine may have caused the increased anticoagulation in these two cases, and suggested that mefloquine should be started several weeks before travel to allow for monitoring of any changes in anticoagulant effects.[1] The manufacturers of mefloquine also recommend that, before departure, travellers also taking anticoagulants should be checked for any alteration in their effect.[2,3] This is probably prudent, although patients should be advised that many other factors to do with travel such as altered diet could contribute to a change in anticoagulant control.

1. Loefler I. Mefloquine and anticoagulant interaction. *J Travel Med* (2003) 10, 194–5.
2. Lariam (Mefloquine hydrochloride). Roche Products Ltd. UK Summary of product characteristics, September 2005.
3. Lariam (Mefloquine hydrochloride). Roche Pharmaceuticals. US Prescribing information, May 2004.

Coumarins + Menthol lozenges

A man had a reduction in the effects of warfarin, which were attributed to the use of menthol cough lozenges during a flu-like illness.

Clinical evidence, mechanism, importance and management

A 57-year-old man taking **warfarin** 49 mg weekly with an INR in the range of 2.28 to 2.68 for the previous 3 weeks was found to have an INR of 1.45. He had been unwell with a flu-like illness over the past week, for which he had been taking about 6 *Halls* menthol cough lozenges (cough drops) per day for 4 days. He said he had not changed his diet or missed any warfarin doses. The **warfarin** dose was increased to 53 mg weekly for a week with an INR rise to 2.2, then the **warfarin** dose was decreased to 52 mg weekly with an INR of 3.06, so the previous dose of 49 mg weekly was resumed with an INR of 2.92.[1]

Whether this case represents an interaction with the menthol lozenges is uncertain. Further study is needed.

1. Kassebaum PJ, Shaw DL, Tomich DJ. Possible warfarin interaction with menthol cough drops. *Ann Pharmacother* (2005) 39, 365–7.

Coumarins + Meprobamate

The anticoagulant effects of warfarin are not altered to a clinically relevant extent by meprobamate.

Clinical evidence, mechanism, importance and management

Meprobamate 400 mg four times daily for 2 weeks was given to 9 patients stabilised on **warfarin**. Three of them showed a small increase in prothrombin times, five a small decrease and one remained unaffected: all the changes were considered to fall within the range of variations normally seen in clinical practice.[1] Moreover, in a later placebo-controlled study in 17 patients taking **warfarin**, the 8 patients who were also given meprobamate 2.4 g daily for 4 weeks showed only a small clinically unimportant reduction in prothrombin times.[2] Similar results were found in another study.[3] No **warfarin** dose adjustments would therefore seem to be needed if meprobamate is added to established treatment with **warfarin**.

1. Udall JA. Warfarin therapy not influenced by meprobamate. A controlled study in nine men. *Curr Ther Res* (1970) 12, 724–8.
2. Gould L, Michael A, Fisch S, Gomprecht RF. Prothrombin levels maintained with meprobamate and warfarin. A controlled study. *JAMA* (1972) 220, 1460–2.
3. deCarolis PP, Gelfand ML. Effect of tranquilizers on prothrombin time response to coumarin. *J Clin Pharmacol* (1975) 15, 557.

Coumarins + Mesalazine (Mesalamine) or Sulfasalazine

A single case report describes reduced warfarin effects in a patient given mesalazine. Another single case report describes a marked reduction in the response to warfarin when mesalazine was switched to sulfasalazine.

Clinical evidence

(a) Mesalazine

A woman stabilised on **warfarin** 5 mg daily, with INRs between 2 and 3, started taking mesalazine 800 mg three times daily for the treatment of a caecal ulcer. Four weeks later she presented to hospital with left leg pain, which was diagnosed as an acute popliteal vein thrombosis, and at the same time it was found that her prothrombin time and INR had fallen to 11.3 seconds and 0.9, respectively. The patient was treated with intravenous heparin. Over the next 10 days INRs of up to 1.7 were achieved by increasing the doses of **warfarin** up to 10 mg daily, but a satisfactory INR of 2.1 was only reached when the mesalazine was stopped. The report says that serum **warfarin** levels were not detectable during the use of mesalazine.[1] For discussion of a patient who had a reduction in the response to warfarin when switched from mesalazine to sulfasalazine, see below.

(b) Sulfasalazine

A 37-year-old woman taking **warfarin** 30 mg weekly with stable INRs between 2 and 3 in the previous 2 years (and also taking beclometasone, salbutamol, aspirin, azathioprine, ethinyloestradiol/norgestrel), had her treatment for arthritis and ulcerative colitis changed from **mesalazine** to sulfasalazine 1 g four times daily. The day after the change her INR was found to be subtherapeutic (1.5) and she needed numerous increases in the **warfarin** doses over the next 6 weeks, eventually needing **warfarin** 75 mg weekly before acceptable INRs were achieved. During this period she developed a new deep vein thrombosis. When the sulfasalazine was later stopped and the mesalazine restarted, her **warfarin** dosage requirements dropped to 45 mg weekly.[2]

Mechanism

Not understood. Sulfasalazine is broken down in the colon to a sulfonamide, sulfapyridine, and 5-aminosalicylic acid (mesalazine). Some 'sulfonamides', (p.376) are known inhibitors of warfarin metabolism, and increase the effects of warfarin. In contrast, in the case with sulfasalazine a marked decrease was noted.

Importance and management

Not established. The case of a reduction in effect of warfarin on starting mesalazine appears to be the first and only report of an interaction, which suggests that it is unlikely to be of general importance. Similarly, the case when mesalazine was switched to sulfasalazine is an unexplained and isolated case, and its validity has been debated.[3,4] There are no other reports in the literature and this possible interaction also seems unlikely to be of general importance. Consider these cases in the event of an unexpected response to treatment.

1. Marinella MA. Mesalamine and warfarin therapy resulting in decreased warfarin effect. *Ann Pharmacother* (1998) 32, 841–2.
2. Teefy AM, Martin JE, Kovacs MJ. Warfarin resistance due to sulfasalazine. *Ann Pharmacother* (2000) 34, 1265–8.
3. Sherman JJ. Comment: other factors should be considered in a possible warfarin and sulfasalazine interaction. *Ann Pharmacother* (2001) 35, 506.
4. Kovacs MJ, Teefy AM. Comment: other factors should be considered in a possible warfarin and sulfasalazine interaction. Author's reply. *Ann Pharmacother* (2001) 35, 506.

Coumarins + Methaqualone

Methaqualone may cause a very small and clinically unimportant reduction in the anticoagulant effects of warfarin.

Clinical evidence, mechanism, importance and management

The average prothrombin time of 10 patients stabilised on **warfarin** was 20.9 seconds before, 20.4 seconds during, and 19.6 seconds after taking methaqualone 300 mg at bedtime for 4 weeks.[1] The plasma **warfarin** levels of another patient were unaffected by methaqualone, although there was some evidence that enzyme induction had occurred.[2] Methaqualone has some enzyme-inducing effects so that any small changes in prothrombin times reflect a limited increase in the metabolism and clearance of **warfarin**, but these appear to be too small to be of clinical significance.[2,3] No special precautions seem to be necessary.

1. Udall JA. Clinical implications of warfarin interactions with five sedatives. *Am J Cardiol* (1975) 35, 67–71.
2. Whitfield JB, Moss DW, Neale G, Orme M, Breckenridge A. Changes in plasma γ-glutamyl transpeptidase activity associated with alterations in drug metabolism in man. *BMJ* (1973) 1, 316–18.
3. Nayak RK, Smyth RD, Chamberlain AP, Polk A, DeLong AF, Herczeg T, Chemburkar PB, Joslin RS, Reavey-Cantwell NH. Methaqualone pharmacokinetics after single- and multiple-dose administration in man. *J Pharmacokinet Biopharm* (1974) 2, 107–21.

Coumarins + Methylphenidate

Methylphenidate appears not to interact with ethyl biscoumacetate.

Clinical evidence, mechanism, importance and management

In one study in 4 healthy subjects, the half-life of a single dose of **ethyl biscoumacetate** was approximately doubled after they took methylphenidate 20 mg daily for 3 to 5 days.[1] However, a later double-blind, placebo-controlled study failed to confirm this interaction: the half-life of **ethyl biscoumacetate** was not altered by methylphenidate 20 mg daily for 4 days in 4 healthy subjects, and was not different to that seen in 4 subjects given placebo.[2] The first authors suggested that methylphenidate inhibits the metabolism of the oral anticoagulant, but this seems unlikely given the findings of the second study.

Although the findings of these 2 studies are at odds with each other, the better-controlled study and the lack of reports of problems in the literature suggest that an interaction is unlikely. There does not seem to be any information about other anticoagulants. Nevertheless the manufacturers recommend caution and suggest that patients taking coumarins should have their INR monitored if methylphenidate is started or stopped.[3]

1. Garrettson LK, Perel JM, Dayton PG. Methylphenidate interaction with both anticonvulsants and ethyl biscoumacetate. *JAMA* (1969) 207, 2053–6.

2. Hague DE, Smith ME, Ryan JR, McMahon FG. The effect of methylphenidate and prolintane on the metabolism of ethyl biscoumacetate. *Clin Pharmacol Ther* (1971) 12, 259–62.
3. Concerta XL (Methylphenidate hydrochloride) Janssen-Cilag Ltd. UK Summary of product characteristics, June 2007.

Coumarins + Metoclopramide

Metoclopramide caused a small decrease in the AUC of phenprocoumon, without altering its anticoagulant effects seemed to occur.

Clinical evidence, mechanism, importance and management

In 12 healthy subjects, metoclopramide 30 mg daily for 10 days slightly reduced the AUC of a single dose of **phenprocoumon** given on day 4 by 16%, but no significant changes were seen in the anticoagulant effects.[1] This suggests that no phenprocoumon dose adjustment would be expected to be necessary if these two drugs are given together. There seems to be no information about any other anticoagulant.

1. Wesermeyer D, Mönig H, Gaska T, Masuch S, Seiler KU, Huss H, Bruhn HD. Der Einfluß von Cisaprid und Metoclopramid auf die Bioverfügbarkeit von Phenprocoumon. *Hamostaseologie* (1991) 11, 95–102.

Coumarins + Metrifonate

Metrifonate did not interact with single-dose warfarin in one study.

Clinical evidence, mechanism, importance and management

A double-blind, placebo-controlled, crossover study in 14 healthy subjects found that metrifonate 50 mg daily for 8 days did not change the pharmacokinetics and pharmacodynamics of a single 25-mg dose of **warfarin** given on day 4. Plasma **warfarin** levels and prothrombin times remained unchanged.[1] This suggests that no **warfarin** dose adjustments are needed if these two drugs are used concurrently. Information about other anticoagulants is lacking.

1. Heinig R, Kitchin N, Rolan P. Disposition of a single dose of warfarin in healthy individuals after pretreatment with metrifonate. *Clin Drug Invest* (1999) 18, 151–9.

Coumarins + Misoprostol

A reduction in the anticoagulant effects of acenocoumarol has been attributed to the use of misoprostol in one patient.

Clinical evidence, mechanism, importance and management

A 39-year-old woman taking **acenocoumarol**, celiprolol, triamterene, cyclothiazide, pravastatin and diosmin had a rise in her prothrombin levels from 0.3 to 1 within 8 days of starting to take diclofenac and misoprostol 400 micrograms daily. A day after these two drugs had been withdrawn her prothrombin level had fallen to 0.67, and after another 3 days to 0.32.[1] The reasons for this reaction are not known, but suspicion falls on the misoprostol because diclofenac, if and when it interacts with anticoagulants, increases rather than reduces their effects (see 'Coumarins + NSAIDs; Diclofenac', p.429). But just why misoprostol should cause these changes is not clear.

This is an isolated case, complicated by the presence of a number of other drugs, which suggests that it is unlikely to be of general importance. More study is needed.

1. Martin MP, Jonville-Bera AP, Bera F, Caillard X, Autret E. Interaction entre le misoprostol et l'acénocoumarol. *Presse Med* (1995) 24, 195.

Coumarins + Moracizine

Moracizine did not alter the pharmacodynamics of single-dose warfarin, and the only pharmacokinetic change was a slight decrease in half-life. An isolated report describes bleeding in a patient taking warfarin with moracizine.

Clinical evidence

In a study in 12 healthy subjects, moracizine 250 mg every 8 hours for 21 days caused little or no change in the pharmacokinetics of a single 25-mg dose of **warfarin** given on day 14. There was only a slight decrease in the **warfarin** elimination half-life, from 37.6 to 34.2 hours, and no change in prothrombin times.[1,2] The manufacturer also noted that clinical experience in 34 patients showed that no significant changes in **warfarin** dosage requirements were needed after moracizine was started.[1]

However, in one case report the prothrombin time of a woman taking **warfarin**, digoxin, captopril and prednisone rose from a range of 15 to 20 seconds up to 41 seconds within 4 days of starting moracizine 300 mg three times daily. She bled (haematemesis, haematuria), but responded rapidly to withdrawal of the **warfarin** and moracizine, and the administration of phytomenadione.[3]

Mechanism

Not understood.

Importance and management

Information appears to be limited to these reports. The study and early clinical experience suggest that no interaction occurs. The case of an increased effect seems to be an isolated report, and therefore unlikely to be of general importance.

1. Siddoway LA, Schwartz SL, Barbey JT, Woosley RL. Clinical pharmacokinetics of moricizine. *Am J Cardiol* (1990) 65, 21D–25D.
2. Benedek IH, King S-YP, Powell RJ, Agra AM, Schary WL, Pieniaszek HJ. Effect of moricizine on the pharmacokinetics and pharmacodynamics of warfarin in healthy volunteers. *J Clin Pharmacol* (1992) 32, 558–63.
3. Serpa MD, Cossolias J, McGreevy MJ. Moricizine-warfarin: a possible interaction. *Ann Pharmacother* (1992) 26, 127.

Coumarins + Nefazodone or Trazodone

In a one study, nefazodone decreased the level of *S*-warfarin by just 12% and did not alter the prothrombin ratio. A handful of case reports describe a moderate reduction in the anticoagulant effects of warfarin caused by trazodone.

Clinical evidence

(a) Nefazodone

In one study, 17 healthy subjects given **warfarin** to achieve a prothrombin ratio of 1.2 to 1.5 for 14 days were then given nefazodone 200 mg or placebo every 12 hours for a further 7 days. The only pharmacokinetic changes were a 12% decrease in the AUC and maximum serum levels of *S*-warfarin. No changes occurred in the prothrombin ratios.[1]

(b) Trazodone

In an early case series, a patient stabilised on **warfarin** was given trazodone 75 mg daily for 8 days without any significant changes in the prothrombin time. Similarly, the same dosage of trazodone had no obvious effect on prothrombin time in a patient who had recently started taking **phenprocoumon** and another who had recently started taking **ethyl biscoumacetate**.[2] However, in another report, a woman needed a small increase in her **warfarin** dose, from 6.4 to 7.5 mg daily, when she was given trazodone 300 mg daily, in order to maintain her prothrombin time at 20 seconds. Her **warfarin** requirements fell when the trazodone was later withdrawn.[3] A retrospective review from June 1998 to June 1999 identified 75 patient taking both trazodone and **warfarin**. Of the patients who had started trazodone during this period (number not stated), at least 3 had a probable interaction. One had a decrease in INR from 2.79 to 1.07 six days after starting trazodone, and needed a 25% increase in the dose of **warfarin**. Another patient had an increase in INR when he ran out of trazodone, and a decrease in INR on restarting the trazodone. A third required a 39% increase in **warfarin** dose after starting trazodone.[4] The manufacturer in the US notes that there have been reports of both increased and decreased prothrombin times in patients taking warfarin with trazodone.[5]

Mechanism

Unknown.

Importance and management

The incidence of this interaction is unknown. All the evidence suggests that some patients require a moderate increase in warfarin dose when starting trazodone. Be aware of this interaction in all patients taking warfarin if trazodone is started or stopped, and adjust the dosage if necessary. The interaction can occur within a few days. The clinical relevance of the 12% decrease in *S*-warfarin levels see with nefazodone is likely to be minor. The authors of the study concluded that no change in warfarin dose is likely to be required on concurrent use.[1]

1. Salazar DE, Dockens RC, Milbrath RL, Raymond RH, Fulmor IE, Chaikin PC, Uderman HD. Pharmacokinetic and pharmacodynamic evaluation of warfarin and nefazodone coadministration in healthy subjects. *J Clin Pharmacol* (1995) 35, 730–8.
2. Cozzolino G, Pazzaglia I, De Gaetano V, Macri M. Clinical investigation on the possible interaction between anti-coagulants and a new psychotropic drug (Trazodone). *Clin Eur* (1972) 11, 593–607.
3. Hardy J-L, Sirois A. Reduction of prothrombin and partial thromboplastin times with trazodone. *Can Med Assoc J* (1986) 135, 1372.
4. Small NL, Giamonna KA. Interaction between warfarin and trazodone. *Ann Pharmacother* (2000) 34, 734–6.
5. Desyrel (Trazodone hydrochloride). Bristol-Myers Squibb Company. US Prescribing information, January 2005.

Coumarins + Nevirapine

One report of 3 cases suggests that warfarin requirements are markedly increased by nevirapine.

Clinical evidence, mechanism, importance and management

A man taking **warfarin** 2.5 mg daily (INR 2.1 to 2.4) needed a doubled **warfarin** dose when his treatment with zidovudine and didanosine was replaced by stavudine, lamivudine and nevirapine. A few days later when his treatment was again changed (to stavudine, lamivudine and saquinavir) his original **warfarin** dosage was found to be adequate. Another patient was resistant to doses of **warfarin** of up to 17 mg daily while taking zidovudine, lamivudine and nevirapine, but he responded to **warfarin** 5 mg daily when the nevirapine was withdrawn. The warfarin dosage had to be raised to 12 mg daily when nevirapine was restarted. Yet another patient showed resistance to **warfarin** while taking nevirapine.[1]

Nevirapine is a known enzyme inducer, and therefore possibly induces the enzymes concerned with the metabolism of the **warfarin**.

Information seems to be limited to these three cases, but it would be prudent to monitor prothrombin times and INRs in any patient if **warfarin** and nevirapine are used concurrently, being alert for the need to increase the **warfarin** dosage (possibly twofold). Information about other oral anticoagulants seems to be lacking, but if the suggested mechanism is correct, all coumarins would be expected to interact to some extent.

1. Dionisio D, Mininni S, Bartolozzi D, Esperti F, Vivarelli A, Leoncini F. Need for increased dose of warfarin in HIV patients taking nevirapine. *AIDS* (2001) 15, 277–8.

Coumarins and related drugs + NSAIDs

Combined use of NSAIDs and coumarin anticoagulants increases the risk of gastrointestinal haemorrhage. Care is needed with the combination. Some individual NSAIDs also alter the pharmacokinetics of warfarin, and these effects are covered in specific monographs that follow.

Clinical evidence

(a) Gastrointestinal bleeding

In a retrospective cohort study of patients hospitalised for peptic ulcer disease, combined current use of both oral anticoagulants and NSAIDs was associated with a marked increase in the risk of haemorrhagic peptic ulcer disease of 12.7 (95% confidence interval 6.3 to 25.7). This was much higher than the risk associated with NSAIDs alone or oral anticoagulants alone (both about a fourfold increased risk). In this study, about 10% of the hospitalisations for haemorrhagic peptic ulcer disease in patients taking anticoagulants were attributed to the concurrent use of NSAIDs. The oral anticoagulants used were the coumarins **warfarin**, **phenprocoumon** and **acenocoumarol**, and the indanediones **phenindione** and **anisindione**. The NSAIDs used were nonacetylated salicylates, **ibuprofen**, **indometacin**, **sulindac**, **naproxen**, **fenoprofen**, **piroxicam**, **tolmetin**, and **meclofenamate**.[1]

In a case-control study, patients taking **warfarin** who were admitted to hospital with upper gastrointestinal haemorrhage were significantly more likely to be taking non-selective NSAIDs (odds ratio 1.9). A similar increased risk was seen with the 'coxibs', (p.428), **celecoxib** and **rofecoxib**.[2] Similarly, in a questionnaire-based study, 12.2% of patients taking **acenocoumarol** or **phenprocoumon** who had a bleeding complication were found to have used an NSAID in the previous month compared with only 2.5% of coumarin users who did not have a bleed (an increased relative risk of bleeding of 5.8). The NSAIDs used in the patients with bleeding complications were **diclofenac** (more than 50% patients), **ibuprofen**, **indometacin**, **naproxen** (all 10 to 12%), **ketoprofen**, **piroxicam**, and **tiaprofenic acid** (all 1 to 6%). The specific NSAIDs and the frequency of their use was similar in the patients without bleeds.[3]

(b) Pharmacokinetic interactions

'Phenylbutazone' (p.434) and related drugs are well known to inhibit the metabolism of **warfarin** by the cytochrome P450 isoenzyme CYP2C9. Few other NSAIDs are known CYP2C9 inhibitors; however; many are CYP2C9 substrates. In one cohort study in patients taking **acenocoumarol** or **phenprocoumon**, use of NSAIDs that are known substrates of CYP2C9 (**celecoxib**, **diclofenac**, **flurbiprofen**, **ibuprofen**, **indometacin**, **ketoprofen**, **meloxicam**, **naproxen** and **piroxicam**) slightly increased the risk of over-anticoagulation (INR greater than 6) in patients with wild-type CYP2C9 (relative risk of 1.69). However, the risk was greater in patients with variant CYP2C9 (relative risk 2.28), and particularly high in those with *3 variant alleles (relative risk 10.8).[4] In another smaller retrospective cohort study, starting the CYP2C9 substrates **diclofenac**, **naproxen**, or **ibuprofen** increased the INR above the therapeutic range in 52 of 112 patients taking **acenocoumarol**. However, in this study CYP2C9 genotype did not influence the interaction between **acenocoumarol** and **diclofenac**, **naproxen**, and **ibuprofen**.[5] For more general information, see 'Genetic factors in drug metabolism', (p.4).

Mechanism

NSAIDs, to a greater or lesser extent irritate the stomach lining, which can result in gastrointestinal bleeding, which will be more severe in anticoagulated patients. Many also have antiplatelet activity, which can affect bleeding times.

Some NSAIDs are inhibitors of the cytochrome P450 isoenzyme CYP2C9, and inhibit the metabolism of warfarin via this isoenzyme. There is also possibly a pharmacokinetic interaction with NSAIDs that are substrates for CYP2C9. People with variant CYP2C9 (about 5 to 11% of Caucasians) have a lower metabolising capacity for warfarin, and require much lower maintenance doses. It is possible that use of an NSAID that is a CYP2C9 substrate may result in reduced warfarin metabolism, although this requires confirmation in controlled studies.

Importance and management

The available data indicate that the risk of bleeding is increased if NSAIDs are used in patients taking coumarin or **indanedione** anticoagulants. For this reason, it would be prudent to avoid the unnecessary concurrent use of NSAIDs when simple analgesics will do. When concurrent use is necessary, extra caution may be appropriate. Further study is required to ascertain whether people with CYP2C9 poor metabolising capacity are at increased risk of an interaction when given NSAIDs that are CYP2C9 substrates.

1. Shorr RI, Ray WA, Daugherty JR, Griffin MR. Concurrent use of nonsteroidal anti-inflammatory drugs and oral anticoagulants places elderly persons at high risk for hemorrhagic peptic ulcer disease. *Arch Intern Med* (1993) 153, 1665–70.
2. Battistella M, Mamdami MM, Juurlink DN, Rabeneck L, Laupacis A. Risk of upper gastrointestinal hemorrhage in warfarin users treated with nonselective NSAIDs or COX-2 inhibitors. *Arch Intern Med* (2005) 165, 189–92.
3. Knijff-Dutmer EAJ, Schut GA, van de Laar MAFJ. Concomitant coumarin-NSAID therapy and risk for bleeding. *Ann Pharmacother* (2003) 37, 12–16.
4. Visser LE, van Schaik RH, van Vliet M, Trienekens PH, De Smet PAGM, Vulto AG, Hofman A, van Duijn CM, Stricker BHC. Allelic variants of cytochrome P450 2C9 modify the interaction between nonsteroidal anti-inflammatory drugs and coumarin anticoagulants. *Clin Pharmacol Ther* (2005) 77, 479–85.
5. van Dijk KN, Plat AW, van Dijk AAC, Piersma-Wichers M, de Vries-Bots AMB, Slomp J, de Jong-van den Berg LTW, Brouwers JRBJ. Potential interaction between acenocoumarol and diclofenac, naproxen and ibuprofen and role of CYP2C9 genotype. *Thromb Haemost* (2004) 91, 95–101.

Coumarins + NSAIDs; Benzydamine

Oral benzydamine did not alter the anticoagulant effects of phenprocoumon. Topical formulations (mouthwash and spray) would not be expected to interact.

Clinical evidence, mechanism, importance and management

In 10 patients stabilised on **phenprocoumon**, the anticoagulant response was not significantly changed by benzydamine 50 mg three times daily for 2 weeks, although there was some evidence of an increase in blood levels of the anticoagulant.[1] This suggests that no **phenprocoumon** dosage adjustments are likely to be needed on concurrent use. Note that benzydamine tends to be used as a topical mouthwash or spray. Neither of these topical formulations would be expected to interact.

1. Duckert F, Widmer LK, Madar G. Gleichzeitige Behandlung mit oralen Antikoagulantien und Benzydamin. *Schweiz Med Wochenschr* (1974) 104, 1069–71.

Coumarins + NSAIDs; Clonixin

Clonixin lysine did not alter the anticoagulant effects of phenprocoumon in a pharmacological study. However, note that all NSAIDs increase the risk of gastrointestinal bleeding, and an increased risk is seen when they are combined with anticoagulants.

Clinical evidence, mechanism, importance and management

In a randomised, crossover study in 12 healthy men, the pharmacokinetics and the anticoagulant activity of a single 18-mg dose of **phenprocoumon** were unchanged by clonixin lysine 125 mg five times daily, given for 3 days before and for 13 days after the **phenprocoumon**.[1] On the basis of this study, no adjustment in coumarin dose would be expected to be needed when clonixin is used. However, care is still needed with every NSAID, because, to a greater or lesser extent, they irritate the stomach lining, which can result in gastrointestinal bleeding, which will be more severe in anticoagulated patients. For more information, see 'NSAIDs', (p.427).

1. Russmann S, Dilger K, Trenk D, Nagyivanyi P, Jänchen E. Effect of lysine clonixinate on the pharmacokinetics and anticoagulant activity of phenprocoumon. *Arzneimittelforschung* (2001) 51, 891–895.

Coumarins and related drugs + NSAIDs; Coxibs

Etoricoxib, lumiracoxib and rofecoxib caused a slight 8% to 15% increase in the INR in response to warfarin, whereas celecoxib and parecoxib had no effect. However, raised INRs accompanied by bleeding, particularly in the elderly, have been attributed to the use of warfarin and celecoxib or rofecoxib in other reports. In addition, in a case-control study in patients taking warfarin, the use of celecoxib or rofecoxib was associated with an increased risk of hospitalisation for upper gastrointestinal haemorrhage, which was of a similar magnitude to that seen with non-selective NSAIDs.

Clinical evidence

(a) Celecoxib

In a placebo-controlled study, **warfarin** 2 to 5 mg daily was given to 24 healthy subjects to maintain a stable prothrombin time of 1.2 to 1.7 times their pretreatment values for at least 3 consecutive days. They were then given placebo or celecoxib 200 mg twice daily for a week. It was found that the steady-state pharmacokinetics of both *S*- and *R*-warfarin and the prothrombin times were unchanged by the presence of the celecoxib.[1]

However, in 16 patients stabilised on **warfarin** and given celecoxib 200 mg daily for 3 weeks, the INR increased by 13%, 6% and 5% at week 1, 2 and 3, respectively, the change at week 1 being statistically significant.[2] In another analysis, of 28 patients taking **warfarin** who were prescribed either celecoxib or rofecoxib, 13 had increases in their INR, of which 7 (5 taking celecoxib) had no other explanation for the INR increase other than the coxib. The average increase in INR in these 7 patients was 1.5, and one patient had bruising and epistaxis and required treatment with phytomenadione.[3]

Case reports of an interaction have also been published.[4-9] In one report, an 88-year-old woman stabilised on **warfarin** had a rise in her INR from 3.1 to 5.8 when celecoxib 200 mg daily was substituted for diclofenac. After several **warfarin** dosage adjustments she was later restabilised on a 25% lower **warfarin** dose.[4] There is a similar case report of a 77-year old patient who required a 10% decrease in **warfarin** dosage to maintain her target INR when celecoxib 100 mg twice daily was also given.[7] In another case, the patient was shown to have a variant of CYP2C9, with lower metabolising capacity, which was thought to explain the interaction,[9] see also 'Mechanism', below. The manufacturers also noted that bleeding events have been reported with this combination, predominantly in the elderly, which led to a change in the product labelling.[10] A 2001 report from the Australian Adverse Drug Reactions Advisory Committee noted they had received 21 reports of increases in the INR in patients taking **warfarin** with celecoxib since the introduction of celecoxib in October 1999. Six of these cases reported bleeding complications. In addition, they had 11 cases of bleeding in patients taking the combination, with no reference to INR, or with an unchanged INR in one case.[11] A review of adverse effects of coxibs mentioned 2 patients taking **warfarin** who had increases in their INR while taking celecoxib.[12]

Moreover, in a case-control study, patients taking **warfarin** and admitted to hospital with upper gastrointestinal haemorrhage were significantly more likely to be also taking celecoxib (odds ratio 1.7). A similar increased risk was seen with rofecoxib and non-selective 'NSAIDs', (p.427).[13] In a retrospective analysis, the relative risk of all bleeding complications was slightly increased (1.34) in 123 patients taking celecoxib with **warfarin** when compared with 1022 control patients taking **warfarin** alone.[14]

(b) Etoricoxib

The manufacturer notes that in healthy subjects stabilised on **warfarin**, etoricoxib 120 mg daily increased the INR by about 13%.[15]

(c) Lumiracoxib

The manufacturer notes that in healthy subjects stabilised on **warfarin**, lumiracoxib 400 mg daily increased the INR by about 15%.[16]

(d) Parecoxib

In a randomised study in healthy subjects given **warfarin**, the use of intravenous parecoxib 10 mg twice daily for 7 days had no significant effects on prothrombin times when compared with placebo. Parecoxib did not affect the pharmacokinetics of *S*- or *R*-warfarin.[17]

(e) Rofecoxib

In a study in 12 healthy subjects,[18] rofecoxib 50 mg daily for 12 days increased the maximum INR after a single 30-mg dose of **warfarin** given on day 7 by about 14%. In a steady-state study, 15 healthy subjects were given **warfarin** 5 mg daily to produce a stable prothrombin time of 1.4 to 1.7 for at least 3 consecutive days. They were then additionally given rofecoxib 25 mg or placebo daily for 3 weeks. It was found that the 24-hour average INR was increased by 8.6% by rofecoxib. Rofecoxib had no effect on the pharmacokinetics of the more potent *S*-warfarin enantiomer, but the AUC of *R*-warfarin was increased by about 40% in both the single dose and steady-state studies.[18] Moreover, in 16 patients stabilised on **warfarin** and given rofecoxib 25 mg daily for 3 weeks, the INR increased by 5%, 9%, and 5% at week 1, 2, and 3, respectively, the change at week 2 being statistically significant.[2] In one case report, an increase in INR was seen in two elderly patients taking **warfarin** and rofecoxib. The INRs were raised, in one case from less than 3 to 4.1 within a month of starting rofecoxib 12.5 mg daily, and in the other case from 3.2 to 4.6 within 2 days of starting rofecoxib. The INRs decreased when the **warfarin** dosage was reduced.[3] In another case, this time in a patient taking **acenocoumarol**, the INR rose from the range of 2 to 3 up to over 8 two weeks after starting rofecoxib 50 mg daily.[19] A 2002 report from the Australian Adverse Drug Reactions Advisory Committee noted that they had received 8 reports of increases in the INR of patients taking **warfarin** with rofecoxib since the introduction of rofecoxib in late 2000. Two of these cases reported bleeding complications. A further patient died of a cerebral haemorrhage, although the INR was stable.[20] A review of the adverse effects of coxibs included 5 patients taking **warfarin** who had increases in their INR while taking rofecoxib and **warfarin**.[12]

Moreover, in a case-control study, patients taking **warfarin** and admitted to hospital with an upper gastrointestinal haemorrhage were significantly more likely to be also taking rofecoxib (odds ratio 2.4).[13] Note that rofecoxib has generally been withdrawn because of adverse cardiovascular effects.

Mechanism

Non-selective 'NSAIDs', (p.427), inhibit platelet aggregation and cause gastrointestinal toxicity, which can result in bleeding, the risk of which is increased in patients taking anticoagulants. Although coxibs are generally considered to be associated with a lower risk of gastrointestinal haemorrhage than non-selective NSAIDs, the only available comparative epidemiological study found a similar increased risk of bleeding when coxibs were given with warfarin.

There is also possibly a pharmacokinetic interaction. Both warfarin and celecoxib are substrates of the cytochrome P450 isoenzyme CYP2C9, and it is possible that people with variants of CYP2C9 with lower metabolising capacity may develop an interaction if given the combination. For more general information, see 'Genetic factors in drug metabolism', (p.4).

Rofecoxib possibly inhibits the metabolism of the less active *R*-warfarin via inhibition of CYP1A2,[18] and the active *R*-acenocoumarol by the same isoenzyme and CYP2C19.[19]

Importance and management

The interaction of coumarin anticoagulants with these coxibs can be clinically significant, but is apparently rare. For example, of the 4 million prescriptions for celecoxib dispensed over the 18-month period from December 1998, about 1% were estimated to be for patients who would have been taking warfarin,[10] and only a handful of cases of an interaction had been reported. However, the manufacturers recommend that anticoagulant activity should be monitored in patients taking warfarin, other coumarins, or indanediones, particularly in the first few days after initiating or changing the dose of a coxib. Others recommend increased monitoring for 3 weeks.[2] Some increased monitoring is certainly appropriate because all NSAIDS, including coxibs, can irritate the gastrointestinal tract and cause bleeding, the risk of which is increased with anticoagulants.

1. Karim A, Tolbert D, Piergies A, Hubbard RC, Harper K, Wallemark C-B, Slater M, Geis GS. Celecoxib does not significantly alter the pharmacokinetics or hypoprothrombinemic effect of warfarin in healthy subjects. *J Clin Pharmacol* (2000) 40, 655–63.
2. Schaefer MG, Plowman BK, Morreale AP, Egan M. Interaction of rofecoxib and celecoxib with warfarin. *Am J Health-Syst Pharm* (2003) 60, 1319–23.
3. Stading JA, Skrabal MZ, Faulkner MA. Seven cases of interaction between warfarin and cyclooxygenase-2 inhibitors. *Am J Health-Syst Pharm* (2001) 58, 2076–80.
4. Haase KK, Rojas-Fernandez CH, Lane L, Frank DA. Potential interaction between celecoxib and warfarin. *Ann Pharmacother* (2000) 34, 666–7.
5. Linder JD, Mönkemüller KE, Davis JV, Wilcox CM. Cyclooxygenase-2 inhibitor celecoxib: a possible cause of gastropathy and hypoprothrombinemia. *South Med J* (2000) 93, 930–2.
6. Mersfedler TL, Stewart LR. Warfarin and celecoxib interaction. *Ann Pharmacother* (2000) 34, 325–7.
7. O'Donnell DC, Hooper JS. Increased international normalized ratio in a patient taking warfarin and celecoxib. *J Pharm Technol* (2001), 17, 3–5.
8. Stoner SC, Lea JW, Dubisar BM, Farrar C. Possible international normalized ratio elevation associated with celecoxib and warfarin in an elderly psychiatric patient. *J Am Geriatr Soc* (2003) 51, 728–9.
9. Malhi H, Atac B, Daly AK, Gupta S. Warfarin and celecoxib interaction in the setting of cytochrome P450 (CYP2C9) polymorphism with bleeding complication. *Postgrad Med J* (2004) 80, 107–9.
10. FDA MedWatch Program, May 1999. Available at: http://www.fda.gov/medwatch/safety/1999/celebr.htm (accessed 17/08/07).
11. ADRAC. Interaction of celecoxib and warfarin. *Aust Adverse Drug React Bull* (2001) 20, 2.
12. Verrico MM, Weber RJ, McKaveney TP, Ansani NT, Towers AL. Adverse drug events involving COX-2 inhibitors. *Ann Pharmacother* (2003) 37, 1203–13.
13. Battistella M, Mamdami MM, Juurlink DN, Rabeneck L, Laupacis A. Risk of upper gastrointestinal hemorrhage in warfarin users treated with nonselective NSAIDs or COX-2 inhibitors. *Arch Intern Med* (2005) 165, 189–92.
14. Chung L, Chakravarty EF, Kearns P, Wang C, Bush TM. Bleeding complications in patients on celecoxib and warfarin. *J Clin Pharm Ther* (2005) 30, 471–7.
15. Arcoxia (Etoricoxib). Merck Sharp & Dohme Ltd. UK Summary of product characteristics, January 2007.
16. Prexige (Lumiracoxib). Novartis Pharmaceuticals UK Ltd. UK Summary of product characteristics, February 2007.
17. Karim A, Bradford D, Qian J, Hubbard R. The COX-2-specific inhibitor parecoxib sodium does not affect warfarin pharmacokinetic and pharmacodynamic parameters. American College of Emergency Physicians. Scientific Assembly, Chicago, Illinois, 15-18 October 2001. Abstract 130.
18. Schwartz JI, Bugianesi KJ, Ebel DL, De Smet M, Haesen R, Larson PJ, Ko A, Verbesselt R, Hunt TL, Lins R, Lens S, Porras AG, Dieck J, Keymeulen B, Gertz BJ. The effect of rofecoxib on the pharmacodynamics and pharmacokinetics of warfarin. *Clin Pharmacol Ther* (2000) 68, 626–36.
19. Girardin F, Siegenthaler M, de Moerloose P, Desmeules J. Rofecoxib interaction with oral anticoagulant acenocoumarol. *Eur J Clin Pharmacol* (2003) 59, 489–90.
20. ADRAC. Interaction of rofecoxib with warfarin. *Aust Adverse Drug React Bull* (2002) 21, 3.

Coumarins + NSAIDs; Diclofenac

Studies suggest that diclofenac does not alter the anticoagulant effect of acenocoumarol, phenprocoumon or warfarin, suggesting dose adjustments are unlikely to be needed. Isolated cases of raised INRs have been described. Note that all NSAIDs increase the risk of gastrointestinal bleeding, and an increased risk is seen when they are combined with anticoagulants.

Clinical evidence

In a crossover study in 29 patients stabilised on **acenocoumarol**, diclofenac 25 mg four times daily for one week did not alter the anticoagulant effect (prothrombin value) of **acenocoumarol**, when compared with placebo.[1] Other studies similarly confirm that diclofenac does not alter the anticoagulant effect of either **phenprocoumon**[2] or **warfarin**.[3]

However, a patient taking **acenocoumarol** developed a pulmonary haemorrhage associated with a very prolonged prothrombin time within 10 days of starting to take diclofenac.[4] Another report mentions a Chinese patient taking **warfarin** who developed an INR of 4 within 4 days of using a 1% diclofenac topical gel for joint pain.[5]

For studies, including the one assessing the effect of CYP2C9 substrates, such as diclofenac, on the risk of bleeding when used with warfarin, see 'Coumarins and related drugs + NSAIDs', p.427.

Mechanism

See 'Coumarins and related drugs + NSAIDs', p.427.

Importance and management

On the basis of the pharmacological studies, no adjustment in coumarin dose would be anticipated to be needed when diclofenac is used. The isolated cases of raised INRs are unexplained. However, care is still needed with every NSAID because, to a greater or lesser extent, they irritate the stomach lining, which can result in gastrointestinal bleeding, which will be more severe in anticoagulated patients. For more information about this and potential CYP2C9-mediated interactions, see 'Coumarins and related drugs + NSAIDs', p.427.

1. Michot F, Ajdacic K, Glaus L. A double-blind clinical trial to determine if an interaction exists between diclofenac sodium and the oral anticoagulant acenocoumarol (nicoumalone). *J Int Med Res* (1975) 3, 153–7.
2. Krzywanek HJ, Breddin K. Beeinflußt Diclofenac die orale Antikoagulantientherapie und die Plättchenaggregation? *Med Welt* (1977) 28, 1843–5.
3. Fitzgerald DE, Russell JG. Voltarol and warfarin, an interaction? In: Chiswell RJ, Birdwood GFB, eds. Current Themes in Rheumatology: Cambridge: Cambridge Medical Publications :p 26–7.
4. Cuadrado Gómez LM, Palau Beato E, Pérez Venegas J, Pérez Moro E. Hemorragia pulmonar debido a la interacción de acenocumarina y diclofenac sódico. *Rev Clin Esp* (1987) 181, 227–8.
5. Chan TYK. Drug interactions as a cause of overanticoagulation and bleedings in Chinese patients receiving warfarin. *Int J Clin Pharmacol Ther* (1998) 36, 403–5.

Coumarins + NSAIDs; Diflunisal

There is limited evidence to suggest that diflunisal might increase the anticoagulant effects of acenocoumarol and possibly warfarin, but probably not phenprocoumon. All NSAIDs increase the risk of gastrointestinal bleeding, and should be used with care in patients taking oral anticoagulants.

Clinical evidence

The total plasma **warfarin** levels of 5 healthy subjects fell by about one-third (from 741 to 533 nanograms/mL) when they were given diflunisal 500 mg twice daily for 2 weeks. Also, unbound **warfarin** increased from 1.02 to 1.34%, but the anticoagulant response was unaffected. When the diflunisal was withdrawn the anticoagulant response was reduced.[1] Another report very briefly describes an increased INR when a patient taking **warfarin** was given diflunisal.[2]

A brief report states that 3 out of 6 subjects taking **acenocoumarol** had significant increases in prothrombin times, but no interaction was seen in 2 subjects on **phenprocoumon**, when they were given diflunisal 750 mg daily.[3]

Mechanism

Uncertain. Diflunisal can displace warfarin from its plasma protein binding sites but this on its own is almost certainly not the full explanation.[1] The fall in anticoagulant response when diflunisal was stopped is possibly linked to a difference in the rates that total and unbound plasma warfarin returned to their original levels.[1]

Importance and management

This interaction is neither well defined nor well documented. Its importance is uncertain. However, the reports cited and the manufacturers suggest that an increased anticoagulant effect should be looked for if diflunisal is added to established treatment with any anticoagulant. A decreased effect might be expected if diflunisal is withdrawn. Note that care is needed with every 'NSAID', (p.427), because, to a greater or lesser extent, they irritate the stomach lining, which can result in gastrointestinal bleeding, which will be more severe in anticoagulated patients.

1. Serlin MJ, Mossman S, Sibeon RG, Tempero KF, Breckenridge AM. Interaction between diflunisal and warfarin. *Clin Pharmacol Ther* (1980) 28, 493–8.
2. Beeley L, Cunningham H, Carmichael A, Brennan A. *Bulletin of the West Midlands Centre for Adverse Drug Reaction Reporting* (1992) 35, 51.
3. Tempero KF, Cirillo VJ, Steelman SL. Diflunisal: a review of pharmacokinetic and pharmacodynamic properties, drug interactions, and special tolerability studies in humans. *Br J Clin Pharmacol* (1977) 4, 31S–36S.

Coumarins + NSAIDs; Etodolac

In a pharmacological study, etodolac did not interact significantly with warfarin, suggesting dose adjustments are unlikely to be needed. Note that all NSAIDs increase the risk of gastrointestinal bleeding, and an increased risk is seen when they are combined with anticoagulants.

Clinical evidence, mechanism, importance and management

In a three-period, crossover study, each period lasting 2.5 days 18 healthy subjects were given **warfarin** 20 mg on day 1, 10 mg on days 2 and 3 and etodolac 200 mg every 12 hours. Although the median peak serum levels of the **warfarin** fell by 19% and the median total clearance rose by 13% in the presence of etodolac, the prothrombin time response remained unchanged.[1,2] On the basis of this study, no adjustment in coumarin dose would be expected to be needed when etodolac is used. However, care is still needed with every 'NSAID', (p.427), because, to a greater or lesser extent, they irritate the stomach lining, which can result in gastrointestinal bleeding, which will be more severe in anticoagulated patients.

1. Ermer JC, Hicks DR, Wheeler SC, Kraml M, Jusko WJ. Concomitant etodolac affects neither the unbound clearance nor the pharmacologic effect of warfarin. *Clin Pharmacol Ther* (1994) 55, 305–16.
2. Zvaifler N. A review of the antiarthritic efficacy and safety of etodolac. *Clin Rheumatol* (1989) 8 (Suppl 1), 43–53.

Coumarins and related drugs + NSAIDs; Fenamates

In pharmacological studies, the anticoagulant effect of acenocoumarol was modestly increased by floctafenine, that of phenprocoumon was increased by floctafenine and glafenine, and that of warfarin was increased to some extent by meclofenamic acid and mefenamic acid. Tolfenamic acid might be expected to interact similarly. However, limited evidence from one small study found glafenine did not alter the response to acenocoumarol, or ethyl biscoumacetate. Note also that all NSAIDs increase the risk of gastrointestinal bleeding, and an increased risk is seen when they are combined with anticoagulants.

Clinical evidence

(a) Floctafenine

In a double-blind study in 20 patients stabilised on **acenocoumarol** or **phenprocoumon** and given either floctafenine 200 mg or placebo four times daily for 3 weeks, floctafenine prolonged their thrombotest times by an average of about one-third, even though the anticoagulant dosage of some of the patients was reduced.[1]

(b) Glafenine

In a double-blind study in 20 patients stabilised on **phenprocoumon** and given either glafenine 200 mg or placebo three times daily it was noted that within a week of starting glafenine there was a significant increase in thrombotest times.[2] In another report, 5 out of 7 patients needed a **phenprocoumon** dose reduction while taking glafenine.[3] Conversely, in another study, 10 patients taking **acenocoumarol**, **ethyl biscoumacetate** or '**indanedione**' had no changes in their anticoagulant response when given glafenine 800 mg daily over a 4-week period.[4]

(c) Meclofenamic acid

After taking sodium meclofenamate 200 to 300 mg daily for 7 days, the average dose of **warfarin** required by 7 patients fell from 6.5 to 4.25 mg daily, and by the end of 4 weeks it was 5.5 mg (a 16% reduction with a 0 to 25% range).[5]

(d) Mefenamic acid

After taking mefenamic acid 500 mg four times daily for a week the mean prothrombin concentrations of 12 healthy subjects stabilised on **warfarin** fell by about 3.5%. Microscopic haematuria was seen in 3 of them, but no overt haemorrhage. Their prothrombin concentrations were 15 to 25% of normal, well within the accepted anticoagulant range.[6]

Mechanism

Uncertain. Mefenamic acid can displace warfarin from its plasma protein binding sites,[7-9] and *in vitro* studies have shown that therapeutic concentrations (equivalent to 4 g daily) can increase the unbound and active warfarin concentrations by 140 to 340%,[7,8] but this interaction mechanism alone is only likely to have a transient effect. See also 'Coumarins and related drugs + NSAIDs', p.427.

Importance and management

The pharmacological studies cited suggest that all the fenamates can cause a small to modest increase in the effects of coumarin anticoagulants. If both drugs are given, increase monitoring and anticipate the need for a small reduction in coumarin dosage. Although there are no data on combined use with the fenamate **tolfenamic acid**, the manufacturer similarly recommends close monitoring of coagulation.[10] Also note that, all 'NSAIDs', (p.427), to a greater or lesser extent irritate the stomach lining, which can result in gastrointestinal bleeding, which will be more severe in anticoagulated patients.

1. Boeijinga JK, van de Broeke RN, Jochemsen R, Breimer DD, Hoogslag MA, Jeletich-Bastiaanse A. De invloed van floctafenine (Idalon) op antistollingsbehandeling met coumarinederivaten. *Ned Tijdschr Geneeskd* (1981) 125, 1931–5.
2. Boeijinga JK, van der Vijgh WJF. Double blind study of the effect of glafenine (Glifanan®) on oral anticoagulant therapy with phenprocoumon (Marcumar®). *Eur J Clin Pharmacol* (1977) 12, 291–6.
3. Boeijinga JK, Bing GT, van der Meer J. De invloed van glafenine (Glifanan) op antistollingsbehandeling met coumarinederivaten. *Ned Tijdschr Geneeskd* (1974) 118, 1895–8.
4. Raby C. Recherches sur une éventuelle potentialisation de l'action des anticoagulants de synthèse par la glafénine. *Therapie* (1977) 32, 293–9.
5. Baragar FD, Smith TC. Drug interaction studies with sodium meclofenamate (Meclomen®). *Curr Ther Res* (1978) 23 (April Suppl), S51–S59.
6. Holmes EL. Pharmacology of the fenamates: IV. Toleration by normal human subjects. *Ann Phys Med* (1966) 9 (Suppl), 36–49.
7. Sellers EM, Koch-Weser J. Displacement of warfarin from human albumin by diazoxide and ethacrynic, mefenamic and nalidixic acids. *Clin Pharmacol Ther* (1970) 11, 524–9.
8. Sellers EM, Koch-Weser J. Kinetics and clinical importance of displacement of warfarin from albumin by acidic drugs. *Ann N Y Acad Sci* (1971) 179, 213–25.
9. McElnay JC, D'Arcy PFD. Displacement of albumin-bound warfarin by anti-inflammatory agents *in vitro*. *J Pharm Pharmacol* (1980) 32, 709–11.
10. Clotam Rapid (Tolfenamic acid). Provalis Healthcare. UK Summary of product characteristics, June 1999.

Coumarins + NSAIDs; Ibuprofen and related drugs

In pharmacological studies, ibuprofen, indoprofen, ketoprofen, naproxen and oxaprozin did not alter the anticoagulant effect of coumarins, but isolated cases of raised INRs have been described with ibuprofen and ketoprofen. A slight increase in anticoagulant effect has been seen with fenbufen, flurbiprofen and tiaprofenic acid, although the clinical relevance is probably small. However, note also that all NSAIDs increase the risk of gastrointestinal bleeding, and an increased risk is seen when they are combined with anticoagulants.

Clinical evidence

(a) Fenbufen

In a study in 10 healthy subjects who were stabilised on **warfarin** then given either fenbufen 400 mg twice daily or placebo for a week, the prothrombin times were increased by 1.9 seconds within 2 days in the fenbufen recipients, and the serum **warfarin** levels fell by 14%.[1]

(b) Flurbiprofen

A small but significant fall in Quick value (from 23.84 and 25.05% to 20.68 and 20.29%) occurred in 19 patients stabilised on **phenprocoumon** when they were given flurbiprofen 50 mg three times daily for 2 weeks. Two patients bled (haematuria, epistaxis, haemorrhoidal bleeding) and the prothrombin times of 3 patients fell below the therapeutic range.[2]

A case report describes two patients taking **acenocoumarol** who had a rise in thrombotest times and bled (haematuria, melaena, haematomas) within 2 to 3 days of starting to take flurbiprofen 150 to 300 mg daily.[3]

(c) Ibuprofen

Ibuprofen 600 mg to 2.4 g daily for 7 to 14 days did not alter the effects of coumarins in studies in: patients stabilised on **phenprocoumon**;[4-6] healthy subjects[7,8] or patients[8] stabilised on **warfarin**; or patients stabilised on **dicoumarol**.[9] However, in one study in 20 patients taking **warfarin**, ibuprofen 600 mg three times daily for 1 week had no effect on prothrombin time; however, it did prolong bleeding time (4 cases above the normal range) and microscopic haematuria and haematoma were seen.[10] Note that, this finding is probably more of a function of the effect of ibuprofen than an interaction *per se*,[11] although it does explain why the combination of an anticoagulants and an 'NSAID', (p.427), has an increased risk of haemorrhage.

A raised INR occurred in one patient on **warfarin** who used topical ibuprofen,[12] and subclinical bleeding with a raised INR occurred in a 74-year-old woman with multiple medical problems taking **warfarin** when she was given ibuprofen.[13] For studies, including one assessing the effect of CYP2C9 substrates, such as diclofenac, on the risk of bleeding, see 'Coumarins and related drugs + NSAIDs', p.427.

(d) Indoprofen

In a placebo-controlled study in 18 patients stabilised on **warfarin** and given indoprofen 600 mg daily for 7 days, no changes occurred in any of the blood coagulation measurements made.[14]

(e) Ketoprofen

In a study in 15 healthy subjects stabilised on **warfarin**, ketoprofen 100 mg twice daily for 7 days had no effect on prothrombin times or coagulation cascade parameters, and there was no evidence of bleeding.[15] This contrasts with an isolated case of bleeding in a patient taking **warfarin** (prothrombin time increased from 18 to 41 seconds) a week after starting ketoprofen 25 mg three times daily.[16]

(f) Naproxen

In a study in 10 healthy subjects, naproxen 375 mg twice daily for 17 days did not alter the pharmacokinetics of a single dose of **warfarin** given on day 10, or its anticoagulant effects.[17] Similar results were found in a study of **warfarin** at steady state.[18] A further study in patients taking **phenprocoumon** showed that naproxen 250 mg twice daily transiently increased the anticoagulant effects and caused an unimportant change in primary bleeding time.[19]

For studies, including one assessing the effect of CYP2C9 substrates, such as diclofenac, on the risk of bleeding, see 'Coumarins and related drugs + NSAIDs', p.427.

(g) Oxaprozin

In a study in 10 healthy subjects stabilised on **warfarin** for an average of 15 days, oxaprozin 1.2 g daily for 7 days did not significantly alter prothrombin times.[20]

(h) Tiaprofenic acid

In a study in 6 healthy subjects, the anticoagulant effects and the pharmacokinetic profile of **phenprocoumon** remained unchanged when they took tiaprofenic acid daily for 2 days.[21] This study is also published elsewhere.[22] No significant interaction occurred in 9 patients stabilised on **acenocoumarol** and given tiaprofenic acid 200 mg three times daily for 2 weeks, but in 4 patients a 'rebound' rise in prothrombin percentages occurred following withdrawal of the NSAID.[23] However, an elderly man taking **acenocoumarol** had severe epistaxis and bruising 4 to 6 weeks after starting to take tiaprofenic acid 300 mg twice daily. His prothrombin time had risen to 129 seconds.[24]

Mechanism

When given alone, ibuprofen and related drugs can prolong bleeding times because of their antiplatelet effects.[11] They may also cause gastrointestinal toxicity. Because of these effects, in patients on anticoagulants, the risk of bleeding is increased by 'NSAIDs', (p.427). Most of the propionic acid derivatives can displace the anticoagulants from plasma protein binding sites to some extent, but this mechanism on its own is rarely, if ever, responsible for clinically important drug interactions.

Importance and management

It is well established that ibuprofen does not alter the anticoagulant effect of warfarin or other coumarins, (although isolated and unexplained cases of bleeding or raised INRs have occurred but only very rarely). On the basis of these studies, no adjustment in coumarin dose would be anticipated to be needed when ibuprofen is used. Pharmacological studies also show no interaction for related propionic acid derivatives including indoprofen, ketoprofen, naproxen and oxaprozin, although the documentation is more limited. A slight increase in anticoagulant effects has been seen with fenbufen, flurbiprofen, and possibly tiaprofenic acid, although this is probably of limited clinical relevance. However, note that some care is still needed with every NSAID, because, to a greater or lesser extent, they irritate the stomach lining, which can result in gastrointestinal bleeding, which will be more severe in anticoagulated patients. For more information about this and potential CYP2C9-mediated interactions, see 'Coumarins and related drugs + NSAIDs', p.427.

1. Savitsky JP, Terzakis T, Bina P, Chiccarelli F, Haynes J. Fenbufen-warfarin interaction in healthy volunteers. *Clin Pharmacol Ther* (1980) 27, 284.
2. Marbet GA, Duckert F, Walter M, Six P, Airenne H. Interaction study between phenprocoumon and flurbiprofen. *Curr Med Res Opin* (1977) 5, 26–31.
3. Stricker BHC, Delhez JL. Interaction between flurbiprofen and coumarins. *BMJ* (1982) 285, 812–13.
4. Thilo D, Nyman F, Duckert F. A study of the effects of the anti-rheumatic drug ibuprofen (Brufen) on patients being treated with the oral anti-coagulant phenprocoumon (Marcoumar). *J Int Med Res* (1974) 2, 276–8.
5. Duckert F. The absence of effect of the antirheumatic drug ibuprofen on oral anticoagulation with phenprocoumon. *Curr Med Res Opin* (1975) 3, 556–7.
6. Boekhout-Mussert MJ, Loeliger EA. Influence of ibuprofen on oral anti-coagulation with phenprocoumon. *J Int Med Res* (1974) 2, 279–83.
7. Penner JA, Abbrecht PH. Lack of interaction between ibuprofen and warfarin. *Curr Ther Res* (1975) 18, 862–71.
8. Goncalves L. Influence of ibuprofen on haemostasis in patients on anticoagulant therapy. *J Int Med Res* (1973) 1, 180–3.
9. Marini U, Cecchi A, Venturino M. Mancanza di interazione tra ibuprofen lisinato e anticoagulanti orali. *Clin Ter* (1985) 112, 25–9.
10. Schulman S, Henriksson K. Interaction of ibuprofen and warfarin on primary haemostasis. *Br J Rheumatol* (1989) 28, 46–9.
11. Pullar T. Interaction of ibuprofen and warfarin on primary haemostasis. *Br J Rheumatol* (1989) 28, 265–6.
12. Beeley L, Cunningham H, Carmichael AE, Brennan A. *Bulletin of the West Midlands Centre for Adverse Drug Reaction Reporting* (1992), 35, 18.
13. Ernst ME, Buys LM. Reevaluating the safety of concurrent warfarin and ibuprofen. *J Pharm Technol* (1997) 13, 244–7.
14. Jacono A, Caso P, Gualtieri S, Raucci D, Bianchi A, Vigorito C, Bergamini N, Iadevaia V. Clinical study of the possible interactions between indoprofen and oral anticoagulants. *Eur J Rheumatol Inflamm* (1981) 4, 32–5.
15. Mieszczak C, Winther K. Lack of interaction of ketoprofen with warfarin. *Eur J Clin Pharmacol* (1993) 44, 205–6.
16. Flessner MF, Knight H. Prolongation of prothrombin time and severe gastrointestinal bleeding associated with combined use of warfarin and ketoprofen. *JAMA* (1988) 259, 353.
17. Slattery JT, Levy G, Jain A, McMahon FG. Effect of naproxen on the kinetics of elimination and anticoagulant activity of a single dose of warfarin. *Clin Pharmacol Ther* (1979) 25, 51–60.
18. Jain A, McMahon FG, Slattery JT, Levy G. Effect of naproxen on the steady-state serum concentration and anticoagulant activity of warfarin. *Clin Pharmacol Ther* (1979) 25, 61–6.
19. Angelkort B. Zum einfluß von Naproxen auf die thrombozytäre Blutstillung und die Antikoagulantien-Behandlung mit Phenprocoumon. *Fortschr Med* (1978) 96, 1249–52.
20. Davis LJ, Kayser SR, Hubscher J, Williams RL. Effect of oxaprozin on the steady-state anticoagulant activity of warfarin. *Clin Pharm* (1984) 3, 295–7.
21. Dürr J, Pfeiffer MH, Wetzelsberger K, Lücker PW. Untersuchung zur Frage einer Interaktion von Tiaprofensäure und Phenprocoumon. *Arzneimittelforschung* (1981) 31, 2163–7.
22. Lücker PW, Penth B, Wetzelsberger K. Pharmacokinetic interaction between tiaprofenic acid and several other compounds for chronic use. *Rheumatology (Oxford)* (1982) 7, 99–106.
23. Meurice J. Interaction of tiaprofenic acid and acenocoumarol. *Rheumatology (Oxford)* (1982) 7, 111–17.
24. Whittaker SJ, Jackson CW, Whorwell PJ. A severe, potentially fatal, interaction between tiaprofenic acid and nicoumalone. *Br J Clin Pract* (1986) 40, 440.

Coumarins + NSAIDs; Indometacin and related drugs

In pharmacological studies, the anticoagulant effects of acenocoumarol, phenprocoumon and warfarin were not affected by indometacin, or phenprocoumon by acemetacin. However, isolated cases of a possible interaction with a raised INR and bleeding complications have been reported. Also, note that, like all NSAIDs, indometacin can irritate the gut thereby increasing the risk of gastrointestinal bleeding, the risk of which is further increased in patients taking anticoagulants.

Clinical evidence

(a) Acemetacin

In a placebo-controlled study in 20 patients stabilised on **phenprocoumon,** acemetacin 60 mg three times daily for 3 weeks did not alter the thromboplastin value.[1]

(b) Indometacin

In a placebo-controlled, double-blind study, indometacin 100 mg daily for 5 days had no effect on the anticoagulant effects of steady-state **warfarin** in 8 healthy subjects.[2] Similarly, when 19 healthy subjects took either indometacin 25 mg four times daily or placebo for 11 days, neither the anticoagulant effects nor the half-life of single doses of **warfarin** were affected.[2]

Other studies in healthy subjects and patients anticoagulated with **acenocoumarol**[3] or **phenprocoumon**[4-6] similarly showed that the anticoagulant effects were not changed by indometacin.

However, isolated cases of possible interactions in patients taking **warfarin** have been reported.[7-10] One patient had a rise in INR from 2 to 5.3,[8] and another had a rise from 2.75 to 3.42, then to 3.6 despite a reduction in **warfarin** dose.[10] However, there are other possible interpretations of this case.[11] In another report a patient taking indometacin appeared to have an enhanced response to **warfarin**, which subsequently improved when ibuprofen was substituted for indometacin.[7] The preliminary report of an analysis of possible drug interactions with **warfarin** stated that indometacin was found to have a clinically relevant effect on the anticoagulant action of warfarin.[12] One patient taking **warfarin** and indometacin died from acute peptic ulceration.[13] Another report includes the interaction in a list, with no details.[9] In a recent report, a patient who was very sensitive to **acenocoumarol** was found to have melaena and an INR of greater than 10 a week after starting indometacin and tetrazepam. He was found to have poor metaboliser phenotype of isoenzyme CYP2C9 (variant *3).[14] For studies, including the one assessing the effect of CYP2C9 substrates, such as diclofenac, on the risk of bleeding, see 'Coumarins and related drugs + NSAIDs', p.427.

Mechanism

None. Indometacin reduces platelet aggregation and thereby prolongs bleeding when it occurs. Acemetacin would act similarly since it is a glycolic acid ester of indometacin and indometacin is the major metabolite.

Importance and management

In pharmacological studies it is well established that indometacin does not normally alter the anticoagulant effects acenocoumarol, phenprocoumon or warfarin. No coumarin dose adjustments would therefore expected to be needed during concurrent use. However, caution is still appropriate, because indometacin, like other NSAIDs, can cause gastrointestinal irritation, ulceration and bleeding, which will be more severe in anticoagulated patients. For more information about this and potential CYP2C9-mediated interactions, see 'Coumarins and related drugs + NSAIDs', p.427.

1. Hess H, Koeppen R. Kontrollierte Doppelblindestudie zur Frage einer möglichen Interferenz von Acemetacin mit einer laufenden Antikoagulanzien-Therapie. *Arzneimittelforschung* (1980) 30, 1421–3.
2. Vesell ES, Passananti GT, Johnson AO. Failure of indomethacin and warfarin to interact in normal human volunteers. *J Clin Pharmacol* (1975) 15, 486–95.
3. Gáspárdy G, Bálint G, Gáspárdy G. Wirkung der Kombination Indomethacin und Syncumar (Acenocumarol) auf den Prothrombinspiegel im Blutplasma. *Z Rheumaforsch* (1967) 26, 332–5.
4. Müller G, Zollinger W. The influence of indomethacin on blood coagulation, particularly with regard to the interference with anticoagulant treatment. In: Heister R, Hofmann HF eds. International Symposium on Inflammation. Munich: Urban and Schwarzenburg, 1966: 1–12.
5. Frost H, Hess H. Concomitant administration of indomethacin and anticoagulants. In: Heister R, Hofmann HF eds. International Symposium on Inflammation. Munich: Urban and Schwarzenburg, 1966: 1–3.
6. Muller KH, Herrmann K. Is simultaneous therapy with anticoagulants and indomethacin feasible? *Med Welt* (1966) 17, 1553–4.
7. Self TH, Soloway MS, Vaughn D. Possible interaction of indomethacin and warfarin. *Drug Intell Clin Pharm* (1978) 12, 580–1.
8. Chan TYK. Prolongation of prothrombin time with the use of indomethacin and warfarin. *Br J Clin Pract* (1997) 51, 177–8.
9. Beeley L, Stewart P. *Bulletin of the West Midlands Centre for Adverse Drug Reaction Reporting* (1987) 25, 28.
10. Chan TYK, Lui SF, Chung SY, Luk S, Critchley JAJH. Adverse interaction between warfarin and indomethacin. *Drug Safety* (1994) 10, 267–9.
11. Day R, Quinn D. Adverse interaction between warfarin and indomethacin. *Drug Safety* (1994) 11, 213–14.
12. Koch-Weser J. Haemorrhagic reactions and drug interactions in 500 warfarin-treated patients. *Clin Pharmacol Ther* (1973) 14, 139.
13. McQueen EG. New Zealand Committee on Adverse Reactions: fourteenth annual report 1979. *N Z Med J* (1980) 91, 226–9.
14. Zarza J, Hermida J, Montes R, Páramo JA, Rocha E. Major bleeding during combined treatment with indomethacin and low doses of acenocoumarol in a homozygous patient for 2C9*3 variant of cytochrome P-450 CYP2C9. *Thromb Haemost* (2003) 90, 161–2.

Coumarins and related drugs + NSAIDs; Ketorolac

Ketorolac did not alter the pharmacokinetics of, or prothrombin time response to, warfarin. However, ketorolac has been associated with serious gastrointestinal bleeding.

Clinical evidence, mechanism, importance and management

In a placebo-controlled, crossover study[1] in 10 healthy subjects, ketorolac 10 mg four times daily for 12 days caused no major changes in the pharmacokinetics of *R*- or *S*-warfarin, nor in the prothrombin time after a single 25-mg dose of **warfarin** given on day 6. This suggests that ketorolac is normally unlikely to affect the anticoagulant response of patients taking **warfarin** chronically, and that no warfarin dose adjustments would be anticipated to be necessary on concurrent use. However, in 1993 the CSM in the UK reported on an analysis of adverse reactions associated with ketorolac: they had received 5 reports of postoperative haemorrhage and four reports of gastrointestinal haemorrhage (one fatal) in patients taking ketorolac.[2] As result of this analysis, the use of ketorolac with anticoagulants was contraindicated in the UK.[2,3] In the US, the manufacturers state that patients taking anticoagulants have an increased risk of bleeding complications if they are also given ketorolac, and therefore they should be used together extremely cautiously. They note that, in particular, there is an increased risk of intramuscular haematoma from intramuscular ketorolac in patients taking anticoagulants.[4] See also 'Coumarins and related drugs + NSAIDs', p.427.

1. Toon S, Holt BL, Mullins FGP, Bullingham R, Aarons L, Rowland M. Investigations into the potential effects of multiple dose ketorolac on the pharmacokinetics and pharmacodynamics of racemic warfarin. *Br J Clin Pharmacol* (1990) 30, 743–50.
2. Committee on the Safety of Medicines/Medicines Control Agency. Ketorolac: new restrictions on dose and duration of treatment. *Current Problems* (1993) 19, 5–6.
3. Toradol (Ketorolac trometamol). Roche Products Ltd. UK Summary of product characteristics, May 2007.
4. Toradol (Ketorolac tromethamine). Roche Pharmaceuticals. US Prescribing information, September 2002.

Coumarins + NSAIDs; Metamizole sodium (Dipyrone)

One report claims that metamizole sodium does not interact with phenprocoumon or ethyl biscoumacetate, whereas another describes a rapid but transient increase in the effects of ethyl biscoumacetate. All NSAIDs increase the risk of gastrointestinal bleeding, and an increased risk is seen when they are combined with anticoagulants.

Clinical evidence, mechanism, importance and management

A single 1-g dose of metamizole sodium did not alter the steady-state anticoagulant effects of either **phenprocoumon** (5 subjects) or **ethyl biscoumacetate** (6 subjects).[1] Conversely, another report describes a short-lived but rapid increase (within 4 hours) in the effects of **ethyl biscoumacetate** caused by single 1-g dose metamizole sodium.[2] The reasons are not understood. However, care is still needed with every 'NSAID', (p.427), because, to a greater or lesser extent, they irritate the stomach lining, which can result in gastrointestinal bleeding, which will be more severe in anticoagulated patients.

1. Badian M, Le Normand Y, Rupp W, Zapf R. There is no interaction between dipyrone (metamizol) and the anticoagulants, phenprocoumon and ethylbiscoumacetate, in normal caucasian subjects. *Int J Pharmaceutics* (1984) 18, 9–15.
2. Mehvar SR, Jamali F. Dipyrone-ethylbiscoumacetate interaction in man. *Indian J Pharm* (1981) 7, 293–9.

Coumarins + NSAIDs; Nabumetone

In pharmacological studies, nabumetone did not alter the anticoagulant effects of acenocoumarol or warfarin. An isolated report describes a raised INR and haemarthrosis in one patient taking warfarin attributed to an interaction with nabumetone. Note that all NSAIDs increase the risk of gastrointestinal bleeding, and an increased risk is seen when they are combined with anticoagulants.

Clinical evidence, mechanism, importance and management

Nabumetone 2 g daily for 2 weeks did not significantly alter the anticoagulant effects of steady-state **warfarin** in healthy subjects.[1] Similarly, nabumetone 1 to 2 g daily for 6 weeks had no effect on the INR in 58 patients stabilised on **warfarin**.[1,2] Another clinical study in osteoarthritis patients also found that there was no difference in the proportion of patients with no INR change and no change in **acenocoumarol** dose in 27 patients given nabumetone 1 to 2 g daily for 4 weeks and 29 patients given placebo.[3] Moreover, nabumetone also appears not to affect bleeding time, platelet aggregation or prothrombin times in the absence of an anticoagulant.[4] However, an isolated and unexplained report describes an increase in INR from 2 to 3.7 and haemarthrosis in a patient taking **warfarin** a week after nabumetone 750 mg twice daily was added.[5]

On the basis of the above studies, no coumarin dose adjustment would be expected to be needed with nabumetone. However, care is still needed with every 'NSAID', (p.427), because, to a greater or lesser extent, they irritate the stomach lining, which can result in gastrointestinal bleeding, which will be more severe in anticoagulated patients.

1. Hilleman DE, Mohiuddin SM, Lucas BD. Nonsteroidal antiinflammatory drug use in patients receiving warfarin: emphasis on nabumetone. *Am J Med* (1993) 95 (Suppl 2A), 30S–34S.
2. Hilleman DE, Mohiuddin SM, Lucas BD. Hypoprothrombinemic effect of nabumetone in warfarin-treated patients. *Pharmacotherapy* (1993) 13, 270–1.
3. Pardo A, García-Losa M, Fernández-Pavón A, del Castillo S, Pascual-García T, García-Méndez E, Dal-Ré R. A placebo-controlled study of interaction between nabumetone and acenocoumarol. *Br J Clin Pharmacol* (1999) 47, 441–4.
4. Al Balla S, Al Momen AK, Al Arfaj H, Al Sugair S, Gader AMA. Interaction between nabumetone — a new non-steroidal anti-inflammatory drug — and the haemostatic system ex vivo. *Haemostasis* (1990) 20, 270–5.
5. Dennis VC, Thomas BK, Hanlon JE. Potentiation of oral anticoagulation and hemarthrosis associated with nabumetone. *Pharmacotherapy* (2000) 20, 234–9.

Coumarins + NSAIDs; Nimesulide

In pharmacological studies, nimesulide did not alter the effects of acenocoumarol or warfarin. Note that all NSAIDs increase the risk of gastrointestinal bleeding, and an increased risk is seen when they are combined with anticoagulants.

Clinical evidence, mechanism, importance and management

In a pilot study in 6 patients stabilised on **acenocoumarol**, a single 100-mg dose of nimesulide did not affect the clotting mechanisms, although the platelet aggregating response to adenosine diphosphate, adrenaline (epinephrine) and collagen was reduced for 2 to 4 hours.[1] Ten patients stabilised on **warfarin** 5 mg daily had no significant changes in their prothrombin times, partial thromboplastin time or bleeding times when they were given nimesulide 100 mg twice daily for a week.[2] However, a few patients showed some increase in anticoagulant activity.[1]

The studies above suggest that no coumarin dose adjustments are expected to be needed when nimesulide is used. However, care is still needed with every 'NSAID', (p.427), because, to a greater or lesser extent, they irritate the stomach lining, which can result in gastrointestinal bleeding, which will be more severe in anticoagulated patients.

1. Perucca E. Drug interactions with nimesulide. *Drugs* (1993) 46 (Suppl 1), 79–82.
2. Auteri A, Bruni F, Blardi P, Di Renzo M, Pasqui AL, Saletti M, Verzuri MS, Scaricabarozzi I, Vargiu G, Di Perri T. Clinical study on pharmacological interaction between nimesulide and

Coumarins + NSAIDs; Oxicam derivatives

Piroxicam increased plasma levels of *R*-acenocoumarol, and a few cases of raised INRs and bleeding have been reported when it was given with acenocoumarol or warfarin. In pharmacological studies, lornoxicam modestly increased the anticoagulant effects of warfarin, and possibly decreased the effect of phenprocoumon, but it did not to interact with acenocoumarol. Studies have indicated that meloxicam does not interact with warfarin, and that tenoxicam does not interact with warfarin or phenprocoumon. Note that all NSAIDs increase the risk of gastrointestinal bleeding, and an increased risk is seen when they are combined with anticoagulants.

Clinical evidence

(a) Lornoxicam

In an open, crossover study in 6 healthy subjects, lornoxicam 8 mg twice daily for 7 days had no effect on the pharmacokinetics or the anticoagulant activity of a single 10-mg dose of **acenocoumarol** given on day 4.[1]

In an open, crossover study in 6 healthy subjects, lornoxicam 8 mg twice daily for 21 days increased the bioavailabilities of *S*- and *R*-phenprocoumon by 14% and 6%, respectively, and decreased their clearances by 15% and 6%, respectively, after a single 9-mg dose of **phenprocoumon** given on day 4. Despite the minor pharmacokinetic changes, statistically significant reductions in the activities of factors II and VII were seen.[2]

Lornoxicam 4 mg twice daily was given to 12 healthy subjects for 5 days, then **warfarin** was added until a stable prothrombin time, averaging about 23.6 seconds, was achieved. The period to achieve this varied from 9 to 24 days, depending on the subject. The **warfarin** was then continued and the lornoxicam withdrawn, whereupon the mean prothrombin time fell to 19.5 seconds, the INR fell from 1.48 to 1.23 and the serum **warfarin** levels fell by 25%.[3]

(b) Meloxicam

Meloxicam 15 mg daily for 7 days did not significantly affect the pharmacokinetics of **warfarin** or INR values[4] in a group of 13 healthy subjects stabilised with INRs of 1.2 to 1.8.

(c) Piroxicam

1. Acenocoumarol. In a single-dose study in healthy subjects, when piroxicam 40 mg was given with acenocoumarol 4 mg the AUC of the more active *R*-isomer was increased by 47% and its maximum plasma level was increased by 28%.[5]

In patients stabilised on acenocoumarol, piroxicam 20 mg daily for 2 weeks increased the effects of acenocoumarol in 4 out of 11 patients: the effect was considered mild in 3 patients, and significant in the fourth, although no specific values were given.[6] An increased prothrombin ratio has been seen in another patient.[7] A further patient taking acenocoumarol developed gastrointestinal bleeding 3 days after starting to take piroxicam 20 mg daily. His INR rose from 2.2 to 6.5.[8]

2. Warfarin. A man stabilised on warfarin had a fall in his prothrombin time from a range of 1.7 to 1.9 times his control value to 1.3 when he stopped taking piroxicam 20 mg daily. The prothrombin times rose and fell when he re-started and then stopped the piroxicam.[9] Another patient taking warfarin had an increase in her prothrombin time (from a range of 16.5 to 18.1 seconds to 24.9 seconds) when piroxicam 20 mg daily was started, and a decrease when it was then stopped.[10] The INR of 2 Chinese patients rose to 4.5 and 4.2 after they were treated with piroxicam 20 mg daily and 0.5% topical piroxicam gel. One of them had bruises over the legs within 3 days.[11]

A woman who spread **warfarin** rat poison with her bare hands developed intracerebral bleeding, possibly exacerbated by piroxicam, which she took occasionally.[12]

(d) Tenoxicam

In single-dose and steady-state studies in a total of 16 healthy subjects, tenoxicam 20 mg daily for 14 days had no significant effect on the anticoagulant effects of **warfarin** or on bleeding times.[13] This report also mentions case studies in a small number of patients and healthy subjects, which similarly found that tenoxicam had no significant effect on the anticoagulant effects of **phenprocoumon**.[13]

Mechanism

Piroxicam inhibits the metabolism of the active *R*-acenocoumarol, but its effect on the metabolism of warfarin is unknown. Lornoxicam inhibited the metabolism of warfarin, but not acenocoumarol, *in vitro*.[14] In addition NSAIDs have antiplatelet effects, which can prolong bleeding if it occurs. They may also cause gastrointestinal toxicity. Because of these effects, in patients taking anticoagulants, the risk of bleeding is increased by 'NSAIDs', (p.427).

Importance and management

The interaction of piroxicam with acenocoumarol would appear to be established, and case reports suggest that warfarin might be similarly affected. Concurrent use need not be avoided, but monitor the outcome well and anticipate the need to reduce the anticoagulant dosage. Lornoxicam appears to have a similar effect with warfarin, although no cases of an interaction have been reported. Meloxicam and tenoxicam appear not to interact. However, care is still needed with every 'NSAID', (p.427), because, to a greater or lesser extent, they irritate the stomach lining, which can result in gastrointestinal bleeding, which will be more severe in anticoagulated patients.

1. Masche UP, Rentsch KM, von Felten A, Meier PJ, Fattinger KE. No clinically relevant effect of lornoxicam intake on acenocoumarol pharmacokinetics and pharmacodynamics. *Eur J Clin Pharmacol* (1999) 54, 865–8.
2. Masche UP, Rentsch KM, von Felten A, Meier PJ, Fattinger KE. Opposite effects of lornoxicam co-administration on phenprocoumon pharmacokinetics and pharmacodynamics. *Eur J Clin Pharmacol* (1999) 54, 857–64.
3. Ravic M, Johnston A, Turner P, Ferber HP. A study of the interaction between lornoxicam and warfarin in healthy volunteers. *Hum Exp Toxicol* (1990) 9, 413–14.
4. Türck D, Su CAPF, Heinzel G, Busch U, Bluhmki E, Hoffmann J. Lack of interaction between meloxicam and warfarin in healthy volunteers. *Eur J Clin Pharmacol* (1997) 51, 421–5.
5. Bonnabry P, Desmeules J, Rudaz S, Leemann T, Veuthey J-L, Dayer P. Stereoselective interaction between piroxicam and acenocoumarol. *Br J Clin Pharmacol* (1996) 41, 525–30.
6. Jacotot B. Interaction of piroxicam with oral anticoagulants. 9th European Congress of Rheumatology, Wiesbaden, September 1979, pp 46–47.
7. Beeley L, Stewart P. *Bulletin of the West Midlands Centre for Adverse Drug Reaction Reporting* (1987) 25, 28.
8. Desprez D, Blanc P, Larrey D, Michel H. Hémorragie digestive favorisée par une hypocoagulation excessive due à une interaction médicamenteuse piroxicam — antagoniste de la vitamine K. *Gastroenterol Clin Biol* (1992) 16, 906–7.
9. Rhodes RS, Rhodes PJ, Klein C, Sintek CD. A warfarin-piroxicam drug interaction. *Drug Intell Clin Pharm* (1985) 19, 556–8.
10. Mallet L, Cooper JW. Prolongation of prothrombin time with the use of piroxicam and warfarin. *Can J Hosp Pharm* (1991) 44, 93–4.
11. Chan TYK. Drug interactions as a cause of overanticoagulation and bleedings in Chinese patients receiving warfarin. *Int J Clin Pharmacol Ther* (1998) 36, 403–5.
12. Abell TL, Merigian KS, Lee JM, Holbert JM, McCall JW. Cutaneous exposure to warfarin-like anticoagulant causing an intracerebral hemorrhage: a case report. *Clin Toxicol* (1994) 32, 69–73.
13. Eichler H-G, Jung M, Kyrle PA, Rotter M, Korn A. Absence of interaction between tenoxicam and warfarin. *Eur J Clin Pharmacol* (1992) 42, 227–9.
14. Kohl C, Steinkellner M. Prediction of pharmacokinetic drug/drug interactions from in vitro data: interactions of the nonsteroidal anti-inflammatory drug lornoxicam with oral anticoagulants. *Drug Metab Dispos* (2000) 28, 161–8.

Coumarins + NSAIDs; Phenazone (Antipyrine)

The anticoagulant effects of warfarin are reduced by phenazone.

Clinical evidence

The plasma **warfarin** concentrations were halved (from 2.93 to 1.41 micrograms/mL) and the anticoagulant effects accordingly reduced after 5 patients took phenazone 600 mg daily for 50 days.[1] The thrombotest percentage of one patient rose from 5 to 50%. In an associated study it was found that phenazone 600 mg daily for 30 days caused a reduction in the **warfarin** half-live from 47 to 27 hours and from 69 to 39 hours, respectively, in 2 patients.[1,2]

Mechanism

Phenazone is an enzyme inducer, which increases the metabolism and clearance of warfarin, thereby reducing its effects.[1,2]

Importance and management

An established interaction. The effects of concurrent use should be monitored and the dosage of warfarin increased appropriately. However, note that phenazone is little used clinically, and an alternative 'NSAID', (p.427), that does not alter the metabolism of coumarins would be more appropriate. Other coumarins might be expected to behave similarly.

1. Breckenridge A, Orme M. Clinical implications of enzyme induction. *Ann N Y Acad Sci* (1971) 179, 421–31.
2. Breckenridge A, Orme ML'E, Thorgeirsson S, Davies DS, Brooks RV. Drug interactions with warfarin: studies with dichloralphenazone, chloral hydrate and phenazone (antipyrine). *Clin Sci* (1971) 40, 351–64.

Coumarins and related drugs + NSAIDs; Phenylbutazone and related drugs

The anticoagulant effects of warfarin are markedly increased by azapropazone, oxyphenbutazone and phenylbutazone. Concurrent use should be avoided because serious bleeding can occur. Feprazone appears to interact similarly.
Bleeding has also been seen in patients taking phenindione or phenprocoumon when given phenylbutazone, but successful concurrent use has been achieved with both phenprocoumon and acenocoumarol, apparently because the anticoagulant dosage was carefully reduced. Note also that all NSAIDs increase the risk of gastrointestinal bleeding, and an increased risk is seen when they are combined with anticoagulants.

Clinical evidence

(a) Azapropazone

A woman taking digoxin, furosemide, spironolactone, allopurinol, and **warfarin** (prothrombin ratio 2.8) developed haematemesis within 4 days of starting to take azapropazone 300 mg four times a day. Her prothrombin ratio was found to have risen to 15.7. Subsequent gastroscopic examination revealed a benign ulcer, the presumed site of the bleeding.[1]

At least 12 other patients are reported to have developed this interaction. Bruising or bleeding (melaena, epistaxis, haematuria) and prolonged prothrombin times have occurred within a few days of starting azapropazone.[2-7] Three patients died.[4-6] Another patient taking **warfarin** and azapropazone, diclofenac and co-proxamol had an increase in prothrombin time.[8]

(b) Feprazone

Five patients stabilised on **warfarin** had a mean prothrombin time rise from 29 to 38 seconds after taking feprazone 200 mg twice daily for 5 days, despite a 40% reduction in the **warfarin** dosage (from 5 to 3 mg daily). Four days after feprazone was stopped, their prothrombin times were almost back to usual. The interaction with feprazone was less marked than that with phenylbutazone.[9]

(c) Oxyphenbutazone

A man stabilised on **warfarin** developed gross haematuria within 9 days of starting to take oxyphenbutazone 400 mg daily. His prothrombin time had increased to 68 seconds.[10] Two similar cases have been described elsewhere.[11,12] A clinical study has also shown that oxyphenbutazone slows the clearance of **dicoumarol**.[13]

(d) Phenylbutazone

In a study in 3 subjects and one patient, phenylbutazone 200 mg three times daily and twice daily, respectively, given for 11 to 19 days before and 11 days after a single dose of **warfarin**, markedly increased the prothrombin time, but *decreased* the half-life of **warfarin**, and the **warfarin** AUC.[14] In another study that gave the enantiomers of **warfarin** separately, it was found that phenylbutazone inhibited the clearance of *S*-warfarin, but increased the clearance of *R*-warfarin.[15] This was confirmed in other studies, were the AUC of *R*-warfarin was decreased by 41% and the AUC of *S*-warfarin increased by 18%.[16]

A number of other studies have shown a markedly increased prothrombin times in patients[9,17] or healthy subjects[18] taking **warfarin** and given phenylbutazone. Moreover, there are a number of case reports demonstrating the clinical importance of this interaction.[14,19-23] In one, a man stabilised on **warfarin** following mitral valve replacement was later given phenylbutazone for back pain by his general practitioner. On admission to hospital a week later he had epistaxis, and his face, legs and arms had begun to swell. He showed extensive bruising of the jaw, elbow and calves, some evidence of gastrointestinal bleeding, and a prothrombin time of 89 seconds. Two similar cases were also reported.[22] A similar interaction occurs between phenylbutazone and **phenprocoumon**. In one study in healthy subjects, phenylbutazone 300 mg daily for 14 days markedly increased the prothrombin time response to a single dose of phenprocoumon given on day 4 by twofold, while decreasing the phenprocoumon AUC by 31%.[24] Cases of a clinically important interaction have also been reported for **phenprocoumon**.[25] In one early report, the required dose of **acenocoumarol** was 25% lower in patients taking phenylbutazone.[26] A single unconfirmed report describes this interaction in two patients taking **phenindione**.[27]

Mechanism

Phenylbutazone very effectively displaces the anticoagulants from their plasma protein binding sites, thereby increasing the concentrations of free and active anticoagulant (an effect easily demonstrated *in vitro*[14,28-32]). By itself, the importance of this mechanism is usually small, since any displaced drug is then available to be cleared, so any effect is usually transient (see 'Protein-binding interactions', (p.3)). However, phenylbutazone also inhibits the metabolism of *S*-warfarin (the more potent of the two warfarin enantiomers) so its effects are increased and prolonged.[15,16,33] In one study, the unbound clearance of *S*-warfarin was decreased fourfold.[33] In contrast, the unbound clearance of *R*-warfarin is not altered, so the total clearance of *R*-warfarin is increased due to displacement.[33] Thus, overall it appears that phenylbutazone decreases total plasma warfarin levels, while increasing its effect.

Azapropazone[34-36] and oxyphenbutazone (the major metabolite of phenylbutazone) probably act similarly.

Importance and management

The pharmacokinetic interaction between warfarin and azapropazone or phenylbutazone is very well established and clinically important. Serious bleeding can result and concurrent use should be avoided. Feprazone and oxyphenbutazone appear to interact similarly. Much less is known about phenindione with phenylbutazone, but they probably interact similarly.[27] Direct evidence of a serious interaction with phenprocoumon seems to be limited to two reports, and there is some evidence (from one paper published in 1957) that successful and apparently uneventful concurrent use is possible, presumably because in the case cited the response and the anticoagulant dosages were carefully controlled.[37] However, the practicalities of such close monitoring outside of a study are unclear. One study found that 25% less acenocoumarol was needed in patients given phenylbutazone.[26] Remember too that phenylbutazone and related drugs affect platelet aggregation and can cause gastrointestinal bleeding, whether an anticoagulant is present or not. It would seem advisable to use an alternative NSAID that interacts to a lesser extent, such as ibuprofen or naproxen, although it should be noted that no 'NSAID', (p.427), is entirely free from interactions with anticoagulants.

1. Powell-Jackson PR. Interaction between azapropazone and warfarin. *BMJ* (1977) 1, 1193–4.
2. Green AE, Hort JF, Korn HET, Leach H. Potentiation of warfarin by azapropazone. *BMJ* (1977) 1, 1532.
3. Beeley L. *Bulletin of the West Midlands Centre for Adverse Drug Reaction Reporting* (1980), 10.
4. Anon. Interactions. Doctors warned on warfarin dangers. *Pharm J* (1983) 230, 676.
5. Win N, Mitchell DC, Jones PAE, French EA. Azapropazone and warfarin. *BMJ* (1991) 302, 969–70.
6. Beeley L, Cunningham H, Carmichael A, Brennan A. *Bulletin of the West Midlands Centre for Adverse Drug Reaction Reporting* (1991) 33, 19.
7. Beeley L, Magee P, Hickey FM. *Bulletin of the West Midlands Centre for Adverse Drug Reaction Reporting* (1989) 28, 34.
8. Beeley L, Stewart P, Hickey FL. *Bulletin of the West Midlands Centre for Adverse Drug Reaction Reporting* (1988) 27, 27.
9. Chierichetti S, Bianchi G, Cerri B. Comparison of feprazone and phenylbutazone interaction with warfarin in man. *Curr Ther Res* (1975) 18, 568–72.
10. Taylor PJ. Hemorrhage while on anticoagulant therapy precipitated by drug interaction. *Ariz Med* (1967) 24, 697–9.
11. Hobbs CB, Miller AL, Thornley JH. Potentiation of anticoagulant therapy by oxyphenylbutazone (a probable case). *Postgrad Med J* (1965) 41, 563–5.
12. Fox SL. Potentiation of anticoagulants caused by pyrazole compounds. *JAMA* (1964) 188, 320–1.
13. Weiner M, Siddiqui AA, Bostanci N, Dayton PG. Drug interactions: the effect of combined administration on the half-life of coumarin and pyrazolone drugs in man. *Fedn Proc* (1965) 24, 153.
14. Aggeler PM, O'Reilly RA, Leong I, Kowitz PE. Potentiation of anticoagulant effect of warfarin by phenylbutazone. *N Engl J Med* (1967) 276, 496–501.
15. Lewis RJ, Trager WF, Chan KK, Breckenridge A, Orme M, Rowland M, Schary W. Warfarin. Stereochemical aspects of its metabolism and the interaction with phenylbutazone. *J Clin Invest* (1974) 53, 1607–17.
16. O'Reilly RA, Trager WF, Motley CH, Howald W. Stereoselective interaction of phenylbutazone with [$^{12}C/^{13}C$] warfarin pseudoracemates in man. *J Clin Invest* (1980) 65, 746–53.
17. Udall JA. Drug interference with warfarin therapy. *Clin Med* (1970) 77, 20–5.
18. Schary WL, Lewis RJ, Rowland M. Warfarin-phenylbutazone interaction in man: a long-term multiple-dose study. *Res Commun Chem Pathol Pharmacol* (1975) 10, 663–72.
19. Eisen MJ. Combined effect of sodium warfarin and phenylbutazone. *JAMA* (1964) 189, 64–5.
20. McLaughlin GE, McCarty DJ, Segal BL. Hemarthrosis complicating anticoagulant therapy. Report of three cases. *JAMA* (1966) 196, 1020–1.
21. Hoffbrand BI, Kininmonth DA. Potentiation of anticoagulants. *BMJ* (1967) 2, 838–9.
22. Bull J, Mackinnon J. Phenylbutazone and anticoagulant control. *Practitioner* (1975) 215, 767–9.
23. Robinson DS. The application of basic principles of drug interaction to clinical practice. *J Urol (Baltimore)* (1975) 113, 100–7.
24. O'Reilly RA. Phenylbutazone and sulfinpyrazone interaction with oral anticoagulant phenprocoumon. *Arch Intern Med* (1982) 142, 1634–7.
25. Sigg A, Pestalozzi H, Clauss A, Koller F. Verstärkung der Antikoagulantienwirkung durch Butazolidin. *Schweiz Med Wochenschr* (1956) 42, 1194–5.
26. Guggisberg W, Montigel C. Erfahrungen mit kombinierter Butazolidin-Sintrom-Prophylaxe und Butazolidin-prophylaxe thromboembolischer Erkrangungen. *Ther Umsch* (1958) 15, 227.
27. Kindermann A. Vaskuläres Allergid nach Butalidon und Gefahren kombinierter Anwendung mit Athrombon (Phenylindandion). *Dermatol Wochenschr* (1961) 143, 172–8.
28. O'Reilly RA. The binding of sodium warfarin to plasma albumin and its displacement by phenylbutazone. *Ann N Y Acad Sci* (1973) 226, 293–308.
29. Seiler K, Duckert F. Properties of 3-(1-phenyl-propyl)-4-oxycoumarin (Marcoumar®) in the plasma when tested in normal cases under the influence of drugs. *Thromb Diath Haemorrh* (1968) 19, 389–96.
30. Tillement J-P, Zini R, Mattei C, Singlas E. Effect of phenylbutazone on the binding of vitamin K antagonists to albumin. *Eur J Clin Pharmacol* (1973) 6, 15–18.
31. Solomon HM, Schrogie JJ. The effect of various drugs on the binding of warfarin-^{14}C to human albumin. *Biochem Pharmacol* (1967) 16, 1219–26.
32. O'Reilly RA. Interaction of several coumarin compounds with human and canine plasma albumin. *Mol Pharmacol* (1971) 7, 209–18.
33. Banfield C, O'Reilly R, Chan E, Rowland M. Phenylbutazone-warfarin interaction in man: further stereochemical and metabolic considerations. *Br J Clin Pharmacol* (1983) 16, 669–75.
34. McElnay JC, D'Arcy PF. Interaction between azapropazone and warfarin. *BMJ* (1977) 2, 773–4.
35. McElnay JC, D'Arcy PF. The effect of azapropazone on the binding of warfarin to human serum proteins. *J Pharm Pharmacol* (1978) 30 (Suppl), 73P.
36. McElnay JC, D'Arcy PF. Interaction between azapropazone and warfarin. *Experientia* (1978) 34, 1320–1.
37. Kaufmann P. Vergleich zwischen einer Thromboembolieprophylaxe mit Antikoagulantien und mit Butazolidin. *Schweiz Med Wochenschr* (1957) 87 (Suppl 24), 755–9.

Coumarins + NSAIDs; Sulindac

In pharmacological studies, sulindac did not significantly alter the anticoagulant effect of warfarin or phenprocoumon. Isolated cases of a modest to marked increase in the anticoagulant effects of warfarin have been reported with sulindac. Note that all NSAIDs increase the risk of gastrointestinal bleeding, and an increased risk is seen when they are combined with anticoagulants.

Clinical evidence

In a study in healthy subjects stabilised on **warfarin**, sulindac 200 mg twice daily for 7 days did not significantly alter the prothrombin time, when compared with placebo, although prothrombin time was slightly higher in the sulindac group.[1] Similarly, in 20 patients stabilised on **phenprocoumon**, sulindac 200 to 400 mg daily for 4 weeks did not alter measures of coagulation or bleeding time.[2]

However, a patient stabilised on **warfarin**, ferrous sulfate, phenobarbital and sulfasalazine had a marked increase in his prothrombin time ratio from about 3.2 to 10 after taking sulindac 100 mg twice daily for 5 days.[3-5] There are 4 similar cases of this interaction on record.[1,5-7] One of the patients had a gastrointestinal bleed after taking only three 100-mg doses of sulindac, although this patient was also taking flurbiprofen.[5] Another patient was stabilised on about a 40% lower dose of **warfarin** with continuation of the sulindac.[6] Another patient had a potassium-losing renal tubular defect, which was thought to contribute to the interaction.[1]

Mechanism

Not understood. In one patient, renal impairment may have caused sulindac accumulation, which in turn may have affected warfarin pharmacokinetics.[1] See also 'Coumarins and related drugs + NSAIDs', p.427.

Importance and management

The pharmacological studies cited suggest that usually no coumarin dose adjustment would be needed in patients given sulindac. However, the isolated cases of an interaction suggest that, rarely, some patients may be affected. Also note that all 'NSAIDs', (p.427) can irritate the gastric mucosa, affect platelet activity and cause gastrointestinal bleeding, which will be more severe in anticoagulated patients.

1. Loftin JP, Vesell ES. Interaction between sulindac and warfarin: different results in normal subjects and in an unusual patient with a potassium-losing renal tubular defect. *J Clin Pharmacol* (1979) 19, 733–42.
2. Schenk H, Klein G, Haralambus J, Goebel R. Coumarintherapie unter dem antirheumaticum sulindac. *Z Rheumatol* (1980) 39, 102–8.
3. Beeley L. *Bulletin of the West Midlands Centre for Adverse Drug Reaction Reporting* (1978) No. 6.

4. Beeley L, Baker S. Personal communication, 1978.
5. Ross JRY, Beeley L. Sulindac, prothrombin time, and anticoagulants. *Lancet* (1979) ii, 1075.
6. Carter SA. Potential effect of sulindac on response of prothrombin-time to oral anticoagulants. *Lancet* (1979) ii, 698–9.
7. McQueen EG. New Zealand Committee on Adverse Drug Reactions. 17th Annual Report 1982. *N Z Med J* (1983) 96, 95–9.

Coumarins + NSAIDs; Tolmetin

In pharmacological studies, tolmetin did not alter the anticoagulant effect of phenprocoumon or warfarin. Isolated cases of raised INRs have been described. Note that all NSAIDs increase the risk of gastrointestinal bleeding, and an increased risk is seen when they are combined with anticoagulants.

Clinical evidence

In a placebo-controlled study, no changes in prothrombin times occurred in 15 healthy subjects stabilised on **warfarin** when they took tolmetin 400 mg three times daily for 14 days.[1] Similarly, no changes in prothrombin times occurred in 15 patients taking **phenprocoumon** when they were given tolmetin 200 mg four times daily for 10 days.[2] Bleeding times were reported to be slightly prolonged though not to a clinically relevant extent.[2] Bleeding times were not significantly altered in healthy subjects given **acenocoumarol** and tolmetin 400 mg twice daily, or patients taking **acenocoumarol** and tolmetin.[3]

However, there is a single published case report of a diabetic patient stabilised on **warfarin**, insulin, digoxin, theophylline, ferrous sulfate, furosemide and sodium polystyrene sulfonate who had a nosebleed after taking three 400-mg doses of tolmetin. His prothrombin time had risen from a range of 15 to 22 seconds up to 70 seconds.[4] The manufacturers of tolmetin and the FDA in the US also have 10 other cases on record,[4,5] received over a 10-year period.[5]

Mechanism

See 'Coumarins and related drugs + NSAIDs', p.427.

Importance and management

The pharmacological studies cited suggest that usually no coumarin dose adjustment would be needed in patients given tolmetin. The isolated cases of an interaction are unexplained.

However, care is needed with every 'NSAID', (p.427) because, to a greater or lesser extent, they irritate the stomach lining, which can result in gastrointestinal bleeding, which will be more severe in anticoagulated patients.

1. Whitsett TL, Barry JP, Czerwinski AW, Hall WH, Hampton JW. Tolmetin and warfarin: a clinical investigation to determine if interaction exists. In 'Tolmetin, A New Non-steroidal Anti-Inflammatory Agent.' Ward JR (ed). Proceedings of a Symposium, Washington DC, April 1975, Excerpta Medica, Amsterdam, New York, p. 160–7.
2. Rüst O, Biland L, Thilo D, Nyman D, Duckert F. Prüfung des Antirheumatikums Tolmetin auf Interaktionen mit oralen Antikoagulantien. *Schweiz Med Wochenschr* (1975) 105, 752–3.
3. Malbach E. Über die Beeinflussung der Blutungszeit durch Tolectin. *Schweiz Rundsch Med Prax* (1978) 67, 161–3.
4. Koren JF, Cochran DL, Janes RL. Tolmetin-warfarin interaction. *Am J Med* (1987) 82, 1278–9.
5. Santopolo AC. Tolmetin-warfarin interaction. *Am J Med* (1987) 82, 1279–80.

Coumarins + Olanzapine

A single dose of olanzapine did not alter the pharmacokinetics or anticoagulant effect of a single dose of warfarin.

Clinical evidence, mechanism, importance and management

In a three-way, randomised, crossover study, 15 healthy subjects were given olanzapine 10 mg, **warfarin** 20 mg or both drugs together as single doses. No significant changes were seen in the pharmacokinetics of either drug, and the adverse effects of the olanzapine and the anticoagulant effects of the **warfarin** were unchanged.[1] Similarly, a 71-year-old woman stabilised on **warfarin** 15 mg/week with an INR of 2.6 had no significant change in INR after taking olanzapine 20 mg daily for 6 weeks (INR 2.6 when taking 15 mg/week and 2 while taking 12.5 mg/week).[2] This evidence suggests that no **warfarin** dose adjustments are anticipated to be needed on concurrent use with olanzapine.

1. Maya JF, Callaghan JT, Bergstrom RF, Cerimele BJ, Kassahun K, Nyhart EH, Brater DC. Olanzapine and warfarin drug interaction. *Clin Pharmacol Ther* (1997) 61, 182.
2. Rogers T, de Leon J, Atcher D. Possible interaction between warfarin and quetiapine. *J Clin Psychopharmacol* (1999) 19, 382–3.

Coumarins + Opioids; Dextropropoxyphene (Propoxyphene)

In one study, dextropropoxyphene did not alter the prothrombin time in patients taking unspecified coumarins. There are isolated cases of patients on warfarin who have shown a marked increase in prothrombin times and/or bleeding when given co-proxamol (dextropropoxyphene with paracetamol).

Clinical evidence

(a) Co-proxamol (Dextropropoxyphene with paracetamol)

A man taking **warfarin** developed marked haematuria within 6 days of starting to take two tablets of co-proxamol three times a day. Thirteen days previously his **warfarin** dose had been increased from 6 mg to 7 mg daily (thrombotest 16%), and then 9 days previously it had been reduced back to 6 mg daily (thrombotest 5%). His plasma **warfarin** levels had risen by one-third (from 1.8 to 2.4 micrograms/mL) despite the reduction in **warfarin** dose.[1] A woman stable for 6 weeks on **warfarin** developed gross haematuria 11 hours after starting co-proxamol. She had taken 6 tablets of co-proxamol over a 6-hour period. Her prothrombin time increased from about 30 to 40 seconds up to 130 seconds.[1]

This interaction has been reported in 5 other patients taking **warfarin**.[2-6] The prothrombin time of one of them rose from 28 to 44 seconds up to 80 seconds within 3 days of substituting paracetamol with two tablets of co-proxamol four times a day.[3] Another developed a prothrombin time of more than 50 seconds after taking 30 tablets of *Darvocet-N 100* (dextropropoxyphene 100 mg, paracetamol 650 mg) and possibly an unknown amount of ibuprofen over a 3-day period.[4] Increased **warfarin** effects leading to severe retroperitoneal haemorrhage have also been briefly reported in a patient taking co-proxamol.[5]

(b) Dextropropoxyphene

A double-blind study in 23 patients anticoagulated with un-named coumarol derivatives and given dextropropoxyphene 450 mg daily for 15 days or ibuprofen did not show any change in prothrombin times with either drug.[7]

Mechanism

Not understood. The effect dextropropoxyphene has on the metabolism of the warfarin enantiomers does not appear to have been studied. Dextropropoxyphene does not interact with other cytochrome P450 isoenzyme CYP2C9 substrates such as 'tolbutamide', (p.486), although it does interact with the CYP3A4 substrate 'carbamazepine', (p.527). There is also the possibility that the paracetamol component had some part to play (see also 'Coumarins + Paracetamol (Acetaminophen)', p.438). Alternatively, these cases may just represent idiosyncratic reactions.

Importance and management

Information about this interaction is very sparse and seems to be limited to the reports cited. The cases cited could just be idiosyncratic reactions. Bear them in mind in the event of an unexpected response to treatment.

1. Orme M, Breckenridge A, Cook P. Warfarin and Distalgesic interaction. *BMJ* (1976) i, 200.
2. Jones RV. Warfarin and Distalgesic interaction. *BMJ* (1976) i, 460.
3. Smith R, Prudden D, Hawkes C. Propoxyphene and warfarin interaction. *Drug Intell Clin Pharm* (1984) 18, 822.
4. Justice JL, Kline SS. Analgesics and warfarin. A case that brings up questions and cautions. *Postgrad Med* (1988) 83, 217-8, 220.
5. Beeley L, Magee P, Hickey FN. *Bulletin of the West Midlands Centre for Adverse Drug Reaction Reporting* (1990) 30, 20.
6. Pilszek FH, Moloney D, Sewell JR. Case report: increased anticoagulant effect of warfarin in patient taking a small dose of co-proxamol. Personal communication, 1994.
7. Franchimont P, Heynen G. Comparative study of ibuprofen and dextropropoxyphene in scapulo-humeral periarthritis following myocardial infarction. 13th International Congress of Rheumatol, Kyoto, Japan. 30th Sept–6th Oct 1973.

Coumarins + Opioids; Hydrocodone

In an isolated report, the anticoagulant effects of warfarin were increased by hydrocodone in one patient and in one healthy subject.

Clinical evidence, mechanism, importance and management

A patient, well stabilised on **warfarin** (and also taking digoxin, propranolol, clofibrate and spironolactone) had a rise in his prothrombin time of about 2 to 3 times his control value when he began to take *Tussionex* (hydrocodone with phenyltoloxamine) for a chronic cough. When the cough syrup was discontinued, his prothrombin time fell again. In a subsequent study in one healthy subject the equivalent dosage of hydrocodone increased the elimination half-life of **warfarin** from 30 to 42 hours.[1] The reason for this interaction is not known, and this case appears to be the only information available. Any interaction is not therefore established. Be aware of the possibility of an interaction in the case of an unexpected increase in the response to **warfarin**.

1. Azarnoff DL. Drug interactions: the potential for adverse effects. *Drug Inf J* (1972) 6, 19–25.

Coumarins + Opioids; Meptazinol

The anticoagulant effects of warfarin were not altered by meptazinol in one study.

Clinical evidence, mechanism, importance and management

Meptazinol 200 mg four times daily for 7 days had no significant effect on the prothrombin indexes of 6 elderly patients stabilised on **warfarin**, nor on the required **warfarin** dose.[1] No **warfarin** dose adjustments would be expected to be needed on concurrent use.

1. Ryd-Kjellen E, Alm A. Effect of meptazinol on chronic anticoagulant therapy. *Hum Toxicol* (1986) 5, 101–2.

Coumarins + Opioids; Tramadol

In one study tramadol did not change the mean INR in response to phenprocoumon, although two patients had increases. Isolated cases of an increase in anticoagulant effects of warfarin and phenprocoumon have been reported. One retrospective cohort study also found an increased risk of bleeding when acenocoumarol or phenprocoumon was given with tramadol.

Clinical evidence

In a double-blind, placebo-controlled, crossover study the mean INRs of 19 patients anticoagulated with **phenprocoumon** were unchanged when they were given tramadol 50 mg three times daily for a week,.[1,2] Although the mean difference was not changed, one patient had an INR rise from 4 to 7.3, and another from a just under 5 to 6, while taking tramadol, but not while taking placebo.

A brief report describes 5 elderly patients (aged 71 to 84 years), anticoagulated with **warfarin** or **phenprocoumon** and taking a range of other drugs, who had clinically important rises in INRs (up to threefold) shortly after starting to take tramadol. One of the patients had gastrointestinal bleeding. Three of the patients were able to continue the tramadol with a reduced anticoagulant dosage.[3]

In another report, a 61-year old woman with a mitral valve replacement stabilised on **warfarin** developed ecchymoses about 2 weeks after starting tramadol 50 mg every 6 hours. Her prothrombin time was found to have risen to 39.6 seconds and her INR was 10.6. These values returned to normal when the tramadol was withdrawn and the **warfarin** temporarily stopped.[4] Other cases have been reported with **warfarin**[5] and **phenprocoumon.**[6] In 2004, the Australian Adverse Drug Reactions Advisory Committee said they had received 11 reports of increases in INR or a haemorrhagic event in patients taking **warfarin** given tramadol. Two patients died of haemorrhagic stroke. They note that this number of cases suggests that the interaction is an uncommon event.[7] Up until March 2003, the Swedish Adverse Drug Reactions Advisory Committee had received reports of 17 cases of a suspected interaction between tramadol and **warfarin** resulting in increases in the INR (to 3.4 to 8.5) and bleeding complications in 35% of patients. One patient who continued tramadol needed the **warfarin** dose to be almost halved.[8]

In a retrospective cohort study of patients taking **acenocoumarol** or **phenprocoumon**, tramadol was found to be associated with a threefold increased risk of bleeding. The study was specifically looking at potentially interacting drugs taken by at least 50 patients and with at least 5 cases of bleeding.[9]

Mechanism

Unknown. It has been suggested that the interaction might be related to a variation in CYP genotype. Seven of 10 patients from the 17 suspected cases of interaction in Sweden had defective CYP2D6 alleles. The authors suggested that since this isoenzyme metabolises tramadol, these patients might have changes in tramadol metabolism that could increase the risk of an interaction with warfarin via CYP3A4. However, CYP3A4 only has a role in the 'metabolism', (p.358), of *R*-warfarin, and inhibition of CYP3A4 usually results in just minor to modest increases in INR. Moreover, defective CYP2D6 alleles have a population prevalence of 42.2%, so if this were the mechanism, many more cases would be expected. Because of the rarity of reports, it could just be that it is not really an interaction, and that there were unknown confounding factors in the suspected cases. Further study is needed.

Importance and management

Not established. One pharmacological study did not show a clear interaction for phenprocoumon and tramadol, although data from 2 patients suggested the possibility. Moreover, isolated cases of an interaction with warfarin and phenprocoumon have been published or reported to regulatory authorities, but the incidence seems to be rare. Because of the uncertainty, it would be prudent to consider monitoring prothrombin times in any patient taking coumarins when tramadol is first added, being aware that a small proportion of patients may need a reduction in the anticoagulant dosage. More study is needed.

1. Boeijinga JK, van Meegen E, van den Ende R, Schook CE, Cohen AF. Lack of interaction between tramadol and coumarins. *J Clin Pharmacol* (1998) 38, 966–70.
2. Boeijinga JK, van Meegen E, van den Ende R, Schook CE, Cohen AF. Is there interaction between tramadol and phenprocoumon? *Lancet* (1997) 350, 1552.
3. Jensen K. Interaktion mellem tramadol og orale antikoagulantia. *Ugeskr Laeger* (1997) 159, 785–6.
4. Sabbe JR, Sims PJ, Sims MH. Tramadol-warfarin interaction. *Pharmacotherapy* (1998) 18, 871–3.
5. Scher ML, Huntington NH, Vitillo JA. Potential interaction between tramadol and warfarin. *Ann Pharmacother* (1997) 31, 646–7.
6. Madsen H, Rasmussen JM, Brøsen K. Interaction between tramadol and phenprocoumon. *Lancet* (1997) 350, 637.
7. ADRAC. Tramadol-warfarin interaction. *Aust Adverse Drug React Bull* (2004) 23, 16.
8. Hedenmalm K, Lindh JD, Säwe J, Rane A. Increased liability of tramadol-warfarin interaction in individuals with mutations in the cytochrome P_{450} 2D6 gene. *Eur J Clin Pharmacol* (2004) 60, 369–72.
9. Penning-van Beest F, Erkens J, Petersen K-U, Koelz HR, Herings R. Main comedications associated with bleeding during anticoagulant therapy with coumarins. *Eur J Clin Pharmacol* (2005) 61, 439–44.

Coumarins and related drugs + Orlistat

Orlistat had no effect on the pharmacodynamics or pharmacokinetics of single-dose warfarin in healthy subjects. However, orlistat reduces fat absorption, and might therefore reduce vitamin K absorption. There is a published report of a patient taking warfarin who developed a modest increase in INR after taking orlistat. Similar cases have been reported to regulatory authorities.

Clinical evidence

In a placebo-controlled, randomised, crossover study, 12 healthy subjects were given orlistat 120 mg three times daily for 16 days, with a single 30-mg dose of **warfarin** on day 11. The pharmacokinetics and pharmacodynamics of the **warfarin** were not altered by the orlistat, and markers of vitamin K nutritional status were not affected.[1] However, regarding this study, the manufacturers US prescribing information states that vitamin K levels did tend to decline in subjects taking orlistat.[2] It is also noted that reports of "decreased prothrombin, increased INR and unbalanced anticoagulant treatment resulting in change of haemostatic parameters" have been reported in patients taking orlistat and anticoagulants.[2] In addition, in 2001 the Canadian regulatory authorities reported that unexpected increases in INR were noted after orlistat was given to patients taking either **warfarin** or **acenocoumarol**. These were managed by dosage adjustments of the coumarin or discontinuation of orlistat.[3]

In a published report, a 66-year-old man stabilised on **warfarin** for 2.5 years who started taking orlistat 120 mg three times daily for weight reduction had a modest increase in his INR, from less than 3, to 4.7 within 18 days. **Warfarin** was withheld and he was later restabilised on approximately two-thirds of the previous dose while continuing the orlistat.[4]

Mechanism

Orlistat may reduce the absorption of fat soluble vitamins including vitamin K,[4,5] and a change to a lower fat diet associated with the use of orlistat may also contribute to changes in the balance between vitamin K and **warfarin**.[4]

Importance and management

The manufacturers say that patients stabilised on anticoagulants and given orlistat should be closely monitored for changes in coagulation parameters.[2,5] Given the reports of changes in INRs, and the fact that changes in dietary 'vitamin K', (p.409) are known to affect warfarin efficacy, this seems prudent in patients taking a coumarin or an **indanedione**.

1. Zhi J, Melia AT, Guerciolini R, Koss-Twardy SG, Passe SM, Rakhit A, Sadowski JA. The effect of orlistat on the pharmacokinetics and pharmacodynamics of warfarin in healthy volunteers. *J Clin Pharmacol* (1996) 36, 659–666.
2. Xenical (Orlistat). Roche Pharmaceuticals. US Prescribing information, January 2007.
3. Canadian Adverse Drug Reaction Monitoring Program. Communiqué. Orlistat (Xenical) interaction with coumarin derivatives: increased INR. *Can Adverse Drug React News* (2001) 11 (Jul), 7.
4. MacWalter RS, Fraser HW, Armstrong KM. Orlistat enhances warfarin effect. *Ann Pharmacother* (2003) 37, 510–12.
5. Xenical (Orlistat). Roche Products Ltd. UK Summary of product characteristics, May 2006.

Coumarins + Oxolamine

Oxolamine markedly increases the effect of warfarin.

Clinical evidence, mechanism, importance and management

In a retrospective study, 11 patients were identified who had been receiving stable **warfarin** therapy and were then given oxolamine in doses of 100 to 600 mg daily for 3 to 10 days. Of six patients who did not have their **warfarin** dose adjusted, the INR increased by 70 to 190% from a range of 1.51 to 2.82 up to a range of 3.24 to 6.45. One patient had a **warfarin** dose reduction of just 14%, with an INR increase from 2.29 to 9.11. Four patients had their **warfarin** dose reduced by 30 to 36%, but one of these still had an INR increase from 2.14 to 4.01. Two of the 11 patients developed a hematoma.[1] In a further prospective study, six patients receiving stable **warfarin** therapy were given oxolamine 300 to 600 mg daily for 4 to 7 days, and the **warfarin** dose was reduced by 50% on starting oxolamine. Three patients had no change in INR, one had a 24% increase and two a 6% and 17% decrease.[1]

The mechanism of this interaction is unknown. Although published information is limited to this study, an interaction seems to be established. If any patient taking **warfarin** requires oxolamine, anticipate the need to roughly halve the **warfarin** dose.

1. Min KA, Zhu X, Oh JM, Shin WG. Effect of oxolamine on anticoagulant effect of warfarin. *Am J Health-Syst Pharm* (2006) 63, 153–6.

Coumarins + Paracetamol (Acetaminophen)

An equal number of randomised studies have found a modest increase in the anticoagulant effect (e.g. an increase in INR of 1) of coumarins as have reported no effect. One retrospective cohort study reported that concurrent use tends to increase the incidence of upper gastrointestinal bleeding, but other cohort studies found no evidence of a change in anticoagulant effect. There are isolated case reports of an increase in anticoagulant effects in patients taking warfarin or acenocoumarol and paracetamol.

Clinical evidence

Over 10 published studies have investigated whether or not paracetamol alters the effect of coumarin anticoagulants, with equal numbers finding no effect or an increased effect, see 'Table 12.5', (p.439). All the randomised, controlled studies showing an interaction have demonstrated a minor to modest effect (e.g. average increase in INR of 1.04 in one well-controlled study[1]). The only study to show a much greater effect (an increased odds ratio of an INR above 6 ranging from 3.5 to 10 for different doses of paracetamol alone or combined with an opioid) was a retrospective case-control study,[2,3] which has the limitations of being non-randomised with all the attendant problems of controlling for possible confounding variables.[4-6] Excluding this study, there appears to be no obvious explanation for the disparate findings between the studies showing an interaction and those not, either by study group, coumarin used, or dose of paracetamol.

There are only 5 published case reports of a possible interaction between paracetamol without opioids and a coumarin (**warfarin** or **acenocoumarol**), which are summarised in 'Table 12.5', (p.439). In addition, there are two reports of a possible interaction with paracetamol combined with codeine or dihydrocodeine listed in 'Table 12.5', (p.439), and 7 others with paracetamol combined with 'dextropropoxyphene (propoxyphene)', (p.436). Note that this incidence is very rare, given the widespread use of paracetamol, and the fact that it is generally considered safe for use with warfarin.

Moreover, in response to one case-control study[2] other clinicians running outpatient anticoagulant clinics have contended that they have not observed an interaction with paracetamol in their experience.[5,6]

Mechanism

Not understood. Paracetamol is mainly metabolised by glucuronidation and sulfation,[7,8] but the cytochrome P450 isoenzymes CYP1A2, CYP3A4 and CYP2E1 metabolise up to 15% of paracetamol under normal conditions.[7] *R*-warfarin is mainly metabolised by CYP3A4 and CYP1A2.[7,8] It has been suggested that in conditions such as ageing, hypoxia or hypertension, the isoenzymes play a more important part in paracetamol metabolism. Consequently paracetamol may then compete with the metabolism of *R*-warfarin to a sufficient degree to provoke an interaction.[8] However, as the *S*-warfarin enantiomer has significantly greater anticoagulant activity than the *R*-warfarin enantiomer, interactions with *R*-warfarin are considered by some to be of questionable significance.[6] Moreover, this explanation might explain rare case reports, but not the slight increases in INR seen in some studies in otherwise healthy subjects and patients.

Another idea is that the toxic metabolite of paracetamol inhibits the enzymes in the vitamin K cycle, and so has additive effects with anticoagulants, but so far this mechanism has only been investigated *in vitro*.[9] Yet another idea is that it is the indications for paracetamol use such as pain or fever that cause the interaction, rather than paracetamol *per se*,[10] but this does not explain why an interaction has been found in otherwise healthy patients or subjects given paracetamol in controlled studies.

Importance and management

Despite the number of studies, an interaction between paracetamol and coumarin anticoagulants is not firmly established, and the importance of the findings remain controversial. Some consider that the dose of paracetamol and its duration of use should be minimised in patients taking coumarins.[7,11] However, in randomised controlled studies, even maximum daily doses of paracetamol (4 g daily) for 2 weeks, had, at most, a modest effect, see 'Table 12.5', (p.439). A dose-related effect has been suggested in a case-controlled study,[2] but a more recent randomised controlled study did not find a dose-response (i.e. there was a slight change in INR of 0.5 with both 1.5 g daily and 3 g daily).[10] Further evidence is therefore required on the possible dose-response effect, and whether there is any value in minimising the dose. Moreover, on the basis of the studies suggesting an interaction, many have advocated increased monitoring in patients starting regular paracetamol. However, others consider that an increase in monitoring is unnecessary, or that increased monitoring during paracetamol use is not necessary unless the underlying illness (e.g. fever) requires increased monitoring. On the basis of the available data, it is not possible to firmly recommend increased monitoring, or dismiss its advisability. Further study is clearly needed.

Table 12.5 Summary of the evidence for and against an interaction between paracetamol (acetaminophen) and coumarins

Study type (year)	*Group*	*Coumarin*	*Paracetamol*	*Outcome*	*Refs*
Studies showing no interaction					
Randomised, crossover (1999)	20 healthy subjects	Warfarin, single-dose	1 g four times daily for one day, and 22 days	No change in warfarin pharmacokinetics or anticoagulant effect with either 1 day or 22 days	1
Clinical (1970)	10 patients	Stable warfarin	3.25 g daily for 2 weeks	No change in average prothrombin time	2
Randomised, placebo-controlled (1969)	20 patients	Phenprocoumon (19 patients) Warfarin (1 patient)	Two doses of 650 mg four hours apart	No change in average prothrombin time over 3 days	3
Randomised, placebo-controlled (2003)	31 patients	Phenprocoumon	Placebo (10 patients), 500 mg three times daily (11 patients), or 1 g three times daily (10 patients) for 2 weeks	Mean rise in INR of 0.46 at day 8 for both doses, which was not considered clinically relevant	4
Cohort (2002)	54 patients taking paracetamol and 180 others not taking paracetamol	Phenprocoumon	2 to 2.5 g per day for 3 days preceding INR determination	No change in anticoagulant effect	5
Cohort (recently started) (2002)	54 patients and 20 controls not given paracetamol	Acenocoumarol or phenprocoumon	Mean of 2.1 g daily	No difference in changes in INR between groups	6
Studies showing an interaction					
Randomised, placebo-controlled, crossover (1968)	50 patients	Stable warfarin, dicoumarol, anisindione,* phenprocoumon	650 mg four times daily for 2 weeks	Average increase in prothrombin time of 3.6 seconds	7
Randomised, placebo-controlled (1982, 1983)	20 patients	Stable acenocoumarol (8 patients) or phenprocoumon (12 patients)	500 mg four times daily for 3 weeks (10 patients); placebo (10 patients)	Average increase in thrombotest value of about 20 seconds (14% increase), which necessitated a reduction in coumarin dose in 5 patients	8, 9
Randomised, placebo-controlled, crossover (1984)	15 healthy subjects	Stable warfarin	4 g daily for 2 weeks	7 of 15 subjects had a prothrombin ratio rise of more than 20% while taking paracetamol compared with 1 of 15 taking placebo	10
Randomised, placebo-controlled, crossover (2005)	11 patients	Stable warfarin	4 g daily for 2 weeks	INR increased by a mean of 1.04 to a mean maximum of 3.47 in patients taking paracetamol, but did not change with placebo	11
Case-control (1998)	93 cases with INR greater than 6 and 196 controls (INR 1.7 to 3.3)	Warfarin	325 mg each week to greater than 1.3 g daily	52 cases (56%) and 70 controls (36%) reported using paracetamol in the preceding week.† The increased risk (3.5 to 10-fold) was related to paracetamol dose	12
Cohort (2001)	4204 patients	Warfarin and/or Phenprocoumon		Standardised incidence ratio of hospitalisation for upper GI bleeding was higher with combined use of paracetamol (4.4) than oral anticoagulants alone (2.8)	13
Case reports of an interaction: paracetamol					
Case report (1999)	72-year-old	Acenocoumarol	1 to 2 g daily long-term	13 days after stopping paracetamol, the INR decreased from a range of 2.5 to 3 down to 1.62. INR gradually increased on restarting paracetamol	14
Case report (2004)	77-year-old	Acenocoumarol	2 to 2.5 g daily for a few weeks	INR 5.4 then 9.1 one week later. Patient restabilised on same acenocoumarol dose and asked not to take more paracetamol than 2 g daily for more than 3 days	15
Case report (2002)	62-year-old	Warfarin	4 to 5 g (duration not stated)	INR of 7.5, with retroperitoneal haematoma. One month previously the INR had been 2.5	16
Case report (2003)	74-year-old	Warfarin	a. 1 g twice daily for 3 days b. 1 g four times daily for 3 days	a. INR of 3.4 then 4 b. INR increased from 2.3 to 6.4	17

Continued

Table 12.5 Summary of the evidence for and against an interaction between paracetamol (acetaminophen) and coumarins (continued)

Study type (year)	Group	Coumarin	Paracetamol	Outcome	Refs
Case report (2004)	76-year-old	Warfarin	Patient recently taking more paracetamol for a flare of arthritis	INR increase from 2.1 to 7, with haematuria and gingival bleeding	18
Paracetamol in combination with opioids‡					
Case report (1991)	66-year-old	Warfarin	Paracetamol/codeine; about 1.6 g daily of paracetamol over 10 days	Increase in prothrombin time from range of 15 to 19 up to 96 seconds. Haematuria and gingival bleeding	19
Case report (1997)	63-year-old	Warfarin	a. Paracetamol/dihydrocodeine 500 mg/10 mg, four daily for 7 days b. Paracetamol/codeine 500 mg/30 mg, three daily for 8 days	a. Increase in INR to 9.6 then 12, with gingival bleeding b. Increase in INR to 8.5	20

*Note that this is an indanedione

†Including 11 cases and 6 controls who reported taking a preparation of paracetamol in combination with an opioid, mostly codeine and oxycodone

‡There are also cases reported with dextropropoxyphene/paracetamol.

1. Kwan D, Bartle WR, Walker SE. The effects of acetaminophen on pharmacokinetics and pharmacodynamics of warfarin. *J Clin Pharmacol* (1999) 39, 68–75.
2. Udall JA. Drug interference with warfarin therapy. *Clin Med* (1970) 77, 20–5.
3. Antlitz AM, Awalt LF. A double blind study of acetaminophen used in conjunction with oral anticoagulant therapy. *Curr Ther Res* (1969) 11, 360–1.
4. Gadisseur APA, van der Meer FJM, Rosendaal FR. Sustained intake of paracetamol (acetaminophen) during oral anticoagulant therapy with coumarins does not cause clinically important INR changes: a randomized double-blind clinical trial. *J Thromb Haemost* (2003) 1, 714–17.
5. Fattinger K, Frisullo R, Masche U, Braunschweig S, Meier PJ, Roos M. No clinically relevant drug interaction between paracetamol and phenprocoumon based on a pharmacoepidemiological cohort study in medical inpatients. *Eur J Clin Pharmacol* (2002) 57, 863–7.
6. van den Bemt PMLA, Geven LM, Kuitert NA, Risselada A, Brouwers JRBJ. The potential interaction between oral anticoagulants and acetaminophen in everyday practice. *Pharm World Sci* (2002) 24, 201–4.
7. Antlitz AM, Mead JA ,Tolentino MA. Potentiation of oral anticoagulant therapy by acetaminophen. *Curr Ther Res* (1968) 10, 501–7.
8. Boeijinga J, Boerstra EE, Ris P, Breimer DD, Jeletich-Bastiaanse A. Interaction between paracetamol and coumarin anticoagulants. *Lancet* (1982) 1, 506.
9. Boeijinga JK, Boerstra EE, Ris P, Breimer DD, Jeletich-Bastiaanse A. De invloed van paracetamol op antistollingsbehandeling met coumarinederivaten. *Pharm Weekbl* (1983) 118, 209–12.
10. Rubin RN, Mentzer RL, Budzynski AZ. Potentiation of anticoagulant effect of warfarin by acetaminophen (TylenolR). *Clin Res* (1984) 32, 698A.
11. Mahé I, Bertrand N, Drouet L, Simoneau G, Mazoyer E, Bal dit Sollier C, Caulin C, Bergmann JF. Paracetamol: a haemorrhagic risk factor in patients on warfarin. *Br J Clin Pharmacol* (2005) 59, 371–4.
12. Hylek EM, Heiman H, Skates SJ, Sheehan MA, Singer DE. Acetaminophen and other risk factors for excessive warfarin anticoagulation. *JAMA* (1998) 279, 657–62.
13. Johnsen SP, Sorensen HT, Mellemkjoer L, Blot WJ, Nielsen GL, McLaughlin JK, Olsen JH. Hospitalisation for upper gastrointestinal bleeding associated with the use of oral anticoagulants. *Thromb Haemost* (2001) 86, 563–8.
14. Bagheri H, Bernhard NB, Montastruc JL. Potentiation of acenocoumarol anticoagulant effect by acetaminophen. *Ann Pharmacother* (1999) 33, 506.
15. Thijssen HH, Soute BA, Vervoort LM, Claessens JG. Paracetamol (acetaminophen) warfarin interaction: NAPQI, the toxic metabolite of paracetamol, is an inhibitor of enzymes in the vitamin K cycle. *Thromb Haemost* (2004) 92, 797–802.
16. Andrews FJ. Retroperitoneal haematoma after paracetamol increased anticoagulation. *Emerg Med J* (2002) 19. 84–5.
17. Gebauer MG, Nyfort-Hansen K, Henschke PJ, Gallus AS. Warfarin and acetaminophen interaction. *Pharmacotherapy* (2003) 23, 109–112.
18. Lesho EP, Saullo L, Udvari-Nagy S. A 76-year-old woman with erratic anticoagulation. *Cleve Clin J Med* (2004) 71, 651–56.
19. Bartle WR, Blakely JA. Potentiation of warfarin anticoagulation by acetaminophen. *JAMA* (1991) 265, 1260.
20. Fitzmaurice DA, Murray JA. Potentiation of anticoagulant effect of warfarin. *Postgrad Med J* (1997) 73, 439–40.

Paracetamol is still considered to be safer than 'aspirin', (p.385) or 'NSAIDs', (p.427), as an analgesic in the presence of an anticoagulant because it does not affect platelets or cause gastric bleeding.

1. Mahé I, Bertrand N, Drouet L, Simoneau G, Mazoyer E, Bal dit Sollier C, Caulin C, Bergmann JF. Paracetamol: a haemorrhagic risk factor in patients on warfarin. *Br J Clin Pharmacol* (2005) 59, 371–4.
2. Hylek EM, Heiman H, Skates SJ, Sheehan MA, Singer DE. Acetaminophen and other risk factors for excessive warfarin anticoagulation. *JAMA* (1998) 279, 657–62
3. Hylek EM. Acetaminophen and risk factors for excess anticoagulation with warfarin. *JAMA* (1998) 280, 697.
4. Gray CD. Acetaminophen and risk factors for excess anticoagulation with warfarin. *JAMA* (1998) 280, 695.
5. Amato MG, Bussey H, Farnett L, Lyons R. Acetaminophen and risk factors for excess anticoagulation with warfarin. *JAMA* (1998) 280, 695–6.
6. Riser J, Gilroy C, Hudson P, McCay L, Willis TA. Acetaminophen and risk factors for excess anticoagulation with warfarin. *JAMA* (1998) 280, 696.
7. Shek KLA, Chan L-N, Nutescu E. Warfarin-acetaminophen drug interaction revisited. *Pharmacotherapy* (1999) 19, 1153–8.
8. Lehmann DF. Enzymatic shunting: resolving the acetaminophen-warfarin controversy. *Pharmacotherapy* (2000) 20, 1464–8.
9. Thijssen HH, Soute BA, Vervoort LM, Claessens JG. Paracetamol (acetaminophen) warfarin interaction: NAPQI, the toxic metabolite of paracetamol, is an inhibitor of enzymes in the vitamin K cycle. *Thromb Haemost* (2004) 92, 797–802.
10. Gadisseur APA, van der Meer FJM, Rosendaal FR. Sustained intake of paracetamol (acetaminophen) during oral anticoagulant therapy with coumarins does not cause clinically important INR changes: a randomized double-blind clinical trial. *J Thromb Haemost* (2003) 1: 714–17.
11. Bell WR. Acetaminophen and warfarin: an undesirable synergy. *JAMA* (1998) 279, 702–3.

Coumarins + Pentoxifylline

Some studies have suggested that pentoxifylline does not alter the anticoagulant effects of phenprocoumon or acenocoumarol; however, one study suggests that there is an increased risk of serious bleeding if pentoxifylline is given with acenocoumarol. Pentoxifylline alone has rarely been associated with bleeding.

Clinical evidence

The anticoagulant effects of **phenprocoumon** were not altered by pentoxifylline 400 mg four times daily for 27 days in 10 patients on stable **phenprocoumon** therapy. Two patients had a slight increase in platelet aggregation.[1]

In a placebo-controlled study of either pentoxifylline 400 mg three times daily, **acenocoumarol** (adjusted to maintain an INR of 2 to 4.5), or both drugs together, 3 major haemorrhagic problems (2 fatal cerebral, 1 gastrointestinal) occurred in the 36 patients taking both drugs. In the 36 patients taking **acenocoumarol** alone, one case of cerebral haemorrhage (resulting in hemiplegia) and another of haematuria with epistaxis occurred. This difference was not statistically significant, but the authors considered that the risk of bleeding was probably increased by the combination.[2] In this study, 69% of patients had an INR within desired range, and 7% had an INR above 4.5. In another randomised study in patients with recurrent venous thrombosis, there was no difference in dose of **acenocoumarol** necessary to reach an INR of 2.5 to 3.5 between 100 patients taking **acenocoumarol** with pentoxifylline 1.2 g daily and 100 patients taking **acenocoumarol** alone. No patients had severe bleeding, and 3 to 4% of patients in both groups had moderate bleeding (haematomas, haematuria).[3]

Mechanism

Pentoxifylline alone has rarely been associated with bleeding,[4] indicating that bleeding may not necessarily be the result of an interaction. The manufacturers say that a causal relationship between pentoxifylline and bleeding has not been established.[5,6]

Importance and management

Information is limited, and an interaction is not established. In the US, the manufacturer recommends that patients taking **warfarin** should have more frequent monitoring of coagulation parameters when given pentoxifylline,[6] and this seems a prudent precaution with this and any other coumarin.

1. Ingerslev J, Mouritzen C, Stenbjerg S. Pentoxifylline does not interfere with stable coumarin anticoagulant therapy: a clinical study. *Pharmatherapeutica* (1986) 4, 595–600.
2. Dettori AG, Pini M, Moratti A, Paolicelli M, Basevi P, Qintavalla R, Manotti C, Di Lecce C and The APIC Study Group. Acenocoumarol and pentoxifylline in intermittent claudication. A controlled clinical study. *Angiology* (1989) 40, 237–48.
3. Moriau M, Lavenne-Pardonge E, Crasborn L, von Frenckell R, Col-Debeys C. The treatment of severe or recurrent deep venous thrombosis. Beneficial effect of the co-administration of antiplatelet agents with or without rheological effects, and anticoagulants. *Thromb Res* (1995) 78, 469–82.
4. Oren R, Yishar U, Lysy J, Livshitz T, Ligumsky M. Pentoxifylline-induced gastrointestinal bleeding. *DICP Ann Pharmacother* (1991) 25, 315–16.
5. Trental 400 (Pentoxifylline). Sanofi-Aventis. UK Summary of product characteristics, September 2004.
6. Trental (Pentoxifylline). Sanofi-Aventis US LLC. US Prescribing information, September 2006.

Coumarins + Phosphodiesterase type-5 inhibitors

In pharmacological studies, sildenafil did not interact with warfarin or acenocoumarol. However, in pulmonary hypertension, there is some evidence of an increased risk of bleeding with concurrent use, and nosebleeds were a common adverse effect of sildenafil alone. There is also a report of two possible cases of rises in INRs in patients taking acenocoumarol or warfarin and sildenafil. Studies suggest that tadalafil and vardenafil do not interact with warfarin.

Clinical evidence

(a) Sildenafil

The manufacturer notes that no significant interaction occurred when sildenafil 50 mg was given with **warfarin** 40 mg,[1-4] or when sildenafil 100 mg was given with **acenocoumarol**.[3] However, in studies in pulmonary hypertension, nosebleeds were a common adverse effect (13%), and concurrent use of vitamin K antagonists and sildenafil resulted in a greater incidence of reports of bleeding (primarily nosebleeds) than placebo.[4] A 68-year-old man taking **acenocoumarol** and enalapril had an increase in his INR from 3.05 to 7.7 without bleeding complications after taking sildenafil. The patient continued to take sildenafil once a week, and the daily dose of **acenocoumarol** was split into two, with a return to stable therapeutic INR values. Another patient taking **warfarin**, ranitidine and pravastatin had a rise in INR on three occasions after taking sildenafil once a week, omitting the dose of ranitidine when he took the sildenafil. On one of these occasions, he had bleeding gums. This rise in INR no longer occurred when he started taking the ranitidine with the sildenafil.[5]

(b) Tadalafil

A double-blind, randomised, crossover study in which a single-dose of **warfarin** was given on day 7 of 12 consecutive days of treatment with either tadalafil 10 mg or placebo found that tadalafil did not affect the AUCs of either *S*-warfarin and *R*-warfarin, and prothrombin times were unchanged.[6]

(c) Vardenafil

No pharmacokinetic interaction was observed when vardenafil was given with **warfarin**,[7,8] and the prothrombin time was unchanged.[8]

Mechanism

The two cases of interactions are unexplained. It is not obvious why dividing the acenocoumarol dose, or using ranitidine, would have reversed an interaction. No interaction via inhibition of coumarin metabolism is likely. Sildenafil alone appears to commonly cause nosebleeds in patients with pulmonary hypertension.[4]

Importance and management

There is no established pharmacokinetic or pharmacodynamic interaction between the phosphodiesterase type-5 inhibitors and warfarin, and no warfarin dose adjustment would therefore be expected to be needed on concurrent use. However, in pulmonary hypertension, sildenafil appears to increase the risk of nosebleeds, and this may be greater in patients taking coumarins. Similarly, the two possible cases with acenocoumarol and warfarin, although not conclusive, do introduce a note of caution.

1. Viagra (Sildenafil citrate). Pfizer Ltd. UK Summary of product characteristics, June 2006.
2. Viagra (Sildenafil citrate). Pfizer Inc. US Prescribing information, October 2006.
3. Revatio (Sildenafil citrate). Pfizer Ltd. UK Summary of product characteristics, March 2007.
4. Revatio (Sildenafil citrate). Pfizer Inc. US Prescribing information, July 2006.
5. Fernández MA, Romá E. International normalized ratio increase in patients taking oral anticoagulant therapy and using sildenafil (Viagra®). *Haematologica* (2003) 88, ELT34.
6. Eli Lilly and Company. Personal communication, March 2003.
7. Levitra (Vardenafil hydrochloride trihydrate). Bayer plc. UK Summary of product characteristics, November 2006.
8. Levitra (Vardenafil hydrochloride). Bayer Pharmaceuticals Corporation. US Prescribing information, March 2007.

Coumarins + Piracetam

In a large clinical study, piracetam did not alter the dose of acenocoumarol required to produce a given INR. A single case report describes a woman stabilised on warfarin who began to bleed within a month of starting to take piracetam. Piracetam has antiplatelet activity, so some caution seems prudent on combined use.

Clinical evidence, mechanism, importance and management

In a randomised study in patients with recurrent venous thrombosis, there was no difference in dose of **acenocoumarol** necessary to reach an INR of 2.5 to 3.5 between 100 patients taking **acenocoumarol** with high-dose piracetam 9.6 g daily and 100 patients taking **acenocoumarol** alone. No patients had severe bleeding, and 3 to 4% of patients in both groups had moderate bleeding (haematomas, haematuria). The addition of piracetam decreased platelet aggregation, levels of fibrinogen, and blood viscosity.[1]

A woman taking **warfarin**, insulin, levothyroxine and digoxin complained of menorrhagia at a routine follow up. Investigations revealed that her British Corrected Ratio had risen to 4.1 (normal range 2.3 to 2.8), and that one month previously she had started to take low-dose piracetam 200 mg three times daily. Within 2 days of withdrawing both the **warfarin** and piracetam her BCR had fallen to 2.07, and the original dose of warfarin was restarted.[2]

Piracetam alone is known to decrease platelet aggregation,[1] and might therefore be expected to increase the risk of bleeding with anticoagulants, similar to other drugs with antiplatelet activity such as 'aspirin', (p.385). The early case appears to be the only report of a possible interaction, but some caution might be prudent on concurrent use.

1. Moriau M, Lavenne-Pardonge E, Crasborn L, von Frenckell R, Col-Debeys C. The treatment of severe or recurrent deep venous thrombosis. Beneficial effect of the co-administration of antiplatelet agents with or without rheological effects, and anticoagulants. *Thromb Res* (1995) 78, 469–82.
2. Pan HYM, Ng RP. The effect of Nootropil in a patient on warfarin. *Eur J Clin Pharmacol* (1983) 24, 711.

Coumarins + Pirmenol

The anticoagulant effects of warfarin are not altered by pirmenol.

Clinical evidence, mechanism, importance and management

The prothrombin time response to a single 25-mg dose of **warfarin** was slightly reduced in most of 12 healthy subjects (reductions ranged from 0.2 to 1.3 seconds) who had taken pirmenol 150 mg twice daily for 14 days, with the warfarin taken on day 8.[1] This suggested that some changes in the dosage of **warfarin** might be required in practice, but a later placebo-controlled study found that the prothrombin times of 10 patients stabilised on **warfarin** were not significantly changed when they were given oral pirmenol 150 mg twice daily for 14 days.[2] No **warfarin** dose adjustments would therefore be expected to be required on concurrent use.

1. Janiczek N, Bockbrader HN, Lebsack ME, Sedman AJ, Chang T. Effect of pirmenol (CI-845) on prothrombin (PT) time following concomitant administration of pirmenol and warfarin to healthy volunteers. *Pharm Res* (1988) 5, S-155.
2. Stringer KA, Switzer DF, Abadier R, Lebsack ME, Sedman A, Chrymko M. The effect of pirmenol administration on the anti-coagulant activity of warfarin. *J Clin Pharmacol* (1991) 31, 607–10.

Coumarins + Probenecid

In healthy subjects, probenecid increased the clearance of single-dose phenprocoumon without altering its anticoagulant effect. The anticoagulant effects of multiple-dose phenprocoumon might be expected to be decreased by probenecid, but this requires confirmation.

Clinical evidence, mechanism, importance and management

In 9 healthy subjects probenecid 500 mg four times daily for 7 days reduced the AUC of a single 0.22-mg/kg dose of **phenprocoumon** given on day one by 47% and reduced the elimination half-life by about one-third. Nevertheless, the reduction in prothrombin time by **phenprocoumon** was not altered by probenecid.[1]

The reasons for this interaction are not understood, but one possibility is that, while probenecid inhibits the glucuronidation of **phenprocoumon** (its normal route of metabolism), it may also increase the formation of hydroxylated metabolites so that its overall loss is increased.[1]

Although the anticoagulant effect of single-dose **phenprocoumon** was not altered in this study, its findings suggests that, in the presence of probenecid, the dosage of phenprocoumon might need to be increased, but this awaits formal clinical confirmation in a multiple-dose study. Nothing further seems to have been published on this potential interaction, so bear its possibility in mind if probenecid is used in a patient taking phenprocoumon. There seems to be nothing documented about other coumarins.

1. Mönig H, Böhm M, Ohnhaus EE, Kirch W. The effects of frusemide and probenecid on the pharmacokinetics of phenprocoumon. *Eur J Clin Pharmacol* (1990) 39, 261–5.

Coumarins + Proguanil

An isolated report describes bleeding in a patient stabilised on warfarin after she took proguanil for about five weeks.

Clinical evidence, mechanism, importance and management

A woman stabilised on **warfarin** developed haematuria, bruising and abdominal and flank discomfort about 5 weeks after starting to take proguanil 200 mg daily. Her prothrombin ratio was found to be 8.6. Within 12 hours of being given fresh frozen plasma and vitamin K her prothrombin ratio had fallen to 2.3. During the 5 weeks she had travelled from Britain to Thailand, Bali, Australia and then New Zealand, and her prothrombin ratio had not been checked during this time. The mechanism of this potential interaction is unknown.[1] Its general importance is uncertain, as factors related to travel (such as a changing diet and changing dose times in different time zones) may have had a part to play in this interaction.

1. Armstrong G, Beg MF, Scahill S. Warfarin potentiated by proguanil. *BMJ* (1991) 303, 789.

Coumarins + Prolintane

The anticoagulant effects of ethyl biscoumacetate are not affected by prolintane.

Clinical evidence, mechanism, importance and management

The response to a single 20-mg/kg dose of **ethyl biscoumacetate** was examined in 4 healthy subjects given prolintane 20 mg daily for 4 days. Assessments were made before prolintane, on day 1 of prolintane, and 8 days after prolintane was stopped. The mean half-life of the anticoagulant and prothrombin times remained unchanged.[1] No **ethyl biscoumacetate** dose adjustments would appear to be required on concurrent use.

1. Hague DE, Smith ME, Ryan JR, McMahon FG. The effect of methylphenidate and prolintane on the metabolism of ethyl biscoumacetate. *Clin Pharmacol Ther* (1971) 12, 259–62.

Coumarins and related drugs + Propafenone

The anticoagulant effects of warfarin, and possibly fluindione and phenprocoumon, are increased by propafenone.

Clinical evidence

The mean steady-state plasma levels of 8 healthy subjects taking **warfarin** 5 mg daily rose by 38% after they took propafenone 225 mg three times daily for a week. Five of the 8 had a distinct prothrombin time increase. The average rise in prothrombin time of the whole group was about 7 seconds, which was considered to be clinically significant.[1] Two case reports describe marked increases in the anticoagulant effects of **fluindione** and **phenprocoumon** in 2 patients taking propafenone.[2,3]

Mechanism

Propafenone may reduce the metabolism of these anticoagulants, thereby increasing their effects. From *in vitro* data, it was concluded that propafenone would affect only *R*-warfarin, whereas both *R*- and *S*-acenocoumarol were affected.[4]

Importance and management

Information seems to be limited to these reports but they suggest that anticoagulant control should be well monitored if propafenone is given to patients taking warfarin, and probably also phenprocoumon and the indanedione fluindione. The anticoagulant dosage should be reduced where necessary. It would be prudent to apply the same precautions with any other coumarin or indanedione anticoagulant.

1. Kates RE, Yee Y-G, Kirsten EB. Interaction between warfarin and propafenone in healthy volunteer subjects. *Clin Pharmacol Ther* (1987) 42, 305–11.
2. Körst HA, Brandes J-W, Littmann K-P. Cave: Propafenon potenziert Wirkung von oralen Antikoagulantien. *Med Klin* (1981) 76, 349–50.
3. Welsch M, Heitz C, Stephan D, Imbs JL. Potentialisation de l'effet anticoagulant de la fluindione par la propafénone. *Therapie* (1991) 46, 254–5.
4. Hermans JJR, Thijssen HHW. Human liver microsomal metabolism of the enantiomers of warfarin and acenocoumarol: P450 isozyme diversity determines the differences in their pharmacokinetics. *Br J Pharmacol* (1993) 110, 482–90.

Coumarins and related drugs + Prostaglandins

Limited evidence suggests that the combined use of intravenous high-dose epoprostenol and warfarin may increase the risk of pulmonary haemorrhage. Continuous subcutaneous treprostinil did not alter the pharmacokinetics or the INR in response to single-dose warfarin, and also did not appear to increase the risk of bleeding when used with warfarin in clinical studies. Because these prostaglandins inhibit platelet aggregation, some caution is appropriate on combined use with anticoagulants.

Clinical evidence

(a) Epoprostenol

In a small retrospective review of 31 patients with primary pulmonary hypertension receiving **warfarin** and continuous intravenous epoprostenol, 9 patients were identified who experienced 11 bleeding episodes (9 cases of pulmonary haemorrhage, 2 of nasal bleeding). Of the 9 cases of pulmonary haemorrhage, 8 were identified clinically by persistent haemoptysis, and 2 cases were associated with severe respiratory distress. Of the 7 patients with an INR available at the time of the first bleeding episode, 6 had an INR under 2 and one had an INR of 3.1. The dose of epoprostenol in patients with bleeds ranged from 28.1 to 164 nanograms/kg per minute, and no patient receiving less than 28 nanograms/kg per minute had a bleed. There was no significant difference in survival in patients with a bleeding episode and those without.[1] In contrast, the manufacturer states that there was no evidence of increased bleeding in patients taking anticoagulants and receiving infusions of epoprostenol in clinical studies.[2]

(b) Treprostinil

In a crossover study in 15 healthy subjects, continuous subcutaneous treprostinil 5 then 10 nanograms/kg every minute for 9 days did not alter the pharmacodynamics (INR) of a single 25-mg oral dose of **warfarin** given on day 3. In addition, there was no change in the pharmacokinetics of *R*- and *S*-warfarin.[3] In the discussion of this study, the authors mention an unpublished retrospective review of data from placebo-controlled clinical studies in patients with pulmonary artery hypertension. From this there was no evidence to suggest that concurrent **warfarin** and treprostinil (155 patients) was associated with increased bleeding or coagulation-related events, when compared with warfarin and placebo (156 patients).[3]

Mechanism

Epoprostenol (prostacyclin) and its long-acting analogue treprostinil are vasodilators that also inhibit platelet aggregation. The related drug iloprost also has these actions. As such, it is anticipated that they might increase the potential for bleeding when given with other anticoagulants.

Importance and management

Anticoagulants such as warfarin are commonly used in patients with pulmonary artery hypertension, a condition for which epoprostenol and now treprostinil have been developed, so the combination is likely to be used frequently. Because these prostaglandins are potent inhibitors of platelet aggregation, they might increase the risk of bleeding with anticoagulants (including coumarins and **indanediones**), although the manufacturers say that there was no evidence of increased bleeding in clinical studies using epoprostenol[2] or treprostinil.[3] Nevertheless, limited evidence from the small survey in Japanese patients given epoprostenol suggests that this may be the case with high-dose epoprostenol. In this study, the authors commented that they no longer use anticoagulant therapy in patients receiving high-dose epoprostenol.[1] However, the manufacturers information states that since almost all patients in clinical studies of epoprostenol were receiving oral anticoagulants, concurrent oral anticoagulation is recommended.[4] although the manufacturers say that there was no evidence of increased bleeding in clinical studies using epoprostenol[2] or treprostinil.[3] There appears to be no direct information about **iloprost** but it seems likely that is will interact similarly. Some caution would be appropriate if any of these prostaglandins is given with a coumarin or **indanedione**. Further study is needed.

1. Ogawa A, Matsubara H, Fujio H, Miyaji K, Nakamura K, Morita H, Saito H, Fukushima Kusano K, Emori T, Date H, Ohe T. Risk of alveolar hemorrhage in patients with primary pulmonary hypertension: anticoagulation and epoprostenol therapy. *Circ J* (2005) 69, 216–20.
2. Flolan (Epoprostenol sodium). GlaxoSmithKline. US Prescribing information, September 2002.
3. Wade M, Hunt TL, Lai AA. Effect of continuous subcutaneous treprostinil therapy on the pharmacodynamics and pharmacokinetics of warfarin. *J Cardiovasc Pharmacol* (2003) 41, 908–15.
4. Flolan (Epoprostenol). GlaxoSmithKline. UK Summary of product characteristics, September 2006.

Coumarins + Protease inhibitors

In pharmacokinetic studies, ritonavir slightly raised *S*-warfarin levels and modestly decreased *R*-warfarin levels, while lopinavir/ritonavir decreased *S*-warfarin levels. In case reports both increased and decreased warfarin effects have been reported with ritonavir. One of these reports also found that indinavir might cause a moderate reduction in anticoagulation. There is also a report of a marked reduction in anticoagulation in a patient taking acenocoumarol, which was associated with the concurrent use of ritonavir or nelfinavir. An isolated report describes a gradual INR rise in an elderly patient taking warfarin when he was given saquinavir.

Clinical evidence

(a) Acenocoumarol

A 46-year-old HIV-positive man with mitraortic valve replacements stabilised on acenocoumarol (INR 2.5 to 3.5) for 5 years and taking zidovudine and didanosine for 17 months was found to have a dramatic decrease in his INR when his drug regimen was changed to stavudine, lamivudine and **ritonavir** 600 mg twice daily. Increasing the acenocoumarol dosage over 5 days from an average of 24 mg to over 70 mg failed to increase the INR to target levels. The INR returned to previous levels within 4 days of stopping **ritonavir**, and the acenocoumarol dosage could be reduced to 3 mg daily. The patient was subsequently given **nelfinavir** and a similar, though less dramatic interaction occurred: while taking **nelfinavir** an INR of 2.5 was achieved with a 210% increase in the acenocoumarol dose.[1]

(b) Warfarin

1. Indinavir. A 50-year-old HIV-positive man, stabilised on warfarin (prothrombin complex activity (PCA) range of 20 to 35%), started taking indinavir 800 mg every 8 hours, but it had to be withdrawn after 12 days because of a generalised skin rash. It was then found that the indinavir had caused a moderate reduction in his level of anticoagulation: 10 and 25 days after indinavir was stopped his PCA was 53% and 43%, respectively. The warfarin dosage was increased to 6.25 and 7.5 mg on alternate days for one week, during which time a PCA of 34% was achieved, and he was then subsequently given warfarin 6.25 mg daily.[2] This patient subsequently needed an increase in warfarin dose when given *ritonavir*, see below.

2. Lopinavir/Ritonavir. In a pharmacokinetic study in healthy subjects,[3] lopinavir/ritonavir 400 mg/100 mg twice daily for 10 days modestly decreased the AUCs of *R*- and *S*-warfarin by 37% and 29%, respectively, after a single 10-mg dose of warfarin and vitamin K were given on day 7. Vitamin K was given to inhibit the pharmacological effect of warfarin without affecting its pharmacokinetics.

3. Ritonavir. The manufacturer reports that, in 12 healthy subjects given ritonavir 400 mg every 12 hours for 12 days, the AUC of *S*-warfarin was increased by 9% (90% confidence interval,17 to 44%) while that of *R*-warfarin was decreased by 33% (-38% to -27%) after a single 5-mg dose of warfarin.[4] The effect of these changes on prothrombin time was not mentioned, but potentially could result in an increased warfarin effect due to the more potent *S*-warfarin, or a decreased effect due to the *R*-warfarin. Both of these outcomes have been reported in individual cases. An increase in warfarin effect was seen in a man taking warfarin 10 mg daily (INRs 2.4 to 3) when his treatment for HIV was changed from efavirenz and abacavir to **ritonavir**, **nelfinavir** and *Combivir* (zidovudine/lamivudine). Within 5 days his INR had risen to 10.4 without any sign of bleeding. It proved difficult to achieve acceptable and steady INRs both while in hospital and after discharge, but eventually it was discovered that the patient could not tolerate liquid ritonavir because of nausea and vomiting, so that he had sometimes skipped or lowered the ritonavir dose or even refused to take it. On the occasions where no ritonavir or low-dose ritonavir was taken, the INRs had been low, whereas when he took the full dose of ritonavir the INRs were high.[5]

In contrast, the INR of a 27-year-old HIV-positive woman taking warfarin fell when she was given **ritonavir**, clarithromycin and zidovudine. It was necessary almost to double the warfarin dosage to maintain satisfactory INRs. Three months later when the **ritonavir** was withdrawn, her INR more than tripled within a week. Her final warfarin maintenance dose was half of that needed before the **ritonavir** was started, and a quarter of the dose needed just before she stopped the **ritonavir**. This case was complicated by the use or withdrawal of a number of other drugs (co-trimoxazole, rifabutin, an oral contraceptive, megestrol), which can also interact with warfarin.[6] Similarly, in another patient taking warfarin 6.25 mg daily with a prothrombin activity complex (PCA) of about 34%, a decrease in warfarin effects (PCA increase to 62%) was noted 20 days after starting **ritonavir** (escalating doses up to 600 mg every 12 hours). The warfarin dosage was then increased to 8.75 mg daily and 24 days later a satisfactory PCA of 33% was achieved.[2] This patient had previously shown a decrease in warfarin effects while taking *indinavir*, see above.

4. Saquinavir. A 73-year-old man who was HIV-positive and who had been taking warfarin, co-trimoxazole, nizatidine, stavudine and lamivudine for 7 months started taking saquinavir 600 mg three times daily. His INR, which had been stable at around 2 for five months, rose to about 2.5 after 4 weeks, and to about 4.2 after 8 weeks, which the author of the report attributed to an interaction with the saquinavir. The situation was solved by reducing the warfarin dosage by 20%.[7]

Mechanism

Protease inhibitors are well known to alter the metabolism of many drugs via inhibition, but sometimes induction of, cytochrome P450 isoenzymes, see 'Table 21.2', (p.773), so it is not surprising that they have altered warfarin effects, although the precise mechanism is unclear. The findings of the two pharmacokinetic studies suggest that, with warfarin, induction predominates, and that the anticoagulant effects are likely to be decreased.

Importance and management

Pharmacokinetic studies have suggested that ritonavir and lopinavir/ritonavir can modestly reduce warfarin levels. Clinical information on an interaction between coumarins and protease inhibitors is limited to the case reports cited, which either show an increase in warfarin effects (ritonavir or saquinavir) or a decrease in warfarin or acenocoumarol effects (indinavir, nelfinavir, or ritonavir). These cases show it would be prudent to monitor the prothrombin times and INRs of any patient if any HIV protease inhibitor is added, being alert for the need to modify the coumarin dosage.

1. Libre JM, Romeu J, López E, Sirera G. Severe interaction between ritonavir and acenocoumarol. *Ann Pharmacother* (2002) 36, 621–3.
2. Gatti G, Alessandrini A, Camera M, Di Biagnio A, Bassetti M, Rizzo F. Influence of indinavir and ritonavir on warfarin anticoagulant activity. *AIDS* (1998) 12, 825–6.
3. Yeh RF, Gaver VE, Patterson KB, Rezk NL, Baxter-Meheux F, Blake MJ, Eron JJ, Klein CE, Rublein JC, Kashuba ADM. Lopinavir/ritonavir induces the hepatic activity of cytochrome P450 enzymes CYP2C9, CYP2C19, and CYP1A2 but inhibits the hepatic and intestinal activity of CYP3A as measured by a phenotyping drug cocktail in healthy volunteers. *J Acquir Immune Defic Syndr* (2006) 42, 52–60.
4. Norvir (Ritonavir). Abbott Laboratories. US Prescribing information, January 2006.
5. Newshan G, Tsang P. Ritonavir and warfarin interaction. *AIDS* (1999) 13, 1788–9.
6. Knoell KR, Young TM, Cousins ES. Potential interaction involving warfarin and ritonavir. *Ann Pharmacother* (1998) 32, 1299–1302.
7. Darlington MR. Hypoprothrombinemia during concomitant therapy with warfarin and saquinavir. *Ann Pharmacother* (1997) 31, 647.

Coumarins + Proton pump inhibitors

In pharmacological studies, omeprazole caused a minor increase in *R*-warfarin levels, with no or a minor increase in anticoagulant effect. Conversely, lansoprazole, pantoprazole and rabeprazole did not alter warfarin pharmacokinetics or anticoagulant effect. Omeprazole does not appear to alter the effects of acenocoumarol and pantoprazole does not appear to later the effects of phenprocoumon. Nevertheless, a number of isolated reports describe increased anticoagulant effects when PPIs are given with coumarins.

Clinical evidence

(a) Esomeprazole

Esomeprazole is the *S*-isomer of omeprazole, and would be expected to behave similarly, see below. The manufacturers say that esomeprazole 40 mg daily did not cause any clinically relevant effects on anticoagulant times in patients stabilised on **warfarin**, but a few isolated cases of raised INRs have been reported post-marketing.[1,2]

(b) Lansoprazole

A study in 24 healthy subjects stabilised on **warfarin** found that lansoprazole 60 mg daily for 9 days had no effect on the pharmacokinetics of either *S*- or *R*-warfarin, and did not alter the effect of **warfarin** on prothrombin times.[3]

However, in 1998 the manufacturers of lansoprazole had on record two reports of possible interactions. An elderly patient taking **warfarin** developed an INR of 7 when lansoprazole was added. Despite a **warfarin** dosage adjustment he had a gastrointestinal haemorrhage, a myocardial infarction and died after 3 weeks. Another man taking **warfarin** (as well as amiodarone, furosemide and lisinopril) became confused, had hallucinations and developed an increased INR (value not known) when given lansoprazole. The lansoprazole was stopped after 4 days, and he then recovered. However, it is uncertain whether this was an interaction or whether he had taken an incorrect **warfarin** dosage because of his confusion.[4]

(c) Omeprazole

1. Acenocoumarol. In a placebo-controlled study in 8 healthy subjects, omeprazole 40 mg daily for 3 days had no effect on the pharmacokinetics of *R*- or *S*-acenocoumarol when a single 10-mg dose of acenocoumarol was given on day 2. In addition, omeprazole did not alter the anticoagulant effects of acenocoumarol.[5] Similarly, there was no evidence of an interaction in a retrospective study of 118 patients given acenocoumarol with omeprazole and 299 patients taking acenocoumarol without omeprazole (matched for age and sex).[6]

However, an isolated case report describes a 78-year-old woman who had been taking acenocoumarol for 60 days and who developed gross haematuria within 5 days of starting omeprazole 20 mg daily. Her INR had risen from a range of 2.5 to 3 up to 5.7, and when the omeprazole was stopped, her INR fell.[7]

2. Warfarin. In 21 healthy subjects who had been stabilised on warfarin, omeprazole 20 mg daily for 2 weeks caused a small but statistically significant decrease in the mean thrombotest percentage, from 21.1 to 18.7%. *S*-warfarin serum levels remained unchanged, but a small 12% rise in *R*-warfarin levels was seen.[8] In a further study, no changes in coagulation times or thrombotest values occurred in 28 patients anticoagulated with warfarin and given omeprazole 20 mg daily for 3 weeks. *S*-warfarin levels were unchanged, while a 9.5% increase in *R*-warfarin levels occurred.[9]

However, a man stabilised on warfarin 5 mg daily developed widespread bruising and haematuria 2 weeks after starting to take omeprazole 20 mg daily. His prothrombin time was found to have risen to 48 seconds. He was later restabilised on omeprazole 20 mg daily with the warfarin dosage reduced to 2 mg daily.[10]

(d) Pantoprazole

In 26 healthy subjects, pantoprazole 40 mg daily for 8 days caused no change in the response to a single 25-mg dose of **warfarin** given on day 2. The pharmacokinetics of *R*- and *S*-warfarin were unaltered, and no changes in the pharmacodynamics of the **warfarin** (prothrombin time, factor VII) were seen.[11] However, the manufacturer notes that there have been reports of increased INR and prothrombin time in patients taking pantoprazole and **warfarin**.[12]

No change in the prothrombin time ratio , was seen in 16 healthy subjects taking individualised maintenance **phenprocoumon** doses when they were given pantoprazole 40 mg daily for 5 days, nor was there any change in the pharmacokinetics of *R*- and *S*-phenprocoumon.[13] However, there is a report of 2 possible cases of an interaction.[14] One patient who was given **phenprocoumon** (loading dose 12 mg on day 1, 9 mg on day 2, 3 mg on day 3, and further as required) and omeprazole 20 mg daily concurrently, had an INR of 3.28 by the fourth day. The **phenprocoumon** was withheld, but the INR remained high for 9 days, when the omeprazole was stopped. Four days later the INR was 1.5 and **phenprocoumon** was restarted at 16.5 mg/week, and stabilised at 9 to 10.5 mg/week. She subsequently had a similar loading dose without problems, in the absence of omeprazole, when **phenprocoumon** was stopped for 3 weeks prior to surgery.[14] Another patient stabilised on **phenprocoumon** 18 mg/week required a slight reduction in dose to 16.5 mg/week after starting omeprazole 20 mg daily.[14]

(e) Rabeprazole

In a placebo-controlled study a single 0.75-mg/kg dose of **warfarin** was given to 21 patients before and after rabeprazole 20 mg daily for 7 days. No significant changes in prothrombin times or in the pharmacokinetics of *R*- or *S*-warfarin were seen.[15] However, the manufacturer notes that there have been reports of increased INR and prothrombin time in patients receiving rabeprazole and **warfarin**.[16]

Mechanism

Studies have shown that omeprazole partially inhibits the metabolism of *R*-warfarin, but not *S*-warfarin,[17,18] which confirms the findings in the pharmacokinetic studies above. It also partially inhibits the metabolism of acenocoumarol.[17] However, these small changes would generally not be expected to be clinically relevant. It has been suggested that the interaction might occur only in patients who are poor metabolisers of the cytochrome P450 isoenzyme CYP2C19 (seen in about 5% of Caucasians), who have five to tenfold higher levels of omeprazole than extensive metabolisers.[5] Other proton pump inhibitors are generally considered to have less potential for pharmacokinetic interactions than omeprazole, but even with these, isolated cases of anticoagulant interactions have been reported. It is possible that the isolated cases of interactions with proton pump inhibitors just represent idiosyncratic effects attributable to other factors, and not to any interaction.

Importance and management

The very minor pharmacokinetic interaction between omeprazole and warfarin, resulting in a less than 15% rise in just the *R*-warfarin levels, is established, but probably of limited clinical relevance. This is borne out by the fact there is only one published case report of an interaction. No pharmacokinetic or pharmacodynamic interaction occurred between warfarin and lansoprazole, pantoprazole or rabeprazole in clinical studies. However, isolated cases of raised INRs have been reported for all the proton pump inhibitors (esomeprazole, lansoprazole, pantoprazole, omeprazole and rabeprazole) and acenocoumarol (one published), phenprocoumon (2 published), and warfarin. When prescribing proton pump inhibitors to patients taking coumarins it would seem prudent to bear in mind that rarely bleeding can occur. Note that the US prescribing information for every proton pump inhibitors states that patients taking a proton pump inhibitor and warfarin may need to be monitored for increases in INR and prothrombin time. The advice in UK varies from recommending monitoring with warfarin and omeprazole[19] or esomeprazole,[1] recommending monitoring with pantoprazole and coumarins on the basis of it being good practice to increase monitoring with any change in concurrent therapy,[20] to no advice with lansoprazole[21] or rabeprazole.[22] Further study is needed to determine whether the risk of an interaction with omeprazole is increased in poor metaboliser phenotypes for CYP2C19, as has been suggested.[5]

1. Nexium Tablets (Esomeprazole magnesium trihydrate). AstraZeneca UK Ltd. UK Summary of product characteristics, May 2007.
2. Nexium (Esomeprazole magnesium). AstraZeneca. US Prescribing information, April 2007.
3. Cavanaugh JH, Winters EP, Cohen A, Locke CS, Braeckman R. Lack of effect of lansoprazole on steady state warfarin metabolism. *Gastroenterology* (1991) 100, A40.
4. Wyeth. Personal communication, January 1998.
5. de Hoon JNJM, Thijssen HHW, Beysens AJMM, Van Bortel LMAB. No effect of short-term omeprazole intake on acenocoumarol pharmacokinetics and pharmacodynamics. *Br J Clin Pharmacol* (1997) 44, 399–401.
6. Vreeburg EM, De Vlaam-Schluter GM, Trienekens PH, Snel P, Tytgat GNJ. Lack of effect of omeprazole on oral acenocoumarol anticoagulant therapy. *Scand J Gastroenterol* (1997) 32, 991–4.
7. García B, Lacambra C, Garrote F, García-Plaza I, Solis J. Possible potentiation of anticoagulant effect of acenocoumarol by omeprazole. *Pharm World Sci* (1994) 16, 231–2.
8. Sutfin T, Balmer K, Boström H, Eriksson S, Höglund P, Paulsen O. Stereoselective interaction of omeprazole with warfarin in healthy men. *Ther Drug Monit* (1989) 11, 176–84.
9. Unge P, Svedberg L-E, Nordgren A, Blom H, Andersson T, Lagerström P-O, Idström J-P. A study of the interaction of omeprazole and warfarin in anticoagulated patients. *Br J Clin Pharmacol* (1992) 34, 509–12.
10. Ahmad S. Omeprazole-warfarin interaction. *South Med J* (1991) 84, 674–5.
11. Duursema L, Müller FO, Schall R, Middle MV, Hundt HKL, Groenewoud G, Steinijans VW, Bliesath H. Lack of effect of pantoprazole on the pharmacodynamics and pharmacokinetics of warfarin. *Br J Clin Pharmacol* (1995) 39, 700–703.
12. Protonix (Pantoprazole sodium). Wyeth Pharmaceuticals Inc. US Prescribing information, June 2007.
13. Ehrlich A, Fuder H, Hartmann M, Wieckhorst G, Timmer W, Huber R, Birkel M, Bliesath H, Steinijans VW, Wurst W, Lücker PW. Lack of pharmacokinetic and pharmacodynamic interaction between pantoprazole and phenprocoumon in man. *Eur J Clin Pharmacol* (1996) 51, 277–281.
14. Enderle C, Müller W, Grass U. Drug interaction: omeprazole and phenprocoumon. *BMC Gastroenterol* (2001) 1, 2. Available at http://www.biomedcentral.com/1471-230X/1/2 (accessed 17/08/07).
15. Humphries TJ, Nardi RV, Spera AC, Lazar JD, Laurent AL, Spanyers SA. Coadministration of rabeprazole sodium (E3810) does not affect the pharmacokinetics of anhydrous theophylline or warfarin. *Gastroenterology* (1996) 110 (Suppl), A138.
16. AcipHex (Rabeprazole sodium). Eisai Inc. US Prescribing information, February 2007.
17. Hermans JJ, Thijssen HH. Human liver microsomal metabolism of the enantiomers of warfarin and acenocoumarol: P450 isozyme diversity determines the differences in their pharmacokinetics. *Br J Pharmacol* (1993) 111, 482–90.
18. Chainuvati S, Nafziger AN, Leeder JS, Gaedigk A, Kearns GL, Sellers E, Zhang Y, Kashuba ADM, Rowland E, Bertino JS. Combined phenotypic assessment of cytochrome P450 1A2, 2C9, 2C19, 2D6, and 3A, *N*-acetyltransferase-2, and xanthine oxidase activities with the "Copperstown 5+1 cocktail". *Clin Pharmacol Ther* (2003) 74, 437–47.
19. Losec Capsules (Omeprazole). AstraZeneca. UK Summary of product characteristics, July 2006.
20. Protium Tablets (Pantoprazole sodium sesquihydrate). Altana Pharma Ltd. UK Summary of product characteristics, December 2005.
21. Zoton FasTab (Lansoprazole). Wyeth Pharmaceuticals. UK Summary of product characteristics, May 2007.
22. Pariet (Rabeprazole sodium). Eisai Ltd. UK Summary of product characteristics, September 2004.

Coumarins + Quetiapine

A case report describes a woman taking warfarin who developed a raised INR when quetiapine was started.

Clinical evidence, mechanism, importance and management

A 71-year old woman receiving long-term treatment with **warfarin**, phenytoin, olanzapine and benztropine had her **warfarin** dosage slightly reduced (from 20 to 19.5 mg weekly) because her INR was raised (from 1.6 to 2.6). Eight days later her treatment with olanzapine was changed to quetiapine 200 mg daily, and after 5 days her INR was 2.7. Two weeks later she was found to have an INR of 9.2. The quetiapine was stopped and she was given two doses of vitamin K by injection. The only clinical symptoms seen were a small amount of bleeding from the injection site and a bruise on her hand. She was eventually later restabilised on phenytoin, olanzapine and **warfarin** 21 mg weekly with an INR of 1.6.

The reasons for this apparent interaction are not known but the authors suggest that the quetiapine may have inhibited the metabolism of the **warfarin** (possibly by competitive inhibition of the cytochrome P450 isoenzymes CYP3A4 and CYP2C9), thereby increasing its effects. They also suggest that the phenytoin may have had some part to play.[1] This is only an isolated case but bear it in mind in the case of an unexpected response to concurrent use.

1. Rogers T, de Leon J, Atcher D. Possible interaction between warfarin and quetiapine. *J Clin Psychopharmacol* (1999) 19, 382–3.

Coumarins + Quinidine

Quinidine did not alter the anticoagulant effect of warfarin in a study in patients, nor in a retrospective analysis of patient data. However, isolated reports of increased warfarin effects and bleeding have been reported, although these stem from over 35 years ago, and nothing further seems to have been reported, suggesting that an interaction is unlikely. Quinidine did not alter the half-life of phenprocoumon in healthy subjects. A small decrease in the effects of dicoumarol and warfarin has also been reported with quinidine, which was attributed to changes in haemodynamic factors following cardioversion.

Clinical evidence

In a controlled study, 10 patients receiving long-term treatment with **warfarin** 2.5 to 12.5 mg daily had no significant alteration in their prothrombin times when they were given quinidine 200 mg four times daily for 2 weeks.[1,2] Similarly, in a retrospective analysis of 8 patients stabilised on **warfarin**, there was no change in anticoagulant control associated with starting or stopping quinidine (600 mg to 1.2 g daily as sulfate or 660 mg daily as gluconate).[3] In the preliminary report of another study in 5 healthy subjects, quinidine 100 mg daily, started 7 days after a single 12-mg dose of **phenprocoumon** did not change the elimination half-life of **phenprocoumon**.[4]

In contrast, another report described 3 patients stabilised on **warfarin**, with Quick values within the range of 15 to 25%, who began to bleed within 7 to 10 days of starting to take quinidine 800 mg to 1.2 g daily. Their Quick values were found to have fallen to 6 to 8%. Bleeding ceased when the warfarin was withdrawn.[5] There is one other case report of haemorrhage associated with the concurrent use of **warfarin** and quinidine,[6] and in an analysis of haemorrhage in patients taking anticoagulants, it was reported that quinidine seemed partly responsible for some cases.[7]

In a further report, 4 patients taking **warfarin** or **dicoumarol** needed dosage *increases* of 8 to 24% to maintain adequate anticoagulation after DC conversion for atrial fibrillation and starting quinidine 400 mg three times daily, an effect that was attributed to haemodynamic factors.[8]

Mechanism

Uncertain. The cases of increased warfarin effects were attributed to quinidine possibly having a direct hypoprothrombinaemic effect of its own.[5] The cases of a slight decrease in anticoagulant effect were attributed to changes in haemodynamic factors as a result of cardioversion.[8]

Importance and management

In one study and one retrospective analysis, quinidine had no effect on the anticoagulant control with warfarin in patients. Therefore, no interaction would normally be anticipated. However, a few isolated cases of increased anticoagulant effect with bleeding have been reported. Nevertheless, the literature is limited, and based solely on evidence from more than 35 years ago. The lack of reports of any further interactions in this time suggests that a clinically relevant interaction is unlikely. Limited evidence suggests that quinidine does not alter phenprocoumon pharmacokinetics.

1. Udall JA. Quinidine and hypoprothrombinemia. *Ann Intern Med* (1968) 69, 403–4.
2. Udall JA. Drug interference with warfarin therapy. *Clin Med* (1970) 77, 20–5.
3. Jones FL. More on quinidine induced hypoprothrombinaemia. *Ann Intern Med* (1968) 69, 1074.
4. Iven H, Lerche L, Kaschube M. Influence of quinine and quinidine on the pharmacokinetics of phenprocoumon in rat and man. *Eur J Pharmacol* (1990) 183, 662.
5. Koch-Weser J. Quinidine-induced hypoprothrombinemic hemorrhage in patients on chronic warfarin therapy. *Ann Intern Med* (1968) 68, 511–17.
6. Gazzaniga AB, Stewart DR. Possible quinidine-induced hemorrhage in a patient on warfarin sodium. *N Engl J Med* (1969) 280, 711–12.
7. Beaumont JL, Tarrit A. Les accidents hémorrhagiques survenus au cours de 1500 traitements anticoagulants. *Sang* (1955) 26, 680–94.
8. Sylvén C, Anderson P. Evidence that disopyramide does not interact with warfarin. *BMJ* (1983) 286, 1181.

Coumarins + Quinine

Isolated reports describe increased anticoagulant effects in two women taking warfarin and a man taking phenprocoumon, which were attributed to the quinine content of tonic water. Limited evidence suggests that quinine does not alter the half-life of phenprocoumon.

Clinical evidence

In the preliminary report of a study in 5 healthy subjects, quinine 100 mg daily started 7 days after a single 12-mg dose of **phenprocoumon** did not change the elimination half-life of **phenprocoumon** in the following 7 days.[1]

However, a patient on long-term **phenprocoumon** treatment repeatedly developed extensive haematuria within 24 hours of drinking 1 litre of Indian tonic water containing 30 mg of quinine.[1]

A woman stabilised on **warfarin** needed a dosage reduction from 6 mg to 4 mg daily when she started to drink 1 to 1.5 litres of tonic water containing quinine each day. Her **warfarin** requirements rose again when the tonic water was stopped. Another woman needed a **warfarin** dosage reduction from 4 mg to 2 mg daily when she started to drink over 2 litres of tonic water daily. They were probably taking about 80 to 180 mg of quinine daily.[2]

Mechanism

Not understood. Two studies[3,4] using the Page method (Russell viper venom)[5] to measure prothrombin times showed that marked increases of up to 12 seconds could occur when 330-mg doses of quinine were given in the absence of an anticoagulant, but other studies[4,6] using the Quick method found that the prothrombin times were only prolonged by up to 2.1 seconds. The changes in prothrombin times could be completely reversed by vitamin K (menadiol sodium diphosphate),[3,4] which suggests that quinine, like the oral anticoagulants, is a competitive inhibitor of vitamin K. However, because the only reports relate to tonic water, it cannot be excluded that some other ingredient is responsible for the effect seen in these patients. Also, they may just represent idiosyncratic reactions.

Importance and management

Not established. The lack of reports relating to the therapeutic use of quinine suggest that no interaction of clinical importance occurs. The isolated cases cited show that very exceptionally decreased anticoagulant requirements and even bleeding can occur when large quantities of tonic water are ingested. However, whether the effect seen was related to the quinine content of this beverage is not established.

1. Iven H, Lerche L, Kaschube M. Influence of quinine and quinidine on the pharmacokinetics of phenprocoumon in rat and man. *Eur J Pharmacol* (1990) 183, 662.
2. Clark DJ. Clinical curio: warfarin and tonic water. *BMJ* (1983) 286, 1258.
3. Pirk LA, Engelberg R. Hypoprothrombinemic action of quinine sulfate. *JAMA* (1945) 128, 1093–5.
4. Pirk LA, Engelberg R. Hypoprothrombinemic action of quinine sulfate. *Am J Med Sci* (1947) 213, 593–7.
5. Page RC, de Beer EJ, Orr ML. Prothrombin studies using Russell viper venom. II. Relation of clotting time to prothrombin concentration in human plasma. *J Lab Clin Med* (1941) 27, 197–201.
6. Quick AJ. Effect of synthetic vitamin K and quinine sulfate on the prothrombin level. *J Lab Clin Med* (1946) 31, 79–84.

Coumarins + Raloxifene

In one study, raloxifene caused a minor increase in warfarin levels, but a 10% decrease in prothrombin time. The manufacturer notes that a small and slow decrease in prothrombin times may occur when raloxifene is given with warfarin, and possibly other coumarins.

Clinical evidence, mechanism, importance and management

In 15 healthy postmenopausal women, raloxifene 120 mg daily for 15 days had minor effects on the pharmacokinetics and pharmacodynamics of a single 20-mg dose of **warfarin** given on day 11. The clearance of both *R*- and *S*-warfarin was slightly decreased (by 7% and 14%, respectively), with similar increases in AUC. Conversely, the maximum prothrombin time was decreased by 10%.[1] As has been suggested for 'lasofoxifene', (p.423), this might be because oestrogenic compounds increase plasma concentrations of vitamin K-dependent clotting factors, so antagonising the effect of **warfarin**.

The manufacturer recommends that because modest decreases in prothrombin times have been seen, which may develop over several weeks, prothrombin times should be checked. They extend this recommendation to cover the use of other coumarins.[2]

1. Miller JW, Skerjanec A, Knadler MP, Ghosh A, Allerheiligen SRB. Divergent effects of raloxifene HCl on the pharmacokinetics and pharmacodynamics of warfarin. *Pharm Res* (2001) 18, 1024–8.
2. Evista (Raloxifene hydrochloride). Eli Lilly and Company Ltd. UK Summary of product characteristics, May 2007.

Coumarins + Retinoids

Case reports describe reduced warfarin effects in a patient given etretinate, and in a patient given isotretinoin. Acitretin did not significantly alter the anticoagulant effects of phenprocoumon in healthy subjects.

Clinical evidence

(a) Phenprocoumon

Acitretin 50 mg daily for 10 days slightly increased the Quick test of 10 healthy subjects stabilised on phenprocoumon, from 22 to 24%, and the corresponding INR value decreased from 2.91 to 2.71. However, these changes were not considered to be significant.[1]

(b) Warfarin

1. Etretinate. A man with T-cell lymphoma who had recently been given chemotherapy (cyclophosphamide, doxorubicin, vincristine and prednisolone) was anticoagulated with warfarin after developing a pulmonary embolism. About three weeks later, he started etretinate 40 mg daily and it was found necessary to increase his warfarin dosage from 7 to 10 mg daily. His liver function tests were normal.[2] This patient had also recently started taking 'co-proxamol', (p.436), 'tolbutamide', (p.380) and 'cimetidine', (p.412)', but all of these have been reported to only rarely *increase* the effect of warfarin.

2. Isotretinoin. A 61-year-old man stabilised on warfarin 2.5 mg daily for 2 to 3 years had a decrease in his INR to below 2.5 after starting oral cefpodoxime proxetil 200 mg twice daily and oral isotretinoin 30 mg daily for inflammatory lesions of the face. He required an increase in warfarin dose to 3.75 mg daily. The cefpodoxime was stopped after 10 days without a further change in warfarin requirement. However, when the isotretinoin was discontinued after 40 days, the INR progressively increased and the warfarin dose was eventually reduced to the pretreatment dose of 2.5 mg daily.[3]

Mechanism

Not understood. It has been suggested that etretinate or isotretinoin may increase the rate of metabolism of warfarin.[2,3]

Importance and management

Information appears to be limited to these reports. The clinical relevance of the two case reports of a modest increase in warfarin requirements on starting etretinate or isotretinoin is uncertain, but, until more is known, consideration could be given to monitoring the INR if patients are given warfarin and these retinoids. The study with acitretin suggests that no phenprocoumon dose adjustments are expected to be needed on starting acitretin.

1. Hartmann D, Mosberg H, Weber W. Lack of effect of acitretin on the hypoprothrombinemic action of phenprocoumon in healthy volunteers. *Dermatologica* (1989) 178, 33–6.
2. Ostlere LS, Langtry JAA, Jones S, Staughton RCD. Reduced therapeutic effect of warfarin caused by etretinate. *Br J Dermatol* (1991) 124, 505–10.
3. Fiallo P. Reduced therapeutic activity of warfarin during treatment with oral isotretinoin. *Br J Dermatol* (2004) 150, 164.

Coumarins + Ribavirin

In a single patient, ribavirin appeared to decrease the effect of warfarin requiring a 40% increase in warfarin dose.

Clinical evidence

A 61-year-old patient who had been taking **warfarin** for a number of years with an INR in the range of 1.8 to 2.7 required a progressive 40% increase in **warfarin** dose (from 45 to 62.5 mg weekly) over the month after starting oral ribavirin 600 mg twice daily and subcutaneous interferon alfa-2b for active hepatitis C infection. During the following 11 months, the **warfarin** dose was stabilised at 57.5 mg weekly. Three weeks after discontinuation of the ribavirin and interferon, his INR had increased from 2.2 to 3.4 requiring a reduction in **warfarin** dose to 47.5 mg weekly. One year later, the patient was rechallenged with ribavirin 1 g daily for 4 weeks alone. At a weekly **warfarin** dose of 52.5 mg, his INR decreased from 2.6 to 1.8.[1]

Mechanism

Unknown. The few cases with 'interferon', (p.422) have suggested that this may *increase* the effect of warfarin. In this case, ribavirin seems to have decreased the effect of warfarin, and overridden any effect of interferon.

Importance and management

This is the only case of this interaction, so it is not established, although the evidence on rechallenge with ribavirin alone lends weight to it being an interaction. The authors recommend increased monitoring of anticoagulant effects in patients taking warfarin requiring ribavirin. Until more is known, this may be prudent.

1. Schulman S. Inhibition of warfarin activity by ribavirin. *Ann Pharmacother* (2002) 36, 72–4.

Coumarins + Ropinirole

A man stabilised on warfarin had an increase in INR necessitating a 25% decrease in his warfarin dose while taking ropinirole.

Clinical evidence, mechanism, importance and management

A frail 63-year-old man taking levodopa/carbidopa daily and **warfarin** 4 mg daily with a stable INR ranging from 1.8 to 2.6 over the past 14 months was evaluated for possible progression of Parkinson's disease. He was then given ropinirole 250 micrograms three times daily with a 25% reduction in his levodopa/carbidopa dose, and 9 days later his INR was noted to have increased to 4.6, but there were no apparent signs of bleeding. **Warfarin** was withheld for 4 days, and then restarted at 2 mg daily, and increased to 3 mg daily 19 days later when his INR was 1.2. After one month the ropinirole was discontinued because of adverse gastrointestinal effects, and 2 months later his INR was 1.4 necessitating an increase in the **warfarin** dose to the original dose of 4 mg daily.[1]

The mechanism of this probable interaction is unknown, and it appears to be the first evidence of such an interaction. No definite conclusions can be drawn from this isolated case.

1. Bair JD, Oppelt TF. Warfarin and ropinirole interaction. *Ann Pharmacother* (2001) 35, 1202–4.

Coumarins + Sevelamer

Sevelamer does not alter the pharmacokinetics of warfarin.

Clinical evidence, mechanism, importance and management

In a study in healthy subjects, the pharmacokinetics of a single 30-mg oral dose of **warfarin** were not statistically changed by sevelamer 2.4 g (equivalent to 6 capsules). Five more doses of sevelamer were given with meals over 2 days to check whether it had any effect on the enterohepatic circulation. No effect was seen.[1-3] Thus it appears that sevelamer does not bind to **warfarin** within the gut to reduce its absorption.

1. Renagel (Sevelamer). Genzyme Therapeutics. UK Summary of product characteristics, June 2007.
2. Renagel Capsules (Sevelamer hydrochloride). Genzyme. US Prescribing information, April 2007.
3. Burke SK, Amin NS, Incerti C, Plone MA, Watson N. Sevelamer hydrochloride (Renagel®), a nonabsorbed phosphate-binding polymer, does not interfere with digoxin or warfarin pharmacokinetics. *J Clin Pharmacol* (2001) 41, 193–8.

Coumarins + SNRIs

In at least six cases venlafaxine appears to have increased the INRs and caused bleeding in patients taking warfarin. A similar case has been seen with duloxetine and warfarin.

Clinical evidence

(a) Duloxetine

A woman taking **warfarin** with a stable INR (mean 2.2 over the previous year) developed petechiae and purpura 55 days after starting duloxetine 30 mg daily, and was found to have an INR of 5. **Warfarin** was stopped on day 58, but the INR continued to rise to greater than 19 on day 85, and she was given vitamin K. On day 94 the duloxetine was stopped. **Warfarin** was restarted on day 110 and by day 140 the INR was 2.2 with the **warfarin** dose stabilised at the original level.[1]

(b) Venlafaxine

The possible interactions of **warfarin** or other anticoagulants with venlafaxine do not appear to have been studied, but, as of May 2000, the manufacturers had on record 6 case reports of increased prothrombin times, raised INRs and bleeding (haematuria, gastrointestinal bleeding, melaena, haemarthrosis) in patients taking **warfarin** with venlafaxine.[2]

Mechanism

Just why these adverse interactions should have occurred is not understood, especially as no pharmacokinetic interaction is thought likely. Venlafaxine alone may uncommonly cause ecchymosis and mucosal bleeding and, rarely, prolonged bleeding time and haemorrhage.[3] However, given the many other factors that can influence anticoagulant control, the reports of possible interactions could just represent idiosyncratic cases.

Importance and management

No interaction is established, and the general relevance of these unpublished cases is uncertain. If one subscribes to the view that increased monitoring is necessary when any drug is started or stopped in a patient on warfarin or related drugs, then it would be prudent to monitor prothrombin times with venlafaxine. More study is needed.

1. Glueck CJ, Khalil Q, Winiarska M, Wang P. Interaction of duloxetine and warfarin causing severe elevation of international normalized ratio. *JAMA* (2006) 295, 1517–18.
2. Wyeth Laboratories. Personal communication, May 2000.
3. Efexor (Venlafaxine hydrochloride). Wyeth Pharmaceuticals. UK Summary of product characteristics, May 2006.

Coumarins + Sodium edetate

A man had a reduction in the effects of warfarin, which was attributed to intravenous chelation therapy that included sodium edetate.

Clinical evidence, mechanism, importance and management

A 64-year-old man who had been taking **warfarin** for 3 weeks, with a gradually increasing dose to 25 mg weekly, had an INR decrease from 2.6 to 1.6 the day after he received intravenous chelation therapy with sodium edetate. He was given a single 10-mg dose of **warfarin** that day, then continued on his 25 mg weekly dose, with an INR in the range of 2.3 to 2.8. The chelation therapy also contained high-dose vitamin C along with various other vitamins and electrolytes.[1]

Whether this case represents an interaction with the chelation therapy is uncertain. Further study is needed.

1. Grebe HB, Gregory PJ. Inhibition of warfarin anticoagulation associated with chelation therapy. *Pharmacotherapy* (2002) 22, 1067–69.

Coumarins and related drugs + SSRIs

In a study, warfarin plasma levels were increased by 65% by fluvoxamine, and raised INRs have been seen in several cases. In another study with warfarin and paroxetine, the majority of patients experienced no interaction, but a few had minor bleeding events. Other studies suggest that citalopram and sertraline do not significantly alter the pharmacokinetics or effects of warfarin. However, isolated reports describe bleeding in patients taking SSRIs and coumarins or fluindione, and SSRIs alone have, rarely, been associated with bleeding.

Clinical evidence

(a) Citalopram

In a study in 12 healthy subjects given a single 25-mg oral dose of **warfarin** either alone or on day 15 of a 21-day course of citalopram 40 mg daily, the pharmacokinetics of both ***R***- and ***S*-warfarin** remained unchanged in the presence of the citalopram, but the maximum prothrombin time was increased by 6.4% (1.6 seconds). This was considered to be clinically irrelevant.[1]

Nevertheless, a 63-year-old patient who had just started **acenocoumarol** 18 mg per week developed spontaneous gingival haemorrhage 10 days after also starting citalopram 20 mg daily for depression. Her INR had increased from a value of 1.8 to greater than 15. She was treated with 2 units of blood and citalopram was withdrawn. Her INR decreased to 1.95 within 5 days and she was able to continue on **acenocoumarol** 18 mg per week.[2]

(b) Escitalopram

Escitalopram is the *S*-isomer of citalopram, and as such would not be expected to interact pharmacokinetically with **warfarin**, see above.

(c) Fluoxetine

In a study in 3 healthy subjects, the half-life of a single 20-mg dose of **warfarin** was not altered by either a single 30-mg dose of fluoxetine given 3 hours before the **warfarin**, or by fluoxetine 30 mg daily for a week with the **warfarin** dose given 3 hours after the last dose of fluoxetine. In addition, fluoxetine had no effect on the warfarin-induced prolongation of prothrombin time.[3] In another study, 6 patients stabilised on **warfarin** had no significant changes in their prothrombin times or INRs while taking fluoxetine 20 mg daily for 21 days. The maximum change was a decrease in prothrombin time of 3.5% (15%) in one patient.[4]

However, there are few reports of increases in INR in patients taking **warfarin** with fluoxetine. In one report, the INR of a man stabilised on **warfarin**, amiodarone, furosemide, digoxin, ciprofloxacin and levothyroxine rose sharply from a range of 1.8 to 2.3 up to 14.9 within 5 days of starting fluoxetine 30 mg daily.[5] The INR of another man with metastatic carcinoma taking **warfarin**, dexamethasone, bisacodyl and lactulose rose from a range of 2.5 to 3.5 up to 15.5 within 2 weeks of starting fluoxetine 20 mg daily. He showed microscopic haematuria but no bleeding.[5] Other reports describe an abdominal haematoma,[5] cerebral haemorrhage,[6] severe bruising[7] and increases in INRs[8] in patients taking fluoxetine and **warfarin**. In 1993, the CSM in the UK was also said to have 4 other similar cases on record.[8] In the preliminary report of one retrospective review of patients records, all of 8 evaluable cases of concurrent use of fluoxetine and **warfarin** had an abnormally prolonged prothrombin time.[9]

Bowel haemorrhage has been reported in a patient taking **warfarin**, fluoxetine and mefenamic acid,[10] but it is likely that mefenamic acid was the contributing factor in this case.[11]

Conversely, in a case-control study in patients stabilised on **warfarin**, the increase in risk of hospitalisation for an upper gastrointestinal bleed after starting either fluvoxamine or fluoxetine was higher than for other SSRIs (relative risk 1.2) but this did not reach statistical significance (95% confidence interval 0.9 to 1.6).[12] Note that these drugs were considered separately, and the number taking each individual SSRI was not stated.

(d) Fluvoxamine

In a study in healthy subjects, fluvoxamine 50 mg three times daily for 12 days increased steady-state plasma **warfarin** levels by about 65% and increased prothrombin times by 27.8%.[13,14] A worldwide literature search by the manufacturers of fluvoxamine identified only 11 reported interactions between **warfarin** and fluvoxamine by 1995, all with clinical signs that included prolonged prothrombin times.[15] An 80-year-old woman who had recently started taking **warfarin**, digoxin and 'colchicine', (p.397), had an increase in her INR from 1.8 to about 10 within a week of starting to take fluvoxamine 25 mg daily. Both the **warfarin** and fluvoxamine were stopped, but her INR only stabilised on the original dose of **warfarin** after the colchicine was withdrawn.[16] Another report describes a 79-year-old woman admitted to hospital because of suicidal thoughts. She was taking **warfarin** (INR 1.6 to 1.8) and citalopram 10 mg at night and other medications including paracetamol with dextropropoxyphene. On the third day in hospital the citalopram dose was increased to 30 mg at bedtime and after 2 days it was discontinued and fluvoxamine 50 mg daily was started to treat depression and possibly obsessive thoughts. Within 4 days the patient's INR had increased to 3.7. Fluvoxamine was replaced with venlafaxine and **warfarin** was omitted for 1 day. The INR gradually decreased to the normal range over about 7 days.[17]

A further isolated report describes a woman stabilised on **fluindione** whose INR rose to 7.13 (from a normal value of about 2.5) within 13 days of starting to take fluvoxamine 100 mg daily. She had received fluoxetine, dosulepin and lorazepam for 15 days before fluvoxamine was started.[18]

Conversely, in a case-control study in patients stabilised on **warfarin**, the increase in risk of hospitalisation for an upper gastrointestinal bleed after starting either fluvoxamine or fluoxetine was higher than for other SSRIs (relative risk 1.2) but this did not reach statistical significance (95% confidence interval 0.9 to 1.6).[12] Note that these drugs were not considered separately, and the number given each individual SSRI was not stated.

(e) Paroxetine

Paroxetine 30 mg daily, given to healthy subjects with **warfarin** 5 mg daily, did not significantly increase mean prothrombin times, but mild, clinically significant bleeding was seen in 5 out of 27 subjects given the combination. Two withdrew from the study because of increased prothrombin times, and another because of haematuria. The pharmacokinetics of the **warfarin** and the paroxetine remained unchanged by concurrent use.[19] In a brief retrospective review, 4 patients taking **warfarin** were said to have had an increase in INR by an average of 3 points (increases of nearly 100% in some cases) associated with the use of paroxetine and sertraline.[20]

A single case report[21] describes severe bleeding (abdominal haematoma) in a patient taking **acenocoumarol** and paroxetine when given phenytoin, but it is by no means clear whether the paroxetine had any part to play in what happened (see 'Phenytoin + Coumarins and related drugs', p.555).

(f) Sertraline

In a placebo-controlled study in healthy subjects, sertraline, in increasing doses up to 200 mg daily for 22 days, increased the prothrombin time AUC in response to a single 0.75-mg/kg dose of **warfarin** by 7.9%. This was statistically significant, but regarded as too small to be clinically relevant.[22]

In a brief retrospective review, 4 patients taking **warfarin** were said to have had an increase in INR by an average of 3 points (increases of nearly 100% in some cases) associated with the use of paroxetine and sertraline.[20]

Mechanism

Pharmacokinetic interactions. Fluvoxamine is a moderate inhibitor of the cytochrome P450 isoenzyme CYP2C9, by which *S*-warfarin is metabolised, and is also a potent inhibitor of CYP1A2 and CYP2C19, by which the less active *R*-warfarin is metabolised Consequently, fluvoxamine would be expected to increase warfarin effects. *In vitro,* fluoxetine, paroxetine, sertraline, and citalopram had little or no inhibitory effect on CYP2C9 mediated *S*-warfarin hydroxylation.[23] In addition, these SSRIs do not inhibit CYP1A2 or

Table 12.6 Summary of pharmacological studies of the effect of statins on warfarin

Study type	*Group*	*Warfarin*	*Statin dose*	*Findings*		*Refs*
				Pharmacokinetics	Anticoagulant effects	
Atorvastatin						
Prospective	12 patients	Stable therapy	80 mg daily for 14 days	NR	Prothrombin time decreased from 18.6 to 17 seconds on days 3 to 5, but was not changed on other days	1
Fluvastatin						
Placebo-controlled	Healthy subjects	Single 30-mg dose	40 mg daily for 8 days	No change in racemic warfarin levels	No change in prothrombin complex activity	2
Crossover	18 Healthy subjects	Single 10-mg dose	40 mg twice daily for 18 days	Increase in AUC of *S*-warfarin of 42% in smokers and 26% in non-smokers	NR	3
Lovastatin						
NR	Patients	Stable therapy	NR	NR	No change in prothrombin time	4
Crossover, placebo-controlled	8 patients	Stable therapy	40 mg daily for 7 days	NR	INR increased from 2.6 to 3 (17%) by day 7	5
Pravastatin						
Prospective	Healthy subjects	5 mg daily	20 mg twice daily	17% increase in warfarin AUC*	No change in prothrombin time on concurrent use for 6 days	6
Crossover, placebo-controlled	8 patients	Stable therapy	20 mg daily for 7 days	NR	No change in INR over the 7 days	5
NR	Elderly healthy subjects	Stable therapy	40 mg	NR	No change in prothrombin time	14
Rosuvastatin						
Placebo-controlled, crossover	18 healthy subjects	Single 25-mg dose	40 mg daily for 10 days	No change in pharmacokinetics of *S*- or *R*-warfarin	INR AUC increased by 10%, and maximum INR increased by 19%	7
Prospective	7 patients	Stable therapy	10 mg daily for up to 14 days then 80 mg daily for up to 14 days	NR	With 10 mg daily, 2 patients had INR increases of 1.5 and 3.7 to values greater than 4. With 80 mg daily, 4 of 5 patients had increases of 1.5 to 2.6 to values greater than 4.	7
Placebo-controlled, crossover	12 healthy subjects	5 mg daily for 14 days	40 mg daily for 7 days	NR	No change in steady-state warfarin pharmacodynamics	8
Simvastatin						
Retrospective analysis of a placebo-controlled study	23 patients	NR	20 mg or 40 mg daily	NR	INR increased from a mean of 2.6 to 3.4 in the simvastatin group without changes in warfarin dose, compared with a decrease from 2.6 to 2.4 in the placebo group	9
NR	Healthy subjects	NR	20 mg or 40 mg daily	NR	INR increased from a mean of 1.7 to 1.8	10, 11
Retrospective cohort	46 patients	Stable with no change	Switch from pravastatin to simvastatin	NR	Mean INR increased from 2.42 to 2.74. Eleven patients had a warfarin dose adjustment after the INR change, 7 a decrease and 4 an increase	12
Retrospective	29 patients	Stable therapy	NR	NR	Warfarin dose decreased from a mean of 4.2 mg daily before to 3.8 mg daily after, while INR increased from a mean of 2.5 to 3.15	13

NR = not reported.
*Atributed to warfarin being nearer steady state by the combined phase of this longitudinal study, in which there was no washout between phases, and sequence of phases was pravastatin alone for 3.5 days, warfarin alone for 6 days, and then both drugs for 6 days.

1. Stern R, Abel R, Gibson GL, Besserer J. Atorvastatin does not alter the anticoagulant activity of warfarin. *J Clin Pharmacol* (1997) 37, 1062–4.
2. Lescol (Fluvastatin sodium). Novartis. US Prescribing information, April 2006.
3. Kim MJ, Nafzinger AN, Kashuba AD, Kirchheiner J, Bauer S, Gaedigk A, Bertino JS. Effects of fluvastatin and cigarette smoking on CYP2C9 activity measured using the probe S-warfarin. *Eur J Clin Pharmacol* (2006) 62, 431–6.

Continued

Table 12.6 Summary of pharmacological studies of the effect of statins on warfarin (continued)

4. Mevacor (Lovastatin). Merck & Co., Inc. US Prescribing information, November 2005.
5. O'Rangers EA, Ford M, Hershey A. The effect of HMG-coA reductase inhibitors on the anticoagulant response to warfarin. *Pharmacotherapy* (1994) 14, 349.
6. Light RT, Pan HY, Glaess SR, Bakry D (ER Squibb). A report on the pharmacokinetic and pharmacodynamic interaction of pravastatin and warfarin in healthy male volunteers. Data on file, (Protocol No 27, 201-59), 1988.
7. Simonson SG, Martin PD, Mitchell PD, Lasseter K, Gibson G, Schneck DW. Effect of rosuvastatin on warfarin pharmacodynamics and pharmacokinetics. *J Clin Pharmacol* (2005) 45, 927–34.
8. Jindal D, Tandon M, Sharma S, Pillai KK. Pharmacodynamic evaluation of warfarin and rosuvastatin co-administration in healthy subjects. *Eur J Clin Pharmacol* (2005) 61, 621–25.
9. Keech A, Collins R, MacMahon S, Armitage J, Lawson A, Wallendszus K, Fatemian M, Kearney E, Lyon V, Mindell J, Mount J, Painter R, Parish S, Slavin B, Sleight P, Youngman L, Peto R for the Oxford Cholesterol Study Group. Three-year follow-up of the Oxford cholesterol study: assessment of the efficacy and safety of simvastatin in preparation for a large mortality study. *Eur Heart J* (1994) 15, 255–69.
10. Zocor (Simvastatin). Merck Sharp & Dohme Ltd. UK Summary of product characteristics, December 2005.
11. Zocor (Simvastatin). Merck & Co., Inc. US Prescribing information, August 2005.
12. Lin JC, Ito MK, Stolley SN, Morreale AP, Marcus DB. The effect of converting from pravastatin to simvastatin on the pharmacodynamics of warfarin. *J Clin Pharmacol* (1999) 39, 86–90.
13. Hickmott H, Wynne H, Kamali F. The effect of simvastatin co-medication on warfarin anticoagulation response and dose requirements. *Thromb Haemost* (2003) 89, 949–50.
14. Pravachol (Pravastatin sodium). Bristol-Myers Squibb Co. US Prescribing information, March 2007.

CYP2C19, therefore they would not be anticipated to increase warfarin levels.

Pharmacodynamic interactions. Serotonin release by platelets plays an important role in haemostasis, and epidemiological studies and case reports suggest that SSRIs alone are rarely associated with bleeding events.[24] There is no firm evidence that the risk of bleeding is increased if SSRIs are given with anticoagulants.

Importance and management

A pharmacokinetic interaction between fluvoxamine and warfarin that leads to increased anticoagulant effects is established. Therefore, the response should be monitored when fluvoxamine is first added, being alert for the need to decrease the anticoagulant dosage.

None of the other SSRIs studied (citalopram, fluoxetine, paroxetine) have been shown to alter the pharmacokinetics of warfarin, and neither fluoxetine nor paroxetine increased the prothrombin time. However, citalopram and sertraline caused a less than 10% increase in prothrombin time, and a few patients taking paroxetine with warfarin had bleeds. However, in general, these effects would generally not be expected to be clinically relevant. Nevertheless, because SSRIs alone can rarely cause bleeding, some predict that this may result in additive effects with coumarins and indanediones, and recommend caution with all SSRIs. Note that there are case reports of interactions with warfarin for many of the SSRIs (citalopram, fluoxetine, paroxetine, sertraline).

1. Priskorn M, Sidhu JS, Larsen F, Davis JD, Khan AZ, Rolan PE. Investigation of multiple dose citalopram on the pharmacokinetics and pharmacodynamics of racemic warfarin. *Br J Clin Pharmacol* (1997) 44, 199–202.
2. Borrás-Blasco J, Marco-Garbayo JL, Bosca-Sanleon B, Navarro-Ruiz A. Probable interaction between citalopram and acenocoumarol. *Ann Pharmacother* (2002) 36, 345.
3. Rowe H, Carmichael R, Lemberger L. The effect of fluoxetine on warfarin metabolism in the rat and man. *Life Sci* (1978) 23, 807–12.
4. Ford MA, Anderson ML, Rindone JP, Jaskar DW. Lack of effect of fluoxetine on the hypoprothrombinemic response of warfarin. *J Clin Psychopharmacol* (1997) 17, 110–12.
5. Hanger HC, Thomas F. Fluoxetine and warfarin interactions. *N Z Med J* (1995), 108, 157.
6. Dent LA, Orrock MW. Warfarin-fluoxetine and diazepam-fluoxetine interaction. *Pharmacotherapy* (1997) 17, 170–2.
7. Claire RJ, Servis ME, Cram DL. Potential interaction between warfarin sodium and fluoxetine. *Am J Psychiatry* (1991) 148, 1604.
8. Woolfrey S, Gammack NS, Dewar MS, Brown PJE. Fluoxetine-warfarin interaction. *BMJ* (1993) 307, 241.
9. Wu J-R, Li P-YY, Yang Y-HK. Concurrent use of fluoxetine and warfarin prolongs prothrombin time: a retrospective survey. *Pharmacotherapy* (1997) 17, 1080.
10. Beeley L, Magee P, Hickey FN. *Bulletin of the West Midlands Centre for Adverse Drug Reaction Reporting* (1990) 30, 32.
11. Dista Products Limited. Personal communication, May 1990.
12. Kurdyak PA, Juurlink DN, Kopp A, Herrmann N, Mamdani MM. Antidepressants, warfarin, and the risk of hemorrhage. *J Clin Psychopharmacol* (2005) 25, 561–4.
13. Benfield P, Ward A. Fluvoxamine. A review of its pharmacodynamic and pharmacokinetic properties, and therapeutic efficacy in depressive illness. *Drugs* (1986) 32, 313–34.
14. Solvay. Personal communication, December 2006.
15. Wagner W, Vause EW. Fluvoxamine. A review of global drug-drug interaction data. *Clin Pharmacokinet* (1995) 29 (Suppl 1), 26–32.
16. Yap KB, Low ST. Interaction of fluvoxamine with warfarin in an elderly woman. *Singapore Med J* (1999) 40, 480–2.
17. Limke KK, Shelton AR, Elliott ES. Fluvoxamine interaction with warfarin. *Ann Pharmacother* (2002) 36, 1890–2.
18. Nezelof S, Vandel P, Bonin B. Fluvoxamine interaction with fluindione: a case report. *Therapie* (1997) 52, 608–9.
19. Bannister SJ, Houser VP, Hulse JD, Kisicki JC, Rasmussen JGC. Evaluation of the potential for interactions of paroxetine with diazepam, cimetidine, warfarin, and digoxin. *Acta Psychiatr Scand* (1989) 80 (Suppl 350), 102–6.
20. Askinazi C. SSRI treatment of depression with comorbid cardiac disease. *Am J Psychiatry* (1996) 153, 135–6.
21. Abad-Santos F, Carcas AJ, Capitán CF, Frias J. Case report. Retroperitoneal haematoma in a patient treated with acenocoumarol, phenytoin and paroxetine. *Clin Lab Haematol* (1995) 17, 195–7.
22. Apseloff G, Wilner KD, Gerber N, Tremaine LM. Effect of sertraline on protein binding of warfarin. *Clin Pharmacokinet* (1997) 32 (Suppl 1), 37–42.
23. Hemeryck A, De Vriendt C, Belpaire FM. Inhibition of CYP2C9 by selective serotonin reuptake inhibitors: in vitro studies with tolbutamide and (S)-warfarin using human liver microsomes. *Eur J Clin Pharmacol* (1999) 54, 947–51.
24. Consumers' Association. Do SSRIs cause gastrointestinal bleeding? *Drug Ther Bull* (2004) 42, 17–18.

Coumarins and related drugs + Statins

Studies have suggested that fluvastatin and rosuvastatin can increase warfarin levels and/or effects. Other studies with atorvastatin, lovastatin, pravastatin, and simvastatin suggest that they do not usually significantly alter the effects of warfarin, although cases of bleeding have been seen when these statins were given with coumarins and fluindione.

Clinical evidence

Pharmacological studies of the effect of statins on **warfarin** are summarised in 'Table 12.6', (p.449), and case reports of interactions between statins and coumarins are summarised in 'Table 12.7', (p.451). An early report, from the first 7 months after lovastatin became available in the USA, notes that the manufacturers had received 10 spontaneous reports of bleeding and/or increased prothrombin times in patients taking **warfarin** with lovastatin.[1,2]

An analysis of the use of simvastatin and warfarin found a 12% lower **warfarin** maintenance dose in patients taking simvastatin,[3] and a trend towards a lower dose with lower 10-hydroxywarfarin (a metabolite of ***R*-warfarin**) levels in patients taking simvastatin or lovastatin.[4] However, an early case report described a patient stabilised on **warfarin** with type III hyperlipoproteinaemia who had no changes in her INR over 20 weeks when treated with simvastatin 10 mg daily for 3 weeks then 20 mg daily.[5] At the other extreme, an isolated report[6] describes rhabdomyolysis with acute renal failure in an 82-year-old man taking simvastatin 20 mg daily within 7 days of starting **warfarin** 5 mg daily; his INR was raised to 4.3.

Mechanism

Fluvastatin is a modest inhibitor of the cytochrome P450 isoenzyme CYP2C9, by which the more potent *S*-warfarin is metabolised. Evidence from an interaction study with the CYP2C9 substrate diclofenac suggests that this interaction is most likely with higher and sustained fluvastatin levels,[7] which might explain why, with warfarin, it was demonstrated in healthy subjects with the maximum recommended daily dose of 80 mg daily, but not the usual clinical dose of 40 mg daily, and why it has not been seen in all patients. Lovastatin and simvastatin appear less likely to interact via CYP2C9,[8] although it is possible they might interact via other

Table 12.7 Summary of the case reports of interactions between statins and coumarins

Year of study	*Patient*	*Coumarin*	*Statin dose (duration before event)*	*INR or PT* before*	*INR or PT after*	*Bleeding complications*	*Longer-term management*	*Refs*
Fluvastatin								
1996	68-year-old	Warfarin	20 mg daily (6 weeks)	3	4.8	None	Warfarin dose decreased by 14%	1
			40 mg daily (2 months)	2.9	3.81	None	Warfarin dose decreased by 12.5%	
	61-year-old	Warfarin	20 mg daily (4 weeks**)	2.29	3.54	None	Warfarin dose decreased by 10%	
	71-year-old	Warfarin	20 mg daily (3 weeks**)	2.92	4.45	None	Warfarin dose decreased by 14%	
1997	68-year-old	Warfarin	20 mg daily (2 weeks)	2.11 to 2.99	4.17	None	Warfarin dose decreased by 18%, then increased back again on withdrawal of fluvastatin	2
	83-year-old	Warfarin	20 mg daily (1 week)	1.84 to 2.73	3.47	None	Warfarin dose decreased by 36%, then increased back again on withdrawal of fluvastatin	
	51-year-old	Warfarin	20 mg daily (1 week)	1.95 to 3.4	4.2	Minor rectal bleeding	Warfarin dose decreased by 13%	
2004	67-year-old	Warfarin	80 mg daily (5 weeks†)	2 to 3	6.6	None	Fluvastatin switched back to atorvastatin, and warfarin restablised at a 14% lower dose	3
Lovastatin								
1990	48-year-old	Warfarin	20 mg daily (3 weeks)	PT 18 to 24 seconds	PT 48 seconds	Minor rectal bleeding	Warfarin dose decreased by 60%	4
	58-year-old	Warfarin	20 mg daily (10 days)	PT 19 to 22 seconds	PT 42 seconds	Epistaxis and haematuria	Warfarin dose decreased by 60%	
1992	85-year-old	Warfarin	20 mg daily (2 weeks)	PT 15 to 17 seconds	PT 24 seconds	None	Lovastatin discontinued	5
1995	78-year-old	Warfarin	40 mg daily (2 months)	1.9 to 3.1	12.3	Gross haematuria, haematoma	Lovastatin discontinued	6
Pravastatin								
1996	64-year-old	Fluindione‡	10 mg daily (5 days)	2.5 to 3.5	10.2	Haematuria	Not reported	7
Rosuvastatin								
2004	74-year-old	Warfarin	Not reported (4 weeks)	2	8	Bruising, haematuria	Not reported	8
2005	36-year-old	Acenocoumarol	10 mg daily (about 45 days)	2 to 3	5.8	Haematoma	Rosuvastatin discontinued	9
Simvastatin								
1996	70-year-old	Acenocoumarol	20 mg daily (3 weeks)	2 to 3.5	9	Not reported	Simvastatin discontinued	10

*Prothrombin time
**Switched from lovastatin
†Switched from atorvastatin
‡Note that this is an indanedione

1. Trilli LE, Kelley CL, Aspinall SL, Kroner BA. Potential interaction between warfarin and fluvastatin. *Ann Pharmacother* (1996) 30, 1399–1402.
2. Kline SS, Harrell CC. Potential warfarin-fluvastatin interaction. *Ann Pharmacother* (1997) 31, 790.
3. Andrus MR. Oral anticoagulant drug interactions with statins: case report of fluvastatin and review of the literature. *Pharmacotherapy* (2004) 24, 285–90.
4. Ahmad S. Lovastatin. Warfarin interaction. *Arch Intern Med* (1990) 150, 2407.
5. Hoffman HS. The interaction of lovastatin and warfarin. *Conn Med* (1992) 56, 107.
6. Iliadis EA, Konwinski MF. Lovastatin during warfarin therapy resulting in bleeding. *PA Medicine* (1995) 98, 31.
7. Trenque T, Choisy H, Germain M-L. Pravastatin: interaction with oral anticoagulant? *BMJ* (1996) 312, 886.
8. Barry M. Rosuvastatin–warfarin drug interaction. *Lancet* (2004) 363, 328.
9. Mondillo S, Ballo P, Galderisi M. Rosuvastatin–acenocoumarol interaction. *Clin Ther* (2005) 27, 782–4.
10. Grau E, Perella M, Pastor E. Simvastatin-oral anticoagulant interaction. *Lancet* (1996) 347, 405–6.

isoenzymes. It may be that because warfarin has multiple routes of metabolism that other isoenzymes can 'pick up' warfarin metabolism if competition for metabolism occurs. Interactions may therefore only occur if other confounding factors are present. Rosuvastatin clearly shows a dose related increase in warfarin effects, but this was not due to an increase in *R*- or *S*-warfarin levels, and the mechanism for this effect is currently unknown.[9]

Importance and management

Data are limited, which is surprising given the widespread use of statins and warfarin, and are sometimes contradictory, all of which complicates making firm recommendations. Recent evidence suggests that a modest pharmacokinetic interaction occurs between **fluvastatin** and warfarin at high doses, and this would explain the case reports of an interaction with this statin. The clinical evidence suggests that only some patients develop an important interaction (3 of 25 evaluable patients in one analysis). In the UK, the manufacturer states that concurrent use of fluvastatin and warfarin may commonly cause significant increases in prothrombin time.[10] Clearly, with **fluvastatin**, increased monitoring is required when starting or stopping the statin, or changing the dose. Similar advice also applies to **rosuvastatin**, which has the best pharmacological data on concurrent use in patients, clearly showing that clinically important increases in INR can occur. In contrast to fluvastatin, this interaction does not appear to have a pharmacokinetic basis.

Data for **simvastatin** appear to be limited to retrospective analyses. In general these show that simvastatin can cause a minor increase in warfarin effects. This would appear to be supported by the fact that there is only one full published report of an interaction in a patient taking acenocoumarol. Some consider that any interaction is of limited clinical importance, and that statin therapy may be switched to simvastatin without any additional monitoring over and above that usually practised for warfarin therapy.[11] However, others,[12] including the manufacturer[13,14] recommend increased monitoring when starting or stopping the statin, or changing the dose, and this may be prudent. There are even less data for **lovastatin**, an analogue of simvastatin, but it appears to interact similarly to simvastatin, and the manufacturer also recommends increased monitoring.[15] There appear to be no data on the effect of lovastatin or simvastatin on the pharmacokinetics of coumarins.

In one pharmacological study, **atorvastatin** did not interact with warfarin, and no cases of an interaction have been published. This suggests that with this statin, no increased monitoring is necessary. In the US, the manufacturer does not give any advice on monitoring,[16] but in the UK, the manufacturer does recommend close monitoring,[17] which seems over-cautious. Limited data for **pravastatin** also suggest that no interaction occurs with warfarin, although there is one isolated case report with the indanedione fluindione. No increased monitoring would appear to be necessary on concurrent use.

1. Tobert JA, Shear CL, Chremos AN, Mantell GE. Clinical experience with lovastatin. *Am J Cardiol* (1990) 65, 23F–26F.
2. Tobert JA. Efficacy and long-term adverse effect pattern of lovastatin. *Am J Cardiol* (1988) 62, 28J–34J.
3. Gage BF, Eby C, Milligan PE, Banet GA, Duncan JR, McLeod HL. Use of pharmacogenetics and clinical factors to predict the maintenance dose of warfarin. *Thromb Haemost* (2004) 91, 87–94.
4. Herman D, Locatelli I, Grabnar I, Peternel P, Stegnar M, Lainščak M, Mrhar A, Breskvar K, Dolžan V. The influence of co-treatment with carbamazepine, amiodarone and statins on warfarin metabolism and maintenance dose. *Eur J Clin Pharmacol* (2006) 62, 291–6.
5. Gaw A, Wosornu D. Simvastatin during warfarin therapy in hyperlipoproteinaemia. *Lancet* (1992) 340, 979–80.
6. Mogyorósi A, Bradley B, Showalter A, Schubert ML. Rhabdomyolysis and acute renal failure due to combination therapy with simvastatin and warfarin. *J Intern Med* (1999) 246, 599–602.
7. Transon C, Leemann T, Vogt N, Dayer P. In vivo inhibition profile of cytochrome P450TB (CYP2C9) by (±)-fluvastatin. *Clin Pharmacol Ther* (1995) 58, 412–17.
8. Transon C, Leemann T, Dayer P. In vitro comparative inhibition profiles of major human drug metabolising cytochrome P450 isozymes (CYP2C9, CYP2D6 and CYP3A4) by HMG-CoA reductase inhibitors. *Eur J Clin Pharmacol* (1996) 50, 209–15.
9. Simonson SG, Martin PD, Mitchell PD, Lasseter K, Gibson G, Schneck DW. Effect of rosuvastatin on warfarin pharmacodynamics and pharmacokinetics. *J Clin Pharmacol* (2005) 45, 927–34.
10. Lescol (Fluvastatin sodium). Novartis Pharmaceuticals UK Ltd. UK Summary of product characteristics, October 2006.
11. Lin JC, Ito MK, Stolley SN, Morreale AP, Marcus DB. The effect of converting from pravastatin to simvastatin on the pharmacodynamics of warfarin. *J Clin Pharmacol* (1999) 39, 86–90.
12. Hickmott H, Wynne H, Kamali F. The effect of simvastatin co-medication on warfarin anticoagulation response and dose requirements. *Thromb Haemost* (2003) 89, 949–50.
13. Zocor (Simvastatin). Merck Sharp & Dohme Ltd. UK Summary of product characteristics, December 2005.
14. Zocor (Simvastatin). Merck & Co., Inc. US Prescribing information, May 2007.
15. Mevacor (Lovastatin). Merck & Co., Inc. US Prescribing information, May 2007.
16. Lipitor (Atorvastatin calcium). Pfizer Inc. US Prescribing information, March 2007.
17. Lipitor (Atorvastatin). Pfizer Ltd. UK Summary of product characteristics, September 2006.

Coumarins + Sucralfate

The simultaneous administration of warfarin and sucralfate did not alter the anticoagulant effect of warfarin in studies in patients on stable therapy. However, case reports describe a marked reduction in the effects of warfarin in four patients taking sucralfate.

Clinical evidence

In an open, crossover study in 8 elderly patients taking **warfarin**, their anticoagulant response (thromboplastin time) and plasma **warfarin** levels remained unchanged while taking sucralfate 1 g three times a day over a 2-week period.[1] Similarly, in a preliminary report of another study, sucralfate 1 g four times daily for 2 weeks had no effect on prothrombin time or plasma **warfarin** levels in 5 patients on stable **warfarin** therapy.[2] In both these studies, the daily **warfarin** dose was taken simultaneously with one of the sucralfate doses.[1,2]

However, there are four case reports of reduced **warfarin** effects with sucralfate. In one of these, a man taking several drugs (digoxin, furosemide, chlorpropamide, potassium chloride) had serum **warfarin** levels that were about two-thirds lower when he was given sucralfate (dose not stated). When the sucralfate was withdrawn, his serum **warfarin** levels rose to their former levels accompanied by a prolongation of prothrombin times.[3] Another patient taking sucralfate had subtherapeutic prothrombin times on starting **warfarin**, despite **warfarin** doses of up to 17.5 mg daily. When the sucralfate was stopped his prothrombin time rose to 1.5 times the control, even though the **warfarin** dose was reduced to 10 mg daily.[4] One other patient appeared to have reduced responses to **warfarin** while taking sucralfate, despite separation of administration.[5] However, another patient taking **warfarin** and sucralfate had a reduced response to **warfarin** only when it was taken simultaneously with sucralfate, but not when administration was separated.[6]

Mechanism

Unknown. It is suggested that the sucralfate may possibly adsorb the warfarin so that its bioavailability is reduced.[4]

Importance and management

The documentation appears to be limited to the reports cited. Any interaction would therefore seem to be uncommon. Concurrent use need not be avoided, but bear this interaction in mind if a patient has a reduced anticoagulant response to warfarin.

1. Neuvonen PJ, Jaakkola A, Tötterman J, Penttilä O. Clinically significant sucralfate-warfarin interaction is not likely. *Br J Clin Pharmacol* (1985) 20, 178–80.
2. Talbert RL, Dalmady-Israel C, Bussey HI, Crawford MH, Ludden TM. Effect of sucralfate on plasma warfarin concentration in patients requiring chronic warfarin therapy. *Drug Intell Clin Pharm* (1985) 19, 456–7.
3. Mungall D, Talbert RL, Phillips C, Jaffe D, Ludden TM. Sucralfate and warfarin. *Ann Intern Med* (1983) 98, 557.
4. Braverman SE, Marino MT. Sucralfate-warfarin interaction. *Drug Intell Clin Pharm* (1988) 22, 913.
5. Rey AM, Gums JG. Altered absorption of digoxin, sustained-release quinidine, and warfarin with sucralfate absorption. *DICP Ann Pharmacother* (1991) 25, 745–6.
6. Parrish RH, Waller B, Gondalia BG. Sucralfate-warfarin interaction. *Ann Pharmacother* (1992) 26, 1015–16.

Coumarins + Sucrose polyesters

Short-term, moderate consumption of potato crisps containing sucrose polyesters (*Olestra, Olean*), which include vitamin K_1, did not alter the INR is response to warfarin.

Clinical evidence

In a randomised, double-blind, placebo-controlled study in 36 patients stabilised on **warfarin**, sucrose polyester 12 g daily (as *Pringles Original Flavor Fat Free Potato Crisps with Olean* 42 g) for one week did not significantly alter the anticoagulant effects of **warfarin** (mean INR increase of 0.02, versus 0.17 for placebo). After one week, greater than expected numbers of patients from both the placebo and sucrose polyester groups had INRs outside the therapeutic range of 2 to 3 (3 sucrose polyester recipients and 3 placebo recipients had an INR above 3 (max 4.1) and 2 in the sucrose polyester group and one in the placebo group had an INR less than 2). Two of each group also withdrew because of diarrhoea: their INRs were therapeutic. Only 22 patients entered the second week of the study, and there was no important effect on INR in these patients after the second week.[1]

Mechanism

Sucrose polyesters are non-absorbable, non-calorific fat replacements. It has been concluded that sucrose polyesters are unlikely to reduce the absorption of oral drugs in general, however, they are known to reduce the absorption of some fat-soluble vitamins, and therefore might lower vitamin K stores.[2] Because of this, snacks containing *Olestra* are supplemented with vitamin K_1 at a level of 8 micrograms per gram of *Olestra*.[3] It is possible that this supplementation could be insufficient to offset the vitamin K-lowering effect and increase patient sensitivity to warfarin, or it could be too much and result in an antagonism of warfarin.

Importance and management

No evidence was found in the above study to suggest that short-term moderate consumption of a snack containing sucrose polyesters (12 g daily, including 96 micrograms of vitamin K daily) altered the anticoagulant effect of warfarin. In 1996, the US FDA considered that the changes in dietary vitamin K intake attributable to eating vitamin-K compensated *Olestra* would likely be within the normal range of dietary variation.[3] However, an intake similar to this of a 'vitamin K_1 supplement', (p.401) has altered coagulation status in some subjects, and pure vitamin K_1 is much more bioavailable than that from 'plant sources', (p.409). Some consider that the snacks may have an impact on serum vitamin K levels.[4] Given these concerns, further study is probably needed.

1. Beckey NP, Korman LB, Parra D. Effect of the moderate consumption of olestra in patients receiving long-term warfarin therapy. *Pharmacotherapy* (1999) 19, 1075–9.
2. Goldman P. Olestra: assessing its potential to interact with drugs in the gastrointestinal tract. *Clin Pharmacol Ther* (1997) 61, 613–18.
3. Department of Health and Human Services. Food and Drug Administration. Food additives permitted for direct addition to food for human consumption; Olestra. *Fed Regist* (1996) 61, 3118–73.
4. Harrell CC, Kline SS. Vitamin K–supplemented snacks containing olestra: implication for patients taking warfarin. *JAMA* (1999), 282, 1133–4.

Coumarins + Sulfinpyrazone

The anticoagulant effects of warfarin are markedly increased by sulfinpyrazone, and there are case reports of moderate to serious bleeding on concurrent use. Acenocoumarol is modestly affected. Phenprocoumon does not appear to be significantly affected. Bear in mind that the antiplatelet effects of sulfinpyrazone might increase the risk of bleeding with coumarins.

Clinical evidence

(a) Acenocoumarol

In a placebo-controlled, crossover study in 22 patients taking acenocoumarol, sulfinpyrazone 800 mg daily for 2 weeks led to a drop in the mean prothrombin time requiring a reduction in anticoagulant dosage by an average of 20%. Four patients withdrew because of bleeding episodes, 3 while taking sulfinpyrazone and one while taking placebo.[1]

(b) Phenprocoumon

In a study in 6 healthy subjects, sulfinpyrazone 400 mg daily for 17 days had little effect on phenprocoumon levels after a single 0.6-mg/kg dose of phenprocoumon given on day 4. The AUC of prothrombin time increased in 4 subjects and decreased in 2, for an overall non-significant mean increase of 16%.[2] Similar findings were reported in another study of similar design.[3]

(c) Warfarin

In a double-blind, placebo-controlled study in 11 patients stabilised on warfarin, sulfinpyrazone 200 mg four times daily for 6 to 12 months reduced the average warfarin dose requirement by 44% from 7.3 to 4.1 mg week, compared with no change in the placebo group. There were 4 episodes of bleeding (haematoma, epistaxes and bleeding gums) in 3 patients receiving sulfinpyrazone and one in the placebo group. The authors noted it was difficult to regulate anticoagulant control in the patients taking sulfinpyrazone.[4,5] Similarly, in another study, the prothrombin ratios of 5 patients taking warfarin rose rapidly over 2 to 3 days after sulfinpyrazone 200 mg every 6 hours was added. The average warfarin requirements fell by 46% and 2 patients needed vitamin K to combat the excessive hypoprothrombinaemia. When the sulfinpyrazone was withdrawn, the warfarin requirements returned to their former levels within 1 to 2 weeks.[6]

A number of case reports have described increased effects of warfarin in patients starting sulfinpyrazone,[7-12] or an exaggerated anticoagulant response in patients taking sulfinpyrazone and then starting warfarin.[13] This interaction has been described in numerous studies and case reports in those taking warfarin.[4,5,7-14] Moderate to severe bleeding occurred in some instances.[8,10,11] An increased anticoagulant effect of warfarin in the first 15 days after starting sulfinpyrazone, followed by an unexplained progressive increased warfarin dose requirement has been described in one report.[14] However, this may have had other explanations, since a constant potentiation of warfarin is usually seen on long-term sulfinpyrazone use.[5]

In subsequent studies in healthy subjects, sulfinpyrazone 200 mg twice daily for 10 days was shown to augment the effect of warfarin (99% or 83% increase in the AUC of the prothrombin time) by inhibiting the clearance of *S*-warfarin (by 51% or 40%) when a single dose of warfarin was given on day 4. In contrast, sulfinpyrazone did not alter the effect of *R*-warfarin, and actually increased its clearance by 30% or 42%.[15,16]

Mechanism

Sulfinpyrazone inhibits the metabolism of the more potent *S*-isomer of warfarin, probably because its sulfide metabolite inhibits the cytochrome P450 isoenzyme CYP2C9.[17] It probably interacts by a similar mechanism with acenocoumarol. It could be speculated that sulfinpyrazone induces the metabolism of *R*-warfarin via CYP1A2, since it modestly induces the metabolism of 'theophylline', (p.1199). Some early *in vitro* evidence[18] suggested that plasma protein binding displacement might explain this interaction, but a study in healthy subjects found that sulfinpyrazone did not alter the free fraction of either *R*- or *S*-warfarin.[19] . Sulfinpyrazone also has antiplatelet effects, so might be expected to increase the risk or severity of bleeding should over-anticoagulation occur.

Importance and management

The increased effect of warfarin with sulfinpyrazone is a well established interaction of clinical importance. If sulfinpyrazone is added, the prothrombin time should be well monitored and suitable anticoagulant dosage reductions made. Halving the dosage of warfarin[4,6,20] has proven to be adequate in patients taking sulfinpyrazone 600 to 800 mg daily. The interaction with acenocoumarol[1] is less marked, and a 20% dose reduction appears adequate in patients taking sulfinpyrazone 600 to 800 mg daily. Phenprocoumon is reported not to have a pharmacokinetic interaction with sulfinpyrazone. Bear in mind that the antiplatelet effects of sulfinpyrazone might increase the risk of bleeding with coumarins.

1. Michot F, Holt NF, Fontanilles F. Über die Beeinflussung der gerinnungshemmenden Wirkung von Acenocoumarol durch Sulfinpyrazon. *Schweiz Med Wochenschr* (1981) 111, 255–60.
2. O'Reilly RA. Phenylbutazone and sulphinpyrazone interaction with oral anticoagulant phenprocoumon. *Arch Intern Med* (1982) 142, 1634–7.
3. Heimark LD, Toon S, Gibaldi M, Trager WF, O'Reilly RA, Goulart DA. The effect of sulfinpyrazone on the disposition of pseudoracemic phenprocoumon in humans. *Clin Pharmacol Ther* (1987) 42, 312–19.
4. Girolami A, Fabris F, Casonato A, Randi ML. Potentiation of anticoagulant response to warfarin by sulphinpyrazone: a double-blind study in patients with prosthetic heart valves. *Clin Lab Haematol* (1982) 4, 23–6.
5. Girolami A, Schivazappa L, Fabris F, Randi ML. Biphasic sulphinpyrazone-warfarin interaction. *BMJ* (1981) 283, 1338.
6. Miners JO, Foenander T, Wanwimolruk S, Gallus AS, Birkett DJ. Interaction of sulphinpyrazone with warfarin. *Eur J Clin Pharmacol* (1982) 22, 327–31.
7. Davis JW, Johns LE. Possible interaction of sulfinpyrazone with coumarins. *N Engl J Med* (1978) 299, 955.
8. Mattingly D, Bradley M, Selley PJ. Hazards of sulphinpyrazone. *BMJ* (1978) 2, 1786–9.
9. Weiss M. Potentiation of coumarin effect by sulfinpyrazone. *Lancet* (1979) i, 609.
10. Gallus A, Birkett D. Sulphinpyrazone and warfarin: a probable drug interaction. *Lancet* (1980) i, 535–6.
11. Thompson PL, Serjeant C. Potentially serious interaction of warfarin with sulphinpyrazone. *Med J Aust* (1981) 1, 41.
12. Jamil A, Reid JM, Messer M. Interaction between sulphinpyrazone and warfarin. *Chest* (1981) 79, 375.
13. Bailey RR, Reddy J. Potentiation of warfarin action by sulphinpyrazone. *Lancet* (1980) i, 254.
14. Nenci GG, Agnelli G, Berrettini M. Biphasic sulphinpyrazone-warfarin interaction. *BMJ* (1981) 282, 1361–2.
15. O'Reilly RA. Stereoselective interaction of sulfinpyrazone with racemic warfarin and its separated enantiomorphs in man. *Circulation* (1982) 65, 202–7.
16. Toon S, Low LK, Gibaldi M, Trager WF, O'Reilly RA, Motley CH, Goulart DA. The warfarin-sulfinpyrazone interaction: stereochemical considerations. *Clin Pharmacol Ther* (1986) 39, 15–24.

17. He M, Kunze KL, Trager WF. Inhibition of (*S*)-warfarin metabolism by sulfinpyrazone and its metabolites. *Drug Metab Dispos* (1995) 23, 659–63.
18. Seiler K, Duckert F. Properties of 3-(1-phenyl-propyl)-4-oxycoumarin (Marcoumar®) in the plasma when tested in normal cases and under the influence of drugs. *Thromb Diath Haemorrh* (1968) 19, 389–96.
19. O'Reilly RA, Goulart DA. Comparative interaction of sulfinpyrazone and phenylbutazone with racemic warfarin: alteration *in vivo* of free fraction of plasma albumin. *J Pharmacol Exp Ther* (1981) 219, 691–4.
20. Tulloch JA, Marr TCK. Sulphinpyrazone and warfarin after myocardial infarction. *BMJ* (1979) ii, 133.

Coumarins + Tamoxifen or Toremifene

In one retrospective analysis, 5 patients taking tamoxifen were very sensitive to warfarin, and, in a second, 5 of 22 patients had problems with over-anticoagulation. Case reports also describe over-anticoagulation in three women taking warfarin and one woman taking acenocoumarol when they also took tamoxifen. It has been suggested that a similar interaction may occur with toremifene.

Clinical evidence

A woman who had been taking **warfarin** for 11 years after a heart valve replacement (prothrombin time of 23 to 34 seconds taking **warfarin** 27 to 28.5 mg weekly), was given tamoxifen 10 mg twice daily as adjuvant therapy after mastectomy for early breast cancer. Three days later her prothrombin time was 39 seconds, and 3 weeks later it was 75.6 seconds, although this was attributed to a 5-day course of co-trimoxazole, and so the warfarin dose was unchanged. Six weeks later she developed haematemesis, abdominal pain and haematuria, and her prothrombin time was found to be 206 seconds. She was restabilised on a little over half the **warfarin** dosage (17.5 mg weekly) while continuing to take the tamoxifen.[1] In another case, a 43-year-old woman was given **warfarin** for a deep vein thrombosis. Seven weeks later tamoxifen 40 mg daily was started, and her prothrombin time increased from 19 to 38 seconds. A warfarin dose reduction from 5 to 1 mg daily was eventually needed to keep her prothrombin time within the range of 20 to 25 seconds. A subsequent retrospective study of the records of women with breast cancer who had been admitted to hospital for serious thromboembolism from 1981 to 1986 revealed 5 other patients taking tamoxifen when **warfarin** was started, and 13 patients not taking tamoxifen. Of the 5 taking tamoxifen, 2 had shown marked increases in prothrombin times, and bleeding, shortly after receiving loading doses of **warfarin** (three daily doses of 10 mg, 10 mg and 5 mg). The other 3 needed daily **warfarin** doses of 2 mg, 2 mg and 3 mg, respectively, which were about one-third of those taken by the 13 other patients not on tamoxifen (mean 6.25 mg).[2]

In another retrospective analysis of hospital admissions from 1980 to 1988, 22 patients were identified who had been given tamoxifen with **warfarin**. Of these, 17 had no problems, but 2 developed grossly elevated British Comparative Ratios and 3 haemorrhaged.[3] In 1987, the manufacturers of tamoxifen had one report of this interaction on their files.[1]

A 53-year-old woman who had been taking **acenocoumarol** for 2 years after a heart valve replacement died after a massive brain haemorrhage about 3 weeks after starting to take tamoxifen 20 mg daily for a benign breast condition.[4]

Mechanism

Unknown.Tamoxifen can *increase* the risk of thrombosis, particularly when it is used with 'antineoplastics', (p.616).

Importance and management

Evidence is limited to the above reports, but it appears that a clinically important interaction between tamoxifen and warfarin can occur, which apparently affects some but not all patients. Monitor the effects closely if tamoxifen is added to treatment with warfarin or acenocoumarol and reduce the dosage as necessary. The reports cited here indicate a reduction of between one-half to two-thirds for warfarin. In the US, when tamoxifen is being used for the primary prevention of breast cancer, the manufacturer specifically contraindicates concurrent use with warfarin or other coumarins.[5]

Consider also that, from a disease perspective, when treating venous thromboembolic disease in patients with cancer, warfarin is generally inferior (higher risk of major bleeds and recurrent thrombosis) to low molecular weight heparins.[6]

Because of the data with tamoxifen, the manufacturers of **toremifene** (indicated for hormone-dependent metastatic breast cancer in postmenopausal women) contraindicate the concurrent use of coumarin anticoagulants in the UK,[7] but just recommend careful monitoring of prothrombin time in the US.[8] However, there appear to be no published reports of any interaction between **toremifene** and warfarin.

1. Lodwick R, McConkey B, Brown AM, Beeley L. Life threatening interaction between tamoxifen and warfarin. *BMJ* (1987) 295, 1141.
2. Tenni P, Lalich DL, Byrne MJ. Life threatening interaction between tamoxifen and warfarin. *BMJ* (1989) 298, 93.
3. Ritchie LD, Grant SMT. Tamoxifen-warfarin interaction: the Aberdeen hospitals drug file. *BMJ* (1989) 298, 1253.
4. Gustovic P, Baldin B, Tricoire MJ, Chichmanian RM. Interaction tamoxifène-acénocoumarol. Une interaction potentiellement dangereuse. *Therapie* (1994) 49, 55–6.
5. Nolvadex (Tamoxifen). AstraZeneca Pharmaceuticals. US Prescribing information, March 2006.
6. Baglin TP, Keeling DM, Watson HG, for the British Committee for Standards in Haematology. Guidelines on oral anticoagulation (warfarin): third edition – 2005 update. *Br J Haematol* (2005) 132, 277–85.
7. Fareston (Toremifene citrate). Orion Pharma UK Ltd. UK Summary of product characteristics, February 2006.
8. Fareston (Toremifene citrate). GTx, Inc. US Prescribing information, December 2004.

Coumarins + Terbinafine

Terbinafine did not interact with warfarin in a study in healthy subjects, and patients have received the combination without apparent problems. However, two isolated cases describe reduced and increased anticoagulation, respectively. A cohort study found no increased risk of over-anticoagulation when acenocoumarol or phenprocoumon were given with terbinafine.

Clinical evidence

In a randomised, placebo-controlled, double-blind study in 16 healthy subjects, terbinafine 250 mg daily for 14 days did not alter the pharmacokinetics or anticoagulant effects of a single 30-mg oral dose of **warfarin** given on day 8.[1] In a post-marketing surveillance study of terbinafine, 26 patients were identified who were also taking **warfarin** and there was no evidence to suggest an interaction in these patients.[2,3] In one cohort study in patients taking **acenocoumarol** or **phenprocoumon**, the concurrent use of oral terbinafine (n=49) or cutaneous terbinafine (n=29) was not associated with an increased risk of over-anticoagulation (INR greater than 6).[4] However, an isolated report describes a 68-year-old woman taking long-term **warfarin** whose INR fell from 2.1 to 1.1 within a month of starting a 3-month course of terbinafine 250 mg daily for tinea unguium. It was necessary to raise her **warfarin** dosage from 5.5 mg daily to a range of 7.5 to 8 mg daily while taking the terbinafine, and to reduce it stepwise to 5.5 mg over the 4 weeks after the terbinafine was stopped.[5] In contrast, another isolated case report describes an elderly woman stabilised on **warfarin** and cimetidine who developed gastrointestinal bleeding about a month after starting to take terbinafine 250 mg daily.[6]

Mechanism

The isolated cases are not understood, and have been questioned.[7]

Importance and management

Normally no interaction occurs between coumarins and terbinafine, while the two isolated cases cited are rarities, and unexplained. There appears therefore to be no reason for avoiding concurrent use, but bear these cases in mind if terbinafine is given to patients taking warfarin.

1. Guerret M, Francheteau P, Hubert M. Evaluation of effects of terbinafine on single oral dose pharmacokinetics and anticoagulant actions of warfarin in healthy volunteers. *Pharmacotherapy* (1997) 17, 767–73.
2. O'Sullivan DP, Needham CA, Bangs A, Atkin K, Kendall FD. Postmarketing surveillance of oral terbinafine in the UK; report of a large cohort study. *Br J Pharmacol* (1996) 42, 559–65.
3. Novartis. Personal communication, February 1998.
4. Visser LE, Penning-van Beest FJA, Kasbergen AAH, De Smet PAGM, Vulto AG, Hofman A, Stricker BHC. Overanticoagulation associated with combined use of antifungal agents and coumarin anticoagulants. *Clin Pharmacol Ther* (2002) 71, 496–502.
5. Warwick JA, Corrall RJ. Serious interaction between warfarin and oral terbinafine. *BMJ* (1998) 316, 440.
6. Gupta AK, Ross GS. Interaction between terbinafine and warfarin. *Dermatology* (1998) 196, 266–7.
7. Gantmacher J, Mills-Bomford J, Williams T. Interaction between warfarin and oral terbinafine. *BMJ* (1998) 317, 205.

Coumarins + Tetracyclic and related antidepressants

In one study mirtazapine caused a slight increase in INR in subjects given warfarin. In studies in patients, maprotiline did not alter the anticoagulant effect of acenocoumarol, and mianserin did not alter the anticoagulant effect of phenprocoumon. In isolated case reports, an increased effect of warfarin and a decreased effect of acenocoumarol was seen when mianserin was given.

Clinical evidence

(a) Maprotiline

The anticoagulant effects of **acenocoumarol** were not affected by maprotiline 50 mg three times daily for 2 weeks in 20 patients stabilised on **acenocoumarol**.[1]

(b) Mianserin

In a randomised, double-blind study in 60 patients taking **phenprocoumon** for 5 weeks, there was no difference in anticoagulant control and **phenprocoumon** dose between placebo recipients and those receiving either mianserin up to 30 mg daily or up to 60 mg daily for 20 days.[2]

A single case report describes a man stabilised on **warfarin** whose British standard ratio rose from 1.8 to 4.6 (prothrombin time rise from 20 to 25 seconds) after taking mianserin 10 mg daily for 7 days.[3] However, another patient taking **warfarin** received mianserin in doses varying between 0 and 120 mg daily for 22 weeks without any change in prothrombin ratio.[4] A further patient stabilised on **acenocoumarol** and amiodarone needed an *increase* in his **acenocoumarol** dosage after starting mianserin, and a decrease when this drug was stopped.[5]

(c) Mirtazapine

In a study in healthy subjects stabilised on individual doses of **warfarin**,[6] mirtazapine 15 mg for 2 days then 30 mg daily for 5 days increased the mean INR from 1.6 to 1.8. This small increase was not considered clinically relevant by the authors of the study or one of the UK manufacturers.[6,7] One UK manufacturer comments that a more pronounced effect cannot be excluded at higher doses of mirtazapine.[8] However, there do not appear to be any published reports of interactions.

Mechanism

Not understood.

Importance and management

Maprotiline does not interact with acenocoumarol and mianserin does not interact with phenprocoumon. The isolated cases of an increase in warfarin effects and a decrease in acenocoumarol effects with mianserin are unexplained, and probably of little general relevance. One UK manufacturer of mirtazapine very cautiously advises that the prothrombin time should be controlled if mirtazapine is given with warfarin.[8] However, there do not appear to be any reports of problems with this combination, and another manufacturer does not consider monitoring to be necessary.[7]

1. Michot F, Glaus K, Jack DB, Theobald W. Antikoagulatorische Wirkung von Sintrom® und Konzentration von Ludiomil® im Blut bei gleichzeitiger Verabreichung beider Präparate. *Med Klin* (1975) 70, 626–9.
2. Kopera H, Schenk H, Stulemeijer S. Phenprocoumon requirement, whole blood coagulation time, bleeding time and plasma γ-GT in patients receiving mianserin. *Eur J Clin Pharmacol* (1978) 13, 351–6.
3. Warwick HMC, Mindham RHS. Concomitant administration of mianserin and warfarin. *Br J Psychiatry* (1983) 143, 308.
4. Shelly RK. Mianserin and warfarin. *Br J Psychiatry* (1984) 145, 97–8.
5. Baettig D, Tillement J-P, Baumann P. Interaction between mianserin and acenocoumarin: a single case study. *Int J Clin Pharmacol Ther* (1994) 32, 165–7.
6. Spaans E, van den Heuvel MW, Chin-Kon-Sung UG, Colbers EPH, Peeters PAM, Sitsen JMA. The effect of mirtazapine on steady state prothrombin time during warfarin therapy. *Pharmacol Toxicol* (2001) 89 (Suppl 1), 80.
7. Zispin (Mirtazapine). Organon Laboratories Ltd. UK Summary of product characteristics, September 2005.
8. Mirtazapine. Genus Pharmaceuticals. UK Summary of product characteristics, May 2005.

Coumarins and related drugs + Thyroid and Antithyroid compounds

Hypothyroidism and hyperthyroidism, respectively, decrease and increase the metabolism of the clotting factors. Correction of these disease states therefore alters anticoagulant requirements. Bleeding has been seen in patients given thyroid hormones without an adjustment of their warfarin dose, and increased warfarin requirements have been seen in a patient given thiamazole. This is more of a drug-disease interaction rather than a direct drug-drug interaction and is therefore likely to occur with any coumarin or indanedione given with any drug that affects thyroid function.

Clinical evidence

(a) Hypothyroidism and Thyroid compounds

In a study in 7 patients with myxoedema (hypothyroidism), the response to a single dose of **warfarin** was increased after 3 months of treatment with **liothyronine** (when euthyroid), when compared with before treatment, without a change in plasma warfarin levels.[1] Various case reports describe similar effects. In one report, brief mention is made of one patient who showed an increased response to **warfarin** after an increase in dose of thyroid replacement therapy, and of another patient on long-term **warfarin** who had a bleeding episode when thyroid replacement therapy was started.[2] Another patient taking **warfarin** developed oral mucosal bleeding with an INR of greater than 11 when her hypothyroidism was overcorrected with **levothyroxine**, although she had no clinical signs of hyperthyroidism.[3] In another case, a subdural haematoma occurred in a child stabilised on **warfarin** when **levothyroxine** was started, and her dose of **warfarin** was eventually reduced from 7.5 mg daily to 5 mg daily.[4]

A patient with myxoedema required a gradual reduction in his dosage of **phenindione** from 200 to 75 mg daily as his thyroid status was corrected by **liothyronine**.[5] A similar patient required a reduction in **acenocoumarol** dose from 16 mg daily to 5 mg daily when hypothyroidism was corrected with **liothyronine**.[5]

(b) Hyperthyroidism and Antithyroid compounds

In 5 patients with hyperthyroidism, the response to a single dose of **warfarin** was decreased 3 months after treatment with **iodine-131** (when euthyroid), when compared with before treatment. In addition, the plasma half-life and levels of **warfarin** were higher after treatment.[6] A hyperthyroid patient taking **warfarin** had a marked increase in his prothrombin times on two occasions when his treatment with **thiamazole** (**methimazole**) was stopped and he became hyperthyroid again.[7] Another similar case has been described where the required dose of **warfarin** increased from 35 mg weekly to 65 mg weekly as the patients hyperthyroid state was corrected with **thiamazole** 30 mg daily. However, the patient then became hypothyroid and required up to 85 mg weekly of **warfarin**. When the **thiamazole** dose was withheld for 5 days and then reduced to 5 mg daily, the patient rapidly developed a markedly raised INR of 7 without bleeding complications.[8] In another report, a patient required just 0.5 mg of **warfarin** daily while hyperthyroid.[3] Another case of possible enhanced response to **warfarin** in a hyperthyroid patient has been reported.[9,10]

Mechanism

In hypothyroid patients the catabolism (destruction) of the blood clotting factors (II, VII, IX and X) is low and this tends to cancel, to some extent, the effects of the anticoagulants, which reduce blood clotting factor synthesis. Conversely, in hyperthyroid patients in whom the catabolism is increased, the net result is an increase in the effects of the anticoagulants.[11] In studies in healthy subjects, **dextrothyroxine** (which has weak thyroid activity compared with levothyroxine) potentiated the anticoagulant effect of **dicoumarol**[12] and warfarin[13] without altering the half-life and plasma levels of the anticoagulants, and without altering vitamin K–dependent clotting activity.[12] Because of this, it was suggested that the thyroid hormones might increase the affinity of the anticoagulants for its receptor sites.[12,13]

Importance and management

A well documented and clinically important interaction occurs if oral anticoagulants and thyroid hormones are taken concurrently.

Hypothyroid patients taking an anticoagulant who are subsequently treated with thyroid hormones as replacement therapy will need a downward adjustment of the anticoagulant dosage as treatment proceeds if excessive hypoprothrombinaemia and bleeding are to be avoided. All of the oral anticoagulants may be expected to behave similarly. Conversely, as the thyroid status of hyperthyroid patients returns to normal by the use of antithyroid drugs (e.g. **carbimazole**, thiamazole, **propylthiouracil**) an increase in the anticoagulant requirements would be expected. Close anticoagulant monitoring and dose adjustment are required, particularly while thyroid hormone levels are being stabilised. Note that, in one case the authors commented that the magnitude and clinical complexity of the interaction between the drugs and disease state was unexpected.[8]

Note that propylthiouracil in the absence of an anticoagulant has very occasionally been reported to cause hypoprothrombinaemia and bleeding.[14,15]

Some drugs can alter thyroid status as an unwanted effect, and this will also alter the response to the oral anticoagulants. For example, 'amiodarone', (p.363) can cause thyrotoxicosis, which decreases warfarin requirements. Also, use of **dextrothyroxine** for hypercholesterolaemia decreased the required dose of warfarin[16,17] and dicoumarol,[18] presumably because it has weak thyroid activity.

1. Rice AJ, McIntosh TJ, Fouts JR, Brunk SF, Wilson WR. Decreased sensitivity to warfarin in patients with myxedema. *Am J Med Sci* (1971) 262, 211–15.
2. Hansten PD. Oral anticoagulants and drugs which alter thyroid function. *Drug Intell Clin Pharm* (1980) 14, 331–4.
3. Chute JP, Ryan CP, Sladek G, Shakir KMM. Exacerbation of warfarin-induced anticoagulation by hyperthyroidism. *Endocr Pract* (1997) 3, 77–9..
4. Costigan DC, Freedman MH, Ehrlich RM. Potentiation of oral anticoagulant effect by L-thyroxine. *Clin Pediatr (Phila)* (1984) 23, 172–4.
5. Walters MB. The relationship between thyroid function and anticoagulant therapy. *Am J Cardiol* (1963) 11, 112–14.
6. McIntosh TJ, Brunk SF, Kölln I. Increased sensitivity to warfarin in thyrotoxicosis. *J Clin Invest* (1970) 49, 63a–64a.
7. Vagenakis AG, Cote R, Miller ME, Braverman LE, Stohlman F. Enhancement of warfarin-induced hypoprothrombinemia by thyrotoxicosis. *Johns Hopkins Med J* (1972) 131, 69–73.
8. Busenbark LA, Cushnie SA. Effect of Graves' disease and methimazole on warfarin anticoagulation. *Ann Pharmacother* (2006) 40, 1200–3.
9. Self TH, Straughn AB, Weisburst MR. Effect of hyperthyroidism on hypoprothrombinemic response to warfarin. *Am J Hosp Pharm* (1976) 33, 387–9.
10. Self T, Weisburst M, Wooton E, Straughn A, Oliver J. Warfarin-induced hypoprothrombinemia. Potentiation by hyperthyroidism. *JAMA* (1975) 231, 1165–6.
11. Loeliger EA, van der Esch B, Mattern MJ, Hemker HC. The biological disappearance rate of prothrombin, factors VII, IX and X from plasma in hypothyroidism, hyperthyroidism and during fever. *Thromb Diath Haemorrh* (1964) 10, 267–77.
12. Schrogie JJ, Solomon HM. The anticoagulant response to bishydroxycoumarin. II. The effect of d-thyroxine, clofibrate and norethandrolone. *Clin Pharmacol Ther* (1967) 8, 70–7.
13. Solomon HM, Schrogie JJ. Change in receptor site affinity: a proposed explanation for the potentiating effect of d-thyroxine on the anticoagulant response to warfarin. *Clin Pharmacol Ther* (1967) 8, 797–9.
14. D'Angelo G, Le Gresley LP. Severe hypoprothrombinæmia after propylthiouracil therapy. *Can Med Assoc J* (1959) 81, 479–81.
15. Gotta AW, Sullivan CA, Seaman J, Jean-Gilles B. Prolonged intraoperative bleeding caused by propylthiouracil-induced hypoprothrombinemia. *Anesthesiology* (1972) 37, 562–3.
16. Owens JC, Neeley WB, Owen WR. Effect of sodium dextrothyroxine in patients receiving anticoagulants. *N Engl J Med* (1962) 266, 76–9.
17. Winters WL, Soloff LA. Observations on sodium d-thyroxine as a hypocholesterolemic agent in persons with hypercholesterolemia with and without ischemic heart disease. *Am J Med Sci* (1962) 243, 458–69.
18. Jones RJ, Cohen L. Sodium dextro-thyroxine in coronary disease and hypercholesterolemia. *Circulation* (1961) 24, 164–70.

Coumarins + Tiabendazole

An isolated case report describes a marked increase in the anticoagulant effects of acenocoumarol in a patient given tiabendazole.

Clinical evidence, mechanism, importance and management

An increase in the anticoagulant effects of **acenocoumarol** occurred in a patient with nephrotic syndrome undergoing dialysis, who was given tiabendazole 8 g daily for 2 days on two occasions about 7 weeks apart.[1] On both occasions, his INR rose from 2.9 to more than 5 without any clinical consequence. The reasons are not understood, nor is the general importance of this interaction known. There seem to be no other reports.

1. Henri P, Mosquet B, Hurault de Ligny B, Lacotte J, Cardinau E, Moulin M, Ryckelinck JP. Imputation d'une hypocoagulabilité à l'interaction tiabendazole-acénocoumarol. *Therapie* (1993) 48, 500–501.

Coumarins + Tobacco

In one study in healthy subjects, stopping smoking caused a minor 13% increase in steady-state warfarin levels. Two cases have been reported of patients who required 14% and 23% reductions in warfarin dose, respectively, on stopping smoking. However, one analysis did not find any significant difference in warfarin dose by smoking status. One patient who stopped chewing tobacco had an increase in INR.

Clinical evidence

(a) Chewing tobacco

In a patient using smokeless tobacco (chewing tobacco) for greater than 85% of waking hours, the INR was found to have increased from 1.1 to 2.3 six days after discontinuation of the tobacco use. This patient had generally had an INR of 1.1 to 1.9 since restarting warfarin 4 months earlier, despite gradually increasing the warfarin dose from 10 mg daily to 25 mg daily alternating with 30 mg daily. However, during this time, he did have two INR spikes of 2.5 and 4.2, which were attributed to dietary changes,[1] but see mechanism below.

(b) Smoking tobacco

In a controlled study in 9 healthy subjects who normally smoked at least one pack of cigarettes daily (size unknown) and who were given **warfarin** to steady-state, smoking abstention for about 6 weeks increased the average steady-state **warfarin** levels by 13%, decreased **warfarin** clearance by 13% and increased the **warfarin** half-life by 23%, but no changes in the prothrombin time occurred.[2] An 80-year-old man taking **warfarin** had a steady rise in his INR (from a range of 2 to 2.8 up to 3.7) over a 3-month period when he gave up smoking. No bleeding occurred. His dose of **warfarin** was reduced by 14%, and the INR stabilised at 2.3 to 2.8 over the next 9 months.[3] Similarly, another patient required a 23% reduction in **warfarin** dose after stopping smoking following recovery from bacterial meningitis.[4]

In contrast, in one retrospective study of patients who had undergone cardiac valve replacement, there was no statistically significant difference between the **warfarin** dosage requirements of 117 non-smokers, 23 light smokers (20 or less cigarettes daily) or 34 heavy smokers (greater than 20 cigarettes daily).[5]

Mechanism

Some of the components of tobacco smoke act as cytochrome P450 isoenzyme inducers, which might cause a small increase in the metabolism of the warfarin. When smoking stops, the enzymes are no longer stimulated, the metabolism of the warfarin falls slightly and its effects are correspondingly slightly increased. Tobacco smoke is known to induce CYP1A2, which has a partial role in the metabolism of the less active *R*-warfarin enantiomer. Note that smoking status had no effect on the *S*-warfarin AUC in one study.[6]

The possible case of an interaction with smokeless tobacco was attributed to the very high 'vitamin-K', (p.458), content of tobacco resulting in relative warfarin resistance. However, there were two previous INR spikes in this patient, which were attributed to dietary changes,[1] an explanation that seems unlikely if there was a high background vitamin K intake from the tobacco. This case is therefore unclear.

Importance and management

The overall picture seems to be that smoking (or giving up smoking) only has a slight to moderate effect on the response to warfarin, and only the occasional patient will need a small dosage alteration. This should easily be detected in the course of routine INR checks. Note that tobacco smoking increases cardiovascular disease risk, and patients requiring anticoagulants should be encouraged and helped to stop smoking.

The isolated case with smokeless tobacco is unclear, but consider the possibility that vitamin K from chewing tobacco may reduce warfarin effects. Further study is needed.

1. Kuykendall JR, Houle MD, Rhodes RS. Possible warfarin failure due to interaction with smokeless tobacco. *Ann Pharmacother* (2004) 38, 595–7.
2. Bachmann K, Shapiro R, Fulton R, Carroll FT, Sullivan TJ. Smoking and warfarin disposition. *Clin Pharmacol Ther* (1979) 25, 309–15.
3. Colucci VJ. Increase in international normalized ratio associated with smoking cessation. *Ann Pharmacother* (2001) 35, 385–6.

4. Evans M, Lewis GM. Increase in international normalized ratio after smoking cessation in a patient receiving warfarin. *Pharmacotherapy* (2005) 25, 1656–9.
5. Weiner B, Faraci PA, Fayad R, Swanson L. Warfarin dosage following prosthetic valve replacement: effect of smoking history. *Drug Intell Clin Pharm* (1984) 18, 904–6.
6. Kim MJ, Nafzinger AN, Kashuba AD, Kirchheiner J, Bauer S, Gaedigk A, Bertino JS. Effects of fluvastatin and cigarette smoking on CYP2C9 activity measured using the probe S-warfarin. *Eur J Clin Pharmacol* (2006) 62, 431–6.

Coumarins + Tolterodine

In healthy subjects, tolterodine did not alter the pharmacokinetics or pharmacodynamics of warfarin, but isolated cases of raised INRs have been reported.

Clinical evidence, mechanism, importance and management

In a placebo-controlled study in healthy subjects, tolterodine 2 mg twice daily for 7 days did not affect the pharmacokinetics of *R*- or *S*-warfarin after a single 25-mg dose of **warfarin** given on day 4, nor were the pharmacokinetics of tolterodine altered by **warfarin**. In addition, the prothrombin time and factor VII activity were not altered by tolterodine.[1]

However, a report describes two patients on stable **warfarin** doses who had elevated INRs shortly after tolterodine 2 mg daily was started and stopped: one had an INR of 6.1 one day after stopping 13 days of tolterodine, and the other had an INR of 7.4 two days after stopping 8 days of tolterodine. In both cases no bleeding occurred and **warfarin** was withheld for three doses and successfully reinstated at the original dose.[2] Another case has been reported of a patient who required a 15% reduction in **warfarin** dose while taking tolterodine 4 mg daily. Her maximum INR had been 3.9. However, she had undergone several warfarin dose increases over the previous 2 months and her INR had been fluctuating.[3]

The controlled study suggests that no **warfarin** dose adjustment would expected to be needed when tolterodine is added to **warfarin** therapy. However, the 3 cases introduce a note of caution. Although additional monitoring would seem over-cautious on the basis of these cases, bear them in mind in the case of an unexpected response to warfarin.

1. Rahimy M, Hallén B, Narang P. Effect of tolterodine on the anticoagulant actions and pharmacokinetics of single-dose warfarin in healthy volunteers. *Arzneimittelforschung* (2002) 52, 890–5.
2. Colucci VJ, Rivey MP. Tolterodine-warfarin drug interaction. *Ann Pharmacother* (1999) 33, 1173–6.
3. Taylor JR. Probable interaction between tolterodine and warfarin. *Pharmacotherapy* (2006) 26, 719–21.

Coumarins + Topical salicylates

Increased warfarin effects have been seen when methyl salicylate or trolamine salicylate were used on the skin.

Clinical evidence

Methyl salicylate, in the form of gels, oil, or ointment applied to the skin, has been found to increase the effects of **warfarin**. Bleeding and bruising and/or raised INRs have been seen with both high[1-3] and low doses[4] of **methyl salicylate**. One report[5] described the possible additive effects of **methyl salicylate oil** (*Kwan Loong Medicated Oil*) and a decoction of *Danshen* (the root of *Salvia miltiorrhiza*) on the response to **warfarin** (see also 'Coumarins and related drugs + Herbal medicines; Danshen (*Salvia miltiorrhiza*)', p.415). A raised prothrombin time has also been reported with topical **trolamine salicylate**.[3]

Mechanism

Methyl and trolamine salicylates possibly interact like high-dose 'aspirin', (p.385), because they are absorbed through the skin.[1]

Importance and management

Although the evidence is limited, it appears that topical methyl salicylate and trolamine salicylate can increase the effect of warfarin.

1. Chow WH, Cheung KL, Ling HM, See T. Potentiation of warfarin anticoagulation by topical methylsalicylate ointment. *J R Soc Med* (1989) 82, 501–2.
2. Yip ASB, Chow WH, Tai YT, Cheung KL. Adverse effect of topical methylsalicylate ointment on warfarin anticoagulation: an unrecognized potential hazard. *Postgrad Med J* (1990) 66, 367–9.
3. Littleton F. Warfarin and topical salicylates. *JAMA* (1990) 263, 2888.
4. Joss JD, LeBlond RF. Potentiation of warfarin anticoagulation associated with topical methyl salicylate. *Ann Pharmacother* (2000) 34, 729–33.
5. Tam LS, Chan TYK, Leung WK, Critchley JAJH. Warfarin interactions with Chinese traditional medicines: danshen and methyl salicylate medicated oil. *Aust N Z J Med* (1995) 25, 258.

Coumarins + Tricyclic antidepressants

Amitriptyline and nortriptyline do not appear to alter the half-life of warfarin, but may possibly increase that of dicoumarol. Limited evidence from analyses of patients taking phenprocoumon or warfarin suggests that use of tricyclics is associated with greater variability in prothrombin times, which can make stable anticoagulation difficult. An isolated case of the potentiation of warfarin by lofepramine has been reported.

Clinical evidence

(a) Dicoumarol

A study in 6 healthy subjects given **nortriptyline** 200 micrograms/kg three times daily for 8 days indicated that the mean half-life of dicoumarol was increased from 35 to 106 hours. In a parallel group, the same dose of **nortriptyline** also increased the half-life of antipyrine.[1] However, in later identical studies by the same research group, **nortriptyline** decreased the half-life of antipyrine in one study, and had no effect in another.[2] The authors were unable to explain these disparate findings with antipyrine,[2] and they cast doubt on the results seen with dicoumarol. In a later study by another group, both **amitriptyline** 75 mg daily and **nortriptyline** 40 mg daily had no consistent effect on the half-life of a single dose of dicoumarol, although there was some evidence of increased bioavailability.[3]

(b) Phenprocoumon

In a retrospective analysis of 7 patients taking phenprocoumon and **amitriptyline**, unpredictable and 'massive fluctuations' in prothrombin times (increases and decreases) were noted, which were not seen in a control group of 7 other patients not taking amitriptyline. Note that the **amitriptyline** dose was not stable. Anticoagulant control improved on stopping the amitriptyline in 5 of the patients.[4] The same authors reported another similar case in a patient taking phenprocoumon and **amitriptyline**.[5]

(c) Warfarin

In a study in 12 healthy subjects,[3] neither **amitriptyline** 75 mg daily nor **nortriptyline** 40 mg daily for 13 days affected the plasma half-life of a single dose of warfarin given on day 9.

However, in the preliminary report of an analysis of 500 patients taking warfarin, a statistically significant difference in the warfarin dose index (prothrombin time prolongation/cumulative warfarin dose) before, during and after therapy was detected for a number of unexpected drugs including **amitriptyline**. However, no further details were given.[6] In another analysis of the stability of anticoagulant control in 277 patients, use of tricyclics (**imipramine, amitriptyline, nortriptyline**) in 16 patients was associated with an increased need for anticoagulant dose modifications (average 3.56 over 6 months). Most of the patients were taking warfarin.[7] Another report briefly lists that potentiation of warfarin occurred in a patient given **lofepramine**.[8]

Mechanism

Not understood. One suggestion is that the tricyclic antidepressants inhibit the metabolism of the anticoagulant (seen in *animals* with nortriptyline or amitriptyline and warfarin,[9] but not with **desipramine** and **acenocoumarol**[10]), but tricyclics are not established known inhibitors of the metabolism of any drug so this seems unlikely. Another idea is that the tricyclics slow gastrointestinal motility thereby increasing the time available for the dissolution and absorption of dicoumarol.[3]

Importance and management

Information about interactions between anticoagulants and tricyclic antidepressant is limited, patchy and inconclusive. It appears that amitriptyline and nortriptyline do not alter the half-life of warfarin, but might increase that of dicoumarol. A greater fluctuation in anticoagulant control was noted in two analyses, one with warfarin and one with phenprocoumon. However, these were uncontrolled studies, and the findings need confirming in a randomised study. Moreover, there do not appear to be any published case reports of an interaction between tricyclics and warfarin. Thus, there is insufficient evidence to recommend any special precautions in patients stabilised on coumarins requiring tricyclics. Bear the possibility of an interaction in mind in the event of unexpected responses to treatment.

1. Vesell ES, Passananti GT, Greene FE. Impairment of drug metabolism in man by allopurinol and nortriptyline. *N Engl J Med* (1970) 283, 1484–8.
2. Vesell ES, Passananti GT, Aurori KC. Anomalous results of studies on drug interaction in man. *Pharmacology* (1975) 13, 101–111.
3. Pond SM, Graham GG, Birkett DJ, Wade DN. Effects of tricyclic antidepressants on drug metabolism. *Clin Pharmacol Ther* (1975) 18, 191–9.
4. Hampel H, Berger C, Kuss H-J, Müller-Spahn F. Unstable anticoagulation in the course of amitriptyline treatment. *Pharmacopsychiatry* (1996) 29, 33–7.
5. Hampel H, Berger C, Müller-Spahn F. Modified anticoagulant potency in an amitriptyline-treated patient? *Acta Haematol (Basel)* (1996) 96, 178–80.
6. Koch-Weser J. Hemorrhagic reactions and drug interactions in 500 warfarin-treated patients. *Clin Pharmacol Ther* (1973) 14, 139.
7. Williams JRB, Griffin JP, Parkins A. Effect of concomitantly administered drugs on the control of long term anticoagulant therapy. *Q J Med* (1976) 45, 63.
8. Beeley L, Stewart P, Hickey FM. *Bulletin of the West Midlands Centre for Adverse Drug Reaction Reporting* (1988) 26, 21.
9. Loomis CW, Racz WJ. Drug interactions of amitriptyline and nortriptyline with warfarin in the rat. *Res Commun Chem Pathol Pharmacol* (1980) 30, 41–58.
10. Weiner M. Effect of centrally active drugs on the action of coumarin anticoagulants. *Nature* (1966) 212, 1599–1600.

Coumarins + Valproate

An isolated case describes a patient who had an increase in her INR the day after starting valproic acid, but was eventually restabilised on the original dose of warfarin while still taking the valproic acid. Valproic acid did not alter the anticoagulant effects of phenprocoumon in one patient. Valproate alone can cause altered bleeding time, bruising, haematoma, epistaxis and haemorrhage.

Clinical evidence

A woman was given **warfarin** for a deep vein thrombosis, and was stabilised on 5 mg alternating with 2.5 mg daily with an INR between 1.8 and 2.6. Valproic acid 250 mg twice daily and fluphenazine 5 mg once daily were then added. The morning after her first dose of valproic acid, the INR increased to 3.9, and **warfarin** dosage was decreased to 2.5 mg daily. Four days later the valproic acid dosage was doubled, and numerous **warfarin** dosage adjustments were needed to keep the INR therapeutic. However, 3 weeks after starting the valproic acid she was discharged on the same **warfarin** dose as before the valproic acid was started.[1]

In one patient taking **phenprocoumon**, valproic acid 500 mg to 1 g daily did not alter the prothrombin time ratio.[2]

Mechanism

There is *in vitro* evidence that the serum binding of warfarin is decreased by sodium valproate so that free warfarin levels rise,[1,3,4] by 32% according to one study.[1] The increase in free warfarin levels is transient until a new equilibrium is reached, but theoretically could result in a transient increase in INR, as is seen with 'cloral hydrate', (p.396).

Valproate inhibits the second stage of platelet aggregation, and a reversible prolongation of bleeding times and thrombocytopenia has been reported, usually with high doses, which can result in spontaneous bruising and bleeding.

Importance and management

There seem to be no other reports of problems associated with concurrent use nor any other direct evidence that an interaction of clinical importance normally occurs. It may be that any interaction occurs only transiently when valproate is added, and the situation rapidly restabilises without any real need to adjust the warfarin dosage. However, some manufacturers recommend closely monitoring the prothrombin time because of the possibility of warfarin protein binding displacement.[5,6] Note that valproate alone can cause spontaneous bruising or bleeding, and if these effects occur, some manufacturers recommend withdrawing valproate pending investigations.[5-7] A reduction of valproate dosage or permanent withdrawal of valproate may be required.[6]

1. Guthrie SK, Stoysich AM, Bader G, Hilleman DE. Hypothesized interaction between valproic acid and warfarin. *J Clin Psychopharmacol* (1995) 15, 138–9.
2. Schlienger R, Kurmann M, Drewe J, Müller-Spahn F, Seifritz E. Inhibition of phenprocoumon anticoagulation by carbamazepine. *Eur Neuropsychopharmacol* (2000) 10, 219–21.
3. Urien S, Albengres E, Tillement J-P. Serum protein binding of valproic acid in healthy subjects and in patients with liver disease. *Int J Clin Pharmacol Ther Toxicol* (1981) 19, 319–25.
4. Panjehshahin MR, Bowmer CJ, Yates MS. Effect of valproic acid, its unsaturated metabolites and some structurally related fatty acids on the binding of warfarin and dansylsarcosine to human albumin. *Biochem Pharmacol* (1991) 41, 1227–33.
5. Epilim (Sodium valproate). Sanofi-Aventis. UK Summary of product characteristics, October 2005.
6. Depakote (Divalproex sodium). Abbott Laboratories. US Prescribing information, October 2006.
7. Orlept (Sodium valproate). Wockhardt UK Ltd. UK Summary of product characteristics, August 2003.

Coumarins and related drugs + Viloxazine

A single report describes three cases where viloxazine possibly increased the anticoagulant effects of acenocoumarol and fluindione.

Clinical evidence

An 82-year-old woman with angina, hypertension and atrial fibrillation, who was taking **acenocoumarol**, molsidomine and flunitrazepam, had a rise in her INR from 3.3 to 7.9 when she started to take viloxazine (dose not stated) for depression. Five days after stopping the viloxazine her INR had fallen to 2.6. This report also briefly describes 2 other cases where viloxazine possibly caused an increase in the anticoagulant effects of **acenocoumarol** and **fluindione**.[1]

Mechanism

Not understood. The authors of the report suggest that viloxazine possibly inhibits cytochrome P450 within the liver, resulting in a reduction in the metabolism and loss of the anticoagulants from the body.[1]

Importance and management

Information seems to be limited to this report so that its general importance is uncertain. Be alert for the need to reduce the dosage of acenocoumarol and fluindione if viloxazine is added to established anticoagulant treatment. Take the same precautions with any of the other coumarin or indanedione anticoagulants, but so far there seems to be no direct evidence that they interact.

1. Chiffoleau A, Delavaud P, Spreux A, Fialip J, Kergueris MF, Chichmanian RM, Lavarenne J, Bourin M, Larousse C. Existe-t-il une interaction métabolique entre la viloxazine et les antivitamines K? *Therapie* (1993) 48, 492–3.

Coumarins + Vinpocetine

In healthy subjects, the anticoagulant effect of warfarin was slightly reduced by vinpocetine, and the warfarin AUC was also slightly reduced.

Clinical evidence, mechanism, importance and management

In a study in 18 healthy subjects taking vinpocetine 10 mg three times daily for 19 days, the anticoagulant effects and pharmacokinetics of a single 25-mg dose of **warfarin** were compared when given before vinpocetine was started, and on day 15.[1] A small 14.6% reduction in the mean prothrombin time occurred, and also an 8.4% reduction in the AUC of **warfarin**. More study is needed to find out whether these small changes are clinically important. Be aware of the small potential for interaction on concurrent use.

1. Hitzenberger G, Sommer W, Grandt R. Influence of vinpocetine on warfarin-induced inhibition of coagulation. *Int J Clin Pharmacol Ther Toxicol* (1990) 28, 323–8.

Coumarins and related drugs + Vitamin K substances

The effects of the coumarin and indanedione anticoagulants can be reduced or abolished by vitamin K_1 (phytomenadione). This is used as an effective antidote for excessive anticoagulation. However, unintentional and unwanted antagonism can occur in patients unknowingly taking vitamin K_1. There is also a case of

antagonism of acenocoumarol in a patient using a proprietary chilblain product containing the vitamin K_4 substance acetomenaphthone.

Clinical evidence

A woman taking **acenocoumarol** had a fall in her British Corrected Ratio to 1.2 (normal range 1.8 to 3) within 2 days of starting to take a non-prescription chilblain preparation (*Gon*) containing **acetomenaphthone** 10 mg per tablet. She took a total of 50 mg of vitamin K_4 over 48 hours.[1]

Mechanism

The coumarin and indanedione oral anticoagulants are vitamin K antagonists, and probably inhibit the enzyme vitamin K epoxide reductase so reducing the synthesis of vitamin K–dependent blood clotting factors by the liver. If the intake of vitamin K_1 increases, the competition swings in favour of the vitamin and the synthesis of the blood clotting factors begins to return to normal. As a result the prothrombin time also begins to fall to its normal value. The role of other vitamin K substances, such as K_4 and K_2, in coagulation is less clear.

Importance and management

The interaction with vitamin K_1 is very well established and clinically important, and is expected to occur with every coumarin and indanedione oral anticoagulant because they have a common mode of action as vitamin K antagonists. The drug intake and diet of any patient who shows 'warfarin resistance' should be investigated for the possibility of this interaction. It can be accommodated either by increasing the anticoagulant dosage, or by reducing the intake of vitamin K_1. However, the role of other vitamin K substances in coagulation is less clear. The case report with acetomenaphthone, a vitamin K_4 substance suggests that this can also antagonise the effect of vitamin K antagonists. It may be prudent for patients to avoid preparations containing this substance. Consider also 'dietary supplements', (p.401), 'enteral feeds', (p.406), 'vitamin K_1–rich foods', (p.409), and 'fermented soya bean', (p.408).

1. Heald GE, Poller L. Anticoagulants and treatment for chilblains. *BMJ* (1974) 1, 455.

Coumarins + Zileuton

Zileuton slightly increases the anticoagulant effects of warfarin and slightly increases *R*-warfarin levels, but this probably has little clinical relevance.

Clinical evidence

In a placebo-controlled study, zileuton 600 mg every 6 hours for 6 days or placebo was given to healthy subjects who had been stabilised on racemic **warfarin** to achieve prothrombin times of 14 to 18 seconds for one week. The zileuton had no effect on the pharmacokinetics of *S*-warfarin, but the *R*-warfarin AUC rose by 22%, and its clearance fell by 15%. The mean prothrombin times increased by 2.3 seconds (morning) and 2 seconds (evening) in the zileuton group. The corresponding increases in the placebo group were 0.7 and 0.2 seconds, respectively.[1]

Mechanism

It seems likely that zileuton inhibits the metabolism of *R*-warfarin, probably by the cytochrome P450 isoenzyme CYP1A2.[2]

Importance and management

Information seems to be limited to this study, but the pharmacokinetic interaction appears to be established. The clinical significance of a 2 second rise in prothrombin times is unclear, but it seems likely to be small. The lack of any published reports of problems with the combination would tend to support this.

1. Awni WM, Hussein Z, Granneman GR, Patterson KJ, Dube LM, Cavanaugh JH. Pharmacodynamic and stereoselective pharmacokinetic interactions between zileuton and warfarin in humans. *Clin Pharmacokinet* (1995) 29 (Suppl 2), 67–76.
2. Lu P, Schrag ML, Slaughter DE, Raab CE, Shou M, Rodrigues AD. Mechanism-based inhibition of human liver microsomal cytochrome P450 1A2 by zileuton, a 5-lipoxygenase inhibitor. *Drug Metab Dispos* (2003) 31, 1352–60.

Drotrecogin alfa + Other drugs that affect coagulation

The manufacturers of drotrecogin alfa contraindicate its use with therapeutic doses of heparin (15 units/kg/hour or more), but state that prophylactic heparin doses may be used concurrently. They also say that the risk benefit ratio of drotrecogin alfa should be carefully assessed in patients who have received thrombolytics in the last 3 days, or oral anticoagulants, aspirin or platelet inhibitors within 7 days.

Clinical evidence, mechanism, importance and management

The manufacturers of drotrecogin alfa note that no formal drug interaction studies have been conducted.[1,2] However, because drotrecogin alfa increases the risk of bleeding, they have a number of cautions and contraindications regarding its use with other drugs affecting haemostasis.[1,2] Nevertheless, they say that in phase III studies of drotrecogin alfa, two-thirds of patients received prophylactic doses of **heparin** or **low-molecular-weight heparin**, and there was no observed increase in the risk of serious bleeding events reported in patients receiving the combination.[1] Therefore, in the US, they specifically state that low-dose **heparin** may be given for the prophylaxis of venous thromboembolic events in patients receiving drotrecogin alfa.[2] However, they state that the increased risk of bleeding should be carefully considered when deciding to use drotrecogin alfa with therapeutic doses of **heparin** for treating an active thromboembolic event.[2] In the UK, the manufacturers specifically contraindicate use with **heparin** at doses of 15 units/kg per hour or more.[1]

Because of the possible increased risk of bleeding, the manufacturers also state that the risks of giving drotrecogin alfa should be weighed against the benefits in patients who have received **thrombolytics** within 3 days, **oral anticoagulants** within 7 days, or **aspirin** (US information specifies greater than 650 mg daily) or other **antiplatelet drugs** within 7 days.[1,2]

1. Xigris (Drotrecogin alfa). Eli Lilly and Company Ltd. UK Summary of product characteristics, April 2007.
2. Xigris (Drotrecogin alfa). Eli Lilly and Company. US Prescribing information, April 2007.

Fondaparinux + Antiplatelet drugs and NSAIDs

Neither aspirin nor piroxicam altered the pharmacokinetics of fondaparinux, and there was no significant change in bleeding time during concurrent use. Nevertheless, the manufacturer recommends close monitoring if antiplatelet drugs or NSAIDs are used with fondaparinux, because of the increased risk of bleeding.

Clinical evidence

A single 975-mg dose of **aspirin** given on day 4 of an 8-day course of subcutaneous fondaparinux 10 mg daily had no effect on fondaparinux pharmacokinetics in 16 healthy subjects. The increase in bleeding time with fondaparinux and **aspirin** was greater than with **aspirin** alone, but this was not statistically significant. **Aspirin** had no effect on the small prolongation of aPTT seen with fondaparinux.[1]

In another study, **piroxicam** 20 mg daily for 10 days was given to 12 healthy subjects with fondaparinux 10 mg daily starting on day 7. Both drugs were also given alone. **Piroxicam** had no effect on fondaparinux pharmacokinetics, and had no effect on the small prolongation of aPTT seen with fondaparinux. There was no difference in bleeding time between the treatments.[1]

Mechanism

Fondaparinux commonly causes bleeding as a consequence of its action.[2] Since antiplatelet drugs and NSAIDs also increase the risk of bleeding, the risk and severity of bleeding is likely to be increased with the combination.

Importance and management

The pharmacological studies described show that the pharmacokinetics of fondaparinux are not changed by aspirin and piroxicam, and that there is only a minor increase in bleeding time. Nevertheless, the manufacturers of fondaparinux say that antiplatelet drugs (**aspirin**, **dipyridamole**, **sulfinpyrazone**, **ticlopidine** or **clopidogrel**) and NSAIDs should be used with caution because of the possible increased risk of haemorrhage. They recommend that if concurrent use is essential, close monitoring is necessary.[2,3] This is considered particularly important in patients undergoing peridural or spinal anaesthesia or spinal puncture, in whom antiplatelet drugs, NSAIDs and fondaparinux are possible risk factors for epidural or spinal haematoma resulting in prolonged or permanent paralysis.[3]

1. Ollier C, Faaij RA, Santoni A, Duvauchelle T, van Haard PMM, Schoemaker RC, Cohen AF, de Greef R, Burggraaf J. Absence of interaction of fondaparinux sodium with aspirin and piroxicam in healthy male volunteers. *Clin Pharmacokinet* (2002) 41 (Suppl 2), 31–37.
2. Arixtra (Fondaparinux sodium). GlaxoSmithKline UK. UK Summary of product characteristics, April 2007.
3. Arixtra (Fondaparinux sodium). GlaxoSmithKline. US Prescribing information, October 2005.

Fondaparinux + Miscellaneous

In the UK, the manufacturer recommends avoiding other drugs that may enhance the risk of haemorrhage with fondaparinux. They specifically name, desirudin, fibrinolytic drugs, glycoprotein IIb/IIIa-receptor antagonists, heparin, heparinoids and low-molecular-weight heparins.[1] Similarly, in the US, the manufacturer states that agents that may enhance the risk of haemorrhage should be discontinued prior to starting fondaparinux. They say that if concurrent use is essential, close monitoring may be appropriate.[2] See also 'warfarin', (p.406), and 'antiplatelet drugs and NSAIDs', (p.459).

1. Arixtra (Fondaparinux sodium). GlaxoSmithKline UK. UK Summary of product characteristics, April 2007.
2. Arixtra (Fondaparinux sodium). GlaxoSmithKline. US Prescribing information, October 2005.

Heparin and LMWHs + Antiplatelet drugs

In a pharmacodynamic study, the dose of heparin did not need changing when clopidogrel was also given, and the antiplatelet effects of clopidogrel were unaltered. Nevertheless concurrent use of heparin or low molecular weight heparins and antiplatelet drugs such as clopidogrel and ticlopidine has the potential to increase the risk of bleeding and increased monitoring would be prudent.

Clinical evidence

(a) Clopidogrel

In a placebo-controlled study in 12 healthy subjects, the dosage of **heparin** given over 4 days did not need modification when clopidogrel 75 mg daily was also given, and the inhibitory effects of clopidogrel on platelet aggregation were unchanged on concurrent use.[1]

The manufacturers of clopidogrel note that in various large clinical studies in patients with acute coronary syndrome or myocardial infarction, most patients received **heparin** or **LMWHs** without an obvious difference in the rate of bleeding or the incidence of major bleeding.[2,3]

In one case the use of **enoxaparin** with clopidogrel was considered to be a contributing factor in a case of spinal epidural haematoma occurring after spinal anaesthesia.[4] Another similar case occurred in a patient taking clopidogrel and given **dalteparin**.[5]

Serious retroperitoneal bleeding occurred in a patient with acute coronary syndrome receiving **enoxaparin**, clopidogrel and aspirin.[6]

(b) Ticlopidine

The manufacturer of ticlopidine notes that it has been used concurrently with **heparin** for about 12 hours in studies of cardiac stenting, but that longer-term safety has not been established.[7]

Mechanism

Antiplatelet drugs increase the risk of bleeding, and the risk is likely to be increased further in patients who are anticoagulated with heparin or LMWHs.

Importance and management

The combined use of heparin or LMWHs with antiplatelet drugs such as clopidogrel has been used in specific situations such as acute coronary syndrome. However, unless specifically indicated, concurrent use of heparin or LMWHs with antiplatelet drugs should probably be avoided because of the likely increase in haemorrhagic risk. If they are used together, the manufacturers of the LMWHs (**bemiparin**, **dalteparin**, **enoxaparin**, **tinzaparin**) recommend caution or careful clinical and laboratory monitoring. Heparin and some LMWHs have rarely caused epidural or spinal haematomas resulting in long-term or permanent paralysis when used for thromboprophylaxis in procedures involving spinal/epidural anaesthesia or spinal puncture. The risk of this may be increased if they are used concurrently with other drugs affecting haemostasis such as antiplatelet drugs, and extreme caution is needed if combined use is considered appropriate in these situations.

Consider also 'Heparin and LMWHs + Aspirin', below and 'Glycoprotein IIb/IIIa antagonists + Drugs that affect coagulation', p.703.

1. Caplain H, D'Honneur G, Cariou R. Prolonged heparin administration during clopidogrel treatment in healthy subjects. *Semin Thromb Hemost* (1999) 25 (Suppl 2), 61–4.
2. Plavix (Clopidogrel hydrogen sulfate). Bristol-Myers Squibb Pharmaceuticals Ltd. UK Summary of product characteristics, June 2007.
3. Plavix (Clopidogrel bisulfate). Sanofi-Aventis/Bristol-Myers Squibb Company. US Prescribing information, February 2007.
4. Litz RJ, Gottschlich B, Stehr SN. Spinal epidural hematoma after spinal anesthesia in a patient treated with clopidogrel and enoxaparin. *Anesthesiology* (2004) 101, 1467–70.
5. Tam NLK, Pac-Soo C, Pretorius PM. Epidural haematoma after a combined spinal-epidural anaesthetic in a patient treated with clopidogrel and dalteparin. *Br J Anaesth* (2006) 96, 262–5.
6. Ernits M, Mohan PS, Fares LG, Hardy H. A retroperitoneal bleed induced by enoxaparin therapy. *Am Surg* (2005) 71, 430–3.
7. Ticlid (Ticlopidine hydrochloride). Roche Pharmaceuticals. US Prescribing information, March 2001.

Heparin + Aprotinin

The activated clotting time (ACT) may not be a reliable method to monitor heparin therapy when aprotinin is used concurrently. This is because aprotinin increases the ACT monitored by some methods, without actually increasing anticoagulation.

Clinical evidence, mechanism, importance and management

Aprotinin prolongs the activated clotting time (ACT) as measured by a celite surface activation method, although the kaolin ACT is much less affected.[1] Therefore, if the ACT is used to monitor the effectiveness of heparin anticoagulation during cardiopulmonary bypass incorporating aprotinin, this may lead to an overestimation of the degree of anticoagulation. This may result in patients not receiving additional necessary heparin during extended extracorporeal circulation, or receiving excess protamine to reverse the effects of heparin at the end of the procedure. The UK manufacturer of aprotinin notes that it is not necessary to adjust the usual heparin/protamine regimen used in cardiopulmonary bypass procedures when aprotinin is also used.[2] The US manufacturer provides additional detailed information on appropriate methods to monitor heparin anticoagulation in the presence of aprotinin.[1]

1. Trasylol (Aprotinin). Bayer HealthCare. US Prescribing information, December 2003.
2. Trasylol (Aprotinin). Bayer plc. UK Summary of product characteristics, September 2006.

Heparin and LMWHs + Aspirin

The combined use of aspirin with heparin or low-molecular-weight heparins slightly increases the risk of haemorrhage. Combined use may be a contributing factor to the very rare complication of epidural or spinal haematoma.

Clinical evidence

(a) Heparin

Eight out of 12 patients with hip fractures developed serious bleeding when they were given heparin 5000 units subcutaneously every 12 hours and aspirin 600 mg twice daily as perioperative prophylaxis for deep vein thrombosis. Haematomas of the hip and thigh occurred in 3 patients, bleeding through the wound in 4, and uterine bleeding in the other patient.[1] In a large, randomised, placebo-controlled study, aspirin 500 mg three times daily, subcutaneous heparin 5000 units twice daily, and the combination were compared for prophylaxis of deep vein thrombosis in 1210 patients undergoing surgery. Haemorrhage severe enough to discontinue the prophylaxis occurred in significantly more patients in the combination group (11 of 402 patients versus 3 of 404 patients in the heparin and aspirin alone groups). In addition, minor haemorrhage occurred more frequently in the combination group (89 patients) compared with aspirin alone (41 patients) or heparin alone (30 patients).[2] In another randomised study in patients with acute unstable angina, the combination of aspirin 325 mg twice daily and an intravenous infusion of heparin 1000 units/hour resulted in slightly greater incidence of serious bleeding than either drug alone (3.3% versus 1.7% and 1.7%).[3]

In an epidemiological study of hospitalised patients receiving heparin, the incidence of bleeding was almost 2.4 times higher in 302 patients also receiving aspirin than in 2354 patients not given aspirin (doses not stated). Surgical patients were excluded from this analysis, as were patients with a discharge diagnosis of cancer or haematological disease.[4]

(b) LMWHs

In a crossover study in 9 healthy subjects, bleeding time was prolonged by the use of aspirin 300 mg daily and subcutaneous **reviparin** 6300 units daily, when compared with either drug alone (9.6 minutes versus 5.5 minutes and 5 minutes, respectively). However, the affect of aspirin on platelet aggregation and the effect of **reviparin** on aPTT were not altered by the combination.[5]

During a 5-year period in one hospital, 3 elderly patients had presented with sudden severe abdominal pain after coughing, which was found to be due to a rectus muscle sheath haematoma. These patients had been receiving subcutaneous **enoxaparin** 40 mg once daily for an average of 6 days with aspirin 100 mg daily.[6] Other cases of retroperitonal haematoma have been reported with **enoxaparin** in which aspirin may have been one of various contributing factors.[7-10] Similarly, the use of aspirin may have been one of a number of contributing factors in a case of spinal epidural haematoma occurring with **enoxaparin**.[11]

Mechanism

Aspirin inhibits platelet aggregation and prolongs bleeding times, and increases the risk of upper gastrointestinal haemorrhage, even at doses of 300 mg daily and less.[12] This risk is likely to be higher in patients also taking anticoagulants. See also 'Coumarins and related drugs + Aspirin', p.385.

Importance and management

The combined use of heparin or LMWHs with aspirin is indicated in specific situations such as the prophylaxis of ischaemic complications of unstable angina.[13] However, unless specifically indicated, it may be prudent to avoid the combined use of aspirin with these drugs, because of the likely increased risk of bleeding. If they are used together, the manufacturers of the LMWHs (**bemiparin**, **dalteparin**, **enoxaparin**, **tinzaparin**) recommend caution or careful clinical and laboratory monitoring. Heparin and some LMWHs have rarely caused epidural or spinal haematomas resulting in long-term or permanent paralysis when used for thromboprophylaxis in procedures involving spinal/epidural anaesthesia or spinal puncture. The risk of this may be increased if they are used concurrently with other drugs affecting haemostasis such as aspirin, and extreme caution is needed if combined use is considered appropriate in these situations.

1. Yett HS, Skillman JJ, Salzman EW. The hazards of aspirin plus heparin. *N Engl J Med* (1978) 298, 1092.
2. Vinazzer H, Loew D, Simma W, Brücke P. Prophylaxis of postoperative thromboembolism by low dose heparin and by acetylsalicylic acid given simultaneously. A double-blind study. *Thromb Res* (1980) 17, 177–84.
3. Théroux P, Ouimet H, McCans J, Latour J-G, Joly P, Lévy G, Pelletier E, Juneau M, Stasiak J, deGuise P, Pelletier GB, Rinzler D, Waters DD. Aspirin, heparin, or both to treat acute unstable angina. *N Engl J Med* (1988) 319, 1105–11.
4. Walker AM, Jick H. Predictors of bleeding during heparin therapy. *JAMA* (1980) 244, 1209–12.
5. Klinkhardt U, Breddin HK, Esslinger HU, Haas S, Kalatzis A, Harder S. Interaction between the LMWH reviparin and aspirin in healthy volunteers. *Br J Clin Pharmacol* (2000) 49, 337–41.
6. Macías-Robles MD, Peliz MG, Gonzalez-Ordonez AJ. Prophylaxis with enoxaparin can produce a giant abdominal wall haematoma when associated with low doses of aspirin among elderly patients suffering cough attacks. *Blood Coagul Fibrinolysis* (2005) 16, 217–19.
7. Melde SL. Enoxaparin-induced retroperitoneal hematoma. *Ann Pharmacother* (2003) 37, 822–4.
8. Kavanagh D, Hill ADK, Martin S, Power C, McDermott EW, O'Higgins N, Murphy K. Life threatening haemorrhagic events associated with the administration of low-molecular-weight-heparin. *Thromb Haemost* (2004) 91, 833–4.
9. Malik A, Capling R, Bastani B. Enoxaparin-associated retroperitoneal bleeding in two patients with renal insufficiency. *Pharmacotherapy* (2005) 25, 769–72.
10. Ernits M, Mohan PS, Fares LG, Hardy H. A retroperitoneal bleed induced by enoxaparin therapy. *Am Surg* (2005) 71, 430–3.
11. Chan L, Bailin MT. Spinal epidural hematoma following central neuraxial blockade and subcutaneous enoxaparin: a case report. *J Clin Anesth* (2004) 16, 382–5.
12. Weil J, Colin-Jones D, Langman M, Lawson D, Logan R, Murphy M, Rawlins M, Vessey M, Wainwright P. Prophylactic aspirin and risk of peptic ulcer bleeding. *BMJ* (1995) 310: 827–30.
13. Harrington RA, Becker RC, Ezekowitz M, Meade TW, O'Connor CM, Vorchheimer DA, Guyatt GH. Antithrombotic therapy for coronary artery disease: the seventh ACCP conference on antithrombotic and thrombolytic therapy. *Chest* (2004) 126 (Suppl), 513S–548S. Available at http://www.chestjournal.org/cgi/content/full/126/3_suppl/513S (accessed 17/08/07).

Heparin + Dextrans

Additive effects on coagulation occur when heparin is given with dextrans.

Clinical evidence, mechanism, importance and management

A study in 9 patients with peripheral vascular disease given 500 mL of dextran showed that the mean clotting time 1 hour after an infusion of 10 000 units of heparin was increased from 36 to 69 minutes. Dextran alone had no effect, but the mean clotting time after 5000 units of heparin with dextran was almost the same as after 10 000 units of heparin alone.[1,2] This study would seem to support two other reports[3,4] of an increase in the incidence of bleeding in those given both heparin and dextran 70. Uneventful concurrent use[5,6] has been described with dextran 40. Note that this is probably of little clinical significance if these drugs are given for their anticoagulant effects; however, increased anticoagulation may be undesirable if dextran 40 is given as a volume expander to a patient already receiving heparin. In this situation some caution is warranted.

1. Atik M. Potentiation of heparin by dextran and its clinical implication. *Thromb Haemost* (1977) 38, 275.
2. Atik M. Personal communication, April 1980.
3. Bloom WL, Brewer SS. The independent yet synergistic effects of heparin and dextran. *Acta Chir Scand* (1968) 387 (Suppl), 53–7.
4. Morrison ND, Stephenson CBS, Maclean D, Stanhope JM. Deep vein thrombosis after femoropopliteal bypass grafting with observations on the incidence of complications following the use of dextran 70. *N Z Med J* (1976) 84, 233–6.
5. Schöndorf TH, Weber U. Prevention of deep vein thrombosis in orthopedic surgery with the combination of low dose heparin plus either dihydroergotamine or dextran. *Scand J Haematol* (1980) 36 (Suppl), 126–40.
6. Serjeant JCB. Mesenteric embolus treated with low-molecular weight dextran. *Lancet* (1965) i, 139–40.

Heparin + LMWHs

There is some evidence that patients receiving enoxaparin preoperatively require more heparin during surgery.

Clinical evidence, mechanism, importance and management

In a clinical study, 30 patients with unstable coronary disease treated preoperatively with **enoxaparin** needed more heparin to maintain an activated clotting time above 480 seconds during surgery than 31 stable control patients not treated with enoxaparin. In addition, the **enoxaparin** recipients had higher heparin levels and lower antithrombin values compared with control patients. All patients were taking low-dose aspirin until the day before surgery, and received tranexamic acid as a bolus dose before cardiopulmonary bypass.[1]

Reasons for these differences are unclear, and their clinical relevance is uncertain. Further study is needed.

1. Pleym H, Videm V, Wahba A, Åsberg A, Amundsen T, Bjella L, Dale O, Stenseth R. Heparin resistance and increased platelet activation in coronary surgery patients treated with enoxaparin preoperatively. *Eur J Cardiothorac Surg* (2006) 29, 933–40.

Heparin + Miscellaneous

Changes in the protein binding of diazepam, propranolol, quinidine and verapamil caused by heparin do not appear to be of clinical importance.

Clinical evidence, mechanism, importance and management

A number of studies have found that heparin reduces the plasma protein binding of several drugs including **diazepam**,[1,2] **propranolol**,[1] **quinidine**[3] and **verapamil**[4] in man and in *animals*. For example, 3 patients taking oral **propranolol** and 5 patients given intramuscular **diazepam** 10 mg were given 3000 units of heparin just before cardiac catheterisation. Five minutes after the heparin was given, the free fraction of **diazepam** was found to have risen fourfold (from 1.8 to 7.9%) while the free **diazepam** levels had risen from 2 to 8.4 nanograms/mL. The free fraction of the **propranolol** rose from 7.4 to 12.5% and the free levels rose from 1.7 to 2.7 nanograms/mL.[1]

It was suggested that these changes occur because heparin displaces these drugs from their binding sites on the plasma albumins and that these changes in protein binding might possibly have some clinical consequences. For example, there could, theoretically, be sudden increases in sedation or respiratory depression because of the rapid increase in the active (free) fraction of **diazepam**.

However, these changes are unlikely to be of clinical importance (see 'Protein-binding interactions', (p.3)). One study even suggested that the heparin-induced protein binding changes are an artefact of the study methods used,[5] and this would seem to be supported by an experimental study, which found that heparin did not have any effect on the beta-blockade caused by **propranolol**.[6] Moreover there seem to be no other reports confirming that these interactions are of real clinical importance. No special precautions would seem to be necessary.

1. Wood AJJ, Robertson D, Robertson RM, Wilkinson GR, Wood M. Elevated plasma free drug concentrations of propranolol and diazepam during cardiac catheterization. *Circulation* (1980) 62, 1119–22.
2. Routledge PA, Kitchell BB, Bjornsson TD, Skinnner T, Linnoila M, Shand DG. Diazepam and *N*-desmethyldiazepam redistribution after heparin. *Clin Pharmacol Ther* (1980) 27, 528–32.
3. Kessler KM, Leech RC, Spann JF. Blood collection techniques, heparin and quinidine protein binding. *Clin Pharmacol Ther* (1979) 25, 204–10.
4. Keefe DL, Yee Y-G, Kates RE. Verapamil protein binding in patients and normal subjects. *Clin Pharmacol Ther* (1981) 29, 21–6.
5. Brown JE, Kitchell BB, Bjornsson TD, Shand DG. The artifactual nature of heparin-induced drug protein-binding alterations. *Clin Pharmacol Ther* (1981) 30, 636–43.
6. DeLeve LD, Piafsky KM. Lack of heparin effect on propranolol-induced β-adrenoceptor blockade. *Clin Pharmacol Ther* (1982) 31, 216.

Heparin + Nitrates

The effects of heparin were reduced by the infusion of glyceryl trinitrate in some studies, but other studies have failed to confirm this interaction. On balance, the evidence favours there being no clinically important interaction. No interaction has been seen with heparin and isosorbide dinitrate or molsidomine.

Clinical evidence

(a) Glyceryl trinitrate (Nitroglycerin)

An interaction between heparin and glyceryl trinitrate was originally reported[1] in 1985. They found a lower aPTT value in patients receiving both intravenous glyceryl trinitrate and heparin, when compared with control patients receiving heparin alone. In a study in healthy subjects, they found the same effect with the propylene glycol diluent alone, so attributed the interaction to the diluent.[1] However, in another study, the same interaction was noted in 2 patients receiving a glyceryl trinitrate preparation without propylene glycol. In this study, while receiving intravenous glyceryl trinitrate, 7 patients with coronary artery disease needed an increased dose of intravenous heparin to achieve satisfactory aPTT ratios of 1.5 to 2.5 on eight occasions. When the glyceryl trinitrate was stopped, in 6 out of 8 occasions there was a marked increase in aPTT values to 3.5. One patient had transient haematuria.[2]

Four other studies have also shown a reduction in the effects of heparin in the presence of intravenous glyceryl trinitrate.[3-6] In one of these, the PT of 27 patients given heparin was more than halved (from 130 to about 60 seconds) when they were given intravenous glyceryl trinitrate 2 to 5 mg/hour. The PT rose again when the glyceryl trinitrate was stopped.[3] In one study, there was some evidence that the effect might occur only at higher doses of intravenous glyceryl trinitrate (above 350 micrograms/minute),[5] whereas in another, an effect was seen at low doses of 25 to 50 micrograms/minute.[6]

In contrast to the above studies, a total of 12 other studies have found no changes in aPTT in patients[7-16] or healthy subjects[17,18] given intravenous glyceryl trinitrate with heparin. In the randomised, placebo-controlled studies in healthy subjects, a 60-minute infusion of glyceryl trinitrate 5 mg had no effect on the aPTT or PT following a 5000 unit intravenous injection of heparin,[17] and a 100 micrograms/minute infusion of glyceryl trinitrate did not alter the anticoagulant effect of a 40 units/kg bolus of heparin in 7 healthy subjects.[18] Two randomised, placebo-controlled studies in patients have also failed to find an effect of intravenous glyceryl trinitrate on a heparin infusion titrated to a given effect,[12] or on an intravenous heparin bolus dose.[14] In the first of these studies, the glyceryl trinitrate preparation contained propylene glycol.[12]

(b) Isosorbide dinitrate

In a randomised, placebo-controlled study in 12 patients receiving a stable infusion of heparin, the use of isosorbide dinitrate 4.8 ± 0.8 mg/hour for 24 hours did not alter the AUC of PT values, when compared with placebo, nor was there any change in PT values in the 5 hours after stopping the nitrate.[12] Similarly, other studies have failed to find an important change in anticoagulation when intravenous isosorbide dinitrate is given with heparin.[8,14,16]

(c) Molsidomine

In a study in 15 patients treated with intravenous heparin then given intravenous molsidomine 2 mg/hour, molsidomine had no effect on the PT.[19]

Mechanism

Not understood. One study suggests that what occurs is related to a glyceryl trinitrate-induced antithrombin III abnormality, and is apparent at doses above 350 micrograms/minute.[5] One study found that heparin levels were lowered,[6] whereas another reported unchanged heparin levels.[3]

Importance and management

The discord between these reports is not understood. However, the best controlled studies in the largest number of patients have failed to find evidence of an interaction. On balance therefore, it appears that a clinically relevant interaction is generally unlikely to be seen. Moreover, given that heparin is routinely monitored, it is likely that if any interaction occurs, it will be rapidly detected and compensated for. No special precautions would appear to be needed if heparin is given with molsidomine or isosorbide dinitrate.

1. Col J, Col-Debeys C, Lavenne-Pardonge E, Meert P, Hericks L, Broze MC, Moriau M. Propylene glycol-induced heparin resistance during nitroglycerin infusion. *Am Heart J* (1985) 110, 171–3.
2. Habbab MA, Haft JI. Heparin resistance induced by intravenous nitroglycerin. A word of caution when both drugs are used concomitantly. *Arch Intern Med* (1987) 147, 857–60.
3. Pizzulli L, Nitsch J, Lüderitz B. Hemmung der Heparinwirkung durch Glyceroltrinitrat. *Dtsch Med Wochenschr* (1988) 113, 1837–40.
4. Dascalov TN, Chaushev AG, Petrov AB, Stancheva LG, Stanachcova SD, Ivanov AA. Nitroglycerin inhibition of the heparin effect in acute myocardial infarction patients. *Eur Heart J* (1990) 11 (Abstract Suppl), 321.
5. Becker RC, Corrao JM, Bovill EG, Gore JM, Baker SP, Miller ML, Lucas FV, Alpert JA. Intravenous nitroglycerin-induced heparin resistance: a qualitative antithrombin III abnormality. *Am Heart J* (1990) 119, 1254–61.
6. Brack MJ, More RS, Hubner PJB, Gerschlick AH. The effect of low dose nitroglycerine on plasma heparin concentrations and activated partial thromboplastin times. *Blood Coag Fibrinol* (1993) 4, 183–6.
7. Lepor NE, Amin DK, Berberian L, Shah PK. Does nitroglycerin induce heparin resistance? *Clin Cardiol* (1989) 12, 432–4.
8. Pye M, Olroyd KG, Conkie J, Hutton I, Cobbe SM. A clinical and in vitro study on the possible interaction of intravenous nitrates with heparin anticoagulation. *Clin Cardiol* (1994) 17, 658–61.
9. Gonzalez ER, Jones HD, Graham S, Elswick RK. Assessment of the drug interaction between intravenous nitroglycerin and heparin. *Ann Pharmacother* (1992) 26, 1512–14.
10. Reich DL, Hammerschlag BC, Rand JH, Perucho-Powell MH, Thys DM. Modest doses of nitroglycerin do not interfere with beef lung heparin anticoagulation in patients taking nitrates. *J Cardiothorac Vasc Anesth* (1992) 6, 677–9
11. Nottestad SY, Mascette AM. Nitroglycerin-induced resistance: absence of interaction at clinically relevant doses. *Mil Med* (1994) 159, 569–71.
12. Bechtold H, Kleist P, Landgraf K, Möser K. Einfluß einer niedrigdosierten intravenösen Nitrattherapie auf die antikoagulatorische Wirkung von Heparin. *Med Klin* (1994) 89, 360–6.
13. Berk SI, Grunwald A, Pal S, Bodenheimer MM. Effect of intravenous nitroglycerin on heparin dosage requirements in coronary artery disease. *Am J Cardiol* (1993) 72, 393–6.
14. Muikku O. Isosorbide dinitrate does not interfere with heparin anticoagulation: a placebo-controlled comparison with nitroglycerin in patients scheduled for coronary artery surgery. *Acta Anaesthesiol Scand* (1994) 38, 583–6.
15. Williams H, Langlosi PF, Kelly JL. The effect of simultaneous intravenous administration of nitroglycerin and heparin on partial thromboplastin time. *Mil Med* (1995) 160, 449–52.
16. Koh KK, Park GS, Song JH, Moon TH, In HH, Kim JJ, Lee HJ, Cho SK, Kim SS. Interaction of intravenous heparin and organic nitrates in acute ischemic syndromes. *Am J Cardiol* (1995) 76, 706–9.
17. Bode V, Welzel D, Franz G, Polensky U. Absence of drug interaction between heparin and nitroglycerin. *Arch Intern Med* (1990) 150, 2117–19.
18. Schoenenberger RA, Ménat L, Weiss P, Marbet GA, Ritz R. Absence of nitroglycerin-induced heparin resistance in healthy volunteers. *Eur Heart J* (1992) 13, 411–14.
19. Wiemer M, Pizzulli L, Reichert H, Lüderitz B. Gibt es eine Wechselwirkung zwischen Heparin und Moldisomin?. *Med Klin* (1994) 89, 45–6.

Heparin and LMWHs + NSAIDs

The bleeding time was prolonged by the concurrent use of dalteparin and ketorolac in healthy subjects, but not by the use of heparin and ketorolac. Parecoxib did not alter the effect of heparin on aPTT. In a small clinical study, intramuscular ketorolac and subcutaneous enoxaparin appeared not to increase measures of postoperative bleeding when compared with opioids. Cases of spinal haematomas have been reported with concurrent use of heparin or low-molecular-weight heparins and NSAIDs. Note that ketorolac may possibly cause serious gastrointestinal bleeding and in the UK it is considered to be contraindicated in patients taking anticoagulants.

Clinical evidence

(a) Ibuprofen

Use of **heparin** and ibuprofen were considered to be contributing factors in a case of spinal haematoma occurring after epidural anaesthesia.[1]

(b) Ketorolac

1. Heparin. In a crossover, placebo-controlled study in healthy subjects, there was no evidence of an interaction between ketorolac and heparin in terms of prolongation of skin bleeding time, platelet aggregation, anti-factor Xa activity, or kaolin-cephalin clotting time. In this study, two doses of oral ketorolac were given (the previous evening, and in the morning), then two 10-mg intramuscular doses of ketorolac were given at 10 am and 2 pm, with simultaneous doses of subcutaneous heparin 5000 units.[2]

2. Low-molecular-weight heparins. In a crossover, placebo-controlled study in healthy subjects, giving ketorolac with **dalteparin** resulted in prolongation of the skin bleeding time, when compared with ketorolac alone (13.95 minutes versus 10.55 minutes). **Dalteparin** alone had no effect on the bleeding time when compared with placebo. In this study, two doses of oral ketorolac 30 mg were given the day before, and one dose an hour after a single 5000-unit subcutaneous dose of **dalteparin**. The combination did not have any greater effect on platelet aggregation, anti-factor Xa activity or aPTT time than the individual drugs alone.[3]

However, a study in hip replacement patients given subcutaneous **enoxaparin** 40 mg once daily found that there were no significant differences in intra-operative blood loss, post-operative drainage, transfusion requirements, bruising, wound oozing, and leg swelling between 34 patients given intramuscular ketorolac 30 mg on induction of anaesthesia then once daily for 4 days postoperatively and 26 patients given unnamed opioids. Patients in this study had any previous NSAID medication stopped 4 weeks before admission, and were not taking aspirin.[4]

The use of **enoxaparin**, ketorolac, and aspirin were considered to be contributing factors in a case of spinal haematoma occurring after lumbar puncture, which resulted in paraplegia.[5] Another case has also been briefly described.[6] In an analysis of reports from the FDA in the US, 16 of 43 patients who developed spinal or epidural haematoma after receiving **enoxaparin** had received concurrent drugs known to prolong bleeding, such as ketorolac or other NSAIDs.[7]

(c) Parecoxib

In an open-label, crossover study in 18 healthy subjects, administration of **heparin** on day 5 of treatment with 40 mg of intravenous parecoxib twice daily for 6 days produced no clinically or statistically significant differences in coagulation parameters (PT, aPTT and platelet counts), when compared with **heparin** alone (bolus dose of heparin 4000 units then a 36-hour infusion of 10 to 14 units/kg). Use of these drugs together was well tolerated. However, prolongation of bleeding time was not assessed.[8]

Mechanism

NSAIDs, to a greater or lesser extent irritate the stomach lining, which can result in gastrointestinal bleeding, which will be more severe in anticoagulated patients. Many also have antiplatelet activity, which can prolong bleeding times.

Importance and management

The CSM in the UK and the UK manufacturers say that ketorolac is contraindicated with anticoagulants, including **low-dose heparin**.[9,10] Conversely, the US manufacturers of ketorolac advise that physicians should carefully weigh the benefits against the risks and use concurrent heparin only extremely cautiously.[11]

If NSAIDs and LMWHs are used together, the manufacturers of the LMWHs (**bemiparin**, **dalteparin**, **enoxaparin**, **tinzaparin**) recommend caution or careful clinical and laboratory monitoring. Heparin and some LMWHs have rarely caused epidural or spinal haematomas resulting in long-term or permanent paralysis when used for thromboprophylaxis in procedures involving spinal/epidural anaesthesia or spinal puncture. The risk of this may be increased if they are used concurrently with other drugs affecting haemostasis such as ketorolac or other NSAIDs, and extreme caution is needed if combined use is considered appropriate in these situations.

1. Litz RJ, Hübler M, Koch T, Albrecht DM. Spinal-epidural hematoma following epidural anesthesia in the presence of antiplatelet and heparin therapy. *Anesthesiology* (2001) 95, 1031–3.
2. Spowart K, Greer IA, McLaren M, Lloyd J, Bullingham RES, Forbes CD. Haemostatic effects of ketorolac with and without concomitant heparin in normal volunteers. *Thromb Haemost* (1988) 60, 382–6.
3. Greer IA, Gibson JL, Young A, Johnstone J, Walker ID. Effect of ketorolac and low-molecular-weight heparin individually and in combination on haemostasis. *Blood Coag Fibrinol* (1999) 10, 367–73.
4. Weale AE, Warwick DJ, Durant N, Prothero D. Is there a clinically significant interaction between low molecular weight heparin and non-steroidal analgesics after total hip replacement? *Ann R Coll Surg Engl* (1995) 77, 35–7.
5. Chan L, Bailin MT. Spinal epidural hematoma following central neuraxial blockade and subcutaneous enoxaparin: a case report. *J Clin Anesth* (2004) 16, 382–5.
6. Price AJ, Obeid D. Is there a clinical interaction between low molecular weight heparin and non-steroidal analgesics after total hip replacement? *Ann R Coll Surg Engl* (1995) 77, 395.
7. Wysowski DK, Talarico L, Bacsanyi J, Botstein P. Spinal and epidural hematoma and low-molecular-weight heparin. *N Engl J Med* (1998) 338, 1774–5.
8. Noveck RJ, Hubbard RC. Parecoxib sodium, an injectable COX-2 specific inhibitor, does not affect unfractionated heparin-regulated blood coagulation parameters. *J Clin Pharmacol* (2004) 44, 474–80.
9. Committee on Safety of Medicines/Medicines Control Agency. Ketorolac: new restrictions on dose and duration of treatment. *Current Problems* (1993) 19, 5–6.
10. Toradol (Ketorolac trometamol). Roche Products Ltd. UK Summary of product characteristics, May 2007.
11. Toradol (Ketorolac tromethamine). Roche Pharmaceuticals. US Prescribing information, September 2002.

Heparin + Probenecid

An isolated case report from the 1950s suggests that the effects of heparin may be possibly increased by probenecid, and bleeding may occur.

Clinical evidence, mechanism, importance and management

In 1950 (but not reported until 1975) a woman with subacute bacterial endocarditis was given probenecid orally and penicillin by intravenous drip, which was kept open with minimal doses of heparin. After a total of about 20 000 units of heparin had been given over a 3-week period, increasing epistaxes developed and the clotting time was found to be 24 minutes (normal 5 to 6 minutes). This was controlled with protamine.[1] However, no reports of this interaction appear to have been made subsequently. This interaction seems unlikely to be of general significance.

1. Sanchez G. Enhancement of heparin effect by probenecid. *N Engl J Med* (1975) 292, 48.

Heparin and LMWHs + SSRIs

Severe bleeding was attributed to the use of tinzaparin in an elderly woman with renal impairment taking fluoxetine.

Clinical evidence, mechanism, importance and management

A 78-year-old woman taking **fluoxetine** was started on once-daily subcutaneous injections of weight-adjusted **tinzaparin** for treatment of deep vein thrombosis. Five days later she suffered a massive intraperitoneal and parietal haematoma. Poor renal function in this patient could have led to accumulation of the low-molecular-weight heparin, but **fluoxetine** was also considered a contributing factor because SSRIs have antiplatelet effects and can contribute to bleeding.[1] Consider also 'Coumarins and related drugs + SSRIs', p.448.

1. de Maistre E, Allart C, Lecompte T, Bollaert P-E. Severe bleeding associated with use of low molecular weight heparin and selective serotonin reuptake inhibitors. *Am J Med* (2002) 113, 530–2.

Heparin + Tobacco

In one study, patients who smoked tobacco had a shorter heparin half-life. However, smoking status is probably not important in predicting heparin dose.

Clinical evidence, mechanism, importance and management

In a study of the factors affecting the sensitivity of individuals to heparin, the heparin half-life in **smokers** was 0.62 hours compared with 0.97 hours in non-smokers. The dosage requirements of the smokers were slightly increased (18.8 compared with 16 units/hour per lean body weight). However, when lean body weight was taken into account, smoking status was no longer related to heparin clearance.[1] Therefore, smoking status is probably not important in predicting heparin dose.

1. Cipolle RJ, Seifert RD, Neilan BA, Zaske DE, Haus E. Heparin kinetics: variables related to disposition and dosage. *Clin Pharmacol Ther* (1981) 29, 387–93.

Heparinoids; Danaparoid + Antiplatelet drugs and NSAIDs

No haemostatic interaction was noted between danaparoid and aspirin in healthy volunteers. However, caution is recommended on combined use because of the possibility of increased bleeding risk.

Clinical evidence

In a randomised, crossover study in healthy subjects, there were no important alterations in coagulation tests and plasma anti-Xa activity when danaparoid (3250 anti-Xa units intravenous bolus followed by 750 units subcutaneously twice daily for 8 days) was given with **aspirin** 500 mg, 14 and 2 hours before the intravenous danaparoid. Similarly, danaparoid did not alter the effects of **aspirin** on platelet function, but the prolongation in bleeding time tended to be longer after the combination.[1]

Mechanism

The manufacturer notes that, in general, combination with antithrombotics that act by other mechanisms, such as aspirin, would be additive.[2]

Importance and management

Any effects in the study with aspirin where not considered to be clinically relevant.[1,2] The manufacturer notes that danaparoid may be used with drugs that interfere with platelet function, such as aspirin and NSAIDs, but considers that caution remains necessary.[2,3] This is considered particularly important in patients undergoing peridural or spinal anaesthesia or spinal puncture, in whom the use of NSAIDs, and probably also danaparoid, are risk factors for epidural or spinal haematoma resulting in prolonged or permanent paralysis.[2,3]

1. de Boer A, Danhof M, Cohen AF, Magnani HN, Breimer DD. Interaction study between Org 10172, a low molecular weight heparinoid, and acetylsalicylic acid in healthy male volunteers. *Thromb Haemost* (1991) 66, 202–7.
2. Orgaran (Danaparoid sodium). Organon Canada Ltd. Canadian product monograph, June 2001.
3. Orgaran (Danaparoid sodium). Organon Laboratories Ltd. UK Summary of product characteristics, July 2003.

Heparinoids; Danaparoid + Diuretics

Chlortalidone had no clinically relevant effect on the anti-Xa activity of danaparoid in healthy volunteers, but caused an increase in the volume of distribution of antithrombin activity of uncertain relevance. Nevertheless, in clinical use danaparoid is frequently used with a number of other drugs including diuretics, and there is no evidence of an interaction.

Clinical evidence, mechanism, importance and management

In a randomised, crossover study in healthy subjects, a slight decrease in clearance (7%) and volume of distribution (19%) of the anti-Xa activity of danaparoid (3250 anti-Xa units intravenous bolus) occurred when it was given about 12 hours after a single 100-mg dose of chlortalidone. Conversely, the apparent volume of distribution of antithrombin activity showed an 80% increase. However, chlortalidone did not change the effect of danaparoid on clotting tests, except for a 4% increase in prothrombin time, which was thought to be a spurious finding.[1] The reasons for these changes are uncertain.

The minor changes in anti-Xa activity are unlikely to be clinically relevant.[1,2] However, the authors considered that relevance of the change in antithrombin activity was uncertain.[1] Nevertheless, the manufacturer notes that in clinical use danaparoid has frequently been used with a variety of drugs, including diuretics, and that there is no evidence of any direct interaction with danaparoid.[2]

1. de Boer A, Stiekema JC, Danhof M, Breimer DD. Influence of chlorthalidone on the pharmacokinetics and pharmacodynamics of Org 10172 (Lomoparan®), a low molecular weight heparinoid, in healthy volunteers. *J Clin Pharmacol* (1991) 31, 611–17.
2. Orgaran (Danaparoid). Organon Canada Ltd. Canadian product monograph, June 2001.

Heparinoids; Danaparoid + Penicillins

Cloxacillin and ticarcillin caused an increase in elimination half-life of anti-Xa activity of danaparoid, which was not considered clinically relevant. Ticarcillin had no effect on haemostasis, but cloxacillin appeared to have some pro-coagulant effects, which were not likely to be due to an interaction with danaparoid. The manufacturer notes that in clinical use danaparoid is frequently used with a number of other drugs, including antibacterials, and there is no evidence of a direct interaction.

Clinical evidence

(a) Cloxacillin

In a randomised, crossover study in 6 healthy subjects, there was a 74% increase in the elimination half-life of the plasma anti-Xa activity of danaparoid (3250 anti-Xa units intravenous bolus) when combined with oral cloxacillin 500 mg four times daily for 3 days beginning 24 hours before the danaparoid. Unexpectedly, there were slight decreased effects on thrombin time and bleeding time, and increased effects on aPTT with the combination, effects that were attributed to cloxacillin alone.[1]

(b) Ticarcillin

In a randomised, crossover study in 12 healthy subjects, there was a 56% increase in the elimination half-life of the plasma anti-Xa activity of danaparoid (3250 anti-Xa units intravenous bolus) when combined with intravenous ticarcillin 4 g four times daily for 2 days beginning immediately before the danaparoid. There were no changes in haemostatic parameters when ticarcillin was given with danaparoid.[1]

Mechanism

Uncertain, but penicillins might compete with danaparoid for renal tubular secretion.[1]

Importance and management

The pharmacokinetic changes seen in the studies with cloxacillin and ticarcillin were not considered clinically relevant.[1,2] In addition, the haemostatic changes seen in the study with cloxacillin were unlikely to be due to an interaction.[1] The manufacturer notes that in clinical use danaparoid has frequently been used with a variety of drugs, including antibacterials, and that there is no evidence of any direct interaction with danaparoid.[2]

1. de Boer A, Stiekema JCJ, Danhof M, van Dinther TG, Boeijinga JK, Cohen AF, Breimer DD. Studies of interaction of a low-molecular-weight heparinoid (Org 10172), with cloxacillin and ticarcillin in healthy male volunteers. *Antimicrob Agents Chemother* (1991) 35, 2110–15.
2. Orgaran (Danaparoid). Organon Canada Ltd. Canadian product monograph, June 2001.

Indanediones + Haloperidol

A single case report describes a marked reduction in the anticoagulant effects of phenindione in a patient given haloperidol.

Clinical evidence, mechanism, importance and management

A man stabilised on **phenindione** 50 mg daily was given haloperidol by injection (5 mg every 8 hours for 24 hours) followed by 3 mg twice daily by mouth. Adequate anticoagulation was not achieved even when the **phenindione** dosage was increased to 150 mg daily. When the haloperidol dosage was halved, the necessary dose of anticoagulant was reduced to 100 mg daily, and only when the haloperidol was withdrawn was it possible to achieve adequate anticoagulation with the original dosage.[1] The reasons for this are not understood. This appears to be the only report of an interaction, and its general importance is therefore limited. Bear it in mind in the event of an unexpected response to treatment.

1. Oakley DP, Lautch H. Haloperidol and anticoagulant treatment. *Lancet* (1963) ii, 1231.

Indanediones + Oxaceprol

An isolated report describes a marked fall in the response to fluindione in a patient given oxaceprol.

Clinical evidence, mechanism, importance and management

A 77-year-old woman with hypertension and atrial fibrillation, taking propafenone, furosemide, enalapril and **fluindione** 15 mg daily, started taking oxaceprol 300 mg daily. Within 2 days her Quick Time had risen from 26 to 57% and by the end of the week to 65%. When the oxaceprol was withdrawn, her Quick value returned to its previous values of 23 to 30%.[1] The mechanism is not understood. The general importance of this interaction is not known but bear it in mind when prescribing oxaceprol and **fluindione**. Be alert for the need to modify the anticoagulant dosage.

1. Bannwarth B, Tréchot P, Mathieu J, Froment J, Netter P. Interaction oxacéprol-fluindione. *Therapie* (1990) 45, 162–3.

Thrombin inhibitors + Antiplatelet drugs and Thrombolytics

Low-dose aspirin did not alter the pharmacokinetics or pharmacodynamic effects of argatroban. Neither abciximab nor eptifibatide appeared to alter argatroban pharmacokinetics. There is no pharmacodynamic interaction between bivalirudin and aspirin, ticlopidine, clopidogrel, abciximab, eptifibatide or tirofiban. Nevertheless, the manufacturers warn of the increased bleeding risks if argatroban, bivalirudin or lepirudin are used with antiplatelet drugs or thrombolytics.

Clinical evidence, mechanism, importance and management

(a) Argatroban

1. Antiplatelet drugs. In a study in healthy subjects, pretreatment with oral **aspirin** 162.5 mg, given 26 and 2 hours prior to argatroban 1 microgram/kg per minute over 4 hours, caused no changes in the pharmacokinetics or pharmacodynamic effects of the argatroban.[1]

In a large clinical study of the combination of argatroban and a glycoprotein IIb/IIIa-receptor antagonist (**abciximab** or **eptifibatide**) in patients undergoing percutaneous coronary intervention, using a population model assessment, the pharmacokinetics of argatroban were similar to those previously seen in healthy subjects. This suggests that neither **abciximab** nor **eptifibatide** alter argatroban pharmacokinetics.[2]

Nevertheless, the manufacturer warns that the use of argatroban with **antiplatelet drugs** may increase the risk of bleeding.[3]

2. Thrombolytics. The manufacturer notes that, in patients with acute myocardial infarction, the incidence of intracranial bleeding was 1% (8 out of 810 patients) in patients receiving both argatroban and thrombolytic therapy (**streptokinase** or **alteplase**).[3] They therefore state that the safety and effectiveness of argatroban with thrombolytics has not been established, and that concurrent use may increase the risk of bleeding.[3]

(b) Bivalirudin

1. Antiplatelet drugs. The UK manufacturer says that no pharmacodynamic interactions were detected when bivalirudin was used with platelet inhibitors, including **aspirin**, **ticlopidine**, **clopidogrel**, **abciximab**, **eptifibatide**, or **tirofiban**.[4] The US manufacturer states that bivalirudin is intended for use with **aspirin** 300 to 325 mg daily, and has been studied only in patients receiving **aspirin**.[5] Both manufacturers state that bivalirudin may be used with a glycoprotein IIb/IIIa-receptor antagonist[4,5] (e.g. **abciximab**, **eptifibatide**, **tirofiban**). Nevertheless, the US manufacturer states that in clinical studies, the concurrent use of bivalirudin with these inhibitors was associated with increased risks of major bleeding events compared to patients not receiving them.[5] The UK manufacturer recommends regular monitoring of haemostasis when bivalirudin is used with platelet inhibitors.[4]

2. Thrombolytics. In the US, the manufacturers state that the concurrent use of bivalirudin with thrombolytics was associated with increased risks of major bleeding events.[5]

(c) Lepirudin

The manufacturers of lepirudin say that no formal interaction studies have been done but they reasonably warn that the concurrent use of lepirudin and other thrombolytics (they name **alteplase** and **streptokinase**) may increase the risk of bleeding complications and considerably enhance the effect of lepirudin on the aPTT. They also warn about the increased risks of bleeding if antiplatelet drugs such as **clopidogrel**, **ticlopidine**, **abciximab**, **eptifibatide** or **tirofiban** are used concurrently.[6,7]

1. Clarke RJ, Mayo G, FitzGerald GA, Fitzgerald DJ. Combined administration of aspirin and a specific thrombin inhibitor in man. *Circulation* (1991) 83, 1510–8.
2. Cox DS, Kleiman NS, Boyle DA, Aluri J, Parchman G, Holdbrook F, Fossler MJ. Pharmacokinetics and pharmacodynamics of argatroban in combination with a platelet glycoprotein IIB/IIIA receptor antagonist in patients undergoing percutaneous coronary intervention. *J Clin Pharmacol* (2004) 44, 981–90.
3. Argatroban. GlaxoSmithKline. US Prescribing information, July 2005.
4. Angiox (Bivalirudin). Nycomed UK Ltd. UK Summary of product characteristics, March 2007.
5. Angiomax (Bivalirudin). The Medicines Company. US Prescribing information, December 2005.
6. Refludan (Lepirudin). Pharmion Ltd. UK Summary of product characteristics, April 2002.
7. Refludan (Lepirudin). Bayer HealthCare Pharmaceuticals Inc. US Prescribing information, November 2006.

Thrombin inhibitors + Other anticoagulants

Use of argatroban with warfarin and related oral anticoagulants has an effect on the measurement of the INR, and the manufacturer provides equations to adjust for this. Argatroban does not alter warfarin pharmacokinetics. The manufacturers warn of the increased bleeding risks if argatroban, bivalirudin or lepirudin are used with other anticoagulants.

Clinical evidence, mechanism, importance and management

(a) Argatroban

In 12 healthy subjects, argatroban 1.25 micrograms/kg per minute was given for 100 hours, with a single 7.5-mg dose of **warfarin** given at hour 4. Neither drug affected the pharmacokinetics of the other. The single dose of **warfarin** in this study did not add to the anticoagulant effect of argatroban.[1] However, a previous study found that the INR and prothrombin time were increased when **warfarin** (7.5 mg on day one, then 3 to 6 mg for 9 days) was used with argatroban (1 to 4 micrograms/kg per minute for 5 hours daily for 11 days), but without any additional effect on vitamin K-dependent factor Xa activity.[2] A similar finding was reported in a study using **acenocoumarol** or **phenprocoumon** and argatroban.[3] This means that the INR reading needs to be corrected before it can be used as a clinical indicator of coagulation status when **warfarin** or other vitamin K antagonists (i.e. the **indanediones**) are used with argatroban. The manufacturer provides detailed information on how this should be done while switching from argatroban to **warfarin**.[4]

Argatroban is currently licensed for use in patients with or at risk of heparin-induced thrombocytopenia, hence it is unlikely to be used with heparin. Nevertheless, the manufacturer states that if **heparin** is to be switched to argatroban, allow sufficient time for heparin's effect on the aPTT to decrease before starting argatroban.[4]

(b) Bivalirudin

In the US, the manufacturers state that concurrent use of bivalirudin with **heparin** or **warfarin** was associated with increased risks of major bleeding events, when compared to patients not receiving these concurrent drugs.[5] In the UK, the manufacturers state that bivalirudin can be started

30 minutes after stopping intravenous **heparin**, but 8 hours should be left after stopping a **low-molecular-weight heparin** given subcutaneously.[6] They recommend regular monitoring of haemostasis when bivalirudin is used with other anticoagulants.[6]

(c) Lepirudin

The manufacturers of lepirudin say that no formal interaction studies have been done but they reasonably warn about the increased risks of bleeding if vitamin K antagonists (i.e. **coumarins** and **indanediones**) are used concurrently.[7,8] Their recommendation[7,8] for changing from lepirudin to an oral anticoagulant is to reduce the lepirudin dosage gradually to reach an aPTT ratio just above 1.5 before beginning the oral anticoagulant, which should be started at the intended maintenance dose without a loading dose. They suggest that parenteral anticoagulation should be continued for 4 to 5 days, and then stopped when the INR stabilises within the target range.

1. Brown PM, Hursting MJ. Lack of pharmacokinetic interactions between argatroban and warfarin. *Am J Health-Syst Pharm* (2002) 59, 2078–83.
2. Sheth SB, DiCicco RA, Hursting MJ, Montague T, Jorkasky DK. Interpreting the international normalized ratio (INR) in individuals receiving argatroban and warfarin. *Thromb Haemost* (2001) 85, 435–40. Correction. ibid. 86, 727.
3. Harder S, Graff J, Klinkhardt U, von Hentig N, Walenga JM, Watanabe H, Osakabe M, Breddin HK. Transition from argatroban to oral anticoagulation with phenprocoumon or acenocoumarol: effects on prothrombin time, activated partial thromboplastin time, and Ecarin clotting time. *Thromb Haemost* (2004) 91, 1137–45.
4. Argatroban. GlaxoSmithKline. US Prescribing information, July 2005.
5. Angiomax (Bivalirudin). The Medicines Company. US Prescribing information, December 2005.
6. Angiox (Bivalirudin). Nycomed UK Ltd. UK Summary of product characteristics, March 2007.
7. Refludan (Lepirudin). Pharmion Ltd. UK Summary of product characteristics, April 2002.
8. Refludan (Lepirudin). Bayer HealthCare Pharmaceuticals Inc. US Prescribing information, November 2006.

Thrombin inhibitors; Argatroban + Erythromycin

Erythromycin has no effect on the pharmacokinetics or activity of argatroban.

Clinical evidence, mechanism, importance and management

In 10 healthy subjects, erythromycin 500 mg four times daily was given for 7 days with a 5-hour intravenous infusion of argatroban 1 microgram/kg per minute given before erythromycin and on day 6. Erythromycin had no effect on the pharmacokinetics of argatroban, and had no effect on the argatroban-induced prolongation of aPTT.[1] No special precautions are likely to be required on concurrent use of argatroban and erythromycin or other inhibitors of the cytochrome P450 isoenzyme CYP3A4 (for a list, see 'Table 1.4', (p.6)).

1. Tran JQ, Di Cicco RA, Sheth SB, Tucci M, Peng L, Jorkasky DK, Hursting MJ, Benincosa LJ. Assessment of the potential pharmacokinetic and pharmacodynamic interactions between erythromycin and argatroban. *J Clin Pharmacol* (1999) 39, 513–19.

Thrombin inhibitors; Argatroban + Lidocaine

There was no pharmacokinetic interaction between argatroban and lidocaine, and no further change in coagulation parameters when both drugs were given together in a study.

Clinical evidence, mechanism, importance and management

In 12 healthy subjects, lidocaine 2 mg/kg per hour was infused for 16 hours (after a loading dose of 1.5 mg/kg over 10 minutes) alone, then in combination with intravenous argatroban 1.5 micrograms/kg per minute for 16 hours. Concurrent use did not affect the pharmacokinetics of either drug. Lidocaine did not alter the effect of argatroban on aPTT.[1]

No special precautions appear likely to be necessary on concurrent use of lidocaine and argatroban.

1. Inglis AML, Sheth SB, Hursting MJ, Tenero DM, Graham AM, DiCicco RA. Investigation of the interaction between argatroban and acetaminophen, lidocaine, or digoxin. *Am J Health-Syst Pharm* (2002) 59, 1257–66.

Thrombin inhibitors; Argatroban + Paracetamol (Acetaminophen)

There was no pharmacokinetic interaction between argatroban and paracetamol, and no further change in coagulation parameters when both drugs were given together in a study.

Clinical evidence, mechanism, importance and management

In 11 healthy subjects, paracetamol 1 g every 6 hours for 5 doses had no effect on the pharmacokinetics of a 19-hour infusion of argatroban 1.5 micrograms/kg per minute, started with the second dose of paracetamol. In addition, argatroban had no effect on paracetamol pharmacokinetics. Paracetamol did not alter the effect of argatroban on aPTT.[1]

No special precautions appear necessary on concurrent use of paracetamol and argatroban.

1. Inglis AML, Sheth SB, Hursting MJ, Tenero DM, Graham AM, DiCicco RA. Investigation of the interaction between argatroban and acetaminophen, lidocaine, or digoxin. *Am J Health-Syst Pharm* (2002) 59, 1257–66.

Thrombin inhibitors; Ximelagatran + Miscellaneous

Aspirin did not alter the pharmacokinetics of melagatran, the active metabolite of ximelagatran, or its effects on the aPTT, but the combination had additive effects on bleeding time. Erythromycin increases the AUC of melagatran, the active metabolite of ximelagatran, and causes a small additional effect on coagulation parameters. The concurrent use of amiodarone and ximelagatran caused a slight increase in the AUC of melagatran and a slight decrease in the AUC of amiodarone, but the clinical relevance of this is unknown.

No pharmacokinetic interaction occurs between ximelagatran and atorvastatin or digoxin, and concurrent use does not change coagulation status. No pharmacokinetic interaction appears to occur between ximelagatran and diazepam, diclofenac or nifedipine. This suggests that ximelagatran has no clinically relevant effect on drugs that are substrates for the cytochrome P450 isoenzymes CYP2C9, CYP2C19, and CYP3A4.

Clinical evidence, mechanism, importance and management

(a) Amiodarone

In a placebo-controlled study in 26 healthy subjects, ximelagatran 36 mg was given every 12 hours for 8 days with a single 600-mg dose of amiodarone on day 4. On combined use there was a slight 21% increase in the AUC of melagatran (the active metabolite of ximelagatran), and a slight 15% decrease in the AUC of amiodarone. Amiodarone did not alter the effect of melagatran on aPTT.[1]

The mechanism of this interaction is unknown. The pharmacokinetic changes seen were not considered to be clinically relevant.

(b) Aspirin

In young healthy subjects, aspirin 450 mg the day before, and 150 mg just before melagatran had no effect on the pharmacokinetics of intravenous melagatran 4.12 mg. In addition, aspirin did not alter the increases seen in aPTT or activated clotting time seen with melagatran. Both aspirin and melagatran increased bleeding time, and the increase with the combination was additive.[2]

(c) Atorvastatin

In 15 healthy subjects, ximelagatran 36 mg twice daily was given for 5 days with a single 40-mg dose of atorvastatin on day 4. There was no change in the pharmacokinetics of either drug or their active metabolites. Atorvastatin did not alter the effect of melagatran on aPTT.[3]

No special precautions are expected to be needed if ximelagatran is used in patients taking atorvastatin.

(d) Diazepam

In 24 healthy subjects, ximelagatran 24 mg twice daily was given for 8 days with a single 100-microgram/kg intravenous dose of diazepam on day 3. There was no change in the pharmacokinetics of either drug or of *N*-desmethyl-diazepam.[4]

Metabolism of diazepam to *N*-desmethyl-diazepam occurs via the cytochrome P450 isoenzyme CYP2C19, and *in vitro* studies had shown that melagatran was a weak inhibitor of this isoenzyme.[4] However, the lack of a pharmacokinetic interaction with diazepam suggests that no clinically relevant interaction occurs, and is also unlikely with other CYP2C19 substrates[4] (for a list see 'Table 1.3', (p.6)).

(e) Diclofenac

In a single-dose study in 24 healthy subjects, simultaneous administration of ximelagatran 24 mg and enteric-coated diclofenac 50 mg caused no change in the pharmacokinetics of either drug. In this study, there was also no additional effect of the combination on activated partial thromboplastin time or capillary bleeding time, suggesting that no pharmacodynamic interaction occurs.[4]

Diclofenac is a substrate for the cytochrome P450 isoenzyme CYP2C9, and *in vitro* study has shown that ximelagatran and melagatran are weak inhibitors of this isoenzyme.[4] However, the lack of a pharmacokinetic interaction with diclofenac suggests that no clinically relevant interaction occurs, and is also unlikely with other CYP2C9 substrates[4] (for a list see 'Table 1.3', (p.6)).

(f) Digoxin

In a double-blind, crossover study, 16 healthy subjects were given oral ximelagatran 36 mg twice daily or placebo for 8 days and a single 500-microgram oral dose of digoxin on day 4. Ximelagatran had no effects on the pharmacokinetics of digoxin. Similarly, digoxin had no effects on the pharmacokinetics of melagatran (the active metabolite) when ximelagatran was given orally. The anticoagulant effect of melagatran (measured as aPTT prolongation) was not altered by digoxin.[5]

(g) Erythromycin

In 16 healthy subjects, erythromycin 500 mg three times daily was given for 5 days with a single 36-mg oral dose of ximelagatran given before erythromycin, and on day 5. Erythromycin increased the AUC of melagatran (the active metabolite of ximelagatran) 1.8-fold, and the maximum plasma level 1.7-fold. This resulted in a small increase in peak aPTT from 41 to 44 seconds.[6]

Ximelagatran is not metabolised by cytochrome P450 isoenzymes, so the known inhibitory effect of erythromycin on CYP3A4 is not thought to be the mechanism for this interaction.

The findings of a pharmacokinetic interaction with a small pharmacodynamic effect indicate that further study is needed. Until more is known, it would certainly be prudent to be cautious if ximelagatran is used in patients taking erythromycin, although note that the pharmacodynamic effect was small and all patients tolerated the combination well.[6]

(h) Nifedipine

In a single-dose study in 34 healthy subjects, giving ximelagatran 24 mg four hours after slow-release nifedipine 60 mg caused no change in the pharmacokinetics of either drug.[4]

Nifedipine is a substrate for the cytochrome P450 isoenzyme CYP3A4, and *in vitro* studies had shown that ximelagatran metabolites might be weak inhibitors of this isoenzyme.[4] However, the lack of a pharmacokinetic interaction with nifedipine suggests that no clinically relevant interaction occurs, and is also unlikely with other CYP3A4 substrates[4] (for a list see 'Table 1.4', (p.6)).

1. Teng R, Sarich TC, Eriksson UG, Hamer JE, Gillette S, Schützer KM, Carlson GF, Knowey PR. A pharmacokinetic study of the combined administration of amiodarone and ximelagatran, an oral direct thrombin inhibitor. *J Clin Pharmacol* (2004) 44, 1063–71.
2. Fager G, Cullberg M, Eriksson-Lepkowska M, Frison L, Eriksson UG. Pharmacokinetics and pharmacodynamics of melagatran, the active form of the oral direct thrombin inhibitor ximelagatran, are not influenced by acetylsalicylic acid. *Eur J Clin Pharmacol* (2003) 59, 283–9.
3. Sarich TC, Schützer K-M, Dorani H, Wall U, Kalies I, Ohlsson L, Eriksson UG. No pharmacokinetic or pharmacodynamic interaction between atorvastatin and the oral direct thrombin inhibitor ximelagatran. *J Clin Pharmacol* (2004) 44, 928–34.
4. Bredberg E, Andersson TB, Frison L, Thuresson A, Johansson S, Eriksson-Lepkowska M, Larsson M, Eriksson UG. Ximelagatran, an oral direct thrombin inhibitor, has a low potential for cytochrome P450-mediated drug-drug interactions. *Clin Pharmacokinet* (2003) 42, 765–77.
5. Sarich TC, Schutzer K-M, Wollbratt M, Wall U, Kessler E, Eriksson UG. No pharmacokinetic or pharmacodynamic interaction between digoxin and ximelagatran, an oral direct thrombin inhibitor. *Blood* (2003) 102, 127b.
6. Dorani H, Schützer K, Sarich TC, Wall U, Ohlsson L, Eriksson UG. Effect of erythromycin on the pharmacokinetics and pharmacodynamics or the oral direct thrombin inhibitor ximelagatran and its active form melagatran. *Clin Pharmacol Ther* (2004) 75, P78.

13

Antidiabetics

The antidiabetics are used to control diabetes mellitus, a disease in which there is total or partial failure of the beta-cells within the pancreas to secrete enough insulin, one of the hormones concerned with the handling of glucose. In some cases there is evidence to show that the disease results from the presence of factors that oppose the activity of insulin.

With insufficient insulin, the body tissues are unable to take up and utilise the glucose that is in circulation in the blood. Because of this, glucose, which is derived largely from the digestion of food, and which would normally be removed and stored in tissues throughout the body, accumulates and boosts the glucose in the blood to such grossly elevated proportions that the kidney is unable to cope with such a load and glucose appears in the urine. Raised blood glucose levels (hyperglycaemia) with glucose and ketone bodies in the urine (glycosuria and ketonuria) are among the manifestations of a serious disturbance in the metabolic chemistry of the body, which, if untreated, can lead to the development of diabetic coma and death.

There are two main types of diabetes: one develops early in life and occurs when the ability of the pancreas suddenly, and often almost totally, fails to produce insulin. This type is called type 1, juvenile, or insulin-dependent diabetes (IDDM), and requires insulin replacement therapy. The other form is type 2, maturity-onset, or non-insulin dependent diabetes mellitus (NIDDM), which is most often seen in those over 40 years old. This occurs when the pancreas gradually loses the ability to produce insulin over a period of months or years and/or resistance to the action of insulin develops. It is often associated with being overweight and can sometimes be satisfactorily controlled simply by losing weight and adhering to an appropriate diet. This may then be augmented with oral antidiabetic drugs, and eventually insulin. A classification of the antidiabetics is given in 'Table 13.1', (p.469).

Modes of action of the antidiabetics

A. Parenteral antidiabetics

(a) Amylin analogues

Pramlintide is a synthetic analogue of amylin, a pancreatic hormone involved in glucose homoeostasis. It slows the rate of gastric emptying and reduces appetite. It is given subcutaneously immediately prior to meals, and is used in patients already receiving insulin.

(b) Incretin mimetics

Exenatide is an incretin mimetic that acts as a glucagon-like peptide-1 (GLP-1) receptor agonist. This increases insulin secretion when glucose levels are high. It is given subcutaneously as an adjunct in type 2 diabetes in patients already receiving metformin, a sulphonylurea, or both.

(c) Insulin

Insulin extracted from the pancreatic tissue of pigs and cattle is so similar to human insulin that it can be used as a replacement. However, human insulin, manufactured by genetically engineered microorganisms, is more commonly used. Insulin is usually given by injection in order to bypass the enzymes of the gut, which would digest and destroy it like any other protein. The onset and duration of action of insulin may be prolonged by complexing with zinc or protamine. More recently, various insulin analogues have been developed, which have specific pharmacokinetic profiles. Insulin aspart and lispro have a faster onset and shorter duration of action than soluble insulin. Insulin glargine and detemir both have a prolonged duration of action.

An inhaled form of insulin has been approved by The European Medicines Agency for use in adult patients with diabetes mellitus.

B. Oral antidiabetics

(a) Aldose reductase inhibitors

Epalrestat inhibits the enzyme aldose reductase, which converts glucose to sorbitol. The accumulation of sorbitol may play a role in some diabetic complications.

(b) Alpha-glucosidase inhibitors

Acarbose, miglitol and voglibose act against alpha glucosidases and specifically against sucrase in the gut to delay the digestion and absorption of monosaccharides from starch and sucrose.

(c) Biguanides

The mode of action of the biguanides, such as metformin, is obscure, but they do not stimulate the pancreas like the sulphonylureas to release insulin, but appear to facilitate the uptake and utilisation of glucose by the cells in some way. Their use is restricted to type 2 diabetes because they are not effective unless insulin is present.

(d) Meglitinides

The meglitinides (e.g. repaglinide) increase endogenous insulin secretion, and so are used in type 2 diabetes.

(e) Sulphonylureas

The sulphonylurea and other sulfonamide-related compounds such as chlorpropamide and tolbutamide were the first synthetic compounds used in medicine as antidiabetics. Among their actions they stimulate the remaining beta-cells of the pancreas to grow and secrete insulin which, with a restricted diet, controls blood glucose levels and permits normal metabolism to occur. Clearly they can only be effective in those diabetics whose pancreas still has the capacity to produce some insulin, so their use is confined to type 2 diabetes.

(f) Thiazolidinediones

The thiazolidinediones (e.g. rosiglitazone) appear to decrease insulin resistance through activation of gamma-PPAR (peroxisome proliferator-activated receptor). They are used in type 2 diabetes.

(g) Other oral antidiabetics

Outside orthodox Western medicine, there are herbal preparations which are used to treat diabetes and which can be given by mouth. Blueberries were traditionally used by the Alpine peasants, and bitter gourd or karela (*Momordica charantia*) is an established part of herbal treatment in the Indian subcontinent and elsewhere. Traditional Chinese medicine also has herbal medicines for diabetes. As yet it is not known how these herbal medicines act and their efficacy awaits formal clinical evaluation.

Interactions

The commonest interactions with antidiabetic drugs are those that result in a rise or fall in blood glucose levels, thereby disturbing the control of diabetes. These are detailed in this section. Other interactions where the antidiabetic drug is the affecting drug are described elsewhere.

Table 13.1 Drugs used in the management of diabetes

Group		*Drugs*
Parenteral antidiabetics		
Amylin analogues		Pramlintide
Incretin mimetics (Glucagon like peptide-1 (GLP-1) receptor agonist)		Exenatide
Insulins	Short-acting	Soluble insulin
	Intermediate- and long-acting	Insulin zinc suspension, Isophane insulin, Protamine zinc insulin
	Short-acting analogues	Insulin aspart, Insulin glulisine, Insulin lispro
	Intermediate to long-acting analogues	Insulin aspart protamine, Insulin detemir, Insulin glargine, Insulin lispro protamine
Oral antidiabetics		
Aldose reductase inhibitors		Epalrestat
Alpha glucosidase inhibitors		Acarbose, Miglitol, Voglibose
Biguanides		Buformin, Metformin, Phenformin
Meglitinides		Nateglinide, Repaglinide
Sulphonylureas		Acetohexamide, Carbutamide, Chlorpropamide, Glibenclamide (Glyburide), Glibornuride, Gliclazide, Glimepiride, Glipizide, Gliquidone, Glisentide, Glisolamide, Glisoxepide, Glycyclamide, Tolazamide, Tolbutamide
Thiazolidinediones (Gamma-PPAR (peroxisome proliferator-activated receptor) agonists)		Pioglitazone, Rosiglitazone
Other drugs		Guar gum

Acarbose + Miscellaneous

Neomycin may increase the efficacy and the gastrointestinal adverse effects of acarbose. There is some indirect evidence that acarbose with alcohol may increase the hepatotoxicity of paracetamol (acetaminophen). Paralytic ileus has been reported in a Japanese patient treated with acarbose and promethazine, an antimuscarinic drug.

Clinical evidence, mechanism, importance and management

(a) Antimuscarinics

A 69-year-old man with a partial gastrectomy and type 2 diabetes, treated with insulin 24 units and acarbose 300 mg daily, was admitted to hospital with diabetic gangrene. After developing cold symptoms he was given *PL granules* (salicylamide, paracetamol, caffeine, **promethazine** methylene disalicylate). The next day he experienced sudden abdominal pain, nausea and vomiting, which was diagnosed as paralytic ileus. He was given intravenous fluids and piperacillin. Oral intake and acarbose were withheld and the ileus resolved after 2 days. The authors note that there are several reports of ileus developing in Japanese patients within 3 months of treatment with alpha-glucosidase inhibitors such as acarbose. The risk seems to be increased with age, a history of abdominal surgery, and a Japanese diet (high in carbohydrates and fibre) rather than Western diet. However, in this case the patient had been taking acarbose for 15 months without problem and it is possible that the antimuscarinic effects of **promethazine** in the *PL granules* may have contributed to the development of ileus.[1] The general clinical relevance of this case is uncertain. However, the authors consider that patients at risk should be monitored if they are given alpha-glucosidase inhibitors, especially if the dose is increased or if antimuscarinics are also given.[1]

(b) Neomycin

Neomycin alone can reduce postprandial blood glucose levels and may enhance the reduction in postprandial glucose levels associated with acarbose.[2] Neomycin 1 g three times daily increased the unpleasant gastrointestinal adverse effects (flatulence, cramps and diarrhoea) of acarbose 200 mg three times daily in 7 healthy subjects.[3] The manufacturers suggest that if these adverse effects are severe the dosage of acarbose should be reduced.[4]

(c) Paracetamol

Studies in *rats* have found that acarbose alone or in combination with alcohol may potentiate the hepatotoxicity of paracetamol.[5] However, it is not known whether this has any clinical relevance.

1. Oba K, Kudo R, Yano M, Watanabe K, Ajiro Y, Okazaki K, Susuki T, Nakano H, Metori S. Ileus after administration of cold remedy in an elderly diabetic patient treated with acarbose. *J Nippon Med Sch* (2001) 68, 61–4.
2. Bayer, Personal Communication, June 1993.
3. Lembcke B, Caspary WF, Fölsch UR, Creutzfeldt W. Influence of neomycin on postprandial metabolic changes and side effects of an α-glucosidehydrolase inhibitor (BAY g 5421). I. Effects on intestinal hydrogen gas production and flatulence. In Frontiers of Hormone Research, vol 7. The Entero-Insular Axis. Satellite Symposium to Xth IDF-Meeting, September 7–8, Göttingen 1979, p 294–5.
4. Glucobay (Acarbose). Bayer plc. UK Summary of product characteristics, October 2006.
5. Wang P-Y, Kaneko T, Wang Y, Sato A. Acarbose alone or in combination with ethanol potentiates the hepatotoxicity of carbon tetrachloride and acetaminophen in rats. *Hepatology* (1999) 29, 161–5.

Alpha-glucosidase inhibitors + Charcoal or Digestive enzymes

The manufacturers of acarbose[1,2] and miglitol[3] reasonably suggest that intestinal adsorbents (e.g. charcoal) or digestive enzyme preparations (such as amylase, pancreatin) should be avoided because, theoretically, they would be expected to reduce the effects of these alpha glucosidase inhibitors.

1. Glucobay (Acarbose). Bayer plc. UK Summary of product characteristics, October 2006.
2. Precose (Acarbose). Bayer Pharmaceuticals Corporation. US Prescribing information, November 2004.
3. Glyset (Miglitol). Pharmacia & Upjohn Company. US Prescribing information, October 2004.

Alpha-glucosidase inhibitors + Other antidiabetics

Some minor decreases in the plasma levels of glibenclamide (glyburide), metformin, and rosiglitazone have been seen with acarbose or miglitol, but these are not clinically relevant. Voglibose had no effect on glibenclamide pharmacokinetics. Alpha glucosidase inhibitors cause a moderate additional blood glucose-lowering effect when used with other antidiabetics, and a possible increased risk of hypoglycaemia should be borne in mind. In patients taking alpha-glucosidase inhibitors, treatment of hypoglycaemia should be with a monosaccharide such as glucose (dextrose) or glucagon, not a disaccharide such as sucrose. The manufacturer of pramlintide recommends that it should not be used in patients taking alpha-glucosidase inhibitors.

Clinical evidence

(a) Glibenclamide (glyburide)

Voglibose had no effect on the pharmacokinetics of glibenclamide in a double-blind crossover trial in 12 healthy male subjects. In this study, subjects were given either **voglibose** 5 mg or a placebo three times daily for 8 days and a single 1.75-mg dose of glibenclamide on the morning of day 8, taken at the same time as the first dose of the **voglibose** or placebo.[1] Similarly, the manufacturers of **acarbose** note that it had no effect on the absorption or disposition of glibenclamide in diabetic patients.[2]

However, in a randomised, double-blind, placebo-controlled study in 28 patients with type 2 diabetes mellitus, **miglitol** reduced the maximum plasma glibenclamide levels and its AUC by 16 and 19%, respectively. The patients were given glibenclamide 2.5 mg twice daily with either **miglitol** 100 mg three times daily or placebo for 2 days. Nevertheless, the average blood glucose levels were reduced more by the drug combination than by the glibenclamide alone: over 5 hours there was a 15% greater reduction, and over 10 hours a 9% greater reduction.[3]

(b) Metformin

A study in 6 healthy subjects found that **acarbose** 50 to 100 mg three times daily reduced the maximum serum levels and the AUC_{0-9} of metformin 1 g by about 35%, but the 24-hour urinary excretion was unchanged.[4]

Another study in 19 diabetic patients given **acarbose** 50 or 100 mg three times daily and metformin 500 mg twice daily, also found that **acarbose** lowered metformin levels (AUC reduced by 12 to 13%, maximum plasma levels reduced by 17 to 20%). Nevertheless, the drug combination reduced the postprandial glucose concentration at 3 hours by 15% more than metformin alone.[5] Similarly, the manufacturer notes that, in a study in healthy subjects, **miglitol** 100 mg three times daily for 7 days reduced the AUC and maximum level of a single 1-g dose of metformin by 12% and 13%, respectively, although this difference was not statistically significant.[6]

(c) Pramlintide

The manufacturer of pramlintide suggests that it should not be used in patients taking drugs that slow the intestinal absorption of nutrients, such as the alpha-glucosidase inhibitors.[7] This is because pramlintide slows gastric emptying (see also 'Pramlintide + Miscellaneous', p.513). Clinical study is needed to see if there is any important effect if the drugs are used together.

(d) Rosiglitazone

A study in 16 healthy subjects found that **acarbose** 100 mg three times daily for a week slightly reduced the absorption of a single 8-mg oral dose of rosiglitazone (AUC reduced by 12%), but this was not considered to be clinically relevant.[8]

Mechanism

The reason for the minor pharmacokinetic changes is uncertain.

Importance and management

The pharmacokinetic changes seen are minor and unlikely to be clinically relevant. The manufacturers say that while alpha glucosidase inhibitors such as acarbose and miglitol do not cause hypoglycaemia when given alone, they may increase the blood glucose-lowering effects of **insulin** and the **sulphonylureas**, for which reason it may be necessary to reduce their dosages. Monitor the outcome when acarbose, miglitol, or voglibose is first given. Any hypoglycaemic episodes should be treated with glucose (dextrose), not sucrose, because alpha glucosidase inhibitors delay the digestion and absorption of disaccharides such as sucrose, but do not affect monosaccharides.[2,6,9] Patients taking alpha-glucosidase inhibitors should not be given pramlintide until the combination has been studied clinically.

1. Kleist P, Ehrlich A, Suzuki Y, Timmer W, Wetzelsberger N, Lücker PW, Fuder H. Concomitant administration of the α-glucosidase inhibitor voglibose (AO-128) does not alter the pharmacokinetics of glibenclamide. *Eur J Clin Pharmacol* (1997) 53, 149–52.
2. Precose (Acarbose). Bayer Pharmaceuticals Corporation. US Prescribing information, November 2004.
3. Sullivan JT, Lettieri JT, Heller AH. Effects of miglitol on pharmacokinetics and pharmacodynamics of glyburide. *Clin Pharmacol Ther* (1998) 63, 155.
4. Scheen AJ, Fierra Alves de Magalhaes AC, Salvatore T, Lefebrve PJ. Reduction of the acute bioavailability of metformin by the α-glucosidase inhibitor acarbose in normal man. *Eur J Clin Invest* (1994) 24 (Suppl 3), 50–4.
5. Lettieri J, Liu MC, Sullivan JT, Heller AH. Pharmacokinetic (PK) and pharmacodynamic (PD) interaction between acarbose (A) and metformin (M) in diabetic (NIDDM) patients. *Clin Pharmacol Ther* (1998) 63, 155.
6. Glyset (Miglitol). Pharmacia & Upjohn Company. US Prescribing information, October 2004.
7. Symlin (Pramlintide acetate). Amylin Pharmaceuticals, Inc. US Prescribing information, June 2005.
8. Miller AK, Inglis AM, Culkin KT, Jorkaksy DK, Freed MI. The effect of acarbose on the pharmacokinetics of rosiglitazone. *Eur J Clin Pharmacol* (2001) 57, 105–9.
9. Glucobay (Acarbose). Bayer plc. UK Summary of product characteristics, October 2006.

Antidiabetics + ACE inhibitors

The concurrent use of ACE inhibitors and antidiabetics normally appears to be uneventful but hypoglycaemia, marked in some instances, has occurred in a small number of diabetics taking insulin or sulphonylureas with captopril, enalapril, lisinopril or perindopril. This has been attributed, but not proved, to be due to an interaction. The United Kingdom Prospective Diabetes Study Group (UKPDS) found no difference in the incidence of hypoglycaemia between patients taking atenolol and those taking captopril. No pharmacokinetic interaction has been found to occur between spirapril and glibenclamide. Subcutaneous exenatide has no important effect on the pharmacokinetics of lisinopril, and does not alter its efficacy.

Clinical evidence

Numerous case reports, small case-control studies, and a pharmacological study in healthy subjects suggest that ACE inhibitors increase the risk of hypoglycaemia in patients receiving insulin or oral antidiabetics, and these are summarised in 'Table 13.2', (p.472). Conversely several larger case-control studies and two randomised controlled studies have not found a significantly increased risk of hypoglycaemia with ACE inhibitors, and these are also summarised in Table 13.2. It is worth highlighting that one of these, the United Kingdom Prospective Diabetes Study Group (UKPDS), found that the number of patients experiencing hypoglycaemic attacks did not differ between patients receiving atenolol 50 to 100 mg daily or **captopril** 25 to 50 mg twice daily for hypertension.[1]

A brief report states that **spirapril** does not have a pharmacokinetic interaction with **glibenclamide**.[2] The manufacturer of exenatide notes that, in a study in hypertensive patients exenatide 10 micrograms twice daily did not alter the steady-state AUC or maximum level of **lisinopril** 5 to 20 mg daily, but it did delay the time to maximum level by 2 hours. However, exenatide did not alter the blood-pressure lowering effect of **lisinopril**.[3]

Mechanism

Not understood. An increase in glucose utilisation and increased insulin sensitivity have been suggested.[4,5] Other possibilities (e.g. altered renal function) are discussed in a series of letters in *The Lancet*.[6-11] There is also an isolated report of persistent severe hypoglycaemia in a non-diabetic patient associated with both **captopril** and **ramipril** therapy.[12] Conversely, high natural ACE activity has been associated with a higher risk of severe hypoglycaemia.[13]

Importance and management

This interaction is not well established nor understood, and it remains the subject of considerable study and debate. However, some cases of severe hypoglycaemia have undoubtedly occurred due to the use of ACE inhibitors by diabetic patients. Nevertheless, some authors consider the risk of severe hypoglycaemia in diabetic patients treated with ACE inhibitors to be very low and negligible compared with the benefits of this class of drugs in diabetes.[14] Moreover, some recent guidelines on the treatment of hypertension in diabetes recommend that all patients with diabetes and hypertension should be treated with an ACE inhibitor.[15,16] To be on the safe side, it would be prudent to warn all patients receiving insulin or oral antidiabetics who are just starting any ACE inhibitors (although only captopril, enalapril, lisinopril and perindopril have been implicated) that excessive hypoglycaemia has been seen very rarely and unpredictably. The problem has been resolved in some patients by reducing the sulphonylurea dosage by a half to three-quarters.[17,18]

Subcutaneous exenatide has no important pharmacokinetic interaction with lisinopril, and would therefore not be expected to have a pharmacokinetic interaction with any other ACE inhibitor, although this needs confirmation.

A false positive urine ketone test can also occur with captopril when using the alkaline-nitroprusside test (*Ketodiastix*), which may affect the monitoring of diabetic control.[19]

1. UK Prospective Diabetes Study Group. Efficacy of atenolol and captopril in reducing risk of macrovascular and microvascular complications in type 2 diabetes: UKPDS 39. *BMJ* (1998) 317, 713–20.
2. Grass P, Gerbeau C, Kutz K. Spirapril: pharmacokinetic properties and drug interactions. *Blood Press Suppl* (1994) 2, 7–13.
3. Byetta (Exenatide). Amylin Pharmaceuticals, Inc. US Prescribing information, February 2007.
4. Ferriere M, Lachkar H, Richard J-L, Bringer J, Orsetti A, Mirouze J. Captopril and insulin sensitivity. *Ann Intern Med* (1985) 102, 134–5.
5. Girardin E, Vial T, Pham E, Evreux J-C. Hypoglycémies induites par les sulfamides hypoglycémiants. *Ann Med Interne (Paris)* (1992) 143, 11–17.
6. van Haeften TW. ACE inhibitors and hypoglycaemia. *Lancet* (1995) 346, 125.
7. Kong N, Bates A, Ryder REJ. ACE inhibitors and hypoglycaemia. *Lancet* (1995) 346, 125.
8. Feher MD, Amiel S. ACE inhibitors and hypoglycaemia. *Lancet* (1995) 346, 125–6.
9. Davie AP. ACE inhibitors and hypoglycaemia. *Lancet* (1995) 346, 126.
10. Wildenborg IHM, Veenstra J, van der Voort PHJ, Verdegaal WP, Silberbusch J. ACE inhibitors and hypoglycaemia. *Lancet* (1995) 346, 126.
11. Herings RMC, de Boer A, Stricker BHC, Leufkens HGM, Porsius AJ. ACE inhibitors and hypoglycaemia. *Lancet* (1995) 346, 126–7.
12. Elorriaga-Sánchez F, Corrales-Bobadilla H, Sosa-Trinidad E, Domínguez-Quezada B. Hipoglucemia severa secundaria a inhibidores de la enzima convertidora de angiotensina en ausencia de diabetes mellitus. Reporte de un caso. *Gac Med Mex* (2001) 137, 249–52.
13. Pedersen-Bjergaard U, Agerholm-Larsen B, Pramming S, Hougaard P, Thorsteinsson B. Prediction of severe hypoglycaemia by angiotensin-converting enzyme activity and genotype in type 1 diabetes. *Diabetologia* (2003) 46, 89–96.
14. Scheen AJ. Drug interactions of clinical importance with antihyperglycaemic agents: an update. *Drug Safety* (2005) 28, 601–31.
15. Kaplan NM. Management of hypertension in patients with type 2 diabetes mellitus: guidelines based on current evidence. *Ann Intern Med* (2001) 135, 1079–83.
16. American Diabetes Association. Hypertension management in adults with diabetes. *Diabetes Care* (2004) 27 (Suppl 1), S65–S67.
17. Arauz-Pacheco C, Ramirez LC, Rios JM, Raskin P. Hypoglycemia induced by angiotensin-converting enzyme inhibitors in patients with non-insulin-dependent diabetes receiving sulfonylurea therapy. *Am J Med* (1990) 89, 811–13.
18. Ahmad S. Drug interaction induces hypoglycemia. *J Fam Pract* (1995) 40, 540–1.
19. Warren SE. False-positive urine ketone test with captopril. *N Engl J Med* (1980) 303, 1003–4.

Antidiabetics + Alcohol

Diabetic patients stabilised with insulin, oral antidiabetics or diet alone need not abstain from alcohol, but they should drink only in moderation and accompanied by food. Epidemiological evidence suggests that heart disease may be less common in diabetic patients who drink in moderation. However, alcohol makes the signs of hypoglycaemia less clear and delayed hypoglycaemia can occur. The CNS depressant effects of alcohol plus hypoglycaemia can make driving or the operation of dangerous machinery much more hazardous. A flushing reaction is common in patients taking chlorpropamide who drink alcohol, but is less common with other sulphonylureas. Limited evidence suggests that alcoholic patients may require above-average doses of tolbutamide.

Clinical evidence

(a) Antidiabetics, general

1. Effect on glucose levels. The blood glucose levels of diabetics may be reduced, remain unchanged, or increased by alcohol, depending on the amount drunk at one time, if it is drunk with food or not, and if use is chronic and excessive.[1] In one early study, 2 out of 7 diabetics receiving **insulin** became severely hypoglycaemic after drinking the equivalent of about 3 measures of spirits.[2] In a hospital study over a 3-year period, 5 type I diabetics were hospitalised with severe hypoglycaemia after binge-drinking. Two of them died without recovery from the initial coma and the other 3

Table 13.2 Interactions between antidiabetics and ACE inhibitors

Patients	*ACE inhibitor*	*Antidiabetic*	*Notes*	*Refs*
Evidence for hypoglycaemia				
1 case	Captopril 50 mg/day	Glibenclamide (glyburide) 10.5 mg/day Metformin 1.7 g/day	Blood glucose 2.2 mmol/L 24 hours after the addition of captopril.	1
1 case	Captopril	Glibenclamide 10.5 mg/day Metformin 1.7 g/day	Blood glucose of 2.9 mmol/L 48 hours after starting captopril. Antidiabetic drugs stopped.	1
3 cases	Captopril	Glibenclamide	Hypoglycaemia reported to a Spanish Regional Pharmacosurveillance centre.	2
1 case	Captopril 12.5 mg/day	Glibenclamide 2.5 mg/day	Hypoglycaemia 7 hours after first dose, blood glucose 2.1 mmol/L, glibenclamide stopped.	3
1 case	Captopril	Unspecified oral antidiabetic	Hypoglycaemia, oral antidiabetic withdrawn.	4
5 cases	Captopril	Unspecified sulphonylureas	Hypoglycaemia reported to Centres Regionaux de Pharmacovigilance in France.	5
3 cases case control study	Captopril	Unspecified oral antidiabetics	Risk of hypoglycaemia increased 3.1-fold.	6
9 cases case control study	Captopril	Insulin	Risk of hypoglycaemia increased 3.7-fold.	6
4 cases	Captopril	Insulin	Hypoglycaemia reported to a Spanish Regional Pharmacosurveillance centre.	2
3 cases	Captopril	Insulin	Unexplained hypoglycaemia.	4
1 case	Enalapril 5 mg/day	Glibenclamide 5 mg/day	Hypoglycaemia, blood glucose 2.3 mmol/L. Dose of glibenclamide reduced to 2.5 mg/day.	3
2 cases	Enalapril 5 mg/day	Glibenclamide 5 mg/day	Hypoglycaemic attacks, glibenclamide reduced to 1.25 mg/day.	7
9 healthy subjects (double-blind, crossover study)	Enalapril 5 mg/day, then 10 mg/day	Glibenclamide 3.5 mg single dose	Hypoglycaemic effects of glibenclamide temporarily enhanced between 2 and 4 hours after enalapril was taken.	8
4 cases	Enalapril	Glibenclamide	Hypoglycaemia reported to a Spanish Regional Pharmacosurveillance centre.	2
1 case	Enalapril	Gliclazide 80 mg/day	Hypoglycaemia when enalapril dose increased from 5 to 10 mg/day.	9
4 cases	Enalapril	Unspecified sulphonylureas	Hypoglycaemia reported to Centres Regionaux de Pharmacovigilance in France.	5
1 case	Enalapril	Unspecified sulphonylurea	Recurrent hypoglycaemia, sulphonylurea withdrawn.	10
10 cases case control study	Enalapril	Unspecified sulphonylurea Insulin	2.4-fold increase in the risk of hypoglycaemia with sulphonylureas. However, no increased risk was seen in insulin users. In addition when all ACE inhibitors were considered together, no significant increase in risk was seen.	11
2 cases case control study	Enalapril	Unspecified oral antidiabetics	Non-significant 5.4-fold increase in the risk of hypoglycaemia.	6
3 cases case control study	Enalapril	Insulin	Non-significant 1.7-fold increase in the risk of hypoglycaemia.	6
1 case	Enalapril	Insulin	Reduced insulin requirements.	10
11 cases	Enalapril	Insulin	Hypoglycaemia reported to a Spanish Regional Pharmacosurveillance centre.	2
1 case	Lisinopril	Glibenclamide and metformin	Hypoglycaemia reported to a Spanish Regional Pharmacosurveillance centre.	2
1 case	Lisinopril 10 mg/day	Gliclazide	Hypoglycaemia resolved on stopping gliclazide.	9
1 case	Perindopril	Glibenclamide	Hypoglycaemia reported to a Spanish Regional Pharmacosurveillance centre.	2
1 case	Ramipril 2.5 mg/day	Glibenclamide 5 mg/day Metformin 1.7 g/day	Patient also on naproxen, renal function deteriorated causing hypoglycaemia due to accumulation of oral antidiabetics.	12

Continued

Table 13.2 Interactions between antidiabetics and ACE inhibitors (continued)

Patients	ACE inhibitor	Antidiabetic	Notes	Refs
7 cases case control study	Unspecified ACE inhibitor	Insulin or oral antidiabetics	3.2-fold increase in the risk of hypoglycaemia leading to hospitalisation.	13
Evidence of no interaction				
8 cases	Captopril 37.5 mg/day	Insulin	No change to daily insulin requirements. No evidence of symptomatic hypoglycaemia.	14
38 cases	Captopril 50 to 100 mg/day or Enalapril 20 to 40 mg/day	Insulin or oral antidiabetics	Antidiabetic treatment unaltered, no evidence of unusual or unexplained hypoglycaemia.	15
18 cases double blind controlled study	Enalapril 20 to 40 mg/day	Insulin	No change to daily insulin requirements. No evidence of unexplained hypoglycaemia.	15
428 patients randomised controlled study	Lisinopril 10 to 20 mg/day or placebo	Insulin	No difference in the number of hypoglycaemic episodes between lisinopril and placebo recipients.	16
22 cases case control study	Captopril or Enalapril	Insulin or oral antidiabetics	Data from Centres Regionaux de Pharmacovigilance in France used. No increased risk of hypoglycaemia detected.	17
598 cases of hypoglycaemia in a retrospective study	Captopril or Enalapril or other classes of antihypertensive	Insulin or oral antidiabetics	No statistically significant increase or decrease in the risk of serious hypoglycaemia among users of ACE inhibitors or any other class of antihypertensives compared with non users of antihypertensives.	18
758 patients randomised controlled study	Captopril 50 to 100 mg/day or atenolol	Insulin or oral antidiabetics or diet alone	The proportion of patients with hypoglycaemic attacks did not differ between the captopril and atenolol groups.	19

1. Rett K, Wicklmayr M, Dietz GJ. Hypoglycemia in hypertensive diabetic patients treated with sulfonylureas, biguanides and captopril. *N Engl J Med* (1988) 319, 1609.
2. Aguirre C, Ayani I, Rodriguez-Sasiain JM. Hypoglycaemia associated with angiotensin converting enzyme inhibitors. *Therapie* (1995) 50 (Suppl), 198.
3. Arauz-Pacheco C, Ramirez LC, Rios JM, Raskin P. Hypoglycemia induced by angiotensin-converting enzyme inhibitors in patients with non-insulin-dependent diabetes receiving sulfonylurea therapy. *Am J Med* (1990) 89, 811-13.
4. Ferriere M, Lachkar H, Richard J-L, Bringer J, Orsetti A, Mirouze J. Captopril and insulin sensitivity. *Ann Intern Med* (1985) 102, 134-5.
5. Girardin E, Vial T, Pham E, Evreux J-C. Hypoglycémies induites par les sulfamides hypoglycémiants. *Ann Med Interne (Paris)* (1992) 143, 11-17.
6. Herings RMC, de Boer A, Stricker BHC, Leufkens HGM, Porsius A. Hypoglycaemia associated with use of inhibitors of angiotensin converting enzyme. *Lancet* (1995) 345, 1195-8.
7. Ahmad S. Drug interaction induces hypoglycemia. *J Fam Pract* (1995) 40, 540-1.
8. Rave K, Flesch S, Kühn-Velten WN, Hompesch BC, Heinemann L, Heise T. Enhancement of blood glucose lowering effect of a sulfonylurea when coadministered with an ACE inhibitor: results of a glucose-clamp study. *Diabetes Metab Res Rev* (2005) 21, 459–64.
9. Veyre B, Ginon I, Vial T, Dragol F, Daumont M. Hypoglycémies par interférence entre un inhibiteur de l'enzyme de conversion et un sulfamide hypoglycémiant. *Presse Med* (1993) 22, 738.
10. McMurray J, Fraser DM. Captopril, enalapril and blood glucose. *Lancet* (1986) i, 1035.
11. Thamer M, Ray NF, Taylor T. Association between antihypertensive drug use and hypoglycemia: a case-control study of diabetic users of insulin or sulfonylureas. *Clin Ther* (1999) 21, 1387-1400.
12. Collin M, Mucklow JC. Drug interactions, renal impairment and hypoglycaemia in a patient with type II diabetes. *Br J Clin Pharmacol* (1999) 48, 134-7.
13. Morris AD, Boyle DIR, McMahon AD, Pearce H, Evans JMM, Newton RW, Jung RT, MacDonald TM, The DARTS/MEMO collaboration. ACE inhibitor use is associated with hospitalization for severe hypoglycaemia in patients with diabetes. *Diabetes Care* (1997) 20, 1363-7.
14. Winocour P, Waldek S, Anderson DC. Captopril and blood glucose. *Lancet* (1986) ii, 461.
15. Passa P, Marre M, Leblanc H. Enalapril, captopril and blood glucose. *Lancet* (1986) i, 1447.
16. The EUCLID study group. Randomised placebo-controlled trial of lisinopril in normotensive patients with insulin-dependent diabetes and normoalbuminuria or microalbuminuria. *Lancet* (1997) 349, 1787-92.
17. Moore N, Kreft-Jais C, Haramburu F, Noblet C, Andrejak M, Ollagnier M, Bégaud B. Reports of hypoglycaemia associated with the use of ACE inhibitors and other drugs: a case/non-case study in the French pharmacovigilance system database. *Br J Clin Pharmacol* (1997) 44, 513-8.
18. Shorr RI, Ray WA, Daugherty JR, Griffin MR. Antihypertensives and the risk of serious hypoglycemia in older persons using insulin or sulfonylureas. *JAMA* (1997) 278, 40–3.
19. UK Prospective Diabetes Study Group. Efficacy of atenolol and captopril in reducing risk of macrovascular and microvascular complications in type 2 diabetes: UKPDS 39. *BMJ* (1998) 317, 713–20.

suffered permanent damage to the nervous system.[3] In another study it was found that alcohol was involved in about 4% of hypoglycaemic episodes requiring hospitalisation.[4] In contrast to these alcohol-induced hypoglycaemic episodes, it was found in two other studies[5,6] that pure alcohol and dry wine had little effect on blood glucose levels. In a recent review of six studies, it was concluded that consumption of a moderate amount of alcohol does not acutely impair glycaemic control in diabetic patients, and may in fact result in a small decrease in plasma glucose concentration.[7] However, another study found that 46 patients with type 2 diabetes and a mean age of 67 years who were regular chronic alcohol users (mean 45 g/day) had a reversible deterioration in metabolic control (higher fasting and postprandial glucose levels and higher glycosylated haemoglobin levels), when compared with 35 non-alcohol users.[8] Another study reported similar findings.[9]

2. Effect on diabetic complications. A review of 4 epidemiological studies concluded that heart disease is less common in people with diabetes who drink moderate amounts of alcohol than in those who do not.[7]

(b) Biguanides

A controlled study in 5 ketosis-resistant patients with type 2 diabetes taking **phenformin** 50 to 100 mg daily found that the equivalent of about 85 mL (3 oz) of whiskey markedly raised their blood lactate and lactate-pyruvate levels. Two of them had blood-lactate levels of more than

50 mg%, and one of these patients had previously experienced nausea, weakness and malaise while taking **phenformin** and alcohol.[10] The ingestion of alcohol is described in other reports as having preceded the onset of **phenformin**-induced lactic-acidosis.[11-13] Some patients have complained that alcohol tastes metallic.

(c) Rosiglitazone

An 8-week study in type 2 diabetics taking rosiglitazone 8 mg daily or a placebo found that 0.6 g/kg of alcohol taken with a meal did not have a clinically relevant effect on plasma glucose levels and no episodes of hypoglycaemia were seen.[14]

(d) Sulphonylureas

About one-third of those taking **chlorpropamide** who drink alcohol, even in quite small amounts, experience a warm, tingling or burning sensation of the face, and sometimes the neck and arms as well. It may also involve the conjunctivae. This can begin within 5 to 20 minutes of drinking, reaching a peak within 30 to 40 minutes, and may persist for 1 to 2 hours. Very occasionally headache occurs, and light-headedness, palpitations, wheezing and breathlessness have also been experienced.[15,16]

This disulfiram-like flushing reaction has been described in numerous reports (far too many to list here) involving large numbers of patients taking **chlorpropamide**. These reports have been extensively reviewed.[15,17-19] A similar reaction can occur, but much less frequently, with other sulphonylureas including **carbutamide**,[20] **glibenclamide (glyburide)**,[16,21] **gliclazide**,[22] **glipizide**,[16] **tolazamide**,[23] and **tolbutamide**.[24,25] In one crossover study, evident flushing phenomenon, after an oral ethanol-loading test, was seen in 6 of 10 patients taking **chlorpropamide**, 3 of 10 taking **tolbutamide**, 2 of 10 taking **glibenclamide**, one of 10 taking **glibornuride** and none of 10 taking **glipizide**.[26]

A study found that the mean half-life of **tolbutamide** in alcoholics was about one-third lower than in control subjects.[27] Alcohol is also reported to prolong but not increase the blood glucose-lowering effects of **glipizide**.[28] Another study found that intravenous infusion of ethanol (equivalent to 1 to 2 units of alcoholic drinks) significantly decreased the nadir plasma glucose level during a fast in 10 elderly patients (age range 60 to 75 years) with type 2 diabetes taking **glibenclamide** 20 mg daily.[29]

Mechanism

The exacerbation of hypoglycaemia by alcohol is not fully understood. However, it is known that if hypoglycaemia occurs when liver glycogen stores are low, the liver turns to the formation of new glucose from amino acids (gluconeogenesis). This gluconeogenesis is inhibited by the presence of alcohol so that the fall in blood glucose levels may not be prevented and a full-scale hypoglycaemic episode can result.

The chlorpropamide-alcohol flush reaction, although extensively studied, is by no means fully understood. It seems to be related to the disulfiram-alcohol reaction, and is accompanied by a rise in blood-acetaldehyde levels (see also 'Alcohol + Disulfiram', p.61). It also appears to be genetically determined[16] and may involve both prostaglandins and endogenous opioids.[30] The decreased half-life of tolbutamide in alcoholics is probably due to the inducing effects of alcohol on liver microsomal enzymes.[27,31,32]

The reasons for the raised blood lactate levels seen during the concurrent use of phenformin and alcohol are not clear, but one suggestion is that it may possibly be related to the competitive demands for isoenzymes by the reactions that convert alcohol to acetaldehyde, and lactate to pyruvate.[10] A study in healthy subjects found that moderate alcohol consumption both improves insulin action, without affecting non-insulin mediated glucose uptake, and decreases lactate clearance. The increase in blood lactate with alcohol is therefore mainly due to inhibition of clearance. Alcohol did not appear to significantly affect beta-cell function.[33]

Importance and management

The documentation of the interactions between antidiabetic drugs and alcohol is surprisingly patchy (with the exception of chlorpropamide and alcohol) but they are of recognised clinical importance.

General comments

The following contains the main recommendations of Diabetes UK (formerly The British Diabetic Association) based on a review of what is currently known:[34,35] Most diabetics need not avoid alcohol totally, but they are advised not to exceed 2 drinks (for women) or 3 drinks (for men) daily. A drink (or unit) is defined in 'Table 3.1', (p.41). The intake of drinks with high-carbohydrate content (sweet sherries, sweet wines, most liqueurs, and low alcohol wines) should be limited. Diabetics should not drink on an empty stomach and they should know that the warning signs of hypoglycaemia may possibly be obscured by the effects of the alcohol. Driving or handling dangerous machinery should be avoided because the CNS depressant effects of alcohol plus hypoglycaemia can be particularly hazardous. Warn patients of the risks of hypoglycaemia occurring several hours after drinking. Those with peripheral neuropathy should be told that alcohol may aggravate the condition and they should not have more than one drink daily. Provided drinking is restricted as suggested, and drinks containing a lot of carbohydrate are avoided, there is no need to include the drink in the dietary allowance. However, diabetics on a weight-reducing diet should try to limit intake to the occasional drink and should include it in their daily calorie allowance.

The advice of the American Diabetes Association is similar: If individuals choose to drink alcohol, daily intake should be limited to 1 drink (for women) or 2 drinks (for men). To reduce the risk of hypoglycaemia, alcohol should be consumed with food.[1]

There is some evidence that heart disease in patients with diabetes may be less common in patients who consume moderate amounts of alcohol, but this is currently not sufficient to recommend that patients who do not drink alcohol should begin to drink in moderation.[7]

Specific comments about oral antidiabetics

The chlorpropamide-alcohol interaction (flushing reaction) is very well documented, but of minimal importance. It is a nuisance and possibly socially embarrassing but normally requires no treatment. Patients should be warned. The incidence is said to lie between 13 and 33%[36,37] although one study claims that it may be as low as 4%.[38] Since it can be provoked by quite small amounts of alcohol (half a glass of sherry or wine) it is virtually impossible for sensitive patients to avoid it if they drink. Most manufacturers issue warnings about the possibility of this reaction with other sulphonylureas, but it is very rarely seen and can therefore almost always be avoided by replacing chlorpropamide with another sulphonylurea. Alcoholic subjects may need above-average doses of tolbutamide.

Metformin does not carry the same risk of lactic acidosis seen with phenformin and it is suggested in a paper[34] prepared for and approved by The British Diabetic Association [now Diabetes UK] that one or two drinks a day are unlikely to be harmful in patients taking **metformin**. However, the drug should not be given to alcoholic patients because of the possibility of liver damage.

1. American Diabetes Association. Nutrition principles and recommendations in diabetes. *Diabetes Care* (2004) 27 (Suppl 1), S36–S46.
2. Walsh CH, O'Sullivan DJ. Effect of moderate alcohol intake on control of diabetes. *Diabetes* (1974) 23, 440–2.
3. Arky RA, Veverbrants E, Abramson EA. Irreversible hypoglycemia. A complication of alcohol and insulin. *JAMA* (1968) 206, 575–8.
4. Potter J, Clarke P, Gale EAM, Dave SH, Tattersall RB. Insulin-induced hypoglycaemia in an accident and emergency department: the tip of an iceberg? *BMJ* (1982) 285, 1180–2.
5. McMonagle J, Felig P. Effects of ethanol ingestion on glucose tolerance and insulin secretion in normal and diabetic subjects. *Metabolism* (1975) 24, 625–32.
6. Lolli G, Balboni C, Ballatore C, Risoldi L, Carletti D, Silvestri L, Pacifici De Tommaso G. Wine in the diets of diabetic patients. *Q J Stud Alcohol* (1963) 24, 412–6.
7. Howard AA, Arnsten JH, Gourevitch MN. Effect of alcohol consumption on diabetes mellitus: a systematic review. *Ann Intern Med* (2004) 140, 211–19.
8. Ben G, Gnudi L, Maran A, Gigante A, Duner E, Iori E, Tiengo A, Avogaro A. Effects of chronic alcohol intake on carbohydrate and lipid metabolism in subjects with type II (non-insulin dependent) diabetes. *Am J Med* (1991) 90, 70–6.
9. Tsai CS, Oke TO, Tam CW, Olubadewo JO, Ochillo RF. The effect of regular alcohol use on the management of non-insulin diabetes mellitus. *Cell Mol Biol (Noisy-le-grand)* (2003) 49, 1327–32.
10. Johnson HK, Waterhouse C. Relationship of alcohol and hyperlactatemia in diabetic subjects treated with phenformin. *Am J Med* (1968) 45, 98–104.
11. Davidson MB, Bozarth WR, Challoner DR, Goodner CJ. Phenformin, hypoglycemia and lactic acidosis. Report of an attempted suicide. *N Engl J Med* (1966) 275, 886–8.
12. Gottlieb A, Duberstein J, Geller A. Phenformin acidosis. *N Engl J Med* (1962) 267, 806–9.
13. Schaffalitzky de Muckadell OB, Køster A, Jensen SL. Fenformin-alkohol interaktion. *Ugeskr Laeger* (1973) 135, 925–7.
14. Culkin KT, Patterson SD, Jorkasky DK, Freed MI. Rosiglitazone (RSG) does not increase the risk of alcohol-induced hypoglycemia in diet-treated type 2 diabetics. *Diabetes* (1999) 48 (Suppl 1), A350.
15. Johnston C, Wiles PG, Pyke DA. Chlorpropamide-alcohol flush: the case in favour. *Diabetologia* (1984) 26, 1–5.
16. Leslie RDG, Pyke DA. Chlorpropamide-alcohol flushing: a dominantly inherited trait associated with diabetes. *BMJ* (1978) 2, 1519–21.
17. Hillson RM, Hockaday TDR. Chlorpropamide-alcohol flush: a critical reappraisal. *Diabetologia* (1984) 26, 6–11.
18. Waldhäusl W. To flush or not to flush? Comments on the chlorpropamide-alcohol flush. *Diabetologia* (1984) 26, 12–14.
19. Groop L, Eriksson CJP, Huupponen R, Ylikarhi R, Pelkonen R. Roles of chlorpropamide, alcohol and acetaldehyde in determining the chlorpropamide-alcohol flush. *Diabetologia* (1984) 26, 34–38.
20. Signorelli S. Tolerance for alcohol in patients on chlorpropamide. *Ann N Y Acad Sci* (1959) 74, 900–903.
21. Stowers JM. Alcohol and glibenclamide. *BMJ* (1971) 3, 533.
22. Conget JI, Vendrell J, Esmatjes E, Halperin I. Gliclazide alcohol flush. *Diabetes Care* (1989) 12, 44.

23. McKendry JBR, Gfeller KF. Clinical experience with the oral antidiabetic compound tolazamide. *Can Med Assoc J* (1967) 96, 531–5.
24. Dolger H. Experience with the tolbutamide treatment of five hundred cases of diabetes on an ambulatory basis. *Ann N Y Acad Sci* (1957) 71, 275–9.
25. Büttner H. Äthanolunverträglichkeit beim Menschen nach Sulfonylharnstoffen. *Dtsch Arch Klin Med* (1961) 207, 1–18.
26. Lao B, Czyzyk A, Szutowski M, Szczepanik Z. Alcohol tolerance in patients with non-insulin-dependent (type 2) diabetes treated with sulphonylurea derivatives. *Arzneimittelforschung* (1994) 44, 727–34.
27. Carulli N, Manenti F, Gallo M, Salvioli GF. Alcohol-drugs interaction in man: alcohol and tolbutamide. *Eur J Clin Invest* (1971) 1, 421–4.
28. Hartling SG, Faber OK, Wegmann M-L, Wahlin-Boll E and Melander A. Interaction of ethanol and glipizide in humans. *Diabetes Care* (1987) 10, 683–6.
29. Burge MR, Zeise T-M, Sobhy TA, Rassam AG, Schade DS. Low-dose ethanol predisposes elderly fasted patients with type 2 diabetes to sulfonylurea-induced low blood glucose. *Diabetes Care* (1999) 22, 2037–43.
30. Johnston C, Wiles PG, Medbak S, Bowcock S, Cooke ED, Pyke DA, Rees LH. The role of endogenous opioids in the chlorpropamide alcohol flush. *Clin Endocrinol (Oxf)* (1984) 21, 489–97.
31. Kater RMH, Roggin G, Tobon F, Zieve P, Iber FL. Increased rate of clearance of drugs from the circulation of alcoholics. *Am J Med Sci* (1969) 258, 35–9.
32. Kater RMH, Tobon F, Iber FL. Increased rate of tolbutamide metabolism in alcoholic patients. *JAMA* (1969) 207, 363–5.
33. Avogaro A, Watanabe RM, Gottardo L, de Kreutzenberg S, Tiengo A, Pacini G. Glucose tolerance during moderate alcohol intake: insights on insulin action from glucose/lactate dynamics. *J Clin Endocrinol Metab* (2002) 87, 1233–8.
34. Connor H, Marks V. Alcohol and diabetes. A position paper prepared by the Nutrition Subcommittee of the British Diabetic Association's Medical Advisory Committee and approved by the Executive Council of the British Diabetic Association. *Hum Nutr Appl Nutr* (1985) 39A, 393–9.
35. Diabetes UK (formerly the British Diabetic Association). Care recommendation: alcohol. Available at: http://www.diabetes.org.uk/Guide-to-diabetes/Food_and_recipes/Alcohol_and_diabetes/ (accessed 17/08/07).
36. Fitzgerald MG, Gaddie R, Malins JM, O'Sullivan DJ. Alcohol sensitivity in diabetics receiving chlorpropamide. *Diabetes* (1962) 11, 40–3.
37. Daeppen JP, Hofstetter JR, Curchod B, Saudan Y. Traitment oral du diabete par un nouvel hypoglycemiant, le P 607 ou Diabinese. *Schweiz Med Wochenschr* (1959) 89, 817–19.
38. De Silva NE, Tunbridge WMG, Alberti KGMM. Low incidence of chlorpropamide-alcohol flushing in diet-treated, non-insulin-dependent diabetics. *Lancet* (1981) i, 128–31.

Antidiabetics + Allopurinol

Allopurinol adversely affected glycaemic control in a patient with type 2 diabetes receiving insulin. Allopurinol caused an increase in the half-life of chlorpropamide, and a minor decrease in the half-life of tolbutamide, but the effect of these changes on the hypoglycaemic response of patients is uncertain. Marked hypoglycaemia and coma occurred in one patient taking gliclazide and allopurinol.

Clinical evidence

A. Insulin

A case report describes improved glycaemic control in a type 2 diabetic patient after allopurinol was stopped. Despite restricted food intake and an increasing dose of insulin, his glycaemic control was poor (fasting blood glucose 14.8 mmol/L) when he took allopurinol 100 mg twice daily. However, within a few days of stopping the allopurinol, an unexpected improvement in glycaemic control was observed (fasting blood glucose reduced to less than 11 mmol/L). He was later rechallenged with allopurinol, which resulted in reduced glucose tolerance, but increased insulin response, suggesting increased insulin resistance. Hyperuricaemia was later controlled with **probenecid,** which did not adversely affect glycaemic control.[1]

B. Sulphonylureas

(a) Chlorpropamide

A brief report describes 6 patients taking chlorpropamide with allopurinol. The half-life of chlorpropamide in one patient with gout and normal renal function exceeded 200 hours (normally 36 hours) after allopurinol had been taken for 10 days, and in 2 others the half-life was extended to 44 and 55 hours. The other 3 patients were given allopurinol for only 1 or 2 days and the half-life of chlorpropamide remained unaltered.[2]

(b) Gliclazide

Severe hypoglycaemia (1.6 mmol/L) and coma occurred in a patient with renal impairment taking gliclazide and allopurinol.[3] Hypoglycaemia has been seen in another patient taking both drugs, but an interaction is less clear, as enalapril and ranitidine, which may also (rarely) interact were also involved.[3]

(c) Tolbutamide

Allopurinol 2.5 mg/kg twice daily for 15 days reduced the half-life of intravenous tolbutamide in 10 healthy subjects by 25%, from 360 to 267 minutes.[4,5]

Mechanism

Not understood. In the case of chlorpropamide it has been suggested that it possibly involves some competition for renal tubular mechanisms.[2]

Importance and management

Information is very limited. Only gliclazide has been implicated in severe hypoglycaemia with allopurinol and there seem to be no reports of either grossly enhanced hypoglycaemia with chlorpropamide and allopurinol, or a reduced effect with tolbutamide and allopurinol. More study is needed to find out whether any of these interactions has general clinical importance, but it seems unlikely.

1. Ohashi K, Ishibashi S, Yazaki Y, Yamada N. Improved glycemic control in a diabetic patient after discontinuation of allopurinol administration. *Diabetes Care* (1998) 21, 192–3.
2. Petitpierre B, Perrin L, Rudhardt M, Herrera A, Fabre J. Behaviour of chlorpropamide in renal insufficiency and under the effect of associated drug therapy. *Int J Clin Pharmacol* (1972) 6, 120–4.
3. Girardin E, Vial T, Pham E, Evreux J-C. Hypoglycémies induites par les sulfamides hypoglycémiants. *Ann Med Interne (Paris)* (1992) 143, 11–17.
4. Gentile S, Porcellini M, Loguercio C, Foglia F, Coltorti M. Modificazioni della depurazione plasmatica di tolbutamide e rifamicina-SV indotte dal trattamento con allopurinolo in volontari sono. *Progr Med (Napoli)* (1979) 35, 637–42.
5. Gentile S, Porcellini M, Foglia F, Loguercio C, Coltorti M. Influenza di allopurinolo sull'emivita plasmatica di tolbutamide e rifamicina-SV in soggetti sani. *Boll Soc Ital Biol Sper* (1979) 55, 345–8.

Antidiabetics + Anabolic steroids

Nandrolone, methandienone, testosterone and stanozolol can enhance the blood glucose-lowering effects of insulin.

Clinical evidence

In a study in 54 diabetics taking **nandrolone phenylpropionate** 25 mg weekly or **nandrolone decanoate** 50 mg given every 3 weeks by intramuscular injection, it was found necessary to reduce the insulin dosage by an average of 36% (reduction range 4 to 56 units) in about one-third of the patients.[1]

Other reports similarly describe an enhanced reduction in blood glucose levels in diabetics receiving insulin and **nandrolone,**[2,3] **methandienone,**[4] **testosterone propionate**[5] or **stanozolol.**[6] A reduction in blood glucose levels has also been seen in healthy subjects given **testosterone propionate.**[7] No changes were seen when **ethylestrenol** was used.[1,2]

Mechanism

Uncertain.

Importance and management

Established interactions but the total picture is incomplete because not all of the anabolic steroids appear to have been studied and they may not necessarily behave identically. A fall in the dosage requirements of insulin may be expected in many patients with the steroids cited. An average reduction of a third is reported.[1] Given these results, and the fact that anabolic steroids have been shown to *impair* glucose tolerance it would seem prudent to closely monitor the concurrent use of any antidiabetic drug.

1. Houtsmuller AJ. The therapeutic applications of anabolic steroids in ophthalmology: biochemical results. *Acta Endocrinol (Copenh)* (1961) 39 (Suppl 63), 154–74.
2. Dardenne U. The therapeutic applications of anabolic steroids in ophthalmology. *Acta Endocrinol (Copenh)* (1961) 39 (Suppl 63), 143–53.
3. Weissel W. Anaboles Hormon bei malignem oder kompliziertem Diabetes mellitus. *Wien Klin Wochenschr* (1962) 74, 234–6.
4. Landon J, Wynn V, Samols E, Bilkus D. The effect of anabolic steroids on blood sugar and plasma insulin levels in man. *Metabolism* (1963) 12, 924–35.
5. Veil WH, Lippross O. 'Unspezifische' wirkungen der Männlichen keimdrücenhormone. *Klin Wochenschr* (1938) 17, 655–8.
6. Pergola F. El estanozolol, nuevo anabolico. *Prensa Med Argent* (1962) 49, 274–90.
7. Talaat M, Habib YA, Habib M. The effect of testosterone on the carbohydrate metabolism in normal subjects. *Arch Int Pharmacodyn Ther* (1957) 111, 215–26.

Antidiabetics + Angiotensin II receptor antagonists

Glibenclamide (glyburide) causes a small reduction in valsartan plasma levels, but this is unlikely to be of any clinical significance. No clinically relevant pharmacokinetic interaction occurs between glibenclamide and candesartan or telmisartan, or between tolbutamide and irbesartan. Eprosartan does not alter the efficacy of glibenclamide. Losartan and possibly eprosartan may reduce awareness of hypoglycaemic symptoms.

Clinical evidence and mechanism

A. Insulin

(a) Eprosartan

A study in 16 healthy subjects found that a single 600-microgram dose of eprosartan did not significantly affect adrenaline (epinephrine) release in response to insulin-induced hypoglycaemia, but the eprosartan tended to blunt some of the haemodynamic responses to hypoglycaemia.[1] Theoretically, therefore, hypoglycaemic symptoms could be reduced in some diabetic patients.

(b) Losartan

Three patients with type 1 diabetes spontaneously reported reduced awareness of hypoglycaemic symptoms (tremor, palpitations, nervousness) after initiation of losartan therapy. A placebo-controlled study in 16 healthy subjects given losartan 50 mg daily for 8 days confirmed an attenuation of the symptomatic and hormonal responses to hypoglycaemia.[2]

B. Glibenclamide (Glyburide)

(a) Candesartan

Glibenclamide 3.5 mg daily did not significantly affect the pharmacokinetics of candesartan 16 mg daily, both given for 7 days, although the maximum plasma concentration of candesartan was slightly increased by 12%. The pharmacokinetics of glibenclamide were not altered by the candesartan.[3]

(b) Eprosartan

Fifteen type 2 diabetics stabilised taking glibenclamide 3.75 to 10 mg daily for at least 30 days had no changes in their 24-hour plasma glucose concentrations when eprosartan 200 mg twice daily was added, for a further 7 days. Concurrent use was safe and well tolerated and it was concluded that there is no clinically relevant interaction between these two drugs.[4]

(c) Valsartan

In a randomised, crossover study, 12 healthy subjects were given single oral doses of valsartan 160 mg and glibenclamide 1.75 mg alone and together.[5] Glibenclamide appeared to decrease the valsartan AUC by 16%, but the plasma concentrations of valsartan showed wide variations between subjects. The pharmacokinetics of glibenclamide were not affected.[5] The changes in valsartan pharmacokinetics seen with glibenclamide appear to have little or no clinical relevance.

C. Tolbutamide

A study in 18 healthy subjects given **irbesartan** 300 mg daily and tolbutamide 1 g daily, either alone or in combination, found that no clinically important pharmacokinetic interactions occurred.[6]

Importance and management

No special precautions would appear to be needed if candesartan, eprosartan, telmisartan or valsartan are given with glibenclamide, or if irbesartan is given with tolbutamide. However, symptoms of hypoglycaemia may be reduced by losartan and possibly other angiotensin II receptor antagonists. Further clinical study is needed, but note that this is similar to the effect of 'ACE inhibitors', (p.471).

1. Christensen M, Ibsen H, Worck R. Effect of eprosartan on catecholamines and peripheral haemodynamics in subjects with insulin-induced hypoglycaemia. *Clin Sci* (2005) 108, 113–19.
2. Deininger E, Oltmanns KM, Wellhoener P, Fruehwald-Schultes B, Kern W, Heuer B, Dominiak P, Born J, Fehm HL, Peters A. Losartan attenuates symptomatic and hormonal responses to hypoglycemia in humans. *Clin Pharmacol Ther* (2001) 70, 362–9.
3. Jonkman JHG, van Lier JJ, van Heiningen PNM, Lins R, Sennewald R, Högemann A. Pharmacokinetic drug interaction studies with candesartan cilexetil. *J Hum Hypertens* (1997) 11 (Suppl 2), S31–S35.
4. Martin DE, DeCherney GS, Ilson BE, Jones BA, Boike SC, Freed MI, Jorasky DK. Eprosartan, an angiotensin II receptor antagonist, does not affect the pharmacodynamics of glyburide in patients with type II diabetes mellitus. *J Clin Pharmacol* (1997) 37, 155–9.
5. Novartis Pharmaceuticals Ltd. Data on file, Protocol 52.
6. Marino MR, Vachharajani NN. Drug interactions with irbesartan. *Clin Pharmacokinet* (2001) 40, 605–14.

Antidiabetics + Antacids

The rate of absorption of some antidiabetics is increased by some antacids, but there appear to be no reports of adverse responses in diabetic patients as a result of any of these interactions.

Clinical evidence

(a) Acarbose

A placebo-controlled study found that 10 mL of *Maalox 70* (**aluminium/magnesium hydroxide**) had no effect on the blood glucose-and insulin-lowering effects of acarbose 100 mg in 24 healthy subjects given a 75-g dose of sucrose. It was concluded that no special precautions are needed if this or similar antacids are used with acarbose.[1]

(b) Chlorpropamide

Magnesium hydroxide 850 mg increased the rate of absorption of chlorpropamide 250 mg in healthy subjects, but the insulin and glucose responses were unaffected.[2]

(c) Glibenclamide (Glyburide)

A single-dose study in healthy subjects found that **magnesium hydroxide** 850 mg had little effect on the rate or extent of absorption of a micronised glibenclamide preparation (*Semi-Euglucon*), but it caused a threefold increase in the peak plasma concentration and the bioavailability of a non-micronised preparation (*Gilemid*).[3] *Maalox* (**aluminium/magnesium hydroxide**) increased the AUC of glibenclamide (given as *Daonil*) by one-third, and its maximum serum level by 50%.[4]

Sodium bicarbonate 1 to 3 g very markedly increased the early bioavailability of non-micronised glibenclamide in healthy subjects, but its activity remained unaltered.[5]

(d) Glipizide

Sodium bicarbonate 3 g significantly increased the absorption of glipizide 5 mg and enhanced its effects to some extent, but the total absorption was unaltered.[6] The AUCs from 0 to 30 minutes, 1-hour, and 2-hours, were increased six-, four- and twofold, respectively, and the time to reach the peak serum level fell from 2.5 to 1 hour. **Aluminium hydroxide** 1 g did not appear to affect the absorption of glipizide 5 mg.[6] **Magnesium hydroxide** 850 mg considerably increased the rate of absorption of glipizide 5 mg, the AUCs from 0 to 30 minutes and 1-hour being increased by 180 and 69%, respectively.[7]

(e) Miglitol

The manufacturer notes that an antacid (not specified) did not alter the pharmacokinetics of miglitol in healthy subjects.[8]

(f) Tolbutamide

Magnesium hydroxide 850 mg increased the 0 to 1-hour and 2-hour AUCs of a single 500-mg dose of tolbutamide 5-fold and 2.5-fold, respectively, in healthy subjects. The total AUC was unaffected. The maximum insulin response was increased fourfold and occurred about an hour earlier, and the glucose responses were also larger and occurred earlier.[2]

Mechanism

Uncertain. The small increase in gastric pH caused by these antacids possibly increases the solubility of these sulphonylureas and therefore increases their absorption.[9]

Importance and management

Although some interactions certainly occur in healthy subjects, their clinical importance in patients with diabetes is uncertain. No reports of adverse reactions appear to have been published, but note that patients taking glipizide with sodium bicarbonate or magnesium hydroxide, or tolbutamide with magnesium hydroxide may experience transient hypoglycaemia. Generally no action seems necessary, but if a problem does occur, separating the dosages as much as possible would probably minimise any effects. Giving glibenclamide half to one hour before the antacid has been suggested.[4]

1. Höpfner M, Durani B, Spengler M, Fölsch UR. Effect of acarbose and simultaneous antacid therapy on blood glucose. *Arzneimittelforschung* (1997) 47, 1108–1111.
2. Kivistö KT, Neuvonen PJ. Effect of magnesium hydroxide on the absorption and efficacy of tolbutamide and chlorpropamide. *Eur J Clin Pharmacol* (1992) 42, 675–80.
3. Neuvonen PJ, Kivistö KT. The effects of magnesium hydroxide on the absorption and efficacy of two glibenclamide preparations. *Br J Clin Pharmacol* (1991) 32, 215–20.
4. Zuccaro P, Pacifici R, Pichini S, Avico U, Federzoni G, Pini LA, Sternieri E. Influence of antacids on the bioavailability of glibenclamide. *Drugs Exp Clin Res* (1989) 15, 165–9.
5. Kivistö KT, Lehto P, Neuvonen PJ. The effects of different doses of sodium bicarbonate on the absorption and activity of non-micronized glibenclamide. *Int J Clin Pharmacol Ther Toxicol* (1993) 31, 236–40.
6. Kivistö KT, Neuvonen PJ. Differential effects of sodium bicarbonate and aluminium hydroxide on the absorption and activity of glipizide. *Eur J Clin Pharmacol* (1991) 40, 383–6.
7. Kivistö KT, Neuvonen PJ. Enhancement of absorption and effect of glipizide by magnesium hydroxide. *Clin Pharmacol Ther* (1991) 49, 39–43.
8. Glyset (Miglitol). Pharmacia & Upjohn Company. US Prescribing information, October 2004.
9. Lehto P, Laine K, Kivistö K, Neuvonen PJ. The effect of pH on the *in vitro* dissolution of sulfonylurea preparations — a mechanism for the antacid-sulfonylurea interaction? *Therapie* (1995) 50 (Suppl), 413.

Antidiabetics + Antimalarials

Hydroxychloroquine may reduce insulin requirements by about 25%, and a case of hypoglycaemia has been reported. Similarly, hypoglycaemia has occurred in a patient taking chloroquine and insulin. Reduced glucose levels or hypoglycaemia have been reported with mefloquine, quinidine, quinine, and sulfadoxine-pyrimethamine. Note that falciparum malaria *per se* can result in severe hypoglycaemia, and quinine in particular may contribute to this.

Clinical evidence, mechanism, importance and management

(a) Effect on diabetic control

1. Chloroquine. A case report describes a patient with type 1 diabetes who had developed insulin resistance and was maintained on intravenous **insulin**, who showed a dramatic return of sensitivity to subcutaneous **insulin**, heralded by a series of hypoglycaemic attacks, within 15 days of starting to take chloroquine phosphate 200 mg every 8 hours.[1] Similarly, chloroquine phosphate (150 mg of chloroquine base) four times daily improved glucose tolerance in 5 out of 6 patients with type 2 diabetes controlled by diet, but had little effect on healthy subjects.[2] It has been suggested that chloroquine might inhibit insulin degradation or increase glucose utilisation in peripheral tissues.[3]

2. Hydroxychloroquine. The effect of hydroxychloroquine on diabetic control with **insulin** or **glibenclamide (glyburide)** was investigated in a randomised, double-blind, placebo-controlled study in 38 patients with poorly controlled type 2 diabetes. The addition of hydroxychloroquine 200 mg three times daily to **insulin** caused a significant improvement in the glycaemic profile and the daily **insulin** dose had to be reduced by about 25%. Patients taking **glibenclamide** with hydroxychloroquine also had a significant improvement in their plasma glucose levels. One patient receiving **insulin** and hydroxychloroquine had severe hypoglycaemia after 2 months of treatment, and it was necessary to drastically reduce the daily dose of **insulin**.[3] The authors suggested that hydroxychloroquine might inhibit insulin degradation or increase glucose utilisation in peripheral tissues.[3]

(b) Treatment of malaria

Hypoglycaemia is a complication of falciparum malaria, which occurs mainly in severe life-threatening disease,[4,5] in pregnant women[4] or children,[6,7] and in patients who are given **quinine** or **quinidine**.[5,7-10] The reasons are not fully understood but renal impairment and poor nutrition, may be contributing factors. In severe malaria, hypoglycaemia may increase as the patient's glucose production becomes insufficient for the host/parasite demand because in this situation glucose utilisation can be increased by 50%.[11]

Additionally, **quinine** reduces plasma glucose by stimulating the release of large amounts of **insulin** from the pancreas,[12] possibly associated with an increase in the sensitivity to **insulin** as the malaria improves,[13] although other factors may also be involved. A study in 32 patients with malaria found that their pre-treatment capillary glucose was below normal in 12.5% of cases. One hour after intravenous **quinine** was given, glucose levels in all patients fell by an average of 11.4% and after 6 hours a further fall of 20.5% was found in 75% of patients (with an increase at 6 hours in the remaining 25% of patients).[10] **Quinidine** has been shown to have a similar effect.[14] Whether these changes can also occur in patients with **quinine**- or **quinidine**-treated malaria and diabetes, despite their pancreatic beta cell impairment, seems not to have been studied, although one isolated report argues against significant **quinine**-mediated mechanisms. Profound and persistent hypoglycaemia was seen in a diabetic patient (type 2 diabetes) with severe falciparum malaria treated with **quinine**, but the hypoglycaemia evolved prior to **quinine** therapy and resolved as the parasitaemia was successfully eradicated, despite continuation of the **quinine**. Subsequently, as she had discontinued antidiabetic medication (chlorpropamide) prior to hospital admission, hyperglycaemia developed (blood glucose ranging from 7.5 to 16 mmol/L) despite continuing to take **quinine**.[15] Any interpretation of disturbances in the control of the diabetes should take into account the severity of the malaria and the possible effects of these drugs.

An isolated report describes life-threatening hypoglycaemia in a 3-year-old boy, with uncomplicated malaria, 90 minutes after he took **sulfadoxine-pyrimethamine** (*Fansidar*).[16] **Mefloquine** has been reported to reduce plasma glucose levels in healthy subjects.[17] **Artemisinin derivatives** such as **artemether** may be associated with fewer episodes of hypoglycaemia than **quinine** in children with severe malaria.[7] **Chloroquine, amodiaquine** and **halofantrine** do not apparently stimulate the release of **insulin**.[14,18]

(c) Treatment of cramps

A study in 12 patients (age 51 to 79 years) with type 2 diabetes taking **gliclazide**, and 10 similar, non-diabetic subjects, found that a single 600-mg dose of **quinine sulphate** at night reduced serum glucose levels in both groups, without affecting serum insulin concentrations.[19] **Quinine** has been responsible for hypoglycaemia in non-diabetic patients, one of whom was taking **quinine sulphate** 325 mg four times daily for leg muscle cramps.[20] Two other non-diabetic patients, one with congestive heart failure and the other with terminal cancer, similarly developed hypoglycaemia when given **quinine** for leg cramps.[21,22]

1. Rees RG, Smith MJ. Effect of chloroquine on insulin and glucose homoeostasis in normal subjects and patients with non-insulin dependent diabetes mellitus. *BMJ* (1987) 294, 900–1.
2. Smith GD, Amos TAS, Mahler R, Peters TJ. Effect of chloroquine on insulin and glucose homoeostasis in normal subjects and patients with non-insulin-dependent diabetes mellitus. *BMJ* (1987) 294, 465–7.
3. Quatraro A, Consoli G, Magno M, Caretta F, Nardozza A, Ceriello A, Giugliano D. Hydroxychloroquine in decompensated, treatment-refractory noninsulin-dependent diabetes mellitus. A new job for an old drug? *Ann Intern Med* (1990) 112, 678–81.
4. Chogle AR. Hypoglycaemia in falciparum malaria. *J Assoc Physicians India* (1998) 46, 921–2.
5. Metha SR, Joshi V, Lazar AI. Unusual acute and chronic complications of malaria. *J Assoc Physicians India* (1996) 44, 451–3.
6. Singh B, Choo KE, Ibrahim J, Johnston W, Davis TME. Non-radioisotopic glucose turnover in children with falciparum malaria end enteric fever. *Trans R Soc Trop Med Hyg* (1998) 92, 532–7.
7. Agbenyega T, Angus BJ, Bedu-Addo G, Baffoe-Bonnie B, Guyton T, Stacpoole PW, Krishna S. Glucose and lactate kinetics in children with severe malaria. *J Clin Endocrinol Metab* (2000) 85, 1569–76.
8. White NJ, Warrell DA, Chanthavanich P, Looareesuwan S, Warrell MJ, Krishna S, Williamson DH, Turner RC. Severe hypoglycemia and hyperinsulinemia in falciparum malaria. *N Engl J Med* (1983) 309, 61–6.
9. Looareesuwan S, Phillips RE, White NJ, Kietinun S, Karbwang J, Rackow C, Turner RC, Warrell DA. Quinine and severe falciparum malaria in late pregnancy. *Lancet* (1985) ii, 4–8.
10. Gupta GB, Varma S. Effect of intravenous quinine on capillary glucose levels in malaria. *J Assoc Physicians India* (2001) 49, 426–9.
11. Binh TQ, Davis TME, Johnston W, Thu LTA, Boston R, Danh PT, Anh TK. Glucose metabolism in severe malaria: minimal model analysis of the intravenous glucose tolerance test incorporating a stable glucose label. *Metabolism* (1997) 46, 1435–40.
12. Davis TME, Binh TQ, Thu LTA, Long TTA, Johnston W, Robertson K, Barrett PHR. Glucose and lactate turnover in adults with falciparum malaria: effect of complications and antimalarial therapy. *Trans R Soc Trop Med Hyg* (2002) 96, 411–17.
13. Davis TME, Pukrittayakamee S, Supanaranond W, Looareesuwan S, Krishna S, Nagachinta B, Turner RC, White NJ. Glucose metabolism in quinine-treated patients with uncomplicated falciparum malaria. *Clin Endocrinol (Oxf)* (1990) 33, 739–49.
14. Phillips RE, Looareesuwan S, White NJ, Chanthavanich P, Karbwang J, Supanaranond W, Turner RC, Warrell DA. Hypoglycaemia and antimalarial drugs: quinidine and release of insulin. *BMJ* (1986) 292, 1319–21.
15. Shalev O, Tsur A, Rahav G. Falciparum malaria-induced hypoglycaemia in a diabetic patient. *Postgrad Med J* (1992) 68, 281–2.
16. Fairhurst RM, Sadou B, Guindo A, Diallo DA, Doumbo OK, Wellems TE. Case report: life-threatening hypoglycaemia associated with sulfadoxine-pyrimethamine, a commonly used antimalarial drug. *Trans R Soc Trop Med Hyg* (2003) 97, 595–6.
17. Davis TM, Dembo LG, Kaye-Eddie SA, Hewitt BJ, Hislop RG, Batty KT. Neurological, cardiovascular and metabolic effects of mefloquine in healthy volunteers: a double-blind, placebo-controlled trial. *Br J Clin Pharmacol* (1996) 42, 415–21.
18. White NJ, Miler KD, Marsh K, Berry CD, Turner RC, Williamson DH, Brown J. Does chloroquine cause hypoglycaemia in the absence of clinical malaria? *Lancet* (1987) 2, 281–2.
19. Dyer JR, Davis TME, Giele C, Annus T, Garcia-Webb P, Robson J. The pharmacokinetics and pharmacodynamics of quinine in the diabetic and non-diabetic elderly. *Br J Clin Pharmacol* (1994) 38, 205–12.
20. Limburg PJ, Katz H, Grant CS, Service FJ. Quinine-induced hypoglycemia. *Ann Intern Med* (1993) 119, 218–19.
21. Harats N, Ackerman Z, Shalit M. Quinine-related hypoglycemia. *N Engl J Med* (1984) 310, 1331.
22. Jones RG, Sue-Ling HM, Kear C, Wiles PG, Quirke P. Severe symptomatic hypoglycaemia due to quinine therapy. *J R Soc Med* (1986) 79, 426–8.

Antidiabetics + Antineoplastics

Asparaginase sometimes induces temporary diabetes mellitus. It seems possible that some diabetics will need changes in the dose of their antidiabetic drugs. There is also evidence that the control of diabetes can be severely disturbed in patients given cyclophosphamide. Capecitabine may cause hyperglycaemia and therefore could aggravate diabetes.

Clinical evidence and mechanism

(a) Asparaginase (Colaspase)

Three patients with acute lymphocytic leukaemia developed diabetes after receiving asparaginase with or without corticosteroids. In two of them this occurred 2 and 4 days after a single dose of asparaginase, and in another patient it occurred 2 days after the fourth dose. Plasma insulin was undetectable. A normal insulin response returned in one patient after 23 days, whereas the other 2 showed a suboptimal response 2 weeks, and 9 months afterwards.[1] In another study, 5 out of 39 patients (3 adults, 2 children) developed hyperglycaemia and glycosuria after treatment with asparaginase. This responded to **insulin**, and blood glucose levels returned to normal in about 2 weeks.[2] In a retrospective analysis, it was found that about 10% of 421 children with leukaemia treated with asparaginase and **prednisone** developed hyperglycaemia, which resolved in all patients. A family history of diabetes and obesity were found to be risk factors.[3] Other cases have been described,[4-6] including one who, unusually, developed persistent hyperglycaemia and required long-term treatment with oral antidiabetics.[5] The reasons for this reaction are not understood but suggestions include inhibition of insulin synthesis,[7] direct damage to the islets of Langerhans,[1] and reduced insulin binding.[7] Hyperglycaemia can be caused by 'corticosteroids' (p.485), and their combined use with asparaginase is probably a contributing factor.

(b) Capecitabine

There appear to be no reports of adverse interactions between antidiabetics and capecitabine, but the manufacturer notes that the control of diabetes mellitus may be affected by capecitabine, for which reason they advise caution.[8]

(c) Cyclophosphamide

Acute hypoglycaemia has been described in 2 diabetic patients receiving **insulin** and **carbutamide** who were also given cyclophosphamide.[9] Three cases of diabetes, apparently induced by the use of cyclophosphamide, have also been reported.[10] The reasons are not understood.

Importance and management

Strictly speaking probably none of these reactions is an interaction, but they serve to underline the importance of monitoring the diabetic control of patients receiving asparaginase, capecitabine or cyclophosphamide.

1. Gailani S, Nussbaum A, Ohnuma T, Freeman A. Diabetes in patients treated with asparaginase. *Clin Pharmacol Ther* (1971) 12, 487–90.
2. Ohnuma T, Holland JF, Freeman A, Sinks LF. Biochemical and pharmacological studies with asparaginase in man. *Cancer Res* (1970) 30, 2297–2305.
3. Pui C-H, Burghen GA, Bowman WP, Aur RJA. Risk factors for hyperglycemia in children with leukemia receiving L-asparaginase and prednisone. *J Pediatr* (1981) 99, 46–50.
4. Wang Y-J, Chu H-Y, Shu S-G, Chi C-S. Hyperglycemia induced by chemotherapeutic agents used in acute lymphoblastic leukemia; report of three cases. *Chin Med J* (1993) 51, 457–61.
5. Hsu Y-J, Chen Y-C, Ho C-L, Kao W-Y, Chao T-Y. Diabetic ketoacidosis and persistent hyperglycemia as long-term complications of L-asparaginase-induced pancreatitis. *Chin Med J* (2002) 65, 441–5.
6. Charan VD, Desai N, Singh AP, Choudhry VP. Diabetes mellitus and pancreatitis as a complication of L-asparaginase therapy. *Indian Pediatr* (1993) 30, 809–10.
7. Burghen G, Pui C-H, Yasuda K and Kitabchi AE. Decreased insulin binding and production: probable mechanism for hyperglycaemia due to therapy with prednisone (PRED) and l-asparaginase (ASP). *Pediatr Res* (1981) 15, 626.
8. Xeloda (Capecitabine). Roche Products Ltd. UK Summary of product characteristics, March 2007.
9. Krüger H-U. Blutzuckersenkende Wirkung von Cyclophosphamid bei Diabetikern. *Med Klin* (1966) 61, 1462–3. Roche Product Limited.
10. Pengelly CR. Diabetes mellitus and cyclophosphamide. *BMJ* (1965) i, 1312–13.

Antidiabetics + Antipsychotics

Chlorpromazine may raise blood glucose levels, particularly in daily doses of 100 mg or more, and disturb the control of diabetes. Clozapine, olanzapine and risperidone are associated with an increased risk of glucose intolerance.

Clinical evidence

(a) Phenothiazines and Butyrophenones

A long-term study was undertaken over the period 1955 to 1966 in a large number of women treated for a year or longer with **chlorpromazine** 100 mg daily or more, or corresponding doses of **perphenazine, thioridazine, trifluoperazine**. This found that about 25% developed hyperglycaemia accompanied by glycosuria, compared with less than 9% in a control group who were not taking phenothiazines. Of those given a phenothiazine, about a quarter had complete remission of the symptoms when the drug was withdrawn or the dosage reduced. **Thioridazine** appeared to be less diabetogenic than the other phenothiazines used.[1]

There are other reports of this response to **chlorpromazine**.[2-11] However, in contrast one study in 850 patients suggests that **chlorpromazine** has no effect on blood glucose levels; 22 diabetic patients in the study had no significant changes in their blood glucose levels. Five patients developed diabetes, but this was believed to be due to factors other than **chlorpromazine** treatment.[12] **Chlorpromazine** 50 to 70 mg daily does not affect blood glucose levels significantly.[11] Further, a more recent analysis discussed in (b) below did not find an increased risk of glucose intolerance with **chlorpromazine** or **haloperidol**, and notes that the number of reports of glucose intolerance with these drugs has remained small.[13]

(b) Atypical antipsychotics

An analysis of reports of glucose intolerance in the adverse reaction database of the WHO Collaborating Centre for International Drug Monitoring found that **clozapine**, **olanzapine** and **risperidone** were associated with an increased risk of glucose intolerance. It is uncertain whether this is a dose-related effect. Additional risk factors with these antipsychotics were an underlying diabetic condition, weight increase, male gender, or the concurrent use of valproic acid, SSRIs or buspirone.[13]

Mechanism

Although some studies found that drugs such as chlorpromazine and haloperidol were not associated with glucose intolerance,[11,13] it seems that chlorpromazine can inhibit the release of insulin, and possibly cause adrenaline release from the adrenals, both of which could result in a rise in blood glucose levels. This may be a dose-related effect.[11] Further, chlorpromazine may cause aggregation and inactivation of insulin by reduction of disulfide bonds.[14] Clozapine may induce insulin resistance and a compensatory increase in insulin secretion. Patients may develop diabetes if this compensatory increase is not achieved. Clozapine and olanzapine may cause weight gain and hypertriglyceridaemia.[13] Schizophrenia itself may be associated with an increased risk of hyperglycaemia.

Importance and management

A long-established reaction first recognised in the early 1950s. The incidence of hyperglycaemia with chlorpromazine in doses of 100 mg or more is about 25%. Increases in the dosage requirements of the antidiabetic should be anticipated during concurrent use.[1] Smaller chlorpromazine doses, of 50 to 70 mg daily do not appear to cause hyperglycaemia. There seems to be little clinical evidence that other phenothiazines or butyrophenones significantly disturb blood glucose levels in diabetics. The atypical antipsychotics, clozapine, olanzapine and risperidone appear to be associated with an increased risk of glucose intolerance and regular monitoring is recommended in the presence of additional risk factors for diabetes mellitus.[13]

1. Thonnard-Neumann E. Phenothiazines and diabetes in hospitalized women. *Am J Psychiatry* (1968) 124, 978–82.
2. Hiles BW. Hyperglycaemia and glycosuria following chlorpromazine therapy. *JAMA* (1956) 162, 1651.
3. Dobkin AB, Lamoureux L, Letienne R, Gilbert RGB. Some studies with Largactil. *Can Med Assoc J* (1954) 70, 626–8.
4. Célice J, Porcher P, Plas F, Hélie J, Peltier A. Action de la chlorpromazine sur la vésicule biliare et le clon droit. *Therapie* (1955) 10, 30–38.
5. Charatan FBE, Bartlett NG. The effect of chlorpromazine ('Largactil') on glucose tolerance. *J Ment Sci* (1955) 101, 351–3.
6. Cooperberg AA, Eidlow S. Haemolytic anemia, jaundice and diabetes mellitus following chlorpromazine therapy. *Can Med Assoc J* (1956) 75, 746–9.
7. Blair D, Brady DM. Recent advances in the treatment of schizophrenia: group training and tranquillizers. *J Ment Sci* (1958) 104, 625–64.
8. Amidsen A. Diabetes mellitus as a side effect of treatment with tricyclic neuroleptics. *Acta Psychiatr Scand* (1964) 40 (Suppl 180), 411–14.
9. Arneson GA. Phenothiazine derivatives and glucose metabolism. *J Neuropsychiatr* (1964) 5, 181–5.
10. Korenyi C, Lowenstein B. Chlorpromazine induced diabetes. *Dis Nerv Syst* (1971) 29, 827–8.
11. Erle G, Basso M, Federspil G, Sicolo N, Scandellari C. Effect of chlorpromazine on blood glucose and plasma insulin in man. *Eur J Clin Pharmacol* (1977) 11, 15–18.
12. Schwarz L, Munoz R. Blood sugar levels in patients treated with chlorpromazine. *Am J Psychiatry* (1968) 125, 253–5.

13. Hedenmalm K, Hägg S, Ståhl M, Mortimer Ö, Spigset O. Glucose intolerance with atypical antipsychotics. *Drug Safety* (2002) 25, 1107–16.
14. Bhattacharyya J, Das KP. Aggregation of insulin by chlorpromazine. *Biochem Pharmacol* (2001) 62, 1293–7.

Antidiabetics + Azoles; Fluconazole

Fluconazole appears not to affect the diabetic control of most patients taking sulphonylureas, but isolated reports describe hypoglycaemic coma in one patient taking glipizide and hypoglycaemia and aggressive behaviour in a patient taking gliclazide. There is some evidence that the blood glucose-lowering effects of both glipizide and glibenclamide (glyburide) may be modestly increased. Fluconazole may cause increases in plasma levels of glimepiride (marked) and nateglinide (modest).

Clinical evidence

(a) Chlorpropamide

After taking fluconazole 100 mg daily for 7 days, the AUC of single 250-mg doses of chlorpropamide was increased by 28% in 18 healthy subjects but the maximum plasma levels and blood glucose levels were unchanged. There was no evidence of hypoglycaemia.[1]

(b) Glibenclamide (Glyburide)

After taking fluconazole 100 mg daily for 7 days, the AUC of a single 5-mg dose of glibenclamide was increased by 44% and maximum plasma levels rose by 19% in 20 healthy subjects. The change in blood glucose levels was not statistically significant but the number of subjects who had symptoms of hypoglycaemia increased.[2] In another study, a group of 14 postmenopausal diabetic women with vulvovaginal candidiasis taking either gliclazide or glibenclamide were given fluconazole 50 mg daily for 14 days. In contrast, none of the patients in this study developed symptoms of hypoglycaemia and their glycosylated haemoglobin and fructosamine concentrations were unchanged. No pharmacokinetic data were reported.[3]

(c) Gliclazide

A group of 14 postmenopausal diabetic women with vulvovaginal candidiasis taking either gliclazide or glibenclamide were given fluconazole 50 mg daily for 14 days. None of the patients developed symptoms of hypoglycaemia and their glycosylated haemoglobin and fructosamine concentrations were unchanged. No pharmacokinetic data were reported.[3]

However, a 56-year-old HIV-positive patient (antiretroviral treatment refused) and type 2 diabetes who had been taking gliclazide for 2 years was given fluconazole 50 mg daily for 2 weeks for oral candidiasis, and prophylactic co-trimoxazole (sulfamethoxazole 400 mg and trimethoprim 80 mg daily). One week after the re-introduction of fluconazole at a higher dose of 200 mg daily he was hospitalised because of weakness and aggressive behaviour. His blood glucose level was 2.2 mmol/L and gliclazide was stopped. He experienced brief loss of consciousness 2 days later while driving his car, but his condition then improved and neurological symptoms did not recur during 3 months follow-up without gliclazide treatment.[4] For the possible contribution of sulfamethoxazole to this interaction, see Mechanism, below.

(d) Glimepiride

A double-blind study in 12 healthy subjects found that fluconazole 400 mg on day one then 200 mg daily for a further 3 days increased the AUC and peak plasma level of a single 0.5-mg dose of glimepiride by about 2.5-fold and 1.5-fold, respectively. Fluconazole increased the mean elimination half-life of glimepiride from 2 to 3.3 hours.[5]

(e) Glipizide

After taking fluconazole 100 mg daily for 7 days, the AUC of a single 2.5-mg dose of glipizide was increased by 49% and their maximum serum levels rose by 17% in 13 healthy subjects. Although blood glucose levels were lowered the change was not statistically significant. However, the number of subjects who had symptoms suggestive of hypoglycaemia increased.[6]

A diabetic patient taking glipizide 2.5 mg three times daily went into a hypoglycaemic coma within 4 days of starting to take fluconazole 200 mg daily. Her blood glucose levels had fallen to less than about 0.05 mmol/L. She rapidly recovered when given glucose.[7]

(f) Nateglinide

In a randomised, double-blind, crossover study, 10 healthy subjects were given a single 30-mg dose of nateglinide on day 4 of a course of fluconazole (given as 400 mg on day one, then 200 mg daily). Fluconazole raised the AUC of nateglinide by 48% (range 20 to 73%) and increased the nateglinide half-life from 1.6 to 1.9 hours. Despite these pharmacokinetic changes fluconazole did not potentiate the blood glucose lowering effects of nateglinide.[8] It was predicted that this interaction may occur with **miconazole** (which inhibits the same isoenzymes as fluconazole), but this needs confirmation.

(g) Tolbutamide

After taking a single 150-mg dose and a further 6 doses of fluconazole 100 mg daily, the AUC of a single 500-mg dose of tolbutamide was increased by about 50%, and the peak plasma levels were raised in 13 healthy subjects. The half-life of the tolbutamide was increased about 40%. Blood glucose levels remained unaltered and none of the subjects showed any evidence of hypoglycaemia.[9,10] However, the authors caution against extrapolating this finding to diabetic patients taking tolbutamide regularly.[9,10]

Mechanism

Fluconazole is an inhibitor of the cytochrome P450 isoenzyme CYP2C9, by which many of the sulphonylureas are metabolised. Inhibition of this isoenzyme leads to an accumulation of the sulphonylurea and therefore an increase in its effects. The hypoglycaemia in the patient taking gliclazide and fluconazole may have been enhanced by sulfamethoxazole, which also inhibits CYP2C9 (see also 'sulfonamides' (p.506)).[4] The moderate pharmacokinetic changes seen when fluconazole is given with nateglinide are also thought to be mediated by CYP2C9.

Importance and management

The almost total absence of adverse reports implies that fluconazole does not usually markedly disturb the control of diabetes in those taking sulphonylureas. For fluconazole the increased plasma levels of glipizide and glimepiride, and the single case of severe hypoglycaemia, as well as the hypoglycaemic symptoms shown by those taking glibenclamide (glyburide) or gliclazide suggest that patients taking these sulphonylureas in particular should be warned to be alert for any evidence of hypoglycaemia. However, there seems to be no reason for avoiding concurrent use. Note that in the study of fluconazole with nateglinide a sub-therapeutic dose was given to healthy subjects, so in clinical practice a greater blood glucose-lowering effect may possibly occur.

1. Anon. A volunteer-blind, placebo-controlled study to assess potential interaction between fluconazole and chlorpropamide in healthy male volunteers. Protocol 238: Pfizer, data on file.
2. Anon. A volunteer-blind, placebo-controlled study to assess potential interaction between fluconazole and glibenclamide in healthy male volunteers. Protocol 236: Pfizer, data on file.
3. Rowe BR, Thorpe J, Barnett A. Safety of fluconazole in women taking oral hypoglycaemic agents. *Lancet* (1992) 339, 255–6.
4. Abad S, Moachon L, Blanche P, Bavoux F, Sicard D, Salmon-Céron D. Possible interaction between gliclazide, fluconazole and sulfamethoxazole resulting in severe hypoglycaemia. *Br J Clin Pharmacol* (2001) 52, 456–7.
5. Niemi M, Backman JT, Neuvonen M, Laitila J, Neuvonen PJ, Kivistö KT. Effects of fluconazole and fluvoxamine on the pharmacokinetics and pharmacodynamics of glimepiride. *Clin Pharmacol Ther* (2001) 69, 194–200.
6. Anon. A volunteer-blind, placebo-controlled study to assess potential interaction between fluconazole and glipizide in healthy male volunteers. Protocol 237: Pfizer, data on file.
7. Fournier JP, Schneider S, Martinez P, Mahagne MH, Ducoeur S, Haffner M, Thiercelin D, Chichmanain RM, Bertrand F. Coma hypoglycémique chez une patiente traitée par glipizide et fluconazole: une possible interaction? *Therapie* (1992) 47, 446–7.
8. Niemi M, Neuvonen M, Juntti-Patinen L, Backman JT, Neuvonen PJ. Effect of fluconazole on the pharmacokinetics and pharmacodynamics of nateglinide. *Clin Pharmacol Ther* (2003) 74, 25–31.
9. Lazar JD, Wilner KD. Drug interactions with fluconazole. *Rev Infect Dis* (1990) 12 (Suppl 3), S327–S333.
10. Anon. A double-blind placebo-controlled study to assess the potential interaction between fluconazole and tolbutamide in healthy male volunteers. Pfizer, data on file.

Antidiabetics + Azoles; Itraconazole or Ketoconazole

Itraconazole also appears not to affect diabetic control in most patients, but there are reports of hypoglycaemia or hyperglycaemia associated with its use. Itraconazole causes modest increases in repaglinide and nateglinide levels, but has no effect on pioglitazone pharmacokinetics. Ketoconazole increases the blood glu-

cose-lowering effects of tolbutamide in healthy subjects and possibly increases the AUC of rosiglitazone and pioglitazone.

Clinical evidence

(a) Itraconazole

Post-marketing surveillance over 10 years indicated that in most patients itraconazole given with either **insulin** or **oral antidiabetics** did not affect diabetic control. However, there were 15 reports suggesting hyperglycaemia and 9 reports suggesting hypoglycaemia when itraconazole was given to patients taking antidiabetics.[1] In clinical trials only one of 189 diabetic patients experienced aggravated diabetes when given itraconazole.[1] The patient in question was also receiving ciclosporin for a renal transplant.

Itraconazole 200 mg then 100 mg twice daily for 4 days did not alter the pharmacokinetics of a single 15-mg dose of **pioglitazone** in 12 healthy subjects.[2]

Itraconazole 200 mg then 100 mg twice daily for 3 days increased the AUC of a single 250-microgram dose of **repaglinide** by 40% in healthy subjects. No change was noted in blood glucose levels, when compared with **repaglinide** alone.[3] However, itraconazole enhanced the pharmacokinetic interaction of gemfibrozil on **repaglinide**; itraconazole plus gemfibrozil increased the AUC of **repaglinide** nearly 20-fold and considerably enhanced the blood glucose-lowering effect of **repaglinide**. In a similar study in healthy subjects, itraconazole plus gemfibrozil increased the AUC of a single 30-mg dose of **nateglinide** by 47%, without causing any significant change in blood glucose response to **nateglinide**.[4]

(b) Ketoconazole

After an overnight fast and breakfast the next morning, 7 healthy subjects were given a single 500-mg dose of **tolbutamide** before and after taking ketoconazole 200 mg daily for a week. Ketoconazole increased the elimination half-life of **tolbutamide** more than threefold (from 3.7 to 12.3 hours) and increased its AUC by 77%. Ketoconazole increased the blood glucose-lowering effects of **tolbutamide** by about 10 to 15%, and 5 of the subjects experienced mild hypoglycaemic symptoms (weakness, sweating and a reeling sensation) at about 2 hours after the dose.[5]

Ketoconazole 200 mg for 5 days increased the AUC and maximum plasma levels of a single 2-mg dose of **repaglinide** by 15 and 8%, respectively, in healthy subjects.[6]

Ketoconazole 200 mg twice daily for 5 days increased the AUC of a single 8-mg dose of **rosiglitazone** by 47% in 10 healthy Korean subjects.[7]

The US manufacturer refers to a 7-day study in which ketoconazole 200 mg twice daily modestly increased the AUC of **pioglitazone**.[8]

Mechanism

The modest changes in repaglinide pharmacokinetics with ketoconazole and itraconazole may be because repaglinide is metabolised by both CYP2C8 and CYP3A4, and one pathway may have the capacity to compensate if the other is inhibited.[9] Similarly, itraconazole modestly affects nateglinide metabolism via CYP3A4.[4]

Although it has been suggested that ketoconazole may inhibit the metabolism of rosiglitazone via CYP2C8 and CYP2C9, ketoconazole is normally only considered to be a significant inhibitor of CYP3A4.

Importance and management

Itraconazole does not usually disturb the control of diabetes, although there are rare reports of hyperglycaemia or hypoglycaemia associated with its use. The effect of itraconazole on repaglinide could potentially be important, especially if a drug which inhibits CYP2C8 such as gemfibrozil is given as well; so increased monitoring of glucose levels is advisable. Similarly, itraconazole may interact with nateglinide to a modest extent. Itraconazole is unlikely to interact with pioglitazone.

Information about ketoconazole and sulphonylureas appears to be limited to one study in healthy subjects. The reaction in diabetics is uncertain, but if ketoconazole is added to tolbutamide, patients should be warned to be alert for any evidence of increased hypoglycaemia. It may become necessary to reduce the tolbutamide dosage. Ketoconazole increases the AUC of rosiglitazone and pioglitazone, and more frequent blood glucose monitoring is recommended. The pharmacokinetic changes with ketoconazole and repaglinide are minor, and unlikely to be of any clinical relevance.

1. Verspeelt J, Marynissen G, Gupta AK, De Doneker P. Safety of itraconazole in diabetic patients. *Dermatology* (1999) 198, 382–4.
2. Jaakkola T, Backman JT, Neuvonen M, Neuvonen PJ. Effects of gemfibrozil, itraconazole, and their combination on the pharmacokinetics of pioglitazone. *Clin Pharmacol Ther* (2005) 77, 404–14.
3. Niemi M, Backman JT, Neuvonen M, Neuvonen PJ. Effects of gemfibrozil, itraconazole, and their combination on the pharmacokinetics and pharmacodynamics of repaglinide: potentially hazardous interaction between gemfibrozil and repaglinide. *Diabetologia* (2003) 46, 347–51.
4. Niemi M, Backman JT, Juntti-Patinen L, Neuvonen M, Neuvonen PJ. Coadministration of gemfibrozil and itraconazole has only a minor effect on the pharmacokinetics of the CYP2C9 and CYP3A4 substrate nateglinide. *Br J Clin Pharmacol* (2005) 60, 208–17.
5. Krishnaiah YSR, Satyanarayana S, Visweswaram D. Interaction between tolbutamide and ketoconazole in healthy subjects. *Br J Clin Pharmacol* (1994) 37, 205–7.
6. Hatorp V, Hansen KT, Thomsen MS. Influence of drugs interacting with CYP3A4 on the pharmacokinetics, pharmacodynamics, and safety of the prandial glucose regulator repaglinide. *J Clin Pharmacol* (2003) 43, 649–60.
7. Park J-Y, Kim K-A, Shin J-G, Lee KY. Effect of ketoconazole on the pharmacokinetics of rosiglitazone in healthy subjects. *Br J Clin Pharmacol* (2004) 58, 397–402.
8. Actos (Pioglitazone hydrochloride). Takeda Pharmaceuticals Company Ltd. US Prescribing information, February 2007.
9. Bidstrup TB, Bjørnsdottir I, Sidelmann UG, Thomsen MS, Hansen KT. CYP2C8 and CYP3A4 are the principal enzymes involved in the human in vitro biotransformation of the insulin secretagogue repaglinide. *Br J Clin Pharmacol* (2003) 56, 305–14.

Antidiabetics + Azoles; Miscellaneous

Hypoglycaemia has been seen in few diabetics taking tolbutamide, glibenclamide or gliclazide when they were given miconazole. Posaconazole slightly enhanced the blood glucose-lowering effects of glipizide in healthy subjects, but did not affect the metabolism of a single dose of tolbutamide. Voriconazole is predicted to increase the levels of the sulphonylureas. Clotrimazole used intravaginally appears not to interact with gliclazide or glibenclamide.

Clinical evidence

(a) Clotrimazole

A group of 15 postmenopausal diabetic women with vulvovaginal candidiasis taking either **gliclazide** or **glibenclamide (glyburide)** were treated with intravaginal clotrimazole 100 mg daily for 14 days. None of the patients developed symptoms of hypoglycaemia and their glycosylated haemoglobin and fructosamine concentrations were unchanged. No pharmacokinetic data were reported.[1]

(b) Miconazole

A diabetic patient taking **tolbutamide** was hospitalised with severe hypoglycaemia about 10 days after starting to take miconazole.[2] In 1983 the French Commission Nationale de Pharmacovigilance reported 6 cases of hypoglycaemia in diabetics taking sulphonylureas (5 with **gliclazide** and one with **glibenclamide (glyburide)**), which occurred within 2 to 6 days of miconazole being started.[2] The same organisation reported a further 8 cases in the 1985 to 1990 period but individual sulphonylureas were not named.[3] Three other cases of hypoglycaemia (two with **gliclazide** and one with **glibenclamide**) are reported elsewhere, in patients given miconazole up to 750 mg daily.[4] Miconazole has been predicted to interact with **nateglinide**, see 'fluconazole', (p.479).

(c) Posaconazole

A study in 12 healthy subjects found that posaconazole 400 mg twice daily for 10 days had no significant effects on the steady-state pharmacokinetics of **glipizide** 10 mg daily, but there was a small significant decrease in blood glucose levels following concurrent use. **Glipizide** did not affect the pharmacokinetics of posaconazole.[5]

In a study using **tolbutamide** as a probe drug for CYP2C9, posaconazole 200 mg once daily for 10 days had no effect on **tolbutamide** metabolism.[6]

(d) Voriconazole

The manufacturers of voriconazole predict that it will raise the levels of the sulphonylureas.[7,8]

Mechanism

Miconazole and voriconazole are inhibitors of the cytochrome P450 isoenzyme CYP2C9, by which many of the sulphonylureas are metabolised. Inhibition of this isoenzyme would therefore be expected to lead to an accumulation of the sulphonylurea and therefore an increase in its effects, as seen with miconazole. Clotrimazole is probably not absorbed in sufficient quantities to cause an interaction.

Importance and management

The interaction between miconazole and the sulphonylureas is established and clinically important, but of uncertain incidence. Concurrent use need not be avoided but it should be monitored and the dosage of the sulphonylurea reduced if necessary. Patients should be warned. Information about other sulphonylureas not cited is lacking but it seems possible that they may interact similarly with miconazole.

Posaconazole slightly enhanced the blood glucose-lowering effects of glipizide in healthy subjects, but the clinical relevance of this is not known. Posaconazole does not appear to affect tolbutamide metabolism.

The manufacturers of voriconazole advise increased blood-glucose monitoring in patients taking sulphonylureas, and until more is known this seems prudent.

Information about intravaginal clotrimazole is very sparse, but it appears not to interact with gliclazide or glibenclamide, and probably not with any of the other oral antidiabetics, not least because its absorption from the vagina is very small.

1. Rowe BR, Thorpe J, Barnett A. Safety of fluconazole in women taking oral hypoglycaemic agents. *Lancet* (1992) 339, 255–6.
2. Meurice JC, Lecomte P, Renard JP, Girard JJ. Interaction miconazole et sulfamides hypoglycémiants. *Presse Med* (1983) 12, 1670.
3. Girardin E, Vial T, Pham E, Evreux J-C. Hypoglycémies induites par les sulfamides hypoglycémiants. *Ann Med Interne (Paris)* (1992) 143, 11–17.
4. Loupi E, Descotes J, Lery N, Evreux JC. Interactions médicamenteuses et miconazole. A propos de 10 observations. *Therapie* (1982) 37, 437–41.
5. Courtney R, Sansone A, Statkevich P, Martinho M, Laughlin M. Assessment of the pharmacokinetic (PK), pharmacodynamic (PD) interaction potential between posaconazole and glipizide in healthy volunteers. *Clin Pharmacol Ther* (2003) 73, P45.
6. Wexler D, Courtney R, Richards W, Banfield C, Lim J, Laughlin M. Effect of posaconazole on cytochrome P450 enzymes: a randomized, open-label, two-way crossover study. *Eur J Pharm Sci* (2004) 21, 645–53.
7. VFEND (Voriconazole). Pfizer Ltd. UK Summary of product characteristics, July 2007.
8. VFEND (Voriconazole). Pfizer Inc. US Prescribing information, November 2006.

Antidiabetics + Benzodiazepines

No adverse interaction normally occurs between antidiabetics and benzodiazepines, but an isolated case of hyperglycaemia has been seen in an insulin-treated patient with type 2 diabetes associated with the use of chlordiazepoxide. The effects of lorazepam were found to be increased in patients given beef/pork insulin rather than human insulin. Pioglitazone caused a minor decrease in the AUC of midazolam, which is probably not clinically relevant.

Clinical evidence, mechanism, importance and management

(a) Insulin

A woman with long-standing type 2 diabetes, which was stabilised with 45 units of **isophane insulin suspension** daily, had a rise in her mean fasting blood glucose from about 12 to 21 mmol/L during a 3-week period while taking **chlordiazepoxide** 40 mg daily.[1] A preliminary report in 8 healthy type 1 diabetics given **lorazepam** 2 mg suggested that while they were taking **human insulin** they were more alert and less sedated than when taking **beef/pork insulin**.[2]

There seems to be nothing in the literature to suggest that a clinically important adverse interaction normally takes place between insulin and the benzodiazepines. No special precautions would appear to be necessary.

(b) Oral antidiabetics

Four patients with type 2 diabetes, two diet-controlled and two taking **tolbutamide**, had no changes in blood glucose levels while taking **chlordiazepoxide**.[1] In another study **diazepam** did not change the half-life of **chlorpropamide**.[3] The manufacturer notes that **pioglitazone** 45 mg once daily for 15 days reduced the AUC and maximum level of a single dose of **midazolam** syrup by 26% in healthy subjects.[4] This is possibly because **pioglitazone** is a weak inducer of the cytochrome P450 isoenzyme CYP3A4,[4] by which **midazolam** is metabolised. The clinical relevance of this small decrease in **midazolam** levels has not been assessed, but it is likely to be minor.

1. Zumoff B, Hellman L. Aggravation of diabetic hyperglycemia by chlordiazepoxide. *JAMA* (1977) 237, 1960–1.
2. Dahlan AA, Vrbancic MI, Hogan TE, Woo D, Herman RI. Greater sedative response to lorazepam in patients with insulin-dependent diabetes mellitus while on treatment with beef/pork versus human insulin. *Clin Invest Med* (1993) 16 (4 Suppl), B18.
3. Petitpierre B, Perrin L, Rudhardt M, Herrera A, Fabre J. Behaviour of chlorpropamide in renal insufficiency and under the effect of associated drug therapy. *Int J Clin Pharmacol* (1972) 6, 120–4.
4. Actos (Pioglitazone hydrochloride). Takeda Pharmaceutical Company Ltd. US Prescribing information, February 2007.

Antidiabetics + Beta blockers

In diabetics using insulin, the normal recovery reaction (blood sugar rise) if hypoglycaemia occurs may be impaired to some extent by propranolol, but serious and severe hypoglycaemia seems rare. Cardioselective beta blockers seem less likely to interact. The blood glucose-lowering effects of the sulphonylureas may possibly be reduced by the beta blockers. Whether insulin or oral antidiabetic drugs are given, patients should be made aware that some of the familiar warning signs of hypoglycaemia (tachycardia, tremor) may not occur, although sweating may be increased. Hypoglycaemia in patients taking beta blockers has been noted to result in significant increases in blood pressure and possibly bradycardia in some studies. Miglitol has been found to reduce the bioavailability of propranolol by 40%.

Clinical evidence

(a) Insulin

1. Hypoglycaemia. Although **propranolol** has occasionally been associated with spontaneous episodes of hypoglycaemia in non-diabetics,[1] and a number of studies in diabetic patients[2] and healthy subjects[3-6] have found that **propranolol** impairs the normal blood sugar rebound if blood sugar levels fall, there appear to be few reports of severe hypoglycaemia or coma in diabetics receiving insulin and **propranolol**. Marked hypoglycaemia and/or coma occurred in 5 diabetic patients receiving insulin due to the use of **propranolol**,[1,7,8] **pindolol**,[8] or **timolol** eye-drops.[9] Other contributory factors (fasting, haemodialysis, etc.) probably had some part to play.[8] **Metoprolol** interacts like **propranolol** but to a lesser extent,[3,5,10] whereas **acebutolol**,[2,5] **alprenolol**,[11] **atenolol**,[2,12,13] **oxprenolol**,[10] **penbutolol**,[6] and **pindolol**[14] have been found to interact minimally or not at all. The situation with **pindolol** is therefore not clear. **Carvedilol** has been associated with the onset of diabetes mellitus in one patient.[15] **Propranolol** (a peripheral vasoconstrictor) has also been found to reduce the rate of absorption of subcutaneous insulin by almost 50%, but the importance of this is uncertain.[16]

However, a large case-control study found no statistically significant increase or decrease in the risk of a serious hypoglycaemic episode in patients over 65 years old receiving insulin and taking either cardioselective beta blockers (**atenolol** and **metoprolol**) or non-selective beta blockers (**propranolol** and **nadolol**) when compared with patients taking no antihypertensive drugs. Overall, of the different antihypertensive drug classes, the risk of hypoglycaemia was lowest with cardioselective beta blockers and highest with non-selective beta blockers, although none of the changes were statistically significant when controlled for demographic factors and markers of comorbidity.[17] Similarly, in 2 other case-control studies, there was no increase in the risk of hypoglycaemia in patients with diabetes receiving insulin and also taking a beta blocker.[18,19]

2. Hypertension. Marked increases in blood pressure and bradycardia may develop if hypoglycaemia occurs in diabetics receiving **insulin** and a beta blocker.[20] In one study in diabetics, insulin-induced hypoglycaemia resulted in blood pressure rises of 38.8/14.3 mmHg in those taking **propranolol** 80 mg twice daily, 27.9/0 mmHg in those taking **atenolol** 100 mg daily and in those taking placebo the systolic blood pressure rose by 15.2 mmHg whereas the diastolic blood pressure fell by 9.9 mmHg.[21] In another study, **insulin**-induced hypoglycaemia resulted in blood pressure rises of 27/14 mmHg in those taking **alprenolol** 200 to 800 mg daily, but no rise occurred in those taking **metoprolol** 100 to 400 mg daily.[22] A report describes a blood pressure rise to 258/144 mmHg in a patient having a hypoglycaemic episode within 2 days of starting **propranolol**.[7] Another patient taking **metoprolol** 50 mg twice daily experienced a rise in blood pressure from 190/96 to 230/112 mmHg during a hypoglycaemic episode.[20]

(b) Oral antidiabetics

1. Effects on blood glucose. The sulphonylurea-induced insulin-release from the pancreas can be inhibited by beta blockers so that the blood glucose-lowering effects are opposed to some extent.

- **Acebutolol** appears to inhibit the effects of **glibenclamide**,[23] but has no effect on **tolbutamide**.[24] Also, two isolated cases of hypoglycaemia have been seen with acebutolol, in one patient taking **gliclazide** and one patient taking **chlorpropamide**.[25]
- **Betaxolol** had no effect on the response to **glibenclamide** or **metformin** in one study.[26]
- **Metoprolol** did not affect the insulin-response to **tolbutamide** in one study.[27]
- **Propranolol** inhibits the effects of **glibenclamide (glyburide)**,[23] and **chlorpropamide**[28] and reduced the insulin-response to **tolbutamide** in one study,[29] but not in another.[27] Also, an isolated report describes hyperosmolar non-ketotic coma in a patient taking **tolbutamide** and propranolol.[30]

It is worth noting that the United Kingdom Prospective Diabetes Study Group (UKPDS) used **atenolol** 50 to 100 mg daily or captopril 25 to 50 mg twice daily for hypertension in diabetics taking a range of antidiabetics. Those given **atenolol** showed a slightly greater increase in glycosylated haemoglobin levels, and gained slightly more weight (3.4 kg for the **atenolol** group compared with 1.6 kg for the captopril group over 9 years). However, both drugs were equally effective in reducing the risk of predefined clinical end points (e.g. diabetic complications, death related to diabetes, heart failure). The number of patients experiencing hypoglycaemic attacks did not differ between the two antihypertensives.[31] This would suggest that beta blockers are generally useful in the treatment of diabetics. Another large case-control study found no statistically significant increase or decrease in the risk of a serious hypoglycaemic episode in elderly patients taking sulphonylureas with either cardioselective beta blockers (**atenolol** and **metoprolol**) or non-selective beta blockers (**propranolol** and **nadolol**) when compared with patients taking no antihypertensive drugs.[17]

2. Pharmacokinetic studies. **Acarbose** 300 mg daily for one week had no effect on the pharmacokinetics or pharmacodynamics of a single 80-mg dose of **propranolol** in healthy subjects.[32] Conversely, the manufacturer of **miglitol** notes that it reduced the bioavailability of **propranolol** by a modest 40%.[33]

No pharmacokinetic interaction was seen in a study in healthy subjects given a single 1.75-mg dose of **glibenclamide** with **carvedilol** 25 mg daily for 6 days.[34]

Mechanism

One of the normal physiological responses to a fall in blood sugar levels is the mobilisation of glucose from the liver under the stimulation of adrenaline from the adrenals. This sugar mobilisation is blocked by non-selective beta blockers (such as propranolol) so that recovery from hypoglycaemia is delayed and may even proceed into a full-scale episode in a hypoglycaemia-prone diabetic. Normally the adrenaline would also increase the heart rate, but with the beta-receptors in the heart already blocked this fails to occur. A rise in blood pressure occurs because the stimulant effects of adrenaline on the beta-2 receptors (vasodilation) are blocked leaving the alpha (vasoconstriction) effects unopposed.

Non-selective beta blockers can also block beta-2 receptors in the pancreas concerned with insulin-release, so that the effects of the sulphonylureas may be blocked.

Importance and management

Extremely well-studied interactions. Concurrent use can be uneventful but there are some risks.

Diabetics receiving insulin may have a prolonged or delayed recovery response to hypoglycaemia while taking a beta blocker, but very severe hypoglycaemia and/or coma is rare. If hypoglycaemia occurs it may be accompanied by a sharp rise in blood pressure. The risk is greatest with propranolol and possibly other non-selective blockers and least with the cardio-selective blockers. The cardioselectivity of a number of beta blockers is given in 'Table 22.1', (p.833). Monitor the effects of concurrent use well, avoid the non-selective beta blockers where possible, and check for any evidence that the insulin dosage needs some adjustment. Warn all patients that some of the normal premonitory signs of a hypoglycaemic attack may not appear, in particular tachycardia and tremors, whereas the hunger, irritability and nausea signs may be unaffected and sweating may even be increased.

Diabetics taking oral sulphonylureas rarely seem to have serious hypoglycaemic episodes caused by beta blockers, and any reductions in the blood glucose-lowering effects of the sulphonylureas normally appear to be of little clinical importance. The selective beta blockers are probably safer than those that are non-selective. Nevertheless, always monitor concurrent use to confirm that diabetic control is well maintained, adjusting the dose of antidiabetic as necessary, and warn all patients (as above) that some of the premonitory signs of hypoglycaemia may not occur.

One experimental study indicated that no interaction occurred between betaxolol and **metformin**,[26] but direct information about other beta blockers seems to be lacking.

There is also a hint from one report that the peripheral vasoconstrictive effects of non-selective beta blockers and the poor peripheral circulation in diabetics could be additive,[7] which is another possible reason for avoiding this type of beta blocker in diabetics.

1. Kotler MN, Berman L, Rubenstein AH. Hypoglycaemia precipitated by propranolol. *Lancet* (1966) 2, 1389–90.
2. Deacon SP, Karunanayake A, Barnett D. Acebutolol, atenolol, and propranolol and metabolic responses to acute hypoglycaemia in diabetics. *BMJ* (1977) 2, 1255–7.
3. Davidson NM, Corrall RJM, Shaw TRD, French EB. Observations in man of hypoglycaemia during selective and non-selective beta-blockade. *Scott Med J* (1976) 22, 69–72.
4. Abramson EA, Arky RA, Woeber KA. Effects of propranolol on the hormonal and metabolic responses to insulin-induced hypoglycaemia. *Lancet* (1966) ii, 1386–9.
5. Newman RJ. Comparison of propranolol, metoprolol, and acebutolol on insulin-induced hypoglycaemia. *BMJ* (1976) 2, 447–9.
6. Sharma SD, Vakil BJ, Samuel MR, Chadha DR. Comparison of penbutolol and propranolol during insulin-induced hypoglycaemia. *Curr Ther Res* (1979) 26, 252–9.
7. McMurtry RJ. Propranolol, hypoglycemia, and hypertensive crisis. *Ann Intern Med* (1974) 80, 669–70.
8. Samii K, Ciancioni C, Rottembourg J, Bisseliches F, Jacobs C. Severe hypoglycaemia due to beta-blocking drugs in haemodialysis patients. *Lancet* (1976) i, 545–6.
9. Angelo-Nielsen K. Timolol topically and diabetes mellitus. *JAMA* (1980) 244, 2263.
10. Viberti GC, Keen H, Bloom SR. Beta blockade and diabetes mellitus: effect of oxprenolol and metoprolol on the metabolic, cardiovascular, and hormonal response to insulin-induced hypoglycemia in insulin-dependent diabetics. *Metabolism* (1980) 29, 873–9.
11. Eisalo A, Heino A, Munter J. The effect of alprenolol in elderly patients with raised blood pressure. *Acta Med Scand* (1974) (Suppl), 554, 23–31.
12. Deacon SP, Barnett D. Comparison of atenolol and propranolol during insulin-induced hypoglycaemia. *BMJ* (1976) 2, 272–3.
13. Waal-Manning HJ. Atenolol and three nonselective β-blockers in hypertension. *Clin Pharmacol Ther* (1979) 25, 8–18.
14. Patsch W, Patsch JR, Sailer S. Untersuchung zur Wirkung von Pindolol auf Kohlehydrat- und Fettstoffwechsel bei Diabetes Mellitus. *Int J Clin Pharmacol Biopharm* (1977) 15, 394–6.
15. Kobayakawa N, Sawaki D, Otani Y, Sekita G, Fukushima K, Takeuchi H, Aoyagi T. A case of severe diabetes mellitus occurred during management of heart failure with carvedilol and furosemide. *Cardiovasc Drugs Ther* (2003) 17, 295.
16. Veenstra J, van der Hulst JP, Wildenborg IH, Njoo SF, Verdegaal WP, Silberbusch J. Effect of antihypertensive drugs on insulin absorption. *Diabetes Care* (1991) 14, 1089–92.
17. Shorr RI, Ray WA, Daugherty JR, Griffin MR. Antihypertensives and the risk of serious hypoglycemia in older persons using insulin or sulfonylureas. *JAMA* (1997) 278, 40–3.
18. Thamer M, Ray NF, Taylor T. Association between antihypertensive drug use and hypoglycemia: a case-control study of diabetic users of insulin or sulfonylureas. *Clin Ther* (1999) 21, 1387–1400.
19. Herings RMC, de Boer A, Stricker BHC, Leufkens HGM, Porsius A. Hypoglycaemia associated with use of inhibitors of angiotensin converting enzyme. *Lancet* (1995) 345, 1195–8.
20. Shepherd AMM, Lin M-S, Keeton TK. Hypoglycemia-induced hypertension in a diabetic patient on metoprolol. *Ann Intern Med* (1981) 94, 357–8.
21. Ryan JR, LaCorte W, Jain A, McMahon FG. Hypertension in hypoglycemic diabetics treated with β-adrenergic antagonists. *Hypertension* (1985) 7, 443–6.
22. Östman J, Arner P, Haglund K, Juhlin-Dannfelt A, Nowak J, Wennlund A. Effect of metoprolol and alprenolol on the metabolic, hormonal, and haemodynamic response to insulin-induced hypoglycaemia in hypertensive, insulin-dependent diabetics. *Acta Med Scand* (1982) 211, 381–5.
23. Zaman R, Kendall MJ, Biggs PI. The effect of acebutolol and propranolol on the hypoglycaemic action of glibenclamide. *Br J Clin Pharmacol* (1982) 13, 507–12.
24. Ryan JR. Clinical pharmacology of acebutolol. *Am Heart J* (1985) 109, 1131–6.
25. Girardin E, Vial T, Pham E, Evreux J-C. Hypoglycémies induites par les sulfamides hypoglycémiants. *Ann Med Interne (Paris)* (1992) 143, 11–17.
26. Sinclair AJ, Davies IB, Warrington SJ. Betaxolol and glucose-insulin relationships: studies in normal subjects taking glibenclamide or metformin. *Br J Clin Pharmacol* (1990) 30, 699–702.
27. Tötterman KJ, Groop LC. No effect of propranolol and metoprolol on the tolbutamide-stimulated insulin-secretion in hypertensive diabetic and non-diabetic patients. *Ann Clin Res* (1982) 14, 190–3.
28. Holt RJ, Gaskins JD. Hyperglycemia associated with propranolol and chlorpropamide coadministration. *Drug Intell Clin Pharm* (1981) 15, 599–600.
29. Massara F, Strumia E, Camanni F, Molinatti GM. Depressed tolbutamide-induced insulin response in subjects treated with propranolol. *Diabetologia* (1971) 7, 287–9.
30. Podolsky S, Pattavina CG. Hyperosmolar nonketotic diabetic coma: a complication of propranolol therapy. *Metabolism* (1973) 22, 685–93.
31. UK Prospective Diabetes Study Group. Efficacy of atenolol and captopril in reducing risk of macrovascular and microvascular complications in type 2 diabetes: UKPDS 39. *BMJ* (1998) 317, 713–20.
32. Hillebrand I, Graefe KH, Bischoff H, Frank G, Raemsch KD, Berchtold P. Serum digoxin-andpropranolol levels during acarbose treatment. *Diabetologia* (1981) 21, 282–3.
33. Glyset (Miglitol). Pharmacia & Upjohn Company. US Prescribing information, October 2004.
34. Harder S, Merz PG, Rietbrock N. Lack of pharmacokinetic interaction between carvedilol and digitoxin, phenprocoumon or glibenclamide. *Cardiovasc Drugs Ther* (1993) 7 (Suppl 2), 447.

Antidiabetics + Bile-acid binding resins

A report suggests that the hypocholesterolaemic effect of colestipol is unaffected in insulin-treated diabetics but it may be ineffective in those taking phenformin and sulphonylureas. Diabetic control was not affected. Colestyramine may enhance the effect of acarbose, and insulin levels may rebound if both drugs are stopped at the same time. There is evidence that the absorption of glipizide may be reduced by about 30% if it is taken at the same time as colestyramine, but tolbutamide does not appear to be affected.

Clinical evidence

(a) Colestipol

The concurrent use of **phenformin** and a sulphonylurea (**chlorpropamide, tolbutamide** or **tolazamide**) inhibited the normal hypocholesterolaemic effects of the colestipol in 12 diabetics with elevated serum cholesterol levels. No such antagonism was seen in two patients with type 2 diabetes receiving **insulin**. The control of diabetes was not affected by the colestipol.[1]

(b) Colestyramine

1. Acarbose. Colestyramine 12 g daily for 6 days, given to 8 healthy subjects taking acarbose 100 mg three times daily, improved the reduction in postprandial insulin levels.[2] The mean serum insulin levels fell by 23% while taking both drugs, but showed a 'rebound' 31% increase above baseline when both were stopped.[2]

2. Glipizide. Colestyramine 8 g in 150 mL of water reduced the absorption of a single 5-mg dose of glipizide in 6 healthy subjects by a mean of 29%. One subject had a 41% reduction in glipizide levels. Peak serum levels were reduced by 33%. The $AUC_{0\text{-}10}$ was used to measure absorption.[3]

3. Tolbutamide. A single-dose study indicated that colestyramine 8 g, given 2 minutes before, and 6 and 12 hours after a 500-mg dose of tolbutamide, did not reduce the amount of tolbutamide absorbed, although the rate of absorption may have changed.[4]

Mechanism

Colestyramine is an anion-exchange resin, intended to bind to bile acids within the gut, but it can also bind with some acidic drugs thereby reducing the amount available for absorption.

Importance and management

Information about glipizide is limited to a single-dose study so that the clinical importance of the reduction in glipizide levels with colestyramine is unknown, but it would seem prudent to monitor the effects of concurrent use in patients. It has been suggested[3] that the glipizide should be taken 1 to 2 hours before the colestyramine to minimise admixture in the gut, but this may only be partially effective because it is believed that glipizide undergoes some entero-hepatic circulation (i.e. after absorption it is excreted in the bile and reabsorbed). The effect of colestyramine on other sulphonylureas is uncertain, with the exception of tolbutamide, which is reported not to interact. The clinical importance of the effects of colestyramine on acarbose in diabetics is uncertain, although the manufacturers note that some enhancement of the effects of acarbose may occur, and they suggest care if both drugs are stopped at the same time because of the possible rebound phenomenon with respect to insulin levels.[5]

The study with colestipol suggests that it may not be suitable for lowering the blood cholesterol levels of diabetics taking chlorpropamide, tolbutamide, or tolazamide or phenformin, but more study is needed to confirm these findings. Phenformin has been withdrawn from many countries because of severe, often fatal, lactic acidosis.

1. Bandisode MS, Boshell BR. Hypocholesterolemic activity of colestipol in diabetes. *Curr Ther Res* (1975) 18, 276–84.
2. Bayer, Personal Communications, June-July 1993.
3. Kivistö K T, Neuvonen P J. The effect of cholestyramine and activated charcoal on glipizide absorption. *Br J Clin Pharmacol* (1990) 30, 733–6.
4. Hunninghake D B, Pollack E. Effect of bile acid sequestering agents on the absorption of aspirin, tolbutamide and warfarin. *Fedn Proc* (1977) 35, 996.
5. Glucobay (Acarbose). Bayer plc. UK Summary of product characteristics, October 2006.

Antidiabetics + Calcium-channel blockers

Calcium-channel blockers are known to have effects on insulin secretion and glucose regulation, but significant disturbances in the control of diabetes appear to be rare. A report describes a patient whose diabetes worsened, requiring an increase in the dose of insulin when diltiazem was given, and a similar case has occurred in a patient taking nifedipine. Deterioration in glucose tolerance has also occurred during nifedipine use. Hypoglycaemia occurred in a patient taking gliclazide and nicardipine. No clinically important changes in nifedipine pharmacokinetics have been seen with acarbose, miglitol, pioglitazone or rosiglitazone; in glibenclamide pharmacokinetics with nimodipine or verapamil; in glipizide or repaglinide pharmacokinetics with nifedipine; or between tolbutamide and diltiazem.

Clinical evidence

A. Dihydropyridines

(a) Effect on glucose tolerance

A study in 20 patients with type 2 diabetes (5 taking **metformin** and 15 diet-controlled) found that both **nifedipine** 10 mg every 8 hours and **nicardipine** 30 mg every 8 hours for 4 weeks did not affect either glucose tolerance tests or the control of the diabetes, but both systolic and diastolic blood pressures were reduced by 4 to 7 mmHg.[1] No important changes in glucose metabolism occurred in six type 2 diabetic patients taking **glibenclamide (glyburide)** when they were given **nifedipine** 20 to 60 mg daily for 12 to 25 weeks.[2] Similarly, other studies have found no important changes in glucose tolerance or control of diabetes in patients taking **chlorpropamide**,[3] **glibenclamide**,[4] **gliclazide**,[5] **glipizide**[3,6] or unspecified antidiabetics[7,8] while also taking **nifedipine**,[3,5-7] **nimodipine**[4] or **nitrendipine**.[8] No change in **insulin** dose was seen in one patient taking **nicardipine**[9] and in 4 patients taking **nitrendipine**.[8]

However, there are reports of a deterioration in glucose tolerance during the use of **nifedipine** in a total of 12 subjects with impaired glucose tolerance.[10,11] A further case report describes a 30% increase in the **insulin** requirements of a diabetic man after he took **nifedipine** 60 mg daily.[12] An isolated case of hypoglycaemia has been described in a patient taking **gliclazide** when **nicardipine** was given.[13] However, a large case-control study found no statistically significant increase or decrease in the risk of a serious hypoglycaemic episode in patients over 65 years old taking insulin or sulphonylureas, who were also taking calcium-channel blockers (**nifedipine** and **verapamil** were the most frequently used), when compared with patients not taking antihypertensive drugs.[14]

(b) Pharmacokinetic studies

1. Alpha-glucosidase inhibitors. The manufacturers of **acarbose** say that in a pilot study of a possible interaction with **nifedipine**, no significant or reproducible changes were seen in plasma **nifedipine** profiles.[15,16] Similarly, the manufacturers of **miglitol** note that it had no effect on the pharmacokinetics and pharmacodynamics of **nifedipine**.[17]

2. Insulin. One study found that **nifedipine** 10 mg increased the rate of absorption of subcutaneous insulin by about 50%.[18]

3. Pioglitazone or Rosiglitazone. Rosiglitazone 8 mg daily for 2 weeks was found to have no clinically relevant effect on the pharmacokinetics of **nifedipine** in 28 healthy subjects.[19] The manufacturer notes that pioglitazone 45 mg once daily for 7 days given with **nifedipine** extended-release 30 mg once daily for 4 days resulted in a small but highly variable change in **nifedipine** pharmacokinetics.[20]

4. Repaglinide. A three-period cross-over open-label study in healthy subjects found that **nifedipine** 10 mg daily decreased the maximum plasma level of repaglinide 2 mg three times daily by 2.7% and increased the bioavailability of repaglinide by 11%, but this was not statistically significant. There was a higher incidence of adverse effects during concurrent use.[21]

5. Sulphonylureas. A study in six type 2 diabetics found that a single 20-mg dose of **nifedipine** had no effect on the pharmacokinetics of **glipizide** 5 to 30 mg daily.[6] Similarly, **nimodipine** caused no change in the pharmacokinetics of **glibenclamide** in 11 patients.[4]

B. Diltiazem

A patient with type 1 diabetes developed worsening and intractable hyperglycaemia (mean serum glucose levels above 13 mmol/L) when given diltiazem 90 mg every 6 hours. Her **insulin** requirements dropped when the diltiazem was withdrawn. When she started taking diltiazem 30 mg every 6 hours her blood glucose levels were still high, but she needed less **insulin** than when taking the higher diltiazem dosage.[22]

A study in 12 healthy subjects found that diltiazem 60 mg three times daily had no effect on the secretion of **insulin** or glucagon, or on plasma glucose levels.[23] Similarly, diltiazem 120 mg three times daily for 3 days had no effect on **insulin** and glucose levels during an oral glucose tolerance test in 10 patients taking **gliclazide**.[5]

A study in 8 healthy subjects found that a single 500-mg dose of **tolbutamide** had no effect on the serum levels of a single 60-mg dose of diltiazem. There was a minor increase of about 10% in the AUC_{0-24} and maximum serum levels of **tolbutamide** in the presence of diltiazem but the blood glucose-lowering effects of **tolbutamide** were not significantly changed.[24]

C. Verapamil

A study in 23 type 2 diabetics, 7 of whom were taking **glibenclamide (glyburide)**, found that verapamil improved the response to an oral glucose tolerance test but did not increase the blood glucose-lowering effects of the **glibenclamide**.[25] Two studies in type 2 diabetics found that verapamil improved the response to glucose tolerance tests,[26,27] but in one of the studies, no alterations in the blood glucose-lowering effects of **glibenclamide** were found.[26] A study in healthy subjects found that verapamil modestly raised the **glibenclamide** AUC by 26% but plasma glucose levels were unchanged.[28] A large case-control study found no statistically significant increase or decrease in the risk of a serious hypoglycaemic episode in patients over 65 years old taking insulin or sulphonylureas, who were also taking calcium-channel blockers (**nifedipine** and **verapamil** were the most frequently used), when compared with patients not taking antihypertensive drugs.[14]

Mechanism

The changes that occur are not fully understood. Suggestions include: inhibition of insulin secretion by the calcium-channel blockers and inhibition of glucagon secretion by glucose; changes in glucose uptake by the liver and other cells; blood glucose rises following catecholamine release after vasodilation, and changes in glucose metabolism. In contrast, one study in non-diabetics suggested that long-acting nifedipine could improve insulin sensitivity.[29]

Importance and management

Very extensively studied, but many of the reports describe single-dose studies or multiple-dose studies in healthy subjects (only a few are cited here), which do not give a clear picture of what may be expected in diabetic patients. Those studies that have concentrated on diabetics indicate that the control of the diabetes is not usually adversely affected by calcium-channel blockers, although isolated cases with diltiazem, nicardipine and nifedipine have been reported.[12,13,22] Similarly, there appear to be no important pharmacokinetic interactions with any of the combinations studied. However, if an otherwise unexplained worsening of diabetic control occurs it may be prudent to consider the use of a calcium-channel blocker as a possible cause. Therefore, in general, no particular precautions normally seem necessary.

1. Collins WCJ, Cullen MJ, Feely J. Calcium channel blocker drugs and diabetic control. *Clin Pharmacol Ther* (1987) 42, 420–3.
2. Kanatsuna T, Nakano K, Mori H, Kano Y, Nishioka H, Kajiyama S, Kitagawa Y, Yoshida T, Kondo M, Nakamura N, Aochi O. Effects of nifedipine on insulin secretion and glucose metabolism in rats and hypertensive type 2 (non-insulin dependent) diabetics. *Arzneimittelforschung* (1985) 35, 514–17.
3. Donnelly T, Harrower ADB. Effect of nifedipine on glucose tolerance and insulin secretion in diabetic and non-diabetic patients. *Curr Med Res Opin* (1980) 6, 690–3.
4. Mück W, Heine PR, Breuel H-P, Niklaus H, Horkulak J, Ahr G. The effect of multiple oral dosing of nimodipine on glibenclamide pharmacodynamics and pharmacokinetics in elderly patients with type-2 diabetes mellitus. *Int J Clin Pharmacol Ther* (1995) 33, 89–94.
5. Monges AM, Pisano P, Aujoulat P, Salducci D, Durand A, Panagides D, Bory M, Crevat A.¹H nuclear magnetic resonance and clinical studies of interaction of calcium antagonists and hypoglycemic sulfonylureas. *Fundam Clin Pharmacol* (1991) 5, 527–38.
6. Connacher AA, El Debani AH, Isles TE, Stevenson IH. Disposition and hypoglycaemic action of glipizide in diabetic patients given a single dose of nifedipine. *Eur J Clin Pharmacol* (1987) 33, 81–3.
7. Abadie E, Passa P. Diabetogenic effects of nifedipine. *BMJ* (1984) 289, 438.
8. Trost BN, Weidmann P. 5 years of antihypertensive monotherapy with the calcium antagonist nitrendipine do not alter carbohydrate homeostasis in diabetic patients. *Diabetes Res Clin Pract* (1988) 5 (Suppl 1), S511.
9. Sakata S, Miura K. Effect of nicardipine in a hypertensive patient with diabetes mellitus. *Clin Ther* (1984) 6, 600–2.
10. Guigliano D, Torella R, Cacciapuoti F, Gentile S, Verza M, Varricchio M. Impairment of insulin secretion in man by nifedipine. *Eur J Clin Pharmacol* (1980) 18, 395–8.
11. Bhatnagar SK, Amin MMA, Al-Yusuf AR. Diabetogenic effects of nifedipine. *BMJ* (1984) 289, 19.
12. Heyman SN, Heyman A, Halperin I. Diabetogenic effect of nifedipine. *DICP Ann Pharmacother* (1989) 23, 236–7.
13. Girardin E, Vial T, Pham E, Evreux J-C. Hypoglycémies induites par les sulfamides hypoglycémiants. *Ann Med Interne (Paris)* (1992) 143, 11–17.
14. Shorr RI, Ray WA, Daugherty JR, Griffin MR. Antihypertensives and the risk of serious hypoglycemia in older persons using insulin or sulfonylureas. *JAMA* (1997) 278, 40–3.
15. Glucobay (Acarbose). Bayer plc. UK Summary of product characteristics, October 2006.
16. Precose (Acarbose). Bayer Pharmaceuticals Corporation. US Prescribing information, November 2004.
17. Glyset (Miglitol). Pharmacia & Upjohn Company. US Prescribing information, October 2004.
18. Veenstra J, van der Hulst JP, Wildenborg IH, Njoo SF, Verdegaal WP, Silberbusch J. Effect of antihypertensive drugs on insulin absorption. *Diabetes Care* (1991) 14, 1089–92.
19. Harris RZ, Inglis AML, Miller AK, Thompson KA, Finnerty D, Patterson S, Jorkasky DK, Freed MI. Rosiglitazone has no clinically significant effect on nifedipine pharmacokinetics. *J Clin Pharmacol* (1999) 39, 1189–94.
20. Actos (Pioglitazone hydrochloride). Takeda Pharmaceutical Company Ltd. US Prescribing information, February 2007.
21. Hatorp V, Hansen KT, Thomsen MS. Influence of drugs interacting with CYP3A4 on the pharmacokinetics, pharmacodynamics, and safety of the prandial glucose regulator repaglinide. *J Clin Pharmacol* (2003) 43, 649–60.
22. Pershadsingh HA, Grant N, McDonald JM. Association of diltiazem therapy with increased insulin resistance in a patient with type I diabetes mellitus. *JAMA* (1987) 257, 930–1.
23. Segrestaa JM, Caulin C, Dahan R, Houlbert D, Thiercelin JF, Herman P, Sauvanet JP, Laurribaud J. Effect of diltiazem on plasma glucose, insulin and glucagon during an oral glucose tolerance test in healthy volunteers. *Eur J Clin Pharmacol* (1984) 26, 481–3.
24. Dixit AA, Rao YM. Pharmacokinetic interaction between diltiazem and tolbutamide. *Drug Metabol Drug Interact* (1999) 15, 269–77.
25. Röjdmark S, Andersson DEH. Influence of verapamil on human glucose tolerance. *Am J Cardiol* (1986) 57, 39D–43D.
26. Röjdmark S, Andersson DEH. Influence of verapamil on glucose tolerance. *Acta Med Scand* (1984) (Suppl), 681, 37–42.
27. Andersson DEH, Röjdmark S. Improvement of glucose tolerance by verapamil in patients with non-insulin-dependent diabetes mellitus. *Acta Med Scand* (1981) 210, 27–33.
28. Semple CG, Omile C, Buchanan KD, Beastall GH, Paterson KR. Effect of oral verapamil on glibenclamide stimulated insulin secretion. *Br J Clin Pharmacol* (1986) 22, 187–90.
29. Koyama Y, Kodama K, Suzuki M, Harano Y. Improvement of insulin sensitivity by a long-acting nifedipine preparation (nifedipine-CR) in patients with essential hypertension. *Am J Hypertens* (2002) 15, 927–31.

Antidiabetics + Cibenzoline (Cifenline)

Hypoglycaemia has been seen in a few patients taking cibenzoline alone, and in one case with gliclazide. The risk factors appear to be age, renal insufficiency, malnutrition and high dosage.

Clinical evidence, mechanism, importance and management

Cibenzoline occasionally and unpredictably causes hypoglycaemia, which may be severe. Marked hypoglycaemia was seen in a 67-year-old non-diabetic patient when cibenzoline was given.[1] A further case report describes hypoglycaemia in an 84-year-old, in whom age, renal impairment and/or malnutrition acted as facilitating factors.[2] The authors of this report noted that hypoglycaemia has been reported in another 20 cases, where the dose was not corrected for age and renal function.[2] A more recent report describes an elderly patient with type 2 diabetes controlled by diet who developed hypoglycaemia and associated dementia-like symptoms during treatment with low dose cibenzoline.[3] Hypoglycaemia also occurred in a 61-year-old patient with renal insufficiency taking **gliclazide** and cibenzoline.[4]

The reasons are not understood. However, in a controlled study in patients with abnormal glucose tolerance and ventricular arrhythmias, cibenzoline exerted a hypoglycaemic effect by facilitating insulin secretion.[5]

This appears to be a drug-disease rather than a drug-drug interaction and diabetic patients do not seem to be more at risk than non-diabetics, but good monitoring is advisable if cibenzoline is given.

1. Hilleman DE, Mohiuddin SM, Ahmed IS, Dahl JM. Cibenzoline-induced hypoglycemia. *Drug Intell Clin Pharm* (1987) 21, 38–40.
2. Houdent C, Noblet C, Vandoren C, Levesque H, Morin C, Moore N, Courtois H, Wolf LM. Hypoglycémia induite par la cibenzoline chez le sujet âgè. *Rev Med Interne* (1991) 12, 143–5.
3. Sakane N, Onishi N, Katamura M, Sato H, Takamasu M, Yoshida T. Cifenline succinate and dementia in an elderly NIDDM patient. *Diabetes Care* (1998) 21, 320–1.
4. Girardin E, Vial T, Pham E, Evreux J-C. Hypoglycémies induites par les sulfamides hypoglycémiants. *Ann Med Interne (Paris)* (1992) 143, 11–17.
5. Saikawa T, Arita M, Yamaguchi K, Ito M. Hypoglycemic effect of cibenzoline in patients with abnormal glucose tolerance and frequent ventricular arrhythmias. *Cardiovasc Drugs Ther* (2000) 14, 665–9.

Antidiabetics + Clonidine

There is evidence that clonidine may possibly suppress the signs and symptoms of hypoglycaemia in diabetic patients. Marked hyperglycaemia occurred in a child using insulin when clonidine was given. However, the effect of clonidine on carbohydrate metabolism appears to be variable, as other reports have described both increases and decreases in blood glucose levels. Clonidine premedication may decrease or increase the hyperglycaemic response to surgery.

Clinical evidence, mechanism, importance and management

(a) Non-diabetic patients

Studies in healthy subjects and patients with hypertension found that their normal response to hypoglycaemia (tachycardia, palpitations, perspiration) caused by a 0.1 unit/kg dose of **insulin** was markedly reduced when they were taking clonidine 450 to 900 micrograms daily.[1,2] In contrast, a study in healthy subjects and non-diabetic patients found that clonidine raises blood glucose levels, apparently by reducing **insulin** secretion,[3] and hypoglycaemia was associated with clonidine testing for growth hormone deficiency in 4 children.[4]

(b) Diabetic patients

A 9-year-old girl with type 1 diabetes stabilised with **insulin** 4 units daily, developed substantial hyperglycaemia and needed up to 56 units of **insulin** daily when she began to take clonidine 50 micrograms daily for Tourette's syndrome. When the clonidine was stopped, she had numerous hypoglycaemic episodes, and within a few days it was possible to reduce her daily dosage of **insulin** to 6 units.[5] A patient with type 2 diabetes and hypertension experienced elevated blood glucose levels and decreased **insulin** secretion when clonidine was given.[6] However, a study in 10 diabetic patients with hypertension found that although clonidine impaired the response to an acute glucose challenge, it did not significantly affect diabetic control over a 10-week period.[7]

In contrast, a placebo-controlled, crossover study in 20 patients with type 2 diabetes found that transdermal clonidine significantly reduced mean fasting plasma glucose levels by 9%.[8]

(c) Hyperglycaemia during surgery

Forty patients with type 2 diabetes (controlled by diet alone, **sulphonylureas**, **biguanides**, or **insulin**), having eye surgery under general anaesthesia, were given either clonidine 225 to 375 micrograms or flunitrazepam as premedication. In diabetic patients there is an increase in blood glucose during stress because of an increase in catecholamine release. Therefore the patients were also given a continuous infusion of **insulin** to maintain blood glucose at 5.5 to 11.1 mmol/L. Clonidine decreased the **insulin** requirement because of improved blood glucose control due to inhibition of catecholamine release.[9] Contrasting results were found in a study in 16 non-diabetic women undergoing abdominal hysterectomy. Eight were given intravenous clonidine 1 microgram/kg and 8 control patients were given saline. Intraoperative plasma glucose levels were higher in the clonidine group and these patients also had lower insulin levels.[10]

Mechanism

The suggested reason for a reduced response to hypoglycaemia is that clonidine depresses the output of the catecholamines (adrenaline, noradrenaline), which are secreted in an effort to raise blood glucose levels, and which are also responsible for these signs.[2] It seems possible that clonidine will similarly suppress the signs and symptoms of hypoglycaemia that can occur in diabetics, but there seem to be no reports confirming this.

Importance and management

The effect of clonidine on carbohydrate metabolism in diabetic patients appears to be variable and the general importance of these interactions is uncertain. In diabetic patients there is an increase in blood glucose during stress because of an increase in catecholamine release. The influence of clonidine on the surgical stress response appears to vary depending on the dose of clonidine and the type of surgery.[10] Thus, clonidine at about 4 micrograms/kg may attenuate the hyperglycaemic response to neurosurgical and non-abdominal procedures, but low-dose clonidine accentuates the hyperglycaemic response to lower abdominal surgery, which results from a decrease in plasma insulin.[9,10]

1. Hedeland H, Dymling J-F, Hökfelt B. The effect of insulin induced hypoglycaemia on plasma renin activity and urinary catecholamines before and following clonidine (Catapresan) in man. *Acta Endocrinol (Copenh)* (1972) 71, 321–30.
2. Hedeland H, Dymling J-F, Hökfelt B. Pharmacological inhibition of adrenaline secretion following insulin induced hypoglycaemia in man: the effect of Catapresan. *Acta Endocrinol (Copenh)* (1971) 67, 97–103.
3. Metz SA, Halter JB, Robertson RP. Induction of defective insulin secretion and impaired glucose tolerance by clonidine. Selective stimulation of metabolic alpha-adrenergic pathways. *Diabetes* (1978) 27, 554–62.
4. Huang C, Banerjee K, Sochett E, Perlman K, Wherrett D, Daneman D. Hypoglycemia associated with clonidine testing for growth hormone deficiency. *J Pediatr* (2001) 139, 323–4.
5. Mimouni-Bloch A, Mimouni M. Clonidine-induced hyperglycemia in a young diabetic girl. *Ann Pharmacother* (1993) 27, 980.
6. Okada S, Miyai Y, Sato K, Masaki Y, Higuchi T, Ogino Y, Ota Z. Effect of clonidine on insulin secretion: a case report. *J Int Med Res* (1986) 14, 299–302.
7. Guthrie GP, Miller RE, Kotchen TA, Koenig SH. Clonidine in patients with diabetes and mild hypertension. *Clin Pharmacol Ther* (1983) 34, 713–17.
8. Giugliano D, Acampora R, Marfella R, La Marca C, Marfella M, Nappo F, D'Onofrio F. Hemodynamic and metabolic effects of transdermal clonidine in patients with hypertension and non-insulin-dependent diabetes mellitus. *Am J Hypertens* (1998) 11, 184–9.
9. Belhoula M, Ciébiéra JP, De La Chapelle A, Boisseau N, Coeurveille D, Raucoules-Aimé M. Clonidine premedication improves metabolic control in type 2 diabetic patients during ophthalmic surgery. *Br J Anaesth* (2003) 90, 434–9.
10. Lattermann R, Schricker T, Georgieff M, Schreiber M. Low dose clonidine premedication accentuates the hyperglycemic response to surgery. *Can J Anesth* (2001) 48, 755–9.

Antidiabetics + Corticosteroids

The blood glucose-lowering effects of the antidiabetics are opposed by corticosteroids with glucocorticoid (hyperglycaemic) activity and significant hyperglycaemia has been seen with systemic corticosteroids. A report also describes deterioration in diabetic control with *inhaled* high-dose fluticasone, then high-dose budesonide, in a patient taking glibenclamide and metformin. High doses of high-potency corticosteroid creams may also, rarely, cause hyperglycaemia.

Clinical evidence, mechanism, importance and management

(a) Local corticosteroids

1. Inhaled. A 67-year-old man with diabetes taking **glibenclamide** 5 mg daily and **metformin** 1.7 g daily had a deterioration in diabetic control (glycosuria and an increase in glycosylated haemoglobin) 3 weeks after starting inhaled **fluticasone** 2 mg daily, by metered dose inhaler with a spacer device, for asthma. The **fluticasone** dose was gradually decreased to 500 micrograms daily after about 3 months, with an improvement in diabetic control. Subsequently, the **fluticasone** dose was increased from 0.5 to 1 mg, and within a week he again developed glycosuria.[1] This same patient was later given inhaled high-dose **budesonide** 2 mg daily and he again developed glycosuria and increased glycated haemoglobin levels, which improved as the dose was gradually decreased to 800 micrograms daily.[2] The adverse effects of *systemic* corticosteroids on glucose tolerance are well known. Although only one case appears to have been reported, it suggests that high-dose inhaled corticosteroids may have a similar effect. It may be prudent to increase monitoring of diabetic control in patients requiring high-dose corticosteroids and consider reducing the dose of the inhaled corticosteroid if possible, or adjusting the dose of the antidiabetic medication as necessary.

2. Topical. Two patients with an abnormal response to the glucose tolerance test, but without overt signs of diabetes mellitus, developed postprandial hyperglycaemia and one developed glycosuria when they used topical corticosteroids for severe psoriasis. These patients were given 15 g of **halcinonide** 0.1% or **betamethasone** 0.1% cream, applied every 12 hours for 15 days under occlusive dressings.[3] These cases appear to be rare, and were associated with high doses of potent or very potent corticosteroids, used under occlusive dressings, which increases systemic absorption. No additional special precautions would generally appear to be necessary in diabetics using moderate amounts of topical corticosteroids.

(b) Systemic corticosteroids

Systemic corticosteroids with glucocorticoid activity can raise blood glucose levels and induce diabetes.[4] This can oppose the blood glucose-lowering effects of the antidiabetics used in the treatment of diabetes mellitus. For example, a disturbance of the control of diabetes is very briefly described in a patient given with **insulin** and **hydrocortisone**.[5] A study in 5 patients with type 2 diabetes taking **chlorpropamide** found that a single 200-mg dose of **cortisone** modified their glucose tolerance. The blood glucose levels of 4 of them rose (3 showed an initial fall), whereas in a previous test with **chlorpropamide** alone the blood glucose levels of 4 of them had fallen.[6] This almost certainly reflects a direct antagonism between the pharmacological effects of the two drugs. Another glucocorticoid, **prednisone**, had no significant effect on the metabolism or clearance of **tolbutamide** in healthy subjects.[7]

There are very few studies of this interaction, probably because the hyperglycaemic activity of the **corticosteroids** has been known for such a long time that the outcome of concurrent use is self-evident. A case-control study found that in patients taking glucocorticoids, the relative risk for development of hyperglycaemia requiring treatment was 2.23, when compared with controls. Risk increased with an increasing daily dose of **hydrocortisone**: doses of 1 to 39 mg were associated with a 1.77-fold increase in risk, doses of 40 to 79 mg were associated with a 3.02-fold increase in risk, doses of 80 to 119 mg were associated with a 5.82-fold increase in risk, and doses of greater than 120 mg were associated with a 10.34-fold increase in risk.[8] Similarly, another study, in healthy subjects, found dose-related decreases in glucose tolerance and higher serum insulin levels associated with single intravenous doses of **hydrocortisone** and **methylprednisolone,** but these changes were more marked with **methylprednisolone** than **hydrocortisone**.[9] **Dexamethasone** has also been shown to induce deterioration in glucose tolerance with an incidence of about 35% in non-diabetic, first-degree relatives of patients with type 2 diabetes, primarily due to reduced insulin secretory capacity.[10]

The effects of systemic corticosteroid treatment in diabetics should be closely monitored and the dosage of the antidiabetic raised as necessary. Antidiabetics are sometimes needed in non-diabetic patients taking **corticosteroids** to reduce blood glucose levels.

1. Faul JL, Tormey W, Tormey V, Burke C. High dose inhaled corticosteroids and dose dependent loss of diabetic control. *BMJ* (1998) 317, 1491.
2. Faul JL, Cormican LJ, Tormey VJ, Tormey WP, Burke CM. Deteriorating diabetic control associated with high-dose inhaled budesonide. *Eur Respir J* (1999) 14, 242–3.
3. Gomez EC, Frost P. Induction of glycosuria and hyperglycemia by topical corticosteroid therapy. *Arch Dermatol* (1976) 112, 1559–62.
4. David DS, Cheigh JS, Braun DW, Fotino M, Stenzel KH, Rubin AL. HLA-A28 and steroid-induced diabetes in renal transplant patients. *JAMA* (1980) 243, 532–3.
5. Manchon ND, Bercoff E, Lemarchand P, Chassagne P, Senant J, Bourreille J. Fréquence et gravité des interactions médicamenteuses dan une population âgée: étude prospective concernant 639 malades. *Rev Med Interne* (1989) 10, 521–5.
6. Danowski TS, Mateer FM, Moses C. Cortisone enhancement of peripheral utilization of glucose and the effects of chlorpropamide. *Ann N Y Acad Sci* (1959) 74, 988–96.
7. Breimer DD, Zilly W, Richter E. Influence of corticosteroid on hexobarbital and tolbutamide disposition. *Clin Pharmacol Ther* (1978) 24, 208–12.
8. Gurwitz JH, Bohn RL, Glynn RJ, Monane M, Mogun H, Avorn J. Glucocorticoids and the risk for initiation of hypoglycemic therapy. *Arch Intern Med* (1994) 154, 97–101.
9. Bruno A, Carucci P, Cassader M, Cavallo-Perin P, Gruden G, Olivetti C, Pagano G. Serum glucose, insulin and C-peptide response to oral glucose after intravenous administration of hydrocortisone and methylprednisolone in man. *Eur J Clin Pharmacol* (1994) 46, 411–15.
10. Henriksen JE, Alford F, Ward GM, Beck-Nielsen H. Risk and mechanism of dexamethasone-induced deterioration of glucose tolerance in non-diabetic first-degree relatives of NIDDM patients. *Diabetologia* (1997) 40, 1439–48.

Antidiabetics + Danazol

Danazol causes insulin resistance. Therefore, on theoretical grounds, danazol would be expected to oppose the effects of antidiabetics, but the practical clinical importance of this is uncertain.

Clinical evidence, mechanism, importance and management

Danazol can disturb glucose metabolism. A study in 14 non-diabetic subjects found that 3 months of treatment with danazol 600 mg daily caused a mild but definite deterioration in glucose tolerance, associated with high insulin levels. Insulin resistance was also seen in 5 subjects taking danazol when they were given intravenous **tolbutamide**.[1] Similarly, another study in 9 non-diabetic women found that danazol 600 mg daily raised insulin levels in response to glucose or intravenous **tolbutamide**.[2] A further study in 9 non-diabetic women also found that danazol caused a mild deterioration in glucose tolerance and a marked increase in the insulin response to glucose loading.[3] Other studies have found that danazol causes marked resistance to both insulin[4-6] and glucagon,[5,6] which could be due to receptor down-regulation resulting from hypersecretion of insulin and glucagon.[5,6]

There is also a report of danazol-associated type 1 diabetes in a patient with endometriosis who took danazol 400 mg twice daily for 8 weeks. The diabetes resolved on withdrawal of danazol, but the development of hyperglycaemia about 5 months later suggested a predisposition to diabetes.[7] However, it has been suggested that the patient probably had type 2 diabetes precipitated by danazol-induced insulin resistance, which would possibly have responded to dietary restriction. Danazol-associated hyperglucagonaemia may have exacerbated the symptoms.[8,9]

For these reasons the manufacturers of danazol advise caution if danazol is given to diabetic patients.[10] Danazol would be expected to oppose the actions of antidiabetics to some extent, but there do not appear to be any studies assessing the clinical relevance of this.

1. Wynn V. Metabolic effects of danazol. *J Int Med Res* (1977) 5 (Suppl 3), 25–35.
2. Goettenberg N, Schlienger J L, Becmeur F, Dellenbach P. Traitement de l'endométriose pelvienne par le danazol. Incidence sur le métabolisme glucidique. *Nouv Presse Med* (1982) 11, 3703–6.
3. Vaughan-Williams C A, Shalet S M. Glucose tolerance and insulin resistance after danazol treatment. *J Obstet Gynaecol* (1989) 9, 229–32.
4. Matalliotakis I, Panidis D, Vlassis G, Neonaki M, Koumantakis E. Decreased sensitivity to insulin during treatment with danazol in women with endometriosis. *Clin Exp Obstet Gynecol* (1997) 24, 160–2.
5. Bruce R, Godsland I, Stevenson J, Devenport M, Borth F, Crook D, Ghatei M, Whitehead M, Wynn V. Danazol induces resistance to both insulin and glucagon in young women. *Clin Sci* (1992) 82, 211–17.
6. Kotzmann H, Linkesch M, Ludvik B, Clodi M, Luger A, Schernthaner G, Prager R, Klauser R. Effect of danazol-induced chronic hyperglucagonaemia on glucose tolerance and turnover. *Eur J Clin Invest* (1995) 25, 942–7.
7. Seifer DB, Freedman LN, Cavender JR, Baker RA. Insulin-dependent diabetes mellitus associated with danazol. *Am J Obstet Gynecol* (1990) 162, 474–5.
8. Williams G. Metabolic effects of danazol. *Am J Obstet Gynecol* (1991) 164, 933–4.
9. Seifer DB. Metabolic effects of danazol. *Am J Obstet Gynecol* (1991) 164, 934.
10. Danol (Danazol). Sanofi-Aventis. UK Summary of product characteristics, April 2006.

Antidiabetics + Dextropropoxyphene (Propoxyphene)

Dextropropoxyphene does not appear to affect the pharmacokinetics of tolbutamide. Hypoglycaemia was seen in a patient taking an unnamed sulphonylurea with co-proxamol, and has also been reported in non-diabetic patients given dextropropoxyphene alone.

Clinical evidence, mechanism, importance and management

After 6 healthy subjects took dextropropoxyphene 65 mg every 8 hours for 4 days, the clearance of a 500-mg intravenous dose of **tolbutamide** was not affected.[1] There is an isolated case of hypoglycaemia in a patient taking an unnamed **sulphonylurea** with **co-proxamol** (dextropropoxyphene with paracetamol (acetaminophen)).[2] There are also several reports of hypoglycaemia in non-diabetic patients taking dextropropoxyphene alone,[3-7] sometimes associated with renal failure,[3,4] advanced age,[5] or with high doses or in overdose.[6] The general importance of these isolated reports is uncertain, and there would normally seem to be little reason for avoiding the concurrent use of antidiabetics and dextropropoxyphene, or for taking particular precautions.

1. Robson RA, Miners JO, Whitehead AG, Birkett DJ. Specificity of the inhibitory effect of dextropropoxyphene on oxidative drug metabolism in man: effects on theophylline and tolbutamide disposition. *Br J Clin Pharmacol* (1987) 23, 772–5.
2. Girardin E, Vial T, Pham E, Evreux J-C. Hypoglycémies induites par les sulfamides hypoglycémiants. *Ann Med Interne (Paris)* (1992) 143, 11–17.
3. Wiederholt IC, Genco M, Foley JM. Recurrent episodes of hypoglycemia induced by propoxyphene. *Neurology* (1967) 17, 703–6.
4. Almirall J, Montoliu J, Torras A, Revert L. Propoxyphene-induced hypoglycemia in a patient with chronic renal failure. *Nephron* (1989) 53, 273–5.
5. Laurent M, Gallinari C, Bonnin M, Soubrie C. Hypoglycémie sous dextropropoxyphène chez des grands vieillards: 7 observations. *Presse Med* (1991) 20, 1628.
6. Karunakara BP, Maiya PP, Hegde SR, Pradeep GCM. Accidental dextropropoxyphene poisoning. *Indian J Pediatr* (2003) 70, 357–8.
7. Santos Gil I, Junquera Crespo M, Sanz Sanz J, Lahulla Pastor F. Hipglucernia secundaria a ingestión de dextropropoxifeno en un paciente adicto a drogas. Med Clin (Barc) 1998, 110, 475–6.

Antidiabetics + Disopyramide

Disopyramide occasionally causes hypoglycaemia, which may be severe. Isolated reports describe severe hypoglycaemia when disopyramide was given to diabetic patients taking gliclazide, or metformin and/or insulin.

Clinical evidence, mechanism, importance and management

Disopyramide occasionally and unpredictably causes hypoglycaemia, which may be severe.[1-7] The reasons are not fully understood, but *in vitro* studies suggest that disopyramide and its main metabolite may enhance insulin release from the pancreas.[8] There is a report of severe hypoglycaemia in an 82-year-old woman with diabetes who was taking **gliclazide**, which occurred 6 months after she started disopyramide 300 mg daily.[9] A further case of hypoglycaemia associated with disopyramide occurred in a 70-year-old woman who had been taking **metformin** 500 mg twice daily and **insulin** 62 units daily. Within 3 months of starting disopyramide 250 mg twice daily her **insulin** dose was reduced to 24 units daily, she stopped taking **metformin** and was eating 'substantial snacks' to avoid hypoglycaemia.[10] The **insulin** requirements of another patient with type 2 diabetes were markedly reduced when disopyramide was started.[11]

The manufacturers note that patients at particular risk for hypoglycaemia are the elderly, the malnourished, and diabetics, and that impaired renal function and impaired cardiac function may be predisposing factors.[12,13] They advise close monitoring of blood glucose levels[12,13] and withdrawal of disopyramide if problems arise.[12] This is not simply a problem for diabetics, but certainly within the context of diabetes the blood glucose-lowering effects of disopyramide may possibly cause particular difficulties. Although not strictly an interaction, the concurrent use of disopyramide and antidiabetics should be well monitored because of the potential for severe hypoglycaemia, as the cases show.

1. Goldberg IJ, Brown LK, Rayfield EJ. Disopyramide (Norpace)-induced hypoglycemia. *Am J Med* (1980) 69, 463–6.
2. Quevdeo SF, Krauss DS, Chazan JA, Crisafulli FS, Kahn CB. Fasting hypoglycemia secondary to disopyramide therapy. Report of two cases. *JAMA* (1981) 245, 2424.
3. Strathman I, Schubert EN, Cohen A, Nitzberg DM. Hypoglycemia in patients receiving disopyramide phosphate. *Drug Intell Clin Pharm* (1983) 17, 635–8.
4. Semel JD, Wortham E, Karl DM. Fasting hypoglycemia associated with disopyramide. *Am Heart J* (1983) 106, 1160–1.
5. Seriès C. Hypoglycémie induite ou favorisée par le disopyramide. *Rev Med Interne* (1988) 9, 528–9.
6. Cacoub P, Deray G, Baumelou A, Grimaldi C, Soubrie C, Jacobs C. Disopyramide-induced hypoglycemia: case report and review of the literature. *Fundam Clin Pharmacol* (1989) 3, 527–35.
7. Stapleton JT, Gillman MW. Hypoglycemic coma due to disopyramide toxicity. *South Med J* (1983) 76, 1453.
8. Horie M, Mizuno N, Tsuji K, Haruna T, Ninomiya T, Ishida H, Seino Y, Sasayama S. Disopyramide and its metabolite enhance insulin release from clonal pancreatic β-cells by blocking K_{ATP} channels. *Cardiovasc Drugs Ther* (2001) 15, 31–9.
9. Wahl D, de Korwin JD, Paille F, Trechot P, Schmitt J. Hypoglycémie sévère probablement induite par le disopyramide chez un diabétique. *Therapie* (1988) 43, 321–2.
10. Reynolds RM, Walker JD. Hypoglycaemia induced by disopyramide in a patient with type 2 diabetes mellitus. *Diabet Med* (2001) 18, 1009–10.
11. Onoda N, Kawagoe M, Shimizu M, Komori T, Takahashi C, Oomori Y, Hirata Y. A case of non-insulin dependent diabetes mellitus whose insulin requirement was markedly reduced after disopyramide treatment for arrhythmia. *Nippon Naika Gakkai Zasshi* (1989) 78, 820–5.
12. Rythmodan Capsules (Disopyramide). Sanofi-Aventis. UK Summary of product characteristics, November 2005.
13. Norpace (Disopyramide). Pharmacia. US Prescribing information, September 2001.

Antidiabetics + Disulfiram

Disulfiram appears not to affect the control of diabetes mellitus. Disulfiram does not appear to affect the pharmacokinetics of tolbutamide and there appears to be no evidence that disulfiram interacts with any other antidiabetics.

Clinical evidence, mechanism, importance and management

The manufacturers of disulfiram say that caution should be exercised if it is used in diabetics,[1] but a reviewer[2] who had given disulfiram to over 20 000 alcoholics said that he had prescribed disulfiram for several hundred patients with diabetes mellitus over 20 years without any apparent adverse effects and therefore any theoretical interaction is rarely, if ever, applicable to clinical practice. It would be reasonable to assume that many of these patients were also taking **insulin** or one of the older oral antidiabetics. There do not appear to be any reported cases in the literature of adverse interactions between disulfiram and any of the antidiabetics. In a study in 5 healthy subjects, disulfiram (400 mg three times daily for one day, then once daily for one day, then 200 mg daily for 2 days) had no significant effect on the half-life or clearance of intravenous **tolbutamide** 500 mg.[3]

The conclusion to be drawn from all of this is that any reaction is very rare (if it ever occurs), and no special precautions would normally appear to be necessary.

1. Antabuse (Disulfiram). Actavis UK Ltd. UK Summary of product characteristics, August 1999.
2. McNichol RW, Ewing JA, Faiman MD, eds. Disulfiram (Antabuse): a unique medical aid to sobriety: history, pharmacology, research, clinical use. Springfield, Ill: Thomas; 1987 pp. 47–90.
3. Svendsen TL, Kristensen MB, Hansen JM, Skovsted L. The influence of disulfiram on the half life and metabolic clearance rate of diphenylhydantoin and tolbutamide in man. *Eur J Clin Pharmacol* (1976) 9, 439–41.

Antidiabetics + Diuretics; Loop

The control of diabetes is not usually disturbed to a clinically relevant extent by etacrynic acid, furosemide, or torasemide. However, there are a few reports showing that etacrynic acid and furosemide can, rarely, raise blood glucose levels.

Clinical evidence

(a) Etacrynic acid

A double-blind study in 24 hypertensive patients, one-third of whom were diabetics, found that etacrynic acid 200 mg daily for 6 weeks impaired their glucose tolerance and raised the blood glucose levels of the diabetics to the same extent as those diabetics and non-diabetics taking hydrochlorothiazide 200 mg daily.[1] In another study no change in carbohydrate metabolism was seen in 6 diabetics given etacrynic acid 150 mg daily for a week.[2]

(b) Furosemide

Although furosemide can elevate blood glucose levels,[3] worsen glucose tolerance[4] and occasionally cause glycosuria or even acute diabetes in individual patients,[5,6] the general picture is that the control of diabetes is not usually affected by furosemide.[7] No clinically relevant changes in the control of diabetes were seen in a 3-month study of 29 patients with type 2 diabetes taking furosemide 40 mg daily and an average of 7 mg of **glibenclamide (glyburide)** daily.[8]

(c) Torasemide

A three-month study in 32 patients with congestive heart failure and type 2 diabetes mellitus taking **glibenclamide** found that torasemide 5 mg daily caused a small but clinically insignificant fall in blood glucose levels.[8]

Mechanism

Uncertain.

Importance and management

Information is limited. Some impairment of glucose tolerance may possibly occur, but there seems to be a lack of evidence in the literature to show that any loop diuretic has much effect on the control of diabetes in most patients.

1. Russell RP, Lindeman RD, Prescott LF. Metabolic and hypotensive effects of ethacrynic acid. Comparative study with hydrochlorothiazide. *JAMA* (1968) 205, 81–5.
2. Dige-Petersen H. Ethacrynic acid and carbohydrate metabolism. *Nord Med* (1966) 75, 123–5.
3. Hutcheon DE, Leonard G. Diuretic and antihypertensive action of frusemide. *J Clin Pharmacol* (1967) 7, 26–33.
4. Breckenridge A, Welborn TA, Dollery CT, Fraser R. Glucose tolerance in hypertensive patients on long-term diuretic therapy. *Lancet* (1967) i, 61–4.
5. Toivonen S, Mustala O. Diabetogenic action of frusemide. *BMJ* (1966) i, 920–21.
6. Kobayakawa N, Sawaki D, Otani Y, Sekita G, Fukushima K, Takeuchi H, Aoyagi T. A case of severe diabetes mellitus occurred during management of heart failure with carvedilol and furosemide. *Cardiovasc Drugs Ther* (2003) 17, 295.
7. Bencomo L, Fyvolent J, Kahana S, Kahana L. Clinical experience with a new diuretic, furosemide. *Curr Ther Res* (1965) 7, 339–45.
8. Lehnert H, Schmitz H, Beyer J, Wilmbusse H, Piesche L. Controlled clinical trial investigating the influence of torasemide and furosemide on carbohydrate metabolism in patients with cardiac failure and concomitant type II diabetes. *Int Congr Ser* (1993) 1023, 271–4.

Antidiabetics + Diuretics; Thiazide and related

By raising blood sugar levels, the thiazide and related diuretics can reduce the effects of the antidiabetics and impair the control of diabetes. However, this effect appears to be dose related, and is less frequent at the low doses now more commonly used for hypertension. Hyponatraemia has rarely been reported when chlorpropamide was given with a thiazide and potassium-sparing diuretic. An isolated report describes severe hypoglycaemia in a patient taking glibenclamide (glyburide) shortly after metolazone was started. Voglibose had no important effect on the pharmacokinetics of hydrochlorothiazide.

Clinical evidence

(a) Effects on glucose control

Chlorothiazide, the first of the thiazide diuretics, was found within a year of its introduction in 1958 to have hyperglycaemic effects.[1] Since then a very large number of reports have described hyperglycaemia, the precipitation of diabetes in prediabetics, and the disturbance of blood sugar control in diabetics taking thiazides. One example from many:

A long-term study in 53 patients with type 2 diabetes found that **chlorothiazide** 500 mg or 1 g daily or **trichlormethiazide** 4 or 8 mg daily caused a mean rise in blood glucose levels from about 6.7 to 7.8 mmol/L. Only 7 patients needed a change in their treatment: 4 required more of their oral antidiabetic, 2 an increase in **insulin** dose, and one was transferred from **tolbutamide** to **insulin**. The oral antidiabetics used included **tolbutamide, chlorpropamide, acetohexamide** and **phenformin**.[2]

A rise in blood sugar levels has been observed with **bendroflumethiazide**,[3,4] **benzthiazide**,[5] **hydrochlorothiazide** 100 to 300 mg daily,[3] and **chlortalidone** 50 to 100 mg daily.[6] A study in hypertensive patients found that **chlortalidone** 50 mg daily increased glucose and insulin levels, but **hydrochlorothiazide** 50 mg daily alone or as part of a potassium and/or magnesium conserving regimen did not.[7]

More recent data suggest that the effects of thiazides on blood glucose may be dose related. In a double-blind randomised study comparing the effects of 1.25 or 5 mg of **bendroflumethiazide** on blood glucose, the lower dose had no effects on insulin action, whereas when the higher dose was given, there was evidence of impaired glucose tolerance.[8] A review of the literature on **hydrochlorothiazide** similarly reports that low doses (6.25 to 12.5 mg) lack significant effects on blood glucose levels.[9]

A man with type 2 diabetes, stabile taking **glibenclamide (glyburide)** 10 mg daily and hospitalised for congestive heart failure, became clinically hypoglycaemic (blood glucose levels unmeasurable by *Labstix*) within 40 hours of starting **metolazone** 5 mg daily. He was treated with intravenous glucose. Although both **glibenclamide** and **metolazone** were stopped, he had 4 further hypoglycaemic episodes over the next 30 hours.[10] The reasons are not understood. *In vitro* studies failed to find any evidence that **metolazone** displaces **glibenclamide** from its protein binding sites, which might possibly have provided some explanation for what happened.[10]

The hypoglycaemic responses of 10 healthy subjects were studied following an intravenous infusion of **tolbutamide** 3 mg/kg, given 3 days before and one hour after the last dose of oral **cicletanine** 100 mg daily for a week.[11] No clinically relevant changes were seen. Note that, studies in *animals* and in non-diabetic hypertensive patients found that, at therapeutic doses, **cicletanine** did not affect glycoregulation.[12] The conclusion to be drawn is that **cicletanine** is unlikely to affect the control of diabetes in patients, but this needs confirmation from longer-term clinical studies.

(b) Hyponatraemia

A hospital report describes 8 cases of low serum sodium concentrations observed over a 5-year period in patients taking **chlorpropamide** and *Moduretic* (**hydrochlorothiazide** 50 mg with amiloride 5 mg).[13]

(c) Pharmacokinetics

A study in 12 healthy subjects given a single 25-mg dose of **hydrochlorothiazide** before and after taking **voglibose** 5 mg three times daily for 11 days found that the **hydrochlorothiazide** plasma levels were slightly increased by the **voglibose** (AUC increased 7.5%, maximum plasma levels increased 15%) but these changes were considered to be clinically irrelevant. The combination was well tolerated and adverse events were unchanged.[14]

Mechanism

Not understood. One study suggested that the hyperglycaemia is due to the inhibition of insulin release by the pancreas.[15] Another suggestion is that the peripheral action of insulin is affected in some way.[5,16] There is also evidence that the effects may be related in part to potassium depletion.[17] The hyponatraemia appears to be due to the additive sodium-losing effects of chlorpropamide, the thiazide and amiloride. Obese patients may be more sensitive to the effects of hydrochlorothiazide on insulin metabolism.[7]

Importance and management

The reduction in hypoglycaemic effect is extremely well documented (not all references are given here) but of only moderate practical importance, particularly since much of the data relates to higher doses of thiazides than are now used clinically for hypertension. Low doses of thiazides have a lesser effect on plasma glucose, and recent guidelines on the treatment of hypertension in diabetes recommend the use of thiazides.[18] If higher doses are used, increased monitoring of diabetic control would seem prudent. There is evidence that the full effects may take many months to develop in some patients.[4] Most patients respond to a modest increase in the dosage of the antidiabetics. This interaction may be expected to occur with all thiazides and possibly related diuretics, such as clopamide and metolazone. Hyponatraemia is a rare but recognised adverse effect of the thiazides and no additional precautions would therefore seem necessary.

1. Wilkins RW. New drugs for the treatment of hypertension. *Ann Intern Med* (1959) 50, 1–10.
2. Kansal PC, Buse J, Buse MG. Thiazide diuretics and control of diabetes mellitus. *South Med J* (1969) 62, 1374–9.
3. Goldner MG, Zarowitz H, Akgun S. Hyperglycemia and glycosuria due to thiazide derivatives administered in diabetes mellitus. *N Engl J Med* (1960) 262, 403–5.
4. Lewis PJ, Kohner EM, Petrie A, Dollery CT. Deterioration of glucose tolerance in hypertensive patients on prolonged diuretic treatment. *Lancet* (1976) i, 564–6.
5. Runyan JW. Influence of thiazide diuretics on carbohydrate metabolism in patients with mild diabetes. *N Engl J Med* (1962) 267, 541–3.
6. Carliner NH, Schelling J-L, Russell RP, Okun R, Davis M. Thiazide- and phthalimidine-induced hyperglycemia in hypertensive patients. *JAMA* (1965) 191, 535–40.
7. Siegel D, Saliba P, Haffner S. Glucose and insulin levels during diuretic therapy in hypertensive men. *Hypertension* (1994) 23, 688–94.
8. Harper R, Ennis CN, Sheridan B, Atkinson AB, Johnston GD, Bell PM. Effects of low dose versus conventional dose thiazide diuretic on insulin action in essential hypertension. *BMJ* (1994) 309, 226–30.
9. Neutel JM. Metabolic manifestations of low-dose diuretics. *Am J Med* (1996) 101 (Suppl 3A), 71S–82S.
10. George S, McBurney A, Cole A. Possible protein binding displacement interaction between glibenclamide and metolazone. *Eur J Clin Pharmacol* (1990) 38, 93–5.
11. Bayés MC, Barbanoj MJ, Vallès J, Torrent J, Obach R, Jané F. A drug interaction study between cicletanine and tolbutamide in healthy volunteers. *Eur J Clin Pharmacol* (1996) 50, 381–4.
12. Mashori GR, Tariq AR, Shahimi MM, Suhaimi H. The effects of cicletanine, a new antihypertensive agent on insulin release in rat isolated pancreas by the perfusion technique. *Singapore Med J* (1996) 37, 278–81.
13. Zalin AM, Hutchinson CE, Jong M, Matthews K. Hyponatraemia during treatment with chlorpropamide and Moduretic (amiloride plus hydrochlorothiazide). *BMJ* (1984) 289, 659.
14. Kleist P, Suzuki Y, Thomsen T, Möller M, Römer A, Hucke HP, Kurowski M, Eckl KM. Voglibose has no effect on the pharmacokinetics of hydrochlorothiazide. *Eur J Clin Pharmacol* (1998) 54, 273–4.
15. Fajans SS, Floyd JC, Knopf RF, Rull J, Guntsche EM, Conn JW. Benzothiadiazine suppression of insulin release from normal and abnormal islet tissue in man. *J Clin Invest* (1966) 45, 481–92.
16. Remenchik AP, Hoover C, Talso PJ. Insulin secretion by hypertensive patients receiving hydrochlorothiazide. *JAMA* (1970) 212, 869.
17. Rapoport MI, Hurd HF. Thiazide-induced glucose intolerance treated with potassium. *Arch Intern Med* (1964) 113, 405–8.
18. American Diabetes Association. Hypertension management in adults with diabetes. *Diabetes Care* (2004) 27 (Suppl 1), S65–7.

Antidiabetics + Fenfluramine

Fenfluramine has inherent blood glucose-lowering activity that can add to, or in some instances replace, the effects of conventional antidiabetic drugs.

Clinical evidence, mechanism, importance and management

A study of the substitution of fenfluramine (initially 40 mg daily, increased to 120 mg daily) for a biguanide antidiabetic found that diabetes was equally well controlled by either drug in 4 of 6 patients.[1] The blood glucose-lowering effects of fenfluramine have also been described elsewhere.[2,3] It seems that fenfluramine increases the uptake of glucose into skeletal muscle, thereby lowering blood glucose levels.[3,4]

This is a well established and, on the whole, an advantageous rather than an adverse reaction, but it would be prudent to check on the extent of the response if fenfluramine is added or withdrawn from the treatment being received by diabetics. However, note that fenfluramine was generally withdrawn in 1997 because its use was found to be associated with a high incidence of abnormal echocardiograms indicating abnormal functioning of heart valves.

1. Jackson WPU. Fenfluramine trials in a diabetic clinic. *S Afr Med J* (1971) 45 (Suppl), 29–30.
2. Turtle JR, Burgess JA. Hypoglycemic action of fenfluramine in diabetes mellitus. *Diabetes* (1973) 22, 858–67.
3. Dykes JRW. The effect of a low-calorie diet with and without fenfluramine, and fenfluramine alone on the glucose tolerance and insulin secretion of overweight non-diabetics. *Postgrad Med J* (1973) 49, 314–17.
4. Kirby MJ, Turner P. Effect of amphetamine, fenfluramine and norfenfluramine on glucose uptake into human isolated skeletal muscle. *Br J Clin Pharmacol* (1974) 1, 340P–341P.

Antidiabetics + Fibrates

A number of reports describe hypoglycaemia and/or an enhancement of the effects of antidiabetic drugs (mostly insulin and sulphonylureas) in patients given fibrates. The combination of gemfibrozil and repaglinide should be avoided, because a marked pharmacokinetic interaction can result in serious hypoglycaemia. Gemfibrozil also causes large increases in the AUCs of pioglitazone and rosiglitazone, and caution is therefore warranted until more is known. Only a modest pharmacokinetic interaction occurs between gemfibrozil and nateglinide. The antidiuretic effects of clofibrate in the treatment of diabetes insipidus are opposed by glibenclamide (glyburide).

Clinical evidence

A. Bezafibrate

(a) Repaglinide

In a study in healthy subjects bezafibrate 400 mg once daily for 5 days had no effect on the pharmacokinetics of a single 250-microgram dose of repaglinide, and did not alter the glucose-lowering effect of repaglinide.[1]

(b) Sulphonylureas and Biguanides

Three elderly patients with type 2 diabetes and mild renal impairment taking **glibenclamide (glyburide)** developed hypoglycaemia when they were given bezafibrate: one of them needed a 60% dosage reduction, another was given **tolbutamide** instead, and the third was able to stop both **glibenclamide** and **buformin**.[2] The French Centres Régionaux de Pharmacovigilance recorded 7 cases of hypoglycaemia during the period 1985 to 1990, which developed in patients taking unnamed sulphonylureas when they were given fibrates (one case with bezafibrate).[3]

B. Ciprofibrate

The French Centres Régionaux de Pharmacovigilance recorded 7 cases of hypoglycaemia during the period 1985 to 1990, which developed in patients taking unnamed **sulphonylureas** when they were given fibrates (3 cases with ciprofibrate).[3]

C. Clofibrate

(a) Hypoglycaemia

Over a 5-day period while taking clofibrate 2 g daily, the control of diabetes was improved in 6 out of 13 patients with type 2 diabetes taking various unnamed sulphonylureas. Hypoglycaemia (blood glucose levels of about 1.7 to 2.2 mmol/L) was seen in 4 patients.[4] Other studies confirm that some, but not all, patients have a fall in blood glucose levels while taking clofibrate and the control of the diabetes can improve.[5-12] In one study[13] the half-life of **chlorpropamide** ranged from 40 to 62 hours in 5 subjects taking clofibrate compared with a mean of about 36 hours in control subjects.

(b) Reduced antidiuretic effects

Clofibrate 2 g daily reduced the volume of urine excreted by 2 patients with pituitary diabetes insipidus, but when **glibenclamide** was also given the volume increased once again. Without treatment they excreted 5.8 and 6.5 litres of urine daily, and this reduced to only 2.4 and 1.7 litres while taking clofibrate, whereas with **glibenclamide** and clofibrate they excreted 3.6 and 3.7 litres daily, respectively.[14]

D. Fenofibrate

(a) Repaglinide

In a study in healthy subjects, fenofibrate 200 mg once daily for 5 days had no effect on the pharmacokinetics of a single 250-microgram dose of repaglinide, and did not alter the glucose-lowering effect of repaglinide.[1]

(b) Sulphonylureas

The French Centres Régionaux de Pharmacovigilance recorded 7 cases of hypoglycaemia during the period 1985 to 1990, which developed in patients taking unnamed sulphonylureas when they were given fibrates (3 with cases fenofibrate).[3]

E. Gemfibrozil

(a) Nateglinide or Repaglinide

In a randomised crossover study, 12 healthy subjects were given gemfibrozil 600 mg twice daily for 3 days, with a 250-microgram dose of repaglinide on day 3. Gemfibrozil raised the AUC of repaglinide eightfold and increased the plasma levels nearly 29-fold.[15] Itraconazole (which may interact, see 'Antidiabetics + Azoles; Itraconazole or Ketoconazole', p.479) given with gemfibrozil and repaglinide further increased these effects. The blood glucose-lowering effects of repaglinide were considerably enhanced and prolonged, both by gemfibrozil alone and in combination with itraconazole.[15] In 2003, the European Agency for the Evaluation of Medicinal Products had received five reports of serious hypoglycaemic episodes with gemfibrozil and repaglinide.[16]

In contrast, in a very similar study by the same research group, the combination of gemfibrozil and itraconazole caused only a modest 47% increase in the AUC of a single dose of nateglinide 30 mg, and did not significantly alter the blood glucose response to nateglinide in healthy subjects.[17]

(b) Pioglitazone or Rosiglitazone

Gemfibrozil 600 mg twice daily for 4 days increased the mean AUC of a single dose of rosiglitazone 4 mg by 2.3-fold, the peak plasma level by 1.2-fold and the 24-hour plasma level by almost tenfold in a study in healthy subjects.[18] In the same way, gemfibrozil increased the mean AUC of a single dose of pioglitazone 3.2-fold without altering its maximum level, but raised the 48-hour plasma level by approximately 15-fold.[19] A similar increase in pioglitazone AUC was reported in another study.[20] In these studies, the effects of these pharmacokinetic changes on the pharmacodynamics of rosiglitazone or pioglitazone were not assessed.[18-20]

(c) Sulphonylureas or Insulin

Fasting blood glucose levels decreased in 10 diabetic patients, and increased in 4 of 14 diabetic patients receiving insulin, **acetohexamide**, **chlorpropamide** or **glipizide** who were given gemfibrozil (800 mg daily initially, reduced later to 400 to 600 mg daily).[21] Another study found that of 20 patients, 9 required a slight increase in the dosage of insulin or sulphonylurea (**glibenclamide** or **chlorpropamide**), and one a decreased dosage, when they were given gemfibrozil 800 mg to 1.6 g daily.[22] A single report describes hypoglycaemia, which occurred in a diabetic taking **glibenclamide** when they were given gemfibrozil 1.2 g daily.[23] The **glibenclamide** dosage was reduced from 5 to 1.25 mg daily with satisfactory diabetic control. When the gemfibrozil was later stopped and restarted, the dosage of the **glibenclamide** had to be increased and then reduced. A placebo-controlled study in 10 healthy subjects found that gemfibrozil 600 mg twice daily for 5 doses increased the AUC of a single 500-microgram dose of **glimepiride** by 23%, but there were no significant changes in serum insulin or blood glucose.[24]

Mechanism

The suggested reasons for the alteration in diabetic control with fibrates include the displacement of the sulphonylureas from their plasma protein binding sites,[7] alterations in their renal excretion,[13] and a decrease in insulin resistance.[6,25] Clofibrate has also been shown to have a blood glucose-lowering action of its own, which improves the glucose tolerance of diabetics.[12] It is thought that gemfibrozil inhibits the metabolism of repaglinide by the cytochrome P450 isoenzyme CYP2C8, and that inhibition of CYP3A4 (its other main route of metabolism) by itraconazole further blocks repaglinide metabolism.[15] Gemfibrozil also inhibits the CYP2C8-mediated metabolism of rosiglitazone and pioglitazone.[18,19] In addition, gemfibrozil may inhibit CYP2C9-mediated metabolism of glimepiride and other sulphonylureas such as glipizide, glibenclamide or **gliclazide**,[24] and also nateglinide.[17] It seems possible that any or all of these mechanisms might contribute towards enhanced hypoglycaemia.

Importance and management

The interaction between the sulphonylureas and clofibrate is established and well documented. The incidence is uncertain, but what is known suggests that between about one-third and one-half of patients may be affected. Alteration in diabetic control, most usually hypoglycaemia, has been seen in diabetics taking sulphonylureas with bezafibrate, ciprofibrate, fenofibrate, and gemfibrozil. There would seem to be no good reason for avoiding the concurrent use of sulphonylureas and fibrates, but be aware that the dosage of the antidiabetic may need adjustment. Patients should be warned that excessive hypoglycaemia occurs occasionally and unpredictably.

Note that on the basis of the study,[15] and following five reports of serious hypoglycaemic episodes with gemfibrozil and repaglinide, the European

Agency for the Evaluation of Medicinal Products decided to contraindicate concurrent use.[16]

Marked increases in the AUC of rosiglitazone and pioglitazone have been demonstrated with gemfibrozil, but the clinical relevance of these has not been assessed. Until further experience is gained, caution is warranted. Only modest increases in plasma levels of nateglinide have been demonstrated with gemfibrozil, but the manufacturer recommends caution if nateglinide is given with CYP2C9 inhibitors including gemfibrozil.[26]

Information about reduced diuretic effects is limited. It would seem prudent to avoid the concurrent use of drugs with actions that are antagonistic.

1. Kajosaari LI, Backman JT, Neuvonen M, Laitila J, Neuvonen PJ. Lack of effect of bezafibrate and fenofibrate on the pharmacokinetics and pharmacodynamics of repaglinide. *Br J Clin Pharmacol* (2004) 58, 390–6.
2. Ohsawa K, Koike N, Takamura T, Nagai Y, Kobayashi KI. Hypoglycaemic attacks after administration of bezafibrate in three cases of non-insulin dependent diabetes mellitus. *J Jpn Diabetes Soc* (1994) 37, 295–300.
3. Girardin E, Vial T, Pham E, Evreux J-C. Hypoglycémies induites par les sulfamides hypoglycémiants. Recensement par les Centres Régionaux de Pharmacovigilance français de 1985 à 1990. *Ann Med Interne (Paris)* (1992) 143, 11–17.
4. Daubresse J-C, Luyckx AS, Lefebvre PJ. Potentiation of hypoglycemic effect of sulfonylureas by clofibrate. *N Engl J Med* (1976) 294, 613.
5. Jain AK, Ryan JR, McMahon FG. Potentiation of hypoglycemic effect of sulfonylureas by halofenate. *N Engl J Med* (1975) 293, 1283–6.
6. Ferrari C, Frezzati S, Testori GP, Bertazzoni A. Potentiation of hypoglycemic response to intravenous tolbutamide by clofibrate. *N Engl J Med* (1976) 294, 1184.
7. Jain AK, Ryan JR, McMahon FG. Potentiation of hypoglycemic effect of sulfonylureas by clofibrate. *N Engl J Med* (1976) 294, 613.
8. Daubresse J-C, Daigneux D, Bruwier M, Luyckx A, Lefebvre PJ. Clofibrate and diabetes control in patients treated with oral hypoglycaemic agents. *Br J Clin Pharmacol* (1979) 7, 599–603.
9. Miller RD. *Atromid* in the treatment of post-climacteric diabetes. *J Atheroscler Res* (1963) 3, 694–700.
10. Csögör SI, Bornemisza P. The effect of clofibrate (Atromid) on intravenous tolbutamide, oral and intravenous glucose tolerance tests. *Clin Trials J* (1977) 14, 15–19.
11. Herriott SC, Percy-Robb IW, Strong JA, Thomson CG. The effect of Atromid on serum cholesterol and glucose tolerance in diabetes mellitus. *J Atheroscler Res* (1963) 3, 679–88.
12. Barnett D, Craig JG, Robinson DS, Rogers MP. Effect of clofibrate on glucose tolerance in maturity-onset diabetes. *Br J Clin Pharmacol* (1977) 4, 455–8.
13. Petitpierre B, Perrin L, Rudhardt M, Herrera A, Fabre J. Behaviour of chlorpropamide in renal insufficiency and under the effect of associated drug therapy. *Int J Clin Pharmacol* (1972) 6, 120–4.
14. Radó JP, Szende L, Marosi J, Juhos E, Sawinsky I, Takó J. Inhibition of the diuretic action of glibenclamide by clofibrate, carbamazepine and 1-deamino-8-D-arginine-vasopressin (DDAVP) in patients with pituitary diabetes insipidus. *Acta Diabetol Lat* (1974) 11, 179–97.
15. Niemi M, Backman JT, Neuvonen M, Neuvonen PJ. Effects of gemfibrozil, itraconazole, and their combination on the pharmacokinetics and pharmacodynamics of repaglinide: potentially hazardous interaction between gemfibrozil and repaglinide. *Diabetologia* (2003) 46, 347–51.
16. EMEA public statement on repaglinide (NovoNorm/Prandin): contraindication of concomitant use of repaglinide and gemfibrozil, 21 May 2003, London. Available at: http://www.emea.eu.int/pdfs/human/press/pus/117003en.pdf (accessed 17/08/07).
17. Niemi M, Backman JT, Juntti-Patinen L, Neuvonen M, Neuvonen PJ. Coadministration of gemfibrozil and itraconazole has only a minor effect on the pharmacokinetics of the CYP2C9 and CYP3A4 substrate nateglinide. *Br J Clin Pharmacol* (2005) 60, 208–17.
18. Niemi M, Backman JT, Granfors M, Laitila J, Neuvonen M, Neuvonen PJ. Gemfibrozil considerably increases the plasma concentrations of rosiglitazone. *Diabetologia* (2003) 46, 1319–23.
19. Jaakkola T, Backman JT, Neuvonen M, Neuvonen PJ. Effects of gemfibrozil, itraconazole, and their combination on the pharmacokinetics of pioglitazone. *Clin Pharmacol Ther* (2005) 77, 404–14.
20. Deng L-J, Wang F, Li H-D. Effect of gemfibrozil on the pharmacokinetics of pioglitazone. *Eur J Clin Pharmacol* (2005) 61, 831–6.
21. de Salcedo I, Gorringe JAL, Silva JL, Santos JA. Gemfibrozil in a group of diabetics. *Proc R Soc Med* (1976) 69 (Suppl 2), 64–70.
22. Konttinen A, Kuisma I, Ralli R, Pohjola S, Ojala K. The effect of gemfibrozil on serum lipids in diabetic patients. *Ann Clin Res* (1979) 11, 240–5.
23. Ahmad S. Gemfibrozil: interaction with glyburide. *South Med J* (1991) 84, 102.
24. Niemi M, Neuvonen PJ, Kivistö KT. Effect of gemfibrozil on the pharmacokinetics and pharmacodynamics of glimepiride. *Clin Pharmacol Ther* (2001) 70, 439–45.
25. Ferrari C, Frezzati S, Romussi M, Bertazzoni A, Testori GP, Antonini S, Paracchi A. Effects of short-term clofibrate administration on glucose tolerance and insulin secretion in patients with chemical diabetes or hypertriglyceridemia. *Metabolism* (1977) 26, 129–39.
26. Starlix (Nateglinide). Novartis Pharmaceuticals UK Ltd. UK Summary of product characteristics, September 2005.

Antidiabetics + Glucosamine ± Chondroitin

In a controlled study, glucosamine supplements with chondroitin had no effect on glycaemic control in patients taking oral antidiabetic drugs but one report notes that unexpected increases in blood glucose levels have occurred.

Clinical evidence, mechanism, importance and management

In 2000, the Canadian Adverse Drug Reaction Monitoring Programme (CADRMP) briefly reported that unexpected increases in blood glucose levels had occurred in diabetic patients taking glucosamine sulfate, or glucosamine with chondroitin.[1] However, in a well controlled study, *Cosamin DS* (glucosamine hydrochloride 1.5 g daily plus chondroitin sulfate sodium 1.2 g) daily for 90 days had no effect on the control of diabetes (glycosylated haemoglobin) in 22 patients with type 2 diabetes, 18 of whom were receiving oral antidiabetics [specific drugs not named] and 4 who were diet controlled.[2]

Endogenous glucosamine has a role in glucose metabolism, and may increase insulin resistance. In one case, glucosamine also reduced hypoglycaemic episodes in a patient with metastatic insulinoma.[3]

The interaction is not established, and the results of the controlled trial suggest that glucosamine supplements are unlikely to affect diabetes control. However, it has been suggested that the results may not be applicable to patients with later stages of diabetes.[4] Therefore, it may be prudent to increase monitoring of blood glucose in these patients if glucosamine supplements are taken. Also, if glucose control unexpectedly deteriorates, bear in mind the possibility of self-medication with supplements such as glucosamine.

1. Canadian Adverse Drug Reaction Monitoring Programme (CADRMP). Communiqué. Glucosamine sulfate: hyperglycemia. *Can Adverse Drug React News* (2000) 10 (Oct), 7.
2. Scroggie DA, Albright A, Harris MD. The effect of glucosamine-chondroitin supplementation on glycosylated hemoglobin levels in patients with type 2 diabetes mellitus: a placebo-controlled, double-blinded, randomized clinical trial. *Arch Intern Med* (2003) 163, 1587–90.
3. Chan NN, Baldeweg SE, Tan TMM, Hurel SJ. Glucosamine sulphate and osteoarthritis. *Lancet* (2001) 357, 1618–19.
4. Jain RK, McCormick JC. Can glucosamine supplements be applied for all patients with type 2 diabetes with osteoarthritis? *Arch Intern Med* (2004) 164, 807.

Antidiabetics + Guanethidine and related drugs

Limited evidence suggests that guanethidine has blood glucose-lowering activity, which may possibly add to the effects of conventional antidiabetics. One case report suggests soluble insulin may exaggerate the hypotensive effects of debrisoquine.

Clinical evidence

(a) Debrisoquine

An man with type 1 diabetes taking debrisoquine 20 mg twice daily developed severe postural hypotension within an hour of receiving 28 units of a short-acting **insulin** (soluble insulin) plus 20 units of **isophane insulin**. He became dizzy and was found to have a standing blood pressure of 97/72 mmHg. The postural fall in systolic pressure was 65 mmHg. He had no evidence of hypoglycaemia and no hypotension when using 48 units of **isophane insulin** without the soluble insulin.[1] **Insulin** can cause hypotension but this is only seen in those with an impaired reflex control of blood pressure.[1]

(b) Guanethidine

A diabetic needed an **insulin** dose increase from 70 to 94 units daily when guanethidine was withdrawn.[2] A later study in 3 patients with type 2 diabetes found that guanethidine 50 to 90 mg daily caused a significant improvement in their glucose tolerance.[3] Two other reports also suggest that guanethidine has blood glucose-lowering effects.[4,5]

Mechanism

It has been suggested that the interaction between insulin and guanethidine occurs because guanethidine can impair the homoeostatic mechanism concerned with raising blood glucose levels, by affecting the release of catecholamines. The balance of the system thus impaired tends to be tipped in favour of a reduced blood glucose level, resulting in a reduced requirement for the antidiabetic. The interaction between debrisoquine and insulin is not understood.

Importance and management

Information about both of these interactions is very limited, and their general importance is uncertain. Increase the frequency of blood glucose monitoring if guanethidine or related drugs are started or stopped. Also check patients given debrisoquine (no longer generally available) and insulin, particularly if they are taking vasodilators, to ensure that excessive hypotension does not develop.

1. Hume L. Potentiation of hypotensive effect of debrisoquine by insulin. *Diabet Med* (1985) 2, 390–1.
2. Gupta KK, Lillicrap CA. Guanethidine and diabetes. *BMJ* (1968) 2, 697–8.
3. Gupta KK. The anti-diabetic action of guanethidine. *Postgrad Med J* (1969) 45, 455–6.
4. Kansal PC, Buse J, Durling FC, Buse MG. Effect of guanethidine and reserpine on glucose tolerance. *Curr Ther Res* (1971) 13, 517–22.
5. Woeber KA, Arky R, Braverman LE. Reversal by guanethidine of abnormal oral glucose tolerance in thyrotoxicosis. *Lancet* (1966) i, 895–8.

Antidiabetics + Guar gum or Glucomannan

Guar gum appeared not to affect the absorption of glipizide or glibenclamide (glyburide) to a clinically relevant extent. Although guar gum modestly reduced the absorption of metformin, it enhanced its postprandial hypoglycaemic effect. Glucomannan appeared to reduce the initial absorption of glibenclamide, but also enhanced its hypoglycaemic effect.

Clinical evidence, mechanism, importance and management

(a) Glucomannan

Glucomannan 3.9 g reduced the plasma levels of a single 2.5-mg dose of **glibenclamide** (**glyburide**) in 9 healthy subjects. Four samples taken over 30 to 150 minutes found that the plasma levels of **glibenclamide** were reduced by about 50%.[1] Despite this, plasma glucose levels were lower with the combination than with **glibenclamide** alone. Because plasma samples were not taken beyond 150 minutes, it is unclear what effect glucomannan has on the extent of **glibenclamide** absorption. The clinical relevance of these changes is unclear, but they seem unlikely to be important.

(b) Guar gum

In one study in 10 healthy subjects guar gum was found to have no effect on the AUC or maximum serum levels of a single 2.5-mg dose of **glipizide**. In this study **glipizide** was given alone, or 30 minutes before breakfast, and this treatment was compared with guar gum granules (4.75 g guar gum) given either with the breakfast or with the **glipizide**.[2]

In one comparative study, guar gum was found to reduce the AUC of **glibenclamide** from one formulation *(Semi-Euglucon)* by about 30%, but not another newer formulation *(Semi-Euglucon-N)*,[3] possibly because the latter preparation is more rapidly and completely absorbed. Similarly, in a double-blind crossover study in 9 patients with type 2 diabetes, guar gum granules 5 g three times daily with meals did not significantly affect the AUC or maximum serum level of **glibenclamide** 3.5 mg twice daily from the newer formulation. In addition, the combination slightly reduced fasting blood glucose when compared with baseline values.[4]

In a single-dose study, guar gum 10 g reduced the absorption rate of **metformin** 1.7 g and reduced the AUC by 39% in healthy subjects, but the total reduction in postprandial blood glucose levels was increased.[5]

It seems doubtful if any of these modest pharmacokinetic interactions has much, if any, clinical relevance because guar gum can improve the metabolic control and decrease serum lipids in patients with type 2 diabetes.[4]

1. Shima K, Tanaka A, Ikegami H, Tabata M, Sawazaki N, Kumahara Y. Effect of dietary fiber, glucomannan, on absorption of sulfonylurea in man. *Horm Metab Res* (1983) 15, 1–3.
2. Huupponen R, Karhuvaara S, Seppälä P. Effect of guar gum on glipizide absorption in man. *Eur J Clin Pharmacol* (1985) 28, 717–9.
3. Neugebauer G, Akpan W, Abshagen U. Interaktion von Guar mit Glibenclamid und Bezafibrat. *Beitr Infusionther Klin Ernahr* (1983) 12, 40–7.
4. Uusitupa M, Södervik H, Silvasti M, Karttunen P. Effects of a gel forming dietary fiber, guar gum, on the absorption of glibenclamide and metabolic control and serum lipids in patients with non-insulin-dependent (type 2) diabetes. *Int J Clin Pharmacol Ther Toxicol* (1990) 28, 153–7.
5. Gin H, Orgerie MB, Aubertin J. The influence of guar gum on absorption of metformin from the gut in healthy volunteers. *Horm Metab Res* (1989) 21, 81–3.

Antidiabetics + H_2-receptor antagonists

On the whole cimetidine and ranitidine do not appear to significantly alter diabetic control with sulphonylureas, although cases of adverse effects have been seen when glibenclamide was given with ranitidine, and when gliclazide or glipizide were given with cimetidine.

Cimetidine appears to reduce the clearance of metformin, and may have contributed to a case of metformin-associated lactic acidosis. Cimetidine did not alter repaglinide pharmacokinetics, and ranitidine did not alter pioglitazone or rosiglitazone pharmacokinetics. Acarbose did not alter ranitidine pharmacokinetics, but miglitol decreased the AUC of ranitidine by 60%.

Clinical evidence

A. Alpha-glucosidase inhibitors

The manufacturer of **acarbose** notes that it had no effect on the pharmacokinetics or pharmacodynamics of **ranitidine** in healthy subjects.[1] Conversely, the manufacturer of **miglitol** notes that it reduced the bioavailability of **ranitidine** by 60%.[2]

B. Biguanides

Cimetidine 800 mg daily was found to reduce the renal clearance of **metformin** in 7 healthy subjects by 27% and increase the AUC by 50%.[3] A 59-year-old woman with type 2 diabetes taking long-term **metformin** 500 mg three times daily developed severe metabolic acidosis with cardiovascular collapse and acute renal failure. Three months previously she had started orlistat 120 mg three times daily, which caused chronic diarrhoea. During the 4 days before hospital admission, she was prescribed **cimetidine** 400 mg twice daily for her abdominal pain. The **metformin**-associated lactic acidosis was considered to have been precipitated by the 'orlistat', (p.498) and **cimetidine**.[4]

C. Sulphonylureas

(a) Chlorpropamide

Cimetidine had no effect on the pharmacokinetics of chlorpropamide in healthy subjects,[5] and in another study the blood glucose-lowering effects of chlorpropamide remained unaltered when **cimetidine** was given.[6]

(b) Glibenclamide (Glyburide)

A study in healthy subjects reported that the blood glucose-lowering effects of glibenclamide were slightly reduced by **cimetidine** and **ranitidine**. This occurred despite the fact that **cimetidine** increased the AUC of glibenclamide by 37% and ranitidine had no significant pharmacokinetic effect on glibenclamide.[7] Marked hypoglycaemia was seen in a patient taking glibenclamide 5 mg daily when **ranitidine** 150 mg twice daily was also taken.[8] Conversely, a study in healthy subjects found that the blood glucose-lowering effects of glibenclamide remained unaltered by **cimetidine**.[6]

(c) Gliclazide

An elderly type 2 diabetic taking gliclazide 160 mg daily developed very low blood glucose levels (1 mmol/L) after starting to take **cimetidine** 800 mg daily.[9]

(d) Glimepiride

In a study in healthy subjects no relevant interactions, either pharmacokinetic or pharmacodynamic, were seen when glimepiride was given with either **cimetidine** or **ranitidine**.[10]

(e) Glipizide

Six patients with type 2 diabetes were given **cimetidine** 400 mg one hour before taking a dose of glipizide (average dose 5.8 mg) and then 3 hours later they were given a standard meal with **cimetidine** 200 mg. The expected rise in blood glucose levels after the meal was reduced by 40% and in two of the patients plasma glucose levels fell to less than 3 mmol/L. Cimetidine increased the glipizide AUC by 23%.[11,12] However, a study in healthy subjects found that the hypoglycaemic activity of glipizide remained unaltered by **cimetidine**.[6]

Two studies in type 2 diabetics found that **ranitidine** 150 mg increased the AUC of glipizide by 29% and 34%,[12,13] and reduced the expected rise in blood sugar levels after a meal by 22%.[12] However, another study by the same research group reported that **ranitidine** 300 mg had no significant effects on either the pharmacokinetics or the effects of glipizide, except that the absorption was delayed.[14]

(f) Tolbutamide

The pharmacokinetics of tolbutamide 250 mg daily for 4 days were not significantly changed in 7 healthy subjects when **cimetidine** 800 mg daily was added for a further 4 days.[15] Other studies also found no pharmacokinetic interaction between tolbutamide and **cimetidine**,[16,17] or between tolbutamide and **ranitidine**,[17] and the hypoglycaemic activity of tolbutamide remained unaltered by **cimetidine**.[6]

In contrast, in another study in healthy subjects, the AUC of tolbutamide was found to be slightly increased by 20% and the elimination half-life decreased by 17% by **cimetidine** 1.2 g daily, but plasma glucose levels were not significantly changed. **Ranitidine** 300 mg had no effect.[18] A later study found effectively the same results.[19]

(g) Unnamed sulphonylureas

A report briefly describes hypoglycaemia in 2 patients on unnamed sulphonylureas given **cimetidine**.[20]

D. Other oral antidiabetics

(a) Pioglitazone

A study in healthy subjects found that when pioglitazone 45 mg daily was given with **ranitidine** 150 mg twice daily the pharmacokinetics of both drugs were not significantly affected.[21]

(b) Repaglinide

An open label crossover trial in 14 healthy subjects found that **cimetidine** 400 mg twice daily had no effect on the pharmacokinetics of repaglinide 2 mg three times daily.[22]

(c) Rosiglitazone

A crossover study in 12 healthy subjects found that pre-treatment with **ranitidine** 150 mg twice daily for 4 days had no effect on the pharmacokinetics of either a single 4-mg oral dose or a single 2-mg intravenous dose of rosiglitazone.[23]

Mechanism

Where an interaction occurs[18] it may be because the cimetidine inhibits the metabolism of the sulphonylurea by the liver, thereby increasing its effects. Cimetidine appears to inhibit the excretion of metformin by the kidneys,[3] and this may have contributed to the case of metformin-associated lactic acidosis described.[4]

Importance and management

The many studies cited here show that cimetidine generally causes no important changes in the pharmacokinetics or pharmacodynamics of the sulphonylureas (chlorpropamide, glimepiride and tolbutamide). Similarly, ranitidine did not interact with glimepiride or tolbutamide. Only a few isolated cases of hypoglycaemia have been reported with ranitidine or cimetidine and sulphonylureas (glibenclamide, gliclazide and unnamed), and only one research group has shown a possible increase in blood glucose lowering effect of glipizide with cimetidine and ranitidine.

It has been suggested that the dosage of metformin may need to be reduced if cimetidine is used, bearing in mind the possibility of lactic acidosis if levels become too high,[3] and there is one case where cimetidine may have contributed to lactic acidosis.

The only other possible interaction of significance appears to be that between miglitol and ranitidine, although the clinical relevance of this has not been assessed.

1. Precose (Acarbose). Bayer Pharmaceuticals Corporation. US Prescribing information, November 2004.
2. Glyset (Miglitol). Pharmacia & Upjohn Company. US Prescribing information, October 2004.
3. Somogyi A, Stockley C, Keal J, Rolan P, Bochner F. Reduction of metformin renal tubular secretion by cimetidine in man. *Br J Clin Pharmacol* (1987) 23, 545–51.
4. Dawson D, Conlon C. Case study: metformin-associated lactic acidosis. Could orlistat be relevant? *Diabetes Care* (2003) 26, 2471–2.
5. Shah GF, Ghandi TP, Patel PR, Patel MR, Gilbert RN, Shridhar PA. Tolbutamide and chlorpropamide kinetics in the presence of cimetidine in human volunteers. *Indian Drugs* (1985) 22, 455–8.
6. Shah GF, Ghandi TP, Patel PR, Patel MR, Gilbert RN, Shridhar PA. The effect of cimetidine on the hypoglycaemic activity of four commonly used sulphonylurea drugs. *Indian Drugs* (1985) 22, 570–2.
7. Kubacka RT, Antal EJ, Juhl RP. The paradoxical effect of cimetidine and ranitidine on glibenclamide pharmacokinetics and pharmacodynamics. *Br J Clin Pharmacol* (1987) 23, 743–51.
8. Lee K, Mize R, Lowenstein SR. Glyburide-induced hypoglycemia and ranitidine. *Ann Intern Med* (1987) 107, 261–2.
9. Archambeaud-Mouveroux F, Nouaille Y, Nadalon S, Treves R, Merle L. Interaction between gliclazide and cimetidine. *Eur J Clin Pharmacol* (1987) 31, 631.
10. Schaaf LJ, Welshman IR, Viveash DM, Carel BJ. The effects of cimetidine and ranitidine on glimepiride pharmacokinetics and pharmacodynamics in normal subjects. *Pharm Res* (1994) 11 (10 Suppl), S-360.
11. Feely J, Peden N. Enhanced sulphonylurea-induced hypoglycaemia with cimetidine. *Br J Clin Pharmacol* (1983) 15, 607P.
12. Feeley J, Collins WCJ, Cullen M, El Debani AH, MacWalter RS, Peden NR, Stevenson IH. Potentiation of the hypoglycaemic response to glipizide in diabetic patients by histamine H_2–receptor antagonists. *Br J Clin Pharmacol* (1993) 35, 321–3.
13. MacWalter RS, El Debani AH, Feeley J, Stevenson IH. Potentiation by ranitidine of the hypoglycaemic response to glipizide in diabetic patients. *Br J Clin Pharmacol* (1985) 19, 121P–122P.
14. Stevenson IH, El Debani AH, MacWalter RS. Glipizide pharmacokinetics and effect in diabetic patients given ranitidine. *Acta Pharmacol Toxicol (Copenh)* (1986) 59 (Suppl 4), 97.
15. Stockley C, Keal J, Rolan P, Bochner F, Somogyi A. Lack of inhibition of tolbutamide hydroxylation by cimetidine in man. *Eur J Clin Pharmacol* (1986) 31, 235–7.
16. Dey NG, Castleden CM, Ward J, Cornhill J, McBurney A. The effect of cimetidine on tolbutamide kinetics. *Br J Clin Pharmacol* (1983) 16, 438–440.
17. Adebayo GI, Coker HAB. Lack of efficacy of cimetidine and ranitidine as inhibitors of tolbutamide metabolism. *Eur J Clin Pharmacol* (1988) 34, 653–6.
18. Cate EW, Rogers JF, Powell JR. Inhibition of tolbutamide elimination by cimetidine but not ranitidine. *J Clin Pharmacol* (1986) 26, 372–7.
19. Toon S, Holt BL, Mullins FGP, Khan A. Effects of cimetidine, ranitidine and omeprazole on tolbutamide pharmacokinetics. *J Pharm Pharmacol* (1995) 47, 85–88.
20. Girardin E, Vial T, Pham E, Evreux J-C. Hypoglycémies induites par les sulfamides hypoglycémiants. *Ann Med Interne (Paris)* (1992) 143, 11–17.
21. Glazer NB, Sanes-Miller C. Pharmacokinetics of coadministration of pioglitazone with ranitidine. *Diabetes* (2001) 50 (suppl 2) A114.
22. Hatorp V, Thomsen MS. Drug interaction studies with repaglinide: repaglinide on digoxin or theophylline pharmacokinetics and cimetidine on repaglinide pharmacokinetics. *J Clin Pharmacol* (2000) 40, 184–92.
23. Miller AK, DiCicco RA, Freed MI. The effect of ranitidine on the pharmacokinetics of rosiglitazone in healthy adult male volunteers. *Clin Ther* (2002) 24, 1062–71.

Antidiabetics + Hormonal contraceptives or HRT

Some women may require small increases or decreases in their dosage of antidiabetic while taking oral contraceptives or HRT, but it is unusual for the control of diabetes to be seriously disturbed. Irrespective of diabetic control, HRT or oral contraceptives should be used with caution in patients with diabetes because of the increased risk of arterial disease. Pioglitazone, rosiglitazone and repaglinide do not appear to alter the pharmacokinetics of contraceptive steroids, and ethinylestradiol/levonorgestrel do not appear to have an important effect on the pharmacokinetics of repaglinide.

Clinical evidence

(a) HRT

1. Insulin. More than half of a group of 30 menopausal diabetics had abnormal glucose tolerance when given **noretynodrel** 5 mg with **mestranol** 75 micrograms, but the changes in their requirements of **insulin** or oral antidiabetic drug were rare and slight.[1] A 3-year, placebo-controlled, randomised study involving 875 postmenopausal women found that HRT (unopposed **conjugated oestrogens**, or **conjugated oestrogens** plus **medroxyprogesterone** or **progesterone**) had little, if any, harmful effect on carbohydrate metabolism.[2]

2. Pioglitazone. The pharmacokinetics of **ethinylestradiol** and **estrone** were not affected when *Premarin* (**conjugated oestrogens**) 0.625 mg and *Provera* (**medroxyprogesterone**) 5 mg was given for 28 days, with pioglitazone 45 mg daily for an additional 14 days.[3]

(b) Oral contraceptives

There are numerous reports of the effect of contraceptive steroids on glucose tolerance in non-diabetics. More recent reports from studies using newer, low-dose oral contraceptives, support the suggestion that changes in glucose metabolism are minimal.[4,5] Problems with glucose metabolism seem very unlikely when the dose of oestrogen is less than 50 micrograms.[6] The progestogen in the oral contraceptive may also be important.[6-9] Progestogens with androgenic properties, such as **norgestrel**, **levonorgestrel** and to a lesser extent **norethisterone (norethindrone)**, may affect carbohydrate metabolism. **Etynodiol (etynodrel)**, which has weak androgenic activity, was found to cause smaller reductions in glucose tolerance, and **noretynodrel** was found to have no effect.[6-8] Studies of healthy, non-diabetic women using oral contraceptives containing **ethinylestradiol** 20 to 40 micrograms with third generation progestogens (**gestodene**, **desogestrel** or **norgestimate**) found no effect on carbohydrate metabolism in women using monophasic oral contraceptives, but impaired glucose tolerance developed in 10% of the women taking triphasic oral contraceptives. It was considered that the clinical consequences of impaired glucose tolerance and reduced **insulin** sensitivity induced by oral contraceptives are probably confined to risk groups e.g. women with ovarian hyperandrogenism, obesity, previous gestational diabetes mellitus, perimenopausal women, or women with a family history of diabetes.[10]

A study in 11 **insulin**-dependent diabetics, free of vascular complications, taking low-dose oral contraceptives (**ethinylestradiol/gestodene** 30/75 micrograms) found that although the plasma levels of most haemostatic variables were comparable to those of non-diabetics using the same oral contraceptive preparation, the rate of fibrin formation was increased and the fibrinolytic response attenuated. This implies that women with diabetes can have a higher sensitivity to the thrombogenic effects of oral contraceptives.[10]

1. Insulin. In one study in 179 diabetic women, 34% needed an increase and 7% needed a decrease in their insulin dose when they were given an oral contraceptive.[11] There are also a few scattered reports of individual diabetics who experienced a marked disturbance of their diabetic control when given an oral contraceptive, some of which were low dose.[12-15]
However, in a study of 38 insulin-dependent diabetics it was found that progestogen-only and combined oral contraceptives had little effect on the control of diabetes,[16] and another report[17] about women taking *Orthonovin* (**norethisterone** with **mestranol**) stated that no insulin dose changes were necessary. Similarly, no change in glycaemic control was found in 22 women with well-regulated insulin-dependent diabetes mellitus who took a monophasic combination of **ethinylestradiol** and **gestodene** for 1 year.[10]

2. Pioglitazone. A randomised double-blind study in 35 healthy women given pioglitazone 45 mg once daily with either a combined oral contraceptive (**ethinylestradiol/norethisterone** 35 micrograms/1 mg) or placebo for 21 days found that pioglitazone does not affect systemic exposure to the oral contraceptive, as measured by AUC.[18] Similar results were reported in another study.[3]

3. Repaglinide. A three-period, cross-over, open-label study in healthy subjects found that a combined oral contraceptive (**ethinylestradiol/levonorgestrel** 30/150 micrograms) increased the maximum plasma level of repaglinide 2 mg three times daily by 17%, although the bioavailability of repaglinide was not altered.[19] Repaglinide did not significantly alter the bioavailability of **ethinylestradiol** or **levonorgestrel**.[19]

4. Rosiglitazone. Rosiglitazone 8 mg daily, given for the first two weeks of two cycles in 32 women taking an oral contraceptive (**ethinylestradiol/norethisterone** 35 micrograms/1 mg, *Ortho-Novum*), was found to have no effect on the pharmacokinetics of either steroid.[20]

Mechanism

The reasons for changes in glucose metabolism are not understood. Many mechanisms have been considered including changes in cortisol secretion, alterations in tissue glucose utilisation, production of excessive amounts of growth hormone, and alterations in liver function.[21]

Importance and management

Moderately well documented. Concurrent use need not be avoided, but some patients may need a small adjustment in their dosage of antidiabetic (increases or decreases). However, it seems likely that routine blood glucose monitoring will identify any problems. Serious disturbances of diabetic control seem extremely rare. Bear in mind that the lowest-strength combined oral contraceptive preparations (20 micrograms of oestrogen) are recommended for patients with risk factors for circulatory disease (such as diabetics), so the potential for interference with their diabetic control will be minimised if this recommendation is followed. The choice of progestogen may also be important, with levonorgestrel having the most detrimental effect.

Similarly, irrespective of control of diabetes, menopausal HRT should be used with caution in diabetics because of the increased risk of arterial disease. See also 'Antidiabetics + Tibolone', p.509.

1. Cochran B, Pote WWH. C-19 nor-steroid effects on plasma lipid and diabetic control of postmenopausal women. *Diabetes* (1963) 12, 366–7.
2. Fineberg SE. Glycaemic control and hormone replacement therapy. Implications of the Postmenopausal Estrogen/Progestogen Intervention (PEPI) study. *Drugs Aging* (2000) 17, 453–61.
3. Carey RA, Liu Y. Pioglitazone does not markedly alter oral contraceptive or hormone replacement therapy pharmacokinetics. *Diabetes* (2000) 49 (Suppl 1), A100.
4. Miccoli R, Orlandi MC, Fruzzetti F, Giampietro O, Melis G, Ricci C, Bertolotto A, Fioretti P, Navalesi R, Masoni A. Metabolic effects of three new low-dose pills: a six-month experience. *Contraception* (1989) 39, 643–52.
5. Troisi RJ, Cowie CC, Harris MI. Oral contraceptive use and glucose metabolism in a national sample of women in the United States. *Am J Obstet Gynecol* (2000) 183, 389–95.
6. Spellacy WN. Carbohydrate metabolism during treatment with estrogen, progestogen, and low-dose oral contraceptives. *Am J Obstet Gynecol* (1982) 142, 732–4.
7. Perlman JA, Russell-Briefel R, Ezzati T, Lieberknecht G. Oral glucose tolerance and the potency of contraceptive progestins. *J Chron Dis* (1985) 38, 857–64.
8. Wynn V. Effect of duration of low-dose oral contraceptive administration on carbohydrate metabolism. *Am J Obstet Gynecol* (1982) 142, 739–46.
9. Knopp RH, Broyles FE, Cheung M, Moore K, Marcovina S, Chandler WL. Comparison of the lipoprotein, carbohydrate, and hemostatic effects of phasic oral contraceptives containing desogestrel or levonorgestrel. *Contraception* (2001) 63, 1–11.
10. Petersen KR. Pharmacodynamic effects of oral contraceptive steroids on biochemical markers for arterial thrombosis. Studies in non-diabetic women and in women with insulin-dependent diabetes mellitus. *Dan Med Bull* (2002) 49, 43–60.
11. Zeller WJ, Brehm H, Schöffling K, Melzer H. Verträglichkeit von hormonalen Ovulationshemmern bei Diabetikerinnen. *Arzneimittelforschung* (1974) 24, 351–7.
12. Kopera H, Dukes MNG, Ijzerman GL. Critical evaluation of clinical data on *Lyndiol*. *Int J Fertil* (1964) 9, 69–74.
13. Peterson WF, Steel MW, Coyne RV. Analysis of the effect of ovulatory suppressants on glucose tolerance. *Am J Obstet Gynecol* (1966) 95, 484–8.
14. Reder JA, Tulgan H. Impairment of diabetic control by norethynodrel with mestranol. *N Y State J Med* (1967) 67, 1073–4.
15. Rennie NJ. Hyperglycaemic episodes in a young woman after taking levonorgestrel-containing oral contraceptives. *N Z Med J* (1994) 107, 440–1.
16. Rådberg T, Gustafson A, Skryten A, Karlsson K. Oral contraception in diabetic women. Diabetes control, serum and high density lipoprotein lipids during low-dose progestogen, combined oestrogen/progestogen and non-hormonal contraception. *Acta Endocrinol (Copenh)* (1981) 98, 246–51.
17. Tyler ET, Olson HJ, Gotlib M, Levin M, Behne D. Long term usage of norethindrone with mestranol preparations in the control of human fertility. *Clin Med* (1964) 71, 997–1024.
18. Karim A, Schwartz L, Perez A, Cao C. Lack of clinically significant drug interaction in the coadministration of pioglitazone with ethinyl estradiol and norethindrone. *Diabetes* (2003) 52 (Suppl 1) A123.
19. Hatorp V, Hansen KT, Thomsen MS. Influence of drugs interacting with CYP3A4 on the pharmacokinetics, pharmacodynamics, and safety of the prandial glucose regulator repaglinide. *J Clin Pharmacol* (2003) 43, 649–60.
20. Inglis AML, Miller AK, Culkin KT, Finnerty D, Patterson SD, Jorkasky DK, Freed MI. Lack of effect of rosiglitazone on the pharmacokinetics of oral contraceptives in healthy female volunteers. *J Clin Pharmacol* (2001) 41, 683–90.
21. Spellacy WN. A review of carbohydrate metabolism and the oral contraceptives. *Am J Obstet Gynecol* (1969) 104, 448–60.

Antidiabetics + Imatinib

An improvement in diabetic control with a reduction in dose of insulin or oral antidiabetics was seen in 6 of 7 diabetics given imatinib for chronic myelogenous leukaemia. A further patient with type 2 diabetes was able to stop all antidiabetic medication during treatment with imatinib.

Clinical evidence, mechanism, importance and management

Use of imatinib 400 or 600 mg daily for the treatment of chronic myelogenous leukaemia was associated with improved glycaemic control in 6 of 7 diabetic patients. This allowed a reduction in **insulin** dose in 2 patients and **oral antidiabetic** drug dosage in 4 patients.[1] A case report describes a 70-year-old woman with type 2 diabetes who needed a reduction in her **insulin** dose when she was given imatinib for chronic myeloid leukaemia. Later, while still taking imatinib, she was able to stop the **insulin** completely.[2]

It was thought that imatinib may have a direct effect on glycaemic control,[1,2] rather than an indirect effect via improvement in leukaemia.[1]

These preliminary findings suggest that diabetic therapy should be well monitored in those given imatinib. Further study is needed.

1. Breccia M, Muscaritoli M, Aversa Z, Mandelli F, Alimena G. Imatinib mesylate may improve fasting blood glucose in diabetic Ph+ chronic myelogenous leukemia patients responsive to treatment. *J Clin Oncol* (2004) 22, 4653–55.
2. Veneri D, Franchini M, Bonora E. Imatinib and regression of type 2 diabetes. *N Engl J Med* (2005) 352, 1049–50.

Antidiabetics + Isoniazid

Some reports suggest that isoniazid causes an increase in blood glucose levels in diabetics, whereas another suggests it causes a decrease.

Clinical evidence

A study in 6 diabetics taking **insulin** found that isoniazid 300 to 400 mg daily increased their fasting blood glucose levels by 40% (from an average of 255 to 357 mg%), and their glucose tolerance curves rose and returned to normal levels more slowly. After 6 days of treatment the average rise was only 20%. Two other patients needed an increased dosage of **insulin** while taking isoniazid 200 mg daily, but this was reduced again when the isoniazid was withdrawn.[1]

Another report describes glycosuria and the development of frank diabetes in 3 out of 50 patients given isoniazid 300 mg daily,[2] and hyperglycaemia has been seen in cases of isoniazid poisoning.[3]

In contrast, another study found that isoniazid had a hypoglycaemic effect in 6 out of 8 diabetics.[4] A 500-mg dose of isoniazid caused an 18% (range 5 to 34%) reduction in blood glucose levels after 4 hours; 3 g of **tolbutamide** caused a 28% (19 to 43%) reduction, and together they caused a 35% (17 to 57%) reduction. However, one patient had a 10% increase in blood glucose levels after taking isoniazid, a 41% decrease after **tolbutamide**, and a 30% decrease after taking both drugs. The diabetic-control of another patient was not affected by either drug.[4]

Mechanism

Not understood.

Importance and management

The major documentation for these reactions dates back to the 1950s, since when the literature has been virtually (and perhaps significantly) silent. The outcome of concurrent use is therefore somewhat uncertain. Nevertheless it would be prudent for diabetics given isoniazid to be monitored for changes in the control of the diabetes. Appropriate dosage adjustments of the antidiabetic should be made where necessary.

1. Luntz GRWN, Smith SG. Effect of isoniazid on carbohydrate metabolism in controls and diabetics. *BMJ* (1953) i, 296–9.
2. Dickson I. Glycosuria and diabetes mellitus following INAH therapy. *Med J Aust* (1962) i, 325–6.
3. Tovaryš A, Šiler Z. Diabetic syndrome and intoxication with INH. *Int Pharm Abstr* (1968) 5, 286.
4. Segarra FO, Sherman DS, Charif BS. Experiences with tolbutamide and chlorpropamide in tuberculous diabetic patients. *Ann N Y Acad Sci* (1959) 74, 656–61.

Antidiabetics + Karela (*Momordica charantia*)

The blood glucose-lowering effects of chlorpropamide and other antidiabetics can be increased by karela.

Clinical evidence

A report of a patient whose diabetes was poorly controlled on diet and **chlorpropamide**, but much better controlled when she ate curry containing karela, provides evidence that the blood glucose-lowering effects of karela and conventional oral antidiabetics can be additive.[1] Other small non-controlled studies have subsequently shown that karela produces a significant improvement in glucose tolerance in patients with type 2 diabetes, both when they are taking **chlorpropamide**,[2] **tolbutamide**,[2] **glibenclamide**,[2,3] **glymidine**[2] or **metformin**,[3] and when they are not taking antidiabetics.[4-6] In these studies, karela was given orally as a juice from the fruit,[2,4] dried powdered fruit,[5,6] fried fruits,[2] aqueous extract,[6] or solvent extract from the fruit.[3]

Hypoglycaemic coma and seizures occurred in two young non-diabetic children after they were given bitter melon (karela) tea.[7]

Mechanism

Karela (also known as bitter melon, bitter gourd, balsam pear, cundeamor) is the fruit of *Momordica charantia* which is indigenous to Asia and South America. The blood glucose-lowering effects of karela may be due to its content of polypeptide P, a blood glucose-lowering peptide,[8] also known as vegetable insulin (v-insulin).[9] This substance is effective when given subcutaneously,[9] but its oral activity is uncertain.[10] Other blood glucose-lowering compounds isolated from karela include charantin (sterol glucoside mixture in the fruit) and vicine a pyrimidine nucleoside found in the seeds). Karela fruit may have both insulin-like effects and stimulate insulin secretion.[10]

Importance and management

Karela is available in the UK and elsewhere, and is used to flavour foods such as curries, and also used as a herbal medicine for the treatment of diabetes mellitus. Its blood glucose-lowering activity is clearly established. Health professionals should therefore be aware that patients may possibly be using karela as well as more orthodox drugs to control their diabetes. Irregular consumption of karela as part of the diet could possibly contribute to unexplained fluctuations in diabetic control.

1. Aslam M, Stockley IH. Interaction between curry ingredient (karela) and drug (chlorpropamide). *Lancet* (1979) i, 607.
2. Leatherdale BA, Panesar KR, Singh G, Atkins TW, Bailey CJ, Bignell AHC. Improvement in glucose tolerance due to Momordica charantia (karela). *BMJ* (1981) 282, 1823–4.
3. Tongia A, Tongia SK, Dave M. Phytochemical determination and extraction of Momordica charantia fruit and its hypoglycemic potentiation of oral hypoglycemic drugs in diabetes mellitus (NIDDM). *Indian J Physiol Pharmacol* (2004) 48, 241–44.
4. Welihinda J, Karunanayake EH, Sheriff MHR, Jaysinghe KSA . Effect of *Momordica charantia* on the glucose tolerance in maturity onset diabetes. *J Ethnopharmacol* (1986) 17, 277–82.
5. Akhtar MS. Trial of Momordica Charantia Linn (Karela) powder in patients with maturity-onset diabetes. *J Pakistan Med Assoc* (1982) 32, 106–7.
6. Srivastava Y, Venkatakrishna-Bhatt H, Verma Y, Venkaiah K, Raval BH. Antidiabetic and adaptogenic properties of *Momordica charantia* extract: an experimental and clinical evaluation. *Phytother Res* (1993) 7, 285–9.
7. Hulin A, Wavelet M, Desbordes JM. Intoxication aiguë par *Momordica charantia* (sorrossi). A propos de deux cas. *Sem Hop Paris* (1988) 64, 2847–8.
8. Khanna P, Jain SC, Panagariya A, Dixit VP. Hypoglycemic activity of polypeptide-p from a plant source. *J Nat Prod* (1981) 44, 648–55.
9. Baldwa VS, Bhandari CM, Pangaria A, Goyal RK. Clinical trial in patients with diabetes mellitus of an insulin-like compound obtained from plant source. *Ups J Med Sci* (1977) 82, 39–41.
10. Raman A, Lau C. Anti-diabetic properties and phytochemistry of *Momordica charantia* (Cucurbitaceae). *Phytomedicine* (1996) 2, 349–62.

Antidiabetics + Ketotifen

The concurrent use of sulphonylureas or biguanides and ketotifen appears to be well tolerated, but a fall in the number of platelets has been seen in one study in patients taking biguanides with ketotifen.

Clinical evidence, mechanism, importance and management

A study in 30 hospitalised diabetics (10 diet controlled, 10 taking unnamed **sulphonylureas**, 10 taking unnamed **biguanides**) found that the concurrent use of ketotifen 4 mg daily for 14 days was generally well tolerated. However, those taking **biguanides** had a significant decrease in platelet counts and 3 had a marked fall on day 14 to slightly below 100×10^9/L, which returned to normal after a few days.[1] This finding underlies the precaution issued by the manufacturers of ketotifen,[2] that the combination should be avoided until this effect is explained. However, no other studies appear to have confirmed the fall in thrombocyte count so that its importance still remains uncertain.[3]

1. Doleček R. Ketotifen in the treatment of diabetics with various allergic conditions. *Pharmatherapeutica* (1981) 2, 568–74.
2. Zaditen (Ketotifen). Novartis Pharmaceuticals UK Ltd. UK Summary of product characteristics, November 2006.
3. Sandoz. Personal communication, 1991.

Antidiabetics + Lithium

An isolated report describes a diabetic patient receiving insulin who developed hyperglycaemia when his serum-lithium levels were high, but not when the lithium dose was reduced. Lithium can raise blood glucose levels and in some instances this has been associated with the development of diabetes mellitus, but the association is unclear and there is little or no evidence that its use normally causes significant changes in diabetic control.

Clinical evidence, mechanism, importance and management

It has been suggested that both lithium and affective disorders may lead to the development of diabetes mellitus or precipitate its appearance, and the incidence of diabetes in manic depressive patients is higher than in the general population; an overall prevalence of 10% has been reported, compared with 3% and 1.8% in other psychiatric patients and the general population, respectively, However, other factors such as weight gain, age, and other medications may also contribute.[1] A study in 10 psychiatric patients found that lithium carbonate for 2 weeks raised their blood glucose levels and impaired their glucose tolerance.[2] There are also a few case reports of hyperglycaemia, impaired glucose tolerance and diabetes mellitus in patients taking lithium.[3-5] However, a long-term investigation over a period of 6 years, involving 460 patients, found that the mean blood glucose levels remained the same before and after treatment with lithium. One patient did develop diabetic ketoacidosis after 4 years of uneventful lithium treatment, but the authors concluded that long-term lithium treatment did not increase the risk of developing diabetes mellitus.[6]

One patient with mania and diabetes developed hyperglycaemia, in the presence of a constant **insulin** dose, when his serum lithium levels were high (approximately 1.4 mmol/L), but reducing the lithium level to 1.1 mmol/L led to a lowering of the fasting blood glucose.[7] However, a study in 6 patients, with type 2 diabetes controlled by diet alone, found that lithium, taken for one week did not alter the metabolic response to a standard 50 g carbohydrate breakfast.[8]

Although there is only the one report of disturbed diabetic control in a diabetic patient taking lithium, it would seem prudent to bear this interaction in mind if lithium is added to the treatment being received by diabetic patients.

1. Russell JD, Johnson GFS. Affective disorders, diabetes mellitus and lithium. *Aust N Z J Psychiatry* (1981) 15, 349–53.

2. Shopsin B, Stern S, Gershon S. Altered carbohydrate metabolism during treatment with lithium carbonate. *Arch Gen Psychiatry* (1972) 26, 566–71.
3. Craig J, Abu-Saleh M, Smith B, Evans I. Diabetes mellitus in patients on lithium. *Lancet* (1977) ii, 1028.
4. Johnstone BB. Diabetes mellitus in patients on lithium. *Lancet* (1977) ii, 935.
5. Martinez-Maldonado M, Terrell J. Lithium carbonate-induced nephrogenic diabetes insipidus and glucose intolerance. *Arch Intern Med* (1973) 132, 881–4.
6. Vestergaard P, Schou M. Does long-term lithium treatment induce diabetes mellitus? *Neuropsychobiology* (1987) 17, 130–2.
7. Waziri R, Nelson J. Lithium in diabetes mellitus: a paradoxical response. *J Clin Psychiatry* (1978) 39, 623–5.
8. Jones GR, Lazarus JH, Davies CJ, Greenwood RH. The effect of short term lithium carbonate in type II diabetes mellitus. *Horm Metab Res* (1983) 15, 422–4.

Antidiabetics + Macrolides

An isolated report describes severe liver damage with prolonged cholestasis in a patient taking chlorpropamide and erythromycin. Isolated cases of hypoglycaemia have been described in patients taking glibenclamide (glyburide) or glipizide with clarithromycin or erythromycin. A study in healthy subjects found that hypoglycaemia may occur if tolbutamide and clarithromycin are given concurrently and another pharmacokinetic study suggests that clarithromycin may enhance the effects of repaglinide.

Clinical evidence, mechanism, importance and management

(a) Effects on the liver

A man with type 2 diabetes taking **chlorpropamide** was given **erythromycin ethylsuccinate** 1 g daily for 3 weeks for a respiratory infection. Two weeks later he complained of increasing fatigue and fever. A short episode of pruriginous skin rash was followed by the appearance of dark urine, jaundice and hepatomegaly. The picture over the next 2 years was that of profound cholestasis, complicated by steatorrhoea and marked hyperlipidaemia with disappearance of interlobular bile ducts. He died of ischaemic cardiomyopathy.[1] The reasons for this serious reaction are not understood, but the authors point out that liver damage occurs in a very small number of patients given sulphonylureas, such as **chlorpropamide**, and also with **erythromycin**. They suggest that there may have been an interaction between the two drugs. This case is also complicated by the prior long-term use of phenformin, which is known to be hepatotoxic.[1] No general conclusions can be drawn from this unusual case.

(b) Hypoglycaemia

1. Repaglinide. **Clarithromycin** 250 mg twice daily given to healthy subjects increased the AUC and maximum plasma concentrations of a single 250-microgram dose of repaglinide, given on day 5, by 40 and 67%, respectively. **Clarithromycin** may inhibit the metabolism of repaglinide by inhibition of cytochrome P450 isoenzyme CYP3A4. There was a similar corresponding rise in circulating insulin levels.[2] The effect of concurrent administration of these drugs should therefore be monitored. Other macrolides that inhibit CYP3A4 (such as erythromycin) would be expected to interact in a similar manner.

2. Sulphonylureas. Two isolated cases of severe hypoglycaemia occurred in elderly, type 2 diabetic patients, with renal impairment, given **glibenclamide** or **glipizide** and **clarithromycin**.[3] A further case of hypoglycaemia occurred when an elderly diabetic patient, with normal renal function, taking **glibenclamide** 5 mg daily also took **clarithromycin** 1 g daily as part of an *Helicobacter pylori* eradication regimen.[4] It was thought that the **clarithromycin** might have displaced **glibenclamide** and **glipizide** from protein binding sites.[3,4]

A case of hypoglycaemia was reported in a patient taking **glibenclamide** and **erythromycin**.[5] However, an earlier single-dose study in 12 **patients** with type 2 diabetes found that **erythromycin** had little effect on **glibenclamide** pharmacokinetics or on its blood glucose-lowering effects.[6] A placebo-controlled study involving 34 patients with type 2 diabetes (most of whom were treated with **glibenclamide** or **glipizide**) found that oral **erythromycin** 400 mg three times daily for a week reduced fructosamine and fasting blood glucose concentrations and increased insulin secretion. Glycaemic control was also improved in a similar study using oral **erythromycin** 200 mg three times daily for 4 weeks.[7] Further studies have shown that **erythromycin** increases gastric motility, which results in better control of blood glucose in patients with type 2 diabetes.[8,9]

A single-dose study in 9 healthy subjects found that **clarithromycin** 250 mg increased the rate of absorption of **tolbutamide** 500 mg by about 20% and increased its bioavailability by 26%. Hypoglycaemia, reported as uneasiness and giddiness, occurred on taking the combination.[10] The general importance of these cases is uncertain, but some caution may be warranted with concurrent use,[3] and the dose of the sulphonylurea may need to be reduced.

1. Geubel AP, Nakad A, Rahier J, Dive C. Prolonged cholestasis and disappearance of interlobular bile ducts following chlorpropamide and erythromycin ethylsuccinate. Case of drug interaction? *Liver* (1988) 8, 350–3.
2. Niemi M, Neuvonen PJ, Kivistö KT. The cytochrome P4503A4 inhibitor clarithromycin increases the plasma concentrations and effects of repaglinide. *Clin Pharmacol Ther* (2001) 70, 58–65.
3. Bussing R, Gende A. Severe hypoglycemia from clarithromycin-sulfonylurea drug interaction. *Diabetes Care* (2002) 25, 1659–60.
4. Leiba A, Leibowitz A, Grossman E. An unusual case of hypoglycemia in a diabetic patient. *Ann Emerg Med* (2004) 44, 427–8.
5. Girardin E, Vial T, Pham E, Evreux J-C. Hypoglycémies induites par les sulfamides hypoglycémiants. *Ann Med Interne (Paris)* (1992) 143, 11–17.
6. Fleishaker JC, Phillips JP. Evaluation of a potential interaction between erythromycin and glyburide in diabetic volunteers. *J Clin Pharmacol* (1991) 31, 259–62.
7. Ueno N, Inui A, Asakawa A, Takao F, Tani S, Komatsu Y, Itoh Z, Kasuga M. Erythromycin improves glycaemic control in patients with type II diabetes mellitus. *Diabetologia* (2000) 43, 411–15.
8. Chang C-T, Shiau Y-C, Lin C-C, Li T-C, Lee C-C, Kao C-H. Improvement of esophageal and gastric motility after 2-week treatment of oral erythromycin in patients with non-insulin-dependent diabetes mellitus. *J Diabetes Complications* (2003) 17, 141–4.
9. Gonlachanvit S, Hsu C-W, Boden GH, Knight LC, Maurer AH, Fisher RS, Parkman HP. Effect of altering gastric emptying on postprandial plasma glucose concentrations following a physiologic meal in type-II diabetic patients. *Dig Dis Sci* (2003) 48, 488–97.
10. Jayasagar G, Dixit AA, Kirshan V, Rao YM. Effect of clarithromycin on the pharmacokinetics of tolbutamide. *Drug Metabol Drug Interact* (2000) 16, 207–15.

Antidiabetics + MAOIs or RIMAs

The blood glucose-lowering effects of insulin and the oral antidiabetics can be increased by MAOIs. This may improve the control of blood glucose levels in most diabetics, but in a few it may cause undesirable hypoglycaemia. Moclobemide appears not to interact.

Clinical evidence

(a) Moclobemide

A study in healthy subjects given **glibenclamide** 2.5 mg daily found that moclobemide 200 mg three times daily for a week had no effect on glucose or insulin concentrations after oral glucose tolerance tests.[1] In clinical trials, 8 diabetics taking **glibenclamide (glyburide)**, **gliclazide**, **metformin** or **chlorpropamide** received moclobemide, and there was no effect on blood glucose levels or any other evidence of an interaction.[1]

(b) Non-selective irreversible MAOIs

A diabetic patient receiving **insulin** experienced postural syncope and hypoglycaemia, which required a reduction in **insulin** dose, when **mebanazine** was also taken.[2] Other reports in diabetics indicate that **mebanazine** increases the blood glucose-lowering effects of **insulin**, **tolbutamide** and **chlorpropamide,** and improves diabetic control.[3-6]

Mechanism

Not fully understood. Mebanazine,[4] iproniazid,[7] isocarboxazid,[8] phenelzine,[4] and tranylcypromine[9] have all been shown to reduce blood glucose levels in the absence of conventional antidiabetics, possibly due to some direct action on the pancreas, which causes the release of insulin.[9] It would seem that this can be additive with the effects of the conventional hypoglycaemics.

Importance and management

The interaction of the non-selective MAOIs is an established interaction of only moderate clinical importance. It can benefit the control of diabetes in many patients, but some individuals may need a reduction in the dose of their antidiabetic to avoid excessive hypoglycaemia. The effects of concurrent use should be monitored. This interaction would seem possible with any antidiabetic/MAOI combination, but this requires confirmation.

No clinically important interaction seems to occur between antidiabetics and moclobemide.

1. Amrein R, Güntert TW, Dingemanse J, Lorscheid T, Stabl M, Schmid-Burgk W. Interactions of moclobemide with concomitantly administered medication: evidence from pharmacological and clinical studies. *Psychopharmacology (Berl)* (1992) 106, S24–S31.
2. Cooper AJ, Keddie KMG. Hypotensive collapse and hypoglycaemia after mebanazine-a monoamine oxidase inhibitor. *Lancet* (1964) i, 1133–5.
3. Wickström L, Pettersson K. Treatment of diabetics with monoamine-oxidase inhibitors. *Lancet* (1964) ii, 995–7.
4. Adnitt PI. Hypoglycemic action of monoamineoxidase inhibitors (MAOI's). *Diabetes* (1968) 17, 628–33.

5. Cooper AJ. The action of mebanazine, a mono amine oxidase inhibitor antidepressant drug in diabetes-part II. *Int J Neuropsychiatry* (1966) 2, 342–5.
6. Adnitt PI, Oleesky S, Schnieden H. The hypoglycaemic action of monoamineoxidase inhibitors (MAOI's). *Diabetologia* (1968) 4, 379.
7. Weiss J, Weiss S, Weiss B. Effects of iproniazid and similar compounds on the gastrointestinal tract. *Ann N Y Acad Sci* (1959) 80, 854–9.
8. van Praag HM, Leijnse B. The influence of some antidepressives of the hydrazine type on the glucose metabolism in depressed patients. *Clin Chim Acta* (1963) 8, 466–75.
9. Bressler R, Vargas-Cordon M, Lebovitz HE. Tranylcypromine: a potent insulin secretagogue and hypoglycemic agent. *Diabetes* (1968) 17, 617–24.

Antidiabetics + Nicotinic acid (Niacin)

Nicotinic acid causes a deterioration in glucose tolerance, which may be dose-related, and can result in the need for an adjustment in antidiabetic medication. Nevertheless, its benefits on lipids may outweigh its effects on glucose tolerance in some diabetics. Concurrent use should be closely monitored.

Clinical evidence

It is well recognised that nicotinic acid can cause deterioration in blood glucose tolerance. For example, in a small randomised crossover study, immediate-release nicotinic acid 1.5 g three times daily caused a 16% increase in mean plasma glucose and a 21% increase in glycosylated haemoglobin levels in 13 patients with type 2 diabetes.[1] In a retrospective study of patients taking controlled-release nicotinic acid (average dose approximately 1.5 g daily), nicotinic acid was discontinued in 106 out of 160 patients who were diabetics; of these, 43 patients (about 40%) had the nicotinic acid discontinued because of poor glycaemic control. Furthermore, 14 patients required the addition of oral antidiabetic drugs to control their diabetes.[2]

In contrast, in another placebo-controlled study including 125 patients with diabetes, immediate-release nicotinic acid 3 g daily (or maximum tolerated dose) only modestly increased plasma glucose levels in patients with diabetes. Moreover, there were no significant differences in antidiabetic medication in diabetics taking nicotinic acid versus placebo, although insulin use was increased by 13% in the nicotinic acid group, when compared with 4% in the placebo group.[3] In a placebo-controlled study in patients with type 2 diabetes taking controlled-release nicotinic acid 1 g or 1.5 g daily, glycosylated haemoglobin marginally increased by 0.29% in the group receiving 1.5 g daily. There was an initial rise in fasting blood glucose between weeks 4 and 8, but this had returned to baseline by week 16. This was probably because some adjustment was made in antidiabetic therapy; 29% of patients taking nicotinic acid 1.5 g required an increase in antidiabetic therapy compared with 16% taking placebo (difference not significant). Only one patient (2%) taking nicotinic acid 1 g and 3 patients (6%) taking nicotinic acid 1.5 g discontinued treatment because of inadequate glucose control.[4] However, it has been noted that patients enrolled in both these studies had good glycaemic control, and that the findings may not be applicable to those with poor glycaemic control.[5]

Mechanism

Nicotinic acid reduces glucose tolerance, possibly by causing or aggravating insulin resistance.

Importance and management

It is well known that nicotinic acid can cause deterioration in glycaemic control in patients with diabetes, but the incidence and clinical relevance of this is more controversial. The beneficial lipid-modifying effects of nicotinic acid directly improve the main lipid disorders observed in diabetes, which are considered an important contributing factor to the high incidence of cardiovascular disease seen in diabetics. The question then is, do the lipid-regulating benefits of nicotinic acid outweigh its adverse effects on glucose homoeostasis? Some consider that they do especially if low doses of nicotinic acid (2 g or less) are used, and recommend the use of nicotinic acid in diabetics in some situations.[6,7] Whenever nicotinic acid is used, diabetic control should be closely monitored, recognising that adjustment of antidiabetics may be needed.

1. Garg A, Grundy SM. Nicotinic acid as therapy for dyslipidemia in non-insulin-dependent diabetes mellitus. *JAMA* (1990) 264, 723–6.
2. Gray DR, Morgan T, Chretien SD, Kashyap ML. Efficacy and safety of controlled-release niacin in dyslipoproteinemic veterans. *Ann Intern Med* (1994) 121, 252–8.
3. Elam MB, Hunninghake DB, Davis KB, Garg R, Johnson C, Egan D, Kostis JB, Sheps DS, Brinton EA. Effect of niacin on lipid and lipoprotein levels and glycemic control in patients with diabetes and peripheral arterial disease. The ADMIT study: a randomized trial. *JAMA* (2000) 284, 1263–70.
4. Grundy SM, Vega GL, McGovern ME, Tulloch BR, Kendall DM, Fitz-Patrick D, Ganda OP, Rosenson RS, Buse JB, Robertson DD, Sheehan JP; Diabetes Multicenter Research Group. Efficacy, safety, and tolerability of once-daily niacin for the treatment of dyslipidemia associated with type 2 diabetes: results of the assessment of diabetes control and evaluation of the efficacy of Niaspan trial. *Arch Intern Med* (2002) 162, 1568–76.
5. Mikhail N. The use of niacin in diabetes mellitus. *Arch Intern Med* (2003) 163, 369–70.
6. Shepherd J, Betteridge J, Van Gaal L; European Consensus Panel. Nicotinic acid in the management of dyslipidaemia associated with diabetes and metabolic syndrome; a position paper developed by a European Consensus Panel. *Curr Med Res Opin* (2005) 21, 665–82.
7. American Diabetes Association. Dyslipidemia management in adults with diabetes. *Diabetes Care* (2004) 27 (Suppl 1), S68–S71.

Antidiabetics + NSAIDs

No adverse interaction normally occurs between most NSAIDs and antidiabetics. However, there are isolated cases of hypoglycaemia in patients given fenclofenac with chlorpropamide and metformin, ibuprofen with glibenclamide, indometacin with chlorpropamide, and naproxen with glibenclamide and metformin. Rofecoxib may have been a precipitating factor in a case of acute renal failure and metformin-associated lactic acidosis. The risk of fluid retention with pioglitazone or rosiglitazone is increased by the NSAIDs.

Consider also 'azapropazone, phenylbutazone, and oxyphenbutazone', (p.498) and the 'salicylates', (p.502) for related drugs that do have adverse interactions with antidiabetics.

Clinical evidence

A. Metformin

A 58-year-old woman with longstanding type 2 diabetes taking metformin 500 mg twice daily developed serious acute renal failure and lactic acidosis one month after starting **rofecoxib**. She made a full recovery. **Rofecoxib** could have precipitated acute renal failure, which would lead to the accumulation of metformin, and metformin-associated lactic acidosis.[1] For a case of hypoglycaemia attributed to ramipril and **naproxen**-induced renal failure in a patient taking metformin and glibenclamide, see Glibenclamide, below.

B. Nateglinide

In a randomised crossover study, 18 healthy subjects were given modified-release **diclofenac** 75 mg on the same day as two 120-mg doses of nateglinide, given 4 hours apart. The pharmacokinetics of both drugs were unaltered by concurrent use.[2]

C. Pioglitazone or Rosiglitazone

The manufacturers say that pioglitazone and rosiglitazone can cause fluid retention, which may exacerbate or precipitate heart failure, particularly in those with limited cardiac reserve.[3,4] Because NSAIDs can also cause fluid retention, the manufacturers issue a warning that concurrent use may possibly increase the risk of oedema.[4]

D. Sulphonylureas

(a) Chlorpropamide

Ibuprofen 1.2 g daily for 4 weeks had no significant effect on the blood glucose levels of ten type 2 diabetic patients taking chlorpropamide 62.5 to 375 mg daily.[5]

A woman whose type 2 diabetes was well controlled with chlorpropamide 500 mg and metformin 1.7 g daily, developed hypoglycaemia within 2 days of exchanging **flurbiprofen** 150 mg daily and **indometacin** 150 mg daily for **fenclofenac** 1.2 g daily. The antidiabetic drugs were withdrawn the next day, but later in the evening she went into a hypoglycaemic coma. The reason for this is not understood, but it was attributed to a protein binding interaction between chlorpropamide and **fenclofenac**.[6] Conversely, another isolated report briefly describes hyperglycaemia with chlorpropamide possibly due to **indometacin**.[7]

(b) Glibenclamide

1. Acemetacin. No changes in the control of diabetes were seen in 20 patients with type 2 diabetes taking glibenclamide when they were given acemetacin 60 mg three times daily.[8]

2. Bromfenac. The blood glucose levels of 12 diabetics taking glibenclamide 10 mg daily were unchanged by bromfenac 50 mg three times daily for 3 days, and the pharmacokinetics of glibenclamide were also unaltered.[9]

3. Diclofenac. The blood glucose levels of 12 diabetics with rheumatic diseases taking glibenclamide were unchanged by diclofenac 150 mg daily for 4 days.[10]

4. Diflunisal. An isolated case of hypoglycaemia has been reported in a patient taking glibenclamide with diflunisal.[11]

5. Etodolac. Etodolac does not appear to affect the pharmacokinetics of glibenclamide.[12]

6. Ibuprofen. A study in 16 healthy subjects found that ibuprofen produced no significant changes in the pharmacokinetics of glibenclamide. However, ibuprofen with glibenclamide caused a greater blood glucose-lowering effect than glibenclamide alone, but the clinical significance of this was uncertain.[13] A 72-year-old man with longstanding type 2 diabetes, well-controlled with glibenclamide 2.5 mg daily took a single 150-mg dose of ibuprofen, and 30 minutes later experienced severe nausea, sweating and palpitations, which were immediately relieved by taking sugar. The symptoms occurred again the next morning after a second dose of ibuprofen and after a further dose in the afternoon he became unconscious and was given intravenous glucose. Ibuprofen was withdrawn and there were no further episodes of hypoglycaemia. It was also noted that hypoglycaemia had not occurred when he had previously taken **aspirin**, **paracetamol** or **diclofenac**.[14]

7. Lornoxicam. Lornoxicam 4 mg twice daily for 6 days had no effect on the pharmacokinetics of a single 5-mg dose of glibenclamide in 15 healthy subjects. The pharmacokinetics of lornoxicam also remained unchanged. However, concurrent use significantly increased plasma insulin levels (AUC 47%) and lowered serum glucose levels (8%), but this is probably not clinically important.[15]

8. Naproxen. A case of severe hypoglycaemia in a diabetic patient was attributed to the accumulation of glibenclamide and **metformin** due to deterioration in renal function caused by the concurrent use of ramipril and naproxen.[16]

9. Nimesulide. Although a preliminary report suggested that nimesulide slightly increased the effects of glibenclamide,[17] a later study using various [unnamed] **sulphonylureas** failed to find that it affected fasting blood glucose levels or the glucose tolerance of diabetic patients.[17]

10. Parecoxib. Valdecoxib, the active metabolite of parecoxib, does not appear to affect either the pharmacokinetics of glibenclamide or its effects on insulin or blood glucose levels.[18]

11. Piroxicam. Healthy subjects and type 2 diabetics had an increased hypoglycaemic response to glibenclamide (blood glucose levels down by 13 to 15%) when they were given piroxicam 10 mg.[19]

12. Tenoxicam. Tenoxicam 20 mg daily was found not to affect the glycoregulation of 8 healthy subjects given glibenclamide 2.5 mg daily.[20]

13. Tolmetin. No changes were seen in the blood glucose levels of 40 diabetics taking glibenclamide when they were given either tolmetin 1.2 g or placebo daily for 5 days.[21]

(c) Glibornuride

A study in healthy subjects found that **tenoxicam** 20 mg daily did not affect the pharmacokinetics of glibornuride or its effect on plasma insulin and blood glucose levels.[22]

(d) Glipizide

In a study in 6 healthy subjects, **indobufen** 200 mg twice daily for 5 days caused a 25% rise in the AUC of a single 5-mg dose of glipizide and a non-significant reduction in their blood glucose levels.[23] No important changes in blood glucose levels occurred in 24 type 2 diabetic patients taking tolbutamide or glipizide when they took **indoprofen** 600 mg daily for 5 days.[24] A study found that although **indoprofen** (200 mg on day 1, then 600 mg daily on days 3 to 8) lowered the plasma levels of a single 5-mg dose of glipizide, the blood glucose levels remained unaffected.[25]

(e) Tolbutamide

A report briefly states that no changes in blood tolbutamide or in fasting blood glucose levels were seen in diabetics given **diflunisal** 375 mg twice daily.[26] In a study in 12 type 2 diabetic patients, **sulindac** 400 mg daily did not affect the half-life, plasma levels, time-to-peak levels or AUC of tolbutamide. An unimportant reduction in fasting blood glucose levels was seen.[27] **Naproxen** 375 mg every 12 hours for 3 days had no effect on the pharmacokinetics or pharmacological effects of tolbutamide in ten type 2 diabetics.[28] The pharmacokinetics of a single 500-mg dose of tolbutamide were unaffected in 7 healthy subjects after they took **tenoxicam** 20 mg daily for 14 days, and blood glucose concentrations were not altered.[29] No important changes in blood glucose levels occurred in 24 type 2 diabetic patients taking tolbutamide or glipizide when they were given **indoprofen** 600 mg daily for 5 days.[24] In other patients taking tolbutamide it was found that **ibuprofen** lowered fasting blood glucose levels, but not below the lower limits of normal.[30]

Mechanism, importance and management

The reports briefly quoted here indicate that no adverse or clinically relevant interaction normally occurs between the oral antidiabetics and the NSAIDs cited. The general silence in the literature would seem to add confirmation. Caution is appropriate with pioglitazone or rosiglitazone and NSAIDs, and patients should be monitored for signs of heart failure. Note that the NSAIDs, including coxibs, can cause renal failure, which can precipitate metformin-associated lactic acidosis. In addition, a reduction in the renal clearance of antidiabetic drugs can result in hypoglycaemia. Adverse interactions can certainly occur between antidiabetics and azapropazone, phenylbutazone, oxyphenbutazone and the salicylates, see 'Antidiabetics + NSAIDs; Phenylbutazone and related drugs', p.498 and 'Antidiabetics + Salicylates', p.502.

1. Price G. Metformin lactic acidosis, acute renal failure and rofecoxib. *Br J Anaesth* (2003) 91, 909–10.
2. Anderson DM, Shelley S, Crick N, Buraglio M. A 3-way crossover study to evaluate the pharmacokinetic interaction between nateglinide and diclofenac in healthy volunteers. *Int J Clin Pharmacol Ther* (2002) 40, 457–64.
3. Actos (Pioglitazone hydrochloride). Takeda UK Ltd. UK Summary of product characteristics, January 2007.
4. Avandia (Rosiglitazone maleate). GlaxoSmithKline UK. UK Summary of product characteristics, May 2007.
5. Shah SJ, Bhandarkar SD, Satoskar RS. Drug interaction between chlorpropamide and non-steroidal anti-inflammatory drugs, ibuprofen and phenylbutazone. *Int J Clin Pharmacol Ther Toxicol* (1984) 22, 470–2.
6. Allen PA, Taylor RT. Fenclofenac and thyroid function tests. *BMJ* (1980) 281, 1642.
7. Beeley L, Beadle F, Elliott D. *Bulletin of the West Midlands Centre for Adverse Drug Reaction Reporting* (1985) 21, 19.
8. Haupt E, Hoppe FK, Rechziegler H, Zündorf P. Zur Frage der Interaktionen von nichtsteroidalen Antirheumatika mit oralen Antidiabetika: Acemetacin-Glibenclamid. *Z Rheumatol* (1987) 46, 170–3.
9. Boni JP, Cevallos WH, DeCleene S, Korth-Bradley JM. The influence of bromfenac on the pharmacokinetics and pharmacodynamic responses to glyburide in diabetic subjects. *Pharmacotherapy* (1997) 17, 783–90.
10. Chlud K. Untersuchungen zur Wechselwirkung von Diclofenac und Glibenclamid. *Z Rheumatol* (1976) 35, 377–82.
11. Girardin E, Vial T, Pham E, Evreux J-C. Hypoglycémies induites par les sulfamides hypoglycémiants. *Ann Med Interne (Paris)* (1992) 143, 11–17.
12. Zvaifler N. A review of the antiarthritic efficacy and safety of etodolac. *Clin Rheumatol* (1989) 8 (Suppl 1), 43–53.
13. Kubacka RT, Antal EJ, Juhl RP, Welshman IR. Effects of aspirin and ibuprofen on the pharmacokinetics and pharmacodynamics of glyburide in healthy subjects. *Ann Pharmacother* (1996) 30, 20–26.
14. Sone H, Takahashi A, Yamada N. Ibuprofen-related hypoglycemia in a patient receiving sulfonylurea. *Ann Intern Med* (2001) 134, 344.
15. Ravic M, Johnston A, Turner P. Clinical pharmacological studies of some possible interactions of lornoxicam with other drugs. *Postgrad Med J* (1990) 66 (Suppl 4), S30–S34.
16. Collin M, Mucklow JC. Drug interactions, renal impairment and hypoglycaemia in a patient with type II diabetes. *Br J Clin Pharmacol* (1999) 48, 134–7.
17. Perucca E. Drug interactions with nimesulide. *Drugs* (1993) 46 (Suppl 1), 79–82.
18. Dynastat injection (Parecoxib sodium). Pfizer Ltd. UK Summary of product characteristics, April 2007.
19. Diwan PV, Sastry MSP, Satyanarayana NV. Potentiation of hypoglycemic response of glibenclamide by piroxicam in rats and humans. *Indian J Exp Biol* (1992) 30, 317–9.
20. Hartmann D, Korn A, Komjati M, Heinz G, Haefelfinger P, Defoin R, Waldhäusl WK. Lack of effect of tenoxicam on dynamic responses to concurrent oral doses of glucose and glibenclamide. *Br J Clin Pharmacol* (1990) 30, 245–52.
21. Chlud K, Kaik B. Clinical studies of the interaction between tolmetin and glibenclamide. *Int J Clin Pharmacol Biopharm* (1977) 15, 409–10.
22. Stoeckel K, Trueb V, Dubach UC, Heintz RC, Ascalone V, Forgo I, Hennes U. Lack of effect of tenoxicam on glibornuride kinetics and response. *Br J Clin Pharmacol* (1985) 19, 249–54.
23. Elvander-Ståhl E, Melander A, Wåhlin-Boll E. Indobufen interacts with the sulphonylurea, glipizide, but not with the β-adrenergic receptor antagonists, propranolol and atenolol. *Br J Clin Pharmacol* (1984) 18, 773–8.
24. Pedrazzi F, Bommartini F, Freddo J, Emanueli A. A study of the possible interaction of indoprofen with hypoglycemic sulfonylureas in diabetic patients. *Eur J Rheumatol Inflamm* (1981) 4, 26–31.
25. Melander A, Wåhlin-Boll E. Interaction of glipizide and indoprofen. *Eur J Rheumatol Inflamm* (1981) 4, 22–5.
26. Tempero KF, Cirillo VJ, Steelman SL. Diflunisal: a review of the pharmacokinetic and pharmacodynamic properties, drug interactions, and special tolerability studies in humans. *Br J Clin Pharmacol* (1977) 4, 31S–36S.
27. Ryan JR, Jain AK, McMahon FG, Vargas R. On the question of an interaction between sulindac and tolbutamide in the control of diabetes. *Clin Pharmacol Ther* (1977) 21, 231–3.
28. Whiting B, Williams RL, Lorenzi M, Varady JC, Robins DS. Effect of naproxen on glucose metabolism and tolbutamide kinetics and dynamics in maturity onset diabetics. *Br J Clin Pharmacol* (1981) 11, 295–302.
29. Day RO, Geisslinger G, Paull P, Williams KM. The effect of tenoxicam on tolbutamide pharmacokinetics and glucose concentrations in healthy volunteers. *Int J Clin Pharmacol Ther* (1995) 33, 308–10.
30. Andersen LA. Ibuprofen and tolbutamide drug interaction study. *Br J Clin Pract* (1980) 34 (Suppl 6), 10–12.

Antidiabetics + NSAIDs; Phenylbutazone and related drugs

The blood glucose-lowering effects of acetohexamide, chlorpropamide, carbutamide, glymidine, glibenclamide (glyburide) and tolbutamide can be increased by phenylbutazone. Severe hypoglycaemia has occurred in a few patients. Similarly, azapropazone can increase the effects of tolbutamide and cause severe hypoglycaemia. Oxyphenbutazone may be expected to behave similarly. Metamizole (dipyrone) and mofebutazone did not interact with glibenclamide.

Clinical evidence

(a) Azapropazone

A woman whose diabetes was well controlled for 3 years with **tolbutamide** 500 mg twice daily, became confused and semi-comatose 4 days after starting to take azapropazone 900 mg daily. She complained of having felt agitated since starting the azapropazone, so it was withdrawn on suspicion of causing hypoglycaemia. Later that evening she became semicomatose and was found to have a plasma glucose level of 2 mmol/L.[1] A subsequent study in 3 healthy subjects found that azapropazone 900 mg daily increased the plasma half-life of **tolbutamide** 500 mg threefold (from 7.7 to 25.2 hours) and reduced its clearance accordingly.[1] Acute hypoglycaemia occurred in another patient taking **tolbutamide** 500 mg three times daily, 5.5 hours after a single 600-mg dose of azapropazone was taken.[2]

(b) Metamizole (Dipyrone)

One randomised, placebo-controlled, crossover study in 12 diabetic patients taking **glibenclamide,** suggested that metamizole 1 g daily for 2 days did not interact with **glibenclamide**; no relevant alteration in blood glucose levels was found.[3]

(c) Mofebutazone

Mofebutazone 900 mg daily has not been found to cause any clinically important changes in blood glucose levels in patients taking **glibenclamide**.[4]

(d) Oxyphenbutazone

Oxyphenbutazone has been found to alter[5] or raise **glymidine** levels[6] and **tolbutamide** levels.[7,8]

(e) Phenylbutazone

A man with type 2 diabetes taking **tolbutamide** experienced an acute hypoglycaemic episode 4 days after starting phenylbutazone 200 mg three times daily, although there was no change in his diet or in the dosage of **tolbutamide**. He was able to control the hypoglycaemia by eating a large bar of chocolate.[9]

There are numerous other case reports and studies of this interaction involving phenylbutazone with **acetohexamide**,[10] **carbutamide**,[11] **chlorpropamide**,[12-14] **glibenclamide (glyburide)**,[15] **glymidine**,[16] and **tolbutamide**,[13,17-23] some of which describe acute hypoglycaemic episodes.[10,12,13,18,20] Several of these interactions have been fatal.[13,23] There is a report suggesting that the interaction between **glibornuride** and phenylbutazone may not be clinically important.[24] In contrast to these reports, a single study describes a paradoxical *rise* in blood glucose levels in 3 African patients taking **tolbutamide** and phenylbutazone.[25] In addition to these reports there is some evidence that **tolbutamide** increases the metabolism of phenylbutazone by 42%,[22] but the extent to which this affects its therapeutic effects is uncertain.

Mechanism

Not fully resolved. Some evidence suggests that phenylbutazone can inhibit the renal excretion of glibenclamide (glyburide),[15] tolbutamide,[19] and the active metabolite of acetohexamide[10] so that they are retained in the body longer and their blood glucose-lowering effects are increased and prolonged. It has also been shown that phenylbutazone can inhibit the metabolism of the sulphonylureas[7,22] as well as causing their displacement from protein binding sites.[26] Azapropazone also possibly inhibits the metabolism of tolbutamide,[1] as well as maybe causing displacement from plasma protein binding sites.[2]

Importance and management

The interactions between the antidiabetics and phenylbutazone are well documented and potentially clinically important. Blood glucose levels may be lowered, but the number of reports of acute hypoglycaemic episodes seems to be small. Concurrent use should therefore be well monitored. A reduction in the dosage of the sulphonylurea may be necessary if excessive hypoglycaemia is to be avoided. Not all sulphonylureas have been shown to interact (glibornuride probably does not do so) but it would be prudent to assume that they all interact until there is good evidence to suggest otherwise. Oxyphenbutazone may be expected to interact like phenylbutazone (it is a metabolite of phenylbutazone) but, unexpectedly, possibly not mofebutazone although more study would be needed to confirm this.

The information regarding an interaction between azapropazone and the sulphonylureas seems to be limited to the cases and small study involving tolbutamide. Nevertheless, the manufacturers of azapropazone say that the concurrent use of sulphonylureas is not recommended.[27]

1. Andreasen PB, Simonsen K, Brocks K, Dimo B, Bouchelouche P. Hypoglycaemia induced by azapropazone-tolbutamide interaction. *Br J Clin Pharmacol* (1981) 12, 581–3.
2. Waller DG, Waller D. Hypoglycaemia due to azapropazone-tolbutamide interaction. *Br J Rheumatol* (1984) 23, 24–5.
3. Haupt E, Hoppe FU, Bamberg E. Zur frage der Wechselwirkungen von Analgetika und oralen Antidiabetika. Metamizol – Glibenclamid. *Med Welt* (1989) 40, 681–3.
4. Speders S. Mofebutazon — Prufung einer moglichen Interaktion mit Glibenclamid. *Fortschr Med* (1993) 111, 366–8.
5. Held H, Scheible G. Interaktion von Phenylbutazon und Oxyphenbutazon mit glymidine. *Arzneimittelforschung* (1981) 31, 1036–8.
6. Held H, Scheible G, von Olderhausen HF. Über Stoffwechsel und Interferenz von Arzneimitteln bei Gesunden und Leberkranken. *Tag Deut Ges Inn Med (Wiesbaden)* (1970) 76, 1153–7.
7. Pond SM, Birkett DJ, Wade DN. Mechanisms of inhibition of tolbutamide metabolism: Phenylbutazone, oxyphenbutazone, sulfaphenazole. *Clin Pharmacol Ther* (1977) 22, 573–9.
8. Kristensen M, Christensen LK. Drug induced changes of the blood glucose lowering effect of oral hypoglycemic agents. *Acta Diabetol Lat* (1969) 6 (Suppl 1), 116–36.
9. Mahfouz M, Abdel-Maguid R, El-Dakhakhny M. Potentiation of the hypoglycaemic action of tolbutamide by different drugs. *Arzneimittelforschung* (1970) 20, 120–2.
10. Field JB, Ohta M, Boyle C, Remer A. Potentiation of acetohexamide hypoglycemia by phenylbutazone. *N Engl J Med* (1967) 277, 889–94.
11. Kaindl F, Kretschy A, Puxkandl H, Wutte J. Zur steigerung des Wirkundseffektes peroraler Antidiabetika durch Pyrazolonderivate. *Wien Klin Wochenschr* (1961) 73, 79–80.
12. Dalgas M, Christiansen I, Kjerulf K. Fenylbutazoninduceret hypoglykaemitilfaelde hos klorpropamidbehandlet diabetiker. *Ugeskr Laeger* (1965) 127, 834–6.
13. Schulz E. Schwere hypoglykämische Reaktionen nach den Sulfonylharnstoffen Tolbutamid, Carbutamid und Chlorpropamid. *Arch Klin Med* (1968) 214, 135–62.
14. Shah SJ, Bhandarkar SD, Satoskar RS. Drug interaction between chlorpropamide and non-steroidal anti-inflammatory drugs, ibuprofen and phenylbutazone. *Int J Clin Pharmacol Ther Toxicol* (1984) 22, 470–2.
15. Schulz E, Koch K, Schmidt FH. Ursachen der Potenzierung der hypoglykämischen Wirkung von Sulfonylharnstoff-derivaten durch Medikamente. II. Pharmakokinetik und Metabolismus von Glibenclamid (HN 419) in Gegenwart von Phenylbutazon. *Eur J Clin Pharmacol* (1971) 4, 32–7.
16. Held H, Kaminski B, von Olderhausen HF. Die beeinflussung der Elimination von Glycodiazin durch Leber-und Nierenfunktionsstorugen und durch eine Behandlung mit Phenylbutazon, Phenprocumarol und Doxycyclin. *Diabetologia* (1970) 6, 386–91.
17. Gulbrandsen R. Økt tolbutamid-effekt ved hjelp av fenylbutazon? *Tidsskr Nor Laegeforen* (1959) 79, 1127–8.
18. Tannenbaum H, Anderson LG, Soeldner JS. Phenylbutazone-tolbutamide drug interaction. *N Engl J Med* (1974) 290, 344.
19. Ober K-F. Mechanism of interaction of tolbutamide and phenylbutazone in diabetic patients. *Eur J Clin Pharmacol* (1974) 7, 291–4.
20. Dent LA, Jue SG. Tolbutamide-phenylbutazone interaction. *Drug Intell Clin Pharm* (1976) 10, 711.
21. Christensen LK, Hansen JM, Kristensen M. Sulphaphenazole-induced hypoglycaemic attacks in tolbutamide-treated diabetics. *Lancet* (1963) ii, 1298–1301.
22. Szita M, Gachályi B, Tornyossy M, Káldor A. Interaction of phenylbutazone and tolbutamide in man. *Int J Clin Pharmacol Ther Toxicol* (1990) 18, 378–80.
23. Slade IH, Iosefa RN. Fatal hypoglycemic coma from the use of tolbutamide in elderly patients: report of two cases. *J Am Geriatr Soc* (1967) 15, 948–50.
24. Eckhardt W, Rudolph R, Sauer H, Schubert WR, Undeutsch D. Zur pharmackologischen Interferenz von Glibornurid mit Sulfaphenazol, Phenylbutazon und Phenprocoumon beim Menschen. *Arzneimittelforschung* (1972) 22, 2212–19.
25. Owusu SK, Ocran K. Paradoxical behaviour of phenylbutazone in African diabetics. *Lancet* (1972) i, 440–41.
26. Hellman B. Potentiating effects of drugs on the binding of glibenclamide to pancreatic beta cells. *Metabolism* (1974) 23, 839–46.
27. Rheumox (Azapropazone dihydrate). Goldshield Pharmaceuticals Ltd. UK Summary of product characteristics, February 2000.

Antidiabetics + Orlistat

Orlistat improved glycaemic control, which resulted in the need to reduce the dose of glibenclamide (glyburide) or glipizide in almost half the patients in one study. In other studies, orlistat also reduced the dose requirement for metformin and for insulin. Orlistat did not alter the pharmacokinetics of glibenclamide or metformin. Orlistat and cimetidine may have contributed to a case of metformin-associated lactic acidosis. The manufacturers recom-

mend avoiding the concurrent use of acarbose and orlistat because of the lack of interaction studies.

Clinical evidence

(a) Acarbose

The manufacturer of orlistat says that in the absence of pharmacokinetic studies its concurrent use with acarbose should be avoided.[1]

(b) Insulin

In a randomised, placebo-controlled, double-blind study in patients with type 2 diabetes receiving insulin with or without metformin or a sulphonylurea, orlistat 120 mg three times daily for one year combined with a reduced-calorie diet improved glycaemic control and allowed a greater reduction in insulin dose (mean reduction of 8.1 units daily versus 1.6 units daily for placebo). Hypoglycaemic episodes occurred in about 17% of orlistat recipients and about 10% of placebo recipients—three orlistat recipients and one placebo recipient required medical intervention due to hypoglycaemia.[2]

(c) Metformin

In a randomised study, 21 healthy subjects were given metformin 500 mg daily for 6 days, with or without orlistat 120 mg three times daily. Orlistat had no effect on the pharmacokinetics of metformin, and the combination was well-tolerated.[3] In a randomised, placebo-controlled, double-blind study in patients with type 2 diabetes taking metformin with or without a sulphonylurea (mainly glibenclamide (glyburide) or glipizide), orlistat 120 mg three times daily for one year improved glycaemic control and allowed a small reduction in the dose of metformin (mean daily reduction of 16 mg versus a mean increase of 49 mg for placebo). Twice as many patients in the orlistat group either reduced or discontinued one or more antidiabetics (17% versus 8% with placebo). Hypoglycaemic episodes (mild to moderate and not requiring treatment) occurred in 10% of orlistat recipients and 4% of placebo recipients.[4] Similarly, improvement in glycaemic control and reduced requirement for oral antidiabetic medication was reported in another study.[5]

A 59-year-old woman with type 2 diabetes taking long-term metformin 500 mg three times daily, developed severe metabolic acidosis with cardiovascular collapse and acute renal failure. Three months previously she had started orlistat 120 mg three times daily, which caused abdominal pain and chronic diarrhoea. During the 4 days before hospital admission, she was prescribed cimetidine 400 mg twice daily for her abdominal pain. The metformin-associated lactic acidosis[6] was considered to have been precipitated by the orlistat and 'cimetidine', (p.491).

(d) Sulphonylureas

A placebo-controlled study in 12 healthy subjects found that orlistat 80 mg three times daily for a little over 4 days had no effect on the pharmacokinetics of a single 5-mg oral dose of **glibenclamide (glyburide)** and the blood glucose lowering effects remained unchanged.[7] A later 1-year, randomised, placebo-controlled, double-blind trial in obese patients with type 2 diabetes in which 139 patients took orlistat found that orlistat reduced fasting blood glucose and glycosylated haemoglobin levels. In addition, 43% of patients taking orlistat 120 mg three times daily were able to decrease their sulphonylurea dosage (**glibenclamide** or **glipizide**), and 11.7% of them were able to discontinue the sulphonylurea. The average dose decrease was 23% compared with 9% in the placebo group.[8]

Mechanism

The benefits of orlistat are likely to be as a result of the beneficial effects of weight reduction on glycaemic control, although in some studies the reduction in glycosylated haemoglobin was not entirely dependent on the magnitude of weight loss.[2]

Importance and management

The benefits of orlistat on glycaemic control in overweight or obese patients with diabetes are established. Antidiabetic treatment should be more closely monitored in patients taking orlistat, and the dose adjusted as necessary.

1. Xenical (Orlistat). Roche Products Ltd. UK Summary of product characteristics, May 2006.
2. Kelly DE, Bray GA, Pi-Sunyer FX, Klein S, Hill J, Miles J, Hollander P. Clinical efficacy of orlistat therapy in overweight and obese patients with insulin-treated type 2 diabetes. A 1-year randomized controlled trial. *Diabetes Care* (2002) 25, 1033–41. Correction. ibid., 2119 and ibid. (2003) 26, 971.
3. Zhi J, Moore R, Kanitra L, Mulligan TE. Pharmacokinetic evaluation of the possible interaction between selected concomitant medications and orlistat at steady state in healthy subjects. *J Clin Pharmacol* (2002) 42, 1011–19.
4. Miles JM, Leiter L, Hollander P, Wadden T, Anderson JW, Doyle M, Foreyt J, Aronne L, Klein S. Effect of orlistat in overweight and obese patients with type 2 diabetes treated with metformin. *Diabetes Care* (2002) 25, 1123–8.
5. Berne C; the Orlistat Swedish Type 2 diabetes Study Group. A randomized study of orlistat in combination with a weight management programme in obese patients with type 2 diabetes treated with metformin. *Diabet Med* (2005) 22, 612–18.
6. Dawson D, Conlon C. Case study: metformin-associated lactic acidosis. Could orlistat be relevant? *Diabetes Care* (2003) 26, 2471–2.
7. Zhi J, Melia AT, Koss-Twardy SG, Min B, Guerciolini R, Freundlich NL, Milla G, Patel IH. The influence of orlistat on the pharmacokinetics and pharmacodynamics of glyburide in healthy volunteers. *J Clin Pharmacol* (1995) 35, 521–5.
8. Hollander PA, Elbein SC, Hirsch IB, Kelley D, McGill J, Taylor T, Weiss SR, Crockett SE, Kaplan RA, Comstock J, Lucas CP, Lodewick PA, Canovatchel W, Chung J, Hauptman J. Role of orlistat in the treatment of obese patients with type 2 diabetes. A 1-year randomized double-blind study. *Diabetes Care* (1998) 21, 1288–94.

Antidiabetics + Pentoxifylline

The manufacturer notes that, rarely, high-dose *injections* of pentoxifylline have intensified the blood glucose-lowering effects of insulin and oral antidiabetic drugs. This effect has not been seen with oral pentoxifylline.[1] For example, in one study oral pentoxifylline 600 mg daily for 9 months did not affect glycosylated haemoglobin levels in type 2 diabetic patients.[2]

1. Trental 400 (Pentoxifylline). Sanofi-Aventis. UK Summary of product characteristics, September 2004.
2. Harmankaya O, Seber S, Yilmaz M. Combination of pentoxifylline with angiotensin converting enzyme inhibitors produces an additional reduction in microalbuminuria in hypertensive type 2 diabetic patients. *Ren Fail* (2003) 25, 465–70.

Antidiabetics + Phenylephrine

Type 1 (insulin-dependent) diabetics can develop elevated blood pressures if they are given phenylephrine eye drops.

Clinical evidence, mechanism, importance and management

A comparative study of 14 type 1 diabetics, who over a period of 2 hours before ocular surgery were given phenylephrine 10% eye drops (a total of 4 doses of one or two drops), found that they had an average blood pressure rise of 34/17 mmHg, whereas another 176 non-diabetic patients similarly treated had no increases in blood pressure.[1] The reason for this pressor reaction is not understood but it would seem that enough phenylephrine is absorbed systemically to stimulate the adrenoceptors of the sympathetic nervous system, which innervates the cardiovascular system. The concentration of phenylephrine in the plasma is a balance between the amount absorbed and rate at which it is then inactivated. The inactivation in diabetics can be reduced (due to sympathetic denervation) so that their phenylephrine levels may rise higher than they would in normal subjects. The authors of this report say that they readily controlled these hypertensive reactions with halothane and by neuroleptanalgesia accompanying regional block with anaesthesia standby. Strictly speaking this is not a drug interaction, but a drug-disease reaction. The mydriatic dosage of phenylephrine should be reduced in type 1 diabetics but whether this is also true for type 2 diabetics is uncertain.

1. Kim JM, Stevenson CE and Mathewson HS. Hypertensive reactions to phenylephrine eyedrops in patients with sympathetic denervation. *Am J Ophthalmol* (1978) 85, 862–8.

Antidiabetics + Quinolones

A number of reports describe severe hypoglycaemia in diabetic patients treated with gatifloxacin and various antidiabetics including insulin, metformin, pioglitazone, repaglinide, rosiglitazone, some sulphonylureas, or voglibose. In contrast, another report describes hyperglycaemia when a diabetic taking metformin and glipizide was given gatifloxacin. A retrospective review reported that almost one quarter of adverse events associated with gatifloxacin involved abnormal glucose homoeostasis, which was at least tenfold higher than with other quinolones. Interaction studies have shown that gatifloxacin may cause hypoglycaemia and hyperglycaemia, whereas studies using cipro-

floxacin and levofloxacin with glibenclamide suggest plasma glucose levels are not usually affected to a clinically relevant extent. However, isolated reports describe hypoglycaemia in diabetic patients taking glibenclamide, when ciprofloxacin, levofloxacin, or norfloxacin was given, and deaths associated with abnormal glucose homoeostasis have been reported in patients taking ciprofloxacin or levofloxacin.

Clinical evidence

A search of the FDA database for adverse drug events associated with **gatifloxacin**, **ciprofloxacin**, **levofloxacin**, and **moxifloxacin** between November 1997 and September 2003 found 10 025 unique adverse events, including 568 involving glucose homoeostasis abnormalities, of which 25 were fatal. **Gatifloxacin** use was associated with 453 (80%) of the adverse events involving glucose homoeostasis, and 17 of these were fatal compared with 3, 5, and 0 fatalities with **ciprofloxacin, levofloxacin,** and **moxifloxacin,** respectively. Of all the adverse events associated with **gatifloxacin**, 24% involved glucose homoeostasis, compared with **ciprofloxacin** (1.3%), **levofloxacin** (1.6%) and **moxifloxacin** (1.3%). The risk of adverse events involving glucose homoeostasis was higher in older patients, in patients taking medications for diabetes (almost 70% of those taking **gatifloxacin** were also using **insulin** or **oral antidiabetics**) and in patients with renal dysfunction whose dosage had not been appropriately adjusted.[1]

(a) Ciprofloxacin

A study in 12 patients with type 2 diabetes mellitus taking **glibenclamide (glyburide)** 10 mg in the morning, plus in some instances 5 mg in the evening, found that ciprofloxacin 1 g daily for a week caused rises in maximum serum **glibenclamide** levels of 20 to 30%, and a rise in the AUC of 25 to 36%. However, none of these changes were statistically significant, and more importantly blood glucose levels were not altered.[2]

Nevertheless, an elderly patient who had been taking **glibenclamide** 5 mg daily for over 2 years was found to be confused, with slurred speech and diaphoresis within a week of starting ciprofloxacin 250 mg twice daily for acute cystitis, and was found to have a serum **glibenclamide** level several times greater than that normally seen.[3] She needed treatment with intravenous glucose to correct the hypoglycaemia. Two further similar cases have been reported, in which hypoglycaemia developed after the first or second dose of ciprofloxacin, for either a wound infection[4] or a urinary tract infection.[5]

(b) Gatifloxacin

In a study in patients with type 2 diabetes controlled by diet and exercise, gatifloxacin 400 mg daily for 10 days had no significant effect on glucose tolerance or most aspects of glucose homoeostasis, but did cause a brief increase in serum insulin levels.[6] In contrast, the manufacturer of gatifloxacin notes that in another study in patents with type 2 diabetes taking **metformin** with or without **glibenclamide**, oral gatifloxacin 400 mg daily for 14 days was associated with initial hypoglycaemia followed by hyperglycaemia.[7]

Moreover, there is a report of 3 cases of hypoglycaemia in elderly type 2 diabetic patients given gatifloxacin. In one of these cases a patient taking **glibenclamide** 5 mg daily and **pioglitazone** 30 mg daily experienced severe, persistent hypoglycaemia within an hour of the first dose of oral gatifloxacin 200 mg. It resolved on withdrawal of all three drugs and she had no further episodes of hypoglycaemia when **glibenclamide** and **pioglitazone** were restarted.[8] Another case describes a patient taking **glimepiride** 2 mg before breakfast and 1 mg before dinner who developed severe hypoglycaemia 12 hours after the first dose of intravenous gatifloxacin 400 mg. Both drugs were discontinued and **glimepiride** was later restarted without further hypoglycaemia.[8] In the remaining case, a patient taking **repaglinide** 500 micrograms every 8 hours was given oral gatifloxacin 400 mg daily for a urinary-tract infection. **Repaglinide** was discontinued 6 hours after the first dose of gatifloxacin because of the patient's lack of appetite. Two hours after the second dose of gatifloxacin, he developed severe hypoglycaemia and also experienced a tonic-clonic seizure. Gatifloxacin was discontinued but hypoglycaemia persisted for 32 hours. **Repaglinide** was restarted 4 days later without further hypoglycaemia.[8] Other case reports have described severe hypoglycaemia when gatifloxacin was given to patients with diabetes taking **insulin** with **repaglinide** and **voglibose**,[9] **glibenclamide**,[10-12] **glibenclamide** with **metformin**,[13] **glibenclamide** with **rosiglitazone**,[12] or **glipizide**.[10]

In contrast, an 82-year-old woman taking **metformin** and **glipizide** who was discharged from hospital taking gatifloxacin 200 mg daily developed severe *hyperglycaemia* within 48 hours. Her serum glucose rapidly reduced with low-dose intravenous **insulin**, but increased again the following day after she took oral gatifloxacin while receiving subcutaneous **insulin**.[10] Hyperglycaemia has also been noted in 2 non-diabetic patients within 48 to 72 hours of starting gatifloxacin.[9,10] See also the FDA findings, above.

(c) Levofloxacin

A study in 24 healthy subjects found that oral levofloxacin had no effect on the pharmacokinetics of a single oral dose of **glibenclamide** nor its effect on plasma glucose levels.[14] No recurrence of hypoglycaemia occurred in a patient taking **gliclazide** and oral levofloxacin who had a severe hypoglycaemic episode while receiving **glibenclamide** and gatifloxacin.[11] However, a fatal case of hypoglycaemia related to intravenous levofloxacin occurred in an elderly patient with diabetes who was taking **glibenclamide**.[15]

(d) Moxifloxacin

The manufacturer notes that the concurrent use of moxifloxacin and **glibenclamide** resulted in an approximate 21% decrease in the peak plasma level of **glibenclamide** in diabetic subjects, but this did not alter blood glucose and endogenous insulin.[16] A pooled analysis from clinical and postmarketing studies suggested that moxifloxacin had no clinically relevant effect on blood glucose homoeostasis, even in patients with diabetes mellitus.[17]

(e) Norfloxacin

The manufacturer notes that the concurrent use of norfloxacin with **glibenclamide** has resulted in severe hypoglycaemia.[18]

Mechanism

Unknown. The authors of one report suggest that the ciprofloxacin may have inhibited the metabolism of the glibenclamide, thereby raising its serum levels.[3] This may possibly be exaggerated in elderly patients whose liver function may be reduced. However, it has also been postulated that quinolones may affect insulin secretion.[5,15] Gatifloxacin can cause disturbances in blood glucose levels;[7] initiation of treatment with gatifloxacin has been associated with increased insulin release and a decrease in blood glucose levels; but from the third day of treatment, an increase in blood glucose levels has also been reported.[1,7] This severe effect of gatifloxacin on glucose homoeostasis does not appear to be a class effect of the quinolones.[8]

Importance and management

Gatifloxacin has been much more frequently associated with disturbances of blood glucose than other fluoroquinolones. The manufacturer notes that when gatifloxacin is used in diabetic patients, blood glucose should be closely monitored. Signs and symptoms of *hypo*glycaemia should be monitored, especially in the first 3 days of therapy, and signs and symptoms of *hyper*glycaemia should be monitored, especially with continued treatment beyond 3 days.[7] Alternatives to gatifloxacin should be considered in patients with diabetes.

Isolated cases of hypoglycaemia in patients with diabetes have also been reported for ciprofloxacin, levofloxacin and norfloxacin. The general clinical relevance of these cases is uncertain but probably minor. However, it may be prudent to consider increasing the frequency of blood glucose monitoring in the elderly, who appear more at risk.

1. Frothingham R. Glucose homeostasis abnormalities associated with use of gatifloxacin. *Clin Infect Dis* (2005) 41, 1269–76.
2. Ludwig E, Szekely E, Graber H, Csiba A. Study of interaction between oral ciprofloxacin and glibenclamide. *Eur J Clin Microbiol Infect Dis* (1991) 10 (Special issue) 378–9.
3. Roberge RJ, Kaplan R, Frank R, Fore C. Glyburide-ciprofloxacin interaction with resistant hypoglycaemia. *Ann Emerg Med* (2000) 36, 160–3.
4. Whitely MS, Worldling J, Patel S, Gibbs KB. Hypoglycaemia in a diabetic patient, associated with ciprofloxacin therapy. *Pract Diabetes* (1993) 10, 35.
5. Lin G, Hays DP, Spillane L. Refractory hypoglycemia from ciprofloxacin and glyburide interaction. *J Toxicol Clin Toxicol* (2004) 42, 295–7.
6. Gajjar DA, LaCreta FP, Kollia GD, Stolz RR, Berger S, Smith WB, Swingle M, Grasela DM. Effect of multiple-dose gatifloxacin or ciprofloxacin on glucose homeostasis and insulin production in patients with noninsulin-dependent diabetes mellitus maintained with diet and exercise. *Pharmacotherapy* (2000) 20, 76S–86S.
7. Tequin (Gatifloxacin). Bristol-Myers Squibb Company. US Prescribing information, January 2006.
8. Menzies DJ, Dorsainvil PA, Cunha BA, Johnson DH. Severe and persistent hypoglycemia due to gatifloxacin interaction with oral hypoglycemic agents. *Am J Med* (2002) 113, 232–4.
9. Khovidhunkit W, Sunthornyothin S. Hypoglycemia, hyperglycemia, and gatifloxacin. *Ann Intern Med* (2004) 141, 969.
10. Biggs WS. Hypoglycemia and hyperglycemia associated with gatifloxacin use in elderly patients. *J Am Board Fam Pract* (2003) 16, 455–7.

11. LeBlanc M, Bélanger C, Cossette P. Severe and resistant hypoglycemia associated with concomitant gatifloxacin and glyburide therapy. *Pharmacotherapy* (2004) 24, 926–31.
12. Bhasin R, Arce FC, Pasmantier R. Hypoglycemia associated with the use of gatifloxacin. *Am J Med Sci* (2005) 330, 250–3.
13. Baker SE, Hangii MC. Possible gatifloxacin-induced hypoglycemia. *Ann Pharmacother* (2002) 36, 1722–6.
14. Hoechst Marion Roussel, Personal Communication, March 1999.
15. Friedrich LV, Dougherty R. Fatal hypoglycemia associated with levofloxacin. *Pharmacotherapy* (2004) 24, 1807–12.
16. Avelox (Moxifloxacin). Bayer plc. UK Summary of product characteristics, July 2006.
17. Gavin JR, Kubin R, Choudhri S, Kubitza D, Himmel H, Gross R, Meyer JM. Moxifloxacin and glucose homeostasis. A pooled-analysis of the evidence from clinical and postmarketing studies. *Drug Safety* (2004) 27, 671–86.
18. Utinor (Norfloxacin). Merck Sharp & Dohme Ltd. UK Summary of product characteristics, November 2005.

Antidiabetics + Rifamycins

Rifampicin (rifampin) reduces the serum levels and blood glucose lowering effects of tolbutamide, gliclazide, chlorpropamide (single case) and glibenclamide (glyburide), and to a lesser extent glimepiride, glipizide and glymidine. Rifampicin also reduces the effects of repaglinide, and possibly also nateglinide. Rifampicin reduces the AUC of rosiglitazone, which could be clinically relevant. An isolated report describes an increased insulin requirement in a patient with type 1 diabetes taking rifampicin.

Clinical evidence

(a) Insulin

A case report describes a 54-year-old woman with type 1 diabetes whose insulin requirements increased from 36 units to 48 units daily when she took **rifampicin**. Immediately on discontinuing her antituberculous therapy, she developed frequent hypoglycaemic attacks, which persisted until her insulin dose was reduced back to 36 units daily.[1]

(b) Nateglinide

In a randomised crossover study, 10 healthy subjects were given a single 60-mg dose of nateglinide the day after a 5-day course of **rifampicin** 600 mg daily. **Rifampicin** reduced the AUC_{0-7} of nateglinide by 24% (range 5 to 53%) and decreased the nateglinide half-life from 1.6 to 1.3 hours. Overall **rifampicin** did not significantly decrease the blood glucose-lowering effects of nateglinide.[2] However, because of the high degree of intersubject variation, the authors suggest that the blood glucose-lowering effects of nateglinide may be reduced in some subjects.[2]

(c) Repaglinide

In one study in healthy subjects, a single 4-mg dose of repaglinide was given one hour after the final dose of **rifampicin** 600 mg daily for 7 days. **Rifampicin** decreased the AUC and the mean maximum plasma concentration of repaglinide by 31% and 26%, respectively, but the blood glucose-lowering effect of repaglinide was not affected.[3] In another study,[4] pretreatment with **rifampicin** 600 mg daily for 5 days increased the AUC and maximum level of a single 500-microgram dose of repaglinide given on day 6 by 57% and 41%, respectively. In this study, **rifampicin** reduced the blood glucose-lowering effect of repaglinide by 35%. A third study investigated the effect of **rifampicin** 600 mg daily for 7 days on a single 4-mg dose of repaglinide given at the same time as the last **rifampicin** dose on day 7 or 24 hours later. When **rifampicin** was given simultaneously, the median AUC of repaglinide was reduced by almost 50%, but when the repaglinide was given 24 hours after the last **rifampicin** dose, the median AUC was reduced by 80%. The size of the effect of **rifampicin** on repaglinide may therefore depend on the administration schedule.[5]

(d) Rosiglitazone

Rifampicin 600 mg daily for 5 days reduced the AUC of a single 4-mg dose of rosiglitazone by 54% and reduced the maximum plasma level by 28%, in a study in healthy subjects. **Rifampicin** increased the formation of *N*-desmethylrosiglitazone.[6] Very similar findings were reported in a study in healthy Korean subjects.[7]

Sulphonylureas

(a) Chlorpropamide

A single case report describes a man with type 2 diabetes who needed an increase in his dosage of chlorpropamide from 250 to 400 mg daily when he was given **rifampicin** 600 mg daily. His serum chlorpropamide levels rose dramatically 12 months later when the **rifampicin** was withdrawn.[8]

(b) Glibenclamide (Glyburide)

A study in 29 type 2 diabetics, stable taking glibenclamide, found that when they were also given **rifampicin** 450 or 600 mg daily for 10 days, their blood glucose levels, both fasting and after meals, were raised. Glibenclamide dosage changes were needed in 15 out of 17 patients in whom the diabetes became uncontrolled. Their blood glucose levels normalised 6 days after stopping the **rifampicin.**[9] Another patient with type 2 diabetes taking glibenclamide had a deterioration in diabetic control, over the 8 months after she started **rifampicin**, which required an increase in glibenclamide dose and the addition of insulin. On stopping **rifampicin**, she had a marked rise in trough serum glibenclamide levels, from 40 to 200 nanograms/mL, but no appreciable change in blood glucose concentrations.[10] A study in 10 healthy subjects found that **rifampicin** 600 mg daily for 5 days decreased the AUC and peak plasma level of a single 1.75-mg dose of glibenclamide given on day 6 by 39% and 22%, respectively. The elimination half-life was shortened from 2 to 1.7 hours. The maximum reduction in blood glucose level was decreased by 36% by **rifampicin.**[11]

(c) Gliclazide

A 65-year-old patient with type 2 diabetes taking gliclazide 80 mg daily for 2 years without problem was given **rifampicin** 450 mg daily, isoniazid, ethambutol and clarithromycin for an atypical mycobacteriosis. Fasting blood glucose levels became elevated requiring an increase in the dose of gliclazide to 120 mg then 160 mg daily. The plasma level of gliclazide on day 75 was 1.4 micrograms/mL, 2 hours after an 80-mg dose. When **rifampicin** was discontinued the gliclazide level increased to 4.7 micrograms/mL and the dose was reduced back to 80 mg daily.[12] A study in 9 healthy subjects found that pre-treatment with **rifampicin** 600 mg for 6 days decreased the AUC of a single 80-mg dose of gliclazide given on day 7 by 70%. The mean elimination half-life of gliclazide was reduced from 9.5 to 3.3 hours and the gliclazide oral clearance was increased by about fourfold. The blood glucose-lowering effects of gliclazide were significantly reduced by **rifampicin.**[13]

(d) Glimepiride

A placebo-controlled study in 10 healthy subjects found that **rifampicin** 600 mg daily for 5 days decreased the AUC of a single 1-mg dose of glimepiride given on day 6 by 34%. **Rifampicin** reduced the elimination half-life of glimepiride by 25%. However, no significant differences in blood glucose were found between the **rifampicin** and placebo regimens.[14]

(e) Glipizide

A placebo-controlled study in 10 healthy subjects found that **rifampicin** 600 mg daily for 5 days decreased the AUC of a single 2.5-mg dose of glipizide given on day 6 by 22%. The elimination half-life was shortened from 3 to 1.9 hours by **rifampicin**. However, no significant differences in blood glucose concentrations were found.[11]

(f) Glymidine

In one study the half-life of glymidine was reduced by about one-third by the concurrent use of **rifampicin.**[15]

(g) Tolbutamide

After treatment for 4 weeks with **rifampicin** the half-life of tolbutamide in 9 diabetic patients with tuberculosis was reduced by 43%, and the serum concentrations measured at 6 hours were halved, when compared with other patients not taking **rifampicin.**[16] Similar results have been found in other studies in patients with cirrhosis or cholestasis,[17] in healthy subjects[18] and in other patients.[19]

Mechanism

Rifampicin is a potent inducer of the liver microsomal enzymes concerned with the metabolism of tolbutamide (cytochrome P450 isoenzyme CYP2C9), which hastens its clearance from the body, thereby reducing its effects.[16-18] The interaction between rifampicin and glibenclamide, gliclazide, glimepiride, glipizide, and nateglinide is probably also due to induction of CYP2C9.[2,11-13] Induction of P-glycoprotein may also play a part.[11,13] The interaction of rifampicin with repaglinide is probably due to induction of CYP3A4,[3,4] and that with rosiglitazone is probably due to induction of CYP2C8 and to a lesser extent CYP2C9.[6,7] The case report with insulin is unexplained.

Importance and management

Information is limited, but the interactions of tolbutamide, glibenclamide (glyburide) and gliclazide with rifampicin appear to be established. Patients taking these sulphonylureas may need an increase in the dosage while taking rifampicin. This also seems possibly true for chlorpropamide, but the documentation for this interaction is even more limited. The effect of rifampicin on the blood glucose-lowering effects of glimepiride, glipizide or glymidine may be of only limited clinical significance, but it should be noted that these were single-dose studies and it is possible that some effect may occur with multiple dosing. Caution is warranted. Similarly although the information regarding nateglinide and repaglinide is limited, a significant interaction is possible, especially with repaglinide, and so an increase in blood glucose monitoring would be prudent. Similarly, the effect on the AUC of rosiglitazone also indicates that diabetic control should be closely monitored if rifampicin is used.

The isolated case of increased insulin requirement suggests that rifampicin may possibly affect the glycaemic control of patients with type 1 diabetes, but this needs further investigation.

There does not seem to be any information regarding the other rifamycins, **rifabutin** (a weak enzyme inducer) and **rifapentine** (a moderate enzyme inducer). However, the manufacturers and the UK Committee on Safety of Medicines warn that rifabutin may possibly reduce the effects of a number of drugs, including oral antidiabetics.[20,21]

1. Atkin SL, Masson EA, Bodmer CW, Walker BA, White MC. Increased insulin requirement in a patient with type 1 diabetes on rifampicin. *Diabet Med* (1993) 10, 392.
2. Niemi M, Backman JT, Neuvonen M, Neuvonen PJ. Effect of rifampicin on the pharmacokinetics and pharmacodynamics of nateglinide in healthy subjects. *Br J Clin Pharmacol* (2003) 56, 427–32.
3. Hatorp V, Hansen KT, Thomsen MS. Influence of drugs interacting with CYP3A4 on the pharmacokinetics, pharmacodynamics, and safety of the prandial glucose regulator repaglinide. *J Clin Pharmacol* (2003) 43, 649–60.
4. Niemi M, Backman JT, Neuvonen M, Neuvonen PJ, Kivistö KT. Rifampin decreases the plasma concentrations and effects of repaglinide. *Clin Pharmacol Ther* (2000) 68, 495–500.
5. Bidstrup TB, Stilling N, Damkier P, Scharling B, Thomsen MS, Brøsen K. Rifampicin seems to act as both an inducer and an inhibitor of the metabolism of repaglinide. *Eur J Clin Pharmacol* (2004) 60, 109–14.
6. Niemi M, Backman JT, Neuvonen PJ. Effects of trimethoprim and rifampin on the pharmacokinetics of the cytochrome P450 2C8 substrate rosiglitazone. *Clin Pharmacol Ther* (2004) 76, 239–49.
7. Park J-Y, Kim K-A, Kang M-H, Kim S-L, Shin J-G. Effect of rifampin on the pharmacokinetics of rosiglitazone in healthy subjects. *Clin Pharmacol Ther* (2004) 75, 157–62.
8. Self TH, Morris T. Interaction of rifampin and chlorpropamide. *Chest* (1980) 77, 800–801.
9. Surekha V, Peter JV, Jeyaseelan L, Cherian AM. Drug interaction: rifampicin and glibenclamide. *Natl Med J India* (1997) 10, 11–12.
10. Self TH, Tsiu SJ, Fowler JW. Interaction of rifampin and glyburide. *Chest* (1989) 96, 1443–4.
11. Niemi M, Backman JT, Neuvonen M, Neuvonen PJ, Kivistö KT. Effects of rifampin on the pharmacokinetics and pharmacodynamics of glyburide and glipizide. *Clin Pharmacol Ther* (2001) 69, 400–6.
12. Kihara Y, Otsuki M. Interaction of gliclazide and rifampicin. *Diabetes Care* (2000) 23, 1204–5.
13. Park J-Y, Kim K-A, Park P-W, Park C-W, Shin J-G. Effect of rifampin on the pharmacokinetics and pharmacodynamics of gliclazide. *Clin Pharmacol Ther* (2003) 74, 334–40.
14. Niemi M, Kivistö KT, Backman JT, Neuvonen PJ. Effect of rifampicin on the pharmacokinetics and pharmacodynamics of glimepiride. *Br J Clin Pharmacol* (2000) 50, 591–5.
15. Held H, Schoene B, Laar HJ, Fleischmann R. Die Aktivität der Benzpyrenhydroxylase im Leberpunktat des Menschen in vitro und ihre Beziehung zur Eliminations-geschwindigkeit von Glycodiazin in vivo. *Verh Dtsch Ges Inn Med* (1974) 80, 501–3.
16. Syvälahti EKG, Pihlajamäki KK, Iisalo EJ. Rifampicin and drug metabolism. *Lancet* (1974) 2, 232–3.
17. Zilly W, Breimer DD, Richter E. Stimulation of drug metabolism by rifampicin in patients with cirrhosis or cholestasis measured by increased hexobarbital and tolbutamide clearance. *Eur J Clin Pharmacol* (1977) 11, 287–93.
18. Zilly W, Breimer DD, Richter E. Induction of drug metabolism in man after rifampicin treatment measured by increased hexobarbital and tolbutamide clearance. *Eur J Clin Pharmacol* (1975) 9, 219–27.
19. Syvälahti E, Pihlajamäki K, Iisalo E. Effect of tuberculostatic agents on the response of serum growth hormone and immunoreactive insulin to intravenous tolbutamide, and on the half-life of tolbutamide. *Int J Clin Pharmacol Biopharm* (1976) 13, 83–9.
20. Mycobutin (Rifabutin). Pharmacia Ltd. UK Summary of product characteristics, October 2006.
21. Committee on the Safety of Medicines/Medicines Control Agency. Revised indication and drug interactions of rifabutin. *Current Problems* (1997) 23, 14.

Antidiabetics + Salicylates

Aspirin and other salicylates can lower blood glucose levels, but small analgesic doses do not normally have an adverse effect on patients taking antidiabetics. Larger doses of salicylates may have a more significant effect, and caution is warranted.

Clinical evidence

(a) Insulin

Twelve children with type 1 diabetes receiving insulin had a reduction in blood glucose levels averaging 15% (from about 10.4 to 8.8 mmol/L) when they were given **aspirin** (patients under 27.2 kg given 1.2 g daily, patients over 27.2 kg given 2.4 g daily) for a week. No significant changes in insulin requirements were necessary.[1]

Eight patients receiving 12 to 48 units of insulin zinc suspension daily required no insulin when they were treated for 2 to 3 weeks with **aspirin** in doses of 3.5 to 7.5 g daily, which were large enough to give maximum therapeutic serum salicylate levels of about 2.5 to 3.3 mmol/L. Six other patients were able to reduce their insulin requirements by between about 20 and 65%.[2]

(b) Chlorpropamide

The blood glucose-lowering effects of chlorpropamide and **sodium salicylate** were found to be additive in 5 healthy subjects. A further study in 6 healthy subjects found that chlorpropamide 100 mg given with **sodium salicylate** 1.5 g lowered blood glucose levels by the same amount as either chlorpropamide 200 mg or **sodium salicylate** 3 g alone.[3]

The blood glucose levels of a patient taking chlorpropamide 500 mg daily were lowered about two-thirds by **aspirin** in doses sufficient to give serum salicylate levels of about 1.9 mmol/L.[4]

(c) Glibenclamide (Glyburide)

Sixteen healthy subjects took a single 5-mg dose of glibenclamide both before and on the fourth day of taking **aspirin** 975 mg four times daily for 4 days. It was found that the **aspirin** reduced the AUC_{0-4} of the glibenclamide by 68% and reduced its mean peak serum levels by 35%. The effects of this on glucose tolerance tests and insulin responses were difficult to interpret, but there was no clear evidence that any clinically relevant changes occurred.[5]

Mechanism

It has been known for over 100 years that aspirin and salicylates have hypoglycaemic properties and in relatively large doses can be used on their own in the treatment of diabetes.[6-10] The simplest explanation for this interaction with antidiabetics is that the blood glucose lowering effects are additive,[3] but there is some evidence that other mechanisms may come into play.[10] In addition aspirin can raise serum chlorpropamide levels, possibly by interfering with renal tubular excretion, and therefore the effects of chlorpropamide are enhanced.[4]

Importance and management

The interaction between the sulphonylureas or insulin and the salicylates is established but of limited importance. Considering the extremely wide use of aspirin it might reasonably be expected that any generally serious interaction would have come to light by now. The data available, coupled with the common experience of diabetics,[11] is that excessive and unwanted hypoglycaemia is very unlikely with small to moderate analgesic doses. Some downward readjustment of the dosage of the antidiabetic may be appropriate if large doses of salicylates are used. Information about other antidiabetics and salicylates appears to be lacking, but they are expected to behave similarly.

1. Kaye R, Athreya BH, Kunzman EE, Baker L. Antipyretics in patients with juvenile diabetes mellitus. *Am J Dis Child* (1966) 112, 52–5.
2. Reid J, Lightbody TD. The insulin equivalence of salicylate. *BMJ* (1959) i, 897–900.
3. Richardson T, Foster J, Mawer GE. Enhancement by sodium salicylate of the blood glucose lowering effect of chlorpropamide - drug interaction or summation of similar effects? *Br J Clin Pharmacol* (1986) 22, 43–48.
4. Stowers JM, Constable LW, Hunter RB. A clinical and pharmacological comparison of chlorpropamide and other sulfonylureas. *Ann N Y Acad Sci* (1959) 74, 689–95.
5. Kubacka RT, Antal EJ, Juhl RP, Welshman IR. Effects of aspirin and ibuprofen on the pharmacokinetics and pharmacodynamics of glyburide in healthy subjects. *Ann Pharmacother* (1996) 30, 20–6.
6. Gilgore SG, Rupp JJ. The long-term response of diabetes mellitus to salicylate therapy. Report of a case. *JAMA* (1962) 180, 65–6.
7. Reid J, Macdougall AI, Andrews MM. Aspirin and diabetes mellitus. *BMJ* (1957) 2, 1071–4.
8. Ebstein W. Zur Therapie des Diabetes mellitus, insbesondere über die Anwendung des salicylsauren Natron bei demselben. Berl Klin Wschr (1876) 13, 337–40.
9. Bartels K. Ueber die therapeutische Verwerthung der Salizylsäure und ihres Nastronsalzes in der inneren Medicin. Dtsch Med Wschr (1878) 4, 423–5.
10. Cattaneo AG, Caviezel F, Pozza G. Pharmacological interaction between tolbutamide and acetylsalicylic acid: study on insulin secretion in man. *Int J Clin Pharmacol Ther Toxicol* (1990) 28, 229–34.
11. Logie AW, Galloway DB, Petrie JC. Drug interactions and long-term antidiabetic therapy. *Br J Clin Pharmacol* (1976) 3, 1027–32.

Antidiabetics + Somatostatin analogues

Octreotide decreases insulin resistance so that the dosage of insulin used by diabetics can be reduced. Fatal diabetic ketoacidosis

occurred in one patient when octreotide was withdrawn. Octreotide appears to have no benefits in those with intact insulin reserves (type 2 diabetes), and it may reduce insulin secretion and affect glucose tolerance in non-diabetic patients. In addition, octreotide has been reported to reduce sulphonylurea-induced hypoglycaemia. Lanreotide may also affect glucose levels in diabetic patients.

Clinical evidence

Changes in glucose tolerance may occur in patients with acromegaly who are given somatostatin analogues. In a prospective study, in 24 acromegalic patients given long-acting **octreotide** or **lanreotide,** insulin resistance was reduced, but insulin secretion was impaired resulting in deterioration of glucose homoeostasis in non-diabetic patients. Of 16 patients with normal glucose tolerance before **octreotide** treatment, 4 developed impaired glucose tolerance, and of 7 patients with impaired glucose tolerance, 4 improved, 1 remained stable and 2 deteriorated to diabetes mellitus; the status of one diabetic patient remained the same.[1] In another study in patients with acromegaly given **octreotide**, impaired glucose tolerance or frank diabetes developed in approximately half of the 55 patients who initially had normal glucose tolerance, but glucose tolerance improved in 3 of the 11 patients who were diabetic.[2] Similar results were reported in a further study, although **octreotide** appeared to be more detrimental to glucose metabolism than **lanreotide**.[3]

(a) Insulin

When 7 patients with type 1 diabetes with poor metabolic control were given **octreotide** 50 micrograms subcutaneously three times daily (at 8, 15 and 23 hours) or by continuous subcutaneous infusion (62.5 or 112.5 micrograms over 24 hours), their blood glucose levels were about 50% lower than when they were given insulin alone. The effects of **octreotide** on blood glucose levels were virtually the same regardless of route of administration or dose.[4] Another study in 6 patients with type 1 diabetes also found that **octreotide** 50 micrograms subcutaneously before meals reduced their daily insulin requirements by about 50%,[5] and other studies confirm that **octreotide** behaves in this way.[6,7] An isolated report describes clinical and biochemical improvement with **lanreotide** 30 mg intramuscularly every 10 days, in a diabetic acromegalic man whose glucose levels were poorly controlled with insulin. However, he experienced hypoglycaemia when the **lanreotide** was replaced with intramuscular **octreotide** 20 mg (depot preparation) and he had to reduce his insulin dose by 30 to 50% for the first week after each **octreotide** injection.[8] Another report describes deterioration in glucose tolerance leading to death from diabetic ketoacidosis when **octreotide** was stopped in a patient with acromegaly and insulin-resistant diabetes mellitus.[9] Eight obese type 2 diabetic patients whose diabetes was not controlled with oral antidiabetics and who needed insulin, had no significant increases in blood glucose levels following a meal when they were given subcutaneous **octreotide** 25 micrograms.[10] **Octreotide** reduced insulin requirements in 6 type 2 diabetic patients with chronic renal failure, but did not significantly affect the glycaemic profile of similar diabetic patients with normal renal function. This effect was thought to be due to a greater reduction in glucagon levels, which are elevated in renal failure.[11]

(b) Oral antidiabetics

Octreotide does not appear to have a clinically relevant beneficial or harmful effect on the blood glucose-lowering effects of oral antidiabetics such as **glibenclamide** (**glyburide**) in patients with type 2 diabetes, although some metabolic changes can occur including suppression of postprandial serum insulin levels.[12,13] A retrospective study of 9 patients with hypoglycaemia occurring as a result of a sulphonylurea overdose (with **glibenclamide** or **glipizide**) found that there was a dramatic and significant reduction in the number of episodes of hypoglycaemia after **octreotide** was given (29 episodes before versus 2 episodes after **octreotide**).[14]

Mechanism

Octreotide is an analogue of the natural hormone somatostatin, and similarly has blood glucose-lowering effects because it inhibits the actions of glucagon and growth hormone (which raise blood glucose levels), and because it also delays the absorption of carbohydrate from the gut. However, somatostatin is also diabetogenic, because it suppresses insulin release. In type 1 diabetes, because there is no endogenous insulin, the blood glucose-lowering effects predominate. In non-diabetics and type 2 diabetics, the actions may cancel out, or there may be poorer glycaemic control. Octreotide is thought to cause less suppression of insulin release than somatostatin, but this may still be important in those with insulin-secreting reserves.

Lanreotide, like somatostatin and its analogues, may produce a transient inhibition of the secretion of insulin and glucagon,[15] but lanreotide may have less affinity for receptors found in the pancreas and so possibly produces a different response to that of octreotide.[1,8]

Sulphonylureas lower blood glucose levels primarily by facilitating preformed insulin release from pancreatic beta cells, and octreotide may oppose this by directly inhibiting insulin secretion from the pancreas.[14]

Importance and management

The interaction between insulin and octreotide is established and hypoglycaemia has been reported. If both drugs are used, anticipate the need to reduce the insulin dosage. The studies cited above[4,5] suggest that about a 50% reduction is possible.

The manufacturers of octreotide say that octreotide may also reduce the requirements of oral antidiabetics in patients with type 1 diabetes mellitus. However, there do not appear to be any studies on this. Conversely, they state that in patients with type 2 diabetes, octreotide may result in prandial *increases* in glycaemia,[16] but two clinical studies in patients with type 2 diabetes given glibenclamide (glyburide) did not show any deterioration (or benefit) in glycaemia.[12,13] However, octreotide has been reported to reduce sulphonylurea-induced hypoglycaemia. Octreotide may affect insulin secretion, and therefore glucose tolerance, and so it would certainly be prudent to monitor the effects of giving octreotide with any of the oral antidiabetics. The manufacturer of lanreotide also recommends that blood glucose levels should be checked in diabetic patients to determine whether antidiabetic treatment needs to be adjusted.[15]

1. Baldelli R, Battista C, Leonetti F, Ghiggi M-R, Ribaudo M-C, Paoloni A, D'Amico E, Ferretti E, Baratta R, Liuzzi A, Trischitta V, Tamburrano G. Glucose homeostasis in acromegaly: effects of long-acting somatostatin analogues treatment. *Clin Endocrinol (Oxf)* (2003) 59, 492–9.
2. Koop BL, Harris AG, Ezzat S. Effect of octreotide on glucose tolerance in acromegaly. *Eur J Endocrinol* (1994) 130, 581–6.
3. Ronchi C, Epaminonda P, Cappiello V, Beck-Peccoz P, Arosio M. Effects of two different somatostatin analogs on glucose tolerance in acromegaly. *J Endocrinol Invest* (2002) 25, 502–7.
4. Lunetta M, Di Mauro M, Le Moli R, Nicoletti F. Effect of octreotide on blood glucose and counterregulatory hormones in insulin-dependent diabetic patients: the role of dose and route of administration. *Eur J Clin Pharmacol* (1996) 51, 139–44.
5. Rios MS, Navascues I, Saban J, Ordoñez A, Sevilla F, Del Pozo E. Somatostatin analog SMS 201–995 and insulin needs in insulin-dependent diabetic patients studied by means of an artificial pancreas. *J Clin Endocrinol Metab* (1986) 63, 1071–4.
6. Candrina R, Giustina G. Effect of a new long-acting somatostatin analogue (SMS 201–995) on glycemic and hormonal profiles in insulin-treated type II diabetic patients. *J Endocrinol Invest* (1988) 11, 501–7.
7. Hadjidakis DJ, Halvatsiotis PG, Ioannou YJ, Mavrokefalos PJ, Raptis SA. The effects of the somatostatin analogue SMS 201–995 on carbohydrate homeostasis of insulin-dependent diabetics as assessed by the artificial endocrine pancreas. *Diabetes Res Clin Pract* (1988) 5, 91–8.
8. Webb SM, Ortega E, Rodríguez-Espinosa J, Mato M-E, Corcoy R. Decreased insulin requirements after LAR-octreotide but not after lanreotide in an acromegalic patient. *Pituitary* (2001) 4, 275–8.
9. Abrahamson MJ. Death from diabetic ketoacidosis after cessation of octreotide in acromegaly. *Lancet* (1990) 336, 318–19.
10. Giustina A, Girelli A, Buffoli MG, Cimino A, Legati F, Valentini U, Giustina G. Low-dose octreotide is able to cause a maximal inhibition of the glycemic responses to a mixed meal in obese type 2 diabetic patients treated with insulin. *Diabetes Res Clin Pract* (1991) 14, 47–54.
11. Di Mauro M, Papalia G, Le Moli R, Nativo B, Nicoletti F, Lunetta M. Effect of octreotide on insulin requirement, hepatic glucose production, growth hormone, glucagon and c-peptide levels in type 2 diabetic patients with chronic renal failure or normal renal function. *Diabetes Res Clin Pract* (2001) 51, 45–50.
12. Davies RR, Miller M, Turner SJ, Watson M, McGill A, Ørskov H, Alberti KGMM, Johnston DG. Effects of somatostatin analogue SMS 201–995 in non-insulin-dependent diabetes. *Clin Endocrinol (Oxf)* (1986) 25, 739–47.
13. Williams G, Füessl HS, Burrin JM, Chilvers E, Bloom SR. Postprandial glycaemic effects of a long-acting somatostatin analogue (octreotide) in non-insulin dependent diabetes mellitus. *Horm Metab Res* (1988) 20, 168–170.
14. McLaughlin SA, Crandall CS, McKinney PE. Octreotide: an antidote for sulfonylurea-induced hypoglycemia. *Ann Emerg Med* (2000) 36, 133–8.
15. Somatuline LA (Lanreotide acetate). Ipsen Ltd. UK Summary of product characteristics, August 2003.
16. Sandostatin (Octreotide). Novartis Pharmaceuticals UK Ltd. UK Summary of product characteristics, March 2004.

Antidiabetics + SSRIs

Hypoglycaemia has occurred in patients with diabetes when given fluoxetine or sertraline and hypoglycaemia unawareness has also been reported with fluoxetine. Conversely, two isolated reports describe hyperglycaemia in patients given fluvoxamine or sertraline. Fluvoxamine slightly reduces the clearance of tolbutamide

and increases the maximum plasma levels of glimepiride, but these changes are unlikely to be clinically relevant in most patients. Fluoxetine did not alter the pharmacokinetics of tolbutamide, and sertraline did not significantly affect the pharmacokinetics of glibenclamide (glyburide) or tolbutamide.

Clinical evidence

(a) Fluoxetine

One study found that single, or multiple doses of fluoxetine for 8 days, did not affect the pharmacokinetics or the blood glucose-lowering effects of **tolbutamide** 1 g.[1] However, studies in obese patients with type 2 diabetes receiving oral antidiabetics have shown that fluoxetine can cause significant weight loss, reduce fasting plasma glucose levels and improve glycaemic control (decrease in glycosylated haemoglobin levels),[2,3] and in those receiving **insulin**, decrease the daily **insulin** dose.[4] The manufacturers of fluoxetine say that hypoglycaemia has occurred in diabetic patients when they took fluoxetine alone, and hyperglycaemia has developed following discontinuation.[5,6]

An **insulin**-dependent diabetic experienced symptoms of hypoglycaemia (nausea, tremor, sweating, anxiety, lightheadedness) after starting to take fluoxetine 20 mg each night. The symptoms disappeared when the fluoxetine was stopped and reappeared when it was restarted. However, blood glucose levels were found to be normal (9 to 11 mmol/L), so it is likely that the effects were purely adverse effects of fluoxetine that were mistaken for symptoms of hypoglycaemia.[7] In contrast, another patient with type 1 diabetes experienced a loss of hypoglycaemic awareness while taking fluoxetine 40 mg daily. Approximately one month after fluoxetine was started, he reported an increased incidence of hypoglycaemia, but these episodes were not accompanied by typical adrenergic symptoms (which he had previously experienced). After 3 grand mal seizures which occurred with blood glucose readings ranging from 1.9 to 2.2 mmol/L, the dose of fluoxetine was gradually decreased. Hypoglycaemic unawareness resolved when the fluoxetine dosage was reduced to 10 mg every second day. Within weeks of discontinuing fluoxetine, blood glucose levels had risen considerably and hypoglycaemia did not recur.[8]

(b) Fluvoxamine

Hyperglycaemia occurred in a 60-year-old woman with type 2 diabetes controlled with **insulin**, 5 days after fluvoxamine was started. Blood glucose levels, which had approximately doubled, decreased when the fluvoxamine was stopped, but increased and then decreased again when the fluvoxamine was restarted and then stopped.[9]

A study in 14 healthy subjects given fluvoxamine 75 or 150 mg daily for 5 days, with a single 500-mg dose of **tolbutamide** on the third day, found that the clearance of **tolbutamide** was modestly reduced by 19% by the 75 mg dose and by 33% by the 150 mg dose of fluvoxamine. The clearance of its metabolites (4-hydroxytolbutamide and carboxytolbutamide) was also significantly decreased.[10]

A randomised, double-blind, crossover study in 12 healthy subjects given fluvoxamine 100 mg or placebo daily for 4 days, with a single 500-microgram dose of **glimepiride** on the fourth day, found the AUC of **glimepiride** was not significantly affected by fluvoxamine. Peak plasma levels of **glimepiride** were increased by 43% and the elimination half-life was prolonged from 2 to 2.3 hours, but there was no significant change in the effects of **glimepiride** on blood glucose concentrations.[11]

(c) Sertraline

After taking sertraline 200 mg daily for 22 days the clearance of a single intravenous dose of **tolbutamide** was decreased by 16% in 25 healthy subjects.[12] In another study in 11 healthy subjects, the pharmacokinetics of a single 5-mg dose of **glibenclamide** (**glyburide**) were found to be unaffected by sertraline, taken in increasing doses up to 200 mg daily over 15 days. Blood glucose levels were also unchanged.[13] However, there is a report of a patient with schizoaffective disorder and type 2 diabetes who developed hypoglycaemia during treatment with sertraline, risperidone and **glibenclamide**.[14] In contrast, another report describes a patient with diet-controlled, type 2 diabetes, whose glucose levels increased after initiation of sertraline treatment.[15]

Mechanism

Fluvoxamine probably decreases the clearance of tolbutamide by inhibition of its metabolism by the cytochrome P450 isoenzyme CYP2C9. This mechanism may also partly explain the increase in plasma levels of glimepiride. However, as the glimepiride AUC was not increased and the half-life was only slightly increased, the increase in plasma levels may also be due to an increased rate of glimepiride absorption caused by the SSRI.[10,11] The effects of other SSRIs may also be associated with enzyme inhibition.[14]

Importance and management

There would seem to be little reason for avoiding concurrent use of fluoxetine, fluvoxamine or sertraline with sulphonylureas, but until more is known it would seem prudent to monitor diabetic control. The manufacturers of fluoxetine, **paroxetine** and sertraline warn that dosages of insulin or oral antidiabetics may need adjustment during concurrent use.[5,6,16,17]

1. Lemberger L, Bergstrom RF, Wolen RL, Farid NA, Enas GG, Aronoff GR. Fluoxetine: clinical pharmacology and physiologic disposition. *J Clin Psychiatry* (1985) 46, 14–19.
2. Breum L, Bjerre U, Bak JF, Jacobsen S, Astrup A. Long-term effects of fluoxetine on glycemic control in obese patients with non-insulin-dependent diabetes mellitus or glucose intolerance: influence on muscle glycogen synthase and insulin receptor kinase activity. *Metabolism* (1995) 44, 1570–6.
3. Daubresse J-C, Kolanowski J, Krzentowski G, Kutnowski M, Scheen A, Van Gaal L. Usefulness of fluoxetine in obese non-insulin-dependent diabetics: a multicenter study. *Obes Res* (1996) 4, 391–6.
4. Gray DS, Fujioka K, Devine W, Bray GA. A randomized double-blind clinical trial of fluoxetine in obese diabetics. *Int J Obes* (1992) 16 (Suppl 4), S67–S72.
5. Prozac (Fluoxetine hydrochloride). Eli Lilly and Company Ltd. UK Summary of product characteristics, March 2007.
6. Prozac (Fluoxetine hydrochloride). Eli Lilly and Company. US Prescribing information, May 2007.
7. Lear J, Burden AC. Fluoxetine side-effects mimicking hypoglycaemia. *Lancet* (1992) 339, 1296.
8. Sawka AM, Burgart V, Zimmerman D. Loss of hypoglycemia awareness in an adolescent with type 1 diabetes mellitus during treatment with fluoxetine hydrochloride. *J Pediatr* (2000) 136, 394–6.
9. Oswald P, Souery D, Mendlewicz J. Fluvoxamine-induced hyperglycaemia in a diabetic patient with comorbid depression. *Int J Neuropsychopharmacol* (2003) 6, 85–7.
10. Madsen H, Enggaard TP, Hansen LL, Klitgaard NA, Brøsen K. Fluvoxamine inhibits the CYP2C9 catalysed biotransformation of tolbutamide. *Clin Pharmacol Ther* (2001) 69, 41–7.
11. Niemi M, Backman JT, Neuvonen M, Laitila J, Neuvonen PJ, Kivistö KT. Effects of fluconazole and fluvoxamine on the pharmacokinetics of glimepiride. *Clin Pharmacol Ther* (2001) 69, 194–200.
12. Tremaine LM, Wilner KD, Preskorn SH. A study of the potential effect of sertraline on the pharmacokinetics and protein binding of tolbutamide. *Clin Pharmacokinet* (1997) 32 (Suppl 1), 31–6.
13. Invicta Pharmaceuticals. A double blind placebo controlled, multiple dose study to assess potential interaction between oral sertraline (200 mg) and glibenclamide (5 mg) in healthy male volunteers. Data on file (Study 223), 1991.
14. Takhar J, Williamson P. Hypoglycemia associated with high doses of sertraline and sulphonylurea compound in a noninsulin-dependent diabetes mellitus patient. *Can J Clin Pharmacol* (1999)6, 12–14.
15. Sansone RA, Sansone LA. Sertraline-induced hyperglycemia: case report. *Int J Psychiatry Med* (2003) 33, 103–5.
16. Lustral (Sertraline hydrochloride). Pfizer Ltd. UK Summary of product characteristics, October 2005.
17. Seroxat (Paroxetine hydrochloride hemihydrate). GlaxoSmithKline UK. UK Summary of product characteristics, April 2007.

Antidiabetics + St John's wort (*Hypericum perforatum*)

St John's wort modestly decreases the AUC of rosiglitazone. Repaglinide is similarly metabolised and may therefore be expected to interact similarly. St John's wort did not affect the metabolism of tolbutamide.

Clinical evidence

(a) Rosiglitazone

A preliminary report of a pharmacokinetic study[1] states that St John's wort 900 mg daily decreased the AUC of a single dose of rosiglitazone by 26% and increased its clearance by 35%.

(b) Tolbutamide

In a study using tolbutamide as a probe drug for CYP2C9 activity, St John's wort 900 mg daily had no effect on the metabolism of a single dose of tolbutamide either after one day or after 2 weeks of use.[2] Similarly, in another study, a St John's wort preparation with low hyperforin content (*Esbericum*) at a dose of 240 mg daily had no effect on tolbutamide metabolism.[3]

Mechanism

Rosiglitazone is known to be metabolised principally by the cytochrome P450 isoenzyme CYP2C8, and it was therefore concluded that St John's wort induces CYP2C8. The magnitude of the effect of St John's wort was not influenced by CYP2C8 genotype.[1] St John's wort has no effect on the metabolism of tolbutamide via CYP2C9.

Importance and management

The clinical relevance of the modest reduction in rosiglitazone levels has not been assessed, but it would seem unlikely to be important. However, the authors state that St John's wort use should be monitored when patients are given CYP2C8 substrates. Of the antidiabetics, in addition to rosiglitazone, this would also include **repaglinide**. Note that **repaglinide** is also a substrate for CYP3A4, of which St John's wort is an established inducer. Further study is needed. No special precautions would appear to be necessary if tolbutamide and St John's wort are used together.

1. Hruska MW, Cheong JA, Langaee TY, Frye RF. Effect of St John's wort administration on CYP2C8 mediated rosiglitazone metabolism. *Clin Pharmacol Ther* (2005) 77, P35.
2. Wang Z, Gorski JC, Hamman MA, Huang S-M, Lesko LJ, Hall SD. The effects of St John's wort *(Hypericum perforatum)* on human cytochrome P450 activity. *Clin Pharmacol Ther* (2001) 70, 317–26.
3. Arold G, Donath F, Maurer A, Diefenbach K, Bauer S, Henneicke-von Zepelin H-H, Friede M, Roots I. No relevant interaction with alprazolam, caffeine, tolbutamide, and digoxin by treatment with a low-hyperforin St John's wort extract. *Planta Med* (2005) 71, 331–7.

Antidiabetics + Statins

No clinically relevant adverse interactions appear to have been reported between the statins and the sulphonylureas. One study reported an increased incidence of adverse effects with repaglinide and simvastatin, the clinical relevance of which is unclear. *Most* studies have shown no pharmacokinetic interaction or increased incidence of adverse effects when pioglitazone or rosiglitazone were used with atorvastatin or simvastatin. Subcutaneous exenatide modestly decreased the AUC of lovastatin, but no clear pattern of altered efficacy of statins was noted in exenatide clinical trials.

Clinical evidence

A. Exenatide

The manufacturer notes[1] that subcutaneous exenatide 10 micrograms twice daily decreased the AUC of a single dose of **lovastatin** by 40%, and the maximum level by 28%. However, they also note that in clinical trials of exenatide, the use of exenatide for 30 weeks in patients already taking statins was not associated with consistent changes in lipid profiles.[1]

B. Repaglinide

A three-period, crossover, open-label study in healthy subjects found that **simvastatin** 20 mg daily increased the maximum plasma level of repaglinide 2 mg three times daily by 26%, although there was high variability and the mean bioavailability of repaglinide was increased by 8%. There was a higher incidence of adverse effects during concurrent use.[2]

C. Sulphonylureas

(a) Chlorpropamide

A study in 7 patients with type 2 diabetes and hypercholesterolaemia, taking chlorpropamide 125 to 750 mg daily, found that **lovastatin** 20 mg twice daily for 6 weeks reduced low-density lipoprotein cholesterol by 28%, total cholesterol by 24% and apolipoprotein B by 24%. The chlorpropamide plasma levels were unchanged, and the diabetic control remained unaltered.[3]

(b) Glibenclamide (Glyburide)

Groups of 16 healthy subjects taking **fluvastatin** 40 mg or **simvastatin** 20 mg daily were given single 3.5-mg oral doses of glibenclamide on days 1, 8 and 15. The maximum plasma concentration and the AUC of glibenclamide were increased by about 20% by the statins. The blood glucose-lowering effects of the glibenclamide remained virtually unchanged by both **fluvastatin** and **simvastatin** in these subjects, and also when **fluvastatin** was tested in a group of 32 patients with type 2 diabetes.[4] The manufacturers of **fluvastatin** report a study in which **fluvastatin** 40 mg twice daily was given to diabetic patients stable taking glibenclamide 5 to 20 mg daily. **Fluvastatin** increased the AUC of glibenclamide by 1.7-fold, and increased the maximum serum levels by 1.6-fold, without causing significant changes in glucose levels.[5]

(c) Tolbutamide

A single 1-g oral dose of tolbutamide was given to two groups of 16 healthy subjects taking **fluvastatin** 40 mg or **simvastatin** 20 mg. The pharmacokinetics of the tolbutamide were affected only to a very minor extent, and the blood glucose-lowering effects of the tolbutamide were unchanged.[4]

D. Thiazolidinediones

One review suggested that patients receiving thiazolidinediones (95% taking **troglitazone**) were more likely to develop hepatotoxicity if taking **atorvastatin** than when taking **simvastatin**.[6] However, **troglitazone** has now been withdrawn due to its hepatotoxic effects. The same authors more recently conducted a similar study. They analysed the FDA adverse event reporting database for reactions affecting muscle, liver, pancreas, or bone marrow where **simvastatin** or **atorvastatin** were implicated. They then looked for events where antidiabetic drugs also featured. Of the 3767 events identified for atorvastatin, 40 also involved rosiglitazone and 20 also involved pioglitazone. Of the 3651 events identified for simvastatin, 10 also involved rosiglitazone and 9 also involved pioglitazone. About half of these events involving pioglitazone or rosiglitazone resulted in hospitalisation or death. Although the data did not allow for an assessment of whether this rate was greater than that expected, the authors say that if simvastatin is used as the control, the data suggest that the number of cases of adverse events with atorvastatin and a thiazolidinedione are greater than would be expected by chance alone.[7]

However, in a study in healthy subjects, **pioglitazone** 45 mg daily did not significantly affect the pharmacokinetics of **simvastatin** 80 mg daily and concurrent use was well tolerated.[8] Similarly, there was no pharmacokinetic interaction between **pioglitazone** 45 mg daily and **atorvastatin** 80 mg daily.[9] Moreover, clinical use of **rosiglitazone** with **atorvastatin** in patients with type 2 diabetes for 16 weeks was well tolerated,[10] as was the clinical use of **rosiglitazone** or **pioglitazone** with **simvastatin**.[11]

Mechanism

The small changes in the pharmacokinetics of glibenclamide caused by fluvastatin and simvastatin are not understood, but they do not appear to be clinically significant. The interaction between atorvastatin or simvastatin and the thiazolidinediones is thought to involve the cytochrome P450 isoenzyme CYP3A4, although this is as yet unconfirmed.

Importance and management

There is little evidence to suggest that special precautions appear to be needed by diabetic patients taking any of the pairs of sulphonylureas and statins cited here (chlorpropamide with lovastatin, or glibenclamide or tolbutamide with fluvastatin or simvastatin). However, the manufacturers of fluvastatin suggest that a serious interaction cannot be ruled out and therefore advise that the use of glibenclamide should be avoided wherever possible.[5]

The clinical significance of the increased incidence of adverse effects with repaglinide and simvastatin is unclear and so an element of caution would seem prudent.

Most studies have shown no pharmacokinetic interaction or increased incidence of adverse effects when pioglitazone or rosiglitazone were used with atorvastatin or simvastatin. The clinical relevance of the apparent increased incidence of adverse muscle and liver effects with the use of pioglitazone or rosiglitazone together with atorvastatin is unclear. Further study is needed. The clinical relevance of the decrease in lovastatin levels with exenatide is also unclear. But experience in clinical studies suggests that it is unlikely to be significant.

Note that a number of the large-scale trials of the use of lipid-regulating drugs in primary or secondary prevention of cardiovascular events included patients with diabetes. A review of these subgroups concluded that statins were the drug of choice for lipid-lowering therapy in patients with type 2 diabetes and known coronary artery disease or other cardiovascular risk factors. There was no evidence to recommend one statin over another.[12]

1. Byetta (Exenatide). Amylin Pharmaceuticals, Inc. US Prescribing information, February 2007.
2. Hatorp V, Hansen KT, Thomsen MS. Influence of drugs interacting with CYP3A4 on the pharmacokinetics, pharmacodynamics, and safety of the prandial glucose regulator repaglinide. *J Clin Pharmacol* (2003) 43, 649–60.
3. Johnson BF, LaBelle P, Wilson J, Allan J, Zupkis RV, Ronca PD. Effects of lovastatin in diabetic patients treated with chlorpropamide. *Clin Pharmacol Ther* (1990) 48, 467–72.

4. Appel S, Rüfenacht T, Kalafsky G, Tetzloff W, Kallay Z, Hitzenberger G, Kutz K. Lack of interaction between fluvastatin and oral hypoglycemic agents in healthy subjects and in patients with non-insulin-dependent diabetes mellitus. *Am J Cardiol* (1995) 76, 29A–32A.
5. Lescol (Fluvastatin sodium). Novartis Pharmaceuticals UK Ltd. UK Summary of product characteristics, October 2006.
6. Alsheikh-Ali AA, Abourjaily HM, Karas RH. Risk of adverse events with concomitant use of atorvastatin or simvastatin and glucose-lowering drugs (thiazolidinediones, metformin, sulfonylurea, insulin, acarbose). *Am J Cardiol* (2002) 89, 1308–10.
7. Alsheikh-Ali AA, Karas RH. Adverse events with concomitant use of simvastatin or atorvastatin and thiazolidinediones. *Am J Cardiol* (2004) 93, 1417–18.
8. Prueksaritanont T, Vega JM, Zhao J, Gagliano K, Kuznetsova O, Musser B, Amin RD, Liu L, Roadcap BA, Dilzer S, Lasseter KC, Rogers JD. Interactions between simvastatin and troglitazone or pioglitazone in healthy subjects. *J Clin Pharmacol* (2001) 41, 573–81.
9. Karim A, Schwartz L, Perez A, Chao C. Lack of clinically significant interaction in coadministration of pioglitazone and atorvastatin calcium. *Diabetes* (2003) 52 (suppl 1) A449.
10. Freed MI, Ratner R, Marcovina SM, Kreider MM, Biswas N, Cohen BR, Brunzell JD; Rosiglitazone Study 108 Investigators. Effects of rosiglitazone alone and in combination with atorvastatin on the metabolic abnormalities in type 2 diabetes mellitus. *Am J Cardiol* (2002) 90, 947–52.
11. Lewin AJ, Kipnes MS, Meneghini LF, Plotkin DJ, Perevozskaya IT, Shah S, Maccubbin DL, Mitchel YB, Tobert JA; Simvastatin/Thiazolidinedione Study Group. Effects of simvastatin on the lipid profile and attainment of low-density lipoprotein cholesterol goals when added to thiazolidinedione therapy in patients with type 2 diabetes mellitus: a multicenter, randomized, double-blind, placebo-controlled trial. *Clin Ther* (2004) 26, 379–89.
12. Snow V, Aronson MD, Hornbake ER, Mottur-Pilson C, Weiss KB, for the Clinical Efficacy Assessment Subcommittee of the American College of Physicians. Lipid control in the management of type 2 diabetes mellitus: a clinical practice guideline from the American College of Physicians. *Ann Intern Med* (2004) 140, 644–9.

Antidiabetics + Sucralfate

Sucralfate appears not to affect the pharmacokinetics of chlorpropamide or rosiglitazone.

Clinical evidence, mechanism, importance and management

(a) Chlorpropamide

A two-way crossover study in 12 healthy subjects found that sucralfate 1 g four times daily, given 1 hour before meals, had no significant effect on the pharmacokinetics of a single 250-mg dose of chlorpropamide.[1] No additional precautions would therefore seem to be necessary on concurrent use.

(b) Rosiglitazone

A single-dose study found that sucralfate 2 g taken 45 minutes before rosiglitazone 8 mg had no significant effect on the pharmacokinetics of rosiglitazone. No special precautions are needed during concurrent use.[2]

1. Letendre PW, Carlson JD, Siefert RD, Dietz AJ, Dimmit D. Effect of sucralfate on the absorption and pharmacokinetics of chlorpropamide. *J Clin Pharmacol* (1986) 26, 622–5.
2. Rao MNVS, Mullangi R, Katneni K, Ravikanth B, Babu AP, Rani UP, Naidu MUR, Srinivas NR, Rajagopalan R. Lack of effect of sucralfate on the absorption and pharmacokinetics of rosiglitazone. *J Clin Pharmacol* (2002) 42, 670–5.

Antidiabetics + Sugar-containing pharmaceuticals

Some pharmaceutical preparations may contain sufficient amounts of sugar to affect the control of diabetes. Diabetics should be warned and advised of sugar-free alternatives where appropriate.

Clinical evidence, mechanism, importance and management

Pharmaceuticals, especially liquid formulations, may contain sugar in significant amounts. The extent to which the use of preparations like these will affect the control of diabetes clearly depends upon the amounts ingested, but the problem is by no means merely theoretical. One report describes the loss of diabetic control (glycosuria) in a woman with type 1 diabetes receiving insulin when given psyllium effervescent powder (*Metamucil* instant-mix), which contains sugar.[1]

The range of other sugar-containing preparations is far too extensive to be listed here. Because of concerns over sugar-containing medicines and dental caries, in children in particular, the number of sugar-free preparations has grown considerably over recent years. In the UK the BNF and MIMS provide guidance as to which preparations are sugar-free. Diabetics should be warned about sugar-containing medicines, and given guidance about the terminology used in labelling. Sweetening agents of note to diabetics include: **invert sugar** (dextrose and fructose), **invert syrup** (67% w/w invert sugar), **syrup BP** (66% w/w sucrose), **glucose liquid** (dextrose content 10 to 20%), **glucose syrup** (33.3% liquid glucose in syrup) and **honey** (70 to 80% glucose and fructose).[2]

1. Catellani J, Collins RJ. Drug labelling. *Lancet* (1978) ii, 98.
2. Greenwood J. Sugar content of liquid prescription medicines. *Pharm J* (1989) 243, 553–7.

Antidiabetics + Sulfinpyrazone

Sulfinpyrazone has no effect on the insulin requirements of diabetics, nor does it affect the control of diabetes in patients taking glibenclamide (glyburide). Increased blood glucose-lowering effects might occur if sulfinpyrazone is given with tolbutamide, but as yet there appear to be no case reports of this interaction. Sulfinpyrazone modestly increased the AUC of nateglinide, but this is unlikely to be clinically relevant.

Clinical evidence

(a) Insulin

A double-blind study in 41 adult diabetics found that sulfinpyrazone 600 to 800 mg daily had no clinically significant effects on insulin requirements over a 12-month period.[1]

(b) Nateglinide

In a crossover study in healthy subjects, sulfinpyrazone 200 mg twice daily for 7 days increased the mean AUC of a single 120-mg dose of nateglinide by 28%, but did not change the mean maximum plasma level.[2]

(c) Sulphonylureas

A study in 19 type 2 diabetics taking **glibenclamide** found that sulfinpyrazone 800 mg daily did not affect diabetic control.[3]

A detailed study of the pharmacokinetics of **tolbutamide** in 6 healthy subjects found that sulfinpyrazone 200 mg every 6 hours for a week, almost doubled the half-life of a 500-mg intravenous dose of **tolbutamide**, from 7.3 to 13.2 hours, and reduced the plasma clearance by 40%.[4]

Mechanism

Sulfinpyrazone is an inhibitor of the cytochrome P450 isoenzyme CYP2C9, by which tolbutamide and nateglinide are metabolised.

Importance and management

Information about an interaction between tolbutamide and sulfinpyrazone appears to be limited to the report cited. So far there appear to be no reports of adverse interactions in patients, but what is known suggests that increased blood glucose-lowering effects, and possibly hypoglycaemia could occur if the dosage of tolbutamide is not reduced. Such an interaction has been described with phenylbutazone, which has a close structural similarity to sulfinpyrazone (see 'Antidiabetics + NSAIDs; Phenylbutazone and related drugs', p.498). Patients should be warned if sulfinpyrazone is added to established treatment with tolbutamide. The modest increase in nateglinide exposure when given with sulfinpyrazone has not been assessed in diabetics, but it seems unlikely to be clinically relevant. There seems to be nothing documented about any other clinically important interactions between antidiabetics and sulfinpyrazone.

1. Pannebakker MAG, den Ottolander GJH, ten Pas JG. Insulin requirements in diabetic patients treated with sulphinpyrazone. *J Int Med Res* (1979) 7, 328–31.
2. Sabia H, Sunkara G, Ligueros-Saylan M, Wang Y, Smith H, McLeod J, Prasad P. Effect of a selective CYP2C9 inhibitor on the pharmacokinetics of nateglinide in healthy subjects. *Eur J Clin Pharmacol* (2004) 60, 407–12.
3. Kritz H, Najemnik C, Irsigler K. Interaktionsstudie mit Sulfinpyrazon (Anturan) und Glibenclamid (Euglucon) bei Typ-II-Diabetikern. *Wien Med Wochenschr* (1983) 133, 237–43.
4. Miners JO, Foenander T, Wanwimolruk S, Gallus AS, Birkett DJ. The effect of sulphinpyrazone on oxidative drug metabolism in man: inhibition of tolbutamide elimination. *Eur J Clin Pharmacol* (1982) 22, 321–6.

Antidiabetics + Sulfonamides

The blood glucose-lowering effects of some of the sulphonylureas are increased by some, but not all, sulfonamides, due to inhibition of their metabolism. However, sulfaphenazole, which was shown to have an important pharmacokinetic interaction with tolbutamide, is no longer used clinically, and other sulfonamides appear less likely to interact. Nevertheless, occasionally and unpredicta-

bly acute hypoglycaemia has occurred in individual patients taking various combinations of sulfonamides and sulphonylureas. There appear to be no reports of a serious adverse interaction between insulin and the sulfonamides. Co-trimoxazole alone may rarely cause hypoglycaemia.

Clinical evidence

'Table 13.3', (p.508) summarises the information on the interactions between sulphonylureas and sulfonamides. For a report of the combined use of co-trimoxazole and fluconazole causing hypoglycaemia with **gliclazide**, see 'Antidiabetics + Azoles; Fluconazole', p.479.

Mechanism

The sulfonamides may inhibit the metabolism of the sulphonylureas so that they accumulate in the body. In this way their serum levels and blood glucose-lowering effects are enhanced.[1-4] Greater understanding of metabolic mechanisms has led to the realisation that some sulfonamides are inhibitors of the cytochrome P450 isoenzyme CYP2C9 by which many of the sulphonylureas are metabolised. Tolbutamide, in particular, is now recognised as an important substrate of CYP2C9.[5,6] Of the sulfonamides, *in vitro* data suggest that sulfaphenazole is a potent inhibitor of CYP2C9, with sulfadiazine, sulfamethizole, sulfafurazole (sulfisoxazole) and sulfamethoxazole being moderate to minor inhibitors, and sulfapyridine, sulfadimethoxine and sulfamonomethoxine having little inhibitory activity.[6] CYP2C9 shows genetic polymorphism, therefore any interaction might only be clinically relevant in a subgroup of the population. There is also some evidence that the sulfonamides can displace the sulphonylureas from their protein binding sites.[4]

Where some of the cases of hypoglycaemia cannot be predicted on pharmacokinetic grounds, it is worth noting that hypoglycaemia induced by co-trimoxazole, in the absence of a conventional antidiabetic,[7-11] and sometimes associated with renal failure,[9] high dose of sulphonamide,[7,11] advanced age,[8,10] or malnutrition,[7] has been described. Note that trimethoprim alone may cause interactions mediated via inhibition of CYP2C8 and CYP2C9, see 'Antidiabetics + Trimethoprim', p.510.

Importance and management

Information is very patchy and incomplete. Most sulfonamides seem to have caused marked problems (acute hypoglycaemia) in only a few patients and serious interactions are uncommon. When a sulfonamide is first added to established treatment with a sulphonylurea, warn the patient that increased blood glucose-lowering effects, sometimes excessive, are a possibility, but that problems appear to be uncommon or rare. Nevertheless, the cautious approach would be to increase the frequency of blood glucose monitoring. In one study, co-trimoxazole did not appear to cause any significant changes in blood glucose or insulin concentrations in patients receiving **insulin**.[12] However, note that co-trimoxazole alone may rarely cause hypoglycaemia (see Mechanism above). For the interactions of trimethoprim alone, see 'Antidiabetics + Trimethoprim', p.510.

1. Lumholtz B, Siersbaek-Nielsen K, Skovsted L, Kampmann J, Hansen JM. Sulphamethizole-induced inhibition of diphenylhydantoin, tolbutamide, and warfarin metabolism. *Clin Pharmacol Ther* (1975) 17, 731–4.
2. Kristensen M, Christensen LK. Drug induced changes of the blood glucose lowering effect of oral hypoglycemic agents. *Acta Diabetol Lat* (1969) 6 (Suppl 1), 116–23.
3. Christensen LK, Hansen JM, Kristensen M. Sulphaphenazole-induced hypoglycaemic attacks in tolbutamide-treated diabetics. *Lancet* (1963) ii, 1298–1301.
4. Hellman B. Potentiating effects of drugs on the binding of glibenclamide to pancreatic beta cells. *Metabolism* (1974) 23, 839–46.
5. Veronese ME, Miners JO, Randles D, Gregov D, Birkett DJ. Validation of the tolbutamide metabolic ratio for population screening with use of sulfaphenazole to produce model phenotypic poor metabolizers. *Clin Pharmacol Ther* (1990) 47, 403–11.
6. Komatsu K, Ito K, Nakajima Y, Kanamitsu S-I, Imaoka S, Funae Y, Green CE, Tyson CA, Shimada N, Sugiyama Y. Prediction of in vivo drug-drug interactions between tolbutamide and various sulfonamides in humans based on in vitro experiments. *Drug Metab Dispos* (2000) 28, 475–81.
7. Hekimsoy Z, Biberoğlu S, Çömleçki A, Tarhan O, Mermut C, Biberoğlu K. Trimethoprim-sulfamethoxazole-induced hypoglycemia in a malnourished patient with severe infection. *Eur J Endocrinol* (1997) 136, 304–6.
8. Mathews WA, Manint JE, Kleiss J. Trimethoprim-sulfamethoxazole-induced hypoglycemia as a cause of altered mental status in an elderly patient. *J Am Board Fam Pract* (2000) 13, 211–12.
9. Lee AJ, Maddix DS. Trimethoprim/sulfamethoxazole-induced hypoglycemia in a patient with acute renal failure. *Ann Pharmacother* (1997) 31, 727–32.
10. Rutschmann OT, Wicki J, Micheli P, Kondo Oestreicher M, Guillermin Spahr ML, Droz M. Co-trimoxazole administration: a rare cause of hypoglycemia in elderly persons. *Schweiz Med Wochenschr* (1998) 128, 1171–4.
11. Johnson JA, Kappel JE, Sharif MN. Hypoglycemia secondary to trimethoprim/sulfamethoxazole administration in a renal transplant patient. *Ann Pharmacother* (1993) 27, 304–6.
12. Mihic M, Mautner LS, Feness JZ, Grant K. Effect of trimethoprim-sulfamethoxazole on blood insulin and glucose concentrations of diabetics. *Can Med Assoc J* (1975), 112, 80S–82S.

Antidiabetics + Terbinafine

Terbinafine is reported not to interact with tolbutamide, and did not affect glucose control in a study in patients treated with insulin or oral antidiabetics.

Clinical evidence

A large-scale post-marketing survey did not find any interaction in patients taking terbinafine with **tolbutamide** [number unknown].[1] In a 154 patient subgroup of this survey no additional risk was noted in patients taking antidiabetics with terbinafine.[2] In a clinical trial in 89 patients with diabetes and toenail fungal infections, oral terbinafine 250 mg daily for 12 weeks had no effect on blood glucose levels in 83% of patients. Eleven (12.4%) of the patients had an elevated blood glucose level at baseline, which was normal at the end of the study, and 4 patients had a normal baseline blood glucose, which became elevated at the end of the study. No episodes of hypoglycaemia were reported. Patients in this study were treated with **insulin** or **oral antidiabetics** (not specified).[3]

Mechanism

On the basis of studies with human liver microsomes, terbinafine is unlikely to alter the metabolism of tolbutamide.[4]

Importance and management

Terbinafine does not appear to interact with tolbutamide or affect glucose control in patients treated with insulin or oral antidiabetics. No special precautions are required on concurrent use.

1. Hall M, Monka C, Krupp P, O'Sullivan D. Safety of oral terbinafine. Results of a postmarketing surveillance study in 25 884 patients. *Arch Dermatol* (1997) 133, 1213–19.
2. O'Sullivan DP, Needham CA, Bangs A, Atkin K, Kendall FD. Postmarketing surveillance of oral terbinafine in the UK: report of a large cohort study. *Br J Clin Pharmacol* (1996) 42, 559–65.
3. Farkas B, Paul C, Dobozy A, Hunyadi J, Horváth A, Fekete G. Terbinafine (Lamisil®) treatment of toenail onychomycosis in patients with insulin-dependent and non-insulin-dependent diabetes mellitus: a multicentre trial. *Br J Dermatol* (2002) 146, 254–60.
4. Back DJ, Stevenson P, Tjia JF. Comparative effects of two antimycotic agents, ketoconazole and terbinafine, on the metabolism of tolbutamide, ethinyloestradiol, cyclosporin and ethoxycoumarin by human liver microsomes *in vitro*. *Br J Clin Pharmacol* (1989) 28, 166–70.

Antidiabetics + Tetracyclines

A few early reports indicated that the blood glucose-lowering effects of insulin and the sulphonylureas may sometimes be increased by oxytetracycline. There is also a case of hypoglycaemia involving insulin and doxycycline. Phenformin-induced lactic acidosis may be precipitated by tetracyclines.

Clinical evidence

(a) Insulin

A diabetic with poorly controlled blood glucose levels needed a marked reduction in his insulin dosage from 208 to 64 units daily in order to control the hypoglycaemia that developed when **oxytetracycline** 250 mg four times daily was given. This reaction was also seen when the patient was given a second course of antibacterials, and in another patient.[1] A report briefly lists a case of hypoglycaemia when a patient receiving insulin was given **doxycycline**,[2] and another case describes doxycycline-induced hypoglycaemia in an elderly diabetic patient treated by diet alone.[3]

(b) Phenformin

There are now at least 6 cases on record of lactic-acidosis in patients taking phenformin that were apparently precipitated by the concurrent use of **tetracycline**.[4-7]

(c) Sulphonylureas

Marked hypoglycaemia occurred in an elderly patient taking **tolbutamide** when **oxytetracycline** was given,[8] and another study in diabetic patients similarly found that **oxytetracycline** could reduce blood glucose levels.[9] The half-life of **glymidine** has been found to be prolonged from 4.6 to 7.6 hours by **doxycycline**,[10] whereas a brief comment in another report

Table 13.3 Interactions between antidiabetics and sulfonamides

Drugs	*Information documented*	*Refs*
Chlorpropamide		
+ sulfafurazole (sulfisoxazole)	1 case of acute hypoglycaemia	1
+ sulfadimidine	1 case of acute hypoglycaemia	2
+ co-trimoxazole	2 cases of acute hypoglycaemia	3, 4
Glibenclamide		
+ co-trimoxazole	In a large review of glibenclamide-associated hypoglycaemia 6 of 57 patients were also taking co-trimoxazole	5
	1 case of hypoglycaemia	6
	No pharmacokinetic interaction in 8 patients	7
Glibornuride		
+ sulfaphenazole	Half-life increased by 34% in 4 subjects (2 diabetic, 2 healthy)	8
Gliclazide		
+ co-trimoxazole	4 cases of acute hypoglycaemia	6
Glipizide		
+ co-trimoxazole	1 case of acute hypoglycaemia	9
	No pharmacokinetic interaction, or change in blood glucose-lowering effects in 8 healthy subjects	10
Insulin		
+ co-trimoxazole	No overall changes in blood glucose or insulin concentrations in 8 patients	11
Tolbutamide		
+ co-trimoxazole	Clearance of intravenous tolbutamide reduced by 25%, half-life increased by 30% in 7 healthy subjects	12
+ sulfafurazole (sulfisoxazole)	3 cases of severe hypoglycaemia	13, 14
	No pharmacokinetic interaction	15, 16
+ sulfamethizole	Half-life of tolbutamide increased 60%. Metabolic clearance reduced by about 40%	17
+ sulfaphenazole	Two cases of severe hypoglycaemia	16
	Half-life of tolbutamide increased three to sixfold	15, 16, 18, 19, 20
+ sulfadiazine	Half-life of tolbutamide increased by about 57%	18
+ sulfadimethoxine	No pharmacokinetic interaction	15, 16
+ sulfamethoxazole	Clearance reduced 14%, half-life increased 20% after intravenous use	12
	Half-life increased by about 65%	15
+ sulfamethoxypyridazine	No pharmacokinetic interaction	16
Unnamed sulphonylurea		
+ co-trimoxazole	1 case of acute hypoglycaemia	11

1. Tucker HSG, Hirsch JI. Sulfonamide-sulfonylurea interaction. *N Engl J Med* (1972) 286, 110–11.
2. Dall JLC, Conway H, McAlpine SG. Hypoglycaemia due to chlorpropamide. *Scott Med J* (1967) 12, 403–4.
3. Ek I. Långvarigt klorpropamidutlöst hypoglykemitillstand Låkemedelsinteraktion? *Lakartidningen* (1974) 71, 2597–8.
4. Baciewicz AM, Swafford WB. Hypoglycemia induced by the interaction of chlorpropamide and co-trimoxazole. *Drug Intell Clin Pharm* (1984) 18, 309–10.
5. Asplund K, Wiholm B-E, Lithner F. Glibenclamide-associated hypoglycaemia: a report on 57 cases. *Diabetologia* (1983) 24, 412–7.
6. Girardin E, Vial T, Pham E, Evreux J-C. Hypoglycémies induites par les sulfamides hypoglycémiants. *Ann Med Interne* (Paris) (1992) 143, 11–17.
7. Sjöberg S, Wiholm BE, Gunnarsson R, Emilsson H, Thunberg E, Christenson I, Östman J. Lack of pharmacokinetic interaction between glibenclamide and trimethoprim-sulphamethoxazole. *Diabet Med* (1987) 4, 245–7.
8. Eckhardt W, Rudolph R, Sauer H, Schubert WR, Undeutsch D. Zur pharmakologischen Interferenz von Glibornurid mit Sulfaphenazol, Phenylbutazon und Phenprocoumon beim Menschen. *Arzneimittelforschung* (1972) 22, 2212–19.
9. Johnson JF, Dobmeier ME. Symptomatic hypoglycemia secondary to a glipizide-trimethoprim/sulfamethoxazole drug interaction. *DICP Ann Pharmacother* (1990) 24, 250–1.
10. Kradjan WA, Witt DM, Opheim KE, Wood FC. Lack of interaction between glipizide and co-trimoxazole. *J Clin Pharmacol* (1994) 34, 997–1002.
11. Mihic M, Mautner LS, Feness JZ, Grant K. Effect of trimethoprim-sulfamethoxazole on blood insulin and glucose concentrations of diabetics. *Can Med Assoc J* (1975), 112, 80S–82S.
12. Wing LMH, Miners JO. Cotrimoxazole as an inhibitor of oxidative drug metabolism: effects of trimethoprim and sulphamethoxazole separately and combined on tolbutamide disposition. *Br J Clin Pharmacol* (1985) 20, 482–5.

Continued

Table 13.3 Interactions between antidiabetics and sulfonamides (continued)

13. Soeldner JS, Steinke J. Hypoglycemia in tolbutamide-treated diabetes. *JAMA* (1965) 193, 148–9.
14. Robinson DS. The application of basic principles of drug interaction to clinical practice. *J Urol* (1975) 113, 100–107.
15. Dubach UC, Buckert A, Raaflaub J. Einfluss von Sulfonamiden auf die blutzuckersenkende Wirkung oraler Antidiabetica. *Schweiz Med Wochenschr* (1966) 96, 1483–6.
16. Christensen LK, Hansen JM, Kristensen M. Sulphaphenazole-induced hypoglycaemic attacks in tolbutamide-treated diabetics. *Lancet* (1963) ii, 1298–1301.
17. Lumholtz B, Siersbaek-Nielsen K, Skovsted L, Kampmann J, Hansen JM. Sulphamethizole-induced inhibition of diphenylhydantoin, tolbutamide, and warfarin metabolism. *Clin Pharmacol Ther* (1975) 17, 731–4.
18. Kristensen M, Christensen LK. Drug induced changes of the blood glucose lowering effect of oral hypoglycemic agents. *Acta Diabetol Lat* (1969) 6 (Suppl 1), 116–23.
19. Back DJ, Tjia J, Mönig H, Ohnhaus EE, Park BK. Selective inhibition of drug oxidation after simultaneous administration of two probe drugs, antipyrine and tolbutamide. *Eur J Clin Pharmacol* (1988) 34, 157–63.
20. Veronese ME, Miners JO, Randles D, Gregov D, Birkett DJ. Validation of the tolbutamide metabolic ratio for population screening with use of sulfaphenazole to produce model phenotypic poor metabolizers. *Clin Pharmacol Ther* (1990) 47, 403–11.

suggests that **demeclocycline** and **doxycycline** may not affect **chlorpropamide** disposition.[11]

Mechanism

Not understood. Several mechanisms have been suggested including prolongation of the half-life of insulin and interference with adrenaline-induced glycaemia.[3]

Importance and management

Information about the interactions between the sulphonylureas or insulin and the tetracyclines is very limited indeed, and clinically important interactions appear to be very uncommon. Concurrent use need not be avoided, but be aware of this interaction in case of an unexpected response to treatment.

Phenformin was withdrawn in some countries because it was associated with a high incidence of lactic acidosis; where available, concurrent use with tetracyclines should be avoided. However, there is nothing to suggest that there is an increased risk if tetracyclines are given with **metformin**.

1. Miller JB. Hypoglycaemic effect of oxytetracycline. *BMJ* (1966) 2, 1007.
2. New Zealand Committee on Adverse Drug Reactions. Ninth Annual Report. *N Z Dent J* (1975) 71, 28–32.
3. Odeh M, Oliven A. Doxycycline-induced hypoglycemia. *J Clin Pharmacol* (2000) 40, 1173–4.
4. Aro A, Korhonen T, Halinen M. Phenformin-induced lacticacidosis precipitated by tetracycline. *Lancet* (1978) 1, 673–4.
5. Tashima CK. Phenformin, tetracycline, and lactic acidosis. *BMJ* (1971) 4, 557–8.
6. Blumenthal SA, Streeten DHP. Phenformin-related lactic acidosis in a thirty-year-old man. *Ann Intern Med* (1976) 84, 55–6.
7. Phillips PJ, Pain RW. Phenformin, tetracycline and lactic acidosis. *Ann Intern Med* (1977) 86, 111.
8. Hiatt N, Bonorris G. Insulin response in pancreatectomized dogs treated with oxytetracycline. *Diabetes* (1970) 19, 307–10.
9. Sen S, Mukerjee AB. Hypoglycaemic action of oxytetracycline. A preliminary study. *J Indian Med Assoc* (1969) 52, 366–9.
10. Held H, Kaminski B, von Olderhausen HF. Die beeinflussung der Elimination von Glycodiazin durch Leber- und Nierenfunctionssorungen und durch eine Behandlung mit Phenylbutazon, Phenprocoumarol und Doxycyclin. *Diabetologia* (1970) 6, 386.
11. Petitpierre B, Perrin L, Rudhardt M, Herrera A, Fabre J. Behaviour of chlorpropamide in renal insufficiency and under the effect of associated drug therapy. *Int J Clin Pharmacol* (1972) 6, 120–24.

Antidiabetics + Thioctic acid

Thioctic acid is reported not to interact with acarbose, metformin or glibenclamide (glyburide).

Clinical evidence, mechanism, importance and management

A study in 24 healthy subjects given tablets containing thioctic acid 200 mg and **metformin** 500 mg found that the pharmacokinetics of the **metformin** were unchanged by the presence of the thioctic acid, and the authors of the report say that there was also no pharmacodynamic interaction.[1] The report gives very few details. A further study in 24 healthy subjects found that a single 600-mg dose of thioctic acid given with **glibenclamide (glyburide)** 3.5 mg did not result in any clinically relevant pharmacokinetic interaction, and thioctic acid did not alter the effect of **glibenclamide** on glucose or insulin levels.[2] Similarly, there was no evidence of a change in thioctic acid pharmacokinetics or pharmacodynamics when it was given to healthy subjects with **acarbose**.[2]

No special precautions seem to be required if thioctic acid is given to patients taking **acarbose**, **metformin** or **glibenclamide**.

1. Schug BS, Schneider E, Elze M, Fieger-Büschges H, Larsimont V, Popescu G, Molz KH, Blume HH, Hermann R. Study of pharmacokinetic interaction of thioctic acid and metformin. *Eur J Clin Pharmacol* (1997) 52 (Suppl), A140.
2. Gleiter CH, Schreeb KH, Freudenthaler S, Thomas M, Elze M, Fieger-Büschges H, Potthast H, Schneider E, Schug BS, Blume HH, Hermann R. Lack of interaction between thioctic acid, glibenclamide and acarbose. *Br J Clin Pharmacol* (1999) 48, 819–25.

Antidiabetics + Tibolone

Tibolone may slightly impair glucose tolerance and therefore possibly reduce the effects of the antidiabetics.

Clinical evidence, mechanism, importance and management

One woman developed diabetes 14 weeks after starting tibolone 2.5 mg daily. However, she had a high normal fasting blood glucose level before starting tibolone, and the diabetes did not resolve on withdrawing the drug.[1] The manufacturers of tibolone noted that on their adverse drug event database they had only 3 cases of diabetes occurring during the use of tibolone, and 3 cases of aggravation of diabetes during its use, which they considered a very low number in relation to the extent of tibolone use.[2]

A metabolic study in 10 women with type 2 diabetes given tibolone 2.5 mg daily and stabilised with diet and oral antidiabetics found there were no changes in glycaemic control, as measured by glycosylated haemoglobin levels.[3] Conversely, a longer 12-month study in 14 women with type 2 diabetes given tibolone found a slight deterioration in glycaemic control (as measured by serum fructosamine),[4] and an early study found that tibolone caused a slight decrease in glucose tolerance in non-diabetic patients.[5]

The manufacturers of tibolone say that patients with diabetes should be closely supervised.[6,7] It would therefore seem prudent to increase the frequency of blood glucose monitoring if tibolone is started or stopped.

1. Konstantopoulos K, Adamides S. A case of diabetes following tibolone therapy. *Maturitas* (1994) 19, 77–8.
2. Atsma WJ. Is Livial diabetogenic? *Maturitas* (1994) 19, 239–40.
3. Feher MD, Cox A, Levy A, Mayne P, Lant AF. Short term blood pressure and metabolic effects of tibolone in postmenopausal women with non-insulin dependent diabetes. *Br J Obstet Gynaecol* (1996) 103, 281–3.
4. Prelevic GM, Beljic T, Balint-Peric L, Ginsburg J. Metabolic effects of tibolone in postmenopausal women with non-insulin dependent diabetes mellitus. *Maturitas* (1998) 28, 271–6.
5. Crona N, Silfverstolpe G, Samsioe G. A double-blind cross-over study on the effects of ORG OD14 compared to oestradiol valerate and placebo on lipid and carbohydrate metabolism in oophorectomized women. *Acta Endocrinol (Copenh)* (1983) 102, 451–5.
6. Livial (Tibolone). Organon Laboratories Ltd. UK Summary of product characteristics, May 2006.
7. Livial (Tibolone). Organon. US Prescribing information, January 2007.

Antidiabetics + Tobacco or Nicotine

Diabetics who smoke tobacco may need more subcutaneous insulin than non-smokers. Smoking or, to a lesser extent, nicotine patches may increase insulin resistance, and stopping smoking can improve glycaemic control in both type 1 and type 2 diabetics. However, the effects of smoking on diabetes appear to be complex, as some studies have reported that smoking does not affect insulin sensitivity or glycaemic control. Preliminary evidence shows that smoking increases the absorption of inhaled insulin.

Clinical evidence, mechanism, importance and management

A study in 163 patients with type 1 diabetes found that, on average, the 114 who smoked needed 15 to 20% more subcutaneous **insulin** than the non-smokers, and up to 30% more **insulin** if they smoked heavily.[1] Possible mechanisms include decreased absorption of **insulin** from the subcutaneous tissue because of peripheral vasoconstriction,[2] and a significant rise (40 to 100%) in the levels of the hormones that oppose the actions of **insulin**.[3,4]

Serum **insulin** levels during the first 6 hours after inhaled **insulin** were 58% higher in smokers than in non-smokers, and peak **insulin** levels were about threefold higher. Minor hypoglycaemia requiring a glucose infusion occurred in 12 smokers but in only one non-smoker. The increased absorption was possibly due to cigarette smoke increasing the permeability of the alveolar-capillary barrier.[5] It should be noted that use of inhaled **insulin** is contraindicated in patients who smoke, or have smoked within the past 6 months.[6]

In a double-blind, crossover study in 12 smokers with type 2 diabetes, stabilised with diet alone or with **oral antidiabetics**, the effect of smoking one cigarette every hour for 6 hours compared with transdermal nicotine (30 cm^2 patch) or a placebo patch. Cigarette smoking and the nicotine patch did not affect endogenous insulin secretion, when compared with placebo, but smoking impaired peripheral insulin action, and resulted in lower rates of glucose utilisation and greater hepatic glucose production. The nicotine patch similarly impaired insulin action, but this was much less pronounced than after cigarette smoking, possibly due to the lower plasma levels of nicotine attained with the patch.[7]

In another study, glycaemic control (as measured by glycosylated haemoglobin) was modestly improved in 7 subjects with type 1 diabetes and 27 subjects with type 2 diabetes, one year after they had stopped smoking. This improved control was considered clinically significant.[8] In a study in patients with type 2 diabetes stabilised with diet alone or diet plus **sulphonylureas** with or without **metformin**, insulin resistance was higher in the 28 smokers than the 12 non-smokers.[9] Further studies have reported that smoking in diabetics is associated with poor glycaemic control,[10] microalbuminuria,[10] and impaired insulin clearance.[11] However, other studies have suggested that smoking does not affect **insulin** requirement in type 1 diabetics[12] or have a significant effect on glycaemic control in type 1 or type 2 diabetics.[3,12,13] There are numerous other studies on the relationship between smoking and diabetes or insulin resistance in non-diabetics, and only a few are cited here as examples. Some studies have indicated that smoking could increase the risk of type 2 diabetes (relative risk of 2.6) and that tobacco use is associated with a low insulin response.[14] However, other studies suggest that a causal relationship between smoking and insulin resistance is unlikely,[15,16] although in one of the studies[16] exposure to environmental tobacco smoke was associated with lower insulin sensitivity.

Glycaemic control is not the only factor of importance with smoking in diabetics. Cigarette smoking may also accelerate progression of atherosclerosis, increase blood pressure, and increase macrovascular complications.[7,16,17] Diabetics who smoke should be given all the help they need to stop smoking.[10,17]

1. Madsbad S, McNair P, Christensen MS, Christiansen C, Faber OK, Binder C, Transbøl I. Influence of smoking on insulin requirement and metabolic status in diabetes mellitus. *Diabetes Care* (1980) 3, 41–3.
2. Klemp P, Staberg B, Madsbad S, Kølendorf K. Smoking reduces insulin absorption from subcutaneous tissue. *BMJ* (1982) 284, 237.
3. Helve E, Yki-Järvinen H, Koivisto VA. Smoking and insulin sensitivity in type I diabetic patients. *Metabolism* (1986) 35, 874–7.
4. Chiodera P, Volpi R, Capretti L, Speroni G, Necchi-Ghiri S, Caffarri G, Colla R, Coiro V. Abnormal effect of cigarette smoking on pituitary hormone secretions in insulin-dependent diabetes mellitus. *Clin Endocrinol (Oxf)* (1997) 46, 351–7.
5. Himmelmann A, Jendle J, Mellén A, Petersen AH, Dahl UL, Wollmer P. The impact of smoking on inhaled insulin. *Diabetes Care* (2003) 26, 677–82.
6. Exubera (Insulin, human) Pfizer Ltd. UK Summary of product characteristics, April 2006.
7. Epifano L, Di Vincenzo A, Fanelli C, Porcellati F, Perriello G, De Feo P, Motolese M, Brunetti P, Bolli GB. Effect of cigarette smoking and of a transdermal nicotine delivery system on glucoregulation in type 2 diabetes mellitus. *Eur J Clin Pharmacol* (1992) 43, 257–63.
8. Gunton JE, Davies L, Wilmshurst E, Fulcher G, McElduff A. Cigarette smoking affects glycemic control in diabetes. *Diabetes Care* (2002) 25, 796–7.
9. Targher G, Alberiche M, Zenere MB, Bonadonna RC, Muggeo M, Bonora E. Cigarette smoking and insulin resistance in patients with noninsulin-dependent diabetes mellitus. *J Clin Endocrinol Metab* (1997) 82, 3619–24.
10. Nilsson PM, Gudbjörnsdottir S, Eliasson B, Cederholm J, for the Steering Committee of the Swedish National Diabetes Register. Smoking is associated with increased HbA_{1c} values and microalbuminuria in patients with diabetes – data from the National Diabetes Register in Sweden. *Diabetes Metab* (2004) 30, 261–8.
11. Bott S, Shafagoj YA, Sawicki PT, Heise T. Impact of smoking on the metabolic action of subcutaneous regular insulin in type 2 diabetic patients. *Horm Metab Res* (2005) 37, 445–9.
12. Mathiesen ER, Søegaard U, Christiansen JS. Smoking and glycaemic control in male insulin dependent (type 1) diabetics. *Diabetes Res* (1984) 1, 155–7.
13. McCulloch P, Lee S, Higgins R, McCall K, Schade DS. Effect of smoking on hemoglobin A_{1c} and body mass index in patients with type 2 diabetes mellitus. *J Investig Med* (2002) 50, 284–7.
14. Persson P-G, Carlsson S, Svanström L, Östenson C-G, Efendic S, Grill V. Cigarette smoking, oral moist snuff use and glucose intolerance. *J Intern Med* (2000) 248, 103–110.
15. Wareham NJ, Ness EM, Byrne CD, Cox BD, Day NE, Hales CN. Cigarette smoking is not associated with hyperinsulinemia: evidence against a causal relationship between smoking and insulin resistance. *Metabolism* (1996) 45, 1551–6.
16. Henkin L, Zaccaro D, Haffner S, Karter A, Rewers M, Sholinsky P, Wagenknecht L. Cigarette smoking, environmental tobacco smoke exposure and insulin sensitivity: the Insulin Resistance Atherosclerosis Study. *Ann Epidemiol* (1999) 9, 290–6.
17. American Diabetes Association. Smoking and diabetes. *Diabetes Care* (2004) 27 (Suppl 1), S74–S75.

Antidiabetics + Tricyclic and related antidepressants

Interactions between antidiabetics and tricyclic or tetracyclic antidepressants appear to be rare, but four isolated cases of hypoglycaemia have been reported.

Clinical evidence, mechanism, importance and management

A study in 4 patients suggested that **amitriptyline** 75 mg daily for 9 days did not affect the half-life of a single 500-mg dose of **tolbutamide**.[1] Although there is some evidence of a change in glucose metabolism during treatment with **mianserin**,[2-4] the alteration failed to affect the control of diabetes in a study in 10 patients and there appear to be no reports of adverse effects caused by concurrent use.[3] In contrast there are four case reports describing interactions:

- A patient taking **tolazamide** became hypoglycaemic 11 days after starting to take **doxepin** 250 mg daily. The patient was eventually stabilised on a daily dose of **tolazamide** that was only 10% of that used before the **doxepin** was given.[5]
- A patient taking **chlorpropamide** (initially 25 mg increased to 75 mg daily) developed marked hypoglycaemia 3 days after starting **nortriptyline** 125 mg daily. The **chlorpropamide** was stopped.[5]
- A patient receiving **insulin** developed violent and agitated behaviour (but no adrenergic symptoms) and hypoglycaemia when she started to take **amitriptyline** 25 mg at bedtime.[6]
- An elderly diabetic woman taking **glibenclamide (glyburide)** and **phenformin** developed hypoglycaemia when given **maprotiline**. She was restabilised on half the dose of **glibenclamide** and **phenformin**.[7]

Apart from these isolated cases[5-7] the literature seems to be silent about interactions between these antidiabetics and the tricyclic or tetracyclic antidepressants. Bearing in mind the length of time these groups of drugs have been available, the risk of a clinically important interaction would seem to be very small.

1. Pond SM, Graham GG, Birkett DJ, Wade DN. Effects of tricyclic antidepressants on drug metabolism. *Clin Pharmacol Ther* (1975) 18, 191–9.
2. Fell PJ, Quantock DC, van der Burg WJ. The human pharmacology of GB94–a new psychotropic agent. *Eur J Clin Pharmacol* (1973) 5, 166–73.
3. Peet M, Behagel H. Mianserin: a decade of scientific development. *Br J Clin Pharmacol* (1978) 5, 5S–9S.
4. Brogden RN, Heel RC, Speight TM, Avery GS. Mianserin: a review of its pharmacological properties and therapeutic efficacy in depressive illness. *Drugs* (1978) 16, 273–301.
5. True BL, Perry PJ, Burns EA. Profound hypoglycemia with the addition of a tricyclic antidepressant to maintenance sulfonylurea therapy. *Am J Psychiatry* (1987) 144, 1220–1.
6. Sherman KE, Bornemann M. Amitriptyline and asymptomatic hypoglycemia. *Ann Intern Med* (1988) 109, 683–4.
7. Zogno MG, Tolfo L, Draghi E. Hypoglycemia caused by maprotiline in a patient taking oral antidiabetics. *Ann Pharmacother* (1994) 28, 406.

Antidiabetics + Trimethoprim

Trimethoprim increases the AUC of repaglinide and would be expected to increase its effects in some patients. The effect of trimethoprim on the AUC of rosiglitazone is more modest and less likely to be clinically relevant. Trimethoprim does not appear to significantly affect the pharmacokinetics of intravenous tolbutamide.

Clinical evidence

(a) Repaglinide

In a study in 9 healthy subjects trimethoprim 160 mg twice daily for 3 days increased the AUC and the maximum plasma level of a single 250-microgram dose of repaglinide by 61% and 41%, respectively. However, the blood glucose-lowering effect of repaglinide was unchanged.[1]

(b) Rosiglitazone

In a study in 10 healthy subjects trimethoprim 160 mg twice daily for 4 days increased the AUC of a single 4-mg dose of rosiglitazone given on day 3 by 37%. The half-life of rosiglitazone was increased by 26% but the peak plasma level was only slightly affected (14% increase).[2] Similarly, in another study, trimethoprim 200 mg twice daily for 5 days increased the AUC of a single 8-mg dose of rosiglitazone by 31% and increased the half-life by 27%.[3]

(c) Tolbutamide

Trimethoprim 150 mg twice daily for 7 days prolonged the elimination half-life of a single intravenous 500-mg dose of tolbutamide by 19% in a study in 7 healthy subjects.[4]

Mechanism

Data suggest that trimethoprim inhibits the metabolism of repaglinide and rosiglitazone by the cytochrome P450 isoenzyme CYP2C8. Tolbutamide is metabolised by CYP2C9, and it is thought possible that trimethoprim may have a slight inhibitory effect on this isoenzyme, although there is very little information about this.[5]

Importance and management

The clinical relevance of the pharmacokinetic changes have not been assessed. However, the changes seen with repaglinide suggest that some patients might experience an increase in the effects of this drug. The UK manufacturers of repaglinide[6] suggest that the concurrent use of trimethoprim should be avoided as the effect of larger doses of both drugs are unknown. The US manufacturers suggest that repaglinide dosage adjustments may be necessary.[7] If both drugs are used it would seem prudent to increase the frequency of blood glucose monitoring until the effects are known.

The more modest increase in AUC of rosiglitazone is less likely to be clinically important, but, until more experience is gained, some caution is warranted. No interaction would be expected between trimethoprim and tolbutamide, although note that co-trimoxazole has rarely caused hypoglycaemia alone or combined with various sulphonylureas, see 'Antidiabetics + Sulfonamides', p.506.

1. Niemi M, Kajosaari LI, Neuvonen M, Backman JT, Neuvonen PJ. The CYP2C8 inhibitor trimethoprim increases the plasma concentrations of repaglinide in healthy subjects. *Br J Clin Pharmacol* (2003) 57, 441–7.
2. Niemi M, Backman JT, Neuvonen PJ. Effects of trimethoprim and rifampin on the pharmacokinetics of the cytochrome P450 2C8 substrate rosiglitazone. *Clin Pharmacol Ther* (2004) 76, 239–49.
3. Hruska MW, Amico JA, Langaee TY, Ferrell RE, Fitzgerald SM, Frye RF. The effect of trimethoprim on CYP2C8 mediated rosiglitazone metabolism in human liver microsomes and healthy subjects. *Br J Clin Pharmacol* (2005) 59, 70–9.
4. Wing LMH, Miners JO. Cotrimoxazole as an inhibitor of oxidative drug metabolism: effects of trimethoprim and sulphamethoxazole separately and combined on tolbutamide disposition. *Br J Clin Pharmacol* (1985) 20, 482–5.
5. Wen X, Wang J-S, Backman JT, Laitila J, Neuvonen PJ. Trimethoprim and sulfamethoxazole are selective inhibitors of CYP2C8 and CYP2C9, respectively. *Drug Metab Dispos* (2002) 30, 631–5.
6. Prandin Tablets (Repaglinide). Daiichi Sankyo UK Ltd. UK Summary of product characteristics, October 2005.
7. Prandin Tablets (Repaglinide). Novo Nordisk Inc. US Prescribing information, June 2006.

Exenatide + Miscellaneous

The rate and extent of paracetamol (acetaminophen) absorption are reduced by exenatide, even when the paracetamol is given up to four hours after the exenatide. The manufacturer therefore recommends that exenatide be used with caution with drugs that require rapid gastrointestinal absorption or drugs that require a threshold level for efficacy (such as the oral contraceptives and some antibacterials). Further study is necessary to establish the clinical relevance of any of these potential interactions.

Clinical evidence, mechanism, importance and management

In a study using **paracetamol** (**acetaminophen**) as a marker of gastric emptying, subcutaneous exenatide 10 micrograms delayed and reduced the maximum plasma levels of **paracetamol** from 0.6 to 4.2 hours and by 37% to 56%, respectively. The overall extent of absorption was slightly reduced (14% to 24% reduction in AUC). This effect was seen when **paracetamol** was given simultaneously with exenatide, or one, two, and four hours after exenatide. It was not seen when **paracetamol** was given one hour *before* exenatide.[1]

This study demonstrates that exenatide slows gastric emptying, and has the potential to delay the absorption of other drugs. The manufacturer recommends that exenatide should be used with caution in patients receiving oral drugs that require rapid gastrointestinal absorption. They do not give any specific examples.[2] However, they do note that exenatide does not affect the absorption of **lisinopril**.

Because exenatide delays gastric emptying and may reduce the rate and extent of absorption of orally administered drugs the manufacturer suggests that it should be used with caution in patients receiving oral drugs that are dependent on threshold concentrations for efficacy. They give **antibacterials** and **oral contraceptives** as an example (but no drugs are specifically named), and recommend that they should be taken at least one hour before exenatide.[2] Whether this is clinically necessary remains to be shown.

1. Blase E, Taylor K, Gao H-y, Wintle M, Fineman M. Pharmacokinetics of an oral drug (acetaminophen) administered at various times in relation to subcutaneous injection of exenatide (exendin-4) in healthy subjects. *J Clin Pharmacol* (2005) 45, 570–7.
2. Byetta (Exenatide). Amylin Pharmaceuticals, Inc. US Prescribing information, February 2007.

Insulin + Naltrexone

The insulin requirements of a patient rose by about 30% when naltrexone was given.

Clinical evidence, mechanism, importance and management

A patient with type 1 diabetes was given naltrexone in an experimental study of the treatment of anorexia nervosa. During two periods of 5 days while taking the naltrexone (dosage not stated), the blood glucose levels of the patient remained unchanged but the **insulin** dosage requirements rose from 52.8 and 61.4 units daily to 71.4 and 76 units daily (a rise of about 30%). The reason is not known but the authors of this report point out that this apparent interaction must have been due to the actions of **insulin** rather than on its release because this patient had no endogenous insulin.[1]

The general clinical importance of this interaction is not known but it would be prudent to be alert for any evidence of increased **insulin** requirements if naltrexone is used in any patient.

1. Marrazzi MA, Jacober S, Luby ED. A naltrexone-induced increase in insulin requirement. *J Clin Psychopharmacol* (1994) 14, 363–5.

Metformin + Cefalexin

Cefalexin modestly increased the serum levels of metformin in a single-dose study.

Clinical evidence, mechanism, importance and management

In a placebo-controlled study in 12 healthy subjects cefalexin 500 mg increased the AUC and maximum serum levels of a single 500-mg dose of metformin by 24% and 34%, respectively. Cefalexin reduced the renal clearance of metformin by 14% by inhibiting metformin tubular secretion via the organic cation system.[1] The clinical relevance of these small changes is uncertain, but they could be greater with longer-term use. The authors recommend that patients receiving metformin with cefalexin should have metformin levels monitored or an alternative antibacterial to cefalexin should be considered.[1] However, based on the available evidence this seems somewhat overcautious.

1. Jayasagar G, Krishna Kumar M, Chandrasekhar K, Madhusudan Rao C, Madhusudan Rao Y. Effect of cephalexin on the pharmacokinetics of metformin in healthy human volunteers. *Drug Metabol Drug Interact* (2002) 19, 41–8.

Metformin + Iodinated contrast media

Parenteral administration of iodinated contrast media may cause renal failure, which could result in lactic acidosis in patients taking metformin.

Clinical evidence, mechanism, importance and management

Parenteral administration of iodinated contrast media to patients taking metformin may result in lactic acidosis. However, the problem is reported to occur only if the contrast media causes renal failure and metformin use is continued. This is because metformin is mainly excreted by the kidneys and in renal failure toxic levels may accumulate,[1] which may result in lactic acidosis. A literature search identified 18 cases of lactic acidosis after the use of contrast media in patients taking metformin.[2] Of these 18 cases, 14 or 15 were associated with pre-existing renal impairment and 2 cases with other contraindications to metformin (sepsis and cirrhosis). The remaining case was in an elderly woman with neurological disease.

The manufacturers of metformin say that it should be stopped before, or at the time of giving the contrast media and not restarted until 48 hours later, and then only after renal function has been re-checked and found to be normal.[3] Guidelines issued by the Royal College of Radiologists are based on this statement and they say that referring clinicians should assess renal function before the test.[4] Similar guidelines have been issued by the European Society for Urogenital medicine.[5,6] Nevertheless, some consider that metformin need not be stopped for 48 hours in those patients with normal renal function.[2] However, a more recent analysis supports the guidelines. Of 97 patients taking metformin who were given intravenous contrast media, 4 developed contrast media-associated nephropathy (all 4 had baseline normal renal function). These patients could have been at increased risk of metformin-associated lactic acidosis had the metformin not been stopped and withheld, as suggested by the guidelines.[7]

1. Rasuli P, Hammond DI. Metformin and contrast media: where is the conflict? *Can Assoc Radiol J* (1998) 49, 161–6.
2. McCartney MM, Gilbert FJ, Murchison LE, Pearson D, McHardy K, Murray AD. Metformin and contrast media – a dangerous combination? *Clin Radiol* (1999) 54, 29–33.
3. Glucophage (Metformin hydrochloride). Merck Pharmaceuticals. UK Summary of product characteristics, October 2004.
4. The Royal College of Radiologists. Guidelines with regard to metformin-induced lactic acidosis and x-ray contrast medium agents. 19th March 1999.
5. Morcos SK, Thomsen HS. European Society of Urogenital Radiology guidelines on administering contrast media. *Abdom Imaging* (2003) 28, 187–190.
6. Thomsen HS, Morcos SK. Contrast media and the kidney: European Society of Urogenital Radiology (ESUR) guidelines. *Br J Radiol* (2003) 76, 513–8.
7. Parra D, Legreid AM, Beckey NP, Reyes S. Metformin monitoring and change in serum creatinine levels in patients undergoing radiologic procedures involving administration of intravenous contrast media. *Pharmacotherapy* (2004) 24, 987–93. Erratum ibid., 1489.

Pioglitazone + Fexofenadine

A study in healthy subjects indicated that the pharmacokinetics of pioglitazone 45 mg daily are not significantly affected by fexofenadine 60 mg twice daily, and that pioglitazone does not affect the pharmacokinetics of fexofenadine.[1]

1. Robert M. Pharmacokinetics of coadministration of pioglitazone with fexofenadine. *Diabetes* (2001) 50 (Suppl 2), A443.

Pioglitazone or Rosiglitazone + Insulin

Pioglitazone and rosiglitazone may cause fluid retention and peripheral oedema, which can worsen or cause heart failure. There is evidence that the incidence of these effects is higher when combined with insulin. The incidence of hypoglycaemia may also be increased.

Clinical evidence

(a) Pioglitazone

It has been noted that in patients receiving insulin the dose may need to be reduced by 10 to 25% if pioglitazone 15 or 30 mg daily is given.[1] In one 16-week, randomised, double-blind, placebo-controlled study,[2] pioglitazone 15 or 30 mg with insulin was compared with insulin alone in 566 patients with long-standing diabetes. Oedema was reported in 15.3% of the patients receiving pioglitazone plus insulin (12.6% and 17.6% with pioglitazone 15 mg and 30 mg, respectively) compared with 7% when insulin was given alone. Four of the 379 patients given with pioglitazone and insulin developed congestive heart failure compared with none of the 187 patients given insulin alone; all 4 had a history of cardiovascular disease. Analysis of this study did not identify specific factors that predict this possible increased risk of congestive heart failure.[1] One case report describes a 57-year-old obese man with type 2 diabetes, no history of heart failure and excellent exercise tolerance, who was given insulin and pioglitazone 30 mg daily. Over the first 4 weeks after starting pioglitazone he developed significant weight gain and subsequently developed heart failure and pulmonary oedema.[3]

(b) Rosiglitazone

A randomised, double-blind, placebo-controlled study in patients with poorly-controlled type 2 diabetes receiving insulin twice daily found that the addition of rosiglitazone 2 or 4 mg twice daily for 26 weeks improved the control of their blood glucose levels and they needed less insulin.[4] Mean total daily insulin reductions were 12% for the 4 mg dose, 5.6% for the 2 mg dose, and 0.6% for placebo. Symptoms consistent with hypoglycaemia also occurred more frequently with the combination; 67% with the 4 mg rosiglitazone dose, 53% with the 2 mg dose, and 38% with placebo. The incidence of oedema was about threefold higher in those patients given insulin and rosiglitazone; 16.2% with the 4 mg dose, and 13.1% with the 2 mg dose, compared with 4.7% in those given placebo. Congestive heart failure occurred in 4 of 209 patients receiving the combination compared with 1 of 104 receiving placebo. However, 2 of the patients receiving rosiglitazone had a prior history of coronary heart disease.[4]

From results of clinical studies, the UK manufacturer has reported an incidence of heart failure of 1.1% with insulin monotherapy and 2.4% when combined with rosiglitazone.[5] In a pilot study in 8 massively obese patients with type 2 diabetes, taking large doses of insulin, the use of rosiglitazone 8 mg daily allowed a 22% reduction in the median insulin dose, and improved glycaemic control. However, 5 of the 8 patients (63%) developed peripheral oedema.[6] One case report described 2 patients receiving insulin who developed congestive heart failure 6 to 12 months after starting rosiglitazone. They recovered when rosiglitazone was withdrawn and diuretic doses increased.[7] Another patient taking metformin, glimepiride, rosiglitazone and insulin unusually developed unilateral oedema 2 years after starting rosiglitazone, which resolved on stopping the rosiglitazone, and reappeared within 5 days of restarting it.[8]

Mechanism

Pioglitazone or rosiglitazone alone can exacerbate or precipitate heart failure because they can cause fluid retention and weight gain.[1,5,9,10] The incidence appears to be greatly increased in patients who are also receiving insulin. An estimated 2 to 5% of patients receiving thiazolidinedione monotherapy and 5 to 15% receiving concurrent insulin therapy experience peripheral oedema.[11] Fluid retention and tissue oedema appear to be part of a vascular 'leak' syndrome but, additionally, thiazolidinediones may potentiate the renal effects of insulin on sodium and water retention. It is conceivable that increased fluid retention caused by thiazolidinediones may alter the already precarious volume status in patients with underlying cardiac or renal dysfunction thus leading to congestive heart failure.[11] However, congestive heart failure has been estimated to occur in as many as 12% of patients who have type 2 diabetes[11] and whether the incidence of heart failure in patients given thiazolidinediones and insulin is simply a reflection of other factors that increase the risk in these patients, or due to some specific interaction with insulin, remains to be established.

Importance and management

The fact that rosiglitazone and pioglitazone can cause weight gain and peripheral oedema, and that the incidence of this is greater in patients who are also using insulin is well established. However, the relevance of this appears to be controversial. In the UK, the manufacturers of the combination product of rosiglitazone with metformin[12] caution the concurrent use of insulin, however rosiglitazone itself is still contraindicated[5] (although note that the summary of product characteristics for rosiglitazone with metformin has been updated more recently. However, in the US both rosiglitazone[10] and pioglitazone[1] are licensed for use with insulin, and in the UK pioglitazone is licensed for use with insulin.[9] The American Heart Association and American Diabetes Association have issued guidelines on the use of thiazolidinediones which take into account risk factors for, or severity of, heart failure. Pioglitazone or rosiglitazone may be used cautiously at low dosage in patients with symptomatic heart disease (New York Heart Association (NYHA) class I or II), but should not be used in patients with class III or IV cardiac functional status. If oedema occurs in a patient taking a thiazolidinedione they recommend that the possible causes be assessed. If symptoms and signs suggest congestive heart failure, they recommend that a dosage change and temporary or permanent discontinuance of the thiazolidinedione should be considered. If there is no evidence of heart failure, they suggest that the thiazolidinedione may be continued, with consideration of dosage reduction or addition of diuretics, and with continued observation of the oedema.[13]

1. Actos (Pioglitazone hydrochloride). Takeda Pharmaceuticals Company Ltd. US Prescribing information, February 2007.
2. Rosenstock J, Einhorn D, Hershon K, Glazer NB, Yu S; Pioglitazone 014 Study Group. Efficacy and safety of pioglitazone in type 2 diabetes: a randomised, placebo-controlled study in patients receiving stable insulin therapy. *Int J Clin Pract* (2002) 56, 251–7.
3. Cheng AYY, Fantus IG. Thiazolidinedione-induced congestive heart failure. *Ann Pharmacother* (2004) 38, 817–20.
4. Raskin P, Rendell M, Riddle MC, Dole JF, Freed MI, Rosenstock J; Rosiglitazone Clinical Trials Study Group. A randomized trial of rosiglitazone therapy in patients with inadequately controlled insulin-treated type 2 diabetes. *Diabetes Care* (2001) 24, 1226–32.
5. Avandia (Rosiglitazone maleate). GlaxoSmithKline UK. UK Summary of product characteristics, May 2007.
6. Buch HN, Baskar V, Barton DM, Kamalakannan D, Akarca C, Singh BM. Combination of insulin and thiazolidinedione therapy in massively obese patients with type 2 diabetes. *Diabet Med* (2002) 19, 572–4.
7. Singh N. Rosiglitazone and heart failure: long-term vigilance. *J Cardiovasc Pharmacol Ther* (2004) 9, 21–5.
8. Bell DSH. Unilateral edema due to a thiazolidinedione. *Diabetes Care* (2003) 26, 2700.
9. Actos (Pioglitazone hydrochloride). Takeda UK Ltd. UK Summary of product characteristics, January 2007.
10. Avandia (Rosiglitazone maleate). GlaxoSmithKline. US Prescribing information, June 2007.
11. Scheen AJ. Combined thiazolidinedione-insulin therapy. Should we be concerned about safety? *Drug Safety* (2004) 27, 841–56.
12. Avandamet (Rosiglitazone/Metformin). GlaxoSmithKline UK. UK Summary of product characteristics, June 2007.
13. Nesto RW, Bell D, Bonow RO, Fonseca V, Grundy SM, Horton ES, Le Winter M, Porte D, Semenkovich CF, Smith S, Young LH, Kahn R. Thiazolidinedione use, fluid retention, and congestive heart failure: a consensus statement from the American Heart Association and American Diabetes Association. *Circulation* (2003) 108, 2941–8.

Pioglitazone or Rosiglitazone + Other oral antidiabetics

The pharmacokinetics of metformin are not altered by pioglitazone or rosiglitazone. Pioglitazone does not alter glipizide pharmacokinetics. Rosiglitazone does not have an important effect on glibenclamide (glyburide) pharmacokinetics, and does not alter glimepiride pharmacokinetics.

Clinical evidence, mechanism, importance and management

(a) Metformin

In healthy subjects, **pioglitazone** 45 mg daily for 7 days did not alter the pharmacokinetics of a single 1-g dose of metformin.[1,2]

The steady-state pharmacokinetics of metformin 500 mg twice daily and **rosiglitazone** 2 mg twice daily were not affected when they were given to healthy subjects for 4 days.[3,4]

No special precautions appear to be needed if metformin is used with the thiazolidinediones.

(b) Sulphonylureas

In healthy subjects, **pioglitazone** 45 mg daily for 7 days did not alter the steady-state pharmacokinetics of **glipizide** 5 mg daily.[1,2]

Rosiglitazone 2 mg twice daily for 7 days did not alter the mean steady-state 24-hour plasma glucose levels in diabetics taking **glibenclamide (glyburide)** 3.75 to 10 mg daily. However, **rosiglitazone** 8 mg daily for 8 days caused a decrease of about 30% in the AUC of **glibenclamide** in healthy Caucasian subjects, and a slight increase in the AUC of **glibenclamide** in Japanese subjects.[3] These changes are not considered clinically relevant.[3,5] No pharmacokinetic interaction appears to occur between **glimepiride** and **rosiglitazone**.[3]

No special precautions appear to be needed if these sulphonylureas are used with the thiazolidinediones.

1. Actos (Pioglitazone hydrochloride). Takeda Pharmaceuticals Company Ltd. US Prescribing information, February 2007.
2. Kortboyer JM, Eckland DJA. Pioglitazone has low potential for drug interactions. *Diabetologia* (1999) 42 (Suppl 1), A228.
3. Avandia (Rosiglitazone maleate). GlaxoSmithKline. US Prescribing information, June 2007.
4. Di Cicco RA, Allen A, Carr A, Fowles S, Jorkasky DK, Freed MI. Rosiglitazone does not alter the pharmacokinetics of metformin. *J Clin Pharmacol* (2000) 40, 1280–5.
5. Avandia (Rosiglitazone maleate). GlaxoSmithKline UK. UK Summary of product characteristics, May 2007.

Pramlintide + Miscellaneous

Pramlintide slows gastric emptying, and therefore the manufacturer recommends that it should not be used with other drugs that alter gastrointestinal motility.

Clinical evidence, mechanism, importance and management

In a study using **paracetamol (acetaminophen)** as a marker of gastric emptying, pramlintide increased the time to maximum plasma **paracetamol** levels by up to 72 minutes and reduced the maximum **paracetamol** level by about 29%, without altering the overall extent of absorption. This effect was seen when **paracetamol** was given simultaneously with pramlintide, or for up to two hours after pramlintide. It was not seen when **paracetamol** was given one to two hours before pramlintide.[1]

This study demonstrates that pramlintide slows gastric emptying, and has the potential to delay the absorption of other drugs. The manufacturer notes that if a rapid onset of action is required (for example when giving an oral **analgesic**), the drug should be given at least one hour before, or two hours after pramlintide.[1]

Furthermore, because of this delay in gastric emptying, the manufacturer recommends that pramlintide should not be used in patients taking drugs that alter gastrointestinal motility. They specifically name **antimuscarinics** such as **atropine**,[1] which delays gastric emptying. Note that pramlintide could, theoretically, oppose the effects of **metoclopramide**, which increases gastric emptying.

1. Symlin (Pramlintide acetate). Amylin Pharmaceuticals, Inc. US Prescribing information, June 2005.

Sitagliptin + Miscellaneous

Single-dose ciclosporin slightly increased the absorption of sitagliptin, although this was not considered clinically relevant. Sitagliptin does not have a clinically relevant effect on the pharmacokinetics of digoxin, oral contraceptives, simvastatin or warfarin.

Clinical evidence, mechanism, importance and management

(a) Ciclosporin

A crossover study in 8 healthy subjects found that when a single 100-mg dose of sitagliptin was given with a single 600-mg dose of ciclosporin there was a 68% increase in the maximum plasma levels of sitagliptin, with a slight increase in overall exposure to sitagliptin (AUC increased by 28%). It is likely that ciclosporin enhances the absorption of sitagliptin via inhibition of P-glycoprotein. However, these changes were considered unlikely to be clinically meaningful, because of the apparent wide therapeutic index of sitagliptin.[1]

(b) Digoxin

The manufacturers describe a study in which digoxin 250 micrograms daily was given with sitagliptin 100 g daily for 10 days. The AUC and maximum plasma levels of digoxin were increased by 11% and 18%, respectively, which was not considered to be clinically significant.[2,3] Therefore it is unlikely that the dose of digoxin will need to be altered on concurrent use.

(c) Hormonal contraceptives

Sitagliptin did not appear to alter the pharmacokinetics of norethisterone (norethindrone) or ethinylestradiol given as part of an oral contraceptive.[2,3]

(d) Simvastatin

Sitagliptin did not appear to alter the pharmacokinetics of a single dose of simvastatin.[2,3]

(e) Warfarin

Sitagliptin did not appear to affect the pharmacokinetics or either *S*- or *R*-warfarin, or the INR in response to warfarin.[2,3]

1. Krishna R, Bergman A, Larson P, Cote J, Lasseter K, Dilzer S, Wang A, Zeng W, Chen L, Wagner J, Herman G. Effect of a single cyclosporine dose on the single-dose pharmacokinetics of sitagliptin (MK-0431), a dipeptidyl peptidase-4 inhibitor, in healthy male subjects. *J Clin Pharmacol* (2007) 47, 165–74.

2. Januvia (Sitagliptin phosphate). Merck and Co., Inc. US Prescribing information, April 2007.
3. Januvia (Sitagliptin phosphate monohydrate). Merck Sharp & Dohme Ltd. UK Summary of product characteristics, March 2007.

Sulphonylureas + Chloramphenicol

The blood glucose-lowering effects of tolbutamide and chlorpropamide can be increased by chloramphenicol and acute hypoglycaemia can occur.

Clinical evidence

A man taking chloramphenicol 2 g daily started taking **tolbutamide** 2 g daily. Three days later he had a typical hypoglycaemic collapse and was found to have serum **tolbutamide** levels three to fourfold higher than expected.[1]

Studies in diabetics have shown that chloramphenicol 2 g daily can increase the serum level and half-life of **tolbutamide** twofold, and two to threefold, respectively.[1,2] Blood glucose levels were reduced by about 25 to 30%.[2,3] Hypoglycaemia, acute in one case, developed in two other patients taking **tolbutamide** with chloramphenicol.[4,5] In another study chloramphenicol 1 to 2 g daily caused an average twofold increase in the half-life of **chlorpropamide**.[6]

Mechanism

Chloramphenicol inhibits the liver enzymes concerned with the metabolism of tolbutamide, and probably chlorpropamide as well, leading to their accumulation in the body. This is reflected in prolonged half-lives, reduced blood glucose levels and occasionally acute hypoglycaemia.[1-4,6]

Importance and management

The interaction between tolbutamide and chloramphenicol is well established and of clinical importance. The incidence is uncertain, but increased blood glucose-lowering effects should be expected if both drugs are given. The interaction between chlorpropamide and chloramphenicol is less well documented. Nevertheless, monitor concurrent use carefully and reduce the dosage of the sulphonylureas as necessary. Some patients may show a particularly exaggerated response. The manufacturers of other sulphonylureas often list chloramphenicol as an interacting drug, based on its interactions with tolbutamide and chlorpropamide, but direct information of an interaction does not appear to be available. No interaction would be expected with chloramphenicol eye drops, because the systemic absorption is likely to be small.

1. Christensen LK, Skovsted L. Inhibition of drug metabolism by chloramphenicol. *Lancet* (1969) ii, 1397–9.
2. Brunová E, Slabochová Z, Platilová H, Pavlík F, Grafnetterová J, Dvořáček K. Interaction of tolbutamide and chloramphenicol in diabetic patients. *Int J Clin Pharmacol Biopharm* (1977) 15, 7–12.
3. Brunová E, Slabochová Z, Platilová H. Influencing the effect of Dirastan (tolbutamide). Simultaneous administration of chloramphenicol in patients with diabetes and bacterial urinary tract inflammation. *Cas Lek Cesk* (1974) 113, 72–5.
4. Ziegelasch H-J. Extreme hypoglykämie unter kombinierter behandlung mit tolbutamid, n-1-butylbiguanidhydrochlorid und chloramphenikol. *Z Gesamte Inn Med* (1972) 27, 63–6.
5. Soeldner JS, Steinke J. Hypoglycemia in tolbutamide-treated diabetes. *JAMA* (1965) 193, 398–9.
6. Petitpierre B, Perrin L, Rudhardt M, Herrera A, Fabre J. Behaviour of chlorpropamide in renal insufficiency and under the effect of associated drug therapy. *Int J Clin Pharmacol* (1972) 6, 120–4.

Sulphonylureas + Heparin

Isolated reports describe hypoglycaemia in two diabetic patients, one taking glipizide, the other taking glibenclamide (glyburide). The effects were attributed to the concurrent use of heparin.

Clinical evidence, mechanism, importance and management

A diabetic, taking **glipizide** 5 mg daily for 6 months, with fair control was hospitalised for the treatment of a foot ulcer. Over a period of 4 days he experienced recurring episodes of hypoglycaemia after taking a routine 5-mg dose of **glipizide**. It was suggested that this might possibly have been due to an interaction with subcutaneous heparin calcium 5000 units every 12 hours which, it is suggested, might have displaced the **glipizide** from its protein binding sites.[1] Another report mentions that hypoglycaemia developed in a patient taking **glibenclamide (glyburide)** and heparin.[2] No other information seems to be available. The general importance of these reports is unknown, but seems likely to be small.

1. McKillop G, Fallon M, Slater SD. Possible interaction between heparin and a sulphonylurea a cause of prolonged hypoglycaemia? *BMJ* (1986) 293, 1073.
2. Beeley L, Daly M, Stewart P. *Bulletin of the West Midlands Centre for Adverse Drug Reaction Reporting* (1987) 24, 24.

Sulphonylureas + Methysergide

A preliminary study indicated that methysergide may enhance the effects of tolbutamide.

Clinical evidence, mechanism, importance and management

Pretreatment with methysergide 2 mg every 6 hours for 2 days increased the amount of insulin secreted in response to a 1-g intravenous dose of **tolbutamide** by almost 40% in 8 patients with type 2 diabetes.[1] Whether in practice the addition or withdrawal of methysergide adversely affects the control of diabetes is uncertain, but the possibility should be borne in mind.

1. Baldridge JA, Quickel KE, Feldman JM and Lebovitz HE. Potentiation of tolbutamide-mediated insulin release in adult onset diabetics by methysergide maleate. *Diabetes* (1974) 23, 21–4.

Sulphonylureas + Probenecid

The clearance of chlorpropamide is reduced by probenecid, but the clinical importance of this is uncertain. Tolbutamide appears not to interact.

Clinical evidence, mechanism, importance and management

A study in 6 patients given single oral doses of **chlorpropamide** found that probenecid 1 to 2 g daily increased the **chlorpropamide** half-life from about 36 to 50 hours.[1] It seems that the probenecid reduces the renal excretion of **chlorpropamide**. Another report in healthy subjects suggested that the half-life of **tolbutamide** was also prolonged by probenecid,[2] but this was not confirmed by a further controlled study.[3]

Information is very limited but it may possibly be necessary to reduce the dosage of **chlorpropamide** in the presence of probenecid. It seems unlikely that a clinically important interaction will occur with **tolbutamide**. Information about other sulphonylureas appears to be lacking.

1. Petitpierre B, Perrin L, Rudhardt M, Herrera A, Fabre J. Behaviour of chlorpropamide in renal insufficiency and under the effect of associated drug therapy. *Int J Clin Pharmacol* (1972) 6, 120–4.
2. Stowers JM, Mahler RF, Hunter RB. Pharmacology and mode of action of the sulphonylureas in man. *Lancet* (1958) i, 278–83.
3. Brook R, Schrogie JJ, Solomon HM. Failure of probenecid to inhibit the rate of metabolism of tolbutamide in man. *Clin Pharmacol Ther* (1968) 9, 314–17.

Sulphonylureas; Chlorpropamide + Urinary acidifiers or alkalinisers

On theoretical grounds the response to chlorpropamide may be decreased if the urine is made alkaline, and increased if urine is acidified.

Clinical evidence, mechanism, importance and management

A study in 6 healthy subjects given a 250-mg oral dose of chlorpropamide found that when the urine was made alkaline (pH 7.1 to 8.2) with **sodium bicarbonate**, the half-life of the chlorpropamide was reduced from 50 to 13 hours, and the 72-hour clearance was increased fourfold. In contrast, when the urine was acidified (pH 5.5 to 4.7) with **ammonium chloride**, the chlorpropamide half-life was increased from 50 to 69 hours and the 72-hour urinary clearance was decreased to 5%, and non-renal (i.e. metabolic) clearance predominated.[1] Another study found that the renal clearance of chlorpropamide was almost 100 times greater at pH 7 than at pH 5.[2] The reasons are that changes in urinary pH affect the ionisation of the chlorpropamide, and this affects the ability of the kidney to reabsorb it from the kidney filtrate (see more details under 'Drug excretion interactions', (p.7)). Thus, urinary pH determines the relative contribution of renal and metabolic clearance.

There appear to be no reports of adverse interactions between chlorpropamide and drugs that can alter urinary pH, but prescribers should be aware of the possibilities: a reduced response if the pH is raised significantly and renal clearance predominates (e.g. with **sodium bicarbonate**, **acetazolamide**, some **antacids**); an increased response if the pH is made more acid than usual and metabolic clearance predominates (e.g. with **ammonium chloride**). Perhaps more importantly, the effects of drugs that alter the hepatic clearance of chlorpropamide are likely to be more significant when its renal clearance is low (i.e. when the urine is acid).[2]

1. Neuvonen PJ, Kärkkäinen S. Effects of charcoal, sodium bicarbonate, and ammonium chloride on chlorpropamide kinetics. *Clin Pharmacol Ther* (1983) 33, 386–93.
2. Neuvonen PJ, Kärkkäinen S, Lehtovaara R. Pharmacokinetics of chlorpropamide in epileptic patients: effects of enzyme induction and urine pH on chlorpropamide elimination. *Eur J Clin Pharmacol* (1987) 32, 297–301.

Sulphonylureas; Glibenclamide (Glyburide) + Bosentan

There appears to be an increased risk of liver toxicity if bosentan is given with glibenclamide, and the combination should probably be avoided. Glibenclamide modestly reduces the plasma levels of bosentan, and bosentan reduces the plasma levels of glibenclamide.

Clinical evidence, mechanism, importance and management

In clinical studies, bosentan was noted to be associated with dose-related asymptomatic elevations in liver enzymes in some patients, and these elevations were higher in patients also receiving glibenclamide.[1] Study in *rats* confirmed that combined use of bosentan and glibenclamide caused increases in serum bile salt levels that were greater than with either drug alone.[1] In addition, *in vitro* study showed bosentan inhibits the bile salt export pump.[1] Glibenclamide also inhibits this pump. Because of the possibility that there may be a pharmacokinetic component to the interaction, the pharmacokinetics of both bosentan and glibenclamide were determined in a crossover study in 12 healthy subjects. However, glibenclamide actually reduced the maximum plasma levels and AUC of bosentan by 24 and 29%, respectively, while bosentan reduced the maximum plasma levels and AUC of glibenclamide by 22 and 40%, respectively. Two subjects had asymptomatic elevated liver enzyme levels while taking bosentan with glibenclamide.[2]

Based on the limited evidence available about the increased risk of liver toxicity, the UK manufacturer of bosentan recommends that it should not be used with drugs that are inhibitors of the bile salt export pump, such as glibenclamide. They suggest that an alternative antidiabetic drug should be used.[3] The US manufacturer contraindicates concurrent use because of the potential for raised liver enzymes.[4] This seems a sensible precaution. Note also that a decrease of 40% in the AUC of glibenclamide may possibly decrease its blood glucose-lowering effects to a clinically relevant extent.[2]

1. Fattinger K, Funk C, Pantze M, Weber C, Reichen J, Stieger B, Meier PJ. The endothelin antagonist bosentan inhibits the canalicular bile salt export pump: a potential mechanism for hepatic adverse reactions. *Clin Pharmacol Ther* (2001) 69, 223–31.
2. van Giersbergen PLM, Treiber A, Clozel M, Bodin F, Dingemanse J. In vivo and in vitro studies exploring the pharmacokinetic interaction between bosentan, a dual endothelin receptor antagonist, and glyburide. *Clin Pharmacol Ther* (2002) 71, 253–62.
3. Tracleer (Bosentan monohydrate). Actelion Pharmaceuticals UK. UK Summary of product characteristics, October 2006.
4. Tracleer (Bosentan). Pantheon, Inc. US Prescribing information, February 2007.

Sulphonylureas; Glibenclamide (Glyburide) + Naftidrofuryl oxalate

One report briefly lists a case of severe hypoglycaemia, which occurred when glibenclamide was given with naftidrofuryl oxalate.[1] No details are given.

1. Beeley L, Magee P, Hickey FM. *Bulletin of the West Midlands Centre for Adverse Drug Reaction Reporting* (1990) 30, 17.

Sulphonylureas; Glibenclamide (Glyburide) + Pantoprazole

There is no pharmacokinetic interaction between glibenclamide (glyburide) and pantoprazole, and pantoprazole does not alter the glucose-lowering effect of glibenclamide.

Clinical evidence, mechanism, importance and management

Pantoprazole 40 mg daily or placebo were given to 20 healthy subjects for 5 days. On day 5 the subjects were additionally given 3.5 mg of a micronised preparation of glibenclamide. The pharmacokinetics of the glibenclamide and the pharmacodynamic profiles of glucose and insulin serum concentrations were not significantly altered, and the pharmacokinetics of pantoprazole were not affected. It was concluded that dosage changes of the micronised preparation of glibenclamide are not needed during treatment with pantoprazole.[1]

1. Walter-Sack IE, Bliesath H, Stötzer F, Huber R, Steinijans VW, Ding R, Mascher H, Wurst W. Lack of pharmacokinetic and pharmacodynamic interaction between pantoprazole and glibenclamide in humans. *Clin Drug Invest* (1998) 15, 253–60.

Sulphonylureas; Glibenclamide (Glyburide) + Vinpocetine

Vinpocetine does not alter the pharmacokinetics or efficacy of glibenclamide.

Clinical evidence, mechanism, importance and management

A study in 18 elderly patients with type 2 diabetes and symptoms of dementia, taking glibenclamide (glyburide), found that 4 days of treatment with vinpocetine 10 mg three times daily did not affect either the pharmacokinetics of the glibenclamide or the control of blood glucose levels.[1] There would seem to be no reason for avoiding concurrent use.

1. Grandt R, Braun W, Schulz H-U, Lührmann B, Frercks H-J. Glibenclamide steady-state plasma levels during concomitant vinpocetine administration in type II diabetic patients. *Arzneimittelforschung* (1989) 39, 1451–4.

Sulfonylureas; Glymidine + Phenobarbital

A study in one subject found that the blood glucose-lowering effects of glymidine were unaffected by phenobarbital.[1] No special precautions would appear necessary on concurrent use.

1. Gerhards E, Kolb KH, Schulze PE. Über 2-Benzolsulfonylamino- 5(β-methoxy-äthoxy) pyrimidin (Glycodiazin). V. In vitro- und in vivo-Versuche zum Einfluß von Phenyläthylbarbitursäure (Luminal) auf den Stoffwechsel und die blutzuckersenkende Wirkung des Glycodiazins. *Naunyn Schmiedebergs Arch Pharmakol Exp Pathol* (1966) 255, 200–20.

Sulphonylureas; Tolbutamide + Aprepitant

Aprepitant slightly reduces tolbutamide levels.

Clinical evidence, mechanism, importance and management

In a study in 12 healthy subjects aprepitant (125 mg on day one, then 80 mg daily on days 2 and 3) decreased the AUC of a single 500-mg dose of tolbutamide by 23%, 28%, 15%, when given on days 4, 8, and 15, respectively, when compared with 12 subjects not given aprepitant.[1]

Aprepitant is an inducer of the cytochrome P450 isoenzyme CYP2C9 by which tolbutamide is metabolised. It therefore increases tolbutamide metabolism, which leads to a reduction in tolbutamide levels. However, the clinical relevance of these small changes has not been assessed. The manufacturer recommends caution when both drugs are given.[2]

1. Shadle CR, Lee Y, Majumdar AK, Petty KJ, Gargano C, Bradstreet TE, Evans JK, Blum RA. Evaluation of potential inductive effects of aprepitant on cytochrome P450 3A4 and 2C9 activity. *J Clin Pharmacol* (2004) 44, 215–23.
2. Emend (Aprepitant). Merck Sharp & Dohme Ltd. UK Summary of product characteristics, February 2007.

Sulphonylureas; Tolbutamide + Echinacea

Echinacea does not have a clinically relevant effect on the pharmacokinetics of tolbutamide.

Clinical evidence, mechanism, importance and management

In a pharmacokinetic study, 12 healthy subjects were given *Echinacea purpurea* root 400 mg four times daily for 8 days with a single 500-mg dose of tolbutamide on day 6. The AUC of tolbutamide was increased by 14%, and the time to maximum levels was increased from 4 to 6 hours.[1] The oral clearance was decreased by a mean of 11%, although 2 subjects had a 25% or greater reduction. These minor to modest changes are unlikely to be clinically relevant.

1. Gorski JC, Huang S-M, Pinto A, Hamman MA, Hilligoss JK, Zaheer NA, Desai M, Miller M, Hall SD. The effect of echinacea (*Echinacea purpurea* root) on cytochrome P450 activity in vivo. *Clin Pharmacol Ther* (2004) 75, 89–100.

Sulphonylureas; Tolbutamide + Tolcapone

Tolcapone did not alter tolbutamide pharmacokinetics in a single-dose study.

Clinical evidence, mechanism, importance and management

In a single-dose study in 12 healthy subjects, tolcapone 200 mg had no effect on the pharmacokinetics of tolbutamide 500 mg, and did not alter the glucose-lowering effect of tolbutamide.[1] This study was conducted since *in vitro* evidence showed that tolcapone inhibits the cytochrome P450 isoenzyme CYP2C9, by which tolbutamide is metabolised. However, the findings in healthy subjects suggest that no clinically relevant changes in pharmacokinetics of tolbutamide are likely.

1. Jorga KM, Fotteler B, Gasser R, Banken L, Birnboeck H. Lack of interaction between tolcapone and tolbutamide in healthy volunteers. *J Clin Pharmacol* (2000) 40, 544–51.

14

Antiepileptics

The antiepileptic drugs find their major application in the treatment of various kinds of epilepsy, although some of them are also used for other conditions, such as pain management.

Drug interactions

The drugs used as antiepileptics are a disparate group, and their interactions need to be considered individually. Carbamazepine and phenytoin have established ranges of therapeutic plasma levels and these are typically fairly narrow. Modest changes in plasma levels may therefore be clinically important.

(a) Carbamazepine or oxcarbazepine

Carbamazepine is extensively metabolised by the cytochrome P450 isoenzyme CYP3A4 to the active metabolite, carbamazepine-10,11-epoxide, which is then further metabolised. Concurrent use of CYP3A4 inhibitors or inducers may therefore lead to toxicity or reduced efficacy. However, importantly, carbamazepine also induces CYP3A4 and so induces its own metabolism (autoinduction). Because of this, it is important that drug interaction studies are multiple-dose and carried out at steady state. Auto-induction also means that moderate inducers of CYP3A4 may have less of an effect on steady-state carbamazepine levels than expected. Oxcarbazepine is a derivative of carbamazepine, but has a lesser effect on CYP3A4. However, both carbamazepine and oxcarbazepine can act as inhibitors of CYP2C19, see 'Phenytoin + Carbamazepine', p.554.

(b) Phenobarbital

Phenobarbital is an inducer of a wide range of cytochrome P450 isoenzymes, and may increase the metabolism of a variety of drugs. It may, itself, also be affected by some enzyme inducers or inhibitors, although these interactions are less established.

(c) Phenytoin

Phenytoin is extensively metabolised by hydroxylation, principally by CYP2C9, although CYP2C19 also plays a role. These isoenzymes show 'genetic polymorphism', (p.4), and CYP2C19 may assume a greater role in individuals who have a poor metaboliser phenotype of CYP2C9. The concurrent use of inhibitors of CYP2C9, and sometimes also CYP2C19, can lead to phenytoin toxicity. In addition, phenytoin metabolism is saturable (it shows non-linear pharmacokinetics), and therefore small changes in metabolism or phenytoin dose can result in marked changes in plasma levels. Moreover, phenytoin is highly protein bound, and drugs that alter its protein binding may alter its levels. Although protein binding interactions are usually not clinically relevant (unless metabolism is also inhibited, see 'Phenytoin + Valproate', p.568), they can be important in interpreting drug levels.

(d) Valproate

Valproate is a generic name that is applied in this section to cover valproic acid and its salts and esters. Valproate undergoes glucuronidation and β-oxidation, and possibly also some metabolism via CYP2C isoenzymes. It can therefore undergo drug interactions via a variety of mechanisms. It acts as an inhibitor of glucuronidation and so may affect other drugs that undergo glucuronidation. Valproate also has non-linear pharmacokinetics due to saturation of plasma protein binding, and so may interact with drugs that alter its protein binding. However, note that, although protein binding interactions are usually not clinically relevant unless metabolism is also inhibited, they can be important in interpreting drug levels.

(e) Newer antiepileptics

Of the newer antiepileptics, both felbamate and topiramate are weak inducers of CYP3A4. They may also inhibit CYP2C19. They are also partially metabolised by the cytochrome P450 isoenzyme system, so may have their metabolism altered by other drugs such as the older enzyme-inducing antiepileptics.

Gabapentin, lamotrigine, levetiracetam, tiagabine, vigabatrin, and zonisamide do not appear to act as inhibitors or inducers of cytochrome P450 isoenzymes, and so appear to cause less drug interactions than the older antiepileptics. Moreover, gabapentin, levetiracetam, and vigabatrin do not appear to be metabolised by the cytochrome P450 system, so appear to be little affected by drug interactions that result from this mechanism. Tiagabine and zonisamide are metabolised by the cytochrome P450 system, so may have their metabolism altered by other drugs such as the older enzyme-inducing antiepileptics. Lamotrigine is metabolised by glucuronidation, and may be affected by inhibitors (e.g. valproate) or inducers (e.g. the older enzyme-inducing antiepileptics) of this process. Lamotrigine may also act as an inducer of glucuronidation.

Antiepileptics + Acetazolamide

Severe osteomalacia and rickets have been seen in a few patients taking phenytoin, phenobarbital, or primidone with acetazolamide. A marked reduction in serum primidone levels with a loss in seizure control, rises in serum carbamazepine levels with toxicity, and rises in phenytoin levels have also been described in a very small number of patients given acetazolamide.

Clinical evidence

(a) Osteomalacia

Severe osteomalacia developed in 2 women taking **phenytoin** or **primidone** and **phenobarbital** when they were given acetazolamide 750 mg daily, despite a normal intake of calcium. When the acetazolamide was withdrawn, the hyperchloraemic acidosis that had been seen in both patients abated and their high urinary excretion of calcium fell by 50%.[1,2]

Similar cases have been described in 3 children given acetazolamide, **phenytoin** and **primidone**, with **phenobarbital** and/or metharbital,[3] who developed rickets.

(b) Reduced serum primidone levels

A patient taking primidone had an increase in seizure-frequency and a virtual absence of primidone (or phenobarbital) in the serum while taking acetazolamide 250 mg daily. Primidone levels rose when the acetazolamide was withdrawn, probably due to improved absorption. A subsequent study in 2 other patients found that acetazolamide had a small effect on primidone absorption in one, and no effect in the other.[4]

(c) Increased serum carbamazepine levels

A 9-year-old girl and two teenage boys, all of them taking the highest dosages of carbamazepine tolerable (without adverse effects), developed signs of toxicity after taking acetazolamide 250 to 750 mg daily. Their serum carbamazepine levels were found to have increased by about 25 to 50%. In one instance toxicity appeared within 48 hours.[5]

The seizure control of 54 children with grand mal and temporal lobe epilepsy was improved when acetazolamide 10 mg/kg daily was added to carbamazepine. Serum carbamazepine levels rose by 1 to 6 mg/L in 60% of the 33 patients sampled. Adverse effects developed in 10 children, and in 8 children this was within 1 to 10 days of starting the acetazolamide. The adverse effects responded to a reduction in the carbamazepine dosage.[6]

(d) Increased serum phenytoin levels

When acetazolamide was added to phenytoin treatment in 6 children, 5 of them had an increase in the phenytoin level (range 20 to 132%, representing an increase of 3 to 12.5 mg/L), and one had a slight decrease (20% or 3 mg/L) [values estimated from figure].[7]

Mechanism

Uncertain. Mild osteomalacia induced by antiepileptics is a recognised phenomenon[8] (see also 'Vitamin D substances + Phenytoin and Barbiturates', p.1291). It seems that this is exaggerated by acetazolamide, which increases urinary calcium excretion, possibly by causing systemic acidosis, which results from the reduced absorption of bicarbonate by the kidney. The changes in the antiepileptic levels are not understood.

Importance and management

The documentation of all of these interactions is very limited, and their incidence is uncertain. Concurrent use should be monitored for the possible development of osteomalacia or altered antiepileptic levels and steps taken to accommodate them. Withdraw the acetazolamide if necessary, or adjust the dosage of the antiepileptic appropriately. In the case of the children with rickets[3] the acetazolamide was withdrawn and high doses of vitamin D was given. It seems possible that other carbonic anhydrase inhibitors may behave like acetazolamide.

1. Mallette LE. Anticonvulsants, acetazolamide and osteomalacia. *N Engl J Med* (1975) 293, 668.
2. Mallette LE. Acetazolamide-accelerated anticonvulsant osteomalacia. *Arch Intern Med* (1977) 137, 1013–17.
3. Matsuda I, Takekoshi Y, Shida N, Fujieda K, Nagai B, Arashima S, Anakura M, Oka Y. Renal tubular acidosis and skeletal demineralization in patients on long-term anticonvulsant therapy. *J Pediatr* (1975) 87, 202–5.
4. Syversen GB, Morgan JP, Weintraub M, Myers GJ. Acetazolamide-induced interference with primidone absorption. *Arch Neurol* (1977) 34, 80–4.
5. McBride MC. Serum carbamazepine levels are increased by acetazolamide. *Ann Neurol* (1984) 16, 393.
6. Forsythe WI, Owens JR, Toothill C. Effectiveness of acetazolamide in the treatment of carbamazepine-resistant epilepsy in children. *Dev Med Child Neurol* (1981) 23, 761–9.
7. Norell E, Lilienbeg G, Gamstorp I. Systematic determination of the serum phenytoin level as an aid in the management of children with epilepsy. *Eur Neurol* (1975) 13, 232–44.
8. Anast CS. Anticonvulsant drugs and calcium metabolism. *N Engl J Med* (1975) 292, 587–8.

Antiepileptics + Aciclovir

Isolated reports describe a marked reduction in serum phenytoin and valproate levels in two children given aciclovir. Seizure frequency increased.

Clinical evidence, mechanism, importance and management

A 7-year-old boy with epilepsy taking **phenytoin, valproate** and nitrazepam was given oral aciclovir 1 g daily for 6 days. After 4 days his trough serum **phenytoin** levels had fallen from 17 to 5 micrograms/mL, and his trough **valproate** levels similarly fell, from 32 to 22 micrograms/mL. When the aciclovir was stopped the serum levels of both antiepileptics rose over a period of 3 to 6 days. During the period when the antiepileptic levels were restabilising, the seizure frequency markedly increased and his EEG worsened. The reason for this apparent interaction is not known, but the authors of the report suggest that the aciclovir may possibly have reduced the absorption of the antiepileptics, in some way not understood.[1] Reduced phenytoin and valproate levels during treatment with aciclovir have been reported in another child.[2]

There appears to be only these isolated reports of an interaction between these drugs. Its general clinical importance is not known. More study is needed.

1. Parmeggiani A, Riva R, Posar A, Rossi PG. Possible interaction between acyclovir and antiepileptic treatment. *Ther Drug Monit* (1995) 17, 312–15.
2. Iglesias Iglesias A-A, Ortega García MP, Guevara Serrano J. Disminución de la concentración sérica de antiepilépticos durante el tratamiento con aciclovir. *Med Clin (Barc)* (2005) 124, 355–6.

Antiepileptics + Antineoplastics; Cytotoxic

Carbamazepine, phenytoin and valproate serum levels can be reduced by several antineoplastic drug regimens and seizures can occur if the antiepileptic dosages are not raised appropriately. In contrast, phenytoin toxicity has occurred when fluorouracil and fluorouracil prodrugs, such as capecitabine, doxifluridine and tegafur, were given. The effects of many antineoplastics are reduced or changed by enzyme-inducing antiepileptics. Increased haematological toxicity may occur if valproate is given with fotemustine and cisplatin.

Clinical evidence

(a) Antiepileptic levels reduced

There are a number of reports (mainly case reports) that implicate a variety of types of chemotherapy in reducing the levels of **carbamazepine**, **phenytoin**, and **valproate**. See 'Table 14.1', (p.519) for details.

(b) Antiepileptic levels raised

Two epileptic patients taking **phenytoin** developed **phenytoin** toxicity when they were given **fluorouracil** to treat colon cancer.[1,2] Three patients with malignant brain tumours developed acute **phenytoin** toxicity associated with raised serum **phenytoin** levels when they were given ***UFT*** (**uracil** and **tegafur**, a prodrug of **fluorouracil**).[3] Another case of **phenytoin** toxicity has been reported with ***UFT***.[4] **Phenytoin** toxicity was also seen in a woman treated with combination therapy that included the fluorouracil prodrug **doxifluridine**.[5] Similarly, **phenytoin** toxicity has occurred in a patient given **capecitabine** (another prodrug of **fluorouracil**).[6] Although in one report,[3] no interaction occurred in one of the patients when the ***UFT*** was replaced by **fluorouracil**, cases of **phenytoin** toxicity have been reported in 3 patients receiving **fluorouracil** with **folinic acid**.[6,7]

Table 14.1 Reduced antiepileptic levels during antineoplastic therapy

Antiepileptic	*Antineoplastic*	*Malignancy*	*Outcome*	*Refs*
Phenytoin	Cisplatin Carmustine	Brain tumours	A retrospective study reviewed the effects of 3 or more cycles of 72 hours of carmustine and cisplatin chemotherapy in 19 patients who did not vomit. A phenytoin dose increase was required in three-quarters of patients, which was, on average, 40% of the original dose (range 20 to 100%). The effect on phenytoin levels persisted after the chemotherapy had finished, with levels returning to normal 2 to 3 weeks later.	1
Phenytoin	Cisplatin Vinblastine Bleomycin	Metastatic germ cell tumour	Estimated phenytoin level 15 micrograms/mL, but level only reached 2 micrograms/mL. Patient fitted.	2
Phenytoin Primidone	Cisplatin Vinblastine Bleomycin	Metastatic embryonal cell cancer	Phenytoin 800 mg daily gave a level of 15 micrograms/mL whilst receiving chemotherapy. After chemotherapy the same dose produced a toxic level of 42.8 micrograms/mL. Phenobarbital levels unaffected.	3
Phenytoin Phenobarbital	Vinblastine Carmustine Methotrexate	Lung cancer with brain metastases	Phenytoin levels fell from 9.4 to 5.6 micrograms/mL 24 hours after vinblastine. Patient fitted. Phenytoin levels returned to normal 2 weeks after chemotherapy. Phenobarbital levels unaffected.	4
Phenytoin Carbamazepine Sodium valproate	Doxorubicin Cisplatin Cyclophosphamide Altretamine	Papillary adenocarcinoma of the ovaries	Seizures occurred 2 to 3 days after starting chemotherapy. All drug levels dropped to one-third or lower. Doses increased to compensate, which led to phenytoin toxicity when the chemotherapy finished.	5
Phenytoin	Carboplatin	Small cell lung cancer with brain metastases	Phenytoin level dropped from 9.7 to 4.6 micrograms/mL 10 days into chemotherapy, resulting in seizures. Phenytoin dose had to be increased by 35% to achieve a level of 10.7 micrograms/mL.	6
Phenytoin	Dacarbazine Carmustine Cisplatin Tamoxifen	Malignant melanoma with brain metastases	Phenytoin level of only 2.5 micrograms/mL despite a loading 1-g dose and a daily dose of 500 mg phenytoin.	7
Phenytoin followed by Carbamazepine	Vincristine Cytarabine Hydroxycarbamide Daunorubicin Methotrexate Tioguanine Cyclophosphamide Carmustine	Stage IV T-cell lymphoma	Phenytoin failed to reach therapeutic levels and so was substituted with carbamazepine. Chemotherapy caused carbamazepine levels to drop below therapeutic levels resulting in seizures. Increasing the dose from 30 to 50 mg/kg per day prevented subtherapeutic levels.	8
Phenytoin	Methotrexate Mercaptopurine Vincristine	Acute lymphoblastic leukaemia	Phenytoin levels dropped from 19.8 micrograms/mL on the day before chemotherapy to 3.6 micrograms/mL on the 6th day of chemotherapy.	9
Phenytoin	Cisplatin Carmustine Etoposide	CNS tumours	Dose of phenytoin had to be increased by 50 to 300% in 10 patients to maintain phenytoin levels in the therapeutic range.	10
Sodium valproate	Methotrexate (high dose)	Acute lymphoblastic leukaemia	A child had a seizure a few hours after methotrexate. Serum valproate levels reduced by 75%. The valproate dose was increased by 50% and clonazepam added.	11
Sodium valproate	Methotrexate Cytarabine Nimustine (by CSF perfusion)	Glioblastoma	CSF valproic acid levels reduced by 70% during the perfusion, but returned to normal levels within 7 hours.	12
Sodium valproate Phenytoin	Cisplatin Etoposide Bleomycin	Testicular cancer	Serum valproate levels reduced by 50% after the first cycle and generalised tonic-clonic seizures occurred. There was no effect on phenytoin levels.	13

1. Grossman SA, Sheidler VR, Gilbert MR. Decreased phenytoin levels in patients receiving chemotherapy. *Am J Med* (1989) 87, 505–10.
2. Sylvester RK, Lewis FB, Caldwell KC, Lobell M, Perri R, Sawchuk RA. Impaired phenytoin bioavailability secondary to cisplatinum, vinblastine, and bleomycin. *Ther Drug Monit* (1984) 6, 302-5.
3. Fincham RW, Schottelius DD. Case report. Decreased phenytoin levels in antineoplastic therapy. *Ther Drug Monit* (1979) 1, 277-83.
4. Bollini P, Riva R, Albani F, Ida N, Cacciari L, Bollini C, Baruzzi A. Decreased phenytoin level during antineoplastic therapy: a case report. *Epilepsia* (1983) 24, 75-8.
5. Neef C, de Voogd-van der Straaten I. An interaction between cytostatic and anticonvulsant drugs. *Clin Pharmacol Ther* (1988) 43, 372-5.
6. Dofferhoff ASM, Berensen HH, Naalt Jvd, Haaxma-Reiche H, Smit EF, Postmus PE. Decreased phenytoin level after carboplatin treatment. *Am J Med* (1990) 89, 247-8.
7. Gattis WA, May DB. Possible interaction involving phenytoin, dexamethasone, and antineoplastic agents: a case report and review. *Ann Pharmacother* (1996) 30, 520-6.
8. Nahum MP, Ben Arush MW, Robinson E. Reduced plasma carbamazepine level during chemotherapy in a child with malignant lymphoma. *Acta Paediatr Scand* (1990) 79, 873-5.

Continued

Table 14.1 Reduced antiepileptic levels during antineoplastic therapy (continued)

9. Jarosinski PF, Moscow JA, Alexander MS, Lesko LJ, Balis FM, Poplack DG. Altered phenytoin clearance during intensive treatment for acute lymphoblastic leukemia. *J Pediatr* (1988) 112, 996-9.
10. Ghosh C, Lazarus HM, Hewlett JS, Creger RJ. Fluctuation of serum phenytoin concentrations during autologous bone marrow transplant for primary central nervous system tumors. *J Neurooncol* (1992) 12, 25-32.
11. Schrøder H, Østergaard JR. Interference of high-dose methotrexate in the metabolism of valproate? *Pediatr Hematol Oncol* (1994) 11, 445-9.
12. Morikawa N, Mori T, Abe T, Kawashima H, Takeyama M, Hori S. Pharmacokinetics of cytosine arabinoside, methotrexate, nimustine and valproic acid in cerebrospinal fluid during cerebrospinal fluid perfusion chemotherapy. *Biol Pharm Bull* (2000) 23, 784-7.
13. Ikeda H, Murakami T, Takano M, Usui T, Kihira K. Pharmacokinetic interaction on valproic acid and recurrence of epileptic seizures during chemotherapy in an epileptic patient. *Br J Clin Pharmacol* (2005) 59, 593-7.

(c) Antineoplastic effects reduced or altered

A number of antiepileptic drugs affect the levels of various antineoplastics. These are discussed elsewhere. See:

- 'Anthracyclines; Doxorubicin + Barbiturates', p.613,
- 'Busulfan + Phenytoin', p.619,
- 'Cyclophosphamide or Ifosfamide + Barbiturates', p.623,
- 'Cyclophosphamide or Ifosfamide + Phenytoin', p.627,
- 'Etoposide + Antiepileptics', p.629,
- 'Imatinib + CYP3A4 inducers', p.637,
- 'Irinotecan + Antiepileptics', p.638,
- 'Methotrexate + Antiepileptics', p.646,
- 'Procarbazine + Antiepileptics', p.656,
- 'Streptozocin + Phenytoin', p.658,
- 'Taxanes; Paclitaxel + Antiepileptics', p.662,
- 'Teniposide + Antiepileptics', p.663,
- 'Topotecan + Phenytoin', p.667,
- 'Toremifene + Antiepileptics', p.667.

(d) Miscellaneous

One report found **valproate** increased haematological toxicity in patients taking **valproate** with **fotemustine** and **cisplatin**.[8]

Mechanism

Not fully understood, but a suggested reason for the fall in serum antiepileptic levels is that these antineoplastics damage the intestinal wall, which reduces the absorption of the antiepileptic. Other mechanisms may also have some part to play. The raised serum phenytoin levels possibly occur because the liver metabolism of the phenytoin is reduced by these antineoplastics. Changes in plasma protein binding may also have been involved.

Importance and management

Information is scattered and incomplete. However, it appears that both altered antiepileptic levels and altered antineoplastic levels can occur, possibly leading to loss of efficacy or toxicity. Where possible, it may be prudent to avoid concurrent use of enzyme-inducing antiepileptics and antineoplastics. If this is not possible, serum antiepileptic levels should be closely monitored during treatment with any of these antineoplastics, making dosage adjustments as necessary, and the efficacy of the antineoplastics should also be closely monitored.

1. Gilbar PJ, Brodribb TR. Phenytoin and fluorouracil interaction. *Ann Pharmacother* (2001) 35, 1367–70.
2. Rosemergy I, Findlay M. Phenytoin toxicity as a result of 5-fluorouracil administration. *N Z Med J* (2002) 115, U124.
3. Wakisaka S, Shimauchi M, Kaji Y, Nonaka A, Kinoshita K. Acute phenytoin intoxication associated with the antineoplastic agent UFT. *Fukuoka Igaku Zasshi* (1990) 81, 192–6.
4. Errea-Abad JM, González-Igual J, Eito-Cativiela JL, Gastón-Añaños J. Intoxicación aguda por fenitoína debida a interacción col el derivado fluoropirimidínico. *Rev Neurol* (1998) 27, 1066–7.
5. Konishi H, Morita K, Minouchi T, Nakajima M, Matsuda M, Yamaji A. Probable metabolic interaction of doxifluridine with phenytoin. *Ann Pharmacother* (2002) 36, 831–4.
6. Brickell K, Parter D, Thompson P. Phenytoin toxicity due to fluoropyrimidines (5FU/capecitabine): three case reports. *Br J Cancer* (2003) 89, 615–16.
7. Gilbar PJ, Brodribb TR. Phenytoin and fluorouracil interaction. *Ann Pharmacother* (2001) 35, 1367–70.
8. Bourg V, Lebrun C, Chichmanian RM, Thomas P, Frenay M. Nitroso-urea–cisplatin-based chemotherapy associated with valproate: increase of haematologic toxicity. *Ann Oncol* (2001) 12, 217–9.

Antiepileptics + Calcium carbimide or Disulfiram

Phenytoin serum levels are markedly and rapidly increased by disulfiram. Phenytoin toxicity can develop. There is evidence that phenobarbital and carbamazepine are not affected by disulfiram, and that phenytoin is not affected by calcium carbimide.

Clinical evidence

The serum **phenytoin** levels of 4 patients rose by 100 to 500% over a 9-day period when they were given disulfiram 400 mg daily. **Phenytoin** levels were still rising even 3 to 4 days after the disulfiram was withdrawn, and had still not returned to normal after 14 days. Two patients developed signs of mild **phenytoin** toxicity.[1] In a follow-up study in two of the patients, one developed ataxia and both had a rise in serum **phenytoin** levels, of 25% and 50%, respectively, during 5 days of disulfiram treatment.[2]

Disulfiram increased the half-life of **phenytoin** from 11 to 19 hours in 10 healthy subjects.[3] There are also other case reports describing this interaction.[4-8]

Phenobarbital levels (from **primidone** in 3 patients and **phenobarbital** in one patient) fluctuated by about 10% (which is unlikely to be clinically significant) when disulfiram was given for 9 days.[1,2]

A case report suggested that **carbamazepine** did not interact with disulfiram,[6] and this has been confirmed in a study of 5 epileptic, non-alcoholic patients.[9]

A study in 4 patients found that calcium carbimide 50 mg daily for a week followed by 100 mg daily for 2 weeks had no effect on serum **phenytoin** levels.[2]

Mechanism

Disulfiram inhibits the liver enzymes concerned with the metabolism of phenytoin (possibly the cytochrome P450 isoenzyme CYP2C9) thereby prolonging its stay in the body and resulting in a rise in its serum levels, to toxic concentrations in some instances. One study concluded that the inhibition was non-competitive.[7]

Importance and management

The interaction between phenytoin and disulfiram is established, moderately well documented, clinically important and potentially serious. It seems to occur in most patients and develops rapidly. Recovery may take 2 to 3 weeks after the disulfiram is withdrawn. It has been suggested that the dosage of phenytoin could be reduced to accommodate the interaction, but it may be difficult to maintain the balance required. Monitor very closely if both drugs are given.[2]

Carbamazepine and phenobarbital do not appear to interact with disulfiram and calcium carbimide does not appear to interact with phenytoin.

1. Olesen OV. Disulfiramum (Antabuse®) as inhibitor of phenytoin metabolism. *Acta Pharmacol Toxicol (Copenh)* (1966) 24, 317–22.
2. Olesen OV. The influence of disulfiram and calcium carbimide on the serum diphenylhydantoin excretion of HPPH in the urine. *Arch Neurol* (1967) 16, 642–4.
3. Svendsen TL, Kristensen MB, Hansen JM, Skovsted L. The influence of disulfiram on the half-life and metabolic clearance rate of diphenylhydantoin and tolbutamide in man. *Eur J Clin Pharmacol* (1976) 9, 439–41.
4. Kiørboe E. Phenytoin intoxication during treatment with Antabuse® (Disulfiram). *Epilepsia* (1966) 7, 246–9.
5. Kiørboe E. Antabus som årsag til forgiftning med fenytoin. *Ugeskr Laeger* (1966) 128, 1531–6.
6. Dry J, Pradalier A. Intoxication par la phénytoïne au cours d'une association thérapeutique avec le disulfirame. *Therapie* (1973) 28, 799–802.

7. Taylor JW, Alexander B, Lyon LW. Mathematical analysis of a phenytoin-disulfiram interaction. *Am J Hosp Pharm* (1981) 38, 93–5.
8. Brown CG, Kaminsky MJ, Feroli ER, Gurley HT. Delirium with phenytoin and disulfiram administration. *Ann Emerg Med* (1983) 12, 310–13.
9. Krag B, Dam M, Angelo H, Christensen JM. Influence of disulfiram on the serum concentration of carbamazepine in patients with epilepsy. *Acta Neurol Scand* (1981) 63, 395–8.

Antiepileptics + Chinese herbal medicines

A study in epileptics found that Saiko-ka-ryukotsu-borei-to enhanced the antiepileptic effects of carbamazepine. Paeoniae Radix does not appear to affect the pharmacokinetics of valproic acid.

Clinical evidence

(a) Carbamazepine

A study in epileptic patients found the antiepileptic effects of carbamazepine were enhanced by concurrent **Saiko-ka-ryukotsu-borei-to**;[1] patients experienced fewer seizures and improved neurological symptoms.[2]

(b) Valproate

The pharmacokinetics of a single 200-mg dose of valproic acid were unaffected by 1.2 g of a powder extract of **Paeoniae Radix** daily for 7 days in 6 healthy subjects.[3]

Mechanism

Not fully understood. As a pharmacokinetic interaction has not been found between Saiko-ka-ryukotsu-borei-to and carbamazepine, the enhanced effects found in the patients with epilepsy may therefore have been due to a pharmacodynamic interaction.[2]

Paeoniae Radix (the dried root of *Paeonia lactiflora*[3]) is reported to reduce the rate of gastric emptying.[4] However, this does not appear to affect the rate of absorption of valproate.

Importance and management

Evidence is limited, but there appears to be no evidence of an adverse effect when using Paeoniae radix with valproate, or Saiko-ka-ryukotsu-borei-to with carbamazepine: concurrent use may even be beneficial. More study is needed to confirm all these findings. Note that adulteration of Chinese medicines with various antiepileptics may lead to unexpected toxicity.[5]

1. Senzaki A, Okubo Y, Matuura M, Kojima T, Toru M. Clinical studies on effects of Saiko-ka-ryukotsu-borei-to (TJ-12) for adult patients with symptomatic localization-related epilepsy. *Rinsho Seishin Igaku* (1993) 22, 641–6.
2. Ohnishi N, Nakasako S, Okada K, Umehara S, Takara K, Nagasawa K, Yoshioka M, Kuroda K, Yokoyama T. Studies on interactions between traditional herbal and Western medicines. IV: Lack of pharmacokinetic interactions between Saiko-ka-ryukotsu-borei-to and carbamazepine in rats. *Eur J Drug Metab Pharmacokinet* (2001) 26, 129–35.
3. Chen LC, Chou MH, Lin MF, Yang LL. Lack of pharmacokinetic interaction between valproic acid and a traditional Chinese medicine, Paeoniae Radix, in healthy volunteers. *J Clin Pharm Ther* (2000) 25, 453–9.
4. Ohnishi N, Yonekawa Y, Nakasako S, Nagasawa K, Yokoyama T, Yoshioka M, Kuroda K. Studies on interactions between traditional herbal and Western medicines. I. Effects of Sho-seiryu-to on the pharmacokinetics of carbamazepine in rats. *Biol Pharm Bull* (1999) 22, 527–31.
5. Lau KK, Lai CK, Chan AYM. Phenytoin poisoning after using Chinese proprietary medicines. *Hum Exp Toxicol* (2000) 19, 385–6.

Antiepileptics + Folates

If folate supplements are given to treat folate deficiency, which can be caused by the use of antiepileptics (phenytoin, phenobarbital, primidone and possibly pheneturide), the serum antiepileptic levels may fall, leading to decreased seizure control in some patients.

Clinical evidence

A study in 50 folate-deficient epileptics (taking **phenytoin, phenobarbital** and **primidone** in various combinations) found that after one month of treatment with folic acid 5 mg daily, the plasma **phenytoin** levels of one group of 10 patients had fallen from 20 to 10 micrograms/mL. In another group of patients taking folic acid 15 mg daily the levels of **phenytoin** fell from 14 to 11 micrograms/mL. Only one patient (in the 5-mg folic acid group) had a marked increase in seizure frequency and severity. No alterations were seen in the **phenobarbital** levels.[1]

Another long-term study was conducted in 26 patients with folic acid deficiency (serum folate less than 5 nanograms/mL), and treated with two or more drugs (**phenytoin, phenobarbital, primidone**). The mental state of 22 of them (as shown by increased alertness, concentration, sociability etc.) improved to a variable degree when they were given folic acid 5 mg three times daily. However, the frequency and severity of seizures in 13 patients (50%) increased to such an extent that the vitamin had to be withdrawn from 9 of them.[2]

Similar results, both of increased seizure activity and decreased serum folate levels, have been described in other studies and reports in patients taking **phenytoin, phenobarbital, primidone** and **pheneturide**.[3-6]

Another report describes lack of **phenytoin** efficacy in a patient receiving ***UFT*** with **folinic acid**, which was attributed to the effect of the **folinic acid** on **phenytoin** levels.[7]

Mechanism

Patients taking antiepileptics may have subnormal serum folic acid levels. Frequencies of 27 to 76% have been reported for phenobarbital, primidone, and phenytoin alone or in various combinations.[8] One possible explanation is that this is due to the enzyme-inducing characteristics of these antiepileptics, which makes excessive demands on folate for the synthesis of the enzymes concerned with drug metabolism. Ultimately drug metabolism becomes limited by the lack of folate, and patients may also develop a reduction in their general mental health[2] and even frank megaloblastic anaemia.[8,9] If folic acid is then given to treat this deficiency, the metabolism of the antiepileptic increases once again,[10] resulting in a reduction in serum antiepileptic levels, which in some instances may become so low that seizure control is partially or totally lost.

Importance and management

A very well documented and clinically important interaction, which has been the subject of review.[11] Reductions in serum phenytoin levels of 16 to 50% have been described in patients taking 5 to 15 mg folic acid daily for 2 to 4 weeks.[1,3,12] If folic acid supplements are given to folate-deficient epileptics taking phenytoin, phenobarbital, primidone and possibly pheneturide, their serum antiepileptic levels should be well monitored so that suitable dosage increases can be made.

1. Baylis EM, Crowley JM, Preece JM, Sylvester PE, Marks V. Influence of folic acid on blood-phenytoin levels. *Lancet* (1971) i, 62–4.
2. Reynolds EH. Effects of folic acid on the mental state and fit-frequency of drug-treated epileptic patients. *Lancet* (1967) i, 1086–9.
3. Strauss RG, Bernstein R. Folic acid and Dilantin antagonism in pregnancy. *Obstet Gynecol* (1974) 44, 345–8.
4. Latham AN, Millbank L, Richens A, Rowe DJF. Liver enzyme induction by anticonvulsant drugs, and its relationship to disturbed calcium and folic acid metabolism. *J Clin Pharmacol* (1973) 13, 337–42.
5. Berg MJ, Fincham RW, Ebert BE, Schottelius DD. Phenytoin pharmacokinetics: before and after folic acid administration. *Epilepsia* (1992) 33, 712–20.
6. Seligmann H, Potasman I, Weller B, Schwartz M, Prokocimer M. Phenytoin-folic acid interaction: a lesson to be learned. *Clin Neuropharmacol* (1999) 5, 268–72.
7. Veldhorst-Janssen NML, Boersma HH, de Krom MCTFM, van Rijswijk REN. Oral tegafur/folinic acid chemotherapy decreases phenytoin efficacy. *Br J Cancer* (2004) 90, 745.
8. Davis RE, Woodliff HJ. Folic acid deficiency in patients receiving anticonvulsant drugs. *Med J Aust* (1971) 2, 1070–2.
9. Ryan GMS, Forshaw JWB. Megaloblastic anaemia due to phenytoin sodium. *BMJ* (1955) 11, 242–3.
10. Berg MJ, Fischer LJ, Rivey MP, Vern BA, Lantz RK, Schottelius DD. Phenytoin and folic acid interaction: a preliminary report. *Ther Drug Monit* (1983) 5, 389–94.
11. Lewis DP, Van Dyke DC, Willhite LA, Stumbo PJ, Berg MJ. Phenytoin-folic acid interaction. *Ann Pharmacother* (1995) 29, 726–35.
12. Furlanut M, Benetello P, Avogaro A, Dainese R. Effects of folic acid on phenytoin kinetics in healthy subjects. *Clin Pharmacol Ther* (1978) 24, 294–7.

Antiepileptics + Mefloquine

A woman whose epilepsy was controlled with sodium valproate developed convulsions when she took mefloquine. Note that mefloquine is normally contraindicated in epilepsy.

Clinical evidence, mechanism, importance and management

An isolated report describes a 20-year-old woman, with a 7-year history of epilepsy (bilateral myoclonus and generalised tonic-clonic seizures) controlled with **sodium valproate** 1.3 g daily, who developed tonic-clonic seizures 8 hours after taking the second of 3 prophylactic doses of mefloquine 250 mg.[1] It is not clear whether this resulted from a drug-drug or a drug-disease interaction. The manufacturers of mefloquine advise its avoidance in those with a history of convulsions as it may increase the risk of convulsions. In these patients mefloquine should be used only for curative treatment if compelling reasons exist.[2]

1. Besser R, Krämer G. Verdacht auf anfallfördernde Wirkung von Mefloquin (Lariam®). *Nervenarzt* (1991) 62, 760–1.
2. Lariam (Mefloquine hydrochloride). Roche Products Ltd. UK Summary of product characteristics, September 2005.

Antiepileptics + Quinine

Preliminary evidence suggests that the effects of carbamazepine and phenobarbital may be increased by quinine, possibly leading to toxicity. An isolated report suggests that phenytoin may reduce the levels of quinine but the levels of phenytoin do not appear to be affected by quinine.

Clinical evidence, mechanism, importance and management

Single doses of **carbamazepine** 200 mg, **phenobarbital** 120 mg or **phenytoin** 200 mg were given to 3 groups of 6 healthy subjects with and without a single 600-mg dose of quinine sulfate. The AUC of **carbamazepine** and **phenobarbital** were increased by 104% and 57%, respectively, and the peak plasma levels were increased by 81% and 53%, respectively. **Phenytoin** was not significantly affected. The reasons for these effects are not known but the authors suggest that quinine inhibits the metabolism of **carbamazepine** and **phenobarbital** (but not **phenytoin**) by the liver, so that their levels become raised.[1]

In an earlier study, **phenobarbital** 125 mg daily for 4 days caused only a small reduction in the plasma half-life of quinine in 2 healthy subjects.[2]

Information seems to be limited to these studies. The importance of the interactions with either **carbamazepine** and **phenobarbital** awaits assessment in a clinically realistic situation (i.e. in patients taking multiple doses) but in the meantime it would seem prudent to monitor the effects of **carbamazepine** or **phenobarbital** for evidence of increased effects and possible toxicity if quinine is also taken.

An isolated report describes a 22-month-old girl treated with **phenytoin**, **sodium valproate** and **topiramate** for epilepsy and then with quinine sulfate (initially intravenously, then orally) followed by a single dose of sulfadoxine/pyrimethamine for malaria. Her malaria film became negative after 4 days of the 7-day quinine course. About 1 month later she was found to have recrudescent falciparum malaria, which was treated with quinine sulfate and then atovaquone/proguanil. Although it is possible that quinine resistance may have occurred, the authors also considered that enzyme induction by **phenytoin** may have led to suboptimal quinine levels.[3]

Although quinine does not appear to affect **phenytoin** levels, the isolated case report suggests that levels of quinine may be reduced in the presence of **phenytoin** and it would seem prudent to monitor carefully concurrent use.

1. Amabeoku GJ, Chikuni O, Akino C, Mutetwa S. Pharmacokinetic interaction of single doses of quinine and carbamazepine, phenobarbitone and phenytoin in healthy volunteers. *East Afr Med J* (1993) 70, 90–3.
2. Saggers VH, Hariratnajothi N, McLean AEM. The effect of diet and phenobarbitone on quinine metabolism in the rat and in man. *Biochem Pharmacol* (1970) 19, 499–503.
3. Fabre C, Criddle J, Nolder D, Klein JL. Recrudescence of imported falciparum malaria after quinine therapy: potential drug interaction with phenytoin. *Trans R Soc Trop Med Hyg* (2005) 99, 871–3.

Antiepileptics + Quinolones

Studies suggest that ciprofloxacin, clinafloxacin, and enoxacin do not usually have a clinically significant effect on phenytoin levels. However, case reports describe both a rise and a fall in phenytoin levels in patients given ciprofloxacin. Quinolones alone very occasionally cause convulsions, therefore they should be used with caution in patients with epilepsy.

Clinical evidence

(a) Ciprofloxacin

In a study in 4 healthy subjects there was no difference in the pharmacokinetics of **phenytoin** 200 mg daily when it was given with ciprofloxacin 500 mg twice daily. However, one of the 4 subjects experienced a 30% decrease in the **phenytoin** maximum serum levels when ciprofloxacin was added.[1] In another study in 7 patients taking **phenytoin**, ciprofloxacin 500 mg twice daily for 10 days caused no significant change in **phenytoin** levels, although there was a tendency for an increase (mean 24% rise).[2] Four case reports describe falls of 50% or more in **phenytoin** serum levels when ciprofloxacin was added, accompanied by seizures in 3 instances.[3-6] Another report describes unexpectedly low **phenytoin** levels (measured after a loading dose) in a woman taking ciprofloxacin.[7] Conversely, **phenytoin** levels rose in an elderly woman, possibly as a result of the ciprofloxacin she was taking.[8] In one report, blood levels of **phenytoin** and **valproic acid** were not affected by ciprofloxacin although a seizure occurred on the fourth day of therapy.[9] Other cases describe seizures in patients taking **phenytoin** when given ciprofloxacin, but with little or no information on **phenytoin** levels.[10]

(b) Clinafloxacin

Phenytoin 300 mg daily was given to healthy subjects for 10 days, then clinafloxacin 400 mg twice daily was added for a further 2 weeks. The maximum serum **phenytoin** levels rose by 18%, from 6.74 to 7.95 mg/L, the AUC rose by 20% and the clearance fell by 17%.[11]

(c) Enoxacin

In a study in healthy subjects, enoxacin did not appear to alter **phenytoin** serum levels, nor were multiple-dose serum enoxacin levels significantly altered by **phenytoin**.[12]

Mechanism

Fluoroquinolones alone rarely cause convulsions both in patients with and without a history of seizures. The mechanism for the effect of ciprofloxacin on phenytoin levels is unknown, and is unlikely to be due to effects on hepatic metabolism or oral absorption.[13,14] However, ciprofloxacin decreased phenytoin levels in an *animal* study, and a suggested reason for this was increased urinary excretion.[15]

Importance and management

The known potential for quinolones to induce seizures suggests that these antibacterials should either be avoided in epileptics, or only used when the benefits of treatment outweigh the potential risks of seizures. Some of the reactions seem to be drug-disease interactions rather than drug-drug interactions, the usual outcome being that the control of epilepsy is worsened. However, it appears that ciprofloxacin may also alter (usually decrease) phenytoin levels, and if this combination is used it would be prudent to consider monitoring phenytoin levels. Enoxacin appears not to alter phenytoin levels.

1. Job ML, Arn SK, Strom JG, Jacobs NF, D'Souza MJ. Effect of ciprofloxacin on the pharmacokinetics of multiple-dose phenytoin serum concentrations. *Ther Drug Monit* (1994) 16, 427–31.
2. Schroeder D, Frye J, Alldredge B, Messing R, Flaherty J. Effect of ciprofloxacin on serum phenytoin concentrations in epileptic patients. *Pharmacotherapy* (1991) 11, 275.
3. Dillard ML, Fink RM, Parkerson R. Ciprofloxacin-phenytoin interaction. *Ann Pharmacother* (1992) 26, 263.
4. Pollak PT, Slayter KL. Hazards of doubling phenytoin dose in the face of an unrecognized interaction with ciprofloxacin. *Ann Pharmacother* (1997) 31, 61–4.
5. Brouwers PJ, DeBoer LE, Guchelaar H-J. Ciprofloxacin-phenytoin interaction. *Ann Pharmacother* (1997) 31, 498.
6. Otero M-J, Morán D, Valverde M-P. Interaction between phenytoin and ciprofloxacin. *Ann Pharmacother* (1999) 33, 251–2.
7. McLeod R, Trinkle R. Comment: unexpectedly low phenytoin concentration in a patient receiving ciprofloxacin. *Ann Pharmacother* (1998) 32, 1110–11.
8. Hull RL. Possible phenytoin-ciprofloxacin interaction. *Ann Pharmacother* (1993) 27, 1283.
9. Slavich IL, Gleffe R, Haas EJ. Grand mal epileptic seizures during ciprofloxacin therapy. *JAMA* (1989) 261, 558–9.
10. Anon. Risk of seizures from concomitant use of ciprofloxacin and phenytoin in patients with epilepsy. *Can Med Assoc J* (1998) 158, 104–5.
11. Randinitis EJ, Koup JR, Bron NJ, Hounslow NJ, Rausch G, Abel R, Vassos AB, Sedman AJ. Drug interaction studies with clinafloxacin and probenecid, cimetidine, phenytoin and warfarin. *Drugs* (1999) 58 (Suppl 2), 254–5.
12. Thomas D, Humphrey G, Kinkel A, Sedman A, Rowland M, Toon S, Aarons L, Hopkins K. A study to evaluate the potential pharmacokinetic interaction between oral enoxacin (ENX) and oral phenytoin (PHE). *Pharm Res* (1986) 3 (Suppl), 99S.
13. Pollak PT, Slayter KL. Comment: ciprofloxacin-phenytoin interaction. *Ann Pharmacother* (1997) 31, 1549–50.
14. Brouwers PJ, de Boer LE, Guchelaar H-J. Comment: ciprofloxacin-phenytoin interaction. *Ann Pharmacother* (1997) 31, 1550.
15. al-Humayyd MS. Ciprofloxacin decreases plasma phenytoin concentrations in the rat. *Eur J Drug Metab Pharmacokinet* (1997) 22, 35–9.

Antiepileptics + St John's wort (*Hypericum perforatum*)

St John's wort modestly increased the clearance of single-dose carbamazepine, but had no effect on multiple-dose carbamazepine pharmacokinetics. Carbamazepine does not appear to significantly affect the pharmacokinetics of hypericin or pseudohypericin (constituents of St John's wort). St John's wort is predicted to reduce the blood levels of phenytoin and phenobarbital, but this awaits clinical confirmation.

Clinical evidence, mechanism, importance and management

In a multiple-dose study, St John's wort had no effect on the pharmacokinetics of **carbamazepine** or its metabolite (carbamazepine-10,11-epoxide) in 8 healthy subjects. In this study, subjects took **carbamazepine** 200 mg increased to 400 mg daily alone for 20 days, then with St John's wort 300 mg (standardised to 0.3% hypericin) three times daily for a further 14 days.[1] In contrast, the AUC of a single 400-mg dose of **carbamazepine** was reduced by 21% after St John's wort 300 mg was given three times daily for 14 days, and the AUC of the 10,11-epoxide metabolite was increased by 26%.[2]

St John's wort is a known enzyme inducer, and the results with single-dose **carbamazepine** are as predicted. However, **carbamazepine** is also an enzyme inducer, which induces its own metabolism (autoinduction). It is suggested that St John's wort is not sufficiently potent an inducer to further induce **carbamazepine** metabolism when autoinduction has occurred,[1] and therefore a small interaction is seen with single doses but no interaction is seen with multiple doses.

A double-blind, placebo-controlled study in healthy subjects found that, apart from a modest 29% decrease in the AUC of pseudohypericin, **carbamazepine** did not significantly affect the pharmacokinetics of either hypericin or pseudohypericin, which are both constituents of St John's wort.[3] The available evidence therefore suggests that a clinically significant interaction between **carbamazepine** and St John's wort is unlikely. Prior to the publication of the above reports, the CSM in the UK had advised that patients taking a number of drugs including the antiepileptics **carbamazepine**, **phenytoin** and **phenobarbital** should not take St John's wort.[4] This advice was based on predicted pharmacokinetic interactions. In the light of the above studies, this advice no longer applies to **carbamazepine**, but until more is known, it should probably still apply to **phenytoin** and **phenobarbital**.

1. Burstein AH, Horton RL, Dunn T, Alfaro RM, Piscitelli SC, Theodore W. Lack of effect of St John's wort on carbamazepine pharmacokinetics in healthy volunteers. *Clin Pharmacol Ther* (2000) 68, 605–12.
2. Burstein AH, Piscitelli SC, Alfaro RM, Theodore W. Effect of St John's wort on carbamazepine single-dose pharmacokinetics. *Epilepsia* (2001) 42 (Suppl 7), 253.
3. Johne A, Perloff ES, Bauer S, Schmider J, Mai I, Brockmöller J, Roots I. Impact of cytochrome P-450 inhibition by cimetidine and induction by carbamazepine on the kinetics of hypericin and pseudohypericin in healthy volunteers. *Eur J Clin Pharmacol* (2004) 60, 617–22.
4. Committee on the Safety of Medicines (UK). Message from Professor A Breckenridge (Chairman of CSM) and Fact Sheet for Health Care Professionals, 29th February 2000.

Antiepileptics + Terbinafine

An isolated report describes the development of fatal toxic epidermal necrolysis shortly after a patient taking phenobarbital and carbamazepine started taking terbinafine.

Clinical evidence, mechanism, importance and management

An isolated report describes a 26-year-old woman with cerebral palsy who had been taking **phenobarbital** 15 mg with **carbamazepine** 400 mg daily for 12 years to control epilepsy, and who developed fatal toxic epidermal necrolysis 2 weeks after starting oral terbinafine 250 mg daily for tinea corporis. The reasons are not understood, but the authors point out that all three drugs can cause adverse skin reactions (erythema multiforme) and suggest that some synergism may have occurred.[1] It is uncertain whether this was a true interaction or a terbinafine adverse effect.

1. White SI, Bowen-Jones D. Toxic epidermal necrolysis induced by terbinafine in a patient on long-term anti-epileptics. *Br J Dermatol* (1996) 134, 188–9.

Antiepileptics + Tobacco

Smoking tobacco appears to have no important effect on the serum levels of phenytoin, phenobarbital or carbamazepine.

Clinical evidence, mechanism, importance and management

A comparative study in 88 epileptic patients taking antiepileptics (**phenobarbital**, **phenytoin** and **carbamazepine** alone or in combination) found that although smoking had a tendency to lower the steady-state serum levels of these drugs, a statistically significant effect on the concentration–dose ratios was only found in the patients taking **phenobarbital**.[1] However, in another study in healthy subjects, there was no difference in the pharmacokinetics of a single 60-mg dose of **phenobarbital** between smokers and non-smokers.[2] In practical terms smoking appears to have only a negligible effect on the serum levels of these antiepileptics and epileptics who smoke are unlikely to need higher doses than non-smokers.

1. Benetello P, Furlanut M, Pasqui L, Carmillo L, Perlotto N, Testa G. Absence of effect of cigarette smoking on serum concentrations of some anticonvulsants in epileptic patients. *Clin Pharmacokinet* (1987) 12, 302–4.
2. Mirfazaelian A, Jahanzad F, Tabatabaei-far M, Farsam H, Mahmoudian M. Effect of smoking on single dose pharmacokinetics of phenobarbital. *Biopharm Drug Dispos* (2001) 22, 403–6.

Antiepileptics + Vitamin B substances

High daily doses of pyridoxine can cause 35% reductions in phenytoin levels and 50% reductions in phenobarbital levels in some patients. Some evidence suggests that high doses of nicotinamide reduce the conversion of primidone to phenobarbital, and increase carbamazepine levels.

Clinical evidence

(a) Nicotinamide

Nicotinamide 41 to 178 mg/kg daily increased the levels of **primidone** and decreased the levels of **primidone**-derived phenobarbital in 3 children. Although two of the children had refractory seizures, seizure frequency decreased while on nicotinamide. Two of the children on **carbamazepine** had increases in their **carbamazepine** levels.[1]

(b) Pyridoxine

Pyridoxine 200 mg daily for 4 weeks reduced the **phenobarbital** serum levels of 5 epileptics by about 50%. Reductions in serum **phenytoin** levels of about 35% (range 17 to 70%) were also seen when patients were given pyridoxine 80 to 400 mg daily for 2 to 4 weeks. However, no interaction occurred in a number of other patients taking these drugs.[2]

Mechanism

It is suggested that the pyridoxine increases and nicotinamide decreases the activity of the liver enzymes concerned with the metabolism of these antiepileptics.[1,2]

Importance and management

Information seems to be limited, but what is known suggests that concurrent use should be monitored if large doses of pyridoxine or nicotinamide are used, being alert for the need to modify the antiepileptic dosage. It seems unlikely that small doses (as in multivitamin preparations) will interact to any great extent.

1. Bourgeois BF, Dodson WE, Ferrendelli JA. Interactions between primidone, carbamazepine, and nicotinamide. *Neurology* (1982) 32, 1122–26.
2. Hansson O, Sillanpaa M. Pyridoxine and serum concentration of phenytoin and phenobarbitone. *Lancet* (1976) i, 256.

Carbamazepine + Allopurinol

There is some evidence to suggest that high-dose allopurinol (15 mg/kg or 600 mg daily) can gradually raise serum carbamazepine levels by about a third. It appears that allopurinol 300 mg daily has no effect on carbamazepine levels.

Clinical evidence

In a 6-month study, 7 epileptic patients taking antiepileptics, which included carbamazepine, were also given allopurinol 100 mg three times daily for 3 months then 200 mg three times daily for 3 months. The mean trough steady-state serum carbamazepine levels of 6 of the patients rose by 30% or more and the carbamazepine clearance fell by 32% during the second 3-month period. A reduction in the carbamazepine dosage was needed in 3 patients because of the symptoms that developed.[1] Similarly, in another study allopurinol 10 mg/kg increased to 15 mg/kg daily for 12 weeks increased carbamazepine levels by 29% in 11 patients taking antiepileptics, which included carbamazepine.[2] Conversely, in another study, allopurinol (150 mg daily in those less than 20 kg, and 300 mg daily for other patients) for 4 months had no effect on carbamazepine levels in 53 patients taking antiepileptics, which included carbamazepine.[3]

Mechanism

Uncertain. A possible explanation is that allopurinol can act as a liver enzyme inhibitor, which reduces the metabolism and clearance of carbamazepine.

Importance and management

Information is limited to these studies, but be alert for the need to reduce the dosage of carbamazepine if high doses of allopurinol are used long-term. This interaction apparently takes several weeks or even months to develop fully. More study is needed.

1. Mikati M, Erba G, Skouteli H, Gadia C. Pharmacokinetic study of allopurinol in resistant epilepsy: evidence for significant drug interactions. *Neurology* (1990) 40 (Suppl 1), 138.
2. Coppola G, Pascotto A. Double-blind, placebo-controlled, cross-over trial of allopurinol as add-on therapy in childhood refractory epilepsy. *Brain Dev* (1996) 18, 50–2.
3. Zagnoni PG, Bianchi A, Zolo P, Canger R, Cornaggia C, D'Alessandro P, DeMarco P, Pisani F, Gianelli M, Verzé L, Viani F, Zaccara G. Allopurinol as add-on therapy in refractory epilepsy: a double-blind placebo-controlled randomized study. *Epilepsia* (1994) 35, 107–12.

Carbamazepine + Amiodarone

Amiodarone does not appear to affect the pharmacokinetics of carbamazepine.

Clinical evidence, mechanism, importance and management

A single 400-mg dose of carbamazepine was given to 9 patients with cardiac disease (premature ventricular contractions, supraventricular tachycardia, sinus arrhythmia) before and after they took amiodarone 200 mg twice daily for a month. The pharmacokinetics of carbamazepine were found to be unchanged by the amiodarone. This certainly suggests that no clinically important interaction occurs, but it needs confirmation in patients who are given both drugs long term. Furthermore, the authors postulate that a higher amiodarone dose may inhibit the metabolism of the carbamazepine by the liver.[1]

1. Leite SAO, Leite PJM, Rocha GA, Routledge PA, Bittencourt PRM. Carbamazepine kinetics in cardiac patients before and during amiodarone. *Arq Neuropsiquiatr* (1994) 52, 210–15.

Carbamazepine + Antipsychotics

An increase in the serum levels of carbamazepine or its epoxide metabolite has been reported in patients given loxapine, haloperidol, quetiapine, risperidone, or chlorpromazine with amoxapine. Toxicity has occurred. Thioridazine appears not to raise carbamazepine-10,11-epoxide levels. Isolated cases of Stevens-Johnson syndrome have occurred in patients taking antipsychotics with carbamazepine. Carbamazepine may reduce levels of many of the antipsychotics. A case of neuroleptic malignant syndrome had been described in a patient taking antipsychotics and carbamazepine. See also 'Antipsychotics + Antiepileptics', p.707.

Clinical evidence, mechanism, importance and management

(a) Raised carbamazepine or carbamazepine-10,11-epoxide levels

Two patients, one taking **loxapine** 500 mg daily and the other taking **chlorpromazine** 350 mg and **amoxapine** 300 mg daily, developed toxicity (ataxia, nausea, anxiety) when given carbamazepine 600 to 900 mg daily, even though their serum carbamazepine levels were low to normal.[1] In another case, neurotoxicity (ataxia, lethargy, visual disturbances) developed in a man given carbamazepine and **loxapine**.[2] In all 3 cases, the toxicity appeared to be due to elevated carbamazepine-10,11-epoxide levels (the metabolite of carbamazepine).[1,2] The problem resolved when the carbamazepine dosages were reduced. Raised carbamazepine-10,11-epoxide levels have also been reported in 2 patients after they were given **quetiapine**, with toxicity in one of the patients.[3] **Risperidone** 1 mg daily for 2 weeks raised carbamazepine levels by about 20% in 8 patients.[4] Raised serum carbamazepine levels have also been seen with 'haloperidol', (p.707).

It is relatively well documented that carbamazepine can reduce the levels of many of the antipsychotics (discussed in individual monographs elsewhere). The above reports show that the effect of the antipsychotic on carbamazepine should also be considered. The levels of both carbamazepine and its metabolite should be monitored if toxicity develops.

(b) No changes to carbamazepine-10,11-epoxide levels

Thioridazine 100 to 200 mg daily was found to have no effect on the steady-state levels of carbamazepine or carbamazepine-10,11-epoxide in 8 epileptic patients,[5] and also carbamazepine had no significant effect on **thioridazine** plasma levels in 6 patients.[6]

(c) Stevens-Johnson syndrome

Three patients treated with various antipsychotics (**fluphenazine**, **haloperidol**, **trifluoperazine**, **chlorpromazine**) developed Stevens-Johnson syndrome within 8 to 14 days of starting to take carbamazepine. All 3 had erythema multiforme skin lesions and at least two mucous membranes were affected. After treatment, all 3 were restarted on all their previous drugs, except carbamazepine, without problems.[7] Another case of Stevens-Johnson syndrome has been reported in a patient taking carbamazepine, **lithium carbonate**, **haloperidol** and **trihexyphenidyl**.[8] The reasons are not understood. Stevens-Johnson syndrome with carbamazepine alone is rare, and the risk appears to be mostly confined to the first 8 weeks of treatment.[9] It may be more common in patients being treated for conditions other than epilepsy.[10] It is not possible to say whether the concurrent use of antipsychotics increases the risk of its development, but until more is known it would be prudent to monitor the outcome, particularly during the first 2 weeks of combined use.

(d) Neuroleptic malignant syndrome

A 54-year old man living in a psychiatric hospital, who had been taking **haloperidol**, **levomepromazine**, **sultopride**, and metixene long-term was prescribed carbamazepine 400 mg daily for impulsive behaviour. The following day he became unstable on his feet, and after 3 days could no longer walk by himself. He had a fever of 40°C, muscle rigidity, diaphoresis, and serum creatine phosphokinase was elevated to 923 units/L. He was diagnosed as having neuroleptic malignant syndrome (NMS), and recovered after body cooling and administration of fluids, with symptoms resolving over 12 days. Before carbamazepine was given, his **haloperidol** level was 19 nanograms/mL and after 3 days of carbamazepine it was reduced to 10.9 nanograms/mL.[11]

Carbamazepine alone is not associated with NMS. It was suggested that carbamazepine may have reduced levels of the antimuscarinic (anticholinergic) antipsychotics (**levomepromazine** and **sultopride**), resulting in cholinergic rebound, and inducing NMS.[11] The general applicability of this case is unknown.

1. Pitterle ME, Collins DM. Carbamazepine-10,11-epoxide evaluation associated with coadministration of loxitane or amoxapine. *Epilepsia* (1988) 29, 654.
2. Collins DM, Gidal BE, Pitterle ME. Potential interaction between carbamazepine and loxapine: case report and retrospective review. *Ann Pharmacother* (1993) 27, 1180–3.
3. Fitzgerald BJ, Okos AJ. Elevation of carbamazepine-10,11-epoxide by quetiapine. *Pharmacotherapy* (2002) 22, 1500–503.
4. Mula M, Monaco F. Carbamazepine–risperidone interactions in patients with epilepsy. *Clin Neuropharmacol* (2002) 25, 97–100.
5. Spina E, Amendola D'Agostino AM, Ioculano MP, Oteri G, Fazio A, Pisani F. No effect of thioridazine on plasma concentrations of carbamazepine and its active metabolite carbamazepine-10,11-epoxide. *Ther Drug Monit* (1990) 12, 511–13.
6. Tiihonen J, Vartiainen H, Hakola P. Carbamazepine-induced changes in plasma levels of neuroleptics. *Pharmacopsychiatry* (1995) 28, 26–8.
7. Wong KE. Stevens-Johnson Syndrome in neuroleptic-carbamazepine combination. *Singapore Med J* (1990) 31, 432–3.
8. Fawcett RG. Erythema multiforme major in a patient treated with carbamazepine. *J Clin Psychiatry* (1987) 48, 416–17.
9. Rzany B, Coreia O, Kelly JP, Naldi L, Auquier A, Stern R. Risk of Stevens-Johnson syndrome and toxic epidermal necrolysis during the first weeks of antiepileptic therapy: a case-control study. *Lancet* (1999) 353, 2190–4.
10. Dhar S, Todi SK. Are carbamazepine-induced Stevens-Johnson syndrome and toxic epidermal necrolysis more common in nonepileptic patients? *Dermatology* (1999) 199, 194.
11. Nisijima K, Kusakabe Y, Ohtuka K, Ishiguro T. Addition of carbamazepine to long-term treatment with neuroleptics may induce neuroleptic malignant syndrome. *Biol Psychiatry* (1998) 44, 930–1.

Carbamazepine + Aspirin or NSAIDs

Carbamazepine levels are unaffected by aspirin or tolfenamic acid.

Clinical evidence, mechanism, importance and management

No changes in carbamazepine serum levels were seen in 10 patients who took aspirin 1.5 g daily for 3 days.[1] It would appear that no precautions are necessary if aspirin is used in patients on carbamazepine.

Tolfenamic acid 300 mg for 3 days had no significant effect on the serum levels of carbamazepine in 11 patients.[1] No special precautions seem necessary if these drugs are taken concurrently.

1. Neuvonen PJ, Lehtovaara R, Bardy A, Elomaa E. Antipyretic analgesics in patients on antiepileptic drug therapy. *Eur J Clin Pharmacol* (1979) 15, 263–8.

Carbamazepine + Azoles

Ketoconazole causes a small to moderate rise in serum carbamazepine levels. A marked rise in carbamazepine levels has been seen in two patients taking fluconazole, with toxicity in one. Adverse effects were seen in another patient when carbamazepine was given with miconazole. Carbamazepine may markedly reduce the levels of itraconazole and possibly voriconazole, and is predicted to lower the levels of posaconazole.

Clinical evidence

(a) Fluconazole

A 33-year-old man whose seizures were stabilised by carbamazepine became extremely lethargic after taking fluconazole 150 mg daily for 3 days. His carbamazepine level was found to have risen from 11.1 to 24.5 micrograms/mL. Symptoms resolved when both drugs were stopped, and carbamazepine was later re-introduced without problem.[1] Another well-documented case report describes a threefold increase in carbamazepine levels (without any signs of toxicity) 10 days after fluconazole 400 mg daily was started.[2]

(b) Itraconazole

About 14 days after starting carbamazepine 400 mg daily, a patient taking itraconazole 200 mg daily was noted to have low itraconazole levels (0.15 mg/L), and about 2 months later they were undetectable. About 3 weeks after stopping the carbamazepine, itraconazole levels had reached the therapeutic range (0.36 mg/L).[3] For mention of 2 patients taking carbamazepine with phenytoin, who had undetectable or very low itraconazole levels, and who relapsed or did not respond to itraconazole therapy, see 'Phenytoin + Azoles', p.552.

(c) Ketoconazole

A study in 8 patients with epilepsy taking carbamazepine found that oral ketoconazole 200 mg daily for 10 days increased their serum carbamazepine levels by 28.6% (from 5.6 to 7.2 micrograms/mL) without affecting carbamazepine-10,11-epoxide levels. When the ketoconazole was stopped the serum carbamazepine levels returned to their former levels.[4]

(d) Miconazole

A patient receiving long-term treatment with carbamazepine 400 mg daily developed malaise, myoclonia and tremor within 3 days of being given oral miconazole 1.125 g. The same reaction occurred on each subsequent occasion that miconazole was given. These toxic effects disappeared when the miconazole was withdrawn.[5]

Mechanism

Carbamazepine levels are thought to rise because azole antifungals inhibit the cytochrome P450 isoenzyme CYP3A4, which is concerned with the metabolism of carbamazepine. Different azoles affect CYP3A4 to varying degrees, see 'azole antifungals', (p.207). Carbamazepine is an enzyme inducer, and appears to decrease the levels of azole antifungals by increasing their metabolism.

Importance and management

Evidence for these interactions is limited and in some cases the effects are only modest. Nevertheless, it would seem prudent to monitor the outcome of adding azole antifungals to established carbamazepine treatment, being alert for any evidence of increased carbamazepine adverse effects.

Note also that carbamazepine may reduce the levels of azole antifungals: a marked reduction in itraconazole levels has been reported, and some manufacturers of itraconazole consequently say that concurrent use of potent enzyme inducers such as carbamazepine is not recommended.[6,7] Based on the interaction with 'phenytoin', (p.552), which results in reduced **posaconazole** levels, the manufacturer of **posaconazole** suggests that concurrent use of **posaconazole** and carbamazepine should be avoided, unless the benefits outweigh the risks.[8] If both drugs are given it would seem sensible to consider increasing the **posaconazole** dose, and increase monitoring of carbamazepine levels. Based on the interaction with 'phenytoin', (p.552), the manufacturers of **voriconazole** also contraindicate the concurrent use of carbamazepine and **voriconazole**.[9,10]

1. Nair DR, Morris HH. Potential fluconazole-induced carbamazepine toxicity. *Ann Pharmacother* (1999) 33, 790–2.
2. Finch CK, Green CA, Self TH. Fluconazole-carbamazepine interaction. *South Med J* (2002) 95, 1099–1100.
3. Bonay M, Jonville-Bera AP, Diot P, Lemarie E, Lavandier M, Autret E. Possible interaction between phenobarbital, carbamazepine and itraconazole. *Drug Safety* (1993) 9, 309–11.
4. Spina E, Arena D, Scordo MG, Fazio A, Pisani F, Perucca E. Elevation of plasma carbamazepine concentrations by ketoconazole in patients with epilepsy. *Ther Drug Monit* (1997) 19, 535–8.
5. Loupi E, Descotes J, Lery N, Evreux JC. Interactions médicamenteuses et miconazole. A propos de 10 observations. *Therapie* (1982) 37, 437–41.
6. Sporanox Capsules (Itraconazole). Janssen-Cilag Ltd. UK Summary of product characteristics, March 2004.
7. Sporanox Capsules (Itraconazole). Janssen. US Prescribing information, June 2006.
8. Noxafil (Posaconazole). Schering-Plough Ltd. UK Summary of product characteristics, October 2006.
9. VFEND (Voriconazole). Pfizer Ltd. UK Summary of product characteristics, July 2007.
10. VFEND (Voriconazole). Pfizer Inc. US Prescribing information, November 2006.

Carbamazepine + Bile-acid binding resins

Colestyramine 8 g did not affect the absorption of carbamazepine 400 mg in 6 healthy subjects, whereas colestipol 10 g reduced it by 10%. Both colestyramine and colestipol were given as a single dose 5 minutes after the carbamazepine.[1] This small reduction is unlikely to be clinically important.

1. Neuvonen PJ, Kivistö K, Hirvisalo EL. Effects of resins and activated charcoal on the absorption of digoxin, carbamazepine and frusemide. *Br J Clin Pharmacol* (1988) 25, 229–33.

Carbamazepine or Oxcarbazepine + Calcium-channel blockers

Both diltiazem and verapamil can increase serum carbamazepine levels causing toxicity. Limited evidence suggests that amlodipine and nifedipine do not affect carbamazepine levels. A single case report describes neurological toxicity in a patient taking phenytoin and carbamazepine with isradipine.
The plasma levels of felodipine, nifedipine, nilvadipine, and nimodipine are reduced by carbamazepine. Felodipine levels are modestly reduced by oxcarbazepine.

Clinical evidence

(a) Diltiazem

An epileptic patient taking carbamazepine 400 mg in the morning and 600 mg in the evening developed symptoms of toxicity (dizziness, nausea, ataxia and diplopia) within 2 days of starting to take diltiazem 60 mg three times daily. His serum carbamazepine levels had risen by about 40% to 21 mg/L, but fell once again when the diltiazem was stopped. No interaction occurred when the diltiazem was replaced by **nifedipine** 20 mg three times daily.[1] Other case reports describe carbamazepine toxicity and a rise in serum levels of up to fourfold in a total of 11 patients given diltiazem.[2-7] One patient required a 62% reduction in the carbamazepine dose.[2] Another patient had a marked fall in serum carbamazepine levels of 54% when diltiazem was stopped.[8] For a further case report involving diltiazem, see *Nifedipine*, below.

(b) Felodipine

After taking felodipine 10 mg daily for 4 days, 10 epileptics (including 4 taking carbamazepine alone and 3 taking carbamazepine with phenytoin) had markedly reduced plasma felodipine levels (peak levels of 1.6 nanomol/L compared with 8.9 nanomol/L in 12 control subjects). The felodipine bioavailability was reduced to 6.6%.[9] A study in 8 subjects found that the AUC of felodipine was reduced by only 28% by oxcarbazepine 600 to 900 mg daily for a week.[10]

(c) Isradipine

A man taking carbamazepine and phenytoin developed neurological toxicity while taking isradipine, which was attributed to an interaction between the phenytoin and isradipine.[11] However, although carbamazepine levels remained within normal limits, a commentator suggested that an interaction between carbamazepine and isradipine was plausible.[12]

(d) Nifedipine

Nifedipine 20 mg twice daily for 2 weeks did not affect the steady-state carbamazepine levels in 12 epileptic patients.[13] Similarly, a retrospective study of 5 patients suggested that nifedipine does not usually raise carbamazepine levels or cause toxicity.[4] A man had a marked rise in serum carbamazepine levels when nifedipine was replaced by **diltiazem**. When **diltiazem** was replaced by **amlodipine**, his carbamazepine levels returned to normal, suggesting that neither nifedipine nor **amlodipine** interact with carbamazepine.[14] Another patient had no change in carbamazepine levels when also given nifedipine.[1]

A study in 12 epileptics receiving long-term treatment with carbamazepine found that the AUC of concurrent nifedipine 20 mg was only 22% of the values seen in 12 healthy subjects not taking carbamazepine.[13]

(e) Nilvadipine

A 59-year-old man taking nilvadipine 8 mg daily for hypertension and haloperidol for psychotic symptoms was given carbamazepine because haloperidol alone did not control symptoms of mania. The carbamazepine dosage was gradually increased from 100 mg to 600 mg daily. Although the manic symptoms were improved, his blood pressure rose to 230/140 mmHg after 3 days of treatment with carbamazepine 600 mg daily. Blood pressure was temporarily controlled by **nifedipine** 10 mg sublingually. Retrospective analyses found that plasma levels of nilvadipine were reduced during the use of carbamazepine 100 and 300 mg daily and undetectable when the carbamazepine dose was increased to 600 mg daily. Plasma levels of nilvadipine rose after carbamazepine was discontinued and blood pressure returned to normal after about 2 weeks.[15]

(f) Nimodipine

A study in 8 epileptic patients receiving long-term treatment (including 2 taking carbamazepine with phenobarbital, 1 taking carbamazepine with clobazam, and 1 taking carbamazepine with phenytoin) found that the AUC of a single 60-mg oral dose of nimodipine was only about 15% of that achieved in a group of healthy subjects,[16] suggesting that carbamazepine lowers nimodipine exposure.

(g) Verapamil

Carbamazepine toxicity developed in 6 epileptic patients within 36 to 96 hours of them starting to take verapamil 120 mg three times daily. The symptoms disappeared when the verapamil was withdrawn. Total carbamazepine plasma levels had risen by 46% (a 33% rise in free plasma carbamazepine levels). Rechallenge of two of the patients who only found mild toxicity with a lower dose of verapamil 120 mg twice a day caused a similar rise in serum verapamil levels, again with mild toxicity. This report also describes another patient who had elevated serum carbamazepine levels while also taking verapamil.[17] Carbamazepine toxicity is described in 3 other patients, again caused by verapamil.[18,19] The verapamil was successfully replaced by **nifedipine** in one patient.[18]

Oxcarbazepine 450 mg twice daily was given to 10 healthy subjects who were then also given verapamil 120 mg twice daily for 5 days. The AUC of the monohydroxy derivative of the oxcarbazepine (the active metabolite) fell by about 20% but oxcarbazepine levels were unaltered.[20]

Mechanism

It would appear that diltiazem and verapamil inhibit the metabolism of carbamazepine by the cytochrome P450 isoenzyme CYP3A4, thereby reducing its loss from the body and increasing serum levels. In contrast, carbamazepine is an enzyme inducer, which increases the metabolism of the calcium-channel blockers by the liver, resulting in a very rapid loss from the body.

Importance and management

Information about the effects of calcium-channel blockers on carbamazepine is limited, but what is known indicates that if carbamazepine is given with verapamil or diltiazem, the carbamazepine dosage may possibly need to be reduced to avoid toxicity. A 50% reduction in the dose of carbamazepine has been suggested if diltiazem is to be used.[5] Nifedipine and amlodipine normally appear to be non-interacting alternatives. Oxcarbazepine appears to be a non-interacting alternative for carbamazepine.

Carbamazepine has been shown to lower the levels of a number of calcium-channel blockers. Given that the majority are metabolised by CYP3A4 (see 'calcium-channel blockers', (p.860)) most calcium-channel blockers would be expected to interact similarly. If a calcium-channel blocker is given to a patient taking carbamazepine expect to need to use a larger dose. If carbamazepine is added to existing treatment with a calcium-channel blocker monitor the blood pressure and expect to need to increase the dose. Note that the manufacturer of nimodipine[21] contraindicates its use with carbamazepine.

Oxcarbazepine interacts to a lesser extent than carbamazepine and it may therefore be a suitable alternative in some patients.

1. Brodie MJ, Macphee GJA. Carbamazepine neurotoxicity precipitated by diltiazem. *BMJ* (1986) 292, 1170–1.
2. Eimer M, Carter BL. Elevated serum carbamazepine concentrations following diltiazem initiation. *Drug Intell Clin Pharm* (1987) 21, 340–2.
3. Ahmad S. Diltiazem-carbamazepine interaction. *Am Heart J* (1990) 120, 1485–6.
4. Bahls FH, Ozuna J, Ritchie DE. Interactions between calcium channel blockers and the anticonvulsants carbamazepine and phenytoin. *Neurology* (1991) 41, 740–2.
5. Shaughnessy AF, Mosley MR. Elevated carbamazepine levels associated with diltiazem use. *Neurology* (1992) 42, 937–8.
6. Maoz E, Grossman E, Thaler M, Rosenthal T. Carbamazepine neurotoxic reaction after administration of diltiazem. *Arch Intern Med* (1992) 152, 2503–4.
7. Wijdicks EFM, Arendt C, Bazzell MC. Postoperative ophthalmoplegia and ataxia due to carbamazepine toxicity facilitated by diltiazem. *J Neuroophthalmol* (2004) 24, 95.
8. Gadde K, Calabrese JR. Diltiazem effect on carbamazepine levels in manic depression. *J Clin Psychopharmacol* (1990) 10, 378–9.
9. Capewell S, Freestone S, Critchley JAJH, Pottage A, Prescott LF. Reduced felodipine bioavailability in patients taking anticonvulsants. *Lancet* (1988) ii, 480–2.
10. Zaccara G, Gangemi PF, Bendoni L, Menge GP, Schwabe S, Monza GC. Influence of single and repeated doses of oxcarbazepine on the pharmacokinetic profile of felodipine. *Ther Drug Monit* (1993) 15, 39–42.
11. Cachat F, Tufro A. Phenytoin/isradipine interaction causing severe neurologic toxicity. *Ann Pharmacother* (2002) 36: 1399–1402.
12. Hauben M. Comment: phenytoin/isradipine interaction causing severe neurologic toxicity. *Ann Pharmacother* (2002) 36: 1974–5.
13. Routledge PA, Soryal I, Eve MD, Williams J, Richens A, Hall R. Reduced bioavailability of nifedipine in patients with epilepsy receiving anticonvulsants. *Br J Clin Pharmacol* (1998) 45, 196P.
14. Cuadrado A, Sánchez MB, Peralta G, González M, Verdejo A, Amat G, Bravo J, Fdez Cortizo MJ, Adín J, De Cos MA, Mediavilla A, Armijo JA. Carbamazepine-amlodipine: a free interaction association? *Methods Find Exp Clin Pharmacol* (1996) 18 (Suppl C), 65.
15. Yasui-Furukori N, Tateishi T. Carbamazepine decreases antihypertensive effect of nilvadipine. *J Clin Pharmacol* (2002) 42, 100–3.
16. Tartara A, Galimberti CA, Manni R, Parietti L, Zucca C, Baasch H, Caresia L, Mück W, Barzaghi N, Gatti G, Perucca E. Differential effects of valproic acid and enzyme-inducing anticonvulsants on nimodipine pharmacokinetics in epileptic patients. *Br J Clin Pharmacol* (1991) 32, 335–40.
17. Macphee GJA, McInnes GT, Thompson GG, Brodie MJ. Verapamil potentiates carbamazepine neurotoxicity: a clinically important inhibitory interaction. *Lancet* (1986) i, 700–3.
18. Beattie B, Biller J, Mehlhaus B, Murray M. Verapamil-induced carbamazepine neurotoxicity. *Eur Neurol* (1988) 28, 104–5.
19. Price WA, DiMarzio LR. Verapamil-carbamazepine neurotoxicity. *J Clin Psychiatry* (1988) 49, 80.
20. Krämer G, Tettenborn B, Flesch G. Oxcarbazepine-verapamil drug interaction in healthy volunteers. *Epilepsia* (1991) 32 (Suppl 1), 70–1.
21. Nimotop (Nimodipine). Bayer plc. UK Summary of product characteristics, August 2005.

Carbamazepine + Danazol

Serum carbamazepine levels can be doubled by danazol and carbamazepine toxicity may occur.

Clinical evidence

The serum carbamazepine levels of 6 epileptic patients approximately doubled within 7 to 30 days of taking danazol 400 to 600 mg daily. Acute carbamazepine toxicity (dizziness, drowsiness, blurred vision, ataxia, nausea) was experienced by 5 out of the 6 patients.[1]

Other reports similarly describe rises in serum carbamazepine levels of 50 to 100% (with toxicity seen in some instances) when danazol was given.[2-4]

Mechanism

Danazol inhibits the metabolism (by the epoxide-trans-diol pathway) of carbamazepine by the liver, thereby reducing its loss from the body.[2,5] During danazol treatment the clearance of carbamazepine has been found to be reduced by 60%.[2]

Importance and management

An established and clinically important interaction. If concurrent use is necessary carbamazepine serum levels should be monitored and the dosage reduced as necessary.

1. Zeilinski JJ, Lichten EM, Haidukewych D. Clinically significant danazol-carbamazepine interaction. *Ther Drug Monit* (1987) 9, 24–7.
2. Krämer G, Theisohn M, von Unruh GE, Eichelbaum M. Carbamazepine-danazol drug interaction: its mechanism examined by a stable isotope technique. *Ther Drug Monit* (1986) 8, 387–92.
3. Hayden M, Buchanan N. Danazol-carbamazepine interaction. *Med J Aust* (1991) 155, 851.
4. Nelson MV. Interaction of danazol and carbamazepine. *Am J Psychiatry* (1988) 145, 768–9.
5. Krämer G, Besser R, Theisohn M, Eichelbaum M. Carbamazepine-danazol drug interaction: mechanism and therapeutic usefulness. *Acta Neurol Scand* (1984) 70, 249.

Carbamazepine + Dantrolene and Oxybutynin

Carbamazepine toxicity has been reported in a patient given oxybutynin and dantrolene.

Clinical evidence

A woman with incomplete tetraplegia who had taken carbamazepine 1 g daily for neuropathic pain for 2 years was given dantrolene in a gradually increasing dose and oxybutynin 5 mg twice daily. Two weeks after staring oxybutynin and while receiving dantrolene 125 mg daily, she experienced dizziness and vomiting, drowsiness, confusion, slurred speech, and nystagmus, and was found to have a raised carbamazepine level of 16 micrograms/mL. All drugs were stopped and the plasma carbamazepine level fell to 8.3 micrograms/mL (therapeutic range 4 to 12 micrograms/mL). Because of pain, urinary frequency and spasticity, daily doses of carbamazepine 600 mg, oxybutynin 10 mg and dantrolene 100 mg were restarted which resulted in a carbamazepine level of 9.2 micrograms/mL. The dantrolene dosage was increased to 125 mg daily because of continuing spasticity, but after one day, symptoms of carbamazepine toxicity occurred and the carbamazepine plasma level was 29 micrograms/mL. Carbamazepine and oxybutynin were discontinued and the dantrolene dose was reduced to 25 mg. In order to relieve the patient's symptoms of pain and spasticity, carbamazepine 400 mg daily and dantrolene 25 mg daily were given (carbamazepine levels of 8.4 micrograms/mL at 7 days). The addition of oxybutynin 5 mg daily was associated with an increase in the carbamazepine level to 32 micrograms/mL and symptoms of toxicity. Carbamazepine was replaced by **valproate** 600 mg daily, which appeared to be beneficial and without an interaction with dantrolene or oxybutynin.[1]

Mechanism, importance and management

In the reported case, oxybutynin was being taken on each occasion when carbamazepine levels increased. This increase was probably due to the inhibition by oxybutynin of the cytochrome P450 isoenzyme CYP3A4-mediated metabolism of carbamazepine. Dantrolene was also being taken and the second episode of carbamazepine toxicity occurred after the dantrolene dose was increased. The exact mechanism of dantrolene metabolism is not known but it may decrease the activity of cytochrome P450 isoenzymes in a dose-dependent manner. Valproate, which is mainly metabolised by glucuronide conjugation, was not affected by concurrent oxybutynin or dantrolene. The authors recommend careful monitoring and, if necessary, dose adjustments if carbamazepine is given with dantrolene and/or oxybutynin.[1]

1. Vander T, Odi H, Bluvstein , Ronen J, Catz A. Carbamazepine toxicity following oxybutynin and dantrolene administration; a case report. *Spinal Cord* (2005) 43, 252–5.

Carbamazepine + Dextromethorphan

Dextromethorphan appears not to affect the serum levels of carbamazepine.

Clinical evidence, mechanism, importance and management

A double-blind, crossover study in 5 epileptic patients with severe complex partial seizures found that dextromethorphan 120 mg daily in liquid form (*Delsym*) over 3 months had no effect on their serum carbamazepine levels. There was a non-significant alteration in the complex partial seizure and tonic-clonic seizure frequency.[1]

1. Fisher RS, Cysyk BJ, Lesser RP, Pontecorvo MJ, Ferkany JT, Schwerdt PR, Hart J, Gordon B. Dextromethorphan for treatment of complex partial seizures. *Neurology* (1990) 40, 547–9.

Carbamazepine or Oxcarbazepine + Dextropropoxyphene (Propoxyphene)

Carbamazepine serum levels can be raised by dextropropoxyphene. Toxicity may develop unless suitable dosage reductions are made. Oxcarbazepine appears not to interact with dextropropoxyphene.

Clinical evidence

(a) Carbamazepine

The observation of toxicity (headache, dizziness, ataxia, nausea, tiredness) in patients taking both carbamazepine and dextropropoxyphene prompted further study. Five carbamazepine-treated patients given dextropropoxyphene 65 mg three times daily had a mean rise in serum carbamazepine levels of 65%, and 3 showed evidence of carbamazepine toxicity. Carbamazepine levels were not taken in a further 2 patients because they withdrew from the study after 2 days of treatment due to adverse effects.[1,2] In a further study a 66% rise in carbamazepine levels was seen after 6 days of treatment with dextropropoxyphene.[3]

Carbamazepine toxicity due to this interaction is reported elsewhere,[4-7] and rises in trough serum carbamazepine levels of 69% to 600% have been described.[8] A study in the elderly compared groups of patients taking either carbamazepine or dextropropoxyphene alone, with patients taking both drugs (21 subjects). The carbamazepine dose was about a third lower in those receiving combined treatment, yet the mean serum carbamazepine levels were still 25% higher than in the patients not taking dextropropoxyphene. The prevalence of adverse effects was also higher in patients taking both drugs.[9]

(b) Oxcarbazepine

Dextropropoxyphene 65 mg three times daily for 7 days did not affect the steady-state levels of the active metabolite of oxcarbazepine in 7 patients with epilepsy or trigeminal neuralgia.[10]

Mechanism

Uncertain. It is suggested that dextropropoxyphene inhibits the metabolism of carbamazepine by the liver, leading to its accumulation in the body.[1,2]

Importance and management

The interaction between carbamazepine and dextropropoxyphene is very well established and clinically important. If concurrent use is necessary reduce the dosage of carbamazepine appropriately to prevent the development of toxicity. In many cases it may be simpler to use a non-interacting analgesic, although the occasional single dose of dextropropoxyphene probably does not matter. No special precautions seem necessary with oxcarbazepine.

1. Dam M, Christiansen J. Interaction of propoxyphene with carbamazepine. *Lancet* (1977) ii, 509.
2. Dam M, Kristensen CB, Hansen BS, Christiansen J. Interaction between carbamazepine and propoxyphene in man. *Acta Neurol Scand* (1977) 56, 603–7.
3. Hansen BS, Dam M, Brandt J, Hvidberg EF, Angelo H, Christensen JM, Lous P. Influence of dextropropoxyphene on steady state serum levels and protein binding of three anti-epileptic drugs in man. *Acta Neurol Scand* (1980) 61, 357–67.
4. Yu YL, Huang CY, Chin D, Woo E, Chang CM. Interaction between carbamazepine and dextropropoxyphene. *Postgrad Med J* (1986) 62, 231–3.
5. Kubacka RT, Ferrante JA. Carbamazepine-propoxyphene interaction. *Clin Pharm* (1983) 2, 104.
6. Risinger MW. Carbamazepine toxicity with concurrent use of propoxyphene: a report of five cases. *Neurology* (1987) 37 (Suppl 1), 87.
7. Allen S. Cerebellar dysfunction following dextropropoxyphene-induced carbamazepine toxicity. *Postgrad Med J* (1994) 70, 764.
8. Oles KS, Mirza W, Penry JK. Catastrophic neurologic signs due to drug interaction: Tegretol and Darvon. *Surg Neurol* (1989) 32, 144–51.

9. Bergendal L, Friberg A, Schaffrath AM, Holmdahl M, Landahl S. The clinical relevance of the interaction between carbamazepine and dextropropoxyphene in elderly patients in Gothenburg, Sweden. *Eur J Clin Pharmacol* (1997) 53, 203–6.
10. Mogensen PH, Jorgensen L, Boas J, Dam M, Vesterager A, Flesch G, Jensen PK. Effects of dextropropoxyphene on the steady-state kinetics of oxcarbazepine and its metabolites. *Acta Neurol Scand* (1992) 85, 14–17.

Carbamazepine + Diuretics

Two patients taking carbamazepine developed hyponatraemia when they were also given hydrochlorothiazide or furosemide. Another patient developed hyponatraemia while taking carbamazepine, hydrochlorothiazide and paroxetine.

Clinical evidence, mechanism, importance and management

Two epileptic patients taking carbamazepine developed symptomatic hyponatraemia while also taking **hydrochlorothiazide** or **furosemide**.[1] Another case has been described in a patient taking carbamazepine when also given **hydrochlorothiazide** and paroxetine.[2] The reasons are uncertain but all these drugs can cause sodium to be lost from the body. This seems to be an uncommon interaction, but be aware that it can occur.

1. Yassa R, Nastase C, Camille Y, Henderson M, Belzile L, Beland F. Carbamazepine, diuretics and hyponatremia: a possible interaction. *J Clin Psychiatry* (1987) 48, 281–3.
2. Kalksma R, Leemhuis MP. Hyponatriëmie bij gebruik van thiazidediuretica: let op combinaties van geneesmiddelen die dit effect versterken. *Ned Tijdschr Geneeskd* (2002) 146, 1521–5.

Carbamazepine + Felbamate

Felbamate modestly reduces serum carbamazepine levels but increases the levels of the active metabolite, carbamazepine-10,11-epoxide. Carbamazepine may reduce felbamate levels. The importance of these changes is uncertain but it is likely to be small.

Clinical evidence

The serum carbamazepine levels of 22 patients, with doses adjusted to keep levels in the range of 4 to 12 micrograms/mL, fell by 25% (range 10 to 42%) when they were given felbamate 3 g daily. The decrease occurred within a week, reaching a plateau after 2 to 4 weeks, and returning to the original levels within 2 to 3 weeks of stopping the felbamate.[1] Other studies in epileptics have found reductions in carbamazepine levels of between 18 and 31% when felbamate was given.[2-7] Some of these studies also found that the serum levels of the active carbamazepine metabolite carbamazepine-10,11-epoxide rose by 33% to 57%.[1,4,5]

Carbamazepine increases the clearance of felbamate by up to 49%.[8-10]

Mechanism

Not established. Felbamate does not induce the cytochrome P450 isoenzyme CYP3A4-mediated metabolism of carbamazepine, but appears to alter the interaction of carbamazepine with CYP3A4.[11]

Importance and management

This interaction is established, but its clinical importance is uncertain because the modest fall in serum carbamazepine levels would seem to be offset by the rise in levels of its metabolite, carbamazepine-10,11-epoxide, which also has anticonvulsant activity. However, monitor carbamazepine levels carefully, reducing the dose as necessary, and be alert for any changes in the anticonvulsant control. The importance of the increased felbamate clearance is uncertain. More study is needed.

1. Albani F, Theodore WH, Washington P, Devinsky O, Bromfield E, Porter RJ, Nice FJ. Effect of Felbamate on plasma levels of carbamazepine and its metabolites. *Epilepsia* (1991) 32, 130–2.
2. Graves NM, Holmes GB,, Fuerst RH, Leppik IE. Effect of felbamate on phenytoin and carbamazepine serum concentrations. *Epilepsia* (1989) 30, 225–9..
3. Fuerst RH, Graves NM, Leppik IE, Brundage RC, Holmes GB, Remmel RP. Felbamate increases phenytoin but decreases carbamazepine concentrations. *Epilepsia* (1988) 29, 488–91.
4. Howard JR, Dix RK, Shumaker RC, Perhach JL. The effect of felbamate on carbamazepine pharmacokinetics. *Epilepsia* (1992) 33 (Suppl 3), 84–5.
5. Wagner ML, Remmel RP, Graves NM, Leppik IE. Effect of felbamate on carbamazepine and its major metabolites. *Clin Pharmacol Ther* (1993) 53, 536–43.
6. Theodore WH, Raubertas RF, Porter RJ, Nice F, Devinsky O, Reeves P, Bromfield E, Ito B, Balish M. Felbamate: a clinical trial for complex partial seizures. *Epilepsia* (1991) 32, 392–7.
7. Leppik IE, Dreifuss FE, Pledger GW, Graves NM, Santilli N, Drury I, Tsay JY, Jacobs MP, Bertram E, Cereghino JJ, Cooper G, Sahlroot JT, Sheridan P, Ashworth M, Lee SI, Sierzant TL. Felbamate for partial seizures: results of a controlled clinical trial. *Neurology* (1991) 41, 1785–9.
8. Wagner ML, Graves NM, Marienau K, Holmes GB, Remmel RP, Leppik IE. Discontinuation of phenytoin and carbamazepine in patients receiving felbamate. *Epilepsia* (1991) 32, 398–406.
9. Kelley MT, Walson PD, Cox S, Dusci LJ. Population pharmacokinetics of felbamate in children. *Ther Drug Monit* (1997) 19, 29–36.
10. Banfield CR, Zhu G-RR, Jen JF, Jensen PK, Schumaker RC, Perhach JL Affrime MB, Glue P. The effect of age on the apparent clearance of felbamate: a retrospective analysis using nonlinear mixed-effects modeling. *Ther Drug Monit* (1996) 18, 19–29.
11. Egnell A-C, Houston B, Boyer S. In vivo CYP3A4 heteroactivation is a possible mechanism for the drug interaction between felbamate and carbamazepine. *J Pharmacol Exp Ther* (2003) 305, 1251–62.

Carbamazepine + Gemfibrozil

Two patients had a modest rise in their carbamazepine serum levels after they took gemfibrozil.

Clinical evidence, mechanism, importance and management

Two patients stable taking carbamazepine had rises in their serum carbamazepine levels when they were given gemfibrozil for type IV hyperlipoproteinaemia. One patient had a rise from 8.8 to 11.4 micrograms/mL within 4 days of starting gemfibrozil 300 mg daily, and the other patient had a rise from 8.3 to 13.7 micrograms/mL three months after gemfibrozil 300 mg twice daily was started.[1] It was suggested that the clearance of carbamazepine is increased in those with elevated cholesterol and total lipids. Thus, when the condition is treated with gemfibrozil, the clearance becomes more normal, which results in a rise in the serum carbamazepine levels.[2] The clinical importance of this interaction is uncertain but be alert for any evidence of carbamazepine toxicity (nausea, vomiting, ataxia and drowsiness) if gemfibrozil is given.

1. Denio L, Drake ME, Pakalnis A. Gemfibrozil-carbamazepine interaction in epileptic patients. *Epilepsia* (1988) 29, 654.
2. Wichlinski LM, Sieradzki E, Gruchala M. Correlation between the total cholesterol serum concentration data and carbamazepine steady-state blood levels in humans. *Drug Intell Clin Pharm* (1983) 17, 812–14.

Carbamazepine + Grapefruit and other fruit juices

Grapefruit juice increases carbamazepine levels. A case of possible carbamazepine toxicity has been seen when a man taking carbamazepine started to eat grapefruit.

Clinical evidence

A 58-year-old man, taking carbamazepine 1 g daily for epilepsy developed visual disturbances with diplopia, and was found to have a carbamazepine level of 11 micrograms/mL (therapeutic range 4 to 10 micrograms/mL). Previous levels had not exceeded 5.4 micrograms/mL. The patient said that one month previously he had started to eat one whole grapefruit each day. The levels restabilised at 5.1 micrograms/mL after the carbamazepine dose was reduced to 800 mg daily.[1]

A randomised, crossover study in 10 epileptic patients taking carbamazepine 200 mg three times daily found that a single 300-mL drink of grapefruit juice increased the plasma levels and AUC of carbamazepine by about 40%.[2]

Mechanism

The cytochrome P450 isoenzyme CYP3A4 is the main enzyme involved in the metabolism of carbamazepine.[3] Components of grapefruit juice are known to inhibit CYP3A4, which in this case would lead to a reduction in the metabolism of carbamazepine, and therefore an increase in levels.[1,2,4] Preliminary *in vitro* and *animal* studies suggest that **pomegranate juice** may also contain components that inhibit the CYP-mediated metabolism of carbamazepine.[5]

Importance and management

Although the information is sparse, the interaction has been predicted, demonstrated in a study, and has also occurred in practice. The authors of the study,[2] suggest that grapefruit juice should be avoided in patients taking carbamazepine. In the case report,[1] the patient continued to eat grapefruit, and this was successfully managed by a reduction in the carbamazepine dose. However, it should be noted that intake of a set amount of grapefruit would need to be maintained for this approach to work. The manufacturers advise carbamazepine dosage adjustment and monitoring of carbamazepine levels in patients taking substances that may raise carbamazepine levels, such as grapefruit juice.[3] If monitoring is not practical, or regular intake of grapefruit is not desired, it would seem prudent to avoid grapefruit/grapefruit juice.

What is of particular interest in the case cited is that the interaction apparently occurred with whole grapefruit, which is not usually considered to be a problem, although it is known that the fruit content of possible active components (e.g. flavonoids) do vary considerably. The juice (as opposed to the whole fruit) more commonly interacts, as the juicing process can increase the flavonoid content.[4] The evidence with **pomegranate juice** is currently too sparse to predict its effects in practice.

1. Bonin B, Vandel P, Vandel S, Kantelip JP. Effect of grapefruit intake on carbamazepine bioavailability: a case report. *Therapie* (2001) 56, 69–71.
2. Garg SK, Kumar N, Bhargava VK, Prabhakar SK. Effect of grapefruit juice on carbamazepine bioavailability in patients with epilepsy. *Clin Pharmacol Ther* (1998) 64, 286–8.
3. Tegretol Chewtabs (Carbamazepine). Novartis Pharmaceuticals UK Ltd. UK Summary of product characteristics, January 2003.
4. Ameer B, Weintraub RA. Drug interactions with grapefruit juice. *Clin Pharmacokinet* (1997) 33, 103–21.
5. Hidaka M, Okumura M, Fujita K-I, Ogikubo T, Yamasaki K, Iwakiri T, Setoguchi N, Arimori K. Effects of pomegranate juice on human cytochrome P450 3A (CYP3A) and carbamazepine pharmacokinetics in rats. *Drug Metab Dispos* (2005) 33, 644–8.

Carbamazepine or Oxcarbazepine + H_2-receptor antagonists

The serum levels of those taking long-term carbamazepine may transiently increase, possibly accompanied by an increase in adverse effects, for the first few days after starting to take cimetidine, but these adverse effects rapidly disappear. Cimetidine does not appear to have this effect on oxcarbazepine levels. Ranitidine appears not to interact with carbamazepine.

Clinical evidence

(a) Carbamazepine

The steady-state carbamazepine levels of 8 healthy subjects taking carbamazepine 300 mg twice daily were increased by 17% within 2 days of them starting to take **cimetidine** 400 mg three times daily. Adverse effects occurred in 6 patients, but after 7 days of treatment the carbamazepine levels had fallen again and the adverse effects disappeared.[1]

Conversely, the steady-state carbamazepine levels of 7 epileptic patients receiving long-term treatment remained unaltered when they were given **cimetidine** 1 g daily for a week.[2] Another study also showed a lack of an interaction in 11 epileptic patients.[3] However, an 89-year-old woman taking carbamazepine 600 mg daily developed symptoms of carbamazepine toxicity within 2 days of starting to take **cimetidine** 400 mg daily, and had a rise in serum carbamazepine levels, which fell when the **cimetidine** was withdrawn.[4] The effects of **cimetidine** may be additive with those of isoniazid, see 'Carbamazepine + Isoniazid or Rifampicin (Rifampin)', below.

The results of these studies in patients and subjects taking carbamazepine long term differ from single-dose studies and short-term studies in healthy subjects. For example, a 33% rise in serum carbamazepine levels,[5] a 20% fall in clearance[6] and a 26% increase in the AUC[7] have been reported, which would indicate that there is some potential for a clinically significant interaction (see 'Mechanism' below).

In 8 healthy subjects **ranitidine** 300 mg daily did not affect the pharmacokinetics of a single 600-mg dose of carbamazepine.[8]

(b) Oxcarbazepine

No changes in the pharmacokinetics of a single 600-mg oral dose of oxcarbazepine were seen in 8 healthy subjects who took **cimetidine** 400 mg twice daily for 7 days.[9]

Mechanism

Not fully understood. It is thought that cimetidine can inhibit the activity of the liver enzymes concerned with the metabolism of carbamazepine (such as the cytochrome P450 isoenzyme CYP3A4), resulting in its reduced clearance from the body, but the effect is short-lived because the auto-inducing effects of the carbamazepine oppose it. This would possibly explain why the single-dose and short-term studies in healthy subjects suggest that a clinically important interaction could occur, but in practice the combination causes few problems in patients receiving long-term treatment.

Importance and management

The interaction between carbamazepine and cimetidine is established but of minimal importance. Patients receiving long-term treatment with carbamazepine should be warned that for the first few days after starting to take cimetidine they may possibly experience some increase in carbamazepine adverse effects (nausea, headache, dizziness, fatigue, drowsiness, ataxia, an inability to concentrate, a bitter taste). However, because the serum levels are only transiently increased, these effects should subside and disappear by the end of a week. Ranitidine appears to be a non-interacting alternative to cimetidine.

1. Dalton MJ, Powell JR, Messenheimer JA, Clark J. Cimetidine and carbamazepine: a complex drug interaction. *Epilepsia* (1986) 27, 553–8.
2. Sonne J, Lühdorf K, Larsen NE and Andreasen PB. Lack of interaction between cimetidine and carbamazepine. *Acta Neurol Scand* (1983) 68, 253–6.
3. Levine M, Jones MW, Sheppard I. Differential effect of cimetidine on serum concentrations of carbamazepine and phenytoin. *Neurology* (1985) 35, 562–5.
4. Telerman-Topet N, Duret ME, Coërs C. Cimetidine interaction with carbamazepine. *Ann Intern Med* (1981) 94, 544.
5. Macphee GJA, Thompson GG, Scobie G, Agnew E, Park BK, Murray T, McColl KEL, Brodie MJ. Effects of cimetidine on carbamazepine auto- and hetero-induction in man. *Br J Clin Pharmacol* (1984) 18, 411–19.
6. Webster LK, Mihaly GW, Jones DB, Smallwood RA, Phillips JA, Vajda FJ. Effect of cimetidine and ranitidine on carbamazepine and sodium valproate pharmacokinetics. *Eur J Clin Pharmacol* (1984) 27, 341–3.
7. Dalton MJ, Powell JR, Messenheimer JA. The influence of cimetidine on single-dose carbamazepine pharmacokinetics. *Epilepsia* (1985) 26, 127–30.
8. Dalton MJ, Powell JR, Messenheimer JA. Ranitidine does not alter single-dose carbamazepine pharmacokinetics in healthy adults. *Drug Intell Clin Pharm* (1985) 19, 941–4.
9. Keränen T, Jolkkonen J, Klosterskov-Jensen P, Menge GP. Oxcarbazepine does not interact with cimetidine in healthy volunteers. *Acta Neurol Scand* (1992) 85, 239–42.

Carbamazepine + Influenza vaccines

In one study carbamazepine levels rose modestly 14 days after an influenza vaccine was given. A case report describes carbamazepine toxicity and markedly increased carbamazepine levels in a teenager 13 days after she was given an influenza vaccine.

Clinical evidence, mechanism, importance and management

The serum carbamazepine levels of 20 children rose by 47% from 6.17 to 9.04 micrograms/mL 14 days after they were given 0.5 mL of influenza vaccine USP, types A and B, whole virus (Squibb). Levels remained elevated on day 28.[1] A teenager taking carbamazepine 400 mg in the morning and 600 mg at night with gabapentin 600 mg three times daily developed signs of carbamazepine toxicity (unsteady, lethargic, slurred speech) 13 days after she was given an influenza vaccination (*Fluzone,* Aventis Pasteur). Her serum carbamazepine level was 27.5 micrograms/mL (previous levels 8.2 to 12.4 micrograms/mL), and she required ventilation for 19 hours. A urine drug screen was positive for tricyclic antidepressants and cocaine, but it was eventually concluded that these were likely to represent false-positive results.[2]

It has been suggested that the vaccine inhibits the liver enzymes concerned with the metabolism of carbamazepine, and therefore raising its levels. The moderate increase in serum carbamazepine levels seen in the first study is unlikely to have much clinical relevance. However, the case report of markedly increased carbamazepine levels introduces a note of caution. Further study is needed.

1. Jann MW, Fidone GS. Effect of influenza vaccine on serum anticonvulsant concentrations. *Clin Pharm* (1986) 5, 817–20.
2. Robertson WC. Carbamazepine toxicity after influenza vaccination. *Pediatr Neurol* (2002) 26, 61–3.

Carbamazepine + Isoniazid or Rifampicin (Rifampin)

Carbamazepine serum levels are markedly and very rapidly increased by isoniazid and toxicity can occur. Rifampicin has been reported both to augment and negate this interaction. There is evidence to suggest that carbamazepine may potentiate isoniazid hepatotoxicity.

Clinical evidence

Disorientation, listlessness, aggression, lethargy and, in one case, extreme drowsiness developed in 10 out of 13 patients taking carbamazepine when they were given isoniazid 200 mg daily. Serum carbamazepine levels were measured in 3 of the patients and they were found to have risen above the normal therapeutic range (initial level not stated).[1]

Carbamazepine toxicity, associated with marked rises in serum carbamazepine levels, has been described in other reports.[2-6] Some of the patients were also taking sodium valproate, which does not seem to be implicated in the interaction, and in one case cimetidine, which was thought to have potentiated the interaction.[6] See also 'Carbamazepine or Oxcarbazepine + H_2-receptor antagonists', p.529.

One report describes carbamazepine toxicity in a patient given isoniazid, but only when rifampicin was present as well. Usually the enzyme-inducing effects of rifampicin would be expected to counteract any enzyme inhibition by isoniazid, so this report is somewhat inexplicable.[7] Conversely, a case report describes reduced carbamazepine levels in a woman given rifampicin and isoniazid, which resulted in reduced carbamazepine efficacy (symptoms of hypomania).[8]

Isoniazid-induced fulminant liver failure occurred in a 16-year-old girl taking carbamazepine and clonazepam, within 5 days of starting isoniazid, rifampicin and pyrazinamide. She recovered with supportive measures and later tolerated the antiepileptics with concurrent rifampicin and pyrazinamide.[9] Isoniazid hepatotoxicity has also occurred in a 74-year-old woman[10] and a 10-year-old boy[11] taking carbamazepine, shortly after treatment with isoniazid, rifampicin, and ethambutol, with or without pyrazinamide, was started.

Mechanism

It seems probable that isoniazid inhibits the activity of the cytochrome P450 isoenzyme CYP3A4, which is concerned with the metabolism of carbamazepine, causing it to accumulate in the body.[12] Rifampicin is a potent enzyme inducer, and would be expected to negate the effects of isoniazid, and to induce the metabolism of carbamazepine. This is supported by one report, but not another.

Importance and management

The documentation is limited, but a clinically important and potentially serious interaction is established between isoniazid and carbamazepine. Toxicity can develop quickly (within 1 to 5 days) and also seems to disappear quickly if the isoniazid is withdrawn. Concurrent use should not be undertaken unless the effects can be closely monitored and suitable downward dosage adjustments made (a reduction to between one-half or one-third was effective in 3 patients[1]). It seems probable that those who are 'slow' metabolisers of isoniazid may show this interaction more quickly and to a greater extent than fast metabolisers.[2]

The effect of concurrent rifampicin on the interaction between isoniazid and carbamazepine is unclear. One report showed negation of the interaction, whereas another showed potential augmentation. Limited evidence suggests that carbamazepine may potentiate isoniazid hepatotoxicity.

1. Valsalan VC, Cooper GL. Carbamazepine intoxication caused by interaction with isoniazid. *BMJ* (1982) 285, 261–2.
2. Wright JM, Stokes EF, Sweeney VP. Isoniazid-induced carbamazepine toxicity and vice versa: a double drug interaction. *N Engl J Med* (1982) 307, 1325–7.
3. Block SH. Carbamazepine-isoniazid interaction. *Pediatrics* (1982) 69, 494–5.
4. Poo Argüelles P, Samarra Riera JM, Gairí Tahull JM, Vernet Bori A. Interacción carbamacepina-tuberculostáticos. *Med Clin (Barc)* (1984) 83, 867–8.
5. Beeley L, Ballantine N. *Bulletin of the West Midlands Centre for Adverse Drug Reaction Reporting* (1981) 13, 8.
6. García B, Zaborras E, Areas V, Obeso G, Jiménez I, de Juana P, Bermejo T. Interaction between isoniazid and carbamazepine potentiated by cimetidine. *Ann Pharmacother* (1992) 26, 841–2.
7. Fleenor ME, Harden JW, Curtis G. Interaction between carbamazepine and antituberculosis agents. *Chest* (1991) 99, 1554.
8. Zolezzi M, Antituberculosis agents and carbamazepine. *Am J Psychiatry* (2002) 159, 874.
9. Campos-Franco J, González-Quintela A, Alende-Sixto MR. Isoniazid-induced hyperacute liver failure in a young patient receiving carbamazepine. *Eur J Intern Med* (2004) 15, 396–7.
10. Barbare JC, Lallement PY, Vorhauer W, Veyssier P. Hépatotoxicité de l'isoniazide: influence de la carbamazépine? *Gastroenterol Clin Biol* (1986) 10, 523–4.
11. Berkowitz FE, Henderson SL, Fajman N, Schoen B, Naughton M. Acute liver failure caused by isoniazid in a child receiving carbamazepine. *Int J Tuberc Lung Dis* (1998) 2, 603–6.
12. Desta Z, Soukhova NV, Flockhart DA. Inhibition of cytochrome P450 (CYP450) isoforms by isoniazid: potent inhibition of CYP2C19 and CYP3A. *Antimicrob Agents Chemother* (2001) 45, 384–92.

Carbamazepine + Isotretinoin

A study in one patient found that isotretinoin modestly reduced the serum levels of both carbamazepine and its active metabolite.

Clinical evidence, mechanism, importance and management

The carbamazepine AUC in an epileptic patient taking carbamazepine 600 mg daily was reduced by 11% when isotretinoin 500 micrograms/kg daily, was taken, and by 24% when 1 mg/kg daily was taken. The AUC of carbamazepine-10,11-epoxide (the active metabolite of carbamazepine) was reduced by 21 and 44% by the small and large doses of isotretinoin, respectively. The patient had no adverse effects.[1] Although the author of the report suggests that monitoring may be necessary in patients given both drugs changes of this magnitude, especially those seen with the lower dose, are not usually clinically significant.

1. Marsden JR. Effect of isotretinoin on carbamazepine pharmacokinetics. *Br J Dermatol* (1988) 119, 403–4.

Carbamazepine + Lamotrigine

Most studies have found that lamotrigine has no effect on the pharmacokinetics of carbamazepine or its epoxide metabolite. However, some studies have found that lamotrigine raises the serum levels of carbamazepine-10,11-epoxide. Carbamazepine reduces lamotrigine levels. Symptoms of toxicity have been seen irrespective of changes in levels.

Clinical evidence

(a) Effects on carbamazepine

The addition of lamotrigine increased the serum levels of carbamazepine-10,11-epoxide, the active metabolite of carbamazepine, in 3 epileptic patients, but carbamazepine levels remained unchanged. One of the patients had carbamazepine-10,11-epoxide serum levels of 2 to 2.2 micrograms/mL while taking carbamazepine 1.1 g daily. The levels rose to 4.7 to 8.7 micrograms/mL when lamotrigine was added. Symptoms of toxicity occurred in 2 patients (dizziness, double vision, sleepiness, nausea).[1] In another study in 9 patients, the addition of lamotrigine 200 mg increased the mean serum carbamazepine-10,11-epoxide levels by 45%. Toxicity was seen in 4 patients (dizziness, nausea, diplopia).[2] The addition of lamotrigine resulted in cerebellar toxicity (nausea, vertigo, nystagmus, ataxia) in 8 out of 9 patients taking subtoxic and just-tolerated doses of carbamazepine when lamotrigine was added. Analysis showed that in all 8 cases at least one of the levels of carbamazepine, carbamazepine-10,11-epoxide or lamotrigine had become unusually high, but the authors concluded the interaction was likely to be pharmacodynamic rather than pharmacokinetic.[3]

In contrast other studies have found that the concurrent use of lamotrigine and carbamazepine does not result in any clinically significant pharmacokinetic changes. Lamotrigine caused no changes in carbamazepine levels in two clinical studies,[4,5] and another pharmacokinetic study found that lamotrigine 200 to 300 mg daily had no effect on the disposition of a single dose of oral carbamazepine-epoxide.[6] Another study in 47 patients taking carbamazepine, to which lamotrigine was added, found no significant changes in carbamazepine or carbamazepine-10,11-epoxide levels. Despite this 9 cases of diplopia or dizziness were recorded, predominantly in those whose carbamazepine levels were already high before the lamotrigine was added, even though there was no change in carbamazepine or carbamazepine-10,11-epoxide levels.[7] A further well-designed study in healthy subjects found that lamotrigine 100 mg twice daily for a week had no effect on the pharmacokinetics of carbamazepine or carbamazepine-10,11-epoxide after a single 200-mg dose of carbamazepine.[8] Similarly, lamotrigine had no effect on mean carbamazepine levels, and actually decreased mean carbamazepine-10,11-epoxide levels by 23% in a study in 14 children. Two children developed diplopia, which was unrelated to drug levels, but responded to a reduction in lamotrigine dose in one, and a reduction in carbamazepine dose in the other.[9]

(b) Effects on lamotrigine

In a retrospective study, the lamotrigine serum concentration-to-dose ratio was much lower in patients also taking carbamazepine than in those taking lamotrigine monotherapy (0.38 versus 0.84).[10] Other studies have reported similar findings.[11,12] In another study, mean increases in lamotrigine levels of about 60% occurred in patients taking lamotrigine with carbamazepine when the carbamazepine was withdrawn.[13] Similarly, a case report describes a rapid increase in lamotrigine levels when carbamazepine was withdrawn.[14] A review of patients taking antiepileptics found that carbamazepine increased the clearance of lamotrigine by 30 to 50%.[15]

Mechanism

The apparent contradiction between the results described is not understood. One suggestion to account for the toxic symptoms seen in some patients is that it occurs at the site of action (a pharmacodynamic interaction) rather than because lamotrigine increases the carbamazepine-10,11-epoxide serum levels.[3,7] Carbamazepine may induce the glucuronidation of lamotrigine.

Importance and management

Overall lamotrigine does not appear to significantly alter carbamazepine levels. However, toxicity has occurred, and therefore patients should be well monitored if lamotrigine is added, and the carbamazepine dose reduced if CNS adverse effects occur. Carbamazepine induces the metabolism of lamotrigine, and the recommended starting dose and long-term maintenance dose of lamotrigine in patients already taking carbamazepine is twice that of patients taking lamotrigine monotherapy.[16] However, if they are also taking valproate in addition to carbamazepine, the lamotrigine dose should be reduced.[16] See 'Lamotrigine + Valproate', p.542.

1. Graves NM, Ritter FJ, Wagner ML, Floren KL, Alexander BJ, Campbell JI, Leppik IE. Effect of lamotrigine on carbamazepine epoxide concentrations. *Epilepsia* (1991) 32 (Suppl 3), 13.
2. Warner T, Patsalos PN, Prevett M, Elyas AA, Duncan JS. Lamotrigine-induced carbamazepine toxicity: an interaction with carbamazepine-10,11-epoxide. *Epilepsy Res* (1992) 11, 147–50.
3. Wolf P. Lamotrigine: preliminary clinical observations on pharmacokinetics and interactions with traditional antiepileptic drugs. *J Epilepsy* (1992) 5, 73–9.
4. Jawad S, Richens A, Goodwin G, Yuen WC. Controlled trial of lamotrigine (Lamictal) for refractory partial seizures. *Epilepsia* (1989) 30, 356–63.
5. Eriksson A-S, Hoppu K, Nergårdh A, Boreus L. Pharmacokinetic interactions between lamotrigine and other antiepileptic drugs in children with intractable epilepsy. *Epilepsia* (1996) 37, 769–73.
6. Pisani F, Xiao B, Fazio A, Spina E, Perucca E, Tomson T. Single dose pharmacokinetics of carbamazepine-10,11-epoxide in patients on lamotrigine monotherapy. *Epilepsy Res* (1994) 19, 245–8.
7. Besag FMC, Berry DJ, Pool F, Newbery JE, Subel B. Carbamazepine toxicity with lamotrigine: a pharmacokinetic or pharmacodynamic interaction? *Epilepsia* (1998) 39, 183–7.
8. Malminiemi K, Keränen T, Kerttula T, Moilanen E, Ylitalo P. Effects of short-term lamotrigine treatment on pharmacokinetics of carbamazepine. *Int J Clin Pharmacol Ther* (2000) 38, 540–5.
9. Eriksson A-S, Boreus LO. No increase in carbamazepine-10,11-epoxide during addition of lamotrigine treatment in children. *Ther Drug Monit* (1997) 19, 499–501.
10. Armijo JA, Bravo J, Cuadrado A, Herranz JL. Lamotrigine serum concentration-to-dose ratio: influence of age and concomitant antiepileptic drugs and dosage implications. *Ther Drug Monit* (1999) 21, 182–190.
11. Böttiger Y, Svensson J-O, Ståhle L. Lamotrigine drug interactions in a TDM material. *Ther Drug Monit* (1999) 21, 171–4.
12. May TW, Rambeck B, Jürgens U. Influence of oxcarbazepine and methsuximide on lamotrigine concentrations in epileptic patients with and without valproic acid comedication: results of a retrospective study. *Ther Drug Monit* (1999) 21, 175–81.
13. Anderson GD, Gidal BE, Messenheimer J, Gilliam FG. Time course of lamotrigine de-induction: impact of step-wise withdrawal of carbamazepine or phenytoin. *Epilepsy Res* (2002) 49, 211–17.
14. Koch HJ, Szecsey A, Vogel M. Clinically relevant reduction of lamotrigine concentrations by carbamazepine. *Eur Psychiatry* (2003) 18, 42.
15. Weintraub D, Buchsbaum R, Resor SR, Hirsch LJ. Effect of antiepileptic drug comedication on lamotrigine clearance. *Arch Neurol* (2005) 62, 1432–6.
16. Lamictal (Lamotrigine). GlaxoSmithKline UK. UK Summary of product characteristics, March 2007.

Carbamazepine + Macrolides

Carbamazepine serum levels are markedly and rapidly increased by erythromycin or troleandomycin, and toxicity can often develop within 1 to 3 days. Telithromycin is predicted to interact similarly. Clarithromycin also raises carbamazepine levels, but to a lesser extent. Studies suggest that azithromycin, flurithromycin, josamycin, midecamycin, and roxithromycin have no interaction, or no clinically significant interaction, with carbamazepine, but note that a case of carbamazepine toxicity has been reported in a patient given roxithromycin.

Clinical evidence

(a) Azithromycin

Azithromycin 500 mg once daily for 3 days had no effect on the pharmacokinetics of carbamazepine 200 mg twice daily or its active metabolite, carbamazepine-10,11-epoxide, in healthy subjects.[1]

(b) Clarithromycin

A pharmacokinetic study[2] in healthy subjects found that clarithromycin 500 mg every 12 hours for 5 days increased the AUC of a single 400-mg dose of carbamazepine by 26%. A retrospective study of 5 epileptic patients found that when they were given clarithromycin (dosage not stated) their serum carbamazepine levels rose by 20 to 50% within 3 to 5 days, despite 30 to 40% reductions in the carbamazepine dosage in 4 of them. Carbamazepine levels in the toxic range were seen in 3 of them, and their carbamazepine dosages were then even further reduced.[3] A number of case reports have described carbamazepine toxicity following the addition of clarithromycin in adults,[4-6] and children.[7,8] Two other epileptic patients had marked rises in serum carbamazepine levels when they were given clarithromycin 500 mg three times daily and omeprazole.[9] It is not clear whether the omeprazole also had some part to play.[10,11] See also 'Carbamazepine + Proton pump inhibitors', p.534.

(c) Erythromycin

An 8-year-old girl taking phenobarbital 50 mg and carbamazepine 800 mg daily was given 500 mg, then later 1 g of erythromycin daily. Within 2 days she began to experience balancing difficulties and ataxia, which were eventually attributed to carbamazepine toxicity. Her serum carbamazepine levels were found to have risen from a little below 10 micrograms/mL to over 25 micrograms/mL (therapeutic range 2 to 10 micrograms/mL). The levels rapidly returned to normal after carbamazepine was withheld for 24 hours and the erythromycin stopped.[12]

A study in 7 healthy subjects confirmed that erythromycin can cause significant increases in carbamazepine levels,[13] and a study in 8 healthy subjects found that the clearance of carbamazepine is reduced by an average of 20% (range 5 to 41%) by erythromycin 1 g daily for 5 days.[14] Another study, in healthy subjects given erythromycin 500 mg three times daily for 10 days, found that the clearance of a single dose of carbamazepine was reduced by about 20% and the maximum serum levels of carbamazepine-10,11-epoxide were reduced by about 40% by erythromycin.[15]

Marked rises in serum carbamazepine levels (up to fivefold in some cases) and/or toxicity (including cases of hepatorenal failure and AV block as well as more typical signs of carbamazepine toxicity) have been described in over 30 cases involving both children and adults. Symptoms commonly began within 24 to 72 hours of starting erythromycin, although in some cases it was as early as 8 hours. In most cases toxicity resolved within 3 to 5 days of stopping the erythromycin.[7,16-34]

(d) Flurithromycin

Flurithromycin 500 mg three times daily for a week increased the AUC of a single 400-mg dose of carbamazepine by about 20% and moderately reduced the production of carbamazepine-10,11-epoxide in healthy subjects.[35]

(e) Josamycin

Josamycin 1 g twice daily for a week reduced the clearance of carbamazepine by about 20% in healthy subjects and in patients.[36-38]

(f) Midecamycin acetate

A single-dose study in 14 subjects found that after taking midecamycin acetate 800 mg twice daily for 8 days the AUC of a single 200-mg dose of carbamazepine was increased by 15%, and the AUC of its active metabolite (carbamazepine-10,11-epoxide) was reduced by 26%.[39] Another study in patients taking carbamazepine found that the addition of midecamycin acetate 600 mg twice daily caused a small increase in the trough serum levels of carbamazepine, and only an 11.6% increase in the AUC.[40]

(g) Roxithromycin

Roxithromycin 150 mg twice daily for 8 days did not affect the pharmacokinetics of a single 200-mg dose of carbamazepine in healthy subjects.[41] However, there is an isolated report of carbamazepine toxicity (levels increased to 21.7 mg/L) in a patient taking carbamazepine and atorvastatin the day after she started to take roxithromycin 150 mg twice daily. Roxithromycin and atorvastatin were stopped and carbamazepine levels fell to 12.5 mg/L within a day. The increased carbamazepine levels were attributed to the concurrent use of roxithromycin.[42]

(h) Telithromycin

The manufacturer predicts that carbamazepine will reduce the levels of telithromycin, with possible loss of efficacy, because carbamazepine induces the cytochrome P450 isoenzyme CYP3A4. Telithromycin is an inhibitor of CYP3A4, and may therefore raise carbamazepine levels.[43]

(i) Troleandomycin

Symptoms of carbamazepine toxicity (dizziness, nausea, vomiting, excessive drowsiness) developed in 8 epileptic patients taking carbamazepine within 24 hours of starting to take troleandomycin. The 2 patients available for examination had a sharp rise in serum carbamazepine levels, from about 5 to 28 micrograms/mL over 3 days, and a rapid fall following withdrawal of the troleandomycin.[44,45]

Another report by the same authors describes a total of 17 similar cases of carbamazepine toxicity caused by troleandomycin.[16] Some of the patients had three or fourfold increases in serum carbamazepine levels. Another case has been described elsewhere.[12] In most instances the serum carbamazepine levels returned to normal within about 3 to 5 days of withdrawing the macrolide.[16]

Mechanism

It seems probable that clarithromycin, erythromycin and troleandomycin, and to a lesser extent some of the other macrolides, slow the rate of metabolism of the carbamazepine by the cytochrome P450 isoenzyme CYP3A4 so that the anticonvulsant accumulates within the body.[46,47] Telithromycin is predicted to interact similarly.[43] It was suggested that the carbamazepine toxicity seen with roxithromycin may have been mediated by P-glycoprotein inhibition, which occurred as a result of an interaction between roxithromycin and atorvastatin.

Importance and management

The interaction between carbamazepine and troleandomycin is established, clinically important and potentially serious. The incidence is high. The rapidity of its development (within 24 hours in some cases) and the extent of the rise in serum carbamazepine levels suggest that it would be difficult to control carbamazepine levels by reducing the dosage. Concurrent use should probably be avoided.

The interaction between carbamazepine and erythromycin is also very well documented, well established and of clinical importance. Concurrent use should be avoided unless the effects can be very closely monitored by measurement of serum carbamazepine levels and suitable dosage reductions made. Toxic symptoms (ataxia, vertigo, drowsiness, lethargy, confusion, diplopia) can develop within 24 hours, but serum carbamazepine levels can return to normal within 8 to 12 hours of withdrawing the antibacterial.[36]

The interaction between carbamazepine and clarithromycin is also established, clinically important and potentially serious. However, the extent of the interaction is less with clarithromycin than with erythromycin or troleandomycin (i.e. the rise in carbamazepine levels is less).[48] It has been recommended that carbamazepine dosages should be reduced by 30 to 50% during treatment with clarithromycin, with monitoring within 3 to 5 days, and patients should be told to tell their doctor of any symptoms of toxicity (dizziness, diplopia, ataxia, mental confusion).

Analysis of the macrolide/carbamazepine interactions has shown that patients requiring high doses of carbamazepine to reach therapeutic levels are likely to have a greater rise in their carbamazepine levels.[48] The extent of the interactions is also correlated with the macrolide dose.[48]

Josamycin, flurithromycin and midecamycin acetate appear to be safer alternatives to either clarithromycin, erythromycin or troleandomycin. Nevertheless a small or moderate reduction in the dosage of the carbamazepine may be needed, with subsequent good monitoring. Pharmacokinetic data suggest that azithromycin and roxithromycin do not interact. However, there is an isolated report of carbamazepine toxicity in a patient taking roxithromycin, but this was complicated by the presence of atorvastatin. Telithromycin is predicted to interact, and the manufacturer advises avoidance of the combination, and suggests that telithromycin should not be used within 2 weeks of stopping carbamazepine.[43]

1. Rapeport WG, Dewland PM, Muirhead DC, Forster PL. Lack of an interaction between azithromycin and carbamazepine. *Br J Clin Pharmacol* (1992) 33, 551P.
2. Richens A, Chu S-Y, Sennello LT, Sonders RC. Effect of multiple doses of clarithromycin (C) on the pharmacokinetics (Pks) of carbamazepine (Carb). *Intersci Conf Antimicrob Agents Chemother* (1990) 30, 213.
3. O'Connor NK, Fris J. Clarithromycin-carbamazepine interaction in a clinical setting. *J Am Board Fam Pract* (1994) 7, 489–92.
4. Albani F, Riva R, Baruzzi A. Clarithromycin-carbamazepine interaction: a case report. *Epilepsia* (1993) 34, 161–2.
5. Yasui N, Otani K, Kaneko S, Shimoyama R, Ohkubo T, Sugawara K. Carbamazepine toxicity induced by clarithromycin coadministration in psychiatric patients. *Int Clin Psychopharmacol* (1997) 12, 225–9.
6. Tatum WO, Gonzalez MA. Carbamazepine toxicity in an epileptic induced by clarithromycin. *Hosp Pharm* (1994) 29, 45–6.
7. Stafstrom CE, Nohria V, Loganbill H, Nahouraii R, Boustany R-M, DeLong GR. Erythromycin-induced carbamazepine toxicity: a continuing problem. *Arch Pediatr Adolesc Med* (1995) 149, 99–101.
8. Carmona Ibáñez G, Guevara Serrano J, Gisbert González S. Toxicidad de carbamacepina inducida por eritromicina. Un problema frencuente. *Farm Clin* (1996) 13, 698–700.
9. Metz DC, Getz HD. *Helicobacter pylori* gastritis therapy with omeprazole and clarithromycin increases serum carbamazepine levels. *Dig Dis Sci* (1995) 40, 912–15.
10. Dammann H-G. Therapy with omeprazole and clarithromycin increases serum carbamazepine levels in patients with *H.pylori* gastritis. *Dig Dis Sci* (1996) 41, 519.
11. Metz DC, Getz HD. Therapy with omeprazole and clarithromycin increases serum carbamazepine levels in patients with *H.pylori* gastritis. *Dig Dis Sci* (1996) 41, 519–20.
12. Amedee-Manesme O, Rey E, Brussieux J, Goutieres F, Aicardi J. Antibiotiques à ne jamais associer à la carbamazépine. *Arch Fr Pediatr* (1982) 39, 126.
13. Miles MV, Tennison MB. Erythromycin effects on multiple-dose carbamazepine kinetics. *Ther Drug Monit* (1989) 11, 47–52.
14. Wong YY, Ludden TM, Bell RD. Effect of erythromycin on carbamazepine kinetics. *Clin Pharmacol Ther* (1983) 33, 460–4.
15. Barzaghi N, Gatti G, Crema F, Monteleone M, Amione C, Leone L, Perucca E. Inhibition by erythromycin of the conversion of carbamazepine to its active 10,11-epoxide metabolite. *Br J Clin Pharmacol* (1987) 24, 836–8.
16. Mesdjian E, Dravet C, Cenraud B, Roger J. Carbamazepine intoxication due to triacetyloleandomycin administration in epileptic patients. *Epilepsia* (1980) 21, 489–96.
17. Straughan J. Erythromycin-carbamazepine interaction? *S Afr Med J* (1982) 61, 420–1.
18. Vajda FJE, Bladin PF. Carbamazepine-erythromycin-base interaction. *Med J Aust* (1984) 140, 81.
19. Hedrick R, Williams F, Morin R, Lamb WA, Cate JC. Carbamazepine-erythromycin interaction leading to carbamazepine toxicity in four epileptic children. *Ther Drug Monit* (1983) 5, 405–7.
20. Miller SL. The association of carbamazepine intoxication and erythromycin use. *Ann Neurol* (1985) 18, 413.
21. Berrettini WH. A case of erythromycin-induced carbamazepine toxicity. *J Clin Psychiatry* (1986) 47, 147.
22. Carranco E, Kareus J, Co S, Peak V, Al-Rajeh S. Carbamazepine toxicity induced by concurrent erythromycin therapy. *Arch Neurol* (1985) 42, 187–8.
23. Goulden KJ, Camfield P, Dooley JM, Fraser A, Meek DC, Renton KW, Tibbles JAR. Severe carbamazepine intoxication after coadministration of erythromycin. *J Pediatr* (1986) 109, 135–8.
24. Wroblewski BA, Singer WD, Whyte J. Carbamazepine-erythromycin interaction. Case studies and clinical significance. *JAMA* (1986) 255, 1165–7.
25. Kessler JM. Erythromycin-carbamazepine interaction. *S Afr Med J* (1985) 67, 1038.
26. Jaster PJ, Abbas D. Erythromycin-carbamazepine interaction. *Neurology* (1986) 36, 594–5.
27. Loiseau P, Guyot M, Pautrizel B, Vincon G, Albin H. Intoxication par la carbamazépine due à l'interaction carbamazépine-érythromycine. *Presse Med* (1985) 14, 162.
28. Zitelli BJ, Howrie DL, Altman H, Marcon TJ. Erythromycin-induced drug interactions. *Clin Pediatr (Phila)* (1987) 26, 117–19.
29. Goldhoorn PB, Hofstee N. Een interactie tussen erytromycine en carbamazepine. *Ned Tijdschr Geneeskd* (1989) 133, 1944.
30. Mitsch RA. Carbamazepine toxicity precipitated by intravenous erythromycin. *DICP Ann Pharmacother* (1989) 23, 878–9.
31. Macnab AJ, Robinson JL, Adderly RJ, D'Orsogna L. Heart block secondary to erythromycin-induced carbamazepine toxicity. *Pediatrics* (1987) 80, 951–3.
32. Woody RC, Kearns GL, Bolyard KJ. Carbamazepine intoxication following the use of erythromycin in children. *Pediatr Infect Dis J* (1987) 6, 578–9.
33. Mota CR, Carvalho C, Mota C, Ferreira P, Vilarinho A, Pereira E. Severe carbamazepine toxicity induced by concurrent erythromycin therapy. *Eur J Pediatr* (1996) 155, 345–8.
34. Viani F, Claris-Appiani A, Rossi LN, Giani M, Romeo A. Severe hepatorenal failure in a child receiving carbamazepine and erythromycin. *Eur J Pediatr* (1992) 151, 715–16.
35. Barzaghi N, Gatti G, Crema F, Faja A, Monteleone M, Amione C, Leone L, Perucca E. Effect of flurithromycin, a new macrolide antibiotic, on carbamazepine disposition in normal subjects. *Int J Clin Pharmacol Res* (1988) 8, 101–5.
36. Albin H, Vinçon G, Pehourcq F, Dangoumau J. Influence de la josamycine sur la pharmacocinétique de la carbamazépine. *Therapie* (1982) 37, 151–6.
37. Vinçon G, Albin H, Demotes-Mainard F, Guyot M, Brachet-Liermain A, Loiseau P. Pharmacokinetic interaction between carbamazepine and josamycin. Proc Eur Congr Biopharmaceutics Pharmacokinetics vol III: Clinical Pharmacokinetics. Edited by Aiache JM and Hirtz J. Published by Imprimerie de l'Université de Clermont-Ferrand. (1984) pp 270–6.
38. Vinçon G, Albin H, Demotes-Mainard F, Guyot M, Bistue C, Loiseau P. Effects of josamycin on carbamazepine kinetics. *Eur J Clin Pharmacol* (1987) 32, 321–3.
39. Couet W, Istin B, Ingrand I, Girault J, Fourtillan J-B. Effect of ponsinomycin on single-dose kinetics and metabolism of carbamazepine. *Ther Drug Monit* (1990) 12, 144–9.
40. Zagnoni PG, DeLuca M, Casini A. Carbamazepine-miocamycin interaction. *Epilepsia* (1991) 32 (Suppl 1), 28.
41. Saint-Salvi B, Tremblay D, Surjus A, Lefebvre MA. A study of the interaction of roxithromycin with theophylline and carbamazepine. *J Antimicrob Chemother* (1987) 20 (Suppl B), 121–9.
42. Corbin C, Mosquet B, Lacotte J, Debruyne D, Denise P, Viader F, Coquerel A. Surdosage en carbamazépine après association à l'atorvastatine et à la roxithromycine. *Therapie* (2004) 59, 267–9.
43. Ketek (Telithromycin). Sanofi-Aventis. UK Summary of product characteristics, May 2007.
44. Dravet C, Mesdjian E, Cenraud B, Roger J. Interaction between carbamazepine and triacetyloleandomycin. *Lancet* (1977) i, 810–11.
45. Dravet C, Mesdjian E, Cenraud B, Roger J. Interaction carbamazépine triacétyloléandomycine: une nouvelle interaction médicamenteuse? *Nouv Presse Med* (1977) 6, 467.
46. Pessayre D, Larrey D, Vitaux J, Breil P, Belghiti J, Benhamou J-P. Formation of an inactive cytochrome P-450 Fe(II)-metabolite complex after administration of troleandomycin in humans. *Biochem Pharmacol* (1982) 31, 1699–1704.
47. Levy RH, Johnson CM, Thummel KE, Kerr BM, Kroetz DL, Korzecwa KR, Gonzales FJ. Mechanism of the interaction between carbamazepine and erythromycin. *Epilepsia* (1993) 34 (Suppl 6), 37–8.
48. Pauwels O. Factors contributing to carbamazepine-macrolide interactions. *Pharmacol Res* (2002) 45, 291–8.

Carbamazepine + MAOIs

Phenelzine, moclobemide and tranylcypromine appear not to interact adversely with carbamazepine.

Clinical evidence, mechanism, importance and management

There appear to be no reports of adverse reactions during the concurrent use of MAOIs and carbamazepine. However, the manufacturers of carbamazepine[1] say that concurrent use should be avoided because of the close structural similarity between carbamazepine and the tricyclic antidepressants (and therefore the theoretical risk of an adverse interaction). They suggest that MAOIs should be discontinued at least 2 weeks before carbamazepine is started. Several reports describe successful use of carbamazepine and MAOIs, namely **tranylcypromine**,[2,3] **phenelzine**,[4] and **moclobemide**.[5] Bearing in mind that the MAOIs and the tricyclics can be given together under certain well controlled conditions (see 'MAOIs or RIMAs + Tricyclic and related antidepressants', p.1149), the warning about the risks may possibly prove to be overcautious. Note that, rarely, the MAOIs have been seen to cause convulsions.

1. Tegretol Chewtabs (Carbamazepine). Novartis Pharmaceuticals UK Ltd. UK Summary of product characteristics, January 2003.
2. Lydiard RB, White D, Harvey B, Taylor A. Lack of pharmacokinetic interaction between tranylcypromine and carbamazepine. *J Clin Psychopharmacol* (1987) 7, 360.
3. Joffe RT, Post RM, Uhde TW. Lack of pharmacokinetic interaction of carbamazepine with tranylcypromine. *Arch Gen Psychiatry* (1985) 42, 738.
4. Yatham LN, Barry S, Mobayed M, Dinan TG. Is the carbamazepine-phenelzine combination safe? *Am J Psychiatry* (1990) 147, 367.
5. Amrein R, Güntert TW, Dingemanse J, Lorscheid T, Stabl M, Schmid-Burgk W. Interactions of moclobemide with concomitantly administered medication: evidence from pharmacological and clinical studies. *Psychopharmacology (Berl)* (1992) 106, S24–S31.

Carbamazepine + Melatonin

Melatonin does not affect the serum levels of carbamazepine or its 10,11-epoxide metabolite.

Clinical evidence, mechanism, importance and management

In a placebo-controlled study on the effects of melatonin on antioxidant enzymes, melatonin 6 to 9 mg/kg daily for 14 days was given with carbamazepine to children with epilepsy. The addition of melatonin increased the antioxidant activity of glutathione reductase, compared with a decrease in the placebo group; similar trends which did not reach statistical significance were found with glutathione peroxidase. Carbamazepine may cause reactive oxygen species (ROS) accumulation and the effect may be antagonised by melatonin. ROS can interact with other molecules within the body, causing damage to cell structures. This results in oxidative stress, which may contribute to the development of some disease states. Serum levels of carbamazepine and its metabolite carbamazepine-10,11-epoxide were not affected by concurrent melatonin which suggests a pharmacokinetic interaction is unlikely.[1]

1. Gupta M, Gupta YK, Agarwal S, Aneja S, Kalaivani M, Kohli K. Effects of add-on melatonin administration on antioxidant enzymes in children with epilepsy taking carbamazepine monotherapy: a randomized, double-blind, placebo-controlled trial. *Epilepsia* (2004) 45, 1636–9.

Carbamazepine + Metronidazole

Increased serum carbamazepine levels and toxicity have been seen in a patient given metronidazole.

Clinical evidence, mechanism, importance and management

A woman taking carbamazepine 1 g daily started taking co-trimoxazole twice daily and metronidazole 250 mg three times daily for diverticulitis. After 2 days the co-trimoxazole was stopped, she was changed to intravenous metronidazole 500 mg three times daily, and cefazolin 500 mg every 8 hours. After 2 days she complained of diplopia, dizziness and nausea, and her serum carbamazepine levels were found to have risen from 9 to 14.3 micrograms/mL. A month later (presumably after the metronidazole had been withdrawn) her serum carbamazepine levels had fallen to 7.1 micrograms/mL. The reasons for this reaction are not understood.[1]

This appears to be the first and only report of an interaction between carbamazepine and metronidazole, so its general importance is uncertain. More study is needed.

1. Patterson BD. Possible interaction between metronidazole and carbamazepine. *Ann Pharmacother* (1994) 28, 1303–4.

Carbamazepine + Nefazodone

Five patients developed elevated serum carbamazepine levels and toxicity when nefazodone was given. A study in healthy subjects using lower carbamazepine doses found only modest increases in carbamazepine levels, and no evidence of toxicity when nefazodone was given. Carbamazepine markedly reduces nefazodone levels.

Clinical evidence

A patient taking carbamazepine 1 g daily developed evidence of toxicity (light-headedness, ataxia) within 15 days of starting to take nefazodone (initially 100 mg twice daily increasing to 150 mg twice daily after a week). Her serum carbamazepine levels had risen from below 8.3 micrograms/mL up to 10.8 micrograms/mL. It was found necessary to reduce the carbamazepine dosage to 600 mg daily to eliminate these adverse effects and to achieve a serum level of 7.4 micrograms/mL.[1] In 4 other patients taking carbamazepine 800 mg or 1 g daily the addition of nefazodone caused up to threefold rises in carbamazepine levels. The carbamazepine dose was reduced by 25 to 60%.[1,2] In a study in 12 healthy subjects no evidence of toxicity was seen when carbamazepine 200 mg twice daily was given with nefazodone 200 mg twice daily for 5 days. However, the levels of carbamazepine were slightly increased (23% increase in AUC) and the levels of nefazodone markedly decreased (93% decrease in AUC). The authors suggest that there may be a greater effect with higher doses of carbamazepine.[3]

Mechanism

Both drugs are metabolised by the cytochrome P450 isoenzyme CYP3A4. Nefazodone is known to inhibit CYP3A4, whereas carbamazepine is a potent inducer of CYP3A4. Hence concurrent use reduces carbamazepine metabolism, leading to raised levels, and increases nefazodone levels, leading to lowered levels.

Importance and management

Information is limited, but it would seem prudent to monitor for signs of carbamazepine toxicity if nefazodone is added to established treatment, especially with doses of carbamazepine above 800 mg. The nefazodone dosage may need to be increased in the presence of carbamazepine, so be alert for a reduced effect. Nefazodone has largely been withdrawn, but the US manufacturer of nefazodone did contraindicate its concurrent use with carbamazepine.[4]

1. Ashton AK, Wolin RE. Nefazodone-induced carbamazepine toxicity. *Am J Psychiatry* (1996) 153, 733.
2. Roth L, Bertschy G. Nefazodone may inhibit the metabolism of carbamazepine: three case reports. *Eur Psychiatry* (2001) 16, 320–1.
3. Laroudie C, Salazar DE, Cosson J-P, Cheuvart B, Istin B, Girault J, Ingrand I, Decourt J-P. Carbamazepine-nefazodone interaction in healthy subjects. *J Clin Psychopharmacol* (2000) 20, 46–53.
4. Nefazodone hydrochloride. Watson Laboratories Inc. US Prescribing information, June 2004.

Carbamazepine + Phenobarbital

Carbamazepine serum levels are reduced to some extent by phenobarbital, and carbamazepine-10,11-epoxide levels are raised. In children, phenobarbital clearance is decreased by carbamazepine.

Clinical evidence

A comparative study found that on average patients taking both carbamazepine and phenobarbital (44 patients) had carbamazepine serum levels that were 18% lower than those taking carbamazepine alone (43 patients).[1] Similar results were found in other studies in both adult and paediatric patients taking both drugs.[2-5] Levels of the active metabolite, carbamazepine-10,11-epoxide, were increased.[3-6] However, one study found that the clearance of a single dose of carbamazepine-10,11-epoxide was higher and the plasma half-life shorter in epileptic patients taking phenobarbital when compared with healthy subjects not taking phenobarbital.[7]

In a prospective study the clearance of phenobarbital in 222 patients receiving monotherapy was compared to that in 63 patients who were also taking carbamazepine. During phenobarbital monotherapy, clearance was highest in the very young, decreased with increasing weight, and was lowest in adults. The pattern was similar for carbamazepine, except that its clearance was decreased by phenobarbital. Further, the effects of carbamazepine on phenobarbital clearance were maximal in young children (about 54%) and minimal in adults.[8]

Mechanism

Phenobarbital and carbamazepine are both known enzyme inducers, and may therefore increase each others metabolism. Phenobarbital may also induce the metabolism of carbamazepine-10,11-epoxide.[7]

Importance and management

An established interaction. It would be prudent to monitor phenobarbital levels in children also given carbamazepine, as changes in clearance may affect dose requirements. The small fall in serum carbamazepine levels probably has little practical importance, especially since the metabolite carbamazepine-10,11-epoxide also has anticonvulsant activity. Consider also 'Carbamazepine + Primidone', below.

1. Christiansen J, Dam M. Influence of phenobarbital and diphenylhydantoin on plasma carbamazepine levels in patients with epilepsy. *Acta Neurol Scand* (1973) 49, 543–6.
2. Cereghino JJ, Brock JT, Van Meter JC, Penry JK, Smith LD, White BG. The efficacy of carbamazepine combinations in epilepsy. *Clin Pharmacol Ther* (1975) 18, 733–41.
3. Rane A, Höjer B, Wilson JT. Kinetics of carbamazepine and its 10,11-epoxide metabolite in children. *Clin Pharmacol Ther* (1976) 19, 276–83.
4. Rambeck B, May T, Juergens U. Serum concentrations of carbamazepine and its epoxide and diol metabolites in epileptic patients: the influence of dose and comedication. *Ther Drug Monit* (1987) 9, 298–303.
5. Liu H, Delgado MR. Interactions of phenobarbital and phenytoin with carbamazepine and its metabolites' concentrations, concentration ratios, and level/dose ratios in epileptic children. *Epilepsia* (1995) 36, 249–54.
6. Dam M, Jensen A, Christiansen J. Plasma level and effect of carbamazepine in grand mal and psychomotor epilepsy. *Acta Neurol Scand* (1975) 75 (Suppl 51), 33–8.
7. Spina E, Martines C, Fazio A, Trio R, Pisani F, Tomson T. Effect of phenobarbital on the pharmacokinetics of carbamazepine-10,11-epoxide, an active metabolite of carbamazepine. *Ther Drug Monit* (1991) 13, 109–12.
8. Yukawa E, To H, Ohdo S, Higuchi S, Aoyama T. Detection of a drug-drug interaction on population-based phenobarbitone clearance using nonlinear mixed-effects modelling. *Eur J Clin Pharmacol* (1998) 54, 69–74.

Carbamazepine + Primidone

A single case report suggests that primidone can reduce the effects of carbamazepine. There is other evidence that carbamazepine may reduce primidone serum levels and increase primidone-derived phenobarbital levels.

Clinical evidence

A 15-year-old boy had complex partial seizures that were not controlled despite treatment with primidone 12 mg/kg daily in three divided doses and carbamazepine 10 mg/kg daily in three divided doses. Even when the carbamazepine dosage was increased to 20 and then 30 mg/kg daily his serum carbamazepine levels only reached 4.8 micrograms/mL, and his seizures continued. When the primidone was gradually withdrawn his serum carbamazepine levels increased to 12 micrograms/mL and his seizures completely disappeared.[1]

An analysis of serum levels of anticonvulsants in children found that the serum levels of primidone tended to be lower in those also taking carbamazepine, but no details were given.[2] Another study found that levels of phenobarbital derived from primidone were 42 micrograms/mL in patients taking primidone, carbamazepine and phenytoin, 24.7 micrograms/mL in patients taking phenytoin and primidone, and just 9.9 micrograms/mL in patients taking primidone alone.[3] A further study found that primidone levels were lower in patients also taking carbamazepine, but there were no significant changes in phenobarbital levels. Carbamazepine-10,11-epoxide levels were increased by primidone.[4] In a retrospective study, the plasma level to dose ratio for primidone was lower in patients also taking carbamazepine than in those taking primidone alone, and the derived phenobarbital levels were higher.[5]

Mechanism

When the primidone was stopped in the single case cited, the clearance of the carbamazepine decreased by about 60%.[1] This is consistent with the known enzyme-inducing effects of primidone (converted in the body to phenobarbital), which can increase the metabolism of other drugs by the liver. There is some evidence to suggest that carbamazepine may increase the metabolism of primidone to phenobarbital.

Importance and management

Direct information seems to be limited to these reports. It may be prudent to monitor combined treatment, and adjust doses if necessary. Consider also 'Carbamazepine + Phenobarbital', p.533.

1. Benetello P, Furlanut M. Primidone-carbamazepine interaction: clinical consequences. *Int J Clin Pharmacol Res* (1987) 7, 165–8.
2. Windorfer A, Sauer W. Drug interactions during anticonvulsant therapy in childhood: diphenylhydantoin, primidone, phenobarbitone, clonazepam, nitrazepam, carbamazepin and dipropylacetate. *Neuropadiatrie* (1977) 8, 29–41.
3. Callaghan N, Feeley M, Duggan F, O'Callaghan M, Seldrup J. The effect of anticonvulsant drugs which induce liver microsomal enzymes on derived and ingested phenobarbitone levels. *Acta Neurol Scand* (1977) 56, 1–6.
4. Callaghan N, Duggan B, O'Hare J, O'Driscoll D. Serum levels of phenobarbitone and phenylethylmalonamide with primidone used as a single drug and in combination with carbamazepine or phenytoin. In Johannessen SI et al. Antiepileptic Therapy: Advances in Drug Monitoring. New York: Raven Press; 1980, 307–13.
5. Battino D, Avanzini G, Bossi L, Croci D, Cusi C, Gomeni C, Moise A. Plasma levels of primidone and its metabolite phenobarbital: effect of age and associated therapy. *Ther Drug Monit* (1983) 5, 73–9.

Carbamazepine + Proton pump inhibitors

Omeprazole markedly raised the levels of a single dose of carbamazepine, but had no significant effect on carbamazepine taken long-term. Some anecdotal reports suggest that carbamazepine serum levels may possibly be reduced by lansoprazole. Pantoprazole did not affect the pharmacokinetics of carbamazepine in one study.

Clinical evidence

(a) Lansoprazole

In 2001 the manufacturers of lansoprazole had on record 5 undetailed case reports of apparent interactions between lansoprazole and carbamazepine. One of them describes the development of carbamazepine toxicity when lansoprazole was added, but there is some doubt about this case because it is thought that the patient may have started to take higher doses of carbamazepine.

The other 4 cases are consistent, in that carbamazepine levels fell shortly after lansoprazole was added, and/or the control of seizures suddenly worsened. One patient had a fall in carbamazepine serum levels from 11.5 to 7.7 mg/L. The carbamazepine levels of another patient returned to normal when the lansoprazole was stopped.[1]

(b) Omeprazole

Omeprazole 20 mg daily for 14 days was found to increase the AUC of a single 400-mg dose of carbamazepine in 7 patients by 75%. The clearance was reduced by 40% and the elimination half-life was more than doubled (from 17.2 to 37.3 hours).[2] However, a retrospective study of the records of 10 patients who had been taking omeprazole 20 mg daily with long-term carbamazepine (rather than a single dose) found a non-significant reduction in carbamazepine serum levels.[3]

(c) Pantoprazole

Pantoprazole 40 mg daily for 5 days had no effect on the AUC of carbamazepine or carbamazepine-10,11-epoxide after a single 400-mg dose of carbamazepine in healthy subjects.[4]

Mechanism

Omeprazole may inhibit the oxidative metabolism of single doses of carbamazepine. However, when carbamazepine is taken continuously it induces its own metabolism by the cytochrome P450 isoenzyme CYP3A4, thereby possibly opposing the effects of this interaction.[3]

Importance and management

It seems that in practice no clinically relevant interaction is likely to occur between omeprazole and carbamazepine. For lansoprazole, information seems to be limited to this handful of reports from which no broad general conclusions can be drawn, but they do suggest that this interaction should be considered if **lansoprazole** is added to established treatment with carbamazepine. Pantoprazole appears not to affect the pharmacokinetics of carbamazepine.

1. Wyeth (UK). Personal communication, September 2001.
2. Naidu MUR, Shoba J, Dixit VK, Kumar A, Kumar TR, Sekhar KR, Sekhar EC. Effect of multiple dose omeprazole on the pharmacokinetics of carbamazepine. *Drug Invest* (1994) 7, 8–12.
3. Böttiger Y, Bertilsson L. No effect on plasma carbamazepine concentration with concomitant omeprazole treatment. *Drug Invest* (1995) 9, 180–1.
4. Huber R, Bliesath H, Hartmann M, Steinijans VW, Koch H, Mascher H, Wurst W. Pantoprazole does not interact with the pharmacokinetics of carbamazepine. *Int J Clin Pharmacol Ther* (1998) 36, 521–4.

Carbamazepine + SSRIs

Some, but not all, reports indicate that carbamazepine serum levels can be increased by fluoxetine and fluvoxamine. Toxicity may develop. Citalopram, paroxetine and sertraline do not normally affect carbamazepine, but there is an isolated case of raised carbamazepine levels with sertraline. Citalopram, paroxetine and sertraline levels may be reduced by carbamazepine. The use of carbamazepine with an SSRI has, rarely, led to effects such as hyponatraemia, the serotonin syndrome, and parkinsonism. Consideration should be given to the fact that SSRIs have been known to cause seizures.

Clinical evidence

(a) Citalopram

In a study in 12 healthy subjects citalopram 40 mg daily for 2 weeks caused no change in the pharmacokinetics of carbamazepine 400 mg once daily.[1] An approximate 30% decrease in citalopram levels occurred in 6 patients taking citalopram 40 to 60 mg daily when they were given carbamazepine 200 to 400 mg daily for 4 weeks. Despite this decrease, the combination was considered clinically useful.[2] Similarly, two patients with epilepsy, major depression, and panic disorder had increased citalopram levels (one had an improved antidepressant response, but the other patient experienced tremor and increased anxiety) when their treatment with carbamazepine was replaced by oxcarbazepine.[3]

(b) Fluoxetine

Two patients developed carbamazepine toxicity (diplopia, blurred vision, tremor, vertigo, nausea, tinnitus etc.) within 7 and 10 days of starting to take fluoxetine 20 mg daily. Their serum carbamazepine levels were found to have risen by about 33% and 60%, respectively. The problem was resolved in one of them by reducing the carbamazepine dosage from 1 g to 800 mg daily, and in the other by stopping the fluoxetine.[4] The effects seen in these cases are supported by a study in 6 healthy patients, where adding fluoxetine 20 mg daily to steady-state carbamazepine caused a rise in the AUC of carbamazepine and carbamazepine-10,11-epoxide (its active metabolite) of about 25 to 50%.[5]

In contrast, fluoxetine 20 mg daily for 3 weeks was found to have no effect on the serum levels of carbamazepine or carbamazepine-10,11-epoxide in 8 epileptic patients stabilised on carbamazepine.[6]

Aside from these pharmacokinetic changes two cases of parkinsonism developed within 3 and 9 days of adding fluoxetine to carbamazepine treatment. In both cases carbamazepine levels were unaffected.[7] A case of the serotonin syndrome (shivering, agitation, myoclonic-like leg contractions, diaphoresis etc.) has also been seen, in a woman taking carbamazepine 200 mg daily and fluoxetine 20 mg daily.[8]

(c) Fluvoxamine

Increased serum levels and signs of carbamazepine toxicity (nausea, vomiting) were seen in 3 patients taking long-term carbamazepine when they were given fluvoxamine. The carbamazepine level almost doubled in one of them within 10 days of starting fluvoxamine 50 to 100 mg daily. The interaction was accommodated by reducing the carbamazepine dosage by 200 mg daily in all three (from 1 g to 800 mg in one of them, and from 800 to 600 mg daily in the other two).[9,10] An approximate doubling of carbamazepine levels has also been seen in other patients given fluvoxamine.[11-14]

In contrast, fluvoxamine 100 mg daily for 3 weeks was found to have no effect on the serum levels of carbamazepine or carbamazepine-10,11-epoxide in 7 epileptic patients stabilised on carbamazepine.[6]

(d) Paroxetine

In epileptic patients, paroxetine 30 mg daily for 16 days caused no changes in the plasma levels or therapeutic effects of carbamazepine. Steady-state paroxetine plasma levels were lower in those taking phenytoin (16 nanograms/mL) than in those taking carbamazepine (27 nanograms/mL) or sodium valproate (73 nanograms/mL).[15]

An elderly patient taking carbamazepine 200 mg daily then 400 mg daily for neuropathic pain associated with herpes zoster infection was given paroxetine 20 mg daily to treat depression. He developed vertigo, bradycardia and syncope and his plasma sodium was found to be low (120 mmol/L). Sodium levels returned to normal (135 mmol/L) over several weeks after carbamazepine was withdrawn.[16]

(e) Sertraline

A double blind, placebo-controlled, parallel group study in 13 healthy subjects (7 taking sertraline, 6 taking placebo) found that sertraline 200 mg daily for 17 days had no effect on the pharmacokinetics of carbamazepine 200 mg twice daily, nor on the pharmacokinetics of carbamazepine-10,11-epoxide. In addition, sertraline did not potentiate the cognitive effects of carbamazepine.[17]

However, an isolated report describes a woman who had taken carbamazepine 600 mg and flecainide 100 mg daily for 2 years, who had a rise in her trough serum carbamazepine levels from 4.7 to 8.5 micrograms/mL within 4 weeks of starting sertraline 100 mg daily. After 3 months of treatment, carbamazepine levels were 11.9 micrograms/mL. At the same time she developed pancytopenia (interpreted as a toxic bone marrow reaction to the increased carbamazepine), which improved when the carbamazepine and sertraline were stopped.[18]

An isolated report describes a woman with schizoaffective disorder successfully treated for 3 years with haloperidol and carbamazepine who was given sertraline 50 mg daily for depression. When she failed to respond, the sertraline dosage was progressively increased to 300 mg daily but her sertraline plasma levels remained low (about 17 to 25% of those predicted). Another patient on carbamazepine similarly failed to respond to the addition of sertraline and had low sertraline levels.[19] In an analysis of plasma sertraline levels the concentration to daily dose ratio of sertraline was significantly lower in patients who had taken sertraline with carbamazepine compared with those who had taken sertraline without carbamazepine,[20] suggesting that carbamazepine lowered sertraline levels.

Mechanism

The evidence suggests that fluoxetine and fluvoxamine inhibit the metabolism of carbamazepine by the liver (presumably by inhibiting the cytochrome P450 isoenzyme CYP3A4) so that its loss from the body is reduced, leading to a rise in its serum levels.[5,12]

Citalopram, sertraline and possibly paroxetine serum levels may be reduced because carbamazepine induces their metabolism by CYP3A4, which results in lower levels of these SSRIs. Oxcarbazepine appears not to interact. Both carbamazepine and paroxetine may cause hyponatraemia so the reduced sodium levels could be due to the effects of both drugs.[16]

Importance and management

Information for fluoxetine and fluvoxamine appears to be limited to these reports. It is not clear why they are inconsistent, but be alert for an increase in carbamazepine serum levels and toxicity if fluoxetine or fluvoxamine is added. The interaction appears rare. A literature search[21] by the manufacturers of fluvoxamine only identified 8 cases of an interaction between fluvoxamine and carbamazepine up until 1995. However, because of the unpredictability of this interaction it would be prudent to monitor concurrent use, particularly in the early stages, so that any patient affected can be quickly identified. Be alert for the need to reduce the carbamazepine dosage. The manufacturers of fluoxetine suggest that carbamazepine should be started at or adjusted towards the lower end of the dosage range in those taking fluoxetine. They additionally suggest caution if fluoxetine has been taken during the previous 5 weeks.[22]

There would seem to be no particular need to monitor carbamazepine levels in patients taking citalopram, paroxetine, or sertraline. However, be aware that the SSRIs may be less effective in the presence of carbamazepine. Consider increasing the dose if necessary.

Note that SSRIs may increase seizure frequency and should therefore be used with caution in patients with epilepsy, and avoided in those with unstable epilepsy.

1. Møller SE, Larsen F, Khan AZ, Rolan PE. Lack of effect of citalopram on the steady-state pharmacokinetics of carbamazepine in healthy male subjects. *J Clin Psychopharmacol* (2001) 21, 493–9.
2. Steinacher L, Vandel P, Zullino DF, Eap CB, Brawand-Amey M, Baumann P. Carbamazepine augmentation in depressive patients non-responding to citalopram: a pharmacokinetic and clinical pilot study. *Eur Neuropsychopharmacol* (2002) 12, 255–60.
3. Leinonen E, Lepola U, Koponen H. Substituting carbamazepine with oxcarbazepine increases citalopram levels. A report on two cases. *Pharmacopsychiatry* (1996) 29, 156–8.
4. Pearson HJ. Interaction of fluoxetine with carbamazepine. *J Clin Psychiatry* (1990) 51, 126.
5. Grimsley SR, Jann MW, Carter JG, D'Mello AP, D'Souza MJ. Increased carbamazepine plasma concentrations after fluoxetine coadministration. *Clin Pharmacol Ther* (1991) 50, 10–15.
6. Spina E, Avenoso A, Pollicino AM, Caputi AP, Fazio A, Pisani F. Carbamazepine coadministration with fluoxetine or fluvoxamine. *Ther Drug Monit* (1993) 15, 247–50.
7. Gernaat HBPE, van de Woude J, Touw DJ. Fluoxetine and parkinsonism in patients taking carbamazepine. *Am J Psychiatry* (1991) 148, 1604–5.
8. Dursun SM, Mathew VM, Reveley MA. Toxic serotonin syndrome after fluoxetine plus carbamazepine. *Lancet* (1993) 342, 442–3.
9. Fritze J, Unsorg B, Lanczik M. Interaction between carbamazepine and fluvoxamine. *Acta Psychiatr Scand* (1991) 84, 583–4.
10. Fritze J, Lanczik M. Pharmacokinetic interactions of carbamazepine and fluvoxamine. *Pharmacopsychiatry* (1993) 26, 153.
11. Bonnet P, Vandel S, Nezelof S, Sechter D, Bizouard P. Carbamazepine, fluvoxamine. Is there a pharmacokinetic interaction? *Therapie* (1992) 47, 165.
12. Martinelli V, Bocchetta A, Palmas AM, del Zompo M. An interaction between carbamazepine and fluvoxamine. *Br J Clin Pharmacol* (1993) 36, 615–16.
13. Debruille C, Robert H, Cottencin O, Regnaut N, Gignac C. Interaction carbamazépine/fluvoxamine: à propos de deux observations. *J Pharm Clin* (1994) 13, 128–30.
14. Cottencin O, Regnaut N, Thevenon Gignac C, Thomas P, Goudemand M, Debruille C, Robert H. Interaction carbamazepine-fluvoxamine sur le taux plasmatique de carbamazepine. *Encephale* (1995) 21, 141–5.
15. Andersen BB, Mikkelsen M, Versterager A, Dam M, Kristensen HB, Pedersen B, Lund J, Mengel H. No influence of the antidepressant paroxetine on carbamazepine, valproate and phenytoin. *Epilepsy Res* (1991) 10, 201–4.
16. Sempere i Verdú E, Bel Reverter M, Palop Larrea V, Hidalgo Mora JJ. Hiponatremia por carbamazepina y paroxetina. *Aten Primaria* (2004) 33, 473.
17. Rapeport WG, Williams SA, Muirhead DC, Dewland PM, Tanner T, Wesnes K. Absence of a sertraline-mediated effect on the pharmacokinetics and pharmacodynamics of carbamazepine. *J Clin Psychiatry* (1996) 57 (Suppl 1), 20–3.
18. Joblin M, Ghose K. Possible interaction of sertraline with carbamazepine. *N Z Med J* (1994) 107, 43.
19. Khan A, Shad MU, Preskorn SH. Lack of sertraline efficacy probably due to an interaction with carbamazepine. *J Clin Psychiatry* (2000) 61, 526–7.
20. Pihlsgård M, Eliasson E.Significant reduction of sertraline plasma levels by carbamazepine and phenytoin. *Eur J Clin Pharmacol* (2002) 57, 915–16.
21. Wagner W, Vause EW. Fluvoxamine. A review of global drug-drug interaction data. *Clin Pharmacokinet* (1995) 29 (Suppl 1), 26–32.
22. Prozac (Fluoxetine hydrochloride). Eli Lilly and Company Ltd. UK Summary of product characteristics, March 2007.

Carbamazepine + Terfenadine

Carbamazepine toxicity, attributed to the use of terfenadine, has been described in one case report but the interaction is not established.

Clinical evidence, mechanism, importance and management

A 18-year-old woman taking carbamazepine after treatment for brain metastases, developed confusion, disorientation, visual hallucinations, nausea and ataxia shortly after starting terfenadine 60 mg twice daily for rhinitis. The symptoms were interpreted as carbamazepine toxicity. However, her total carbamazepine serum levels of 8.9 mg/L were within the normal range. An interaction due to protein binding displacement was suspected and measurement of free carbamazepine revealed levels of 6 mg/L, almost three times the upper limit of normal. All the symptoms disappeared when the terfenadine was stopped. The authors speculate that the terfenadine had displaced the carbamazepine from its plasma protein binding sites, thereby increasing the levels of free and active carbamazepine.[1] The report is very brief and does not say whether any other drugs were being taken concurrently, so that this interaction is not established.

1. Hirschfeld S, Jarosinski P. Drug interaction of terfenadine and carbamazepine. *Ann Intern Med* (1993) 118, 907–8.

Carbamazepine + Ticlopidine

One case report suggests that ticlopidine may have caused increased carbamazepine levels, with associated toxicity.

Clinical evidence, mechanism, importance and management

A 67-year-old man taking carbamazepine 600 mg twice daily developed symptoms of carbamazepine toxicity (drowsiness, dizziness, ataxia) within a week of starting to take ticlopidine 250 mg twice daily. His carbamazepine level one week after starting the ticlopidine was 17.7 [micrograms/mL], but it had been only 10.1 [micrograms/mL] five weeks earlier. The carbamazepine dose was reduced to 500 mg twice daily, with resolution of symptoms, and producing a level of 12.5 [micrograms/mL] one week later. After stopping the ticlopidine, carbamazepine levels fell to 9.9 [micrograms/mL]. It was suggested that ticlopidine may interfere with carbamazepine metabolism.[1] However, carbamazepine is principally metabolised by the cytochrome P450 isoenzyme CYP3A4, and ticlopidine is not usually considered an inhibitor of this isoenzyme. This is the only report so far, and its general relevance is uncertain.

1. Brown RIG, Cooper TG. Ticlopidine-carbamazepine interaction in a coronary stent patient. *Can J Cardiol* (1997) 13, 853–4.

Carbamazepine + Trazodone

A single case report describes a moderate rise in serum carbamazepine levels in a patient given trazodone. Carbamazepine may moderately decrease trazodone levels.

Clinical evidence, mechanism, importance and management

A 53-year-old man who had been taking carbamazepine 700 mg daily for 7 months (serum levels 7.2 and 7.9 mg/L) started taking trazodone 100 mg daily. Two months later his serum carbamazepine levels were 10 mg/L and the concentration/dose ratio had increased by about 26%, but no signs or symptoms of carbamazepine toxicity were seen. The reasons for this interaction are not known but the authors suggest that it might occur because trazodone inhibits the cytochrome P450 isoenzyme CYP3A4 resulting in a reduction in the metabolism of the carbamazepine.[1]

This seems to be the first and only report of raised carbamazepine levels with trazodone, and its general importance is unknown. The rise was only moderate and in this case was clinically irrelevant, but a carbamazepine serum rise of 26% might possibly be of importance in those patients with serum levels already near the top end of the therapeutic range.

In 6 patients taking trazodone 150 or 300 mg daily, the addition of carbamazepine 400 mg daily for 4 weeks decreased the plasma levels of trazodone by 24%, and of the active metabolite of trazodone by 40%.[2] However, the combination was considered clinically useful in three of the cases.[2] In another study, when carbamazepine 400 mg daily was given with trazodone 100 to 300 mg daily, the plasma levels of trazodone and its active metabolite were reduced by 76% and 60%, respectively.[3] The FDA in the US and the manufacturer of trazodone recommend that patients should be closely monitored and trazodone doses increased if necessary when both drugs are given.[4]

1. Romero AS, Delgado RG, Peña MF. Interaction between trazodone and carbamazepine. *Ann Pharmacother* (1999) 33, 1370.
2. Otani K, Ishida M, Kaneko S, Mihara K, Ohkubo T, Osanai T, Sugawara K. Effects of carbamazepine coadministration on plasma concentrations of trazodone and its active metabolite, *m*-chlorophenylpiperazine. *Ther Drug Monit* (1996) 18, 164–7.
3. Desyrel (Trazodone hydrochloride). Bristol-Myers Squibb Company. US Prescribing information, January 2005.
4. Molipaxin (Trazodone hydrochloride). Sanofi-Aventis. UK Summary of product characteristics, July 2005.

Carbamazepine + Valnoctamide

Carbamazepine toxicity may develop if valnoctamide is also taken.

Clinical evidence

A study in 6 epileptic patients taking carbamazepine 800 to 1200 mg daily found that valnoctamide 200 mg three times daily for 7 days caused a 1.5 to 6.5-fold increase in the serum levels of carbamazepine-10,11-epoxide (an active metabolite). Clinical signs of carbamazepine toxicity (drowsiness, ataxia, nystagmus) were seen in 4 of them. Two patients were also taking phenobarbital or phenytoin, and the serum levels of these drugs were unaffected by valnoctamide.[1] A further study in 6 healthy subjects found that valnoctamide 600 mg daily for 8 days increased the half-life of a single 100-mg dose of carbamazepine-10,11-epoxide threefold, from 6.7 to 19.7 hours, and decreased its oral clearance fourfold.[2]

Mechanism

Valnoctamide inhibits the enzyme epoxide hydrolase, which is concerned with the metabolism and elimination of carbamazepine and its active epoxide metabolite.[1,2]

Importance and management

Information is limited but the interaction appears to be established. Patients taking carbamazepine who also take valnoctamide could rapidly develop carbamazepine toxicity because the metabolism of its major metabolite, carbamazepine-10,11-epoxide, is inhibited. This interaction is very similar to the interaction that occurs between carbamazepine and valpromide (an isomer of valnoctamide), see 'Carbamazepine + Valproate', below. Concurrent valnoctamide should be avoided unless the carbamazepine dosage can be reduced appropriately.

1. Pisani F, Fazio A, Artesi C, Oteri G, Spina E, Tomson T, Perucca E. Impairment of carbamazepine-10,11-epoxide elimination by valnoctamide, a valpromide isomer, in healthy subjects. *Br J Clin Pharmacol* (1992) 34, 85–7.
2. Pisani F, Haj-Yehia A, Fazio A, Artesi C, Oteri G, Perucca E, Kroetz DL, Levy RH, Bialer M. Carbamazepine-valnoctamide interaction in epileptic patients: in vitro/in vivo correlation. *Epilepsia* (1993) 34, 954–9.

Carbamazepine + Valproate

The serum levels of carbamazepine are usually only slightly affected by sodium valproate, valproic acid or valpromide but a moderate to marked rise in the levels of its active metabolite, carbamazepine-10,11-epoxide may occur.
Carbamazepine may reduce the serum levels of sodium valproate by 60% or more. Concurrent use may possibly increase the incidence of sodium valproate-induced hepatotoxicity.

Clinical evidence

(a) Carbamazepine

1. Sodium valproate or valproic acid. A study in 7 adult epileptic patients who had been taking carbamazepine 8.3 to 13.3 mg/kg for more than 2 months found that their steady-state serum carbamazepine levels fell by an average of 24% (range 3 to 59%) over a 6-day period when they were given sodium valproate 1 g twice daily. The carbamazepine levels were reduced in 6 of the patients and remained unchanged in one. The levels of the active metabolite, carbamazepine-10,11-epoxide, increased by a mean of 38%, with small decreases or no change in 4 patients and 24 to 150% increases in the remaining 3 patients.[1,2]
Other reports state that falls,[3,4] no changes[3,5-7] and even a slight rise[4] in carbamazepine levels have been seen in some patients also taking sodium valproate or valproic acid. The serum levels of carbamazepine-10,11-epoxide are reported to be increased by about 50 to 100%.[6,8-10] This active metabolite may cause the development of marked adverse effects such as blurred vision, dizziness, vomiting, tiredness and even nystagmus.[6-8,11] Acute psychosis, tentatively attributed to elevated epoxide levels, occurred in one patient when carbamazepine was added to sodium valproate treatment.[12]

2. Valpromide. Symptoms of carbamazepine toxicity developed in 5 out of 7 epileptic patients taking carbamazepine when concurrent treatment with sodium valproate was replaced by valpromide, despite the fact that their serum carbamazepine levels did not increase.[13] The toxicity appeared to be connected with a fourfold increase in the serum levels of the metabolite of carbamazepine, carbamazepine-10,11-epoxide, which rose to 8.5 micrograms/mL.[13]
In another study in 6 epileptic patients the serum levels of carbamazepine-10,11-epoxide rose by 330% (range 110 to 864%) within a week of starting valpromide, and two of the patients developed confusion, dizziness and vomiting. The symptoms disappeared and serum carbamazepine-10,11-epoxide levels fell when the valpromide dosage was reduced by one-third.[6]
A study in healthy subjects given a single 100-mg oral dose of carbamazepine-10,11-epoxide confirmed that valpromide 300 mg twice daily for 8 days reduced carbamazepine-10,11-epoxide clearance by 73%, and increased peak levels by 62%.[14]

(b) Valproate levels

A pharmacokinetic study in 6 healthy subjects found that carbamazepine, 200 mg daily, over a 17-day period increased the sodium valproate clearance by 30%.[15]
Other reports have described reductions in serum sodium valproate levels of 34 to 38% when carbamazepine was added,[16-18] and rises of 50 to 65% when the carbamazepine was withdrawn.[19,20] The rise appears to reach a plateau after about 4 weeks.[20] A pharmacokinetic model has been devised to estimate valproate clearance when given with carbamazepine.[21]

(c) Other effects

Evidence from epidemiological studies suggests that the risk of fatal hepatotoxicity is higher when sodium valproate is given with other antiepileptics than when it is given alone, especially in infants.[22,23] A single case report describes hepatocellular and cholestatic jaundice and a reversible Parkinsonian syndrome in a woman taking sodium valproate and carbamazepine, which reversed when the carbamazepine was withdrawn. Levels of both drugs did not exceed the therapeutic range at any stage. The Parkinsonian syndrome was attributed to a drug interaction, whereas the hepatotoxicity was considered most likely to be due to the carbamazepine, although the valproate may have contributed.[24]

Mechanism

The evidence suggests that carbamazepine increases the metabolism of valproate, so that it is cleared from the body more quickly. Carbamazepine may also possibly increase the formation of a minor but hepatotoxic metabolite of sodium valproate (2-propyl-4-pentenoic acid or 4-ene-VPA).[25,26]
The latter stages of carbamazepine metabolism appear to be inhibited by both valproate and its amide derivative, valpromide.[27] The levels of the metabolite carbamazepine-,10,11-epoxide increase during concurrent use, probably by inhibition of its metabolism to carbamazepine-10,11-trans-diol,[28-30] by epoxide hydrolase. Valpromide was found to be about 100 times more potent an inhibitor of this enzyme than sodium valproate *in vitro*[31] and caused a threefold higher rise in epoxide levels than valproate in one study.[6] The carbamazepine-10,11-epoxide metabolite has anticonvulsant activity, but it may also cause toxicity if its serum levels become excessive.[6,32]
It has also been suggested that valproate is not a selective inhibitor of epoxide hydrolase but that it inhibits all the steps of the epoxide-diol pathway.[33] The trans-diol metabolite is then further converted by glucuronidation, and it seems that this step is also inhibited.[30]

Importance and management

Moderately well documented interactions, which are established.
A minor to modest fall in carbamazepine levels may occur, but there may be a moderate to marked rise in the active epoxide metabolite. Therefore, be alert for signs of toxicity, which may indicate high levels of carbamazepine-10,11-epoxide and a need to reduce the carbamazepine dose.
Be alert for falls in the serum levels of valproate if carbamazepine is added, and rises if carbamazepine is withdrawn. Sodium valproate has been associated with serious hepatotoxicity, especially in children aged less than 3 years, and this has been more common in those receiving other antiepileptics. Sodium valproate monotherapy is to be preferred in this group.
There is also some debate about whether the combination of valproate (especially valpromide) and carbamazepine should be avoided, not only because of the risk of toxicity but also because inhibition of epoxide hydrolase may be undesirable.[13] This enzyme is possibly important for the detoxification of a number of teratogenic, mutagenic and carcinogenic epoxides.[6,13] More study is needed.

1. Levy RH, Morselli PL, Bianchetti G, Guyot M, Brachet-Liermain A, Loiseau P. Interaction between valproic acid and carbamazepine in epileptic patients. In: RH Levy, (ed). Metabolism of Antiepileptic Drugs. New York: Raven Press, 1984: 45–51.
2. Levy RH, Moreland TA, Morselli PL, Guyot M, Brachet-Liermain A, Loiseau P. Carbamazepine/valproic acid interaction in man and rhesus monkey. *Epilepsia* (1984) 25, 338–45.
3. Wilder BJ, Willmore LJ, Bruni J, Villarreal HJ. Valproic acid: interaction with other anticonvulsant drugs. *Neurology* (1978) 28, 892–6.
4. Varma R, Michos GA, Varma RS, Hoshino AY. Clinical trials of Depakene (valproic acid) coadministered with other anticonvulsants in epileptic patients. *Res Commun Psychol Psychiatr Behav* (1980) 5, 265–73.

5. Fowler GW. Effects of dipropylacetate on serum levels of anticonvulsants in children. *Proc West Pharmacol Soc* (1978) 21, 37–40.
6. Pisani F, Fazio A, Oteri G, Ruello C, Gitto C, Russo R, Perucca E. Sodium valproate and valpromide: differential interactions with carbamazepine in epileptic patients. *Epilepsia* (1986) 27, 548–52.
7. Sunaoshi W, Miura H, Takanashi S, Shira H, Hosoda N. Influence of concurrent administration of sodium valproate on the plasma concentrations of carbamazepine and its epoxide and diol metabolites. *Jpn J Psychiatry Neurol* (1991) 45, 474–7.
8. Kutt H, Solomon G, Peterson H, Dhar A, Caronna J. Accumulation of carbamazepine epoxide caused by valproate contributing to intoxication syndromes. *Neurology* (1985) 35 (Suppl 1), 286.
9. Liu H, Delgado MR. Improved therapeutic monitoring of drug interactions in epileptic children using carbamazepine polytherapy. *Ther Drug Monit* (1994) 16, 132–8.
10. Macphee GJA, Mitchell JR, Wiseman L, McLellan AR, Park BK, McInnes GT, Brodie MJ. Effect of sodium valproate on carbamazepine disposition and psychomotor profile in man. *Br J Clin Pharmacol* (1988) 25, 59–66.
11. Rambeck B, Sälke-Treumann A, May T, Boenigk HE. Valproic acid-induced carbamazepine-10,11-epoxide toxicity in children and adolescents. *Eur Neurol* (1990) 30, 79–83.
12. McKee RJW, Larkin JG, Brodie MJ. Acute psychosis with carbamazepine and sodium valproate. *Lancet* (1989) i, 167.
13. Meijer JWA, Binnie CD, Debets RMChr, Van Parys JAP and de Beer-Pawlikowski NKB. Possible hazard of valpromide-carbamazepine combination therapy in epilepsy. *Lancet* (1984) i, 802.
14. Perucca E, Pisani F, Spina E, Oteri G, Fazio A, Bertilsson L. Effects of valpromide and viloxazine on the elimination of carbamazepine-10,11-epoxide, an active metabolite of carbamazepine. *Pharm Res* (1989) 21, 111–12.
15. Bowdle TA, Levy RH, Cutler RE. Effects of carbamazepine on valproic acid kinetics in normal subjects. *Clin Pharmacol Ther* (1979) 26, 629–34.
16. Reunanen MI, Luoma P, Myllylä VV, Hokkanen E. Low serum valproic acid concentrations in epileptic patients on combination therapy. *Curr Ther Res* (1980) 28, 456–62.
17. May T, Rambeck B. Serum concentrations of valproic acid: influence of dose and comedication. *Ther Drug Monit* (1985) 7, 387–90.
18. Panesar SK, Orr JM, Farrell K, Burton RW, Kassahun K, Abbott FS. The effect of carbamazepine on valproic acid disposition in adult volunteers. *Br J Clin Pharmacol* (1989) 27, 323–8.
19. Henriksen O, Johannessen SI. Clinical and pharmacokinetic observations on sodium valproate — a 5 year follow-up study in 100 children with epilepsy. *Acta Neurol Scand* (1982) 65, 504–23.
20. Jann MW, Fidone GS, Israel MK, Bonadero P. Increased valproate serum concentrations upon carbamazepine cessation. *Epilepsia* (1988) 29, 578–81.
21. Yukawa E, Honda T, Ohdo S, Higuchi S, Aoyama T. Detection of carbamazepine-induced changes in valproic acid relative clearance in man by simple pharmacokinetic screening. *J Pharm Pharmacol* (1997) 49, 751–6.
22. Dreifuss FE, Santilli N, Langer DH, Sweeney KP, Moline KA, Menander KB. Valproic acid hepatic fatalities: a retrospective review. *Neurology* (1987) 37, 379–85.
23. Dreifuss FE, Langer DH, Moline KA, Maxwell DE. Valproic acid hepatic fatalities. II. US experience since 1984. *Neurology* (1989) 39, 201–7.
24. Froomes PR, Stewart MR. A reversible Parkinsonian syndrome and hepatotoxicity following addition of carbamazepine to sodium valproate. *Aust N Z J Med* (1994) 24, 413–14.
25. Levy RH, Rettenmeier AW, Anderson GD, Wilensky AJ, Friel PN, Baillie TA, Acheampong A, Tor J, Guyot M, Loiseau P. Effects of polytherapy with phenytoin, carbamazepine, and stiripentol on formation of 4-ene-valproate, a hepatotoxic metabolite of valproic acid. *Clin Pharmacol Ther* (1990) 48, 225–35.
26. Kondo T, Otani K, Hirano T, Kaneko S, Fukushima Y. The effects of phenytoin and carbamazepine on serum concentrations of mono-unsaturated metabolites of valproic acid. *Br J Clin Pharmacol* (1990) 29, 116–9.
27. Pisani F, Fazio A, Oteri G, Spina E, Perucca E and Bertilsson L. Effect of valpromide on the pharmacokinetics of carbamazepine-10,11-epoxide. *Br J Clin Pharmacol* (1988) 25, 611–13.
28. Pisani F, Caputo M, Fazio A, Oteri G, Russo M, Spina E, Perucca E, Bertilsson L. Interaction of carbamazepine-10,11-epoxide, an active metabolite of carbamazepine, with valproate: a pharmacokinetic study. *Epilepsia* (1990) 31, 339–42.
29. Robbins DK, Wedlund PJ, Kuhn R, Baumann RJ, Levy RH, Chang S-L. Inhibition of epoxide hydrolase by valproic acid in epileptic patients receiving carbamazepine. *Br J Clin Pharmacol* (1990) 29, 759–62.
30. Bernus I, Dickinson RG, Hooper WD, Eadie MJ. The mechanism of the carbamazepine-valproate interaction in humans. *Br J Clin Pharmacol* (1997) 44, 21–27.
31. Kerr BM, Rettie AE, Eddy AC, Loiseau P, Guyot M, Wilensky AJ, Levy RH. Inhibition of human liver microsomal epoxide hydrolase by valproate and valpromide: in vitro/in vivo correlation. *Clin Pharmacol Ther* (1989) 46, 82–93. Correction. ibid. 343.
32. Levy RH, Kerr BM, Loiseau P, Guyot M and Wilensky AJ. Inhibition of carbamazepine epoxide elimination by valpromide and valproic acid. *Epilepsia* (1986) 27, 592.
33. Svinarov DA, Pippenger CE. Valproic acid-carbamazepine interaction: is valproic acid a selective inhibitor of epoxide hydrolase? *Ther Drug Monit* (1995) 17, 217–20.

Carbamazepine + Vigabatrin

Vigabatrin does not normally alter carbamazepine levels, although one study has shown a modest increase, and one a modest decrease.

Clinical evidence

In an early clinical study, vigabatrin 2 to 3 g daily did not change the serum levels of carbamazepine in 12 patients.[1] Similarly, other studies found that carbamazepine levels were not significantly altered by the addition of vigabatrin.[2,3] However, in one study in which 59 patients taking carbamazepine received vigabatrin, 34 patients had an increase in carbamazepine levels, 3 had no change, and 22 had a decrease, resulting in a mean overall increase of 6%, which was not significant.[4] Similarly, in another study 46 out of 66 patients had an increase in carbamazepine level of at least 10% (mean increase about 24%), and in 24 of these patients the carbamazepine level exceeded the therapeutic level.[5] In this study, the increase in carbamazepine level was greater the lower the initial carbamazepine level.[5] In contrast, one study in 15 patients reported a mean 18% decrease in carbamazepine levels when vigabatrin was added.[6]

Mechanism

Not understood.

Importance and management

The studies seem to suggest that any change in carbamazepine levels with vigabatrin is of borderline clinical significance and therefore the majority of patients will not be affected. Any change is likely to be more important in patients at the top of the therapeutic carbamazepine range. It would therefore seem prudent to be alert for any increase in carbamazepine adverse effects (such as nausea and vomiting, ataxia, and drowsiness) and consider taking carbamazepine levels if these develop.

1. Tassinari CA, Michelucci R, Ambrosetto G, Salvi F. Double-blind study of vigabatrin in the treatment of drug-resistant epilepsy. *Arch Neurol* (1987) 44, 907–10.
2. Rimmer EM, Richens A. Interaction between vigabatrin and phenytoin. *Br J Clin Pharmacol* (1989) 27, 27S–33S.
3. Bernardina BD, Fontana E, Vigevano F, Fusco L, Torelli D, Galeone D, Buti D, Cianchetti C, Gnanasakthy A, Iudice A. Efficacy and tolerability of vigabatrin in children with refractory partial seizures: a single-blind dose-increasing study. *Epilepsia* (1995) 36, 687–91.
4. Browne TR, Mattson RH, Penry JK, Smith DB, Treiman DM, Wilder BJ, Ben-Menachem E, Napoliello MJ, Sherry KM, Szabo GK. Vigabatrin for refractory complex partial seizures: multicenter single-blind study with long-term follow up. *Neurology* (1987) 37, 184–9.
5. Jędrzejczak J, Dławichowska E, Owczarek K, Majkowski J. Effect of vigabatrin addition on carbamazepine blood serum levels in patients with epilepsy. *Epilepsy Res* (2000) 39, 115–20.
6. Sánchez-Alcaraz A, Quintana B, López E, Rodríguez I, Llopis P. Effect of vigabatrin on the pharmacokinetics of carbamazepine. *J Clin Pharm Ther* (2002) 27, 427–30.

Carbamazepine + Viloxazine

Viloxazine can cause a marked rise in serum carbamazepine levels and toxicity has been seen, but it does not appear to alter oxcarbazepine levels.

Clinical evidence

(a) Carbamazepine

The serum carbamazepine levels of 7 patients rose by 50%, from 8.1 to 12.1 micrograms/mL, after they took viloxazine 100 mg three times daily for 3 weeks.[1] Signs of mild toxicity (dizziness, ataxia, fatigue, drowsiness) developed in 5 of them. These symptoms disappeared and the serum carbamazepine levels fell when the viloxazine was withdrawn.[1] Another report found a 2.5-fold increase in serum carbamazepine levels in one patient within 2 weeks of starting to take viloxazine 300 mg daily.[2] Another report found an average 55% rise in plasma carbamazepine levels and toxicity in 4 of 7 patients taking viloxazine.[3] Yet another patient developed choreoathetosis and increased serum carbamazepine levels, which was attributed to the use of viloxazine.[4] In one study, the pharmacokinetics of a single dose of viloxazine were reported to be unaffected by carbamazepine,[5] but in the case report cited above, which was at steady-state, the viloxazine levels were found to be reduced.[2]

(b) Oxcarbazepine

In 6 patients with simple or partial seizures the steady-state serum levels of oxcarbazepine (average dose 1500 mg daily) were unaffected by the addition of viloxazine 100 mg twice daily for 10 days. No adverse effects were seen.[6]

Mechanism

Uncertain. What is known suggests that viloxazine inhibits the metabolism of carbamazepine, thereby reducing its clearance and raising its serum levels.

Importance and management

Information seems to be limited to the reports cited. If concurrent use is undertaken, serum carbamazepine levels should be monitored closely and suitable dosage reductions made as necessary to avoid possible toxicity. No special precautions seem necessary with oxcarbazepine.

1. Pisani F, Narbone MC, Fazio A, Crisafulli P, Primerano G, Amendola D'Angostino A, Oteri G, Di Perri R. Effect of viloxazine on serum carbamazepine levels in epileptic patients. *Epilepsia* (1984) 25, 482–5.
2. Odou P, Geronimi-Ferret D, Degen P, Robert H. Viloxazine-carbamazépine. Double interaction dangereuse? A propos d'un cas. *J Pharm Clin* (1996) 15, 157–60.

3. Pisani F, Fazio A, Oteri G, Perucca E, Russo M, Trio R, Pisani B, Di Perri R. Carbamazepine-viloxazine interaction in patients with epilepsy. *J Neurol Neurosurg Psychiatry* (1986) 49, 1142–5.
4. Mosquet B, Starace J, Madelaine S, Simon JY, Lacotte J, Moulin M. Syndrome choréo-athétosique sous carbamazépine et viloxazine. *Therapie* (1994) 49, 513–14.
5. Pisani F, Fazio A, Spina E, Artesi C, Pisani B, Russo M, Trio R, Perucca E. Pharmacokinetics of the antidepressant drug viloxazine in normal subjects and in epileptic patients receiving chronic anticonvulsant treatment. *Psychopharmacology (Berl)* (1986) 90, 295–8.
6. Pisani F, Fazio A, Oteri G, Artesi C, Xiao B, Perucca E, Di Perri R. Effects of the antidepressant drug viloxazine on oxcarbazepine and its hydroxylated metabolites in patients with epilepsy. *Acta Neurol Scand* (1994) 90, 130–2.

Ethosuximide + Isoniazid

A single report describes a patient who developed psychotic behaviour and signs of ethosuximide toxicity when given isoniazid.

Clinical evidence, mechanism, importance and management

An epileptic patient, who had been stable taking ethosuximide and sodium valproate for 2 years, developed persistent hiccuping, nausea, vomiting, anorexia and insomnia within a week of starting to take isoniazid 300 mg daily. Psychotic behaviour gradually developed over the next 5 weeks and so the isoniazid was stopped. The appearance of these symptoms appeared to be related to the sharp rise in serum ethosuximide levels (from about 50 up to 198 micrograms/mL).[1] It is suggested that the isoniazid may have inhibited the metabolism of the ethosuximide, leading to accumulation and toxicity. The general importance of this case is uncertain.

1. van Wieringen A, Vrijlandt CM. Ethosuximide intoxication caused by interaction with isoniazid. *Neurology* (1983) 33, 1227–8.

Ethosuximide + Other antiepileptics

Minor to modest falls in serum ethosuximide levels may occur if carbamazepine, primidone or phenytoin are also given, whereas methylphenobarbital or sodium valproate may cause a rise in ethosuximide levels. The effect of all these changes on seizure control is uncertain. Lamotrigine appears not to affect ethosuximide levels.
Ethosuximide is reported to have caused phenytoin toxicity in a few cases, and it appears that ethosuximide can reduce valproate serum levels.

Clinical evidence

(a) Barbiturates

In a retrospective analysis, the level to dose ratio of ethosuximide was 33% lower in 29 epileptic patients taking ethosuximide and **primidone** than in 39 patients taking ethosuximide alone,[1] suggesting that primidone reduces ethosuximide levels.

Similarly, in another study, which compared the pharmacokinetics of a single dose of ethosuximide in 10 epileptic patients taking **phenobarbital**, phenytoin and/or carbamazepine with 12 healthy controls, the epileptic group had markedly shorter (about halved) ethosuximide half-lives.[2] Conversely, another report stated that ethosuximide levels tended to rise [amount not stated] when **methylphenobarbital** was used (the opposite effect to that which would be expected), but did not appear to be affected by **phenobarbital** or **primidone**.[3] Phenobarbital levels (from **primidone**) do not appear to be affected by ethosuximide.[4]

(b) Carbamazepine

A study in 6 healthy subjects taking ethosuximide 500 mg daily found that the mean plasma levels of ethosuximide were reduced by 17%, from 32 to 27 mg/mL by carbamazepine 200 mg daily for 18 days. One individual had a 35% reduction in ethosuximide levels.[5] Another study, which compared 10 epileptic patients (taking enzyme-inducing antiepileptic drugs, including 4 taking carbamazepine) with 12 healthy controls found that the epileptic group had markedly shorter (about halved) ethosuximide half-lives.[2]

In contrast, the concurrent use of carbamazepine did not affect the correlation between ethosuximide dose and levels in another study.[3]

(c) Lamotrigine

Five children taking ethosuximide and various other antiepileptics had no change in their plasma ethosuximide levels when lamotrigine was also given.[6]

(d) Phenytoin

A study compared the pharmacokinetics of a single dose of ethosuximide in 10 epileptic patients taking phenobarbital, phenytoin and/or carbamazepine with 12 healthy controls. The epileptic group had markedly shorter (about halved) ethosuximide half-lives.[2] In contrast, the concurrent use of phenytoin did not affect the correlation between ethosuximide levels and dose in another study.[3]

Three cases have occurred in which ethosuximide appeared to have been responsible for increasing phenytoin levels,[7-9] leading to the development of phenytoin toxicity in 2 patients.[8,9]

(e) Sodium valproate

Four out of 5 patients taking ethosuximide (average dose 27 mg/kg) had an increase in their serum levels of about 50% (from 73 to 112 micrograms/mL), within 3 weeks of starting to take sodium valproate (adjusted to the maximum tolerated dose). Sedation occurred and ethosuximide dose reductions were necessary.[10] In a single-dose study in 6 healthy subjects, treatment with sodium valproate for 9 days was reported to have increased the ethosuximide half-life and reduced the clearance by 15%.[11] However, other studies have described no changes[12,13] or even lower serum ethosuximide levels (level to dose ratio reduced by 36%).[1]

One study in 13 children found that ethosuximide can lower valproate serum levels. In the presence of ethosuximide the valproate levels were lower than with valproate alone (87 versus 120 micrograms/mL). After stopping ethosuximide the valproate levels rose by about 40%.[14]

Mechanism

The most probable explanation for the fall in ethosuximide levels is that the carbamazepine and the other enzyme-inducing antiepileptics increase the metabolism and clearance of ethosuximide, which is known to be metabolised by the cytochrome P450 isoenzyme CYP3A.[2]

Importance and management

The concurrent use of antiepileptics is common and often advantageous. Information on these interactions is sparse and even contradictory and their clinical importance is uncertain. Nevertheless, good monitoring would clearly be appropriate if these drugs are used with ethosuximide to monitor for potential toxicity and to ensure adequate seizure control.

1. Battino D, Cusi C, Franceschetti S, Moise A, Spina S, Avanzini G. Ethosuximide plasma concentrations: influence of age and associated concomitant therapy. *Clin Pharmacokinet* (1982) 7, 176–80.
2. Giaccone M, Bartoli A, Gatti G, Marchiselli R, Pisani F, Latella MA, Perucca E. Effect of enzyme inducing anticonvulsants on ethosuximide pharmacokinetics in epileptic patients. *Br J Clin Pharmacol* (1996) 41, 575–9.
3. Smith GA, McKauge L, Dubetz D, Tyrer JH, Eadie MJ. Factors influencing plasma concentrations of ethosuximide. *Clin Pharmacokinet* (1979) 4, 38–52.
4. Schmidt D. The effect of phenytoin and ethosuximide on primidone metabolism in patients with epilepsy. *J Neurol* (1975) 209, 115–23.
5. Warren JW, Benmaman JD, Wannamaker BB, Levy RH. Kinetics of a carbamazepine-ethosuximide interaction. *Clin Pharmacol Ther* (1980) 28, 646–51.
6. Eriksson A-S, Hoppu K, Nergårdh A, Boreus L. Pharmacokinetic interactions between lamotrigine and other antiepileptic drugs in children with intractable epilepsy. *Epilepsia* (1996) 37, 769–73.
7. Lander CM, Eadie MJ, Tyrer JH. Interactions between anticonvulsants. *Proc Aust Assoc Neurol* (1975) 12, 111–16.
8. Dawson GW, Brown HW, Clark BG. Serum phenytoin after ethosuximide. *Ann Neurol* (1978) 4, 583–4.
9. Frantzen E, Hansen JM, Hansen OE, Kristensen M. Phenytoin (Dilantin) intoxication. *Acta Neurol Scand* (1967) 43, 440–6.
10. Mattson RH, Cramer JA. Valproic acid and ethosuximide interaction. *Ann Neurol* (1980) 7, 583–4.
11. Pisani F, Narbone MC, Trunfio C, Fazio A, La Rosa G, Oteri G, Di Perri R. Valproic acid-ethosuximide interaction: a pharmacokinetic study. *Epilepsia* (1984) 25, 229–33.
12. Fowler GW. Effect of dipropylacetate on serum levels of anticonvulsants in children. *Proc West Pharmacol Soc* (1978) 21, 37–40.
13. Bauer LA, Harris C, Wilensky AJ, Raisys VA, Levy RH. Ethosuximide kinetics: possible interaction with valproic acid. *Clin Pharmacol Ther* (1982) 31, 741–5.
14. Sälke-Kellermann RA, May T, Boenigk HE. Influence of ethosuximide on valproic acid serum concentrations. *Epilepsy Res* (1997) 26, 345–349.

Felbamate + Antacids

An aluminium/magnesium hydroxide-containing antacid had no effect on the absorption of felbamate.

Clinical evidence, mechanism, importance and management

Felbamate 2.4 g daily was given to 9 epileptic women for 2 weeks. For a third week the felbamate was taken with an antacid containing **aluminium/magnesium hydroxide** (*Maalox Plus*). No significant changes in the plasma levels or AUC were seen.[1] No special precautions would seem to be needed if felbamate is taken with this or any other similar antacid.

1. Sachdeo RC, Narang-Sachdeo SK, Howard JR, Dix RK, Shumaker RC, Perhach JL, Rosenberg A. Effect of antacid on the absorption of felbamate in subjects with epilepsy. *Epilepsia* (1993) 34 (Suppl 6), 79–80.

Felbamate + Erythromycin

Erythromycin does not alter felbamate pharmacokinetics.

Clinical evidence, mechanism, importance and management

In a randomised, crossover study, 12 epileptic patients were given felbamate 3 g or 3.6 g daily, either alone or with erythromycin 333 mg every 8 hours for 10 days. The pharmacokinetics of felbamate were unchanged by erythromycin.[1] There would therefore seem no reason for avoiding erythromycin in patients taking felbamate.

1. Sachdeo RJ, Narang-Sachdeo SK, Montgomery PA, Shumaker RC, Perhach JL, Lyness WH, Rosenberg A. Evaluation of the potential interaction between felbamate and erythromycin in patients with epilepsy. *J Clin Pharmacol* (1998) 38, 184–90.

Felbamate + Gabapentin

There is some evidence that the half-life of felbamate may be prolonged by gabapentin.

Clinical evidence, mechanism, importance and management

In a retrospective examination of clinical data from patients taking felbamate, its half-life was found to be 24 hours in 40 patients taking felbamate alone, whereas in 18 other patients also taking gabapentin (including 7 taking a third drug), the half-life was extended to 32.7 hours.[1] The practical clinical importance of this is uncertain but be alert for the need to reduce the felbamate dosage. More study is needed.

1. Hussein G, Troupin AS, Montouris G. Gabapentin interaction with felbamate. *Neurology* (1996) 47, 1106.

Fosphenytoin + Miscellaneous

Fosphenytoin is a prodrug of phenytoin, which is rapidly and completely hydrolysed to phenytoin in the body. It is predicted to interact with other drugs in the same way as phenytoin.[1,2] No drugs are known to interfere with the conversion of fosphenytoin to phenytoin.[2]

1. Fierro LS, Savulich DH, Benezra DA. Safety of fosphenytoin sodium. *Am J Health-Syst Pharm* (1996) 53, 2707–12.
2. Pro-Epanutin (Fosphenytoin sodium). Pfizer Ltd. UK Summary of product characteristics, May 2005.

Gabapentin + Antacids

Aluminium/magnesium hydroxide slightly reduces the absorption of gabapentin.

Clinical evidence, mechanism, importance and management

An **aluminium/magnesium hydroxide** antacid (*Maalox TC*) reduced the bioavailability of gabapentin 400 mg by about 20% when given either at the same time or 2 hours after gabapentin. When the antacid was given 2 hours before the gabapentin, the bioavailability was reduced by about 10%.[1] These small changes are unlikely to be of clinical importance. However, the manufacturer does recommend that gabapentin is taken about 2 hours after **aluminium/magnesium-containing antacids**.[2]

1. Busch JA, Radulovic LL, Bockbrader HN, Underwood BA, Sedman AJ, Chang T. Effect of *Maalox TC®* on single-dose pharmacokinetics of gabapentin capsules in healthy subjects. *Pharm Res* (1992) 9 (10 Suppl), S-315.
2. Neurontin (Gabapentin). Pfizer Ltd. UK Summary of product characteristics, August 2006.

Gabapentin + Cimetidine

A brief report notes that cimetidine decreased the renal clearance of gabapentin by 12%, which was not expected to be clinically important. No study details were given.[1]

1. Busch JA, Bockbrader HN, Randinitis EJ, Chang T, Welling PG, Reece PA, Underwood B, Sedman AJ, Vollmer KO, Türck D. Lack of clinically significant drug interactions with Neurontin (Gabapentin). 20th International Epilepsy Congress. Oslo, Norway, July 1993. Abstract 013958.

Gabapentin + Food

Food, including protein and enteral feeds, does not have a clinically important effect on the absorption of gabapentin.

Clinical evidence, mechanism, importance and management

A high-protein meal (80 g of total protein) increased the maximum serum levels of a single 800-mg dose of gabapentin by 36% in healthy subjects. The AUC was increased by 11%, which was not statistically significant. These findings were the opposite of those expected, since L-amino acids compete for gabapentin intestinal transport *in vitro*.[1]

In another single-dose study, the absorption of gabapentin capsules did not differ when opened and mixed with either **apple sauce** or **orange juice**, but tended to be higher (AUC increased by 26%) when mixed with a protein-containing vehicle (**chocolate pudding**).[2] Similarly, no change in absorption was found when gabapentin syrup was mixed with tap water, **grape juice**, or an **enteral feed** (*Sustacal*), but a modest 31% increase in AUC was seen when it was mixed with **chocolate milk**.[3]

These small changes are unlikely to be of clinical importance, so it does not matter when gabapentin is taken in relation to food.

1. Gidal BE, Maly MM, Budde J, Lensmeyer GL, Pitterle ME, Jones JC. Effect of a high-protein meal on gabapentin pharmacokinetics. *Epilepsy Res* (1996) 23, 71–6.
2. Gidal BE, Maly MM, Kowalski JW, Rutecki PA, Pitterle ME, Cook DE. Gabapentin absorption: effect of mixing with foods of varying macronutrient composition. *Ann Pharmacother* (1998) 32, 405–9.
3. Parnell J, Sheth R, Limdi N, Gidal BE. Oral absorption of gabapentin syrup is not impaired by concomitant administration with various beverages or enteral nutrition supplement. *Epilepsia* (2001) 42 (Suppl 7), 91.

Gabapentin + Other antiepileptics

Gabapentin does not normally affect the pharmacokinetics of carbamazepine, phenytoin, phenobarbital or sodium valproate, and no dosage adjustments are needed on concurrent use. However, isolated reports describe increased phenytoin levels and toxicity in two patients given gabapentin.

Clinical evidence, mechanism, importance and management

The pharmacokinetics of both **phenytoin** and gabapentin remained unchanged in 8 epileptics who were given gabapentin 400 mg three times daily for 8 days, in addition to **phenytoin**, which they had been taking for at least 2 months.[1] Other studies confirm that the steady-state pharmacokinetics of **phenytoin** are unaffected by gabapentin, and that the pharmacokinetics of gabapentin are similarly unaffected by **phenytoin**.[2,3] These reports contrast with an isolated report of a patient taking **phenytoin**, **carbamazepine** and **clobazam** whose serum **phenytoin** levels increased three to fourfold, with symptoms of toxicity, on two occasions when gabapentin 300 to 600 mg daily was given. **Carbamazepine** serum levels remained unchanged. The author suggests that this differing reaction may be because the patient was taking more than one antiepileptic, unlike previous studies where only single drugs had been used.[4] However, another case of **phenytoin** toxicity possibly attributable to gabapentin has been described in a patient who was not taking any other antiepileptics.[5]

Gabapentin does not affect **phenobarbital** levels, nor is it affected by **phenobarbital**.[2,3,6] Other studies confirm that the steady-state pharmacokinetics of **carbamazepine** and **sodium valproate** are unaffected by gabapentin, and that the pharmacokinetics of gabapentin are similarly unaffected by these antiepileptics.[2,3,7]

It would seem therefore that no dosage adjustments are normally needed if gabapentin is added to treatment with most of these antiepileptics. However, if gabapentin is added to **phenytoin** it may be wise to bear the possibility of raised **phenytoin** levels in mind. For mention that gabapentin may prolong the half-life of **felbamate**, see 'Felbamate + Gabapentin', p.540. For mention of the lack of interaction between **levetiracetam** and gabapentin, see 'Levetiracetam + Other antiepileptics', p.543.

1. Anhut H, Leppik I, Schmidt B, Thomann P. Drug interaction study of the new anticonvulsant gabapentin with phenytoin in epileptic patients. *Naunyn Schmiedebergs Arch Pharmacol* (1988) 337 (Suppl), R127.
2. Brockbrader HN, Radulovic LL, Loewen G, Chang T, Welling PG, Reece PA, Underwood B, Sedman AJ. Lack of drug-drug interactions between Neurontin (gabapentin) and other antiepileptic drugs. 20th International Epilepsy Congress, Oslo, Norway. July 1993 (Abstract).
3. Richens A. Clinical pharmacokinetics of gabapentin. New Trends in Epilepsy Management: The Role of Gabapentin International Congress and Symposium Series No 198, Royal Society of Medicine Services, London, NY 1993, 41–6.
4. Tyndel F. Interaction of gabapentin with other antiepileptics. *Lancet* (1994) 343, 1363–4.
5. Sánchez-Romero A, Durán-Quintana JA, García-Delgado R, Margariot-Rangel C, Proveda-Andrés JL. Posible interacción gabapentina-fenitoína. *Rev Neurol* (2002) 34, 952–3.
6. Hooper WD, Kavanagh MC, Herkes GK, Eadie MJ. Lack of a pharmacokinetic interaction between phenobarbitone and gabapentin. *Br J Clin Pharmacol* (1991) 31, 171–4.
7. Radulovic LL, Wilder BJ, Leppik IE, Bockbrader HN, Chang T, Posvar EL, Sedman AJ, Uthman BM, Erdman GR. Lack of interaction of gabapentin with carbamazepine or valproate. *Epilepsia* (1994) 35, 155–61.

Gabapentin + Probenecid

A brief report notes that probenecid had no effect on the renal clearance of gabapentin. No study details were given.[1]

1. Busch JA, Bockbrader HN, Randinitis EJ, Chang T, Welling PG, Reece PA, Underwood B, Sedman AJ, Vollmer KO, Türck D. Lack of clinically significant drug interactions with Neurontin (Gabapentin). 20th International Epilepsy Congress. Oslo, Norway, July 1993. Abstract 013958.

Lamotrigine + Antimycobacterials

Rifampicin markedly increased the clearance of lamotrigine in a pharmacokinetic study. A case report has described a similar finding, and also included some limited evidence suggesting that isoniazid may inhibit lamotrigine metabolism.

Clinical evidence

Rifampicin 600 mg daily for 5 days increased the clearance of a single 25-mg dose of lamotrigine by 97% and decreased the AUC by 44% in 10 healthy subjects. The amount of lamotrigine glucuronide recovered in the urine was increased by 36%.[1] Similarly, a case report[2] describes a 56-year-old woman taking lamotrigine 150 mg daily who had unexpectedly low serum lamotrigine levels of 1.3 mg/L after starting **rifampicin, isoniazid** and pyrazinamide. The lamotrigine dosage was therefore increased to 250 mg daily. After treatment was changed to **isoniazid** and ethambutol, the lamotrigine serum levels rose to 12.4 mg/L. Levels less than 10 mg/L are associated with less toxicity; however, in this patient no toxicity was seen.

Mechanism

Rifampicin increases the loss of lamotrigine from the body, probably by inducing glucuronidation via UDP-glucuronyl transferases.[1] It was suggested that isoniazid may have inhibited lamotrigine metabolism.[2]

Importance and management

Information appears to be limited to these reports, but the interaction between lamotrigine and rifampicin would appear to be established. Be aware that rifampicin could reduce the efficacy of lamotrigine, and that increased lamotrigine doses are likely to be required.

The case report also raises the possibility of an interaction between lamotrigine and isoniazid. If isoniazid is added to or withdrawn from lamotrigine treatment, be alert for the need to adjust the lamotrigine dosage.

1. Ebert U, Thong NQ, Oertel R, Kirch W. Effects of rifampicin and cimetidine on pharmacokinetics and pharmacodynamics of lamotrigine in healthy subjects. *Eur J Clin Pharmacol* (2000) 56, 299–304.
2. Armijo JA, Sánchez B, Peralta FG, Cuadrado A, Leno C. Lamotrigine interaction with rifampicin and isoniazid. A case report. *Methods Find Exp Clin Pharmacol* (1996) 18 (Suppl C), 59.

Lamotrigine + Cimetidine

Cimetidine 400 mg twice daily for 5 days had no effect on the pharmacokinetics of a single 25-mg dose of lamotrigine in 10 healthy subjects. No change in lamotrigine dose appears to be needed during concurrent use.[1]

1. Ebert U, Thong NQ, Oertel R, Kirch W. Effects of rifampicin and cimetidine on pharmacokinetics and pharmacodynamics of lamotrigine in healthy subjects. *Eur J Clin Pharmacol* (2000) 56, 299–304.

Lamotrigine + Felbamate

Felbamate appears not to affect the pharmacokinetics of lamotrigine.

Clinical evidence, mechanism, importance and management

In 21 healthy subjects felbamate 1.2 g twice daily had minimal effects on the pharmacokinetics of lamotrigine 100 mg twice daily when they were given together for 10 days. A 14% increase in the lamotrigine AUC was seen, which was not considered clinically relevant.[1] Similarly, there was no difference between lamotrigine pharmacokinetics in 6 patients receiving lamotrigine and felbamate and 5 patients taking lamotrigine alone.[2] Therefore the dose of lamotrigine does not need to be adjusted if felbamate is given.

1. Colucci R, Glue P, Holt B, Banfield C, Reidenberg P, Meehan JW, Pai S, Nomeir A, Lim J, Lin C-C, Affrime MB. Effect of felbamate on the pharmacokinetics of lamotrigine. *J Clin Pharmacol* (1996) 36, 634–8.
2. Gidal BE, Kanner A, Maly M, Rutecki P, Lensmeyer GL. Lamotrigine pharmacokinetics in patients receiving felbamate. *Epilepsy Res* (1997) 27, 1–5.

Lamotrigine + Phenobarbital or Primidone

Phenobarbital has been associated with reduced lamotrigine serum levels. Phenobarbital and primidone levels were unchanged.

Clinical evidence, mechanism, importance and management

In a retrospective study, the lamotrigine serum concentration-to-dose ratio was lower in patients also taking phenobarbital than in those receiving lamotrigine monotherapy (0.52 versus 0.99),[1] suggesting that phenobarbital lowers lamotrigine levels. Similar findings have been reported in another study.[2] No changes in the serum levels of phenobarbital or primidone were seen in a study in 12 patients given lamotrigine 75 to 400 mg daily.[3]

Phenobarbital induces the metabolism of lamotrigine, and the recommended starting dose and long-term maintenance dose of lamotrigine in patients already taking phenobarbital or primidone is twice that of patients receiving lamotrigine monotherapy.[4,5] However, note that if they are also taking valproate in addition to phenobarbital, the lamotrigine dose should be reduced, see 'Lamotrigine + Valproate', p.542. The lamotrigine dosage may need to be reduced if phenobarbital is withdrawn.

1. May TW, Rambeck B, Jürgens U. Serum concentrations of lamotrigine in epileptic patients: the influence of dose and comedication. *Ther Drug Monit* (1996) 18, 523–31.
2. Armijo JA, Bravo J, Cuadrado A, Herranz JL. Lamotrigine serum concentration-to-dose ratio: influence of age and concomitant antiepileptic drugs and dosage implications. *Ther Drug Monit* (1999) 21, 182–190.
3. Jawad S, Richens A, Goodwin G, Yuen WC. Controlled trial of lamotrigine (Lamictal) for refractory partial seizures. *Epilepsia* (1989) 30, 356–63.
4. Lamictal (Lamotrigine). GlaxoSmithKline UK. UK Summary of product characteristics, March 2007.
5. Lamictal (Lamotrigine). GlaxoSmithKline. US Prescribing information, May 2007.

Lamotrigine + Phenytoin

Phenytoin has been associated with reduced lamotrigine serum levels. Lamotrigine has no effect on phenytoin levels.

Clinical evidence, mechanism, importance and management

In a retrospective study, the lamotrigine serum concentration-to-dose ratio was much lower in patients receiving concomitant phenytoin than in those taking lamotrigine monotherapy (0.32 versus 0.98),[1] suggesting that phenytoin lowers lamotrigine levels. Other studies in patients taking lamotrigine with phenytoin have reported similar findings.[2,3] In another study, the mean lamotrigine levels were approximately doubled when phenytoin was withdrawn.[4] In contrast one study suggests that the serum level of phenytoin was unchanged in patients given lamotrigine 75 to 400 mg daily.[5]

Phenytoin is a known hepatic enzyme inducer, which increases lamotrigine metabolism. The recommended starting dose and long-term maintenance dose of lamotrigine in patients already taking phenytoin is twice that of patients receiving lamotrigine monotherapy.[6,7]

However, note that if they are also taking valproate in addition to phenytoin, the lamotrigine dose should be reduced, see 'Lamotrigine + Valproate', below. The lamotrigine dosage may need to be reduced if phenytoin is withdrawn.

1. May TW, Rambeck B, Jürgens U. Serum concentrations of lamotrigine in epileptic patients: the influence of dose and comedication. *Ther Drug Monit* (1996) 18, 523–31.
2. Armijo JA, Bravo J, Cuadrado A, Herranz JL. Lamotrigine serum concentration-to-dose ratio: influence of age and concomitant antiepileptic drugs and dosage implications. *Ther Drug Monit* (1999) 21, 182–190.
3. Böttiger Y, Svensson J-O, Ståhle L. Lamotrigine drug interactions in a TDM material. *Ther Drug Monit* (1999) 21, 171–4.
4. Anderson GD, Gidal BE, Messenheimer J, Gilliam FG. Time course of lamotrigine de-induction: impact of step-wise withdrawal of carbamazepine or phenytoin. *Epilepsy Res* (2002) 49, 211–17.
5. Jawad S, Richens A, Goodwin G, Yuen WC. Controlled trial of lamotrigine (Lamictal) for refractory partial seizures. *Epilepsia* (1989) 30, 356–63.
6. Lamictal (Lamotrigine). GlaxoSmithKline UK. UK Summary of product characteristics, March 2007.
7. Lamictal (Lamotrigine). GlaxoSmithKline. US Prescribing information, May 2007.

Lamotrigine + Sertraline

A report describes two cases, which suggest that sertraline may increase lamotrigine levels and cause toxicity.

Clinical evidence, mechanism, importance and management

A patient's lamotrigine levels were found to have doubled and symptoms of toxicity were noted (confusion, cognitive impairment) 6 weeks after sertraline 25 mg daily was started.[1] The lamotrigine dose was halved, and the sertraline dose titrated to 50 mg daily. Symptoms of toxicity resolved, but the lamotrigine levels were still 24% higher than before sertraline was started. In another patient taking sertraline and lamotrigine with signs of lamotrigine toxicity, a 33% reduction in sertraline dose resulted in a halving of the lamotrigine level even though the lamotrigine dose was increased by 33%.

The authors suggest that sertraline may competitively inhibit the glucuronidation of lamotrigine. Evidence so far appears limited to this case report. In view of the increased risk of rash with increased lamotrigine levels (see also 'Lamotrigine + Valproate', below), it may be prudent to monitor the combination. Further study is needed.

1. Kaufman KR, Gerner R. Lamotrigine toxicity secondary to sertraline. *Seizure* (1998) 7, 163–5.

Lamotrigine + Topiramate

Topiramate does not appear to alter the pharmacokinetics of lamotrigine, although one study suggested that it reduced lamotrigine levels. Lamotrigine has no effect on topiramate levels.

Clinical evidence, mechanism, importance and management

In the preliminary report of one study, it was found that serum lamotrigine levels decreased by 40 to 50% in 4 of 7 patients stable taking lamotrigine 350 to 800 mg daily when they were given topiramate, titrated to 800 mg daily.[1] In contrast, other authors reported that the addition of topiramate 75 to 800 mg daily had little effect on the steady state serum levels of lamotrigine 100 to 950 mg daily in 24 patients. The mean lamotrigine level before topiramate was 10.4 mg/L and during topiramate was 9.7 mg/L. Only 2 of the patients had reductions of greater than 30% (40% and 43%).[2] A further study by the same research group confirmed the lack of effect of topiramate on lamotrigine pharmacokinetics.[3] The authors of the second study[2] note that there is some evidence that peak-to-trough variations of as much as 30 to 40% can occur during lamotrigine therapy, and therefore timing of blood sampling might be a factor in the findings of the first study.[1]

Lamotrigine had no effect on topiramate pharmacokinetics in one study in 13 patients. The oral clearance of topiramate 400 mg daily was 2.6 L/hour when given alone, and 2.7 L/hour when given with lamotrigine, and the AUC and plasma levels of topiramate were also similar.[3]

The balance of the evidence suggests that there is no important pharmacokinetic interaction between topiramate and lamotrigine. No special precautions appear to be necessary during concurrent use.

1. Wnuk W, Volanski A, Foletti G. Topiramate decreases lamotrigine concentrations. *Ther Drug Monit* (1999) 21, 449.
2. Berry DJ, Besag FMC, Pool F, Natarajan J, Doose D. Lack of an effect of topiramate on lamotrigine serum concentrations. *Epilepsia* (2002) 43, 818–23.
3. Doose DR, Brodie MJ, Wilson EA, Chadwick D, Oxbury J, Berry DJ, Schwabe S, Bialer M. Topiramate and lamotrigine pharmacokinetics during repetitive monotherapy and combination therapy in epilepsy patients. *Epilepsia* (2003) 44, 917–22.

Lamotrigine + Valproate

The serum levels of lamotrigine can be markedly increased by valproate. Concurrent use has been associated with skin rashes, tremor and other toxic reactions. Lamotrigine has been found to cause small increases, decreases or no changes in valproate levels.

Clinical evidence

(a) Effects on lamotrigine levels

In 6 healthy subjects sodium valproate 200 mg every 8 hours reduced the clearance of lamotrigine by 20%, and increased its AUC by 30%.[1] In another study, in 18 healthy subjects receiving valproate 500 mg twice daily, the clearance of lamotrigine 50, 100 or 150 mg daily was also markedly reduced, and the half-life increased.[2] In a retrospective study, the lamotrigine serum concentration-to-dose ratio was markedly higher in patients also taking valproate than in those receiving lamotrigine monotherapy (3.57 versus 0.98), suggesting that valproate increases lamotrigine levels. In patients also taking phenytoin, the effects of valproate on lamotrigine were offset (0.99 versus 0.98). However, the effects of valproate on lamotrigine were not completely offset by either carbamazepine or phenobarbital (1.67 or 1.8, respectively versus 0.98).[3] Other studies have reported broadly similar findings.[4-6] Three studies have found that the effect of valproate on lamotrigine was independent of the valproate dose or serum level (that is, it is maximal within the usual therapeutic dose range of valproate).[6-8] Another study has shown that the inhibition of lamotrigine clearance by valproate begins at very low valproate dosages (less than 125 mg daily), and is maximal at doses of about 500 mg daily.[9]

(b) Effects on valproate levels

In one study, 18 healthy subjects taking valproate 500 mg twice daily were also given lamotrigine 50, 100 or 150 mg daily. The lamotrigine caused a 25% decrease in valproate serum levels and a 25% increase in valproate oral clearance.[2] A study in 11 children taking valproate and other antiepileptics noted that no clinically important changes in valproate serum levels occurred when lamotrigine was added.[10] A retrospective analysis found that lamotrigine was associated with only a 7% reduction in valproate levels, which would not be expected to be clinically significant.[11]

(c) Toxic reactions

1. Tremor. In 3 patients severe and disabling tremor (sometimes preventing them from feeding themselves) occurred when they were given lamotrigine and sodium valproate. The problem resolved when the dosages were reduced.[12] In a study of 13 adult patients, all developed upper limb tremor when given lamotrigine with valproate, which could be minimised by reducing the dosage of either or both drugs.[13] Other studies have found similar effects.[7,14,15]

2. Rash. In a survey of adult epileptics who had lamotrigine added to their existing treatment, 33 were also taking valproate. Of these, 10 patients (30%) developed a rash, whereas only 6 of the 70 (8%) not taking valproate did so.[16] In another analysis of skin rash in patients taking lamotrigine, 11 of 12 patients with serious rash were also taking sodium valproate, and all but one had a lamotrigine starting dose that is higher than currently recommended.[17] However, in another study in which patients taking valproate were given lower initial doses of lamotrigine, there was no difference in incidence of rash in those taking lamotrigine and valproate, when compared with those taking lamotrigine and other antiepileptics (13% versus 14.2%).[18]

3. Other. Severe multiorgan dysfunction and disseminated intravascular coagulation was seen in 2 children when they took lamotrigine with valproate.[19] Three patients taking lamotrigine developed neurotoxicity (confusion, lethargy) after starting to take valproate (an intravenous bolus dose of valproic acid then oral therapy). Lamotrigine levels had risen by 2.9 to 6.9 times those before valproic acid.[14] Confusion, disorientation, visual disturbances and behavioural changes were reported in another patient 4 days after valproate was added to her treatment with lamotrigine. Lamotrigine levels were found to be 22.9 micrograms/mL (normal range 1 to 13 micrograms/mL). She recovered within 2 days of the discontinuation of both drugs.[20]
One study reported that the formation of hepatotoxic metabolites of valproate was unaffected by lamotrigine.[2]

Mechanism

Not fully understood. It is thought that valproate reduces lamotrigine glucuronidation by competitive inhibition, which results in a decreased lamotrigine clearance.[1,2,21] Raised lamotrigine levels have been implicated in the development of rash.[18,22] Increased valproate clearance may be due to enzyme induction. Tremor may be the result of a pharmacodynamic interaction.[7,13]

Importance and management

A well documented interaction. Concurrent use can be therapeutically valuable, but the lamotrigine dosage should be reduced by about half when valproate is added to avoid possible toxicity (sedation, tremor, ataxia, fatigue, rash).[2,7-9,12,18,23] In patients already taking valproate, the manufacturer of lamotrigine recommends a lamotrigine starting dose that is half that of lamotrigine monotherapy, irrespective of whether they are also receiving enzyme-inducing anticonvulsants, and a very gradual dose-escalation rate.[24] The outcome should be very well monitored. The CSM in the UK has suggested that the concurrent use of sodium valproate is one of the main risk factors for the development of serious skin reactions to lamotrigine, because it prolongs the half-life of lamotrigine.[22] Rashes are potentially serious and should be evaluated promptly.[18,24,25] The reports cited above[12,19] also suggest that sometimes other serious reactions (disabling tremor, multiorgan dysfunction) can occur.

1. Yuen AWC, Land G, Weatherley BC, Peck AW. Sodium valproate acutely inhibits lamotrigine metabolism. *Br J Clin Pharmacol* (1992) 33, 511–13.
2. Anderson GD, Yau MK, Gidal BE, Harris SJ, Levy RH, Lai AA, Wolf KB, Wargin WA, Dren AT. Bidirectional interaction of valproate and lamotrigine in healthy subjects. *Clin Pharmacol Ther* (1996) 60, 145–56.
3. May TW, Rambeck B, Jürgens U. Serum concentrations of lamotrigine in epileptic patients: the influence of dose and comedication. *Ther Drug Monit* (1996) 18, 523–31.
4. Armijo JA, Bravo J, Cuadrado A, Herranz JL. Lamotrigine serum concentration-to-dose ratio: influence of age and concomitant antiepileptic drugs and dosage implications. *Ther Drug Monit* (1999) 21, 182–190.
5. Böttiger Y, Svensson J-O, Ståhle L. Lamotrigine drug interactions in a TDM material. *Ther Drug Monit* (1999) 21, 171–4.
6. Gidal BE, Anderson GD, Rutecki PR, Shaw R, Lanning A. Lack of effect of valproate concentration on lamotrigine pharmacokinetics in developmentally disabled patients with epilepsy. *Epilepsy Res* (2000) 42, 23–31.
7. Kanner A, Frey M. Adding valproate to lamotrigine: a study of their pharmacokinetic interaction. *Neurology* (2000) 55, 588–91.
8. Decerce J, McJilton JS, Nadkarni MA, Ramsay RE. Lamotrigine-valproate interaction: relationship to the dose of valproate. *Epilepsia* (2000) 41(Suppl. 7), 220–1.
9. Gidal BE, Sheth R, Parnell J, Maloney K, Sale M. Evaluation of VPA dose and concentration effects on lamotrigine pharmacokinetics: implications for conversion to monotherapy. *Epilepsy Res* (2003) 57, 85–93.
10. Eriksson A-S, Hoppu K, Nergårdh A, Boreus L. Pharmacokinetic interactions between lamotrigine and other antiepileptic drugs in children with intractable epilepsy. *Epilepsia* (1996) 37, 769–73.
11. Mataringa M-I, May TW, Rambeck B. Does lamotrigine influence valproate concentrations? *Ther Drug Monit* (2002) 24, 631–6.
12. Reutens DC, Duncan JS, Patsalos PN. Disabling tremor after lamotrigine with sodium valproate. *Lancet* (1993) 342, 185–6.
13. Pisani F, Oteri G, Russo MF, Di Perri R, Perucca E, Richens A. The efficacy of valproate-lamotrigine comedication in refractory complex partial seizures: evidence for a pharmacodynamic interaction. *Epilepsia* (1999) 40, 1141–6.
14. Voudris K, Mastroyianni S, Skardoutsou A, Katsarou E, Mavrommatis P. Disabling tremor in epileptic children receiving sodium valproate after addition of lamotrigine. P2197. *Eur J Neurol* (2003) 10 (Suppl. 1), 180.
15. Burneo JG, Limdi N, Kuzniecky RI, Knowlton RC, Mendez M, Lawn N, Faught E, Welty TE, Prasad A. Neurotoxicity following addition of intravenous valproate to lamotrigine therapy. *Neurology* (2003) 60, 1991–2.
16. Li LM, Russo M, O'Donoghue MF, Duncan JS, Sander JWAS. Allergic skin rash and concomitant valproate therapy: evidence for an increased risk. *Arq Neuropsiquiatr* (1996) 54, 47–9.
17. Wong ICK, Mawer GE, Sander JWAS. Factors influencing the incidence of lamotrigine-related skin rash. *Ann Pharmacother* (1999) 33, 1037–42.
18. Faught E, Morris G, Jacobson M, French J, Harden C, Montouris G, Rosenfeld W. Adding lamotrigine to valproate: incidence of rash and other adverse effects. Postmarketing antiepileptic drug survey (PADS) Group. *Epilepsia* (1999) 40, 1135–40.
19. Chattergoon DS, McGuigan M, Koren G, Hwang P, Ito S. Multiorgan dysfunction and disseminated intravascular coagulation in children receiving lamotrigine and valproic acid. *Neurology* (1997) 49, 1442–4.
20. Mueller TH, Beeber AR. Delirium from valproic acid with lamotrigine. *Am J Psychiatry* (2004) 161, 1128–9.
21. Panayiotopoulos CP, Ferrie CD, Knott C, Robinson RO. Interaction of lamotrigine with sodium valproate. *Lancet* (1993) 341, 445.
22. Committee on the Safety of Medicines/Medicines Control Agency. *Current Problems* (1996) 22, 12.
23. Pisani F, Di Perri R, Perucca E, Richens A. Interaction of lamotrigine with sodium valproate. *Lancet* (1993) 341, 1224.
24. Lamictal (Lamotrigine). GlaxoSmithKline UK. UK Summary of product characteristics, March 2007.
25. Lamictal (Lamotrigine). GlaxoSmithKline. US Prescribing information, May 2007.

Levetiracetam + Food

The oral absorption of levetiracetam is not significantly affected by food.

Clinical evidence, mechanism, importance and management

In a study, 10 healthy subjects were given a 500-mg levetiracetam tablet with 120 mL of water or crushed and mixed with either 4 oz apple sauce or 120 mL of an enteral nutrition formulation (*Sustacal*). The overall rate and extent of absorption of oral levetiracetam were not significantly affected by crushing and mixing the tablet with either apple sauce or an enteral nutrition preparation, although the peak serum level of levetiracetam may be slightly reduced if it is mixed with enteral nutrition.[1]

1. Fay MA, Sheth RD, Gidal BE. Oral absorption kinetics of levetiracetam: the effect of mixing with food or enteral nutrition formulas. *Clin Ther* (2005) 27, 594–8.

Levetiracetam + Other antiepileptics

There is some evidence that the enzyme-inducing antiepileptics (carbamazepine, phenobarbital, phenytoin and primidone) may modestly reduce levetiracetam levels, but this is not thought to be clinically relevant. Levetiracetam does not usually alter the levels of these antiepileptics. However, some studies have found modestly raised phenytoin levels, and cases of possible carbamazepine toxicity have also been reported. There appears to be no pharmacokinetic interaction between levetiracetam and gabapentin, lamotrigine, or valproate.

Clinical evidence, mechanism, importance and management

(a) Carbamazepine

Evidence from clinical studies suggests that levetiracetam does not affect the serum levels of carbamazepine.[1-3] There is also some evidence that patients taking levetiracetam and also receiving enzyme-inducing antiepileptics such as carbamazepine had modestly (24%) lower levetiracetam levels than those also receiving antiepileptics not considered to be enzyme-inducers, but this was not considered clinically relevant, see (d) below.[4] Similarly, another retrospective analysis of patient data found that the serum levetiracetam level to dose ratio was modestly lower in patients also receiving carbamazepine than those receiving monotherapy (0.32 versus 0.52),[5] suggesting that carbamazepine moderately lowers levetiracetam levels. One report describes 4 patients who experienced disabling symptoms compatible with carbamazepine toxicity when levetiracetam was added. The symptoms resolved after a decrease in the carbamazepine dosage or withdrawal of the levetiracetam. A pharmacodynamic interaction was suggested, because levels of carbamazepine and its metabolite, carbamazepine-10,11-epoxide, were not affected.[6]

In general, there is no need to modify the dose of either carbamazepine or levetiracetam when used together. However, the report of possible toxicity suggests that some caution is warranted.

(b) Phenytoin

There is some evidence that patients taking levetiracetam with enzyme-inducing antiepileptics such as phenytoin had modestly (24%) lower levetiracetam levels than those taking other antiepileptics not considered to be enzyme inducers, but this was not considered clinically relevant, see (d) below.[4] Similarly, another retrospective analysis of patient data found that the serum levetiracetam level-to-dose ratio was modestly lower in patients also receiving phenytoin than those receiving monotherapy (0.32 versus 0.52),[5] suggesting that phenytoin modestly lowers levetiracetam levels.

However, evidence from clinical studies suggests that levetiracetam does not affect the serum levels of phenytoin.[1-3] Similarly, in another study, levetiracetam 1.5 g twice daily for 12 weeks had no effect on the steady-state pharmacokinetics of phenytoin in 6 subjects with epilepsy who were taking stable doses of phenytoin.[7] In one clinical study the addition of levetiracetam increased phenytoin levels by 27% to 52% in 4 patients. A further patient had a 75% increase in phenytoin levels [estimated from figure] and experienced signs of toxicity (sedation, ataxia) and required a reduction in his phenytoin dose. Another patient with raised phenytoin levels [estimated increase of 47%] had the dose of levetiracetam reduced.[8]

In general therefore, there is no need to modify the dose of either phenytoin or levetiracetam when they are used together. However, the report of raised phenytoin levels suggests that some caution is warranted.

(c) Valproate

There was no difference in the pharmacokinetics of a single 1.5-g dose of levetiracetam given to healthy subjects before or after sodium valproate 500 mg twice daily for 8 days. In addition, levetiracetam did not affect the pharmacokinetics of valproate.[9] In an analysis of clinical study data, the AUC of levetiracetam in 57 patients also taking valproic acid was slightly (11%) higher than in 28 patients also taking antiepileptics not thought to affect microsomal enzymes (gabapentin, lamotrigine, vigabatrin), but this was not thought to be clinically relevant.[4] In another retrospective analysis of patient data, the serum levetiracetam level-to-dose ratio was the same in patients also receiving valproic acid than those receiving monotherapy (0.53 versus 0.52),[5] suggesting that valproate does not alter levetiracetam levels. Furthermore, evidence from clinical studies suggests that levetiracetam does not affect the serum levels of valproate.[1,3] There appears to be no need to adjust the doses of either sodium valproate or levetiracetam if these drugs are used together.

(d) Other antiepileptics

The AUC of levetiracetam tended to be lower in 436 patients also taking enzyme-inducing antiepileptics (carbamazepine, phenobarbital, phenytoin, **primidone**) than in 28 patients also taking antiepileptics not thought to affect microsomal enzymes (**gabapentin**, **lamotrigine**, **vigabatrin**), but the difference was modest (24%).[4] Another retrospective analysis of patient data found that the serum levetiracetam level-to-dose ratio did not differ significantly between patients also taking **lamotrigine** and those taking levetiracetam alone (0.45 versus 0.52), but was modestly lower in those taking **oxcarbazepine** (0.34 versus 0.52).[5]

Furthermore, evidence from clinical studies suggests that levetiracetam does not affect the serum levels of **gabapentin**, **lamotrigine**, **phenobarbital**, or **primidone**.[1-3] In general therefore, no dosage adjustments would seem to be needed if levetiracetam is used as add-on therapy with any of these drugs.

1. Keppra (Levetiracetam). UCB Pharma Ltd. UK Summary of product characteristics, January 2007.
2. Patsalos PN. Pharmacokinetic profile of levetiracetam: towards ideal characteristics. *Pharmacol Ther* (2000) 85, 77–85.
3. Keppra (Levetiracetam). UCB Inc. US Prescribing information, March 2007.
4. Perucca E, Gidal BE, Baltès E. Effects of antiepileptic comedication on levetiracetam pharmacokinetics: a pooled analysis of data from randomized adjunctive therapy trials. *Epilepsy Res* (2003) 53, 47–56.
5. May TW, Rambeck B, Jürgens U. Serum concentrations of levetiracetam in epileptic patients: the influence of dose and co-medication. *Ther Drug Monit* (2003) 25, 690–9.
6. Sisodiya SM, Sander JWAS, Patsalos PN. Carbamazepine toxicity during combination therapy with levetiracetam: a pharmacodynamic interaction. *Epilepsy Res* (2002) 48, 217–19.
7. Browne TR, Szabo GK, Leppik IE, Josephs E, Paz J, Baltes E, Jensen CM. Absence of pharmacokinetic drug interaction of levetiracetam with phenytoin in patients with epilepsy determined by new technique. *J Clin Pharmacol* (2000) 40, 590–5.
8. Sharief MK, et al. Efficacy and tolerability study of ucb L059 in patients with refractory epilepsy. *J Epilepsy* (1996) 9, 106–12.
9. Coupez R, Nicolas J-M, Browne TR. Levetiracetam, a new antiepileptic agent: lack of in vitro and in vivo pharmacokinetic interaction with valproic acid. *Epilepsia* (2003) 44, 171–8.

Levetiracetam + Probenecid

Probenecid increased the plasma levels of an inactive metabolite of levetiracetam.

Clinical evidence, mechanism, importance and management

Probenecid 500 mg four times daily did not affect the renal excretion of levetiracetam. However, the renal excretion of its primary and pharmacologically inactive metabolite (ucb L057) was reduced by 61%, and plasma concentrations increased 2.5-fold,[1] although the manufacturer notes that these levels were still low.[2] The clinical relevance of elevated levels of ucb L057 is not known, therefore some have suggested caution is warranted.[1] The effect of levetiracetam on probenecid has not been studied.[2,3]

1. Patsalos PN. Pharmacokinetic profile of levetiracetam: toward ideal characteristics. *Pharmacol Ther* (2000) 85, 77–85.
2. Keppra (Levetiracetam). UCB Pharma Ltd. UK Summary of product characteristics, January 2007.
3. Keppra (Levetiracetam). UCB Inc. US Prescribing information, March 2007.

Mesuximide + Other antiepileptics

Phenobarbital, phenytoin, and possibly felbamate increase the levels of the active metabolite of mesuximide, *N*-desmethylmesuximide. Mesuximide increases the serum levels of phenobarbital and phenytoin, and decreases the levels of lamotrigine, and to a lesser extent, valproate.

Clinical evidence

(a) Felbamate

Three adolescent epileptic patients taking mesuximide developed mild adverse effects within 3 days of starting to take felbamate, which became more serious after one month (decreased appetite, nausea, weight loss, insomnia, dizziness, hiccups, slurred speech). During this time the levels of the active metabolite of mesuximide, *N*-desmethylmesuximide, rose by 26% and 46% in two patients, respectively. The adverse effects disappeared and *N*-desmethylmesuximide levels fell when the mesuximide dosage was reduced. Other antiepileptics being taken were carbamazepine, ethotoin and valproate.[1]

(b) Lamotrigine

In 6 patients taking mesuximide, lamotrigine levels were 53% lower (range 36 to 72%), when compared with lamotrigine levels before starting or after stopping mesuximide. In some patients deterioration in seizure control was seen while taking mesuximide, and an improvement in seizure control occurred after mesuximide was stopped.[2] In another study, lamotrigine levels were about 70% lower in 13 patients also taking mesuximide than in 64 patients taking lamotrigine alone, when corrected for dose. Note that in patients also taking valproate, the reduction in lamotrigine levels caused by mesuximide was compensated for by the increase caused by valproate, see also 'Lamotrigine + Valproate', p.542.[3]

(c) Phenobarbital or primidone

A study in hospitalised patients with petit mal epilepsy found that when mesuximide was given to 8 patients taking phenobarbital and 13 patients taking primidone, the mean serum levels of phenobarbital rose by 38% and 40%, respectively. Dose reductions were needed in 50% and 62% of patients, respectively. It was also found that the concurrent use of phenobarbital increased the serum levels of the active metabolite of mesuximide, *N*-desmethylmesuximide.[4]

(d) Phenytoin

Mesuximide was given to 17 patients taking phenytoin, which resulted in a 78% rise in the phenytoin serum levels requiring dose reductions in about 30% of the patients. It was also found that the concurrent use of phenytoin increased the serum levels of the active metabolite of mesuximide, *N*-desmethylmesuximide.[4]

(e) Valproate

A retrospective analysis of serum valproate levels was carried out in 17 patients who started and/or stopped taking mesuximide and whose concurrent medication remained unaltered. In the 14 patients starting mesuximide, a mean decrease in valproate levels of 32% was seen. In the 8 patients who stopped mesuximide a 30% increase in valproate levels occurred.[5] Note that the related drug, ethosuximide, has also been reported to lower valproate levels, see 'Ethosuximide + Other antiepileptics', p.539.

Mechanism

It has been suggested that phenobarbital, phenytoin and felbamate compete with mesuximide for the same metabolic mechanisms (hydroxylation) in the liver. As a result each one is metabolised more slowly and therefore their levels increase. Mesuximide appears to increase the clearance of valproate, and lamotrigine (which is principally via glucuronidation).

Importance and management

Information about these interactions is limited. Nevertheless, concurrent use should be monitored. Anticipate the need to reduce the dose of phenytoin, phenobarbital or primidone if mesuximide is given. The dose of lamotrigine may need to be increased if mesuximide is given. There is also some evidence that the dose of valproate may need to be increased.

The activity of mesuximide is thought to be due to its active metabolite, *N*-desmethylmesuximide. Therefore, it has been suggested that levels of this metabolite should also be monitored. Anticipate the need to reduce the dose of mesuximide if felbamate is added. Other antiepileptics such as phenobarbital and phenytoin may also increase levels of *N*-desmethylmesuximide.[4]

1. Patrias J, Espe-Lillo J, Ritter FJ. Felbamate-methsuximide interaction. *Epilepsia* (1992) 33 (Suppl 3) 84.
2. Besag FM, Berry DJ, Pool F. Methsuximide lowers lamotrigine blood levels: a pharmacokinetic antiepileptic drug interaction. *Epilepsia* (2000) 41, 624–7.
3. May TW, Rambeck B, Jürgens U. Influence of oxcarbazepine and methsuximide on lamotrigine concentrations in epileptic patients with and without valproic acid comedication: results of a retrospective study. *Ther Drug Monit* (1999) 21, 175–81.
4. Rambeck B. Pharmacological interactions of mesuximide with phenobarbital and phenytoin in hospitalized epileptic patients. *Epilepsia* (1979) 20, 147–56.
5. Besag FMC, Berry DJ, Vasey M. Methsuximide reduces valproic acid serum levels. *Ther Drug Monit* (2001) 23, 694–7.

Oxcarbazepine + Erythromycin

Erythromycin does not appear to affect the pharmacokinetics of oxcarbazepine.

Clinical evidence, mechanism, importance and management

In a study in 8 healthy subjects the pharmacokinetics of a single 600-mg dose of oxcarbazepine was unaffected by erythromycin 500 mg twice daily for 7 days.[1] Erythromycin appears not to interact with oxcarbazepine, and no special precautions therefore seem to be required during concurrent use.

1. Keränen T, Jolkkonen J, Jensen PK, Menge GP, Andersson P. Absence of interaction between oxcarbazepine and erythromycin. *Acta Neurol Scand* (1992) 86, 120–3.

Oxcarbazepine + Felbamate

Felbamate has no clinically relevant effect on the pharmacokinetics of oxcarbazepine, but concurrent use appears to increase the incidence of adverse effects.

Clinical evidence, mechanism, importance and management

A double-blind, randomised study in 8 healthy subjects found that oxcarbazepine 300 to 600 mg every 12 hours, given with felbamate 600 to 1200 mg every 12 hours for 10 days had no effect on the plasma levels of the major active metabolite of oxcarbazepine (monohydroxyoxcarbazepine). However, the levels of dihydroxyoxcarbazepine (a minor, inactive metabolite) were reduced, and the maximum serum levels of oxcarbazepine were reduced, by about 20%. Although these changes were considered to be clinically irrelevant, the incidence of some adverse effects (dizziness, somnolence, nausea, diplopia) rose during concurrent use.[1]

1. Hulsman JARJ, Rentmeester TW, Banfield CR, Reidenberg P, Colucci RD, Meehan JW, Radwanski E, Mojaverian P, Lin C-C, Nezamis J, Affrime MB, Glue P. Effects of felbamate on the pharmacokinetics of the monohydroxy and dihydroxy metabolites of oxcarbazepine. *Clin Pharmacol Ther* (1995) 58, 383–9.

Oxcarbazepine + Other antiepileptics

Oxcarbazepine appears not to affect the pharmacokinetics of carbamazepine, phenobarbital or valproate to a clinically relevant extent, but may modestly reduce lamotrigine levels. High doses of oxcarbazepine increase phenytoin levels, and a reduction in the phenytoin dose may be required. Phenytoin and phenobarbital can increase the loss of the active metabolite of oxcarbazepine, monohydroxyoxcarbazepine, although this is probably not clinically relevant. Lamotrigine may increase levels of monohydroxyoxcarbazepine, although one study found no pharmacokinetic interaction.

Clinical evidence

(a) Effects of oxcarbazepine on other antiepileptics

A double-blind, crossover comparison of oxcarbazepine and **carbamazepine** in 42 epileptic patients found that when **carbamazepine** was replaced by oxcarbazepine, the serum levels of **valproate** rose by 32%, and the serum levels of **phenytoin** rose by 23%. In patients taking both **valproate** and **phenytoin** together, oxcarbazepine caused a rise in the serum levels of 21% and 25% respectively. The study extended over 12 weeks to establish steady-state levels.[1] Another study in 4 young epileptic patients (aged 13 to 17) found that the level to dose ratio of free **valproate** rose when switched from concurrent **carbamazepine** to oxcarbazepine, with an increase in valproate adverse effects, which resolved when the valproate dose was decreased.[2]

A later study in 35 epileptic patients found that when oxcarbazepine 300 mg three times daily was added to treatment with **carbamazepine, sodium valproate** or **phenytoin** for 3 weeks there were no clinically relevant changes in the pharmacokinetics of any of these anticonvulsants.[3] However, analysis of data from clinical studies found that oxcarbazepine decreased **carbamazepine** levels by about 15 to 22%, increased **phenobarbital** levels by about 14%, and at high doses increased **phenytoin** levels by up to 40%.[4,5] In another analysis, **lamotrigine** levels were about 34% lower in 14 patients also taking oxcarbazepine than in 64 patients taking **lamotrigine** alone, when corrected for dose. In this study, the effect of oxcarbazepine was less than that of **carbamazepine** (34% versus 47%).[6] Similarly, in another analysis, the addition of oxcarbazepine to **lamotrigine** reduced **lamotrigine** levels by 15 to 75%.[7] However in contrast to these findings, one study in healthy subjects found that oxcarbazepine had no effect on the pharmacokinetics of **lamotrigine**, although adverse effects were reported to be more frequent and severe during concurrent treatment.[8]

(b) Effects of other antiepileptics on oxcarbazepine

The AUCs of oxcarbazepine and its active metabolite (monohydroxyoxcarbazepine) were reduced by **phenobarbital**, by 43% and 25%, respectively. There were no other significant effects on the pharmacokinetics of oxcarbazepine.[9] Another study found that **phenytoin** caused a 29% reduction in the AUC of monohydroxyoxcarbazepine.[3] Another study found that the serum levels of monohydroxyoxcarbazepine were not affected by **phenobarbital** or **phenytoin** but its further conversion to dihydroxyoxcarbazepine was increased.[10] Since the conversion to dihydroxyoxcarbazepine is a minor step in the metabolism of monohydroxyoxcarbazepine, the overall antiepileptic action of oxcarbazepine is unlikely to be altered. Correspondingly, a study found that **phenytoin** 100 to 375 mg daily increased the clearance of the active metabolite, monohydroxyoxcarbazepine by almost 40%.[11] The AUC of monohydroxyoxcarbazepine was also 40% lower in the presence of **carbamazepine.**[3] Similarly, **carbamazepine**, **phenobarbital**, and **phenytoin** were found to increase the apparent clearance of monohydroxyoxcarbazepine by 31 to 35% in a study in children.[12]

A retrospective analysis found that monohydroxyoxcarbazepine levels to oxcarbazepine dose ratios were higher in 7 patients also taking **lamotrigine** than in those taking oxcarbazepine alone,[13] suggesting that lamotrigine decreased oxcarbazepine metabolism. However in contrast to these findings, one study in healthy subjects found that **lamotrigine** had no effect on the pharmacokinetics of oxcarbazepine or monohydroxyoxcarbazepine although adverse effects were reported to be more frequent and more severe during concurrent treatment.[8]

Mechanism

Unlike carbamazepine, oxcarbazepine appears not to have marked enzyme-inducing properties so that it would not be expected to have as great an effect on the metabolism of other antiepileptics. However, oxcarbazepine does appear to act as an inhibitor of the cytochrome P450 isoenzyme CYP2C19 at high concentrations and therefore may raise phenytoin levels (see 'Phenytoin + Carbamazepine', p.554, for more on this mechanism). Other antiepileptics can increase the metabolism of the active metabolite of oxcarbazepine, monohydroxyoxcarbazepine. The situation with lamotrigine is not clear. In one study lamotrigine appeared to decrease the metabolism of oxcarbazepine but another study found no pharmacokinetic interaction.

Importance and management

Information about the concurrent use of oxcarbazepine and other antiepileptics is limited, but growing. The overall picture seems to be that, oxcarbazepine is a less potent enzyme inducer than carbamazepine, and therefore it does not markedly affect the serum levels of other antiepileptics. If oxcarbazepine is substituted for carbamazepine, be aware that drug levels of some other antiepileptics may rise. High oxcarbazepine doses may increase phenytoin levels, and the manufacturer notes that a decrease in the phenytoin dose may be required.[4] The clinical relevance of the modest reductions in lamotrigine levels is uncertain. For mention of modestly reduced levetiracetam levels, see 'Levetiracetam + Other antiepileptics', p.543.

Any changes in the pharmacokinetics of oxcarbazepine brought about by other antiepileptics seem to be of minimal clinical relevance. However, the clinical relevance of the increase in the active metabolite monohydroxyoxcarbazepine with lamotrigine requires further study. In addition, there is the theoretical risk that monohydroxyoxcarbazepine levels might rise to toxic levels if carbamazepine or phenytoin were withdrawn.[3] For mention that there may be an increase in adverse effects if oxcarbazepine is used with felbamate, see 'Oxcarbazepine + Felbamate', p.545.

1. Houtkooper MA, Lammertsma A, Meyer JWA, Goedhart DM, Meinardi H, van Oorschot CAEH, Blom GF, Höppener RJEA, Hulsman JARJ. Oxcarbazepine (GP 47.680): a possible alternative to carbamazepine? *Epilepsia* (1987) 28, 693–8.
2. Battino D, Croci D, Granata T, Bernadi G, Monza G. Changes in unbound and total valproic acid concentrations after replacement of carbamazepine with oxcarbazepine. *Ther Drug Monit* (1992) 14, 376–9.
3. McKee PJW, Blacklaw J, Forrest G, Gillham RA, Walker SM, Connelly D, Brodie MJ. A double blind, placebo-controlled interaction study between oxcarbazepine and carbamazepine, sodium valproate and phenytoin in epileptic patients. *Br J Clin Pharmacol* (1994) 37, 27–32.
4. Trileptal (Oxcarbazepine). Novartis Pharmaceuticals UK Ltd. UK Summary of product characteristics. October 2005.
5. Hossain M, Sallas W, D'Souza J. Drug-drug interaction profile of oxcarbazepine in children and adults. *Neurology* (1999) 52 (Suppl 2), A525.
6. May TW, Rambeck B, Jürgens U. Influence of oxcarbazepine and methsuximide on lamotrigine concentrations in epileptic patients with and without valproic acid comedication: results of a retrospective study. *Ther Drug Monit* (1999) 21, 175–81.
7. Krämer G, Dorn T, Etter H. Oxcarbazepine: clinically relevant drug interaction with lamotrigine. *Epilepsia* (2003) 44 (Suppl 9), 95–6.
8. Theis JGW, Sidhu J, Palmer J, Job S, Bullman J, Ascher J. Lack of pharmacokinetic interaction between oxcarbazepine and lamotrigine. *Neuropsychopharmacology* (2005) 30, 2269–74.
9. Tartara A, Galimberti CA, Manni R, Morini R, Limido G, Gatti G, Bartoli A, Strad G, Perucca E. The pharmacokinetics of oxcarbazepine and its active metabolite 10-hydroxy-carbazepine in healthy subjects and in epileptic patients taking phenobarbitone or valproic acid. *Br J Clin Pharmacol* (1993) 36, 366–8.
10. Kumps A, Wurth C. Oxcarbazepine disposition: preliminary observations in patients. *Biopharm Drug Dispos* (1990) 11, 365–70.
11. Arnoldussen W, Hulsman J, Rentmeester T. Interaction between oxcarbazepine and phenytoin. *Epilepsia* (1993) 34 (Suppl 6), 37.
12. Sallas WM, Milosavljev S, D'Souza J, Hossain M. Pharmacokinetic drug interactions in children taking oxcarbazepine. *Clin Pharmacol Ther* (2003) 74, 138–49.
13. Guénault N, Odou P, Robert H. Increase in dihydroxycarbamazepine serum levels in patients co-medicated with oxcarbazepine and lamotrigine. *Eur J Clin Pharmacol* (2003) 59, 781–2.

Paraldehyde + Disulfiram

***Animal* data suggest that disulfiram can increase paraldehyde levels and prolong its effects. There is a theoretical potential for a disulfiram reaction.**

Clinical evidence, mechanism, importance and management

It is thought that paraldehyde is depolymerised in the liver to acetaldehyde, and then oxidised by acetaldehyde dehydrogenase.[1] Since disulfiram inhibits this enzyme, concurrent use would be expected to result in the accumulation of acetaldehyde and result in a modified disulfiram reaction.[2] However, studies in *animals* given disulfiram and paraldehyde found increases in paraldehyde levels and hypnotic effect, with only small increases in acetaldehyde and no increase in toxicity.[2,3] In addition, there appear to be no reports of a disulfiram reaction involving paraldehyde in humans. Three cases of mental confusion have been reported in patients receiving disulfiram and paraldehyde.[4] Note that, patients with liver disease are at greater risk of adverse effects of paraldehyde, and the addition of disulfiram results in a further risk. Therefore it may be prudent to avoid concurrent use.

1. Hitchcock P, Nelson EE. The metabolism of paraldehyde: II. *J Pharmacol Exp Ther* (1943) 79, 286–94.
2. Keplinger ML, Wells JA. Effect of Antabuse on the action of paraldehyde in mice and dogs. *Fedn Proc* (1956) 15, 445–6.
3. Keplinger ML, Wells JA. The effect of disulfiram on the action and metabolism of paraldehyde. *J Pharmacol Exp Ther* (1957), 119: 19–25.
4. Christie GL. Three cases of transient confusional psychosis in patients receiving con-current antabuse and paraldehyde therapy. *Med J Aust* (1956) May 12: 789–91.

Phenobarbital or Primidone + Allopurinol

Allopurinol appears not to alter phenobarbital levels, including those derived from primidone.

Clinical evidence, mechanism, importance and management

In a study of add-on therapy, allopurinol (150 mg daily in those less than 20 kg, and 300 mg daily for other patients) for 4 months, had no effect on phenobarbital levels in 46 patients taking antiepileptics including phenobarbital.[1] In another similar study, allopurinol 10 mg/kg increased to 15 mg/kg daily for 12 weeks had no effect on serum phenobarbital levels in 11 patients taking primidone or phenobarbital with or without other antiepileptics.[2] Therefore phenobarbital or primidone dosage alterations are unlikely to be required if allopurinol is used.

1. Zagnoni PG, Bianchi A, Zolo P, Canger R, Cornaggia C, D'Alessandro P, DeMarco P, Pisani F, Gianelli M, Verzé L, Viani F, Zaccara G. Allopurinol as add-on therapy in refractory epilepsy: a double-blind placebo-controlled randomized study. *Epilepsia* (1994) 35, 107–12.
2. Coppola G, Pascotto A. Double-blind, placebo-controlled, cross-over trial of allopurinol as add-on therapy in childhood refractory epilepsy. *Brain Dev* (1996) 18, 50–2.

Phenobarbital + Azoles

Limited evidence suggests phenobarbital causes a marked decrease in itraconazole levels, and might decrease ketoconazole levels. Phenobarbital is also predicted to decrease posaconazole levels and markedly decrease voriconazole levels.

Clinical evidence, mechanism, importance and management

(a) Itraconazole

The serum levels of itraconazole 200 mg daily were very low (0.01 to 0.03 mg/L, therapeutic range 0.25 to 2 mg/L) in a patient taking **phenobarbital**. Two months after stopping the **phenobarbital** they were higher (0.15 mg/L), but still below the therapeutic range, apparently because carbamazepine had been recently started.[1] For mention of two other patients who had very low itraconazole levels while taking both phenytoin and phenobarbital, see 'Phenytoin + Azoles', p.552. Some makers of itraconazole say that concurrent use of potent enzyme inducers such as phenobarbital is not recommended.[2,3]

(b) Ketoconazole

Low ketoconazole levels in a patient with leukaemia receiving various antineoplastics was attributed to the concurrent use of phenytoin and phenobarbital therapy.[4] It may be prudent to monitor the effects of ketoconazole if phenobarbital is also given.

(c) Posaconazole

Based on the evidence with 'phenytoin', (p.552), the manufacturer of posaconazole predicts that phenobarbital will reduce posaconazole levels, and therefore suggests avoiding the combination unless the benefits outweigh the risks.[5] If concurrent use is necessary monitor for posaconazole efficacy.

(d) Voriconazole

Based on the evidence with 'phenytoin', (p.552), the manufacturer of voriconazole predicts that phenobarbital will reduce voriconazole levels, and therefore contraindicates their concurrent use.[6,7] In the US the manufacturer extends this contraindication to all long-acting barbiturates.[7]

1. Bonay M, Jonville-Bera AP, Diot P, Lemarie E, Lavandier M, Autret E. Possible interaction between phenobarbital, carbamazepine and itraconazole. *Drug Safety* (1993) 9, 309–11.
2. Sporanox Capsules (Itraconazole). Janssen-Cilag Ltd. UK Summary of product characteristics, March 2004.
3. Sporanox Capsules (Itraconazole). Janssen. US Prescribing information, June 2006.
4. Stockley RJ, Daneshmend TK, Bredow MT, Warnock DW, Richardson MD, Slade RR. Ketoconazole pharmacokinetics during chronic dosing in adults with haematological malignancy. *Eur J Clin Microbiol* (1986) 5, 513–17.
5. Noxafil (Posaconazole). Schering-Plough Ltd. UK Summary of product characteristics, October 2006.
6. VFEND (Voriconazole). Pfizer Ltd. UK Summary of product characteristics, July 2007.
7. VFEND (Voriconazole). Pfizer Inc. US Prescribing information, November 2006.

Phenobarbital + Dextropropoxyphene (Propoxyphene)

An average 20% rise was seen in the serum phenobarbital levels of 4 epileptic patients after they took dextropropoxyphene 65 mg three times a day for a week.[1] This rise is unlikely to be clinically significant in most patients.

1. Hansen BS, Dam M, Brandt J, Hvidberg EF, Angelo H, Christensen JM, Lous P. Influence of dextropropoxyphene on steady state serum levels and protein binding of three anti-epileptic drugs in man. *Acta Neurol Scand* (1980) 61, 357–67.

Phenobarbital or Primidone + Felbamate

Felbamate causes a moderate increase in plasma phenobarbital levels (including those derived from primidone), which has resulted in phenobarbital toxicity.

Clinical evidence

When 24 healthy subjects taking phenobarbital 100 mg daily were also given felbamate 1.2 g twice daily for 10 days, the AUC and the maximum plasma levels of phenobarbital were raised by 22% and 24%, respectively. Concurrent use was said to be safe and well tolerated.[1] A 30% increase in phenobarbital plasma concentrations was seen in another 19 patients taking phenobarbital or primidone (which is metabolised to phenobarbital) when given felbamate (average dose 2458 mg daily).[2] A phenobarbital dosage reduction of about 30% was needed in another 6 patients when they started to take felbamate.[3] A man taking sodium valproate and phenobarbital had an almost 50% increase in phenobarbital serum levels over a 5-week period after felbamate 50 mg/kg was added, despite an initial phenobarbital dosage reduction from 230 mg to 200 mg daily. He was hospitalised because of increased lethargy, anorexia and ataxia and was eventually discharged on a phenobarbital dosage of 150 mg daily.[4]

It was noted that felbamate levels were lower in patients taking phenobarbital than in historical control patients who were not taking phenobarbital.[1] However, in a modelling study, phenobarbital apparently had little or no effect on the pharmacokinetics of felbamate.[5]

Mechanism

Not established. It seems possible that the felbamate may inhibit more than one pathway in the metabolism of the phenobarbital, resulting in a reduction in its loss from the body. The cytochrome P450 isoenzyme CYP2C19 may be involved.[1,6]

Importance and management

An established interaction. If felbamate is added to established treatment with phenobarbital or primidone, particularly in patients already taking substantial doses, monitor well for any evidence of increased adverse effects (drowsiness, lethargy, anorexia, ataxia) and reduce the dosages of the phenobarbital or primidone if necessary.

1. Reidenberg P, Glue P, Banfield CR, Colucci RD, Meehan JW, Radwanski E, Mojavarian P, Lin C-C, Nezamis J, Guillaume M, Affime MB. Effects of felbamate on the pharmacokinetics of phenobarbital. *Clin Pharmacol Ther* (1995) 58, 279–87.
2. Kerrick JM, Wolff DL, Risinger MW, Graves NM. Increased phenobarbital plasma concentrations after felbamate initiation. *Epilepsia* (1994) 35 (Suppl 8), 96.
3. Sachdeo RC, Padela MF. The effect of felbamate on phenobarbital serum concentrations. *Epilepsia* (1994) 35 (Suppl 8), 94.
4. Gidal BE, Zupanc ML. Potential pharmacokinetic interaction between felbamate and phenobarbital. *Ann Pharmacother* (1994) 28, 455–8.
5. Kelley MT, Walson PD, Cox S, Dusci LJ. Population pharmacokinetics of felbamate in children. *Ther Drug Monit* (1997) 19, 29–36.
6. Glue P, Banfield CR, Perhach JL, Mather GG, Racha JK, Levy RH. Pharmacokinetic interactions with felbamate. *Clin Pharmacokinet* (1997) 33, 214–24.

Phenobarbital + Influenza vaccines

Influenza vaccine can cause a moderate rise in serum phenobarbital levels.

Clinical evidence, mechanism, importance and management

Serum phenobarbital levels rose by about 30% in 11 out of 27 children when given 0.5 mL of a whole virus influenza vaccine USP, types A and B, (Squibb). Levels remained elevated 28 days after vaccination.[1]

It was suggested that the vaccine inhibits the liver enzymes concerned with the metabolism of phenobarbital, thereby reducing its loss from the body. Information is very limited. Note that, a similar 30% increase in phenobarbital levels with felbamate has eventually required a dosage adjustment; however with this interaction the increase will eventually be self-limiting. Therefore it seems unlikely that this moderate increase in phenobarbital levels will be of clinical significance..

1. Jann MW, Fidone GS. Effect of influenza vaccine on serum anticonvulsant concentrations. *Clin Pharm* (1986) 5, 817–20.

Phenobarbital + Troleandomycin

Troleandomycin caused a modest fall in the plasma phenobarbital levels of one patient.

Clinical evidence, mechanism, importance and management

A patient phenobarbital and carbamazepine had a modest fall in plasma phenobarbital levels from about 40 to 31 micrograms/mL, and a rise in carbamazepine levels, when given troleandomycin.[1] The general importance of this single report is uncertain, but this modest is probably of limited clinical importance. For a discussion of the rise in carbamazepine levels with troleandomycin, see 'Carbamazepine + Macrolides', p.531.

1. Dravet C, Mesdjian E, Cenraud B and Roger J. Interaction between carbamazepine and triacetyloleandomycin. *Lancet* (1977) i, 810–11.

Phenobarbital + Valproate

Serum phenobarbital levels can be increased by valproate, which may result in excessive sedation and lethargy. Small reductions in valproate levels have also been reported. Combined use of phenobarbital and valproate may cause an increase in serum liver enzymes.

Clinical evidence

A 6-month study in 11 epileptic patients taking phenobarbital 90 to 400 mg daily found that when they were also given valproic acid 11.2 to 42.7 mg/kg daily sedation developed. On average the dosage of phenobarbital was reduced to 54% of the original dose with continued good seizure control. Another 2 patients who did not have their phenobarbital dose reduced had an increase in their phenobarbital levels of 12% and 48%, respectively, when valproic acid was added.[1]

Another study found that sodium valproate 1.2 g daily raised serum phenobarbital levels in 20 patients by an average of 27%. Signs of toxicity occurred in 13 patients, but the dose only needed to be reduced in 3 patients.[2] This interaction has been described in numerous other reports, and dose reductions of the phenobarbital were almost always necessary to avoid excessive drowsiness.[3-17] In one study the rise in phenobarbital levels was much greater in children (over 100%) than in adults (about 50%).[18]

A reduction in sodium valproate levels of about 25% has also been reported, but the effect on seizure control was not mentioned.[19] A reduction in valproate levels caused by phenobarbital has also been reported elsewhere.[20]

The incidence of increased liver enzyme activity was found to be higher in 41 patients receiving phenobarbital with valproate than in 40 patients taking valproate alone (ALT 7.3% versus 0%). When phenytoin was also given an even greater incidence of increases (ALT 26.1% and AST 28.3% versus about 20%) occurred. However, the increases were mild and were not considered clinically important.[21]

Mechanism

The evidence indicates that valproate inhibits three steps in the metabolism of phenobarbital by the liver, leading to its accumulation in the body. The inhibited steps are the formation of *p*-hydroxyphenobarbital by the cytochrome P450 isoenzyme CYP2C9,[22] the *N*-glucosidation of phenobarbital[23] and the *O*-glucuronidation of *p*-hydroxyphenobarbital.[23]

Importance and management

An extremely well documented and well established interaction of clinical importance. The incidence seems to be high. The effects of concurrent use should be well monitored and suitable phenobarbital dosage reductions made as necessary to avoid toxicity. The dosage may need to be reduced by a third to a half.[1] The significance of the modest reduction in valproate levels is not clear, especially as valproate levels do not correlate well with efficacy of treatment. Valproate has been associated with serious hepatotoxicity, especially in children aged less than 3 years, and this has been more common in those receiving other anticonvulsants. Valproate monotherapy is to be preferred in this group.

1. Wilder BJ, Willmore LJ, Bruni J, Villarreal HJ. Valproic acid: interaction with other anticonvulsant drugs. *Neurology* (1978) 28, 892–6.
2. Richens A, Ahmad S. Controlled trial of sodium valproate in severe epilepsy. *BMJ* (1975) 4, 255–6.
3. Schobben F, van der Kleijn E and Gabreëls FJM. Pharmacokinetics of di-n-propylacetate in epileptic patients. *Eur J Clin Pharmacol* (1975) 8, 97–105.
4. Gram L, Wulff K, Rasmussen KE, Flachs H, Würtz-Jørgensen A, Sommerbeck KW, Løhren V. Valproate sodium: a controlled clinical trial including monitoring of drug levels. *Epilepsia* (1977) 18, 141–8.
5. Jeavons PM, Clark JE. Sodium valproate in treatment of epilepsy. *BMJ* (1974) 2, 584–6.
6. Völzke E, Doose H. Dipropylacetate (Dépakine®, Ergenyl®) in the treatment of epilepsy. *Epilepsia* (1973) 14, 185–93.
7. Millet Y, Sainty JM, Galland MC, Sidoine R, Jouglard J. Problèmes posés par l'association thérapeutique phénobarbital-dipropylacétate de sodium. A propos d'un cas. *Eur J Toxicol Environ Hyg* (1976) 9, 381–3.
8. Jeavons PM, Clark JE, Maheshwari MC. Treatment of generalized epilepsies of childhood and adolescence with sodium valproate ('Epilim'). *Dev Med Child Neurol* (1977) 19, 9–25.
9. Vakil SD, Critchley EMR, Phillips JC, Fahim Y, Haydock C, Cocks A, Dyer T. The effect of sodium valproate (Epilim) on phenytoin and phenobarbitone blood levels. Clinical and Pharmacological Aspects of Sodium Valproate (Epilim) in the Treatment of Epilepsy. Proceedings of a Symposium held at Nottingham University, September 1975, 75–7.
10. Scott DF, Boxer CM, Herzberg JL. A study of the hypnotic effects of Epilim and its possible interaction with phenobarbitone. Clinical and Pharmacological Aspects of Sodium Valproate (Epilim) in the Treatment of Epilepsy. Proceedings of a Symposium held at Nottingham University, September 1975, 155–7.
11. Richens A, Scoular IT, Ahmad S, Jordan BJ. Pharmacokinetics and efficacy of Epilim in patients receiving long-term therapy with other antiepileptic drugs. Clinical and Pharmacological Aspects of Sodium Valproate (Epilim) in the Treatment of Epilepsy. Proceedings of a Symposium held at Nottingham University, September 1975, 78–88.
12. Loiseau P, Orgogozo JM, Brachet-Liermain A, Morselli PL. Pharmacokinetic studies on the interaction between phenobarbital and valproic acid. In Adv Epileptol Proc Cong Int League Epilepsy 13th. Edited by Meinardi H and Rowan A. (1977/8) p 261–5.
13. Fowler GW. Effect of dipropylacetate on serum levels of anticonvulsants in children. *Proc West Pharmacol Soc* (1978) 21, 37–40.
14. Patel IH, Levy RH, Cutler RE. Phenobarbital-valproic acid interaction. *Clin Pharmacol Ther* (1980) 27, 515–21.
15. Coulter DL, Wu H, Allen RJ. Valproic acid therapy in childhood epilepsy. *JAMA* (1980) 244, 785–8.
16. Kapetanovic IM, Kupferberg HJ, Porter RJ, Theodore W, Schulman E, Penry JK. Mechanism of valproate-phenobarbital interaction in epileptic patients. *Clin Pharmacol Ther* (1981) 29, 480–6.
17. Yukara E, To H, Ohdo S, Higuchi S, Aoyama T. Detection of a drug-drug interaction on population based phenobarbitone clearance using nonlinear mixed-effects modeling. *Eur J Clin Pharmacol* (1998) 54, 69–74.
18. Fernandez de Gatta MR, Alonso Gonzalez AC, Garcia Sanchez MJ, Dominguez-Gil Hurle A, Santos Borbujo J, Monzon Corral L. Effect of sodium valproate on phenobarbital serum levels in children and adults. *Ther Drug Monit* (1986) 8, 416–20.
19. May T, Rambeck B. Serum concentrations of valproic acid: influence of dose and comedication. *Ther Drug Monit* (1985) 7, 387–90.
20. Meinardi H, Bongers E. Analytical data in connection with the clinical use of di-n-propylacetate. In: Schneider H, (ed). Clinical Pharmacology of Antiepileptic Drugs. New York and Berlin: Springer-Verlag; 1975 pp. 235–41.
21. Haidukewych D, John G. Chronic valproic acid and coantiepileptic drug therapy and incidence of increases in serum liver enzymes. *Ther Drug Monit* (1986) 8, 407–410.
22. Hurst SI, Hargreaves JA, Howald WN, Racha JK, Mather GG, Labroo R, Carlson SP, Levy RH. Enzymatic mechanism for the phenobarbital-valproate interaction. *Epilepsia* (1997) 38 (Suppl 8), 111–12.
23. Bernus I, Dickinson RG, Hooper WD, Eadie MJ. Inhibition of phenobarbitone *N*-glucosidation by valproate. *Br J Clin Pharmacol* (1994) 38, 411–16.

Phenytoin + Allopurinol

A case report describes phenytoin toxicity in a boy given allopurinol. Another study found raised phenytoin levels in 2 of 18 patients given allopurinol.

Clinical evidence, mechanism, importance and management

A 13-year-old boy with Lesch-Nyhan syndrome who was taking phenobarbital, clonazepam, valproic acid and phenytoin 200 mg daily became somnolent within 7 days of starting to take allopurinol 150 mg daily. His serum phenytoin levels were found to have increased from 7.5 to 20.8 micrograms/mL.[1] In another study, 2 patients had a marked increase in phenytoin levels when given allopurinol (150 mg daily in those less than 20 kg, and 300 mg daily for other patients) for 4 months, which in one case led to withdrawal from the study, and in the other to a phenytoin dosage reduction. However, 16 other patients had no change in phenytoin levels while taking this dose of allopurinol.[2]

The reason for this reaction is not known. An *animal* study confirmed that 50 mg/kg, but not 20 mg/kg, of allopurinol reduced phenytoin elimination, but was unable to work out the mechanism.[3]

Although information is limited, it appears that allopurinol may raise phenytoin levels in some patients. It would therefore be prudent to monitor for phenytoin toxicity (e.g. blurred vision, nystagmus, ataxia or drowsiness) when allopurinol is added.

1. Yokochi K, Yokochi A, Chiba K, Ishizaki T. Phenytoin-allopurinol interaction: Michaelis-Menten kinetic parameters of phenytoin with and without allopurinol in a child with Lesch-Nyhan syndrome. *Ther Drug Monit* (1982) 4, 353–7.
2. Zagnoni PG, Bianchi A, Zolo P, Canger R, Cornaggia C, D'Alessandro P, DeMarco P, Pisani F, Gianelli M, Verzé L, Viani F, Zaccara G. Allopurinol as add-on therapy in refractory epilepsy: a double-blind placebo-controlled randomized study. *Epilepsia* (1994) 35, 107–12.
3. Ogiso T, Ito Y, Iwaki M, Tsunekawa K. Drug interaction between phenytoin and allopurinol. *J Pharmacobiodyn* (1990) 13, 36–43.

Phenytoin + Amiodarone

Serum phenytoin levels can be raised by amiodarone, markedly so in some individuals, and phenytoin toxicity may occur. Amiodarone serum levels are reduced by phenytoin.

Clinical evidence

(a) Phenytoin serum levels increased

Three patients had a marked rise in serum phenytoin levels 10 days to 4 weeks after being given amiodarone 400 mg to 1.2 g daily. One of them developed phenytoin toxicity (ataxia, lethargy, vertigo) within 4 weeks of starting to take amiodarone and had a serum phenytoin level of 40 micrograms/mL, representing a three to fourfold rise. Levels restabilised when the phenytoin dosage was withheld and then reduced from 300 to 200 mg daily. The serum phenytoin levels of the other 2 patients were approximately doubled by the amiodarone.[1]

A study in healthy subjects found that amiodarone 200 mg daily for 3 weeks increased the AUC of a single 5-mg/kg intravenous dose of phenytoin by 40%.[2] Another pharmacokinetic study found that amiodarone 200 mg daily for 6 weeks raised the AUC and steady-state peak serum levels of phenytoin by 40% and 33%, respectively. Phenytoin 2 to 4 mg/kg daily was given orally for 14 days before and during the last 2 weeks of amiodarone therapy.[3] Other case reports describe 3 patients who had two to threefold rises in serum phenytoin levels, and toxicity, 2 to 6 weeks after starting amiodarone.[4-6]

(b) Amiodarone serum levels reduced

A study in 5 healthy subjects given amiodarone 200 mg daily found that over a 5-week period the serum amiodarone levels gradually increased. When phenytoin 3 to 4 mg/kg daily was added for a period of 2 weeks, the serum amiodarone levels fell to concentrations that were between about 50 and 65% of those predicted.[7]

Mechanism

Uncertain. It seems possible that amiodarone inhibits the liver enzymes concerned with the metabolism of phenytoin, resulting in a rise in its serum levels.[3] It seems unlikely that drug displacement from protein binding sites had a part to play as free and bound levels of phenytoin remained constant.[3]

Phenytoin is an enzyme-inducing drug that possibly increases the metabolism of the amiodarone by the liver.

Importance and management

Information seems to be limited to the reports cited, but both interactions appear to be clinically important. Concurrent use should not be undertaken unless the effects can be well monitored.

The phenytoin dosage should be reduced as necessary. A 25 to 30% reduction has been recommended for those taking phenytoin 2 to 4 mg/kg daily, but it should be remembered that small alterations in phenytoin dose may result in a large change in phenytoin levels, as phenytoin kinetics are non-linear.[3,8,9] Note that the phenytoin levels in some individuals were doubled after only 10 days of concurrent use.[1] Amiodarone has a long half-life so that this interaction will persist for weeks after its withdrawal. Continued monitoring is important. Be aware that ataxia due to phenytoin toxicity (e.g. blurred vision, nystagmus, ataxia or drowsiness) may be confused with amiodarone-induced ataxia.[1,5]

It is not clear whether or not the amiodarone dosage should be increased to accommodate this interaction because the metabolite of amiodarone (*N*-desethylamiodarone) also has important antiarrhythmic effects.[7]

1. McGovern B, Geer VR, LaRaia PJ, Garan H, Ruskin JN. Possible interaction between amiodarone and phenytoin. *Ann Intern Med* (1984) 101, 650–1.
2. Nolan PE, Marcus FI, Hoyer GL, Bliss M, Gear K. Pharmacokinetic interaction between intravenous phenytoin and amiodarone in healthy volunteers. *Clin Pharmacol Ther* (1989) 46, 43–50.
3. Nolan PE, Erstad BL, Hoyer GL, Bliss M, Gear K, Marcus FI. Steady-state interaction between amiodarone and phenytoin in normal subjects. *Am J Cardiol* (1990) 65, 1252–7.
4. Gore JM, Haffajee CI, Alpert JS. Interaction of amiodarone and diphenylhydantoin. *Am J Cardiol* (1984) 54, 1145.
5. Shackleford EJ, Watson FT. Amiodarone-phenytoin interaction. *Drug Intell Clin Pharm* (1987) 21, 921.
6. Ahmad S. Amiodarone and phenytoin: interaction. *J Am Geriatr Soc* (1995) 43, 1449–50.
7. Nolan PE, Marcus FI, Karol MD, Hoyer GL, Gear K. Effect of phenytoin on the clinical pharmacokinetics of amiodarone. *J Clin Pharmacol* (1990) 30, 1112–19.
8. Nolan PE, Erstad BL, Hoyer GL, Bliss M, Gear K, Marcus FI. Interaction between amiodarone and phenytoin. *Am J Cardiol* (1991) 67, 328–9.
9. Duffal SB, McKenzie SK. Interaction between amiodarone and phenytoin. *Am J Cardiol* (1991) 67, 328.

Phenytoin + Antacids

Some studies have shown that antacids can reduce phenytoin serum levels and this may have been responsible for some loss of seizure control in a few patients. However other studies have shown no interaction, and it seems that usually no clinically important interaction occurs.

Clinical evidence

(a) Evidence of an interaction

A review briefly mentions that 3 patients taking phenytoin were found to have low serum phenytoin levels of 2 to 4 micrograms/mL when they were given phenytoin at the same time as antacids (unnamed), but when the antacid administration was delayed by 2 to 3 hours the serum phenytoin levels rose two to threefold.[1]

Elsewhere, 2 epileptic patients are reported to have had inadequate seizure control, which coincided with the ingestion of **aluminium/magnesium hydroxide** antacids for dyspepsia.[2] The AUC of a single dose of phenytoin was reduced by about 25% in 8 healthy subjects given either **aluminium/magnesium hydroxide** or **calcium carbonate**.[3]

(b) Evidence of no interaction

A study in 6 healthy subjects given **aluminium** or **magnesium hydroxide** failed to show any change in the rate or extent of absorption of a single dose of phenytoin,[2] and a similar study found **calcium carbonate** also had no effect on the absorption of phenytoin.[4] A controlled study in 6 epileptic patients found that a **magnesium trisilicate** and **aluminium hydroxide** antacid (*Gelusil*) caused a slight 12% reduction in steady-state serum phenytoin levels, which would not be expected to be clinically significant. Seizure frequency was not affected.[4] A study in 2 subjects found that the absorption of phenytoin was not altered by a mixture of **aluminium/magnesium hydroxide** and **magnesium trisilicate**, or **calcium carbonate**.[5] In another study, no statistically significant decrease in absorption was seen in 6 healthy subjects given a **dimeticone**, **aluminium hydroxide** and **magnesium oxide** antacid (*Asilone*).[6]

Mechanism

Not understood. One suggestion is that diarrhoea and a general increase in peristalsis caused by some antacids may cause a reduction in phenytoin absorption. Another is that antacids may cause changes in gastric acid secretion, which could affect phenytoin solubility.

Importance and management

This possible interaction is fairly well documented, but the results are conflicting. In practice it appears not to be important in most patients, although some loss of seizure control has been seen to occur in isolated cases. The interaction is unpredictable because it seems to depend on the individual patient and the antacid being taken. Concurrent use need not be avoided but if there is any hint that phenytoin levels are reduced, separation of the dosages by 2 to 3 hours may, as with other interactions caused by antacids, minimise the effects.

1. Pippinger L. Personal communication quoted by Kutt H in Interactions of antiepileptic drugs. *Epilepsia* (1975) 16, 393–402.
2. O'Brien LS, Orme ML'E, Breckenridge AM. Failure of antacids to alter the pharmacokinetics of phenytoin. *Br J Clin Pharmacol* (1978) 6, 176–7.
3. Carter BL, Garnett WR, Pellock JM, Stratton MA, Howell JR. Effect of antacids on phenytoin bioavailability. *Ther Drug Monit* (1981) 3, 333–40.
4. Kulshreshtha VK, Thomas M, Wadsworth J, Richens A. Interaction between phenytoin and antacids. *Br J Clin Pharmacol* (1978) 6, 177–9.
5. Chapron DJ, Kramer PA, Mariano SL, Hohnadel DC. Effect of calcium and antacids on phenytoin bioavailability. *Arch Neurol* (1979) 36, 436–8.
6. McElnay JC, Uprichard G, Collier PS. The effect of activated dimethicone and a proprietary antacid preparation containing this agent on the absorption of phenytoin. *Br J Clin Pharmacol* (1982) 13, 501–5.

Phenytoin + Antidiabetics

Large and toxic doses of phenytoin have been observed to cause hyperglycaemia, but normal therapeutic doses do not usually affect the control of diabetes. Two isolated cases of phenytoin toxicity have been attributed to the use of tolazamide or tolbutamide. Miglitol does not affect the bioavailability of phenytoin.

Clinical evidence

(a) Response to antidiabetics

Phenytoin has been shown in a number of reports[1-6] to raise the blood glucose levels of both diabetics and non-diabetics. However, in all but one of these cases the phenytoin dosage was large (at least 8 mg/kg) or even in the toxic range (70 to 80 mg/kg). There is little evidence that a hyperglycaemic response to usual doses of phenytoin is normally large enough to interfere with the control of diabetes, either with diet alone or with conventional antidiabetic drugs. In the one case where the interaction occurred with a therapeutic dose of phenytoin (1.2 g in the 24 hours following status epilepticus), the situation was complicated by the use of many other drugs and by renal impairment.[2]

(b) Response to phenytoin

Tolbutamide 500 mg two or three times daily was given to 17 patients taking phenytoin 100 to 400 mg daily.[7] The patients had a transient 45% rise in the amount of non-protein-bound phenytoin by day 2, which had disappeared by day 4. The introduction to this report briefly mentions a man given phenytoin and **tolazamide** who developed phenytoin toxicity, which disappeared when the **tolazamide** was replaced by **insulin**.[7] A woman previously uneventfully treated with phenytoin and **tolbutamide** developed toxicity on a later occasion when she took **tolbutamide** with twice the previous dose of phenytoin.[8] One study in healthy subjects found that **miglitol** 100 mg three times daily for 5 days did not affect the bioavailability of a single 400-mg dose of phenytoin.[9]

Mechanism

Studies in *animals* and man[10-12] suggest that phenytoin-induced hyperglycaemia occurs because the release of insulin from the pancreas is impaired. This implies that no interaction is possible without functional pancreatic tissue. Just why the phenytoin appeared to interact with tolazamide and tolbutamide is uncertain, but it is possible that these antidiabetics competitively inhibit phenytoin hydroxylation[13] by the cytochrome P450 isoenzyme CYP2C9.[14]

Importance and management

The weight of evidence shows that no interaction of clinical importance normally occurs between phenytoin and the antidiabetic drugs (most of the studies involved sulphonylureas). No special precautions seem normally to be necessary.

1. Klein JP. Diphenylhydantoin intoxication associated with hyperglycaemia. *J Pediatr* (1966) 69, 463–5.
2. Goldberg EM, Sanbar SS. Hyperglycaemic, nonketotic coma following administration of Dilantin (diphenylhydantoin). *Diabetes* (1969) 18, 101–6.
3. Peters BH, Samaan NA. Hyperglycaemia with relative hypoinsulinemia in diphenylhydantoin toxicity. *N Engl J Med* (1969) 281, 91–2.
4. Millichap JG. Hyperglycemic effect of diphenylhydantoin. *N Engl J Med* (1969) 281, 447.
5. Fariss BL, Lutcher CL. Diphenylhydantoin-induced hyperglycaemia and impaired insulin release. *Diabetes* (1971) 20, 177–81.
6. Treasure T, Toseland PA. Hyperglycaemia due to phenytoin toxicity. *Arch Dis Child* (1971) 46, 563–4.
7. Wesseling H, Mols-Thürkow I. Interaction of diphenylhydantoin (DPH) and tolbutamide in man. *Eur J Clin Pharmacol* (1975) 8, 75–8.
8. Beech E, Mathur SVS, Harrold BP. Phenytoin toxicity produced by tolbutamide. *BMJ* (1988) 297, 1613–14.
9. Richardt D, Rosmarin C, Havlik I, Schall R. No effect of miglitol on the oral bioavailability of single-dose phenytoin in healthy males. *Clin Drug Invest* (1997) 13, 171–4.
10. Kizer JS, Vargas-Cordon M, Brendel K, Bressler R. The *in vitro* inhibition of insulin secretion by diphenylhydantoin. *J Clin Invest* (1970) 49, 1942–8.
11. Levin SR, Booker J, Smith DF, Grodsky M. Inhibition of insulin secretion by diphenylhydantoin in the isolated perfused pancreas. *J Clin Endocrinol Metab* (1970) 30, 400–1.
12. Malherbe C, Burrill KC, Levin SR, Karam JH, Forsham PH. Effect of diphenylhydantoin on insulin secretion in man. *N Engl J Med* (1972) 286, 339–42.
13. Wesseling H, Thurkow I and Mulder GJ. Effect of sulphonylureas (tolazamide, tolbutamide and chlorpropamide) on the metabolism of diphenylhydantoin in the rat. *Biochem Pharmacol* (1973) 22, 3033–40.
14. Tassaneeyakul W, Veronese ME, Birkett DJ, Doecke CJ, McManus ME, Sansom LN, Miners JO. Co-regulation of phenytoin and tolbutamide metabolism in humans. *Br J Clin Pharmacol* (1992) 34, 494–8.

Phenytoin + Antimycobacterials

Serum phenytoin levels are markedly reduced by rifampicin, but can be raised by isoniazid. Those who are slow acetylators (slow metabolisers) of isoniazid may develop phenytoin toxicity if the dosage of phenytoin is not reduced appropriately. If rifampicin and isoniazid are given together, serum phenytoin levels may fall in patients who are fast acetylators of isoniazid, but may occasionally rise in those who are slow acetylators. Clofazimine may reduce serum phenytoin levels.

Clinical evidence

(a) Isoniazid

A study in 32 patients given phenytoin 300 mg daily found that within a week of starting to take isoniazid 300 mg daily and **aminosalicylic acid** 15 g daily, 6 of them had phenytoin levels almost 5 micrograms/mL higher than the rest of the group. On the following days when the phenytoin levels of these 6 patients rose above 20 micrograms/mL the typical signs of phenytoin toxicity were seen. All 6 had unusually high serum isoniazid levels and were identified as slow acetylators of isoniazid.[1]

Rises in serum phenytoin levels and toxicity induced by the concurrent use of isoniazid has been described in numerous other reports,[2-15] involving large numbers of patients, one of which describes a fatality.[8]

(b) Rifampicin

A study in 6 patients found that the clearance of intravenous phenytoin 100 mg doubled, from 46.7 to 97.8 mL/minute, when rifampicin 450 mg daily was taken for 2 weeks.[16]

A man taking phenytoin 400 mg daily experienced a seizure 3 days after starting rifampicin 600 mg daily. His phenytoin level was low (5.1 micrograms/mL) so the rifampicin was stopped and the phenytoin dose increased to 500 mg daily. His level increased slowly over the next 2 weeks, eventually ranging between 16 and 25 micrograms/mL.[17] Another man taking phenytoin needed a dosage reduction from 375 to 325 mg daily to keep his serum phenytoin levels within the therapeutic range when he stopped taking rifampicin.[18] See also, *Rifampicin and Clofazimine*, below.

(c) Rifampicin and Clofazimine

A man with AIDS taking a large number of drugs (rifampicin, clofazimine, ciprofloxacin, ethambutol, clarithromycin, diphenoxylate, bismuth, octreotide, co-trimoxazole, amphotericin, flucytosine, amikacin, zalcitabine) was also given phenytoin to control a right-sided seizure disorder. Despite taking phenytoin 1.6 g daily, and a trial of intravenous treatment, his trough phenytoin plasma levels remained almost undetectable until the rifampicin was withdrawn, when they rose to 5 micrograms/mL with the oral dose. When the clofazimine was withdrawn the levels rose even further to 10 micrograms/mL.[19]

(d) Rifampicin and Isoniazid

A patient taking phenytoin 300 mg daily developed progressive drowsiness (a sign of phenytoin toxicity) during the first week of taking isoniazid, rifampicin and ethambutol. His serum phenytoin levels rose to 46.1 micrograms/mL. He slowly recovered when the phenytoin was stopped, and he was later stabilised taking only 200 mg of phenytoin daily. He proved to be a slow acetylator of isoniazid.[20] Another patient taking phenytoin 300 mg daily was also given isoniazid, rifampicin and ethambutol but, in anticipation of the response seen in the previous patient, his phenytoin dosage was reduced to 200 mg daily. Within 3 days he developed seizures because his serum phenytoin levels had fallen to only 8 micrograms/mL. He needed a daily dosage of 400 mg of phenytoin to keep the serum levels within the therapeutic range. He was a fast acetylator of isoniazid.[20]

The clearance of phenytoin was doubled in 14 patients given rifampicin 450 mg, isoniazid 300 mg and ethambutol 900 mg to 1.2 g daily for 2 weeks. No further changes occurred in the pharmacokinetics of phenytoin after 3 months of antimycobacterial treatment. In this study, the interaction was of a similar magnitude in both the 8 slow and the 6 fast acetylators.[16]

Mechanism

Rifampicin (a known potent liver enzyme inducer) increases the metabolism and clearance of the phenytoin from the body so that a larger dose is needed to maintain adequate serum levels. Isoniazid inhibits the liver microsomal enzymes that metabolise phenytoin, and as a result the phenytoin accumulates and its serum levels rise.[21] Only those who are slow acetylators (slow metabolisers) of isoniazid normally attain blood levels of isoniazid that are sufficiently high to cause extensive inhibition of the phenytoin metabolism. Fast acetylators (fast metabolisers) remove the isoniazid too quickly for this to occur. Acetylator status is genetically determined. Thus some individuals will show a rapid rise in phenytoin levels, which eventually reaches toxic concentrations, whereas others will show only a relatively slow and unimportant rise to a plateau within, or only slightly above the therapeutic range.

If isoniazid and rifampicin are given together, the enzyme inhibitory effects of isoniazid may oppose the effects of rifampicin in those who are slow acetylators of isoniazid, but in those who are fast acetylators, the isoniazid will be cleared too quickly for it effectively to oppose the rifampicin effects. However, in one study isoniazid did not counter the effects of rifampicin in slow acetylators.[16]

The interaction involving clofazimine is not understood.

Importance and management

Direct information seems to be limited to these reports, but the interactions appear to be of clinical importance. Monitor the serum phenytoin levels and increase the dosage appropriately if rifampicin alone is started. Reduce the dosage if the rifampicin is stopped. If both rifampicin and isoniazid are given, the outcome may depend on the isoniazid acetylator status of the patient. Those who are fast acetylators will probably also need an increased phenytoin dosage. Those who are slow acetylators may need a smaller phenytoin dosage if toxicity is to be avoided. All patients should be monitored very closely as, unless acetylator status is known, the outcome is unpredictable.

The interaction with phenytoin and isoniazid alone is well documented, well established, clinically important and potentially serious. About 50% of the population are slow or relatively slow metabolisers of isoniazid,[1] but not all of them develop serum phenytoin levels in the toxic range. The reports indicate that somewhere between 10 and 33% of patients are at risk.[1-4,10] This adverse interaction may take only a few days to develop fully in some patients, but several weeks in others. Therefore concurrent use should be very closely monitored, making suitable dosage reductions as necessary. One patient was reported to have had better seizure control with fewer adverse effects while taking both drugs than with phenytoin alone.[22]

Information about clofazimine seems to be limited to one report. Monitor concurrent use, anticipating the need to increase the phenytoin dosage.

1. Brennan RW, Dehejia H, Kutt H, Verebely K, McDowell F. Diphenylhydantoin intoxication attendant to slow inactivation of isoniazid. *Neurology* (1970) 20, 687–93.
2. Kutt H, Brennan R, Dehejia H, Verebely K. Diphenylhydantoin intoxication. A complication of isoniazid therapy. *Am Rev Respir Dis* (1970) 101, 377–84.
3. Murray FJ. Outbreak of unexpected reactions among epileptics taking isoniazid. *Am Rev Respir Dis* (1962) 86, 729–32.
4. Kutt H, Winters W, McDowell FH. Depression of parahydroxylation of diphenylhydantoin by antituberculosis chemotherapy. *Neurology* (1966) 16, 594–602.
5. Manigand G, Thieblot P, Deparis M. Accidents de la diphénylhydantoïne induits par les traitements antituberculeux. *Presse Med* (1971) 79, 815–16.
6. Beauvais P, Mercier D, Hanoteau J, Brissand H-E. Intoxication a la diphenylhydantoine induite par l'isoniazide. *Arch Fr Pediatr* (1973) 30, 541–6.
7. Johnson J. Epanutin and isoniazid interaction. *BMJ* (1975) 1, 152.
8. Johnson J, Freeman HL. Death due to isoniazid (INH) and phenytoin. *Br J Psychiatry* (1975) 129, 511.
9. Geering JM, Ruch W, Dettli L. Diphenylhydantoin-Intoxikation durch Diphenylhydantoin-Isoniazid-Interaktion. *Schweiz Med Wochenschr* (1974) 104, 1224–8.
10. Miller RR, Porter J, Greenblatt DJ. Clinical importance of the interaction of phenytoin and isoniazid. A report from the Boston Collaborative Drug Surveillance Program. *Chest* (1979) 75, 356–8.
11. Witmer DR, Ritschel WA. Phenytoin-isoniazid interaction: a kinetic approach to management. *Drug Intell Clin Pharm* (1984) 18, 483–6.
12. Perucca E and Richens A. Anticonvulsant drug interactions. In: Tyrer J (ed) The treatment of epilepsy. MTP Lancaster. (1980) pp 95–128.
13. Sandyk R. Phenytoin toxicity induced by antituberculosis drugs. *S Afr Med J* (1982) 61, 382.
14. Yew WW, Lau KS, Ling MHM. Phenytoin toxicity in a patient with isoniazid-induced hepatitis. *Tubercle* (1991) 72, 309–10.
15. Walubo A, Aboo A. Phenytoin toxicity due to concomitant antituberculosis therapy. *S Afr Med J* (1995) 85, 1175–6.
16. Kay L, Kampmann JP, Svendsen TL, Vergman B, Hansen JEM, Skovsted L, Kristensen M. Influence of rifampicin and isoniazid on the kinetics of phenytoin. *Br J Clin Pharmacol* (1985) 20, 323–6.
17. Wagner JC, Slama TG. Rifampin-phenytoin drug interaction. *Drug Intell Clin Pharm* (1984) 18, 497.
18. Abajo FJ. Phenytoin interaction with rifampicin. *BMJ* (1988) 297, 1048.
19. Cone LA, Woodard DR, Simmons JC, Sonnenshein MA. Drug interactions in patients with AIDS. *Clin Infect Dis* (1992) 15, 1066–8.
20. O'Reilly D, Basran GS, Hourihan B, Macfarlane JT. Interaction between phenytoin and antituberculous drugs. *Thorax* (1987) 42, 736.
21. Desta Z, Soukhova NV, Flockhart DA. Inhibition of cytochrome P450 (CYP450) isoforms by isoniazid: potent inhibition of CYP2C19 and CYP3A. *Antimicrob Agents Chemother* (2001), 45, 384–92.
22. Thulasimnay M, Kela AK. Improvement of psychomotor epilepsy due to interaction of phenytoin-isoniazid. *Tubercle* (1984) 65, 229–30.

Phenytoin + Aspirin or NSAIDs

Serum phenytoin levels can be markedly increased by azapropazone and toxicity can develop rapidly. It is inadvisable for patients to take these drugs together. Phenytoin serum levels can also be increased by phenylbutazone and phenytoin toxicity may occur. It seems likely that oxyphenbutazone will interact similarly. Phenytoin toxicity has been seen in one patient taking ibuprofen, although no pharmacokinetic interaction was found in a study. Phenytoin toxicity occurred in a patient taking celecoxib. High-dose aspirin can cause protein-binding displacement of phenytoin, but this does not usually seem to be clinically important. No clinically significant interaction occurs between phenytoin and bromfenac, etodolac or tolfenamic acid.

Clinical evidence, mechanism, importance and management

(a) Aspirin

It has been suggested that if a patient has been taking large quantities of aspirin, phenytoin is 'potentiated'.[1] This comment remains unconfirmed, although a study in 10 healthy subjects did find that aspirin 975 mg every 4 hours caused protein binding displacement of phenytoin, resulting in a 16% rise in free salivary phenytoin levels and a 24% decrease in serum levels. However, these changes were considered unlikely to be clinically significant, and aspirin doses of 325 and 650 mg every 4 hours had no appreciable effect on phenytoin.[2] Similar effects on protein binding displacement have been seen in other studies.[3-7] However, although the ratios of free and bound phenytoin may change, there does not appear to be a clinical effect, possibly because the extra free phenytoin is metabolised by the liver.[6] A study in 10 epileptics taking phenytoin found that when they were also given aspirin 500 mg three times daily for 3 days, no significant changes in serum phenytoin levels or antiepileptic effects occurred.[8] The extremely common use of aspirin, and the almost total silence in the literature about an adverse interaction between phenytoin and aspirin implies that no special precautions are likely to be needed.

(b) Azapropazone

A patient taking phenytoin developed phenytoin toxicity within 2 weeks of starting azapropazone 600 mg twice daily. Further study in 5 healthy subjects given phenytoin 125 to 250 mg daily found that azapropazone 600 mg twice daily, briefly decreased their mean serum phenytoin levels from 5 to 3.7 micrograms/mL before they rose steadily over the next 7 days to 10.5 micrograms/mL.[9,10] An extension of this study is described elsewhere.[11]

Another report describes phenytoin toxicity in a woman taking phenytoin and primidone when fenclofenac was replaced by azapropazone 1.2 g daily.[12]

The most likely explanation is that azapropazone inhibits the liver enzymes concerned with the metabolism of phenytoin, resulting in its accumulation. It also seems possible that azapropazone displaces phenytoin from its plasma protein binding sites so that levels of unbound (and active) phenytoin are increased. Information seems to be limited to the reports cited, but it appears to be a clinically important interaction. The incidence is uncertain, but an interaction occurred in all 5 of the subjects in the study cited.[9,11] The manufacturers contraindicate azapropazone in patients taking phenytoin.[13]

(c) Bromfenac

Twelve healthy subjects were given bromfenac 50 mg three times daily for 4 days and then phenytoin 300 to 330 mg for up to 14 days (to achieve stable levels), and then both drugs for 8 days. It was found that the peak phenytoin serum levels and AUC were increased by 9% and 11%, respectively, while the bromfenac peak levels and AUC were reduced by 42%. The suggested reason for the reduction in bromfenac levels is that the phenytoin increases its metabolism by the liver.[14] In practical terms these results indicate that there is no need to adjust the dosage of phenytoin if bromfenac is added, nor any need to increase the bromfenac dosage unless there is any evidence that its efficacy is diminished.

(d) Celecoxib

An elderly woman taking phenytoin 300 mg daily who had also been taking celecoxib for the previous 6 months, developed signs of phenytoin toxicity. She was found to have a phenytoin level of 42 micrograms/mL, and a very slow rate of elimination.[15] It was thought that celecoxib may have competed with phenytoin for elimination via the cytochrome P450 isoenzyme CYP2C9. Further study is needed. Until then, it may be prudent to warn patients to monitor for signs of phenytoin toxicity (e.g. blurred vision, nystagmus, ataxia or drowsiness). if celecoxib is started, or consider monitoring phenytoin levels.

(e) Etodolac

A three-way crossover study in 16 healthy subjects found that etodolac 200 mg every 12 hours for 3 days had no effect on the pharmacokinetics or the pharmacological effects of phenytoin (100 mg twice daily for 2 days, 100 mg on day three).[16] There would seem to be no reason for avoiding the concurrent use of these drugs.

(f) Ibuprofen

Studies in healthy subjects found that the pharmacokinetics of single 300- or 900-mg doses of phenytoin were not significantly altered by ibuprofen 300 or 400 mg every 6 hours.[17,18] However, a single report describes a woman stabilised on phenytoin 300 mg daily who developed phenytoin toxicity within a week of starting to take ibuprofen 400 mg four times daily.[19] Her serum phenytoin levels had risen to about 25 micrograms/mL. The phenytoin was stopped for 3 days and the ibuprofen withdrawn, and within 10 days the phenytoin level had dropped to about 17 micrograms/mL. The reasons for this interaction are not understood.

Both phenytoin and ibuprofen have been available for many years and this case seems to be the first and only report of an adverse interaction. No special precautions would normally seem to be necessary.

(g) Oxyphenbutazone or Phenylbutazone

Six epileptic patients taking phenytoin 200 to 350 mg daily who were then also given phenylbutazone 100 mg three times daily had a mean fall in their phenytoin serum levels from 15 to 13 micrograms/mL over the first 3 days, after which the levels rose steadily to 19 micrograms/mL over the next 11 days. One patient developed symptoms of toxicity. His levels of free phenytoin more than doubled.[8] Another study found that phenylbutazone increased the steady state half-life of phenytoin from 13.7 to 22 hours.[20]

The predominant effect of phenylbutazone seems to be the inhibition of the enzymes concerned with the metabolism of phenytoin,[20] leading to its accumulation in the body and a rise in its serum levels. The initial transient fall may possibly be related in some way to the displacement by the phenylbutazone of the phenytoin from its plasma protein binding sites.[21] An established interaction, although the documentation is very limited. Monitor the outcome of adding phenylbutazone and reduce the phenytoin dosage as necessary. There is no direct evidence that oxyphenbutazone interacts like phenylbutazone, but since it is the main metabolic product of phenylbutazone in the body and has been shown to prolong the half-life of phenytoin in *animals*[22] it would be expected to interact similarly.

(h) Tolfenamic acid

Tolfenamic acid 300 mg daily for 3 days had no significant effect on the serum levels of phenytoin in 11 patients.[8] No special precautions seem necessary if these drugs are taken concurrently.

1. Toakley JG. Dilantin overdosage. *Med J Aust* (1968) 2, 640.
2. Leonard RF, Knott PJ, Rankin GO, Robinson DS, Melnick DE. Phenytoin-salicylate interaction. *Clin Pharmacol Ther* (1981) 29, 56–60.
3. Ehrnebo M, Odar-Cederlöf I. Distribution of pentobarbital and diphenylhydantoin between plasma and cells in blood: effect of salicylic acid, temperature and total drug concentration. *Eur J Clin Pharmacol* (1977) 11, 37–42.
4. Fraser DG, Ludden TM, Evens RP, Sutherland EW. Displacement of phenytoin from plasma binding sites by salicylate. *Clin Pharmacol Ther* (1980) 27, 165–9.
5. Paxton JW. Effects of aspirin on salivary and serum phenytoin kinetics in healthy subjects. *Clin Pharmacol Ther* (1980) 27, 170–8.
6. Olanow CW, Finn A, Prussak C. The effect of salicylate on phenytoin pharmacokinetics. *Trans Am Neurol Assoc* (1979) 104, 109–10.
7. Inoue F, Walsh RJ. Folate supplements and phenytoin-salicylate interaction. *Neurology* (1983) 33, 115–16.
8. Neuvonen PJ, Lehtovaara R, Bardy A, Elomaa E. Antipyretic analgesics in patients on antiepileptic drug therapy. *Eur J Clin Pharmacol* (1979) 15, 263–8.
9. Geaney DP, Carver JG, Aronson JK, Warlow CP. Interaction of azapropazone with phenytoin. *BMJ* (1982) 284, 1373.
10. Aronson JK, Hardman M, Reynolds DJM. ABC of monitoring drug therapy. Phenytoin. *BMJ* (1992) 305, 1215–18.
11. Geaney DP, Carver JG, Davies CL, Aronson JK. Pharmacokinetic investigation of the interaction of azapropazone with phenytoin. *Br J Clin Pharmacol* (1983) 15, 727–34.
12. Roberts CJC, Daneshmend TK, Macfarlane D, Dieppe PA. Anticonvulsant intoxication precipitated by azapropazone. *Postgrad Med J* (1981) 57, 191–2.
13. Rheumox (Azapropazone dihydrate). Goldshield Pharmaceuticals Ltd. UK Summary of product characteristics, February 2000.
14. Gumbhir-Shah K, Cevallos WH, DeCleene SA, Korth-Bradley JM. Evaluation of pharmacokinetic interaction between bromfenac and phenytoin in healthy males. *J Clin Pharmacol* (1997) 37, 160–8.
15. Keeling KL, Jortani SA, Linder MW, Valdes R. Prolonged elimination half-life of phenytoin in an elderly patient also on celecoxib. *Clin Chem* (2002) 48 (Suppl.), A52–A53.
16. Zvaifler N. A review of the antiarthritic efficacy and safety of etodolac. *Clin Rheumatol* (1989) 8 (Suppl 1), 43–53.
17. Bachmann KA, Schwartz JI, Forney RB, Jauregui L, Sullivan TJ. Inability of ibuprofen to alter single dose phenytoin disposition. *Br J Clin Pharmacol* (1986) 21, 165–9.
18. Townsend RJ, Fraser DG, Scavone JM, Cox SR. The effects of ibuprofen on phenytoin pharmacokinetics. *Drug Intell Clin Pharm* (1985) 19, 447–8.
19. Sandyk R. Phenytoin toxicity induced by interaction with ibuprofen. *S Afr Med J* (1982) 62, 592.
20. Andreasen PB, Frøland A, Skovsted L, Andersen SA, Hague M. Diphenylhydantoin half-life in man and its inhibition by phenylbutazone: the role of genetic factors. *Acta Med Scand* (1973) 193, 561–4.
21. Lunde PKM, Rane A, Yaffe SJ, Lund L, Sjöqvist F. Plasma protein binding of diphenylhydantoin in man. Interaction with other drugs and the effect of temperature and plasma dilution. *Clin Pharmacol Ther* (1970) 11, 846–55.
22. Soda DM, Levy G. Inhibition of drug metabolism by hydroxylated metabolites: cross-inhibition and specificity. *J Pharm Sci* (1975) 64, 1928–31.

Phenytoin + Atovaquone

In 12 healthy subjects, atovaquone (1 g, given both twelve hours before and with a single 600-mg dose of phenytoin) did not affect the pharmacokinetics of phenytoin. It was concluded that a clinically important pharmacokinetic interaction is unlikely.[1]

1. Davis JD, Dixon R, Khan AZ, Toon S, Rolan PE, Posner J. Atovaquone has no effect on the pharmacokinetics of phenytoin in healthy male volunteers. *Br J Clin Pharmacol* (1996) 42, 246–8.

Phenytoin + Azoles

Phenytoin levels are raised by fluconazole (toxicity seen). Posaconazole, voriconazole and possibly miconazole interact similarly. Itraconazole (and therefore probably ketoconazole) have little effect on phenytoin levels.

Phenytoin decreases itraconazole and possibly ketoconazole levels (treatment failures seen). Posaconazole and voriconazole are similarly affected. Fluconazole levels are not usually affected by phenytoin, although there is one report of reduced efficacy.

Clinical evidence

(a) Fluconazole

In a randomised, placebo-controlled study, 10 subjects given phenytoin 200 mg daily for the last 3 days of a 14-day course of fluconazole 200 mg daily were compared with 10 other subjects taking phenytoin alone. Fluconazole caused the phenytoin AUC to rise by 75%, and the trough phenytoin levels to rise by 128%. Phenytoin appeared not to affect fluconazole trough levels.[1] Two other studies reported similar findings.[2,3]

There are reports describing at least 7 cases of phenytoin toxicity caused by fluconazole.[4-7]

A brief report noted that 3 of 9 patients taking fluconazole and phenytoin required an increase in fluconazole dose or the substitution of another antifungal due to a lack of efficacy. It was suggested that phenytoin may reduce fluconazole levels in some patients.[8] However, in the controlled studies cited above,[1,3] fluconazole serum levels were unaltered by phenytoin.

(b) Itraconazole

After taking oral phenytoin 300 mg daily for 15 days, the AUC of a single 200-mg dose of itraconazole was reduced more than 90% in 13 healthy subjects. The half-life of itraconazole fell from 22.3 to 3.8 hours. A parallel study[9] in another group found that itraconazole 200 mg for 15 days increased the phenytoin AUC by 10.3%.

Two patients taking phenytoin and two taking phenytoin with carbamazepine either did not respond to treatment with itraconazole 400 mg daily for aspergillosis, coccidioidomycosis or cryptococcosis, or suffered a relapse. All of them had undetectable or substantially reduced serum itraconazole levels compared with other patients taking itraconazole alone.[10] Two other patients also had very low itraconazole serum levels while taking phenytoin and phenobarbital.[11]

(c) Ketoconazole

A study in 9 healthy subjects found that ketoconazole 200 mg twice daily for 6 days did not significantly alter the $AUC_{0\text{-}48h}$ of a single 250-mg dose of phenytoin.[2]

A man being treated for coccidioidal meningitis with ketoconazole 400 mg daily relapsed when he was given phenytoin 300 mg daily. A pharmacokinetic study found that his peak serum ketoconazole levels and AUC were reduced compared with the values seen before the phenytoin was started. Even though the ketoconazole dose was increased to 600 mg, and later 1.2 g, his serum levels remained low compared with other patients taking only 400 or 600 mg of ketoconazole.[12] Coccidioidomycosis progressed in another patient taking phenytoin despite the use of ketoconazole.[10] Low serum ketoconazole levels were seen in one patient taking phenytoin and phenobarbital.[13]

(d) Miconazole

A man with epilepsy, well controlled with phenytoin, developed symptoms of phenytoin toxicity within one day of starting *intravenous* miconazole 500 mg every 8 hours and flucytosine. After one week of concurrent treatment his serum phenytoin levels had risen by 50%, from 29 to 43 micrograms/mL. He had some symptoms of very mild phenytoin toxicity before the antifungal treatment was started.[14] Another patient developed symptoms of toxicity (nystagmus, ataxia) within 5 days of starting to take oral miconazole 500 mg daily. His serum phenytoin level rose to 40.8 micrograms/mL. After discontinuation of the miconazole the same dose of phenytoin resulted in a level of 14.5 micrograms/mL.[15]

(e) Posaconazole

In a study in healthy subjects the concurrent use of posaconazole 200 mg daily and phenytoin 200 mg daily for 10 days decreased the AUC of posaconazole by 50%, when compared to controls. Although there was no statistically significant change in phenytoin pharmacokinetics, some subjects had increases in phenytoin levels that could be clinically relevant.[16]

(f) Voriconazole

Studies in healthy subjects found that phenytoin 300 mg daily decreased the maximum serum levels and AUC of voriconazole by 49% and 69%, respectively. Also, voriconazole 400 mg twice daily increased the maximum serum levels and AUC of phenytoin 300 mg daily by 67% and 81%, respectively.[17]

Mechanism

Fluconazole inhibits the cytochrome P450 isoenzymes responsible for phenytoin metabolism (probably CYP2C9).[2] Voriconazole and miconazole probably act similarly, but ketoconazole and itraconazole do not affect this isoenzyme and therefore do not significantly affect phenytoin levels. Phenytoin is an enzyme inducer, and appears to induce the metabolism of these azoles to varying degrees.

Importance and management

The increase in serum phenytoin levels with **fluconazole** is established and clinically important. Toxicity can develop within 2 to 7 days unless the phenytoin dosage is reduced. Monitor serum phenytoin levels closely and reduce the dosage appropriately. Also be alert for any evidence of reduced fluconazole effects.

The decrease in **itraconazole** levels with phenytoin is established, clinically important and its incidence appears to be high. Because such a marked fall in itraconazole levels occurs, it is difficult to predict by how much its dosage should be increased, for which reason the authors of one report advise using another antifungal instead.[9] Similarly, the UK manufacturer of itraconazole says that use with potent enzyme inducers such as phenytoin is not recommended.[18] The small rise in serum phenytoin levels caused by itraconazole is unlikely to be clinically important.

Information on the interaction between **ketoconazole** and phenytoin appears to be limited to these reports, but be alert for any signs of a reduced antifungal response. It may be necessary to increase the dosage of the ketoconazole. Ketoconazole probably does not have an important effect on phenytoin levels.

Evidence for increased phenytoin levels with **miconazole** is limited, even so it would be prudent to monitor serum phenytoin levels, including when the oral gel is used at a dose of 5 to 10 mL four times daily (15 mg/kg per day).[19]

Phenytoin halves **posaconazole** levels, and posaconazole might increase phenytoin levels. The manufacturer of posaconazole suggests that concurrent use should be avoided unless the benefits outweigh the risks.[20] If used together it would seem sensible to consider increasing the posaconazole dose, and increase monitoring of phenytoin adverse effects, taking levels as necessary, and adjusting the phenytoin dose as appropriate.

The interaction between phenytoin and **voriconazole** is established. The UK manufacturers say that concurrent use of voriconazole and phenytoin should be avoided unless the benefits outweigh the risks.[21] If used together, the manufacturers recommend careful monitoring of phenytoin levels and adverse effects, and doubling the dose of oral **voriconazole** (from 200 to 400 mg twice daily and from 100 mg to 200 mg twice daily in patients less than 40 kg) or increasing the dose of intravenous **voriconazole** (from 4 to 5 mg/kg twice daily).[21,22]

1. Blum RA, Wilton JH, Hilligoss DM, Gardner MJ, Henry EB, Harrison NJ, Schentag JJ. Effect of fluconazole on the disposition of phenytoin. *Clin Pharmacol Ther* (1991) 49, 420–5.
2. Touchette MA, Chandrasekar PH, Millad MA, Edwards DJ. Contrasting effects of fluconazole and ketoconazole on phenytoin and testosterone disposition in man. *Br J Clin Pharmacol* (1992) 34, 75–8.
3. Lazar JD, Wilner KD. Drug interactions with fluconazole. *Rev Infect Dis* (1990) 12 (Suppl 3), S327–S333.
4. Mitchell AS, Holland JT. Fluconazole and phenytoin: a predictable interaction. *BMJ* (1989) 298, 1315.
5. Howitt KM, Oziemski MA. Phenytoin toxicity induced by fluconazole. *Med J Aust* (1989) 151, 603–4.
6. Sugar AM. Quoted as Personal Communication by Grant SM, Clissold SP. Fluconazole. A review of its pharmacodynamic and pharmacokinetic properties, and therapeutic potential in superficial and system mycoses. *Drugs* (1990) 39, 877–916.
7. Cadle RM, Zenon GJ, Rodriguez-Barradas MC, Hamill RJ. Fluconazole-induced symptomatic phenytoin toxicity. *Ann Pharmacother* (1994) 28, 191–5.
8. Tett S, Carey D, Lee H-S. Drug interactions with fluconazole. *Med J Aust* (1992) 156, 365.
9. Ducharme MP, Slaughter RL, Warbasse LH, Chandrasekar PH, Van der Velde V, Mannens G, Edwards DJ. Itraconazole and hydroxyitraconazole serum concentrations are reduced more than tenfold by phenytoin. *Clin Pharmacol Ther* (1995) 58, 617–24.
10. Tucker RM, Denning DW, Hanson LH, Rinaldi MG, Graybill JR, Sharkey PK, Pappagianis D, Stevens DA. Interaction of azoles with rifampin, phenytoin, and carbamazepine: in vitro and clinical observations. *Clin Infect Dis* (1992) 14, 165–74.
11. Hay RJ, Clayton YM, Moore MK, Midgely G. An evaluation of itraconazole in the management of onychomycosis. *Br J Dermatol* (1988) 119, 359–66.
12. Brass C, Galgiani JN, Blaschke TF, Defelice R, O'Reilly RA, Stevens DA. Disposition of ketoconazole, an oral antifungal, in humans. *Antimicrob Agents Chemother* (1982) 21, 151–8.
13. Stockley RJ, Daneshmend TK, Bredow MT, Warnock DW, Richardson MD, Slade RR. Ketoconazole pharmacokinetics during chronic dosing in adults with haematological malignancy. *Eur J Clin Microbiol* (1986) 5, 513–17.
14. Rolan PE, Somogyi AA, Drew MJR, Cobain WG, South D, Bochner F. Phenytoin intoxication during treatment with parenteral miconazole. *BMJ* (1983) 287, 1760.
15. Loupi E, Descotes J, Lery N, Evreux JC. Interactions medicamenteuses et miconazole. A propos de 10 observations. *Therapie* (1982) 37, 437–41.
16. Courtney RD, Statkevich P, Laughlin M, Pai S, Lim J, Clement RP, Batra VK. Potential for a drug interaction between posaconazole and phenytoin. *Intersci Conf Antimicrob Agents Chemother* (2001) 41, 4.
17. Purkins L, Wood N, Ghahramani P, Love ER, Eve MD, Fielding A. Coadministration of voriconazole and phenytoin: pharmacokinetic interaction, safety, and toleration. *Br J Clin Pharmacol* (2003) 56, 37–44.
18. Sporanox Capsules (Itraconazole). Janssen-Cilag Ltd. UK Summary of product characteristics, March 2004.
19. Daktarin Oral Gel (Miconazole). Janssen-Cilag Ltd. UK Summary of product characteristics, May 2006.
20. Noxafil (Posaconazole). Schering-Plough Ltd. UK Summary of product characteristics, October 2006.
21. VFEND (Voriconazole). Pfizer Ltd. UK Summary of product characteristics, July 2007.
22. VFEND (Voriconazole). Pfizer Inc. US Prescribing information, November 2006.

Phenytoin + Bile-acid binding resins

Neither colestyramine nor colestipol affect the absorption of phenytoin from the gut.

Clinical evidence, mechanism, importance and management

Neither colestyramine 5 g nor colestipol 10 g had a significant effect on the absorption of a single 500-mg dose of phenytoin in 6 healthy subjects. The resins were given 2 minutes before and 6 and 12 hours after the phenytoin.[1] Another study in 6 healthy subjects found that colestyramine 4 g four times daily for 5 days had no significant effect on the extent of the absorption of a single 400-mg dose of phenytoin (given on day 3, two minutes after the colestyramine).[2] No special precautions would seem to be necessary if either of these drugs and phenytoin is taken concurrently.

1. Callaghan JT, Tsuru M, Holtzman JL, Hunningshake DB. Effect of cholestyramine and colestipol on the absorption of phenytoin. *Eur J Clin Pharmacol* (1983) 24, 675–8.
2. Barzaghi N, Monteleone M, Amione C, Lecchini S, Perucca E, Frigo GM. Lack of effect of cholestyramine on phenytoin bioavailability. *J Clin Pharmacol* (1988) 28, 1112–14.

Phenytoin + Calcium-channel blockers

Diltiazem can increase serum phenytoin levels. A single case report describes phenytoin toxicity with nifedipine and another case report describes neurological toxicity when a patient taking phenytoin and carbamazepine was given isradipine.
The plasma levels of felodipine and nisoldipine are very markedly reduced by phenytoin (either alone or with carbamazepine). Case reports suggest that nimodipine and verapamil levels may be reduced by phenytoin, and that phenytoin levels may be raised by nifedipine.

Clinical evidence

(a) Diltiazem

Elevated serum phenytoin levels and signs of toxicity developed in 2 out of 14 patients taking phenytoin when they were also given diltiazem.[1] A patient taking phenytoin 250 mg twice daily developed signs of toxicity within 2 weeks of starting to take diltiazem 240 mg every 8 hours.[2]

(b) Felodipine

After taking felodipine 10 mg daily for 4 days, 10 epileptic patients (including 2 taking phenytoin alone and 3 taking phenytoin with carbamazepine) had markedly reduced plasma felodipine levels (peak levels of 1.6 nanomol/L compared with 8.9 nanomol/L in 12 control subjects). The felodipine bioavailability was reduced to 6.6%.[3]

(c) Isradipine

A man taking carbamazepine and phenytoin developed neurological toxicity while also taking isradipine, which the authors attributed to a pharmacokinetic or pharmacodynamic interaction between the phenytoin and isradipine.[4] However, a commentator considered that an interaction between the carbamazepine and isradipine was more plausible.[5]

(d) Nifedipine

An isolated report describes phenytoin toxicity in a man taking phenytoin, 3 weeks after he started to take nifedipine 30 mg daily. His serum phenytoin level was 30.4 micrograms/mL. The nifedipine was stopped, and over the next 2 weeks his serum phenytoin levels fell to 10.5 micrograms/mL. A further 2 weeks later all the symptoms had resolved.[6] However, a retrospective study of 8 patients suggested that nifedipine does not usually interact.[1] One of the manufacturers of nifedipine notes that the bioavailability of nifedipine may be reduced by concurrent phenytoin.[7]

(e) Nimodipine

A study in 8 epileptic patients one of whom was taking phenytoin with carbamazepine found that the AUC of a single 60-mg oral dose of nimodipine was only about 15% of that obtained from a group of healthy subjects.[8]

(f) Nisoldipine

Twelve epileptic patients receiving long-term phenytoin treatment and 12 healthy subjects were given single 40- or 20-mg doses of nisoldipine. The mean nisoldipine AUCs (normalised for a 20-mg dose) were 1.6 micrograms/L per hour for the epileptics, and 15.2 micrograms/L per hour for the healthy subjects.[9]

(g) Verapamil

A woman taking phenytoin who was then also given verapamil had persistently subnormal plasma verapamil levels (less than 50 nanograms/mL) despite increases in the verapamil dosage from 80 mg twice daily to 160 mg three times daily. When the phenytoin was stopped, her plasma verapamil levels rose to the expected concentrations.[10]

Mechanism

Diltiazem may inhibit the metabolism of phenytoin. In contrast, the antiepileptics are well recognised as enzyme inducers, which can increase the metabolism of the calcium-channel blockers by the liver, resulting in a very rapid loss from the body.

Importance and management

Information about the effects of calcium-channel blockers on phenytoin is limited, but what is known indicates that if diltiazem is given with phenytoin, the dosage of phenytoin may possibly need to be reduced to avoid toxicity. The case report of phenytoin toxicity with nifedipine is isolated, and of unknown importance. Phenytoin markedly reduces felodipine, verapamil and possibly nifedipine levels. Although not all calcium-channel blockers have been studied, most would be expected to interact with phenytoin similarly, as they are metabolised by the same isoenzymes (see 'Calcium-channel blockers', (p.860)). A considerable increase in the dosage of any calcium-channel blocker will probably be needed in the presence of phenytoin. Note that the manufacturers of nimodipine[11] and nisoldipine[12] contraindicate the concurrent use of phenytoin because of the possibility of a large reduction in their levels.

1. Bahls FH, Ozuna J, Ritchie DE. Interactions between calcium channel blockers and the anticonvulsants carbamazepine and phenytoin. *Neurology* (1991) 41, 740–2.
2. Clarke WR, Horn JR, Kawabori I, Gurtel S. Potentially serious drug interactions secondary to high-dose diltiazem used in the treatment of pulmonary hypertension. *Pharmacotherapy* (1993) 13, 402–5.
3. Capewell S, Freestone S, Critchley JAJH, Pottage A, Prescott LF. Reduced felodipine bioavailability in patients taking anticonvulsants. *Lancet* (1988) ii, 480–2.
4. Cachat F, Tufro A. Phenytoin/isradipine interaction causing severe neurologic toxicity. *Ann Pharmacother* (2002) 36: 1399–1402.
5. Hauben M. Comment: phenytoin/isradipine interaction causing severe neurologic toxicity. *Ann Pharmacother* (2002) 36: 1974–5.
6. Ahmad S. Nifedipine-phenytoin interaction. *J Am Coll Cardiol* (1984) 3, 1582.
7. Adalat Retard (Nifedipine). Bayer plc. UK Summary of product characteristics, September 2006
8. Tartara A, Galimberti CA, Manni R, Parietti L, Zucca C, Baasch H, Caresia L, Mück W, Barzaghi N, Gatti G, Perucca E. Differential effects of valproic acid and enzyme-inducing anticonvulsants on nimodipine pharmacokinetics in epileptic patients. *Br J Clin Pharmacol* (1991) 32, 335–40.
9. Michelucci R, Cipolla G, Passarelli D, Gatti G, Ochan M, Heinig R, Tassinari CA, Perucca E. Reduced plasma nisoldipine concentrations in phenytoin-treated patients with epilepsy. *Epilepsia* (1996) 37, 1107–10.
10. Woodcock BG, Kirsten R, Nelson K, Rietbrock S, Hopf R, Kaltenbach M. A reduction in verapamil concentrations with phenytoin. *N Engl J Med* (1991) 325, 1179.
11. Nimotop (Nimodipine). Bayer plc. UK Summary of product characteristics, August 2005.
12. Syscor MR (Nisoldipine). Forest Laboratories UK Ltd. UK Summary of product characteristics. August 1998.

Phenytoin + Carbamazepine

Some reports describe rises in serum phenytoin levels, with toxicity, whereas others describe falls in phenytoin levels. Genetic differences in the metabolism of these drugs may be an explanation for the differences. Falls in carbamazepine serum levels, sometimes with rises in carbamazepine-10,11-epoxide levels, have been described.

Clinical evidence

(a) Reduced serum phenytoin levels

Carbamazepine 600 mg daily for 4 to 14 days reduced the serum phenytoin levels of 3 out of 7 patients, from 15 to 7 micrograms/mL, from 18 to 12 micrograms/mL and from 16 to 10 micrograms/mL, respectively. Phenytoin serum levels rose again 10 days after carbamazepine was withdrawn.[1]

Reduced serum phenytoin levels in patients given carbamazepine have been described in other reports.[2-5]

(b) Raised serum phenytoin levels

A study in 6 epileptic patients taking phenytoin 350 to 600 mg daily found that over a 12-week period the addition of carbamazepine 600 to 800 mg daily increased the phenytoin serum levels by 35%, increased its half-life by 41% and reduced its clearance by 36.5%. Neurotoxicity increased by 204%, with additional symptoms of toxicity (sedation, ataxia, nystagmus, etc.) developing in 5 of the 6 patients. The phenytoin dosage remained unchanged throughout the period of the study.[6]

Other reports have also described increases in serum phenytoin levels,[7-12] which were as large as 81%, and even up to 100% in some cases.[8,10]

(c) Reduced serum carbamazepine levels

A series of multiple regression analyses on data from a large number of patients [the precise number is not clear from the report], showed that phenytoin reduced plasma carbamazepine, by, on average, 0.9 micrograms/mL for each 2 mg/kg per day of phenytoin.[7]

Reduced serum carbamazepine levels have been described in other studies and reports.[3,11,13-16] Two studies found that phenytoin markedly increased the levels of the active metabolite of carbamazepine, carbamazepine-10,11-epoxide.[17,18]

Mechanism

Not understood. Both carbamazepine and phenytoin are enzyme inducers, and might therefore be expected to decrease the metabolism of each other. However, more recently it has been shown that carbamazepine can inhibit the cytochrome P450 isoenzyme CYP2C19, which is one of the enzymes involved in phenytoin metabolism.[19] Carbamazepine might therefore cause increases in phenytoin levels by this mechanism. Moreover, CYP2C19 shows genetic polymorphism (see 'Genetic factors in drug metabolism', (p.4), for a general discussion), so an interaction via this mechanism would not occur in all patients.

Importance and management

Phenytoin may decrease carbamazepine levels, but carbamazepine has variable effects on phenytoin levels, with both increases and decreases described. Monitor antiepileptic levels during concurrent use (where possible including the active metabolite of carbamazepine, carbamazepine-10,11-epoxide) so that steps can be taken to avoid the development of toxicity or lack of efficacy. Not all patients appear to have an adverse interaction, and, at present, it does not seem possible to identify those potentially at risk. The risk of carbamazepine-induced water intoxication is reported to be reduced in patients also taking phenytoin.[14]

1. Hansen JM, Siersbæk-Nielsen K, Skovsted L. Carbamazepine-induced acceleration of diphenylhydantoin and warfarin metabolism in man. *Clin Pharmacol Ther* (1971) 12, 539–43.
2. Cereghino JJ, Van Meter JC, Brock JT, Penry JK, Smith LD, White BG. Preliminary observations of serum carbamazepine concentration in epileptic patients. *Neurology* (1973) 23, 357–66.
3. Hooper WD, Dubetz DK, Eadie MJ, Tyrer JH. Preliminary observations on the clinical pharmacology of carbamazepine ('Tegretol'). *Proc Aust Assoc Neurol* (1974) 11, 189–98.
4. Lai M-L, Lin T-S, Huang JD. Effect of single- and multiple-dose carbamazepine on the pharmacokinetics of diphenylhydantoin. *Eur J Clin Pharmacol* (1992) 43, 201–3.
5. Windorfer A, Sauer W. Drug interactions during anticonvulsant therapy in childhood: diphenylhydantoin, primidone, phenobarbitone, clonazepam, nitrazepam, carbamazepin and dipropylacetate. *Neuropadiatrie* (1977) 8, 29–41.
6. Browne TR, Szabo GK, Evans JE, Evans BA, Greenblatt DJ, Mikati MA. Carbamazepine increases phenytoin serum concentration and reduces phenytoin clearance. *Neurology* (1988) 38, 1146–50.
7. Lander CM, Eadie MJ, Tyrer JH. Interactions between anticonvulsants. *Proc Aust Assoc Neurol* (1975) 12, 111–16.
8. Gratz ES, Theodore WH, Newmark ME, Kupferberg HJ, Porter RJ, Qu Z. Effect of carbamazepine on phenytoin clearance in patients with complex partial seizures. *Neurology* (1982) 32, A223.
9. Leppik IE, Pepin SM, Jacobi J, Miller KW. Effect of carbamazepine on the Michaelis-Menten parameters of phenytoin. In Metabolism of Antiepileptic Drugs (ed Levy RH et al) Raven Press, New York. (1984) pp 217–22.
10. Zielinski JJ, Haidukewych D, Leheta BJ. Carbamazepine-phenytoin interaction: elevation of plasma phenytoin concentrations due to carbamazepine comedication. *Ther Drug Monit* (1985) 7, 51–3.
11. Hidano F, Obata N, Yahaba Y, Unno K, Fukui R. Drug interactions with phenytoin and carbamazepine. *Folia Psychiatr Neurol Jpn* (1983) 37, 342–4.
12. Zielinski JJ, Haidukewych D. Dual effects of carbamazepine-phenytoin interaction. *Ther Drug Monit* (1987) 9, 21–3.
13. Cereghino JJ, Brock JT, Van Meter JC, Penry JK, Smith LD, White BG. The efficacy of carbamazepine combinations in epilepsy. *Clin Pharmacol Ther* (1975) 18, 733–41.
14. Perucca E, Richens A. Reversal by phenytoin of carbamazepine-induced water intoxication: a pharmacokinetic interaction. *J Neurol Neurosurg Psychiatry* (1980) 43, 540–5.
15. Ramsay RE, McManus DQ, Guterman A, Briggle TV, Vazquez D, Perchalski R, Yost RA, Wong P. Carbamazepine metabolism in humans: effect of concurrent anticonvulsant therapy. *Ther Drug Monit* (1990) 12, 235–41.

16. Chapron DJ, LaPierre BA, Abou-Elkair M. Unmasking the significant enzyme-inducing effects of phenytoin on serum carbamazepine concentrations during phenytoin withdrawal. *Ann Pharmacother* (1993) 27, 708–11.
17. Hagiwara M, Takahashi R, Watabe M, Amanuma I, Kan R, Takahashi Y, Kumashiro H. Influence of phenytoin on metabolism of carbamazepine. *Neurosciences* (1989) 15, 303–9.
18. Dam M, Jensen A, Christiansen J. Plasma level and effect of carbamazepine in grand mal and psychomotor epilepsy. *Acta Neurol Scand* (1975) 75 (Suppl 51), 33–8.
19. Lakehal F, Wurden CJ, Kalhorn TF, Levy RH. Carbamazepine and oxcarbazepine decrease phenytoin metabolism through inhibition of CYP2C19. *Epilepsy Res* (2002) 52, 79–83.

Phenytoin + Chloramphenicol

Serum phenytoin levels can be raised by intravenous chloramphenicol and phenytoin toxicity may occur. Other evidence indicates that phenytoin may increase or decrease serum chloramphenicol levels in children.

Clinical evidence

(a) Effect on chloramphenicol

A child given a 6-week course of intravenous chloramphenicol 100 mg/kg daily in four divided doses had a reduction in chloramphenicol peak and trough serum levels of 46% and 74%, respectively, within 2 days of starting phenytoin 4 mg/kg daily. Levels were further reduced by 63% and 87%, respectively, by the addition of phenobarbital 4 mg/kg daily.[1] Consider also 'Chloramphenicol + Phenobarbital', (p.300). In contrast, 6 children (aged 1 month to 12 years) developed raised, toxic chloramphenicol levels while receiving phenytoin.[2]

(b) Effect on phenytoin

A man taking phenytoin 100 mg four times daily developed signs of toxicity within a week of also receiving intravenous chloramphenicol (1 g every 6 hours for 4 doses then 2 g every 6 hours). His serum phenytoin levels had risen by about threefold, from about 7 to 24 micrograms/mL.[3]

This interaction has been described in a number of other reports.[4-12] One study found that intravenous chloramphenicol more than doubled the half-life of phenytoin.[4] The AUC of phenytoin after a single intravenous dose of **fosphenytoin** was 23% higher (not significant) in children also given intravenous chloramphenicol when compared with those given intravenous cefotaxime. In addition, the phenytoin half-life was significantly prolonged by chloramphenicol (23.7 hours versus 15.5 hours).[13]

Mechanism

It seems probable that chloramphenicol, a known enzyme inhibitor,[14] affects the liver enzymes (possibly cytochrome P450 isoenzyme CYP2C19[15]) concerned with the metabolism of phenytoin thereby reducing its rate of clearance from the body. The changes in the pharmacokinetics of chloramphenicol in children are not understood.

Importance and management

The rise in serum phenytoin levels with intravenous chloramphenicol in adults is well documented and clinically important. A two to fourfold rise can occur within a few days. Concurrent use should be avoided unless the effects can be closely monitored and appropriate phenytoin dosage reductions made as necessary. The use of a single prophylactic dose of phenytoin or fosphenytoin may be an exception to this.[13] It seems very doubtful if enough chloramphenicol is absorbed from eye drops or ointments for an interaction to occur.

The general clinical importance of the changes in serum chloramphenicol levels in children is uncertain, but the effects of concurrent use should certainly be monitored. More study is needed.

1. Powell DA, Nahata M, Durrell DC, Glazer JP and Hilty MD. Interactions among chloramphenicol, phenytoin and phenobarbitone in a pediatric patient. *J Pediatr* (1981) 98, 1001.
2. Krasinski K, Kusmiesz H, Nelson JD. Pharmacologic interactions among chloramphenicol, phenytoin and phenobarbital. *Pediatr Infect Dis* (1982) 1, 232–5.
3. Ballek RE, Reidenberg MM, Orr L. Inhibition of diphenylhydantoin metabolism by chloramphenicol. *Lancet* (1973) i, 150.
4. Christensen LK, Skovsted L. Inhibition of drug metabolism by chloramphenicol. *Lancet* (1969) ii, 1397–9.
5. Houghton GW, Richens A. Inhibition of phenytoin metabolism by other drugs used in epilepsy. *Int J Clin Pharmacol Biopharm* (1975) 12, 210–16.
6. Rose JQ, Choi HK, Schentag JJ, Kinkel WR, Jusko WJ. Intoxication caused by interaction of chloramphenicol and phenytoin. *JAMA* (1977) 237, 2630–1.
7. Koup JR, Gibaldi M, McNamara P, Hilligoss DM, Colburn WA, Bruck E. Interaction of chloramphenicol with phenytoin and phenobarbital. *Clin Pharmacol Ther* (1978) 24, 571–5.
8. Vincent FM, Mills L, Sullivan JK. Chloramphenicol-induced phenytoin intoxication. *Ann Neurol* (1978) 3, 469.
9. Harper JM, Yost RL, Stewart RB, Ciezkowski J. Phenytoin-chloramphenicol interaction. *Drug Intell Clin Pharm* (1979) 13, 425–9.
10. Greenlaw CW. Chloramphenicol-phenytoin drug interaction. *Drug Intell Clin Pharm* (1979) 13, 609–10.
11. Saltiel M, Stephens NM. Phenytoin-chloramphenicol interaction. *Drug Intell Clin Pharm* (1980) 14, 221.
12. Cosh DG, Rowett DS, Lee PC, McCarthy PJ. Case report — phenytoin therapy complicated by concurrent chloramphenicol and enteral nutrition. *Aust J Hosp Pharm* (1987) 17, 51–3.
13. Ogutu BR, Newton CRJC, Muchohi SN, Otieno GO, Kokwaro GO. Phenytoin pharmacokinetics and clinical effects in African children following fosphenytoin and chloramphenicol coadministration. *Br J Clin Pharmacol* (2002) 54, 635–42.
14. Dixon RL, Fouts JR. Inhibition of microsomal drug metabolic pathways by chloramphenicol. *Biochem Pharmacol* (1962) 11, 715–20.
15. Park J-Y, Kim K-A, Kim S-L. Chloramphenicol is a potent inhibitor of cytochrome P450 isoforms CYP2C19 and CYP3A4 in human liver microsomes. *Antimicrob Agents Chemother* (2003) 47, 3464–9.

Phenytoin + Chlorphenamine

In two patients phenytoin toxicity was attributed to the concurrent use of chlorphenamine.

Clinical evidence, mechanism, importance and management

A week or so after starting to take chlorphenamine 4 mg three times daily, a woman taking phenytoin and phenobarbital developed phenytoin toxicity with serum phenytoin levels of about 65 micrograms/mL. The toxic symptoms disappeared and phenytoin levels fell when the chlorphenamine was withdrawn.[1] Another woman taking antiepileptics, including phenytoin, developed slight grimacing of the face and involuntary jaw movements (but no speech slurring, ataxia or nystagmus) within 12 days of starting to take chlorphenamine 12 to 16 mg daily. Her serum phenytoin level had risen to 30 micrograms/mL but it fell when the chlorphenamine was withdrawn.[2]

The reason for these reactions is not clear but it has been suggested that chlorphenamine may have inhibited the metabolism of phenytoin by the liver. These are isolated cases, and their general relevance is uncertain, but it seems likely to be small.

1. Pugh RNH, Geddes AM, Yeoman WB. Interaction of phenytoin with chlorpheniramine. *Br J Clin Pharmacol* (1975) 2, 173–5.
2. Ahmad S, Laidlaw J, Houghton GW, Richens A. Involuntary movements caused by phenytoin intoxication in epileptic patients. *J Neurol Neurosurg Psychiatry* (1975) 38, 225–31.

Phenytoin + Coumarins and related drugs

The serum levels of phenytoin can be increased by dicoumarol (toxicity seen) and phenprocoumon, but they are usually unchanged by warfarin and phenindione. However, a single case of phenytoin toxicity has been seen with warfarin. Phenytoin would be expected to reduce the anticoagulant effects of coumarin anticoagulants, and this has been demonstrated for dicoumarol and warfarin. However, cases of increased effects of warfarin have been reported, and one study showed the effects of phenprocoumon were generally unaltered. A single case of severe bleeding has been described in a patient taking acenocoumarol, paroxetine and phenytoin.

Clinical evidence

The reports of interactions between phenytoin and various anticoagulants are summarised in 'Table 14.2', (p.556), and discussed in further detail below.

(a) Acenocoumarol

A 68-year-old woman with a double mitral valve lesion, atrial fibrillation and hypertension, taking digoxin and diuretics, was stabilised on acenocoumarol 17 mg per week in divided doses and paroxetine. Phenytoin 400 mg daily for 3 days then 300 mg daily was started because of a seizure, and 11 days later she developed ataxia, lethargy and nystagmus (free phenytoin levels of 12.5 micromol/L). At the same time her INR was found to have risen from a range of 2 to 4, up to 14.5 and a huge retroperitoneal haematoma was discovered. After appropriate treatment she was discharged taking acenocoumarol 13 mg per week in divided doses and half the phenytoin dosage.[1]

(b) Dicoumarol

Phenytoin 300 mg daily was given to 6 subjects taking dicoumarol 40 to 160 mg daily for a week. No significant changes in the prothrombin-pro-

Table 14.2 Summary of interactions between phenytoin and anticoagulants

Concurrent treatment with phenytoin and anticoagulant	*Effect on anticoagulant*	*Effect on serum phenytoin levels*
Dicoumarol	Reduced[1]	Markedly increased[10-12]
Phenprocoumon	Usually unchanged[2]	Increased[11]
Acenocoumarol	Single case of increase[3]	Uncertain
Warfarin	Increased[4-9,14] Single case of increase followed by decrease[7]	Usually unchanged[11] Increased in two cases[9,13]
Phenindione	Not documented	Usually unchanged[10,11]

1. Hansen JM, Siersbæk-Nielsen K, Kristensen M, Skovsted L,Christensen LK. Effect of diphenylhydantoin on the metabolism of dicoumarol in man. *Acta Med Scand* (1971) 189, 15-19.
2. Chrishe HW, Tauchert M, Hilger HH. Effect of phenytoin on the metabolism of phenprocoumon. *Eur J Clin Invest* (1974) 4, 331.
3. Abad-Santos F, Carcas AJ, F-Capitán C, Frias J. Case report. Retroperitoneal haematoma in a patient treated with acenocoumarol, phenytoin and paroxetine. *Clin Lab Haematol* (1995) 17, 195-7.
4. Nappi JM. Warfarin and phenytoin interaction. *Ann Intern Med* (1979) 90, 852.
5. Koch-Weser J. Haemorrhagic reactions and drug interactions in 500 warfarin treated patients. *Clin Pharmacol Ther* (1973) 14, 139.
6. Taylor JW, Alexander B, Lyon LW. A comparative evaluation of oral anticoagulant-phenytoin interactions. *Drug Intell Clin Pharm* (1980) 14, 669-73.
7. Levine M, Sheppard I. Biphasic interaction of phenytoin with warfarin. *Clin Pharm* (1984) 3, 200-3.
8. Panegyres PK, Rischbieth RH. Fatal phenytoin warfarin interaction. *Postgrad Med J* (1991) 67, 98.
9. Meisheri YV. Simultaneous phenytoin and warfarin toxicity on chronic concomitant therapy. *J Assoc Physicians India* (1996) 44, 661-2.
10. Hansen JM, Kristensen M, Skovsted L, Christensen LK. Dicoumarol-induced diphenylhydantoin intoxication. *Lancet* (1966) ii, 265-6.
11. Skovsted L, Kristensen M, Hansen JM, Siersbæk-Nielsen K. The effect of different oral anticoagulants on diphenylhydantoin (DPH) and tolbutamide metabolism. *Acta Med Scand* (1976) 199, 513-15.
12. Franzten E, Hansen JM, Hansen OE, Kristensen M. Phenytoin (Dilantin®) intoxication. *Acta Neurol Scand* (1967) 43, 440-6.
13. Rothermich NO. Diphenylhydantoin intoxication. *Lancet* (1966) ii, 640.
14. Hassan Y, Awaisu A, Aziz NA, Ismail O. The compexity of achieving anticoagulation control in the face of warfarin-phenytoin interaction. *Pharm World Sci* (2005) 27, 16-19.

convertin concentration occurred until 3 days after stopping the phenytoin. In the following 5 days it climbed from 20 to 50%, with an accompanying drop in the serum dicoumarol levels.[2] Four other subjects taking dicoumarol 60 mg daily were also given phenytoin 300 mg daily for the first week of treatment, and then 100 mg daily for 5 more weeks. The prothrombin-proconvertin concentration had risen from 20 to 70% after 2 weeks of concurrent treatment, representing an antagonism of the anticoagulant effect, and only fell to previous levels 5.5 weeks after stopping the phenytoin.[2]

A study in 6 subjects taking phenytoin 300 mg daily found that when they were also given dicoumarol (doses adjusted to give prothrombin values of about 30%) their serum phenytoin levels rose on average by almost 10 micrograms/mL (126%) over 7 days.[3] In another study the half-life of phenytoin in 3 patients increased by about fivefold during dicoumarol treatment.[4]

A patient taking dicoumarol developed phenytoin toxicity within a few days of starting to take phenytoin 300 mg daily (dose based on a weight of 62 kg). Phenytoin was withdrawn, and re-introduced at 200 mg daily, which gave satisfactory phenytoin levels.[5]

(c) Phenindione

A study in 4 patients taking phenytoin 300 mg daily found that phenindione did not affect their serum phenytoin levels.[4]

(d) Phenprocoumon

An investigation in patients taking long-term phenprocoumon treatment found that in the majority of cases phenytoin had no significant effect on either serum phenprocoumon levels or the anticoagulant control, although a few patients had a fall and others a rise in serum anticoagulant levels, with consequent decreased or increased effect.[6]

A study in 4 patients taking phenytoin 300 mg daily found that when they were given phenprocoumon their serum phenytoin levels rose from about 10 micrograms/mL to 14 micrograms/mL over 7 days.[4] The phenytoin half-life increased from 9.9 to 14 hours.

(e) Warfarin

The prothrombin time of a patient taking warfarin increased from 21 to 32 seconds over a month when phenytoin 300 mg daily was also given, despite a 22% reduction in the warfarin dosage. He was restabilised on the original warfarin dosage when the phenytoin was withdrawn. Six other reports describe this interaction.[7-12] One of them describes a patient who had an increased anticoagulant response to warfarin for the first 6 days after phenytoin was added. The anticoagulant effect then declined to less than the level seen before the addition of phenytoin.[10] Conversely, a population pharmacokinetic analysis reported that the clearance of warfarin was *increased* by 30% in 6 patients taking phenytoin or phenobarbital.[13] However, the findings were not reported separately for the two drugs, and are therefore difficult to interpret (phenobarbital is a known inducer of warfarin clearance, see 'Coumarins + Barbiturates', p.390).

A study in 2 patients taking phenytoin 300 mg daily found that their serum phenytoin levels were unaffected by warfarin given for 7 days, and the half-life of phenytoin in 4 other patients was unaffected.[4] However, a patient taking phenytoin 300 mg daily developed symptoms of toxicity shortly after starting to take warfarin.[14] Another patient developed phenytoin toxicity 6 months after starting to take phenytoin with warfarin.[12]

Mechanism

Multiple, complex and poorly understood. Dicoumarol and phenprocoumon (but not normally warfarin) appear to inhibit the metabolism of phenytoin by the liver, so that its loss from the body is reduced. Phenytoin is an inducer of the cytochrome P450 isoenzyme CYP2C9, which is involved in metabolism of the coumarin anticoagulants. Phenytoin would therefore be expected to decrease the levels and effect of some coumarins, and this has been shown for dicoumarol. However, increased effects of warfarin have been noted, suggesting reduced metabolism of warfarin. Why this occurs is uncertain, but poor CYP2C9 metaboliser phenotype (see 'Genetic factors', (p.4)) may provide an explanation.[15] Phenytoin possibly also has a diverse depressant effect on the liver, which lowers blood clotting factor production.[16]

Importance and management

None of these interactions has been extensively studied nor are they well established, but what is known suggests that the use of dicoumarol with phenytoin should be avoided or monitored very closely. Serum phenytoin levels and anticoagulant control should be well monitored if acenocoumarol, phenprocoumon or warfarin is given with phenytoin. Dosage adjustments may be needed to accommodate any interactions. Information about other anticoagulants (apart from phenindione, which had no effect on phenytoin levels) appears to be lacking, but it would clearly be prudent to monitor the effects of concurrent use.

1. Abad-Santos F, Carcas AJ, F-Capitán C, Frias J. Case report. Retroperitoneal haematoma in a patient treated with acenocoumarol, phenytoin and paroxetine. *Clin Lab Haematol* (1995) 17, 195–7.
2. Hansen JM, Siersbæk-Nielsen K, Kristensen M, Skovsted L,Christensen LK. Effect of diphenylhydantoin on the metabolism of dicoumarol in man. *Acta Med Scand* (1971) 189, 15–19.
3. Hansen JM, Kristensen M, Skovsted L, Christensen LK. Dicoumarol-induced diphenylhydantoin intoxication. *Lancet* (1966) ii, 265–6.
4. Skovsted L, Kristensen M, Hansen JM, Siersbæk-Nielsen K. The effect of different oral anticoagulants on diphenylhydantoin (DPH) and tolbutamide metabolism. *Acta Med Scand* (1976) 199, 513–15.
5. Franzten E, Hansen JM, Hansen OE, Kristensen M. Phenytoin (Dilantin®) intoxication. *Acta Neurol Scand* (1967) 43, 440–6.
6. Chrishe HW, Tauchert M, Hilger HH. Effect of phenytoin on the metabolism of phenprocoumon. *Eur J Clin Invest* (1974) 4, 331.
7. Nappi JM. Warfarin and phenytoin interaction. *Ann Intern Med* (1979) 90, 852.
8. Koch-Weser J. Haemorrhagic reactions and drug interactions in 500 warfarin treated patients. *Clin Pharmacol Ther* (1973) 14, 139.
9. Taylor JW, Alexander B, Lyon LW. A comparative evaluation of oral anticoagulant-phenytoin interactions. *Drug Intell Clin Pharm* (1980) 14, 669–73.
10. Levine M, Sheppard I. Biphasic interaction of phenytoin with warfarin. *Clin Pharm* (1984) 3, 200–3.
11. Panegyres PK, Rischbieth RH. Fatal phenytoin warfarin interaction. *Postgrad Med J* (1991) 67, 98.
12. Meisheri YV. Simultaneous phenytoin and warfarin toxicity on chronic concomitant therapy. *J Assoc Physicians India* (1996) 44, 661–2.
13. Mungall DR, Ludden TM, Marshall J, Hawkins DW, Talbert RL, Crawford MH. Population pharmacokinetics of racemic warfarin in adult patients. *J Pharmacokinet Biopharm* (1985) 13, 213–27.
14. Rothermich NO. Diphenylhydantoin intoxication. *Lancet* (1966) ii, 640.
15. Rettie AE, Haining RL, Bajpai M, Levy RH. A common genetic basis for idiosyncratic toxicity of warfarin and phenytoin. *Epilepsy Res* (1999) 35, 253–5.
16. Solomon GE, Hilgartner MW, Kutt H. Coagulation defects caused by diphenylhydantoin. *Neurology* (1972) 22, 1165–71.

Phenytoin + Dextromethorphan

Dextromethorphan appears not to affect the serum levels of phenytoin.

Clinical evidence, mechanism, importance and management

A double-blind, crossover study in 4 epileptic patients with severe complex partial seizures found that dextromethorphan 120 mg daily in liquid form (*Delsym*) over 3 months had no effect on their serum phenytoin levels. There was a non-significant alteration in the complex partial seizure and tonic-clonic seizure frequency.[1]

1. Fisher RS, Cysyk BJ, Lesser RP, Pontecorvo MJ, Ferkany JT, Schwerdt PR, Hart J, Gordon B. Dextromethorphan for treatment of complex partial seizures. *Neurology* (1990) 40, 547–9.

Phenytoin + Dextropropoxyphene (Propoxyphene)

Although no interaction generally appears to occur between phenytoin and dextropropoxyphene, a case report describes phenytoin toxicity in a patient given both drugs.

Clinical evidence, mechanism, importance and management

Only a very small rise in serum phenytoin levels occurred in 6 patients who took dextropropoxyphene 65 mg three times daily for 6 to 13 days.[1] In contrast, a review briefly mentions one patient who developed toxic serum phenytoin levels while taking dextropropoxyphene in doses of up to 600 mg daily on an as-required basis.[2]

Concurrent use need not be avoided, but since rises in the serum levels of phenytoin can occur it would be prudent to monitor the outcome. It is probably sufficient just to monitor for increased adverse effects (blurred vision, nystagmus, ataxia or drowsiness).

1. Hansen BS, Dam M, Brandt J, Hvidberg EF, Angelo H, Christensen JM, Lous P. Influence of dextropropoxyphene on steady state serum levels and protein binding of three anti-epileptic drugs in man. *Acta Neurol Scand* (1980) 61, 357–67.
2. Kutt H. Biochemical and genetic factors regulating Dilantin metabolism in man. *Ann N Y Acad Sci* (1971) 179, 704–22.

Phenytoin + Diazoxide

Three children and one adult had very marked reductions in serum phenytoin levels when diazoxide was given, and in one case seizure control was lost. There is some evidence that the effects of diazoxide may also be reduced.

Clinical evidence

A child receiving phenytoin 29 mg/kg daily and an adult receiving phenytoin 1 g daily were unable to achieve therapeutic phenytoin serum levels while taking diazoxide. When the diazoxide was withdrawn, satisfactory serum phenytoin levels were achieved with dosages of only 6.6 mg/kg and 400 mg daily, in the child and the adult, respectively. When diazoxide was restarted experimentally in the adult, the serum phenytoin levels became undetectable after 4 days, and seizures occurred.[1] Two other reports describe this interaction.[2,3] In addition it appears that the effects of the diazoxide can also be reduced.[2,4]

Mechanism

What is known suggests that diazoxide increases the metabolism and the clearance of phenytoin from the body.[1,2] The half-life of diazoxide is possibly reduced by phenytoin.[4]

Importance and management

Information is limited to these reports, but the interaction would appear to be established. Monitor the effects of concurrent use, being alert for the need to increase the phenytoin dosage. The clinical importance of the reduced diazoxide effects is uncertain.

1. Roe TF, Podosin RL, Blaskovics ME. Drug Interaction: diazoxide and diphenylhydantoin. *J Pediatr* (1975) 87, 480–4.
2. Petro DJ, Vannucci RC, Kulin HE. Diazoxide-diphenylhydantoin interaction. *J Pediatr* (1976) 89, 331–2.
3. Turck D, Largilliere C, Dupuis B, Farriaux JP. Interaction entre le diazoxide et la phénytoïne. *Presse Med* (1986) 15, 31.
4. Pruitt AW, Dayton PG, Patterson JH. Disposition of diazoxide in children. *Clin Pharmacol Ther* (1973) 14, 73–82.

Phenytoin + Dichloralphenazone

There is some evidence that serum phenytoin levels may be reduced by dichloralphenazone.

Clinical evidence, mechanism, importance and management

After taking dichloralphenazone 1.3 g each night for 13 nights the total body clearance of a single intravenous dose of phenytoin was doubled in 5 healthy subjects.[1] The phenazone component of dichloralphenazone is a known enzyme inducer and the increased clearance of phenytoin is probably due to an enhancement of its metabolism by the liver. There seem to be no additional reports of adverse effects in patients given both drugs, so that the clinical importance of this interaction is uncertain. However, it would seem prudent to watch for a reduction in serum phenytoin levels if dichloralphenazone is added to established treatment with phenytoin.

1. Riddell JG, Salem SAM, McDevitt DG. Interaction between phenytoin and dichloralphenazone. *Br J Clin Pharmacol* (1980) 9, 118P.

Phenytoin + Felbamate

Felbamate causes a moderate increase in plasma phenytoin levels. Felbamate plasma levels are reduced, but the importance of this is uncertain.

Clinical evidence

A pilot study in 4 patients noted that felbamate increased plasma phenytoin levels.[1] Therefore, in a further study the phenytoin dose was automatically reduced by 20% when felbamate was given. Of 5 patients, one needed a slight increase in phenytoin dosage, whereas 2 others needed a further reduction in their phenytoin dosage.[2] In a later full report of this study, it was noted that phenytoin dosage decreases of 10 to 30% were required to maintain stable levels.[3] Another study in epileptic patients found that felbamate 1.2 or 1.8 g daily increased the maximum plasma phenytoin levels by 31% and 69%, respectively. Higher felbamate doses necessitated phenytoin dose reductions of 20 to 40%.[4]

Studies in children and adults have found that phenytoin increased the clearance of felbamate by about 40%,[5,6] and decreased maximum felbamate levels by 56 to 60%, when compared with patients receiving felbamate alone.[4] Another report suggested that this effect was dose-dependent.[7]

Mechanism

Uncertain but felbamate probably acts as a competitive inhibitor of phenytoin metabolism, thereby reducing its loss from the body and increasing its serum levels,[2,8] whereas phenytoin induces felbamate metabolism, thereby increasing its clearance.[7]

Importance and management

Established interactions. The phenytoin dosage may need to be reduced (a 20 to 40% reduction seems to be about right[2,4,8]) if felbamate is added, and to increase it if felbamate is withdrawn. However, note that as phenytoin pharmacokinetics are non-linear any dosage adjustments will need to be assessed in individual patients. The importance of the reduced felbamate levels is uncertain, but is probably less important because felbamate has a wide therapeutic range.[4]

1. Sheridan PH, Ashworth M, Milne K, White BG, Santilli N, Lothman EW, Dreifuss FE, Jacobs MP, Martinez P, Leppik IE. Open pilot study of felbamate (ADD 03055) in partial seizures. *Epilepsia* (1986) 27, 649.
2. Fuerst RH, Graves NM, Leppik IE, Remmel RP, Rosenfeld WE, Sierzant TL. A preliminary report on alteration of carbamazepine and phenytoin metabolism by felbamate. *Drug Intell Clin Pharm* (1986) 20, 465–6.
3. Leppik IE, Dreifuss FE, Pledger GW, Graves NM, Santilli N, Drury I, Tsay JY, Jacobs MP, Bertram E, Cereghino JJ, Cooper G, Sahlroot JT, Sheridan P, Ashworth M, Lee SI, Sierzant TL. Felbamate for partial seizures: results of a controlled clinical trial. *Neurology* (1991) 41, 1785–9.
4. Sachdeo R, Wagner M, Sachdeo S, Schumaker RC, Lyness WH, Rosenberg A, Ward D, Perhach JL. Coadministration of phenytoin and felbamate: evidence of additional phenytoin dose-reduction requirements based on pharmacokinetics and tolerability with increasing doses of felbamate. *Epilepsia* (1999) 40, 1122–8.
5. Kelley MT, Walson PD, Cox S, Dusci LJ. Population pharmacokinetics of felbamate in children. *Ther Drug Monit* (1997) 19, 29–36.
6. Banfield CR, Zhu G-RR, Jen JF, Jensen PK, Schumaker RC, Perhach JL Affrime MB, Glue P. The effect of age on the apparent clearance of felbamate: a retrospective analysis using nonlinear mixed-effects modeling. *Ther Drug Monit* (1996) 18, 19–29.
7. Wagner ML, Graves NM, Marienau K, Holmes GB, Remmel RP, Leppik IE. Discontinuation of phenytoin and carbamazepine in patients receiving felbamate. *Epilepsia* (1991) 32, 398–406.
8. Fuerst RH, Graves NM, Leppik IE, Brundage RC, Holmes GB, Remmel RP. Felbamate increases phenytoin but decreases carbamazepine concentrations. *Epilepsia* (1988) 29, 488–91.

Phenytoin + Food

The absorption of phenytoin can be affected by some foods. A very marked reduction in phenytoin absorption has been described when it was given with enteral feeds (e.g. *Isocal, Osmolite*), by nasogastric or jejunostomy tubes.

Clinical evidence

(a) Food by mouth

A study found that serum drug levels were lower than expected when phenytoin was disguised in **vanilla pudding** and given to children. However, when the phenytoin was mixed with **apple sauce**, 3 out of 10 patients developed serum phenytoin levels within the toxic range, and the mean levels were twice those seen when the tablets were mixed with the **vanilla pudding**.[1] The absorption of phenytoin as the acid in a micronised form (*Fenantoin*, ACO, Sweden) was faster and the peak serum levels were on average 40% higher when it was given after a **standardised breakfast**.[2] In a further study to investigate the effects of component parts of the **standardised breakfast**, the same authors found that **fat** had no measurable effect, but **carbohydrate** may enhance and **protein** reduce the absorption of phenytoin.[3]

Another study in 5 subjects found that the bioavailability of a single dose of phenytoin was enhanced when it was given immediately after a '**balanced**' **meal**. Administration after a **high-lipid meal** resulted in large inter-patient variability in phenytoin bioavailability.[4] One single dose study found that, when taken with a **high-protein meal**, the total absorption of phenytoin was not affected, although it was slightly delayed.[5]

An epileptic had a marked fall in his serum phenytoin levels accompanied by an increased seizure frequency when phenytoin was given at bedtime with 8 oz of a food supplement (***Ensure***).[6] Another patient had reduced phenytoin serum levels when phenytoin was given as an oral suspension with oral ***Fresubin liquid food concentrate***.[7]

However, in contrast, a study in 10 healthy subjects found that when ***Ensure*** or ***Vivonex TEN*** was given every 4 hours for 24 hours, the absorption of a single 400-mg dose of phenytoin was unaffected.[8] Similarly, a single-dose study in healthy subjects found that the bioavailability of phenytoin sodium 400 mg in a capsule formulation (*Dilantin Kapseals*) was not affected by concurrent enteral feeds (***Ensure***).[9]

A study in healthy subjects found phenytoin levels were reduced by enteral feeds, but that it was easier to attain therapeutic levels of phenytoin in those also receiving a **meat-based** formulation (***Compleat Modified***) rather than a **protein hydrolysate** formulation (***Osmolite***).[10]

(b) Food by nasogastric tube

A patient taking phenytoin 300 mg daily who was being fed with ***Fortison*** through a nasogastric tube, following a brain injury sustained in a road traffic accident, had a phenytoin serum level of only 1 mg/L. When phenytoin 420 mg was given diluted in water and separated from the food by 2 hours, a serum level of 6 mg/L was achieved.[11] This report describes a similar reaction in another patient with a cerebral tumour.[11]

A study in 20 patients and 5 healthy subjects found that phenytoin absorption was reduced by about 70% when it was given by nasogastric tube with an **enteral feed** product (***Isocal***) at a rate of 100 to 125 mL/hour.[12] Other reports describe the same interaction in patients given ***Ensure***,[13] ***Isocal***,[14,15] or ***Osmolite***.[13,16-18]

However, another study in healthy subjects found the absolute bioavailability of phenytoin suspension or phenytoin sodium solution given by nasogastric tube was not affected by an enteral feed product (***Isocal***).[19]

(c) Food by jejunostomy tube

A woman with a history of seizures had acceptable serum phenytoin levels when phenytoin was given intravenously, but they fell from 19.1 micrograms/mL to less than 2.5 micrograms/mL when a comparable dose of phenytoin suspension was given in the presence of an **enteral feed** product (***Jevity***), given by jejunostomy tube.[20]

Mechanism

Not fully resolved. Phenytoin can bind to some food substances, which reduces its absorption.[21,22] One study in healthy subjects failed to find any difference in phenytoin bioavailability after fasting or with *Ensure* (given hourly or every 4 hours), suggesting that factors other than direct contact of phenytoin and feed contribute to decreased phenytoin bioavailability.[23] Phenytoin can also become bound to the nasogastric tubing[24] and may also be poorly absorbed if the tubing empties into the duodenum rather than the stomach.[24] Delivery into the jejunum appears to have an even greater detrimental effect on phenytoin absorption, because there is even less time for adequate absorption.[20] Other factors that could contribute to the interaction are gastrointestinal transit time, the nitrogen source in the feed, the calcium content and pH of the feed, the dose form of phenytoin or its dilution before administration.[25]

Importance and management

Phenytoin is often taken orally with food to reduce gastric irritation. This normally appears not to have a marked effect on absorption, but the studies cited above show that some formulations and some foods can interact. If there are problems with the control of seizures or evidence of toxicity, review how and when the patient is taking the phenytoin.

Some studies in healthy subjects failed to find an interaction between phenytoin and enteral feeding.[8,9,19,23] However, many studies in patients have found a clinically important interaction between phenytoin and enteral feeds given orally or by nasogastric tube. The markedly reduced bioavailability associated with the nasogastric route has been successfully managed by giving the phenytoin diluted in water 2 hours after stopping the feed, flushing with 60 mL of water, and waiting another 2 hours before restarting the feed,[11,12] However, one limited study failed to confirm that this method is successful,[13] and some sources suggest waiting 1 hour[26] or 6 hours[14] after the phenytoin dose before restarting the feed. Some increase in the phenytoin dosage may also be needed. Monitor concurrent use closely. The same problem can clearly also occur when enteral feeds are given by jejunostomy tube. Approaches on how to minimise any potential interaction have been reported,[25,27] including the development and use of an algorithm.[25]

1. Jann MW, Bean J, Fidone G. Interaction of dietary pudding with phenytoin. *Pediatrics* (1986) 78, 952–3.
2. Melander A, Brante G, Johansson Ö, Lindberg T, Wåhlin-Boll E. Influence of food on the absorption of phenytoin in man. *Eur J Clin Pharmacol* (1979) 15, 269–74.

3. Johansson Ö, Wahlin-Boll E, Lindberg T, Melander A. Opposite effects of carbohydrate and protein on phenytoin absorption in man. *Drug Nutr Interact* (1983) 2, 139–44.
4. Sekikawa H, Nakano M, Takada M, Arita T. Influence of dietary components on the bioavailability of phenytoin. *Chem Pharm Bull (Tokyo)* (1980) 28, 2443–9.
5. Kennedy MC, Wade DN. The effect of food on the absorption of phenytoin. *Aust N Z J Med* (1982) 12, 258–61.
6. Longe RL, Smith OB. Phenytoin interaction with an oral feeding results in loss of seizure control. *J Am Geriatr Soc* (1988) 36, 542–4.
7. Taylor DM, Massey CA, Willson WG, Dhillon S. Lowered serum phenytoin concentrations during therapy with liquid food concentrates. *Ann Pharmacother* (1993) 27, 369.
8. Marvel ME, Bertino JS. Comparative effects of an elemental and a complex enteral feeding formulation on the absorption of phenytoin suspension. *J Parenter Enteral Nutr* (1991) 15, 316–8.
9. Nishimura LY, Armstrong EP, Plezia PM, Iacono RP. Influence of enteral feedings on phenytoin sodium absorption from capsules. *Drug Intell Clin Pharm* (1988) 22, 130–3.
10. Guidry JR, Eastwood TF, Curry SC. Phenytoin absorption in volunteers receiving selected enteral feedings. *West J Med* (1989) 150, 659–61.
11. Summers VM, Grant R. Nasogastric feeding and phenytoin interaction. *Pharm J* (1989) 243, 181.
12. Bauer LA. Interference of oral phenytoin absorption by continuous nasogastric feedings. *Neurology* (1982) 32, 570–2.
13. Ozuna J, Friel P. Effect of enteral tube feeding on serum phenytoin levels. *J Neurosurg Nurs* (1984) 16, 289–91.
14. Pearce GA. Apparent inhibition of phenytoin absorption by an enteral nutrient formula. *Aust J Hosp Pharm* (1988) 18, 289–92.
15. Worden JP, Wood CA, Workman CH. Phenytoin and nasogastric feedings. *Neurology* (1984) 34, 132.
16. Hatton RC. Dietary interaction with phenytoin. *Clin Pharm* (1984) 3, 110–11.
17. Weinryb J, Cogen R. Interaction of nasogastric phenytoin and enteral feeding solution. *J Am Geriatr Soc* (1989) 37, 195–6.
18. Maynard GA, Jones KM, Guidry JR. Phenytoin absorption from tube feedings. *Arch Intern Med* (1987) 147, 1821.
19. Doak KK, Haas CE, Dunnigan KJ, Reiss RA, Reiser JR, Huntress J, Altavela JL. Bioavailability of phenytoin acid and phenytoin sodium with enteral feedings. *Pharmacotherapy* (1998) 18, 637–45.
20. Rodman DP, Stevenson TL, Ray TR. Phenytoin malabsorption after jejunostomy tube delivery. *Pharmacotherapy* (1995) 15, 801–5.
21. Miller SW, Strom JG. Stability of phenytoin in three enteral nutrient formulas. *Am J Hosp Pharm* (1988) 45, 2529–32.
22. Hooks MA, Longe RL, Taylor AT, Francisco GE. Recovery of phenytoin from an enteral nutrient formula. *Am J Hosp Pharm* (1986) 43, 685–8.
23. Krueger KA, Garnett WR, Comstock TJ, Fitzsimmons WE, Karnes HT, Pellock JM. Effect of two administration schedules of an enteral nutrient formula on phenytoin bioavailability. *Epilepsia* (1987) 28, 706–12.
24. Fleisher D, Sheth N, Kou JH. Phenytoin interaction with enteral feedings administered through nasogastric tubes. *J Parenter Enteral Nutr* (1990) 14, 513–16.
25. Gilbert S. How to minimize interaction between phenytoin and enteral feedings: two approaches. A Strategic approach. *Nutr Clin Pract* (1996) 11, 28–30.
26. Faraji B, Yu P-P. Serum phenytoin levels of patients on gastrostomy tube feeding. *J Neurosci Nurs* (1998) 30, 55–9.
27. Hatton J, Magnuson B. How to minimize interaction between phenytoin and enteral feedings: two approaches. B Therapeutic options. *Nutr Clin Pract* (1996) 11, 30–1.

Phenytoin + H_2-receptor antagonists

Phenytoin serum levels are raised by the use of cimetidine and toxicity has occurred. Limited evidence suggests that low (non-prescription) doses of cimetidine may not interact. Very rarely bone marrow depression develops on concurrent use. Famotidine, nizatidine and ranitidine do not normally interact with phenytoin, although, rarely, cases of elevated phenytoin levels have been reported.

Clinical evidence

(a) Cimetidine

The serum phenytoin levels of 9 patients rose by 60% (from 5.7 to 9.1 micrograms/mL) when they were given cimetidine 200 mg three times daily and 400 mg at night for 3 weeks. The serum phenytoin level returned to its former levels within 2 weeks of stopping the cimetidine.[1]

This interaction has been described in many reports and studies involving patients[2-7] and healthy subjects.[8-11] Phenytoin toxicity has developed in some individuals. The extent of the rise in serum levels is very variable being quoted as 13 to 33% over about 6 days in one report[2] and 22 to 280% over 3 weeks in others.[4,12] There is some evidence that the effect may be dependent on cimetidine dose. One study found that the effect of cimetidine 2.4 g daily was greater than that of 1.2 g daily or 400 mg daily, which did not differ from each other.[9] In another study, cimetidine 200 mg twice daily for 2 weeks had no effect on serum phenytoin levels in 9 patients taking stable doses of phenytoin.[13]

Severe and life-threatening agranulocytosis in 2 patients[14,15] and thrombocytopenia in 6 other patients[16-18] have been attributed to the concurrent use of phenytoin and cimetidine. Severe skin reactions have also been reported in 3 patients treated with phenytoin, cimetidine, and dexamethasone after resection of brain tumours, which resolved on discontinuing phenytoin.[19] See also 'Corticosteroids + Phenytoin', p.1059 for the effects of dexamethasone on phenytoin levels.

(b) Famotidine

A study in 10 subjects found that famotidine 40 mg daily for 7 days did not alter the pharmacokinetics of a single dose of phenytoin.[20] However, a single case report describes phenytoin toxicity and an almost doubled serum level (increase from 18 to 33 micrograms/mL) in a patient given famotidine. This was managed by a reduction in the phenytoin dose.[21]

(c) Nizatidine

Nizatidine 150 mg twice daily for 9 doses had no effects on the pharmacokinetics of a single dose of phenytoin in 18 healthy subjects.[22]

(d) Ranitidine

A study in 4 patients found that ranitidine 150 mg twice daily for 2 weeks did not alter phenytoin levels.[4,12] Similarly, a double-blind, crossover study in healthy subjects found that ranitidine 150 mg twice daily for 6 days had no significant effect on steady state phenytoin levels.[23] However, one patient had a 40% increase in serum phenytoin levels over a month when ranitidine 150 mg twice daily was given,[24] and two others also developed elevated serum phenytoin levels and signs of toxicity, which were attributed to the use of ranitidine.[25,26] Another patient developed a severe skin reaction when treated with phenytoin, ranitidine and dexamethasone after resection of a brain tumour, which resolved on discontinuing phenytoin.[19]

Mechanism

Cimetidine inhibits the activity of the liver enzymes concerned with the metabolism of phenytoin, thus allowing it to accumulate in the body and, in some instances, to reach toxic concentrations. Famotidine, nizatidine and ranitidine normally do not affect these enzymes. Agranulocytosis and thrombocytopenia are relatively rare manifestations of bone marrow depression caused by both phenytoin and the H_2-receptor antagonists.

Importance and management

The interaction between phenytoin and cimetidine is well documented and clinically important. It is not possible to identify individuals who will show the greatest response, but those with serum levels at the top end of the therapeutic range are most at risk. Do not give cimetidine to patients already taking phenytoin unless the serum levels can be monitored and suitable dosage reductions made as necessary. The results from one small study suggest that low doses of cimetidine (such as those available without a prescription in the UK) may not interact.[13] Since there are only rare cases cited for famotidine, nizatidine, and ranitidine extra monitoring beyond that usually carried out in patients receiving phenytoin does not appear to be warranted but be alert for signs of phenytoin toxicity (e.g. blurred vision, nystagmus, ataxia or drowsiness) when these H_2-receptor antagonists are first added to established treatment with phenytoin.

1. Neuvonen PJ, Tokola R, Kaste M. Cimetidine-phenytoin interaction: effect on serum phenytoin concentration and antipyrine test. *Eur J Clin Pharmacol* (1981) 21, 215–20.
2. Hetzel DJ, Bochner F, Hallpike JF, Shearman DJC, Hann CS. Cimetidine interaction with phenytoin. *BMJ* (1981) 282, 1512.
3. Algozzine GJ, Stewart RB, Springer PK. Decreased clearance of phenytoin with cimetidine. *Ann Intern Med* (1981) 95, 244–5.
4. Watts RW, Hetzel DJ, Bochner F, Hallpike JF, Hann CS, Shearman DJC. Lack of interaction between ranitidine and phenytoin. *Br J Clin Pharmacol* (1983) 15, 499–500.
5. Phillips P, Hansky J. Phenytoin toxicity secondary to cimetidine administration. *Med J Aust* (1984) 141, 602.
6. Griffin JW, May JR, DiPiro JT. Drug interactions: theory versus practice. *Am J Med* (1984) 77 (Suppl 5B), 85–9.
7. Salem RB, Breland BD, Mishra SK, Jordan JE. Effect of cimetidine on phenytoin serum levels. *Epilepsia* (1983) 24, 284–8.
8. Iteogu MO, Murphy JE, Shleifer N, Davis R. Effect of cimetidine on single-dose phenytoin kinetics. *Clin Pharm* (1983) 2, 302–4.
9. Bartle WR, Walker SE, Shapero T. Dose-dependent effect of cimetidine on phenytoin kinetics. *Clin Pharmacol Ther* (1983) 33, 649–55.
10. Frigo GM, Lecchini S, Caravaggi M, Gatti G, Tonini M, D'Angelo L, Perucca E, Crema A. Reduction of phenytoin clearance caused by cimetidine. *Eur J Clin Pharmacol* (1983) 25, 135–7.
11. Hsieh Y-Y, Huang J-D, Lai M-L, Lin M-S, Liu R-T, Wan EC-J. The complexity of cimetidine-phenytoin interaction. *Taiwan Yi Xue Hui Za Zhi* (1986) 85, 395–402.
12. Hetzel DJ, Watts RW, Bochner F, Shearman DJC. Ranitidine, unlike cimetidine, does not interact with phenytoin. *Aust N Z J Med* (1983) 13, 324.
13. Rafi JA, Frazier LM, Driscoll-Bannister SM, O'Hara KA, Garnett WR, Pugh CB. Effect of over-the-counter cimetidine on phenytoin concentrations in patients with seizures. *Ann Pharmacother* (1999) 33, 769–74.
14. Sazie E, Jaffe JP. Severe granulocytopenia with cimetidine and phenytoin. *Ann Intern Med* (1980) 93, 151–2.
15. Al-Kawas FH, Lenes BA, Sacher RA. Cimetidine and agranulocytosis. *Ann Intern Med* (1979) 90, 992–3.
16. Wong YY, Lichtor T, Brown FD. Severe thrombocytopenia associated with phenytoin and cimetidine therapy. *Surg Neurol* (1985) 23, 169–72.
17. Yue CP, Mann KS, Chan KH. Severe thrombocytopenia due to combined cimetidine and phenytoin therapy. *Neurosurgery* (1987) 20, 963–5.

18. Arbiser JL, Goldstein AM, Gordon D. Thrombocytopenia following administration of phenytoin, dexamethasone and cimetidine: a case report and a potential mechanism. *J Intern Med* (1993) 234, 91–4.
19. Cohen AD, Reichental E, Halevy S. Phenytoin-induced severe cutaneous drug reactions: suspected interactions with corticosteroids and H2-blockers. *Isr Med Assoc J* (1999) 1, 95–7.
20. Sambol NC, Upton RA, Chremos AN, Lin ET, Williams RL. A comparison of the influence of famotidine and cimetidine on phenytoin elimination and hepatic blood flow. *Br J Clin Pharmacol* (1989) 27, 83–7.
21. Shinn AF. Unrecognized drug interactions with famotidine and nizatidine. *Arch Intern Med* (1991) 151, 810, 814.
22. Bachmann KA, Sullivan TJ, Jauregui L, Reese JH, Miller K, Levine L. Absence of an inhibitory effect of omeprazole and nizatidine on phenytoin disposition, a marker of CYP2C activity. *Br J Clin Pharmacol* (1993) 36, 380–2.
23. Mukherjee S, Wicks JFC, Dixon JS, Richens A. Absence of a pharmacokinetic interaction between ranitidine and phenytoin. *Gastroenterology* (1996) 110 (Suppl), A202.
24. Bramhall D, Levine M. Possible interaction of ranitidine with phenytoin. *Drug Intell Clin Pharm* (1988) 22, 979–80.
25. Tse CST, Akinwande KI, Biallowons K. Phenytoin concentration elevation subsequent to ranitidine administration. *Ann Pharmacother* (1993) 27, 1448–51.
26. Tse CST, Iagmin P. Phenytoin and ranitidine interaction. *Ann Intern Med* (1994) 120, 892–3.

Phenytoin + Immunoglobulins

An isolated report describes an epileptic patient taking phenytoin who died, probably from hypersensitivity myocarditis, two days after receiving immunoglobulins for Guillain-Barré syndrome.

Clinical evidence, mechanism, importance and management

A man who had been taking phenytoin for 8 years was diagnosed as having Guillain-Barré syndrome for which intravenous immunoglobulin was started at 400 mg/kg daily. On day 2 the patient complained of abdominal pain, aching shoulders and backache. He subsequently developed hypotension and died, despite resuscitation attempts. A post-mortem suggested that he had died from hypersensitivity myocarditis, which the authors of the report suggest might have resulted from the long-term use of the phenytoin.[1] This hypersensitivity with phenytoin has been reported before.[2] Because this complication is so serious, the authors of this report suggest that leukocyte counts, in particular eosinophils, should be monitored if immunoglobulins and phenytoin are given concurrently.[1] The general importance of this alleged interaction is not known. However, note that subsequent to this report, intravenous immunoglobulin has successfully been used to treat a few cases of hypersensitivity syndrome to phenytoin,[3-5] one including eosinophilia.[3] Intravenous immunoglobulin alone has also been associated with causing myocarditis.[6]

1. Koehler PJ, Koudstaal J. Lethal hypersensitivity myocarditis associated with the use of intravenous gammaglobulin for Guillain-Barré syndrome, in combination with phenytoin. *J Neurol* (1996) 243, 366–7.
2. Fenoglio JJ, McAllister HA, Mullick FG. Drug related myocarditis.I. Hypersensitivity myocarditis. *Hum Pathol* (1981) 12, 900–7.
3. Scheuerman O, Nofech-Moses Y, Rachmel A, Ashkenazi S. Successful treatment of antiepileptic drug hypersensitivity syndrome with intravenous immune globulin. *Pediatrics* (2001) 107, E14.
4. Salzman MB, Smith EM. Phenytoin-induced thrombocytopenia treated with intravenous immune globulin. *J Pediatr Hematol Oncol* (1998) 20, 152–3.
5. Mostella J, Pieroni R, Jones R, Finch CK. Anticonvulsant hypersensitivity syndrome: treatment with corticosteroids and intravenous immunoglobulin. *South Med J* (2004) 97, 319–21.
6. Akhtar I, Bastani B. Acute renal failure and myocarditis associated with intravenous immunoglobulin therapy. *Ann Intern Med* (2003) 139, W65.

Phenytoin + Influenza vaccines

Influenza vaccine is reported to increase, decrease or to have no effect on phenytoin serum levels. The efficacy of the vaccine remains unchanged.

Clinical evidence

(a) Phenytoin levels

The serum phenytoin levels of 8 epileptic children were increased by about 50%, from 9.5 to 15.16 micrograms/mL, 7 days after they were given 0.5 mL of an influenza virus vaccine USP, types A and B, whole virus (Squibb). The phenytoin levels returned to baseline over the following 7 days.[1] Temporary rises in the serum phenytoin levels of 3 patients, apparently caused by influenza vaccination, are briefly described in another report.[2]

In contrast, another study in 16 patients given 0.5 mL of an inactivated whole-virion trivalent influenza vaccine found that 7 and 14 days later their mean serum phenytoin levels were not significantly altered, although 4 of them showed a trend towards raised levels. Subsequently, these 4 patients had serum phenytoin increases ranging from 46 to 170%, which returned to baseline between week 4 and 17 after immunisation.[3]

In yet another study, within 4 days of receiving 0.5 mL of a subvirion, trivalent influenza vaccine, the serum phenytoin levels of 7 patients were reduced by 11 to 14%, which is unlikely to have much clinical significance.[4] A further study[5] measured both free and total phenytoin levels in 8 patients receiving phenytoin alone. Two days after receiving 0.5 mL of a trivalent influenza vaccine, the total phenytoin level had increased by 10%, and this then returned to baseline levels by day 7. However, the free phenytoin level gradually decreased after vaccination to a maximum of 25% less at day 14.

(b) Vaccine efficacy

The efficacy of influenza vaccine is reported to be unchanged by phenytoin.[6]

Mechanism

Where an interaction occurs it is suggested that it may be due to the inhibitory effect of the vaccine on the liver enzymes concerned with the metabolism of the phenytoin, resulting in a reduced clearance from the body.[1]

Importance and management

The outcome of immunisation with influenza vaccine on phenytoin levels is uncertain. Concurrent use need not be avoided but it would be prudent to monitor the effects closely. Be aware that any alteration in levels may take a couple of weeks to develop and usually resolves spontaneously.

1. Jann MW, Fidone GS. Effect of influenza vaccine on serum anticonvulsant concentrations. *Clin Pharm* (1986) 5, 817–20.
2. Mooradian AD, Hernandez L, Tamai IC, Marshall C. Variability of serum phenytoin concentrations in nursing home patients. *Arch Intern Med* (1989) 149, 890–2.
3. Levine M, Jones MW, Gribble M. Increased serum phenytoin concentration following influenza vaccination. *Clin Pharm* (1984) 3, 505–9.
4. Sawchuk RJ, Rector TS, Fordice JJ, Leppik IE. Case report. Effect of influenza vaccination on plasma phenytoin concentrations. *Ther Drug Monit* (1979) 1, 285–8.
5. Smith CD, Bledsoe MA, Curran R, Green L, Lewis J. Effect of influenza vaccine on serum concentrations of total and free phenytoin. *Clin Pharm* (1988) 7, 828–32.
6. Levine M, Beattie BL, McLean DM, Corman D. Phenytoin therapy and immune response to influenza vaccine. *Clin Pharm* (1985) 4, 191–4.

Phenytoin + Isotretinoin

A study in 7 healthy subjects taking phenytoin 300 mg daily found that the addition of isotretinoin 40 mg twice daily for 11 days had no effect on the steady-state pharmacokinetics of phenytoin.[1] No special precautions would seem to be needed if these drugs are given concurrently.

1. Oo C, Barsanti F, Zhang R. Lack of effect of isotretinoin on the pharmacokinetics of phenytoin at steady-state. *Pharm Res* (1997) 14 (11 Suppl), S-561.

Phenytoin + Loxapine

A single case report describes decreased serum phenytoin levels in a patient given loxapine.

Clinical evidence, mechanism, importance and management

The serum phenytoin levels of an epileptic patient were reduced by loxapine, and showed a marked rise when it was withdrawn.[1] The general importance of this case is uncertain, but bear this interaction in mind, particularly as loxapine can lower the convulsive threshold.

1. Ryan GM, Matthews PA. Phenytoin metabolism stimulated by loxapine. *Drug Intell Clin Pharm* (1977) 11, 428.

Phenytoin + Macrolides

Erythromycin appears not to interact with phenytoin. Limited evidence suggests that clarithromycin may possibly raise serum phenytoin levels.

Clinical evidence

(a) Clarithromycin

A retrospective study of serum phenytoin levels in a group of 21 patients with AIDS and a large control group of 557 subjects suggested that the concurrent use of clarithromycin (a total of 22 samples from at least 10 patients) was associated with higher serum phenytoin levels. The concentration/dose ratio of the phenytoin was 1.6 without clarithromycin and 3.9 with clarithromycin.[1]

(b) Erythromycin

A single-dose study found that the mean clearance of phenytoin was unchanged by erythromycin 333 mg every 8 hours for 7 days in 8 healthy subjects. However, there were occasional large changes in phenytoin clearance.[2] Similarly, in another study erythromycin 250 mg every 6 hours for 7 days had no effect on the pharmacokinetics of a single dose of phenytoin in 8 healthy subjects.[3]

Mechanism

Not known, but it could be that clarithromycin inhibits the metabolism of the phenytoin by the liver. An *animal* study found that erythromycin, clarithromycin, and **roxithromycin** reduced the metabolism and increased levels of phenytoin.[4]

Importance and management

This seems to be the first and only evidence that clarithromycin possibly interacts like this. Given that the interaction was identified retrospectively any interaction seems unlikely to cause an acute problem. Erythromycin appears not to interact with phenytoin, but nevertheless caution has been recommended.[2]

1. Burger DM, Meenhorst PL, Mulder JW, Kraaijeveld CL, Koks CHW, Bult A, Beijnen JH. Therapeutic drug monitoring of phenytoin in patients with the acquired immunodeficiency syndrome. *Ther Drug Monit* (1994) 16, 616–20.
2. Bachmann K, Schwartz JI, Forney RB, Jauregui L. Single dose phenytoin clearance during erythromycin treatment. *Res Commun Chem Pathol Pharmacol* (1984) 46, 207–17.
3. Milne RW, Coulthard K, Nation RL, Penna AC, Roberts G, Sansom LN. Lack of effect of erythromycin on the pharmacokinetics of single oral doses of phenytoin. *Br J Clin Pharmacol* (1988) 26, 330–3.
4. Al-Humayyd MS. Pharmacokinetic interactions between erythromycin, clarithromycin, roxithromycin and phenytoin in the rat. *Chemotherapy* (1997) 43, 77–85.

Phenytoin + Methylphenidate

Although two small studies found that methylphenidate did not alter phenytoin levels, raised serum phenytoin levels and phenytoin toxicity have been seen in three patients given methylphenidate.

Clinical evidence

A 5-year-old hyperkinetic epileptic boy taking phenytoin 8.9 mg/kg and **primidone** 17.7 mg/kg daily, developed ataxia without nystagmus when he was also given methylphenidate 40 mg daily. Serum levels of both the antiepileptics were found to be at toxic levels and only began to fall when the methylphenidate dosage was reduced.[1]

A further case of phenytoin toxicity occurred in another child given methylphenidate.[2] Only one other case has been reported, but this patient was later rechallenged with the two drugs and phenytoin toxicity was not seen.[3]

Furthermore, this interaction has not been seen in clinical studies and observations of 3 healthy subjects[3] and more than 11 patients[4] taking phenytoin and methylphenidate.

Mechanism

Not fully understood. The suggestion is that methylphenidate acts as an enzyme inhibitor, slowing the metabolism of the phenytoin by the liver and leading to its accumulation in those individuals whose drug metabolising system is virtually saturated by phenytoin.

Importance and management

These appear to be the only reports, and any interaction is not established. Concurrent use of phenytoin need not be avoided but be alert for any evidence of toxicity, particularly if the phenytoin dosage is high. It would seem prudent to monitor for symptoms of phenytoin toxicity (e.g. blurred vision, nystagmus, ataxia or drowsiness) and take levels if necessary.

1. Garrettson LK, Perel JM, Dayton PG. Methylphenidate interaction with both anticonvulsants and ethyl biscoumacetate. A new action of methylphenidate. *JAMA* (1969) 207, 2053–6.
2. Ghofrani M. Possible phenytoin-methylphenidate interaction. *Dev Med Child Neurol* (1988) 30, 267–8.
3. Mirkin BL, Wright F. Drug interactions: effect of methylphenidate on the disposition of diphenylhydantoin in man. *Neurology* (1971) 21, 1123–8.
4. Kupferberg HJ, Jeffery W, Hunninghake DB. Effect of methylphenidate on plasma anticonvulsant levels. *Clin Pharmacol Ther* (1972) 13, 201–4.

Phenytoin + Metronidazole

One study found that the half-life of phenytoin was modestly prolonged by metronidazole, whereas another found no change in phenytoin pharmacokinetics. An anecdotal report describes a few patients who developed toxic phenytoin levels when given metronidazole.

Clinical evidence, mechanism, importance and management

A pharmacokinetic study[1] in 7 healthy subjects found that metronidazole 250 mg three times daily increased the half-life of a single 300-mg intravenous dose of phenytoin by about 40% (from 16 to 23 hours) and reduced the clearance by 15%. In contrast, another study in 5 healthy subjects found that the pharmacokinetics of a single 300-mg oral dose of phenytoin were unaffected by metronidazole 400 mg twice daily for 6 days.[2] An anecdotal report describes several patients (exact number not stated) who developed toxic phenytoin serum levels when given metronidazole.[3] These appear to be the only reports of this potential interaction, and the reason for their discordant findings is not clear. It seems likely that few patients are likely to experience a clinically significant interaction.

1. Blyden GT, Scavone JM, Greenblatt DJ. Metronidazole impairs clearance of phenytoin but not of alprazolam or lorazepam. *J Clin Pharmacol* (1988) 28, 240–5.
2. Jensen JC, Gugler R. Interaction between metronidazole and drugs eliminated by oxidative metabolism. *Clin Pharmacol Ther* (1985) 37, 407–10.
3. Picard EH. Side effects of metronidazole. *Mayo Clin Proc* (1983) 58, 401.

Phenytoin + Nefazodone

Nefazodone did not affect the pharmacokinetics of phenytoin in healthy subjects.

Clinical evidence, mechanism, importance and management

Nefazodone 200 mg twice daily for 7 days had no effect on the pharmacokinetics of a single 300-mg dose of phenytoin in healthy subjects, and no changes in vital signs, ECGs or other physical measurements were seen. There was no evidence that a clinically significant interaction was likely.[1]

1. Marino MR, Langenbacher KM, Hammett JL, Nichola P, Uderman HD. The effect of nefazodone on the single-dose pharmacokinetics of phenytoin in healthy male subjects. *J Clin Psychopharmacol* (1997) 17, 27–33.

Phenytoin + Nitrofurantoin

An isolated report describes a reduction in serum phenytoin levels and poor seizure control in a patient given nitrofurantoin.

Clinical evidence, mechanism, importance and management

A patient with seizures due to a brain tumour was taking phenytoin 300 mg daily. He had a seizure within a day of being given nitrofurantoin 200 mg for a urinary-tract infection and, despite a recent increase in the phenytoin dose to 350 mg, his serum phenytoin levels were found to be modestly reduced (from about 9 to 7.6 micrograms/mL). They continued to fall to 6.3 micrograms/mL despite a further increase in the phenytoin dosage to 400 mg daily. When the nitrofurantoin was stopped he was restabilised on his original dosage of phenytoin. The reasons are not understood but, on the basis of a noted rise in serum gamma glutamyltransferase levels during the use of the nitrofurantoin, the authors speculate that it increased the metabolism of the phenytoin by the liver.[1] The general importance of this interaction is uncertain, but probably small.

1. Heipertz R, Pilz H. Interaction of nitrofurantoin with diphenylhydantoin. *J Neurol* (1978) 218, 297–301.

Phenytoin + Orlistat

Orlistat does not alter the pharmacokinetics of phenytoin.

Clinical evidence, mechanism, importance and management

In a placebo-controlled, randomised, crossover study, 12 healthy subjects were given a single 300-mg dose of phenytoin on day 4 of a 7-day course of orlistat 120 mg three times daily. The pharmacokinetics of phenytoin were unchanged by orlistat,[1] and no special precautions are therefore thought to be needed if these two drugs are given concurrently.

1. Melia AT, Mulligan TE, Zhi J. The effect of orlistat on the pharmacokinetics of phenytoin in healthy volunteers. *J Clin Pharmacol* (1996) 36, 654–8.

Phenytoin + Penicillins

An isolated case describes a marked reduction in serum phenytoin levels, resulting in seizures, which was attributed to the use of oxacillin.

Clinical evidence, mechanism, importance and management

An epileptic woman taking phenytoin 400 mg daily, hospitalised for second degree burns sustained during a generalised seizure, experienced brief clonic seizures and was found to have an marked reduction in her serum phenytoin levels, from 16.3 to 3.5 micrograms/mL, which was attributed to the concurrent use of oral **oxacillin** 500 mg every 6 hours. The phenytoin dose was increased, but seizures continued and progressed to status epilepticus, and intravenous phenytoin was given. Doses of oral phenytoin of about 600 mg daily were required to maintain minimum therapeutic levels, sometimes with supplementation of small intravenous doses. Just before the **oxacillin** was withdrawn the serum phenytoin level was 22.3 micrograms/mL, but 6 months later it had risen to 39.9 micrograms/mL, and the phenytoin dose was reduced.[1] Other studies have shown that penicillins such as **oxacillin**, **cloxacillin** and **dicloxacillin** can displace phenytoin from plasma protein binding, decreasing total serum levels but increasing the free fraction of phenytoin. If anything, this would be predicted to increase phenytoin toxicity.[2,3] This seems to be only report of an adverse interaction between phenytoin and a penicillin. Its general importance is probably small.

1. Fincham RW, Wiley DE, Schottelius DD. Use of phenytoin levels in a case of status epilepticus. *Neurology* (1976) 26, 879–81.
2. Arimori K, Nakano M, Otagiri M, Uekama K. Effects of penicillins on binding of phenytoin to plasma proteins *in vitro* and *in vivo*. *Biopharm Drug Dispos* (1984) 5, 219–27.
3. Dasgupta A, Sperelakis A, Mason A, Dean R. Phenytoin-oxacillin interactions in normal and uremic sera. *Pharmacotherapy* (1997) 17, 375–8.

Phenytoin + Pheneturide

Phenytoin serum levels can be increased by about 50% by pheneturide.

Clinical evidence, mechanism, importance and management

In 9 patients the steady-state half-life of phenytoin was prolonged from 32 to 47 hours by pheneturide. Mean serum levels were raised by about 50% but fell rapidly over the 2 weeks after pheneturide was withdrawn.[1] This study confirms a previous report of this interaction.[2] The reason for this interaction is uncertain, but since the two drugs have a similar structure it is possible that they compete for the same metabolising enzymes in the liver, thereby resulting, at least initially, in a reduction in the metabolism of the phenytoin. If concurrent use is undertaken the outcome should be well monitored. Reduce the phenytoin dosage as necessary.

1. Houghton GW, Richens A. Inhibition of phenytoin metabolism by other drugs used in epilepsy. *Int J Clin Pharmacol Biopharm* (1975) 12, 210–16.
2. Hulsman JW, van Heycop Ten Ham MW and van Zijl CHW. Influence of ethylphenacemide on serum levels of other anticonvulsant drugs. *Epilepsia* (1970) 11, 207.

Phenytoin + Phenobarbital

The concurrent use of phenytoin and phenobarbital is normally advantageous and uneventful. Changes in serum phenytoin levels (often decreases but sometimes increases) can occur if phenobarbital is added, but seizure control is not usually affected. Phenytoin toxicity following phenobarbital withdrawal has been seen. Increased phenobarbital levels and possibly toxicity may result if phenytoin is given to patients taking phenobarbital.

Clinical evidence

A study in 10 epileptic patients taking phenytoin 2.8 to 6.8 mg/kg daily found that while taking phenobarbital 1.1 to 2.5 mg/kg daily their serum phenytoin levels were reduced. Five patients had a mean reduction of about 65%, from 15.7 to 5.7 micrograms/mL. In most cases phenytoin levels rose again when the phenobarbital was withdrawn. In one patient this was so rapid and steep that he developed ataxia and a cerebellar syndrome with phenytoin levels of up to 60 micrograms/mL, despite a reduction in the phenytoin dosage.[1]

This reduction in phenytoin levels by phenobarbital has been described in other reports.[2-7] However, some of these also described a very transient and small rise[4] or no alteration[4,5] in serum phenytoin levels in individual patients. Three other studies have found that phenobarbital does not alter phenytoin levels.[8-10]

Elevated serum phenobarbital levels occurred in epileptic children when they were also given phenytoin. In 5 patients the phenobarbital levels were approximately doubled. In some cases mild ataxia was seen but the relatively high barbiturate levels were well tolerated.[1] A long-term study in 6 adult epileptics found that when phenytoin was added to phenobarbital, the level/dose ratio of the phenobarbital gradually rose by about 60% over one year, and then gradually fell again over the next 2 years.[11] This suggests that initially, phenytoin reduces phenobarbital metabolism. In another patient taking phenobarbital 100 mg and phenytoin 160 mg daily, serum levels of phenobarbital increased by about 53% within about 2 days when the dose of phenytoin was increased to 490 mg daily.[12]

Mechanism

Phenobarbital can have a dual effect on phenytoin metabolism: it may cause enzyme induction, which results in a more rapid clearance of the phenytoin from the body, or with large doses it may inhibit metabolism by competing for enzyme systems. The total effect will depend on the balance between the two drugs. The reason for the elevation of serum phenobarbital levels is not fully understood, but the extent may be dependent on the serum level of phenytoin.[12,13]

Importance and management

Concurrent use can be therapeutically valuable. Changes in dosage or the addition or withdrawal of either drug need to be monitored to ensure that toxicity does not occur, or that seizure control is not worsened. The contradictory reports cited here do not provide a clear picture of what is likely to happen. Consider also 'Primidone + Phenytoin', p.570.

1. Morselli PL, Rizzo M, Garattini S. Interaction between phenobarbital and diphenylhydantoin in animals and in epileptic patients. *Ann N Y Acad Sci* (1971) 179, 88–107.
2. Cucinell SA, Conney AH, Sansur M, Burns JJ. Drug interactions in man. I. Lowering effect of phenobarbital on plasma levels of bishydroxycoumarin (Dicumarol) and diphenylhydantoin (Dilantin). *Clin Pharmacol Ther* (1965) 6, 420–9.
3. Buchanan RA, Heffelfinger JC, Weiss CF. The effect of phenobarbital on diphenylhydantoin metabolism in children. *Pediatrics* (1969) 43, 114–16.
4. Kutt H, Haynes J, Verebely K, McDowell F. The effect of phenobarbital on plasma diphenylhydantoin level and metabolism in man and rat liver microsomes. *Neurology* (1969) 19, 611–16.
5. Garrettson LK, Dayton PG. Disappearance of phenobarbital and diphenylhydantoin from serum of children. *Clin Pharmacol Ther* (1970) 11, 674–9.
6. Abarbanel J, Herishanu Y, Rosenberg P, Eylath U. In vivo interaction of anticonvulsant drugs. *J Neurol* (1978) 218, 137–44.
7. Kristensen M, Hansen JM, Skovsted L. The influence of phenobarbital on the half-life of diphenylhydantoin in man. *Acta Med Scand* (1969) 185, 347–50.
8. Diamond WD, Buchanan RA. A clinical study of the effect of phenobarbital on diphenylhydantoin plasma levels. *J Clin Pharmacol* (1970) 10, 306–11.
9. Booker HE, Tormey A, Toussaint J. Concurrent administration of phenobarbital and diphenylhydantoin: lack of an interference effect. *Neurology* (1971) 21, 383–5.
10. Browne TR, Szabo GK, Evans J, Evans BA, Greenblatt DJ, Mikati MA. Phenobarbital does not alter phenytoin steady-state serum concentration or pharmacokinetics. *Neurology* (1988) 38, 639–42.
11. Encinas MP, Santos Buelga D, Alonso González AC, García Sánchez MJ, Domínguez-Gil Hurlé A. Influence of length of treatment on the interaction between phenobarbital and phenytoin. *J Clin Pharm Ther* (1992) 17, 49–50.

12. Kuranari M, Tatsukawa H, Seike M, Saikawa T, Ashikari Y, Kodama Y, Sakata T, Takeyama M. Effect of phenytoin on phenobarbital pharmacokinetics in a patient with epilepsy. *Ann Pharmacother* (1995) 29, 83–4.
13. Lambie DG, Johnson RH. The effects of phenytoin on phenobarbitone and primidone metabolism. *J Neurol Neurosurg Psychiatry* (1981) 44, 148–51.

Phenytoin + Phenothiazines

The serum levels of phenytoin can be raised or lowered by the use of chlorpromazine, prochlorperazine or thioridazine. Phenytoin may reduce levels of the active metabolite of thioridazine.

Clinical evidence

(a) Chlorpromazine

The serum phenytoin levels of a patient taking phenytoin, primidone and sulthiame doubled after chlorpromazine 50 mg daily was taken for a month.[1] However, another 4 patients taking chlorpromazine 50 to 100 mg daily showed no interaction.[1] In another report, one out of 3 patients taking phenytoin and phenobarbital had a fall in their serum phenytoin levels when they were also given chlorpromazine.[2] A further very brief report states that in rare instances chlorpromazine has been noted to impair phenytoin metabolism.[3]

In a large study in patients taking phenytoin with various phenothiazines (chlorpromazine, **thioridazine** or **mesoridazine**), phenytoin levels were decreased by 44% when the phenothiazines were started, and by 33% when the phenothiazine dose was increased. A number of patients experienced an increased frequency of seizures. In patients who had these phenothiazines discontinued or the dosage *decreased*, the phenytoin levels increased by 55% and 71%, respectively, and toxic levels occurred in some patients.[4]

(b) Prochlorperazine

A single very brief report states that in rare instances prochlorperazine has been noted to impair phenytoin metabolism.[3]

(c) Thioridazine

One out of 6 patients taking phenytoin and phenobarbital had a marked rise in serum phenytoin levels when thioridazine was added, whereas 4 others had a fall in phenytoin levels.[2] Phenytoin toxicity has also been described in 2 patients after about 2 weeks of concurrent treatment with thioridazine.[5] A retrospective study in 27 patients taking phenytoin found that when they were given thioridazine their serum phenytoin levels were increased by at least 4 micrograms/mL (4 patients), decreased by at least 4 micrograms/mL (2), or were unchanged (21).[6] Another retrospective study comparing 28 patients taking both phenytoin and thioridazine with patients taking either drug alone found no evidence that thioridazine increased the risk of phenytoin toxicity.[7] A further study found no changes in serum phenytoin or thioridazine levels in patients given both drugs, but serum levels of mesoridazine (the active metabolite of thioridazine) were reduced, suggesting higher doses of thioridazine may be necessary to achieve the same effect.[8] See also the study[4] in section (a), which found a decrease in phenytoin levels and an increase in seizure frequency when patients took phenothiazines including thioridazine.

Mechanism

Uncertain. Phenothiazines such as thioridazine are inhibitors of the cytochrome P450 isoenzyme CYP2D6, and as such would not be expected to affect phenytoin metabolism, at least by this mechanism.

Importance and management

A confusing situation as the results are inconsistent. The concurrent use of phenytoin and the phenothiazines cited need not be avoided, but it would be prudent to watch for any signs of changes in serum phenytoin levels that would affect antiepileptic control. It is also worth remembering that phenothiazines may decrease the seizure threshold. In one study a trend towards increased seizure frequency was noted after phenothiazines were added, or doses increased.[4] Also note that phenytoin may reduce levels of some phenothiazines. Whether all phenothiazines interact similarly is uncertain.

1. Houghton GW, Richens A. Inhibition of phenytoin metabolism by other drugs used in epilepsy. *Int J Clin Pharmacol Biopharm* (1975) 12, 210–16.
2. Siris JH, Pippenger CE, Werner WL, Masland RL. Anticonvulsant drug-serum levels in psychiatric patients with seizure disorders. Effects of certain psychotropic drugs. *N Y State J Med* (1974) 74, 1554–6.
3. Kutt H, McDowell F. Management of epilepsy with diphenylhydantoin sodium. Dosage regulation for problem patients. *JAMA* (1968) 203, 969–72.
4. Haidukewych D, Rodin EA. Effect of phenothiazines on serum antiepileptic drug concentrations in psychiatric patients with seizure disorder. *Ther Drug Monit* (1985) 7, 401–4.
5. Vincent FM. Phenothiazine-induced phenytoin intoxication. *Ann Intern Med* (1980) 93, 56–7.
6. Sands CD, Robinson JD, Salem RB, Stewart RB, Muniz C. Effect of thioridazine on phenytoin serum concentration: a retrospective study. *Drug Intell Clin Pharm* (1987) 21, 267–72.
7. Gotz VP, Yost RL, Lamadrid ME, Buchanan CD. Evaluation of a potential interaction: thioridazine-phenytoin — negative findings. *Hosp Pharm* (1984) 19, 555–7.
8. Linnoila M, Viukari M, Vaisanen K, Auvinen J. Effect of anticonvulsants on plasma haloperidol and thioridazine levels. *Am J Psychiatry* (1980) 137, 819–21.

Phenytoin + Proton pump inhibitors

A study in epileptic patients found that omeprazole 20 mg daily did not affect the serum levels of phenytoin, whereas earlier studies in healthy subjects suggested that phenytoin levels might be modestly raised by omeprazole 40 mg daily. A study with esomeprazole also suggests it may cause a minor rise in phenytoin levels. Lansoprazole does not normally affect phenytoin levels, but an isolated case report of toxicity is tentatively attributed to an interaction. Pantoprazole and rabeprazole appear not to interact.

Clinical evidence

(a) Esomeprazole

Esomeprazole inhibits the cytochrome P450 isoenzyme CYP2C19 so that the plasma levels of drugs metabolised by this enzyme might be expected to be increased by concurrent use. This is true for phenytoin, which the manufacturers say showed a 13% increase in trough plasma levels in patients given esomeprazole 40 mg.[1]

(b) Lansoprazole

In a group of 12 healthy subjects lansoprazole 60 mg daily for 7 days caused only a very small and clinically irrelevant rise (less than 3%) in the AUC of a single intravenous dose of phenytoin.[2,3] In contrast the manufacturer has received an isolated report of the development of blurred vision, diarrhoea, muscle pain, dizziness, abdominal pain, salivary hypersecretion, increased sweating and incoordination in a man taking phenytoin, which occurred within a day of stopping sustained-release propranolol 80 mg and starting lansoprazole.[4] The phenytoin serum levels were not measured but the symptoms might possibly have been due to phenytoin toxicity, although it should be said that if an interaction with lansoprazole was responsible, it developed unusually quickly.

(c) Omeprazole

Omeprazole 20 mg daily for 3 weeks caused no changes in the mean steady-state serum phenytoin levels in 8 epileptic patients.[5] Four patients had unchanged levels, 2 had falls and 2 had rises, but none of them was adversely affected by the omeprazole treatment.[5]

After taking omeprazole 40 mg daily for 7 days the AUC of a single 300-mg dose of phenytoin was increased by 25% in 10 healthy subjects.[6] In another study the clearance of a 250-mg intravenous dose of phenytoin was reduced by 15% by omeprazole 40 mg given for 7 days.[7] A further study found that 3 doses of omeprazole 40 mg had no effect on the pharmacokinetics of a single dose of phenytoin.[8]

(d) Pantoprazole

In a randomised, crossover study in 23 healthy subjects it was found that pantoprazole 40 mg daily for 7 days did not alter the pharmacokinetics (AUC, maximum serum levels, half-life) of a single 300-mg dose of phenytoin.[9] This study has also been published elsewhere.[10]

(e) Rabeprazole

A preliminary report, which gives no details, states that when rabeprazole was used with phenytoin, no significant changes in the pharmacokinetics of phenytoin were seen.[11]

Mechanism

Not understood. A possible explanation is that if the dosage of omeprazole is high enough, it may possibly reduce the metabolism of phenytoin by CYP2C19. However, CYP2C19 has only a minor role in phenytoin metabolism.[12] Esomeprazole may interact similarly. With lansoprazole, the overall picture is that it does not act as an enzyme inducer or inhibitor[13] (or it is only very weak) so that it would not be expected to interact with phenytoin to a clinically relevant extent (confirmed by the study cited above[2]). The same appears to be true for pantoprazole and rabeprazole.

Importance and management

Information is very limited but it seems that omeprazole 20 mg daily does not affect serum phenytoin levels, whereas 40 mg daily may possibly cause a slight increase. No special precautions would normally seem necessary if lansoprazole or omeprazole is given with phenytoin, but until more is known it would be prudent to be aware of this possible interaction if concurrent use is necessary. Similarly, the manufacturers of esomeprazole suggest concurrent use should be monitored,[1] although the elevation in levels seen in the study would not usually be expected to be clinically significant. More study is needed. No special precautions would seem to be necessary if rabeprazole or pantoprazole and phenytoin are given concurrently.

1. Nexium Tablets (Esomeprazole magnesium trihydrate). AstraZeneca UK Ltd. UK Summary of product characteristics, May 2007.
2. Karol MD, Mukherji D, Cavanaugh JH. Lack of effect of concomitant multi-dose lansoprazole on single-dose phenytoin pharmacokinetics in subjects. *Gastroenterology* (1994) 106, A103.
3. Karol MD, Locke CS, Cavanaugh JH. Lack of a pharmacokinetic interaction between lansoprazole and intravenously administered phenytoin. *J Clin Pharmacol* (1999) 39, 1283–9.
4. Wyeth, personal communication, January 1998.
5. Andersson T, Lagerström P-O, Unge P. A study of the interaction between omeprazole and phenytoin in epileptic patients. *Ther Drug Monit* (1990) 12, 329–33.
6. Prichard PJ, Walt RP, Kitchingman GK, Somerville KW, Langman MJS, Williams J, Richens A. Oral phenytoin pharmacokinetics during omeprazole therapy. *Br J Clin Pharmacol* (1987) 24, 543–5.
7. Gugler R, Jensen JC. Omeprazole inhibits oxidative drug metabolism. Studies with diazepam and phenytoin in vivo and 7-ethoxycoumarin in vitro. *Gastroenterology* (1985) 89, 1235–41.
8. Bachmann KA, Sullivan TJ, Jauregui L, Reese JH, Miller K, Levine L. Absence of an inhibitory effect of omeprazole and nizatidine on phenytoin disposition, a marker of CYP2C activity. *Br J Clin Pharmacol* (1993) 36, 380–2.
9. Middle MV, Müller FO, Schall R, Groenewoud G, Hundt HKL, Huber R, Bliesath H, Steinijans VW. No influence of pantoprazole on the pharmacokinetics of phenytoin. *Int J Clin Pharmacol Ther* (1995) 33, 304–7.
10. Middle MV, Müller FO, Schall R, Groenewoud G, Hundt HKL, Huber R, Bliesath H, Steinijans VW. No influence of pantoprazole on the pharmacokinetics of phenytoin. *Int J Clin Pharmacol Ther* (1996) 34 (Suppl 1), S72–S75.
11. Humphries TJ, Nardi RV, Lazar JD, Spanyers SA. Drug-drug interaction evaluation of rabeprazole sodium: a clean/expected slate? *Gut* (1996) 39 (Suppl 3), A47.
12. Giancarlo GM, Venkatakrishnan K, Granda BW, von Moltke LL, Greenblatt DJ. Relative contributions of CYP2C9 and 2C19 to phenytoin 4-hydroxylation in vitro: inhibition by sulfaphenazole, omeprazole, and ticlopidine. *Eur J Clin Pharmacol* (2001) 57, 31–36.
13. Cavanaugh JH, Park YK, Awni WM, Mukherjee DX, Karol MD, Granneman GR. Effect of lansoprazole on antipyrine and ICG pharmacokinetics. *Gastroenterology* (1991) 100, A40.

Phenytoin + *Shankhapushpi* (SRC)

A case report, and an *animal* study, indicate that an antiepileptic Ayurvedic herbal preparation, *Shankhapushpi* (*SRC*), can markedly reduce plasma phenytoin levels, leading to an increased seizure frequency.

Clinical evidence

An epileptic man taking **phenobarbital** 120 mg daily and **phenytoin** 500 mg daily developed an increase in seizure frequency when *Shankhapushpi* (*SRC*) three times a day was given. His plasma **phenytoin** levels were found to have fallen from 18.2 to 9.3 micrograms/mL, whereas his **phenobarbital** levels were little changed. When the *SRC* was stopped the **phenytoin** plasma levels rose to 30.3 micrograms/mL, and toxicity was seen. A reduction in the dose of **phenytoin** to 400 mg daily resulted in levels of 16.2 micrograms/mL. Another possible case has also been reported.[1,2]

Subsequent studies in *rats* found that *SRC* reduces the plasma levels of **phenytoin** by about half.[3] These pharmacokinetic effects were only seen after multiple doses, not single doses of **phenytoin**. A pharmacodynamic interaction, resulting in reduced antiepileptic activity was also noted.[1,3,4]

Mechanism

Not understood. There is evidence from *animal* studies that *SRC* may affect the pharmacokinetics of the phenytoin and possibly its pharmacodynamics as well,[1,3] thereby reducing its antiepileptic activity. It is also suggested that one of the ingredients of *SRC* may have some antiepileptic activity.[3]

Importance and management

Information about this interaction appears to be limited to these reports. *Shankhapushpi* (*SRC*) is given because it has some antiepileptic activity (demonstrated in *animal* studies[3,4]), but there is little point in combining it with phenytoin if the outcome is a fall in plasma phenytoin levels, accompanied by an increase in seizure frequency. For this reason concurrent use should be avoided. *SRC* is a syrup prepared from *Convolvulus pluricaulis* leaves, *Nardostachys jatamansi* rhizomes, *Onosma bracteatum* leaves and flowers and the whole plant of *Centella asiatica, Nepeta hindostana* and *Nepeta elliptica*.[3] The first two of these plants appear to contain compounds with antiepileptic activity.[5]

It has been suggested that adulteration of traditional medicines with various antiepileptics[6,7] may be an unexpected factor in these interactions.

1. Kshirsagar NA, Personal communication 1991.
2. Kshirsagar NA, Dalvi SS, Joshi MV, Sharma SS, Sant HM, Shah PU, Chandra RS. Phenytoin and ayurvedic preparation – clinically important interaction in epileptic patients. *J Assoc Physicians India* (1992) 40, 354–5.
3. Dandekar UP, Chandra RS, Dalvi SS, Joshi MV, Gokhale PC, Sharma AV, Shah PU, Kshirsagar NA. Analysis of a clinically important interaction between phenytoin and Shankhapushpi, an Ayurvedic preparation. *J Ethnopharmacol* (1992) 35, 285–8.
4. Kshirsagar NA, Chandra RS, Dandekar UP, Dalvi SS, Sharma AV, Joshi MV, Gokhale PC, Shah PU. Investigation of a novel clinically important interaction between phenytoin and Ayurvedic preparation. *Eur J Pharmacol* (1990) 183, 519.
5. Sharma VN, Barar FSK, Khanna NK, Mahawar MM. Some pharmacological actions of *convolvulus pluricaulis* chois: an Indian indigenous herb. *Indian J Med Res* (1965) 53, 871–6.
6. Bharucha NE. Co-prescription of conventional and 'alternative' medicines. *J R Coll Physicians Lond* (1999) 33, 285.
7. Gogtay NJ, Dalvi SS, Rane CT, Pawar HS, Narayana RV, Shah PU, Kshirsagar NA. A story of "ayurvedic" tablets and misled epileptic patients. *J Assoc Physicians India* (1999) 47, 1116.

Phenytoin + SSRIs

Phenytoin serum levels can be increased in some patients by fluoxetine and toxicity may occur. There are also isolated reports of phenytoin toxicity in patients taking fluvoxamine. Phenytoin and sertraline do not normally interact, but two patients have shown increased serum phenytoin levels. Sertraline and possibly paroxetine levels may be reduced by phenytoin. Note that SSRIs should be avoided in unstable epilepsy and used with care in other epileptics.

Clinical evidence

(a) Fluoxetine

A woman taking phenytoin 370 mg, diazepam 4 mg, and clonazepam 6 mg daily was given fluoxetine 20 mg for depression.[1] Five days later her serum phenytoin levels had risen from 18 to 26.5 mg/L, and a further 9 days later to 30 mg/L, accompanied by signs of toxicity (tremor, headache, abnormal thinking, increased partial seizure activity). Seven days after stopping the phenytoin the serum levels had fallen to 22 mg/L.

Two other patients, taking phenytoin 300 and 400 mg daily, respectively, had marked rises in serum phenytoin levels (from 15 to 35 micrograms/mL and from 11.5 to 47 micrograms/mL), accompanied by signs of phenytoin toxicity, within 5 to 10 days of starting fluoxetine 20 or 40 mg daily. The problem resolved when the fluoxetine was stopped or the phenytoin dosage reduced.[2] Another patient only developed this interaction after taking fluoxetine for about 9 months.[3]

A review initiated by the US Food and Drug Administration and the manufacturers of fluoxetine briefly describes another 23 anecdotal observations of suspected phenytoin/fluoxetine interactions (most of them incompletely documented). These suggest that a marked 1.5-fold increase in serum phenytoin levels, with accompanying toxicity, can occur within 1 to 42 days (mean onset time of 2 weeks) after starting fluoxetine.[4] Another case describes raised phenytoin levels with improved efficacy when fluoxetine was started, and reduced levels and possible loss of efficacy when fluoxetine was stopped.[5] Conversely, a retrospective review of 7 patients taking phenytoin and fluoxetine found no cases of an interaction.[6]

(b) Fluvoxamine

About one month after starting to take fluvoxamine 50 mg daily, a woman taking phenytoin 300 mg daily experienced ataxia and was found to have a threefold increase in her phenytoin levels (from 16.6 to 49.1 micrograms/mL). Fluvoxamine was subsequently discontinued, and the phenytoin dose reduced, with gradual recovery.[7] Another report describes phenytoin toxicity (serum levels of 48 mg/L) in an 86-year-old woman after she took fluvoxamine 100 to 200 mg daily for 10 days.[8]

However the fluvoxamine was started only 2 days after the phenytoin, in a dose of 200 mg twice daily, had been started, and the serum phenytoin levels were not checked until the toxicity had actually developed. Both drugs were then stopped and the phenytoin later successfully reinstated without the fluvoxamine. A worldwide analysis of data up to 1995 by the manufacturers of fluvoxamine identified only 2 reported cases of interactions (clinical symptoms only) between phenytoin and fluvoxamine.[9]

(c) Paroxetine

In a group of epileptic patients, paroxetine 30 mg daily for 16 days caused no changes in the plasma levels or therapeutic effects of phenytoin. Steady-state paroxetine plasma levels were lower in those also taking phenytoin (16 nanograms/mL) than in those taking carbamazepine (27 nanograms/mL) or valproate (73 nanograms/mL).[10]

(d) Sertraline

A double-blind, randomised, placebo-controlled study in 30 healthy subjects taking phenytoin 100 mg three times daily, found that sertraline 50 to 200 mg daily did not affect the steady-state trough serum levels of phenytoin, nor was there any evidence that concurrent use impaired cognitive function.[11] However, another report describes 2 elderly patients whose serum phenytoin levels rose when they were given sertraline, but there was no evidence of toxicity. One of them had an almost fourfold rise in serum phenytoin levels whereas the other had a rise of only about one-third.[12]

In an analysis of plasma sertraline levels the concentration to daily dose ratio of sertraline was significantly lower in patients who had taken sertraline with phenytoin compared to those who had taken sertraline without phenytoin,[13] which suggested that phenytoin increases sertraline metabolism

Mechanism

An *in vitro* investigation found that fluoxetine and fluvoxamine inhibited the metabolism of phenytoin by the cytochrome P450 isoenzyme CYP2C9 in human liver tissue.[14] This would presumably lead to a rise in serum phenytoin levels. In this study, sertraline was a weaker inhibitor of CYP2C9, and was considered less likely to interact with phenytoin.[14] A similar study also suggested that the risk of interaction was greatest for fluoxetine, and less likely with sertraline and paroxetine.[15] Sertraline plasma levels may be reduced because of enzyme induction by phenytoin which would increase its metabolism and clearance from the body.[13]

Importance and management

The interaction between phenytoin and fluoxetine appears to be established but its incidence is not known. Because of the unpredictable nature of this interaction, if fluoxetine is added to treatment with phenytoin in any patient be alert for the need to reduce the phenytoin dosage. Ideally the phenytoin serum levels should be monitored. Similarly, to be on the safe side phenytoin levels should be monitored when fluvoxamine is first added to treatment with phenytoin so that any patient affected can be quickly identified. Although an interaction with sertraline appears less likely, be alert for any evidence of an increase in phenytoin adverse effects (e.g. blurred vision, nystagmus, ataxia or drowsiness) if sertraline is given. More study of these interactions is needed. Note that SSRIs should be avoided in patients with unstable epilepsy, and those with controlled epilepsy should be carefully monitored, because of the potential increased seizure risk.

1. Woods DJ, Coulter DM, Pillans P. Interaction of phenytoin and fluoxetine. *N Z Med J* (1994) 107, 19.
2. Jalil P. Toxic reaction following the combined administration of fluoxetine and phenytoin: two case reports. *J Neurol Neurosurg Psychiatry* (1992) 55, 412–13.
3. Darley J. Interaction between phenytoin and fluoxetine. *Seizure* (1994) 3, 151–2.
4. Shader RI, Greenblatt DJ, von Moltke LL. Fluoxetine inhibition of phenytoin metabolism. *J Clin Psychopharmacol* (1994) 14, 375–6.
5. Shad MU, Preskorn SH. Drug-drug interaction in reverse: possible loss of phenytoin efficacy as a result of fluoxetine discontinuation. *J Clin Psychopharmacol* (1999) 19, 471–2.
6. Bécares J, Puente M, De Juana P, García B, Bermego T. Fluoxetina y fenitoína: interacción o interpretación errónea de los niveles séricos? *Farm Clin* (1997) 14, 474–8.
7. Mamiya K, Kojima K, Yukawa E, Higuchi S, Ieiri I, Ninomiya H, Tashiro N. Case report. Phenytoin intoxication induced by fluvoxamine. *Ther Drug Monit* (2001) 23, 75–7.
8. Feldman D, Claudel B, Feldman F, Allilaire JF, Thuillier A. Cas clinique d'interaction médicamenteuse entre phénytoïne et fluvoxamine. *J Pharm Clin* (1995) 14, 296–7.
9. Wagner W, Vause EW. Fluvoxamine. A review of global drug-drug interaction data. *Clin Pharmacokinet* (1995) 29 (Suppl 1), 26–32.
10. Andersen BB, Mikkelsen M, Versterager A, Dam M, Kristensen HB, Pedersen B, Lund J, Mengel H. No influence of the antidepressant paroxetine on carbamazepine, valproate and phenytoin. *Epilepsy Res* (1991) 10, 201–4.
11. Rapeport WG, Muirhead DC, Williams SA, Cross M, Wesnes K. Absence of effect of sertraline on the pharmacokinetics and pharmacodynamics of phenytoin. *J Clin Psychiatry* (1996) 57 (Suppl 1), 24–8.
12. Haselberger MB, Freedman LS, Tolbert S. Elevated serum phenytoin concentrations associated with coadministration of sertraline. *J Clin Psychopharmacol* (1997) 17, 107–9.
13. Pihlsgård M, Eliasson E. Significant reduction of sertraline plasma levels by carbamazepine and phenytoin. *Eur J Clin Pharmacol* (2002) 57, 915–6.
14. Schmider J, Greenblatt DJ, von Moltke LL, Karsov D, Shader RI. Inhibition of CYP2C9 by selective serotonin reuptake inhibitors *in vitro*: studies of phenytoin *p*-hydroxylation. *Br J Clin Pharmacol* (1997) 44, 495–8.
15. Nelson MH, Birnbaum AK, Remmel RP. Inhibition of phenytoin hydroxylation in human liver microsomes by several selective serotonin re-uptake inhibitors. *Epilepsy Res* (2001) 44, 71–82.

Phenytoin + Sucralfate

The absorption of single-dose phenytoin can be reduced by about 7 to 20% by sucralfate, but this effect was not seen in a multiple-dose study. The interaction is unlikely to be clinically relevant.

Clinical evidence

Sucralfate 1 g was found to reduce the absorption (measured over a 24-hour period) of a single 300-mg dose of phenytoin in 8 healthy subjects by 20%.[1] Peak serum phenytoin levels were also reduced, but this was not statistically significant. Another single-dose study found a reduction in phenytoin absorption of 7.7 to 9.5%.[2] However, sucralfate 1 g four times daily for 7 days had no effect on the steady-state levels of phenytoin 5 to 7 mg/kg daily in 6 healthy subjects. The fourth daily dose of sucralfate was taken simultaneously with the daily phenytoin dose at bedtime. After 7 days, all phenytoin levels were within 15% of the baseline values (range, 6% decrease to 15% increase).[3]

Mechanism

Uncertain. Reduced bioavailability has been demonstrated in a single-dose study in *dogs* when the drugs were used simultaneously, and this did not occur if the phenytoin was given 2 hours after the sucralfate.[4]

Importance and management

Information is limited. The reduction in absorption shown in single-dose studies was quite small, and was not seen in a multiple-dose study, suggesting it is unlikely to be clinically relevant.

1. Smart HL, Somerville KW, Williams J, Richens A, Langman MJS. The effects of sucralfate upon phenytoin absorption in man. *Br J Clin Pharmacol* (1985) 20, 238–40.
2. Hall TG, Cuddy PG, Glass CJ, Melethil S. Effect of sucralfate on phenytoin bioavailability. *Drug Intell Clin Pharm* (1986) 20, 607–11.
3. Malli R, Jones WN, Rindone JP, Labadie EL. The effect of sucralfate on the steady-state serum concentrations of phenytoin. *Drug Metabol Drug Interact* (1989) 7, 287–93.
4. Lacz JP, Groschang AG, Giesing DH, Browne RK. The effect of sucralfate on drug absorption in dogs. *Gastroenterology* (1982) 82, 1108.

Phenytoin + Sulfinpyrazone

Some limited evidence indicates that phenytoin serum levels may be markedly increased by sulfinpyrazone.

Clinical evidence

A review of the drug interactions of sulfinpyrazone identified two studies that found interactions with phenytoin.[1] In the first, the serum phenytoin levels of 2 out of 5 patients taking phenytoin 250 to 350 mg daily were doubled from about 10 to 20 micrograms/mL within 11 days of starting to take sulfinpyrazone 800 mg daily. One of the remaining patients had a small increase in phenytoin levels, but the other two had no changes at all. When the sulfinpyrazone was withdrawn, the serum phenytoin concentrations fell to their former levels. The second study was a clinical study in epileptic patients that found that sulfinpyrazone 800 mg daily for a week increased the phenytoin half-life from 10 to 16.5 hours and reduced the metabolic clearance from 59 to 32 mL/minute.

Mechanism

Uncertain. It seems probable that sulfinpyrazone inhibits the metabolism of the phenytoin by the liver, thereby allowing it to accumulate in the body and leading to a rise in its serum levels. Displacement of phenytoin from its plasma protein binding sites may also have a small part to play.

Importance and management

Information seems to be limited to these studies, which await confirmation. A similar interaction with phenytoin has been reported with phenylbutazone, which has a very close chemical relationship with sulfinpyrazone (see 'Phenytoin + Aspirin or NSAIDs', p.551). Thus what is known suggests that concurrent use should be monitored and suitable phenytoin dosage reductions made where necessary.

1. Pedersen AK, Jacobsen P, Kampmann JP, Hansen JM. Clinical pharmacokinetics and potentially important drug interactions of sulphinpyrazone. *Clin Pharmacokinet* (1982) 7, 42–56.

Phenytoin + Sulfonamides and/or Trimethoprim

Phenytoin serum levels can be raised by co-trimoxazole, sulfamethizole, sulfamethoxazole, sulfadiazine and trimethoprim. Phenytoin toxicity may develop in some cases. A single case of liver failure has been described in a patient taking phenytoin with co-trimoxazole. Sulfamethoxypyridazine, and sulfafurazole (sulfisoxazole) are reported not to interact.

Clinical evidence

(a) Co-trimoxazole or Trimethoprim

A patient taking phenytoin 400 mg daily developed signs of toxicity (ataxia, nystagmus, loss of balance) within 2 weeks of starting to take co-trimoxazole 960 mg twice daily. His serum levels were found to have risen to about 38 micrograms/mL (normal range about 10 to 20 micrograms/mL).[1]

A child who was stable taking phenytoin and sultiame developed phenytoin toxicity within 48 hours of starting co-trimoxazole. Toxicity resolved when the antibacterial was changed to amoxicillin.[2] A clinical study found that co-trimoxazole and trimethoprim can increase the phenytoin half-life by 39% and 51%, respectively, and decrease the mean metabolic clearance by 27% and 30%, respectively.[3] Sulfamethoxazole alone had only a small effect on the half-life and did not affect the clearance of phenytoin.[3] A case report describes fatal acute hepatic failure in a 60-year-old woman 10 days after starting co-trimoxazole and 14 days after starting phenytoin.[4] This patient was also given cimetidine, which may raise phenytoin levels (see 'Phenytoin + H_2-receptor antagonists', p.559).

(b) Sulfadiazine

After taking sulfadiazine 4 g daily for a week, the half-life of a single intravenous dose of phenytoin was found to have increased by 80% in 8 patients. The mean metabolic clearance decreased by 45%.[3]

(c) Sulfamethizole

The development of phenytoin toxicity in a patient taking sulfamethizole prompted a study of this interaction in 8 patients given phenytoin. After the concurrent use of sulfamethizole 1 g four times daily for 7 days the phenytoin half-life had lengthened from 11.8 to 19.6 hours. Of the 4 patients receiving long-term treatment with phenytoin, 3 had rises in serum phenytoin levels from 22 to 33 micrograms/mL, from 19 to 23 micrograms/mL and from 4 to 7 micrograms/mL respectively. The phenytoin levels of the fourth patient were not affected.[5,6] Another single-dose study found that the half-life of phenytoin was increased and the mean metabolic clearance reduced by 36%.[3]

(d) Other sulfonamides

Pretreatment for one week with **sulfamethoxypyridazine** or **sulfadimethoxine** did not significantly alter the pharmacokinetics of a single dose of phenytoin.[3]

Mechanism

The sulfonamides that interact appear to do so by inhibiting the metabolism of the phenytoin by the liver (possibly by the cytochrome P450 isoenzyme CYP2C9)[7], resulting in its accumulation in the body. This would also seem to be true for trimethoprim. Depletion of glucuronic acid by phenytoin may have increased the hepatotoxicity of co-trimoxazole.[4]

Importance and management

The documentation seems to be limited to the reports cited, but the interaction is established. Co-trimoxazole, sulfamethizole, sulfadiazine and trimethoprim can increase serum phenytoin levels. The interaction probably occurs in most patients, but the small number of adverse reaction reports suggests that the risk of toxicity is small. It is clearly most likely in those with serum phenytoin levels at the top end of the range. If concurrent use is thought appropriate, the serum phenytoin levels should be closely monitored and the phenytoin dosage reduced if necessary. Alternatively, if appropriate, use a non-interacting antibacterial (in some circumstances 'penicillins', (p.562), or 'macrolides', (p.560), may be appropriate). There seems to be no information about other sulfonamides but it would be prudent to be alert for this interaction with any of them.

1. Wilcox JB. Phenytoin intoxication and co-trimoxazole. *N Z Med J* (1981) 94, 235–6.
2. Gillman MA, Sandyk R. Phenytoin toxicity and co-trimoxazole. *Ann Intern Med* (1985) 102, 559.
3. Hansen JM, Kampmann JP, Siersbæk-Nielsen K, Lumholtz B, Arrøe M, Abildgaard U, Skovsted L. The effect of different sulfonamides on phenytoin metabolism in man. *Acta Med Scand* (1979) (Suppl 624), 106–10.
4. Ilario MJ-M, Ruiz JE, Axiotis CA. Acute fulminant hepatic failure in a woman treated with phenytoin and trimethoprim-sulfamethoxazole. *Arch Pathol Lab Med* (2000) 124, 1800–3.
5. Lumholtz B, Siersbaek-Nielsen K, Skovsted L, Kampmann J, Hansen JM. Sulfamethizole-induced inhibition of diphenylhydantoin, tolbutamide and warfarin metabolism. *Clin Pharmacol Ther* (1975) 17, 731–4.
6. Siersbaek-Nielsen K, Hansen JM, Skovsted L, Lumholtz B, Kampmann J. Sulphamethizole-induced inhibition of diphenylhydantoin and tolbutamide metabolism in man. *Clin Pharmacol Ther* (1973) 14, 148.
7. Giancarlo GM, Venkatakrishnan K, Granda BW, von Moltke LL, Greenblatt DJ. Relative contributions of CYP2C9 and 2C19 to phenytoin 4-hydroxylation in vitro: inhibition by sulfaphenazole, omeprazole, and ticlopidine. *Eur J Clin Pharmacol* (2001) 57, 31–36.

Phenytoin + Sultiame

Serum phenytoin levels can be approximately doubled by sultiame and phenytoin toxicity may occur.

Clinical evidence

The serum phenytoin levels in 6 out of 7 epileptic patients approximately doubled within about 5 to 25 days of starting to take sultiame 400 mg daily. All experienced an increase in adverse effects and definite phenytoin toxicity occurred in 2 of them. In most of the patients, phenytoin serum levels fell back to baseline over the 2 months following the withdrawal of sultiame.[1] All of the patients were also taking **phenobarbital** and although greater variations in serum **phenobarbital** were seen, they were not considered to be clinically significant.[1]

A number of other reports confirm this interaction,[2-8] some of which describe the development of phenytoin toxicity.

Mechanism

The evidence suggests that sultiame interferes with the metabolism of the phenytoin by the liver, leading to its accumulation in the body.

Importance and management

A reasonably well-documented, established and clinically important interaction. The incidence seems to be high. If sultiame is added to established treatment with phenytoin, increases in serum phenytoin levels of up to 75% or more may be expected.[3,7] Phenytoin serum levels should be closely monitored and appropriate dosage reductions made to prevent the development of toxicity. The changes in phenobarbital levels appear to be unimportant.

1. Olesen OV, Jensen ON, Drug-interaction between sulthiame (Ospolot (R)) and phenytoin in the treatment of epilepsy. *Dan Med Bull* (1969) 16, 154–8.
2. Houghton GW, Richens A. Inhibition of phenytoin metabolism by sulthiame. *Br J Pharmacol* (1973) 49, 157P–158P.
3. Houghton GW, Richens A. Inhibition of phenytoin metabolism by sulthiame in epileptic patients. *Br J Clin Pharmacol* (1974) 1, 59–66.
4. Richens A, Houghton GW. Phenytoin intoxication caused by sulthiame. *Lancet* (1973) ii, 1442–3.
5. Houghton GW, Richens A. Inhibition of phenytoin metabolism by other drugs used in epilepsy. *Int J Clin Pharmacol Biopharm* (1975) 12, 210–16.
6. Frantzen E, Hansen JM, Hansen OE, Kristensen M. Phenytoin (Dilantin®) intoxication. *Acta Neurol Scand* (1967) 43, 440–6.

7. Houghton GW, Richens A. Phenytoin intoxication induced by sulthiame in epileptic patients. *J Neurol Neurosurg Psychiatry* (1974) 37, 275–81.
8. Hansen JM, Kristensen M, Skovsted L. Sulthiame (Ospolot®) as inhibitor of diphenylhydantoin metabolism. *Epilepsia* (1968) 9, 17–22.

Phenytoin + Tamoxifen

Some preliminary evidence suggests that high-dose tamoxifen can cause the serum levels of phenytoin to rise, causing toxicity. Phenytoin may lower tamoxifen levels.

Clinical evidence, mechanism, importance and management

A man who had undergone an operation 10 years previously for a brain tumour and had since remained seizure-free while taking phenytoin 200 mg twice daily began to have breakthrough seizures. It was established that his brain tumour had recurred and so tamoxifen was started as experimental treatment. The dose of tamoxifen was slowly titrated to 200 mg daily over a 6-week period. He continued to receive phenytoin and was also given **carbamazepine** as his seizures were not controlled, but when the maximum dosage of tamoxifen (200 mg daily) was reached he began to develop symptoms of phenytoin toxicity with a serum level of 28 micrograms/mL. The toxicity disappeared and the phenytoin levels decreased when the phenytoin dosage was reduced. The **carbamazepine** serum levels remained unchanged throughout.[1]

The authors of this report say that other patients of theirs similarly treated with tamoxifen also developed phenytoin toxicity, which disappeared when the phenytoin dosage was reduced by 15 to 20%. Another study of the pharmacokinetics of high dose tamoxifen in patients with brain tumours found that the mean tamoxifen levels in 15 patients taking phenytoin were about 60% lower than in patients not taking phenytoin, although this did not reach statistical significance due to high inter-patient variability.[2] The reasons for these possible interactions are not known, but it could be that tamoxifen and phenytoin both compete for the same metabolising enzymes.

The evidence for this interaction is very slim indeed and it may possibly only occur with high dose tamoxifen. Consider monitoring phenytoin levels if high-dose tamoxifen is added and monitor the efficacy of the tamoxifen. More study is needed.

1. Rabinowicz AL, Hinton DR, Dyck P, Couldwell WT. High-dose tamoxifen in treatment of brain tumors: interaction with antiepileptic drugs. *Epilepsia* (1995) 36, 513–15.
2. Ducharme J, Fried K, Shenouda G, Leyland-Jones B, Wainer IW. Tamoxifen metabolic patterns within a glioma patient population treated with high-dose tamoxifen. *Br J Clin Pharmacol* (1997) 43: 189–93.

Phenytoin + Terfenadine

A 1-day and a 2-week course of terfenadine 60 mg twice daily had no effect on the pharmacokinetics of phenytoin in 12 patients with epilepsy.[1] No special precautions are needed if both drugs are used.

1. Coniglio AA, Garnett WR, Pellock JH, Tsidonis O, Hepler CD, Serafin R, Small RE, Driscoll SM, Karnes HT. Effect of acute and chronic terfenadine on free and total serum phenytoin concentrations in epileptic patients. *Epilepsia* (1989) 30, 611–16.

Phenytoin + Ticlopidine

Ticlopidine reduces the metabolism of phenytoin. A number of case reports describe patients who developed phenytoin toxicity when ticlopidine was added.

Clinical evidence

A 65-year-old man taking phenytoin 200 mg daily and clobazam developed signs of phenytoin toxicity (vertigo, ataxia, somnolence) within a week of starting ticlopidine 250 mg daily. His serum phenytoin levels had risen from 18 mg/L to 34 mg/L. When the phenytoin dosage was reduced to 200 mg daily the toxic symptoms disappeared within a few days and his serum phenytoin levels fell to 18 mg/L. To test whether an interaction had occurred, the ticlopidine was stopped, whereupon the serum phenytoin levels fell, within about 3 weeks, to 8 mg/L, during which time the patient experienced his first seizure in 2 years. When the ticlopidine was restarted, his serum phenytoin levels rose again, within a month, to 19 mg/L.[1] A number of other case reports describe phenytoin toxicity, which occurred within 2 to 6 weeks of starting ticlopidine 250 mg once or twice daily.[2-7] These were usually managed by reducing the phenytoin dose. One patient then experienced breakthrough seizures after the ticlopidine was stopped without re-adjusting the phenytoin dose.[6] One case in a patient also taking **phenobarbital** reported that no change in **phenobarbital** levels occurred.[4]

A study in 6 patients taking phenytoin alone found that ticlopidine 250 mg twice daily approximately halved the steady-state phenytoin clearance.[8]

Mechanism

The metabolism of phenytoin to 5-(4-hydroxyphenyl)-5-phenylhydantoin (HPPH) by the cytochrome P450 isoenzyme CYP2C19, and to a lesser extent by CYP2C9, in the liver is inhibited by ticlopidine.[1,3,4,9] Further metabolism of HPPH to dihydroxylated products is mediated mainly by CYP2C19 and this may also be inhibited by ticlopidine.[9]

Importance and management

The interaction is established and clinically important, but its incidence is unknown. It would now be prudent to monitor serum phenytoin levels very closely in any patient if ticlopidine is added to established treatment, being alert for the need to reduce the phenytoin dosage. If ticlopidine is discontinued, the phenytoin dose may need to be increased.

1. Riva R, Cerullo A, Albani F, Baruzzi A. Ticlopidine impairs phenytoin clearance: a case report. *Neurology* (1996) 46, 1172–3.
2. Rindone JP, Bryan G. Phenytoin toxicity associated with ticlopidine administration. *Arch Intern Med* (1996) 156, 1113.
3. Privitera M, Welty TE. Acute phenytoin toxicity followed by seizure breakthrough from a ticlopidine-phenytoin interaction. *Arch Neurol* (1996) 53, 1191–2.
4. Donahue SR, Flockhart DA, Abernethy DR, Ko J-W. Ticlopidine inhibition of phenytoin metabolism mediated by potent inhibition of CYP2C19. *Clin Pharmacol Ther* (1997) 62, 572–7.
5. López-Ariztegui N, Ochoa M, Sánchez-Migallón, Nevado C, Martín M, Intoxicación aguda por fenitoína secundaria a interacción con ticlopidina. *Rev Neurol* (1998) 26, 1017–18.
6. Klaassen SL. Ticlopidine-induced phenytoin toxicity. *Ann Pharmacother* (1998) 32, 1295–8.
7. Dahm AEA, Brørs O. Fenytoinforgiftning forårsaket av interaksjon med tiklopidin. *Tidsskr Nor Laegeforen* (2002) 122, 278–80.
8. Donahue S, Flockhart DA, Abernethy DR. Ticlopidine inhibits phenytoin clearance. *Clin Pharmacol Ther* (1999) 66, 563–8.
9. Giancarlo GM, Venkatakrishnan K, Granda BW, von Moltke LL, Greenblatt DJ. Relative contributions of CYP2C9 and 2C19 to phenytoin 4-hydroxylation in vitro: inhibition by sulfaphenazole, omeprazole, and ticlopidine. *Eur J Clin Pharmacol* (2001) 57, 31–36.

Phenytoin + Tizanidine

An isolated report describes a modest increase in serum phenytoin levels caused by tizanidine.

Clinical evidence, mechanism, importance and management

An isolated report describes a 59-year-old man whose phenytoin levels rose by one-third, from about 19 to 25.5 micrograms/mL, and who experienced drowsiness within a week of starting tizanidine 6 mg daily. The phenytoin was stopped for 3 days and restarted at a reduced dose, but the drowsiness recurred in 3 weeks (phenytoin level 20.5 micrograms/mL). Therefore, the tizanidine was withdrawn.[1] The general importance of this interaction is unclear, but it would seem prudent to remain aware of this interaction in case of an unusual response to treatment.

1. Ueno K, Miyai K, Mitsuzane K. Phenytoin-tizanidine interaction. *DICP Ann Pharmacother* (1991) 25, 1273.

Phenytoin + Trazodone

An isolated case report describes phenytoin toxicity in a patient given trazodone.

Clinical evidence, mechanism, importance and management

A patient taking phenytoin 300 mg daily developed progressive signs of phenytoin toxicity after taking trazodone 500 mg daily for 4 months. His serum phenytoin levels had risen from 17.8 to 46 micrograms/mL.[1] Therapeutic phenytoin serum levels were restored by reducing the phenytoin dosage to 200 mg daily and the trazodone dosage to 400 mg daily. The reasons for this apparent interaction are not understood, and this appears to be the only reported case of an interaction. No general conclusions can be drawn.

1. Dorn JM. A case of phenytoin toxicity possibly precipitated by trazodone. *J Clin Psychiatry* (1986) 47, 89–90.

Phenytoin + Tricyclic antidepressants

Evidence from two patients suggests that imipramine can raise serum phenytoin levels but nortriptyline and amitriptyline appear not to do so. Phenytoin possibly reduces serum desipramine levels. Note that the tricyclics also lower the convulsive threshold.

Clinical evidence

(a) Phenytoin levels

The serum phenytoin levels of 2 patients rose over a 3-month period when they were given **imipramine** 75 mg daily. One of them had an increase in phenytoin levels from about 7.6 to 15 micrograms/mL and developed mild toxicity (drowsiness and uncoordination). These signs disappeared and the phenytoin serum levels of both patients fell when the **imipramine** was withdrawn. One of them was also taking nitrazepam and clonazepam, and the other sodium valproate and carbamazepine, but were stable on these combinations before the addition of **imipramine**.[1]

Other studies have shown that **nortriptyline** 75 mg daily had an insignificant effect on the serum phenytoin levels of 5 patients,[2] and that **amitriptyline** had no effect on the elimination of phenytoin in 3 subjects.[3]

(b) Tricyclic antidepressant levels

A report describes 2 patients who had low serum **desipramine** levels, despite taking standard dosages, while they were also taking phenytoin.[4]

Mechanism

One suggestion is that imipramine inhibits the metabolism of the phenytoin by the liver, which results in its accumulation in the body. *In vitro* study[5] has shown that the tricyclics can inhibit the cytochrome P450 isoenzyme CYP2C19, but this isoenzyme usually has only a minor role in phenytoin metabolism (see 'Antiepileptics', (p.517)). The reduced desipramine levels may be a result of enzyme induction by the phenytoin.

Importance and management

The documentation is very limited indeed and none of these interactions is adequately established. The results of the *in vitro* study suggest that the interaction may only assume importance in those who are deficient in CYP2C9, the enzyme usually responsible for phenytoin metabolism.[5] The tricyclic antidepressants as a group lower the seizure threshold,[6] which suggests extra care should be taken if deciding to use them in epileptic patients. If concurrent use is undertaken the effects should be very well monitored.

1. Perucca E, Richens A. Interaction between phenytoin and imipramine. *Br J Clin Pharmacol* (1977) 4, 485–6.
2. Houghton GW, Richens A. Inhibition of phenytoin metabolism by other drugs used in epilepsy. *Int J Clin Pharmacol Biopharm* (1975) 12, 210–16.
3. Pond SM, Graham GG, Birkett DJ, Wade DN. Effects of tricyclic antidepressants on drug metabolism. *Clin Pharmacol Ther* (1975) 18, 191–9.
4. Fogel BS, Haltzman S. Desipramine and phenytoin: a potential drug interaction of therapeutic relevance. *J Clin Psychiatry* (1987) 48, 387–8.
5. Shin J-G, Park J-Y, Kim M-J, Shon J-H, Yoon Y-R, Cha I-J, Lee S-S, Oh S-W, Kim S-W, Flockhart DA. Inhibitory effects of tricyclic antidepressants (TCAs) on human cytochrome P450 enzymes in vitro: mechanism of drug interaction between TCAs and phenytoin. *Drug Metab Dispos* (2002) 30, 1102–7.
6. Dallos V, Heathfield K. Iatrogenic epilepsy due to antidepressant drugs. *BMJ* (1969) 4, 80–2.

Phenytoin + Valproate

The concurrent use of phenytoin and valproate is common and usually uneventful. Initially total serum phenytoin levels may fall but this is offset by a rise in the levels of free (and active) phenytoin, which may very occasionally cause some toxicity. After continued use the total serum phenytoin levels rise once again, and there might be sustained increases in free phenytoin levels. There is also some very limited evidence to suggest that concurrent use possibly increases the incidence of valproate hepatotoxicity.

Clinical evidence

(a) Phenytoin levels

A number of reports clearly show that total serum levels of phenytoin fall during the early concurrent use of valproate, while the concentrations of free phenytoin rise.[1-5] In one report it was noted that within 4 to 7 days the total serum phenytoin levels had fallen from 19.4 to 14.6 micrograms/mL.[1] A study extending over a year in 8 patients taking phenytoin and valproate found that by the end of 8 weeks the total serum phenytoin levels of 6 of them had fallen by almost as much as 50%, but had returned to their original levels in all but one patient by the end of the year.[6] Similar results were found in another study.[7] However, in a further study, some patients had a sustained increase in the free fraction of phenytoin.[4] Another regression analysis showed that valproate increased the free fraction of phenytoin.[8] The occasional patient may have symptoms of phenytoin toxicity and the dosage may need to be reduced.[9] Delirium and an increased seizure frequency were seen in one patient taking valproic acid with phenytoin.[10]

(b) Valproate levels

Valproate levels are reduced by the presence of phenytoin.[11,12] Valproate levels increased by 30 to 200% when phenytoin was discontinued in 12 patients taking both drugs, which allowed dosage reductions in 6 patients. In these patients, there was no change in seizure control when phenytoin was stopped.[13]

(c) Hepatotoxicity

Epidemiological studies suggest that the risk of fatal hepatotoxicity is higher when valproate is given as polytherapy with enzyme inducers such as phenytoin than when it is given as monotherapy, especially in infants.[14,15] For mention of raised liver enzymes with concurrent use of valproate, phenobarbital and phenytoin, see 'Phenobarbital + Valproate', p.547.

Mechanism

The initial fall in total serum phenytoin levels appears to result from the displacement of phenytoin from its protein binding sites by valproate,[1-5,10] the extent being subject to the diurnal variation in valproate levels.[16] This allows more of the unbound drug to be exposed to metabolism by the liver and the total phenytoin levels fall. After several weeks the metabolism of the phenytoin is inhibited by the valproate and phenytoin levels rise.[2,4] This may result in sustained elevation of free (active) phenytoin levels.[17] Phenytoin reduces valproate levels, probably because it increases its metabolism by the liver. Because phenytoin is an enzyme inducer it may also possibly increase the formation of a minor but hepatotoxic metabolite of valproate (2-propyl-4-pentenoic acid or 4-ene-VPA).[18]

Importance and management

An extremely well-documented interaction (only a selection of the references being listed here). Concurrent use is common and usually advantageous, the adverse effects of the interactions between the drugs usually being of only minor practical importance. However, the outcome should still be monitored. A few patients may experience mild toxicity if valproate is started, but most patients taking phenytoin do not need a dosage change. During the first few weeks total serum phenytoin levels may fall by 20 to 50%, but usually no increase in the dosage is needed, because it is balanced by an increase in the levels of free (active) phenytoin levels. In the following period, the total phenytoin levels may rise again. This may result in a sustained rise in free phenytoin levels.

When monitoring concurrent use it is important to understand fully the implications of changes in 'total' and 'free' or 'unbound' serum phenytoin concentrations. Where monitoring of free phenytoin levels is not available, various nomograms have been designed for predicting unbound phenytoin concentrations during the use of valproate.[17,19] Bear in mind the evidence that the incidence of valproate induced liver toxicity may be increased, especially in infants.

1. Mattson RH, Cramer JA, Williamson PD, Novelly RA. Valproic acid in epilepsy: clinical and pharmacological effects. *Ann Neurol* (1978) 3, 20–5.
2. Perucca E, Hebdige S, Frigo GM, Gatti G, Lecchini S, Crema A. Interaction between phenytoin and valproic acid: plasma protein binding and metabolic effects. *Clin Pharmacol Ther* (1980) 28, 779–89.
3. Tsanaclis LM, Allen J, Perucca E, Routledge PA, Richens A. Effect of valproate on free plasma phenytoin concentrations. *Br J Clin Pharmacol* (1984) 18, 17–20.
4. Bruni J, Gallo JM, Lee CS, Pershalski RJ, Wilder BJ. Interactions of valproic acid with phenytoin. *Neurology* (1980) 30, 1233–6.
5. Friel PN, Leal KW, Wilensky AJ. Valproic acid-phenytoin interaction. *Ther Drug Monit* (1979) 1, 243–8.

6. Bruni J, Wilder BJ, Willmore LJ, Barbour B. Valproic acid and plasma levels of phenytoin. *Neurology* (1979) 29, 904–5.
7. Vakil SD, Critchley EMR, Philips JC, Fahim Y, Haydock D, Cocks A, Dyer T. The effect of sodium valproate (Epilim) on phenytoin and phenobarbitone blood levels. In 'Clinical and Pharmacological Aspects of Sodium Valproate (Epilim) in the Treatment of Epilepsy'. Proceedings of a symposium held at Nottingham University, September 1975, MCS Consultants, England, p 75–7.
8. Mamiya K, Yukawa E, Matsumoto T, Aita C, Goto S. Synergistic effect of valproate coadministration and hypoalbuminemia on the serum-free phenytoin concentration in patients with severe motor and intellectual disabilities. *Clin Neuropharmacol* (2002) 25, 230–3.
9. Haigh D, Forsythe WI. The treatment of childhood epilepsy with sodium valproate. *Dev Med Child Neurol* (1975) 17, 743–8.
10. Tollefson GD. Delirium induced by the competitive interaction between phenytoin and dipropylacetate. *J Clin Psychopharmacol* (1981) 1, 154–8.
11. May T, Rambeck B. Serum concentrations of valproic acid: influence of dose and co-medication. *Ther Drug Monit* (1985) 7, 387–90.
12. Sackellares JC, Sato S, Dreifuss FE, Penry JK. Reduction of steady-state valproate levels by other antiepileptic drugs. *Epilepsia* (1981) 22, 437–41.
13. McNew CD, Michel NC, McCabe PH. Pharmacokinetic interaction between valproic acid and phenytoin: is combination of these drugs "rational" polypharmacy. *Epilepsia* (1998) 39 (Suppl 6), abstract 4.100.
14. Dreifuss FE, Santilli N, Langer DH, Sweeney KP, Moline KA, Menander KB. Valproic acid fatalities: a retrospective review. *Neurology* (1987) 37, 379–85.
15. Dreifuss FE, Langer DH, Moline KA, Maxwell JE. Valproic acid hepatic fatalities. II. US experience since 1984. *Neurology* (1989) 39, 201–7.
16. Riva R, Albani F, Contin M, Perucca E, Ambrosetto G, Gobbi G, Santucci M, Procaccianti G, Baruzzi A. Time-dependent interaction between phenytoin and valproic acid. *Neurology* (1985) 35, 510–15.
17. Kerrick JM, Wolff DL, Graves NM. Predicting unbound phenytoin concentrations in patients receiving valproic acid: a comparison of two predicting methods. *Ann Pharmacother* (1995) 29, 470–4.
18. Levy RH, Rettenmeier AW, Anderson GD, Wilensky AJ, Friel PN, Baillie TA, Acheampong A, Tor J, Guyot M, Loiseau P. Effects of polytherapy with phenytoin, carbamazepine, and stiripentol on formation of 4-ene-valproate, a hepatotoxic metabolite of valproic acid. *Clin Pharmacol Ther* (1990) 48, 225–35.
19. May TW, Rambeck B, Nothbaum N. Nomogram for the prediction of unbound phenytoin concentrations in patients on a combined treatment of phenytoin and valproic acid. *Eur Neurol* (1991) 31, 57–60.

Phenytoin + Vigabatrin

Vigabatrin causes a small to moderate fall in serum phenytoin levels.

Clinical evidence

In one early clinical study, the mean plasma phenytoin levels in 19 patients were about 30% lower when they were given vigabatrin 2 to 3 g daily: in 2 patients they fell below the therapeutic range. However, the change in phenytoin levels was not correlated with the change in seizure frequency.[1] Another clinical study found that vigabatrin reduced the mean serum phenytoin levels by 20% in 53 patients; 41 patients had a decrease in phenytoin levels and 12 had an increase. In this study, some of the patients (number not stated) with decreased phenytoin levels had an increase in seizure frequency and required a phenytoin dosage increase.[2,3] In another analysis, the decrease in phenytoin levels did not occur until the fifth week of vigabatrin therapy.[4] Three other studies have shown roughly similar decreases in phenytoin levels when vigabatrin was added.[5-7]

Mechanism

Not understood. The decrease in phenytoin levels does not appear to be due to reduced metabolism or altered plasma protein binding.[4] Similarly, it is not due to altered bioavailability, since the interaction occurred with intravenous phenytoin.[5]

Importance and management

The interaction between phenytoin and vigabatrin would appear to be established. Vigabatrin causes a modest decrease in phenytoin levels in some patients, which takes a number of weeks to become apparent. A small increase in the dosage of phenytoin may possibly be needed in some patients.

1. Tassinari CA, Michelucci R, Ambrosetto G, Salvi F. Double-blind study of vigabatrin in the treatment of drug-resistant epilepsy. *Arch Neurol* (1987) 44, 907–10.
2. Browne TR, Mattson RH, Penry JK, Smith DB, Treiman DM, Wilder BJ, Ben-Menachem E, Miketta RM, Sherry KM, Szabo GK. A multicentre study of vigabatrin for drug-resistant epilepsy. *Br J Clin Pharmacol* (1989) 95S–100S.
3. Browne TR, Mattson RH, Penry JK, Smith DB, Treiman DM, Wilder BJ, Ben-Menachem E, Napoliello MJ, Sherry KM, Szabo GK. Vigabatrin for refractory complex partial seizures: multicenter single-blind study with long-term follow up. *Neurology* (1987) 37, 184–9.
4. Rimmer EM, Richens A. Double-blind study of γ-vinyl GABA in patients with refractory epilepsy. *Lancet* (1984) i, 189–90.
5. Gatti G, Bartoli A, Marchiselli R, Michelucci R, Tassinari CA, Pisani F, Zaccara G, Timmings P, Richens A, Perucca E. Vigabatrin-induced decrease in serum phenytoin concentration does not involve a change in phenytoin bioavailability. *Br J Clin Pharmacol* (1993) 36, 603–6.
6. Rimmer EM, Richens A. Interaction between vigabatrin and phenytoin. *Br J Clin Pharmacol* (1989) 27, 27S–33S.
7. Bernardina BD, Fontana E, Vigevano F, Fusco L, Torelli D, Galeone D, Buti D, Cianchetti C, Gnanasakthy A, Iudice A. Efficacy and tolerability of vigabatrin in children with refractory partial seizures: a single-blind dose-increasing study. *Epilepsia* (1995) 36, 687–91.

Phenytoin + Viloxazine

Viloxazine can cause a marked rise in serum carbamazepine levels and toxicity has been seen. Viloxazine can also raise serum phenytoin to toxic levels, but appears not to alter oxcarbazepine levels.

Clinical evidence

The serum phenytoin levels of 10 epileptic patients rose by 37%, from 18.8 to 25.7 micrograms/mL over the 3 weeks following the addition of viloxazine 150 to 300 mg daily. The rise ranged from 7 to 94%. Signs of toxicity (ataxia, nystagmus) developed in 4 of the patients 12 to 16 days after starting the viloxazine. Their serum phenytoin levels had risen to between 32.3 and 41 micrograms/mL.[1] When viloxazine was withdrawn the symptoms disappeared and phenytoin levels fell.[1] The pharmacokinetics of viloxazine were unaffected by phenytoin.[2]

Mechanism

Uncertain. What is known suggests that viloxazine inhibits the metabolism of phenytoin, thereby reducing its clearance and raising its serum levels.

Importance and management

Information seems to be limited to the reports cited. If concurrent use is undertaken, serum phenytoin levels should be monitored closely and suitable dosage reductions made as necessary to avoid possible toxicity.

1. Pisani F, Fazio A, Artesi C, Russo M, Trio R, Oteri G, Perucca E, Di Perri R. Elevation of plasma phenytoin by viloxazine in epileptic patients: a clinically significant interaction. *J Neurol Neurosurg Psychiatry* (1992) 55, 126–7.
2. Pisani F, Fazio A, Spina E, Artesi C, Pisani B, Russo M, Trio R, Perucca E. Pharmacokinetics of the antidepressant drug viloxazine in normal subjects and in epileptic patients receiving chronic anticonvulsant treatment. *Psychopharmacology (Berl)* (1986) 90, 295–8.

Phenytoin + Zidovudine

Although one study found that zidovudine did not alter the pharmacokinetics of phenytoin, there is other evidence suggesting that some changes possibly occur, although these may actually be due to HIV infection.

Clinical evidence, mechanism, importance and management

Although there are said to have been 13 cases of a possible interaction between zidovudine and phenytoin, the details are not described in the report.[1] No significant changes in the pharmacokinetics of phenytoin 300 mg daily were seen in 12 asymptomatic HIV-positive patients who were taking zidovudine 200 mg every 4 hours.[1] Another study found that the mean phenytoin dose was higher in HIV-positive patients, when compared to epileptic subjects without the virus, while the mean phenytoin levels in the HIV-positive group were lower (i.e. a higher phenytoin dose resulted in lower serum levels in HIV-positive subjects). Zidovudine did not appear to affect the levels.[2,3] The current evidence would suggest that it is HIV infection, rather than zidovudine that affects phenytoin levels, but more study is needed to confirm this.

1. Sarver P, Lampkin TA, Dukes GE, Messenheimer JA, Kirby MG, Dalton MJ, Hak LJ. Effect of zidovudine on the pharmacokinetic disposition of phenytoin in HIV positive asymptomatic patients. *Pharmacotherapy* (1991) 11, 108–9.
2. Burger DW, Meerhorst PL, Koks CHW, Beijnen JH. Phenytoin (PH) monitoring in HIV (+) individuals: is there an interaction with zidovudine (ZDV)? 9th International Conference on AIDS & 5th World Congress on Sexually Transmitted Diseases, Berlin. June 6–11, 1993. Abstract PO-B31-2214.
3. Burger DM, Meenhorst PL, Mulder JW, Kraaijeveld CL, Koks CHW, Bult A, Beijnen JH. Therapeutic drug monitoring of phenytoin in patients with the acquired immunodeficiency syndrome. *Ther Drug Monit* (1994) 16, 616–20.

Phenytoin + Zileuton

The pharmacokinetics of phenytoin are unchanged by zileuton.

Clinical evidence, mechanism, importance and management

A controlled study in 20 healthy subjects found that the pharmacokinetics of a single 300-mg dose of phenytoin were unaltered by zileuton 600 mg every 6 hours for 5 days.[1] An *in vitro* study found that zileuton had little effect on the isoenzymes responsible for the metabolism of phenytoin.[2] These studies suggest that zileuton is unlikely to affect phenytoin levels in clinical use.

1. Samara E, Cavanaugh JH, Mukherjee D, Granneman GR. Lack of pharmacokinetic interaction between zileuton and phenytoin in humans. *Clin Pharmacokinet* (1995) 29 (Suppl 2), 84–91.
2. Lu P, Schrag ML, Slaughter DE, Raab CE, Shou M, Rodrigues AD. Mechanism-based inhibition of human liver microsomal cytochrome P450 1A2 by zileuton, a 5-lipoxygenase inhibitor. *Drug Metab Dispos* (2003) 31, 1352–60.

Piracetam + Other antiepileptics

Piracetam does not appear to alter the levels of sodium valproate or primidone. No interaction has been found between piracetam and carbamazepine, clonazepam, phenobarbital, or phenytoin.

Clinical evidence, mechanism, importance and management

The addition of piracetam (2 to 4 g three times daily, increased to a maximum of 18 to 24 g daily) did not affect plasma levels of **sodium valproate** or **primidone** in patients with myoclonus. The exact number of patients taking these drugs is unclear, since the report just states that 28 patients were taking **clonazepam**, **sodium valproate**, or **primidone**, alone or in combination.[1] Another similar report, briefly noted the same finding.[2] The manufacturer notes that, although based on a small number of patients, no interaction has been found between piracetam and **clonazepam**, **carbamazepine**, **phenytoin**, **phenobarbital** and **sodium valproate**.[3] No special precautions appear to be required if piracetam is used with these antiepileptics.

1. Obeso JA, Artieda J, Quinn N, Rothwell JC, Luquin MR, Vaamonde J, Marsden CD. Piracetam in the treatment of different types of myoclonus. *Clin Neuropharmacol* (1988) 11, 529–36.
2. Raychev I. Piracetam (pyramem) in the treatment of cortical myoclonus. 5th European Congress of Epileptology, Madrid 2002. P382.
3. Nootropil (Piracetam). UCB Pharma Ltd. UK Summary of product characteristics, May 2005.

Pregabalin + Miscellaneous

There appears to be no pharmacokinetic interaction between pregabalin and carbamazepine, gabapentin, lamotrigine, phenobarbital, phenytoin, topiramate, valproate, alcohol, lorazepam, or oxycodone. However, the impairment of cognitive and gross motor function caused by oxycodone was additive with pregabalin, and pregabalin may potentiate the effects of alcohol and lorazepam.

Clinical evidence, mechanism, importance and management

(a) Alcohol or Lorazepam

The manufacturer notes that there was no clinically relevant pharmacokinetic interaction between pregabalin and lorazepam or alcohol, and that concurrent use caused no clinically important effect on respiration. However, they note that pregabalin may potentiate the effects of lorazepam and alcohol.[1]

(b) Other antiepileptics

Pregabalin 200 mg three times daily for 7 days was added to monotherapy with various antiepileptics in patients with partial epilepsy. Pregabalin did not alter the steady-state levels of **phenytoin**, **carbamazepine** (and its active metabolite, carbamazepine-10,11-epoxide), **valproate** or **lamotrigine**. In addition, the steady-state pharmacokinetics of pregabalin were not different to those seen previously in healthy subjects taking pregabalin alone, suggesting that these antiepileptics do not alter pregabalin pharmacokinetics.[2] Similarly, population pharmacokinetic analyses of clinical studies found no important changes in the pharmacokinetics of **lamotrigine**, **phenobarbital**, **phenytoin**, **topiramate** or **valproate** when they were given with pregabalin, and the pharmacokinetics of pregabalin were unaffected by these drugs.[3] The manufacturer also notes that there is no pharmacokinetic interaction between pregabalin and **gabapentin**.[1]

(c) Oxycodone

The manufacturer notes that there was no clinically relevant pharmacokinetic interaction between pregabalin and oxycodone, and that there was no clinically important effect on respiration. However, pregabalin appeared to cause an additive impairment in cognitive and gross motor function when given with oxycodone.[1] This suggests caution is warranted during combined use.

1. Lyrica (Pregabalin). Pfizer Ltd. UK Summary of product characteristics, June 2007.
2. Brodie MJ, Wilson EA, Wesche DL, Alvey CW, Randinitis EJ, Posvar EL, Hounslow NJ, Bron NJ, Gibson GL, Bockbrader HN. Pregabalin drug interaction studies: lack of effect on the pharmacokinetics of carbamazepine, phenytoin, lamotrigine, and valproate in patients with partial epilepsy. *Epilepsia* (2005) 46, 1407–13.
3. Bockbrader HN, Burger PJ, Corrigan BW, Kugler AR, Knapp LE, Garofalo EA, Lalonde RL. Population pharmacokinetic analyses of commonly prescribed antiepileptic drugs coadministered with pregabalin in adult patients with refractory partial seizures. *Epilepsia* (2001) 42 (Suppl 7), 84.

Primidone + Isoniazid

A single case report describes elevated serum primidone levels and reduced phenobarbital levels when primidone was given with isoniazid.

Clinical evidence, mechanism, importance and management

A patient taking primidone had raised serum primidone levels and reduced serum phenobarbital levels. This was attributed to the concurrent use of isoniazid, which inhibited the metabolism of the primidone by the liver. The half-life of primidone rose from 8.7 to 14 hours while taking isoniazid and steady-state primidone levels rose by 83%.[1] The importance of this interaction is uncertain but prescribers should bear this interaction in mind in case of an unexpected response to primidone.

1. Sutton G, Kupferberg HJ. Isoniazid as an inhibitor of primidone metabolism. *Neurology* (1975) 25, 1179–81.

Primidone + Miscellaneous

Primidone is substantially converted to phenobarbital within the body and it is therefore expected to interact with other drugs in the same way as phenobarbital. Some drugs may increase the conversion of primidone to phenobarbital.

Clinical evidence, mechanism, importance and management

Primidone is substantially converted to phenobarbital within the body. For example, a group of patients taking long-term primidone developed serum primidone levels of 9 micrograms/mL and serum phenobarbital levels of 31 micrograms/mL.[1] Primidone would therefore be expected to interact with other drugs in the same way as phenobarbital. Some enzyme-inducing drugs might increase the conversion of primidone to phenobarbital, and this has been demonstrated for 'phenytoin', below, and 'carbamazepine', (p.534). Some patients have been treated with a combination of phenobarbital and primidone. In this situation higher phenobarbital levels might be expected.

1. Booker HE, Hosokowa K, Burdette RD, Darcey B. A clinical study of serum primidone levels. *Epilepsia* (1970) 11, 395–402.

Primidone + Phenytoin

Primidone-derived serum phenobarbital levels are increased by phenytoin. This is normally an advantageous interaction, but phenobarbital toxicity occasionally occurs.

Clinical evidence

A study in 44 epileptic patients taking primidone and phenytoin found that their serum phenobarbital to primidone ratio was high (4.35) when compared with that in 15 other patients who were only taking primidone

(1.05).[1] This suggests that in the presence of phenytoin, primidone-derived phenobarbital levels are higher than when primidone is given alone. Similar results are described in other studies.[2-7] A few patients may develop barbiturate toxicity.[8]

An initial marked decrease in phenytoin levels, then an increase to half the initial phenytoin level, was seen in the first few weeks after withdrawing primidone in an infant. Derived phenobarbital levels before discontinuing the primidone were very high, and were associated with marked sedation.[9]

Mechanism

Phenytoin increases the metabolic conversion of primidone to phenobarbital, while possibly depressing the subsequent metabolic destruction (hydroxylation) of the phenobarbital. The net effect is a rise in phenobarbital levels.[10] Phenobarbital may increase or decrease phenytoin levels, see 'Phenytoin + Phenobarbital', p.562.

Importance and management

Well documented. This is normally an advantageous interaction since phenobarbital is itself an active antiepileptic. However, it should be borne in mind that phenobarbital serum levels could sometimes reach toxic concentrations,[8] even if only a small dose of phenytoin is added. Changes in phenytoin levels may also occur (see 'Phenytoin + Phenobarbital', p.562).

1. Fincham RW, Schottelius DD, Sahs AL. The influence of diphenylhydantoin on primidone metabolism. *Arch Neurol* (1974) 30, 259–62.
2. Fincham RW, Schottelius DD, Sahs AL. The influence of diphenylhydantoin on primidone metabolism. *Trans Am Neurol Assoc* (1973) 98, 197–9.
3. Schmidt D. The effect of phenytoin and ethosuximide on primidone metabolism in patients with epilepsy. *J Neurol* (1975) 209, 115–23.
4. Reynolds EH, Fenton G, Fenwick P, Johnson AL, Laundy M. Interaction of phenytoin and primidone. *BMJ* (1975) 2, 594–5.
5. Callaghan N, Feeley M, Duggan F, O'Callaghan M, Seldrup J. The effect of anticonvulsant drugs which induce liver microsomal enzymes on derived and ingested phenobarbitone levels. *Acta Neurol Scand* (1977) 56, 1–6.
6. Battino D, Avanzini G, Bossi L, Croci D, Cusi C, Gomeni C, Moise A. Plasma levels of primidone and its metabolite phenobarbital: effect of age and associated therapy. *Ther Drug Monit* (1983) 5, 73–9.
7. Garrettson LK, Gomez M. Phenytoin-primidone interaction. *Br J Clin Pharmacol* (1977) 4, 693–5.
8. Galdames D, Ortiz M, Saavedra I, Aguilera L. Interaccion fenitoina-primidona: intoxicacion por fenobarbital, en un adulto tratado con ambas drogas. *Rev Med Chil* (1980) 108, 716–20.
9. Wilson JT, Wilkinson GR. Chronic and severe phenobarbital intoxication in a child treated with primidone and diphenylhydantoin. *J Pediatr* (1973) 83, 484–9.
10. Porro MG, Kupferberg HJ, Porter RJ, Theodore WH, Newmark ME. Phenytoin: an inhibitor and inducer of primidone metabolism in an epileptic patient. *Br J Clin Pharmacol* (1982) 14, 294–7.

Primidone + Valproate

Valproate has been reported to cause increases, decreases, and no change in serum primidone levels. Primidone-derived phenobarbital levels appear to be increased by valproate.

Clinical evidence

In a number of cases, patients taking primidone required a decrease in the primidone dosage after valproate was added.[1-4] In 6 cases this was due to an increase in the primidone-derived phenobarbital level,[1] and in the other cases phenobarbital levels were not measured, but the dosage reduction was needed to overcome the sedation that occurred when the valproate was added.[2-4] Primidone levels were not measured in any of these cases.[1-4] In two other studies, primidone levels either decreased,[5] or did not change when valproate was added.[6] However, phenobarbital levels, where measured, had increased.[6]

In 7 children the serum levels of primidone 10 to 18 mg/kg daily rose two to threefold when valproate (dosage not stated) was also given. After 1 to 3 months of continued therapy the serum primidone levels fell in 3 of the patients but persisted in one. Follow-up primidone levels were not taken in the other 3 patients, and no patient had phenobarbital levels measured.[7]

In contrast, in a further study, neither phenobarbital levels nor primidone levels were significantly altered when valproate was given.[8]

Mechanism

It has been suggested that valproate decreases the conversion of primidone to phenobarbital, and decreases the metabolism of phenobarbital (see also 'Phenobarbital + Valproate', p.547). This would result in increased primidone and phenobarbital levels. However, increased renal clearance of primidone may occur, resulting in no overall change to the primidone levels. Depending on the balance between these various effects a variety of levels may result.[8] The results of one study suggest that this proposed inhibition of primidone metabolism caused by valproate may diminish over the first few months of concurrent use.[7]

Importance and management

There seems to be little consistency about the effect of valproate on primidone levels. However, in the majority of cases phenobarbital levels seem to be raised (see also 'Phenobarbital + Valproate', p.547). It would seem prudent not to measure primidone levels without corresponding phenobarbital levels. Monitor the patient for increased signs of sedation, which may be resolved by a reduction in the primidone dose.

1. Wilder BJ, Willmore LJ, Bruni J, Villarreal HJ. Valproic acid: interaction with other anticonvulsant drugs. *Neurology* (1978) 28, 892–6.
2. Haigh D, Forsythe WI. The treatment of childhood epilepsy with sodium valproate. *Dev Med Child Neurol* (1975) 17, 743–8.
3. Richens A, Ahmad S. Controlled trial of sodium valproate in severe epilepsy. *BMJ* (1975) 4, 255–6.
4. Völzke E, Doose H. Dipropylacetate (Dépakine®, Ergenyl®) in the treatment of epilepsy. *Epilepsia* (1973) 14, 185–93.
5. Varma R, Michos GA, Varma RS, Hoshino AY. Clinical trials of Depakene (valproic acid) coadministered with other anticonvulsants in epileptic patients. *Res Commun Psychol Psychiatr Behav* (1980) 5, 265–73.
6. Yukawa E, Higuchi S, Aoyama T. The effect of concurrent administration of sodium valproate on serum levels of primidone and its metabolite phenobarbital. *J Clin Pharm Ther* (1989) 14, 387–92.
7. Windorfer A, Sauer W, Gädeke R. Elevation of diphenylhydantoin and primidone serum concentration by addition of dipropylacetate, a new anticonvulsant drug. *Acta Paediatr Scand* (1975) 64, 771–2.
8. Bruni J. Valproic acid and plasma levels of primidone and derived phenobarbital. *Can J Neurol Sci* (1981) 8, 91–2.

Progabide + Other antiepileptics

Progabide may raise phenytoin levels and alter the serum levels of carbamazepine, clonazepam, phenobarbital. The effect of these antiepileptics on progabide levels appears to be only moderate or small.

Clinical evidence

(a) Phenytoin

Marked increases in serum phenytoin levels have been seen in a few patients also given progabide,[1-4] while smaller changes have been described in some studies,[5,6] and negligible changes in others.[7]

In one study, 17 out of 26 epileptics needed a reduction in their phenytoin dosage to keep the levels within 25% of the serum levels achieved in the absence of progabide. Over half the patients needed a dose reduction within 4 weeks of starting concurrent treatment. Most of those needing a dosage reduction had a maximum increase in the serum level of 40% or more, which was sometimes accompanied by toxicity.[2,8] In a later report of this study, of a total of 32 epileptic patients taking carbamazepine with phenytoin and then given progabide, 22 needed a reduction in phenytoin dosage to maintain serum levels within 25% of those achieved in the absence of progabide. In addition, it appeared this effect on phenytoin serum levels continued for a while after progabide was withdrawn.[4]

(b) Other antiepileptics

Information about antiepileptics other than phenytoin is limited, but progabide is reported to minimally reduce,[1,9,10] minimally increase[1] or not to change **carbamazepine**[2,3,5-7] serum levels. An increase of up to 24% in the levels of carbamazepine-10,11-epoxide (the active metabolite of **carbamazepine**) has also been reported.[6,10] **Valproate**,[3,5-7] and **clonazepam**[11] serum levels were not significantly affected by progabide. Progabide appears to cause a small increase in serum **phenobarbital** levels, which is of little clinical importance.[1,5-7]

Mechanism

Uncertain.

Importance and management

Some small to moderate changes in the serum levels of carbamazepine, phenobarbital, valproate and clonazepam can apparently occur in the presence of progabide, but only the interaction with phenytoin appears to be clinically relevant. Be alert for the need to reduce the dosage of phenytoin if progabide is used concurrently. The slight effects of the antiepileptics on progabide levels are of unknown, but probably minor, significance.

1. Schmidt D, Utech K. Progabide for refractory partial epilepsy: a controlled add-on trial. *Neurology* (1986) 36, 217–221.
2. Cloyd JC, Brundage RC, Leppik IE, Graves NM, Welty TE. Effect of progabide on serum phenytoin and carbamazepine concentrations: a preliminary report. In: LERS Monograph series, volume 3. Edited by Bartholini G et al. Epilepsy and GABA receptor agonists: basic and therapeutic research. Meeting, Paris, March 1984. Raven Press, New York. (1985) pp 271–8. ISBN: 0881671061
3. Crawford P, Chadwick D. A comparative study of progabide, valproate and placebo as add-on therapy in patients with refractory epilepsy. *J Neurol Neurosurg Psychiatry* (1986) 49, 1251–7.
4. Brundage RC, Cloyd JC, Leppik IE, Graves NM and Welty TE. Effect of progabide on serum phenytoin and carbamazepine concentrations. *Clin Neuropharmacol* (1987) 10, 545–54.
5. Bianchetti G, Thiercelin JF, Thenot JP, Feuerstein J, Lambert D, Rulliere R, Thebault JJ, Morselli PL. Effect of progabide on the pharmacokinetics of various antiepileptic drugs. *Neurology* (1984) 34 (Suppl 1), 213.
6. Bianchetti G, Padovani P, Thénot JP, Thiercelin JF, Morselli PL. Pharmacokinetic interactions of progabide with other antiepileptic drugs. *Epilepsia* (1987) 28, 68–73.
7. Thénot JP, Bianchetti G, Abriol C, Feuerstein J, Lambert D, Thébault JJ, Warrington SJ, Rowland M. Interactions between progabide and antiepileptic drugs. In: LERS Monograph series, volume 3. Edited by Bartholini G et al. Epilepsy and GABA receptor agonists: basic and therapeutic research. Meeting, Paris, March 1984. Raven Press, New York. (1985) pp 259–69. ISBN: 0881671061
8. Brundage RC, Leppik IE, Cloyd JC, Graves NM. Effect of progabide on phenytoin pharmacokinetics. *Epilepsia* (1984) 25, 656–7.
9. Dam M, Gram L, Philbert A, Hansen BS, Blatt Lyon B, Christensen JM, Angelo HR. Progabide: a controlled trial in partial epilepsy. *Epilepsia* (1983) 24, 127–34.
10. Graves NM, Fuerst RH, Cloyd JC, Brundage RC, Welty TE, Leppik IE. Progabide-induced changes in carbamazepine metabolism. *Epilepsia* (1988) 29, 775–80.
11. Warrington SJ, O'Brien C, Thiercelin JF, Orofiamma B and Morselli PL. Evaluation of pharmacodynamic interaction between progabide and clonazepam in healthy men. In: LERS Monograph series, volume 3. Edited by Bartholini G et al. Epilepsy and GABA receptor agonists: basic and therapeutic research. Meeting, Paris, March 1984. Raven Press, New York. (1985) pp 279–86. ISBN: 0881671061

Remacemide + Other antiepileptics

Remacemide causes modest increases in carbamazepine and phenytoin serum levels. Carbamazepine, phenobarbital and phenytoin moderately reduce remacemide serum levels. Valproate and lamotrigine do not appear to interact with remacemide.

Clinical evidence

(a) Carbamazepine

When a group of 10 patients taking carbamazepine were also given up to 300 mg of remacemide twice daily for 2 weeks the minimum serum levels and AUC of carbamazepine were increased by 20% and 22%, respectively. No patients had symptoms of carbamazepine toxicity.[1] Another study of 11 patients taking carbamazepine found that remacemide caused a similar 20 to 30% increase in the AUC of carbamazepine, again without signs of toxicity. No consistent changes in the AUC of carbamazepine-10,11-epoxide, the main metabolite of carbamazepine, were seen.[2] Another study has reported a slight inhibitory effect of remacemide on carbamazepine metabolism, which is in line with these other findings.[3] One of these studies also reported that the AUC of remacemide was decreased by 40 to 50% and the AUC of its main metabolite by about 70% in the presence of carbamazepine, when compared with healthy subjects (presumably not taking carbamazepine).[2]

However, a further study of the efficacy of remacemide and carbamazepine in combination found that about two-thirds of the 120 patients treated needed 14 to 50% reductions in their carbamazepine dose, to ensure levels remained in the therapeutic range.[4]

(b) Lamotrigine

There was no clinically relevant pharmacokinetic interaction between remacemide (200 mg daily increased to 200 mg three times daily) and lamotrigine (200 mg twice daily decreased to 100 mg daily) in healthy subjects.[5]

(c) Phenobarbital

Phenobarbital 30 mg daily increased to 90 mg daily increased the clearance of remacemide 200 mg twice daily by 67%, and slightly increased the plasma levels of phenobarbital (by 9%) in a study in healthy subjects.[6]

(d) Phenytoin

A group of 10 patients taking phenytoin were also given up to 300 mg remacemide twice daily for 2 weeks. On average remacemide did not affect phenytoin pharmacokinetics but 5 patients had an increase in minimum serum levels of 30% or more. No patients had symptoms of phenytoin toxicity.[1] In another study 10 epileptics, who had been taking phenytoin for at least 3 months, were given remacemide 300 mg twice daily for 12 days. Phenytoin maximum plasma levels were increased by 13.7% and the AUC was raised by 11.5%. Average concentrations of remacemide and its main metabolite were around only 40% and 30%, respectively, of those achieved in healthy subjects taking remacemide alone, at the same dosage.[7] Another study reported a slight inhibitory effect of remacemide on phenytoin metabolism, which is in line with these other findings.[3]

(e) Sodium valproate

A group of 10 patients taking valproate were also given remacemide up to 300 mg twice daily for 14 days. The pharmacokinetics of valproate remained unchanged.[1] Another study in 17 patients confirmed these findings,[8] and an earlier study by the same authors also noted no effect of remacemide on valproate metabolism.[3]

Mechanism

Not fully understood, but *in vitro* studies indicate that remacemide inhibits the cytochrome P450 isoenzyme CYP3A4, which in practice would be expected to result in a reduction in the metabolism of the carbamazepine resulting in an increase in its serum levels. Remacemide appears to inhibit CYP2C9 to a lesser extent, which is reflected in a smaller interaction with phenytoin. Valproate is metabolised by glucuronidation and is therefore unaffected.[1]

Carbamazepine and phenytoin, known enzyme inducers, also seem to increase the metabolism of the remacemide.[7]

Importance and management

Information is limited, but the interactions of remacemide with carbamazepine, phenobarbital and phenytoin appear to be established, but so far only the carbamazepine interaction seems to have been shown to be of clinical importance. Even so, until more experience has been gained, monitor the effects of concurrent use with phenytoin or phenobarbital. No interaction occurs between remacemide and valproate or lamotrigine.

1. Riley RJ, Slee D, Martin CA, Webborn PJH, Wattam DG, Jones T, Logan CJ. *In vitro* evaluation of pharmacokinetic interactions between remacemide hydrochloride and established anticonvulsants. *Br J Clin Pharmacol* (1996) 41, 461P.
2. Leach JP, Blacklaw J, Stewart M, Jamieson V, Jones T, Oxley R, Richens A, Brodie MJ. Mutual pharmacokinetic interactions between remacemide hydrochloride and carbamazepine. *Epilepsia* (1995) 36 (Suppl 3), S163.
3. Leach JP, Blacklaw J, Stewart M, Jamieson V, Oxley R, Richens A, Brodie MJ. Interactions between remacemide and the established antiepileptic drugs. *Epilepsia* (1994) 35 (Suppl 7), 75.
4. Mawer GE, Jamieson V, Lucas SB, Wild JM. Adjustment of carbamazepine dose to offset the effects of the interaction with remacemide hydrochloride in a double-blind, multicentre, add-on drug trial (CR2237) in refractory epilepsy. *Epilepsia* (1999) 40, 190–6.
5. Blakey GE, Lockton JA, Rolan IP. The effect of lamotrigine on the disposition of remacemide hydrochloride. *Epilepsia* (1999) 40 (Suppl 2), 251.
6. Hooper WD, Eadie MJ, Blakey GE, Lockton JA, Manun'Ebo M. Evaluation of a pharmacokinetic interaction between remacemide hydrochloride and phenobarbitone in healthy males. *Br J Clin Pharmacol* (2001) 51, 249–55.
7. Leach JP, Girvan J, Jamieson V, Jones T, Richens A, Brodie MJ. Mutual interaction between remacemide hydrochloride and phenytoin. *Epilepsy Res* (1997) 26, 381–8.
8. Leach JP, Girvan J, Jamieson V, Jones T, Richens A, Brodie MJ. Lack of pharmacokinetic interaction between remacemide hydrochloride and sodium valproate in epileptic patients. *Seizure* (1997) 6, 179–84.

Retigabine + Other antiepileptics

The clearance of retigabine is increased by carbamazepine and phenytoin, but not by phenobarbital, topiramate, or valproate. Retigabine does not alter the pharmacokinetics of any of these antiepileptics. There is a modest pharmacokinetic interaction between retigabine and lamotrigine.

Clinical evidence, mechanism, importance and management

(a) Enzyme-inducing antiepileptics

The preliminary report of a study notes that the clearance of retigabine was increased (amount not stated) by **carbamazepine** and **phenytoin**, whereas retigabine did not alter **carbamazepine** or **phenytoin** pharmacokinetics in patients with epilepsy.[1] This is consistent with the known enzyme-inducing properties of **carbamazepine** and **phenytoin**, and the fact that retigabine has not been shown to induce hepatic enzymes. In contrast, in a study in healthy subjects, **phenobarbital** 90 mg daily did not affect the pharmacokinetics of retigabine 200 mg every 8 hours, and the pharmacokinetics of **phenobarbital** were not altered by retigabine.[2] The clinical relevance of the effect of **carbamazepine** and **phenytoin** on retigabine remains to be assessed. No dosage adjustments seem to be necessary with **phenobarbital**.

(b) Lamotrigine

In a study in 14 healthy subjects lamotrigine 25 mg daily for 5 days increased the AUC of a single 200-mg dose of retigabine by 15% and decreased the clearance by 13%.[3] In another 15 subjects, retigabine 200 mg twice daily increased to 300 mg twice daily over 15 days decreased the AUC of a single 200-mg dose of lamotrigine by 18% and increased clearance by 22%. It was suggested that lamotrigine competes for renal elimination with retigabine, but the mechanism behind the decreased lamotrigine levels is unknown.[3] These modest changes are unlikely to be clinically important for most patients, but the authors suggest that the effects need to be assessed at the upper recommended dose ranges, and therefore advise caution.

(c) Topiramate

The preliminary report of a study notes that the pharmacokinetics of retigabine and topiramate were not altered by concurrent use in patients with epilepsy.[1] No special dosing precautions are necessary.

(d) Valproate

The preliminary report of a study notes that the pharmacokinetics of retigabine and valproic acid were not altered by concurrent use in patients with epilepsy.[1] No special dosing precautions are necessary.

1. Sachdeo RC, Ferron GM, Partiot AM, Biton V, Rosenfeld WB, Porter RJ, Fritz T, Althouse S, Troy SM. An early determination of drug-drug interaction between valproic acid, phenytoin, carbamazepine or topiramate, and retigabine in epileptic patients. *Neurology* (2001) 56 (Suppl 3). A331–A332.
2. Ferron GM, Patat A, Parks V, Rolan P, Troy SM. Lack of pharmacokinetic interaction between retigabine and phenobarbitone at steady state in healthy subjects. *Br J Clin Pharmacol* (2003) 56, 39–45.
3. Hermann R, Knebel NG, Niebch G, Richards L, Borlak J, Locher M. Pharmacokinetic interaction between retigabine and lamotrigine in healthy subjects. *Eur J Clin Pharmacol* (2003) 58, 795–802.

Stiripentol + Other antiepileptics

Stiripentol causes marked rises in the serum levels of carbamazepine, phenobarbital and phenytoin. Stiripentol causes only a small rise in the serum levels of valproate.

Clinical evidence

Epileptic patients taking two or three antiepileptics (**phenytoin**, **phenobarbital**, **carbamazepine**, **clobazam**, **primidone**, **nitrazepam**) were also given stiripentol, increasing from 600 mg to 2.4 g daily. The 5 patients taking **phenytoin** had an average 37% reduction in the **phenytoin** clearance when they took stiripentol 1.2 g daily, and a 78% reduction when they took stiripentol 2.4 g daily. These changes in clearance were reflected in marked rises in the steady-state serum levels of **phenytoin**: for example the serum **phenytoin** levels of one patient rose from 14.4 to 27.4 mg/L over 30 days while he was taking stiripentol, despite a 50% reduction in his **phenytoin** dosage. **Phenytoin** toxicity was seen in another two subjects.[1] The clearance of **carbamazepine** in one subject fell by 39% when stiripentol 1.2 g daily was taken and by 71% when stiripentol 2.4 g daily was taken. **Phenobarbital** clearance in two subjects fell by about 30 to 40% when they took stiripentol 2.4 g daily.[1] Three other studies in adults and children confirmed that stiripentol reduces the clearance of **carbamazepine** by between about 50% and 65%,[2-4] and significantly increases carbamazepine levels.[5] Another study found that the formation of carbamazepine-10,11-epoxide, the active metabolite of **carbamazepine** was markedly reduced in children taking **carbamazepine** with stiripentol.[6]

Valproate 1 g daily was given to 8 subjects with or without stiripentol 1.2 g daily. The stiripentol caused a 14% increase in the peak serum levels of **valproate**.[7] In another 11 patients no adverse effects on motor, perceptual or attention tests were seen when stiripentol was given with other antiepileptic drugs, but the doses of **phenobarbital**, **phenytoin** and **carbamazepine** were reduced before the combination was taken.[8]

Mechanism

Stiripentol inhibits the activity of various cytochrome P450 liver isoenzymes including CYP1A2, CYP2C9, CYP2C19, CYP2D6 and CYP3A4, some of which are concerned with the metabolism of other antiepileptics. As a result the loss of the antiepileptic from the body is reduced and the serum levels rise accordingly.[3,9] In the case of valproate, cytochrome P450-mediated metabolism is only involved in minor valproate metabolic pathways and therefore only a small rise in serum levels occurs.[7] However, there is evidence that stiripentol may reduce the formation of a minor but hepatotoxic metabolite of valproate (2-propyl-4-pentenoic acid or 4-ene-VPA).[10]

Importance and management

Established and clinically important interactions. The phenytoin, phenobarbital and carbamazepine dosages should be reduced to avoid the development of elevated serum levels and possible toxicity during the concurrent use of stiripentol. One study[3] suggests that the carbamazepine dosage should be decreased incrementally over 7 to 10 days, beginning as soon as the stiripentol is started and, regardless of age, the maintenance dose of carbamazepine should aim to give serum levels of 5 to 10 micrograms/mL. Stiripentol causes only small changes in the serum levels of valproate and dosage adjustments are unlikely to be needed with this combination.

1. Levy RH, Loiseau P, Guyot M, Blehaut HM, Tor J, Morland TA. Stiripentol kinetics in epilepsy: nonlinearity and interactions. *Clin Pharmacol Ther* (1984) 36, 661–9.
2. Levy RH, Kerr BM, Farwell J, Anderson GD, Martinez-Lage JM, Tor J. Carbamazepine/stiripentol interaction in adult and pediatric patients. *Epilepsia* (1989) 30, 701.
3. Kerr BM, Martinez-Lage JM, Viteri C, Tor J, Eddy AC, Levy RH. Carbamazepine dose requirements during stiripentol therapy: influence of cytochrome P-450 inhibition by stiripentol. *Epilepsia* (1991) 32, 267–74.
4. Levy RH, Martinez-Lage JM, Tor J, Blehaut H, Gonzalez I, Bainbridge B. Stiripentol level-dose relationship and interaction with carbamazepine in epileptic patients. *Epilepsia* (1985) 26, 544–5.
5. Tran A, Vauzelle-Kervroedan F, Rey E, Pons G. d'Athis P, Chiron C, Dulac O, Renard F, Olive G. Effect of stiripentol on carbamazepine plasma concentration and metabolism in epileptic children. *Eur J Clin Pharmacol* (1996) 50, 497–500.
6. Cazali N, Tran A, Treluyer JM, Rey E, d'Athis P, Vincent J, Pons G. Inhibitory effect of stiripentol on carbamazepine and saquinavir metabolism in human. *Br J Clin Pharmacol* (2003) 56, 526–36.
7. Levy RH, Loiseau P, Guyot M, Acheampong A, Tor J, Rettenmeier AW. Effects of stiripentol on valproate plasma level and metabolism. *Epilepsia* (1987) 28, 605.
8. Loiseau P, Strube E, Tor J, Levy RH, Dodrill C. Evaluation neuropsychologique et thérapeutique du stiripentol dans l'épilepsie. *Rev Neurol (Paris)* (1988) 144, 165–72.
9. Mather GG, Bishop FE, Trager WF, Kunze KK, Thummel KE, Shen DD, Roskos LK, Lepage F, Gillardin JM, Levy RH. Mechanisms of stiripentol interactions with carbamazepine and phenytoin. *Epilepsia* (1995) 36 (Suppl 3), S162.
10. Levy RH, Rettenmeier AW, Anderson GD, Wilensky AJ, Friel PN, Baillie TA, Acheampong A, Tor J, Guyot M, Loiseau P. Effects of polytherapy with phenytoin, carbamazepine, and stiripentol on formation of 4-ene-valproate, a hepatotoxic metabolite of valproic acid. *Clin Pharmacol Ther* (1990) 48, 225–35.

Tiagabine + Miscellaneous

The pharmacokinetics of tiagabine were not altered by cimetidine or erythromycin. No clinically relevant pharmacokinetic interactions occur between tiagabine and theophylline or warfarin.

Clinical evidence, mechanism, importance and management

Cimetidine 400 mg twice daily for 5 days increased the steady-state AUC of tiagabine 4 mg twice daily by just 5% in a study in 12 healthy subjects.[1,2] This change would not be clinically relevant.

Erythromycin 500 mg twice daily had no clinically relevant effect on the steady-state pharmacokinetics of tiagabine 4 mg twice daily in a study in 14 healthy subjects.[3] No dose adjustment would be required during concurrent use.

Multiple dose studies in healthy subjects have also excluded any clinically relevant pharmacokinetic interactions between tiagabine and **theophylline** or **warfarin** but no further study details were given.[1]

1. Mengel H, Jansen JA, Sommerville K, Jonkman JHG, Wesnes K, Cohen A, Carlson GF, Marshall R, Snel S, Dirach J, Kastberg H. Tiagabine: evaluation of the risk of interaction with theophylline, warfarin, digoxin, cimetidine, oral contraceptives, triazolam, or ethanol. *Epilepsia* (1995) 36 (Suppl 3), S160.
2. Snel S, Jonkman JHG, van Heiningen PNM, Jansen JA, Mengel HB. Tiagabine: evaluation of risk of interaction with cimetidine in healthy male volunteers. *Epilepsia* (1994) 35 (Suppl 7), 74.
3. Thomsen MS, Groes L, Agersø H, Kruse T. Lack of pharmacokinetic interaction between tiagabine and erythromycin. *J Clin Pharmacol* (1998) 38, 1051–6.

Tiagabine + Other antiepileptics

Tiagabine plasma levels are reduced by enzyme-inducing antiepileptics (carbamazepine, phenytoin, phenobarbital and primi-

done). Tiagabine doses may need to be lower in patients *not* taking these drugs. Tiagabine may cause a slight reduction in valproate levels (not clinically relevant), but has no effect on carbamazepine, phenytoin or vigabatrin levels.

Clinical evidence, mechanism, importance and management

In an early clinical study, tiagabine was reported to have no significant effect on the plasma levels of **carbamazepine**, **phenytoin**, **valproate**, and **vigabatrin**.[1] Similarly, tiagabine (titrated from 8 mg up to a maximum of 48 mg daily over 18 days) did not alter the steady-state pharmacokinetics of **phenytoin** or **carbamazepine** in 12 patients with epilepsy.[2] However, in another similar study, it reduced the AUC of **valproate** by 10%, but this reduction is not expected to be clinically significant.[3]

A study in patients taking 1 to 3 other enzyme-inducing antiepileptics (**phenobarbital**, **phenytoin**, **carbamazepine**, **primidone**) found that tiagabine half-lives were shorter (3.8 to 4.9 hours) when compared with historical values in healthy subjects taking tiagabine alone (7.1 hours).[4] The manufacturers say that the plasma concentrations of tiagabine may be reduced 1.5 to 3-fold by these enzyme-inducing antiepileptics.[5] Based on this, they recommend that the initial maintenance dose of tiagabine in patients *not* taking enzyme-inducing drugs should be lower (15 to 30 mg daily) than in those taking these drugs (30 to 45 mg daily).[5]

1. Richens A, Chadwick DW, Duncan JS, Dam M, Gram L, Mikkelsen M, Morrow J, Mengel H, Shu V, McKelvy JF, Pierce MW. Adjunctive treatment of partial seizures with tiagabine: a placebo-controlled trial. *Epilepsy Res* (1995) 21, 37–42.
2. Gustavson LE, Cato A, Boellner SW, Cao GX, Qian JX, Guenther HJ, Sommerville KW. Lack of pharmacokinetic drug interactions between tiagabine and carbamazepine or phenytoin. *Am J Ther* (1998) 5, 9–16.
3. Gustavson LE, Sommerville KW, Boellner SW, Witt GF, Guenther HJ, Granneman GR. Lack of a clinically significant pharmacokinetic drug interaction between tiagabine and valproate. *Am J Ther* (1998) 5, 73–79.
4. So EL, Wolff D, Graves NM, Leppik IE, Cascino GD, Pixton GC, Gustavson LE. Pharmacokinetics of tiagabine as add-on therapy in patients taking enzyme-inducing drugs. *Epilepsy Res* (1995) 22, 221–6.
5. Gabitril (Tiagabine). Cephalon UK Ltd. UK Summary of product characteristics, November 2003.

Topiramate + Carbamazepine

Topiramate plasma levels may be reduced by carbamazepine. Carbamazepine levels are not affected by topiramate. However, one report suggests that the toxicity seen when topiramate is added to maximum tolerated doses of carbamazepine may respond to a reduction in the carbamazepine dose.

Clinical evidence

(a) Carbamazepine levels

In a study in 12 epileptic patients topiramate titrated up to a maximum of 400 mg twice daily had no effect on the steady-state plasma levels of carbamazepine 300 to 800 mg every 8 hours or on its main metabolite, carbamazepine-10,11-epoxide.[1] An earlier study in epileptic patients also reported that topiramate does not affect the pharmacokinetics of carbamazepine.[2] In contrast, another report describes 2 patients taking a maximum tolerated dose of carbamazepine who started treatment with topiramate and subsequently developed symptoms suggestive of carbamazepine toxicity. In both these cases, the symptoms resolved when the carbamazepine dose was reduced, and this enabled continued titration of the topiramate dose in one. A review of the clinical use of these two drugs found another 23 cases that fitted this pattern. Carbamazepine levels were not reported.[3]

(b) Topiramate levels

The topiramate plasma levels and AUC were found to be about 40% lower in the presence of carbamazepine in a study in 12 epileptic patients.[1] A population pharmacokinetic study reported that patients taking carbamazepine had 32% lower morning topiramate level than patients not taking enzyme-inducing antiepileptics.[4] In a study in healthy subjects carbamazepine 600 mg daily was found to cause a twofold increase the clearance of a single 200-mg dose of topiramate. The mean half-life of topiramate decreased from 29 to 19 hours. There was also a two- to threefold increase in the formation of the 2 major metabolites of topiramate (2,3-diol-TPM and 10-OH-TPM), although 41% of topiramate was excreted unchanged in the urine in the presence of carbamazepine.[5] In contrast, an earlier study reported that carbamazepine did not have a major effect on the pharmacokinetics of topiramate.[2]

Mechanism

Carbamazepine appears to induce the metabolism of topiramate. Although topiramate can weakly induce CYP3A4 this does not usually appear to have a clinically relevant effect on carbamazepine metabolism, unless carbamazepine is already at the maximum tolerated dose.

Importance and management

Carbamazepine possibly results in a moderate reduction in topiramate plasma levels, but this is probably of limited clinical importance. There is some evidence that the toxicity seen when topiramate is added to maximum tolerated doses of carbamazepine may respond to a reduction in the carbamazepine dose.

1. Sachdeo RC, Sachdeo SK, Walker SA, Kramer LD, Nayak RK, Doose DR. Steady-state pharmacokinetics of topiramate and carbamazepine in patients with epilepsy during monotherapy and concomitant therapy. *Epilepsia* (1996) 37, 774–80.
2. Wilensky AJ, Ojemann LM, Chemelir T, Margul BL, Doose DR. Topiramate pharmacokinetics in epileptic patients receiving carbamazepine. *Epilepsia* (1989) 30, 645–6.
3. Mack CJ, Kuc S, Mulcrone SA, Pilley A, Grünewald RA. Interaction of topiramate with carbamazepine: two case reports and a review of clinical experience. *Seizure* (2002) 11, 464–7.
4. May TW, Jürges U. Serum concentrations of topiramate in epileptic patients: the influence of dose and comedication. *Epilepsia* (1999) 40 (Suppl 2), 249.
5. Britzi M, Perucca E, Soback S, Levy RH, Fattore C, Crema F, Gatti G, Doose DR, Maryanoff BE, Bialer M. Pharmacokinetic and metabolic investigation of topiramate disposition in healthy subjects in the absence and in the presence of enzyme induction by carbamazepine. *Epilepsia* (2005) 46, 378–84.

Topiramate + Phenobarbital or Primidone

Topiramate appears not to alter the pharmacokinetics of phenobarbital or primidone. Phenobarbital reduces topiramate levels.

Clinical evidence, mechanism, importance and management

A review of data from double blind, placebo-controlled studies found that over periods of 8 to 12 weeks the plasma levels of phenobarbital or primidone in patients (number not stated) with partial seizures remained unchanged when they were also given topiramate.[1]

A population pharmacokinetic study reported that patients taking phenobarbital had 31% lower morning topiramate levels than patients not taking enzyme-inducing antiepileptics.[2] Another study that grouped carbamazepine, phenobarbital and phenytoin reported that patients taking one or more of these drugs had 1.5-fold greater topiramate clearance than patients taking lamotrigine or valproate.[3] Phenobarbital probably induces the metabolism of topiramate thereby reducing its levels.

When topiramate is added to existing treatment with phenytoin or phenobarbital its dose should be titrated to effect. If phenobarbital or primidone are withdrawn or added, be aware that the dose of topiramate may need adjustment.

1. Doose DR, Walker SA, Pledger G, Lim P, Reife RA. Evaluation of phenobarbital and primidone/phenobarbital (primidone's active metabolite) plasma concentrations during administration of add-on topiramate therapy in five multicenter, double-blind, placebo-controlled trials in outpatients with partial seizures. *Epilepsia* (1995) 36 (Suppl 3), S158.
2. May TW, Jürges U. Serum concentrations of topiramate in epileptic patients: the influence of dose and comedication. *Epilepsia* (1999) 40 (Suppl 2), 249.
3. Contin M, Riva R, Albani F, Avoni P, Baruzzi A. Topiramate therapeutic monitoring in patients with epilepsy: effect of concomitant antiepileptic drugs. *Ther Drug Monit* (2002) 24, 332–7.

Topiramate + Phenytoin

In some patients the plasma levels of phenytoin are slightly raised by topiramate, and topiramate plasma levels may be reduced by phenytoin.

Clinical evidence

Topiramate, titrated to a maximum of 400 mg twice daily, was given to 12 epileptic patients taking phenytoin 260 to 600 mg daily. When the maximum tolerated dose of topiramate was reached, the phenytoin dose was then reduced, and in some cases the phenytoin was subsequently discontinued. Topiramate clearance was assessed in 2 patients and was found to be increased two to threefold by phenytoin.[1] Similarly, a population pharmacokinetic study reported that patients taking phenytoin and topiramate had 50% lower morning topiramate levels than patients not taking enzyme-inducing antiepileptics.[2]

In the first study above, 3 of the 12 patients had a decrease in phenytoin clearance and an increase of 25 to 55% in the AUC of phenytoin when taking topiramate: the other 9 had no changes.[1] This slight increase is said not to be clinically significant based on analyses from six add-on studies.[3]

Mechanism

An *in vitro* study using human liver microsomes found that topiramate does not inhibit most hepatic cytochrome P450 isoenzymes, except for CYP2C19 at high concentrations.[1] This isoenzyme plays a minor role in phenytoin metabolism, but it has been suggested this may become important at high doses of topiramate in patients who are poor CYP2C9 metabolisers,[1] (see 'genetic factors in drug metabolism', (p.4), for more information). Phenytoin appears to induce the metabolism of topiramate.

Importance and management

The interaction between topiramate and phenytoin appears to be established, and topiramate dose adjustments may be required if phenytoin is added or discontinued. No reduction in the phenytoin dosage seems necessary in the majority of patients, but be aware that a few patients may have increased phenytoin levels, particularly at high topiramate doses. Monitor phenytoin levels.

1. Sachdeo RC, Sachdeo SK, Levy RH, Streeter AJ, Bishop FE, Kunze KL, Mather GG, Roskos LK, Shen DD, Thummel KE, Trager WF, Curtin CR, Doose DR, Gisclon LG, Bialer M. Topiramate and phenytoin pharmacokinetics during repetitive monotherapy and combination therapy to epileptic patients. *Epilepsia* (2002) 43: 691–6.
2. May TW, Jürges U. Serum concentrations of topiramate in epileptic patients: the influence of dose and comedication. *Epilepsia* (1999) 40 (Suppl, 2), 249.
3. Johannessen SI. Pharmacokinetics and interaction profile of topiramate: review and comparison with other newer antiepileptic drugs. *Epilepsia* (1997) 38 (Suppl 1), S18–S23.

Topiramate + Valproate

Encephalopathy has been reported in patients given topiramate with or without valproate. One study found no clinically relevant pharmacokinetic interaction between topiramate and valproate.

Clinical evidence, mechanism, importance and management

Six patients with severe epilepsy developed stuporous encephalopathy with marked cognitive impairment when taking topiramate with valproate (5 patients) or when taking topiramate alone (1 patient). Four of the patients had hyperammonaemia which resolved when topiramate or valproate were withdrawn. The toxicity was possibly due to a synergistic effect of valproate and topiramate on liver ornithine metabolism resulting in hyperammonaemia. It was also possible that the encephalopathy was due to topiramate toxicity in at-risk patients such as those with pre-existing chronic encephalopathy.[1]

In a study in 12 epileptic patients, the pharmacokinetics of both topiramate, titrated to 400 mg twice daily, and valproate 1 to 4.5 g daily were slightly changed by concurrent use. The topiramate AUC was raised by about 18%, and the valproate AUC was reduced by 11.3%, but these changes were not considered to be clinically relevant.[2] However, the proportion of various metabolites of valproate was altered by topiramate: metabolism to 4-ene-valproate (a putative hepatotoxin) and metabolism by oxidation increased, whereas conjugation decreased.[2] Similar changes have been seen with other enzyme-inducing antiepileptics (see Mechanism in 'Phenytoin + Valproate', p.568).

The pharmacokinetic study suggests that dosage adjustments and special precautions are not required during concurrent use.[2] However, the report of encephalopathy with topiramate and valproate indicates that particularly for at-risk patients such as those with pre-existing encephalopathy careful monitoring is advised in these patients.[1]

1. Latour P, Biraben A, Polard E, Bentué-Ferrer D, Beauplet A, Tribut O, Allain H. Drug induced encephalopathy in six epileptic patients: topiramate? valproate? or both? *Hum Psychopharmacol Clin Exp* (2004) 19, 193–203.
2. Rosenfeld WE, Liao S, Kramer LD, Anderson G, Palmer M, Levy RH, Nayak RK. Comparison of the steady-state pharmacokinetics of topiramate and valproate in patients with epilepsy during monotherapy and concomitant therapy. *Epilepsia* (1997) 38, 324–33.

Valproate + Acarbose

An isolated case report describes reduced valproate levels in a patient taking acarbose.

Clinical evidence, mechanism, importance and management

An epileptic patient taking sodium valproate for 10 years had a 40% fall in his normally stable plasma levels from 67 to 40.5 micrograms/mL when acarbose was added. No other drugs were being taken. When the acarbose was stopped and then restarted, the valproate levels rose and then fell once again. The reason is not understood but the authors of the report suggest that the acarbose possibly reduces the absorption of valproate.[1] This is an isolated report and its general importance is unknown, but it would seem prudent to be alert for any evidence of reduced effects if acarbose is added to valproate treatment.

1. Serrano JS, Jiménez CM, Serrano MI, Garrido H, Balboa B. May acarbose impair valproate bioavailability? *Methods Find Exp Clin Pharmacol* (1996) 18 (Suppl C), 98.

Valproate + Allopurinol

Allopurinol appears not to alter valproate levels.

Clinical evidence, mechanism, importance and management

A study investigating allopurinol in refractory epilepsy found that allopurinol (150 mg daily in those less than 20 kg, and 300 mg daily for other patients for 4 months) had no effect on valproate levels in 28 patients taking antiepileptics including valproate.[1] In another similar study, allopurinol 10 mg/kg increased to 15 mg/kg daily for 12 weeks had no effect on serum valproate levels in 6 patients taking antiepileptics including valproate.[2] Therefore valproate dosage alterations are unlikely to be required if allopurinol is used.

1. Zagnoni PG, Bianchi A, Zolo P, Canger R, Cornaggia C, D'Alessandro P, DeMarco P, Pisani F, Gianelli M, Verzé L, Viani F, Zaccara G. Allopurinol as add-on therapy in refractory epilepsy: a double-blind placebo-controlled randomized study. *Epilepsia* (1994) 35, 107–12.
2. Coppola G, Pascotto A. Double-blind, placebo-controlled, cross-over trial of allopurinol as add-on therapy in childhood refractory epilepsy. *Brain Dev* (1996) 18, 50–2.

Valproate + Antacids

The absorption of valproate was slightly, but not significantly, increased by an aluminium/magnesium hydroxide suspension but not by magnesium trisilicate or a calcium carbonate suspension.

Clinical evidence, mechanism, importance and management

In 7 healthy subjects the AUC of a single 500-mg dose of valproic acid, given 1 hour after breakfast, was increased by 12% (range 3 to 28%) by 62 mL of an **aluminium/magnesium hydroxide** suspension (*Maalox*) given with and 2 hours after valproate. Neither **magnesium trisilicate** suspension (*Trisogel*) nor **calcium carbonate** suspension (*Titralac*) had a significant effect on absorption.[1] No special precautions would seem necessary during concurrent use.

1. May CA, Garnett WR, Small RE, Pellock JM. Effects of three antacids on the bioavailability of valproic acid. *Clin Pharm* (1982) 1, 244–7.

Valproate + Aspirin or NSAIDs

Valproate toxicity developed in three patients given large and repeated doses of aspirin. Increased levels of free valproate were found in 5 children within hours of them taking aspirin. Conversely, a slightly reduced valproate level was reported in one patient who took ibuprofen. Modestly altered protein binding has been shown when sodium valproate was given with diflunisal or naproxen, but this appears unlikely to be clinically important.

Clinical evidence, mechanism, importance and management

(a) Aspirin

A 17-year-old girl taking valproate 21 mg/kg daily was prescribed aspirin 18 mg/kg daily for lupus arthritis. Within a few days she developed a disabling tremor which disappeared when the aspirin was stopped. Total serum valproate levels were not significantly changed, but the free fraction fell from 24% to 14% when the aspirin was withdrawn. Similar toxic reactions (tremor, nystagmus, drowsiness, ataxia) were seen in 2 children, aged 6 and 4 years, given 12 and 20 mg/kg aspirin every 4 hours while taking valproate.[1] In 5 epileptic children taking valproate, free valproate levels increased by 31 to 66% (average 49%) 17 hours after starting aspirin 11.5 to 16.9 mg/kg four times daily.[2] One case report of fatal hyperammonaemia was speculated to have been induced by valproate, and the authors also considered that concurrent use of aspirin and 'cimetidine', (p.578) may have contributed.[3]

Aspirin displaces valproate from its protein binding sites[2,4] and also alters its metabolism by the liver[5] so that the levels of free (and pharmacologically active) valproate rise. This could temporarily increase both the therapeutic and toxic effects of the valproate. However, there is evidence that increased hepatic elimination of valproate counterbalances this effect.

Direct information seems to be limited to the studies cited. Clinically relevant interactions appear rare, probably because in most cases the effects of aspirin on free valproate levels cancel each other out. The combination need not necessarily be avoided, but it would seem prudent to be aware of this interaction if valproate and high-dose aspirin are used.

(b) Diflunisal

Diflunisal 250 mg twice daily for 7 days given with sodium valproate 200 mg twice daily caused a 20% increase in the unbound fraction of valproate in 7 healthy subjects. There was a 35% increase in the AUC of one of the oxidation metabolites of valproate, and a small decrease in the AUC of some of the diflunisal glucuronide metabolites. This was shown to be due to changes in renal clearance of these metabolites.[6] Whether any of these modest changes have any clinical relevance remains to be seen, but it appears unlikely.

(c) Ibuprofen

A 15-year-old boy was found to have a subtherapeutic valproate level (43 micrograms/mL) 3 days after starting to take ibuprofen 600 mg every 6 hours for post-fracture analgesia. The ibuprofen was stopped, and after one week the valproate levels were within the therapeutic range (60 micrograms/mL).[7] The general importance of this isolated case is unknown. More study is needed.

(d) Naproxen

A study in 6 healthy subjects found that naproxen 500 mg twice daily moderately decreased the AUC of a single 800-mg dose of sodium valproate by 11%.[8] Similarly, in another study, when naproxen 500 mg twice daily was given with sodium valproate 500 mg twice daily the AUC of valproate was decreased by 20% and the AUC of naproxen was increased by 7%.[9] It is suggested that naproxen and sodium valproate displace each other from their protein binding sites.[8,9] The clinical relevance of these modest changes is uncertain, but is likely to be small.[8]

1. Goulden KJ, Dooley JM, Camfield PR, Fraser AD. Clinical valproate toxicity induced by acetylsalicylic acid. *Neurology* (1987) 37, 1392–4.
2. Farrell K, Orr JM, Abbott FS, Ferguson S, Sheppard I, Godolphin W, Bruni J. The effect of acetylsalicylic acid on serum free valproate concentrations and valproate clearance in children. *J Pediatr* (1982) 101, 142–4.
3. Ichikawa H, Amano T, Kawabata K, Kushiro M, Wada J, Nagake Y, Makino H. Fatal hyperammonemia in a patient with systemic lupus erythematosus. *Intern Med* (1998) 37, 700–3.
4. Orr JM, Abbott FS, Farrell K, Ferguson S, Sheppard I, Godolphin W. Interaction between valproic acid and aspirin in epileptic children: serum protein binding and metabolic effects. *Clin Pharmacol Ther* (1982) 31, 642–9.
5. Abbott FS, Kassam J, Orr JM, Farrell K. The effect of aspirin on valproic acid metabolism. *Clin Pharmacol Ther* (1986) 40, 94–100.
6. Addison RS, Parker-Scott SL, Eadie MJ, Hooper WD, Dickinson RG. Steady-state dispositions of valproate and diflunisal alone and coadministration to healthy volunteers. *Eur J Clin Pharmacol* (2000) 56, 715–21.
7. Mankin KP, Scanlon M. Side effect of ibuprofen and valproic acid. *Orthopedics* (1998) 21, 264, 270.
8. Grimaldi R, Lecchini S, Crema F, Perucca E. *In vivo* plasma protein binding interaction between valproic acid and naproxen. *Eur J Drug Metab Pharmacokinet* (1984) 9, 359–63.
9. Addison RS, Parker-Scott SL, Hooper WD, Eadie MJ, Dickinson RG. Effect of naproxen coadministration on valproate disposition. *Biopharm Drug Dispos* (2000) 21, 235–42.

Valproate + Bile-acid binding resins

Colestyramine causes a very small reduction in the absorption of valproate. No interaction occurs if administration of the drugs is separated by 3 hours. Colesevelam does not interact.

Clinical evidence

(a) Colesevelam

Colesevelam 4.5 g had no effect on the pharmacokinetics of valproic acid 250 mg in a single-dose study in 26 healthy subjects.[1]

(b) Colestyramine

A single 250-mg dose of valproic acid was given to 6 healthy subjects either alone, at the same time as colestyramine 4 g twice daily, or with the colestyramine taken 3 hours after the valproic acid. The bioavailability of valproate taken alone and when separated from the colestyramine by 3 hours remained the same. When the valproate was taken at the same time as the colestyramine the valproate AUC fell by 15% and the maximum serum levels fell by 21%.[2,3]

Mechanism

Colestyramine is an ion-exchange resin intended to bind with bile acids in the gut, but it can also bind with drugs as well, leading to a reduction in their absorption. This apparently occurs to a limited extent with valproate.

Importance and management

Direct information about colestyramine and valproate appears to be limited to this single study, but what happened is consistent with the way colestyramine interacts with a number of other drugs. The fall in the bioavailability is small and probably of very limited clinical importance, but the interaction can be totally avoided by separating the dosages by 3 hours so that admixture in the gut is minimised. Colesevelam does not interact.

1. Donovan JM, Stypinski D, Stiles MR, Olson TA, Burke SK. Drug interactions with colesevelam hydrochloride, a novel, potent lipid-lowering agent. *Cardiovasc Drugs Ther* (2000) 14, 681–90.
2. Pennell AT, Ravis WR, Malloy MJ, Sead A, Diskin C. Cholestyramine decreases valproic acid serum concentrations. *J Clin Pharmacol* (1992) 32, 755.
3. Malloy MJ, Ravis WR, Pennell AT, Diskin CJ. Effect of cholestyramine resin on single dose valproate pharmacokinetics. *Int J Clin Pharmacol Ther* (1996) 34, 208–11.

Valproate + Carbapenems

Panipenem/betamipron dramatically reduced the valproate serum levels of 6 patients. Imipenem and meropenem have similar effects and seizures have occurred when they were given to patients taking valproate. Ertapenem is predicted to interact similarly.

Clinical evidence

(a) Imipenem

A report describes a reduction in valproate levels from 80 micrograms/mL to 24 then 33 micrograms/mL in an epileptic patient 4 and 11 days after imipenem was given to treat a *Pseudomonas aeruginosa* infection.[1]

(b) Meropenem

A report describes two patients whose valproate levels fell when meropenem and amikacin were given. The first patient had been maintained on intravenous valproate 1.2 to 1.6 g daily with valproate levels of between 50 and 100 mg/L. Two days after the addition of the antibacterials the levels had halved, and after 3 days of subtherapeutic levels, phenytoin was substituted for valproate. The other patient experienced a drop in valproate levels from 44 mg/L to 5 mg/L within 24 hours of being given meropenem, despite being given greater doses of valproic acid.[2] Other reports[1,3-8] describe reductions in valproate levels in several other patients when they were also given meropenem: three of them developed seizures.[1,7,8]

(c) Panipenem

A report describes 3 cases of Japanese children taking antiepileptic drugs who had marked reductions in valproate serum levels while receiving panipenem/betamipron for serious chest infections.[9] An increased seizure-frequency occurred in 2 of the patients. In one case the serum valproate levels fell from 30.1 to 1.53 mg/L within 4 days of starting panipenem, and rose again when it was stopped. All 3 patients were also taking carbamazepine but its serum levels were unchanged by the panipenem/betamipron. In a further 3 cases, 60 to 100% reductions in valproate levels were reported, which occurred within 2 days of starting concurrent treatment. Increased seizure frequency occurred in 2 cases.[10]

Mechanism

Unknown, but the speed of the interaction is said to be inconsistent with enzyme induction, and accelerated renal excretion has been suggested.[2] Altered protein binding has been shown in *animal* and *in vitro* studies.[11]

Importance and management

Although there is only an isolated report of an interaction between valproate and imipenem, there are now several reports of the interaction between valproate and meropenem or panipenem. Seizures or increased seizure frequency have been reported. It would therefore seem prudent to monitor the valproate levels in any patient also given carbapenems, being alert for the need to increase the valproate dosage, or to use another antibacterial, or an alternative to valproate. Carbamazepine[9] and phenytoin[2] did not interact in the above reports. The manufacturers of **ertapenem** have no reports of an interaction on their files,[12] but prudently warn about a possible interaction with valproate[13] because of the interactions seen with other carbapenems.

1. Llinares Tello F, Bosacoma Ros N, Hernández Prats C, Climent Grana E, Selva Otaolaurruchi J, Ordovás Baines JP. Interacción farmacocinética entre ácido valproico y antibióticos carbapenémicos: descripción de tres casos. *Farm Hosp* (2003) 27, 258–63.
2. De Turck BJG, Diltoer MW, Cornelis PJWW, Maes V, Spapen HDM, Camu F, Huyghens LP. Lowering of plasma valproic acid concentrations during concomitant therapy with meropenem and amikacin. *J Antimicrob Chemother* (1998) 42, 563–4.
3. Plasencia AP, Soy D, Nicolas JM. Interacción farmacocinética entre el ácido valproico y el meropenem. *Med Clin (Barc)* (2004) 123, 38–9.
4. Nacarkucuk E, Saglam H, Okan M. Meropenem decreases serum level of valproic acid. *Pediatr Neurol* (2004) 31, 232–4.
5. Clause D, Decleire P-Y, Vanbinst R, Soyer A, Hantson P. Pharmacokinetic interaction between valproic acid and meropenem. *Intensive Care Med* (2005) 31, 1293–4.
6. Sala Piñol F, Padullés Zamora N, Hidalgo Albert E, Clemente Bautista S, Cabañas Poy MJ, Oliveras Arenas M, Balcells Ramírez J. Interacción farmacocinética entre ácido valproico y meropenem. *An Pediatr (Barc)* (2006) 64, 93–5.
7. Coves-Orts FJ, Borrás-Blasco J, Navarro-Ruiz A, Murcia-López A, Palacios-Ortega F. Acute seizures due to a probable interaction between valproic acid and meropenem. *Ann Pharmacother* (2005) 39, 533–7.
8. Santucci M, Parmeggiani A, Riva R. Seizure worsening caused by decreased serum valproate during meropenem therapy. *J Child Neurol* (2005) 20, 456–7.
9. Nagai K, Shimizu T, Togo A, Takeya M, Yokomizo Y, Sakata Y, Matsuishi T, Kato H. Decrease in serum levels of valproic acid during treatment with a new carbapenem, panipenem/betamipron. *J Antimicrob Chemother* (1997) 39, 295–6.
10. Yamagata T, Momoi MY, Murai K, Ikematsu K, Suwa K, Sakamoto K, Fujimura A. Panipenem—Betamipron and decreases in serum valproic acid concentration. *Ther Drug Monit* (1998) 20, 396–400.
11. Hobara N, Hokama N, Ohshiro S, Kameya H, Sakanashi M. Possible mechanisms of low levels of plasma valproate concentration following simultaneous administration of sodium valproate and meropenem. *Biog Amines* (2003) 17, 409–20.
12. Merck Sharp & Dohme. Personal communication, September 2003.
13. Invanz (Ertapenem). Merck Sharp & Dohme Ltd. UK Summary of product characteristics, May 2007.

Valproate + Chlorpromazine

Valproate serum levels are slightly raised in patients given chlorpromazine, but this appears to be of minimal clinical importance. An isolated report describes severe hepatotoxicity on concurrent use.

Clinical evidence, mechanism, importance and management

The steady-state trough serum levels of valproate 400 mg daily rose by 22% when 6 patients taking valproate were given chlorpromazine 100 to 300 mg daily. The half-life increased by 14% and the clearance fell by 14% (possibly due to some reduction in its liver metabolism)[1]. This interaction would normally seem to be of minimal importance. Severe hepatotoxicity occurred in another patient given both drugs,[2] but remember that both drugs independently can be hepatotoxic.

1. Ishizaki T, Chiba K, Saito M, Kobayashi K, Iizuka R. The effects of neuroleptics (haloperidol and chlorpromazine) on the pharmacokinetics of valproic acid in schizophrenic patients. *J Clin Psychopharmacol* (1984) 4, 254–61.
2. Bach N, Thung SN, Schaffner F, Tobias H. Exaggerated cholestasis and hepatic fibrosis following simultaneous administration of chlorpromazine and sodium valproate. *Dig Dis Sci* (1989) 34, 1303–7.

Valproate + Erythromycin

Two isolated reports describe valproate toxicity in a woman and a child given erythromycin. Another report describes vitamin K deficiency in a child given valproate and erythromycin.

Clinical evidence, mechanism, importance and management

A woman taking lithium and valproate 3.5 g daily developed fatigue and walking difficulties a day after starting to take erythromycin 250 mg four times daily. Within a week she had also developed slurred speech, confusion, difficulty in concentrating and a worsening gait. Her serum valproate levels had risen from 88 mg/L (measured 2 months before) to 260 mg/L. She recovered within 24 hours of the valproate and erythromycin being withdrawn. Her serum lithium levels remained unchanged.[1] A child taking sodium valproate had a threefold increase in serum valproate levels after taking erythromycin 150 mg every 8 hours and aspirin 250 mg every 6 hours for 3 days.[2] These case reports contrast with another study in a 10-year-old boy taking valproic acid 375 mg twice daily who had only very small and clinically unimportant changes in the pharmacokinetics of valproate, consistent with inhibition of cytochrome P450 metabolism, when given erythromycin 250 mg four times daily.[3]

Another child taking valproic acid developed a deficiency of prothrombin complex after taking erythromycin 300 mg three times daily. This resolved when the patient was given oral vitamin K. It was suggested that the effect was because the numbers of vitamin-K producing intestinal bacteria were reduced.[4]

The general relevance of these isolated reports is unclear, but probably small. Further study is needed.

1. Redington K, Wells C, Petito F. Erythromycin and valproate interaction. *Ann Intern Med* (1992) 116, 877–8.
2. Sanchez-Romero A, Pamirez IO. Interacción ácido valproico-eritromicina. *An Esp Pediatr* (1990) 32, 78–9.
3. Gopaul SV, Farrell K, Rakshi K, Abbott FS. A case study of erythromycin interaction with valproic acid. *Pharm Res* (1996) 13 (9 Suppl), S434.
4. Cordes I, Buchmann S, Scheffner D. Vitamin K-mangel unter Erythromycin. Beobachtung bei einem mit Valproat behandelten Jungen. *Monatsschr Kinderheilkd* (1990) 138, 85–7.

Valproate + Felbamate

Felbamate can raise valproate serum levels causing toxicity. Valproate may slightly decrease the clearance of felbamate.

Clinical evidence

(a) Effect on sodium valproate

The average steady-state valproate serum levels in 7 epileptics were raised by 28%, from 66.9 to 85.4 micrograms/mL, by felbamate 1.2 g daily, and by 54%, from 66.9 to 103 micrograms/mL by felbamate 2.4 g daily. The AUC of valproate was raised by 28% and 54% by felbamate 1.2 and 2.4 g, respectively.[1] Valproate clearance was correspondingly reduced by felbamate.[1] Similar effects were seen in another study.[2,3] It was suggested that in children the interaction may be more marked.[3] Many of the patients experienced nausea. Other toxic effects included lethargy, drowsiness, headaches, cognitive disturbances and low platelet counts.[1,2]

(b) Effect on felbamate

The clearance of felbamate was decreased 21% by valproate in one study,[4] and another reported a significantly lower felbamate clearance in the presence of valproate.[5] Yet another study noted only a minimal effect of valproate on felbamate clearance.[6]

Mechanism

Uncertain. Altered plasma protein binding of valproate is unlikely to be important.[7] Felbamate may cause inhibition of the oxidative pathway of valproate metabolism.[8]

Importance and management

An established interaction. It may be necessary to reduce the valproate dosage to avoid toxicity if felbamate is given. The authors of one report suggest a 30 to 50% reduction. It may also be necessary to reduce the felbamate dosage as well. If both drugs are given monitor closely, particularly during the initial stages of treatment.

1. Wagner ML, Graves NM, Leppik IE, Remmel RP, Shumaker RC, Ward DL, Perhach JL. The effect of felbamate on valproic acid disposition. *Clin Pharmacol Ther* (1994) 56, 494–502.
2. Liu H, Delgado MR. Significant drug interaction between valproate and felbamate in epileptic children. *Epilepsia* (1995) 36 (Suppl 3), S160.
3. Delgado MR. Changes in valproic acid concentrations and dose/level ratios by felbamate coadministration in children. *Ann Neurol* (1994) 36, 538.
4. Kelley MT, Walson PD, Cox S, Dusci LJ. Population pharmacokinetics of felbamate in children. *Ther Drug Monit* (1997) 19, 29–36.

5. Wagner ML, Leppik IE, Graves NM, Remme RP, Campbell JI. Felbamate serum concentrations: effect of valproate, carbamazepine, phenytoin and phenobarbital. *Epilepsia* (1990) 31, 642.
6. Banfield CR, Zhu G-RR, Jen JF, Jensen PK, Schumaker RC, Perhach JL Affrime MB, Glue P. The effect of age on the apparent clearance of felbamate: a retrospective analysis using nonlinear mixed-effects modeling. *Ther Drug Monit* (1996) 18, 19–29.
7. Bernus I, Dickinson RG, Hooper WD, Franklin ME, Eadie MJ. Effect of felbamate on the plasma protein binding of valproate. *Clin Drug Invest* (1995) 10, 288–95.
8. Hooper WD, Franklin ME, Glue P, Banfield CR, Radwanski E, McLaughlin DB, McIntyre ME, Dickinson RG, Eadie MJ. Effect of felbamate on valproic acid disposition in healthy volunteers: inhibition of β-oxidation. *Epilepsia* (1996) 37, 91–7.

Valproate + Fluoxetine

Isolated reports describe marked increases or modest decreases in valproate levels in a small number of patients given fluoxetine. Valproate toxicity occurred in one patient.

Clinical evidence

A woman with an atypical bipolar disorder and 'severe mental retardation' taking semisodium valproate (divalproex sodium) 3 g daily had a rise in her serum valproic acid levels from 93.5 to 152 mg/L within 2 weeks of starting to take fluoxetine 20 mg daily. The valproate dosage was reduced to 2.25 g daily and 2 weeks later the serum valproic acid levels had fallen to 113 mg/L. No adverse effects were seen.[1] Another woman taking valproic acid developed elevated serum valproate levels (a rise from 78 to 126 mg/L) without any accompanying clinical symptoms within 1 month of starting to take fluoxetine 20 mg daily. Valproate levels fell again when the fluoxetine was stopped.[2] Similarly, a 17-year-old taking valproic acid and felbamate developed drowsiness and difficulty in being roused 2 weeks after starting fluoxetine 20 mg daily. His valproate level had increased to 141 micrograms/mL from a previous range of 100 to 110 micrograms/mL. His valproate dose was reduced by about 15%, and his consciousness improved.[3]

In contrast 2 cases of *reduced* valproate levels have also been reported in patients taking fluoxetine. In the first case, a 67-year-old woman taking valproic acid 2 g daily and fluoxetine 20 mg daily had a serum valproate level of 51.9 mg/L. This increased to 64.9 mg/L 9 days after fluoxetine was discontinued and fell to 32.6 mg/L 6 days after fluoxetine was restarted. In the second case, an 81-year-old woman was taking valproic acid 1 g with fluoxetine 20 mg daily and had serum valproate levels of 41.9 mg/L. The fluoxetine was stopped, and 6 days later valproate serum levels had risen to 56.2 mg/L. After re-introduction of fluoxetine her valproate levels fell to 45.6 mg/L.[4]

Mechanism

Not understood.

Importance and management

These reports are somewhat confusing and inconsistent, but the overall picture is that concurrent use need not be avoided, but that the outcome should probably be monitored (indicators of valproate toxicity include nausea, vomiting, and dizziness). More study is needed.

1. Sovner R, Davis JM. A potential drug interaction between fluoxetine and valproic acid. *J Clin Psychopharmacol* (1991) 11, 389.
2. Lucena MI, Blanco E, Corrales MA, Berthier ML. Interaction of fluoxetine and valproic acid. *Am J Psychiatry* (1998) 155, 575.
3. Cruz-Flores S, Hayat GR, Mirza W. Valproic toxicity with fluoxetine therapy. Missouri Med 1995 Jun 92 (6) 296–7.
4. Droulers A, Bodak N, Oudjhani M, Lefevre des Noettes V, Bodak A. Decrease of valproic acid concentration in the blood when coprescribed with fluoxetine. *J Clin Psychopharmacol* (1997) 17, 139–40.

Valproate + Food

A study in 12 healthy subjects found that dietary fibre (citrus pectin 14 g) did not affect the rate or extent of absorption of a single 500-mg dose of valproate.[1]

1. Issy AM, Lanchote VL, de Carvalho D, Silva HC. Lack of kinetic interaction between valproic acid and citrus pectin. *Ther Drug Monit* (1997) 19, 516–20.

Valproate + H_2-receptor antagonists

Aside from one tentative case report, cimetidine and ranitidine do not appear to have a clinically significant interaction with valproate.

Clinical evidence, mechanism, importance and management

The clearance of a single oral dose of sodium valproate was reduced in 6 patients by 2 to 17% after a 4-week course of **cimetidine**, but was not affected by **ranitidine**.[1] It seems doubtful if the interaction between valproate and **cimetidine** is of clinical importance. However, a case of fatal hyperammonaemia in a patient with systemic lupus erythematosus was speculated to have been induced by valproate, and the authors also considered that the concurrent use of **cimetidine** and aspirin (see 'Valproate + Aspirin or NSAIDs', p.575) may have contributed.[2] The general importance of this case is unknown.

1. Webster LK, Mihaly GW, Jones DB, Smallwood RA, Phillips JA, Vajda FJ. Effect of cimetidine and ranitidine on carbamazepine and sodium valproate pharmacokinetics. *Eur J Clin Pharmacol* (1984) 27, 341–3.
2. Ichikawa H, Amano T, Kawabata K, Kushiro M, Wada J, Nagake Y, Makino H. Fatal hyperammonemia in a patient with systemic lupus erythematosus. *Intern Med* (1998) 37, 700–3.

Valproate + Isoniazid

An isolated report describes the development of raised serum valproate levels and toxicity in a child given isoniazid while taking valproate. Another report describes raised hepatic enzymes and drowsiness in a patient taking both drugs.

Clinical evidence, mechanism, importance and management

A 5-year-old girl with left partial seizures, successfully treated with valproate 600 mg daily and clonazepam for 7 months, developed signs of valproate toxicity (drowsiness, asthenia) shortly after starting to take isoniazid 200 mg daily (because of a positive tuberculin reaction). Her serum valproate levels were found to have risen to around 121 to 139 mg/L (normal therapeutic range 50 to 100 mg/L).[1] Over the next few months various changes were made in her treatment, the most significant being a 62% reduction in the dosage of valproate, which was needed to maintain satisfactory therapeutic levels. Later when the isoniazid was stopped her valproate levels fell below therapeutic levels and seizures recurred. It was then found necessary to increase the valproate to its former dosage. The suggested explanation for this interaction is that the isoniazid inhibited the metabolism (oxidation) of valproate by the liver so that it accumulated. The child was found to be a very slow acetylator of isoniazid.[1]

Another child who had been treated with valproate for several years was prescribed isoniazid for the treatment of tuberculosis. At the same time, seizures recurred, and the valproate was stopped and primidone 750 mg daily started. Seven months later seizures persisted, and she was admitted to hospital. Liver enzyme values were normal. Valproate 300 mg daily increased to 600 mg daily was added, and within 2 days she was vomiting and drowsy. After 5 days she had increased liver enzymes and her prothrombin time had fallen, so the valproate was stopped. Valproate levels were 81 micrograms/mL. It was speculated that the CNS effects and hepatic impairment were due to an interaction between the valproate and isoniazid.[2]

The general importance of these cases is uncertain, but bear them in mind in the event of an unexpected response to treatment.

1. Jonville AP, Gauchez AS, Autret E, Billard C, Barbier P, Nsabiyumva F, Breteau M. Interaction between isoniazid and valproate: a case of valproate overdosage. *Eur J Clin Pharmacol* (1991) 40, 197–8.
2. Dockweiler U. Isoniazid-induced valproic-acid toxicity, or vice versa. *Lancet* (1987) ii, 152.

Valproate + Methylphenidate

Two children taking valproic acid rapidly developed severe dyskinesias and bruxism after the first and second dose of methylphenidate, respectively. Valproate appears to potentiate the effects of methylphenidate, possibly by a pharmacokinetic mechanism, or because of additive dopaminergic effects. The authors of the re-

port advise clinical observation while the dose of methylphenidate is being established.[1]

1. Gara L, Roberts W. Adverse response to methylphenidate in combination with valproic acid. *J Child Adolesc Psychopharmacol* (2000) 10, 39–43.

Valproate + Propranolol

One patient had a reduction in valproate clearance when also given propranolol, but 12 other patients had no changes.

Clinical evidence, mechanism, importance and management

An isolated report describes a 28% reduction in valproate clearance in a patient taking valproate semisodium with propranolol 40 mg, and a 35% reduction with propranolol 80 mg. However, 12 other patients taking valproate had no changes in clearance, serum levels or half-life when given propranolol 60 or 120 mg daily for 3 weeks.[1] This interaction would therefore not appear to be of general importance. No special precautions would seem necessary.

1. Nemire RE, Toledo CA, Ramsay RE. A pharmacokinetic study to determine the drug interaction between valproate and propranolol. *Pharmacotherapy* (1996) 16, 1059–62.

Valproate + Theophylline

A study in 6 healthy subjects found that oral aminophylline 200 mg every 6 hours for 3 doses did not affect the pharmacokinetics of a single 400-mg dose of sodium valproate.[1]

1. Kulkarni C, Vaz J, David J, Joseph T. Aminophylline alters pharmacokinetics of carbamazepine but not that of sodium valproate — a single dose pharmacokinetic study in human volunteers. *Indian J Physiol Pharmacol* (1995) 39, 122–6.

Vigabatrin + Clomipramine

An isolated case report describes mania in an epileptic patient taking vigabatrin and clomipramine.

Clinical evidence, mechanism, importance and management

An isolated report describes an epileptic man taking carbamazepine and clobazam who started taking clomipramine 35 mg daily for depression. About one month later, vigabatrin 2 g daily was added for better seizure control. After about a week, the patient then progressively showed signs of mania, requiring hospitalisation after about 10 weeks. The clomipramine was stopped, the vigabatrin continued (because of its efficacy), and haloperidol started. Within a week the patient's mood had stabilised. The authors of the report attributed the mania to an interaction between the vigabatrin and the clomipramine.[1] Note that both clomipramine and vigabatrin can cause psychiatric disorders including mania, and vigabatrin should be used with caution in patients with depression. No general conclusions can be based on this single report.

1. Sastre-Garau P, Thomas P, Beaussart M, Goudemand M. Accès maniaque consécutif à une association vigabatrin-clomipramine. *Encephale* (1993) 19, 351–2.

Vigabatrin + Felbamate

No clinically relevant pharmacokinetic interactions appear to occur between vigabatrin and felbamate.

Clinical evidence, mechanism, importance and management

In a study of 16 subjects, felbamate 2.4 g daily increased the AUC of vigabatrin 2 g daily by 13%, which is unlikely to be clinically significant. In a second study in a further 18 subjects, vigabatrin did not affect felbamate pharmacokinetics.[1] There would therefore seem to be no reason for avoiding concurrent use.

1. Reidenberg P, Glue P, Banfield C, Colucci R, Meehan J, Rey E, Radwanski E, Nomeir A, Lim J, Lin C, Guillaume M, Affrime MB. Pharmacokinetic interaction studies between felbamate and vigabatrin. *Br J Clin Pharmacol* (1995) 40, 157–60.

Vigabatrin + Phenobarbital or Primidone

Vigabatrin causes a trivial decrease in phenobarbital and primidone levels. There is some evidence that phenobarbital may reduce the efficacy of vigabatrin in infantile spasms.

Clinical evidence

In an early clinical study, vigabatrin 2 to 3 g daily did not change the serum levels of phenobarbital in 26 patients.[1] Similarly, another study found that phenobarbital levels were not significantly altered by vigabatrin.[2] Another study found that vigabatrin caused serum level reductions of 7% with phenobarbital and 11% with primidone.[3,4] Alterations of this size would not be expected to be clinically significant.

There is some evidence that the efficacy of vigabatrin for infantile seizures may be reduced in those taking phenobarbital. The median time to response after starting vigabatrin was 3 days in 3 infants not taking phenobarbital and 34 days in 6 patients taking phenobarbital. Three patients did not respond to vigabatrin until after phenobarbital was withdrawn.[5]

Mechanism

Not understood.

Importance and management

There appears to be no change in phenobarbital levels with vigabatrin, but some suggestion that vigabatrin may be less effective for infantile spasms in the presence of phenobarbital. Bear this possibility in mind.

1. Tassinari CA, Michelucci R, Ambrosetto G, Salvi F. Double-blind study of vigabatrin in the treatment of drug-resistant epilepsy. *Arch Neurol* (1987) 44, 907–10.
2. Bernardina BD, Fontana E, Vigevano F, Fusco L, Torelli D, Galeone D, Buti D, Cianchetti C, Gnanasakthy A, Iudice A. Efficacy and tolerability of vigabatrin in children with refractory partial seizures: a single-blind dose-increasing study. *Epilepsia* (1995) 36, 687–91.
3. Browne TR, Mattson RH, Penry JK, Smith DB, Treiman DM, Wilder BJ, Ben-Menachem E, Miketta RM, Sherry KM, Szabo GK. A multicentre study of vigabatrin for drug-resistant epilepsy. *Br J Clin Pharmacol* (1989) 95S–100S.
4. Browne TR, Mattson RH, Penry JK, Smith DB, Treiman DM, Wilder BJ, Ben-Menachem E, Napoliello MJ, Sherry KM, Szabo GK. Vigabatrin for refractory complex partial seizures: multicenter single-blind study with long-term follow up. *Neurology* (1987) 37, 184–9.
5. Spence SJ, Nakagawa J, Sankar R, Shields WD. Phenobarbital interferes with the efficacy of vigabatrin in treating infantile spasms in patients with tuberous sclerosis. *Epilepsia* (2000) 41 (Suppl 7), 189.

Vigabatrin + Valproate

No pharmacokinetic interaction appears to occur between vigabatrin and valproate, but one retrospective study found a correlation between valproate levels and vigabatrin levels.

Clinical evidence, mechanism, importance and management

Vigabatrin 40 to 80 mg/kg daily did not change the serum levels of sodium valproate in 11 children.[1] The combined use of vigabatrin and sodium valproate in 16 children with refractory epilepsy was found not to affect the steady-state serum levels of either drug and the combination reduced the frequency of seizures.[2] However, a retrospective analysis of serum samples from 53 patients found that the vigabatrin concentration-to-dose ratio was increased as the valproate trough steady state levels increased,[3] suggesting that valproate slightly raises vigabatrin levels. However, no dosage adjustments usually appear to be necessary on combined use.

1. Bernardina BD, Fontana E, Vigevano F, Fusco L, Torelli D, Galeone D, Buti D, Cianchetti C, Gnanasakthy A, Iudice A. Efficacy and tolerability of vigabatrin in children with refractory partial seizures: a single-blind dose-increasing study. *Epilepsia* (1995) 36, 687–91.
2. Armijo JA, Arteaga R, Valdizán EM, Herranz JL. Coadministration of vigabatrin and valproate in children with refractory epilepsy. *Clin Neuropharmacol* (1992) 15, 459–69.
3. Armijo JA, Cuadrado A, Bravo J, Arteaga R. Vigabatrin serum concentration to dosage ratio: influence of age and associated antiepileptic drugs. *Ther Drug Monit* (1997) 19, 491–8

Zonisamide + Miscellaneous

Cimetidine does not alter zonisamide pharmacokinetics. Food has no effect on the absorption of zonisamide. A case of reduced zonisamide levels possibly caused by risperidone has been described.

Potent inhibitors of CYP3A4 are predicted to modestly decrease zonisamide clearance.

Clinical evidence, mechanism, importance and management

(a) Cimetidine

When a single 300-mg oral dose of zonisamide was given to healthy subjects, it was found that cimetidine 300 mg four times daily for 13 days did not affect the zonisamide clearance, half-life, apparent volume of distribution or the amount of drug recovered from the urine. The drugs were well tolerated.[1,2] No special precautions would seem to be needed if both drugs are used.

(b) Food

There was no difference in the pharmacokinetics of a single 300- or 400-mg dose of zonisamide when given in the fasted state or after breakfast in a study in healthy subjects. Zonisamide may be taken without regard to the timing of meals.[3]

(c) Risperidone

A 57-year-old man taking zonisamide was prescribed risperidone 2 mg daily, which was gradually increased to 10 mg daily. About 2 months after starting the risperidone, the zonisamide level had fallen from 23.7 to 10.7 micrograms/mL. The risperidone was stopped, and the zonisamide level had slightly increased again to 12.4 micrograms/mL about one month later. It was suggested that a metabolic interaction occurred.[4] More study is needed to establish any interaction.

(d) Cytochrome P450 isoenzyme CYP3A4 inhibitors

In vitro studies have shown that the cytochrome P450 isoenzyme CYP3A4 is the principal enzyme involved in the metabolism of zonisamide.[5] Based on *in vitro* data, it is predicted that **ketoconazole**, **ciclosporin**, **miconazole** and **fluconazole** may cause a modest to minor decrease in the clearance of zonisamide. Conversely, **itraconazole** and **triazolam** are not predicted to have an effect.[5] *In vitro* predictions do not always mirror what happens in clinical use, therefore, further study is needed.

1. Schentag JJ, Gengo FM, Wilton JH, Sedman AJ, Grasela TH, Brockbrader HN. Influence of phenobarbital, cimetidine, and renal disease on zonisamide kinetics. *Pharm Res* (1987) 4 (Suppl), S-79.
2. Groves L, Wallace J, Shellenberger K. Effect of cimetidine on zonisamide pharmacokinetics in healthy volunteers. *Epilepsia* (1998) 39 (Suppl 6), 191.
3. Shellenberger K, Wallace J, Groves L. Effect of food on pharmacokinetics of zonisamide in healthy volunteers. *Epilepsia* (1998) 39 (Suppl 6), 191.
4. Okumura K. Decrease in plasma zonisamide concentrations after coadministration of risperidone in a patient with schizophrenia receiving zonisamide therapy. *Int Clin Psychopharmacol* (1999) 14, 55.
5. Nakasa H, Nakamura H, Ono S, Tsutsui M, Kiuchi M, Ohmori S, Kitada M. Prediction of drug-drug interactions of zonisamide metabolism in humans from in vitro data. *Eur J Clin Pharmacol* (1998) 54, 177–83.

Zonisamide + Other antiepileptics

Phenobarbital, phenytoin and carbamazepine can cause a small to moderate reduction in the serum levels of zonisamide, while lamotrigine may increase zonisamide levels. Clonazepam and valproate have little or no effect. Zonisamide shows variable effects (a modest decrease, an increase, or no effect) on carbamazepine serum levels, but has no important effect on lamotrigine, phenobarbital, primidone or valproate levels. Most studies also suggest that zonisamide has no effect on phenytoin levels, but two showed a modest increase.

Clinical evidence

(a) Carbamazepine

In one study the ratio of plasma level to zonisamide dose was 39% lower in 17 patients taking carbamazepine than in 28 patients taking zonisamide alone, suggesting that carbamazepine modestly reduces zonisamide levels.[1] Similarly, in another study in 12 epileptic children taking zonisamide 8.6 to 13.6 mg/kg daily, carbamazepine 12.1 to 18.1 mg/kg daily reduced zonisamide plasma levels by about 35 to 37%.[2] In an early study in 2 groups of patients, one taking carbamazepine and the other phenytoin, it was noted that the zonisamide AUC following a single 400-mg dose was 40% higher in the carbamazepine group than the phenytoin group.[3] However, in the first study, the plasma concentration-to-dose ratio was the same in patients taking carbamazepine as in those taking phenytoin.[1] Therefore the comparative effects of carbamazepine and phenytoin on zonisamide levels are unclear.

In one study, the ratio of carbamazepine-10,11-epoxide (the major active metabolite of carbamazepine) to carbamazepine in the plasma was 50% lower in patients also taking zonisamide, suggesting that zonisamide reduces carbamazepine metabolism. However, the plasma concentration-to-dose ratio of carbamazepine was only 20% higher, which was not significant.[1] An early pilot study had noted a consistent rise in carbamazepine plasma levels following initiation of zonisamide therapy in 7 patients (range 26 to 270%).[4] The opposite effect was seen in a study of 16 paediatric patients in whom zonisamide reduced the ratio of carbamazepine serum levels to dose by up to 22% and increased the relative amount of its major metabolite in the serum by up to 100%, suggesting that zonisamide increases the metabolism of carbamazepine. However, the free fraction of carbamazepine remained unaltered.[5]

Contrasting with these three studies are four others that found no changes in the serum levels of carbamazepine or carbamazepine-10,11-epoxide when zonisamide was used,[2,6-8] although in one of the studies, the renal clearance of carbamazepine-10,11-epoxide was significantly reduced by zonisamide.[8] A further study similarly found no change in the plasma level of carbamazepine in 41 patients also given zonisamide (7.5 versus 7.4 micrograms/mL).[9]

(b) Clonazepam

In one study the ratio of plasma level to dose of zonisamide did not differ between 8 patients also taking clonazepam and 28 patients taking zonisamide alone, suggesting clonazepam has no effect on zonisamide levels.[1]

(c) Lamotrigine

Zonisamide 100 mg daily increased to 200 mg twice daily did not alter the steady-state pharmacokinetics of lamotrigine in 18 patients.[10,11] Further, the pharmacokinetics of zonisamide were unaffected by lamotrigine.[11] However, in 2 patients who were stable taking zonisamide 600 mg daily or 800 mg daily, the addition of lamotrigine (incremental doses up to 400 mg daily) caused about twofold increases in their zonisamide levels, with symptoms of toxicity that were maximal 40 to 60 minutes after taking a zonisamide dose.[12]

(d) Phenobarbital or Primidone

In one study the ratio of plasma level to dose of zonisamide was 29% lower in 11 patients also taking phenobarbital than in 28 patients taking zonisamide alone, suggesting that phenobarbital reduces zonisamide levels.[1] Similarly, another study in healthy subjects found that pretreatment with phenobarbital increased the clearance of a single dose of zonisamide by about twofold.[13] A further study found no changes in the serum levels of phenobarbital or primidone in 34 and 13 patients, respectively, who were also given zonisamide.[9]

(e) Phenytoin

In one study the ratio of plasma level to dose of zonisamide was 39% lower in 14 patients also taking phenytoin than in 28 patients taking zonisamide alone, suggesting phenytoin modestly reduces zonisamide levels.[1] In an early study in 2 groups of patients, one taking carbamazepine and the other phenytoin, it was noted that the zonisamide AUC following a single 400-mg dose was 40% higher in the carbamazepine group than the phenytoin group.[3] However, in the first study, the reduction in zonisamide level-to-dose ratio was the same for phenytoin as for carbamazepine.[1] Therefore the comparative effect of phenytoin and carbamazepine on zonisamide levels is unclear.

Zonisamide 300 to 600 mg daily did not affect the phenytoin serum levels in 10 patients.[6] Another study found that zonisamide did not affect the serum levels of phenytoin in 9 children.[14] A further study similarly found no change in the plasma level of phenytoin in 33 patients also given zonisamide.[9] In contrast to these three studies, in a population pharmacokinetic analysis, the clearance of phenytoin at a given dose was 14% lower and the serum level 16% higher in 39 patients also taking zonisamide.[15] Similarly, the preliminary results from 9 patients in another study showed that there was a 28% increase in the steady-state AUC of phenytoin when zonisamide 100 mg daily increased to 200 mg twice daily was given.[16] However, a later study by the same authors, in 19 patients, found that zonisamide did not affect the pharmacokinetics of phenytoin to a clinically relevant extent.[17]

(f) Valproate

In one study the ratio of plasma level to dose of zonisamide was about 20% lower in 24 patients also taking valproate than in 28 taking zonisamide alone, suggesting that valproate has little effect on zonisamide levels.[1] Similarly, another study in 16 patients found that valproate did not affect the pharmacokinetics of zonisamide.[18] Further, the steady-state pharmacokinetics of valproate did not change when zonisamide 100 mg daily increased to 200 mg twice daily was added to the therapy of 16 patients.[18,19]

Another study found that zonisamide did not affect the serum levels of sodium valproate in 12 children.[14] A further study similarly found no marked changes in the plasma level of valproic acid in 7 patients also given zonisamide.[9]

Mechanism

Uncertain. It seems possible that phenobarbital, phenytoin and carbamazepine can induce the metabolism of zonisamide thereby reducing its serum levels. The plasma protein binding of zonisamide is unaffected by other antiepileptics (phenobarbital, phenytoin, carbamazepine, valproate).[20]

Importance and management

None of these studies reported any major problems during concurrent use of zonisamide and these other antiepileptic drugs. Zonisamide serum levels are lower with phenobarbital, phenytoin and carbamazepine, and there is the possibility of carbamazepine or phenytoin level changes, so it would be prudent to monitor patients taking any of these combinations.

1. Shinoda M, Akita M, Hasegawa M, Hasegawa T, Nabeshima T. The necessity of adjusting the dosage of zonisamide when coadministered with other anti-epileptic drugs. *Biol Pharm Bull* (1996) 19, 1090–2.
2. Abo J, Miura H, Takanashi S, Shirai H, Sunaoshi W, Hosoda N, Abo K, Takei K. Drug interaction between zonisamide and carbamazepine: a pharmacokinetic study in children with cryptogenic localization-related epilepsies. *Epilepsia* (1995) 36 (Suppl 3), S162.
3. Ojemann LM, Shastri RA, Wilensky AJ, Friel PN, Levy RH, McLean JR, Buchanan RA. Comparative pharmacokinetics of zonisamide (CI-912) in epileptic patients on carbamazepine or phenytoin monotherapy. *Ther Drug Monit* (1986) 8, 293–6.
4. Sackellares JC, Donofrio PD, Wagner JG, Abou-Khalil B, Berent S, Aasved-Hoyt K. Pilot study of zonisamide (1,2-Benzisoxazole-3-methanesulfonamide) in patients with refractory partial seizures. *Epilepsia* (1985) 26, 206–11.
5. Minami T, Ieiri I, Ohtsubo K, Hirakawa Y, Ueda K, Higuchi S, Aoyama T. Influence of additional therapy with zonisamide (Excegran) on protein binding and metabolism of carbamazepine. *Epilepsia* (1994) 35, 1023–5.
6. Browne TR, Szabo GK, Kres J, Pylilo RJ. Drug interactions of zonisamide (CI–912) with phenytoin and carbamazepine. *J Clin Pharmacol* (1986) 26, 555.
7. Rosenfeld WE, Bergen D, Garnett W, Shah J, Floren LC, Gross J, Tupper R, Shellenberger K. Steady-state drug interaction study of zonisamide and carbamazepine in patients with epilepsy. *Neurology* (2001) 56 (Suppl 3), A336.
8. Ragueneau-Majlessi I, Levy RH, Bergen D, Garnett W, Rosenfeld W, Mather G, Shah J, Grundy JS. Carbamazepine pharmacokinetics are not affected by zonisamide: in vitro mechanistic study and in vivo clinical study in epileptic patients. *Epilepsy Res* (2004) 62, 1–11.
9. Schmidt D, Jacob R, Loiseau P, Deisenhammer E, Klinger D, Despland A, Egli M, Bauer G, Stenzel E, Blankenhorn V. Zonisamide for add-on treatment of refractory partial epilepsy: a European double-blind trial. *Epilepsy Res* (1993) 15, 67–73.
10. Brodie M, Wilson E, Smith D, Dunkley D, Shah J, Floren L, Shellenberger K. Steady-state drug interaction study of zonisamide and lamotrigine in epileptic patients. *Neurology* (2001) 56 (Suppl 3), A337.
11. Levy RH, Ragueneau-Majlessi I, Brodie MJ, Smith DF, Shah J, Pan W-J. Lack of clinically significant pharmacokinetic interactions between zonisamide and lamotrigine at steady state in patients with epilepsy. *Ther Drug Monit* (2005) 27, 193–8.
12. McJilton J, DeToledo J, DeCerce J, Huda S, Abubakr A, Ramsay RE. Cotherapy of lamotrigine/zonisamide results in significant elevation of zonisamide levels. *Epilepsia* (1996) 37 (Suppl 5), 173.
13. Schentag JJ, Gengo FM, Wilton AJ, Sedman AJ, Grasela TH, Bockbrader HN. Influence of phenobarbital, cimetidine, and renal disease on zonisamide kinetics. *Pharm Res* (1987) 4 (Suppl), S-79.
14. Tasaki K, Minami T, Ieiri I, Ohtsubo K, Hirakawa Y, Ueda K, Higuchi S. Drug interactions of zonisamide with phenytoin and sodium valproate: serum concentrations and protein binding. *Brain Dev* (1995) 17, 182–5.
15. Odani A, Hashimoto Y, Takayanagi K, Otsuki Y, Koue T, Takano M, Yasuhara M, Hattori H, Furusho K, Inui K-I. Population pharmacokinetics of phenytoin in Japanese patients with epilepsy: analysis with a dose-dependent clearance model. *Biol Pharm Bull* (1996) 19, 444–8.
16. Garnett WR, Towne AR, Rosenfeld WE, Shah J, Floren LC, Gross J, Tupper R, Shellenberger K. Steady-state pharmacokinetic interaction study of zonisamide (Zonegran) and phenytoin in subjects with epilepsy. *Neurology* (2001) 56 (Suppl 3), A336.
17. Levy RH, Ragueneau-Majlessi I, Garnett WR, Schmerler M, Rosenfeld W, Shah J, Pan W-J. Lack of a clinically significant effect of zonisamide on phenytoin steady-state pharmacokinetics in patients with epilepsy. *J Clin Pharmacol* (2004) 44, 1230–4.
18. Ragueneau-Majlessi I, Levy RH, Brodie M, Smith D, Shah J, Grundy JS. Lack of pharmacokinetic interactions between steady-state zonisamide and valproic acid in patients with epilepsy. *Clin Pharmacokinet* (2005) 44, 517–23.
19. Smith D, Brodie M, Dunkley D, Shah J, Floren L, Shellenberger K. Steady-state drug interaction study of zonisamide and sodium valproate in epileptic patients. *Neurology* (2001) 56 (Suppl 3), A338.
20. Kimura M, Tanaka N, Kimura Y, Miyake K, Kitaura T, Fukuchi H, Harada Y. Factors influencing serum concentration of zonisamide in epileptic patients. *Chem Pharm Bull (Tokyo)* (1992) 40, 193–5.

15

Antihistamines

Antihistamines (histamine H_1-antagonists) vary in their interaction profiles by sedative potential, route of metabolism, and cardiotoxicity (QT interval prolongation) .

(a) Additive sedative effects

The older antihistamines (e.g. chlorphenamine, diphenhydramine and hydroxyzine) are also referred to as sedating antihistamines or first-generation antihistamines. As the former name suggests they have the potential to cause additive sedative effects with other sedating drugs. This type of interaction is discussed elsewhere, see 'CNS depressants + CNS depressants', p.1253. The sedating antihistamines also tend to have antimuscarinic (also called anticholinergic) adverse effects and so therefore may interact additively with other antimuscarinic-type drugs. This is also discussed elsewhere, see 'Antimuscarinics + Antimuscarinics', p.674.

The newer (non-sedating antihistamines or second-generation antihistamines) have a low potential to cause sedative effects. This appears to be because they are substrates for P-glycoprotein, an efflux transporter found in many organs, which would have the effect of actively ejecting any drug molecules that crossed the blood-brain barrier. Nevertheless, sedation may occur on rare occasions and patients should be advised to be alert to the possibility of drowsiness if they have not taken the drug before. Any drowsiness is likely to become apparent after the first few doses, and would indicate that additive sedative effects with other sedating drugs might be expected. The antihistamines are listed, by sedative potential, in 'Table 15.1', (below).

(b) Metabolism

Some of the sedating antihistamines, such as diphenhydramine, are inhibitors of the cytochrome P450 isoenzyme CYP2D6. None of the non-sedating antihistamines are known to inhibit cytochrome P450 isoenzymes, but some are substrates for CYP3A4 including astemizole, desloratadine, ebastine, loratadine, mizolastine, and terfenadine, see 'Table 15.2', (p.583). This has important consequences for the potential cardiotoxicity of astemizole and terfenadine, see (c) below. Loratadine and desloratadine are also substrates for CYP2D6, and mizolastine is also metabolised by glucuronidation. Cetirizine, levocetirizine and fexofenadine are minimally metabolised. Where pharmacokinetic interactions occur with fexofenadine, these appear to be mediated via drug transporters such as P-glycoprotein and/or organic anion transport polypeptide (OATP). For more information see 'Drug transporter proteins', (p.8).

(c) QT interval prolongation and cardiac arrhythmias

Important drug interactions occur with the non-sedating antihistamines astemizole and terfenadine. Raised serum levels of these two antihistamines can block potassium channels, lengthening the QT interval and increasing the risk of potentially fatal cardiac arrhythmias (torsade de pointes). Therefore, dangerous interactions may result when other drugs reduce the metabolism of astemizole or terfenadine, usually by inhibition of the cytochrome P450 isoenzyme CYP3A4. Such drugs include the 'macrolides', (p.589) and the 'azoles', (p.584). Adverse interactions are also predicted when astemizole or terfenadine are used with drugs that prolong the QT interval, see 'Antihistamines + Drugs that prolong the QT interval', p.587. Due to these potentially fatal interactions, astemizole has been withdrawn from many countries, while terfenadine has been withdrawn in the US and reclassified as a prescription-only medicine in the UK. Apart from possibly ebastine, loratadine and mizolastine, where information is inconclusive, none of the other non-sedating antihistamines have been clearly shown to be associated with QT prolongation (see 'Table 15.2', (p.583)). Therefore, even when pharmacokinetic interactions result in increased levels, these are unlikely to be clinically important in terms of cardiotoxicity.

Table 15.1 Systemic antihistamines (classified by sedative potential) and topical antihistamines

Sedative potential	*Antihistamine*
Non-sedative	Acrivastine, Astemizole,* Cetirizine, Desloratadine, Ebastine,* Fexofenadine, Levocetirizine, Loratadine, Mizolastine,* Rupatadine, Terfenadine*
Sedating	Azatadine, Brompheniramine, Buclizine, Chlorphenamine, Cinnarizine, Clemastine, Cyclizine, Cyproheptadine, Dexchlorpheniramine, Flunarizine, Meclozine, Mepyramine, Mequitazine, Pheniramine, Tripelennamine, Triprolidine
Significantly sedating	Alimemazine, Bromazine, Carbinoxamine, Dimenhydrinate, Diphenhydramine, Doxylamine, Hydroxyzine, Promethazine, Trimeprazine
Topical use (mainly)	Antazoline, Azelastine, Emedastine, Epinastine, Levocabastine, Olopatadine

*Important QT prolongation known to occur (astemizole, terfenadine), or may possibly occur (ebastine, mizolastine), see Table 15.2, p. 583

Table 15.2 Metabolism and cardiac effects of non-sedating antihistamines

Drug	*Drug blocks the HERG†* *potassium channel in vitro*	*QTc interval prolongation shown in pharmacological studies with drug alone*	*QTc interval prolongation shown in pharmacological studies with CYP3A4 inhibitors*	*Case reports of torsade de pointes with drug alone*	*Case reports of torsade de pointes with CYP3A4 inhibitors*
Metabolised by CYP3A4					
Astemizole	Yes[1]	Yes[2]	Yes. See Azoles, p. 584	Several[2-8]	Yes. See Azoles, p. 584, or Macrolides, p. 589
Desloratadine	No	No	No	No	No
Ebastine	Yes[9]	Uncertain	Yes. See Azoles, p. 584, or Macrolides, p. 589	No	No
Loratadine	Yes, in one study[10]	No	Yes. See Azoles, p. 584, or Nefazodone, p. 592	Possible case[11-13]	Yes. See Azoles, p. 584, or Macrolides, p. 589
Mizolastine	Yes[14]	Uncertain	Yes. See Azoles, p. 584	No	No
Terfenadine	Yes[10,15]	Yes	Yes. See Azoles, p. 584, Macrolides, p. 589, or Nefazodone, p. 592	A few[16,17]	Yes. See Azoles, p. 584, or Macrolides, p. 589
Not metabolised by CYP3A4					
Cetirizine	No	No	No	Possible case[18]	No
Fexofenadine	No	No	No	Possible case[19,20]	No
Levocetirizine	No	No	No	No	No

†The HERG (human ether-a-go-go related gene) channel is involved in cardiac action potential repolarisation and is known to be blocked by certain drugs. Blocking HERG channels results in prolongation of the QT interval.

1. Zhou Z, Vorperian VR, Gong Q, Zhang S, January CT. Block of HERG potassium channels by the antihistamine astemizole and its metabolites desmethylastemizole and norastemizole. *J Cardiovasc Electrophysiol* (1999) 10, 836–43.
2. Craft TM. Torsade de pointes after astemizole overdose. *BMJ* (1986) 292, 660.
3. Snook J, Boothman-Burrell D, Watkins J, Colin-Jones D. Torsade de pointes ventricular tachycardia associated with astemizole overdose. *Br J Clin Pract* (1988) 42, 257–9.
4. Simons FER, Kesselman MS, Giddins NG, Pelech AN, Simons KJ. Astemizole-induced torsade de pointes. *Lancet* (1988) ii, 624.
5. Bishop RO, Gaudry PL. Prolonged Q-T interval following astemizole overdose. *Arch Emerg Med* (1989) 6, 63–5.
6. Hasan RA, Zureikat GY, Nolan BM. Torsade de pointes associated with astemizole overdose treated with magnesium sulfate. *Pediatr Emerg Care* (1993) 9, 23–5.
7. Gowardman J. QT prolongation on the standard dose of astemizole. *N Z Med J* (1996) 109, 38.
8. Vorperian VR, Zhou Z, Mohammad S, Hoon TJ, Studenik C, January CT. Torsade de pointes with an antihistamine metabolite: potassium channel blockade with desmethylastemizole. *J Am Coll Cardiol* (1996) 28, 1556–61.
9. Ko CM, Ducic I, Fan J, Shuba YM, Morad M. Suppression of mammalian K+ channel family by ebastine. *J Pharmacol Exp Ther* (1997) 281, 233–44.
10. Crumb WJ. Loratadine blockade of K+ channels in human heart: comparison with terfenadine under physiological conditions. *J Pharmacol Exp Ther* (2000) 292, 261–4.
11. Kuchar DL, Walker BD, Thorburn CW. Ventricular tachycardia following ingestion of a commonly used antihistamine, *Med J Aust* (2002) 176, 429–30.
12. Sager PT, Veltri EP. Ventricular tachycardia following ingestion of a commonly used antihistamine. *Med J Aust* (2003) 178, 245–6.
13. Kuchar DL, Walker BD, Thorburn CW. In reply. *Med J Aust* (2003) 178, 246.
14. Taglialatela M, Pannaccione A, Castaldo P, Giorgio G, Annunziato L. Inhibition of HERG1 K(+) channels by the novel second-generation antihistamine mizolastine. *Br J Pharmacol* (2000) 131, 1081–8.
15. Woosley RL, Chen Y, Freiman JP, Gillis RA. Mechanism of the cardiotoxic actions of terfenadine. *JAMA* (1993) 269, 1532–6.
16. MacConnell TJ, Stanners AJ. Torsades de pointes complicating treatment with terfenadine. *Br Med J* (1991) 302, 1469.
17. June RA, Nasr I. Torsades de pointes with terfenadine ingestion. *Am J Emerg Med* (1997) 15, 542–3.
18. Renard S, Ostorero M, Yvorra S, Zerrouk Z, Bargas E, Bertocchio P, Pracchia S, Ebagosti A. Torsades de pointes caused by cetirizine overdose. *Arch Mal Coeur Vaiss* (2005) 98; 157–61.
19. Pinto YM, van Gelder IC, Heeringa M, Crijns HJ. QT lengthening and life-threatening arrhythmias associated with fexofenadine. *Lancet* (1999), 353, 980.
20. Scherer CR, Lerche C, Decher N, Dennis AT, Maier P, Ficker E, Busch AE, Wollnik B, Steinmeyer K. The antihistamine fexofenadine does not affect Ikr currents in a case report of drug-induced cardiac arrhythmia. *Br J Pharmacol* (2002) 137, 892–900.

Antihistamines + Azoles

The azole antifungals raise the levels of astemizole and terfenadine, which can result in life-threatening arrhythmias. Arrhythmias have been reported for astemizole with ketoconazole, and terfenadine with itraconazole, ketoconazole, and even topical oxiconazole. Consequently all azoles are contraindicated with astemizole and terfenadine.

Ketoconazole increases mizolastine levels, which resulted in some QT prolongation in one study, therefore all azoles are contraindicated. The manufacturers of ebastine advise caution with ketoconazole and itraconazole as ketoconazole raises ebastine levels. The manufacturers of acrivastine advise caution with azoles due to a lack of data.

The situation with loratadine and ketoconazole is unclear as one study found that concurrent use caused a small increase in the QT interval.

Ketoconazole raises the levels of desloratadine, emedastine, fexofenadine but as no adverse cardiac effects were seen these combinations are considered safe. No interaction occurs between ketoconazole and azelastine, cetirizine, intranasal levocabastine, and none is expected with levocetirizine.

Clinical evidence

The effect of various azole antifungals on the plasma levels of the non-sedating antihistamines, and their cardiac effects from controlled studies are summarised in 'Table 15.3', (p.585). The subsections below include data from case reports and further studies.

A. Astemizole

(a) Ketoconazole

A 63-year old woman developed torsade de pointes arrhythmia and was found to have a prolonged QT interval after taking astemizole and ketoconazole. These two drugs were withdrawn and she was successfully treated with a temporary pacemaker, magnesium sulphate and lidocaine. She was later discharged with a normal ECG.[1]

(b) Miconazole

An *in vitro* study using human liver microsomal enzymes and ^{14}C-labelled compounds found that miconazole inhibits the metabolism of astemizole. On the basis of the values obtained it has been predicted that a clinically relevant interaction could occur *in vivo*.[2]

B. Desloratadine

A chemotherapy patient developed severe pruritus and was given desloratadine and clemastine. Because of a pyrexia of unknown origin she was treated with meropenem and then 48 hours later **fluconazole** was added. After about 36 hours severe hepatotoxicity was detected, and apart from the anti-infectives the other drugs were stopped. Liver parameters recovered over the following week. Because the patient had previously received clemastine and **fluconazole** without problems, this case was attributed to a possible interaction between **fluconazole** and desloratadine.[3]

C. Ebastine

One *animal* study showed that ebastine given with **ketoconazole** had a similar potential for QTc prolongation as **terfenadine** given with **ketoconazole**. The potential was greater than that for **loratadine**, which was not considered to have a significant effect.[4] A review of the safety of ebastine cites two studies assessing the potential interaction between ebastine and **ketoconazole**. One, a single dose study, found that the combination did not affect the QTc interval, whereas in a multiple dose study the QTc interval was prolonged by 18.1 milliseconds by the combination.[5]

D. Fexofenadine

(a) Itraconazole

In a single dose study, administration of itraconazole 200 mg one hour prior to fexofenadine 180 mg increased the AUC of fexofenadine 2.3-fold, and 3-fold in two groups of subjects of different genotypes for the gene encoding P-glycoprotein. Itraconazole pretreatment increased the effect of fexofenadine on histamine-induced wheal and flare reaction.[6]

(b) Ketoconazole

Fexofenadine has no effect on the pharmacokinetics of ketoconazole.[7]

E. Loratadine

In one study[8] the cardiac effects of loratadine were found to be similar to those of ebastine (see C. above), which caused a small increase in the QT interval. However, loratadine alone, given at 4 times the recommended dose for 90 days, had no effect on the QTc interval when compared with placebo,[9] and *animal* studies suggest that the combination of ketoconazole and loratadine does not significantly affect the QTc interval.[4] As at 1993, there had been no cases of torsade de pointes reported during worldwide clinical use of loratadine,[9] but see also 'Table 15.2', (p.583).

F. Terfenadine

(a) Fluconazole

By January 1993 no clinically significant interactions between terfenadine and fluconazole had been reported to the FDA.[10]

(b) Itraconazole

A 26-year-old woman taking 60 mg terfenadine twice daily began to have fainting episodes on the third evening after starting to take itraconazole 100 mg twice daily for vaginitis. When admitted to hospital the next morning her ECG showed a QT interval of 580 milliseconds and her heart rate was 67 bpm. Several episodes of torsade de pointes were recorded, and she fainted during two of them. No arrhythmias were seen 20 hours after the last itraconazole dose, and her QT interval returned to normal after 3 days. She was found to have terfenadine levels of 28 nanograms/mL in the first sample of serum taken (normally less than 5 nanograms/mL) and she still had levels of 12 nanograms/mL about 60 hours after taking the last tablet.[11,12] Two other similar cases have been reported,[13,14] and the FDA has received four well-documented cases of severe cardiac complications due to this interaction.[15]

(c) Ketoconazole

A 39-year-old woman taking terfenadine 60 mg twice daily developed a number of episodes of syncope and light-headedness, preceded by palpitations, dyspnoea and diaphoresis, within 2 days of starting to take ketoconazole 200 mg twice daily. ECG monitoring revealed torsade de pointes and a QTc interval of 655 milliseconds. Her terfenadine serum levels were 57 nanograms/mL (levels expected to be 10 nanograms/mL or less). Other drugs being taken were cefaclor (stopped 3 to 4 days before the problems started) and medroxyprogesterone acetate. She had taken terfenadine and cefaclor on two previous occasions in the absence of ketoconazole without problems.[16,17] Other cases of an interaction between terfenadine and ketoconazole have also been reported.[18,19]

(d) Oxiconazole

A 25-year-old woman complained of palpitations and chest pain radiating down her left arm, and was also found to be having frequent ventricular premature beats in a pattern of bigeminy. On questioning it turned out that she was taking terfenadine and using topical oxiconazole for ringworm on her arm. Both drugs were stopped and her symptoms disappeared the following week.[20]

Mechanism

In vitro studies have shown that ketoconazole inhibits the metabolism of astemizole.[21] Ketoconazole, and to a lesser extent itraconazole and miconazole,[2,21] also appear to reduce the metabolism of terfenadine by inhibition of the cytochrome P450 isoenzyme CYP3A.[21-23] High serum levels of astemizole and terfenadine (but not its metabolites) block cardiac potassium channels leading to prolongation of the QT interval, which may precipitate the development of torsade de pointes arrhythmia (see 'Table 15.2', (p.583)). The risk of cardiac arrhythmias with other non-sedating antihistamines appears to be non-existent or very much lower (see 'Table 15.2', (p.583)), so any pharmacokinetic interactions do not result in clinically relevant cardiac toxicity. In fact, studies have shown that desloratadine at nine times the recommended dose,[24] fexofenadine in overdose,[7,25] and mizolastine at four times the recommended dose[26] do not affect the QT interval. However, some questions remain about loratadine and ebastine. Additionally, some studies have reported that ketoconazole alone is associated with a small increase in QT interval,[8] and at least one case of torsade de pointes has been reported for ketoconazole alone.[27] Therefore the cardiac effects of ketoconazole may be additive with those of the antihistamines, and this may be important for ebastine and loratadine.

Table 15.3 Summary of the effects of azoles on the pharmacokinetics and cardiovascular effects of non-sedating antihistamines

Antihistamine (Oral unless specified)	*Azole (Oral unless specified)*	*Duration of combined use (days)*	*Subjects*	*Cmax increase*[‡]	*AUC increase*	*Effect on QTc*	*Refs*
Astemizole[*] 10 mg single dose	Itraconazole 200 mg twice daily	Single dose	12 healthy subjects	No change	82%	No change	1
Azelastine[*] 4 mg twice daily	Ketoconazole 200 mg twice daily	7	12 healthy subjects	Not determined. In vitro tests suggest no change likely.	Not determined. In vitro tests suggest no change likely.	No change	2
Cetirizine 20 mg daily	Ketoconazole 400 mg daily	10	Healthy subjects	No change	No change	No change	3
Desloratadine 7.5 mg daily	Ketoconazole 200 mg twice daily	10	24 healthy subjects	27%	21%	No change	4
Ebastine 20 mg daily	Ketoconazole 400 mg daily	8	55 healthy subjects	16-fold	42-fold	Mean increase of 5.25 milliseconds when antihistamine added to ketoconazole. Mean increase of 12.21 milliseconds from baseline. QTc did not exceed 500 milliseconds in any subject.[†]	5
Emedastine 4 mg daily	Ketoconazole 200 mg twice daily	5	12 healthy subjects	37%	34%	No change	6
Fexofenadine 120 mg twice daily	Ketoconazole 400 mg daily	7	24 healthy subjects	135%	164%	No change	7
Levocabastine 200 micrograms twice daily intranasal	Ketoconazole 200 mg single dose	Single dose	37 subjects	No change	No change	No change	8
Loratadine 20 mg single dose	Ketoconazole 200 mg twice daily	Single dose	12 healthy subjects	144% Loratadine 33% Desloratadine	184% Loratadine 54% Desloratadine		9
Loratadine 10 mg daily	Ketoconazole 200 mg twice daily	10	24 healthy subjects	172% Loratadine 76% Desloratadine	247% Loratadine 82% Desloratadine	No change	10
Loratadine 10 mg daily	Ketoconazole 400 mg daily	8	62 healthy subjects	248% Loratadine 82% Desloratadine	346% Loratadine 94% Desloratadine	Mean increase of 3.16 milliseconds when antihistamine added to ketoconazole. Mean increase of 10.68 milliseconds from baseline. QTc did not exceed 500 milliseconds in any subject.[†]	5
Mizolastine 10 mg single dose	Ketoconazole 100 mg, 200 mg, 400 mg single doses	Single dose	12 healthy subjects		45%, 61% and 95% respectively		11
Mizolastine 10 mg daily	Ketoconazole 200 mg twice daily	5				Mean increase of 7 milliseconds over mizolastine or placebo alone. None exceeded 500 milliseconds	12
Terfenadine[*] 60 mg twice daily	Fluconazole 200 mg daily	6	6 healthy subjects		No change Terfenadine 34% Terfenadine acid metabolite	No change	13
Terfenadine[*] 60 mg twice daily	Fluconazole 800 mg daily	7	Note - 6 subjects previously found to have measurable terfenadine levels at steady state		52% Terfenadine 5% Terfenadine acid metabolite	Increase	14

Continued

Table 15.3 Summary of the effects of azoles on the pharmacokinetics and cardiovascular effects of non-sedating antihistamines (continued)

Antihistamine (Oral unless specified)	*Azole (Oral unless specified)*	*Duration of combined use (days)*	*Subjects*	*Cmax increase*‡	*AUC increase*	*Effect on QTc*	*Refs*
Terfenadine* 120 mg single dose	Itraconazole 200 mg daily	Single dose	6 healthy subjects	Terfenadine 25%, 115%, 156% in the 3 subjects who had measurable levels prior to itraconazole	30% Terfenadine acid metabolite	Mean increase of 27 milliseconds when compared to terfenadine alone	15
Terfenadine* 120 mg single dose	Ketoconazole 400 mg daily	Single dose	12 healthy subjects	≥170% Terfenadine ↓71% Terfenadine acid metabolite		Prolongation by 10 to 20 milliseconds	16,17
Terfenadine* 60 mg twice daily	Ketoconazole 200 mg twice daily	4 to 7	6 healthy subjects	<5 to 7 nanograms/mL Terfenadine levels increased to 81 nanograms/mL in one subject	57% Terfenadine acid metabolite	Mean increase of 74 milliseconds	18

*Cases of torsade de pointes have been reported for this antihistamine
†QTc intervals calculated using the Fridericia cube route formula, rather than the more commonly used Bazett square root formula, which the authors suggest would lead to a 5 to 6 millisecond overestimation
‡Note that terfenadine levels are normally undetectable

1. Lefebvre RA, Van Peer A, Woestenborghs R. Influence of itraconazole on the pharmacokinetics and electrocardiographic effects of astemizole. *Br J Clin Pharmacol* (1997) 43, 319–22.
2. Morganroth J, Lyness WH, Perhach JL, Mather GG, Harr JE, Trager WF, Levy RH, Rosenberg A. Lack of effect of azelastine and ketoconazole coadministration on electrocardiographic parameters in healthy volunteers. *J Clin Pharmacol* (1997) 37, 1065–72.
3. UCB Pharma. Personal communication, September 1994.
4. Banfield C, Herron JM, Keung A, Pahdi D, Affrime M. Desloratadine has no clinically relevant electrocardiographic or pharmacodynamic interactions with ketoconazole. *Clin Pharmacokinet* (2002) 41 (Suppl 1), 37–44.
5. Chaikin P, Gillen MS, Malik M, Pentikis H, Rhodes GR, Roberts DJ. Co-administration of ketoconazole with H1-antagonists ebastine and loratadine in healthy subjects: pharmacokinetic and pharmacodynamic effects. *Br J Clin Pharmacol* (2005) 59, 346–54.
6. Herranz U, Rusca A, Assandri A. Emedastine-ketoconazole: pharmacokinetic and pharmacodynamic interactions in healthy volunteers. *Int J Clin Pharmacol Ther* (2001) 39, 102–9.
7. Allegra (Fexofenadine hydrochloride). Aventis Pharmaceuticals Inc. US Prescribing Information, May 2003.
8. Pesco-Koplowitz L, Hassell A, Lee P, Zhou H, Hall N, Wiesinger B, Mechlinski W, Grover M, Hunt T, Smith R, Travers S. Lack of effect of erythromycin and ketoconazole on the pharmacokinetics of steady-state intranasal levocobastine. *J Clin Pharmacol* (1999) 39, 76–85.
9. Van Peer A, Crabbé R, Woestenborghs R, Heykants J, Janssens M. Ketoconazole inhibits loratadine metabolism in man. *Allergy* (1993) 48 (Suppl 16), 34.
10. Kosoglou T, Salfi M, Lim JM, Batra VK, Cayen MN, Affrime MB. Evaluation of the pharmacokinetics and electrocardiographic pharmacodynamics of loratadine with concomitant administration of ketoconazole or cimetidine. *Br J Clin Pharmacol* (2000) 50, 581–9.
11. Dubruc C, Gillet G, Chaufour S, Holt B, Jensen R, Maurel P, Thenot JP. Metabolic interaction studies of mizolastine with ketoconazole and erythromycin in rat, dog and man. *Clin Pharmacol Ther* (1998) 63, 228.
12. Delauche-Cavallier MC, Chaufour S, Guérault E, Lacroux A, Murrieta M, Wajman A. QT interval monitoring during clinical studies with mizolastine, a new H1 antihistamine. *Clin Exp Allergy* (1999) 29 (Suppl 3), 206–11.
13. Honig PK, Wortham DC, Zamani K, Mullin JC, Conner DP, Cantilena LR. The effect of fluconazole on the steady-state pharmacokinetics and electrographic pharmacodynamics of terfenadine in humans. *Clin Pharmacol Ther* (1993) 53, 630–6.
14. Cantilena LR, Sorrels S, Wiley T, Wortham D. Fluconazole alters terfenadine pharmacokinetics and electrocardiographic pharmacodynamics. *Clin Pharmacol Ther* (1995) 57, 185.
15. Honig PK, Wortham DC, Hull R, Zamani K, Smith JE, Cantilena LR. Itraconazole affects single-dose terfenadine pharmacokinetics and cardiac repolarization pharmacodynamics. *J Clin Pharmacol* (1993) 33, 1201–6.
16. Mathews DR, McNutt B, Okerholm R, Flicker M, McBride G. Torsades de pointes occurring in association with terfenadine use. *JAMA* (1991) 266, 2375–6.
17. Eller MG, Okerholm RA. Pharmacokinetic interaction between terfenadine and ketoconazole. *Clin Pharmacol Ther* (1991) 49, 130.
18. Honig PK, Wortham DC, Zamani K, Conner DP, Mullin JC, Cantilena LR. Terfenadine-ketoconazole interaction. Pharmacokinetic and electrocardiographic consequences. *JAMA* (1993) 269, 1513–18.

Fexofenadine is not metabolised by CYP3A4, but it is a substrate for P-glycoprotein and OATP,[28] therefore azole antifungals may increase its levels by inhibiting drug transporter proteins.

Importance and management

The interactions of astemizole with ketoconazole, and terfenadine with itraconazole or ketoconazole are established and clinically important, although much of the evidence for them is indirect. Astemizole would also be expected to interact similarly with itraconazole. The risk of an interaction with terfenadine or astemizole and other azole antifungals seems smaller.

The incidence of an interaction is probably low, but because of the potential severity and unpredictability of this interaction, the concurrent use of astemizole and terfenadine is contraindicated with all azole antifungals in all patients. This is a recommendation of the manufacturers[29,30] and the CSM in the UK.[31] The manufacturer of terfenadine extends this contraindication to the concurrent use of topical azoles.[30]

The use of azole antifungals with mizolastine is also contraindicated,[32] and the manufacturer of ebastine advises against the concurrent use of ketoconazole and itraconazole.[33] Because there are no data on **acrivastine** with ketoconazole, the manufacturer advises caution.[34]

Ketoconazole markedly raises loratadine levels. In one study, this was associated with a small increase in QT interval, but no obvious alteration in adverse event profile. No special precautions appear to have been recommended for the use of loratadine with azoles.

Desloratadine, emedastine and fexofenadine levels are raised by ketoconazole but because this does not result in adverse cardiac effects concurrent use is considered safe. Azelastine, cetirizine (and therefore probably its isomer **levocetirizine**) and levocabastine seem to be free from clinically significant pharmacokinetic interactions, and have no cardiac effects, and so may therefore provide suitable alternatives if a non-sedating antihistamine is needed in a patient taking azole antifungals.

1. Tsai W-C, Tsai L-M, Chen J-H. Combined use of astemizole and ketoconazole resulting in torsade de pointes. *J Formos Med Assoc* (1977) 96, 144–6.
2. Lavrijsen K, Heykants J. Interaction potential of miconazole with the metabolism of astemizole and desmethylastemizole in human liver microsomes. Data on file, Janssen Research Foundation, N 102975/1, December 1993.
3. Schöttker B, Dösch A, Kraemer DM. Severe hepatotoxicity after application of desloratadine and fluconazole. *Acta Haematol (Basel)* (2003) 110, 43–44.
4. Hey JA, del Prado M, Kreutner W, Egan RW. Cardiotoxic and drug interaction profile of the second generation antihistamines ebastine and terfenadine in an experimental animal model of torsade de pointes. *Arzneimittelforschung* (1996) 46, 159–63.
5. Moss AJ, Morganroth J. Cardiac effects of ebastine and other antihistamines in humans. *Drug Safety* (1999) 21 (Suppl 1), 69–80.
6. Shon J-H, Yoon Y-R, Hong W-S, Nguyen PM, Lee S-S, Choi Y-G, Cha I-J, Shin J-G. Effect of itraconazole on the pharmacokinetics and pharmacodynamics of fexofenadine in relation to the *MDR1* genetic polymorphism. *Clin Pharmacol Ther* (2005) 78, 191–201.
7. Allegra (Fexofenadine hydrochloride). Sanofi-Aventis US LLC. US Prescribing Information, January 2007.
8. Chaikin P, Gillen MS, Malik M, Pentikis H, Rhodes GR, Roberts DJ. Co-administration of ketoconazole with H1-antagonists ebastine and loratadine in healthy subjects: pharmacokinetic and pharmacodynamic effects. *Br J Clin Pharmacol* (2005) 59, 346–54.
9. Affrime MB, Lorber R, Danzig M, Cuss F, Brannan MD. Three month evaluation of electrocardiographic effects of loratadine in humans. *J Allergy Clin Immunol* (1993) 91, 259.
10. Honig PK, Wortham DC, Zamani K, Mullin JC, Conner DP, Cantilena LR. The effect of fluconazole on the steady-state pharmacokinetics and electrographic pharmacodynamics of terfenadine in humans. *Clin Pharmacol Ther* (1993) 53, 630–6.
11. Pohjola-Sintonen S, Viitasalo M, Toivonen L, Neuvonen P. Torsades de pointes after terfenadine-itraconazole interaction. *BMJ* (1993) 306, 186.
12. Pohjola-Sintonen S, Viitasalo M, Toivonen L, Neuvonen P. Itraconazole prevents terfenadine metabolism and increases risk of torsades de pointes ventricular tachycardia. *Eur J Clin Pharmacol* (1993) 45, 191–3.
13. Crane JK, Shih H-T. Syncope and cardiac arrhythmia due to an interaction between itraconazole and terfenadine. *Am J Med* (1993) 95, 445–6.
14. Romkes JH, Froger CL, Wever EFD, Westerhof PW. Wegrakingen tijdens simultaan gebruik van terfenadine en itraconazol. *Ned Tijdschr Geneeskd* (1997) 141, 950–3.
15. Honig PK, Wortham DC, Hull R, Zamani K, Smith JE, Cantilena LR. Itraconazole affects single-dose terfenadine pharmacokinetics and cardiac repolarization pharmacodynamics. *J Clin Pharmacol* (1993) 33, 1201–6.
16. Monahan BP, Ferguson CL, Killeavy ES, Lloyd BK, Troy J, Cantilena LR. Torsades de pointes occurring in association with terfenadine use. *JAMA* (1990) 264, 2788–90.
17. Cantilena LR, Ferguson CL, Monahan BP. Torsades de pointes occurring in association with terfenadine use. *JAMA* (1991) 266, 2375–6.
18. Zimmermann M, Duruz H, Guinand O, Broccard O, Levy P, Lacatis D, Bloch A. Torsades de pointes after treatment with terfenadine and ketoconazole. *Eur Heart J* (1992) 13, 1002–3.
19. Peck CC, Temple R, Collins JM. Understanding consequences of concurrent therapies. *JAMA* (1993) 269, 1550–2.
20. Griffith JS. Interaction between terfenadine and topical antifungal agents. *Am Fam Physician* (1995) 51, 1396–7.
21. Lavrijsen K, Van Houdt J, Meuldermans W, Janssens M, Heykants J. The interaction of ketoconazole, itraconazole and erythromycin with the in vitro metabolism of antihistamines in human liver microsomes. *Allergy* (1993) 48 (Suppl 16), 34.
22. Jurima-Romet M, Crawford K, Cyr T, Inaba T. Terfenadine metabolism in human liver. In vitro inhibition by macrolide antibiotics and azole antifungals. *Drug Metab Dispos* (1994) 22, 849–57.
23. von Moltke LL, Greenblatt DJ, Duan SX, Harmatz JS, Shader RI. *In vitro* prediction of the terfenadine-ketoconazole pharmacokinetic interaction. *J Clin Pharmacol* (1994) 34, 1222–7.
24. Neoclarityn (Desloratadine). Schering-Plough Ltd. UK Summary of product characteristics, September 2006.
25. Telfast (Fexofenadine hydrochloride). Aventis Pharma Ltd. UK Summary of product characteristics, September 2004.
26. Delauche-Cavallier MC, Chaufour S, Guérault E, Lacroux A, Murrieta M, Wajman A. QT interval monitoring during clinical studies with mizolastine, a new H1 antihistamine. *Clin Exp Allergy* (1999) 29 (Suppl 3), 206–11.
27. Mok NS, Lo YK, Tsui PT, Lam CW. Ketoconazole induced torsade de pointes without concomitant use of QT-interval-prolonging drug. *J Cardiovasc Electrophysiol* (2005) 16, 1375–7.
28. Tannergren C, Knutson T, Knutson L, Lennernäs H. The effect of ketoconazole on the *in vivo* intestinal permeability of fexofenadine using a regional perfusion technique. *Br J Clin Pharmacol* (2003) 55, 182–90.
29. Hismanal (Astemizole). Janssen-Cilag Ltd. UK Summary of product characteristics, June 1998.
30. Histafen (Terfenadine). Approved Prescription Services Ltd. UK Summary of product characteristics, December 1999.
31. Committee on Safety of Medicines. Ventricular arrhythmias due to terfenadine and astemizole. *Current Problems* (1992) 35, 1–2.
32. Mizollen (Mizolastine). Schwarz Pharma Ltd. UK Summary of product characteristics, May 2006.
33. Kestin (Ebastine). Almirall SAS. French prescribing information, August 2003.
34. Benadryl Allergy Relief (Acrivastine). Pfizer. UK Summary of product characteristics, February 2005.

Antihistamines + Benzodiazepines and related drugs

Benzodiazepines impair psychomotor performance, but neither ebastine nor mizolastine (both non-sedating antihistamines) further impair this. An enhanced sedative effect would be expected if known sedative antihistamines are given with benzodiazepines. Diphenhydramine did not alter the pharmacokinetics of zaleplon.

Clinical evidence

(a) Diphenhydramine

A randomised single dose three-period crossover study in healthy subjects found that diphenhydramine 50 mg had no significant effect on the pharmacokinetics of a single 10-mg dose of **zaleplon**, despite the fact diphenhydramine is a moderate inhibitor of the primary metabolic pathway [aldehyde oxidase] of **zaleplon**.[1]

(b) Ebastine

Ebastine 20 mg daily did not impair the performance of a number of psychomotor tests in 12 healthy subjects, although body sway and flicker fusion tests were altered. When ebastine was given with a single 15-mg dose of **diazepam**, it did not further impair performance compared with diazepam alone, and did not alter plasma **diazepam** levels.[2]

(c) Mizolastine

Mizolastine appears to lack sedative effects, and does not have a detrimental effect on psychomotor performance.[3] A single 2-mg dose of oral **lorazepam** was found to impair the performance of psychomotor tests in 16 healthy subjects, and caused some sedation and amnesia, but these effects were not changed when the subjects also took mizolastine 10 mg daily for 8 days.[3]

Mechanism, importance and management

A number of older antihistamines cause sedation, and this would be expected to be increased by some of the benzodiazepines by the simple addition of their CNS depressant effects. Non-sedating antihistamines would not be expected to have this effect (but see also 'Antihistamines', (p.582)), and this has been confirmed for ebastine and mizolastine.

1. Darwish M. Overview of drug interaction studies with zaleplon. Poster presented at 13th Annual Meeting of Associated Professional Sleep Studies (APSS), Orlando, Florida, June 23rd, 1999.
2. Mattila MJ, Aranko K, Kuitunen T. Diazepam effects on the performance of healthy subjects are not enhanced by treatment with the antihistamine ebastine. *Br J Clin Pharmacol* (1993) 35, 272–7.
3. Patat A, Perault MC, Vandel B, Ulliac N, Zieleniuk I, Rosenzweig P. Lack of interaction between a new antihistamine, mizolastine, and lorazepam on psychomotor performance and memory in healthy volunteers. *Br J Clin Pharmacol* (1995) 39, 31–8.

Antihistamines + Drugs that prolong the QT interval

Astemizole and terfenadine should generally not be used with other drugs that can also prolong the QT interval. The manufacturer of mizolastine issues the same advice. One early study found that hydroxyzine caused ECG abnormalities in high doses. The authors suggested that its use with other drugs that can cause cardiac abnormalities might increase the likelihood of arrhythmias and sudden death, but there is no published evidence of this.

Clinical evidence, mechanism, importance and management

(a) Non-sedating antihistamines

The manufacturers of **astemizole**[1] and **terfenadine**[2] contraindicate the concurrent use of any other drugs that can also prolong the QT interval (for a list, see 'Table 9.2', (p.257)). However, note that the primary risk of QT prolongation and torsade de pointes arrhythmia with **astemizole** and **terfenadine** appears to be from drugs that significantly inhibit their metabolism (e.g. 'azoles', (p.584) and 'macrolides', (p.589)). Clinically relevant QT prolongation has not yet been shown conclusively for any of the other antihistamines (see 'Table 15.2', (p.583)), although the manufacturers of **mizolastine**[3] still contraindicate its use with drugs that prolong the QT interval. Isolated cases have been described with other antihistamines: a case of torsade de pointes has been attributed to the concurrent use of amiodarone and '**loratadine**', (p.246); a case report of torsade de pointes with sotalol and '**terfenadine**', (p.859) was attributed solely to additive effects of QT prolongation with these drugs; and a small additional QT-prolonging effect has also been shown when **terfenadine** was given with 'sparfloxacin', (p.593).

Consider also 'Drugs that prolong the QT interval + Other drugs that prolong the QT interval', p.257.

(b) Sedating antihistamines

A study, conducted in 1958, in 25 elderly psychotic patients taking high-dose **hydroxyzine** 300 mg daily over a 9-week period found that ECG changes were mild, except for an alteration in T waves, which were definite in 9 patients. In each case the T waves were lower in altitude, broadened and flattened and sometimes notched. The QT interval was usually prolonged. A repeat of the study in a few patients, at least one given **hydroxyzine** 400 mg, found similar effects, the most pronounced change being a marked attenuation of cardiac repolarisation. On the basis of these observations the authors suggest that other drugs that cause ECG abnormalities such as thioridazine might aggravate and exaggerate these **hydroxyzine**-induced changes and increase the risk of sudden death.[4] However, note that in the decades of use of **hydroxyzine** since this study was conducted there appear to be only a few isolated reports of arrhythmias (tachycardia) associated with its use.[5,6] Note also that some manufacturers do not give any warnings regarding the use of **hydroxyzine** in patients with cardiac disorders, nor are any cardiac adverse effects mentioned, even for overdose.[7,8] However, one manufacturer does suggest that caution is necessary in patients pre-disposed to arrhythmias, or on drugs that may cause arrhythmias.[9]

1. Hismanal (Astemizole). Janssen-Cilag Ltd. UK Summary of product characteristics, June 1998.
2. Histafen (Terfenadine). Approved Prescription Services Ltd. UK Summary of product characteristics, December 1999.
3. Mizollen (Mizolastine). Schwarz Pharma Ltd. UK Summary of product characteristics, May 2006.
4. Hollister LE. Hydroxyzine hydrochloride: possible adverse cardiac interactions. *Psychopharmacol Comm* (1975) 1, 61–5.
5. Wong AR, Rasool AH. Hydroxyzine-induced supraventricular tachycardia in a nine-year-old child. *Singapore Med J* (2004) 45, 90–2.
6. Magera BE, Betlach CJ, Sweatt AP, Derrick CW. Hydroxyzine intoxication in a 13-month-old child. *Pediatrics* (1981) 67, 280–3.
7. Atarax (Hydroxyzine hydrochloride). Alliance Pharmaceuticals. UK Summary of product characteristics, January 2007.
8. Vistaril (Hydroxyzine pamoate). Pfizer Inc. US Prescribing information, April 2004.
9. Ucerax (Hydroxyzine hydrochloride). UCB Pharma Ltd. UK Summary of product characteristics, February 2006.

Antihistamines + Grapefruit and other fruit juices

Grapefruit juice raises terfenadine levels, increasing the risk of QT interval prolongation and torsade de pointes arrhythmias. Grapefruit juice does not appear to alter the pharmacokinetics of astemizole and desloratadine. The absorption of fexofenadine is modestly reduced by grapefruit juice, orange juice and apple juice.

Clinical evidence

(a) Astemizole

In a study in 12 healthy subjects the steady-state pharmacokinetics of astemizole (30 mg daily for 4 days, then 10 mg daily for the next 20 days), were unaffected by 800 mL of **grapefruit juice** (given as 200 mL every 4 hours).[1]

(b) Desloratadine

The bioavailability of a single 5-mg dose of desloratadine was unaffected by 8 oz (240 mL) of double-strength **grapefruit juice**, which was given three times daily for 2 days preceding the desloratadine and then 5 minutes before and 2 hours after the dose.[2]

(c) Fexofenadine

In a study in 23 healthy subjects the AUC of fexofenadine 60 mg was reduced by 30% by double-strength **grapefruit juice** (8 oz or 240 mL), which was given three times daily for 2 days before the fexofenadine and then 5 minutes before and 2 hours after the dose.[2] Similarly, another study found that **grapefruit juice** at normal strength decreased the AUC of a single 120-mg dose of fexofenadine by 67%. Dilute **grapefruit juice** (25%) caused a smaller reduction of 23%. Normal strength **orange juice** and **apple juice** similarly decreased the AUC of fexofenadine by 72% and 77% respectively.[3] In this study, 300 mL of juice was given with the fexofenadine, followed by 150 mL every half an hour to a total volume of 1.2 L. A subsequent study found that a single 300 mL dose of normal strength **grapefruit juice** reduced the AUC of a single 120-mg dose of fexofenadine by 42% when they were given simultaneously.[4] An effect was apparent for 300 mL of **grapefruit juice** given up to 10 hours prior to fexofenadine 120 mg in at least some of 12 subjects involved in this study.[5]

(d) Terfenadine

Terfenadine 60 mg was given to 6 healthy subjects every 12 hours for 14 days, given simultaneously with 240 mL of double-strength **grapefruit juice** every 12 hours for the final 7 days. Terfenadine was only detectable in the plasma when **grapefruit juice** was taken. The mean QTc interval was found to have risen from 420 to 434 milliseconds,[6] which is not of a magnitude usually considered to be clinically significant. The effects were less pronounced in a further 6 subjects who took the **grapefruit juice** 2 hours after the terfenadine.[6] Several other reports confirm these pharmacokinetics findings, although some did not find any changes in the QTc interval.[7-9]

Mechanism

Not fully understood, but it seems likely that some component of grapefruit juice inhibits the metabolism of the terfenadine to its active metabolite (by the cytochrome P450 isoenzyme CYP3A4), so that the parent drug accumulates.[8] Terfenadine, but not its metabolite, causes QTc prolongation. Increased QTc intervals are associated with the development of ventricular tachycardia and torsade de pointes arrhythmias, which are potentially life-threatening.

Fexofenadine is a substrate for P-glycoprotein, and organic anion transporting polypeptide (OATP), both of which affect fexofenadine uptake. OATP in particular may be inhibited by grapefruit juice, apple juice, and orange juice, so these juices may reduce fexofenadine levels by preventing its absorption.[3]

Importance and management

The interaction between terfenadine and grapefruit juice is established and potentially clinically important. However, the serious cardiac effects may only occur in a small subset of individuals. As of 1996 neither the FDA nor the CSM appeared to have reports of problems in patients that were attributable to the use of antihistamines and grapefruit juice,[7,10] although in 1997 the CSM had one report of a probable interaction with terfenadine.[11] Nevertheless because of the risk of serious cardiotoxicity (however small) it would be prudent for all patients taking terfenadine to avoid grapefruit juice. At least one manufacturer of terfenadine contraindicates grapefruit juice.[12]

The evidence from healthy subjects suggests that astemizole does not interact, but it is possible that individuals predisposed to cardiac conduction disorders are at risk.

Further study is required to determine the clinical relevance, if any, of the reductions in fexofenadine bioavailability in the presence of grapefruit juice, orange juice, and apple juice. Consider this interaction as the cause if fexofenadine seems less effective than expected.

Desloratadine appears to be a safe alternative.

1. Janssen-Cilag Ltd, Data on file (Study AST-BEL-7 + Amendment) 1995.
2. Banfield C, Gupta S, Marino M, Lim J, Affrime M. Grapefruit juice reduces the oral bioavailability of fexofenadine but not desloratadine. *Clin Pharmacokinet* (2002) 41, 311–18.
3. Dresser GK, Bailey DG, Leake BF, Schwarz UI, Dawson PA, Freeman DJ, Kim RB. Fruit juices inhibit organic anion transporting polypeptide–mediated drug uptake to decrease the oral availability of fexofenadine. *Clin Pharmacol Ther* (2002) 71, 11–20.
4. Dresser GK, Kim RB, Bailey DG. Effect of grapefruit juice volume on the reduction of fexofenadine bioavailability: possible role of organic anion transporting polypeptides. *Clin Pharmacol Ther* (2005) 77, 170–7.
5. Dresser GK, Kim RB, Bailey DG. Duration of grapefruit juice effect on fexofenadine interaction. *Clin Pharmacol Ther* (2003) 73, P48.
6. Benton RE, Honig PK, Zamani K, Cantilena LR, Woosley RL. Grapefruit juice alters terfenadine pharmacokinetics, resulting in prolongation of repolarization on the electrocardiogram. *Clin Pharmacol Ther* (1996) 59, 383–8.
7. Honig PK, Wortham DC, Lazarev A, Cantilena LR. Grapefruit juice alters the systemic bioavailability and cardiac repolarization of terfenadine in poor metabolizers of terfenadine. *J Clin Pharmacol* (1996) 36, 345–51.
8. Clifford CP, Adams DA, Murray S, Taylor GW, Wilkins MR, Boobis AR, Davies DS. The cardiac effects of terfenadine after inhibition of its metabolism by grapefruit juice. *Eur J Clin Pharmacol* (1997) 52, 311–15.
9. Rau SE, Bend JR, Arnold JMO, Tran LT, Spence JD, Bailey DG. Grapefruit juice–terfenadine single-dose interaction: magnitude, mechanism, and relevance. *Clin Pharmacol Ther* (1997) 61, 401–9.
10. Committee on Safety of Medicines/Medicines Control Agency. Drug interactions with grapefruit juice. *Current Problems* (1997) 23, 2.
11. Anon. Grapefruit juice and terfenadine: the "final straw". *Pharm J* (1997) 258, 618.
12. Histafen (Terfenadine). Approved Prescription Services Ltd. UK Summary of product characteristics, December 1999.

Antihistamines + H_2-receptor antagonists

No pharmacokinetic interaction appears to occur when cimetidine is given with cetirizine, desloratadine, ebastine or terfenadine, or when ranitidine is given with terfenadine or chlorphenamine. However, an isolated case report describes torsade de pointes in one patient taking terfenadine with cimetidine. Cimetidine moderately raises hydroxyzine levels and considerably raises loratadine levels, but this is not thought to be of clinical significance. The renal clearance of fexofenadine was reduced by cimetidine in one study although there was no change in plasma pharmacokinetics.

Clinical evidence

A. Non-sedating antihistamines

(a) Cetirizine

Cetirizine 10 mg was given to 8 patients with chronic urticaria before and after they took **cimetidine** 600 mg every 12 hours for 10 days. The pharmacokinetics of cetirizine were statistically unaltered and its effects remained unchanged.[1]

(b) Desloratadine

In a parallel study in 18 healthy subjects, **cimetidine** 600 mg every 12 hours had little effect on the pharmacokinetics of desloratadine 5 mg daily. The desloratadine AUC increased by about 20% and the maximum level by about 10%,[2,3] but there was no change in ECG parameters including the QTc interval.[2]

(c) Ebastine

In a study in 12 healthy subjects **cimetidine** had no significant effect on the conversion of single 20-mg doses of ebastine to its active metabolite carebastine, and there was no evidence of sedation or other adverse effects. In this study **cimetidine** was given as 2 g in divided doses the day before the ebastine dose and 400 mg four times daily both on the day of and the day after the ebastine dose.[4]

(d) Fexofenadine

Cimetidine 400 mg twice daily for 6 days did not cause any changes in the plasma pharmacokinetics of a single 120-mg dose of fexofenadine in 12 healthy subjects. However, the renal clearance of fexofenadine was decreased by 39%.[5]

(e) Loratadine

Loratadine 10 mg and **cimetidine** 300 mg every 6 hours were given alone and together to 24 healthy subjects for 10 days. The AUCs of loratadine and its metabolite were increased by 103% and 6% respectively, but the safety profile of the loratadine (clinical laboratory tests, vital signs and adverse events) were unchanged. Cardiac repolarisation and all other ECG measurements were unaltered, and no sedation or syncope were seen.[6]

(f) Terfenadine

Cimetidine 1.2 g daily for 5 days had no effect on the pharmacokinetics of a single 120-mg dose of terfenadine in 12 healthy subjects.[7] Another study in two groups of 6 healthy subjects confirmed that **cimetidine** 600 mg every 12 hours or **ranitidine** 150 mg every 12 hours had no effect on the pharmacokinetics of terfenadine 60 mg every 12 hours. No adverse ECG changes were seen.[8] However, an isolated case report describes a 63-year-old woman who had 8 episodes of syncope (later identified as being due to torsade de pointes) and a convulsion 2 days after starting terfenadine 60 mg twice daily and **cimetidine** 400 mg twice daily. She was also taking chlorphenamine and co-proxamol (paracetamol (acetaminophen) and dextropropoxyphene (propoxyphene)).[9]

B. Sedating antihistamines

(a) Chlorphenamine

A study in healthy subjects found that the pharmacokinetics of a single 4-mg dose of racemic chlorphenamine were unaffected by **ranitidine** 75 mg twice daily for 6 days.[10]

(b) Hydroxyzine

In one study, 8 patients with chronic urticaria were given hydroxyzine 25 mg before and after taking **cimetidine** 600 mg every 12 hours for 10 days. The **cimetidine** increased the AUC of hydroxyzine by 33% and also increased its suppression of the wheal and flare response (although this was not statistically significant).[1] A previous study in 7 patients found that **cimetidine** raised serum hydroxyzine levels.[11]

Mechanism

Cimetidine is a non-specific cytochrome P450 isoenzyme inhibitor, but it would seem that in most cases, with the exception of loratadine, these enzyme inhibitory effects do not significantly affect the metabolism of antihistamines. More recent evidence has shown cimetidine can also affect drug transporter proteins, in particular it may inhibit organic cation transporters. However, it probably does not affect anion transporter proteins since it does not affect the plasma pharmacokinetics of fexofenadine, which is a substrate of these transporters.[5]

Importance and management

There would seem to be no good reason for avoiding the concurrent use of either cetirizine, ebastine, fexofenadine, hydroxyzine, or loratadine with cimetidine, or chlorphenamine with ranitidine, nor would any of the other H_2-receptor antagonists be expected to interact with any of these antihistamines.

The situation with terfenadine and cimetidine is not totally clear because of the isolated case report of toxicity cited here, but currently there is not enough evidence to advise against the use of these two drugs. The manufacturer of **mizolastine** recommends caution with concurrent cimetidine on the basis that cimetidine might increase **mizolastine** levels and prolong the QT interval.[12] This is a cautious approach since a link between **mizolastine** and cardiac arrhythmias has not been proven.

1. Simons FER, Sussman GL, Simons KJ. Effect of the H_2-antagonist cimetidine on the pharmacokinetics and pharmacodynamics of the H_1-antagonists hydroxyzine and cetirizine in patients with chronic urticaria. *J Allergy Clin Immunol* (1995) 95, 685–93.
2. Clarinex (Desloratadine). Schering Corporation. US Prescribing information, February 2007.
3. Krishna G, Khalilieh S, Ezzet F, Marino M, Kantesaria B, Lim J, Batra V. Effect of cimetidine on the pharmacokinetics of desloratadine. *AAPS PharmSci* (2001) 3, 3. Available at: http://www.aapspharmaceutica.com/search/abstract_view.asp?id=824&ct=01Abstracts (accessed 20/08/07).
4. van Rooij J, Schoemaker HC, Bruno R, Reinhoudt JF, Breimer DD, Cohen AF. Cimetidine does not influence the metabolism of the H_1-receptor antagonist ebastine to its active metabolite carebastine. *Br J Clin Pharmacol* (1993) 35, 661–3.
5. Yasui-Furukori N, Uno T, Sugawara K, Tateishi T. Different effects of three transporting inhibitors, verapamil, cimetidine, and probenecid, on fexofenadine pharmacokinetics. *Clin Pharmacol Ther* (2005) 77, 17–23.
6. Kosoglou T, Salfi M, Lim JM, Batra VK, Cayen MN, Affrime MB. Evaluation of the pharmacokinetics and electrocardiographic pharmacodynamics of loratadine with concomitant administration of ketoconazole or cimetidine. *Br J Clin Pharmacol* (2000) 50, 581–9.
7. Eller MG, Okerhold RA. Effect of cimetidine on terfenadine and terfenadine metabolite pharmacokinetics. *Pharm Res* (1991) 8 (10 Suppl), S-297.
8. Honig PK, Wortham DC, Zamani K, Conner DP, Mullin JC, Cantilena LR. Effect of concomitant administration of cimetidine and ranitidine on the pharmacokinetics and electrocardiographic effects of terfenadine. *Eur J Clin Pharmacol* (1993) 45, 41–6.
9. Ng PW, Chan WK, Chan TYK. Torsade de pointes during concomitant use of terfenadine and cimetidine. *Aust N Z J Med* (1996) 26, 120–1.
10. Koch KM, O'Connor-Semmes RL, Davis IM, Yin Y. Stereoselective pharmacokinetics of chlorpheniramine and the effect of ranitidine. *J Pharm Sci* (1998) 87, 1097–1100.
11. Salo OP, Kauppinen K, Männistö PT. Cimetidine increases the plasma concentration of hydroxyzine. *Acta Derm Venereol (Stockh)* (1986), 66, 349–50.
12. Mizollen (Mizolastine). Schwarz Pharma Ltd. UK Summary of product characteristics, May 2006.

Antihistamines + Macrolides

Erythromycin causes terfenadine and astemizole to accumulate in a few individuals, which can prolong the QT interval and lead to life-threatening torsade de pointes arrhythmias. Cases of torsade de pointes have been reported for astemizole with erythromycin, and terfenadine with erythromycin or troleandomycin. Other macrolides are believed to interact similarly, with the exception of azithromycin and possibly dirithromycin.

Erythromycin modestly raises mizolastine levels, although this had no effect on the QT interval. Nevertheless, the manufacturers of mizolastine contraindicate erythromycin. Erythromycin markedly raised ebastine levels, which caused a modest prolongation of the QT interval. The manufacturers of ebastine advise against the

concurrent use of erythromycin, clarithromycin and josamycin. Because there is no information for acrivastine, the manufacturer advises caution.

There is a case of torsade de pointes possibly due to spiramycin with the sedating antihistamine mequitazine. The situation with erythromycin and loratadine is unclear as one study found that the combination caused a very slight increase in QT interval.

Both azithromycin and erythromycin raise fexofenadine levels, but this had no effect on the QT interval, or on adverse events. Azelastine, cetirizine, desloratadine, and intranasal levocabastine seem to be free of clinically relevant interactions with macrolides.

Clinical evidence

The effect of various macrolides on the plasma levels of the non-sedating antihistamines, and their cardiac effects from controlled studies are summarised in 'Table 15.4', (p.591). The subsections below include data from case reports and other studies.

(a) Astemizole

1. Azithromycin. The manufacturers of astemizole report that an *in vivo* study has shown that azithromycin had a negligible effect on the bioavailability of astemizole.[1]

2. Erythromycin. An 87-year-old woman collapsed suddenly in her kitchen 4 days after starting to take astemizole 10 mg daily and erythromycin twice daily [dose unknown]. An ECG showed her to be having multiple episodes of torsade de pointes arrhythmias, the longest of which lasted 17 seconds. Her QTc was 720 milliseconds and she was mildly hypokalaemic. She was given a temporary pacemaker and when she was eventually discharged with a normal sinus rhythm, her QTc had fallen to 475 milliseconds.[2]

(b) Loratadine

A study of loratadine alone in 50 healthy subjects found that 40 mg of loratadine daily (four times the recommended dose) for 90 days caused no changes in the ECG measurements, no episodes of dizziness or syncope, and no arrhythmias,[3] but see also 'Table 15.2', (p.583).

(c) Mequitazine

A 21-year-old woman with a congenital long QT syndrome had several syncopal attacks, one at least of which was caused by torsade de pointes. This was attributed to the concurrent use of mequitazine and **spiramycin** over a 2-day period. The problem resolved when the drugs were withdrawn.[4]

(d) Terfenadine

1. Erythromycin. A 18-year-old girl who was taking terfenadine 60 mg twice daily and erythromycin 250 mg every 6 hours, fainted while at school and, when later hospitalised, was seen to have repeated episodes of ventricular tachycardia and ventricular fibrillation requiring resuscitation. Later she was also noted to have torsade de pointes. Her QTc interval was found to be prolonged at 630 milliseconds. The drugs were withdrawn and 9 days later, after a period in intensive care, she was discharged symptom-free with a normal QTc interval.[5]

In contrast, a retrospective report found no documented cardiac adverse events in 92 patients who had received erythromycin and terfenadine.[6]

2. Troleandomycin. The manufacturers of terfenadine have on record a case of a woman, with a history of aortic valve disease, who had an episode of torsade de pointes arrhythmia while taking troleandomycin. She had taken more than the maximum recommended dose of terfenadine.[7] Another woman taking terfenadine 60 mg three times daily developed torsade de pointes arrhythmia and a prolonged QTc interval when troleandomycin 500 mg three times daily was added. She recovered when both were stopped, but again developed a significantly prolonged QTc interval when both were restarted.[8]

Mechanism

Some macrolides (particularly erythromycin and clarithromycin) appear to reduce the metabolism of terfenadine and astemizole by inhibition of the cytochrome P450 isoenzyme CYP3A.[9,10] High serum levels of astemizole and terfenadine cause a prolongation of the QT interval and may precipitate the development of torsade de pointes arrhythmia, see 'Table 15.2', (p.583). The risk of cardiac arrhythmias with other non-sedating antihistamines appears to be non-existent or very much lower (see 'Table 15.2', (p.583)), so any pharmacokinetic interactions do not result in clinically relevant cardiac toxicity. In fact, studies have shown that fexofenadine in overdose,[11,12] and mizolastine at four times the recommended dose[13] do not affect the QT interval. However, some questions remain about mizolastine and ebastine.

The increased levels of fexofenadine with erythromycin may be due to increased absorption and decreased biliary secretion,[12] via an effect on drug transporters.

Importance and management

The interactions of terfenadine with erythromycin, clarithromycin, and troleandomycin; and astemizole with erythromycin are established, clinically important and potentially hazardous. From the reports above it does seem that only a very few individuals develop a clinically important adverse interaction with these macrolides, but identifying them in advance is not often practical or possible. Because of the unpredictability and potential severity of this interaction, the FDA,[6] the CSM[14] in the UK and the manufacturers of terfenadine[15] and astemizole[1] now contraindicate macrolides in anyone taking terfenadine or astemizole. The only exception to this is azithromycin with astemizole.[1] The manufacturer of terfenadine extends this contraindication to the concurrent use of topical macrolides.[15]

The manufacturers of mizolastine also contraindicate the concurrent use of the macrolides,[16] despite any evidence of a significant interaction. Erythromycin markedly raises ebastine levels causing a modest increase in QT interval. The manufacturer of ebastine advises against concurrent use of the macrolides erythromycin, clarithromycin and **josamycin**.[17] Erythromycin also raises loratadine levels, which caused a very slight increase in QTc interval in one study. However, no special precautions appear to have been recommended for the use of loratadine with macrolides. Because there are no data on **acrivastine** with erythromycin, the manufacturer advises caution.[18]

Fexofenadine levels are raised by both azithromycin and erythromycin but because this does not result in adverse cardiac effects concurrent use is considered safe. Azelastine, cetirizine (and therefore probably its isomer **levocetirizine**) desloratadine and levocabastine seem to be free from clinically significant pharmacokinetic interactions, and have no cardiac effects, and so may therefore provide suitable alternatives if a non-sedating antihistamine is needed in a patient taking macrolides.

The isolated case with mequitazine is unlikely to be of general importance, since this sedating antihistamine is not usually associated with causing ventricular arrhythmias.

1. Hismanal (Astemizole). Janssen-Cilag Ltd. UK Summary of product characteristics, June 1998.
2. Goss JE, Ramo BW, Blake K. Torsades de pointes associated with astemizole (Hismanal) therapy. *Arch Intern Med* (1993) 153, 2705.
3. Affrime MB, Lorber R, Danzig M, Cuss F, Brannan MD. Three month evaluation of electrocardiographic effects of loratadine in humans. *J Allergy Clin Immunol* (1993) 91, 259.
4. Verdun F, Mansourati J, Jobic Y, Bouquin V, Munier S, Guillo P, Pagès Y, Boschat J, Blanc J-J. Torsades de pointes sous traitement par spiramycine et méquitazine. À propos d'un cas. *Arch Mal Coeur Vaiss* (1997) 90, 103–6.
5. Biglin KE, Faraon MS, Constance TD, Lieh-Lai M. Drug-induced torsades de pointes: a possible interaction of terfenadine and erythromycin. *Ann Pharmacother* (1994) 28, 282.
6. Schoenwetter WF, Kelloway JS, Lindgren D. A retrospective evaluation of potential cardiac side-effects induced by concurrent use of terfenadine and erythromycin. *J Allergy Clin Immunol* (1993) 91, 259.
7. Marion Merrell Dow. Personal Communication, August 1993.
8. Fournier P, Pacouret G, Charbonnier B. Une nouvelle cause de torsades de pointes: association terfénadine et troléandomycine. *Ann Cardiol Angeiol (Paris)* (1993) 42, 249–52.
9. Yun C-H, Okerholm RA, Guengerich FP. Oxidation of the antihistaminic drug terfenadine in human liver microsomes. Role of cytochrome P-450 3A(4) in *N*-dealkylation and C-hydroxylation. *Drug Metab Dispos* (1993) 21, 403–9.
10. Jurima-Romet M, Crawford K, Cyr T, Inaba T. Terfenadine metabolism in human liver. In vitro inhibition by macrolide antibiotics and azole antifungals. *Drug Metab Dispos* (1994) 22, 849–57.
11. Allegra (Fexofenadine hydrochloride). Sanofi-Aventis US LLC. US Prescribing information, January 2007.
12. Telfast (Fexofenadine hydrochloride). Aventis Pharma Ltd. UK Summary of product characteristics, September 2004.
13. Chaufour S, Caplain H, Lilienthal N, L'Héritier C, Deschamps C, Rosenzweig P. Mizolastine, a new H_1 antagonist, does not affect the cardiac repolarisation in healthy volunteers. *Clin Pharmacol Ther* (1998) 63, 214.
14. Committee on Safety of Medicines. Ventricular arrhythmias due to terfenadine and astemizole. *Current Problems* (1992) 35, 1–2.
15. Histafen (Terfenadine). Approved Prescription Services Ltd. UK Summary of product characteristics, December 1999.
16. Mizollen (Mizolastine). Schwarz Pharma Ltd. UK Summary of product characteristics, May 2006.
17. Kestin (Ebastine). Almirall SAS. French prescribing information, August 2003.
18. Benadryl Allergy Relief (Acrivastine). Pfizer. UK Summary of product characteristics, February 2005.

Table 15.4 Summary of the effect of macrolides on the pharmacokinetics and cardiovascular effects of non-sedating antihistamines

Antihistamine	*Macrolide*	*Duration of combined use (days)*	*Subjects*	*Cmax increase*[†]	*AUC increase*	*Effect on QTc*	*Refs*
Astemizole[*] 30 mg single dose	Dirithromycin 500 mg daily	Single dose of antihistamine	18 healthy subjects	No change	36%	No change	1
Azelastine[*] 4 mg twice daily	Erythromycin 500 mg three times daily	7	8 healthy subjects	No change	No change	No change	2
Cetirizine 20 mg daily	Erythromycin 500 mg three times daily	10	Healthy subjects	No change	No change	No change	3
Desloratadine 5 mg daily	Azithromycin 500 mg, then 250 mg daily	5	18 healthy subjects	No change	No change	No change	4
Desloratadine 7.5 mg daily	Erythromycin 500 mg three times daily	10	24 healthy subjects	20%	10%	No change	5
Ebastine 20 mg daily	Erythromycin 2.4 g daily	10	30 healthy subjects	119% Similar changes found for carebastine	164% Similar changes found for carebastine	Mean increase of 19.6 milliseconds	6
Fexofenadine 60 mg twice daily	Azithromycin 500 mg, then 250 mg daily	5	18 healthy subjects	69%	67%	No change	4
Fexofenadine 120 mg twice daily	Erythromycin 500 mg three times daily	7	24 healthy subjects	82%	109%	No change	7
Levocabastine 200 micrograms twice daily intranasal	Erythromycin 333 mg single dose	Single dose of macrolide	38 healthy subjects	No change	No change	No change	8
Loratadine 10 mg daily	Clarithromycin 500 mg twice daily	10	24 healthy subjects	36% Loratadine 69% Descarbo-ethoxyloratadine	76% Loratadine 49% Descarbo-ethoxyloratadine	Mean increase of 4 milliseconds. Maximum QTc 439 milliseconds	9
Loratadine 10 mg daily	Erythromcyin 500 mg three times daily	10	24 healthy subjects	53% Loratadine 61% Descarbo-ethoxyloratadine	40% Loratadine 46% Descarbo-ethoxyloratadine	No change	10
Mizolastine 10 mg daily	Erythromycin 1 g twice daily	6	12 healthy subjects	40%	53%	No change	11
Terfenadine[*] 60 mg twice daily	Azithromycin 500 mg then 250 mg daily	5	Healthy subjects	Terfenadine undetectable No change in terfenadine acid metabolite	No change in terfenadine acid metabolite	No change	12, 13
Terfenadine[*] 60 mg twice daily	Clarithromycin 500 mg twice daily	7	6 healthy subjects	4 of 6 subjects with measurable terfenadine levels 110% Terfenadine acid metabolite	156% Terfenadine acid metabolite	Mean increase of 20 milliseconds	12
Terfenadine[*] 60 mg twice daily	Clarithromycin 500 mg twice daily	5	14 healthy subjects	2 of 14 subjects with measurable terfenadine levels 119% Terfenadine acid metabolite	181% Terfenadine acid metabolite	Not documented	14
Terfenadine[*] 60 mg twice daily	Dirithromycin 500 mg daily	10	6 healthy subjects	No change in terfenadine acid metabolite	No change in terfenadine acid metabolite	No change	15

Continued

Table 15.4 Summary of the effect of macrolides on the pharmacokinetics and cardiovascular effects of non-sedating antihistamines (continued)

Antihistamine	*Macrolide*	*Duration of combined use (days)*	*Subjects*	*Cmax increase*†	*AUC increase*	*Effect on QTc*	*Refs*
Terfenadine* 60 mg twice daily	Erythromycin 500 mg three times daily	7	9 subjects	3 of 9 subjects with measurable terfenadine levels 107% Terfenadine acid metabolite	170% Terfenadine acid metabolite	64 milliseconds in the 3 subjects with measurable terfenadine levels. No significant change in the other 6 subjects	16
Terfenadine* 60 mg twice daily	Erythromycin 500 mg three times daily	7	6 healthy subjects	4 of 6 subjects with measurable terfenadine levels 87% Terfenadine acid metabolite	109% Terfenadine acid metabolite	Mean increase of 34 milliseconds	12
Terfenadine* 60 mg twice daily	Erythromycin 333 mg three times daily	7		22% Terfenadine acid metabolite	42% Terfenadine acid metabolite	Mean increase of 4 to 10 milliseconds with erythromycin alone. No further increase with terfenadine	17, 18

*Cases of torsade de pointes have been reported for this antihistamine, see Macrolides, p. 589.
†Note that terfenadine levels are normally undetectable.

1. Bachmann K, Sullivan TJ, Reese JH, Jauregui L, Miller K, Scott M, Stotka J, Harris J. A study of the interaction between dirithromycin and astemizole in healthy adults. *Am J Ther* (1997) 4, 73–9.
2. Sale M, Lyness W, Perhach J, Woosley R, Rosenberg A. Lack of effect of coadministration of erythromycin (ERY) with azelastine (AZ) on pharmacokinetics (PK) or ECG parameters. *Ann Allergy Asthma Immunol* (1996) 74, 91.
3. UCB Pharma. Personal communication, September 1994.
4. Gupta S, Banfield C, Kantesaria B, Marino M, Clement R, Affrime M, Batra V. Pharmacokinetic and safety profile of desloratadine and fexofenadine when coadministered with azithromycin: a randomized, placebo-controlled, parallel-group study. *Clin Ther* (2001) 23, 451–66.
5. Banfield C, Hunt T, Reyderman L, Statkevich P, Padhi D, Affrime M. Lack of clinically relevant interaction between desloratadine and erythromycin. *Clin Pharmacokinet* (2002) 41 (Suppl 1), 29–35.
6. Gillen M, Pentikis H, Rhodes G, Chaikin P, Morganroth J. Pharmacokinetic (PK) and pharmacodynamic (PD) interaction of ebastine (EBA) and erythromycin (ERY). *Clin Invest Med* (1998) (Suppl), S20.
7. Allegra (Fexofenadine hydrochloride). Aventis Pharmaceuticals Inc. US Prescribing information, May 2003.
8. Pesco-Koplowitz L, Hassell A, Lee P, Zhou H, Hall N, Wiesinger B, Mechlinski W, Grover M, Hunt T, Smith R, Travers S. Lack of effect of erythromycin and ketoconazole on the pharmacokinetics and pharmacodynamics of steady-state intranasal levocabastine. *J Clin Pharmacol* (1999) 39, 76–85.
9. Carr RA, Edmonds A, Shi H, Locke CS, Gustavson LE, Craft JÇ, Harris SI, Palmer R. Steady-state pharmacokinetics and electrocardiographic pharmacodynamics of clarithromycin and loratadine after individual or concomitant administration. *Antimicrob Agents Chemother* (1998) 42, 1176–80.
10. Brannan MD, Reidenberg P, Radwanski E, Shneyer L, Lin C-C, Cayen MN, Affrime MB. Loratadine administered concomitantly with erythromycin: pharmacokinetic and electrocardiographic evaluations. *Clin Pharmacol Ther* (1995) 58, 269–78.
11. Chaufour S, Holt B, Jensen R, Dubruc C, Deschamp C, Rosenzweig R. Interaction study between mizolastine, a new H1 antihistamine, and erythromycin. *Clin Pharmacol Ther* (1998) 63, 214.
12. Honig PK, Wortham DC, Zamani K, Cantilena LR. Comparison of the effect of the macrolide antibiotics erythromycin, clarithromycin and azithromycin on terfenadine steady-state pharmacokinetics and electrocardiographic parameters. *Drug Invest* (1994) 7, 148–56.
13. Harris S, Hilligoss DM, Colangelo PM, Eller M, Okerholm R. Azithromycin and terfenadine: lack of drug interaction. *Clin Pharmacol Ther* (1995) 58, 310–15.
14. Gustavson LE, Blahunka KS, Witt GF, Harris SI, Palmer RN. Evaluation of the pharmacokinetic drug interaction between terfenadine and clarithromycin. *Pharm Res* (1993) 10 (10 Suppl), S-311.
15. Goldberg MJ, Ring B, DeSante K, Cerimele B, Hatcher B, Sides G, Wrighton S. Effect of dirithromycin on human CYP3A in vitro and on pharmacokinetics and pharmacodynamics of terfenadine in vivo. *J Clin Pharmacol* (1996) 36, 1154–60.
16. Honig PK, Woosley RL, Zamani K, Conner DP, Cantilena LR. Changes in the pharmacokinetics and electrocardiographic pharmacodynamics of terfenadine with concomitant administration of erythromycin. *Clin Pharmacol Ther* (1992) 52, 231–8.
17. Eller M, Russell T, Ruberg S, Okerholm R, McNutt B. Effect of erythromycin on terfenadine metabolite pharmacokinetics. *Clin Pharmacol Ther* (1993) 53, 161.
18. Mathews DR, McNutt B, Okerholm R, Flicker M, McBride G. Torsades de pointes occurring in association with terfenadine use. *JAMA* (1991) 266, 2375–6.

Antihistamines + Nefazodone

Nefazodone inhibits the metabolism of terfenadine and thereby prolongs the QT interval. This combination should be avoided. There is also some evidence that the combination of nefazodone and loratadine increases the QT interval, although to a lesser extent than terfenadine. *In vitro* evidence suggests nefazodone will also inhibit the metabolism of astemizole.

Clinical evidence, mechanism, importance and management

(a) Astemizole

The manufacturers of nefazodone and astemizole say that an *in vitro* study suggests that nefazodone may increase astemizole levels, and so concurrent use is contraindicated.[1,2] The advice to avoid the combination would seem prudent since raised levels of astemizole with other inhibitors of CYP3A4 such as the 'macrolides', (p.589), have been rarely associated with life-threatening torsade de pointes arrhythmias.

(b) Loratadine

A randomised, placebo-controlled study in healthy subjects found that when they were given nefazodone 300 mg twice daily with loratadine 20 mg once daily, the loratadine AUC was increased by 39%. Similarly, the QTc interval was increased by 21.6 milliseconds by the combination, which was about half the increase seen with terfenadine 60 mg twice daily given with the same dose of nefazodone. Neither nefazodone, loratadine nor terfenadine alone prolonged the QTc interval.[3] The findings for loratadine in this study were unexpected, since this antihistamine was considered to have no clinically relevant effect on the QT interval (but see also 'Table 15.2', (p.583)). The use of the Bazett formula to calculate QTc has been questioned,[4] but this is the most commonly used formula, and any overestimation would also apply to terfenadine. This appears to be the only study to have directly compared loratadine with terfenadine, and although it shows that loratadine at twice the recommended dose has half the QT-prolonging effect of terfenadine (at the maximum recommended dose), it nevertheless raises questions about the cardiac safety of loratadine.[4,5] Further study is needed.

(c) Terfenadine

In a randomised, placebo-controlled study, healthy subjects were given nefazodone 300 mg twice daily and terfenadine 60 mg twice daily, given alone and in combination. Nefazodone increased the AUC of terfenadine by about fivefold, which was associated with a mean increase in the QTc interval of 42.4 milliseconds. This was considered to result in a clinically significant, increase in the risk of torsade de pointes arrhythmias.[3] Studies using human liver microsomes found that nefazodone is a moderately weak inhibitor of the CYP3A4-mediated *N*-dealkylation and *C*-hydroxylation of terfenadine.[6] Nefazodone is contraindicated with terfenadine,[1,7] and it has been suggested that this explains the lack of clinical reports.[6]

1. Robinson DS, Roberts DL, Smith JM, Stringfellow JC, Kaplita SB, Seminara JA, Marcus RN. The safety profile of nefazodone. *J Clin Psychiatry* (1996) 57 (Suppl 2), 31–8.
2. Hismanal (Astemizole). Janssen-Cilag Ltd. UK Summary of product characteristics, June 1998.
3. Abernethy DR, Barbey JT, Franc J, Brown KS, Feirrera I, Ford N, Salazar DE. Loratadine and terfenadine interaction with nefazodone; both antihistamines are associated with QTc prolongation. *Clin Pharmacol Ther* (2001) 69; 96–103.
4. Barbey JT. Loratadine/nefazodone interaction. *Clin Pharmacol Ther* (2002) 71, 403.
5. Abernethy DR. Reply. *Clin Pharmacol Ther* (2002) 71, 403.
6. Jurima-Romet M, Wright M, Neigh S. Terfenadine-antidepressant interactions: an *in vitro* inhibition study using human liver microsomes. *Br J Clin Pharmacol* (1998) 45, 318–21.
7. Histafen (Terfenadine). Approved Prescription Services Ltd. UK Summary of product characteristics, December 1999.

Antihistamines + Protease inhibitors

Nelfinavir markedly increases terfenadine levels, which is expected to increase the risk of QT prolongation and torsade de pointes arrhythmias. Other protease inhibitors are predicted to interact similarly with both terfenadine and astemizole, and concurrent use is contraindicated. Ritonavir modestly increases cetirizine levels, and *in vitro* data suggests that saquinavir will have a similar effect, but this is not considered to be clinically relevant. Based on in vitro data, ritonavir is predicted to markedly raise fexofenadine levels, but this may not be of any clinical relevance.

Clinical evidence, mechanism, importance and management

(a) Astemizole

Protease inhibitors are inhibitors of the cytochrome P450 isoenzyme CYP3A4, by which astemizole is metabolised. On the basis of the interaction of astemizole with other CYP3A4 inhibitors, such as the 'azoles', (p.584), the concurrent use of astemizole with any protease inhibitor is contraindicated.[1] This seems a sensible precaution.

(b) Cetirizine

In a study in 16 healthy subjects the concurrent use of cetirizine 10 mg daily and **ritonavir** 600 mg twice daily for 4 days (after reaching steady-state **ritonavir** levels), increased the AUC of cetirizine by 42% with a slight 9% increase in maximum plasma levels. It was suggested that **ritonavir** may have decreased the renal excretion of cetirizine. The increase in cetirizine levels was not considered to be clinically relevant. **Ritonavir** pharmacokinetics were minimally affected by cetirizine.[2]

(c) Fexofenadine

An *in vitro* study showed that **ritonavir** markedly reduced the transport of fexofenadine, thought to be via inhibition of P-glycoprotein.[3] This would be predicted to markedly increase the bioavailability of fexofenadine, as occurs with verapamil, see 'Calcium-channel blockers + Antihistamines', p.861. However, the similar marked increases in fexofenadine levels that occurred with 'erythromycin', (p.589) and 'ketoconazole', (p.584) did not increase adverse effects and were not associated with any prolongation of the QT interval. This suggests that a clinically relevant interaction between **ritonavir** and fexofenadine is not expected.

(d) Terfenadine

Nelfinavir 750 mg every 8 hours for 5 days raised the levels of a single 60-mg dose of terfenadine from less than 5 nanograms/mL to a range of 5 to 15 nanograms/mL. The pharmacokinetics of **nelfinavir** were unaffected.[4] This rise in terfenadine levels is predicted to prolong the QT interval, and to increase the risk of torsade de pointes arrhythmias. In an *in vitro* study, **saquinavir** was a potent inhibitor of the metabolism of **terfenadine**.[5] Note that **saquinavir** is the least potent CYP3A4 inhibitor of the protease inhibitors. On the basis of *in vitro* study, and what is known about interactions with other inhibitors of CYP3A4 such as the 'azoles', (p.584), all protease inhibitors are predicted to raise terfenadine levels and consequently concurrent use is contraindicated.[6] Because of the seriousness of this reaction, and the fact that it is not possible to predict which individuals will be affected, this seems a sensible precaution.

1. Hismanal (Astemizole). Janssen-Cilag Ltd. UK Summary of product characteristics, June 1998.
2. Peytavin G, Gautran C, Otoul C, Cremieux AC, Moulaert B, Delatour F, Melac M, Strolin-Benedetti M, Farinotti R. Evaluation of pharmacokinetic interaction between cetirizine and ritonavir, an HIV-1 protease inhibitor, in healthy male volunteers. *Eur J Clin Pharmacol* (2005) 61, 267–73.
3. Perloff MD, von Moltke LL, Greenblatt DJ. Fexofenadine transport in caco-2 cells: inhibition with verapamil and ritonavir. *J Clin Pharmacol* (2002) 42, 1269–74.
4. Kerr B, Yuep G, Daniels R, Quart B, Kravcik S, Sahai J, Anderson R. Strategic approach to nelfinavir mesylate (NFV) drug interactions involving CYP3A metabolism. 6th European Conference on Clinical Aspects and Treatment of HIV-infection, Hamburg, October 11–15th 1997. Abstracts.
5. Fitzsimmons ME, Collins JM. Selective biotransformation of the human immunodeficiency virus protease inhibitor saquinavir by human small-intestinal cytochrome P4503A4. *Drug Metab Dispos* (1997) 25, 256–6.
6. Histafen (Terfenadine). Approved Prescription Services Ltd. UK Summary of product characteristics, December 1999.

Antihistamines + Quinolones

Studies in healthy subjects showed that there was a small additive effect on the QT interval when terfenadine was given with sparfloxacin.

Clinical evidence, mechanism, importance and management

In a single-dose, placebo-controlled study in 8 healthy subjects, **sparfloxacin** 400 mg increased the QT interval by 14 milliseconds, **terfenadine** 60 mg increased the QT interval by 7.5 milliseconds (not statistically significant), and the combination caused an additive increase of 24.7 milliseconds.[1]

The effects of the combination in this study were shown to be purely additive.[1]

In a placebo-controlled study 22 patients were given **sparfloxacin** 400 mg on day 1 and 200 mg on days 2 to 4 with **terfenadine** 60 mg twice a day for 7 doses. The increase in the QT interval when the two drugs were given together was additive, and no pharmacokinetic interaction was found.[2]

Since the effects of therapeutic doses of **terfenadine** on the QT interval are minimal, any additional effect with **sparfloxacin** would be small. Nevertheless, since torsade de pointes can cause sudden death, the combination of two drugs with the potential to prolong the QT interval is generally considered contraindicated (see 'Drugs that prolong the QT interval + Other drugs that prolong the QT interval', p.257) and the manufacturer of **terfenadine** specifically contraindicates **sparfloxacin**.[3] If an antihistamine is required in a patient taking **sparfloxacin**, one that has no effect on the QT interval should be used, for example, **cetirizine**, see 'Table 15.2', (p.583). Other quinolones that cause QT prolongation include **gatifloxacin** and **moxifloxacin**, see 'Table 9.2', (p.257), and it would also be prudent to avoid use of antihistamines that prolong the QT interval (e.g. **astemizole** and **terfenadine**) with these quinolones.

1. Akhtar M, Saha N, Roy A, Pillai KK. Effect of sparfloxacin and terfenadine combination on QT-intervals at various RR-intervals. *Indian J Pharmacol* (2002) 34, 264–8.
2. Morganroth J, Hunt T, Dorr MB, Magner D, Talbot GH. The effect of terfenadine on the cardiac pharmacodynamics of sparfloxacin. *Clin Ther* (1999) 21, 1514–24.
3. Histafen (Terfenadine). Approved Prescription Services Ltd. UK Summary of product characteristics, December 1999.

Antihistamines + SSRIs

Two isolated reports describe cardiotoxicity, which was attributed to the concurrent use of terfenadine and fluoxetine, although other evidence suggests that an interaction is unlikely. Terfenadine does not appear to interact with paroxetine or sertraline. Nonetheless, the manufacturers of both astemizole and terfenadine contraindicate the concurrent use of SSRIs. There does not

appear to be a significant interaction between desloratadine and fluoxetine. An interaction between fluoxetine and loratadine is theoretically possible, but the clinical significance of this is unclear.

Clinical evidence

A. Astemizole

The manufacturer of astemizole contraindicates the concurrent use of SSRIs because there is a risk that they will inhibit astemizole metabolism, leading to a rise in its serum levels, which could result in QT interval prolongation and the development of torsade de pointes arrhythmias.[1]

B. Desloratadine

The concurrent use of desloratadine 5 mg daily and **fluoxetine** 20 mg daily for 7 days (after attainment of **fluoxetine** steady-state) had no clinically relevant effects on the pharmacokinetics of desloratadine or **fluoxetine** (changes in maximum levels and AUC were less than 15%). There was no change in ECG parameters including the QTc interval, and the combination did not increase the incidence of adverse effects.[2] This study was placebo-controlled and in healthy subjects who were of extensive metaboliser phenotype for CYP2D6.

C. Loratadine

Fluoxetine is an inhibitor of the cytochrome P450 isoenzymes CYP3A4 (weak inhibitor) and CYP2D6 (moderate inhibitor), by which loratadine is metabolised. Fluoxetine may therefore moderately raise loratadine levels. One study suggests that high-dose loratadine does not cause adverse cardiac adverse effects.[3] However, more recent case reports and studies have cast some doubt over the cardiac safety of loratadine (see 'Table 15.2', (p.583)).

D. Terfenadine

(a) Fluoxetine

A 41-year-old man with no previous history of heart disease awoke one night short of breath, with a sensation of his heart missing beats and beating irregularly. He also experienced orthostatic hypotension on a number of occasions. However, a later ECG showed a normal sinus rhythm. He was taking daily doses of terfenadine 120 mg, fluoxetine 20 mg (started a month previously), ibuprofen 2.4 g, misoprostol 400 micrograms, *Midrin* (paracetamol (acetaminophen), dichloralphenazone, isometheptene mucate) and ranitidine 300 mg. This reaction was attributed to an interaction between fluoxetine and terfenadine. However, a few days after stopping the terfenadine, and 12 days after this episode, his cardiac rhythm as recorded by a 24-hour Holter monitor showed some minor abnormalities (intermittent sinus tachycardia, isolated premature beats), although nothing approaching the previous alarming episode.[4] A woman taking several drugs (topical aciclovir, beclometasone, pseudoephedrine, ibuprofen) had a prolonged QTc interval of 550 milliseconds two weeks after starting terfenadine and fluoxetine, but she remained asymptomatic. Within a week of stopping the terfenadine her QTc interval had returned to normal.[5]

In contrast, 12 healthy subjects who were given a single 60-mg dose of terfenadine before and after taking fluoxetine 60 mg daily for 8 days showed no significant changes in the pharmacokinetics of terfenadine or its acid metabolite.[6] Other *in vitro* studies with human liver microsomal enzymes confirmed that fluoxetine has only a very slight inhibitory effect on the metabolism of terfenadine, which was considered to be clinically irrelevant.[7]

(b) Paroxetine

A two-period crossover study in 11 healthy subjects given terfenadine 60 mg twice daily found that paroxetine 20 mg daily for 8 days had no effect on the AUC of terfenadine or the QTc interval. A small, clinically unimportant reduction in the levels of carboxyterfenadine was seen. It was concluded that there is no clinically relevant interaction between terfenadine and paroxetine.[8] *In vitro* studies with human liver microsomal enzymes confirmed that paroxetine has only a very slight inhibitory effect on the metabolism of terfenadine, which is not considered to be clinically significant.[7]

(c) Sertraline

Although the CSM in the UK initially stated that terfenadine should not be used with sertraline, they subsequently reviewed the data and now consider that an interaction is unlikely.[9]

Mechanism

Not understood. An *in vitro* model study using human liver microsomal enzymes, which accurately predicted a large and potentially hazardous interaction between terfenadine and ketoconazole or itraconazole (now clinically proven–see 'Antihistamines + Azoles', p.584), found that six SSRIs (desmethylsertraline, fluoxetine, fluvoxamine, norfluoxetine, paroxetine, sertraline) at usual clinical doses were at least 20 times less potent than ketoconazole at inhibiting terfenadine metabolism.[7] This suggests that all of these SSRIs are very unlikely to interact with terfenadine clinically, although the authors of the study warn that if high doses of SSRIs are used (particularly fluoxetine) some caution is appropriate.[7] Astemizole is metabolised in part by the cytochrome P450 isoenzyme CYP2D6, which is inhibited to a variable extent by the SSRIs, and therefore interactions involving this isoenzyme are possible.

Importance and management

The interaction between the SSRIs and terfenadine is not adequately established, and there is little evidence regarding interactions between the SSRIs and astemizole, although it is possible that the contraindication with astemizole has contributed to minimal usage of the combination and therefore a lack of reported interactions. In addition to fluoxetine and paroxetine, the manufacturers of terfenadine list **fluvoxamine** and **citalopram** as drugs that are expected to increase terfenadine serum levels,[10] but direct evidence of this seems to be lacking. Nonetheless, the manufacturer contraindicates the use of all these SSRIs with terfenadine.[10] Due to the severity of the potential interaction, it would appear prudent to use caution if terfenadine is used with any SSRI (excepting perhaps sertraline), and consider an alternative antihistamine without cardiac effects (see 'Table 15.2', (p.583)), wherever possible. Desloratadine appears to be a non-interacting alternative.

The situation with loratadine is unclear, and currently all the evidence is theoretical.

1. Hismanal (Astemizole). Janssen-Cilag Ltd. UK Summary of product characteristics, June 1998.
2. Gupta S, Banfield C, Kantesaria B, Flannery B, Herron J. Pharmacokinetics/pharmacodynamics of desloratadine and fluoxetine in healthy volunteers. *J Clin Pharmacol* (2004) 44, 1252–9.
3. Affrime MB, Lorber R, Danzig M, Cuss F, Brannan MD. Three month evaluation of electrocardiographic effects of loratadine in humans. *J Allergy Clin Immunol* (1993) 91, 259.
4. Swims MP. Potential terfenadine-fluoxetine interaction. *Ann Pharmacother* (1993) 27, 1404–5.
5. Marchiando RJ, Cook MD, Jue SG. Probable terfenadine-fluoxetine-associated cardiac toxicity. *Ann Pharmacother* (1995) 29, 937–8.
6. Bergstrom RF, Goldberg MJ, Cerimele BJ, Hatcher BL. Assessment of the potential for a pharmacokinetic interaction between fluoxetine and terfenadine. *Clin Pharmacol Ther* (1997) 62, 643–51.
7. von Moltke LL, Greenblatt DJ, Duan SX, Harmatz JS, Wright CE, Shader RI. Inhibition of terfenadine metabolism *in vitro* by azole antifungal agents and by selective serotonin reuptake inhibitor antidepressants: relation to pharmacokinetic interactions *in vivo*. *J Clin Psychopharmacol* (1996) 16, 104–112.
8. Martin DE, Zussman BD, Everitt DE, Benincosa LJ, Etheredge RC, Jorkasky DK. Paroxetine does not affect the cardiac safety and pharmacokinetics of terfenadine in healthy adult men. *J Clin Psychopharmacol* (1997) 17, 451–9.
9. Committee on Safety of Medicines/Medicines Control Agency. Sertraline and terfenadine. *Current Problems* (1998) 24, 4.
10. Histafen (Terfenadine). Approved Prescription Services Ltd. UK Summary of product characteristics, December 1999.

Antihistamines + Terbinafine

Terbinafine does not interact with astemizole or terfenadine to a clinically relevant extent.

Clinical evidence, mechanism, importance and management

In a large scale post-marketing survey of 25,884 patients taking terbinafine, over 40% were taking at least one other drug. From amongst this group, an unknown number of patients were taking **astemizole** or **terfenadine**. No adverse interactions were reported.[1] A cross-over study in 26 healthy subjects given terbinafine 250 mg daily or placebo with **terfenadine** 60 mg twice daily for 7 days found that terbinafine reduced the trough levels of terfenadine acid metabolite by about 20% on the last day of concurrent use. Other **terfenadine** acid metabolite pharmacokinetic parameters were not affected. The AUC, and peak and trough plasma levels of terbinafine were increased by about 16%, 6.6%, and 22%, respectively, after 7 days of concurrent use. Although the incidence of ECG abnormalities was not significantly higher in any group, a 10% prolongation of the QT interval was found in those receiving **terfenadine** either alone or with terbinafine. Concurrent use was well-tolerated and it was concluded that terbinafine could safely be given with **terfenadine**.[2]

1. Hall M, Monka C, Krupp P, O'Sullivan D. Safety of oral terbinafine. Results of a postmarketing surveillance study in 25 884 patients. *Arch Dermatol* (1997) 133, 1213–19.
2. Robbins B, Chang C-T, Cramer JA, Garreffa S, Hafkin B, Hunt TL, Meligeni J. Safe coadministration of terbinafine and terfenadine: a placebo-controlled crossover study of pharmacokinetic and pharmacodynamic interactions in healthy volunteers. *Clin Pharmacol Ther* (1996) 59, 275–83.

Antihistamines; Ocular + Miscellaneous

No specific interaction studies have been performed with eye-drop formulations of the antihistamines azelastine, emedastine, epinastine, or olopatadine. However, interactions are not anticipated since very little drug is expected to reach the systemic circulation.

Clinical evidence, mechanism, importance and management

The UK manufacturer of **azelastine** eye drops notes that interaction studies with high oral doses of **azelastine** bear no relevance to the eye drops, as systemic levels are only in the picogram range after administration of eye drops.[1] Similarly, the manufacturer of **epinastine** eye drops notes that no drug interactions are anticipated since systemic **epinastine** levels are extremely low after ocular use. They note that **epinastine** is also excreted mostly unchanged.[2] The manufacturer of **olopatadine** eye drops notes that *in vitro* studies showed that it was not an inhibitor of the common cytochrome P450 isoenzymes.[3] No drug interactions would be anticipated between these, or any other, antihistamine eye drops and systemically administered drugs.

The manufacturer of **emedastine** eye drops notes that an interval of 10 minutes should be allowed after the administration of the eye drops and other ophthalmically administered medicines,[4] which is good practice for any ocular drugs.

1. Optilast Eye Drops (Azelastine). Viatris Pharmaceuticals. UK Summary of product characteristics, September 2006.
2. Relestat (Epinastine). Allergan Ltd. UK Summary of product characteristics, February 2005.
3. Opatanol (Olopatadine). Alcon Laboratories (UK) Ltd. UK Summary of product characteristics, May 2002.
4. Emadine (Emedastine). Alcon Laboratories (UK) Ltd. UK Summary of product characteristics, January 1999.

Astemizole + Quinine

Quinine causes a marked but transient increase in plasma astemizole levels, and to avoid the possible risk of cardiac arrhythmias the manufacturers contraindicate this combination. Three case reports confirm that this is a clinically important interaction.

Clinical evidence

Astemizole 30 mg daily for 4 days followed by 10 mg daily for the next 20 days, was given to 12 healthy subjects. The steady-state pharmacokinetics of the astemizole were then examined after the subjects took quinine 20 mg every 4 hours for 12 hours (a total of 80 mg quinine), and after a single 430-mg dose of quinine. The smaller dose of quinine caused only a slight increase in the maximum plasma astemizole levels and AUC, but the larger single dose of quinine resulted in a transient threefold increase in both maximum plasma levels and AUC, especially of desmethylastemizole, the metabolite of astemizole.[1]

A patient who had been taking astemizole 10 mg daily for 10 months with fluoxetine, alprazolam, isradipine, and diuretics with potassium had a syncopal episode one hour after taking the first dose of quinine sulphate 260 mg for leg cramp. The ECG showed recurrent episodes of torsade de pointes with a QT interval of greater than 680 milliseconds. The only electrolyte abnormality was slight hypomagnesaemia. Intravenous magnesium was given and the patient's QT interval shortened to 420 milliseconds over 3 days.[2] The manufacturers have on record two other case reports[3] of cardiac arrhythmias possibly attributable to an interaction between astemizole and quinine.

Mechanism

Uncertain. One suggestion is that the interaction is not primarily due to inhibition of the metabolism of astemizole by the quinine, but rather to a transient quinine-induced displacement of both astemizole and its metabolite from its tissue binding sites.[1] Note that the desmethyl metabolite of astemizole causes QTc prolongation.

Importance and management

Information is very limited, but on the basis of the evidence cited above the manufacturers of astemizole contraindicate the concurrent use of quinine in order to avoid the risk of cardiac arrhythmias.[4] The case report that is cited here confirms that this is a potentially clinically hazardous drug combination.[2]

The larger single dose of 430 mg of quinine used in the study approached the dosage used for the treatment of malaria, whereas the smaller dose of 80 mg was equivalent to the amount contained in 2 litres of a quinine-containing soft drink.[1] There would therefore appear to be no reason for those on astemizole to avoid moderate quantities of these quinine-containing drinks. See also 'Drugs that prolong the QT interval + Other drugs that prolong the QT interval', p.257.

1. Janssen-Cilag Ltd, Data on file (Study AST-BEL-7 + Amendment) 1995.
2. Martin ES, Rogalski K, Black JN. Quinine may trigger torsades de pointes during astemizole therapy. *Pacing Clin Electrophysiol* (1997) 20, 2024–5.
3. Janssen-Cilag Ltd. Personal Communication, May 1997.
4. Hismanal (Astemizole). Janssen-Cilag Ltd. UK Summary of product characteristics, June 1998.

Cinnarizine + Phenylpropanolamine

Phenylpropanolamine 50 mg counteracted the mild sedation caused by cinnarizine 25 or 50 mg, and improved the performance of some skills related to driving in 12 healthy subjects.[1]

1. Savolainen K, Mattila MJ, Mattila ME. Actions and interactions of cinnarizine and phenylpropanolamine on human psychomotor performance. *Curr Ther Res* (1992) 52, 160–8.

Fexofenadine + Antacids or Omeprazole

An aluminium/magnesium hydroxide-containing antacid modestly reduced fexofenadine levels, and it is recommended that dosing should be separated by 2 hours. Omeprazole does not appear to interact with fexofenadine.

Clinical evidence, mechanism, importance and management

(a) Antacids

The manufacturer[1] notes that when a single 120-mg dose of fexofenadine was given within 15 minutes of an aluminium/magnesium hydroxide antacid *(Maalox)*, the fexofenadine AUC was decreased by 41% and the maximum level was decreased by 43%. Although the effect of these reductions on possible efficacy has not been assessed, the manufacturer recommends that it is advisable to leave 2 hours between the administration of fexofenadine and antacids containing aluminium and magnesium hydroxide.[2]

(b) Omeprazole

The manufacturer notes that no interaction has been seen between fexofenadine and omeprazole.[2]

1. Allegra (Fexofenadine hydrochloride). Sanofi-Aventis US LLC. US Prescribing Information, January 2007.
2. Telfast (Fexofenadine hydrochloride). Aventis Pharma Ltd. UK Summary of product characteristics, September 2004.

Fexofenadine + Rifampicin (Rifampin)

Rifampicin increases the oral clearance of fexofenadine, but the clinical significance of this is unclear.

Clinical evidence, mechanism, importance and management

A single 60-mg dose of fexofenadine was given to 24 healthy subjects 2 days before and on the last day of a 6-day course of rifampicin 600 mg daily. The oral clearance of fexofenadine was increased 1.3- to 5.3-fold, with no effect on renal clearance or half-life. This was thought to be due to the effect of rifampicin on P-glycoprotein, which is involved in the uptake of fexofenadine.[1] The clinical significance of this interaction is unclear, but until more is known it would seem prudent to monitor the efficacy of fexofenadine if it is given in combination with rifampicin.

1. Hamman MA, Bruce MA, Haehner-Daniels BD, Hall SD. The effect of rifampin administration on the disposition of fexofenadine. *Clin Pharmacol Ther* (2001) 69, 114–21.

Fexofenadine + St John's wort (*Hypericum perforatum*)

Pretreatment with St John's wort (*Hypericum perforatum*) had no clinically relevant effect on the plasma levels of single-dose fexofenadine in one study, but markedly reduced them in another.

Clinical evidence, mechanism, importance and management

A single 900-mg dose of St John's wort (*Hypericum perforatum*) increased the maximum plasma level of a single 60-mg dose of fexofenadine by 45% and increased the AUC by 31% in 12 healthy subjects. Conversely, St John's wort 300 mg three times daily for 14 days caused a slight 5 to 10% decrease in the maximum level and AUC of a single dose of fexofenadine 60 mg in the same subjects.[1] In contrast, in another study, 12 days of pretreatment with St John's wort increased the oral clearance of a single dose of fexofenadine by about 1.6-fold in healthy subjects.[2] In both these studies St John's wort was thought to be interacting via its effects on P-glycoprotein.

The findings from these two studies for multiple dose St John's wort suggest that either no clinically relevant decrease in fexofenadine levels occurs, or that a decrease occurs that is possibly clinically important. Further study is needed. If fexofenadine becomes less effective in a patient taking regular St John's wort, consider the St John's wort as a possible cause.

1. Wang Z, Hamman MA, Huang S-M, Lesko LJ, Hall SD. Effect of St John's wort on the pharmacokinetics of fexofenadine. *Clin Pharmacol Ther* (2002) 71, 414–20.
2. Dresser GK, Schwarz UI, Wilkinson GR, Kim RB. Coordinate induction of both cytochrome P4503A and MDR1 by St John's wort in healthy subjects. *Clin Pharmacol Ther* (2003) 73, 41–50.

Terfenadine + Atorvastatin

Atorvastatin does not appear to alter the pharmacokinetics of terfenadine.

Clinical evidence, mechanism, importance and management

A group of healthy subjects were given a single 120-mg dose of terfenadine on day 8 of a 10-day course of atorvastatin 80 mg daily. It was found that the atorvastatin caused some small to moderate changes in the pharmacokinetics of the terfenadine and its metabolite fexofenadine (AUC increased by 35% and decreased by 2% respectively, maximum serum levels decreased by 8% and decreased by 16% respectively), none of which reached statistical significance. More importantly there were no changes in the QTc interval, which indicates that atorvastatin does not increase the cardiotoxicity of the terfenadine.[1] There would therefore appear to be no reason for avoiding concurrent use.

1. Stern RH, Smithers JA, Olson SC. Atorvastatin does not produce a clinically significant effect on the pharmacokinetics of terfenadine. *J Clin Pharmacol* (1998) 38, 753–7.

Terfenadine + Paracetamol (Acetaminophen)

An isolated report describes the development of torsade de pointes arrhythmia in an elderly man on very large doses of paracetamol (acetaminophen) and amitriptyline when he began to take terfenadine.

Clinical evidence, mechanism, importance and management

An 86-year-old man taking **amitriptyline** 25 mg at night, prednisone 3 mg daily and excessive amounts of paracetamol (up to 1 g every 2 hours over a 6-month period) developed breathlessness and bradycardia shortly after starting to take terfenadine 60 mg twice daily. In hospital he became unconscious and was initially pulseless but recovered spontaneously. An ECG showed that he had AV block and a prolonged QT interval, which resulted in runs of self-limiting torsade de pointes arrhythmia.[1] The reasons for this reaction are not known, but a suggested explanation is that overdosage with paracetamol produced large amounts of a metabolite (*N*-acetyl-p-benzoquinoneimine). This metabolite could have inhibited the metabolism of the terfenadine by the cytochrome P450 isoenzyme CYP3A4, thereby resulting in terfenadine accumulation and the development of its cardiotoxic effects.[1] The **amitriptyline** may additionally have had some part to play because it can also (although rarely) cause torsade de pointes.

This is an isolated case and unlikely to be of general importance. There would seem to be little reason on the basis of this report for patients on terfenadine to avoid normal therapeutic doses of paracetamol (acetaminophen). There appear to be no other reports of this interaction.

1. Matsis PP, Easthope RN. Torsades de pointes ventricular tachycardia associated with terfenadine and paracetamol self medication. *N Z Med J* (1994) 107, 402–403.

Terfenadine + Venlafaxine

Venlafaxine does not appear to significantly alter the pharmacokinetics of terfenadine.

Clinical evidence, mechanism, importance and management

A study in 24 subjects given a single 120-mg oral dose of terfenadine before and after taking venlafaxine 75 mg every 12 hours for 9 days found that the pharmacokinetic profile of terfenadine was unchanged, although its acid metabolite concentrations were slightly decreased by about 25%.[1] This study was undertaken to confirm that venlafaxine lacks inhibitory activity on the cytochrome P450 isoenzyme CYP3A4, but at the same time it also indicates that venlafaxine does not raise the serum levels of terfenadine, which are associated with serious cardiotoxicity. There would therefore seem to be no reason for avoiding concurrent use.

1. Amchin J, Zarycranski W, Taylor K, Albano D, Klockowski PM. Effect of venlafaxine on the pharmacokinetics of terfenadine. *Psychopharmacol Bull* (1998) 34,383–9.

Terfenadine + Zileuton

In one study zileuton modestly increased terfenadine levels, without altering the QTc interval. Nevertheless, the combination is contraindicated.

Clinical evidence, mechanism, importance and management

Terfenadine 60 mg every 12 hours for 7 days was given to 15 healthy subjects with either zileuton 600 mg every 6 hours or a placebo. The mean AUC_{0-6} and the maximum plasma concentrations of terfenadine increased by 35% in the presence of zileuton, but the levels were still very low (less than 5 nanograms/mL). The maximum plasma concentration and AUC of carboxyterfenadine (a terfenadine metabolite) were increased by about 15% by zileuton. ECG measurements showed that the addition of zileuton did not increase the QTc interval nor cause any other significant changes.[1] The authors concluded that the interaction was unlikely to be of clinical significance. However, the manufacturers of terfenadine currently contraindicate zileuton, on the basis that any drug that inhibits terfenadine metabolism may result in accumulation of terfenadine and prolongation of the QT interval with the risk of life-threatening arrhythmias.[2] Because of the unpredictability of these interactions, this seems a sensible precaution.

1. Awni WM, Cavanaugh JH, Leese P, Kasier J, Cao G, Locke CS, Dube LM. The pharmacokinetic and pharmacodynamic interaction between zileuton and terfenadine. *Eur J Clin Pharmacol* (1997) 52, 49–54.
2. Histafen (Terfenadine). Approved Prescription Services Ltd. UK Summary of product characteristics, December 1999.

16

Antimigraine drugs

The drugs dealt with in this section are the ergot derivatives and the triptans (or more properly the serotonin 5-HT_1 agonists), whose main use is in the treatment of migraine. 'Table 16.1', (below) lists some of the drugs commonly used in migraine. Drugs such as propranolol, which are more commonly used in other conditions, are discussed elsewhere in the publication.

(a) Ergot derivatives

The main problem with the use of the ergot derivatives is that of ergotism. Drug interactions may result in additive effects or cause raised levels of ergot derivatives, which may result in the symptoms of ergot poisoning. This may include severe circulatory problems e.g. the extremities may become numb, cold to the touch, tingle, and muscle pain may result. In extreme cases there may be no palpable pulse. Ultimately gangrene may develop, and amputation may be required. Chest pain can also occur, and in some cases myocardial infarction has been reported. Since ergotamine and dihydroergotamine are metabolised in the liver by CYP3A4, drugs which inhibit this isoenzyme, particularly potent inhibitors, such as the 'protease inhibitors', (p.600), should generally be avoided due to the risk of precipitating ergotism.

(b) Triptans

Although the triptans would be expected to share a number of pharmacodynamic drug interactions, due to their differing metabolic pathways they will not all necessarily share the same pharmacokinetic interactions. For example, sumatriptan, which is metabolised mainly by monoamine oxidase A, is unlikely to interact with macrolide antibacterials, which are inhibitors of the cytochrome P450 isoenzyme CYP3A4. However, eletriptan, which is metabolised by CYP3A4 and possibly CYP2D6 could potentially interact (see 'Triptans + Macrolides', p.604, for full details). Frovatriptan and zolmitriptan are substrates for CYP1A2, and are affected by CYP1A2 inhibitors such as fluvoxamine, but zolmitriptan also inhibits CYP1A2 and may therefore be expected to have additional interactions. The picture with zolmitriptan becomes more complicated since it is also metabolised by monoamine oxidase A. Naratriptan appears unlikely to undergo significant pharmacokinetic interactions since half the dose is excreted unchanged and the rest metabolised by a variety of isoenzymes. A summary of the metabolic pathways of the triptans can be found in 'Table 16.2', (below).

Early in the development of triptans it was theorised that they might possibly add to the increased levels of serotonin caused by other serotonergic drugs, leading to excess serotonergic activity and increasing the risk of 'the serotonin syndrome', (p.9). Therefore sumatriptan was contraindicated in patients taking SSRIs, MAOIs, and lithium, but note, there is little evidence that this occurs in practice. However, there is also a pharmacokinetic interaction between some triptans and 'MAOIs', see (p.604) or 'SSRIs', (p.605).

Table 16.1 Antimigraine drugs

Group	*Drugs*
Antihistamines	Flunarizine, Pizotifen
Beta blockers	Atenolol, Metoprolol, Nadolol, Propranolol, Timolol
Ergot derivatives	Codergocrine, Ergotamine, Dihydroergotamine, Methysergide
Triptans (Serotonin (5-HT_1) agonists)	Almotriptan, Eletriptan, Frovatriptan, Naratriptan, Rizatriptan, Sumatriptan, Zolmitriptan

Table 16.2 Interactions between drug metabolising enzymes and the triptans†

	MAO-A	*CYP1A2*	*CYP2C9*	*CYP2C19*	*CYP2D6*	*CYP3A4*
Almotriptan	Substrate				Substrate	Substrate
Eletriptan						Substrate
Frovatriptan		Substrate			Possible substrate	
Naratriptan		Substrate (minor)	Substrate (minor)	Substrate (minor)	Substrate (minor)	Substrate (minor)
Rizatriptan	Substrate	Substrate (minor)				
Sumatriptan	Substrate					
Zolmitriptan	Substrate	Substrate				Substrate

†Other isoenzymes have been implicated, but not at clinically relevant concentrations of the triptans

Ergot derivatives + Antidepressants

One isolated report describes three cases in which patients developed symptoms indicative of the serotonin syndrome when they took amitriptyline, paroxetine/imipramine, or sertraline with dihydroergotamine.

Clinical evidence

A woman taking **imipramine**, **paroxetine** and lithium, who had a 3-week continuous headache, was treated with 300 micrograms of **dihydroergotamine** intravenously. Within 5 minutes of a subsequent 500-microgram dose she developed dysarthria, dilated pupils, diaphoresis, diffuse weakness, and barely responded to commands. She was diffusely hyperreflexic and showed occasional myoclonic jerks. She recovered after 90 minutes.[1]

A woman with a history of migraine headaches responded well to **amitriptyline**, metoclopramide, and **dihydroergotamine**. Six weeks after the **amitriptyline** was replaced by **sertraline**, she was again successfully treated for acute migraine with 10 mg of intravenous metoclopramide and 1 mg of intravenous **dihydroergotamine**. However, 2 hours later she developed nausea, emesis, agitation, weakness, diaphoresis, salivation, chills, and fever. All of the symptoms subsided after 24 hours.[1]

A woman with a history of migraines (treated prophylactically with **amitriptyline** and propranolol) was admitted to hospital in status migrainosus. She was given 1 mg of **dihydroergotamine**, 10 mg of prochlorperazine and 10 mg of metoclopramide (all intravenously). Within 20 minutes she became diaphoretic, tachycardic, diffusely hyperreflexic, agitated, confused, and briefly lost consciousness twice. Diazepam 8 mg given intramuscularly calmed her agitation, and all the symptoms resolved after 6 hours. A year later she was given 6 mg of subcutaneous sumatriptan while taking **nortriptyline** daily with no ill effects.[1]

Mechanism

Not understood. All of these patients appeared to have developed symptoms similar to those of the serotonin syndrome, which is thought to be due to hyperstimulation of 5-HT receptors in the brain. Dihydroergotamine is a 5-HT agonist while paroxetine and sertraline are both serotonin (5-HT) reuptake inhibitors, all of which might be expected to increase 5-HT concentrations in the CNS, and thereby increase receptor stimulation.

Importance and management

These appear to be isolated cases and not of general importance, nevertheless they illustrate the potential for the development of the serotonin syndrome in patients given multidrug regimens that affect 5-HT receptors. The syndrome is rare and it may (so it has been suggested[1]) sometimes be an idiosyncratic reaction.

1. Mathew NT, Tietjen GE, Lucker C. Serotonin syndrome complicating migraine pharmacotherapy. *Cephalalgia* (1996) 16, 323–7.

Ergot derivatives + CYP3A4 inhibitors

The azole antifungals are predicted to raise the levels of ergot derivatives, which may lead to ergotism. Concurrent use is contraindicated. Methysergide is also contraindicated with cimetidine and NNRTIs such as delavirdine. Caution is also advised with other CYP3A4 inhibitors, including grapefruit juice and quinupristin/dalfopristin.

Clinical evidence, mechanism, importance and management

The ergot alkaloids are mainly metabolised by the cytochrome P450 isoenzyme CYP3A4. The manufacturers of ergotamine dihydroergotamine and methysergide therefore logically predict that their levels will be raised by CYP3A4 inhibitors and advise against their concurrent use. They specifically contraindicate 'macrolides', (p.599), and 'protease inhibitors', (p.600), which are potent CYP3A4 inhibitors[1-3] and which have been shown to interact with these ergot derivatives in a number of cases. They also contraindicate the **azole antifungals** and the **NNRTIs** (**delavirdine, efavirenz**).[1,4] Although there appear to be no studies or case reports, given the way other potent CYP3A4 inhibitors interact, this seems prudent. Note that, of the azoles, **ketoconazole**, **itraconazole** are the most potent CYP3A4 inhibitors, and would therefore be expected to interact to the greatest extent. The US manufacturers of ergotamine and dihydroergotamine specifically contraindicate these azoles, but advise caution with **fluconazole** and **clotrimazole**, which are less potent CYP3A4 inhibitors.[2,3] The manufacturers of ergotamine also advise caution with the use of less potent CYP3A4 inhibitors including **grapefruit juice**,[2] **quinupristin/dalfopristin** and **cimetidine**.[1] The manufacturers of dihydroergotamine[3] and methysergide[4] give a similar list.

Given the rarity of cases of an adverse effect with the potent CYP3A4 inhibitors any clinically significant interaction with these drugs would be expected to be extremely rare indeed, but concurrent use should be well monitored so any adverse effect can be identified swiftly and appropriate treatment given.

1. Cafergot Suppositories (Ergotamine tartrate and caffeine). Alliance Pharmaceuticals. UK Summary of product characteristics, January 2007.
2. Cafergot Suppositories (Ergotamine tartrate and caffeine). Novartis. US Prescribing information, March 2003.
3. Migranal (Dihydroergotamine mesylate). Valeant Pharmaceuticals International. US Prescribing information, March 2006.
4. Deseril (Methysergide). Alliance Pharmaceuticals. UK Summary of product characteristics, December 2006.

Ergot derivatives + Glyceryl trinitrate (Nitroglycerin)

The ergot derivatives such as dihydroergotamine would be expected to oppose the anti-anginal effects of glyceryl trinitrate. Nevertheless, an *animal* study has not borne out this expectation.

Clinical evidence, mechanism, importance and management

There seem to be no clinical reports of adverse interactions between the ergot derivatives and glyceryl trinitrate, but since **ergot** causes vasoconstriction and can provoke angina it would be expected to oppose the effects of glyceryl trinitrate when used as a vasodilator for the treatment of angina.[1] Nevertheless, a study in *animals* suggests that **dihydroergotamine** will not worsen exercise-induced angina pectoris, and that the antianginal efficacy of glyceryl trinitrate will not be neutralised by pretreatment with **dihydroergotamine**.[2]

However, glyceryl trinitrate has also been shown to increase the bioavailability of **dihydroergotamine** (by up to 370% in one case) in subjects with orthostatic hypotension, which would increase its vasoconstrictor effects.[1] The clinical outcome of concurrent use is therefore uncertain. Note that ergot derivatives are generally regarded as contraindicated in those with ischaemic heart disease.

1. Bobik A, Jennings G, Skews H, Esler M, McLean A. Low oral bioavailability of dihydroergotamine and first-pass extraction in patients with orthostatic hypotension. *Clin Pharmacol Ther* (1981) 30, 673–9.
2. Schneider W, Krumpl G, Mayer N, Raberger G. The effects of nitroglycerin on exercise-induced regional myocardial contractile dysfunction are not diminished by pretreatment with dihydroergotamine. *Br J Pharmacol* (1987) 92, 87–95.

Ergot derivatives + Heparin

The use of dihydroergotamine with heparin has resulted in ergotism. In some cases, amputation of the affected limb was necessary. The rate of absorption and peak levels of subcutaneous dihydroergotamine are reduced by heparin.

Clinical evidence, mechanism, importance and management

There have been several reports of ergotism following the combined use of **dihydroergotamine** and heparin for thromboembolic prophylaxis. In a retrospective review of 61 092 Austrian patients attending trauma units who received **dihydroergotamine** and heparin prophylaxis, complications attributable to ergotism were seen in 142 patients. In 7 patients amputation was necessary and in a further 7 cases immediate opening of the vessel and catheter dilatation was successful.[1] Other published reports support this interaction,[2,3] including a report of two patients who experienced fatal myocardial infarctions, attributed to coronary artery spasm as a complication of prophylaxis with **dihydroergotamine** and heparin.[4]

It has been found that the use of heparin results in a 25% increase in the AUC of subcutaneously administered **dihydroergotamine**. Giving the two drugs at the same site reduced the rate of dihydroergotamine absorption by 63%, the time to peak levels by 110%, and the peak levels by 15%. **Dihydroergotamine** had no effect on the pharmacokinetics of heparin.[5]

Because of the risk of peripheral ischaemia, the combination of **dihydroergotamine** and heparin is no longer widely used for thromboembolic prophylaxis. If the combination is used, the patient must be closely observed for any sign of vascular spasm.

1. Gatterer R. Ergotism as complication of thromboembolic prophylaxis with heparin and dihydroergotamine. *Lancet* (1986) II, 638–639.
2. Warmuth-Metz M. Ergotismus der unteren Extremität als Folge einer DHE-Heparin-Thromboseprophylaxe. *Radiologe* (1988) 28, 491–3.
3. Jahn R. Ergotismus – ein Risiko bei der Thromboseprophylaxe? *Zentralbl Chir* (1985) 110, 482–5.
4. Rem JA, Gratzl O, Follath F, Pult I. Ergotism as complication of thromboembolic prophylaxis with heparin-dihydroergotamine. *Lancet* (1987) I, 219.
5. Schran HF, Bitz DW, DiSerio FJ, Hirsh J. The pharmacokinetics and bioavailability of subcutaneously administered dihydroergotamine, heparin and the dihydroergotamine-heparin combination. Thromb Res. (1983) 31, 51–67.

Ergot derivatives + Macrolides

Ergot toxicity can develop rapidly in patients taking ergotamine or dihydroergotamine if they are given erythromycin or troleandomycin. Three possible cases of toxicity have occurred with clarithromycin, and one case has been reported with each of josamycin and oleandomycin. Toxicity is predicted to occur with midecamycin. No cases of toxicity appear to have been described with spiramycin, and none would be expected. There is no direct information about azithromycin but it would not be expected to interact.

Clinical evidence

(a) Clarithromycin

A 59-year-old woman took **ergotamine tartrate** 2 mg for a typical migraine headache. After 2 hours her tongue became swollen, painful and bluish in colour. She showed some hypertension (BP 200/110 mmHg) and her fingers and toes were cold and cyanotic (blue). She had taken this dose of **ergotamine** many times previously without problems, but on this occasion she had been taking clarithromycin 500 mg twice daily for the last 5 days. This adverse reaction was diagnosed as ergotism. Other evidence suggests that this patient may possibly have been unusually sensitive to vascular occlusion.[1] The authors of this report briefly quote another case, originating from the manufacturers of clarithromycin, of a possible interaction with **dihydroergotamine**, although this was complicated by the concurrent use of other medications (not named) used in the management of AIDS.[1] A woman who had previously uneventfully taken *Cafergot* (**ergotamine tartrate** 1 mg, caffeine 100 mg) for migraine developed ergotism (leg pain, cold and cyanosed limbs, and impalpable pulses) within 3 days of starting to take clarithromycin (dosage not stated). The authors postulated that **smoking** and the use of **oxymetazoline** (both of which have vasoconstrictor effects) may also have had some part to play.[2]

(b) Erythromycin

A woman who had regularly and uneventfully taken *Migral* (**ergotamine tartrate** 2 mg, cyclizine hydrochloride 50 mg, caffeine 100 mg) on a number of previous occasions, took one tablet during a course of treatment with erythromycin 250 mg every 6 hours. Within 2 days she developed severe ischaemic pain in her arms and legs during exercise, with a burning sensation in her feet and hands. When admitted to hospital 10 days later, her extremities were cool and cyanosed. Her pulse could not be detected in the lower limbs.[3]

Eight other cases of acute ergotism have been reported[4-11] in which patients were taking **ergotamine tartrate** or **dihydroergotamine** and erythromycin. The reaction has been reported to develop within a few hours,[7] but it may take several days to occur.[10] One case appeared to occur when the erythromycin was started 3 days after the last dose of **dihydroergotamine**.[5]

(c) Josamycin

An isolated report describes a 33-year-old woman who developed severe ischaemia of the legs within 3 days of starting to take josamycin 2 g daily and **ergotamine tartrate** 300 micrograms. Her legs and feet were cold, white and painful, and most of her peripheral pulses were impalpable.[12]

(d) Midecamycin diacetate (Miocamycin)

After 12 healthy subjects took midecamycin diacetate 800 mg twice daily for 8 days, the peak concentrations of a single 9-mg dose of **dihydroergotamine** were raised 3 to 40-fold.[13]

(e) Oleandomycin

A case of ergotism has been reported in a 45-year-old woman who had been taking **ergotamine** 4 mg daily for 5 years and recently also oleandomycin.[14]

(f) Troleandomycin

A 40-year-old woman who had been taking **dihydroergotamine**, 90 drops daily, for 3 years without problems, developed cramp in her legs within a few hours of starting to take troleandomycin 250 mg four times a day. Five days later she was admitted to hospital as an emergency, with severe ischaemia of her arms and legs. Her limbs were cold and all her peripheral pulses were impalpable.[15]

There are reports of several other patients who had taken normal doses of **ergotamine tartrate** or **dihydroergotamine** for months or years without problems, who then developed severe ergotism within hours or days of starting to take normal doses of troleandomycin.[16-23] This resulted in a myocardial infarction in one patient.[24]

Mechanism

Erythromycin and troleandomycin are potent inhibitors of the cytochrome P450 isoenzyme CYP3A4, an enzyme involved in the metabolism of ergot derivatives.[25] Clarithromycin and oleandomycin are also known to inhibit CYP3A4. As a result the ergot is poorly metabolised and accumulates in the body. This leads to increased vasoconstriction and ultimately ischaemia. **Spiramycin**, and josamycin normally do not inhibit CYP3A4 and are therefore not expected to interact,[25] although a case has been reported.[12]

Importance and management

The interactions of ergot derivatives with erythromycin and troleandomycin are well documented, well established, and clinically important, whereas information about clarithromycin appears to be confined to three possible cases and that relating to oleandomycin to one case. There are no adverse reports about midecamycin, but it is expected to interact similarly. The concurrent use of all of these macrolides and ergot derivatives should be avoided. Some of the cases cited were effectively treated with sodium nitroprusside or naftidrofuryl oxalate, with or without heparin.[1,5,7-9,21] Spiramycin, and josamycin would not be expected to interact because they do not inhibit CYP3A4. However, there is one unexplained and unconfirmed report of an interaction with josamycin.[12]

It has been suggested that ergot alkaloids should be avoided with **azithromycin**, because clinically important interactions have been seen between these drugs and other macrolide antibacterials related to **azithromycin**,[26,27] and the UK manufacturers of both ergotamine and **azithromycin** contraindicate the combination.[28,29] However, there seems so far to be no direct evidence of any adverse interactions between ergot alkaloids and **azithromycin**, and the US manufacturers say that concurrent use can be undertaken with careful monitoring.[30]

1. Horowitz RS, Dart RC, Gomez HF. Clinical ergotism with lingual ischemia induced by a clarithromycin-ergotamine interaction. *Arch Intern Med* (1996) 156, 456–8.
2. Ausband SC, Goodman PE. An unusual case of clarithromycin associated ergotism. *J Emerg Med* (2001) 21, 411–13.
3. Francis H, Tyndall A, Webb J. Severe vascular spasm due to erythromycin-ergotamine interaction. *Clin Rheumatol* (1984) 3, 243–6.
4. Lagier G, Castot A, Riboulet G, Boesh C. Un cas d'ergotisme mineur semblant en rapport avec une potentialisation de l'ergotamine par l'éthylsuccinate d'érythromycine. *Therapie* (1979) 34, 515–21.
5. Neveux E, Lesgourgues B, Luton J-P, Guilhaume B, Bertagna, Picard J. Ergotisme aigu par association proprionate d'érythromycine-dihydroergotamine. *Nouv Presse Med* (1981) 10, 2830.
6. Collet AM, Moncharmont D, San Marco JL, Eissinger F, Pinot JJ, Laselve L. Ergotisme iatrogène: rôle de l'association tartrate d'ergotamine-propionate d'érythromycine. *Sem Hop Paris* (1982) 58, 1624–6.
7. Boucharlat J, Franco A, Carpentier P, Charignon Y, Denis B, Hommel M. Ergotisme en milieu psychiatrique par association D.H.E. propionate d'erythromycine. A propos d'une observation. *Ann Med Psychol (Paris)* (1980) 138, 292–6.
8. Leroy F, Asseman P, Pruvost P, Adnet P, Lacroix D, Thery C. Dihydroergotamine-erythromycin-induced ergotism. *Ann Intern Med* (1988) 109, 249.
9. Ghali R, De Léan J, Douville Y, Noël H-P, Labbé R. Erythromycin-associated ergotamine intoxication: arteriographic and electrophysiologic analysis of a rare cause of severe ischemia of the lower extremities and associated ischemic neuropathy. *Ann Vasc Surg* (1993) 7, 291–6.
10. Bird PA, Sturgess AD. Clinical ergotism with severe bilateral upper limb ischaemia precipitated by an erythromycin-ergotamine interaction. *Aust N Z J Med* (2000) 30, 635–6.
11. Karam B, Farah E, Ashoush R, Jebara V, Ghayad E. Ergotism precipitated by erythromycin: a rare case of vasospasm. *Eur J Vasc Endovasc Surg* (2000) 19, 96–8.
12. Grolleau JY, Martin M, de la Guerrande B, Barrier J, Peltier P. Ergotism aigu lors d'une association josamycine/tartrate d'ergotamine. *Therapie* (1981) 36, 319–21.

13. Couet W, Mathieu HP, Fourtillan JB. Effect of ponsinomycin on the pharmacokinetics of dihydroergotamine administered orally. *Fundam Clin Pharmacol* (1991) 5, 47–52.
14. Monsarrat M, Lefebvre D, Parraguette J, Vaysse C, Bastide G. Ergotisme aigu par association ergotamine-oleandomycine. *Nouv Presse Med* (1982) 11, 603.
15. Franco A, Bourlard P, Massot C, Lecoeur J, Guidicelli H, Bessard G. Ergotisme aigu par association dihydroergotamine-triacétyloléandomycine. *Nouv Presse Med* (1978) 7, 205.
16. Lesca H, Ossard D, Reynier P. Les risques de l'association tri-acétyl-oléandomycine et tartrate d'ergotamine. *Nouv Presse Med* (1976) 5, 1832–3.
17. Hayton AC. Precipitation of acute ergotism by triacetyloleandomycin. *N Z Med J* (1969) 69, 42.
18. Dupuy JC, Lardy P, Seaulau P, Kervoelen P, Paulet J. Spasmes artériels systémiques. Tartrate d'ergotamine. *Arch Mal Coeur* (1979) 72, 86–91.
19. Bigorie B, Aimez P, Soria RJ, Samama F di Maria G, Guy-Grand B, Bour H. L'association triacétyl oléandomycin-tartrate d'ergotamine est-elle dangereuse? *Nouv Presse Med* (1975) 4, 2723–5.
20. Vayssairat M, Fiessinger J-N, Becquemin M-H, Housset E. Association dihydroergotamine et triacétyloléandomycine. Rôle dans une nécrose digitale iatrogène. *Nouv Presse Med* (1978) 7, 2077.
21. Matthews NT, Havill JH. Ergotism with therapeutic doses of ergotamine tartrate. *N Z Med J* (1979) 89, 476–7.
22. Chignier E, Riou R, Descotes J, Meunier P, Courpron P, Vignon G. Ergotisme iatrogène aigu par association médicamenteuse diagnostiqué par exploration non invasive (vélocimétrie à effet Doppler). *Nouv Presse Med* (1978) 7, 2478.
23. Bacourt F, Couffinhal J-C. Ischémie des membres par association dihydroergotamine-triacétyloléandomycine. Nouvelle observation. *Nouv Presse Med* (1978) 7, 1561.
24. Baudouy PY, Mellat M, Velleteau de Moulliac M. Infarctus du myocarde provoqué par l'association tartrate d'ergotamine-troléandomycine. *Rev Med Interne* (1988) 9, 420–2.
25. Pessayre D, Larrey D, Funck-Brentano C, Benhamou JP. Drug interactions and hepatitis produced by some macrolide antibiotics. *J Antimicrob Chemother* (1985) 16 (Suppl A), 181–94.
26. Hopkins S. Clinical toleration and safety of azithromycin. *Am J Med* (1991) 91 (Suppl 3A), 40S–45S.
27. Lode H. The pharmacokinetics of azithromycin and their clinical significance. *Eur J Clin Microbiol Infect Dis* (1991) 10, 807–12.
28. Zithromax (Azithromycin). Pfizer Ltd. UK Summary of product characteristics, July 2006.
29. Migril (Ergotamine tartrate, cyclizine hydrochloride and caffeine hydrate). Wockhardt UK Ltd. Summary of product characteristics, December 2003.
30. Zithromax (Azithromycin). Pfizer Inc. US Prescribing information, March 2007.

Ergot derivatives + Methysergide

The concurrent use of methysergide and other ergot derivatives can increase the risk of severe and persistent spasm of major arteries in some patients.

Clinical evidence

A man developed loss of temperature sensitivity over the right side of his face and arm, as well as vertigo, dysphagia and hoarseness 7 days after starting combined treatment with methysergide 2 mg three times daily and 500 micrograms of subcutaneous **ergotamine tartrate** at night. Continued use resulted in impaired pain, touch and temperature sensation over the right side of his face, shoulder and arm. Arteriography demonstrated left vertebral artery occlusion and right vertebral arterial spasm. These symptoms, apart from the loss of temperature sensitivity, resolved when the drugs were stopped.[1] Another man treated for cluster headaches with methysergide 2 mg, intramuscular **ergotamine tartrate** and pizotifen developed ischaemia of the right foot, with impalpable popliteal and pedal pulses. Arteriography showed that blood flow to the arteries of the right leg was reduced.[1]

Another report describes prolonged myocardial ischaemia in a patient with cluster headaches when a single 2-mg dose of **ergotamine tartrate** was added to methysergide 2 mg three times daily. Sublingual glyceryl trinitrate relieved the pain,[2] (but see also 'Ergot derivatives + Glyceryl trinitrate (Nitroglycerin)', p.598)

A further case is reported of a woman who developed gangrene of both big toes following surgical treatment of bilateral hallux valgus (bone swellings). Before the time of operation, and for 20 days afterwards she took 6 tablets of *Bellergal* (total of **ergotamine tartrate** 1.8 mg, alkaloids of belladonna 0.6 mg, phenobarbital 120 mg daily) and methysergide maleate 6 mg daily. One toe was subsequently removed by amputation, the other recovered slowly following cessation of the **ergotamine** and methysergide.[3]

Mechanism

Cluster headaches are associated with abnormal dilatation of the carotid arteries, which can be constricted by ergot derivatives. In the cases cited it would seem that combined vasoconstrictor effects caused arterial spasm elsewhere in the body, resulting in serious tissue ischaemia. Parenteral ergotamine increases the risk of arterial spasm.

Importance and management

Direct information seems to be limited to these cases. Cardiovascular complications can occur with ergot derivatives given alone, but these cases suggest that their concurrent use may unpredictably increase the risk in some patients. Clearly they should be used together with great caution, or avoided.

1. Joyce DA, Gubbay SS. Arterial complications of migraine treatment with methysergide and parenteral ergotamine. *BMJ* (1982) 285, 260–1.
2. Galer BS, Lipton RB, Solomon S, Newman LC, Spierings ELH. Myocardial ischemia related to ergot alkaloids: a case report and literature review. *Headache* (1991) 31, 446–50.
3. Vaughan-Lane T. Gangrene induced by methysergide and ergotamine. J Bone Joint Surg Br. (1979) 61–B, 213–14.

Ergot derivatives + Protease inhibitors

A patient receiving indinavir rapidly developed ergotism after taking normal doses of ergotamine. At least ten other patients taking ritonavir and ergotamine have had the same interaction. A patient taking nelfinavir developed peripheral arterial vasoconstriction after also taking ergotamine. Other ergot derivatives are predicted to interact similarly.

Clinical evidence

(a) Indinavir

An HIV-positive man who had been taking lamivudine, stavudine, co-trimoxazole and indinavir (2.4 g daily) for more than a year was given *Gynergene caféiné* (**ergotamine tartrate** 1 mg with caffeine 100 mg) for migraine. He took two doses on two consecutive days, and 5 days later presented in hospital with numbness and cyanosis of the toes of his left foot. The next day he complained of intermittent claudication of his left leg, and 6 days later was admitted to hospital because of worsening symptoms and night cramps. Examination showed a typical picture of ergotism, with vasospasm and reduced blood flow in the popliteal, tibial and femoral arteries. He was treated with heparin and buflomedil, and recovered after 3 days.[1]

See (c) ritonavir below for details regarding a fatality involving indinavir, ritonavir and ergotamine.

(b) Nelfinavir

A 40-year-old HIV-positive woman twice took **ergotamine** 2 mg for a migraine while also taking nelfinavir, zidovudine and lamivudine. On the first occasion she developed pain and cyanosis in her toes, and on the second occasion she developed cyanosis and oedema in her hands and feet, causing pain so severe that she was unable to walk. On both occasions peripheral arterial pulses were not palpable. Although she recovered spontaneously on both occasions, the authors caution concurrent use due to the extremely severe potential effects.[2]

(c) Ritonavir

A 63-year-old man with AIDS, who had taken **ergotamine tartrate** 1 to 2 mg daily for migraine headaches over the last 5 years, had his treatment with zidovudine, zalcitabine and co-trimoxazole changed to zidovudine, didanosine and ritonavir (600 mg every 12 hours). Within 10 days he developed paraesthesias, coldness, cyanosis and skin paleness of both arms, and when admitted to hospital his axillary, brachial, radial and ulnar pulses were found to be absent. An arterial doppler test showed the absence of blood flow in both his radial and ulnar arteries and he was diagnosed as having ergotism. The **ergotamine** and ritonavir were stopped, and he recovered when treated with prostaglandin E1 and calcium nadroparin.[3]

Another man, aged 31 years, taking ritonavir 400 mg twice daily (and also taking pizotifen, nelfinavir, stavudine, lamivudine, co-trimoxazole and venlafaxine) developed severe burning and numbness in both feet, and paraesthesias in his hands after taking 4 tablets of **ergotamine** 1 mg and caffeine 100 mg, over 10 days. He was diagnosed as having ergotism. The drugs were stopped and he was treated effectively with intravenous alprostadil and heparin.[4]

A case report describes irreversible coma in a 34-year-old woman who was taking ritonavir 600 mg twice daily, lamivudine and stavudine. She presented with dizziness, loss of vision, headache, vomiting, diarrhoea and a feeling of cold in her left foot after having taken three tablets of **ergotamine** 1 mg in the preceding 4 days. Peripheral pulses were absent in her extremities. After an initial period of recovery she again experienced a loss of consciousness, with signs of stenosis and vasospasm with cerebral hypoperfusion. Despite treatment with alprostadil, and discontinuation of ritonavir her condition deteriorated, and 2 years after the initial presentation, she remained in coma vigil (a state of altered consciousness).[5]

A fatality has been reported in a 49-year-old man taking ritonavir 200 mg twice daily and indinavir 800 mg twice daily in addition to stavudine and lamivudine. After taking three tablets of *Cafergot* (**ergotamine tartrate** 1 mg and caffeine 100 mg) his headache worsened, he developed progressive lower extremity weakness, severe peripheral vasoconstriction, labile hypertension and livedo reticularis (skin discolouration due to underlying capillary changes). He lapsed into coma and on day 5 was declared "brain dead".[6]

At least 6 other cases of ergotism have been reported in patients taking ritonavir after taking ergot derivatives,[7-12] and one required surgical amputation of the toes.[8] The ergotism developed in three of the patients within a few hours to 24 hours of taking a single 1- or 2-mg dose of **ergotamine tartrate**,[7,9,11] and in the others within about 4 to 15 days.[8,10,12] One was taking a combination drug (**ergotamine tartrate** 300 micrograms, belladonna extract 200 micrograms and phenobarbital 20 mg) twice daily for gastric discomfort,[8] another took up to 2 mg of **ergotamine** daily,[10] and a third received 10 mg of ergotamine rectally over 4 consecutive days.[12]

Mechanism

Protease inhibitors reduce the metabolism of ergotamine by inhibiting the cytochrome P450 isoenzyme CYP3A4 to varying degrees. Therefore ergotamine levels are increased, which may result in toxicity. Ergotamine poisoning causes arterial spasm, which reduces and even shuts down the flow of blood in arteries.

Importance and management

Information appears to be limited to these reports, but what happened is consistent with the way other drugs that are potent inhibitors of CYP3A4 can interact with ergot derivatives (see 'Ergot derivatives + Macrolides', p.599). This interaction would appear to be established, and is clearly clinically important. It would now be prudent for any patient taking indinavir or ritonavir, and probably nelfinavir, to avoid the concurrent use of ergotamine or any other ergot derivative, such as **dihydroergotamine** or **methysergide**. Information about possible interactions between ergot derivatives and other protease inhibitors seems to be lacking. Even so to be on the safe side the manufacturers of most of the other protease inhibitors contraindicate concurrent use with ergot derivatives.

1. Rosenthal E, Sala F, Chichmanian R-M, Batt M, Cassuto J-P. Ergotism related to concurrent administration of ergotamine tartrate and indinavir. *JAMA* (1999) 281, 987.
2. Mortier E, Pouchot J, Vinceneux P, Lalande M. Ergotism related to interaction between nelfinavir and ergotamine. *Am J Med* (2001) 110, 594.
3. Caballero-Granado FJ, Viciana P, Cordero E, Gómez-Vera MJ, del Nozal M, López-Cortés LF. Ergotism related to concurrent administration of ergotamine tartrate and ritonavir in an AIDS patient. *Antimicrob Agents Chemother* (1997), 41,1207.
4. Phan TG, Agaliotis D, White G, Britton WJ. Ischaemic peripheral neuritis secondary to ergotism associated with ritonavir therapy. *Med J Aust* (1999) 171, 502, 504.
5. Pardo Rey C, Yebra M, Borrallo M, Vega A, Ramos A, Montero MC. Irreversible coma, ergotamine and ritonavir. *Clin Infect Dis* (2003) 37, e72–3.
6. Tribble MA, Gregg CR, Margolis DM, Amirkhan R, Smith JW. Fatal ergotism induced by an HIV protease inhibitor. *Headache* (2002) 42, 694–5.
7. Montero A, Giovannoni AG, Tvrde PL. Leg ischemia in a patient receiving ritonavir and ergotamine. *Ann Intern Med* (1999) 130, 329–30.
8. Liaudet L, Buclin T, Jaccard C, Eckert P. Severe ergotism associated with interaction between ritonavir and ergotamine. *BMJ* (1999) 318, 771.
9. Blanche P, Rigolet A, Gombert B, Ginsburg C, Salmon D, Sicard D. Ergotism related to a single dose of ergotamine tartrate in an AIDS patient treated with ritonavir. *Postgrad Med J* (1999) 75, 546–7.
10. Vila A, Mykietiuk A, Bonvehì P, Temporiti E, Urueña A, Herrera F. Clinical ergotism induced by ritonavir. *Scand J Infect Dis* (2001) 33, 788–9.
11. Baldwin ZK, Ceraldi C. Ergotism associated with HIV antiviral protease inhibitor therapy. *J Vasc Surg* (2003) 37, 676–8
12. Spiegel M, Schmidauer C, Kampfl A, Sarcletti M, Poewe W. Cerebral ergotism under treatment with ergotamine and ritonavir. *Neurology* (2001) 57, 743–4.

Ergot derivatives + Tetracyclines

Five patients taking ergotamine or dihydroergotamine developed ergotism when they also took doxycycline or tetracycline.

Clinical evidence

A woman who had previously taken **ergotamine tartrate** successfully and uneventfully for 16 years was given **doxycycline** and **dihydroergotamine** 30 drops three times a day. Five days later her hands and feet became cold and reddened, and she was diagnosed as having a mild form of ergotism.[1]

Other cases of ergotism, some of them more severe, have been described in two patients taking **ergotamine tartrate** and **doxycycline**,[2,3] and in 3 patients taking **tetracycline**-containing preparations.[2,4,5]

Mechanism

Unknown. One suggestion is that these antibacterials may inhibit the activity of the liver enzymes concerned with the metabolism and clearance of ergotamine, thereby prolonging its stay in the body and enhancing its activity.[1] One of the patients had a history of alcoholism[2] and two of them were in their eighties,[5] so impaired liver function may have played a part.

Importance and management

Information is very limited indeed. The incidence and general importance of this interaction is uncertain, but it would clearly be prudent to be on the alert for signs of ergotism in any patient given ergot derivatives and a tetracycline. However, note that one of the manufacturers of ergotamine[6] actually recommends that the concurrent use of 'tetracycline' should be avoided. Impairment of liver function may possibly be a contributory factor in this interaction.

1. Amblard P, Reymond JL, Franco A, Beani JC, Carpentier P, Lemonnier D, Bessard G. Ergotisme. Forme mineure par association dihydroergotamine-chlorhydrate de doxycycline, étude capillaroscopique. *Nouv Presse Med* (1978) 7, 4148–9.
2. Dupuy JC, Lardy P, Seaulau P, Kervoelen P, Paulet J. Spasmes artériels systémiques. Tartrate d'ergotamine. *Arch Mal Coeur* (1979) 72, 86–91.
3. Van Gestel R, Noirhomme Ph. Ergotism aigu par association de tartrate d'ergotamine et de doxycycline. *Louvain Med* (1984) 103, 207–208.
4. L'Yvonnet M, Boillot A, Jacquet AM, Barale F, Grandmottet P, Zurlinden B, Gillet JY. A propos d'un cas exceptionnel d'intoxication aigue par un dérivé de l'ergot de seigle. *Gynecologie* (1974) 25, 541–3.
5. Sibertin-Blanc M. Les dangers de l'ergotisme a propos de deux observations. *Arch Med Ouest* (1977) 9, 265–6.
6. Cafergot Suppositories (Ergotamine tartrate and caffeine). Alliance Pharmaceuticals. UK Summary of product characteristics, January 2007.

Flunarizine + Antiepileptics

Limited evidence suggests that phenytoin and carbamazepine can reduce serum flunarizine levels. Flunarizine does not appear to alter phenytoin or carbamazepine levels.

Clinical evidence, mechanism, importance and management

A study found that flunarizine levels were lower in patients receiving multiple antiepileptics than in those receiving only one antiepileptic (statistically significant only for flunarizine 10 mg). The antiepileptics taken were **carbamazepine**, **phenytoin**, and **sodium valproate**. Flunarizine did not affect the serum levels of these antiepileptics.[1] Similarly, in another study involving 12 patients, four of whom were taking **phenytoin**, four **carbamazepine** and four both **phenytoin** and **carbamazepine**, there was no difference in the pharmacokinetics of a single 30-mg dose of flunarizine or of multiple-dose flunarizine between the three groups. However, the apparent clearance values of flunarizine were several fold greater in these patients than previously observed in healthy volunteers. There were no differences identified in the mean steady-state levels of the antiepileptics before and during flunarizine therapy.[2]

Although not conclusive, these data suggest that enzyme-inducing antiepileptics increase the metabolism of flunarizine. There would seem to be no reason for avoiding concurrent use, but the outcome should be monitored.

1. Binnie CD, de Beukelaar F, Meijer JWA, Meinardi H, Overweg J, Wauquier A, van Wieringen A. Open dose-ranging trial of flunarizine as add-on therapy in epilepsy. *Epilepsia* (1985) 26, 424–8.
2. Kapetanovic IM, Torchin CD, Kupferberg HJ, Treiman DM, Di Giorgio C, Barber K, Norton L, Lau M, Whitley L, Cereghino JJ. Pharmacokinetic profile of flunarizine after single and multiple dosing in epileptic patients receiving comedication. *Epilepsia* (1988) 29, 770–4.

Triptans + Azoles

Ketoconazole and fluconazole increase the AUC of eletriptan by about sixfold and twofold, respectively. Almotriptan is less affected, and ketoconazole only raises its AUC by about 60%. Itraconazole is predicted to interact in the same way as ketoconazole.

Clinical evidence

(a) Almotriptan

In a randomised, open label, crossover study, 16 healthy subjects were given **ketoconazole** 400 mg daily on days 1 to 3, with a single 12.5-mg dose of almotriptan on day 2. Ketoconazole increased the AUC and maximum plasma levels of almotriptan by 57% and 61%, respectively. The renal clearance of almotriptan was also reduced by approximately 16%.[1]

(b) Eletriptan

A pharmacokinetic study by the manufacturers of eletriptan found that **ketoconazole** 400 mg increased the maximum serum levels of eletriptan 2.7-fold, the AUC 5.9-fold and prolonged its half-life from 4.8 to 8.3 hours. **Fluconazole** caused a lesser 1.4-fold increase in the maximum serum levels of eletriptan, and a twofold increase in its AUC.[2]

Mechanism

Ketoconazole is a potent inhibitor of the cytochrome P450 isoenzyme CYP3A4, by which eletriptan is metabolised. Fluconazole is a less potent inhibitor of CYP3A4, and therefore has a more modest effect. Almotriptan is also metabolised by CYP3A4, but as this is not the only route of metabolism, and therefore inhibition of CYP3A4 by ketoconazole has a less dramatic effect on its levels.

Importance and management

Although studies are limited these interactions are established. In the study with almotriptan and ketoconazole adverse events were not significantly altered, and so no almotriptan dosage adjustment is considered necessary when using this combination.[1] Ketoconazole dramatically raises eletriptan levels, and therefore the manufacturers advise that concurrent use should be avoided.

Itraconazole, which is also a potent inhibitor of CYP3A4, has been predicted to interact in the same way as ketoconazole.[2-4] In addition, the US manufacturers recommend that eletriptan should not be given within 72 hours of itraconazole and ketoconazole.[2] Fluconazole is a less potent inhibitor of CYP3A4 and therefore may be used with caution. Other triptans would be expected to have little or no interaction with the azoles as they are not predominantly metabolised by CYP3A4 (see 'Table 16.2', (p.597)).

1. Fleishaker JC, Herman BD, Carel BJ, Azie NE. Interaction between ketoconazole and almotriptan in healthy volunteers. *J Clin Pharmacol* (2003) 43, 423–7.
2. Relpax (Eletriptan hydrobromide). Pfizer Inc. US Prescribing information, April 2007.
3. Relpax (Eletriptan hydrobromide). Pfizer Ltd. UK Summary of product characteristics, March 2006.
4. Axert (Almotriptan malate). Ortho-McNeil Pharmaceutical Inc. US Prescribing Information, May 2007.

Triptans + Beta blockers

No clinically important interaction occurs between most triptans and propranolol, but the plasma levels of rizatriptan are almost doubled by propranolol.

Clinical evidence, mechanism, importance and management

(a) Almotriptan

Twelve healthy subjects were given **propranolol** 80 mg twice daily for 7 days followed by a single 12.5-mg dose of almotriptan. Although some small changes were noted in the pharmacokinetics of almotriptan, these were not considered to be clinically significant and concurrent use of the combination was well tolerated.[1]

(b) Eletriptan

In an interaction study, 12 healthy subjects were given a single 80-mg dose of eletriptan following pre-treatment with **propranolol** 80 mg twice daily for 7 days. It was found that the eletriptan AUC was increased 1.3-fold and the half-life increased from 4.9 to 5.2 hours. However, these changes were not considered to be clinically significant. No significant blood pressure changes or any adverse events were seen, when compared with taking eletriptan alone.[2]

The manufacturers say that in clinical trials where eletriptan was taken with beta blockers, no evidence of an interaction was seen.[3]

(c) Frovatriptan

A single 2.5-mg oral dose of frovatriptan was given to 12 healthy subjects after they had received pre-treatment with **propranolol** 80 mg twice daily for 7 days. The AUC and maximum levels of frovatriptan were increased by 25% and 23%, respectively. However, no changes occurred in the ECGs and vital signs of the subjects, and so the pharmacokinetic interaction was not thought to be of clinical significance.[4]

(d) Naratriptan

The manufacturers of naratriptan report that there is no evidence of interactions with **beta blockers** (none specifically named)[5] so there would appear to be no problems with the concurrent use of **propranolol** with any other beta blocker.

(e) Rizatriptan

A series of double-blind, placebo-controlled studies were conducted in a total of 51 patients who were given a single 10-mg dose of rizatriptan after 7 days of pre-treatment with **propranolol** 60 or 120 mg twice daily, **nadolol** 80 mg daily, **metoprolol** 100 mg daily, or placebo.[6] **Nadolol** and **metoprolol** had no effect on the pharmacokinetics of rizatriptan. However, **propranolol** raised the AUC and the maximum plasma concentration of rizatriptan by 1.67 and 1.75-fold, respectively. Adjusting the dose of **propranolol** and separating the administration by 2 hours had little effect on this interaction.[6] *In vitro* studies have shown that **propranolol** markedly inhibits the metabolism of rizatriptan, whereas **atenolol**, **nadolol** and **timolol** do not affect the metabolism of rizatriptan.[6] The manufacturers recommend that a 5-mg dose of rizatriptan (rather than the more usual 10 mg) should be used in the presence of **propranolol**, with a maximum of two[7] or three doses in 24 hours.[8] In the UK, they also state that administration should be separated by at least 2 hours,[7] although the rationale for this is less clear given the findings of the above study.[6] No reduction in the rizatriptan dosage would seem to be needed in the presence of **nadolol**, **metoprolol**, **atenolol** or **timolol**.

(f) Sumatriptan

In a study in 10 healthy subjects, **propranolol** 80 mg twice daily for 7 days did not alter the pharmacokinetics of a single 300-mg dose of sumatriptan given on day 7. There was no significant effect on pulse rate or blood pressure.[9]

(g) Zolmitriptan

In a double-blind, randomised, crossover study, 12 healthy subjects were given **propranolol** 160 mg or a placebo daily for 7 days, with a single 10-mg oral dose of zolmitriptan on day 7. The **propranolol** increased the maximum serum levels and the AUC of the zolmitriptan by 56% and 37%, respectively, and reduced the extent of its conversion to its active metabolite, probably due to inhibition of, or competition for metabolism by, cytochrome P450 isoenzymes. However, it was concluded that no clinically important changes in the therapeutic effects of zolmitriptan are likely, nor are any adjustments in its dosage needed.[10]

1. Fleishaker JC, Sisson TA, Carel BJ, Azie NE. Lack of pharmacokinetic interaction between the antimigraine compound, almotriptan, and propranolol in healthy volunteers. *Cephalalgia* (2001) 21, 61–65.
2. Milton KA, Tan L, Love R. The pharmacokinetic and pharmacodynamic interactions of oral eletriptan and propranolol in healthy volunteers. *Cephalalgia* (1998) 18, 412.
3. Relpax (Eletriptan hydrobromide). Pfizer Ltd. UK Summary of product characteristics, March 2006.
4. Buchan P, Ward C, Stewart AJ. The effect of propranolol on the pharmacokinetic and safety profiles of frovatriptan. *Headache* (1999) 39, 345.
5. Naramig (Naratriptan hydrochloride). GlaxoSmithKline UK. UK Summary of product characteristics, November 2005.
6. Goldberg MR, Sciberras D, De Smet M, Lowry R, Tomasko L, Lee Y, Olah TV, Zhao J, Vyas KP, Halpin R, Kari PH, James I. Influence of β-adrenoceptor antagonists on the pharmacokinetics of rizatriptan, a 5-$HT_{1B/1D}$ agonist: differential effects of propranolol, nadolol and metoprolol. *Br J Clin Pharmacol* (2001) 52, 69–76.
7. Maxalt (Rizatriptan benzoate). Merck Sharp & Dohme Ltd. UK Summary of product characteristics, April 2003.
8. Maxalt (Rizatriptan benzoate). Merck & Co., Inc. US Prescribing information, April 2007.
9. Scott AK, Walley T, Breckenridge AM, Lacey LF, Fowler PA. Lack of an interaction between propranolol and sumatriptan. *Br J Clin Pharmacol* (1991) 32, 581–4.
10. Peck RW, Seaber EJ, Dixon R, Gillotin CG, Weatherley BC, Layton G, Posner J. The interaction between propranolol and the novel antimigraine agent zolmitriptan (311C90). *Br J Clin Pharmacol* (1997) 44, 595–9.

Triptans + Ergot derivatives

Simultaneous use of the ergot derivatives is contraindicated with all the triptans because of the theoretical risk of additive vasoconstriction, although this has been demonstrated only in one study with sumatriptan, and there is one isolated case of myocardial in-

farction in a woman taking sumatriptan and methysergide. No important additive effect has been seen in pharmacodynamic studies with almotriptan, eletriptan, frovatriptan, naratriptan, rizatriptan or zolmitriptan. Some of the manufacturers of the triptans give recommendations for the number of hours that should be allowed between administration of triptans and ergot derivatives.

Clinical evidence

(a) Almotriptan

The manufacturers of almotriptan say that no additive vasospastic effects were seen in a clinical study in 12 healthy subjects given almotriptan and **ergotamine**.[1] However, they do note that such effects are theoretically possible.

(b) Eletriptan

The manufacturers report that when oral **ergotamine** with caffeine was given 1 hour and 2 hours after eletriptan, minor additive increases in blood pressure were seen.[2]

(c) Frovatriptan

In a randomised, crossover study, 12 healthy subjects were given a single 5-mg dose of oral frovatriptan, a single 2-mg sublingual dose of **ergotamine**, or both drugs together. The **ergotamine** reduced the maximum levels and AUC of frovatriptan by about 25%. However, the frovatriptan had no effect on **ergotamine** pharmacokinetics, and no clinically significant changes in the haemodynamics or the ECGs of the subjects were noted.[3]

(d) Naratriptan

A study in 12 healthy subjects found that 1 mg of intramuscular **dihydroergotamine** reduced the AUC and the maximum serum levels of a single 2.5-mg dose of naratriptan by 15% and 20%, respectively, but this was considered to be clinically irrelevant. Concurrent use was well tolerated and no clinically significant blood pressure, heart rate or ECG effects were seen.[4]

(e) Rizatriptan

Additive vasospastic effects were not observed in a pharmacodynamic study in 16 healthy subjects given oral rizatriptan 10 mg and intravenous **ergotamine** 250 micrograms.[5,6]

(f) Sumatriptan

A study in 38 migraine sufferers found that 1 mg of intravenous **dihydroergotamine** alone caused maximum increases in blood pressure of 13/9 mmHg, while 2 or 4 mg of subcutaneous sumatriptan alone caused a smaller rise in blood pressure of 7/6 mmHg. When given together the blood pressure rises were no greater than with **dihydroergotamine** alone.[7] A clinical study of subcutaneous sumatriptan in patients taking oral **dihydroergotamine** found that the adverse event profile of sumatriptan was not affected by concurrent use.[8] However, another pharmacodynamic study found that subcutaneous sumatriptan and intravenous **ergotamine** had additive vasoconstrictive effects (as assessed by decreases in toe-arm systolic blood pressure gradients).[9]

Myocardial infarction has been reported in a 43-year-old woman after she took two 2-mg doses of **methysergide** 12 hours apart, followed by sumatriptan 6 mg subcutaneously. Severe chest pain and tightness with breathlessness began 15 minutes later, and results of various tests were consistent with 'coronary spasm on an area of atherosclerosis'.[10]

(g) Zolmitriptan

In a randomised, double-blind, placebo-controlled study, 12 healthy subjects were given 5 mg of oral **dihydroergotamine** or a placebo twice daily for 10 days, with oral zolmitriptan 10 mg (four times the usual dose) on day 10. No significant changes in blood pressure, ECGs, or zolmitriptan pharmacokinetics were seen. Concurrent use was well tolerated.[11] Another randomised, double-blind, placebo-controlled study in 12 healthy subjects looked at the effects of oral zolmitriptan 20 mg (eight times the usual dose) given with oral **ergotamine** 2 mg (contained in *Cafergot* tablets; **ergotamine** 1 mg with caffeine 100 mg). Using a very detailed and thorough range of techniques, no clinically relevant cardiovascular changes were found, even at this large dose of zolmitriptan, and concurrent use was generally well tolerated. No important changes in the zolmitriptan pharmacokinetics were seen.[12]

Mechanism

Vasoconstriction is a well known adverse effect of ergot derivatives, and coronary vasoconstriction may also occur rarely with the triptans. (Note that in 1992, soon after the marketing of sumatriptan, the CSM in the UK had received 34 reports of pain or tightness in the chest caused by sumatriptan, possibly due to coronary vasoconstriction.[13]) It is therefore theoretically possible that the drugs may have additive vasoconstrictive effects, although there is little evidence of this in practice.

Importance and management

Due to the theoretical risk of additive vasoconstriction, and possible significant coronary vasoconstriction (see sumatriptan above) ergot derivatives are generally contraindicated with the triptans (the exception being naratriptan,[14] where concurrent use is not recommended). The UK manufacturers of sumatriptan say that ergotamine should not be given less than 6 hours after taking the triptan, and recommend that the triptan should not be taken less than 24 hours after taking ergotamine.[15] The same recommendations are made by the UK manufacturers of almotriptan,[1] rizatriptan,[5] and zolmitriptan,[16] whereas the UK manufacturers of eletriptan,[2] and frovatriptan,[17] recommend that ergot derivatives are not given for a minimum of 24 hours (not just 6 hours) after these triptans. In general, in the US, it is recommended that triptans should not be taken within 24 hours of any ergotamine or ergot-type medication.

1. Almogran (Almotriptan hydrogen malate). Organon Laboratories Ltd. UK Summary of product characteristics, April 2007.
2. Relpax (Eletriptan hydrobromide). Pfizer Ltd. UK Summary of product characteristics, March 2006.
3. Buchan P, Ward C, Oliver SD. Lack of clinically significant interactions between frovatriptan and ergotamine. *Cephalalgia* (1999) 19, 364.
4. Kempsford RD, Nicholls B, Lam R, Wintermute S. A study to investigate the potential interaction of naratriptan and dihydroergotamine. 8th International Headache Congress, Amsterdam, June 1997.
5. Maxalt (Rizatriptan benzoate). Merck Sharp & Dohme Ltd. UK Summary of product characteristics, April 2003.
6. Tfelt-Hansen P, Siedelin K, Stepanavage M. Lines C. The effect of rizatriptan, ergotamine, and their combination on human peripheral arteries: a double-blind, placebo-controlled, crossover study in normal subjects. Br J Clin Pharmacol. (2002) 54, 38–44.
7. Fowler PA, Lacey LF, Thomas M, Keene ON, Tanner RJN, Baber NS. The clinical pharmacology, pharmacokinetics and metabolism of sumatriptan. *Eur Neurol* (1991) 31, 291–4.
8. Henry P, d'Allens H and the French Migraine Network Bordeaux-Lyon-Grenoble. Subcutaneous sumatriptan in the acute treatment of migraine in patients using dihydroergotamine as prophylaxis. *Headache* (1993) 33, 432–5.
9. Tfelt-Hansen P, Sperling B, Winter PDO'B. Transient additional effect of sumatriptan on ergotamine-induced constriction of peripheral arteries in man. *Clin Pharmacol Ther* (1992) 51, 149.
10. Liston H, Bennett L, Usher B, Nappi J. The association of the combination of sumatriptan and methysergide in myocardial infarction in a premenopausal woman. *Arch Intern Med* (1999) 159, 511–13.
11. Veronese L, Gillotin C, Marion-Gallois R, Weatherley BC, Thebault JJ, Guillaume M, Peck RW. Lack of interaction between oral dihydroergotamine and the novel antimigraine compound zolmitriptan in healthy volunteers. *Clin Drug Invest* (1997) 14, 217–20.
12. Dixon RM, Meire HB, Evans DH, Watt H, On N, Posner J, Rolan PE. Peripheral vascular effects and pharmacokinetics of the antimigraine compound, zolmitriptan, in combination with oral ergotamine in healthy volunteers. *Cephalalgia* (1997) 17, 639–46.
13. Committee on Safety of Medicines. Sumatriptan (Imigran) and chest pain. *Current Problems* (1992) 34, 2.
14. Naramig (Naratriptan hydrochloride). GlaxoSmithKline UK. UK Summary of product characteristics, November 2005.
15. Imigran Radis (Sumatriptan succinate). GlaxoSmithKline UK. UK Summary of product characteristics, May 2006.
16. Zomig (Zolmitriptan). AstraZeneca UK Ltd. UK Summary of product characteristics, September 2006.
17. Migard (Frovatriptan succinate monohydrate). A. Menarini Pharma UK SRL. UK Summary of product characteristics, February 2005.

Triptans + Flunarizine

Flunarizine did not alter the pharmacokinetics or pharmacodynamics of sumatriptan in one study. Flunarizine does not appear to interact with eletriptan.

Clinical evidence, mechanism, importance and management

(a) Eletriptan

The manufacturer notes that although no formal interaction studies have been carried out, there was no evidence of an interaction between eletriptan and flunarizine in clinical trials.[1]

(b) Sumatriptan

A double-blind study found that flunarizine 10 mg daily for 8 days had no effect on the pharmacokinetics of a single dose of sumatriptan, and the combination caused no significant changes in blood pressure, ECG or heart rate.[2]

1. Relpax (Eletriptan hydrobromide). Pfizer Ltd. UK Summary of product characteristics, March 2006.
2. Van Hecken AM, Depré M, De Schepper PJ, Fowler PA, Lacey LF, Durham JM. Lack of effect of flunarizine on the pharmacokinetics and pharmacodynamics of sumatriptan in healthy volunteers. *Br J Clin Pharmacol* (1992) 34, 82–4.

Triptans + Macrolides

Erythromycin markedly raises the plasma levels of eletriptan. Clarithromycin, josamycin and troleandomycin are predicted to interact similarly. Almotriptan levels may be raised by erythromycin. Clarithromycin does not significantly alter the pharmacokinetics of sumatriptan.

Clinical evidence

(a) Eletriptan

A clinical pharmacokinetic study by the manufacturers of eletriptan[1] found that **erythromycin** 1 g increased the maximum serum levels of eletriptan 2-fold, the AUC 3.6-fold and prolonged its half-life from 4.6 to 7.1 hours.

(b) Sumatriptan

A study in which 24 healthy subjects were given sumatriptan 50 mg on the morning of the fourth day of a course of **clarithromycin** 500 mg twice daily, found that **clarithromycin** did not significantly affect the pharmacokinetics of sumatriptan.[2]

Mechanism

The macrolides are, to varying degrees, inhibitors of the cytochrome P450 isoenzyme CYP3A4, by which eletriptan is metabolised. Therefore giving erythromycin raises eletriptan plasma levels. Sumatriptan is not metabolised by CYP3A4 and therefore does not interact.

Importance and management

Information is limited but an interaction between eletriptan and erythromycin appears to be established. Because of the elevated levels seen, the manufacturers advise against their concurrent use.[1,3] Other drugs that are potent CYP3A4 inhibitors are predicted to raise serum eletriptan levels similarly. Such drugs include **clarithromycin**[1,3] **josamycin**,[1] and **troleandomycin**.[3] In addition, the US manufacturers recommend that eletriptan should not be given within 72 hours of **clarithromycin** or **troleandomycin**.[3]

Other triptans would be expected to have little or no interaction with the azoles as they are not predominantly metabolised by CYP3A4 (see 'Table 16.2', (p.597)). The exception to this is **almotriptan**, which is metabolised in part by CYP3A4. The US manufacturers[4] therefore predict that its levels may be raised by erythromycin. However, note that, based on its interaction with 'ketoconazole', (p.601), dosage adjustments would not be expected to be necessary.

1. Relpax (Eletriptan hydrobromide). Pfizer Ltd. UK Summary of product characteristics, March 2006.
2. Moore KHP, Leese PT, McNeal S, Gray P, O'Quinn S, Bye C, Sale M. The pharmacokinetics of sumatriptan when administered with clarithromycin in healthy volunteers. *Clin Ther* (2002) 24, 583–94.
3. Relpax (Eletriptan hydrobromide). Pfizer Inc. US Prescribing information, April 2007.
4. Axert (Almotriptan malate). Ortho-McNeil Pharmaceutical Inc. US Prescribing Information, May 2007.

Triptans + MAOIs

Moclobemide markedly inhibits the metabolism of rizatriptan, and approximately doubles the bioavailability of sumatriptan. The manufacturers contraindicate these triptans with moclobemide and non-selective MAOIs. Moclobemide modestly inhibited the metabolism of zolmitriptan but had no clinically significant effect on almotriptan or frovatriptan.

Selegiline does not interact with sumatriptan or zolmitriptan, and would not be expected to interact with any of the other triptans.

Non-selective MAOIs (e.g. phenelzine) are not expected to interact with eletriptan, frovatriptan, or naratriptan. Nevertheless, the manufacturer of frovatriptan contraindicates the concurrent use of MAOIs, based on a theoretical increased risk of serotonin syndrome.

Clinical evidence, mechanism, importance and management

(a) Almotriptan

In a study in 12 healthy subjects, **moclobemide** 150 mg twice daily for 8 days increased the AUC of a single 12.5-mg dose of almotriptan given on day 8 by 37%, decreased its clearance by 27% and increased the half-life by 24%, which was not considered clinically significant.[1] These findings are consistent with the fact that less than half of a dose of almotriptan is metabolised by monoamine oxidase A,[2] and it would seem therefore that concurrent use need not be avoided. There appears to be no direct clinical information about the use of non-selective MAOIs but it seems unlikely that a clinically relevant interaction will occur.

(b) Eletriptan

The manufacturer of eletriptan notes that it is not a substrate for monoamine oxidase, and therefore no interaction with MAOIs is expected.[3,4] Because of this, they have not undertaken a formal interaction study.[3]

(c) Frovatriptan

The manufacturer of frovatriptan notes that it is not a substrate for, or an inhibitor of, monoamine oxidase.[5,6] Nevertheless, they say that a potential risk of serotonin syndrome or hypertension cannot be excluded when it is used with MAOIs, so concomitant use is not recommended[5] (but see also 'Antimigraine drugs', (p.597)). A study in 9 healthy subjects given a single 2.5-mg oral dose of frovatriptan following pre-treatment with **moclobemide** 150 mg twice daily for 7 days did not find any pharmacokinetic changes, or any changes in the vital signs and ECGs of the subjects. Therefore no adverse interaction would be expected with concurrent use.[7]

(d) Naratriptan

The manufacturer of naratriptan notes that it does not inhibit monoamine oxidase. Therefore interactions with MAOIs are not anticipated.[8]

(e) Rizatriptan

In a double blind, randomised, crossover study, 12 healthy subjects were given **moclobemide** 150 mg or a placebo three times daily for 4 days, with a single 10-mg dose of rizatriptan on day 4. The **moclobemide** increased the AUCs of rizatriptan and its active (but minor) metabolite by 2.2- and 5.3-fold, respectively, and increased their maximum serum levels by 1.4- and 2.6-fold, respectively. MAO-A is the principal enzyme concerned with the metabolism of rizatriptan. **Moclobemide** inhibits this enzyme and therefore raises rizatriptan levels. Despite these rises, the concurrent use of these drugs was well tolerated and any adverse effects were mild and similar to those seen when rizatriptan was given with the placebo. However, because of the magnitude of the rises, the authors recommend avoiding the combination.[9] The manufacturers of rizatriptan contraindicate its use both during, and 2 weeks after stopping an MAOI, the stated reasons being that similar or greater rises in serum levels may be expected with irreversible non-selective MAOIs than with moclobemide.[10,11] In addition, the US manufacturers[11] note that no interaction would be expected with selective inhibitors of MAO-A (namely **selegiline** and **rasagiline**).

(f) Sumatriptan

Three groups of 14 subjects were given a placebo, **moclobemide** 150 mg three times daily, or **selegiline** 5 mg twice daily for 8 days, with subcutaneous sumatriptan 6 mg on day 8. No statistically significant differences in pulse rates or in blood pressures were seen between any of the groups following the injection of the sumatriptan. However, the sumatriptan AUC of the **moclobemide**-treated group was approximately doubled (129% increase), its clearance was reduced by 56% and its half-life increased by 52%. The pharmacokinetic changes seen in the **selegiline** group were not consistent. There were no differences in the adverse events experienced by any of the three groups.[12] An *in vitro* study of the metabolism of sumatriptan confirms that it is the MAO-A enzyme, not MAO-B, that is the major enzyme involved in the metabolism of sumatriptan.[13]

A comprehensive search of the literature and reports from proprietary manufacturers, identified published reports of 31 patients taking sumatriptan and MAOIs concurrently, but no adverse events were reported,[14] and a patient taking **moclobemide** 300 mg three times daily had no adverse effects when given oral sumatriptan 100 mg on six occasions.[15]

However, a patient who had taken an overdose of **moclobemide**, together with sumatriptan, sertraline, and citalopram developed the serotonin syndrome.[16]

The interaction between moclobemide and sumatriptan appears to be established. The same interaction seems likely to occur with any RIMA or non-selective MAOI, but not with the selective MAO-B inhibitors like **selegiline**. However, the increased sumatriptan bioavailability appears not to be clinically important because, in the study cited, those subjects taking moclobemide did not experience any more adverse effects than those taking the selegiline or placebo. Despite this the UK manufacturers of sumatriptan quite clearly say that the concurrent use of sumatriptan and MAOIs is contraindicated both during and for 2 weeks after stopping an MAOI.[17]

(g) Zolmitriptan

In a series of three-period, crossover, randomised studies, 12 healthy subjects were given **selegiline** 10 mg daily or **moclobemide** 150 mg twice daily for 7 days, with a single 10-mg oral dose of zolmitriptan on day 7.[18] It was found that the AUC of the zolmitriptan was increased by 26% by the **moclobemide**. A threefold increase in the AUC of the active metabolite also occurred.[19] It is likely that moclobemide inhibited the metabolism of zolmitriptan via monoamine oxidase A. Despite these increases, because of the good tolerability profile of zolmitriptan, no dosage reductions are thought to be needed if given with **moclobemide**, but a maximum intake of 5 mg in 24 hours is recommended by the UK manufacturers.[19] However, the US manufacturers contraindicate the use of zolmitriptan both during and for 2 weeks after the use of RIMAs.[20]

Selegiline on the other hand had no effect on the pharmacokinetics of zolmitriptan or its metabolites, apart from a small (7%) reduction in its renal clearance.[18] This finding was expected, since **selegiline** is specific for monoamine oxidase B (but note that this specificity is lost at higher doses). No special precautions would therefore seem to be necessary if **selegiline** is given with sumatriptan.

1. Fleishaker JC, Ryan KK, Jansat JM, Carel BJ, Bell DJA, Burke MT, Azie NE. Effect of MAO-A inhibition on the pharmacokinetics of almotriptan, an antimigraine agent in humans. *Br J Clin Pharmacol* (2001) 51, 437–41.
2. Almogran (Almotriptan hydrogen malate). Organon Laboratories Ltd. UK Summary of product characteristics, April 2007.
3. Relpax (Eletriptan hydrobromide). Pfizer Ltd. UK Summary of product characteristics, March 2006.
4. Relpax (Eletriptan hydrobromide). Pfizer Inc. US Prescribing information, April 2007.
5. Migard (Frovatriptan succinate monohydrate). A. Menarini Pharma UK SRL. UK Summary of product characteristics, February 2005.
6. Frova (Frovatriptan succinate). Endo Pharmaceuticals Inc. US Prescribing information, March 2007.
7. Buchan P, Ward C, Freestone S. Lack of interaction between frovatriptan and monoamine oxidase inhibitor. *Cephalalgia* (1999) 19, 364.
8. Naramig (Naratriptan hydrochloride). GlaxoSmithKline UK. UK Summary of product characteristics, November 2005.
9. van Haarst AD, van Gerven JMA, Cohen AF, De Smet M, Sterrett A, Birk KL, Fisher AL, De Puy ME, Goldberg MR, Musson DG. The effects of moclobemide on the pharmacokinetics of the 5-$HT_{1B/1D}$ agonist rizatriptan in healthy volunteers. *Br J Clin Pharmacol* (1999) 48, 190–96.
10. Maxalt (Rizatriptan benzoate). Merck Sharp & Dohme Ltd. UK Summary of product characteristics, April 2003.
11. Maxalt (Rizatriptan benzoate). Merck & Co., Inc. US Prescribing information, April 2007.
12. Glaxo Pharmaceuticals UK Limited. A study to determine whether the pharmacokinetics, safety or tolerability of subcutaneously administered sumatriptan (6 mg) are altered by interaction with concurrent oral monoamine oxidase inhibitors. Data on file (Protocol C92–050), 1993.
13. Dixon CM, Park GR, Tarbit MH. Characterization of the enzyme responsible for the metabolism of sumatriptan in human liver. *Biochem Pharmacol* (1994) 47, 1253–7.
14. Gardner DM, Lynd LD. Sumatriptan contraindications and the serotonin syndrome. *Ann Pharmacother* (1998) 32, 33–38.
15. Blier P, Bergeron R. The safety of concomitant use of sumatriptan and antidepressant treatments. *J Clin Psychopharmacol* (1995) 15, 106–9.
16. Höjer J, Personne M, Skagius A-S, Hansson O. Serotoninergt syndrom: flera allvarliga fall med denna ofta förbisedda diagnos. *Lakartidningen* (2002) 99, 2054–5, 2058–60.
17. Imigran Radis (Sumatriptan succinate). GlaxoSmithKline UK. UK Summary of product characteristics, May 2006.
18. Rolan P. Potential drug interactions with the novel antimigraine compound zolmitriptan (Zomig™, 311C90). *Cephalalgia* (1997) 17 (Suppl 18), 21–7.
19. Zomig (Zolmitriptan). AstraZeneca UK Ltd. UK Summary of product characteristics, September 2006.
20. Zomig (Zolmitriptan). AstraZeneca Pharmaceuticals LP. US Prescribing information, January 2007.

Triptans + Pizotifen

Pizotifen did not alter the pharmacokinetics or pharmacodynamics of sumatriptan or zolmitriptan, and did not alter the efficacy of acute sumatriptan for migraine. It seems unlikely that any of the other triptans will interact.

Clinical evidence

(a) Sumatriptan

Pizotifen 500 micrograms three times daily for 8 days in 14 healthy subjects was found to have no significant effect on the pharmacokinetics of sumatriptan. In addition, there were no significant changes in blood pressure or heart rate.[1] In a clinical study, the addition of pizotifen prophylaxis did not alter the efficacy of acute sumatriptan for migraine relief. In this study, the combination was associated with more weight gain than sumatriptan alone, an effect which was attributed solely to the pizotifen.[2]

(b) Zolmitriptan

In a double-blind, randomised study, 12 healthy subjects were given pizotifen 1.5 mg or a placebo once daily for 8 days, with oral zolmitriptan 10 mg on day 8. Pizotifen did not significantly alter the pharmacokinetics of zolmitriptan, and no clinically relevant changes in heart rates or ECGs or blood pressures were seen as a result of concurrent use.[3]

Mechanism, importance and management

Although the information is limited, it shows that no sumatriptan or zolmitriptan dosage adjustments are expected to be needed if used with pizotifen. On the basis of the information on sumatriptan and zolmitriptan it seems unlikely that any of the other triptans will interact.

1. Fowler PA, Lacey LF, Thomas M, Keene ON, Tanner RJN, Baber NS. The clinical pharmacology, pharmacokinetics and metabolism of sumatriptan. *Eur Neurol* (1991) 31, 291–4.
2. Cleland PG, Barnes D, Elrington GM, Loizou LA, Rawes GD. Studies to assess if pizotifen prophylaxis improves migraine beyond the benefit offered by acute sumatriptan therapy alone. *Eur Neurol* (1997) 38, 31–8.
3. Seaber EJ, Gillotin C, Mohanlal R, Layton G, Posner J, Peck R. Lack of interaction between pizotifen and the novel antimigraine compound zolmitriptan in healthy volunteers. *Clin Drug Invest* (1997) 14, 221–5.

Triptans + Protease inhibitors

The manufacturers state that the concurrent use of eletriptan and ritonavir, indinavir, or nelfinavir should be avoided, because these protease inhibitors are potent inhibitors of the cytochrome P450 isoenzyme CYP3A4, an enzyme involved in the metabolism of eletriptan. Concurrent use would therefore be expected to markedly increase levels of eletriptan.[1,2] In addition, the US manufacturers recommend that eletriptan should not be given within 72 hours of ritonavir and nelfinavir.[2] This predicted interaction is based on the known interaction with 'erythromycin', (p.604) and 'ketoconazole', (p.601). Similar predictions are made by the manufacturers of almotriptan, and they advise caution with the use of ritonavir.[3]

1. Relpax (Eletriptan hydrobromide). Pfizer Ltd. UK Summary of product characteristics, March 2006.
2. Relpax (Eletriptan hydrobromide). Pfizer Inc. US Prescribing information, April 2007.
3. Axert (Almotriptan malate). Ortho-McNeil Pharmaceutical Inc. US Prescribing Information, May 2007.

Triptans + SSRIs and related antidepressants

The SSRIs normally appear not to interact with the triptans, but there are a few rare cases of dyskinesias when sumatriptan was given with an SSRI, and there is some evidence to suggest that the serotonin syndrome may occasionally develop. Venlafaxine and duloxetine are predicted to interact similarly. Fluvoxamine modestly inhibits the metabolism of frovatriptan, and may inhibit the metabolism of zolmitriptan.

Clinical evidence

(a) Almotriptan

Fluoxetine 60 mg daily was given to 14 healthy subjects for 8 days, with a single 12.5-mg dose of almotriptan on day 8. **Fluoxetine** raised the maximum plasma levels of almotriptan by about 18%. The combination was well tolerated and caused no ECG changes, so no dose alterations were considered necessary.[1]

(b) Eletriptan

The manufacturer notes that although no formal interaction studies have been done, there was no evidence of an interaction between eletriptan and SSRIs in clinical trials, and that SSRIs appeared unlikely to alter the pharmacokinetics of eletriptan.[2]

(c) Frovatriptan

Fluvoxamine has been shown to increase the blood levels of frovatriptan by 27 to 49%.[3] The manufacturer recommends caution with concurrent use of frovatriptan and **fluvoxamine** or other SSRIs.[4]

(d) Naratriptan

The UK manufacturer of naratriptan notes that there is no evidence of interactions with SSRIs.[5]

(e) Rizatriptan

A single 10-mg dose of rizatriptan was given to 12 healthy subjects after they took **paroxetine** 20 mg or a placebo daily for 14 days. The plasma levels of rizatriptan and its active metabolite were not altered by **paroxetine**, and no adverse effects were seen. Safety evaluations included blood pressure, heart rate, temperature and a visual analogue assessment of mood. There was no evidence of the serotonin syndrome.[6]

(f) Sumatriptan

A study in 11 healthy subjects found that **paroxetine** 20 mg daily for 16 days had no effect on the response to a 6-mg dose of subcutaneous sumatriptan, as measured by prolactin levels. The sumatriptan levels remained unaltered, its cardiovascular effects were unchanged and no clinically significant adverse effects occurred.[7] Other studies report that the concurrent use of sumatriptan and SSRIs (**fluoxetine** 20 to 60 mg daily, **fluvoxamine** 200 mg daily, **paroxetine** 20 to 50 mg daily, **sertraline** 50 to 100 mg daily) was successful and uneventful.[8,9] No adverse effects have been noted in 148 other patients.[10] However, a case report describes a 65-year-old woman who had been taking **paroxetine** 20 mg [daily] for a number of years, who developed confusion, strange behaviour, sinus tachycardia, hypertension and hyperthermia shortly after starting sumatriptan. The serotonin syndrome was diagnosed, and she recovered completely on withdrawal of the two drugs.[11]

Additionally, in Canada, post-marketing surveillance of the voluntary reports received by the manufacturers of **fluoxetine**, identified 2 cases that showed good evidence, and another 4 cases that showed some, but not strong evidence, of reactions consistent with the serotonin syndrome in patients also taking sumatriptan.[12] Other cases describe a decrease in the efficacy of sumatriptan with **fluoxetine**,[13] dyskinesias and dystonias with sumatriptan and **paroxetine**,[14] and twenty possible cases of the serotonin syndrome with sumatriptan and SSRIs.[10,15]

The manufacturers of sumatriptan also say that they have rare post-marketing reports of weakness, hyperreflexia and incoordination following the use of sumatriptan and SSRIs.[16]

A prospective study of 12 339 individuals receiving sumatriptan by injection identified 14.5% of these (1784) who were also taking SSRIs (**fluoxetine** 8.3%, **sertraline** 5.5%, **paroxetine** 3.9%, other 0.4%) or **venlafaxine** 1.7%. Patients taking SSRIs were found to have a higher absolute frequency of adverse neurological effects compared with those not taking antidepressants (0.8% and 0.25%, respectively). However, the authors concluded that there was no evidence of an interaction since the adverse events occurred more than 24 hours after the administration of sumatriptan.[17] One case of intractable migraine was reported in a patient taking an SSRI and sumatriptan. The authors report that this infers a lack of effect of the sumatriptan.[17]

(g) Zolmitriptan

A two-period crossover, double-blind study in 20 subjects given **fluoxetine** 20 mg or a placebo daily for 28 days, with zolmitriptan 10 mg on day 28, found that the pharmacokinetics of zolmitriptan were unaffected by **fluoxetine**.[18] Only very slight changes were seen in the pharmacokinetics of its active metabolite.[18] **Sertraline**, **paroxetine**, and **citalopram** are also not expected to alter the pharmacokinetics of zolmitriptan. However, **fluvoxamine**, a CYP1A2 inhibitor, is predicted to increase levels of zolmitriptan,[19] based on the known interaction with cimetidine (see 'Triptans; Zolmitriptan + Cimetidine', p.608).

Mechanism

Not understood. SSRIs increase the levels of 5-HT (serotonin) at post-synaptic receptors. In theory the triptans (5-HT_1 agonists) might possibly add to the effects of these increased levels of serotonin, but in practice it is questionable whether this is normally clinically relevant (see also 'Antimigraine drugs', (p.597)). Fluvoxamine probably inhibits the metabolism of frovatriptan[4] by cytochrome P450 isoenzyme CYP1A2, and is predicted to interact with zolmitriptan[19] by the same mechanism.

Importance and management

The weight of evidence suggests that the concurrent use of the triptans and SSRIs is normally uneventful, but adverse reactions do occur occasionally. The authors of some of the references above concluded that their findings do not imply that concurrent use should be avoided, but that caution and close monitoring should be used.[10,12] Many of the US manufacturers of the triptans generally advise that patients receiving a triptan and an SSRI or an SNRI (i.e duloxetine or venlafaxine) should be monitored for any signs of weakness, hyperreflexia, and incoordination. However, see also 'Antimigraine drugs', (p.597). Since fluvoxamine is predicted to have a pharmacokinetic interaction with zolmitriptan the manufacturers recommend a maximum dosage of 5 mg in 24 hours in the presence of fluvoxamine.[19]

1. Fleishaker JC, Ryan KK, Carel BJ, Azie NE. Evaluation of the potential pharmacokinetic interaction between almotriptan and fluoxetine in healthy volunteers. *J Clin Pharmacol* (2001) 41, 217–23.
2. Relpax (Eletriptan hydrobromide). Pfizer Ltd. UK Summary of product characteristics, March 2006.
3. Wade A, Buchan P, Mant T, Ward C. Frovatriptan has no clinically significant interaction with fluvoxamine. *Cephalalgia* (2001) 21, 427.
4. Migard (Frovatriptan succinate monohydrate). A. Menarini Pharma UK SRL. UK Summary of product characteristics, February 2005.
5. Naramig (Naratriptan hydrochloride). GlaxoSmithKline UK. UK Summary of product characteristics, November 2005.
6. Goldberg MR, Lowry RC, Musson DG, Birk KL, Fisher A, DePuy ME, Shadle CR. Lack of pharmacokinetic and pharmacodynamic interaction between rizatriptan and paroxetine. *J Clin Pharmacol* (1999) 39, 192–9.
7. Wing Y-K, Clifford EM, Sheehan BD, Campling GM, Hockney RA, Cowen PJ. Paroxetine treatment and the prolactin response to sumatriptan. *Psychopharmacology (Berl)* (1996) 124, 377–9.
8. Blier P, Bergeron R. The safety of concomitant use of sumatriptan and antidepressant treatments. *J Clin Psychopharmacol* (1995) 15, 106–9.
9. Leung M, Ong M. Lack of an interaction between sumatriptan and selective serotonin reuptake inhibitors. *Headache* (1995) 35, 488–9.
10. Gardner DM, Lynd LD. Sumatriptan contraindications and the serotonin syndrome. *Ann Pharmacother* (1998) 32, 33–8.
11. Hendrix Y, van Zagten MSG. Het serotoninesyndroom bij gelijktijdig gebruik van paroxetine en sumatriptan. *Ned Tijdschr Geneeskd* (2005) 149, 888–90.
12. Joffe RT, Sokolov STH. Co-administration of fluoxetine and sumatriptan: the Canadian experience. *Acta Psychiatr Scand* (1997) 95, 551–2.
13. Szabo CP. Fluoxetine and sumatriptan: possibly a counterproductive combination. *J Clin Psychiatry* (1995) 56, 37–8.
14. Abraham JT, Brown R, Meltzer HY. Clozapine treatment of persistent paroxysmal dyskinesia associated with concomitant paroxetine and sumatriptan use. *Biol Psychiatry* (1997) 42, 144–6.
15. Mathew NT. Serotonin syndrome complicating migraine pharmacotherapy. *Cephalalgia* (1996) 16, 323–7.
16. GlaxoWellcome. Personal communication, August 1997.
17. Putnam GP, O'Quinn S, Bolden-Watson CP, Davis RL, Gutterman DL, Fox AW. Migraine polypharmacy and the tolerability of sumatriptan: a large-scale, prospective study. *Cephalalgia* (1999) 19, 668–75.
18. Smith DA, Cleary EW, Watkins S, Huffman CS, Polvino WJ. Zolmitriptan (311C90) does not interact with fluoxetine in healthy volunteers. *Int J Clin Pharmacol Ther* (1998) 36, 301–5.
19. Zomig (Zolmitriptan). AstraZeneca UK Ltd. UK Summary of product characteristics, September 2006.

Triptans + St John's wort (*Hypericum perforatum*)

The CSM in the UK noted that pharmacodynamic (potentiation) interactions have been identified between triptans and St John's wort (*Hypericum perforatum*) leading to an increased risk of adverse effects. They suggest that patients taking triptans should not take St John's wort preparations.[1]

1. Committee on Safety of Medicines/Medicines Control Agency. Reminder: St John's Wort (*Hypericum perforatum*) interactions. *Current Problems* (2000) 26, 6–7.

Triptans + Tobacco

The clearance of naratriptan and possibly frovatriptan is modestly increased by smoking. However, this is unlikely to be clinically relevant. There was no evidence of an interaction between smoking and sumatriptan.

Clinical evidence

(a) Frovatriptan

In a retrospective analysis of pharmacokinetic data from phase I studies, there was a trend for a lower frovatriptan AUC and maximum plasma level in smokers when compared with non-smokers. The clearance tended to be higher but the half-life did not differ.[1]

(b) Naratriptan

The manufacturer notes that smoking increased the clearance of naratriptan by 30%.[2]

(c) Sumatriptan

A prospective study of 12 339 individuals receiving sumatriptan by injection identified 18.3% of these (2262) who were current smokers. There was no evidence of an interaction between sumatriptan and tobacco smoking.[3]

Mechanism

Tobacco smoke is known to induce the cytochrome P450 isoenzyme CYP1A2, which metabolises both naratriptan and frovatriptan to some extent. **Zolmitriptan** is also a substrate of CYP1A2, but the effect of smoking does not appear to have been studied.

Importance and management

Although data are limited, the possible small changes in the pharmacokinetics of frovatriptan and naratriptan with smoking are unlikely to be clinically relevant. It should be noted that smoking is a recognised risk factor for cardiovascular disease. Patients with such risk factors should only use the triptans after careful evaluation.

1. Buchan P. Effects of alcohol, smoking and oral contraceptives on the pharmacokinetics of frovatriptan. *Eur J Neurol* (2000) 7 (Suppl 3), 67–105.
2. Amerge (Naratriptan hydrochloride). GlaxoSmithKline. US Prescribing information, April 2007.
3. Putnam GP, O'Quinn S, Bolden-Watson CP, Davis RL, Gutterman DL, Fox AW. Migraine polypharmacy and the tolerability of sumatriptan: a large-scale, prospective study. *Cephalalgia* (1999) 19, 668–75.

Triptans + Verapamil

Verapamil inhibits the metabolism of eletriptan (AUC increased 2.7-fold) and almotriptan (AUC increased by 20%) but neither of these changes are considered to be clinically significant.

Clinical evidence, mechanism, importance and management

(a) Almotriptan

In a crossover study, 12 healthy subjects were given a single 12.5-mg dose of almotriptan, either alone or following a week of treatment with sustained-release verapamil 120 mg twice daily. The AUC and maximum plasma level of almotriptan were raised by about 20% and 24%, respectively, by verapamil. However, the only effect this caused was a slight increase in systolic BP (8 mmHg) 2 hours after the dose. It was suggested that verapamil may inhibit the metabolism of almotriptan via the cytochrome P450 isoenzyme CYP3A4. The authors suggest that changes of this magnitude do not warrant dosage adjustments.[1]

(b) Eletriptan

In a clinical study with verapamil 480 mg, the maximum plasma levels and AUC of eletriptan were markedly increased by 2.2-fold and 2.7-fold, respectively.[2,3] However, the UK manufacturers state that these increases were not clinically significant as there were no associated increases in blood pressure or adverse events compared to eletriptan alone.[2]

1. Fleishaker JC, Sisson TA, Carel BJ, Azie NE. Pharmacokinetic interaction between verapamil and almotriptan in healthy volunteers. *Clin Pharmacol Ther* (2000) 67, 498–503.
2. Relpax (Eletriptan hydrobromide). Pfizer Ltd. UK Summary of product characteristics, March 2006.
3. Relpax (Eletriptan hydrobromide). Pfizer Inc. US Prescribing information, April 2007.

Triptans; Sumatriptan + Butorphanol

Sumatriptan given by injection appears not to interact with butorphanol nasal spray, but if both drugs are given sequentially by nasal spray a modest reduction in butorphanol absorption may occur.

Clinical evidence, mechanism, importance and management

No pharmacokinetic interactions or change in adverse effects were found to occur between single 1-mg doses of butorphanol tartrate nasal spray and a 6-mg subcutaneous dose of sumatriptan succinate in 24 healthy subjects. It was concluded that concurrent use during acute migraine attacks need not be avoided.[1]

In another study, 19 healthy subjects were given a 1-mg dose of butorphanol nasal spray either 1 or 30 minutes following a 20-mg dose of sumatriptan nasal spray. When butorphanol was given 1 minute after sumatriptan the AUC and maximum plasma levels of butorphanol were reduced by about 29% and 38%, respectively. When butorphanol was given 30 minutes after sumatriptan no significant pharmacokinetic interaction was noted. It was suggested that sumatriptan may cause a transient vasoconstriction of nasal blood vessels, leading to reduced butorphanol absorption. It would therefore seem wise to separate administration to ensure the full effects of butorphanol are achieved.[2]

1. Srinivas NR, Shyu WC, Upmalis D, Lee JS, Barbhaiya RH. Lack of pharmacokinetic interaction between butorphanol tartrate nasal spray and sumatriptan succinate. *J Clin Pharmacol* (1995) 35, 432–7.
2. Vachharajani NN, Shyu W-C, Nichola PS, Boulton DW. A pharmacokinetic interaction study between butorphanol and sumatriptan nasal sprays in healthy subjects: importance of the timing of butorphanol administration. *Cephalalgia* (2002) 22, 282–7.

Triptans; Sumatriptan + Loxapine

An isolated report describes a woman taking loxapine who developed a severe dystonic reaction when she was given sumatriptan.

Clinical evidence, mechanism, importance and management

A woman was taking loxapine 10 mg twice daily for psychotic target symptoms, benzatropine for the prophylaxis of extrapyramidal effects, carbamazepine for mood stabilisation, and *Fiorcet* (paracetamol (acetaminophen), caffeine, and butalbital) for migraine headaches. Two days after the loxapine dosage was raised to 35 mg daily she was given a single 6-mg subcutaneous dose of sumatriptan for a migraine headache. Within 15 minutes she developed torticollis, which was treated with intramuscular benzatropine and intravenous diphenhydramine.

The authors of the report suggest that this reaction was possibly caused by the additive dystonic effects of the loxapine and sumatriptan, despite the presence of the benzatropine. Dystonia is not an uncommon extrapyramidal reaction associated with antipsychotics, and neck stiffness and dystonia are recognised adverse effects of sumatriptan, but of low incidence.[1] This seems to be the first and only report of this apparent interaction, and therefore its general significance is unclear.

1. Garcia G, Kaufman MB, Colucci RD. Dystonic reaction associated with sumatriptan. *Ann Pharmacother* (1994) 28, 1199.

Triptans; Sumatriptan + Naproxen

A study in 12 healthy subjects found that a single 500-mg dose of naproxen had no significant effect on the pharmacokinetics of a single 100-mg oral dose of sumatriptan.[1]

1. Srinivasu P, Rambhau D, Rao BR, Rao YM. Lack of pharmacokinetic interaction between sumatriptan and naproxen. *J Clin Pharmacol* (2000) 40, 99–104.

Triptans; Sumatriptan + Topiramate

Topiramate does not significantly affect the pharmacokinetics of oral or subcutaneous sumatriptan.

Clinical evidence, mechanism, importance and management

In a study 24 healthy subjects were given topiramate 50 mg every 12 hours increased to 100 mg every 12 hours for a total of 7 days, with a single 100-mg oral dose of sumatriptan on day 7. It was found that topiramate reduced the AUC of sumatriptan by 10%, but this was not considered to be clinically relevant. Topiramate had no effect on the AUC of sumatriptan given as a 6 mg subcutaneous dose. The clearance of topiramate appeared to be reduced, when data from this study was compared with that from historical controls, but the magnitude of the effect was not stated.[1] The clinical significance of this effect is unclear.

1. Bialer M, Doose DR, Murthy B, Curtin C, Wang S-S, Twyman RE, SchwabeS. Pharmacokinetic interactions of topiramate. Clin Pharmacokinet. (2004) 43, 763–80.

Triptans; Zolmitriptan + Cimetidine

Cimetidine raises the plasma levels of zolmitriptan.

Clinical evidence, mechanism, importance and management

The manufacturer of zolmitriptan notes that the half-life of zolmitriptan was increased by 44% and the AUC by 48% when it was given after the use of cimetidine. They suggest that this may be because of the inhibitory effect of cimetidine on the cytochrome P450 isoenzyme CYP1A2, an enzyme involved in the metabolism of zolmitriptan. The UK manufacturer recommends a zolmitriptan dose reduction to a maximum of 5 mg in 24 hours in patients taking cimetidine.[1] The US manufacturer makes no recommendation on dose.[2]

1. Zomig (Zolmitriptan). AstraZeneca UK Ltd. UK Summary of product characteristics, September 2006.
2. Zomig (Zolmitriptan). AstraZeneca Pharmaceuticals LP. US Prescribing information, January 2007.

Triptans; Zolmitriptan + Metoclopramide

Metoclopramide does not affect the pharmacokinetics of zolmitriptan.

Clinical evidence, mechanism, importance and management

In a randomised, crossover study, 15 healthy subjects were given single 10-mg doses of zolmitriptan alone or with metoclopramide 10 mg. Metoclopramide had no effect on the pharmacokinetics of zolmitriptan, so there would appear to be no reason for avoiding concurrent use of these two drugs.[1]

1. Seaber EJ, Ridout G, Layton G, Posner J, Peck RW. The novel anti-migraine zolmitriptan (Zomig 311C90) has no clinically significant interactions with paracetamol or metoclopramide. *Eur J Clin Pharmacol* (1997) 53, 229–34.

Triptans; Zolmitriptan + Paracetamol (Acetaminophen)

Paracetamol causes a slight increase in zolmitriptan levels and zolmitriptan causes a slight reduction in the rate and extent of paracetamol absorption, but this does not appear to be clinically relevant.

Clinical evidence, mechanism, importance and management

In a randomised, crossover study, 15 healthy subjects were given single 10-mg doses of zolmitriptan, alone or with 1 g paracetamol. The paracetamol increased the zolmitriptan maximum plasma levels and AUC by 11%, while reducing its renal clearance by 9%. The paracetamol maximum plasma levels and AUC were reduced by 31% and 11%, and absorption was delayed (time to achieve maximum levels 3 versus 0.75 hours). The presence of oral metoclopramide 10 mg did not affect the interaction between zolmitriptan and paracetamol.[1] It was suggested that zolmitriptan might have some inhibitory effect on gastric emptying thereby slowing the absorption of paracetamol.The authors considered that the small changes in pharmacokinetics seen were of no clinical relevance.[1]

1. Seaber EJ, Ridout G, Layton G, Posner J, Peck RW. The novel anti-migraine compound zolmitriptan (Zomig 311C90) has no clinically significant interactions with paracetamol or metoclopramide. *Eur J Clin Pharmacol* (1997) 53, 229–34.

Triptans; Zolmitriptan + Quinolones

The UK manufacturer recommends a dose reduction of zolmitriptan to a maximum of 5 mg in 24 hours in patients taking quinolone antibacterials such as ciprofloxacin. This is because these antibacterials are predicted to increase levels of zolmitriptan by inhibiting the cytochrome P450 isoenzyme CYP1A2, an enzyme involved in the metabolism of zolmitriptan.[1] This is based on the known interaction with 'cimetidine', (above). However, the US manufacturer makes no comment on this theoretical interaction.[2]

1. Zomig (Zolmitriptan). AstraZeneca UK Ltd. UK Summary of product characteristics, September 2006.
2. Zomig (Zolmitriptan). AstraZeneca Pharmaceuticals LP. US Prescribing information, January 2007.

Triptans; Zolmitriptan + Xylometazoline

In a clinical study in 18 healthy subjects, there was no change in the rate or extent of absorption of intranasal zolmitriptan 5 mg given 30 minutes after xylometazoline nasal spray.[1] This suggests that nasal vasoconstriction does not affect absorption of intranasal zolmitriptan.

1. Nairn K, Kemp JV, Dane AL, Roberts DW, Dixon R. Evaluation of the effect of xylometazoline on the absorption of zolmitriptan nasal spray. *Clin Drug Invest* (2002) 22, 703–7.

17

Antineoplastics

The antineoplastic drugs (also called cytotoxics or sometimes cytostatics) are used in the treatment of malignant disease alone or in conjunction with radiotherapy, surgery or immunosuppressants. They also find application in the treatment of a number of autoimmune disorders such as rheumatoid arthritis and psoriasis, and a few are used with other immunosuppressant drugs (ciclosporin, corticosteroids) to prevent transplant rejection. These other drugs are dealt with under the section on 'immunosuppressants', (p.1009).

Of all the drugs discussed in this publication, the antineoplastic drugs are amongst the most toxic and have a low therapeutic index. This means that quite small increases in their levels can lead to the development of serious and life-threatening toxicity. A list of the antineoplastic drugs that are featured in this section appears in 'Table 17.1', (below), grouped by their primary mechanism of action. This table also includes a number of hormone antagonists that are used in the treatment of cancer.

Unlike most of the other interaction monographs in this publication, some of the information on the antineoplastic drugs is derived from *animal* experiments and *in vitro* studies, so that confirmation of their clinical relevance is still needed. The reason for including these data is that the antineoplastic drugs as a group do not lend themselves readily to the kind of clinical studies that can be undertaken with many other drugs, and there would seem to be justification in this instance for including indirect evidence of this kind. The aim is not to make definite predictions, but to warn users of the interaction possibilities.

Table 17.1 Antineoplastics used in the treatment of cancer

Action	*Drugs*
Alkylating agents, and drugs that appear to have an alkylating action	
Nitrosoureas	Carmustine, Lomustine, Streptozocin
Platinum derivatives	Carboplatin, Cisplatin, Oxaliplatin
Others	Altretamine, Busulfan, Chlorambucil, Chlormethine (Mechlorethamine), Cyclophosphamide, Dacarbazine, Estramustine, Ifosfamide, Melphalan, Temozolomide, Thiotepa
Antimetabolites	
Folate antagonists	Methotrexate, Pemetrexed, Raltitrexed
Podophylotoxin derivatives	Etoposide, Teniposide
Purine analogues	Azathioprine, Cladribine, Fludarabine, Mercaptopurine, Tioguanine
Pyridmidine analogues	Capecitabine, Carmofur, Cytarabine, Fluorouracil, Gemcitabine, Tegafur
Mitotic inhibitors	
Vinca alkaloids	Vinblastine, Vincristine, Vindesine, Vinorelbine
Taxanes	Docetaxel, Paclitaxel
Topoisomerase inhibitors	Irinotecan, Topotecan, 9-Aminocamptothecin
Cytotoxic antibiotics	
Anthracyclines	Aclarubicin, Daunorubicin, Doxorubicin, Epirubicin, Idarubicin, Mitoxantrone
Others	Bleomycin, Dactinomycin, Mitomycin, Plicamycin
Anti-androgens	Bicalutamide, Flutamide, Nilutamide
Anti-oestrogens	
Oestrogen-receptor antagonists	Fulvestrant, Tamoxifen, Toremifene
Aromatase inhibitors	Aminoglutethimide, Anastrozole, Exemestane, Formestane, Letrozole
Miscellaneous	Amsacrine, Asparaginase (Colaspase, Crisantaspase, Pegaspargase), Bexarotene, Erlotinib, Hydroxycarbamide, Imatinib, Mitotane, Pentostatin, Procarbazine, Sorafenib, Thalidomide, Trastuzumab, Tretinoin

Altretamine (Hexamethylmelamine) + Antidepressants

Severe orthostatic hypotension has been described in patients given altretamine with either phenelzine, amitriptyline or imipramine.

Clinical evidence, mechanism, importance and management

Four patients experienced very severe orthostatic hypotension (described by the authors as potentially life-threatening) when they were given altretamine 150 to 250 mg/m² with either **phenelzine** 60 mg daily, **amitriptyline** 50 mg daily or **imipramine** 50 to 150 mg daily.[1] They experienced incapacitating dizziness, severe lightheadedness, and/or fainting within a few days of taking both drugs concurrently. Standing blood pressures as low as 50/30 and 60/40 mmHg were recorded. The reasons are not known. One of the patients had no problems when **imipramine** was replaced by **nortriptyline** 50 mg daily. One other patient who had also taken altretamine with antidepressants reported dizziness, while another noted non-specific discomfort. The incidence of this interaction is unknown, but it is clear that the concurrent use of altretamine and **tricyclics** or **MAOIs** should be closely monitored.

1. Bruckner HW, Schleifer SJ. Orthostatic hypotension as a complication of hexamethylmelamine antidepressant interaction. *Cancer Treat Rep* (1983) 67, 516.

Altretamine (Hexamethylmelamine) + Pyridoxine (Vitamin B$_6$)

Pyridoxine reduced the neurotoxicity associated with altretamine, but also reduced its effectiveness.

Clinical evidence, mechanism, importance and management

In a large randomised study in women with advanced ovarian cancer the neurotoxicity associated with altretamine and cisplatin chemotherapy was reduced by pyridoxine, but the response duration was also reduced.[1] In this study, cisplatin was given on day 1 (37.5 or 75 mg/m²) and altretamine 200 mg/m² daily was given on days 8 to 21, and half the patients also received pyridoxine 100 mg three times daily on days 1 to 21. It is unclear how pyridoxine reduced the activity of this regimen, but the use of pyridoxine (vitamin B$_6$) should probably be avoided in patients receiving altretamine.

1. Wiernik PH, Yeap B, Vogel SE, Kaplan BH, Comis RL, Falkson G, Davis TE, Fazzini E, Cheuvart B, Horton J. Hexamethylmelamine and low or moderate dose cisplatin with or without pyridoxine for treatment of advanced ovarian carcinoma: a study of the Eastern Cooperative Oncology Group. *Cancer Invest* (1992) 10, 1–9.

9-Aminocamptothecin + Antiepileptics

Enzyme-inducing antiepileptics can lower the serum levels of 9-aminocamptothecin.

Clinical evidence, mechanism, importance and management

A study in 59 patients with glioblastoma multiforme or recurrent high grade astrocytomas found that the steady-state plasma levels of 9-aminocamptothecin were reduced to about one-third in 29 of the patients also taking antiepileptics (**carbamazepine**, **phenobarbital**, **phenytoin**, sodium valproate). The incidence of myelosuppression was greater in those not taking antiepileptics.[1] A further study also found that the clearance of 9-aminocamptothecin was increased by **carbamazepine** and **phenytoin**.[2] The reason for the reduced 9-aminocamptothecin levels is not known, but it seems likely that it was due to the enzyme-inducing activity of **carbamazepine**, **phenobarbital** and **phenytoin**. These results suggest that higher than usual doses of 9-aminocamptothecin are possibly needed in the presence of enzyme-inducing antiepileptics. Related topoisomerase inhibitors are similarly affected, see 'Irinotecan + Antiepileptics', p.638, and 'Topotecan + Phenytoin', p.667.

1. Grossman SA, Hochberg F, Fisher J, Chen T-L, Kim L, Gregory R, Grochow LB, Piantadosi S. Increased 9-aminocamptothecin dose requirements in patients on anticonvulsants. *Cancer Chemother Pharmacol* (1998) 42, 118–26.
2. Minami H, Lad TE, Nicholas MK, Vokes EE, Ratain MJ. Pharmacokinetics and pharmacodynamics of 9-aminocamptothecin infused over 72 hours in phase II studies. *Clin Cancer Res* (1999) 5, 1325–30.

Aminoglutethimide + Danazol

Danazol may reduce the efficacy of aminoglutethimide.

Clinical evidence, mechanism, importance and management

In a randomised clinical study, giving danazol with aminoglutethimide in women with breast cancer, reduced the response rate compared with aminoglutethimide alone. It was found that danazol suppresses sex hormone binding globulin leading to increased free oestradiol, which counteracts the oestradiol suppressive effect of aminoglutethimide.[1] Danazol should probably not be combined with anti-oestrogenic treatments.

1. Dowsett M, Murray RML, Pitt P, Jeffcoate SL. Antagonism of aminoglutethimide and danazol in the suppression of serum free oestradiol in breast cancer patients. *Eur J Cancer Clin Oncol* (1985) 21, 1063–8.

Aminoglutethimide + Diuretics

A single case report describes hyponatraemia, which occurred after a patient had taken aminoglutethimide and bendroflumethiazide for 10 months.

Clinical evidence, mechanism, importance and management

A woman who, for several years, had been taking **bendroflumethiazide** 10 mg daily and **potassium chloride** 578 mg for hypertension and mild cardiac decompensation, was given aminoglutethimide 1 g daily, and hydrocortisone 60 mg daily, for breast cancer. After 10 months of treatment she was hospitalised with severe hyponatraemia, which resolved on withdrawal of all the drugs. No significant change in electrolytes occurred over 3 months when the aminoglutethimide and hydrocortisone were used alone, but serum sodium fell again when the diuretic was restarted. The serum sodium levels were subsequently maintained by the addition of fludrocortisone 100 micrograms daily.[1] The hyponatraemia was thought to be caused by the combined inhibitory effect of the aminoglutethimide on aldosterone production (which normally retains sodium in the body) and the sodium loss caused by the diuretic. Plasma electrolytes should be monitored when aminoglutethimide is used, and this would seem particularly important if it is given with any diuretic.

1. Bork E, Hansen M. Severe hyponatremia following simultaneous administration of aminoglutethimide and diuretics. *Cancer Treat Rep* (1986) 70, 689–90.

5-Aminolevulinic acid + St John's wort (*Hypericum perforatum*)

An isolated case report describes a severe phototoxic reaction attributed to a synergistic effect of 5-aminolevulinic acid and St John's wort.

Clinical evidence, mechanism, importance and management

A 47-year-old woman experienced a phototoxic reaction on skin areas exposed to light 6 hours after receiving 5-aminolevulinic acid 40 mg/kg. She developed a burning erythematous rash and severe swelling of the face, neck and hands. Treatment with oral corticosteroids resulted in complete resolution after skin desquamation. She was also taking St John's wort (*Hyperiforce*), and it was suggested that there was a synergistic photosensitivity reaction between the two drugs. *In vitro* studies confirmed this.[1] This appears to be the only report of such an effect, but bear it in mind in the event of an unexpected adverse reaction to 5-aminolevulinic acid.

1. Ladner DP, Klein SD, Steiner RA, Walt H. Synergistic toxicity of δ-aminolaevulinic acid-induced protoporphyrin IX used for photodiagnosis and hypericum extract, a herbal antidepressant. *Br J Dermatol* (2001) 144, 901–22.

Anastrozole + Miscellaneous

Anastrozole does not appear to interact with aspirin, cimetidine, digoxin, oral antidiabetics or quinapril. It also appears to have no effect on cytochrome P450 enzymes, so it is unlikely to interact with drugs that are affected by enzyme inducers or inhibitors.

Clinical evidence, mechanism, importance and management

In a pharmacokinetic study, 10 elderly women with breast cancer were given anastrozole 1 mg daily for 10 weeks and 5 of them who also had hypertension were additionally given **quinapril**, after week 4, for 28 days. **Quinapril** did not affect plasma anastrozole levels and dose modification is not required during concurrent use.[1] A clinical study with **cimetidine** has shown that it does not affect the pharmacokinetics of anastrozole,[2] which suggests that anastrozole is unlikely to be affected by other drugs that inhibit cytochrome P450. Another clinical study showed that anastrozole does not affect the pharmacokinetics of **antipyrine (phenazone)**,[3] so that it is unlikely to interact with those drugs which are known to be affected by enzyme inducers and inhibitors.

The UK manufacturers also say that in clinical studies there was no evidence of any interactions between anastrozole and commonly used drugs;[4] **aspirin**, **digoxin**, and **oral antidiabetics** were specifically mentioned in the early product information.[5]

1. Repetto L, Vannozzi O, Hazini A, Sestini A, Pietropaolo M, Rosso R. Anastrozole and quinapril can be safely coadministered to elderly women with breast cancer and hypertension: a pharmacokinetic study. *Ann Oncol* (2003) 14, 1587–90.
2. Zeneca. Effect of cimetidine on anastrozole pharmacokinetics. Data on file, 1995.
3. Zeneca. Effect of anastrozole treatment on antipyrine pharmacokinetics in postmenopausal female volunteers. Data on file, 1995.
4. Arimidex (Anastrozole). AstraZeneca UK Ltd. UK Summary of product characteristics, June 2006.
5. Arimidex (Anastrozole) Monograph. Zeneca. September 1995.

Anthracyclines + Calcium-channel blockers

Verapamil can increase the efficacy of doxorubicin in tissue culture systems and increase doxorubicin levels in patients. D-verapamil can alter the pharmacokinetics of epirubicin and possibly increase its bone marrow depressant effects.

Clinical evidence, mechanism, importance and management

(a) Doxorubicin

The efficacy of doxorubicin can be increased by **verapamil** and **nicardipine** in doxorubicin-resistant tissue culture systems,[1] while **nifedipine** has only minimal activity. A study in five patients with small cell lung cancer given doxorubicin, vincristine, etoposide and cyclophosphamide showed that when they were given **verapamil** 240 to 480 mg daily the AUC of doxorubicin was doubled, its peak serum levels were raised and its clearance was reduced. No increased toxicity was seen in this study.[2] However, although another study found no increase in non-cardiac toxicities, **verapamil** caused an unacceptable degree of cardiac toxicity.[3] Be alert for this possibility if both drugs are used.

(b) Epirubicin

When used to reduce multidrug resistance in patients with advanced colorectal cancer receiving epirubicin, the **D-isomer of verapamil** appears to increase the bone marrow depressant toxicity of epirubicin.[4] Another study found that **D-verapamil** halved the AUC and half-life of epirubicin, and increased its clearance,[5] while yet another did not find these changes but found that the production of the metabolites of epirubicin was increased.[6] These changes should be taken into account if both drugs are used. More study is needed to evaluate the possible advantages and disadvantages of giving these drugs together.

1. Ramu A, Spanier R, Rahamimoff H, Fuks Z. Restoration of doxorubicin responsiveness in doxorubicin-resistant P388 murine leukaemia cells. *Br J Cancer* (1984) 50, 501–7.
2. Kerr DJ, Graham J, Cummings J, Morrison JG, Thompson GG, Brodie MJ, Kaye SB. The effect of verapamil on the pharmacokinetics of adriamycin. *Cancer Chemother Pharmacol* (1986) 18, 239–42.
3. Ozols RF, Cunnion RE, Klecker RW, Hamilton TC, Ostchega Y, Parrillo JE, Young RC. Verapamil and adriamycin in the treatment of drug-resistant ovarian cancer patients. *J Clin Oncol* (1987) 5, 641–7.
4. Scheithauer W, Kornek G, Kastner J, Raderer M, Locker G, Depisch D, Pidlich J, Tetzner C. Phase II study of d-verapamil and doxorubicin in patients with metastatic colorectal cancer. *Eur J Cancer* (1993) 29A, 2337–8.
5. Scheithauer W, Schenk T, Czejka M. Pharmacokinetic interaction between epirubicin and the multidrug resistance reverting agent D-verapamil. *Br J Cancer* (1993) 68, 8–9.
6. Mross K, Hamm K, Hossfeld DK. Effects of verapamil on the pharmacokinetics and metabolism of epirubicin. *Cancer Chemother Pharmacol* (1993) 31, 369–75.

Anthracyclines + Ciclosporin

High-dose ciclosporin increases the serum levels and the myelotoxicity of doxorubicin. An isolated report describes severe neurotoxicity and coma in a patient who had taken ciclosporin and was then subsequently given doxorubicin. Ciclosporin can also increase daunorubicin, epirubicin, idarubicin and mitoxantrone serum levels.

Clinical evidence

(a) Daunorubicin

In a randomised study in patients treated with daunorubicin, ciclosporin significantly reduced the frequency of resistance to induction therapy (31% versus 47%) and increased relapse-free and overall survival. Ciclosporin recipients had higher steady-state serum levels of daunorubicin and its active metabolite daunorubicinol.[1]

(b) Doxorubicin

Eight patients with small cell lung cancer were given an initial course of doxorubicin (25 to 70 mg/m^2 over 1 hour) and a subsequent ciclosporin-modulated doxorubicin course (ciclosporin 6 mg/kg bolus, then 16 mg/kg daily for 2 days) for multidrug resistant tumour modulation. All of the patients were also given cyclophosphamide and vincristine. Ciclosporin increased the AUC of doxorubicin by 48%, and that of its active metabolite doxorubicinol by 443%. The myelotoxicity was increased by concurrent use: the leucocyte count fell by 84% after doxorubicin and by 91% after doxorubicin with ciclosporin, and the platelet counts fell by 36% and 73%, respectively. The patients showed significant weight loss and severe myalgias.[2]

Three preliminary phase I studies[3-5] are consistent with this report. In these studies, ciclosporin was found to increase the doxorubicin AUC by 40 to 73%, and the doxorubicinol AUC by 250 to 285%. However, no evidence of increased cardiotoxicity was found in a study of 23 patients given ciclosporin and doxorubicin.[6]

A cardiac transplant patient was given ciclosporin 2 mg/kg daily for 22 months. The ciclosporin was stopped and he was given doxorubicin 60 mg, vincristine 2 mg, cyclophosphamide 600 mg and prednisone 80 mg to treat Burkitt's lymphoma stage IVB. Eight hours later he developed disturbances of consciousness which lead to stage I coma, from which he spontaneously recovered 12 hours later. A week later a similar course of chemotherapy was started, and 10 to 15 minutes later he lost consciousness and generalised tonic clonic seizures progressively developed. He died 8 days later without recovering consciousness.[7]

(c) Epirubicin

Preliminary evidence suggests that ciclosporin can markedly increase the AUC of epirubicin (up to about fourfold) and increase the bone marrow suppression.[5] Ciclosporin did not increase the cardiotoxicity of epirubicin in 20 patients in one study.[6]

(d) Idarubicin

The concurrent use of ciclosporin and idarubicin increased the AUC of idarubicin and its active metabolite idarubicinol by 77% and 181%, respectively, in 9 patients, when compared with 11 patients receiving idarubicin alone.[8] Unacceptable toxicity occurred when idarubicin 9 or 12 mg/m^2 daily was combined with ciclosporin 16 mg/kg daily, when compared with idarubicin 12 mg/m^2 alone: 3 of 7 patients treated with the combination died. Increases in the AUC of idarubicin and idarubicinol produced by ciclosporin have also been reported elsewhere.[9]

(e) Mitoxantrone

The pharmacokinetics of mitoxantrone 10 mg/m^2 daily were compared with mitoxantrone 6 mg/m^2 (a 40% reduction in dose) with high-dose ciclosporin in children. The ciclosporin recipients had a 42% reduction in mitoxantrone clearance, a 12% increase in mitoxantrone AUC, and similar toxicity.[10]

Mechanism

Uncertain. One reason may be that the ciclosporin affects the P-glycoprotein of the biliary tract so that the clearance of these anthracyclines in the bile is reduced. An additional reason may be that ciclosporin inhibits the metabolism of metabolites, such as doxorubicinol, so that they accumulate.[2] The increased levels of both would explain the increases in toxicity. It is not clear why such severe neurotoxicity was seen in one patient.

Importance and management

An established and clinically important interaction. Ciclosporin alters the pharmacokinetics of the anthracyclines resulting in increased serum levels. This pharmacokinetic interaction has complicated study into the value of using ciclosporin to modulate multidrug resistance in tumours and thereby improve the response to chemotherapy. In the case of anthracyclines and 'etoposide', (p.630), any benefit could just be attributed to dose intensification. Consequently, some have suggested reducing the dose of the anthracycline.[10] The use of high-dose ciclosporin for multidrug resistant tumour modulation remains experimental and should only be used in clinical studies. Concurrent use should be very well monitored. More study is needed to find out the possible effects of low-dose ciclosporin.

1. List AF, Kopecky KL, Willman CL, Head DR, Persons DL, Slovak ML, Dorr R, Karanes C, Hynes HE, Doroshow JH, Shurafa M, Appelbaum FR. Benefit of cyclosporine modulation of drug resistance in patients with poor-risk acute myeloid leukemia: a Southwest Oncology Group study. *Blood* (2001) 98, 3212–20.
2. Rushing DA, Raber SR, Rodvold KA, Piscitelli SC, Plank GS, Tewksbury DA. The effects of cyclosporine on the pharmacokinetics of doxorubicin in patients with small cell lung cancer. *Cancer* (1994) 74, 834–41.
3. Scheulen ME, Budach W, Skorzec M, Wiefelspütz JK, Seeber S. Influence of cyclosporin A on the pharmacokinetics and pharmacodynamics of doxorubicin. *Proc Am Assoc Cancer Res* (1993) 34, 213.
4. Bartlett NL, Lum BL, Fisher GA, Brophy NA, Ehsan MN, Halsey J, Sikic BI. Phase I trial of doxorubicin with cyclosporine as a modulator of multidrug resistance. *J Clin Oncol* (1994) 12, 835–42.
5. Eggert J, Scheulen ME, Schütte J, Budach W, Annweiler HM, Mengelkolch B, Skorzec M, Wiefelspütz J, Sack H, Seeber S. Influence of cyclosporin A on the pharmacokinetics and pharmacodynamics of doxorubicin and epirubicin. *Ann Hematol* (1994) 68, A26.
6. Eising EG, Gries P, Eggert J, Scheulen ME. Does the multi-drug resistance modulator cyclosporin A increase the cardiotoxicity of high-dose anthracycline chemotherapy. *Acta Oncol* (1997) 36, 735–40.
7. Barbui T, Rambaldi A, Parenzan L, Zucchelli M, Perico N, Remuzzi G. Neurological symptoms and coma associated with doxorubicin administration during chronic cyclosporin therapy. *Lancet* (1992) 339, 1421.
8. Pea F, Damiani D, Michieli M, Ermacora A, Baraldo M, Russo D, Fanin R, Baccarani M, Furlanut M. Multidrug resistance modulation in vivo: the effect of cyclosporin A alone or with dexverapamil on idarubicin pharmacokinetics in acute leukemia. *Eur J Clin Pharmacol* (1999) 55, 361–8.
9. Smeets M, Raymakers R, Muus P, Vierwinden G, Linssen P, Masereeuw R, de Witte T. Cyclosporin increases cellular idarubicin and idarubicinol concentrations in relapsed or refractory AML mainly due to reduced systemic clearance. *Leukemia* (2001) 15, 80–8.
10. Lacayo NJ, Lum BL, Becton DL, Weinstein H, Ravindranath Y, Chang MN, Bomgaars L, Lauer SJ, Sikic BI. Pharmacokinetic interactions of cyclosporine with etoposide and mitoxantrone in children with acute myeloid leukemia. *Leukemia* (2002) 16, 920–7.

Anthracyclines + Taxanes

Toxicity associated with combinations of paclitaxel with doxorubicin or epirubicin depends on the order of administration. Some modest pharmacokinetic changes may occur when paclitaxel and epirubicin are given together. The combination of doxorubicin and paclitaxel is more cardiotoxic than doxorubicin alone: paclitaxel increases doxorubicin levels but doxorubicin does not alter paclitaxel levels. Docetaxel may modestly affect the pharmacokinetics of epirubicin and doxorubicin.

Clinical evidence

(a) Doxorubicin

Early studies in patients with breast cancer found a higher frequency of toxicity (particularly mucositis) when **paclitaxel** was given before doxorubicin (given as 24-hour and 48-hour infusions, respectively).[1] A subsequent study with similar effects revealed that doxorubicin clearance was reduced by one-third if **paclitaxel** was given first.[2] In another study the peak plasma levels of doxorubicin were increased when it was given by bolus injection 15 minutes after a 3-hour infusion of **paclitaxel**. The effect was non-linear and dependent on the dose of **paclitaxel**.[3] The same authors had already shown that this regimen produced a higher than expected incidence of cardiac toxicity.[4] Subsequent studies[5,6] have shown this schedule to result in unacceptable cardiotoxicity when the total cumulative doxorubicin dose exceeds 340 to 380 mg/m^2. However, when **paclitaxel** and doxorubicin were given together as a 3-hour infusion the levels of doxorubicin were lower than when it was given before **paclitaxel**,[3] and in another study the pharmacokinetics of each drug were found to be unchanged when they were given simultaneously as a 72-hour infusion.[7]

In 10 patients the AUC of intravenous pegylated liposomal doxorubicin (*Caelyx*) 30 to 35 mg/m^2 was increased by a mean of 80% when it was given with intravenous **paclitaxel** 70 or 175 mg/m^2. Peak plasma levels of doxorubicin were also increased and clearance was reduced by 71%. In 9 other patients given *Caelyx* with **docetaxel** 30 or 60 mg/m^2, the AUC of doxorubicin was increased by 12% and clearance reduced by only 16%.[8]

In a study, 627 patients with breast cancer were given either doxorubicin 50 mg/m^2 with **docetaxel** 75 mg/m^2, or doxorubicin 60 mg/m^2 with cyclophosphamide 600 mg/m^2 postoperatively for 4 courses to assess disease-free survival at 5 years. The study was terminated prematurely because of the high risk of life-threatening complications in those given doxorubicin with **docetaxel** (2 deaths associated with drug toxicity and one case of perforated peritonitis in patients with febrile neutropenia). The incidence of febrile neutropenia was 40.8% and 7.1% in the doxorubicin-**docetaxel** and doxorubicin-cyclophosphamide groups, respectively.[9]

A woman with recurrence of breast cancer developed pseudomembranous colitis (non-*Clostridium difficile*) and cholestatic jaundice 6 days after completing her first cycle of treatment with doxorubicin and **docetaxel** and again 4 days after the second cycle about one month later.[10]

(b) Epirubicin

The pharmacokinetics of epirubicin were compared in 4 patients with breast cancer given intravenous epirubicin 90 mg/m^2 alone and 16 patients given the same dose followed immediately either by **paclitaxel** 175 mg/m^2 as a 3-hour infusion or **docetaxel** 70 mg/m^2 as a 1-hour infusion. No effect on epirubicin levels was detected, but the concentrations of epirubicin metabolites (epirubicinol and deoxydoxorubicinone) were increased by both **paclitaxel** and **docetaxel**.[11] In a subsequent study 21 patients were given the same regimen of epirubicin followed immediately by **paclitaxel** and 18 patients were given the drugs in the reverse order. Non-haematological toxicity was unaffected by the order of administration but when **paclitaxel** was given first the neutrophil and platelet nadir was lower and neutrophil recovery was slower. The AUC for epirubicin was also higher when **paclitaxel** was given first but the pharmacokinetics of **paclitaxel** were unaffected.[12] In one study, 21 women with breast cancer were given intravenous epirubicin 90 mg/m^2 followed 15 minutes later by a 3-hour intravenous infusion of **paclitaxel** 175 mg/m^2 (6 patients), 200 mg/m^2 (9 patients), or 225 mg/m^2 (6 patients). Six women were given **paclitaxel** 200 mg/m^2 30 hours after epirubicin. A significant increase in the AUC of epirubicin occurred with **paclitaxel** 200 mg/m^2 (23%) and 225 mg/m^2 (34%) and increases in the AUC of the metabolite of epirubicin (epirubicinol) occurred at all dose levels of **paclitaxel** compared with those found when epirubicin was given 30 hours before **paclitaxel**.[13] In another study, exposure to epirubicin metabolites, but not epirubicin itself, was increased when it was given 15 minutes before a 3-hour infusion of **paclitaxel**, when compared to a regimen using a 24-hour interval between the two drugs. In addition, the neutrophil nadir was lower, and clearance of **paclitaxel** was 30% slower with the former regimen, but cardiac toxicity was uncommon.[14]

Conversely, a study of the combination of **docetaxel** and epirubicin did not find that the sequence of drug administration affected the pharmacokinetics of epirubicin, nor was there any difference in toxicity.[15] In another study, 16 patients with breast cancer had a transient but significant increase in epirubicin plasma levels during the subsequent infusion (after an interval of 1 hour) of **docetaxel** 75 mg/m^2, which was not seen if the **docetaxel** was given within 10 minutes of epirubicin.[16]

Mechanism

Studies in *mice* have found that the taxanes docetaxel and paclitaxel, and the vehicle used for paclitaxel *Cremophor*, may all modify the distribution and metabolism of doxorubicin increasing its levels in the heart, liver and kidneys. This may contribute to the cardiac toxicity seen during use with paclitaxel.[17] Similarly, *in vitro* studies in human myocardium showed that paclitaxel and docetaxel increased the conversion of doxorubicin to doxorubicinol, the metabolite that is thought to be responsible for cardiotoxicity.[18] An *in vitro* study on the effect of paclitaxel and *Cremophor* on epirubicin metabolism in human blood found that paclitaxel slightly decreased production of epirubicinol. A marked inhibition of epirubicinol production occurred in the presence of *Cremophor*, but because of the low volume of distribution of *Cremophor* this is not likely to be of clinical significance.[13] In addition, *in vitro* studies have shown that the taxanes may reduce the biliary excretion of doxorubicin and epirubicin by inhibiting P-glycoprotein,[3] and inhibition of epirubicinol excretion via competition for P-glycoprotein by paclitaxel and *Cremophor* may be significant.[13]

The case of pseudomembranous colitis and cholestatic jaundice in one patient was attributed to the combination of docetaxel and doxorubicin, but the patient was also receiving long-term treatment with erythromycin and omeprazole which may have contributed to the interaction by inhibiting docetaxel metabolism by the cytochrome P450 isoenzyme CYP3A.[10]

Importance and management

The effect of paclitaxel on doxorubicin appears to be established. It has been noted that when paclitaxel or docetaxel are given with pegylated doxorubicin, exposure to doxorubicin is increased by at least 50% and less than 20%, respectively and that this should be taken into account during concurrent use.[8] Various strategies have been suggested to reduce the cardiotoxicity of the combination of doxorubicin and taxanes. These include giving doxorubicin at least 24 hours before paclitaxel; reducing the cumulative dose of doxorubicin; or adding the cytoprotective drug dexrazoxane.[19] Epirubicin is considered less cardiotoxic than doxorubicin, and may be an alternative in some situations. However, it still appears preferable to give the anthracycline before the taxane. Docetaxel appears to have little clinically relevant effect on epirubicin, but this requires confirmation. Further study is needed on the optimum scheduling of anthracyclines and taxanes to maximise efficacy and minimise toxicity.

1. Sledge GW, Robert N, Sparano JA, Cogleigh M, Goldstein LJ, Neuberg D, Rowinsky E, Baughman C, McCaskill-Stevens W. Eastern Cooperative Oncology Group studies of paclitaxel and doxorubicin in advanced breast cancer. *Semin Oncol* (1995) 22, 105–8.
2. Holmes FA, Madden T, Newman RA, Valero V, Theriault RL, Fraschini G, Walters RS, Booser DJ, Buzdar AU, Willey J, Hortobagyi GN. Sequence-dependent alteration of doxorubicin pharmacokinetics by paclitaxel in a phase I study of paclitaxel and doxorubicin in patients with metastatic breast cancer. *J Clin Oncol* (1996) 14, 2713–21.
3. Gianni L, Viganò L, Locatelli A, Capri G, Giani A, Tarenzi E, Bonadonna G. Human pharmacokinetic characterization and in vitro study of the interaction between doxorubicin and paclitaxel in patients with breast cancer. *J Clin Oncol* (1997) 15, 1906–15.
4. Gianni L, Munzone E, Capri G, Fulfaro F, Tarenzi E, Villani F, Spreafico C, Laffranchi A, Caraceni A, Martini C, Stefanelli M, Valagussa P, Bonadonna G. Paclitaxel by 3-hour infusion in combination with bolus doxorubicin in women with untreated metastatic breast cancer: high antitumor efficacy and cardiac effects in a dose-finding and sequence-finding study. *J Clin Oncol* (1995) 13, 2688–99.
5. Gianni L, Dombernowsky P, Sledge G, Martin M, Amadori D, Arbuck SG, Ravdin P, Brown M, Messina M, Tuck D, Weil C, Winograd B. Cardiac function following combination therapy with paclitaxel and doxorubicin: an analysis of 657 women with advanced breast cancer. *Ann Oncol* (2001) 12, 1067–73.
6. Giordano SH, Booser DJ, Murray JL, Ibrahim NK, Rahman ZU, Valero V, Theriault RL, Rosales MF, Rivera E, Frye D, Ewer M, Ordonez NG, Buzdar AU, Hortobagyi GN. A detailed evaluation of cardiac toxicity: a phase II study of doxorubicin and one- or three-hour-infusion paclitaxel in patients with metastatic breast cancer. *Clin Cancer Res* (2002) 8, 3360–8.
7. Berg SL, Cowan KH, Balis FM, Fisherman JS, Denicoff AM, Hillig M, Poplack DG, O'Shaughnessy JA. Pharmacokinetics of Taxol and doxorubicin administered alone and in combination by continuous 72-hour infusion. *J Natl Cancer Inst* (1994) 86, 143–5.
8. Briasoulis E, Karavasilis V, Tzamakou E, Rammou D, Soulti K, Piperidou C, Pavlidis N. Interaction pharmacokinetics of pegylated liposomal doxorubicin (Caelyx) on coadministration with paclitaxel or docetaxel. *Cancer Chemother Pharmacol* (2004) 53, 452–7.
9. Brain EGC, Bachelot T, Serin D, Kirscher S, Graic Y, Eymard J-C, Extra J-M, Combe M, Fourme E, Noguès C, Rouëssé J, RAPP-01 Trial Investigators. Life-threatening sepsis associated with adjuvant doxorubicin plus docetaxel for intermediate-risk breast cancer. *JAMA* (2005) 293, 2367–71.
10. Sundar S, Chan SY. Cholestatic jaundice and pseudomembranous colitis following combination therapy with doxorubicin and docetaxel. *Anticancer Drugs* (2003) 14, 327–9.
11. Eposito M, Venturini M, Vannozzi MO, Tolino G, Lunardi G, Garrone O, Angiolini C, Viale M, Bergaglio M, Del Mastro L, Rosso R. Comparative effects of paclitaxel and docetaxel on the metabolism and pharmacokinetics of epirubicin in breast cancer patients. *J Clin Oncol* (1999) 17, 1132–40.
12. Venturini M, Lunardi G, Del Mastro L, Vannozzi MO, Tolino G, Numico G, Viale M, Pastrone I, Angiolini C, Bertelli G, Straneo M, Rosso R, Esposito M. Sequence effect of epirubicin and paclitaxel treatment on pharmacokinetics and toxicity. *J Clin Oncol* (2000) 18, 2116–25.
13. Danesi R, Innocenti F, Fogli S, Gennari A, Baldini E, Di Paolo A, Salvadori B, Bocci G, Conte PF, Del Tacca M. Pharmacokinetics and pharmacodynamics of combination chemotherapy with paclitaxel and epirubicin in breast cancer patients. *Br J Clin Pharmacol* (2002) 53, 508–18.
14. Grasselli G, Viganò L, Capri G, Locatelli A, Tarenzi E, Spreafico C, Bertuzzi A, Giani A, Materazzo C, Cresta S, Perotti A, Valagussa P, Gianni L. Clinical and pharmacologic study of the epirubicin and paclitaxel combination in women with metastatic breast cancer. *J Clin Oncol* (2001) 19, 2222–31.
15. Lunardi G, Venturini M, Vannozzi MO, Tolino G, Del Mastro L, Bighin C, Schettini G, Esposito M. Influence of alternate sequences of epirubicin and docetaxel on the pharmacokinetic behaviour of both drugs in advanced breast cancer. *Ann Oncol* (2002) 13, 280–5.
16. Ceruti M, Tagini V, Recalenda V, Arpicco S, Cattel L, Airoldi M, Bumma C. Docetaxel in combination with epirubicin in metastatic breast cancer: pharmacokinetic interactions. *Farmaco* (1999) 54, 733–9.
17. Colombo T, Parisi I, Zucchetti M, Sessa C, Goldhirsch A, D'Incalci M. Pharmacokinetic interactions of paclitaxel, docetaxel and their vehicles with doxorubicin. *Ann Oncol* (1999) 10, 391–5.
18. Minotti G, Saponiero A, Licata S, Menna P, Calafiore AM, Teodori G, Gianni L. Paclitaxel and docetaxel enhance the metabolism of doxorubicin to toxic species in human myocardium. *Clin Cancer Res* (2001) 7, 1511–15.
19. Sparano JA. Use of dexrazoxane and other strategies to prevent cardiomyopathy associated with doxorubicin-taxane combinations. *Semin Oncol* (1998) 25 (Suppl 10), 66–71.

Anthracyclines; Aclarubicin + Other antineoplastics

The bone marrow depressant effects of aclarubicin can be particularly severe in patients who have previously been treated with nitrosoureas or mitomycin. Aclarubicin appears not to interact with cyclophosphamide, cytarabine, enocitabine (behenoyl cytarabine), fluorouracil, mercaptopurine, tioguanine or vincristine.

Clinical evidence, mechanism, importance and management

Myelosuppression is among the adverse effects of aclarubicin. The concurrent use of other drugs with similar myelosuppressant actions may be expected to have additive effects. Previous treatment with **nitrosoureas** (not specifically named) or **mitomycin** has been shown to increase the severity of the myelosuppression.[1,2]

1. Van Echo DA, Whitacre MY, Aisner J, Applefeld MM, Wiernik PH. Phase I trial of aclacinomycin A. *Cancer Treat Rep* (1982) 66, 1127–32.
2. Bedikian AY, Karlin D, Stroehlein J, Valdivieso M, Korinek J, Bodey G. Phase II evaluation of aclacinomycin A (ACM-A, NSC208734) in patients with metastatic colorectal cancer. *Am J Clin Oncol* (1983) 6, 187–190.

Anthracyclines; Doxorubicin + Barbiturates

The effects of doxorubicin may be reduced by the barbiturates.

Clinical evidence, mechanism, importance and management

A comparative study in patients given doxorubicin found that those also taking barbiturates had a plasma clearance that was 50% higher than those who were not (318 mL/minute compared with 202 mL/minute).[1] This clinical study is in agreement with previous studies in *mice*.[2] A possible explanation is that the barbiturate increases the metabolism of the doxorubicin. It seems possible that the dosage of doxorubicin will need to be increased in barbiturate-treated patients to achieve maximal therapeutic effects.

1. Riggs CE, Engel S, Wesley M, Wiernik PH, Bachur NR. Doxorubicin pharmacokinetics, prochlorperazine and barbiturate effects. *Clin Pharmacol Ther* (1982) 31, 263.
2. Reich SD, Bachur NR. Alterations in adriamycin efficacy by phenobarbital. *Cancer* (1976) 36, 3803–6.

Anthracyclines; Doxorubicin + Tamoxifen

Tamoxifen appears to have no significant effect on the pharmacokinetics of doxorubicin.

Clinical evidence, mechanism, importance and management

A pharmacokinetic study in patients with non-Hodgkin's lymphoma receiving CHOP (cyclophosphamide, vincristine, prednisone and doxorubicin 37.5 to 50 mg/m^2) found that the addition of tamoxifen 480 mg daily for 5 days had no significant effect on the AUC or total clearance of doxorubicin.[1] For the possible additive thromboembolic effect of doxorubicin and tamoxifen, see 'Antineoplastics + Tamoxifen', p.616.

1. El-Yazigi A, Berry J, Ezzat A, Wahab FA. Effect of tamoxifen on the pharmacokinetics of doxorubicin in patients with non-Hodgkin's lymphoma. *Ther Drug Monit* (1997) 19, 632–6.

Anthracyclines; Epirubicin + Cimetidine

Cimetidine can increase epirubicin serum levels.

Clinical evidence, mechanism, importance and management

In a study in 8 patients, cimetidine 400 mg twice daily increased the AUC of epirubicin by 50%. At the same time the AUCs of two metabolites of epirubicin, epirubicinol and 7-deoxydoxorubicinol aglycone, increased by 41% and 357%, respectively. Liver blood flow also increased by 17%.[1] The mechanism is unknown. More study of this interaction is needed but be aware of the possibility of cimetidine increasing the exposure to epirubicin; monitor the patient closely and adjust epirubicin dosage if needed. Cimetidine is available without a prescription in some countries so that patients may unwittingly increase the toxicity of epirubicin. Cimetidine has also increased the levels or toxicity of some other antineoplastics, see 'Nitrosoureas + Cimetidine', p.655, 'Cyclophosphamide + H_2-receptor antagonists', p.626 and 'Fluorouracil + H_2-receptor antagonists', p.633.

1. Murray LS, Jodrell DI, Morrison JG, Cook A, Kerr DJ, Whiting B, Kaye SB, Cassidy J. The effect of cimetidine on the pharmacokinetics of epirubicin in patients with advanced breast cancer: preliminary evidence of a potentially common drug interaction. *Clin Oncol* (1998) 10, 35–8.

Antineoplastics + Aprepitant

Aprepitant had no effect on the pharmacokinetics of a single dose of docetaxel. The activation of cyclophosphamide and thiotepa was slightly lower in patients receiving aprepitant, but this was not clinically relevant. However, because of the possibility of increased toxicity the manufacturer recommends caution with antineoplastics principally metabolised by the cytochrome P450 isoenzyme CYP3A4, particularly irinotecan, and also etoposide, vinorelbine, paclitaxel, ifosfamide, imatinib, vinblastine and vincristine, although there appears to be some limited evidence of safe concurrent use.

Clinical evidence

(a) Cyclophosphamide

The rate of auto-induction of cyclophosphamide was 23% lower and exposure to the active metabolite 4-hydroxycyclophosphamide was 5% lower in 6 patients receiving aprepitant with a 4-day course of high-dose CTC (cyclophosphamide, thiotepa, carboplatin) when compared with 49 patients receiving high-dose CTC without aprepitant.[1]

(b) Docetaxel

Aprepitant 125 mg given one hour before docetaxel on day one, then 80 mg daily on days 2 and 3 had no effect on the pharmacokinetics of a single 60- to 100-mg/m^2 infusion of docetaxel in 10 cancer patients, and did not alter the toxicity profile. Each subject acted as their own control.[2]

(c) Thiotepa

The formation clearance of thiotepa was 33% lower and exposure to the active metabolite TEPA (triethylenephosphamide) was 20% lower in 6 patients receiving aprepitant with a 4-day course of high-dose CTC (cyclophosphamide, thiotepa, carboplatin) when compared with 49 patients receiving high-dose CTC without aprepitant.[1]

Mechanism

In the short-term, aprepitant is an inhibitor of the cytochrome P450 isoenzyme CYP3A4, and might therefore reduce the activation of antineoplastics activated by this isoenzyme (cyclophosphamide, thiotepa), or increase the toxicity of antineoplastics metabolised by this enzyme (docetaxel, irinotecan).

Importance and management

The UK manufacturer of aprepitant recommends caution when it is used with antineoplastics that are metabolised by CYP3A4, particularly **irinotecan**, because of the possibility of increased toxicity with this drug.[3] They also mention that **etoposide**, **vinorelbine**, docetaxel, **paclitaxel**,[3,4] **ifosfamide**, **imatinib**, **vinblastine** and **vincristine**,[4] were given without dosage adjustment for potential interactions, but as this was not a formal interaction study they recommend caution. However, with intravenous docetaxel, it appears that no important changes in pharmacokinetics occur, and therefore dosage adjustments are unlikely to be needed for this drug, and possibly also other intravenous antineoplastics metabolised by CYP3A4.[2] Similarly, the minor reductions in the activation of cyclophosphamide and thiotepa were considered small compared to total variability, and therefore unlikely to be clinically important.

1. de Jonge ME, Huitaema AD, Holtkamp MJ, van Dam SM, Beijnen JH, Rodenhuis S. Aprepitant inhibits cyclophosphamide bioactivation and thiotepa metabolism. *Cancer Chemother Pharmacol* (2005) 56, 370–8. Epub 2005, Apr 19.
2. Nygren P, Hande K, Petty KJ, Fedgchin M, van Dyck K, Majumdar A, Panebianco D, de Smet M, Ahmed T, Murphy MG, Gottesdiener KM, Cocquyt V, van Belle S. Lack of effect of aprepitant on the pharmacokinetics of docetaxel in cancer patients. *Cancer Chemother Pharmacol* (2005) 55, 609–16.
3. Emend (Aprepitant). Merck Sharp & Dohme Ltd. UK Summary of product characteristics, February 2007.
4. Emend (Aprepitant). Merck & Co., Inc. US Prescribing information, June 2006.

Antineoplastics + Colony-stimulating factors

Because of the increased risk of myelosuppression, colony-stimulating factors such as filgrastim, lenograstim, and molgramostim should not be given at the same time as myelosuppressive cytotoxic antineoplastics.

Clinical evidence, mechanism, importance and management

Colony-stimulating factors such as filgrastim, lenograstim, and molgramostim promote the growth of myeloid cell lines. Since rapidly dividing myeloid cells have increased sensitivity to cytotoxic chemotherapy the manufacturers have advised that these drugs should not be used from 24 hours before until 24 hours after cytotoxic chemotherapy.[1-3] In support of this, the manufacturer of filgrastim notes that preliminary evidence confirmed that the severity of neutropenia could be exacerbated when patients were treated concurrently with **fluorouracil** and filgrastim.[2]

Note also that there is some evidence that colony-stimulating factors may potentiate the pulmonary toxicity of 'bleomycin', (p.618) and 'cyclophosphamide', (p.625).

1. Granocyte (Lenograstim). Chugai Pharma UK Ltd. UK Summary of product characteristics, October 2004.
2. Neupogen (Filgrastim). Amgen Ltd. UK Summary of product characteristics, January 2007.
3. Leucomax (Molgramostim). Schering-Plough Ltd. UK Summary of product characteristics, June 2000.

Antineoplastics + 5-HT$_3$-receptor antagonists

Some evidence suggests ondansetron may modestly affect the pharmacokinetics of cyclophosphamide and cisplatin but it does not appear to affect those of carmustine. Ondansetron did not affect the *in vitro* activity of epirubicin, bleomycin, cisplatin or estramustine. Cisplatin and fluorouracil do not affect the pharmacokinetics of ondansetron. In *in vitro* studies granisetron potentiated the cytotoxic effects of epirubicin, had an additive effect on bleomycin and estramustine activity and appeared not to affect the metabolism of docetaxel and paclitaxel.

Clinical evidence, mechanism, importance and management

(a) Granisetron

In an *in vitro* study, granisetron significantly potentiated the cytotoxic effects of **epirubicin** on fibroblasts, and the effect of granisetron on the cytotoxic effects of **bleomycin** and **estramustine** in lung cancer cells appeared to be additive. The clinical relevance of the effects of granisetron on **epirubicin** is not known.[1] Another *in vitro* study found that granisetron did not affect the metabolism of **docetaxel** or **paclitaxel**.[2]

(b) Ondansetron

The pharmacokinetics of high-dose **cyclophosphamide**, **cisplatin** and **carmustine** in 23 patients given ondansetron, lorazepam and diphenhydramine as antiemetics were compared with those in 129 patients who received prochlorperazine instead of ondansetron. It was found that the AUCs of **cyclophosphamide** and **cisplatin**, but not that of **carmustine**, were significantly lower (by 15% and 19%, respectively) in the ondansetron group.[3] Similarly, in another study, the pharmacokinetics of antineoplastics were analysed in 54 patients with breast cancer who were receiving high-dose **cyclophosphamide**, **cisplatin** and **carmustine** with lorazepam and ondansetron with or without prochlorperazine and compared with 75 matched control patients whose had been given prochlorperazine and lorazepam. In those given ondansetron the median AUC of **cyclophosphamide** was 17% lower, the **cisplatin** AUC was about 10% higher and the **carmustine** AUC was unchanged.[4] In contrast, a study in 10 patients who received intravenous **cyclophosphamide** 600 mg/m^2 and **epirubicin** 90 mg/m^2 and either oral ondansetron 16 mg or placebo found that the pharmacokinetic parameters of **cyclophosphamide** or its metabolite were not significantly altered by ondansetron although there was considerable variation between subjects. It was concluded that ondansetron can be safely given with **cyclophosphamide.**[5] No significant changes in the pharmacokinetics of ondansetron occurred in 20 cancer patients taking **cisplatin** 20 to 40 mg/m^2 and/or **fluorouracil** 1 g/m^2 for 5 days but the clearance was lower than in healthy subjects.[6]

An *in vitro* study found that ondansetron did not affect the cytotoxic effects of **bleomycin, epirubicin, estramustine** or **cisplatin** in fibroblasts and lung cancer cells.[1]

Information seems to be limited to these studies, and the interaction is not established. The clinical relevance of these possible modest changes in AUC of cyclophosphamide (0 to 17% reduction) and cisplatin (19% reduction or 10% increase) remain to be determined.

1. Behnam Motlagh P, Henriksson R, Grankvist K. Interaction of the antiemetics ondansetron and granisetron with the cytotoxicity induced by irradiation, epirubicin, bleomycin, estramustine, and cisplatin in vitro. *Acta Oncol* (1995) 34, 871–5.
2. Watanabe Y, Nakajima K, Nozaki K, Hoshiai H, Noda K. The effect of granisetron on in vitro metabolism of paclitaxel and docetaxel. *Cancer J* (2003) 9, 67–70.
3. Cagnoni PJ, Matthes S, Day TC, Bearman SI, Shpall EJ, Jones RB. Modification of the pharmacokinetics of high-dose cyclophosphamide and cisplatin by antiemetics. *Bone Marrow Transplant* (1999) 24, 1–4.
4. Gilbert CJ, Petros WP, Vredenburgh J, Hussein A, Ross M, Rubin P, Fehdrau R, Cavanaugh C, Berry D, McKinstry C, Peters WP. Pharmacokinetic interaction between ondansetron and cyclophosphamide during high-dose chemotherapy for breast cancer. *Cancer Chemother Pharmacol* (1998) 42, 497–503.
5. Lorenz C, Eickhoff C, Baumann F, Sehouli J, Preiss R, Schunack W, Jaehde U. Does ondansetron affect the metabolism of cyclophosphamide? *Int J Clin Pharmacol Ther* (2000) 38, 143–4.
6. Hsyu P-H, Bozigian HP, Pritchard JF, Kernodle A, Panella J, Hansen LA, Griffin RH. Effect of chemotherapy on the pharmacokinetics of oral ondansetron. *Pharm Res* (1991) 8 (Suppl 10), S-257.

Antineoplastics + Megestrol

There is some *in vitro* evidence to suggest that megestrol acetate may antagonise the antitumour activity of cisplatin. In one clinical study megestrol reduced the response rates to etoposide with cisplatin but in another had no effect on response rates to alternating cycles of cyclophosphamide, doxorubicin and vincristine, and etoposide with cisplatin.

Clinical evidence

A study in 243 patients with advanced small-cell lung cancer (SCLC) treated with **etoposide** and **cisplatin** found that those who also received megestrol acetate 800 mg daily had increased non-fluid body-weight and significantly less nausea and vomiting. Although the 1-year survival rate was similar in both groups those who received megestrol had a significantly worse response rate to **cisplatin** (68% compared with 80%) and a higher incidence of thromboembolic events. However the megestrol recipients did have poorer quality of life (a prognostic factor) at the beginning of the study and this may have influenced the findings.[1] In a similar study, megestrol acetate had no effect on response rates, symptom profile or overall survival in patients with SCLC receiving chemotherapy (alternating cycles of **cyclophosphamide**, **doxorubicin** and **vincristine**, and **etoposide** with **cisplatin** for a maximum of 6 cycles). In this study, megestrol acetate was given at a dose of 160 mg three times daily for 8 days starting 3 days before each cycle of chemotherapy.[2]

Mechanism

An *in vitro* study found that megestrol may antagonise the antineoplastic activity of cisplatin by up-regulating cellular detoxification mechanisms.[3]

Importance and management

The authors of the first study suggest that megestrol acetate should not be used routinely at the time of chemotherapy.[1] Be aware that the use of megestrol may antagonise the antitumour activity of cisplatin. More study is needed.

1. Rowland KM, Loprinzi CL, Shaw EG, Maksymiuk AW, Kuross SA, Jung S-H, Kugler JW, Tschetter LK, Ghosh C, Schaefer PL, Owen D, Washburn JH, Webb TA, Mailliard JA, Jett JR. Randomized double-blind placebo-controlled trial of cisplatin and etoposide plus megestrol acetate/placebo in extensive-stage small-cell lung cancer: a North Central Cancer Treatment Group Study. *J Clin Oncol* (1996) 14, 135–41.
2. Wood L, Palmer M, Hewitt J, Urtasun R, Bruera E, Rapp E, Thaell JF. Results of a phase III, double-blind, placebo-controlled trial of megestrol acetate modulation of P-glycoprotein-mediated drug resistance in the first-line management of small-cell lung carcinoma. *Br J Cancer* (1998) 77, 627–31.
3. Pu Y-S, Cheng A-L, Chen J, Guan J-Y, Lu S-H, Lai M-K, Hsieh C-Y. Megestrol acetate antagonizes cisplatin cytotoxicity. *Anticancer Drugs* (1998) 9, 733–8.

Antineoplastics + Propofol

There are two isolated reports of severe pain occurring when patients who had previously received intravenous chemotherapy were given intravenous propofol via hand veins.

Clinical evidence, mechanism, importance and management

Although pain on injection of propofol is well known one group of workers noted that on a number of occasions patients previously treated with intravenous chemotherapy had marked pain, both at the site of injection and up the arm, when given propofol via hand veins.[1] This would seem to link with a report of a 15-year-old girl with acute lymphoblastic leukaemia who had been treated with several injections of **cyclophosphamide**, **methotrexate** and **vincristine** during the previous 6 months, and who was cannulated in her hand and given an infusion of *Plasmalyte B*. An injection of 60 micrograms of fentanyl via this cannula was painful and 20 mg of lidocaine helped, but 20 mg of propofol caused extreme pain. A further 20 mg of lidocaine was given and the propofol administration was stopped, but the pain continued. The whole hand became blue and congested, and blood began to move backwards up the drip tubing. The venous congestion gradually subsided over the next 15 minutes.[2] The authors recommended that propofol should be avoided in patients who have recently had intravenous chemotherapy.[2] The general applicability of these reports remains to be determined. The use of propofol alone may cause pain and it should be noted that the manufacturers of propofol recommend that local pain associated with propofol during the induction phase can be minimised by the use of the larger veins on the forearm and antecubital fossa.[3]

1. Whitlock JE, Nicol ME, Pattison J. Painful injection of propofol. *Anaesthesia* (1989) 44, 618.
2. Butt AD, James MFM. Venospasm due to propofol after chemotherapy. *S Afr Med J* (1990) 77, 168.
3. Diprivan (Propofol). AstraZeneca UK Ltd. UK Summary of product characteristics, May 2007.

Antineoplastics + Protease inhibitors

Use of protease inhibitor-based regimens has been found to be associated with a higher incidence of infections and neutropenia in patients receiving cyclophosphamide, doxorubicin and etoposide (CDE) than use of a NNRTI-based regimen.

Clinical evidence, mechanism, importance and management

A study to compare the incidence of neutropenia and infection resulting from protease inhibitor or NNRTI-based antiretroviral regimen given with **cyclophosphamide**, **doxorubicin** and **etoposide** (**CDE**) chemotherapy for AIDS-related non-Hodgkin's lymphoma was carried out in 46 patients with AIDS-related non-Hodgkin's lymphoma. Eleven patients were taking protease inhibitor-based antiretroviral treatment. There was a higher incidence of infections requiring hospitalisation in the group taking a protease inhibitor than in the NNRTI-based treatment group (48% compared with 25%). There was a similar difference in the incidence of grade 4 neutropenia (54% compared with 38%) and day 10 and day 14 neutrophil counts were significantly lower in patients receiving protease inhibitors, resulting in delays in giving chemotherapy in 16% of cycles (compared with 9% when no protease inhibitor was given). Overall, however, there was no difference in response rate, disease-free survival or overall survival between the two groups. The authors suggested that the increase in myelosuppression may be caused by the protease inhibitors reducing the metabolism of CDE via inhibition of cytochrome P450 enzymes, or inhibition of P-glycoprotein.[1] Inhibitors of CYP3A4 may increase toxicity with etoposide, see 'Etoposide + CYP3A4 inhibitors', p.631.

1. Bower M, McCall-Peat N, Ryan N, Davies L, Young AM, Gupta S, Nelson M, Gazzard B, Stebbing J. Protease inhibitors potentiate chemotherapy-induced neutropenia. *Blood* (2004) 104, 2943–46.

Antineoplastics + Semaxanib

The combination of semaxanib, cisplatin and gemcitabine has caused an unexpectedly high incidence of thromboembolic events.

Clinical evidence, mechanism, importance and management

The pharmacokinetics of semaxanib (SU5416), **cisplatin** and **gemcitabine** were unaltered when they were given together in a phase I study but investigation of the combination was terminated after 8 of the 19 patients had thromboembolic events (transient ischaemic attacks, cerebrovascular accidents, deep vein thromboses). **Gemcitabine** 1250 mg/m^2 was given on day 1, immediately followed by **cisplatin** 80 mg/m^2, then semaxanib 85 mg/m^2 (escalated to 145 mg/m^2 in some patients). **Gemcitabine** then semaxanib were given on day 8, and semaxanib alone on days 4, 11, 15, and 18. The cycle was repeated every 3 weeks.[1] The incidence of thromboembolic events in this study (42%) was much higher than that seen with **cisplatin** and **gemcitabine** (0%) or semaxanib alone (2.2%), and was thought to be a result of the drug combination.[1] **Cisplatin** in particular, due to its effects on platelets and its vasoconstrictive effects, may be the drug interacting with the semaxanib.[2] Preliminary results of other studies of semaxanib with: **irinotecan**; **fluorouracil** and folinic acid; **irinotecan, fluorouracil** and folinic acid; or **paclitaxel** and **carboplatin** did not report this complication.[3-6] The authors of the first study[1] caution against further clinical trials of antineoplastics with angiogenesis inhibitors such as semaxanib until the exact cause of the thromboembolic events has been elucidated.

1. Kuenen BC, Rosen L, Smit EF, Parson MRN, Levi M, Ruijter R, Huisman H, Kedde MA, Noordhuis P, van der Vijgh WJF, Peters GJ, Cropp GF, Scigalla P, Hoekman K, Pinedo HM, Giaccone G. Dose-finding and pharmacokinetic study of cisplatin, gemcitabine, and SU5416 in patients with solid tumors. *J Clin Oncol* (2002) 20, 1657–67.
2. Marx GM, Steer CB, Harper P, Pavlakis N, Rixe O, Khayat D. Unexpected serious toxicity with chemotherapy and antiangiogenic combinations: time to take stock. *J Clin Oncol* (2002) 20, 1446–8.
3. Rosen PJ, Amado R, Hecht JR, Chang D, Mulay M, Parson M Laxa B, Brown J, Cropp G, Hannah A, Rosen L. A phase I/II study of SU5416 in combination with 5-FU/leucovorin in patients with metastatic colorectal cancer. *Proc Am Soc Clin Oncol* (2000) 19, 3A.
4. Rothenberg ML, Berlin JD, Cropp GF, Fleischer AC, Schumaker RD, Hande KR, Culley A, Dorminy C, Donnelly E, Chen J, Schaaf L, Hannah AL. A phase I/II study of SU5416 in combination with irinotecan/5-FU/LV (IFL) in patients with metastatic colorectal cancer. *Proc Am Soc Clin Oncol* (2001) 20, 75A.
5. Rosen P, Kabbinavar F, Figlin RA, Parson M, Laxa B, Hernandez L, Mayers A, Cropp GF, Hannah AL, Rosen LS. A phase I/II trial and pharmacokinetic (PK) study of SU5416 in combination with paclitaxel/carboplatin. *Proc Am Soc Clin Oncol* (2001) 20, 98A.
6. Hoff PM, Wolff RA, Bogaard K, Waldrum S, Abbruzzese JL. A phase I study of escalating doses of the tyrosine kinase inhibitor semaxanib (SU5416) in combination with irinotecan in patients with advanced colorectal cancer. *Jpn J Clin Oncol* (2006) 36, 100–3.

Antineoplastics + Tamoxifen

Antineoplastics and tamoxifen are associated with an increased risk of thrombosis and there is the possibility that their combined use may further increase this risk.

Clinical evidence, mechanism, importance and management

A retrospective analysis of data from various Eastern Cooperative Oncology Group studies, suggested that venous thromboembolic complications were more common in women given tamoxifen with adjuvant chemotherapy (**CMF**; **cyclophosphamide, methotrexate, fluorouracil**) than women given **CMF** alone (3.8% versus 0% in one study).[1] In another study of patients given tamoxifen 30 mg daily for 2 years the incidence of thromboembolic events was 2.6% compared with 13.6% in those also given 8 cycles of **CMF**. The authors of this study considered the rate of thromboembolic events with the combination to be higher than that usually seen with **CMF**, and suggested that this occurred as a result of an interaction between tamoxifen and **CMF**.[2] In contrast, in another study, in the first 12 weeks of therapy, thrombosis occurred in 5 of 103 patients given tamoxifen with chemotherapy (**cyclophosphamide, methotrexate, fluorouracil, vincristine**, prednisone, **doxorubicin**) compared with 4 of 102 given the same chemotherapy alone, suggesting that tamoxifen made no significant contribution to the rate of thromboembolic events.[3]

Tamoxifen alone is known to carry a small risk of thromboembolic events when used for primary prevention of breast cancer.[4] Antineoplastic chemotherapy also increases the risk of thrombosis,[3] and cancer *per se* increases the risk, as does surgery for cancer.[5]

To what extent, if any, tamoxifen further increases the risk of thrombosis with antineoplastic therapy is unclear from the above studies. However, some authors recommend that serious consideration be given to the use of prophylactic anticoagulants if adjuvant CMF is given with tamoxifen in women with breast cancer,[2] and the UK manufacturers endorse this.[6] This may be prudent with antineoplastic chemotherapy in any case.

1. Saphner T, Tormey DC, Gray R. Venous and arterial thrombosis in patients who received adjuvant therapy for breast cancer. *J Clin Oncol* (1991) 9, 286–94.
2. Pritchard KI, Paterson AHG, Paul NA, Zee B, Fine S, Pater J. Increased thromboembolic complications with concurrent tamoxifen and chemotherapy in a randomized trial of adjuvant therapy for women with breast cancer. National Cancer Institute of Canada Clinical Trials Group Breast Cancer Site Group. *J Clin Oncol* (1996) 14, 2731–7.
3. Levine MN, Gent M, Hirsh J, Arnold A, Goodyear MD, Hryniuk W, De Pauw S. The thrombogenic effect of anticancer drug therapy in women with stage II breast cancer. *N Engl J Med* (1988) 318; 404–7.
4. Fischer B, Constantino JP, Wickerham DL, Redmond CK, Kavanah M, Cronin WM, Vogel V, Robidoux A, Dimitrov N, Atkins J, Daly M, Wieand S, Tan-Chiu E, Ford L, Wolmark N. Tamoxifen for prevention of breast cancer: report of the National Surgical Adjuvant Breast and Bowel Project P-1 Study. *J Natl Cancer Inst* (1998) 90, 1371–88.
5. Rickles FR, Levine MN. Venous thromboembolism in malignancy and malignancy in venous thromboembolism. *Haemostasis* (1998) 28 (Suppl 3), 43–9.
6. Nolvadex D (Tamoxifen). AstraZeneca UK Ltd. UK Summary of product characteristics, July 2005.

Antineoplastics + Vaccines

The immune response of the body is suppressed by cytotoxic antineoplastics. The effectiveness of vaccines may be poor and generalised infection may occur in patients immunised with live vaccines.

Clinical evidence, mechanism, importance and management

Since cytotoxic antineoplastics are immunosuppressant, they reduce the response of the body to immunisation. A study[1] in 53 patients with Hodgkin's disease showed that chemotherapy reduced the antibody response to a **pneumococcal vaccine** by 60% when measured 3 weeks after immunisation. The patients were taking **chlormethine** (mechlorethamine), **vincristine**, prednisone and **procarbazine**. A few of them had also been given **bleomycin, vinblastine** or **cyclophosphamide**. Subtotal radiotherapy reduced the response by a further 15%. The response to **influenza immunisation** in children with various malignancies was also markedly suppressed by chemotherapy. The regimen included prednisone and the cytotoxic drugs **mercaptopurine, methotrexate**, and **vincristine**. Some of them were also given **dactinomycin** and **cyclophosphamide**.[2] In another study only 9 out of 17 children with leukaemia or other malignant diseases and taking **methotrexate, cyclophosphamide, mercaptopurine** and prednisone developed a significant response to immunisation with **inactivated measles vaccine**.[3] Furthermore, immunisation with **live vaccines** may result in a potentially life-threatening infection. For example, a woman taking **methotrexate** 15 mg once a month for psoriasis developed a generalised vaccinial infection after vaccination against **smallpox**.[4] Studies in *animals* given **smallpox vaccine** confirmed that they were more susceptible to infection if they had been given **methotrexate, mercaptopurine** or **cyclophosphamide**.[5]

Extreme care should therefore be exercised when using live vaccines for immunisation of patients who are receiving cytotoxics or other immunosuppressant drugs (see also 'Corticosteroids + Vaccines; Live', p.1061, and 'Immunosuppressants + Vaccines', p.1064).

1. Siber GR, Weitzman SA, Aisenberg AC, Weinstein HJ, Schiffman G. Impaired antibody response to pneumococcal vaccine after treatment for Hodgkins disease. *N Engl J Med* (1978) 299, 442–8.
2. Gross PA, Lee H, Wolff JA, Hall CB, Minnefore AB, Lazicki ME. Influenza immunization in immunosuppressed children. *J Pediatr* (1978) 92, 30–5.
3. Stiehm ER, Ablin A, Kushner JH, Zoger S. Measles vaccination in patients on immunosuppressive drugs. *Am J Dis Child* (1966) 111, 191–4.
4. Allison J. Methotrexate and smallpox vaccination. *Lancet* (1968) ii, 1250.
5. Rosenbaum EH, Cohen RA, Glatstein HR. Vaccination of a patient receiving immunosuppressive therapy for lymphosarcoma. *JAMA* (1966) 198, 737–40.

Bexarotene + Miscellaneous

Gemfibrozil raises bexarotene plasma levels. The manufacturers warn that, theoretically, inhibitors of CYP3A4 (azoles, grapefruit juice, protease inhibitors and some macrolides) may possibly raise bexarotene levels, whereas CYP3A4 inducers (phenytoin, phenobarbital, rifampicin (rifampin)) may possibly reduce them. They also suggest that the efficacy of oral contraceptives may be reduced, and increased blood glucose-lowering effects may occur with insulin or oral antidiabetic drugs. No interaction seems to occur between bexarotene and atorvastatin or levothyroxine.

Clinical evidence, mechanism, importance and management

(a) Effects of enzyme inducers and inhibitors

Because it is known that bexarotene is metabolised by the cytochrome P450 isoenzyme CYP3A4, the manufacturers point out that there is a theoretical risk that drugs that inhibit CYP3A4 might increase bexarotene levels. They list **clarithromycin**, **erythromycin**, **itraconazole**, **ketoconazole**, **protease inhibitors** and **grapefruit juice** as possible interacting drugs because of their known inhibitory effects on CYP3A4. They also list a number of known CYP3A4 inducers, namely **dexamethasone**, **phenytoin**, **phenobarbital** and **rifampicin** (**rifampin**), because they may theoretically increase the metabolism of bexarotene and reduce its levels.[1,2]

The manufacturers also say that because bexarotene can induce liver enzymes, it may theoretically increase the metabolism of other substances metabolised by CYP3A4 such as **tamoxifen** and the steroids in oral or other systemic **contraceptives**, thereby reducing both their serum levels and their efficacy. For this reason they advise the use of additional non-hormonal contraception (e.g. a barrier method) to avoid the risk of contraceptive failure. They point out that this is particularly important because if failure were to occur, the foetus might be exposed to the teratogenic effects of bexarotene.[1,2]

(b) Other possible drug interactions

A population analysis of patients with cutaneous T-cell lymphoma found that the concurrent use of **gemfibrozil** substantially increased the plasma levels of bexarotene. The reasons for this effect are unknown, although inhibition of CYP3A4 by **gemfibrozil** may be partially responsible.[3] The US manufacturers state concurrent use is not recommended,[2] but note that fibrates are not generally recognised as inhibitors of this isoenzyme, see 'Lipid regulating drugs', (p.1086). Under similar conditions, they say that bexarotene levels were not affected by **atorvastatin** or **levothyroxine**. Changes in thyroid function caused by bexarotene have been successfully treated with **thyroid hormone supplements**.[1-3]

The manufacturers recommend that because bexarotene is related to **vitamin A**, any **vitamin A supplements** should be limited to 15 000 units or less daily to avoid potentially additive toxic effects. They also say that although no cases of hypoglycaemia have been seen, because of the known mode of action of bexarotene it should be used with caution if given with **insulin** or drugs that enhance insulin secretion (e.g. **sulfonylureas**) or insulin sensitisers (e.g. **thiazolidinediones**).[1,2] For a list of these drugs see 'Table 13.1', (p.469).

1. Targretin (Bexarotene). Cephalon Ltd. UK Summary of product characteristics, April 2007.
2. Targretin (Bexarotene). Ligand Pharmaceuticals, Inc. US Prescribing information, April 2003.
3. Talpur R, Ward S, Apisarnthanarax N, Breuer-McHam J, Duvic M. Optimizing bexarotene therapy for cutaneous T-cell lymphoma. *J Am Acad Dermatol* (2002) 47, 672–84.

Bicalutamide + Phenazone (Antipyrine)

The results of an interaction study between bicalutamide and phenazone suggest that bicalutamide is unlikely to interact with other drugs through enzyme induction.

Clinical evidence, mechanism, importance and management

The pharmacokinetics and metabolism of phenazone (largely used as an investigational marker drug of enzyme induction or inhibition) were studied in two groups of patients with prostate cancer before and after they took either bicalutamide 50 mg daily (7 patients) or 150 mg daily (11 patients) for 12 weeks. Small changes in the phenazone pharmacokinetics were found (half-life reduced by 16.3% with the 50 mg bicalutamide dosage, AUC reduced by 18.6% with the 150 mg bicalutamide dosage). Nevertheless it was considered that bicalutamide does not significantly induce the liver enzymes responsible for the metabolism of phenazone and is therefore unlikely to interact with any other drugs by causing enzyme induction.[1]

1. Kaisary A, Klarskov P, McKillop D. Absence of hepatic enzyme induction in prostate cancer patients receiving 'Casodex' (bicalutamide). *Anticancer Drugs* (1996) 7, 54–9.

Bleomycin + Cisplatin

Cisplatin can increase the pulmonary toxicity of bleomycin by reducing its renal excretion. Digital ischaemia and arterial thrombosis have also been described in patients receiving both drugs.

Clinical evidence

Thirty patients with carcinoma of the cervix and 15 patients with germ cell tumours were given combination chemotherapy including bleomycin and cisplatin. Cisplatin was given by infusion on day 1, followed by bleomycin given intramuscularly every 12 hours for 4 days or by continuous infusion over 72 hours. Nine of the patients with normal renal function and no previous pulmonary disease developed serious pulmonary toxicity and 6 died from respiratory failure.[1]

In a study of 18 patients given cisplatin and bleomycin for the treatment of disseminated testicular non-seminoma, 2 patients developed pneumonitis, and it was found that the cisplatin-induced reduction in renal function was paralleled by an increase in bleomycin-induced pulmonary toxicity.[2] Similar results were found in a much larger study of 54 patients by the same group.[3] A study in 2 children showed that the total plasma clearance of bleomycin was halved (from 39 to 18 $mL/minute/m^2$) when they were also given cisplatin in cumulative doses exceeding 300 mg/m^2. The renal clearance in one of the children fell from 30 to 8.2 $mL/minute/m^2$ although there was no evidence of severe bleomycin toxicity in either child.[4] Two cases of fatal bleomycin toxicity have been described in patients with cisplatin-induced renal impairment.[5,6]

A case report describes arterial thrombosis associated with pathological vascular changes in the arteries of a man treated with cisplatin, bleomycin and etoposide.[7] Another man developed fatal thrombotic microangiopathy (characterised by microangiopathic haemolytic anaemia, thrombocytopenia, renal impairment), which was attributed to the use of bleomycin and cisplatin.[8]

In an earlier study, digital ischaemia occurred in 41% of patients treated with cisplatin, bleomycin and vinblastine compared with 21% of patients treated with only cisplatin and vinblastine.[9]

Mechanism

Renal excretion accounts for almost half of the total body clearance of bleomycin. Cisplatin is nephrotoxic and reduces the glomerular filtration rate so that the clearance of bleomycin is reduced. The accumulating bleomycin apparently causes the pulmonary toxicity.

Importance and management

Pulmonary toxicity with bleomycin is an established reaction with a potentially serious, sometimes fatal, outcome. Concurrent use should be very closely monitored and renal function checked. One of the problems is that levels of creatinine may not accurately indicate the extent of renal damage both during and after cisplatin treatment. The renal toxicity of cisplatin may also develop rapidly. Other toxic effects on the vascular system can also occur.

1. Rabinowits M, Souhami L, Gil RA, Andrade CAV, Paiva HC. Increased pulmonary toxicity with bleomycin and cisplatin chemotherapy combinations. *Am J Clin Oncol* (1990) 13, 132–8.
2. van Barneveld PWC, Sleijfer D Th, van der Mark Th W, Mulder NH, Donker AJM, Meijer S, Schraffordt Koops H, Sluiter HJ, Peset R. Influence of platinum-induced renal toxicity on bleomycin-induced pulmonary toxicity in patients with disseminated testicular carcinoma. *Oncology* (1984) 41, 4–7.
3. Sleijfer S, van der Mark TW, Schraffordt Koops H, Mulder NH. Enhanced effects of bleomycin on pulmonary function disturbances in patients with decreased renal function due to cisplatin. *Eur J Cancer* (1996) 32A, 550–2.
4. Yee GC, Crom WR, Champion JE, Brodeur GM, Evans WE. Cisplatin-induced changes in bleomycin elimination. *Cancer Treat Rep* (1983) 67, 587–9.
5. Bennett WM, Pastore L, Houghton DC. Fatal pulmonary bleomycin toxicity in cisplatin-induced acute renal failure. *Cancer Treat Rep* (1980) 64, 921–4.
6. Perry DJ, Weiss RB, Taylor HG. Enhanced bleomycin toxicity during acute renal failure. *Cancer Treat Rep* (1982) 66, 592–3.
7. Garstin IWH, Cooper GG, Hood JM. Arterial thrombosis after treatment with bleomycin and cisplatin. *BMJ* (1990) 300, 1018.

8. Fields SM, Lindley CM. Thrombotic microangiopathy associated with chemotherapy: case report and review of the literature. *DICP Ann Pharmacother* (1989) 23, 582–8.
9. Vogelzang NJ, Bosl GJ, Johnson K, Kennedy BJ. Raynaud's phenomenon : a common toxicity after combination chemotherapy for testicular cancer. *Ann Intern Med* (1981) 95, 288–92.

Bleomycin + Colony-stimulating factors

The concurrent use of granulocyte colony-stimulating factor or granulocyte-macrophage colony-stimulating factor has been linked with an increased occurrence of bleomycin-induced pulmonary toxicity.

Clinical evidence, mechanism, importance and management

Pulmonary toxicity that developed at low cumulative bleomycin doses (70 to 130 units/m^2) in at least 3 of 5 patients given standard ABVD treatment (doxorubicin, bleomycin, vinblastine, and dacarbazine) was attributed by the author of the report to the synergistic action of concurrent treatment with **G-CSF** (granulocyte colony-stimulating factor).[1] In another report 8 out of 40 patients with malignant non-Hodgkin's lymphoma given **G-CSF** developed drug-induced pneumonia. Three of these patients were treated with chemotherapy regimens including bleomycin (MACOB-B, COP-BLAM III), and all 3 died of respiratory failure. None of 35 other patients, similarly treated but without **G-CSF**, developed pneumonia.[2] Non-infectious interstitial pneumonitis developed in a patient given doxorubicin, cyclophosphamide, bleomycin, vinblastine, methotrexate and prednisone with **GM-CSF** (granulocyte-macrophage colony-stimulating factor).[3] Five further reports have identified a total of 23 other patients who developed bleomycin-pulmonary toxicity probably potentiated by **G-CSF** or **GM-CSF**, including at least 7 fatalities.[4-8]

In contrast, analysis of two placebo-controlled studies of the use of adjuvant **G-CSF** (**filgrastim** or **lenograstim**) with combination chemotherapy including bleomycin found no evidence of an increase in pulmonary complications. Overall 7 of 139 patients treated with placebo and 9 of 139 treated with the **G-CSF** had pulmonary complications possibly related to bleomycin.[9,10] Similarly, another retrospective analysis found that 34% of patients treated with bleomycin and **G-CSF** developed pulmonary toxicity, compared with 33% of those treated with bleomycin alone.[11]

These interactions are not firmly established, but good pulmonary function monitoring appears to be advisable when colony-stimulating factors are used with antineoplastics causing pulmonary toxicity, such as bleomycin. If interstitial pneumonia occurs, the drugs should be discontinued and high-dose corticosteroids started immediately.[7] More study is needed.

Consider also 'Cyclophosphamide + Colony-stimulating factors', p.625.

1. Matthews JH. Pulmonary toxicity of ABVD chemotherapy and G-CSF in Hodgkin's disease: possible synergy. *Lancet* (1993) 342, 988.
2. Iki S, Yoshinaga K, Ohbayashi Y, Urabe A. Cytotoxic drug-induced pneumonia and possible augmentation by G-CSF — clinical attention. *Ann Hematol* (1993) 66, 217–18.
3. Philippe B, Couderc LJ, Balloul-Delclaux E, Janvier M, Caubarrere I. Pulmonary toxicity of chemotherapy and GM-CSF. *Respir Med* (1994) 88, 715.
4. Dirix LY, Schrijvers D, Druwè P, Van Den Brande J, Verhoeven D, Van Oosterom AT. Pulmonary toxicity and bleomycin. *Lancet* (1994) 344, 56.
5. Lei KIK, Leung WT, Johnson PJ. Serious pulmonary complications in patients receiving recombinant granulocyte colony-stimulating factor during BACOP chemotherapy for aggressive non-Hodgkin's lymphoma. *Br J Cancer* (1994) 70, 1009–13.
6. Katoh M, Shikoshi K, Takada M, Umeda M, Tsukahara T, Kitagawa S, Shirai T. Development of interstitial pneumonitis during treatment with granulocyte colony-stimulating factor. *Ann Hematol* (1993) 67, 201–2.
7. Niitsu N, Iki S, Muroi K, Motomura S, Murakami M, Takeyama H, Ohsaka A, Urabe A. Interstitial pneumonia in patients receiving granulocyte colony-stimulating factor during chemotherapy: survey in Japan 1991–96. *Br J Cancer* (1997) 76, 1661–6.
8. Couderc L-J, Stelianides S, Franchon I, Stern M, Epardeau B, Baumelou E, Caubarrere I, Hermine O. Pulmonary toxicity of chemotherapy and G/GM-CSF: a report of five cases. *Respir Med* (1999) 93, 65–8.
9. Bastion Y, Reyes F, Bosly A, Gisselbrecht C, Yver A, Gilles E, Maral J, Coiffier B. Possible toxicity with the association of G-CSF and bleomycin. *Lancet* (1994) 343, 1221–2.
10. Bastion Y, Coiffier B. Pulmonary toxicity of bleomycin: is G-CSF a risk factor? *Lancet* (1994) 344, 474.
11. Saxman SB, Nichols CR, Einhorn LH. Pulmonary toxicity in patients with advanced-stage germ cell tumors receiving bleomycin with and without granulocyte colony stimulating factor. *Chest* (1997) 111, 657–60.

Bleomycin + Oxygen

Serious and potentially fatal pulmonary toxicity can develop in patients treated with bleomycin who are exposed to conventional oxygen concentrations during anaesthesia.

Clinical evidence

Five patients treated with bleomycin, exposed to oxygen concentrations of 35 to 42% during and immediately following anaesthesia, developed a severe respiratory distress syndrome and died. Bleomycin-induced pneumonitis and lung fibrosis were diagnosed at post-mortem. Another group of 12 matched patients who underwent the same procedures but with lower oxygen concentrations (22 to 25%) had an uneventful postoperative course.[1]

Another comparative study[2] similarly demonstrated that adult respiratory distress syndrome (ARDS) in patients receiving bleomycin was reduced by a technique allowing the use of lower oxygen concentrations of 22 to 30%. Bleomycin-induced pulmonary toxicity, apparently related to oxygen concentrations, has also been described in other case reports.[3-7] Studies in *animals* have also confirmed that the severity of bleomycin-induced pulmonary toxicity is increased by oxygen.[8-10] However, in two other series of patients treated with bleomycin and undergoing surgery there was no obvious increase in pulmonary complications despite the use of usual concentrations of oxygen.[11,12]

Mechanism

Not understood. One suggestion is that bleomycin-injured lung tissue is less able to scavenge free oxygen radicals, which may be present, and damage occurs as a result.[3]

Importance and management

An established, well-documented, serious and potentially fatal interaction. It is advised that any patient receiving bleomycin and undergoing general anaesthesia should have their inspired oxygen concentrations limited to less than 30%, and the fluid replacement should be carefully monitored to minimise the crystalloid load. This is clearly very effective because one author has treated 700 patients following these guidelines without a single case of pulmonary failure.[13] It has also been suggested that reduced oxygen levels should be continued during the recovery period and at any time during hospitalisation.[3] If an oxygen concentration equal to or greater than 30% has to be used, the short-term use of prophylactic corticosteroids should be considered. Intravenous corticosteroids should be given at once if bleomycin toxicity is suspected.[3]

1. Goldiner PL, Carlon GC, Cvitkovic E, Schweizer O, Howland WS. Factors influencing postoperative morbidity and mortality in patients treated with bleomycin. *BMJ* (1978) 1, 1664–7.
2. El-Baz N, Ivankovich AD, Faber LP, Logas WG. The incidence of bleomycin lung toxicity after anesthesia for pulmonary resection: a comparison between HFV and IPPV. *Anesthesiology* (1984) 61, A107.
3. Gilson AJ, Sahn SA. Reactivation of bleomycin lung toxicity following oxygen administration. A second response to corticosteroids. *Chest* (1985) 88, 304–6.
4. Cersosimo RJ, Matthews SJ, Hong WK. Bleomycin pneumonitis potentiated by oxygen administration. *Drug Intell Clin Pharm* (1985) 19, 921–3.
5. Hulbert JC, Grossman JE, Cummings KB. Risk factors of anesthesia and surgery in bleomycin-treated patients. *J Urol (Baltimore)* (1983) 130, 163–4.
6. Donohue JP, Rowland RG. Complications of retroperitoneal lymph node dissection. *J Urol (Baltimore)* (1981) 125, 338–40.
7. Ingrassia TS, Ryu JH, Trastek VF, Rosenow EC. Oxygen-exacerbated bleomycin pulmonary toxicity. *Mayo Clin Proc* (1991) 66, 173–8.
8. Toledo CH, Ross WE, Hood I, Block ER. Potentiation of bleomycin toxicity by oxygen. *Cancer Treat Rep* (1982) 66, 359–62.
9. Berend N. The effect of bleomycin and oxygen on rat lung. *Pathology* (1984) 16, 136–9.
10. Rinaldo J, Goldstein RH, Snider GL. Modification of oxygen toxicity after lung injury by bleomycin in hamsters. *Am Rev Respir Dis* (1982) 126, 1030–3.
11. Douglas MJ, Coppin CML. Bleomycin and subsequent anesthesia: a retrospective study at Vancouver General Hospital. *Can Anaesth Soc J* (1980) 27, 449–52.
12. Mandelbaum I, Williams SD, Einhorn LH. Aggressive surgical management of testicular carcinoma metastatic to lungs and mediastinum. *Ann Thorac Surg* (1980) 30, 224–9.
13. Goldiner PL. Editorial comment. *J Urol (Baltimore)* (1983) 130, 164.

Busulfan + Azoles

Itraconazole, but not fluconazole, modestly reduces the clearance of busulfan. There is some limited evidence to suggest that the use of busulfan with ketoconazole may increase the risk of hepatic veno-occlusive disease.

Clinical evidence, mechanism, importance and management

The pharmacokinetics of busulfan in 26 bone marrow transplant patients, who had received busulfan without concurrent antifungal therapy, were compared with those in 13 similar patients given busulfan with **itraconazole** and in 13 given busulfan with **fluconazole**. The busulfan clearance was decreased by 20% by **itraconazole** (probably because **itraconazole** inhibits the metabolism of busulfan by the liver) but busulfan clearance was not affected by the **fluconazole**.[1]. The expected rise in serum busulfan levels is only likely to be moderate, but until more information is available it would be prudent to monitor for any signs of increased busulfan toxicity if **itraconazole** is used, but no special precautions seem to be needed with **fluconazole**. Concurrent **ketoconazole** has been identified as a possible risk factor for hepatic veno-occlusive disease after high-dose busulfan.[2] Further study is needed to confirm or refute this.

1. Buggia I, Zecca N, Alessandrino EP, Locatelli F, Rosti G, Bosi A, Pession A, Rotoli B, Majolino I, Dallorso A, Regazzi MB. Itraconazole can increase systemic exposure to busulfan in patients given bone marrow transplantation. *Anticancer Res* (1996) 16, 2083–8.
2. Méresse V, Hartmann O, Vassal G, Benhamou E, Valteau-Couanet D, Brugieres L, Lemerie J. Risk factors for hepatic veno-occlusive disease after high-dose busulfan-containing regimens followed by autologous bone marrow transplantation: a study in 136 children. *Bone Marrow Transplant* (1992) 10, 135–41.

Busulfan + Benzodiazepines

Diazepam and lorazepam do not appear to alter the pharmacokinetics of busulfan.

Clinical evidence, mechanism, importance and management

In a study in patients receiving high-dose busulfan, no pharmacokinetic changes were seen in 8 patients given **diazepam**, apart from a steady decline in steady-state serum levels in just one.[1] Similarly, in another study, **lorazepam** did not alter the absorption and clearance of high-dose busulfan in children undergoing stem-cell transplantation.[2] Benzodiazepines may therefore be a suitable alternative to 'phenytoin', (below) for seizure prophylaxis during high-dose busulfan treatment.[2]

1. Hassan M, Öberg G, Björkholm M, Wallin I, Lindgren M. Influence of prophylactic anticonvulsant therapy on high-dose busulphan kinetics. *Cancer Chemother Pharmacol* (1993) 33, 181–6.
2. Chan KW, Mullen CA, Worth LL, Choroszy M, Koontz S, Tran H, Slopis J. Lorazepam for seizure prophylaxis during high-dose busulfan administration. *Bone Marrow Transplant* (2002) 29, 963–5.

Busulfan + Ketobemidone

Ketobemidone may increase plasma levels of busulfan.

Clinical evidence, mechanism, importance and management

A patient with acute myeloid leukaemia started treatment with a 4-day course of busulfan 1 mg/kg four times daily followed by cyclophosphamide for 2 days before bone marrow transplantation. At the time he was also receiving ketobemidone 1 g daily for a rectal fissure. Busulfan plasma levels after the first dose were elevated (AUC increased by about one-third). Later, when the dose of ketobemidone was reduced and morphine substituted, busulfan levels decreased.[1] The authors suggest that ketobemidone should not be used with high-dose busulfan unless monitoring is possible: dose adjustments may be required to prevent busulfan toxicity. An alternative analgesic should be considered.

1. Hassan M, Svensson J-O, Nilsson C, Hentschke P, AL-Shurbaji A, Aschan J, Ljungman P, Ringdén O. Ketobemidone may alter busulfan pharmacokinetics during high-dose therapy. *Ther Drug Monit* (2000) 22, 383–5.

Busulfan + Phenytoin

Phenytoin modestly increases the clearance of busulfan and lowers its serum levels. Subtherapeutic levels of phenytoin may occur in the presence of busulfan.

Clinical evidence

Seven patients given high-dose busulfan (1 mg/kg four times daily for 4 days) before bone marrow transplantation had a 19% increase in clearance, a 16% lower AUC and a shorter half-life (reduced from 3.94 to 3.03 hours) when they were given phenytoin 2.5 to 5 mg/kg daily. A continuous decline in the steady-state plasma levels of busulfan was also seen in 4 of the patients.[1]

In a study in 51 patients given busulfan and prophylactic phenytoin 300 mg daily for 5 days, 3 patients developed convulsions and plasma levels analysed in 2 of them were found to be subtherapeutic.[2]

Mechanism

It seems likely that the phenytoin (a well recognised enzyme inducer) increases the metabolism of the busulfan by the liver, thereby decreasing its levels. In an *animal* study, phenytoin was found to reduce the myelosuppressive effects of busulfan.[3]

Importance and management

The authors of one study suggest that antiepileptics with fewer enzyme-inducing properties than phenytoin should be used as prophylaxis if busulfan is given for bone marrow transplant pretreatment.[1] One UK manufacturer recommends prophylaxis with a benzodiazepine rather than phenytoin if high-dose busulfan is given.[4] 'Clobazam', (p.619), has been suggested as a possible alternative to phenytoin.[5]

The UK manufacturer of parenteral busulfan found no evidence that phenytoin increased its clearance.[6] However, the US manufacturer of parenteral busulfan gives a dose assuming that phenytoin will also be given, and notes that if other antiepileptics are used instead, the busulfan plasma levels may be increased and monitoring is recommended.[7]

To overcome the problem of reduced phenytoin levels, the authors recommended a loading dose of phenytoin 18 mg/kg on the day before the first dose of busulfan, then 300 mg daily until 48 hours after the last busulfan dose. A further loading dose was given if the phenytoin level was subtherapeutic 48 hours after the initial dose (required in 35% of patients).[2]

1. Hassan M, Öberg G, Björkholm M, Wallin I, Lindgren M. Influence of prophylactic anticonvulsant therapy on high-dose busulphan kinetics. *Cancer Chemother Pharmacol* (1993) 33, 181–6.
2. Grigg AP, Shepherd JD, Phillips GL. Busulphan and phenytoin. Ann Intern Med (1989) 111, 1049–50. Correction. *Ann Intern Med* (1989) 112, 313.
3. Fitzsimmons WE, Ghalie R, Kaizer H. The effect of hepatic enzyme inducers on busulfan neurotoxicity and myelotoxicity. *Cancer Chemother Pharmacol* (1990) 27, 226–8.
4. Myleran Tablets (Busulfan). GlaxoSmithKline UK. UK Summary of product characteristics, October 2006.
5. Schwarer AP, Opat SS, Watson AL, Cole-Sinclair MF. Clobazam for seizure prophylaxis during busulfan chemotherapy. *Lancet* (1995) 346, 1238.
6. Busilvex (Busulfan). Pierre Fabre Ltd. UK Summary of product characteristics, March 2007.
7. Busulfex (Busulfan). PDL BioPharma, Inc. US Prescribing information, July 2007.

Busulfan + Tioguanine

There is evidence that the long-term use of busulfan with tioguanine increases the risk of nodular regenerative hyperplasia of the liver, portal hypertension and oesophageal varices.

Clinical evidence, mechanism, importance and management

Five patients receiving continuous busulfan 2 mg and tioguanine 80 mg five days weekly for chronic myeloid leukaemia (CML) developed oesophageal varices and abnormal liver function tests. Three of them had gastrointestinal haemorrhages and one died. Liver biopsy of 4 of the patients showed nodular regenerative hyperplasia, which was the cause of portal hypertension and varices.[1] A later analysis of the Medical Research Council study comparing busulfan with busulfan and tioguanine in 675 patients with CML, revealed a total of 18 cases of portal hypertension and oesophageal varices (including 4 described in the first report[1]), all 18 of which occurred in patients receiving both drugs. In addition, there was no survival advantage with the combination.[2] The risk of portal hypertension may be related to long-term use of tioguanine, or to its combination with busulfan. This drug combination should not be routinely used for long-term maintenance therapy of CML.[2]

1. Key NS, Kelly PMA, Emerson PM, Chapman RWG, Allan NC, McGee JO'D. Oesophageal varices associated with busulphan-thioguanine combination therapy for chronic myeloid leukaemia. *Lancet* (1987) 2, 1050–2.
2. Shepherd, PCA, Fooks J, Gray R, Allan NC. Thioguanine used in maintenance therapy of chronic myeloid leukaemia causes non-cirrhotic portal hypertension. *Br J Haematol* (1991) 79, 185–92.

Cetuximab + Irinotecan

No pharmacokinetic interaction occurs between cetuximab and irinotecan.

Clinical evidence, mechanism, importance and management

Cetuximab is used with irinotecan in the treatment of metastatic colorectal cancer. In a study 14 patients with advanced EGFR (epidermal growth factor responsive) positive adenocarcinoma were given either irinotecan 350 mg/m^2 every 3 weeks and cetuximab 400 mg/m^2 at week 2 then 250 mg/m^2 each week or cetuximab each week starting at week 1 and irinotecan starting at week 4. There was at least a 1 hour period between the end of the cetuximab infusion and the start of the irinotecan infusion. No evidence was found of a pharmacokinetic interaction between cetuximab and irinotecan, nor was there any significant increase in serious toxicities for the combination, when compared with treatment with either drug alone.[1]

1. Delbaldo C, Pierga J-Y, Dieras V, Faivre S, Laurence V, Vedovato J-C, Bonnaay M, Mueser M, Nolting A, Kovar A, Raymond E. *Eur J Cancer* (2005) 41, 1739–45.

Chlorambucil + Prednisone

An isolated report describes seizures in a patient, which were possibly caused by the use of chlorambucil with prednisone.

Clinical evidence, mechanism, importance and management

A patient with non-Hodgkin's lymphoma experienced a syncopal episode with generalised tonic-clonic seizures 8 days after completing an initial 5-day course of treatment with chlorambucil 12 mg daily and prednisone 50 mg daily. The seizures were controlled with intravenous clonazepam. Four weeks later, on the third day of a second course, she again had generalised tonic-clonic seizures, which resolved spontaneously.

Chlorambucil-induced seizures have occurred in children with nephrotic syndrome. Cases in adults usually involve high-dose chlorambucil or are in patients with a history of seizures. The seizures in this patient may have been due to the additive effects of both drugs in reducing the seizure threshold.[1]

Note that chlorambucil and prednisone or prednisolone have been widely used together.

1. Jourdan E, Topart D, Pinzani V, Jourdan J. Chlorambucil/prednisone-induced seizures in a patient with non-Hodgkin's lymphoma. *Am J Hematol* (2001) 67, 147.

Cisplatin + Aminoglycosides

The renal toxicity of cisplatin is potentiated by aminoglycoside antibacterials such as gentamicin and tobramycin. Extra care is required in patients treated with cisplatin requiring these antibacterials. In one retrospective analysis in patients taking cisplatin, hearing loss was not associated with the concurrent use of ototoxic drugs, including tobramycin.

Clinical evidence

(a) Hypomagnesaemia

Both cisplatin and the aminoglycosides can cause excessive loss of magnesium, and it has been suggested that combined use increases this loss.[1]

(b) Nephrotoxicity

Early after the introduction of cisplatin it became apparent that aminoglycosides could increase the nephrotoxicity of this drug. In one report, 4 patients treated with cisplatin, in dosages ranging from low to very high (eight doses of 0.5 mg/kg, one or two doses of 3 mg/kg or a single-dose of 5 mg/kg), and who were subsequently given **gentamicin** and cefalotin developed acute and fatal renal failure. Autopsy revealed extensive renal tubular necrosis.[2]

Two similar cases of severe renal toxicity, attributed to the use of **gentamicin** and cefalotin in patients who had previously been given cisplatin, are described elsewhere.[3,4] Another patient treated with cisplatin and **gentamicin** developed acute renal failure.[5] A further 3 patients treated with cisplatin then **gentamicin** or **tobramycin** had greater decreases in creatinine levels than 12 others receiving cisplatin alone.[5] A retrospective comparative study confirmed that the incidence of abnormal renal function was higher in patients who had received cisplatin and an aminoglycoside than in patients who had received cisplatin alone (12 of 17 versus 19 of 50 patients, respectively), but the renal impairment was described as usually mild and not clinically significant.[6] Similarly, a brief report stated that aminoglycoside use was associated with a greater decline in renal function in children receiving high-dose cisplatin.[7] Conversely, in another study aminoglycosides were not found to be a significant factor in the development of renal impairment after the use of high-dose cisplatin-based therapy, and use of appropriate supportive care (hydration and mannitol diuresis) probably played a part in this.[8]

There is also evidence from a study in children to show that previous treatment with cisplatin is a risk factor for the delayed elimination of aminoglycosides (**gentamicin**, **amikacin**, **tobramycin**).[9]

(c) Ototoxicity

In one small retrospective analysis of cancer patients, the risk of developing hearing loss after low-dose, slow-infusion cisplatin did not correlate significantly with the concurrent use of other ototoxic drugs, such as furosemide or **tobramycin**.[10] Enhanced renal toxicity and ototoxicity have been reported in *guinea pigs* given cisplatin and **kanamycin** for 2 weeks.[11] In another *animal* study **gentamicin** was given for 14 days. A single dose of cisplatin given early in the course enhanced the ototoxic effects of **gentamicin** but no increase in ototoxicity occurred when cisplatin was given at the end of the **gentamicin** course.[12]

Mechanism

Cisplatin is nephrotoxic and it would appear that its damaging effects on the kidney are additive with the nephrotoxic effects of the aminoglycoside antibacterials. Both gentamicin and cisplatin may cause ototoxicity.[13] Previous exposure to cisplatin caused a significant decrease in gentamicin clearance in *rats*.[14]

Importance and management

An established and potentially serious interaction. However, aminoglycosides remain an important group of antibacterials for the empirical treatment of febrile neutropenia in patients receiving chemotherapy,[15,16] including cisplatin-based regimens. However, in selecting an initial antibacterial regimen, it has been suggested that concurrent use of some drugs, including cisplatin and aminoglycosides, should be avoided if possible because of additive renal toxicity.[17] Good supportive care is required (e.g. pre and post-treatment hydration with mannitol diuresis), and renal function should be well monitored. Audiometric tests should be carried out when cisplatin is used, particularly when other ototoxic drugs are also given.

1. Flombaum CD. Hypomagnesemia associated with cisplatin combination chemotherapy. *Arch Intern Med* (1984) 144, 2336–7.
2. Gonzalez-Vitale JC, Hayes DM, Cvitkovic E, Sternberg SS. Acute renal failure after *cis*-Dichlorodiammineplatinum (II) and gentamicin-cephalothin therapies. *Cancer Treat Rep* (1978) 62, 693–8.
3. Salem PA, Jabboury KW, Khalil MF. Severe nephrotoxicity: a probable complication of cis-dichlorodiammineplatinum (II) and cephalothin-gentamicin therapy. *Oncology* (1982) 39, 31–2.
4. Leite JBF, De Campelo Gentil F, Burchenal J, Marques A, Teixeira MIC, Abrão FA. Insuficiênza renal aguda após o uso de cis-diaminodicloroplatina, gentamicina e cefalosporina. *Rev Paul Med* (1981) 97, 75–7.
5. Dentino M, Luft FC, Yum MN, Williams SD, Einhorn LH. Long term effect of cis-diamminedichloride platinum (CDDP) on renal function and structure in man. *Cancer* (1978) 41, 1274–81.
6. Haas A, Anderson L, Lad T. The influence of aminoglycosides on the nephrotoxicity of *cis*-diamminedichloroplatinum in cancer patients. *J Infect Dis* (1983) 147, 363.
7. Pearson ADJ, Kohli M, Scott GW, Craft AW. Toxicity of high dose cisplatinum in children — the additive role of aminoglycosides. *Proc Am Assoc Cancer Res* (1987) 28, 221.
8. Cooper BW, Creger RJ, Soegiarso W, Mackay WL, Lazarus HM. Renal dysfunction during high-dose cisplatin therapy and autologous hematopoietic stem cell transplantation: effect of aminoglycoside therapy. *Am J Med* (1993) 94, 497–504.
9. Christensen ML, Stewart CF, Crom WR. Evaluation of aminoglycoside disposition in patients previously treated with cisplatin. *Ther Drug Monit* (1989) 11, 631–6.
10. Hallmark RJ, Snyder JM, Jusenius K, Tamimi HK. Factors influencing ototoxicity in ovarian cancer patients treated with Cis-platinum based chemotherapy. *Eur J Gynaecol Oncol* (1992) 13, 35–44.
11. Schweitzer VG, Hawkins JE, Lilly DJ, Litterst CJ, Abrams G, Davis JA, Christy M. Ototoxic and nephrotoxic effects of combined treatment with *cis*-diamminedichloroplatinum and kanamycin in the guinea pig. *Otolaryngol Head Neck Surg* (1984) 92, 38–49.
12. Riggs LC, Brummett RE, Guitjens SK, Matz GJ. Ototoxicity resulting from combined administration of cisplatin and gentamicin. *Laryngoscope* (1996) 106, 401–6.
13. Lautermann J, Dehne N, Schacht J, Jahnke K. Aminoglykosid- und cisplatin-Ototoxizität: von der Grundlagenforschung zur Klinik. *Laryngorhinootologie* (2004) 83, 317–23.
14. Engineer MS, Bodey GP, Newman RA, Ho DH. Effects of cisplatin-induced nephrotoxicity on gentamicin pharmacokinetics in rats. *Drug Metab Dispos* (1987) 15, 329–34.
15. Ziglam HM, Gelly K, Olver W. A survey of the management of neutropenic fever in oncology units in the UK. *Int J Antimicrob Agents* (2007) 29, 430–3.
16. Tamura K. Initial empirical antimicrobial therapy: duration and subsequent modifications. *Clin Infect Dis* (2004) 39 (Suppl 1) S59–S64.
17. Hughes WT, Armstrong D, Bodey GP, Bow EJ, Brown AE, Calandra T, Feld R, Pizzo PA, Rolston KVI, Shenep JL, Young LS, for the Infectious Diseases Society of America. 2002 Guidelines for the use of antimicrobial agents in neutropenic patients with cancer. *Clin Infect Dis* (2002) 34, 730–51.

Cisplatin + Diuretics

A single report describes the development of renal failure in a patient treated with furosemide and other antihypertensives during cisplatin therapy. However, note that furosemide can be used to promote diuresis during cisplatin therapy to reduce the risk of nephrotoxicity. Although *animal* studies show that the damaging effects of cisplatin on the ear can be markedly increased by the concurrent use of etacrynic acid or furosemide a retrospective analysis in patients did not find this effect.

Clinical evidence, mechanism, importance and management

(a) Nephrotoxicity

Three hours after receiving intravenous cisplatin 70 mg/m^2 a patient experienced severe nausea and vomiting and his blood pressure rose from 150/90 to 248/140 mmHg. This was managed with **furosemide** 40 mg intravenously, **hydralazine** 10 mg intramuscularly, **diazoxide** 300 mg intravenously and **propranolol** 20 mg orally twice daily for 2 days. Nine days later the patient showed evidence of renal impairment (creatinine raised from about 88 micromol/L to 283 micromol/L), which resolved within 3 weeks. The patient was subsequently similarly treated on two occasions with cisplatin and again developed hypertension, but no treatment was given and there was no evidence of renal impairment.[1] The reasons for the renal impairment are not known, but a study in *rats*[2] indicate that kidney damage may possibly be related to the concentrations of cisplatin, and that **furosemide** can increase cisplatin levels in the kidney. However, another study in patients found that there was no difference in the toxicity or pharmacokinetics of cisplatin when **furosemide** was used to induce diuresis, compared with mannitol.[3] Two other studies have also found that **furosemide** does not alter cisplatin pharmacokinetics.[4,5] Another study showed that sodium chloride solution with or without **furosemide** was associated with less cisplatin nephrotoxicity than sodium chloride solution with mannitol.[6]

Information seems to be limited to the case cited and its general clinical importance is uncertain. Although mannitol is by far the more usual drug used to induce diuresis during the use of cisplatin in order to reduce the risk of nephrotoxicity, **furosemide** may also be used for this indication.[7]

(b) Ototoxicity

Both cisplatin and loop diuretics such as **etacrynic acid** and **furosemide** given alone can be ototoxic in man. A study[8] in *guinea pigs* showed that when cisplatin 7 mg/kg or **etacrynic acid** 50 mg/kg were given alone their ototoxic effects were reversible, but when given together the damaging effects on the ear were profound, prolonged and possibly permanent. Similarly, while cisplatin-induced ototoxicity was potentiated by **furosemide** in *guinea pigs* in one study[9] in another this was only seen when a very high dose of **furosemide** was used.[10] In one small retrospective analysis of cancer patients, the risk of developing hearing loss after low-dose slow-infusion cisplatin did not correlate significantly with concurrent use of other ototoxic drugs, such as **furosemide**.[11] Audiometric tests should be carried out when cisplatin is used, and this is of particular importance when other ototoxic drugs are also given.

1. Markman M, Trump DL. Nephrotoxicity with cisplatin and antihypertensive medications. *Ann Intern Med* (1982) 96, 257.
2. Pera MF, Zook BC, Harder HC. Effects of mannitol or furosemide diuresis on the nephrotoxicity and physiological disposition of *cis*-dichlorodiammineplatinum-(II) in rats. *Cancer Res* (1979) 39, 1269–79.
3. Ostrow S, Egorin MJ, Hahn D, Markus S, Aisner J, Chang P, LeRoy A, Bachur NR, Wiernik PH. High-dose cisplatin therapy using mannitol versus furosemide diuresis: comparative pharmacokinetics and toxicity. *Cancer Treat Rep* (1981) 65, 73–8.
4. Dumas M, d'Athis P, de Gislain C, Lautissier JL, Autissier N, Escousse A, Guerrin J. Influence of frusemide on cis-dichlorodiammineplatinum (II) pharmaco-kinetics. *Eur J Drug Metab Pharmacokinet* (1987) 12, 203–6.
5. Dumas M, de Gislain C, d'Athis P, Chadoint-Noudeau V, Escousse A, Guerrin J, Autissier N. Evaluation of the effect of furosemide on ultrafilterable platinum kinetics in patients treated with *cis*-diamminedichloroplatinium. *Cancer Chemother Pharmacol* (1989) 23, 37–40.
6. Santoso JT, Lucci JA, Coleman RL, Schafer I, Hannigan EV. Saline, mannitol, and furosemide hydration in acute cisplatin nephrotoxicity: a randomised trial. *Cancer Chemother Pharmacol* (2003) 52, 13–18.
7. Numico G, Benasso M, Vannozzi MO, Merlano M, Rosso R, Viale M, Esposito M. Hydration regimen and hematological toxicity of a cisplatin-based chemotherapy regimen. Clinical observations and pharmacokinetic analysis. *Anticancer Res* (1998) 18, 1313–18.
8. Komune S, Snow JB. Potentiating effects of cisplatin and ethacrynic acid in ototoxicity. *Arch Otolaryngol* (1981) 107, 594–7.
9. McAlpine D, Johnstone BM. The ototoxic mechanism of cisplatin. *Hear Res* (1990) 47, 191–203.
10. Laurell G, Engström B. The combined effect of cisplatin and furosemide on hearing function in guinea pigs. *Hear Res* (1989) 38, 19–26.
11. Hallmark RJ, Snyder JM, Jusenius K, Tamimi HK. Factors influencing ototoxicity in ovarian cancer patients treated with Cis-platinum based chemotherapy. *Eur J Gynaecol Oncol* (1992) 13, 35–44.

Cisplatin + H_2-receptor antagonists

Cimetidine and ranitidine probably do not have a clinically relevant effect on the renal clearance of cisplatin.

Clinical evidence, mechanism, importance and management

Some *animal* studies have shown that organic cations such as **cimetidine** and **ranitidine** may compete with the renal tubular transport of cisplatin and thus could be useful in reducing cisplatin nephrotoxicity.[1,2] However, in a study of 10 children receiving cisplatin, **ranitidine** had no effect on the total body disposition or renal clearance of cisplatin. This finding and further studies in *dogs* showed that cisplatin may not share transport systems with organic cations to a clinically relevant extent.[3] Although information is limited, it appears that there is no interaction between cisplatin and **cimetidine** or **ranitidine**. Note that **cimetidine** has increased the levels or toxicity of some other antineoplastics, see 'Nitrosoureas + Cimetidine', p.655, 'Cyclophosphamide + H_2-receptor antagonists', p.626, 'Anthracyclines; Epirubicin + Cimetidine', p.613, and 'Fluorouracil + H_2-receptor antagonists', p.633.

1. Klein J, Bentur Y, Cheung D, Moselhy G, Koren G. Renal handling of cisplatin: interactions with organic anions and cations in the dog. *Clin Invest Med* (1991) 14, 388–94.
2. Haragsim L, Zima T, Něměček K. Nephrotoxic effects of platinum cytostatics–preventive effects of nifedipine and cimetidine. *Sb Lek* (1994) 95, 173–83.
3. Ito S, Weitzman S, Klein J, Greenberg M, Lau R, Atanakovic G, Koren G. Lack of cisplatin-ranitidine kinetic interactions: *in vivo* study in children, and *in vitro* study using dog renal brush border membrane vesicles. *Life Sci* (1998) 62, PL387–PL392.

Cisplatin + Probenecid

The available clinical data suggest that the nephrotoxicity of cisplatin is reduced by probenecid, but uncertainty remains.

Clinical evidence, mechanism, importance and management

In a randomised study in cancer patients, probenecid 2 to 4 g daily reduced the fractional clearance of free platinum after a single 60- to 100-mg/m^2 dose of cisplatin given as a 24-hour infusion, and no cases of renal impairment were seen.[1] Similarly, in a further phase I dose-escalation study no renal impairment was seen in patients given cisplatin at doses from 100 to 160 mg/m^2 when they were also given probenecid 1 g every 6 hours for 12 doses (beginning 24 hours before the cisplatin infusion, and continuing for 24 hours after).[2] It was concluded that probenecid may protect against cisplatin-induced renal toxicity. An earlier study in *rats* had also suggested that giving probenecid before cisplatin reduced nephrotoxicity, as assessed by blood urea levels and serum creatinine.[3] Subsequently, a study in *dogs* has found that probenecid decreases the renal clearance of free cisplatin,[4] and another in *mice* found that probenecid reduces the renal tubular damage seen with cisplatin alone.[5]

Conversely, some researchers have suggested that the combination of probenecid and cisplatin is potentially more toxic than cisplatin alone. They found that probenecid increased the fractional clearance of free platinum from cisplatin in *rats*, and that pretreatment with probenecid increased nephrotoxicity, as assessed by blood urea levels.[6] Other authors similarly reported that probenecid increased cisplatin clearance in *rats*.[7]

It is unclear why some *animal* studies show that probenecid increases cisplatin-induced nephrotoxicity whereas others show a decrease. Although the available clinical data suggest that there is a decrease, some uncertainty remains. The combination should be used with caution.

1. Jacobs C, Coleman CN, Rich L, Hirst K, Weiner MW. Inhibition of *cis*-diamminedichloroplatinum secretion by the human kidney with probenecid. *Cancer Res* (1984) 44, 3632–5.
2. Jacobs C, Kaubisch S, Halsey J, Lum BL, Gosland M, Coleman CN, Sikic BI. The use of probenecid as a chemoprotector against cisplatin nephrotoxicity. *Cancer* (1991) 67, 1518–24.
3. Ross DA, Gale GR. Reduction of the renal toxicity of *cis*-dichlorodiammineplatinum (II) by probenecid. *Cancer Treat Rep* (1979) 63, 781–7.
4. Klein J, Bentur Y, Cheung D, Moselhy G, Koren G. Renal handling of cisplatin: interactions with organic anions and cations in the dog. *Clin Invest Med* (1991) 14, 388–94.
5. Ban M, Hettich D, Huguet N. Nephrotoxicity mechanism of *cis*-platinum (II) diamine dichloride in mice. *Toxicol Lett* (1994) 71, 161–8.

6. Daley-Yates PT, McBrien DCH. Enhancement of cisplatin nephrotoxicity by probenecid. *Cancer Treat Rep* (1984) 68, 445–6.
7. Osman NM, Litterst CL. Effect of probenecid and *N'*-methylnicotinamide on renal handling of *cis*-dichlorodiammineplatinum-II in rats. *Cancer Lett* (1983) 19, 107–11.

Cyclophosphamide + Allopurinol

There is some evidence to suggest that the incidence of serious bone marrow depression caused by cyclophosphamide can be increased by allopurinol, but this was not confirmed in a controlled study. Allopurinol may prolong the half-life of cyclophosphamide and increase the levels of its cytotoxic metabolites.

Clinical evidence

A retrospective epidemiological survey of patients in four hospitals who, over a 4-year period, had been treated with cyclophosphamide, found that the incidence of serious bone marrow depression was 57.7% in 26 patients who had also received allopurinol, and 18.8% in 32 patients who had not.[1] A pharmacokinetic study in 9 patients with malignant disease and 2 healthy subjects showed that while taking allopurinol 600 mg daily the concentration of the cytotoxic metabolites of cyclophosphamide increased by an average of 37.5% (range 1.5 to 110%).[2] Another pharmacokinetic study reported that the half-life of cyclophosphamide was more than twofold longer in 3 children also receiving allopurinol 300 mg/m^2, when compared with that in children not given allopurinol.[3] However, another study found that although allopurinol pre-treatment increased the half-life of cyclophosphamide, the plasma alkylating activity and urinary metabolite and cyclophosphamide excretion were unchanged.[4] Moreover, a randomised controlled study,[5] designed as a follow-up to the survey cited above,[1] failed to confirm that allopurinol increased the toxicity of cyclophosphamide in 81 patients with Hodgkin's or non-Hodgkin's lymphoma. In this study, there was no difference in nadirs for white blood cells and platelets during 3 cycles of cyclophosphamide-containing chemotherapy in 44 patients receiving allopurinol and in 37 patients not receiving allopurinol.

Mechanism

Not understood. Cyclophosphamide itself is inactive, but it is converted by the liver into cytotoxic metabolites.[4] Allopurinol or its metabolite oxypurinol may inhibit their renal excretion, or may alter hepatic metabolism.[2,3]

Importance and management

This interaction is not established with any certainty. The authors of the randomised study consider that, if necessary, allopurinol can be used safely to prevent hyperuricaemia with the chemotherapy regimens used for lymphomas.[5] However, the other data introduce a note of caution. Be alert for increased cyclophosphamide toxicity if allopurinol is given.

1. Boston Collaborative Drug Surveillance Programme. Allopurinol and cytotoxic drugs. Interaction in relation to bone marrow depression. *JAMA* (1974) 227, 1036–40.
2. Witten J, Frederiksen PL, Mouridsen HT. The pharmacokinetics of cyclophosphamide in man after treatment with allopurinol. *Acta Pharmacol Toxicol (Copenh)* (1980) 46, 392–4.
3. Yule SM, Boddy AV, Cole M, Price L, Wyllie R, Tasso MJ, Pearson ADJ, Idle JR. Cyclophosphamide pharmacokinetics in children. *Br J Clin Pharmacol* (1996) 41, 13–19.
4. Bagley CM, Bostick FW, DeVita VT. Clinical pharmacology of cyclophosphamide. *Cancer Res* (1973) 33, 226–33.
5. Stolbach L, Begg C, Bennett JM, Silverstein M, Falkson G, Harris DT, Glick J. Evaluation of bone marrow toxic reaction in patients treated with allopurinol. *JAMA* (1982) 247, 334–6.

Cyclophosphamide + Amiodarone

Early-onset pulmonary toxicity occurred in one patient taking amiodarone after high-dose cyclophosphamide was given. Fatal pulmonary toxicity occurred in another patient taking amiodarone after a single dose of cyclophosphamide.

Clinical evidence

A patient with dendritic cell carcinoma who had been taking amiodarone for 18 months, and who had received 6 cycles of chemotherapy including cyclophosphamide over the previous 12 months, was admitted to hospital with progressive shortness of breath 18 days after being given a single 4000-mg/m^2 dose of cyclophosphamide. He was found to have interstitial pneumonitis and a lung biopsy indicated drug-induced pulmonary toxicity. The patient's condition improved rapidly over the following 10 days with discontinuation of amiodarone and treatment with prednisolone 60 mg daily. Over the previous year he had also received vincristine, etoposide and prednisone, cisplatin, cytarabine and dexamethasone as part of his chemotherapy.[1] A patient with non-Hodgkin's lymphoma who had been taking amiodarone 300 mg twice daily for 4 years, developed acute respiratory distress 2 days after being given a single dose of cyclophosphamide. This was eventually fatal. Autopsy revealed lung damage consistent with the effects of amiodarone and cyclophosphamide, with the cyclophosphamide the major cause. Other drugs used as part of the chemotherapy regimen were rituximab, doxorubicin, vincristine and prednisone.[2]

Mechanism

Pulmonary toxicity may occur in about 10% of patients given amiodarone.[3,4] Pulmonary toxicity due to cyclophosphamide may occur between 1 to 6 months after exposure or occur as a more insidious form after about 6 months. The early onset of symptoms in the patients described above suggests accelerated mechanisms of pulmonary toxicity. Both cyclophosphamide and amiodarone pulmonary toxicity appear to be enhanced by oxygen and the combination of cyclophosphamide with amiodarone may enhance oxidative stress and therefore pulmonary toxicity.

Importance and management

Although information seems to be limited to the two case reports cited, the potential for both cyclophosphamide and amiodarone to cause pulmonary toxicity is established. Be alert to the possibility of enhanced pulmonary toxicity if these drugs are given together.

1. Bhagat R, Sporn TA, Long GD, Folz RJ. Amiodarone and cyclophosphamide: potential for enhanced lung toxicity. *Bone Marrow Transplant* (2001) 27, 1109–1111.
2. Gupta S, Mahipal A. Fatal pulmonary toxicity after a single dose of cyclophosphamide. *Pharmacotherapy* (2007) 27, 616–18.
3. Martin WJ, Rosenow EC. Amiodarone pulmonary toxicity. Recognition and pathogenesis (Part 1). *Chest* (1988) 93, 1067–75.
4. Martin WJ, Rosenow EC. Amiodarone pulmonary toxicity. Recognition and pathogenesis (Part 2). *Chest* (1988) 93, 1242–8.

Cyclophosphamide + Azathioprine

A report describes liver damage in four patients given cyclophosphamide and who had previously taken azathioprine. However, another study found that liver function improved when cyclophosphamide was substituted for azathioprine in 29 patients.

Clinical evidence, mechanism, importance and management

Four patients (two with systemic lupus erythematosus, one with Sjogren's syndrome, and one with Wegener's granulomatosis) developed liver injury when given cyclophosphamide and 3 of them had liver cell necrosis. All had previously been treated with azathioprine and 2 of them had received cyclophosphamide previously without apparent liver damage. It was suggested that azathioprine and cyclophosphamide may have interacted.[1] However, in a retrospective study of cardiac transplant recipients, substitution of cyclophosphamide for azathioprine was associated with improvement in liver function tests in 29 patients with suspected azathioprine-induced liver impairment.[2]

1. Shaunak S, Munro JM, Weinbren K, Walport MJ, Cox TM. Cyclophosphamide-induced liver necrosis: a possible interaction with azathioprine. *Q J Med* (1988) New Series 67, 309–17.
2. Wagoner LE, Olsen SL, Bristow MR, O'Connell JB, Taylor DO, Lappe DL, Renlund DG. Cyclophosphamide as an alternative to azathioprine in cardiac transplant recipients with suspected azathioprine-induced hepatotoxicity. *Transplantation* (1993) 56, 1415–18.

Cyclophosphamide or Ifosfamide + Azoles

Fluconazole and itraconazole inhibit the metabolism of cyclophosphamide. There is some evidence that, compared with fluconazole, itraconazole might increase cyclophosphamide toxicity. Ketoconazole inhibits the metabolism of ifosfamide. This did not improve the ratio of active to inactive-toxic metabolites, and the possibility remains that ifosfamide efficacy could be reduced.

Clinical evidence, mechanism, importance and management

(a) Cyclophosphamide

Twenty-two children with established cyclophosphamide metabolism profiles and who were not receiving other treatment known to affect drug metabolism were included in a retrospective case series investigation. The clearance of cyclophosphamide was reduced by 43% in 9 children who were given oral or intravenous **fluconazole** 5 mg/kg daily compared to the remaining 13 children who did not receive **fluconazole**.[1] A study in patients given either intravenous or oral **fluconazole** 400 mg daily or **itraconazole** (either 200 mg daily intravenously or 2.5 mg/kg three times daily orally) for prophylaxis after allogenic stem cell transplantation found that those given **itraconazole** developed higher bilirubin and creatinine levels in the first 20 days after transplantation than those given **fluconazole**. Highest values were in patients who received **itraconazole** with cyclophosphamide. In this study, analysis of cyclophosphamide pharmacokinetics in 9 **itraconazole** recipients and 140 **fluconazole** recipients revealed that **itraconazole** recipients had a 20% greater clearance of cyclophosphamide, leading to greater exposure to the active metabolite of cyclophosphamide, 4-hydroxycyclophosphamide (HCY), and its metabolites.[2]

Cyclophosphamide is oxidised to HCY by the cytochrome P450 isoenzymes CYP2B6, CYP3A4, CYP2C9, and CYP2A6 and then HCY undergoes further metabolism to produce several toxic metabolites. It is also metabolised by CYP3A4 to an inactive metabolite, deschloroethylcyclophosphamide (DCCP). **Itraconazole** is a more potent inhibitor of CYP3A4 than **fluconazole**, but unlike **itraconazole**, **fluconazole** can also inhibit CYP2C9. It has been suggested that inhibition of CYP2C9 by **fluconazole** may decrease the formation of HCY and result in increased levels of DCCP and fewer toxic metabolites.[2] Further study is required to determine whether the inhibition of active metabolite formation by **fluconazole** reduces the therapeutic effect of cyclophosphamide.[1] Until more is known it may be prudent to encourage caution when azoles are used in patients receiving cyclophosphamide, other than therapies established in randomised clinical studies, being alert for unexpected toxicity or reduced efficacy.

(b) Ifosfamide

Eight patients undergoing chemotherapy were also given (for the first or second cycle of treatment) **ketoconazole** 200 mg twice daily for 4 days starting one day before treatment with ifosfamide. Concurrent treatment with **ketoconazole** modestly decreased the clearance of ifosfamide by 11%, increased its AUC by 14%, and increased urinary elimination by 26%. The fraction of ifosfamide metabolised to the inactive-neurotoxic, dechloroethylated metabolite was not affected, whereas the fraction metabolised to the active, hydroxylated metabolite was modestly decreased.[3]

Ketoconazole is an inhibitor of the cytochrome P450 isoenzyme CYP3A4, an enzyme that is involved in the production of active and inactive-toxic metabolites of ifosfamide (see also 'Cyclophosphamide or Ifosfamide + Barbiturates', below). In the clinical study cited, **ketoconazole** modestly decreased the proportion of ifosfamide undergoing activation. It was suggested that concurrent use should be avoided, as it might result in decreased ifosfamide efficacy,[3] although this remains to be shown.

1. Yule SM, Walker D, Cole M, Mcsorley L, Cholerton S, Daly AK, Pearson ADJ, Boddy AV. The effect of fluconazole on cyclophosphamide metabolism in children. *Drug Metab Dispos* (1999) 27, 417–21.
2. Marr KA, Leisenring W, Crippa F, Slattery JT, Corey L, Boeckh M, McDonald GB. Cyclophosphamide metabolism is affected by azole antifungals. *Blood* (2004) 103, 1557–9.
3. Kerbusch T, Jansen RLH, Mathôt RAA, Huitema ADR, Jansen M, van Rijswijk REN, Beijnen JH. Modulation of the cytochrome P450–mediated metabolism of ifosfamide by ketoconazole and rifampin. *Clin Pharmacol Ther* (2001) 70, 132–41.

Cyclophosphamide or Ifosfamide + Barbiturates

Evidence suggests that neither the toxicity nor the therapeutic effects of cyclophosphamide and ifosfamide are significantly altered by the concurrent use of barbiturates. However, an isolated report describes a girl taking phenobarbital who developed encephalopathy when given ifosfamide.

Clinical evidence

(a) Cyclophosphamide

In 4 patients **phenobarbital** 180 mg daily in divided doses for 10 days increased the mean plasma levels of cyclophosphamide total metabolites by 50% and increased their rate of urinary excretion.[1] Similarly, another study in 11 patients given cyclophosphamide reported that the peak level of normustard-like substances was 1.5 times higher after pretreatment with **phenobarbital**.[2] Similar changes in cyclophosphamide pharmacokinetics have been described in *animal* studies, and these have generally also shown that **phenobarbital** has no effect on the antitumour activity of cyclophosphamide[3] although some have shown a reduction in its effects.[4]

Cyclophosphamide was reported to inhibit the clearance and increase the effects of **pentobarbital** in a study in *rats*.[5] Another study found auto-induction of cyclophosphamide clearance in a patient taking **phenobarbital** with subsequent chemotherapy courses similar to that in patients not taking **phenobarbital**.[6]

(b) Ifosfamide

A 15-year-old girl who had been taking **phenobarbital** for epilepsy since infancy developed confusion and gradually became unconscious 6 hours after being given a first dose of ifosfamide for metastatic rhabdomyosarcoma. Her chemotherapy regimen was ifosfamide 3 g/m^2, mesna 3.6 g/m^2, vincristine 2 mg and dactinomycin. An EEG revealed signs of severe diffuse encephalopathy. She remained unconscious for 24 hours but was asymptomatic after 48 hours.[7] In a pharmacokinetic study, **phenobarbital** 60 mg daily for 3 days had no effect on the pharmacokinetics of high-dose ifosfamide (4 g/m^2 over 1 hour each day for 3 days). The AUC for ifosfamide decreased from day one to day 3 irrespective of **phenobarbital** administration.[8]

Mechanism

Cyclophosphamide and ifosfamide are prodrugs that undergo hepatic metabolism, and it seems that they are able to induce their own metabolism. Cyclophosphamide appears to be hydroxylated by the cytochrome P450 subfamilies CYP2B and CYP2C, in particular, to form active metabolites, whereas ifosfamide appears to be principally hydroxylated by CYP3A. Both drugs also undergo dechloroethylation to produce inactive but neurotoxic metabolites, which can cause encephalopathy. For cyclophosphamide, this seems to be primarily catalysed by CYP3A, whereas for ifosfamide both CYP3A and CYP2B appear to be involved. Ifosfamide has a higher incidence of encephalopathy than cyclophosphamide.[9] Phenobarbital and other barbiturates are inducers of both CYP2B and CYP3A. Therefore it is unlikely that barbiturates will generally alter the balance between dechloroethylation and hydroxylation for cyclophosphamide,[3] although there is some evidence from *animal* studies they may do so for ifosfamide.[10]

Importance and management

The relationship between the case of encephalopathy and the use of ifosfamide with phenobarbital is not established, but it serves to emphasise the need for particular caution and good monitoring if concurrent use is undertaken. More study is needed. Although barbiturates can cause an increase in the rate of metabolism of cyclophosphamide, this does not appear to alter the AUC and the efficacy of this drug.

1. Jao JY, Jusko WJ, Cohen JL. Phenobarbital effects on cyclophosphamide pharmacokinetics in man. *Cancer Res* (1972) 32, 2761–4.
2. Maezawa S, Ohira S, Sakauma M, Matsuoka S, Wakui A, Saito T. Effects of inducer of liver drug-metabolizing enzyme on blood level of active metabolites of cyclophosphamide in rats and in cancer patients. *Tohoku J Exp Med* (1981) 134, 45–53.
3. Yu LJ, Drewes P, Gustafsson K, Brain EGC, Hecht JED, Waxman DJ. In Vivo modulation of alternative pathways of P-450-catalyzed cyclophosphamide metabolism: impact on pharmacokinetics and antitumor activity. *J Pharmacol Exp Ther* (1999) 288, 928–37.
4. Alberts DS, van Daalen Wetters T. The effect of phenobarbital on cyclophosphamide antitumour activity. *Cancer Res* (1976) 36, 2785–9.
5. Donelli MG, Colombo T, Garattini S. Effect of cyclophosphamide on the activity and distribution of pentobarbital in rats. *Biochem Pharmacol* (1973) 22, 2609–14.
6. Chen T-L, Passos-Coelho JL, Noe DA, Kennedy MJ, Black KC, Colvin M, Grochow LB. Nonlinear pharmacokinetics of cyclophosphamide in patients with metastatic breast cancer receiving high-dose chemotherapy followed by autologous bone marrow transplantation. *Cancer Res* (1995) 55, 810–16. Correction. ibid. 1600.
7. Ghosn M, Carde P, Leclerq B, Flamant F, Friedman S, Droz JP, Hayat M. Ifosfamide/mesna related encephalopathy: a case report with a possible role of phenobarbital in enhancing neurotoxicity. *Bull Cancer* (1988) 75, 391–2.
8. Lokiec F, Santoni J, Weill S, Tubiana-Hulin M. Phenobarbital administration does not affect high-dose ifosfamide pharmacokinetics in humans. *Anticancer Drugs* (1996) 7, 893–6.
9. Goren MP, Wright RK, Pratt CB, Pell FE. Dechloroethylation of ifosfamide and neurotoxicity. *Lancet* (1986) ii, 1219–20.
10. Brain EGC, Yu LJ, Gustafsson K, Drewes P, Waxman DJ. Modulation of P450-dependent ifosfamide pharmacokinetics: a better understanding of drug activation in vivo. *Br J Cancer* (1998) 77, 1768–76.

Cyclophosphamide or Ifosfamide + Benzodiazepines

***Animal* studies suggest that the benzodiazepines may possibly increase the metabolic activation and the toxicity of high doses of cyclophosphamide and ifosfamide. However, diazepam did not alter the pharmacokinetics of high-dose cyclophosphamide in a clinical study. Note also that lorazepam is widely used for chemotherapy-induced nausea and vomiting.**

Clinical evidence, mechanism, importance and management

Studies in *mice* found that pretreatment with benzodiazepines (**chlordiazepoxide, diazepam, oxazepam**) increased the levels of the active metabolites and the lethality of high-dose cyclophosphamide[1] and similarly increased the levels of active metabolites and enhanced the toxicity of high-dose ifosfamide.[2] However, a clinical study found that the prophylactic use of **diazepam** 5 mg daily as an antiepileptic had no effect on the pharmacokinetics of very high-dose cyclophosphamide (60 mg/kg intravenously over 2 hours for 2 days) or its neurotoxic (dechloroethylated) metabolites in 3 patients receiving cyclophosphamide and busulfan before bone marrow transplantation.[3] In the *animal* studies, it was suggested that benzodiazepines may induce the liver enzymes concerned with the metabolism of cyclophosphamide and ifosfamide to its active cytotoxic products. There are very limited data on this potential interaction. The widespread use of the benzodiazepine **lorazepam** in antiemetic regimens for chemotherapy-induced nausea and vomiting suggest that a significant increase in toxicity or alteration in efficacy of cyclophosphamide and ifosfamide does not occur clinically, but there do not appear to be any studies directly addressing this question.

1. Sasaki K-I, Furusawa S, Takayanagi G. Effects of chlordiazepoxide, diazepam and oxazepam on the antitumour activity, the lethality and the blood level of active metabolites of cyclophosphamide and cyclophosphamide oxidase activity in mice. *J Pharmacobiodyn* (1983) 6, 767–72.
2. Furusawa S, Fujimura T, Sasaki K, Takayanagi Y. Potentiation of ifosfamide toxicity by chlordiazepoxide, diazepam, and oxazepam. *Chem Pharm Bull (Tokyo)* (1989) 73, 3420–2.
3. Williams ML, Wainer IW, Embree L, Barnett M, Granvil CL, Ducharme MP. Enantioselective induction of cyclophosphamide metabolism by phenytoin. *Chirality* (1999) 11, 569–74.

Cyclophosphamide + Busulfan

The levels of cyclophosphamide may be increased, and those of its active metabolite decreased, if it is given within 24 hours of busulfan treatment.

Clinical evidence, mechanism, importance and management

In one study, the ratio of the AUC of cyclophosphamide and that of its active metabolite hydroxycyclophosphamide was higher in patients also receiving phenytoin and busulfan than in those receiving irradiation (suggesting reduced cyclophosphamide activation), but variability between patients was high.[1] In a similar study, 23 bone marrow transplant patients were pretreated with busulfan 4 mg/kg/day for 4 days, followed by cyclophosphamide 60 mg/kg/day for 2 days. The interval between the last dose of busulfan and starting cyclophosphamide was 24 to 50 hours in 12 patients [group A] and 7 to 15 hours in the remaining 11 [group B]. Nine others pretreated with cyclophosphamide and total body irradiation acted as the controls. In group A the AUCs of cyclophosphamide and hydroxycyclophosphamide were similar to those in the controls but in group B the AUC of cyclophosphamide was more than doubled and the AUC of hydroxycyclophosphamide significantly lower (representing a reduced ratio of hydroxycyclophosphamide to cyclophosphamide). In addition group B had greater toxicity.[2] Busulfan may directly inhibit the hepatic activation of cyclophosphamide or may act indirectly by depleting glutathione. Phenytoin induces the metabolism of cyclophosphamide (see 'Cyclophosphamide or Ifosfamide + Phenytoin', p.627).

It seems therefore that if the cyclophosphamide is given at least 24 hours after the last busulfan dose, its serum levels will not be greatly affected, whereas if the interval is short, activation may be decreased and toxicity increased. Further study is required to determine the optimum timing to achieve maximum efficacy and minimum drug toxicity while taking into account other concurrent medication such as phenytoin.

1. Slattery JT, Kalhorn TF, McDonald GB, Lambert K, Buckner CD, Bensinger WI, Anasetti C, Appelbaum FR. Conditioning regimen-dependent disposition of cyclophosphamide and hydroxycyclophosphamide in human marrow transplantation patients. *J Clin Oncol* (1996) 14, 1484–94.
2. Hassan M, Ljungman P, Ringdén O, Hassan Z, Öberg G, Nilsson C, Békassy A, Bielenstein M, Abdel-Rehim M, Georén S, Astner L. The effect of busulphan on the pharmacokinetics of cyclophosphamide and its 4-hydroxy metabolite: time interval influence on the therapeutic efficacy and therapy-related toxicity. *Bone Marrow Transplant* (2000) 25, 915–24.

Cyclophosphamide + Chloramphenicol

Some limited evidence suggests that chloramphenicol may reduce the production of the active metabolites of cyclophosphamide. Whether this reduces its therapeutic efficacy remains to be determined.

Clinical evidence, mechanism, importance and management

Cyclophosphamide itself is inactive, but after administration it is metabolised to active alkylating metabolites. A study in *animals*[1] found that pretreatment with chloramphenicol reduced the effects of cyclophosphamide and reduced the production of its active metabolites. Although another *animal* study also found a reduction in lethality of cyclophosphamide with chloramphenicol, the immunosuppressive effect of cyclophosphamide was unchanged.[2] A study in 4 patients found that chloramphenicol 1 g twice daily for 12 days prolonged the mean serum half-life of a single intravenous dose of cyclophosphamide from 7.5 to 11.5 hours, but did not significantly affect the AUC of the metabolites.[3]

Chloramphenicol is an inhibitor of the cytochrome P450 isoenzyme subfamily CYP2B, which is partially responsible for the activation of cyclophosphamide. It therefore seems possible that a reduction in the activity of cyclophosphamide may occur, but the extent to which this affects treatment with cyclophosphamide is uncertain. Concurrent use need not be avoided, but be alert for evidence of a reduced response. More study is needed.

1. Dixon RL. Effect of chloramphenicol on the metabolism and lethality of cyclophosphamide in rats. *Proc Soc Exp Biol Med* (1968) 127, 1151–5.
2. Berenbaum MC, Cope WA, Double JA. The effect of microsomal enzyme inhibition on the immunosuppressive and toxic effects of cyclophosphamide. *Clin Exp Immunol* (1973) 14, 257–70.
3. Faber OK, Mouridsen HT, Skovsted L. The effect of chloramphenicol and sulphaphenazole on the biotransformation of cyclophosphamide in man. *Br J Clin Pharmacol* (1975) 2, 281–5.

Cyclophosphamide or Ifosfamide + Cisplatin

The renal toxicity of ifosfamide may be greater when used with cisplatin or in those who have had prior treatment with cisplatin. Ifosfamide may increase the hearing loss due to cisplatin.

Clinical evidence

(a) Nephrotoxicity

A comparative study in 36 children with malignant solid tumours taking a range of drugs including some known to be potentially nephrotoxic (high dose methotrexate, aminoglycosides, cyclophosphamide), indicated that previous treatment with cisplatin increased their susceptibility to ifosfamide toxicity (neurotoxicity, severe leucopenia or acute tubular damage).[1] Similarly, in another study the cumulative cisplatin dose given before high-dose ICE (ifosfamide, carboplatin, and etoposide) was found to be a strong risk factor for the development of nephrotoxicity.[2] The nephrotoxicity may not be reversible; 3 cases requiring long-term haemodialysis have been described.[3]

Other studies also suggested that the concurrent use of ifosfamide with cisplatin appeared to increase nephrotoxicity; one showed an increase in depletion of phosphate reabsorption,[4] whereas the other showed increased microglobulin excretion.[5]

(b) Ototoxicity

A retrospective comparative study found that when ifosfamide was added to cisplatin, the hearing loss caused by cisplatin was exacerbated.[6]

Mechanism

Both cisplatin and ifosfamide are commonly associated with nephrotoxicity. It is thought that concurrent or possibly previous treatment with cisplatin damages the kidney tubules so that the clearance of the ifosfamide metabolites is reduced and their toxic effects are thereby increased. Damaged kidney tubules may also be less capable of converting mesna to its active kidney-protecting form. The increase in the hearing loss is not understood.

Importance and management

These interactions appear to be established. The authors of the paper cited[1] point out that the majority of patients who develop toxicity have persistently high urinary NAG concentrations (*N*-acetyl-*β*-D-glucosaminidase, an enzyme released by renal tubular cells), even though serum creatinine levels remain within the acceptable range for ifosfamide treatment. They suggest that evidence of subclinical tubular damage should be sought for by monitoring the excretion of urinary NAG. Note that cisplatin and ifosfamide are widely used in combination, and the related drug **cyclophosphamide** is also routinely used with cisplatin. Amifostine may be useful in reducing the nephrotoxicity of this combination.[7] The authors who reported on hearing loss advised that serial audiograms should be done in patients treated with both drugs.[6]

1. Goren MP, Wright RK, Pratt CB, Horowitz ME, Dodge RK, Viar MJ, Kovnar EH. Potentiation of ifosfamide neurotoxicity, hematotoxicity, and tubular nephrotoxicity by prior *cis*-diamminedichloroplatinum(II) therapy. *Cancer Res* (1987) 47, 1457–60.
2. Caglar K, Kinalp C, Arpaci F, Turan M, Saglam K, Ozturk B, Komurcu Ş, Yavuz I, Yenicesu M, Ozet A, Vural A. Cumulative prior dose of cisplatin as a cause of the nephrotoxicity of high-dose chemotherapy followed by autologous stem-cell transplantation. *Nephrol Dial Transplant* (2002) 17, 1931–5.
3. Martinez F, Deray G, Cacoub P, Beaufils H, Jacobs C. Ifosfamide nephrotoxicity: deleterious effect of previous cisplatin administration. *Lancet* (1996) 348, 1100–1.
4. Rossi R, Danzebrink S, Hillebrand D, Linnenbürger K, Ullrich K, Jürgens H. Ifosfamide-induced subclinical nephrotoxicity and its potentiation by cisplatinum. *Med Pediatr Oncol* (1994) 22, 27–32.
5. Hacke M, Schmoll H-J, Alt JM, Baumann K, Stolte H. Nephrotoxicity of *cis*-diamminedichloroplatinum with or without ifosfamide in cancer treatment. *Clin Physiol Biochem* (1983) 1, 17–26.
6. Meyer WH, Ayers D, McHaney VA, Roberson P, Pratt CB. Ifosfamide and exacerbation of cisplatin-induced hearing loss. *Lancet* (1993) 341, 754–5.
7. Hartmann JT, Fels LM, Knop S, Stolte H, Kanz L, Bokemeyer C. A randomized trial comparing the nephrotoxicity of cisplatin/ifosfamide-based combination chemotherapy with or without amifostine in patients with solid tumors. *Invest New Drugs* (2000) 18, 281–9.

Cyclophosphamide + Colony-stimulating factors

Granulocyte colony-stimulating factor (G-CSF) used with cyclophosphamide has been associated with an increased occurrence of pulmonary toxicity.

Clinical evidence, mechanism, importance and management

A 1-year-old boy with a neuroblastoma Evans stage III died of respiratory failure following treatment with **filgrastim** (a **G-CSF**) and normal doses of cyclophosphamide and doxorubicin. The authors of the report suggest that the pulmonary toxicity of the cyclophosphamide (normally only seen with high cumulative doses) is potentiated by **filgrastim**.[1] Six of 53 patients treated with CHOP (cyclophosphamide, doxorubicin, vincristine and prednisolone) and **G-CSF** developed pulmonary toxicity, which was considered a much higher incidence than usually seen with CHOP alone. The development of toxicity correlated with the mean peak leucocyte count.[2] Another 10 cases of interstitial pneumonitis have occurred with cyclophosphamide-based regimens (not including bleomycin or methotrexate) and **G-CSF**.[3,4] There is some evidence that the pulmonary toxicity of bleomycin might possibly also be increased by colony-stimulating factors (see 'Bleomycin + Colony-stimulating factors', p.618). These interactions are not firmly established, but good pulmonary function monitoring appears to be advisable when colony-stimulating factors are used with antineoplastics causing pulmonary toxicity. If interstitial pneumonitis occurs, the drugs should be discontinued and high-dose corticosteroids started immediately.[2] More study is needed.

1. van Woensel JBM, Knoester H, Leeuw JA, van Aalderen WMC. Acute respiratory insufficiency during doxorubicin, cyclophosphamide, and G-CSF therapy. *Lancet* (1994) 344, 759–60.
2. Yokose N, Ogata K, Tamura H, An E, Nakamura K, Kamikubo K, Kudoh S, Dan K, Nomura T. Pulmonary toxicity after granulocyte colony-stimulating factor-combined chemotherapy for non-Hodgkin's lymphoma. *Br J Cancer* (1998) 77, 2286–90.
3. Niitsu N, Iki S, Muroi K, Motomura S, Murakami M, Takeyama H, Ohsaka A, Urabe A. Interstitial pneumonia in patients receiving granulocyte colony-stimulating factor during chemotherapy: survey in Japan 1991–96. *Br J Cancer* (1997) 76, 1661–6.
4. Hasegawa Y, Ninomiya J, Kamoshita M, Ohtani K, Kobayashi T, Kojima J, Nagasawa T, Abe T. Interstitial pneumonitis related to granulocyte colony-stimulating factor administration following chemotherapy for elderly patients with non-Hodgkin's lymphoma. *Intern Med* (1997) 36, 360–4.

Cyclophosphamide or Ifosfamide + Corticosteroids

There is limited and conflicting evidence on the effect of prednisone and prednisolone on the metabolic activation of cyclophosphamide. Synergistic increases in enzyme induction may occur if cyclophosphamide is given with dexamethasone. Dexamethasone does not appear to alter ifosfamide metabolism.

Clinical evidence

(a) Dexamethasone

In an *in vitro* study it was noted that the combination of cyclophosphamide with dexamethasone resulted in a greater induction of the cytochrome P450 isoenzyme CYP3A4 than with cyclophosphamide alone; the extent of induction being dependent on baseline CYP3A4 activity.[1] In *rats*,[2] dexamethasone pretreatment caused a fourfold increase in the AUC of the inactive, neurotoxic, dechloroethylated metabolite of cyclophosphamide, and caused a 60% decrease in the AUC of the active, hydroxylated metabolite. In an earlier study in patients receiving high-dose cyclophosphamide and dexamethasone for 2 days, total clearance of both cyclophosphamide and dexamethasone were higher on the second than the first day, with higher concentrations of cyclophosphamide metabolites.[3]

In *rats*, dexamethasone pretreatment had no net impact on the fraction of ifosfamide undergoing activation.[4] Similarly, in a clinical study, ifosfamide metabolism was no different when patients were given dexamethasone 4 mg every 8 hours with ifosfamide for 3 days than when they received ifosfamide alone.[5]

(b) Prednisone or Prednisolone

In an early study, single doses of prednisone were shown to inhibit the metabolic activation of cyclophosphamide,[6,7] whereas another study briefly mentioned that massive single doses of prednisolone given just before cyclophosphamide did not inhibit cyclophosphamide metabolism.[8] Longer-term prednisone treatment (50 mg daily for 1 to 2 weeks) increased the rate of activation of cyclophosphamide in the first study.[6,7] Conversely, another study in 7 patients with systemic vasculitis given prednisone 1 mg/kg daily and cyclophosphamide 600 mg/m^2 intravenously every 3 weeks for 6 cycles found that, by the last cycle, the AUC of cyclophosphamide had significantly increased while that of its active metabolites had significantly decreased.[9]

Mechanism

Cyclophosphamide and ifosfamide are prodrugs that undergo hepatic metabolism to active and inactive-neurotoxic metabolites, and it appears they induce their own metabolism (see also 'Cyclophosphamide or Ifosfamide + Barbiturates', p.623). Corticosteroids are inducers of the cytochrome P450 isoenzymes CYP3A4. For cyclophosphamide, the CYP3A subfamily is thought to be principally involved in production of inactive-neurotoxic metabolites, whereas, for ifosfamide, CYP3A catalyses both the production of active and inactive-neurotoxic metabolites. On this basis, corticosteroids might be expected to decrease the efficacy and increase the neurotoxicity of cyclophosphamide (although this does not take account of auto-induction), whereas for ifosfamide they would not be expected to alter the balance between efficacy and toxicity.

Importance and management

The documentation is very limited. It appears that dexamethasone does not have any appreciable effect on the metabolism of ifosfamide. The information on cyclophosphamide is conflicting, and the clinical importance of any changes remains to be established. However, it should be noted that prednisone and prednisolone have a long established use as part of chemotherapy regimens including cyclophosphamide and are also often combined in various autoimmune diseases, and dexamethasone is widely used as an antiemetic with cancer chemotherapy.

1. Lindley C, Hamilton G, McCune JS, Faucette S, Shord SS, Hawke RL, Wang H, Gilbert D, Jolley S, Yan B, LeCluyse EL. The effect of cyclophosphamide with and without dexamethasone on cytochrome P450 3A4 and 2B6 in human hepatocytes. *Drug Metab Dispos* (2002) 30, 814–22.
2. Yu LJ, Drewes P, Gustafsson K, Brain EGC, Hecht JED, Waxman DJ. In vivo modulation of alternative pathways of P-450-catalyzed cyclophosphamide metabolism: impact on pharmacokinetics and antitumor activity. *J Pharmacol Exp Ther* (1999) 288, 928–37.
3. Moore MJ, Hardy RW, Thiessen JJ, Soldin SJ, Erlichman C. Rapid development of enhanced clearance after high-dose cyclophosphamide. *Clin Pharmacol Ther* (1988) 44, 622–8.
4. Brain EGC, Yu LJ, Gustafsson K, Drewes P, Waxman DJ. Modulation of P450-dependent ifosfamide pharmacokinetics: a better understanding of drug activation in vivo. *Br J Cancer* (1998) 77, 1768–76.
5. Singer JM, Hartley JM, Brennan C, Nicholson PW, Souhami RL. The pharmacokinetics and metabolism of ifosfamide during bolus and infusional administration: a randomized cross-over study. *Br J Cancer* (1998) 77, 978–84.
6. Faber OK, Mouridsen HT. Cyclophosphamide activation and corticosteroids. *N Engl J Med* (1974) 291, 211.
7. Faber OK, Mouridsen HT, Skovsted L. The biotransformation of cyclophosphamide in man: influence of prednisone. *Acta Pharmacol Toxicol (Copenh)* (1974) 35, 195–200.
8. Bagley CM, Bostick FW, DeVita VT. Clinical pharmacology of cyclophosphamide. *Cancer Res* (1973) 33, 226–33.
9. Belfayol-Pisanté L, Guillevin L, Tod M, Fauvelle F. Possible influence of prednisone on the pharmacokinetics of cyclophosphamide in systemic vasculitis. *Clin Drug Invest* (1999) 18, 225–31.

Cyclophosphamide + H_2-receptor antagonists

Ranitidine, and probably famotidine, appear not to increase the bone marrow toxicity of cyclophosphamide. *Animal* studies suggest that cimetidine might.

Clinical evidence, mechanism, importance and management

A study in 7 cancer patients found that although oral **ranitidine** 300 mg daily significantly prolonged the half-life and increased the AUC of intravenous cyclophosphamide 600 mg/m^2, it did not significantly affect the AUCs of the two major alkylating metabolites of cyclophosphamide, nor did it affect its bone marrow toxicity (leucopenia, granulocytopenia). The authors of the study conclude that **ranitidine** can safely be given with cyclophosphamide.[1] The same authors previously reported that **cimetidine**, when given with cyclophosphamide, increased the AUC of total alkylating metabolites of cyclophosphamide, and resulted in greater toxicity to normal bone marrow, but increased survival in leukaemia-bearing *mice*.[2,3] Other studies in *mice* have shown that **cimetidine**, but not **famotidine**, increases the toxicity of cyclophosphamide to normal bone marrow cells.[4]

Cimetidine inhibits the cytochrome P450 isoenzyme CYP2C9, which has a minor role in the activation of cyclophosphamide (see 'Cyclophosphamide or Ifosfamide + Barbiturates', p.623). These results suggest that no special precautions are likely to be needed when **ranitidine** or **famotidine** are given with cyclophosphamide. The relevance of the findings with **cimetidine** is uncertain. **Cimetidine** has also increased the levels or toxicity of some other antineoplastics, see 'Nitrosoureas + Cimetidine', p.655, 'Anthracyclines; Epirubicin + Cimetidine', p.613, and 'Fluorouracil + H_2-receptor antagonists', p.633.

1. Alberts DS, Mason-Liddil N, Plezia PM, Roe DJ, Dorr RT, Struck RF, Phillips JG. Lack of ranitidine effects on cyclophosphamide bone marrow toxicity or metabolism: a placebo-controlled clinical trial. *J Natl Cancer Inst* (1991) 83, 1739–43.
2. Dorr RT, Alberts DS. Cimetidine enhancement of cyclophosphamide antitumour activity. *Br J Cancer* (1982) 45, 35–43.
3. Dorr RT, Soble MJ, Alberts DS. Interaction of cimetidine but not ranitidine with cyclophosphamide in mice. *Cancer Res* (1986) 46, 1795–9.
4. Lerza RA, Bogliolo GV, Mecoboni MP, Saviane AG, Pannacciulli IM. Effect of H2 antagonists cimetidine and famotidine on the hemotoxicity of cyclophosphamide. *Anticancer Res* (1988) 8, 1241–5.

Cyclophosphamide + Indometacin

A single case report describes acute water intoxication when a patient taking indometacin was given low-dose intravenous cyclophosphamide.

Clinical evidence, mechanism, importance and management

A patient with multiple myeloma taking indometacin 50 mg every 8 hours, developed acute water intoxication and salt retention after being given a single bolus intravenous injection of cyclophosphamide 500 mg (less than 10 mg/kg). The reasons are not understood, but it is suggested that it was due to the additive or synergistic effects of the two drugs, since water intoxication had not been noted before with this low-dose of cyclophosphamide.[1] There do not appear to be any further reports or studies on this potential interaction but water intoxication has subsequently been reported with low-dose intravenous cyclophosphamide alone.[2] The evidence does not justify any special precautions when both drugs are used.

1. Webberley M J, Murray J A. Life-threatening acute hyponatraemia induced by low dose cyclophosphamide and indomethacin. *Postgrad Med J* (1989) 65, 950–2.
2. McCarron MO, Wright GD, Roberts SD. Water intoxication after low dose cyclophosphamide. *BMJ* (1995) 311, 292.

Cyclophosphamide + Metronidazole

A case report describes encephalopathy in a girl treated with cyclophosphamide and metronidazole.

Clinical evidence, mechanism, importance and management

After the fourth dose of pulse intravenous cyclophosphamide, a 9-year-old girl developed pancytopenia and gastrointestinal bleeding. She was then given metronidazole for presumptive *Clostridium difficile* colitis. Within 6 hours she developed encephalopathy with seizures and visual hallucinations, requiring antipsychotic therapy. Metronidazole is thought to cause disulfiram-like reactions by inhibiting aldehyde dehydrogenase (see 'Alcohol + Antibacterials; Metronidazole', p.44), and it was suggested that inhibition of this enzyme may cause toxic metabolites of cyclophosphamide to accumulate (see also 'Cyclophosphamide or Ifosfamide + Barbiturates', p.623).[1] This appears to be the only report of this potential interaction, and its general relevance is unclear. Further study is required.

1. Pinsk MN, Renton K, Crocker JFS, Acott PD. A proposed drug interaction leading to cyclophosphamide-induced encephalopathy. *Pediatr Res* (2002) 51, 437A.

Cyclophosphamide + Pentostatin

Acute and fatal cardiovascular collapse developed in two patients when pentostatin was added to high-dose cyclophosphamide treatment. Some recent studies have found the combination to be effective and safe in patients with chronic lymphocytic leukaemia.

Clinical evidence, mechanism, importance and management

A clinical study that was started to find out if pentostatin would improve the immunosuppressive effects of cyclophosphamide, carmustine and etoposide in bone marrow transplant patients was stopped when acute and fatal cardiovascular collapse developed in the first 2 patients. Both patients had been given cyclophosphamide 800 mg/m^2 and etoposide 200 mg/m^2, both every 12 hours for 8 doses, and carmustine 112 mg/m^2 daily for 4 doses. On day 3 pentostatin 4 mg/m^2, given over 4 hours, was added. Within 8 to 18 hours after completion of chemotherapy both patients developed confusion, hypothermia, hypotension, respiratory distress, pulmonary oedema, and eventually fatal ventricular fibrillation within 45 to 120 minutes of the first symptoms. A later study in *rats* similarly found that pentostatin markedly increased the acute toxicity of cyclophosphamide. The reasons for this cardiotoxicity are not understood. Neither of the 2 patients had previously shown any evidence of cardiac abnormalities.[1]

However, in a more recent study in patients with previously treated chronic lymphocytic leukaemia (CLL), pentostatin 4 mg/m^2 with cyclophosphamide 600 mg/m^2 was found to be safe and effective.[2] Another study found that pentostatin 4 mg/m^2 and cyclophosphamide 600 mg/m^2 with or without rituximab 375 mg/m^2 was safe and effective for patients with Waldenstrom's macroglobinaemia.[3] Other studies in patients with previously treated or untreated CLL found that cyclophosphamide 600 mg/m^2 with pentostatin 4 or 2 mg/m^2 and rituximab 375 mg/m^2 was effective and was either well-tolerated or had only modest toxicity.[4,5]

1. Gryn J, Gordon R, Bapat A, Goldman N, Goldberg J. Pentostatin increases the acute toxicity of high dose cyclophosphamide. *Bone Marrow Transplant* (1993) 12, 217–20.

2. Weiss MA, Maslak PG, Jurcic JG, Scheinberg DA, Aliff TB, Lamanna N, Frankel SR, Kossman SE, Horgan D. Pentostatin and cyclophosphamide: an effective new regimen in previously treated patients with chronic lymphocytic leukemia. J Clin Oncol (2003 21, 1278–84.
3. Hensel M, Villalobos M, Kornacker M, Krasniqi F, Ho AD. Pentostatin/cyclophosphamide with or without rituximab: an effective regimen for patients with Waldenström's macroglobulinaemia/lymphoplasmacytic lymphoma. *Clin Lymphoma Myeloma* (2005) 6, 131–5.
4. Lamanna N, Kalaycio M, Maslak P, Jurcic JG, Heaney M, Brentjens R, Zelenetz AD, Horgan D, Gencarelli A, Panageas KS, Scheinberg DA, Weiss MA. Pentostatin, cyclophosphamide, and rituximab is an active, well-tolerated regimen for patients with previously treated chronic lymphocytic leukaemia. *J Clin Oncol* (2006) 24, 1575–81.
5. Kay NE, Geyer SM, Call TG, Shanafelt TD, Zent CS, Jelinek DF, Tschumper R, Bone ND, Dewald GW, Lin TS, Heerema NA, Smith L, Grever MR, Byrd JC. Combination chemoimmunotherapy with pentostatin, cyclophosphamide, and rituximab shows significant clinical activity with low accompanying toxicity in previously untreated B chronic lymphocytic leukaemia. Blood 2007, 109, 405–11.

Cyclophosphamide or Ifosfamide + Phenytoin

Phenytoin increases the metabolism of cyclophosphamide and ifosfamide, but the clinical relevance of this is uncertain. Both unchanged and increased efficacy has been suggested.

Clinical evidence

A child taking phenytoin and also given ifosfamide and etoposide had a neurotoxic reaction. The plasma levels of the dechloroethylated metabolites of ifosfamide were subsequently found to be markedly altered compared with those previously seen in 14 other children receiving the same chemotherapy but not taking phenytoin. The child recovered uneventfully after 3 days, and achieved clinical remission (she had not responded to first-line chemotherapy).[1] In a subsequent study, the use of prophylactic phenytoin increased the formation of *S*-dechloroethylated cyclophosphamide in 3 patients receiving cyclophosphamide and busulfan.[2] In yet another study, the ratio of the AUC of active hydroxycyclophosphamide to cyclophosphamide was higher in patients receiving phenytoin and busulfan than in those receiving irradiation.[3] It is likely that phenytoin was responsible for this effect since busulfan alone decreases cyclophosphamide metabolism (see 'Cyclophosphamide + Busulfan', p.624). In an earlier study, in patients receiving enzyme-inducing drugs (2 of whom received phenytoin), the peak plasma levels of the alkylating metabolites of cyclophosphamide were raised, but declined rapidly, so that overall exposure was not different from those not taking these drugs.[4] Another study reported that a patient taking phenytoin had a high clearance rate for cyclophosphamide during her first chemotherapy course, and that auto-induction of cyclophosphamide clearance was not apparent during her second course.[5]

Mechanism

The alteration in the pattern of ifosfamide metabolites suggested that phenytoin had induced the activity of the cytochrome P450 isoenzyme CYP2B6, and to a lesser extent CYP3A4.[1] The pattern of the increase in cyclophosphamide clearance is also consistent with induction of CYP2B and CYP3A.[2] See also 'Cyclophosphamide or Ifosfamide + Barbiturates', p.623.

Importance and management

The alteration in the metabolism of cyclophosphamide and ifosfamide caused by phenytoin is not surprising, but the clinical importance of any changes remains to be established. The authors of the study from the 1970s concluded that phenytoin was unlikely to have much effect on the antitumour and toxic effects of cyclophosphamide.[4] Conversely, the authors of the more recent studies suggest that phenytoin may increase the therapeutic efficacy of cyclophosphamide and ifosfamide.[1,2] Further study is needed.

Note that reduced phenytoin levels and seizures have been reported in a patient receiving chemotherapy including cyclophosphamide, see 'Table 14.1', (p.519).

1. Ducharme MP, Bernstein ML, Granvil CP, Gehrcke B, Wainer IW. Phenytoin-induced alteration in the *N*-dechloroethylation of ifosfamide stereoisomers. *Cancer Chemother Pharmacol* (1997) 40, 531–3.
2. Williams ML, Wainer IW, Embree L, Barnett M, Granvil CL, Ducharme MP. Enantioselective induction of cyclophosphamide metabolism by phenytoin. *Chirality* (1999) 11, 569–74.
3. Slattery JT, Kalhorn TF, McDonald GB, Lambert K, Buckner CD, Bensinger WI, Anasetti C, Appelbaum FR. Conditioning regimen-dependent disposition of cyclophosphamide and hydroxycyclophosphamide in human marrow transplantation patients. *J Clin Oncol* (1996) 14, 1484–94.
4. Bagley CM, Bostick FW, DeVita VT. Clinical pharmacology of cyclophosphamide. *Cancer Res* (1973) 33, 226–33.
5. Chen T-L, Passos-Coelho JL, Noe DA, Kennedy MJ, Black KC, Colvin M, Grochow LB. Nonlinear pharmacokinetics of cyclophosphamide in patients with metastatic breast cancer receiving high-dose chemotherapy followed by autologous bone marrow transplantation. *Cancer Res* (1995) 55, 810–16. Correction. ibid. 1600.

Cyclophosphamide or Ifosfamide + Rifampicin (Rifampin)

Rifampicin induced the metabolism of cyclophosphamide and ifosfamide. For ifosfamide, this did not improve the ratio of active to inactive-toxic metabolites, and the possibility remains that efficacy could be reduced.

Clinical evidence, mechanism, importance and management

In a clinical study, rifampicin increased the clearance of ifosfamide by about 100%. In this study, patients were given rifampicin 300 mg twice daily for 3 days before ifosfamide and for 3 days concurrently for one cycle, then for another cycle they were given the ifosfamide alone. The fraction of ifosfamide metabolised to the inactive-neurotoxic, dechloroethylated metabolite was increased, but elimination of this metabolite was also increased resulting in reduced exposure. The fraction metabolised to the active, hydroxylated metabolite, and its exposure, were not altered appreciably.[1]

An *in vitro* study in human liver cells showed that rifampicin was a potent inducer of the activation (hydroxylation) of cyclophosphamide and ifosfamide.[2]

Rifampicin is an inducer of the cytochrome P450 isoenzymes CYP3A4 and CYP2B6, which are involved in the metabolism of cyclophosphamide and ifosfamide (see also 'Cyclophosphamide or Ifosfamide + Barbiturates', p.623). In the clinical study cited,[1] rifampicin did not have a positive effect on the proportion of ifosfamide undergoing activation. In addition, since rifampicin increased metabolism overall, there is the possibility of decreased efficacy,[1] although this remains to be shown.

1. Kerbusch T, Jansen RLH, Mathôt RAA, Huitema ADR, Jansen M, van Rijswijk REN, Beijnen JH. Modulation of the cytochrome P450–mediated metabolism of ifosfamide by ketoconazole and rifampin. *Clin Pharmacol Ther* (2001) 70, 132–41.
2. Chang TKH, Yu L, Maurel P, Waxman DJ. Enhanced cyclophosphamide and ifosfamide activation in primary human hepatocyte cultures: response to cytochrome P-450 inducers and autoinduction by oxazaphosphorines. *Cancer Res* (1997) 57, 1946–54.

Cyclophosphamide + Sulfonamides

Some very limited evidence suggests that sulfaphenazole may modestly inhibit the metabolism of cyclophosphamide to its active metabolite, but the clinical importance of this is uncertain.

Clinical evidence, mechanism, importance and management

A study in 7 patients given a 50-mg dose of cyclophosphamide with **sulfaphenazole** 1 g twice daily for 9 to 14 days showed that the half-life of cyclophosphamide was unchanged in 3 patients, longer in 2 and shorter in the remaining 2 patients.[1] **Sulfaphenazole** and **sulfamethoxazole** are inhibitors of the cytochrome P450 isoenzyme CYP2C9, which shows genetic polymorphism (i.e. some people produce very little, while others produce larger quantities). This enzyme has a minor role in the metabolism (and therefore activation) of cyclophosphamide, and the extent of its involvement varies between patients. For example, an *in vitro* study showed that **sulfaphenazole** inhibited cyclophosphamide activation by 17 to 27% in one human liver sample, but insignificant inhibition occurred in two others.[2] Thus, sulfonamides such as **sulfaphenazole** and **sulfamethoxazole** may moderately inhibit the activation of cyclophosphamide in some patients, but the clinical relevance of this is uncertain. Note that **co-trimoxazole** is sometimes used for prophylaxis of infection in patients receiving chemotherapy. One study showed that this use did not *increase* the myelotoxicity of CAE (cyclophosphamide, doxorubicin, and etoposide).[3]

1. Faber OK, Mouridsen HT, Skovsted L. The effect of chloramphenicol and sulphaphenazole on the biotransformation of cyclophosphamide in man. *Br J Clin Pharmacol* (1975) 2, 281–5.

2. Roy P, Yu LJ, Crespi CL, Waxman DJ. Development of a substrate-activity based approach to identify the major human liver P-450 catalysts of cyclophosphamide and ifosfamide activation based on cDNA-expressed activities and liver microsomal P-450 profiles. *Drug Metab Dispos* (1999) 27, 655–66.
3. de Jongh CA, Wade JC, Finley RS, Joshi JH, Aisner J, Wiernik PH, Schimpff SC. Trimethoprim/sulfamethoxazole versus placebo: a double-blind comparison of infection prophylaxis in patients with small cell carcinoma of the lung. *J Clin Oncol* (1983) 1, 302–7.

Cyclophosphamide or Ifosfamide + Taxanes

The clearance of ifosfamide is higher when it is given after docetaxel. This results in less toxicity, but the effect on efficacy is unknown. Ifosfamide did not alter the pharmacokinetics of docetaxel. The sequence of ifosfamide followed by paclitaxel was antagonistic *in vitro*.

Clinical evidence, mechanism, importance and management

(a) Docetaxel

The AUCs of ifosfamide and its metabolites were lower when ifosfamide was given immediately after docetaxel than when it was given 24 hours before docetaxel, due to increased clearance. Docetaxel pharmacokinetics were unaltered by ifosfamide.[1] This supports the evidence that the maximum tolerated dose is greater when ifosfamide is given after docetaxel.[2] The mechanism is unknown, but it has been suggested[3] that docetaxel may competitively inhibit the activation of ifosfamide by the cytochrome P450 isoenzyme CYP3A4. These results show that the toxicity, and possibly efficacy, of the combination are schedule dependent. More study is needed. Cyclophosphamide does not appear to alter docetaxel pharmacokinetics. For full details see also 'Taxanes + Cyclophosphamide', p.661.

(b) Paclitaxel

In vitro studies in human liver microsomes found that additive or synergistic cytotoxicity occurred when activated ifosfamide (hydroxyifosfamide) and paclitaxel were given together or when paclitaxel was given first followed by hydroxyifosfamide. In contrast pronounced antagonism was seen when hydroxyifosfamide was given before paclitaxel.[4] The mechanism is unknown. These results suggest that the scheduling of this combination may be important for efficacy. More study is needed. There is some evidence that toxicity associated with combinations of paclitaxel and cyclophosphamide is sequence-dependent. For full details see also 'Taxanes + Cyclophosphamide', p.661.

1. Schrijvers D, Pronk L, Highley M, Bruno R, Locci-Tonelli D, De Bruijn E, Van Oosterom AT, Verweij J. Pharmacokinetics of ifosfamide are changed by combination with docetaxel. *Am J Clin Oncol* (2000) 23, 358–63.
2. Pronk L, Schrijvers D, Schellens JHM, De Bruijn EA, Planting ASTh, Locci-Tonelli D, Groult V, Verweij J, Van Oosterom AT. Phase I study on docetaxel and ifosfamide in patients with advanced solid tumours. *Br J Cancer* (1998) 77, 153–8.
3. Ando Y. Possible metabolic interaction between docetaxel and ifosfamide. *Br J Cancer* (2000) 82, 497.
4. Vanhoefer U, Schleucher N, Klaassen U, Seeber S, Harstrick A. Ifosfamide-based drug combinations: preclinical evaluation of drug interactions and translation into the clinic. *Semin Oncol* (2000) 27 (Suppl 1), 8–13.

Cyclophosphamide + Thiotepa

Pretreatment with thiotepa may inhibit the metabolism of cyclophosphamide to its active metabolite and decrease both its efficacy and toxicity. Cyclophosphamide appears not to affect the metabolism of thiotepa.

Clinical evidence, mechanism, importance and management

(a) Effect on cyclophosphamide

The proportion of cyclophosphamide excreted unchanged in the urine (i.e. never metabolically activated) was found to be higher when cyclophosphamide was given as a 96-hour infusion with thiotepa and novobiocin than when it was given alone. The authors suggested that the possibility that thiotepa inhibited the metabolism of cyclophosphamide should be investigated.[1] Later, other authors observed that the concentration of the active metabolite of cyclophosphamide, 4-hydroxycyclophosphamide, decreased sharply after thiotepa was given to 20 patients.[2] In a study to investigate this effect further, 3 patients were given high-dose cyclophosphamide 1000 or 1500 mg/m^2 as a 1-hour infusion, followed by carboplatin and thiotepa for 4 days. The order of infusion was reversed on one treatment day in each of 4 courses. Giving thiotepa 1 hour before cyclophosphamide resulted in decreases in the peak plasma levels and AUC of 4-hydroxycyclophosphamide of 62% and 26%, respectively, when compared with thiotepa given 1 hour after cyclophosphamide.[2] In human microsomes, thiotepa was found to inhibit the conversion of cyclophosphamide to hydroxycyclophosphamide.[2] These results suggest that thiotepa can decrease both the efficacy and toxicity of cyclophosphamide, and that the order of administration may be of critical importance. The authors question the practice of giving cyclophosphamide and thiotepa simultaneously.[2]

(b) Effect on thiotepa

In an *in vitro* study using human microsomes, cyclophosphamide had no effect on the metabolism of thiotepa to TEPA (triethylenephosphamide) by cytochrome P450 at therapeutic concentrations.[2,3]

1. Chen T-L, Passos-Coelho JL, Noe DA, Kennedy MJ, Black KC, Colvin M, Grochow LB. Nonlinear pharmacokinetics of cyclophosphamide in patients with metastatic breast cancer receiving high-dose chemotherapy followed by autologous bone marrow transplantation. *Cancer Res* (1995) 55, 810–16. Correction. ibid.1600.
2. Huitema ADR, Kerbusch T, Tibben MM, Rodenhuis S, Beijnen JH. Reduction of cyclophosphamide bioactivation by thioTEPA: critical sequence-dependency in high-dose chemotherapy regimens. *Cancer Chemother Pharmacol* (2000) 46, 119–27.
3. Van Maanen MJ, Huitema ADR, Beijnen JH. Influence of co-medicated drugs on the biotransformation of thioTEPA to TEPA and thioTEPA-mercapturate. *Anticancer Res* (2000) 20, 1711–16.

Erlotinib + Miscellaneous

The metabolism of erlotinib is markedly affected by other drugs that are potent inhibitors (e.g. ketoconazole) or inducers (e.g. rifampicin) of the cytochrome P450 isoenzyme CYP3A4. Alternatives to these drugs should be used where possible; if not, alteration of the dose of erlotinib is required. The concurrent use of temozolomide may either reduce or increase erlotinib levels, depending on the dose of erlotinib. Smoking increases the metabolism of erlotinib.

Clinical evidence, mechanism, importance and management

(a) Antiepileptics, enzyme-inducing

As part of a study in 33 patients with glioma, the pharmacokinetics of erlotinib 100 mg daily increasing to 500 mg daily was compared between patients taking enzyme-inducing antiepileptics and those not. There was a 33 to 71% lower exposure to erlotinib when it was given with an enzyme-inducing antiepileptic drug, thought to be due to increased activity of the cytochrome P450 enzymes. Antiepileptic drugs taken were **carbamazepine**, **oxcarbazepine**, **phenytoin**, **fosphenytoin**, **phenobarbital** and **primidone**. Patients taking these drugs tolerated a higher dose of erlotinib, and for further studies in this disease it was recommended that the dose of erlotinib should be at least 500 mg daily in those taking enzyme-inducing antiepileptics and 200 mg daily in those patients not taking these drugs.[1] However, note that the manufacturer of erlotinib recommends using alternatives to these enzyme-inducing antiepileptics if possible, see *CYP3A4 inducers*, below.

(b) CYP3A4 Inhibitors

The AUC of erlotinib has been found to be increased by 66% when given with **ketoconazole** 200 mg twice daily for 5 days. The manufacturers advise caution with concurrent use, and recommend that the dose of erlotinib should be reduced if severe adverse reactions occur when given with strong CYP3A4 inhibitors. They specifically name **atazanavir**, **clarithromycin**, **erythromycin**, **grapefruit** and **grapefruit juice**, **indinavir**, **itraconazole**, **ketoconazole**, **nefazodone**, **nelfinavir**, **ritonavir**, **saquinavir**, **telithromycin**, **troleandomycin** and **voriconazole**.[2,3]

(c) CYP3A4 inducers

Pretreatment with **rifampicin** 600 mg once daily for 7 days reduced the AUC of erlotinib by about 66%.[3] In another study, the AUC of a single 450-mg dose of erlotinib, taken after 11 days treatment with **rifampicin** was about 57% of that of erlotinib 150 mg taken without rifampicin.[2,3] The manufacturers advise that alternative treatments with no cytochrome P450 enzyme-inducing activity should be considered. If this is not possible, the starting dose of erlotinib should be adjusted to 300 mg (UK) with close monitoring, and, if tolerated, further increased after 2 weeks, in 50 mg increments, to 450 mg.[3] They also advise caution with other CYP3A4 inducers, and specifically name **barbiturates**, **carbamazepine**, **phenobarbital**, **phenytoin**, **rifabutin**, **rifapentine**, and **St John's wort**, and recommend the use of alternative non-inducing drugs when possible.[2,3] For enzyme-inducing antiepileptics, see also (a) above.

(d) Drugs that affect gastrointestinal pH

Drugs, such as **antacids**, **H_2-receptor antagonists** or **proton pump inhibitors**, that increase the pH of the gastrointestinal tract may reduce the solubility of erlotinib, which the manufacturers[2,3] state has a decreased solubility above pH 5. The manufacturers therefore recommend caution with concurrent use of these drugs during treatment with erlotinib as they cannot exclude that these drugs will reduce erlotinib efficacy.[2]

(e) Gemcitabine

There was no change in the pharmacokinetics of gemcitabine or erlotinib on concurrent use in a phase 1 study.[2]

(f) Temozolomide

As part of a phase 1 study, 16 patients with glioma were given erlotinib 100 mg daily increasing to 250 mg daily alone, and 14 were given erlotinib and temozolomide 150 mg/m^2 increasing to 200 mg/m^2 for 5 days in each 28 day cycle. At the lowest dose of erlotinib, the group also taking temozolomide had a 49% lower maximum plasma level of erlotinib, and almost 50% lower AUC of both erlotinib and its metabolite OSI-420. As the dose of erlotinib increased to 250 mg daily, this difference was reversed with temozolomide group showing a 45% higher AUC of erlotinib. The reason for these paradoxical findings is unclear, and their clinical relevance is uncertain.[1]

(g) Tobacco

Twelve cigarette smokers and 14 non-smokers were given oral erlotinib 150 mg on day 1 and 300 mg on day 15 of a study. The subjects who smoked had lower maximum plasma levels of erlotinib; 35% lower after the 150 mg dose and 20% lower after the 300 mg dose. The AUC was also reduced by 65% and 57%, respectively. Cigarette smoking induces CYP1A1 and 1A2, which are involved in the metabolism of erlotinib. Consideration should therefore be given to the smoking status of a patient when planning treatment with erlotinib.[4] The manufacturer says that these decreases are likely to be clinically important, and that patients should be encouraged to stop smoking.[2,3]

(h) Warfarin

Raised INRs and infrequent bleeding have been reported in patients taking warfarin with erlotinib. Patients taking these drugs, and other coumarins, should be closely monitored for INR changes.[2,3]

1. Prados MD, Lamborn KR, Chang S, Burton E, Butowski N, Malec M, Kapadia A, Rabbitt J, Page MS, Fedoroff A, Xie D, Kelley SK. Phase 1 study of erlotinib HCl alone and combined with temozolomide in patients with stable or recurrent malignant glioma. *Neuro-oncol* (2006) 8, 67–78.
2. Tarceva (Erlotinib) Genetech, Inc. US Prescribing information, May 2007.
3. Tarceva (Erlotinib) Roche Products Ltd. UK Summary of product characteristics, February 2007.
4. Hamilton M, Wolf JL, Rusk J, Beard SE, Clark GM, Witt K, Cagnoni PJ. Effects of smoking on the pharmacokinetics of erlotinib. *Clin Cancer Res* (2006) 12, 2166–71.

Estramustine + Clodronate

Clodronate markedly increases the serum levels of estramustine.

Clinical evidence, mechanism, importance and management

Estramustine bioavailability in 12 patients was increased by about 80% when clodronate 800 mg four times daily was given with estramustine 280 mg twice daily for 5 days. The serum levels and AUC of clodronate were not changed by estramustine.[1] Documentation appears to be limited to this study. However, the efficacy and toxicity of estramustine should be monitored if clodronate is also given. The effects of other bisphosphonates do not appear to have been studied.

1. Kylmälä T, Castrén-Kortekangas P, Seppänen J, Ylitalo P, Tammela TLJ. Effect of concomitant administration of clodronate and estramustine phosphate on their bioavailability in patients with metastasized prostate cancer. *Pharmacol Toxicol* (1996) 79, 157–60.

Estramustine + Food and Calcium compounds

The absorption of estramustine is reduced by milk, foods, and drugs containing calcium.

Clinical evidence

A randomised three-way crossover study in 6 patients with prostate cancer showed that the absorption of single-doses of estramustine disodium (equivalent to 140 mg of estramustine) was reduced by 59% when taken with 200 mL of **milk**, and by 33% when taken with a standardised **breakfast** (2 pieces of white bread with margarine, ham, tomato, marmalade and water). Peak serum estramustine levels were reduced by 68% and 43%, respectively.[1]

Mechanism

In vitro studies suggest that estramustine combines with calcium ions in milk and food to form a poorly-soluble complex that is not as well absorbed as the parent compound.[1]

Importance and management

An established interaction although the information is limited. The manufacturers recommend that estramustine should be taken not less than 1 hour before or 2 hours after meals, and that it should not be taken with milk, milk products, calcium-rich foods,[2,3] or drugs (such as **calcium-containing antacids**).[3]

1. Gunnarsson P O, Davidsson T, Andersson S-B, Backman C, Johansson S-Å. Impairment of estramustine phosphate absorption by concurrent intake of milk and food. *Eur J Clin Pharmacol* (1990) 38, 189–93.
2. Estracyt (Estramustine sodium phosphate). Pharmacia Ltd. UK Summary of product characteristics, July 2007.
3. Emcyt (Estramustine phosphate sodium). Pharmacia & Upjohn Co. US Prescribing information, February 2006.

Etoposide + Antiepileptics

Etoposide clearance appears to be increased by phenobarbital, phenytoin, and probably carbamazepine, and this may result in reduced efficacy.

Clinical evidence, mechanism, importance and management

The clearance of etoposide was found to be highly variable in children given etoposide 320 to 500 mg/m^2 over 6 hours on alternate days for a total of 3 doses. However, it was 77% higher in 7 children taking antiepileptics (**phenobarbital**, **phenytoin** or both) than in 22 others not taking antiepileptics.[1] In a retrospective survey, long-term antiepileptic use (**phenytoin**, **phenobarbital**, **carbamazepine**, or a combination) was associated with worse event-free survival, and greater haematological and/or CNS relapse in children receiving chemotherapy for B-lineage acute lymphoblastic leukaemia. The authors considered that the increased clearance of etoposide induced by the antiepileptics was a likely factor in these findings.[2] Be alert for the possible need to give larger doses of etoposide if these antiepileptics are used. More study is needed.

1. Rodman JH, Murry DJ, Madden T, Santana VM. Altered etoposide pharmacokinetics and time to engraftment in pediatric patients undergoing autologous bone marrow transplantation. *J Clin Oncol* (1994) 12, 2390–7.
2. Relling MV, Pui C-H, Sandlund JT, Rivera GK, Hancock ML, Boyett JM, Schuetz EG, Evans WE. Adverse effect of anticonvulsants on efficacy of chemotherapy for acute lymphoblastic leukaemia. *Lancet* (2000) 356, 285–90.

Etoposide + Atovaquone

The concurrent use of atovaquone with etoposide may modestly increase exposure to etoposide catechol. The clinical relevance of this is unclear.

Clinical evidence, mechanism, importance and management

A study in 9 children with acute lymphoblastic leukaemia or non-Hodgkin's lymphoma found that the AUC of etoposide and its metabolite etoposide catechol were slightly increased, by 8.6% and 28.4%, respectively, following atovaquone 45 mg/kg daily, when compared with co-trimoxazole 150/750 mg/m^2 daily. The mechanism by which this occurs is unclear, but atovaquone may affect the metabolism of etoposide by the cytochrome P450 isoenzyme CYP3A4 or its transport by P-glycoprotein.[1] The authors considered that an interaction with co-trimoxazole was unlikely, so used it as a control, however, ideally this requires confirmation. The relevance of the minor changes seen is unclear. The authors note that the risk of etoposide-related secondary acute myeloid leukaemia has been linked to minor changes in therapy, therefore, they advise caution if atovaquone is given with etoposide, particularly if it is used with other substrates of CYP3A4 or P-glycoprotein.[1] They also say it may be possible to avoid the interaction by separating the administration by 1 to 2 days,[1] but this requires confirmation.

1. van de Poll MEC, Relling MV, Schuetz EG, Harrison PL, Hughes W, Flynn PM. The effect of atovaquone on etoposide pharmacokinetics in children with acute lymphoblastic leukemia. *Cancer Chemother Pharmacol* (2001) 47, 467–72.

Etoposide + Ciclosporin

High-dose ciclosporin markedly raises etoposide serum levels and increases the suppression of white blood cell production. Severe toxicity has been reported in one patient.

Clinical evidence

In a comparative study,16 patients with multidrug resistant advanced cancer were given 20 paired courses of etoposide, alone or with ciclosporin. Ciclosporin levels were measured at the end of a 2-hour infusion: ciclosporin levels of greater than 2000 nanograms/mL were defined as high-dose and those less than 2000 nanograms/mL as low-dose. High and low-dose ciclosporin, respectively, increased the etoposide AUC by 80% and 50%, decreased the total clearance by 38% and 28%, increased its half-life by 108% and 40%, reduced the leucocyte count nadir by 64% and 37% and altered the volume of distribution at steady state by 46% and 1.4%.[1] The patients were given 150 to 200 mg/m^2 of etoposide daily as a 2-hour intravenous infusion for 3 consecutive days and ciclosporin in doses ranging from 5 to 21 mg/kg daily as a 3-day continuous infusion.[1] In another study, 18 children with recurrent or refractory tumours who had previously received etoposide were given high-dose ciclosporin (either a continuous infusion of 15 mg/kg per 24 hours for 60 hours (13 patients) or 30 mg/kg over 3 hours on 3 consecutive days (5 patients) and etoposide 150 mg/m^2 over 1 hour for 3 days, starting 1 hour after the beginning of the ciclosporin infusion. The AUC and half-life of etoposide were increased by 89% and 78%, respectively, and the clearance was decreased by 48%.[2] In a further study in children, the pharmacokinetics of etoposide 100 mg/m^2 daily were compared with etoposide 60 mg/m^2 (a 40% reduction in dose) with high-dose ciclosporin. Despite the dose reduction, recipients of ciclosporin had a 71% reduction in etoposide clearance and a 47% increase in the etoposide AUC, although toxicity was similar.[3]

The leukaemic cells in the bone marrow of a patient with acute T-lymphocyte leukaemia were totally cleared when ciclosporin 8.3 mg/kg orally twice daily was given with etoposide 100 to 300 mg daily for 2 to 5 days, but the adverse effects were severe (mental confusion, renal and hepatic toxicity). The patient died from respiratory failure precipitated by a chest infection.[4]

A patient with chronic myeloid leukaemia who had responded poorly to treatment with etoposide, mitoxantrone and cytarabine for blast crisis, returned to the chronic phase when given etoposide with ciclosporin.[5] An *in vitro* study by the same authors showed that etoposide was partially toxic to blast cells but that its effect on blast cells was increased sixfold when it was given with ciclosporin.[5]

Mechanism

It is suggested that the ciclosporin decreases the metabolism of the etoposide by inhibiting its metabolism by cytochrome P450 isoenzymes[6] and inhibiting P-glycoprotein mediated efflux from the hepatocyte, as well as inhibiting some unknown non-renal clearance mechanism.[1] The total effect is to cause the retention of etoposide in the body, thereby increasing its effects.

Importance and management

An established interaction. Ciclosporin alters the pharmacokinetics of etoposide resulting in increased serum levels. This pharmacokinetic interaction has complicated the study of the value of using ciclosporin to modulate multidrug resistance in tumours to improve the response to chemotherapy. In the case of 'anthracyclines', (p.611) and etoposide, any benefit could just be attributed to dose intensification. Consequently, some,[1-3] including one manufacturer,[7] have suggested reducing the dose of etoposide by 40% or 50% in the presence of ciclosporin.[1-3] In one study, a continuous infusion of ciclosporin was better tolerated than an intermittent regimen, but it was associated with similar hepatic and renal impairment as the short schedule (transient hyperbilirubinaemia, and elevated creatinine or urea).[2] The use of high-dose ciclosporin for multidrug resistant tumour modulation remains experimental and should only be undertaken in clinical studies. Concurrent use should be very well monitored. More study is needed to find out the possible effects of low-dose ciclosporin.

1. Lum BL, Kaubisch S, Yahanda AM, Adler KM, Jew L, Ehsan MN, Brophy NA, Halsey J, Gosland MP, Sikic BI. Alteration of etoposide pharmacokinetics and pharmacodynamics by cyclosporine in a phase I trial to modulate multidrug resistance. *J Clin Oncol* (1992) 10, 1635–42.
2. Bisogno G, Cowie F, Boddy A, Thomas HD, Dick G, Pinkerton CR. High-dose cyclosporin with etoposide—toxicity and pharmacokinetic interaction in children with solid tumours. *Br J Cancer* (1998) 77, 2304–9.
3. Lacayo NJ, Lum BL, Becton DL, Weinstein H, Ravindranath Y, Chang MN, Bomgaars L, Lauer SJ, Sikic BI. Pharmacokinetic interactions of cyclosporine with etoposide and mitoxantrone in children with acute myeloid leukemia. *Leukemia* (2002) 16, 920–7.
4. Kloke O, Osieka R. Interaction of cyclosporin A with antineoplastic agents. *Klin Wochenschr* (1985) 63, 1081–2.
5. Maia RC, Noronha H, Vasconcelos FC, Rumjanek VM. Interaction of cyclosporin A and etoposide. Clinical and *in vitro* assessment in blast phase of chronic myeloid leukaemia. *Clin Lab Haematol* (1997) 19, 215–7.
6. Kawashiro T, Yamashita K, Zhao X-J, Koyama E, Tani M, Chiba K, Ishizaki T. A study on the metabolism of etoposide and possible interaction with antitumor or supporting agents by human liver microsomes. *J Pharmacol Exp Ther* (1998) 386, 1294–1300.
7. Eposin (Etoposide). Medac GmbH. UK Summary of product characteristics, January 2005.

Etoposide + Cisplatin or Carboplatin

The clearance of etoposide may be modestly reduced by carboplatin and cisplatin, but this is probably unlikely to be clinically relevant.

Clinical evidence, mechanism, importance and management

(a) Carboplatin

In one study in 4 patients, the pharmacokinetics of etoposide were unchanged when carboplatin was also given.[1] However, in another study of 14 young patients receiving etoposide and carboplatin the clearance of etoposide was lower than in previous reports in adults and children. They had been given an escalating dosage regimen starting with etoposide 960 mg/m^2, and increasing to 1200, and 1500 mg/m^2, given in three divided doses on alternate days, with carboplatin 400 to 700 mg/m^2 given on the other days, followed by autologous marrow rescue. The authors point out that the dose and the timing of carboplatin may be important determinants for any interaction.[2] In yet another study,[3] carboplatin did not affect the pharmacokinetics of etoposide during the first cycle of chemotherapy (etoposide was given on days 1, 2 and 3, and carboplatin on day 2, and the AUC of etoposide was compared for days 1 and 2). However, during a second cycle of chemotherapy, the etoposide AUC was 8% higher on day 2 than day 1. These changes were considered unlikely to be clinically important.[3]

(b) Cisplatin

A study in 17 children with neuroblastoma found that when intravenous cisplatin 90 mg/m^2 was given immediately before etoposide, the clearance of etoposide 780 mg/m^2 fell by 20% and the serum levels rose. But after a cumulative dose of cisplatin of 360 mg/m^2 it had no effect on the clearance of etoposide.[4] In another study, cisplatin did not affect the pharmacokinetics of etoposide during the first cycle of chemotherapy (etoposide was given on days 1, 2 and 3, and cisplatin on day 2, and the AUC of etoposide was compared for days 1 and 2). However, during a second cycle of chemotherapy, the etoposide AUC was 28% higher on day 3 than day 1. These changes were considered unlikely to be clinically important.[3]

1. Newell DR, Eeles RA, Gumbrell LA, Boxall FE, Horwich A, Calvert AH. Carboplatin and etoposide pharmacokinetics in patients with testicular teratoma. *Cancer Chemother Pharmacol* (1989) 23, 376–72.
2. Rodman JH, Murry DJ, Madden T, Santana VM. Altered etoposide pharmacokinetics and time to engraftment in pediatric patients undergoing autologous bone marrow transplantation. *J Clin Oncol* (1994) 12, 2390–7.
3. Thomas HD, Porter DJ, Bartelink I, Nobbs JR, Cole M, Elliott S, Newell DR, Calvert AH, Highley M, Boddy AV. Randomized cross-over clinical trial to study potential pharmacokinetics interactions between cisplatin or carboplatin and etoposide. *Br J Clin Pharmacol* (2002) 53, 83–91.
4. Relling MV, McLeod HL, Bowman LC, Santana VM. Etoposide pharmacokinetics and pharmacodynamics after acute and chronic exposure to cisplatin. *Clin Pharmacol Ther* (1994) 56, 503–11.

Etoposide + CYP3A4 inhibitors

***In vitro* studies show that some CYP3A4 inhibitors may possibly increase the effects and toxicity of etoposide. In one clinical study, etoposide clearance was increased by prednisone.**

Clinical evidence, mechanism, importance and management

In vitro studies using human liver microsomes show that **ketoconazole**, **prednisolone**, **troleandomycin**, **verapamil** and **vincristine** can inhibit the metabolism (3′-demethylation) of etoposide by the cytochrome P450 isoenzyme CYP3A4. The implications of this are that concurrent use with these drugs might increase both the efficacy and the toxicity of etoposide.[1]

However in a study, 102 children with acute lymphoblastic leukaemia were given **prednisone** 40 mg/m² daily for 28 days with etoposide 300 mg/m² on day 29. Forty-eight of them with high risk disease were given continuation therapy and received etoposide 300 mg/m² at week 54, two weeks or more after the last **prednisone** dose. Etoposide clearance was 62% higher on day 29 than at week 54 and the AUC for the catechol metabolite was significantly lower (27%) on day 29 compared with week 54.[2]

There seems to be little clinical confirmation that the potential interactions with the drugs listed above, other than corticosteroids (which found the opposite of the predicted effect) have clinical relevance, but good monitoring would be a prudent precaution. See also 'Antineoplastics + Protease inhibitors', p.615.

1. Kawashiro T, Yamashita K, Zhao X-J, Koyama E, Tani M, Chiba K, Ishizaki T. A study on the metabolism of etoposide and possible interactions with antitumor or supporting agents by human liver microsomes. *J Pharmacol Exp Ther* (1998) 386, 1294–1300.
2. Kishi S, Yang W, Boureau B, Morand S, Das S, Chen P, Cook EH, Rosner GL, Schuetz E, Pui C-H, Relling MV. Effects of prednisone and genetic polymorphisms on etoposide disposition in children with acute lymphoblastic leukaemia. *Blood* (2004) 103, 67–72.

Etoposide + Food

In 8 patients with extensive small cell lung carcinoma the pharmacokinetics of a 100-mg oral dose of etoposide were unaffected when it was taken with a full breakfast, when compared with the fasting state.[1] However, the manufacturer recommends that etoposide should be taken on an empty stomach.[2]

1. Harvey VJ, Slevin ML, Joel SP, Johnston A, Wrigley PFM. The effect of food and concurrent chemotherapy on the bioavailability of oral etoposide. *Br J Cancer* (1985) 52, 363–7.
2. Vepesid Capsules (Etoposide). Bristol-Myers Pharmaceuticals. UK Summary of product characteristics, July 2005.

Etoposide + Other antineoplastics

Doxorubicin and cyclophosphamide have no clinically relevant effects on the pharmacokinetics of oral or intravenous etoposide. Methotrexate and procarbazine do not affect the pharmacokinetics of oral etoposide.

Clinical evidence, mechanism, importance and management

A pharmacokinetic study in 7 patients with small-cell lung cancer (SCLC) treated with **cyclophosphamide** 800 mg/m², **doxorubicin** 40 mg/m² and etoposide 100 mg/m² (all given intravenously) found that the protein binding, metabolism and renal clearance of etoposide were unaffected by the other antineoplastics.[1] Similarly, another study found only modest changes in the pharmacokinetics of intravenous etoposide when it was given with **cyclophosphamide** and **doxorubicin**, compared with use alone, and these changes were considered unlikely to be clinically relevant. Specifically, the AUC of etoposide was 9% higher and the clearance was 10% lower on day 1 of the CAE cycle (**cyclophosphamide**, **doxorubicin**, and etoposide) compared with days 2 and 3 (etoposide alone).[2] This is a commonly used regimen, and these data suggest there is no pharmacokinetic interaction.

Similarly, no changes in etoposide pharmacokinetics were seen when oral etoposide 100 mg was given immediately after oral **cyclophosphamide** 100 mg/m² and **methotrexate** 12.5 mg/m² in 8 patients with SCLC. In addition, no changes were seen when the same dose of oral etoposide was given 15 minutes after intravenous **doxorubicin** 35 mg/m² and oral **procarbazine** 60 mg/m².[3] Oral etoposide pharmacokinetics appear not to be affected by these antineoplastics.

For the lack of effect of platinum derivatives, see 'Etoposide + Cisplatin or Carboplatin', p.630.

1. Van Hoogenhuijze J, Lankelma J, Stam J, Pinedo HM. Unchanged pharmacokinetics of VP-16-213 (etoposide, NSC 141540) during concomitant administration of doxorubicin and cyclophosphamide. *Eur J Cancer Clin Oncol* (1987) 23, 807–11.
2. Busse D, Würthwein G, Hinske C, Hempel G, Fromm MF, Eichelbaum M, Kroemer HK, Busch FW. Pharmacokinetics of intravenous etoposide in patients with breast cancer: influence of dose escalation and cyclophosphamide and doxorubicin coadministration. *Naunyn Schmiedebergs Arch Pharmacol* (2002) 366, 218–25.
3. Harvey VJ, Slevin ML, Joel SP, Johnston A, Wrigley PFM. The effect of food and concurrent chemotherapy on the bioavailability of oral etoposide. *Br J Cancer* (1985) 52, 363–7.

Etoposide + St John's wort (*Hypericum perforatum*)

***In vitro* studies suggest that hypericin, a component of St John's wort may antagonise the effects of etoposide. It may also stimulate the hepatic metabolism of etoposide by the cytochrome P450 isoenzyme CYP3A4. Information is very limited but it seems that it would be prudent to avoid St John's wort in patients taking etoposide or related drugs.[1] More study is needed.**

1. Peebles KA, Baker RK, Kurz EU, Schneider BJ, Kroll DJ. Catalytic inhibition of human DNA topoisomerase IIα by hypericin, a naphthodianthrone from St. John's wort (*Hypericum perforatum*). *Biochem Pharmacol* (2001) 62, 1059–70.

Exemestane + CYP3A4 inducers and inhibitors

Ketoconazole appears not to interact with exemestane, whereas rifampicin reduces exemestane levels.

Clinical evidence, mechanism, importance and management

The manufacturers say that *in vitro* evidence shows that while exemestane is metabolised by both the cytochrome P450 isoenzyme CYP3A4 and aldoketoreductases, a clinical study found that **ketoconazole** (a specific inhibitor of CYP3A4) had no significant effects on the pharmacokinetics of exemestane. The manufacturers therefore suggest that interactions with CYP3A4 enzyme inhibitors are unlikely.[1,2]

However, in an interaction study the potent enzyme inducer **rifampicin** reduced the AUC and maximum plasma levels of exemestane by 54% and 41%, respectively.

The manufacturers therefore caution the use of exemestane with CYP3A4 inducers such as **carbamazepine**, **phenobarbital**, **phenytoin** and **St John's wort**.[1,2] The clinical relevance of these potential interactions is unknown, but it would seem prudent to monitor the outcome of concurrent use to ensure exemestane efficacy.

1. Aromasin (Exemestane). Pharmacia Ltd. UK Summary of product characteristics, August 2005.
2. Aromasin (Exemestane). Pharmacia & Upjohn Company. US Prescribing information, February 2007.

Fludarabine + Dipyridamole

Because fludarabine phosphate is an analogue of adenine, the UK manufacturers warn that drugs that are adenosine uptake inhibitors, such as dipyridamole, may prevent the uptake of fludarabine into cells and reduce its efficacy.[1,2] Dipyridamole should probably therefore be avoided in patients receiving fludarabine.

1. Schering Health Care Ltd. Personal communication, February 1995.
2. Fludara Tablets (Fludarabine phosphate). Schering Health Care Ltd. UK Summary of product characteristics, September 2005.

Fludarabine + Pentostatin

When fludarabine phosphate and pentostatin were used in the treatment of chronic lymphoid leukaemia, 4 out of 6 patients de-

veloped pulmonary toxicity consistent with interstitial pneumonitis, and 3 of them died.[1] Pentostatin should therefore not be used concurrently with fludarabine.[2,3]

1. Schering Health Care Ltd. Personal communication, February 1995.
2. Fludara Tablets (Fludarabine phosphate). Schering Health Care Ltd. UK Summary of product characteristics, September 2005.
3. Fludara (Fludarabine phosphate). Bayer HealthCare Pharmaceuticals Inc. US Prescribing information, October 2003.

Fluorouracil + Allopurinol

Allopurinol has been studied as a modulator of the effects of fluorouracil, but has not gained an established clinical use in this setting.

Clinical evidence, mechanism, importance and management

Some early studies showed that allopurinol 300 mg two to four times daily allowed the usual maximum tolerated dose of fluorouracil to be increased by up to twofold.[1-3] The hope was that allopurinol would prove useful to decrease the toxicity and/or improve the activity of fluorouracil. However, most studies have shown no increase in response rates in colorectal cancer with allopurinol,[4,5] even when the fluorouracil dose was escalated,[2,4] and some have also shown no reduction in toxicity.[5-7] These are by no means all the studies, and are just cited as examples. Allopurinol mouthwash has also been investigated to reduce the incidence of stomatitis with fluorouracil. Some controlled studies have shown a benefit,[8] whereas others have not.[9] Allopurinol clearly modulates some of the effects of fluorouracil; however, this has not been shown to be obviously beneficial or harmful in the clinical setting.

1. Howell SB, Wung WE, Taetle R, Hussain F, Romine JS. Modulation of 5-fluorouracil toxicity by allopurinol in man. *Cancer* (1981) 48, 1281–9.
2. Fox RM, Woods RL, Tattersall MHN, Piper AA, Sampson D. Allopurinol modulation of fluorouracil toxicity. *Cancer Chemother Pharmacol* (1981) 5, 151–5.
3. Woolley PV, Ayoob MJ, Smith FP, Lokey JL, DeGreen P, Marantz A, Schein PS. A controlled trial of the effect of 4-hydroxypyrazolopyrimidine (allopurinol) on the toxicity of a single bolus dose of 5-fluorouracil. *J Clin Oncol* (1985) 3, 103–9.
4. Tsavaris N, Bacoyannis C, Milonakis N, Sarafidou M, Zamanis N, Magoulas D, Kosmidis P. Folinic acid plus high-dose 5-fluorouracil with allopurinol protection in the treatment of advanced colorectal carcinoma. *Eur J Cancer* (1990) 26, 1054–6.
5. Merimsky O, Inbar M, Chaitchik S. Treatment of advanced colorectal cancer by 5-fluorouracil–leucovorin combination with or without allopurinol: a prospective randomized study. *Anticancer Drugs* (1991) 2, 447–51.
6. Howell SB, Pfeifle CE, Wung WE. Effect of allopurinol on the toxicity of high-dose 5-fluorouracil administered by intermittent bolus injection. *Cancer* (1983) 51, 220–5.
7. Garewal H, Ahmann FR. Failure of allopurinol to provide clinically significant protection against the hematologic toxicity of a bolus 5-FU schedule. *Oncology* (1986) 43, 216–18.
8. Porta C, Moroni M, Nastasi G. Allopurinol mouthwashes in the treatment of 5-fluorouracil-induced stomatitis. *Am J Clin Oncol* (1994) 17, 246–7.
9. Loprinzi CL, Cianflone SG, Dose AM, Etzell PS, Burnham NL, Therneau TM, Hagen L, Gainey DK, Cross M, Athmann LM, Fischer T, O'Connell MJ. A controlled evaluation of an allopurinol mouthwash as prophylaxis against 5-fluorouracil-induced stomatitis. *Cancer* (1990) 65, 1879–82.

Fluorouracil + Aminoglycosides; Oral

Neomycin can delay the gastrointestinal absorption of fluorouracil, but the clinical importance of this is uncertain.

Clinical evidence, mechanism, importance and management

Some preliminary information from a study in 12 patients treated for metastatic adenocarcinoma found that with the use of oral **neomycin** 500 mg four times daily for a week delayed the absorption of fluorouracil, but the effects were generally too small to reduce the therapeutic response, except possibly in one patient.[1] It seems probable that this interaction occurs because **neomycin** can induce a malabsorption syndrome. If **neomycin**, and most probably **paromomycin** or **kanamycin** are used in patients receiving fluorouracil, the possibility of this interaction should be borne in mind.

1. Bruckner HW, Creasey WA. The administration of 5-fluorouracil by mouth. *Cancer* (1974) 33, 14–18.

Fluorouracil + Cisplatin or Oxaliplatin

Giving low-dose cisplatin with a fluorouracil infusion markedly increased toxicity in one study. Cardiotoxicity may possibly be increased if higher doses of cisplatin are given with fluorouracil. Oxaliplatin appears to moderately raise fluorouracil levels, without increasing its toxicity.

Clinical evidence, mechanism, importance and management

(a) Cisplatin

Giving low-dose cisplatin 20 mg/m² once a week with continuous ambulatory fluorouracil infusions of 300 mg/m² daily considerably increased the toxicity (nausea, vomiting, anorexia, diarrhoea, stomatitis, myelosuppression) in 18 patients with advanced cancers. More than half developed multiple toxicities, and severe toxicity occurred in two-thirds. Leucopenia occurred in 28% given both drugs whereas it was virtually nonexistent with fluorouracil alone. Toxicity requiring treatment interruption or dose reduction was seen in 55% of patients receiving fluorouracil alone, and this rose to 94% in the presence of cisplatin.[1] In another study, signs of cardiotoxicity (chest pain, ST-T wave changes, arrhythmias) were seen in 12 of 80 patients given fluorouracil with cisplatin for carcinoma of the head, neck, oesophagus and stomach.[2] Studies in humans and *rats* have shown that there is prolonged elevation of filterable platinum levels associated with concurrent use of cisplatin and fluorouracil.[3]

The combination of a platinum derivative and fluorouracil is widely used, but the optimum schedule to improve activity and reduce toxicity is not firmly established. In one study of bolus cisplatin and continuous infusion fluorouracil, modifying the dose of fluorouracil based on AUC reduced toxicity while still maintaining response rates.[4] In another study, cisplatin pharmacokinetics were said to be optimum when it was given as a continuous infusion with a continuous infusion of fluorouracil.[5] Further study is needed.

(b) Oxaliplatin

In one study, 28 patients with advanced or metastatic colorectal cancer were given fluorouracil alone, or immediately following an 85 mg/m² dose of oxaliplatin given over 2 hours. Oxaliplatin did not significantly affect the pharmacokinetics of fluorouracil (either 2 cycles of a 400 mg/m² bolus followed by a 46-hour infusion of 2400 mg/m² given to 10 patients, with pharmacokinetic sampling over 46 hours, or a single cycle of a 400 mg/m² bolus followed by 600 mg/m² over 22 hours given to 18 patients, with pharmacokinetic sampling over 22 hours).[6] However, in another study 29 patients with advanced colorectal cancer were given fluorouracil in a dose adjusted to give levels of between 2.5 and 3 mg/L (dose range 750 to 3500 mg/m² per week) either alone, or immediately following a 2-hour infusion of oxaliplatin 130 mg/m². In this study pharmacokinetic samples were taken on days 1, 8 and 15. Oxaliplatin raised the plasma levels of fluorouracil by about one-third, with the effect appearing to last for 15 days, however, fluorouracil toxicity was not increased.[7]

The combination of fluorouracil and oxaliplatin is widely used, but one of the studies cited here suggest that the schedules could still be adjusted to optimise efficacy and minimise toxicity.[7]

1. Jeske J, Hansen RM, Libnoch JA, Anderson T. 5-Fluorouracil infusion and low-dose weekly cisplatin: an analysis of increased toxicity. *Am J Clin Oncol* (1990) 13, 485–8.
2. Jeremic B, Jevremovic S, Djuric L, Mijatovic L. Cardiotoxicity during chemotherapy treatment with 5-fluorouracil and cisplatin. *J Chemother* (1990) 2, 264–7.
3. Belliveau JF, Posner MR, Crabtree GW, Weitberg AB, Wiemann MC, Cummings FJ, O'Leary GP, Ingersoll E, Calabresi P. Clinical pharmacokinetics of 3-day continuous infusion cisplatin and daily bolus 5-fluorouracil. *Eur J Clin Pharmacol* (1991) 40, 115–17.
4. Fety R, Rolland F, Barberi-Heyob M, Hardouin A, Campion L, Conroy T, Merlin J-L, Riviére A, Perrocheau G, Etienne MC, Milano G. Clinical impact of pharmacokinetically-guided dose adaptation of 5-fluorouracil: results from a multicentric randomized trial in patients with locally advanced head and neck carcinomas. *Clin Cancer Res* (1998) 4, 2039–45.
5. Ikeda K, Terashima M, Kawamura H, Takiyama I, Koeda K, Takagane A, Sato N, Ishida K, Iwaya T, Maesawa C, Yoshinari H, Saito K. Pharmacokinetics of cisplatin in combined cisplatin and 5-fluorouracil therapy: a comparative study of three different schedules of cisplatin administration. *Jpn J Clin Oncol* (1998) 28, 168–75.
6. Joel SP, Papamichael D, Richards F, Davis T, Aslanis V, Chatelut E, Locke K, Slevin ML, Seymour MT. Lack of pharmacokinetic interaction between 5-fluorouracil and oxaliplatin. *Clin Pharmacol Ther* (2004) 76, 45–54.
7. Boisdron-Celle M, Craipeau MC, Brienza S, Delva R, Guérin-Meyer V, Cvitkovic E, Gamelin E. Influence of oxaliplatin on 5-fluorouracil plasma clearance and clinical consequences. *Cancer Chemother Pharmacol* (2002) 49, 235–43.

Fluorouracil + Dipyridamole

One study suggested that intravenous dipyridamole may reduce the steady-state plasma levels of fluorouracil, whereas others found that oral dipyridamole caused no important changes in fluorouracil pharmacokinetics.

Clinical evidence, mechanism, importance and management

Numerous preclinical studies found that dipyridamole enhanced the activity of fluorouracil, leading to its investigation as a biomodulator.[1] However, unexpectedly, in one phase I study of the combination, the use of dipyridamole was associated with lower steady state plasma level of fluorouracil, suggesting an approximately 30% increase in total body clearance or volume of distribution of fluorouracil.[2] In this study, 47 patients with advanced cancer were given fluorouracil in escalating doses ranging from 185 mg/m^2 daily to 3600 mg/m^2 daily with or without dipyridamole as a continuous infusion of 7.7 mg/kg per day for 72 hours.[2] In contrast, in a later randomised study, oral dipyridamole 75 mg three times daily for 5 days did not significantly alter the pharmacokinetics of fluorouracil, except for prolonging the half-life and slightly increasing the dose-intensity: over 5 cycles the average dose of fluorouracil was 479 mg/m^2 alone, compared with 533 mg/m^2 in the presence of dipyridamole. In this study, oral dipyridamole did not improve the antineoplastic activity of fluorouracil and folinic acid.[3] Similarly, another clinical study found that oral dipyridamole did not significantly alter the pharmacokinetics of fluorouracil.[4] Thus, despite the promise of preclinical studies, the benefits of combining dipyridamole with fluorouracil have not been realised clinically.

1. Grem JL. Biochemical modulation of fluorouracil by dipyridamole: preclinical and clinical experience. *Semin Oncol* (1992) 19 (Suppl 3), 56–65.
2. Trump DL, Egorin MJ, Forrest A, Willson JKV, Remick S, Tutsch KD. Pharmacokinetic and pharmacodynamic analysis of fluorouracil during 72-hour continuous infusion with and without dipyridamole. *J Clin Oncol* (1991) 9, 2027–35.
3. Köhne C-H, Hiddemann W, Schüller J, Weiss J, Lohrmann H-P, Schmitz-Hüber U, Bodenstein H, Schöber C, Wilke H, Grem J, Schmoll H-J. Failure of orally administered dipyridamole to enhance the antineoplastic activity of fluorouracil in combination with leucovorin in patients with advanced colorectal cancer: a prospective randomized trial. *J Clin Oncol* (1995) 13, 1201–8.
4. Czejka MJ, Jäger W, Schüller J, Fogl U, Weiss C, Schernthaner G. Clinical pharmacokinetics of fluorouracil: influence of the biomodulating agents interferon, dipyridamole and folinic acid alone and in combination. *Arzneimittelforschung* (1993) 43, 387–90.

Fluorouracil + Folic acid

Two patients developed severe fluorouracil toxicity while taking multivitamin preparations containing folic acid.

Clinical evidence

A woman who underwent surgery for carcinoma of the rectum was, a month later, given intravenous fluorouracil 500 mg/m^2 daily for 5 days. At the end of this chemotherapy she was admitted to hospital with anorexia, severe mouth ulceration, bloody diarrhoea and vaginal bleeding, which was interpreted as fluorouracil toxicity. Her concurrent medication included folic acid 5 mg daily (in *Multi-B forte*) along with loperamide, sulfasalazine, vitamins B_{12} and K, and HRT. A month later, when she was again given fluorouracil, but without the folic acid, her treatment was well tolerated and without toxicity. A man similarly treated with fluorouracil for colonic cancer was admitted to hospital 2 days later with severe mouth ulceration and bloody diarrhoea. He too was found to be taking a multivitamin preparation, containing folic acid 500 micrograms (amount taken daily not known). Subsequent courses of fluorouracil at the same dosage but without the folic acid were well tolerated.[1] For a report of fatal toxicity associated with the concurrent use of folic acid and capecitabine, see 'Fluorouracil prodrugs; Capecitabine + Folinates', p.635.

Mechanism

It would seem that folic acid increases fluorouracil inhibition of thymidine formation which is important for DNA synthesis, and thereby increases fluorouracil toxicity.

Importance and management

Direct information seem to be limited to these two cases and a case of fatal toxicity associated with concurrent folic acid and capecitabine, a prodrug of fluorouracil (see 'Fluorouracil prodrugs; Capecitabine + Folinates', p.635) but the interaction would appear to be established. What happened is consistent with the way **folinic acid**, another source of folate, is used therapeutically to increase the potency of fluorouracil. Patients treated with fluorouracil should therefore not be given folic acid, and should be told to avoid multivitamin preparations containing folic acid to prevent the development of severe fluorouracil adverse effects.

1. Mainwaring P, Grygiel JJ. Interaction of 5-fluorouracil with folates. *Aust N Z J Med* (1995) 25, 60.

Fluorouracil + Gemcitabine

Pharmacokinetic analysis has shown that gemcitabine enhances systemic exposure to fluorouracil in patients with pancreatic carcinoma given folinic acid, fluorouracil, and gemcitabine.[1,2] In addition, *in vitro*, gemcitabine increases the accumulation of fluorouracil and its cytotoxicity.[1] Further study is needed.

1. Francini G, Correale P, Cetta F, Zuckermann M, Cerretani D, Micheli V, Bruni G, Clerici M, Pozzessere D, Petrioli R, Marsili S, Messinese S, Sabatino M, Giorgio G. Effects of gemcitabine on 5-fluorouracil activity, pharmacokinetics and pharmacodynamics in vitro and in cancer patients. *Gastroenterology* (2002) 122 (Suppl 1), A308.
2. Correale P, Cerretani D, Marsili S, Pozzessere D, Petrioli R, Messinese S, Sabatino M, Roviello F, Pinto E, Francini G, Giorgi G. Gemcitabine increases systemic 5-fluorouracil exposure in advanced cancer patients. *Eur J Cancer* (2003) 39, 1547–51.

Fluorouracil + H_2-receptor antagonists

Some data indicate that 4 weeks, but not 1 week, of treatment with cimetidine can markedly increase plasma fluorouracil levels. The combination may have increased activity in colorectal cancer.

Clinical evidence, mechanism, importance and management

A study in 6 patients with carcinoma given fluorouracil (15 mg/kg daily for 5 days, repeated every 4 weeks) found that **cimetidine** 1 g daily for 4 weeks increased the peak plasma fluorouracil levels by 74% and the AUC by 72% when fluorouracil was given orally. When fluorouracil was given intravenously the AUC was increased by 27% and the total body clearance was reduced by 28% by **cimetidine**. In this small group, no increased toxicity was noted. The pharmacokinetics of fluorouracil were unaltered when **cimetidine** was given for only one week.[1] **Cimetidine** had similar effects in *animal* studies but **ranitidine** had no effect on fluorouracil metabolism.[2] It is suggested that **cimetidine** reduces the hepatic metabolism of fluorouracil.[1,2] At least three clinical studies have shown some treatment benefits from giving fluorouracil with long-term **cimetidine** in colorectal cancer.[3-5] However, this benefit has been attributed to immunomodulation[3] or inhibition of adhesion,[4] rather than any pharmacokinetic interaction. Whatever the mechanism, it appears that **cimetidine** can increase the activity of fluorouracil. Concurrent treatment should be undertaken with care. **Cimetidine** can be obtained without a prescription in some countries so that patients may unwittingly increase the toxicity of fluorouracil. **Ranitidine** does not appear to interact.

1. Harvey VJ, Slevin ML, Dilloway MR, Clark PI, Johnston A, Lant AF. The influence of cimetidine on the pharmacokinetics of 5-fluorouracil. *Br J Clin Pharmacol* (1984) 18, 421–30.
2. Dilloway MR, Lant AF. Effect of H_2-receptor antagonists on the pharmacokinetics of 5-fluorouracil in the rat and monkey. *Biopharm Drug Dispos* (1991) 12, 17–28.
3. Links M, Clingan PR, Phadke K, O'Baugh J, Legge J, Adams WJ, Ross WB, Morris DL. A randomized trial of cimetidine with 5-fluorouracil and folinic acid in metastatic colorectal cancer. *Eur J Surg Oncol* (1995) 21, 523–5.
4. Matsumoto S, Imaeda Y, Umemoto S, Kobayashi K, Suzuki H, Okamoto T. Cimetidine increases survival of colorectal cancer patients with high levels of sialyl Lewis-X and sialyl Lewis-A epitope expression on tumour cells. *Br J Cancer* (2002) 86, 159–60.
5. Yoshimatsu K, Ishibashi K, Hashimoto M, Umehara A, Yokomizo H, Yoshida K, Fujimoto T, Iwasaki K, Ogawa K. Effect of cimetidine with chemotherapy on stage IV colorectal cancer. *Gan To Kagaku Ryoho* (2003) 30, 1794–7.

Fluorouracil + Interferon alfa

Interferon alfa has increased plasma fluorouracil levels in some, but not other, studies.

Clinical evidence, mechanism, importance and management

In a pharmacokinetic study 26 patients with colorectal cancer were given a 5-day continuous infusion of fluorouracil 750 mg/m^2 daily repeated in week 4 followed by a bolus intravenous injection of 750 mg/m^2 once a week with or without subcutaneous interferon alfa-2a (*Roferon*) 9 million units three times a week. There was considerable within-patient variation but no significant differences in steady-state plasma levels were found between the two groups.[1] Similarly, others have also reported that interferon alfa does not significantly alter fluorouracil pharmacokinetics;[2,3] however, other studies[4-8] have found a significant increase in peak fluorouracil levels and/or AUC when interferon alfa is given. Despite promising early pre-clinical and clinical data indicating that interferon may improve the response to fluorouracil, this has not yet been demonstrated in randomised studies.[9] A study in 27 patients with metastatic melanoma treated with fluorouracil 1000 mg/m^2 every 28 days and interferon alfa 2a in doses of up to 9 million units daily for 70 days and then 3 million units three times a week for up to a year, found that the response rate was similar to that obtained in other studies using interferon alone. The most frequent adverse effects were related to the interferon, and no patients were withdrawn from the study due to toxicity.[10]

1. Pittman K, Perren T, Ward U, Primrose J, Slevin M, Patel N, Selby P. Pharmacokinetics of 5-fluorouracil in colorectal cancer patients receiving interferon. *Ann Oncol* (1993) 4, 515–6.
2. Seymour MT, Patel N, Johnston A, Joel SP, Slevin ML. Lack of effect of interferon α2a upon fluorouracil pharmacokinetics. *Br J Cancer* (1994) 70, 724–8.
3. Kim J, Zhi J, Satoh H, Koss-Twardy SG, Passe SM, Patel IH, Pazdur R. Pharmacokinetics of recombinant human interferon-α2a combined with 5-fluorouracil in patients with advanced colorectal carcinoma. *Anticancer Drugs* (1998) 9, 689–96.
4. Schüller J, Czejka MJ, Schernthaner G, Fogl U, Jäger W, Micksche M. Influence of interferon alfa-2b with or without folinic acid on pharmacokinetics of fluorouracil. *Semin Oncol* (1992) 19 (2 suppl 3) 93–7.
5. Grem JL, McAtee N, Murphy RF, Balis FM, Steinberg SM, Hamilton JM, Sorensen JM, Sartor O, Kramer BS, Goldstein LJ, Gay LM, Caubo KM, Goldspiel B, Allegra CJ. A pilot study of interferon alfa-2a in combination with fluorouracil plus high dose leucovorin in metastatic gastrointestinal carcinoma. *J Clin Oncol* (1991) 9, 1811–20.
6. Danhauser LL, Freimann JH, Gilchrist TL, Gutterman JU, Hunter CY, Yeomans AC, Markowitz AB. Phase I and plasma pharmacokinetic study of infusional fluorouracil combined with recombinant interferon alfa-2b in patients with advanced cancer. *J Clin Oncol* (1993) 11, 751–61.
7. Larsson P-A, Glimelius B, Jeppsson B, Jönsson P-E, Malmberg M, Gustavsson B, Carlsson G, Svedberg M. A pharmacokinetic study of 5-FU/leucovorin and alpha-interferon in advanced cancer. *Acta Oncol* (2000) 39, 59–63.
8. Schüller J, Czejka M. Pharmacokinetic interaction of 5-fluorouracil and interferon alpha-2b with or without folinic acid. *Med Oncol* (1995) 12, 47–53.
9. Makower D, Wadler S. Interferons as biomodulators of fluoropyrimidines in the treatment of colorectal cancer. *Semin Oncol* (1999) 26, 663–71.
10. Walpole ET, Hersey P, Thomson D, McLeod GRC. Recombinant interferon-α2a plus 5-fluorouracil for the treatment of metastatic melanoma. *Melanoma Res* (1997) 7, 513–16.

Fluorouracil + Metronidazole

The toxicity, but not the efficacy of fluorouracil, is increased by metronidazole.

Clinical evidence

A marked increase in fluorouracil toxicity was noted in 27 patients with metastatic colorectal cancer when they were given intravenous metronidazole 750 mg/m^2 one hour before receiving intravenous fluorouracil 600 mg/m^2 5 days per week, every 4 weeks. Granulocytopenia occurred in 74% of patients, nausea and vomiting in 48%, anaemia in 41%, stomatitis and oral ulceration in 34%, and thrombocytopenia in 19%.[1] A pharmacokinetic study in 10 patients found that metronidazole reduced the clearance of fluorouracil by 27% over the 5-day period and increased the AUC by 34%. *In vitro* studies with human colon cancer cells failed to show any increased efficacy.[1]

Studies using another nitroimidazole, misonidazole, in patients with colorectal cancer also found an increased incidence and severity of gastrointestinal toxicity with concurrent use,[2,3] a slightly increased incidence of leucopenia[2] and a reduction in the clearance of fluorouracil.[3]

Mechanism

Metronidazole reduces the clearance of fluorouracil, thereby increasing its toxic effects.

Importance and management

Information is limited but the interaction between fluorouracil and metronidazole appears to be established. It was hoped that metronidazole or misonidazole (no longer in clinical use) might increase the efficacy of fluorouracil. However, the studies above show that the toxicity of fluorouracil is increased without an obvious increase in its therapeutic efficacy. Care should be taken if metronidazole is required for its antimicrobial effects in a patient receiving fluorouracil. Whether other nitroimidazoles (e.g. tinidazole) behave similarly appears not to have been studied.

1. Bardakji Z, Jolivet J, Langelier Y, Besner J-G, Ayoub J. 5-Fluorouracil-metronidazole combination therapy in metastatic colorectal cancer. *Cancer Chemother Pharmacol* (1986) 18, 140–44.
2. Spooner D, Bugden RD, Peckham MJ, Wist EA. The combination of 5-fluorouracil with misonidazole in patients with advanced colorectal cancer. *Int J Radiat Oncol Biol Phys* (1982) 8, 387–9.
3. McDermott BJ, Van den Berg HW, Martin WMC, Murphy RF. Pharmacokinetic rationale for the interaction of 5-fluorouracil and misonidazole in humans. *Br J Cancer* (1983) 48, 705–10.

Fluorouracil + Miscellaneous

A retrospective analysis of studies in a total of 250 patients given fluorouracil for the treatment of gastrointestinal cancer found that chlorprothixene, cinnarizine, prochlorperazine, sodium pentobarbital, thiethylperazine, trimethobenzamide (in antiemetic doses) did not significantly increase toxicity or decrease therapeutic effects, when compared with a placebo.[1]

1. Moertel CG, Reitemeier RJ, Hahn RG. Effect of concomitant drug treatment on toxic and therapeutic activity of 5-fluorouracil (5-FU; NSC-19893). *Cancer Chemother Rep* (1972) 56, 245–7.

Fluorouracil prodrugs + Sorivudine

Marked and rapidly fatal toxicity, attributed to fluorouracil toxicity, has been seen in patients given tegafur or other fluorouracil prodrugs with sorivudine. Fluorouracil is expected to interact similarly.

Clinical evidence

In 1993, the Japanese Ministry of Health reported that 15 Japanese patients with cancer and a viral disease died several days after being given a fluorouracil prodrug (e.g. **tegafur**) and sorivudine. Before death most of them developed severe toxicity including severe anorexia, marked damage to the bone marrow with decreases in white cell and platelet counts, and marked atrophy of the intestinal membrane, with diarrhoea and loss of blood. Eight other patients given both drugs developed symptoms of severe toxicity.[1,2]

Mechanism

Sorivudine appears to be converted in the gut into a metabolite (BVU or bromovinyluracil) that is a potent inhibitor of dihydropyrimidine dehydrogenase (DPD), an enzyme involved in the metabolism of fluorouracil (which is derived from tegafur and other fluorouracil prodrugs).[1,3] There is some evidence that DPD activity is genetically determined, and that there are poor fluorouracil metabolisers with low DPD activity, who would be expected to be more susceptible to this interaction.[4]

Importance and management

Information appears to be limited to these reports but the interaction appears to be established and of clinical importance. The concurrent use of inhibitors of DPD (such as sorivudine and **brivudine**) and oral fluorouracil prodrugs such as **capecitabine**[5] and tegafur is contraindicated. Note that sorivudine was withdrawn from the market following confirmation of this interaction.

1. Okuda H, Nishiyama T, Ogura Y, Nagayama S, Ikeda K, Yamaguchi S, Nakamura Y, Kawaguchi K, Watabe T. Lethal drug interactions of sorivudine, a new antiviral drug, with oral 5-fluorouracil prodrugs. *Drug Metab Dispos* (1997) 25, 270–3.
2. Diasio RB. Sorivudine and 5-fluorouracil; a clinically significant drug-drug interaction due to inhibition of dihydropyrimidine dehydrogenase. *Br J Clin Pharmacol* (1998) 46, 1–4.
3. Watabe T, Okuda H, Ogura K. Lethal drug interactions of the new antiviral, sorivudine, with anticancer prodrugs of 5-fluorouracil. *Yakugaku Zasshi* (1997) 117, 910–21. (In Japanese).
4. Watabe T, Ogura K, Nishiyama T. Molecular toxicological mechanism of the lethal interactions of the new antiviral drug, sorivudine, with 5-fluorouracil prodrugs and genetic deficiency of dihydropyrimidine dehydrogenase. *Yakugaku Zasshi* (2002) 122, 527–35.
5. Xeloda (Capecitabine). Roche Products Ltd. UK Summary of product characteristics, March 2007.

Fluorouracil prodrugs; Capecitabine + Allopurinol

The activity of capecitabine is predicted to be decreased by allopurinol.

Clinical evidence, mechanism, importance and management

Capecitabine is a prodrug, which is activated by several enzymatic steps to produce active fluorouracil within the body. Because allopurinol is reported to modulate fluorouracil, with possible decreased efficacy (see

'Fluorouracil + Allopurinol', p.632), the UK manufacturers of capecitabine say that allopurinol should be avoided.[1]

1. Xeloda (Capecitabine). Roche Products Ltd. UK Summary of product characteristics, March 2007.

Fluorouracil prodrugs; Capecitabine + Antacids

The absorption of capecitabine was not affected by an aluminium/magnesium hydroxide antacid.

Clinical evidence, mechanism, importance and management

A study in 12 patients found that 20 mL of an **aluminium/magnesium hydroxide** antacid (*Maalox*) caused a small increase in the plasma levels of a single 1250-mg/m^2 oral dose of capecitabine and one metabolite (5′-DFCR) but it had no effect on the other 3 major metabolites (5′DFUR, 5-FU and FBAL).[1] There would therefore seem to be no reason for taking special precautions if capecitabine and an antacid of this type are used concurrently.

1. Reigner B, Clive S, Cassidy J, Jodrell D, Schulz R, Goggin T, Banken L, Roos B, Utoh M, Mulligan T, Weidekamm E. Influence of the antacid Maalox on the pharmacokinetics of capecitabine in cancer patients. *Cancer Chemother Pharmacol* (1999) 43, 309–15.

Fluorouracil prodrugs; Capecitabine + Folinates

A patient died after treatment with capecitabine possibly because the concurrent use of folic acid enhanced capecitabine toxicity. The maximum tolerated dose of capecitabine is decreased by folinic acid.

Clinical evidence, mechanism, importance and management

(a) Folic acid

A 51-year-old woman with metastatic breast cancer started treatment with capecitabine 2500 mg/m^2 daily for 14 days every 21 days. Treatment was stopped after 8 days because she developed diarrhoea, vomiting and hand-foot syndrome. She improved with parenteral hydration and symptomatic treatment, but 3 weeks later still had diarrhoea, leg oedema and hand-foot syndrome. She was found to have been taking folic acid 15 mg daily for several weeks before starting capecitabine and had continued to take it during and after capecitabine treatment. The patient's condition improved when the folic acid was stopped, but she then developed diarrhoea and fever followed by necrotic colitis and she died from septic shock and vascular collapse. It is possible that the concurrent use of folic acid enhanced the toxicity of capecitabine.[1]

(b) Folinic acid

Studies in patients with refractory advanced cancer have shown that folinic acid 30 mg twice daily does not have a major effect on the pharmacokinetics of capecitabine.[2] However, the pharmacodynamics of capecitabine were affected as determined by the more frequent occurrence of dose-limiting gastrointestinal disorders or hand-foot syndrome.[2] The UK manufacturers say that the maximum tolerated capecitabine dose when used alone in the intermittent regimen is 3000 mg/m^2, but it is reduced to 2000 mg/m^2 if folinic acid 30 mg twice daily is also given.[3]

1. Clippe C, Freyer G, Milano G, Trillet-Lenoir V. Lethal toxicity of capecitabine due to abusive folic acid prescription? *Clin Oncol* (2003) 15, 1–2.
2. Cassidy J, Dirix L, Bissett D, Reigner B, Griffin T, Allman D, Osterwalder B, Van Oosterom AT. A phase I study of capecitabine in combination with oral leucovorin in patients with intractable solid tumours. *Clin Cancer Res* (1998) 4, 2755–61.
3. Xeloda (Capecitabine). Roche Products Ltd. UK Summary of product characteristics, March 2007.

Fluorouracil prodrugs; Capecitabine + Interferon alfa

The maximum tolerated dose of capecitabine is decreased by interferon alfa.

Clinical evidence, mechanism, importance and management

The UK manufacturers[1] say that the maximum tolerated capecitabine dose when used alone is 3000 mg/m^2, but when combined with interferon alfa-2a (3 million units/m^2 daily) the maximum tolerated dose is 2000 mg/m^2. Capecitabine is a prodrug of fluorouracil, which is thought to be modulated by interferon alfa. See also 'Fluorouracil + Interferon alfa', p.633.

1. Xeloda (Capecitabine). Roche Products Ltd. UK Summary of product characteristics, March 2007.

Fluorouracil prodrugs; Capecitabine + Taxanes

There are no clinically significant pharmacokinetic interactions between capecitabine and paclitaxel, and probably not between capecitabine and docetaxel.

Clinical evidence, mechanism, importance and management

A study in patients with advanced solid tumours found that the use of capecitabine with **docetaxel**, resulted in an almost twofold decrease in the maximum plasma concentration and AUC of fluorouracil. The authors suggest that more study is needed to assess the significance of this finding. Other pharmacokinetic parameters of capecitabine were not affected by **docetaxel**, and the pharmacokinetics of **docetaxel** were not significantly affected by capecitabine or its metabolites.[1]

Other studies in similar patients also found that capecitabine did not alter the pharmacokinetics of **docetaxel**[2] and that the concurrent use of **paclitaxel** and capecitabine did not significantly alter the pharmacokinetics of either drug.[3]

1. Pronk LC, Vasey P, Sparreboom A, Reigner B, Planting AST, Gordon RJ, Osterwalder B, Verweij J. A phase I and pharmacokinetic study of the combination of capecitabine and docetaxel in patients with advanced solid tumours. *Br J Cancer* (2000) 83, 22–9.
2. Ramanathan RK, Ramalingam S, Egorin MJ, Belani P, Potter DM, Fakih M, Jung LL, Strychor S, Jacobs SA, Friedland DM, Shin DM, Chatta GS, Tutchko S, Zamboni WC. Phase I study of weekly (day 1 and 8) docetaxel in combination with capecitabine in patients with advanced solid malignancies. *Cancer Chemother Pharmacol* (2005) 55, 354–60.
3. Villalona-Calero MA, Weiss GR, Burris HA, Kraynak M, Rodrigues G, Drengler RL, Eckhardt SG, Reigner B, Moczygemba J, Burger HU, Griffin T, Von Hoff DD, Rowinsky EK. Phase I and pharmacokinetic study of the oral fluoropyrimidine capecitabine in combination with paclitaxel in patients with advanced solid malignancies. *J Clin Oncol* (1999) 17, 1915–25.

Fulvestrant + Miscellaneous

The pharmacokinetics of intravenous fulvestrant were not affected by rifampicin, an inducer of the cytochrome P450 isoenzyme CYP3A4, or ketoconazole, an inhibitor of CYP3A4. In addition, intramuscular fulvestrant did not affect the pharmacokinetics of midazolam, a substrate of CYP3A4. It is therefore unlikely that fulvestrant will be affected by drug interactions involving this isoenzyme.[1]

1. Robertson JFR, Harrison M. Fulvestrant: pharmacokinetics and pharmacology. *Br J Cancer* (2004) 90 (Suppl. 1), S7–S10.

Gemcitabine + Anthracyclines

The concurrent use of gemcitabine and doxorubicin or epirubicin does not appear to affect the pharmacokinetics of either drug. An *in vitro* study found that the efficacy of the combination of gemcitabine and epirubicin may be schedule-dependent.

Clinical evidence, mechanism, importance and management

The pharmacokinetics of gemcitabine and **doxorubicin** did not differ when they were given on the same day, when compared with when they were given alone in patients with breast cancer.[1] Similarly, gemcitabine pharmacokinetics were unchanged by the concurrent use of **epirubicin** and paclitaxel in patients with breast cancer,[2] and gemcitabine did not alter the interaction between **epirubicin** and paclitaxel (see 'Anthracyclines + Taxanes', p.612).

An *in vitro* study using human bladder cancer cells found that both gemcitabine and **epirubicin** alone exerted a cytotoxic effect but the efficacy of the combination of **epirubicin** and gemcitabine depended on the schedule used. When the drugs were used concurrently or if gemcitabine was used before **epirubicin**, there was an antagonistic interaction. There was synergistic cytotoxic activity when **epirubicin** was used before gemcitabine. This schedule is being investigated in clinical studies.[3]

1. Pérez-Manga G, Lluch A, Alba E, Moreno-Nogueira JA, Palomero M, García-Conde J, Khayat D, Rivelles N. Gemcitabine in combination with doxorubicin in advanced breast cancer: final results of a phase II pharmacokinetic trial. *J Clin Oncol* (2000) 18, 2545–52.
2. Conte PF, Gennari A, Donati S, Salvadori B, Baldini E, Bengala C, Pazzagli I, Orlandini C, Danesi R, Fogli S, Del Tacca M. Gemcitabine plus epirubicin plus taxol (GET) in advanced breast cancer: a phase II study. *Breast Cancer Res Treat* (2001) 68, 171–9.
3. Zoli W, Ricotti L, Tesei A, Ulivi P, Campani AG, Fabbri F, Gunelli R, Frassineti GL, Amadori D. Schedule-dependent cytotoxic interaction between epidoxorubicin and gemcitabine in human bladder cancer cells *in vitro*. *Clin Cancer Res* (2004) 10, 1500–1507.

Gemcitabine + Platinum derivatives

The toxicity and pharmacokinetics of gemcitabine combined with platinum drugs such as cisplatin is dependent upon the order in which they are given.

Clinical evidence, mechanism, importance and management

(a) Carboplatin

Gemcitabine 1000 mg/m^2 on days 1, 8, and 15 has been given with carboplatin (maximum tolerated dose, giving an AUC of 5.2 mg/mL per minute) on day 1, in a monthly cycle. No difference was detected in toxicity or tolerated dose when the gemcitabine was given before or after the carboplatin.[1] However, subsequent authors reported that this same dose schedule, with carboplatin given immediately after the gemcitabine, caused unexpected and severe thrombocytopenia, and could not be recommended.[2]

(b) Cisplatin

When gemcitabine was given 4 hours before or after cisplatin there were no major differences in the plasma pharmacokinetics of gemcitabine, deaminated gemcitabine and platinum. Similarly, cisplatin given 24 hours before gemcitabine did not significantly change gemcitabine and deaminated gemcitabine levels, although there was a trend towards an increased AUC of gemcitabine triphosphate.[3] Gemcitabine given 24 hours before cisplatin decreased the platinum AUC twofold,[3] and caused the least leucopenia of the schedules.[4] Anaemia, thrombocytopenia, nausea and vomiting, and fatigue were not sequence dependent.[4] On the basis of these findings, the authors are further evaluating the schedule of cisplatin given 24 hours before gemcitabine.[3,4] Note that the combination of cisplatin and gemcitabine is commonly used for the treatment of various cancers, usually with the drugs given concurrently or sequentially on the same day.[5]

(c) Oxaliplatin

The pharmacokinetics of gemcitabine 800 to 1500 mg/m^2 and its main metabolite did not appear to be affected by oxaliplatin 70 to 100 mg/m^2 when oxaliplatin was given immediately after gemcitabine once every two weeks.[6]

1. Langer CJ, Claver P, Ozols RF. Gemcitabine and carboplatin in combination: phase I and phase II studies. *Semin Oncol* (1998) 25 (Suppl 9), 51–4.
2. Ng EW, Sandler AB, Robinson L, Einhorn LH. A phase II study of carboplatin plus gemcitabine in advanced non-small-cell lung cancer (NSCLC): a Hoosier Oncology Group study. *Am J Clin Oncol* (1999) 22, 550–3.
3. van Moorsel CJ, Kroep JR, Pinedo HM, Veerman G, Voorn DA, Postmus PE, Vermorken JB, van Groeningen CJ, van der Vijgh WJ, Peters GJ. Pharmacokinetic schedule finding study of the combination of gemcitabine and cisplatin in patients with solid tumors. *Ann Oncol* (1999) 10, 441–8.
4. Kroep JR, Peters GJ, van Moorsel CJA, Catik A, Vermorken JB, Pinedo HM, van Groeningen CJ. Gemcitabine-cisplatin: a schedule finding study. *Ann Oncol* (1999) 10, 1503–10.
5. Gemzar (Gemcitabine). Eli Lilly and Co Ltd. UK Summary of product characteristics, October 2005.
6. Faivre S, Le Chevalier T, Monnerat C, Lokiec F, Novello S, Taieb J, Pautier P, Lhommé C, Ruffié P, Kayitalire L, Armand J-P, Raymond E. Phase I-II and pharmacokinetic study of gemcitabine combined with oxaliplatin in patients with advanced non-small-cell lung cancer and ovarian carcinoma. *Ann Oncol* (2002) 13, 1479–89.

Gemcitabine + Taxanes

One study found that giving paclitaxel before gemcitabine increased the gemcitabine levels by 25%, but other studies did not find a pharmacokinetic interaction. Gemcitabine distribution may be altered by docetaxel, but docetaxel pharmacokinetics are not affected. The clinical response to the combination of gemcitabine and a taxane may depend on the sequence of administration.

Clinical evidence, mechanism, importance and management

(a) Docetaxel

In a study of gemcitabine and docetaxel, given on days 1 and 8 of a 21-day cycle, drug toxicity and pharmacokinetics were unaffected by the relative order of their administration.[1] However, in another study, it appeared that while docetaxel pharmacokinetics were unaffected, the distribution of gemcitabine was altered by docetaxel, although there was no clear relationship between this and toxicity.[2]

A response rate of 43% was reported in a study in which 35 patients with sarcomas were given gemcitabine 675 mg/m^2 over 90 minutes on day 1 and 8, followed by docetaxel 100 mg/m^2, given over 60 minutes, on day 8. The possible synergistic antitumour effect may have been secondary to both the prolonged gemcitabine infusion and the sequence of drug administration.[3] More study is needed.

(b) Paclitaxel

A study in 18 patients with non-small-cell lung cancer found that when they were given gemcitabine 1000 mg/m^2 on days 1 and 8 and paclitaxel 150 to 200 mg/m^2 on day one as a 3-hour infusion immediately before the gemcitabine, the plasma levels of gemcitabine and the AUC of its deaminated metabolite were unchanged, as was the AUC of paclitaxel. However, paclitaxel increased gemcitabine triphosphate levels, potentially improving efficacy.[4] In a study in 14 patients with non-small cell lung cancer, gemcitabine 800 mg/m^2 was administered on day 1 and 8 of a 21 day cycle and paclitaxel 110 mg/m^2 was given 3 hours before the second dose of gemcitabine on day 8. When paclitaxel was given first the clearance, volume of distribution and interpatient pharmacokinetic variability of gemcitabine were decreased. Plasma levels of gemcitabine were increased by 25%, but there was no correlation between these changes and toxicity, and the clinical significance of the interaction is uncertain.[5] In another study, no pharmacokinetic interactions were detected between gemcitabine and paclitaxel given once weekly, although gemcitabine showed saturation kinetics at higher doses.[6,7] Another study in patients with advanced breast cancer given gemcitabine, epirubicin and paclitaxel also found no pharmacokinetic interaction between gemcitabine and paclitaxel.[8]

The high overall response rate of 71% in a phase II study[9] in patients with advanced breast cancer treated with gemcitabine and paclitaxel, prompted an *in vitro* study[10] which found that administration of paclitaxel followed by gemcitabine resulted in synergistic cytotoxic activity, whereas gemcitabine followed by paclitaxel had antagonistic activity. Phase III studies are being carried out to further evaluate the effects of order of administration of these drugs in patients with metastatic breast cancer.[11]

1. Bhargava P, Marshall JL, Fried K, Williams M, Lefebvre P, Dahut W, Hanfelt J, Gehan E, Figuera M, Hawkins MJ, Rizvi NA. Phase I and pharmacokinetic study of two sequences of gemcitabine and docetaxel administered weekly to patients with advanced cancer. *Cancer Chemother Pharmacol* (2001) 48, 95–103.
2. Dumez H, Louwerens M, Pawinsky A, Planting AST, de Jonge MJA, Van Oosterom AT, Highley M, Guetens G, Mantel M, De Boeck G, de Bruijn E, Verweij J. The impact of drug administration sequence and pharmacokinetic interaction in a phase I study of the combination of docetaxel and gemcitabine in patients with advanced solid tumors. *Anticancer Drugs* (2002) 13, 583–93.
3. Leu KM, Ostruszka LJ, Shewach D, Zalupski M, Sondak V, Biermann JS, Lee JS-J, Couwlier C, Palazzolo K, Baker LH. Laboratory and clinical evidence of synergistic cytotoxicity of sequential treatment with gemcitabine followed by docetaxel in the treatment of sarcoma. *J Clin Oncol* (2004) 22, 1706–12.
4. Kroep JR, Giaccone G, Voorn DA, Smit EF, Beijnen JH, Rosing H, van Moorsel CJA, van Groeningen CJ, Postmus PE, Pinedo HM, Peters GJ. Gemcitabine and paclitaxel: pharmacokinetic and pharmacodynamic interactions in patients with non-small-cell lung cancer. *J Clin Oncol* (1999) 17, 2190–7.
5. Shord SS, Faucette SR, Gillenwater HH, Pescatore SL, Hawke RL, Socinski MA, Lindley C. Gemcitabine pharmacokinetics and interaction with paclitaxel in patients with advanced non-small-cell lung cancer. *Cancer Chemother Pharmacol* (2003) 51, 328–36.
6. De Pas T, de Braud F, Danesi R, Sessa C, Catania C, Curigliano G, Fogli S, del Tacca M, Zampino G, Sbanotto A, Rocca A, Cinieri S, Marrocco E, Milani A, Goldhirsch A. Phase I and pharmacologic study of weekly gemcitabine and paclitaxel in chemo-naïve patients with advanced non-small-cell lung cancer. *Ann Oncol* (2000) 11, 821–7.
7. Fogli S, Danesi R, De Braud F, De Pas T, Curigliano G, Giovannetti G, Del Tacca M. Drug distribution and pharmacokinetic/pharmacodynamic relationship of paclitaxel and gemcitabine in patients with non-small-cell lung cancer. *Ann Oncol* (2001) 12, 1553–9.
8. Fogli S, Danesi R, Gennari A, Donati S, Conte PF, Del Tacca M. Gemcitabine, epirubicin and paclitaxel: pharmacokinetic and pharmacodynamic interactions in advanced breast cancer. *Ann Oncol* (2002) 13, 919–27.
9. Colomer R, Llombart-Cussac A, Lluch A, Barnadas A, Ojeda B, Carañana V, Fernández Y, García-Conde J, Alonso S, Montero S, Hornedo J, Guillem V. Biweekly paclitaxel plus gemcitabine in advanced breast cancer: phase II trial and predictive value of HER2 extracellular domain. *Ann Oncol* (2004) 15, 201–206.
10. Oliveras C, Vázquez-Martin A, Ferrer L, de Llorens R, Colomer R. Gemcitabine plus paclitaxel, is there a better schedule for treatment? *Breast Cancer Res Treat* (2004) 88 (Suppl 1) S205.
11. Colomer R. What is the best schedule for administration of gemcitabine-taxane? *Cancer Treat Rev* (2005) 31 (Suppl 4) S23–S28.

Imatinib + CYP3A4 inducers

Rifampicin (rifampin) and St John's wort (*Hypericum perforatum*) lower serum imatinib levels; other CYP3A4 inducers (such as carbamazepine, phenobarbital and phenytoin) are predicted to do the same.

Clinical evidence

(a) Rifampicin (Rifampin)

A study reported that pretreatment with rifampicin 600 mg daily for 11 days decreased the maximum serum levels and AUC of a 400 mg dose of imatinib by 54% and 74%, respectively.[1]

(b) St John's wort (Hypericum perforatum)

In a study in 12 healthy subjects, the pharmacokinetics of a single dose of imatinib was determined before and on day 12 of two weeks of treatment with St John's wort (*Hypericum perforatum*) extract (Kira [LI 160], Lichtwer Pharma) 300 mg three times daily. The AUC and maximum plasma level of imatinib was decreased by 30% and 15%, respectively. Imatinib clearance was increased by 43% and its half-life was decreased from 12.8 to 9 hours.[2] Similar results were found in another study.[3]

Mechanism

Rifampicin is a known potent inducer of many cytochrome P450 isoenzymes, including CYP3A4, by which imatinib is metabolised. Therefore rifampicin increases imatinib metabolism and decreases its levels. St John's wort induces intestinal CYP3A4 and it therefore also reduces imatinib levels.

Importance and management

Subtherapeutic levels of imatinib may occur if rifampicin is given. The manufacturers therefore reasonably recommend caution, and suggest that concurrent use with potent enzyme-inducing drugs should be avoided.[4,5] St John's wort has smaller effects, but they may be sufficient to impair the effects of imatinib, and it has therefore been suggested that concurrent use should also be avoided.[2]

No specific studies have been carried out with imatinib and other CYP3A4-inducing drugs, but the manufacturers suggest that **carbamazepine**, **dexamethasone**, **phenobarbital**, and **phenytoin**, may also reduce imatinib serum levels, and they have a possible case on file with phenytoin.[6] The manufacturers therefore reasonably recommend caution, and suggest that concurrent use with these drugs should be avoided.[4,5] However, if this is not possible it would be prudent to monitor the outcome of concurrent use, and increase the imatinib dose as necessary.

1. Bolton AE, Peng B, Hubert M, Krebs-Brown A, Capdeville R, Keller U, Seiberling M. Effect of rifampicin on the pharmacokinetics of imatinib mesylate (Gleevec, STI571) in healthy subjects. *Cancer Chemother Pharmacol* (2004) 53, 102–6.
2. Frye RF, Fitzgerald SM, Lagattuta TF, Hruska MW, Egorin MJ. Effect of St John's wort on imatinib mesylate pharmacokinetics. *Clin Pharmacol Ther* (2004) 76, 323–9.
3. Smith P. The influence of St John's wort on the pharmacokinetics and protein binding of imatinib mesylate. *Pharmacotherapy* (2004) 24, 1508–14.
4. Glivec (Imatinib mesilate). Novartis Pharmaceuticals UK Ltd. UK Summary of product characteristics, November 2006.
5. Gleevec (Imatinib mesylate). Novartis Pharmaceuticals Corporation. US Prescribing information, November 2006.
6. Novartis Pharmaceuticals UK Limited. Personal communication, December 2001.

Imatinib + CYP3A4 inhibitors

Ketoconazole raises serum imatinib levels; other cytochrome P450 isoenzyme CYP3A4 inhibitors (such as other azoles and macrolides) are predicted to do the same.

Clinical evidence

(a) Ketoconazole

An open-label, randomised, crossover study in 14 healthy subjects found that the maximum serum levels and AUC of imatinib rose by 26% and 40%, respectively, when they were given a single 400-mg dose of ketoconazole with a single 200-mg dose of imatinib.[1]

(b) Voriconazole

A patient with chronic myeloid leukaemia developed a pustular eruption while taking imatinib 400 mg daily, increased to 800 mg daily 12 weeks after starting to take voriconazole for pulmonary aspergillosis. His imatinib plasma levels were approximately twice the predicted levels while taking both drugs. His condition improved within 3 weeks of stopping both voriconazole and imatinib, and did not recur with voriconazole treatment alone.[2]

Mechanism

Ketoconazole is a potent inhibitor of the cytochrome P450 isoenzyme CYP3A4, which is involved in the metabolism of imatinib. Therefore ketoconazole reduces the metabolism and clearance of imatinib and its serum levels rise accordingly. Adverse skin reactions occur frequently with imatinib and may be associated with high does of imatinib and/or increased levels due to an interaction with CYP3A4 inhibitors, such as voriconazole.[2]

Importance and management

The manufacturers therefore advise caution with ketoconazole and with other CYP3A4 inhibitors (examples listed are **clarithromycin**, **erythromycin** and **itraconazole**),[3,4] but it is not entirely clear what action should be taken because information about excessive serum levels is very limited. The authors of one report suggest monitoring plasma levels of imatinib to identify patients at risk of severe toxicity.[2]

1. Novartis Pharmaceuticals UK Limited. Personal communication, December 2001.
2. Gambillara E, Laffitte E, Widmer N, Decosterd LA, Duchosal MA, Kovacsovics T, Panizzon RG. Severe pustular eruption associated with imatinib and voriconazole in a patient with chronic myeloid leukaemia. *Dermatology* (2005) 211, 363–5.
3. Glivec (Imatinib mesilate). Novartis Pharmaceuticals UK Ltd. UK Summary of product characteristics, November 2006.
4. Gleevec (Imatinib mesylate). Novartis Pharmaceuticals Corporation. US Prescribing information, November 2006.

Imatinib + Miscellaneous

Imatinib increases serum tacrolimus levels and is therefore predicted to increase ciclosporin levels. Imatinib may also increases the levels of some benzodiazepines (e.g. midazolam), some calcium-channel blockers (e.g. nifedipine), oestrogens, paracetamol, pimozide, and warfarin. In one case lansoprazole was suspected to have raised imatinib levels.

Clinical evidence, mechanism, importance and management

(a) Calcium-channel blockers

The manufacturers suggest that the levels of the dihydropyridine calcium-channel blockers may be increased by imatinib.[1,2] This suggestion is supported by the case of a patient taking **nifedipine** who developed nausea, vomiting and abdominal pain 8 weeks after starting to take imatinib 400 mg [daily]. Ultrasound showed a thickened gallbladder wall, dilatation of the principal bile ducts and a gallstone. He had not previously had any gall bladder disease. Imatinib was stopped until the abdominal pain was resolved and then restarted at half the initial dose. It was suggested that imatinib may inhibit the metabolism of **nifedipine**, leading to an increase in its effects on lipids, leading to an increase in biliary secretion and gallstone development.[3] This needs confirmation.

(b) Ciclosporin or Tacrolimus

One study in patients with leukaemia who had undergone stem cell transplantation found that the levels of tacrolimus were increased by 25 to 33% within 72 hours of starting imatinib. An empiric tacrolimus dose reduction of 25% at the start of imatinib treatment was found to prevent further serum level fluctuations.[4] The manufacturers suggest that ciclosporin levels may also be increased by imatinib, via its effects on the cytochrome P450 isoenzyme CYP3A4.[1,2]

(c) Lansoprazole

A patient with a recurrence of a gastrointestinal stromal tumour was given imatinib 400 mg daily without adverse effect. However, after 2 months, lansoprazole 15 mg daily was also given for dyspepsia and the patient developed bilateral eyelid oedema with hyperaemic conjunctivae and labial oedema. Both drugs were stopped, but on reintroduction the symptoms reappeared and she developed Stevens-Johnson syndrome. Both drugs were again stopped and she recovered after treatment with methylprednisolone and desloratadine for one month. Two months later, she took a single dose of lansoprazole on the day before treatment with imatinib 300 mg daily (with prednisone and desloratadine) was started. One day later she developed eyelid and labial oedema and a generalised rash. She recovered after imatinib was stopped. Although the adverse effects could be attributed to either imatinib or lansoprazole alone, it was possible that the effects may have been the result of an interaction in which levels of imatinib were increased by lansoprazole, which is a weak inhibitor of CYP3A4.[5] This needs confirmation.

(d) Oestrogens

A patient taking a low-dose oestrogen contraceptive developed nausea and abdominal pain after taking imatinib 400 mg daily for 4 months. Ultrasound showed multiple gallstones and increased gallbladder wall thickness.[3] Imatinib is reported to increase plasma oestrogen levels by inhibiting its metabolism by the cytochrome P450 isoenzyme CYP3A4, possibly leading to increased cholesterol excretion, reduced bile salt excretion and gallstone development. This needs confirmation.

(e) Paracetamol (Acetaminophen)

During clinical studies one patient regularly taking paracetamol for fever, died of acute liver failure 11 days after starting to take imatinib.[6] The manufacturers report that imatinib inhibits paracetamol O-glucuronidation *in vitro*. Although this potential interaction has not been studied in humans, the manufacturers recommend caution during concurrent use, especially with high doses of paracetamol.[1,2]

(f) Warfarin

The manufacturers say that because warfarin is metabolised by CYP2C9, patients needing anticoagulation should be given low-molecular-weight or standard **heparin** instead. This recommendation is based on an observation in one patient[7] and *in vitro* studies[1,2] that show that imatinib can inhibit CYP2C9. There seems to be no other evidence that a clinically relevant interaction is likely to occur.

(g) Other drugs

The manufacturers of imatinib predict that it may raise the levels of **pimozide** with potentially serious consequences [arrhythmias] because of CYP3A4 inhibition. They also suggest that imatinib may raise the levels of the **triazolo-benzodiazepines** (e.g. **triazolam**, **midazolam**).[1,2] This could lead to increased and prolonged sedation.

1. Glivec (Imatinib mesilate). Novartis Pharmaceuticals UK Ltd. UK Summary of product characteristics, November 2006.
2. Gleevec (Imatinib mesylate). Novartis Pharmaceuticals Corporation. US Prescribing information, November 2006.
3. Breccia M, D'Andrea M, Alimena G. Can nifedipine and estrogen interaction with imatinib be responsible for gallbladder stone development? *Eur J Haematol* (2005) 75, 89–90.
4. Sheth SR, Hicks K, Ippoliti C, Giralt , Champlin RE, Anderlini P. Safety, tolerability, and drug interactions of adjuvant imatinib mesylate (Gleevec) within the first 100 days following stem cell transplantation (SCT) in patients with Ph+ CML and PH+ ALL at high risk for recurrence. *Blood* (2002) 100, Abstract 2500.
5. Severino G, Chillotti C, De Lisa R, Del Zompo M, Ardau R. Adverse reactions during imatinib and lansoprazole treatment in gastrointestinal stromal tumors. Ann Pharmacother 2005) 39, 162–4.
6. Talpaz M, Silver RT, Druker B, Paquette R, Goldman JM, Reese SF, Capdeville R. A phase II study of STI 571 in adult patients with Philadelphia chromosome positive chronic myeloid leukaemia in accelerated phase. *Blood* (2000) 96 (Suppl 1), 469a.
7. Novartis Pharmaceuticals UK Limited. Personal communication, December 2001.

Irinotecan + Antiepileptics

In patients with malignant gliomas, enzyme-inducing antiepileptics (carbamazepine, phenobarbital, phenytoin) and, to a lesser extent, non-enzyme inducing antiepileptics (gabapentin, valproate) increased the clearance of irinotecan. The clearance of the active metabolite of irinotecan was also increased by phenytoin. A number of case reports support these suggestions.

Clinical evidence, mechanism, importance and management

(a) Carbamazepine

In a preliminary report of studies in patients with malignant glioma, the clearance of irinotecan was increased almost twofold in the presence of carbamazepine. Peak plasma levels and AUC of irinotecan and SN-38 were significantly decreased.[1]

(b) Phenobarbital

Preclinical data from *rats*[2] indicate that phenobarbital may lead to a reduction in the AUC of both irinotecan and its active metabolite SN-38. This is thought to be because phenobarbital induces the enzymes responsible for glucuronidation of SN-38. In a preliminary report of studies in patients with malignant glioma, clearance of irinotecan was increased by about 1.7-fold in the presence of phenobarbital. The AUC and peak plasma levels of irinotecan and SN-38 were significantly decreased.[1] In a phase I study in patients given ciclosporin and irinotecan, giving phenobarbital 90 mg daily for 2 weeks before irinotecan allowed a dose escalation of irinotecan from 75 mg/m^2 to 144 mg/m^2. Phenobarbital increased irinotecan clearance by 27% and reduced the AUC of SN-38 by 75%, when compared to irinotecan pharmacokinetics in patients given irinotecan with ciclosporin. Further clinical studies are needed to assess the effects of phenobarbital (with ciclosporin; see also, 'Irinotecan + Ciclosporin', p.639) on the antitumour response and toxicity of irinotecan.[3]

(c) Phenytoin

A 14-year-old girl with glioblastoma was given irinotecan 20 to 60 mg/m^2 daily for 5 days on 2 consecutive weeks every 21 days for 2 cycles. During the first cycle she also received phenytoin 300 mg and dexamethasone 6 mg daily. Irinotecan clearance was increased 2.5-fold compared with that in other patients receiving irinotecan alone, and there was decreased exposure to the active metabolite of irinotecan, SN-38. The effect on clearance decreased slowly over 8 days after stopping phenytoin.[4] Another patient taking phenytoin and irinotecan was found to have much lower AUCs for irinotecan and SN-38 compared with data from patients not taking phenytoin.[5] Similarly, a third patient had a threefold increase in irinotecan clearance and about a 60% reduction in the AUCs of irinotecan and SN-38 after starting phenytoin.[6] In a comparative study, the AUC of the lactone forms of irinotecan and SN-38 were 27% and 51% lower, respectively, in 10 children taking enzyme-inducing antiepileptics (7 receiving phenytoin) than in 21 children not taking these antiepileptics.[7] A preliminary report of studies in patients with malignant glioma, clearance of irinotecan was increased by about twofold in the presence of phenytoin. Peak plasma levels and AUC of irinotecan and SN-38 were significantly decreased.[1]

It is thought that phenytoin increases the metabolism of irinotecan to an inactive metabolite by inducing the cytochrome P450 isoenzyme CYP3A, leading to decreased exposure to the active metabolite.[5]

The information is limited but serves to emphasise the need for caution and monitoring if irinotecan is given with phenytoin, which may reduce the availability of its active metabolite. Note that phenytoin has also been shown to increase the clearance of a related topoisomerase inhibitor, topotecan (see 'Topotecan + Phenytoin', p.667) and 9-aminocamptothecin (see '9-Aminocamptothecin + Antiepileptics', p.610).

(d) Non-enzyme-inducing antiepileptics

Preclinical data from *rats*[2] suggests that **sodium valproate** increases the AUC of the active metabolite of irinotecan, SN-38. This is because **valproate** inhibits its subsequent glucuronidation. The clinical relevance of this remains to be determined. A preliminary report of studies in patients with malignant gliomas found that in patients also taking non-enzyme-inducing antiepileptics (**gabapentin**, **lamotrigine**, **levetiracetam**, **tiagabine**, **topiramate**, **valproate**, or **zonisamide**) there was a small but statistically significant increase (about 1.4-fold) in irinotecan clearance.[1]

1. Kuhn JG. Influence of anticonvulsants on the metabolism and elimination of irinotecan: A North American Brain Tumor Consortium Preliminary Report. *Oncology* (2002) 16 (Suppl) 33–40.
2. Gupta E, Wang X, Ramirez J, Ratain MJ. Modulation of the glucuronidation of SN-38, the active metabolite of irinotecan, by valproic acid and phenobarbital. *Cancer Chemother Pharmacol* (1997) 39, 440–4.
3. Innocenti F, Undevia SD, Ramírez J, Mani S, Schilsky RL, Vogelzang NJ, Prado M, Ratain MJ. A phase I trial of pharmacologic modulation of irinotecan with cyclosporine and phenobarbital. *Clin Pharmacol Ther* (2004) 76, 490–502.
4. Radomski KM, Gajjar AJ, Kirstein MN, Ma MK, Wimmer P, Thompson SJ, Houghton PJ, Stewart CF. Irinotecan clearance is increased after concomitant administration of enzyme inducers in a patient with glioblastoma multiforme. *Pharmacotherapy* (2000) 20, 353.
5. Mathijssen RHJ, Sparreboom A, Dumez J, van Oosterom AT, de Bruijn EA. Altered irinotecan metabolism in a patient receiving phenytoin. *Anticancer Drugs* (2002) 13, 139–40.
6. Murry DJ, Cherrick I, Salama V, Berg S, Bernstein M, Kuttesch N, Blaney SM. Influence of phenytoin on the disposition of irinotecan: a case report. *J Pediatr Hematol Oncol* (2002) 24, 130–3.
7. Crews KR, Stewart CF, Jones-Wallace D, Thompson SJ, Houghton PJ, Heideman RL, Fouladi M, Bowers DC, Chintagumpala MM, Gajjar A. Altered irinotecan pharmacokinetics in pediatric high-grade glioma patients receiving enzyme-inducing anticonvulsant therapy. *Clin Cancer Res* (2002) 8, 2202–9.

Irinotecan + Cannabis

The pharmacokinetics of irinotecan are not altered by a herbal tea containing cannabis.

Clinical evidence, mechanism, importance and management

In a crossover study 24 patients were given intravenous **irinotecan** 600 mg before and 12 days after starting a 15-day course of 200 mL daily of a herbal tea containing cannabis 1 g/L. This was prepared from medicinal-grade cannabis (*Cannabis sativa* L. Flos, variety Bedrocan®) containing the cannabinoids Δ^9-tetrahydrocannabinol 18% and cannabidiol 0.8%. The clearance and the AUC of **irinotecan** and its metabolites, SN-38 and SN-38G, were not significantly altered by the presence of cannabis. No dosage adjustments are likely to be needed if **irinotecan** is given with cannabis.[1]

1. Engels FK, de Jong FA, Sparreboom A, Mathot RA, Loos WJ, Kitzen JJEM, de Bruijn P, Verweij J, Mathijssen RHJ. Medicinal cannabis does not influence the clinical pharmacokinetics of irinotecan and docetaxel. *Oncologist* (2007) 12, 291–300.

Irinotecan + Ciclosporin

Ciclosporin reduces the clearance of irinotecan and increases exposure to its active metabolite, SN-38.

Clinical evidence, mechanism, importance and management

In a phase I study in patients with refractory solid tumours or lymphomas, ciclosporin 5 to 10 mg/kg was given as a 6-hour infusion beginning 3 hours before administration of irinotecan (initial dose 25 mg/m² increased to 72 mg/m² weekly). Ciclosporin increased the AUC of SN-38 (the active metabolite of irinotecan) by 23 to 630% and reduced irinotecan clearance by 39 to 64%, when compared with historical controls. The effects of ciclosporin on irinotecan may be due to inhibition of irinotecan- and SN-38-related biliary transporters,[1] and this suggestion is supported by a study in *rats*.[2] Further clinical studies are needed to assess the effects of ciclosporin on the antitumour response and toxicity of irinotecan.

1. Innocenti F, Undevia SD, Ramírez J, Mani S, Schilsky RL, Vogelzang NJ, Prado M, Ratain MJ. A phase I trial of pharmacologic modulation of irinotecan with cyclosporine and phenobarbital. *Clin Pharmacol Ther* (2004) 76, 490–502.

2. Gupta E, Safa AR, Wang X, Ratain MJ. Pharmacokinetic modulation of irinotecan and metabolites by cyclosporin A. *Cancer Res* (1996) 56, 1309–14.

Irinotecan + Fluorouracil

While some studies suggest that giving fluorouracil after irinotecan reduces the conversion of irinotecan to its active metabolite, others do not.

Clinical evidence, mechanism, importance and management

A study in 33 patients with metastatic colorectal cancer found that the toxicity and pharmacokinetics of irinotecan given with fluorouracil depended upon the order of administration of the two drugs.[1] When irinotecan was given before fluorouracil, the AUC of the major active metabolite of irinotecan, SN-38, was about 40% lower, and toxicity was lower. In this study, patients were randomised to receive a 60-minute infusion of irinotecan (150 mg/m² starting dose, escalated by 50 mg/m² increments) immediately before or after a 48-hour infusion of fluorouracil 3500 mg/m² modulated by folinic acid in cycle 1, then given in the reverse sequence in cycle 2. Similarly, in a study using historical controls, the AUC of SN-38 was about 28% lower and the AUC of irinotecan about 35% higher when irinotecan was given over 90 minutes immediately before a 7-day fluorouracil infusion, compared with irinotecan alone.[2] Similar findings were reported in a study in *rats*.[3] In contrast, another study found that fluorouracil did not substantially affect the metabolism of irinotecan to SN-38. The AUC of irinotecan and SN-38 did not differ between irinotecan alone, irinotecan immediately followed by folinic acid and fluorouracil, and irinotecan immediately after folinic acid and fluorouracil. In this study, irinotecan 100 to 150 mg/m² was given as a 90-minute infusion, and fluorouracil 210 to 500 mg/m² by rapid intravenous injection.[4] Similarly, preliminary reports from another research group found that the clearance of irinotecan did not differ when it was given one day before or one day after 5 daily bolus doses of fluorouracil.[5,6]

From these data it is unclear whether or not fluorouracil alters the pharmacokinetics of irinotecan. A key difference between the main studies is the use of bolus[4] or continuous infusion[1] fluorouracil. The combination is in established clinical usage, where the recommendation is to give irinotecan before fluorouracil and folinic acid.[7,8] This combination has been shown to be more effective than fluorouracil and folinic acid alone.[7,8] Whether this is the optimal schedule remains to be determined.

1. Falcone A, Di Paolo A, Masi G, Allegrini G, Danesi R, Lencioni M, Pfanner E, Comis S, Del Tacca M, Conte P. Sequence effect of irinotecan and fluorouracil treatment on pharmacokinetics and toxicity in chemotherapy-naive metastatic colorectal cancer patients. *J Clin Oncol* (2001) 19, 3456–62.

2. Sasaki Y, Ohtsu A, Shimada Y, Ono K, Saijo N. Simultaneous administration of CPT-11 and fluorouracil: alteration of the pharmacokinetics of CPT-11 and SN-38 in patients with advanced colorectal cancer. *J Natl Cancer Inst* (1994) 86 1096–8.

3. Umezawa T, Kiba T, Numata K, Saito T, Nakaoka M, Shintani S, Sekihara H. Comparisons of the pharmacokinetics and the leukopenia and thrombocytopenia grade after administration of irinotecan and 5-fluorouracil in combination to rats. *Anticancer Res* (2000) 20, 4235–42.

4. Salz LB, Kanowitz J, Kemeny NE, Schaaf L, Spriggs D, Staton BA, Berkery R, Steger C, Eng M, Dietz A, Locker P, Kelsen DP. Phase I clinical and pharmacokinetic study of irinotecan, fluorouracil, and leucovorin in patients with advanced solid tumors. *J Clin Oncol* (1996) 14, 2959–67.

5. Grossin F, Barbault H, Benhammouda A, Rixe O, Antoine E, Auclerc G, Weil M, Nizri D, Farabos C, Mignard D, Mahjoubi M, Khayat D, Bastian G. A phase I pharmacokinetics study of concomitant CPT-11 and 5FU combination. *Proc Am Assoc Cancer Res* (1996) 37, 168.

6. Benhammouda A, Bastian G, Rixe O, Antoine E, Gozy M, Auclerc G, Grossin F, Nizri D, Gil-Delgado M, Weil M, Bismuth H, Mignard DM, Mahjoubi M, Lenseigne S, Khayat D. A phase I pharmacokinetic study of CPT-11 and 5-FU combination. *Proc Am Soc Clin Oncol* (1997) 16, 202a.

7. Campto (Irinotecan). Pfizer Ltd. UK Summary of product characteristics, January 2007.

8. Camptosar (Irinotecan hydrochloride). Pfizer Inc. US Prescribing information, June 2006.

Irinotecan + Ketoconazole

Ketoconazole, and therefore probably itraconazole, decreases irinotecan levels and increases the levels of its active metabolite.

Clinical evidence, mechanism, importance and management

A study found that ketoconazole decreased the AUC of irinotecan by 87% and increased the AUC of the active metabolite, SN-38, by 109%. This probably occurred because ketoconazole is a potent inhibitor of the cytochrome P450 isoenzyme CYP3A4 by which irinotecan is metabolised. The manufacturers of irinotecan recommend that the concurrent use of ketoconazole should be avoided.[1,2] The US manufacturers recommend stopping ketoconazole at least one week before starting irinotecan and contraindicate concurrent use.[2] It is likely that other azoles that are strong inhibitors of CYP3A4, such as **itraconazole**, may also affect the metabolism of irinotecan.

1. Campto (Irinotecan hydrochloride trihydrate). Pfizer Ltd. UK Summary of product characteristics, January 2007.

2. Camptosar (Irinotecan hydrochloride). Pfizer Inc. US Prescribing information, June 2006.

Irinotecan + Milk thistle

Milk thistle does not affect the pharmacokinetics of irinotecan.

Clinical evidence, mechanism, importance and management

A pharmacokinetic study was undertaken in 6 patients who were being treated with intravenous irinotecan 125 mg/m² once weekly for 4 weeks, followed by a 2 week rest period. Four days before the second dose of irinotecan, a 14-day course of 200 mg milk thistle seed extract (containing silymarin 80%) three times daily was started. The pharmacokinetics of irinotecan and its metabolites did not differ between week 1 (no milk thistle), week 2 (4 days of milk thistle) or week 3 (12 days of milk thistle).[1] No dosage alterations would therefore be expected to be needed if milk thistle (standardised with silymarin 80%) is given with irinotecan.

1. van Erp NPH, Baker SD, Zhao M, Rudek MA, Guchelaar H-J, Nortier JWR, Sparreboom A, Gelderblom H. Effect of milk thistle (*Silybum marianum*) on the pharmacokinetics of irinotecan. *Clin Cancer Res* (2005) 11, 7800–6.

Irinotecan + Miscellaneous

Preclinical data suggest that vinorelbine and physostigmine may decrease the formation of the active metabolite of irinotecan, SN-38.

Clinical evidence, mechanism, importance and management

In studies in human liver microsomes, **nifedipine**, **clonazepam**, **methylprednisolone**, **omeprazole**, and **vinorelbine** had significant effects on the metabolism of irinotecan. However, only the effect of **vinorelbine** occurred at a concentration considered clinically relevant.[1] Similarly, of various potential carboxylesterase inhibitors, only **physostigmine** was considered sufficiently potent to possibly inhibit irinotecan activation.[2] Further study is needed to assess the clinical relevance of these findings.

1. Charasson V, Haaz M-C, Robert J. Determination of drug interactions occurring with the metabolic pathways of irinotecan. *Drug Metab Dispos* (2002) 30, 731–3.
2. Slatter JG, Su P, Sams JP, Schaaf LJ, Wienkers LC. Bioactivation of the anticancer agent CPT-11 to SN-38 by human hepatic microsomal carboxylesterases and the *in vitro* assessment of potential drug interactions. *Drug Metab Dispos* (1997) 25, 1157–64.

Irinotecan + Oxaliplatin

An isolated report suggests that the cholinergic toxicity associated with irinotecan may be enhanced by oxaliplatin.

Clinical evidence, mechanism, importance and management

One of 15 patients given a 1-hour infusion of irinotecan 80 mg/m² following an 2-hour infusion of oxaliplatin 85 mg/m² experienced hypersalivation and abdominal pain, which was treated successfully with atropine. In this patient, symptoms did not recur during subsequent treatment with irinotecan alone, nor when drugs were separated by one day, but rechallenge with the original combined regimen produced cholinergic toxicity.[1] The combination of irinotecan with oxaliplatin did not alter the pharmacokinetics of either drug in one study[2] therefore it was suggested that the observed effects in the patient may have been due to a pharmacodynamic interaction.[3] It has been suggested that the cholinergic effects of irinotecan, which is a potent inhibitor of acetylcholinesterase,[4] may be enhanced by oxaliplatin, which may like other alkylating drugs also inhibit acetylcholinesterase.[3] The clinical relevance of this report is unknown. The combination of irinotecan and oxaliplatin has been extensively evaluated in clinical studies, and this appears to be the only report of this problem. However, it has been noted that the prophylactic use of atropine with irinotecan could mask any increased cholinergic toxicity.[3,5] Further study is needed.

1. Valencak J, Raderer M, Kornek GV, Henja MH, Scheithauer W. Irinotecan-related cholinergic syndrome induced by coadministration of oxaliplatin. *J Natl Cancer Inst* (1998) 90, 160.
2. Wasserman E, Cuvier C, Lokiec F, Goldwasser F, Kalla S, Méry-Mignard D, Ouldkaci M, Besmaine A, Dupont-André G, Mahjoubi M, Marty M, Misset JL, Cvitkovic E. Combination of oxaliplatin plus irinotecan in patients with gastrointestinal tumors: results of two independent phase I studies with pharmacokinetics. *J Clin Oncol* (1999) 17, 1751–9.
3. Dodds HM, Bishop JF, Rivory LP. More about: irinotecan-related cholinergic syndrome induced by coadministration of oxaliplatin. *J Natl Cancer Inst* (1999) 91, 91–2.
4. Dodds HM, Rivory LP. The mechanism of the inhibition of acetylcholinesterase by irinotecan (CPT-11)–a lead in explaining the cholinergic toxicity of CPT-11 and its time-course. *Proc Am Assoc Cancer Res* (1998) 39, 327.
5. Cvitkovic E, Marty M, Wasserman E, Cuvier C, Goldwasser F, Misset JL. Re: irinotecan-related cholinergic syndrome induced by coadministration of oxaliplatin. *J Natl Cancer Inst* (1998) 90, 1016–17.

Irinotecan + Rifampicin (Rifampin)

A single case report found that rifampicin reduced the formation of two active metabolites of irinotecan. The clinical significance of this finding is unclear.

Clinical evidence, mechanism, importance and management

A case report describes a 54-year-old man with small cell lung cancer and *Mycobacterium* infection who was uneventfully treated with rifampicin 450 mg daily, isoniazid, streptomycin and pyrazinamide. After 2 weeks of antimycobacterial treatment he was given irinotecan, 75 mg/m² on days 1 and 8, and cisplatin 60 mg/m² on day 1 for 4 cycles, for one of which rifampicin treatment was interrupted for a 4-day period. There was no difference in the pharmacokinetic profile of irinotecan with or without concurrent rifampicin, but the AUC of two active metabolites of irinotecan were reduced by 20% and 58%.[1]

Further study is required to assess the significance of this finding. Also note that the effects of rifampicin can persist for some time after it is stopped and therefore a 4-day period may not have been sufficient for any effect to become apparent.

1. Yonemori K, Takeda Y, Toyota E, Kobayashi N, Kudo K. Potential interactions between irinotecan and rifampin in a patient with small-cell lung cancer. *Int J Clin Oncol* (2004) 9, 206–9.

Irinotecan + Selenium

Selenium at a dose of 2.2 mg daily does not appear to alter the pharmacokinetics of irinotecan, nor does it attenuate the toxicity of irinotecan.

Clinical evidence, mechanism, importance and management

In a study in 13 patients with metastatic or unresectable solid tumours **selenomethionine**, at a dose of elemental selenium 2.2 mg daily, was given with irinotecan weekly, in escalating doses from 125 mg/m² to 160 mg/m² for 4 weeks of a 6-week cycle. Irinotecan doses above the previously recommended maximum tolerated dose were still considered intolerable, with 3 of 4 patients receiving a dose of 160 mg/m² developing dose-limiting diarrhoea. There were no significant alterations in the pharmacokinetics of irinotecan or its metabolites, SN-38 and SN-38G. It was suggested that higher doses of selenomethionine should be investigated to see if they protect against irinotecan toxicity.[1]

1. Fakih MG, Pendyala L, Smith PF, Creaven PJ, Reid ME, Badmaev V, Azrak RG, Prey JD, Lawrence D, Rustum YM. A phase I and pharmacokinetic study of fixed-dose selenomethionine and irinotecan in solid tumors. *Clin Cancer Res* (2006) 12, 1237–44.

Irinotecan + Sorafenib

Sorafenib might increase levels of irinotecan and its major metabolite.

Clinical evidence, mechanism, importance and management

A study in 3 groups of 6 patients given sorafenib in doses of 200 mg, 400 mg or 800 mg daily, and irinotecan 125 mg/m² as an intravenous infusion found that the pharmacokinetics of irinotecan and its major active metabolite, SN-38, were not affected by sorafenib. In addition, sorafenib pharmacokinetics were not affected by irinotecan.[1]

In contrast, the manufacturers note that when sorafenib was given with irinotecan there was a 26 to 42% increase in the AUC of irinotecan, and a 67 to 120% increase in the AUC of SN-38. They suggest that this occurs because sorafenib inhibits glucuronidation of SN-38. The clinical significance of this finding is unknown, but they recommend caution on concurrent use.[2,3]

1. Mross K, Steinbild S, Baas F, Reil M, Buss P, Mersmann S, Voliotis D, Schwartz B, Brendel E. Drug-drug interaction pharmacokinetic study with the Raf kinase inhibitor (RKI) BAY 43-9006 administered in combination with irinotecan (CPT-11) in patients with solid tumors. *Int J Clin Pharmacol Ther* (2003) 41, 618–19.
2. Nexavar (Sorafenib tosylate). Bayer plc. UK Summary of product characteristics, January 2007.
3. Nexavar (Sorafenib tosylate). Bayer Pharmaceuticals Corp. US Prescribing information, February 2007.

Irinotecan + St John's wort (*Hypericum perforatum*)

St John's wort increases the metabolism of irinotecan, which may decrease its activity.

Clinical evidence

In a randomised, crossover study St John's wort decreased the plasma levels of the active metabolite of irinotecan, SN-38, by 42%. Myelosuppression was also reduced; with irinotecan alone the leucocyte and neutrophil counts decreased by 56% and 63%, respectively, but in the presence of St

John's wort the decreases were only 8.6% and 4.3%, respectively. In this study, irinotecan was given as a single 350-mg/m^2 intravenous dose every 3 weeks, and during one cycle a St John's wort preparation was given three times daily, beginning 14 days before and stopping 4 days after the irinotecan.[1]

Mechanism

St John's wort induces the cytochrome P450 isoenzyme CYP3A4 and P-glycoprotein, which are both involved in the metabolism of irinotecan. The evidence suggests that St John's wort increases the metabolism of irinotecan to an unknown inactive metabolite, rather than the active SN-38, thereby reducing its effects.[1]

Importance and management

The evidence appears to be limited to this study. Irinotecan has a narrow therapeutic range, and the lower levels of SN-38 suggest that its activity will be reduced in the presence of St John's wort. It would therefore seem sensible to warn patients who are about to receive irinotecan to avoid St John's wort. It seems likely that **topotecan**, a related drug that is also a substrate for CYP3A4, will be similarly affected, but evidence for this is currently lacking.

1. Mathijssen RHJ, Verweij J, de Bruijn P, Loos WJ, Sparreboom A. Effects of St John's wort on irinotecan metabolism. *J Natl Cancer Inst* (2002) 94, 1247–9.

Irinotecan + Thalidomide

Thalidomide slightly increases irinotecan levels, but the clinical significance of this is uncertain.

Clinical evidence, mechanism, importance and management

Patients with solid tumours treated with irinotecan 350 mg/m^2 on day 1 of a 3 week cycle were also given thalidomide 400 mg daily from days 1 to 14 of the first cycle. Thalidomide slightly increased the AUC of irinotecan by 21% (not significant) and its SN-38-glucuronide metabolite by 28%, but decreased the AUC of the SN-38 metabolite by 26%. There was no difference in the toxicities seen when irinotecan was given with or without thalidomide.[1] Further study is required in larger groups of patients to establish if these changes in irinotecan pharmacokinetics are clinically relevant.

1. Allegrini G, Di Paolo A, Cerri E, Cupini S, Amatori F, Masi G, Danesi R, Marcucci L, Bocci G, Del Tacca M, Falcone A. Irinotecan in combination with thalidomide in patients with advanced solid tumors: a clinical study with pharmacodynamic and pharmacokinetic evaluation. *Cancer Chemother Pharmacol* (2006) 58, 585–93.

Irinotecan + Tobacco

Retrospective data suggests that tobacco smoking might increase the clearance of irinotecan and reduce its toxicity, and presumably therefore, its efficacy.

Clinical evidence

In a retrospective analysis, the pharmacokinetics of irinotecan were compared between 49 patients who were smokers and 141 who were non-smokers, and who had received intravenous irinotecan 175 to 350 mg/m^2 (or a fixed dose of 600 mg) once every 3 weeks. Clearance of irinotecan was 18% faster in the group of patients who smoked, and these patients also showed more extensive conversion of the active metabolite SN-38 to the inactive glucuronide (SN-38G). Smokers experienced significantly less haematological toxicity than non-smokers (grade 3 to 4 neutropenia 6% versus 38%), possibly as a result of the increased rate of clearance.[1]

Mechanism

Irinotecan is metabolised by the cytochrome P450 CYP3A isoenzymes, which, although not the most commonly implicated isoenzyme in interactions involving tobacco smoking, may be induced by some of the components of tobacco smoke, resulting in increased clearance of irinotecan. In addition, smoking might induce glucuronyltransferases (which are responsible for glucuronidation).[1]

Importance and management

The findings of this retrospective analysis suggest that smoking might reduce the efficacy of irinotecan. However, the evidence is insufficient to make recommendations regarding smoking cessation or an increased irinotecan dose.[1] Further study is required.

1. van der Bol JM, Mathijssen RHJ, Loos WJ, Friberg LE, van Schaik RHN, de Jonge MJA, Planting AST, Verweij J, Sparreboom A, de Jong FA. Cigarette smoking and irinotecan treatment: pharmacokinetic interaction and effects on neutropenia. *J Clin Oncol* (2007) 25. Published ahead of print at http://jco.ascopubs.org/cgi/reprint/JCO.2006.09.6115v1.

Letrozole + Cimetidine

The pharmacokinetics of a single 2.5-mg dose of letrozole were unchanged by cimetidine 400 mg every 12 hours in 17 healthy subjects.[1]

1. Morgan JM, Palmisano M, Spencer S, Hirschhorn W, Piraino AJ, Rackley RJ, Choi L. Pharmacokinetic effect of cimetidine on a single 2.5-mg dose of letrozole in healthy subjects. *J Clin Pharmacol* (1996) 36, 852.

Letrozole + Miscellaneous

The UK manufacturers report that in interaction clinical studies there was no evidence of clinically relevant interactions between letrozole and other commonly prescribed drugs, namely benzodiazepines such as diazepam, barbiturates, diclofenac, furosemide, ibuprofen, omeprazole, and paracetamol (acetaminophen).[1]

1. Femara (Letrozole). Novartis Pharmaceuticals UK Ltd. UK Summary of product characteristics, May 2007.

Melphalan + Cimetidine

Cimetidine modestly reduces the bioavailability of melphalan.

Clinical evidence, mechanism, importance and management

A study in 8 patients with multiple myeloma or monoclonal gammopathy showed that pretreatment with cimetidine 1 g daily for 6 days reduced the bioavailability of a 10-mg oral dose of melphalan by 30%. The melphalan half-life was reduced from 1.94 to 1.57 hours. The interindividual variation in melphalan pharmacokinetics was high.[1] Note that, because of the variability in melphalan absorption, the dose of oral melphalan is usually cautiously increased until myelosuppression is seen, to ensure therapeutic levels. Therefore, this modest interaction with cimetidine is unlikely to have many clinical consequences.

1. Sviland L, Robinson A, Proctor SJ, Bateman DN. Interaction of cimetidine with oral melphalan. *Cancer Chemother Pharmacol* (1987) 20, 173–5.

Melphalan + Food

The absorption of oral melphalan can be reduced by food.

Clinical evidence, mechanism, importance and management

A study in 10 patients with multiple myeloma showed that the half-life of oral melphalan 5 mg/m^2 was unaffected when it was taken with a standardised **breakfast**, but the AUC was reduced by 39%. In one patient, no melphalan was detectable in the plasma when it was given with food. In 8 of the patients who had also been given intravenous melphalan at the same dose, the bioavailability of oral melphalan was calculated to be 85% (range 26% to 96%) when fasting and 58% (7% to 99%) when given with food. The authors recommend that melphalan should not be taken with food.[1] The manufacturer notes that absorption after oral administration is highly variable, and that the dosage should be adjusted based on frequent monitoring of blood counts. They make no specific recommendations about intake in relation to food.[2,3]

1. Reece PA, Kotasek D, Morris RG, Dale BM, Sage RE. The effect of food on oral melphalan absorption. *Cancer Chemother Pharmacol* (1986) 16, 194–7.

2. Alkeran Tablets (Melphalan). GlaxoSmithKline UK. UK Summary of product characteristics, July 2007.
3. Alkeran (Melphalan). GlaxoSmithKline. US Prescribing information, November 2004.

Melphalan + Interferon alfa

Interferon alfa modestly decreases the AUC of melphalan, but melphalan cytotoxicity is possibly increased because of the interferon-induced fever.

Clinical evidence, mechanism, importance and management

In 10 myeloma patients the AUC of melphalan 250 microgram/kg was reduced by 13% when it was given 5 hours after the administration of human interferon alfa (7 x 10^6 units/m^2), possibly due to the fever caused by the interferon.[1] The clinical importance of this is uncertain but the authors of the report suggest that despite this small reduction in the AUC, the cytotoxicity of the melphalan is increased by the fever. The use of interferon alfa with melphalan and prednisone in multiple myeloma has been associated with more adverse effects.[2-4]

1. Ehrsson H, Eksborg S, Wallin I, Österborg A, Mellstedt H. Oral melphalan pharmacokinetics: influence of interferon-induced fever. *Clin Pharmacol Ther* (1990) 47, 86–90.
2. Österborg A, Björkholm M, Björeman M, Brenning G, Carlson K, Celsing F, Gahrton G, Grimfors G, Gyllenhammar J, Hast R. Natural interferon-α in combination with melphalan/prednisone versus melphalan/prednisone in the treatment of multiple myeloma stages II and III: a randomized study from the Myeloma Group of Central Sweden. *Blood* (1993) 81, 1428–34.
3. Cooper MR, Dear K, McIntyre OR, Ozer H, Ellerton J, Canellos G, Bernhardt B, Duggan D, Faragher D, Schiffer C. A randomized clinical trial comparing melphalan/prednisone with or without interferon alfa-2b in newly diagnosed patients with multiple myeloma: a Cancer and Leukemia Group B study. *J Clin Oncol* (1993) 11, 155–60.
4. The Nordic Myeloma Study Group. Interferon-α 2b added to melphalan-prednisone for initial and maintenance therapy in multiple myeloma: a randomized, controlled trial. *Ann Intern Med* (1996) 124, 212–22.

Methotrexate + Amiodarone

An isolated case report tentatively attributes the development of methotrexate toxicity with the concurrent use of amiodarone.

Clinical evidence, mechanism, importance and management

An elderly woman, whose psoriasis was effectively controlled for 2 years with methotrexate, developed ulceration of the psoriatic plaques within 2 weeks of starting treatment with amiodarone. The reason is not understood. A modest increase in her dosage of furosemide is a suggested contributory factor because it might have interfered with the excretion of the methotrexate.[1]

1. Reynolds NJ, Jones SK, Crossley J, Harman RRM. Methotrexate induced skin necrosis: a drug interaction with amiodarone? *BMJ* (1989) 299, 980–1.

Methotrexate + Amphotericin B

Amphotericin B may delay the clearance of methotrexate.

Clinical evidence, mechanism, importance and management

Two children had delayed clearance of pulse methotrexate (1 g/m^2 over 24 hours) while they were receiving amphotericin B. Methotrexate levels were about 300 to 500% higher 48 hours after methotrexate when they were receiving amphotericin B, compared with methotrexate alone.[1] In a study, methotrexate clearance in 18 children given high-dose methotrexate (1 g/m^2 intravenously) was significantly correlated with the glomerular filtration rate (GFR). Concurrent amphotericin B in 6 of the children significantly decreased the GFR.[2] A history of heavy amphotericin B treatment (greater than 30 mg/kg) correlated with decreased methotrexate clearance in 24 children with relapsed leukaemia.[3] Amphotericin B may cause renal impairment, which can result in delayed methotrexate clearance. The adverse effects of methotrexate should be carefully monitored (e.g. patient reported symptoms, LFTs, blood counts) in patients taking amphotericin B or those previously extensively treated with the drug. In patients taking large doses of methotrexate (e.g. not the weekly doses given for conditions such as rheumatoid arthritis) the monitoring of methotrexate levels is recommended.

1. Parker RI, Mahan RM, Giugliano DA. Delayed methotrexate clearance during treatment with amphotericin B. *Pediatr Res* (2002) 51 (4 part 2), 258A.
2. Murry DJ, Synold TW, Pui C-H, Rodman JH. Renal function and methotrexate clearance in children with newly diagnosed leukemia. *Pharmacotherapy* (1995) 15, 144–9.
3. Wall AM, Gajjar A, Link A, Mahmoud H, Pui C-H, Relling MV. Individualized methotrexate dosing in children with relapsed acute lymphoblastic leukemia. *Leukemia* (2000) 14, 221–5.

Methotrexate + Antibacterials; Aminoglycosides, oral

There is evidence that the gastrointestinal absorption of methotrexate can be reduced by paromomycin, neomycin and possibly other oral aminoglycosides, but increased by kanamycin.

Clinical evidence

A study in 10 patients with small cell bronchogenic carcinoma taking methotrexate found that when they were also given a range of oral anti-infectives (**paromomycin**, vancomycin, polymyxin B, nystatin) the urinary recovery of methotrexate was reduced by over one-third (from 69% to 44%).[1] The **paromomycin** was believed to have been responsible. In another study the concurrent use of **neomycin** 500 mg four times a day for 3 days reduced the methotrexate AUC and the 72-hour cumulative excretion by 50%.[2] In contrast, the same report suggests that **kanamycin** can increase the absorption of methotrexate, but no details are given.

Mechanism

Oral aminoglycosides reduce the activity of the gut flora, which metabolise methotrexate so that more is available for absorption. However, paromomycin[3] and neomycin, in common with other oral aminoglycosides, can cause a malabsorption syndrome, which reduces drug absorption and presumably negates any effect altering the gut flora has. Kanamycin may possibly be different because it causes less malabsorption.

Importance and management

The documentation of these interactions is sparse, but it would seem prudent to be on the alert for a reduction in the response to methotrexate if patients are given oral aminoglycosides such as paromomycin or neomycin. An increased response may possibly occur with kanamycin. No interaction would be expected if aminoglycosides are given parenterally.

1. Cohen MH, Creaven PJ, Fossieck BE, Johnston AV, Williams CL. Effect of oral prophylactic broad spectrum nonabsorbable antibiotics on the gastrointestinal absorption of nutrients and methotrexate in small cell bronchogenic carcinoma patients. *Cancer* (1976) 38, 1556–9.
2. Shen DD, Azarnoff D. Clinical pharmacokinetics of methotrexate. *Clin Pharmacokinet* (1978) 3, 1–13.
3. Keusch GT, Troncale FJ, Buchanan RD. Malabsorption due to paromomycin. *Arch Intern Med* (1970) 125, 273–6.

Methotrexate + Antibacterials; Cefotiam

Pancytopenia and pseudomembraneous colitis occurred when a patient treated with low-dose methotrexate and loxoprofen was given cefotiam.

Clinical evidence, mechanism, importance and management

An elderly woman who had been treated with low-dose methotrexate 5 mg weekly and loxoprofen for one month developed acute pyelonephritis. Intravenous cefotiam was started, and on day 7 she developed severe watery diarrhoea. Analysis showed pancytopenia and *Clostridium difficile* infection. Methotrexate and cefotiam were stopped, and vancomycin started, and the patient recovered.[1] It was suggested that the combination of the antineoplastic drug and antibacterial increased the risk of *Clostridium difficile* diarrhoea. In addition, the NSAID (see 'Methotrexate + NSAIDs', p.649) and renal impairment from the pyelonephritis could have contributed to the methotrexate toxicity.[1] This appears to be an isolated case, and any interaction with cefotiam is not established.

1. Nanke Y, Kotake S, Akama H, Tomii M, Kamatani N. Pancytopenia and colitis with *Clostridium difficile* in a rheumatoid arthritis patient taking methotrexate, antibiotics and non-steroidal anti-inflammatory drugs. *Clin Rheumatol* (2001) 20, 73–5.

Methotrexate + Antibacterials; Ciprofloxacin

A report describes two patients who developed methotrexate toxicity when they were given ciprofloxacin.

Clinical evidence

When 2 patients with osteosarcoma, treated with high-dose methotrexate 12 g/m^2 per course, were given ciprofloxacin 500 mg twice daily, either during or 2 days before the start of the methotrexate course, methotrexate elimination was delayed, resulting in raised serum levels, severe cutaneous toxicity and renal impairment. The first patient also had hepatic injury and haematological toxicity. Following increased folinic acid rescue, methotrexate levels normalised after several days. In earlier courses without ciprofloxacin in the first patient and subsequent courses without ciprofloxacin in the second patient, methotrexate elimination was normal.[1] This preliminary report[1] has subsequently been published in full.[2,3]

Mechanism

Not fully understood. Ciprofloxacin may displace methotrexate from its plasma-protein binding sites resulting in a rise in levels of unbound methotrexate. Ciprofloxacin may also cause a decrease in renal clearance of methotrexate.

Importance and management

Information appears to be limited to one report, but it would seem prudent to monitor for raised methotrexate levels if concurrent use is necessary. More study is needed.

1. Dalle JH, Auvrignon A, Vassal G, Leverger G. Possible ciprofloxacin-methotrexate interaction: a report of 2 cases. *Intersci Conf Antimicrob Agents Chemother* (2000) 40, 477.
2. Dalle JH, Auvrignon A, Vassal G, Leverger G, Kalifa C. Interaction méthotrexate–ciprofloxacine: à propos de deux cas d'intoxication sévère. *Arch Pediatr* (2001) 8, 1078–81.
3. Dalle J-H, Auvrignon A, Vassal G, Leverger G. Interaction between methotrexate and ciprofloxacin. *J Pediatr Hematol Oncol* (2002) 24, 321–2.

Methotrexate + Antibacterials; Co-trimoxazole or Trimethoprim

Eleven cases of severe bone marrow depression have been reported, three of them fatal, caused by the concurrent use of low-dose methotrexate and treatment doses of trimethoprim or co-trimoxazole (sulfamethoxazole and trimethoprim). Pancytopenia has also been reported in a few patients given treatment doses of co-trimoxazole shortly after stopping methotrexate.

Clinical evidence

A 61-year-old patient with rheumatoid arthritis, taking methotrexate 7.5 mg weekly, developed generalised bone marrow hypoplasia over 2 months after a 10-day course of treatment with co-trimoxazole for a urinary tract infection. She had taken a total of 775 mg of methotrexate when the hypoplasia appeared.[1] Eleven other cases of severe bone marrow depression, three of them fatal,[2,3] have been described in patients taking low-dose weekly methotrexate with given co-trimoxazole[2,4-8] or trimethoprim.[3,6,9,10] Life-threatening complications (no details given) are said to have occurred in two other patients taking low-dose methotrexate with **unnamed sulfonamides**.[11] A 10-year (1981 to 1991) regional survey in Ottawa identified co-trimoxazole as one of four factors associated with serious pancytopenia in patients taking low-dose methotrexate. The other factors were elevated BUN or creatinine levels, increased mean corpuscular volumes and increasing age.[12]

Three cases of severe pancytopenia, one of them fatal, have been reported in patients given treatment dose co-trimoxazole for pneumocystis pneumonia shortly after stopping low-dose methotrexate therapy.[13-15] A fatal case of severe agranulocytosis and toxic epidermal necrolysis occurred in a patient receiving co-trimoxazole for prophylaxis of pneumocystis pneumonia after high-dose methotrexate therapy.[16]

Mechanism

Not fully understood. Both drugs can suppress the activity of dihydrofolate reductase and it seems possible that they can act additively to produce folate deficiency, which could lead to some of the bone marrow changes seen. There may also be a pharmacokinetic mechanism. An early study found that the concurrent use of co-trimoxazole had no effect on the pharmacokinetics of methotrexate in children;[17] however, another study reported that co-trimoxazole caused an increase in 'free' methotrexate from about 37% to 52% while the renal clearance was more than halved.[18] This was calculated to increase the exposure to methotrexate by 66%.[18] Another sulfonamide, **sulfafurazole** (sulfisoxazole),[19] has been found to cause a small reduction in the clearance of methotrexate by the kidneys.

Importance and management

Information seems to be limited to the reports cited but the interactions between methotrexate and co-trimoxazole or trimethoprim are established. Low-dose co-trimoxazole is commonly given to patients taking methotrexate as prophylaxis of pneumocystis pneumonia without problem. This type of patient should be having regular blood monitoring as a matter of course. However, the situation with higher doses of either drug is potentially more hazardous. Some have recommended avoiding the combination. If both drugs must be used, the haematological picture should be very closely monitored because the outcome can be life-threatening.

1. Thomas MH, Gutterman LA. Methotrexate toxicity in a patient receiving trimethoprim-sulfamethoxazole. *J Rheumatol* (1986) 13, 440–1.
2. Groenendal H, Rampen FHJ. Methotrexate and trimethoprim-sulphamethoxazole — a potentially hazardous combination. *Clin Exp Dermatol* (1990) 15, 358–60.
3. Steuer A, Gumpel JM. Methotrexate and trimethoprim: a fatal interaction. *Br J Rheumatol* (1998) 37, 105–6.
4. Thevenet JP, Ristori JM, Cure H, Mizony MH, Bussiere JL. Pancytopénie au cours due traitement d'une polyarthrite rheumatoïde par méthotrexate après administration de triméthoprime-sulfaméthoxazole. *Presse Med* (1987) 16, 1487.
5. Maricic M, Davis M, Gall EP. Megaloblastic pancytopenia in a patient receiving concurrent methotrexate and trimethoprim-sulphamethoxazole treatment. *Arthritis Rheum* (1986) 29, 133–5.
6. Jeurissen ME, Boerbooms AM, van de Putte LB. Pancytopenia and methotrexate with trimethoprim-sulfamethoxazole. *Ann Intern Med* (1989) 111, 261.
7. Liddle BJ, Marsden JR. Drug interactions with methotrexate. *Br J Dermatol* (1989) 120, 582–3.
8. Govert JA, Patton S, Fine RL. Pancytopenia from using trimethoprim and methotrexate. *Ann Intern Med* (1992) 117, 877–8.
9. Ng HWK, Macfarlane AW, Graham RM, Verbov JL. Near fatal drug interactions with methotrexate given for psoriasis. *BMJ* (1987) 295, 752–3.
10. Saravana S, Lalukotta K. Myelotoxicity due to methotrexate—an iatrogenic cause. *Eur J Haematol* (2003) 71, 315–16.
11. Zachariae H. Methotrexate and non-steroidal anti-inflammatory drugs. *Br J Dermatol* (1992) 126, 95.
12. Al-Awadhi A, Dale P, McKendry RJR. Pancytopenia associated with low dose methotrexate therapy. A regional survey. *J Rheumatol* (1993) 20, 1121–5.
13. Dan M, Shapira I. Possible role of methotrexate in trimethoprim- sulfamethoxazole-induced acute megaloblastic anemia. *Isr J Med Sci* (1984) 20, 262–3.
14. Kobrinsky NL, Ramsay NKC. Acute megaloblastic anemia induced by high-dose trimethoprim-sulfamethoxazole. *Ann Intern Med* (1981) 94, 780–1.
15. Chevrel G, Brantus JF, Sainte-Laudy, Miossec P. Allergic pancytopenia to trimethoprim-sulphamethoxazole for *Pneumocystis carinii* pneumonia following methotrexate treatment for rheumatoid arthritis. *Rheumatology (Oxford)* (1999) 38, 475–6.
16. Yang CH, Yang LJ, Jaing TH, Chan HL. Toxic epidermal necrolysis following combination of methotrexate and trimethoprim-sulfamethoxazole. *Int J Dermatol* (2000) 39, 621–3.
17. Beach BJ, Woods WG, Howell SB. Influence of co-trimoxazole on methotrexate pharmacokinetics in children with acute lymphoblastic leukemia. *Am J Pediatr Hematol Oncol* (1981) 3, 115–19.
18. Ferrazzini G, Klein J, Sulh H, Chung D, Griesbrecht E, Koren G. Interaction between trimethoprim-sulfamethoxazole and methotrexate in children with leukemia. *J Pediatr* (1990) 117, 823–6.
19. Liegler DG, Henderson ES, Hahn MA, Oliverio VT. The effect of organic acids on renal clearance of methotrexate in man. *Clin Pharmacol Ther* (1969) 10, 849–57.

Methotrexate + Antibacterials; Penicillins

Reduced clearance and acute methotrexate toxicity has been attributed to the concurrent use of various penicillins (amoxicillin, benzylpenicillin, carbenicillin, dicloxacillin, flucloxacillin, mezlocillin, oxacillin, penicillin, phenoxymethylpenicillin, piperacillin, ticarcillin) in a small number of case reports.

Clinical evidence

Reduced methotrexate clearance and acute methotrexate toxicity has been attributed to the concurrent use of various penicillins in a number of patients. See 'Table 17.2', (p.644) for details.

A survey of the Wyeth/Lederle safety database in 1996 identified two additional unpublished cases of methotrexate toxicity (aplastic anaemia, thrombocytopenia, pneumonitis) in patients who had recently started penicillins.[1]

Table 17.2 Reports of reduced methotrexate clearance during penicillin use

Methotrexate	*Penicillin (dose)*	*Indication (number of patients)*	*Outcome*	*Refs*
High-dose regimen (with folinic acid rescue)				
Intravenous infusion 8 g/m^2 over 6 hours	Amoxicillin (1 g every 6 hours orally)	Osteogenic sarcoma (1)	56% reduction in methotrexate clearance; prolonged and marked enhancement of methotrexate plasma levels; acute and subacute methotrexate toxicity	1
Intravenous infusion 6 g/m^2 (10.8 g) over one hour, then 1.2 g/m^2 per hour for 23 hours	Carbenicillin (30 g daily)	Acute lymphoblastic leukaemia (1)	Elevated plasma methotrexate levels and decreased methotrexate clearance	2
Intravenous bolus 15 to 60 mg/m^2, then 15 to 60 mg/m^2 intravenous infusion over 36 hours	Dicloxacillin (not stated) (Indometacin also given)	Oesophageal cancer (1)	93% reduction in methotrexate clearance; prolonged folinic acid rescue necessary	3
Intravenous infusion 12 g/m^2 over 4 hours	Mezlocillin (330 mg/kg daily)	Osteogenic sarcoma (1)	Reduced methotrexate clearance; increased gastrointestinal toxicity	4
Intravenous infusion 15 g over 6 hours	Oxacillin (1 g every 8 hours starting 6 hours after methotrexate infusion)	Osteogenic sarcoma (1)	Plasma methotrexate levels 53-fold higher than in previous cycles without oxacillin; fatal acute toxicity (renal failure and aplastic anaemia)	5
Intravenous bolus 15 to 60 mg/m^2, then 15 to 60 mg/m^2 intravenous infusion over 36 hours	Penicillin [sic] (not stated)	Breast cancer (1)	36% reduction in methotrexate clearance; prolonged folinic acid rescue necessary	3
Intravenous bolus 15 to 60 mg/m^2, then 15 to 60 mg/m^2 intravenous infusion over 36 hours	Piperacillin (not stated)	Chronic Myeloid Leukaemia (1)	67% reduction in methotrexate clearance; prolonged folinic acid rescue necessary	3
Intravenous infusion 3 g/m^2 over 6 hours	Piperacillin (1 g every 6 hours intravenously)	Non-Hodgkin's lymphoma (1)	Reduced methotrexate clearance	6
Intravenous bolus 15 to 60 mg/m^2, then 15 to 60 mg/m^2 intravenous infusion over 36 hours	Ticarcillin (not stated)	Acute Myeloid Leukaemia (1)	60% reduction in methotrexate clearance; prolonged folinic acid rescue necessary	3
Low-dose regimen				
7.5 mg weekly	Amoxicillin 500 mg orally three times daily for 7 days; from day 17, intravenous flucloxacillin 2 g every 4 hours, plus intravenous benzylpenicillin 2 million units every 4 hours	Rheumatoid arthritis	Neutropenia and thrombocytopenia probably as a result of reduced methotrexate clearance; folinic acid given, but patient died	7
7.5 mg weekly orally	Co-amoxiclav (amoxicillin + clavulanic acid)	Psoriasis (1)	Neutropenia and thrombocytopenia, probably as a result of reduced methotrexate clearance	7
5 mg weekly orally	Flucloxacillin (4 g four times daily, intravenously then orally)	Rheumatoid arthritis (1)	Suspected methotrexate-induced pneumonitis	8
5 to 15 mg weekly orally	Flucloxacillin (500 mg four times daily orally)	Rheumatoid arthritis (10, and 10 not given flucloxacillin)	No significant effect on methotrexate pharmacokinetics	8
2.5 mg three times each week orally	Flucloxacillin (1 g every 6 hours intravenously) plus piperacillin (2 g every 6 hours intravenously)	Psoriasis (1)	Neutropenia and thrombocytopenia, probably as a result of reduced methotrexate clearance; folinic acid given, but patient died	7
5 mg twice weekly orally	Piperacillin (intravenous; dose not stated)	Psoriasis (1)	Neutropenia and thrombocytopenia, probably as a result of reduced methotrexate clearance; folinic acid given, but patient died	7
Other regimen				
Intravenous 50 mg weekly	Phenoxymethylpenicillin 250 mg on alternate days	Dermatomyositis (also treated with prednisone; and prostatic cancer treated with diethylstilbestrol (stilboestrol); also treated with furosemide)	Methotrexate toxicity within week of starting phenoxymethylpenicillin; treated with folinic acid and fluid replacement (and nafcillin and tobramycin)	9

1. Ronchera CL, Hernández T, Peris JE, Torres F, Granero L, Jiménez NV, Plá JM. Pharmacokinetic interaction between high-dose methotrexate and amoxycillin. *Ther Drug Monit* (1993) 15, 375–9.
2. Gibson DL, Bleyer AW, Savitch JL. Carbenicillin potentiation of methotrexate plasma concentration during high dose methotrexate therapy. American Society of Hospital Pharmacists. Mid year clinical meeting abstracts, New Orleans, Dec 1981. p. 111.

Continued

Table 17.2 Reports of reduced methotrexate clearance during penicillin use (continued)

3. Bloom EJ, Ignoffo RJ, Reis CA, Cadman E. Delayed clearance (CL) of methotrexate (MTX) associated with antibiotics and anti-inflammatory agents. *Clin Res* (1986) 34, 560A.
4. Dean R, Nachman J, Lorenzana AN. Possible methotrexate-mezlocillin interaction. *Am J Pediatr Hematol Oncol* (1992) 14, 88–9.
5. Titier K, Lagrange F, Péhourcq F, Moore N, Molimard M. Pharmacokinetic interaction between high-dose methotrexate and oxacillin. *Ther Drug Monit* (2002) 24, 570–2.
6. Yamamoto K, Sawada Y, Matsushita U, Moriwaki K, Bessho F, Iga T. Delayed elimination of methotrexate associated with piperacillin administration. *Ann Pharmacother* (1997) 31, 1261–2.
7. Mayall B, Poggi G, Parkin JD. Neutropenia due to low-dose methotrexate therapy for psoriasis and rheumatoid arthritis may be fatal. *Med J Aust* (1991) 155, 480–4.
8. Herrick AL, Grennan DM, Griffen K, Aarons L, Gifford LA. Lack of interaction between flucloxacillin and methotrexate in patients with rheumatoid arthritis. *Br J Clin Pharmacol* (1996) 41, 223–7.
9. Nierenberg DW, Mamelok RD. Toxic reaction to methotrexate in a patient receiving penicillin and furosemide: a possible interaction. *Arch Dermatol* (1983) 119, 449–50.

Mechanism

It is thought that weak acids such as the penicillins can possibly successfully compete with methotrexate in the kidney tubules for excretion so that the methotrexate is retained, thereby increasing its effects and its toxicity.[2] However, this was not demonstrated in a study with flucloxacillin,[3] and the mechanism has been disputed.[4]

Importance and management

Information seems to be limited to the reports given here, which would seem to indicate that serious interactions between methotrexate and penicillins are uncommon. It is not known why only a few patients have been affected and what other factors may have contributed, but the problem does not seem to be confined to patients receiving high-dose methotrexate. There is not enough evidence to forbid concurrent use (although some do advise against it[5]), but close monitoring is obviously advisable. One published recommendation is to carry out twice-weekly platelet and white cell counts for 2 weeks initially, with the measurement of methotrexate levels if toxicity is suspected. Folinic acid (leucovorin) rescue should be available.[6] For the general guidelines given by the CSM in the UK on the use of methotrexate see *Importance and management* in 'Methotrexate + NSAIDs', p.649.

1. Wyeth/Lederle. Personal communication, July 1996.
2. Iven H, Brasch H. Influence of the antibiotics piperacillin, doxycycline, and tobramycin on the pharmacokinetics of methotrexate in rabbits. *Cancer Chemother Pharmacol* (1986) 17, 218–22.
3. Herrick AL, Grennan DM, Giriffen K, Aarons L, Gifford LA. Lack of interaction between flucloxacillin and methotrexate in patients with rheumatoid arthritis. *Br J Clin Pharmacol* (1996) 41, 223–7.
4. Herrick AL, Grennan DM, Aarons L. Lack of interaction between methotrexate and penicillins. *Rheumatology (Oxford)* (1999) 38, 284–5.
5. Dawson JK, Abernethy VE, Lynch MP. Methotrexate and penicillin interaction. *Br J Rheumatol* (1998) 37, 807.
6. Mayall B, Poggi G, Parkin JD. Neutropenia due to low-dose methotrexate therapy for psoriasis and rheumatoid arthritis may be fatal. *Med J Aust* (1991) 155, 480–4.

Methotrexate + Antibacterials; Pristinamycin

An isolated report describes severe methotrexate toxicity when a patient was also given pristinamycin.

Clinical evidence

A 13-year-old boy with acute lymphoblastic leukaemia had a relapse and began a series of regimens with high-dose methotrexate in combination with other drugs, including dexamethasone, mercaptopurine, vincristine, cytarabine and asparaginase, tioguanine and ifosfamide. During a late cycle when he was also taking pristinamycin 2 g daily for a staphylococcal infection, the clearance of methotrexate was markedly decreased (half-life prolonged from 6 to 203 hours). He developed severe methotrexate toxicity (oral mucositis, anusitis, balanitis, neutropenia and thrombocytopenia) and was given folinic acid rescue and haemodialysis.[1]

Mechanism

Not understood, but on the basis of experimental evidence the authors of the report excluded the possibilities of kidney impairment or reduction by the pristinamycin of liver metabolism.[1]

Importance and management

This appears to be the first and only report of an interaction between methotrexate and pristinamycin. Its general importance is unknown but the authors strongly advise the avoidance of pristinamycin in patients taking methotrexate.[1]

1. Thyss A, Milano G, Renée N, Cassuto-Viguier E, Jambou P, Soler C. Severe interaction between methotrexate and a macrolide-like antibiotic. *J Natl Cancer Inst* (1993) 85, 582–3.

Methotrexate + Antibacterials; Tetracyclines

Two case reports describe the development of methotrexate toxicity in patients also given tetracycline or doxycycline.

Clinical evidence, mechanism, importance and management

A man being successfully and uneventfully treated for psoriasis with methotrexate 25 mg weekly was also given **tetracycline** 500 mg four times daily for a mycoplasmal infection. Within 5 days he developed recurrent fever, ulcerative stomatitis and diarrhoea. His white cell count fell to 1000 and his platelet count to 30 000 (units not stated, previous counts not given), all signs of methotrexate toxicity. The problem resolved when the methotrexate was withdrawn, but the psoriasis returned.[1] A 17-year-old girl with osteosarcoma of the femur was given **doxycycline** 100 mg every 12 hours for an abscess in her left eye at the same time as her eleventh cycle of high-dose methotrexate with folinic acid rescue. Elevated plasma methotrexate levels were observed and she developed haematological toxicity and severe vomiting, requiring antiemetics, continued folinic acid, a prolonged stay in hospital and postponement of her next dose of methotrexate. **Doxycycline** had not been taken during the first 10 cycles of methotrexate and the pharmacokinetic changes and symptoms seen in the eleventh cycle were attributed to the concurrent use of **doxycycline**.[2] This interaction has also been observed in *mice,*[3] but not *rabbits.*[4] Displacement of the methotrexate from its binding sites may be part of the explanation. There appears to be the only two clinical reports of this interaction on record. Concurrent use need not be avoided, but it should be well monitored.

1. Turck M. Successful psoriasis treatment then sudden 'cytotoxicity'. *Hosp Pract* (1984) 19, 175–6.
2. Tortajada-Ituren JJ, Ordovás-Baines JP, Llopis-Salvia P, Jiménez-Torres NV. High-dose methotrexate-doxycycline interaction. *Ann Pharmacother* (1999) 33, 804–8.
3. Dixon RL. The interaction between various drugs and methotrexate. *Toxicol Appl Pharmacol* (1968) 12, 308.
4. Iven H, Brasch H. Influence of the antibiotics piperacillin, doxycycline, and tobramycin on the pharmacokinetics of methotrexate in rabbits. *Cancer Chemother Pharmacol* (1986) 17, 218–22.

Methotrexate + Antibacterials; Vancomycin

Delayed excretion and toxicity was seen when high-dose methotrexate was given to two patients recently treated with vancomycin. No significant interaction was found in eight other patients.

Clinical evidence, mechanism, importance and management

Two patients treated with a chemotherapy regimen containing high-dose methotrexate, cisplatin, doxorubicin and ifosfamide had delayed methotrexate excretion and methotrexate toxicity during a cycle soon after they had received vancomycin. Methotrexate levels took 170 to 231 hours to fall to 200 micromol/mL, and toxicity (mucositis) occurred. Subclinical renal impairment was found, which subsequently improved. In previous and subsequent cycles, where vancomycin was not given, serum methotrexate levels in both patients fell to 200 micromol/mL within 48 to 96 hours.[1] It was suggested that vancomycin caused subclinical nephrotoxicity, which resulted in delayed excretion of methotrexate, which is primarily renally excreted.[1]

However, in another report of 8 patients who had received high-dose methotrexate following the use of vancomycin (all but one within 10 days) for previous neutropenia, there was no significant interaction in the absence of overt renal impairment. It was suggested that the difference in outcome may be due to slightly lower methotrexate doses and the fact that the drug regimen in the 8 patients did not include ifosfamide, which particularly in combination with cisplatin may cause cumulative renal tubular damage.[2]

Vancomycin is commonly used in oncology patients with febrile neutropenia, and this appears to be the first report of this interaction. The authors of this report[1] suggest that it would be prudent to measure glomerular filtration rate with an EDTA renal scan before giving high-dose methotrexate to patients recently treated with vancomycin, to allow modification of the methotrexate dose if necessary.[1] However, the authors of the second report disagree and suggest such monitoring cannot be supported by their findings.[2] Further study is needed.

1. Blum R, Seymour JF, Toner G. Significant impairment of high-dose methotrexate clearance following vancomycin administration in the absence of overt renal impairment. *Ann Oncol* (2002) 13, 327–30.

2. Shamash J, Joel S, Lundholm L, Millard L, Oliver T. High-dose methotrexate clearance following prior vancomycin administration: no significant interaction in the absence of overt renal impairment. *Ann Oncol* (2003) 14, 169–70.

Methotrexate + Antiepileptics

Enzyme-inducing antiepileptics appear to increase the clearance of methotrexate given as a 24-hour infusion, and their use is associated with lower efficacy of combination therapy for B-lineage leukaemia.

Clinical evidence, mechanism, importance and management

In a retrospective survey, long-term antiepileptic use (**phenytoin, phenobarbital, carbamazepine**, or a combination) was associated with worse event-free survival, and greater haematological relapse and CNS relapse in children receiving chemotherapy for B-lineage acute lymphoblastic leukaemia. Faster clearance of high-dose methotrexate given as a 24-hour infusion was found in those receiving these enzyme-inducing antiepileptics, but clearance of short 4 to 6-hour methotrexate infusions did not appear to be affected, neither was weekly low-dose methotrexate.[1] Further study is needed.

Note that reduced phenytoin and carbamazepine levels, but unaltered phenobarbital levels, have been reported in various case reports of patients receiving chemotherapy including methotrexate, see 'Table 14.1', (p.519).

1. Relling MV, Pui C-H, Sandlund JT, Rivera GK, Hancock ML, Boyett JM, Schuetz EG, Evans WE. Adverse effect of anticonvulsants on efficacy of chemotherapy for acute lymphoblastic leukaemia. *Lancet* (2000) 356, 285–90.

Methotrexate + Ascorbic acid (Vitamin C)

A study in a single patient showed that the urinary excretion of methotrexate was not significantly changed by the concurrent use of large amounts of vitamin C.

Clinical evidence, mechanism, importance and management

Vitamin C 1 g three times daily was found to have no effect on the urinary excretion of methotrexate 45 mg given intravenously to a woman with breast cancer, despite the urine becoming more acidic at pH 5.9 (compare 'Methotrexate + Urinary alkalinisers', p.654). She was also receiving oral cyclophosphamide, propranolol, amitriptyline, perphenazine and prochlorperazine.[1] No special precautions appear to be necessary.

1. Sketris IS, Farmer PS, Fraser A. Effect of vitamin C on the excretion of methotrexate. *Cancer Treat Rep* (1984) 68, 446–7.

Methotrexate + Caffeine

Although caffeine may theoretically reduce the efficacy of methotrexate, the clinical significance of a high caffeine intake is unclear.

Clinical evidence

A study in 39 patients who had recently started treatment with methotrexate 7.5 mg weekly found that patients with a self reported high caffeine intake (more than 180 mg caffeine per day, 13 patients) had less relief in their symptoms of rheumatoid arthritis, such as swollen joints and joint pain, and smaller reductions from baseline in their erythrocyte sedimentation rate (ESR), a marker for inflammation, than patients with a low caffeine intake (less than 120 mg caffeine per day, 13 patients).[1] A survey of 91 patients taking methotrexate 5 to 15 mg weekly for rheumatoid arthritis found that those who were regular coffee drinkers (more than 7 cups a week) had a higher rate of methotrexate discontinuation (due to treatment failure in 80% of cases).[2]

In contrast, an analysis of data in 264 patients taking long-term methotrexate for rheumatoid arthritis found that the consumption of caffeinated beverages did not appear to affect the efficacy of methotrexate for rheumatoid arthritis in either low, moderate or high consumers of caffeinated drinks. The average dose of methotrexate was 16 mg weekly and the average intake of caffeine from caffeinated drinks was 212 mg daily. No difference in inflammatory markers or worsening of rheumatoid arthritis was found between the low-caffeine intake group and the high-caffeine intake group.[3] A survey in 64 patients taking methotrexate (mean dose of 13 mg weekly) for psoriasis and psoriatic arthritis found no effect on the efficacy or dosage requirements of methotrexate between low caffeine intake (less than 120 mg daily) and high caffeine intake (more than 180 mg daily).[4]

Mechanism

It is not known exactly how methotrexate produces its effects in rheumatoid arthritis, but one theory is that it possibly increases levels of adenosine by blocking a step in purine biosynthesis, leading to accumulation of adenosine, which results in anti-inflammatory effects.[1] It also inhibits the enzyme 5-aminoimidazole-4-carboxamide ribonucleotide (AICAR) transformylase, raising levels of AICAR, which in turn increases adenosine levels. It may also contribute to the phosphorylation of adenosine nucleotides creating an accumulation of adenosine in tissues.[1,3] Caffeine is an adenosine receptor antagonist and therefore could reverse the effects of methotrexate.

Importance and management

There is limited information available regarding a potential interaction between caffeine consumption and methotrexate. The data collection results and patient survey seem to indicate that caffeine intake is not an issue, even with a high intake, although one study and another survey did find a reduced efficacy in those with a higher caffeine intake. However, these results, particularly the surveys, were limited by a number of factors, including subjective reporting of caffeine consumption, lack of caffeine blood levels, and uncontrolled ingestion of both drugs. One UK manufacturer of intravenous methotrexate (licenced for rheumatoid arthritis) recommends avoiding the excessive consumption of caffeine and theophylline-containing drinks.[5] There do not appear to be any case reports or studies indicating treatment failure with a high caffeine intake in patients receiving chemotherapy with high-dose methotrexate. More study is needed but bear in mind that a high caffeine intake may be a factor in a reduced benefit from methotrexate given for psoriasis or rheumatoid arthritis.

1. Nesher G, Mates M, Zevin S. Effect of caffeine consumption on efficacy of methotrexate in rheumatoid arthritis. *Arthritis Rheum* (2003) 48, 571–2.

2. Silke C, Murphy MS, Buckley T, Busteed S, Molloy MG, Phelan M. The effect of caffeine ingestion on the efficacy of methotrexate. *Rheumatology (Oxford)* (2001) 40, 34.

3. Benito-Garcia E, Heller JE, Chibnik LB, Maher NE, Matthews HM, Bilics JA, Weinblatt ME, Shadick NA. Dietary caffeine intake does not affect methotrexate efficacy in patients with rheumatoid arthritis. *J Rheumatol* (2006) 33, 1275–81.

4. Swanson DL, Barnes SA, Mengden Koon SJ, el-Azhary RA. Caffeine consumption and methotrexate dosing requirement in psoriasis and psoriatic arthritis. *Int J Dermatol* (2007) 46, 157–9.

5. Metoject (Methotrexate). Medac GmbH. UK Summary of product characteristics, July 2006.

Methotrexate + Chloroquine or Hydroxychloroquine

Chloroquine caused a moderate reduction in the AUC of methotrexate in one study. Conversely, hydroxychloroquine caused a minor increase in the AUC of methotrexate in another study.

Clinical evidence, mechanism, importance and management

Eleven patients with rheumatoid arthritis taking methotrexate 15 mg weekly were studied after they took a single dose of methotrexate alone and after they took methotrexate with chloroquine 250 mg. The chloroquine reduced the maximum plasma levels of methotrexate by 20% and its AUC by 28%. It is suggested that this occurs because the absorption of the methotrexate from the gut is reduced in some way.[1] These reductions are only modest, but they may reduce both the toxicity and the efficacy of the methotrexate: the clinical importance of this interaction awaits assessment.

In contrast, in a randomised crossover study in 10 healthy subjects, hydroxychloroquine 200 mg *increased* the AUC of methotrexate 15 mg by 52%, while still slightly decreasing the maximum methotrexate level (by 17%),.[2] The authors considered that the increased AUC could explain the increased efficacy of the combination in rheumatoid arthritis, while the decreased maximum level could explain the reduction in acute liver toxicity.[2] Further study is needed.

1. Seideman P, Albertioni F, Beck O, Eksborg S, Peterson C. Chloroquine reduces the bioavailability of methotrexate in patients with rheumatoid arthritis. A possible mechanism of reduced hepatotoxicity. *Arthritis Rheum* (1994) 37, 830–3.
2. Carmichael SJ, Beal J, Day RO, Tett SE. Combination therapy with methotrexate and hydroxychloroquine for rheumatoid arthritis increases exposure to methotrexate. *J Rheumatol* (2002) 29, 2077–83.

Methotrexate + Cisplatin

The risk of methotrexate toxicity appears to be markedly increased by the previous use of cisplatin. Methotrexate may inhibit the clearance of cisplatin.

Clinical evidence, mechanism, importance and management

Six out of 106 patients developed clinical signs of methotrexate toxicity and died 6 to 13 days after receiving standard doses of methotrexate (20 to 50 mg/m^2) in the absence of signs of renal impairment, and despite having previously been given methotrexate without serious toxicity. On this occasion all had previously been given cisplatin. Four of the patients were regarded as good-risk (i.e. methotrexate toxicity was not considered likely as they did not have renal or hepatic impairment, and their general condition was good).[1] A study in children and adolescents suggested that those who had received a cumulative dose of cisplatin greater than 360 mg/m^2 had delayed methotrexate clearance and a greater risk of methotrexate toxicity.[2] Similarly, a further report by the same authors, in 14 patients receiving high-dose methotrexate,[3] indicated that prior treatment with one course of cisplatin sharply increased the serum levels of methotrexate, particularly if the cumulative cisplatin dose exceeded 400 mg/m^2.

The picture is not totally clear but it seems possible that the previous use of cisplatin causes kidney damage that may not necessarily be detectable with the usual creatinine clearance tests. The effect is to cause a marked reduction in the clearance of the methotrexate. The serum methotrexate levels of such patients should be closely monitored so that any delay in its clearance is detected early and folinic acid rescue therapy can be given.[2] This appears to prevent serious toxicity.[1-3]

There is also a report that suggests that methotrexate inhibits the renal clearance of cisplatin. The renal clearance of platinum in 4 of 5 patients with non-small-cell lung cancer given cisplatin 50 mg/m^2 and methotrexate 40 mg/m^2 was reduced in the first 6 hours after administration (50% lower in the first 3 hours). Apart from a transient increase in serum urea nitrogen and creatinine in one patient, there was no sign of nephrotoxicity with concurrent use.[4]

1. Haim N, Kedar A, Robinson E. Methotrexate-related deaths in patients previously treated with *cis*-diamminedichloride platinum. *Cancer Chemother Pharmacol* (1984) 13, 223–5.
2. Crom WR, Pratt CB, Green AA, Champion JE, Crom DB, Stewart CF, Evans WE. The effect of prior cisplatin therapy on the pharmacokinetics of high-dose methotrexate. *J Clin Oncol* (1984) 2, 655–61.
3. Crom WR, Teresi ME, Meyer WH, Green AA, Evans WE. The intrapatient effect of cisplatin therapy on the pharmacokinetics of high-dose methotrexate. *Drug Intell Clin Pharm* (1985) 19, 467.
4. Preiss R, Brovtsyn VK, Perevodchikova NI, Bychkov MB, Hüller H, Belova LA, Michailov P. Effect of methotrexate on the pharmacokinetics and renal clearance of cisplatin. *Eur J Clin Pharmacol* (1988) 34, 139–44.

Methotrexate + Colestyramine

The serum methotrexate levels of three patients given methotrexate by infusion were markedly reduced by colestyramine.

Clinical evidence

An 11-year-old girl with osteosarcoma who developed colitis when treated with high-dose intravenous methotrexate, was subsequently given colestyramine 2 g every 6 hours from 6 to 48 hours after the methotrexate. Serum methotrexate levels at 24 hours were approximately halved. A marked fall in serum methotrexate levels was seen in another patient similarly treated.[1] Colestyramine similarly reduced methotrexate levels in cases of toxicity in another two patients.[2,3]

Mechanism

Methotrexate undergoes enterohepatic recirculation, that is to say it is excreted into the gut in the bile and re-absorbed further along the gut. If colestyramine is given orally, it can bind strongly to the methotrexate in the gut, thereby preventing its reabsorption and, as a result, the serum levels fall.[1,4]

Importance and management

The documentation seems to be limited. In the cases cited[1-3] the colestyramine was deliberately used to reduce serum methotrexate levels. However, in some circumstances it might represent an unwanted interaction. Since methotrexate is excreted into the gut in the bile, separating the oral dosages of the colestyramine and methotrexate may not necessarily prevent their coming into contact and interacting together. Monitor concurrent use.

1. Erttmann R, Landbeck G. Effect of oral cholestyramine on the elimination of high-dose methotrexate. *J Cancer Res Clin Oncol* (1985) 110, 48–50.
2. Shinozaki T, Watanabe H, Tomidokoro R, Yamamoto K, Horiuchi R, Takagishi K. Successful rescue by oral cholestyramine of a patient with methotrexate nephrotoxicity: nonrenal excretion of serum methotrexate. *Med Pediatr Oncol* (2000) 34, 226–8.
3. Fernández Megía MJ, Alós Almiñana M, Terol Castera MJ. Manejo de la intoxicación por metotrexato: a propósito de un caso. *Farm Hosp* (2004) 28, 371–4.
4. McAnena OJ, Ridge JA, Daly JM. Alteration of methotrexate metabolism in rats by administration of an elemental liquid diet. II. Reduced toxicity and improved survival using cholestyramine. *Cancer* (1987) 59, 1091–7.

Methotrexate + Corticosteroids

Methotrexate clearance may be modestly reduced by the long-term use of prednisolone, but methotrexate does not alter prednisolone pharmacokinetics. Limited evidence suggests methotrexate may alter prednisone levels. Dexamethasone may increase the acute hepatotoxicity of high-dose methotrexate.

Clinical evidence, mechanism, importance and management

There is some evidence that **prednisolone** may reduce the clearance of methotrexate: patients taking long-term **prednisolone** 15 mg daily had a 20% lower clearance of intramuscular methotrexate 10 mg and a 30% higher AUC than patients given **prednisolone** 15 mg daily for just 4 days before the methotrexate, or those not given corticosteroids.[1] In another study, methotrexate had no effect on **prednisolone** pharmacokinetics in 7 patients, or **methylprednisolone** pharmacokinetics in one patient.[2] Preliminary findings of another study suggested that methotrexate may increase plasma methylprednisone levels in response to a dose of **prednisone**; in 2 of 4 patients given methotrexate, plasma methylprednisone levels remained stable despite a decrease in the **prednisone** dose.[3] These findings require confirmation. Their clinical relevance is uncertain.

Dexamethasone may increase the acute hepatotoxicity of high-dose methotrexate. A retrospective comparison in children with brain tumours given methotrexate alone (24 patients), or with **dexamethasone** (33 patients), found that no serious brain oedema occurred in either of the groups and there were no differences in bone marrow toxicity or mucositis, but liver enzymes were significantly higher in the **dexamethasone** group indicating liver toxicity. AST levels were 76 units/L compared with 19 units/L, and ALT levels were 140 units/L compared with 39 units/L. This effect was not due to differences in serum methotrexate levels.[4] The authors recommend that **dexamethasone** should not be included in high-dose methotrexate protocols for children with brain tumours when they are not glucocorticoid dependent.[4]

1. Lafforgue P, Monjanel-Mouterde S, Durand A, Catalin J, Acquaviva PC. Is there an interaction between low doses of corticosteroids and methotrexate in patients with rheumatoid arthritis? A pharmacokinetic study in 33 patients. *J Rheumatol* (1993) 20, 263–7.
2. Glynn-Barnhart AM, Erzurum SC, Leff JA, Martin RJ, Cochran JE, Cott GR, Szefler SJ. Effect of low-dose methotrexate on the disposition of glucocorticoids and theophylline. *J Allergy Clin Immunol* (1991) 88, 180–6.
3. Sockin SM, Ostro MG, Goldman MA, Bloch KJ. The effect of methotrexate on plasma prednisolone levels in steroid dependent asthmatics. *J Allergy Clin Immunol* (1992) 89, 286.
4. Wolff JEA, Hauch H, Kühl J, Egeler RM, Jürgens H. Dexamethasone increases hepatotoxicity of MTX in children with brain tumours. *Anticancer Res* (1998) 18, 2895–9.

Methotrexate + Diuretics

Some very limited evidence suggests that triamterene may possibly increase the bone marrow suppressive effects of methotrexate. It seems doubtful if thiazides interact adversely.

Clinical evidence, mechanism, importance and management

A 57 year-old woman who had been treated for several years with daily doses of diclofenac 150 mg, atenolol 50 mg and **triamterene** with **hydrochlorothiazide** 50/25 mg, for rheumatoid arthritis and hypertension, additionally started treatment with methotrexate 5 mg weekly. After 2 months she was admitted to hospital with pancytopenia, extensive mucosal ulceration and renal impairment. The authors point out that **triamterene** is structurally similar to folate and has anti-folate activity, which may therefore have been additive with the effects of methotrexate,[1] but the diclofenac may also have contributed (see 'Methotrexate + NSAIDs', p.649). In 1998, the manufacturer noted there were two other reports of pancytopenia in patients taking methotrexate and **triamterene**, but again the patients were also taking NSAIDs.[2]

A study in 9 patients found that neither **furosemide** nor **hydroflumethiazide** had any effect on the clearance of methotrexate in the urine.[3] However, a study in women with breast cancer, treated with methotrexate, **cyclophosphamide** and **fluorouracil** found that the concurrent use of a **thiazide diuretic** appeared to increase the myelosuppressant effects, but it is not clear which of the antineoplastics might have been affected.[4]

1. Richmond R, McRorie ER, Ogden DA, Lambert CM. Methotrexate and triamterene — a potentially fatal combination. *Ann Rheum Dis* (1997) 56, 209–10.
2. Wyeth/Lederle. Data on file, September 1998.
3. Kristensen LØ, Weismann K, Hutters L. Renal function and the rate of disappearance of methotrexate from serum. *Eur J Clin Pharmacol* (1975) 8, 439–44.
4. Orr LE. Potentiation of myelosuppression from cancer chemotherapy and thiazide diuretics. *Drug Intell Clin Pharm* (1981) 15, 967–70.

Methotrexate + Fluorouracil

Two patients taking low-dose methotrexate had a toxic skin reaction when they started to use a cream containing fluorouracil. The activity of systemic treatment with methotrexate and fluorouracil are said to be dependent on the order in which the two drugs are given, but this does not appear to be important in the commonly used CMF regimen.

Clinical evidence, mechanism, importance and management

(a) Topical fluorouracil

Two patients with rheumatoid arthritis treated with low-dose methotrexate 7.5 to 12.5 mg weekly for 6 to 14 months were given 2% fluorouracil cream for actinic keratosis. Within 2 to 3 days both patients developed erythema, blister formation and necrosis. The cream was stopped and the lesions healed over the next 2 to 3 weeks.[1] It would seem that concurrent use should be avoided.

(b) Systemic fluorouracil

In vitro and *animal* data indicate that methotrexate and fluorouracil can be mutually antagonistic under certain conditions.[2-4] Other studies indicate that the sequence (methotrexate first)[5,6] is important for additive or synergistic activity. However, the combination of cyclophosphamide, methotrexate and fluorouracil (CMF) has been the most commonly used adjuvant therapy in breast cancer, and the sequence of administration is said not to be important.[7]

1. Blackburn WD, Alarcón GS. Toxic response to topical fluorouracil in two rheumatoid arthritis patients receiving low dose weekly methotrexate. *Arthritis Rheum* (1990) 33, 303–4.
2. Tattersall MHN, Jackson RC, Connors TA, Harrap KR. Combination chemotherapy: the interaction of methotrexate and 5-fluorouracil. *Eur J Cancer* (1973) 9, 733–9.
3. Maugh TH. Cancer chemotherapy: an unexpected drug interaction. *Science* (1976) 194, 310.
4. Waxman S, Bruckner H. Antitumour drug interactions: additional data. *Science* (1976) 194, 672.
5. Bertino JR, Sawicki WL, Lindquist CA, Gupta VS. Schedule-dependent antitumor effects of methotrexate and 5-fluorouracil. *Cancer Res* (1977) 37, 327–8.
6. Brown I, Ward HWC. Therapeutic consequences of antitumour drug interactions: methotrexate and 5-fluorouracil in the chemotherapy of C3H mice with transplanted mammary adenocarcinoma. *Cancer Lett* (1978) 5, 291–7.
7. Summerhayes M, Daniels S, eds. Practical Chemotherapy: A Multidisciplinary Guide. 1st ed. UK: Radcliffe Medical Press; 2003 P. 91.

Methotrexate + Folinates

Folic acid or folinic acid are sometimes added to low-dose methotrexate treatment for rheumatoid arthritis or psoriasis to reduce adverse effects. Folinic acid is frequently used as an antidote to high-dose methotrexate in cancer therapy. Patients taking methotrexate should avoid the inadvertent use of folates in multivitamin preparations.

Clinical evidence, mechanism, importance and management

Methotrexate acts as a folic acid antagonist by reversibly binding to the enzyme dihydrofolate reductase so blocking the conversion of folic acid to tetrahydrofolate. Therefore folic acid and folinic acid (a derivative of tetrahydrofolate) would be expected to interfere with both the toxic and therapeutic effects of methotrexate.

Folic acid or folinic acid are commonly used to reduce the adverse effects of low-dose methotrexate used for rheumatoid arthritis and psoriasis, although the optimum doses and schedules to maximise tolerability and efficacy remain to be determined.

Similarly, folinic acid is used in conjunction with high-dose methotrexate for various cancers to minimise toxicity, when it is typically started 24 hours after methotrexate administration (folinic acid or 'leucovorin' rescue). In this setting, the antidote effect is clearly influenced by the dose of folinate in relation to the dose of methotrexate, and the timing of folinate administration in relation to methotrexate administration.

Patients taking methotrexate for any indication should avoid the inadvertent or unsupervised use of folates, which are commonly found in multivitamin preparations.

Methotrexate + Food

The absorption of low-dose oral methotrexate appears not to be significantly affected by food.

Clinical evidence, mechanism, importance and management

In 10 children with lymphoblastic leukaemia the peak serum levels of a 15-mg/m^2 oral dose of methotrexate (measured at 1.5 hours) were reduced by about 40% when the methotrexate was taken with a **milky meal** (milk, cornflakes, sugar, white bread and butter). The AUC_{0-4} was reduced by about 25%. A smaller reduction in methotrexate absorption was seen when it was taken after a **'citrus meal'** (orange juice, fresh orange, white bread, butter and jam).[1] However, a 4-hour study is too short to assess the extent of the total absorption. Another study in 16 other children given methotrexate 8 to 22.7 mg/m^2 found that the peak levels and AUC were not significantly affected if methotrexate was given before a meal.[2] Yet another study in 12 healthy subjects found that a **high fat-content breakfast** delayed the absorption of methotrexate 7.5 mg orally by about 30 minutes but the extent of the absorption was unchanged.[3] It would therefore appear that methotrexate may be taken without regard to meals.

1. Pinkerton CR, Welshman SG, Glasgow JFT, Bridges JM. Can food influence the absorption of methotrexate in children with acute lymphoblastic leukaemia? *Lancet* (1980) 2, 944–6.
2. Madanat F, Awidi A, Shaheen O, Ottman S, Al-Turk W. Effects of food and gender on the pharmacokinetics of methotrexate in children. *Res Commun Chem Pathol Pharmacol* (1987) 55, 279–82.
3. Kozloski GD, De Vito JM, Kisicki JC, Johnson JB. The effect of food on the absorption of methotrexate sodium tablets in healthy volunteers. *Arthritis Rheum* (1992) 35, 761–4.

Methotrexate + Miscellaneous

Animal **studies suggested that the toxicity of methotrexate might be increased by the use of chloramphenicol, aminosalicylic acid, sodium salicylate, sulfamethoxypyridazine, tetracycline or tolbutamide, but confirmation of this in man has only been seen with the salicylates, sulphonamides and possibly tetracycline.**

Clinical evidence, mechanism, importance and management

Some lists, reviews and books on interactions say that **chloramphenicol**, aminosalicylic acid, sodium salicylate, **sulfamethoxypyridazine**, tetracycline or **tolbutamide** interact with methotrexate, apparently based largely on the preliminary findings of a study in which male *mice* were treated for 5 days with each of 4 doses of methotrexate (1.53 to 12.25 mg/kg intravenously) and immediately afterwards with non-toxic intraperitoneal doses of the drugs listed. These drugs were said to decrease the lethal dose and/or decrease the survival time of the *mice*.[1] That is to say, the toxicity of the methotrexate was increased. The reasons are not understood, but it is suggested that displacement of the methotrexate from its plasma protein binding sites could result in a rise in the levels of unbound and active methotrexate, and in the case of sodium salicylate to a decrease in renal clearance.

These *animal* studies were done in 1968. Since then the clinical importance of the interaction with salicylates has been confirmed (see 'Methotrexate + NSAIDs', p.649); there are a few cases involving 'sulfonamides', (p.643)); and there are two isolated case report of an interaction with 'tetracyclines', (p.645), but there appears to be no direct clinical evidence of interactions between methotrexate and **chloramphenicol** or **tolbutamide**. The results of *animal* experiments cannot be applied directly and uncritically to man and it now seems probable that some of these suggested or alleged interactions are more theoretical than real.

1. Dixon RL. The interaction between various drugs and methotrexate. *Toxicol Appl Pharmacol* (1968) 12, 308.

Methotrexate + Nitrous oxide

Methotrexate-induced stomatitis and other toxic effects may be increased by the use of nitrous oxide.

Clinical evidence, mechanism, importance and management

A study in which intravenous methotrexate, cyclophosphamide and fluorouracil (CMF) were used within 36 hours of mastectomy suggested that stomatitis may be caused by a toxic interaction between methotrexate and nitrous oxide used during anaesthesia. Stomatitis was much more common in those receiving CMF within 6 hours of surgery.[1-3] A possible reason is that the effects of methotrexate on tetrahydrofolate metabolism are increased by nitrous oxide, and this has been confirmed in *animals*.[4] It was found that the incidence of stomatitis, severe leucopenia, thrombocytopenia, and of severe systemic and local infections could be reduced by giving calcium folinate (leucovorin) and intravenous hydration.[2,3] Alternatively, the use of nitrous oxide shortly before methotrexate administration should be avoided.[4]

1. Ludwig Breast Cancer Study Group. Toxic effects of early adjuvant chemotherapy for breast cancer. *Lancet* (1983) ii, 542–4.
2. Goldhirsch A, Gelber RD, Tattersall MNH, Rudenstam C-M, Cavalli F. Methotrexate/nitrous-oxide toxic interaction in perioperative chemotherapy for early breast cancer. *Lancet* (1987) ii, 151.
3. Ludwig Breast Cancer Study Group. On the safety of perioperative adjuvant chemotherapy with cyclophosphamide, methotrexate and 5-fluorouracil in breast cancer. *Eur J Cancer Clin Oncol* (1988) 24, 1305–8.
4. Ermens AAM, Schoester M, Spijkers LJM, Lindemans J, Abels J. Toxicity of methotrexate in rats preexposed to nitrous oxide. *Cancer Res* (1989) 49, 6337–41.

Methotrexate + NSAIDs

Increased methotrexate toxicity, sometimes life-threatening, has been seen in a few patients also taking NSAIDs whereas other patients have been treated uneventfully. The pharmacokinetics of methotrexate can also be changed by some NSAIDs (aspirin, choline magnesium trisalicylate, etodolac, etoricoxib, ibuprofen, metamizole sodium, naproxen, rofecoxib, sodium salicylate, tolmetin). The development of toxicity may be dose related and the risk appears to be lowest in those taking low-dose methotrexate for psoriasis or rheumatoid arthritis who have normal renal function.

Clinical evidence

(a) Aminophenazone

Megaloblastic pancytopenia occurred in a woman with rheumatoid arthritis who took methotrexate 15 mg weekly with aminophenazone 1 to 1.5 g daily.[1]

(b) Aspirin and other salicylates

A study in 15 patients with rheumatoid arthritis given a single 10-mg bolus dose of methotrexate, either with or without aspirin 975 mg four times daily, found that the methotrexate clearance was reduced by aspirin (systemic clearance about 16%, renal clearance of unbound methotrexate about 30%). Also the unbound fraction of methotrexate was higher during aspirin use. Despite these changes no acute toxicity was seen.[2] Another study found that aspirin did not affect the pharmacokinetics of methotrexate.[3] Yet another study found that, although aspirin did not alter the pharmacokinetics of methotrexate, it did increase the AUC of the metabolite 7-hydroxymethotrexate.[4]

A study in 4 patients found that the renal clearance of methotrexate was reduced by 35% by an infusion of **sodium salicylate** (2 g initially, then 33 mg/minute).[5] A further study found that **choline magnesium trisalicylate** reduced methotrexate clearance by 24 to 41%, and increased the unbound fraction by 28%, when compared with paracetamol (acetaminophen).[6]

Lethal pancytopenia in 2 patients given methotrexate and aspirin prompted a retrospective survey of the records of other patients given intra-arterial infusions of methotrexate 50 mg daily for 10 days, for epidermoid carcinoma of the oral cavity. Six out of 7 who developed rapid and serious pancytopenia were found to have taken aspirin or other salicylates.[7] There are other case reports[8,9] of methotrexate toxicity in patients taking salicylates but whether a causal relationship exists is uncertain. It has been suggested that pneumonitis in patients receiving low-dose methotrexate may have resulted from the concurrent use of aspirin 4 to 5 g daily.[10]

See also the report about the comparative use of aspirin and other NSAIDs in section (w), below, on NSAIDs in general.

(c) Azapropazone

A woman who had been taking methotrexate 25 mg weekly for 4 years for psoriasis had acute toxicity (oral and genital ulceration, bone marrow failure) shortly after starting to take azapropazone (reducing from a dose of 2.4 g on the first day, 1.8 g on the second day to 1.2 g daily for a week). She was also taking aspirin 300 mg daily.[11,12]

(d) Bromfenac

In a short-term study, 10 patients taking methotrexate weekly were given bromfenac 50 mg three times daily for 6 days. No significant changes were seen in either the pharmacokinetics of bromfenac or methotrexate. However, the AUC of the major metabolite of methotrexate, 7-hydroxymethotrexate, was increased by 30% and its renal clearance was reduced by 16%. Eight of the patients had mild to moderate adverse effects and one patient had to withdraw because of moderate hypertension. No patient had any clinically important abnormal laboratory test results.[13] Note that systemic bromfenac has been withdrawn from the market because of reports of hepatic failure.

(e) Celecoxib

Fourteen female patients with rheumatoid arthritis taking methotrexate 5 to 20 mg weekly for at least 3 months were also given celecoxib 200 mg or a placebo twice daily for a week. It was found that the maximum serum levels of the methotrexate, its AUC, renal clearance, and other pharmacokinetic parameters were unchanged by the celecoxib.[14] The authors note that, in clinical studies, celecoxib was taken in combination with low-dose methotrexate for up to 12 weeks by over 450 patients, and the incidence of adverse effects was similar to that in patients taking methotrexate with placebo.[14]

(f) Diclofenac

A study found that diclofenac 100 mg daily did not affect the pharmacokinetics of methotrexate;[3] however, 5 patients taking low-dose methotrexate 7.5 to 12.5 mg weekly for psoriasis or rheumatoid arthritis developed serious/fatal neutropenias. These cases probably involved other drug interactions, but diclofenac may have been an additional factor in two of them.[15] Other cases involving diclofenac are mentioned in the sections on *indometacin* (k) and *ketoprofen* (l).

(g) Etodolac

A pharmacokinetic study in patients with rheumatoid arthritis found that etodolac 600 mg daily did not affect the AUC of methotrexate, but the duration of exposure was lengthened (mean residence time increased from 8.5 to 11.4 hours). No clinical toxicity was seen.[16]

(h) Etoricoxib

A study in patients taking methotrexate 7.5 to 20 mg weekly for rheumatoid arthritis found that the addition of etoricoxib 60, 90 or 120 mg daily had no effect on the methotrexate AUC or on its renal clearance. However, another similar study found that etoricoxib 120 mg daily increased the methotrexate AUC by 28% and reduced its clearance by 13%.[17]

(i) Flurbiprofen

A study in 6 patients taking low doses of methotrexate 10 to 25 mg weekly found no important changes in methotrexate levels when they were given flurbiprofen 100 mg three times daily.[18] In another study of 10 patients with rheumatoid arthritis taking methotrexate 7.5 to 17.5 mg weekly and flurbiprofen 3 mg/kg daily, methotrexate oral and renal clearance were similarly unaffected by flurbiprofen.[19]

In contrast to these pharmacokinetic studies, a case report describes an elderly woman who had been taking methotrexate 2.5 mg three times a week for 3 years for rheumatoid arthritis, who developed haematemesis, neutropenia and thrombocytopenia (diagnosed as methotrexate toxicity) within 1 to 2 weeks of starting to take flurbiprofen 100 mg daily.[20]

(j) Ibuprofen

A study in 7 patients found that the clearance of oral methotrexate 7.5 to 15 mg was halved by ibuprofen 40 mg/kg per day, when compared with paracetamol (acetaminophen).[21] In a related study the clearance of methotrexate was reduced by 40% by ibuprofen.[6] Another study in 6 patients with rheumatoid arthritis taking methotrexate 10 to 25 mg weekly found that ibuprofen 800 mg three times daily had no effect on the pharmacokinetics of methotrexate.[18] Similar findings have been reported by other workers.[3] A patient taking methotrexate who was given ibuprofen required prolonged folinic acid rescue because the clearance of methotrexate had fallen by two-thirds.[22] Another patient receiving high-dose methotrexate (7.5 g/m^2) had severe methotrexate-induced nephrotoxicity and delayed excretion of methotrexate while taking ibuprofen 400 mg every 4 hours.[23] A report attributes pancytopenia and resulting pneumocystis pneumonia in a 16-year-old patient taking methotrexate 5 to 10 mg weekly to the concurrent use of ibuprofen 600 mg twice daily (and also 1 mg prednisolone daily).[24]

(k) Indometacin

The AUC of child taking methotrexate 7.5 mg/m^2 weekly for 9 months was increased by 140% when indometacin and **aspirin** were also given.[25] Another study found that indometacin did not affect the pharmacokinetics of methotrexate.[3]

Two patients given sequential intermediate-dose methotrexate and fluorouracil who were also taking indometacin 75 to 100 mg daily died from acute drug toxicity, which the authors of the report attributed to indometacin-associated renal failure.[26] Another case of acute renal failure has been described,[27] but there were no cases of toxicity in 4 other patients taking methotrexate with either paracetamol (acetaminophen) or indometacin.[9] An elderly woman taking indometacin 50 mg daily rectally and **diclofenac** 100 mg daily intravenously died after being given single 10-mg intramuscular dose of methotrexate.[28]

(l) Ketoprofen

In a study in 10 patients with rheumatoid arthritis taking methotrexate 7.5 to 17.5 mg weekly and ketoprofen 3 mg/kg daily, the methotrexate oral and renal clearance and the fraction of methotrexate unbound were unaffected by ketoprofen.[19] Similarly, in another study in 18 patients with rheumatoid arthritis who were given intravenous methotrexate 15 mg weekly, ketoprofen had no significant effect on the AUC, half-life, or clearance of methotrexate and its major metabolite, 7-hydroxymethotrexate.[29] However, a retrospective study of 118 cycles of *high-dose* methotrexate treatment (800 to 8300 mg/m^2; mean 3200 mg/m^2) in 36 patients found that 4 out of the 9 patients who developed severe methotrexate toxicity had also taken ketoprofen 150 to 200 mg daily for 2 to 15 days. Three of them died. A marked and prolonged rise in serum methotrexate levels was observed. Another patient who had methotrexate toxicity had also been given **diclofenac** 150 mg (in one day).[30] The authors of this report state that ketoprofen should not be given at the same time as high-dose methotrexate, but it may be safe to give it 12 to 24 hours after the methotrexate because 50% of the methotrexate is excreted by the kidneys within 6 to 12 hours. This was tried in two patients without adverse effects.[30]

(m) Lumiracoxib

In a double-blind, placebo-controlled study in patients with rheumatoid arthritis given low-dose methotrexate 7.5 to 15 mg weekly, lumiracoxib 400 mg daily for 7 days had no significant effects on the pharmacokinetics of methotrexate.[31]

(n) Meloxicam

Thirteen patients with rheumatoid arthritis were given intravenous methotrexate 15 mg before and after taking meloxicam 15 mg daily for a week. The pharmacokinetics of the methotrexate were unaffected by the meloxicam and no increase in toxicity was seen.[32]

(o) Metamizole sodium (Dipyrone)

A study in a patient with osteosarcoma found that metamizole sodium 4 g daily more than doubled the methotrexate AUC during the first cycle of high-dose methotrexate treatment.[33]

(p) Naproxen

Naproxen had no significant effect on the AUC, half-life, or clearance of methotrexate and its major metabolite 7-hydroxymethotrexate in 18 patients with rheumatoid arthritis given intravenous methotrexate 15 mg weekly.[29] Other studies have found that naproxen did not affect the pharmacokinetics of methotrexate.[3] In a study in 27 patients with rheumatoid arthritis who had taken oral methotrexate 7.5 to 15 mg weekly for at least 3 months, the concurrent use of naproxen 600 mg twice daily with lansoprazole did not affect the pharmacokinetics of methotrexate or 7-hydroxymethotrexate.[34] Another study in patients with rheumatoid arthritis with normal renal function found that no toxicity was caused when naproxen 500 mg twice daily was given with methotrexate 15 mg given orally or intravenously, nor was the methotrexate clearance altered.[35]

In contrast, a study found that the clearance of methotrexate was decreased by 22% by naproxen.[6,21] In addition, two children taking methotrexate for 1 and 2 years had increases in the AUC of methotrexate of 22% and 71% when given naproxen with **aspirin** or **indometacin**, respectively.[25] A further study in 9 children taking methotrexate 0.22 to 1.02 mg/kg per week found that the clearance was increased in 4 children by more than 30% when they were given naproxen 14.6 to 18.8 mg/kg daily. There was also a 30% or more change in the pharmacokinetics of naproxen in 6 of the patients, but as both increases and decreases in clearance occurred, the significance of these findings are uncertain.[36] A woman died of gross methotrexate toxicity apparently exacerbated by the concurrent use of naproxen,[37] and a report attributes pneumonitis in a patient taking methotrexate 7.5 to 10 mg weekly to the concurrent use of naproxen (initially 1 g then 500 mg) daily.[38]

(q) Parecoxib

Studies in patients with rheumatoid arthritis found that oral valdecoxib 40 mg twice daily had no clinically significant effect on the plasma levels of methotrexate given weekly by the intramuscular route [dose not stated].[39] Even so the manufacturers suggest that careful monitoring should be considered, probably because of the problems seen with other NSAIDs. Note that valdecoxib is the main metabolite of parecoxib.

(r) Phenylbutazone

Two patients taking methotrexate for psoriasis developed methotrexate toxicity and skin ulceration shortly after starting to take phenylbutazone 200 to 600 mg daily. One of them died from septicaemia following bone marrow depression.[40]

(s) Piroxicam

No effect on the pharmacokinetics of either free or bound methotrexate was seen in 20 patients with rheumatoid arthritis taking methotrexate 10 mg weekly when they were given piroxicam 20 mg daily for at least 15 days.[41] In another study in 10 patients with rheumatoid arthritis taking methotrexate 7.5 to 17.5 mg weekly, methotrexate oral and renal clearance were similarly unaffected by piroxicam 20 mg daily.[19]

(t) Rofecoxib

Rofecoxib 12.5 to 50 mg once daily had no effect on the AUC and renal clearance of methotrexate or 7-hydroxymethotrexate in 19 patients taking methotrexate 7.5 to 20 mg once weekly.[42] However, the authors note that in previous evaluations (data on file), higher than therapeutic doses of rofecoxib (75 mg and 250 mg) were associated with a 23% and 40% increase in the AUC of methotrexate, and an 11% and 40% decrease in its renal clearance, respectively.[42]

(u) Sulindac

Sulindac (mean dose 400 mg daily) had no effect on the pharmacokinetics of a single 10-mg/m^2 intravenous dose of methotrexate, but it slightly increased the AUC of the 7-hydroxymethotrexate metabolite.[4]

(v) Tolmetin

Three children taking methotrexate for between 6 months and 1 year had increases in the AUC of methotrexate of 42% when given tolmetin, and of 18% and 25% when given tolmetin with **aspirin**.[25]

(w) NSAIDs in general

In a study of 34 patients with rheumatoid arthritis taking methotrexate 5 or 10 mg/m^2 (to nearest 2.5 mg) weekly, 12 patients also took **aspirin** (average 4.5 g daily) and 22 took other NSAIDs. Twenty-one of the 34 also took prednisone. Toxicity, sometimes serious (5 patients withdrawn), was common, but no clinical differences between **aspirin** or other NSAIDs with respect to this toxicity was seen during 12 months of concurrent use.[43]

A preliminary report of a study in 87 patients receiving long-term treatment with methotrexate (mean weekly dose 8.19 mg), most of whom were also taking unspecified NSAIDs, found that the majority (72%) experienced no untoward effects and in the rest adverse effects were only relatively mild.[44] The concurrent use of methotrexate and NSAIDs in more than 450 patients with psoriatic arthritis or rheumatoid arthritis was said to be without clinical interaction problems.[45]

A literature review of interactions between methotrexate and NSAIDs found that low-dose methotrexate pharmacokinetics were unaltered by NSAIDs, with the exception of salicylates.[46]

In a review of the records of 315 patients with rheumatoid arthritis taking low-dose methotrexate, 13 patients had low platelet counts. The thrombocytopenia was believed to have resulted from an interaction with an NSAID or in some patients a multiple drug interaction. If multiple drug interactions were not involved, the authors found that if the NSAID was given on a separate day, or dosages spaced according to the NSAID half-life, therapy could be re-introduced avoiding the problems of thrombocytopenia.[47]

Mechanism

Methotrexate is largely cleared unchanged from the body by renal excretion. The NSAIDs as a group inhibit the synthesis of the prostaglandins (PGE_2) resulting in a fall in renal perfusion, which could lead to a rise in serum methotrexate levels, accompanied by increased toxicity. In addition, salicylates competitively inhibit the tubular secretion of methotrexate, which would further reduce its clearance.[5] NSAIDs can also cause renal impairment, which would allow the methotrexate to accumulate. The pyrazolone derivatives and related drugs (e.g. azapropazone, metamizole sodium, phenylbutazone, aminophenazone), in particular, can cause bone marrow depression, which could be additive with that of methotrexate. Protein binding displacement of methotrexate or its metabolite (7-hydroxymethotrexate) have also been suggested as possible additional mechanisms.[48,49] There is also some evidence that 7-hydroxymethotrexate is cleared more slowly in the presence of NSAIDs.[4]

Importance and management

The evidence presented here clearly shows that a few patients taking methotrexate have developed very serious toxicity, apparently due to the concurrent use of NSAIDs whereas many other patients have experienced no problems at all. There is also other evidence that the pharmacokinetics of the methotrexate are changed (in particular reduced clearance) by some NSAIDs (aspirin, choline magnesium trisalicylate, etodolac, ibuprofen, metamizole sodium, rofecoxib (at higher than therapeutic doses), sodium salicylate, tolmetin), which might be expected to increase its toxicity.

The consensus of opinion seems to be that the risks are greatest with high-dose methotrexate (150 mg or more daily to treat neoplastic diseases) and in patients with impaired renal function, but less in those given low doses (5 to 25 mg weekly) for psoriasis or rheumatoid arthritis and with normal kidney function. The manufacturers of methotrexate and the CSM do not advise the avoidance of NSAIDs (except azapropazone and non-prescription aspirin and ibuprofen), even though their use is a recognised additional risk factor for toxicity. Instead their advice is that the methotrexate dosage should be well monitored, which implies that the precautions for methotrexate use should be stepped up. The advice of the CSM in the UK is that any patient given methotrexate alone should have a full blood count, renal and liver function tests before starting treatment. These should be repeated weekly until therapy is stabilised, and thereafter every 2 to 3 months. Patients should be told to report any sign or symptom suggestive of infection, particularly sore throat (which might possibly indicate that white cell counts have fallen) or dyspnoea or cough (suggestive of pulmonary toxicity).[50] Aminophenazone or metamizole sodium can cause agranulocytosis on their own (and they consequently have limited use) so their use with methotrexate should also be avoided.

Some of the NSAIDs cited here have not been reported to interact (celecoxib, lumiracoxib, meloxicam, piroxicam), and information about some other NSAIDs seems to be lacking, but the same general precautions indicated above should be followed with all NSAIDs just to be on the safe side.

1. Noskov SM. Megaloblastic pancytopenia in a female patient with rheumatoid arthritis given methotrexate and amidopyrine. *Ter Arkh* (1990) 62, 122–3.
2. Stewart CF, Fleming RA, Germain BF, Seleznick MJ, Evans WE. Aspirin alters methotrexate disposition in rheumatoid arthritis patients. *Arthritis Rheum* (1991) 34, 1514–20.
3. Iqbal MP, Baig JA, Ali AA, Niazi SK, Mehboobali N, Hussain MA. The effects of non-steroidal anti-inflammatory drugs on the disposition of methotrexate in patients with rheumatoid arthritis. *Biopharm Drug Dispos* (1998) 19, 163–7.
4. Furst DE, Herman RA, Koehnke R, Erickson N, Hash L, Riggs CE, Porras A, Veng-Pedersen P. Effect of aspirin and sulindac on methotrexate clearance. *J Pharm Sci* (1990) 79, 782–6.
5. Liegler DG, Henderson ES, Hahn MA, Oliverio VT. The effect of organic acids on renal clearance of methotrexate in man. *Clin Pharmacol Ther* (1969) 10, 849–57.
6. Tracy TS, Krohn K, Jones DR, Bradley JD, Hall SD, Brater DC. The effects of salicylate, ibuprofen, and naproxen on the disposition of methotrexate in patients with rheumatoid arthritis. *Eur J Clin Pharmacol* (1992) 42, 121–5.
7. Zuik M, Mandel MA. Methotrexate-salicylate interaction: a clinical and experimental study. *Surg Forum* (1975) 26, 567–9.
8. Dubin HV, Harrell ER. Liver disease associated with methotrexate treatment of psoriatic patients. *Arch Dermatol* (1970) 102, 498–503.
9. Baker H. Intermittent high dose oral methotrexate therapy in psoriasis. *Br J Dermatol* (1970) 82, 65–9.
10. Maier WP, Leon-Perez R, Miller SB. Pneumonitis during low-dose methotrexate therapy. *Arch Intern Med* (1986) 146, 602–3.
11. Daly HM, Scott GL, Boyle J, Roberts CJC. Methotrexate toxicity precipitated by azapropazone. *Br J Dermatol* (1986) 114, 733–35.
12. Burton JL. Drug interactions with methotrexate. *Br J Dermatol* (1991) 124, 300–1.
13. Gumbhir-Shah K, Cevallos WH, Decleene SA, Korth-Bradley JM. Lack of interaction between bromfenac and methotrexate in patients with rheumatoid arthritis. *J Rheumatol* (1996) 23, 984–9.
14. Karim A, Tolbert DS, Hunt TL, Hubbard RC, Harper KM, Geis GS. Celecoxib, a specific COX-2 inhibitor, has no significant effect on methotrexate pharmacokinetics in patients with rheumatoid arthritis. *J Rheumatol* (1999) 26, 2539–43.
15. Mayall B, Poggi G, Parkin JD. Neutropenia due to low-dose methotrexate therapy for psoriasis and rheumatoid arthritis may be fatal. *Med J Aust* (1991) 155, 480–4.
16. Anaya J-M, Fabre D, Bressolle F, Bologna C, Alric R, Cocciglio M, Dropsy R, Sany J. Effect of etodolac on methotrexate pharmacokinetics in patients with rheumatoid arthritis. *J Rheumatol* (1994) 21, 203–8.
17. Arcoxia (Etoricoxib). Merck Sharp & Dohme Ltd. UK Summary of product characteristics, January 2007.
18. Skeith KJ, Russell AS, Jamali F, Coates J, Friedman H. Lack of significant interaction between low dose methotrexate and ibuprofen or flurbiprofen in patients with arthritis. *J Rheumatol* (1990) 17, 1008–10.
19. Tracy TS, Worster T, Bradley JD, Greene PK, Brater DC. Methotrexate disposition following concomitant administration of ketoprofen, piroxicam and flurbiprofen in patients with rheumatoid arthritis. *Br J Clin Pharmacol* (1994) 37, 453–6.
20. Frenia ML, Long KS. Methotrexate and nonsteroidal antiinflammatory drug interactions. *Ann Pharmacother* (1992) 26, 234–7.
21. Tracy TS, Jones DR, Hall SD, Brater DC, Bradley JD, Krohn K. The effect of NSAIDs on methotrexate disposition in patients with rheumatoid arthritis. *Clin Pharmacol Ther* (1990) 47, 138.
22. Bloom EJ, Ignoffo RJ, Reis CA, Cadman E. Delayed clearance (CL) of methotrexate (MTX) associated with antibiotics and antiinflammatory agents. *Clin Res* (1986) 34, 560A.
23. Cassano WF. Serious methotrexate toxicity caused by interaction with ibuprofen. *Am J Pediatr Hematol Oncol* (1989) 11, 481–2.
24. Carmichael AJ, Ryatt KS. *Pneumocystis carinii* pneumonia following methotrexate. *Br J Dermatol* (1990) 122, 291.
25. Dupuis LL, Koren G, Shore A, Silverman ED, Laxer RM. Methotrexate-nonsteroidal antiinflammatory drug interaction in children with arthritis. *J Rheumatol* (1990) 17, 1469–73.
26. Ellison NM, Servi RJ. Acute renal failure and death following sequential intermediate-dose methotrexate and 5-FU: a possible adverse effect due to concomitant indomethacin administration. *Cancer Treat Rep* (1985) 69, 342–3.
27. Maiche AG. Acute renal failure due to concomitant action of methotrexate and indomethacin. *Lancet* (1986) i, 1390.

28. Gabrielli A, Leoni P, Danieli G. Methotrexate and non-steroidal anti-inflammatory drugs. *BMJ* (1987) 294, 776.
29. Christophidis N, Dawson TM, Angelis P, Ryan PFJ. A double-blind, randomised, placebo controlled pharmacokinetic and clinical study of the interaction of ketoprofen and naproxen with methotrexate in rheumatoid arthritis. *Arthritis Rheum* (1994) 37 (9 Suppl), S252.
30. Thyss A, Milano G, Kubar J, Namer M, Schneider M. Clinical and pharmacokinetic evidence of a life-threatening interaction between methotrexate and ketoprofen. *Lancet* (1986) i, 256–8.
31. Hartmann SN, Rordorf CM, Milosavljev S, Branson JM, Chales GH, Juvin RR, Lafforgue P, Le Parc JM, Tavernier CG, Meyer OC. Lumiracoxib does not affect methotrexate pharmacokinetics in rheumatoid arthritis patients. *Ann Pharmacother* (2004) 38, 1582–7.
32. Hübner G, Sander D, Degner FL, Türck D, Rau R. Lack of pharmacokinetic interaction of meloxicam with methotrexate in patients with rheumatoid arthritis. *J Rheumatol* (1997) 24, 845–51.
33. Hernández de la Figuera y Gómez T, Torres NVJ, Ronchera Oms CL, Ordovás Baines JP. Interacción farmacocinética entre metotrexato a altas dosis y dipirona. *Rev Farmacol Clin Exp* (1989) 6, 77–81.
34. Vakily M, Amer F, Kukulka MJ, Andhivarothai N. Coadministration of lansoprazole and naproxen does not affect the pharmacokinetic profile of methotrexate in adult patients with rheumatoid arthritis. *J Clin Pharmacol* (2005) 45, 1179–86.
35. Stewart CF, Fleming RA, Arkin CR, Evans WE. Coadministration of naproxen and low-dose methotrexate in patients with rheumatoid arthritis. *Clin Pharmacol Ther* (1990) 47, 540–6.
36. Wallace CA, Smith AL, Sherry DD. Pilot investigation of naproxen/methotrexate interaction in patients with juvenile rheumatoid arthritis. *J Rheumatol* (1993) 20, 1764–8.
37. Singh RR, Malaviya AN, Pandey JN, Guleria JS. Fatal interaction between methotrexate and naproxen. *Lancet* (1986) i, 1390.
38. Englebrecht JA, Calhoon SL, Scherrer JJ. Methotrexate pneumonitis after low-dose therapy for rheumatoid arthritis. *Arthritis Rheum* (1983) 26, 1275–8.
39. Dynastat Injection (Parecoxib sodium). Pfizer Ltd. UK Summary of product characteristics, April 2007.
40. Adams JD, Hunter GA. Drug interaction in psoriasis. *Aust J Dermatol* (1976) 17, 39–40.
41. Combe B, Edno L, Lafforgue P, Bologna C, Bernard J-C, Acquaviva P, Sany J, Bressolle F. Total and free methotrexate pharmacokinetics, with and without piroxicam, in rheumatoid arthritis patients. *Br J Rheumatol* (1995) 34, 421–8.
42. Schwartz JI, Agrawal NGB, Wong PH, Bachmann KA, Porras AG, Miller JL, Ebel DL, Sack MR, Holmes GB, Redfern JS, Gertz BJ. Lack of pharmacokinetic interaction between rofecoxib and methotrexate in rheumatoid arthritis patients. *J Clin Pharmacol* (2001) 41, 1120–30.
43. Rooney TW, Furst DE, Koehnke R, Burmeister L. Aspirin is not associated with more toxicity than other nonsteroidal antiinflammatory drugs in patients with rheumatoid arthritis treated with methotrexate. *J Rheumatol* (1993) 20, 1297–1302.
44. Wilke WS, Calabrese LH, Segal AM. Incidence of untoward reactions in patients with rheumatoid arthritis treated with methotrexate. *Arthritis Rheum* (1983) 26 (Suppl), S56.
45. Zachariae H. Methotrexate and non-steroidal anti-inflammatory drugs. *Br J Dermatol* (1992) 126, 95.
46. Carpentier N, Ratsimbazafy V, Bertin P, Vergne P, Bonnet C, Bannwarth B, Dehais J, Treves R. Interaction méthotrexate/anti-inflammatoires non stéroïdiens: importance de la dose. *J Pharm Clin* (1999) 18, 295–9.
47. Franck H, Rau R, Herborn G. Thrombocytopenia in patients with rheumatoid arthritis on long-term treatment with low dose methotrexate. *Clin Rheumatol* (1996) 15, 163–7.
48. Slørdal L, Sager G, Aarbakke J. Pharmacokinetic interactions with methotrexate: is 7-hydroxy-methotrexate the culprit? *Lancet* (1988) i, 591–2.
49. Parish RC, Johnson V. Effect of salicylate on plasma protein binding of methotrexate. *Clin Pharmacol Ther* (1996) 59, 162.
50. The Committee on Safety of Medicines/Medicines Control Agency. Blood dyscrasias and other ADRs with low-dose methotrexate. *Current Problems* (1997) 23, 12.

Methotrexate + Paracetamol (Acetaminophen)

Paracetamol appears not to interact with methotrexate.

Clinical evidence, mechanism, importance and management

A study in patients with rheumatoid arthritis found that the clearance of oral methotrexate 7.5 to 15 mg was unaffected by the concurrent use of paracetamol.[1] In a study of patients with psoriasis taking methotrexate in doses up to 25 mg weekly, no cases of toxicity occurred in 4 patients also taking paracetamol or indometacin.[2] In one study, methotrexate clearance was reduced by NSAIDs but not by paracetamol, which was included in the study as a control.[3]

1. Tracy TS, Jones DR, Hall SD, Brater DC, Bradley JD, Krohn K. The effect of NSAIDs on methotrexate disposition in patients with rheumatoid arthritis. *Clin Pharmacol Ther* (1990) 47, 138.
2. Baker H. Intermittent high dose oral methotrexate therapy in psoriasis. *Br J Dermatol* (1970) 82, 65–9.
3. Tracy TS, Krohn K, Jones DR, Bradley JD, Hall SD, Brater DC. The effects of salicylate, ibuprofen, and naproxen on the disposition of methotrexate in patients with rheumatoid arthritis. *Eur J Clin Pharmacol* (1992) 42, 121–5.

Methotrexate + Probenecid

Probenecid markedly increases serum methotrexate levels (three to fourfold).

Clinical evidence

The concurrent use of oral or intravenous probenecid 500 mg to 1 g and methotrexate 200 mg/m^2 as an intravenous bolus resulted in serum methotrexate levels in 4 patients that were more than four times higher than in 4 others who had not been given probenecid (400 micrograms/L compared with 90 micrograms/L, measured 24-hours post-dose).[1]

A three to fourfold increase in serum methotrexate levels at 24 hours was also seen in 4 patients given probenecid.[2] Pretreatment with probenecid (500 mg every 6 hours for 5 doses) doubled the serum methotrexate levels of another 4 patients.[3] Severe and life-threatening pancytopenia occurred when a woman taking low-dose methotrexate 7.5 mg weekly for rheumatoid arthritis was given probenecid. She also had renal impairment, hypoalbuminaemia and was taking salsalate (a salicylic acid derivative).[4]

Mechanism

Probenecid inhibits the renal excretion of methotrexate in both *monkeys* and *rats*[5,6] and this probably also happens in man. Changes in the protein binding of methotrexate may also have some part to play.[7] The increased methotrexate levels increase the risk of serious bone marrow depression.

Importance and management

An established and clinically important interaction. A marked increase in both the therapeutic and toxic effects of methotrexate can occur, apparently even with low doses if other risk factors are present.[4] Anticipate the need to reduce the dosage of the methotrexate and monitor the effects well if probenecid is used concurrently, or avoid the combination.

1. Aherne GW, Piall E, Marks V, Mould G, White WF. Prolongation and enhancement of serum methotrexate concentrations by probenecid. *BMJ* (1978) 1, 1097–99.
2. Howell SB, Olshen RA, Rice JA. Effect of probenecid on cerebrospinal fluid methotrexate kinetics. *Clin Pharmacol Ther* (1979) 26, 641–6.
3. Lilly MB, Omura GA. Clinical pharmacology of oral intermediate-dose methotrexate with or without probenecid. *Cancer Chemother Pharmacol* (1985) 15, 220–2.
4. Basin KS, Escalante A, Beardmore TD. Severe pancytopenia in a patient taking low dose methotrexate and probenecid. *J Rheumatol* (1991) 18, 609–10
5. Bourke RS, Chheda G, Bremer A, Watanabe O, Tower DB. Inhibition of renal tubular transport of methotrexate by probenecid. *Cancer Res* (1975) 35, 110–6.
6. Kates RE, Tozer TN, Sorby DL. Increased methotrexate toxicity due to concurrent probenecid administration. *Biochem Pharmacol* (1976) 25, 1485–8.
7. Paxton JW. Interaction of probenecid with the protein binding of methotrexate. *Pharmacology* (1984) 28, 86–9.

Methotrexate + Proton pump inhibitors

The excretion of methotrexate is reported to have been reduced in twelve patients given omeprazole and three patients given lansoprazole. However, similar elevations in methotrexate levels in another patient were independent of omeprazole use. One patient had myalgia and elevated 7-hydroxymethotrexate levels when given methotrexate with pantoprazole.

Clinical evidence

(a) Lansoprazole

In a study in 76 patients with solid tumours treated with high-dose methotrexate infusions (300 mg/m^2 to 12 g/m^2 over 1 to 24 hours), the clearance of methotrexate and its metabolite 7-hydroxymethotrexate was significantly decreased and plasma levels significantly increased in the 3 patients who were also given lansoprazole 30 mg daily.[1]

(b) Omeprazole

In a study in 76 patients with solid tumours treated with high-dose methotrexate infusions (300 mg/m^2 to 12 g/m^2 over 1 to 24 hours), the clearance of methotrexate and its metabolite 7-hydroxymethotrexate was significantly decreased and the plasma levels significantly increased in the 10 patients who had also been given omeprazole 20 to 40 mg daily.[1] A man with Hodgkin's disease developed osteosarcoma and was treated with cyclophosphamide, bleomycin, dactinomycin and methotrexate, followed by folinic acid rescue. He was also taking senna, levothyroxine, omeprazole, baclofen, aciclovir, ferrous sulfate and docusate sodium. During the first cycle of treatment his serum methotrexate levels remained elevated for several days, and suspicion fell on the omeprazole, which was stopped. The patient's serum methotrexate levels then fell rapidly, and during the following three cycles the methotrexate pharmacokinetics were normal.[2] An 11-year-old boy with osteoblastic osteosarcoma was given high-dose methotrexate 15 g as a 4-hour infusion. He was also given omeprazole 20 mg twice daily (for about one week prior to methotrexate), megestrol acetate, sucralfate and folinic acid rescue. Methotrexate elimination was delayed and so further folinic acid was given. When later cycles of methotrexate were given, with ranitidine instead of omeprazole, the elimination of methotrexate was normal. The elimination half-life of the initial phase after the first dose given with omeprazole was 65% longer, when compared with that of the second dose without omeprazole.[3]

In contrast to these findings, a case is reported in which a man with chondroblastic osteosarcoma, who had been taking omeprazole, was treated with high-dose methotrexate 20 g over 6 hours with hydration, urinary alkalinisation and, after 24 hours, folinic acid rescue. The folinic acid dose was adjusted in response to elevated methotrexate levels and omeprazole was stopped. A second dose of methotrexate 2 weeks later, this time without omeprazole, resulted in similar elevated methotrexate levels. Thus the elevated methotrexate levels in this patient could not be attributed to co-administered omeprazole.[4]

(c) Pantoprazole

Severe generalised myalgia occurred in a man taking pantoprazole 20 mg daily after he received intramuscular methotrexate 15 mg weekly. The symptoms subsided and eventually disappeared when the pantoprazole was replaced with ranitidine. The symptoms reappeared in response to rechallenge with pantoprazole, and the AUC of 7-hydroxymethotrexate was found to be increased by about 70%, although the AUC of methotrexate was unchanged.[5]

Mechanism

Proton pump inhibitors may affect renal, and possibly hepatic, clearance of methotrexate by inhibition of methotrexate transporter proteins.[1,6] It has been suggested that omeprazole may inhibit the activity of a hydrogen-ion dependent mechanism in the kidney, on which methotrexate depends for its excretion, so that its loss is diminished.[2] It has also been suggested that the situation with lansoprazole may be similar, but that pantoprazole may differ since at about the pH found in the renal tubules (pH 5), pantoprazole is more slowly activated than omeprazole.[3] However, a case of an interaction with pantoprazole has also been reported.[5]

Importance and management

Information seems to be limited to these few reports and with the exception of one case report, they all found that proton pump inhibitors reduced the clearance of methotrexate. Any changes in methotrexate kinetics are important in terms of the potential for increased toxicity. Further study is required. The authors of one study in which the levels of methotrexate and its active metabolite were increased during the concurrent use of omeprazole or lansoprazole advise against concurrent use.[1] Further, the authors of one report recommend that if omeprazole is necessary for a patient about to receive methotrexate, then omeprazole should be discontinued 4 to 5 days before methotrexate administration.[3] The situation with other proton pump inhibitors may be similar. Ranitidine was found to be a suitable alternative in two of the cases.[3,5] Note that the risks would appear to be most significant with high-dose methotrexate, but the case report involving a 15 mg weekly dose of methotrexate introduces a note of caution in all patients.

1. Joerger M, Huitema ADR, van den Bongard HJGD, Baas P, Schornagel JH, Schellens JHM, Beijnen JH. Determinants of the elimination of methotrexate and 7-hydroxy-methotrexate following high-dose infusional therapy to cancer patients. *Br J Clin Pharmacol* (2005) 62, 71–80.
2. Reid T, Yuen A, Catolico M, Carlson RW. Impact of omeprazole on the plasma clearance of methotrexate. *Cancer Chemother Pharmacol* (1993) 33, 82–4.
3. Beorlegui B, Aldaz A, Ortega A, Aquerreta I, Sierrasesúmega L, Giráldez J. Potential interaction between methotrexate and omeprazole. *Ann Pharmacother* (2000) 34, 1024–7.
4. Whelan J, Hoare D, Leonard P. Omeprazole does not alter plasma methotrexate clearance. *Cancer Chemother Pharmacol* (1999) 44, 88–9.
5. Tröger U, Stötzel B, Martens-Lobenhoffer J, Gollnick H, Meyer FP. Severe myalgia from an interaction between treatments with pantoprazole and methotrexate. *BMJ* (2002) 324, 1497.
6. Breedveld P, Zelcer N, Pluim D, Sönmezer Ö, Tibben MM, Beijnen JH, Schinkel AH, van Tellingen O, Borst P, Schellens JHM. Mechanisms of the pharmacokinetic interaction between methotrexate and benzimidazoles: potential role for breast cancer resistance protein in clinical drug-drug interactions. *Cancer Res* (2004) 64, 5804–11.

Methotrexate + Retinoids

Although the concurrent use of methotrexate with etretinate can be successful, the incidence of severe liver toxicity appears to be considerably increased. The serum levels of methotrexate may be increased by etretinate.

Clinical evidence

A man was given a 48-hour infusion of methotrexate 10 mg every week, for chronic discoid psoriasis but when he was also given **etretinate** 30 mg daily his serum methotrexate levels almost doubled. Concentrations at 12 and 24 hours during the infusion were 0.11 mmol/L, compared with 0.07 and 0.05 mmol/L before the **etretinate**.[1] A later study[2] in psoriatic patients found that those receiving **etretinate** had 38% higher maximum plasma levels of methotrexate, but no difference in clearance or elimination half-life (i.e. no methotrexate accumulation).

Severe toxic hepatitis has been reported in a number of cases when both **etretinate** and methotrexate were given.[3-5] It may take several months to develop.[5] In one clinic, signs of liver toxicity were seen in 2 out of 10 patients given both drugs, but there was no evidence of liver toxicity in 531 patients given methotrexate alone or in 110 patients given **etretinate** alone.[3]

Mechanism

Not understood. The increased incidence of toxic hepatitis may possibly be related to the increased maximum methotrexate plasma levels.

Importance and management

Although methotrexate and etretinate have been used together with success for psoriasis,[6-8] the risk of severe drug-induced hepatitis seems to be very considerably increased. One author says that he has decided not to use this combination in future.[3] Concurrent use should clearly be undertaken with great care. Etretinate has been largely superseded by **acitretin** (a metabolite of etretinate, which has a shorter half-life) but some consider that the combination of methotrexate and **acitretin** should also be avoided.[9]

1. Harrison PV, Peat M, James R, Orrell D. Methotrexate and retinoids in combination for psoriasis. *Lancet* (1987) ii, 512.
2. Larsen FG, Nielsen-Kudsk F, Jakobsen P, Schrøder H, Kragballe K. Interaction of etretinate with methotrexate pharmacokinetics in psoriatic patients. *J Clin Pharmacol* (1990) 30, 802–7.
3. Zachariae H. Dangers of methotrexate/etretinate combination therapy. *Lancet* (1988) i, 422.
4. Zachariae H. Methotrexate and etretinate as concurrent therapies in the treatment of psoriasis. *Arch Dermatol* (1984) 120, 155.
5. Beck H-I, Foged EK. Toxic hepatitis due to combination therapy with methotrexate and etretinate in psoriasis. *Dermatologica* (1983) 167, 94–6.
6. Vanderveen EE, Ellis CN, Campbell JP, Case PC, Voorhees JJ. Methotrexate and etretinate as concurrent therapies in severe psoriasis. *Arch Dermatol* (1982) 118, 660–2.
7. Adams JD. Concurrent methotrexate and etretinate therapy for psoriasis. *Arch Dermatol* (1983) 119, 793.
8. Rosenbaum MM, Roenigk HH. Treatment of generalized pustular psoriasis with etretinate (Ro 10-9359) and methotrexate. *J Am Acad Dermatol* (1984) 10, 357–61.
9. van de Kerkhof PCM. Therapeutic strategies: rotational therapy and combinations. *Clin Exp Dermatol* (2001) 26, 356–61.

Methotrexate + Sulfasalazine

The pharmacokinetics of methotrexate are unaffected by sulfasalazine. Clinical studies in patients with rheumatoid arthritis suggest that the combination of methotrexate and sulfasalazine may not improve therapeutic efficacy and may result in folate-deficiency anaemias.

Clinical evidence, mechanism, importance and management

A study in 15 patients with rheumatoid arthritis found that when sulfasalazine 2 g was given with methotrexate 7.5 mg weekly, the pharmacokinetics of the methotrexate remained unchanged. Similarly, methotrexate did not alter the trough levels of sulfasalazine.[1] Although this study suggests there is no reason to avoid the concurrent use of sulfasalazine and methotrexate, clinical studies in patients with rheumatoid arthritis have found that concurrent use does not significantly increase therapeutic efficacy and seems to increase the development of folate-deficiency anaemias.[2] The results of an *in vitro* study suggest this may be because sulfasalazine is a potent inhibitor of the reduced folate carrier- (RFC-) mediated cellular uptake of methotrexate and folinate.[3] An alternative explanation is that both sulfasalazine and methotrexate promote enhanced adenosine release which may suppress inflammation and the combination of two drugs with the same mechanism of action may not improve the therapeutic response of either.[4]

1. Haagsma CJ, Russel FGM, Vree TB, van Riel PLCM, van de Putte LBA. Combination of methotrexate and sulphasalazine in patients with rheumatoid arthritis: pharmacokinetic analysis and relationship to clinical response. *Br J Clin Pharmacol* (1996) 42, 195–200.
2. O'Dell JR, Leff R, Paulsen G, Haire C, Mallek J, Eckhoff PJ, Fernandez A, Blakely K, Wees S, Stoner J, Hadley S, Felt J, Palmer W, Waytz P, Churchill M, Klassen L, Moore G. Treatment of rheumatoid arthritis with methotrexate and hydroxychloroquine, methotrexate and sulfasalazine, or a combination of the three medications: results of a two-year, randomized, double-blind, placebo-controlled trial. *Arthritis Rheum* (2002) 46, 1164–70.

3. Jansen G, van der Heijden J, Oerlemans R, Lems WF, Ifergan I, Scheper RJ, Assaraf YG, Dijkmans BAC. Sulfasalazine is a potent inhibitor of the reduced folate carrier: implications for combination therapies with methotrexate in rheumatoid arthritis. *Arthritis Rheum* (2004) 50, 2130–9.
4. Cronstein BN. Therapeutic cocktails for rheumatoid arthritis: the mixmaster's guide. *Arthritis Rheum* (2004) 50, 2041–3.

Methotrexate + Tacrolimus

No adverse interaction appears to occur between methotrexate and tacrolimus.

Clinical evidence, mechanism, importance and management

A study in 3 bone marrow transplant patients taking tacrolimus 30 micrograms/kg per day found that low-dose methotrexate (15 mg/m^2 on day 1, and 10 mg/m^2 on days 3, 6 and 11) did not significantly affect clinical care and no interaction of clinical significance was seen.[1] A further study in 40 patients given methotrexate (15 mg/m^2 on day 1 followed by 10 mg/m^2 on days 3, 6 and 11 after a transplant) with 30 micrograms/kg of intravenous tacrolimus daily, similarly found no evidence of an adverse interaction.[2]

1. Dix S, Devine SM, Geller RB, Wingard JR. Re: severe interaction between methotrexate and a macrolide-like antibiotic. *J Natl Cancer Inst* (1995) 87, 1641–2.
2. Wingard JR, Nash RA, Ratanatharathorn V, Fay JW, Klein JL, Przepiorka D, Maher RM, Devine SM, Boswell G, Bekersky I, Fitzsimmons W. Lack of interaction between tacrolimus (FK506) and methotrexate in bone marrow transplant recipients. *Bone Marrow Transplant* (1997) 20, 49–51.

Methotrexate + Theophylline

Methotrexate causes a modest reduction in the theophylline clearance. Theophylline may reduce methotrexate-induced neurotoxicity, but there is the possibility that it may also reduce methotrexate efficacy.

Clinical evidence

(a) Effects on theophylline

The apparent clearance of theophylline (given as oral aminophylline, choline theophyllinate or theophylline) was reduced by 19% in 8 patients with severe, steroid-dependent asthma after 6 weeks of treatment with intramuscular methotrexate 15 mg weekly. Three patients complained of nausea and the theophylline dosage was reduced in one of them as the theophylline level was more than 20 micrograms/mL.[1]

(b) Effects on methotrexate

Four of 6 patients aged 3 to 16 years with acute lymphoblastic leukaemia and high-dose methotrexate-induced neurotoxicity had a complete resolution of their symptoms when they were given a 2.5-mg/kg aminophylline infusion over 1 hour. The other 2 had some improvement in symptoms. One patient also had symptom relief with rapid-release theophylline.[2] Similar results were reported for another child who developed neurotoxicity after receiving high-dose methotrexate. In this case, aminophylline was reported not to alter methotrexate levels.[3] A patient with methotrexate-induced leukoencephalopathy recovered after being given a combination of intravenous folinic acid with intravenous aminophylline 145 mg daily for 7 days.[4]

Mechanism

It is not known why theophylline clearance is altered. Methotrexate neurotoxicity may be linked with increased levels of adenosine. Theophylline is a competitive antagonist for adenosine receptors at serum concentrations within the therapeutic range used in respiratory disease.[2]

Importance and management

The clinical importance of the small reduction in theophylline clearance is uncertain, although it may be worth bearing this in mind in patients maintained at the higher end of the therapeutic levels for theophylline, as they may be more likely to develop toxicity. Aminophylline may reduce methotrexate-induced neurotoxicity, and, although there is some evidence that theophylline does not alter the cytotoxic effects of methotrexate, this requires confirmation.[2] One UK manufacturer of methotrexate (licenced for rheumatoid arthritis) recommends avoiding excessive consumption of caffeine and theophylline-containing drinks, however this recommendation appears to be based on studies and surveys which looked at the effects of caffeine intake in patients taking low-dose, weekly methotrexate for rheumatoid arthritis or psoriasis,[5,6] see 'Methotrexate + Caffeine', p.646.

1. Glynn-Barnhart AM, Erzurum SC, Leff JA, Martin RJ, Cochran JE, Cott GR, Szefler SJ. Effect of low-dose methotrexate on the disposition of glucocorticoids and theophylline. *J Allergy Clin Immunol* (1991) 88, 180–6.
2. Bernini JC, Fort DW, Griener JC, Kane BJ, Chappell WB, Kamen BA. Aminophylline for methotrexate-induced neurotoxicity. *Lancet* (1995) 345, 544–7.
3. Peyriere H, Poiree M, Cociglio M, Margueritte G, Hansel S, Hillaire-Buys D. Reversal of neurologic disturbances related to high-dose methotrexate by aminophylline. *Med Pediatr Oncol* (2001) 36, 662–4.
4. Jaksic W, Veljkovic D, Pozza C, Lewis I. Methotrexate-induced leukoencephalopathy reversed by aminophylline and high-dose folinic acid. *Acta Haematol (Basel)* (2004) 111, 230–2.
5. Metoject (Methotrexate). Medac GmbH. UK Summary of product characteristics, July 2006.
6. Medac UK. Personal Communication, March 2007.

Methotrexate + Urinary alkalinisers

Alkalinisation increases the solubility of methotrexate in the urine and also increases its excretion.

Clinical evidence, mechanism, importance and management

Methotrexate is much more soluble in alkaline than in acid fluids, therefore urinary alkalinisers such as **sodium bicarbonate** and **acetazolamide** (and ample fluids) are often given to patients receiving high-dose methotrexate to prevent the precipitation of methotrexate in the renal tubules, which would cause damage. However alkalinisation also increases the loss of methotrexate in the urine because at high pH values more of the drug exists in the ionised form, which is not readily reabsorbed by the tubules. This increased loss was clearly shown in about 70 patients in whom alkalinisation of the urine (to pH greater than 7) with **sodium bicarbonate** and hydration reduced the serum methotrexate levels at 48 hours by 73% and at 72 hours by 76%.[1] In this instance the interaction was being exploited therapeutically to avoid toxicity. This interaction has also been shown by others.[2] The possible consequences should be recognised if concurrent use is undertaken.

For the effects of acidic urine on methotrexate excretion see 'Methotrexate + Ascorbic acid (Vitamin C)', p.646.

1. Nirenberg A, Mosende C, Mehta BM, Gisolfi AL, Rosen G. High dose methotrexate with citrovorum factor rescue: predictive value of serum methotrexate concentrations and corrective measures to avert toxicity. *Cancer Treat Rep* (1977) 61, 779–83.
2. Sand TE, Jacobsen S. Effect of urine pH and flow on renal clearance of methotrexate. *Eur J Clin Pharmacol* (1981) 19, 453–6.

Mitomycin + Doxorubicin

An increased incidence of cardiotoxicity has been seen in patients treated with mitomycin who were previously or simultaneously given doxorubicin.

Clinical evidence, mechanism, importance and management

Fourteen out of 91 (15.3%) patients with advanced breast cancer who had previously failed to respond to doxorubicin developed congestive heart failure when later treated with a combination of intravenous mitomycin 20 mg/m^2 every 4 to 6 weeks and megestrol acetate 160 mg daily. None of them had any pre-existing heart disease. This compares with only 3 out of 89 (3.5%) of another group of patients who had received doxorubicin but no mitomycin. The maximum cumulative dose of doxorubicin was 450 mg/m^2 and all of the patients had also been given cyclophosphamide. Some of them also received other drugs during the doxorubicin phase of treatment. These included fluorouracil, methotrexate, tegafur and vincristine. The heart failure developed slowly (mean time of 8.5 months) compared with those in the control group (1.5 months).[1]

Other studies have also suggested that the combination of mitomycin and doxorubicin may increase cardiotoxicity.[2,3] In a randomised study, 2 of 39 patients treated with doxorubicin 45 mg/m^2 once every 3 weeks and mitomycin 10 mg/m^2 once every 6 weeks developed cardiomyopathy, compared with none of 42 patients treated with doxorubicin 75 mg/m^2 once every 3 weeks alone.[4]

The reasons for this apparent synergistic cardiotoxicity are not understood, but it may be related to free radical generation. This interaction is not established with certainty. The authors of one report suggest that its incidence is probably less than 10%, and that it does not occur until a cumulative mitomycin dose of 30 mg/m² or more.[3] It may be prudent to monitor patients treated with mitomycin closely if they have previously received anthracycline drugs.[1] Note that the combination (FAM, fluorouracil, doxorubicin and mitomycin) has been widely used for gastric cancer.

1. Buzdar AU, Legha SS, Tashima CK, Hortobagyi GN, Yap HY, Krutchik AN, Luna MA, Blumenschein GR. Adriamycin and mitomycin C: possible synergistic cardiotoxicity. *Cancer Treat Rep* (1978) 62, 1005–8.
2. Villani F, Comazzi R, Lacaita G, Guindani A, Genitoni V, Volonterio A, Brambilla MC. Possible enhancement of the cardiotoxicity of doxorubicin when combined with mitomycin C. *Med Oncol Tumor Pharmacother* (1985) 2, 93–7.
3. Verweij J, Funke-Küpper AJ, Teule GJJ, Pinedo HM. A prospective study on the dose dependency of cardiotoxicity induced by mitomycin C. *Med Oncol Tumor Pharmacother* (1988) 5, 159–63.
4. Andersson M, Daugaard S, von der Maase H, Mouridsen HT. Doxorubicin versus mitomycin versus doxorubicin plus mitomycin in advanced breast cancer: a randomized study. *Cancer Treat Rep* (1986) 70, 1181–6.

Mitomycin + Fluorouracil

Serious and potentially life-threatening intravascular haemolysis and renal failure may develop rarely after the long-term use of mitomycin and fluorouracil.

Clinical evidence, mechanism, importance and management

Two patients developed chronic haemolysis and progressive renal impairment after long-term treatment with mitomycin and fluorouracil following partial or total gastrectomy for gastric cancer. The haemolysis was exacerbated by blood transfusions. The authors of the report[1] say that these two cases are "... the extreme of a syndrome we are finding increasingly in our pretransfusion patients, after 6 months or more of maintenance therapy." A similar syndrome occurred in 2 other patients, one with gastric carcinoma and one without, when treated with these two drugs.[2,3] This severe and potentially fatal syndrome has also been seen with mitomycin alone.[4,5] Its incidence is not known, but note that a regimen of fluorouracil, doxorubicin and mitomycin (FAM) has been widely used in gastric cancer and there are only a few reports of this syndrome. The authors of one report suggest that the drugs should be stopped at the first sign of intravascular haemolysis, persistent proteinuria and rising urea levels (two consecutive values above 8 mmol/L).[1] The syndrome has also occurred when tamoxifen was given to patients who had been treated with mitomycin, see 'Mitomycin + Tamoxifen', below.

1. Jones BG, Fielding JW, Newman CE, Howell A, Brookes VS. Intravascular haemolysis and renal impairment after blood transfusion in two patients on long-term 5-fluorouracil and mitomycin-C. *Lancet* (1980) i, 1275–7.
2. Krauss S, Sonoda T, Solomon A. Treatment of advanced gastrointestinal carcinoma with 5-fluorouracil and mitomycin C. *Cancer* (1979) 43, 1598–1603.
3. Lempert KD. Haemolysis and renal impairment syndrome in patients on 5-fluorouracil and mitomycin-C. *Lancet* (1980) ii, 369–70.
4. Rumpf KW, Reiger J, Lankisch PG, von Heyden HW, Nagel GA, Scheler F. Mitomycin-induced haemolysis and renal failure. *Lancet* (1980) ii, 1037–8.
5. Schiebe ME, Hoffmann W, Belka C, Bamberg M. Mitomycin C-related hemolytic uremic syndrome in cancer patients. *Anticancer Drugs* (1998) 9, 433–5.

Mitomycin + Furosemide

A study in 5 patients with advanced solid tumours treated with mitomycin C 10 mg/m² showed that furosemide given as a 40 mg intravenous bolus either 120 or 200 minutes after the mitomycin had no effect on its pharmacokinetics.[1]

1. Verweij J, Kerpel-Fronius S, Stuurman M, de Vries J, Pinedo HM. Absence of interaction between furosemide and mitomycin C. *Cancer Chemother Pharmacol* (1987) 19, 84–6.

Mitomycin + Tamoxifen

Haemolytic anaemia, thrombocytopenia and renal impairment, leading to potentially fatal haemolytic uraemic syndrome, has occurred in a few patients given tamoxifen with, or shortly after, mitomycin.

Clinical evidence, mechanism, importance and management

After a woman with metastatic breast cancer who had previously been treated with mitomycin, mitoxantrone and methotrexate, developed rapidly fatal acute renal failure 21 days after starting tamoxifen, a retrospective survey was undertaken of other patients who had also received all of these drugs.[1] Nine out of 94 (9.6%) patients developed anaemia, thrombocytopenia and renal impairment, compared with none in another group of 45 patients not given tamoxifen. One of the 9 died from renal failure. The doses used were mitomycin 7 mg/m² intravenously every 42 days for four courses; mitoxantrone 7 mg/m² and methotrexate 35 mg/m² intravenously every 21 days for eight courses; tamoxifen 20 mg orally daily.[1] A few other reports describe cases of haemolytic uraemic syndrome in patients given mitomycin and tamoxifen.[2-4]

The authors of the first study suggested that this haemolytic uraemic syndrome was due to a combination of subclinical endothelial damage induced by mitomycin C, and a thrombotic effect on platelets caused by tamoxifen.[1] They advise the avoidance of tamoxifen with or shortly after mitomycin C unless concurrent use can be carefully monitored. Erythropoietin may be useful in managing the syndrome.[4] This syndrome has also occurred rarely with mitomycin alone, or when combined with fluorouracil, see 'Mitomycin + Fluorouracil', above.

1. Montes A, Powles TJ, O'Brien MER, Ashley SE, Luckit J, Treleaven J. A toxic interaction between mitomycin C and tamoxifen causing the haemolytic uraemic syndrome. *Eur J Cancer* (1993) 29A, 1854–7.
2. Ellis PA, Luckitt J, Treleaven J, Smith IE. Haemolytic uraemic syndrome in a patient with lung cancer: further evidence for a toxic interaction between mitomycin-C and tamoxifen. *Clin Oncol (R Coll Radiol)* (1996) 8, 402–3.
3. Arola O, Aho H, Asola M, Kauppila M, Nikkanen V, Voipio-Pulkki LM. Hemolyyttis-ureeminen oireyhytmä-mitomysiinihoidon vakava komplikaatio. *Duodecim* (1997) 113, 1923–9.
4. O'Brien MER, Casey S, Treleaven J, Powles TJ. Use of erythropoietin in the management of the haemolytic uraemic syndrome induced by mitomycin C/tamoxifen. *Eur J Cancer* (1994) 30A, 894–5.

Mitotane + Spironolactone

In an isolated report, the effects of mitotane appeared to be inhibited by spironolactone in a patient with Cushing's disease.

Clinical evidence, mechanism, importance and management

A woman with Cushing's disease taking chlorpropamide, digoxin and furosemide was given spironolactone 50 mg four times daily to control hypokalaemia. She was also given mitotane 3 g daily for 5 months to control the elevated cortisol levels, but this had no effect.[1] When an interaction was suspected (on the basis of *animal* studies[1]) it was decided to withdraw the spironolactone, whereupon severe nausea and profuse diarrhoea developed within 24 to 48 hours, suggesting mitotane toxicity. This subsided, and then redeveloped when the mitotane was stopped, and then restarted a week later. The mechanism of this apparent interaction is not understood. It would seem that mitotane can become ineffective in the management of Cushing's syndrome in the presence of spironolactone.

1. Wortsman J, Soler NG. Mitotane. Spironolactone antagonism in Cushing's syndrome. *JAMA* (1977) 238, 2527.

Nitrosoureas + Cimetidine

The bone marrow depressant effects of carmustine and lomustine are possibly increased by cimetidine.

Clinical evidence

Nine patients treated with **carmustine** 80 mg/m² daily for 3 days, cimetidine 300 mg four times daily for 1 to 4 weeks, steroids, and cranial irradiation over 6 weeks, demonstrated marked leucopenia during the first cycle. Bone marrow aspirates confirmed the marked decrease in granulocytic elements in 2 patients. In comparison, 31 patients treated similarly, but without cimetidine, had no significant white cell depression.[1,2]

Neutropenia was found in a man taking regular cimetidine, phenytoin, phenobarbital, and dexamethasone, 53 days after he was given **lomustine** 120 mg, and 16 days after he was given **lomustine** 160 mg. The cimetidine was discontinued and the neutropenia rapidly reversed within 14 days. The neutrophil nadir from the **lomustine** 160 mg dose occurred after a further 16 to 19 days and was much less severe.[3]

Mechanism

Studies in *animals* suggest that cimetidine impairs the clearance of carmustine.[4] Cimetidine has also increased the levels or toxicity of some other antineoplastics, see 'Cyclophosphamide + H_2-receptor antagonists', p.626, 'Anthracyclines; Epirubicin + Cimetidine', p.613, and 'Fluorouracil + H_2-receptor antagonists', p.633.

Importance and management

Information appears to be limited to the reports cited, but it seems to be an established reaction. Patients given both drugs should be closely monitored for changes in blood cell counts. Because of its immunomodulatory effects, cimetidine has been used as an adjunct to carmustine in the treatment of malignant melanoma, but this did not improve outcomes.[5]

1. Selker RG, Moore P, LoDolce D. Bone-marrow depression with cimetidine plus carmustine. *N Engl J Med* (1978) 299, 834.
2. Volkin RL, Shadduck RK, Winkelstein A, Zeigler ZR, Selker RG. Potentiation of carmustine-cranial irradiation-induced myelosuppression by cimetidine. *Arch Intern Med* (1982) 142, 243–5.
3. Hess WA, Kornblith PL. Combination of lomustine and cimetidine in the treatment of a patient with malignant glioblastoma: a case report. *Cancer Treat Rep* (1985) 69, 733.
4. Dorr RT, Soble MJ. H_2-Antagonists and carmustine. *J Cancer Res Clin Oncol* (1989) 115, 41–6.
5. Morton RF, Creagan ET, Schaid DJ, Kardinal CG, McCormack GW, McHale MS, Wiesenfeld M. Phase II trial of recombinant leukocyte A interferon (IFN-α2A) plus 1,3-bis(2-chloroethyl)-1-nitrosourea (BCNU) and the combination cimetidine with BCNU in patients with disseminated malignant melanoma. *Am J Clin Oncol* (1991) 14, 152–5.

Nitrosoureas; Lomustine + Theophylline

A single case report describes thrombocytopenia and bleeding attributed to the concurrent use of lomustine and theophylline.

Clinical evidence, mechanism, importance and management

An asthmatic woman taking theophylline and treated for medulloblastoma with lomustine, prednisone and vincristine, developed severe nose bleeding and thrombocytopenia 3 weeks after the third cycle of chemotherapy.[1] This was attributed to the concurrent use of lomustine and theophylline. The suggested explanation for this effect is that theophylline inhibited the activity of phosphodiesterase within the platelets, thereby increasing cyclic AMP levels and disrupting normal platelet function, which seems to be supported by an experimental study,[2] while lomustine causes thrombocytopenia. What is known is far too limited to act as more than a warning of the possibility of increased thrombocytopenia during the concurrent use of theophylline and lomustine.

1. Zeltzer PM, Feig SA. Theophylline-induced lomustine toxicity. *Lancet* (1979) ii, 960–1.
2. DeWys WD, Bathina S. Synergistic anti-tumour effect of cyclic AMP elevation (induced by theophylline) and cytotoxic drug treatment. *Proc Am Assoc Cancer Res* (1978) 19, 104.

Pemetrexed + Miscellaneous

Aspirin and ibuprofen had little effect on pemetrexed clearance in patients with normal renal function, but they, and other short-acting NSAIDs, should be withheld in patients with mild to moderate renal function. NSAIDs with longer half-lives such as piroxicam should be withheld in all patients. Caution is recommended if pemetrexed is given with nephrotoxic drugs such as the aminoglycosides, loop diuretics, and ciclosporin, and drugs that are secreted by the renal tubules, such as probenecid and penicillin.

Clinical evidence, mechanism, importance and management

(a) Cisplatin

The US manufacturers state that there is no pharmacokinetic interaction between pemetrexed and cisplatin,[1] but there is the possibility that cisplatin-induced nephrotoxicity could decrease pemetrexed clearance and increase its toxicity.[1,2] However, it should be noted that the use of pemetrexed with cisplatin is indicated for mesothelioma.[1,2]

(b) Folic acid and vitamin B_{12}

Oral folic acid and intramuscular vitamin B_{12} has been reported to not alter the pharmacokinetics of pemetrexed[1] and because these vitamins were found to decrease pemetrexed toxicity, it is recommended that all patients receiving pemetrexed should receive folic acid and B_{12} supplements.[1,2]

(c) Nephrotoxic drugs

The manufacturers consider that the concurrent use of nephrotoxic drugs could potentially decrease the clearance of pemetrexed and therefore increase its toxicity.[1,2] In the UK, the manufacturer specifically mentions **aminoglycosides**, **loop diuretics**, **platinum compounds** (see also (a) cisplatin above) and **ciclosporin**, and recommends caution with combined use, and, if necessary, close monitoring of creatinine clearance.[2]

(d) NSAIDs and Aspirin

In a study in 27 patients with advanced cancer, aspirin 325 mg every 6 hours for 9 doses, starting 2 days before and with the last dose 1 hour before an infusion of pemetrexed 500 mg/m^2, did not alter the pharmacokinetics of pemetrexed.[3] In a similar study **ibuprofen** 400 mg four times daily caused a slight 16% decrease in the clearance of pemetrexed, and increased its AUC by 20%.[3] The effects of higher doses of aspirin or **ibuprofen** are not known, but they could be greater. Because of this, in patients with normal renal function, the manufacturer recommends caution when pemetrexed is used with high doses of NSAIDs (e.g. **ibuprofen** greater than 1.6 g daily) or high-dose aspirin (greater than 1.3 g daily).[2] Moreover, in patients with mild to moderate renal impairment, the manufacturer recommends that NSAIDs and higher dose aspirin be avoided for 2 days before, the day of, and for 2 days after pemetrexed use.[1,2]

Because of the lack of data on pemetrexed clearance with NSAIDs with longer half-lives [e.g. **piroxicam**], the manufacturer recommends that all patients taking these NSAIDs stop them for 5 days before pemetrexed, on the day, and for at least 2 days afterwards.[1,2]

(e) Probenecid and other drugs secreted by the renal tubules

It is possible that drugs that are secreted by the renal tubules (e.g. probenecid, **penicillin**) could decrease the clearance of pemetrexed, which is also secreted by this mechanism. For this reason, the manufacturer recommends caution with combined use, and, if necessary, close monitoring of creatinine clearance.[2]

1. Alimta (Pemetrexed). Eli Lilly and Company. US Prescribing information, February 2007.
2. Alimta (Pemetrexed disodium). Eli Lilly and Company Ltd. UK Summary of product characteristics, March 2007.
3. Sweeney CJ, Takimoto CH, Latz JE, Baker SD, Murry DJ, Krull JH, Fife K, Battiato L, Cleverly A, Chaudhary AK, Chaudhuri T, Sandler A, Mita AC, Rowinsky EK. Two drug interaction studies evaluating the pharmacokinetics and toxicity of pemetrexed when coadministered with aspirin or ibuprofen in patients with advanced cancer. *Clin Cancer Res* (2006) 12, 536–42.

Procarbazine + Antiepileptics

The use of enzyme-inducing antiepileptics seems to increase the risk of procarbazine hypersensitivity reactions.

Clinical evidence, mechanism, importance and management

A study of the records of 83 patients with primary brain tumours who were treated with procarbazine between 1981 and 1996 showed that 20 of them had procarbazine hypersensitivity reactions. Of these 20, 95% had also taken antiepileptics compared with 71% of those not developing hypersensitivity. In addition, there was a significant dose-response association between the development of hypersensitivity reactions and the serum levels of the antiepileptics used (**phenytoin**, **phenobarbital**, or **carbamazepine**, with or without valproate).[1] It was suggested that the enzyme-inducing antiepileptics may increase the metabolism of procarbazine to metabolites causing hypersensitivity. This may also explain why the incidence of procarbazine-induced hypersensitivity is higher in patients with brain tumours, who commonly receive seizure-prophylaxis therapy.[1]

1. Lehmann DF, Hurteau TE, Newman N, Coyle TE. Anticonvulsant usage is associated with an increased risk of procarbazine hypersensitivity reactions in patients with brain tumours. *Clin Pharmacol Ther* (1997) 62, 225–9.

Procarbazine + Chlormethine (Mechlorethamine)

A report on two patients suggests that the use of high doses of procarbazine with chlormethine may result in neurological toxicity.

Clinical evidence, mechanism, importance and management

Two patients with acute myelogenous leukaemia admitted to hospital for marrow transplantation and who were given *high doses* of procarbazine 12.5 and 15 mg/kg and chlormethine 0.75 and 1 mg/kg on the same day became lethargic, somnolent and disorientated for about a week. Two other patients who received the same drugs on different days had no neurological complications. In addition, only one of 45 patients treated with high-dose procarbazine alone had similar persistent lethargy. Although no interaction has been proved, the authors suggest that the chlormethine may have enhanced the neurotoxic effects of the procarbazine, and advise that it would be prudent to avoid high-doses of these drugs on the same day.[1] Note that lower doses of the combination have been widely used in the MOPP regimen (mechlorethamine, vincristine, procarbazine, and prednisone) without problems.

1. Weiss GB, Weiden PL, Thomas ED. Central nervous system disturbances after combined administration of procarbazine and mechlorethamine. *Cancer Treat Rep* (1977) 61, 1713–14.

Procarbazine + Miscellaneous

The effects of drugs that can cause CNS depression or lower blood pressure may possibly be increased by the presence of procarbazine.

Clinical evidence, mechanism, importance and management

(a) Antihypertensives

In one early clinical study, 4 of 48 patients developed postural hypotension when treated with procarbazine. In addition, another patient with hypertension (180/110 mmHg) had a progressive fall in blood pressure (to 110/80 mmHg) while being treated with procarbazine.[1] Additive hypotensive effects may therefore be expected if procarbazine is given to patients taking antihypertensives.

(b) CNS depressants

Procarbazine can cause CNS depression ranging from mild drowsiness to profound stupor. In early clinical studies, the incidence was variously reported as 8%, 14%, and 31% (when combined with prochlorperazine, see also (c) below).[1-3] Additive CNS depression may therefore be expected if other drugs possessing CNS-depressant activity are given with procarbazine.

(c) Prochlorperazine

An isolated report describes an acute dystonic reaction (difficulty in speaking or moving, intermittent contractions of muscles on the left side of the neck) in a patient taking procarbazine with prochlorperazine.[4] Prochlorperazine was thought to have contributed to the sedative effects of procarbazine in one early clinical study.[3]

1. Samuels ML, Leary WV, Alexanian R, Howe CD, Frei E. Clinical trials with N-isopropyl-α-(2-methylhydrazino)-p-toluamide hydrochloride in malignant lymphoma and other disseminated neoplasia. *Cancer* (1967) 20. 1187–94.
2. Stolinsky DC, Solomon J, Pugh RP, Stevens AR, Jacobs EM, Irwin LE, Wood DA, Steinfeld JL, Bateman JR. Clinical experience with procarbazine in Hodgkin's disease, reticulum cell sarcoma, and lymphosarcoma. *Cancer* (1970) 26, 984–90.
3. Brunner KW, Young CW. A methylhydrazine derivative in Hodgkin's disease and other malignant neoplasms: therapeutic and toxic effects studied in 51 patients. *Ann Intern Med* (1965) 63, 69–86.
4. Poster DS. Procarbazine-prochlorperazine interaction: an underreported phenomenon. *J Med* (1978) 9, 519–24.

Procarbazine + Sympathomimetics

Despite warnings, it seems doubtful that the weak MAO-inhibitory properties of procarbazine can under normal circumstances cause a hypertensive reaction with tyramine or other sympathomimetics.

Clinical evidence, mechanism, importance and management

The manufacturers say that procarbazine is a weak inhibitor of MAO and therefore predict that interactions with certain foods and drugs may occur in rare cases.[1] This is apparently based on the results of *animal* experiments, which show that the monoamine oxidase inhibitory properties of procarbazine are weaker than pheniprazine.[2] There seem to be no formal reports of hypertensive reactions in patients taking procarbazine who have eaten tyramine-containing foods (e.g. cheese) or after using indirectly-acting sympathomimetic amines (e.g. **phenylpropanolamine**, **amfetamines**, etc.). The only account traced is purely anecdotal and unconfirmed: "... I recall one patient who described vividly reactions to wine and chicken livers which had occurred while he was taking MOPP chemotherapy (mechlorethamine, vincristine, procarbazine, and prednisone) several years earlier. Since he had not been forewarned, the reactions had been a frightening experience."[3] A practical way to deal with this interaction problem has been suggested by a practitioner in an Oncology unit:[3] patients taking procarbazine should ideally be given a list of the potentially interacting foodstuffs (see 'MAOIs or RIMAs + Tyramine-rich foods', p.1153), with a warning about the nature of the possible reaction but also with the advice that it very rarely occurs. The foods may continue to be eaten, but patients should start with small quantities to ensure that they still agree with them. Those taking MOPP should also be told that any reaction is most likely to occur during the second week of a 14-day course of treatment with procarbazine, and during the week after it has been stopped.

1. Procarbazine Capsules (Procarbazine hydrochloride). Cambridge Laboratories. UK Summary of product characteristics, August 2006.
2. De Vita VT, Hahn MA, Oliverio VT. Monoamine oxidase inhibition by a new carcinostatic agent. N-isopropyl-α-(2-methylhydrazino)-p-toluamide (MIH). *Proc Soc Exp Biol Med* (1965) 120, 561–5.
3. Maxwell MB. Reexamining the dietary restrictions with procarbazine (an MAOI). *Cancer Nurs* (1980) 3, 451–7.

Raltitrexed + Miscellaneous

On theoretical grounds the manufacturers say that folinic acid and folic acid may possibly interfere with the action of raltitrexed. Warfarin and NSAIDs do not appear to interact with raltitrexed.

Clinical evidence, mechanism, importance and management

(a) Folinates

The antimetabolite, raltitrexed, is a folate analogue and is a potent and specific inhibitor of the enzyme thymidylate synthase. Inhibition of this enzyme ultimately interferes with the synthesis of deoxyribonucleic acid (DNA) leading to cell death. The intracellular polyglutamation of raltitrexed leads to the formation within cells of even more potent inhibitors of thymidylate synthase. Folate (methylene tetrahydrofolate) is a co-factor required by thymidylate synthase and therefore theoretically folinic acid or folic acid may interfere with the action of raltitrexed. Clinical interaction studies have not yet been undertaken to confirm these predicted interactions.[1]

(b) Warfarin, NSAIDs

The manufacturers say that no specific clinical interaction studies have been conducted but a review of the clinical study database did not reveal any evidence of interactions between raltitrexed and warfarin, NSAIDs or other drugs.[1]

1. Tomudex (Raltitrexed). AstraZeneca UK Ltd. UK Summary of product characteristics, October 2001.

Sorafenib + Miscellaneous

Sorafenib levels may be reduced by inhibitors of CYP3A4. Antacids may reduce the absorption of sorafenib. Sorafenib may increase docetaxel and doxorubicin levels. Isolated cases of raised INRs and bleeding have been reported in patients taking warfarin with sorafenib.

Clinical evidence, mechanism, importance and management

(a) Cytochrome P450 inducers

A 5 day course of **rifampicin** (**rifampin**) reduced the AUC of a single dose of sorafenib by an average of 37%. Other inducers of the cytochrome P450 isoenzyme CYP3A4, such as **St John's wort**, **carbamazepine**, **phenytoin**, **phenobarbital** and **dexamethasone**, may also reduce sorafenib levels.[1]

(b) Docetaxel

Sorafenib 200 mg or 400 mg twice daily on days 2 to 19 of a 21-day cycle increased the AUC and maximum concentration of docetaxel 75 or

100 mg/m^2 every 21 days were increased by 36 to 80%, and 16 to 32%, respectively.[1] The manufacturer therefore recommends caution with concurrent use of these drugs.[1]

(c) Doxorubicin

A 21% increase in the AUC of doxorubicin occurred when it was given with sorafenib. The manufacturers therefore recommend caution with concurrent use of these drugs.[1,2]

(d) Drugs that affect gastrointestinal pH

Drugs, such as **antacids**, **H_2-receptor antagonists** or **proton pump inhibitors**, that raise the pH of the gastrointestinal tract may reduce the solubility of sorafenib, although this has not been specifically studied. The manufacturers therefore recommend avoiding chronic treatment with these drugs during treatment with sorafenib as they cannot exclude the possibility that these drugs will reduce sorafenib efficacy.[1]

(e) Warfarin

A study in patients given sorafenib and taking warfarin found that the INR did not differ between those patients taking sorafenib and those not taking sorafenib, despite previous *in vitro* evidence that sorafenib inhibits the cytochrome P450 isoenzyme CYP2C9, the main isoenzyme involved in the metabolism of warfarin.

However, raised INRs and infrequent bleeding have been reported in patients taking warfarin with sorafenib. The manufacturers therefore advise close monitoring of the INR patients taking these drugs together.[1,2]

1. Nexavar (Sorafenib tosylate). Bayer plc. UK Summary of product characteristics, January 2007.
2. Nexavar (Sorafenib tosylate). Bayer Pharmaceuticals Corp. US Prescribing information, February 2007.

Streptozocin + Phenytoin

A single case report indicates that phenytoin can reduce or abolish the effects of streptozocin.

Clinical evidence, mechanism, importance and management

A patient with an organic hypoglycaemic syndrome, due to a metastatic apud cell carcinoma of the pancreas, who was taking streptozocin 2 g daily with phenytoin 400 mg daily for 4 days, failed to show the expected response until the phenytoin was withdrawn.[1] It would seem that the phenytoin inhibited the effects of the streptozocin by some mechanism as yet unknown. Although this is an isolated case report its authors recommend that concurrent use should be avoided.

1. Koranyi L, Gero L. Influence of diphenylhydantoin on the effect of streptozotocin. *BMJ* (1979) 1, 127.

Tamoxifen + Aromatase inhibitors

Aminoglutethimide, but not anastrozole, exemestane, or letrozole, markedly increases tamoxifen clearance and reduces its serum levels. Tamoxifen modestly reduces anastrozole and letrozole levels, but it does not alter aminoglutethimide levels, or exemestane levels and effects.

Clinical evidence

(a) Effect on tamoxifen

In 6 menopausal women with breast cancer **aminoglutethimide** 250 mg four times daily for 6 weeks markedly reduced the serum levels of tamoxifen 20 to 80 mg daily and most of its metabolites. The clearance of the tamoxifen was increased by 3.2-fold and the tamoxifen AUC was reduced by 73% (range 56 to 80%).[1] Conversely, the concurrent use of **anastrozole** 1 mg daily for 28 days did not affect the pharmacokinetics of tamoxifen in a double-blind, placebo-controlled study in 34 women with breast cancer who had been taking tamoxifen 20 mg daily for at least 10 weeks.[2] Similarly, **letrozole** 2.5 mg daily had no effect on the pharmacokinetics of tamoxifen in 18 women taking tamoxifen 20 mg daily.[3] Further, a study in 32 women clinically disease-free following primary treatment for breast cancer and who had been taking tamoxifen 20 mg daily for at least 4 months found that **exemestane** 25 mg daily for 8 weeks had no effect on the pharmacokinetics of tamoxifen or the formation of tamoxifen metabolites and the combination was well-tolerated.[4]

(b) Effect on aromatase inhibitors

Tamoxifen 20 to 80 mg daily did not alter the pharmacokinetics of **aminoglutethimide** 250 mg four times daily.[1] In a pilot study, 18 postmenopausal women with breast cancer were given **exemestane** 25 mg daily for 14 days, then **exemestane** and tamoxifen 20 mg daily for 4 weeks. Tamoxifen did not affect the pharmacokinetics (plasma levels) or pharmacodynamics (estrone, estrone sulfate and estradiol suppression) of **exemestane** and the combination was well-tolerated.[5] In 12 women **letrozole** levels were reduced by 38% (range 0 to 70%) 6 weeks after tamoxifen 20 mg daily was added to **letrozole** 2.5 mg daily. This reduction persisted after 4 to 8 months; however, the estradiol suppressant effects of **letrozole** did not appear to be affected.[6] Similarly, although the estradiol suppressant effects of **anastrozole** 1 mg daily did not appear to be affected by tamoxifen 20 mg daily in two studies,[2,7] in one of these studies, **anastrozole** levels were decreased by 27% by tamoxifen.[7]

Mechanism

It is likely that aminoglutethimide, an enzyme inducer, increases the metabolism of the tamoxifen by the liver, thereby increasing its loss from the body. It is not known how tamoxifen reduces anastrozole and letrozole levels, although it may also be via enzyme induction.[6]

Importance and mechanism

Theoretically, the combination of an oestrogen antagonist such as tamoxifen and an aromatase inhibitor should provide additional benefit in the treatment of hormone-dependent cancers, however, no clinical studies have yet found this to be so. The pharmacokinetic interactions described above may partly explain this. It may be preferable to use these drugs sequentially rather than concurrently.[6]

1. Lien EA, Anker G, Lønning PE, Solheim E, Ueland PM. Decreased serum concentrations of tamoxifen and its metabolites induced by aminoglutethimide. *Cancer Res* (1990) 50, 5851–7.
2. Dowsett M, Tobias JS, Howell A, Blackman GM, Welch H, King N, Ponzone R, von Euler M, Baum M. The effect of anastrozole on the pharmacokinetics of tamoxifen in post-menopausal women with early breast cancer. *Br J Cancer* (1999) 79, 311–15.
3. Ingle JN, Suman VJ, Johnson PA, Krook JE, Mailliard JA, Wheeler RH, Loprinzi CL, Perez EA, Jordan VC, Dowsett M. Evaluation of tamoxifen plus letrozole with assessment of pharmacokinetic interaction in postmenopausal women with metastatic breast cancer. *Clin Cancer Res* (1999) 5, 1642–9.
4. Hutson PR, Love RR, Havighurst TC, Rogers E, Cleary JF. Effect of exemestane on tamoxifen pharmacokinetics in postmenopausal women treated for breast cancer. *Clin Cancer Res* (2005) 11, 8722–7.
5. Rivera E, Valero V, Francis D, Asnis AG, Schaaf LJ, Duncan B, Hortobagyi GN. Pilot study evaluating the pharmacokinetics, pharmacodynamics, and safety of the combination of exemestane and tamoxifen. *Clin Cancer Res* (2004) 10, 1943–8.
6. Dowsett M, Pfister C, Johnston SRD, Miles DW, Houston SJ, Verbeek JA, Gundacker H, Sioufi A, Smith IE. Impact of tamoxifen on the pharmacokinetics and endocrine effects of the aromatase inhibitor letrozole in postmenopausal women with breast cancer. *Clin Cancer Res* (1999) 5, 2238–43.
7. Dowsett M, on behalf of the ATAC Trialists' Group. Pharmacokinetics of 'Arimidex' and tamoxifen alone and in combination in the ATAC adjuvant breast cancer trial. *Breast Cancer Res Treat* (2000) 64, 64.

Tamoxifen and other anti-oestrogens + Herbal medicines

Indirect evidence hints at the possibility that some herbal medicines that possess oestrogenic activity may oppose the actions of anti-oestrogens, such as tamoxifen, used in the treatment of breast cancer.

Clinical evidence, mechanism, importance and management

A letter in the Medical Journal of Australia[1] draws attention to fact that some women with breast cancer receiving chemotherapy or hormone antagonists who develop menopausal symptoms have found relief from hot flushes by taking a Chinese herb **'dong quai'** (or **'danggui'** root), which has been identified as *Angelica sinensis*. A possible explanation is that this and some other herbs (**vitex berry** (***Agnus castus***), **hops flower** (**lupulus**), **ginseng root**, **black cohosh** (**cimicifuga**)) have significant oestrogen-binding activity and physiological oestrogenic actions.[2] The concern expressed in the letter is that the oestrogenic activity of these herbs might directly stimulate breast cancer growth and oppose the actions of competitive oestrogen receptor antagonists such as tamoxifen. Consider also, 'Tamoxifen and other anti-oestrogens + HRT', p.659.

Although this is largely speculative at the moment, the writer of the letter suggests that such herbal medicines are undesirable in patients with breast cancer. In addition to tamoxifen, there are now a number of other drugs used for breast cancer that in one way or another reduce the stimulation of oestrogen receptors (**anastrozole**, **exemestane**, **letrozole**, **toremifene**). More study is needed.

1. Boyle FM. Adverse interaction of herbal medicine with breast cancer treatment. *Med J Aust* (1997) 167, 286.
2. Eagon CL, Elm MS, Teepe AG, Eagon PK. Medicinal botanicals: estrogenicity in rat uterus and liver. *Proc Am Assoc Cancer Res* (1997) 38, 293.

Tamoxifen and other anti-oestrogens + HRT

Contrary to expectations HRT may not increase the risk of recurrent breast cancer in women taking tamoxifen. HRT is reported to oppose the lipid-lowering effects of tamoxifen.

Clinical evidence, mechanism, importance and management

(a) Anti-oestrogenic effects

In a cohort study of the use of HRT in the management of menopausal symptoms in women treated for breast cancer, the use of continuous combined HRT (an oestrogen plus a progestogen) was not associated with an increased risk of breast cancer recurrence in women taking tamoxifen.[1] This is of interest since HRT might be expected to oppose the effects of anti-oestrogens such as tamoxifen in the treatment and prevention of breast cancer. For this reason, HRT and other oestrogens are often considered to be contraindicated in women taking anti-oestrogens such as **anastrozole**,[2] **exemestane**,[3,4] **letrozole**, tamoxifen and **toremifene** (see also 'Tamoxifen and other anti-oestrogens + Herbal medicines', p.658). The cohort study described[1] suggests that there need not be a complete restriction on their concurrent use, but ideally randomised prospective studies are required to confirm this.

(b) Cardiovascular effects

A large-scale comparative study was undertaken over a 12-month period in groups of women taking tamoxifen alone, HRT alone, or tamoxifen with transdermal HRT to see whether the cardiovascular risk factors (low-density lipoprotein cholesterol, high-density lipoprotein-cholesterol levels, platelet counts) were changed by concurrent use. It was found that the decrease in total and LDL-cholesterol levels due to the tamoxifen was unchanged in current HRT users, but reduced by two-thirds in women taking tamoxifen who then started HRT.[5] It would therefore seem important to check the outcome of concurrent use. More study is needed.

1. Dew JE, Wren BG, Eden JA. Tamoxifen, hormone receptors, and hormone replacement therapy in women previously treated for breast cancer: a cohort study. *Climacteric* (2002) 5, 151–5.
2. Arimidex (Anastrozole). AstraZeneca UK Ltd. UK Summary of product characteristics, June 2006.
3. Aromasin (Exemestane). Pharmacia Ltd. UK Summary of product characteristics, August 2005.
4. Aromasin (Exemestane). Pharmacia & Upjohn Company. US Prescribing information, February 2007.
5. Decensi A, Robertson C, Rotmensz N, Severi G, Maisonneuve P, Sacchini V, Boyle P, Costa A, Veronesi U. Effect of tamoxifen and transdermal hormone replacement therapy on cardiovascular risk factors in a prevention trial. *Br J Cancer* (1998) 78, 572–8.

Tamoxifen + Medroxyprogesterone acetate

Medroxyprogesterone affects the metabolism of tamoxifen but the clinical importance of this is uncertain.

Clinical evidence, mechanism, importance and management

In 20 women with breast cancer taking tamoxifen 20 mg twice daily, the addition of medroxyprogesterone acetate 500 mg twice daily only slightly reduced the tamoxifen serum levels over a 6-month period, but considerably reduced the levels of the desmethyl metabolite of tamoxifen, presumably because of some effect on the metabolism of the tamoxifen by the liver.[1] The clinical importance of this interaction awaits assessment.

1. Reid AD, Horobin JM, Newman EL, Preece PE. Tamoxifen metabolism is altered by simultaneous administration of medroxyprogesterone acetate in breast cancer patients. *Breast Cancer Res Treat* (1992) 22, 153–6.

Tamoxifen + Rifampicin (Rifampin)

Rifampicin increased the metabolism of tamoxifen.

Clinical evidence, mechanism, importance and management

In 10 healthy *men* rifampicin 600 mg daily for 5 days reduced the AUC of a single 80-mg dose of tamoxifen by 86%, reduced the peak plasma levels by 55%, and reduced the half-life by 44%. Similarly, the AUC of *N*-demethyltamoxifen was reduced by 62%.[1]

It is likely that rifampicin induces the metabolism of tamoxifen by the cytochrome P450 isoenzyme CYP3A4, thereby reducing its levels. These findings suggest that the efficacy of tamoxifen may be reduced by rifampicin. However, there is some *in vitro* evidence that suggests that tamoxifen and rifampicin have additive antineoplastic effects in pancreatic carcinoma cell lines.[2] Also, tamoxifen induces its own metabolism on long-term use.[3] Thus, further study is needed to assess the clinical impact of the long-term combined use of these drugs.

1. Kivistö KT, Villikka K, Nyman L, Anttila M, Neuvonen PJ. Tamoxifen and toremifene concentrations in plasma are greatly decreased by rifampin. *Clin Pharmacol Ther* (1998) 64, 648–54.
2. West CML, Reeves SJ, Brough W. Additive interaction between tamoxifen and rifampicin in human biliary tract carcinoma cells. *Cancer Lett* (1990) 55, 159–63.
3. Desai PB, Nallani SC, Sane RS, Moore LB, Goodwin BJ, Buckley DJ, Buckley AR. Induction of cytochrome P450 3A4 in primary human hepatocytes and activation of the human pregnane X receptor by tamoxifen and 4-hydroxytamoxifen. *Drug Metab Dispos* (2002) 30, 608–12.

Tamoxifen + SSRIs

Paroxetine reduces the metabolism of tamoxifen to one of its active metabolites. The clinical relevance of this is unknown, although one small case-control study found that inhibitors of CYP2D6 such as the SSRIs did not increase the recurrence of breast cancer in tamoxifen users.

Clinical evidence

Twelve women taking tamoxifen 20 mg daily were also given **paroxetine** 10 mg daily for 4 weeks, and plasma levels of tamoxifen and its metabolites were measured.[1] Before **paroxetine**, the plasma levels of the 4-hydroxy-*N*-desmethyl-tamoxifen metabolite (endoxifen) were about 12 times higher than those of the 4-hydroxy-tamoxifen metabolite. **Paroxetine** reduced endoxifen levels by 56%, but those of *N*-desmethyl-tamoxifen, and 4-hydroxy-tamoxifen were unchanged. The reduction in endoxifen levels was greatest in those who were extensive metabolisers of the cytochrome P450 isoenzyme CYP2D6 (see 'Genetic factors', (p.4)). In a further study by the same research group, 80 women starting tamoxifen 20 mg daily had plasma levels of tamoxifen measured after 1 and 4 months of therapy.[2] These were then correlated with CYP2D6 metaboliser phenotype and the concurrent use of CYP2D6 inhibitors (taken by 24 women). In women who were CYP2D6 extensive metabolisers, use of CYP2D6 inhibitors was associated with a 58% lower endoxifen level, which was substantially lower in those taking **paroxetine**, but only slightly reduced by venlafaxine, and intermediate in those taking **sertraline**.[2]

However, a case-control study of 28 women taking tamoxifen with recurrences of oestrogen receptor positive breast cancer found that there was no difference in the number of women taking CYP2D6 inhibitors (**fluoxetine**, **paroxetine**, **sertraline**) between cases and controls (women taking tamoxifen with no recurrence). Similarly, there was no differences for CYP2C9 inhibitors (including **paroxetine** and **sertraline**).[3]

Mechanism

Endoxifen and 4-hydroxy-tamoxifen are more active anti-oestrogens than tamoxifen.[1] Tamoxifen is metabolised to 4-hydroxy-tamoxifen and *N*-desmethyl-tamoxifen principally by CYP3A,[1] although others have found that other isoenzymes are involved,[4] and to endoxifen by CYP2D6.[1] Of the SSRIs, paroxetine is the most potent inhibitor of CYP2D6. However, tamoxifen resistance may be more to do with altered oestrogen receptor sensitivity than reduced levels of tamoxifen metabolites.[3] Further it has been suggested that the plasma levels of tamoxifen and metabolites found in one study[1] would be sufficient to block oestrogen binding to oestrogen receptors so that a decrease in endoxifen levels would not substantially affect anti-oestrogen activity.[5]

Importance and management

Although information is limited, it is established that potent inhibitors of CYP2D6 such as paroxetine can alter the metabolism of tamoxifen to its active metabolites. However, the effect this has on the clinical efficacy of tamoxifen remains to be established. The one small case-control study suggests the effect is not great. At present, there is insufficient evidence to recommend caution when giving SSRIs with tamoxifen, but further study is clearly needed. Any interaction would apply equally to other CYP2D6 inhibitors, see 'Table 1.3', (p.6) for a list.

1. Stearns V, Johnson MD, Rae JM, Morocho A, Novielli A, Bhargava P, Hayes DF, Desta Z, Flockhart DA. Active tamoxifen metabolite plasma concentrations after coadministration of tamoxifen and the selective serotonin reuptake inhibitor paroxetine. *J Natl Cancer Inst* (2003) 95, 1758–64.
2. Jin Y, Desta Z, Stearns V, Ward B, Ho H, Lee K-H, Skaar T, Storniolo AM, Li L, Araba A, Blanchard R, Nguyen A, Ullmer L, Hayden J, Lemler S, Weinshilboum RM, Rae JM, Hayes DF, Flockhart DA. CYP2D6 genotype, antidepressant use, and tamoxifen metabolism during adjuvant breast cancer treatment. *J Natl Cancer Inst* (2005) 97, 30–9.
3. Lehmann D, Nelsen J, Ramanath V, Newman N, Duggan D, Smith A. Lack of attenuation in the antitumor effect of tamoxifen by chronic CYP isoform inhibition. *J Clin Pharmacol* (2004) 44, 861–5.
4. Coller JK, Krebsfaenger N, Klein K, Endrizzi K, Wolbold R, Lang T, Nüssler A, Neuhaus P, Zanger UM, Eichelbaum M, Mürdter TE. The influence of CYP2B6, CYP2C9 and CYP2D6 genotypes on the formation of the potent antioestrogen Z-4-hydroxy-tamoxifen in human liver. *Br J Clin Pharmacol* (2002) 54, 157–67.
5. Ratliff B, Dietze EC, Bean GR, Moore C, Wanko S, Seewaldt VL. RE: Active tamoxifen metabolite plasma concentrations after coadministration of tamoxifen and the selective serotonin reuptake inhibitor paroxetine. *J Natl Cancer Inst* (2004) 96, 883.

Taxanes + Amifostine

Amifostine had no effect on docetaxel and paclitaxel pharmacokinetics, except in one study which found that amifostine extended paclitaxel plasma circulation time. Amifostine appears not to reduce the toxicity of these taxanes.

Clinical evidence, mechanism, importance and management

In a randomised study, amifostine did not alter the response to, or the pharmacokinetics of, **paclitaxel**, neither did it protect against **paclitaxel**-related neurotoxicity or myelotoxicity.[1] Another study in 8 patients has confirmed that amifostine (750 mg/m^2 as a 15-minute infusion 30 minutes beforehand) had no effect on the pharmacokinetics of **paclitaxel** 135 to 200 mg/m^2. Six of the patients were also taking epirubicin and cisplatin.[2] Although the preliminary findings of an earlier study had suggested that pre-treatment with amifostine reduced the AUC of **paclitaxel** by 29%,[3] the full report of this study concluded that amifostine had no clinically relevant effect on **paclitaxel** pharmacokinetics.[4] In a study in which patients were given amifostine 500 mg as an infusion over 15 minutes just before low-dose **paclitaxel** 80 mg/m^2 as a one-hour infusion, amifostine reduced maximum plasma levels by about 20%. However, the AUC of paclitaxel was not affected, but the paclitaxel plasma circulation time was prolonged.[5]

Amifostine had no effect on the pharmacokinetics of **docetaxel**, nor did it reduce **docetaxel**-induced myelotoxicity.[6]

The finding in two of these studies[1,6] that the toxicity of taxanes was not reduced by amifostine does not support earlier *in vitro* data where amifostine protected normal tissue from **paclitaxel** toxicity.[7]

Most studies show no beneficial or adverse consequences from giving amifostine with the taxanes. Further study is needed to evaluate the possible effects of amifostine on taxane plasma circulation time.

1. Gelmon K, Eisenhauer E, Bryce C, Tolcher A, Mayer L, Tomlinson E, Zee B, Blackstein M, Tomiak E, Yau J, Batist G, Fisher B, Iglesias J. Randomized phase II study of high-dose paclitaxel with or without amifostine in patients with metastatic breast cancer. *J Clin Oncol* (1999) 17, 3038–47.
2. Van den Brande J, Nannan Panday VR, Hoekman K, Rosing H, Huijskes RVHP, Verheijen RHM, Beijnen JH, Vermorken JB. Pharmacologic study of paclitaxel administered with or without the cytoprotective agent amifostine, and given as a single agent or in combination with epirubicin and cisplatin in patients with advanced solid tumours. *Am J Clin Oncol* (2001) 24, 401–3.
3. Schüller J, Czejka M, Pietrzak C, Springer B, Wirth M, Schernthaner G. Influence of the cytoprotective agent amifostine (AMI) on pharmacokinetics (PK) of paclitaxel (PAC) and Taxotere® (TXT). *Proc Am Soc Clin Oncol* (1997) 16, 224a.
4. Czejka M, Schueller J, Eder I, Reznicek G, Kraule C, Zeleni U, Freitag R. Clinical pharmacokinetics and metabolism of paclitaxel after polychemotherapy with the cytoprotective agent amifostine. *Anticancer Res* (2000) 20, 3871–7.
5. Juan O, Rocher A, Sánchez A, Sánchez JJ, Alberola V. Influence of the cyto-protective agent amifostine on the pharmacokinetics of low-dose paclitaxel. *Chemotherapy* (2005) 51, 200–5.
6. Freyer G, Hennebert P, Awada A, Gil T, Kerger J, Selleslags J, Brassinne C, Piccart M, de Valeriola D. Influence of amifostine on the toxicity and pharmacokinetics of docetaxel in metastatic breast cancer patients: a pilot study. *Clin Cancer Res* (2002) 8, 95–102.
7. Taylor CW, Wang LM, List AF, Fernandes D, Paine-Murrieta GD, Johnson CS, Capizzi RL. Amifostine protects normal tissues from paclitaxel toxicity while cytotoxicity against tumour cells is maintained. *Eur J Cancer* (1997) 33, 1693–8.

Taxanes + Ciclosporin

Ciclosporin increases the levels of docetaxel and paclitaxel after *oral* administration.

Clinical evidence, mechanism, importance and management

(a) Docetaxel

One study has demonstrated that the bioavailability of *oral* docetaxel may be increased from 8% to 90% by ciclosporin due to inhibition of both P-glycoprotein transport and the metabolism of docetaxel by the cytochrome P450 isoenzyme CYP3A4.[1] In another study, the AUC of ciclosporin was increased by about 1.5-fold when it was given with *oral* docetaxel, probably because of competitive inhibition of CYP3A4-mediated ciclosporin metabolism.[2]

(b) Paclitaxel

Oral paclitaxel has poor bioavailability because of a high affinity for P-glycoprotein in the gastrointestinal tract. Studies in *mice* have shown that the combination of ciclosporin with oral paclitaxel produced a tenfold increase in systemic exposure to paclitaxel. Plasma levels of paclitaxel were below therapeutic concentrations in 5 patients when they were given an oral dose (intravenous formulation) of paclitaxel 60 mg/m^2 followed by intravenous doses of 175 mg/m^2 for subsequent courses. However, therapeutic levels above 100 micromol/mL (a ninefold increase) were achieved in 9 patients who received the same regimen with ciclosporin 15 mg/kg. The combination was well-tolerated, but further study is required to determine whether paclitaxel treatment via the oral route is as active as that by the intravenous route.[3]

1. Malingré MM, Richel DJ, Beijnen JH, Rosing H, Koopman FJ, Ten Bokkel Huinink WW, Schot ME, Schellens JHM. Coadministration of cyclosporine strongly enhances the oral bioavailability of docetaxel. *J Clin Oncol* (2001) 19, 1160–6.
2. Malingré MM, Ten Bokkel Huinink WW, Mackay M, Schellens JHM, Beijnen JH. Pharmacokinetics of oral cyclosporin A when co-administered to enhance the absorption of orally administered docetaxel. *Eur J Clin Pharmacol* (2001) 57, 305–7.
3. Meerum Terwogt JM, Beijnen JH, ten Bokkel Huinink WW, Rosing H, Schellens JHM. Coadministration of cyclosporin enables oral therapy with paclitaxel. *Lancet* (1998) 352, 285.

Taxanes + Cisplatin or Carboplatin

The toxicity of paclitaxel given with cisplatin appears to be dependent on the order of administration, with more severe myelosuppression occurring if cisplatin is given first. There does not appear to be any sequence dependent interaction for the combination of docetaxel with carboplatin or docetaxel with cisplatin. Paclitaxel may reduce the thrombocytopenia associated with carboplatin. The combination of carboplatin with paclitaxel appears to be more neurotoxic than carboplatin with docetaxel.

Clinical evidence, mechanism, importance and management

(a) Carboplatin

Several clinical studies have found that the severity of thrombocytopenia with the combination of **paclitaxel** and carboplatin was less than that expected with carboplatin alone.[1-5] This does not appear to be due to any changes in carboplatin pharmacokinetics. In one study, patients were given carboplatin as a 30-minute infusion, either alone or immediately following **paclitaxel** 175 mg/m^2 as a 3-hour infusion, and it was found that the pharmacokinetics of carboplatin were not significantly affected by **paclitaxel**.[6] Similarly, a pharmacokinetic interaction was not noted when **paclitaxel** and carboplatin were given in either order in another study.[1] Other studies found the AUC of carboplatin to be similar to that predicted, despite the presence of paclitaxel.[2,5] Although one study found the AUC of carboplatin to be about 12% lower in the presence of **paclitaxel**,[4] the same researchers also found that the AUC associated with a 50% decrease in platelet count increased by 68% (i.e. more carboplatin is needed to cause the same degree of thrombocytopenia), which suggests a pharmacodynamic basis for the attenuated toxicity of the combination.[7] Other researchers also reported that the AUC of carboplatin causing a 50% reduction in platelets was about 6.3 mg/mL per minute when given with **paclitaxel** compared with historical data of 4 mg/mL per minute when given alone.[8] Although thrombocytopenia may be lower than expected, myelosuppression (in the form of neutropenia) is a dose-limiting toxicity of the combination of carboplatin and **paclitaxel**.[1-4] In one study, patients given **paclitaxel** with carboplatin experienced significantly greater neurotoxicity than those given **docetaxel** with carboplatin, but the regimens were similar in efficacy.[9] Further, there appear to be no pharmacokinetic interactions between carboplatin and **docetaxel**.[10,11]

(b) Cisplatin

Early studies of the combination of cisplatin and **paclitaxel** showed that the degree of myelosuppression was sequence dependent. When cisplatin was given first, a greater degree of myelosuppression was seen.[12] Pharmacokinetic studies suggest that sequence-dependent differences in myelosuppression may be due to a 25% reduction in **paclitaxel** clearance when cisplatin is given first.[12] For this reason, the manufacturers recommend that **paclitaxel** is given before cisplatin.[13,14] There is also some evidence that *myelosuppression* is greater for the combination when **paclitaxel** is given over 24 hours as opposed to 3 hours.[13] When **paclitaxel** is given with cisplatin, *neurotoxicity* (peripheral neuropathy) is common,[13] and there is some evidence that this is more severe if the **paclitaxel** is given over 3 hours as opposed to over 24 hours.[15] In one study,[16] neurotoxicity was unexpectedly severe when **paclitaxel** alone was used in patients who had relapsed after treatment with cisplatin; however, this was not the case in another similar study.[17]

In contrast to **paclitaxel**, early studies did not reveal any obvious sequence dependent toxicity for the combination of **docetaxel** and cisplatin.[18] In addition, cisplatin did not cause any significant changes in **docetaxel** pharmacokinetics.[18,19]

1. Huizing MT, Giaccone G, van Warmerdam LJC, Rosing H, Bakker PJM, Vermorken JB, Postmus PE, van Zandwijk, Koolen MGJ, ten Bokkel Huinink, van der Vijgh WJF, Bierhorst FJ, Lai A, Dalesio O, Pinedo HM, Veenhof CHN, Beijnen JH. Pharmacokinetics of paclitaxel and carboplatin in a dose-escalating and dose-sequencing study in patients with non-small-cell lung cancer. *J Clin Oncol* (1997) 15, 317–29.
2. Bookman MA, McGuire WP, Kilpatrick D, Keenan E, Hogan WM, Johnson SW, O'Dwyer P, Rowinsky E, Gallion HH, Ozols RF. Carboplatin and paclitaxel in ovarian carcinoma: a phase I study of the Gynecologic Oncology Group. *J Clin Oncol* (1996) 14, 1895–1902.
3. Huizing MT, van Warmerdam LJC, Rosing H, Schaefers MCW, Lai A, Helmerhorst TJM, Veenhof CHN, Birkhofer MJ, Rodenhuis S, Beijnen JH, ten Bokkel Huinink WW. Phase I and pharmacologic study of the combination paclitaxel and carboplatin as first-line chemotherapy in stage III and IV ovarian cancer. *J Clin Oncol* (1997) 15, 1953–64.
4. Belani CP, Kearns CM, Zuhowski EG, Erkmen K, Hiponia D, Zacharski D, Engstrom C, Ramanathan RK, Capozzoli MJ, Aisner J, Egorin MJ. Phase I trial, including pharmacokinetics and pharmacodynamic correlations, of combination paclitaxel and carboplatin in patients with metastatic non-small-cell lung cancer. *J Clin Oncol* (1999) 17, 676–84.
5. Siddiqui N, Boddy AV, Thomas HD, Bailey NP, Robson L, Lind MJ, Calvert AH. A clinical and pharmacokinetic study of the combination of carboplatin and paclitaxel for epithelial ovarian cancer. *Br J Cancer* (1997) 75, 287–94.
6. Obasaju CK, Johnson SW, Rogatko A, Kilpatrick D, Brennan JM, Hamilton TC, Ozols RF, O'Dwyer PJ, Gallo JM. Evaluation of carboplatin pharmacokinetics in the absence and presence of paclitaxel. *Clin Cancer Res* (1996) 2, 549–52.
7. Kearns CM, Belani CP, Erkmen K, Zuhowski M, Hiponia D, Ergstrom C, Ramanthan R, Trenn M, Aisner J, Ergorin MJ. Reduced platelet toxicity with combination carboplatin & paclitaxel: pharmacodynamic modulation of carboplatin associated thrombocytopenia. *Proc Am Soc Clin Oncol* (1995) 14, 170.
8. van Warmerdam LJC, Huizing MT, Giaccone G, Postmus PE, ten Bokkel Huinink WW, van Zandwijk N, Koolen MGJ, Helmerhorst TJM, van der Vijgh WJF, Veenhof CHN, Beijnen JH. Clinical pharmacology of carboplatin administered in combination with paclitaxel. *Semin Oncol* (1997) 24 (Suppl 2), S2-97–S2-104.
9. Kaye SB, Vasey PA. Docetaxel in ovarian cancer: phase III perspectives and future development. *Semin Oncol* (2002) 29 (3 Suppl 12) 22–7.
10. Oka M, Fukuda M, Nagashima S, Fukuda M, Kinoshita A, Soda H, Doi S, Narasaki F, Suenaga M, Takatani H, Nakamura Y, Kawabata S, Tsurutani J, Kanda T, Kohno S. Phase I study of second-line chemotherapy with docetaxel and carboplatin in non-small-cell lung cancer. *Cancer Chemother Pharmacol* (2001) 48, 446–50.
11. Ando M, Saka H, Ando Y, Minami H, Kuzuya T, Yamamoto M, Watanabe A, Sakai S, Shimokata K, Hasegawa Y. Sequence effect of docetaxel and carboplatin on toxicity, tumor response and pharmacokinetics in non-small-cell lung cancer patients: a phase I study of two sequences. *Cancer Chemother Pharmacol* (2005) 55, 552–8.
12. Rowkinsky EK, Gilbert M, McGuire WP, Noe DA, Grochow LB, Forastiere AA, Ettinger DS, Lubejko BG, Clarke B, Sartorius SE, Cornblath DR, Hendricks CB, Donehower RC. Sequences of taxol and cisplatin: a phase I and pharmacologic study. *J Clin Oncol* (1991) 9, 1692–1703.
13. Taxol (Paclitaxel). Bristol-Myers Squibb Pharmaceuticals Ltd. UK Summary of product characteristics, August 2005.
14. Taxol (Paclitaxel). Bristol-Myers Squibb Company. US Prescribing information, March 2003.
15. Connelly E, Markman M, Kennedy A, Webster K, Kulp B, Peterson G, Belinson J. Paclitaxel delivered as a 3-hr infusion with cisplatin in patients with gynecologic cancers: unexpected incidence of neurotoxicity. *Gynecol Oncol* (1996) 62, 166–8.
16. Cavaletti G, Bogliun G, Marzorati L, Zincone A, Marzola M, Colombo N, Tredici G. Peripheral neurotoxicity of taxol in patients previously treated with cisplatin. *Cancer* (1995) 75, 1141–50.
17. McGuire WP, Rowinsky EK, Rosenhein NB, Grumbine FC, Ettinger DS, Armstrong DK, Donehower RC. Taxol: a unique antineoplastic agent with significant activity in advanced ovarian epithelial neoplasms. *Ann Intern Med* (1989) 111, 273–9.
18. Pronk LC, Schellens JHM, Planting AST, van den Bent MJ, Hilkens PHE, van der Burg MEL, de Boer-Dennert M, Ma J, Blanc C, Harteveld M, Bruno R, Stoter G, Verweij J. Phase I and pharmacologic study of docetaxel and cisplatin in patients with advanced solid tumors. *J Clin Oncol* (1997) 15, 1071–9.
19. Millward MJ, Zalcberg J, Bishop JF, Webster LK, Zimet A, Rischin D, Toner GC, Laird J, Cosolo W, Urch M, Bruno R, Loret C, James R, Blanc C. Phase I trial of docetaxel and cisplatin in previously untreated patients with advanced non-small-cell lung cancer. *J Clin Oncol* (1997) 15, 750–8.

Taxanes + Cyclophosphamide

There is some evidence to suggest that the toxicity associated with combinations of paclitaxel and cyclophosphamide is dependent on the order of administration. Results from one study indicate that docetaxel pharmacokinetics are unaltered by cyclophosphamide.

Clinical evidence, mechanism, importance and management

(a) Docetaxel

The pharmacokinetics of docetaxel were not altered by pretreatment with an intravenous bolus dose of cyclophosphamide in a phase I study.[1] For a report that the pharmacokinetics of docetaxel are not affected by **ifosfamide**, see 'Cyclophosphamide or Ifosfamide + Taxanes', p.628.

(b) Paclitaxel

A study in patients given paclitaxel as a 24-hour infusion and cyclophosphamide as an infusion over 1 hour found that neutropenia and thrombocytopenia were more severe when paclitaxel preceded cyclophosphamide.[2] Similarly, in another study, concurrent use of a continuous 72-hour infusion of paclitaxel and a daily bolus of cyclophosphamide had acceptable toxicity. However, when the cyclophosphamide was given as a single intravenous dose after the end of the 72-hour paclitaxel infusion, severe haematological and gastrointestinal toxicity occurred.[3] Whether the clinical efficacy of this combination is also altered by the schedule and sequence has not been determined. See also 'Cyclophosphamide or Ifosfamide + Taxanes', p.628.

1. Vasey PA, Roché H, Bisset D, Terret C, Vernillet L, Riva A, Ramazeilles C, Azli N, Kaye SB, Twelves CJ. Phase I study of docetaxel in combination with cyclophosphamide as first-line chemotherapy for metastatic breast cancer. *Br J Cancer* (2002) 87, 1072–8.
2. Kennedy MJ, Zahurak ML, Donehower RC, Noe DA, Sartorius S, Chen T-L, Bowling K, Rowinsky EK. Phase I and pharmacologic study of sequences of paclitaxel and cyclophosphamide supported by granulocyte colony-stimulating factor in women with previously treated metastatic breast cancer. *J Clin Oncol* (1996) 14, 783–91.
3. Tolcher AW, Cowan KH, Noone MH, Denicoff AM, Kohler DR, Goldspiel BR, Barnes CS, McCabe M, Gossard MR, Zujewski J, O'Shaughnessy J. Phase I study of paclitaxel in combination with cyclophosphamide and granulocyte colony-stimulating factor in metastatic breast cancer patients. *J Clin Oncol* (1996) 14, 95–102.

Taxanes + Protease inhibitors

Life-threatening haematological toxicities have been reported in a few patients taking protease inhibitors when given paclitaxel or docetaxel. Nelfinavir and ritonavir appear to inhibit the clearance of paclitaxel and are predicted to inhibit the metabolism of docetaxel by CYP3A4.

Clinical evidence

(a) Docetaxel

A HIV-positive 64-year-old woman taking **nelfinavir** was given trastuzumab and docetaxel 36 mg/m^2 for breast cancer. Three days later she was hospitalised with early, severe myelosuppression, which was attributed to an interaction between the nelfinavir and docetaxel, and she died from sepsis.[1]

(b) Paclitaxel

A 39-year-old woman taking **lopinavir** was given **carboplatin** and paclitaxel 175 mg/m^2 for adenocarcinoma. Five days later she was hospitalised with early, severe myelosuppression, which was attributed to an interaction between lopinavir and paclitaxel, and she later died.[1] In another report, an HIV-positive patient who was taking **lopinavir/ritonavir**, delavirdine and didanosine was also given paclitaxel 100 mg/m^2 to treat Kaposi's sarcoma. Within 3 days he developed myalgia and arthralgia, and 8 days after treatment developed fever, tachycardia and a productive cough. He was treated with antibacterials and G-CSF, but later died. Findings at post mortem included severe oesophageal mucositis, *Streptococcus viridans* pneumonia and a massive saddle embolism (an embolism that sits across two vessels).[2] A second patient taking **indinavir**, **ritonavir**, lamivudine and stavudine developed severe leucopenia and thrombocytopenia within 7 days of being given paclitaxel 100 mg/m^2 for Kaposi's sarcoma, and again after a second course of paclitaxel. Further courses of paclitaxel were tolerated by giving a reduced dose of 60 mg/m^2 together with G-CSF.[2]

The UK manufacturer of paclitaxel briefly mentions that studies in patients with Kaposi's sarcoma, who were taking multiple concomitant medications, suggest that the systemic clearance of paclitaxel was significantly lower in the presence of **nelfinavir** and **ritonavir**, but not with **indinavir**.[3]

Mechanism

Paclitaxel is metabolised by the cytochrome P450 enzymes CYP2C8 and CYP3A4. Docetaxel is metabolised by CYP3A4. Protease inhibitors such as ritonavir and indinavir are known to inhibit CYP3A4, which might result in increased taxane levels and toxicity.

Importance and management

Evidence is limited, nevertheless the UK manufacturers advise that paclitaxel should be given to patients also receiving protease inhibitors with caution.[3] The manufacturers of docetaxel also advise that it should be used with caution with drugs that inhibit CYP3A4, see 'Taxanes; Docetaxel + Miscellaneous', below, which would include the protease inhibitors.

1. Parameswaran R, Sweeney C, Einhorn LH. Interaction between highly active antiretroviral therapy (HAART) and taxanes: a report of two cases. *Proc Am Soc Clin Oncol* (2002) 21, abstract 2194.
2. Bundow D, Aboulafia DM. Potential drug interaction with paclitaxel and highly active antiretroviral therapy in two patients with AIDS-associated Kaposi sarcoma. *Am J Clin Oncol* (2004) 27, 81–4.
3. Taxol (Paclitaxel). Bristol-Myers Squibb Pharmaceuticals Ltd. UK Summary of product characteristics, August 2005.

Taxanes; Docetaxel + Cannabis

The pharmacokinetics of docetaxel are not altered by a herbal tea containing cannabis.

Clinical evidence, mechanism, importance and management

In a crossover study 24 patients were given **docetaxel** 180 mg before and on day 12 of a 15-day course of 200 mL daily of a herbal tea containing cannabis 1 g/L. This was prepared from medicinal-grade cannabis (*Cannabis sativa* L. Flos, variety Bedrocan®) containing the cannabinoids Δ^9-tetrahydrocannabinol 18% and cannabidiol 0.8%. The clearance and the AUC of **docetaxel** were not significantly altered by the cannabis. No dosage adjustments are likely to be needed if **docetaxel** is given with cannabis.[1]

1. Engels FK, de Jong FA, Sparreboom A, Mathot RA, Loos WJ, Kitzen JJEM, de Bruijn P, Verweij J, Mathijssen RHJ. Medicinal cannabis does not influence the clinical pharmacokinetics of irinotecan and docetaxel. *Oncologist* (2007) 12, 291–300.

Taxanes; Docetaxel + Miscellaneous

Based on *in vitro* studies, the manufacturers suggest that CYP3A inhibitors (such as ketoconazole and erythromycin) will raise docetaxel levels, whereas CYP3A inducers (such as rifampicin (rifampin) and the barbiturates) will reduce docetaxel levels. This has been seen for ketoconazole.

Clinical evidence, mechanism, importance and management

The manufacturers[1,2] say that no formal clinical drug interaction studies have been carried out with docetaxel, but because it is known from *in vitro* studies that the metabolism of docetaxel is mainly mediated by the cytochrome P450 isoenzyme CYP3A family,[3] they say that drugs that are inhibitors of CYP3A might possibly increase its serum levels and increase its toxicity. Caution is advised. The drugs named include **erythromycin**, **ketoconazole**, **terfenadine**, **troleandomycin** and **nifedipine**,[1,2] although note that some of these drugs (such as **terfenadine** and **nifedipine**) are more usually considered to be competitive inhibitors of CYP3A4 (that is, they share the same metabolic pathway) rather than actually inhibiting the isoenzyme. This prediction is supported by a study in 7 patients, in which **ketoconazole** 200 mg daily for 3 days reduced the clearance of docetaxel 10 mg/m^2 by 49%, which could increase the risk of neutropenia.[4]

An *in vitro* study found that **hyperforin**, a constituent of **St John's wort** induced docetaxel metabolism in a dose-dependent manner by 2.6 to 7-fold when compared to controls. In the same study, **rifampicin (rifampin)** increased docetaxel metabolism by 6.8 to 32-fold when compared to controls.[5]

Microsomes prepared from patients treated with **pentobarbital** and/or **phenobarbital** are reported to have stimulated docetaxel metabolism strikingly whereas those prepared from a patient taking **prednisone** did not.[6] In a study in patients with metastatic prostatic cancer, **prednisone** did not significantly affect the pharmacokinetics of docetaxel.[1]

None of these drugs, with the exception of **ketoconazole**, **pentobarbital**, **phenobarbital** and **prednisone**, appear to have been studied in patients, so that the clinical importance of these predicted interactions awaits formal clinical evaluation.

1. Taxotere (Docetaxel). Sanofi-Aventis. UK Summary of product characteristics, October 2006.
2. Taxotere (Docetaxel). Sanofi-Aventis US LLC. US Prescribing information, December 2006.
3. Clarke SJ, Rivory LP. Clinical pharmacokinetics of docetaxel. *Clin Pharmacokinet* (1999) 36, 99–114.
4. Engels FK, ten Tije AJ, Baker SD, Lee CKK, Loos WJ, Vulto AG, Verweij J, Sparreboom A. Effect of cytochrome P450 3A4 inhibition on the pharmacokinetics of docetaxel. *Clin Pharmacol Ther* (2004) 75, 448–54.
5. Komoroski BJ, Parise RA, Egorin MJ, Strom SC, Venkataramanan R. Effect of the St. John's wort constituent hyperforin on docetaxel metabolism by human hepatocyte cultures. *Clin Cancer Res* (2005) 11, 6972–9.
6. Royer I, Monsarrat B, Sonnier M, Wright M, Cresteil T. Metabolism of docetaxel by human cytochromes P450: Interactions with paclitaxel and other antineoplastic drugs. *Cancer Res* (1996) 56, 58–65.

Taxanes; Paclitaxel + Antiepileptics

Enzyme-inducing antiepileptics (phenytoin, carbamazepine, and phenobarbital) increase the clearance of paclitaxel and increase its maximum tolerated dose.

Clinical evidence, mechanism, importance and management

In a study in patients with glioblastoma multiforme the maximum tolerated dose (MTD) of paclitaxel was 43% higher in patients receiving antiepileptics (**phenytoin**, **carbamazepine**, and **phenobarbital**) than in those not receiving them.[1] Another study in patients with recurrent malignant gliomas reported the same finding: a 50% increase in MTD coupled with a 104% increase in plasma clearance of paclitaxel in those taking antiepileptics. In addition, this study reported that the dose-limiting toxicity differed: central neurotoxicity in those taking antiepileptics and myelosuppression and/or gastrointestinal toxicity in those not.[2]

It is probable that enzyme-inducing antiepileptics increase the metabolism of paclitaxel, and therefore it is likely that patients taking these antiepileptics will require an increase in paclitaxel dose. Further study is needed. Note that barbiturates are predicted to increase the metabolism of docetaxel, see 'Taxanes; Docetaxel + Miscellaneous', above.

1. Fetell MR, Grossman SA, Fisher JD, Erlanger B, Rowinsky E, Stockel J, Piantadosi S. Preirradiation paclitaxel in glioblastoma multiforme: efficacy, pharmacology, and drug interactions. New approaches to Brain Tumor Therapy Central Nervous System Consortium. *J Clin Oncol* (1997) 15, 3121–8.
2. Chang SM, Kuhn JG, Rizzo J, Robins HI, Schold SC, Spence AM, Berger MS, Mehta MP, Bozik ME, Pollack I, Gilbert M, Fulton C, Rankin C, Malec M, Prados MD. Phase I study of paclitaxel in patients with recurrent malignant glioma: a North American Brain Tumor Consortium report. *J Clin Oncol* (1998) 16, 2188–94.

Taxanes; Paclitaxel + Ketoconazole

Ketoconazole does not appear to affect the pharmacokinetics of paclitaxel.

Clinical evidence, mechanism, importance and management

Women with ovarian cancer were treated with 3-hour infusions of paclitaxel 175 mg/m^2 once every 21 days. It was found that when single oral doses of ketoconazole were given 3 hours before or 3 hours after the paclitaxel, the serum levels of the paclitaxel and its principal metabolite (6-alpha-hydroxypaclitaxel) remained unchanged. These findings confirmed those of *in vitro* studies. The conclusion was reached that these two drugs can therefore be given together safely without any dosage adjustments.[1,2]

1. Jamis-Dow CA, Pearl ML, Watkins PB, Blake DS, Klecker RW, Collins JM. Predicting drug interactions in vivo from experiments in vitro: human studies with paclitaxel and ketoconazole. *Am J Clin Oncol* (1997) 20, 592–99.
2. Taxol (Paclitaxel). Bristol-Myers Squibb Pharmaceuticals Ltd. UK Summary of product characteristics, August 2005.

Taxanes; Paclitaxel + Miscellaneous

***In vitro* studies with human liver tissue suggest that no metabolic interactions are likely to occur between paclitaxel and cimetidine, dexamethasone or diphenhydramine. *Cremophor* may inhibit the intracellular uptake and metabolism of paclitaxel.**

Clinical evidence, mechanism, importance and management

(a) Cimetidine, Dexamethasone, Diphenhydramine

On the basis of an *in vitro* study using human liver slices and human liver microsomes it has been concluded that the metabolism of paclitaxel is unlikely to be altered by cimetidine, dexamethasone or diphenhydramine, all of which are frequently given to prevent the hypersensitivity reactions associated with paclitaxel or its vehicle, *Cremophor* (see b, below).[1] The UK manufacturers say that paclitaxel clearance in patients is not affected by cimetidine premedication,[2] although some authors[3] have advised caution when using cimetidine with docetaxel or paclitaxel since cimetidine is known to affect the cytochrome P450 isoenzyme CYP3A4, which is responsible, in part, for the metabolism of these taxanes.

(b) Cremophor

In vitro, *Cremophor* was found to inhibit the metabolism of paclitaxel in human liver microsomes,[1] which might be expected to increase its toxicity. The concentration used in the *in vitro* study may be achieved clinically in patients given paclitaxel with *Cremophor* as the vehicle.[4] This may be worth bearing in mind if other drugs formulated with *Cremophor* are given with paclitaxel.

(c) Methotrexate

An *in vitro* study in human bladder cancer cells found that the antineoplastic effect of paclitaxel in combination with methotrexate was dependent on the order of exposure to the two drugs.[5]

1. Jamis-Dow CA, Klecker RW, Katki AG, Collins JM. Metabolism of taxol by humans and rat liver in vitro: a screen for drug interactions and interspecies differences. *Cancer Chemother Pharmacol* (1995) 36, 107–14.
2. Taxol (Paclitaxel). Bristol-Myers Squibb Pharmaceuticals Ltd. UK Summary of product characteristics, August 2005.
3. Clouse T, Geisler JP, Manahan KJ, Gudenkauf TJ, Linnemeier G, Wiemann MC. Should we be using cimetidine to premedicate patients receiving docetaxel or paclitaxel? *Gynecol Oncol* (2004) 95, 270–1.
4. Rischin D, Webster LK, Millward MJ, Linahan BM, Toner GC, Woollett AM, Morton CG, Bishop JF. Cremophor pharmacokinetics in patients receiving 3-, 6-, and 24-hour infusions of paclitaxel. *J Natl Cancer Inst* (1996) 88, 1297–1301.
5. Cos J, Bellmunt J, Soler C, Ribas A, Lluis JM, Murio JE, Margarit C. Comparative study of sequential combinations of paclitaxel and methotrexate on a human bladder cancer cell line. *Cancer Invest* (2000) 18, 429–35.

Temozolomide + Miscellaneous

Valproic acid may reduce the clearance of temozolomide. Carbamazepine, H_2-receptor antagonists, dexamethasone, phenobarbital, phenytoin, prochlorperazine and ondansetron did not affect the clearance. Food, but not ranitidine slightly reduced extent of absorption of temozolomide.

Clinical evidence, mechanism, importance and management

The manufacturer notes that concurrent use of **carbamazepine**, **dexamethasone**, **H_2-receptor antagonists**, **ondansetron**, **phenobarbital**, **phenytoin** or **prochlorperazine** did not affect the clearance of temozolomide, based on an analysis of population pharmacokinetics from phase II studies.[1,2] However, **valproic acid** modestly reduced the clearance of temozolomide.[1,2]

Ranitidine 150 mg twice daily had no effect on the absorption or plasma pharmacokinetics of temozolomide, or that of its active metabolite in a study in 12 patients given temozolomide 150 mg/m^2 daily.[3] The manufacturer notes that **food** slightly reduces the temozolomide AUC by 9% and maximum plasma concentration by 33%. They recommend that it should be given without **food**.[1,2]

1. Temodal (Temozolomide). Schering-Plough Ltd. UK Summary of product characteristics, April 2007.
2. Temodar (Temozolomide). Schering Corporation. US Prescribing information, March 2007.
3. Beale P, Judson I, Moore S, Statkevich P, Marco A, Cutler D, Reidenberg P, Brada M. Effect of gastric pH on the relative oral bioavailability and pharmacokinetics of temozolomide. *Cancer Chemother Pharmacol* (1999) 44, 389–94.

Teniposide + Antiepileptics

Carbamazepine, phenytoin and phenobarbital markedly increase the clearance of teniposide. A reduction in its effects has been noted in B-lineage leukaemia.

Clinical evidence, mechanism, importance and management

The clearance of teniposide was increased two to threefold (from 13 to 32 mL/minute per m^1) in 6 children with acute lymphocytic leukaemia when they also took **phenytoin** or **phenobarbital**.[2] Another patient had a twofold increase in teniposide clearance when **carbamazepine** was given.[2] In a retrospective survey, long-term antiepileptic use (**phenytoin**, **phenobarbital**, **carbamazepine**, or a combination) was associated with worse event-free survival, and greater haematological relapse and CNS relapse in children receiving chemotherapy for B-lineage acute lymphoblastic leukaemia. In this study, faster clearance of teniposide was found in those receiving antiepileptics.[1]

These effects probably occur because these antiepileptics are potent liver enzyme inducers, which may increase the metabolism of teniposide by the liver and thereby reduce its levels. The authors of these reports therefore conclude that an increased dosage of teniposide will be needed in the presence of these antiepileptics to achieve systemic exposure to the drug comparable to that achievable in their absence.[2] It may be preferable to use alternative antiepileptics (that are not enzyme inducers) in patients requiring teniposide.[1] More study is needed.

1. Relling MV, Pui C-H, Sandlund JT, Rivera GK, Hancock ML, Boyett JM, Schuetz EG, Evans WE. Adverse effect of anticonvulsants on efficacy of chemotherapy for acute lymphoblastic leukaemia. *Lancet* (2000) 356, 285–90.
2. Baker DK, Relling MV, Pui C-H, Christensen ML, Evans WE, Rodman JH. Increased teniposide clearance with concomitant anticonvulsant therapy. *J Clin Oncol* (1992) 10, 311–5.

Thalidomide + Doxorubicin

The concurrent use of thalidomide and doxorubicin is associated with an increased risk of deep-vein thrombosis in patients with multiple myeloma.

Clinical evidence, mechanism, importance and management

In a study in 100 patients with newly diagnosed multiple myeloma given induction chemotherapy (dexamethasone, vincristine, doxorubicin, cyclophosphamide, etoposide and cisplatin) with or without thalidomide, deep vein thrombosis developed in 14 of the 50 patients (28%) given thalidomide compared with 2 of 50 patients (4%) not given thalidomide.[1] Deep vein thrombosis has been reported to occur in 10% of patients treated for multiple myeloma but is reported to occur in about 2% in patients with multiple myeloma treated with thalidomide alone.[1]

In a further study by the same authors, 232 patients with multiple myeloma were treated with DT-PACE (dexamethasone, thalidomide, cisplatin, doxorubicin, cyclophosphamide, etoposide) if they had preceding standard dose therapy but no prior autotransplantation, or with DCEP-T (dexamethasone, cyclophosphamide, etoposide, cisplatin, thalidomide) for relapse after transplantation. Deep-vein thrombosis developed in 31 of 192 patients (16%) treated with the doxorubicin-containing regimen (DT-PACE) and only 1 of 40 (2.5%) treated with DCEP-T (no doxorubicin).[2]

In patients with multiple myeloma, the risk of deep-vein thrombosis appears to be increased when thalidomide is given with combination chemotherapy containing doxorubicin. It has been suggested that, until more information is available, the concurrent use of thalidomide and doxorubicin should probably be limited to patients in monitored investigational studies.[2]

1. Zangari M, Anaissie E, Barlogie B, Badros A, Desikan R, Gopal AV, Morris C, Toor A, Siegel E, Fink L, Tricot G. Increased risk of deep-vein thrombosis in patients with multiple myeloma receiving thalidomide and chemotherapy. *Blood* (2001) 98, 1614–5.
2. Zangari M, Siegel E, Barlogie B, Anaissie E, Saghafifar F, Fassas A, Morris C, Fink L, Tricot G. Thrombogenic activity of doxorubicin in myeloma patients receiving thalidomide: implications for therapy. *Blood* (2002) 100, 1168–71.

Thalidomide + Epoetins

A higher than expected incidence of thromboembolic events occurred in patients with myelodysplastic syndrome treated with thalidomide and darbepoetin-alfa, but not in patients with multiple myeloma given thalidomide with epoetin.

Clinical evidence, mechanism, importance and management

A phase II study to investigate the efficacy and tolerability of the concurrent use of thalidomide 100 mg daily and **darbepoetin-alfa** 2.25 micrograms/kg per week subcutaneously in patients with myelodysplastic syndrome was discontinued because of an unexpectedly high incidence of thromboembolic events. Of the first 7 patients enrolled in the study, two developed deep vein thrombosis and one died of pulmonary embolism. The authors recommended careful monitoring and possibly thromboprophylaxis (heparin or warfarin) in patients with myelodysplastic syndrome given both thalidomide and epoetin.[1]

In contrast to these findings, in a study in patients with multiple myeloma treated with thalidomide, thromboses were reported in 4 of 49 patients (8.1%) also treated with epoetin and in 14 of 150 patients not treated with epoetin (9.3%). These results suggest that epoetin does not increase the risk of thrombosis in patients with multiple myeloma receiving thalidomide.[2]

The differences in findings have not been explained, but may be due to differences in both the disease states and the actions of darbepoetin alfa and epoetin in different regimens.

1. Steurer M, Sudmeier I, Stauder R, Gastl G. Thromboembolic events in patients with myelodysplastic syndrome receiving thalidomide in combination with darbepoietin-alpha. *Br J Haematol* (2003) 121, 101–3.
2. Galli M, Elice F, Crippa C, Comotti B, Rodeghiero F, Barbui T. Recombinant human erythropoietin and the risk of thrombosis in patients receiving thalidomide for multiple myeloma. *Haematologica* (2004) 89, 1141–2.

Thalidomide + Interferons

Severe bone marrow depression is reported in a patient given thalidomide with peginterferon alfa.

Clinical evidence, mechanism, importance and management

A patient with multiple myeloma in remission after an autologous stem cell transplantation was given thalidomide 200 mg daily. Five weeks after also being given **peginterferon alfa-2b** severe reversible bone marrow hypoplasia developed. **Peginterferon** was probably responsible for the bone marrow depression. However, thalidomide may also cause bone marrow depression and it was suggested that the severe suppression in this patient may have been due to the combined effects of the **peginterferon** and thalidomide.[1]

1. Gómez-Rangel JD, Ruiz-Delgado GJ, Ruiz-Argüelles GJ. Pegylated-interferon induced severe bone marrow hypoplasia in a patient with multiple myeloma receiving thalidomide. *Am J Hematol* (2003) 74, 290–1.

Thalidomide + Miscellaneous

Rifampicin and phenobarbital did not appear to alter thalidomide clearance in one study. Thalidomide increases the effect of other CNS depressants, and its CNS depressant activity is reduced by CNS stimulants. Thalidomide does not alter the pharmacokinetics of oral contraceptive steroids.

Clinical evidence, mechanism, importance and management

(a) CNS depressants

Animal studies have shown an increase in CNS depressant activity when thalidomide was given with **alcohol**, **barbiturates**, **chlorpromazine** and **reserpine**.[1]

(b) CNS stimulants

The depressant effect of thalidomide is reduced by the concurrent use of CNS stimulants such as **metamfetamine** and **methylphenidate**.[1]

(c) Cytochrome P450 isoenzyme inducers

There was no clear relationship between thalidomide clearance and the concurrent use of enzyme inducers such as **rifampicin (rifampin)**, or **phenobarbital** in a study in patients with glioma.[2] For the possible additive CNS depressant effect with barbiturates, see *CNS depressants*, above.

(d) Hormonal contraceptives

Thalidomide 200 mg daily for 3 weeks did not alter the pharmacokinetics of single doses of **ethinylestradiol/norethisterone** in two studies in healthy women.[3,4] Thalidomide is not therefore expected to alter the clinical efficacy of oral contraceptives. Note that, because thalidomide is an established human teratogen, it is very important that women taking it do not become pregnant. In the USA, it is standard practice to recommend that two forms of contraception should be used, of which hormonal contraceptives can be one.[5] This is because, even though hormonal methods of contraception are highly effective, they do, on rare occasions, fail.

1. Teo SK, Colburn WA, Tracewell WG, Kook KA, Stirling DI, Jaworsky MS, Scheffler MA, Thomas SD, Laskin OL. Clinical pharmacokinetics of thalidomide. *Clin Pharmacokinet* (2004) 43, 311–27.
2. Fine HA, Figg WD, Jaeckle K, Wen PY, Kyritsis AP, Loeffler JS, Levin VA, Black PM, Kaplan R, Pluda JM, Yung WK. Phase II trial of the antiangiogenic agent thalidomide in patients with recurrent high-grade gliomas. *J Clin Oncol* (2000) 18, 708–15.
3. Trapnell CB, Donahue SR, Collins JM, Flockhart DA, Thacker D, Abernethy DR. Thalidomide does not alter the pharmacokinetics of ethinyl estradiol and norethindrone. *Clin Pharmacol Ther* (1998) 64, 597–602.
4. Scheffler MR, Colburn W, Kook KA, Thomas SD. Thalidomide does not alter estrogen-progesterone hormone single-dose pharmacokinetics. *Clin Pharmacol Ther* (1999) 65, 483–90.
5. Thalomid (Thalidomide). Calgene Corp. US Prescribing information, February 2007.

Thalidomide + Zoledronic acid

The pharmacokinetics of zoledronic acid are not affected by thalidomide.

Clinical evidence, mechanism, importance and management

In a study intravenous zoledronic acid 4 mg every 4 weeks with alternate day prednisolone was given with or without thalidomide 200 mg daily for up to 1 year. The zoledronic acid pharmacokinetics were not affected by thalidomide and based on renal function no clinically adverse interaction occurred during concurrent use. The subjects in this study were patients with multiple myeloma with no disease progression 6 weeks after autologous stem-cell transplantation and conditioning with melphalan.[1]

1. Spencer A, Roberts A, Bailey M, Schran H, Lynch K. No evidence for an adverse interaction between zoledronic acid and thalidomide: preliminary safety analysis from the Australasian Leukaemia and Lymphoma Group (ALLG) MM6 Myeloma Trial. *Blood* (2003) 102, 383–4.

Thiopurines + Allopurinol

The haematological effects of azathioprine and mercaptopurine are markedly increased by allopurinol.

Clinical evidence

(a) Azathioprine

A patient taking allopurinol 300 mg daily for gout was also given azathioprine 100 mg daily to treat autoimmune haemolytic anaemia. Within 10 weeks his platelet count fell from 236 to 45 x 10^9/L, his white cell count fell from 9.4 to 0.8 x 10^9/L and his haemoglobin concentration fell from 11.5 to 5.3 g/dL.[1]

A number of other reports similarly describe reversible bone marrow toxicity associated with anaemia, pancytopenia, leucocytopenia and thrombocytopenia in patients given azathioprine with allopurinol,[1-9] and in one case a fatality occurred as a result of neutropenia and septicaemia.[8] In a retrospective analysis of 24 patients who had received both azathioprine and allopurinol, 11 developed leucopenia, 7 developed moderate anaemia, and 5 developed thrombocytopenia. Only 14 of the patients had received a greater than two-thirds reduction in their azathioprine dose when allopurinol was started, but despite this, some of these patients still developed haematological toxicity.[10]

(b) Mercaptopurine

In early studies, allopurinol 200 to 300 mg reduced the effective dose of mercaptopurine by approximately fourfold in 7 patients with chronic granulocytic leukaemia or variants.[11]

Profound pancytopenia developed in the first 3 of 13 children given maintenance treatment with mercaptopurine 2.5 mg/kg daily and allopurinol 10 mg/kg daily, but when the mercaptopurine dosage was halved, toxicity was manageable in the remaining 9 children.[12] Severe leucopenia and thrombocytopenia occurred in another patient given allopurinol with standard dose mercaptopurine.[13]

A pharmacokinetic study found that allopurinol caused a fivefold increase in the AUC and in peak plasma mercaptopurine levels when the mercaptopurine was given *orally*. The bioavailability increased from 12% to 59%.[14] This did not occur when the mercaptopurine was given *intravenously*.[14,15]

Mechanism

Azathioprine is firstly metabolised in the liver to mercaptopurine and then enzymatically oxidised in the liver and intestinal wall by xanthine oxidase to an inactive compound (6-thiouric acid), which is excreted. Allopurinol inhibits first-pass metabolism by xanthine oxidase so that mercaptopurine accumulates, blood levels rise and its toxic effects develop (leucopenia, thrombocytopenia, etc.).

Importance and management

A well documented, well established, clinically important and potentially life-threatening interaction. The dosages of azathioprine and mercaptopurine should be reduced by about two-thirds or three-quarters when given orally to reduce the development of toxicity. Despite taking these precautions toxicity may still be seen[10] and very close haematological monitoring is advisable if concurrent use is necessary. On the basis of two studies[14,15] it would seem that this precaution might not be necessary if mercaptopurine is given intravenously, but note that parenteral mercaptopurine is not routinely available.

1. Boyd IW. Allopurinol-azathioprine interaction. *J Intern Med* (1991) 229, 386.
2. Garcia-Ortiz RE, De Los Angeles Rodriguez M. Pancytopenia associated with the interaction of allopurinol and azathioprine. *J Pharm Technol* (1991) 7, 224–6.
3. Glogner P, Heni N. Panzytopenie nach Kombinationsbehandlung mit Allopurinol und Azathioprin. *Med Welt* (1976) 27, 1545–6.
4. Brooks RJ, Dorr RT, Durie BGM. Interaction of allopurinol with 6-mercaptopurine and azathioprine. *Biomedicine* (1982) 36, 217–22.
5. Klugkist H, Lincke HO. Panzytopenie unter Behandlung mit Azathioprin durch Interaktion mit Allopurinol bei Myasthenia gravis. *Akt Neurol* (1987) 14, 165–7.
6. Zazgornik J, Kopsa H, Schmidt P, Pils P, Kuschan K, Deutsch E. Increased danger of bone marrow damage in simultaneous azathioprine-allopurinol therapy. *Int J Clin Pharmacol Ther Toxicol* (1981) 19, 96–7.
7. Venkat Raman G, Sharman VL, Lee HA. Azathioprine and allopurinol: a potentially dangerous combination. *J Intern Med* (1990) 228, 69–71.
8. Adverse Drug Reactions Advisory Committee. Allopurinol and azathioprine. Fatal interaction. *Med J Aust* (1980) 2, 130.
9. Kennedy DT, Hayney MS, Lake KD. Azathioprine and allopurinol: the price of an avoidable drug interaction. *Ann Pharmacother* (1996) 30, 951–4.
10. Cummins D, Sekar M, Halil O, Banner N. Myelosuppression associated with azathioprine-allopurinol interaction after heart and lung transplantation. *Transplantation* (1996) 61, 1661–2.
11. Rundles RW, Wyngaarden JB, Hitchings GH, Elion GB, Silberman HR. Effects of xanthine oxidase inhibitor on thiopurine metabolism, hyperuricaemia and gout. *Trans Assoc Am Physicians* (1963) 76, 126–40.
12. Levine AS, Sharp HL, Mitchell J, Krivit W, Nesbit ME. Combination therapy with 6-mercaptopurine (NSC-755) and allopurinol (NSC-1390) during induction and maintenance of remission of acute leukaemia in children. *Cancer Chemother Rep* (1969) 53, 53–7.
13. Berns A, Rubenfeld S, Rymzo WI, and Calabro JJ. Hazard of combining allopurinol and thiopurine. *N Engl J Med* (1972) 286, 730–1.
14. Zimm S, Collins JM, O'Neill D, Chabner BA, Poplak DG. Inhibition of first-pass metabolism in cancer chemotherapy: interaction of 6-mercaptopurine and allopurinol. *Clin Pharmacol Ther* (1983) 34, 810–17.
15. Coffey JJ, White CA, Lesk AB, Rogers WI, Serpick AA. Effect of allopurinol on the pharmacokinetics of 6–mercaptopurine (NSC 755) in cancer patients. *Cancer Res* (1972) 32, 1283–9.

Thiopurines + 5-Aminosalicylates

The haematological toxicity of azathioprine and mercaptopurine may be increased by mesalazine, olsalazine or sulfasalazine. Balsalazide may be less likely to interact but this requires confirmation.

Clinical evidence

(a) Balsalazide

The frequency of clinically important neutropenia did not increase significantly in 10 patients with Crohn's disease receiving **azathioprine** or **mercaptopurine** when they were given balsalazide 6.75 g daily for 8 weeks, but significant increases in whole blood 6-thioguanine nucleotide concentrations were seen.[1]

(b) Mesalazine

A 13-year old boy with severe ulcerative pancolitis and cholangitis was treated with prednisone 60 mg daily, ursodeoxycholic acid 15 mg/kg daily and mesalazine 25 mg/kg daily. When **azathioprine** 2 mg/kg daily was added in an attempt to reduce the prednisone dosage, he developed marked and prolonged **azathioprine** toxicity (severe pancytopenia), which was attributed to an interaction resulting from abnormally high, persistent levels of an **azathioprine** metabolite.[2] In another study, there was a trend towards an increased rate of clinically important neutropenia in 10 patients with Crohn's disease receiving **azathioprine** or **mercaptopurine** when they were given mesalazine 4 g daily for 8 weeks. One patient was withdrawn from the study after 6 weeks because of leucopenia. Significant increases in whole blood 6-thioguanine nucleotide concentrations were also seen.[1]

(c) Olsalazine

A case report describes a patient with Crohn's disease who had two separate episodes of bone marrow suppression while receiving **mercaptopurine** 50 to 75 mg daily and olsalazine 1 to 1.75 g daily. It was found necessary to reduce the **mercaptopurine** dosage on the first occasion and to withdraw both drugs on the second.[3]

(d) Sulfasalazine

A decrease in leucocyte counts was seen in 4 patients taking **azathioprine** (2.1 to 3.3 mg/kg daily) after the addition of sulfasalazine. This lasted several months in one patient, and was transitory in two. The fourth patient developed agranulocytosis after 4 days, which required treatment discontinuation. When the drugs were later resumed at a lower dose, no reduction in leucocyte counts occurred.[4] Another report describes 38 patients taking **azathioprine** (mean dose 92.8 mg) and sulfasalazine (mean dose 2.1 g) for rheumatoid or psoriatic arthritis. Some patients did well, but in general the combination was poorly tolerated, and only 45% continued treatment after 6 months. Reasons for withdrawal included rash (3 patients), gastrointestinal upset (7), leucopenia (1) and nephrotic syndrome (1).[5] In another study, there was a trend towards an increased rate of clinically important neutropenia in 12 patients with Crohn's disease receiving **azathioprine** or **mercaptopurine** when they were given sulfasalazine 4 g daily for 8 weeks. One patient withdrew from the study after 6 weeks because of leucopenia. Significant increases in whole blood 6-thioguanine nucleotide concentrations were also found.[1]

Mechanism

The metabolism of azathioprine and mercaptopurine depends on *S*-methylation by thiopurine methyltransferase (TPMT) and oxidation by xanthine oxidase. An *in vitro* study using recombinant TPMT found that both sulfasalazine and its metabolites inhibit the activity of TPMT.[6] Therefore if these drugs are used together, the clearance of azathioprine and mercaptopurine may be reduced by the sulfasalazine, resulting in an increase in their toxicity (there is only a small margin between their therapeutic and toxic levels). About 11% of patients may be at particular risk because of genetic polymorphism whereby they have TPMT enzyme activity that is only half that of the rest of the population.[1,6] *In vitro* studies confirmed that mesalazine,[7] olsalazine and its metabolite olsalazine-*O*-sulfate[3,7] and balsalazide[7] are inhibitors of recombinant TPMT. In patients, increased levels of 6-thioguanine nucleotide are probably due to inhibition of TPMT.[1] It is suggested that the reported *in vitro* concentration (IC_{50}) of balsalazide required to halve the TPMT activity is about 1000 times higher than peak plasma levels after therapeutic doses and therefore an interaction is unlikely. Mesalazine and olsalazine peak levels may also be less than the IC_{50} concentrations, but peak plasma levels of sulfasalazine are close to IC_{50} concentrations.[8]

Importance and management

These reports underline the importance of taking particular care if azathioprine or mercaptopurine are used with balsalazide, mesalazine, olsalazine, or sulfasalazine. Balsalazide may be less likely to interact, but this requires confirmation.[1] Some have postulated that the interaction may actually benefit patients, as increased whole blood 6-thioguanine nucleotide or mild leucopenia is associated with a greater chance of remission in those taking azathioprine or mercaptopurine.[1,9] Extra monitoring of white blood cell counts is required when starting therapy with the combination.[9] More study is needed.

1. Lowry PW, Franklin CL, Weaver AL, Szumlanski CL, Mays DC, Loftus EV, Tremaine WJ, Lipsky JJ, Weinshilboum RM, Sandborn WJ. Leucopenia resulting from a drug interaction between azathioprine or 6-mercaptopurine and mesalamine, sulphasalazine, or balsalazide. *Gut* (2001) 49, 656–64.
2. Chouraqui JP, Serre-Debeauvais F, Armari C, Savariau N. Azathioprine toxicity in a child with ulcerative colitis: interaction with mesalazine. *Gastroenterology* (1996) 110 (4 Suppl), A883.
3. Lewis LD, Benin A, Szumlanski CL, Otterness DM, Lennard L, Weinshilboum RM, Nierenberg DW. Olsalazine and 6-mercaptopurine-related bone marrow suppression: a possible drug-drug interaction. *Clin Pharmacol Ther* (1997) 62, 464–75.
4. Bliddal H, Helin P. Leucopenia in adult Still's disease during treatment with azathioprine and sulphasalazine. *Clin Rheumatol* (1987) 6, 244–50.
5. Helliwell PS. Combination therapy with sulphasalazine and azathioprine. *Br J Rheumatol* (1996) 35, 493–4.
6. Szumlanski CL, Weinshilboum RM. Sulphasalazine inhibition of thiopurine methyltransferase: possible mechanism for interaction with 6-mercaptopurine and azathioprine. *Br J Clin Pharmacol* (1995) 39, 456–9.
7. Lowry PW, Szumlanski CL, Weinshilboum RM, Sandborn WJ. Balsalazide and azathioprine or 6-mercaptopurine: evidence for a potentially serious drug interaction. *Gastroenterology* (1999) 116, 1505–6.
8. Green JRB. Balsalazide and azathioprine or 6-mercaptopurine. *Gastroenterology* (1999) 117, 1513–14.
9. Present DH. Interaction of 6-mercaptopurine and azathioprine with 5-aminosalicylic acid agents. *Gastroenterology* (2000) 119, 276–7.

Thiopurines; Azathioprine + Co-trimoxazole or Trimethoprim

There is some evidence that the risk of haematological toxicity may be increased in renal transplant patients taking azathioprine if they are given co-trimoxazole or trimethoprim, particularly if they are given for extended periods. However, other evidence suggests that the drugs may be used together safely, and the combination is commonly used in practice.

Clinical evidence

The observation that haematological toxicity often seemed to occur in renal transplant patients given azathioprine and co-trimoxazole, prompted a retrospective survey of the records of 40 patients. It was found that there was no difference in the incidence of thrombocytopenia and neutropenia in those given azathioprine, either alone, or with co-trimoxazole, (trimethoprim 160 to 320 mg and sulfamethoxazole 800 mg to 1.6 g daily) for a short time (6 to 16 days), but a significant increase occurred in the incidence and duration of thrombocytopenia and neutropenia if both drugs were given together for 22 days or more.[1]

Another report describes a marked fall in white cell counts in renal transplant recipients during concurrent treatment with either co-trimoxazole (described as frequent) or trimethoprim (3 cases).[2] In one case the fall occurred within 5 days and was managed by temporarily withdrawing the azathioprine and reducing the trimethoprim dosage from 300 to 100 mg daily.[2]

Conversely, in an early study, there was no difference in the incidence of leucopenia when renal transplant recipients were given co-trimoxazole or other antibacterials.[3] Similarly, in 252 renal transplant patients given continuous prophylaxis with co-trimoxazole or **sulfafurazole** for 12 to 25 months, toxicity was minimal: leucopenia occurred only occasionally and was reversed by temporarily withholding azathioprine. This was needed in a similar number of patients with each antibacterial.[4] In another placebo-controlled study in cardiac transplant recipients taking triple therapy including azathioprine, co-trimoxazole prophylaxis for 4 months did not alter total white blood cell counts: leucopenia did not occur and no change in azathioprine dose was required.[5]

Mechanism

Not understood. It seems possible that the bone marrow depressant effects of all three drugs may be additive. In addition, in some patients impaired renal function may allow co-trimoxazole levels to become elevated, and haemodialysis may deplete folate levels, which could exacerbate the antifolate effects of the co-trimoxazole. Trimethoprim has been shown to inhibit renal tubular creatinine secretion.[6]

Importance and management

Information appears to be limited and the interaction is not established. Although there is some evidence of increased risk of haematological toxicity in renal transplant patients taking azathioprine if they are treated with co-trimoxazole or trimethoprim, this has not been shown in all studies. Two of the early studies suggested that the incidence of leucopenia with co-trimoxazole was related to the time after transplantation, and it improved if the dose of azathioprine was decreased or temporarily suspended.[3,7] Prophylaxis with co-trimoxazole post-transplant is commonly used in some centres.

1. Bradley PP, Warden GD, Maxwell JG, Rothstein G. Neutropenia and thrombocytopenia in renal allograft recipients treated with trimethoprim-sulfamethoxazole. *Ann Intern Med* (1980) 93, 560–2.
2. Bailey RR. Leukopenia due to a trimethoprim-azathioprine interaction. *N Z Med J* (1984) 97, 739.
3. Hall CL. Co-trimoxazole and azathioprine: a safe combination. *BMJ* (1974) 4, 15–16.
4. Peters C, Peterson P, Marabella P, Simmons RL, Najarian JS. Continuous sulfa prophylaxis for urinary tract infection in renal transplant recipients. *Am J Surg* (1983) 146, 589–93.
5. Olsen SL, Renlund DG, O'Connell JB, Taylor DO, Lassetter JE, Eastburn TE, Hammond EH, Bristow MR. Prevention of *Pneumocystis carinii* pneumonia in cardiac transplant recipients by trimethoprim sulfamethoxazole. *Transplantation* (1993) 56, 359–62.
6. Berg KJ, Gjellestad A, Nordby G, Rootwelt K, Djoseland O, Fauchald P, Mehl A, Narverud J, Talseth T. Renal effects of trimethoprim in ciclosporin- and azathioprine-treated kidney-allografted patients. *Nephron* (1989) 53, 218–22.
7. Hulme B, Reeves DS. Leucopenia associated with trimethoprim-sulphamethoxazole after renal transplantation. *BMJ* (1971) 3, 610–12.

Thiopurines; Mercaptopurine + Doxorubicin

One study postulated that the hepatotoxicity of *intravenous* mercaptopurine can be increased by doxorubicin.

Clinical evidence, mechanism, importance and management

One report describes 11 patients who developed liver damage after being given *intravenous* mercaptopurine 500 mg/m^2 daily for 5 days, with doxorubicin 50 mg/m^2 on the first day. The frequency and severity of liver damage was greater than the authors had previously seen with mercaptopurine alone. They postulated that doxorubicin potentiated the hepatotoxicity of mercaptopurine.[1] Mercaptopurine is no longer commonly used *intravenously*, and the dose given in this study is much higher than that currently used *orally*. The general applicability of this study is therefore unknown.

1. Minow RA, Stern MH, Casey JH, Rodriguez V, Luna MA. Clinico-pathological correlation of liver damage in patients treated with 6-mercaptopurine and adriamycin. *Cancer* (1976) 38, 1524–8.

Thiopurines; Mercaptopurine + Food

Food may reduce and delay the absorption of mercaptopurine.

Clinical evidence

A study in 17 children with acute lymphoblastic leukaemia showed that the absorption of mercaptopurine 5 mg/m^2 was reduced if it was given 15 minutes after a standard **breakfast** of 250 mL of milk and 50 g of biscuits, when compared with fasting. The AUC was reduced by 26%, the maximum plasma levels by 36%, and the time to maximum plasma levels delayed from 1.2 to 2.3 hours.[1] Some individuals showed more marked effects than others; 11 subjects had a decrease in absorption, whereas 6 subjects had no change or a small increase.[1] Similarly, in another study in 7 children, peak plasma mercaptopurine levels were lower and were delayed when it was given with a **standard breakfast** compared with those after an overnight fast.[2] However, in a third study in 10 children, mercaptopurine levels varied widely between individuals and there was no clear effect of food. The peak plasma levels were increased only 11% (range 67% decrease to 81% increase), and the AUC was increased by a mean of 3% (range 53% decrease to 86% increase) when given in the fasting state compared with after food.[3]

Mechanism

Not understood. Delayed gastric emptying is a suggested reason.[1]

Importance and management

The documentation is limited, and the interaction is not established. Mercaptopurine levels vary widely, and it is not established whether food is a clear factor in this variation. Some have suggested that mercaptopurine should be taken before food to optimise its absorption,[2] whereas others do not consider the evidence sufficient to make a recommendation.[3]

1. Riccardi R, Balis FM, Ferrara P, Lasorella A, Poplak DG, Mastrangelo R. Influence of food intake on bioavailability of oral 6-mercaptopurine in children with acute lymphoblastic leukaemia. *J Pediatr Hematol Oncol* (1986) 3, 319–24.
2. Burton NK, Barnett MJ, Aherne GW, Evans J, Douglas I, Lister TA. The effect of food on the oral administration of 6-mercaptopurine. *Cancer Chemother Pharmacol* (1986) 18, 90–1.
3. Lönnerholm G, Kreuger A, Lindström B, Myrdal U. Oral mercaptopurine in childhood leukemia: influence of food intake on bioavailability. *Pediatr Hematol Oncol* (1989) 6, 105–12.

Thiopurines; Mercaptopurine + Methotrexate

Methotrexate can increase the bioavailability of mercaptopurine, but the contribution this makes to their synergistic action in leukaemia is unclear. One report suggests the combination may not be synergistic.

Clinical evidence, mechanism, importance and management

In 14 children receiving maintenance therapy for leukaemia oral low-dose methotrexate 20 mg/m^2 increased the AUC and peak plasma levels of mercaptopurine 75 mg/m^2 by 31% and 26%, respectively.[1] In another study, 10 children with acute lymphoblastic leukaemia in remission were treated with mercaptopurine 25 mg/m^2 daily and intravenous infusions of high-dose methotrexate 2 or 5 g/m^2 once every other week for consolidation therapy. It was found that methotrexate 2 or 5 g/m^2 increased the AUC of mercaptopurine by 69% and 93% , respectively, and raised the maximum serum levels of mercaptopurine by 108% and 121%, respectively.[2] The reasons for this pharmacokinetic interaction are not understood, although it is thought that methotrexate is a xanthine oxidase inhibitor, which may therefore inhibit the metabolism of mercaptopurine.[1,2]

The combination of methotrexate and mercaptopurine has an established place in the therapy of leukaemia and has been found to be synergistic. These pharmacokinetic findings may be part of the explanation for this, although biochemical mechanisms may be more important.[3] The risk of relapse of leukaemia did not appear to be related to the pharmacokinetics of methotrexate or mercaptopurine, which showed considerable inter and intrapatient variability, in one study in children.[4]

In contrast, one report suggests that, in certain circumstances at least, the combination of mercaptopurine and methotrexate may not be synergistic. In a study, children with newly diagnosed acute lymphoblastic leukaemia were given intravenous mercaptopurine 1 g/m^2 over 6 hours, either alone, or after low-dose oral methotrexate (6 doses of 30 mg/m^2) or high-dose intravenous methotrexate (1 g/m^2 over 24 hours). Methotrexate increased the plasma levels of mercaptopurine, but, unexpectedly, it was also found that thioguanine nucleotide levels in bone marrow leukaemic lymphoblasts were 13-fold lower during methotrexate use. It is not known whether methotrexate would reduce thiopurine metabolite levels in leukaemic lymphoblasts when mercaptopurine is given as continuation therapy where the leukaemic burden is less substantial than in newly diagnosed cases. In addition, the changes in leukocyte counts over 3 days suggested mercaptopurine alone had little effect, and although methotrexate caused a reduction in intracellular thiopurine metabolite levels, it produced a greater decrease in leukocytes than mercaptopurine alone. It was concluded that in this particular study, the antileukaemic effect was primarily due to methotrexate.[5]

1. Balis FM, Holcenberg JS, Zimm S, Tubergen D, Collins JM, Murphy RF, Gilchrist GS, Hammond D, Poplack DG. The effect of methotrexate on the bioavailability of oral 6-mercaptopurine. *Clin Pharmacol Ther* (1987) 41, 384–7.
2. Innocenti F, Danesi R, Di Paolo A, Loru B, Favre C, Nardi M, Bocci G, Nardini D, Macchia P, Del Tacca M. Clinical and experimental pharmacokinetic interaction between 6-mercaptopurine and methotrexate. *Cancer Chemother Pharmacol* (1996) 37, 409–14.
3. Giverhaug T, Loennechen T, Aarbakke J. The interaction of 6-mercaptopurine (6-MP) and methotrexate (MTX). *Gen Pharmacol* (1999) 33, 341–6.
4. Balis FM, Holcenberg JS, Poplack DG, Ge J, Sather HN, Murphy RF, Ames MM, Waskerwitz MJ, Tubergen DG, Zimm S, Gilchrist GS, Bleyer WA. Pharmacokinetics and pharmacodynamics of oral methotrexate and mercaptopurine in children with lower risk acute lymphoblastic leukemia: a joint Children's Cancer Group and Pediatric Oncology Branch study. *Blood* (1998) 92, 3569–77.
5. Dervieux T, Hancock ML, Pui C-H, Rivera GK, Sandlund JT, Ribeiro RC, Boyett J, Evans WE, Relling MV. Antagonism by methotrexate on mercaptopurine disposition in lymphoblasts during up-front treatment of acute lymphoblastic leukemia. *Clin Pharmacol Ther* (2003) 73, 506–16.

Topotecan + Amifostine

In 10 women with ovarian cancer amifostine (given daily, before topotecan, for 5 days) did not significantly affect the pharmacokinetics of topotecan.[1]

1. Zackrisson A-L, Malmström H, Peterson C. No evidence that amifostine influences the plasma pharmacokinetics of topotecan in ovarian cancer patients. *Eur J Clin Pharmacol* (2002) 58, 103–8.

Topotecan + Phenytoin

Phenytoin may possibly increase topotecan clearance.

Clinical evidence, mechanism, importance and management

A 5-year-old child with medulloblastoma received a course of topotecan, firstly with phenytoin and then without. Phenytoin increased the total topotecan clearance by 47%.[1] This suggests that an increased topotecan dosage may possibly be needed in the presence of phenytoin in other patients. For a similar effect of antiepileptics on related topoisomerase inhibitors, see 'Irinotecan + Antiepileptics', p.638 and '9-Aminocamptothecin + Antiepileptics', p.610.

1. Zamboni WC, Gajjar AJ, Heideman RL, Beijnen JH, Rosing H, Houghton PJ, Stewart CF. Phenytoin alters the disposition of topotecan and *N*-desmethyl topotecan in a patient with medulloblastoma. *Clin Cancer Res* (1998) 4, 783–9.

Topotecan + Probenecid

In *mice,* probenecid markedly inhibited the renal tubular secretion of topotecan, which led to an increase in topotecan systemic exposure.[1]

1. Zamboni WC, Houghton PJ, Johnson RK, Hulstein JL, Crom WR, Cheshire PJ, Hanna SK, Richmond LB, Luo X, Stewart CL. Probenecid alters topotecan systemic and renal disposition by inhibiting renal tubular secretion. *J Pharmacol Exp Ther* (1998) 284, 89–94.

Topotecan + Ranitidine

Ranitidine does not alter the pharmacokinetics of topotecan.

Clinical evidence, mechanism, importance and management

In 18 patients with solid tumours, the pharmacokinetics of topotecan (given in initial doses of 2.3 mg/m^2 daily for 5 days and repeated every 3 weeks) and its active metabolite, topotecan lactone, were not affected by the previous use of ranitidine 150 mg twice daily for 4 days.[1] No special precautions would seem necessary if ranitidine or other drugs that increase gastric pH are given with oral topotecan.

1. Akhtar S, Beckman RA, Mould DR, Doyle E, Fields SZ, Wright J. Pretreatment with ranitidine does not reduce the bioavailability of orally administered topotecan. *Cancer Chemother Pharmacol* (2000) 46, 204–10.

Toremifene + Antiepileptics

Carbamazepine, phenobarbital and possibly phenytoin can reduce the serum levels of toremifene.

Clinical evidence, mechanism, importance and management

A pharmacokinetic study of toremifene in two groups of 10 patients (a control group and a group of patients taking antiepileptics) found that the AUC of a single 120-mg dose of toremifene and its half-life was approximately halved in the antiepileptic group. The antiepileptics used were **carbamazepine** alone (3 patients) or with clonazepam (3 patients), or **phenobarbital** alone (3 patients) or with **phenytoin** (1 patient). This interaction is thought to occur because these antiepileptics induce the liver enzymes (almost certainly the cytochrome P450 isoenzyme CYP3A4) by which toremifene is metabolised, resulting in increased toremifene clearance.[1] The UK manufacturers of toremifene have therefore reasonably suggested that the toremifene dosage may need to be doubled in the presence of these antiepileptics.[2]

1. Anttila M, Laakso S, Nyländen P, Sotaniemi EA. Pharmacokinetics of the novel antiestrogenic agent toremifene in subjects with altered liver and kidney function. *Clin Pharmacol Ther* (1995) 57, 628–35.
2. Fareston (Toremifene citrate). Orion Pharma UK Ltd. UK Summary of product characteristics, February 2006.

Toremifene + Miscellaneous

Based on theoretical considerations, the manufacturers advise care when toremifene is given with thiazides and with CYP3A inhibitors such as erythromycin, ketoconazole, and troleandomycin.

Clinical evidence, mechanism, importance and management

The manufacturers of toremifene note that it is mainly metabolised by the cytochrome P450 isoenzymes CYP3A4, CYP3A5, and CYP3A6 so it is suggested that drugs that can inhibit these enzymes (such as **erythromycin, troleandomycin, ketoconazole**) may possibly increase its effects.[1,2]

Hypercalcaemia is a recognised adverse effect of toremifene, and it is suggested that drugs such as the **thiazides**, which decrease renal calcium excretion, may increase the risk of hypercalcaemia.[1,2] These warnings are based on indirect evidence and theoretical considerations so that their clinical importance awaits confirmation.

1. Fareston (Toremifene citrate). Orion Pharma UK Ltd. UK Summary of product characteristics, February 2006.
2. Fareston (Toremifene citrate). GTx, Inc. US Prescribing information, December 2004.

Toremifene + Rifampicin (Rifampin)

Rifampicin increases the metabolism of toremifene, and might be expected to reduce its efficacy.

Clinical evidence, mechanism, importance and management

A study in 9 healthy men found that rifampicin 600 mg daily for 5 days reduced the AUC, peak plasma levels, and half-life of a single 120-mg dose of toremifene by 87%, 55%, and 44%, respectively. Similarly, the AUC of *N*-demethyltoremifene was reduced by 80%.[1] Rifampicin may therefore reduce the efficacy of toremifene.[1]

1. Kivistö KT, Villikka K, Nyman L, Anttila M, Neuvonen PJ. Tamoxifen and toremifene concentrations in plasma are greatly decreased by rifampin. *Clin Pharmacol Ther* (1998) 64, 648–54.

Tretinoin + Antifibrinolytics

In acute promyelocytic leukaemia the combination of tretinoin and antifibrinolytics such as tranexamic acid and aprotinin has been associated with fatal thrombotic complications.

Clinical evidence, mechanism, importance and management

In an analysis of 31 patients with acute promyelocytic leukaemia (APL) treated over a 7-year period, **tranexamic acid** 1 to 2 g daily for 6 days was given for prophylaxis of haemorrhage to 15 of 24 patients receiving tretinoin and chemotherapy, 4 of 4 receiving tretinoin only and 2 of 3 receiving chemotherapy only. Seven of the patients treated with tretinoin died during the study period and 4 of them, who had received only the combination of tretinoin and **tranexamic acid**, died within 42 days (early deaths). Three of the early deaths were attributed to thrombotic complications.[1] Another earlier report describes a similar fatal case of thromboembolism in a patient treated with tretinoin and **tranexamic acid**,[2] and another in a patient treated with tretinoin and **aprotinin**.[3] A further report describes acute renal cortex necrosis as a result of arterial thrombosis in a patient treated with tretinoin and **tranexamic acid**.[4] Tretinoin alone causes a procoagulant tendency in APL, and this may be exacerbated by use of antifibrinolytics. Although antifibrinolytics and chemotherapy may be safely used concurrently in APL, the combination of tretinoin and antifibrinolytics can cause fatal thrombotic complications and should be used with caution. The use of blood, platelets and plasma rather than **tranexamic acid** for prophylaxis of haemorrhage has been advocated for APL patients.[1]

1. Brown JE, Olujohungbe A, Chang J, Ryder WDJ, Chopra R, Scarffe JH. All-*trans* retinoic acid (ATRA) and tranexamic acid: a potentially fatal combination in acute promyelocytic leukaemia. *Br J Haematol* (2000) 110, 1010–12.
2. Hashimoto S, Koike T, Tatewaki W, Seki Y, Sato N, Azegami T, Tsukada N, Takahashi H, Kimura H, Ueno M, Arakawa M, Shibata A. fatal thromboembolism in acute promyelocytic leukemia during all-*trans* retinoic acid therapy combined with antifibrinolytic therapy for prophylaxis of hemorrhage. *Leukemia* (1994) 8, 1113–15.
3. Mahendra P, Keeling DM, Hood IM, Baglin TP, Marcus RE. Fatal thromboembolism in acute promyelocytic leukaemia treated with a combination of all-trans retinoic acid and aprotinin. *Clin Lab Haematol* (1996) 18, 51–2.
4. Levin M-D, Betjes MGH, v d Kwast TH, Wenberg BL, Leebeek FWG. Acute renal cortex necrosis caused by arterial thrombosis during treatment for acute promyelocytic leukemia. *Haematologica* (2003) 88, ECR21.

Tretinoin + Azoles

The metabolism of tretinoin can be inhibited by fluconazole, and a case report describes tretinoin toxicity as a result of this interaction. Ketoconazole may interact similarly.

Clinical evidence, mechanism, importance and management

A 4-year-old boy with acute promyelocytic leukaemia was given induction chemotherapy consisting of cytarabine, daunorubicin and tretinoin 45 mg/m^2 daily in two divided doses. Febrile neutropenia was treated with meropenem and amphotericin B for periods up to day 20. On day 20 he started antifungal prophylaxis with **fluconazole** 100 mg daily. The next day he complained of headache and a week later he had headache, vomiting and papilloedema. His CT scan was normal. Pseudotumor cerebri was diagnosed and symptoms of increased intracranial pressure resolved within a day of stopping tretinoin. Restarting tretinoin on day 30 at 75% of the previous dose resulted in headache and vomiting, and the treatment was continued from day 35 with an even lower dose (30%), which caused headache but only one episode of vomiting. **Fluconazole** was stopped on day 41 and within 24 hours the patient had improved clinically with the headache and vomiting fully resolved. He was then able to tolerate the full dose of tretinoin without adverse effects.[1]

Fluconazole inhibits the cytochrome P450 isoenzymes CYP3A4 and CYP2C9, which are amongst those involved in the oxidative metabolism of tretinoin, and it was suggested that this resulted in increased plasma levels of tretinoin.[1] Another study has also shown that **fluconazole** may inhibit the ADPH-dependent cytochrome P450-mediated metabolism of tretinoin.[2] **Ketoconazole** may similarly affect the pharmacokinetics of tretinoin.[3]

Although it has been suggested that drugs such as **fluconazole** may be useful in overcoming clinical resistance to tretinoin,[2] it has also been suggested that the concurrent use of tretinoin with drugs that affect its metabolism should be avoided if possible, or patients should be carefully monitored.[1]

1. Vanier KL, Mattiussi AJ, Johnston DL. Interaction of all-trans-retinoic acid with fluconazole in acute promyelocytic leukaemia. *J Pediatr Hematol Oncol* (2003) 25, 403–4.
2. Schwartz EL, Hallam S, Gallagher RE, Wiernik PH. Inhibition of all-trans retinoic acid metabolism by fluconazole in vitro and in patients with acute promyelocytic leukaemia. *Biochem Pharmacol* (1995) 50, 923–8.
3. Rigas JR, Francis PA, Muindi JRF, Kris MG, Huselton C, DeGrazia F, Orazem JP, Young CW, Warrell RP. Constitutive variability in the pharmacokinetics of the natural retinoid, all-trans-retinoic acid, and its modulation by ketoconazole. *J Natl Cancer Inst* (1993) 85, 1921–6.

Vinca alkaloids + Azoles

Itraconazole can increase the toxicity of vincristine and vinblastine; posaconazole and voriconazole may interact similarly. There is a theoretical possibility that itraconazole and ketoconazole may increase the toxicity of vinorelbine.

Clinical evidence, mechanism, importance and management

Four out of 14 patients with ALL given induction chemotherapy with weekly injections of **vincristine** (with prednisone, daunorubicin and asparaginase) and antifungal prophylaxis with **itraconazole** 400 mg daily, developed severe and early **vincristine**-induced neurotoxicity (paraesthesia and muscle weakness of the hands and feet, paralytic ileus, mild laryngeal nerve paralysis). The degree and early onset of these neurotoxic reactions were unusual, and were all reversible except for mild paraesthesia in one patient. The complications were more serious than in a previous series of 460 patients given **vincristine** without **itraconazole** (29% compared to 6%).[1] Five children with ALL developed severe **vincristine** toxicity attributed to the concurrent use of **itraconazole**. They were also receiving 'nifedipine', (p.671), which is known to reduce the clearance of **vincristine**, and which may have made things worse.[2] Severe **vincristine** neurotoxicity developed in four other children[3-5] and two adults[6] with ALL when they were given **itraconazole**. Another study similarly indicates that greater **vincristine** toxicity may occur in patients given **itraconazole**.[7]

The reasons for this interaction are not understood, but among the suggestions are that the **itraconazole** inhibits the metabolism of **vincristine** by the cytochrome P450 enzyme system, so that it is cleared from the body less quickly.[1] Another possible explanation is that **itraconazole** inhibits P-glycoprotein,[1] and increased **vincristine** neurotoxicity may be the result of the inhibition of this pump in endothelial cells of the blood-brain barrier.[7]

The authors of one report[1] suggest that **itraconazole** should be avoided in patients taking **vincristine**, and the manufacturers of **vincristine** also issue a warning about the increased risks of concurrent use.[8]

Acute neurotoxicity and myelotoxicity occurred in a boy with Hodgkin's lymphoma treated with **vinblastine**, doxorubicin and methotrexate when he was also given **itraconazole**. The toxicity did not occur when he was given the same chemotherapy without itraconazole.[9]

Some UK[10] and US[11] manufacturers advise caution if **vinorelbine**, which is metabolised by CYP3A4, is given with inhibitors of this isoenzyme such as **itraconazole** and **ketoconazole** because of the theoretical risk of increased neurotoxicity. The manufacturers of **vindesine** note that concurrent administration with CYP3A inhibitors may result in early onset or increased severity of vindesine side-effects.[12]

The manufacturers of **posaconazole** advise avoidance of concurrent use with vinca alkaloids (**vincristine** and **vinblastine** are named), but if they are given, then dose adjustments of the vinca alkaloids should be considered.[13]

The manufacturers of **voriconazole** advise caution if it is given to patients treated with the vinca alkaloids (**vincristine** and **vinblastine** are named) because of the risk of neurotoxicity.[14,15] The US manufacturer recommends that dose adjustments of the vinca alkaloids should be considered.[15]

1. Böhme A, Ganser A, Hoelzer D. Aggravation of vincristine-induced neurotoxicity by itraconazole in the treatment of adult ALL. *Ann Hematol* (1995) 71, 311–12.
2. Murphy JA, Ross LM, Gibson BES. Vincristine toxicity in five children with acute lymphoblastic leukaemia. *Lancet* (1995) 346, 443.
3. Ariffin H, Omar KZ, Ang EL, Shekhar K. Severe vincristine neurotoxicity with concomitant use of itraconazole. *J Paediatr Child Health* (2003) 39, 638–9.
4. Jeng MR, Feusner J. Itraconazole-enhanced vincristine neurotoxicity in a child with acute lymphoblastic leukemia. *Pediatr Hematol Oncol* (2001) 18, 137–42.
5. Sathiapalan RK, Al-Nasser A, El-Sohl H, Al-Mohsen I, Al-Jumaah S. Vincristine-itraconazole interaction: cause for increasing concern. *J Pediatr Hematol Oncol* (2002) 24, 591.
6. Gillies J, Hung KA, Fitzsimons E, Soutar R. Severe vincristine toxicity in combination with itraconazole. *Clin Lab Haematol* (1998) 20, 123–4.
7. Muenchow N, Janka G, Erttmann R, Looft G, Bielack S, Winkler K. Increased vincristine neurotoxicity during treatment with itraconazole in 3 pediatric patients with acute myelogenous leukaemia. *Blood* (1999) 94 (Suppl 1, part 2) 234b.
8. Vincristine sulphate. Mayne Pharma plc. UK Summary of product characteristics, April 2004.
9. Bashir H, Motl S, Metzger ML, Howard SC, Kaste S, Krasin MP, Hudson MM. Itraconazole-enhanced chemotherapy toxicity in a patient with Hodgkin lymphoma. *J Pediatr Hematol Oncol* (2006) 28, 33–5.
10. Vinorelbine. Mayne Pharma plc. UK Summary of product characteristics, June 2006.
11. Navelbine (Vinorelbine tartrate). Pierre Fabre Pharmaceuticals Inc. US Prescribing information, August 2005.
12. Eldisine (Vindesine). Eli Lilly and Company Ltd. UK Summary of product characteristics, September 1998.
13. Noxafil (Posaconazole). Schering-Plough Ltd. UK Summary of product characteristics, October 2006.
14. VFEND (Voriconazole). Pfizer Ltd. UK Summary of product characteristics, July 2007.
15. VFEND (Voriconazole). Pfizer Inc. US Prescribing information, November 2006.

Vinca alkaloids + Macrolides

Erythromycin increased the toxicity of vinblastine in three patients. Clarithromycin possibly does not interact with vinca alkaloids.

Clinical evidence

Three patients with renal cell carcinoma given ciclosporin 10 or 13 mg/kg daily and **erythromycin** 1 g daily for 3 days developed severe toxicity when given **vinblastine** 7 to 10 mg/m^2 on the third day. Ciclosporin was used as a modifier of multidrug resistance and **erythromycin** was given to achieve higher ciclosporin levels at a lower dose (see 'Ciclosporin + Antibacterials; Macrolides', p.1016). To rule out increased ciclosporin toxicity, one patient was given **erythromycin** without ciclosporin but he still developed **vinblastine** toxicity (severe neutropenia, constipation, myositis, severe myalgia) typical of much higher doses of **vinblastine**. Of the other 2 patients, only negligible toxicity developed in one when he was later given **vinblastine** alone, and the other had received ciclosporin and **vinblastine** on two previous occasions without problems.[1] Other authors report that they have used **clarithromycin** with standard doses of vinca alkaloids in at least 6 patients without any evidence of increased toxicity.[2]

Mechanism

Uncertain, but erythromycin inhibits the cytochrome P450 isoenzyme CYP3A4, which is concerned with the metabolism of vinblastine.[3] This would be expected to reduce the metabolism of vinblastine resulting in an increase in its toxicity.

Importance and management

Information seems to be limited to this report. On the basis of their findings the authors suggest that erythromycin should be avoided at the time of vinblastine infusion.[1] Use with clarithromycin may be safe.[2] The UK manufacturers of **vincristine** and **vindesine** have warned that caution should be exercised in patients taking any drugs known to inhibit the CYP3A subfamily because of the risk of an earlier onset and/or increased severity of adverse effects.[4,5] One manufacturer of vinblastine states that erythromycin may increase vinblastine toxicity.[6] Note that itraconazole, another CYP3A4 inhibitor, is known to increase the toxicity of vincristine, see 'Vinca alkaloids + Azoles', p.668.

1. Tobe SW, Siu LL, Jamal SA, Skorecki KL, Murphy GF, Warner E. Vinblastine and erythromycin: an unrecognized serious drug interaction. *Cancer Chemother Pharmacol* (1995) 35, 188–190.
2. Torresin A, Cassola G, Penco G, Crisalli MP, Piersantelli N. Vinca alkaloids and macrolides in human immunodeficiency virus-related malignancies: a safe association. *Cancer Chemother Pharmacol* (1996) 39, 176–7.
3. Zhou-Pan X-R, Sérée E, Zhou X-J, Placidi M, Maurel P, Barra Y, Rahmani R. Involvement of human liver cytochrome P450 3A in vinblastine metabolism: drug interactions. *Cancer Res* (1993) 53, 5121–6.
4. Eldisine (Vindesine). Eli Lilly and Company Ltd. UK Summary of product characteristics, September 1998.
5. Vincristine sulphate. Mayne Pharma plc. UK Summary of product characteristics, April 2004.
6. Vinblastine sulphate. Mayne Pharma plc. Summary of product characteristics, January 2003.

Vinca alkaloids + Mitomycin

A syndrome of acute pulmonary toxicity, characterised by severe shortness of breath, can occur when vinblastine, vindesine or vinorelbine is given with mitomycin. Fatalities have occurred.

Clinical evidence, mechanism, importance and management

There are now numerous reports describing acute lung disease in patients given mitomycin with vinca alkaloids, which appears to be different to the chronic pulmonary fibrosis seen with mitomycin alone. Sudden onset of acute shortness of breath has been described shortly after administration of the vinca alkaloid as part of a vinca alkaloid and mitomycin-containing regimen. Chest radiographs have shown diffuse lung damage characterised by interstitial infiltrates and pulmonary oedema. The acute syndrome has usually improved over 24 hours, although some patients have chronic respiratory impairment (60% in one case series[1]). Fatalities have occurred.[2-4] The syndrome has been reported with mitomycin and **vinblastine**,[1-9] **vindesine**[1,8,10-12] and **vinorelbine**.[12-15] The incidence is reported to be about 3 to 6%.[1,7,12]

The potential hazards of combining these drugs should be recognised, and in view of the unpredictability of the reaction, close observation of patients receiving this combination is recommended.[1,3] If the reaction occurs, supportive measures such as supplemental oxygen and mechanical ventilation may be needed. Corticosteroids are also often used in an attempt to treat the acute symptoms, and to possibly decrease the risk of chronic respiratory impairment.[1] In patients who have developed acute pulmonary toxicity, the use of both mitomycin and vinca alkaloids should subsequently be avoided.[1]

1. Rivera MP, Kris MG, Gralla RJ, White DA. Syndrome of acute dyspnea related to combined mitomycin plus vinca alkaloid chemotherapy. *Am J Clin Oncol* (1995) 18, 245–50.
2. Ozols RF, Hogan WM, Ostchega T, Young RC. MVP (mitomycin, vinblastine, progesterone): a second-line regimen in ovarian cancer with a high incidence of pulmonary toxicity. *Cancer Treat Rep* (1983) 67, 721–2.
3. Rao SX, Ramaswamy G, Levin M, McCravey JW. Fatal acute respiratory failure after vinblastine-mitomycin therapy in lung carcinoma. *Arch Intern Med* (1985) 145, 1905–7.

4. Ballen KK, Weiss ST. Fatal acute respiratory failure following vinblastine and mitomycin administration for breast cancer. *Am J Med Sci* (1988) 295, 558–60.
5. Israel RH, Olsen JP. Pulmonary edema associated with intravenous vinblastine. *JAMA* (1978) 240, 1585.
6. Konits PH, Aisner J, Sutherland JC, Wiernik PH. Possible pulmonary toxicity secondary to vinblastine. *Cancer* (1982) 50, 2771–4.
7. Hoelzer KL, Harrison BR, Luedke SW, Luedke DW. Vinblastine-associated pulmonary toxicity in patients receiving combination therapy with mitomycin and cisplatin. *Drug Intell Clin Pharm* (1986) 20, 287–9.
8. Kris MG, Pablo D, Gralla J, Burke MT, Prestifillippo J, Lewin D. Dyspnea following vinblastine or vindesine administration in patients receiving mitomycin plus vinca alkaloid combination therapy. *Cancer Treat Rep* (1984) 68, 1029–31.
9. Lagler U, Gattiker HH. Akute Dyspnoe nach intravenöser Gabe von Vinblastin/Mitomycin. *Schweiz Med Wochenschr* (1989) 119, 290–2.
10. Dyke RW. Acute bronchospasm after a vinca alkaloid in patients previously treated with mitomycin. *N Engl J Med* (1984) 310, 389.
11. Luedke D, McLaughlin TT, Daughaday C, Luedke S, Harrison B, Reed G, Martello O. Mitomycin C and vindesine associated pulmonary toxicity with variable clinical expression. *Cancer* (1985) 55, 542–5.
12. Thomas P, Pradal M, Le Caer H, Montcharmont D, Vervolet D, Kleisbauer JP. Bronchospasme aigu dû à l'association alcaloïde de la pervenche-mitomycine. *Rev Mal Respir* (1993) 10, 268–70.
13. Raderer M, Kornek G, Hejna M, Vorbeck F, Weinlaender G, Scheithauer W. Acute pulmonary toxicity associated with high-dose vinorelbine and mitomycin C. *Ann Oncol* (1996) 7, 973–5.
14. Rouzaud P, Estivals M, Pujazon MC, Carles P, Lauque D. Complications respiratoires de l'association vinorelbine-mitomycine. *Rev Mal Respir* (1999) 16, 81–4.
15. Uoshima N, Yoshioka K, Tegoshi J, Wada S, Fujiwara Y. Acute respiratory failure caused by vinorelbine tartrate in a patient with non-small cell lung cancer. *Intern Med* (2001) 40, 779–82.

Vinca alkaloids; Vinblastine + Bleomycin

The combination of vinblastine and bleomycin with or without cisplatin commonly causes Raynaud's phenomenon. Rarely, it also appears to cause serious life-threatening cardiovascular toxicity.

Clinical evidence, mechanism, importance and management

Five patients (aged 23 to 58) treated for germ cell tumours died from unexpected acute life-threatening vascular events (myocardial infarction, rectal infarction, cerebrovascular accident) after treatment with VBP (vinblastine, bleomycin, cisplatin). A survey of the literature by the authors of this paper revealed 14 other cases of both acute and long-term cardiovascular problems (myocardial infarction, coronary heart disease, cerebrovascular accident) in patients given VBP.[1]

Raynaud's phenomenon is common, occurring in one-third to half of those treated with vinblastine and bleomycin or VBP,[2,3] and there is evidence that blood vessels are pathologically altered.[2] Cisplatin may contribute to the effect.[3] Analysis of late vascular toxicity after chemotherapy for testicular cancer revealed that the use of VBP carried a higher risk of Raynaud's phenomenon than bleomycin with etoposide and cisplatin (BEP).[4]

The use of the VBP (PVB) regimen has largely been replaced by the BEP (PEB) regimen, because of its reduced toxicity.

1. Samuels BL, Vogelzang NJ, Kennedy BJ. Severe vascular toxicity associated with vinblastine, bleomycin and cisplatin chemotherapy. *Cancer Chemother Pharmacol* (1987) 19, 253–6.
2. Vogelzang NJ, Bosl GJ, Johnson K, Kennedy BJ. Raynaud's phenomenon: a common toxicity after combination chemotherapy for testicular cancer. *Ann Intern Med* (1981) 95, 288–92.
3. Hansen SW. Late-effects after treatment for germ-cell cancer with cisplatin, vinblastine, and bleomycin. *Dan Med Bull* (1992) 39, 391–9.
4. Berger CC, Bokemeyer C, Schneider M, Kuczyk MA, Schmoll H-J. Secondary Raynaud's phenomenon and other late vascular complications following chemotherapy for testicular cancer. *Eur J Cancer* (1995) 31A, 2229–38.

Vinca alkaloids; Vinblastine + Protease inhibitors

Severe neutropenia has been seen in two patients given vinblastine and antiretroviral regimens including lopinavir/ritonavir.

Clinical evidence, mechanism, importance and management

A 55-year-old HIV-positive man who was taking zidovudine, lamivudine, abacavir, nevirapine and **ritonavir**-boosted **lopinavir** experienced unexpected severe gastrointestinal and haematological toxicities and moderate renal failure after the second and third intravenous injections of vinblastine 10 mg given to treat multicentric Castleman's disease (MCD). Subsequently, the antiretrovirals were stopped and the patient did not experience these toxicities when vinblastine was given alone. When the MCD was under control, the antiretrovirals were then restarted, and the vinblastine dose reduced to 3 mg every three weeks without problems.[1] A second HIV-positive patient who was taking a **lopinavir/ritonavir** based antiretroviral regimen developed life-threatening neutropenia when given ABVD chemotherapy, consisting of doxorubicin, bleomycin, vinblastine and dacarbazine for Hodgkin's lymphoma. Further vinblastine treatment was successfully given by interrupting the protease inhibitors around the time the chemotherapy was given.[2]

It was suggested that the metabolism of vinblastine by the cytochrome P450 isoenzyme CYP3A was inhibited by ritonavir, resulting in increased toxicity.

These appear to be the only cases so far of a possible interaction. Nevertheless, it would now be prudent to carefully monitor any patient taking a ritonavir-based antiretroviral regimen who receives vinblastine. Further study is needed.

1. Kotb R, Vincent I, Dulioust A, Peretti D, Taburet A-M, Delfraissy J-F, Goujard C. Life-threatening interaction between antiretroviral therapy and vinblastine in HIV-associated multicentric Castleman's disease. *Eur J Haematol* (2006) 76, 269–71.
2. Makinson A, Martelli N, Peyrière H, Turriere C, Le Moing V, Reynes J. Profound neutropenia resulting from interaction between antiretroviral therapy and vinblastine in a patient with HIV-associated Hodgkin's disease. *Eur J Haematol* (2007) 78, 358–60.

Vinca alkaloids; Vincristine + Antiepileptics

Carbamazepine and phenytoin appear to reduce the plasma levels of vincristine, and may reduce its efficacy. A number of case reports have described reduced phenytoin levels in patients receiving chemotherapy including vinca alkaloids.

Clinical evidence, mechanism, importance and management

The systemic clearance of vincristine 2 mg was 63% higher and the AUC was 43% lower in 9 patients receiving **carbamazepine** or **phenytoin** than in 6 patients not taking antiepileptics. In this study, patients were being treated with procarbazine, lomustine and vincristine for brain tumours.[1] In a retrospective survey, long-term antiepileptic use (**phenytoin**, **phenobarbital**, **carbamazepine**, or a combination) was associated with worse event-free survival, and greater haematological relapse and CNS relapse in children receiving chemotherapy for B-lineage acute lymphoblastic leukaemia. The authors considered that the increased clearance of vincristine induced by the antiepileptics was a likely factor in these findings.[2]

These enzyme-inducing antiepileptics increase the metabolism of vincristine by the cytochrome P450 isoenzyme CYP3A4. However, *in vitro* studies have shown that **phenytoin** may potentiate the antineoplastic (antimitotic) effects of the vinca alkaloids.[3,4] Thus, further study is required to determine the overall effect of **phenytoin** on the efficacy and toxicity of vincristine and other **vinca alkaloids**. **Carbamazepine** would be expected to reduce the efficacy of vincristine.

Note that a number of case reports have described reduced **phenytoin** levels in patients receiving chemotherapy including **vinca alkaloids**, see 'Table 14.1', (p.519).

1. Villikka K, Kivistö KT, Mäenpää H, Joensuu H, Neuvonen PJ. Cytochrome P450-inducing antiepileptics increase the clearance of vincristine in patients with brain tumors. *Clin Pharmacol Ther* (1999) 66, 589–93.
2. Relling MV, Pui CH, Sandlund JT, Rivera GK, Hancock ML, Boyett JM, Schuetz EG, Evans WE. Adverse effect of anticonvulsants on efficacy of chemotherapy for acute lymphoblastic leukaemia. *Lancet* (2000) 356, 285–90.
3. Ganapathi R, Hercbergs A, Grabowski D, Ford J. Selective enhancement of vincristine cytotoxicity in multidrug-resistant tumor cells by dilantin (phenytoin). *Cancer Res* (1993) 53, 3262–5. Correction. ibid. 6079.
4. Lobert S, Ingram JW, Correia JJ. Additivity of dilantin and vinblastine inhibitory effects on microtubule assembly. *Cancer Res* (1999) 59, 4816–22.

Vinca alkaloids; Vincristine + Asparaginase

An isolated case report suggests that vincristine neurotoxicity may possibly have been increased by subsequent asparaginase therapy.[1,2] The UK manufacturer recommends that vincristine should be given 12 to 24 hours before asparaginase.[3] Regimens including both drugs are commonly used in treating leukaemia.

1. Hildebrand J, Kenis Y. Vincristine neurotoxicity. *N Engl J Med* (1972) 287, 517.
2. Hildebrand J, Kenis Y. Additive toxicity of vincristine and other drugs for the peripheral nervous system. *Acta Neurol Belg* (1971) 71, 486–91.
3. Vincristine sulphate. Mayne Pharma plc. UK Summary of product characteristics, April 2004.

Vinca alkaloids; Vincristine + Isoniazid

Some limited evidence suggests that vincristine neurotoxicity may possibly be increased by isoniazid.

Clinical evidence, mechanism, importance and management

An 85-year-old woman with Hodgkin's disease was given COPP/ABVD, alternating every 28 days. She started COPP (cyclophosphamide and 2 mg vincristine on day 1, with procarbazine and prednisone days 1 to 14) and was also given isoniazid 300 mg daily as prophylaxis of tuberculosis. Five days after the start of this treatment she experienced tingling in her fingers and weakness in her legs, which was interpreted by the authors of this report as being vincristine toxicity brought about by the concurrent use of isoniazid (paraesthesia of the feet and/or hands being a recognised early manifestation of vincristine toxicity). Their reasoning was that such a small dosage of vincristine dosage on its own was unlikely to cause severe neurotoxicity of this kind, but it is not clear why isoniazid should apparently interact like this. The authors suggest that the age of this patient and her diabetes (well controlled) may have contributed to this increase in vincristine neurotoxicity.[1]

This report is consistent with another much earlier report of two patients who also developed peripheral neurotoxicity when they were given vincristine after starting to take isoniazid and pyridoxine, the cumulative doses of vincristine being 11 mg and 11.2 mg, respectively,[2,3] and of a case of severe neurotoxicity with an overdose of isoniazid and high-dose vincristine.[4]

These reports appear to be the only ones implicating isoniazid in an increase in vincristine toxicity, but they serve to emphasise the importance of very close neurological supervision in anyone given both drugs.

1. Carrión C, Espinosa E, Herrero A, García B. Possible vincristine-isoniazid interaction. *Ann Pharmacother* (1995) 29, 201.
2. Hildebrand J, Kenis Y. Vincristine neurotoxicity. *N Engl J Med* (1972) 287, 517.
3. Hildebrand J, Kenis Y. Additive toxicity of vincristine and other drugs for the peripheral nervous system. *Acta Neurol Belg* (1971) 71, 486–91.
4. Frappaz D, Biron P, Biron E, Amrane A, Philip T, Brunat-Mentigny M. Toxicite neurologique severe (coma, convulsions, neuropathie motrice distale) secondaire a l'association d'une intoxication accidentelle a l'isoniazide (INH) et d'un protocole comportant de fortes doses de vincristine (VCR). *Pediatrie* (1984) 39, 133–40.

Vinca alkaloids; Vincristine + Nifedipine

Nifedipine reduces the clearance of vincristine.

Clinical evidence, mechanism, importance and management

In a study in 12 patients nifedipine reduced the clearance of a single 2-mg intravenous dose of vincristine by 68%, and increased the AUC threefold, when compared with 14 patients receiving vincristine alone. Nifedipine was given at a dose of 10 mg three times daily for 3 days before and 7 days after vincristine was given. However, no important adverse effects were noted in either group of patients, suggesting that these pharmacokinetic changes did not markedly increase vincristine toxicity.[1] Further study is needed. Note that increased vincristine-related neurotoxicity has been seen in a child taking nifedipine and itraconazole (see 'Vinca alkaloids + Azoles', p.668).

1. Fedeli L, Colozza M, Boschetti E, Sabalich I, Aristei C, Guerciolini R, Del Favero A, Rossetti R, Tonato M, Rambotti P, Davis S. Pharmacokinetics of vincristine in cancer patients treated with nifedipine. *Cancer* (1989) 64, 1805–11.

18

Antiparkinsonian and related drugs

The drugs in this section are considered together because their major therapeutic application is in the treatment of Parkinson's disease, although some of the related antimuscarinic (anticholinergic) drugs included here are also used for other conditions. Parkinson's disease is named after Dr James Parkinson who originally described the four main signs of the disease, namely rigidity, tremor, dystonias and dyskinesias (movement disorders). Similar symptoms may also be displayed as the unwanted adverse effects of therapy with certain drugs.

The basic cause of the disease lies in the basal ganglia of the brain, particularly the striatum and the substantia nigra, where the normal balance between dopaminergic nerve fibres (those that use dopamine as the chemical transmitter) and cholinergic nerve fibres (those that use acetylcholine as the transmitter) is lost, because the dopaminergic fibres degenerate. As a result the cholinergic fibres end up in relative excess. Much of the treatment of Parkinson's disease is based on an attempt to redress the balance, and there are several groups of drugs that can be used to this end. These are listed in 'Table 18.1', (below), and discussed below.

Levodopa

Levodopa can pass the blood-brain barrier (unlike dopamine), where it is converted into dopamine, and thus acts by 'topping up' the CNS dopaminergic system. Levodopa is most usually given with **carbidopa** or **benserazide** (dopa-decarboxylase inhibitors), which prevent the 'wasteful' peripheral metabolism of levodopa. This allows lower doses of levodopa to be given, which results in fewer adverse effects.

Amantadine (and memantine)

These drugs may augment dopaminergic activity in the brain.

Dopamine agonists

Bromocriptine, cabergoline, pergolide, ropinirole and similar drugs act as dopamine agonists and so also have the effect of increasing dopaminergic activity in the brain.

Entacapone and tolcapone

The catechol-*O*-methyltransferase (COMT) inhibitors work by inhibiting the peripheral metabolism of levodopa by COMT. Note that this enzyme is the major metabolising enzyme for levodopa when a decarboxylase inhibitor (e.g. benserazide) is being used.

Rasagiline and selegiline

The selective irreversible MAO-B inhibitors enhance dopamine activity by preventing dopamine degradation. These drugs sometimes interact like older non-selective MAOIs, and the reader is cross-referred to the information under MAOIs when appropriate. Selegiline undergoes rapid first-pass metabolism to produce amfetamine metabolites. A buccal tablet has been developed, which markedly reduces this first-pass metabolism, and is consequently given as a smaller dose.

Antimuscarinics

Benzhexol, orphenadrine, procyclidine and other antimuscarinic (anticholinergic) drugs work by correcting the relative cholinergic excess.

The interactions that affect the antimuscarinic effects of these drugs are discussed in this section. However, the antimuscarinics also affect the actions of other drugs (such as the centrally-acting anticholinesterases) and these are therefore discussed elsewhere in the publication.

Table 18.1 Antiparkinsonian drugs

Group	*Drugs*
Dopaminergic drugs	
Amino-acid precursor of dopamine	Levodopa
Levodopa combined with a peripheral dopa-decarboxylase inhibitor	Co-beneldopa (levodopa + benserazide) Co-careldopa (levodopa + carbidopa)
COMT-inhibitors	Entacapone, Tolcapone
Dopamine agonists	
Ergot derivatives	Bromocriptine, Cabergoline, Lisuride, Pergolide
Non-ergot dopamine agonists	Piribedil, Pramipexole, Quinagolide, Ropinirole, Rotigotine
Other dopamine agonists	Apomorphine
MAO-B inhibitors	Rasagiline, Selegiline
Other	Amantadine
Other	
Peripheral dopa-decarboxylase inhibitors	Benserazide, Carbidopa
Antimuscarinics	Benzatropine, Biperiden, Bornaprine, Dexetimide, Metixene, Orphenadrine, Procyclidine, Profenamine, Trihexyphenidyl, Tropatepine

Amantadine + Co-trimoxazole

An interaction between amantadine and co-trimoxazole is thought to have caused acute confusion in an elderly man and amantadine toxicity in a patient with end-stage renal disease. However, in both cases other factors could have been responsible for the adverse reactions.

Clinical evidence, mechanism, importance and management

An 84-year-old man with parkinsonism, COPD and chronic atrial fibrillation, had been taking amantadine 100 mg twice daily and digoxin 125 micrograms daily for at least 2 years. Within 72 hours of starting co-trimoxazole twice daily for bronchitis he became mentally confused, incoherent and combative. He also showed cogwheel rigidity and a resting tremor. Within 24 hours of stopping the amantadine and co-trimoxazole, the patient's mental status returned to normal.[1] The reasons for this reaction are not understood, but on the basis of *animal* studies, the authors suggest that the **trimethoprim** component of the co-trimoxazole may have competed with the amantadine for renal secretion. This resulted in an accumulation of amantadine and led to the adverse effects seen.[1] This interaction is more likely in the elderly because ageing results in a decrease in the clearance of these and many other drugs. However, it should be noted that both drugs can cause some mental confusion, and also that mental confusion is not an uncommon symptom of infection in the elderly. Another case of amantadine toxicity has been reported in a 27-year-old woman with end-stage renal disease who was also taking co-trimoxazole. As in the other case the authors suggest that the **trimethoprim** component of the co-trimoxazole may have competed with the amantadine for renal secretion. However, they also note that amantadine toxicity occurred 5 days after the amantadine dose was increased, and during an episode of acute renal failure, which could both account for the toxicity.[2]

These seem to be the only reports of a possible interaction, so the general importance of this interaction remains uncertain.

1. Speeg KV, Leighton JA, Maldonado AL. Case report: toxic delirium in a patient taking amantadine and trimethoprim-sulfamethoxazole. *Am J Med Sci* (1989) 298, 410–12.
2. Michalski LS, Hantsch CE, Hou SH. Amantadine toxicity in a renal transplant patient. Abstracts of the 2003 North American Congress of Clinical Toxicology Annual Meeting, 93.

Amantadine + Diuretics

A patient has been described who developed amantadine toxicity when given hydrochlorothiazide-triamterene.

Clinical evidence

Amantadine toxicity (ataxia, agitation, hallucinations) developed in a patient within a week of starting to take two tablets of *Dyazide* (**hydrochlorothiazide** with **triamterene**) daily. The symptoms rapidly disappeared when all the drugs were withdrawn. In a later study this patient showed about a 50% rise in amantadine plasma levels (from 156 to 243 nanograms/mL) after taking the diuretic for 7 days.[1]

Mechanism

Uncertain. Amantadine is largely excreted unchanged in the urine and it seems probable that these diuretics reduce the renal clearance.[1]

Importance and management

Published information about an adverse interaction appears to be limited. There seems to be little reason for avoiding concurrent use, but bear this case in mind in the event of an unexpected response to treatment.

1. Wilson TW, Rajput AH. Amantadine–Dyazide interaction. *Can Med Assoc J* (1983) 129, 974–5.

Amantadine + MAOIs or MAO-B inhibitors

An isolated report describes a rise in blood pressure in a patient on amantadine within 72 hours of taking phenelzine. One manufacturer suggests that the use of selegiline with amantadine may increase adverse effects.

Clinical evidence, mechanism, importance and management

(a) Older non-selective MAOIs

A 49-year-old woman was taking amantadine 200 mg daily, haloperidol 5 mg daily and flurazepam 30 mg at night was given **phenelzine** 15 mg twice daily for depression. Within 72 hours her blood pressure rose from 140/90 to 160/110 mmHg. The **phenelzine** was withdrawn, and 24 hours later, the amantadine and haloperidol were withdrawn. The blood pressure remained elevated for a further 72 hours.[1] In contrast, a woman is reported to have been successfully and uneventfully treated with amantadine 200 mg daily for Parkinson's disease and **phenelzine** 45 mg daily for depression.[2]

The first case appears to be the only reported interaction with amantadine. Its general importance is uncertain, but bear it in mind in case of an unusual response to treatment.

(b) Selective MAO-B inhibitors

One manufacturer of **selegiline** states that concurrent use of amantadine can increase the occurrence of adverse effects (e.g. dizziness, tremor, orthostatic hypotension).[3]

1. Jack RA, Daniel DG. Possible interaction between phenelzine and amantadine. *Arch Gen Psychiatry* (1984) 41, 726.
2. Greenberg R, Meyers BS. Treatment of major depression and Parkinson's disease with combined phenelzine and amantadine. *Am J Psychiatry* (1985) 142, 273–4.
3. Zelapar (Selegiline hydrochloride). Zeneus Pharma Ltd. UK summary of product characteristics, January 2006.

Amantadine + Phenylpropanolamine

The use of amantadine in a patient also taking phenylpropanolamine resulted in psychosis, and concurrent use in another patient resulted in intense and recurrent déjà vu experiences.

Clinical evidence, mechanism, importance and management

A case report describes the development of severe psychosis in a woman within 7 to 8 days of starting amantadine 100 mg [frequency unclear but possibly twice daily] and phenylpropanolamine 80 mg daily. The reasons are not known, but both drugs alone, and in high doses sometimes cause psychosis, and concurrent use may enhance this effect.[1] Another report describes intense and recurrent déjà vu experiences in a 39-year-old man taking amantadine 100 mg twice daily and phenylpropanolamine 25 mg twice daily during a viral infection. These experiences stopped the day he discontinued the drugs. He had previously taken phenylpropanolamine without this effect. The authors considered the déjà vu experiences to be related to increased dopamine activity caused by both drugs.[2]

Concurrent use need not be avoided, but remain aware of the potential for this interaction.

1. Stroe AE, Hall J, Amin F. Psychotic episode related to phenylpropanolamine and amantadine in a healthy female. *Gen Hosp Psychiatry* (1995) 17, 457–8.
2. Taiminen T, Jääskeläinen SK. Intense and recurrent déjà vu experiences related to amantadine and phenylpropanolamine in a healthy male. *J Clin Neurosci* (2001) 8, 460–2.

Amantadine + Quinidine or Quinine

In a single-dose study, quinidine and quinine modestly reduced the loss of amantadine in the urine in men, but not women. However, the absence of any clinical reports suggest that a significant interaction is unlikely.

Clinical evidence, mechanism, importance and management

Single-dose studies into the renal excretion of amantadine in healthy subjects found that quinine sulfate 200 mg and quinidine sulfate 200 mg reduced the renal clearance of oral amantadine 3 mg/kg by about 30%, but only in male subjects.[1] Whether long-term use of these drugs would therefore cause a clinically relevant rise in serum amantadine levels is uncertain. However, the absence of any clinical reports suggests it is unlikely.

Nevertheless, be aware that amantadine toxicity (e.g. headache, nausea, or dizziness) could possibly result from the concurrent use of quinine or quinidine.

1. Gaudry SE, Sitar DS, Smyth DD, McKenzie JK, Aoki FY. Gender and age as factors in the inhibition of renal clearance of amantadine by quinine and quinidine. *Clin Pharmacol Ther* (1993) 54, 23–7.

Amantadine + Tobacco

Amantadine clearance was not altered by tobacco smoking in one study.

Clinical evidence, mechanism, importance and management

The elimination of a single 3-mg/kg dose of amantadine was compared between heavy smokers (20 or more cigarettes daily) and non-smokers.

Although a higher apparent volume of distribution was noted in the heavy smokers, renal and plasma clearances were unchanged, suggesting that no interaction of note occurs.[1]

1. Wong LTY, Sitar DS, Aoki FY. Chronic tobacco smoking and gender as variables affecting amantadine disposition in healthy subjects. *Br J Clin Pharmacol* (1995) 39, 81–4.

Antimuscarinics + Antimuscarinics

Additive antimuscarinic effects, both peripheral and central, can develop if two or more drugs with antimuscarinic effects are used together. The outcome may be harmful.

Clinical evidence, mechanism, importance and management

The antimuscarinic (sometimes called anticholinergic) effects of some drugs are exploited therapeutically. These include antimuscarinic bronchodilators, gastrointestinal antispasmodics, mydriatics, urological antimuscarinics, and drugs such as **trihexyphenidyl** and **benzatropine** (see 'Table 18.1', (p.672)), which are used for the control of parkinsonian symptoms. Other drugs, such as some antiemetics, sedating antihistamines, antipsychotics, and tricyclic antidepressants, (see 'Table 18.2', (below)), may also possess some antimuscarinic effects that are unwanted and troublesome, but usually not serious, unless they are worsened by the addition of another drug with similar properties.

The easily recognised and common peripheral antimuscarinic effects are blurred vision, dry mouth, constipation, difficulty in urination, reduced sweating and tachycardia. Central effects include confusion, disorientation, visual hallucinations, agitation, irritability, delirium, memory problems, belligerence and even aggressiveness. Problems are most likely to arise in patients with particular physical conditions such as glaucoma, prostatic hypertrophy or constipation, in whom antimuscarinic drugs should be used with caution, if at all. It has been pointed out that the antimuscarinic adverse effects can mimic the effects of normal ageing.

'Table 18.1', (p.672) and 'Table 18.2', (below) list many of the drugs with antimuscarinic effects, which may be expected to be additive if used together, but apart from some reports describing life-threatening reactions (see 'Antipsychotics + Antimuscarinics', p.708) there are very few reports describing this simple additive interaction, probably because the outcome is so obvious. Many of these interactions are therefore 'theoretical' but their probability is high.

Some drugs with only minimal antimuscarinic properties sometimes cause difficulties if given with other antimuscarinics. A patient taking **isopropamide iodide** developed urinary retention needing catheterisation, only when **trazodone** 75 mg daily was also taken, but not when either drug was taken alone.[1] **Trazodone** is usually regarded as having minimal antimuscarinic effects. Another case describes acute psychosis in an elderly woman taking **hyoscine** and **meclozine**, both of which have antimuscarinic effects.[2]

If the central antimuscarinic effects caused by the use of antimuscarinic drugs are not clearly recognised for what they are, there is the risk that antipsychotics may be prescribed to treat them. Many antipsychotics also have antimuscarinic adverse effects so that matters are simply made worse. If the patient then demonstrates dystonias, akathisia, tremor and rigidity, even more antimuscarinics may be added to control the extrapyramidal effects, which merely adds to the continuing downward cycle of drug-induced problems.

In addition to the obvious and very well recognised drugs with antimuscarinic effects, a study of the 25 drugs most commonly prescribed for the elderly identified detectable antimuscarinic activity (using an antimuscarinic radioreceptor assay) in 14 of them, 9 of which (**codeine**, **digoxin**, **dipyridamole**, **isosorbide dinitrate**, **nifedipine**, **prednisolone**, **ranitidine**, **theophylline**, and **warfarin**) produced levels of antimuscarinic activity that have been shown to cause significant impairment in tests of memory and attention in the elderly.[3] Thus the problem may not necessarily be confined to those drugs that have well recognised antimuscarinic properties.

1. Chan CH, Ruskiewicz RJ. Anticholinergic side effects of trazodone combined with another pharmacologic agent. *Am J Psychiatry* (1990) 147, 533.
2. Osterholm RK, Camoriano JK. Transdermal scopolamine psychosis. *JAMA* (1982) 247, 3081.
3. Tune L, Carr S, Hoag E, Cooper T. Anticholinergic effects of drugs commonly prescribed for the elderly: potential means for assessing risk of delirium. *Am J Psychiatry* (1992) 149, 1393–4.

Antimuscarinics + Areca (Betel nuts)

The control of the extrapyramidal (parkinsonian) adverse effects of fluphenazine and flupenthixol with procyclidine was lost in two patients when they began to chew areca.

Clinical evidence

An Indian patient receiving depot fluphenazine (50 mg every three weeks) for schizophrenia, and with mild parkinsonian tremor controlled with **procyclidine** 5 mg twice daily, developed marked rigidity, bradykinesia and jaw tremor when he began to chew areca. The symptoms were so severe he could barely speak. When he stopped chewing areca his stiffness and abnormal movements disappeared. Another patient receiving depot flupenthixol developed marked stiffness, tremor and akathisia, despite taking

Table 18.2 Drugs with antimuscarinic effects (main or adverse effects)

Group	*Drugs*
Antiarrhythmics	Disopyramide, Propafenone
Antiemetics	Cyclizine, Dimenhydrinate, Meclozine, Hyoscine (Scopolamine)
Antihistamines	Brompheniramine, Chlorphenamine, Cyproheptadine, Diphenhydramine, Hydroxyzine, Triprolidine
Antiparkinsonian drugs (Antimuscarinics)	see Table 18.1, p. 672
Antipsychotics	Chlorpromazine, Chlorprothixene, Clozapine, Loxapine, Perphenazine, Pimozide, Mesoridazine, Trifluoperazine, Thioridazine
Antispasmodics	Anisotropine, Atropine, Belladonna alkaloids, Dicycloverine (Dicyclomine), Flavoxate, Hyoscine (Scopolamine), Hyoscyamine, Isopropamide, Oxybutynin, Propantheline, Tolterodine
Antiulcer drugs	Clidinium, Hexocyclium, Isopropamide, Mepenzolate, Methanthelinium, Oxyphencyclimine, Pirenzepine, Tridihexethyl
Cycloplegic mydriatics	Atropine, Cyclopentolate, Homatropine, Hyoscine (Scopolamine), Tropicamide
Muscle relaxants	Baclofen, Cyclobenzaprine, Orphenadrine
Peripheral vasodilator	Papaverine
Tricyclic and related antidepressants	Amitriptyline, Amoxapine, Clomipramine, Desipramine, Doxepin, Imipramine, Maprotiline, Protriptyline, Nortriptyline, Trimipramine

After Barkin RL, Stein ZLG. *South Med J* (1989) 82, 1547, and others.
The categorization is not exclusive; some of these drugs are used for a range of effects. There are many other antimuscarinic drugs.

up to 20 mg of **procyclidine** daily, when he began to chew areca. The symptoms vanished within 4 days of stopping the areca.[1]

Mechanism

Areca contains arecoline, an alkaloid with cholinergic activity, which could therefore oppose the antimuscarinic (anticholinergic) actions of procyclidine. As the procyclidine was being used to control the extrapyramidal adverse effects of the two antipsychotics, opposing its action allowed the adverse effects to re-emerge and worsen.

Importance and management

Direct information seems to be limited to this report but the interaction would seem to be established and clinically important. Patients taking antimuscarinic drugs for the control of drug-induced extrapyramidal (parkinsonian) adverse effects, or Parkinson's disease, should avoid areca. The authors of this report suggest that a dental inspection for the characteristic red stains of the areca may possibly provide a simple explanation for the sudden and otherwise mysterious deterioration in the symptoms of patients. Betel is traditionally chewed by those from the continent of Asia, and the East Indies. Symptoms seem to develop over a period of 2 weeks, and resolve fairly rapidly (within a week).

1. Deahl M. Betel nut-induced extrapyramidal syndrome: an unusual drug interaction. *Mov Disord* (1989) 4, 330–3.

Antimuscarinics + SSRIs

Eight patients developed delirium when given fluoxetine, paroxetine or sertraline with benzatropine, in the presence of an antipsychotic (usually perphenazine or haloperidol). Other patients taking the combination remained symptom free.

Clinical evidence, mechanism, importance and management

Five patients became confused and developed delirium when given an antipsychotic, an SSRI (4 taking **fluoxetine** and one taking **paroxetine**) and **benzatropine**. No peripheral antimuscarinic toxicity was seen. The delirium developed within 2 days in two cases, but took several weeks to appear in another. The authors of the report attributed this to an interaction between the SSRIs and **benzatropine**, speculating that the SSRIs may have inhibited the metabolism of the **benzatropine** thereby increasing its toxicity. Alternatively they suggest a possible additive central antimuscarinic effect. They also very briefly mention two other patients who became delirious when given an unnamed antipsychotic and either **sertraline** or **paroxetine** with **benzatropine**.[1] It is noteworthy that 4 of the first group of patients were given perphenazine and one haloperidol,[1] both of which have been involved in additive antimuscarinic interactions (see 'Antipsychotics + Antimuscarinics', p.708). Also note that adverse interactions have been reported with the use of 'antipsychotics and SSRIs', (p.712). Another case describes delirium in a 17-year-old boy, 8 days after **paroxetine** was added to his medication which included **benzatropine** and haloperidol. Serum levels of **benzatropine** were markedly increased.[2]

In contrast, another report describes 12 patients on **fluoxetine** and perphenazine who also received **benzatropine** 1 mg daily without showing signs of delirium.[3,4] The general clinical importance of this interaction is therefore very uncertain indeed, but it would now seem prudent to be alert for evidence of confusion and possible delirium in patients given SSRIs with **benzatropine**, particularly if they are also taking other psychotropics that may have antimuscarinic actions. The authors of the first report say that they have not seen delirium with combinations of SSRIs (not named) and other antimuscarinic drugs such as **biperiden** and **diphenhydramine**.[1]

1. Roth A, Akyol S, Nelson JC. Delirium associated with the combination of a neuroleptic, an SSRI, and benztropine. *J Clin Psychiatry* (1994) 55, 492–5.
2. Armstrong SC, Schweitzer SM. Delirium associated with paroxetine and benztropine combination. *Am J Psychiatry* (1997) 154, 581–2.
3. Rothschild AJ, Samson JA, Bessette MP, Carter-Campbell JT. Efficacy of the combination of fluoxetine and perphenazine in the treatment of psychotic depression. *J Clin Psychiatry* (1993) 54, 338–42.
4. Rothschild AJ. Delirium: an SSRI-benztropine adverse effect? *J Clin Psychiatry* (1995) 56, 537.

Apomorphine + Antihypertensives

The hypotensive adverse effects of apomorphine may possibly be increased by nitrates, calcium-channel blockers and alpha blockers. There is some evidence that ACE inhibitors, beta blockers and diuretics do not increase the risk of hypotension. Nevertheless, caution is advised with all antihypertensives, and patients should be told about the symptoms of orthostatic hypotension and what to do should they occur.

Clinical evidence

(a) ACE inhibitors

A single 5-mg sublingual dose of apomorphine produced no clinically relevant changes in heart rate or blood pressure in 25 patients taking ACE inhibitors [not specifically named]. One patient experienced symptomatic hypotension.[1]

(b) Alpha blockers

A single 5-mg sublingual dose of apomorphine caused a greater decrease in systolic blood pressure from supine to standing in 24 patients taking alpha blockers [not specifically named] when compared with placebo (decrease in systolic BP of 23 versus 13 mmHg at 40 minutes post dose). One patient experienced symptomatic hypotension.[1]

(c) Beta blockers

A single 5-mg sublingual dose of apomorphine produced no clinically relevant changes in heart rate or blood pressure in 26 patients taking beta blockers [not specifically named]. One patient experienced syncope and one had symptomatic hypotension.[1]

(d) Calcium-channel blockers

A single 5-mg sublingual dose of apomorphine caused a greater decrease in systolic blood pressure from supine to standing in 26 patients taking calcium-channel blockers [not specifically named] when compared with placebo (decreased in systolic BP of 17 versus 11 mmHg at 20 minutes post dose).[1]

(e) Diuretics

A single 5-mg sublingual dose of apomorphine produced no clinically relevant changes in heart rate or blood pressure in 21 patients taking diuretics [not specifically named]. One patient experienced symptomatic hypotension.[1]

(f) Nitrates

1. Short-acting. A single 5-mg sublingual dose of apomorphine produced no clinically relevant changes in heart rate or blood pressure in 20 patients taking short-acting nitrates. The apomorphine was given 30 minutes before the patient took their short-acting nitrate. Two patients experienced symptomatic hypotension after their sublingual glyceryl trinitrate.[1]

2. Long-acting. A single 5-mg sublingual dose of apomorphine caused a greater decrease in systolic blood pressure from supine to standing in 20 patients taking long-acting nitrates when compared with placebo (decrease in systolic BP of 12 versus 6 mmHg at 50 minutes post dose). Two patients experienced symptomatic hypotension.[1]

Mechanism

Apomorphine alone may cause postural hypotension, and this is potentially additive with the effects of vasoactive antihypertensives and nitrates.

Importance and management

A potentially clinically relevant interaction resulting in orthostatic hypotension may occur when sublingual apomorphine is given to patients on calcium channel blockers or alpha blockers. Similarly symptomatic hypotension on standing may be more common in patients taking nitrates. Note that the 5-mg dose used in the study was slightly higher than the recommended 2- to 3-mg sublingual dose commonly used for erectile dysfunction. All the patients who had symptomatic hypotension experienced a prodrome of symptoms such as nausea, dizziness, pallor, and/or sweating.[1] On the basis of this study the manufacturers suggest caution in patients on antihypertensives and particularly nitrates, which in practice means telling patients what may possibly happen and what to do if adverse effects occur (i.e. do not attempt to stand up, but lie down and raise their legs until the symptoms resolve).[2] Note that the cardiovascular conditions contraindicating or cautioning either the use of sublingual apomorphine for erectile dysfunction or subcutaneous apomorphine in parkinsonism should be observed.[2,3]

1. Fagan TC, Buttler S, Marbury T, Taylor A, Edmonds A, and the SL APO study group. Cardiovascular safety of sublingual apomorphine in patients on stable doses of oral antihypertensive agents and nitrates. *Am J Cardiol* (2001) 88, 760–6.
2. Uprima (Apomorphine). Abbott Laboratories Ltd. UK Summary of product characteristics, September 2004.
3. APO-go ampoules (Apomorphine hydrochloride). Britannia Pharmaceuticals Ltd. UK Summary of product characteristics, March 2007.

Apomorphine + COMT inhibitors

Entacapone had no effect on the pharmacokinetics or efficacy of apomorphine in a single-dose study. Similarly, tolcapone had no relevant effect on single-dose apomorphine.

Clinical evidence

(a) Entacapone

In a placebo-controlled crossover study in 24 patients with Parkinson's disease a single dose of entacapone 200 mg or 400 mg given 30 minutes before a subcutaneous injection of apomorphine had no effect on the pharmacokinetics of apomorphine. In addition, entacapone had no effect on measures of apomorphine efficacy (tapping test and incidence of dyskinesias).[1]

(b) Tolcapone

Tolcapone 200 mg three times daily for 5 days then 200 mg one hour before sublingual apomorphine 40 mg caused a non-significant increase in the AUC of apomorphine of about 13% in 5 patients with Parkinson's disease.[2]

Mechanism

In vitro and *animal* data suggested that the enzyme catechol-*O*-methyl transferase (COMT) is involved in the metabolism of apomorphine[3] and that COMT inhibitors might increase apomorphine bioavailability. However, the single dose studies above suggest that this metabolic pathway for apomorphine may not be important in humans.

Importance and management

The evidence from these single-dose studies suggest that there is no pharmacokinetic interaction between entacapone or tolcapone and apomorphine, and that the drugs can be used together without alteration of the apomorphine dose. However, further data are required from longer-term concurrent use to confirm this. Until more is known, increased monitoring during concurrent use of COMT inhibitors and apomorphine may be prudent, as is recommended by the manufacturers.[4-6]

1. Zijlmans JCM, Debilly B, Rascol O, Lees AJ, Durif F. Safety of entacapone and apomorphine coadministration in levodopa-treated Parkinson's disease patients: pharmacokinetic and pharmacodynamic results of a multicenter, double-blind, placebo-controlled, cross-over study. *Mov Disord* (2004) 19, 1006–11.
2. Ondo WG, Hunter C, Vuong KD, Jankovic VJ. The pharmacokinetic and clinical effects of tolcapone on a single dose of apomorphine in Parkinson's disease. *Parkinsonism Relat Disord* (2000) 6, 237–40.
3. Coudoré F, Durif F, Duroux E, Eschalier A, Fialip J. Effect of tolcapone on plasma and striatal apomorphine disposition in rats. *Neuroreport* (1997) 8, 877–80.
4. Tasmar (Tolcapone). Valeant Pharmaceuticals Ltd. UK Summary of product characteristics, August 2006.
5. Tasmar (Tolcapone). Valeant Pharmaceuticals International. US Prescribing information, December 2006.
6. Comtess (Entacapone). Orion Pharma (UK) Ltd. UK Summary of product characteristics, February 2007.

Apomorphine + Hormonal contraceptives

The sedative effects of apomorphine were decreased by a combined oral contraceptive in one study.

Clinical evidence, mechanism, importance and management

A study[1] in a group of 9 women found that the sedative effects of a single 5-micrograms/kg subcutaneous dose of apomorphine were decreased when they were taking a combined oral contraceptive (**ethinylestradiol** 30 micrograms, **levonorgestrel** 150 or 250 micrograms). The clinical importance of this is uncertain.

1. Chalmers JS, Fulli-Lemaire I, Cowen PJ. Effects of the contraceptive pill on sedative responses to clonidine and apomorphine in normal women. *Psychol Med* (1985) 15, 363–7.

Apomorphine + Miscellaneous

The hypotensive adverse effects of apomorphine may possibly be increased by alcohol. The concurrent use of other drugs used for erectile dysfunction or dopamine agonists or antagonists is not recommended. However, domperidone, and prochlorperazine are said not to interact when apomorphine is used for erectile dysfunction, and domperidone is the recommended antiemetic when apomorphine is used for Parkinson's disease. There is evidence that antidepressants, antiepileptics, and ondansetron do not interact adversely.

Clinical evidence, mechanism, importance and management

(a) Alcohol

The manufacturers say that interaction studies in subjects given apomorphine (for erectile dysfunction) found that alcohol increased the incidence and extent of hypotension (one of the adverse effects of apomorphine). They also point out that alcohol can diminish sexual performance.[1]

(b) Antidepressants

The manufacturers say that no studies about interactions between apomorphine and antidepressants have been undertaken, but clinical experience in erectile dysfunction suggests that no interaction occurs.[1]

(c) Antiemetics

The small doses of apomorphine used for erectile dysfunction (2 to 3 mg) do not normally cause vomiting, but nausea does occur in about 7% of patients and the manufacturers say that interaction studies and/or clinical experience show that **domperidone**, **ondansetron** or **prochlorperazine** may safely be given as antiemetics in this patient group.[1] Studies with other antiemetics have not been carried out, so at the moment concurrent use is not recommended.[1]

Note that **prochlorperazine** should not be given if apomorphine is used for Parkinson's disease, as its dopamine antagonist actions can worsen the disease (see also 'Levodopa + Antiemetics', p.682). Because apomorphine is highly emetogenic at the doses required for the treatment of Parkinson's disease (1 to 4 mg/hour by subcutaneous infusion), patients with Parkinson's disease requiring apomorphine should be pretreated with **domperidone** 20 mg three times daily for at least 2 days.[2] Rare reports of extrapyramidal adverse effects have been reported with **ondansetron**,[3] which may be of relevance in patients with Parkinson's Disease.

(d) Antiepileptics

The manufacturers say that no studies about interactions between apomorphine and antiepileptics have been undertaken, but clinical experience in erectile dysfunction suggests that no interaction occurs.[1]

(e) Dopamine antagonists

The manufacturers say that apomorphine should not be given with centrally-acting dopamine antagonists[1] because potentially they may antagonise the effects of apomorphine. Such drugs would include some **antipsychotics**. Some manufacturers recommend that if neuroleptics are necessary in patients with Parkinson's disease receiving dopamine agonists, the dopamine agonist should be progressively reduced (and then stopped[4]), as sudden withdrawal may cause neuroleptic malignant syndrome.[2,4]

The manufacturer of *APO-go* specifically notes that there is a potential interaction between **clozapine** and apomorphine, although they say that **clozapine** may also be used to reduce the symptoms of neuropsychiatric complications of Parkinson's disease.[2] See also prochlorperazine in (c) above, and 'Levodopa + Antipsychotics', p.683.

(f) Other dopamine agonists

The manufacturers say that apomorphine should not be given with other centrally-acting dopamine agonists.[1] See 'Table 18.1', (p.672) for a list of these drugs.

(g) Other drugs used for erectile dysfunction

The manufacturers say that no formal studies have been done with a combination of apomorphine and other drugs used for erectile dysfunction but there seems to be no evidence of problems, nevertheless they do not recommend concurrent use.[1] Other drugs used for this condition include **alprostadil, moxisylyte, papaverine, phentolamine**, and the **phosphodiesterase inhibitors** such as **sildenafil**.

1. Uprima (Apomorphine). Abbott Laboratories Ltd. UK Summary of product characteristics, September 2004.
2. APO-go ampoules (Apomorphine hydrochloride). Britannia Pharmaceuticals Ltd. UK Summary of product characteristics, March 2007.
3. Zofran (Ondansetron). GlaxoSmithKline UK. UK Summary of product characteristics, October 2006.
4. Britannia Pharmaceuticals Ltd. Personal Communication, March 2006.

Bromocriptine and other dopamine agonists + Antiemetics

Domperidone and metoclopramide would be expected to reduce the prolactin-lowering effect of bromocriptine. Metoclopramide, but not domperidone, would be expected to reduce the effect of any dopamine agonist.

Clinical evidence, mechanism, importance and management

(a) Antiemetic effect

Dopamine agonists frequently cause nausea and vomiting on starting treatment. The manufacturers of **bromocriptine**,[1] **lisuride**,[2] and **pergolide**[3] state that if necessary this may be reduced by taking a peripheral dopamine antagonist such as **domperidone**. **Metoclopramide** is not considered a suitable antiemetic for use in Parkinson's disease because it crosses the blood brain barrier and has central dopamine antagonist effects, and may therefore reduce the efficacy of dopamine agonists in this condition, see also 'Levodopa + Antiemetics', p.682. The manufacturers of **cabergoline**,[4] **ropinirole**,[5] and **rotigotine**[6] advise against the use of metoclopramide for this reason.

(b) Prolactin-lowering effect

Both **domperidone** and **metoclopramide** are dopamine antagonists and can raise prolactin levels, sometimes causing galactorrhoea, gynaecomastia or mastalgia.[7,8] They would therefore be expected to reduce the prolactin-lowering effect of **bromocriptine**.[1] However, an early study in 10 patients with Parkinson's disease given single doses of **bromocriptine** 12.5 to 100 mg found that pretreatment with a single 60-mg dose of **metoclopramide** had no consistent effect on plasma bromocriptine levels or on the clinical or hormonal response[9] [although this does not seem to have been studied in a multiple dose study]. Nevertheless, it would be prudent to monitor the efficacy of **bromocriptine** if **domperidone** or **metoclopramide** are required.

1. Parlodel (Bromocriptine). Novartis Pharmaceuticals UK Ltd. UK Summary of product characteristics, September 2006.
2. Lisuride. Cambridge Laboratories. UK Summary of product characteristics, January 2001.
3. Celance (Pergolide mesilate). Eli Lilly and Company Ltd. UK Summary of product characteristics, July 2007.
4. Cabaser (Cabergoline). Pharmacia Ltd. UK Summary of product characteristics, March 2007.
5. Requip (Ropinirole hydrochloride). GlaxoSmithKline UK. UK Summary of product characteristics, March 2007.
6. Neupro (Rotigotine). Schwarz Pharma Ltd. UK Summary of product characteristics, January 2007.
7. Motilium (Domperidone). Sanofi-Aventis. UK Summary of product characteristics, June 2004.
8. Maxolon Tablets (Metoclopramide). Shire Pharmaceuticals Ltd. UK Summary of product characteristics, December 2006.
9. Price P, Debono A, Parkes JD, Marsden CD, Roenthaler J. Plasma bromocriptine levels, clinical and growth hormone responses in parkinsonism. *Br J Clin Pharmacol* (1978) 6: 303–9.

Bromocriptine and other dopamine agonists + Antipsychotics

Some antipsychotics have dopamine antagonist actions, which would be expected to inhibit the efficacy of dopamine agonists such as bromocriptine. Careful monitoring is required if combined use is considered necessary.

Clinical evidence, mechanism, importance and management

Many antipsychotics have dopamine antagonist properties and can cause movement disorders (extrapyramidal effects). For this reason, these drugs can reduce the efficacy of dopamine agonists used in Parkinson's disease, and exacerbate the disorder. This interaction is well established for levodopa: see 'Antipsychotics', (p.683), which discusses the relative tendency for various classical and atypical antipsychotics to cause this effect. It would equally well be anticipated for any dopamine agonist. Therefore, the manufacturers of **bromocriptine**,[1] **cabergoline**,[2] **lisuride**,[3] **pergolide**,[4] **pramipexole**,[5] **ropinirole**[6] and **rotigotine**[7] all caution against concurrent use with dopamine antagonist antipsychotics. If an antipsychotic is required for psychosis in Parkinson's disease, the risk-benefit ratio should be carefully assessed, and an antipsychotic chosen that has a lower risk of extrapyramidal effects such as an atypical antipsychotic. Similarly, the prolactin-lowering effects of **bromocriptine**,[1] **cabergoline**[8] and **quinagolide**[9] are expected to be reduced by dopamine antagonist antipsychotics.

Dopamine agonists may also lessen some of the effects of antipsychotics: for a case of reduced efficacy see 'Antipsychotics + Bromocriptine', p.710.

1. Parlodel (Bromocriptine). Novartis Pharmaceuticals UK Ltd. UK Summary of product characteristics, September 2006.
2. Cabaser (Cabergoline). Pharmacia Ltd. UK Summary of product characteristics, March 2007.
3. Lisuride. Cambridge Laboratories. UK Summary of product characteristics, January 2001.
4. Celance (Pergolide mesilate). Eli Lilly and Company Ltd. UK Summary of product characteristics, July 2007.
5. Mirapexin (Pramipexole). Boehringer Ingelheim Ltd. UK Summary of product characteristics, August 2006.
6. Requip (Ropinirole hydrochloride). GlaxoSmithKline UK. UK Summary of product characteristics, March 2007.
7. Neupro (Rotigotine). Schwarz Pharma Ltd. UK Summary of product characteristics, January 2007.
8. Dostinex (Cabergoline). Pharmacia Ltd. UK Summary of product characteristics, June 2007.
9. Norpolac (Quinagolide). Ferring Pharmaceuticals Ltd. UK summary of product characteristics, December 2004.

Bromocriptine and other dopamine agonists + Ergot derivatives

Because cabergoline is an ergot derivative, the manufacturers have looked at what happens if other ergot derivatives are used concurrently, but have so far found no evidence of changes in the efficacy or safety of cabergoline. Nevertheless they do not recommend their concurrent use.[1] Similarly, the manufacturers of bromocriptine do not recommend concurrent use of other ergot derivatives.[2]

1. Dostinex (Cabergoline). Pharmacia Ltd. UK Summary of product characteristics, June 2007.
2. Parlodel (Bromocriptine). Novartis Pharmaceuticals UK Ltd. UK Summary of product characteristics, September 2006.

Bromocriptine and other dopamine agonists + Food

Food did not alter the pharmacokinetics of bromocriptine, cabergoline or lisuride. These dopamine agonists are usually taken with food to try and improve their tolerability.

Clinical evidence

(a) Bromocriptine

Taking a single dose of bromocriptine 7.5 mg after breakfast did not alter the bromocriptine AUC compared with the fasted state, although it slightly reduced the maximum plasma level in a study in 7 healthy subjects.[1]

(b) Cabergoline

The pharmacokinetics of cabergoline did not change when a single dose of cabergoline 1 mg was taken after breakfast compared with the fasting state in a study in healthy subjects.[2]

(c) Lisuride

Thirty healthy subjects were given lisuride 200 micrograms orally while fasting or with food. It was found that food did not significantly modify either the pharmacokinetics or the pharmacodynamics of the lisuride.[3]

Mechanism

None.

Importance and management

Food had no effect on the pharmacokinetics of the ergot dopamine agonists studied, and as **rotigotine** is given transdermally, food is not expected to affect its pharmacokinetics.[4] The manufacturers of bromocriptine, cabergoline and lisuride recommend that they are taken with food.[5-7] They commonly cause nausea and vomiting, especially on starting therapy, and taking them with food may improve tolerability.[6,7]

1. Kopitar Z, Vrhovac B, Povšič L, Plavšić F, Francetić I, Urbančič J. The effect of food and metoclopramide on the pharmacokinetics and side effects of bromocriptine. *Eur J Drug Metab Pharmacokinet* (1991) 16, 177–81.
2. Persiani S, Rocchetti M, Pacciarini MA, Holt B, Toon S, Strolin-Benedetti M. The effect of food on cabergoline pharmacokinetics and tolerability in healthy volunteers. *Biopharm Drug Dispos* (1996) 17, 443–55.
3. Gandon JM, Le Coz F, Kühne G, Hümpel M, Allain H. PK/PD interaction studies of lisuride with erythromycin and food in healthy volunteers. *Clin Pharmacol Ther* (1995) 57, 191.
4. Neupro (Rotigotine). Schwarz Pharma Ltd. UK Summary of product characteristics, January 2007.
5. Lisuride. Cambridge Laboratories. UK Summary of product characteristics, January 2001.
6. Parlodel (Bromocriptine). Novartis Pharmaceuticals UK Ltd. UK Summary of product characteristics, September 2006.
7. Cabaser (Cabergoline). Pharmacia Ltd. UK Summary of product characteristics, March 2007.

Bromocriptine + Griseofulvin

Evidence from a single patient, who was taking bromocriptine for acromegaly, suggests that its effects can be opposed by griseofulvin.

Clinical evidence, mechanism, importance and management

In a study of the effects of bromocriptine used for the treatment of acromegaly, one patient who initially had a good response to bromocriptine developed resistance to the drug. After a number of months it was found that this patient had subsequently been given griseofulvin 500 mg daily for the treatment of a fungal nail infection. When the griseofulvin was stopped, the bromocriptine was again effective.[1] The mechanism of this interaction and its general importance are unknown, but prescribers should be aware of it when treating patients with bromocriptine.

1. Schwinn G, Dirks H, McIntosh C, Köbberling J. Metabolic and clinical studies on patients with acromegaly treated with bromocriptine over 22 months. *Eur J Clin Invest* (1977) 7, 101–7.

Bromocriptine and other dopamine agonists + Macrolides

Erythromycin markedly increases bromocriptine plasma levels, and a case of toxicity has been reported. Bromocriptine toxicity also occurred in a patient given josamycin. Clarithromycin increases cabergoline levels, and erythromycin would be expected to interact similarly. Erythromycin had no effect on lisuride levels.

Clinical evidence

(a) Bromocriptine

1. Erythromycin. Erythromycin estolate 250 mg four times daily for 4 days increased the peak plasma levels and the AUC of a single 5-mg oral dose of bromocriptine by about 360% and 268%, respectively in 5 healthy subjects.[1] Another report describes 2 women taking levodopa/carbidopa and bromocriptine for parkinsonism in whom the disease was better controlled when erythromycin was added. Bromocriptine plasma levels were found to be 40 to 50% higher while they were taking erythromycin.[2] An elderly woman taking levodopa and bromocriptine 15 mg developed psychotic symptoms when she took erythromycin, which were attributed to bromocriptine toxicity.[3]

2. Josamycin. An elderly man with Parkinson's disease, well-controlled for 10 months with daily levodopa/benserazide, bromocriptine 70 mg and domperidone, was additionally given josamycin 2 g daily for a respiratory infection. Shortly after the first dose he became drowsy with visual hallucinations, and began to show involuntary movements of his limbs, similar to the dystonic and dyskinetic movements seen in choreoathetosis. These adverse effects (interpreted as bromocriptine toxicity) disappeared within a few days of withdrawing the josamycin.[4]

(b) Cabergoline

The concurrent use of cabergoline 1 mg daily and **clarithromycin** 400 mg daily increased the AUC of cabergoline by 163% and increased the maximum level by 176% in healthy subjects. Preliminary results from a study in patients with Parkinson's disease also showed that **clarithromycin** increased the bioavailability of cabergoline by about 2 to 4-fold.[5]

(c) Lisuride

Twelve healthy subjects were given lisuride 200 micrograms orally or 50 micrograms as a 30 minute intravenous infusion after taking **erythromycin** [dose unknown] twice daily for 4 days. Preliminary results showed that **erythromycin** did not significantly modify either the pharmacokinetics or the pharmacodynamics of the lisuride.[6]

Mechanism

The ergot dopamine agonists bromocriptine and cabergoline undergo extensive metabolism, most likely by the cytochrome P450 isoenzyme CYP3A4. Erythromycin and clarithromycin (and potentially other macrolides, with the exception of azithromycin) inhibit this metabolism, thus significantly elevating bromocriptine and cabergoline plasma levels.[1]

Importance and management

Information seems to be limited to these reports, but the pharmacokinetic interaction would appear to be established. Concurrent use should be well monitored if any of these macrolides (clarithromycin, erythromycin, josamycin) is added to bromocriptine or cabergoline treatment. Note that azithromycin does not normally cause enzyme inhibition and so may not interact. Moderately increased levels may be therapeutically advantageous, but grossly elevated levels can be toxic. The authors of one report[1] suggest reducing the bromocriptine dose, while in another case the dose was reduced by 50% to avoid toxicity.[3] Preliminary data suggest that dosage adjustments are not needed if lisuride is given with erythromycin.

1. Nelson MV, Berchou RC, Kareti D, LeWitt PA. Pharmacokinetic evaluation of erythromycin and caffeine administered with bromocriptine. *Clin Pharmacol Ther* (1990) 47, 694–7.
2. Sibley WA, Laguna JF. Enhancement of bromocriptine clinical effect and plasma levels with erythromycin. *Excerpta Med* (1981) 548, 329–30.
3. Alegre M, Noé E, Martínez Lage JM. Psicosis por interacción de eritromicina con bromocriptina en enfermedad de Parkinson. *Neurologia* (1997) 12, 429.
4. Montastruc JL, Rascol A. Traitement de la maladie de Parkinson par doses élevées de bromocriptine. Interaction possible avec la josamycine. *Presse Med* (1984) 13, 2267–8.
5. Nomoto M, Nomura T, Nakatsuka A, Nagai M, Yabe U. Pharmacokinetic study on the interaction between cabergoline and clarithromycin in healthy volunteers and patients with Parkinson's disease. *Clin Pharmacol Ther* (2004) 75, P79.
6. Gandon JM, Le Coz F, Kühne G, Hümpel M, Allain H. PK/PD interaction studies of lisuride with erythromycin and food in healthy volunteers. *Clin Pharmacol Ther* (1995) 57, 191.

Bromocriptine + Octreotide

Octreotide modestly increases the bioavailability of bromocriptine, whereas bromocriptine does not appear to alter octreotide pharmacokinetics.

Clinical evidence, mechanism, importance and management

The combined use of bromocriptine 5 mg twice daily and subcutaneous octreotide 200 micrograms twice daily increased the bioavailability of bromocriptine by about 40%, without altering its clearance or half-life. The pharmacokinetics of octreotide were unchanged.[1] This effect may contribute to the increased efficacy of combined treatment in acromegaly shown in some studies. Bear it in mind when considering combined therapy.

1. Fløgstad AK, Halse J, Grass P, Abisch E, Djøseland O, Kutz K, Bodd E, Jervell J. A comparison of octreotide, bromocriptine, or a combination of both drugs in acromegaly. *J Clin Endocrinol Metab* (1994) 79, 461–5.

Bromocriptine + Proton pump inhibitors

A single case describes worsening mobility, which was attributed to an interaction between lansoprazole and bromocriptine. The

same patient later received bromocriptine and omeprazole without problems.

Clinical evidence, mechanism, importance and management

A 73-year-old man taking levodopa/benserazide and bromocriptine for Parkinson's disease was given **lansoprazole** 15 mg daily to treat reflux oesophagitis. Two days later, the patient exhibited akinesia (more motor difficulties and slowness in movements) associated with frequent falls. **Lansoprazole** was discontinued, with disappearance of the symptoms the day after. About 3 months later the patient was prescribed **omeprazole** 20 mg daily, which caused no aggravation of Parkinson's disease over the following 6 months.

The authors attribute this case to a possible interaction between **lansoprazole** and bromocriptine,[1] although any mechanism is unclear, especially as **omeprazole** was given without problems.

This single unexplained case seems unlikely to be of clinical significance.

1. Anglès A, Bagheri H, Saivin S, Montastruc JL. Interaction between lansoprazole and bromocriptine in a patient with Parkinson's disease. *Therapie* (2002) 57, 408–10.

Bromocriptine + Sympathomimetics

A healthy postpartum woman taking bromocriptine developed very severe headache and marked hypertension after also taking phenylpropanolamine. Similarly another woman developed seizures with cerebral vasospasm, and a third developed a severe headache, hypertension and severe cardiac dysfunction after also taking isometheptene. A further patient taking bromocriptine developed psychosis when pseudoephedrine was added.

Clinical evidence

Two healthy women who had given birth 3 to 4 days previously, developed severe headaches while taking bromocriptine 2.5 mg twice daily for milk suppression. After additionally taking three 65-mg doses of **isometheptene mucate**, the headache of one of them markedly worsened, and hypertension with life-threatening ventricular tachycardia and cardiac dysfunction developed. The other woman took two 75-mg doses of **phenylpropanolamine**, and developed grand mal seizures and cerebral vasospasm.[1]

A 32-year-old woman took two 5-mg doses of bromocriptine for milk suppression without any adverse effects following the birth of a child. Within 2 hours of taking a third dose with **phenylpropanolamine** 50 mg she awoke with a very severe headache and was found to have a blood pressure of 240/140 mmHg. She was given 5 mg of intramuscular morphine and her blood pressure became normal within 24 hours. Another 5-mg dose of bromocriptine taken 48 hours after the original dose of **phenylpropanolamine** had the same effect, but the blood pressure rise was less severe (160/120 mmHg).[2]

A woman who had recently given birth and who had taken bromocriptine 2.5 mg twice daily for 9 days without problems became psychotic shortly after starting to take **pseudoephedrine** 60 mg four times daily.[3]

Mechanism

Not understood. Severe hypertension occasionally occurs with either bromocriptine or phenylpropanolamine given alone. Shortly after giving birth some individuals show increased vascular reactivity, and it could be that all of these factors conspired together to cause these adverse effects.[2] Psychosis occasionally occurs after giving birth or on bromocriptine alone, so that in the latter case the addition of pseudoephedrine may have been coincidental.[3]

Importance and management

Direct information seems to be limited to these four cases, but the severity of the reactions suggests that it might be prudent for postpartum patients to avoid sympathomimetics like these while taking bromocriptine. Note that bromocriptine is not recommended for the routine suppression of lactation postpartum.

1. Kulig K, Moore LL, Kirk M, Smith D, Stallworth J, Rumack B. Bromocriptine-associated headache: possible life-threatening sympathomimetic interaction. *Obstet Gynecol* (1991) 78, 941–3.
2. Chan JCN, Critchley JAJH, Cockram CS. Postpartum hypertension, bromocriptine and phenylpropanolamine. *Drug Invest* (1994) 8, 254–6.
3. Reeves RR, Pinkofsky HB. Postpartum psychosis induced by bromocriptine and pseudoephedrine. *J Fam Pract* (1997) 45, 164–6.

Cabergoline + Itraconazole

Two patients taking cabergoline had improvements in their Parkinson's disease symptoms while taking itraconazole. In one case a 300% increase in cabergoline levels occurred, and the other patient reduced the dose of her medications without adversely affecting disease control.

Clinical evidence

A man with Parkinson's disease taking cabergoline 4 mg once daily and selegiline 5 mg twice daily was prescribed pulse itraconazole therapy (200 mg twice daily for one week out of four) for a fungal nail infection. At the end of the first week the patient reported improvements in his parkinsonism, which was confirmed by clinical investigation. The improvement gradually decreased during the weeks without itraconazole therapy, and re-emerged while taking the itraconazole. Analysis of cabergoline blood levels found a 300% increase in levels after he had taken itraconazole for a week.[1]

Another similar patient taking cabergoline 2 mg twice daily, selegiline, entacapone, and levodopa/carbidopa, experienced symptoms of overdose (hyperkinesia of the extremities) 3 days after starting itraconazole 200 mg twice daily. She reduced the dose of her Parkinson's medication, and had marked improvement in her usual Parkinson's symptoms, which then gradually reduced after stopping the itraconazole. This was repeated following two additional periods of itraconazole therapy.[1]

Mechanism

Cabergoline is an ergot derivative that is metabolised by the cytochrome P450 isoenzyme CYP3A4 (see also 'Bromocriptine and other dopamine agonists + Macrolides', p.678). Itraconazole is a potent inhibitor of this isoenzyme, and would therefore be expected to increase cabergoline levels.

Importance and management

Although evidence is limited, this interaction would be predicted on the basis of the known pharmacokinetics of cabergoline. It would be prudent to monitor toxicity and efficacy in any patient on cabergoline requiring itraconazole, or similar potent inhibitors of CYP3A4 (see 'Table 1.4', (p.6) for a list).

1. Christensen J, Dupont E, Østergaard K. Cabergoline plasma concentration is increased during concomitant treatment with itraconazole. *Mov Disord* (2002) 17, 1360–2.

COMT inhibitors + MAOIs

In a single dose study, there was no adverse effect on heart rate or blood pressure when entacapone was given with moclobemide (a RIMA), but caution is recommended until further clinical experience is gained. The COMT inhibitors may be used with the MAO-B inhibitors (such as selegiline). However, the manufacturers of entacapone and tolcapone contraindicate concurrent use of non-selective MAOIs or a combination of both a RIMA and a MAO-B inhibitor.

Clinical evidence

In a single-dose, placebo-controlled study, **moclobemide** 150 mg did not change the heart rate or blood pressure at rest or during exercise, when given **entacapone** 200 mg, compared with either drug alone or placebo. In addition, the plasma concentrations of endogenous noradrenaline (norepinephrine) and adrenaline (epinephrine) were not altered.[1]

Mechanism

Monoamine oxidase and COMT are the two major enzyme systems involved in the metabolism of catecholamines. Therefore it is theoretically possible that the combination of a COMT inhibitor and a non-selective MAOI would result in inhibition of the normal metabolism of catecholamines, with an increase in their effects (e.g. hypertension). Using an MAO-B inhibitor with a RIMA is similar to giving a non-selective MAOI and therefore using these two drugs with a COMT inhibitor would also be likely to inhibit the normal metabolism of catecholamines.

Importance and management

The results of the single-dose study of entacapone and the RIMA moclobemide suggest that no adverse haemodynamic interaction occurs. Nevertheless, this finding needs confirmation in a clinical setting. Until further information is available, caution would be advisable on combined use. The manufacturers of entacapone and **tolcapone** contraindicate or advise against the use of non-selective MAOIs (e.g. **phenelzine, tranylcypromine**)[2-5] and combinations of both a RIMA (e.g. moclobemide) plus an MAO-B inhibitor (e.g. **selegiline**).[2,4] However, they state that **selegiline** alone is compatible with the COMT inhibitors provided not more than 10 mg daily is used.[2,4] At this dose, **selegiline** is likely to remain selective for MAO-B.

1. Illi A, Sundberg S, Ojala-Karlsson P, Scheinin M, Gordin A. Simultaneous inhibition of catechol-*O*-methyltransferase and monoamine oxidase A: effects on hemodynamics and catecholamine metabolism in healthy volunteers. *Clin Pharmacol Ther* (1996) 59, 450–7.
2. Tasmar (Tolcapone). Valeant Pharmaceuticals Ltd. UK Summary of product characteristics, August 2006.
3. Tasmar (Tolcapone). Valeant Pharmaceuticals International. US Prescribing information, December 2006.
4. Comtess (Entacapone). Orion Pharma (UK) Ltd. UK Summary of product characteristics, February 2007.
5. Comtan (Entacapone). Novartis. US Prescribing information, March 2000.

COMT inhibitors + Sympathomimetics; Directly-acting

Entacapone potentiated the increase in heart rate and arrhythmogenic effects of isoprenaline (isoproterenol) and epinephrine (adrenaline) in a study in healthy subjects. Therefore, the manufacturers of entacapone and tolcapone issue a caution about the concurrent use of adrenaline (epinephrine), isoprenaline (isoproterenol), and a number of other sympathomimetics.

Clinical evidence

The maximal increase in heart rate during an infusion of **adrenaline (epinephrine)** was about 80% greater (25 *versus* 14 bpm) after pretreatment with a single 400-mg dose of **entacapone** in a study in healthy subjects. Similarly, the maximal increase in heart rate during **isoprenaline (isoproterenol)** infusion was about 50% greater (40 *versus* 27 bpm) after pretreatment with the same dose of **entacapone**. Moreover, more subjects experienced palpitations when pretreated with **entacapone**, and this study was terminated early because of two cases of ventricular arrhythmias, one requiring treatment with propranolol. There was no change in blood pressure, nor any increase in plasma levels of the sympathomimetics.[1]

Mechanism

Tolcapone and entacapone inhibit the enzyme catechol-*O*-methyl transferase (COMT), which is concerned with the metabolism of drugs such as adrenaline (epinephrine) and isoprenaline (isoproterenol). There is therefore a possibility of increased serum levels and related adverse effects of these drugs.

Importance and management

The evidence from this single-dose study confirms the theoretical prediction that COMT inhibitors might potentiate the effects of directly-acting sympathomimetics such as adrenaline (epinephrine). Because of this, the manufacturers of entacapone and tolcapone suggest caution if drugs known to be metabolised by COMT are given to patients on COMT inhibitors.[2-5] Of the sympathomimetics, adrenaline (epinephrine), **dobutamine**, **dopamine**, isoprenaline (isoproterenol) and **noradrenaline (norepinephrine)**, are specifically named in one or more of the lists,[2-5] and one manufacturer of entacapone also lists **bitolterol** and **isoetarine (isoetharine)**, and specifically includes the inhaled route of administration.[5] See also 'COMT inhibitors + Sympathomimetics; Indirectly-acting', below.

1. Illi A, Sundberg S, Ojala-Karlsson P, Korhonen P, Scheinin M, Gordin A. The effect of entacapone on the disposition and hemodynamic effects of intravenous isoproterenol and epinephrine. *Clin Pharmacol Ther* (1995) 58, 221–7.
2. Tasmar (Tolcapone). Valeant Pharmaceuticals Ltd. UK Summary of product characteristics, August 2006.
3. Tasmar (Tolcapone). Valeant Pharmaceuticals International. US Prescribing information, December 2006.
4. Comtess (Entacapone). Orion Pharma (UK) Ltd. UK Summary of product characteristics, February 2007.
5. Comtan (Entacapone). Novartis. US Prescribing information, March 2000.

COMT inhibitors + Sympathomimetics; Indirectly-acting

A single case report describes severe hypertension in a patient given entacapone and intravenous ephedrine. Tolcapone did not alter the effect of ephedrine in one study.

Clinical evidence

(a) Entacapone

A 76-year-old woman with Parkinson's disease taking levodopa/carbidopa and entacapone 200 mg five times daily, was given 3 mg of intravenous ephedrine during cataract surgery to correct a low blood pressure of 85/35 mmHg. Her blood pressure immediately rose to 225/125 mmHg. The patient needed several doses of hydralazine over the following 140 minutes before her blood pressure returned to normal.[1]

(b) Tolcapone

The manufacturer notes that tolcapone did not alter the effect of ephedrine (route of administration not stated) on haemodynamic parameters or plasma catecholamine levels, either at rest or during exercise.[2,3]

Mechanism

COMT inhibitors may inhibit the normal metabolism of ephedrine (and the catecholamines it releases at adrenergic nerve endings), which could result in a marked exaggeration of its normal effects.[1] See also 'COMT inhibitors + Sympathomimetics; Directly-acting', above.

Importance and management

The single case report with entacapone and intravenous ephedrine appears to be the only evidence that COMT inhibitors could potentiate the effect of indirectly-acting sympathomimetics such as ephedrine. The manufacturer of tolcapone states that ephedrine and tolcapone can be used concurrently.[2,3] Nevertheless, some caution may be warranted with intravenous ephedrine.

1. Renfrew C, Dickson R, Schwab C. Severe hypertension following ephedrine administration in a patient receiving entacapone. *Anesthesiology* (2000) 93, 1562.
2. Tasmar (Tolcapone). Valeant Pharmaceuticals Ltd. UK Summary of product characteristics, August 2006.
3. Tasmar (Tolcapone). Valeant Pharmaceuticals International. US Prescribing information, December 2006.

COMT inhibitors + Tricyclic and related antidepressants

Entacapone and imipramine did not interact adversely in a single-dose study. Similarly, tolcapone and desipramine did not interact adversely. Nevertheless, the manufacturers of entacapone and tolcapone recommend caution if they are used with tricyclic antidepressants or other drugs that inhibit noradrenaline (norepinephrine) uptake, such as maprotiline or venlafaxine.

Clinical evidence

(a) Entacapone

In a single-dose crossover study 12 healthy women were given entacapone 200 mg with imipramine 75 mg, either drug alone, or placebo. Although both drugs can impair the inactivation of catecholamines the study found no evidence that combined drug use had any relevant effect on haemodynamics or on free adrenaline (epinephrine) or noradrenaline (norepinephrine) plasma levels. The combination was well tolerated in all subjects.[1]

(b) Tolcapone

In one study, healthy subjects were given **desipramine** 25 mg three times daily for 3 days then 50 mg three times daily for 10 days. For the last 5 days they were also given levodopa/carbidopa 100/25 mg three times daily and either a placebo or tolcapone 200 mg three times daily. The addition of tolcapone to combined treatment with levodopa/carbidopa and **desipramine** did not lead to any changes in haemodynamics or catecholamine levels, nor to any changes in **desipramine** pharmacokinetics.[2]

Mechanism

Both COMT inhibitors and drugs with noradrenaline re-uptake inhibitory activity can impair the inactivation of catecholamines, so in theory the effects of catecholamines may be increased by concurrent use. However, this did not appear to occur in the above studies.

Importance and management

In these pharmacological studies, no important interaction between entacapone and imipramine or between tolcapone and desipramine was detected. Nevertheless, the manufacturer of entacapone says there is limited clinical experience of the use of entacapone with tricyclic antidepressants, and they therefore recommend caution.[3] Similarly, the manufacturers of tolcapone suggest that caution should be exercised with desipramine[4,5] and any drugs that are potent noradrenaline (norepinephrine) uptake inhibitors such as **maprotiline** and **venlafaxine**.[4]

1. Illi A, Sundberg S, Ojala-Karlsson P, Scheinin M, Gordin A. Simultaneous inhibition of catecholamine-*O*-methylation by entacapone and neuronal uptake by imipramine: lack of interactions. *Eur J Clin Pharmacol* (1996) 51, 273–6.
2. Jorga KM, Fotteler B, Modi M, Rabbia M. Effect of tolcapone on the haemodynamic effects and tolerability of desipramine. *Eur Neurol* (2000) 44, 94–103.
3. Comtess (Entacapone). Orion Pharma (UK) Ltd. UK Summary of product characteristics, February 2007.
4. Tasmar (Tolcapone). Valeant Pharmaceuticals Ltd. UK Summary of product characteristics, August 2006.
5. Tasmar (Tolcapone). Valeant Pharmaceuticals International. US Prescribing information, December 2006.

COMT inhibitors; Entacapone + Iron compounds

Entacapone formed chelates with iron *in vitro*. The manufacturer recommends that iron preparations and entacapone are given 2 to 3 hours apart.

Clinical evidence, mechanism, importance and management

An *in vitro* study[1] found that entacapone formed chelates with iron. Although the clinical relevance of this does not appear to have been assessed, the manufacturers recommend that entacapone and iron preparations should be taken at least 2 to 3 hours apart.[2]

1. Orama M, Tilus P, Taskinen J, Lotta T. Iron (III)-chelating properties of the novel catechol *O*-methyltransferase inhibitor entacapone in aqueous solution. *J Pharm Sci* (1997) 86, 827–31.
2. Comtess (Entacapone). Orion Pharma (UK) Ltd. UK Summary of product characteristics, February 2007.

Levodopa + Antacids

Antacids do not appear to interact significantly with immediate-release levodopa, but they may reduce the bioavailability of modified-release preparations of levodopa.

Clinical evidence

(a) Immediate-release preparations

One study found that 15 mL of an **aluminium/magnesium hydroxide** antacid, given 30 minutes before levodopa, to a patient with a prolonged gastric emptying time, caused a threefold increase in levodopa serum levels, which was associated with a marked improvement in symptoms.[1] Another patient was able to reduce his levodopa dose when taking antacids, without affecting symptom control.[1] A further study found that the maximum plasma concentration of levodopa was raised by 20% when 20 mL of an antacid was given before the levodopa.[2]

However, when 8 patients (only 3 with Parkinson's disease) were given *Mylanta* (containing **aluminium/magnesium hydroxide** and simeticone), 30 minutes before, and/or with levodopa, only occasional increases in bioavailability were seen. One of the 3 patients with Parkinson's disease who had shown improved bioavailability while on antacids had his levodopa dose lowered and continued to take *Mylanta*, but the parkinsonian symptoms worsened and the levodopa was increased back to the original dose.[3] Another study, in 15 parkinsonian patients taking dopamine agonists (e.g. bromocriptine) and levodopa/carbidopa who were given six 30-mL doses of **aluminium hydroxide** daily, inferred that the antacid had no significant effect on levodopa bioavailability, because of the lack of clinical fluctuations in effect.[4]

(b) Sustained-release preparations

In a study using *Madopar HBS*, a sustained-release preparation of levodopa and benserazide, the concurrent use of an unnamed antacid reduced the levodopa bioavailability by about one-third in healthy subjects.[5] The manufacturers of *Madopar CR* state that antacids reduce the bioavailability of levodopa from the controlled-release preparation in comparison with conventional *Madopar*.[6]

Mechanism

The small intestine is the major site of absorption for levodopa, and delayed gastric emptying appears to result in low plasma levodopa levels, probably because levodopa can be metabolised in the stomach. In theory, antacids may reduce gastric emptying time, and increase levodopa absorption.[1] It is not known why antacids reduced absorption from the slow-release preparation.[5]

Importance and management

The overall picture is that concurrent use need not be avoided with standard preparations, although some individuals may be affected so the outcome should be monitored. With modified-release preparations it would seem advisable to avoid concurrent administration (1 to 2 hours is usually enough in other similar cases of interactions with antacids). Again, the outcome should be monitored.

1. Rivera-Calimlim L, Dujovne CA, Morgan JP, Lasagna L, Bianchine JR. Absorption and metabolism of L-dopa by the human stomach. *Eur J Clin Invest* (1971) 1, 313–20.
2. Pocelinko R, Thomas GB, Solomon HM. The effect of an antacid on the absorption and metabolism of levodopa. *Clin Pharmacol Ther* (1972) 13, 149.
3. Leon AS, Spiegel HE. The effect of antacid administration on the absorption and metabolism of levodopa. *J Clin Pharmacol* (1972) 12, 263–7.
4. Lau E, Waterman K, Glover R, Schulzer M, Calne DB. Effect of antacid on levodopa therapy. *Clin Neuropharmacol* (1986) 9, 477–9.
5. Malcolm SL, Allen JG, Bird H, Quinn NP, Marion MH, Marsden CD, O'Leary CG. Single-dose pharmacokinetics of Madopar HBS in patients and effect of food and antacid on the absorption of Madopar HBS in volunteers. *Eur Neurol* (1987) 27 (Suppl 1), 28–35.
6. Madopar CR (Levodopa/benserazide hydrochloride). Roche Products Ltd. UK Summary of product characteristics, January 2006.

Levodopa + Anticholinesterases; Centrally acting

Reports describe cases of a worsening of Parkinson's disease in patients given donepezil or tacrine. Other centrally acting anticholinesterases may exacerbate or induce extrapyramidal symptoms, including worsening of Parkinson's disease. In contrast, one study found that donepezil did not affect the control of Parkinson's disease, and actually caused a non-significant increase in levodopa levels.

Clinical evidence

(a) Donepezil

Donepezil 5 mg daily for 15 days caused a modest 30% increase in the AUC_{0-4} of levodopa in a placebo-controlled study in 23 patients with Parkinson's disease taking levodopa/carbidopa. There was no change in carbidopa pharmacokinetics, and the pharmacokinetics of donepezil did not differ between the patients with Parkinson's disease and a control group of healthy subjects. There was no obvious difference in adverse effects between patients with Parkinson's disease and the control subjects, and no evidence that donepezil significantly altered motor activity in those treated with levodopa/carbidopa.[1] This latter finding is in contrast to a report which found a worsening of Parkinson's disease, which responded to levodopa/carbidopa, in 3 of 9 patients who had taken donepezil for 24 weeks.[2]

(b) Tacrine

The mild parkinsonism of an elderly woman with Alzheimer's disease worsened, leading to severe tremor, stiffness and gait dysfunction within 2 weeks of doubling her tacrine dosage from 10 mg to 20 mg four times daily. This improved when levodopa/carbidopa was started, but the tremor returned when tacrine was increased to 30 mg four times daily. The symptoms disappeared when the tacrine dosage was reduced to 20 mg four times daily.[3]

Mechanism

Parkinsonism is due to an imbalance between two neurotransmitters, dopamine and acetylcholine, in the basal ganglia of the brain. Centrally acting anticholinesterases increase the amount of acetylcholine in the brain, which could lead to an exacerbation of parkinsonian symptoms. Levodopa improves the situation by increasing the levels of dopamine. It is not known why donepezil modestly increased the levels of levodopa.

Importance and management

Direct information seems to be limited, but the reports of worsening Parkinson's disease are consistent with the known pharmacology of these drugs and the biochemical pathology of Parkinson's disease. Be aware that if donepezil or tacrine is given to any patient with parkinsonism, whether taking levodopa or any other anti-parkinson drug, the disease may possibly worsen. The antiparkinson drug dosage may need increasing and/or the dosage of the anticholinesterase may need reducing. Other centrally acting anticholinesterases (**galantamine**, **rivastigmine**) may also worsen Parkinson's disease.

1. Okereke CS, Kirby L, Kumar D, Cullen EI, Pratt RD, Hahne WA. Concurrent administration of donepezil HCl and levodopa/carbidopa in patients with Parkinson's disease: assessment of pharmacokinetic changes and safety following multiple oral doses. *Br J Clin Pharmacol* (2004) 58 (Suppl 1): 41–9.
2. Shea C, MacKnight C, Rockwood K. Donepezil for treatment of dementia with Lewy bodies: a case series of nine patients. *Int Psychogeriatr* (1998) 10, 229–38.
3. Ott BR, Lannon MC. Exacerbation of parkinsonism by tacrine. *Clin Neuropharmacol* (1992) 15, 322–5.

Levodopa + Antiemetics

Although metoclopramide can increase the rate of levodopa absorption, it may also antagonise its effects by aggravating symptoms of Parkinson's disease, so metoclopramide should generally be avoided in patients with Parkinson's disease. However, two studies found no evidence that metoclopramide altered the efficacy of levodopa. Phenothiazine antiemetics such as prochlorperazine are also generally considered to be contraindicated in Parkinson's disease. See also 'Levodopa + Antipsychotics', p.683. In one small study, promethazine did not affect the control of Parkinson's disease in patients taking levodopa. Domperidone is the antiemetic of choice to prevent and treat nausea and vomiting caused by levodopa. Other antiemetics that are generally considered useful include cyclizine and 5-HT$_3$ antagonists.

Clinical evidence, mechanism, importance and management

(a) Domperidone

Domperidone is a dopamine antagonist similar to metoclopramide.[1] However, since it acts on the dopamine receptors in the stomach wall, and unlike metoclopramide, it does not readily cross the blood-brain barrier, it does not appear to oppose the effects of levodopa within the brain, although some extrapyramidal symptoms have been observed. It may even slightly increase the bioavailability and effects of levodopa (by stimulating gastric emptying).[2] Domperidone can therefore be used to control the nausea and vomiting associated with levodopa treatment of Parkinson's disease.

(b) Metoclopramide

Metoclopramide is a dopamine antagonist that can cause extrapyramidal disturbances (parkinsonian symptoms), especially in children and young adults, and possibly also in the elderly, where the effects may be misdiagnosed as Parkinson's disease.[3] On the other hand, metoclopramide stimulates gastric emptying, which can result in an increase in the bioavailability of levodopa.[4,5] The outcome of these two effects (possible antagonism resulting in aggravation of Parkinson's disease, or potentiation resulting in increased bioavailability) is uncertain, and it is generally considered that metoclopramide should be avoided in Parkinson's disease. However, in one open study, metoclopramide 30 to 60 mg daily in divided doses for a range of 4 to 16 weeks caused no change in mean total disability scores in 10 patients with Parkinson's disease taking levodopa.[6] Similarly, in a controlled trial in 7 patients, the incidence and severity of levodopa-induced involuntary movements was unchanged and additional acute dyskinesias did not appear when metoclopramide was also given.[6] Nevertheless, if alternative antiemetics are unsuitable for a patient with Parkinson's disease and consequently metoclopramide is given, it would seem prudent to monitor the outcome closely.

(c) Phenothiazine antiemetics

Phenothiazines block the dopamine receptors in the brain and can therefore upset the balance between cholinergic and dopaminergic components within the striatum and substantia nigra. As a consequence they may not only induce the development of extrapyramidal (parkinsonian) symptoms, but they can aggravate parkinsonism and antagonise the effects of levodopa used in its treatment. See 'Levodopa + Antipsychotics', p.683. Phenothiazines, used in smaller doses as antiemetics, such as **prochlorperazine**,[7,8] can also behave in this way. For this reason drugs of this kind are generally regarded as contraindicated in patients with Parkinson's disease, and there are other more suitable alternatives, see (d) below. However, one small controlled study found that **promethazine** (a phenothiazine derivative with few extrapyramidal effects) did not change the total disability score or alter the incidence or severity of levodopa-induced involuntary movements in 4 patients with Parkinson's disease taking levodopa.[6]

(d) Non-interacting antiemetics

Antiemetics that are generally considered useful in patients with Parkinson's disease include **cyclizine** and 5-HT$_3$ antagonists such as **granisetron** and **ondansetron**,[3] which do not affect dopamine, and **domperidone** as discussed above. However, note that rare cases of extrapyramidal adverse effects have been reported with **ondansetron**, which may be of relevance in patients with Parkinson's disease.[9]

1. Bradbrook ID, Gillies HC, Morrison PJ, Rogers HJ. The effects of domperidone on the absorption of levodopa in normal subjects. *Eur J Clin Pharmacol* (1986) 29, 721–3.
2. Shindler JS, Finnerty GT, Towlson K, Dolan AL, Davies CL, Parkes JD. Domperidone and levodopa in Parkinson's disease. *Br J Clin Pharmacol* (1984) 18, 959–62.
3. Avorn J, Gurwitz JH, Bohn RL, Mogun H, Monane M, Walker A. Increased incidence of levodopa therapy following metoclopramide usage. *JAMA* (1995) 274, 1780–2.
4. Berkowitz DM, McCallum RW. Interaction of levodopa and metoclopramide on gastric emptying. *Clin Pharmacol Ther* (1980) 27, 414–20.
5. Mearrick PT, Wade DN, Birkett DJ, Morris J. Metoclopramide, gastric emptying and L-dopa absorption. *Aust N Z J Med* (1974) 4, 144–8.
6. Tarsy D, Parkes JD, Marsden CD. Metoclopramide and pimozide in Parkinson's disease and levodopa-induced dyskinesias. *J Neurol Neurosurg Psychiatry* (1975) 38, 331–5.
7. Duvoisin R.C. Diphenidol for levodopa induced nausea and vomiting. *JAMA* (1972) 221, 1408.
8. Campbell JB. Long-term treatment of Parkinson's disease with levodopa. *Neurology* (1970) 20, 18–22.
9. Zofran (Ondansetron). GlaxoSmithKline UK. UK Summary of product characteristics, October 2006.

Levodopa + Antimuscarinics

Antimuscarinics and other drugs with antimuscarinic effects, such as the tricyclics, may modestly reduce the rate, and possibly the extent, of absorption of levodopa. One case describes levodopa toxicity, which occurred after the withdrawal of an antimuscarinic.

Clinical evidence

A study[1] in 6 healthy subjects and 6 patients with Parkinson's disease found that **trihexyphenidyl** 2 mg twice daily for 3 days lowered the peak plasma levels of a 500-mg dose of levodopa by 42% in the healthy subjects and 17% in the patients, although the interaction was present in only about half of the subjects. The AUC was reduced in both groups by less than 20%.[1]

A study in 6 patients with Parkinson's disease taking levodopa plus carbidopa or benserazide found that **orphenadrine** caused either a delay, a reduction, or an increase in levodopa absorption in 3 patients.[2] Another study in 4 healthy subjects[3] found that **imipramine** 25 mg four times daily for 3 days reduced the peak plasma concentration of a single 500-mg dose of levodopa by about 50%, but did not appear to alter the extent of absorption. See also 'Levodopa + Tricyclic antidepressants', p.690 for other non-antimuscarinic interactions of the tricyclics.

A patient who needed 7 g of levodopa daily while taking **homatropine** developed levodopa toxicity when the **homatropine** was withdrawn, and he was subsequently restabilised on only 4 g of levodopa daily.[4]

Mechanism

The small intestine is the major site of absorption for levodopa. Delayed gastric emptying, which can be caused by antimuscarinics, appears to result in lower plasma levodopa levels and thus lower brain levodopa levels. This is because the gastric mucosa has more time to metabolise the levodopa to dopamine and therefore less is available for absorption.[5]

Importance and management

Antimuscarinics are commonly given with levodopa, and they are of established benefit. However, limited evidence suggests they might sometimes reduce levodopa efficacy. Levodopa preparations are now more usually given in conjunction with a dopa decarboxylase inhibitor to minimise metabolism in the gastric mucosa. This would be expected to minimise the effects of any interaction. However, note that one of the above studies included a dopa-decarboxylase inhibitor, yet still found an effect on levodopa absorption. There is certainly no need to avoid concurrent use, but it would be prudent to be alert for any evidence of a reduced levodopa response if antimuscarinics are added, or for levodopa toxicity if they are withdrawn.

1. Algeri S, Cerletti C, Curcio M, Morselli PL, Bonollo L, Buniva G, Minazzi M, Minoli G. Effect of anticholinergic drugs on gastro-intestinal absorption of L-dopa in rats and in man. *Eur J Pharmacol* (1976) 35, 293–9.
2. Contin M, Riva R, Martinelli P, Procaccianti G, Albani F, Baruzzi A. Combined levodopa-anticholinergic therapy in the treatment of Parkinson's disease. *Clin Neuropharmacol* (1991) 14, 148–55.
3. Morgan JP, Rivera-Calimlim L, Messiha F, Sundaresan PR, Trabert N. Imipramine-mediated interference with levodopa absorption from the gastrointestinal tract in man. *Neurology* (1975) 25, 1029–34.
4. Fermaglich J, O'Doherty DS. Effect of gastric motility on levodopa. *Dis Nerv Syst* (1972) 33, 624–5.
5. Rivera-Calimlim L, Dujovne CA, Morgan JP, Lasagna L, Bianchine JR. Absorption and metabolism of L-dopa by the human stomach. *Eur J Clin Invest* (1971) 1, 313–20.

Levodopa + Antipsychotics

Phenothiazines, butyrophenones, diphenylbutylpiperidines and thioxanthenes can oppose the effects of levodopa because of their dopamine antagonist properties, causing deterioration of motor function in Parkinson's disease. The antipsychotic effects and extrapyramidal adverse effects of these drugs can be opposed by levodopa. Of the atypical antipsychotics, risperidone and olanzapine cause deterioration in motor function in Parkinson's disease. Ziprasidone may act similarly, and there have been reports with quetiapine. Clozapine does not have this effect.

Clinical evidence, mechanism, importance and management

(a) Classical antipsychotics

Phenothiazines (e.g. fluphenazine, perphenazine, prochlorperazine, and trifluoperazine), **butyrophenones** (e.g. haloperidol, droperidol) **diphenylbutylpiperidines** (e.g. pimozide) and **thioxanthenes** (e.g. flupentixol and zuclopenthixol) block the dopamine receptors in the brain and can therefore upset the balance between cholinergic and dopaminergic components within the striatum and substantia nigra. As a consequence they may not only induce the development of extrapyramidal (parkinsonian) symptoms, but they can aggravate parkinsonism and antagonise the effects of levodopa used in its treatment.[1-5] For this reason drugs of this kind are generally regarded as contraindicated in patients being treated for Parkinson's disease, or only used with great caution in carefully controlled conditions. The extrapyramidal symptoms that frequently occur with the **phenothiazines** have in the past been treated without much success with levodopa. However, the levodopa may also antagonise the antipsychotic effects of the **phenothiazines**,[6] and other dopamine-antagonist antipsychotics. Consider also 'Levodopa + Antiemetics', p.682.

(b) Atypical antipsychotics

Of the atypical antipsychotics, both **risperidone** and **olanzapine** have caused deterioration of motor function in patients with Parkinson's disease. There have also been reports of deterioration in motor function with **quetiapine**. There is far less experience with **ziprasidone**, but it may have a propensity to cause extrapyramidal adverse effects that is similar to **olanzapine.**

Low-dose **clozapine** appears to cause little deterioration in motor function, and may improve tremor. It therefore remains the preferred antipsychotic for patients with Parkinson's disease and levodopa-induced psychosis. Note that individual reports and studies of the use of these antipsychotics in patients with Parkinson's disease are numerous. The reader is referred to a recent review on the topic.[7]

1. Duvoisin RC. Diphenidol for levodopa induced nausea and vomiting. *JAMA* (1972) 221, 1408.
2. Klawans HL, Weiner WJ. Attempted use of haloperidol in the treatment of L-dopa induced dyskinesias. *J Neurol Neurosurg Psychiatry* (1974) 37, 427–30.
3. Hunter KR, Stern GM, Laurence DR. Use of levodopa and other drugs. *Lancet* (1970) ii, 1283–5.
4. Lipper S. Psychosis in a patient on bromocriptine and levodopa with carbidopa. *Lancet* (1976) ii, 571–2.
5. Tarsy D, Parkes JD, Marsden CD. Metoclopramide and pimozide in Parkinson's disease and levodopa-induced dyskinesias. *J Neurol Neurosurg Psychiatry* (1975) 38, 331–5.
6. Yaryura-Tobias JA, Wolpert A, Dana L, Merlis S. Action of L-dopa in drug induced extrapyramidalism. *Dis Nerv Syst* (1970) 1, 60–3.
7. Fernandez HH, Trieschmann ME, Friedman JH. Treatment of psychosis in Parkinson's disease. *Drug Safety* (2003) 26, 643–59.

Levodopa + Baclofen

Unpleasant adverse effects (hallucinations, confusion, headache, nausea) and worsening of the symptoms of parkinsonism have occurred in patients on levodopa who were given baclofen.

Clinical evidence

Twelve patients with parkinsonism on levodopa plus a dopa-decarboxylase inhibitor were additionally given baclofen. The eventual baclofen dosage was intended to be 90 mg daily, but the adverse effects were considerable (visual hallucinations, a toxic confusional state, headaches, nausea) so that only 2 patients reached this dosage, and 2 patients withdrew because they could not tolerate these adverse effects. The mean dosage for those who continued was 45 mg daily. Rigidity was aggravated by an average of 46% and functional capacity deteriorated by 21%.[1]

A patient with Parkinson's disease taking levodopa/carbidopa, orphenadrine and diazepam became acutely confused, agitated, incontinent and hallucinated when given a third dose of baclofen (in all 15 mg). The baclofen was stopped, but on the following night she again hallucinated and became confused. The next day she was given two 2.5-mg doses of baclofen but she became anxious and hallucinated with paranoid ideas.[2]

Mechanism

Not understood. The toxicity seen appears to be an exaggeration of the known adverse effects of baclofen.

Importance and management

Information appears to be limited to these reports, but they suggest that baclofen should be used very cautiously in patients taking levodopa.

1. Lees AJ, Shaw KM, Stern GM. Baclofen in Parkinson's disease. *J Neurol Neurosurg Psychiatry* (1978) 41, 707–8.
2. Skausig OB, Korsgaard S. Hallucinations and baclofen. *Lancet* (1977) 1, 1258.

Levodopa + Benzodiazepines and related drugs

On rare occasions it seems that the therapeutic effects of levodopa can be reduced by chlordiazepoxide, diazepam or nitrazepam.

Clinical evidence

Various benzodiazepines [dose unstated] were given to 8 patients with Parkinson's disease in addition to their levodopa treatment. In 5 of the patients (3 taking **chlordiazepoxide**, 1 taking **nitrazepam**, 1 taking **oxazepam**) no interactions were seen. However, the other 3 patients (1 taking **diazepam**, 2 taking **nitrazepam**) experienced transient disturbances in the control of their Parkinson's disease, which lasted up to

3 weeks in the case of the patient taking **diazepam**.[1] Other cases of a reversible loss of control of Parkinson's disease have been seen in 3 patients taking **diazepam**[2] and 4 patients taking **chlordiazepoxide**.[3,4] In one further case, a patient taking **chlordiazepoxide** experienced falls associated with a worsening of parkinsonian symptoms while taking **chlordiazepoxide**. She recovered 5 days after the **chlordiazepoxide** was withdrawn.[5]

In contrast, a case-control study of patients with Parkinson's disease taking levodopa therapy did not find a statistically significant increase in the required dose of antiparkinsonian drug treatment in the 180 days after starting a benzodiazepine.[6]

Mechanism

Not understood, although *animal* studies have shown that benzodiazepines can decrease the levels of dopamine in the striatum.[6]

Importance and management

Not established. Given the widespread use of benzodiazepines in patients taking levodopa,[7] any major or common interaction would be expected to have come to light by now. It would therefore seem that this interaction is fairly rare, and on the basis of one of the reports cited above, possibly only transient. There is no need to avoid concurrent use, but bear these reports in mind in the case of an unexpected response to treatment.

1. Hunter KR, Stern GM, Laurence DR. Use of levodopa with other drugs. *Lancet* (1970) ii, 1283–5.
2. Wodak J, Gilligan BS, Veale JL, Dowty BJ. Review of 12 months' treatment with L-dopa in Parkinson's disease, with remarks on unusual side effects. *Med J Aust* (1972) 2, 1277–82.
3. Mackie L. Drug antagonism. *BMJ* (1971) 2, 651.
4. Schwarz GA, Fahn S. Newer medical treatments in parkinsonism. *Med Clin North Am* (1970) 54, 773–85.
5. Yosselson-Superstine S, Lipman AG. Chlordiazepoxide interaction with levodopa. *Ann Intern Med* (1982) 96, 259–60.
6. van de Vijver DAMC, Roos RAC, Jansen PAF, Porsius AJ, de Boer A. Influence of benzodiazepines on antiparkinsonian drug treatment in levodopa users. *Acta Neurol Scand* (2002) 105, 8–12.
7. van de Vijver DAMC, de Boer A, Herings RMC, Roos RAC, Porsius AJ. Increased use of psychotropic drugs by patients with Parkinson's disease. *Br J Clin Pharmacol* (1999) 47, 476P.

Levodopa + Beta blockers

The concurrent use of levodopa and beta blockers normally appears to be favourable, but be aware that, as with all antihypertensives, additive hypotensive effects can occur.

Clinical evidence, mechanism, importance and management

Most of the effects of the combined use of levodopa and beta blockers seem to be favourable, although additive hypotension can be a problem. Dopamine derived from levodopa stimulates beta-receptors in the heart, which can cause arrhythmias.[1] These receptors are blocked by **propranolol** and other beta blockers. An enhancement of the effects of levodopa and a reduction in tremor has been described in 23 out of 25 patients taking **propranolol**,[2] but not in 9 patients taking **oxprenolol**,[3] or in another placebo-controlled study in 18 patients taking **propranolol**.[4] Early evidence showed that growth hormone levels were substantially raised by **propranolol**[5,6] or **practolol**[6] [now withdrawn due to fatal reactions] in conjunction with levodopa, but no clinical relevance for this has been demonstrated.

1. Goldberg LI, Whitsett TL. Cardiovascular effects of levodopa. *Clin Pharmacol Ther* (1971) 12, 376–82.
2. Kissel P, Tridon P, André JM. Levodopa-propranolol therapy in parkinsonian tremor. *Lancet* (1974) ii, 403–4.
3. Sandler M, Fellows LE, Calne DB, Findley LJ. Oxprenolol and levodopa in parkinsonian patients. *Lancet* (1975) i, 168.
4. Marsden CD, Parkes JD, Rees JE. Propranolol in Parkinson's disease. *Lancet* (1974) ii, 410.
5. Camanni F, Massara F. Enhancement of levodopa-induced growth-hormone stimulation by propranolol. *Lancet* (1974) i, 942.
6. Lotti G, Delitala G, Masala A. Enhancement of levodopa-induced growth-hormone stimulation by practolol. *Lancet* (1974) 2, 1329.

Levodopa + Bromocriptine and other dopamine agonists

The combined use of levodopa and dopamine agonists can increase efficacy and adverse effects in Parkinson's disease, therefore doses of both drugs should be slowly adjusted to optimise therapy. A study suggests that bromocriptine can moderately alter levodopa levels whereas there was no pharmacokinetic interaction between levodopa and cabergoline, pramipexole or ropinirole. An isolated report describes the development of the serotonin syndrome when levodopa/carbidopa was added to treatment with bromocriptine.

Clinical evidence

(a) Bromocriptine

A study in 20 patients with Parkinson's disease taking levodopa/carbidopa found that overall there was no difference in plasma levodopa levels after bromocriptine was also taken, although some patients had either significant elevations or significant reductions in levels. However, the only adverse clinical change found was an increase in dyskinesias in the patients with elevated levodopa levels.[1] An earlier study found no pharmacokinetic interaction between levodopa/carbidopa and bromocriptine, but it should be noted that this was a single-dose study and may not reflect long-term concurrent use.[2]

A patient with parkinsonism, who had been taking bromocriptine 60 mg daily for nearly 3 years, was also given levodopa/carbidopa (25/250 mg daily increasing over a week to 75/750 mg) while the bromocriptine dose was reduced to 20 mg daily. On the seventh day he started shivering, and developed myoclonus of the trunk and limbs, hyperreflexia, patellar clonus, tremor, diaphoresis, anxiety, diarrhoea, tachycardia and had a temperature of 37.9°C with a blood pressure of 180/100 mmHg. The serotonin syndrome was suspected. The patient responded to treatment with the 5-HT antagonist methysergide.[3]

A case of pathological gambling was attributed to the combined use of bromocriptine and levodopa/carbidopa in a 54-year-old woman.[4]

(b) Cabergoline

Levodopa/carbidopa 25/250 mg daily did not cause a clinically significant change in the pharmacokinetics of cabergoline 2 mg daily when the combination was given to patients newly diagnosed with Parkinson's disease. Similarly, cabergoline (in increasing doses up to 4 mg once daily) for 8 weeks had no effect on the absorption, AUC or elimination half-life of levodopa in another group of patients with fluctuating Parkinson's disease who were taking levodopa/carbidopa.[5]

(c) Pergolide

The manufacturer notes that the use of pergolide in patients on levodopa may cause and/or exacerbate pre-existing states of dyskinesia, confusion, and hallucinations. Also, they say that stopping pergolide abruptly in patients on levodopa may precipitate the onset of hallucinations and confusion.[6]

(d) Pramipexole

Patients on a stable dose of levodopa/carbidopa were given increasing doses of pramipexole or placebo for 7 weeks. Pramipexole 1.5 mg daily and 4.5 mg daily had no effect on levodopa bioavailability.[7] As pramipexole enhances the actions of levodopa the manufacturer suggests reducing the dose of levodopa as the dose of pramipexole is increased.[8]

(e) Ropinirole

In patients on a stable dose of levodopa with a dopa-decarboxylase inhibitor, ropinirole had no effect on the pharmacokinetics of levodopa, except for a small clinically irrelevant 16% increase in maximum level. Similarly, levodopa had no effect on the pharmacokinetics of ropinirole in another group of patients.[9] As the dose of ropinirole is increased, the dose of levodopa may be reduced gradually, by around 20% in total.[10]

(f) Rotigotine

The manufacturer of rotigotine reports that levodopa and carbidopa had no effect on the pharmacokinetics of rotigotine and similarly, rotigotine had no effect on the pharmacokinetics of either levodopa or carbidopa. However, as with other dopamine agonists, rotigotine may cause and/or exacerbate dyskinesia in patients taking levodopa and may potentiate the dopaminergic adverse reactions of levodopa.[11]

Mechanism

Additive dopaminergic effects would be expected. The serotonin syndrome is thought to occur because of increased stimulation of the 5-HT receptors in the brainstem and spinal cord. A syndrome resembling neuroleptic malignant syndrome (which has similar symptoms to the serotonin syndrome) can occur when a dopamine agonist like bromocriptine is withdrawn abruptly. It is therefore possible that the effects of reducing the bromocriptine dose were additive with those of levodopa, which can displace serotonin from the nerve endings.[3] Pathological gambling has been associated with the misuse of levodopa and dopamine agonists alone, but an association is not clearly established.

Importance and management

The combined use of levodopa and ergot dopamine agonists can increase efficacy in Parkinson's disease, but adverse effects such as hallucinations and dyskinesias may also be increased, and the dose of both drugs should be gradually adjusted to optimise therapy. If the decision is made to withdraw the dopamine agonist, this should be done slowly, over several days.

The serotonin syndrome described with levodopa and bromocriptine appears to be an isolated incident and not of general importance. Similarly, the case of gambling with levodopa/bromocriptine is probably not of general importance, except to say that use of dopaminergic drugs should be considered as a possible contributing factor in a patient with pathological gambling.

1. Rabey JM, Schwartz M, Graff E, Harsat A, Vered Y. The influence of bromocriptine on the pharmacokinetics of levodopa in Parkinson's disease. *Clin Neuropharmacol* (1991) 14, 514–22.
2. Bentué-Ferrer D, Allain H, Reymann JM, Sabouraud O, Van den Driessche J. Lack of pharmacokinetic influence on levodopa by bromocriptine. *Clin Neuropharmacol* (1988) 11, 83–6.
3. Sandyk R. L-Dopa induced "serotonin syndrome" in a parkinsonian patient on bromocriptine. *J Clin Psychopharmacol* (1986) 6, 194–5.
4. Polard E, Trioux E, Flet L, Colin F, Allain H. Ludopathie induite par la lévodopa associée à la bromocriptine. *Presse Med* (2003) 32, 1223.
5. Del Dotto P, Colzi A, Musatti E, Benedetti MS, Persiani S, Fariello R, Bonuccelli U. Clinical and pharmacokinetic evaluation of L-dopa and cabergoline cotreatment in Parkinson's disease. *Clin Neuropharmacol* (1997) 20, 455–65.
6. Celance (Pergolide mesilate). Eli Lilly and Company Ltd. UK Summary of product characteristics, July 2007.
7. Kompoliti K, Adler CH, Raman R, Pincus JH, Leibowitz MT, Ferry JJ, Blasucci L, Caviness JN, Leurgans S, Chase WM, Yones LC, Tan E, Carvey P, Goetz CG. Gender and pramipexole effects on levodopa pharmacokinetics and pharmacodynamics. *Neurology* (2002) 58, 1418–22.
8. Mirapexin (Pramipexole). Boehringer Ingelheim Ltd. UK Summary of product characteristics, August 2006.
9. Taylor AC, Beerahee A, Citerone DR, Cyronak MJ, Leigh TJ, Fitzpatrick KL, Lopez-Gil A, Vakil SD, Burns E, Lennox G. Lack of a pharmacokinetic interaction at steady state between ropinirole and L-dopa in patients with Parkinson's disease. *Pharmacotherapy* (1999) 19, 150–6.
10. Requip (Ropinirole hydrochloride). GlaxoSmithKline UK. UK Summary of product characteristics, March 2007.
11. Neupro (Rotigotine). Schwarz Pharma Ltd. UK Summary of product characteristics, January 2007.

Levodopa + Clonidine

Limited evidence suggests that clonidine may oppose the effects of levodopa. Be aware that, as with all antihypertensives, additive hypotensive effects may occur.

Clinical evidence

A study in 2 patients taking levodopa with carbidopa found that concurrent treatment with clonidine (up to 1.5 mg daily for 10 to 24 days) caused a worsening of the parkinsonism (an exacerbation of rigidity and akinesia). The concurrent use of antimuscarinic drugs reduced the effects of this interaction.[1]

Another report on 10 hypertensive and 3 normotensive patients with Parkinson's disease, 9 of them taking levodopa and 4 of them not, claimed that concurrent treatment with clonidine did not affect the control of the parkinsonism. However, 2 patients stopped taking the clonidine because of an increase in tremor and gait disturbance.[2]

Mechanism

Not understood. A suggestion is that clonidine opposes the antiparkinson effects by stimulating alpha-receptors in the brain. Another idea is that clonidine directly stimulates post-synaptic dopaminergic receptors.

Importance and management

Information seems to be limited to these reports. Be alert for a reduction in the control of the Parkinson's disease during concurrent use. The effects of this interaction appear to be reduced if antimuscarinic drugs are also being used.[1] Also note, that as with all antihypertensives, additive hypotensive effects may occur.

1. Shoulson I, Chase TN. Clonidine and the anti-parkinsonian response to L-dopa or piribedil. *Neuropharmacology* (1976) 15, 25–7.
2. Tarsy D, Parkes JD, Marsden CD. Clonidine in Parkinson disease. *Arch Neurol* (1975) 32, 134–6.

Levodopa + COMT inhibitors

Entacapone and tolcapone increase the AUC of levodopa given with benserazide or carbidopa. This may require a reduction in the levodopa dose to avoid symptoms of dopamine excess when first starting the COMT inhibitor. Tolcapone increases the levels of benserazide, but neither entacapone nor tolcapone alters carbidopa pharmacokinetics.

Clinical evidence

(a) Levodopa

Entacapone[1,2] and **tolcapone**[3,4] have been shown to increase the AUC and prolong the elimination half-life of levodopa (as levodopa/benserazide or levodopa/carbidopa) without altering the maximum levodopa level. COMT inhibitors can therefore improve the clinical condition of patients with Parkinson's disease, which is mainly seen as a decrease in 'off' time.[5] However, as levodopa levels are raised, there may be an accompanying increase in the adverse effects of levodopa (e.g. dyskinesias, nausea, vomiting, orthostatic hypotension, hallucinations).[6-8]

(b) Benserazide or carbidopa

The effects of COMT inhibitors on the pharmacokinetics of dopa-decarboxylase inhibitors has also been studied. Neither **entacapone**[2] nor **tolcapone**[9] altered the pharmacokinetics of carbidopa. However, **tolcapone** increased the serum levels of benserazide in patients with Parkinson's disease.[10] The benserazide levels remained within the usual range in patients taking levodopa products containing benserazide 25 mg and **tolcapone** 200 mg three times daily. However, with a 50-mg dose of benserazide the AUC of benserazide was increased 4.8-fold with standard-release preparation and 2.3-fold with a controlled-release preparation.[10]

Mechanism

When levodopa is given with a dopa-decarboxylase inhibitor such as carbidopa or benserazide, COMT becomes the major enzyme for metabolising levodopa, so inhibiting COMT delays the breakdown of levodopa.

Importance and management

When starting a COMT inhibitor, all patients should be informed of the symptoms of excess levodopa, and what to do if they occur. The manufacturers of entacapone suggest that if entacapone is started, the daily dose of levodopa should be reduced by about 10 to 30% (within the first few days or weeks) to accommodate these potential adverse effects.[7,11] This can be done by either extending the dosing intervals and/or by reducing the amount of levodopa per dose. Patients on levodopa/benserazide may require a greater dose reduction than those on levodopa/carbidopa because entacapone increases the bioavailability of standard levodopa/benserazide preparations by 5 to 10% more than standard levodopa/carbidopa.[7] The manufacturers of tolcapone say that the average reduction in the daily dose of levodopa required on starting tolcapone was 30%, and that greater than 70% of patients on levodopa doses above 600 mg daily required such a reduction.[8,12] The clinical significance of the increase in benserazide levels is unknown, but the manufacturers advise good monitoring for benserazide adverse effects.[12]

1. Myllylä VV, Sotaniemi KA, Illi A, Suominen K, Keränen T. Effect of entacapone, a COMT inhibitor, on the pharmacokinetics of levodopa and on cardiovascular responses in patients with Parkinson's disease. *Eur J Clin Pharmacol* (1993) 45, 419–23.
2. Keränen T, Gordin A, Harjola V-P, Karlsson M, Korpela K, Pentikäinen PJ, Rita H, Seppälä L, Wikberg T. The effect of catechol-*O*-methyl transferase inhibition by entacapone on the pharmacokinetics and metabolism of levodopa in healthy volunteers. *Clin Neuropharmacol* (1993) 16, 145–56.
3. Dingemanse J, Jorga K, Zürcher G, Schmitt M, Sedek G, da Prada M, van Brummelen P. Pharmacokinetic-pharmacodynamic interaction between the COMT inhibitor tolcapone and single-dose levodopa. *Br J Clin Pharmacol* (1995) 40, 253–62.

4. Sêdek G, Jorga K, Schmitt M, Burns RS, Leese P. Effect of tolcapone on plasma levodopa concentrations after coadministration with levodopa/carbidopa to healthy volunteers. *Clin Neuropharmacol* (1997) 20, 531–41.
5. Heikkinen H, Nutt JG, LeWitt PA, Koller WC, Gordin A. The effects of different repeated doses of entacapone on the pharmacokinetics of L-dopa and on the clinical response to L-dopa in Parkinson's disease. *Clin Neuropharmacol* (2001) 24, 150–7.
6. Ruottinen HM, Rinne UK. Entacapone prolongs levodopa response in a one month double blind study in parkinsonian patients with levodopa related fluctuations. *J Neurol Neurosurg Psychiatry* (1996) 60, 36–40.
7. Comtess (Entacapone). Orion Pharma (UK) Ltd. UK Summary of product characteristics, February 2007.
8. Tasmar (Tolcapone). Valeant Pharmaceuticals International. US Prescribing information, December 2006.
9. Jorga KM, Nicholl DJ. COMT inhibition with tolcapone does not affect carbidopa pharmacokinetics in parkinsonian patients in levodopa/carbidopa (Sinemet). *Br J Clin Pharmacol* (1999) 48, 449–52.
10. Jorga KM, Larsen JP, Beiske A, Schleimer M, Fotteler B, Schmitt M, Moe B. The effect of tolcapone on the pharmacokinetics of benserazide. *Eur J Neurol* (1999) 6, 211–19.
11. Comtan (Entacapone). Novartis. US Prescribing information, March 2000.
12. Tasmar (Tolcapone). Valeant Pharmaceuticals Ltd. UK Summary of product characteristics, August 2006.

Levodopa + Dacarbazine

An isolated report describes a reduction in the effects of levodopa caused by dacarbazine.

Clinical evidence, mechanism, importance and management

A patient who had been treated surgically for melanoma, continued to have intermittent dacarbazine treatment (200 mg intravenously daily) for sporadic positive melanuria. He later developed Parkinson's disease, and was started on levodopa, which had no effect on his melanoma. However, each time he was treated with dacarbazine he complained that the effects of the levodopa/benserazide were reduced and his Schwab and England score (measures of activities of daily living) fell by as much as 25%. A subsequent double-blind study on the patient using a modified Columbia Score confirmed this.[1] The reasons are not understood, but since the serum dopamine levels remained unchanged it is suggested that competition between the two drugs at the blood-brain barrier may be the explanation.[1] Be alert for the need to modify levodopa treatment if dacarbazine is used concurrently. However, note also that the manufacturers contraindicate levodopa in those with a history of malignant melanoma because there is some suggestion that levodopa may activate this malignancy,[2] although some consider that this is unlikely from the available evidence.[3]

1. Merello M, Esteguy M, Perazzo F, Leiguarda R. Impaired levodopa response in Parkinson's disease during melanoma therapy. *Clin Neuropharmacol* (1992) 15, 69–74.
2. Madopar Capsules (Levodopa/Benserazide hydrochloride). Roche Products Ltd. UK Summary of product characteristics, January 2006.
3. Siple JF, Schneider DC, Wanlass WA, Rosenblatt BK. Levodopa therapy and the risk of malignant melanoma. *Ann Pharmacother* (2000) 34, 382–5.

Levodopa + Food

The fluctuations in response to levodopa experienced by some patients may be due to the timing of meals and the type of diet, particularly the protein content, both of which can reduce the effects of levodopa. The effects of levodopa can be reduced by the amino acid methionine, and the blood levels of levodopa can be reduced by the amino acid tryptophan.

Clinical evidence

(a) Effects of meals

A study in patients with Parkinson's disease taking levodopa found that if taken with a meal, the mean absorption of levodopa from the gut and the peak plasma levels were reduced by 27 and 29% respectively, and the peak plasma level was delayed by 34 minutes.[1] Another study found that peak plasma levodopa levels were reduced if the levodopa was taken with food rather than when fasting.[2]

(b) Effects of protein

A study in healthy subjects found that a **low-protein meal** (protein 10.5 g) caused a small reduction in levodopa absorption when compared with the fasting state, but also found that a **high-protein meal** (protein 30.5 g) was no different to the fasting state.[3] Other studies have found that a high daily intake of protein reduces the effects of levodopa (with or without a dopa-decarboxylase inhibitor), compared with a lower intake of protein.[4-6]

(c) Effects of specific amino acids

A study found that the clinical response to a constant intravenous infusion of levodopa in 4 patients was unchanged by **glycine** and **lysine** but was reduced by **phenylalanine**, **leucine** and **isoleucine**, although the plasma levodopa levels remained unchanged.[1]

Fourteen patients treated with levodopa for Parkinson's disease were given a **low-methionine** diet (0.5 g daily) for a period of 8 days. Seven patients were given additional **methionine** (4.5 g daily), while the other 7 were given placebo. Five out of the 7 given **methionine** 4.5 g daily showed a definite worsening of the symptoms (gait, tremor, rigidity, etc.). The symptoms subsided when the **methionine** was withdrawn, although this took 7 to 10 days in one patient. Three out of the 7 given placebo (while on the low-methionine diet) showed some subjective improvement.[7]

The blood levels of levodopa were markedly reduced in normal healthy subjects when levodopa 500 mg was taken with 1 g of **tryptophan**.[8] The clinical importance of this was not assessed.

Mechanism

(a) Meals that delay gastric emptying increase the potential for peripheral metabolism of levodopa in the gut, which reduces the amount available for absorption. In addition (b) some large neutral amino acids arising from the digestion of proteins can compete with levodopa for transport into the brain so that the therapeutic response may be reduced, whereas other amino acids (c) do not have this effect.[1,3,5,9]

Importance and management

An established interaction, but unpredictable. Since the fluctuations in the response of patients to levodopa may be influenced by what is eaten and when, a change in the pattern of drug and food administration on a trial-and-error basis may be helpful. Note that the manufacturers of *Madopar* recommend taking with food or slowly increasing the dose in the early stages of treatment to control anorexia, nausea, vomiting, and diarrhoea.[10] Multiple small doses of levodopa and distributing the intake of proteins may also diminish the effects of these interactions. Diets that conform to the recommended daily allowance of protein (said to be 800 mg/kg in this report) are reported to reduce this adverse drug-food interaction.[5]

The amino acid methionine is used therapeutically, and although information about its interaction with levodopa is very limited, it indicates that large doses of methionine should be avoided in patients being treated with levodopa.

1. Anon. Timing of meals may affect clinical response to levodopa. *Am Pharm* (1985) 25, 34–5.
2. Morgan JP, Bianchine JR, Spiegel HE, Nutley NJ, Rivera-Calimlim L, Hersey RM. Metabolism of levodopa in patients with Parkinson's disease. *Arch Neurol* (1971) 25, 39–44.
3. Robertson DRC, Higginson I, Macklin BS, Renwick AG, Waller DG, George CF. The influence of protein containing meals on the pharmacokinetics of levodopa in healthy volunteers. *Br J Clin Pharmacol* (1991) 31, 413–17.
4. Gillespie NG, Mena I, Cotzias GC, Bell MA. Diets affecting treatment of parkinsonism with levodopa. *J Am Diet Assoc* (1973) 62, 525–8.
5. Juncos JL, Fabbrini G, Mouradian MM, Serrati C, Chase TN. Dietary influences on the antiparkinsonian response to levodopa. *Arch Neurol* (1987) 44, 1003–1005.
6. Carter JH, Nutt JG, Woodward WR, Hatcher LF, Trotman TL. Amount and distribution of dietary protein affects clinical response to levodopa in Parkinson's disease. *Neurology* (1989) 39, 552–6.
7. Pearce LA, Waterbury LD. L-methionine: a possible levodopa antagonist. *Neurology* (1974) 24, 640–1.
8. Weitbrecht W-U, Weigel K. Der einfluß von L-tryptophan auf die L-dopa-resorption. *Dtsch Med Wochenschr* (1976) 101, 20–2.
9. Daniel PM, Moorhouse SR, Pratt OE. Do changes in blood levels of other aromatic aminoacids influence levodopa therapy? *Lancet* (1976) i, 95.
10. Madopar Capsules (Levodopa/Benserazide hydrochloride). Roche Products Ltd. UK Summary of product characteristics, January 2006.

Levodopa + Indinavir

An isolated report describes a man taking levodopa who developed severe dyskinesias when given indinavir.

Clinical evidence, mechanism, importance and management

A 66-year-old man with idiopathic Parkinson's disease and AIDS was free of dyskinesias when taking levodopa with a dopa-decarboxylase inhibitor, although he had unpredictable fluctuations. After 1 month of starting indinavir 2400 mg daily, lamivudine and zidovudine, he developed severe peak-dose dyskinesias, and the 'on' periods lasted all day, with no flectuations. The antivirals were stopped and the dyskinesias improved within 5 days. Each antiviral was then given separately for 2 weeks. Only indinavir induced dyskinesias, which started after 3 days of treatment.[1]

The mechanism of this interaction is uncertain, but may be related to the inhibition of cytochrome P450 by protease inhibitors such as indinavir.[1]

This appears to be the only report of this possible interaction. Bear in mind the possibility that the levodopa dose may need to be decreased if a protease inhibitor such as indinavir is required.

1. Caparros-Lefebvre D, Lannuzel A, Tiberghien F, Strobel M. Protease inhibitors enhance levodopa effects in Parkinson's disease. *Mov Disord* (1999) 14, 535.

Levodopa + Iron compounds

Ferrous sulfate can reduce the bioavailability of levodopa and carbidopa, and may possibly reduce the control of Parkinson's disease.

Clinical evidence

A study in 9 patients with Parkinson's disease found that a single 325-mg dose of **ferrous sulfate** reduced the AUC of levodopa by 30% and reduced the AUC of carbidopa by more than 75%. There was a trend towards an increase in disability, suggesting a worsening of disease, but this did not reach statistical significance. Some, but not all of the patients had some deterioration in the control of their disease[1]

In another study, 8 healthy subjects were given a single 250-mg dose of levodopa, with and without a single 325-mg dose of **ferrous sulfate**, and the plasma levodopa levels were measured for the following 6 hours. Peak plasma levodopa levels and the levodopa AUC were reduced by 55% and the AUC was reduced by 51%. Those subjects who had the highest peak levels and greatest absorption when given levodopa alone, showed the greatest reductions when additionally given **ferrous sulfate**.[2]

Mechanism

Ferrous iron rapidly oxidises to ferric iron at the pH values found in the gastrointestinal tract. Ferric iron binds strongly to carbidopa and levodopa to form chelation complexes that are poorly absorbed.[2-4]

Importance and management

Information appears to be limited to these single-dose and *in vitro* studies. The importance of this interaction in patients taking both drugs long-term awaits further study but the extent of the reductions in absorption (30 to 50%), and the hint of worsening control,[1] suggests that this interaction may be of clinical importance. Be alert for any evidence of this. Separating the administration of the iron and levodopa as much as possible is likely to prove effective, as this appears to be an absorption interaction. More study is needed.

1. Campbell NRC, Rankine D, Goodridge AE, Hasinoff BB, Kara M. Sinemet-ferrous sulphate interaction in patients with Parkinson's disease. *Br J Clin Pharmacol* (1990) 30, 599–605.
2. Campbell NRC, Hasinoff B. Ferrous sulfate reduces levodopa bioavailability: chelation as a possible mechanism. *Clin Pharmacol Ther* (1989) 45, 220–5.
3. Campbell RRA, Hasinoff B, Chernenko G, Barrowman J, Campbell NRC. The effect of ferrous sulfate and pH on L-dopa absorption. *Can J Physiol Pharmacol* (1990) 68, 603–7.
4. Greene RJ, Hall AD, Hider RC. The interaction of orally administered iron with levodopa and methyldopa therapy. *J Pharm Pharmacol* (1990) 42, 502–4.

Levodopa + Isoniazid

There is evidence that isoniazid can reduce the control of Parkinson's disease in patients taking levodopa. An isolated case report describes hypertension, tachycardia, flushing and tremor in a patient attributed to concurrent use of levodopa and isoniazid.

Clinical evidence

Following the observation that levodopa-induced dyskinesias were reduced by isoniazid in one patient, a further study was undertaken in 20 others taking levodopa plus a dopa-decarboxylase inhibitor. It was found that isoniazid (average dose 290 mg daily, range 100 to 800 mg daily) reduced the dyskinesias of 18 of the 20 patients. However, the reduction in dyskinesias was accompanied by an intolerable worsening of parkinsonism, shown by decreased mobility and greater 'off' periods. The reduction in mobility was so severe that the isoniazid had to be stopped immediately in several cases and was discontinued after an average of 5.2 weeks in all the patients. Control of parkinsonism was then restored.[1] Another patient taking levodopa/carbidopa similarly had a deterioration in the control of parkinsonism within 1 to 2 weeks of starting isoniazid/rifampicin (*Rifinah*). When the antitubercular drugs were stopped, the patient's motor performance improved ('on' period lengthened by 75%), the levodopa AUC rose by 37%, its half-life doubled, and the maximum plasma levels fell by 33%.[2]

An isolated report describes a patient on levodopa who developed hypertension, agitation, tachycardia, flushing and severe non-parkinsonian tremor after starting to take isoniazid. He recovered when the isoniazid was stopped.[3]

Mechanism

Not understood. Metabolic studies in one patient suggest that isoniazid inhibits dopa-decarboxylase,[2] although other mechanisms have been proposed.[1,2] The isolated case of hypertension and tachycardia is also not understood, but it has been suggested that it may have been due to a weak monoamine oxidase inhibitory effect of the isoniazid metabolites. See 'MAOIs or RIMAs + Levodopa', p.1136, for further explanation.

Importance and management

Information seems to be limited to the reports cited. If concurrent use is thought to be necessary, be alert for any evidence of a reduction in the control of the parkinsonism, and be aware that drug treatment may need to be modified. One of the reports suggests that it may take 15 to 20 days or more for the deterioration in parkinsonian symptoms to occur.[1] More study is needed. The isolated case seems not to be of general importance.

1. Gershanik OS, Luquin MR, Scipioni O, Obeso JA. Isoniazid therapy in Parkinson's disease. *Mov Disord* (1988) 3, 133–9.
2. Wenning GK, O'Connell MT, Patsalos PN, Quinn NP. A clinical and pharmacokinetic case study of an interaction of levodopa and antituberculous therapy in Parkinson's disease. *Mov Disord* (1995) 10, 664–7.
3. Morgan JP. Isoniazid and levodopa. *Ann Intern Med* (1980) 92, 434.

Levodopa + MAO-B inhibitors

No serious interaction occurs between levodopa and selegiline, although the dose of levodopa may need to be reduced when selegiline is added. Levodopa does not affect rasagiline clearance.

Clinical evidence

(a) Rasagiline

The manufacturer notes that levodopa had no effect on rasagiline clearance.[1]

(b) Selegiline

The combination of levodopa and selegiline has been very extensively used. No serious hypertensive reactions of the kind seen with 'non-selective MAOIs and levodopa', (p.1136) seem to occur. No adverse pharmacokinetic interactions have been reported,[2,3] and serious adverse interactions are said to be lacking.[4,5] Many studies have reported beneficial effects of this combination,[6-11] but one has suggested that it may result in increased mortality.[12] Urinary retention has also been suggested as being associated with this drug combination.[13] Selegiline potentiates the effects of levodopa, so the usual adverse effects (dyskinesias, nausea, agitation, confusion, hallucinations, headache, postural hypotension, cardiac arrhythmias, and vertigo) may be increased, particularly if the levodopa dose is too high.[14]

Mechanism

MAO-B inhibitors prevent the metabolism of dopamine, therefore additive dopaminergic effects occur with levodopa.

Importance and management

No adverse interactions occur if levodopa and selegiline are given concurrently. However, the manufacturers say that after adding selegiline a reduction in the dose of levodopa is usually required to avoid symptoms of levodopa excess (about 10 to 30% is suggested).[14-16] Reduction of the levodopa dose should be gradual, in steps of 10% every 3 to 4 days.[15]

1. Azilect (Rasagiline mesilate). Teva Pharmaceuticals Ltd. UK Summary of product characteristics, April 2007.
2. Roberts J, Waller DG, O'Shea N, Macklin BS, Renwick AG. The effect of selegiline on the peripheral pharmacokinetics of levodopa in young volunteers. *Br J Clin Pharmacol* (1995) 40, 404–6.
3. Cedarbaum JM, Silvestri M, Clark M, Harts A, Kutt H. L-Deprenyl, levodopa pharmacokinetics, and response fluctuations in Parkinson's disease. *Clin Neuropharmacol* (1990) 13, 29–35.
4. Birkmayer W, Riederer P, Ambrozi L, Youdim MBH. Implications of combined treatment with 'Madopar' and L-deprenil in Parkinson's disease. *Lancet* (1977) i, 439–43.
5. Elsworth JD, Glover V, Reynolds GP, Sandler M, Lees AJ, Phuapradit P, Shaw KM, Stern GM, Kumar P. Deprenyl administration in man: a selective monoamine oxidase B inhibitor without the 'cheese effect'. *Psychopharmacology (Berl)* (1978) 57, 33–8.
6. Shan DE, Yeh SI. An add-on study of selegiline to Madopar in the treatment of parkinsonian patients with dose-related fluctuations: comparison between Jumexal and Parkryl. *Zhonghua Yi Xue Za Zhi (Taipei)* (1996), 58, 264–8.
7. Brannan T, Yahr MD. Comparative-study of selegiline plus L-dopa–carbidopa versus L-dopa–carbidopa alone in the treatment of Parkinson's disease. *Ann Neurol* (1995) 37, 95–8.
8. Golbe LI, Lieberman AN, Muenter MD, Ahlslog JE, Gopinathan G, Neophytides AN, Foo SH, Duvoisin RC. Deprenyl in the treatment of symptom fluctuations in advanced Parkinson's disease. *Clin Neuropharmacol* (1988) 11, 45–55.
9. Presthus J, Berstad J, Lien K. Selegiline (l-deprenyl) and low-dose levodopa treatment of Parkinson's disease. *Acta Neurol Scand* (1987) 76, 200–3.
10. Birkmayer W, Birkmayer GD. Effect of (–)deprenyl in long-term treatment of Parkinson's disease. A 10-years experience. *J Neural Transm* (1986) 22 (Suppl), 219–25.
11. Birkmayer W, Knoll J, Riederer P, Youdim MBH, Hars V, Marton J. Increased life expectancy resulting from addition of L-deprenyl to Madopar® treatment in Parkinson's disease: a longterm study. *J Neural Transm* (1985) 64, 113–127.
12. Parkinson's Disease Research Group of the United Kingdom. Comparison of therapeutic effects and mortality data of levodopa and levodopa combined with selegiline in patients with early, mild Parkinson's disease. *BMJ* (1995) 311, 1602–7.
13. Waters CH. Side effects of selegiline (Eldepryl). *J Geriatr Psychiatry Neurol* (1992) 5, 31–34.
14. Eldepryl (Selegiline hydrochloride). Orion Pharma (UK) Ltd. UK Summary of product characteristics, July 2006.
15. Zelapar (Selegiline hydrochloride). Cephalon Ltd. UK Summary of product characteristics, November 2006.
16. Selegiline hydrochloride tablets USP. Endo Generic Products. US Prescribing information, November 2001.

Levodopa + Methyldopa

Methyldopa can increase the effects of levodopa and permit a reduction in the dosage in some patients taking levodopa alone, but it can also worsen dyskinesias in others. This interaction would not be expected to be significant in a patient taking levodopa with benserazide or carbidopa but this does not appear to have been studied. A small increase in the hypotensive actions of methyldopa may also occur.

Clinical evidence

(a) Effects on the response to levodopa

A double-blind crossover study in 10 patients with Parkinson's disease who had been taking levodopa alone for 12 to 40 months, found that the optimum daily dose of levodopa fell by 68% with methyldopa 1920 mg daily, and by 50% with methyldopa 800 mg daily.[1]

Other reports in patients taking levodopa alone describe reductions in the levodopa dosage of up to 30%[2] and 70%[3] during concurrent treatment with methyldopa. Another report states that the control of Parkinson's disease improved during the concurrent use of methyldopa in some patients taking levodopa alone, but the dyskinesias were worsened in others.[4] Methyldopa on its own can cause a reversible parkinsonian-like syndrome.[5-7]

(b) Effects on the response to methyldopa

A study in 18 patients with Parkinson's disease taking levodopa alone found that combined use of levodopa and methyldopa lowered the blood pressure. The doses used did not affect the systolic blood pressure when given alone. Daily doses of 1 to 2.5 g of levodopa with methyldopa 500 mg caused a 12/6 mmHg fall in blood pressure. No change in the control of the Parkinson's disease was seen, but the study lasted only a few days.[8]

Mechanism

(a) Methyldopa inhibits the breakdown of levodopa outside the brain (by dopa decarboxylase) so that more is available to exert its therapeutic effects.

(b) The increased hypotension may simply be due to the additive effects of the two drugs.

Importance and management

Well documented. Concurrent use need not be avoided but the outcome should be well monitored. In patients on levodopa alone, the use of methyldopa may allow a reduction in the dosage of the levodopa (the reports cited[1-3] quote figures of between 30 and 70%) and may enhance the control of Parkinson's disease, but it should also be borne in mind that in some patients dyskinesias may be worsened. However, in the presence of carbidopa or benserazide the dopa decarboxylase effects of methyldopa would be expected to be less significant and so it seems unlikely that a dose reduction of levodopa would be required. The increased hypotensive effects seem to be small, but they too should be checked.

1. Fermaglich J, Chase TN. Methyldopa or methyldopahydrazine as levodopa synergists. *Lancet* (1973) i, 1261–2.
2. Mones RJ. Evaluation of alpha methyl dopa and alpha methyl dopa hydrazine with L-dopa therapy. *N Y State J Med* (1974) 74, 47–51.
3. Fermaglich J, O'Doherty DS. Second generation of L-dopa therapy. *Neurology* (1971) 21, 408–9.
4. Sweet RD, Lee JE, McDowell FH. Methyldopa as an adjunct to levodopa treatment of Parkinson's disease. *Clin Pharmacol Ther* (1972) 13, 23–7.
5. Groden BM. Parkinsonism occurring with methyldopa treatment. *BMJ* (1963) 1, 1001.
6. Peaston MJT. Parkinsonism associated with alpha-methyldopa therapy. *BMJ* (1964) 2, 168.
7. Strang RR. Parkinsonism occurring during methyldopa therapy. *Can Med Assoc J* (1966) 95, 928–9.
8. Gibberd FB, Small E. Interaction between levodopa and methyldopa. *BMJ* (1973) 2, 90–1.

Levodopa + Mirtazapine

An isolated report describes the development of serious psychosis, which was attributed to an interaction between levodopa and mirtazapine.

Clinical evidence, mechanism, importance and management

A 44-year-old woman taking levodopa/carbidopa, pergolide, selegiline and memantine for Parkinson's disease, was started on mirtazapine in increasing doses rising from 15 to 60 mg daily over 24 days, for depression, labile mood, anxiety, social withdrawal and sleep disturbance. She initially improved, but then major depression and psychosis developed, and on day 26 she attempted self-strangulation. She recovered when the mirtazapine, memantine and selegiline were stopped and low-dose clozapine started. The authors concluded that the reaction was attributable to dopamine-induced psychosis triggered by the addition of mirtazapine to levodopa.[1]

1. Normann C, Hesslinger B, Frauenknecht S, Berger M, Walden J. Psychosis during chronic levodopa therapy triggered by the new antidepressive drug mirtazapine. *Pharmacopsychiatry* (1997) 30, 263–5.

Levodopa + Papaverine

Case reports describe a deterioration in the control of parkinsonism in patients taking levodopa when given papaverine, but a controlled trial failed to confirm this interaction.

Clinical evidence

(a) Levodopa effects reduced

A woman with long-standing parkinsonism, well controlled on levodopa (with the later addition of carbidopa), began to show a steady worsening of her parkinsonism within a week of additionally starting papaverine 100 mg daily for cerebral vascular insufficiency. The deterioration continued until the papaverine was withdrawn. The normal response to levodopa returned within a week. Four other patients had a similar response.[1] Two other similar cases have been described in another report.[2]

(b) Levodopa effects unchanged

A double-blind crossover trial in 9 patients with parkinsonism taking levodopa (range 100 to 750 mg daily) plus a dopa-decarboxylase inhibitor did not find any changes in disease control when they also took papaverine hydrochloride 150 mg daily for 3 weeks. Two patients were also taking bromocriptine 40 mg daily and two trihexyphenidyl 15 mg daily.[3]

Mechanism

Not understood. One suggestion is that papaverine blocks the dopamine receptors in the striatum of the brain, thereby inhibiting the effects of the levodopa.[1,4] Another is that papaverine may have a reserpine-like action on the vesicles of adrenergic neurones[1,5] (i.e. it can deplete dopamine stores).

Importance and management

Direct information seems to be limited to the reports cited. Concurrent use can apparently be uneventful. However, in the light of the reports of adverse interactions it would be prudent to monitor the outcome closely. Carefully controlled trials can provide a good picture of the general situation, but may not necessarily identify the occasional patient who may be affected by an interaction.

1. Duvoisin RC. Antagonism of levodopa by papaverine. *JAMA* (1975) 231, 845.
2. Posner DM. Antagonism of levodopa by papaverine. *JAMA* (1975) 233, 768.
3. Montastruc JL, Rascol O, Belin J, Ane M, Rascol A. Does papaverine interact with levodopa in Parkinson's disease? *Ann Neurol* (1987) 22, 558–9.
4. Gonzalez-Vegas JA. Antagonism of dopamine-mediated inhibition in the nigro-striatal pathway: a mode of action of some catatonia-inducing drugs. *Brain Res* (1974) 80, 219–28.
5. Cubeddu L, Weiner N. Relationship between a granular effect and exocytotic release of norepinephrine by nerve stimulation. *Pharmacologist* (1974) 16, 190.

Levodopa + Penicillamine

Penicillamine can raise plasma levodopa levels in a few patients. This may improve the control of the parkinsonism but the adverse effects of levodopa may also be increased.

Clinical evidence, mechanism, importance and management

A patient with Parkinson's disease taking levodopa with a dopa-decarboxylase inhibitor [probably carbidopa] had a 60% increase in his levodopa plasma levels after taking penicillamine 600 mg daily. This resulted in improved control of symptoms but with an increase in dyskinesia. It was noted that this patient had slightly low serum copper and ceruloplasmin levels.[1] Another study also saw improvements in 2 patients with Parkinson's disease taking levodopa when they also took penicillamine, but levodopa levels were apparently not measured. Again it was noted that the patients had slightly low copper and ceruloplasmin levels. In another 4 similar patients the effects of penicillamine seemed absent in the presence of normal copper and ceruloplasmin levels.[2] The authors of this report[2] attribute the improvement in parkinsonism to the copper chelating properties of penicillamine. However, the authors of the other report[1] suggest that as the effect of penicillamine would not be this rapid, penicillamine must be affecting levodopa pharmacokinetics.

This limited evidence suggests that the concurrent use of levodopa and penicillamine need not be avoided, and in some patients parkinsonian symptoms may be improved. However, if both drugs are given, monitor the effects as an increase in the adverse effects of levodopa is also possible.

1. Mizuta E, Kuno S. Effect of D-penicillamine on pharmacokinetics of levodopa in Parkinson's disease. *Clin Neuropharmacol* (1993) 16, 448–50.
2. Sato M, Yamane K, Oosawa Y, Tanaka H, Shirata A, Nagayama T, Maruyama S. Two cases of Parkinson's disease whose symptoms were markedly improved by D-penicillamine. A study with emphasis on cases displaying a slightly low level of serum copper and ceruloplasmin. *Neurol Ther Chiba* (1992) 9, 555–9.

Levodopa + Phenylbutazone

A single case report describes antagonism of the effects of levodopa by phenylbutazone.

Clinical evidence, mechanism, importance and management

A patient (who was very sensitive to levodopa) found that he was only able to prevent the involuntary movements of his tongue, jaw, neck and limbs caused by levodopa, by taking frequent small doses (125 mg) of levodopa. He was able to suppress the levodopa adverse effects with phenylbutazone. However, the phenylbutazone also lessened the therapeutic effect of the levodopa.[1] The reason is not understood. This interaction has not been confirmed, and its general importance is not known.

1. Wodak J, Gilligan BS, Veale JL, Dowty BJ. Review of 12 months' treatment with L-dopa in Parkinson's disease, with remarks on unusual side effects. *Med J Aust* (1972) 2, 1277–82.

Levodopa + Phenytoin

The therapeutic effects of levodopa can be reduced or abolished by phenytoin.

Clinical evidence, mechanism, importance and management

A study in 5 patients taking levodopa 630 to 4600 mg (four also taking carbidopa 150 to 225 mg daily) for Parkinson's disease, found that when they also took phenytoin in doses of up to 500 mg daily for 5 to 19 days the levodopa-induced dyskinesias were relieved, but the beneficial effects of the levodopa on parkinsonism were reduced or abolished. The patients became slow, rigidity re-emerged, and some of them became unable to get out of a chair. Within 2 weeks of stopping the phenytoin, their parkinsonism was again well controlled by the levodopa.[1] Despite many suggestions, the mechanism of this interaction is not understood. Information seems to be limited to this study, nevertheless it would seem prudent to monitor concurrent use for any evidence of reduced levodopa efficacy.

1. Mendez JS, Cotzias GC, Mena I, Papavasiliou PS. Diphenylhydantoin blocking of levodopa effects. *Arch Neurol* (1975) 32, 44–6.

Levodopa + Pyridoxine (Vitamin B_6)

The effects of levodopa are reduced or abolished by pyridoxine, but this interaction does not occur when levodopa is given with the dopa-decarboxylase inhibitors carbidopa or benserazide, as is usual clinical practice.

Clinical evidence

(a) Levodopa

A study in 25 patients taking levodopa alone found that if they were given high doses of pyridoxine (750 to 1000 mg daily), the effects of the levodopa were reduced within 24 hours, and were completely abolished within 3 to 4 days. Daily doses of pyridoxine 50 to 100 mg also reduced or abolished the effects of levodopa, and an increase in the signs and symptoms of parkinsonism occurred in 8 out of 10 patients taking only 5 to 10 mg of pyridoxine daily.[1]

The antagonism of the effects of levodopa (given without a dopa-decarboxylase inhibitor) by pyridoxine has been described in numerous other reports.[1-6]

(b) Levodopa/carbidopa

A study in 15 patients with Parkinson's disease taking long-term levodopa found that a single 250-mg oral dose of levodopa produced a peak dopa level of 600 nanograms/mL. When pyridoxine 50 mg was also given, the peak plasma levels of dopa fell by almost 70%. When the levodopa was given with carbidopa 50 mg the peak plasma dopa levels were 1300 nanograms/mL, and were not significantly affected by pyridoxine.[6] The results from a subset of these patients have been reported elsewhere.[7] The absence of an interaction in the presence of a dopa-decarboxylase inhibitor is confirmed in another report.[8]

Mechanism

The conversion of levodopa to dopamine within the body requires the presence of pyridoxal-5-phosphate (derived from pyridoxine) as a co-factor. When dietary amounts of pyridoxine are high, the peripheral metabolism of levodopa by dopa-decarboxylase is increased so that less is available for entry into the CNS, and its effects are reduced accordingly. Pyridoxine may also alter levodopa metabolism by Schiff-base formation. However, in the presence of dopa-decarboxylase inhibitors such as carbidopa or benserazide, this peripheral metabolism of levodopa is reduced and much larger amounts are available for entry into the CNS, even if quite small doses are given. So even in the presence of large amounts of pyridoxine, the peripheral metabolism remains unaffected and the serum levels of levodopa are virtually unaltered.

Importance and management

A clinically important, well documented and well established interaction, but principally of historical interest now since levodopa is rarely used alone. The problem of this interaction can be totally solved by using levodopa with a dopa-decarboxylase inhibitor such as carbidopa or benserazide. In the rare cases that levodopa is used alone, pyridoxine in doses as low as 5 mg daily can reduce the effects of levodopa and should therefore be avoided. Warn patients about proprietary pyridoxine-containing preparations such as multivitamins and supplements. Some breakfast cereals are fortified with pyridoxine and other vitamins, but the amounts are usually too small to matter (e.g. a 30 g serving of Kellogg's Corn Flakes or Rice Krispies (UK products) contains only about 0.6 mg of pyridoxine). There is no good clinical evidence to suggest that a low-pyridoxine diet is desirable, and indeed it may be harmful since the normal dietary requirements are about 2 mg daily.

1. Duvoisin RC, Yahr MD, Coté LD. Pyridoxine reversal of L-dopa effects in parkinsonism. *Trans Am Neurol Assoc* (1969) 94, 81–4.
2. Celesia GG, Barr AN. Psychosis and other psychiatric manifestations of levodopa therapy. *Arch Neurol* (1970) 23, 193–200.
3. Carter AB. Pyridoxine and parkinsonism. *BMJ* (1973) 4, 236.
4. Cotzias GC, Papavasiliou PS. Blocking the negative effects of pyridoxine on patients receiving levodopa. *JAMA* (1971) 215, 1504–5.
5. Leon AS, Spiegel HE, Thomas G, Abrams WB. Pyridoxine antagonism of levodopa in parkinsonism. *JAMA* (1971) 218, 1924–7.
6. Mars H. Levodopa, carbidopa, and pyridoxine in Parkinson disease: metabolic interactions. *Arch Neurol* (1974) 30, 444–7.
7. Mars H. Metabolic interactions of pyridoxine, levodopa, and carbidopa in Parkinson's disease. *Trans Am Neurol Assoc* (1973) 98, 241–5.
8. Papavasiliou PS, Cotzias GC, Düby SE, Steck AJ, Fehling C, Bell MA. Levodopa in parkinsonism: potentiation of central effects with a peripheral inhibitor. *N Engl J Med* (1972) 285, 8–14.

Levodopa + Rauwolfia alkaloids

The effects of levodopa are opposed by rauwolfia alkaloids such as reserpine.

Clinical evidence, mechanism, importance and management

Reserpine and other rauwolfia alkaloids deplete the brain of monoamines, including dopamine, thereby reducing their effects.[1] This can lead to parkinsonian-like symptoms, and may oppose the actions of administered levodopa. There are not only sound pharmacological reasons for believing this to be an interaction of clinical importance, but a reduction in the antiparkinsonian activity of levodopa has been observed in patients given **reserpine**.[2] The rauwolfia alkaloids should be avoided in patients with Parkinson's disease, whether or not they are taking levodopa.

1. Bianchine JR, Sunyapridakul L. Interactions between levodopa and other drugs: significance in the treatment of Parkinson's disease. *Drugs* (1973) 6, 364–88.
2. Yahr MD. Personal communication, February 1977.

Levodopa + Spiramycin

The plasma levels of levodopa (given with carbidopa) are reduced by spiramycin, thereby reducing its therapeutic effects.

Clinical evidence

The observation of a patient with Parkinson's disease taking levodopa/carbidopa whose condition became less well-controlled when treated with spiramycin, prompted further study. Levodopa/carbidopa 250/25 mg was given to 7 healthy subjects after they had taken spiramycin 1 g twice daily for 3 days. The spiramycin reduced the AUC of levodopa by 57%, and maximum plasma levels fell from 2162 to 1680 nanograms/mL (not significant). The relative bioavailability of levodopa was only 43%. The plasma levels of the carbidopa were barely detectable.[1]

Mechanism

Not fully established. In some way spiramycin markedly reduces the absorption of carbidopa, possibly by forming a non-absorbable complex in the gut or by accelerating its transit through the gut. As a result, not enough carbidopa is absorbed to inhibit the peripheral metabolism of the levodopa by dopa-decarboxylase, so that the effects of the levodopa are reduced.[1]

Importance and management

Information is very limited, but the interaction appears to be established and of clinical importance. The management of this interaction is unclear, but since it appears to be due to an effect on absorption it would seem prudent to try to separate the dosing of these two drugs by as much as possible, although this may be difficult with some levodopa regimens. Monitor the outcome of concurrent use on the control of Parkinson's disease. It is not known whether other macrolide antibacterials behave in a similar way, or whether spiramycin affects levodopa/benserazide preparations. More study is needed.

1. Brion N, Kollenbach K, Marion MH, Grégoire A, Advenier C, Pays M. Effect of a macrolide (spiramycin) on the pharmacokinetics of L-dopa and carbidopa in healthy volunteers. *Clin Neuropharmacol* (1992) 15, 229–35.

Levodopa + SSRIs

The use of an SSRI is often beneficial in parkinsonian patients taking levodopa to treat the depression associated with the disease. However, sometimes parkinsonian symptoms are worsened.

Clinical evidence

Four patients taking levodopa 375 to 990 mg daily, a dopa-decarboxylase inhibitor [drug and dose not stated] and amantadine [dose not stated], had a deterioration in the control of their parkinsonism when they were also given **fluoxetine** 20 mg daily for 8 to 11 weeks. The **fluoxetine** was withdrawn and their motor performance was restored. The antidepressant efficacy of **fluoxetine** was not found to be substantial in any of the 4 patients.[1] Another patient taking levodopa developed frequent hallucinations after the addition of **fluoxetine**. They resolved when the **fluoxetine** was withdrawn.[2] In a retrospective study of 23 parkinsonian patients who were given **fluoxetine** up to 40 mg daily, 20 patients had no change in the control of their parkinsonism but 3 others experienced a worsening in their Parkinson's disease signs.[3] These are just a few of the reports on the onset or worsening of Parkinson's with SSRIs, and a number of reviews have been published about the extrapyramidal effects of SSRIs.[4,5]

Mechanism

Not understood. Extrapyramidal effects are rare but recognised adverse effects of SSRIs.[4,5]

Importance and management

Although the information is limited, it seems that in some cases parkinsonism can be worsened by SSRIs. Concurrent use is valuable and need not be avoided, but monitor the outcome and withdraw the SSRI if necessary.

1. Jansen Steur ENH. Increase of Parkinson disability after fluoxetine medication. *Neurology* (1993) 43, 211–13.
2. Lauterbach EC. Dopaminergic hallucinosis with fluoxetine in Parkinson's disease. *Am J Psychiatry* (1993) 150, 1750.
3. Caley CF, Friedman JH. Does fluoxetine exacerbate Parkinson's disease? *J Clin Psychiatry* (1992) 53, 278–282.
4. Anonymous. Extrapyramidal effects of SSRI antidepressants. *Prescrire Int* (2001) 10, 118–19.
5. Gerber PE, Lynd LD. Selective serotonin-reuptake inhibitor-induced movement disorders. *Ann Pharmacother* (1998) 32, 692–8.

Levodopa + Tricyclic antidepressants

The concurrent use of levodopa and the tricyclics is usually uneventful although two unexplained hypertensive crises have occurred when imipramine or amitriptyline was used with levodopa/carbidopa. See also 'Levodopa + Antimuscarinics', p.682 for interactions due to the antimuscarinic effects of tricyclic antidepressants.

Clinical evidence

A hypertensive crisis (blood pressure 210/110 mmHg) associated with agitation, tremor and generalised rigidity developed in a woman taking 6 tablets of levodopa/carbidopa 100/10 mg daily the day after she started to take **imipramine** 25 mg three times daily. The **imipramine** was stopped and she recovered over the following 24 hours. The same reaction occurred again when she was later accidentally given **amitriptyline** 25 mg three times daily.[1] A similar hypertensive reaction (a rise from 190/110 to 270/140 mmHg) occurred over 34 hours in another woman taking **amitriptyline** 20 mg at night when she was given levodopa/carbidopa 50/5 mg and metoclopramide 10 mg, both three times a day. This resolved when all three drugs were stopped.[2]

Mechanism

Not understood.

Importance and management

Information seems to be limited to these reports. Concurrent use is normally successful and uneventful.[3-5] However, be alert for the possibility of a hypertensive reaction, which resolves if the tricyclic antidepressant is withdrawn. See also 'Levodopa + Antimuscarinics', p.682 for interactions due to the antimuscarinic adverse effects of tricyclic antidepressants.

1. Edwards M. Adverse interaction of levodopa with tricyclic antidepressants. *Practitioner* (1982) 226, 1447 and 1449.
2. Rampton DS. Hypertensive crisis in a patient given Sinemet, metoclopramide, and amitriptyline. *BMJ* (1977) 3, 607–8.
3. Yahr MD. The treatment of Parkinsonism. Current concepts. *Med Clin North Am* (1972) 56, 1377–92.
4. Calne DB, Reid JL. Antiparkinsonian drugs: pharmacological and therapeutic aspects. *Drugs* (1972) 4, 49–74.
5. van Wieringen A, Wright J. Observations on patients with Parkinson's disease treated with L-dopa. I. Trial and evaluation of L-dopa therapy. *S Afr Med J* (1972) 46, 1262–6.

MAO-B inhibitors + Antidepressants

A few cases of the serotonin syndrome and other serious CNS disturbances have been seen when selegiline was given with tricyclic antidepressants, fluoxetine or venlafaxine. One of the manufacturers of selegiline contraindicates its use with any antidepressant drug, while another advises avoiding SSRIs and venlafaxine, and using caution with tricyclics. See also 'MAO-B inhibitors + MAOIs or RIMAs', p.692 for information on selegiline and MAOIs. The manufacturer of rasagiline specifically recommends avoiding the concurrent use of fluoxetine or fluvoxamine and recommends caution on the concurrent use of any antidepressant.

Clinical evidence

A. SSRIs

(a) Citalopram

In a double-blind randomised study 18 healthy subjects were given citalopram 20 mg or a placebo daily for 10 days followed by 4 days with concurrent **selegiline** 10 mg daily. There was no evidence of changes in vital signs or in the frequency of adverse events, but the bioavailability of the **selegiline** was slightly reduced by about 30% in the presence of citalopram. The authors of this report concluded that no clinically relevant interaction occurred between **selegiline** and citalopram.[1]

(b) Fluoxetine

A woman with Parkinson's disease taking **selegiline**, bromocriptine and levodopa/carbidopa was also given fluoxetine 20 mg. Several days later she developed episodes of shivering and sweating in the mid-afternoon, which lasted several hours. Her hands became blue, cold and mottled and her blood pressure was elevated (200/120 mmHg). These episodes disappeared when both fluoxetine and **selegiline** were stopped, and did not reappear when the fluoxetine alone was restarted.[2] A case of mild serotonin syndrome has been described in a woman taking levodopa and **selegiline** a few days after starting fluoxetine,[3] and a possible case of the serotonin syndrome has been described in another patient taking **selegiline** and fluoxetine.[4]

Other patients have become hyperactive and apparently manic,[2] have developed ataxia,[5] or developed a tonic-clonic seizure and headache, flushes, palpitations, and a blood pressure of 250/130 mmHg (a pseudophaeochromocytoma syndrome),[6] all after the concurrent use of fluoxetine and **selegiline**. These reports contrast with a retrospective study of 23 patients with parkinsonism, who received both **selegiline** and fluoxetine without any serious adverse effects occurring, although worsening confusion was noted in 5 patients.[7]

(c) Fluvoxamine

The manufacturer of **selegiline** notes that serious reactions similar to those seen with fluoxetine have occurred in patients receiving **selegiline** and fluvoxamine.[8]

(d) Paroxetine

A retrospective study of patients with Parkinson's disease taking **selegiline** 5 to 10 mg daily (and other antiparkinsonian drugs such as levodopa/carbidopa, bromocriptine, amantadine, pergolide, and antimuscarinics) noted that the addition of paroxetine 10 to 40 mg daily caused no adverse effects and the patients appeared to obtain overall benefit, including some improvement in parkinsonian symptoms.[9] However, the manufacturers of **selegiline** note that serious reactions similar to those seen with fluoxetine have occurred in patients receiving **selegiline** and paroxetine.[8,10]

(e) Sertraline

A retrospective study of patients with Parkinson's disease taking **selegiline** 5 to 10 mg daily (and other antiparkinsonian drugs such as levodopa/carbidopa, bromocriptine, amantadine, pergolide, and antimuscarinics) noted that the addition of sertraline 25 to 100 mg daily caused no adverse effects and the patients appeared to obtain overall benefit, including some improvement in parkinsonian symptoms.[9] However, the manufacturers of **selegiline** note that serious reactions similar to those seen with concurrent fluoxetine have occurred in patients receiving **selegiline** and sertraline.[8,10]

B. Tetracyclic antidepressants

For a case report of a hypertensive crisis, which was attributed to the concurrent use of **maprotiline**, **selegiline** and ephedrine, see 'MAO-B inhibitors + Sympathomimetics; Indirectly-acting', p.693.

C. Tricyclic antidepressants

Between 1989 and 1994 the FDA in the USA received 16 reports of adverse interactions between **selegiline** and tricyclic antidepressants, which were attributed to the serotonin syndrome.[11]

The manufacturers very briefly describe severe CNS toxicity in one patient given **selegiline** and **amitriptyline** (hyperpyrexia and death), and in another given **protriptyline** (tremor, agitation, restlessness, followed by unresponsiveness and death).[8,10,12] They state that related adverse events including hypertension, syncope, asystole, diaphoresis, seizures, changes in behavioural and mental status, and muscular rigidity have also been reported in some patients receiving **selegiline** and various tricyclics.[8,10] A further report describes the serotonin syndrome in a woman given **nortriptyline** and **selegiline** concurrently.[13]

However, these warnings need to be balanced by other reports indicating that these reactions are uncommon. One study based on the findings of 45 investigators treating 4,568 patients with **selegiline** and antidepressants [not specifically named but possibly including the tricyclics] found that only 11 patients (0.24%) experienced symptoms considered to represent the serotonin syndrome, and only 2 patients (0.04%) experienced symptoms considered to be serious.[14] Another small retrospective study designed to evaluate the tolerability and efficacy of combining **selegiline** and tricyclic antidepressants [not specifically named] identified 28 patients who had taken both drugs.[11] In total, 17 patients definitely benefited and 6 patients possibly benefited from taking the combination. Another retrospective study of 25 occasions of combined tricyclic-**selegiline** use found no cases of the serotonin syndrome.[4]

D. Miscellaneous antidepressants

(a) Trazodone

A retrospective study of patients with Parkinson's disease taking **selegiline** 5 to 10 mg daily (and other anti-parkinson drugs such as levodopa/carbidopa, bromocriptine, amantadine, pergolide, and antimuscarinics) noted that the addition of trazodone 25 to 150 mg daily caused no adverse effects and the patients appeared to obtain overall benefit, including some improvement in parkinsonian symptoms.[9]

(b) Venlafaxine

A man developed the serotonin syndrome 15 days after stopping **selegiline** 50 mg [daily] and within 30 minutes of starting venlafaxine 37.5 mg.[15]

Mechanism

Not fully understood. In some cases the symptoms seen appear to be consistent with the serotonin syndrome, which is typified by CNS irritability, increased muscle tone, shivering, altered consciousness and myoclonus, and appears to be associated with the use of more than one serotonergic drug, see 'The serotonin syndrome', (p.9). This syndrome has also occurred with non-selective MAOIs and 'SSRIs', (p.1142), 'tricyclics', (p.1149), and 'venlafaxine', (p.1156). Note that selegiline may have some non-selective MAOI activity.

Importance and management

The possibility of the serotonin syndrome or similar (signs and symptoms may include diaphoresis, flushing, ataxia, tremor, hyperthermia, hyper/hypotension, seizures, palpitation, dizziness and mental changes that include agitation, confusion and hallucinations progressing to delirium and coma)[8,12] occurring with selegiline and SSRIs or venlafaxine would appear to be established, although the incidence is very rare. The manufacturers of selegiline recommend that these drug combinations should be avoided.[8,10,12] In addition, selegiline should not be started for 5 weeks after stopping fluoxetine, 2 weeks after stopping sertraline, and one week after stopping other SSRIs, and SSRIs should not be started for 2 weeks after stopping selegiline.[8,12]

Similarly, the manufacturers of **rasagiline** recommend avoiding combined use with fluoxetine and fluvoxamine. **Rasagiline** should not be started for 5 weeks after stopping fluoxetine or 2 weeks after starting fluvoxamine, and fluoxetine should not be started for 2 weeks after stopping **rasagiline**.[16]

If the decision is made to combine selegiline and any of the tricyclic antidepressants, the outcome should be well monitored, but the likelihood of problems seems to be small. Nevertheless, some manufacturers of selegiline advise avoiding the combination of tricyclic antidepressants and selegiline.[10,12] Similarly, the manufacturers of **rasagiline** advise caution if it is given with antidepressants.[16]

Limited evidence suggests that trazodone is unlikely to interact with selegiline.[9] However, interactions with other antidepressants are rare. Therefore if trazodone is given with either selegiline or **rasagiline** some caution would seem prudent.

1. Laine K, Anttila M, Heinonen E, Helminen A, Huupponen R, Mäki-Ikola O, Reinikainen K, Scheinin M. Lack of adverse interactions between concomitantly administered selegiline and citalopram. *Clin Neuropharmacol* (1997) 20, 419–33.
2. Suchowersky O, deVries JD. Interaction of fluoxetine and selegiline. *Can J Psychiatry* (1990) 35, 571–2.
3. Garcia-Monco JC, Padierna A, Gomez Beldarrain M. Selegiline, fluoxetine, and depression in Parkinson's disease. *Mov Disord* (1995) 10, 352–8.
4. Ritter JL, Alexander B. Retrospective study of selegiline-antidepressant drug interactions and a review of the literature. *Ann Clin Psychiatry* (1997) 9, 7–13.
5. Jermain DM, Hughes PL, Follender AB. Potential fluoxetine-selegiline interaction. *Ann Pharmacother* (1992) 26, 1300.
6. Montastruc JL, Chamontin B, Senard JM, Tran MA, Rascol O, Llau ME, Rascol A. Pseudophaeochromocytoma in parkinsonian patient treated with fluoxetine plus selegiline. *Lancet* (1993) 341, 555.
7. Waters CH. Fluoxetine and selegiline — lack of significant interaction. *Can J Neurol Sci* (1994) 21, 259–61.
8. Eldepryl (Selegiline hydrochloride). Orion Pharma (UK) Ltd. UK Summary of product characteristics, July 2006.
9. Toyama SC, Iacono RP. Is it safe to combine a selective serotonin reuptake inhibitor with selegiline? *Ann Pharmacother* (1994) 28, 405–6.
10. Selegiline hydrochloride tablets, USP. Endo Generic Products. US prescribing information, November 2001.
11. Yu LJ, Zweig RM. Successful combination of selegiline and antidepressants in Parkinson's disease. *Neurology* (1996) 46 (2 Suppl), A374.
12. Zelapar (Selegiline hydrochloride). Cephalon Ltd. UK Summary of product characteristics, November 2006.
13. Hinds NP, Hillier CEM, Wiles CM. Possible serotonin syndrome arising from an interaction between nortriptyline and selegiline in a lady with parkinsonism. *J Neurol* (2000) 247, 811.
14. Richard I, Kurlan R, Tanner C. Serotonin syndrome and the combined use of Deprenyl and an antidepressant in Parkinson's disease. *Neurology* (1996) 46 (2 Suppl), A374.
15. Gitlin MJ. Venlafaxine, monoamine oxidase inhibitors, and the serotonin syndrome. *J Clin Psychopharmacol* (1997) 17, 66–67.
16. Azilect (Rasagiline mesilate). Teva Pharmaceuticals Ltd. UK Summary of product characteristics, April 2007.

MAO-B inhibitors + Dextromethorphan

The manufacturer of rasagiline[1] suggests that its use with dextromethorphan should be avoided. Similarly, some consider that patients taking selegiline should try to avoid dextromethorphan.[2] These warnings are based on the serious adverse reactions (the serotonin syndrome or similar) that have rarely occurred when dextromethorphan has been used with 'non-selective MAOIs or RIMAs', (p.1134). The likelihood of any interaction with MAO-B inhibitors would appear to be very small, but because of the potential severity, some caution would appear to be prudent.

1. Azilect (Rasagiline mesilate). Teva Pharmaceuticals Ltd. UK Summary of product characteristics, April 2007.
2. Jacob JE, Wagner ML, Sage JI. Safety of selegiline with cold medications. *Ann Pharmacother* (2003) 37, 438–41.

MAO-B inhibitors + MAOIs or RIMAs

Marked orthostatic hypotension has been seen in two patients taking iproniazid or tranylcypromine/trifluoperazine when given selegiline. When the RIMA moclobemide is given with selegiline, restriction of dietary tyramine is necessary, and there may be an increased risk of hypotensive reactions. Some manufacturers of MAO-B inhibitors contraindicate the concurrent use of MAOIs or RIMAs.

Clinical evidence, mechanism, importance and management

(a) MAOIs

In a pilot study, one patient taking **iproniazid** 150 mg daily developed severe orthostatic hypotension on two occasions within an hour of taking **selegiline** 5 mg. Two other patients (one on **tranylcypromine**/trifluoperazine and one on **tranylcypromine**/trifluoperazine plus **isocarboxazid**) did not have this reaction to **selegiline** 5 mg twice daily. The authors mention another patient who similarly developed postural hypotension on two occasions within 2 hours of taking **selegiline** 5 mg. He had stopped taking **tranylcypromine**/trifluoperazine, 4 weeks previously.[1] The reasons are not understood. This evidence suggests that **selegiline** should be given with caution to patients taking, or who have recently stopped, non-selective MAOIs. One UK manufacturer of **selegiline**[2] and the manufacturer of **rasagiline**[3] actually contraindicate the concurrent use of non-selective MAOIs. At least 14 days should elapse between stopping rasagiline and starting an MAOI.[3]

(b) RIMAs

A study in 24 healthy subjects, designed to assess the safety and tolerability of giving **moclobemide** 100 to 400 mg and **selegiline** 5 mg twice daily, sequentially or combined, found that the adverse effects were no greater under steady-state conditions than with either drug alone, but the sensitivity to tyramine was considerably increased. The mean tyramine sensitivity factor for **moclobemide** alone was 2 to 3, **selegiline** alone was 1.4, and **moclobemide** plus **selegiline** was 8 to 9 (and even 18 in one subject).[4,5] The reason is, that when taken together, the **moclobemide** inhibits MAO-A while **selegiline** inhibits MAO-B, so that little or no MAO activity remains available to metabolise the tyramine. However, unexpectedly, the combined effect was more than additive.[5] **Selegiline** had no effect on the pharmacokinetics of **moclobemide**.[6] In a clinical trial using tyramine restriction, one of 5 **selegiline** recipients and one of 5 **selegiline/moclobemide** recipients reported symptomatic hypotension, and there was no increase in blood pressure in any patient.[7]

In practical terms this means that patients taking **moclobemide** with **selegiline** should be given the same dietary restrictions for tyramine-rich foods and drinks (see 'tyramine-rich drinks', (p.1151) and 'tyramine-rich foods', (p.1153)), that relate to the non-selective MAOIs such as phenelzine and tranylcypromine.[5] However, because of the potential risks the manufacturer of **moclobemide**[8] contraindicate this combination. On the basis of work done on the *pig* it is suggested that if **selegiline** is replaced by **moclobemide**, the dietary restrictions can be relaxed after a wash-out period of about 2 weeks. If switching from **moclobemide** to **selegiline**, a wash-out period of 1 to 2 days is sufficient.[4]

1. Pare CMB, Al Mousawi M, Sandler M, Glover V. Attempts to attenuate the 'cheese effect'. Combined drug therapy in depressive illness. *J Affect Disord* (1985) 9, 137–41.
2. Zelapar (Selegiline hydrochloride). Cephalon Ltd. UK Summary of product characteristics, November 2006.
3. Azilect (Rasagiline mesilate). Teva Pharmaceuticals Ltd. UK Summary of product characteristics, April 2007.
4. Dingemanse J. An update of recent moclobemide interaction data. *Int Clin Psychopharmacol* (1993) 7, 167–80.
5. Korn A, Wagner B, Moritz E, Dingemanse J. Tyramine pressor sensitivity in healthy subjects during combined treatment with moclobemide and selegiline. *Eur J Clin Pharmacol* (1996) 49, 273–8.
6. Dingemanse J, Kneer J, Wallnöfer A, Kettler R, Zürcher G, Koulu M, Korn A. Pharmacokinetic-pharmacodynamic interactions between two selective monoamine oxidase inhibitors: moclobemide and selegiline. *Clin Neuropharmacol* (1996) 19, 399–414.

7. Jansen Steur ENH, Ballering LAP. Moclobemide and selegiline in the treatment of depression in Parkinson's disease. *J Neurol Neurosurg Psychiatry* (1997) 63, 547.
8. Manerix (Moclobemide). Roche Products Ltd. UK Summary of product characteristics, September 2005.

MAO-B inhibitors + Pethidine (Meperidine)

A case of fluctuating stupor and agitation, with muscle rigidity, sweating and a raised temperature has been reported when pethidine was used with selegiline. This case is similar to cases reported with the older non-selective MAOIs or RIMAs and pethidine. The manufacturers say that selegiline and rasagiline should not be used with pethidine.

Clinical evidence, mechanism, importance and management

A patient taking **selegiline** 5 mg twice daily, pergolide, levodopa/carbidopa, imipramine and desipramine was treated with pethidine beginning on postoperative day one for 4 days in doses of 75 to 150 mg daily. On the second day he became increasingly restless and irritable, progressing to delirium on the fourth day, with fluctuations between stupor and severe agitation associated with muscular rigidity, sweating and a raised temperature. The patient remained normotensive. Both pethidine and then **selegiline** were stopped, with full recovery.[1] This case is similar to various cases described with 'older nonselective MAOI inhibitors and pethidine', see (p.1140). US information states that other serious reactions including death have occurred with the combination of **selegiline** and pethidine.[2]

On the basis of this evidence the manufacturers of **selegiline**[2,3] and **rasagiline**[4] contraindicate concurrent use with **pethidine**, which is a prudent precaution. The manufacturers of **rasagiline** additionally say that pethidine should not be given until 14 days after stopping **rasagiline**,[4] which makes sense since it is an irreversible inhibitor of MAO-B. One manufacturer of **selegiline** also cautions that **tramadol** may potentially interact with **selegiline**,[5] which seems a possibility based on evidence of an interaction between 'tramadol and non-selective MAOIs', (p.1141). Another manufacturer of **selegiline** contraindicates concurrent use with all opioids,[3] which is probably unnecessary, based on the evidence with non-selective MAOIs, see 'MAOIs or RIMAs + Opioids; Pethidine (Meperidine)', p.1140.

1. Zornberg GL, Bodkin JA, Cohen BM. Severe adverse interaction between pethidine and selegiline. *Lancet* (1991) 337, 246.
2. Selegiline hydrochloride tablets USP. Endo Generic Products. US Prescribing information, November 2001.
3. Zelapar (Selegiline hydrochloride). Cephalon Ltd. UK Summary of product characteristics, November 2006.
4. Azilect (Rasagiline mesilate). Teva Pharmaceuticals Ltd. UK Summary of product characteristics, April 2007.
5. Eldepryl (Selegiline hydrochloride). Orion Pharma (UK) Ltd. UK Summary of product characteristics, July 2006.

MAO-B inhibitors + Sympathomimetics; Indirectly-acting

An isolated report describes a hypertensive crisis, which was attributed to an interaction between selegiline, ephedrine, and maprotiline.

Clinical evidence

An isolated case report describes a man taking **selegiline** 10 mg daily, levodopa/carbidopa, lisuride, maprotiline 75 mg daily, and theophylline/**ephedrine** 180 mg/32 mg daily who developed hypertensive crises (blood pressure up to 300/150 mmHg), intense vasoconstriction, confusion, abdominal pain, sweating, and tachycardia (110 bpm) within 2 days of raising the dose of theophylline/**ephedrine** to 270 mg/48 mg daily. All of the drugs were stopped, and the patient was treated with intravenous nicardipine. He recovered uneventfully.[1]

Mechanism

It is thought that this reaction occurred as a result of excess sympathomimetic amines: ephedrine is an indirectly-acting sympathomimetic that causes increased release of noradrenaline; selegiline has some MAO-A inhibitory activity and may therefore inhibit noradrenaline metabolism; and maprotiline inhibits reuptake of noradrenaline.[1] Compare also 'MAOIs or RIMAs + Sympathomimetics; Indirectly-acting', p.1147 and 'MAOIs or RIMAs + Tricyclic and related antidepressants', p.1149.

Importance and management

This appears to be the only report of a hypertensive reaction in a patient taking selegiline and ephedrine, and concurrent maprotiline was also implicated. In general, if selegiline is used at recommended doses it is selective for MAO-B and no restrictions are required in the use of indirectly-acting sympathomimetics such as ephedrine and **pseudoephedrine**. Nevertheless, this report suggests that, rarely, interactions are still possible, and some consider that patients taking selegiline should try to avoid **pseudoephedrine**.[2] The manufacturer of **rasagiline** also recommends against the concurrent use of sympathomimetics such as those present in decongestants or cold medications containing ephedrine or **pseudoephedrine**.[3]

1. Lefebvre H, Noblet C, Moore N, Wolf LM. Pseudo-phaeochromocytoma after multiple drug interactions involving the selective monoamine oxidase inhibitor selegiline. *Clin Endocrinol (Oxf)* (1995) 42, 95–9.
2. Jacob JE, Wagner ML, Sage JI. Safety of selegiline with cold medications. *Ann Pharmacother* (2003) 37, 438–41.
3. Azilect (Rasagiline mesilate). Teva Pharmaceuticals Ltd. UK Summary of product characteristics, April 2007.

MAO-B inhibitors + Tyramine-rich foods

No dietary restrictions are required with the doses of rasagiline and selegiline recommended for use in Parkinson's disease. An isolated report describes the cheese reaction in a patient taking selegiline 20 mg daily. Thus, at higher doses of selegiline, restriction of the amount of tyramine in the diet may be necessary.

Clinical evidence

(a) Rasagiline

The manufacturer notes that the results of four tyramine challenge studies, together with the results of home monitoring of blood pressure after meals (from 464 patients treated with rasagiline 0.5 or 1 mg daily or placebo without tyramine restrictions), and the lack of reported problems in clinical trials without tyramine restriction, indicate that no dietary restrictions are necessary with rasagiline.[1] No specific details were provided of any of the studies.

(b) Selegiline

1. Oral selegiline. The pressor response to oral tyramine was not altered by pretreatment with selegiline 10 mg daily in healthy volunteers and patients with Parkinson's disease.[2] However, another study[3] found that selegiline 5 mg daily for at least 14 days reduced the dose of oral tyramine required to achieve the cardiovascular threshold (increase in systolic BP of greater than 30 mmHg, a diastolic BP greater than 100 mmHg or a fall in heart rate of greater than 20%) by a factor of 2.8. Nevertheless, this reduction was less than the RIMA moclobemide (4.3) and the MAOI phenelzine (10.3).[3] In other studies, higher doses of selegiline (20 or 30 mg daily) increased the sensitivity to oral tyramine by 2- to 4.5-fold.[4,5] A patient taking selegiline 20 mg daily was reported to have had a hypertensive reaction (severe headache and rise in blood pressure) after eating macaroni and **cheese**,[6] but this appears to be the only published report of the 'cheese reaction' with selegiline.

2. Buccal and transdermal selegiline. The dose of tyramine required to elicit a pressor effect was not altered by pretreatment with buccal selegiline 1.25 mg in healthy subjects.[7] Similarly, the pressor response to tyramine up to 200 mg was not significantly altered by pretreatment with a single 24-hour application of transdermal selegiline 7.8 mg/24 hour in healthy subjects.[8]

Mechanism

Rasagiline and selegiline specifically inhibit MAO-B, which leaves MAO-A still available to metabolise any tyramine in foodstuffs. However, at higher doses the selectivity of selegiline diminishes, and inhibition of the metabolism of tyramine is more likely. Nevertheless, the 2- to 4.5-fold increase in effect of tyramine seen with selegiline 5 to 30 mg daily is still less than that seen with older non-selective MAOIs, see 'MAOIs or RIMAs + Tyramine-rich foods', p.1153.

Importance and management

The manufacturer states that no dietary tyramine restrictions are necessary with rasagiline.[1] Similarly, at the recommended doses of conventional or buccal selegiline used in Parkinson's disease the manufacturers say that no dietary restrictions are necessary,[9-11] and this is supported by the scarcity of any published reports of reactions. If higher doses of selegiline are used, patients should be advised to avoid large amounts of tyramine-rich foods. For a list of the possible tyramine-content of some foods, see 'Table 32.3', (p.1154).

1. Azilect (Rasagiline mesilate). Teva Pharmaceuticals Ltd. UK Summary of product characteristics, April 2007.
2. Elsworth JD, Glover V, Reynolds GP, Sandler M, Lees AJ, Phuapradit P, Shaw KM, Stern GM, Kumar P. Deprenyl administration in man: a selective monoamine oxidase B inhibitor without the 'cheese effect'. *Psychopharmacology (Berl)* (1978) 57, 33–8.
3. Warrington SJ, Turner P, Mant TGK, Morrison P, Haywood G, Glover V, Goodwin BL, Sandler M, St John-Smith P, McClelland GR. Clinical pharmacology of moclobemide, a new reversible monoamine oxidase inhibitor. *J Psychopharmacol* (1991) 5, 82–91.
4. Prasad A, Glover V, Goodwin BL, Sandler M, Signy M, Smith SE. Enhanced pressor sensitivity to oral tyramine challenge following high dose selegiline treatment. *Psychopharmacology (Berl)* (1988) 95, 540–3.
5. Bieck PR, Antonin KH. Tyramine potentiation during treatment with MAO inhibitors: brofaromine and moclobemide vs irreversible inhibitors. *J Neural Transm* (1989) (Suppl 28), 21–31.
6. McGrath PJ, Stewart JW, Quitkin FM. A possible l-deprenyl induced hypertensive reaction. *J Clin Psychopharmacol* (1989) 9, 310–11.
7. Clarke A, Johnson ES, Mallard N, Corn TH, Johnston A, Boyce M, Warrington S, MacMahon DG. A new low-dose formulation of selegiline: clinical efficacy, patient preference and selectivity for MAO-B inhibition. *J Neural Transm* (2003) 110, 1273–8.
8. Barrett JS, Hochadel TJ, Morales RJ, Rohatagi S, DeWitt KE, Watson SK, Darnow J, Azzaro AJ, DiSanto AR. Pressor response to tyramine after single 24-hour application of a selegiline transdermal system in healthy males. *J Clin Pharmacol* (1997) 37, 238–47.
9. Eldepryl (Selegiline hydrochloride). Orion Pharma (UK) Ltd. UK Summary of product characteristics, July 2006.
10. Zelapar (Selegiline hydrochloride). Cephalon Ltd. UK Summary of product characteristics, November 2006.
11. Eldepryl (Selegiline hydrochloride). Somerset Pharmaceuticals Inc. US Prescribing information, July 1998.

MAO-B inhibitors; Rasagiline + CYP1A2 inhibitors

Ciprofloxacin increases the AUC of rasagiline. Other inhibitors of cytochrome P450 isoenzyme CYP1A2 are predicted to interact similarly.

Clinical evidence, mechanism, importance and management

The manufacturer notes that concurrent use of rasagiline and **ciprofloxacin** increased the AUC of rasagiline by 83%.[1] **Ciprofloxacin** inhibits the cytochrome P450 isoenzyme CYP1A2, which is the major enzyme responsible for the metabolism of rasagiline. The clinical relevance of this increase has not been assessed, but until more is known caution is warranted. This caution should be extended to other potent inhibitors of CYP1A2. For a list see 'Table 1.2', (p.4).

1. Azilect (Rasagiline mesilate). Teva Pharmaceuticals Ltd. UK Summary of product characteristics, April 2007.

MAO-B inhibitors; Selegiline + Cocaine

Cocaine and selegiline appear not to interact adversely.

Clinical evidence, mechanism, importance and management

In a study to establish the safety of using selegiline to prevent relapse in cocaine addiction, 5 otherwise healthy intravenous cocaine users were given 0, 20 and 40 mg intravenous doses of cocaine one hour apart following treatment with selegiline 10 mg or placebo orally. The cocaine increased the heart rate, blood pressure, pupil diameter and subjective indices of euphoria as expected. However, the presence of selegiline reduced pupillary diameter, but did not alter the pupil dilation or other effects normally caused by cocaine. It was concluded that concurrent use is safe and unlikely to increase the reinforcing effects of cocaine.[1] In another study, transdermal selegiline did not alter the pharmacokinetics of intravenous cocaine in cocaine-dependent subjects. Some physiological effects (blood pressure and heart rate) and subjective effects of cocaine were attenuated by selegiline.[2]

1. Haberny KA, Walsh SL, Ginn DH, Wilkins JN, Garner JE, Setoda D, Bigelow GE. Absence of acute cocaine interactions with the MAO-B inhibitor selegiline. *Drug Alcohol Depend* (1995) 39, 55–62.
2. Houtsmuller EJ, Notes LD, Newton T, van Sluis N, Chiang N, Elkashef A, Bigelow GE. Transdermal selegiline and intravenous cocaine: safety and interactions. *Psychopharmacology (Berl)* (2004) 172, 31–40.

MAO-B inhibitors; Selegiline + Dopamine agonists

No significant pharmacokinetic interaction occurs between selegiline and cabergoline, pramipexole or ropinirole.

Clinical evidence, mechanism, importance and management

(a) Cabergoline

No pharmacokinetic interaction was found to occur between cabergoline 1 mg daily and selegiline 10 mg daily after 22 days of concurrent use in a study in 6 subjects with Parkinson's disease.[1]

(b) Pramipexole

The manufacturers of pramipexole say that no pharmacokinetic interaction occurs with selegiline.[2]

(c) Ropinirole

The manufacturers of ropinirole note that a population pharmacokinetic analysis showed a lack of effect of selegiline on ropinirole.[3]

1. Dostert P, Benedetti MS, Persiani S, La Croix R, Bosc M, Fiorentini F, Deffond D, Vernay D, Dordain G. Lack of pharmacokinetic interaction between the selective dopamine agonist cabergoline and the MAO-B inhibitor selegiline. *J Neural Transm* (1995) 45 (Suppl), 247–57.
2. Mirapexin (Pramipexole). Boehringer Ingelheim Ltd. UK Summary of product characteristics, August 2006.
3. SmithKline Beecham. Personal Communication, September 1996.

MAO-B inhibitors; Selegiline + Hormonal contraceptives or HRT

In a small study, the bioavailability of selegiline was markedly higher (mean of about 20-fold) in women taking combined oral contraceptives than in those not taking contraceptives. In a controlled study, the AUC of selegiline was modestly increased by HRT (60%) and the change was not considered clinically relevant.

Clinical evidence

(a) Combined oral contraceptives

The AUCs of single doses of selegiline 5 to 40 mg were 16 to 45-fold higher in 4 women taking combined oral contraceptives than in 4 women who were not taking contraceptives. Three subjects were taking ethinylestradiol/gestodene 30/75 micrograms, and one was taking a triphasic preparation of ethinylestradiol/levonorgestrel.[1]

(b) HRT

The AUC of a single 10-mg dose of selegiline was increased by 60% (which was not statistically significant) following 10 days of HRT (containing estradiol valerate/levonorgestrel 2 mg/250 micrograms) in a crossover study in 12 young healthy women. There was marked variability in selegiline levels with two women having a threefold increase in AUC, and 3 having a decrease. Other changes in pharmacokinetics of selegiline or its metabolites were small.[2]

Mechanism

It was suggested that the combined oral contraceptive inhibited the first pass metabolism of selegiline and so markedly increased its bioavailability.[1] However, this was not found for HRT containing a different estrogenic hormone.

Importance and management

Although data are limited, it appears that combined oral contraceptives may markedly increase the bioavailability of selegiline. One UK manufacturer advises caution with combined use,[3] and the other suggests the combination should be avoided.[4] Although short-term use of menopausal HRT also increased the AUC of selegiline, the changes were modest and were not considered clinically relevant. Nevertheless, the results perhaps need confirming with longer term combined use. One UK manufacturer of selegiline also advises the avoidance of concurrent HRT.[4]

1. Laine K, Anttila M, Helminen A, Karnani H, Huupponen R. Dose linearity study of selegiline pharmacokinetics after oral administration: evidence for strong drug interaction with female sex steroids. *Br J Clin Pharmacol* (1999) 47, 249–54.
2. Palovaara S, Anttila M, Nyman L, Laine K. Effect of concomitant hormone replacement therapy containing estradiol and levonorgestrel on the pharmacokinetics of selegiline. *Eur J Clin Pharmacol* (2002) 58: 259–63.
3. Eldepryl (Selegiline hydrochloride). Orion Pharma (UK) Ltd. UK Summary of product characteristics, July 2006.
4. Zelapar (Selegiline hydrochloride). Cephalon Ltd. UK Summary of product characteristics, November 2006.

MAO-B inhibitors; Selegiline + Itraconazole

The concurrent use of selegiline and itraconazole does not appear to alter the pharmacokinetics of either drug.

Clinical evidence, mechanism, importance and management

In a randomised placebo-controlled crossover study, 12 healthy subjects were given selegiline 10 mg after taking itraconazole 200 mg daily for 4 days. Itraconazole did not have any significant effects on the pharmacokinetics of selegiline, although the AUC of desmethylselegiline, a primary metabolite, was increased by 11%. The pharmacokinetics of itraconazole were also unaffected. There would appear to be no reason for avoiding concurrent use.[1]

1. Kivistö KT, Wang J-S, Backman JT, Nyman L, Taavitsainen P, Anttila M, Neuvonen PJ. Selegiline pharmacokinetics are unaffected by the CYP3A4 inhibitor itraconazole. *Eur J Clin Pharmacol* (2001) 57, 37–42.

Memantine + Miscellaneous

Drugs that make the urine alkaline (e.g. sodium bicarbonate, carbonic anhydrase inhibitors) will reduce the elimination of memantine. Memantine should be used with caution with other NMDA antagonists, such as amantadine, ketamine and dextromethorphan, or concurrent use should be avoided, because of the theoretical increased risk of adverse effects. Memantine is predicted to interact with other drugs eliminated by the same renal secretion mechanism, but no important interaction was seen with glibenclamide, hydrochlorothiazide, metformin or triamterene.

Clinical evidence, mechanism, importance and management

(a) Antidiabetics

The use of memantine with a combined product containing **glibenclamide** and **metformin** did not result in any changes in the pharmacokinetics of either of the three drugs. Memantine did not reduce the glucose-lowering effects of either drug.[1]

(b) Antispasmodic drugs

Memantine might modify the effects of antispasmodic drugs such as **dantrolene** or **baclofen** and dosage adjustment might be required.[2]

(c) Barbiturates and Antipsychotics

Memantine is predicted to reduce the effects of barbiturates and antipsychotics.[2]

(d) Dopaminergics

Memantine is predicted to enhance the effects of dopaminergic drugs.[2]

(e) Drugs that make the urine alkaline

The clearance of memantine was markedly reduced (by about 80%) when the urine was alkaline (pH 8).[1] This would be expected to lead to memantine accumulation and an increase in adverse effects. Drugs that could interact via this mechanism include **sodium bicarbonate** and **carbonic anhydrase inhibitors** (such as acetazolamide).[1]

(f) Interactions via cytochrome P450 isoenzymes

The results of *in vitro* studies indicate that memantine is not likely to cause interactions via induction or inhibition of the major cytochrome P450 isoenzymes involved in drug metabolism (CYP1A2, CYP2C9, CYP3A4).[1,2] In addition, memantine is not metabolised by this enzyme system, and is therefore not expected to undergo interactions via this mechanism.[1]

(g) Other drugs eliminated by renal tubular secretion

Memantine is predicted to interact with other drugs that use the same renal cationic transport system leading to increased levels of memantine and/or the other drug. The manufacturer lists **cimetidine**, **ranitidine**, **hydrochlorothiazide**, **metformin**, **procainamide**, **quinidine**, **quinine** and **triamterene** as possible examples.[1,2] However, in an interaction study, the concurrent use of memantine and **hydrochlorothiazide/triamterene** did not result in any change in the steady-state AUC of memantine or **triamterene**, and the AUC of **hydrochlorothiazide** showed a modest *reduction* of about 20%.[1] This degree of change is unlikely to be clinically relevant. Therefore, whether any clinically important interactions occur via this mechanism remains to be established.

(h) Other NMDA-antagonists

Memantine is chemically related to **amantadine**, and the manufacturer advises that concurrent use should be avoided[2] or undertaken with caution[1] because of the increased risk of adverse CNS-related drug reactions such as psychosis.[2] Although there are no data, an increased risk is also predicted for **ketamine** and **dextromethorphan**, which are also NMDA antagonists. Avoidance of,[2] or caution with,[1] concurrent use is advised.

(i) Warfarin

The manufacturer of memantine notes that, although no causal relationship has been established, isolated cases of INR increases have been reported in patients treated with warfarin. They suggest close monitoring of anticoagulant effects.[1,2]

1. Namenda (Memantine). Forest Pharmaceuticals, Inc. US Prescribing information, April 2007.
2. Ebixa (Memantine). Lundbeck Ltd. UK Summary of product characteristics, November 2006.

Piribedil + Clonidine

Clonidine is reported to oppose the effects of piribedil.

Clinical evidence, mechanism, importance and management

A study in 5 patients taking piribedil found that concurrent treatment with clonidine (up to 1.5 mg daily for 10 to 24 days) caused a worsening of the parkinsonism (an exacerbation of rigidity and akinesia). The concurrent use of antimuscarinic drugs reduced the effects of this interaction.[1] The reason is uncertain.

1. Shoulson I, Chase TN. Clonidine and the anti-parkinsonian response to L-dopa or piribedil. *Neuropharmacology* (1976) 15, 25–7.

Pramipexole + Drugs altering its renal clearance

Cimetidine, and possibly amantadine modestly reduce the clearance of pramipexole from the body, and some caution is advised on concurrent use. Probenecid had a minor effect on pramipexole clearance, which is not clinically relevant.

Clinical evidence, mechanism, importance and management

A study in 12 healthy subjects found that multiple doses of **cimetidine** reduced the total oral clearance of a single 250-microgram dose of pramipexole by about 35% and increased its half-life by 40%. A similar reduction in the renal clearance of pramipexole was noted. The authors suggest that **cimetidine** reduces the renal excretion of pramipexole by inhibiting the active renal organic cation transport system.[1] The manufacturers say that **cimetidine** and other drugs that are eliminated by this route such as **amantadine** may interact with pramipexole to reduce excretion of either or both drugs.[2] The clinical significance of these interactions is uncertain, and as yet there appear to be no reports of any adverse interactions. Nevertheless, the manufacturers suggest a reduction of the pramipexole dose should be considered when **amantadine** or **cimetidine** are given with pramipexole.[2]

Multiple doses of **probenecid** given to 12 healthy subjects reduced the clearance of a single 250-microgram dose of pramipexole by 10.3%.[1] This change is not clinically relevant.

1. Wright CE, Lasher Sisson T, Ichhpurani AK, Peters GR. Influence of probenecid (PR) and cimetidine (C) on pramipexole (PX) pharmacokinetics. *Clin Pharmacol Ther* (1996) 59, 183.
2. Mirapexin (Pramipexole). Boehringer Ingelheim Ltd. UK Summary of product characteristics, August 2006.

Ropinirole + CYP1A2 inhibitors

Ciprofloxacin increased the AUC of ropinirole by 84%, and other CYP1A2 inhibitors are predicted to interact similarly. Ropinirole dose adjustment may be required if potent CYP1A2 inhibitors are started or stopped.

Clinical evidence

Ciprofloxacin 500 mg twice daily increased the AUC of ropinirole 2 mg three times daily by 84% and increased the maximum plasma level by 60% in a study in 12 patients.[1]

Mechanism

Ropinirole is principally metabolised by the cytochrome P450 isoenzyme CYP1A2, of which ciprofloxacin is a known inhibitor.

Importance and management

Although the clinical relevance of this pharmacokinetic interaction has not been assessed, it would seem possible that the effects of ropinirole may be increased. The manufacturers suggest that if therapy with a known potent inhibitor of CYP1A2 is stopped or started during therapy with ropinirole, adjustment of the ropinirole dose may be required.[1,2] The UK manufacturer specifically mentions **cimetidine** and **fluvoxamine** in addition to ciprofloxacin.[2] For a full list of CYP1A2 inhibitors, see 'Table 1.2', (p.4).

1. Requip (Ropinirole hydrochloride). GlaxoSmithKline. US Prescribing information, October 2006.
2. Requip (Ropinirole hydrochloride). GlaxoSmithKline UK. UK Summary of product characteristics, March 2007.

Ropinirole + Miscellaneous

Estrogens (HRT) and tobacco smoking may reduce the clearance of ropinirole. Amantadine and trihexyphenidyl appear not to alter the pharmacokinetics of ropinirole.

Clinical evidence, mechanism, importance and management

(a) Amantadine

The manufacturer notes that population analysis revealed that amantadine did not have any relevant effects on ropinirole pharmacokinetics.[1,2]

(b) Estrogens

Population pharmacokinetic analysis of clinical study data showed that estrogens (mainly ethinylestradiol[2]) used in HRT reduced ropinirole clearance by one-third.[1-4] In another analysis it was found that women taking HRT received a slightly lower daily dose of ropinirole than those not on HRT, with no difference in adverse effects.[4] Therefore, in women already receiving HRT, ropinirole treatment may be started using the usual dose titration.[2,3] However, it is suggested that a reduction in the ropinirole dosage may be needed if HRT is started, and an increase if it is withdrawn.[2,3]

(c) Tobacco

The manufacturer notes that 7 tobacco smokers were found to have a 38% lower ropinirole AUC and a 30% lower maximum level than 11 non-smokers in a study in patients with restless leg syndrome.[2] Tobacco induces the cytochrome P450 isoenzyme CYP1A2, by which ropinirole is extensively metabolised. Because the dose of ropinirole is titrated to effect, this interaction is unlikely to be clinically relevant, except perhaps if patients stop or start smoking while taking ropinirole.

(d) Trihexyphenidyl

The manufacturer notes that population analysis revealed that trihexyphenidyl did not have any relevant effects on ropinirole pharmacokinetics.[1]

1. SmithKline Beecham. Personal Communication, September 1996.
2. Requip (Ropinirole hydrochloride). GlaxoSmithKline. US Prescribing information, October 2006.
3. Requip (Ropinirole hydrochloride). GlaxoSmithKline UK. UK Summary of product characteristics, March 2007.
4. SmithKline Beecham. Personal Communication, May 1999.

19

Antiplatelet drugs and Thrombolytics

Platelets usually circulate in the plasma in an inactive form, but following injury to blood vessels they become activated and adhere to the site of injury. Platelet aggregation then occurs, which contributes to the haemostatic plug. Platelet aggregation involves the binding of fibrinogen with a glycoprotein IIb/IIIa receptor on the platelet surface. The activated platelets secrete substances such as adenosine diphosphate (ADP) and thromboxane A_2 that result in additional platelet aggregation and also cause vasoconstriction. Finally a number of platelet derived factors stimulate production of thrombin and hence fibrin through the coagulation cascade (see 'The blood clotting process', (p.358)). Opposing this process is the fibrinolysis pathway, which is initiated during clot formation by a number of mediators such as tissue plasminogen activator (tPA) and urokinase. These proteins convert plasminogen to plasmin, which in turn degrades fibrin, the main component of the clot.

Antiplatelet drugs (see 'Table 19.1', (below)) reduce platelet aggregation and are used to prevent thromboembolic events. They act through a wide range of mechanisms including:

- prevention of thromboxane A_2 synthesis or inhibition of thromboxane receptors e.g. aspirin inhibits platelet cyclo-oxygenase, preventing synthesis of thromboxane A_2
- interference with adenosine diphosphate mediated platelet activation e.g. thienopyridines; inhibition of adenosine reuptake e.g. dipyridamole; interference with adenosine metabolism by inhibiting cyclic adenosine monophosphate (cAMP) phosphodiesterase e.g. cilostazol
- interference in the final step in platelet aggregation by stopping fibrinogen binding with the glycoprotein IIb/IIIa receptor on the platelet surface

Therefore some antiplatelet drugs can have beneficial additive effects with other antiplatelet drugs that act via different mechanisms. Furthermore, other drugs such as dextrans, heparin, some prostaglandins and sulfinpyrazone also have some antiplatelet activity.

Thrombolytics (see 'Table 19.1', (below)) are used in the treatment of thromboembolic disorders. Thrombolytics activate plasminogen to form plasmin, which is a proteolytic enzyme that degrades fibrin and therefore produces clot dissolution.

This section is primarily concerned with those interactions where the activities of antiplatelet drugs or thrombolytics are changed by the presence of another drug. Note that the interactions of high-dose aspirin are covered under analgesics.

Table 19.1 Antiplatelet drugs and thrombolytics

Group	*Drugs*
Antiplatelet drugs	
Adenosine reuptake inhibitors/Phosphodiesterase inhibitors	Cilostazol, Dipyridamole
Cyclo-oxygenase inhibitors	Aspirin, Indobufen, Triflusal
Glycoprotein IIb/IIIa-receptor antagonists	Abciximab, Eptifibatide, Tirofiban
Thienopyridines (inhibitors of adenosine diphosphate mediated platelet aggregation)	Clopidogrel, Ticlopidine
Thromboxane receptor antagonists	Picotamide
Miscellaneous	Ditazole, Trapidil
Thrombolytics	
Thrombolytics	Alteplase, Anistreplase, Defibrotide, Reteplase, Streptokinase, Tenecteplase, Urokinase

Alteplase + Glyceryl trinitrate (Nitroglycerin)

Glyceryl trinitrate may reduce the thrombolytic efficacy of alteplase, but this is not thought to be clinically relevant.

Clinical evidence, mechanism, importance and management

In a randomised study, 60 patients with acute anterior myocardial infarction were given intravenous alteplase 100 mg over 3 hours, as well as heparin and aspirin. In addition, 27 of the patients were also given intravenous glyceryl trinitrate 100 micrograms/minute for 8 hours. Patients receiving both alteplase and glyceryl trinitrate had signs of reperfusion less often (56%) than the patients who received alteplase alone (76%). In the combined treatment group time to reperfusion was also longer (37.8 versus 19.6 minutes) and the incidence of coronary artery re-occlusion was higher (53% versus 24%). Giving alteplase with glyceryl trinitrate produced plasma levels of tissue plasminogen activator (tPA) antigen that were about two-thirds lower than when alteplase was given alone.[1] Impaired thrombolysis has been found in another study[2] and also in an earlier study in *dogs*.[3]

It was postulated that glyceryl trinitrate increased hepatic blood flow and therefore increased the metabolism of alteplase, which resulted in reduced plasma tPA levels.[1] However, an *in vitro* study found that glyceryl trinitrate enhanced the degradation of alteplase, and therefore a mechanism other than increased hepatic blood flow seems likely to be involved.[4] It has been suggested that this interaction may not be clinically important,[5] and the current evidence is too sparse to warrant changing current practice.

1. Romeo F, Rosano GMC, Martuscelli E, De Luca F, Bianco C, Colistra C, Comito M, Cardona N, Miceli F, Rosano V, Mehta JL. Concurrent nitroglycerin administration reduces the efficacy of recombinant tissue-type plasminogen activator in patients with acute anterior wall myocardial infarction. *Am Heart J* (1995) 130, 692–7.
2. Nicolini FA, Ferrini D, Ottani F, Galvani M, Ronchi A, Behrens PH, Rusticali F, Mehta JL. Concurrent nitroglycerin therapy impairs tissue-type plasminogen activator-induced thrombolysis in patients with acute myocardial infarction. *Am J Cardiol* (1994) 74, 662–6.
3. Mehta JL, Nicolini FA, Nichols WW, Saldeen TGP. Concurrent nitroglycerin administration decreases thrombolytic potential of tissue-type plasminogen activator. *J Am Coll Cardiol* (1991) 17, 805–11.
4. White CM, Fan C, Chen BP, Kluger J, Chow MSS. Assessment of the drug interaction between alteplase and nitroglycerin: an in vitro study. *Pharmacotherapy* (2000) 20, 380–2.
5. Boehringer Ingelheim. Personal communication, March 1999.

Anagrelide + Miscellaneous

Anagrelide should not be used with other phosphodiesterase III inhibitors (e.g. milrinone) because of the potential for increased inotropic effects. Inhibitors of CYP1A2 (e.g. fluvoxamine) are predicted to increase anagrelide levels. Some caution might be required with concurrent aspirin and other platelet inhibitors. Whether anagrelide inhibits theophylline metabolism to a clinically relevant extent is not known. No pharmacokinetic interaction occurs with digoxin or warfarin.

Clinical evidence, mechanism, importance and management

(a) Aspirin

Based on *in vitro* data, anagrelide could have additive effects with drugs that inhibit platelet function, such as aspirin; although in clinical development no such effects were observed. Nevertheless, the manufacturer recommends that the risk/benefit ratio should be assessed before aspirin in used with anagrelide in patients with a high platelet count (greater than 1500 x 10^9/L) and/or a history of haemorrhage.[1]

(b) CYP1A2 inhibitors and substrates

Anagrelide is principally metabolised by the cytochrome P450 isoenzyme CYP1A2. Drugs that are inhibitors of this isoenzyme are therefore predicted to reduce the clearance of anagrelide, and the manufacturer specifically names **fluvoxamine** and **omeprazole**.[1] Be aware that increased effects, both beneficial and adverse, might occur. However, note that **omeprazole** is only a weak CYP1A2 inhibitor, and would not be expected to have much effect on anagrelide. **Grapefruit juice** has also been predicted to interact via this mechanism,[1] but again, it has little clinically relevant effect on CYP1A2. For a list of CYP1A2 inhibitors, see 'Table 1.2', (p.4).

Anagrelide is a weak inhibitor of CYP1A2, therefore be aware that it might interact with CYP1A2 substrates, such as **theophylline**.[1]

(c) Digoxin

The manufacturer briefly mentions that there was no pharmacokinetic interaction between digoxin and anagrelide.[1]

(d) Food

Food delays the absorption of anagrelide, but does not alter the overall amount absorbed. The interaction is not clinically relevant.[1]

(e) Hydroxycarbamide

In a preclinical study in *dogs*, there was no pharmacokinetic interaction between hydroxycarbamide and anagrelide, therefore no clinical pharmacokinetic interaction is expected.[1]

(f) Other phosphodiesterase inhibitors

Anagrelide is a cyclic AMP phosphodiesterase III inhibitor, and consequently has positive inotropic effects. The manufacturer recommends against its concurrent use with other phosphodiesterase III inhibitors, because of the potential increased inotropic effects, and they specifically mention **amrinone**, **cilostazol**, **enoximone**, **milrinone**, and **olprinone**.[1]

(g) Warfarin

The manufacturer briefly mentions that there was no pharmacokinetic interaction between warfarin and anagrelide.[1]

1. Xagrid (Anagrelide hydrochloride). Shire Pharmaceuticals, Ltd. UK Summary of product characteristics, March 2007.

Antiplatelet drugs + Aspirin

There is an increased risk of bleeding if clopidogrel is given with aspirin, but the use of low-dose aspirin and clopidogrel can be beneficial. Ticlopidine increases the antiaggregant effects of aspirin and there is an increased risk of bleeding on concurrent use. Cilostazol appears not to interact to a clinically relevant extent with low-dose aspirin, and the addition of dipyridamole to aspirin does not appear to increase the incidence of bleeding.

Clinical evidence, mechanism, importance and management

(a) Cilostazol

In a randomised, double-blind, placebo-controlled study involving 11 healthy subjects, cilostazol 100 mg twice daily given with aspirin 325 mg daily for 5 days increased the inhibition of ADP-induced platelet aggregation by 23 to 35% when compared with the use of cilostazol alone, but there were no statistically significant additive effects on arachidonic acid-induced platelet aggregation. In addition, no clinically relevant effects on prothrombin times, aPTT or bleeding times occurred when cilostazol was given with or without aspirin. However, there was a minor 22% increase in the AUC of cilostazol when it was given with aspirin.[1] The US manufacturers report that in 8 randomised, placebo-controlled trials, in a total of 201 patients receiving cilostazol and aspirin, the incidence of bleeding was no greater than that seen with aspirin and placebo. The most frequent doses and mean duration of aspirin therapy were 75 to 81 mg daily for 137 days (107 patients) and 325 mg daily for 54 days (85 patients).[2]

These studies suggest that no special precautions are needed if cilostazol is used concurrently with low-dose aspirin, although note that the UK manufacturer of cilostazol recommends that, when given with cilostazol, the daily dose of aspirin should not exceed 80 mg.[3]

(b) Clopidogrel

A variety of studies have investigated the beneficial effects of using the combination of aspirin with clopidogrel. Although these studies were primarily designed to assess the benefits of concurrent use they did also report on bleeding events. The key findings were:

- In patients with recent acute coronary syndrome (CURE): an increase in major bleeding events following the use of clopidogrel 75 mg daily with aspirin 75 to 325 mg daily compared with aspirin alone (3.7% versus 2.7%, respectively).[4]
- In patients with recent stroke or transient ischaemic attack (MATCH): an increase in life-threatening bleeding events following the use of clopidogrel 75 mg daily with aspirin 75 mg daily compared with aspirin alone (2.6% versus 1.3%, respectively).[5]
- In patients with clinically evident cardiovascular disease or multiple atherosclerotic risk factors (CHARISMA): an increase in the risk of moderate and severe bleeding following the use of clopidogrel 75 mg

daily with aspirin 75 to 162 mg daily compared with aspirin alone (moderate 2.1% and 1.3%, respectively, severe 1.7% and 1.3%, respectively).[6]

A study in 7 healthy subjects found that clopidogrel 75 mg and aspirin 150 mg daily for 2 days caused a significant 3.4-fold increase in bleeding time relative to baseline, and when the clopidogrel dose was increased to 300 mg there was a 5-fold increase in bleeding time.[7] Spontaneous haemarthrosis of the knee has been associated with the concurrent use of aspirin and clopidogrel in one patient.[8] A report describes two surgical cases, which were complicated by bleeding associated with the combination of aspirin and clopidogrel. In both cases the bleeding was delayed, in that it was not obvious until the end of surgery, causing unanticipated surgical re-exploration.[9] Further reports describe increased perioperative bleeding in patients taking both aspirin and clopidogrel.[10,11]

The manufacturer of clopidogrel warns that the concurrent use of clopidogrel and aspirin should be undertaken with caution because of the increased risk of bleeding, although the two drugs have been given together for up to one year. They recommend that, in patients taking clopidogrel, the dose of aspirin should not exceed 100 mg daily as higher doses are associated with higher bleeding risks.[12] For patients undergoing surgery, it has been suggested that, if possible, the combined use of clopidogrel and aspirin should be discontinued about 5 days before the surgery to minimise the risks of bleeding.[4,10,13] The manufacturer says that if an antiplatelet effect is not necessary, clopidogrel should be discontinued 5 to 7 days prior to surgery,[12,14] although note that this needs to be balanced against the possible adverse effects of stopping such treatment.

(c) Dipyridamole

A study in 10 healthy subjects found that dipyridamole 50 mg three times daily given with a single 180-mg dose of aspirin, or dipyridamole 75 mg three times daily given with aspirin 120 mg maximally inhibited platelet functions but did not prolong the bleeding time.[15] The manufacturer of dipyridamole states that the addition of dipyridamole to aspirin does not increase the incidence of bleeding events.[16]

(d) Ticlopidine

Aspirin combined with ticlopidine appears to inhibit platelet aggregation more than either drug alone.[17,18] The UK manufacturer of ticlopidine[19] warns that combined use increases the risk of bleeding because there is an increase in platelet antiaggregant activity and aspirin also damages the gastro-duodenal lining, which can cause bleeding. They recommend that clinical monitoring is advisable.[19]

1. Mallikaarjun S, Forbes WP, Bramer SL. Interaction potential and tolerability of the coadministration of cilostazol and aspirin. *Clin Pharmacokinet* (1999) 37 (Suppl 2), 87–93.
2. Pletal (Cilostazol). Otsuka America Pharmaceutical, Inc. US Prescribing information, August 2006.
3. Pletal (Cilostazol). Otsuka Pharmaceuticals (UK) Ltd. UK Summary of product characteristics, May 2006.
4. Yusuf S, Zhao F, Mehta SR, Chrolavicius S, Tognoni G, Fox KK; The Clopidogrel in Unstable Angina to Prevent Recurrent Events (CURE) Trial Investigators. Effects of clopidogrel in addition to aspirin in patients with acute coronary syndromes without ST-segment elevation. *N Engl J Med* (2001) 345, 494–502.
5. Diener H-C, Bogousslavsky J, Brass LM, Cimminiello C, Csiba L, Kaste M, Leys D, Matias-Guiu J, Rupprecht H-J, on behalf of the MATCH investigators. Aspirin and clopidogrel compared with clopidogrel alone after recent ischaemic stroke or transient ischaemic attack in high-risk patients (MATCH): randomised, double-blind, placebo-controlled trial. *Lancet* (2004) 364, 331–7.
6. Bhatt DL, Fox KAA, Hacke W, Berger PB, Black HR, Boden WE, Cacoub P, Cohen EA, Creager MA, Easton JD, Flather MD, Haffner SM, Hamm CW, Hankey GJ, Johnston SC, Mak K-H, Mas J-L, Montalescot G, Pearson TA, Steg PG, Steinhubl SR, Weber MA, Brennan DM, Fabry-Ribaudo L, Booth J, Topol EJ for the CHARISMA Investigators. Clopidogrel and aspirin versus aspirin alone for the prevention of atherothrombotic events. *N Engl J Med* (2006) 354, 1706–17.
7. Payne DA, Hayes PD, Jones CI, Belham P, Naylor AR, Goodall AH. Combined therapy with clopidogrel and aspirin significantly increases the bleeding time through a synergistic antiplatelet action. *J Vasc Surg* (2002) 35, 1204–9.
8. Gille J, Bernotat J, Böhm S, Behrens P, Löhr JF. Spontaneous hemarthrosis of the knee associated with clopidogrel and aspirin treatment. *Z Rheumatol* (2003) 62, 80–1.
9. Moore M, Power M. Perioperative hemorrhage and combined clopidogrel and aspirin therapy. *Anesthesiology* (2004) 101, 792–4.
10. Yende S, Wunderink RG. Effect of clopidogrel on bleeding after coronary artery bypass surgery. *Crit Care Med* (2001) 29, 2271–5.
11. Chapman TWL, Bowley DMG, Lambert AW, Walker AJ, Ashley SA, Wilkins DC. Haemorrhage associated with combined clopidogrel and aspirin therapy. *Eur J Vasc Endovasc Surg* (2001) 22, 478–9.
12. Plavix (Clopidogrel hydrogen sulfate). Bristol-Myers Squibb Pharmaceuticals Ltd. UK Summary of product characteristics, June 2007.
13. Yusuf S, Mehta S. Treatment of acute coronary syndromes. Reply. *N Engl J Med* (2002) 346, 207–8.
14. Plavix (Clopidogrel bisulfate). Sanofi-Aventis/Bristol-Myers Squibb Company. US Prescribing information, February 2007.
15. Rajah SM, Penny AF, Crow MJ, Pepper MD, Watson DA. The interaction of varying doses of dipyridamole and acetyl salicylic acid on the inhibition of platelet functions and their effect on bleeding time. *Br J Clin Pharmacol* (1979) 8, 483–9.
16. Persantin (Dipyridamole). Boehringer Ingelheim Ltd. UK Summary of product characteristics, July 2004.
17. Splawinska B, Kuzniar J, Malinga K, Mazurek AP, Splawinski J. The efficacy and potency of antiplatelet activity of ticlopidine is increased by aspirin. *Int J Clin Pharmacol Ther* (1996) 34, 352–6.
18. Gryglewski RJ, Uracz W, Świês J. Unusual effects of aspirin on ticlopidine induced thrombolysis. *Thorax* (2000) 55 (Suppl 2) S17–S19.
19. Ticlid (Ticlopidine). Sanofi Synthelabo. UK Summary of product characteristics, May 2000.

Antiplatelet drugs + Bupropion

Clopidogrel and ticlopidine appear to inhibit the metabolism of bupropion. Dosage adjustments may be necessary.

Clinical evidence

(a) Clopidogrel

A study in healthy subjects given clopidogrel 75 mg once daily for 4 days found that the AUC of a single 150-mg dose of bupropion was increased by 60% and the AUC of its active metabolite, hydroxybupropion was reduced by 52%.[1]

(b) Ticlopidine

A study in healthy subjects given ticlopidine 250 mg twice daily for 4 days found that the AUC of a single 150-mg dose of bupropion was increased by 85% and the AUC of its active metabolite, hydroxybupropion was reduced by 84%.[1]

Mechanism

The reduction in bupropion hydroxylation is due to inhibition of its cytochrome P450 isoenzyme CYP2B6-mediated metabolism by clopidogrel or ticlopidine.[1,2]

Importance and management

Patients taking bupropion may require dose adjustments if they also take clopidogrel or ticlopidine.[1] Until more is known about this interaction it would seem prudent to monitor for increased bupropion adverse effects (lightheadedness, gastrointestinal effects) and efficacy.

1. Turpeinen M, Tolonen A, Uusitalo J, Jalonen J, Pelkonen O, Laine K. Effect of clopidogrel and ticlopidine on cytochrome P450 2B6 activity as measured by bupropion hydroxylation. *Clin Pharmacol Ther* (2005) 77, 553–9.
2. Richter T, Mürdter TE, Heinkele G, Pleiss J, Tatzel S, Schwab M, Eichelbaum M, Zanger UM. Potent mechanism-based inhibition of human CYP2B6 by clopidogrel and ticlopidine. *J Pharmacol Exp Ther* (2004) 308, 189–97.

Antiplatelet drugs + Herbal medicines

***Ginkgo biloba* has been associated with platelet, bleeding and clotting disorders and there are isolated reports of serious adverse reactions after its concurrent use with antiplatelet drugs such as aspirin, clopidogrel and ticlopidine. An *animal* study suggests that *Kangen-Karyu* may also enhance the antiplatelet and antithrombotic effects of ticlopidine.**

Clinical evidence

(a) Ginkgo biloba

A 70-year-old man developed spontaneous bleeding from the iris into the anterior chamber of his eye within a week of starting to take a *Ginkoba* tablet twice daily. He experienced recurrent episodes of blurred vision in one eye lasting about 15 minutes, during which he could see a red discoloration through his cornea. Each *Ginkoba* tablet contained 40 mg of concentrated (50:1) extract of *Ginkgo biloba*. He was also taking **aspirin** 325 mg daily, which he had taken uneventfully for 3 years since having coronary bypass surgery. He stopped taking the *Ginkoba* but continued with the **aspirin**, and 3 months later had experienced no recurrence of the bleeding.[1] In an analysis of supplement use, 23% of 123 patients were currently taking supplements, and 4 patients were found to be taking ginkgo and aspirin. However, no problems from this use were found on review of the patients' notes.[2]

A search of Health Canada's database of spontaneous adverse reactions for the period January 1999 to June 2003 found 21 reports of suspected adverse reactions associated with ginkgo. Most of these involved platelet, bleeding and clotting disorders. One report of a fatal gastrointestinal haemorrhage was associated with **ticlopidine** and ginkgo, both taken over

2 years along with other medications. Another report was of a stroke in a patient taking multiple drugs including **clopidogrel**, aspirin and a herbal product containing ginkgo.[3]

(b) Kangen-Karyu

Kangen-Karyu is a Chinese traditional herbal medicine used for 'blood stasis'. A study in *animals* suggested that *Kangen-Karyu* may augment the antiplatelet and antithrombotic effects of **ticlopidine** and that the dosage of ticlopidine should be reduced to prevent adverse effects such as thrombotic thrombocytopenic purpura or haemorrhage.[4]

Mechanism

The reason for the bleeding is not known, but *Ginkgo biloba* extract contains ginkgolide B, which is a potent inhibitor of platelet-activating factor, which is needed for arachidonate-independent platelet aggregation. On their own, *Ginkgo biloba* supplements have been associated with prolonged bleeding times,[5,6] left and bilateral subdural haematomas,[5,7] a right parietal haematoma,[8] post-laparoscopic cholecystectomy bleeding,[9] and subarachnoid haemorrhage.[6] The authors of the first report[1] suggest that the use of aspirin, which is also an inhibitor of platelet aggregation, may have had an additional part to play in what happened.

Importance and management

The evidence from these reports is too slim to forbid patients taking aspirin, clopidogrel or ticlopidine and *Ginkgo biloba* concurrently, but some do recommend caution,[10] which seems prudent. Medical professionals should be aware of the possibility of increased bleeding tendency with *Ginkgo biloba*, and report any suspected cases.[8] Consider also 'NSAIDs + *Ginkgo biloba*', p.148. Similarly caution would seem prudent if *Kangen-karyu* is used with any antiplatelet drug.

1. Rosenblatt M, Mindel J. Spontaneous hyphema associated with ingestion of *Ginkgo biloba* extract. *N Engl J Med* (1997) 336, 1108.
2. Ly J, Percy L, Dhanani S. Use of dietary supplements and their interactions with prescription drugs in the elderly. *Am J Health-Syst Pharm* (2002) 59, 1759–62.
3. Natural health products and adverse reactions. *Can Adverse React News* (2004) 14, 2–3.
4. Makino T, Wakushima H, Okamoto T, Okukubo Y, Deguchi Y, Kano Y. Pharmacokinetic and pharmacological interactions between ticlopidine hydrochloride and *Kangen-Karyu* – Chinese traditional herbal medicine. *Phytother Res* (2003) 17, 1021–4.
5. Rowin J, Lewis SL. Spontaneous bilateral subdural hematomas associated with chronic *Ginkgo biloba* ingestion. *Neurology* (1996) 46, 1775–6.
6. Vale S. Subarachnoid haemorrhage associated with *Ginkgo biloba*. *Lancet* (1998) 352, 36.
7. Gilbert GJ. *Ginkgo biloba*. *Neurology* (1997) 48, 1137.
8. Benjamin J, Muir T, Briggs K, Pentland B. A case of cerebral haemorrhage – can *Ginkgo biloba* be implicated? *Postgrad Med J* (2001) 77, 112–13.
9. Fessenden JM, Wittenborn W, Clarke L. Gingko biloba: a case report of herbal medicine and bleeding postoperatively from a laparoscopic cholecystectomy. *Am Surg* (2001) 67, 33–5.
10. Griffiths J, Jordan S, Pilon S. Natural health products and adverse reactions. *Can Adverse React News* (2004) 14, 2–3.

Antiplatelet drugs + NSAIDs

The manufacturers of clopidogrel warn about possible gastrointestinal bleeding if it is used with naproxen or other NSAIDs. There is also an increased risk of bleeding if ticlopidine is given with NSAIDs.

Clinical evidence, mechanism, importance and management

(a) Clopidogrel

A double-blind, placebo-controlled study in 30 healthy subjects given **naproxen** 250 mg twice daily, found that the addition of clopidogrel 75 mg daily increased faecal blood loss compared with **naproxen** alone. Six subjects receiving both drugs had bleeding time prolongation factors above 5, which was greater than expected (clopidogrel alone prolongs bleeding by a factor of about 2) and one subject had subcutaneous haemorrhages of moderate intensity after taking clopidogrel with **naproxen**.[1] A report describes intracerebral haemorrhage in an 86-year-old woman after taking **celecoxib** 200 mg daily with clopidogrel 75 mg daily for 3 weeks. The authors comment that there may possibly have been a pharmacokinetic interaction between clopidogrel and **celecoxib** mediated via the cytochrome P450 isoenzyme CYP2C9, although the haemorrhage could have been secondary to other factors such as age or the individual drugs.[2]

Due to the lack of interaction studies with other NSAIDs, it is unclear whether there is an increased risk of gastrointestinal bleeding with all NSAIDs. The manufacturers advise caution if NSAIDs and clopidogrel are given together.[3,4]

(b) Ticlopidine

The UK manufacturer of ticlopidine warns that concurrent use of NSAIDs increases the risk of bleeding because there is an increase in platelet antiaggregant activity and because NSAIDs damage the gastro-duodenal lining, which can cause bleeding. They recommend that if NSAIDs are necessary, close clinical monitoring is advisable.[5]

1. Van Hecken A, Depré M, Wynants K, Vanbilloen H, Verbruggen A, Arnout J, Vanhove P, Cariou R, De Schepper PJ. Effect of clopidogrel on naproxen-induced gastrointestinal blood loss in healthy volunteers. *Drug Metabol Drug Interact* (1998) 14, 193–205 .
2. Fisher AA, Le Couteur DG. Intracerebral hemorrhage following possible interaction between celecoxib and clopidogrel. *Ann Pharmacother* (2001) 35, 1567–9.
3. Plavix (Clopidogrel hydrogen sulfate). Bristol-Myers Squibb Pharmaceuticals Ltd. UK Summary of product characteristics, June 2007.
4. Plavix (Clopidogrel bisulfate). Sanofi-Aventis/Bristol-Myers Squibb Company. US Prescribing information, February 2007.
5. Ticlid (Ticlopidine). Sanofi Synthelabo. UK Summary of product characteristics, May 2000.

Cilostazol + Clopidogrel

In one study clopidogrel slightly increased levels of cilostazol, without altering platelet count, aPTT, or prothrombin time. However, the effect of concurrent use on bleeding time was not assessed.

Clinical evidence, mechanism, importance and management

The concurrent use of cilostazol 150 mg twice daily and clopidogrel 75 mg daily for 5 days increased the AUC of cilostazol by only 9%, but increased the AUC of the dehydro metabolite of cilostazol by 24% (this metabolite has 3 to 4 times the potency of cilostazol in inhibiting platelet aggregation). No changes in platelet count, prothrombin time or aPTT were seen. However, clopidogrel alone prolonged bleeding time, and it was not possible to determine whether there was an additive effect with cilostazol.[1]

The UK manufacturer suggests caution if cilostazol is given with any drug that inhibits platelet aggregation, and say that consideration should be given to monitoring the bleeding time at intervals.[1]

1. Pletal (Cilostazol). Otsuka Pharmaceuticals (UK) Ltd. UK Summary of product characteristics, May 2006.

Cilostazol + Food

Food increases the bioavailability of cilostazol, which may increase adverse effects.

Clinical evidence, mechanism, importance and management

A randomised, single-dose, crossover study in 15 healthy subjects found that giving cilostazol 100 mg within 10 minutes of a high fat meal caused an increase in the rate and extent of cilostazol absorption. The maximum plasma concentration of cilostazol was increased by about 95%, the AUC was increased by 25%, and the half-life decreased from 15.1 to 5.4 hours, when compared with the fasted state.[1] The manufacturer recommends that cilostazol should be taken 30 minutes before or 2 hours after food, because the increase in maximum plasma concentrations of cilostazol when taken with food may be associated with an increased incidence of adverse effects.[2,3]

1. Bramer SL, Forbes WP. Relative bioavailability and effects of a high fat meal on single dose cilostazol pharmacokinetics. *Clin Pharmacokinet* (1999) 37 (Suppl 2), 13–23.
2. Pletal (Cilostazol). Otsuka Pharmaceuticals (UK) Ltd. UK Summary of product characteristics, May 2006.
3. Pletal (Cilostazol). Otsuka America Pharmaceutical, Inc. US Prescribing information, August 2006.

Cilostazol + Miscellaneous

Erythromycin, diltiazem and ketoconazole, all inhibitors of the cytochrome P450 isoenzyme CYP3A4, increase the plasma levels of cilostazol. Other inhibitors of CYP3A4 are predicted to interact similarly, but grapefruit juice does not appear to interact significantly. Cilostazol may increase the levels of lovastatin and other substrates of CYP3A4 (and possibly CYP2C19).
Omeprazole, an inhibitor of CYP2C19, increases the bioavailabil-

ity of cilostazol and its active metabolite; other CYP2C19 inhibitors are predicted to interact similarly.
Quinidine, an inhibitor of CYP2D6, does not appear to affect the pharmacokinetics of cilostazol and it is therefore suggested that other CYP2D6 inhibitors or substrates will not interact. Cilostazol appears not to interact to a clinically relevant extent with tobacco smoke.

Clinical evidence, mechanism, importance and management

(a) CYP2C19 inhibitors

In a crossover study[1] in 20 healthy subjects **omeprazole** 40 mg daily for one week increased the AUC of a single 100-mg dose of cilostazol by a modest 26%. More importantly, the AUC of 3,4-dehydro-cilostazol (a metabolite with 4 to 7 times the activity of cilostazol) was increased by 69%.[2,3] **Omeprazole** inhibits the cytochrome P450 isoenzyme CYP2C19, which is involved in the metabolism of cilostazol, and may possibly also affect the elimination of the active metabolite. For this reason the US manufacturers suggest that the dose of cilostazol should be halved when given with **omeprazole**,[2] while the UK manufacturers contraindicate concurrent use.[3] Other CYP2C19 inhibitors such as **lansoprazole** may also interact, and therefore concurrent use is contraindicated by the UK manufacturers.[3] The manufacturers also recommend caution with drugs that are substrates of CYP2C19.[3]

(b) CYP3A4 inhibitors

A study in 16 healthy subjects found that **erythromycin** 500 mg three times daily increased the maximum plasma level and the AUC of a single 100-mg oral dose of cilostazol by 47% and 73%, respectively. **Erythromycin** inhibits the cytochrome P450 isoenzyme CYP3A4, by which cilostazol is metabolised, thereby raising its plasma levels.[4] Other macrolide antibacterials e.g. **clarithromycin** (but not **azithromycin**) would be expected to have a similar effect.[2]

Diltiazem is also a moderate inhibitor of CYP3A4. When **diltiazem** 180 mg daily was given with cilostazol 100 mg twice daily the AUC of cilostazol was increased by about 40%.[2,3]

In a single-dose study, **ketoconazole** 400 mg caused a greater than two-fold increase in the AUC of cilostazol.[3] Other potent CYP3A4 inhibitors such as **itraconazole** are expected to interact similarly.[2]

In view of these effects the US manufacturers suggest halving the dose of cilostazol in the presence of CYP3A4 inhibitors such as **erythromycin**, **diltiazem**, **itraconazole**, and **ketoconazole**.[2] However, the UK manufacturers contraindicate CYP3A4 inhibitors, and they specifically name **erythromycin**, **diltiazem**, **ketoconazole**, **cimetidine**, and the **protease inhibitors**.[3] Just why these recommendations differ is not clear. The US manufacturers suggest that other CYP3A4 inhibitors, such as **azole antifungals** (**fluconazole**, **miconazole**), **SSRIs** (**fluoxetine**, **fluvoxamine**, **sertraline**) and **nefazodone**, may also interact.[2]

(c) Grapefruit juice

Grapefruit juice has been predicted to increase the levels of cilostazol by inhibiting CYP3A4.[2] However, the UK manufacturers note that 240 mL of grapefruit juice did not have a notable effect on the pharmacokinetics of a single 100-mg dose of cilostazol.[3] No special precautions seem necessary on concurrent use.

(d) Lovastatin and other substrates of CYP3A4

In a study in 13 healthy subjects, a single 80-mg oral dose of lovastatin was given before, and then on the final day of a 7-day treatment period with cilostazol 100 mg twice daily. The AUCs of lovastatin and its beta-hydroxy acid metabolite were increased by about 60 and 70%, respectively by cilostazol, but the maximum plasma levels were unaffected.[5] At the end of this study (day 9), 12 subjects were given lovastatin 80 mg with a larger 150-mg dose of cilostazol. It was found that the maximum level and the AUC of the lovastatin metabolite were increased by about twofold, suggesting that larger cilostazol doses may have a greater effect.[5] Lovastatin is metabolised by the cytochrome P450 isoenzyme CYP3A4 and although cilostazol can inhibit this enzyme, *in vitro* studies indicate that this occurs only at concentrations several times greater than those found therapeutically. The increases in lovastatin levels described here are lower than those seen with potent CYP3A4 inhibitors (e.g. see 'Statins + Azoles', p.1093) but the authors of the study still suggest that the dose of lovastatin may need to be reduced if cilostazol is also taken. Lovastatin decreased the absorption of cilostazol by about 15%, but this was not considered to be clinically relevant.[5]

The UK manufacturers advise caution when cilostazol is given with drugs that are substrates of CYP3A4, especially those with a narrow therapeutic index. They specifically mention **cisapride**, **midazolam**, **nifedipine** and **verapamil**.[3] Further study is needed to establish these predicted interactions.

(e) Quinidine

A crossover study in 22 healthy subjects found that the pharmacokinetics of a single 100-mg dose of cilostazol were unaffected by pretreatment with two 200-mg doses of quinidine sulfate, one taken 25 hours previously and the other taken one hour previously. Quinidine inhibits the activity of the cytochrome P450 isoenzyme CYP2D6, and it appears that this enzyme does not play a significant role in the metabolism of cilostazol or its primary metabolites.[6]

(f) Tobacco smoking

The manufacturers report that population pharmacokinetic analysis suggests that tobacco smoking reduces the exposure to cilostazol by about 20%,[2] but this is unlikely to have much, if any, clinical relevance.

1. Suri A, Bramer SL. Effect of omeprazole on the metabolism of cilostazol. *Clin Pharmacokinet* (1999) 37, (Suppl 2), 53–9.
2. Pletal (Cilostazol). Otsuka America Pharmaceutical, Inc. US Prescribing information, August 2006.
3. Pletal (Cilostazol). Otsuka Pharmaceuticals (UK) Ltd. UK Summary of product characteristics, May 2006.
4. Suri A, Forbes WP, Bramer SL. Effects of CYP3A inhibition on the metabolism of cilostazol. *Clin Pharmacokinet* (1999) 37 (Suppl 2), 61–8.
5. Bramer SL, Brisson J, Corey AE, Mallikaarjun S. Effect of multiple cilostazol doses on single dose lovastatin pharmacokinetics in healthy volunteers. *Clin Pharmacokinet* (1999) 37 (Suppl 2), 69–77.
6. Bramer SL, Suri A. Inhibition of CYP2D6 by quinidine and its effects on the metabolism of cilostazol. *Clin Pharmacokinet* (1999) 37 (Suppl 2), 41–51.

Clopidogrel + Miscellaneous

No adverse interactions appear to occur with clopidogrel and aluminium/magnesium hydroxide, atenolol, cimetidine, digoxin, food, insulin, nifedipine, oestrogens, phenobarbital, phenytoin or tolbutamide.

Clinical evidence, mechanism, importance and management

Two studies, one in 12 healthy subjects (average age 67 years) and the other in 12 healthy subjects (average age 23 years), found that the bioavailability of a single 75-mg dose of clopidogrel remained unchanged when it was taken with food or 1-hour after two 400-mg tablets of **aluminium/magnesium hydroxide**.[1] No clinically significant pharmacodynamic interactions were seen when clopidogrel was given with **atenolol**, **nifedipine** or a combination of **atenolol** and **nifedipine**,[2] and the activity of clopidogrel was not altered by the concurrent use of **cimetidine**,[3] **oestrogen**[3] or **phenobarbital**.[3] Another study found that clopidogrel does not alter the plasma levels of **digoxin** and that the pharmacodynamics of clopidogrel do not appear to be affected by **digoxin**.[4] One study found that the inhibition of platelet aggregation by clopidogrel was not reduced by **acetylcysteine**.[5] Data from the CAPRIE study and other clinical studies showed that **ACE inhibitors**, **antidiabetics** (**insulin**, **tolbutamide** named),[3] **antiepileptics** (**phenytoin** named),[3] **beta blockers**, **calcium-channel blockers**, **coronary or peripheral vasodilators**, **diuretics** and **HRT** have been safely given with clopidogrel.[6]

No special precautions would therefore seem necessary when clopidogrel is given with any of these drugs.

1. McEwen J, Strauch G, Perles P, Pritchard G, Moreland TE, Necciari J, Dickinson JP. Clopidogrel bioavailability: absence of influence of food or antacids. *Semin Thromb Hemost* (1999) 25 (Suppl 2), 47–50.
2. Forbes CD, Lowe GDO, Maclaren M, Shaw BG, Dickinson JP, Kieffer G. Clopidogrel compatibility with concomitant cardiac co-medications: a study of its interactions with a beta-blocker and a calcium uptake antagonist. *Semin Thromb Hemost* (1999) 25 (Suppl 2), 55–9.
3. Plavix (Clopidogrel hydrogen sulfate). Bristol-Myers Squibb Pharmaceuticals Ltd. UK Summary of product characteristics, June 2007.
4. Peeters PAM, Crijns HJMJ, Tamminga WJ, Jonkman JHG, Dickinson JP, Necciari J. Clopidogrel, a novel antiplatelet agent, and digoxin: absence of pharmacodynamic and pharmacokinetic interaction. *Semin Thromb Hemost* (1999) 25 (Suppl 2), 51–4.

5. Campbell CL, Berger PB, Nuttall GA, Orford JL, Santrach PJ, Oliver WC, Ereth MH, Thompson CM, Murphy MK, McGlassen DL, Schrader LM, Steinhubl SR. Can N-acetylcysteine reverse the antiplatelet effects of clopidogrel? An in vivo and vitro study. *Am Heart J* (2005) 150, 796–9.
6. Morais J, on behalf of the CAPRIE investigators. Use of concomitant medications in the CAPRIE trial: clopidogrel is unlikely to be associated with clinically significant drug interactions. *Eur Heart J* (1998) 19 (Abstract Suppl) 5.

Clopidogrel + Statins

Some evidence suggests that atorvastatin, and possibly other CYP3A4-metabolised statins (e.g. simvastatin) may interfere with the antiplatelet actions of clopidogrel, but the data is conflicting and there is currently insufficient evidence to warrant changing practice.

Clinical evidence

Some studies have shown that statins metabolised by CYP3A4 (most notably atorvastatin) can cause a reduction in the antiplatelet activity of clopidogrel, especially during the initial stages of treatment (following the loading dose of clopidogrel), whereas other, mainly retrospective, studies have found no clinical evidence of reduced efficacy. However, the studies are difficult to compare as some have measured platelet function using different techniques and other studies are based on clinical outcome using varying lengths of treatment and end points. Furthermore, up to 25% of patients may not respond at all to clopidogrel and this seems unrelated to treatment with a statin.[1]

Dose may be an important factor as to whether or not a significant clinical interaction occurs. One study found that a high loading dose of clopidogrel (600 mg) was not affected by statins,[2] but there is increased risk of serious bleeding with this dose. Lower doses of statins (e.g. atorvastatin 10 mg daily)[3] also appear to be less likely to interact, and one study found that the effect was dose-dependent.[4]

Some studies have found that **atorvastatin** attenuates the antiplatelet activity of clopidogrel in patients undergoing coronary artery stenting,[4-6] or balloon angioplasty.[6] However, other studies have found no evidence of an interaction.[1-3,7-12] Furthermore, one of the studies reporting an interaction[4] has been criticised for, among other things, being small, non-randomised, and using poorly defined study groups.[1]

Simvastatin has also been found to reduce the effects of clopidogrel in patients undergoing coronary artery stenting or balloon angioplasty,[6] although other studies have found no interaction.[2,11] The situation with **pravastatin** is clearer, as several studies have reported a lack of an interaction,[2-5,7,8,11,12] and there do not appear to be any studies suggesting that an interaction occurs. Similarly, studies including **cerivastatin**,[7] **lovastatin**,[2,7] **fluvastatin**,[2,5,7,8,11] or **rosuvastatin**[12] suggest that they do not interact with clopidogrel. Furthermore, a prospective single centre cohort study in 1651 patients with acute coronary syndromes found that clopidogrel plus a statin was associated with *lower* 6-month mortality and morbidity compared with the use of clopidogrel alone. There was no significant difference in clinical benefit between a statin predominantly metabolised by the cytochrome P450 isoenzyme CYP3A4 (said to be **atorvastatin**, **cerivastatin**, **lovastatin**, **simvastatin**) or a statin not predominantly metabolised by CYP3A4 (**fluvastatin**, **pravastatin**, **rosuvastatin**).[13] Similarly, a retrospective examination of data from the CREDO trial suggested that there was no difference in 1-year outcomes in patients given **atorvastatin** or **pravastatin**.[8] Despite this, some commentators have suggested that there were actually differences at the 28-day endpoint[14] and a trend towards differences in the 1-year outcome,[15] and suggest that an interaction may therefore have occurred.

Mechanism

Clopidogrel is an inactive prodrug that is metabolised mainly in the liver. The cytochrome P450 isoenzyme CYP3A4 appears to be primarily responsible for the metabolism and activation of clopidogrel, although other isoenzymes are also involved. Several statins, including atorvastatin, are also metabolised by CYP3A4 and it has been suggested that these statins may competitively inhibit the activation of clopidogrel.[4,16] However, it has been suggested that the expression and/or activity of CYP3A4 can vary widely between individuals and this, rather than an interaction, may conceivably lead to individual variation in metabolism.[14] The effect of CYP3A4-metabolised statins on the antiplatelet effects of clopidogrel may occur only in the loading phase of therapy (within the first 24 hours). It has been suggested that the lack of an interaction in maintenance treatment may be due an adaptation of platelet function or the metabolic capability of the liver or possibly due to upregulation of CYP3A4 in the liver.[17]

Importance and management

The picture is quite confused and by no means conclusive. Even though the statins metabolised by CYP3A4 appear to reduce the antiplatelet effect of clopidogrel, the overall clinical effect is unclear. The beneficial properties of statins may offset any attenuating effects on the antiplatelet action of clopidogrel.[18] Nevertheless, it has been suggested that higher doses of atorvastatin, and perhaps simvastatin, should not be prescribed for patients taking clopidogrel, particularly patients recovering from acute coronary syndrome, stent implantation (particularly a drug-eluting stent), or brachytherapy; pravastatin or rosuvastatin may be preferred in these patients.[15] However, other workers have said, given the marginal interference and high variability, until there is evidence to change clinical practice, there is no need to discontinue the statin use during clopidogrel treatment or to prefer hydrophilic statins in patients with clopidogrel comedication.[1,19,20] Further prospective studies are needed to determine whether a clinically significant interaction exists. Until then, a change in practice does not seem justified.

1. Serebruany VL, Steinhubl SR, Hennekens CH. Are antiplatelet effects of clopidogrel inhibited by atorvastatin? A research question formulated but not yet adequately tested. *Circulation* (2003) 107, 1568–9.
2. Müller I, Besta F, Schulz C, Li Z, Massberg S, Gawaz M. Effects of statins on platelet inhibition by a high loading dose of clopidogrel. *Circulation* (2003) 108, 2195–7.
3. Mitsios JV, Papathanasiou AI, Rodis FI, Elisaf M, Goudevenos JA, Tselepis AD. Atorvastatin does not affect the antiplatelet potency of clopidogrel when it is administered concomitantly for 5 weeks in patients with acute coronary syndromes. *Circulation* (2004) 109, 1335–8.
4. Lau WC, Waskell LA, Watkins PB, Neer CJ, Horowitz K, Hopp AS, Tait AR, Carville DGM, Guyer KE, Bates ER. Atorvastatin reduces the ability of clopidogrel to inhibit platelet aggregation. A new drug–drug interaction. *Circulation* (2003) 107, 32–7.
5. Günesdogan B, Neubauer H, Mügge A. Is the clopidogrel effect by patients treated with statins diminished? A flow cytometric evaluation of a possible interaction. *Eur Heart J* (2002) 23 (Abstract Suppl) 725.
6. Neubauer H, Günesdogan B, Hanefeld C, Spiecker M, Mügge A. Lipophilic statins interfere with the inhibitory effects of clopidogrel on platelet function – a flow cytometry study. *Eur Heart J* (2003) 24, 1744–9.
7. Serebruany VL, Malinin AI, Callahan KP, Gurbel PA, Steinhubl SR. Statins do not affect platelet inhibition with clopidogrel during coronary stenting. *Atherosclerosis* (2001) 159, 239–41.
8. Saw J, Steinhubl SR, Berger PB, Kereiakes DJ, Serebruany VL, Brennan D, Topol EJ; for the Clopidogrel for the Reduction of Events During Observation (CREDO) Investigators. Lack of adverse clopidogrel–atorvastatin clinical interaction from secondary analysis of a randomized, placebo-controlled clopidogrel trial. *Circulation* (2003) 108, 921–4.
9. Wienbergen H, Gitt AK, Schiele R, Juenger C, Heer T, Meisenzahl C, Limbourg P, Bossaller C, Senges J, for the MITRA PLUS Study Group. Comparison of clinical benefits of clopidogrel therapy in patients with acute coronary syndromes taking atorvastatin versus other statin therapies. *Am J Cardiol* (2003) 92, 285–8.
10. Serebruany VL, Midei MG, Malinin AI, Oshrine BR, Lowry DR, Sane DC, Tanguay J-F, Steinhubl SR, Berger PB, O'Connor CM, Hennekens CH. Absence of interaction between atorvastatin or other statins and clopidogrel: results from the interaction study. *Arch Intern Med* (2004) 164, 2051–7.
11. Smith SM, Judge HM, Peters G, Storey RF. Multiple antiplatelet effects of clopidogrel are not modulated by statin type in patients undergoing percutaneous coronary intervention. *Platelets* (2004) 15, 465–74.
12. Mach F, Senouf D, Fontana P, Boehlen F, Reber G, Daali Y, de Moerloose P, Sigwart U. Not all statins interfere with clopidogrel during antiplatelet therapy. *Eur J Clin Invest* (2005) 35, 476–81.
13. Mukherjee D, Kline-Rogers E, Fang J, Munir K, Eagle KA. Lack of clopidogrel-CYP3A4 statin interaction in patients with acute coronary syndrome. Heart 2005, 91, 23–6.
14. Ford I, Williams D. Does the use of statins compromise the effectiveness of platelet inhibition by clopidogrel? *Platelets* (2004) 15, 201–5.
15. Bates ER, Mukherjee D, Lau WC. Drug–drug interactions involving antiplatelet agents. *Eur Heart J* (2003) 24, 1707–9.
16. Clarke TA, Waskell LA. The metabolism of clopidogrel is catalyzed by human cytochrome P450 3A and is inhibited by atorvastatin. *Drug Metab Dispos* (2003) 31, 53–9.
17. Tselepis AD, Goudevenos JA. Lipophilic statins do not affect the antiplatelet potency of clopidogrel. *Platelets* (2005) 16, 225–6.
18. Schafer AI. Genetic and acquired determinants of individual variability of response to antiplatelet drugs. *Circulation* (2003) 108, 910–11.
19. Neubauer H, Mugge A. Do statins really interfere with clopidogrel-induced platelet function?: Reply. *Circulation* (2003) 108, 448–9.
20. Shechter M. Do statins really interfere with clopidogrel-induced platelet function? *Circulation* (2003) 108, 448.

Dipyridamole + Beta blockers

No adverse reactions normally occur in patients taking beta blockers who undergo dipyridamole–thallium-201 scintigraphy and echocardiography, but case reports suggest that very rarely bradycardia and asystole can occur.

Clinical evidence

A 71-year-old woman taking **nadolol** 120 mg daily and bendroflumethiazide, with a 3-week history of chest pain, was given a 300-mg dose of oral dipyridamole as part of a diagnostic dipyridamole-thallium imaging test for coronary artery disease. She was given thallium-201 intravenously, 50 minutes after the dipyridamole, but 3 minutes later, while exercising, she complained of chest pain and then had a cardiac arrest. She was given cardiopulmonary resuscitation and a normal cardiac rhythm was obtained after she was given intravenous aminophylline.[1]

Adverse interactions occurred in another 2 patients taking beta blockers during diagnostic dipyridamole-thallium stress testing. One patient, who was taking **atenolol**, developed bradycardia then asystole, which was treated with aminophylline and atropine, and the other patient, who was taking **metoprolol**, developed bradycardia, which resolved after she was given aminophylline.[2]

These reports need to be set in a broad context. A very extensive study of high-dose dipyridamole echocardiography (10 451 tests in 9 122 patients) noted significant adverse effects in only 96 patients, with major adverse reactions occurring in just 7 patients. Three of the 7 developed asystole and two of these patients were taking unnamed beta blockers.[3]

Mechanism

Not established. One possible explanation is that both drugs have negative chronotropic effects on the heart.

Importance and management

The value and safety of dipyridamole perfusion scintigraphy and echocardiography have been very extensively studied in very large numbers of patients, and reports of bradycardia and asystole, attributed to an interaction between dipyridamole and beta blockers, are sparse. It would therefore appear to be a relatively rare interaction (if such it is).

1. Blumenthal MS, McCauley CS. Cardiac arrest during dipyridamole imaging. *Chest* (1988) 93, 1103–4.
2. Roach PJ, Magee MA, Freedman SB. Asystole and bradycardia during dipyridamole stress testing in patients receiving beta blockers. *Int J Cardiol* (1993) 42, 92–4.
3. Picano E *et al.* on behalf of the Echo-Persantine International Cooperative Study Group. Safety of intravenous high-dose dipyridamole echocardiography. *Am J Cardiol* (1992) 70, 252–8.

Dipyridamole + Drugs that affect gastric pH

The effective disintegration, dissolution and eventual absorption of dipyridamole in tablet form depends upon having a low pH in the stomach. Drugs that raise the gastric pH significantly are expected to reduce the bioavailability of dipyridamole.

Clinical evidence, mechanism, importance and management

The solubility of dipyridamole depends very much on the pH. It is very soluble at low pH values and almost insoluble at neutral pH.[1] This indicates that dipyridamole needs a low pH in the stomach if solid formulations of the drug are to disintegrate and dissolve adequately. A study in 11 healthy elderly subjects (6 control subjects with a low fasting gastric pH and 5 achlorhydric subjects with fasting gastric pH greater than 5) found that elevated gastric pH reduced the absorption of a single 50-mg oral dose of dipyridamole. In addition, pretreatment with **famotidine** 40 mg increased the gastric pH to above 5 for at least 3 hours, which resulted in reduced dipyridamole absorption. The dipyridamole AUC was reduced by 37% (not statistically significant) and the maximum serum levels were significantly delayed and reduced.[2] In another study 20 healthy subjects were given **lansoprazole** 30 mg daily for 5 days and then either:

- a single dose of an extended release preparation of dipyridamole 200 mg with aspirin 25 mg (formulated with tartaric acid to improve bioavailability of dipyridamole if the gastric pH is elevated)
- or a conventional dipyridamole formulation (100 mg given with 81 mg of aspirin, followed 6 hours later by another dose of dipyridamole).

In the presence of **lansoprazole** (gastric pH greater than 4) the relative bioavailability of dipyridamole with conventional tablets was about 50% of that with the buffered extended release tablets.[3]

A consequential conclusion is that any drug that raises the stomach pH significantly would be likely to reduce the dissolution and absorption of dipyridamole. It would therefore be reasonable to expect that proton pump inhibitors, H_2-receptor antagonists and possibly antacids, which can raise the gastric pH, would interact to reduce the bioavailability of dipyridamole. Further study is needed to find out whether this is a clinically relevant interaction or not.

1. Boehringer Ingelheim. Data on file (Study 1482B).
2. Russell TL, Berardi RR, Barnett JL, O'Sullivan TL, Wagner JG, Dressman JB. pH-related changes in the absorption of dipyridamole in the elderly. *Pharm Res* (1994) 11 136–43.
3. Derendorf H, VanderMaelen CP, Brickl R-S, MacGregor TR, Eisert W. Dipyridamole bioavailability in subjects with reduced gastric acidity. *J Clin Pharmacol* (2005) 45, 845–50.

Dipyridamole + Irbesartan

A study in 13 patients with coronary artery disease found that irbesartan 150 mg daily reduced the extent and severity of perfusion defects after dipyridamole-induced stress.[1]

1. Altun GD, Altun A, Yildiz M, Firat MF, Hacimahmutoglu S, Berkarda S. Irbesartan has a masking effect on dipyridamole stress induced myocardial perfusion defects. *Nucl Med Commun* (2004) 25, 195–9.

Dipyridamole + Xanthines

Caffeine (in tea, coffee, cola, etc.) may interfere with dipyridamole–thallium-201 scintigraphy tests. Similarly, theophylline can also reduce some of the effects of dipyridamole.

Clinical evidence, mechanism, importance and management

Caffeine 4 mg/kg intravenously (roughly equivalent to 2 to 3 cups of coffee), given before dipyridamole–thallium-201 myocardial scintigraphy, caused a false-negative test result in a patient.[1] A further study in 8 healthy subjects confirmed that **caffeine** inhibits the haemodynamic response to an infusion of dipyridamole.[2] Similarly, oral **theophylline** markedly reduced the diagnostic accuracy of myocardial imaging using dipyridamole.[3] In addition, intravenous **aminophylline** accelerated the myocardial washout rate of thallium-201 after a dipyridamole infusion.[4]

It appears that xanthine derivatives such as **caffeine** and **theophylline** might antagonise some of the haemodynamic effects of dipyridamole because they act as competitive antagonists of adenosine (an endogenous vasodilator involved in the action of dipyridamole).[1,2] Due to these opposing effects, parenteral **aminophylline** has been used to treat adverse events associated with intravenous dipyridamole,[5,6] and it is recommended that **aminophylline** should be made available before beginning dipyridamole echocardiography.[6,7]

Patients should therefore abstain from **caffeine** (tea, coffee, chocolate, cocoa, cola, caffeine-containing analgesics etc.)[1,2,7] and other xanthine derivatives such as **theophylline**[3] for 24 hours[2,6] before dipyridamole testing, and if during the test the haemodynamic response is low (e.g. no increase in heart rate) the presence of **caffeine** should be suspected.[2]

1. Smits P, Aengevaeren WRM, Corstens FHM, Thien T. Caffeine reduces dipyridamole-induced myocardial ischemia. *J Nucl Med* (1989) 30, 1723–6.
2. Smits P, Straatman C, Pijpers E, Thien T. Dose-dependent inhibition of the hemodynamic response to dipyridamole by caffeine. *Clin Pharmacol Ther* (1991) 50, 529–37.
3. Daley PJ, Mahn TH, Zielonka JS, Krubsack AJ, Akhtar R, Bamrah VS. Effect of maintenance oral theophylline on dipyridamole–thallium-201 myocardial imaging using SPECT and dipyridamole-induced hemodynamic changes. *Am Heart J* (1988) 115, 1185–92.
4. Takeishi Y, Tono-oka I, Kubota I, Ikeda K, Masakane I, Chiba J, Abe S, Tsuiki K, Tomoike H. Intravenous aminophylline affects myocardial washout of thallium-201 after dipyridamole infusion. *Am J Noninvasive Cardiol* (1992) 6, 116–21.
5. Ranhosky A, Kempthorne-Rawson J, and the Intravenous Dipyridamole Thallium Imaging Study Group. The safety of intravenous dipyridamole thallium myocardial perfusion imaging. *Circulation* (1990) 81, 1205–9.
6. Persantin Ampoules (Dipyridamole). Boehringer Ingelheim Ltd. UK Summary of product characteristics, July 2004.
7. Picano E *et al.* on behalf of the Echo-Persantine International Cooperative Study Group. Safety of intravenous high-dose dipyridamole echocardiography. *Am J Cardiol* (1992) 70, 252–8.

Glycoprotein IIb/IIIa antagonists + Drugs that affect coagulation

The risk of bleeding with glycoprotein IIb/IIIa antagonists may be increased by heparin and thrombolytics, but low-dose thrombolytic therapy appears less likely to cause a problem.

Clinical evidence, mechanism, importance and management

(a) Abciximab

Although the manufacturers of abciximab recommend concurrent therapy with **heparin**, they also report that there is an increase in the incidence of bleeding.[1,2] In one study in patients with acute coronary syndrome without early revascularisation, the concurrent use of **low-molecular-weight heparin** was considered to be one of the factors that increased the risk of bleeding events with abciximab.[3]

Limited experience of abciximab in patients who have received **thrombolytics** suggests an increase in the risk of bleeding.[1,2] A retrospective analysis of 103 patients who presented with acute myocardial infarction and underwent angioplasty with adjunctive abciximab therapy, found that there was a significant increase in major bleeding complications when abciximab was used with full-dose **alteplase**. A major bleed occurred in 5 of 22 (23%) patients who underwent angioplasty within 15 hours of receiving thrombolytic therapy compared with 0 of 36 patients who underwent elective angioplasty more than 15 hours after fibrinolysis, and 1 of 45 (2%) without prior fibrinolysis.[4] However, the combination of abciximab with low-dose **reteplase** appeared not to result in the haemorrhagic complications associated with full-dose fibrinolytic therapy,[5] and no increase in bleeding complications were reported in studies using reduced-dose thrombolytic therapy with full-dose abciximab.[5,6]

The manufacturer of abciximab recommends caution when it is used with other drugs that affect haemostasis, such as **heparin**, **warfarin**, **thrombolytics** and antiplatelet drugs other than aspirin, such as **dipyridamole** and **ticlopidine**.[1,2]

(b) Eptifibatide

In an acute myocardial infarction study involving 181 patients, eptifibatide at the highest infusion rates studied (1.3 and 2 micrograms/kg per minute) appeared to increase the risk of bleeding when given with **streptokinase** 1.5 million units over 60 minutes. However, the manufacturers state that data on the use of eptifibatide in patients receiving thrombolytics are limited, and in a percutaneous coronary intervention study and an acute myocardial infarction study there was no consistent evidence that eptifibatide increased the risk of major or minor bleeding associated with **alteplase**.[7,8]

The UK manufacturer of eptifibatide reports that concurrent use with **warfarin** and **dipyridamole** did not appear to increase the risk of major and minor bleeding, and the use of **heparin** is recommended, but they warn that if eptifibatide is given with **heparin**, there must be careful monitoring including the aPTT.

Caution must be employed when eptifibatide is used with other drugs that affect haemostasis, including **clopidogrel**, **ticlopidine**, **dipyridamole**, **oral anticoagulants** or **thrombolytics** and concurrent or planned use of another **glycoprotein IIb/IIIa inhibitor** is contraindicated.[7,8]

1. ReoPro (Abciximab). Eli Lilly and Company Ltd. UK Summary of product characteristics, June 2005.
2. ReoPro (Abciximab). Centocor. US Prescribing information, November 2005.
3. Lenderink T, Boersma E, Ruzyllo W, Widimsky P, Ohman EM, Armstrong PW, Wallentin L, Simoons ML; GUSTO IV-ACS Investigators. Bleeding events with abciximab in acute coronary syndromes without early revascularization: an analysis of GUSTO IV-ACS. *Am Heart J* (2004) 147, 865–73.
4. Sundlof DW, Rerkpattanapitat P, Wongpraparut N, Pathi P, Kotler MN, Jacobs LE, Ledley GS, Yazdanfar S. Incidence of bleeding complications associated with *abciximab* use in conjunction with thrombolytic therapy in patients requiring percutaneous transluminal coronary angioplasty. *Am J Cardiol* (1999) 83, 1569 – 71.
5. Califf RM. Glycoprotein IIb/IIIa blockade and thrombolytics: early lessons from the SPEED and GUSTO IV trials. *Am Heart J* (1999) 138, S12–S15.
6. Gibson CM. Primary angioplasty compared with thrombolysis: new issues in the era of glycoprotein IIb/IIIa inhibition and intracoronary stenting. *Ann Intern Med* (1999) 130, 841–7.
7. Integrilin (Eptifibatide). GlaxoSmithKline UK. UK Summary of product characteristics, March 2007.
8. Integrilin (Eptifibatide). Millennium Pharmaceuticals Inc. US Prescribing information, June 2006.

Streptokinase + Aspirin

Patients with acute ischaemic stroke treated with streptokinase have an increased risk of early death due to cerebral haemorrhage if they are also given aspirin.

Clinical evidence, mechanism, importance and management

A post hoc analysis of 313 patients with acute ischaemic stroke given intravenous streptokinase 1.5 million units found that the addition of oral aspirin 300 mg daily for 10 days increased the risk of early death. The combined regimen significantly increased early fatalities (from day 3 to 10) with 53 deaths occurring out of 156 patients (34%) compared with 30 of 157 (19%) who received streptokinase alone. Early death was mainly due to cerebral causes (42 versus 24) and associated with intracranial haemorrhage (25 versus 11).[1]

If streptokinase is given to acute ischaemic stroke patients, it would seem sensible to avoid giving aspirin until thrombolysis is accomplished.[1]

1. Ciccone A, Motto C, Aritzu E, Piana A, Candelise L, on behalf of the MAST-I Collaborative Group. Negative interaction of aspirin and streptokinase in acute ischemic stroke: further analysis of the Multicenter Acute Stroke Trial-Italy. *Cerebrovasc Dis* (2000) 10, 61–4.

Streptokinase + Other thrombolytics

The thrombolytic effects of streptokinase or anistreplase are likely to be reduced or abolished if they are given some time after a dose of streptokinase because of persistently high levels of streptokinase antibodies. There is also an increased risk of hypersensitivity reactions. This may also be true for urokinase.

Clinical evidence

A study in 25 patients who had been given streptokinase for the treatment of acute myocardial infarction, found that 12 weeks later, 24 patients had enough anti-streptokinase antibodies in circulation to neutralise an entire 1.5 million unit dose of streptokinase. After 4 to 8 months, 18 out of 20 still had enough antibodies to neutralise half of a 1.5 million unit dose of streptokinase.[1] Further study has suggested that after streptokinase use, anti-streptokinase antibodies fall within 24 hours, but then increase gradually and are significantly raised by 4 days after treatment. The antibody titres reach a peak (approximately 200 times that of pretreatment levels) after 2 weeks and then subsequently decline, but remain above baseline values for at least one year.[2] Antibody titres may remain high enough to neutralise the effects of streptokinase for several years after a dose,[3,4] and high titres persisting for up to 7.5 years have been reported.[5] However, in contrast, another study found that the neutralising antibody titres had returned to control levels by 2 years.[6] Increased titres of streptokinase antibodies have also been seen in patients receiving topical streptokinase for wound care,[7] intrapleural streptokinase for pleural effusions,[8] and following streptococcal infections.[9] Apart from the reduced thrombolytic effect, repeated dosing[10] or high pre-treatment anti-streptokinase antibody titres[11] may increase the risk of allergic reactions.

Anistreplase, like its parent drug streptokinase, has been shown to be neutralised by anti-streptokinase antibodies.[12,13]

Of 6 patients given **urokinase** 1.5 million units infused over 30 minutes for recurrent myocardial infarction, rigors occurred in 4 patients and 2 of these also had bronchospasm; they had all previously received streptokinase.[14]

Mechanism

Streptokinase use causes the production of anti-streptokinase antibodies. These persist in the circulation so that the clot-dissolving effects of another dose of streptokinase given many months later may be ineffective, or less effective, because it becomes bound and neutralised by the antibodies. Many people already have a very low titre of antibodies resulting from previous streptococcal infections, yet this does not usually appear to influence thrombolysis.[15]

Importance and management

The interaction that results in neutralisation of the thrombolytics is established and clinically important. One author[16] says that clinically, therapy is not repeated within a year as it would not work. Given that it has been suggested that the effects may be very persistent, it would seem prudent, if a second use is needed, to use a thrombolytic with less antigenic effects such as alteplase. The British National Formulary says that streptokinase should not be used again beyond 4 days of the first use of either streptokinase or anistreplase.[17] In addition, the manufacturer recommends avoidance of streptokinase in patients who have had recent streptococcal infections that have produced high anti-streptokinase titres, such as acute rheumatic fever or acute glomerulonephritis.[9]

Little is known about the increased risk of hypersensitivity reactions.

1. Jalihal S, Morris GK. Antistreptokinase titres after intravenous streptokinase. *Lancet* (1990) 335, 184–5.

2. Lynch M, Littler WA, Pentecost BL, Stockley RA. Immunoglobulin response to intravenous streptokinase in acute myocardial infarction. *Br Heart J* (1991) 66, 139–42.
3. Elliott JM, Cross DB, Cederholm-Williams SA, White HD. Neutralizing antibodies to streptokinase four years after intravenous thrombolytic therapy. *Am J Cardiol* (1993) 71, 640–5.
4. Lee HS, Cross S, Davidson R, Reid T, Jennings K. Raised levels of antistreptokinase antibody and neutralization titres from 4 days to 54 months after administration of streptokinase or anistreplase. *Eur Heart J* (1993) 14, 84–9.
5. Squire IB, Lawley W, Fletcher S, Holme E, Hillis WS, Hewitt C, Woods KL. Humoral and cellular immune responses up to 7.5 years after administration of streptokinase for acute myocardial infarction. *Eur Heart J* (1999) 20, 1245–52.
6. McGrath K, Hogan C, Hunt D, O'Malley C, Green N, Dauer R, Dalli A. Neutralising antibodies after streptokinase treatment for myocardial infarction: a persisting puzzle. *Br Heart J* (1995) 74, 122–3.
7. Green C. Antistreptokinase titres after topical streptokinase. *Lancet* (1993) 341, 1602–3.
8. Laisaar T, Pullerits T. Effect of intrapleural streptokinase administration on antistreptokinase antibody level in patients with loculated pleural effusions. *Chest* (2003) 123, 432–5.
9. Streptase (Streptokinase). CSL Behring UK Ltd. UK Summary of product characteristics, March 2007.
10. White HD, Cross DB, Williams BF, Norris RM. Safety and efficacy of repeat thrombolytic treatment after acute myocardial infarction. *Br Heart J* (1990) 64, 177–81.
11. Lee HS, Yule S, McKenzie A, Cross S, Reid T, Davidson R, Jennings K. Hypersensitivity reactions to streptokinase in patients with high pre-treatment antistreptokinase antibody and neutralisation titres. *Eur Heart J* (1993) 14, 1640–3.
12. Binette MJ, Agnone FA. Failure of APSAC thrombolysis. *Ann Intern Med* (1993) 119, 637.
13. Brugemann J, van der Meer J, Bom VJJ, van der Schaaf W, de Graeff PA, Lie KI. Anti-streptokinase antibodies inhibit fibrinolytic effects of anistreplase in acute myocardial infarction. *Am J Cardiol* (1993) 72, 462–4.
14. Matsis P, Mann S. Rigors and bronchospasm with urokinase after streptokinase. *Lancet* (1992) 340, 1552.
15. Fears R, Hearn J, Standring R, Anderson JL, Marder VJ. Lack of influence of pretreatment antistreptokinase antibody on efficacy in a multicenter patency comparison of intravenous streptokinase and anistreplase in acute myocardial infarction. *Am Heart J* (1992) 124, 305–14.
16. Moriarty AJ. Anaphylaxis and streptokinase. *Hosp Update* (1987) 13, 342.
17. British National Formulary. 53rd ed. London: The British Medical Association and The Pharmaceutical Press; 2007. p. 132.

Ticlopidine + Antacids or Food

Food causes a moderate increase, and *Maalox* causes a moderate decrease, in the absorption of ticlopidine.

Clinical evidence, mechanism, importance and management

In a study in 12 healthy subjects the extent of absorption of a single 250-mg dose of ticlopidine was increased by 20% and occurred more rapidly when ticlopidine was taken after food, when compared with the fasting state. In contrast, 30 mL of *Maalox* [**aluminium/magnesium hydroxide**] reduced the extent of ticlopidine absorption by about 20%.[1] These modest changes are unlikely to be of much clinical importance.

It is suggested that ticlopidine is taken with food, but this is to minimise gastric intolerance.[1]

1. Shah J, Fratis A, Ellis D, Murakami S, Teitelbaum P. Effect of food and antacid on absorption of orally administered ticlopidine hydrochloride. *J Clin Pharmacol* (1990) 30, 733–6.

Ticlopidine + Miscellaneous

Ticlopidine-induced increases in bleeding times are opposed by methylprednisolone and prednisolone but its effects on platelet function are not affected. Ticlopidine decreases the clearance of phenazone (antipyrine), which suggests that it has mild enzyme-inhibiting effects. Beta blockers, calcium-channel blockers and diuretics are reported not to interact with ticlopidine.

Clinical evidence, mechanism, importance and management

(a) Corticosteroids

A study involving 14 healthy subjects found that a single 20-mg intravenous injection of **methylprednisolone** or oral **prednisolone** 15 mg twice daily for 7 days decreased the prolongation of bleeding times caused by ticlopidine 250 to 500 mg twice daily for 7 days. However, the antiplatelet effects of ticlopidine were not affected.[1] The clinical importance of this interaction is uncertain.

(b) Phenazone (Antipyrine)

A study in 10 healthy subjects found that ticlopidine 250 mg twice daily for 3 weeks decreased the clearance of phenazone (a marker of enzyme inhibition or induction). The AUC increased by 14% and the half-life increased by 27%, suggesting that ticlopidine has some mild enzyme-inhibiting effects.[2] This is consistent with the way ticlopidine appears to inhibit the metabolism of 'theophylline', (p.1177), but so far no other drugs seem to be affected to a clinically important extent.

(c) Non-interacting drugs

The manufacturers of ticlopidine report that in clinical studies in which ticlopidine was given with **beta blockers**, **calcium-channel blockers** and **diuretics** [none of the individual drugs named], no clinically significant adverse interactions were reported.[3,4]

1. Thébault J, Blatrix C, Blanchard J, Panak E. A possible method to control prolongations of bleeding time under antiplatelet therapy with ticlopidine. *Thromb Haemost* (1982) 48, 6–8.
2. Knudsen JB, Bastain W, Sefton CM, Allen JG, Dickinson JP. Pharmacokinetics of ticlopidine during chronic oral administration to healthy volunteers and its effects on antipyrine pharmacokinetics. *Xenobiotica* (1992) 22, 579–89.
3. Ticlid (Ticlopidine). Sanofi Synthelabo. UK Summary of product characteristics, May 2000.
4. Ticlid (Ticlopidine hydrochloride). Roche Pharmaceuticals. US Prescribing information, March 2001.

20

Antipsychotics, Anxiolytics and Hypnotics

The interactions where the effects of antipsychotic, anxiolytic and hypnotic drugs are affected are covered in this section but there are other monographs elsewhere in this publication where the effects of other drugs are altered by a benzodiazepine or antipsychotic.

(a) Antipsychotics

The antipsychotics are represented by chlorpromazine (and other phenothiazines), haloperidol (and other butyrophenones) and thioxanthenes, and the atypical, or newer, antipsychotic drugs, such as clozapine and risperidone. Their major use is in the treatment of psychoses such as schizophrenia and mania. These are listed in 'Table 20.1', (below). Some of the antipsychotics are also used as antiemetics, and for motor tics and hiccups.

The majority of interactions between the older antipsychotics are pharmacodynamic, relating to their effect on dopamine, whilst several of the newer atypical antipsychotics are metabolised to a significant extent by the cytochrome P450 isoenzymes. The concurrent use of other drugs which are inhibitors or inducers of these isoenzymes may result in large changes in plasma levels. In particular, tobacco smoking and caffeine can have an effect on the pharmacokinetics of some of these drugs, leading to adverse effects or lack of therapeutic effect following lifestyle changes.

(b) Benzodiazepines

The anxiolytics include the benzodiazepines and related drugs, cloral hydrate and other drugs used to treat psychoneuroses such as anxiety and tension, and are intended to induce calm without causing drowsiness and sleep. Some of the benzodiazepines and related drugs are also used as antiepileptics and hypnotics. 'Table 20.1', (below) contains a list of the benzodiazepines and related drugs. Many benzodiazepines undergo phase I metabolism by *N*-dealkylation and hydroxylation and many of the metabolites are active. They may then undergo phase II conjugation, mainly to form glucuronides before being excreted. For example, diazepam is metabolised to nordazepam (desmethyldiazepam), temazepam and oxazepam. The metabolism of diazepam in the liver is also mediated by cytochrome P450 isoenzymes, particularly CYP2C19, and diazepam is excreted mainly as free or conjugated metabolites.

The triazolo-and related benzodiazepines, such as alprazolam, midazolam and triazolam, are mainly metabolised by hydroxylation, mediated by CYP3A4, to active compounds, which then rapidly undergo glucuronide conjugation.

Therefore drugs that affect CYP2C19 may interact with benzodiazepines such as diazepam and those that affect CYP3A4 may interact with midazolam or triazolam.

Benzodiazepines such as lorazepam, oxazepam and temazepam, which are mainly conjugated without prior phase I metabolism, are unlikely to be involved in interactions with inhibitors or inducers of cytochrome P450. Benzodiazepines themselves do not significantly induce cytochrome P450 isoenzymes, so interactions involving enhanced metabolism of other drugs are not usual.

(c) Non-benzodiazepine hypnotics

Zaleplon, **zolpidem** and **zopiclone** are metabolised by several cytochrome CYP450 isoenzymes and it has been suggested that because of this, other drugs which affect a particular isoenzyme such as CYP3A4, may have less effect on their metabolism. However, their pharmacokinetics are affected by potent inducers such as rifampicin and by inhibitors such as the azole antifungals. **Buspirone** undergoes CYP3A4-mediated metabolism in the liver.

Table 20.1 Antipsychotics, anxiolytics, and hypnotics

Group	*Drugs*
Antipsychotics	
Atypical antipsychotics	Amisulpride, Aripiprazole, Clozapine, Olanzapine, Quetiapine, Risperidone, Sertindole, Ziprasidone, Zotepine
Phenothiazines	Butaperazine, Chlorpromazine, Fluphenazine, Levomepromazine, Mesoridazine, Pericyazine, Perphenazine, Prochlorperazine, Promazine, Thioridazine, Trifluoperazine
Butyrophenones	Benperidol, Bromperidol, Droperidol, Haloperidol
Thioxanthenes	Chlorprothixene, Flupentixol, Tiotixene, Zuclopenthixol
Miscellaneous	Loxapine, Molindone, Pimozide, Sulpiride
Anxiolytics and hypnotics	
Benzodiazepines	Alprazolam, Bromazepam, Brotizolam, Chlordiazepoxide, Clobazam, Clonazepam, Clorazepate, Clotiazepam, Diazepam, Flunitrazepam, Flurazepam, Ketazolam, Loprazolam, Lorazepam, Lormetazepam, Medazepam, Midazolam, Nitrazepam, Oxazepam, Oxazolam, Quazepam, Temazepam, Triazolam
Miscellaneous	Buspirone, Clomethiazole, Cloral betaine, Cloral hydrate, Eszopiclone, Glutethimide, Hydroxyzine, Meprobamate, Promethazine, Triclofos, Zaleplon, Zolpidem, Zopiclone

Amisulpride + Lithium

Amisulpride does not appear to affect the pharmacokinetics of lithium. However, limited evidence suggests that lithium may increase the plasma levels of amisulpride.

Clinical evidence, mechanism, importance and management

In a study in 24 healthy subjects, lithium carbonate 500 mg twice daily was given for 7 days to obtain stable lithium serum levels, and then amisulpride 100 mg twice daily or placebo was added for a further 7 days. Amisulpride appeared to have no effect on lithium pharmacokinetics.[1] In a pharmacokinetic analysis of amisulpride levels in patients with schizophrenia or schizoaffective disorder, dose-corrected amisulpride plasma levels were 1.8-fold higher in 3 patients taking lithium than in 13 patients taking amisulpride alone.[2] Further study is needed to confirm this finding and establish its clinical significance.

1. Canal M, Legangneux E, van Lier JJ, van Vliet AA, Coulouvrat C. Lack of effect of amisulpride on the pharmacokinetics and safety of lithium. *Int J Neuropsychopharmacol* (2003) 6, 103–9.
2. Bergemann N, Kopitz J, Kress KR, Frick A. Plasma amisulpride levels in schizophrenia or schizoaffective disorder. *Eur Neuropsychopharmacol* (2004) 14, 245–50.

Antipsychotics + Antacids or Sucralfate

Antacids containing aluminium/magnesium hydroxide or magnesium trisilicate can reduce the serum levels of chlorpromazine which would be expected to reduce the therapeutic response. Sucralfate and an aluminium/magnesium hydroxide antacid can reduce the absorption of sulpiride. *In vitro* studies suggest that this interaction may possibly also occur with other antacids and phenothiazines. There seem to be no clinical studies or reports confirming the anecdotal evidence of a possible reduction in the effects of haloperidol by antacids.

Clinical evidence

(a) Haloperidol

In 1982 a questioner in a letter asked whether haloperidol interacts with antacids because he had a patient responding well to treatment with haloperidol who had begun to deteriorate when *Amphojel* (**aluminium hydroxide**) was added. In a written answer it was stated[1] that there are no reports of this interaction but several clinicians had said that based on clinical impressions oral haloperidol and antacids should not be given together.

(b) Phenothiazines

A study in 10 patients taking **chlorpromazine** 600 mg to 1.2 g daily showed that 30 mL of *Aludrox* (**aluminium/magnesium hydroxide gel**) reduced their urinary excretion of **chlorpromazine** by 10 to 45%.[2]

A study was prompted by the observation of one psychiatric patient, taking **chlorpromazine** who relapsed within 3 days of starting to take an unnamed antacid. When 30 mL of *Gelusil* (**aluminium hydroxide** with **magnesium trisilicate**) was given with **chlorpromazine** suspension to 6 patients, the serum **chlorpromazine** levels measured 2 hours later were reduced by about 20% (from 168 to 132 nanograms/mL).[3] *In vitro* studies have also found that other phenothiazines (**trifluoperazine**, **fluphenazine**, **perphenazine**, **thioridazine**) are adsorbed to a considerable extent onto a number of antacids (**magnesium trisilicate**, **bismuth subnitrate**, **aluminium hydroxide** with **magnesium carbonate**) but there do not appear to be any clinical studies of the possible clinical effects of these interactions.[4]

(c) Sulpiride

A study in 6 healthy subjects found that the bioavailability of a single 100-mg dose of sulpiride was reduced by 40% by **sucralfate** 1 g and by 32% by 30 mL of *Simeco* (**aluminium/magnesium hydroxide** and **simeticone**). When either the **sucralfate** or the antacid were taken 2 hours before sulpiride the reduction in bioavailability was only about 25%, and no change in bioavailability was seen in one subject when the **sucralfate** was given 2 hours after the sulpiride.[5]

Mechanism

Chlorpromazine and other phenothiazines become adsorbed onto these antacids,[3,6] which would seem to account for the reduced bioavailability. It is possible that adsorption also occurs with sulpiride, but this has not been proven.

Importance and management

Clinical information seems to be limited to the reports cited. Reductions of up to 45% in serum antipsychotic levels would be expected to be clinically important, but so far only one case seems to have been reported.[3] Separating the doses as much as possible (1 to 2 hours) to avoid admixture in the gut should minimise any effects. This may also prove of use in the interactions with haloperidol and sulpiride (although note; the haloperidol interaction is not confirmed). In the case of chlorpromazine an alternative would be to use calcium carbonate-glycine or magnesium hydroxide gel, which seem to affect its gastrointestinal absorption to a lesser extent.[6] Other phenothiazines and antacids are known to interact *in vitro*,[4] but the clinical importance of these interactions awaits further study.

1. Goldstein BJ. Interaction of antacids with psychotropics. *Hosp Community Psychiatry* (1982) 33, 96.
2. Forrest FM, Forrest IS, Serra MT. Modification of chlorpromazine metabolism by some other drugs frequently administered to psychiatric patients. *Biol Psychiatry* (1970) 2, 53–8.
3. Fann WE, Davis JM, Janowsky DS, Sekerke HJ, Schmidt DM. Chlorpromazine: effects of antacids on its gastrointestinal absorption. *J Clin Pharmacol* (1973) 13, 388–90.
4. Moustafa MA, Babhair SA, Kouta HI. Decreased bioavailability of some antipsychotic phenothiazines due to interactions with adsorbent antacid and antidiarrhoeal mixtures. *Int J Pharmaceutics* (1987) 36, 185–9.
5. Gouda MW, Hikal AH, Babhair SA, ElHofy SA, Mahrous GM. Effect of sucralfate and antacids on the bioavailability of sulpiride in humans. *Int J Pharmaceutics* (1984) 22, 257–63.
6. Pinell OC, Fenimore DC, Davis CM, Moreira O, Fann WE. Drug-drug interaction of chlorpromazine and antacid. *Clin Pharmacol Ther* (1978) 23, 125.

Antipsychotics + Antiepileptics

Haloperidol plasma levels are roughly halved by carbamazepine, phenobarbital and phenytoin. Bromperidol, fluphenazine and tiotixene levels are also reduced by carbamazepine. The plasma levels of chlorpromazine and haloperidol do not appear to be affected by oxcarbazepine. Neurotoxicity has been seen with haloperidol and carbamazepine and haloperidol can raise serum carbamazepine levels. Valproate or valproic acid appear not to interact.

Clinical evidence

(a) Carbamazepine

For mention of carbamazepine toxicity and other adverse reactions following the concurrent use of antipsychotics, see 'Carbamazepine + Antipsychotics', p.524.

1. Bromperidol. When 13 schizophrenic patients taking bromperidol 12 or 24 mg daily were given carbamazepine 200 mg twice daily for 4 weeks, the plasma levels of bromperidol and reduced bromperidol (a metabolite) were decreased by 37% and 23%, respectively. Despite this fall in levels, the Clinical Global Impression scores (a measure of severity of illness) fell slightly.[1]

2. Chlorpromazine. **Oxcarbazepine** was substituted for carbamazepine in 4 difficult to treat schizophrenic patients. All patients were also taking chlorpromazine, and in 3 cases other antipsychotic medication (lithium, zuclopenthixol or clozapine). After 3 weeks of taking the **oxcarbazepine** all the 4 patients had rises in their chlorpromazine levels, of 28%, 63%, 76%, and 90%, respectively. In one case this rise was associated with increased extrapyramidal adverse effects.[2]

3. Fluphenazine. A patient receiving intramuscular fluphenazine decanoate 37.5 mg weekly had a rise in serum levels from 0.6 to 1.17 nanograms/mL 6 weeks after stopping carbamazepine 800 mg daily. A moderate improvement in his schizophrenic condition occurred.[3]

4. Haloperidol. A study in 9 schizophrenics taking haloperidol (average dose 30 mg daily) found a 55% reduction in plasma haloperidol levels (a mean fall from 45.5 to 21.2 nanograms/mL) when they were given carbamazepine for 5 weeks (precise dose not stated). They also took trihexyphenidyl 10 mg daily and oxazepam 30 mg at night as necessary. Carbamazepine serum levels and the control of the disease remained unchanged.[4]

Other studies have similarly found 40 to 60% falls in plasma haloperidol levels in patients taking carbamazepine,[5-7] with the occasional patient having undetectable levels.[6,8] Decreases in plasma haloperidol levels of unspecified amounts have also been described.[9-12] A study in 9 patients taking haloperidol 6 mg twice daily who were then given carbamazepine, with the daily dose increased at fortnightly intervals from 100 to 300 and to 600 mg, found a dose-dependent reduction in haloperidol levels. Mean plasma haloperidol levels were reduced by 25%, 61%, and 82%, respectively.[13] A few patients have had clinical worsening or increased adverse effects.[6-8] Three patients had two to fivefold increases in plasma haloperidol levels and clinical improvement when carbamazepine 1.2 to 1.4 g daily was stopped, but extrapyramidal adverse effects developed within 1 to 30 days.[14] Three cases of neurotoxicity (drowsiness, slurred speech, confusion) have also been described in patients taking haloperidol and carbamazepine.[9,15,16]

A case report describes 3 schizophrenic patients taking haloperidol whose treatment was changed from carbamazepine to **oxcarbazepine**. After 2 weeks their plasma haloperidol levels had dramatically risen (from 6 to 18 nanomol/L, from 6 to 14 nanomol/L and from 17 to 27 nanomol/L). This was accompanied by severe extrapyramidal adverse effects, which necessitated dose reductions in 2 patients.[2]

A fall of 45% in haloperidol levels was noted in a study of 7 patients taking haloperidol and carbamazepine, and patients also experienced a worsening of clinical symptoms.[17]

A study in Japanese schizophrenic patients found that carbamazepine reduced the serum haloperidol levels by an unstated amount, while at the same time the serum carbamazepine levels were raised by about 30%, despite a 25% dose reduction.[10] An associated study by the same group of workers found that concurrent use increased the incidence of QTc lengthening.[18]

5. Tiotixene. A retrospective study in 42 patients found that the mean clearance of tiotixene in those taking liver enzyme inducer drugs (carbamazepine, phenytoin, primidone) was threefold greater than in the control group. Of the group taking enzyme inducers, 5 patients had non-detectable serum tiotixene levels, and not surprisingly showed no clinical response.[19]

(b) Phenobarbital and/or Phenytoin

A study in epileptic patients, 2 taking phenobarbital, 3 taking phenytoin, and 4 taking both drugs, found that after taking **haloperidol** 10 mg three times daily for 6 weeks their serum **haloperidol** levels were about half of those in a control group who were not taking anticonvulsants (19.4 compared to 36.6 nanograms/mL). Antiepileptic levels remained unchanged.[20]

A patient had a marked rise in serum **haloperidol** levels and clinical improvement when phenytoin 300 mg daily was stopped.[14] A retrospective study found that phenobarbital reduced the **haloperidol** concentration/dose ratio, suggesting that phenobarbital may affect the metabolism of **haloperidol**.[12] See also *Tiotixene* above.

A case-control, retrospective review of patients taking **thioridazine** 100 to 200 mg daily with either phenytoin, phenobarbital or both drugs found a reduction in both phenobarbital (approximately 25%) and **thioridazine** levels when taken together. Inconsistent effects were seen on the pharmacokinetics of phenytoin, with a possible trend towards a reduction in phenytoin levels. These results, together with the seizure threshold-lowering effect of phenothiazines, highlights the need to carefully monitor antiepileptic drug levels if phenothiazines are added to, or removed from therapy.[21] See 'Phenothiazines + Barbiturates', p.759, for the interaction of phenobarbital with chlorpromazine.

(c) Valproic acid or Valproate

A study in 6 patients given **haloperidol** 6 to 10 mg daily found no significant interaction with valproic acid.[22] Similarly, **haloperidol** was not found to interact with valproate in two further studies,[17,23] although in one of these studies an increase of 64% in **haloperidol** plasma levels was seen, which was considered not significant.[17] For the interaction of valproic acid with chlorpromazine, see 'Valproate + Chlorpromazine', p.577.

Mechanism

Carbamazepine, phenobarbital and phenytoin are recognised enzyme inducers, therefore it seems highly likely that the reduced plasma bromperidol, chlorpromazine and haloperidol levels occur because their metabolism by the liver is markedly increased by these antiepileptics. Oxcarbazepine does not appear to interact, probably because it is not an enzyme inducer.

Importance and management

The interactions of haloperidol with carbamazepine, phenytoin and phenobarbital are moderately well documented and appear to be clinically important, but only a few patients have been reported to show clinical worsening. Although there are advantages in adding carbamazepine to haloperidol in treating some patients[24] be alert for the need to increase the haloperidol dosage if any of these antiepileptics is also given. The authors of one study with phenobarbital and phenytoin suggest a two to threefold increase in the haloperidol dosage may be needed.[20] Another study, in which intramuscular haloperidol was used, recommended shortening the interval between injections rather than raising the dosage, but it was not stated by how much.[25] Remember too that if the anticonvulsants are withdrawn it may be necessary to reduce the haloperidol dosage. Also be alert for the development of dystonic reactions and for a rise in serum carbamazepine levels. Similar precautions seem necessary with tiotixene, and may be needed with bromperidol and chlorpromazine, but this needs confirmation. Limited evidence suggest that no special precautions are necessary with oxcarbazepine, or if sodium valproate is used with haloperidol.

1. Otani K, Ishida M, Yasui N, Kondo T, Mihara K, Suzuki A, Furukori H, Kaneko S, Inoue Y. Interaction between carbamazepine and bromperidol. *Eur J Clin Pharmacol* (1997) 53, 219–22.
2. Raitasuo V, Lehtovaara R, Huttunen MO. Effect of switching carbamazepine to oxcarbazepine on the plasma levels of neuroleptics. A case report. *Psychopharmacology (Berl)* (1994) 116, 115–16.
3. Jann MW, Fidone GS, Hernandez JM, Amrung S, Davis CM. Clinical implications of increased antipsychotic plasma concentrations upon anticonvulsant cessation. *Psychiatry Res* (1989) 28, 153–9.
4. Kidron R, Averbuch I, Klein E, Belmaker RH. Carbamazepine-induced reduction of blood levels of haloperidol in chronic schizophrenia. *Biol Psychiatry* (1985) 20, 219–22.
5. Jann MW, Ereshefsky L, Saklad SR, Seidel DR, Davis CM, Burch NR, Bowden CL. Effects of carbamazepine on plasma haloperidol levels. *J Clin Psychopharmacol* (1985) 5, 106–9.
6. Arana GW, Goff DC, Friedman H, Ornsteen M, Greenblatt DJ, Black B, Shader RI. Does carbamazepine-induced reduction of plasma haloperidol levels worsen psychotic symptoms? *Am J Psychiatry* (1986) 143, 650–1.
7. Kahn EM, Schulz SC, Perel JM, Alexander JE. Change in haloperidol level due to carbamazepine—a complicating factor in combined medication for schizophrenia. *J Clin Psychopharmacol* (1990) 10, 54–7.
8. Fast DK, Jones BD, Kusalic M, Erickson M. Effect of carbamazepine on neuroleptic plasma levels and efficacy. *Am J Psychiatry* (1986) 143, 117–18.
9. Brayley J, Yellowlees P. An interaction between haloperidol and carbamazepine in a patient with cerebral palsy. *Aust N Z J Psychiatry* (1987) 21, 605–7.
10. Iwahashi K, Miyatake R, Suwaki H, Hosokawa K, Ichikawa Y. The drug–drug interaction effects of haloperidol on plasma carbamazepine levels. *Clin Neuropharmacol* (1995) 18, 233–6.
11. Jann MW, Chang W-H, Lane H-Y. Differences in haloperidol epidemiologic pharmacokinetic studies. *J Clin Psychopharmacol* (2001) 21, 628–30.
12. Hirokane G, Someya T, Takahashi S, Morita S, Shimoda K. Interindividual variation of plasma haloperidol concentrations and the impact of concomitant medications: the analysis of therapeutic drug monitoring data. *Ther Drug Monit* (1999) 21, 82–6.
13. Yasui-Furukori N, Kondo T, Mihara K, Suziki A, Inoue Y, Kaneko S. Significant dose effect of carbamazepine on reduction of steady-state plasma concentration of haloperidol in schizophrenic patients. *J Clin Psychopharmacol* (2003) 23, 435–40.
14. Jann MW, Fidone GS, Hernandez JM, Amrung S, Davis CM. Clinical implications of increased antipsychotic plasma concentrations upon anticonvulsant cessation. *Psychiatry Res* (1989) 28, 153–9.
15. Kanter GL, Yerevanian BI, Ciccone JR. Case report of a possible interaction between neuroleptics and carbamazepine. *Am J Psychiatry* (1984) 141, 1101–2.
16. Yerevanian BI, Hodgman CH. A haloperidol-carbamazepine interaction in a patient with rapid-cycling bipolar disorder. *Am J Psychiatry* (1985) 142, 785–6.
17. Hesslinger B, Normann C, Langosch JM, Klose P, Berger M, Walden J. Effects of carbamazepine and valproate on haloperidol plasma levels and on psychopathologic outcome in schizophrenic patients. *J Clin Psychopharmacol* (1999) 19, 310–15.
18. Iwahashi K, Nakamura K, Miyatake R, Suwaki H, Hosokawa K. Cardiac effects of haloperidol and carbamazepine treatment. *Am J Psychiatry* (1996) 153, 135.
19. Ereshefsky L, Saklad SR, Watanabe MD, Davis CM, Jann MW. Thiothixene pharmacokinetic interactions: a study of hepatic enzyme inducers, clearance inhibitors, and demographic variables. *J Clin Psychopharmacol* (1991) 11, 296–301.
20. Linnoila M, Viukari M, Vaisanen K, Auvinen J. Effect of anticonvulsants on plasma haloperidol and thioridazine levels. *Am J Psychiatry* (1980) 137, 819–21.
21. Gay PE, Madsen JA. Interaction between phenobarbital and thioridazine. *Neurology* (1983) 33, 1631–2.
22. Ishizaki T, Chiba K, Saito M, Kobayashi K, Iizuka R. The effects of neuroleptics (haloperidol and chlorpromazine) on the pharmacokinetics of valproic acid in schizophrenic patients. *J Clin Psychopharmacol* (1984) 4, 254–61.
23. Normann C, Klose P, Hesslinger B, Langosch JM, Berger M, Walden J. Haloperidol plasma levels and psychopathology in schizophrenic patients with antiepileptic co-medication: a clinical trial. *Pharmacopsychiatry* (1997) 30, 204.
24. Klein E, Bental E, Lerer B, Belmaker RH. Carbamazepine and haloperidol *v* placebo and haloperidol in excited psychoses: a controlled study. *Arch Gen Psychiatry* (1984) 41, 165–70.
25. Pupeschi G, Agenet C, Levron J-C, Barges-Bertocchio M-H. Do enzyme inducers modify haloperidol decanoate rate of release? *Prog Neuropsychopharmacol Biol Psychiatry* (1994) 18, 1323–32.

Antipsychotics + Antimuscarinics

Antipsychotics and antimuscarinics are very often given together advantageously and uneventfully, but occasionally serious and even life-threatening interactions occur. These include heat stroke in hot and humid conditions, severe constipation and adynamic ileus, and atropine-like psychoses. Antimuscarinics used to

counteract the extrapyramidal adverse effects of antipsychotics may also reduce or abolish their therapeutic effects.

Clinical evidence

The use of antipsychotics with antimuscarinics can result in a generalised, low grade, but not usually serious, additive increase in the antimuscarinic effects of these drugs (blurred vision, dry mouth, constipation, difficulty in urination, see 'Antimuscarinics + Antimuscarinics', p.674). However, sometimes serious intensification takes place. For the sake of clarity these have been subdivided here into (a) heat stroke, (b) constipation and adynamic ileus, (c) atropine-like psychoses, (d) antagonism of antipsychotic effects and (e) miscellaneous effects.

(a) Heat stroke in hot and humid conditions

Three patients were admitted to hospital in Philadelphia for drug-induced hyperpyrexia during a hot and humid period. In each case their skin and mucous membranes were dry and they were tachycardic (120 bpm). There was no evidence of infection.[1]

Drug combinations implicated in reports of heat stroke, some of them fatal, include:[1-5]

- **chlorpromazine** and **benzatropine**
- **chlorpromazine** and **trifluoperazine**
- **chlorpromazine**, **amitriptyline** and **benzatropine**
- **chlorpromazine**, **chlorprothixene** and **benzatropine**
- **chlorpromazine**, **fluphenazine**, **trihexyphenidyl** and **benzatropine**
- **chlorpromazine**, **trifluoperazine** and **benzatropine**
- **haloperidol** and **benzatropine**
- **promazine** and **benzatropine**.

The danger of heat stroke in patients taking **atropine** or **atropine-like compounds** was recognised in the 1920s, and the warning has been repeated many times.[6,7]

(b) Constipation and adynamic ileus

Paralytic ileus with faecal impaction (fatal in 6 cases) has been reported in a number of patients taking:

- **chlorpromazine** and **amitriptyline**,[8] **imipramine**,[9] **nortriptyline**,[10] or **trihexyphenidyl**[9]
- **haloperidol** and **benzatropine**[11]
- **levomepromazine** and **imipramine** with **benzatropine**[9]
- **levomepromazine** and **trihexyphenidyl**[9]
- **mesoridazine** and **benzatropine**[12]
- **thioridazine** and **imipramine** with **trihexyphenidyl**[9]
- **trifluoperazine** and **benzatropine**[13] or **trihexyphenidyl**[9]
- **trifluoperazine** and **benzatropine** with **methylphenidate**.[14]

Severe constipation also occurred in a woman given **thioridazine**, **biperiden** and **doxepin**.[15]

(c) Atropine-like psychoses

In a double-blind study 3 patients given a **phenothiazine** and **benzatropine** for the parkinsonian adverse effects, developed an intermittent toxic confusional state (marked disturbance of short-term memory, impaired attention, disorientation, anxiety, visual and auditory hallucinations) with peripheral antimuscarinics signs.[16] Similar reactions occurred in 3 elderly patients given **imipramine** or **desipramine**, with **trihexyphenidyl**,[17] and in another man given **chlorpromazine**, **benzatropine** and **doxepin**.[15]

(d) Antagonism of the antipsychotic effects

A study in psychiatric patients given **chlorpromazine** 300 to 800 mg daily found that when **trihexyphenidyl** 6 to 10 mg daily was added, the plasma **chlorpromazine** levels were reduced from a range of 100 to 300 nanograms/mL to less than 30 nanograms/mL. When the **trihexyphenidyl** was withdrawn the plasma **chlorpromazine** levels rose again and clinical improvement was seen.[18,19]

Other studies confirm that **trihexyphenidyl**[20,21] and **orphenadrine**[22] reduce the plasma levels and effects of **chlorpromazine**. In contrast to these reports, another found that **trihexyphenidyl** increased **chlorpromazine** levels by 41% in 20 young schizophrenics, but no clinical change was seen. The levels dropped again over the first 4 weeks of treatment.[23] Some of the beneficial actions of **haloperidol** on social avoidance behaviour are lost during concurrent treatment with **benzatropine**, but cognitive integrative function is unaffected.[24]

A study to investigate any possible interaction between **procyclidine** 5 to 15 mg daily and **chlorpromazine**, **fluphenazine** or **haloperidol** found that the addition of **procyclidine** caused a transient fall in the serum levels of **chlorpromazine**, whilst the fall in levels of **fluphenazine** and **haloperidol** was maintained for the 4 week treatment period with **procyclidine**. Two patients in the **haloperidol** group experienced a worsening of symptoms whilst taking **procyclidine**.[25]

(e) Miscellaneous effects

A study in psychotic patients found that the addition of **biperiden** 2 mg three times daily or **orphenadrine** 50 mg three times daily for 3 weeks had no effect on the steady-state levels of **perphenazine** 24 to 48 mg daily.[26]

An isolated report describes the development of a hypoglycaemic coma in a non-diabetic patient given **chlorpromazine** and **orphenadrine**.[27]

Mechanism

Antimuscarinic (anticholinergic) drugs inhibit the parasympathetic nervous system, which innervates the sweat glands, so that when the ambient temperature rises the major body heat-losing mechanism can be partially or wholly lost.[28] Phenothiazines, thioxanthenes and butyrophenones may also have some antimuscarinic effects, but additionally they impair to a varying extent the hypothalamic thermoregulatory mechanisms that control the body's ability to keep a constant temperature when exposed to heat or cold. Thus, when the ambient temperature rises, the body temperature also rises. The tricyclics can similarly disrupt temperature control. Therefore in very hot and humid conditions, when the need to reduce the temperature is great, the additive effects of these drugs can make patients unable to control their temperature,[4] which can be fatal.

Antimuscarinic drugs also reduce peristalsis, which in the extreme can result in total gut stasis. Additive effects can occur if two or more antimuscarinic drugs are taken.

The toxic psychoses described resemble the CNS effects of atropine or belladonna poisoning and appear to result from the additive effects of the drugs used.

The mechanism for antipsychotic antagonism is not understood. *Animal* studies suggest that the site of interaction is in the gut.[19]

Importance and management

Established and well-documented interactions. While these drugs have been widely used together with apparent advantage and without problems, prescribers should be aware that an unspectacular low-grade antimuscarinic toxicity can easily go undetected, particularly in the elderly because the symptoms can be so similar to the general complaints of this group. Also be aware of the serious problems that can sometimes develop, particularly if high doses are used.

- Warn patients to minimise outdoor exposure and/or exercise in hot and humid climates, particularly if they are taking high doses of antipsychotic/antimuscarinic drugs.
- Be alert for severe constipation and for the development of complete gut stasis, which can be fatal.
- Be aware that the symptoms of central antimuscarinic psychosis can be confused with the basic psychotic symptoms of the patient. Withdrawal of one or more of the drugs, or a dosage reduction and/or appropriate symptomatic treatment can be used to control these interactions.
- Ensure that the concurrent use of antimuscarinics to control the extrapyramidal adverse effects of neuroleptics is necessary[29,30] and be aware that the therapeutic effects may possibly be reduced as a result.

Note that tricyclic antidepressants have antimuscarinic adverse effects and may therefore interact similarly. The tricyclics also have other interactions with antipsychotics, see 'Phenothiazines + Tricyclic antidepressants', p.760. Some antipsychotics and antimuscarinics prolong the QT interval. Consider also 'Antimuscarinics + Antimuscarinics', p.674.

1. Westlake RJ, Rastegar A. Hyperpyrexia from drug combinations. *JAMA* (1973) 225, 1250.
2. Zelman S, Guillan R. Heat stroke in phenothiazine-treated patients: a report of three fatalities. *Am J Psychiatry* (1970) 126, 1787–90.
3. Sarnquist F, Larson CP. Drug-induced heat stroke. *Anesthesiology* (1973) 39, 348–50.
4. Reimer DR, Mohan J, Nagaswami S. Heat dyscontrol syndrome in patients receiving antipsychotic, antidepressant and antiparkinson drug therapy. *J Fla Med Assoc* (1974) 61, 573–4.
5. Mirtello JM. Drug-induced heat stroke. *DICP Ann Pharmacother* (1978) 12, 652–7.
6. Willcox WH. The nature, prevention, and treatment of heat hyperpyrexia: the clinical aspect. *BMJ* (1920) 1, 392–7.
7. Litman RE. Heat sensitivity due to autonomic drugs. *JAMA* (1952) 149, 635–6.
8. Burkitt EA, Sutcliffe CK. Paralytic ileus after amitriptyline ("Tryptizol"). *BMJ* (1961) 2, 1648–9.
9. Warnes H, Lehmann HE, Ban TA. Adynamic ileus during psychoactive medication: a report of three fatal and five severe cases. *Can Med Assoc J* (1967) 96, 1112–13.
10. Milner G, Hills NF. Adynamic ileus and nortriptyline. *BMJ* (1966) 1, 841–2.
11. Sheikh RA, Prindiville T, Yasmeen S. Haloperidol and benztropine interaction presenting as acute intestinal pseudo-obstruction. *Am J Gastroenterol* (2001) 96, 934–5.

12. Wade LC, Ellenor GL. Combination mesoridazine- and benztropine mesylate- induced paralytic ileus. Two case reports. *DICP Ann Pharmacother* (1980) 14, 17–22.
13. Giordano J, Huang A, Canter JW. Fatal paralytic ileus complicating phenothiazine therapy. *South Med J* (1975) 68, 351–3.
14. Spiro RK, Kysilewskyj RM. Iatrogenic ileus secondary to medication. *J Med Soc New Jers* (1973) 70, 565–7.
15. Ayd FJ. Doxepin with other drugs. *South Med J* (1973) 66, 465–71.
16. Davis JM. Psychopharmacology in the aged. Use of psychotropic drugs in geriatric patients. *J Geriatr Psychiatry* (1974) 7, 145.
17. Rogers SC. Imipramine and benzhexol. *BMJ* (1967) 1, 500.
18. Rivera-Calimlim L, Castañeda L, Lasagna L. Effect of mode of management on plasma chlorpromazine in psychiatric patients. *Clin Pharmacol Ther* (1973) 14, 978–86.
19. Rivera-Calimlim L, Castañeda L, Lasagna L. Chlorpromazine and trihexyphenidyl interaction in psychiatric patients. *Pharmacologist* (1973) 15, 212.
20. Chan TL, Sakalis G, Gershon S. Some aspects of chlorpromazine metabolism in humans. *Clin Pharmacol Ther* (1973) 14, 133.
21. Rivera-Calimlim L, Nasrallah H, Strauss J, Lasagna L. Clinical response and plasma levels: effect of dose, dosage schedules, and drug interactions on plasma chlorpromazine levels. *Am J Psychiatry* (1976) 133, 646–52.
22. Loga S, Curry S, Lader M. Interactions of orphenadrine and phenobarbitone with chlorpromazine: plasma concentrations and effects in man. *Br J Clin Pharmacol* (1975) 2, 197–208.
23. Rockland L, Cooper T, Schwartz F, Weber D, Sullivan T. Effects of trihexyphenidyl on plasma chlorpromazine in young schizophrenics. *Can J Psychiatry* (1990) 35, 604–7.
24. Singh MM, Smith JM. Reversal of some therapeutic effects of an antipsychotic agent by an antiparkinsonism drug. *J Nerv Ment Dis* (1973) 157, 50–8.
25. Bamrah JS, Kumar V, Krska J Soni SD. Interactions between procyclidine and neuroleptic drugs. Some pharmacological and clinical aspects. *Br J Psychiatry* (1986) 149, 726–733.
26. Hansen LB, Elley J, Christensen TR, Larsen N-E, Naestoft J, Hvidberg EF. Plasma levels of perphenazine and its major metabolites during simultaneous treatment with anticholinergic drugs. *Br J Clin Pharmacol* (1979) 7, 75–80.
27. Buckle RM, Guillebaud J. Hypoglycaemic coma occurring during treatment with chlorpromazine and orphenadrine. *BMJ* (1967) 4, 599–600.
28. Kollias J, Bullard RW. The influence of chlorpromazine on physical and chemical mechanisms of temperature regulation in the rat. *J Pharmacol Exp Ther* (1964) 145, 373–81.
29. Prien RF. Unpublished surveys from the NIMH Collaborative Project on Drug Therapy in Chronic Schizophrenia and the VA Collaborative Project on Interim Drug Therapy in Chronic Schizophrenia. *Int Drug Ther Newslett* (1974) 9, 29–32.
30. Klett CJ, Caffey EM. Evaluating the long-term need for antiparkinson drugs by chronic schizophrenics. *Arch Gen Psychiatry* (1972) 26, 374–9.

Antipsychotics + Bromocriptine

The concurrent use of bromocriptine with antipsychotics can be successful. However, one report describes the re-emergence of schizophrenic symptoms in a patient when bromocriptine was added to treatment with molindone and imipramine. Another case reports a rise in prolactin levels and deterioration of vision when thioridazine was given with bromocriptine.

Clinical evidence, mechanism, importance and management

Single 2-mg doses of bromocriptine have been found to improve the psychopathology of chronic schizophrenia in patients taking antipsychotics[1] and a case report describes a reduction in psychopathology when bromocriptine 2.5 mg daily was given with **haloperidol**.[2]

A case of reduced prolactin levels has been reported in a man treated with **fluphenazine** and **benzatropine** who took bromocriptine to treat a pituitary tumour. His prolactin level became undetectable, and his psychiatric status was unchanged, although no reduction in tumour size was seen with the bromocriptine.[3] However, the prolactin levels of a patient with a prolactin-secreting pituitary adenoma fell from almost 8,000 nanograms/mL to 400 nanograms/mL when bromocriptine was started, but increased again to 1,000 nanograms/mL when he started to take **thioridazine** 25 mg twice daily. As the **thioridazine** dose was increased to 200 mg daily, his prolactin level increased further to 2,000 nanograms/mL and his visual fields deteriorated. Normal vision returned within 5 days of stopping the **thioridazine**, and his prolactin levels fell to below 500 nanograms/mL.[4] A woman with schizoaffective schizophrenia, taking **molindone** 100 mg and imipramine 200 mg daily, relapsed within 5 days of starting treatment with bromocriptine 2.5 mg three times daily for amenorrhoea and galactorrhoea.[5] Within 3 days of stopping the bromocriptine the symptoms of relapse (agitation, delusions, and auditory hallucinations) vanished. The reason suggested by the authors of the report is that the bromocriptine (a dopamine agonist) opposed the actions of the antipsychotic medication (dopamine antagonists) thereby allowing the schizophrenia to re-emerge. Limited evidence suggests that 'levodopa', (p.683), and other 'dopamine agonists', (p.677), also may antagonise the effects of antipsychotics, which adds weight to this theory.

1. Cutler NR, Jeste DV, Kaufmann CA, Karoum F, Schran HF, Wyatt RJ. Low dose bromocriptine: a study of acute effects in chronic medicated schizophrenics. *Prog Neuropsychopharmacol Biol Psychiatry* (1984) 8, 277–83.
2. Gattaz WF, Köllisch M. Bromocriptine in the treatment of neuroleptic-resistant schizophrenia. *Biol Psychiatry* (1986) 21, 519–21.
3. Kellner C, Harris P, Blumhardt C. Concurrent use of bromocriptine and fluphenazine. *J Clin Psychiatry* (1985) 46, 455.
4. Robbins RK, Kern PA, Thompson TL. Interactions between thioridazine and bromocriptine in a patient with a prolactin-secreting pituitary adenoma. *Am J Med* (1984) 76, 921–3.
5. Frye PE, Pariser SF, Kim MH, O'Shaughnessy RW. Bromocriptine associated with symptom exacerbation during neuroleptic treatment of schizoaffective schizophrenia. *J Clin Psychiatry* (1982) 43, 252–3.

Antipsychotics + Coffee or Tea

Tea and coffee can cause some drugs to precipitate out of solution *in vitro*, but so far there is no clinical evidence to show that this normally affects the bioavailability of the drugs nor that it has a detrimental effect on treatment.

Clinical evidence, mechanism, importance and management

A single report describes 2 patients whose schizophrenia was said to have been exacerbated by an increased consumption of tea and coffee.[1] Subsequent *in vitro* studies[2-6] showed that a number of drugs (**chlorpromazine, promethazine, fluphenazine, orphenadrine, promazine, prochlorperazine, trifluoperazine, thioridazine, loxapine, haloperidol, droperidol**) form a precipitate with tea or coffee due to the formation of a drug-tannin complex, which was thought might possibly lower the absorption of these drugs in the gut. Studies with *rats* also showed that tea abolished the cataleptic effects of **chlorpromazine**, which did not appear to be related to the presence of caffeine.[7] However, the drug-tannin complex gives up the drug into solution if it becomes acidified, as in the stomach.[6] Moreover, a clinical study of this interaction showed that the plasma levels of **chlorpromazine**, **fluphenazine**, **trifluoperazine** and **haloperidol** in a group of 16 patients were unaffected by the consumption of tea or coffee.[8] Their behaviour also remained unchanged.[8] A study in 12 healthy subjects also concluded that there was no significant decrease in plasma levels of a single 5-mg dose of **fluphenazine** given with either tea, coffee, or water.[9] So there appears to be little or no direct evidence that this physicochemical interaction is normally of any clinical importance.

1. Mikkelsen EJ. Caffeine and schizophrenia. *J Clin Psychiatry* (1978) 39, 732–5.
2. Kulhanek F, Linde OK, Meisenberg G. Precipitation of antipsychotic drugs in interaction with coffee or tea. *Lancet* (1979) ii, 1130.
3. Hirsch SR. Precipitation of antipsychotic drugs in interaction with tea or coffee. *Lancet* (1979) ii, 1130–1.
4. Lasswell WL, Wilkins JM, Weber SS. In vitro interaction of selected drugs with coffee, tea, and gallotannic acid. *Drug Nutr Interact* (1984) 2, 235–41.
5. Lasswell WL, Weber SS, Wilkins JM. *In vitro* interaction of neuroleptics and tricyclic antidepressants with coffee, tea, and gallotannic acid. *J Pharm Sci* (1984) 73, 1056–8.
6. Curry ML, Curry SH, Marroum PJ. Interaction of phenothiazine and related drugs and caffeinated beverages. *DICP Ann Pharmacother* (1991) 25, 437–8.
7. Cheeseman HJ, Neal MJ. Interaction of chlorpromazine with tea and coffee. *Br J Clin Pharmacol* (1981) 12, 165–9.
8. Bowen S, Taylor KM, Gibb IAM. Effect of coffee and tea on blood levels and efficacy of antipsychotic drugs. *Lancet* (1981) i, 1217–18.
9. Wallace SM, Suveges LG, Blackburn JL, Korchinski ED, Midha KK. Oral fluphenazine and tea and coffee drinking. *Lancet* (1981) ii, 691.

Antipsychotics + Lithium

Chlorpromazine levels can be reduced to subtherapeutic concentrations by lithium. The development of severe extrapyramidal adverse effects or severe neurotoxicity has been seen in one or more patients given lithium with various antipsychotics Sleepwalking has been described in some patients taking chlorpromazine-like drugs and lithium.

Clinical evidence

(a) Chlorpromazine

In a double-blind study in psychiatric patients it was found that chlorpromazine 400 to 800 mg daily, a dose that normally produced plasma levels of 100 to 300 nanograms/mL, only produced levels of 0 to 70 nanograms/mL when lithium carbonate was also given.[1]

Other studies confirm that normal therapeutic levels of lithium carbonate reduce plasma chlorpromazine levels.[2,3] The peak serum levels and AUC of chlorpromazine were reduced by 40% and 26%, respectively, in healthy subjects given lithium carbonate.[2]

A paranoid schizophrenic taking chlorpromazine 200 to 600 mg daily for 5 years with no extrapyramidal symptoms developed stiffness of his face, arms and legs, and parkinsonian tremor of both hands within one day of starting to take lithium 900 mg daily. His lithium blood level after 3 days was 0.5 mmol/L. He was later given lithium 1.8 g daily (blood level

1.17 mmol/L), chlorpromazine 200 mg daily and benzatropine 2 mg daily, which improved his condition, but he still complained of stiffness and had a persistent hand tremor.[4]

A number of other reports describe the emergence of severe extrapyramidal adverse effects when chlorpromazine was given with lithium.[5-7] Ventricular fibrillation, thought to be caused by chlorpromazine toxicity, occurred in a patient taking lithium when both drugs were suddenly withdrawn.[8] Severe neurotoxicity has also been seen in a handful of other patients taking lithium and chlorpromazine.[9,10]

(b) Haloperidol

A large-scale retrospective study of the literature over the period 1966 to 1996 using the Medline database identified 41 cases of neurotoxic adverse effects in 41 patients with low therapeutic concentrations of lithium. Of these patients, 10 were taking haloperidol.[9]

Another retrospective study using both Medline and the spontaneous reporting system of the FDA in the US, over the period 1969 to 1994, identified 237 cases of severe neurotoxicity involving lithium, of which 59 also involved the concurrent use of haloperidol.[11,12]

Other reports describe encephalopathic syndromes (lethargy, fever, tremulousness, confusion, extrapyramidal and cerebellar dysfunction),[13] neuromuscular symptoms, impaired consciousness and hyperthermia,[14] delirium, severe extrapyramidal symptoms and organic brain damage in patients taking haloperidol with lithium.[15-26] In one study it was found that of the 13 patients who were taking haloperidol, 5 developed neurotoxic reactions, and they were receiving higher doses of haloperidol (average dose was 59 mg) than the 8 patients who did not develop such symptoms (average dose was 34.9 mg).[27] The sudden emergence of extrapyramidal or other adverse effects with lithium and haloperidol has also been described in other studies.[9,15,28]

In contrast to the reports cited above, there are others describing successful and uneventful use.[13,29-32] A retrospective search of Danish hospital records found that 425 patients had taken both drugs and none of them had developed serious adverse reactions.[33]

A small rise in serum lithium levels occurs in the presence of haloperidol, but it is almost certainly of little or no clinical significance.[34]

(c) Other antipsychotics

A large-scale retrospective study of the literature over the period 1966 to 1996 using the Medline database identified 41 cases of neurotoxic adverse effects in 41 patients with low, therapeutic concentrations of lithium. Of these patients, 51.2% were also taking at least one antipsychotic drug.[9] Another retrospective study using both Medline and the spontaneous reporting system of the FDA in the US, over the period 1969 to 1994, identified 237 cases of severe neurotoxicity involving lithium, with 188 involving lithium with antipsychotics.[11,12] The sudden emergence of extrapyramidal or other adverse effects has also been described in other studies. The antipsychotics implicated in this interaction with lithium are **amoxapine**,[11,12] **bromperidol**,[11,12] **chlorprothixene**,[11,12] **clopenthixol**,[9] **clozapine**,[9,11,12] **flupentixol**,[15,28,35] **fluphenazine**,[9,11,12,15,28,36] **levomepromazine**,[9,11,12] **loxapine**,[11,12,37,38] **mesoridazine**,[11,12] **molindone**,[11,12] **perphenazine**,[11,12,28] **pipotiazine**,[39] **prochlorperazine**,[11,12] **sulpiride**,[40] **thioridazine**,[9,11,12,28,41,42] **tiotixene**,[9,11,12,16,28] **trifluoperazine**,[11,12] and **zuclopenthixol**.[9] Examples of some cases are cited in a little more detail below.

A study of 10 patients taking **fluphenazine**, **haloperidol** or **tiotixene** found that the addition of lithium worsened their extrapyramidal symptoms.[43] Neurotoxicity (tremor, rigidity, ataxia, tiredness, vomiting, confusion) attributed to an interaction between lithium and **fluphenazine** has been described in another patient. He previously took **haloperidol** and later took **chlorpromazine** with lithium, without problem.[44] Irreversible brain damage has been reported in a patient taking **fluphenazine decanoate** and lithium.[45] Severe neurotoxic complications (seizures, encephalopathy, delirium, abnormal EEGs) developed in 4 patients taking **thioridazine** 400 mg daily or more and lithium. Serum lithium levels remained below 1 mmol/L. Lithium and other phenothiazines had been taken by 3 of them for extended periods without problems, and the fourth subsequently took lithium and **fluphenazine** without problems.[46] In one study the concurrent use of lithium and **chlorpromazine**, **perphenazine**, or **thioridazine** was associated with sleep-walking episodes in 9% of patients.[47] **Somnolence**, confusion, delirium, creatinine phosphokinase elevation and fever occurred in a man taking lithium when **risperidone** was given.[48] A retrospective review of 39 patients with a diagnosis of neurotoxicity caused by treatment with lithium and an antipsychotic, found that the onset of symptoms varied from 24 hours to 3 months after taking the two drugs together, with an average delay of 12.7 days.[28]

A study in 8 patients found a fourfold increase in half life of **molindone** when given with lithium.[49]

Mechanism

Not understood. One suggestion to account for the reduced serum levels of chlorpromazine, which is based on *animal* studies,[50,51] is that chlorpromazine can be metabolised in the gut. Therefore, if lithium delays gastric emptying, more chlorpromazine will be metabolised before it reaches the circulation. Just why severe neurotoxicity and other adverse effects sometimes develop in patients taking lithium and antipsychotics is not understood. It is the subject of considerable discussion and debate.[9,11,12,52,53]

Importance and management

Information about the reduction in chlorpromazine levels caused by lithium is limited, but it would seem to be an established interaction of clinical importance. Serum chlorpromazine levels below 30 nanograms/mL have been shown to be ineffective, whereas clinical improvement is usually associated with levels within the 150 to 300 nanogram/mL range.[54] Thus a fall in levels to below 70 nanograms/mL, as described in one study, would be expected to result in a reduced therapeutic response to chlorpromazine. Therefore the effects of concurrent use should be closely monitored and the chlorpromazine dosage increased if necessary.

The development of severe neurotoxic or severe extrapyramidal adverse effects with combinations of antipsychotics and lithium appears to be uncommon and unexplained but be alert for any evidence of toxicity if lithium is given with any of these drugs. One recommendation is that the onset of neurological manifestations, such as excessive drowsiness or movement disorders, warrants electroencephalography without delay and withdrawal of the drugs, especially as irreversible effects have been seen. A review[55] suggests that the concurrent use of haloperidol seems to be safe if lithium levels are below 1 mmol/L. It is not known whether this also applies to other antipsychotics.

At the moment there seems to be no way of identifying the apparently small number of patients who are particularly at risk, but possible likely factors include a previous history of extrapyramidal reactions with antipsychotics and the use of large doses of the antipsychotic.

For interactions of **atypical antipsychotics** with lithium see 'amisulpride', (p.707); 'aripiprazole', (p.714); 'clozapine', (p.748); 'olanzapine', (p.756); 'quetiapine', (p.763); and 'ziprasidone', (p.770).

1. Kerzner B, Rivera-Calimlim L. Lithium and chlorpromazine (CPZ) interaction. *Clin Pharmacol Ther* (1976) 19, 109.
2. Rivera-Calimlim L, Kerzner B, Karch FE. Effect of lithium on plasma chlorpromazine levels. *Clin Pharmacol Ther* (1978) 23, 451–5.
3. Rivera-Calimlim L, Nasrallah H, Strauss J, Lasagna L. Clinical response and plasma levels: effect of dose, dosage schedules, and drug interactions on plasma chlorpromazine levels. *Am J Psychiatry* (1976) 133, 646–52.
4. Addonizio G. Rapid induction of extrapyramidal side effects with combined use of lithium and neuroleptics. *J Clin Psychopharmacol* (1985) 5, 296–8.
5. McGennis AJ. Hazards of lithium and neuroleptics in schizo-affective disorder. *Br J Psychiatry* (1983) 142, 99–100.
6. Yassa R. A case of lithium-chlorpromazine interaction. *J Clin Psychiatry* (1986) 47, 90–1.
7. Habib M, Khalil R, Le Pensec-Bertrand D, Ali-Cherif A, Bongrand MC, Crevat A. Syndrome neurologique persistant après traitement par les sels de lithium: toxicité de l'association lithium-neuroleptiques? *Rev Neurol (Paris)* (1986) 142, 1, 61–4.
8. Stevenson RN, Blanshard C, Patterson DLH. Ventricular fibrillation due to lithium withdrawal – an interaction with chlorpromazine? *Postgrad Med J* (1989) 65, 936–8.
9. Emilien G, Maloteaux JM. Lithium neurotoxicity at low therapeutic doses: hypotheses for causes and mechanism of action following a retrospective analysis of published case reports. *Acta Neurol Belg* (1996) 96, 281–93.
10. Boudouresques G, Poncet M, Ali Cherif A, Tafani B, Boudouresques. Encéphalopathie aiguë, au cours d'un traitement associant phenothiazine et lithium. Une nouvelle observation avec lithémie basse. *Nouv Presse Med* (1980) 9, 2580.
11. Goldman SA. Lithium and neuroleptics in combination: is there enhancement of neurotoxicity leading to permanent sequelae? *J Clin Pharmacol* (1996) 36, 951–62.
12. Goldman SA. FDA MedWatch Report: lithium and neuroleptics in combination: the spectrum of neurotoxicity. *Psychopharmacol Bull* (1996) 32, 299–309.
13. Cohen WJ, Cohen NH. Lithium carbonate, haloperidol, and irreversible brain damage. *JAMA* (1974) 230, 1283–7.
14. Thornton WE, Pray BJ. Lithium intoxication: a report of two cases. *Can Psychiatr Assoc J* (1975) 20, 281–2.
15. Kamlana SH, Kerry RJ, Khan IA. Lithium: some drug interactions. *Practitioner* (1980) 224, 1291–2.
16. Fetzer J, Kader G, Danahy S. Lithium encephalopathy: a clinical, psychiatric, and EEG evaluation. *Am J Psychiatry* (1981) 138, 1622–3.
17. Marhold J, Zimanová J, Lachman M, Král J, Vojtěchovský M. To the incompatibility of haloperidol with lithium salts. *Act Nerv Super (Praha)* (1974) 16, 199–200.
18. Wilson WH. Addition of lithium to haloperidol in non-affective antipsychotic non-responsive schizophrenia: a double blind, placebo controlled, parallel design clinical trial. *Psychopharmacology (Berl)* (1993) 111, 359–66.
19. Loudon JB, Waring H. Toxic reactions to lithium and haloperidol. *Lancet* (1976) ii, 1088.
20. Juhl RP, Tsuang MT, Perry PJ. Concomitant administration of haloperidol and lithium carbonate in acute mania. *Dis Nerv Syst* (1977) 38, 675.

21. Spring G, Frankel M. New data on lithium and haloperidol incompatibility. *Am J Psychiatry* (1981) 138, 818–21.
22. Menes C, Burra P, Hoaken PCS. Untoward effects following combined neuroleptic-lithium therapy. *Can J Psychiatry* (1980) 25, 573–6.
23. Keitner GI, Rahman S. Reversible neurotoxicity with combined lithium-haloperidol administration. *J Clin Psychopharmacol* (1984) 4, 104–5.
24. Thomas CJ. Brain damage with lithium/haloperidol. *Br J Psychiatry* (1979) 134, 552.
25. Thomas C, Tatham A, Jakubowski S. Lithium/haloperidol combinations and brain damage. *Lancet* (1982) i, 626.
26. Sandyk R, Hurwitz MD. Toxic irreversible encephalopathy induced by lithium carbonate and haloperidol. A report of 2 cases. *S Afr Med J* (1983) 64, 875–6.
27. Miller F, Menninger J. Correlation of neuroleptic dose and neurotoxicity in patients given lithium and a neuroleptic. *Hosp Community Psychiatry* (1987) 38, 1219–21.
28. Prakash R, Kelwala S, Ban TA. Neurotoxicity with combined administration of lithium and a neuroleptic. *Compr Psychiatry* (1982) 23, 567–71.
29. Garfinkel PE, Stancer HC, Persad E. A comparison of haloperidol, lithium carbonate and their combination in the treatment of mania. *J Affect Disord* (1980) 2, 279–88.
30. Baptista T. Lithium-neuroleptics combination and irreversible brain damage. *Acta Psychiatr Scand* (1986) 73, 111.
31. Goldney RD, Spence ND. Safety of the combination of lithium and neuroleptic drugs. *Am J Psychiatry* (1986) 143, 882–4.
32. Biederman J, Lerner Y, Belmaker H. Combination of lithium and haloperidol in schizo-affective disorder. A controlled study. *Arch Gen Psychiatry* (1979) 36, 327–33.
33. Baastrup PC, Hollnagel P, Sørensen R, Schou M. Adverse reactions in treatment with lithium carbonate and haloperidol. *JAMA* (1976) 236, 2645–6.
34. Schaffer CB, Batra K, Garvey MJ, Mungas DM, Schaffer LC. The effect of haloperidol on serum levels of lithium in adult manic patients. *Biol Psychiatry* (1984) 19, 1495–9.
35. West A. Adverse effects of lithium treatment. *BMJ* (1977) 2, 642.
36. Sachdev PS. Lithium potentiation of neuroleptic-related extrapyramidal side effects. *Am J Psychiatry* (1986) 143, 942.
37. de la Gandara J, Dominguez RA. Lithium and loxapine: a potential interaction. *J Clin Psychiatry* (1988) 49, 126.
38. Fuller MA, Sajatovic M. Neurotoxicity resulting from a combination of lithium and loxapine. *J Clin Psychiatry* (1989) 50, 187.
39. Abbar M, Petit P, Castelnau D, Blayac JP. Encéphalopathie toxique lors d'une association lithium-neuroleptiques. *Psychiatr Psychobiol* (1989) 4, 239–40.
40. Dinan TG, O'Keane V. Acute extrapyramidal reactions following lithium and sulpiride co-administration: two case reports. *Hum Psychopharmacol* (1991) 6, 67–9.
41. Bailine SH, Doft M. Neurotoxicity induced by combined lithium–thioridazine treatment. *Biol Psychiatry* (1986) 21, 834–7.
42. Cantor CH. Encephalopathy with lithium and thioridazine in combination. *Med J Aust* (1986) 144, 164–5.
43. Addonizio G, Roth SD, Stokes PE, Stoll PM. Increased extrapyramidal symptoms with addition of lithium to neuroleptics. *J Nerv Ment Dis* (1988) 176, 682–5.
44. Alevizos B. Toxic reactions to lithium and neuroleptics. *Br J Psychiatry* (1979) 135, 482.
45. Singh SV. Lithium carbonate/fluphenazine decanoate producing irreversible brain damage. *Lancet* (1982) ii, 278.
46. Spring GK. Neurotoxicity with combined use of lithium and thioridazine. *J Clin Psychiatry* (1979) 40, 135–8.
47. Charney DS, Kales A, Soldatos CR, Nelson JC. Somnambulistic-like episodes secondary to combined lithium-neuroleptic treatment. *Br J Psychiatry* (1979) 135, 418–24.
48. Swanson CL, Price WA, McEvoy JP. Effects of concomitant risperidone and lithium treatment. *Am J Psychiatry* (1995) 152, 1096.
49. Wolf ME, Mosnaim AD. Lithium and molindone interactions: pharmacokinetic studies. *Res Commun Psychol Psychiatr Behav* (1986) 11, 23–28.
50. Sundaresan PR, Rivera-Calimlim L. Distribution of chlorpromazine in the gastrointestinal tract of the rat and its effects on absorptive function. *J Pharmacol Exp Ther* (1975) 194, 593–602.
51. Curry SH, D'Mello A, Mould GP. Destruction of chlorpromazine during absorption in the rat *in vivo* and *in vitro*. *Br J Pharmacol* (1971) 42, 403–11.
52. Geisler A, Klysner R. Combined effect of lithium and flupenthixol on striatal adenylate cyclase. *Lancet* (1977) i, 430–1.
53. von Knorring L. Possible mechanisms for the presumed interaction between lithium and neuroleptics. *Hum Psychopharmacol* (1990) 5, 287–92.
54. Rivera-Calimlim L, Castañeda L, Lasagna L. Significance of plasma levels of chlorpromazine. *Clin Pharmacol Ther* (1973) 14, 144.
55. Batchelor DH, Lowe MR. Reported neurotoxicity with the lithium/haloperidol combination and other neuroleptics—a literature review. *Hum Psychopharmacol* (1990) 5, 275–80.

Antipsychotics + Orlistat

No changes in the plasma levels of haloperidol or clozapine were seen when orlistat was also given.

Clinical evidence, mechanism, importance and management

In a study, 8 patients who had experienced weight gain as a result of treatment with **haloperidol** (2), **clozapine** (2), clomipramine (3), desipramine (1), or carbamazepine (2), and were given orlistat 120 mg three times daily for 8 weeks. There was no significant changes in the plasma levels of the antipsychotic drugs, and steatorrhoea, which occurred in three patients, had no effect on their bioavailability.[1] Although an interaction appears to be unlikely, due to the small numbers involved in this study, it would be advisable to monitor patients for reduced absorption of antipsychotic drugs until more data is available.

1. Hilger E. Quiner S, Ginzel I, Walter H, Saria L, Barnas C. The effect of orlistat on plasma levels of psychotropic drugs in patients with long-term psychopharmacotherapy. *J Clin Psychopharmacol* (2002) 22, 68–70.

Antipsychotics + SSRIs

On the whole no significant adverse interactions appear to occur between the antipsychotics and the SSRIs. However, a number of case reports describe extrapyramidal adverse effects following the use of fluoxetine or paroxetine with an antipsychotic, and galactorrhoea and amenorrhoea developed in one patient given loxapine and fluvoxamine. Fluoxetine and fluvoxamine appear to raise haloperidol levels, which may increase adverse effects. Thioridazine levels are expected to be increased with fluoxetine, fluvoxamine, or paroxetine treatment with a risk of QT interval prolongation.

Clinical evidence, mechanism, importance and management

(a) Chlorpromazine

A study in schizophrenic patients found that over a 12-week period the serum levels of chlorpromazine were not significantly altered by **citalopram** 40 mg daily.[1]

(b) Cyamemazine

A study in patients taking cyamemazine found that **fluvoxamine** 150 mg daily had no effect on its serum levels, but the authors of the report also say that no firm conclusions should be drawn from this finding because the number of patients was too small.[2]

(c) Flupentixol

Parkinson-like symptoms developed in a patient taking amitriptyline and flupenthixol when **fluoxetine** was given.[3]

(d) Fluphenazine

A severe dystonic reaction (painful jaw tightness and throat 'closing up') occurred in a man taking **fluoxetine** 40 mg daily when he took fluphenazine 2.5 mg on two consecutive nights.[4]

(e) Haloperidol

1. Citalopram. A study in schizophrenic patients found that over a 12-week period the serum levels of haloperidol were not significantly altered by citalopram 40 mg daily.[1]

2. Escitalopram. Escitalopram is an inhibitor of the cytochrome P450 isoenzyme CYP2D6, and may therefore inhibit haloperidol metabolism The manufacturers say that consideration should be given to reducing the dose of haloperidol.[5]

3. Fluoxetine. A woman taking haloperidol 2 to 5 mg daily for 2 years with only occasional mild extrapyramidal symptoms began to experience severe extrapyramidal symptoms (tongue stiffness, parkinsonism, akathisia) shortly after starting to take fluoxetine 40 mg twice daily and was virtually incapacitated for 3 days. Both drugs were stopped and she recovered over a period of one week.[6] Three other patients developed movement disorders after receiving both drugs,[7-9]
In one case severe antimuscarinic adverse effects also occurred.[8]
A report describes 8 patients who had a 20% rise in plasma haloperidol levels when fluoxetine 20 mg daily was added. Although no overall increase in extrapyramidal effects was seen, one patient developed tremor, and another developed akathisia.[10] Similarly 15 patients showed an increase of nearly 30% in haloperidol plasma levels after fluoxetine was given, and 5 of 17 patients had aggravated parkinsonian symptoms.[11] Another report describes a more than 100% rise in plasma haloperidol levels accompanied by clinical improvement in 7 patients given fluoxetine 20 to 40 mg with haloperidol.[12]

4. Fluvoxamine. A study in 12 schizophrenic patients found that haloperidol levels were increased by 20%, 39%, and 60% by fluvoxamine 25, 75, and 150 mg daily, respectively, which suggested the extent of the interaction was related to the dose of fluvoxamine.[13] A study in 3 schizophrenic patients found that the addition of fluvoxamine caused their serum haloperidol levels to rise, and when the fluvoxamine was stopped the levels fell. This was not a formal pharmacokinetic study, but while taking fluvoxamine 150 to 200 mg daily the haloperidol serum levels of one patient rose from 17 to 38 nanograms/mL. The fluvoxamine was then stopped and 54 days later his serum haloperidol levels had fallen to 9 nanograms/mL. This patient became lethargic and showed worsening of all of the clinical and cognitive functions assessed while taking these drugs.[14] It should be noted that all three patients were also taking benzatropine (see 'Antimuscarinics + SSRIs', p.675). Another limited study also observed that fluvoxamine caused a rise in the serum levels of haloperidol.[2]

5. Paroxetine. In one study the sedative effects and impairment of psychomotor performance caused by haloperidol 3 mg were not increased by paroxetine 30 mg.[15]

6. Sertraline. In a randomised, placebo-controlled study, 21 healthy subjects were given a single 2-mg dose of haloperidol on days 2 to 25. On days 9 to 25 the subjects were given sertraline, increased over 7 days to 200 mg daily. All subjects took psychomotor tests on days 1, 2 and 25 to assess the effect of haloperidol. Their cognitive function was impaired for 6 to 8 hours after taking the haloperidol, but this effect had disappeared after 23 hours. Overall, sertraline did not appear to worsen the cognitive impairment caused by haloperidol.[16] Another study found similar pharmacodynamic results, and also found that the pharmacokinetics of haloperidol are unaffected by sertraline.[17] In contrast, a study in 16 hospitalised patients who were taking haloperidol found that the addition of sertraline 50 mg daily for 2 weeks resulted in an increase in plasma haloperidol concentrations, and a reduction in the plasma concentrations of the metabolite, reduced haloperidol.[18]

(f) Levomepromazine

A study in patients taking levomepromazine found that **fluvoxamine** 150 mg daily did not affect its serum levels, but the authors of the report also say that no firm conclusions should be drawn from this finding because the number of patients was too small.[2] A further study in 15 patients also found that there was no significant change in the pharmacokinetics of **fluvoxamine** when given with levomepromazine in doses of 5 to 25 mg daily. Additionally, patients in this study found that the levomepromazine counteracted the insomnia caused by **fluvoxamine**.[19]

A study in three groups of 8 healthy subjects taking **citalopram** 40 mg daily for 10 days found that a single 50-mg oral dose of levomepromazine increased the initial steady-state levels of the primary metabolite of **citalopram** (desmethylcitalopram) by 10 to 20%, which was not considered to be clinically significant.[20]

A study in schizophrenic patients found that over a 12-week period the serum levels of levomepromazine were not significantly altered by **citalopram** 40 mg daily.[1]

(g) Loxapine

A 38-year-old woman developed amenorrhoea, followed shortly by galactorrhoea, about 6 weeks after starting to take fluvoxamine and loxapine. The galactorrhoea resolved within 3 weeks of stopping the **fluvoxamine**, and menstruation occurred one week later. Her prolactin levels were found to be 80 micrograms/L (normal 4 to 30 micrograms/L).[21]

(h) Metopimazine

A French regional pharmacovigilance centre reported 37 cases of extrapyramidal adverse effects linked to concurrent use of an SSRI and a neuroleptic. In 2 cases **metopimazine** was given.[22]

(i) Molindone

An elderly woman taking molindone 10 mg twice daily developed severe and disabling extrapyramidal symptoms (severe bradykinesia, tremor, inability to feed herself, delirium) within about 2 weeks of starting **paroxetine** 10 mg daily. The symptoms resolved when molindone was stopped, and no problems occurred when **fluoxetine** alone was started.[23]

(j) Pericyazine

A New Zealand study describes a patient who developed extrapyramidal symptoms when given pericyazine and **fluoxetine**.[7]

(k) Perphenazine

1. Citalopram. A study in schizophrenic patients found that over a 12-week period the serum levels of perphenazine were not significantly altered by citalopram 40 mg daily.[1]

2. Fluoxetine. The combination of perphenazine and fluoxetine was found to be effective in the treatment of psychotic depression in 30 patients, and the adverse effects (which included dry mouth, blurred vision, constipation, tremor or rigidity, orthostasis and hypotension) were thought to be easier to tolerate than an antipsychotic with a tricyclic antidepressant.[24] However, one woman developed marked extrapyramidal symptoms within 2 weeks of starting perphenazine 4 mg twice daily and fluoxetine 20 mg daily.[25]

3. Paroxetine. The effects of a single 100-microgram/kg oral dose of perphenazine on the performance of psychomotor tests were assessed after 4, 6, 8 and 10 hours in 5 subjects. The tests were then repeated after the subjects also took paroxetine 20 mg daily for 10 days. The scores for these tests were worsened by the perphenazine when compared with a placebo and further worsened by the presence of the paroxetine. In addition to over-sedation and impairment of the performance of psychomotor tests and memory, 2 of the subjects developed akathisia 10 hours after taking both drugs. The AUC of the perphenazine was increased sevenfold and the maximum plasma levels sixfold.[26]

(l) Pimozide

See 'Pimozide + SSRIs', p.762.

(m) Sulpiride

Parkinson-like symptoms developed in a patient taking sulpiride and maprotiline when **fluoxetine** was also given.[27]

(n) Thioridazine

A study in schizophrenic patients found that over a 12-week period the serum levels of thioridazine were not significantly altered by **citalopram** 40 mg daily.[1]

A study in 10 schizophrenic patients found that when **fluvoxamine** 50 mg daily was added to established treatment with thioridazine 30 to 200 mg daily, thioridazine plasma levels were increased by 225%. There were no reported changes in either clinical status or adverse effects.[28]

(o) Tiotixene

A study in 10 healthy subjects found that **paroxetine** 20 mg daily for 3 days did not significantly affect the pharmacokinetics of a single 20-mg dose of tiotixene.[29]

(p) Trifluoperazine

A New Zealand study describes a patient who developed extrapyramidal symptoms when given trifluoperazine and **fluoxetine**.[7]

(q) Zuclopenthixol

A study in schizophrenic patients found that over a 12-week period the serum levels of zuclopenthixol were not significantly altered by **citalopram** 40 mg daily.[1]

Mechanism

Movement disorders and raised antipsychotic serum levels seem most common with fluoxetine and paroxetine, possibly because they inhibit the metabolism of some antipsychotics by the cytochrome P450 isoenzyme CYP2D6.[26] However, the movement disorders may just be a result of the additive adverse effects of antipsychotics and SSRIs. Fluoxetine alone has been shown to occasionally cause movement disorders.[7,30]

Galactorrhoea is a known adverse effect of loxapine, but just why fluvoxamine apparently increased this effect is not understood.[21]

Importance and management

On the whole significant interactions between the antipsychotics and SSRIs appear rare (although see thioridazine, below). The combination can be useful and so the isolated cases of extrapyramidal adverse effects should not prevent concurrent use. However, if extrapyramidal effects become troublesome bear this interaction in mind as a possible cause. The significance of the rise in haloperidol levels caused by fluoxetine and fluvoxamine is unclear, be aware that haloperidol adverse effects may be increased in some patients and consider reducing the haloperidol dose if problems occur. The rise in perphenazine levels caused by paroxetine seems to result in a greater number of more serious adverse effects and so consideration should be given to reducing the dose of perphenazine if paroxetine is started. Citalopram may be a suitable alternative as it does not appear to affect perphenazine levels.

Note that, although the studies with thioridazine did not appear to show any clinically significant interaction the US manufacturers of fluoxetine,[31] fluvoxamine,[32] and paroxetine,[33] contraindicate the concurrent use of thioridazine as they suggest that its metabolism (by CYP2D6) may be inhibited by these SSRIs, leading to raised levels and the risk of QT prolongation The use of thioridazine is also contraindicated for 5 weeks after fluoxetine has been stopped.[31] Similarly, it has been suggested that the dose of thioridazine may need to be reduced when it is given with escitalopram.[5]

SSRI antidepressants may lower the seizure threshold, and therefore concomitant use with other drugs, which can also lower the seizure threshold, such as phenothiazines, should be undertaken with caution.

1. Syvälahti EKG, Taiminen T, Saarijärvi S, Lehto H, Niemi H, Ahola V, Dahl M-L, Salokangas RKR. Citalopram causes no significant alterations in plasma neuroleptic levels in schizophrenic patients. *J Int Med Res* (1997) 25, 24–32.
2. Vandel S, Bertschy G, Baumann P, Bouquet S, Bonin B, Francois T, Sechter D, Bizouard P. Fluvoxamine and fluoxetine: Interaction studies with amitriptyline, clomipramine and neuroleptics in phenotyped patients. *Pharmacol Res* (1995) 31, 347–53.
3. Touw DJ, Gernaat HBPE, van der Woude J. Parkinsonisme na toevoeging van fluoxetine aan behandeling met neuroleptica of carbamazepine. *Ned Tijdschr Geneeskd* (1992) 136, 332–4.
4. Ketai R. Interaction between fluoxetine and neuroleptics. *Am J Psychiatry* (1993) 150, 836–7.
5. Cipralex (Escitalopram oxalate). Lundbeck Ltd. UK Summary of product characteristics, December 2005.
6. Tate JL. Extrapyramidal symptoms in a patient taking haloperidol and fluoxetine. *Am J Psychiatry* (1989) 146, 399–400.
7. Coulter DM, Pillans PI. Fluoxetine and extrapyramidal side effects. *Am J Psychiatry* (1995) 152, 122–5.
8. Benazzi F. Urinary retention with fluoxetine–haloperidol combination in a young patient. *Can J Psychiatry* (1996) 41, 606–7.
9. D'Souza DC, Bennett A, Abi-Dargham A, Krystal JH. Precipitation of a psychoneuromotor syndrome by fluoxetine in a haloperidol-treated schizophrenic patient. *J Clin Psychopharmacol* (1994) 14, 361–3.
10. Goff DC, Midha KK, Brotman AW, Waites M, Baldessarini RJ. Elevation of plasma concentrations of haloperidol after the addition of fluoxetine. *Am J Psychiatry* (1991) 148, 790–2.
11. Shim J-C, Kelly DL, Kim Y-H, Yoon Y-R, Park J-H, Shin J-G, Conley RR. Fluoxetine augmentation of haloperidol in chronic schizophrenia. *J Clin Psychopharmacol* (2003) 23, 520–2.
12. Viala A, Aymard N, Leyris A, Caroli F. Corrélations pharmacocliniques lors de l'administration de fluoxétine chez des patients schizophrènes déprimés traités par halopéridol décanoate. *Therapie* (1996) 51, 19–25.
13. Yasui-Furukori N, Kondo T, Mihara K, Inoue Y, Kaneko S. Fluvoxamine dose-dependent interaction with haloperidol and the effects on negative symptoms in schizophrenia. *Psychopharmacology (Berl)* (2004) 171, 223–7.
14. Daniel DG, Randolph C, Jaskiw G, Handel S, Williams T, Abi-Dargham A, Shoaf S, Egan M, Elkashef A, Liboff S, Linnoila M. Coadministration of fluvoxamine increases serum concentrations of haloperidol. *J Clin Psychopharmacol* (1994) 14, 340–3.
15. Cooper SM, Jackson D, Loudon JM, McClelland GR, Raptopoulos P. The psychomotor effects of paroxetine alone and in combination with haloperidol, amylobarbitone, oxazepam, or alcohol. *Acta Psychiatr Scand* (1989) 80 (Suppl 350), 53–5.
16. Williams SA, Wesnes K, Oliver SD, Rapeport WG. Absence of effect of sertraline on time-based sensitization of cognitive impairment with haloperidol. *J Clin Psychiatry* (1996) 57 (Suppl 1), 7–11.
17. Lee MS, Kim YK, Lee SK, Suh KY. A double-blind study of adjunctive sertraline in haloperidol-stabilized patients with chronic schizophrenia. *J Clin Psychopharmacol* (1998) 18, 399–403.
18. Lee M-S, Han C-S, You Y-W, Kim S-H. Co-administration of sertraline and haloperidol. *Psychiatry Clin Neurosci* (1998) 52, S193–8.
19. Yoshimura R, Ueda N, Nakamura J. Low dosage of levomepromazine did not increase plasma concentrations of fluvoxamine. *Int Clin Psychopharmacol* (2000) 15, 233–5.
20. Gram LF, Hansen MG, Sindrup SH, Brøsen K, Poulsen JH, Aaes-Jørgensen T, Overø KF. Citalopram: interaction studies with levomepromazine, imipramine and lithium. *Ther Drug Monit* (1993) 15, 18–24.
21. Jeffries J, Bezchlibnyk-Butler K, Remington G. Amenorrhea and galactorrhea associated with fluvoxamine in a loxapine-treated patient. *J Clin Psychopharmacol* (1992) 12, 296–7.
22. Anon. Extrapyramidal reactions to SSRI antidepressant + neuroleptic combinations. *Prescrire Int* (2004) 13, 57.
23. Malek-Ahmadi P, Allen SA. Paroxetine-molindone interaction. *J Clin Psychiatry* (1995) 56, 82–3.
24. Rothchild AJ, Samson JA, Bessette MP, Carter-Campbell JT. Efficacy of the combination of fluoxetine and perphenazine in the treatment of psychotic depression. *J Clin Psychiatry* (1993) 54, 338–42.
25. Lock JD, Gwirtsman HE, Targ EF. Possible adverse drug interactions between fluoxetine and other psychotropics. *J Clin Psychopharmacol* (1990) 10, 383–4.
26. Özdemir V, Naranjo CA, Herrmann N, Reed K, Sellers EM, Kalow W. Paroxetine potentiates the central nervous system side effects of perphenazine: contribution of cytochrome P4502D6 inhibition in vivo. *Clin Pharmacol Ther* (1997) 62, 334–47.
27. Touw DJ, Gernaat HBPE, van der Woude J. Parkinsonisme na toevoeging van fluoxetine aan behandeling met neuroleptica of carbamazepine. *Ned Tijdschr Geneeskd* (1992) 136, 332–3.
28. Carrillo JA, Ramos SI, Herraiz AG, Llerena A, Agundez JAG, Berecz R, Duran M, Benítez J. Pharmacokinetic interaction of fluvoxamine and thioridazine in schizophrenic patients. *J Clin Psychopharmacol* (1999) 19, 494–9.
29. Guthrie SK, Hariharan M, Kumar AA, Bader G, Tandon R. The effect of paroxetine on thiothixene pharmacokinetics. *J Clin Pharm Ther* (1997) 22, 221–6.
30. Bouchard RH, Pourcher E, Vincent P. Fluoxetine and extrapyramidal side effects. *Am J Psychiatry* (1989) 146, 1352–3.
31. Prozac (Fluoxetine hydrochloride). Eli Lilly and Company. US Prescribing information, May 2007.
32. Fluvoxamine maleate tablets. Apotex Corp. US Prescribing information, January 2001.
33. Paxil (Paroxetine hydrochloride). GlaxoSmithKline. US Prescribing information, July 2006.

Antipsychotics + Tobacco or Cannabis

Smokers of tobacco or cannabis may possibly need larger doses of chlorpromazine, fluphenazine, haloperidol or tiotixene than non-smokers.

Clinical evidence

(a) Chlorpromazine

A comparative study found that the frequency of drowsiness in 403 patients taking chlorpromazine was 16% in non-smokers, 11% in light smokers, and 3% in heavy smokers (more than 20 cigarettes daily).[1] Another report describes a patient taking chlorpromazine who experienced increased sedation and dizziness and higher plasma chlorpromazine levels when he gave up smoking.[2] A study in 31 patients found that the clearance of chlorpromazine was increased by 38% by tobacco smoking, by 50% by cannabis smoking, and by 107% when both tobacco and cannabis were smoked.[3]

(b) Fluphenazine

A retrospective study in 40 psychiatric inpatients found that the plasma fluphenazine levels of non-smokers were more than double those of smokers (1.83 nanograms/mL compared with 0.89 nanograms/mL) when they were given fluphenazine hydrochloride by mouth. The clearance of both oral and intramuscular fluphenazine was 1.67-fold and 2.33-fold greater, respectively, in the smokers than in the non-smokers.[4] No behavioural differences were seen.[4]

(c) Haloperidol

Steady-state haloperidol levels were found to be lower in a group of 23 cigarette smokers than in another group of 27 non-smokers (16.83 nanograms/mL compared with 28.8 nanograms/mL) and the clearance was increased by 44%.[5] Other studies have broadly confirmed these findings.[6,7]

(d) Tiotixene

Tobacco smoking increased the clearance of tiotixene in patients taking enzyme inhibitors or no other drugs, but not in patients taking enzyme inducers. Those who smoked were found to need on average 45% more tiotixene than the non-smokers taking no other interacting drugs.[8]

Mechanism

Not established. The probable reason is that some of the components of tobacco smoke act as enzyme inducers, which increase the rate at which the liver metabolises these antipsychotics, thereby reducing their serum levels and clinical effects.

Importance and management

Established interactions but of uncertain clinical importance. Be alert for the need to increase the dosages of these antipsychotics in patients who smoke, and reduce the dosages if smoking is stopped.

1. Swett C. Drowsiness due to chlorpromazine in relation to cigarette smoking: a report from the Boston Collaborative Drug Surveillance Program. *Arch Gen Psychiatry* (1974) 31, 211–13.
2. Stimmel GL, Falloon IRH. Chlorpromazine plasma levels, adverse effects, and tobacco smoking: case report. *J Clin Psychiatry* (1983) 44, 420–2.
3. Chetty M, Miller R, Moodley SV. Smoking and body weight influence the clearance of chlorpromazine. *Eur J Clin Pharmacol* (1994) 46, 523–6.
4. Ereshefsky L, Jann MW, Saklad SR, Davis CM, Richards AL, Burch NR. Effects of smoking on fluphenazine clearance in psychiatric inpatients. *Biol Psychiatry* (1985) 20, 329–32.
5. Jann MW, Saklad SR, Ereshefsky L, Richards AL, Harrington CA, Davis CM. Effects of smoking on haloperidol and reduced haloperidol plasma concentrations and haloperidol clearance. *Psychopharmacology (Berl)* (1986) 90, 468–70.
6. Perry PJ, Miller DD, Arndt SV, Smith DA, Holman TL. Haloperidol dosing requirements: the contribution of smoking and nonlinear pharmacokinetics. *J Clin Psychopharmacol* (1993) 13, 46–51.
7. Pan L, Vander Stichele R, Rosseel MT, Berlo JA, De Schepper N, Belpaire FM. Effects of smoking, CYP2D6 genotype, and concomitant drug intake on the steady state plasma concentrations of haloperidol and reduced haloperidol in schizophrenic inpatients. *Ther Drug Monit* (1999) 21, 489–97.
8. Ereshefsky L, Saklad SR, Watanabe MD, Davis CM, Jann MW. Thiothixene pharmacokinetic interactions: a study of hepatic enzyme inducers, clearance inhibitors, and demographic variables. *J Clin Psychopharmacol* (1991) 11, 296–301.

Aripiprazole + Lithium

Lithium does not affect the pharmacokinetics of aripiprazole to a clinically significant extent.

Clinical evidence, mechanism, importance and management

Aripiprazole 30 mg daily was given to 7 healthy subjects for 5 weeks, with lithium carbonate slow-release tablets 1.2 to 1.8 g daily (to give a plasma level of 1 to 1.4 mmol/L) for weeks 3 to 5 of the study. The mean AUC and maximum plasma concentrations of aripiprazole were found to increase by 15% and 19%, respectively, but these changes were not considered to be clinically significant.[1]

1. Citrome L, Josiassen R, Bark N, Salazar DE, Mallikaarjun S. Pharmacokinetics of aripiprazole and concomitant lithium and valproate. *J Clin Pharmacol* (2005) 45, 89–93.

Aripiprazole + Miscellaneous

Aripiprazole plasma levels are increased by inhibitors, and decreased by inducers, of CYP3A4. Quinidine increases aripiprazole levels. The manufacturers advise caution with drugs that can prolong the QT interval. Food and famotidine do not have a clinically relevant effect on the pharmacokinetics of aripiprazole, and aripiprazole does not affect the pharmacokinetics of dextromethorphan, omeprazole, and warfarin.

Clinical evidence, mechanism, importance and management

(a) CYP3A4 inducers

The manufacturers report that **carbamazepine** reduced the mean maximum plasma concentration and AUC of aripiprazole 30 mg by 68% and 73%, respectively. They recommend that the dose of aripiprazole is doubled when taken with **carbamazepine**.[1,2] Other potent inducers of CYP3A4, such as **efavirenz**, **nevirapine**, **phenytoin**, **phenobarbital**, **primidone**, **rifabutin**, **rifampicin** and **St John's wort** are expected to have similar effects and an increase in the dose of aripiprazole may also be necessary if these drugs are given.[1]

(b) CYP3A4 inhibitors

Ketoconazole, an inhibitor of CYP3A4, increased the AUC and maximum plasma concentration of aripiprazole by 63% and 37%, respectively.[1,2] Other potent inhibitors of CYP3A4, such as **itraconazole** and **protease inhibitors** would be expected to produce similar or greater increases in aripiprazole levels, and the manufacturers recommend that the dose of aripiprazole should be halved with these drugs. The dose of aripiprazole should also be increased again if the drug is stopped. Moderate inhibitors of CYP3A4, such as diltiazem, may produce more modest increases in aripiprazole levels,[1] and patients should be closely monitored for signs of aripiprazole toxicity, although an initial dose reduction of aripiprazole may not be required.

(c) Famotidine

Famotidine reduces the rate of absorption of aripiprazole but this effect is not clinically significant.[1]

(d) Food

A study in 39 healthy subjects who received 15 mg aripiprazole either after fasting, or 5 minutes after a high-fat breakfast, found no significant changes in the pharmacokinetics of aripiprazole.[3]

(e) QT prolongation

The manufacturers report that in clinical studies the incidence of QT prolongation with aripiprazole was comparable to placebo. Nevertheless, they recommend caution when prescribing aripiprazole with other drugs that may prolong the QT interval or cause electrolyte disturbances, see 'drugs that prolong the QT interval', (p.257).

(f) Quinidine

Quinidine, an inhibitor of CYP2D6, has been found to increase the AUC of aripiprazole by 107%, although the maximum concentration was unchanged. It is recommended that the dose of aripiprazole is halved if given concomitantly with quinidine.[1,2]

(g) Miscellaneous

Aripiprazole 10 to 30 mg daily had no significant effects on the metabolism of **dextromethorphan** (CYP2D6 and CYP3A4 substrate), **warfarin** (CYP2C9 substrate) and **omeprazole** (CYP2C19 substrate). Aripiprazole is not expected to affect CYP1A2-mediated metabolism. The manufacturers therefore conclude that aripiprazole is unlikely to have clinically significant interactions with drugs that are substrates for these isoenzymes.[1]

1. Abilify (Aripiprazole). Bristol-Myers Squibb Pharmaceuticals Ltd. UK Summary of product characteristics, June 2007.
2. Abilify (Aripiprazole). Bristol-Myers Squibb Company. US Prescribing information, November 2006.
3. Mallikaarjun S, Riesgo Y, Salazar F, Bramer S, Xie J, Weston I. Time of dosing and food effect on aripiprazole pharmacokinetics. *Eur Neuropsychopharmacol* (2003) S332.

Aripiprazole + SSRIs and related antidepressants

Fluoxetine and probably paroxetine may cause clinically significant increases in aripiprazole levels. The concurrent use of aripiprazole with SSRIs or venlafaxine has led to adverse effects such as the neuroleptic malignant syndrome and extrapyramidal symptoms.

Clinical evidence, mechanism, importance and management

A study analysing routing samples sent for aripiprazole monitoring noted that the plasma levels of aripiprazole were 44% higher in 5 patients taking inhibitors of the cytochrome P450 isoenzyme CYP2D6, which included 2 patients taking **fluoxetine**. However, note that they also included levomepromazine in this group, which is not known to be a potent CYP2D6 inhibitor, and may therefore have reduced the true increase seen with **fluoxetine**. Further, in 6 patients taking **escitalopram** or **citalopram** the plasma levels of aripiprazole were found to be 39% and 34% higher, respectively, when compared with patients taking aripiprazole alone.[1]

The manufacturers suggest that potent inhibitors of CYP2D6, such as **fluoxetine** and **paroxetine** would be expected to increase aripiprazole levels, and they recommend that the dose of aripiprazole should be halved if these drugs are given.[2,3] The UK manufacturer suggests that weaker inhibitors of this isoenzyme (they name **escitalopram**) would only be expected to cause modest increases in aripiprazole levels, and therefore no dosage adjustment would expected to be required.[2]

Two case reports of extrapyramidal effects in association with aripiprazole treatment have been attributed to an interaction with antidepressants. In the first case the patient, who was taking **venlafaxine**, trazodone and clonazepam, developed parkinsonian symptoms a few days after starting to take aripiprazole 15 mg daily. Her symptoms resolved on stopping the aripiprazole. The second patient was taking **sertraline** 200 mg daily, and after starting to take aripiprazole 10 mg daily he developed akathisia. This did not respond to a reduction of aripiprazole dose, but gradually resolved when the aripiprazole was withdrawn.[4] Neuroleptic malignant syndrome developed in a patient within 2 weeks of starting aripiprazole 30 mg daily and **fluoxetine** 20 mg daily. The patient had stopped taking the aripiprazole 2 days before admission, fluoxetine was stopped on admission, and he recovered within one week with symptomatic treatment. The authors suggested that **fluoxetine** may have increased the risk of this syndrome developing by raising aripiprazole levels.[5]

The concurrent use of aripiprazole and SSRIs can be useful, but it is important to remember to adjust the dose if **paroxetine** or **fluoxetine** are started or stopped, and be aware that, rarely, adverse effects such as extrapyramidal symptoms and the neuroleptic malignant syndrome may develop.

1. Castberg I, Spigset O. Effects of comedication on the serum levels of aripiprazole: evidence from routine therapeutic drug monitoring service. *Pharmacopsychiatry* (2007) 40, 107–10.
2. Abilify (Aripiprazole). Bristol-Myers Squibb Pharmaceuticals Ltd. UK Summary of product characteristics, June 2007.
3. Abilify (Aripiprazole). Bristol-Myers Squibb Company. US Prescribing information, November 2006.
4. Cohen ST, Rulf D, Pies R. Extrapyramidal side effects associated with aripiprazole coprescription in 2 patients. *J Clin Psychiatry* (2005) 66, 135–6.
5. Duggal HS, Kithas J. Possible neuroleptic malignant syndrome with aripiprazole and fluoxetine. *Am J Psychiatry* (2005) 162, 397–8.

Aripiprazole + Valproate

Valproate causes a reduction in aripiprazole levels which is not considered to be clinically significant.

Clinical evidence, mechanism, importance and management

Aripiprazole 30 mg daily was given to 6 healthy subjects for 5 weeks, with **valproate semisodium (divalproex sodium)** daily in doses to achieve a serum valproate level of 50 to 125 mg/L, for weeks 3 to 5 of the study. The mean AUC and maximum plasma concentrations of aripiprazole were found to decrease by 24% and 26%, respectively, and the time to maximum aripiprazole levels was extended by 2 hours. Since aripiprazole and valproate share the same protein binding sites, it was considered likely that the valproate displaced bound aripiprazole leading to increased oral clearance. The change in levels was not considered to be clinically significant.[1]

1. Citrome L, Josiassen R, Bark N, Salazar DE, Mallikaarjun S. Pharmacokinetics of aripiprazole and concomitant lithium and valproate. *J Clin Pharmacol* (2005) 45, 89–93.

Barbiturates + Miscellaneous

Miconazole increases serum pentobarbital levels. The hypnotic effects of pentobarbital are reduced or abolished by the concurrent use of caffeine.

Clinical evidence, mechanism, importance and management

(a) Caffeine

In a placebo-controlled study caffeine 250 mg and **pentobarbital** 100 mg were given together and alone to 34 patients. It was found that the hypnotic effects of the **pentobarbital** given with caffeine were reduced, and indistinguishable from those of the placebo.[1] Caffeine stimulates the cerebral cortex and impairs sleep, whereas pentobarbital depresses the cortex and promotes sleep. These mutually opposing actions would seem to explain this interaction. This seems to be only direct study of this interaction, but it is well supported by common experience and the numerous studies of the properties of each of these compounds. Patients given barbiturate hypnotics should avoid caffeine-containing drinks (tea, coffee, cola drinks, etc.) or analgesics at or near bedtime if the hypnotic is to be effective.

(b) Miconazole

High-dose intravenous **pentobarbital** was given to 5 patients in intensive care to decrease intracranial pressure. When miconazole was also given, all patients had marked rises in plasma **pentobarbital** levels, and a 50 to 90% reduction in total plasma clearance. This is thought to occur because miconazole inhibits the liver enzymes concerned with the metabolism of the barbiturate, thereby reducing its clearance from the body.[2] It would be prudent to monitor the effects of concurrent use to ensure that plasma barbiturate levels do not rise too high. Note that miconazole oral gel can be absorbed in sufficient amounts to potentially interact. There seems to be no information about other barbiturates.

1. Forrest WH, Bellville JW, Brown BW. The interaction of caffeine with pentobarbital as a nighttime hypnotic. *Anesthesiology* (1972) 36, 37–41.
2. Heinemeyer G, Roots I, Schulz H, Dennhardt R. Hemmung der Pentobarbital-Elimination durch Miconazol bei Intesivtherapie des erhöhten intracraniellen Druckes. *Intensivmed* (1985) 22, 164–7.

Benzodiazepines + Acetazolamide

Although acetazolamide can be used to treat acute mountain sickness at very high altitudes, a case report suggests that it may potentiate the respiratory depressant effects of benzodiazepines such as triazolam. Acetazolamide did not improve symptoms of sleep apnoea worsened by flurazepam.

Clinical evidence, mechanism, importance and management

A study in elderly subjects found that sleep apnoea worsened in 4 of 10 subjects given a single 30-mg dose of **flurazepam** at night. These 4 subjects were then pretreated with acetazolamide 500 mg twice daily for 3 days, as acetazolamide has been found to improve sleep apnoea. A further dose of **flurazepam** 30 mg was given on the fourth night.[1] Treatment with acetazolamide did not block the benzodiazepine-associated increase of sleep apnoea in these subjects, possibly because the acetazolamide treatment period was not long enough.[1]

Acetazolamide is sometimes used by climbers at very high altitudes as a prophylactic against acute mountain sickness. Benzodiazepines are used in this situation to treat insomnia, which is common at high altitude. Benzodiazepines are believed to depress breathing because they reduce the normal respiratory response to hypoxia. This was demonstrated by a Japanese climber in the Himalayas who took acetazolamide 500 mg daily and **triazolam** 500 micrograms, and then needed to be reminded to hyperventilate in order to relieve his hypoxia while returning from a climb. The acetazolamide did not prevent, and may possibly have increased, the central ventilatory depression of the **triazolam**, possibly by increasing its delivery to the brain. The authors of the report advise against taking these two drugs together at high altitudes,[2] thus confirming a previous warning about the risks of taking benzodiazepines at high altitude.[3]

1. Guilleminault C, Silvestri R, Mondini S, Coburn S. Aging and sleep apnea: action of benzodiazepine, acetazolamide, alcohol, and sleep deprivation in a healthy elderly group. *J Gerontol* (1984) 39, 655–61.
2. Masuyama S, Hirata K, Saito A. 'Ondine's curse': side effect of acetazolamide? *Am J Med* (1989) 86, 637.
3. Sutton JR, Powles ACP, Gray GW, Houston CS. Insomnia, sedation, and high altitude cerebral oedema. *Lancet* (1979) i, 165.

Benzodiazepines + Alosetron

Alosetron 1 mg twice daily for 2 days had no significant effect on the pharmacokinetics of a single 1-mg dose of alprazolam in 12 healthy subjects. No increase in adverse effects was noted with the combination.[1] No special precautions therefore seem necessary on concurrent use.

1. D'Souza DL, Levasseur LM, Nezamis J, Robbins DK, Simms L, Koch KM. Effect of alosetron on the pharmacokinetics of alprazolam. *J Clin Pharmacol* (2001) 41, 452–4.

Benzodiazepines + Amiodarone

An isolated report describes clonazepam toxicity, which was attributed to the concurrent use of amiodarone.

Clinical evidence, mechanism, importance and management

A 78-year-old man with congestive heart failure and coronary artery disease was taking furosemide, potassium, and calcium supplements, a multivitamin preparation, and amiodarone 200 mg daily for sustained ventricular tachycardia. Two months after **clonazepam** 500 micrograms at night was added to treat restless leg syndrome he developed slurred speech, confusion, difficulty in walking, dry mouth and urinary incontinence. This was interpreted as **clonazepam** toxicity. The problems cleared when the **clonazepam** was stopped. The authors of the report suggest that the amiodarone may have inhibited the oxidative metabolism of the **clonazepam** by the liver, thereby allowing it to accumulate. They also point out that this patient may have been more sensitive to these effects because of a degree of hypothyroidism caused by the amiodarone. Hypothyroidism is known to decrease the metabolism of drugs that undergo oxidative metabolism by the liver.[1]

This is an unconfirmed and isolated case of doubtful general importance.

1. Witt DM, Ellsworth AJ, Leversee JH. Amiodarone–clonazepam interaction. *Ann Pharmacother* (1993) 27, 1463–4.

Benzodiazepines + Antacids

Although antacids can moderately change the rate of absorption of chlordiazepoxide, clorazepate and diazepam, no adverse interaction of clinical importance has been reported.

Clinical evidence

In a three-period study 10 healthy subjects were given **clorazepate** 7.5 mg at night, with either water, or with ***Maalox*** 30 mL, or with ***Maalox*** 30 mL three times daily before meals. The mean steady-state serum levels of the active metabolite of clorazepate, desmethyldiazepam, were not affected by ***Maalox***, although they varied widely between individuals.[1] This is in line with another report,[2] but contrasts with a single-dose study, in which the peak plasma concentration of desmethyldiazepam was delayed and reduced by about one-third by the use of ***Maalox***. The AUC_{0-48} was reduced by about 10%.[3]

In another study the absorption of a single dose of **chlordiazepoxide** was delayed by ***Maalox***, though the total amount of drug absorbed was not significantly affected.[4] Similar results have been found with **diazepam** and aluminium hydroxide-containing antacids.[5] Another study found that 40 mL of **Aluminium Hydroxide Gel BP** and 30 mL of **sodium citrate** (0.3 mmol/L) marginally hastened the sedative effect of **diazepam** 10 mg when used as an oral premedication before minor surgery. **Magnesium Trisilicate Mixture BPC** 30 mL tended to delay sedation.[6]

Mechanism

The delay in the absorption of chlordiazepoxide and diazepam is attributed to the effect of the antacid on gastric emptying. Clorazepate on the other hand is a prodrug, which needs acid conditions in the stomach for conversion by hydrolysis and decarboxylation to its active form. Antacids are presumed to inhibit this conversion by raising the pH of the stomach contents.[7]

Importance and management

Most of the reports describe single-dose studies, but what is known suggests that no adverse interaction of any clinical importance is likely if antacids are given with chlordiazepoxide, clorazepate or diazepam. Whether the delay in absorption has an undesirable effect in those who only take benzodiazepines during acute episodes of anxiety, and who need rapid relief is uncertain. Information about other benzodiazepines is lacking. However, no special precautions would seem to be necessary.

1. Shader RI, Ciraulo DA, Greenblatt DJ, Harmatz JS. Steady-state plasma desmethyldiazepam during long-term clorazepate use: effect of antacids. *Clin Pharmacol Ther* (1982) 31, 180–3.
2. Chun AHC, Carrigan PJ, Hoffman DJ, Kershner RP, Stuart JD. Effect of antacids on absorption of clorazepate. *Clin Pharmacol Ther* (1977) 22, 329–35.
3. Shader RI, Georgotas A, Greenblatt DJ, Harmatz JS, Allen MD. Impaired absorption of desmethyldiazepam from clorazepate by magnesium aluminum hydroxide. *Clin Pharmacol Ther* (1978) 24, 308–15.
4. Greenblatt DJ, Shader RI, Harmatz JS, Franke K, Koch-Weser J. Influence of magnesium and aluminum hydroxide mixture on chlordiazepoxide absorption. *Clin Pharmacol Ther* (1976) 19, 234–9.
5. Greenblatt DJ, Allen MD, MacLaughlin DS, Harmatz JS, Shader RI. Diazepam absorption: effect of antacids and food. *Clin Pharmacol Ther* (1978) 24, 600–9.
6. Nair SG, Gamble JAS, Dundee JW, Howard PJ. The influence of three antacids on the absorption and clinical action of oral diazepam. *Br J Anaesth* (1976) 48, 1175–80.
7. Abruzzo CW, Macasieb T, Weinfeld R, Rider JA, Kaplan SA. Changes in the oral absorption characteristics in man of dipotassium clorazepate at normal and elevated gastric pH. *J Pharmacokinet Biopharm* (1977) 5, 377–90.

Benzodiazepines and related drugs + Antiepileptics; Carbamazepine

The use of benzodiazepines with carbamazepine is common, although some evidence suggests that the effects of the benzodiazepines are sometimes reduced. Levels of alprazolam were reduced by almost 50% and levels of midazolam were markedly reduced and its effects almost abolished by carbamazepine. Single-dose studies have shown that the sedative effects of zopiclone and carbamazepine are additive, however it has been predicted that when taken long-term carbamazepine will reduce the effects of zopiclone.

Clinical evidence

A. Benzodiazepines

(a) Alprazolam

A patient with atypical bipolar disorder and panic attacks, given alprazolam 7.5 mg daily, had a reduction of more than 50% in plasma alprazolam levels, from 43 to 19.3 nanograms/mL when given carbamazepine. This was accompanied by a deterioration in his clinical condition, which was managed with haloperidol.[1]

(b) Clobazam

A study found that carbamazepine reduces the plasma levels of clobazam and increases the levels of norclobazam (the principal metabolite).[2] Similarly, a reduction in steady-state clobazam levels, with a rise in norclobazam levels, is described in another study in 6 healthy subjects taking carbamazepine.[3]

A 66-year-old man taking carbamazepine and topiramate experienced fatigue, ataxia, impairment of gait and clumsiness while taking clobazam 10 mg daily. His symptoms resolved when the clobazam was stopped. When he was later given carbamazepine, topiramate, and clobazam 20 mg daily his carbamazepine level rose from 36.8 to 41.9 micromol/L. The carbamazepine level returned to 35.5 micromol/L 5 days after the clobazam was stopped.[4] However, another study in 15 epileptic patients taking carbamazepine alone and another 7 patients taking carbamazepine with clobazam, found that carbamazepine levels were similar in both groups, but levels of carbamazepine metabolites, including the active carbamazepine-10,11-epoxide, were higher in those also taking clobazam. It was suggested that clobazam increased the metabolism of carbamazepine by about 1.5-fold.[5]

(c) Clonazepam

Clonazepam, in slowly increasing doses up to a maximum of 4 to 6 mg/day given over a 6-week period, had no effect on carbamazepine serum levels. Some patients were also taking phenobarbital.[6] A study in 7 healthy subjects found that carbamazepine 200 mg daily given over a 3-week period reduced the plasma levels of clonazepam 1 mg daily from a range of 4 to 7 nanograms/mL down to 2.5 to 4 nanograms/mL, and reduced the half-life by about one-third.[7] A retrospective analysis of the this interaction in 183 patients found that clonazepam clearance was increased by 22% and carbamazepine clearance was decreased by 20.5% by concurrent use.[8]

(d) Diazepam

A study found that the plasma clearance of a single 10-mg intravenous dose of diazepam was threefold greater, and the half-life shorter in a group of 9 epileptics when compared to 6 healthy subjects. Seven of the epileptics were taking carbamazepine.[9]

(e) Midazolam

The pharmacokinetics and pharmacodynamics of a single 15-mg oral dose of midazolam was studied in 6 epileptic patients taking either carbamazepine, phenytoin or both drugs together, and in 7 control subjects not taking either antiepileptic. The AUC of midazolam in the epileptics was reduced to 5.7%, and the peak serum levels to 7.4% of the value in the control subjects. The pharmacodynamic effects of the midazolam (subjective drowsiness, body sway with eyes closed and open, as well as more formal tests) were also reduced. Most of the epileptics did not notice any effects from taking midazolam, while the control subjects were clearly sedated for 2 to 4 hours, and also experienced amnesia after taking the midazolam.[10]

B. Non-benzodiazepine hypnotics

A crossover study in 12 healthy subjects given a single 7.5-mg dose of **zopiclone** and carbamazepine 600 mg found only minor changes in the plasma levels of both drugs. **Zopiclone** levels were higher and carbamazepine levels slightly lower. Psychomotor tests confirmed that both drugs had sedative effects, which were additive, and in a simulated driving test it was found that co-ordination was impaired and reaction times prolonged.[11] However, there do not appear to be any multiple-dose studies. Carbamazepine is a strong inducer of the cytochrome P450 isoenzyme CYP3A4 (by which **zopiclone** is metabolised) and it is therefore predicted that the effect of long-term carbamazepine treatment would be a reduction in **zopiclone** serum levels and hypnotic effects.[12]

Mechanism, importance and management

The midazolam and possibly alprazolam interactions with carbamazepine appear to be of greatest clinical significance. Alprazolam and midazolam are both metabolised by the cytochrome P450 isoenzyme CYP3A4, of which carbamazepine is a known inducer. Much larger doses of midazolam are likely to be needed in the presence of carbamazepine. An alternative sedative may be needed. **Triazolam** is predicted to interact like midazolam.[10]

Since norclobazam retains some of the activity of clobazam the effects of carbamazepine probably have little clinical significance, and the case of carbamazepine toxicity appears to be isolated and is therefore probably of limited importance. The pharmacokinetic changes seen with clonazepam seem likely to be too small to be clinically significant, but this needs confirmation.

The evidence for an interaction between zopiclone and carbamazepine is slim, and the effects of long-term use unclear. However, it would seem prudent to be alert for the need to increase the zopiclone dosage in patients taking carbamazepine. More study of this potential interaction is needed.

1. Arana GW, Epstein S, Molloy M, Greenblatt DJ. Carbamazepine-induced reduction of plasma alprazolam concentrations: a clinical case report. *J Clin Psychiatry* (1988) 49, 448–9.
2. Bun H, Monjanel-Mouterde S, Noel F, Durand A, Cano J-P. Effects of age and antiepileptic drugs on plasma levels and kinetics of clobazam and N-desmethylclobazam. *Pharmacol Toxicol* (1990) 67, 136–40.
3. Levy RH, Lane EA, Guyot M, Brachet-Liermain A, Cenraud B, Loiseau P. Analysis of parent drug-metabolite relationship in the presence of an inducer: application to the carbamazepine-clobazam interaction in normal man. *Drug Metab Dispos* (1983) 11, 286–92.
4. Genton P, Nguyen VH, Mesdjian E. Carbamazepine intoxication with negative myoclonus after the addition of clobazam. *Epilepsia* (1998) 39, 1115–18.
5. Muñoz JJ, De Salamanca RE, Diaz-Obregón C, Timoneda FL. The effect of clobazam on steady state plasma concentrations of carbamazepine and its metabolites. *Br J Clin Pharmacol* (1990) 29, 763–5.

6. Johannessen SI, Strandjord RE, Munthe-Kaas AW. Lack of effect of clonazepam on serum levels of diphenylhydantoin, phenobarbital and carbamazepine. *Acta Neurol Scand* (1977) 55, 506–12.
7. Lai AA, Levy RH, Cutler RE. Time-course of interaction between carbamazepine and clonazepam in normal man. *Clin Pharmacol Ther* (1978) 24, 316–23.
8. Yukawa E, Nonaka T, Yukawa M, Ohdo S, Higuchi S, Kuroda T, Goto Y. Pharmacoepidemiologic investigation of a clonazepam-carbamazepine interaction by mixed effect modeling using routine clinical pharmacokinetic data in Japanese patients. *J Clin Psychopharmacol* (2001) 21, 588–93.
9. Dhillon S, Richens A. Pharmacokinetics of diazepam in epileptic patients and normal volunteers following intravenous administration. *Br J Clin Pharmacol* (1981) 12, 841–4.
10. Backman JT, Olkkola KT, Ojala M, Laaksovirta H, Neuvonen PJ. Concentrations and effects of oral midazolam are greatly reduced in patients treated with carbamazepine or phenytoin. *Epilepsia* (1996) 37, 253–7.
11. Kuitunen T, Mattila MJ, Seppälä T, Aranko K, Mattila ME. Actions of zopiclone and carbamazepine, alone and in combination, on human skilled performance in laboratory and clinical tests. *Br J Clin Pharmacol* (1990) 30, 453–61.
12. Villikka K, Kivistö KT, Lamberg TS, Kantola T, Neuvonen PJ. Concentrations and effects of zopiclone are greatly reduced by rifampicin. *Br J Clin Pharmacol* (1997) 43, 471–4.

Benzodiazepines + Antiepileptics; Miscellaneous

The use of benzodiazepines with antiepileptics is common and possibly accompanied by some changes in serum levels, which are normally of limited clinical importance. However, isolated interactions have been reported between chlordiazepoxide or clobazam and phenobarbital; between clonazepam and lamotrigine or primidone; and between clorazepate and primidone.

Clinical evidence

(a) Felbamate

A retrospective study compared norclobazam level to dose ratios in patients taking **clobazam** and enzyme-inducing antiepileptics, without felbamate (group B, 28 patients) or with felbamate (group C, 16 patients). When compared with 22 patients (group A) receiving **clobazam** alone or with non-enzyme-inducing antiepileptics, the norclobazam level to dose ratio of group B was increased twofold and the norclobazam level to dose ratio of group C was increased fivefold,[1] suggesting that felbamate further increased the effect of enzyme-inducing antiepileptics on **clobazam** metabolism. However, in 18 healthy subjects, the pharmacokinetics of **clonazepam** 1 mg every 12 hours were not significantly altered by felbamate 1.2 g every 12 hours for 10 days.[2] No serious adverse reactions were reported.

(b) Lamotrigine

The plasma **clonazepam** levels in 4 of 8 patients fell by about 38% when they were also given lamotrigine.[3]

(c) Phenobarbital and Primidone

A single case report describes a man given phenobarbital and **chlordiazepoxide** who became drowsy, unsteady, and developed slurred speech, nystagmus, poor memory and hallucinations, all of which disappeared once the phenobarbital was withdrawn and the **chlordiazepoxide** dose reduced from 80 to 60 mg daily.[4]

Phenobarbital slightly reduces the levels of both **clobazam** and its active metabolite, norclobazam.[5]

Clonazepam, in slowly increasing doses up to a maximum of 4 to 6 mg daily, given over a 6-week period to patients taking phenobarbital with or without carbamazepine, had no effect on phenobarbital levels.[6] A study in patients receiving various combinations of phenytoin, phenobarbital and primidone, found that their serum levels were not significantly altered by the addition of **clonazepam** 3 mg daily for 4 weeks, but the levels of **clonazepam** were reduced in the presence of the other antiepileptics, particularly phenobarbital and primidone. Depression was reported in one patient and personality changes with irritability and violent behaviour was reported in another.[7] A study found that phenobarbital caused some small changes in the pharmacokinetics of a single dose of **clonazepam** but only the small increase in clearance was statistically significant.[8] In contrast, an analysis of the serum levels of antiepileptics in children found that those taking **clonazepam** had markedly higher levels of primidone, and toxicity was seen.[9]

A report suggested that the concurrent use of primidone and **clorazepate** may have been responsible for the development of irritability, aggression and depression in 6 of 8 patients.[10]

Phenobarbital 100 mg daily for 8 days had no effect on the metabolism of **diazepam** in a group of healthy subjects.[11] Some modest additive CNS depression may possibly be expected, but the authors of this report make no comment about this.

(d) Tiagabine

Studies in healthy subjects have excluded any pharmacodynamic interaction between tiagabine and **triazolam.**[12]

Mechanism

Uncertain. Changes in the drug metabolism in some cases or simple additive effects in others seem likely. It has been suggested that felbamate inhibits the clearance of norclobazam.[1]

Importance and management

None of the interactions between the benzodiazepines and antiepileptics described here appear to be of major clinical importance, with the possible exception of the interaction between clobazam and felbamate. If both drugs are given be aware that additive sedative or other adverse effects may occur. This may also be possible in some rare cases with chlordiazepoxide or clobazam and phenobarbital; clonazepam and lamotrigine or primidone; and clorazepate and primidone.

1. Contin M, Riva R, Albani F, Baruzzi A. Effect of felbamate on clobazam and its metabolite kinetics in patients with epilepsy. *Ther Drug Monit* (1999) 21, 604–8.
2. Colucci R, Glue P, Banfield C, Reidenberg P, Meehan J, Radwanski E, Korduba C, Lin C, Dogterom P, Ebels T, Hendricks G, Jonkman JHG, Affrime M. Effect of felbamate on the pharmacokinetics of clonazepam. *Am J Ther* (1996) 3, 294–7.
3. Eriksson A-S, Hoppu K, Nergårdh A, Boreus L. Pharmacokinetic interactions between lamotrigine and other antiepileptic drugs in children with intractable epilepsy. *Epilepsia* (1996) 37, 769–73.
4. Kane FJ, McCurdy RL. An unusual reaction to combined Librium-barbiturate therapy. *Am J Psychiatry* (1964) 120, 816.
5. Bun H, Monjanel-Mouterde S, Noel F, Durand A, Cano J-P. Effects of age and antiepileptic drugs on plasma levels and kinetics of clobazam and N-desmethylclobazam. *Pharmacol Toxicol* (1990) 67, 136–40.
6. Johannessen SI, Strandjord RE, Munthe-Kaas AW. Lack of effect of clonazepam on serum levels of diphenylhydantoin, phenobarbital and carbamazepine. *Acta Neurol Scand* (1977) 55, 506–12.
7. Nanda RN, Johnson RH, Keogh HJ, Lambie DG, Melville ID. Treatment of epilepsy with clonazepam and its effect on other anticonvulsants. *J Neurol Neurosurg Psychiatry* (1977) 40, 538–43.
8. Khoo K-C, Mendels J, Rothbart M, Garland WA, Colburn WA, Min BH, Lucek R, Carbone JJ, Boxen baum HG, Kaplan SA. Influence of phenytoin and phenobarbital on the disposition of a single oral dose of clonazepam. *Clin Pharmacol Ther* (1980) 28, 368–75.
9. Windorfer A, Sauer W. Drug interactions during anticonvulsant therapy in childhood: diphenylhydantoin, primidone, phenobarbitone, clonazepam, nitrazepam, carbamazepin and dipropylacetate. *Neuropadiatrie* (1977) 8, 29–41.
10. Feldman RG. Chlorazepate in temporal lobe epilepsy. *JAMA* (1976) 236, 2603.
11. Brockmeyer N, Dylewicz P, Habicht H, Ohnhaus EE. The metabolism of diazepam following different enzyme inducing agents. *Br J Clin Pharmacol* (1985) 19. 544P.
12. Richens A, Marshall RW, Dirach J, Jansen JA, Snel S, Pedersen PC. Absence of interaction between tiagabine, a new antiepileptic drug, and the benzodiazepine triazolam. *Drug Metabol Drug Interact* (1998) 14, 159–77.

Benzodiazepines + Antiepileptics; Phenytoin

Reports are inconsistent: benzodiazepines can cause serum phenytoin levels to increase (toxicity has been seen), decrease, or remain unaltered. In addition phenytoin may reduce clonazepam, diazepam, midazolam and oxazepam serum levels.

Clinical evidence

(a) Phenytoin levels increased

The observation that toxicity developed in patients taking phenytoin when they were given **chlordiazepoxide** or **diazepam** prompted a more detailed study. The serum phenytoin levels of 25 patients taking phenytoin 300 or 400 mg daily and **chlordiazepoxide** or **diazepam** were 80 to 90% higher than those of 99 subjects taking phenytoin without a benzodiazepine.[1]

Further reports attribute increased phenytoin serum levels and phenytoin toxicity to **chlordiazepoxide**[2], **clobazam,**[3] **clonazepam,**[4-7] and **diazepam.**[8-10]

(b) Phenytoin levels decreased

The serum phenytoin levels of 12 patients fell by about 30% over a 2-month period while they were taking **clonazepam** 1.5 to 12 mg daily. When data from another 12 patients were combined, the mean fall was only 18%.[11] Other studies describe similar findings with **clonazepam**[5,12] and **diazepam.**[13,14]

(c) Phenytoin levels unchanged

In one study **alprazolam** did not affect the serum phenytoin levels in healthy subjects.[15] **Clonazepam** did not alter serum phenytoin levels in one study,[16] and another concluded that it produced no predictable change in phenytoin levels.[5] A single-dose study in healthy subjects found no significant pharmacokinetic interaction between intravenous **diazepam** 10 mg and intravenous **fosphenytoin** 1.125 g (or the phenytoin formed by the hydrolysis of fosphenytoin).[17]

(d) Benzodiazepine levels reduced

A study in 5 patients given phenytoin 250 to 400 mg daily found that serum **clonazepam** levels were reduced by more than 50%,[18] and another study found that phenytoin decreased the clearance of **clonazepam** by about 50%.[19] In a further study phenytoin reduced the plasma levels of **clobazam** and increased the levels of norclobazam (the principal metabolite).[20] **Diazepam**[21] and **oxazepam**[22] may be similarly affected in epileptic patients given phenytoin.

The pharmacokinetics and pharmacodynamics of a single 15-mg oral dose of **midazolam** was studied in 6 epileptic patients taking either carbamazepine, phenytoin or both drugs together, and in 7 control subjects not taking either of these antiepileptics. The AUC of **midazolam** in the epileptic patients was reduced to 5.7%, and the peak serum levels to 7.4% of their value in the control subjects. The pharmacodynamic effects (subjective drowsiness, body sway with eyes closed and open, as well as more formal tests) were also reduced. Most of the epileptic patients did not notice any effects of the **midazolam**, while the control subjects were clearly sedated for 2 to 4 hours after taking the **midazolam**, and also experienced amnesia.[23]

Mechanism

The inconsistency of these reports is not understood. Benzodiazepine-induced changes in the metabolism of phenytoin[2,8,10,14] as well as alterations in the apparent volume of distribution have been suggested as possible mechanisms. Enzyme induction by phenytoin may possibly account for the reduction in serum benzodiazepine levels.

Importance and management

A confusing picture. Concurrent use certainly need not be avoided (it has proved to be valuable in many cases) but monitor the outcome of concurrent use and consider monitoring serum phenytoin levels so that undesirable changes can be detected. Only diazepam, chlordiazepoxide and clonazepam have been implicated, but it seems possible that other benzodiazepines could also interact.

1. Vajda FJE, Prineas RJ, Lovell RRH. Interaction between phenytoin and the benzodiazepines. *Lancet* (1971) i, 346.
2. Kutt H, McDowell F. Management of epilepsy with diphenylhydantoin sodium. *JAMA* (1968) 203, 969–72.
3. Zifkin B, Sherwin A, Andermann F. Phenytoin toxicity due to interaction with clobazam. *Neurology* (1991) 41, 313–14.
4. Eeg-Olofsson O. Experiences with Rivotril in treatment of epilepsy — particularly minor motor epilepsy — in mentally retarded children. *Acta Neurol Scand* (1973) 49 (Suppl 53), 29–31.
5. Huang CY, McLeod JG, Sampson D, Hensley WJ. Clonazepam in the treatment of epilepsy. *Med J Aust* (1974) 2, 5–8.
6. Janz D, Schneider H. Bericht über Wodadiboff II (Workshop on the determination of antiepileptic drugs in body fluids). In 'Antiepileptische Langzeitmedikation'. *Bibl Psychiatr* (1975) 151, 55–7.
7. Windorfer A, Sauer W. Drug interactions during anticonvulsant therapy in childhood: diphenylhydantoin, primidone, phenobarbitone, clonazepam, nitrazepam, carbamazepin and dipropylacetate. *Neuropadiatrie* (1977) 8, 29–41.
8. Rogers HJ, Haslam RA, Longstreth J, Lietman PS. Phenytoin intoxication during concurrent diazepam therapy. *J Neurol Neurosurg Psychiatry* (1977) 40, 890–5.
9. Kariks J, Perry SW, Wood D. Serum folic acid and phenytoin levels in permanently hospitalized patients receiving anticonvulsant therapy. *Med J Aust* (1971) 2, 368–71.
10. Murphy A, Wilbur K. Phenytion–diazepam interaction. *Ann Pharmacother* (2003) 37, 659–63.
11. Edwards VE, Eadie MJ. Clonazepam — a clinical study of its effectiveness as an anticonvulsant. *Proc Aust Assoc Neurol* (1973) 10, 61–6.
12. Saavedra IN, Aguilera LI, Faure E, Galdames DG. Case report. Phenytoin/clonazepam interaction. *Ther Drug Monit* (1985) 7, 481–4.
13. Siris JH, Pippenger CE, Werner WL, Masland RL. Anticonvulsant drug-serum levels in psychiatric patients with seizure disorders. *N Y State J Med* (1974) 74, 1554–6.
14. Houghton GW, Richens A. The effect of benzodiazepines and pheneturide on phenytoin metabolism in man. *Br J Clin Pharmacol* (1974) 1, P344–P345.
15. Patrias JM, DiPiro JT, Cheung RPF, Townsend RJ. Effect of alprazolam on phenytoin pharmacokinetics. *Drug Intell Clin Pharm* (1987) 21, 2A.
16. Johannessen SI, Strandjord RE, Munthe-Kaas AW. Lack of effect of clonazepam on serum levels of diphenylhydantoin, phenobarbital and carbamazepine. *Acta Neurol Scand* (1977) 55, 506–12.
17. Hussey EK, Dukes GE, Messenheimer JA, Brouwer KLR, Donn KH, Krol TF, Hak LJ. Evaluation of the pharmacokinetic interaction between diazepam and ACC-9653 (a phenytoin prodrug) in healthy male volunteers. *Pharm Res* (1990) 7, 1172–6.
18. Sjö O, Hvidberg EF, Naestoft J, Lund M. Pharmacokinetics and side-effects of clonazepam and its 7-amino metabolite in man. *Eur J Clin Pharmacol* (1975) 8, 249–54.
19. Khoo K-C, Mendels J, Rothbart M, Garland WA, Colburn WA, Min BH, Lucek R, Carbone JJ, Boxen baum HG, Kaplan SA. Influence of phenytoin and phenobarbital on the disposition of a single oral dose of clonazepam. *Clin Pharmacol Ther* (1980) 28, 368–75.
20. Bun H, Monjanel-Mouterde S, Noel F, Durand A, Cano J-P. Effects of age and antiepileptic drugs on plasma levels and kinetics of clobazam and N-desmethylclobazam. *Pharmacol Toxicol* (1990) 67, 136–40.
21. Hepner GW, Vesell ES, Lipton A, Harvey HA, Wilkinson GR, Schenker S. Disposition of aminopyrine, antipyrine, diazepam, and indocyanine green in patients with liver disease or on anticonvulsant therapy: diazepam breath test and correlations in drug elimination. *J Lab Clin Med* (1977) 90, 440–56.
22. Scott AK, Khir ASM, Steele WH, Hawksworth GM, Petrie JC. Oxazepam pharmacokinetics in patients with epilepsy treated long-term with phenytoin alone or in combination with phenobarbitone. *Br J Clin Pharmacol* (1983) 16, 441–4.
23. Backman JT, Olkkola KT, Ojala M, Laaksovirta H, Neuvonen PJ. Concentrations and effects of oral midazolam are greatly reduced in patients treated with carbamazepine or phenytoin. *Epilepsia* (1996) 37, 253–7.

Benzodiazepines + Antiepileptics; Valproate

Valproate appears to increase the serum levels of diazepam lorazepam and possibly midazolam, while clobazam appears to raise valproate levels. Clonazepam clearance may increase and valproate clearance decrease during concurrent use, and increased adverse effects have been seen. An isolated case describes sleepwalking in a patient taking valproate and zolpidem.

Clinical evidence

A. Benzodiazepines

(a) Clobazam

In one study sodium valproate was reported to have no marked effect on clobazam,[1] but a study in children found that clobazam caused an 11% increase in the serum levels of valproate, despite a reduction of at least 10% in the valproate dosage.[2]

(b) Clonazepam

The addition of clonazepam to sodium valproate increased the unwanted effects (drowsiness, absence status) in 9 out of 12 paediatric and adolescent patients.[3] An analysis of the clonazepam-valproate interaction in 317 epileptic patients found that concurrent use increased clonazepam clearance by 14% and decreased valproate clearance by 17.9%.[4]

(c) Diazepam

Sodium valproate increased the serum levels of free diazepam twofold in 6 healthy subjects.[5]

(d) Lorazepam

In healthy subjects, lorazepam 1 mg every 12 hours for 3 days had no effect on the pharmacokinetics of valproate semisodium 500 mg every 12 hours. However, valproate semisodium increased the AUC and maximum serum levels of lorazepam by 20% and 8%, respectively. Sedation scores were not affected by concurrent treatment, suggesting that the interaction is not clinically significant.[6]

A 40% decrease in the clearance of a 2-mg intravenous bolus dose of lorazepam was seen in 6 out of 8 healthy subjects while they were taking valproate 250 mg twice daily.[7] A woman taking valproate, phenytoin, and carbamazepine went into a coma after she received a total of 6 mg of intravenous lorazepam. She promptly recovered on stopping the valproate.[8]

(e) Midazolam

An *in vitro* study in which midazolam was added to serum found that the free fraction of midazolam in the serum from valproate-treated epileptic patients was almost double that found in serum from untreated healthy subjects. It was suggested that displacement of midazolam by valproate could result in an increase in midazolam effects.[9] *Animal* studies suggest that pre-treatment with valproate may increase the levels of midazolam in the brain.[9]

B. Non-benzodiazepine hypnotic

A report describes sleepwalking in a patient when valproate 250 mg twice daily was added to treatment with **zolpidem** 5 mg at night and citalopram 30 mg daily. The patient stopped the valproate and the sleepwalking episodes resolved. Later, the valproate was restarted causing the sleepwalking to recur. This time the symptoms resolved when the **zolpidem** was stopped.[10]

Mechanism

It seems that valproate reduces the glucuronidation of lorazepam,[6,7] and therefore benzodiazepines that are mainly metabolised by glucuronide conjugation, such as **oxazepam** and **temazepam** are also likely to be affected. It is also thought that valproate may displace midazolam from its plasma binding sites.[9] However, this mechanism alone rarely results in clinically significant interactions.

Importance and management

Evidence of an adverse interaction between valproate and the benzodiazepines and related hypnotics is sparse, and concurrent use is generally beneficial. However, on rare occasions potentially clinically significant effects have been seen. It has been suggested that the combination of clonazepam and sodium valproate should be avoided.[3] However, a very brief letter points out that neither drug affects the serum concentrations of the other and that clonazepam and valproate can be given together in patients with absence seizures since some patients have an excellent response to the combination.[11]

It has been recommended that if clobazam is added to valproate it would be prudent to monitor for any increases in valproate serum levels.[2]

Enhanced sedation has been briefly described during the concurrent use of valproate and unnamed benzodiazepines.[12]

1. Bun H, Monjanel-Mouterde S, Noel F, Durand A, Cano J-P. Effects of age and antiepileptic drugs on plasma levels and kinetics of clobazam and N-desmethylclobazam. *Pharmacol Toxicol* (1990) 67, 136–40.
2. Theis JGW, Koren G, Daneman R, Sherwin AL, Menzano E, Cortez M, Hwang P. Interactions of clobazam with conventional antiepileptics in children. *J Child Neurol* (1997) 12, 208–13.
3. Jeavons PM, Clark JE, Maheshwari MC. Treatment of generalized epilepsies of childhood and adolescence with sodium valproate ('Epilim'). *Dev Med Child Neurol* (1977) 19, 9–25.
4. Yukawa E, Nonaka T, Yukawa M, Higuchi S, Kuroda T, Goto Y. Pharmacoepidemiologic investigation of a clonazepam-valproic acid interaction by mixed effect modeling using routine clinical pharmacokinetic data in Japanese patients. *J Clin Pharm Ther* (2003) 28, 497–504.
5. Dhillon S, Richens A. Valproic acid and diazepam interaction *in vivo*. *Br J Clin Pharmacol* (1982) 13, 553–60.
6. Samara EE, Granneman RG, Witt GF, Cavanaugh JH. Effect of valproate on the pharmacokinetics and pharmacodynamics of lorazepam. *J Clin Pharmacol* (1997) 37, 442–50.
7. Anderson GD, Gidal BE, Kantor ED, Wilensky AJ. Lorazepam-valproate interaction: studies in normal subjects and isolated perfused rat liver. *Epilepsia* (1994) 35, 221–5.
8. Lee S-A, Lee JK, Heo K. Coma probably induced by lorazepam–valproate interaction. *Seizure* (2002) 11, 124–5.
9. Calvo R, Suárez E, Rodríguez-Sasiaín JM, Aguilera L. Effect of sodium valproate on midazolam distribution. *J Pharm Pharmacol* (1988) 40, 150–2.
10. Sattar SP, Ramaswamy S, Bhatia SC, Petty F. Somnambulism due to probable interaction of valproic acid and zolpidem. *Ann Pharmacother* (2003) 37, 1429–33.
11. Browne TR. Interaction between clonazepam and sodium valproate. *N Engl J Med* (1979) 300, 679.
12. Völzke E, Doose H. Dipropylacetate (Dépakine®, Ergenyl®) in the treatment of epilepsy. *Epilepsia* (1973) 14, 185–93.

Benzodiazepines and related drugs + Antimuscarinics

Atropine and hyoscine do not affect the absorption or the sedative effects of diazepam but atropine may slow the absorption of zopiclone.

Clinical evidence, mechanism, importance and management

(a) Diazepam

A study in 8 healthy subjects given a single 10-mg oral dose of diazepam showed that serum diazepam levels were not significantly changed by the concurrent use of **atropine** 1 mg or **hyoscine hydrobromide** 1 mg, nor were the sedative effects of diazepam altered.[1]

(b) Zopiclone

In 12 healthy subjects the absorption of a single 7.5-mg dose of zopiclone was reduced by intravenous **atropine** 600 micrograms. Mean plasma zopiclone levels at 1 hour were reduced from 22.7 nanograms/mL to 6.5 nanograms/mL and at 2 hours from 49.3 nanograms/mL to 31.9 nanograms/mL by **atropine**. This was presumably due to altered gut motility.[2] The clinical importance of these findings is not known.

1. Gregoretti SM, Uges DRA. Influence of oral atropine or hyoscine on the absorption of oral diazepam. *Br J Anaesth* (1982) 54, 1231–4.
2. Elliott P, Chestnutt WN, Elwood RJ, Dundee JW. Effect of atropine and metoclopramide on the plasma concentrations of orally administered zopiclone. *Br J Anaesth* (1983) 55, 1159P–1160P.

Benzodiazepines + Antipsychotics

Marked respiratory depression has been reported in three patients when they were given lorazepam with loxapine, and neuroleptic malignant syndrome has been reported in another three patients taking benzodiazepines and antipsychotics. The effects of lorazepam on psychomotor tests and memory was not affected by concurrent amisulpride. Airways obstruction has been reported in patients given intramuscular levomepromazine with intravenous benzodiazepines. Additive sedative effects appear to occur with zaleplon, zolpidem or zopiclone and some antipsychotics.

Clinical evidence, mechanism, importance and management

A. Benzodiazepines

(a) Lorazepam

1. Loxapine. A woman with a manic bipolar affective disorder was admitted to hospital and given lorazepam 2 mg with loxapine 25 mg. After 2 hours she was found to be lethargic with sonorous respirations, occasional episodes of apnoea and an irregular respiration as low as 4 breaths per minute. She was given oxygen and recovered spontaneously within 12 hours. She had experienced no previous problems with lorazepam, and had none when it was later given while she was taking perphenazine.[1] Two other cases have been reported where patients given intramuscular lorazepam 1 to 2 mg and oral loxapine 50 mg developed prolonged stupor, a significantly lowered respiration rate (8 breaths per minute), and in one case hypotension. Both showed signs of recovery within 3 to 5 hours and both had taken each of these drugs alone without problems.[2]

2. Amisulpride. A single-dose study in 18 healthy subjects found that amisulpride 50 mg or 200 mg did not potentiate or antagonise the effects of a single 2-mg dose of lorazepam on psychomotor performance or memory.[3]

(b) Other benzodiazepines

1. Neuroleptic malignant syndrome. Three cases of neuroleptic malignant syndrome have been reported following the use of **diazepam** with **risperidone**, **clorazepate** with **zuclopenthixol** and **tiapride** with **clonazepam**. In 2 cases this followed the abrupt withdrawal of long-term benzodiazepines. All 3 patients recovered, one without any treatment.[4] These reports are isolated and unexplained. There appears to be no clear reason for avoiding concurrent use, but it should be well monitored.

2. Obstruction of airways. A patient with catatonic schizophrenia was given intravenous **diazepam** 20 mg followed by intramuscular haloperidol 10 mg and **levomepromazine** 50 mg. Because of combative behaviour about 50 minutes later, he was given intravenous **flunitrazepam** 2 mg, and about 2 hours later another dose of both intravenous haloperidol 12 mg and **flunitrazepam** 5 mg. An hour after the last injection he became mildly cyanotic due to collapse of glossopharyngeal structures and excessive oral and nasal secretions, causing airways obstruction. Four other cases of airways obstruction associated with the combination of intramuscular **levomepromazine** in doses of 0.52 mg/kg or more and intravenous **flunitrazepam** or **diazepam** are also described. A subsequent review of all cases found that there were no cases of airways obstruction in patients who received haloperidol with either **levomepromazine** or a benzodiazepine. The interaction occurred immediately after the last intravenous injection in one patient and about 25 minutes after intramuscular **levomepromazine** but onset may be delayed up to 2 hours or more.[5]

B. Non-benzodiazepine hypnotics

(a) Zaleplon

A single 50-mg dose of **thioridazine**[6] had no effect on the pharmacokinetics of zaleplon 20 mg, and the psychomotor tests showed only short term additive effects lasting 1 to 4 hours. These short-term CNS additive effects are small and unlikely to be clinically relevant, and so there would seem to be no reason for avoiding concurrent use.

(b) Zolpidem

Single-dose studies found that the pharmacokinetics of 20-mg doses of zolpidem were unaffected by 50 mg of **chlorpromazine**[7,8] or 2 mg of **haloperidol**.[7] The pharmacokinetics of both of these antipsychotics were unaffected by zolpidem, except that in one study the elimination half-life of **chlorpromazine** was increased from about 5 to 8 hours.[8] **Chlorpromazine** increased the sedative effects of zolpidem (as indicated by impaired performances of manual dexterity and Stroop's tests).[7,8] It seems likely that additive sedation will be seen with other sedative drugs.

(c) Zopiclone

No pharmacokinetic interaction was found when 12 healthy subjects were given a single 7.5-mg oral dose of zopiclone with **chlorpromazine** 50 mg. However, the overall performance in a number of psychomotor tests (including digit symbol substitution and simulated driving) was definitely impaired more by the combination of the drugs than by **chlorpromazine** alone. Zopiclone with **chlorpromazine** impaired memory and learning, and caused a marked impairment of the performance of the tests.[9] In practical terms this means that patients given **chlorpromazine** with either of these drugs should be warned that they will almost certainly feel drowsy and be less able to drive or handle potentially hazardous machinery safely.

1. Cohen S, Khan A. Respiratory distress with the use of lorazepam in mania. *J Clin Psychopharmacol* (1987) 7, 199–200.
2. Battaglia J, Thornton L, Young C. Loxapine-lorazepam-induced hypotension and stupor. *J Clin Psychopharmacol* (1989) 9, 227–8.
3. Perault MC, Bergougnan L, Paillat A, Zieleniuk I, Rosenzweig P, Vandel B. Lack of interaction between amisulpride and lorazepam on psychomotor performance and memory in healthy volunteers. *Hum Psychopharmacol* (1998) 13, 493–500.
4. Bobolakis I. Neuroleptic malignant syndrome after antipsychotic drug administration during benzodiazepine withdrawal. *J Clin Psychopharmacol* (2000) 20, 281–3.
5. Hatta K, Takahashi T, Nakamura H, Yamashiro H, Endo H, Kito K, Saeki T, Masui K, Yonezawa Y. A risk for obstruction of the airways in the parenteral use of levomepromazine with benzodiazepine. *Pharmacopsychiatry* (1998) 31, 126–30.
6. Hetta J, Broman J-E, Darwish M, Troy SM. Psychomotor effects of zaleplon and thioridazine coadministration. *Eur J Clin Pharmacol* (2000) 56, 211–17.
7. Sauvanet JP, Langer SZ Morselli PL, eds. Imidazopyridines in Sleep Disorders. New York: Raven Press; 1988 p. 165–73.
8. Desager JP, Hulhoven R, Harvengt C, Hermann P, Guillet P, Thiercelin JF. Possible interactions between zolpidem, a new sleep inducer and chlorpromazine, a phenothiazine neuroleptic. *Psychopharmacology (Berl)* (1988) 96, 63–6.
9. Mattila MJ, Vanakoski J, Matilla-Evenden ME, Karonen S-L. Suriclone enhances the actions of chlorpromazine on human psychomotor performance but not on memory or plasma prolactin in healthy subjects. *Eur J Clin Pharmacol* (1994) 46, 215–20.

Benzodiazepines + Aprepitant

Aprepitant inhibits the metabolism of oral midazolam resulting in increased plasma levels. It appears to have less effect on intravenous midazolam. A few days after aprepitant treatment is stopped a transient slight reduction in midazolam plasma levels may occur due to induction of its metabolism. Alprazolam and triazolam are expected to be affected similarly.

Clinical evidence

In a randomised study 16 healthy subjects took either aprepitant 125 mg on day 1 followed by 80 mg daily for 4 days, or 40 mg on day 1 followed by 25 mg daily for 4 days, with a single 2-mg oral dose of midazolam on days 1 and 5. The aprepitant 40/25 mg dosing schedule had no significant effect on the pharmacokinetics of midazolam. However, the aprepitant 125/80 mg dosing schedule increased the AUC of oral midazolam by 126% and 229% on days 1 and 5, respectively, and increased the maximum plasma levels of midazolam by 46% and 94% on days 1 and 5, respectively.[1]

In a randomised, placebo-controlled study, 24 healthy subjects were given aprepitant 125 mg on day one then 80 mg daily for a further 2 days. A single 2-mg intravenous dose of midazolam was given on days 4, 8 and 15. The 3-day aprepitant regimen increased midazolam levels slightly on day 4 (AUC increased by 25% and clearance reduced by 20%), decreased midazolam levels slightly on day 8 (AUC decreased by 19% and clearance increased by 24%) and had almost no effect by day 15, when compared to placebo.[2]

Mechanism

Aprepitant inhibits the cytochrome P450 isoenzyme CYP3A4 by which midazolam is metabolised, resulting in increased midazolam levels. The pharmacokinetic effect on intravenous midazolam indicate the effects of aprepitant on systemic rather than on intestinal CYP3A4 activity. Aprepitant is also a mild inducer of CYP3A4,[2,3] however the induction is transient, with maximal effect 3 to 5 days after the end of treatment.

Importance and management

Based on the way midazolam interacts with similarly potent inhibitors of CYP3A4, aprepitant may be expected to increased the drowsiness and length of sedation and amnesia in patients given midazolam. Consider reducing the midazolam dose in patients given aprepitant and monitor the outcome of concurrent use carefully. The manufacturer notes that the potential effects of increased levels of other benzodiazepines metabolised via CYP3A4, such as **alprazolam** and **triazolam**, should be considered if they are given with aprepitant. They also state that the effects of aprepitant on plasma levels of intravenously administered CYP3A4 substrates are expected to be less than the effects on orally administered substrates.[3]

1. Majumdar AK, McCrea JB, Panebianco DL, Hesney M, Dru J, Constanzer M, Goldberg MR, Murphy G, Gottesdiener KM, Lines CR, Petty KJ, Blum RA. Effects of aprepitant on cytochrome P450 3A4 activity using midazolam as a probe. *Clin Pharmacol Ther* (2003) 74, 150–6.
2. Shadle CR, Lee Y, Majumdar AK, Petty KJ, Gargano C, Bradstreet TE, Evans JK, Blum RA. Evaluation of potential inductive effects of aprepitant on cytochrome P450 3A4 and 2C9 activity. *J Clin Pharmacol* (2004) 44, 215–23.
3. Emend (Aprepitant). Merck Sharp & Dohme Ltd. UK Summary of product characteristics, February 2007.

Benzodiazepines + Aspirin

The induction of anaesthesia with midazolam is more rapid in patients who have been pretreated with aspirin.

Clinical evidence

A study in patients about to undergo surgery found that pretreatment with aspirin 1 g (given as intravenous **lysine acetylsalicylate**) one minute before induction shortened the induction time with intravenous midazolam 300 micrograms/kg. Only 60% were 'asleep' within 3 minutes of receiving midazolam alone, but 80 to 81% were 'asleep' within 3 minutes of receiving midazolam given after the aspirin pretreatment.[1]

Mechanism

Not understood. It has been suggested that aspirin increases the amount of free (and active) midazolam in the plasma since they compete for the binding sites on the plasma albumins.[1,2]

Importance and management

Information is limited but what is known shows that the effects of midazolam are increased by aspirin. Be alert for the need to reduce the dosage. However, note also that regular aspirin use may increase the risk of bleeding during surgery, and in some situations this may justify avoidance of aspirin in the week before surgery.[3]

1. Dundee JW, Halliday NJ, McMurray TJ. Aspirin and probenecid pretreatment influences the potency of thiopentone and the onset of action of midazolam. *Eur J Anaesthesiol* (1986) 3, 247–51.
2. Halliday NJ, Dundee JW, Collier PS, Howard PJ. Effects of aspirin pretreatment on the *in vitro* serum binding of midazolam. *Br J Clin Pharmacol* (1985) 19, 581P–582P.
3. Anon. Drugs in the peri-operative period: 4 – Cardiovascular drugs. *Drug Ther Bull* (1999) 37, 89–92.

Benzodiazepines and related drugs + Azoles

Fluconazole, itraconazole and ketoconazole very markedly increase the serum levels of midazolam and triazolam, thereby increasing and prolonging their sedative and amnesic effects. Similar but smaller effects are seen with itraconazole or ketoconazole and alprazolam and with itraconazole and brotizolam. Even less effect is seen with etizolam and itraconazole and no important interaction occurs between estazolam and itraconazole. Small effects are found with the non-benzodiazepine hypnotic, zolpidem, with ketoconazole and even less effects with zopiclone and itraconazole.
No important interaction occurs between bromazepam and fluconazole, temazepam and itraconazole, zolpidem and fluconazole and probably chlordiazepoxide and ketoconazole.

Clinical evidence

A. Benzodiazepines

(a) Alprazolam

1. Itraconazole. A single 800-microgram dose of alprazolam was given to 10 healthy subjects before and after a 6-day course of itraconazole 200 mg daily. The itraconazole increased the AUC and the half-life of alprazolam nearly threefold, and psychomotor function was impaired.[1]

2. Ketoconazole. A study in healthy subjects found that ketoconazole 200 mg twice daily decreased the clearance of alprazolam 1 mg by about two-thirds, and prolonged its half-life fourfold, but the maximum serum levels remained unchanged.[2]

(b) Bromazepam

Fluconazole 100 mg daily for 4 days had no effect on the pharmacokinetics or pharmacodynamics of bromazepam in 12 healthy subjects.[3]

(c) Brotizolam

A placebo-controlled study in 10 healthy subjects found that **itraconazole** 200 mg daily for 4 days increased the AUC_{0-24} and maximum plasma levels of a single 500-microgram dose of brotizolam given on day 4 by about 2.5-fold and 25%, respectively. The elimination half-life of brotizolam was also increased, from 4.51 to 23.27 hours, and sedation was increased.[4]

(d) Chlordiazepoxide

After taking **ketoconazole** 400 mg daily for 5 days the clearance of chlordiazepoxide 600 micrograms/kg was decreased by 38% in 12 healthy subjects.[5]

(e) Estazolam

A placebo-controlled study[6] found that **itraconazole** 100 mg daily for 7 days did not affect the pharmacokinetics or pharmacodynamics of a single 4-mg dose of estazolam given to 10 healthy subjects on day 4.

(f) Etizolam

A placebo-controlled study in healthy subjects found that **itraconazole** 100 mg twice daily for 7 days increased the AUC of a single 1-mg dose of etizolam given on day 6 by about 50%. The elimination half-life of etizolam was also increased, from 12 to 17.3 hours.[7]

(g) Midazolam

1. Fluconazole. A study in 12 healthy subjects found that fluconazole 200 mg daily for 5 days reduced the clearance of a single 7.5-mg oral dose of midazolam by 51%, and increased the AUC of midazolam 3.5-fold. It was found that the subjects could hardly be wakened during the first hour after taking the midazolam.[8] Another study found that a single 150-mg dose of fluconazole increased the serum levels of a single 10-mg dose of midazolam by about 30%.[9] Yet another study found that the route of administration of fluconazole (i.e. whether oral or intravenous) made little or no difference to the pharmacodynamic effects of midazolam.[10] Fluconazole caused a fourfold increase in plasma midazolam levels in intensive care unit patients receiving midazolam infusions. The interaction was most marked in patients with renal failure.[11] These reports contrast with another, which found that fluconazole 150 mg only slightly increased the effects of a single 10-mg dose of midazolam.[12]

2. Itraconazole. When 9 healthy subjects were given oral midazolam 7.5 mg, before and after taking itraconazole 200 mg daily for 4 days, the itraconazole was found to have increased the AUC of midazolam by about tenfold, increased the peak plasma levels about threefold, and prolonged the half-life from 2.8 to 7.9 hours. The subjects could hardly be wakened during the first hour after taking the midazolam and most of them experienced amnesia lasting several hours.[13] A later study found that itraconazole 100 mg daily for 4 days increased the AUC of midazolam sixfold and the peak plasma levels 2.5-fold.[14] A further study confirmed the marked effect of itraconazole on oral midazolam, but found that the effects of bolus doses of intravenous midazolam were not increased to a clinically significant extent, although their results suggested that long-term, high-dose infusions of midazolam need to be titrated according to effect to avoid overdosage.[8]

3. Ketoconazole. When 9 healthy subjects were given oral midazolam 7.5 mg before and after taking ketoconazole 400 mg daily for 4 days, the ketoconazole was found to have increased the AUC of midazolam by almost 17-fold, increased the peak plasma levels about fourfold, and prolonged the half-life from 2.8 to 8.7 hours. The subjects could hardly be wakened during the first hour after taking the midazolam and most of them experienced amnesia lasting several hours.[13] Ketoconazole has been shown to reduce the metabolism of midazolam and greatly prolong its effects in another study.[15]

(h) Temazepam

Itraconazole 200 mg daily was given to 10 healthy subjects for 4 days, with a single 20-mg dose of temazepam on day 4. A very small increase in the temazepam AUC was seen, but the psychomotor tests carried out were unchanged.[16]

(i) Triazolam

1. Fluconazole. Eight healthy subjects were given fluconazole or a placebo daily for 4 days, with a single 250-microgram oral dose of triazolam on day 4. The AUC of triazolam was increased by 1.6-fold, 2.1-fold, and 4.4-fold by 50, 100, and 200 mg fluconazole, respectively, and the maximum plasma triazolam levels were more than doubled by the 200-mg fluconazole dose. The 100- and 200-mg fluconazole doses both produced significant changes in the psychomotor tests of triazolam, but the 50-mg dose did not.[17]

2. Itraconazole. The AUC of a single 250-microgram dose of triazolam was increased by about 28-fold after 9 healthy subjects were given itraconazole 200 mg daily for 4 days. Peak plasma levels were increased threefold. Marked changes in psychomotor and other responses were also seen. The subjects had amnesia and were still very tired and confused as long as 17 hours after taking the triazolam.[18] Another study found that the interaction persists for several days after taking the itraconazole.[19]

3. Ketoconazole. A study in healthy subjects found that when they were given triazolam 125 micrograms, after ketoconazole 200 mg taken 17 hours and 1 hour earlier, the triazolam half-life was prolonged (from 4 to almost 18 hours in one subject) and the clearance was increased ninefold. Pharmacodynamic testing found an increase in the impairment of a digit-symbol substitution test, and increased effects on EEG beta activity.[20] The AUC of a single 250-microgram dose of triazolam was increased by about 23-fold by ketoconazole 400 mg daily for 4 days. Peak plasma levels were increased threefold. Marked changes in psychomotor and other responses were seen. The subjects had amnesia and were still very tired and confused as long as 17 hours after taking the triazolam.[18] Another study similarly found that ketoconazole inhibited the metabolism of triazolam leading to an increase in its sedative effects.[21]

B. Non-benzodiazepine hypnotics

(a) Zolpidem

1. Fluconazole. In a placebo-controlled study in healthy subjects **itraconazole** 100 mg twice daily for 2 days had no significant effect on the pharmacokinetics of a single 5-mg dose of zolpidem given with the third dose of fluconazole.[22]

2. Itraconazole. Itraconazole 200 mg daily or a placebo was given to 10 healthy subjects for 4 days. On day 4 they were also given a single 10-mg oral dose of zolpidem. The mean peak serum levels of the zolpidem were increased by 12.5% and the AUC was increased by 35%, but the performance of a number of psychomotor tests (digit symbol substitution, critical flicker fusion, subjective drowsiness, postural sway) remained unaltered.[23] Another study similarly found that itraconazole did not interact significantly with zolpidem.[22]

3. Ketoconazole. A study in 12 healthy subjects found that following three 200-mg doses of ketoconazole given every 12 hours, the AUC of zolpidem 5 mg was increased 1.7-fold and the subjects were more sedated, as shown by the digit symbol substitution test.[22]

(b) Zopiclone

Itraconazole 200 mg daily or a placebo was given to 10 healthy young subjects for 4 days. On day 4 they were also given a single 7.5-mg oral dose of zopiclone. The **itraconazole** increased the maximum plasma levels of the zopiclone by 29% (from 49 to 63 nanograms/mL), increased its AUC by 73%, and prolonged its half-life from 5 to 7 hours. But despite these increases, there were no statistical or clinical differences between the performance of the psychomotor tests carried out during the placebo and **itraconazole** phases of the study.[24]

Mechanism

Itraconazole, ketoconazole, and to a lesser extent fluconazole are potent inhibitors of the cytochrome P450 isoenzyme CYP3A4. The benzodiazepines and zopiclone and zolpidem are, to varying degrees, metabolised by CYP3A4, with the extent of the interaction related to how significant CYP3A4 is in their metabolism. So, for example midazolam, which is predominantly metabolised by CYP3A4 is greatly affected, whereas CYP3A4 is not a significant metabolic route in the metabolism of temazepam, so it is only slightly affected. Other isoenzymes are also involved in the metabolism of zopiclone and zolpidem so they are only moderately affected. The azoles inhibit CYP3A4 in the liver (hence intravenous benzodiazepines can be affected) but studies have also suggested that ketoconazole inhibits metabolism of midazolam[15] and triazolam[21] by CYP3A4 in the gut wall, which explains why oral benzodiazepines are most affected.

Ketoconazole appears to inhibit the oxidation of chlordiazepoxide by the liver.[5]

Importance and management

The interactions between midazolam or triazolam and itraconazole or ketoconazole are established and clinically important. In very broad terms the dosage of midazolam would need to be reduced by about 75% or more in the presence of these antifungals to avoid excessive sedation, and even then the effects would still be expected to be prolonged. Unless appropriate precautions are taken (very reduced dosages) these interactions can be dangerous. Patients taking itraconazole or ketoconazole are unlikely to be able to drive (for example) for at least 6 hours after receiving midazolam. Patients should also be warned about the likelihood of increased sedation. There is some evidence that bolus doses of intravenous midazolam given in the presence of itraconazole or fluconazole are not increased to a clinically significant degree, and normal doses can be used.[14] However, where high doses of intravenous midazolam are used long term (e.g. during intensive care treatment) it has been suggested that the dosage will need to be titrated to avoid long-lasting hypnotic effects.[8] These precautions are equally applicable to triazolam with itraconazole or ketoconazole and midazolam with ketoconazole. Fluconazole interacts less significantly but even so, the midazolam or triazolam dosage probably needs to be reduced, possibly by as much as half.

The effects of alprazolam and brotizolam are increased and prolonged by ketoconazole and itraconazole, but the extent of this is less than that seen with midazolam or triazolam. However, some dosage reductions may still be necessary.

The effects of itraconazole on temazepam or zopiclone and ketoconazole on chlordiazepoxide or zolpidem are small and seem unlikely to be clinically significant in most patients.

1. Yasui N, Kondo T, Otani K, Furukori H, Kaneko S, Ohkubo T, Nagasaki T, Sugawara K. Effect of itraconazole on the single oral dose pharmacokinetics and pharmacodynamics of alprazolam. *Psychopharmacology (Berl)* (1998) 139, 269–73.
2. Greenblatt DJ, Wright CE, von Moltke LL, Harmatz JS, Ehrenberg BL, Harrel LM, Corbett K, Counihan M, Tobias S, Shader RI. Ketoconazole inhibition of triazolam and alprazolam clearance: differential kinetic and dynamic consequences. *Clin Pharmacol Ther* (1998) 64, 237–47.
3. Ohtani Y, Kotegawa T, Tsutsumi K, Morimoto T, Hirose Y, Nakano S. Effect of fluconazole on the pharmacokinetics and pharmacodynamics of oral and rectal bromazepam: an application of electroencephalography as the pharmacodynamic method. *J Clin Pharmacol* (2002) 42, 183–91.
4. Osanai T, Ohkubo T, Yasui N, Kondo T, Kaneko S. Effect of itraconazole on the pharmacokinetics and pharmacodynamics of a single dose of brotizolam. *Br J Clin Pharmacol* (2004) 58, 476–81.
5. Brown MW, Maldonado AL, Meredith CG, Speeg KV. Effect of ketoconazole on hepatic oxidative drug metabolism. *Clin Pharmacol Ther* (1985) 37, 290–7.
6. Otsuji Y, Okuyama N, Aoshima T, Fukasawa T, Kato K, Gerstenberg G, Miura M, Ohkubo T, Sugawara K, Otani K. No effect of itraconazole on the single oral dose pharmacokinetics and pharmacodynamics of estazolam. *Ther Drug Monit* (2002) 24, 375–8.
7. Araki K, Yasui-Furukori N, Fukasawa T, Aoshima T, Suzuki A, Inoue Y, Tateishi T, Otani K. Inhibition of the metabolism of etizolam by itraconazole in humans: evidence for the involvement of CYP3A4 in etizolam metabolism. *Eur J Clin Pharmacol* (2004) 60, 427–30.
8. Olkkola KT, Ahonen J, Neuvonen PJ. The effect of the systemic antimycotics, itraconazole and fluconazole, on the pharmacokinetics and pharmacodynamics of intravenous and oral midazolam. *Anesth Analg* (1996) 82, 511–16.
9. Mattila MJ, Vainio P, Vanakoski J. Fluconazole moderately increases midazolam effects on performance. *Br J Clin Pharmacol* (1995) 39, 567P.
10. Ahonen J, Olkkola KT, Neuvonen PJ. Effect of route of administration of fluconazole on the interaction between fluconazole and midazolam. *Eur J Clin Pharmacol* (1997) 51, 415–19.
11. Ahonen J, Olkkola KT, Takala A, Neuvonen PJ. Interaction between fluconazole and midazolam in intensive care patients. *Acta Anaesthesiol Scand* (1999) 43, 509–14.
12. Vanakoski J, Mattila MJ, Vainio P, Idänpään-Heikkilä JJ, Törnwall M. 150 mg fluconazole does not substantially increase the effects of 10 mg midazolam or the plasma midazolam concentrations in healthy subjects. *Int J Clin Pharmacol Ther* (1995) 33, 518–23.
13. Olkkola KT, Backman JT, Neuvonen PJ. Midazolam should be avoided in patients receiving systemic antimycotics ketoconazole or itraconazole. *Clin Pharmacol Ther* (1994) 55, 481–5.
14. Ahonen J, Olkkola KT, Neuvonen PJ. Effect of itraconazole and terbinafine on the pharmacokinetics and pharmacodynamics of midazolam in healthy volunteers. *Br J Clin Pharmacol* (1995) 40, 270–2.
15. Lam YWF, Alfaro CL, Ereshefsky L, Miller M. Pharmacokinetic and pharmacodynamic interactions of oral midazolam with ketoconazole, fluoxetine, fluvoxamine, and nefazodone. *J Clin Pharmacol* (2003) 43, 1274–82.
16. Ahonen J, Olkkola KT, Neuvonen PJ. Lack of effect of antimycotic itraconazole on the pharmacokinetics or pharmacodynamics of temazepam. *Ther Drug Monit* (1996) 18, 124–7.
17. Varhe A, Olkkola KT, Neuvonen PJ. Effect of fluconazole dose on the extent of fluconazole-triazolam interaction. *Br J Clin Pharmacol* (1996) 42, 465–70.
18. Varhe A, Olkkola KT, Neuvonen PJ. Oral triazolam is potentially hazardous to patients receiving systemic antimycotics ketoconazole or itraconazole. *Clin Pharmacol Ther* (1994) 56, 601–7.
19. Neuvonen PJ, Varhe A, Olkkola KT. The effect of ingestion time interval on the interaction between itraconazole and triazolam. *Clin Pharmacol Ther* (1996) 60, 326–31.
20. Greenblatt DJ, von Moltke LL, Harmatz JS, Harrel LM, Tobias S, Shader RI, Wright CE. Interaction of triazolam and ketoconazole. *Lancet* (1995) 345, 191.
21. von Moltke LL, Greenblatt DJ, Harmatz JS, Duan SX, Harrel LM, Cotreau-Bibbo MM, Pritchard GA, Wright CE, Shader RI. Triazolam biotransformation by human liver microsomes *in vitro*: effects of metabolic inhibitors and clinical confirmation of a predicted interaction with ketoconazole. *J Pharmacol Exp Ther* (1996) 276, 370–9.
22. Greenblatt DJ, von Moltke LL, Harmatz JS, Mertzanis P, Graf JA, Durol ALB, Counihan M, Roth-Schechter B, Shader RI. Kinetic and dynamic interaction study of zolpidem with ketoconazole, itraconazole, and fluconazole. *Clin Pharmacol Ther* (1998) 64, 661–71.
23. Luurila H, Kivistö KT, Neuvonen PJ. Effect of itraconazole on the pharmacokinetics and pharmacodynamics of zolpidem. *Eur J Clin Pharmacol* (1998) 54, 163–6.
24. Jalava K-M, Olkkola KT, Neuvonen PJ. Effect of itraconazole on the pharmacokinetics and pharmacodynamics of zopiclone. *Eur J Clin Pharmacol* (1996) 51, 331–4.

Benzodiazepines and related drugs + Beta blockers

Only small and clinically unimportant pharmacokinetic interactions occur between most benzodiazepines and beta blockers, but there is some evidence that patients taking diazepam may possibly be more accident-prone while taking metoprolol. An isolated report describes marked bradycardia when an elderly woman taking propranolol started to take clomethiazole.

Clinical evidence and mechanism

(a) Benzodiazepines

No significant *pharmacokinetic* interaction occurs between:

- **alprazolam** and **propranolol**[1]
- **clorazepate** and **propranolol**[2]
- **diazepam** and **atenolol**[3] or **propranolol**[3]
- **lorazepam** and **metoprolol**[4] or **propranolol**[1]
- **oxazepam** and **labetalol**[5] or **propranolol**.[5]

Moderate changes, which seem unlikely to be clinically significant, were found between:

- **diazepam** and **propranolol** (diazepam clearance reduced by 17%)[1] or **metoprolol** (diazepam clearance reduced by 18%,[6] AUC increased by 25%[3])
- **bromazepam** and **metoprolol** (**bromazepam** AUC increased by 35%)[4] or **propranolol** (**bromazepam** half-life increased by 22%).[7]

However, studies of psychomotor performance have shown that simple reaction times with **oxazepam** combined with either **propranolol** or **labetalol** are increased,[5] and those taking **diazepam** and **metoprolol** have a reduced kinetic visual acuity,[3,8] which is related to driving ability.[9] Moreover, choice reaction times at 2 hours were also found to be lengthened when taking **diazepam** and **metoprolol**, **propranolol** or **atenolol**, but at 8 hours they only persisted with **diazepam** and **metoprolol**.[8]

(b) Clomethiazole

An 84-year-old woman taking **propranolol** 40 mg twice daily for hypertension underwent skin grafting. Her pulse was stable (54 to 64 bpm) until the thirteenth day after the operation when she took two oral doses of clomethiazole 192 mg, 9 hours apart. Three hours after taking the second dose her heart rate fell to 43 bpm with a PR interval of 0.24 seconds, and by 5 hours after the dose her pulse rate was down to 36 bpm. Her pulse had risen to 70 bpm twelve hours after stopping both drugs, and had restabilised 2 days later at about 60 bpm with a PR interval of 0.2 seconds. At this time the **propranolol** was restarted, with haloperidol.[10]

Importance and management

Information about interactions between the benzodiazepines and beta blockers is very limited indeed. The current evidence does not seem to justify any additional caution, but bear this interaction in mind in the case of an unexpected response to treatment. The interaction between propranolol and clomethiazole appears to be an isolated case and therefore probably of limited clinical significance.

1. Ochs HR, Greenblatt DJ, Verburg-Ochs B. Propranolol interactions with diazepam, lorazepam, and alprazolam. *Clin Pharmacol Ther* (1984) 36, 451–5.
2. Ochs HR, Greenblatt DJ, Locniskar A, Weinbrenner J. Influence of propranolol coadministration or cigarette smoking on the kinetics of desmethyldiazepam following intravenous clorazepate. *Klin Wochenschr* (1986) 64, 1217–21.
3. Hawksworth G, Betts T, Crowe A, Knight R, Nyemitei-Addo I, Parry K, Petrie JC, Raffle A, Parsons A. Diazepam/β-adrenoceptor antagonist interactions. *Br J Clin Pharmacol* (1984) 17, 69S–76S.
4. Scott AK, Cameron GA, Hawksworth GM. Interaction of metoprolol with lorazepam and bromazepam. *Eur J Clin Pharmacol* (1991) 40, 405–9.
5. Sonne J, Døssing M, Loft S, Olesen KL, Vollmer-Larsen A, Victor MA, Hamberg O, Thyssen H. Single dose pharmacokinetics and pharmacodynamics of oral oxazepam during concomitant administration of propranolol and labetalol. *Br J Clin Pharmacol* (1990) 29, 33–7.
6. Klotz U, Reimann IW. Pharmacokinetic and pharmacodynamic interaction study of diazepam and metoprolol. *Eur J Clin Pharmacol* (1984) 26, 223–6.

7. Ochs HR, Greenblatt DJ, Friedman H, Burstein ES, Locniskar A, Harmatz JS, Shader RI. Bromazepam pharmacokinetics: influence of age, gender, oral contraceptives, cimetidine, and propranolol. *Clin Pharmacol Ther* (1987) 41, 562–70.
8. Betts TA, Crowe A, Knight R, Raffle A, Parsons A, Blake A, Hawksworth G, Petrie JC. Is there a clinically relevant interaction between diazepam and lipophilic β-blocking drugs? *Drugs* (1983) 25 (Suppl 2), 279–80.
9. Betts TA, Knight R, Crowe A, Blake A, Harvey P, Mortiboy D. Effect of β-blockers on psychomotor performance in normal volunteers. *Eur J Clin Pharmacol* (1985) 28 (Suppl), 39–49.
10. Adverse Drug Reactions Advisory Committee. Chlormethiazole/propranolol interaction? *Med J Aust* (1979) 2, 553.

Benzodiazepines + Black cohosh

The pharmacokinetics of midazolam are unaffected by the use of black cohosh (*Cimicifuga*).

Clinical evidence, mechanism, importance and management

In a study in 19 healthy subjects given black cohosh extract (standardised to triterpene glycosides 2.5%) 40 mg twice daily for 28 days with a single 8-mg oral dose of **midazolam** on day 28, there was no change in the pharmacokinetics of **midazolam**. In addition, black cohosh had no effect on the duration of midazolam-induced sleep.[1] Similarly, in another study in 12 non-smoking healthy subjects given black cohosh root extract (standardised to triterpene glycosides 0.2%) 1090 mg twice daily for 28 days, there was no significant change in the pharmacokinetics of a single 8-mg oral dose of **midazolam**.[2]

As black cohosh extract does not appear to alter the pharmacokinetics of **midazolam**, a probe substrate for the cytochrome P450 isoenzyme CYP3A4, it is therefore unlikely that it will alter the pharmacokinetics of other substrates of this isoenzyme, see 'Table 1.4', (p.6), for a list.

1. Gurley B, Hubbard MA, Williams DK, Thaden J, Tong Y, Gentry WB, Breen P, Carrier DJ, Cheboyina S. Assessing the clinical significance of botanical supplementation on human cytochrome P450 3A activity: comparison of a milk thistle and black cohosh product to rifampin and clarithromycin. *J Clin Pharmacol* (2006) 46, 201–13.
2. Gurley BJ, Gardner SF, Hubbard MA, Williams DK, Gentry WB, Khan IA, Shah A. In vivo effects of goldenseal, kava kava, black cohosh, and valerian on human cytochrome P450 1A2, 2D6, 2E1, and 3A4/5 phenotypes. *Clin Pharmacol Ther* (2005) 77, 415–26.

Benzodiazepines + Buspirone

No adverse interaction appears to occur if buspirone and alprazolam are given together. When buspirone is given with diazepam the adverse effects appear to be mild and short-lived.

Clinical evidence, mechanism, importance and management

In 12 healthy subjects buspirone 15 mg every 8 hours had no effect on the plasma levels of **diazepam** 5 mg daily for 10 days, but the levels of the metabolite nordiazepam were raised by about 20%. All subjects experienced some mild adverse effects (headache, nausea, dizziness, and in two cases muscle twitching). These symptoms subsided after a few days.[1]

In 12 healthy subjects buspirone 10 mg every 8 hours increased the maximum plasma levels and AUC of **alprazolam** 1 mg every 8 hours by 7% and 8%, respectively. The maximum plasma levels of buspirone were not altered, but the AUC of buspirone was increased by 29%. However, these changes were within the normal pharmacokinetic variability of these drugs. No unexpected adverse effects were seen.[2]

There would seem to be no reason for avoiding the concurrent use of either diazepam or alprazolam and buspirone.

1. Gammans RE, Mayol RF, Labudde JA. Metabolism and disposition of buspirone. *Am J Med* (1986) 80 (Suppl 3B), 41–51.
2. Buch AB, Van Harken DR, Seidehamel RJ, Barbhaiya RH. A study of pharmacokinetic interaction between buspirone and alprazolam at steady state. *J Clin Pharmacol* (1993) 33, 1104–9.

Benzodiazepines + Calcium-channel blockers

Of the calcium-channel blockers diltiazem and verapamil are known to inhibit CYP3A4, the route by which benzodiazepines such as midazolam and triazolam are metabolised. Increased effects, such as sedation, which have been marked in some cases, have been seen in patients given these drugs. Alprazolam would be expected to interact similarly. There appear to be no clinically significant interactions between other calcium-channel blockers and benzodiazepines.

Clinical evidence

(a) Diazepam

1. Diltiazem. When single doses of diazepam 5 mg and diltiazem 60 mg were given to 6 subjects it was found that the plasma levels of each drug were not significantly altered by the presence of the other drug.[1] In another study, poor and extensive metabolisers of the cytochrome P450 isoenzyme CYP2C19 (see 'Genetic factors in drug metabolism', (p.4)) were given diltiazem 200 mg daily for 3 days before and 7 days after a single 2-mg dose of diazepam. It was found that there were no differences in the interaction between the phenotypes, and both groups showed an increase in the AUC and half-life of diazepam. However, the clinical effects of the pharmacokinetic changes were not assessed.[2]

2. Felodipine. The pharmacokinetics of a 10-mg intravenous dose of diazepam were unchanged in 12 healthy subjects after they took felodipine 10 mg daily for 12 days but the AUC and peak serum levels of the diazepam metabolite, desmethyldiazepam, were raised by 14% and 16%, respectively.[3]

3. Nimodipine. The serum levels of diazepam 10 mg daily and nimodipine 30 mg three times daily were unaffected by concurrent use in 24 healthy, elderly subjects, and no clinically relevant changes in haemodynamics, ECG recordings, clinical chemistry or haematology occurred.[4]

(b) Midazolam

1. Diltiazem. After taking diltiazem 60 mg three times daily for 2 days, 9 healthy female subjects were given midazolam 15 mg orally. The AUC of midazolam was increased fourfold, the maximum serum levels doubled, and the half-life increased by 49%. It was almost impossible for the subjects to stay awake for 90 minutes after taking the midazolam. They suffered several hours of amnesia and there was a marked decrease in the performance of pharmacodynamic tests (digit symbol substitution, Maddox wing test).[5] Diltiazem 60 mg, given to 15 patients 2 hours before induction of anaesthesia with midazolam and alfentanil, increased the AUC and half-life of midazolam by 15% and 43%, respectively. Tracheal extubation was performed on average 2.5 hours later, when compared with placebo.[6]

2. Lercanidipine. Midazolam appears to increase the absorption of lercanidipine by 40%.[7] The clinical relevance of this interaction is as yet unclear.

3. Nitrendipine. A study in 9 healthy subjects found that the pharmacokinetics and pharmacodynamics of midazolam were unaffected by a single 20-mg dose of nitrendipine.[8]

4. Verapamil. After taking verapamil 80 mg three times daily for 2 days, 9 healthy female subjects were given midazolam 15 mg orally. The AUC of the midazolam was increased threefold, the maximum serum levels were doubled, and the half-life increased by 41%. It was almost impossible for the subjects to stay awake for 90 minutes after taking the midazolam. They suffered several hours of amnesia and there was a marked decrease in the performance of pharmacodynamic tests (digit symbol substitution, Maddox wing test).[5]

(c) Temazepam

Diltiazem 40 mg had no little or no effect on the hypnotic effects of temazepam in 16 healthy insomniacs.[9]

(d) Triazolam

1. Diltiazem. A study in 7 healthy subjects found that diltiazem 60 mg three times daily for 3 days increased the AUC of a single 250-microgram dose of triazolam 2.3-fold and almost doubled its peak serum levels. Pharmacodynamic tests showed an increase in the sedative effects of triazolam.[10] Another study in 10 healthy subjects found that diltiazem 60 mg three times daily for 2 days increased the AUC of a single 250-microgram dose of triazolam 3.4-fold, and approximately doubled its maximum plasma level and half-life. The pharmacodynamic changes were briefly described as profound and prolonged.[11] In contrast, diltiazem 40 mg was found to have little or no effect on the hypnotic effects of triazolam in 16 healthy insomniacs in another study.[9]

2. Isradipine. Isradipine 5 mg daily reduced the AUC of a single 250-microgram dose of triazolam by 20% in 9 healthy subjects, but no difference in the pharmacodynamic effects of triazolam were seen.[12]

Mechanism

The evidence suggests that diltiazem and verapamil inhibit the metabolism of midazolam and triazolam, by the cytochrome P450 isoenzyme CYP3A4, leading to increased serum levels and increased effects.

Importance and management

The interactions between midazolam and diltiazem, midazolam and verapamil, and triazolam and diltiazem are established and clinically important. The authors of one report say that patients on either of these calcium-channel blockers are probably incapable of doing skilled tasks (e.g. car driving) for up to 6 hours after taking midazolam 15 mg, and possibly even after 8 to 10 hours. They suggest that the usual dose of midazolam should be reduced at least 50% to avoid unnecessary deep sleep and prolonged hypnosis, and they also point out that since the half-life of the midazolam is prolonged, the effects will persist regardless of the dose.[5] The same seems likely to be true for triazolam and diltiazem, and the interaction is also predicted to occur with triazolam and verapamil.[11] As alprazolam is also metabolised by CYP3A4, this interaction would be expected to occur although there do not appear to be any clinical reports of an interaction.

No special precautions appear to be necessary when other calcium-channel blockers are given with a benzodiazepine.

1. Etoh A, Kohno K. Studies on the drug interaction of diltiazem. IV. Relationship between first pass metabolism of various drugs and the absorption enhancing effect of diltiazem. *Yakugaku Zasshi* (1983) 103, 581–8.
2. Kosuge K, Jun Y, Watanabe H, Kimura M, Nishimoto M, Ishizaki T, Ohashi K. Effects of CYP3A4 inhibition by diltiazem on pharmacokinetics and dynamics of diazepam in relation to CYP2C19 genotype status. *Drug Metab Dispos* (2001) 29, 1284–9.
3. Meyer BH, Müller FO, Hundt HKL, Luus HG, de la Rey N, Röthig H-J. The effects of felodipine on the pharmacokinetics of diazepam. *Int J Clin Pharmacol Ther Toxicol* (1992) 30, 117–21.
4. Heine PR, Weyer G, Breuel H-P, Mück W, Schmage N, Kuhlmann J. Lack of interaction between diazepam and nimodipine during chronic oral administration to healthy elderly subjects. *Br J Clin Pharmacol* (1994) 38, 39–43.
5. Backman JT, Olkkola KT, Aranko K, Himberg J-J, Neuvonen PJ. Dose of midazolam should be reduced during diltiazem and verapamil treatments. *Br J Clin Pharmacol* (1994) 37, 221–5.
6. Ahonen J, Olkkola KT, Salmenperä M, Hynynen M, Neuvonen PJ. Effect of diltiazem on midazolam and alfentanil disposition in patients undergoing coronary artery bypass grafting. *Anesthesiology* (1996) 85, 1246–52.
7. Zanidip (Lercanidipine hydrochloride). Recordati Pharmaceuticals Ltd. UK Summary of product characteristics, October 2004.
8. Handel J, Ziegler G, Gemeinhardt A, Stuber H, Fischer C, Klotz U. Lack of effect of nitrendipine on the pharmacokinetics and pharmacodynamics of midazolam during steady state. *Br J Clin Pharmacol* (1988) 25, 243–50.
9. Scharf MB, Sachais BA, Mayleben DW, Jennings SW. The effects of a calcium channel blocker on the effects of temazepam and triazolam. *Curr Ther Res* (1990) 48, 516–23.
10. Kosuge K, Nishimoto M, Kimura M, Umemura K, Nakashima M, Ohashi K. Enhanced effect of triazolam with diltiazem. *Br J Clin Pharmacol* (1997) 43, 367–72.
11. Varhe A, Olkkola KT, Neuvonen PJ. Diltiazem enhances the effects of triazolam by inhibiting its metabolism. *Clin Pharmacol Ther* (1996) 59, 369–75.
12. Backman JT, Wang J-S, Wen X, Kivistö KT, Neuvonen PJ. Mibefradil but not isradipine substantially elevates the plasma concentrations of the CYP3A4 substrate triazolam. *Clin Pharmacol Ther* (1999) 66, 401–7.

Benzodiazepines + Colestyramine and Neomycin

The clearance of lorazepam is increased by colestyramine with neomycin.

Clinical evidence, mechanism, importance and management

A study in 7 healthy subjects found that neomycin 1 g every 6 hours with colestyramine 4 g every 4 hours reduced the half-life of oral **lorazepam** from 15.8 to 11.7 hours, and increased the clearance of free **lorazepam** by 34%.[1] The reasons for these changes are not clear but parallel studies using intravenous **lorazepam**[1] suggested that neomycin and colestyramine may interfere with the possible enterohepatic circulation of **lorazepam**.

The clinical importance of this interaction is uncertain but probably small. Other benzodiazepines do not appear to have been studied.

1. Herman RJ, Duc Van Pham J, Szakacs CBN. Disposition of lorazepam in human beings: enterohepatic recirculation and first-pass effect. *Clin Pharmacol Ther* (1989) 46, 18–25.

Benzodiazepines + Corticosteroids

The metabolism of oral midazolam may be increased in patients receiving long-term treatment with corticosteroids.

Clinical evidence, mechanism, importance and management

Intravenous **midazolam** 200 micrograms/kg was given to 8 patients receiving long-term treatment with corticosteroids (6 taking **prednisolone** 2.5 mg to 15 mg daily; 1 taking **betamethasone** 0.5 mg daily; 1 taking **methylprednisolone** 48 mg daily) and to 10 other patients not taking corticosteroids. In the patients taking corticosteroids the AUC of **midazolam** was decreased and the clearance increased, when compared with the patients not taking corticosteroids; however the differences were not significant. The onset of anaesthesia between the two groups was also not different. It was suggested that the trend towards increased **midazolam** metabolism may be due to induction of the cytochrome P450 isoenzyme CYP3A4 and/or UDP-glucuronosyltransferase. Although the results with intravenous metabolism were not significant the authors note that it is possible that the metabolism of oral **midazolam** may be more markedly affected.[1]

1. Nakajima M, Suzuki T, Sasaki T, Yokoi T, Hosoyamada A, Yamamoto T, Kuroiwa Y. Effects of chronic administration of glucocorticoid on midazolam pharmacokinetics in humans. *Ther Drug Monit* (1999) 21, 507–13.

Benzodiazepines + Dexamfetamine

Dexamfetamine reverses the sedative effects and some of the memory-impairing effects of triazolam.

Clinical evidence, mechanism, importance and management

A placebo-controlled study in 20 healthy subjects found that a single 20-mg/70 kg dose of dexamfetamine sulfate reversed the sedative effects of a single 250-micrograms/70 kg dose of **triazolam**. The study also found that dexamfetamine selectively reversed some of the memory-impairing effects of **triazolam**.[1]

1. Mintzer MZ, Griffiths RR. Triazolam-amphetamine interaction: dissociation of effects on memory versus arousal. *J Psychopharmacol* (2003) 17, 17–29.

Benzodiazepines + Disulfiram

An isolated report describes temazepam toxicity due to disulfiram. The serum levels of chlordiazepoxide and diazepam are increased by the use of disulfiram and some patients may possibly experience increased drowsiness. Alprazolam, oxazepam and lorazepam are either not affected, or only minimally affected, by disulfiram.

Clinical evidence

A man taking disulfiram 200 mg daily developed confusion, drowsiness, slurred speech and an unsteady gait within a few days of starting to take **temazepam** 20 mg at night. This was interpreted as **temazepam** toxicity. The symptoms disappeared when both drugs were stopped.[1]

After taking disulfiram 500 mg daily for 14 to 16 days, the plasma clearance of single doses of **chlordiazepoxide** and **diazepam** were reduced by 54% and 41%, respectively, and the half-lives were increased by 84% and 37%, respectively. The plasma levels of **chlordiazepoxide** were approximately doubled. **Oxazepam** was also given following disulfiram treatment but changes in **oxazepam** pharmacokinetics were minimal. There was no difference in the interaction between alcoholic subjects (without hepatic cirrhosis) and healthy subjects.[2]

Other studies show that the pharmacokinetics of **lorazepam** and **alprazolam** are unaffected by disulfiram.[3,4]

Mechanism

Disulfiram inhibits the initial metabolism (*N*-demethylation and oxidation) of both chlordiazepoxide and diazepam by the liver so that an alternative but slower metabolic pathway is used. This results in the accumulation of these benzodiazepines in the body. In contrast, the metabolism (glucuronidation) of oxazepam and lorazepam is minimally affected by disulfiram so that their clearance from the body remains largely unaffected.[2,3] The possible interaction between disulfiram and temazepam is not understood, as temazepam is also mainly eliminated in the urine as the inactive glucuronide metabolite, and so its metabolism would not be expected to be affected by disulfiram.

Importance and management

There seems to be only one report (with temazepam) of a clinically significant interaction between disulfiram and the benzodiazepines, and this report is unconfirmed, as the patient did not take temazepam alone. The other reports only describe potential interactions that have been identified by single-dose studies. These do not necessarily reliably predict what will happen in practice. However, it seems possible that some patients will experience increased drowsiness, possibly because of this interaction, and because drowsiness is a very common adverse effect of disulfiram. Reduce the dosage of the benzodiazepine if necessary. Benzodiazepines that are metabolised by similar pathways to diazepam and chlordiazepoxide, may possibly interact in the same way (e.g. bromazepam, clonazepam, clorazepate, prazepam, ketazolam, clobazam, flurazepam, nitrazepam, medazepam) but this needs confirmation. Alprazolam, oxazepam and lorazepam appear to be non-interacting alternatives.

1. Hardman M, Biniwale A, Clarke CE. Temazepam toxicity precipitated by disulfiram. *Lancet* (1994) 344, 1231–2.
2. MacLeod SM, Sellers EM, Giles HG, Billings BJ, Martin PR, Greenblatt DJ, Marshman JA. Interaction of disulfiram with benzodiazepines. *Clin Pharmacol Ther* (1978) 24, 583–9.
3. Sellers EM, Giles HG, Greenblatt DJ, Naranjo CA. Differential effects on benzodiazepine disposition by disulfiram and ethanol. *Arzneimittelforschung* (1980) 30, 882–6.
4. Diquet B, Gujadhur L, Lamiable D, Warot D, Hayoun H, Choisy H. Lack of interaction between disulfiram and alprazolam in alcoholic patients. *Eur J Clin Pharmacol* (1990) 38, 157–60.

Benzodiazepines + Echinacea

Echinacea does not appear to alter the AUC and clearance of oral midazolam, although the bioavailability may be increased. Clearance of intravenous midazolam may be increased in patients taking echinacea.

Clinical evidence, mechanism, importance and management

In a pharmacokinetic study, 12 healthy subjects were given *Echinacea purpurea* root 400 mg four times daily for 28 days, with a single 50-microgram/kg *intravenous* dose of **midazolam** on day 6, and, 24 hours later, a single 5-mg *oral* dose of **midazolam**. The clearance of intravenous midazolam was increased by 42%, and the AUC was reduced by 23%, but there were no significant changes in these parameters after oral dosing. However, the oral bioavailability of midazolam was increased by 50% by echinacea. The authors suggested that the echinacea may have exerted opposing effects on the cytochrome P450 isoenzyme CYP3A in the liver and the intestine, which resulted in this apparent anomaly.[1] In another study in 12 healthy subjects given *Echinacea purpurea* 800 mg twice daily for 28 days with a single 8-mg oral dose of **midazolam**, there was no difference in the ratio of midazolam to its 1-hydroxy metabolite.[2]

The findings of the first study with oral and intravenous midazolam suggest that the effect of echinacea on CYP3A4 substrates might depend on the whether they have high or low oral bioavailability and whether they have high or low hepatic clearance. Further study is needed.

1. Gorski JC, Huang S-M, Pinto A, Hamman MA, Hilligoss JK, Zaheer NA, Desai M, Miller M, Hall SD. The effect of echinacea (*Echinacea purpurea* root) on cytochrome P450 activity in vivo. *Clin Pharmacol Ther* (2004) 75, 89–100.
2. Gurley BJ, Gardner SF, Hubbard MA, Williams DK, Gentry WB, Carrier J, Khan IA, Edwards DJ, Shah A. In vivo assessment of botanical supplementation on human cytochrome P450 phenotypes: *Citrus aurantium*, *Echinacea purpurea*, milk thistle, and saw palmetto. *Clin Pharmacol Ther* (2004) 76, 428–40.

Benzodiazepines + Ethambutol

Ethambutol appears not to interact with diazepam.

Clinical evidence, mechanism, importance and management

A study in 6 patients, newly diagnosed with tuberculosis and taking ethambutol 25 mg/kg, found that although some of the pharmacokinetic parameters of **diazepam** were different to those obtained in healthy control subjects not taking ethambutol, the differences were not significant.[1] There seems to be nothing in the literature to suggest that ethambutol interacts with other benzodiazepines.

1. Ochs HR, Greenblatt DJ, Roberts G-M, Dengler HJ. Diazepam interaction with antituberculosis drugs. *Clin Pharmacol Ther* (1981) 29, 671–8.

Benzodiazepines + Food

Food can delay and reduce the hypnotic effects of flunitrazepam and loprazolam. Food can markedly enhance the absorption of quazepam.

Clinical evidence, mechanism, importance and management

A study in 2 groups of 8 healthy subjects found that when they took single 2-mg doses of **flunitrazepam** or **loprazolam** 2 hours after an evening meal (spaghetti, meat, salad, an apple and wine) and 1 hour before going to bed, the peak plasma levels of **flunitrazepam** and **loprazolam** were reduced by 63% and 41%, respectively. The time to reach these levels were delayed by 2.5 hours and 3.6 hours, respectively, and the absorption half-lives of the drugs were considerably prolonged.[1] It seems probable therefore that the onset of sleep with these benzodiazepines may be delayed by food.

In a crossover study 9 healthy subjects were given single 20-mg dose of **quazepam** after fasting, 30 minutes after a standard meal, and 3 hours after a standard meal. The peak plasma levels and $AUC_{0\text{-}8h}$ for **quazepam** were increased by 3-fold and 2.4-fold, respectively, when given 30 minutes after food, and by 2.5-fold and 2.1-fold, respectively, when given 3 hours after food, when compared with the fasting state. The CNS-depressant effects of **quazepam** were enhanced to a similar extent by administration 30 minutes or 3 hours after food.[2] Another study found similar increases in the bioavailability when **quazepam** was taken 2 hours after food, but did not find any significant difference in the subjective effects of **quazepam**, such as drowsiness, malaise, and calmness, when compared with fasting.[3] In another study by the same authors, it was found that both low-fat and high-fat meals increased the absorption of **quazepam**.[4] Some authorities contraindicate the administration of **quazepam** with food,[4] and it would be prudent to advise patients taking **quazepam** to avoid taking it at the same time or for about 2 to 3 hours after eating.

1. Bareggi SR, Pirola R, Truci G, Leva S, Smirna S. Effect of after-dinner administration on the pharmacokinetics of oral flunitrazepam and loprazolam. *J Clin Pharmacol* (1988) 28, 371–5.
2. Yasui-Furukori N, Takahata T, Kondo T, Mihara K, Kaneko S, Tateishi T. Time effects of food intake on the pharmacokinetics and pharmacodynamics of quazepam. *Br J Clin Pharmacol* (2003) 55, 382–8.
3. Kim Y, Morikawa M, Ohsawa H, Kou M, Ishida E, Igarashi J, Kajimoto T, Danno T, Nakata M, Yokoyama T, Tokuyama A, Nakamura Y, Kishimoto T. Effects of food on the pharmacokinetics and clinical efficacy of quazepam. *Jpn J Neuropsychopharmacol* (2003) 23, 205–10.
4. Yasui-Furukori N, Kondo T, Takahata T, Mihara K, Ono S, Kaneko S, Tateishi T. Effect of dietary fat content in meals on pharmacokinetics of quazepam. *J Clin Pharmacol* (2002) 42, 1335–40.

Benzodiazepines + *Gingko biloba*

***Ginkgo biloba* does not significantly affect the pharmacokinetics of alprazolam.**

Clinical evidence, mechanism, importance and management

Ginkgo biloba leaf extract 120 mg twice daily for 16 days was given to 12 healthy subjects before and with a single 2-mg dose of alprazolam on day 14. The *Ginkgo biloba* preparation (*Ginkgold*) was standardised to ginkgo flavonol glycosides 24% and terpene lactones 6%. The alprazolam AUC was reduced by 17%, and the maximum concentration was not significantly affected: these findings are unlikely to be of clinical significance.[1]

Alprazolam is a probe substrate for the cytochrome P450 isoenzyme CYP3A4 activity, and the findings of this study suggest that Ginkgo biloba is unlikely to have clinically relevant effects on substrates of this isoenzyme, see 'Table 1.4', (p.6).

1. Markowitz JS, Donovan JL, DeVane CL, Sipkes L, Chavin KD. Multiple-dose administration of *Ginkgo biloba* did not affect cytochrome P-450 2D6 or 3A4 activity in normal volunteers. *J Clin Psychopharmacol* (2003) 23, 576–81.

Benzodiazepines + Grapefruit juice

Grapefruit juice can increase the bioavailability of oral diazepam and quazepam but there is evidence that this may be of little practical importance. Midazolam and triazolam levels are also raised by grapefruit juice, and this may be of some clinical significance.

Clinical evidence

A study in 8 healthy subjects found that 250 mL of grapefruit juice increased the AUC and maximum plasma levels of a single 5-mg oral dose of **diazepam** by 3.2-fold and 1.5-fold, respectively.[1] Another study in 9 healthy subjects found that grapefruit juice increased the AUC of **quazepam** and its active metabolite, 2-oxoquazepam, by 38% and 28%, respectively, after a single 15-mg oral dose of **quazepam**, although these increases were not statistically significant. The pharmacodynamic effects of **quazepam**, such as sedation, were not enhanced by grapefruit juice.[2]

Grapefruit juice 200 mL was given to 8 healthy subjects followed 60 minutes later by 5 mg of **intravenous midazolam** or 15 minutes later by 15 mg of **oral midazolam**. The pharmacokinetics of **intravenous midazolam** remained unchanged, but the AUC of the **oral midazolam** was increased by 52%, and its maximum plasma levels rose by 56%. These changes were also reflected in the psychometric measurements made.[3]

A large scale placebo-controlled study in a total of 120 healthy young medical students used psychomotor tests to measure the effect of benzodiazepines with and without grapefruit juice. Subjects were given **midazolam** 10 mg or **triazolam** 250 micrograms with 300 mL of grapefruit juice. Only a minor increase in the benzodiazepine effects occurred with grapefruit juice, and these effects were of little or no practical importance.[4]

A single oral 250-microgram dose of **triazolam** was given to 10 healthy subjects with either 250 mL grapefruit juice or water. The mean AUC of the **triazolam** was increased 1.5-fold by the grapefruit juice, the peak plasma levels were increased 1.3-fold, and the time when the plasma levels peaked was prolonged from 1.5 to 2.5 hours. A slight decrease in psychomotor performance occurred (more drowsiness and tiredness).[5] Similar increases in the AUC of **triazolam** were found in another single-dose study, and although grapefruit juice was not found to enhance the sedative effects of **triazolam**, it did result in deterioration of performance in the digit symbol substitution test.[2]

Another study of the interaction between **triazolam** and grapefruit juice found that the effects of grapefruit juice were much more pronounced when multiple doses of grapefruit juice were given. The **triazolam** AUC and half-life were increased by about 50% and 6%, respectively, when single doses of grapefruit juice were given, and by about 150% and 50%, respectively, by multiple doses of grapefruit juice. The effect of grapefruit juice on psychomotor tests was also greater after multiple dosing.[6]

Mechanism

The evidence suggests that grapefruit juice inhibits the metabolism of these benzodiazepines by the cytochrome P450 isoenzyme CYP3A4, so that more is left to enter the circulation.[3] In one study grapefruit juice was found to have a greater effect on the bioavailability and pharmacodynamics of triazolam than on quazepam. This was considered to be because triazolam is metabolised by CYP3A4, while quazepam is metabolised by CYP2C9 as well as by CYP3A4.[2]

Importance and management

Established interactions. These increases in bioavailability might be expected to increase the extent of the sedation and amnesia due to these benzodiazepines, but in young healthy adults this is apparently of little importance. The clinical effects of the interaction with diazepam appear not to have been investigated. The effects of midazolam and triazolam may be more enhanced than those of other benzodiazepines, because these drugs are more dependent on CYP3A4 for their metabolism (see *Mechanism*, above).What is not clear is whether other factors such as old age or liver cirrhosis might increase the risk of adverse effects with concurrent use.

1. Özdemir M, Aktan Y, Boydağ BS, Cingi MI, Musmul A. Interaction between grapefruit juice and diazepam in humans. *Eur J Drug Metab Pharmacokinet* (1998) 23, 55–9.
2. Sugimoto K-I, Araki N, Ohmori M, Harada K-I, Cui Y, Tsuruoka S, Kawaguchi A, Fujimura A. Interaction between grapefruit juice and hypnotic drugs: comparison of triazolam and quazepam. *Eur J Clin Pharmacol* (2006) 62, 209–15.
3. Kupferschmidt HHT, Ha HR, Ziegler WH, Meier PJ, Krähenbühl S. Interaction between grapefruit juice and midazolam in humans. *Clin Pharmacol Ther* (1995) 58, 20–8.
4. Vanakoski J, Mattila MJ, Seppälä T. Grapefruit juice does not enhance the effects of midazolam and triazolam in man. *Eur J Clin Pharmacol* (1996) 50, 501–8.
5. Hukkinen SK, Varhe A, Olkkola KT, Neuvonen PJ. Plasma concentrations of triazolam are increased by concomitant ingestion of grapefruit juice. *Clin Pharmacol Ther* (1995) 58, 127–31.
6. Lilja JJ, Kivistö KT, Backman JT, Neuvonen PJ. Effect of grapefruit juice dose on grapefruit juice–triazolam interaction: repeated consumption prolongs triazolam half-life. *Eur J Clin Pharmacol* (2000) 56, 411–15.

Benzodiazepines and related drugs + H_2-receptor antagonists

The serum levels of many of the benzodiazepines and related drugs are raised by cimetidine, but normally this appears to be of little or no clinical importance and only the occasional patient may experience an increase in the effects (sedation). The interactions with midazolam, zaleplon, and zolpidem may be more significant, but this is not established. Famotidine, nizatidine and ranitidine do not normally appear to interact with most benzodiazepines. Increased sedation appears to occur with clomethiazole and cimetidine.

Clinical evidence

A. Benzodiazepines

(a) Cimetidine

The combined serum level of **diazepam** and its active metabolite, desmethyldiazepam, was found to be increased by 75% in 10 patients who took cimetidine 300 mg four times daily for 2 weeks, but reaction times and other motor and intellectual tests remained unaffected.[1] Other reports describe a rise in the plasma levels and/or AUC of **diazepam** (associated with increased sedation in one report[2]) due to cimetidine,[3-9] and generalised incoordination has also been described in one individual.[10]

Cimetidine also raises the serum levels of **adinazolam**,[11] **alprazolam**,[12,13] **chlordiazepoxide**,[14] **clobazam**,[15] **clorazepate**,[16] **flurazepam**,[17] **nitrazepam**,[18] and **triazolam**,[12,13,19,20] and reduces the clearance of **bromazepam**.[21]

Liver cirrhosis increases the effects of cimetidine on the loss of **chlordiazepoxide**.[22] Confusion has been reported in a 50-year-old man taking **clorazepate** when he was given cimetidine,[23] and increased sedation has been seen in some patients taking **adinazolam** and cimetidine.[11] Prolonged hypnosis in an elderly woman[24] and CNS toxicity (including lethargy and hallucinations)[25] in a 49-year-old woman have been attributed to an interaction between **triazolam** and cimetidine but this remains unconfirmed.

In contrast, cimetidine does not normally interact with **clobazam**,[26] **clotiazepam**,[27] **lormetazepam**,[28] **oxazepam**[17,29,30] or **temazepam**,[31,32] although prolonged post-operative sedation was seen in one patient given **oxazepam** and cimetidine.[33]

There is some controversy about whether or not **midazolam** is affected by cimetidine. An increase in sedation,[34,35] an increase in **midazolam** levels[35-37] and no pharmacokinetic interaction[38] have been reported with the combination.

Similarly, one study found an increase in **lorazepam** levels with a 400 mg dose of cimetidine, but no effect with 200 mg:[3] other studies suggest that no interaction occurs between **lorazepam** and cimetidine.[17,29]

(b) Famotidine

Famotidine does not interact with **bromazepam**,[39] **clorazepate**,[39] **chlordiazepoxide**,[39] **diazepam**[9,40,41] or **triazolam**.[39]

(c) Nizatidine

Nizatidine does not interact significantly with **diazepam**.[42-44]

(d) Ranitidine

Ranitidine does not interact significantly with **adinazolam**,[45] **diazepam**,[42,46,47] **lorazepam**,[47] or **temazepam**,[32,48] but it can modestly increase the bioavailability (by about 10 to 30%) of oral **triazolam**.[49,50] There is some controversy about whether or not **midazolam** is affected by ranitidine. Increases in sedation have been reported on a number of occasions,[34,36,48,51] but a lack of effect has also been documented.[37,38]

(e) Roxatidine

Roxatidine does not interact with **diazepam** or its active metabolite, desmethyldiazepam.[52]

B. Non-benzodiazepine hypnotics

(a) Cimetidine

Cimetidine increases plasma levels of **zaleplon**[53] and slightly increases sleep duration with **zolpidem**.[54] Cimetidine reduces the clearance of **clomethiazole** and increases sleep duration from a range of 30 to 60 minutes up to at least 2 hours.[55]

(b) Ranitidine

Ranitidine does not interact significantly with **clomethiazole**.[56]

Mechanism

Cimetidine inhibits the liver enzymes concerned with the metabolism of diazepam, alprazolam, chlordiazepoxide, clomethiazole, clorazepate, flurazepam, nitrazepam, triazolam, and zaleplon. As a result their clearance from the body is reduced and their serum levels rise.

Lorazepam, oxazepam and temazepam are metabolised by a different metabolic pathway involving glucuronidation, which is not affected by cimetidine, and so they do not usually interact.

Ranitidine, famotidine and nizatidine appear not to inhibit liver microsomal enzymes. There is some evidence that ranitidine increases the absorption of triazolam, and possibly other benzodiazepines, due to changes in gastric pH,[50] although it has been suggested that this effect is negligible.[20] Cimetidine has been said to similarly affect the absorption of diazepam and lorazepam.[3]

Importance and management

The interactions between the benzodiazepines or related drugs and cimetidine are well documented (not all the references are listed here) but normally they appear to be of little clinical importance, although a few patients may be adversely affected (increased effects, drowsiness, etc.) and this may be more common with the non-benzodiazepine hypnotic, clomethiazole, and possibly, midazolam. If symptoms occur in any patient taking a benzodiazepine or related drug and cimetidine, reduce the benzodiazepine dose, or alternatively, use a non-interacting benzodiazepine, such as lorazepam, lormetazepam, oxazepam or temazepam, or a non-interacting H_2-receptor antagonist such as ranitidine, famotidine, nizatidine or roxatidine, although note that the effects of oral triazolam are possibly very slightly increased.

1. Greenblatt DJ, Abernethy DR, Morse DS, Harmatz JS and Shader RI. Clinical importance of the interaction of diazepam and cimetidine. *Anesth Analg* (1986) 65, 176–80.
2. Klotz U, Reimann I. Delayed clearance of diazepam due to cimetidine. *N Engl J Med* (1980) 302, 1012–13.
3. McGowan WAW, Dundee JW. The effect of intravenous cimetidine on the absorption of orally administered diazepam and lorazepam. *Br J Clin Pharmacol* (1982) 14, 207–11.
4. Klotz U, Reimann I. Elevation of steady-state diazepam levels by cimetidine. *Clin Pharmacol Ther* (1981) 30, 513–17.
5. Gough PA, Curry SH, Araujo OE, Robinson JD, Dallman JJ. Influence of cimetidine on oral diazepam elimination with measurement of subsequent cognitive change. *Br J Clin Pharmacol* (1982) 14, 739–42.
6. Klotz U, Antilla V-J. Drug interactions with cimetidine: pharmacokinetic studies to evaluate its mechanism. *Naunyn Schmiedebergs Arch Pharmacol* (1980) 311, R77.
7. Bressler R, Carter D, Winters L. Enprostil, in contrast to cimetidine, does not affect diazepam pharmacokinetics. *Adv Therapy* (1988) 5, 306–12.
8. Lima DR, Santos RM, Werneck E, Andrade GN. Effect of orally administered misoprostol and cimetidine on the steady state pharmacokinetics of diazepam and nordiazepam in human volunteers. *Eur J Drug Metab Pharmacokinet* (1991) 16, 161–70.
9. Lockniskar A, Greenblatt DJ, Harmatz JS, Zinny MA, Shader RI. Interaction of diazepam with famotidine and cimetidine, two H_2-receptor antagonists. *J Clin Pharmacol* (1986) 26, 299–303.
10. Anon. Court warns on interaction of drugs. *Doctor* (1979) 9, 1.
11. Hulhoven R, Desager JP, Cox S, Harvengt C. Influence of repeated administration of cimetidine on the pharmacokinetics and pharmacodynamics of adinazolam in healthy subjects. *Eur J Clin Pharmacol* (1988) 35, 59–64.
12. Pourbaix S, Desager JP, Hulhoven R, Smith RB, Harvengt C. Pharmacokinetic consequences of long term coadministration of cimetidine and triazolobenzodiazepines, alprazolam and triazolam, in healthy subjects. *Int J Clin Pharmacol Ther Toxicol* (1985) 23, 447–51.
13. Abernethy DR, Greenblatt DJ, Divoll M, Moschitto LJ, Harmatz JS, Shader RI. Interaction of cimetidine with the triazolobenzodiazepines alprazolam and triazolam. *Psychopharmacology (Berl)* (1983) 80, 275–8.
14. Desmond PV, Patwardhan RV, Schenker S, Speeg KV. Cimetidine impairs elimination of chlordiazepoxide (Librium) in man. *Ann Intern Med* (1980) 93, 266–8.
15. Pullar T, Edwards D, Haigh JRM, Peaker S, Feeley MP. The effect of cimetidine on the single dose pharmacokinetics of oral clobazam and *N*-desmethylclobazam. *Br J Clin Pharmacol* (1987) 23, 317–21.
16. Divoll M, Abernethy DR, Greenblatt DJ. Cimetidine impairs drug oxidizing capacity in the elderly. *Clin Pharmacol Ther* (1982) 31, 218.
17. Greenblatt DJ, Abernethy DR, Koepke HH, Shader RI. Interaction of cimetidine with oxazepam, lorazepam, and flurazepam. *J Clin Pharmacol* (1984) 24, 187–93.
18. Ochs HR, Greenblatt DJ, Gugler R, Müntefering G, Locniskar A, Abernethy DR. Cimetidine impairs nitrazepam clearance. *Clin Pharmacol Ther* (1983) 34, 227–30.
19. Friedman H, Greenblatt DJ, Burstein ES, Scavone JM, Harmatz JS, Shader RI. Triazolam kinetics: interaction with cimetidine, propranolol, and the combination. *J Clin Pharmacol* (1988) 28, 228–33.
20. Cox SR, Kroboth PD, Anderson PH, Smith RB. Mechanism for the interaction between triazolam and cimetidine. *Biopharm Drug Dispos* (1986) 7, 567–75.
21. Ochs HR, Greenblatt DJ, Friedman H, Burstein ES, Locniskar A, Harmatz JS, Shader RI. Bromazepam pharmacokinetics: influence of age, gender, oral contraceptives, cimetidine and propranolol. *Clin Pharmacol Ther* (1987) 41, 562–70.
22. Nelson DC, Schenker S, Hoyumpa AM, Speeg KV, Avant GR. The effects of cimetidine on chlordiazepoxide elimination in cirrhosis. *Clin Res* (1981) 29, 824A.
23. Bouden A, El Hechmi Z, Douki S. Cimetidine-benzodiazepine association confusiogene: a propros d'une observation. *Tunis Med* (1990) 68, 63–4.
24. Parker WA, MacLachlan RA. Prolonged hypnotic response to triazolam-cimetidine combination in an elderly patient. *Drug Intell Clin Pharm* (1984) 18, 980–1.
25. Britton ML, Waller ES. Central nervous system toxicity associated with concurrent use of triazolam and cimetidine. *Drug Intell Clin Pharm* (1985) 19, 666–8.
26. Grigoleit H-G, Hajdú P, Hundt HKL, Koeppen D, Malerczyk V, Meyer BH, Müller FO, Witte PU. Pharmacokinetic aspects of the interaction between clobazam and cimetidine. *Eur J Clin Pharmacol* (1983) 25, 139–42.
27. Ochs HR, Greenblatt DJ, Verburg-Ochs B, Harmatz JS, Grehl H. Disposition of clotiazepam: influence of age, sex, oral contraceptives, cimetidine, isoniazid and ethanol. *Eur J Clin Pharmacol* (1984) 26, 55–9.
28. Doenicke A, Dorow R, Täuber U. Die Pharmakokinetik von Lormetazepam nach Cimetidin. *Anaesthesist* (1991) 40, 675–9.
29. Patwardhan RV, Yarborough GW, Desmond PV, Johnson RF, Schenker S, Speeg KV. Cimetidine spares the glucuronidation of lorazepam and oxazepam. *Gastroenterology* (1980) 79, 912–16.
30. Klotz U, Reimann I. Influence of cimetidine on the pharmacokinetics of desmethyldiazepam and oxazepam. *Eur J Clin Pharmacol* (1980) 18, 517–20.
31. Greenblatt DJ, Abernethy DR, Divoll M, Locniskar A, Harmatz JS, Shader RI. Noninteraction of temazepam and cimetidine. *J Pharm Sci* (1984) 73, 399–401.
32. Elliott P, Dundee JW, Collier PS, McClean E. The influence of two H_2-receptor antagonists, cimetidine and ranitidine, on the systemic availability of temazepam. *Br J Anaesth* (1984) 56, 800P–801P.
33. Lam AM, Parkin JA. Cimetidine and prolonged post-operative somnolence. *Can Anaesth Soc J* (1981) 28, 450–2.
34. Sanders LD, Whitehead C, Gildersleve CD, Rosen M, Robinson JO. Interaction of H_2-receptor antagonists and benzodiazepine sedation. *Anaesthesia* (1993) 48, 286–92.
35. Salonen M, Aantaa E, Aaltonen L, Kanto J. Importance of the interaction of midazolam and cimetidine. *Acta Pharmacol Toxicol (Copenh)* (1986) 58, 91–5.
36. Fee JPH, Collier PS, Howard PJ, Dundee JW. Cimetidine and ranitidine increase midazolam bioavailability. *Clin Pharmacol Ther* (1987) 41, 80–4.
37. Klotz U, Arvela P, Rosenkranz B. Effect of single doses of cimetidine and ranitidine on the steady-state plasma levels of midazolam. *Clin Pharmacol Ther* (1985) 38, 652–5.
38. Greenblatt DJ, Locniskar A, Scavone JM, Blyden GT, Ochs HR, Harmatz JS, Shader RI. Absence of interaction of cimetidine and ranitidine with intravenous and oral midazolam. *Anesth Analg* (1986) 65, 176–80.
39. Chichmanian RM, Mignot G, Spreux A, Jean-Girard C, Hofliger P. Tolérance de la famotidine. Étude due réseau médecins sentinelles en pharmacovigilance. *Therapie* (1992) 47, 239–43.
40. Locniskar A, Greenblatt DJ, Harmatz JS, Zinny MA. Influence of famotidine and cimetidine on the pharmacokinetic properties of intravenous diazepam. *J Clin Pharmacol* (1985) 25, 459–60.
41. Klotz U, Arvela P, Rosenkranz B. Famotidine, a new H_2-receptor antagonist, does not affect hepatic elimination of diazepam or tubular secretion of procainamide. *Eur J Clin Pharmacol* (1985) 28, 671–5.
42. Klotz U, Gottlieb W, Keohane PP, Dammann HG. Nocturnal doses of ranitidine and nizatidine do not affect the disposition of diazepam. *J Clin Pharmacol* (1987) 27, 210–12.
43. Klotz U, Dammann HG, Gottlieb WR, Walter TA, Keohane P. Nizatidine (300 mg nocte) does not interfere with diazepam pharmacokinetics in man. *Br J Clin Pharmacol* (1987) 23, 105–6.
44. Klotz U. Lack of effect of nizatidine on drug metabolism. *Scand J Gastroenterol* (1987) 22 (Suppl 136), 18–23.
45. Suttle AB, Songer SS, Dukes GE, Hak LJ, Koruda M, Fleishaker JC, Brouwer KLR. Ranitidine does not alter adinazolam pharmacokinetics or pharmacodynamics. *Clin Pharmacol Ther* (1991) 49, 178.
46. Klotz U, Reimann IW, Ohnhaus EE. Effect of ranitidine on the steady state pharmacokinetics of diazepam. *Eur J Clin Pharmacol* (1983) 24, 357–60.
47. Abernethy DR, Greenblatt DJ, Eshelman FN, Shader RI. Ranitidine does not impair oxidative or conjugative metabolism: noninteraction with antipyrine, diazepam, and lorazepam. *Clin Pharmacol Ther* (1984) 35, 188–92.
48. Wilson CM, Robinson FP, Thompson EM, Dundee JW, Elliott P. Effect of pre-treatment with ranitidine on the hypnotic action of single doses of midazolam, temazepam and zopiclone. *Br J Anaesth* (1986) 58, 483–6.
49. Vanderveen RP, Jirak JL, Peters GR, Cox SR, Bombardt PA. Effect of ranitidine on the disposition of orally and intravenously administered triazolam. *Clin Pharm* (1991) 10, 539–43.
50. O'Connor-Semmes RL, Kersey K, Williams DH, Lam R, Koch KM. Effect of ranitidine on the pharmacokinetics of triazolam and á-hydroxytriazolam in both young (19-60 years) and older (61-78 years) people. *Clin Pharmacol Ther* (2001) 70, 126–31.
51. Elwood RJ, Hildebrand PJ, Dundee JW, Collier PS. Ranitidine influences the uptake of oral midazolam. *Br J Clin Pharmacol* (1983) 15, 743–5.
52. Labs RA. Interaction of roxatidine acetate with antacids, food and other drugs. *Drugs* (1988) 35 (Suppl 3), 82–9.
53. Darwish M. Analysis of potential drug interactions with zaleplon. *J Am Geriatr Soc* (1999) 47, S62.
54. Hulhoven R, Desager JP, Harvengt C, Herman P, Guillet P, Thiercelin JF. Lack of interaction between zolpidem and H_2 antagonists, cimetidine and ranitidine. *Int J Clin Pharmacol Res* (1988) 8, 471–6.
55. Shaw G, Bury RW, Mashford ML, Breen KJ, Desmond PV. Cimetidine impairs the elimination of chlormethiazole. *Eur J Clin Pharmacol* (1981) 21, 83–5.
56. Mashford ML, Harman PJ, Morphett BJ, Breen KJ, Desmond PV. Ranitidine does not affect chlormethiazole or indocyanine green disposition. *Clin Pharmacol Ther* (1983) 34, 231–3.

Benzodiazepines and related drugs + Hormonal contraceptives

Hormonal contraceptives can increase the effects of alprazolam, chlordiazepoxide, diazepam, nitrazepam and triazolam, and reduce the effects of oxazepam, lorazepam and temazepam, but whether in practice there is a need for dosage adjustments has not been determined. Chlordiazepoxide, diazepam, nitrazepam and meprobamate can possibly increase the incidence of breakthrough bleeding.

Clinical evidence

(a) Effects on benzodiazepines and related drugs

A controlled study found that the mean half-life of intravenous **chlordiazepoxide** 600 micrograms/kg was virtually doubled (11.6 hours compared with 20.6 hours) and the total clearance was almost two-thirds lower in 6 women taking oral contraceptives when compared with 6 women not taking oral contraceptives.[1]

Similar but less marked effects were found in other studies in women taking oral contraceptives given **chlordiazepoxide**,[2] **diazepam**,[3,4] **alprazolam**[5] and to an even lesser extent with **triazolam**[5] and **nitrazepam**.[6] No clinically significant pharmacokinetic changes were seen with **bromazepam**,[7] **clotiazepam**,[8] **midazolam** (given orally[9] intramuscularly[10] or intravenously[9]) or **zolpidem**.[11]

A controlled study, comparing 7 women taking an oral contraceptive with 8 women not taking oral contraceptives found that the mean half-life of intravenous **lorazepam** 2 mg was over 50% shorter in the oral contraceptive group (6 hours compared to 14 hours) and the total clearance was over threefold greater.[1]

A smaller increase in the elimination rate was seen in other controlled studies in women taking oral contraceptives and **lorazepam**,[5,12] or **temazepam**,[5] and in two other studies small decreases in the half-life of **oxazepam** were observed.[1,12]

(b) Effects on contraceptives

A study in 72 patients taking combined oral contraceptives (*Rigevidon*, *Anteovin*) found that breakthrough bleeding occurred in 36.1% of patients while taking **chlordiazepoxide** 10 to 20 mg daily, **diazepam** 5 to 15 mg daily, **nitrazepam** 5 to 10 mg daily or **meprobamate** 200 to 600 mg daily, but no pregnancies occurred. Only three cases of bleeding occurred with **diazepam** or **nitrazepam**.[13] The average values for breakthrough bleeding with these two oral contraceptives were 9.1% for *Rigevidon* and 3.3% for *Anteovin* in the absence of other drugs. It was possible to establish a causal relationship between the bleeding and the use of the hypnotic in 77% of the cases either by stopping the drug or by changing it for another.[13]

Mechanism

Oral contraceptives affect the metabolism of the benzodiazepines by the liver in different ways: oxidative metabolism is reduced (alprazolam, chlordiazepoxide, diazepam, etc.), whereas metabolism by glucuronide conjugation is increased (lorazepam, oxazepam, temazepam, etc.). Just why these hypnotics should cause breakthrough bleeding is not understood.

Importance and management

Established interactions but of uncertain clinical importance. Long-term use of benzodiazepines that are highly oxidised (alprazolam, chlordiazepoxide, diazepam, nitrazepam, etc.) in women taking oral contraceptives should be monitored to ensure that the dosage is not too high. Those taking benzodiazepines that are metabolised to glucuronides (lorazepam, oxazepam, temazepam, etc.) may possibly need a dosage increase but this is not proven. Bromazepam, clotiazepam, midazolam and zolpidem appear not to interact. No firm conclusions could be drawn from the results of one study, which set out to evaluate the importance of this interaction.[14]

The increased incidence of breakthrough bleeding (more than one-third) due to these hypnotics, is an unpleasant reaction and it suggests that the contraceptive is possibly unreliable, but no outright contraceptive failures have been reported.[13] Limited evidence from the study suggests that changing the hypnotic or the contraceptive might avoid breakthrough bleeding. Note that the UK Family Planning Association[15] did not consider that additional contraceptive precautions were necessary with clonazepam or clobazam and it seems unlikely that they will be necessary with any benzodiazepine.

1. Patwardhan RV, Mitchell MC, Johnson RF, Schenker S. Differential effects of oral contraceptive steroids on the metabolism of benzodiazepines. *Hepatology* (1983) 3, 248–53.
2. Roberts RK, Desmond PV, Wilkinson GR, Schenker S. Disposition of chlordiazepoxide: sex differences and effects of oral contraceptives. *Clin Pharmacol Ther* (1979) 25, 826–31.
3. Giles HG, Sellers EM, Naranjo CA, Frecker RC, Greenblatt DJ. Disposition of intravenous diazepam in young men and women. *Eur J Clin Pharmacol* (1981) 20, 207–13.
4. Abernethy DR, Greenblatt DJ, Divoll M, Arendt R, Ochs HR, Shader RI. Impairment of diazepam metabolism by low-dose estrogen-containing oral-contraceptive steroids. *N Engl J Med* (1982) 306, 791–2.
5. Stoehr GP, Kroboth PD, Juhl RP, Wender DB, Phillips P, Smith RB. Effect of oral contraceptives on triazolam, temazepam, alprazolam, and lorazepam kinetics. *Clin Pharmacol Ther* (1984) 36, 683–90.
6. Jochemsen R, Van der Graff M, Boejinga JK, Breimer DD. Influence of sex, menstrual cycle and oral contraception on the disposition of nitrazepam. *Br J Clin Pharmacol* (1982) 13, 319–24.
7. Ochs HR, Greenblatt DJ, Friedman H, Burstein ES, Locniskar A, Harmatz JS, Shader RI. Bromazepam pharmacokinetics: influence of age, gender, oral contraceptives, cimetidine, and propranolol. *Clin Pharmacol Ther* (1987) 41, 562–70.
8. Ochs HR, Greenblatt DJ, Verburg-Ochs B, Harmatz JS, Grehl H. Disposition of clotiazepam: influence of age, sex, oral contraceptives, cimetidine, isoniazid and ethanol. *Eur J Clin Pharmacol* (1984) 26, 55–9.
9. Belle DJ, Callaghan JT, Gorski JC, Maya JF, Mousa O, Wrighton SA, Hall SD. The effects of an oral contraceptive containing ethinyloestradiol and norgestrel on CYP3A activity. *Br J Clin Pharmacol* (2002) 53, 67–74.
10. Holazo AA, Winkler MB, Patel IH. Effects of age, gender and oral contraceptives on intramuscular midazolam pharmacokinetics. *J Clin Pharmacol* (1988) 28, 1040–5.
11. Olubodun JO, Ochs HR, Trüten V, Klein A, von Moltke LL, Harmatz JS, Shader RI, Greenblatt DJ. Zolpidem pharmacokinetic properties in young females: influence of smoking and oral contraceptive use. *J Clin Pharmacol* (2002) 42, 1142–6.
12. Abernethy DR, Greenblatt DJ, Ochs HR, Weyers D, Divoll M, Harmatz JS, Shader RI. Lorazepam and oxazepam kinetics in women on low-dose oral contraceptives. *Clin Pharmacol Ther* (1983) 33, 628–32.
13. Somos P. Interaction between certain psychopharmaca and low-dose oral contraceptives. *Ther Hung* (1990) 38, 37–40.
14. Kroboth PD, Smith RB, Stoehr GP, Juhl RP. Pharmacodynamic evaluation of the benzodiazepine–oral contraceptive interaction. *Clin Pharmacol Ther* (1985) 38, 525–32.
15. Belfield T, ed. FPA Contraceptive Handbook: a guide for family planning and other health professionals. 3rd ed. London: Family Planning Association, 1999.

Benzodiazepines + 5-HT_3-receptor antagonists

Lorazepam does not appear to interact with granisetron, and temazepam does not appear to interact with ondansetron.

Clinical evidence, mechanism, importance and management

Lorazepam 2.5 mg, given to 12 healthy subjects, clearly affected the performance of a number of psychometric tests. Statistically significant increases occurred in drowsiness, feebleness, muzziness, clumsiness, lethargy, mental slowness, relaxation, dreaminess, incompetence, sadness, and withdrawal. However, there was very little evidence that **granisetron** 160 micrograms/kg alone had any effect on the performance of these tests except that clumsiness and inattentiveness were increased, nor was there evidence that **granisetron** added to the effects of **lorazepam** when both drugs were taken concurrently.[1]

In a placebo-controlled, crossover study in 24 healthy subjects **ondansetron** 8 mg did not affect the pharmacokinetics of **temazepam** 20 mg. The psychomotor performances of the subjects (subjective and objective sedation, memory and other measurements) were not influenced by the presence of the **ondansetron**.[2]

No additional special precautions would seem to be necessary if either of these pairs of drugs are given.

1. Leigh TJ, Link CGG, Fell GL. Effects of granisetron and lorazepam, alone and in combination, on psychometric performance. *Br J Clin Pharmacol* (1991) 31, 333–6.
2. Preston GC, Keene ON, Palmer JL. The effect of ondansetron on the pharmacokinetics and pharmacodynamics of temazepam. *Anaesthesia* (1996) 51, 827–30.

Benzodiazepines + Influenza vaccines

The pharmacokinetics of alprazolam, chlordiazepoxide and lorazepam are not affected by influenza vaccination.

Clinical evidence, mechanism, importance and management

The pharmacokinetics of single doses of oral **alprazolam** 1 mg, or intravenous **lorazepam** 2 mg remained unaffected in healthy subjects when the benzodiazepines were given 7 and 21 days after 0.5 mL of an intramuscular trivalent influenza vaccine.[1] Similarly, in another study, neither **lorazepam** nor **chlordiazepoxide** metabolism was altered when they were given 1 and 7 days after a trivalent influenza vaccine.[2] There would seem to be no reason for avoiding the concurrent use of these drugs.

1. Scavone JM, Blyden GT, Greenblatt DJ. Lack of effect of influenza vaccine on the pharmacokinetics of antipyrine, alprazolam, paracetamol (acetaminophen) and lorazepam. *Clin Pharmacokinet* (1989) 16, 180–5.
2. Meredith CG, Christian CD, Johnson RF, Troxell R, Davis GL, Schenker S. Effects of influenza virus vaccine on hepatic drug metabolism. *Clin Pharmacol Ther* (1985) 37, 396–401.

Benzodiazepines + Isoniazid

Isoniazid reduces the clearance of both diazepam and triazolam. Some increase in their effects would be expected. No interaction occurs with oxazepam or clotiazepam.

Clinical evidence

(a) Interacting benzodiazepines

A study in 9 healthy subjects found that isoniazid 90 mg twice daily for 3 days increased the half-life of a single 5- or 7.5-mg dose of **diazepam** from about 34 to 45 hours, and reduced the total clearance by 26%.[1] A study in 6 healthy subjects found that isoniazid 90 mg twice daily for 3 days, increased the half-life of a single 500 microgram dose of **triazolam** from 2.5 to 3.3 hours, increased the AUC by 46% and reduced the clearance by 43%.[2]

(b) Non-interacting benzodiazepines

A study in 9 healthy subjects found that isoniazid 90 mg twice daily for 3 days had no effect on the pharmacokinetics of a single 30-mg oral dose of **oxazepam**.[2] Similarly, in another study, the pharmacokinetics of **clotiazepam** were not altered by isoniazid.[3]

Mechanism

What is known suggests that isoniazid acts as an enzyme inhibitor, decreasing the metabolism and loss of diazepam and triazolam from the body, thereby increasing and prolonging their effects. Oxazepam which is metabolised by glucuronidation would be unlikely to interact.

Importance and management

Information is limited but the interactions appear to be established. Their clinical importance is uncertain but be alert for the need to decrease the dosages of diazepam and triazolam if isoniazid is started. There seems to be no direct information about other benzodiazepines, but those undergoing high first-pass extraction and/or liver microsomal metabolism may interact similarly. Oxazepam and clotiazepam appear not to interact.

1. Ochs HR, Greenblatt DJ, Roberts G-M, Dengler HJ. Diazepam interaction with antituberculosis drugs. *Clin Pharmacol Ther* (1981) 29, 671–8.
2. Ochs HR, Greenblatt DJ, Knüchel M. Differential effect of isoniazid on triazolam oxidation and oxazepam conjugation. *Br J Clin Pharmacol* (1983) 16, 743–6.
3. Ochs HR, Greenblatt DJ, Verburg-Ochs B, Harmatz JS, Grehl H. Disposition of clotiazepam: influence of age, sex, oral contraceptives, cimetidine, isoniazid and ethanol. *Eur J Clin Pharmacol* (1984) 26, 55–9.

Benzodiazepines + Kava

A man taking alprazolam became semicomatose a few days after starting to take kava, which was suggested to be due to additive sedation. The pharmacokinetics of midazolam were unaffected by kava.

Clinical evidence, mechanism, importance and management

(a) Alprazolam

A 54-year-old man taking alprazolam, cimetidine and terazosin was hospitalised in a lethargic and disorientated state 3 days after starting to take kava, which he had bought from a local health food store. He denied having overdosed with any of these drugs. The patient became alert again after several hours.[1] The reason for what happened is not known, but the suggested explanation is that the kava α-pyrones might have had additive sedative effects with those of the alprazolam.[1,2] This is an isolated case and its general importance is not known.

(b) Midazolam

In a study in 6 subjects who regularly took 7 to 27 g of kavalactones weekly as an aqueous kava extract, there was no change in the metabolism of a single 8-mg oral dose of midazolam before or after they stopped kava for 30 days.[3] Similar results were found in a study in 12 healthy subjects given kava kava root extract 1 g twice daily for 28 days before receiving a single 8-mg dose of oral midazolam.[4] In contrast to some *in vitro* data, these studies show that kava has no effect on the cytochrome P450 isoenzyme CYP3A4, of which midazolam is a probe substrate.[4] It is possible that the kava levels achieved clinically are insufficient to affect CYP3A4. The findings of these studies suggest that it is unlikely that kava will alter the pharmacokinetics of other substrates of CYP3A4 (see 'Table 1.4', (p.6), for a list).

1. Almeida JC, Grimsley EW. Coma from the health food store: interaction between kava and alprazolam. *Ann Intern Med* (1996) 125, 940–1.
2. Jussofie A, Schmiz A, Hiemke C. Kavapyrone enriched extract from *Piper methysticum* as modulator of GABA binding site in different regions of rat brain. *Psychopharmacology (Berl)* (1994) 116, 469–74.
3. Russman S, Lauterburg BH, Barguil Y, Choblet E, Cabalion P, Rentsch K, Wenk M. Traditional aqueous kava extracts inhibit cytochrome P450 1A2 in humans: protective effect against environmental carcinogens? *Clin Pharmacol Ther* (2005) 77, 453–4.
4. Gurley BJ, Gardner SF, Hubbard MA, Williams DK, Gentry WB, Khan IA, Shah A. In vivo effects of goldenseal, kava kava, black cohosh, and valerian on human cytochrome P450 1A2, 2D6, 2E1, and 3A4/5 phenotypes. *Clin Pharmacol Ther* (2005) 77, 415–26.

Benzodiazepines and related drugs + Macrolides

The serum levels and effects of midazolam, triazolam and zopiclone are markedly increased and prolonged by erythromycin. The same interaction has been seen with clarithromycin, josamycin, or troleandomycin but not azithromycin. Alprazolam would be expected to be similarly affected. Other benzodiazepines, and the related hypnotic zaleplon, appear not to interact with the macrolides to a clinically significant extent.

Clinical evidence

A. Benzodiazepines

(a) Alprazolam

In a randomised study 12 healthy subjects were given **erythromycin** 400 mg three times daily for 10 days with a single 800-microgram dose of alprazolam on day 8. The alprazolam AUC_{0-48} was increased by 61% and the half-life increased from 16 to 40.3 hours. However, no increase in sedation was seen.[1] The manufacturers predict that other macrolides will interact similarly, and they specifically name **erythromycin** and **troleandomycin**.[2]

(b) Brotizolam

A randomised study in healthy subjects found that **erythromycin** 400 mg three times daily for 7 days increased AUC of a single 500-microgram dose of brotizolam by 2.5-fold. The elimination half-life was also increased from 9.4 hours to 20.7 hours. However, **erythromycin** did not affect the affect the changes in psychomotor function associated with brotizolam.[3]

(c) Diazepam

In a crossover study, 6 healthy subjects were given a single 5-mg oral dose of diazepam after taking **erythromycin** 500 mg three times daily for one week. The diazepam AUC was increased by a modest 15%, but its pharmacodynamic effects were unchanged.[4]

(d) Flunitrazepam

In a crossover study, 5 healthy subjects were given a single 1-mg oral dose of flunitrazepam after taking **erythromycin** 500 mg three times daily for one week. The flunitrazepam AUC was increased by 25% but its pharmacodynamic effects were unchanged.[4]

(e) Midazolam

1. Azithromycin. A study in 64 healthy medical students found that azithromycin 750 mg had no effect on the metabolism of a 10- or 15-mg dose of midazolam, and did not alter the performance of a number of psychomotor tests.[5] A study in 10 healthy subjects given azithromycin 250 mg daily found that some small changes in pharmacokinetics of midazolam 15 mg (a possible small delay in its onset of action), but its pharmacodynamic effects were unaltered.[6] Other studies confirm that azithromycin does not interact with midazolam.[7,8]

2. Clarithromycin. Oral 4 mg and intravenous 50 microgram/kg doses of midazolam were given simultaneously to 16 healthy subjects, before and after they took clarithromycin 500 mg twice daily for 7 days. It was found that clarithromycin reduced the systemic clearance of midazolam by about 64%, which resulted in a doubling of the midazolam-induced sleeping time.[9] Similar results were found in another study.[8]

3. Erythromycin. A study in 12 healthy subjects found that erythromycin 500 mg three times daily for 6 days almost tripled the peak plasma levels of a single 15-mg dose of midazolam, more than doubled its half-life and increased the AUC by more than fourfold. The subjects could hardly be wakened during the first hour after being given the midazolam, and most experienced amnesia lasting several hours.[10]

The serum levels of a 500-microgram/kg oral dose of midazolam, given to an 8-year-old boy as pre-medication before surgery, were approximately doubled when he was given intravenous erythromycin. He developed nausea and tachycardia, and after 40 minutes (by which point he had received 200 mg of erythromycin) he lost consciousness.[11] A patient in a coronary care unit given 300 mg of intravenous midazolam over 14 hours slept for about 6 days (apart from brief wakening when given flumazenil). The midazolam half-life was increased by about tenfold. This was attributed to an interaction due to the combined effects of erythromycin 4 g daily and amiodarone 1.7 g over 3 days.[12,13] Other studies and reports have also described this interaction.[5,7,14,15]

4. Roxithromycin. In 10 healthy subjects roxithromycin 300 mg daily for 6 days increased the AUC of a single 15-mg dose of midazolam by about 47%, and lengthened the half-life from 1.7 to 2.2 hours. Only minor psychomotor changes were seen.[16] A modest increase in the effects of midazolam were seen in another study in subjects given roxithromycin 300 mg, but the effects were very much weaker than those seen with erythromycin.[15]

(f) Nitrazepam

When 10 healthy subjects were given **erythromycin** 500 mg three times daily for 4 days, the AUC of a single 5-mg dose of nitrazepam was increased by 25%, the peak plasma levels were increased by 30% and the concentration peak time was reduced by over 50%. However, hardly any changes were seen in the psychomotor tests undertaken.[17]

(g) Temazepam

A randomised, study in 10 healthy subjects found that **erythromycin** 500 mg three times daily for 6 days had no significant effect on the pharmacokinetics or psychomotor effects of a single 20-mg dose of temazepam.[18]

(h) Triazolam

1. Azithromycin. A clinical study in 12 healthy subjects found that azithromycin did not affect the pharmacokinetics of a single 125-microgram dose of triazolam.[19] These results were supported by an *in vitro* study, which confirmed that azithromycin was only a weak inhibitor of triazolam metabolism.[19]

2. Clarithromycin. An *in vitro* study found clarithromycin to be a relatively potent inhibitor of triazolam metabolism. These results were confirmed in practice with 12 healthy subjects, who were given both drugs. The oral clearance of triazolam was reduced by 77% by clarithromycin, when compared with placebo.[19]

3. Erythromycin. A study in 16 healthy subjects found that erythromycin 333 mg three times daily for 3 days, reduced the clearance of a single 500-microgram dose of triazolam by about 50%, doubled the AUC, and increased the maximum plasma levels by about one-third (from 2.8 to 4.1 nanograms/mL).[20] Other reports confirm the marked decrease in clearance and an increase in peak levels.[19,21] Repeated visual hallucinations and abnormal body sensations occurred in one patient with acute pneumonia and chronic renal failure taking erythromycin 600 mg daily after each dose of triazolam and **nitrazepam**. These symptoms had not occurred before the addition of erythromycin.[22]

4. Josamycin. Josamycin has been reported to increase triazolam levels causing an increase in its effects.[23]

5. Roxithromycin. A study found that roxithromycin 300 mg had only a slight effect on the effects of triazolam.[15]

6. Troleandomycin. Troleandomycin 2 g daily given to 7 healthy subjects for 7 days increased the peak triazolam levels by 107%, the AUC by 275% and the half-life from 1.81 to 6.48 hours. Apparent oral clearance was reduced by 74%. Marked psychomotor impairment and amnesia was seen.[24] Troleandomycin has been reported to interact similarly in a patient on triazolam, causing an increase in its effects.[23] An *in vitro* study has shown troleandomycin to be a potent inhibitor of triazolam metabolism.[19]

B. Non-benzodiazepine hypnotics

(a) Zaleplon

The manufacturers say that a single 800-mg dose of **erythromycin** increased the plasma levels of zaleplon by 34%.[25]

(b) Zolpidem

In a study in healthy subjects **clarithromycin** had no effects on the pharmacokinetics of zolpidem or on its sedative effects.[26]

(c) Zopiclone

Zopiclone 7.5 mg was given to 10 healthy subjects before and after taking **erythromycin** 500 mg three times daily for 6 days. The **erythromycin** increased the plasma concentration of the zopiclone fivefold at 30 minutes and twofold at one hour. Peak plasma levels rose by about 40% and occurred at 1 hour instead of 2 hours. The 1-hour and 2-hour AUCs were increased threefold and twofold, respectively, while the total AUC was increased by nearly 80%.[27] These pharmacokinetic changes were reflected in some small changes in a number of psychomotor tests.[27]

Mechanism

Some of the macrolides (notably erythromycin and troleandomycin) are potent inhibitors of the cytochrome P450 isoenzyme CYP3A4. Benzodiazepines, such as midazolam, that are predominantly metabolised by CYP3A4 are affected more than those such as diazepam, where CYP3A4 plays only a minor part in the metabolism. Further, CYP3A4-mediated metabolism occurs in the liver and also in the intestines. Midazolam and triazolam undergo extensive first-pass metabolism (low bioavailability of about 40%) but alprazolam and brotizolam undergo less first-pass metabolism (bioavailabilities of about 90% and 70%, respectively). Erythromycin causes greater increases in the levels and AUC of midazolam and triazolam than in those of alprazolam and brotizolam, and this may be related to the extent of first-pass metabolism.[3] The non-benzodiazepine hypnotics, zaleplon and zopiclone are, to varying degrees, also metabolised by CYP3A4. The macrolides can therefore reduce the metabolism of some of the benzodiazepines and related drugs, raising their serum levels and increasing and prolonging their effects.

Importance and management

The interactions of midazolam with erythromycin and triazolam with clarithromycin, erythromycin or troleandomycin appear to be established, and of clinical importance. The dosages of the midazolam and triazolam should be reduced 50 to 75% when these antibacterials are used if excessive effects (marked drowsiness, memory loss) are to be avoided. Remember too that the hypnotic effects are also prolonged so that patients should be warned about hangover effects the following morning if they intend to drive. Much less is known about the use of midazolam with clarithromycin but similar precautions may be necessary. The manufacturers of zaleplon say that patients should be advised that increased sedation is possible with erythromycin, although a dose adjustment is usually not required.[25]

Limited information from single-dose studies suggests that erythromycin may increase levels of alprazolam and brotizolam but no pharmacodynamic changes were found. Nevertheless, the manufacturers advise caution if alprazolam is used with a macrolide.[2]

Azithromycin does not interact with midazolam or triazolam, and the effects of roxithromycin on midazolam and triazolam, and of erythromycin on diazepam, flunitrazepam, nitrazepam, temazepam and zopiclone or clarithromycin on zolpidem appear to be small and unimportant, or the effects negligible, so that no special precautions seem to be necessary.

1. Yasui N, Otani K, Kaneko S, Ohkubo T, Osanai T, Sugawara K, Chiba K, Ishizaki T. A kinetic and dynamic study of oral alprazolam with and without erythromycin in humans: in vivo evidence for the involvement of CYP3A4 in alprazolam metabolism. *Clin Pharmacol Ther* (1996) 59, 514–19.
2. Xanax Tablets (Alprazolam). Pharmacia Ltd. UK Summary of product characteristics, June 2003.
3. Tokairin T, Fukasawa T, Ysaui-Fukukori N, Aoshima T, Suzuki A, Inoue Y, Tateishi T, Otani K. Inhibition of the metabolism of brotizolam by erythromycin in humans: *in vivo* evidence for the involvement of CYP3A4 in brotizolam metabolism. *Br J Clin Pharmacol* (2005) 60, 172–5.
4. Luurila H, Olkkola KT, Neuvonen PJ. Interaction between erythromycin and the benzodiazepines diazepam and flunitrazepam. *Pharmacol Toxicol* (1996) 78, 117–22..
5. Mattila MJ, Vanakoski J, Idänpään-Heikkilä JJ. Azithromycin does not alter the effects of oral midazolam on human performance. *Eur J Clin Pharmacol* (1994) 47, 49–52.
6. Backman JT, Olkkola KT, Neuvonen PJ. Azithromycin does not increase plasma concentrations of oral midazolam. *Int J Clin Pharmacol Ther* (1995) 33, 356–9.
7. Zimmermann T, Yeates RA, Laufen H, Scharpf F, Leitold M, Wildfeuer A. Influence of the antibiotics erythromycin and azithromycin on the pharmacokinetics and pharmacodynamics of midazolam. *Arzneimittelforschung* (1996) 46, 213–17.
8. Yeates RA, Laufen H, Zimmermann T. Interaction between midazolam and clarithromycin: comparison with azithromycin. *Int J Clin Pharmacol Ther* (1996) 34, 400–5.
9. Gorski JC, Jones DR, Haehner-Daniels BD, Hamman MA, O'Mara EM, Hall SD. The contribution of intestinal and hepatic CYP3A to the interaction between midazolam and clarithromycin. *Clin Pharmacol Ther* (1998) 64, 133–43.
10. Olkkola KT, Aranko K, Luurila H, Hiller A, Saarnivaara L, Himberg J-J, Neuvonen PJ. A potentially hazardous interaction between erythromycin and midazolam. *Clin Pharmacol Ther* (1993) 53, 298–305.
11. Hiller A, Olkkola KT, Isohanni P, Saarnivaara L. Unconsciousness associated with midazolam and erythromycin. *Br J Anaesth* (1990) 65, 826–8.
12. Gascon M-P, Dayer P, Waldvogel F. Les interactions médicamenteuses du midazolam. *Schweiz Med Wochenschr* (1989) 119, 1834–6.
13. Gascon M-P, Dayer P. In vitro forecasting of drugs which may interfere with the biotransformation of midazolam. *Eur J Clin Pharmacol* (1991) 41, 573–8.
14. Byatt CM, Lewis LD, Dawling S, Cochrane GM. Accumulation of midazolam after repeated dosage in patients receiving mechanical ventilation in an intensive care unit. *BMJ* (1984) 289, 799–800.
15. Mattila MJ, Idänpään-Heikkilä JJ, Törnwall M, Vanakoski J. Oral single doses of erythromycin and roxithromycin may increase the effects of midazolam on human performance. *Pharmacol Toxicol* (1993) 73, 180–5.
16. Backman JT, Aranko K, Himberg J-J, Olkkola KT. A pharmacokinetic interaction between roxithromycin and midazolam. *Eur J Clin Pharmacol* (1994) 46, 551–5.

17. Luurila H, Olkkola KT, Neuvonen PJ. Interaction between erythromycin and nitrazepam in healthy volunteers. *Pharmacol Toxicol* (1995) 76, 255–8.
18. Luurila H, Olkkola KT, Neuvonen PJ. Lack of interaction of erythromycin and temazepam. *Ther Drug Monit* (1994) 16, 548–51.
19. Greenblatt DJ, von Moltke LL, Harmatz JS, Counihan M, Graf JA, Durol ALB, Mertzanis P, Duan SX, Wright CE, Shader RI. Inhibition of triazolam clearance by macrolide antimicrobial agents: in vitro correlates and dynamic consequences. *Clin Pharmacol Ther* (1998) 64, 278–85.
20. Phillips JP, Antal EJ, Smith RB. A pharmacokinetic drug interaction between erythromycin and triazolam. *J Clin Psychopharmacol* (1986) 6, 297–9.
21. Hugues FC, Le Jeunne C, Munera Y. Conséquences en thérapeutique de l'inhibition microsomiale hépatique par les macrolides. *Sem Hop Paris* (1987) 63, 2280–3.
22. Tokinaga N, Kondo T, Kaneko S, Otani K, Mihara K, Morita S. Hallucinations after a therapeutic dose of benzodiazepine hypnotics with co-administration of erythromycin. *Psychiatry Clin Neurosci* (1996) 50, 337–9.
23. Carry PV, Ducluzeau R, Jourdan C, Bourrat C, Vigneou C, Descotes J. De nouvelles interactions avec les macrolides? *Lyon Med* (1982) 248, 189–90.
24. Warot D, Bergougnan L, Lamiable D, Berlin I, Bensimon G, Danjou P, Puech AJ. Troleandomycin-triazolam interaction in healthy volunteers: pharmacokinetic and psychometric evaluation. *Eur J Clin Pharmacol* (1987) 32, 389–93.
25. Sonata (Zaleplon). Wyeth Pharmaceuticals. UK Summary of product characteristics, June 2006.
26. Greenblatt DJ, von Moltke LL, Harmatz JS. Clarithromycin impairs the clearance and potentiates clinical effects of trazodone but not of zolpidem. *Clin Pharmacol Ther* (2005) 77, P28.
27. Aranko K, Luurila H, Backman JT, Neuvonen PJ, Olkkola KT. The effect of erythromycin on the pharmacokinetics and pharmacodynamics of zopiclone. *Br J Clin Pharmacol* (1994) 38, 363–7.

Benzodiazepines and related drugs + Metoclopramide

Intravenous, but not oral, metoclopramide increases the rate of absorption of diazepam and raises its maximum plasma levels. Metoclopramide increases the rate of absorption of zopiclone.

Clinical evidence, mechanism, importance and management

(a) Diazepam

Intravenous metoclopramide increased the peak plasma levels of diazepam by 38% and increased the rate of absorption (peak levels occurred at 30 minutes instead of 60 minutes),[1] but in 6 healthy subjects oral metoclopramide 10 mg did not increase the rate of absorption of oral diazepam 0.2 mg/kg.[2] The reason is not understood. The clinical importance of this interaction is not known, but it is probably small.

(b) Zopiclone

The rate of absorption of a single 7.5-mg dose of oral zopiclone was increased by metoclopramide 10 mg given intravenously to 12 healthy subjects. This was presumably because these drugs alter gut motility. Metoclopramide increased the mean plasma levels of zopiclone, from 22.7 to 44.4 nanograms/mL at 1 hour, and from 49.3 to 59.6 nanograms/mL at 2 hours.[3] The clinical importance of these findings is not known.

1. Gamble JAS, Gaston JH, Nair SG, Dundee JW. Some pharmacological factors influencing the absorption of diazepam following oral administration. *Br J Anaesth* (1976) 48, 1181–5.
2. Chapman MH, Woolner DF, Begg EJ, Atkinson HC, Sharman JR. Co-administered oral metoclopramide does not enhance the rate of absorption of oral diazepam. *Anaesth Intensive Care* (1988) 16, 202–5.
3. Elliott P, Chestnutt WN, Elwood RJ, Dundee JW. Effect of atropine and metoclopramide on the plasma concentrations of orally administered zopiclone. *Br J Anaesth* (1983) 55, 1159P–1160P.

Benzodiazepines + Metronidazole

Metronidazole does not interact with alprazolam, diazepam, lorazepam, or midazolam.

Clinical evidence, mechanism, importance and management

A study in healthy subjects found that metronidazole 400 mg twice daily for 5 days had no effect on the pharmacokinetics of a single 100-microgram/kg intravenous dose of **diazepam**.[1] Another study in healthy subjects found that metronidazole 750 mg had no effect on the pharmacokinetics of **alprazolam** or **lorazepam**.[2] *In vivo* and *in vitro* studies have shown that metronidazole has no effect on the pharmacokinetics or pharmacodynamics of **midazolam**.[3] Interactions with other benzodiazepines seem unlikely.

1. Jensen JC, Gugler R. Interaction between metronidazole and drugs eliminated by oxidative metabolism. *Clin Pharmacol Ther* (1985) 37, 407–10.
2. Blyden GT, Greenblatt DJ, Scavone JM. Metronidazole impairs clearance of phenytoin but not of alprazolam or lorazepam. *Clin Pharmacol Ther* (1986) 39, 181.
3. Wang J-S, Backman JT, Kivistö KT, Neuvonen PJ. Effects of metronidazole on midazolam metabolism in vitro and in vivo. *Eur J Clin Pharmacol* (2000) 56, 555–9.

Benzodiazepines + Milk thistle

Milk thistle does not alter the pharmacokinetics of midazolam.

Clinical evidence, mechanism, importance and management

In a study 19 healthy subjects were given milk thistle 300 mg three times daily for 14 days (standardised to silymarin 80%) with a single 8-mg oral dose of **midazolam** on the last day. There was no change in the pharmacokinetics of **midazolam**, and milk thistle had no effect on the duration of midazolam-induced sleep.[1] Similarly, in another study in 12 healthy subjects, milk thistle 175 mg (standardised to silymarins 80%) given twice daily for 28 days had no significant effects on the metabolism of a single 8-mg dose of **midazolam**.[2]

These studies show that the pharmacokinetics of **midazolam**, a probe substrate for the cytochrome P450 isoenzyme CYP3A4, are not affected by the concurrent use of milk thistle. This suggests that milk thistle is unlikely to affect the metabolism of other drugs that are substrates of CYP3A4, see 'Table 1.4', (p.6), for a list.

1. Gurley B, Hubbard MA, Williams DK, Thaden J, Tong Y, Gentry WB, Breen P, Carrier DJ, Cheboyina S. Assessing the clinical significance of botanical supplementation on human cytochrome P450 3A activity: comparison of a milk thistle and black cohosh product to rifampin and clarithromycin. *J Clin Pharmacol* (2006) 46, 201–13.
2. Gurley BJ, Gardner SF, Hubbard MA, Williams DK, Gentry WB, Carrier J, Khan IA, Edwards DJ, Shah A. In vivo assessment of botanical supplementation on human cytochrome P450 phenotypes: *Citrus aurantium*, *Echinacea purpurea*, milk thistle, and saw palmetto. *Clin Pharmacol Ther* (2004) 76, 428–40.

Benzodiazepines + Misoprostol

A study in 12 subjects found that misoprostol 200 micrograms four times daily for 7 days had no effect on the steady-state plasma levels of diazepam 10 mg daily or on the plasma levels of the metabolite, nordiazepam.[1] No special precautions would therefore seem to be necessary if misoprostol is given with diazepam.

1. Lima DR, Santos RM, Werneck E, Andrade GN. Effect of orally administered misoprostol and cimetidine on the steady state pharmacokinetics of diazepam and nordiazepam in human volunteers. *Eur J Drug Metab Pharmacokinet* (1991) 16, 161–70.

Benzodiazepines + Modafinil

Modafinil reduces triazolam levels. It may therefore also affect the metabolism of other similarly metabolised benzodiazepines such as alprazolam and midazolam. Conversely, modafinil might increase diazepam levels.

Clinical evidence, mechanism, importance and management

In a single-dose study, 34 healthy women (all taking an oral contraceptive containing ethinylestradiol and norgestimate) were given a single 125-microgram dose of **triazolam**, both before and on the last day of taking modafinil (200 mg daily for 7 days then 400 mg daily for 21 days) or placebo. The AUC of **triazolam** was reduced by almost 60%, its maximum plasma level was reduced by 42% and its elimination half-life was reduced by about 1 hour by modafinil, when compared with placebo.[1]

Modafinil is known to induce the cytochrome P450 isoenzyme CYP3A4, by which triazolam is metabolised, and it is therefore likely to reduce triazolam levels by this mechanism. It seems possible that other benzodiazepines metabolised by CYP3A4 (**alprazolam**, **midazolam**) may be similarly affected. It would therefore seem prudent to monitor for a reduction in the sedative effects and a reduced duration of action of these benzodiazepines in patients taking modafinil: increase the dose if necessary.[2]

Conversely, modafinil inhibits the cytochrome P450 isoenzyme CYP2C19. The manufacturers therefore predict that the elimination of **diazepam**, which is metabolised by this isoenzyme, may be reduced. They suggest that a dosage reduction may be necessary on concurrent use.[2,3]

1. Robertson P, Hellreigel ET, Arora S, Nelson M. Effect of modafinil on the pharmacokinetics of ethinyl estradiol and triazolam in healthy volunteers. *Clin Pharmacol Ther* (2002) 71, 46–56.
2. Provigil (Modafinil), Cephalon, Inc. US Prescribing information, December 2004.
3. Provigil (Modafinil). Cephalon Ltd. UK Summary of product characteristics, July 2007.

Benzodiazepines and related drugs + Nefazodone

Nefazodone increases the plasma levels and effects of alprazolam, midazolam, triazolam and zopiclone, but not lorazepam.

Clinical evidence

A. Benzodiazepines

(a) Alprazolam

A placebo-controlled study in 12 healthy subjects found that nefazodone 200 mg twice daily caused an almost twofold increase in the plasma levels of alprazolam 1 mg twice daily taken for 7 days.[1] Another study found that impairment of psychomotor performance and increased sedation occurred when nefazodone was given with alprazolam.[2] A case report describes benzodiazepine withdrawal symptoms in a woman taking alprazolam after nefazodone was withdrawn following several years of concurrent use. She needed an alprazolam dosage increase from 500 micrograms to 4 mg daily to control her symptoms.[3]

(b) Lorazepam

A placebo-controlled study in healthy subjects given nefazodone 200 mg twice daily found no changes in the pharmacokinetics of lorazepam 2 mg twice daily.[1] Another study showed that psychomotor performance was not further impaired and no additional sedation occurred when nefazodone was given with lorazepam.[2]

(c) Midazolam

A study in 10 healthy subjects found that both the AUC and the maximum plasma level of a single 10-mg dose of midazolam were increased about fivefold and twofold, respectively, when they took nefazodone 200 mg twice daily.[4]

(d) Triazolam

A study in 12 healthy subjects found that the maximum plasma levels, the half-life and the AUC of a single 250-microgram dose of triazolam were increased 1.7-fold, 4.6-fold, and 4-fold, respectively, by nefazodone 200 mg twice daily.[5] Another study showed that impairment of psychomotor performance and increased sedation occurred when nefazodone was given with triazolam.[2]

B. Non-benzodiazepine hypnotics

An 86-year-old woman taking diltiazem, irbesartan, lorazepam, and pravastatin started taking nefazodone 50 mg twice daily, increasing to 500 mg daily in divided doses, for the treatment of a major depressive episode. Because of associated insomnia, **zopiclone** was added, starting at 15 mg each night, but this was reduced after 5 days to 7.5 mg because of morning drowsiness. Plasma levels of *S*-zopiclone and *R*-zopiclone were 107 nanograms/mL and 20.6 nanograms/mL, respectively, at this time. After several months, nefazodone was replaced by venlafaxine. The *S*-zopiclone and *R*-zopiclone levels were again measured and found to be only 16.9 nanograms/mL and 1.45 nanograms/mL, respectively.[6]

Mechanism

Nefazodone appears to inhibit the oxidative metabolism of alprazolam, midazolam, triazolam and zopiclone by the cytochrome P450 isoenzyme CYP3A4 so that they accumulate in the body. Lorazepam is unaffected because it is primarily excreted as a conjugate.

Importance and management

The interactions of nefazodone with alprazolam, midazolam, triazolam and zopiclone are established and clinically important. The practical consequences are that the effects of alprazolam, midazolam and triazolam are expected to be increased but the extent is uncertain. Be alert for any evidence of any psychomotor impairment, drowsiness etc. and reduce the benzodiazepine dosage if necessary. More study is needed. Lorazepam does not interact with nefazodone. There seems to be no direct information about other benzodiazepines and related drugs.

1. Greene DS, Salazar DE, Dockens RC, Kroboth P, Barbhaiya RH. Coadministration of nefazodone and benzodiazepines: III. A pharmacokinetic interaction study with alprazolam. *J Clin Psychopharmacol* (1995) 15, 399–408.
2. Kroboth P, Folan M, Lush R, Chaikin PC, Barbhaiya RH, Salazar DE. Coadministration of nefazodone and benzodiazepines II: pharmacodynamic assessment. *Clin Pharmacol Ther* (1994) 55, 142.
3. Ninan T. Pharmacokinetically induced benzodiazepine withdrawal. *Psychopharmacol Bull* (2001) 35, 94–100.
4. Lam YWF, Alfaro CL, Ereshefsky L, Miller M. Pharmacokinetic and pharmacodynamic interactions of oral midazolam with ketoconazole, fluoxetine, fluvoxamine, and nefazodone. *J Clin Pharmacol* (2003) 43, 1274–82.
5. Barbhaiya RH, Shukla UA, Kroboth PD, Greene DS. Coadministration of nefazodone and benzodiazepines: II. A pharmacokinetic interaction study with triazolam. *J Clin Psychopharmacol* (1995) 15, 320–6.
6. Alderman CP, Gebauer MG, Gilbert AL, Condon JT. Possible interaction of zopiclone and nefazodone. *Ann Pharmacother* (2001) 35, 1378–80.

Benzodiazepines and related drugs + NSAIDs

Diclofenac reduces the dose of midazolam needed to produce sedation and hypnosis. Diazepam has a small effect on the pharmacokinetics of diclofenac, ibuprofen and naproxen. Diazepam and indometacin appear not to interact adversely, although feelings of dizziness may be increased. Zaleplon and ibuprofen appear not to interact.

Clinical evidence, mechanism, importance and management

(a) Diazepam

1. Diclofenac. In a study in 8 healthy subjects, diazepam increased the AUC of diclofenac by 60% while the clearance was reduced by 36%.[1] The effects of diazepam on diclofenac appeared to depend on the time of administration and may reflect time-dependent effects of diazepam on gastrointestinal function. More study is needed.

2. Ibuprofen. A study in 8 healthy subjects investigating the effects of diazepam on ibuprofen pharmacokinetics found that the ibuprofen half-life was increased from 2.39 to 3.59 hours and the clearance was reduced by about one-third when diazepam and ibuprofen were given at 10 pm, but no effect was seen with morning dosing.[2] The clinical importance of this is uncertain.

3. Indometacin. Diazepam 10 to 15 mg impaired the performance of a number of psychomotor tests (digit symbol substitution, letter cancellation, tracking and flicker fusion) in 119 healthy medical students. It also caused subjective drowsiness, mental slowness and clumsiness. When indometacin 50 or 100 mg was given the effects were little different from diazepam alone, except that the feeling of dizziness (common to both drugs) was increased and caused subjective clumsiness.[3]

4. Naproxen. A double-blind, crossover study failed to find any clinically important changes in mood or attention in healthy subjects given naproxen and diazepam.[4] A single-dose study in 10 healthy subjects found that peak serum concentrations of naproxen 500 mg were reduced by 23%, the time to peak concentration was increased (1.36 to 2 hours) and the absorption rate constant was decreased (4.07 to 2.42 h^{-1}) by diazepam 10 mg. Other pharmacokinetic parameters were not affected.[5] No special precautions appear to be necessary.

(b) Midazolam

A clinical study found that **diclofenac** 75 mg given intravenously to 10 patients reduced the dose of intravenous midazolam needed to produce sedation and hypnosis by 35%, when compared with 10 control subjects not given **diclofenac**.[6] The clinical importance of this is uncertain.

For the interactions of parecoxib with midazolam see 'NSAIDs; Parecoxib + Miscellaneous', p.160.

(c) Zaleplon

A randomised, single-dose study in 17 healthy subjects found that **ibuprofen** 600 mg had no effect on the pharmacokinetics of zaleplon 10 mg.[7]

1. Mahender VN, Rambhau D, Rao BR, Rao VVS, Venkateshwarlu G. Time-dependent influence of diazepam on the pharmacokinetics of orally administered diclofenac sodium in human subjects. *Clin Drug Invest* (1995) 10, 296–301.
2. Bapuji AT, Rambhau D, Srinivasu P, Rao BR, Apte SS. Time dependent influence of diazepam on the pharmacokinetics of ibuprofen in man. *Drug Metabol Drug Interact* (1999) 15, 71–81.
3. Nuotto E, Saarialho-Kere U. Actions and interactions of indomethacin and diazepam on performance in healthy volunteers. *Pharmacol Toxicol* (1988) 62, 293–7.
4. Stitt FW, Latour R, Frane JW. A clinical study of naproxen-diazepam drug interaction on tests of mood and attention. *Curr Ther Res* (1977) 21, 149–56.
5. Rao BR, Rambhau D. Influence of diazepam on the pharmacokinetic properties of orally administered naproxen. *Drug Invest* (1992) 4, 416–21.
6. Carrero E, Castillo J, Bogdanovich A, Nalda MA. El diclofenac reduce las dosis sedante e hipnótica de midazolam. *Rev Esp Anestesiol Reanim* (1991) 38, 127.
7. Garcia PS, Carcas A, Zapater P, Rosendo J, Paty I, Leister CA, Troy SM. Absence of an interaction between ibuprofen and zaleplon. *Am J Health-Syst Pharm* (2000) 57, 1137–41.

Benzodiazepines + Paracetamol (Acetaminophen)

Paracetamol reduces the urinary excretion of diazepam but diazepam plasma levels are little affected.

Clinical evidence, mechanism, importance and management

The 96-hour urinary excretion of a single 10-mg oral dose of **diazepam** and its metabolite, nordiazepam, were reduced from 44% to 12% and from 27% to 8%, respectively, in 2 female subjects, and from 11% to 4.5%, respectively, in a male subject, by a single 500-mg dose of paracetamol. The reasons are not understood. Plasma levels of **diazepam** and its metabolite were not significantly affected.[1] There would seem to be no reason for avoiding concurrent use. There seems to be no information about other benzodiazepines.

1. Mulley BA, Potter BI, Rye RM, Takeshita K. Interactions between diazepam and paracetamol. *J Clin Pharm* (1978) 3, 25–35.

Benzodiazepines + Probenecid

Probenecid reduces the clearance of adinazolam, lorazepam and nitrazepam. Increased effects (e.g. sedation) may be expected. Probenecid does not appear to interact with temazepam.

Clinical evidence

(a) Adinazolam

In a single-dose study in 16 healthy subjects, probenecid 2 g increased the psychomotor effects of sustained-release adinazolam 60 mg. The tests used were symbol-digit substitution, digit span forwards and continuous performance tasks.[1] The peak serum levels of adinazolam and its active metabolite, *N*-desmethyladinazolam, were increased by 37% and 49%, respectively, and the clearances were reduced by 16% and 53%, respectively, by probenecid. Both drugs have uricosuric actions, but when used together the effects appear not to be additive.[1]

(b) Lorazepam

Probenecid 500 mg every 6 hours approximately halved the clearance of a single 2-mg intravenous dose of lorazepam in 9 healthy subjects. The elimination half-life was more than doubled, from 14.3 hours to 33 hours.[2]

(c) Nitrazepam

Probenecid 500 mg daily for 7 days reduced the clearance of nitrazepam by 25% in healthy subjects.[3]

(d) Temazepam

Probenecid 500 mg daily for 7 days but did not significantly affect the clearance of temazepam in healthy subjects.[3]

Mechanism

Probenecid inhibits the renal tubular clearance of many drugs and their metabolites, including some of the benzodiazepines. It also inhibits the glucuronidation of nitrazepam and lorazepam by the liver.[2,3] The overall result is that these benzodiazepines accumulate and their effects are increased. Temazepam, which also undergoes glucuronidation, was not affected, possibly as increased sulfation compensated.[3]

Importance and management

Established interactions but of uncertain clinical importance. Be alert for increases in the effects (sedation, antegrade amnesia) of adinazolam, lorazepam and possibly nitrazepam. Reduce the dosage as necessary. Note that adinazolam is no longer available.There seems to be no direct information about other benzodiazepines, but those that are metabolised like lorazepam and nitrazepam (e.g. oxazepam) may also interact. Temazepam does not appear to interact with probenecid.

1. Golden PL, Warner PE, Fleishaker JC, Jewell RC, Millikin S, Lyon J, Brouwer KLR. Effects of probenecid on the pharmacokinetics and pharmacodynamics of adinazolam in humans. *Clin Pharmacol Ther* (1994) 56, 133–41.
2. Abernethy DR, Greenblatt DJ, Ameer B, Shader RI. Probenecid impairment of acetaminophen and lorazepam clearance: direct inhibition of ether glucuronide formation. *J Pharmacol Exp Ther* (1985) 234, 345–9.
3. Brockmeyer NH, Mertins L, Klimek K, Goos M, Ohnhaus EE. Comparative effects of rifampin and/or probenecid on the pharmacokinetics of temazepam and nitrazepam. *Int J Clin Pharmacol Ther Toxicol* (1990) 28, 387–93.

Benzodiazepines and related drugs + Protease inhibitors

A study and a case report show that saquinavir markedly decreases midazolam metabolism, resulting in a significant increase in sedation. Ritonavir similarly affects triazolam and, to a lesser extent, alprazolam, but appears not to affect zolpidem levels.

Clinical evidence, mechanism, importance and management

A. Benzodiazepines

(a) Alprazolam

A crossover study in 10 healthy subjects found that **ritonavir** 200 mg for 4 doses decreased the clearance of a single 1-mg dose of alprazolam by 59%. The half-life of alprazolam was increased from 13.3 to 29.6 hours and the subjects experienced increased and prolonged sedation.[1]

(b) Midazolam

A randomised study in 12 healthy subjects found that **saquinavir** (soft-gel formulation) 1.2 g three times daily increased the bioavailability of oral midazolam from 41 to 90% and increased the AUC fivefold. Psychomotor tests showed impaired skills and greater sedation in the presence of **saquinavir**.[2] When intravenous midazolam was given, the sedative effects were only marginally altered.[2] However, a 32-year-old with advanced HIV, taking zidovudine, lamivudine, co-trimoxazole and **saquinavir** 600 mg three times daily, did not wake spontaneously from a 5 mg intravenous dose of midazolam. He was given 300 micrograms of intravenous flumazenil to revert the prolonged sedation, but he was not free from sedation until 5 hours later. On a previous occasion, in the absence of **saquinavir**, he woke spontaneously 2 hours after the dose of midazolam.[3] The manufacturers of saquinavir note that in 16 healthy subjects, saquinavir/ritonavir 1000/100 mg twice daily for 2 weeks increased the maximum levels and AUC of a single 7.5-mg oral dose of midazolam by 4.3-fold and 12.4-fold, respectively.[4]

(c) Triazolam

In a crossover study in 6 healthy subjects **ritonavir** 200 mg for 4 doses reduced the clearance of triazolam 125 micrograms to less than 4% of control values and increased the half-life from 3 to 41 hours, which resulted in increased and prolonged sedation.[5] A very brief case report also describes prolonged sedation in a patient given **ritonavir** and triazolam.[6]

B. Non-benzodiazepine hypnotics

A crossover study in 6 healthy subjects found that **ritonavir** 200 mg twice daily for 4 doses resulted in only a small and clinically unimportant reduction in the clearance of a single 5-mg dose of **zolpidem**.[5]

Mechanism

Alprazolam, midazolam and triazolam are metabolised by the cytochrome P450 isoenzyme CYP3A4, which is inhibited, to varying degrees, by the protease inhibitors. Benzodiazepine levels and effects are therefore increased by saquinavir and ritonavir. Zolpidem metabolism depends on several isoenzymes so inhibition of CYP3A4 alone may not produce clinically significant changes in its clearance.

Importance and management

This interaction is of clinical importance: be alert for the need to reduce the midazolam dosage in the presence of saquinavir. The authors of the study[2] suggest that continuous intravenous midazolam doses should be reduced by 50%, but do not consider dose adjustments to single intravenous doses necessary.[2] The same precautions would seem appropriate with triazolam. However, the manufacturer of saquinavir contraindicates the concurrent use of oral midazolam and triazolam.[4,7] They note that no studies have been conducted with ritonavir-boosted saquinavir but that a 3 to 4-fold increase in intravenous midazolam levels would be expected.[4] Use of intravenous midazolam with saquinavir is not contraindicated but they advise that its use be restricted to an intensive care unit or similar setting so that the appropriate management of respiratory depression is available.[4]

The UK manufacturer of ritonavir contraindicates its use with **clorazepate**, **diazepam**, **estazolam**, **flurazepam**, midazolam and triazolam as they are highly metabolised by the cytochrome P450 isoenzymes and therefore may cause extreme sedation and respiratory depression in the presence of ritonavir.[8] The US manufacturer of ritonavir contraindicates its use with triazolam and midazolam.[9] This interaction is likely to occur at least to some extent with all protease inhibitors and any of these highly metabolised benzodiazepines, and the use of (oral) midazolam and triazolam is largely contraindicated.

The manufacturer of ritonavir notes that zolpidem and ritonavir may be given concurrently with careful monitoring for excessive sedative effects.[8]

1. Greenblatt DJ, von Moltke LL, Harmatz JS, Durol ALB, Daily JP, Graf JA, Mertzanis P, Hoffman JL, Shader RI. Alprazolam-ritonavir interaction: implications for product labeling. *Clin Pharmacol Ther* (2000) 67, 335–41.
2. Palkama VJ, Ahonen J, Neuvonen PJ, Olkkola KT. Effect of saquinavir on the pharmacokinetics and pharmacodynamics of oral and intravenous midazolam. *Clin Pharmacol Ther* (1999) 66, 33–9.
3. Merry C, Mulcahy F, Barry M, Gibbons S, Back D. Saquinavir interaction with midazolam: pharmacokinetic considerations when prescribing protease inhibitors for patients with HIV disease. *AIDS* (1997) 11, 268–9.
4. Invirase Hard Capsules (Saquinavir mesilate). Roche Products Ltd. UK Summary of product characteristics, May 2007.
5. Greenblatt DJ, von Moltke LL, Harmatz JS, Durol AL, Daily JP, Graf JA, Mertzanis P, Hoffman JL, Shader RI. Differential impairment of triazolam and zolpidem clearance by ritonavir. *J Acquir Immune Defic Syndr* (2000) 24, 129–36.
6. Shader RI, Greenblatt DJ. Protease inhibitors and drug interaction—an alert. *J Clin Psychopharmacol* (1996) 16, 343–4.
7. Invirase (Saquinavir mesilate). Roche Laboratories Inc. US prescribing information, September 2005.
8. Norvir (Ritonavir). Abbott Laboratories Ltd. UK Summary of product characteristics, May 2007.
9. Norvir (Ritonavir). Abbott Laboratories. US Prescribing information, January 2006.

Benzodiazepines + Proton pump inhibitors

Gait disturbances (attributed to benzodiazepine toxicity) occurred in two patients given triazolam and lorazepam or flurazepam with omeprazole, and another patient taking diazepam and omeprazole became wobbly and sedated. Lansoprazole, pantoprazole, or rabeprazole appear not to interact to a clinically relevant extent with diazepam. Diazepam serum levels are increased by esomeprazole but the clinical relevance of this is unknown.

Clinical evidence

(a) Esomeprazole

Esomeprazole inhibits the cytochrome P450 isoenzyme CYP2C19 so the plasma levels of drugs that are metabolised by this isoenzyme might be expected to be increased by concurrent use. This is true for **diazepam**, which showed a 45% decrease in clearance (which would be expected to result in some increase in its levels) when given with esomeprazole 40 mg.[1]

(b) Lansoprazole

Lansoprazole 60 mg daily for 10 days was found to have no effect on the pharmacokinetics of a single 100-microgram/kg intravenous dose of **diazepam**.[2]

(c) Omeprazole

Two elderly patients, both smokers, taking **triazolam** with **lorazepam** or **flurazepam**, developed gait disturbances when they were given omeprazole 20 mg daily. They rapidly recovered when either the benzodiazepines or the omeprazole were stopped.[3] A brief report describes a patient taking omeprazole who became wobbly and sedated by small, unspecified doses of **diazepam**,[4] and another report describes a patient who developed toxic levels of nordiazepam and remained unconscious for 13 days after receiving a high dose of **clorazepate** (1500 mg over about 29 hours) and omeprazole 80 mg daily.[5]

One study in 8 healthy subjects found that omeprazole 40 mg daily for one week reduced the clearance of a single 100-microgram/kg intravenous dose of **diazepam** by 54%,[6] while another study found that omeprazole 20 mg reduced **diazepam** clearance by 27%.[7]

A further study found that omeprazole 40 mg reduced the oral clearance of **diazepam** by 42% in white American subjects but only by 21% in Chinese subjects.[8] Metaboliser status (see 'Genetic factors', (p.4)) was also found to be important in another study of this interaction: only extensive metabolisers of CYP2C19 showed a significant decrease in **diazepam** clearance when given omeprazole.[9]

(d) Pantoprazole

In a placebo-controlled study in 12 healthy subjects, intravenous pantoprazole 240 mg for 7 days did not change the half-life, clearance and AUC of a 100-microgram/kg intravenous bolus dose of **diazepam**.[10]

(e) Rabeprazole

Rabeprazole 20 mg daily or placebo was given to 15 patients (in 3 groups) for 23 days with a single 100-microgram/kg dose of **diazepam** on day 8. Each group contained at least two poor metabolisers and three extensive metabolisers of the cytochrome P450 isoenzyme CYP2C19 (see 'Genetic factors', (p.4)). No significant changes in the pharmacokinetics of the **diazepam** were seen.[11] Another study similarly found that rabeprazole does not affect the pharmacokinetics of **diazepam** in both poor and extensive metabolisers of CYP2C19.[9]

Mechanism

In vitro studies with human liver microsomes suggest that omeprazole inhibits diazepam metabolism because it inhibits the cytochrome P450 isoenzymes CYP3A, and CYP2C19.[12] Studies in humans suggest that CYP2C19 may be the most important isoenzyme in this interaction.[8] The reaction with lorazepam (and other glucuronidated benzodiazepines) may possibly not be an interaction (so it is suggested) but an adverse effect of giving sedating medications to markedly anaemic patients.[4]

Importance and management

Information is limited, but what is currently known suggests that patients given omeprazole, and possibly esomeprazole, with diazepam may experience increased benzodiazepine effects (sedation, unstable gait etc). If this occurs the benzodiazepine dosage should be reduced. Lansoprazole, pantoprazole and rabeprazole do not appear to interact with diazepam.

Further, an *in vitro* study suggests that omeprazole may possibly interact similarly with **midazolam**,[13] although this needs confirmation. There seems to be no information regarding other benzodiazepines.

1. Nexium Tablets (Esomeprazole magnesium trihydrate). AstraZeneca UK Ltd. UK Summary of product characteristics, May 2007.
2. Lefebvre RA, Flouvat B, Karolac-Tamisier S, Moerman E, Van Ganse E. Influence of lansoprazole treatment on diazepam plasma concentrations. *Clin Pharmacol Ther* (1992) 52, 458–63.
3. Martí-Massó JF, López de Munain A, López de Dicastillo G. Ataxia following gastric bleeding due to omeprazole–benzodiazepine interaction. *Ann Pharmacother* (1992) 26, 429–30.
4. Shader RI. Question the experts. *J Clin Psychopharmacol* (1993) 13, 459.
5. Konrad A. Protracted episode of reduced consciousness following co-medication with omeprazole and clorazepate. *Clin Drug Invest* (2000) 19, 307–11.
6. Gugler R, Jensen JC. Omeprazole inhibits elimination of diazepam. *Lancet* (1984) i, 969.
7. Andersson T, Andrén K, Cederberg C, Edvardsson G, Heggelund A, Lundborg P. Effect of omeprazole and cimetidine on plasma diazepam levels. *Eur J Clin Pharmacol* (1990) 39, 51–4.
8. Caraco Y, Tateishi T, Wood AJ. Interethnic difference in omeprazole's inhibition of diazepam metabolism. *Clin Pharmacol Ther* (1995) 58, 62–72.
9. Ishizaki T, Chiba K, Manabe K, Koyama E, Hayashi M, Yasuda S, Horai Y, Tomono Y, Yamato C, Toyoki T. Comparison of the interaction potential of a new proton pump inhibitor, E3810, versus omeprazole with diazepam in extensive and poor metabolizers of *S*-mephenytoin 4′-hydroxylation. *Clin Pharmacol Ther* (1995) 58, 155–64.
10. Gugler R, Hartmann M, Rudi J, Brod I, Huber R, Steinijans VW, Bliesath H, Wurst W, Klotz U. Lack of pharmacokinetic interaction of pantoprazole and diazepam in man. *Br J Clin Pharmacol* (1996) 42, 249–52.
11. Merritt GJ, Humphries TJ, Spera AC, Hale JA, Laurent AL. Effect of rabeprazole sodium on the pharmacokinetics of diazepam in healthy male volunteers. *Pharm Res* (1997) 14 (Suppl 11), S-566.
12. Zomorodi K, Houston JB. Diazepam–omeprazole inhibition interaction: an *in vitro* investigation using human liver microsomes. *Br J Clin Pharmacol* (1996) 42, 157–62.
13. Li G, Klotz U. Inhibitory effect of omeprazole on the metabolism of midazolam in vitro. *Arzneimittelforschung* (1990) 40, 1105–7.

Benzodiazepines + Quinolones

Ciprofloxacin causes a marked reduction in the clearance of diazepam, but this does not appear to be clinically important in most individuals. Ciprofloxacin appears not to interact with temazepam, and gatifloxacin appears not to interact with midazolam.

Clinical evidence, mechanism, importance and management

(a) Ciprofloxacin

Ciprofloxacin 500 mg twice daily for 3 days was found to have no effect on the pharmacokinetics of **diazepam** in a study in 10 healthy subjects.[1] However, a later study in 12 healthy subjects found that ciprofloxacin 500 mg twice daily for 5 days increased the AUC of a single 5-mg intravenous dose of **diazepam** by 50%, reduced its clearance by 37% and doubled its half-life. These changes caused no significant alteration in the performance of a number of psychometric tests. It was suggested that the clearance of diazepam was reduced because ciprofloxacin inhibited the cytochrome P450-mediated metabolism of diazepam.[2] Another study by the same group found that ciprofloxacin does not interact with **temazepam**.[3]

It seems unlikely that any marked increases in **diazepam** effects (drowsiness etc.) will occur in most patients, but it may possibly be significant in those who have reduced renal or hepatic clearance (e.g. the elderly).[2] This needs confirmation.

(b) Gatifloxacin

Gatifloxacin 400 mg daily for 5 days had no effect on the pharmacokinetics of **midazolam** in 14 healthy subjects. The pharmacokinetics of gatifloxacin were also unaffected by concurrent use.[4]

1. Wijnands WJA, Trooster JFG, Teunissen PC, Cats HA, Vree TB. Ciprofloxacin does not impair the elimination of diazepam in humans. *Drug Metab Dispos* (1990) 18, 954–7.
2. Kamali F, Thomas SHL, Edwards C. The influence of steady-state ciprofloxacin on the pharmacokinetics and pharmacodynamics of a single dose of diazepam in healthy volunteers. *Eur J Clin Pharmacol* (1993) 44, 365–7.
3. Kamali F, Nicholson E, Edwards C. Ciprofloxacin does not influence temazepam pharmacokinetics. *Br J Clin Pharmacol* (1994) 37, 118P.
4. Grasela DM, LaCreta FP, Kollia GD, Randall DM, Uderman HD. Open-label, nonrandomized study of the effects of gatifloxacin on the pharmacokinetics of midazolam in healthy male volunteers. *Pharmacotherapy* (2000) 20, 330–5.

Benzodiazepines and related drugs + Rifampicin (Rifampin)

Rifampicin causes a very marked increase in the metabolism and/or clearance of diazepam and nitrazepam. Rifampicin also causes a marked increase in the clearance of midazolam and triazolam and the non-benzodiazepine hypnotics, zaleplon, zolpidem and zopiclone. Benzodiazepines and related drugs that are metabolised similarly are expected to interact in the same way.

Clinical evidence

A. Benzodiazepines

(a) Diazepam

The mean half-life of diazepam was reduced from 58 to 14 hours and the clearance was increased fourfold in 7 patients with tuberculosis who were given daily doses of isoniazid 500 mg to 2.2 g, rifampicin 450 to 600 mg and ethambutol 25 mg/kg, when compared with healthy control subjects.[1] In 21 healthy subjects rifampicin 600 mg or 1.2 g daily for 7 days increased the clearance of diazepam by about threefold.[2]

(b) Midazolam

A pharmacokinetic study in 10 healthy subjects found that rifampicin 600 mg daily for 5 days reduced the AUC of a single 15-mg oral dose of midazolam by 96%, and reduced the half-life by almost two-thirds. The psychomotor effects of the midazolam (as measured by the digit symbol substitution test, Maddox wing test, postural sway and drowsiness) were almost totally lost.[3]

(c) Nitrazepam

A study in healthy subjects found that rifampicin 600 mg daily for 7 days increased the total body clearance of nitrazepam by 83%.[4]

(d) Temazepam

A study found that the pharmacokinetics of temazepam were unchanged by rifampicin.[4]

(e) Triazolam

Triazolam 500 micrograms orally was given to 10 healthy subjects before and after rifampicin 600 mg daily or a placebo for 5 days. Rifampicin reduced the triazolam AUC by 95% and decreased the maximum plasma triazolam levels by 88% when compared with the placebo group. The elimination half-life was reduced from 2.8 to 1.3 hours. Pharmacodynamic tests (drowsiness, sway, Maddox wing, etc.) showed that rifampicin abolished the effects of triazolam.[5]

B. Non-benzodiazepine hypnotics

(a) Zaleplon

A non-randomised, crossover study in healthy subjects found that rifampicin 600 mg daily for 14 days increased the clearance of a 10-mg dose of zaleplon by 5.4-fold, decreasing its maximum serum levels and AUC by 80%.[6]

(b) Zolpidem

In a randomised, placebo-controlled, study, 8 healthy subjects were given rifampicin 600 mg daily for 5 days and then on day 6 they were given a single 20-mg oral dose of zolpidem. It was found that the rifampicin reduced the zolpidem AUC by 73%, reduced the maximum plasma level by about 60% and reduced its half-life from 2.5 to 1.6 hours. A significant reduction in the effects of zolpidem was also seen, as measured by a number of psychomotor tests (digital symbol substitution, critical flicker fusion, subjective drowsiness, etc.).[7]

(c) Zopiclone

In a two-phase study, 8 healthy subjects were given rifampicin 600 mg or a placebo daily for 5 days, with a single 10-mg oral dose of zopiclone on day 6. The rifampicin reduced the zopiclone AUC by 82%, decreased the peak serum levels by 71% and reduced its half-life from 3.8 to 2.3 hours. A significant reduction in the effects of zopiclone was also seen, as measured by the performance of psychomotor tests.[8]

Mechanism

Rifampicin is a potent liver enzyme inducer, which increases the metabolism of several benzodiazepines and the non-benzodiazepine hypnotics, zaleplon, zolpidem and zopiclone, thereby decreasing their levels. The metabolism of midazolam by the cytochrome P450 isoenzyme CYP3A4 in both liver and gut is affected.[3] The enzyme inducing effects of rifampicin seem to predominate if isoniazid (an enzyme inhibitor) is also present. Temazepam undergoes glucuronidation and is therefore unaffected by rifampicin.

Importance and management

The documentation of these interactions is limited but what has been reported is consistent with the way rifampicin interacts with many other drugs. The clinical importance of some of these interactions between the benzodiazepines and related drugs and rifampicin has not yet been assessed but what is known suggests that the dosage of diazepam and nitrazepam may need to be increased if rifampicin is given. Be alert for a reduction in the effects of other similarly metabolised benzodiazepines (e.g. chlordiazepoxide, flurazepam).

The effect of rifampicin on oral midazolam, triazolam, zaleplon, zolpidem and zopiclone is so large that they are likely to become ineffective and an alternative should be used instead. Alprazolam is also predicted to interact because CYP3A is involved with its metabolism.[9]

Those benzodiazepines that, like temazepam, undergo glucuronidation (e.g. lorazepam, oxazepam) are not expected to be affected by rifampicin and may be useful alternatives.

1. Ochs HR, Greenblatt DJ, Roberts G-M, Dengler HJ. Diazepam interaction with antituberculosis drugs. *Clin Pharmacol Ther* (1981) 29, 671–8.
2. Ohnhaus EE, Brockmeyer N, Dylewicz P, Habicht H. The effect of antipyrine and rifampin on the metabolism of diazepam. *Clin Pharmacol Ther* (1987) 42, 148–56.
3. Backman JT, Olkkola KT, Neuvonen PJ. Rifampin drastically reduces plasma concentrations and effects of oral midazolam. *Clin Pharmacol Ther* (1996) 59, 7–13.
4. Brockmeyer NH, Mertins L, Klimek K, Goos M, Ohnhaus EE. Comparative effects of rifampin and/or probenecid on the pharmacokinetics of temazepam and nitrazepam. *Int J Clin Pharmacol Ther Toxicol* (1990) 28, 387–93.
5. Villikka K, Kivistö KT, Backman JT, Olkkola KT, Neuvonen PJ. Triazolam is ineffective in patients taking rifampin. *Clin Pharmacol Ther* (1997) 61, 8–14.
6. Darwish M. Overview of drug interaction studies with zaleplon. Poster presented at 13th Annual Meeting of Associated Professional Sleep Studies (APSS), Orlando, Florida, June 23rd, 1999.
7. Villikka K, Kivistö KT, Luurila H, Neuvonen PJ. Rifampicin reduces plasma concentrations and effects of zolpidem. *Clin Pharmacol Ther* (1997) 62, 629–34.
8. Villikka K, Kivistö KT, Lamberg TS, Kantola T, Neuvonen PJ. Concentrations and effects of zopiclone are greatly reduced by rifampicin. *Br J Clin Pharmacol* (1997) 43, 471–4.
9. Greenblatt DJ, von Moltke LL, Harmatz JS, Ciraulo DA, Shader RI. Alprazolam pharmacokinetics, metabolism, and plasma levels: clinical implications. *J Clin Psychiatry* (1993) 54, 10 (Suppl), 4–11.

Benzodiazepines + Saw palmetto

No pharmacokinetic interaction is expected between saw palmetto and alprazolam or midazolam.

Clinical evidence, mechanism, importance and management

Saw palmetto 320 mg daily, given to 12 subjects for 16 days, did not affect the pharmacokinetics of a single 2-mg dose of **alprazolam** given on day 14 day.[1] In another study in 12 healthy subjects who took saw palmetto,160 mg twice daily for 28 days, there was no change in metabolic ratio of a single 8-mg dose of **midazolam**.[2] These findings suggest that saw palmetto does not alter the activity of the cytochrome P450 isoenzyme CYP3A4, and no dosage adjustments of these benzodiazepines would be expected to be needed on concurrent use.

1. Markowitz JS, Donovan JL, DeVane L, Taylor RM, Ruan Y, Wang J-S, Chavin KD. Multiple doses of saw palmetto (*Serenoa repens*) did not alter cytochrome P450 2D6 and 3A4 activity in normal volunteers. *Clin Pharmacol Ther* (2003) 74, 536–42.

2. Gurley BJ, Gardner SF, Hubbard MA, Williams DK, Gentry WB, Carrier J, Khan IA, Edwards DJ, Shah A. In vivo assessment of botanical supplementation on human cytochrome P450 phenotypes: *Citrus aurantium*, *Echinacea purpurea*, milk thistle, and saw palmetto. *Clin Pharmacol Ther* (2004) 76, 428–40.

Benzodiazepines and related drugs + SNRIs

Visual hallucinations have been seen in one patient given zolpidem and venlafaxine. No important interaction normally appears to occur between venlafaxine and alprazolam or diazepam. The pharmacokinetics of duloxetine were not affected by lorazepam or temazepam.

Clinical evidence

A 27-year-old woman who had been taking **venlafaxine** 37.5 mg at night for a week and terfenadine for a few years started taking **zolpidem** 10 mg daily. After 2 days, and within 45 minutes of the **zolpidem** dose, she developed visual hallucinations, which lasted for 2 to 4 hours. A similar episode occurred 2 weeks later when she had discontinued the terfenadine.[1]

A double-blind study in 18 healthy subjects taking **venlafaxine** 50 mg every 8 hours found that the concurrent use of **diazepam** 10 mg did not have a clinically significant effect on the pharmacokinetics of either drug, or their major active metabolites (*O*-desmethylvenlafaxine and desmethyldiazepam). **Diazepam** affected the performance of a battery of pharmacodynamic tests, but the addition of **venlafaxine** had no further effects.[2]

A study in 16 healthy subjects found that **venlafaxine** 75 mg twice daily reduced the AUC of a single 2-mg oral dose of **alprazolam** by 29% and reduced its half-life by 21%, but the performance of psychometric tests were only minimally changed.[3]

Mechanism

Uncertain. It has been suggested that a pharmacodynamic interaction between serotonin reuptake inhibition and zolpidem may lead to prolonged zolpidem-associated hallucinations in susceptible individuals.[1]

Importance and management

The studies suggest that no special precautions are necessary during the concurrent use of venlafaxine and diazepam or alprazolam, or between **duloxetine** and lorazepam or temazepam. Similarly, the manufacturer of **duloxetine** reports that its pharmacokinetics were not affected by lorazepam or temazepam under steady state conditions.[4]

However, a pharmacodynamic interaction may occur. Hallucinations have been seen with zolpidem alone, and they have also occurred, rarely, when zolpidem and some benzodiazepines were given with the 'SSRIs', (below), which are related to venlafaxine. However, adverse effects such as these seem rare and the concurrent use of these drugs need not be avoided, but bear this possible interaction in mind if hallucinations occur.

1. Elko CJ, Burgess JL, Robertson WO. Zolpidem-associated hallucinations and serotonin reuptake inhibition: a possible interaction. *Clin Toxicol* (1998), 36, 195–203.

2. Troy SM, Lucki I, Peirgies AA, Parker VD, Klockowski PM, Chiang ST. Pharmacokinetic and pharmacodynamic evaluation of the potential drug interaction between venlafaxine and diazepam. *J Clin Pharmacol* (1995) 35, 410–19.

3. Amchin J, Zarycranski W, Taylor KP, Albano D, Klockowski PM. Effect of venlafaxine on the pharmacokinetics of alprazolam. *Psychopharmacol Bull* (1998) 34, 211–19.

4. Cymbalta (Duloxetine hydrochloride). Eli Lilly and Company. US Prescribing information, May 2007.

Benzodiazepines and related drugs + SSRIs

There is some evidence to suggest that the metabolism of some benzodiazepines (such as alprazolam, bromazepam, diazepam, and also possibly midazolam, nitrazepam and triazolam) may be reduced by some SSRIs (such as fluoxetine and fluvoxamine). On the whole, no clinically significant interaction appears to occur between other SSRIs and the benzodiazepines or related drugs such as cloral hydrate or zaleplon. There is some evidence to support the suggestion that sedation is likely to be increased by the concurrent use of SSRIs and benzodiazepines. Rare cases of hallucinations have been seen with zolpidem and some SSRIs. Symptoms of the serotonin syndrome have been reported in two patients taking paroxetine and a benzodiazepine.

Clinical evidence

(a) Citalopram

The UK manufacturer of citalopram says that no pharmacodynamic interactions have been noted in clinical studies in which citalopram was given with benzodiazepines,[1] although the US manufacturer points out that caution should be used with citalopram and any CNS active drug.[2]

A general study in psychiatric patients found that when data on benzodiazepines was pooled, they caused a modest 23% increase in serum citalopram levels, which is almost certainly too small to be clinically relevant. **Alprazolam** was the only benzodiazepine to cause an elevation of citalopram levels (by 13%) when analysed alone.[3] In another study, citalopram was found to have no effect on **alprazolam** plasma levels, although the time to maximum **alprazolam** concentration was increased by 30 minutes.[4] Similarly, a study in 17 healthy subjects found no pharmacokinetic interaction between **triazolam** and citalopram, and it was suggested that **triazolam** and other substrates of the cytochrome P450 isoenzyme CYP3A4 are unlikely to have pharmacokinetic interactions with citalopram.[5]

(b) Fluoxetine

The concurrent use of fluoxetine 60 mg daily has been found to reduce the clearance of **alprazolam** 1 mg four times daily by about 21% and to increase its plasma levels by about 30%. These changes were accompanied by increased psychomotor impairment.[6] This appears to be due to reduced **alprazolam** metabolism.[7] Another study also reported impaired **alprazolam** metabolism, considered to be due to the inhibition of cytochrome P450 isoenzyme CYP3A4 by fluoxetine, although no significant changes in **alprazolam** pharmacodynamics were found.[4]

Fluoxetine 30 mg, given daily for 1 or 8 days, had no effect on the pharmacokinetics of **diazepam** 10 mg.[8] A later study by the same group, using 60 mg of fluoxetine suggested that the **diazepam** half-life and AUC were increased, possibly because the fluoxetine decreased the metabolism of **diazepam**. However, they concluded that this was not of any clinical significance.[9] Another study found that fluoxetine 60 mg alone did not affect psychomotor performance but fluoxetine 60 mg plus **diazepam** 5 mg significantly impaired the divided attention tracking test and vigilance test more than with **diazepam** 5 mg alone.[10] Other studies found that the pharmacokinetics of **clonazepam**,[11] **estazolam**,[12] **midazolam**,[13,14] **triazolam**,[15] and **zolpidem**[16,17] were not significantly affected by fluoxetine.

In contrast, isolated cases of visual hallucinations lasting up to 7 hours have been reported in patients taking **zolpidem** who were also taking fluoxetine.[18] Marked drowsiness occurred for a whole day in a patient taking fluoxetine 20 mg daily after being given **cloral hydrate** 500 mg the night before. She later tolerated **cloral hydrate** 1 g in the absence of fluoxetine without adverse effects.[19]

(c) Fluvoxamine

In 60 healthy subjects fluvoxamine 50 mg daily for 3 days then 100 mg daily for 7 days, doubled the plasma levels of **alprazolam** 1 mg four times daily given on days 7 to 10. The **alprazolam** clearance was more than halved. Psychomotor performance and memory were found to be significantly worsened, even after only one day.[20] A study in 23 Japanese patients found that fluvoxamine increased the plasma levels of **alprazolam** by 58%. There was wide interpatient variability, possibly associated with differences in the cytochrome P450 isoenzyme CYP2C19 levels in these patients (see 'Genetic factors', (p.4)), although it is unclear exactly what impact this isoenzyme has on the interaction.[21]

Fluvoxamine 50 mg twice daily increased the plasma levels of a single 12-mg dose of **bromazepam** in 12 healthy subjects by 36% and increased the AUC almost 2.5-fold. Some increased impairment in cognitive function was seen.[22]

Fluvoxamine has been found not to interact adversely with **cloral hydrate**.[23] Fluvoxamine (50 mg on day one, 100 mg on day 2, then 150 mg daily thereafter) for 16 days decreased the clearance of a single 10-mg dose of **diazepam** given on day 4 in 8 healthy subjects by about 65%. The half-life was increased from 51 to 118 hours, and the AUC was increased threefold.[24]

Fluvoxamine 50 mg twice daily caused a very small, non-significant, increase in the serum levels and AUC of a single 4-mg dose of **lorazepam** in 12 healthy subjects.[22]

A study in 10 healthy subjects[14] found that fluvoxamine 50 mg twice daily for 8 days then 100 mg twice daily for 6 days had minimal effects on the pharmacokinetics of a single 10-mg dose of **midazolam** given on day 12.

In a placebo-controlled study in 12 healthy subjects it was found that fluvoxamine 25 mg twice daily for 14 days had no effect on the pharmacokinetics of a single 20-mg dose of **quazepam**. However, formation of the metabolite 2-oxoquazepam was decreased, and there was a minor decrease in the sedative effects of **quazepam** at 4 hours, although these changes were considered to be of little clinical significance.[25]

(d) Paroxetine

No important changes in the pharmacokinetics of paroxetine were seen when 12 healthy subjects given paroxetine 30 mg daily were also given **diazepam** 5 mg three times a day. Adverse events were not increased by the combination.[26] In another study it was found that paroxetine did not increase the impairment of a number of psychomotor tests caused by **oxazepam**.[27] *In vitro* studies using human liver microsomal enzymes have shown that paroxetine is a relatively weak inhibitor of **alprazolam** metabolism mediated by the cytochrome P450 subfamily CYP3A.[28,29] Furthermore, a randomised, placebo-controlled study in 22 healthy subjects reported no evidence for a pharmacokinetic or pharmacological interaction between paroxetine and **alprazolam**.[30]

An isolated report describes worsening anxiety, agitation, mild abdominal cramps and diaphoresis in a woman taking paroxetine, shortly after starting **clonazepam** (dosage stated as one tablet). This toxic response was suggested as being the serotonin syndrome, although in fact many of the usual signs were absent and moreover, **clonazepam** has actually been used to treat the myoclonus that occurs in the serotonin syndrome. She was effectively treated with **lorazepam**.[31] Another report describes a patient who was admitted to hospital with symptoms of the serotonin syndrome within 6 days of starting daily treatment with paroxetine 20 mg, **etizolam** 1 mg and **brotizolam** 250 micrograms. Paroxetine was discontinued on day 6. The serotonin syndrome usually resolves within 24 hours of discontinuing the causative medication but symptoms in this patient continued for a total of 10 days.[32]

In a double-blind study in healthy subjects it was found that paroxetine 20 mg for 9 days had no effect on the pharmacokinetics of **zaleplon** 20 mg, and psychomotor performance was unaffected by concurrent use.[33]

An isolated report describes a healthy 16-year-old girl with depression who took paroxetine 20 mg daily for 3 days, and then on the evening of the third night a single 10-mg dose of **zolpidem**. Within 1 hour she began to hallucinate, then became disorientated and was unable to recognise members of her family. She recovered spontaneously within 4 hours.[34]

(e) Sertraline

No clinically relevant effects were found in interaction studies in which sertraline was given with a single intravenous dose of **diazepam**.[35,36] One *in vitro* study in human liver microsomes suggested that sertraline inhibits the metabolism of **alprazolam**,[7] whereas another suggested no interaction occurred.[37] *In vivo* studies largely demonstrate a lack of interaction. For example, a pharmacokinetic study in 10 healthy subjects found that sertraline 50 to 150 mg daily had no effect on the pharmacokinetics of **alprazolam**, although some small decreases in a driving simulation score were seen at the 100- and 150-mg doses of sertraline.[38] Similarly, sertraline 50 mg daily had no effect on the pharmacokinetics of **alprazolam** 1 mg daily in 12 healthy subjects, after 2 weeks of concurrent use.[37]

A study in 13 subjects given daily doses of **clonazepam** 1 mg with sertraline 100 mg for 10 days found no evidence that the addition of sertraline to clonazepam made the subjects more sedated or less able to carry out simple psychometric tests.[39]

Sertraline appears to have no clinically significant effects on the pharmacokinetics of **zolpidem**,[40] but isolated cases of visual hallucinations lasting up to 7 hours have been reported in patients on **zolpidem** who were taking sertraline.[18]

Mechanism

The evidence suggests that fluvoxamine inhibits the metabolism of those benzodiazepines that undergo oxidation (e.g. alprazolam,[29] bromazepam, diazepam) thereby increasing and prolonging their effects, but not those that are metabolised by glucuronidation (e.g. lorazepam). Zaleplon is metabolised by aldehyde oxidase and therefore does not interact.

Importance and management

Evidence is limited, but what is known suggests that the dosages of alprazolam, bromazepam, diazepam and other similarly metabolised benzodiazepines such as nitrazepam should be reduced, probably by half, in the presence of fluvoxamine to avoid adverse effects (drowsiness, reduced psychomotor performance and memory). The US manufacturer recommends avoiding the use of fluvoxamine with diazepam as substantial diazepam accumulation could occur. They also note that as fluvoxamine has non-linear kinetics, the effects of higher doses of fluvoxamine such as 300 mg could be substantially greater, particularly with long-term diazepam use.[41] The UK manufacturer also includes midazolam and triazolam.[42] Fluvoxamine is unlikely to affect lorazepam and other benzodiazepines metabolised by glucuronidation (e.g. lormetazepam, oxazepam, temazepam).[41] It seems unlikely that sertraline will affect any of the benzodiazepines and it may therefore be a useful alternative to fluvoxamine. Nevertheless, the manufacturers of sertraline say that it should not be given with benzodiazepines or other tranquillisers in patients who drive or operate machinery.[43]

The hallucinations seen with the SSRIs and zolpidem appear rare, and reactions of this kind have been seen with zolpidem alone. The concurrent use of these drugs need not be avoided, but bear this possible interaction in mind if hallucinations occur.

1. Cipramil (Citalopram hydrobromide). Lundbeck Ltd. UK Summary of product characteristics, January 2007.
2. Celexa (Citalopram hydrobromide). Forest Pharmaceuticals, Inc. US Prescribing information, May 2007.
3. Leinonen E, Lepola U, Koponen H, Kinnunen I. The effect of age and concomitant treatment with other psychoactive drugs on serum concentrations of citalopram measured with a non-enantioselective method. *Ther Drug Monit* (1996) 18, 111–17.
4. Hall J, Naranjo CA, Sproule BA, Herrmann N. Pharmacokinetic and pharmacodynamic evaluation of the inhibition of alprazolam by citalopram and fluoxetine. *J Clin Psychopharmacol* (2003) 23, 349–57.
5. Nolting A, Abramowitz W. Lack of interaction between citalopram and the CYP3A4 substrate triazolam. *Pharmacotherapy* (2000) 20, 750–5.
6. Lasher TA, Fleishaker JC, Steenwyk RC, Antal EJ. Pharmacokinetic pharmacodynamic evaluation of the combined administration of alprazolam and fluoxetine. *Psychopharmacology (Berl)* (1991) 104, 323–7.
7. von Moltke LL, Greenblatt DJ, Cotreau-Bibbo MM, Harmatz JS, Shader RI. Inhibitors of alprazolam metabolism *in vitro*: effect of serotonin-reuptake-inhibitor antidepressants, ketoconazole and quinidine. *Br J Clin Pharmacol* (1994) 38, 23–31.
8. Lemberger L, Bergstrom RF, Wolen RL, Farid NA, Enas GG, Aronoff GR. Fluoxetine: clinical pharmacology and physiologic disposition. *J Clin Psychiatry* (1985) 46, 3 (Sec 2), 14–19.
9. Lemberger L, Rowe H, Bosomworth JC, Tenbarge JB, Bergstrom RF. The effect of fluoxetine on the pharmacokinetics and psychomotor responses of diazepam. *Clin Pharmacol Ther* (1988) 43, 412–19.
10. Moskowitz H, Burns M. The effects on performance of two antidepressants, alone and in combination with diazepam. *Prog Neuropsychopharmacol Biol Psychiatry* (1988) 12, 783–92.
11. Greenblatt DJ, Preskorn SH, Cotreau MM, Horst WD, Harmatz JS. Fluoxetine impairs clearance of alprazolam but not of clonazepam. *Clin Pharmacol Ther* (1992) 52, 479–86.
12. Cavanaugh J, Schneck D, Eason C, Hansen M, Gustavson L. Lack of effect of fluoxetine on the pharmacokinetics (PK) and pharmacodynamics (PD) of estazolam. *Clin Pharmacol Ther* (1994) 55, 141.
13. Lam YWF, Alfaro CL, Ereshefsky L, Miller M. Effect of antidepressants and ketoconazole on oral midazolam pharmacokinetics. *Clin Pharmacol Ther* (1998) 63, 229.
14. Lam YWF, Alfaro CL, Ereshefsky L, Miller M. Pharmacokinetics and pharmacodynamic interactions of oral midazolam with ketoconazole, fluoxetine, fluvoxamine, and nefazodone. *J Clin Pharmacol* (2003) 43, 1274–82.
15. Wright CE, Lasher-Sisson TA, Steenwyk RC, Swanson CN. A pharmacokinetic evaluation of the combined administration of triazolam and fluoxetine. *Pharmacotherapy* (1992) 12, 103–6.
16. Piergies AA, Sweet J, Johnson M, Roth-Schechter BF, Allard S. The effect of co-administration of zolpidem with fluoxetine: pharmacokinetics and pharmacodynamics. *Int J Clin Pharmacol Ther* (1996) 34, 178–83.
17. Allard S, Sainati S, Roth-Schechter B, Macintyre J. Minimal interaction between fluoxetine and multiple-dose zolpidem in healthy women. *Drug Metab Dispos* (1998) 26, 617–22.
18. Elko CJ, Burgess JL, Robertson WO. Zolpidem-associated hallucinations and serotonin reuptake inhibition: a possible interaction. *J Toxicol Clin Toxicol* (1998) 36, 195–203.

19. Devarajan S. Interaction of fluoxetine and chloral hydrate. *Can J Psychiatry* (1992) 37, 590–1.
20. Fleishaker JC, Hulst LK. A pharmacokinetic and pharmacodynamic evaluation of the combined administration of alprazolam and fluvoxamine. *Eur J Clin Pharmacol* (1994) 46, 35–9.
21. Suzuki Y, Shioiri T, Muratake T, Kawashima Y, Sato S, Hagiwara M, Inoue Y, Shimoda K, Someya T. Effects of concomitant fluvoxamine on the metabolism of alprazolam in Japanese psychiatric patients: interaction with CYP2C19 mutated alleles. *Eur J Clin Pharmacol* (2003) 58, 829–33.
22. Van Harten J, Holland RL, Wesnes K. Influence of multiple-dose administration of fluvoxamine on the pharmacokinetics of the benzodiazepines bromazepam and lorazepam: a randomised, cross-over study. *Eur Neuropsychopharmacol* (1992) 2, 381.
23. Benfield P, Ward A. Fluvoxamine, a review of its pharmacodynamic and pharmacokinetic properties and therapeutic efficacy in depressive illness. *Drugs* (1986) 32, 313–34.
24. Perucca E, Gatti G, Cipolla G, Spina E, Barel S, Soback S, Gips M, Bialer M. Inhibition of diazepam metabolism by fluvoxamine: a pharmacokinetic study in normal volunteers. *Clin Pharmacol Ther* (1994) 56, 471–6.
25. Kanda H, Yasui-Furukori N, Fukasawa T, Aoshima T, Suzuki A, Otani K. Interaction study between fluvoxamine and quazepam. *J Clin Pharmacol* (2003) 43, 1392–7.
26. Bannister SJ, Houser VP, Hulse JD, Kisicki JC, Rasmussen JGC. Evaluation of the potential for interactions of paroxetine with diazepam, cimetidine, warfarin, and digoxin. *Acta Psychiatr Scand* (1989) 80 (Suppl 350), 102–6.
27. Cooper SM, Jackson D, Loudon JM, McClelland GR, Raptopoulos P. The psychomotor effects of paroxetine alone and in combination with haloperidol, amylobarbitone, oxazepam, or alcohol. *Acta Psychiatr Scand* (1989) 80 (Suppl 350), 53–55.
28. Greenblatt DJ, von Moltke LL, Harmatz JS, Ciraulo DA, Shader RI. Alprazolam pharmacokinetics, metabolism, and plasma levels: clinical implications. *J Clin Psychiatry* (1993) 54 (Suppl), 4–11.
29. von Moltke LL, Greenblatt DJ, Court MH, Duan SX, Harmatz JS, Shader RI. Inhibition of alprazolam and desipramine hydroxylation *in vitro* by paroxetine and fluvoxamine: comparison with other selective serotonin reuptake inhibitor antidepressants. *J Clin Psychopharmacol* (1995) 15, 125–31.
30. Calvo G, García-Gea C, Luque A, Morte A, Dal-Ré R, Barbanoj M. Lack of pharmacologic interaction between paroxetine and alprazolam at steady state in healthy volunteers. *J Clin Psychopharmacol* (2004) 24, 268–76.
31. Rella JG, Hoffman RS. Possible serotonin syndrome from paroxetine and clonazepam. *Clin Toxicol* (1998) 36, 257–8.
32. Ochiai Y, Katsu H, Okino S, Wakutsu N, Nakayama K. A prolongation case of the serotonin syndrome by paroxetine – about the recovery process. *Seishin Shinkeigaku Zasshi* (2003) 105, 1532–8.
33. Darwish M. Overview of drug interaction studies with zaleplon. Poster presented at 13th Annual Meeting of Associated Professional Sleep Studies (APSS), Orlando, Florida, June 23rd, 1999.
34. Katz SE. Possible paroxetine-zolpidem interaction. *Am J Psychiatry* (1995) 152, 1689.
35. Warrington SJ. Clinical implications of the pharmacology of sertraline. *Int Clin Psychopharmacol* (1991) 6 (Suppl 2), 11–21.
36. Gardner MJ, Baris BA, Wilner KD, Preskorn SH. Effect of sertraline on the pharmacokinetics and protein binding of diazepam in healthy volunteers. *Clin Pharmacokinet* (1997) 32 (Suppl 1), 43–9.
37. Preskorn SH, Greenblatt DJ, Harvey AT. Lack of effect of sertraline on the pharmacokinetics of alprazolam. *J Clin Psychopharmacol* (2000) 20, 585–6.
38. Hassan PC, Sproule BA, Herrmann N, Reed K, Naranjo CA. Dose-response evaluation of sertraline-alprazolam interaction in humans. *Clin Pharmacol Ther* (1998) 63, 185.
39. Kroboth PD, Bonate PL, Smith RB, Suarez E. Clonazepam (Klonopin®) and sertraline (Zoloft®): absence of drug interaction in a multiple dose study. *Clin Pharmacol Ther* (1997), 61, 178.
40. Allard S, Sainati S, Roth-Schechter BF. Coadministration of short-term zolpidem with sertraline in healthy women. *J Clin Pharmacol* (1999) 39, 184–91.
41. Fluvoxamine maleate tablets. Apotex Corp. US Prescribing information, January 2001.
42. Faverin (Fluvoxamine). Solvay Healthcare Ltd. UK Summary of product characteristics, June 2006.
43. Lustral (Sertraline hydrochloride). Pfizer Ltd. UK Summary of product characteristics, October 2005.

Benzodiazepines + St John's wort *(Hypericum perforatum)*

St John's wort decreases the plasma levels of quazepam, although this did not reduce its effects in one study. Alprazolam appears not to interact, although this needs confirmation. The bioavailability of midazolam was reduced by long-term but not single doses of St John's wort.

Clinical evidence, mechanism, importance and management

(a) Alprazolam

Alprazolam 1 or 2 mg was given to 7 healthy subjects on the third day of a 3-day treatment period with St John's wort (*Solaray*; hypericin content standardised at 0.3%) 300 mg three times daily. The pharmacokinetics of alprazolam were unchanged by the St John's wort, but the authors note that 3 days may have been an insufficient time for St John's wort to fully induce cytochrome P450 isoenzymes.[1] In another study, 16 healthy subjects were given St John's wort extract 120 mg (*Esbericum* capsules; corresponding to 0.5 mg total hypericins and 1.76 mg hyperforin) twice daily for 10 days. A single 1-mg dose of alprazolam was given on the day before treatment with St John's wort and on the last day of treatment. St John's wort extract at this low dosage and low hyperforin content had no clinically relevant effects on the pharmacokinetics of alprazolam, when compared with 12 subjects given placebo.[2]

(b) Midazolam

An open-label study in 12 healthy subjects found that a single 900-mg dose of St John's wort had no significant effect on the pharmacokinetics of single doses of either oral midazolam 5 mg or intravenous midazolam 0.05 mg/kg, although there was a trend for increased oral clearance. However, St John's wort 300 mg three times daily for 14 or 15 days decreased the AUC and maximum plasma concentration of oral midazolam by about 50% and 40%, respectively. Intravenous midazolam was not significantly affected. St John's wort appears to increase the metabolism of oral midazolam by induction of the cytochrome P450 isoenzyme CYP3A4 in the gut, resulting in reduced midazolam bioavailability.[3] Similar results were found in another study.[4]

(c) Quazepam

In a placebo-controlled study, 13 healthy subjects were given St John's wort (*TruNature*; hypericin content standardised at 0.3%) 300 mg three times daily for 14 days with a single 15-mg dose of quazepam on day 14. Although St John's wort did not affect the pharmacodynamic effects of quazepam it did decrease the quazepam AUC by 26% and the maximum plasma levels by 29%.This was attributed to the effects of St John's wort on the cytochrome P450 isoenzyme CYP3A4, by which quazepam is metabolised.[5]

1. Markowitz JS, DeVane CL, Boulton DW, Carson SW, Nahas Z, Risch SC. Effect of St John's wort (*Hypericum perforatum*) on cytochrome P-450 2D6 and 3A4 activity in healthy volunteers. *Life Sci* (2000) 66, 133–9.
2. Arold G, Donath F, Maurer A, Diefenbach K, Bauer S, Henneike-von Zepelin H-H, Friede M, Roots I. No relevant interaction with alprazolam, caffeine, tolbutamide, and digoxin by treatment with a low hyperforin St John's wort extract. *Planta Med* (2005) 71, 331–7.
3. Wang Z, Gorski C, Hamman MA, Huang S-M, Lesko LJ, Hall SD. The effects of St John's wort (*Hypericum perforatum*) on human cytochrome P450 activity. *Clin Pharmacol Ther* (2001) 70, 317–26.
4. Dresser GK, Schwarz UI, Wilkinson GR, Kim RB. Coordinate induction of both cytochrome P4503A and MDR1 by St John's wort in healthy subjects. *Clin Pharmacol Ther* (2003) 73, 41–50.
5. Kawaguchi A, Ohmori M, Tsuruoka S, Harada K, Miyamori I, Yano R, Nakamura T, Masada M, Fujimura A. Drug interaction between St John's wort and quazepam. *Br J Clin Pharmacol* (2004) 58, 403–10.

Benzodiazepines + Sucrose polyesters

Sucrose polyesters (e.g. *Olestra*) do not appear to interact with diazepam.

Clinical evidence, mechanism, importance and management

A single 5-mg dose of **diazepam** was given to 8 healthy subjects with 18 g of sucrose polyester (*Olestra*). Sucrose polyester had no effect on the pharmacokinetics of **diazepam**.[1] Sucrose polyesters, are non-absorbable, non-calorific fat replacements. It has been concluded that sucrose polyesters are unlikely to reduce the absorption of oral drugs in general.[2]

1. Roberts RJ, Leff RD. Influence of absorbable and nonabsorbable lipids and lipidlike substances on drug availability. *Clin Pharmacol Ther* (1989) 45, 299–304.
2. Goldman P. Olestra: assessing its potential to interact with drugs in the gastrointestinal tract. *Clin Pharmacol Ther* (1997) 61, 613–18.

Benzodiazepines + Tadalafil

Tadalafil does not alter the pharmacokinetics of midazolam.

Clinical evidence, mechanism, importance and management

An open label study in 12 healthy subjects found that while taking tadalafil 10 mg daily for 14 consecutive days, the pharmacokinetics of a single 15-mg oral dose of midazolam were unchanged.[1] Since midazolam is metabolised by the cytochrome P450 isoenzyme CYP3A4, it was concluded that the absence of any interaction shows that tadalafil does not inhibit or induce the activity of this isoenzyme.[2] No special precautions are therefore needed if midazolam is given with tadalafil.

1. Ring BJ, Patterson BE, Mitchell MI, Vandenbranden M, Gillespie J, Bedding AW, Jewell H, Payne CD, Forgue ST, Eckstein J, Wrighton SA, Phillips DL. Effect of tadalafil on cytochrome P450 3A4-mediated clearance: studies in vitro and in vivo. *Clin Pharmacol Ther* (2005) 77, 63–75.
2. Eli Lilly and Company. Personal communication, March 2003.

Benzodiazepines + Terbinafine

Terbinafine does not interact with midazolam or triazolam to a clinically relevant extent.

Clinical evidence, mechanism, importance and management

Terbinafine 250 mg daily for 4 days had no effect on the pharmacokinetics of a single 7.5-mg dose of **midazolam**[1] or a single 250-microgram dose of **triazolam**[2] in 12 healthy subjects. The performance of a number of psychomotor tests was unaffected by concurrent use. No special precautions would seem to be necessary if terbinafine is given with either of these drugs.

1. Ahonen J, Olkkola KT, Neuvonen PJ. Effect of itraconazole and terbinafine on the pharmacokinetics and pharmacodynamics of midazolam in healthy volunteers. *Br J Clin Pharmacol* (1995) 40, 270–2.
2. Varhe A, Olkkola KT, Neuvonen PJ. Fluconazole, but not terbinafine, enhances the effects of triazolam by inhibiting its metabolism. *Br J Clin Pharmacol* (1996) 41, 319–23.

Benzodiazepines and related drugs + Tobacco

Smokers may possibly need larger doses of some benzodiazepines and zolpidem than non-smokers.

Clinical evidence, mechanism, importance and management

Some studies have suggested that smoking does not affect the pharmacokinetics of **diazepam**,[1,2] **chlordiazepoxide**,[3] **clorazepate**,[4] **lorazepam**,[2] **midazolam**,[2] or **triazolam**,[5] but others have found that the clearance of **alprazolam**,[6] **clorazepate**,[7] **diazepam**,[8] **lorazepam**[9] and **oxazepam**[10,11] is increased by smoking, but not all the changes were significant.[8] The Boston Collaborative Drug Surveillance Program reported a decreased frequency of drowsiness in smokers who took **diazepam** or **chlordiazepoxide**,[12] which confirmed the findings of a previous study.[13] It has also been noted that two heavy smokers had a very high clearance and did not experience any sedative effects following the use of **zolpidem**.[14]

The probable reason for the reduction in sedative effects with these drugs is that some of the components of tobacco smoke are enzyme inducers, which increase the rate at which the liver metabolises these benzodiazepines, thereby reducing their effects. The inference to be drawn is that smokers may possibly need larger doses than non-smokers to achieve the same therapeutic effects. Smoking also possibly reduces the drowsiness that the benzodiazepines and non-benzodiazepine hypnotics, such as **zolpidem**, can cause. However, one study suggested that caffeine intake,[13] and others suggest age, may affect the response to benzodiazepines, so the picture is not altogether clear. Whether any of these interactions has much clinical relevance awaits assessment.

1. Klotz U, Avant GR, Hoyumpa A, Schenker S, Wilkinson GR. The effects of age and liver disease on the disposition and elimination of diazepam in adult man. *J Clin Invest* (1975) 55, 347–59.
2. Ochs HR, Greenblatt DJ, Knüchel M. Kinetics of diazepam, midazolam, and lorazepam in cigarette smokers. *Chest* (1985) 87, 223–6.
3. Desmond PV, Roberts RK, Wilkinson GR, Schenker S. No effect of smoking on metabolism of chlordiazepoxide. *N Engl J Med* (1979) 300, 199–200.
4. Ochs HR, Greenblatt DJ, Locniskar A, Weinbrenner J. Influence of propranolol coadministration or cigarette smoking on the kinetics of desmethyldiazepam following intravenous clorazepate. *Klin Wochenschr* (1986) 64, 1217–21.
5. Ochs HR, Greenblatt DJ, Burstein ES. Lack of influence of cigarette smoking on triazolam pharmacokinetics. *Br J Clin Pharmacol* (1987) 23, 759–63.
6. Smith RB, Gwilt PR, Wright CE. Single- and multiple-dose pharmacokinetics of oral alprazolam in healthy smoking and nonsmoking men. *Clin Pharm* (1983) 2, 139–43.
7. Norman TR, Fulton A, Burrows GD, Maguire KP. Pharmacokinetics of N-desmethyldiazepam after a single oral dose of clorazepate: the effect of smoking. *Eur J Clin Pharmacol* (1981) 21, 229–33.
8. Greenblatt DJ, Allen MD, Harmatz JS, Shader RI. Diazepam disposition determinants. *Clin Pharmacol Ther* (1980) 27, 301–12.
9. Greenblatt DJ, Allen MD, Locniskar A, Harmatz JS, Shader RI. Lorazepam kinetics in the elderly. *Clin Pharmacol Ther* (1979) 26, 103–13.
10. Greenblatt DJ, Divoll M, Harmatz JS, Shader RI. Oxazepam kinetics: effects of age and sex. *J Pharmacol Exp Ther* (1980) 215, 86–91.
11. Ochs HR, Greenblatt DJ, Otten H. Disposition of oxazepam in relation to age, sex, and cigarette smoking. *Klin Wochenschr* (1981) 59, 899–903.
12. Boston Collaborative Drug Surveillance Program. Clinical depression of the central nervous system due to diazepam and chlordiazepoxide in relation to cigarette smoking and age. *N Engl J Med* (1973) 288, 277–80.
13. Downing RW, Rickels K. Coffee consumption, cigarette smoking and reporting of drowsiness in anxious patients treated with benzodiazepines or placebo. *Acta Psychiatr Scand* (1981) 64, 398–408.
14. Harvengt C, Hulhoven R, Desager JP, Coupez JM, Guillet P, Fuseau E, Lambert D, Warrington SJ. Drug interactions investigated with zolpidem. In: Sauvanet JP, Langer SZ, Morselli PL, eds. Imidazopyridines in Sleep Disorders. New York: Raven Press; 1988: pp. 165–73.

Benzodiazepines + Vinpocetine

Vinpocetine does not appear to interact adversely with oxazepam. Vinpocetine may improve short-term memory impairment induced by flunitrazepam.

Clinical evidence, mechanism, importance and management

No changes in the steady-state plasma levels of **oxazepam** 10 mg three times daily were seen in 16 healthy subjects who took vinpocetine 10 mg three times daily for 7 days.[1] There would therefore seem to be no reason for taking special precautions if these two drugs are given together.

A study in 8 healthy subjects found that vinpocetine 40 mg three times daily for 2 days did not significantly improve **flunitrazepam**-induced impairment of memory, although the combination did appear to significantly improve patients ability to sleep.[2]

1. Storm G, Oosterhuis, Sollie FAE, Visscher HW, Sommer W, Beitinger H, Jonkman JHG. Lack of pharmacokinetic interaction between vinpocetine and oxazepam. *Br J Clin Pharmacol* (1994) 38, 143–6.
2. Bhatti JZ, Hindmarch I. Vinpocetine effects on cognitive impairments produced by flunitrazepam. *Int Clin Psychopharmacol* (1987) 2, 325–31.

Benzodiazepines and related drugs + Xanthines

Aminophylline, theophylline and caffeine appear to antagonise the effects of the benzodiazepines (mainly sedative effects, but possibly also anxiolytic effects), and aminophylline and theophylline appear to reduce the levels of alprazolam. The effects of zopiclone may be similarly antagonised.

Clinical evidence

A. Benzodiazepines

In a comparative study, two groups of patients were given **alprazolam** 500 micrograms twice daily for 7 days. One of the patient groups had 6 patients who had chronic obstructive pulmonary disease (COPD) and were taking **theophylline**, and the other group had 7 patients with chronic heart failure or atherosclerotic disease (one patient also with COPD) and were not taking **theophylline**. On day 7, those taking the **theophylline** were found to have lower trough serum **alprazolam** levels of 13.25 nanograms/mL, while in the other group the levels were 43.92 nanograms/mL.[1]

A patient who was unrousable and unresponsive having been given **diazepam** 60 mg given over 10 minutes and nitrous oxide/oxygen anaesthesia, rapidly returned to consciousness when given **aminophylline** 56 mg intravenously.[2] Other reports confirm this antagonism of **diazepam**, by low doses of **aminophylline** (60 mg to 4.5 mg/kg intravenously).[3-5] Caffeine, and to a lesser extent **theophylline** and **aminophylline**, counteract the drowsiness and mental slowness induced by a single 10- to 20-mg dose of **diazepam**.[6-9] **Flunitrazepam**,[10] **lorazepam**,[11] and **midazolam**[12] also appear to be affected; however, there is some controversy about whether or not **theophylline** and **aminophylline** antagonise the effects of **midazolam**.[13,14]

There is also some evidence to suggest that **caffeine** and **clonazepam**[15] or **triazolam**[16] have mutually opposing effects.

B. Non-benzodiazepine hypnotics

Zopiclone appears to counter the stimulant effects of **caffeine** more easily than **caffeine** counters the sedative effects of **zopiclone**.[16] No pharmacokinetic interaction occurred between **zolpidem** and **caffeine** (given as one cup of **coffee** containing **caffeine** 300 mg), and the hypnotic effects of **zolpidem** were unchanged.[17]

Mechanism

Uncertain. One suggestion is that the xanthines can block adenosine receptors.[3] Another is that the xanthines induce the metabolism of the benzodiazepines by the liver so that levels, and therefore effects, are reduced.[18]

Importance and management

The documentation is somewhat sparse and there is a need for more study over the range of benzodiazepines and related drugs, but the overall picture is that these interactions are established. The extent to which these xanthines actually reduce the anxiolytic effects of the benzodiazepines remains uncertain (it needs assessment) but be alert for reduced benzodiazepine effects if both are used. Caffeine in tea or coffee appears to reduce the sedative effects of triazolam and zopiclone. This would appear to be a disadvantage at night, but may possibly be useful the next morning.

1. Tuncok Y, Akpinar O, Guven H, Akkoclu A. The effects of theophylline on serum alprazolam levels. *Int J Clin Pharmacol Ther* (1994) 32, 642–5.
2. Stirt JA. Aminophylline is a diazepam antagonist. *Anesth Analg* (1981) 60, 767–8.
3. Niemand D, Martinell S, Arvidsson S, Svedmyr N, Ekström-Jodal B. Aminophylline inhibition of diazepam sedation: is adenosine blockade of GABA-receptors the mechanism? *Lancet* (1984) i, 463–4.
4. Arvidsson SB, Ekström-Jodal B, Martinell SAG, Niemand D. Aminophylline antagonises diazepam sedation. *Lancet* (1982) 2, 1467.
5. Kleindienst G, Usinger P. Diazepam sedation is not antagonised completely by aminophylline. *Lancet* (1984) 1, 113.
6. Mattila MJ, Nuotto E. Caffeine and theophylline counteract diazepam effects in man. *Med Biol* (1983) 61, 337–43.
7. Mattila MJ, Palva E, Savolainen K. Caffeine antagonizes diazepam effects in man. *Med Biol* (1982) 60, 121–3.
8. Henauer SA, Hollister LE, Gillespie HK, Moore F. Theophylline antagonizes diazepam-induced psychomotor impairment. *Eur J Clin Pharmacol* (1983) 25, 743–7.
9. Meyer BH, Weis OF, Müller FO. Antagonism of diazepam by aminophylline in healthy volunteers. *Anesth Analg* (1984) 63, 900–2.
10. Gürel A, Elevli M, Hamulu A. Aminophylline reversal of flunitrazepam sedation. *Anesth Analg* (1987) 66, 333–6.
11. Wangler MA, Kilpatrick DS. Aminophylline is an antagonist of lorazepam. *Anesth Analg* (1985) 64, 834–6.
12. Kanto J, Aaltonen L, Himberg J-J, Hovi-Viander M. Midazolam as an intravenous induction agent in the elderly: a clinical and pharmacokinetic study. *Anesth Analg* (1986) 65, 15–20.
13. Gallen JS. Aminophylline reversal of midazolam sedation. *Anesth Analg* (1989) 69, 268.
14. Sleigh JW. Failure of aminophylline to antagonize midazolam sedation. *Anesth Analg* (1986) 65, 540.
15. Gaillard J-M, Sovilla J-Y, Blois R. The effects of clonazepam, caffeine and the combination of the two drugs on human sleep. In: Koella WP, Rüther E, Schulz H, eds. Sleep '84. New York: Gustav Fischer Verlag; 1985: pp. 314–15.
16. Mattila ME, Mattila MJ, Nuotto E. Caffeine moderately antagonizes the effects of triazolam and zopiclone on the psychomotor performance of healthy subjects. *Pharmacol Toxicol* (1992) 70, 286–9.
17. Salvà P, Costa J. Clinical pharmacokinetics and pharmacodynamics of zolpidem: therapeutic implications. *Clin Pharmacokinet* (1995) 29, 142–53.
18. Ghoneim MM, Hinrichs JV, Chiang C-K, Loke WH. Pharmacokinetic and pharmacodynamic interactions between caffeine and diazepam. *J Clin Psychopharmacol* (1986) 6, 75–80.

Buspirone + Azoles

The plasma levels of buspirone are markedly increased by itraconazole. Ketoconazole is predicted to interact similarly.

Clinical evidence

In a placebo-controlled study, 8 healthy subjects were given buspirone 10 mg, before and after taking **itraconazole** 100 mg twice daily for 4 days. It was found that the buspirone maximum plasma levels and its AUC were increased 13-fold and 19-fold, respectively, by **itraconazole**. These increased buspirone levels caused a moderate impairment of psychomotor performance (digital symbol substitution, body sway, drowsiness, etc.) and an increase in adverse effects.[1]

Mechanism

Itraconazole is a potent inhibitor of the cytochrome P450 isoenzyme CYP3A4, by which buspirone is metabolised. Itraconazole therefore increases buspirone levels and effects.

Importance and management

Direct information appears to be limited to this study but the interaction would seem to be established. The dosage of buspirone should be greatly reduced if itraconazole is given concurrently. The manufacturers recommend 2.5 mg daily[2] or twice daily.[3] **Ketoconazole** is predicted to interact similarly because it is also a potent CYP3A4 inhibitor.[1]

1. Kivistö KT, Lamberg TS, Kantola T, Neuvonen PJ. Plasma buspirone concentrations are greatly increased by erythromycin and itraconazole. *Clin Pharmacol Ther* (1997) 62, 348–54.
2. BuSpar (Buspirone hydrochloride). Bristol-Myers Squibb Company. US Prescribing information, March 2007.
3. Buspar (Buspirone hydrochloride). Bristol-Myers Pharmaceuticals. UK Summary of product characteristics, March 2007.

Buspirone + Calcium-channel blockers

Diltiazem and verapamil can markedly raise the plasma levels of buspirone, increasing the likelihood of adverse effects.

Clinical evidence, mechanism, importance and management

In a randomised study in 9 healthy subjects, **diltiazem** 60 mg three times daily for 5 doses increased the AUC of a single 10-mg dose of buspirone by 5.5-fold and increased its maximum plasma levels by 4.1-fold.

When **verapamil** 80 mg three times daily was similarly given with buspirone, the buspirone AUC and maximum plasma levels were both increased by 3.4-fold.

The increased buspirone levels are thought to occur because both **diltiazem** and **verapamil** inhibit the cytochrome P450 isoenzyme CYP3A4, which is concerned with the metabolism of the buspirone.[1]

The practical consequences of this interaction are that the effects of buspirone are likely to be increased by **diltiazem** and **verapamil**. Concurrent use need not be avoided but be alert for the need to reduce the buspirone dosage. The US manufacturer suggests adjusting according to response,[2] while the UK manufacturer suggests starting with buspirone 2.5 mg twice daily.[3] Information about other calcium-channel blockers appears to be lacking, but they do not commonly appear to interact by inhibiting CYP3A4 (see 'Calcium-channel blockers', (p.860)).

1. Lamberg TS, Kivistö KT, Neuvonen PJ. Effects of verapamil and diltiazem on the pharmacokinetics and pharmacodynamics of buspirone. *Clin Pharmacol Ther* (1998) 63, 640–5.
2. BuSpar (Buspirone hydrochloride). Bristol-Myers Squibb Company. US Prescribing information, March 2007.
3. Buspar (Buspirone hydrochloride). Bristol-Myers Pharmaceuticals. UK Summary of product characteristics, March 2007.

Buspirone + Grapefruit juice

Grapefruit juice can significantly increase plasma levels of buspirone.

Clinical evidence, mechanism, importance and management

In a randomised, crossover study, 10 healthy subjects were given either double-strength grapefruit juice 200 mL or water 200 mL three times daily for 2 days, with a single 10-mg dose of buspirone, given at the same time as the grapefruit juice or water, on the third day, with additional grapefruit juice or water 30 and 90 minutes later. Grapefruit juice increased the peak plasma level and AUC of buspirone by 4.3-fold and 9.2-fold, respectively. The time to peak buspirone level was increased from 0.75 to 3 hours. An increase in the effects of buspirone was seen only in the subjective overall drug effect. Grapefruit juice probably delayed gastric emptying and inhibited the metabolism of buspirone by the cytochrome P450 isoenzyme CYP3A4. The authors of this study recommended that the concurrent use of buspirone and grapefruit juice should be avoided.[1] However the UK manufacturer recommends that a lower dose of buspirone 2.5 mg twice daily should be used with potent inhibitors of CYP3A4 such as grapefruit juice:[2] the US manufacturer suggests that patients should avoid drinking large quantities of grapefruit juice.[3]

1. Lilja JJ, Kivistö KT, Backman JT, Lamberg TS, Neuvonen PJ. Grapefruit juice substantially increases plasma concentrations of buspirone. *Clin Pharmacol Ther* (1998) 64, 655–60.
2. Buspar (Buspirone hydrochloride). Bristol-Myers Pharmaceuticals. UK Summary of product characteristics, March 2007.
3. BuSpar (Buspirone hydrochloride). Bristol-Myers Squibb Company. US Prescribing information, March 2007.

Buspirone + Herbal medicines

Two patients taking buspirone developed marked CNS effects after starting to take herbal medicines including St John's wort and ginkgo biloba.

Clinical evidence, mechanism, importance and management

A 27-year-old woman who had been taking buspirone 30 mg daily for over one month started to take **St John's wort** (*Hypericum 2000 Plus*, Herb Valley, Australia) three tablets daily. After 2 months she complained of nervousness, aggression, hyperactivity, insomnia, confusion and disorientation, which was attributed to the serotonin syndrome. The **St John's wort** was stopped, the buspirone was increased to 50 mg daily and her symptoms resolved over a week.[1] A 42-year-old woman who was taking fluoxetine 20 mg twice daily and buspirone 15 mg twice daily started to develop symptoms of anxiety, with episodes of over-sleeping and memory deficits. It was discovered that she had been self-medicating with **St John's wort**, **ginkgo biloba** and melatonin. She was asked to stop the non-prescribed medication and her symptoms resolved.[2]

The exact mechanism of these interactions are not clear, but it seems most likely they were due to the additive effects of the buspirone and the herbal medicines, either through their effects on elevating mood or through excess effects on serotonin. Fluoxetine may have had a part to play in one of the cases, see 'SSRIs + St John's wort (*Hypericum perforatum*)', p.1224. The clinical significance of these cases is unclear, but they highlight the importance of considering adverse effects from herbal medicines when they are used with conventional medicines.

1. Dannawi M. Possible serotonin syndrome after combination of buspirone and St John's wort. *J Psychopharmacol* (2002) 16, 401.
2. Spinella M, Eaton LA. Hypomania induced by herbal and pharmaceutical psychotropic medicines following mild traumatic brain injury. *Brain Inj* (2002) 16, 359–67.

Buspirone + Macrolides

The plasma levels of buspirone are markedly increased by erythromycin.

Clinical evidence

In a placebo-controlled study buspirone 10 mg was given to 8 healthy subjects before and after they took **erythromycin** 500 mg three times daily for 4 days. It was found that the buspirone maximum plasma levels and its AUC were increased fivefold and sixfold, respectively, by the **erythromycin**. These increased buspirone levels caused a moderate impairment of psychomotor performance (digital symbol substitution, body sway, drowsiness, etc.) and an increase in adverse effects.[1]

Mechanism

Erythromycin is a potent inhibitor of the cytochrome P450 isoenzyme CYP3A4, by which buspirone is metabolised. Erythromycin therefore increases buspirone levels and hence its effects.

Importance and management

Direct information appears to be limited to this study but the interactions would seem to be established. The dosage of buspirone should be reduced if erythromycin is given concurrently. The manufacturers suggest using buspirone 2.5 mg twice daily,[2,3] adjusted according to response.[3]

Other macrolides (such as **clarithromycin**) are also inhibitors of CYP3A4 and may therefore interact similarly.

1. Kivistö KT, Lamberg TS, Kantola T, Neuvonen PJ. Plasma buspirone concentrations are greatly increased by erythromycin and itraconazole. *Clin Pharmacol Ther* (1997) 62, 348–54.
2. Buspar (Buspirone hydrochloride). Bristol-Myers Pharmaceuticals. UK Summary of product characteristics, March 2007.
3. BuSpar (Buspirone hydrochloride). Bristol-Myers Squibb Company. US Prescribing information, March 2007.

Buspirone + Miscellaneous

Buspirone does not appear to interact with amitriptyline, cimetidine or terfenadine. An isolated report describes mania when an alcoholic patient taking buspirone was given disulfiram. Nefazodone greatly increases buspirone levels.

Clinical evidence, mechanism, importance and management

(a) Amitriptyline

Buspirone 15 mg every 8 hours given with amitriptyline 25 mg every 8 hours for 10 days had no significant effect on the steady-state serum levels of amitriptyline or its metabolite, nortriptyline, in healthy subjects. No evidence of a pharmacodynamic interaction was seen.[1] There would seem to be no reason for avoiding concurrent use.

(b) Cimetidine

In 10 healthy subjects, cimetidine 1 g daily for 7 days had no effect on the plasma levels of buspirone 15 mg three times daily. Some small pharmacokinetic changes were seen, but the performance of three psychomotor function tests remained unaltered.[2] There would seem to be no reason for avoiding concurrent use.

(c) Disulfiram

An isolated report describes mania in an alcoholic patient taking buspirone 20 mg daily, possibly due to an interaction with disulfiram 400 mg daily,[3] but buspirone on its own has also apparently caused mania.[4,5] The reasons for this reaction are not understood, and the general significance of this isolated case is unknown.

(d) Nefazodone

Nefazodone 250 mg twice daily caused a 20-fold increase in the maximum plasma levels of buspirone 2.5 or 5 mg twice daily and a 50-fold increase in its AUC. Buspirone 5 mg twice daily raised the AUC of nefazodone by 23%, which is unlikely to be clinically significant. The manufacturer recommended that buspirone 2.5 mg daily should be used if nefazodone is given.[6]

(e) Terfenadine

A single 10-mg dose of buspirone was given to 10 healthy subjects after they had taken terfenadine 120 mg daily for 3 days. There were no significant effects on the pharmacokinetics or pharmacodynamics of buspirone.[7]

1. Gammans RE, Mayol RF, Labudde JA. Metabolism and disposition of buspirone. *Am J Med* (1986) 80 (Suppl 3B), 41–51.
2. Gammans RE, Pfeffer M, Westrick ML, Faulkner HC, Rehm KD, Goodson PJ. Lack of interaction between cimetidine and buspirone. *Pharmacotherapy* (1987) 7, 72–9.
3. McIvor RJ, Sinanan K. Buspirone-induced mania. *Br J Psychiatry* (1991) 158, 136–7.
4. Price WA, Bielefeld M. Buspirone-induced mania. *J Clin Psychopharmacol* (1989) 9, 150–1.
5. McDaniel JS, Ninan PT, Magnuson JV. Possible induction of mania by buspirone. *Am J Psychiatry* (1990) 147, 125–6.
6. Serzone (Nefazodone). Bristol-Myers Squibb Company. US Prescribing information, April 2004.
7. Lamberg TS, Kivistö KT, Neuvonen PJ. Lack of effect of terfenadine on the pharmacokinetics of the CYP3A4 substrate buspirone. *Pharmacol Toxicol* (1999) 84, 165–9.

Buspirone + Protease inhibitors

Ritonavir, and possibly indinavir, are predicted to reduce the metabolism of buspirone. A single case report describes Parkinson-like symptoms attributed to concurrent use of buspirone with ritonavir and also possibly indinavir.

Clinical evidence, mechanism, importance and management

A 54-year-old man who had been taking high-dose buspirone (40 mg every morning and 30 mg every evening) developed Parkinson-like symptoms about 6 weeks after starting to take **ritonavir** 400 mg and **indinavir** 400 mg, both twice daily. The dose of buspirone was reduced to 15 mg three times daily, **ritonavir** and **indinavir** were discontinued, and amprenavir 1.2 g twice daily was started. The Parkinson-like symptoms were reduced after about one week and completely resolved after 2 weeks. Buspirone is metabolised by the cytochrome P450 isoenzyme CYP3A4, and it is probable that **ritonavir**, and possibly, but to a lesser extent, **indinavir**, inhibited the metabolism of buspirone resulting in toxic levels.[1] This appears to be an isolated case report however, the manufacturer of buspirone usually recommends that a lower dose of buspirone (2.5 mg twice daily in the UK) should be used with potent inhibitors of CYP3A4,[2] such as **ritonavir**.

1. Clay PG, Adams MM. Pseudo-Parkinson disease secondary to ritonavir-buspirone interaction. *Ann Pharmacother* (2003) 37, 202–5.
2. Buspar (Buspirone hydrochloride). Bristol-Myers Pharmaceuticals. UK Summary of product characteristics, March 2007.

Buspirone + Rifampicin (Rifampin)

Rifampicin can cause a marked reduction in the plasma levels and effects of buspirone.

Clinical evidence

In a randomised, study, buspirone 30 mg daily was given to 10 healthy subjects, before and after they took rifampicin 600 mg daily for 5 days. It was found that rifampicin reduced the total AUC of buspirone by almost 90% and reduced its peak plasma levels by 87%. The pharmacodynamic effects of buspirone were reduced accordingly (as measured by digit symbol substitution, critical flicker fusion, body sway and visual analogue scales for subjective drowsiness).[1]

Mechanism

Not fully established, but it is almost certain that rifampicin induces the cytochrome P450 isoenzyme CYP3A4 in the gut and liver, which metabolises buspirone. Therefore the metabolism and clearance of buspirone are increased.

Importance and management

Direct information appears to be limited to this study but it is consistent with the way rifampicin interacts with many other drugs. This interaction would appear to be clinically important. If both drugs are used be alert for the need to use an increased buspirone dosage.

1. Lambert TS, Kivistö KT, Neuvonen PJ. Concentrations and effects of buspirone are considerably reduced by rifampicin. *Br J Clin Pharmacol* (1998) 45, 381–5.

Buspirone + SSRIs

An isolated report describes the development of the serotonin syndrome when buspirone was given with citalopram. The combination of buspirone and fluoxetine can be effective, but seizures and worsening of symptoms have been reported. Fluvoxamine may possibly reduce the effects of buspirone.

Clinical evidence, mechanism, importance and management

(a) Citalopram

An isolated report describes the development of the serotonin syndrome and hyponatraemia, thought to be caused by an interaction between citalopram and buspirone.[1] The general importance of this interaction is unknown.

(b) Fluoxetine

A 35-year-old man with a long history of depression, anxiety and panic started taking buspirone 60 mg daily. His anxiety abated, but, because of worsening depression he was also given trazodone 200 mg daily for 3 weeks. This had little effect, so fluoxetine 20 mg daily was added. Within 48 hours his usual symptoms of anxiety had returned and persisted even when the dose of buspirone was raised to 80 mg daily. Stopping the buspirone did not increase his anxiety.[2] Another patient with obsessive-compulsive disorder taking fluoxetine experienced a marked worsening of his symptoms when buspirone 5 mg twice daily was added.[3] A patient taking fluoxetine 80 mg daily had a grand mal seizure 3 weeks after buspirone 30 mg daily was added. The drugs were stopped and an EEG showed no signs of epilepsy, so the seizure was attributed to a drug interaction.[4] Other reports describe the effective concurrent use of fluoxetine and buspirone in patients with treatment-resistant depression[5] and with obsessive-compulsive disorder.[6,7]

The reasons for these adverse reactions are not understood, but there would seem to be little reason for avoiding concurrent use, however bear these case reports of interactions in mind when both drugs are used.

(c) Fluvoxamine

A double-blind study in 9 healthy subjects found that after taking fluvoxamine (mean dose 127 mg daily, range 100 to 150 mg daily) for 3 weeks, the plasma levels of a single 30-mg dose of buspirone were increased almost threefold. Even so, the psychological responses to the buspirone were reduced.[8] However, a study in 10 healthy subjects given a single 10-mg dose of buspirone after taking fluvoxamine 100 mg daily for 5 days, found that although the pharmacokinetics of buspirone were altered (AUC increased 2.4-fold) the pharmacodynamic tests remained unchanged.[9]

It has been suggested that fluvoxamine inhibits the liver enzymes concerned with the metabolism of buspirone. Concurrent use need not be avoided but it would be wise to remain alert to the possibility of reduced buspirone effects until more is known.

1. Spigset O, Adielsson G. Combined serotonin syndrome and hyponatraemia caused by a citalopram–buspirone interaction. *Int Clin Psychopharmacol* (1997) 12, 61–3.
2. Bodkin JA, Teicher MH. Fluoxetine may antagonize the anxiolytic action of buspirone. *J Clin Psychopharmacol* (1989) 9, 150.
3. Tanquary J, Masand P. Paradoxical reaction to buspirone augmentation of fluoxetine. *J Clin Psychopharmacol* (1990) 10, 377.
4. Grady TA, Pigott TA, L'Heureux F, Murphy DL. Seizure associated with fluoxetine and adjuvant buspirone therapy. *J Clin Psychopharmacol* (1992) 12, 70–1.
5. Bakish D. Fluoxetine potentiation by buspirone: three case histories. *Can J Psychiatry* (1991) 36, 749–50.
6. Markovitz PJ, Stagno SJ, Calabrese JR. Buspirone augmentation of fluoxetine in obsessive-compulsive disorder. *Am J Psychiatry* (1990) 147, 798–800.
7. Jenike MA, Baer L, Buttolph L. Buspirone augmentation of fluoxetine in patients with obsessive compulsive disorder. *J Clin Psychiatry* (1991) 52, 13–14.
8. Anderson IM, Deakin JFW, Miller HEJ. The effect of chronic fluvoxamine on hormonal and psychological responses to buspirone in normal volunteers. *Psychopharmacology (Berl)* (1996) 128, 74–82.
9. Lamberg TS, Kivistö KT, Laitila J, Mårtensson K, Neuvonen PJ. The effect of fluvoxamine on the pharmacokinetics and pharmacodynamics of buspirone. *Eur J Clin Pharmacol* (1998) 54, 761–6.

Chlorpromazine + Cimetidine

One study found that chlorpromazine serum levels are reduced by cimetidine, while another study suggested that cimetidine can increase chlorpromazine levels.

Clinical evidence, mechanism, importance and management

A study in 8 patients taking chlorpromazine 75 to 450 mg daily found that cimetidine 1 g daily in divided doses for one week decreased their steady-state chlorpromazine levels by one-third, from 37 to 24 micrograms/mL. A two-thirds *reduction* was noted in one patient.[1] The reasons for this effect are not understood but a decrease in absorption from the gut has been suggested.[1]

In contrast, another report describes 2 schizophrenic patients taking chlorpromazine 100 mg four times daily who became excessively sedated when they were given cimetidine 400 mg twice daily. The sedation disappeared when the chlorpromazine dosage was halved. When the cimetidine was later withdrawn it was found necessary to give the original chlorpromazine dosage.[2] Chlorpromazine serum levels were not measured.

There is no simple explanation for these discordant reports, but they emphasise the need to monitor the concurrent use of chlorpromazine and cimetidine. More study is needed. There seems to be no information about other phenothiazines.

1. Howes CA, Pullar T, Sourindhrin I, Mistra PC, Capel H, Lawson DH, Tilstone WJ. Reduced steady-state plasma concentrations of chlorpromazine and indomethacin in patients receiving cimetidine. *Eur J Clin Pharmacol* (1983) 24, 99–102.
2. Byrne A, O'Shea B. Adverse interaction between cimetidine and chlorpromazine in two cases of chronic schizophrenia. *Br J Psychiatry* (1989) 155, 413–15.

Chlorpromazine + Tetrabenazine

An isolated report describes severe Parkinson-like symptoms when a woman with Huntington's chorea was given tetrabenazine and chlorpromazine.

Clinical evidence, mechanism, importance and management

A woman with Huntington's chorea, successfully treated with tetrabenazine 100 mg daily for 9 years, became motionless, rigid, mute and only able to respond by blinking her eyes within one day of being given two intramuscular injections of chlorpromazine 25 mg. This was diagnosed as severe drug-induced parkinsonism, which rapidly responded to the withdrawal of both drugs and treatment with benzatropine mesilate given intramuscularly and orally. She had previously tolerated chlorpromazine well.[1] The reason for this reaction is not understood, and, as tetrabenazine is used to treat movement disorders its clinical significance is unclear.

1. Moss JH, Stewart DE. Iatrogenic parkinsonism in Huntington's chorea. *Can J Psychiatry* (1986) 31, 865–6.

Clomethiazole + Diazoxide

Clomethiazole and diazoxide, given to pregnant women in labour, can cause marked respiratory depression in their infants for up to 36 hours after birth.

Clinical evidence

An infusion of 0.8% clomethiazole, in a dose of 4 to 24 g, was given during labour to 21 pregnant women of 28 to 40 weeks gestation for eclampsia or pre-eclamptic toxaemia. Diazoxide 75 to 150 mg was also given intravenously to 14 of the women for hypertension. All 21 babies were born alive but 13 suffered hypotonia, hypoventilation or apnoea for 24 to 36 hours after birth. All of the neonates affected, apart from one, came from the group of mothers who had been given diazoxide. Three of them died of respiratory distress syndrome; one was only 28 weeks' gestation.[1]

Mechanism

Clomethiazole has some respiratory depressant effects, and is contraindicated in patients with respiratory deficiency, but it is not clear why, having passed across the placenta into the foetus, its effects should apparently be so markedly increased by diazoxide.

Importance and management

Although use of this drug combination in eclampsia is historical, the interaction is included on account of its severity. The author of the report says that the respiratory depression was managed successfully with intermittent positive pressure ventilation, provided that respiratory distress syndrome was not also present.[1]

1. Johnson RA. Adverse neonatal reaction to maternal administration of intravenous chlormethiazole and diazoxide. *BMJ* (1976) 1, 943.

Clomethiazole + Furosemide

Ten female patients aged 66 to 90 years were given clomethiazole edisilate syrup 500 mg each evening and 250 mg each morning as a sedative, with furosemide 20 to 80 mg. No significant changes in the serum levels or effects of clomethiazole or furosemide were detected, and no other significant adverse reactions were seen.[1]

1. Reid J, Judge TG. Chlormethiazole night sedation in elderly subjects receiving other medications. *Practitioner* (1980) 224, 751–3.

Clozapine + Antiepileptics

Clozapine serum levels are approximately halved by carbamazepine and possibly by phenobarbital and phenytoin. An isolated case of fatal pancytopenia has been seen in one patient taking clozapine and carbamazepine, and neuroleptic malignant syndrome occurred in another. Sodium valproate can apparently lower serum clozapine levels, and an isolated case report suggests that lamotrigine may raise them.

Clinical evidence

(a) Carbamazepine

A study by a therapeutic drug monitoring service for clozapine found that the concentration/dose ratio of 17 patients taking carbamazepine was 50% of that found in 124 other patients taking clozapine alone.[1] A 47% decrease in the serum levels of clozapine were seen in another 12 patients when they were given carbamazepine. **Oxcarbazepine** did not interact.[2] The plasma clozapine levels of 2 patients who had been taking clozapine 600 or 800 mg daily and carbamazepine 600 or 800 mg daily for several months were increased from 1.4 to 2.4 micromol/L and from 1.5 to 3 micromol/L, respectively, within 2 weeks of stopping the carbamazepine.[3]

A man with mania taking carbamazepine 1.2 g daily and lithium developed muscle rigidity, mild hyperpyrexia, tachycardia, sweating and somnolence (diagnosed as neuroleptic malignant syndrome) 3 days after his lithium was stopped and clozapine 25 mg daily started. The symptoms immediately improved when the clozapine was stopped.[4]

A patient taking carbamazepine, lithium, benzatropine and clonazepam developed fatal pancytopenia about 10 weeks after starting clozapine 400 mg daily.[5] A retrospective study of the records of other patients given clozapine and carbamazepine found a significant increase in granulopenia.[6] A previous report had not found this, due to a statistical error.[7]

A case report describes 2 schizophrenic patients taking clozapine whose treatment was changed from carbamazepine to **oxcarbazepine**. After 3 weeks their plasma clozapine levels had risen from 1.4 to 1.7 micromol/L and from 1.5 to 2.5 micromolmol/L, respectively.[8]

(b) Lamotrigine

A 35-year-old man, who had been taking clozapine for 3 years, became dizzy and sedated about one month after starting to take lamotrigine. His plasma clozapine levels were found to have increased to 1020 micrograms/L. When the lamotrigine was stopped his levels fell to 450 micrograms/L.[9]

A study in 11 patients taking clozapine in doses of 200 mg to 500 mg daily, and who were also given lamotrigine in increasing doses over 8 weeks to 200 mg daily found no significant changes in the pharmacokinetics of clozapine.[10]

(c) Phenobarbital

Mean clozapine plasma levels in 7 patients taking clozapine and phenobarbital were 35% lower than those of 15 patients taking clozapine alone.[11]

(d) Phenytoin

Two patients developed reduced clozapine levels (falls of 65 to 85%) and worsening psychoses when phenytoin was added to their treatment.[12] Another patient developed neutropenia, which was attributed to concurrent use of phenytoin and clozapine. When the phenytoin was stopped clozapine levels rose from 114 to 137 nanograms/mL, suggesting a pharmacokinetic interaction,[13] rather than just additive adverse effects.

(e) Valproate

A controlled study in 11 patients found that when sodium valproate (at an average dose of 1.06 g daily) was added to clozapine, the steady-state serum clozapine levels were increased by 39% and the levels of the demethylated metabolite increased by 23%. However, correction of these levels for dose and weight reduced the total clozapine metabolite values to only 6% above those of the controls. No increase in clozapine adverse effects was seen.[14] Another study found that sodium valproate and clozapine had no significant effect on the pharmacokinetics of each other.[15] In contrast, a study in 4 schizophrenics treated with clozapine 550 to 650 mg daily found that when valproate semisodium 750 mg to 1 g daily was added, the serum clozapine levels began to fall, and by 3 weeks had dropped by an average of 41%. No deterioration in clinical condition occurred.[16] A 15% decrease in clozapine levels was seen in another study in 7 patients given clozapine and sodium valproate.[17] Clozapine levels were doubled in a patient after valproic acid treatment was stopped, suggesting that the valproate had increased the metabolism of clozapine. An alternative explanation suggested was that the valproate may have reduced the absorption of clozapine.[18] An isolated report describes sedation, confusion, slurred speech and impaired functioning on two occasions when semisodium valproate was added to clozapine treatment in a 37-year-old man.[19]

Mechanism

Not established, but it seems likely that carbamazepine, phenobarbital and phenytoin (recognised potent enzyme inducers) increase the metabolism of clozapine by the liver, thereby reducing its effects. It has been suggested that this is because these drugs induce the activity of the cytochrome P450 isoenzyme CYP1A2.[1,13] Carbamazepine and phenobarbital may also have an effect via CYP3A4. The case of pancytopenia may possibly have been due to the additive bone marrow depressant effects of the clozapine and carbamazepine.

Importance and management

The interaction between clozapine and carbamazepine is much more firmly established than that between clozapine and phenobarbital or phenytoin, but they appear to be clinically important. Monitor symptoms and be alert for the need to increase the clozapine dosage if any of these drugs are given concurrently, and reduce the dosage if they are withdrawn. However, because of the substantial risk of bone marrow suppression the manufacturers of clozapine advise that carbamazepine should not be given concurrently.[20,21]

As yet there only appears to be one case report with lamotrigine, so the situation is unclear. There appears to be no pharmacokinetic mechanism for this interaction, so it awaits confirmation.

The situation with sodium valproate is not entirely clear. There are cases of successful concurrent use,[19] but in the light of the reports cited here it would clearly be prudent to monitor concurrent use closely. A subgroup analysis of 20 patients who received clozapine and carbamazepine, clonazepam, phenobarbital, phenytoin, or valproate suggested that this group of patients showed less clinical improvement than patients who were not also taking an antiepileptic. However, the indication for the antiepileptic drug was not always clear and combined treatment may have been used in patients who were more severely ill, or less responsive to clozapine alone.[22]

1. Jerling M, Lindström L, Bondesson U, Bertilsson L. Fluvoxamine inhibition and carbamazepine induction of the metabolism of clozapine: evidence from a therapeutic drug monitoring service. *Ther Drug Monit* (1994) 16, 368–74.
2. Tiihonen J, Vartiainen H, Hakola P. Carbamazepine-induced changes in plasma levels of neuroleptics. *Pharmacopsychiatry* (1995) 28, 26–8.
3. Raitasuo V, Lehtovaara R, Huttunen MO. Carbamazepine and plasma levels of clozapine. *Am J Psychiatry* (1993) 150, 169.
4. Müller T, Becker T, Fritze J. Neuroleptic malignant syndrome after clozapine plus carbamazepine. *Lancet* (1988) 2, 1500.
5. Gerson SL, Lieberman JA, Friedenberg WR, Lee D, Marx JJ, Meltzer H. Polypharmacy in fatal clozapine-associated agranulocytosis. *Lancet* (1991) 338, 262–3.
6. Langbehm DR, Alexander B. Increased risk of side-effects in psychiatric patients treated with clozapine and carbamazepine: a reanalysis. *Pharmacopsychiatry* (2000) 33,196.
7. Junghan U, Albers M, Woggon B. Increased risk of hematological side-effects in psychiatric patients treated with clozapine and carbamazepine? *Pharmacopsychiatry* (1993) 26, 262.
8. Raitasuo V, Lehtovaara R, Huttunen MO. Effect of switching carbamazepine to oxcarbazepine on the plasma levels of neuroleptics: a case report. *Psychopharmacology (Berl)* (1994) 116, 115–16.
9. Kossen M, Selten JP, Kahn RS. Elevated clozapine plasma level with lamotrigine. *Am J Psychiatry* (2001) 158, 1930.
10. Spina W, D'Arrigo C, Migliardi G, Santoro V, Muscatello MR, Micò U, D'Amico G, Perucca E. Effect of adjunctive lamotrigine treatment on the plasma concentrations of clozapine, risperidone and olanzapine in patients with schizophrenia or bipolar disorder. *Ther Drug Monit* (2006) 28, 599–602.
11. Facciolà G, Avenoso A, Spina E, Perucca E. Inducing effect of phenobarbital on clozapine metabolism in patients with chronic schizophrenia. *Ther Drug Monit* (1998) 20, 628–30.
12. Miller DD. Effect of phenytoin on plasma clozapine concentrations in two patients. *J Clin Psychiatry* (1991) 52, 23–5.
13. Shad MU. A complex interaction between clozapine and phenytoin. *J Pharm Technol* (2004) 20, 280–2.
14. Centorrino F, Baldessarini RJ, Kando J, Frankenburg FR, Volpicelli SA, Puopolo PR, Flood JG. Serum concentrations of clozapine and its major metabolites: effects of cotreatment with fluoxetine or valproate. *Am J Psychiatry* (1994) 151, 123–5.
15. Facciolà G, Avenoso A, Scordo MG, Madia AG, Ventimiglia A, Perucca E, Spina E. Small effects of valproic acid on the plasma concentrations of clozapine and its major metabolites in patients with schizophrenic or affective disorders. *Ther Drug Monit* (1999) 21, 341–5.
16. Finley P, Warner D. Potential impact of valproic acid therapy on clozapine disposition. *Biol Psychiatry* (1994) 36, 487–8.
17. Longo LP, Salzman C. Valproic acid effects on serum concentrations of clozapine and norclozapine. *Am J Psychiatry* (1995) 152, 650.
18. Conca A, Beraus W, König P, Waschgler R. A case of pharmacokinetic interference in comedication of clozapine and valproic acid. *Pharmacopsychiatry* (2000) 33, 234–5.
19. Costello LE, Suppes T. A clinically significant interaction between clozapine and valproate. *J Clin Psychopharmacol* (1995) 15, 139–141.
20. Clozaril (Clozapine). Novartis Pharmaceuticals UK Ltd. UK Summary of product characteristics, September 2005.
21. Clozaril (Clozapine). Novartis Pharmaceuticals Corporation. US Prescribing information, May 2005.
22. Wilson WH. Do anticonvulsants hinder clozapine treatment? *Biol Psychiatry* (1995) 37, 132–3.

Clozapine + Antihypertensives

There are isolated cases of apparent hypotensive interactions between clozapine, and enalapril, lisinopril or propranolol. Additive hypotensive effects are possible with clozapine and any antihypertensive drug.

Clinical evidence, mechanism, importance and management

A patient taking **enalapril** 5 mg twice daily fainted within an hour of being given an initial 25-mg dose of clozapine. Later he was stabilised without problems taking **enalapril** 2.5 mg twice daily and clozapine, initially 12.5 mg daily, later rising to 800 mg daily. Another patient taking **enalapril** 5 mg daily fainted within 5 hours of being given clozapine 25 mg. He needed resuscitation, but was later treated with clozapine in doses up to 600 mg daily.[1] The clozapine blood levels of a 39-year-old man rose from 490 to 966 nanograms/mL after the addition of **lisinopril** 5 mg daily. When the **lisinopril** dose was increased to 10 mg daily, the levels further rose to 1092 nanograms/mL. The dose of clozapine was reduced, and **lisinopril** replaced by diltiazem, after which his levels began to return to normal.[2]

Coma developed in a woman taking **propranolol** 40 mg daily 1.5 to 2 hours after she was given a single 150-mg dose of clozapine. She had stopped taking fluphenazine 24 hours earlier. The patient recovered, and was subsequently slowly titrated up to a daily clozapine dose of 100 mg in addition to the **propranolol**, without any problems. Although the authors state that an interaction between **propranolol** and clozapine was the likely cause of the coma, the effects of fluphenazine cannot be wholly ruled out.[3]

Clozapine has alpha-blocking effects and therefore may cause orthostatic hypotension. The manufacturers note that this is more likely in the presence of other antipsychotics or benzodiazepines and during initial titration with rapid dose increases. Because of the potential for additive effects they recommend caution when giving clozapine to patients taking any hypotensive drug.[4,5]

1. Aronowitz JS, Chakos MH, Safferman AZ, Lieberman JA. Syncope associated with the combination of clozapine and enalapril. *J Clin Psychopharmacol* (1994) 14, 429–30.
2. Abraham G, Grunberg B, Gratz S. Possible interaction of clozapine and lisinopril. *Am J Psychiatry* (2001) 158, 969.
3. Vetter PH, Proppe DG. Clozapine-induced coma. *J Nerv Ment Dis* (1992) 180, 58–9.
4. Clozaril (Clozapine). Novartis Pharmaceuticals UK Ltd. UK Summary of product characteristics, September 2005.
5. Clozaril (Clozapine). Novartis Pharmaceuticals Corporation. US Prescribing information, May 2005.

Clozapine + Antimuscarinics

The antimuscarinic effects of clozapine are additive with those of other antimuscarinic drugs, which has led to urinary retention and delirium.

Clinical evidence, mechanism, importance and management

The manufacturers of clozapine warn that the antimuscarinic effects of some drugs may be additive with those of clozapine, which may lead to adverse effects such as dry mouth and constipation.[1,2] Confirmation of the clinical relevance of this proposed interaction was seen in a patient who developed severe urinary retention while taking clozapine and **meclozine**.[3]

A man with a schizoaffective disorder taking **nortriptyline**, **perphenazine** and propranolol was also given clozapine 150 mg daily. Some improvement was seen after 8 days, and over the next week the propranolol was gradually discontinued while the clozapine dosage was raised to 225 mg daily. The patient then began to complain of extreme fatigue and slurred speech, and by day 17 was delirious and confused. His serum **nortriptyline** levels were found to have doubled (from 93 to 185 nanograms/mL) from the time the clozapine was started. He recovered within 5 days of stopping all of the drugs, after which the clozapine was restarted.[4] The authors of the report interpreted the symptoms as an antimuscarinic delirium arising from the additive antimuscarinic effects of the clozapine, **nortriptyline** and **perphenazine**, made worse by the increased levels of **nortriptyline**.[4] Just why the **nortriptyline** levels rose is not clear, but one possible explanation is that the **nortriptyline** and clozapine compete for metabolism by the same liver enzymes, resulting in a reduction in the clearance of the **nortriptyline**. 'Table 18.1', (p.672) and 'Table 18.2', (p.674) give lists of drugs that have antimuscarinic activity.

Consider also 'Antipsychotics + Antimuscarinics', p.708.

1. Clozaril (Clozapine). Novartis Pharmaceuticals UK Ltd. UK Summary of product characteristics, September 2005.
2. Clozaril (Clozapine). Novartis Pharmaceuticals Corporation. US Prescribing information, May 2005.
3. Cohen MAA, Alfonso CA, Mosquera M. Development of urinary retention during treatment with clozapine and meclizine. *Am J Psychiatry* (1994) 151, 619–20.
4. Smith T, Riskin J. Effect of clozapine on plasma nortriptyline concentration. *Pharmacopsychiatry* (1994) 27, 41–2.

Clozapine + Azoles

Itraconazole and ketoconazole do not interact with clozapine.

Clinical evidence, mechanism, importance and management

A double-blind study in 7 schizophrenic patients taking clozapine found that when **itraconazole** 200 mg daily was given for a week, no changes in the levels of clozapine or its desmethylclozapine metabolite were seen.[1]

A single 50-mg dose of clozapine was given to 5 schizophrenic patients before and after a 7-day course of **ketoconazole** 400 mg daily. The **ketoconazole** had no significant effect on the pharmacokinetics of the clozapine.[2]

The conclusion is that the cytochrome P450 isoenzyme CYP3A4 is of only minor importance in clozapine metabolism, and that because no interaction takes place between clozapine and **itraconazole** or **ketoconazole**, both it and other inhibitors of CYP3A4 can be used with clozapine.[1,2] However, note that raised clozapine levels have been attributed to treatment with the CYP3A4 inhibitor, erythromycin, see 'Clozapine + Erythromycin', p.747.

1. Raaska K, Neuvonen PJ. Serum concentrations of clozapine and *N*-desmethylclozapine are unaffected by the potent CYP3A4 inhibitor itraconazole. *Eur J Clin Pharmacol* (1998) 54, 167–70.
2. Lane H-Y, Chiu C-C, Kazmi Y, Desai H, Lam YWF, Jann MW, Chang W-H. Lack of CYP3A4 inhibition by grapefruit juice and ketoconazole upon clozapine administration *in vivo*. *Drug Metabol Drug Interact* (2001) 18, 263–78.

Clozapine + Benzodiazepines

A handful of reports describe severe hypotension, respiratory depression, unconsciousness and potentially fatal respiratory arrest in patients taking benzodiazepines and clozapine. One case of fatal respiratory arrest has been reported with lorazepam and clozapine. Dizziness and sedation are also increased.

Clinical evidence

A schizophrenic patient failed to respond to fluphenazine, **diazepam**, **clobazam** and **lormetazepam** having taken the combination for several weeks. The fluphenazine was stopped and clozapine started at a dose of 25 mg at noon and 100 mg at night. Toxic delirium and severe hypersalivation developed 3 hours later. The patient collapsed (systolic blood pressure 50 mmHg, diastolic blood pressure unrecordable) and stopped breathing. Resuscitation was started, and the patient remained unconscious for 30 minutes. After a few drug-free days clozapine 12.5 mg was successfully re-introduced, and very slowly titrated upwards; a low benzodiazepine dosage was also given.[1]

Another patient taking clozapine died suddenly and unexpectedly during the night, apparently due to respiratory arrest, after being given three 2-mg intravenous doses of **lorazepam** the previous day.[2]

There are at least 6 other cases of severe hypotension, respiratory depression or loss of consciousness in patients taking clozapine and **flurazepam**, **lorazepam** or **diazepam**,[1,3-5] as well as other cases of marked sedation, hypersalivation, ataxia and delirium in patients taking **lorazepam** and clozapine.[6,7] Two of these reports[1,3] are from the same group of workers and it is not clear whether they are about the same or different patients.

Mechanism

Not understood. Clozapine on its own very occasionally causes respiratory arrest and hypotension.

Importance and management

The authors of the first of these reports[1] say that the relative risk of the cardiovascular/respiratory reaction is only 2.1%. Another report[2] says that the death cited above is the only life-threatening event among 162 patients given clozapine and benzodiazepines between 1986 and 1991 so that the incidence of serious problems is quite low. Even so, concurrent use should be very well monitored because of the severity of the reaction, even if it is rare.

1. Grohmann R, Rüther E, Sassim N, Schmidt LG. Adverse effects of clozapine. *Psychopharmacology (Berl)* (1989) 99, S101–S104.
2. Klimke A, Klieser E. Sudden death after intravenous application of lorazepam in a patient treated with clozapine. *Am J Psychiatry* (1994) 151, 780.
3. Sassim N, Grohmann R. Adverse drug reactions with clozapine and simultaneous application of benzodiazepines. *Pharmacopsychiatry* (1988) 21, 306–7.
4. Friedman LJ, Tabb SE, Worthington JJ, Sanchez CJ, Sved M. Clozapine – a novel antipsychotic agent. *N Engl J Med* (1991) 325, 518–9.
5. Tupala E, Niskanen L, Tiihonen J. Transient syncope and ECG changes associated with the concurrent administration of clozapine and diazepam. *J Clin Psychiatry* (1999) 60, 619–20.
6. Cobb CD, Anderson CB, Seidel DR. Possible interaction between clozapine and lorazepam. *Am J Psychiatry* (1991) 148, 1606–7.
7. Jackson CW, Markowitz JS, Brewerton TD. Delirium associated with clozapine and benzodiazepine combinations. *Ann Clin Psychiatry* (1995) 7, 139–41.

Clozapine + Caffeine

Caffeine increases serum clozapine levels, which may increase the incidence of its adverse effects.

Clinical evidence

In a crossover study, 6 coffee-drinking patients taking clozapine were given decaffeinated or caffeine-containing instant coffee for 7 days. The plasma levels of clozapine were 26% higher while the patients were taking caffeine.[1] A study in 12 healthy subjects[2] found that caffeine 400 mg to 1 g daily, raised the AUC and decreased the clearance of a single 12.5-mg dose of clozapine by 19% and 14%, respectively. A previous study in 7 patients had found that clozapine levels decreased by 47% when the subjects avoided caffeine for 5 days, and increased again when caffeine consumption was resumed.[3]

A 66-year-old woman taking clozapine 300 mg daily developed supraventricular tachycardia (180 bpm) when she was given 500 mg of intravenous caffeine sodium benzoate to increase seizure length during an ECT session. Verapamil was needed to revert the arrhythmia. Before taking clozapine she had received caffeine sodium benzoate in doses of up to 1 g during ECT sessions without problems.[4] Another patient taking clozapine for schizophrenia had an exacerbation of his psychotic symptoms, which was attributed to caffeinated coffee (5 to 10 cups daily). The problem resolved when the patient stopped drinking caffeine. He had previously not had any problems with caffeine while taking haloperidol 30 mg and procyclidine 30 mg daily.[5] A 31-year-old woman taking clozapine 550 mg daily developed increased daytime sleepiness, sialorrhoea and withdrawn behaviour after taking about 1.2 g of caffeine daily (as drinks and tablets). Her plasma clozapine levels fell from 1500 to 630 nanograms/mL when her caffeine intake was stopped.[6]

Mechanism

Caffeine is a competitive inhibitor of the cytochrome P450 isoenzyme CYP1A2, which is one of the major isoenzymes involved in the metabolism of caffeine. Consequently clozapine serum levels and effects increase.[2,3,7]

Importance and management

This would appear to be an established and clinically important interaction, but unlikely to be a problem if clozapine serum levels are established and well monitored, and caffeine intake remains fairly stable and moderate. Possible exceptions are if large doses of caffeine are given during ECT treatment or if for some other reason the caffeine intake suddenly increases or decreases markedly.

1. Raaska K, Raitasuo V, Laitila J, Neuvonen PJ. Effect of caffeine-containing versus decaffeinated coffee on serum clozapine concentrations in hospitalised patients. *Basic Clin Pharmacol Toxicol* (2004) 94, 13–18.
2. Hägg S, Spigset O, Mjörndal T, Dahlqvist R. Effect of caffeine on clozapine pharmacokinetics in healthy volunteers. *Br J Clin Pharmacol* (2000) 49, 59–63.
3. Carrillo JA, Herraiz AG, Ramos SI, Benitez J. Effects of caffeine withdrawal from the diet on the metabolism of clozapine in schizophrenic patients. *J Clin Psychopharmacol* (1998) 18, 311–16.
4. Beale MD, Pritchett JT, Kellner CH. Supraventricular tachycardia in a patient receiving ECT, clozapine, and caffeine. *Convuls Ther* (1994) 10, 228–31.
5. Vainer JL, Chouinard G. Interaction between caffeine and clozapine. *J Clin Psychopharmacol* (1994) 14, 284–5.
6. Odom-White A, de Leon J. Clozapine levels and caffeine. *J Clin Psychiatry* (1996) 57, 175–6.
7. Carrillo JA, Jerling M, Bertilsson L. Comments to "Interaction between caffeine and clozapine". *J Clin Psychopharmacol* (1995) 15, 376–7.

Clozapine + Drugs that suppress bone marrow

The manufacturers caution the use of clozapine with other drugs that can cause bone marrow suppression. Low white cells counts have been seen in patients taking clozapine and chloroquine, co-trimoxazole, methazolamide, nitrofurantoin, olanzapine, or thiamazole.

Clinical evidence, mechanism, importance and management

Clozapine can cause blood dyscrasias and potentially fatal agranulocytosis, therefore the manufacturers say that it should not be given with other drugs that have a well-known potential to cause agranulocytosis.[1,2] The

UK manufacturer lists **carbamazepine** (see also 'Clozapine + Antiepileptics', p.744), **chloramphenicol**, **cytotoxics**, **penicillamine**, pyrazolone analgesics (e.g. **phenylbutazone**), **sulphonamides** (e.g. **co-trimoxazole**) and, because they cannot be stopped if an adverse reaction occurs, they advise against the use of **depot antipsychotics**.[1] There are several cases that confirm the clinical significance of these predicted interactions.

A woman was taking **thiamazole** for Graves' disease, at times with various different antipsychotics including haloperidol, flupentixol, zuclopenthixol and perphenazine for schizophrenia. Because of the severe extrapyramidal reactions and failure to control the schizophrenia, clozapine, increased over 5 days to 250 mg daily, was started instead. Within 5 days her white cell count had fallen to 2200/mm^3, which rose to 4000/mm^3, one month after both drugs were stopped. Later, after the **thiamazole** was stopped she was given the same dose of clozapine without these adverse effects.[3]

A patient who had been taking clozapine 500 mg daily for 8 months developed granulocytopenia within 8 days of starting **nitrofurantoin** 200 mg daily.[4]

An 86-year old woman taking clozapine developed neutropenia 2 weeks after **methazolamide** for glaucoma was added. Both drugs were stopped and her white cell count recovered. She later restarted clozapine without problem and so the toxic effect was attributed to the combined use of two drugs.[5]

Neutropenia developed 4 days after **co-trimoxazole** was started in a 47-year-old woman who had been uneventfully taking clozapine for 5 years. **Co-trimoxazole** was stopped and the white cell counts returned to normal over the next 2 weeks.[6]

Three patients have been described who showed a delay in recovery from clozapine-induced agranulocytosis when given **olanzapine**, and it has been suggested that **olanzapine** should therefore be avoided until the patient's haematological status has normalised.[7]

However, in contrast, a patient taking clozapine 25 mg daily had no significant changes in his white cell count after taking **chloroquine** for malaria prophylaxis, over the course of one month.[8]

1. Clozaril (Clozapine). Novartis Pharmaceuticals UK Ltd. UK Summary of product characteristics, September 2005.
2. Clozaril (Clozapine). Novartis Pharmaceuticals Corporation. US Prescribing information, May 2005.
3. Rocco PL. Concurrent treatment with clozapine and methimazole inducing granulocytopenia: a case report. *Hum Psychopharmacol* (1993) 8, 445–6.
4. Juul Povlsen U, Noring U, Fog R, Gerlach J. Tolerability and therapeutic effect of clozapine. *Acta Psychiatr Scand* (1985) 71, 176–85.
5. Burke WJ, Ranno AE. Neutropenia with clozapine and methazolamide. *J Clin Psychopharmacol* (1994) 14, 357–8.
6. Henderson DC, Borba CP. Trimethoprim-sulfamethoxazole and clozapine. *Psychiatr Serv* (2001) 52, 111–12.
7. Flynn SW, Altman S, MacEwan GW, Black LL, Greenidge LL, Honer WG. Prolongation of clozapine-induced granulocytopenia associated with olanzapine. *J Clin Psychopharmacol* (1997) 17, 494–5.
8. König P, Künz A. Compatibility of clozapine and chloroquine. *Lancet* (1991) 338, 948.

Clozapine + Erythromycin

A study in healthy subjects found no evidence of an interaction between clozapine and erythromycin, but three case reports describe clozapine toxicity (seizures in one patient, drowsiness, incoordination and incontinence in another and neutropenia in the third) when the patients were given erythromycin.

Clinical evidence

A randomised, crossover study in 12 healthy subjects found that erythromycin 500 mg three times daily did not affect the pharmacokinetics of a single 12.5-mg dose of clozapine.[1]

In contrast, a schizophrenic man taking clozapine 800 mg daily, was given erythromycin 250 mg four times daily for a fever and sore throat caused by pharyngitis. After a week he had a single tonic-clonic seizure and his serum clozapine levels were found to be 1300 micrograms/mL. Both drugs were stopped, and the clozapine restarted 2 days later, initially at only 400 mg daily, but after several weeks had increased to 800 mg daily, giving serum clozapine levels of 700 micrograms/mL.[2] Another schizophrenic taking clozapine 600 mg daily became drowsy, with slurred speech, incontinence, difficulty in walking and incoordination within 2 to 3 days of starting to take erythromycin 333 mg three times daily. His serum clozapine level was found to be 1150 micrograms/L and he had leucocytosis. He recovered when both drugs were stopped. When he later restarted treatment with the same clozapine dosage, but without the erythromycin, his steady-state trough clozapine serum level was 385 micrograms/L.[3] Another case also describes a reduced white cell count when erythromycin was added to established clozapine therapy, but no clozapine levels were available.[4]

Mechanism

Uncertain. One suggestion is that erythromycin might have inhibited the cytochrome P450 isoenzyme CYP3A4, which has a minor role in the metabolism of clozapine, leading to a reduced clearance, which resulted in increased serum clozapine levels and toxicity.[2,3] Clozapine is mainly metabolised by CYP1A2, which is not known to be affected by the macrolides.

Importance and management

Information appears to be limited to this study and the three case reports, but clozapine has not been found to interact with other potent inhibitors of CYP3A4, see 'Clozapine + Azoles', p.745. An interaction seems unlikely, although the case reports do suggest that rarely some patients may be affected. Bear this interaction in mind in the case of an unexpected response to treatment. Note that infection may be a sign of clozapine-induced agranulocytosis.

1. Hägg S, Spigset O, Mjörndal T, Granberg K, Persbo-Lundqvist G, Dahlqvist R. Absence of interaction between erythromycin and a single dose of clozapine. *Eur J Clin Pharmacol* (1999) 55, 221–6.
2. Funderburg LG, Vertrees JE, True JE, Miller AL. Seizure following addition of erythromycin to clozapine treatment. *Am J Psychiatry* (1994) 151, 1840–1.
3. Cohen LG, Chesley S, Eugenio L, Flood JG, Fisch J, Goff DC. Erythromycin-induced clozapine toxic reaction. *Arch Intern Med* (1996) 156, 675–7.
4. Usiskin SI, Nicolson R, Lenane M, Rapoport JL. Retreatment with clozapine after erythromycin-induced neutropenia. *Am J Psychiatry* (2000) 157, 1021.

Clozapine + H_2-receptor antagonists

A single case report describes increased serum clozapine levels and toxicity due to cimetidine, but not ranitidine.

Clinical evidence, mechanism, importance and management

A man with chronic paranoid schizophrenia was taking atenolol and clozapine 900 mg daily. When **cimetidine** 400 mg twice daily was added for gastritis, his serum clozapine levels rose by almost 60% (from a range of 992 to 1081 nanograms/mL to a range of 1559 to 1701 nanograms/mL) but this did not result in any adverse effects. Within 3 days of raising the dosage of **cimetidine** to 400 mg three times daily he developed evidence of clozapine toxicity (marked diaphoresis, dizziness, vomiting, weakness, orthostatic hypotension), all of which resolved over 5 days when the clozapine dosage was lowered to 200 mg daily, and the **cimetidine** was stopped. The serum clozapine levels during this period were not reported. When **cimetidine** was replaced by **ranitidine** 150 mg twice daily his clozapine serum levels were not affected.[1]

The suggested reason for this interaction is that the **cimetidine** (a potent non-specific enzyme inhibitor) reduces the metabolism of clozapine by the liver so that it accumulates, causing toxicity. **Ranitidine** does not cause enzyme inhibition and therefore does not interact.

Information appears to be limited to this report but it is consistent with the way **cimetidine** interacts with many other drugs. **Ranitidine**, and possibly other H_2-receptor antagonists such as **famotidine** or **nizatidine**, which do not inhibit liver enzymes, would seem to be preferable and safer alternatives; however, this needs confirmation.

1. Szymanski S, Lieberman JA, Picou D, Masiar S, Cooper T. A case report of cimetidine-induced clozapine toxicity. *J Clin Psychiatry* (1991) 52, 21–2.

Clozapine + Hormonal contraceptives

A case report describes raised clozapine levels with associated adverse effects when a patient also took a combined oral contraceptive.

Clinical evidence, mechanism, importance and management

A 47-year-old smoker with paranoid schizophrenia taking clozapine 550 mg daily had a good therapeutic response at this dose, but also reported drowsiness, weakness and dizziness. The patient was also taking a combined oral contraceptive containing **norethisterone** 500 micrograms and **ethinylestradiol** 35 micrograms. Clozapine plasma levels ranged from 736 to 792 nanograms/mL (therapeutic range 300 to 700 nanograms/mL). After 2 months she stopped taking her combined oral contraceptive and noted that the adverse effects of clozapine resolved, and clozapine levels were found to be 378 to 401 nanograms/mL. The patient did not stop smoking during this time. It was suggested that the oral contraceptive inhibited the cytochrome P450 isoenzymes CYP1A2, CYP2C19 and CYP3A4 resulting in raised clozapine plasma levels. The authors note that slower titration and smaller doses of clozapine may be needed in patients taking hormonal contraceptives.[1] Further study is needed as this appears to be the only published case report of this interaction.

1. Gabbay V, O'Dowd MA, Mamamtavrishvili M, Asnis GM. Clozapine and oral contraceptives: a possible drug interaction. *J Clin Psychopharmacol* (2002) 22, 621–2.

Clozapine + Lithium

A few patients given lithium carbonate and clozapine have experienced adverse reactions including myoclonus, neuroleptic malignant syndrome, seizures, delirium and psychoses.

Clinical evidence

A man with poorly controlled schizophrenia, taking clozapine 750 mg daily for 6 weeks, was given lithium, initially 900 mg and then subsequently 1.2 g daily. His serum lithium level was 0.86 mmol/L. Within one week he began to experience paroxysmal jerky movements of his upper and lower extremities lasting about 30 minutes. This myoclonus resolved when both drugs were stopped, and did not recur when clozapine was restarted alone.[1] Another patient developed neuroleptic malignant syndrome (stiffness, rigidity, tachycardia, diaphoresis, hypertension) 3 to 4 weeks after clozapine was added to his lithium treatment. The symptoms disappeared within 2 to 3 days of stopping the clozapine.[2] An elderly man also developed neuroleptic malignant syndrome 3 days after starting to take clozapine 25 mg daily. He was also taking carbamazepine, and had stopped taking lithium 3 days earlier.[3]

Four out of 10 patients taking lithium carbonate (mean dose of 1.4 g daily) and clozapine (mean maximum dose 900 mg daily) developed reversible neurological symptoms including involuntary jerking of the limbs and tongue, facial spasm, tremor, confusion, generalised weakness, stumbling gait, leaning and falling to the right. One of them also became delirious. Serum lithium levels remained unchanged, and the problems resolved when the lithium was stopped. Three of the four had a recurrence of the symptoms when rechallenged with the drug combination.[4] A man taking clozapine and lithium carbonate developed psychosis with delusions and visual hallucinations over a 5-day period when clozapine was tapered off and stopped. This was accompanied by a doubling in his serum lithium levels. He recovered completely when the drugs were stopped.[5] Two patients taking clozapine developed seizures: one developed a tonic clonic seizure within 4 days of adding lithium carbonate 900 mg to clozapine 600 mg daily, and the other a grand mal seizure within 6 days of adding lithium carbonate 900 mg to clozapine 900 mg daily.[6]

A review of the medical records of 44 patients taking clozapine and lithium identified 28 patients who had experienced an adverse effect, three of which were possibly associated with the drug combination. There were two reports of myoclonus and one of a grand mal seizure.[7]

Lithium is thought to have masked a clozapine-induced agranulocytosis in a 59-year-old woman who developed leucopenia and subsequently agranulocytosis after 40 days of treatment with lithium and clozapine.[8] It has been suggested that lithium may help to protect patients from adverse effects of clozapine, in particular agranulocytosis, although a clozapine rechallenge in a patient who has previously experienced a blood dyscrasia with clozapine should only be undertaken with great caution.[9]

Mechanism

Not understood.

Importance and management

Some patients develop a toxic reaction when given both drugs, and others do not, for reasons that are not understood. Concurrent use should therefore be extremely well monitored including close monitoring of full blood counts as well as lithium levels. One group of workers suggest that lithium levels of no more than 0.5 mmol/L may give therapeutic benefits while minimising adverse effects.[4]

1. Lemus CZ, Lieberman JA, Johns CA. Myoclonus during treatment with clozapine and lithium: the role of serotonin. *Hillside J Clin Psychiatry* (1989) 11, 127–30.
2. Pope HG, Cole JO, Choras PT, Fulwiler CE. Apparent neuroleptic malignant syndrome with clozapine and lithium. *J Nerv Ment Dis* (1986) 174, 493–5.
3. Müller T, Becker T, Fritze J. Neuroleptic malignant syndrome after clozapine plus carbamazepine. *Lancet* (1988) ii, 1500.
4. Blake LM, Marks RC, Luchins DJ. Reversible neurologic symptoms with clozapine and lithium. *J Clin Psychopharmacol* (1992) 12, 297–9.
5. Hellwig B, Hesslinger B, Walder J. Tapering off clozapine in a clozapine-lithium co-medication may cause an acute organic psychosis. A case report. *Pharmacopsychiatry* (1995) 28, 187.
6. Garcia G, Crismon ML, Dorson PG. Seizures in two patients after the addition of lithium to a clozapine regimen. *J Clin Psychopharmacol* (1994) 14, 426–7.
7. Bender S, Linka T, Wolstein J, Gehendges S, Paulus H-J, Schall U, Gastpar M. Safety and efficacy of combined clozapine-lithium pharmacotherapy. *Int J Neuropsychopharmacol* (2004) 7,59–63.
8. Valevski A, Modai I, Lahav M, Weizman A. Clozapine-lithium combined treatment and agranulocytosis. *Int Clin Psychopharmacol* (1993) 8, 63–5.
9. Kanaan RA, Kerwin RW. Lithium and clozapine rechallenge: a retrospective case analysis. *J Clin Psychiatry* (2006) 67, 756–60.

Clozapine + Miscellaneous

There are isolated cases of apparent interactions between clozapine, and ampicillin, buspirone, caffeine, haloperidol, loperamide, modafinil, nefazodone, nicotinic acid, tryptophan, or vitamin C. Grapefruit juice, influenza vaccine mirtazapine, reboxetine, or venlafaxine do not appear to interact. Cocaine levels may increase when taken with clozapine.

Clinical evidence, mechanism, importance and management

(a) Ampicillin

An isolated report describes a 17-year-old taking clozapine (12.5 mg increased to 50 mg three times daily) who was given ampicillin 500 mg four times daily, starting on day 15 of clozapine treatment. On the next day the patient became easily distracted, very drowsy and salivated excessively. These adverse reactions stopped when the ampicillin was replaced by doxycycline.[1]

(b) Buspirone

A man who had been taking clozapine for a year developed acute and potentially lethal gastrointestinal bleeding and marked hyperglycaemia about 5 weeks after starting buspirone, and one week after the buspirone dosage was raised to 20 mg daily. No gut pathology (e.g. ulceration) was detected and there were no problems when he was subsequently given clozapine alone, so the reaction was attributed to the drug combination.[2]

(c) Cocaine

A single-dose study in 8 cocaine addicts found that there was a dose-dependent rise in cocaine levels of 6%, 49% and 67% after clozapine was given in doses of 12.5, 25 or 50 mg, respectively, with intranasal cocaine 2 mg/kg. Subjective questioning revealed a reduction in the positive effects of cocaine. One subject also experienced a near-syncopal attack which required medical attention.[3]

(d) Grapefruit juice

Grapefruit juice did not affect the metabolism of clozapine in two studies in a total of 36 schizophrenic patients.[4,5]

(e) Haloperidol

A 68-year-old man taking clozapine 600 mg daily and venlafaxine, lorazepam, aspirin, vitamin E and multivitamins, was given haloperidol 4 mg daily to control persistent paranoid delusions and hallucinations. After 27 days he was found collapsed and was lethargic, tachycardic, feverish and delirious. Neuroleptic malignant syndrome was suspected so the antipsychotics were withheld, and the patient recovered over the following 7 days. Clozapine was later re-started without a recurrence of symptoms.[6] A case of elevated haloperidol levels has been reported in a 40-year-old man who was given haloperidol intramuscular injections 50 mg every 4 weeks. He was also given clozapine in increasing doses from 50 to 250 mg daily. Over this time his haloperidol levels increased from 12 nanogram/mL to 166 nanogram/mL, although it is not clear whether he had attained steady-state levels when the first measurement was reported.[7]

(f) Influenza vaccine

In an open-label study in 14 patients the metabolism of clozapine was not altered following a single intramuscular dose of influenza vaccine (*Influvac* 2001 to 2002 formula, Solvay).[8]

(g) Loperamide

A patient taking clozapine 500 mg daily died after taking loperamide 6 mg daily during an episode of food poisoning. The authors of the report attribute the death to toxic megacolon brought on by the additive effects of clozapine and loperamide on gut transit.[9] Toxic megacolon can sometimes occur with loperamide alone, especially in the presence of an infection. Also, the manufacturers of clozapine say that care is necessary in patients given clozapine with drugs known to cause constipation (see also 'Clozapine + Antimuscarinics', p.745) because on rare occasions clozapine alone has been shown to cause significant impairment of intestinal function (such as paralytic ileus).[10,11]

(h) Mirtazapine

A study in 9 patients taking clozapine in doses ranging from 100 to 650 mg daily found no significant change in the pharmacokinetics of clozapine after the addition of mirtazapine 30 mg daily.[12]

(i) Modafinil

A 42-year-old man taking clozapine 450 mg daily was given modafinil, titrated up to 300 mg daily, to combat sedation. After about one month of concurrent use he developed dizziness and an unsteady gait, and his clozapine level was found to be 1400 nanograms/mL. His clozapine level had been 761 nanograms/mL while taking clozapine 400 mg daily, and because the 50 mg clozapine dose increase was not thought large enough to almost double his clozapine level, an interaction with modafinil was suspected.[13]

(j) Nefazodone

A 40-year-old man who had been successfully treated with risperidone and clozapine 425 to 475 mg daily started taking nefazodone 200 mg daily, increasing to 300 mg daily, for the treatment of persistent depression. After one week on the higher dose he became dizzy and hypotensive and it was noted that his clozapine level had risen from 133 to 233 nanograms/mL. This was thought to be due to an inhibitory effect of nefazodone on the cytochrome P450 isoenzyme CYP3A4,[14] although note that other potent inhibitors of CYP3A4 (such as 'erythromycin', (p.747) or the 'azoles', (p.745)) rarely appear to increase clozapine levels. In contrast, a small study in 6 patients taking clozapine and who were then additionally prescribed nefazodone found no significant effects on the pharmacokinetics of clozapine.[15]

A possible case of neutropenia caused by the addition of nefazodone to treatment with sodium valproate and clozapine has been reported. The patient had been receiving treatment with sodium valproate and clozapine for many months when nefazodone was started in increasing doses up to 200 mg twice daily. Within one week her neutrophil count had dropped to 1.8×10^9/L, and remained low until the nefazodone was discontinued. The patient's serum level of clozapine was reported to remain stable during this time and the patient had not had any previous episodes of leucopenia during treatment with clozapine.[16]

(k) Nicotinic acid/Tryptophan/Vitamin C

A man with schizophrenia taking tryptophan, lorazepam, vitamin C, benzatropine and nicotinic acid, developed a severe urticarial rash covering his face, neck and trunk 3 days after starting clozapine 150 mg daily. All of the drugs except lorazepam were stopped, and the rash subsided. It did not recur when clozapine was restarted, even at a dose of 600 mg daily, nor when small doses of benzatropine and fluphenazine were briefly added. The authors draw the inference that tryptophan, vitamin C and nicotinic acid may have been responsible for this alleged interaction with clozapine.[17]

(l) Reboxetine

A small study in 7 patients found that reboxetine 8 mg daily had no effect on the metabolism of clozapine or its major metabolite.[18]

(m) Ritonavir

Ritonavir is a potent inhibitor of the cytochrome P450 isoenzymes CYP3A4 and CYP2D6, and is therefore expected to increase plasma levels of clozapine. This may result in serious haematologic abnormalities, although there appear to be no published studies or case reports of this effect. The UK manufacturers therefore contraindicate combined use.[19]

(n) Venlafaxine

In 11 patients venlafaxine in doses of up to 150 mg daily did not affect the pharmacokinetics of established clozapine treatment in doses up to 950 mg daily.[20]

1. Csík V, Molnár J. Possible adverse interaction between clozapine and ampicillin in an adolescent with schizophrenia. *J Child Adolesc Psychopharmacol* (1994) 4, 123–8.
2. Good MI. Lethal interaction of clozapine and buspirone? *Am J Psychiatry* (1997) 154, 1472–3.
3. Farren CK, Hameedi FA, Rosen MA, Woods S, Jatlow P, Kosten TR. Significant interaction between clozapine and cocaine in cocaine addicts. *Drug Alcohol Depend* (2000) 59, 153–63.
4. Lane H-Y, Chiu C-C, Kazmi Y, Desai H, Lam YWF, Jan MW, Chang W-H. Lack of CYP3A4 inhibition by grapefruit juice and ketoconazole upon clozapine administration *in vivo*. *Drug Metabol Drug Interact* (2001) 18, 263–78.
5. Lane H-Y, Jann MW, Chang Y-C, Chiu C-C, Huang M-C, Lee S-H, Chang W-H. Repeated ingestion of grapefruit juice does not alter clozapine's steady-state plasma levels, effectiveness, and tolerability. *J Clin Psychiatry* (2001) 62, 812–17.
6. Garcia G, Ghani S, Poveda RA, Dansky BL. Neuroleptic malignant syndrome with antidepressant/antipsychotic drug combination. *Ann Pharmacother* (2001) 35, 784–5.
7. Allen SA. Effect of chlorpromazine and clozapine on plasma concentrations of haloperidol in a patient with schizophrenia. *J Clin Pharmacol* (2000) 40, 1296–7.
8. Raaska K, Raitasuo V, Neuvonen PJ. Effect of influenza vaccination on serum clozapine and its main metabolite concentrations in patients with schizophrenia. *Eur J Clin Pharmacol* (2001) 57, 705–8.
9. Eronen M, Putkonen H, Hallikainen T, Vartiainen H. Lethal gastroenteritis associated with clozapine and loperamide. *Am J Psychiatry* (2003) 160, 2242–3.
10. Clozaril (Clozapine). Novartis Pharmaceuticals UK Ltd. UK Summary of product characteristics, September 2005.
11. Clozaril (Clozapine). Novartis Pharmaceuticals Corporation. US Prescribing information, May 2005.
12. Zoccali R, Muscatello MR, La Torre D, Malara G, Canale A, Crucitti D, D'Arrigo C, Spina E. Lack of a pharmacokinetic interaction between mirtazapine and the newer antipsychotics clozapine, risperidone and olanzapine in patients with chronic schizophrenia. *Pharm Res* (2003) 48, 411–14.
13. Dequardo JR. Modafinil-associated clozapine toxicity. *Am J Psychiatry* (2002) 159, 1243–4.
14. Khan AY, Preskorn SH. Increase in plasma levels of clozapine and norclozapine after administration of nefazodone. *J Clin Psychiatry* (2001) 62, 375–6.
15. Taylor D, Bodani M, Hubbeling A, Murray R. The effect of nefazodone on clozapine plasma concentrations. *Int Clin Psychopharmacol* (1999) 14, 185–7.
16. Macdonald J, Rawlins S. Neutropenia due to nefazodone, interaction or coincidence? *Aust N Z J Psychiatry* (2000) 34, 1031–2.
17. Goumeniouk AD, Ancill RJ, MacEwan GW, Koczapski AB. A case of drug-drug interaction involving clozapine. *Can J Psychiatry* (1991) 36, 234–5.
18. Spina E, Avenoso A, Scordo MG, Ancione M, Madia A, Levita A. No effect of reboxetine on plasma concentrations of clozapine, risperidone, and their active metabolites. *Ther Drug Monit* (2001) 23, 675–8.
19. Norvir (Ritonavir). Abbott Laboratories Ltd. UK Summary of product characteristics, May 2007.
20. Repo-Tiihonen E, Eloranta A, Hallikainen T, Tiihonen J. Effects of venlafaxine treatment on clozapine plasma levels in schizophrenic patients. *Neuropsychobiology* (2005) 51, 173–6.

Clozapine + Proton pump inhibitors

Omeprazole appears to reduce the serum levels of clozapine.

Clinical evidence, mechanism, importance and management

A retrospective study identified 13 patients taking clozapine and **omeprazole** in who the proton pump inhibitor was subsequently changed to **pantoprazole**. This resulted in an increase in the mean clozapine serum level from 445 to 579 nanograms/mL in 3 non-smokers, but in the 10 smokers there was a slight *reduction* in levels, from 364 to 323 nanograms/mL. Both **omeprazole** and smoking are known to induce the cytochrome P450 isoenzyme CYP1A2, which is the major isoenzyme involved in the metabolism of clozapine. The authors suggest that when **omeprazole** was stopped in the non-smokers there was no CYP1A2 induction, hence clozapine levels rose, whereas CYP1A2 induction continued in the smokers, so their levels were only slightly affected.[1]

A case report describes two patients (both smokers) whose clozapine levels were reduced, from 762 to 443 nanograms/mL and from 369 to 204 nanograms/mL, respectively, after **omeprazole** was started. However, no changes in clinical condition were noted.[2]

Other proton pump inhibitors do not appear to have been studied.

1. Mookhoek EJ, Loonen AJM. Retrospective evaluation of the effect of omeprazole on clozapine metabolism. *Pharm World Sci* (2004) 26, 180–2.
2. Frick A, Kopitz J, Bergemann N. Omeprazole reduces clozapine plasma concentrations. *Pharmacopsychiatry* (2003) 36, 121–3.

Clozapine + Quinolones

An isolated report describes the development of agitation in an elderly man taking clozapine, which was tentatively attributed to an interaction with ciprofloxacin. A study supports this observation.

Clinical evidence, mechanism, importance and management

An elderly man with multi-infarct dementia and behavioural disturbances, taking clozapine, glibenclamide (glyburide), trazodone and melatonin, was hospitalised for agitation on the last day of a 10-day course of ciprofloxacin 500 mg twice daily. When the ciprofloxacin course was completed, his plasma clozapine serum levels fell from 90 nanograms/mL to undetectable levels (lower limit of detection being 50 nanograms/mL).[1]

Ciprofloxacin 250 mg twice daily for 7 days was given to 7 schizophrenic patients taking clozapine. The mean serum clozapine and *N*-desmethylclozapine levels were increased by 29% and 31%, respectively, but no additional adverse effects were reported. Interindividual variation in serum levels was high, so it seems likely that some patients may demonstrate a clinically significant interaction.[2] This interaction probably occurs because ciprofloxacin inhibits the cytochrome P450 isoenzyme CYP1A2, the major isoenzyme involved in the metabolism of clozapine, resulting in elevated clozapine levels. Monitor the outcome carefully if ciprofloxacin is added to clozapine treatment. There seem to be no other reports of an interaction between clozapine and other quinolones, but as they all inhibit CYP1A2 to a varying extent (see 'Theophylline + Quinolones', p.1192) some interaction seems possible.

1. Markowitz JS, Gill HS, Devane CL, Mintzer JE. Fluoroquinolone inhibition of clozapine metabolism. *Am J Psychiatry* (1997) 153, 881.
2. Raaska K, Neuvonen PJ. Ciprofloxacin increases serum clozapine and *N*-desmethylclozapine: a study in patients with schizophrenia. *Eur J Clin Pharmacol* (2000) 56, 585–9.

Clozapine + Rifampicin (Rifampin)

The serum clozapine levels of a patient were greatly reduced when rifampicin was also given.

Clinical evidence, mechanism, importance and management

A schizophrenic patient taking clozapine developed tuberculosis and was given rifampicin, isoniazid and pyrazinamide. Within 2 to 3 weeks his trough serum clozapine levels had fallen dramatically from about 250 nanograms/mL to 40 nanograms/mL, but rose again rapidly when the rifampicin was replaced by ciprofloxacin. It was suggested that rifampicin (a potent non-specific enzyme inducer) increased the metabolism of clozapine, probably by the cytochrome P450 isoenzymes CYP1A2 and CYP3A, thereby reducing its levels.[1]

This appears to be an isolated case but it is consistent with the way rifampicin interacts with other drugs. Clozapine serum levels should be well monitored if rifampicin is added, being alert for the need to increase its dosage. An alternative (as in this case) is to use another antibacterial. However, note that there are reports of an interaction between 'clozapine and ciprofloxacin', (p.749).

1. Joos AAB, Frank UG, Kaschka WP. Pharmacokinetic interaction of clozapine and rifampicin in a forensic patient with an atypical mycobacterial infection. *J Clin Psychopharmacol* (1998) 18, 83–5.

Clozapine + Risperidone

The concurrent use of clozapine and risperidone can be effective and well tolerated but two isolated reports describe a rise in serum clozapine levels when risperidone was added and the development of atrial ectopics. Dystonia has been seen when clozapine was replaced by risperidone.

Clinical evidence

A man with a schizoaffective disorder taking clozapine started to take risperidone, firstly 500 micrograms twice daily, and then after a week 1 mg twice daily. Clinical improvement was seen and it was found that after 2 weeks his serum clozapine levels had risen by 74%, from 344 to 598 nanograms/mL, without any adverse effects.[1] The serum clozapine levels of another patient more than doubled when risperidone was given. No signs of clozapine toxicity were seen, but mild oculogyric crises were reported.[2] A schizophrenic patient taking clozapine and trihexyphenidyl who developed tachycardia of 120 bpm, which was controlled with propranolol, developed atrial ectopics when risperidone 1.5 mg daily was added. The ectopics stopped when the risperidone was withdrawn and started again when it was re-introduced. Clozapine plasma levels were normal throughout the duration of risperidone treatment.[3] Four patients have been described who developed dystonia after their treatment was changed from clozapine to risperidone.[4] A single case of agranulocytosis has been seen 6 weeks after risperidone was added to stable clozapine treatment. The patient needed 3 doses of G-CSF before the white cell count returned to normal.[5] Another case report describes neuroleptic malignant syndrome in a 20-year-old man within 2 days of clozapine being added to risperidone treatment. The drugs were stopped and he recovered over the following 10 days. He subsequently received clozapine alone without problem.[6]

Contrasting with these reports is a study in 12 schizophrenic patients, which found that the addition of risperidone to clozapine was both effective and well tolerated, although 4 patients complained of mild akathisia. Serum clozapine levels were not significantly changed.[7] A retrospective study in 18 patients also found that risperidone did not alter clozapine serum levels.[8]

Mechanism, importance and management

The suggested reason for the raised clozapine levels is that both drugs compete for metabolism by the cytochrome P450 isoenzyme CYP2D6 resulting in a reduction in the metabolism of the clozapine.[1,2] The dystonias are attributed to cholinergic rebound and ongoing dopamine blockade caused by a rapid switch of medication. The recommendation is that withdrawal of clozapine should be tapered and possibly that an antimuscarinic drug should be given.[4] The raised clozapine levels seem to be isolated cases and therefore of doubtful general significance.

1. Tyson SC, Devane LC, Risch SC. Pharmacokinetic interaction between risperidone and clozapine. *Am J Psychiatry* (1995) 152, 1401–2.
2. Koreen AR, Lieberman JA, Kronig M, Cooper TB. Cross-tapering clozapine and risperidone. *Am J Psychiatry* (1995) 152, 1690.
3. Chong SA, Tan CH, Lee HS. Atrial ectopics with clozapine-risperidone combination. *J Clin Psychopharmacol* (1997) 17, 130–1.
4. Simpson GM, Meyer JM. Dystonia while changing from clozapine to risperidone. *J Clin Psychopharmacol* (1996) 16, 260–1.
5. Godleski LS, Sernyak MJ. Agranulocytosis after addition of risperidone to clozapine treatment. *Am J Psychiatry* (1996) 153, 735–6.
6. Kontaxakis VP, Havaki-Kontaxaki BJ, Stamouli SS, Christodoulou GN. Toxic interaction between risperidone and clozapine: a case report. *Prog Neuropsychopharmacol Biol Psychiatry* (2002) 26, 407–9.
7. Henderson DC, Goff DC. Risperidone as an adjunct to clozapine therapy in chronic schizophrenics. *J Clin Psychiatry* (1996) 57, 395–7.
8. Raaska K, Raitasuo V, Neuvonen PJ. Therapeutic drug monitoring data: risperidone does not increase serum clozapine concentration. *Eur J Clin Pharmacol* (2002) 58, 587–91.

Clozapine + SSRIs

Fluoxetine, paroxetine, sertraline and possibly citalopram can raise serum clozapine levels. Escitalopram is predicted to interact similarly. Particularly large increases in clozapine levels can occur with fluvoxamine. Clozapine toxicity has been seen in some patients.

Clinical evidence

(a) Citalopram

Preliminary studies in 5 patients found that their mean plasma clozapine levels were unchanged by citalopram.[1] Another study in 8 patients found similar results.[2] However, a patient who was stable taking clozapine developed sedation, hypersalivation and confusion shortly after he started to take citalopram 40 mg daily. When total clozapine serum levels were measured they were found to be 1097 nanograms/mL. The citalopram dose was reduced to 20 mg daily, the symptoms resolved over the following 2 weeks, and the total clozapine level dropped to 792 nanograms/mL.[3]

(b) Fluoxetine

Several studies and case reports have found increased clozapine levels of 30 to 75%, and increased levels of the metabolite norclozapine of 34 to 52% after fluoxetine was added to established clozapine treatment.[4-6] In one case the levels of clozapine and norclozapine were raised over fivefold, accompanied by hypertension. Clozapine levels became subtherapeutic 2 weeks after fluoxetine was withdrawn, necessitating an increase in dosage.[7]

A patient who had been taking clozapine 500 mg and lorazepam 3 mg daily, developed myoclonic jerks of his whole body 79 days after fluoxetine 20 mg was added. These decreased over the next 2 days when the fluoxetine and lorazepam were stopped.[8] A case report describes a patient taking clozapine, who developed severe SSRI withdrawal within a day of stopping treatment with fluoxetine 40 mg daily, which had been taken for 4 months. The symptoms resolved when treatment with fluvoxamine was started. Although it was suggested that clozapine may have been involved in this effect[9] its role is unclear.

The death of a 44-year old patient who was taking clozapine and fluoxetine was felt to be due to an increase in clozapine levels caused by fluoxetine.[10]

In contrast, there are reports of successful use,[11] and no pharmacokinetic changes[12] when clozapine and fluoxetine were used together.

A case has also been reported of a patient with schizophrenia and depression, whose cognitive symptoms improved when he took clozapine and fluoxetine, but when treatment was changed to sertraline, this improvement was not sustained. The authors tentatively suggested that the fluoxetine elevated plasma clozapine levels by inhibition of CYP2D6, whereas this effect was not seen with sertraline as it is a much weaker inhibitor of this enzyme.[13] However, this explanation has been questioned, since the role of other drug metabolising enzymes was not considered.[14]

(c) Fluvoxamine

Up to tenfold elevations in plasma clozapine levels have been seen in several studies and case reports when clozapine was given with fluvoxamine.[15-25] These elevations occurred as early as 14 days after combined treatment was started,[25] but were often not associated with any significant adverse effects, even after treatment had continued for a year in one patient.[18] Another study, which compared 12 patients taking clozapine with 11 patients taking clozapine and fluvoxamine, found that in the combined treatment group, clozapine doses were about half those used when clozapine was given alone. A trend towards decreased granulocyte levels was also seen in the clozapine/fluvoxamine group, but not when clozapine was used alone.[26]

Another patient had extremely high plasma clozapine levels of up to 4160 micrograms/L as a result of taking fluvoxamine.[27]

Other cases have also demonstrated worsening psychosis[28] or extrapyramidal adverse effects[29] (including, rigidity, tremors and akathisia) and sedation within days of giving fluvoxamine with clozapine.

A study in 68 patients taking either clozapine alone or clozapine and fluvoxamine found a trend towards less weight increase after 12 weeks of treatment in the group of patients also taking fluvoxamine. Those patients taking clozapine alone were found to have significantly higher glucose and triglyceride levels.[30] Note that fluvoxamine treatment alone can result in weight loss.

(d) Paroxetine

The serum levels of clozapine and norclozapine rose by 57% and 50%, respectively, in 16 schizophrenic patients after they took an average of 31.2 mg of paroxetine daily. One patient taking clozapine 300 mg daily developed reversible cerebral intoxication when given paroxetine 40 mg daily.[5] Another patient with a delusional disorder developed an antimuscarinic syndrome with doubled serum clozapine levels within about 3 weeks of the addition of paroxetine.[31] A further study in 9 patients found that the serum levels of clozapine and norclozapine rose by 31% and 20%, respectively, when paroxetine 20 to 40 mg daily was given for 3 weeks. Two patients experienced mild and transient sedation 2 to 3 days after starting paroxetine. The rise in clozapine levels was not associated with an increase in efficacy and was well tolerated.[32] In contrast, a study in 14 patients taking clozapine 2.5 to 3 mg/kg daily found that the addition of paroxetine 20 mg daily had no effect on the serum levels of clozapine.[23] This, or similar work, has been published elsewhere.[33]

An increase in the plasma levels of clozapine, thought to be due to concurrent treatment with paroxetine, has been suggested as the causative factor in the development of a fatal venous thromboembolism in a 47-year-old woman.[34]

A fatal case of neuroleptic malignant syndrome which started to develop two days after the introduction of clozapine 25 mg daily to established treatment with paroxetine 20 mg daily has been reported. The patient had previously taken clozapine alone with no problem.[35]

(e) Sertraline

In 10 schizophrenic patients the serum levels of clozapine and norclozapine increased by 30% and 52%, respectively, when they started to take an average of 92.5 mg of sertraline daily.[5] Another patient taking clozapine 600 mg daily had a 40% reduction in total clozapine serum levels within one month of stopping sertraline 300 mg daily.[36]

The serum clozapine levels of a schizophrenic patient doubled within a month of adding sertraline 50 mg daily and her psychosis worsened. When the sertraline was stopped she improved and her serum clozapine levels fell once again.[28] In contrast, a study in 8 patients who were taking clozapine 200 to 400 mg daily and were also given sertraline 50 to 100 mg per day for 3 weeks, found no significant changes in the levels of clozapine and its major metabolites.[32]

A case report describes sudden cardiac death in a 26-year-old man, which the authors attributed to an interaction between clozapine and sertraline.[37] However, this interaction has been questioned as it is said that the patient had other risk factors that were more likely to have caused the fatality.[38]

Mechanism

The SSRIs (including **escitalopram**) are known to inhibit the cytochrome P450 isoenzyme CYP2D6 to a varying extent. Fluvoxamine is also a potent inhibitor of CYP1A2. Both of these isoenzymes are involved in the metabolism of clozapine, the most significant being CYP1A2, so their inhibition causes clozapine levels to rise. The levels of clozapine and norclozapine rise together, and so it has been suggested that the metabolic step inhibited is after the *N*-dealkylation step.[5]

Importance and management

These interactions are established. Concurrent use need not be avoided, but it would be prudent to monitor the outcome closely when any is used with clozapine because of the rises in serum clozapine and norclozapine levels that can occur, and because of the rare potential for deterioration in clinical status. Adjust the clozapine dosage as necessary. The authors of one study suggest particularly close monitoring if the daily clozapine dosage exceeds 300 mg or 3.5 mg/kg.[5] The interaction is greatest with fluvoxamine, so other SSRIs may be a more prudent choice, although close monitoring is still required.

1. Taylor D, Ellison Z, Ementon Shaw L, Wickham H, Murray R. Co-administration of citalopram and clozapine: effect on plasma clozapine levels. *Int Clin Psychopharmacol* (1998) 13, 19–21.
2. Avenoso A, Facciolà G, Scordo MG, Gitto C, Ferrante GD, Madia AG, Spina E. No effect of citalopram on plasma levels of clozapine, risperidone and their active metabolites in patients with chronic schizophrenia. *Clin Drug Invest* (1998) 16, 393–8.
3. Borba CP, Henderson DC. Citalopram and clozapine: potential drug interaction. *J Clin Psychiatry* (2000) 61, 301–2.
4. Centorrino F, Baldessarini RJ, Kando J, Frankenburg FR, Volpicelli SA, Puopolo PR, Flood JG. Serum concentrations of clozapine and its major metabolites: effects of cotreatment with fluoxetine or valproate. *Am J Psychiatry* (1994) 151, 123–5.
5. Centorrino F, Baldessarini RJ, Frankenburg FR, Kando J, Volpicelli SA, Flood JG. Serum levels of clozapine and norclozapine in patients treated with selective serotonin reuptake inhibitors. *Am J Psychiatry* (1996) 153, 820–2.
6. Spina E, Avenoso A, Facciolà G, Fabrazzo M, Monteleone P, Maj M, Perucca E, Caputi AP. Effect of fluoxetine on the plasma concentrations of clozapine and its major metabolites in patients with schizophrenia. *Int Clin Psychopharmacol* (1998) 13, 141–5.
7. Sloan D, O'Boyle J. Hypertension and increased serum clozapine associated with clozapine and fluoxetine in combination. *Ir J Psychol Med* (1977) 14, 149–51.
8. Kingsbury SJ, Puckett KM. Effects of fluoxetine on serum clozapine levels. *Am J Psychiatry* (1995) 152, 473–4.
9. Lu M-L, Lane H-Y, Chang W-H. Selective serotonin reuptake inhibitor syndrome: precipitated by concomitant clozapine? *J Clin Psychopharmacol* (1999) 19, 386–7.
10. Ferslew KE, Hagardorn AN, Harlan GC, McCormick WF. A fatal drug interaction between clozapine and fluoxetine. *J Forensic Sci* (1998) 43, 1082–5.
11. Cassady SL, Thaker GK. Addition of fluoxetine to clozapine. *Am J Psychiatry* (1992) 149, 1274.
12. Eggert AE, Crismon ML, Dorson PG. Lack of effect of fluoxetine on plasma clozapine concentrations. *J Clin Psychiatry* (1994) 55, 454–5.
13. Purdon SE, Snaterse M. Selective serotonin reuptake inhibitor modulation of clozapine effects on cognition in schizophrenia. *Can J Psychiatry* (1998) 43, 84–5.
14. Chong S-A, Remington G. Re: Sertraline-clozapine interaction. *Can J Psychiatry* (1998) 43, 856–7.
15. Hiemke C, Weigmann H, Müller H, Dahmen N, Wetzel H, Fuchs E. Elevated clozapine plasma levels after addition of fluvoxamine. *Abstr Soc Neurosci* (1993) 19, 382.
16. Weigmann H, Müller H, Dahmen N, Wetzel H, Hiemke C. Interactions of fluvoxamine with the metabolism of clozapine. *Pharmacopsychiatry* (1993) 26, 209.
17. Jerling M, Lindström L, Bondesson U, Bertilsson L. Fluvoxamine inhibition and carbamazepine induction of the metabolism of clozapine: evidence from a therapeutic drug monitoring service. *Ther Drug Monit* (1994) 16, 368–74.
18. Dumortier G, Lochu A, Colen de Melo P, Ghribi O, Roche Rabreau D, Degrassat K, Desce JM. Elevated clozapine plasma concentrations after fluvoxamine initiation. *Am J Psychiatry* (1996) 153, 738–9.
19. Olesen OV, Starup G, Linnet K. Alvorlig lægmiddelinteraktion mellem clozapin – Leponex og fluvoxamin – Fevarin. *Ugeskr Laeger* (1996) 158, 6931–2.
20. Dequardo JR, Roberts M. Elevated clozapine levels after fluvoxamine initiation. *Am J Psychiatry* (1996) 153, 840–1.
21. Koponen HJ, Leinonen E, Lepola U. Fluvoxamine increases the clozapine serum levels significantly. *Eur Neuropsychopharmacol* (1996) 6, 69–71.
22. Hiemke C, Weigmann H, Härtter S, Dahmen N, Wetzel H, Müller H. Elevated levels of clozapine in serum after addition of fluvoxamine. *J Clin Psychopharmacol* (1994) 14, 279–81.

23. Wetzel H, Anghelescu I, Szegedi A, Wiesner J, Weigmann H, Hörtter S, Hiemke C. Pharmacokinetic interactions of clozapine with selective serotonin reuptake inhibitors: differential effects of fluvoxamine and paroxetine in a prospective study. *J Clin Psychopharmacol* (1998) 18, 2–9.
24. Wang C-Y, Zhang Z-J, Li W-B, Zhai Y-M, Cai Z-J, Weng Y-Z, Zhu R-H, Zhao J-P, Zhou H-H. The differential effects of steady-state fluvoxamine on the pharmacokinetics of olanzapine and clozapine in healthy volunteers. *J Clin Pharmacol* (2004) 44, 785–92.
25. Lu M-L, Lane H-Y, Chen K-P, Jann MW, Su M-H, Chang W-H. Fluvoxamine reduces the clozapine dosage needed in refractory schizophrenic patients. *J Clin Psychiatry* (2000) 61, 594–9.
26. Hinze-Selch D, Deuschle M, Weber B, Heuser I, Pollmächer T. Effect of coadministration of clozapine and fluvoxamine versus clozapine monotherapy on blood cell counts, plasma levels of cytokines and body weight. *Psychopharmacology (Berl)* (2000) 149, 163–9.
27. Heeringa M, Beurskens R, Schouten W, Verduijn MM. Elevated plasma levels of clozapine after concomitant use of fluvoxamine. *Pharm World Sci* (1999) 21, 243–4.
28. Chong SA, Tan CH, Lee HS. Worsening of psychosis with clozapine and selective serotonin reuptake inhibitor combination: two case reports. *J Clin Psychopharmacol* (1997) 17, 68–9.
29. Kuo F-J, Lane H-Y, Chang W-H. Extrapyramidal symptoms after addition of fluvoxamine to clozapine. *J Clin Psychopharmacol* (1998) 18, 483–4.
30. Lu M-L, Lane H-S, Lin S-K, Chen K-P, Chang W-H. Adjunctive fluvoxamine inhibits clozapine-related weight gain and metabolic disturbances. *J Clin Psychiatry* (2004) 65, 766–71.
31. Joos AAB, König F, Frank UG, Kaschka WP, Mörike KE, Ewald R. Dose-dependent pharmacokinetic interaction of clozapine and paroxetine in an extensive metabolizer. *Pharmacopsychiatry* (1997) 30, 266–70.
32. Spina E, Avenoso A, Salemi M, Facciolá G, Scordo MG, Ancione M, Madia A. Plasma concentrations of clozapine and its major metabolites during combined treatment with paroxetine or sertraline. *Pharmacopsychiatry* (2000) 33, 213–17.
33. Anghelescu I, Szegedi A, Schlegel S, Weigmann H, Hiemke C, Wetzel H. Combination treatment with clozapine and paroxetine in schizophrenia: safety and tolerability data from a prospective open clinical trial. *Eur Neuropsychopharmacol* (1998) 8, 315–320.
34. Farah RE, Makhoul NM, Farah RE, Shai MD. Fatal venous thromboembolism associated with antipsychotic therapy. *Ann Pharmacother* (2004) 38, 1435–8.
35. Gambassi G, Capurso S, Tarsitani P, Liperito R, Bernabei R. Fatal neuroleptic malignant syndrome in a previously long-term user of clozapine following its reintroduction in combination with paroxetine. *Aging Clin Exp Res* (2006) 18, 266–70.
36. Pinniniti NR, De Leon J. Interaction of sertraline with clozapine. *J Clin Psychopharmacol* (1997) 17, 119.
37. Hoehns JD, Fouts MM, Kelly MW, Tu KB. Sudden cardiac death with clozapine and sertraline combination. *Ann Pharmacother* (2001) 35, 862–6.
38. Gillespie JA. Comment: sudden cardiac death with clozapine and sertraline combination. *Ann Pharmacother* (2001) 35, 1671.

Clozapine + Tobacco

Smoking tobacco appears to decrease clozapine levels, although not all studies have found an effect.

Clinical evidence, mechanism, importance and management

Tobacco smoking might be expected to lower serum clozapine levels because the smoke contains aromatic hydrocarbons that are potent inducers of the cytochrome P450 isoenzyme CYP1A2, but studies of this likely interaction have been equivocal. One group of workers found no differences in clozapine levels with smoking,[1] while another group found that smokers had lower clozapine levels.[2] In addition, a case report describes clozapine-induced seizures in a man when he gave up smoking, although no levels were available so the authors point out it is difficult to be sure that smoking cessation was the cause.[3] Two further case reports describe elevations in clozapine plasma levels when the patients stopped smoking abruptly.[4] A retrospective study found that the clozapine clearance was 86% higher in 9 smokers than in 3 non-smokers, although it should be noted that this study was not specifically looking at the effects of smoking.[5] A suggestion has been made that in a patient who started to smoke, a 1.5-fold increase in clozapine dose should be anticipated. Likewise, a patient who stops smoking may experience a 1.5-fold increase in clozapine levels within 2 to 4 weeks of stopping smoking. In all cases, dose adjustments should be guided by the clinical status of the patient, and clozapine levels where available.[6]

1. Hasegawa M, Gutierrez-Esteinou R, Way L, Meltzer HY. Relationship between clinical efficacy and clozapine concentrations in plasma in schizophrenia: effect of smoking. *J Clin Psychopharmacol* (1993) 13, 383–90.
2. Haring C, Meise U, Humpel C, Fleischhacker WW, Hinterhuber H. Dose-related plasma effects of clozapine: influence of smoking behaviour, sex and age. *Psychopharmacology (Berl)* (1989) 99, S38–S40.
3. McCarthy RH. Seizures following smoking cessation in a clozapine responder. *Pharmacopsychiatry* (1994) 27, 210–11.
4. Bondolfi G, Morel F, Crettol S, Rachid F, Baumann P, Eap CB. Increased clozapine plasma concentrations and side effects induced by smoking cessation in 2 *CYP1A2* genotyped patients. *Ther Drug Monit* (2005) 27, 539–43.
5. Mookhoek EJ, Loonen AJM. Retrospective evaluation of the effect of omeprazole on clozapine metabolism. *Pharm World Sci* (2004) 26, 180–2.
6. de Leon J. Atypical antipsychotic dosing: the effect of smoking and caffeine. *Psychiatr Serv* (2004) 55, 491–3.

Droperidol + MAOIs

An isolated report describes hypotension in a patient given droperidol shortly after the withdrawal of phenelzine.

Clinical evidence, mechanism, importance and management

Four days after the withdrawal of **phenelzine** and perphenazine, a patient was given operative premedication of droperidol 20 mg and hyoscine 400 micrograms, orally. About 2 hours later he was observed to be pale, sweating profusely and slightly cyanosed, with a blood pressure of 75/60 mmHg and a pulse rate of 60 bpm. He was not excitable, and no changes in respiration were seen. The blood pressure gradually rose to 115/80 mmHg over the next 45 minutes, but did not return to his normal level of 160/100 mmHg for 36 hours. The same premedication was given 11 days later without any adverse effects.[1] The response was attributed to the residual effects of **phenelzine** treatment. Its general significance is unclear.

1. Penlington GN. Droperidol and monoamine-oxidase inhibitors. *BMJ* (1966) 1, 483–4.

Fluphenazine + Ascorbic acid (Vitamin C)

A single case report describes a reduction in serum fluphenazine levels and signs of a reduction in its effects when a patient was also given ascorbic acid.

Clinical evidence, mechanism, importance and management

A man with a history of manic behaviour, taking fluphenazine 15 mg daily, had a 25% reduction in his plasma fluphenazine levels, from 0.93 to 0.705 nanograms/mL, over a 13-day period while taking ascorbic acid 500 mg twice daily. This was accompanied by a deterioration in his behaviour.[1] The reason for this effect is not understood. There seem to be no other reports of this interaction with fluphenazine or any other phenothiazine so that this interaction would not appear to be of general importance.

1. Dysken MW, Cumming RJ, Channon RA, Davis JM. Drug interaction between ascorbic acid and fluphenazine. *JAMA* (1979) 241, 2008.

Fluphenazine + Spiramycin

Acute dystonia occurred when a man taking fluphenazine was also given spiramycin.

Clinical evidence, mechanism, importance and management

A man with a schizoaffective disorder taking lorazepam, orphenadrine, fluvoxamine and fluphenazine decanoate 12.5 mg every 2 weeks, developed acute and painful dystonia of the trunk, neck, right arm and leg about one week after his last fluphenazine injection and on the fourth day of taking spiramycin 6 million units daily for gingivitis. The problem resolved when he was given biperiden.[1] The reasons for this adverse reaction are not understood, nor is it entirely clear whether this was an interaction between fluphenazine and spiramycin, although the author suggested that a causal link existed. This seems to be the only report of an alleged interaction between fluphenazine and a macrolide antibacterial and it is therefore of little or no general importance.

1. Benazzi F. Spiramycin-associated acute dystonia during neuroleptic treatment. *Can J Psychiatry* (1997) 42, 665–6.

Glutethimide + Tobacco

A study in 7 subjects found that glutethimide worsened psychomotor performance in smokers more than in non-smokers, possibly due to an increase in glutethimide absorption.[1] However there

would seem to be no need for particular caution if smokers take glutethimide.

1. Crow JW, Lain P, Bochner F, Shoeman DW, Azarnoff DL. Glutethimide and 4-OH glutethimide: pharmacokinetics and effect on performance in man. *Clin Pharmacol Ther* (1978) 22, 458–64.

Haloperidol + Alosetron

A placebo-controlled study in 10 patients taking haloperidol found that alosetron 1 mg daily given during weeks 2 and 3 of the 8-week study period caused no change in haloperidol pharmacokinetics.[1]

1. Gupta SK, Kunka RL, Metz A, Lloyd T, Rudolph G, Perel JM. Effect of alosetron (a new 5-HT_3 receptor antagonist) on the pharmacokinetics of haloperidol in schizophrenic patients. *J Clin Pharmacol* (1995) 35, 202–7.

Haloperidol + Antimycobacterials

The serum levels of haloperidol can be reduced by rifampicin (rifampin), and possibly raised by isoniazid.

Clinical evidence

A study in schizophrenic patients taking haloperidol, 7 of whom were also taking a range of antimycobacterial drugs (**ethambutol**, **isoniazid**, **rifampicin**), and 18 of whom were taking **isoniazid** only, showed that those receiving multiple drugs, which included **rifampicin** had significantly lower haloperidol serum levels. The half-life of haloperidol in 2 patients taking **rifampicin** was 4.9 hours compared with 9.4 hours in 3 other patients not taking **rifampicin**.[1] Three of the patients taking **isoniazid** (without rifampicin or ethambutol) had *increased* serum haloperidol levels.[1]

The trough serum haloperidol levels of 15 schizophrenics fell to 37.4% of the expected level after they took **rifampicin** 600 mg daily for 7 days.[2] After 28 days the serum level had dropped further to 30% of the expected level. In another group of 5 patients taking haloperidol and **rifampicin**, the serum haloperidol levels rose to 229% of the previous level 7 days after **rifampicin** was stopped, and to 329% 28 days after **rifampicin** was stopped.[2] The clinical effects of the haloperidol appeared to be reduced by the **rifampicin**.[2]

Mechanism

The likeliest explanation is that the rifampicin, a recognised enzyme inducer, increases the metabolism and loss of the haloperidol from the body.

Importance and management

The interaction between haloperidol and rifampicin would appear to be established and clinically important. Be alert for any evidence of reduced haloperidol effects if rifampicin alone is used, and possibly increased effects if isoniazid alone is used. Adjust the haloperidol dosage if necessary.

1. Takeda M, Nishinuma K, Yamashita S, Matsubayashi T, Tanino S, Nishimura T. Serum haloperidol levels of schizophrenics receiving treatment for tuberculosis. *Clin Neuropharmacol* (1986) 9, 386–97.
2. Kim Y-H, Cha I-J, Shim J-C, Shin J-G, Yoon Y-R, Kim Y-K, Kim J-I, Park G-H, Jang I-J, Woo J-I, Shin S-G. Effect of rifampin on the plasma concentration and the clinical effect of haloperidol concomitantly administered to schizophrenic patients. *J Clin Psychopharmacol* (1996) 16, 247–52.

Haloperidol + Buspirone

Two studies found that buspirone can cause a rise in plasma haloperidol levels, while another study found that no interaction occurred.

Clinical evidence, mechanism, importance and management

A pharmacokinetic study in 27 schizophrenic patients taking haloperidol 10 to 40 mg daily found that buspirone 5 mg three times daily for 2 weeks, followed by 10 mg three times daily for 4 weeks, did not significantly affect the steady-state plasma haloperidol levels.[1]

These findings contrast with those of a 6-week study, in which 6 out of 7 schizophrenics had 15 to 122% rises in their plasma haloperidol levels when they were given buspirone.[2] The authors also mention a single-dose study in healthy subjects, which found a 30% rise in haloperidol levels when subjects were given buspirone.[2]

It is not known why these findings differ, but since no adverse reactions have been reported, there would seem to be no reason for avoiding concurrent use. However, be aware that some patients seem to experience large rises in haloperidol levels, so consider this potential interaction if the effects of haloperidol seem excessive.

1. Huang HF, Jann MW, Wei F-C, Chang T-P, Chen J-S, Juang D-J, Lin S-K, Lam YFW, Chien C-P, Chang W-H. Lack of pharmacokinetic interaction between buspirone and haloperidol in patients with schizophrenia. *J Clin Pharmacol* (1996) 36, 963–9.
2. Goff DC, Midha KK, Brotman AW, McCormick S, Waites M, Amico ET. An open trial of buspirone added to neuroleptics in schizophrenic patients. *J Clin Psychopharmacol* (1991) 11, 193–7.

Haloperidol + Chlorpromazine

Some patients may show a large increase in haloperidol levels when they are given chlorpromazine.

Clinical evidence, mechanism, importance and management

Haloperidol was given to 43 patients in doses of 2 to 21 mg daily for 2 months, and then chlorpromazine 50 mg to 300 mg daily was added for a further 2 months. Haloperidol plasma levels were found to increase by an average of 28.5%, and levels of the metabolite, reduced haloperidol, were increased by 161%. However, the variation in effect was large. Chlorpromazine was thought to raise haloperidol levels by inhibiting haloperidol metabolism by the cytochrome P450 isoenzyme CYP2D6. The large inter-individual variation suggested that differences in cytochrome P450 genotypes may affect haloperidol metabolism,[1] and therefore some patients may be at risk of developing adverse effects related to high haloperidol levels.

1. Suzuki Y, Someya T, Shimoda K, Hirokane G, Morita S, Yokono A, Inoue Y, Takahashi S. Importance of the cytochrome P450 2D6 genotype for the drug metabolic interaction between chlorpromazine and haloperidol. *Ther Drug Monit* (2001) 23, 363–8.

Haloperidol + Dexamfetamine

Acute dystonia occurred in two healthy subjects when they were given haloperidol with dexamfetamine.

Clinical evidence, mechanism, importance and management

Two healthy young women were given haloperidol 5 mg and dexamfetamine 5 mg as part of a neuropharmacological study. After 29 hours one of them developed stiffness of neck and limbs, parkinsonian facies, her tongue protruded, and she had oropharyngeal spasm. After 34 hours the other woman developed an oculogyric crisis and acute dystonia of the neck with her back slightly arched. Both recovered rapidly after being given 10 mg of intramuscular procyclidine.[1]

The reasons for this interaction are not fully understood, but the authors of the study suggest that the acute dystonia was due to a potentiation of dopamine release. The clinical significance of this interaction is unclear.

1. Capstick C, Checkley S, Gray J, Dawe S. Dystonia induced by amphetamine and haloperidol. *Br J Psychiatry* (1994) 165, 276.

Haloperidol + Granisetron

Granisetron appears not to increase the adverse effects of haloperidol.

Clinical evidence, mechanism, importance and management

A study in 12 healthy subjects found that while haloperidol 3 mg alone caused some impaired psychometric performance (increased drowsiness, muzziness, lethargy, mental slowness, etc.), the addition of granisetron 160 micrograms/kg did not seem to make performance significantly worse.[1] If both drugs are used, no additional precautions would seem necessary.

1. Leigh TJ, Link CGG, Fell GL. Effects of granisetron and haloperidol, alone and in combination, on psychometric performance and the EEG. *Br J Clin Pharmacol* (1992) 34, 65–70.

Haloperidol + Grapefruit juice

Ingestion of 200 mL of regular-strength grapefruit juice three times a day for 7 days was found not to affect the pharmacokinetics of haloperidol in 12 schizophrenic patients receiving haloperidol 6 mg twice daily.[1]

1. Yasui N, Kondo T, Suzuki A, Otani K, Mihara K, Furukori H, Kaneko S, Inoue Y. Lack of significant pharmacokinetic interaction between haloperidol and grapefruit juice. *Int Clin Psychopharmacol* (1999) 14, 113–8.

Haloperidol + Imipenem

Marked but transient hypotension was seen when three patients receiving intravenous imipenem were given low dose intravenous haloperidol.

Clinical evidence, mechanism, importance and management

Three patients in intensive care who were being treated with intravenous imipenem 500 mg (with cilastatin) every 6 hours for 2, 3, and 7 days, respectively, developed a rapid and short-lived episode of hypotension when they were given a 2.5-mg dose of intravenous haloperidol. For example, the blood pressure of one of the patients fell from 117/75 mmHg to 91/49 mmHg. After 30 minutes her blood pressure had risen to 100/57 mmHg. No treatment for hypotension was given to any of the patients and the reaction was brief and self-limiting. Two of them were also taking famotidine and erythromycin. No acute ECG changes were seen.[1]

The reason for this fall in blood pressure is not understood, but the authors attribute what happened to the concurrent use of haloperidol and imipenem, although they point out that intravenous haloperidol alone can cause orthostatic hypotension. One suggestion is that competitive protein binding displacement might have transiently increased the levels of free haloperidol,[1] although this has been questioned, and a suggestion made that the clinical condition of the patients may have had a greater part to play in the development of hypotension than a drug-drug interaction.[2]

The authors advise that if haloperidol is used, low doses should be given, and the outcome well monitored. They say that no pressor agent was needed in these cases, but they suggest the possible use of metaraminol, phenylephrine or noradrenaline (norepinephrine) rather than dopamine, the vasopressor effects of which might be blocked or reversed by haloperidol.[1]

1. Franco-Bronson K, Gajwani P. Hypotension associated with intravenous haloperidol and imipenem. *J Clin Psychopharmacol* (1999) 19, 480–1.
2. Hauben M. Comments on "Hypotension associated with intravenous haloperidol and imipenem". *J Clin Psychopharmacol* (2001) 21, 345–7.

Haloperidol + Indometacin

Profound drowsiness and confusion have been described in patients given haloperidol with indometacin.

Clinical evidence, mechanism, importance and management

A crossover study in 20 patients, designed to find out the possible advantages of combining haloperidol 5 mg daily with indometacin 25 mg three times daily, was eventually abandoned because 13 patients (11 taking haloperidol and 2 taking placebo) failed to complete the study. Profound drowsiness or tiredness caused 6 of the haloperidol-treated patients to withdraw. The authors of this paper said that the combined treatment produced drowsiness and confusion greater than anything expected with haloperidol alone, and sufficiently severe that in some cases independent functioning was affected.[1]

Evidence of this interaction appears to be very limited. If concurrent use is thought appropriate, warn patients about this potentially severe effect. It might be wiser to avoid concurrent use because many patients requiring this type of treatment may not be hospitalised and under the day-to-day scrutiny of the prescriber.

1. Bird HA, Le Gallez P, Wright V. Drowsiness due to haloperidol/indomethacin in combination. *Lancet* (1983) i, 830–1.

Haloperidol and related drugs + Itraconazole

Itraconazole increases the plasma levels of haloperidol, and its metabolite, reduced haloperidol. Bromperidol may be similarly affected.

Clinical evidence

(a) Bromperidol

A study in 8 patients found that plasma levels of bromperidol 12 or 24 mg daily, were increased by itraconazole 200 mg daily for 7 days. The average increase was approximately 87%, but there was wide variation between patients, with some being unaffected and others having increases of up to 302%. Levels of the metabolite of bromperidol, reduced bromperidol, were similarly increased, by up to 415%.[1]

(b) Haloperidol

A study in 13 schizophrenic patients taking haloperidol 6 mg or 12 mg twice daily found an increase in the levels of haloperidol and its metabolite, reduced haloperidol, when itraconazole 200 mg daily was given for 7 days. Haloperidol levels increased by 30%, and levels of the metabolite, reduced haloperidol, were increased by 24%. There was also an increase in neurological adverse effects during itraconazole treatment.[2] In a randomised study 15 healthy subjects were given itraconazole 200 mg twice daily for 10 days with a single 5-mg dose of haloperidol on day 7. Itraconazole increased the AUC of haloperidol by 55% in the 8 subjects with normal CYP2D6 and by 81% in those with unstable CYP2D6. No significant changes in QT prolongation were seen.[3]

Mechanism, importance and management

It is likely that itraconazole inhibited the metabolism of bromperidol and haloperidol by CYP3A4. The wide variation in results may be attributed to interindividual variation in CYP3A4 activity.

The clinical significance of the raised levels is unclear, although one study found an increase in neurological adverse effects with haloperidol. It may be prudent to monitor concurrent use, decreasing the haloperidol or bromperidol dose if adverse effects become troublesome. This interaction may be of more importance in those patients have less active CYP2D6, the predominant isoenzyme involved in the metabolism of haloperidol, as CYP3A4, which is inhibited by itraconazole, will then become more important. It is likely that other azoles that are potent inhibitors of CYP3A4, such as ketoconazole, would interact similarly, but this needs confirmation.

1. Furukori H, Kondo T, Yasui N, Otani K, Tokinaga N, Nagashima U, Kaneko S, Inoue Y. Effects of itraconazole on the steady-state plasma concentrations of bromperidol and reduced bromperidol in schizophrenic patients. *Psychopharmacology (Berl)* (1999) 145, 189–92.
2. Yasui N, Kondo T, Otani K, Furukori H, Mihara K, Suzuki A, Kaneko S, Inoue Y. Effects of itraconazole on the steady-state plasma concentrations of haloperidol and its reduced metabolite in schizophrenic patients: in vivo evidence of the involvement of CYP3A4 for haloperidol metabolism. *J Clin Psychopharmacol* (1999) 19, 149–54.
3. Park J-Y, Shon J-H, Kim K-A, Jung H-J, Shim J-C, Yoon Y-R, Cha I-J, Shin J-G. Combined effects of itraconazole and CYP2D6*10 genetic polymorphism on the pharmacokinetics and pharmacodynamics of haloperidol in healthy subjects. *J Clin Psychopharmacol* (2006) 26, 135–42.

Haloperidol + Nefazodone

Nefazodone does not appear to significantly affect the pharmacokinetics of haloperidol.

Clinical evidence, mechanism, importance and management

After taking nefazodone 200 mg twice daily for about 7 days to achieve steady-state pharmacokinetics, the AUC of haloperidol 5 mg in 12 healthy subjects was found to be increased by 36% but the maximum plasma levels of haloperidol were unaltered. The pharmacokinetics of the nefazodone were unaltered.[1] It seems fairly unlikely that this change is enough to be of clinical relevance.

1. Barbhaiya RH, Shukla UA, Greene DS, Breuel H-P, Midha KK. Investigation of pharmacokinetic and pharmacodynamic interactions after coadministration of nefazodone and haloperidol. *J Clin Psychopharmacol* (1996) 16, 26–34.

Haloperidol + Quinidine

Haloperidol levels can be markedly increased by quinidine.

Clinical evidence, mechanism, importance and management

An experimental study in 13 healthy subjects found quinidine bisulfate 250 mg, taken about 1 hour before a single 5-mg dose of haloperidol approximately doubled the maximum plasma levels and the AUC of haloperidol. The reasons for this effect are not understood.[1] The clinical importance of this interaction has not been assessed, but it seems likely that the effects and adverse effects of haloperidol will be increased if quinidine is added. Be alert for this interaction if both drugs are given.

See also 'Drugs that prolong the QT interval + Other drugs that prolong the QT interval', p.257.

1. Young D, Midha KK, Fossler MJ, Hawes EM, Hubbard JW, McKay G, Korchinski ED. Effect of quinidine on the interconversion kinetics between haloperidol and reduced haloperidol in humans: implications for the involvement of cytochrome P450IID6. *Eur J Clin Pharmacol* (1993) 44, 433–8.

Haloperidol + Risperidone

A case report describes neuroleptic malignant syndrome in a patient taking risperidone and haloperidol.

Clinical evidence, mechanism, importance and management

A case report describes a 57-year-old man who had been taking haloperidol 4 mg three times daily uneventfully for several years. At a review, his treatment was changed to risperidone, in increasing doses to 3 g twice daily, and mirtazapine 15 mg at night. Despite being advised to stop haloperidol when he started risperidone, the patient continued to take haloperidol, and by the third day of concurrent use he had become pyrexial, and exhibited rigidity of his trunk and extremities. He was diagnosed as having the neuroleptic malignant syndrome, was given dantrolene, bromocriptine and lorazepam, and recovered over the next 2 months. The effects seen in this patient were thought to be due to the additive dopamine antagonism from both the haloperidol and risperidone. Mirtazapine may have also contributed, although the patient only took two doses before he was admitted. The authors suggest that if antipsychotic treatment is to be changed, it is advisable to slowly reduce the dose of the old antipsychotic and, simultaneously, slowly increase the dose of the new drug to avoid the risk of a psychotic relapse, and the patient should be closely monitored during this time for signs of neuroleptic malignant syndrome.[1]

1. Reeves RR, Mack JE, Torres RA. Neuroleptic malignant syndrome during a change from haloperidol to risperidone. *Ann Pharmacother* (2001) 35, 698–701.

Haloperidol + Venlafaxine

Venlafaxine can increase the serum levels of haloperidol. This is consistent with an isolated report, which describes a man who developed urinary retention when venlafaxine was added to a previously well-tolerated regimen of haloperidol and alprazolam.

Clinical evidence, mechanism, importance and management

A study in 24 healthy subjects found that steady-state venlafaxine 75 mg every 12 hours reduced the renal clearance of a single 2-mg dose of haloperidol by 42%, resulting in a 70% rise in the AUC and an 88% rise in its maximum serum levels.[1-3] This rise in haloperidol levels would seem to be consistent with an isolated report of a 75-year-old man taking haloperidol 1 mg and alprazolam 500 micrograms daily, who suddenly developed urinary retention when venlafaxine 37.5 mg daily was added. Urinary retention resolved spontaneously when all the drugs were stopped.[4]

It was suggested that venlafaxine inhibits the cytochrome P450 isoenzyme CYP2D6, which is concerned with the metabolism of haloperidol. As a result the serum levels of the haloperidol rise, thereby increasing its antimuscarinic effects,[4] which in this case resulted in urinary retention.

The evidence is very limited but be aware that increased haloperidol adverse effects may occur if venlafaxine is also given. It may be necessary to reduce the haloperidol dosage.

1. Efexor XL (Venlafaxine hydrochloride). Wyeth Pharmaceuticals. UK Summary of product characteristics, May 2006.
2. Wyeth, Personal communication, April 2001.
3. Effexor XR (Venlafaxine hydrochloride). Wyeth Pharmaceuticals Inc. US Prescribing information, June 2007.
4. Benazzi F. Urinary retention with venlafaxine-haloperidol combination. *Pharmacopsychiatry* (1997) 30, 27.

Olanzapine + Antiepileptics

Carbamazepine and valproate appear to lower olanzapine levels. The combination of olanzapine and valproate appears to increase the risk of hepatic injury in children. Olanzapine reduces lamotrigine levels and lamotrigine may increase olanzapine levels, although these changes are not expected to be clinically significant in the majority of patients. Oxcarbazepine dose not appear to affect the pharmacokinetics of olanzapine.

Clinical evidence, mechanism, importance and management

(a) Carbamazepine

Multiple-dose studies in healthy subjects have shown that carbamazepine increases the metabolism of olanzapine (by induction of the cytochrome P450 isoenzyme CYP1A2). The clearance of olanzapine was increased by 44% and its elimination half-life was reduced 20%, but these changes were not considered significant enough to necessitate dosage adjustments of either drug.[1] Another study found that 5 patients taking olanzapine and carbamazepine had a concentration/dose ratio 36% lower than 22 patients taking olanzapine alone.[2] A later study by the same authors found similar results, and also found that this increased olanzapine metabolism was probably due to an increase in glucuronidation, which was induced by the carbamazepine.[3]

A retrospective study identified 10 patients taking olanzapine and carbamazepine. The patients taking carbamazepine were taking olanzapine doses that were double those of subjects taking olanzapine alone. When corrected for dose it was found that the concentration/dose ratio of olanzapine was 71% lower in those also taking carbamazepine.[4] A 23 year-old woman required an olanzapine dose reduction from 15 mg daily to 10 mg daily to maintain similar serum olanzapine concentrations after discontinuing treatment with carbamazepine 600 mg per day.[5]

It would seem prudent to closely monitor the outcome of concurrent use and adjust the olanzapine dose as necessary.

(b) Lamotrigine

A study in 43 healthy subjects found that steady-state olanzapine pharmacokinetics were not affected by lamotrigine 200 mg daily. However, the AUC and maximum plasma concentrations of lamotrigine were reduced by 24% and 20%, respectively. Although this reduction was not considered to be clinically significant, interpatient variation indicated that some patients may require adjustment of their lamotrigine dose if olanzapine is started or discontinued.[6]

A further study in 14 healthy subjects given lamotrigine 50 mg daily, and a single 5-mg dose of olanzapine found no significant changes in the AUC and maximum plasma concentrations of lamotrigine when given with olanzapine, although the time to maximum plasma levels of lamotrigine was increased from 1.8 hours to 4.2 hours. This may be due to antimuscarinic effects of olanzapine slowing the gastrointestinal absorption of lamotrigine.[7] As only a single dose of olanzapine, and low doses of both drugs were used, the clinical significance of this finding is unclear.

A study in 14 patients taking olanzapine in doses of 10 mg to 20 mg daily, and who were also given lamotrigine in increasing doses over 8 weeks to 200 mg daily found no changes in the pharmacokinetics of olanzapine with a lamotrigine dose of 100 mg daily, but when the dose was increased to 200 mg daily, an increase of 16% in olanzapine plasma levels occurred. This increase would not be expected to have clinical significance.[8]

(c) Oxcarbazepine

A study in 13 patients taking olanzapine 5 to 20 mg daily found that the addition of oxcarbazepine for 5 weeks, at an initial dose of 300 mg daily increased to 900 mg to 1.2 g after one week, had no significant effects on the pharmacokinetics of olanzapine. Concurrent use was generally well tolerated.[9] No special consideration or monitoring therefore appears necessary with oxcarbazepine and olanzapine treatment.

(d) Valproate

A retrospective study identified 52 children (under 18 years old) who were treated with olanzapine alone (17), semisodium valproate alone (23) or both drugs together (12). At least one peak liver enzyme level (ALT, AST or lactate dehydrogenase) was found to be above the normal range in 59% of those taking olanzapine alone, 26% of those taking valproate alone, and 100% of patients receiving the combination. Liver enzymes were persistently elevated in 42% of the patients receiving combination treatment, and 2 of these patients had levels that were three times the upper limit of normal. Treatment was discontinued due to pancreatitis in one and steatohepatitis in the other. The authors recommend measuring liver enzymes every 3 to 4 months for the first year of treatment, thereafter monitoring every 6 months if no adverse effects are detected.[10]

A significant reduction in olanzapine plasma levels of between 32.3% and 78.8% was found in 4 patients who were additionally given valproate, thought to be due to the valproate inducing the enzymes involved in the metabolism of olanzapine.[11]

1. Zyprexa (Olanzapine). Eli Lilly. Clinical and Laboratory Experience A Comprehensive Monograph, August 1996.
2. Olesen OV, Linnet K. Olanzapine serum concentrations in psychiatric patients given standard doses: the influence of comedication. *Ther Drug Monit* (1999) 21, 87–90.
3. Linnet K, Olesen OV. Free and glucuronidated olanzapine serum concentrations in psychiatric patients: influence of carbamazepine comedication. *Ther Drug Monit* (2002) 24, 512–17.
4. Skogh E, Reis M, Dahl M-L, Lundmark J, Bengtsson F. Therapeutic drug monitoring data on olanzapine and its N-demethyl metabolite in the naturalistic clinical setting. *Ther Drug Monit* (2002) 24, 518–26.
5. Licht RW, Olesen OV, Friis P, Laustsen T. Olanzapine serum concentrations lowered by concomitant treatment with carbamazepine. *J Clin Psychopharmacol* (2000) 20, 110–12.
6. Sidhu J, Job S, Bullman J, Francis E, Abbott R, Ascher J, Theis JGW. Pharmacokinetics and tolerability of lamotrigine and olanzapine coadministered to healthy subjects. *Br J Clin Pharmacol* (2006) 61, 420–6.
7. Jann MW, Hon YY, Shamsi SA, Zheng J, Awad EA, Spratlin V. Lack of pharmacokinetic interaction between lamotrigine and olanzapine in healthy volunteers. *Pharmacotherapy* (2006) 26, 627–633.
8. Spina E, D'Arrigo C, Migliardi G, Santoro V, Muscatello MR, Micò U, D'Amico G, Perucca E. Effect of adjunctive lamotrigine treatment on the plasma concentrations of clozapine, risperidone and olanzapine in patients with schizophrenia or bipolar disorder. *Ther Drug Monit* (2006) 28, 599–602.
9. Muscatello MR, Pacetti M, Cacciola M, La Torre D, Zoccali R, D'Arrigo C, Migliardi G, Spina E. Plasma concentrations of risperidone and olanzapine during coadministration with oxcarbazepine. *Epilepsia* (2005) 46, 771–4.
10. Gonzalez-Heydrich J, Raches D, Wilens TE, Leichtner A, Mezzacappa E. Retrospective study of hepatic enzyme elevations in children treated with olanzapine, divalproex, and their combination. *J Am Acad Child Adolesc Psychiatry* (2003) 12, 1227–33.
11. Bergemann N, Kress KR, Abu-Tair F, Frick A, Kopitz J. Valproate lowers plasma concentrations of olanzapine. *Pharmacopsychiatry* (2005) 38, 44.

Olanzapine + Lithium

Several case reports suggest that some patients taking olanzapine and lithium may develop adverse reactions (neuroleptic malignant syndrome or serotonin syndrome, encephalopathy, priapism) without raised serum lithium levels. One study found no pharmacokinetic interaction between the drugs, but another analysis suggested that lithium may reduce olanzapine plasma levels.

Clinical evidence, mechanism, importance and management

A 16-year-old boy taking lithium 1.2 g daily with a therapeutic serum lithium level, developed neuroleptic malignant syndrome (generalised rigidity, urinary retention, fever, tachycardia) about 2 weeks after his olanzapine dose was increased from 10 to 20 mg daily. Both drugs were stopped, and the symptoms resolved over 8 days. He had previously taken olanzapine and lithium separately without problem.[1]

A 59-year-old man who had been diagnosed with encephalopathy and confusion while taking a combination of carbamazepine, haloperidol and lithium (therapeutic lithium level), developed similar symptoms when he was later given lithium with olanzapine.[2] Another elderly patient who had taken lithium for 7 years, developed severe delirium and extrapyramidal symptoms after the addition of olanzapine. Serum lithium levels were found to be 3 mmol/L.[3] The serotonin syndrome developed in a patient with bipolar affective disorder taking lithium and citalopram after olanzapine was also given. She became increasingly irritable 3 months after starting the combination and one month later (4 days after increasing the dose of olanzapine from 15 to 20 mg and stopping the citalopram) she became severely agitated, confused and was sweating profusely with hyperreflexia, tremor and a low-grade fever. The symptoms resolved on cessation of her medication.[4] Citalopram may have contributed to this reaction, as the serotonin syndrome has been reported with 'lithium and SSRIs', (p.1115).

A case of non-ketotic hyperosmolar syndrome has been reported in a non-diabetic patient taking olanzapine, lithium and valproic acid. Symptoms began only 5 days after the olanzapine was started.[5] Priapism, which was reversed by surgical detumescence, occurred when a 30-year-old man took olanzapine with lithium.[6]

In an open-label study, 12 healthy subjects took a single 32.4-mmol dose of lithium with olanzapine 10 mg, and after a washout period, olanzapine 10 mg daily for 8 days, with a single 32.4-mmol dose of lithium on the last day. No pharmacokinetic interactions were detected.[7] However, an analysis of olanzapine levels in schizophrenic patients found that concurrent lithium was associated with lower olanzapine plasma levels.[8]

The case reports detailed above suggest that some patients may develop a pharmacodynamic interaction. Concurrent use of lithium and olanzapine need not be avoided but be aware that there is some risk of developing adverse reactions to the combination. The presence of other serotonergic drugs (e.g. antidepressants such as SSRIs) or dopamine antagonists (e.g. antipsychotics such as haloperidol) is likely to increase the risk of an interaction.

1. Berry N, Pradhan S, Sagar R, Gupta SK. Neuroleptic malignant syndrome in an adolescent receiving olanzapine-lithium combination therapy. *Pharmacotherapy* (2003) 23, 255–9.
2. Swartz CM. Olanzapine-lithium encephalopathy. *Psychosomatics* (2001) 42, 370.
3. Tuglu C, Erdogan E, Abay E. Delirium and extrapyramidal symptoms due to a lithium-olanzapine combination therapy: a case report. *J Korean Med Sci* (2005) 20, 691–4.
4. Haslett CD, Kumar S. Can olanzapine be implicated in causing serotonin syndrome? *Psychiatry Clin Neurosci* (2002) 56, 533–5.
5. Chen PS, Yang YK, Yeh TL, Lo YC, Wang YT. Nonketotic hyperosmolar syndrome from olanzapine, lithium, and valproic acid cotreatment. *Ann Pharmacother* (2003) 37, 919–20.
6. Jagadheesan K, Thakur A, Akhtar S. Irreversible priapism during olanzapine and lithium therapy. *Aust N Z J Psychiatry* (2004) 38, 381.
7. Demolle D, Onkelinx C, Müller-Oerlinghausen B. Interaction between olanzapine and lithium in healthy male volunteers. *Therapie* (1995) 50 (Suppl), 486.
8. Bergemann N, Frick A, Parzer P, Kopitz J. Olanzapine plasma concentration, average daily dose, and interaction with co-medication in schizophrenic patients. *Pharmacopsychiatry* (2004) 37, 63–8.

Olanzapine + Miscellaneous

Activated charcoal causes a fall in olanzapine levels and venlafaxine moderately raise olanzapine levels. Additive dopaminergic effects have been seen in one patient taking olanzapine and haloperidol. Olanzapine appears not to interact to a clinically relevant extent with aluminium/magnesium hydroxide antacids, cimetidine or diazepam. However, excessive sedation and hypotension may occur with parenteral benzodiazepines and intramuscular olanzapine.

Clinical evidence, mechanism, importance and management

(a) Antacids

The manufacturers of olanzapine say that single doses of an **aluminium/magnesium-containing antacid** had no effect on the pharmacokinetics of olanzapine.[1] No special precautions would seem to be needed during concurrent use.

(b) Benzodiazepines

In vivo studies have found that no pharmacokinetic interaction occurs between olanzapine and **diazepam**.[1] This confirms *in vitro* studies using human liver microsomes,[1] which demonstrated that olanzapine did not inhibit the cytochrome P450 isoenzymes CYP3A4 or CYP2C19, which are concerned with the metabolism of **diazepam**. It was noted that mild increases in heart rate, sedation and dry mouth were seen in patients taking both drugs, but no dosage adjustments were thought to be necessary.[2] There would therefore appear to be no reason for avoiding concurrent use.

Intramuscular **lorazepam** 2 mg, given 1 hour after intramuscular olanzapine 5 mg increased the drowsiness seen with either drug alone. The pharmacokinetics of both drugs were not affected.[3,4] One case report describes hypotension occurring following the intramuscular use of a single 2-mg dose of **lorazepam** to a patient receiving treatment with intramuscular olanzapine 10 mg, the most recent dose being given 30 minutes before the **lorazepam**. His blood pressure dropped from 124/74 to 66/30 mm Hg; 12 hours later his blood pressure had returned to normal.[5] Intramuscular olanzapine has been associated with hypotension, bradycardia, respiratory depression, and rarely death, particularly in patients who have also received benzodiazepines. The manufacturers therefore say that concurrent use is not recommended. If both drugs are needed, parenteral benzodiazepines should not be given for 1 hour after intramuscular olanzapine. If a parenteral benzodiazepine has already been given, intramuscular olanzapine should only be given with careful consideration and monitoring of sedation and respiration.[4]

(c) Charcoal, activated

The manufacturers report that activated charcoal reduces the bioavailability of oral olanzapine by 50 to 60%,[1,3] and recommend that administration be separated by 2 hours.[1]

(d) Cimetidine

The manufacturers say that cimetidine has no effect on the bioavailability of olanzapine.[3] No special precautions would seem to be needed during concurrent use.

(e) Haloperidol

A 67-year-old man with a long history of bipolar disorder was taking haloperidol 10 mg daily, with valproate and benzatropine. Because he had previously had parkinsonian symptoms, olanzapine was started, to be increased as the haloperidol was decreased. On day 6 his parkinsonian symptoms became particularly marked. The haloperidol was stopped and 2 days later the symptoms had resolved. It is thought that either the small amount of dopaminergic activity of olanzapine combined with that of the haloperidol brought on these symptoms, or that olanzapine affected the metabolism of haloperidol, caused increased levels and therefore greater dopaminergic activity.[6] The significance of this interaction is not clear, but it would be wise to be aware of this interaction if both drugs are used.

(f) Venlafaxine

A retrospective study found that venlafaxine caused a 27% increase in olanzapine plasma levels. The clinical significance of this finding is unclear.[7]

1. Zyprexa (Olanzapine). Eli Lilly and Company Ltd. UK Summary of product characteristics, September 2006.
2. Zyprexa (Olanzapine). Eli Lilly. Clinical and Laboratory Experience A Comprehensive Monograph. August 1996.
3. Zyprexa (Olanzapine). Eli Lilly and Company. US Prescribing information, November 2006.
4. Zyprexa Powder for Solution for Injection (Olanzapine). Eli Lilly and Company Ltd. UK Summary of product characteristics, September 2006.
5. Zacher JL, Roche-Desilets J. Hypotension secondary to the combination of intramuscular olanzapine and intramuscular lorazepam. *J Clin Psychiatry* (2005) 66, 1614–15.
6. Gomberg RF. Interaction between olanzapine and haloperidol. *J Clin Psychopharmacol* (1999) 19, 272–3.
7. Gex-Fabry M, Balant-Gorgia AE, Balant LP. Therapeutic drug monitoring of olanzapine: the combined effect of age, gender, smoking, and comedication. *Ther Drug Monit* (2003) 25, 46–53.

Olanzapine + Probenecid

Probenecid may increase the AUC and maximum plasma levels of olanzapine, but the clinical significance of this finding is unclear.

Clinical evidence, mechanism, importance and management

Twelve healthy subjects were given a single 5-mg dose of olanzapine alone, or on day 2 of a 4 day course of probenecid 500 mg twice daily. The AUC and maximum plasma levels of olanzapine were significantly increased by about 20%, but overall bioavailability was not affected. The probenecid is thought to have caused these small effects by reducing the glucuronidation of olanzapine.[1] As this was a single dose study, the clinical implications of this interaction when olanzapine is taken regularly, are unclear, but probably small

1. Markowitz JS, DeVane CL, Liston HL, Bouton DW, Risch SC. The effects of probenecid on the disposition of risperidone and olanzapine in healthy volunteers. *Clin Pharmacol Ther* (2002) 71, 30–8.

Olanzapine + Quinolones

The olanzapine levels of a patient were reduced when ciprofloxacin was stopped.

Clinical evidence, mechanism, importance and management

The olanzapine levels of a patient were rapidly reduced, by more than 50%, when ciprofloxacin 250 mg twice daily was stopped. On the day of the last dose of a 7 day course of ciprofloxacin her olanzapine plasma level was 32.6 nanograms/mL, but within 3 days it had fallen to 14.6 nanograms/mL. It is thought that elevated levels occurred because ciprofloxacin inhibits the cytochrome P450 isoenzyme CYP1A2, which is involved in the metabolism of olanzapine.[1] The UK manufacturers of olanzapine recommend that a lower dose of olanzapine should be given to patients taking ciprofloxacin.[2] Note that other quinolones can inhibit CYP1A2 to varying degrees (for an example see 'Theophylline + Quinolones', p.1192) and may therefore be expected to interact similarly.

1. Markowitz JS, DeVane CL. Suspected ciprofloxacin inhibition of olanzapine resulting in increased plasma concentration. *J Clin Psychopharmacol* (1999) 19, 289–90.
2. Zyprexa (Olanzapine). Eli Lilly and Company Ltd. UK Summary of product characteristics, September 2006.

Olanzapine + Ritonavir

Ritonavir almost halves olanzapine levels.

Clinical evidence, mechanism, importance and management

A single 10-mg dose of olanzapine was given to 14 healthy, non-smoking subjects after they had taken ritonavir for 11 days (initially 300 mg twice daily, escalating to 500 mg twice daily). Ritonavir decreased the AUC and maximum plasma levels of olanzapine by 53% and 40%, respectively, and reduced the half-life from 32 to 16 hours.[1]

The authors suggest that ritonavir increased the metabolism of olanzapine by inducing the cytochrome P450 isoenzyme CYP1A2, which is the main metabolic route of olanzapine. They also suggest that increased glucuronidation, mediated by glucuronyltransferases induced by ritonavir, may have contributed.

It seems likely that increased olanzapine doses may be needed in the presence of ritonavir. If concurrent use is necessary monitor for olanzapine efficacy and increase the dose if necessary.

1. Penzak SR, Hon YY, Lawhorn WD, Shirley KL, Spratlin V, Jann MW. Influence of ritonavir on olanzapine pharmacokinetics in healthy volunteers. *J Clin Psychopharmacol* (2002) 22, 366–70.

Olanzapine + SSRIs

Fluvoxamine causes a rise in serum olanzapine levels, which is associated with increased adverse effects. Fluoxetine, paroxetine and sertraline appear to moderately raise olanzapine levels while citalopram appears to have no effect. A case of retarded ejaculation has been seen in one patient taking olanzapine and paroxetine, and the serotonin syndrome has been reported in patients taking citalopram or fluoxetine with olanzapine.

Clinical evidence, mechanism, importance and management

(a) Fluvoxamine

In a placebo-controlled study, fluvoxamine 50 to 100 mg daily was given to 10 male smokers daily for 11 days, with olanzapine 2.5 to 7.5 mg daily on days 4 to 11. During the initial 4 days of concurrent use somnolence was increased by 19 to 115%, when compared to the group taking olanzapine and placebo, but the subjects accommodated to this over the next 4 days. Fluvoxamine increased the olanzapine maximum plasma levels and AUC by 84% and 119%, respectively, and the olanzapine clearance fell by 50%.[1] A retrospective study found that in patients taking fluvoxamine and olanzapine the concentration/dose ratio was 2.3-fold higher than those taking olanzapine alone.[2] In another study 10 schizophrenic patients were given fluvoxamine 50 mg daily from days 1 to 14 followed by fluvoxamine 100 mg daily from days 15 to 28. A single 10-mg dose of olanzapine was given on day 10 and again on day 24. The maximum plasma levels of olanzapine were raised by 12% and 64% and the clearance was reduced by about 25% and 35%, by 50 and 100 mg of fluvoxamine, respectively. Increased sedation was also seen, which was more frequent with fluvoxamine 100 mg daily.[3] Other studies have found 50 to 81% increases in olanzapine levels with fluvoxamine 100 mg daily, which took up to 8 weeks to occur. There was a marked variation between individuals in the extent of the interaction.[4-6] In one study, plasma levels of olanzapine were maintained when the dose of olanzapine was reduced by an average of 4.5 mg daily following the addition of fluvoxamine 25 mg daily.[7]

The olanzapine plasma levels of a 21-year-old woman were 6 times the recommended upper limit while she was taking fluvoxamine. During this time she developed rigidity and tremor. After the olanzapine dose was reduced from 15 mg to 5 mg daily the levels were still almost double the recommended level.[8]

(b) Other SSRIs

The manufacturers say that **fluoxetine** 60 mg daily for 8 days caused an increase of 16% in olanzapine maximum serum levels and a 16% decrease in clearance. These differences were considered to be too small to necessitate dosage adjustments.[9] Similar results were found in a published study.[10] A case report describes a patient who had been taking **fluoxetine** 80 mg daily for several weeks with no adverse effects who developed the serotonin syndrome within 3 weeks of starting to take olanzapine 5 mg daily. His symptoms resolved after discontinuing the **fluoxetine**, and he was later able to tolerate a 20 mg daily dose of **fluoxetine** and olanzapine with no further adverse effects.[11] The serotonin syndrome has also been reported in a patient taking olanzapine, **citalopram** and lithium, see 'Olanzapine + Lithium', p.756.

A patient taking fluvoxamine had olanzapine levels double the upper recommended limit; when **paroxetine** was substituted for fluvoxamine the olanzapine levels became almost normal.[8] Another patient taking **paroxetine** developed retarded ejaculation 2 months after he started to take olanzapine 15 mg daily. This adverse effect resolved when the olanzapine was given in divided doses.[12]

A retrospective study found that **sertraline** had no effect on the concentration/dose ratio of olanzapine, suggesting that it does not interact.[2]

Another study found that **paroxetine**, **fluoxetine** and **sertraline** increased olanzapine levels by about 32%, but **citalopram** had no effect.[6]

Mechanism

Fluvoxamine inhibits the cytochrome P450 isoenzyme CYP1A2, which is the major isoenzyme involved in the metabolism of olanzapine,[1] resulting in increased olanzapine levels and adverse effects. All SSRIs affect CYP2D6 (to differing extents). This isoenzyme has a minor role in olanzapine metabolism, and therefore SSRIs other than fluvoxamine have only a small effect on olanzapine levels.

Importance and management

The manufacturers of olanzapine suggest that lower olanzapine doses may be needed if fluvoxamine is given.[9,13] Monitor for fluvoxamine adverse effects. Other SSRIs appear not to interact significantly, although the case report with paroxetine suggests that additive adverse effects are a possibility.

1. Mäenpää J, Wrighton S, Bergstrom R, Cerimele B, Tatum D, Hatcher B, Callaghan JT. Pharmacokinetic (PK) and pharmacodynamic (PD) interactions between fluvoxamine and olanzapine. *Clin Pharmacol Ther* (1997) 61, 225.
2. Weigmann H, Gerek S, Zeisig A, Müller M, Härtter S, Heimke C. Fluvoxamine but not sertraline inhibits the metabolism of olanzapine: evidence from a therapeutic drug monitoring service. *Ther Drug Monit* (2001) 23, 410–13.
3. Chiu C-C, Lane H-Y, Huang M-C, Liu H-C, Jann MW, Hon Y-Y, Chang W-H, Lu M-L. Dose-dependent alterations in the pharmacokinetics of olanzapine during coadministration of fluvoxamine in patients with schizophrenia. *J Clin Pharmacol* (2004) 44, 1385–90.
4. Wang C-Y, Zhang Z-J, Li W-B, Zhai Y-M, Cai Z-J, Weng Y-Z, Zhu R-H, Zhao J-P, Zhou H-H. The differential effects of steady-state fluvoxamine on the pharmacokinetics of olanzapine and clozapine in healthy volunteers. *J Clin Pharmacol* (2004) 44, 785–92.
5. Hiemke C, Peled A, Jabarin M, Hadjez J, Weigmann H, Härtter S, Ilan M, Ritsner M, Silver H. Fluvoxamine augmentation of olanzapine in chronic schizophrenia: pharmacokinetic interactions and clinical effects. *J Clin Psychopharmacol* (2002) 22, 502–6.
6. Gex-Fabry M, Balant-Gorgia AE, Balant LP. Therapeutic drug monitoring of olanzapine: the combined effect of age, gender, smoking, and comedication. *Ther Drug Monit* (2003) 25, 46–53.
7. Albers LJ, Ozdemir V, Marder SR, Raggi MA, Aravagiri M. Endrenyi L. Reist C. Low-dose fluvoxamine as an adjunct to reduce olanzapine therapeutic dose requirements. A prospective dose-adjusted drug interaction strategy. *J Clin Psychopharmacol* (2005) 25, 170–4.
8. de Jong J, Hoogenboom B, van Troostwijk LD, de Haan L. Interaction of olanzapine with fluvoxamine. *Psychopharmacology (Berl)* (2001) 155, 219–20.
9. Zyprexa (Olanzapine). Eli Lilly and Company. US Prescribing information, November 2006.
10. Gossen D, de Suray J-M, Vandenhende F, Onkelinx C, Gangji D. Influence of fluoxetine on olanzapine pharmacokinetics. *AAPS PharmSci* (2002) 4, E11.
11. Chopra P, Ng C, Schweitzer I. Serotonin syndrome associated with fluoxetine and olanzapine. *World J Biol Psychiatry* (2004) 5, 114–15.
12. Bizouard P, Vandel S, Kantelip JP. Olanzapine-induced retarded ejaculation: role of paroxetine comedication? A case report. *Therapie* (2001) 56, 443–5.
13. Zyprexa (Olanzapine). Eli Lilly and Company Ltd. UK Summary of product characteristics, September 2006.

Olanzapine + Tobacco

Smoking tobacco increases the clearance of olanzapine.

Clinical evidence, mechanism, importance and management

A retrospective study found that cigarette smoking reduced olanzapine levels,[1-3] in one study by 12%[1] and by about 50% in another,[3] and that smokers needed higher doses of olanzapine than non-smokers (10 mg compared with 12.5 mg) yet had lower olanzapine levels (60 nanomol/L compared with 92 nanomol/L).[4]

A study in 17 psychiatric patients found that the olanzapine concentration dose ratio was directly related to CYP1A2 activity: both CYP1A2 activity and olanzapine levels were sixfold higher in smokers than non-smokers.[5] A case report describes a patient who was successfully treated with olanzapine 15 mg daily whilst in hospital and smoking up to 12 cigarettes a day. However, on discharge his cigarette consumption increased to 80 per day, and his schizophrenic symptoms worsened. Olanzapine plasma levels reduced from 52 nanograms/mL to 30 nanograms/mL as his cigarette consumption increased to 80 per day.[6]

The manufacturers say that smokers have a 40% greater clearance of olanzapine than non-smokers.[7] The consequences are that the effects of olanzapine will be reduced to some extent by smoking. The manufacturers say that dosage adjustments are not routinely recommended in smokers because of the overall variability in dosing between individuals.[7,8]

1. Gex-Fabry M, Balant-Gorgia AE, Balant LP. Therapeutic drug monitoring of olanzapine: the combined effect of age, gender, smoking, and comedication. *Ther Drug Monit* (2003) 25, 46–53.
2. Theisen FM, Haberhausen M, Schulz E, Fleischhaker C, Clement H-W, Heinzel-Gutenbrunner M, Remschmidt H. Serum levels of olanzapine and its N-desmethyl and 2-hydroxymethyl metabolites in child and adolescent psychiatric disorders: effects of dose, diagnosis, age, sex, smoking, and comedication. *Ther Drug Monit* (2006) 28, 750–9.
3. Haslemo T, Eikeseth PH, Tanum L, Molden E, Refsum H. The effect of variable cigarette consumption on the interaction with clozapine and olanzapine. *Eur J Clin Pharmacol* (2006) 62, 1049–53.
4. Skogh E, Reis M, Dahl M-L, Lundmark J, Bengtsson F. Therapeutic drug monitoring data on olanzapine and its N-demethyl metabolite in the naturalistic clinical setting. *Ther Drug Monit* (2002) 24, 518–26.
5. Carillo JA, Herráiz AG, Ramos SI, Gervasini G, Vizcaíno S, Benítez J. Role of the smoking-induced cytochrome P450 (CYP)1A2 and polymorphic CYP2D6 in steady-state concentration of olanzapine. *J Clin Psychopharmacol* (2003) 23, 119–27.
6. Chiu C-C, Lu M-L, Huang M-C, Chen K-P. Heavy smoking, reduced olanzapine levels, and treatment effects. A case report. *Ther Drug Monit* (2004) 26, 579–81.
7. Zyprexa (Olanzapine). Eli Lilly and Company. US Prescribing information, November 2006.
8. Zyprexa (Olanzapine). Eli Lilly and Company Ltd. UK Summary of product characteristics, September 2006.

Olanzapine + Tricyclic and related antidepressants

No pharmacokinetic interaction occurs between imipramine or mirtazapine and olanzapine, but the additive effects of clomipramine and olanzapine was thought to have caused a seizure in one patient.

Clinical evidence, mechanism, importance and management

(a) Mirtazapine

In a study in 7 patients, mirtazapine 30 mg daily did not significantly affect the pharmacokinetics of olanzapine, taken in doses ranging from 10 to 20 mg daily.[1]

(b) Tricyclic antidepressants

A randomised, crossover study in 9 healthy men given single doses of olanzapine 5 mg and **imipramine** 75 mg found no clinically relevant pharmacokinetic or pharmacodynamic interactions between the two drugs.[2] This would seem to confirm *in vitro* studies using human liver microsomes,[3] which demonstrated that olanzapine causes minimal inhibition of the cytochrome P450 isoenzyme CYP2D6, an enzyme involved in the metabolism of the tricyclic antidepressants. However, one case report describes seizures, thought to be caused by the additive effects of olanzapine and **clomipramine**. Neither drug alone had produced this reaction in the patient.[4] No special precautions would seem to be necessary if both drugs are used concurrently, but be aware that they both have the potential to lower the seizure threshold and that the effect may be additive.

1. Zoccali R, Muscatello MR, La Torre D, Malara G, Canale A, Crucitti D, D'Arrigo C, Spina E. Lack of a pharmacokinetic interaction between mirtazapine and the newer antipsychotics clozapine, risperidone and olanzapine in patients with chronic schizophrenia. *Pharm Res* (2003) 48, 411–14.
2. Callaghan JT, Cerimele BJ, Kassahun KJ, Nyhart EH, Hoyes-Beehler PJ, Kondraske GV. Olanzapine: interaction study with imipramine. *J Clin Pharmacol* (1997) 37, 971–8.
3. Zyprexa (Olanzapine). Eli Lilly and Company Ltd. UK Summary of product characteristics, September 2006.
4. Deshauer D, Albuquerque J, Alda M, Grof P. Seizures caused by possible interaction between olanzapine and clomipramine. *J Clin Psychopharmacol* (2000) 20, 283–4.

Perospirone + Miscellaneous

Carbamazepine reduces, and itraconazole increases, perospirone levels.

Clinical evidence, mechanism, importance and management

(a) Carbamazepine

Carbamazepine reduced the plasma levels of a single 8-mg dose of perospirone to below the detection limit.[1] This is likely to be as a result of carbamazepine-induced induction of perospirone metabolism by CYP3A4.

(b) Itraconazole

Administration of itraconazole 200 mg daily for 5 days, with a single 8-mg dose of perospirone given on day 6 resulted in a 6-fold increase in perospirone maximum plasma levels. A similar increase in the AUC and the half-life of perospirone was also seen.[2] As itraconazole is a potent inhibitor of CYP3A4, the increase in levels is likely to be due to inhibition of metabolism of perospirone.

1. Masui T, Kusumi I, Takahashi Y, Koyama T. Effect of carbamazepine on the single oral dose pharmacokinetics of perospirone and its active metabolite. *Prog Neuropsychopharmacol Biol Psychiatry* (2006) 30, 1330–3.
2. Masui T, Kusumi I, Takahashi Y, Koyama T. Effects of itraconazole and tandospirone on the pharmacokinetics of perospirone. *Ther Drug Monit* (2006) 28, 73–5.

Perphenazine + Disulfiram

A single case report describes a man taking perphenazine whose psychotic symptoms re-emerged when he started to take disulfiram.

Clinical evidence, mechanism, importance and management

A man taking perphenazine 8 mg twice daily developed marked psychosis soon after starting to take disulfiram 100 mg daily.[1] His serum perphenazine levels had fallen from a range of 2 to 3 nanomol/L to less than 1 nanomol/L. Doubling the dosage of perphenazine had little effect, and no substantial clinical improvement or rise in serum levels occurred until he was given intramuscular perphenazine enantate 50 mg weekly, at which point the levels rose to about 4 nanomol/L. The results of clinical biochemical tests suggested that the disulfiram was acting as an enzyme inducer, resulting in increased metabolism and clearance of the perphenazine. However, disulfiram normally acts as an enzyme *inhibitor*. Too little is known to assess the general importance of this interaction, and there seems to be no information about an interaction with other phenothiazines.

1. Hansen LB, Larsen N-E. Metabolic interaction between perphenazine and disulfiram. *Lancet* (1982) ii, 1472.

Phenothiazines + Antimalarials

Chloroquine, amodiaquine and *Fansidar* (sulfadoxine/pyrimethamine) can markedly increase serum chlorpromazine levels.

Clinical evidence

A total of 15 schizophrenic patients (in three groups of five) taking **chlorpromazine** 400 or 500 mg daily for at least 2 weeks were given single doses of either **chloroquine sulphate** 400 mg, **amodiaquine hydrochloride** 600 mg or three tablets of *Fansidar* (**pyrimethamine** 25 mg with **sulfadoxine** 500 mg) one hour before the **chlorpromazine**. Serum **chlorpromazine** levels 3 hours later were found to be raised about threefold by the **chloroquine** and **amodiaquine**, and almost fourfold by the *Fansidar*. The plasma level of 7-hydroxychlorpromazine, one of the major metabolites of **chlorpromazine**, was also elevated, but not those of the other metabolite, chlorpromazine sulphoxide. The serum **chlorpromazine** levels of the patients given **chloroquine** or *Fansidar* were, to some extent, still elevated 4 days later. There was subjective evidence that the patients were more heavily sedated when given the antimalarials.[1]

Mechanism

Not understood. Both chloroquine and *Fansidar* have relatively long half-lives compared with amodiaquine, which may explain the persistence of their effects.

Importance and management

Direct information about this interaction seems to be limited to this study. Its clinical importance is uncertain but it seems possible that these antimalarials could cause chlorpromazine toxicity. Monitor the effects of concurrent use closely and anticipate the need to reduce the chlorpromazine dosage. More study is needed. See also 'Drugs that prolong the QT interval + Other drugs that prolong the QT interval', p.257. For mention that promethazine may increase chloroquine levels, see 'Chloroquine + Promethazine', p.223.

1. Makanjuola ROA, Dixon PAF, Oforah E. Effects of antimalarial agents on plasma levels of chlorpromazine and its metabolites in schizophrenic patients. *Trop Geogr Med* (1988) 40, 31–3.

Phenothiazines + Barbiturates

The levels of chlorpromazine, and possibly thioridazine, are decreased by phenobarbital. Phenothiazines also appear to reduce barbiturate levels. However, the clinical importance of these reductions is uncertain. Pentobarbital, promethazine and hyoscine in combination are said to increase the incidence of peri-operative agitation.

Clinical evidence

(a) Phenothiazine levels reduced

A study in 12 schizophrenic patients taking **chlorpromazine** 100 mg three times daily found that **phenobarbital** 50 mg three times daily reduced plasma **chlorpromazine** levels by 25 to 30%, which was accompanied by changes in certain physiological measurements, which clearly reflected a reduced response. The conclusion was made that there was no advantage to be gained by concurrent use.[1]

In another study in 7 patients, the plasma levels of **thioridazine** were reduced by **phenobarbital**, but the clinical effects of this were uncertain.[2] However, another study found that **phenobarbital** caused no changes in serum **thioridazine** levels, but the levels of its active metabolite (mesoridazine) were reduced.[3]

(b) Phenobarbital levels reduced

A study in epileptic patients found that their serum phenobarbital levels fell by 29% when they were given phenothiazines, which included **chlorpromazine**, **thioridazine** or **mesoridazine**, and increased when the phenothiazine was withdrawn.[4]

This study confirms another, in which **thioridazine** 100 to 200 mg daily was found to reduce serum phenobarbital levels by about 25%.[5] There is also some limited evidence that the concurrent use of pentobarbital, **promethazine** and hyoscine increases the incidence of pre-operative, peri-operative and postoperative agitation, and it has been suggested that this triple combination should be avoided.[6]

Mechanism

Uncertain. The barbiturates are potent liver enzyme inducers, and so it is presumed that they increase the metabolism of the phenothiazines by the liver.

Importance and management

These interactions appear to be established, but the documentation is limited. Their importance is uncertain, but be alert for evidence of reductions in response to both drugs if a phenothiazine and a barbiturate are given, and to increased responses if one of the drugs is withdrawn. So far only chlorpromazine, mesoridazine, phenobarbital and thioridazine are implicated, but it seems possible that other phenothiazines and barbiturates will behave similarly.

1. Loga S, Curry S, Lader M. Interactions of orphenadrine and phenobarbitone with chlorpromazine: plasma concentrations and effects in man. *Br J Clin Pharmacol* (1975) 2, 197–208.
2. Ellenor GL, Musa MN, Beuthin FC. Phenobarbital-thioridazine interaction in man. *Res Commun Chem Pathol Pharmacol* (1978) 21, 185–8.
3. Linnoila M, Viukari M, Vaisanen K, Auvinen J. Effect of anticonvulsants on plasma haloperidol and thioridazine levels. *Am J Psychiatry* (1980) 137, 819–21.
4. Haidukewych D, Rodin EA. Effect of phenothiazines on serum antiepileptic drug concentrations in psychiatric patients with seizure disorder. *Ther Drug Monit* (1985) 7, 401–4.
5. Gay PE, Madsen JA. Interaction between phenobarbital and thioridazine. *Neurology* (1983) 33, 1631–2.
6. Macris SG, Levy L. Preanesthetic medication: untoward effects of certain drug combinations. *Anesthesiology* (1965) 26, 256.

Phenothiazines + Hormonal contraceptives or HRT

Oestrogens can increase the plasma levels of butaperazine. A case report describes a marked rise in serum chlorpromazine levels in a woman taking a combined oral contraceptive.

Clinical evidence, mechanism, importance and management

A severe dystonic reaction to a single dose of **prochlorperazine** in a pregnant woman (presumed to be due to increased plasma levels resulting from high oestrogen levels), prompted further study. Four postmenopausal schizophrenic women. **Conjugated oestrogens** (*Premarin*) 1.25 mg daily increased the plasma **butaperazine** levels by 48% (from 231 to 343 nanograms/mL) and increased the AUC by 92%.[1]

A case report describes a woman who had been taking **chlorpromazine** 100 mg three times daily for one week without problems when a combined oral contraceptive (**ethinylestradiol/norgestrel**) was started. Four days later she developed severe dyskinesias and tremor, and her **chlorpromazine** levels were found to have increased by about sixfold.[2] This case was briefly mentioned in an earlier report by the same authors.[3]

The reasons are not understood but increased absorption or reduced liver metabolism of the phenothiazines are suggested.[1,2] The general clinical importance of these findings is not known, and documentation is very limited. There seem to be no other reports of adverse reactions, and the available data are insufficient to justify any general precautions. Further study is needed.

1. El-Yousef MK, Manier DH. Estrogen effects on phenothiazine derivative blood levels. *JAMA* (1974) 228, 827–8.
2. Chetty M, Miller R. Oral contraceptives increase the plasma concentrations of chlorpromazine. *Ther Drug Monit* (2001) 23, 556–8.
3. Chetty M, Miller R, Moodley SV. Smoking and body weight influence the clearance of chlorpromazine. *Eur J Clin Pharmacol* (1994) 46, 523–6.

Phenothiazines + Trazodone

Undesirable hypotension occurred in two patients taking chlorpromazine or trifluoperazine with trazodone. Thioridazine causes a moderate rise in trazodone plasma levels. A fatal case of jaundice and hepatic encephalopathy has been reported with the use of trifluoperazine, thioridazine and trazodone.

Clinical evidence, mechanism, importance and management

A depressed patient taking **chlorpromazine** began to complain of dizziness and unstable gait within 2 weeks of starting to take trazodone 100 mg one to three times daily. His blood pressure had fallen to between 92/58 and 126/72 mmHg. Within 2 days of stopping the trazodone his blood pressure had restabilised.[1] A patient taking **trifluoperazine** was given trazodone 100 mg daily and within 2 days she complained of dizziness and was found to have a blood pressure of 86/52 mmHg. Within one day of stopping the trazodone her blood pressure was back to 100/65 mmHg.[1] It would seem that the hypotensive adverse effects of the two drugs can be additive.

A study, undertaken to confirm the involvement of the cytochrome P450 isoenzyme CYP2D6 in the metabolism of trazodone, found that when 11 depressed patients were given trazodone 150 to 300 mg at bedtime for 18 weeks, and then with **thioridazine** 20 mg twice daily for one week, the plasma levels of the trazodone and its active metabolite, *m*-chlorophenylpiperazine, rose by 36% and 54%, respectively.[2] No adverse reactions were described. In contrast, a case of fatal hepatic necrosis with cholestasis has been attributed to the concurrent use of trazodone and phenothiazines. A 72-year-old woman taking trifluoperazine, trazodone and lithium carbonate developed an elevated alanine aminotransferase level. Trifluoperazine was replaced with **thioridazine**, but 9 weeks later she became jaundiced and developed hepatic encephalopathy, and died 6 weeks after the onset of jaundice. The authors consider that the combination of the phenothiazines and trazodone were the cause of her hepatic necrosis: both phenothiazines and trazodone have been reported to individually cause hepatic adverse effects.[3]

Patients given phenothiazines and trazodone should be monitored for signs of excessive hypotension and should have their liver function tests closely monitored.

1. Asayesh K. Combination of trazodone and phenothiazines: a possible additive hypotensive effect. *Can J Psychiatry* (1986) 31, 857–8.
2. Yasui N, Otani K, Kaneko S, Ohkubo T, Osanai T, Ishida M, Mihara K, Kondo T, Sugawara K, Fukushima Y. Inhibition of trazodone metabolism by thioridazine in humans. *Ther Drug Monit* (1995) 17, 333–5.
3. Hull M, Jones R, Bendall M. Fatal hepatic necrosis associated with trazodone and neuroleptic drugs. *BMJ* (1994) 309, 378.

Phenothiazines + Tricyclic antidepressants

The concurrent use of tricyclic antidepressants and phenothiazines is common, but the tricyclic levels are increased by many of the phenothiazines, and the levels of some phenothiazines are also increased by the tricyclics. It has been suggested that concurrent use might contribute to an increased incidence of tardive dyskinesia. Nevertheless, fixed-dose combined preparations are available. Tricyclics have also been shown to reverse the therapeutic effects of chlorpromazine.

Clinical evidence

(a) Effect of phenothiazines on tricyclic antidepressants

An extended study of 4 patients given intramuscular **fluphenazine decanoate** 12.5 mg weekly, with benzatropine 2 mg three times daily and **imipramine** 300 mg daily, found that the mean combined plasma concentrations of **imipramine** and its metabolite, desipramine, were 850 nanograms/mL. This appeared high, when compared with 60 other patients who were taking **imipramine** 225 mg daily and had levels of 180 nanograms/mL.[1]

A comparative study of 99 patients taking **amitriptyline** or **nortriptyline** alone, and 60 other patients also taking **perphenazine** 10 mg daily, found that although the tricyclic antidepressant dosages were the same, the plasma tricyclic antidepressant levels of the **perphenazine** group were up to 70% higher.[2]

Other studies have described increased tricyclic antidepressant levels with phenothiazines. There is currently evidence for this interaction between:

- **imipramine**,[3-5] and **chlorpromazine**
- **nortriptyline**,[6] and **levomepromazine**
- **amitriptyline**,[7] **imipramine**,[5,8,9] **desipramine**[10] or **nortriptyline**,[6,11-13] and **perphenazine**
- **desipramine**,[14] **imipramine**[15] or **nortriptyline**,[6] and **thioridazine**.

However, other studies have found no interaction between:

- **amitriptyline**[6,11,16] or **nortriptyline**,[17] and **perphenazine**
- **amitriptyline**[6] and **thioridazine**
- **amitriptyline**[6] and **levomepromazine**
- **amitriptyline**[11] or **nortriptyline**,[11] and **zuclopenthixol**.

It should be noted that in the case of **amitriptyline**, although the levels were not affected, levels of nortriptyline, its metabolite, were raised.[6]

(b) Effect of tricyclic antidepressant on phenothiazines

In a controlled study in 8 schizophrenic patients taking **butaperazine** 20 mg daily, 6 of them taking **desipramine** 150 mg or more daily had a rise in serum **butaperazine** levels of between 50 and 300%. The other

2 patients, taking **desipramine** 100 mg or less, had no changes in **butaperazine** levels.[18] Other studies have found a rise in phenothiazine levels when tricyclic antidepressants are added. So far, interactions with **chlorpromazine** and **amitriptyline**,[19] **imipramine**[19] or **nortriptyline**[20] have been documented.

One study in 7 chronic schizophrenics also reported that giving **nortriptyline** 50 mg three times daily to patients taking **chlorpromazine** 100 mg three times daily resulted in profound worsening of the clinical state, with marked increases in agitation and tension, despite the fact that the **chlorpromazine** levels were actually raised. The **nortriptyline** was withdrawn.[20] A temporary reversion to a disruptive behaviour pattern has been seen in other patients taking **chlorpromazine** when **amitriptyline** was given.[21] One patient experienced a severe catatonic reaction that was attributed to the use of **thioridazine** and **amitriptyline**,[22] and the case of a woman who became anxious with widely staring eyes, a persistent jerking of her head and at times the inability to speak was thought to be due to the use of **imipramine** and **chlorpromazine**.[23] Ventricular tachycardia has also been reported in a 38-year-old woman taking **desipramine** and **thioridazine**, which responded to treatment with lidocaine.[24]

Mechanism

The rise in the serum levels of both drugs is thought to be due to a mutual inhibition of the liver enzymes concerned with the metabolism of both drugs, which results in their accumulation.[3,4,8,18,20]

Importance and management

Established interactions, but the advantages and disadvantages of concurrent use are still the subject of debate. These two groups of drugs are widely used together in the treatment of schizophrenic patients who show depression, and for mixed anxiety and depression. A number of fixed-dose combinations have been marketed, e.g. amitriptyline with perphenazine), and nortriptyline with fluphenazine. However, the safety of using both drugs together has been questioned.

One of the problems of phenothiazine treatment is the development of tardive dyskinesias, and some evidence suggests that the higher the dosage, the greater the incidence.[25] The symptoms can be transiently masked by increasing the dosage,[26] and so it has been suggested that the presence of a tricyclic antidepressant might not only be a factor causing tardive dyskinesia to develop, but might also mask the condition.[18,27] It has been recommended that the addition of full antidepressant doses of nortriptyline to average antipsychotic doses of chlorpromazine should be avoided because the therapeutic actions of the chlorpromazine may be reversed.[20] See also 'Antipsychotics + Antimuscarinics', p.708.

Attention has also been drawn to excessive weight gain associated with several months use of amitriptyline with thioridazine for the treatment of chronic pain,[28] but note that excessive weight gain is a recognised adverse effect of the antipsychotics alone.

The tricyclic antidepressants and many antipsychotics increase the QT interval, see 'Drugs that prolong the QT interval + Other drugs that prolong the QT interval', p.257, for further information.

1. Siris SG, Cooper TB, Rifkin AE, Brenner R, Lieberman JA. Plasma imipramine concentrations in patients receiving concomitant fluphenazine decanoate. *Am J Psychiatry* (1982) 139, 104–6.
2. Linnoila M, George L, Guthrie S. Interaction between antidepressants and perphenazine in psychiatric patients. *Am J Psychiatry* (1982) 139, 1329–31.
3. Gram LF, Overø KF. Drug interaction: inhibitory effect of neuroleptics on metabolism of tricyclic antidepressants in man. *BMJ* (1972) 1, 463–5.
4. Crammer JL, Rolfe B. Interaction of imipramine and chlorpromazine in man. *Psychopharmacologia* (1972) 26 (Suppl), 81.
5. Gram LF. Lægemiddelinteraktion: hæmmende virkning af neurolepltica på tricycliske antidepressivas metabolisering. *Nord Psykiatr Tidsskr* (1971) 25, 357–60.
6. Jerling M, Bertilsson L, Sjöqvist F. The use of therapeutic drug monitoring data to document kinetic drug interactions: an example with amitriptyline and nortriptyline. *Ther Drug Monit* (1994) 16, 1–12.
7. Perel JM, Stiller RL, Feldman BL, Lin FC, Narayanan S. Therapeutic drug monitoring (TDM) of the amitriptyline (AT)/perphenazine (PER) interaction in depressed patients. *Clin Chem* (1985) 31, 939–40.
8. Gram LF, Overø KF, Kirk L. Influence of neuroleptics and benzodiazepines on metabolism of tricyclic antidepressants in man. *Am J Psychiatry* (1974) 131, 863–6.
9. Gram LF. Effects of perphenazine on imipramine metabolism in man. *Psychopharmacol Comm* (1975) 1, 165–75.
10. Nelson JC, Jatlow PI. Neuroleptic effect on desipramine steady-state plasma concentrations. *Am J Psychiatry* (1980) 137, 1232–4.
11. Linnet K. Comparison of the kinetic interactions of the neuroleptics perphenazine and zuclopenthixol with tricyclic antidepressives. *Ther Drug Monit* (1995) 17, 308–11.
12. Mulsant BH, Foglia JP, Sweet RA, Rosen J, Lo KH, Pollock BG. The effects of perphenazine on the concentration of nortriptyline and its hydroxymetabolites in older patients. *J Clin Psychopharmacol* (1997) 17, 318–21.
13. Overø KF, Gram LF, Hansen V. Interaction of perphenazine with the kinetics of nortriptyline. *Acta Pharmacol Toxicol (Copenh)* (1977) 40, 97–105.
14. Hirschowitz J, Bennett JA, Zemlan FP, Garver DL. Thioridazine effect on desipramine plasma levels. *J Clin Psychopharmacol* (1983) 3, 376–9.
15. Maynard GL, Soni P. Thioridazine interferences with imipramine metabolism and measurement. *Ther Drug Monit* (1996) 18, 729–31.
16. Cooper SF, Dugal R, Elie R, Albert J-M. Metabolic interaction between amitriptyline and perphenazine in psychiatric patients. *Prog Neuropsychopharmacol* (1979) 3, 369–76.
17. Kragh-Sørensen P, Borgå O, Garle M, Bolvig Hansen L, Hansen CE, Hvidberg EF, Larsen N-E, Sjöqvist F. Effect of simultaneous treatment with low doses of perphenazine on plasma and urine concentrations of nortriptyline and 10-hydroxynortriptyline. *Eur J Clin Pharmacol* (1977) 11, 479–83.
18. El-Yousef MK, Manier DH. Tricyclic antidepressants and phenothiazines. *JAMA* (1974) 229, 1419.
19. Rasheed A, Javed MA, Nazir S, Khawaja O. Interaction of chlorpromazine with tricyclic antidepressants in schizophrenic patients. *J Pakistan Med Assoc* (1994) 44, 233–4.
20. Loga S, Curry S, Lader M. Interaction of chlorpromazine and nortriptyline in patients with schizophrenia. *Clin Pharmacokinet* (1981) 6, 454–62.
21. O'Connor JW. Personal communication, February 1983.
22. Witton K. Severe toxic reaction to combined amitriptyline and thioridazine. *Am J Psychiatry* (1965) 121, 812–13.
23. Kane FJ. An unusual reaction to combined imipramine-thorazine therapy. *Am J Psychiatry* (1963) 120, 186–7.
24. Wilens TE, Stern TA. Ventricular tachycardia associated with desipramine and thioridazine. *Psychosomatics* (1990) 31, 100–3.
25. Crane GE. Persistent dyskinesia. *Br J Psychiatry* (1973), 122, 395–405.
26. Crane GE. Tardive dyskinesia in patients treated with major neuroleptics: a review of the literature. *Am J Psychiatry* (1968) 124 (Suppl), 40–8.
27. Ayd FJ. Pharmacokinetic interaction between tricyclic antidepressants and phenothiazine neuroleptics. *Int Drug Ther Newslett* (1974) 9, 31–2.
28. Pfister AK. Weight gain from combined phenothiazine and tricyclic therapy. *JAMA* (1978) 239, 1959.

Pimozide + CYP3A4 inhibitors

Inhibition of CYP3A4 results in markedly increased pimozide levels and increases the risk of QT interval prolongation and the development of life-threatening arrhythmias.

Clinical evidence, mechanism, importance and management

The sudden death of a patient taking pimozide and **clarithromycin** prompted a study of a possible interaction between the two drugs. Using human liver microsomes it was found that pimozide is partly metabolised by the cytochrome P450 isoenzyme CYP3A, and that 2 micromol of **clarithromycin** inhibits this enzyme by at least 80%.[1] The practical consequences of this were seen in a later study in 12 healthy subjects, which found that **clarithromycin** 500 mg twice daily for 5 days more than doubled the AUC of a single 6-mg oral dose of pimozide and raised its maximum serum levels by almost 50%. The QTc interval was prolonged by about 17 milliseconds with pimozide alone and by 24 milliseconds when **clarithromycin** was added.[2] The results were the same in both poor and extensive CYP2D6 metabolisers (see 'Genetic factors', (p.4)). CYP2D6 status was considered as this is the other main metabolic route of pimozide. The authors of this study concluded that **clarithromycin** can therefore increase the cardiotoxicity of pimozide during chronic use, irrespective of the CYP2D6 status of the patient.[2] Pimozide alone has been associated with ventricular arrhythmias, prolongation of the QT interval, T-wave changes and sudden and unexpected death, even in the young with no previous evidence of cardiac disease.[3,4] Due to the severity of this interaction the UK manufacturers contraindicate the use of macrolides with pimozide,[5] whereas the US manufacturers contraindicate pimozide with **azithromycin**, **clarithromycin**, **dirithromycin**, **erythromycin** and **troleandomycin**.[6] However, note that azithromycin does not usually interact with other drugs by inhibiting CYP3A4.

The use of many inhibitors of the cytochrome P450 isoenzyme CYP3A4 with pimozide is contraindicated since they are expected to increase plasma levels of pimozide, which is likely to result in QT prolongation and associated arrhythmias. The manufacturers specifically mention **azole antifungals**, **fluvoxamine**, **grapefruit juice**, **nefazodone**, **protease inhibitors**, and **zileuton**.[5,6] Drugs that are known to cause clinically relevant CYP3A4 inhibition are listed in 'Table 1.4', (p.6).

1. Flockhart DA, Richard E, Woosely RL, Pearle PL, Drici M-D. A metabolic interaction between clarithromycin and pimozide may result in cardiac toxicity. *Clin Pharmacol Ther* (1996) 59, 189.
2. Desta Z, Kerbusch T, Flockhart DA. Effect of clarithromycin on the pharmacokinetics and pharmacodynamics of pimozide in healthy poor and extensive metabolizers of cytochrome P450 2D6 (CYP2D6). *Clin Pharmacol Ther* (1999) 65, 10–20.
3. Committee on Safety of Medicines. Cardiotoxic effects of pimozide. *Current Problems* (1990) 29.
4. Flockhart DA, Drici M-D, Kerbusch T, Soukhova N, Richard E, Pearle PL, Mahal SK, Babb VJ. Studies on the mechanism of a fatal clarithromycin-pimozide interaction in a patient with Tourette syndrome. *J Clin Psychopharmacol* (2000) 20, 317–24.
5. Orap (Pimozide). Janssen-Cilag Ltd. UK Summary of product characteristics, May 2007.
6. Orap (Pimozide). Gate Pharmaceuticals. US Prescribing information, August 2005.

Pimozide + SSRIs

Pimozide levels are expected to rise when used with fluoxetine, fluvoxamine, paroxetine, or sertraline, which would increase the risk of potentially fatal torsade de pointes arrhythmias. The use of SSRIs and pimozide has also led to extrapyramidal adverse effects, oculogyric crises and sedation in rare cases.

Clinical evidence, mechanism, importance and management

(a) Fluoxetine

A patient taking fluoxetine and pimozide had a worsening of extrapyramidal symptoms, and another developed marked sinus bradycardia of 35 to 44 bpm with somnolence.[1] This case was the subject of later discussion on the mechanism of the interaction.[2,3] One patient also developed extrapyramidal symptoms,[4] while another became stuporous when given both drugs.[5]

(b) Paroxetine

A boy of about 10 years, with various disorders (motor tics, enuresis, attention deficit hyperactivity disorder, Tourettes's disorder, impulsivity, albinism) was treated for a year with pimozide 2 mg twice, and later three times daily.[6] Within 3 days of starting paroxetine 10 mg in the morning, he began to complain of his eyes hurting and his mother noted that about 4 hours after taking the paroxetine his eyes were rolled back in his head but the problem had resolved by the evening. This oculogyric crisis occurred on a further occasion, and so the paroxetine was stopped. There was no other evidence of either extrapyramidal or hyperserotonergic reactions. This case needs to be viewed in its particular context (oculogyric crises are associated with albinism) so that it may not be of general importance. In a study of a single 2-mg dose of pimozide given with paroxetine 60 mg daily, a 151% rise in pimozide AUC and a 62% rise in maximum plasma levels occurred.[7]

(c) Sertraline

A study found that sertraline 200 mg daily caused a 40% rise in the AUC and maximum plasma levels of a single 2-mg dose of pimozide. No ECG changes were seen.[8,9]

A fatality has been reported with an overdose of moclobemide, sertraline and pimozide, with blood levels suggesting that none of the drugs individually would have been fatal.[10]

Mechanism

The SSRIs can, to varying degrees inhibit the cytochrome P450 isoenzyme CYP2D6 (and fluvoxamine possibly also inhibits CYP3A4) by which pimozide is metabolised. Concurrent use would therefore be expected to lead to raised pimozide levels.

Importance and management

Evidence is limited, however the interaction is potentially severe as raised pimozide levels can cause torsade de pointes arrhythmias, which can be fatal. The manufacturers of pimozide contraindicate its use with SSRIs, and in the UK they specifically name sertraline, paroxetine, and citalopram; which has been seen to cause QT prolongation with pimozide, and its isomer, escitalopram.[7] The US manufacturers additionally contraindicate fluvoxamine.[11] Neither manufacturer mentions fluoxetine (except with regard to the possibility of additive bradycardia[11]), but as it is known to have greater effects on CYP2D6 than either sertraline or citalopram, it would seem prudent to also consider it as contraindicated.

1. Ahmed I, Dagincourt PG, Miller LG, Shader RI. Possible interaction between fluoxetine and pimozide causing sinus bradycardia. *Can J Psychiatry* (1993) 38, 62–3.
2. Friedman EH. Re: bradycardia and somnolence after adding fluoxetine to pimozide regimen. *Can J Psychiatry* (1994) 39, 634.
3. Ahmed I. Re: bradycardia and somnolence after adding fluoxetine to pimozide regimen. *Can J Psychiatry* (1994) 39, 634.
4. Coulter DM, Pillans PI. Fluoxetine and extrapyramidal side effects. *Am J Psychiatry* (1995) 152, 122–5.
5. Hansen-Grant S, Silk KR, Guthrie S. Fluoxetine-pimozide interaction. *Am J Psychiatry* (1993) 150, 1751–2.
6. Horrigan JP, Barnhill LJ. Paroxetine–pimozide drug interaction. *J Am Acad Child Adolesc Psychiatry* (1994) 33, 1060–1.
7. Orap (Pimozide). Janssen-Cilag Ltd. UK Summary of product characteristics, May 2007.
8. Zoloft (Sertraline hydrochloride). Pfizer Inc. US Prescribing information, June 2007.
9. Lustral (Sertraline hydrochloride). Pfizer Ltd, UK Summary of product characteristics, October 2005.
10. McIntyre IM, King CV, Staikos V, Gall J, Drummer OH. A fatality involving moclobemide, sertraline, and pimozide. *J Forensic Sci* (1997) 42, 951–3.
11. Orap (Pimozide). Gate Pharmaceuticals. US Prescribing information, August 2005.

Prochlorperazine + Metoclopramide

A single case report describes tongue swelling and respiratory obstruction in a patient given prochlorperazine and then metoclopramide.

Clinical evidence, mechanism, importance and management

A 19-year-old woman experienced progressive swelling of the tongue, partial upper-airways obstruction and a sensation of choking over a period of 12 hours after she was given intramuscular doses of metoclopramide to a total of 30 mg. She had received a 12.5-mg intramuscular dose of prochlorperazine for nausea 24 hours earlier. On examination her tongue was strikingly blue, but within 15 minutes of receiving benzatropine 2 mg it returned to its normal size and colour. The respiratory distress also disappeared.[1] The authors of the report

suggested that the dystonic adverse effects of both drugs were additive, leading to the effects seen.[1] However, it should be noted that oedema of the tongue has also been described with metoclopramide alone.[2] Young patients, especially women, are particularly susceptible to the adverse effects of metoclopramide, and this patient received the standard total daily dose over just 12 hours, so an interaction is by no means established.

1. Alroe C, Bowen P. Metoclopramide and prochlorperazine: ''the blue-tongue sign''. *Med J Aust* (1989) 150, 724–5.
2. Robinson OPW. Metoclopramide—side effects and safety. *Postgrad Med J* (1973) 49 (Suppl July), 77–80.

Promazine + Attapulgite-pectin

An attapulgite-pectin antidiarrhoeal preparation caused a small reduction in the absorption of promazine in one subject.

Clinical evidence, mechanism, importance and management

A study in one healthy subject found that attapulgite-pectin reduced the absorption of a single 50-mg dose of promazine by about 25%, possibly due to adsorption of the phenothiazine onto the attapulgite.[1] The clinical importance of this interaction and whether other phenothiazines behave similarly does not appear to have been studied. If a problem does occur, separating administration as much as possible (2 hours or more) to avoid admixture in the gut has been shown to minimise the effects of this type of interaction with other drugs.

1. Sorby DL, Liu G. Effects of adsorbents on drug absorption II. Effect of an antidiarrhea mixture on promazine absorption. *J Pharm Sci* (1966) 55, 504–10.

Quetiapine + Antipsychotics

Quetiapine does not appear to interact with haloperidol or risperidone. Thioridazine moderately reduces quetiapine levels and a case report describes a seizure in a patient taking olanzapine and quetiapine.

Clinical evidence, mechanism, importance and management

In patients with schizophrenia or bipolar disorder given quetiapine 300 mg twice daily, **thioridazine** 200 mg twice daily reduced the steady-state quetiapine AUC and its maximum and minimum plasma levels by about 41%, 48% and 33%, respectively. It was suggested that this was due to an increased metabolism of quetiapine, although the mechanism for this effect was unclear.[1] These reductions are only moderate and their importance is not known, but until more information is available it would seem prudent to monitor concurrent use, being alert for the need to raise the quetiapine dosage.

Haloperidol 7.5 mg twice daily and **risperidone** 3 mg twice daily for 9 days had no significant effect on the pharmacokinetics of quetiapine 300 mg twice daily in the same study.[1] However, there is a case report describing considerable QT prolongation in a patient who took quetiapine 2 g whilst also taking **risperidone**. The authors consider this significant as the overdose was small, and because no QT prolongation was seen in toxicity studies of quetiapine when doses as large as 9.6 g were used,[2] although there is a single case of prolonged QTc interval associated with an overdose of 9.6 g.[3] No special precautions would therefore appear to be routinely necessary if either of these drugs and quetiapine are used concurrently.

A case report describes a seizure lasting 30 to 60 seconds in a 27-year-old woman one day after quetiapine 100 mg daily was added to treatment with **olanzapine** 15 mg daily and sertraline 100 mg daily. The seizure was attributed to an interaction between quetiapine and **olanzapine**, although it seems possible that the sertraline also may have contributed.[4]

Concurrent use need not be avoided, but this case highlights the importance of considering seizure potential when prescribing multiple antipsychotic medications.

1. Potkin SG, Thyrum PT, Alva G, Bera R, Yeh C, Arvanitis LA. The safety and pharmacokinetics of quetiapine when coadministered with haloperidol, risperidone, or thioridazine. *J Clin Psychopharmacol* (2002) 22, 121–30.
2. Beelen AP, Yeo K-TJ, Lewis LD. Asymptomatic QTc prolongation associated with quetiapine fumarate overdose in a patient being treated with risperidone. *Hum Exp Toxicol* (2001) 20, 215–19.
3. Gajwani P, Pozuelo L, Tesar GE. QT interval prolongation associated with quetiapine (Seroquel) overdose. *Psychosomatics* (2000) 41, 63–5.
4. Hedges DW, Jeppson KG. New-onset seizure associated with quetiapine and olanzapine. *Ann Pharmacother* (2002) 36, 437–9.

Quetiapine + CYP3A4 inducers

The plasma levels of quetiapine are reduced by phenytoin and carbamazepine, and are predicted to be reduced by barbiturates and rifampicin.

Clinical evidence, mechanism, importance and management

When 17 patients taking quetiapine 250 mg three times daily were given **phenytoin** 100 mg three times daily for 10 days, the oral clearance of quetiapine was increased fivefold.[1] This increased clearance appears to occur because **phenytoin** is an inducer of the cytochrome P450 isoenzyme CYP3A4, which is also concerned with the metabolism of quetiapine. In a study 14 patients took quetiapine 300 mg twice daily for 28 days, with **carbamazepine** 200 mg three times daily for 20 days. It was found that the AUC and maximum plasma levels of quetiapine were reduced by 87% and 80%, respectively.[2] **Carbamazepine** is also an inducer of CYP3A4, and therefore probably reduces quetiapine levels by this mechanism.

The manufacturers of quetiapine suggest that dosage adjustments [increases] may be necessary if quetiapine is given with **carbamazepine**, **phenytoin** or other enzyme inducers (such as **barbiturates** or **rifampicin (rifampin)**.[3,4] This is a reasonable prediction but no direct clinical evidence is yet available. However, be alert for the need to use an increased quetiapine dosage in patients given any of these drugs.

See 'Carbamazepine + Antipsychotics', p.524 for comment on the effect of quetiapine on carbamazepine.

1. Wong YWJ, Yeh C, Thyrum PT. The effects of concomitant phenytoin administration on the steady-state pharmacokinetics of quetiapine. *J Clin Psychopharmacol* (2001) 21, 89–93.
2. Grimm SW, Richtand NM, Winter HR, Stams KR, Reele SB. Effects of cytochrome P450 3A modulators ketoconazole and carbamazepine on quetiapine pharmacokinetics. *Br J Clin Pharmacol* (2006), 61, 58–69.
3. Seroquel (Quetiapine fumarate). AstraZeneca UK Ltd. UK Summary of product characteristics, November 2006.
4. Seroquel (Quetiapine fumarate). AstraZeneca. US Prescribing information, July 2007.

Quetiapine + CYP3A4 inhibitors

The plasma levels of quetiapine are increased by erythromycin and ketoconazole. Azoles, macrolides, and protease inhibitors are expected to interact similarly.

Clinical evidence, mechanism, importance and management

Twelve healthy subjects received a single 25-mg dose of quetiapine on day 4 of a 4 day course of **ketoconazole** 200 mg daily. The AUC and maximum plasma levels of quetiapine were increased by 522% and 235%, respectively, and the mean half-life of quetiapine was increased from 2.61 to 6.76 hours.[1] **Ketoconazole** is a potent inhibitor of the cytochrome P450 isoenzyme CYP3A4 by which quetiapine is metabolised. Concurrent use therefore reduced quetiapine metabolism and increased its levels.

A study in 19 Chinese patients who received quetiapine 200 mg twice daily and **erythromycin** 500 mg three times daily found that **erythromycin** increased the maximum plasma concentration, half-life and AUC of quetiapine by 68%, 92%, and 129%, respectively.[2] These increases probably occurred because **erythromycin** inhibited the metabolism of quetiapine by CYP3A4.

The UK manufacturers[3] advise caution if quetiapine is given with **macrolides** and **azole antifungals**, and suggest that lower quetiapine doses should be considered. The US manufacturers also advise caution, and specifically name **itraconazole** and **fluconazole**, **erythromycin** and **protease inhibitors**,[4] all of which are inhibitors of CYP3A4.

1. Grimm SW, Richtand NM, Winter HR, Stams KR, Reele SB. Effects of cytochrome P450 3A modulators ketoconazole and carbamazepine on quetiapine pharmacokinetics. *Br J Clin Pharmacol* (2006), 61, 58–69.
2. Li K-Y, Li X, Cheng Z-N, Zhang B-K, Peng W-X, Li H-D. Effect of erythromycin on metabolism of quetiapine in Chinese suffering from schizophrenia. *Eur J Clin Pharmacol* (2005) 60, 791–5.
3. Seroquel (Quetiapine fumarate). AstraZeneca UK Ltd. UK Summary of product characteristics, November 2006.
4. Seroquel (Quetiapine fumarate). AstraZeneca. US Prescribing information, July 2007.

Quetiapine + Lithium

Quetiapine slightly raised serum lithium levels in one study, but this was not statistically significant. Combined use did not increase the incidence of extrapyramidal symptoms in another study.

Clinical evidence, mechanism, importance and management

The steady-state serum lithium levels of 10 patients with schizophrenia, or schizoaffective or bipolar disorders were studied before, during, and after the concurrent use of quetiapine 250 mg three times daily. The lithium AUC_{0-12} and the maximum serum levels were raised by 12% and 4.5%, respectively, by quetiapine, and concurrent use was well tolerated.[1] This small rise was not statistically or clinically significant.

A randomised, placebo-controlled study in 191 patients found that quetiapine, combined with either lithium or valproate semisodium (divalproex sodium), was superior to lithium or valproate semisodium alone for treating bipolar mania. The incidence of extrapyramidal symptoms in patients receiving quetiapine with lithium or valproate semisodium was similar to those receiving placebo with lithium or valproate semisodium.[2] No special precautions would therefore appear to be necessary on concurrent use.

1. Potkin SG, Thyrum PT, Bera R, Carreon D, Alva G, Kalali AH, Yeh C. Open-label study of the effect of combination quetiapine/lithium therapy on lithium pharmacokinetics and tolerability. *Clin Ther* (2002) 24, 1809–23.
2. Sachs G, Chengappa KNR, Suppes T, Mullen JA, Brecher M, Devine NA, Sweitzer DE. Quetiapine with lithium or divalproex for the treatment of bipolar mania: a randomized, double-blind, placebo-controlled study. *Bipolar Disord* (2004) 6, 213–23.

Quetiapine + Miscellaneous

Quetiapine dose not appear to interact to a clinically relevant extent with cimetidine, fluoxetine, imipramine or lorazepam. Isolated cases of adverse outcomes have been reported with diphenhydramine, lovastatin and mirtazapine.

Clinical evidence, mechanism, importance and management

(a) Antidepressants

Fluoxetine 60 mg daily or **imipramine** 75 mg twice daily for 5 days had no clinically significant effect on the steady-state plasma levels of quetiapine 300 mg twice daily.[1] No special precautions would therefore appear to be necessary if either of these drugs and quetiapine are used concurrently.

A falsely elevated **imipramine** level was recorded when HPLC was used to determine serum **imipramine** levels in a patient taking **imipramine**, quetiapine, fluvoxamine, lithium and docusate. The abnormal readings were found to have been caused by a metabolite of quetiapine, and normal readings were obtained by altering the wavelength for detection of **imipramine**.[2] **Nortriptyline** levels have been found to be falsely elevated in a patient also taking quetiapine when blood was analysed using fluorescence polarisation immunoassay, but were normal when an HPLC analysis was undertaken.[3] Other immunoassay methods for identifying tricyclic antidepressants in blood and urine have also given false positive results in the presence of quetiapine.[4]

An isolated case of increased prolactin levels after the introduction of **mirtazapine** 15 mg daily has been reported in a woman who was taking quetiapine 400 mg daily. Her prolactin level normalised when the **mirtazapine** was stopped, but rechallenge again produced an increase in prolactin levels, although this was transient and appeared to resolve within one month. The authors suggest that the mirtazapine may have caused an increase in quetiapine-induced dopamine receptor blockade, or alternatively an agonist action at opioid receptors altered dopamine receptor function.[5]

(b) Cimetidine

Quetiapine 150 mg three times daily was given to 7 psychotic men with cimetidine 400 mg three times daily for 4 days. There were some slight alterations in the pharmacokinetics of the quetiapine, but these were within the intraindividual changes seen and so were not considered significant.[6] There would therefore appear to be no reason for avoiding concurrent use.

(c) Diphenhydramine

A patient taking diphenhydramine 100 mg daily developed urinary retention when she increased her dose of quetiapine from 900 mg daily to 2.4 g daily. When the dose of quetiapine was reduced back to 900 mg daily, her urinary retention resolved. A further episode occurred when the patient again increased her quetiapine dose. Although quetiapine does not normally have antimuscarinic adverse effects at usual therapeutic doses, it is suggested by the authors that the likelihood of these adverse effects is increased at doses of quetiapine greater than 900 mg daily. This effect may have occurred as a result of additive antimuscarinic activity of both diphenhydramine and high-dose quetiapine.[7]

(d) Lorazepam

The pharmacokinetics and pharmacodynamic effects of a single 2-mg dose of lorazepam were studied in 10 men taking quetiapine 250 mg three times daily. It was found that the maximum serum lorazepam levels were not significantly changed by quetiapine, and the alterations in the performance of a number of psychometric tests were small and considered not to be clinically relevant.[8]

(e) Lovastatin

A patient taking quetiapine 800 mg daily and sertraline 100 mg daily developed a prolonged QTc interval of 569 milliseconds after starting to take lovastatin 10 mg daily. Following a reduction in the lovastatin dose to 5 mg daily, her QTc interval returned to her baseline of 424 milliseconds. It is suggested that lovastatin competitively inhibited the metabolism of quetiapine by CYP3A4, as both drugs are substrates for this enzyme, resulting in increased quetiapine levels.[9] However, the full contribution of sertraline to this case was only briefly considered, and full details relating to the cardiac effects and calculation of the QTc interval are not given.[10]

(f) Valproate

Analysis of plasma quetiapine levels of 94 patients, 9 of whom were also taking valproate, found a 77% increase in the concentration dose ratio compared with those patients not taking valproate.[11] The US manufacturers[12] report that valproate semisodium (divalproex sodium) increases the maximum plasma levels of quetiapine by 17%, and the UK manufacturers state that these changes are not clinically relevant.[13]

1. Potkin SG, Thyrum PT, Alva G, Carreon D, Yeh C, Kalali A, Arvanitis LA. Effect of fluoxetine and imipramine on the pharmacokinetics and tolerability of the antipsychotic quetiapine. *J Clin Psychopharmacol* (2002) 22, 174–82.
2. Al-Mateen CS, Wolf CE. Falsely elevated imipramine levels in a patient taking quetiapine. *J Am Acad Child Adolesc Psychiatry* (2002) 41, 5–6.
3. Schussler JM, Juenke JM, Schussler I. Quetiapine and falsely elevated nortriptyline level. *Am J Psychiatry* (2003) 160, 589.
4. Hayes KM. Law , Burns MM. Quetiapine (Seroquel®) produces false positive tricyclic antidepressant screen. *Pediatr Res* (2003) 53, 104A.
5. Orlandi V, Speca A, Salviati M, Biondi M. Abnormal prolactin elevation in a schizophrenic patient in treatment with quetiapine and mirtazapine. The role of the opioid system. *J Clin Psychopharmacol* (2003) 23, 677–9.
6. Strakowski SM, Keck PE, Wong YWJ, Thyrum PT, Yeh C. The effect of multiple doses of cimetidine on the steady-state pharmacokinetics of quetiapine in men with selected psychotic disorders. *J Clin Psychopharmacol* (2002) 22, 201–5.
7. Sokolski KN, Brown BJ, Melden M. Urinary retention following repeated high-dose quetiapine. *Ann Pharmacother* (2004) 38, 899–900.
8. Potkin SG. The pharmacokinetics and pharmacodynamics of lorazepam given before and during treatment with ICI 204,636 (Seroquel) in men with selected psychotic disorders. (5077IL/0027). Zeneca Pharma. Data on file (Study 27).
9. Furst BA, Champion KM, Pierre JM, Wirshing DA, Wirshing WC. Possible association of QTc interval prolongation with co-administration of quetiapine and lovastatin. *Biol Psychiatry* (2002) 51, 264–5.
10. Geller W, Smith M, Winter H, Brecher M. Response: possible association of QTc interval prolongation with co-administration of quetiapine and lovastatin. *Biol Psychiatry* (2002) 52, 911–15.
11. Aichhorn W, Marksteiner J, Walch T, Zernig G, Saria A, Kemmler G. Influence of age, gender, body weight and valproate comedication on quetiapine plasma concentrations. *Int Clin Psychopharmacol* (2006) 21, 81–5.
12. Seroquel (Quetiapine fumarate). AstraZeneca. US Prescribing information, July 2007.
13. Seroquel (Quetiapine fumarate). AstraZeneca UK Ltd. UK Summary of product characteristics, November 2006.

Risperidone + Carbamazepine or Oxcarbazepine

Carbamazepine increases the metabolism of risperidone, resulting in reduced risperidone levels. Oxcarbazepine dose not significantly affect the pharmacokinetics of risperidone.

Clinical evidence

(a) Carbamazepine

A 22-year-old man taking risperidone 4 mg daily and carbamazepine 600 mg daily for schizophrenia had lower than expected risperidone levels, so his dose was doubled and the carbamazepine tailed off. Ten days after carbamazepine had been discontinued it was noted that his plasma 9-hydroxyrisperidone level was 49 micrograms/L; it had only been 19 micrograms/L when he was taking carbamazepine.[1] There are 4 other cases of this interaction between risperidone and carbamazepine.[2-4] In one case, the addition of carbamazepine to established risperidone treatment resulted in a reduction in the risperidone and 9-hydroxyrisperidone levels of about 75% and 65%, respectively, accompanied by the return of the patients psychotic symptoms.[4] In 2 other cases, a 20-year-old and an 81-year-old man developed parkinsonian symptoms when carbamazepine was stopped. The symptoms resolved when the doses of risperidone were reduced by about two-thirds.[2]

These cases are supported by a study in 5 patients taking carbamazepine and risperidone for schizophrenia or bipolar disorders. The dose-normalised plasma level of risperidone and its active metabolite, 9-hydroxyrisperidone, were 68% and 64% lower, respectively, with carbamazepine, when compared to those with risperidone alone.[5] Another study in 11 patients who had been taking risperidone for 2 to 68 weeks found that carbamazepine 200 mg twice daily for a week approximately halved the plasma levels of risperidone and its active moiety (risperidone plus 9-hydroxyrisperidone).[6]

(b) Oxcarbazepine

A study in 12 patients taking risperidone 2 to 6 mg daily found that the addition of oxcarbazepine for 5 weeks, at an initial dose of 300 mg daily increased to 900 mg to 1.2 g after one week, had no significant effects on the pharmacokinetics of risperidone. Concurrent use was generally well tolerated.[7]

Mechanism

Carbamazepine is a known potent enzyme inducer, which appears to increase the metabolism of risperidone by the cytochrome P450 isoenzyme CYP2D6 (although other isoenzymes may play a part). The extent of the interaction appears to be related to CYP2D6 genotype (see 'Genetic factors', (p.4)). Oxcarbazepine is not known to affect CYP2D6-mediated metabolism.

Importance and management

It would seem important to monitor the levels of risperidone and 9-hydroxyrisperidone in patients given carbamazepine, being alert for the need to raise the risperidone dosage, possibly by as much as two-thirds.

For mention that risperidone may moderately increase carbamazepine levels see 'Carbamazepine + Antipsychotics', p.524.

No special consideration or monitoring appears necessary with concurrent oxcarbazepine and risperidone treatment.

1. de Leon J, Bork J. Risperidone and cytochrome P450 3A. *J Clin Psychiatry* (1997) 58, 450.

2. Takahashi H, Yoshida K, Higuchi H, Shimizu T. Development of parkinsonian symptoms after discontinuation of carbamazepine in patients concurrently treated with risperidone: two case reports. *Clin Neuropharmacol* (2001) 24, 358–60.
3. Alfaro CL, Nicolson R, Lenane M, Rapoport JL. Carbamazepine and/or fluvoxamine drug interaction with risperidone in a patient on multiple psychotropic medications. *Ann Pharmacother* (2000) 34, 122–3.
4. Spina E, Scordo MG, Avenoso A, Perucca E. Adverse drug interaction between risperidone and carbamazepine in a patient with chronic schizophrenia and deficient CYP2D6 activity. *J Clin Psychopharmacol* (2001) 21, 108–9.
5. Spina E, Avenoso A, Facciolà G, Salemi M, Scordo MG, Giacobello T, Madia AG, Perucca E. Plasma concentrations of risperidone and 9-hydroxyrisperidone: effect of comedication with carbamazepine or valproate. *Ther Drug Monit* (2000) 22, 481–5.
6. Ono S, Mihara K, Suzuki A, Kondo T, Yasui-Furukori N, Furukori H, de Vries R, Kaneko S. Significant pharmacokinetic interaction between risperidone and carbamazepine: its relationship with CYP2D6 genotypes. *Psychopharmacology (Berl)* (2002) 162, 50–54.
7. Muscatello MR, Pacetti M, Cacciola M, La Torre D, Zoccali R, D'Arrigo C, Migliardi G, Spina E. Plasma concentrations of risperidone and olanzapine during coadministration with oxcarbazepine. *Epilepsia* (2005) 46, 771–4.

Risperidone + Itraconazole

Itraconazole increases the plasma levels of both risperidone and its active metabolite, 9-hydroxyrisperidone.

Clinical evidence

A study in 19 patients who were taking risperidone 2 to 8 mg daily found that the addition of itraconazole 200 mg daily for a week increased the plasma levels of risperidone and its active metabolite, 9-hydroxyrisperidone, by 82% and 70%, respectively. The levels returned to pre-treatment values one week after the itraconazole was stopped.[1] There was a small difference in the increase in the levels of risperidone between CYP2D6 extensive and poor metabolisers of risperidone, with extensive metabolisers showing a rise of 67% and poor metabolisers a rise of 70%.

Mechanism

Inhibition of metabolism of risperidone by the cytochrome P450 isoenzyme CYP3A is thought to have caused the increase in levels. The difference in the increase in levels of the extensive and poor metabolisers indicates that CYP2D6 has a minor part in the metabolism of risperidone.

Importance and management

Risperidone levels are expected to increase if itraconazole is given concurrently. Be aware for any signs of increased adverse effects, and consider reducing the dosage as necessary.

1. Jung SM, Kim KA, Cho HK, Jung IG, Park PW, Byun WT, Park JY. Cytochrome P450 3A inhibitor itraconazole affects plasma concentrations of risperidone and 9-hydroxyrisperidone in schizophrenic patients. *Clin Pharmacol Ther* (2005) 78, 520–8.

Risperidone + Lamotrigine

One small study found no interaction between risperidone and lamotrigine, although a case report describes increased risperidone levels on concurrent use, and a retrospective study suggests that lamotrigine increases the variability on risperidone levels.

Clinical evidence

An isolated case report describes markedly increased risperidone levels in a patient given increasing doses of lamotrigine. When the lamotrigine dose was increased from 175 mg daily to 200 mg daily, the risperidone level increased from 69 nanogram/mL to 263 nanogram/mL. A further increase in the lamotrigine dose to 225 mg daily, while maintaining the risperidone dose of 8 mg daily resulted in a risperidone plasma level of 412 nanogram/mL, and the patient complained of dizziness and tiredness.[1] A retrospective review of 5 patients taking risperidone and lamotrigine, for whom there was pharmacokinetic data available both before and after the addition of lamotrigine, revealed a wide variation in alterations of risperidone levels, from a reduction of 40.5% to a rise of 73.6% after the addition of lamotrigine, with an average decrease of 7%.[2] A study in 10 patients taking risperidone 3 mg to 6 mg daily, and who were also given lamotrigine in increasing doses over 8 weeks to 200 mg daily also found no changes in the pharmacokinetics of risperidone.[3]

Mechanism, importance and management

Risperidone is metabolised by CYP2D6, but since lamotrigine is not a known inhibitor of this enzyme, a pharmacokinetic interaction was not thought to explain the change in levels.[1] The retrospective review and small study above failed to find any evidence of a consistent effect of lamotrigine on risperidone pharmacokinetics. However in view of the case report above, and also the fact that some individuals in the review demonstrated large changes in their risperidone levels, it would seem prudent to monitor patients for an increase in adverse effects, or a lack of therapeutic effect, if lamotrigine is given with risperidone.

1. Bienentreu SD, Kronmüller K-TH. Increase in risperidone plasma level with lamotrigine. *Am J Psychiatry* (2005) 162, 811–2.
2. Castberg I, Spigset O. Risperidone and lamotrigine: no evidence of a drug interaction. *J Clin Psychiatry* (2006) 67, 1159.
3. Spina W, D'Arrigo C, Migliardi G, Santoro V, Muscatello MR, Micò U, D'Amico G, Perucca E. Effect of adjunctive lamotrigine treatment on the plasma concentrations of clozapine, risperidone and olanzapine in patients with schizophrenia or bipolar disorder. *Ther Drug Monit* (2006) 28, 599–602.

Risperidone + Levomepromazine

Twenty patients receiving risperidone for at least 2 weeks were also given levomepromazine, in doses of 5 mg to 75 mg daily. There were no changes in the pharmacokinetics of risperidone or its active metabolite, 9-hydroxyrisperidone, and there was no aggravation of extrapyramidal effects.[1]

1. Yoshimura R, Shinkai K, Kakihara S, Goto M, Yamada Y, Kaji K, Ueda N, Nakamura J. Little effects of low dosage of levomepromazine on plasma risperidone levels. *Pharmacopsychiatry* (2005) 38, 98–100.

Risperidone + Lithium

Extrapyramidal adverse effects have been seen in a patient taking risperidone and lithium. No changes in lithium pharmacokinetics are expected.

Clinical evidence, mechanism, importance and management

A case report describes a 42-year-old woman who developed extrapyramidal adverse effects of the mouth after the addition of risperidone to established lithium treatment of 800 mg daily. Three days after her risperidone dose had reached 5 mg daily, she experienced an abrupt onset of abnormal perioral movements. Her serum lithium level was 0.7 mmol/L. Symptoms resolved after intravenous promethazine was given.[1] A non-diabetic patient developed diabetic ketoacidosis, 2 years after starting treatment with risperidone and lithium. During this acute illness he also experienced neuroleptic malignant syndrome and a myocardial infarction. The authors consider the combination of these two drugs was a causative factor, as the patient was able to continue treatment with lithium alone with no recurrence of this condition, or the need for antidiabetic medication.[2] The manufacturers of risperidone state that there was no significant change in the AUC and maximum plasma concentration of lithium when it was taken with risperidone.[3,4] In general no particular caution would seem necessary on concurrent use, but be aware that, in rare cases, adverse effects may occur.

1. Mendhekar DN. Rabbit syndrome induced by combined lithium and risperidone. *Can J Psychiatry* (2005) 50, 369.
2. Ananth J, Johnson KM, Levander EM, Harry JL. Diabetic ketoacidosis, neuroleptic malignant syndrome, and myocardial infarction in a patient taking risperidone and lithium carbonate.
3. Risperdal (Risperidone). Janssen-Cilag Ltd. UK Summary of product characteristics, July 2007.
4. Risperdal Consta (Risperidone) Janssen Pharmaceutical Ltd. US Prescribing information, April 2007.

Risperidone + Probenecid

Twelve healthy subjects were given a single 1-mg dose of risperidone alone, or on day 2 of a 4 day course of probenecid 500 mg

twice daily. There were no significant changes in the pharmacokinetics of risperidone.[1]

1. Markowitz JS, DeVane CL, Liston HL, Bouton DW, Risch SC. The effects of probenecid on the disposition of risperidone and olanzapine in healthy volunteers. *Clin Pharmacol Ther* (2002) 71, 30–8.

Risperidone + Protease inhibitors

The neuroleptic malignant syndrome, ataxia and severe lethargy leading to a coma, and extrapyramidal adverse effects have been seen in patients given risperidone with indinavir and ritonavir.

Clinical evidence, mechanism, importance and management

A 35-year-old man with AIDS was diagnosed with a Tourette's-like disorder and given risperidone 1 mg twice daily. After 2 weeks the risperidone was increased to 2 mg twice daily and he was also given **indinavir** 800 mg twice daily with **ritonavir** 200 mg twice daily. He discontinued the antiretrovirals after 5 days due to nausea, but started them again 1 month later when the tic disorder had improved. After 1 week he became short of breath and fatigued with worsening tremor and other extrapyramidal adverse effects. The antiretrovirals were stopped and the risperidone dose increased to 3 mg twice daily. Over the next 3 days his symptoms worsened and began to interfere with daily living. Risperidone was discontinued and clonazepam started, and his symptoms resolved.[1] Another patient developed neuroleptic malignant syndrome 3 days after starting to take risperidone with **indinavir** and **ritonavir**. This patient also recovered when the risperidone was stopped.[2] A third patient taking **indinavir** and **ritonavir** was given risperidone 3 mg twice daily to treat symptoms of mania. After 2 doses he became ataxic, drowsy and disorientated, which further developed into lethargy and coma. He recovered 24 hours after stopping all medication.[3]

Indinavir inhibits the cytochrome P450 isoenzyme CYP3A4 and **ritonavir** inhibits CYP2D6 and CYP3A4, which are the main isoenzymes involved in the metabolism of risperidone. Therefore concurrent use would be expected to raise risperidone levels. The symptoms reported in the cases above may have all been due to increased risperidone levels.[1,3]

These appear to be the only reports of an interaction between risperidone and protease inhibitors, and their general significance is unclear. Until more is known it would be prudent to monitor patients taking risperidone who are given these protease inhibitors, particularly **ritonavir**, for risperidone adverse effects.

1. Kelly DV, Béïque LC, Bowmer MI. Extrapyramidal symptoms with ritonavir/indinavir plus risperidone. *Ann Pharmacother* (2002) 36, 827–30.
2. Lee SI, Klesmer J, Hirsch BE. Neuroleptic malignant syndrome associated with the use of risperidone, ritonavir and indinavir: a case report. *Psychosomatics* (2000) 41, 453–4.
3. Jover F, Cuadrado J-M, Andreu L, Merino J. Reversible coma caused by risperidone-ritonavir interaction. *Clin Neuropharmacol* (2002) 25, 251–3.

Risperidone + Reboxetine

No clinically relevant pharmacokinetic interaction appears to occur between risperidone and reboxetine.

Clinical evidence, mechanism, importance and management

Reboxetine 8 mg daily was given to 7 schizophrenic patients taking risperidone 8 mg daily for a period of 3 weeks. Reboxetine had no significant effects on the pharmacokinetics of either risperidone or its active metabolite, 9-hydroxyrisperidone, suggesting that no additional precautions are necessary if reboxetine and risperidone are used together.[1]

1. Spina E, Avenoso A, Scordo MG, Ancione M, Madia A, Levita A. No effect of reboxetine on plasma concentrations of clozapine, risperidone, and their active metabolites. *Ther Drug Monit* (2001) 23, 675–8.

Risperidone + SSRIs

Fluoxetine, fluvoxamine, and paroxetine appear to raise risperidone levels. Sertraline appears to only moderately increase risperidone levels at high doses. The combination of SSRIs and risperidone is generally useful, but has resulted in a number of adverse effects including priapism, extrapyramidal effects and the serotonin syndrome.

Clinical evidence

(a) Citalopram

A study in 7 patients found that citalopram had no effect on the plasma levels of risperidone or its active metabolite 9-hydroxyrisperidone.[1] A 29-year-old man with idiopathic priapism, about one 4-hour erection every 1 to 2 months, which typically woke him up, began to experience much longer bouts lasting 6 to 8 hours when he was given risperidone 4 mg daily. Within about 4 weeks of adding citalopram 40 mg daily to a slightly reduced risperidone dose (3 mg daily), he began to have almost daily erections lasting 12 hours. Three days after his dosages were changed to risperidone 3 mg twice daily with citalopram 20 mg daily he had an episode of such persistent priapism that emergency detumescence was needed. When both drugs were stopped he improved markedly and then only had occasional 4-hour erections, as before.[2]

(b) Fluoxetine

A pharmacokinetic study in 10 patients found that fluoxetine 20 mg daily raised the levels of risperidone 2 or 3 mg twice daily from 12 to 19 nanograms/mL after 3 weeks and to 56 nanograms/mL after 4 weeks. All patients experienced a rise in risperidone levels, but this varied from two to tenfold. One patient withdrew from the study because of severe akathisia and another two patients needed treatment with biperiden to control parkinsonian adverse effects.[3] Similar findings were found in another study.[4]

A 30-year-old woman taking valproate, clonazepam, and risperidone 3 mg daily for schizophrenia was also given fluoxetine 5 mg daily for a depressive disorder. The depression improved, but she noticed painful bilateral breast enlargement, which resolved when risperidone was stopped. Similar symptoms were noted when the risperidone was later restarted.[5]

An 18-year old developed extrapyramidal adverse effects, and later persistent dyskinetic tongue movements when given fluoxetine and risperidone,[6] and a 46-year-old man taking risperidone 2 mg daily developed urinary retention, extrapyramidal adverse effects, sedation and constipation, which developed over 10 days after fluoxetine 20 mg daily was started.[7] A 26-year-old man developed severe tardive dyskinesia during treatment with risperidone and fluoxetine.[8] A deterioration in obsessive-compulsive disorder has been seen when risperidone 3 mg daily was started in a patient who was partially successfully treated with fluoxetine 60 mg daily. After the addition of risperidone his condition returned to his pre-fluoxetine state. His condition gradually improved over a 3-month period once the risperidone was stopped. It was suggested that inhibition of metabolism of risperidone by fluoxetine may have resulted in elevated risperidone levels, leading to a deterioration in his condition.[9]

(c) Fluvoxamine

A 24-year-old woman taking risperidone 3 mg twice daily developed fever, limb rigidity, and confusion 3 days after starting fluvoxamine 50 mg daily. She required ventilation after her condition worsened and was eventually diagnosed as having either the serotonin syndrome or neuroleptic malignant syndrome. Both drugs were stopped and her condition resolved. She was later successfully treated with fluvoxamine 100 mg twice daily.[10] A study, 6 patients who had been taking risperidone 3 to 6 mg daily for at least 4 weeks, with fluvoxamine 100 mg daily for a further 8 weeks, found no changes in the pharmacokinetics of risperidone or its metabolite. However. 5 patients also enrolled into this study were increased to fluvoxamine 200 mg daily for weeks 5 to 8, and there was an 85% increase in plasma risperidone levels by the end of week 8. There was no change in the pharmacokinetics of the active metabolite, 9-hydroxyrisperidone and no adverse reactions to risperidone were noted.[11]

(d) Paroxetine

Paroxetine 20 mg daily was given to 10 patients taking risperidone 2 to 4 mg twice daily. After 4 weeks paroxetine had increased the levels of risperidone and its active metabolite, 9-hydroxyrisperidone, by 45%. Although the combination was generally well-tolerated one patient developed parkinsonian adverse effects.[12] Another study was undertaken in 12 patients taking risperidone 2 mg twice daily and paroxetine in doses increasing from 10 mg daily to 20 mg and 40 mg at 4 week intervals. The plasma levels of risperidone were increased 3.8-fold, 7.1-fold and 9.7-fold when given with paroxetine 10 mg, 20 mg and 40 mg daily, respectively. There was no change in the pharmacokinetics of the active metabolite,

9-hydroxyrisperidone. Negative symptoms of schizophrenia were improved, but there was an increased incidence of extrapyramidal adverse effects when patients took paroxetine 20 mg or 40 mg daily.[13]

A case report describes two elderly patients taking paroxetine who developed the serotonin syndrome within a couple of days of a risperidone dose increase. One patient's treatment had recently been changed from venlafaxine to paroxetine, which may have contributed to the reaction[14] (see 'SNRIs; Venlafaxine + Antidepressants', p.1212). A further case report describes a 53-year-old man who developed symptoms suggestive of the serotonin syndrome 10 weeks after starting to take risperidone 3 mg daily and paroxetine 20 mg daily. A deterioration in his condition occurred within 2 hours of doubling the dose of both drugs. His symptoms resolved 2 days after stopping both drugs.[15]

(e) Sertraline

A study in 11 patients taking risperidone 4 to 6 mg daily found that patients given sertraline 50 to 100 mg daily for 8 weeks had no significant changes in the pharmacokinetics of risperidone. However, 2 patients required a dose increase to 150 mg by week 8, and in these patients the risperidone levels were increased by 36% and 52%, respectively. No significant adverse effects were reported in any of the patients and no signs of risperidone toxicity were seen in the 2 patients with raised risperidone levels.[16]

Mechanism

Fluoxetine and paroxetine inhibit the cytochrome P450 isoenzyme CYP2D6 by which risperidone is metabolised, hence risperidone levels rise. This can lead to extrapyramidal adverse effects and, it has been suggested, the increased prolactin levels and gynaecomastia seen in one patient.[5] Sertraline is thought to have a dose-dependent effects on CYP2D6 inhibition.[16]

Many of the other reactions (sedation, urinary retention, priapism) appear to be a result of additive adverse effects of the SSRIs and risperidone. The serotonin syndrome can result when two drugs with serotonin effects are given together, see 'Additive or synergistic interactions', (p.9).

Importance and management

The elevated risperidone levels seen with fluoxetine and paroxetine appear to be well-documented and clinically significant. The manufacturers of risperidone[17,18] say that when adding either of these SSRIs the risperidone dose should be re-evaluated (presumably decreased). A one-third reduction in the risperidone dose has been suggested with fluoxetine.[4] The concurrent use of risperidone and sertraline in usual therapeutic doses appears to be safe and well-tolerated. The significance of the raised risperidone levels in the two patients taking high-dose sertraline is unclear, however neither patient developed risperidone toxicity. The case reports of the serotonin syndrome appear to be rare, but they should be borne in mind when prescribing SSRIs and risperidone together.

1. Avenoso A, Facciolà G, Scordo MG, Gitto C, Ferrante GD, Madia AG, Spina E. No effect of citalopram on plasma levels of clozapine, risperidone and their active metabolites in patients with chronic schizophrenia. *Clin Drug Invest* (1998) 16, 393–8.
2. Freudenreich O. Exacerbation of idiopathic priapism with risperidone-citalopram combination. *J Clin Psychiatry* (2002) 63, 249–50.
3. Spina E, Avenoso A, Scordo MG, Ancione M, Madia A, Gatti G, Perucca E. Inhibition of risperidone metabolism by fluoxetine in patients with schizophrenia: a clinically relevant pharmacokinetic interaction. *J Clin Psychopharmacol* (2002) 22, 419–23.
4. Bondolfi G, Eap CB, Bertschy G, Zullino D, Vermeulen A, Baumann P. The effect of fluoxetine on the pharmacokinetics and safety of risperidone in psychotic patients. *Pharmacopsychiatry* (2002) 35, 50–56.
5. Benazzi F. Gynecomastia with risperidone-fluoxetine combination. *Pharmacopsychiatry* (1999) 32, 41.
6. Daniel DG, Egan M, Hyde T. Probable neuroleptic induced tardive dyskinesia in association with combined SSRI and risperidone treatment. *Schizophr Res* (1996) 18, 149.
7. Bozikas V, Petrikis P, Karavatos A. Urinary retention caused after fluoxetine-risperidone combination. *J Psychopharmacol* (2001) 15, 142–3.
8. Dubbelman YD, Thung FH, Heeringa M. Ernstige tardieve dyskinesieën tijdens behandeling met risperidon en fluoxetine. *Ned Tijdschr Geneeskd* (1998) 142, 1508–11.
9. Andrade C. Risperidone may worsen fluoxetine-treated OCD. *J Clin Psychiatry* (1998) 59, 255–6.
10. Reeves RR, Mack JE, Bedingfield JJ. Neurotoxic syndrome associated with risperidone and fluvoxamine. *Ann Pharmacother* (2002) 36, 440–3.
11. D'Arrigo C, Migliardi G, Santoro V, Morgante L, Muscatello MR, Ancione M, Spina E. Effect of fluvoxamine on plasma risperidone concentrations in patients with schizophrenia. *Pharmacol Res* (2005) 52, 497–501.
12. Spina E, Avenoso A, Facciolà G, Scordo MG, Ancione M, Madia AG. Plasma concentrations of risperidone and 9-hydroxyrisperidone during combined treatment with paroxetine. *Ther Drug Monit* (2001) 23, 223–7.
13. Saito M, Yasui-Furukori M, Nakagami T, Furukori H, Kaneko S. Dose-dependent interaction of paroxetine with risperidone in schizophrenic patients. *J Clin Psychopharmacol* (2005) 25, 527–32.
14. Karki SD, Masood G-R. Combination risperidone and SSRI-induced serotonin syndrome. *Ann Pharmacother* (2003) 37, 388–91.
15. Hamilton S, Malone K. Serotonin syndrome during treatment with paroxetine and risperidone. *J Clin Psychopharmacol* (2000) 20, 103–5.
16. Spina E, D'Arrigo C, Migliardi G, Morgante L, Zoccali R, Ancione M, Madia A. Plasma risperidone concentrations during combined treatment with sertraline. *Ther Drug Monit* (2004) 26, 386–90.
17. Risperdal (Risperidone). Janssen-Cilag Ltd. UK Summary of product characteristics, July 2007.
18. Risperdal (Risperidone). Janssen Pharmaceutica Products. US Prescribing information, February 2007.

Risperidone + Tetracycline

A patient experienced a worsening of his tics when tetracycline was added to treatment with risperidone and sertraline.

Clinical evidence, mechanism, importance and management

A 15-year-old boy taking risperidone 1.5 mg twice daily and sertraline 100 mg daily was given tetracycline 250 mg twice daily. His tics worsened, and did not respond to an increase in his sertraline dosage from 100 mg to 150 mg daily. After stopping the tetracycline, his tics improved within a few weeks. The exact mechanism of this interaction is unclear, but it has been suggested that the tetracycline somehow reduced the activity of the risperidone. Induction of CYP2D6 by tetracycline was thought unlikely, and inactivation of the risperidone or its active metabolite was considered a possible explanation.[1] This appears to be the only reported case of this interaction and its general significance is unknown.

1. Steele M, Couturier J. A possible tetracycline-risperidone-sertraline interaction in an adolescent. *Can J Clin Pharmacol* (1999) 6, 15–17.

Risperidone + Tricyclic and related antidepressants

No pharmacokinetic interaction normally occurs between risperidone and amitriptyline or mirtazapine, but extrapyramidal reactions have been reported in one patient taking amitriptyline with risperidone.

Clinical evidence, mechanism, importance and management

(a) Amitriptyline

A study in 12 schizophrenic patients found that amitriptyline 50 to 100 mg daily had no effect on the serum levels of risperidone 3 mg twice daily.[1] However, a 26-year-old man taking amitriptyline 25 mg daily developed extrapyramidal reactions after his dosage of risperidone was increased from 2 to 4 mg daily.[2] On another occasion extrapyramidal adverse effects developed after risperidone 2 mg daily was added to treatment with amitriptyline 25 mg and fluoxetine 20 mg daily.[2] Both pharmacokinetic and pharmacodynamic reasons for this reaction have been suggested.[3] The cases illustrate that there is the potential for an adverse interaction between these drugs , which should be borne in mind when prescribing both drugs.

(b) Mirtazapine

A study in 8 patients taking risperidone in doses ranging from 3 to 8 mg daily found no significant change in the pharmacokinetics of risperidone and its metabolite, 9-hydroxyrisperidone when they were also given mirtazapine 30 mg daily.[4]

1. Sommers DK, Snyman JR, van Wyk M, Blom MW, Huang ML, Levron JC. Lack of effect of amitriptyline on risperidone pharmacokinetics in schizophrenic patients. *Int Clin Psychopharmacol* (1997) 12, 141–5.
2. Brown ES. Extrapyramidal side effects with low-dose risperidone. *Can J Psychiatry* (1997) 42, 325–6.
3. Caley CF. Extrapyramidal reactions from concurrent SSRI and atypical antipsychotic use. *Can J Psychiatry* (1998) 43, 307–8.
4. Zoccali R, Muscatello MR, La Torre D, Malara G, Canale A, Crucitti D, D'Arrigo C, Spina E. Lack of a pharmacokinetic interaction between mirtazapine and the newer antipsychotics clozapine, risperidone and olanzapine in patients with chronic schizophrenia. *Pharm Res* (2003) 48, 411–14.

Risperidone + Valproate

There are case reports describing oedema in patients taking risperidone and sodium valproate. Studies suggest that risperidone does not alter the pharmacokinetics of sodium valproate or valp-

roic acid, although cases of increased and decreased levels have been reported.

Clinical evidence, mechanism, importance and management

A study comparing 10 patients taking **sodium valproate** and risperidone with 23 patients taking risperidone alone found no significant difference between the two groups, suggesting that **sodium valproate** and risperidone can be safely used together.[1] A study in 21 patients with bipolar disorder who were given **valproate semisodium** 1 g daily with risperidone 2 mg daily for 2 days increasing to 4 mg daily for 12 days found no significant changes in the pharmacokinetics of valproate. Adverse effects were unaltered.[2] However, the valproate levels of a 10-year-old boy increased from 143 to 191 mg/L 5 days after he started to take risperidone (initially 2 mg daily, then later 3 mg daily). This was attributed to an interaction, the exact mechanism of which is unclear.[3,4] Conversely, a 15-year-old girl experienced a reduction in her valproate levels, from 80 to 57 microgram/mL when risperidone 1 mg three times daily was added to established treatment with **valproic acid**.[5] Another case report describes the development of generalised acute oedema in a schizophrenic patient when risperidone (titrated to 10 mg daily) was added to established **sodium valproate** treatment. The oedema was unresponsive to diuretics, but resolved when the risperidone dose was reduced to 2 mg. When the risperidone dose was later increased to 8 mg the oedema reappeared, so the risperidone was withdrawn.[6] A second case of oedema has been reported in a 35-year-old man who had taken **valproate semisodium** uneventfully for over 6 years. After treatment with risperidone for 2.5 weeks, significant oedema developed, which responded to treatment with hydrochlorothiazide and triamterene.[7] Note that both drugs can cause oedema alone.[8,9]

No special precautions seem necessary on concurrent use, but it is worth bearing these cases in mind when these two drugs are used together.

1. Spina E, Avenoso A, Facciolà G, Salemi M, Scordo MG, Giacobello T, Madia AG, Perucca E. Plasma concentrations of risperidone and 9-hydroxyrisperidone: effect of comedication with carbamazepine or valproate. *Ther Drug Monit* (2000) 22, 481–5.
2. Ravindran A, Silverstone P, Lacroix D, von Schaick E, Vermeulen A, Alexander J. Risperidone does not affect steady-state pharmacokinetics of divalproex sodium in patients with bipolar disorder. *Clin Pharmacokinet* (2004) 43, 733–40.
3. van Wattum PJ. Valproic acid and risperidone. *J Am Acad Child Adolesc Psychiatry* (2001) 40, 866–7.
4. Sund JK, Aamo T, Spigset O. Valproic acid and risperidone: a drug interaction? *J Am Acad Child Adolesc Psychiatry* (2003) 42, 1–2.
5. Bertoldo M. Valproic acid and risperidone. *J Am Acad Child Adolesc Psychiatry* (2002) 41, 632.
6. Sanders RD, Lehrer DS. Edema associated with addition of risperidone to valproate treatment. *J Clin Psychiatry* (1998) 59, 689–90.
7. Baldassano CF, Ghaemi SN. Generalized edema with risperidone: divalproex sodium treatment. *J Clin Psychiatry* (1996) 57, 422.
8. Risperdal (Risperidone). Janssen-Cilag Ltd. UK Summary of product characteristics, July 2007.
9. Depakote (Valproate semisodium). Sanofi-Aventis. UK Summary of product characteristics, September 2005.

Risperidone + Venlafaxine

No clinically relevant pharmacokinetic interaction appears to occur between risperidone and venlafaxine.

Clinical evidence, mechanism, importance and management

Steady-state venlafaxine 75 mg every 12 hours was found to increase the AUC of a single 1-mg oral dose of risperidone by about 32%, but the pharmacokinetic profile of the risperidone plus its active metabolite (9-hydroxyrisperidone) was not significantly changed, nor were any adverse events seen.[1] There would seem to be no reason for avoiding concurrent use.

1. Amchin J, Zarycranski W, Taylor KP, Albano D, Klockowski PM. Effect of venlafaxine on the pharmacokinetics of risperidone. *J Clin Pharmacol* (1999) 39, 297–309.

Ritanserin + Miscellaneous

Ritanserin does not interact with alcohol, cimetidine or ranitidine.

Clinical evidence, mechanism, importance and management

A study in 20 healthy subjects given ritanserin 10 mg with and without **alcohol** 0.5 g/kg found no pharmacokinetic or pharmacodynamic interactions between these drugs.[1] **Cimetidine** 800 mg daily or **ranitidine** 300 mg daily given to 9 healthy subjects for 11 days caused only small changes in the pharmacokinetics of a single 10-mg dose of ritanserin given on day 3. These changes were attributed to altered absorption,[2] but were of little or no clinical significance.

1. Estevez F, Parrillo S, Giusti M, Monti JM. Single-dose ritanserin and alcohol in healthy volunteers: a placebo-controlled trial. *Alcohol* (1995) 12, 541–5.
2. Trenk D, Seiler K-U, Buschmann M, Szathmary S, Benn H-P, Jähnchen E. Effect of concomitantly administered cimetidine or ranitidine on the pharmacokinetics of the 5-HT_2-receptor antagonist ritanserin. *J Clin Pharmacol* (1993) 33, 330–4.

Sertindole + Miscellaneous

The manufacturers of sertindole contraindicate the concurrent use of cimetidine, diltiazem, erythromycin, itraconazole, ketoconazole, terfenadine and verapamil because of an increased risk of cardiac arrhythmias. Carbamazepine and phenytoin reduce plasma sertindole levels whereas fluoxetine and paroxetine increase them. No clinically relevant interactions occur with alprazolam, antacids, food or tobacco smoking.

Clinical evidence, mechanism, importance and management

(a) Antacids or Food

A **standardised breakfast** or ***Maalox*** 45 mL had no significant effect on the AUC of a single 4-mg dose of sertindole in 16 healthy subjects, and only minor and unimportant changes occurred in maximum serum levels.[1,2] No special precautions are needed if sertindole is given with ***Maalox***, and it may be given without regard to meals.

(b) Antiepileptics

The metabolism of sertindole is markedly increased by enzyme inducers, such as **phenytoin** and **carbamazepine**, and plasma sertindole levels may be reduced by 2 to 3-fold. The manufacturers therefore say that the daily dosage of sertindole may need to be increased towards the upper end of the maximum dosage range to accommodate this interaction.[3,4]

(c) Azoles

No formal studies have been carried out on the use of sertindole with either **itraconazole** or **ketoconazole**, but because both of these antifungals are potent inhibitors of CYP3A it is expected that a marked rise in serum sertindole levels may occur if they are given. The manufacturers therefore say that concurrent use is contraindicated[3] because elevated serum levels are associated with a prolongation of the QTc interval and an increased risk of cardiac arrhythmias.

(d) Benzodiazepines

A pharmacokinetic study in 14 healthy subjects found only minor changes in pharmacokinetics of a single 1-mg dose of **alprazolam** due to the presence of sertindole 12 mg daily. The changes were considered to be clinically unimportant.[5]

(e) Calcium-channel blockers

Studies in patients found that **diltiazem**, **nifedipine** or **verapamil** resulted in a 20% reduction in the sertindole clearance, attributed to inhibition of CYP3A metabolism.[4] The manufacturers contraindicate concurrent use (**diltiazem** and **verapamil** are specifically named) as raised sertindole levels may prolong the QT interval.[3]

(f) Cimetidine

Because cimetidine is a potent inhibitor of the cytochrome P450 isoenzyme CYP3A it is expected that sertindole levels may be increased. The manufacturers therefore contraindicate concurrent use as raised sertindole levels may prolong the QT interval.[3]

(g) Erythromycin

A single 4-mg dose of sertindole was given to 10 healthy subjects before and after a course of erythromycin 250 mg every 6 hours for 10 days. The mean maximum serum levels were increased by 15%, probably because erythromycin inhibits the cytochrome P450 isoenzyme CYP3A4, but this was not considered to be clinically significant. The incidence of adverse events also rose (diarrhoea, abdominal pain, dizziness) but no ECG changes were seen.[6,7] Nevertheless the manufacturers contraindicate erythromycin because raised sertindole levels may prolong the QT interval.[3] Also note that intravenous erythromycin is itself associated with prolongation of the QT interval, see 'drugs that prolong the QT interval', (p.257).

(h) Protease inhibitors

The protease inhibitor are all, to varying degrees, inhibitors of the cytochrome P450 isoenzyme CYP3A4 by which sertindole is metabolised. The manufacturers therefore contraindicate concurrent use, as raised sertindole levels may lead to torsade de pointes arrhythmias, which are potentially life-threatening.[3]

(i) SSRIs

Fluoxetine and **paroxetine** are inhibitors of the cytochrome P450 isoenzyme CYP2D6. Concurrent use results in a two- to three-fold increase in sertindole plasma levels. The manufacturers advise that low maintenance doses of sertindole may be needed and recommend close ECG monitoring when doses are adjusted.[3] An isolated case report describes a man with paranoid psychosis and unipolar depression whose condition unexpectedly seriously worsened when **paroxetine** was stopped while continuing to take sertindole.[8]

(j) Terfenadine

A single 120-mg dose of terfenadine was given to 14 healthy subjects who had taken sertindole 20 mg daily for 5 days. The pharmacokinetics of neither drug was significantly changed, nor that of the metabolite of terfenadine (carboxyterfenadine), although it was concluded that sertindole may be a modest inhibitor of the first pass metabolism of terfenadine.[9,10] However, it was found that the combination caused an additive increase of 49 milliseconds in the QTc interval and therefore these two drugs are contraindicated by the manufacturer.[3]

(k) Tobacco

The clearance of sertindole is increased by tobacco smoking (probably because of the induction of cytochrome P450 isoenzymes) but no sertraline dosage alteration is thought necessary.[4]

1. Granneman GR, Wozniak P, Ereshefsky L, Silber C, Mack R. Effect of food and antacid on the bioavailability of sertindole (M94–164). Poster presentation at the American College of Neuropsychopharmacology Annual Meeting, San Juan, Puerto Rico, December 1996.
2. Wong S, Linnen P, Mack R, Granneman GR. Effects of food, antacid, and dosage form on the pharmacokinetics and relative bioavailability of sertindole in healthy volunteers. *Biopharm Drug Dispos* (1997) 18, 533–41.
3. Serdolect (Sertindole). Lundbeck Ltd. UK Summary of product characteristics, June 2003.
4. Granneman GR, Wozniak P, Ereshefsky L, Silber C, Mack R. Population pharmacokinetics of sertindole during long-term treatment of patients with schizophrenia. Poster presentation at the American College of Neuropsychopharmacology Annual Meeting, San Juan, Puerto Rico, December 1996.
5. Wong SL, Locke C, Staser J, Granneman GR. Lack of multiple dosing effect of sertindole on the pharmacokinetics of alprazolam in healthy volunteers. *Psychopharmacology (Berl)* (1998) 135, 236–41.
6. Granneman GR, Wozniak P, Ereshefsky L, Silber C, Mack R. Effect of erythromycin on the pharmacokinetics of sertindole (M94–145). Poster presentation at the American College of Neuropsychopharmacology Annual Meeting, San Juan, Puerto Rico, December 1996.
7. Wong SL, Cao G, Mack RJ, Granneman GR. The effect of erythromycin on the CYP3A component of sertindole clearance in healthy volunteers. *J Clin Pharmacol* (1997) 37, 1056–61.
8. Walker-Kinnear M, McnNaughton S. Paroxetine discontinuation syndrome in association with sertindole therapy. *Br J Psychiatry* (1997) 170, 389.
9. Granneman GR, Wozniak P, Ereshefsky L, Silber C, Mack R. Effect of sertindole on the pharmacokinetics of terfenadine (M94–146). Poster presentation at the American College of Neuropsychopharmacology Annual Meeting, San Juan, Puerto Rico, December 1996.
10. Wong SL, Cao G, Mack R, Granneman GR. Lack of CYP3A inhibition effects of sertindole on terfenadine in healthy volunteers. *Int J Clin Pharmacol Ther* (1998) 36, 146–51.

Thioridazine + Naltrexone

Extreme lethargy occurred when two patients taking thioridazine were given naltrexone.

Clinical evidence, mechanism, importance and management

Two schizophrenic patients taking thioridazine 50 to 200 mg three times daily for at least one year took part in a pilot project to assess the efficacy of naltrexone for the treatment of tardive dyskinesias. Both patients tolerated the first challenge dose of intravenous naltrexone 800 micrograms without problems, but experienced extreme lethargy and slept almost continuously after the second naltrexone dose of 50 to 100 mg orally. The severe lethargy resolved within 12 hours of stopping the naltrexone.[1] The reasons for this reaction are not understood. Information seems to be limited to this report and the general importance of this interaction is unknown. There seems to be nothing documented about other phenothiazines. Note that a case report has described excessive sleepiness and lethargy in a 58-year-old man who took a single 100-mg dose of naltrexone alone,[2] so an interaction is by no means established.

1. Maany I, O'Brien CP, Woody G. Interaction between thioridazine and naltrexone. *Am J Psychiatry* (1987) 144, 966.
2. Malcolm R, Gabel T, Morton A. Idiosyncratic reaction to naltrexone augmented by thioridazine. *Am J Psychiatry* (1988) 145, 773–4.

Thioridazine + Phenylpropanolamine

A single case report describes fatal ventricular fibrillation, which was attributed to the use of thioridazine with phenylpropanolamine.

Clinical evidence, mechanism, importance and management

A 27-year-old schizophrenic woman who was taking thioridazine 100 mg daily and procyclidine 2.5 mg twice daily was found dead in bed 2 hours after taking a single capsule of *Contac C* (phenylpropanolamine 50 mg with chlorphenamine 4 mg). The principal cause of death was attributed to ventricular fibrillation.[1] Just why this happened is not understood but it is suggested that it may have been due to the combined effects of the thioridazine (known to be cardiotoxic and to cause T-wave abnormalities) and the phenylpropanolamine (possibly able to cause ventricular arrhythmias).

The general importance of this alleged interaction is uncertain but the authors of the report suggest that ephedrine-like drugs such as phenylpropanolamine should not be given to patients taking thioridazine or **mesoridazine**.

1. Chouinard G, Ghadirian AM, Jones BD. Death attributed to ventricular arrhythmia induced by thioridazine in combination with a single Contac C capsule. *Can Med Assoc J* (1978) 119, 729–31.

Tiotixene + Enzyme inhibitors

A group of patients taking enzyme inhibitors (cimetidine, doxepin, isoniazid, nortriptyline, propranolol) had a tiotixene clearance of 9.51 L/minute, which was 71% less than that seen in patients taking tiotixene alone.[1] It seems possible that the tiotixene dose will need to be reduced in those taking these drugs but this needs confirmation. Monitor concurrent use for tiotixene adverse effects and adjust the dose accordingly.

1. Ereshefsky L, Saklad SR, Watanabe MD, Davis CM, Jann MW. Thiothixene pharmacokinetic interactions: a study of hepatic enzyme inducers, clearance inhibitors, and demographic variables. *J Clin Psychopharmacol* (1991) 11, 296–301.

Trifluoperazine + Venlafaxine

A case of neuroleptic malignant syndrome has been reported in a patient taking trifluoperazine 1 mg daily who then took one dose of venlafaxine 75 mg. This may have occurred as a result of dopamine inhibition by the two drugs.[1] A suggestion that the symptoms seen may have been due to 'the serotonin syndrome', (p.9), has also been made.[2]

1. Nimmagadda SR, Ryan DH, Atkin SL. Neuroleptic malignant syndrome after venlafaxine. *Lancet* (2000) 354, 289–90.
2. Cassidy EM, O'Kearne V. Neuroleptic malignant syndrome after venlafaxine. *Lancet* (2000) 355, 2164–5.

Ziprasidone + Carbamazepine

Low doses of carbamazepine do not appear to affect the pharmacokinetics of ziprasidone.

Clinical evidence, mechanism, importance and management

In a randomised study, healthy subjects were given ziprasidone 20 mg twice daily with either placebo (10 subjects), or carbamazepine 200 mg twice daily for 5 doses (9 subjects). It was found that the AUC_{0-12} and maximum serum levels of ziprasidone were reduced by 36% and 27%, respectively, in the carbamazepine group. It was concluded that while induction of the cytochrome P450 isoenzyme CYP3A4 by carbamazepine is responsible for this modest reduction in the steady-state levels of ziprasidone, the extent is not clinically relevant.[1] No special precautions would seem to be needed with this dosage of carbamazepine,[1] but there is the possibility that higher doses may interact to a greater extent. In this situation it would be prudent to monitor concurrent use to ensure ziprasidone is effective.

1. Miceli JJ, Anziano RJ, Robarge L, Hansen RA. Laurent A. The effect of carbamazepine on the steady-state pharmacokinetics of ziprasidone in healthy volunteers. *Br J Clin Pharmacol* (2000) 49 (Suppl 1), 65S–70S.

Ziprasidone + Ketoconazole

Ketoconazole moderately increases ziprasidone levels but this is not expected to be clinically relevant.

Clinical evidence, mechanism, importance and management

In a randomised, placebo-controlled study, 14 healthy subjects were given a 40-mg dose of ziprasidone before and after taking ketoconazole 400 mg daily for 6 days. It was found that ketoconazole increased the AUC and maximum serum levels of ziprasidone by 33% and 34%, respectively. This modest rise in levels probably occurs because ketoconazole inhibits the cytochrome P450 isoenzyme CYP3A4 by which ziprasidone is metabolised. However, it was concluded that the increase is not clinically relevant.[1] No special precautions would therefore seem to be needed on concurrent use.

1. Miceli JJ, Smith M, Robarge L, Morse T, Laurent A. The effects of ketoconazole on ziprasidone pharmacokinetics – a placebo-controlled crossover study in healthy volunteers. *Br J Clin Pharmacol* (2000) 49 (Suppl 1), 71S–76S.

Ziprasidone + Lithium

Ziprasidone does not appear to alter the pharmacokinetics of lithium.

Clinical evidence, mechanism, importance and management

A randomised, placebo-controlled study in 25 healthy subjects taking lithium carbonate 450 mg twice daily for 15 days, found that ziprasidone 20 mg twice daily on days 9 to 11, followed by 40 mg twice daily on days 12 to 15 caused only a small increase in the steady-state serum-lithium levels (14% compared with 11% in the placebo group). A 5% reduction in renal clearance was seen in the ziprasidone group and a 9% reduction was seen in the placebo group. These differences were neither statistically nor clinically significant.[1] No special precautions would therefore seem to be necessary if ziprasidone is given to patients taking lithium.

1. Apseloff G, Mullet D, Wilner KD, Anziano RJ, Tensfeldt TG, Pelletier SM, Gerber N. The effects of ziprasidone on steady-state lithium levels and renal clearance of lithium. *Br J Clin Pharmacol* (2000) 49 (Suppl 1), 61S–64S.

Ziprasidone + Miscellaneous

The manufacturers warn of the possible risks of giving ziprasidone with drugs that prolong the QT interval, and of the possible antagonism that may occur with levodopa and other dopamine agonists. Ziprasidone appears not to interact to a clinically relevant extent with an aluminium/magnesium hydroxide antacid, benzatropine, cimetidine, lorazepam, propranolol or tobacco smoking.

Clinical evidence, mechanism, importance and management

(a) Antacids or Cimetidine

A single 40-mg oral dose of ziprasidone were given to 10 healthy subjects either alone, with cimetidine 800 mg daily for 2 days, or with three 30-mL doses of ***Maalox*** (**aluminium/magnesium hydroxide**). The only change in the pharmacokinetics of ziprasidone was a 6% increase in the AUC with cimetidine. It was concluded that no special precautions are needed if either of these drugs and ziprasidone are given concurrently, and that any inhibition of the cytochrome P450 isoenzyme CYP3A4 is irrelevant because alternative metabolic pathways are available. The results of the study with cimetidine also suggest that other non-specific inhibitors of cytochrome P450 are unlikely to alter the ziprasidone pharmacokinetics.[1]

(b) Drugs that prolong the QT interval

Studies in healthy subjects found that ziprasidone 160 mg increased the QTc interval by about 10 milliseconds. While only a relatively moderate increase in the QT interval actually occurs with ziprasidone, because of the possibility of additive effects with some other drugs (and the attendant risk of torsade de pointes), to be on the safe side the manufacturers of ziprasidone contraindicate its use with other drugs that can prolong the QT interval.[2] A list of QT-prolonging drugs is to be found in 'Table 9.2', (p.257). A case has been reported of a 70-year-old man who took **quetiapine** and ziprasidone and who developed cardiac arrhythmias with extrasystoles, and a prolonged QTc interval of 482 milliseconds, an increase of 65 milliseconds from his value with **quetiapine** alone. On stopping **quetiapine** and reducing the dose of ziprasidone, his QTc interval normalised.[3]

(c) Levodopa and dopamine agonists

The mechanism by which ziprasidone acts to control schizophrenia is not understood, but it is known to be an antagonist of dopamine type 2 (D_2) receptors and therefore it may possibly oppose the effects of levodopa and other dopamine agonists. There seem to be no clinical reports of problems during concurrent use, but good monitoring would be advisable if ziprasidone is given with any dopamine agonist.

(d) Miscellaneous drugs

The manufacturers say that population pharmacokinetic analysis of schizophrenic patients who were enrolled in clinical studies showed that no significant pharmacokinetic interactions occurred with **benzatropine**, **lorazepam** or **propranolol**.[2] The manufacturers also point out that since ziprasidone is not metabolised by the cytochrome P450 isoenzyme CYP1A2, smoking should not affect its pharmacokinetics. This is borne out by studies in patients, which did not reveal any differences in the pharmacokinetics of ziprasidone between **tobacco smokers** and non-smokers.[2]

1. Wilner KD, Hansen RA, Folger CJ, Geoffroy P. The pharmacokinetics of ziprasidone in healthy volunteers treated with cimetidine or antacid. *Br J Clin Pharmacol* (2000) 49 (Suppl 1), 57S–60S.
2. Geodon (Ziprasidone). Pfizer Inc. US prescribing information, May 2005.
3. Minov C. QTc-Zeitverlängerung unter ziprasidon in kombination mit quetiapin. *Psychiatr Prax* (2004) 31, S142–4.

Zotepine + Miscellaneous

There appears to be little or no information about adverse interactions between zotepine and other drugs, but the manufacturers warn about the concurrent use of antihypertensives, anaesthetics, antipsychotics, and drugs that prolong the QTc interval. Two cases of deep vein thrombosis have been reported in patients taking zotepine with paroxetine.

Clinical evidence, mechanism, importance and management

(a) Antihypertensives

Zotepine has alpha-adrenergic blocking properties, which may cause orthostatic hypotension, especially when treatment is first started or if the dosage is increased. The manufacturers advise caution when it is given with hypotensive agents, including some **anaesthetics**, the implication being that any orthostatic hypotension may possibly be worsened. If patients feel faint and dizzy when they stand up, they should be advised to get up more slowly, and if necessary, a smaller dosage should be used.[1]

(b) Antimuscarinics

Biperiden 6 mg daily for 2 weeks was found not to affect the pharmacokinetics of zotepine in a study in 21 patients.[2]

(c) Antipsychotics

The manufacturers point out that, as with some other antipsychotics, zotepine has clear pro-convulsive effects, which may be additive with other antipsychotics, particularly if high doses of either or both drugs are used.

They therefore recommend that zotepine doses above 300 mg daily or the concurrent use of high doses of other antipsychotics should be avoided.[1]

(d) Desipramine

No pharmacokinetic interaction was seen when zotepine was given with desipramine, indicating that the cytochrome P450 isoenzyme CYP2D6 is not involved in the metabolism of zotepine.[1]

(e) Diazepam or Fluoxetine

In a clinical interaction study, fluoxetine and diazepam increased the plasma concentrations of zotepine and norzotepine. The manufacturers advise caution if these drugs are given concurrently.[1]

(f) Drugs that prolong the QT interval

The manufacturers of zotepine advise caution when treating patients taking drugs known to prolong the QTc interval (or those with coronary heart disease or at risk of hypokalaemia) because zotepine also shows a dose-related QTc interval prolongation,[1] the implication being that the effects may be additive. See also 'Drugs that prolong the QT interval + Other drugs that prolong the QT interval', p.257.

(g) Paroxetine

Two case reports have described mobile, elderly male patients who developed deep vein thrombosis when taking paroxetine and zotepine. In the first case the patient was taking paroxetine 40 mg daily, and zotepine was added to his treatment 3 weeks later, initially at a dose of 75 mg daily, then increased to 150 mg daily. After 17 days of treatment with zotepine 150 mg daily the patient developed significant swelling of the right leg, and a deep vein thrombosis was diagnosed by Doppler studies and venography. The second patient also received paroxetine 40 mg daily to which was added zotepine 150 mg daily, and within 3 days of starting zotepine, the patient had developed painful swelling of the right calf, dyspnoea and tachycardia. A deep vein thrombosis was confirmed. They were part of a review of 150 patients consecutively admitted to a psychiatric ward. They were the only two patients who received this combination of drugs, and the only two who developed a thromboembolism. The mechanism of this interaction is unclear.[3]

1. Zoleptil (Zotepine). Orion Pharma UK Ltd. UK Summary of product characteristics, April 2002.
2. Otani K, Hirano T, Kondo T, Kaneko S, Fukushima Y, Noda K, Tashiro Y. Biperiden and piroheptine do not affect the serum level of zotepine, a new antipsychotic drug. *Br J Psychiatry* (1990) 157, 128–30.
3. Pantel J, Schröder J, Eysenbach, K, Mundt Ch. Two cases of deep vein thrombosis associated with a combined paroxetine and zotepine therapy. *Pharmacopsychiatry* (1997) 30, 109–11.

21

Antivirals

This section is concerned with the drugs used to treat viral infections. These drugs may be grouped by the viral infections they are used to treat, and also by drug class (see 'Table 21.1', (p.773)). Where antivirals affect other drugs the interactions are generally covered elsewhere.

Antivirals active against herpes

(a) Nucleoside analogues

The nucleoside analogues are principally eliminated unchanged by the kidneys by a process of active tubular secretion as well as glomerular filtration. The few interactions with these drugs mainly involve altered renal clearance (e.g. probenecid), but since they have a wide therapeutic range, even these interactions are of debatable clinical relevance. Cytochrome P450-mediated interactions are not important for this group of drugs.

Antiretrovirals active against HIV

Treatment of HIV infection commonly requires a combination of 3 to 4 antiretrovirals, termed highly active antiretroviral therapy (HAART). In addition, patients often receive a large number of other drugs for comorbid conditions. This markedly increases the risk of drug interactions and complicates their assessment.

(a) CCR5 antagonists

CCR5 antagonists are a new class of entry inhibitors currently under development. Maraviroc is the nearest to marketing, and is a substrate of CYP3A4. Because of this, CYP3A4 inducers (e.g. efavirenz) lower its levels and CYP3A4 inhibitors (e.g. protease inhibitors) increase its levels.

(b) Fusion inhibitors

The fusion inhibitor, enfuvirtide, is a peptide. It does not cause cytochrome P450-mediated drug interactions, and is not affected by potent enzyme inducers (rifampicin) or inhibitors (ritonavir).

(c) Non-nucleoside reverse transcriptase inhibitors (NNRTIs)

The NNRTIs are extensively metabolised by the cytochrome P450 isoenzyme system, particularly by CYP3A4. They are also inducers (nevirapine, efavirenz) or inhibitors (delavirdine) of CYP3A4. NNRTIs would therefore be expected to interact with each other, and with protease inhibitors, but not with NRTIs (see below). They also have the potential to interact with other drugs metabolised by CYP3A4, and are affected by CYP3A4 inhibitors and inducers. Delavirdine and efavirenz may also inhibit some other P450 isoenzymes. For a summary, see 'Table 21.2', (p.773).

(d) Nucleoside reverse transcriptase inhibitors (NRTIs)

NRTIs are prodrugs, which need to be activated by phosphorylation within cells to a triphosphate anabolite. Drugs may therefore interact with NRTIs by increasing or decreasing intracellular activation. NRTIs may also interact with each other by this mechanism. This interaction mechanism is studied *in vitro*, and clinical data are often not available, or the clinical relevance is unclear. Nevertheless, it is generally recommended that drugs inhibiting the intracellular activation of NRTIs are not used concurrently (e.g. 'doxorubicin and stavudine', (p.808), or 'zidovudine and stavudine', (p.800)). 'Hydroxycarbamide', (p.799), may increase the intracellular activation of NRTIs.

NRTIs are water soluble, and are mainly eliminated by the kidneys (didanosine, lamivudine, stavudine, and zalcitabine) or undergo hepatic glucuronidation (abacavir, zidovudine). The few important interactions with these drugs primarily involve altered renal clearance. For zidovudine (and possibly abacavir) some interactions occur via altered glucuronidation, but the clinical relevance of these are less clear (e.g. 'rifampicin', (p.792)). Cytochrome P450-mediated interactions are not important for this class of drugs.

Some of the didanosine preparations (e.g. chewable tablets) are formulated with antacid buffers that are intended to facilitate didanosine absorption by minimising acid-induced hydrolysis in the stomach. These preparations can therefore alter the absorption of other drugs that are affected by antacids (e.g. azole antifungals, quinolone antibacterials, tetracyclines). This interaction may be minimised by separating administration by at least 2 hours. Alternatively, the enteric-coated preparation of didanosine (gastro-resistant capsules) may be used.

(e) Protease Inhibitors

The protease inhibitors are extensively metabolised by the cytochrome P450 isoenzyme system, particularly by CYP3A4. All of them inhibit CYP3A4, with ritonavir being the most potent inhibitor, followed by indinavir, nelfinavir, amprenavir, and saquinavir. The protease inhibitors therefore have the potential to interact with other drugs metabolised by CYP3A4, and are also affected by CYP3A4 inhibitors and inducers. Ritonavir and nelfinavir also affect some other cytochrome P450 isoenzymes, as summarised in 'Table 21.2', (p.773). In addition, protease inhibitors are substrates as well as inhibitors of P-glycoprotein. Protease inhibitors therefore have the potential to interact with each other, and with NNRTIs, but are not likely to interact with NRTIs.

The plasma level of protease inhibitors is thought to be critical in maintaining efficacy and minimising the potential for development of viral resistance. Therefore even modest reductions in levels are potentially clinically important.

General references

1. Barry M, Mulcahy F, Merry C, Gibbons S, Back D. Pharmacokinetics and potential interactions amongst antiretroviral agents used to treat patients with HIV infection. *Clin Pharmacokinet* (1999) 36, 289–304.
2. de Maat MMR, Ekhart GC, Huitema ADR, Koks CHW, Mulder JW, Beijnen JH. Drug interactions between antiretroviral drugs and comedicated agents. *Clin Pharmacokinet* (2003) 42, 223–82.

Table 21.1 Classification of Antivirals

Group	*Drugs*
Antivirals for hepatitis viruses	
Nucleoside analogues	Entecavir, Lamivudine, Telbivudine
Nucleotide analogues	Adefovir
Miscellaneous	Interferon alfa, Peginterferon alfa, Ribavirin
Antivirals for herpes viruses	
Guanine nucleoside analogues	Aciclovir, Famciclovir, Ganciclovir, Penciclovir, Valaciclovir, Valganciclovir
Other nucleoside analogues	Idoxuridine, Trifluridine, Vidarabine
Nucleotide analogues	Cidofovir, Fomivirsen
Miscellaneous	Foscarnet sodium, Inosine pranobex
Antivirals for HIV infection (antiretrovirals)	
CCR5 antagonists	Maraviroc
HIV-fusion inhibitors	Enfuvirtide
Non-nucleoside reverse transcriptase inhibitors (NNRTIs)	Delavirdine, Efavirenz, Nevirapine
Nucleoside reverse transcriptase inhibitors (NRTIs)	Abacavir, Didanosine, Emtricitabine, Lamivudine, Stavudine, Zalcitabine, Zidovudine
Nucleotide reverse transcriptase inhibitors	Tenofovir
Protease inhibitors	Amprenavir, Atazanavir, Darunavir, Fosamprenavir, Indinavir, Lopinavir, Nelfinavir, Ritonavir, Saquinavir, Tipranavir
Antivirals for influenza	
Neuraminidase inhibitors	Oseltamivir, Zanamivir
Others	Amantadine, Rimantadine

Table 21.2 Summary of the effect of the protease inhibitors and NNRTIs on cytochrome P450 isoenzymes

Antiviral	*Substrate*	*Inhibits*	*Induces*
Protease inhibitors			
Amprenavir or Fosamprenavir	CYP3A4	CYP3A4	
Atazanavir	CYP3A4	CYP3A4	
Darunavir	CYP3A4	CYP3A4	
Indinavir	CYP3A4	CYP3A4	
Lopinavir	CYP3A4	CYP3A4	
Nelfinavir	CYP3A4, CYP2C19, CYP2C9, CYP2D6	CYP3A4	
Ritonavir	CYP3A4, CYP2D6	CYP3A4, CYP2D6	CYP3A4
Saquinavir	CYP3A4	CYP3A4	
Tipranavir	CYP3A4	CYP3A4, CYP2D6	CYP3A4
NNRTIs (Non-nucleoside reverse transcriptase inhibitors)			
Delavirdine	CYP3A4, CYP2D6	CYP3A4, CYP2C9, CYP2D6, CYP2C19	
Efavirenz	CYP3A4, CYP2B6	CYP3A4, CYP2C9, CYP2C19	CYP3A4
Nevirapine	CYP3A4		CYP3A4

Aciclovir and related drugs + Antacids

Valaciclovir does not interact with an aluminium/magnesium hydroxide antacid.

Clinical evidence, mechanism, importance and management

On three separate occasions, 18 healthy subjects were given a single 1-g oral dose of valaciclovir, either alone, 65 minutes before, or 30 minutes after they took 30 mL of *Maalox* (**aluminium/magnesium hydroxide**). The pharmacokinetics of aciclovir (the active metabolite of valaciclovir) remained unchanged. It was concluded that no special precautions are needed if these drugs are taken together, and the authors of the report also suggest that it is unlikely that other antacids will interact.[1]

1. de Bony F, Bidault R, Peck R, Posner J. Lack of interaction between valaciclovir, the L-valyl ester of acyclovir, and Maalox antacid. *J Antimicrob Chemother* (1996) 37, 383–7.

Aciclovir and related drugs + Cephalosporins

Retrospective data from children suggest that ceftriaxone might have increased the renal toxicity of intravenous aciclovir. Cefalexin does not appear to alter the absorption of valaciclovir to a clinically relevant extent.

Clinical evidence, mechanism, importance and management

(a) Cefalexin

In a single-dose, crossover study involving 16 healthy subjects, the concurrent use of cefalexin 500 mg and **valaciclovir** 500 mg caused only a minimal mean 7.1% reduction in the AUC of aciclovir (the metabolite of **valaciclovir**). However, this reduction was only seen if one subject who had an increase in aciclovir AUC was excluded. Furthermore, there was considerable interindividual variability in the effects of cefalexin.

Both cefalexin and valaciclovir are substrates for human peptide transporter 1 (hPEPT1), and *in vitro* and *animal* data indicated that cefalexin might markedly reduce valaciclovir absorption.[1] However, the findings in this clinical study show a minimal interaction. No special precautions appear to be needed on concurrent use.

(b) Ceftriaxone

A retrospective analysis of 17 children who had received intravenous aciclovir and ceftriaxone for suspected meningo-encephalitis revealed that 12 developed a significant increase in serum creatinine, and three of these developed acute renal failure. This rate of renal toxicity is higher than that seen with aciclovir alone, and was attributed to the concurrent use of ceftriaxone. The dose of aciclovir correlated with nephrotoxicity. The authors concluded that caution is required with the combination, and that renal function should be monitored if both drugs are needed.[2]

1. Phan DD, Chin-Hong P, Lin ET, Anderle P, Sadee W, Guglielmo BJ. Intra- and interindividual variabilities of valacyclovir oral bioavailability and effect of coadministration of an hPEPT1 inhibitor. *Antimicrob Agents Chemother* (2003) 47, 2351–3.
2. Vomiero G, Carpenter B, Robb I, Filler G. Combination of ceftriaxone and acyclovir - an underestimated nephrotoxic potential? *Pediatr Nephrol* (2002) 17, 633–7.

Aciclovir and related drugs + Cimetidine

Single-dose studies have found that cimetidine increases the AUC of aciclovir and valaciclovir, but this is thought unlikely to be clinically important. No clinically important interaction appears to occur if famciclovir is given with cimetidine.

Clinical evidence

(a) Aciclovir or Valaciclovir

Twelve healthy subjects were given a 1-g dose of valaciclovir alone or with cimetidine 800 mg, taken 10 hours and 1 hour before. The AUC_{0-3} for the prodrug valaciclovir was increased by 73% by cimetidine, and the AUC_{0-24} for the active metabolite of valaciclovir, aciclovir, was increased by 27%. The renal clearance of aciclovir was reduced by 22%, although the total urinary recovery of aciclovir was unchanged.[1]

(b) Famciclovir

In a study, 12 healthy subjects were given cimetidine 400 mg twice daily for 8 days with a single 500-mg dose of famciclovir, a prodrug for penciclovir, on the last day. The AUC of penciclovir was increased by about 18% by cimetidine, but there was no change in renal clearance.[2,3]

Mechanism

The increase in aciclovir AUC with cimetidine is attributable to a reduction in its renal excretion, probably due to competition for secretion by the kidney tubules.[1] When 'probenecid', (p.775), a renal tubular secretion competitor, and cimetidine were both given the effects on aciclovir were greater than either drug alone.[1] Cimetidine does not significantly alter the pharmacokinetics of famciclovir/penciclovir.[3]

Importance and management

These interactions are established but, because aciclovir has such a wide therapeutic index,[4] the authors of the study suggest that its interaction with cimetidine is probably clinically unimportant.[1] It seems likely that no changes in the usual dosages of aciclovir or valaciclovir will be needed in patients also taking cimetidine. However, the UK manufacturer states that caution is required with high doses of valaciclovir, and that alternatives to cimetidine could be considered in this situation.[4] No special precautions would seem necessary if cimetidine is used with famciclovir.

1. De Bony F, Tod M, Bidault R, On NT, Posner J, Rolan P. Multiple interactions of cimetidine and probenecid with valaciclovir and its metabolite acyclovir. *Antimicrob Agents Chemother* (2002) 46, 458–63.
2. Pratt SK, Fowles SE, Pierce DM, Prince WT. An investigation of the potential interaction between cimetidine and famciclovir in non-patient volunteers. *Br J Clin Pharmacol* (1991) 32, 656P–657P.
3. Daniels S, Schentag JJ. Drug interaction studies and safety of famciclovir in healthy volunteers: a review. *Antiviral Chem Chemother* (1993) 4 (Suppl 1), 57–64.
4. Valtrex (Valaciclovir). GlaxoSmithKline UK. UK Summary of product characteristics, September 2005.

Aciclovir and related drugs + Hydrochlorothiazide

Hydrochlorothiazide does not affect the pharmacokinetics or safety profile of valaciclovir.

Clinical evidence, mechanism, importance and management

A study in a group of elderly subjects (65 to 83 years old) given valaciclovir 500 mg or 1 g three times daily for 8 days found that its safety profile was unchanged in the presence of hydrochlorothiazide, and was similar to that in young healthy subjects.[1] The pharmacokinetics of the active metabolite of valaciclovir, aciclovir, were not significantly different.[1] There would seem to be no reason for avoiding the concurrent use of either valaciclovir or aciclovir and hydrochlorothiazide.

1. Wang LH, Schultz M, Weller S, Smiley ML, Blum MR. Pharmacokinetics and safety of multiple-dose valaciclovir in geriatric volunteers with and without concomitant diuretic therapy. *Antimicrob Agents Chemother* (1996) 40, 80–5.

Aciclovir and related drugs + Mycophenolate

The concurrent use of aciclovir or ganciclovir and mycophenolate mofetil does not appear to significantly affect the pharmacokinetics of either drug, but the manufacturers recommend care in renal impairment. There are reports of neutropenia in patients taking mycophenolate with valaciclovir or ganciclovir.

Clinical evidence, mechanism, importance and management

(a) Aciclovir or Valaciclovir

In a three-period crossover study healthy subjects were given a single dose of oral aciclovir 800 mg and mycophenolate mofetil 1 g, both together and alone. The renal clearances of both drugs were not significantly altered by concurrent use. The AUC of aciclovir was increased by about 17% (not statistically significant), that of mycophenolic acid by about 9% (not significant), and that of the glucuronide metabolite of mycophenolate by about 9%. It was concluded that none of these changes was likely to be clinically significant.[1,2] In another single-dose study in healthy subjects, a bigger 31% increase in the AUC of aciclovir was seen when it was given with mycophenolate mofetil: there were no changes to mycophenolic acid pharmacokinetics. The concurrent use of valaciclovir 2 g with mycophenolate mofetil 1 g did not alter aciclovir pharmacokinetics, and the only change in mycophenolate pharmacokinetics was a 12% decrease in AUC of its glucuronide metabolite.[3] None of these changes are likely to be clinically important in patients with normal renal function. The manufacturers of mycophenolate state that, in renal impairment there may be competition for tubular secretion and that further increases in concentrations of both aciclovir and mycophenolate may occur.[4,5]

Note that some data suggest that mycophenolate potentiates the antiherpes virus activity of aciclovir, which may be clinically useful.[6] There is a case report of a renal transplant patient taking, amongst other drugs, mycophenolate mofetil 1 g twice daily who developed neutropenia after starting valaciclovir 6 g daily for prophylactic treatment of a cytomegalovirus infection after successful treatment with ganciclovir. The neutropenia resolved on stopping the valaciclovir. The authors suggested that mycophenolate may increase the haematotoxic effect of valaciclovir especially at high doses.[7] Neutropenia is a rare adverse effect of valaciclovir alone. Bear the possibility of an interaction in mind should neutropenia occur with the combination.

(b) Ganciclovir or Valganciclovir

A crossover study in 12 transplant patients found no pharmacokinetic interaction between a single 1.5-g oral dose of mycophenolate mofetil and intravenous ganciclovir 5 mg/kg, but the renal clearance of ganciclovir was slightly reduced, by 12%.[8] However, the manufacturers note that it is anticipated that the concurrent use of these two drugs will result in increases in ganciclovir levels, and levels of the inactive metabolite of mycophenolate, due to competition for renal tubular secretion. They suggest careful monitoring in patients with renal impairment given both drugs.[4,5,9] These cautions are also applied to the ganciclovir prodrug valganciclovir.[10,11]

Five cases of neutrophil dysplasia in transplant patients appeared to be related to the combination of ganciclovir and mycophenolate, rather than mycophenolate alone.[12] This emphasises the need for caution with concurrent use. The manufacturer of valganciclovir says that since both mycophenolate mofetil and ganciclovir have the potential to cause neutropenia and leucopenia, patients should be monitored for additive toxicity.[10]

Note that some data suggests that mycophenolate potentiates the antiherpes virus activity of ganciclovir, which may be clinically useful.[6]

1. Shah J, Juan D, Bullingham R, Wong B, Wong R, Fu C. A single dose drug interaction study of mycophenolate mofetil and acyclovir in normal subjects. *J Clin Pharmacol* (1994) 34, 1029.
2. Syntex. A single-dose, pharmacokinetic drug interaction study of oral mycophenolate mofetil and oral acyclovir in normal subjects. Data on file, 1994.
3. Gimenez F, Foeillet E, Bourdon O, Weller S, Garret C, Bidault R, Singlas E. Evaluation of pharmacokinetic interactions after oral administration of mycophenolate mofetil and valaciclovir or aciclovir to healthy subjects. *Clin Pharmacokinet* (2004) 43, 685–92.
4. CellCept (Mycophenolate mofetil). Roche Products Ltd. UK Summary of product characteristics, March 2006.
5. CellCept (Mycophenolate mofetil). Roche Laboratories Inc. US Prescribing information, October 2005.
6. Neyts J, Andrei G, De Clercq E. The novel immunosuppressive agent mycophenolate mofetil markedly potentiates the antiherpesvirus activities of acyclovir, ganciclovir, and penciclovir in vitro and in vivo. *Antimicrob Agents Chemother* (1998) 42, 216–22.
7. Royer B, Zanetta G, Bérard M, Davani S, Tanter Y, Rifle G, Kantelip J-P. A neutropenia suggesting an interaction between valacyclovir and mycophenolate mofetil. *Clin Transplant* (2003) 17, 158–61.
8. Wolfe EJ, Mathur V, Tomlanovich S, Jung D, Wong R, Griffy K, Aweeka FT. Pharmacokinetics of mycophenolate mofetil and intravenous ganciclovir alone and in combination in renal transplant recipients. *Pharmacotherapy* (1997) 17, 591–8.
9. Cymevene IV (Ganciclovir sodium). Roche Products Ltd. UK Summary of product characteristics, February 2006.
10. Valcyte (Valganciclovir hydrochloride). Roche Products Ltd. UK Summary of product characteristics, April 2006.
11. Valcyte (Valganciclovir hydrochloride). Roche Pharmaceuticals. US Prescribing information, January 2006.
12. Kennedy GA, Kay TD, Johnson DW, Hawley CM, Campbell SB, Isbel NM, Marlton P, Cobcroft R, Gill D, Cull G. Neutrophil dysplasia characterised by a pseudo-Pelger–Huet anomaly occurring with the use of mycophenolate mofetil and ganciclovir following renal transplantation: a report of five cases. *Pathology* (2002) 34, 263–6.

Aciclovir and related drugs + Probenecid

Probenecid reduces the renal excretion and increases the plasma levels of aciclovir, valaciclovir, and ganciclovir. Famciclovir and valganciclovir are predicted to interact similarly.

Clinical evidence

(a) Aciclovir or Valaciclovir

Twelve healthy subjects were given valaciclovir 1 g alone, or with probenecid 1 g, taken 2 hours earlier. Probenecid increased the AUC_{0-3} for the prodrug valaciclovir by 22%, and the AUC_{0-24} for its active metabolite, aciclovir, by 48%. The renal clearance of aciclovir was reduced by 33%, although the total urinary recovery of aciclovir was unchanged.[1] An earlier study had found that oral probenecid 1 g caused a similar increase in the AUC of intravenous aciclovir.[2]

(b) Ganciclovir

A pharmacokinetic study[3] in HIV-positive patients found that probenecid 500 mg every 6 hours increased the AUC of oral ganciclovir 1 g every 8 hours by 53.1%, and reduced the renal clearance by 12.3%.

Mechanism

The increases in aciclovir and ganciclovir AUCs are attributable to a reduction in their renal excretion by probenecid, probably due to competition for secretion by the kidney tubules.[1,3] The effects on aciclovir of combining probenecid and 'cimetidine', (p.774) were greater than either drug alone.[1]

Importance and management

These interactions are established, but because aciclovir has such a wide therapeutic index,[4] the authors of the study suggest that its interaction with *cimetidine* is probably clinically unimportant.[1] Therefore it seems likely that no changes in the usual dosages of aciclovir or valaciclovir will be needed in patients taking probenecid. However, the UK manufacturer states that caution is required with high doses of valaciclovir, and that alternatives to probenecid could be considered in this situation.[4] The US manufacturer suggests that the dosage of valaciclovir does not need to be altered in patients with normal renal function taking probenecid.[5]

It may be prudent to be alert for increased ganciclovir effects and toxicity if probenecid is used concurrently. **Valganciclovir** is a prodrug of ganciclovir, and the manufacturers recommend that patients taking valganciclovir with probenecid should be closely monitored for ganciclovir toxicity.[6,7] The manufacturers of **famciclovir** suggest that a similar interaction might also occur with probenecid and famciclovir, resulting in an increase in the plasma levels of penciclovir (the active metabolite of famciclovir).[8,9]

1. De Bony F, Tod M, Bidault R, On NT, Posner J, Rolan P. Multiple interactions of cimetidine and probenecid with valaciclovir and its metabolite acyclovir. *Antimicrob Agents Chemother* (2002) 46, 458–63.
2. Laskin OL, de Miranda P, King DH, Page DA, Longstreth JA, Rocco L, Lietman PS. Effects of probenecid on the pharmacokinetics and elimination of acyclovir in humans. *Antimicrob Agents Chemother* (1982) 21, 804–7.
3. Gaines K, Wong R, Jung D, Cimoch P, Lavelle J, Pollard R. Pharmacokinetic interactions with oral ganciclovir: zidovudine, didanosine, probenecid. 10th Int Conf AIDS, Yokohama (Japan), 1994. Abstract p7.
4. Valtrex (Valaciclovir). GlaxoSmithKline UK. UK Summary of product characteristics, September 2005.
5. Valtrex (Valacyclovir hydrochloride). GlaxoSmithKline. US Prescribing information, July 2006.
6. Valcyte (Valganciclovir hydrochloride). Roche Products Ltd. UK Summary of product characteristics, April 2006.
7. Valcyte (Valganciclovir hydrochloride). Roche Pharmaceuticals. US Prescribing information, January 2006.
8. Famvir (Famciclovir). Novartis Pharmaceuticals UK Ltd. UK Summary of product characteristics, December 2004.
9. Famvir (Famciclovir). Novartis Pharmaceuticals Corp. US Prescribing information, December 2006.

Adefovir + Miscellaneous

No clinically significant interaction appears to occur between adefovir and co-trimoxazole, didanosine, delavirdine, efavirenz, ibuprofen, indinavir, lamivudine, nelfinavir, nevirapine, paracetamol, tenofovir, or zidovudine. Adefovir possibly reduces saquinavir levels.

Clinical evidence, mechanism, importance and management

(a) Antiretrovirals

The UK manufacturer notes that at doses 6 to 12 times higher than the 10-mg dose of adefovir recommended for hepatitis B infection, there was no interaction with the NRTIs **lamivudine** or **zidovudine**, the NNRTIs

delavirdine, **efavirenz** or **nevirapine**, or the protease inhibitors **indinavir** or **nelfinavir**.[1] The concurrent use of adefovir 60 mg with **saquinavir** soft capsules increased the adefovir AUC by 20%, which is not clinically relevant.[1] In a population pharmacokinetic analysis, combination of **saquinavir** with adefovir appeared to result in a 49% increase in the clearance of saquinavir.[2] The concurrent use of adefovir 60 mg with **didanosine** buffered tablets increased the **didanosine** AUC by 29%, which is not clinically relevant.[1] See also *Lamivudine* and *Tenofovir*, below.

(b) Drugs undergoing, or affecting, tubular secretion

Adefovir is excreted by the kidneys, by a combination of glomerular filtration and active secretion via the renal transporter, human Organic Anion Transporter 1 (hOAT1). The potential for pharmacokinetic interactions with **co-trimoxazole**, **ibuprofen**, **lamivudine**, **paracetamol** and **tenofovir** (other drugs that also undergo, or may affect tubular secretion) has been investigated.[1,3]

1. Co-trimoxazole (Trimethoprim/Sulfamethoxazole). The manufacturers note that there was no pharmacokinetic interaction between adefovir 10 mg once daily and **co-trimoxazole** 960 mg twice daily in 18 healthy subjects.[1,3]

2. Ibuprofen. The concurrent use of adefovir 10 mg and ibuprofen 800 mg three times daily modestly increased the AUC and maximum level of adefovir by 23% and 33%, respectively. These changes were considered to be due to higher bioavailability rather than a reduction in renal clearance, and are not considered clinically relevant. Adefovir did not alter ibuprofen pharmacokinetics.[1,3]

3. Lamivudine. The manufacturers note that there was no pharmacokinetic interaction between adefovir 10 mg once daily and lamivudine 100 mg once daily in healthy subjects.[1,3]

4. Paracetamol. The manufacturers note that there was no pharmacokinetic interaction between adefovir 10 mg once daily and paracetamol 1 g four times daily in healthy subjects.[1,3]

5. Tenofovir. In 24 healthy subjects there was no pharmacokinetic interaction between a single 10-mg dose of adefovir dipivoxil given alone and on day 7 of tenofovir disoproxil fumarate 300 mg daily for 7 days. In particular, renal clearances of both drugs were not changed on concurrent use.[4] However, the manufacturers still advise close monitoring during concurrent use, since the clinical safety, including renal effects, has not yet been assessed.[1,3]

1. Hepsera (Adefovir dipivoxil). Gilead Sciences International Ltd. UK Summary of product characteristics, September 2006.
2. Fletcher CV, Jiang H, Brundage RC, Acosta EP, Haubrich R, Katzenstein D, Gulick RM. Sex-based differences in saquinavir pharmacology and virologic response in AIDS Clinical Trials Group Study 359. *J Infect Dis* (2004) 189, 1176–84.
3. Hepsera (Adefovir dipivoxil). Gilead Sciences, Inc. US Prescribing information, October 2006.
4. Kearney BP, Ramanathan S, Cheng AK, Ebrahimi R, Shah J. Systemic and renal pharmacokinetics of adefovir and tenofovir upon coadministration. *J Clin Pharmacol* (2005) 45, 935–40. Erratum. Ibid., 1206.

Cidofovir + Miscellaneous

Cidofovir with probenecid modestly decreased levels of trimethoprim and sulfamethoxazole (co-trimoxazole), and caused moderate increases in didanosine levels, but did not alter fluconazole pharmacokinetics. None of these drugs altered cidofovir pharmacokinetics.

Clinical evidence

(a) Co-trimoxazole (Trimethoprim/Sulfamethoxazole)

In a study, 6 HIV-positive subjects were given co-trimoxazole 960 mg daily with a single 3-mg/kg dose of cidofovir with probenecid given on day 7. The AUC and maximum plasma concentrations of both trimethoprim and sulfamethoxazole were decreased by about 30% and renal clearance was significantly increased. The pharmacokinetics of cidofovir were not affected.[1]

(b) Didanosine

In a study, 6 HIV-positive subjects were given didanosine 100 or 200 mg twice daily for 7 days with a single 3-mg/kg dose of cidofovir with probenecid given on day 7. The AUC of didanosine was increased 1.6-fold, but the pharmacokinetics of cidofovir were not affected.[1]

(c) Fluconazole

In a study, 6 HIV-positive subjects were given fluconazole 100 mg daily for 13 days with a single 3-mg/kg dose of cidofovir with probenecid given on day 13. The pharmacokinetics of both drugs were unaffected.[1]

Mechanism

It was suggested that cidofovir/probenecid might alter the renal elimination of these drugs.[1]

Importance and management

The modest decreases in trimethoprim and sulfamethoxazole levels, and moderate increases in didanosine levels caused by cidofovir are considered unlikely to be clinically relevant because of the infrequent dosing schedule of cidofovir/probenecid. No dose adjustments are considered necessary.[1]

1. Luber A, Lalezari J, Rooney J, Jaffe H, Flaherty J. Drug-drug interaction study with intravenous cidofovir (CDV) and either trimethoprim/sulfamethoxazole (TMP/SMX), didanosine (DDI), or fluconazole (FLU) in HIV-infected individuals. *Intersci Conf Antimicrob Agents Chemother* (2002) 42, 27.

Cidofovir + Probenecid

Probenecid reduces the nephrotoxicity of cidofovir, and it is recommended it should always be used concurrently.[1,2] Therefore, when using cidofovir/probenecid the interactions of probenecid should be considered. Of particular note, zidovudine should be temporarily discontinued or the dosage halved when cidofovir/probenecid is used,[1,2] see 'NRTIs + Probenecid', p.803.

1. Vistide (Cidofovir). Pharmacia Ltd. UK Summary of product characteristics, September 2004.
2. Vistide (Cidofovir). Gilead Sciences, Inc. US Prescribing information, September 2000.

Enfuvirtide + Cytochrome P450 isoenzyme substrates

Enfuvirtide had no effect on the metabolism of dapsone or debrisoquine, and had little effect on the metabolism of caffeine, chlorzoxazone, and mephenytoin. Thus, it is not anticipated that enfuvirtide would cause clinically important drug interactions with drugs metabolised by the cytochrome P450 isoenzymes.

Clinical evidence, mechanism, importance and management

A single oral dose of five drugs (**caffeine** 100 mg, **chlorzoxazone** 250 mg, **dapsone** 100 mg, **debrisoquine** 10 mg and **mephenytoin** 100 mg) was given to 12 HIV-positive subjects, before, and after they were given subcutaneous enfuvirtide 90 mg twice daily for 6 days. Enfuvirtide had no effect on the urinary **dapsone** recovery ratio (a measure of the activity of the cytochrome P450 isoenzyme CYP3A4), plasma monoacetyldapsone-to-**dapsone** ratio (a measure of *N*-acetyltransferase (NAT) activity) or urinary **debrisoquine** recovery ratio (a measure of CYP2D6 activity). Enfuvirtide had little effect (less than 30% change) on the plasma paraxanthine-to-**caffeine** ratio (a measure of CYP1A2 activity), the plasma 6-hydroxychlorzoxazone-to-**chlorzoxazone** ratio (a measure of CYP2E1 activity) and urinary recovery of 4-hydroxy**mephenytoin** (a measure of CYP2C19 activity). Subjects in this study were taking up to 3 NRTIs in stable doses, and were not taking any NNRTIs or protease inhibitors.[1]

This type of study is being increasingly used to assess the potential for new drugs to cause clinically important cytochrome P450-mediated drug interactions. The results indicate that enfuvirtide is unlikely to cause clinically important changes in the pharmacokinetics of drugs metabolised by CYP3A4, NAT and CYP2D6. They also give some reassurance that drugs metabolised by CYP1A2, CYP2E1 and CYP2C19 are unlikely to be significantly affected, although the modest changes seen introduce some caution. No substrate for CYP2C9 was included in this study, but enfuvirtide does not affect CYP2C9 *in vitro*.[1]

1. Zhang X, Lalezari JP, Badley AD, Dorr A, Kolis SJ, Kinchelow T, Patel IH. Assessment of drug-drug interaction potential of enfuvirtide in human immunodeficiency virus type 1–infected patients. *Clin Pharmacol Ther* (2004) 75, 558–68.

Enfuvirtide + Protease inhibitors

Ritonavir caused a minor increase in enfuvirtide exposure, which is not clinically relevant. Saquinavir/ritonavir had little effect on enfuvirtide.

Clinical evidence, mechanism, importance and management

Subcutaneous enfuvirtide 90 mg twice daily was given for 7 days to 24 HIV-positive subjects with either **ritonavir** 200 mg twice daily or **saquinavir/ritonavir** 1 g/100 mg twice daily given for the last 4 days. **Ritonavir** caused a minor 24% increase in the AUC of enfuvirtide, and **saquinavir/ritonavir** caused a 14% increase in the AUC of enfuvirtide. Such small increases in enfuvirtide exposure are not clinically relevant. No special precautions appear warranted during concurrent use.[1]

1. Ruxrungtham K, Boyd M, Bellibas SE, Zhang X, Dorr A, Kolis S, Kinchelow T, Buss N, Patel IH. Lack of interaction between enfuvirtide and ritonavir or ritonavir-boosted saquinavir in HIV-1-infected patients. *J Clin Pharmacol* (2004) 44, 793–802.

Enfuvirtide + Rifampicin (Rifampin)

Rifampicin has no effect on the pharmacokinetics of enfuvirtide.

Clinical evidence, mechanism, importance and management

Subcutaneous enfuvirtide 90 mg twice daily for 3 days was given to 12 HIV-positive subjects before, and during, the last 3 days of a 10-day course of rifampicin 600 mg daily. The AUC of enfuvirtide and its metabolite were not significantly altered by rifampicin.[1]

Enfuvirtide is a peptide, and would not be expected to be affected by enzyme inducers such as rifampicin. The findings of this study support this. No special precautions are required during concurrent use.

1. Boyd MA, Zhang X, Dorr A, Ruxrungtham K, Kolis S, Nieforth K, Kinchelow T, Buss N, Patel IH. Lack of enzyme-inducing effect of rifampicin on the pharmacokinetics of enfuvirtide. *J Clin Pharmacol* (2003) 43, 1382–91.

Entecavir + Miscellaneous

There appears to be no pharmacokinetic interaction between entecavir and adefovir, lamivudine or tenofovir. However, interactions with other renally excreted drugs cannot be excluded. No interactions mediated by cytochrome P450 isoenzymes are expected with entecavir.

Clinical evidence, mechanism, importance and management

(a) Renally excreted drugs

Since entecavir is predominantly eliminated by the kidney, the concurrent use of drugs that reduce renal function or compete for active tubular secretion may increase serum concentrations of either entecavir or the concurrent drug. However, the manufacturers note that there was no pharmacokinetic interaction between entecavir and **lamivudine**, **adefovir** or **tenofovir** at steady state.[1,2] They say that, apart from these drugs, the effects of concurrent use of entecavir with drugs that are excreted renally or affect renal function have not been evaluated, and they therefore recommend that patients should be monitored closely for adverse reactions when entecavir is given.[1]

(b) Cytochrome P450-mediated interactions

The manufacturers say that entecavir is not a substrate, an inducer or an inhibitor of cytochrome P450 isoenzymes. Therefore drug interactions are unlikely to occur with entecavir by this mechanism.[1,2]

1. Baraclude (Entecavir). Bristol-Myers Squibb Pharmaceuticals Ltd. UK Summary of product characteristics, July 2007.
2. Baraclude (Entecavir). Bristol-Myers Squibb Company. US Prescribing information, March 2007.

Famciclovir + Miscellaneous

No clinically important pharmacokinetic interactions appear to occur when famciclovir is given with allopurinol, digoxin or theophylline.

Clinical evidence, mechanism, importance and management

When 12 healthy subjects were given famciclovir 500 mg after taking **allopurinol** 300 mg daily for 5 days there were no clinically relevant changes in the pharmacokinetics of either drug.[1] It was concluded that xanthine oxidase does not play an important role in the metabolism of famciclovir to penciclovir.[1,2]

Similarly, no clinically significant changes in the pharmacokinetics of famciclovir were seen in healthy subjects given famciclovir with **theophylline**[3] or **digoxin**. The pharmacokinetics of **theophylline** and **digoxin** were also unaffected.[4,5]

No special precautions would therefore seem necessary if any of these drugs is given with famciclovir.

1. Fowles SE, Pratt SK, Laroche J, Prince WT. Lack of a pharmacokinetic interaction between oral famciclovir and allopurinol in healthy volunteers. *Eur J Clin Pharmacol* (1994) 46, 355–9.
2. Daniels S, Schentag JJ. Drug interaction studies and safety of famciclovir in healthy volunteers: a review. *Antiviral Chem Chemother* (1993) 4 (Suppl 1), 57–64.
3. Fairless AJ, Pratt SK, Pue MA, Fowles SE, Wolf D, Daniels S, Prince WT. An investigation into the potential interaction between theophylline and oral famciclovir in healthy male volunteers. *Br J Clin Pharmacol* (1992) 34, 171P–172P.
4. Pue MA, Saporito M, Laroche J, Lua S, Bygate E, Daniels S, Broom C. An investigation of the potential interaction between digoxin and oral famciclovir in healthy male volunteers. *Br J Clin Pharmacol* (1993) 36, 177P.
5. Siederer S, Scott S, Fowles S, Haveresch L, Hust R. Lack of interaction between steady-state digoxin and famciclovir. *Intersci Conf Antimicrob Agents Chemother* (1996) 36, A33.

Foscarnet + Ciprofloxacin

Two patients developed tonic-clonic seizures when they were given foscarnet with ciprofloxacin.

Clinical evidence

An HIV-positive patient taking multiple drugs (including ciprofloxacin 750 mg twice daily, clarithromycin, cimetidine, fluconazole, morphine, rifampicin and vancomycin) was also given intravenous foscarnet 60 mg/kg every 8 hours for a cytomegalovirus infection. He was only given half of the first dose, but 9 hours later he developed a tonic-clonic seizure. On completion of infusion of the first dose he again experienced similar seizure activity. About 45 minutes after the start of the second foscarnet dose, he had a third grand mal seizure. No further seizures occurred when the foscarnet was stopped.[1] Another HIV-positive patient was given foscarnet 60 mg/kg every 8 hours for 10 days without problem, until he started ciprofloxacin 750 mg twice daily, clofazimine, ethambutol, pyrazinamide and rifampicin for mycobacterial sepsis. Within 2 days, a few minutes after the start of the foscarnet infusion, he developed a seizure. This resolved when the foscarnet was stopped, and recurred when the foscarnet was restarted.[1]

Mechanism

Both foscarnet and ciprofloxacin have the potential to cause seizures and it seems that some enhancement of this activity occurs if they are used in combination. Subsequent study in *mice* has shown that the combination of ciprofloxacin and foscarnet does increase the likelihood of seizures, and that the interaction is likely to be due to altered GABA-receptor binding. An interaction was not found for **enoxacin** and foscarnet.[2]

Importance and management

Direct information seems to be limited to these two cases. It is impossible to know for certain if the seizures were due to the combined effects of these two drugs or not, but the evidence seems to point in that direction. The general importance of this interaction is uncertain, but it would seem prudent to monitor very closely if these drugs are used together.

1. Fan-Havard P, Sanchorawala V, Oh J, Moser EM, Smith SP. Concurrent use of foscarnet and ciprofloxacin may increase the propensity for seizures. *Ann Pharmacother* (1994) 28, 869–72.
2. Matsuo H, Ryu M, Nagata A, Uchida T, Kawakami J-I, Yamamoto K, Iga T, Sawada Y. Neurotoxicodynamics of the interaction between ciprofloxacin and foscarnet in mice. *Antimicrob Agents Chemother* (1998) 42, 691–4.

Foscarnet + NRTIs

No pharmacokinetic interactions occur between foscarnet and didanosine, zalcitabine or zidovudine. The UK manufacturer does not recommend the concurrent use of lamivudine and foscarnet.

Clinical evidence, mechanism, importance and management

(a) Didanosine

In a three-phase study, 12 HIV-positive patients were given 4 doses of intravenous foscarnet 90 mg/kg, 4 doses of oral didanosine 200 mg, and 4 doses of both drugs together. Based on the data obtained from these patients (drug clearance, volume of distribution, half-life, mean residence time), no pharmacokinetic interactions were said to occur between these two drugs. This suggests that no dosage adjustments will be needed during concurrent use.[1] The antiretroviral effects of foscarnet and didanosine were synergistic.[2]

(b) Lamivudine

The UK manufacturer says that lamivudine should not be given with foscarnet,[3] presumably because of possible interference with renal excretion. Note that the US manufacturer does not make any recommendation.[4] Foscarnet does not affect lamivudine intracellular activation.[5]

(c) Stavudine

Foscarnet does not affect stavudine intracellular activation.[6]

(d) Zalcitabine

Intravenous foscarnet 90 mg/kg every 12 hours and oral zalcitabine 750 micrograms every 8 hours were given to 12 HIV-positive subjects for 2 days. There were no clinically significant alterations in the pharmacokinetics of either drug.[7] However, the manufacturers of zalcitabine[8,9] suggested that the concurrent use of zalcitabine and foscarnet should be well monitored, because foscarnet may possibly decrease the renal clearance of the zalcitabine, thereby increasing its serum levels and its toxicity, particularly peripheral neuropathy. The antiretroviral effects of foscarnet and zalcitabine were synergistic.[2]

(e) Zidovudine

The antiviral effects of foscarnet and zidovudine appear to be additive or synergistic. No significant alteration in the pharmacokinetics of either drug was seen in a 14-day study in 5 AIDS patients given both drugs.[10] Foscarnet does not appear to affect zidovudine intracellular activation,[11] and the manufacturer notes that there was no evidence of increased myelotoxicity when foscarnet was used with zidovudine.[12] No special precautions are required on concurrent use.

1. Aweeka FT, Mathur V, Dorsey R, Jacobson MA, Martin-Munley S, Pirrung D, Franco J, Lizak P, Johnson J, Gambertoglio J. Concomitant foscarnet and didanosine; a pharmacokinetic (PK) evaluation in patients with HIV disease. American Society of Microbiology 2nd National Conference on Human Retroviruses and Related infections, Washington DC, 1995. Abstract 492.
2. Palmer S, Harmenberg J, Cox S. Synergistic inhibition of human immunodeficiency virus isolates (including 3'-azido-3'-deoxythymidine-resistant isolates) by foscarnet in combination with 2',3'-dideoxyinosine or 2',3'-dideoxycytidine. *Antimicrob Agents Chemother* (1996) 40, 1285–8.
3. Epivir (Lamivudine). GlaxoSmithKline UK. UK Summary of product characteristics, March 2007.
4. Epivir (Lamivudine). GlaxoSmithKline. US Prescribing information, October 2006.
5. Kewn S, Hoggard PG, Sales SD, Johnson MA, Back DJ. The intracellular activation of lamivudine (3TC) and determination of 2'-deoxycytidine-5'-triphosphate (dCTP) pools in the presence and absence of various drugs in HepG2 cells. *Br J Clin Pharmacol* (2000) 50, 597–604.
6. Hoggard PG, Kewn S, Barry MG, Khoo SH, Back DJ. Effects of drugs on 2',3'-dideoxy-2',3'-didehydrothymidine phosphorylation in vitro. *Antimicrob Agents Chemother* (1997) 41, 1231–6.
7. Aweeka FT, Brody SR, Jacobson M, Botwin K, Martin-Munley S. Is there a pharmacokinetic interaction between foscarnet and zalcitabine during concomitant administration? *Clin Ther* (1998) 20, 232–43.
8. Hivid (Zalcitabine). Roche Products Ltd. UK Summary of product characteristics, November 2004.
9. Hivid (Zalcitabine). Roche Pharmaceuticals. US Prescribing information, September 2002.
10. Aweeka FT, Gambertoglio JG, van der Horst C, Raasch R, Jacobson MA. Pharmacokinetics of concomitantly administered foscarnet and zidovudine for treatment of human immunodeficiency virus infection (AIDS clinical trials group protocol 053). *Antimicrob Agents Chemother* (1992) 36, 1773–8.
11. Brody SR, Aweeka FT. Pharmacokinetics of intracellular zidovudine and its phosphorylated anabolites in the absence and presence of other antiviral agents using an in vitro human PBMC model. *Clin Pharmacol Ther* (1997) 61, 149.
12. Foscavir (Foscarnet). AstraZeneca UK Ltd. UK Summary of product characteristics, May 2007.

Foscarnet + Pentamidine

Four patients had marked hypocalcaemia when they were given foscarnet with intravenous pentamidine. One of them died.

Clinical evidence, mechanism, importance and management

Four patients with suspected AIDS-related cytomegaloviral infections of the chest developed signs of hypocalcaemia within 10 days of starting treatment with foscarnet and intravenous pentamidine (dosages not stated). All 4 had paraesthesia of the hands and feet, and 3 of them had Chvostek's and Trousseau's signs (signs of tetany). The serum calcium levels of 3 of them fell but normalised when one of the drugs was stopped. The fourth patient died with severe hypocalcaemia of 1.42 mmol/L.[1]

Both drugs have been associated with hypocalcaemia in HIV-positive patients, and in these 4 patients their effects appear to have been additive. Very close monitoring of calcium levels is advised if foscarnet is used with parenteral pentamidine.

1. Youle MS, Clarbour J, Gazzard B, Chanas A. Severe hypocalcaemia in AIDS patients treated with foscarnet and pentamidine. *Lancet* (1988) 1, 1455–6.

Foscarnet + Probenecid

Probenecid does not alter the pharmacokinetics of foscarnet.

Clinical evidence, mechanism, importance and management

A study in 10 HIV-positive patients found that probenecid 1 g twice daily for 3 days had no effect on the pharmacokinetics of foscarnet 90 mg/kg given intravenously over 2 hours. The authors conclude that, because of the lack of interaction with probenecid, almost all of the renal elimination of foscarnet is by glomerular filtration, with only a minimal contribution of active tubular secretion.[1] No special precautions seem to be necessary.

1. Noormohamed FH, Youle MS, Higgs CJ, Gazzard BG, Lant AF. Renal excretion and pharmacokinetics of foscarnet in HIV sero-positive patients: effect of probenecid pretreatment. *Br J Clin Pharmacol* (1997) 43, 112–15.

Ganciclovir or Valganciclovir + Imipenem

Based on an early possible report,[1] the manufacturer notes that generalised seizures have been reported in patients who received ganciclovir with imipenem-cilastatin. They recommend that ganciclovir and its prodrug valganciclovir should not be used with imipenem unless the benefits outweigh the risks.[2-4] No further reports of this interaction appear to have been published, or reported to the manufacturer.[1] Note that both ganciclovir and imipenem alone may cause seizures.

1. Roche Products Ltd. Personal communication, March 2007.
2. Cymevene IV (Ganciclovir sodium). Roche Products Ltd. UK Summary of product characteristics, February 2006.
3. Valcyte (Valganciclovir hydrochloride). Roche Products Ltd. UK Summary of product characteristics, April 2006.
4. Cytovene-IV (Ganciclovir sodium). Roche Pharmaceuticals. US Prescribing information, January 2006.

Ganciclovir + Trimethoprim

There is no clinically relevant pharmacokinetic interaction between ganciclovir and trimethoprim.

Clinical evidence, mechanism, importance and management

Ganciclovir 1 g every 8 hours was given to 12 HIV-positive subjects with trimethoprim 200 mg daily for 7 days. Ganciclovir clearance was decreased by 13%, and the half-life was increased by 18%, while the trimethoprim minimum plasma concentration was raised by 13%. The combination was well tolerated and none of these changes were considered clinically significant, so no dose alteration appears necessary on concurrent use.[1] Both ganciclovir and trimethoprim are known to be myelosuppressive,[2] and the manufacturer of ganciclovir and its prodrug

valganciclovir notes that there is the possibility that the risk of this toxicity may be increased when they are used together. Therefore, they recommend that the combination should only be used if the benefits outweigh the risks of treatment.[3-5]

1. Jung D, AbdelHameed MH, Hunter J, Teitelbaum P, Dorr A, Griffy K. The pharmacokinetics and safety profile of oral ganciclovir in combination with trimethoprim in HIV- and CMV-seropositive patients. *Br J Clin Pharmacol* (1999) 47, 255–9.
2. Meynard J-L, Guiguet M, Arsac S, Frottier J, Meyohas M-C. Frequency and risk factors of infectious complications in neutropenic patients infected with HIV. *AIDS* (1997) 11, 995–8.
3. Cymevene IV (Ganciclovir sodium). Roche Products Ltd. UK Summary of product characteristics, February 2006.
4. Valcyte (Valganciclovir hydrochloride). Roche Products Ltd. UK Summary of product characteristics, April 2006.
5. Cytovene-IV (Ganciclovir sodium). Roche Pharmaceuticals. US Prescribing information, January 2006.

Idoxuridine + Miscellaneous

The topical solution of idoxuridine, *Herpid*, contains the solvent dimethyl sulfoxide as an absorption enhancer. This can increase the absorption of many substances, and therefore no other topical medications should be used concurrently on the same areas as *Herpid*.[1]

1. Herpid (Idoxuridine). Astellas Pharma Ltd. UK Summary of product characteristics, November 2005.

Influenza vaccines + Paracetamol (Acetaminophen)

Paracetamol does not affect antibody production in response to influenza vaccination and appears to reduce its adverse effects. The pharmacokinetics of paracetamol do not appear to be affected by influenza vaccine.

Clinical evidence, mechanism, importance and management

The pharmacokinetics of a single 650-mg dose of intravenous paracetamol were unaffected in healthy subjects when it was given 7 and 21 days after 0.5 mL of trivalent influenza vaccine given intramuscularly.[1] Paracetamol 1 g four times daily for 2 days had no effect on the production of influenza virus antibodies in a group of 39 elderly patients given an inactivated influenza virus vaccine, and the paracetamol appeared to reduce the adverse effects of the vaccine (e.g. fever), although this was not statistically significant.[2] There would seem to be no reason for avoiding the concurrent use of paracetamol and influenza vaccine.

1. Scavone JM, Blyden GT, Greenblatt DJ. Lack of effect of influenza vaccine on the pharmacokinetics of antipyrine, alprazolam, paracetamol (acetaminophen) and lorazepam. *Clin Pharmacokinet* (1989) 16, 180–5.
2. Gross PA, Levandowski RA, Russo C, Weksler M, Bonelli J, Dran S, Munk G, Deichmiller S, Hilsen R, Panush RF. Vaccine immune response and side effects with the use of acetaminophen with influenza vaccine. *Clin Diagn Lab Immunol* (1994) 1, 134–8.

Influenza vaccine, live + Antivirals active against influenza

The manufacturers advise that antivirals active against influenza such as oseltamivir and rimantadine should not be given until 2 weeks after the administration of *live* influenza virus vaccines, and that these vaccines should not be given until 48 hours after stopping the antiviral.[1-3] This is because of the theoretical concern that these antiviral drugs will inhibit replication of live vaccine virus, and therefore reduce its effect. Note that most influenza vaccines are inactivated (split virion or surface antigen), and that these would not be expected to be affected by antivirals active against influenza.

1. FluMist (Influenza virus vaccine live, intranasal). MedImmune Vaccines, Inc. US Prescribing information, January 2007.
2. Tamiflu (Oseltamivir phosphate). Roche Pharmaceuticals. US Prescribing information, July 2007.
3. Flumadine (Rimantadine hydrochloride). Forest Pharmaceuticals, Inc. US Prescribing information, June 2006.

Interferons + ACE inhibitors

A case series suggests that severe granulocytopenia can develop if ACE inhibitors and interferon are given concurrently.

Clinical evidence

Patients with cryoglobulinaemia were treated with 3 million units of recombinant **interferon alfa-2a** (35 patients) or natural **interferon beta** (3 patients), usually given daily for 3 months, then on alternate days for periods of 6 to 17 months. Severe toxicity developed in 3 patients, who were the only ones amongst the group to also be taking ACE inhibitors. Granulocytopenia developed in 2 patients within a few days of starting **enalapril** 10 mg daily or **captopril** 50 mg daily, and subsided 1 to 2 weeks after both drugs were stopped. Another patient, already taking **enalapril** 5 mg daily, developed severe granulocytopenia when interferon was started, and again when re-challenged with both drugs. None of the other 35 patients receiving interferon alone developed any significant haematological problems. The reasons for this severe reaction are not understood but the authors of the report suggest that it may be an autoimmune response.[1]

A follow-up letter commenting on this report described 2 further patients with hepatitis C infection, cryoglobulinaemia and glomerulonephritis, who took **captopril** 75 mg or **enalapril** 20 mg daily for several weeks, and who had granulocytopenia within 9 days of being given 3 million units of recombinant **interferon alfa-2a**, daily or on alternate days. However, this resolved without any change in treatment. Another patient with multiple myeloma given **interferon alfa-2a** 3 million units 3 times weekly and long-term **benazepril** 10 mg daily had a normal granulocyte count after 3 months.[2]

Mechanism

Interferons alone are associated with myelosuppression, particularly granulocytopenia. ACE inhibitors have, rarely, caused neutropenia and agranulocytosis.

Importance and management

These two reports appear to be the only information suggesting an interaction. Regular full blood counts are generally recommended when interferons are used, and therefore, no extra precautions would appear to be required if ACE inhibitors are also given. Bear the possibility of an interaction in mind.

1. Casato M, Pucillo LP, Leoni M, di Lullo L, Gabrielli A, Sansonno D, Dammacco F, Danieli G, Bonomo L. Granulocytopenia after combined therapy with interferon and angiotensin-converting enzyme inhibitors: evidence for a synergistic hematologic toxicity. *Am J Med* (1995) 99, 386–91.
2. Jacquot C, Caudwell V, Belenfant X. Granulocytopenia after combined therapy with interferon and angiotensin-converting enzyme inhibitors: evidence for a synergistic hematologic toxicity. *Am J Med* (1996) 101, 235–6.

Interferons + Analgesics or Corticosteroids

Prednisone and paracetamol have disparate effects on some measures of the antiviral activity of interferon, but the clinical relevance of this is unclear. Isolated cases of acute hepatitis have been seen when interferon was given with paracetamol.

Clinical evidence, mechanism, importance and management

A single intramuscular dose of recombinant human **interferon alfa-2a** 18 million units was given to 8 healthy subjects alone, or after one day of either **aspirin** 650 mg every 4 hours, **paracetamol** 650 mg every 4 hours or **prednisone** 40 mg daily, for a total of 8 days. None of these additional drugs reduced the interferon adverse effects of fever, chills, headache, or myalgia. Only **prednisone** appeared to reduce one of the two measures of interferon activity.[1] In a later similar study by the same research group, the effect of the same drugs and doses (started 3 days before the interferon) was evaluated with a lower dose of **interferon alfa-2a** (3 million units). When data for **aspirin**, **paracetamol** or **prednisone** was combined the subjects had a 47% reduction in symptom score, when compared with control subjects not taking any of these three drugs. The **prednisone** group also had fewer hours of fever. In this study, neither **prednisone** nor **aspirin** consistently altered measures of the antiviral activity of interferon, but **paracetamol** appeared to enhance them.[2]

Taken together, the results of these two studies suggest that these drugs may reduce the flu-like adverse effects of interferon, perhaps more so at lower doses of interferon. The clinical relevance of the measures of antiviral activity of interferon is uncertain, so the disparate effects found with **paracetamol** and **prednisone** are unclear.

The authors of a report describing an unusual acute form of hepatitis, occurring in 3 patients receiving **interferon alfa-2a**, vinblastine and **paracetamol**, suggested that this might have been due to a drug interaction.[3] Another two similar cases have been reported with **interferon alfa-2b** and **paracetamol**, but no liver toxicity occurred when one of these patients was given **indometacin** with interferon instead.[4] The general relevance of these isolated reports is unclear.

1. Witter FR, Woods AS, Griffin MD, Smith CR, Nadler P, Lietman PS. Effects of prednisone, aspirin and acetaminophen on an *in vivo* biologic response to interferon in humans. *Clin Pharmacol Ther* (1988) 44, 239–43.
2. Hendrix CW, Petty BG, Woods A, Kuwahara SK, Witter FR, Soo W, Griffin DE, Lietman PS. Modulation of α-interferon's antiviral and clinical effects by aspirin, acetaminophen, and prednisone in healthy volunteers. *Antiviral Res* (1995) 28, 121–31.
3. Kellokumpu-Lehtinen P, Iisalo E, Nordman E. Hepatotoxicity of paracetamol in combination with interferon and vinblastine. *Lancet* (1989) 1, 1143.
4. Fabris P, Dalla Palma M, de Lalla F. Idiosyncratic acute hepatitis caused by paracetamol in two patients with melanoma treated with high-dose interferon-α. *Ann Intern Med* (2001) 134, 345.

Interferons + Ribavirin

There was no evidence of any changes in pharmacokinetic parameters when ribavirin and interferon alfa-2b were given together.[1] Another study using peginterferon alfa-2b also found no pharmacokinetic interactions with ribavirin.[2] The combination of interferon alfa and ribavirin has enhanced efficacy against hepatitis C.

1. Khakoo S, Glue P, Grellier L, Wells B, Bell A, Dash C, Murray-Lyon I, Lypnyj D, Flannery B, Walters K, Dusheiko GM. Ribavirin and interferon alfa-2b in chronic hepatitis C: assessment of possible pharmacokinetic and pharmacodynamic interactions. *Br J Clin Pharmacol* (1998) 46, 563–70.
2. Glue P, Rouzier-Panis R, Raffanel C, Sabo R, Gupta SK, Salfi M, Jacobs S, Clement RP. A dose-ranging study of pegylated interferon alfa-2b and ribavirin in chronic hepatitis C. The Hepatitis C Intervention Therapy Group. *Hepatology* (2000) 32, 647–53.

Maraviroc + CYP3A4 inducers

Efavirenz reduces the plasma levels of maraviroc by about 50% and rifampicin reduces them by about two-thirds. A regimen containing nevirapine appeared to have little effect on the levels of a single dose of maraviroc.

Clinical evidence

(a) Efavirenz

In a placebo-controlled study in healthy subjects, efavirenz 600 mg once daily for 14 days reduced the steady-state AUC and maximum plasma level of maraviroc 100 mg twice daily by about 50%. Doubling the dose of maraviroc to 200 mg twice daily overcame this increase in metabolism, resulting in a minor 10% increase in AUC and 20% increase in maximum level, when compared with maraviroc 100 mg twice daily alone.[1] Similarly, in another study, the AUC of a single 300-mg dose of maraviroc was about 50% lower in two groups of 8 patients; one group taking efavirenz, lamivudine and zidovudine and the other taking efavirenz, didanosine and tenofovir.[2] When efavirenz 600 mg daily was added to lopinavir/ritonavir 400/100 mg twice daily with maraviroc 300 mg twice daily, the increase in maraviroc AUC seen with these 'protease inhibitors', (p.780), was reduced from about 300% to about 150%, when compared with the AUC for maraviroc alone.[3] Similarly, when efavirenz 600 mg daily was added to saquinavir/ritonavir 1000/100 mg twice daily with maraviroc 100 mg twice daily, the increase in maraviroc AUC seen with these protease inhibitors was reduced from 877% to 400%, when compared with the AUC for maraviroc alone.[3]

(b) Nevirapine

In 8 patients taking nevirapine, lamivudine and tenofovir the AUC of a single 300-mg dose of maraviroc was unchanged and its maximum plasma level was about 50% higher, when compared with HIV-positive subjects taking maraviroc alone.[2]

(c) Rifampicin (Rifampin)

In a placebo-controlled study in healthy subjects, rifampicin 600 mg once daily for 14 days reduced the steady-state AUC and maximum and minimum plasma levels of maraviroc 100 mg twice daily by about two-thirds. Doubling the dose of maraviroc to 200 mg twice daily overcame this increased metabolism, resulting in an AUC comparable to that of maraviroc 100 mg twice daily alone.[1]

Mechanism

Maraviroc is a substrate of the cytochrome P450 isoenzyme CYP3A4, and its levels would therefore be expected to be reduced by inducers of this enzyme, such as efavirenz and rifampicin. For a list of CYP3A4 inducers, see 'Table 1.4', (p.6).

Importance and management

The pharmacokinetic interactions with efavirenz and rifampicin are likely to be clinically important. The reduction in maraviroc plasma levels seen could result in decreased efficacy and the development of viral resistance. Doubling the dose of maraviroc overcame this interaction, and this is the suggested approach of the manufacturer when maraviroc is used in the absence of protease inhibitors.[4] Efavirenz appears to halve the increase in maraviroc levels seen with ritonavir-boosted protease inhibitors.

1. Jenkins T, Abel S, Russell D, Boucher M, Whitlock L, Weissgerber G, Muirhead G. The effect of P450 inducers on the pharmacokinetics of CCR5 antagonist, UK-427,857, in healthy volunteers. 5th International Workshop on Clinical Pharmacology of HIV Therapy. Rome, 1–3 April, 2004. Poster 5.4. Available at: http://www.hivpresentation.com/assets/5FAD1272-C09F-296A-61F3127678938120.pdf (accessed 21/08/07).
2. Muirhead G, Pozniak A, Gazzard B, Nelson M, Moyle G, Ridgway C, Taylor-Worth R, Russell D. A novel probe drug interaction study to investigate the effect of selected ARV combinations on the pharmacokinetics of a single oral dose of maraviroc (UK-427,857) in HIV +ve subjects. 12th Conference on Retroviruses and Opportunistic Infections, Boston MA, February 22–25, 2005. Available at: http://www.retroconference.org/2005/cd/Abstracts/24409.htm (accessed 21/08/07).
3. Muirhead G, Ridgway C, Leahy D, Mills C, van der Merwe R, Russell D. A study to investigate the combined co-administration of P450 CYP3A4 inhibitors and inducers on the pharmacokinetics of the novel CCR5 inhibitor UK-427,857. 7th International Congress on Drug Therapy in HIV infection, Glasgow, UK, 14-18 November 2004.
4. Abel S, Russell D, Ridgway C, Muirhead G. Overview of the drug-drug interaction data for maraviroc (UK-427,857). 6th International Workshop on Clinical Pharmacology of HIV Therapy. Québec, 28–30 April, 2005. Abstract 76. Available at: http://www.hivpresentation.com/assets/85C8CA27-E0C4-D510-0840664A09B59518.PDF (accessed 21/08/07).

Maraviroc + CYP3A4 inhibitors

Atazanavir, atazanavir/ritonavir, lopinavir/ritonavir and saquinavir markedly increased the AUC of maraviroc by about three to fivefold in healthy subjects. Ritonavir-boosted saquinavir had an even greater effect (about tenfold). In contrast, tipranavir/ritonavir had no effect. Ketoconazole caused a fivefold increase. The manufacturer suggests that the dose of maraviroc should be halved when used with protease inhibitors.

Clinical evidence

(a) Protease inhibitors

Saquinavir 1.2 g three times daily increased the AUC and maximum level of maraviroc 100 mg twice daily by 4.2-fold and 3.3-fold, respectively, in healthy subjects.[1] Furthermore, combining **saquinavir** 1 g with **ritonavir** 100 mg twice daily, increased the AUC of maraviroc by almost tenfold.[2] **Lopinavir/ritonavir** 400/100 mg twice daily increased the AUC and maximum level of maraviroc 300 mg twice daily by almost fourfold and twofold, respectively.[2]

Atazanavir 400 mg daily increased the AUC and maximum level of maraviroc by 257% and 109%, respectively.[3] **Atazanavir/ritonavir** 300/100 mg increased the AUC of maraviroc by almost fivefold.[3] In a study in HIV-positive patients, the AUC of a single 300-mg oral dose of maraviroc was doubled in 5 patients taking **lopinavir/ritonavir** 400/100 mg twice daily, stavudine and lamivudine when compared with that after one dose in a study in HIV-positive subjects taking maraviroc 300 mg daily alone.[4] Adding 'efavirenz', (p.780) halved the effect of **lopinavir/ritonavir** and **saquinavir/ritonavir** on the maraviroc AUC.[2]

In contrast, **tipranavir/ritonavir** 500/200 mg twice daily had no clinically significant effect on the AUC or maximum level of maraviroc 150 mg twice daily in healthy subjects.[5]

(b) Ketoconazole

Ketoconazole 400 mg once daily increased the AUC and maximum level of maraviroc 100 mg twice daily by fivefold and 3.4-fold, respectively, in healthy subjects.[1]

Mechanism

Maraviroc is a substrate of the cytochrome P450 isoenzyme CYP3A4 of which most protease inhibitors and ketoconazole are potent inhibitors.

Importance and management

Established and clinically important interactions. Increases of this magnitude are likely to result in increased adverse effects. The manufacturer has suggested that the dose of maraviroc is halved when it is used with protease inhibitors.[6] For a list of other inhibitors of CYP3A4, which might be expected to interact similarly, see 'Table 1.4', (p.6).

1. Abel S, Russell D, Ridgway C, Medhurst C, Weissgerber G, Muirhead G. Effect of CYP3A4 inhibitors on the pharmacokinetics of CCR5 antagonist UK-427,857 in healthy volunteers. 5th International Workshop on Clinical Pharmacology of HIV Therapy,1-3 April, 2004 Rome. Available at: http://www.hivpresentation.com/assets/5FAD12A1-C09F-296A-615C5C1DBA535EE6.pdf (accessed 21/08/07)
2. Muirhead G, Ridgway C, Leahy D, Mills C, van der Merwe R, Russell D. A study to investigate the combined co-administration of P450 CYP3A4 inhibitors and inducers on the pharmacokinetics of the novel CCR5 inhibitor UK-427,857. 7th International Congress on Drug Therapy in HIV infection, Glasgow, UK, 14-18 November 2004.
3. Muirhead G, Abel S, Russell D, Hackman F, Taylor-Worth R, Toh M, Tan LH. An investigation of the effects of atazanavir and ritonavir boosted atazanavir on the pharmcokinetics of the novel CCR5 inhibitor UK-427,857. 7th International Congress on Drug Therapy in HIV infection, Glasgow, UK, 14-18 November 2004.
4. Muirhead G, Pozniak A, Gazzard B, Nelson M, Moyle G, Ridgway C, Taylor-Worth R, Russell D. A novel probe drug interaction study to investigate the effect of selected ARV combinations on the pharmacokinetics of a single oral dose of maraviroc (UK-427,857) in HIV + ve subjects. 12th Conference on Retroviruses and Opportunistic Infections, Boston MA, February 22–25, 2005. Available at: http://www.retroconference.org/2005/cd/Abstracts/24409.htm (accessed 21/08/07).
5. Abel S, Taylor-Worth R, Ridgway C, Weissgerber G, Kraft M. Effect of tipranavir/ritonavir on the pharmacokinetics of maraviroc (MVC, UK-427,857). 7th International Workshop on Clinical Pharmacology of HIV Therapy; April 20-22, 2006; Lisbon, Portugal.
6. Abel S, Russell D, Ridgway C, Muirhead G. Overview of the drug-drug interaction data for maraviroc (UK-427,857). 6th International Workshop on Clinical Pharmacology of HIV Therapy. Québec, 28-30 April, 2005. Abstract 76. Available at: http://www.hivpresentation.com/assets/85C8CA27-E0C4-D510-0840664A09B59518.PDF (accessed 21/08/07).

Maraviroc + Drugs that affect renal clearance

Neither co-trimoxazole nor tenofovir had any important effect on maraviroc levels.

Clinical evidence

(a) Co-trimoxazole

Co-trimoxazole (sulfamethoxazole/trimethoprim 800/160 mg) twice daily had no clinically relevant effect on the pharmacokinetics of maraviroc 300 mg twice daily (a 10% increase in AUC and a 19% increase in maximum level).[1]

(b) Tenofovir

In a placebo-controlled, crossover study in healthy subjects, the concurrent use of maraviroc 300 mg twice daily and tenofovir disoproxil fumarate 300 mg once daily had no effect on the pharmacokinetics of maraviroc.[1,2]

Mechanism

Maraviroc undergoes some renal clearance (about 20% of total clearance).[1] Co-trimoxazole affects renal tubular transport, and tenofovir is predominantly excreted renally, so it was of interest to see if these had any effect on maraviroc levels.[1]

Importance and management

The pharmacokinetic data suggest that no maraviroc dose adjustment is likely to be needed if it is given with tenofovir or co-trimoxazole.

1. Pfizer Inc. Maraviroc Tablets NDA 22-128. Antiviral Drugs Advisory Committee (AVDAC) briefing document. April 24, 2007. Available at: http://www.fda.gov/ohrms/dockets/ac/07/briefing/2007-4283b1-01-Pfizer.pdf (accessed 21/08/07).
2. Muirhead G, Russell D, Abel S, Turner K, Taylor-Worth R, Tan LH, Toh M. An investigation of the effects of tenofovir on the pharmacokinetics of the novel CCR5 inhibitors UK-427,857. 7th International Congress on Drug Therapy in HIV Infection, 14–18 November 2004, Glasgow. Available at: http://www.aegis.com/conferences/hiv-glasgow/2004/P282.html (accessed 21/08/07).

Maraviroc + Miscellaneous

Maraviroc had no clinically relevant effect on the pharmacokinetics of lamivudine, zidovudine, or a combined oral contraceptive containing ethinylestradiol and levonorgestrel. No clinically important effect was seen with the CYP3A4 substrate midazolam. Food may reduce the absorption of maraviroc, but this is probably not clinically relevant.

Clinical evidence, mechanism, importance and management

(a) Food

In healthy male subjects, food significantly reduced the rate and extent of absorption of maraviroc.[1] However, the manufacturer reported that food appeared to have little effect on the antiviral activity of maraviroc, and so food restriction was not considered necessary.[2]

(b) Hormonal contraceptives

Maraviroc 100 mg twice daily had no effect on contraceptive steroid levels after administration of the combined oral contraceptive **ethinylestradiol/levonorgestrel** 30/150 micrograms daily for 7 days in a placebo-controlled crossover study in 15 healthy women.[3]

(c) Midazolam

In a placebo-controlled study in 12 healthy subjects maraviroc 300 mg twice daily for 7 days slightly increased the AUC of a single 7.5-mg dose of midazolam given on day 7 by 18%, after to. This increase is unlikely to be clinically relevant.[4] Midazolam is a probe substrate of the cytochrome P450 isoenzyme CYP3A4, and the findings suggest that maraviroc is unlikely to have an important effect on other CYP3A4 substrates. For a list see 'Table 1.4', (p.6).

(d) NRTIs

In a placebo-controlled, crossover study in healthy subjects maraviroc 300 mg twice daily had no clinically relevant effect on the pharmacokinetics of **zidovudine/lamivudine** (*Combivir*) 300/150 mg twice daily, when they were given together for one week.[5] For the effect of other NRTIs in combination with protease inhibitors or NNRTIs on maraviroc, see 'CYP3A4 inhibitors', (p.780) and 'CYP3A4 inducers', (p.780), and for the effect of tenofovir, see 'Drugs that affect renal clearance', (above).

1. Abel S, Van der Ryst E, Muirhead GJ, Rosario M, Edgington A, Weissgerber G. Pharmacokinetics of single and multiple oral doses of UK-427,857—a novel CCR5 antagonist in healthy volunteers. 10th Conference on Retroviruses and Opportunistic Infections, Boston MA, Feb 10–14, 2003. Available at: http://www.retroconference.org/2003/cd/Abstract/547.htm (accessed 21/08/07).
2. Pfizer Inc. Maraviroc Tablets NDA 22-128. Antiviral Drugs Advisory Committee (AVDAC) briefing document. April 24, 2007. Available at: http://www.fda.gov/ohrms/dockets/ac/07/briefing/2007-4283b1-01-Pfizer.pdf (accessed 21/08/07).
3. Abel S, Whitlock L, Ridgway C, Saifulanwar A, Bakhtyari A, Russell D. Effect of UK-427,857 on the pharmacokinetics of oral contraceptive steroids, and the pharmacokinetics of UK-427,857 in healthy young women. Intersci Conf Antimicrob Agents Chemother, Chicago 14–17 September, 2003.
4. Abel S, Russell D, Ridgway C, Medhurst C. Whitlock L, Weissgerber G, Muirhead G. The effect of CCR5 antagonist UK-427,857, on the pharmacokinetics of CYP3A4 substrates in healthy volunteers. 5th International Workshop on Clinical Pharmacology of HIV Therapy. Rome, 1–3 April, 2004. Poster 5.7. Available at: http://www.hivpresentation.com/assets/5FAD1291-C09F-296A-61DA447701A7C603.pdf (accessed 21/08/07).
5. Russell D, Abel S, Hackman F, Whitlock L, van der Merwe R, Muirhead G. The effect of maraviroc (UK-427,857) on the pharmacokinetics of 3TC/AZT (Combivir™) in healthy subjects. 6th International Workshop on Clinical Pharmacology of HIV Therapy. Québec, 28–30 April, 2005. Abstract 30. Available at: http://www.hivpresentation.com/assets/85C4305C-E0C4-D510-02B06CE974717ADB.PDF (accessed 21/08/07).

NNRTIs + Antiepileptics; Enzyme-inducing

The concurrent use of carbamazepine and efavirenz leads to a modest reduction in the plasma levels of both drugs; similar effects may be expected with phenytoin and phenobarbital. The use of nevirapine and carbamazepine may also result in decreased levels of both drugs.

Clinical evidence

The manufacturer notes that there was a pharmacokinetic interaction between **efavirenz** 600 mg daily and **carbamazepine** 400 mg daily in a study in healthy subjects. The steady-state AUC, and maximum and minimum plasma concentrations of **carbamazepine** decreased by 27%, 20% and 35%, respectively, while the steady-state AUC, and maximum and minimum plasma concentrations of **efavirenz** decreased by 36%, 21%, and 47%, respectively. The steady-state levels of the active carbamazepine epoxide metabolite remained unchanged.[1,2]

Mechanism

Efavirenz and carbamazepine are both inducers and substrates of the cytochrome P450 isoenzyme CYP3A4, and so they can both increase the metabolism of the other drug. **Nevirapine** would be expected to interact similarly (see 'Table 21.2', (p.773)).

Importance and management

The manufacturers of efavirenz note that an alternative to carbamazepine should be considered (especially with doses of greater than 400 mg daily, the study dose).[1,2] The US manufacturer of nevirapine recommends caution with the concurrent use of carbamazepine.[3]

In the UK, the manufacturer states that no data are available on the potential interactions of efavirenz with **phenytoin** or **phenobarbital**. They say that when efavirenz is given with these drugs, there is a potential for reduction or increase in the plasma concentrations of each drug. They therefore recommend periodic monitoring of plasma levels.[1]

1. Sustiva (Efavirenz). Bristol-Myers Squibb Pharmaceuticals Ltd. UK Summary of product characteristics, May 2007.
2. Sustiva (Efavirenz). Bristol-Myers Squibb Company. US Prescribing information, January 2007.
3. Viramune (Nevirapine). Boehringer Ingelheim Pharmaceuticals, Inc. US Prescribing information, June 2007.

NNRTIs + Antiepileptics; Valproate

Efavirenz levels were not altered by valproic acid in one study in HIV-positive patients, and valproic acid levels were not different to those in a control group not taking efavirenz. However, one patient had a marked decrease in valproate levels after starting efavirenz. A case of hepatotoxicity has occurred in a patient taking valproic acid with nevirapine and saquinavir/ritonavir.

Clinical evidence

In a study in 11 HIV-positive patients taking **efavirenz** 600 mg once daily with various NRTIs, there was no change in the pharmacokinetics of **efavirenz** after they took valproic acid 250 mg twice daily for 7 days. Valproic acid levels achieved in these patients were not significantly different from those in 11 HIV-positive control patients mainly taking NRTI antiretrovirals, even when the 3 control patients taking a protease inhibitor or NNRTI (amprenavir, indinavir, or nelfinavir plus nevirapine) were excluded.[1]

However, a bipolar patient with multidrug addiction had a decrease in plasma valproic acid levels of more than 50% shortly after starting an antiretroviral regimen including **efavirenz**. Even though the valproate dose was increased to 4 g daily, it was found difficult to achieve a target plasma level of 50 mg/dL. About 3 months later, following a valproate dose reduction to 1.5 g daily due to adverse effects, his level was unaltered, at 52 mg/dL.[2]

A case of valproate-associated hepatotoxicity occurred in a 51-year-old man about 3 weeks after he started **nevirapine** 200 mg twice daily, saquinavir/ritonavir 400/400 mg twice daily, and stavudine. Serum valproic acid levels remained therapeutic.[3]

Mechanism

Uncertain.

Importance and management

The findings of the study[1] suggest that valproate can be used with efavirenz-based regimens without any anticipated pharmacokinetic drug interaction. However, the case report introduces a note of caution. It may be appropriate to monitor valproate levels in patients taking efavirenz. It is unclear whether the case of hepatotoxicity was a result of a drug interaction. Note that there has been some concern about using valproate in HIV infection but there seems to be no established reason to avoid or specifically promote the use of valproate in HIV-infection *per se*.

1. DiCenzo R, Peterson D, Cruttenden K, Morse G, Riggs G, Gelbard H, Schifitto G. Effects of valproic acid coadministration on plasma efavirenz and lopinavir concentrations in human immunodeficiency virus-infected adults. *Antimicrob Agents Chemother* (2004) 48, 4328–31.
2. Saraga M, Preisig M, Zullino DF. Reduced valproate plasma levels possible after introduction of efavirenz in a bipolar patient. *Bipolar Disord* (2006) 8, 415–17.
3. Cozza KL, Swanton EJ, Humphreys CW. Hepatotoxicity with combination of valproic acid, ritonavir, and nevirapine: a case report. *Psychosomatics* (2000) 41, 452–3.

NNRTIs + Azoles; Fluconazole

Fluconazole doubles nevirapine exposure, and the combination should be used with caution. Fluconazole causes a minor rise in efavirenz steady-state levels, and does not alter delavirdine levels. Fluconazole levels are not altered by these NNRTIs.

Clinical evidence, mechanism, importance and management

(a) Delavirdine

Delavirdine mesilate 300 mg three times daily was given to 13 HIV-positive subjects for 30 days. Fluconazole 400 mg daily was given to 8 of them on days 16 to 30. No differences in the pharmacokinetics of either drug were noted between the two groups.[1] On the basis of these results, it would appear that no dosage adjustments are needed if these drugs are used together.

(b) Efavirenz

Fluconazole 400 mg daily for one day, then 200 mg daily for 6 days was given to 20 healthy subjects with efavirenz 400 mg daily. The pharmacokinetics of fluconazole were not affected, and although the AUC of efavirenz was raised by 15%, no clinically significant effects are anticipated.[2]

(c) Nevirapine

The concurrent use of fluconazole and nevirapine doubled the exposure to nevirapine compared with historical control data, although nevirapine did not have any clinically relevant effect on fluconazole pharmacokinetics.[3,4] The manufacturer suggests that patients should be closely monitored for nevirapine-associated adverse effects if fluconazole and nevirapine are used concurrently.[3,4] However, in a retrospective study of patients who had received a nevirapine-based HAART regimen, there was no increase in the incidence of clinical hepatitis, elevated aminotransferases or skin rashes, when the outcomes of 225 patients not receiving fluconazole, 392 patients treated with fluconazole 400 mg weekly, and 69 patients receiving fluconazole 200 mg daily with nevirapine were compared.[5]

1. Borin MT, Cox SR, Herman BD, Carel BJ, Anderson RD, Freimuth WW. Effect of fluconazole on the steady-state pharmacokinetics of delavirdine in human immunodeficiency virus-positive patients. *Antimicrob Agents Chemother* (1997) 41, 1892–7.
2. Benedek IH, Fiske WD, White SJ, Kornhauser DM. Plasma levels of fluconazole (FL) are not altered by coadministration of DMP 266 in healthy volunteers. *Intersci Conf Antimicrob Agents Chemother* (1997) 37, 1.
3. Viramune (Nevirapine anhydrate). Boehringer Ingelheim Ltd. UK Summary of product characteristics, January 2007.
4. Viramune (Nevirapine). Boehringer Ingelheim Pharmaceuticals, Inc. US Prescribing information, June 2007.
5. Manosuthi W, Chumpathat N, Chaovavanich A, Sungkanuparph S. Safety and tolerability of nevirapine-based antiretroviral therapy in HIV-infected patients receiving fluconazole for cryptococcal prophylaxis: a retrospective cohort study. *BMC Infect Dis* (2005) 5, 67.

NNRTIs + Azoles; Itraconazole

Itraconazole had no effect on efavirenz levels, whereas efavirenz modestly decreased itraconazole levels. Nevirapine may also decrease itraconazole levels.

Clinical evidence

In a study in healthy subjects, **efavirenz** 600 mg daily decreased the steady-state maximum plasma levels and the AUC of itraconazole 200 mg twice daily by 37% and 39%, respectively, and caused a similar decrease in hydroxyitraconazole levels. The steady-state maximum plasma levels and the AUC of **efavirenz** were not affected by itraconazole.[1,2]

Mechanism

The metabolism of itraconazole by the cytochrome P450 isoenzyme CYP3A4 is induced by efavirenz. Nevirapine might interact similarly as it also induces CYP3A4.

Importance and management

On the basis of the pharmacokinetic study, the manufacturers of efavirenz say that alternatives to itraconazole should be considered.[1,2] If there are no appropriate alternatives, it might be prudent to increase the dose of itraconazole, with increased monitoring for efficacy and toxicity of the combination.

Nevirapine might be expected to interact similarly to efavirenz, therefore monitor itraconazole efficacy carefully and anticipate the need to increase the dose.

1. Sustiva (Efavirenz). Bristol-Myers Squibb Pharmaceuticals Ltd. UK Summary of product characteristics, May 2007.
2. Sustiva (Efavirenz). Bristol-Myers Squibb Company. US Prescribing information, January 2007.

NNRTIs + Azoles; Ketoconazole

Nevirapine markedly reduces the AUC of ketoconazole. In theory, efavirenz may interact similarly, whereas delavirdine may increase ketoconazole levels. The NNRTI plasma levels may be raised by ketoconazole.

Clinical evidence

(a) Delavirdine

The manufacturer notes that the minimum level of delavirdine was 50% higher than population pharmacokinetic data in 26 patients taking ketoconazole.[1]

(b) Nevirapine

The manufacturers of nevirapine quote a study in which nevirapine 200 mg twice daily was given with ketoconazole 400 mg daily. The ketoconazole AUC was markedly reduced by 72% and its maximum plasma levels were reduced by 44%.[2,3] In addition, the nevirapine plasma levels were raised by 15 to 28% compared with historical control data.[2]

Mechanism

Ketoconazole is likely to inhibit the metabolism of the NNRTIs by the cytochrome P450 isoenzyme CYP3A4. Nevirapine induces the metabolism of ketoconazole by CYP3A4, and, in theory, **efavirenz** is likely to interact similarly, whereas delavirdine is likely to inhibit ketoconazole metabolism by CYP3A4 (see 'Table 21.2', (p.773)).

Importance and management

The manufacturer of nevirapine states that ketoconazole and nevirapine should not be used together, because of the likely reduced efficacy of ketoconazole.[2,3] Efavirenz might be expected to interact similarly although the manufacturer of efavirenz says that the potential for an interaction has not been studied.[4] NNRTI levels might be raised by ketoconazole, which might increase adverse effects. Cautious monitoring of efficacy and adverse effects would be prudent if concurrent use is necessary.

1. Rescriptor (Delavirdine mesylate). Pfizer Inc. US Prescribing information, June 2006.
2. Viramune (Nevirapine anhydrate). Boehringer Ingelheim Ltd. UK Summary of product characteristics, January 2007.
3. Viramune (Nevirapine). Boehringer Ingelheim Pharmaceuticals, Inc. US Prescribing information, June 2007.
4. Sustiva (Efavirenz). Bristol-Myers Squibb Pharmaceuticals Ltd. UK Summary of product characteristics, May 2007.

NNRTIs + Azoles; Posaconazole

The manufacturer of posaconazole predicts that it will increase the plasma levels of the NNRTIs because it inhibits the cytochrome P450 isoenzyme CYP3A4, by which they are metabolised. They recommend patients should be carefully monitored for any occurrence of toxicity during concurrent use.[1]

1. Noxafil (Posaconazole). Schering-Plough Ltd. UK Summary of product characteristics, October 2006.

NNRTIs + Azoles; Voriconazole

Efavirenz markedly decreases voriconazole levels and voriconazole modestly increases efavirenz levels. Voriconazole is predicted to increase levels of both delavirdine and nevirapine. Like efavirenz, nevirapine is predicted to decrease voriconazole levels, whereas delavirdine is predicted to increase voriconazole levels.

Clinical evidence

In a study in healthy subjects, **efavirenz** 400 mg daily decreased the steady-state maximum plasma levels and the AUC of voriconazole 200 mg twice daily by 61% and 77%, respectively. At the same time, the steady-state maximum plasma levels and the AUC of **efavirenz** were increased by 38% and 44%, respectively.[1] In a dose-adjustment study, when voriconazole 300 mg twice daily and **efavirenz** 300 mg daily were used together, the AUC of voriconazole was 55% lower than that seen with the standard dose of voriconazole 200 mg twice daily alone, and the **efavirenz** AUC was equivalent to that seen with efavirenz 600 mg daily alone.[2-4] In a further dose-adjustment study, when voriconazole 400 mg twice daily was given with **efavirenz** 300 mg once daily, the AUC of voriconazole was just 7% lower than that seen with voriconazole 200 mg twice daily alone. The AUC of **efavirenz** was increased by 17% and the maximum plasma concentration was equivalent, when compared with efavirenz 600 mg once daily alone.[2-4]

There is one case of a patient taking a variety of antiretrovirals and antibacterials who developed oral candidiasis while taking voriconazole 200 mg twice daily, which was attributed to an interaction with **efavirenz**. The dose of voriconazole was titrated upwards to 350 mg twice daily to achieve higher trough levels. The candidiasis was eventually found to be resistant to voriconazole, and it was postulated that this developed because of under-dosing in the presence of **efavirenz**.[5]

Mechanism

The metabolism of voriconazole by the cytochrome P450 isoenzyme CYP3A4 is induced by efavirenz. **Nevirapine** is predicted to interact similarly, whereas **delavirdine** is predicted to inhibit the metabolism of voriconazole. All the NNRTIs are substrates of CYP3A4, which is inhibited by voriconazole.

Importance and management

On the basis of the pharmacokinetic studies the manufacturers contraindicate the concurrent use of efavirenz and voriconazole,[6] unless the doses of both drugs are adjusted.[2-4] The recommendation is to double the usual dose of voriconazole to 400 mg twice daily, and to halve the usual efavirenz dose to 300 mg once daily.[2-4]

Nevirapine might be expected to interact similarly to efavirenz, whereas delavirdine might increase voriconazole levels. The manufacturers of voriconazole suggest that patients given delavirdine or nevirapine should be carefully monitored for evidence of drug toxicity and/or loss of efficacy during concurrent use.[2,3]

1. Liu P, Foster G, Labadie R, Gutierrez MJ, Sharma A. Pharmacokinetic interaction between voriconazole and efavirenz at steady state in healthy subjects. *Clin Pharmacol Ther* (2005) 77, P40.
2. VFEND (Voriconazole). Pfizer Ltd. UK Summary of product characteristics, July 2007.
3. VFEND (Voriconazole). Pfizer Inc. US Prescribing information, November 2006.
4. Sustiva (Efavirenz). Bristol-Myers Squibb Company. US Prescribing information, January 2007.
5. Gerzenshtein L, Patel SM, Scarsi KK, Postelnick MJ, Flaherty JP. Breakthrough *Candida* infections in patients receiving voriconazole. *Ann Pharmacother* (2005) 39, 1342–5.
6. Sustiva (Efavirenz). Bristol-Myers Squibb Pharmaceuticals Ltd. UK Summary of product characteristics, May 2007.

NNRTIs + Drugs that affect gastric pH

Antacids roughly halve the AUC of delavirdine, and the H_2-receptor antagonists or proton pump inhibitors would be expected to interact similarly. Aluminium/magnesium antacids do not interact to a clinically relevant extent with efavirenz or nevirapine, and famotidine does not alter the absorption of efavirenz.

Clinical evidence, mechanism, importance and management

(a) Delavirdine

Delavirdine is poorly soluble at pHs greater than 3, so the effect of giving delavirdine 300 mg ten minutes after an antacid was studied in 12 healthy subjects. The AUC and maximum serum levels of delavirdine were reduced by 48% and 57%, respectively, suggesting that delavirdine should not be given with antacids.[1] The manufacturer recommends separating administration by at least one hour.[2] Although it has not been studied, it is predicted that other drugs that reduce gastric acidity, such as H_2-receptor antagonists and proton pump inhibitors, will also reduce the absorption of delavirdine, and their long-term use with delavirdine is not recommended.[2]

(b) Efavirenz

The manufacturer notes that neither **aluminium/magnesium hydroxide** antacids nor **famotidine** had any effect on the absorption of efavirenz.[3] No efavirenz dosage adjustment is expected to be necessary with these drugs.[4] Other drugs that reduce gastric acidity are not expected to affect efavirenz absorption.[3]

(c) Nevirapine

In a study in 24 healthy subjects it was found that 30 mL of *Maalox* (**aluminium/magnesium hydroxide**) caused some moderate changes in the pharmacokinetics of nevirapine 200 mg, but none of them was considered to be clinically relevant.[5] No special precautions would seem to be necessary.

1. Cox SR, Della-Coletta AA, Turner SW, Freimuth WW. Single-dose pharmacokinetic (PK) studies with delavirdine (DLV) mesylate: dose proportionality and effects of food and antacid. *Intersci Conf Antimicrob Agents Chemother* (1994) 34, 82.
2. Rescriptor (Delavirdine mesylate). Pfizer Inc. US Prescribing information, June 2006.
3. Sustiva (Efavirenz). Bristol-Myers Squibb Pharmaceuticals Ltd. UK Summary of product characteristics, May 2007.
4. Sustiva (Efavirenz). Bristol-Myers Squibb Company. US Prescribing information, January 2007.
5. Lamson M, Cort S, Macy H, Love J, Korpalski D, Pav J, Keirns J. Effects of food or antacid on the bioavailability of nevirapine 200 mg tablets. 11th International Conference on AIDS, Vancouver, 1996. Abstract Tu.B.2323.

NNRTIs + Food

Food has no clinically relevant effect on the levels of delavirdine or nevirapine. Food modestly increases efavirenz levels, and the manufacturer suggests that this might increase the frequency of adverse effects.

Clinical evidence, mechanism, importance and management

(a) Delavirdine

In a randomised, crossover study in 13 HIV-positive patients taking delavirdine 400 mg daily, there were no changes in the steady-state serum levels of delavirdine taken with or without food for 2 weeks.[1] This differed from a previous single-dose study, in which there was a 26% fall in the AUC of delavirdine given with food.[2] There would appear to be no need to avoid taking delavirdine with food. For mention that orange juice increased the absorption of delavirdine in patients with gastric hypoacidity, see 'NNRTIs; Delavirdine + Acids', p.791.

(b) Efavirenz

The manufacturer of efavirenz notes that taking a 600-mg efavirenz *tablet* with a **high-fat meal** increased its AUC by 28%, when compared with fasting conditions, and increased its maximum concentration by 79%.[3,4] After a similar meal, the AUC and maximum level of the *capsule* formulation was increased by 22% and 39%, respectively, and after a **low-fat meal** the increases were 17% and 51%, respectively.[4] The manufacturer says that these increases might increase the frequency of adverse effects. They recommend that efavirenz is taken without food, preferably at bedtime.[3,4]

(c) Nevirapine

In a study in 24 healthy subjects, a **high-fat breakfast** caused some moderate changes in the pharmacokinetics of oral nevirapine 200 mg, but the AUC was not affected and none of the changes were considered to be clinically relevant.[5] Nevirapine may be taken with or without food.

1. Morse GD, Fischl MA, Cox SR, Thompson L, Della-Coletta AA, Freimuth WW. Effect of food on the steady-state (SS) pharmacokinetics of delavirdine mesylate (DLV) in HIV+ patients. *Intersci Conf Antimicrob Agents Chemother* (1995) 35, 210.
2. Cox SR, Della-Coletta AA, Turner SW, Freimuth WW. Single-dose pharmacokinetic (PK) studies with delavirdine (DLV) mesylate: dose proportionality and effects of food and antacid. *Intersci Conf Antimicrob Agents Chemother* (1994) 34, 82.
3. Sustiva (Efavirenz). Bristol-Myers Squibb Pharmaceuticals Ltd. UK Summary of product characteristics, May 2007.
4. Sustiva (Efavirenz). Bristol-Myers Squibb Company. US Prescribing information, January 2007.
5. Lamson MJ, Cort S, Sabo JP, MacGregor TR, Keirns JJ, Effects of food or antacid on the bioavailability of nevirapine 200 mg in 24 healthy volunteers. *Pharm Res* (1995) 12 (9 Suppl), S-101.

NNRTIs + Macrolides

Delavirdine may increase the levels of clarithromycin, whereas efavirenz and nevirapine may reduce clarithromycin levels, and increase those of its hydroxy metabolite. Clarithromycin does not appear to affect the pharmacokinetics of delavirdine, efavirenz or nevirapine to a clinically relevant extent. There is no pharmacokinetic interaction between azithromycin and efavirenz. A case of a neuropsychiatric reaction has been attributed to the use of clarithromycin in a man taking nevirapine.

Clinical evidence

(a) Delavirdine

In 7 HIV-positive patients **clarithromycin** 500 mg twice daily for 15 days did not cause a clinically significant change in the pharmacokinetics of delavirdine 300 mg three times daily, when compared with 4 other HIV-positive patients taking only delavirdine. The combination was well tolerated and no serious adverse events occurred.[1] However, although delavirdine levels are unaffected, the manufacturer notes that the AUC of **clarithromycin** was doubled by delavirdine.[2]

(b) Efavirenz

The manufacturer notes that the concurrent use of **clarithromycin** 500 mg twice daily and efavirenz 400 mg daily for 7 days reduced the AUC of **clarithromycin** by 39% and increased the AUC of its hydroxy metabolite by 34%. Moreover, 46% of subjects receiving the combination developed a rash.[3,4] Clarithromycin had minimal effect on the pharmacokinetics of efavirenz.[4]

The manufacturer also notes that there was no clinically significant pharmacokinetic interaction when a single 600-mg dose of **azithromycin** was given to healthy subjects who had been taking efavirenz 400 mg daily for 7 days.[3,4]

(c) Nevirapine

The manufacturer notes that the AUC of nevirapine was increased by 26% by **clarithromycin**, when compared with historical controls. The AUC of **clarithromycin** was reduced by 31% and the AUC of its hydroxy metabolite was increased by 42%.[5,6] A man developed hyperactivity (poor concentration, anxiety, suicidal and homicidal ideation) when taking **clarithromycin** and antiretroviral drugs, including nevirapine. This was thought to be due to accumulation of the hydroxy metabolite of **clarithromycin**.[7]

Mechanism

The NNRTIs are substrates of the cytochrome P450 isoenzyme CYP3A4, which is inhibited by clarithromycin. Delavirdine is also reported to inhibit CYP3A4, whereas efavirenz and nevirapine induce CYP3A4. Therefore alterations in the metabolism of these drugs by CYP3A4 results in the altered levels seen.

Importance and management

It appears that clarithromycin has minimal effects on the pharmacokinetics of the NNRTIs. However, delavirdine may increase levels of clarithromycin. The manufacturer of **delavirdine** recommends that when the drugs are used concurrently the dose of clarithromycin should be reduced in patients with renal impairment.[2] In contrast, efavirenz and nevirapine may decrease clarithromycin levels and increase the levels of the hydroxy metabolite of clarithromycin. The manufacturer of **nevirapine** suggests that no dose adjustment of clarithromycin is needed; however, they say that alternatives to clarithromycin should be considered for the treatment of Mycobacterium-avium complex, as the hydroxy metabolite is not as active against this bacterium.[5,6] The manufacturer of **efavirenz** says that the clinical significance of the changes to clarithromycin pharmacokinetics is not known, but they suggest alternatives to clarithromycin should be considered.[3,4] Further study and experience of these combinations is needed.

1. Cox SR, Borin MT, Driver MR, Levy B, Freimuth WW. Effect of clarithromycin on the steady-state pharmacokinetics of delavirdine in HIV-1 patients. American Society for Microbiology, 2nd National Conference on Human Retroviruses, 1995. Abstract 487.
2. Rescriptor (Delavirdine mesylate). Pharmacia & Upjohn Company. US prescribing information, February 2006.
3. Sustiva (Efavirenz). Bristol-Myers Squibb Pharmaceuticals Ltd. UK Summary of product characteristics, May 2007.
4. Sustiva (Efavirenz). Bristol-Myers Squibb Company. US Prescribing information, January 2007.
5. Viramune (Nevirapine anhydrate). Boehringer Ingelheim Ltd. UK Summary of product characteristics, January 2007.
6. Viramune (Nevirapine). Boehringer Ingelheim Pharmaceuticals, Inc. US Prescribing information, June 2007.
7. Prime K, French P. Neuropsychiatric reaction induced by clarithromycin in a patient on highly active antiretroviral therapy (HAART). *Sex Transm Infect* (2001) 77, 297–8.

NNRTIs + NNRTIs

Nevirapine modestly reduces the levels of efavirenz, whereas efavirenz has no effect on nevirapine levels.

Clinical evidence, mechanism, importance and management

In a study in HIV-positive patients taking efavirenz 600 mg daily, the addition of **nevirapine** 400 mg daily resulted in a median decrease in the AUC of **efavirenz** of 22%, and a decrease in its minimum plasma concentration of 36%. The steady-state pharmacokinetics of **nevirapine** were not altered by **efavirenz**, when compared with historical control data.[1] However, the UK manufacturer does not recommend this combination as concurrent use of **efavirenz** and **nevirapine** could lead to a higher risk of adverse effects. Moreover they say that concurrent use does not improve efficacy over either NNRTI alone.[2]

1. Veldkamp AI, Harris M, Montaner JSG, Moyle G, Gazzard B, Youle M, Johnson M, Kwakkelstein MO, Carlier H, van Leeuwen R, Beijnen JH, Lange JMA, Reiss P, Hoetelmans RMW. The steady-state pharmacokinetics of efavirenz and nevirapine when used in combination in human immunodeficiency virus type 1-infected persons. *J Infect Dis* (2001) 184, 37–42.
2. Viramune (Nevirapine anhydrate). Boehringer Ingelheim Ltd. UK Summary of product characteristics, January 2007.

NNRTIs + NRTIs

Delavirdine absorption is reduced by the buffered preparation of didanosine. This interaction would not be expected with the enteric-coated preparation of didanosine. Delavirdine does not affect the pharmacokinetics of zidovudine. There is no pharmacokinetic interaction between efavirenz and zidovudine or lamivudine. There is no clinically relevant pharmacokinetic interaction between nevirapine and didanosine, lamivudine, stavudine, zalcitabine or zidovudine.

Clinical evidence, mechanism, importance and management

(a) Delavirdine

A study in 34 HIV-positive patients taking **zidovudine** 200 mg three times daily found that delavirdine mesilate 400 mg to 1.2 g daily for 9 days had no clinically significant effect on the pharmacokinetics of **zidovudine**.[1]

In a steady-state study, 9 HIV-positive patients taking **didanosine** 200 mg twice daily were also given delavirdine mesilate 400 mg three times daily for 14 days. **Didanosine** caused a 37% reduction in the maximum delavirdine serum levels, but when the drugs were given 1 hour apart no significant effect occurred.[2] A single-dose study in 12 HIV-positive patients found similar results.[3] The buffered preparation of **didanosine** contains antacids to increase its absorption, and antacids decrease the absorption of delavirdine (see 'NNRTIs + Drugs that affect gastric pH', p.784). The authors of one report suggest that separating the doses by about one hour is preferable.[2] The enteric-coated preparation of **didanosine**, which does not contain antacids, would not be expected to reduce the absorption of delavirdine.

(b) Efavirenz

The manufacturer notes that there were no clinically significant pharmacokinetic interactions between efavirenz and **zidovudine** or **lamivudine** in patients with HIV.[4,5] No dosage adjustments are required on concurrent use.[5] No pharmacokinetic interactions are anticipated with other NRTIs.[4,5]

(c) Nevirapine

The pharmacokinetics of **didanosine** and **zidovudine** with or without nevirapine were assessed in 175 HIV-positive subjects. The bioavailability of **didanosine** was not affected, but the bioavailability of **zidovudine** was decreased by about one-third by nevirapine.[6] In a steady-state study in 24 HIV-positive patients, nevirapine 200 mg every 12 hours was added to regimens of **didanosine**, **didanosine** with **zidovudine**, or **zidovudine** with **zalcitabine** for a 4-week period. No significant changes in the pharmacokinetics of **didanosine** or **zalcitabine** were seen. However, in the **didanosine/zidovudine** group the peak **zidovudine** plasma levels and AUC were reduced by 27% and 32%, respectively. The **zidovudine** pharmacokinetics in the **zidovudine/zalcitabine** group were not affected.[7] The reasons for these changes are not clear, but the clinical consequences are thought to be small, and the safety data indicate that the concurrent use of these drugs is safe and well tolerated. In another study, the simultaneous administration of nevirapine with **didanosine** tablets containing antacids had no effect on nevirapine absorption in 4 patients.[8] The manufacturer says that no dosage adjustments are needed if **didanosine**, **zalcitabine** or **zidovudine** is taken with nevirapine.[9]

Nevirapine 200 mg once daily for 2 weeks then 200 mg twice daily had no effect on the AUC of **stavudine** 30 to 40 mg twice daily in a study in 22 patients.[10,11] Nevirapine appears to have no effect on **lamivudine** clearance, based on a population pharmacokinetic study.[12]

1. Morse GD, Cox SR, DeRemer MF, Batts DH, Freimuth WW. Zidovudine (ZDV) pharmacokinetics (PK) during an escalating, multiple-dose study of delavirdine (DLV) mesylate. *Intersci Conf Antimicrob Agents Chemother* (1994) 34, 132.
2. Cox SR, Cohn SE, Greisberger C, Reichman RC, Della-Coletta AA, Freimuth WW, Morse GD. Evaluation of the steady-state (SS) pharmacokinetic interaction between didanosine (ddI) and delavirdine mesylate (DLV) in HIV+ patients. *Intersci Conf Antimicrob Agents Chemother* (1995) 35, 210.
3. Morse GD, Fischl MA, Shelton MJ, Cox SR, Driver M, DeRemer M, Freimuth WW. Single-dose pharmacokinetics of delavirdine mesylate and didanosine in patients with human immunodeficiency virus infection. *Antimicrob Agents Chemother* (1997) 41, 169–74.
4. Sustiva (Efavirenz). Bristol-Myers Squibb Pharmaceuticals Ltd. UK Summary of product characteristics, May 2007.
5. Sustiva (Efavirenz). Bristol-Myers Squibb Company. US Prescribing information, January 2007.
6. Zhou XJ, Sheiner LB, D'Aquila RT, Hughes MD, Hirsch MS, Fischl MA, Johnson VA, Myers M, Sommadossi JP and the NIAID ACTG241 Investigators. Population pharmacokinetics of nevirapine, zidovudine and didanosine after combination therapy in HIV-infected patients. *Clin Pharmacol Ther* (1998) 63,182.
7. MacGregor TR, Lamson MJ, Cort S, Pav JW, Saag MS, Elvin AT, Sommadossi J-P, Myers M, Keirns JJ. Steady state pharmacokinetics of nevirapine, didanosine, zalcitabine, and zidovudine combination therapy in HIV-1 positive patients. *Pharm Res* (1995) 12 (9 Suppl), S-101.
8. van Heeswijk RPG, Veldkamp AI, Mulder JW, Meenhorst PL, Wit FWNM, Reiss P, Lange JMA, Kwakkelstein MO, Beijnen JH, Hoetelmans RMW. Nevirapine plus didanosine: once or twice daily combination? *J Acquir Immune Defic Syndr* (2000) 25, 93–5.
9. Viramune (Nevirapine anhydrate). Boehringer Ingelheim Ltd. UK Summary of product characteristics, January 2007.
10. Skowron G, Leoung G, Hall DB, Robinson P, Lewis R, Grosso R, Jacobs M, Kerr B, MacGregor T, Stevens M, Fisher A, Odgen R, Yen-Lieberman B. Pharmacokinetic evaluation and short-term activity of stavudine, nevirapine, and nelfinavir therapy in HIV-1-infected adults. *J Acquir Immune Defic Syndr* (2004) 35, 351–8.
11. Viramune (Nevirapine). Boehringer Ingelheim Pharmaceuticals, Inc. US Prescribing information, June 2007.
12. Sabo JP, Lamson MJ, Leitz G, Yong C-L, MacGregor TR. Pharmacokinetics of nevirapine and lamivudine in patients with HIV-1 infection. AAPS PharmSci. (2000) 2, E1–E7.

NNRTIs + Protease inhibitors

In general, efavirenz and nevirapine decrease the levels of protease inhibitors, whereas delavirdine increases them. Ritonavir is sometimes used to elevate the levels of other protease inhibitors when efavirenz or nevirapine are required. Amprenavir and nelfinavir decrease the levels of delavirdine. Most protease inhibitors do not appear to affect the levels of efavirenz or nevirapine. There is some evidence of increased adverse effects with antiviral doses of ritonavir and efavirenz, or saquinavir and delavirdine, including raised liver enzymes. Note that NNRTIs are not given with protease inhibitors in current first-line regimens for HIV infection: either an NNRTI or protease inhibitors are combined with dual NRTIs.

Table 21.3 Summary of the pharmacokinetic interactions of NNRTIs and protease inhibitors

Drug combination	*No. of healthy subjects (unless specified)*	*Change in AUC (unless specified)*		*Refs*
		NNRTI	Protease inhibitor	
Delavirdine studies (usually 400 mg three times daily or 600 mg twice daily)				
Amprenavir	6 HIV-positive children		3-fold increase in Cmax* 5 to 10-fold increase in Cmin*	1
Amprenavir 1200 mg Amprenavir 1200 mg twice daily alone then 600 mg twice daily in combination	12 11	21% increase 47% decrease	4-fold increase 32% increase versus twice the dose given alone	2
Amprenavir 600 mg twice daily	18	61% decrease	130% increase	3
Indinavir 800 mg alone then 600 mg in combination	14	No change	44% increase versus higher dose given alone	4, 5
Nelfinavir 750 mg three times daily	24	42% decrease	92% increase	6
Ritonavir 300 mg twice daily		No change in steady state level	No change in steady state level	4
Ritonavir 600 mg twice daily	12 HIV-positive subjects	No change*	64% increase 81% increase in Cmin	7
Ritonavir 100 mg twice daily	19	No change	80% increase	8
Saquinavir 600 mg three times daily		No change in steady state level	5-fold increase in steady state level	4
Efavirenz studies (600 mg once daily)				
Amprenavir	2 HIV-positive children		Undetectable levels in less than 4 hours†	1
Amprenavir 1200 mg twice daily	7 HIV-positive subjects		About an 80% decrease in trough levels†	9
Amprenavir 1200 mg twice daily	11 HIV-positive subjects	No change*	24% decrease 43% decrease in Cmin	10
Atazanavir 400 mg once daily			74% decrease	11
Atazanavir/Ritonavir 300/100 mg once daily			39% increase	11
Darunavir/Ritonavir 300/100 mg twice daily		21% increase	31% decrease in Cmin (darunavir)	12
Fosamprenavir/Ritonavir 1395 mg/200 mg once daily	11		31% decrease in Cmin (amprenavir)	13
Fosamprenavir/Ritonavir 700 mg/100 mg twice daily	14		Slight decrease in Cmin (amprenavir)	13
Fosamprenavir/Ritonavir 1395 mg/300 mg once daily	11		Amprenavir levels comparable to that seen with 1395 mg/200 mg alone	13
Indinavir 800 mg three times daily alone then 1000 mg three times daily in combination			33% to 46% decrease versus lower dose given alone	14
Indinavir/Ritonavir 800/100 mg twice daily	14	No change*	25% decrease (indinavir) 36% decrease (ritonavir)	15
Indinavir/Ritonavir 800/100 mg twice daily	20 HIV-positive subjects	31% increase in Cmin*	Cmin halved* (indinavir)	16
Lopinavir/Ritonavir 400/100 mg twice daily	24 HIV-positive subjects		44% decrease in Cmin* (lopinavir)	17
Lopinavir/Ritonavir 533/133 mg twice daily	26 HIV-positive subjects		No significant change in Cmin versus lower dose given without efavirenz* (lopinavir)	17
Lopinavir/Ritonavir 600/150 mg twice daily			28 to 44% increase (lopinavir), 62 to 95% increase (ritonavir) compared with standard dose alone	18

Continued

Table 21.3 Summary of the pharmacokinetic interactions of NNRTIs and protease inhibitors (continued)

Drug combination	*No. of healthy subjects (unless specified)*	*Change in AUC (unless specified)*		*Refs*
		NNRTI	Protease inhibitor	
Lopinavir/Ritonavir 300/75 mg/m^2 twice daily	15 HIV-positive children	No change*	No change*	19
Nelfinavir 750 mg three times daily		No change	20% increase (nelfinavir), 37% decrease in M8 metabolite	20
Nelfinavir/Ritonavir 1875/200 mg once daily	24	No change*	30% increase (nelfinavir) 20% decrease (ritonavir)	21
Ritonavir 500 mg twice daily		21% increase	17% increase	22
Saquinavir 1200 mg three times daily			62% decrease	14
Saquinavir/Ritonavir 400/400 mg twice daily	12	No change*	No change in Cmin (ritonavir) 10% decrease in Cmin (saquinavir)	23
Tipranavir/Ritonavir 500/100 mg twice daily	24/21	No change	About a 40% decrease in Cmin (tipranavir)*	24
Nevirapine studies (200 mg once daily increased to twice daily)				
Darunavir/Ritonavir 400/100 mg twice daily		27% increase	No change in Cmin* (darunavir)	12
Fosamprenavir 1400 mg twice daily		29% increase	35% decrease in Cmin (amprenavir)	25
Fosamprenavir/Ritonavir 700/100 mg twice daily		14% increase	19% decrease in Cmin (amprenavir)	25
Indinavir 800 mg three times daily	19 HIV-positive subjects	No change*	28% decrease 48% decrease in Cmin	26
Indinavir 800 mg three times daily alone or 1000 mg three times daily in combination	124 HIV-positive subjects	No change	27% decrease in Cmin versus therapy alone at lower dose	27
Indinavir/Ritonavir 800/100 mg twice daily	21 HIV-positive subjects		57% decrease in Cmin (indinavir)‡	28
Lopinavir/ritonavir 300/75 mg/m^2 twice daily	27 HIV-positive children		22% decrease, 55% decrease in Cmin (lopinavir)	29
Nelfinavir 750 mg three times daily	7 HIV-positive subjects	No change*	50% decrease possibly due to sampling before nelfinavir steady state was reached	30, 31
Nelfinavir 750 mg three times daily	23 HIV-positive positive	No change*	No change	32
Nelfinavir 750 mg three times daily	13 HIV-positive subjects		No change	33
Nelfinavir 750 mg three times daily	23		No change; 32% decrease in Cmin 62% decrease in M8 metabolite	34
Ritonavir 600 mg twice daily	18 HIV-positive subjects	No change	No change	34, 35
Saquinavir 600 mg three times daily	21 HIV-positive subjects	No change	27% decrease	36
Saquinavir/ritonavir	20 HIV-positive subjects	No change*	No change	35
Tipranavir/ritonavir 250/200 mg twice daily	26 HIV-positive subjects	No change	No data	24

*Versus historical control data
†Therapeutic levels subsequently achieved by the addition of low-dose ritonavir
‡Versus data from 139 patients not taking nevirapine
Cmax = maximum serum concentration, Cmin = minimum serum concentration

1. Wintergerst U, Engelhorn C, Kurowski M, Hoffmann F, Notheis G, Belohradsky BH. Pharmacokinetic interaction of amprenavir in combination with efavirenz or delavirdine in HIV-infected children. *AIDS* (2000) 14, 1866–8.
2. Tran JQ, Petersen C, Garrett M, Hee B, Kerr BM. Pharmacokinetic interaction between amprenavir and delavirdine: evidence of induced clearance by amprenavir. *Clin Pharmacol Ther* (2002) 72, 615–26.
3. Justesen US, Klitgaard NA, Brosen K, Pedersen C. Pharmacokinetic interaction between amprenavir and delavirdine after multiple-dose administration in healthy volunteers. *Br J Clin Pharmacol* (2003) 55, 100–6.
4. Cox SR, Ferry JJ, Batts DH, Carlson GF, Schneck DW, Herman BD, Della-Coletta AA, Chambers JH, Carel BJ, Stewart F, Buss N, Brown A. Delavirdine (D) and marketed protease inhibitors (PIs): pharmacokinetic (PK) interaction studies in healthy volunteers. 4th Conference on Retroviruses and Opportunistic Infections, Washington, 1997. Abstract 372.

Continued

Table 21.3 Summary of the pharmacokinetic interactions of NNRTIs and protease inhibitors (continued)

5. Ferry JJ, Herman BD, Carel BJ, Carlson GF, Batts DH. Pharmacokinetic drug-drug interaction study of delavirdine and indinavir in healthy volunteers. *J Acquir Immune Defic Syndr Hum Retrovirol* (1998) 18, 252–9.
6. Cox SR, Schneck DW, Herman BD, Carel BJ, Gullotti BR, Kerr BM, Freimuth WW. Delavirdine (DLV) and nelfinavir (NFV): A pharmacokinetic (PK) drug-drug interaction study in healthy adult volunteers. 5th Conference on Retroviruses and Opportunistic Infections, Chicago, 1998. Abstract 345.
7. Shelton MJ, Hewitt RG, Adams J, Della-Coletta A, Cox S, Morse GD. Pharmacokinetics of ritonavir and delavirdine in human immunodeficiency virus-infected patients. *Antimicrob Agents Chemother* (2003) 47, 1694–9.
8. Tran JQ, Petersen C, Garrett M, Smith M, Hee B, Lillibridge J, Kerr B. Delavirdine significantly increases exposure of low dose ritonavir in healthy volunteers. *Intersci Conf Antimicrob Agents Chemother* (2001) 41, 15.
9. Duval X, Le Moing V, Longuet P, Leport C, Vildé J-L, Lamotte C, Peytavin G, Farinotti R. Efavirenz-induced decrease in plasma amprenavir levels in human immunodeficiency virus-infected patients and correction by ritonavir. *Antimicrob Agents Chemother* (2000) 44, 2593.
10. Falloon J, Piscitelli S, Vogel S, Sadler B, Mitsuya H, Kavlick MF, Yoshimura K, Rogers M, LaFon S, Manion DJ, Lane HC, Masur H. Combination therapy with amprenavir, abacavir, and efavirenz in human immunodeficiency virus (HIV)-infected patients failing a protease-inhibitor regimen: pharmacokinetic drug interactions and antiviral activity. *Clin Infect Dis* (2000) 30, 313–18.
11. Reyataz (Atazanavir sulfate). Bristol-Myers Squibb Company. US Prescribing information, March 2007.
12. Prezista (Darunavir). Tibotec, Inc. US Prescribing information, June 2006.
13. Wire MB, Ballow C, Preston SL, Hendrix CW, Piliero PJ, Lou Y, Stein DS. Pharmacokinetics and safety of GW433908 and ritonavir, with and without efavirenz, in healthy volunteers. *AIDS* (2004) 18, 897–907.
14. Sustiva (Efavirenz). Bristol-Myers Squibb Pharmaceuticals Ltd. UK Summary of product characteristics, March 2005.
15. Aarnoutse RE, Grintjes KJT, Telgt DSC, Stek M, Hugen PWH, Reiss P, Koopmans PP, Hekster YA, Burger DM. The influence of efavirenz on the pharmacokinetics of a twice-daily combination of indinavir and low-dose ritonavir in healthy volunteers. *Clin Pharmacol Ther* (2002) 71, 57–67.
16. Boyd MA, Aarnoutse RE, Ruxrungtham K, Stek M, van Heeswijk RPG, Lange JMA, Cooper DA, Phanuphak P, Burger DM. Pharmacokinetics of indinavir/ritonavir (800/100 mg) in combination with efavirenz (600 mg) in HIV-1-infected subjects. *J Acquir Immune Defic Syndr* (2003) 34, 134–9.
17. Hsu A, Isaacson J, Brun S, Bernstein B, Lam W, Bertz R, Foit C, Rynkiewicz K, Richards B, King M, Rode R, Kempf DJ, Granneman GR, Sun E. Pharmacokinetic-pharmacodynamic analysis of lopinavir-ritonavir in combination with efavirenz and two nucleoside reverse transcriptase inhibitors in extensively pretreated human immunodeficiency virus-infected patients. *Antimicrob Agents Chemother* (2003) 47, 350–9.
18. Kaletra Tablets (Lopinavir/Ritonavir). Abbott Laboratories Ltd. UK Summary of product characteristics, March 2007.
19. Bergshoeff AS, Fraaij PL, Ndagijimana J, Verweel G, Hartwig NG, Niehues T, De Groot R, Burger DM. Increased dose of lopinavir/ritonavir compensates for efavirenz-induced drug-drug interaction in HIV-1-infected children. *J Acquir Immune Defic Syndr* (2005) 39, 63–8.
20. Fiske WD, Benedek IH, White SJ, Pepperess KA, Joseph JL, Kornhauser DM. Pharmacokinetic interaction between efavirenz (EFV) and nelfinavir mesylate (NFV) in healthy volunteers. 5th Conference on Retroviruses and Opportunistic Infections, Chicago, 1998. Abstract 349.
21. la Porte CJL, de Graaff-Teulen MJA, Colbers EPH, Voncken DS, Ibanez SM, Koopmans PP, Hekster YA, Burger DM. Effect of efavirenz treatment on the pharmacokinetics of nelfinavir boosted by ritonavir in healthy volunteers. *Br J Clin Pharmacol* (2004) 58, 632–40.
22. Norvir (Ritonavir). Abbott Laboratories Ltd. UK Summary of product characteristics, May 2007.
23. Piliero PJ, Preston SL, Japour A, Stevens RC, Morvillo C, Drusano GL. Pharmacokinetics of the combination of ritonavir plus saquinavir, with and without efavirenz, in healthy volunteers. *Intersci Conf Antimicrob Agents Chemother* (2001) 41, 15.
24. Aptivus (Tipranavir). Boehringer Ingelheim. US Prescribing information, February 2007.
25. Lexiva (Fosamprenavir). GlaxoSmithKline. US Prescribing information, June 2007.
26. Murphy RL, Sommadossi J-P, Lamson M, Hall DB, Myers M, Dusek A. Antiviral effect and pharmacokinetic interaction between nevirapine and indinavir in persons infected with human immunodeficiency virus type 1. *J Infect Dis* (1999) 179, 1116–23.
27. Launay O, Peytavin G, Flandre P, Gerard L, Levy C, Joly V, Aboulker JP, Yeni P. Pharmacokinetic (PK) interaction between nevirapine (NVP) and indinavir (IDV) in ANRS 081 trial. *Intersci Conf Antimicrob Agents Chemother* (2000) 40, 331.
28. Burger DM, Prins JM, van der Ende ME, Aarnoutse RE. The effect of nevirapine on the pharmacokinetics of indinavir/ritonavir 800/100 mg BID. *J Acquir Immune Defic Syndr* (2004) 35, 97–8.
29. Hsu A, Bertz R, Renz C, Lam W, Rode R, Deetz C, Schweitzer SM, Berstein B, Brun S, Granneman GR, Sun E. Assessment of the pharmacokinetic interaction between lopinavir/ritonavir (ABT-378/r) and nevirapine (NVP) in HIV-infected pediatric subjects. *AIDS* (2000) 14 (Suppl. 4), S100.
30. Merry C, Barry MG, Mulcahy F, Ryan M, Tjia JF, Halifax KL, Breckenridge AM, Back DJ. The pharmacokinetics of combination therapy with nelfinavir plus nevirapine. *AIDS* (1998) 12, 1163–7.
31. Skowron G, Leoung G, Kerr B, Dusek A, Anderson R, Beebe S, Grosso R. Lack of pharmacokinetic interaction between nelfinavir and nevirapine. *AIDS* (1998) 12, 1243–4.
32. Skowron G, Leoung G, Hall DB, Robinson P, Lewis R, Grosso R, Jacobs M, Kerr B, MacGregor T, Stevens M, Fisher A, Odgen R, Yen-Lieberman B. Pharmacokinetic evaluation and short-term activity of stavudine, nevirapine, and nelfinavir therapy in HIV-1-infected adults. *J Acquir Immune Defic Syndr* (2004) 35, 351–8.
33. Vilaro J, Mascaro J, Colomer J, Cucurull J, Garcia D, Yanez A. The pharmacokinetics of combination therapy with nelfinavir (NFV) plus nevirapine (NVP) in HIV positive patients. *Intersci Conf Antimicrob Agents Chemother* (2001) 41, 16.
34. Viramune (Nevirapine). Boehringer Ingelheim. US Prescribing information, June 2007.
35. Viramune (Nevirapine). Boehringer Ingelheim Ltd. UK Summary of product characteristics, January 2007.
36. Sahai J, Cameron W, Salgo M, Stewart F, Myers M, Lamson M, Gagnier P. Drug interaction study between saquinavir (SQV) and nevirapine (NVP). 4th Conference on Retroviruses and Opportunistic Infections, Washington, 1997. Abstract 613.

Clinical evidence, mechanism, importance and management

(a) Delavirdine

For a summary of the studies of the pharmacokinetic interactions of delavirdine and various protease inhibitors, see 'Table 21.3', (p.786). In general, these studies show that delavirdine can markedly increase protease inhibitor exposure. In addition, **amprenavir** and **nelfinavir** have been shown to approximately halve the AUC of delavirdine.

Delavirdine and the protease inhibitors are known to be both inhibitors of, and substrates for the cytochrome P450 isoenzyme CYP3A4, see 'Table 21.2', (p.773).

It has been suggested that delavirdine could be used clinically to boost the exposure to protease inhibitors, and this has been tried in at least one study.[1] However, this combination is complicated by the reduction in delavirdine levels with some protease inhibitors, and the combination may not be appropriate if the antiviral effect of delavirdine is required.[2] Moreover, if the combination is used, patients should be closely monitored for toxicity since in one study of **nelfinavir** and delavirdine, 4 out of 24 subjects had to stop both drugs before completing the study because of neutropenia, which resolved over several days.[3] The UK manufacturer of **saquinavir** says that liver function should be monitored frequently if delavirdine is also given, because in a small preliminary study hepatic enzymes were raised in 13% of subjects (grade 3 or 4 in 6%) receiving the combination.[4]

(b) Efavirenz

For a summary of the studies of the pharmacokinetic interactions of efavirenz and various protease inhibitors, see 'Table 21.3', (p.786). Most of the protease inhibitors did not affect efavirenz levels, although **ritonavir** caused a 20% increase in levels. Efavirenz is an inducer of the cytochrome P450 isoenzyme CYP3A4, by which the protease inhibitors are metabolised. With the exceptions of **nelfinavir** and **ritonavir**, which showed minor to modest increases in levels, efavirenz reduces the levels of the protease inhibitors, often to levels likely to lead to reduced antiviral efficacy. Ways to overcome this include the addition of low-dose **ritonavir** to boost the levels of the protease inhibitor (recommended for **amprenavir**, **atazanavir**, **fosamprenavir**, **saquinavir**) or increasing the dose for protease inhibitors already boosted by **ritonavir** (recommended for **lopinavir/ritonavir**). For a summary of the manufacturers' recommended regimens for use with efavirenz 600 mg daily see 'Table 21.4', (below). However, the manufacturers of efavirenz note that increased adverse effects, including dizziness, nausea, paraesthesia and elevated liver enzyme levels occurred with the combination of efavirenz and **ritonavir** 500 or 600 mg twice daily (antiretroviral dosage), and the combination was not well tolerated.[5,6] They recommend monitoring liver enzyme levels with this combination.[6] The UK manufacturer says that the tolerability of low-dose **ritonavir** with efavirenz has not been assessed, and they caution that the possibility of an increase in the incidence of efavirenz-associated adverse events should be considered with any **ritonavir**-boosted regimen used with efavirenz, due to a possible interaction.[5]

With **lopinavir/ritonavir**, although an increased dose of 533/133 mg twice daily with efavirenz or nevirapine produced similar plasma levels of lopinavir to those seen with the lower dose of 400/100 mg twice daily without an NNRTI, the proportion of patients with a suboptimal minimum lopinavir level tended to be higher in those patients receiving the NNRTI.[7] This suggests that some patients may need a further increase in lopinavir/ritonavir dose. Another study with **atazanavir/ritonavir** also found that the increased dose of atazanavir for use with NNRTIs did not appear to overcome the inducer effect of NNRTIs (efavirenz or nevirapine) and led to a 43% lower median minimum atazanavir level, and a greater proportion of patients with suboptimal minimum levels (25% versus 7%).[8]

(c) Nevirapine

For a summary of the studies of the pharmacokinetic interactions of nevirapine and various protease inhibitors, see 'Table 21.3', (p.786). Most protease inhibitors do not appear to affect the levels of nevirapine, although some caused a minor to modest increase. Nevirapine is an inducer of the cytochrome P450 isoenzyme CYP3A4, and so would be expected to reduce the levels of some of the protease inhibitors (see 'Table 21.2', (p.773)), sometimes to levels that are unlikely to be effective. Low-dose **ritonavir** has been used to boost the levels of some protease inhibitors when they were given with nevirapine. For a summary of the manufacturers' recommended regimens for use with nevirapine see 'Table 21.4', (below). If nevirapine is used with protease inhibitors, therapy should be closely monitored. For studies suggesting that increased doses of lopina-

Table 21.4 Summary of the manufacturers' dosage recommendations (unless stated otherwise) for combined use of protease inhibitors and NNRTIs

	Dose of protease inhibitor to be used with standard dose of the NNRTI		
	Delavirdine 400 mg three times daily	**Efavirenz 600 mg daily**	**Nevirapine 200 mg twice daily**
Amprenavir	Appropriate dose not established. Care (potentially subtherapeutic)	Appropriate dose not established (amprenavir levels reduced)	Appropriate dose not established (amprenavir levels may be decreased)
Amprenavir/Nelfinavir		No dosage adjustments required	
Amprenavir/Ritonavir*	Appropriate dose not established. Care (unpredictable effect)	600/100 mg twice daily	
Amprenavir/Saquinavir		Avoid	
Atazanavir		Avoid	In the absence of data, avoid
Atazanavir/Ritonavir*		400/100 mg once daily† (UK) 300/100 mg once daily (US)	In the absence of data, avoid
Darunavir/Ritonavir*		Care	No dose adjustments required
Fosamprenavir	Caution (delavirdine potentially subtherapeutic)	Appropriate dose not established	Avoid
Fosamprenavir/Ritonavir*		700/100 mg twice daily or 1400/300 mg once daily	700/100 mg twice daily
Indinavir	Consider reducing dose to 400 to 600 mg three times daily. Optimum dose not established	Optimum dose not known. Increasing the dose to 1 g three times daily does not compensate for induced metabolism	Consider increasing to 1 g three times daily. Optimum dose not known
Indinavir/Ritonavir*		Appropriate dose not established. 800/100 mg twice daily has been tried	
Lopinavir/Ritonavir*	Appropriate dose not established	533/133 mg twice daily† or 600/150 mg twice daily. Avoid once daily regimens	533/133 mg twice daily† or 600/150 mg twice daily. Avoid once daily regimens
Nelfinavir	Avoid	No dose adjustments required	No dose adjustment likely (UK). Appropriate dose not established (US)
Ritonavir*	Ritonavir dose reductions might be appropriate	No dose adjustments required, but not well tolerated. Monitor liver function	No dose adjustments required
Saquinavir	Appropriate dose not established. Monitor liver function	Avoid	Appropriate dose not established
Saquinavir/Ritonavir*		No dose adjustments required. Monitor liver function	Dose adjustments unlikely to be needed
Tipranavir/Ritonavir*		Appropriate dose not established. Care	Appropriate dose not established. Care

*The UK manufactuer of efavirenz advises caution, because the possibility of an increase in the incidence of efavirenz-associated adverse events should be considered with any ritonavir-boosted regimen used with efavirenz, due to a possible interaction. This is because the combination of efavirenz with ritonavir at antiviral doses caused increased dizziness, nausea, paraesthesia and elevated transaminase levels.

†This dose increase may not be sufficient in some patients, so some caution is required.

vir/ritonavir and atazanavir/ritonavir may not be sufficient in all patients given NNRTIs (including nevirapine), see *Efavirenz*, above.

1. Harris M, Alexander C, O'Shaughnessy M, Montaner JSG. Delavirdine increases drug exposure of ritonavir-boosted protease inhibitors. *AIDS* (2002) 16, 798–9.
2. Justesen US, Klitgaard NA, Brosen K, Pedersen C. Pharmacokinetic interaction between amprenavir and delavirdine after multiple-dose administration in healthy volunteers. *Br J Clin Pharmacol* (2003) 55, 100–6.
3. Cox SR, Schneck DW, Herman BD, Carel BJ, Gullotti BR, Kerr BM, Freimuth WW. Delavirdine (DLV) and nelfinavir (NFV): A pharmacokinetic (PK) drug-drug interaction study in healthy adult volunteers. 5th Conference on Retroviruses and Opportunistic Infections, Chicago, 1998. Abstract 345.
4. Invirase Hard Capsules (Saquinavir mesilate). Roche Products Ltd. UK Summary of product characteristics, May 2007.
5. Sustiva (Efavirenz). Bristol-Myers Squibb Pharmaceuticals Ltd. UK Summary of product characteristics, May 2007.
6. Sustiva (Efavirenz). Bristol-Myers Squibb Company. US Prescribing information, January 2007.
7. Solas C, Poizot-Martin I, Drogoul M-P, Ravaux I, Dhiver C, Lafeuillade A, Allegre T, Mokhtari M, Moreau J, Lepeu G, Petit N, Durand A, Lacarelle B. Therapeutic drug monitoring of lopinavir/ritonavir given alone or with a non-nucleoside reverse transcriptase inhibitor. *Br J Clin Pharmacol* (2004) 57, 436–40.
8. Poirier J-M, Guiard-Schmid J-B, Meynard J-L, Bonnard P, Zouai O, Lukiana T, Jaillon P, Girard P-M, Pialoux G. Critical drug interaction between ritonavir-boosted atazanavir regimen and non-nucleoside reverse transcriptase inhibitors. *AIDS* (2006) 20, 1087–9.

NNRTIs + Rifamycins

Rifabutin and rifampicin (rifampin) cause a very marked fall in delavirdine plasma levels: rifabutin levels are raised when the delavirdine dose is increased to compensate for this. Rifabutin does not affect efavirenz levels, whereas efavirenz decreases rifabutin levels. There is usually no important interaction between rifabutin and nevirapine, although some patients may have a higher risk of rifabutin adverse effects.

Neither efavirenz nor nevirapine affect rifampicin levels, but rifampicin modestly reduces the levels of these NNRTIs, and there is some debate about whether it is necessary to increase their dose.

Clinical evidence, mechanism, importance and management

(a) Delavirdine

In a controlled study in 7 HIV-positive patients taking delavirdine mesilate 400 mg three times daily for 30 days, the addition of **rifabutin** 300 mg daily from days 16 to 30 caused a fivefold increase in the delavirdine clearance, and an 84% fall in the steady-state plasma levels.[1] This was presumably due to the enzyme-inducing effects of the **rifabutin**. A similar study using **rifampicin** in place of **rifabutin** found that **rifampicin** caused a 27-fold increase in clearance of delavirdine, and the steady-state plasma levels became almost undetectable.[2]

In another study,[3] where the dose of delavirdine was titrated to achieve a trough level of at least 5 micromol/L, the AUC of **rifabutin** was found to increase by 242%.

It has been recommended that the combination of delavirdine and **rifampicin** should be considered as contraindicated because the effects of the interaction are so large.[2] The CDC in the US and the manufacturer recommend that neither **rifabutin** nor **rifampicin** should be used with delavirdine.[4,5]

(b) Efavirenz

1. Rifabutin. In a study in healthy subjects the concurrent use of efavirenz 600 mg once daily and rifabutin 300 mg once daily for 2 weeks resulted in a modest 38% decrease in the AUC of rifabutin and a 45% decrease in the minimum levels, but no change in efavirenz levels.[6]

The CDC in the US state that the combination is probably clinically useful, and they suggest increasing the dose of rifabutin to 450 mg or 600 mg daily, or 600 mg two to three times weekly.[4] In one study doubling the rifabutin dose from 300 mg twice weekly to 600 mg twice weekly when starting efavirenz resulted in rifabutin AUCs that were 20% higher than baseline values.[7] However, in one analysis, 8 of 35 patients (23%) taking efavirenz and given rifabutin 450 mg once daily were found to have subtherapeutic rifabutin levels, and they were switched to isoniazid.[8] Concurrent use should therefore be closely monitored.

2. Rifampicin (Rifampin). In patients with HIV and tuberculosis the concurrent use of HAART including efavirenz 600 mg once daily with antitubercular therapy including rifampicin 480 to 720 mg daily decreased the AUC of efavirenz by 22% and decreased the trough concentration by 25% (although large interpatient variability was observed). Overall the pharmacokinetics of efavirenz 800 mg daily with rifampicin were similar to those of efavirenz 600 mg daily without rifampicin. The pharmacokinetics of rifampicin were not substantially altered by efavirenz.[9] A similar 26% reduction in efavirenz AUC was reported in a study in healthy subjects.[10] The CDC in the US suggest that it may be advisable to increase the efavirenz dose to 800 mg daily when used with rifampicin,[4] and the UK manufacturer also recommends this.[11] However, in one analysis 7 of 9 patients receiving rifampicin and efavirenz 800 mg daily developed significant clinical toxicity and were found to have efavirenz levels markedly higher than the therapeutic range.[12] In another study in Thai patients taking rifampicin, median efavirenz plasma levels were comparable between those receiving 600 mg daily and 800 mg daily and similar virological outcomes were seen.[13,14] Therefore, a 600 mg dose of efavirenz may be sufficient in some patients. Concurrent use should be well monitored.

(c) Nevirapine

1. Rifabutin. In one study, the pharmacokinetics of nevirapine were only minimally affected by rifabutin in 19 patients, when compared with historical data.[15] The manufacturer notes that the concurrent use of rifabutin with nevirapine caused a minor 9% increase in nevirapine clearance and a 17% increase in its AUC, and a 28% increase in maximum steady-state rifabutin levels.[16,17] They say that because of the high intersubject variability, some patients may experience large increases in rifabutin exposure and may be at higher risk of adverse effects. Concurrent use should be well monitored and undertaken cautiously. The CDC in the US state that the combination of nevirapine and rifabutin can be used.[4]

2. Rifampicin (Rifampin). The manufacturer states that the AUC of nevirapine was reduced by 58% by rifampicin in 14 subjects, when compared with historical data. There was no change in steady-state rifampicin pharmacokinetics.[16,17] Based on these pharmacokinetic data, the manufacturer suggests that the concurrent use of rifampicin with nevirapine is not recommended, and that rifabutin may be considered instead, with close monitoring of adverse effects.[16,17]

A further study in HIV-positive patients with tuberculosis found that the rifampicin caused a 31% decrease in the AUC of nevirapine and a non-significant 21% decrease in its trough concentration.[18] The authors of this study suggested that there is probably no need to increase the nevirapine dose, since the trough levels were still sufficiently above the level needed for antiviral activity.[18] Moreover, subsequent observational data supported the continued efficacy of standard dose nevirapine when it was used with rifampicin.[19] Similarly, others have reported the successful use of nevirapine with twice weekly rifampicin with little effect on trough nevirapine levels.[20] In yet another study, the concurrent use of rifampicin and nevirapine reduced nevirapine levels by about 18% with no reduction in virological response, although the proportion of patients with trough levels below the recommended level was much higher (29.7% versus 6.8%) at 8 weeks.[21] In contrast, in another study in 13 patients taking nevirapine 200 mg twice daily, the addition of rifampicin 450 mg or 600 mg daily caused a 46% reduction in the AUC of nevirapine, and a 53% reduction in the minimum levels, with 8 of the patients having a nevirapine trough level below the therapeutic range (3 micrograms/mL). In 7 of the patients who had a reduction in the minimum levels to less than the therapeutic range, increasing the dose of nevirapine to 300 mg twice daily for 2 weeks increased the levels to above the therapeutic range in all patients without increasing adverse effects.[22] The CDC in the US state that the combination of nevirapine and rifampicin should only be used if clearly indicated and with careful monitoring, because of insufficient data on whether dose adjustments are necessary.[4] Further study is needed.

1. Borin MT, Chambers JH, Carel BJ, Freimuth WW, Aksentijevich S, Piergies AA. Pharmacokinetic study of the interaction between rifabutin and delavirdine mesylate in HIV-1 infected patients. *Antiviral Res* (1997) 35, 53–63.
2. Borin MT, Chambers JH, Carel BJ, Gagnon S, Freimuth WW. Pharmacokinetic study of the interaction between rifampin and delavirdine mesylate. *Clin Pharmacol Ther* (1997) 61, 544–53.
3. Cox SR, Herman BD, Batts DH, et al. Delavirdine and rifabutin: pharmacokinetic evaluation in HIV-1 patients with concentration-targeting of delavirdine [abstract no. 344]. 5th Conference on Retroviruses and Opportunistic Infections, Chicago, 1998.
4. Centers for Disease Control and Prevention. Updated guidelines for the use of rifamycins for the treatment of tuberculosis among HIV-infected patients taking protease inhibitors or non-nucleoside reverse transcriptase inhibitors. *MMWR* (2004) 53, 37.
5. Rescriptor (Delavirdine mesylate). Pfizer Inc. US Prescribing information, June 2006.
6. Benedek IH, Fiske WD, White SJ, Stevenson D, Joseph JL, Kornhauser DM. Pharmacokinetic interaction between multiple doses of efavirenz and rifabutin in healthy volunteers [abstract no. 461]. *Clin Infect Dis* (1998) 27, 1008.
7. Weiner M, Benator D, Peloquin CA, Burman W, Vernon A, Engle M, Khan A, Zhao Z; the Tuberculosis Trials Consortium. Evaluation of the drug interaction between rifabutin and efavirenz in patients with HIV infection and tuberculosis. *Clin Infect Dis* (2005) 41, 1343–9.
8. Spradling P, Drociuk D, McLaughlin S, Lee LM, Peloquin CA, Gallicano K, Pozsik C, Onorato I, Castro KG, Ridzon R. Drug-drug interactions in inmates treated for human immunodeficiency virus and *Mycobacterium tuberculosis* infection or disease: an institutional tuberculosis outbreak. *Clin Infect Dis* (2002) 35, 1106–12.

9. López-Cortés LF, Ruiz-Valderas R, Viciana P, Alarcón-González A, Gómez-Mateos J, León-Jimenez E, Sarasa-Nacenta M, López-Pua Y, Pachón J. Pharmacokinetic interactions between efavirenz and rifampicin in HIV-infected patients with tuberculosis. *Clin Pharmacokinet* (2002) 41, 681–90.
10. Benedek I, Joshi A, Fiske WD, et al. Pharmacokinetic interaction between efavirenz and rifampin in healthy volunteers. 12th World AIDS Conference, Geneva, June 28-Jul 3 1998. 829.
11. Sustiva (Efavirenz). Bristol-Myers Squibb Pharmaceuticals Ltd. UK Summary of product characteristics, May 2007.
12. Brennan-Benson P, Lyus R, Harrison T, Pakianathan M, Macallan D. Pharmacokinetic interactions between efavirenz and rifampicin in the treatment of HIV and tuberculosis: one size does not fit all. *AIDS* (2005) 19, 1541–3.
13. Manosuthi W, Sungkanuparph S, Thakkinstian A, Vibhagool A, Kiertiburanakul S, Rattanasiri S, Prasithsirikul W, Sankote J, Mahanontharit A, Ruxrungtham K. Efavirenz levels and 24-week efficacy in HIV-infected patients with tuberculosis receiving highly active antiretroviral therapy and rifampicin. *AIDS* (2005) 19, 1481–6.
14. Manosuthi W, Kiertiburanakul S, Sungkanuparph S, Ruxrungtham K, Vibhagool A, Rattanasiri S, Thakkinstian A. Efavirenz 600 mg/day versus efavirenz 800 mg/day in HIV-infected patients with tuberculosis receiving rifampicin: 48 weeks results. *AIDS* (2006) 20, 131–2.
15. Maldonado S, Lamson M, Gigliotti M, Pav JW, Robinson P. Pharmacokinetic interaction between nevirapine and rifabutin. *Intersci Conf Antimicrob Agents Chemother* (1999) 39, 21.
16. Viramune (Nevirapine anhydrate). Boehringer Ingelheim Ltd. UK Summary of product characteristics, January 2007.
17. Viramune (Nevirapine). Boehringer Ingelheim Pharmaceuticals, Inc. US Prescribing information, June 2007.
18. Ribera E, Pou L, Lopez RM, Crespo M, Falco V, Ocaña I, Ruiz I, Pahissa A. Pharmacokinetic interaction between nevirapine and rifampicin in HIV-infected patients with tuberculosis. *J Acquir Immune Defic Syndr* (2001) 28, 450–3.
19. Oliva J, Moreno S, Sanz J, Ribera E, Pérez Molina JAÒ, Rubio R, Casas E, Mariño A. Co-administration of rifampin and nevirapine in HIV-infected patients with tuberculosis. *AIDS* (2003) 17, 637–8.
20. Dean GL, Back DJ, de Ruiter A. Effect of tuberculosis therapy on nevirapine trough plasma concentrations. *AIDS* (1999) 13, 2489–90.
21. Manosuthi W, Sungkanuparph S, Thakkinstian A, Rattanasiri S, Chaovavanich A, Prasithsirikul W, Likanonsakul S, Ruxrungtham K. Plasma nevirapine levels and 24-week efficacy in HIV-infected patients receiving nevirapine-based highly active antiretroviral therapy with or without rifampicin. *Clin Infect Dis* (2006) 43, 253–5.
22. Ramachandran G, Hemanthkumar AK, Rajasekaran S, Padmapriyadarsini C, Narendran G, Sukumar B, Sathishnarayan S, Raja K, Kumaraswami V, Swaminathan S. Increasing nevirapine dose can overcome reduced bioavailability due to rifampicin coadministration. *J Acquir Immune Defic Syndr* (2006) 42, 36–41.

NNRTIs + St John's wort (*Hypericum perforatum*)

There is some evidence to suggest that St John's wort may decrease the levels of nevirapine. Delavirdine and efavirenz would be expected to be similarly affected.

Clinical evidence, mechanism, importance and management

Nevirapine levels, obtained by routine monitoring, were noted to be lower in 5 men who were also taking St John's wort. Based on a pharmacokinetic modelling analysis, it was estimated that St John's wort increased the oral clearance of **nevirapine** by about 35%.[1] This finding supports predictions based on the known metabolism of the NNRTIs by the cytochrome P450 isoenzyme CYP3A4 (see 'Table 21.2', (p.773)), of which St John's wort is a known inducer. It confirms advice issued by the CSM in the UK,[2] that St John's wort may decrease blood levels of the NNRTIs with possible loss of HIV suppression, so combined use should be avoided.

1. de Maat MMR, Hoetelmans RMW, Mathôt RAA, van Gorp ECM, Meenhorst PL, Mulder JW, Beijnen JH. Drug interaction between St John's wort and nevirapine. *AIDS* (2001) 15, 420–1.
2. Committee on Safety of Medicines. Message from Professor A Breckenridge (Chairman of CSM) and Fact Sheet for Health Care Professionals, 29th February 2000.

NNRTIs + Tenofovir

No pharmacokinetic interaction appears to occur between tenofovir and efavirenz or nevirapine. Some clinical data have shown a high rate of treatment failure when tenofovir is given with enteric-coated didanosine and either efavirenz or nevirapine.

Clinical evidence, mechanism, importance and management

In a pharmacokinetic study, there was no interaction between **efavirenz** 600 mg daily and tenofovir disoproxil fumarate 300 mg daily.[1,2] Similarly, in a retrospective analysis, plasma levels of **nevirapine** 200 mg twice daily or 400 mg once daily did not differ between patients taking tenofovir disoproxil fumarate 300 mg once daily and those not. Also, **efavirenz** plasma levels did not differ between patients taking tenofovir and patients not taking tenofovir. It appeared that neither **nevirapine** nor **efavirenz** altered tenofovir levels.[3]

Some clinical data have shown a high rate of treatment failure with a once daily combination of tenofovir disoproxil fumarate 300 mg, enteric-coated didanosine 200 or 250 mg and either **efavirenz** 600 mg daily or **nevirapine** 400 mg daily.[4] These specific combinations should probably not be used. However, there are clinical data supporting the use of other tenofovir and **efavirenz**-based regimens, and the manufacturers specifically caution against the use of tenofovir with didanosine,[1,2] see 'NRTIs + Tenofovir', p.806.

1. Viread (Tenofovir disoproxil fumarate). Gilead Sciences International Ltd. UK Summary of product characteristics, May 2007.
2. Viread (Tenofovir disoproxil fumarate). Gilead Sciences, Inc. US prescribing information, May 2007.
3. Droste JA, Kearney BP, Hekster YA, Burger DM. Assessment of drug-drug interactions between tenofovir disoproxil fumarate and the nonnucleoside reverse transcriptase inhibitors nevirapine and efavirenz in HIV-infected patients. *J Acquir Immune Defic Syndr* (2006) 41, 37–43.
4. Hodder SL. Re: Important new clinical data. Potential early virologic failure associated with the combination antiretroviral regimen of tenofovir disoproxil fumarate, didanosine, and either efavirenz or nevirapine in HIV treatment-naïve patients with high baseline viral loads. Bristol-Myers Squibb Company, November 2004. Available at: www.fda.gov/oashi/aids/listserv/bms.pdf (accessed 21/08/07).

NNRTIs; Delavirdine + Acids

In patients with poor gastric acid production, orange juice and glutamic acid increase the absorption of delavirdine.

Clinical evidence, mechanism, importance and management

When **glutamic acid** 1.36 g three times daily was given with delavirdine 400 mg three times daily to 8 HIV-positive subjects with gastric hypoacidity, the AUC of delavirdine was increased by 50%.[1] Similarly, **orange juice** increased delavirdine absorption by 50% to 70% in subjects with gastric hypoacidity, but had less effect (0 to 30%) in those with normal gastric acidity. However, despite the use of **orange juice**, the AUC of delavirdine was still about 50% lower in patients with gastric hypoacidity than those without.[2]

Delavirdine is a weak base that is poorly soluble at neutral pH (note that antacids reduce its absorption, see 'NNRTIs + Drugs that affect gastric pH', p.784). Therefore, in subjects with gastric hypoacidity, the absorption of delavirdine is reduced, and substances that lower gastric pH increase its absorption.

The clinical value of using **glutamic acid** or acidic beverages with delavirdine is unknown. Nevertheless, the manufacturer recommends that, in patients with achlorhydria, delavirdine should be taken with an **acidic beverage** such as **orange** or **cranberry juice**.[3]

1. Morse GD, Adams JM, Shelton MJ, Hewitt RG, Cox SR, Chambers JH. Gastric acidification increases delavirdine mesylate (DLV) exposure in HIV+ subjects with gastric hypoacidity (GH). *Clin Pharmacol Ther* (1996) 59, 141.
2. Shelton MJ, Hewitt RG, Adams JM, Cox SR, Chambers JH, Morse GD. Delavirdine malabsorption in HIV-infected subjects with spontaneous gastric hypoacidity. *J Clin Pharmacol* (2003) 43, 171–9.
3. Rescriptor (Delavirdine mesylate). Pfizer Inc. US Prescribing information, June 2006.

NRTIs + Aciclovir and related drugs

The concurrent use of zidovudine and aciclovir normally appears to be uneventful, but an isolated report describes overwhelming fatigue in one patient given zidovudine and intravenous aciclovir. Famciclovir did not alter the pharmacokinetics of zidovudine or emtricitabine.

Clinical evidence, mechanism, importance and management

(a) Aciclovir

A study in 20 HIV-positive men found no pharmacokinetic interaction between **zidovudine** 100 mg and aciclovir 400 or 800 mg, both given every 4 hours, 5 times a day, and the combination was well tolerated over a 6-month period.[1] When 41 HIV-positive patients taking **zidovudine** were given aciclovir, no changes in the pharmacokinetics of the **zidovudine** occurred and the adverse effects were unchanged.[2] In a group of AIDS patients taking **zidovudine**, some of whom were also given aciclovir, no obvious problems developed that could be attributed to the use of the aciclovir.[3]

In contrast, a man with herpes who had been treated with intravenous aciclovir 250 mg every 8 hours for 3 days, developed overwhelming fatigue and lethargy within about an hour of starting oral **zidovudine** 200 mg every 4 hours. This lessened slightly on changing from intravenous to oral aciclovir, which was continued for 3 days, and symptoms resolved when the aciclovir was withdrawn. The symptoms developed again when intravenous aciclovir was given as a test.[4] This isolated case of fatigue is not understood, and no other cases appear to have been reported. There would seem to be no reason for avoiding concurrent use.

(b) Famciclovir

Only minimal changes in **zidovudine** pharmacokinetics were seen when 12 HIV-positive patients taking **zidovudine** 400 mg to 1 g daily were given a single 500-mg dose of famciclovir.[5]

In a study in 12 healthy subjects there was no important pharmacokinetic interaction between single doses of **emtricitabine** 200 mg and famciclovir 500 mg.[6]

1. Hollander H, Lifson AR, Maha M, Blum R, Rutherfod GW, Nusinoff-Lehrman S. Phase I study of low-dose zidovudine and acyclovir in asymptomatic human immunodeficiency virus seropositive individuals. *Am J Med* (1989) 87, 628–32.
2. Tartaglione TA, Collier AC, Opheim K, Gianola FG, Benedetti J, Corey L. Pharmacokinetic evaluations of low- and high-dose zidovudine plus high-dose acyclovir in patients with symptomatic human immunodeficiency virus infection. *Antimicrob Agents Chemother* (1991) 35, 2225–31.
3. Richman DD, Fischl MA, Grieco MH, Gottlieb MS, Volberding PA, Laskin OL, Leedom JM, Groopman JE, Mildvan D, Hirsch MS, Jackson GG, Durack DT, Nusinoff-Lehrman S and the AZT Collaborative Working Group. The toxicity of azidothymidine (AZT) in the treatment of patients with AIDS and AIDS-related complex. A double-blind, placebo-controlled trial. *N Engl J Med* (1987) 317, 192–7.
4. Bach MC. Possible drug interaction during therapy with azidothymidine and acyclovir for AIDS. *N Engl J Med* (1987) 316, 547.
5. Rousseau F, Scott S, Pratt S, Fowles S, Sparrow P, Lascoux C, Lehner V, Sereni D. Safe coadministration of famciclovir and zidovudine. *Intersci Conf Antimicrob Agents Chemother* (1994) 34, 83.
6. Wang LH, Blum MR, Hui J, Hulett L, Chittick GE, Rousseau F. Lack of significant pharmacokinetic interactions between emtricitabine and other nucleoside antivirals in healthy volunteers. *Intersci Conf Antimicrob Agents Chemother* (2001) 41, 18.

NRTIs + Antacids

Aluminium/magnesium hydroxide caused a 25% reduction in the bioavailability of zalcitabine. Antacids would not be expected to have any additional pharmacokinetic effect on buffered didanosine preparations.

Clinical evidence, mechanism, importance and management

(a) Didanosine

Didanosine is acid labile. To increase its absorption, some didanosine preparations (e.g. buffered tablets) have been formulated with antacids.[1] Additional concurrent antacids would not be expected to have any further clinically relevant effect on didanosine pharmacokinetics, although the US manufacturers of the oral powder for solution[2] suggest that additional antacids may increase the adverse effects of the components of this preparation (presumably both the antacid and didanosine components).

(b) Zalcitabine

A study in 12 HIV-positive patients given a single 1.5-g dose of zalcitabine found that 30 mL of *Maalox* [**aluminium/magnesium hydroxide**] caused a 25% reduction in the bioavailability of the zalcitabine.[3] The changes are moderate and of uncertain clinical importance. The manufacturer recommended that zalcitabine should not be taken at the same time as **aluminium/magnesium**-containing antacids.[4,5]

1. Videx Tablets (Didanosine). Bristol-Myers Squibb Pharmaceuticals Ltd. UK Summary of product characteristics, December 2006.
2. Videx Pediatric Powder for Oral Solution (Didanosine). Bristol-Myers Squibb Company. US Prescribing information, August 2006.
3. Massarella JW, Holazo AA, Koss-Twardy S, Min B, Smith B, Nazareno LA. The effects of cimetidine and Maalox® on the pharmacokinetics of zalcitabine in HIV-positive patients. *Pharm Res* (1994) 11 (10 Suppl), S-415.
4. Hivid (Zalcitabine). Roche Products Ltd. UK Summary of product characteristics, November 2004.
5. Hivid (Zalcitabine). Roche Pharmaceuticals. US Prescribing information, September 2002.

NRTIs + Antiepileptics

Valproate increases the bioavailability of zidovudine, and one case of severe anaemia was attributed to the interaction. A case of liver toxicity with combined use has also been reported. Phenytoin and phenobarbital are predicted to slightly decrease abacavir levels.

Clinical evidence

(a) Abacavir

The UK manufacturer of abacavir says that **phenobarbital** and **phenytoin** may slightly decrease abacavir concentrations by affecting glucuronyltransferases.[1] There appears to be no other information on this.

(b) Zidovudine

The AUC and mean plasma levels of zidovudine 100 mg every 8 hours were increased by 80% in 6 HIV-positive subjects when they were given **valproic acid** 250 or 500 mg every 8 hours for 4 days. No adverse reactions, changes in hepatic or renal function, or alterations in the blood picture were reported.[2] A case report describes an AIDS patient taking zidovudine 100 mg five times daily who had a two- to threefold increase in trough and peak serum zidovudine levels, and a 74% increase in the CSF zidovudine levels while taking **valproic acid** 500 mg three times daily.[3] In another report, a patient taking **carbamazepine**, **clobazam** and **gabapentin** was given zidovudine, **lamivudine** and **abacavir**. Nine months later, **valproic acid** 500 mg twice daily was added because of a seizure frequency of greater than one per month. At this time, his haemoglobin level was normal. About 2 months later, he was found to have severe anaemia, requiring a blood transfusion. **Stavudine** was substituted for zidovudine in his antiretroviral therapy, and 4 months later his haemoglobin was normal. The adverse haematological effects were attributed to an interaction between the valproate and zidovudine.[4] Another HIV-positive patient, who had been taking valproate for 2 years and , zidovudine, developed severe encephalopathy, adult respiratory distress syndrome and liver failure (steatosis). Both valproate and zidovudine were stopped, and the patient gradually recovered.[5]

For the possible effect of zidovudine on phenytoin levels, see 'Phenytoin + Zidovudine', p.569.

Mechanism

The evidence indicates that the metabolism (glucuronidation) of zidovudine is inhibited by valproate so that its bioavailability is increased.[2,3] It was suggested that this caused zidovudine haematological toxicity in the case reported.[4] The glucuronidation of abacavir is predicted to be increased by drugs that can induce UDP-glucuronyltransferase, such as phenobarbital and phenytoin.[1]

Importance and management

Information seems to be limited to the papers cited, but an interaction between zidovudine and valproate would appear to be established. It would therefore seem prudent to monitor for any evidence of increased zidovudine effects and possible toxicity if valproate is added. The other NRTIs do not undergo significant glucuronidation (see 'Antivirals', (p.772)), and would therefore not be expected to interact with valproate. For a discussion of drug-disease considerations when using valproate in HIV infection, see under Importance and management in 'protease inhibitors', (p.812).

1. Ziagen (Abacavir sulfate). GlaxoSmithKline UK. UK Summary of product characteristics, May 2007.
2. Lertora JJL, Rege AB, Greenspan DL, Akula S, George WJ, Hyslop NE, Agrawal KC. Pharmacokinetic interaction between zidovudine and valproic acid in patients infected with human immunodeficiency virus. *Clin Pharmacol Ther* (1994) 56, 272–8.
3. Akula SK, Rege AB, Dreisbach AW, Dejace PMJT, Lertora JJL. Valproic acid increases cerebrospinal fluid zidovudine levels in a patient with AIDS. *Am J Med Sci* (1997) 313, 244–6.
4. Antoniou T, Gough K, Yoong D, Arbess G. Severe anemia secondary to a probable drug interaction between zidovudine and valproic acid. *Clin Infect Dis* (2004) 38, e38–40.
5. Leppik IE, Gapany S, Walczak T. An HIV-positive patient with epilepsy. *Epilepsy Behav* (2003) 4 (Suppl 1), S17–S19.

NRTIs + Antimycobacterials

Didanosine, stavudine and zalcitabine are not expected to interact with rifabutin, but rifabutin may modestly increase the clearance of zidovudine. An isolated case describes undetectable rifabutin levels in a patient taking antiretrovirals including buffered didanosine.

Rifampicin (rifampin) appears to modestly increase the clearance of zidovudine, and is predicted to interact similarly with abacavir.

Isoniazid, pyrazinamide and ethambutol appear not to interact with zidovudine.
The clearance of isoniazid is increased by zalcitabine, and there is a theoretical increased risk of peripheral neuropathy.

Clinical evidence, mechanism, importance and management

(a) Abacavir

The UK manufacturer of abacavir[1] says that potent enzyme inducers such as **rifampicin** (**rifampin**) may slightly decrease abacavir plasma concentrations due to their ability to induce UDP-glucuronyltransferases (see also *Zidovudine*, below). As yet, there appears to be no other information on this.

(b) Didanosine

Rifabutin 300 to 600 mg daily for 12 days did not significantly affect the pharmacokinetics of [buffered] didanosine 167 to 250 mg twice daily in 12 patients with AIDS.[2] The steady-state pharmacokinetics of **rifabutin** were not affected by didanosine (buffered sachet preparation),[3] which suggests that the buffer used in the didanosine preparation had no effect on **rifabutin** absorption.[3] However, a case has been reported of a patient taking lopinavir/ritonavir, efavirenz, lamivudine and buffered didanosine who had impaired **rifabutin** absorption. When **rifabutin** was taken 30 minutes after didanosine, **rifabutin** levels were undetectable, but when **rifabutin** was taken 3 hours after didanosine, **rifabutin** levels were apparent.[4]

The controlled study[3] suggests that no special precautions are necessary if both drugs are given. However, the case report[4] introduces an element of caution, especially if other drugs that may affect **rifabutin** pharmacokinetics are used. If indeed **rifabutin** absorption is affected by antacids (there appear to be no clinical data on this), then giving the drugs at least 2 hours apart, or using the enteric-coated didanosine preparation should avoid the interaction.[4]

(c) Stavudine

A study in 10 HIV-positive subjects found that **rifabutin** 300 mg daily had no significant effects on the pharmacokinetics of the stavudine 30 or 40 mg twice daily and the incidence of adverse effects did not increase.[5] No special precautions would seem necessary if both drugs are given.

(d) Zalcitabine

A study in 12 HIV-positive patients found that when zalcitabine 1.5 mg three times daily was given with **isoniazid** 300 mg daily the pharmacokinetics of the zalcitabine remained unchanged but the clearance of the **isoniazid** was approximately doubled.[6] The UK manufacturer of zalcitabine[7] recommended caution with the combination because of the possibility of an increased risk of peripheral neuropathy; the US manufacturer recommended that the combination should be avoided where possible.[8]

The UK manufacturer of **rifabutin** suggests that no significant interaction would be expected between **rifabutin** and zalcitabine.[9]

(e) Zidovudine

The pharmacokinetics of **rifabutin** are not affected by the concurrent use of zidovudine in AIDS patients,[10,11] and **rifabutin** does not affect the pharmacokinetics of zidovudine in HIV-positive patients,[12] although one review found a trend towards increased zidovudine clearance.[13] No increase in adverse effects appears to occur when **rifabutin** is given with zidovudine.[11]

In a retrospective study of healthy subjects and HIV-positive individuals, the clearance of zidovudine was increased by 132% by **rifampicin** and by 50% by **rifabutin**, suggesting that the enzyme-inducing effects of **rifabutin** are less than those of **rifampicin**, so less significant interactions would be expected.[14]

A comparative study in HIV-positive patients given zidovudine and antitubercular treatment (**isoniazid**, **rifampicin**, **pyrazinamide**, **ethambutol** initially, then **isoniazid** and **rifampicin**) for 8 months found no evidence of an adverse interaction. However, marked anaemia occurred in those subjects given both groups of drugs, but it was not necessary to permanently stop zidovudine in any patient. The authors advise careful monitoring for haematological toxicity.[15] Another study in 4 HIV-positive patients found that **rifampicin** lowered the AUC and increased the clearance of zidovudine in all patients, probably due to the enzyme-inducing activity of the **rifampicin**, which increases the glucuronidation of zidovudine. When the **rifampicin** was stopped in one patient, his zidovudine AUC doubled.[16] A later study of the same interaction in 8 HIV-positive men found that **rifampicin** significantly induced the glucuronidation of zidovudine and suggested that the effect wore off 14 days after stopping the **rifampicin**. The authors of this study suggest that dosage alterations may not be necessary on concurrent use.[17]

1. Ziagen (Abacavir sulfate). GlaxoSmithKline UK. UK Summary of product characteristics, May 2007.
2. Sahai J, Foss N, Li R, Narang PK, Cameron DW. Rifabutin and didanosine interaction in AIDS patients. *Clin Pharmacol Ther* (1993) 53, 197.
3. Li RC, Narang PK, Sahai J, Cameron W, Bianchine JR. Rifabutin absorption in the gut unaltered by concomitant administration of didanosine in AIDS patients. *Antimicrob Agents Chemother* (1997) 41, 1566–70.
4. Marzolini C, Chave J-P, Telenti A, Brenas-Chinchon L, Biollaz J. Impaired absorption of rifabutin by concomitant administration of didanosine. *AIDS* (2001) 15, 2203–4.
5. Piscitelli SC, Kelly G, Walker RE, Kovacs J, Falloon J, Davey RT, Raje S, Masur H, Polis MA. A multiple drug interaction study of stavudine with agents for opportunistic infections in human immunodeficiency virus-infected patients. *Antimicrob Agents Chemother* (1999) 43, 647–50.
6. Lee BL, Täuber MG, Chambers HF, Gambertoglio J, Delahunty T. The effect of zalcitabine on the pharmacokinetics of isoniazid in HIV-infected patients. *Intersci Conf Antimicrob Agents Chemother* (1994) 34, 3.
7. Hivid (Zalcitabine). Roche Products Ltd. UK Summary of product characteristics, November 2004.
8. Hivid (Zalcitabine). Roche Pharmaceuticals. US Prescribing information, September 2002.
9. Mycobutin (Rifabutin). Pharmacia Ltd. UK Summary of product characteristics, October 2006.
10. Narang PK, Nightingale S, Lewis RC, Colborn D, Wynne B, Li R. Concomitant zidovudine (ZDV) dosing does not affect rifabutin (RIF) disposition in AIDS patients. 9th International Conference AIDS & 4th STD World Congress, Berlin, June 6–11, 1993. Abstract PO-B31-2216.
11. Li RC, Nightingale S, Lewis RC, Colburn DC, Narang PK. Lack of effect of concomitant zidovudine on rifabutin kinetics in patients with AIDS-related complex. *Antimicrob Agents Chemother* (1996) 40, 1397–1402.
12. Gallicano K, Sahai J, Swick L, Seguin I, Pakuts A, Cameron DW. Effect of rifabutin on the pharmacokinetics of zidovudine in patients infected with human immunodeficiency virus. *Clin Infect Dis* (1995) 21, 1008–11.
13. Narang PK, Sale M. Population based assessment of rifabutin (R) effect on zidovudine (ZDV) disposition in AIDS patients. *Clin Pharmacol Ther* (1993) 53, 219.
14. Narang PK, Gupta S, Li RC, Strolin-Benedetti M, Della Bruna C, Bianchine JR. Assessing dosing implications of enzyme inducing potential: rifabutin (RIF) vs. rifampin (RFM). *Intersci Conf Antimicrob Agents Chemother* (1993) 33, 228.
15. Antoniskis D, Easley AC, Espina BM, Davidson PT, Barnes PF. Combined toxicity of zidovudine and antituberculosis chemotherapy. *Am Rev Respir Dis* (1992) 145, 430–4.
16. Burger DM, Meenhorst PL, Koks CHW, Beijnen JH. Pharmacokinetic interaction between rifampin and zidovudine. *Antimicrob Agents Chemother* (1993) 37, 1426–31.
17. Gallicano KD, Sahai J, Shukla VK, Seguin I, Pakuts A, Kwok D, Foster BC, Cameron DW. Induction of zidovudine glucuronidation and amination pathways by rifampicin in HIV-infected patients. *Br J Clin Pharmacol* (1999) 48, 168–79.

NRTIs + Atovaquone

Moderate increases in the AUC of zidovudine, not usually requiring dose adjustments, have been seen with atovaquone. However, it may be prudent to regularly monitor for adverse effects. Atovaquone decreased the AUC of didanosine. Neither didanosine nor zidovudine affected atovaquone pharmacokinetics.

Clinical evidence

(a) Didanosine

The manufacturer of atovaquone notes that it decreased the AUC of didanosine by 24% in a multiple dose interaction study. There was no change in the pharmacokinetics of atovaquone.[1]

(b) Zidovudine

A study in 14 HIV-positive patients given atovaquone 750 mg every 12 hours and zidovudine 200 mg every 8 hours found that under steady-state conditions the zidovudine had no effect on the pharmacokinetics of atovaquone.[2] This confirmed the findings of a previous analysis of pharmacokinetic data from a small number of patients enrolled in clinical studies.[3] However, the AUC of the zidovudine was increased by about 30%, and its clearance was reduced by 25% by the concurrent use of atovaquone.[2]

Mechanism

Atovaquone might inhibit the metabolism (glucuronidation) of zidovudine.[2]

Importance and management

The manufacturer of atovaquone notes that the decrease in didanosine levels is unlikely to be clinically relevant.[1] They also say that the increased plasma levels of zidovudine likely with a 3-week course of atovaquone for acute Pneumocystis pneumonia are unlikely to increase the adverse effects of zidovudine,[1] and routine dose adjustments are not required.[4] Nevertheless, the manufacturers of atovaquone and zidovudine do recommend regular monitoring for zidovudine-associated adverse effects when the drugs are used together, particularly if atovaquone suspension is used, as this achieves higher atovaquone levels, which might have a greater effect.[1,5] The authors of the study with zidovudine[2] suggest that increases could possibly be important in patients also taking other drugs causing bone marrow toxicity (such as ganciclovir, amphotericin B, flucytosine). If bone marrow toxicity is seen, it is suggested that the zidovudine dosage may need to be reduced by a third.[2]

1. Wellvone Oral Suspension (Atovaquone). GlaxoSmithKline UK. UK Summary of product characteristics, May 2006.
2. Lee BL, Täuber MG, Sadler B, Goldstein D, Chambers HF. Atovaquone inhibits the glucuronidation and increases the plasma concentrations of zidovudine. *Clin Pharmacol Ther* (1996) 59, 14–21.
3. Sadler BM, Blum MR. Relationship between steady-state plasma concentrations of atovaquone (C_{ss}) and the use of various concomitant medications in AIDS patients with *Pneumocystis carinii* pneumonia. 9th International Conference AIDS & 4th STD World Congress, Berlin, June 6–11 1993. Abstract PO-B31-2213.
4. Retrovir (Zidovudine). GlaxoSmithKline. US Prescribing information, November 2006.
5. Retrovir (Zidovudine). GlaxoSmithKline UK. UK Summary of product characteristics, December 2006.

NRTIs + Azoles

Fluconazole has no significant effect on the pharmacokinetics of didanosine or stavudine, but it may cause an increase in serum zidovudine levels although the clinical importance of this is uncertain. Fluconazole serum levels remain unchanged.

Itraconazole appears not to affect the pharmacokinetics of zidovudine. Serum levels of itraconazole are markedly reduced when buffered didanosine is given at the same time, but itraconazole and ketoconazole are not affected if buffered didanosine is given 2 hours later. Enteric-coated didanosine has no clinically relevant effect on the pharmacokinetics of fluconazole, itraconazole or ketoconazole. The frequency of haematological toxicity with zidovudine was not increased by ketoconazole.

Clinical evidence

(a) Didanosine

1. Buffered preparation. A 35-year-old patient with AIDS was given **itraconazole** capsules 200 mg twice daily following an episode of cryptococcal meningitis. When he relapsed it was noted that he had been taking the **itraconazole** at the same time as his buffered didanosine. Subsequent study in this patient indicated a marked delay in **itraconazole** absorption when it was taken with didanosine. Two hours after the dose, plasma **itraconazole** concentrations of 1.6 micrograms/mL were observed without didanosine, but were undetectable with didanosine. A peak **itraconazole** level of 1.4 micrograms/mL was observed when it was given 8 hours after a dose of didanosine.[1] In 6 healthy subjects when [buffered] didanosine was given with a single 200-mg oral dose of **itraconazole**, the peak levels of **itraconazole** were undetectable; in the absence of didanosine, **itraconazole** levels were 0.9 micrograms/mL.[2] A later study in 12 HIV-positive patients found that the AUC of **itraconazole** after a single 200-mg dose was not significantly different when buffered didanosine 200 mg was given 4 hours before or 2 hours after **itraconazole**.[3]

Twelve HIV-positive patients were given buffered didanosine 375 mg twice daily either alone or 2 hours after **ketoconazole** 200 mg daily, for 4 days. Didanosine maximum plasma levels were slightly reduced by 12% and no significant changes in the pharmacokinetics of the **ketoconazole** were seen when dosing was separated in this way.[4]

A group of 12 HIV-positive subjects taking buffered didanosine 100 to 250 mg twice daily were also given **fluconazole** for 7 days (two 200-mg doses on the first day, followed by 200 mg daily). The pharmacokinetics of the didanosine remained unchanged in the presence of the **fluconazole**, and concurrent use was well tolerated. **Fluconazole** pharmacokinetics were not assessed.[5]

2. Enteric-coated preparation. Enteric-coated didanosine 400 mg had no significant effect on the pharmacokinetics of **fluconazole** 200 mg in 14 healthy subjects, and no clinically relevant effect on the pharmacokinetics of **itraconazole** 200 mg in 25 healthy subjects.[6] Similarly, enteric-coated didanosine 400 mg had no clinically relevant effect on the pharmacokinetics of **ketoconazole** 200 mg in 24 healthy subjects. Three of the subjects had increased concentrations of **ketoconazole** with didanosine, but their values for **ketoconazole** alone appeared unusually low. When their data were excluded, no effect on AUC was seen in the remaining 21 subjects.[7]

(b) Stavudine

A study in 10 HIV-positive subjects taking stavudine 40 mg twice daily, found that the addition of **fluconazole** 200 mg daily for one week had no significant effect on the pharmacokinetics of the stavudine.[8]

(c) Zidovudine

On two occasions, 12 HIV-positive men were given zidovudine 200 mg every 8 hours with and without **fluconazole** 400 mg daily for 7 days. While taking **fluconazole** the AUC of the zidovudine increased by 74%, the maximum serum levels increased by 84%, the terminal half-life was increased by 128% and the clearance was reduced by 43%.[9] In contrast, another study in 10 HIV-positive patients found only a very small change in the pharmacokinetics of a single 500-mg dose of zidovudine given before and after 7 days treatment with **fluconazole** (e.g. a 7% increase in zidovudine AUC). In another 10 patients, zidovudine had no effect on the pharmacokinetics of a single dose of **fluconazole**.[10]

Itraconazole 200 mg daily for 2 weeks was reported to have no effect on the pharmacokinetics of zidovudine in 7 patients, but the serum levels in 2 patients were higher.[11]

A study of zidovudine use in 282 AIDS patients found that haematological abnormalities (anaemia, leucopenia, neutropenia) were very common, but this was not increased by the concurrent use of **ketoconazole** in some of these patients.[12]

Mechanism

Itraconazole capsules and ketoconazole depend on stomach acidity for absorption. A raised gastric pH, caused by the antacids in the buffered didanosine formulation appears to reduce itraconazole absorption (consider, 'Azoles + Antacids', p.215). The didanosine itself appears to have no part to play in this interaction. The enteric-coated preparation of didanosine does not contain any antacids and therefore does not interact.

In vitro data suggest that the altered zidovudine pharmacokinetics may, in part, occur because fluconazole inhibits zidovudine glucuronidation.[13]

Importance and management

The most significant interaction occurs between the buffered preparation of didanosine and itraconazole. Patients should avoid taking both drugs at the same time, but giving the itraconazole at least 2 hours before the didanosine appears to solve any problem. Any possible interaction with ketoconazole can similarly be avoided by giving ketoconazole at least 2 hours before didanosine. Alternatively, the interaction may be avoided by using the enteric-coated preparation of didanosine.

There is no pharmacokinetic interaction between stavudine and fluconazole. No interaction would be expected with other similar NRTIs such as **lamivudine** and **zalcitabine** (see 'Antivirals', (p.772)).

There is evidence of a minor interaction between zidovudine and fluconazole, but this is unlikely to be clinically significant.

1. Moreno F, Hardin TC, Rinaldi MG, Graybill JR. Itraconazole-didanosine excipient interaction. *JAMA* (1993) 269, 1508.
2. May DB, Drew RH, Yedinak KC, Bartlett JA. Effect of simultaneous didanosine administration on itraconazole absorption in healthy volunteers. *Pharmacotherapy* (1994) 14, 509–13.
3. Hardin TC, Sharkey-Mathis PK, Rinaldi MG, Graybill JR. Evaluation of the pharmacokinetic interaction between itraconazole and didanosine in HIV-infected subjects. *Intersci Conf Antimicrob Agents Chemother* (1995) 35, 6.
4. Knupp CA, Brater DC, Relue J, Barbhaiya RH. Pharmacokinetics of didanosine and ketoconazole after coadministration to patients seropositive for the human immunodeficiency virus. *J Clin Pharmacol* (1993) 33, 912–17.
5. Bruzzese VL, Gillum JG, Israel DS, Johnson GL, Kaplowitz LG, Polk RE. Effect of fluconazole on pharmacokinetics of 2′,3′-dideoxyinosine in persons seropositive for human immunodeficiency virus. *Antimicrob Agents Chemother* (1995) 39, 1050–53.
6. Damle B, Hess H, Kaul S, Knupp C. Absence of clinically relevant drug interactions following simultaneous administration of didanosine-encapsulated, enteric-coated bead formulation with either itraconazole or fluconazole. *Biopharm Drug Dispos* (2002) 23, 59–66.
7. Damle BD, Mummaneni V, Kaul S, Knupp C. Lack of effect of simultaneously administered didanosine encapsulated enteric bead formulation (Videx EC) on oral absorption of indinavir, ketoconazole, or ciprofloxacin. *Antimicrob Agents Chemother* (2002) 46, 385–91.
8. Piscitelli SC, Kelly G, Walker RE, Kovacs J, Falloon J, Davey RT, Raje S, Masur H, Polis MA. A multiple drug interaction study of stavudine with agents for opportunistic infections in human immunodeficiency virus-infected patients. *Antimicrob Agents Chemother* (1999) 43, 647–50.
9. Sahai J, Gallicano K, Pakuts A, Cameron DW. Effect of fluconazole on zidovudine pharmacokinetics in patients infected with human deficiency virus. *J Infect Dis* (1994) 169, 1103–7.
10. Brockmeyer NH, Tillmann I, Mertins L, Barthel B, Goos M. Pharmacokinetic interaction of fluconazole and zidovudine in HIV-positive patients. *Eur J Med Res* (1997) 2, 377–83.
11. Henrivaux P, Fairon Y, Fillet G. Pharmacokinetics of AZT among HIV infected patients treated by itraconazole. 5th Int Conf AIDS, Montreal. 1989, Abstract M.B.P.340.

12. Richman DD, Fischl MA, Grieco MH, Gottlieb MS, Volberding PA, Laskin OL, Leedom JM, Groopman JE, Mildvan D, Hirsch MS, Jackson GG, Durack DT, Nusinoff-Lehrman S and the AZT Collaborative Working Group. The toxicity of azidothymidine (AZT) in the treatment of patients with AIDS and AIDS-related complex. A double-blind, placebo-controlled trial. *N Engl J Med* (1987) 317, 192–7.
13. Asgari M, Back DJ. Effect of azoles on the glucuronidation of zidovudine by human liver UDP-glucuronyltransferase. *J Infect Dis* (1995) 172, 1634–5.

NRTIs + Co-trimoxazole or Trimethoprim

Trimethoprim, both alone and as co-trimoxazole (trimethoprim with sulfamethoxazole) reduces the renal clearance of lamivudine, zalcitabine and zidovudine, and therefore raises their plasma levels. However, the extent of the interaction does not usually appear to be clinically significant in patients with normal renal function. No clinically significant adverse pharmacokinetic interaction occurs if didanosine is given with co-trimoxazole or trimethoprim.

Clinical evidence

(a) Didanosine

A study in 10 HIV-positive subjects investigated the pharmacokinetics of didanosine 200 mg, trimethoprim 200 mg and sulfamethoxazole 1 g in combination. Most pharmacokinetic parameters were unchanged. However, didanosine clearance was reduced by 35%, trimethoprim clearance was decreased by 32% and sulfamethoxazole clearance was increased by 39%, when all 3 drugs were given together. When only 2 of the 3 drugs were given, trimethoprim caused a 27% decrease in the clearance of didanosine, and didanosine caused an 82% increase in the clearance of sulfamethoxazole.[1] Despite these alterations in clearance, the maximum serum concentration, AUC and half-life of each of the three drugs were minimally affected.[1]

(b) Lamivudine

In a study of 14 HIV-positive patients taking co-trimoxazole 960 mg daily for 5 days, it was found that the AUC of a single 300-mg dose of lamivudine given on day 4 was increased by 43% and the renal clearance was decreased by 35%. The pharmacokinetics of the trimethoprim and the sulfamethoxazole were unaffected.[2] Similarly, in a population pharmacokinetic analysis, the concurrent use of lamivudine and co-trimoxazole was associated with a 31% reduction in the apparent oral clearance of lamivudine, and an estimated 43% increase in steady-state lamivudine levels.[3] The UK manufacturer notes that the interaction is due to trimethoprim, and that sulfamethoxazole did not interact.[4]

(c) Stavudine

The UK manufacturer notes that an interaction with trimethoprim is possible, since both drugs are actively secreted by the renal tubules.[5]

(d) Zalcitabine

In a steady-state study, 8 HIV-positive patients received zalcitabine 1.5 mg three times daily with and without trimethoprim 200 mg twice daily. The trimethoprim increased the AUC and decreased the clearance of zalcitabine by about 35%.[6]

(e) Zidovudine

A study in 9 HIV-positive patients given zidovudine 3 mg/kg by infusion over 1 hour found that neither trimethoprim 150 mg nor co-trimoxazole 960 mg affected the metabolic clearance of the zidovudine. However, the renal clearances of zidovudine were reduced by 48% and 58%, by trimethoprim and co-trimoxazole respectively, and the renal clearances of its glucuronide metabolite were reduced by 20% and 27%, respectively.[7] Another study also found that co-trimoxazole did not alter zidovudine pharmacokinetics.[8] A further 5 HIV-positive patients had a 30% increase in the AUC of zidovudine when they were given trimethoprim [dosages not stated].[9] Zidovudine renal clearance was reduced by 58% in 8 HIV-positive subjects when they were also given trimethoprim 200 mg, but the AUC_{0-6} of the zidovudine glucuronide/zidovudine ratio was unchanged, suggesting that the metabolism was unaffected.[10]

Increases in the half-lives of trimethoprim, sulfamethoxazole and N-acetyl sulfamethoxazole of 72%, 39%, and 115%, respectively, were seen when co-trimoxazole was given to 4 patients with AIDS taking zidovudine 250 mg every 8 hours for 8 days.[11]

A study of zidovudine use in 282 AIDS patients found that haematological abnormalities (anaemia, leucopenia, neutropenia) were common. However, the frequency was not increased in the patients [number unknown] also taking co-trimoxazole.[12]

Mechanism

A likely reason is that the trimethoprim inhibits the secretion of both zidovudine and its glucuronide by the kidney tubules. It is not known why the half-life of co-trimoxazole is increased. The other NRTIs that interact are likely to do so by the same mechanism.

Importance and management

Established interactions. With the NRTIs that are actively excreted via the kidneys (e.g. lamivudine, stavudine, and zalcitabine), it is unlikely that dosage alterations are necessary unless the patient has renal impairment. However, when both drugs are needed, patients should be closely monitored for signs of toxicity. Moreover, the UK manufacturer of lamivudine recommends that the use of lamivudine with high-dose co-trimoxazole for the treatment of Pneumocystis pneumonia and toxoplasmosis should be avoided.[4] Since renal clearance represents only 20 to 30% of the total clearance of zidovudine, the authors of two of these reports[7,10] suggest that this interaction is unlikely to be clinically important for zidovudine unless the glucuronidation by the liver is impaired by liver disease or other drugs. Didanosine also does not appear to interact to a clinically relevant extent.

Nevertheless concurrent use should be well monitored, especially because co-trimoxazole alone has been associated with a high incidence of adverse effects in patients with AIDS.[13]

1. Srinivas NR, Knupp CA, Batteiger B, Smith RA, Barbhaiya RH. A pharmacokinetic interaction study of didanosine coadministered with trimethoprim and/or sulphamethoxazole in HIV seropositive asymptomatic male patients. *Br J Clin Pharmacol* (1996) 41, 207–15.
2. Moore KHP, Yuen GJ, Raasch RH, Eron JJ, Martin D, Mydlow PK, Hussey EK. Pharmacokinetics of lamivudine administered alone and with trimethoprim-sulfamethoxazole. *Clin Pharmacol Ther* (1996) 59, 550–8.
3. Sabo JP, Lamson MJ, Leitz G, Yong C-L, MacGregor TR. Pharmacokinetics of nevirapine and lamivudine in patients with HIV-1 infection. AAPS PharmSci. (2000) 2, E1–E7.
4. Epivir (Lamivudine). GlaxoSmithKline UK. UK Summary of product characteristics, March 2007.
5. Zerit (Stavudine). Bristol-Myers Squibb Pharmaceuticals Ltd. UK Summary of product characteristics, January 2007.
6. Lee BL, Täuber MG, Chambers HF, Gambertoglio J, Delahunty T. The effect of trimethoprim (TMP) on the pharmacokinetics (PK) of zalcitabine (ddC) in HIV-infected patients. *Intersci Conf Antimicrob Agents Chemother* (1995) 35, 6.
7. Chatton JY, Munafo A, Chave JP, Steinhäuslin F, Roch-Ramel F, Glauser MP, Biollaz J. Trimethoprim, alone of in combination with sulphamethoxazole, decreases the renal excretion of zidovudine and its glucuronide. *Br J Clin Pharmacol* (1992) 34, 551–4.
8. Cañas E, Pachon J, Garcia-Pesquera F, Castillo JR, Viciana P, Cisneros JM, Jimenez-Mejias M. Absence of effect of trimethoprim-sulfamethoxazole on pharmacokinetics of zidovudine in patients infected with human immunodeficiency virus. *Antimicrob Agents Chemother* (1996) 40, 230–33.
9. Lee BL, Safrin S, Makrides V, Benowitz NL, Gambertoglio JG, Mills J. Trimethoprim decreases the renal clearance of zidovudine. *Clin Pharmacol Ther* (1992) 51,183.
10. Lee BL, Safrin S, Makrides V, Gambertoglio JG. Zidovudine, trimethoprim, and dapsone pharmacokinetic interactions in patients with human immunodeficiency virus infection. *Antimicrob Agents Chemother* (1996) 40, 1231–6.
11. Berson A, Happy K, Rousseau F, Grateau G, Farinotti R, Séréni D. Effect of zidovudine (AZT) on cotrimoxazole (TMP-SMX) kinetics: preliminary results. 9th International Conference on AIDS & 5th STD World Congress, Berlin, June 6-11 1993. Abstract PO-B30-2193.
12. Richman DD, Fischl MA, Grieco MH, Gottlieb MS, Volberding PA, Laskin OL, Leedom JM, Groopman JE, Mildvan D, Hirsch MS, Jackson GG, Durack DT, Nusinoff-Lehrman S and the AZT Collaborative Working Group. The toxicity of azidothymidine (AZT) in the treatment of patients with AIDS and AIDS-related complex. A double-blind, placebo-controlled trial. *N Engl J Med* (1987) 317, 192–7.
13. Medina I, Mills J, Leoung G, Hopewell PC, Lee B, Modin G, Benowitz N, Wofsy CB. Oral therapy for Pneumocystis carinii pneumonia in the acquired immunodeficiency syndrome: a controlled trial of trimethoprim-sulfamethoxazole versus trimethoprim-dapsone. *N Engl J Med* (1990) 323, 776–82.

NRTIs + Cytokines

Interferon alfa does not alter the pharmacokinetics of didanosine or lamivudine to a clinically relevant extent. Interferon alfa and, particularly, interferon beta can cause an increase in the serum levels of zidovudine. HIV-positive patients infected with hepatitis C and treated with interferon alfa and ribavirin may be at special risk of NRTI-associated lactic acidosis. Interleukin-2 appears not to interact significantly with zidovudine.

Clinical evidence

(a) Interferon

AIDS patients who had been taking **zidovudine** 200 mg every 4 hours for 8 weeks were also given subcutaneous **recombinant beta interferon** 45 million units daily. After 3 and 15 days the **zidovudine** metabolism was reduced by 75% and 97%, respectively. By day 15 the **zidovudine** half-life was increased by about twofold.[1] Another study in 6 children aged 3 months to 17 years found that after 5 weeks of concurrent use **interferon alfa** increased the AUC of **zidovudine** by 36%, increased its maximum serum level by 69% and reduced its clearance by 20%.[2]

Interferon alfa 1 to 15 million units daily was given to 26 HIV-positive patients taking **didanosine** sachets 100 to 375 mg twice daily. The interferon appeared to have no clinically significant effects on the pharmacokinetics of the **didanosine**.[3] Similarly, a single subcutaneous injection of **interferon alfa** 10 million units had no clinically significant effects on the pharmacokinetics of **lamivudine** 100 mg daily, given to 19 healthy subjects for 7 days (the **lamivudine** AUC was decreased by about 10%). **Lamivudine** did not appear to alter the pharmacokinetics of **interferon alfa**.[4]

(b) Interleukin-2

A study found that a 4-week course of interleukin-2 (0.25 million units/m^2 daily) by continuous infusion had no clinically significant effect on the pharmacokinetics of a 100-mg intravenous dose of **zidovudine**.[5] Another study in 8 HIV-positive men given oral **zidovudine** 200 mg every 4 hours found similar results.[3] No special precautions would seem necessary.

Mechanism

Interferon beta appears to inhibit the metabolism (glucuronidation) of the zidovudine by the liver.

Importance and management

Information seems to be limited to these reports. The results of the first report suggest that the zidovudine dosage may need to be reduced if interferon beta is added in order to avoid increased zidovudine toxicity. A dosage reduction of two-thirds, or even more, may be necessary. More study is needed to confirm these observations. Interferon alfa appears to interact to a lesser extent. The manufacturers warn that the risk of haematological toxicity may be increased if zidovudine and interferon are used together, and combined use in hepatitis C may increase the risk of NRTI-associated lactic acidosis: patients at risk should be carefully monitored.[6,7] Interferon alfa does not appear to affect the pharmacokinetics of didanosine or lamivudine. Nevertheless, all manufacturers note that, because of the risk of NRTI-associated lactic acidosis, caution should be exercised when giving NRTIs (**abacavir**, didanosine, **emtricitabine**, lamivudine, **stavudine**, zidovudine) to any patient with hepatomegaly, hepatitis or other known risk factors for liver disease and hepatic steatosis, and that HIV-positive patients infected with hepatitis C and treated with interferon alfa and ribavirin may constitute a special risk. Patients at increased risk should be monitored closely.

1. Nokta M, Loh JP, Douidar SM, Ahmed AE, Pollard RB. Metabolic interaction of recombinant interferon-β and zidovudine in AIDS patients. *J Interferon Res* (1991) 11, 159–64.
2. Diaz C, Yogev R, Rodriguez J, Rege A, George W, Lertora J. ACTG-153: Zidovudine pharmacokinetics when used in combination with interferon alpha. *Intersci Conf Antimicrob Agents Chemother* (1994) 34, 79.
3. Piscitelli SC, Amantea MA, Vogel S, Bechtel C, Metcalf JA, Kovacs JA. Effects of cytokines on antiviral pharmacokinetics: an alternative approach to assessment of drug interactions using bioequivalence guidelines. *Antimicrob Agents Chemother* (1996) 40, 161–5.
4. Johnson MA, Jenkins JM, Bye C. A study of the pharmacokinetic interaction between lamivudine and alpha interferon. *Eur J Clin Pharmacol* (2000) 56, 289–92.
5. Skinner MH, Pauloin D, Schwartz D, Merigan TC, Blaschke TF. IL-2 does not alter zidovudine kinetics. *Clin Pharmacol Ther* (1989) 45, 128.
6. Retrovir (Zidovudine). GlaxoSmithKline UK. UK Summary of product characteristics, December 2006.
7. Retrovir (Zidovudine). GlaxoSmithKline. US Prescribing information, November 2006.

NRTIs + Dapsone

Buffered didanosine does not alter the pharmacokinetics of dapsone, but there is some circumstantial evidence to suggest that it may reduce the prophylactic effects of dapsone in preventing Pneumocystis pneumonia. Dapsone has no effect on the pharmacokinetics of zalcitabine, whereas zalcitabine causes a small rise in the serum levels of dapsone, and there is a theoretical increased risk of peripheral neuropathy with the combination. Dapsone appears not to affect the pharmacokinetics of zidovudine, although concurrent use may be associated with increased blood dyscrasias.

Clinical evidence, mechanism, importance and management

(a) Didanosine

An early report of the use of buffered didanosine described the development of Pneumocystis pneumonia in 11 out of 28 HIV-positive patients taking dapsone prophylaxis, compared with only 1 of 12 taking aerosolised pentamidine, and none of 17 taking co-trimoxazole. Of the 11 patients where prophylaxis failed, 4 died from respiratory failure.[1] The authors suggested that the most likely explanation of the high failure rate of dapsone with didanosine, was reduced dapsone absorption due to the citrate-phosphate buffer in the didanosine formulation.[1] This has led to some recommending that the drugs be taken at least 2 hours apart.

However, in a controlled study in 6 HIV-positive subjects, dapsone pharmacokinetics were not altered when a dose of buffered didanosine was taken within 5 minutes.[2] Similarly, in 6 healthy subjects, dapsone pharmacokinetics were not altered by the aluminium/magnesium antacids and other excipients contained in didanosine tablets.[2] Another study in healthy subjects also failed to confirm that a marked rise in gastric pH affects the absorption of dapsone, see 'Dapsone + Antacids', p.303. Furthermore, low dapsone levels have been found in patients receiving a weekly dapsone regimen who took dapsone at least 2 hours before or 6 hours after didanosine, and in patients taking zidovudine or no antiretrovirals (although this study did not look at whether dapsone levels were correlated with efficacy).[3] In a retrospective analysis, other authors found no evidence to confirm a correlation between failure of Pneumocystis pneumonia prophylaxis with dapsone and use of drugs that increase gastric pH (didanosine, H_2-receptor antagonists, antacids).[4]

It has therefore been adequately demonstrated that the buffered preparation of didanosine and antacids do not affect dapsone absorption. The explanation for the apparent failure of Pneumocystis pneumonia prophylaxis in the original report[1] is unresolved. Despite the use of both didanosine and dapsone in the management of HIV and opportunistic infections there do not appear to be any further reports of problems with the combination.

(b) Zalcitabine

A pharmacokinetic study in 12 HIV-positive patients who were given zalcitabine 1.5 mg three times daily and dapsone 100 mg daily, alone or together, found that dapsone did not significantly affect the kinetics of the zalcitabine. However, zalcitabine decreased the clearance of dapsone by 21%, increased its maximum serum levels by 19% and increased its half-life by 34%.[5] These changes are relatively small and seem unlikely to have much clinical relevance, but until this is confirmed it would seem prudent to monitor the concurrent use of these two drugs. The UK manufacturer[6] recommended caution with the combination because of the possibility of an increased risk of peripheral neuropathy; the US manufacturer advised avoiding the combination where possible.[7]

(c) Zidovudine

Dapsone 100 mg daily had no effect on the pharmacokinetics of a single 200-mg dose of zidovudine in 8 HIV-positive subjects.[8] In a further study, which considered the safety of dapsone in combination with zidovudine, dapsone was shown to increase the risk of zidovudine-related blood dyscrasias.[9] Therefore it would seem that dapsone and zidovudine can be given concurrently, but monitoring for an increase in adverse events would seem advisable.

1. Metroka CE, McMechan MF, Andrada R, Laubenstein LJ, Jacobus DP. Failure of prophylaxis with dapsone in patients taking dideoxyinosine. *N Engl J Med* (1992) 325, 737.
2. Sahai J, Garber G, Gallicano K, Oliveras L, Cameron DW. Effects of the antacids in didanosine tablets on dapsone pharmacokinetics. *Ann Intern Med* (1995) 123, 584–7.
3. Opravil M, Joos B, Lüthy R. Levels of dapsone and pyrimethamine in serum during once-weekly dosing for prophylaxis of *Pneumocystis carinii* pneumonia and toxoplasmic encephalitis. *Antimicrob Agents Chemother* (1994) 38, 1197–9.
4. Huengsberg M, Castelino S, Sherrard J, O'Farrell N, Bingham J. Does drug interaction cause failure of PCP prophylaxis with dapsone? *Lancet* (1993) 341, 48.
5. Lee BL, Tauber MG, Chambers HF, Gambertoglio J, Delahunty T. Zalcitabine (DDC) and dapsone (DAP) pharmacokinetic (PK) interaction in HIV-infected patients. *Clin Pharmacol Ther* (1995) 57, 186.
6. Hivid (Zalcitabine). Roche Products Ltd. UK Summary of product characteristics, November 2004.
7. Hivid (Zalcitabine). Roche Pharmaceuticals. US Prescribing information, September 2002.

8. Lee BL, Safrin S, Makrides V, Gambertoglio JG. Zidovudine, trimethoprim, and dapsone pharmacokinetic interactions in patients with human immunodeficiency virus infection. *Antimicrob Agents Chemother* (1996) 40, 1231–6.
9. Pinching AJ, Helbert M, Peddle B, Robinson D, Janes K, Gor D, Jeffries DJ, Stoneham C, Mitchell D, Kocsis AE, Mann J, Forster SM, Harris JRW. Clinical experience with zidovudine for patients with acquired immune deficiency syndrome and acquired immune deficiency syndrome-related complex. *J Infect* (1989) 18 (Suppl 1), 33–40.

NRTIs + Drugs that cause pancreatitis

Additive pancreatic toxicity has been described with zalcitabine and intravenous pentamidine, and is expected when didanosine or stavudine are given with other drugs that can cause pancreatitis. An isolated case describes pancreatitis with lamivudine and azathioprine.

Clinical evidence

(a) Lamivudine

A single case report describes a 51-year-old woman with a kidney transplant who developed pancreatitis after starting lamivudine. **Azathioprine** had been discontinued only 3 days before and it is possible (although the evidence is weak) that the residual serum **azathioprine** had interacted with lamivudine to cause the pancreatitis.[1]

(b) Zalcitabine

Fatal fulminant pancreatitis occurred in a patient given zalcitabine and intravenous **pentamidine**.[2]

Mechanism

Possible additive toxicity.

Importance and management

Of the NRTIs, **didanosine**, **stavudine** and zalcitabine have been associated with fatal pancreatitis.[2-7]

The manufacturers of zalcitabine recommended that if a drug that has the potential to cause pancreatitis is required, treatment with zalcitabine should be interrupted.[2,7] They specifically applied this to the use of pentamidine to treat Pneumocystis pneumonia.[2,7]

The manufacturers of **didanosine** have a similar recommendation and state that, if concurrent use is unavoidable, there should be close observation.[3,4] Similarly, other authors recommend temporarily discontinuing didanosine in patients needing systemic pentamidine or **sulfonamide**-containing regimens.[8] The UK manufacturer of **stavudine** recommends that patients receiving concurrent treatment with drugs known to cause pancreatitis should be carefully observed,[5] and the US manufacturer specifically recommends caution with combined use of **didanosine** and **stavudine**,[6] see 'NRTIs + NRTIs', p.800. Note that **hydroxycarbamide (hydroxyurea)** may increase the risk of pancreatitis with didanosine and stavudine, and the combination should probably be avoided, see 'NRTIs + Hydroxycarbamide', p.799.

The UK manufacturer states that lamivudine is rarely associated with pancreatitis, but recommend that treatment with lamivudine should be stopped if there is any suspicion of pancreatitis:[9] no firm conclusions can be drawn from the case discussed above.

1. Van Vlierberghe H, Elewaut A. Development of a necrotising pancreatitis after starting lamivudine in a kidney transplant patient with fibrosing cholestatic hepatitis: A possible role of the interaction lamivudine and azathioprine. *Gastroenterology* (1997) 112 (4 Suppl), A1407.
2. Hivid (Zalcitabine). Roche Products Ltd. UK Summary of product characteristics, November 2004.
3. Videx Tablets (Didanosine). Bristol-Myers Squibb Pharmaceuticals Ltd. UK Summary of product characteristics, December 2006.
4. Videx (Didanosine). Bristol-Myers Squibb Company. US Prescribing information, August 2006.
5. Zerit (Stavudine). Bristol-Myers Squibb Pharmaceuticals Ltd. UK Summary of product characteristics, January 2007.
6. Zerit (Stavudine). Bristol-Myers Squibb Company. US Prescribing information, August 2006.
7. Hivid (Zalcitabine). Roche Pharmaceuticals. US Prescribing information, September 2002.
8. Yarchoan R, Mitsuya H, Pluda JM, Marczyk KS, Thomas RV, Hartman NR, Brouwers P, Perno C-F, Allain J-P, Johns DG, Broder S. The National Cancer Institute phase I study of 2',3'-dideoxyinosine administration in adults with AIDS or AIDS-related complex: analysis of activity and toxicity profiles. *Rev Infect Dis* (1990) 12 (Suppl 5), S522–S533.
9. Epivir (Lamivudine). GlaxoSmithKline UK. UK Summary of product characteristics, March 2007.

NRTIs + Food

Food can reduce the extent of absorption of didanosine, possibly causing a loss in efficacy. The extent of absorption of zalcitabine and zidovudine is reduced slightly by food. Food does not affect the extent of absorption of abacavir, emtricitabine, lamivudine, and stavudine.

Clinical evidence, mechanism, importance and management

(a) Abacavir

The manufacturer of abacavir notes that food delayed its rate, but not extent, of absorption. Therefore, abacavir can be taken with or without food.[1,2]

(b) Didanosine

1. Buffered preparations. Didanosine (as two 150-mg chewable tablets) was given to 10 HIV-positive subjects on four occasions: 30 minutes before breakfast, 1 hour before breakfast, 1 hour after breakfast, and 2 hours after breakfast. When the dose was given before breakfast the results were very similar to those obtained for subjects in the fasting state. When given after a breakfast, the didanosine AUC and maximum plasma concentration were both decreased by about 50%.[3] Similar results were found in another study.[4] A further study[5] using sachets containing didanosine, sucrose and citrate-phosphate buffer, similarly found that food reduced the bioavailability by 41% (a reduction from 29% to 17%). The reason would appear to be that food delays gastric emptying so that the didanosine is exposed to prolonged contact with gastric acid, which causes decomposition (see 'Antivirals', (p.772)), with a resultant fall in bioavailability.[6] To achieve maximum bioavailability the didanosine buffered preparations should be taken on an empty stomach at least 30 minutes before food[6,7] or 2 hours after food.[7]

2. Enteric-coated preparation. Giving didanosine gastro-resistant capsules with a high-fat meal or a light meal reduced the AUC by 19% and 27%, respectively, compared with the fasting state. A similar 24% decrease in the AUC was also seen when didanosine was taken 1 hour before a light meal. However, the effect on the AUC was negligible when it was taken 1.5 to 3 hours before a light meal.[8] Sprinkling the capsule contents on yoghurt or apple sauce also decreased the AUC by 20% or 18%, respectively.[8] Despite these modest changes in AUC, the manufacturer recommends that didanosine gastro-resistant capsules are taken intact on an empty stomach,[8,9] at least 2 hours before or 2 hours after a meal.[8]

(c) Emtricitabine

The manufacturer says that giving emtricitabine hard capsules with a high-fat meal did not affect the AUC of emtricitabine but slightly reduced the maximum level by 29%. Similarly, giving emtricitabine oral solution with a low-fat or high-fat meal did not affect the AUC or maximum level of emtricitabine. Therefore, both these formulations of emtricitabine may be given with or without food.[10,11]

(d) Lamivudine

The manufacturer notes that food delayed the rate and reduced the maximum plasma concentration (by about 45%), but not the extent (AUC), of lamivudine absorption. Therefore, lamivudine can be taken with or without food.[12,13]

(e) Stavudine

The UK manufacturer of stavudine notes that a standardised high-fat meal reduced, and delayed the time to reach the maximum plasma concentration (specific details not given), but did not alter the extent of systemic exposure of stavudine, when compared with the fasting state. Nevertheless, they recommend that, for optimal absorption, stavudine should be taken on an empty stomach at least 1 hour before meals. However, if this is not possible, they suggest giving stavudine with a light meal; in addition the contents of the capsule may be mixed with food.[14] The US manufacturer states that stavudine can be taken with food or on an empty stomach.[15]

(f) Zalcitabine

The manufacturers of zalcitabine[16,17] noted that food decreased the maximum plasma concentration by 39% and prolonged the time to achieve maximum concentrations from 0.8 to 1.6 hours compared with the fasting state. The extent of absorption was decreased by 14%. The UK manufacturer stated that zalcitabine could be taken with or without food.[16]

(g) Zidovudine

Zidovudine was given to 13 AIDS patients either with breakfast or when fasting. The maximum plasma level of zidovudine was 2.8-fold greater in the fasted patients, and the AUC was reduced by 22% when zidovudine was given with food.[18] Zidovudine rate and extent of absorption was reduced in another study by a standard breakfast (14% decrease in AUC with a 200-mg dose and 33% with a 100-mg dose).[19] In a study[20] of 8 patients, a high-fat meal reduced the maximum zidovudine serum levels by about 50%. In all these cases inter-individual variation in zidovudine absorption was high.[18-20] However, when a sustained-release formulation of zidovudine was used, the absorption was delayed, but the AUC was increased by 28% by a high-fat meal.[21] In contrast zidovudine AUC was not affected by 25 g of a **protein supplement**.[22]

Inter-individual variation appears high and the practical consequences of the changes caused are uncertain. Some have suggested that zidovudine should be taken on an empty stomach;[19,20] the US manufacturer states that zidovudine can be taken with or without food,[23] but the UK manufacturer gives no specific recommendations regarding its administration in relation to food.[24]

1. Ziagen (Abacavir sulfate). GlaxoSmithKline UK. UK Summary of product characteristics, May 2007.
2. Ziagen (Abacavir sulfate). GlaxoSmithKline. US Prescribing information, July 2002.
3. Knupp CA, Milbrath R, Barbhaiya RH. Effect of time of food administration on the bioavailability of didanosine from a chewable tablet formulation. *J Clin Pharmacol* (1993) 33, 568–73.
4. Shyu WC, Knupp CA, Pittman KA, Dunkle L, Barbhaiya RH. Food-induced reduction in bioavailability of didanosine. *Clin Pharmacol Ther* (1991) 50, 503–7.
5. Hartman NR, Yarchoan R, Pluda JM, Thomas RV, Wyvill KM, Flora KP, Broder S, Johns DG. Pharmacokinetics of 2′,3′-dideoxyinosine in patients with severe human immunodeficiency infection. II. The effects of different oral formulations and the presence of other medications. *Clin Pharmacol Ther* (1991) 50, 278–85.
6. Videx Tablets (Didanosine). Bristol-Myers Squibb Pharmaceuticals Ltd. UK Summary of product characteristics, December 2006.
7. Videx Pediatric Powder for Oral Solution (Didanosine). Bristol-Myers Squibb Company. US Prescribing information, August 2006.
8. Videx EC (Didanosine). Bristol-Myers Squibb Pharmaceuticals Ltd. UK Summary of product characteristics, December 2006.
9. Videx EC (Didanosine). Bristol-Myers Squibb Company. US Prescribing information, March 2007.
10. Emtriva (Emtricitabine). Gilead Sciences International Ltd. UK Summary of product characteristics, April 2007.
11. Emtriva (Emtricitabine). Gilead Sciences, Inc. US Prescribing information, December 2006.
12. Epivir (Lamivudine). GlaxoSmithKline UK. UK Summary of product characteristics, March 2007.
13. Epivir (Lamivudine). GlaxoSmithKline. US Prescribing information, October 2006.
14. Zerit (Stavudine). Bristol-Myers Squibb Pharmaceuticals Ltd. UK Summary of product characteristics, January 2007.
15. Zerit (Stavudine). Bristol-Myers Squibb Company. US Prescribing information, August 2006.
16. Hivid (Zalcitabine). Roche Products Ltd. UK Summary of product characteristics, November 2004.
17. Hivid (Zalcitabine). Roche Pharmaceuticals. US Prescribing information, September 2002.
18. Lotterer E, Ruhnke M, Trautmann M, Beyer R, Bauer FE. Decreased and variable systemic availability of zidovudine in patients with AIDS if administered with a meal. *Eur J Clin Pharmacol* (1991) 40, 305–8.
19. Ruhnke M, Bauer FE, Seifert M, Trautmann M, Hille H, Koeppe P. Effects of standard breakfast on pharmacokinetics of oral zidovudine in patients with AIDS. *Antimicrob Agents Chemother* (1993) 37, 2153–8.
20. Unadkat JD, Collier AC, Crosby SS, Cummings D, Opheim KE, Corey L. Pharmacokinetics of oral zidovudine (azidothymidine) in patients with AIDS when administered with and without a high-fat meal. *AIDS* (1990) 4, 229–32.
21. Hollister AS, Frazer HA. The effects of a high fat meal on the serum pharmacokinetics of sustained-release zidovudine. *Clin Pharmacol Ther* (1994) 55, 193.
22. Sahai J, Gallicano K, Garber G, McGilveray I, Hawley-Foss N, Turgeon N, Cameron DW. The effect of a protein meal on zidovudine pharmacokinetics in HIV-infected patients. *Br J Clin Pharmacol* (1992) 33, 657–60.
23. Retrovir (Zidovudine). GlaxoSmithKline. US Prescribing information, November 2006.
24. Retrovir (Zidovudine). GlaxoSmithKline UK. UK Summary of product characteristics, December 2006.

NRTIs + Ganciclovir

The concurrent use of zidovudine and ganciclovir produces a very marked increase in haematological toxicity, without any apparent increase in efficacy. Didanosine serum levels are raised by ganciclovir, but there is some evidence suggesting that the efficacy of ganciclovir prophylaxis is reduced. Ganciclovir does not appear to interact with stavudine, and there is no clinically important pharmacokinetic interaction between ganciclovir and zalcitabine. Until further information is available, the manufacturers of lamivudine advise the avoidance of intravenous ganciclovir.

Clinical evidence

(a) Didanosine

Buffered didanosine 200 mg twice daily was given to 12 HIV-positive patients with oral ganciclovir 1 g three times daily. When the didanosine was given 2 hours before ganciclovir, the maximum serum levels and AUC of didanosine were raised by about 47% and 83%, respectively, and those of ganciclovir were decreased by about 26% and 22%, respectively. When the didanosine was given simultaneously with ganciclovir, the maximum serum levels and AUC of didanosine were similarly raised, by about 53% and 77%, respectively, but those of ganciclovir were unchanged. The renal clearance of didanosine was not significantly changed by ganciclovir.[1] Similar increases in didanosine levels with ganciclovir given intravenously[2] and high-dose oral ganciclovir 2 g every 8 hours have also been reported.[3] However, in contrast, an earlier study found that the pharmacokinetics of didanosine (sachet preparation) were not altered by intravenous ganciclovir.[4]

Rates of dose-limiting intolerance to the combination of didanosine and ganciclovir were reported to be similar to those seen with didanosine alone in one small study (15 of 32 patients tolerated usual doses of didanosine with the ganciclovir).[5] Analysis of the results of a large randomised study unexpectedly suggested that there was an increased risk of cytomegalovirus infection in those patients taking ganciclovir and didanosine, when compared with those not taking didanosine.[6]

(b) Lamivudine

The UK manufacturer of lamivudine says that concurrent use with intravenous ganciclovir is not recommended until further information becomes available,[7] although they give no reason for this advice. They do not mention oral ganciclovir.[7]

(c) Stavudine

In a study of 11 HIV-positive patients, oral ganciclovir 1 g three times daily had no significant effect on the pharmacokinetics of stavudine 40 mg twice daily, nor were the pharmacokinetics of ganciclovir affected by the stavudine.[8] There were no serious or severe adverse events attributed to the combination.

(d) Zalcitabine

In a study in 10 HIV-positive patients, zalcitabine 750 micrograms every 8 hours increased the AUC of oral ganciclovir 1 g three times daily by 22%. There was no change in zalcitabine pharmacokinetics. There were no serious or severe adverse events attributed to the combination.[8]

(e) Zidovudine

The efficacy of zidovudine 100 or 200 mg every 4 hours, given alone or with intravenous ganciclovir 5 mg/kg twice daily for 14 days, then once daily for 5 days of each week, was assessed in 40 patients for the treatment of cytomegalovirus (CMV). Severe haematological toxicity occurred in all of the first 10 patients given zidovudine 1.2 g daily and ganciclovir. Consequently the dose of zidovudine was reduced to 600 mg daily. Overall 82% of the 40 patients enrolled experienced profound and rapid toxicity (anaemia, neutropenia, leucopenia, gastrointestinal disturbances). Zidovudine dosage reductions to 300 mg daily were needed in many patients. No change in the pharmacokinetics of zidovudine or ganciclovir was noted.[9]

Another study in 6 AIDS patients with CMV retinitis given zidovudine and ganciclovir found increased bone marrow toxicity but no improved efficacy over ganciclovir alone.[10] Increased toxicity (myelotoxicity and pancytopenia) following the use of both drugs has also been reported elsewhere.[11,12]

In contrast to the first study,[9] a specific study on the pharmacokinetics of zidovudine and ganciclovir in HIV-positive subjects reported that oral ganciclovir increased the maximum levels and AUC of zidovudine by 38% and 15%, respectively, without altering renal clearance. Zidovudine did not alter ganciclovir pharmacokinetics.[1]

Mechanism

It is not known why ganciclovir increases the levels of didanosine and zidovudine: it does not appear to be due to competition for active secretion by the kidney tubules.[1]

The toxicity of the zidovudine/ganciclovir combination may be simply additive,[9] but *in vitro* studies with three human cell lines found synergistic cytotoxicity when both drugs were used.[13]

There is some *in vitro* evidence to suggest that ganciclovir antagonises the anti-HIV activity of zidovudine and didanosine.[14]

Importance and management

The interactions between ganciclovir and didanosine or zidovudine would appear to be established, but the clinical importance is uncertain. Zidovudine seems to be associated with greater toxicity than didanosine. However, there is also some evidence suggesting reduced ganciclovir efficacy in the presence of didanosine, and this requires further study. Close and careful monitoring is required if either combination is used.

Ganciclovir does not appear to alter the pharmacokinetics of stavudine or zalcitabine. Zalcitabine increased ganciclovir levels to a minor extent, although this is probably not clinically important.

1. Cimoch PJ, Lavelle J, Pollard R, Griffy KG, Wong R, Tarnowski TL, Casserella S, Jung D. Pharmacokinetics of oral ganciclovir alone and in combination with zidovudine, didanosine, and probenecid in HIV-infected subjects. *J Acquir Immune Defic Syndr Hum Retrovirol* (1998) 17, 227–34.
2. Frascino RJ, Anderson RD, Griffy KG, Jung D, Yu S. Two multiple dose crossover studies of IV ganciclovir (GCV) and didanosine (ddI) in HIV infected persons. *Intersci Conf Antimicrob Agents Chemother* (1995) 35, 6.
3. Jung D, Griffy K, Dorr A, Raschke R, Tarnowski TL, Hulse J, Kates RE. Effect of high-dose oral ganciclovir on didanosine disposition in human immunodeficiency virus (HIV)-positive patients. *J Clin Pharmacol* (1998) 38, 1057–62.
4. Hartman NR, Yarchoan R, Pluda JM, Thomas RV, Wyvill KM, Flora KP, Broder S, Johns DG. Pharmacokinetics of 2′,3′-dideoxyinosine in patients with severe human immunodeficiency infection. II. The effects of different oral formulations and the presence of other medications. *Clin Pharmacol Ther* (1991) 50, 278–85.
5. Jacobson MA, Owen W, Campbell J, Brosgart C, Abrams DI. Tolerability of combined ganciclovir and didanosine for the treatment of cytomegalovirus disease associated with AIDS. *Clin Infect Dis* (1993) 16 (Suppl 1), S69–S73.
6. Brosgart CL, Louis TA, Hillman DW, Craig CP, Alston B, Fisher E, Abrams DI, Luskin-Hawk RL, Sampson JH, Ward DJ, Thompson MA, Torres RA. A randomized, placebo-controlled trial of the safety and efficacy of oral ganciclovir for prophylaxis of cytomegalovirus disease in HIV-infected individuals. *AIDS* (1998) 12, 269–77.
7. Epivir (Lamivudine). GlaxoSmithKline UK. UK Summary of product characteristics, March 2007.
8. Jung D, AbdelHameed MH, Teitelbaum P, Dorr A, Griffy K. The pharmacokinetics and safety profile of oral ganciclovir combined with zalcitabine or stavudine in asymptomatic HIV- and CMV-seropositive patients. *J Clin Pharmacol* (1999) 39, 505–12.
9. Hochster H, Dieterich D, Bozzette S, Reichman RC, Connor JD, Liebes L, Sonke RL, Spector SA, Valentine F, Pettinelli C, Richman DD. Toxicity of combined ganciclovir and zidovudine for cytomegalovirus disease associated with AIDS. An AIDS clinical trials group study. *Ann Intern Med* (1990) 113, 111–17.
10. Millar AB, Miller RF, Patou G, Mindel A, Marsh R, Semple SJG. Treatment of cytomegalovirus retinitis with zidovudine and ganciclovir in patients with AIDS: outcome and toxicity. *Genitourin Med* (1990) 66, 156–8.
11. Jacobson MA, de Miranda P, Gordon SM, Blum MR, Volberding P, Mills J. Prolonged pancytopenia due to combined ganciclovir and zidovudine therapy. *J Infect Dis* (1988) 158, 489–90.
12. Pinching AJ, Helbert M, Peddle B, Robinson D, Janes K, Gor D, Jeffries DJ, Stoneham C, Mitchell D, Kocsis AE, Mann J, Forster SM, Harris JRW. Clinical experience with zidovudine for patients with acquired immune deficiency syndrome and acquired immune deficiency syndrome-related complex. *J Infect* (1989) 18 (Suppl 1), 33–40.
13. Prichard MN, Prichard LE, Baguley WA, Nassiri MR, Shipman C. Three-dimensional analysis of the synergistic cytotoxicity of ganciclovir and zidovudine. *Antimicrob Agents Chemother* (1991) 35, 1060–5.
14. Medina DJ, Hsiung GD, Mellors JW. Ganciclovir antagonizes the anti-human immunodeficiency virus type 1 activity of zidovudine and didanosine in vitro. *Antimicrob Agents Chemother* (1992) 36, 1127–30.

NRTIs + H_2-receptor antagonists

The concurrent use of buffered didanosine and ranitidine results in a minor increase in the serum levels of didanosine, and a minor decrease in the serum levels of ranitidine. Both changes seem to be clinically unimportant. Cimetidine raises serum zalcitabine levels, but this is of uncertain importance. Cimetidine and ranitidine do not have a clinically significant effect on zidovudine or lamivudine serum levels.

Clinical evidence, mechanism, importance and management

(a) Didanosine

Didanosine 375 mg (buffered sachet preparation) was given to 12 HIV-positive subjects either alone, or 2 hours after a single 150-mg dose of **ranitidine**. The didanosine AUC was increased by 14% by the **ranitidine**.[1] The reason for this effect is not known but the **ranitidine** possibly enhanced the effects of the citrate-phosphate buffer with which the didanosine sachet was formulated. The **ranitidine** AUC was reduced by 16% for reasons that are not understood, but it is possible that antacids (such as the citrate-phosphate buffer) reduce the absorption of **ranitidine**[1] (see 'H_2-receptor antagonists + Antacids', p.966).

These bioavailability changes appear to be too small to matter clinically, and no particular precautions would seem necessary if the drugs are taken in this way. It is not known whether other H_2-receptor antagonists behave similarly.

(b) Lamivudine

Lamivudine is cleared predominantly from the body by the kidneys using the organic cationic transport system; however, **cimetidine** and **ranitidine**, which partly use this mechanism, do not interact with lamivudine.[2]

(c) Zalcitabine

A study in 12 HIV-positive patients given a single 1.5-mg dose of zalcitabine found that **cimetidine** 800 mg caused a 24% reduction in the renal clearance of zalcitabine (assumed to be due to a reduction in renal tubular secretion) and a 36% increase in the AUC of zalcitabine.[3] These changes are relatively moderate and of uncertain clinical importance. Monitor concurrent use for possible toxicity.

(d) Zidovudine

In a randomised crossover study zidovudine 600 mg daily was given to 5 HIV-positive men and one man with AIDS. The zidovudine was given either alone, with **cimetidine** 300 mg four times daily, or with **ranitidine** 150 mg twice daily, each for 7 days. **Cimetidine** reduced the renal elimination of the zidovudine by 56%, but had no effect on its AUC. It was suggested that the reduction in clearance was due to inhibition of tubular secretion. **Ranitidine** had no effect on zidovudine pharmacokinetics. No clinical toxicity occurred and the immunological parameters measured (CD4 and CD8) were not significantly altered. The authors concluded that no change in the dosage of zidovudine is needed if either of these H_2-receptor antagonists is given concurrently.[4] Information about other H_2-receptor antagonists seems to be lacking.

1. Knupp CA, Graziano FM, Dixon RM, Barbhaiya RH. Pharmacokinetic-interaction study of didanosine and ranitidine in patients seropositive for human immunodeficiency virus. *Antimicrob Agents Chemother* (1992) 36, 2075–9.
2. Epivir (Lamivudine). GlaxoSmithKline UK. UK Summary of product characteristics, March 2007.
3. Massarella JW, Holazo AA, Koss-Twardy S, Min B, Smith B, Nazareno LA. The effects of cimetidine and Maalox® on the pharmacokinetics of zalcitabine in HIV-positive patients. *Pharm Res* (1994) 11 (10 Suppl), S-415.
4. Fletcher CV, Henry WK, Noormohamed SE, Rhame FS, Balfour HH. The effect of cimetidine and ranitidine administration with zidovudine. *Pharmacotherapy* (1995) 15, 701–8.

NRTIs + Hydroxycarbamide

Hydroxycarbamide appears to increase the antiviral activity of NRTIs, particularly didanosine. However, the combination of hydroxycarbamide and didanosine may carry a higher risk of adverse effects including neuropathy and pancreatitis, especially if stavudine is also given.

Clinical evidence, mechanism, importance and management

Data from *in vitro* studies have shown that hydroxycarbamide increases the antiviral activity of NRTIs, particularly **didanosine**, possibly by increasing their intracellular activation (phosphorylation).[1,2] The combination is therefore under clinical investigation. Some randomised studies[3,4] have shown that the addition of hydroxycarbamide to reverse transcriptase inhibitors improves virologic response, whereas others have not demonstrated this.[5]

Of concern is that a number of studies have shown increased toxicity. One study reported that the relative risk of neuropathy when **didanosine** was given with hydroxycarbamide was 2.35, compared with **didanosine** alone, and increased to 7.8 when **stavudine** was also added.[6] Another study reported an increased incidence of neuropathy, and an increased incidence of fatigue and nausea and vomiting.[7] The risk of pancreatitis may also be increased. In one study, 3 patients randomised to indinavir, **didanosine**, **stavudine** and hydroxycarbamide developed pancreatitis and died, compared with no deaths in those receiving the same antivirals without hydroxycarbamide.[8] Another case of pancreatitis (non-fatal) has been reported when hydroxycarbamide was given with **stavudine**, **didanosine** and nevirapine.[9] Hepatotoxicity and hepatic failure resulting in death have also been reported in patients given hydroxycarbamide, **didanosine** and **stavudine**.[10,11] In response to these data, the manufacturers of **didanosine** and **stavudine** specifically state that use of these two NRTIs with hydroxycarbamide should be avoided.[10-13] Moreover, the UK manufacturers go as far as to say that hydroxycarbamide should not be used in the treatment of HIV infection.[12,13]

Further studies are needed to define the role of hydroxycarbamide in combination with NRTIs in HIV infection.[14]

1. Palmer S, Cox S. Increased activation of the combination of 3'-azido-3'-deoxythymidine and 2'-deoxy-3'-thiacytidine in the presence of hydroxyurea. *Antimicrob Agents Chemother* (1997) 41, 460–4.

2. Rana KZ, Simmons KA, Dudley MN. Hydroxyurea reduces the 50% inhibitory concentration of didanosine in HIV-infected cells. *AIDS* (1999) 13, 2186–8.
3. Lafeuillade A, Hittinger G, Chadapaud S, Maillefet S, Rieu A, Poggi C. The HYDILE trial: efficacy and tolerance of a quadruple combination of reverse transcriptase inhibitors versus the same regimen plus hydroxyurea or hydroxyurea and interleukin-2 in HIV-infected patients failing protease inhibitor–based combinations. *HIV Clin Trials* (2002) 3, 263–71.
4. Rodriguez CG, Vila J, Capurro AF, Maidana MM, Boffo Lissin LD. Combination therapy with hydroxyurea versus without hydroxyurea as first line treatment options for antiretroviral-naive patients. *HIV Clin Trials* (2000) 1, 1–8.
5. Zala C, Salomon H, Ochoa C, Kijak G, Federico A, Perez H, Montaner JSG, Cahn P. Higher rate of toxicity with no increased efficacy when hydroxyurea is added to a regimen of stavudine plus didanosine and nevirapine in primary HIV infection. *J Acquir Immune Defic Syndr* (2002) 29, 368–73.
6. Moore RD, Wong W-ME, Keruly JC, McArthur JC. Incidence of neuropathy in HIV-infected patients on monotherapy versus those on combination therapy with didanosine, stavudine and hydroxyurea. *AIDS* (2000) 14, 273–8.
7. Rutschmann OT, Vernazza PL, Bucher HC, Opravil M, Ledergerber B, Telenti A, Malinverni R, Bernasconi E, Fagard C, Leduc D, Perrin L, Hirschel B. Long-term hydroxyurea in combination with didanosine and stavudine for the treatment of HIV-1 infection. *AIDS* (2000) 14, 2145–51.
8. Havlir DV, Gilbert PB, Bennett K, Collier AC, Hirsch MS, Tebas P, Adams EM, Wheat LJ, Goodwin D, Schnittman S, Holohan MK, Richman DD; ACTG 5025 Study Team. Effects of treatment intensification with hydroxyurea in HIV-infected patients with virologic suppression. *AIDS* (2001) 1379–88.
9. Longhurst HJ, Pinching AJ. Pancreatitis associated with hydroxyurea in combination with didanosine. *BMJ* (2001) 322, 81.
10. Videx (Didanosine). Bristol-Myers Squibb Company. US Prescribing information, August 2006.
11. Zerit (Stavudine). Bristol-Myers Squibb Company. US Prescribing information, August 2006.
12. Videx Tablets (Didanosine). Bristol-Myers Squibb Pharmaceuticals Ltd. UK Summary of product characteristics, December 2006.
13. Zerit (Stavudine). Bristol-Myers Squibb Pharmaceuticals Ltd. UK Summary of product characteristics, January 2007.
14. Lisziewicz J, Foli A, Wainberg M, Lori F. Hydroxyurea in the treatment of HIV infection: clinical efficacy and safety concerns. *Drug Safety* (2003) 26, 605–24.

NRTIs + Macrolides

Clarithromycin causes some reduction in the bioavailability of zidovudine, but this is minimised if the two drugs are given at least 2 hours apart. Clarithromycin does not appear to interact with didanosine, stavudine or zalcitabine, and azithromycin does not interact with didanosine or zidovudine.

Clinical evidence

(a) Didanosine

When **azithromycin** 1.2 g daily for 14 days was given to 12 HIV-positive subjects with didanosine 200 mg twice daily there was no significant change in the pharmacokinetics of either drug.[1]

Clarithromycin 1 g twice daily for 7 days was given to 4 HIV-positive patients and 8 AIDS patients already taking oral didanosine. For the group as a whole the pharmacokinetics of the didanosine remained unchanged, but there were large differences in the AUC between subjects that could have hidden an interaction.[2]

(b) Stavudine

A study in 10 HIV-positive subjects found that the addition of **clarithromycin** 500 mg twice daily to stavudine 30 or 40 mg twice daily had no significant effects on the pharmacokinetics of the stavudine and the incidence of adverse effects did not increase.[3] No special precautions would seem necessary if both drugs are given.

(c) Zalcitabine

A 7-day course of **clarithromycin** 500 mg twice daily was given to 12 HIV-positive subjects already taking zalcitabine. The addition of **clarithromycin** caused no change to the pharmacokinetics of zalcitabine.[4]

(d) Zidovudine

Azithromycin 600 mg to 1.2 g daily for 14 days did not affect the pharmacokinetics of zidovudine 100 mg five times daily in 12 HIV-positive subjects.[1] Similarly, **azithromycin** 1 g given weekly to 9 HIV-positive subjects caused no change in the pharmacokinetics of zidovudine 10 mg/kg daily. The **azithromycin** pharmacokinetics also remained unchanged.[5]

Fifteen HIV-positive patients were given zidovudine 100 mg every 4 hours 5 times a day and oral **clarithromycin** 500 mg, 1 g or 2 g every 12 hours, both together and alone. The pharmacokinetics of the **clarithromycin** were not substantially changed but the zidovudine levels and AUCs were reduced by 23 to 58% and 12 to 36%, respectively. However, these effects were not seen in all patients.[6,7] Another study similarly found that **clarithromycin** caused a moderate reduction in the AUC of oral zidovudine (by up to 27%). No changes were seen when the zidovudine was given 4 or more hours after the **clarithromycin**.[8] Zidovudine and **clarithromycin** were given to 16 AIDS patients 2 hours apart for 4 days. The maximum plasma levels of the zidovudine rose by about 50%, but the minimum levels and the AUC over 8 hours did not change.[9]

Mechanism

Not understood but the interaction between clarithromycin and zidovudine may possibly be due to some changes in absorption.

Importance and management

The overall picture is slightly confusing, but it seems that some reductions in zidovudine levels are likely if clarithromycin is taken at the same time, but no important changes seem to occur if the administration of the drugs is separated. The authors of one study recommend that the clarithromycin is given at least 2 hours before or after the zidovudine.[7] The UK manufacturer of zidovudine includes this recommendation,[10] but the US manufacturer does not include any information on use with clarithromycin.[11]

The authors of the report on didanosine conclude that clarithromycin may safely be given with didanosine,[2] and it also seems likely that didanosine or zidovudine and azithromycin; stavudine and clarithromycin; and zalcitabine and clarithromycin can be used safely together.

1. Amsden G, Flaherty J, Luke D. Lack of an effect of azithromycin on the disposition of zidovudine and dideoxyinosine in HIV-infected patients. *J Clin Pharmacol* (2001) 41, 210–16.
2. Gillum JG, Bruzzese VL, Israel DS, Kaplowitz LG, Polk RE. Effect of clarithromycin on the pharmacokinetics of 2′,3′-dideoxyinosine in patients who are seropositive for human immunodeficiency virus. *Clin Infect Dis* (1996) 22, 716–18.
3. Piscitelli SC, Kelly G, Walker RE, Kovacs J, Falloon J, Davey RT, Raje S, Masur H, Polis MA. A multiple drug interaction study of stavudine with agents for opportunistic infections in human immunodeficiency virus-infected patients. *Antimicrob Agents Chemother* (1999) 43, 647–50.
4. Pastore A, van Cleef G, Fisher EJ, Gillum JG, LeBel M, Polk RE. Dideoxycytidine (ddC) pharmacokinetics and interaction with clarithromycin in patients seropositive for HIV. 4th Conference on Retroviruses and Opportunistic Infections, Washington DC, January 22nd-26th 1997. Abstract 613.
5. Chave J-P, Munafo A, Chatton J-Y, Dayer P, Glauser MP, Biollaz J. Once-a-week azithromycin in AIDS patients: tolerability, kinetics, and effects on zidovudine disposition. *Antimicrob Agents Chemother* (1992) 36, 1013–18.
6. Gustavson LE, Chu S-Y, Mackenthun A, Gupta SD, Craft JC. Drug interaction between clarithromycin and oral zidovudine in HIV-1 infected patients. *Clin Pharmacol Ther* (1993) 53, 163.
7. Polis MA, Piscitelli SC, Vogel S, Witebsky FG, Conville PS, Petty B, Kovacs JA, Davey RT, Walker RE, Falloon J, Metcalf JA, Craft C, Lane HC, Masur H. Clarithromycin lowers plasma zidovudine levels in persons with human immunodeficiency virus infection. *Antimicrob Agents Chemother* (1997) 41, 1709–14.
8. Petty B, Polis M, Haneiwich S, Dellerson M, Craft JC, Chaisson R. Pharmacokinetic assessment of clarithromycin plus zidovudine in HIV patients. *Intersci Conf Antimicrob Agents Chemother* (1992) 32, 114.
9. Vance E, Watson-Bitar M, Gustavson L, Kazanjian P. Pharmacokinetics of clarithromycin and zidovudine in patients with AIDS. *Antimicrob Agents Chemother* (1995) 39, 1355–60.
10. Retrovir (Zidovudine). GlaxoSmithKline UK. UK Summary of product characteristics, December 2006.
11. Retrovir (Zidovudine). GlaxoSmithKline. US Prescribing information, November 2006.

NRTIs + NRTIs

Some combinations of NRTIs are potentially antagonistic (stavudine with zidovudine, lamivudine with zalcitabine) and some are expected to result in additive toxicity (didanosine with stavudine or zalcitabine, and possibly stavudine with zalcitabine). Some do not appear to result in additional benefits (emtricitabine with lamivudine), and some are considered inferior to other combinations (stavudine with lamivudine, zidovudine with zalcitabine or didanosine). None of these combinations are recommended. Combinations that are specifically recommended (with other antiretrovirals) include lamivudine with abacavir, didanosine or zidovudine, or didanosine with emtricitabine. Sole use of all triple NRTI regimens should generally be avoided, with the possible exception of abacavir or 'tenofovir', (p.806) with zidovudine and lamivudine.

Clinical evidence, mechanism, importance and management

A. Abacavir

(a) Lamivudine

A single 150-mg dose of lamivudine was given with abacavir 600 mg to 13 HIV-positive subjects. The pharmacokinetics of abacavir were not significantly affected, but the lamivudine maximum plasma levels and AUC were decreased by 35% and 15%, respectively. These changes were considered to be consistent with a change in absorption. The extent of the change is not thought to be clinically significant and so no dose alteration would seem necessary on concurrent use.[1] In UK and US guidelines, the combination of abacavir plus lamivudine is currently a recommended dual NRTI option for use with an NNRTI or a protease inhibitor for the treatment of HIV-infection in treatment naïve patients.[2,3] The triple NRTI combination of abacavir, lamivudine and zidovudine may also be considered if protease inhibitors or NNRTIs cannot be used.[3]

(b) Zidovudine

A single 300-mg dose of zidovudine was given with abacavir 600 mg to 13 HIV-positive subjects. The pharmacokinetics of abacavir were not significantly affected. The zidovudine maximum plasma level decreased by 20%, but the AUC was unchanged. This change is not thought to be clinically significant and so no dose alteration would seem necessary on concurrent use.[1] These results were confirmed in a steady-state study in which 79 HIV-positive subjects received 8 weeks of treatment with abacavir 600 mg to 1.8 g daily, in divided doses, and zidovudine 600 mg daily, in divided doses.[4] The triple NRTI combination of abacavir, lamivudine and zidovudine may also be considered if protease inhibitors or NNRTIs cannot be used.[3]

B. Didanosine

(a) Emtricitabine

In UK and US guidelines, the combination of didanosine with emtricitabine is currently a recommended alternative dual NRTI option for use with an NNRTI or a protease inhibitor, for the treatment of HIV-infection in treatment naïve patients.[2,3]

(b) Lamivudine

Lamivudine is cleared predominantly from the body by the kidneys using the organic cationic transport system. Didanosine is not cleared by this mechanism and so is unlikely to interact with lamivudine by this mechanism.[5] Didanosine does not affect the intracellular activation of lamivudine *in vitro*.[6] In UK and US guidelines, the combination of didanosine with lamivudine is currently a recommended alternative dual NRTI option for use with an NNRTI or a protease inhibitor, for the treatment of HIV-infection in treatment naïve patients.[2,3]

(c) Stavudine

Didanosine does not interfere with the intracellular activation of stavudine *in vitro*.[7] Didanosine 100 mg twice daily was given to 10 HIV-positive subjects with stavudine 40 mg twice daily for 9 doses. The didanosine pharmacokinetics were unchanged by concurrent use. The half-life of the stavudine increased from 1.56 to 1.96 hours, but the AUC was unchanged and adverse effects were minimal. The authors of the report concluded that no clinically significant pharmacokinetic interaction, and no change in acute safety and tolerance, are likely if both drugs are given concurrently.[8]

However, both didanosine and stavudine can cause peripheral neuropathy and pancreatitis, and there is some evidence that this risk may be additive. In one early study, combination treatment with stavudine and didanosine was given to 13 HIV-positive subjects for 8 weeks. Neuropathy occurred in 3 patients, with only 2 restarting treatment.[9] In another study, the relative risk of neuropathy was 1.39 for stavudine alone relative to didanosine alone, and 3.5 for combined use of both drugs.[10] In 1999, the manufacturer of didanosine issued a stronger warning about the risk of pancreatitis with didanosine, and noted this risk was higher in patients also taking stavudine,[11] see also 'NRTIs + Hydroxycarbamide', p.799. Combined use should be carefully monitored. See also 'NRTIs + Drugs that cause pancreatitis', p.797.

A case of symptomatic hyperlactataemia occurred in a patient after changing his antiretroviral therapy to didanosine, stavudine and nevirapine.[12] The combination of stavudine and didanosine has been associated with a high incidence of toxicity, particularly peripheral neuropathy, pancreatitis, and lactic acidosis. The development of lactic acidosis has resulted in fatalities in pregnant women.[3] It has been suggested that this combination of NRTIs is associated with the greatest toxicity.[12] US guidelines say that the combination of didanosine and stavudine should not be recommended at any time, with the exception of when no other antiretroviral options are available, and only if the potential benefits outweigh the risks.[3] UK guidelines say that stavudine is not recommended for use as one of the NRTIs for initial therapy of HIV because of its toxicity.[2]

(d) Zalcitabine

In vitro, didanosine had no significant effect on the intracellular activation of zalcitabine.[13] A 29-year-old man with persistent mild neuropathy due to zalcitabine developed severe neuropathy when given didanosine 3 weeks after discontinuing zalcitabine. As the didanosine neuropathy developed so rapidly it was suggested that it was caused by additive toxicity with zalcitabine.[14] Note also that both drugs are associated with pancreatitis. The manufacturers advise caution and careful monitoring if drugs that share these serious adverse effects are used concurrently. See also 'NRTIs + Drugs that cause pancreatitis', p.797. US guidelines say that the combination of didanosine and zalcitabine should not be recommended at any time because of additive peripheral neuropathy.[3]

(e) Zidovudine

A study in 8 HIV-positive patients found that when they were given zidovudine 250 mg with didanosine 250 mg (buffered sachet formulation), the pharmacokinetics of the didanosine were unaltered but the zidovudine AUC was raised by 35%, possibly due to altered absorption.[15] Conversely, in another study zidovudine plasma levels were lower in 4 out of 5 HIV-positive patients when given didanosine (chewable tablets) and there was an average 14% reduction in the zidovudine AUC. The zidovudine clearance was increased by 29% but the didanosine pharmacokinetics were unchanged.[16] A study in over 50 young subjects ranging in age from 3 months to 21 years found that when compared with day 3 (start of concurrent use), no significant changes in AUCs occurred after 4 or 12 weeks of them taking zidovudine 60 to 180 mg/m^2 every 6 hours with didanosine 60 to 180 mg/m^2 every 12 hours (given 2 minutes after an antacid).[17] Several other studies have not found a pharmacokinetic interaction or evidence of increased toxicity when didanosine and zidovudine are used concurrently.[18-21]

The reports are slightly contradictory, but the weight of evidence seems to be that no clinically relevant interaction occurs. UK guidelines say there are no data on the use of zidovudine with enteric-coated didanosine as part of HAART, and that the combination cannot be recommended.[2]

C. Emtricitabine

(a) Lamivudine

US guidelines state that the combination of emtricitabine and lamivudine should not be offered at any time because of the similar resistance profile of the two drugs and there being no potential benefit.[3]

(b) Stavudine

There was no important pharmacokinetic interaction between single doses of emtricitabine 200 mg and stavudine 40 mg in 6 healthy subjects.[22] UK guidelines say that stavudine is not recommended for use as one of the NRTIs for initial therapy of HIV because of its toxicity.[2]

(c) Zidovudine

In a single-dose study in 6 healthy subjects the AUC and maximum level of zidovudine 300 mg were increased by 26% and 66%, respectively, by emtricitabine 200 mg. The pharmacokinetics of emtricitabine were not altered.[22] The authors suggest that these increases in zidovudine levels are unlikely to be clinically relevant based on experience of using the two drugs together for 48 weeks in a phase III clinical study.[22] Further experience is needed.

D. Lamivudine

(a) Stavudine

Nucleoside reverse transcriptase inhibitors such as lamivudine need to be activated by phosphorylation within cells to a triphosphate anabolite. Since stavudine does not affect this phosphorylation *in vitro*[6] it is predicted that no interaction is likely to occur by this mechanism. The manufacturer briefly states that no clinically relevant pharmacokinetic interaction was noted between stavudine 40 mg and lamivudine 150 mg in a single-dose study.[23,24] Nevertheless, current US guidelines state that the combination of stavudine and lamivudine is not a preferred or alternative dual NRTI combination for use in initial antiretroviral regimens because of significant toxicities including lipoatrophy, peripheral neuropathy and serious, life-threatening lactic acidosis with hepatic steatosis, with or without pancreatitis, and rapidly progressive neuromuscular weakness.[3] Similarly, UK guidelines say that stavudine is not recommended for use as one of the NRTIs for initial therapy of HIV because of its toxicity.[2]

(b) Zalcitabine

Lamivudine is cleared predominantly from the body by the kidneys using the organic cationic transport system. Zalcitabine is not cleared in this way and so is unlikely to interact with lamivudine by this mechanism.[5] However, the manufacturers[5,13,25,26] and US guidelines[3] say that lamivudine is not recommended to be used with zalcitabine, since lamivudine may inhibit the intracellular activation of zalcitabine.

(c) Zidovudine

Lamivudine 300 mg twice daily was given to 12 HIV-positive patients for 5 doses, with a 200-mg dose of zidovudine with the last dose. No major changes in the pharmacokinetics of the zidovudine occurred and it was concluded that dosage adjustments are not needed if these two drugs are given concurrently.[27] Another study found the same results,[1] and an extensive study in over 200 patients has shown that combined use can be safe and effective.[28]

However there are case reports of blood dyscrasias occurring with concurrent use. Zidovudine 500 to 600 mg daily was given with lamivudine 300 mg daily to 8 HIV-positive men. Zidovudine or lamivudine alone had previously been given to 6 of these 8 without problem. However, when the drugs were combined, blood dyscrasias occurred in all patients within 7 weeks. Anaemia, with a 50% fall in haemoglobin, occurred in 7 patients, while the other patient developed leucopenia and thrombocytopenia. The drug combination was stopped, blood transfusions were given, and all patients improved or recovered over 5 weeks. Zidovudine or lamivudine alone was later started in 5 patients without further haematological problems.[29] Similar precipitous falls in haemoglobin occurred in another 2 patients when lamivudine 300 mg daily was added to their long-term zidovudine treatment. Again both recovered when the drugs were stopped and blood was given.[30] Anaemia is a common adverse effect of zidovudine, but these patients had no problems until the lamivudine was added. The available evidence indicates that concurrent use can be safe and effective, with the adverse interactions cited here being uncommon. It has been suggested that a complete baseline blood count should be done, both when combined treatment is started, and every month for the first 3 months of treatment.[30] In UK and US guidelines, the combination of zidovudine with lamivudine is currently a preferred dual NRTI option for use with an NNRTI or a protease inhibitor for the treatment of HIV-infection in treatment naïve patients.[2,3] The triple NRTI combination of abacavir, lamivudine and zidovudine may also be considered if protease inhibitors or NNRTIs cannot be used.[3]

E. Stavudine

(a) Zalcitabine

In vitro, stavudine had no significant effect on the intracellular activation of zalcitabine.[13] Both stavudine and zalcitabine have the potential to cause peripheral neuropathy and pancreatitis. Combined use of drugs causing these serious adverse effects should be closely monitored (see also 'NRTIs + Drugs that cause pancreatitis', p.797). US guidelines say that the combination of stavudine and zalcitabine should not be recommended at any time because of additive peripheral neuropathy.[3]

(b) Zidovudine

Nucleoside reverse transcriptase inhibitors such as stavudine need to be phosphorylated within cells to a triphosphate anabolite before they become effective. *In vitro* studies using mononucleated blood cells found that zidovudine significantly inhibited this phosphorylation.[7] Antagonism between zidovudine and stavudine has also been seen in a clinical study.[31] The manufacturers[23,24] and US guidelines[3] currently do not recommend the combination.

F. Zalcitabine

In vitro, zalcitabine had no significant effect on the intracellular activation of **zidovudine**.[13] In a study in 56 patients with advanced HIV infection, taking zidovudine 50 to 200 mg every 8 hours and zalcitabine 5 to 10 micrograms/kg every 8 hours, neither drug affected the pharmacokinetics of the other nor was toxicity increased.[32] No special precautions would appear to be necessary. Nevertheless, current US guidelines state that the combination of zalcitabine and zidovudine is not recommended as a dual NRTI combination for use in initial antiretroviral regimens because of inferior virological activity and a higher rate of adverse effects than other dual NRTI alternatives.[3]

1. Wang LH, Chittick GE, McDowell JA. Single-dose pharmacokinetics and safety of abacavir (1592U89), zidovudine, and lamivudine administered alone and in combination in adults with human immunodeficiency virus infection. *Antimicrob Agents Chemother* (1999) 43, 1708–15.
2. Gazzard B, Bernard EJ, Boffito M, Churchill D, Edwards S, Fisher M, Geretti AM, Johnson M, Leen C, Peters B, Pozniak A, Ross J, Walsh J, Wilkins E, Youle M; BHIVA Writing Committee. British HIV Association (BHIVA) guidelines for the treatment of HIV-infected adults with antiretroviral therapy (2006). *HIV Med* (2006) 7, 487–503. Available at: http://www.bhiva.org/files/file1001303.pdf (accessed 21/08/07).
3. US Department of Health and Human Services; Panel on Antiretroviral Guidelines for Adults and Adolescents. Guidelines for the use of antiretroviral agents in HIV-1-infected adults and adolescents. October 10, 2006; 1–113. Available at: http://aidsinfo.nih.gov/contentfiles/AdultandAdolescentGL.pdf (accessed 21/08/07).
4. McDowell JA, Lou Y, Symonds WS, Stein DS. Multiple-dose pharmacokinetics and pharmacodynamics of abacavir alone and in combination with zidovudine in human immunodeficiency virus-infected adults. *Antimicrob Agents Chemother* (2000) 44, 2061–7.
5. Epivir (Lamivudine). GlaxoSmithKline UK. UK Summary of product characteristics, March 2007.
6. Kewn S, Veal GJ, Hoggard PG, Barry MG, Back DJ. Lamivudine (3TC). Phosphorylation and drug interactions *in vitro*. *Biochem Pharmacol* (1997) 54, 589–95.
7. Hoggard PG, Kewn S, Barry MG, Khoo SH, Back DJ. Effects of drugs on 2',3'-dideoxy-2',3'-didehydrothymidine phosphorylation in vitro. *Antimicrob Agents Chemother* (1997) 41, 1231–6.
8. Seifert RD, Stewart MB, Sramek JJ, Conrad J, Kaul S, Cutler NR. Pharmacokinetics of co-administered didanosine and stavudine in HIV-seropositive male patients. *Br J Clin Pharmacol* (1994) 38, 405–10.
9. Kalathoor S, Sinclair J, Andron L, Sension MG, High K. Combination therapy with stavudine and didanosine. 4th Conference on Retroviruses and Opportunistic Infections, Washington DC, Jan 22-26 1997. Abstract 552.
10. Moore RD, Wong W-ME, Keruly JC, McArthur JC. Incidence of neuropathy in HIV-infected patients on monotherapy versus those on combination therapy with didanosine, stavudine, and hydroxyurea. *AIDS* (2000) 14, 273–8.
11. Anon. ddI, d4T, hydroxyurea: new pancreatitis warning. *AIDS Treat News* (1999) Nov 19 (No. 331), 1–3.
12. Antoniou T, Weisdorf T, Gough K. Symptomatic hyperlactatemia in an HIV-positive patient: a case report and discussion. *Can Med Assoc J* (2003) 168, 195–8.
13. Hivid (Zalcitabine). Roche Products Ltd. UK Summary of product characteristics, November 2004.
14. LeLacheur SF, Simon GL. Exacerbation of dideoxycytidine-induced neuropathy with dideoxyinosine. *J Acquir Immune Defic Syndr* (1991) 4, 538–9.
15. Barry M, Howe JL, Ormesher S, Back DJ, Breckenridge AM, Bergin C, Mulcahy F, Beeching N, Nye F. Pharmacokinetics of zidovudine and dideoxyinosine alone and in combination in patients with acquired immunodeficiency syndrome. *Br J Clin Pharmacol* (1994) 37, 421–6.
16. Burger DM, Meenhorst PL, Kroon FP, Mulder JW, Koks CHW, Bult A, Beijnen JH. Pharmacokinetic interaction study of zidovudine and didanosine. *J Drug Dev* (1994) 6, 187–94.
17. Mueller BU, Pizzo PA, Farley M, Husson RN, Goldsmith J, Kovacs A, Woods L, Ono J, Church JA, Brouwers P, Jarosinski P, Venzon D, Balis FM. Pharmacokinetic evaluation of the combination of zidovudine and didanosine in children with human immunodeficiency virus infection. *J Pediatr* (1994) 125, 142–6.
18. Collier AC, Coombs RW, Fischl MA, Skolnik PR, Northfelt D, Boutin P, Hooper CJ, Kaplan LD, Volberding PA, Davis LG, Henrard DR, Weller S, Corey L. Combination therapy with zidovudine and didanosine compared with zidovudine alone in HIV-1 infection. *Ann Intern Med* (1993) 119, 786–93.
19. Sahai J, Gallicano K, Seguin I, Garber G, Cameron W. Interaction between zidovudine (ZDV) and didanosine (ddI). *Intersci Conf Antimicrob Agents Chemother* (1994) 34, 82.
20. Sahai J, Gallicano K, Garber G, Pakuts A, Cameron W. Pharmacokinetics of simultaneously administered zidovudine and didanosine in HIV-seropositive male patients. *J Acquir Immune Defic Syndr Hum Retrovirol* (1995) 10, 54–60.
21. Gibb D, Barry M, Ormesher S, Nokes L, Seefried M, Giaquinto C, Back D. Pharmacokinetics of zidovudine and dideoxyinosine alone and combination in children with HIV infection. *Br J Clin Pharmacol* (1995) 39, 527–30.
22. Wang LH, Blum MR, Hui J, Hulett L, Chittick GE, Rousseau F. Lack of significant pharmacokinetic interactions between emtricitabine and other nucleoside antivirals in healthy volunteers. *Intersci Conf Antimicrob Agents Chemother* (2001) 41, 18.
23. Zerit (Stavudine). Bristol-Myers Squibb Pharmaceuticals Ltd. UK Summary of product characteristics, January 2007.
24. Zerit (Stavudine). Bristol-Myers Squibb Company. US Prescribing information, August 2006.
25. Hivid (Zalcitabine). Roche Pharmaceuticals. US Prescribing information, September 2002.
26. Epivir (Lamivudine). GlaxoSmithKline. US Prescribing information, October 2006.
27. Rana KZ, Horton CM, Yuen GJ, Pivarnik PE, Mikolich DM, Fisher AE, Mydlow PK, Dudley MN. Effect of lamivudine on zidovudine pharmacokinetics in asymptomatic HIV-infected individuals. *Intersci Conf Antimicrob Agents Chemother* (1994) 34, 83.
28. Staszewski S, Loveday C, Picazo JJ, Dellamonica P, Skinhøj P, Johnson MA, Danner SA, Harrigan PR, Hill AM, Verity L, McDade H; for the Lamivudine European HIV Working Group. Safety and efficacy of lamivudine-zidovudine combination therapy in zidovudine-experienced patients. A randomized controlled comparison with zidovudine monotherapy. *JAMA* (1996) 276, 111–17.
29. Tseng A, Fletcher D, Gold W, Conly J, Keystone D, Walmsley S. Precipitous declines in hemoglobin with combination AZT/3TC. 4th Conference on Retroviruses and Opportunistic Infections, Washington, Jan 22-26, 1997. Abstract 559.
30. Hester EK, Peacock JE. Profound and unanticipated anemia with lamivudine-zidovudine combination therapy in zidovudine-experienced patients with HIV infection. *AIDS* (1998) 12, 439–51.
31. Havlir DV, Tierney C, Friedland GH, Pollard RB, Smeaton L, Sommadossi JP, Fox L, Kessler H, Fife KH, Richman DD. In vivo antagonism with zidovudine plus stavudine combination therapy. *J Infect Dis* (2000) 182, 321–5.
32. Meng T-C, Fischl MA, Boota AM, Spector SA, Bennett D, Bassiakos Y, Lai S, Wright B, Richman DD. Combination therapy with zidovudine and dideoxycytidine in patients with advanced human immunodeficiency virus infection. *Ann Intern Med* (1992) 116, 13–20.

NRTIs + Paracetamol (Acetaminophen)

Limited and unconfirmed evidence suggests that paracetamol possibly increases the bone marrow suppressant effects of zidovudine. Single case reports describe severe liver toxicity when patients were given paracetamol with either zidovudine or didanosine.

Clinical evidence

(a) Didanosine

Increasing abdominal pain occurred in a 47-year-old HIV-positive man one month after he started didanosine (his other medications included nevirapine, hydroxycarbamide, aciclovir and lorazepam). He had been treating the pain with paracetamol, and had taken 4 g over 3 days. Severe hepatitis and pancreatitis was diagnosed, which slowly resolved over the following 3 weeks.[1]

(b) Zidovudine

An early study of zidovudine use in 282 AIDS patients found that haematological abnormalities (anaemia, leucopenia, neutropenia) were very common and 21% needed multiple red cell transfusions. Some of the patients also received paracetamol, which increased the haematological toxicity (neutropenia) by an unstated amount.[2]

Short-term clinical studies using paracetamol 650 mg up to every 4 hours found that it had no clinically significant effects on the pharmacokinetics of zidovudine,[3-6] although in one case clearance was slightly increased.[7] An 8-month study in a single patient suggested that long-term concurrent use did not affect the pharmacokinetics of either drug. However, in this individual very rapid absorption and a high peak serum level of zidovudine were seen, so for safety the zidovudine dosage was reduced from 200 mg every 4 hours to 100 mg every 6 hours.[8]

A patient taking zidovudine and co-trimoxazole took 3.3 g of paracetamol over 36 hours. Within 2 days he developed severe hepatotoxicity, and as other causes were excluded, the reaction was attributed to the paracetamol. The authors suggested that zidovudine may have augmented the paracetamol toxicity.[9] However, in a single-dose study, reduced paracetamol glucuronidation and increased formation of hepatotoxic metabolites was seen in patients with advanced HIV infection compared with healthy HIV-positive subjects and those without HIV, and this effect was independent of zidovudine use.[10] In contrast, in another study, disease state (AIDS versus healthy HIV-positive subjects) was not found to alter paracetamol metabolism, and zidovudine was found to *increase* paracetamol glucuronidation in some patients.[11]

Mechanism

Not understood. Paracetamol does not increase the serum levels of zidovudine,[3-5,7] which might have provided an explanation for the apparent increased toxicity. One *in vitro* study found that paracetamol does not affect the glucuronidation of zidovudine,[12] whereas another found that paracetamol did inhibit zidovudine metabolism to the glucuronide.[13] The effect of zidovudine on paracetamol metabolism is also unclear.

Didanosine may cause pancreatitis or hepatic disease, and zidovudine may also rarely cause hepatic disease. It has been suggested that the hepatotoxicity of didanosine and paracetamol are augmented when they are given together.[1]

Importance and management

The authors suggest extreme caution when potentially hepatotoxic drugs such as paracetamol are used with didanosine.[1] Note that paracetamol is a widely used non-prescription analgesic, and this appears to be an isolated report of potential combined toxicity with didanosine. Further study is needed to assess any association of combined use of these drugs with hepatotoxicity.

The short-term use of zidovudine and paracetamol does not appear to alter the pharmacokinetics of either drug. Whether paracetamol can increase the haematological toxicity of zidovudine and whether the drugs have combined hepatotoxicity is unclear from the available data. More study is needed.

1. Lederman JC, Nawaz H. Toxic interaction of didanosine and acetaminophen leading to severe hepatitis and pancreatitis: a case report and review of the literature. *Am J Gastroenterol* (2001) 96, 3474–5.
2. Richman DD, Fischl MA, Grieco MH, Gottlieb MS, Volberding PA, Laskin OL, Leedom JM, Groopman JE, Mildvan D, Hirsch MS, Jackson GG, Durack DT, Nusinoff-Lehrman S and the AZT Collaborative Working Group. The toxicity of azidothymidine (AZT) in the treatment of patients with AIDS and AIDS-related complex. A double-blind, placebo-controlled trial. *N Engl J Med* (1987) 317, 192–7.
3. Steffe EM, King JH, Inciardi JF, Flynn NF, Goldstein E, Tonjes TS, Benet LZ. The effect of acetaminophen on zidovudine metabolism in HIV-infected patients. *J Acquir Immune Defic Syndr* (1990) 3, 691–4.
4. Ptachcinski J, Pazin G, Ho M. The effect of acetaminophen on the pharmacokinetics of zidovudine. *Pharmacotherapy* (1989) 9, 190.
5. Pazin GJ, Ptachcinski RJ, Sheehan M, Ho M. Interactive pharmacokinetics of zidovudine and acetaminophen. 5th International Conference on AIDS, Montreal, 1989. Abstract M.B.P.338.
6. Burger DM, Meenhorst PL, Underberg WJM, van der Heijde JF, Koks CHW, Beijnen JH. Short-term, combined use of paracetamol and zidovudine does not alter the pharmacokinetics of either drug. *Neth J Med* (1994) 44, 161–5.
7. Sattler FR, Ko R, Antoniskis D, Shields M, Cohen J, Nicoloff J, Leedom J, Koda R. Acetaminophen does not impair clearance of zidovudine. *Ann Intern Med* (1991) 114, 937–40.
8. Burger DM, Meenhorst PL, Koks CHW, Beijnen JH. Pharmacokinetics of zidovudine and acetaminophen in a patient on chronic acetaminophen therapy. *Ann Pharmacother* (1994) 28, 327–30.
9. Shriner K, Goetz MB. Severe hepatotoxicity in a patient receiving both acetaminophen and zidovudine. *Am J Med* (1992) 93, 94–6.
10. Esteban A, Pérez-Mateo M, Boix V, González M, Portilla J, Mora A. Abnormalities in the metabolism of acetaminophen in patients infected with the human immunodeficiency virus (HIV). *Methods Find Exp Clin Pharmacol* (1997) 19, 129–32.
11. O'Neil WM, Pezzullo JC, Di Girolamo A, Tsoukas CM, Wainer IW. Glucuronidation and sulphation of paracetamol in HIV-positive patients and patients with AIDS. *Br J Clin Pharmacol* (1999) 48, 811–18.
12. Kamali F, Rawlins MD. Influence of probenecid and paracetamol (acetaminophen) on zidovudine glucuronidation in human liver *in vitro*. *Biopharm Drug Dispos* (1992) 13, 403–9.
13. Schumann L, Unadkat JD. Does acetaminophen potentiate the hematotoxicity of zidovudine (ZDV or AZT) by inhibition of its metabolism to the glucuronide? *Pharm Res* (1988) 5 (Suppl), S-177.

NRTIs + Probenecid

Probenecid reduces the loss of zalcitabine and zidovudine, increasing their serum levels. The combination of zalcitabine and probenecid is well tolerated, but the incidence of adverse effects appears to be greatly increased with the combination of probenecid and zidovudine.

Clinical evidence

(a) Zalcitabine

In a single-dose study, 12 HIV-positive or AIDS patients were given zalcitabine 1.5 mg alone or with probenecid 500 mg, given 8 and 2 hours before then 4 hours after. The renal clearance of the zalcitabine was decreased 42% by probenecid, its half-life was increased by 47% and its AUC was increased by 54%.[1]

(b) Zidovudine

In 12 patients with AIDS or AIDS-related complex the concurrent use of zidovudine and probenecid 500 mg every 8 hours for 3 days increased the AUC of zidovudine by an average of 80% (range 14 to 192%).[2]

Other studies in patients[3-5] and healthy subjects[6] found that probenecid roughly doubled the AUC of zidovudine when given in a variety of dosing schedules.[3,4] However, the effects on zidovudine pharmacokinetics were minimal if the two drugs were given 6 hours apart.[5] Another report describes a very high incidence of rashes in 6 out of 8 HIV-positive men given zidovudine with probenecid 500 mg every 6 hours. The rash and other symptoms (such as malaise, fever and myalgia) were sufficiently severe for the probenecid to be withdrawn in 4 of them.[7] A later study found that when using only 250 mg of probenecid every 8 hours the AUC of zidovudine was increased by 70% but the adverse effects still occurred, although the incidence was possibly somewhat lower.[8] Conversely, others reported the successful use of probenecid 500 mg three times daily with a reduced dose of zidovudine (600 mg daily) in 7 patients without any occurrence of rash.[9]

Mechanism

Experimental clinical evidence indicates that probenecid reduces metabolism (glucuronidation) of zidovudine by the liver enzymes, and inhibits renal secretion of the zidovudine glucuronide metabolite.[2-4,6,10,11] The interaction with zalcitabine is presumably due to inhibition of zalcitabine secretion in the renal tubules.[1]

Importance and management

The concurrent use of zidovudine and probenecid should be well monitored to ensure that zidovudine levels do not rise excessively. Reduce the zidovudine dosage as necessary. However, the apparent increase in adverse effects during concurrent use seen by one group of researchers[7,8] should be borne in mind.

The concurrent use of zalcitabine and probenecid was well tolerated, and because the zalcitabine half-life is short compared to its dosing schedule significant accumulation would not be expected.

It would seem prudent to monitor for any signs of toxicity if either drug combination is used long-term. The safety of combined use needs further assessment.

1. Massarella JW, Nazareno LA, Passe S, Min B. The effect of probenecid on the pharmacokinetics of zalcitabine in HIV-positive patients. *Pharm Res* (1996) 13, 449–52.
2. Kornhauser DM, Petty BG, Hendrix CW, Woods AS, Nerhood LJ, Bartlett JG, Lietman PS. Probenecid and zidovudine metabolism. *Lancet* (1989) 2, 473–5.
3. Hedaya MA, Elmquist WF, Sawchuk RJ. Probenecid inhibits the metabolic and renal clearances of zidovudine (AZT) in human volunteers. *Pharm Res* (1990) 7, 411–17.
4. de Miranda P, Good SS, Yarchoan R, Thomas RV, Blum MR, Myers CE, Broder S. Alteration of zidovudine pharmacokinetics by probenecid in patients with AIDS or AIDS-related complex. *Clin Pharmacol Ther* (1989) 46, 494–500.

5. McDermott J, Kennedy J, Ellis-Pegler RB, Thomas MG. Pharmacokinetics of zidovudine plus probenecid. *J Infect Dis* (1992) 166, 687–8.
6. Campion JJ, Bawdon RE, Baskin LB, Barton CI. Effect of probenecid on the pharmacokinetics of zidovudine and zidovudine glucuronide. *Pharmacotherapy* (1990) 10, 235.
7. Petty BG, Kornhauser DM, Lietman PS. Zidovudine with probenecid: a warning. *Lancet* (1990) 1, 1044–5.
8. Petty BG, Barditch-Crovo PA, Nerhood L, Kornhauser DM, Kuwahara S, Lietman PS. Unexpected clinical toxicity of probenecid (P) with zidovudine (Z) in patients with HIV infection. *Intersci Conf Antimicrob Agents Chemother* (1991) 31, 323.
9. Duckworth AS, Duckworth GW, Henderson G, Contreras G. Zidovudine with probenecid. *Lancet* (1990) 336, 441.
10. Sim SM, Back DJ, Breckenridge AM. The effect of various drugs on the glucuronidation of zidovudine (azidothymidine; AZT) by human liver microsomes. *Br J Clin Pharmacol* (1991) 32, 17–21.
11. Kamali F, Rawlins MD. Influence of probenecid and paracetamol (acetaminophen) on zidovudine glucuronidation in human liver *in vitro*. *Biopharm Drug Dispos* (1992) 13, 403–9.

NRTIs + Protease inhibitors

Buffered didanosine decreases the AUC of indinavir, and the drugs should be given one hour apart. Buffered didanosine interacts similarly with atazanavir. Tipranavir with low-dose ritonavir modestly reduced the AUC of abacavir and zidovudine, and such combinations are not recommended in the UK. The changes in pharmacokinetics seen when giving other combinations of protease inhibitors with NRTIs do not appear to be clinically significant. Protease inhibitors do not affect the intracellular activation of NRTIs.

Clinical evidence, mechanism, importance and management

The protease inhibitors **indinavir**, **ritonavir**, and **saquinavir** had no effect on intracellular activation of various NRTIs (**didanosine**, **lamivudine**, **stavudine**, **zalcitabine** and **zidovudine**).[1] No interaction would be expected by this mechanism. Other potential interactions are discussed below.

(a) Abacavir

1. Amprenavir. A phase I study in HIV-positive patients given amprenavir 900 mg twice daily with abacavir 300 mg twice daily for 3 weeks found that neither drug had any clinically significant effect on the pharmacokinetics of the other.[2] The manufacturer of amprenavir notes that its AUC, and minimum and maximum levels were increased by 29%, 27%, and 47%, respectively, by abacavir,[3,4] without any change in abacavir pharmacokinetics, but no dosage adjustments are considered necessary.[3]

2. Lopinavir/Ritonavir. The manufacturer of lopinavir/ritonavir notes that it induces glucuronidation and therefore has the potential to reduce abacavir plasma levels. However this, and its clinical relevance, have yet to be studied.[5,6]

3. Tipranavir with Ritonavir. Tipranavir given with low-dose ritonavir decreased the AUC of abacavir by approximately 40%. The clinical relevance of this reduction has not been established,[7,8] but it may decrease the efficacy of abacavir.[7] Therefore the UK manufacturer states that the concurrent use of tipranavir and low-dose ritonavir with abacavir is not recommended unless there are no other available NRTIs suitable for patient management.[7]

(b) Didanosine

1. Amprenavir. The AUC and the minimum level of amprenavir 600 mg twice daily were not altered to a clinically relevant extent when it was given simultaneously with, or one hour before, buffered didanosine; or simultaneously with the enteric-coated preparation of didanosine. The only notable change was a 15% decrease in the maximum levels of amprenavir when it was given with buffered didanosine, which was not considered clinically significant.[9] Nevertheless, the manufacturers of amprenavir suggest that it should be given at least one hour apart from didanosine,[3,4] and this has also be recommended for regimens containing amprenavir and ritonavir.[9]

2. Atazanavir. The manufacturer of atazanavir found that buffered didanosine markedly decreased atazanavir plasma levels, with little change in didanosine levels,[10] and they recommend that administration should be separated.[10,11] Conversely, although enteric-coated didanosine did not alter atazanavir levels, simultaneous administration with food reduced didanosine levels, and therefore administration should be separated.[10] Note that 'didanosine', (p.797), is preferably taken on an empty stomach, whereas 'atazanavir', (p.818), should be taken with food.

3. Indinavir. The concurrent use of [buffered] didanosine and indinavir reduced the AUC of indinavir by 80%, but when indinavir was given one hour before didanosine its pharmacokinetics were not significantly affected.[12] Similarly, another study found that the pharmacokinetics of indinavir 800 mg were unchanged when it was given one hour after buffered didanosine 400 mg.[13] An enteric-coated preparation of didanosine had no effect on the pharmacokinetics of indinavir in a single-dose study in 23 healthy subjects.[14] Indinavir may require a normal acidic gastric pH for optimal absorption, whereas some didanosine preparations are formulated with buffering agents to raise gastric pH. Any increase in pH would therefore be expected to reduce indinavir absorption.[15] The manufacturers of indinavir recommend that indinavir and didanosine should be given at least one hour apart.[15,16] This recommendation would not apply to the enteric-coated preparation of didanosine.[14] Note that both 'didanosine', (p.797), and 'indinavir', (p.818), are preferably taken on an empty stomach.

4. Nelfinavir. The pharmacokinetics of nelfinavir were not significantly altered after concurrent use with didanosine.[17] Note that 'nelfinavir', (p.818), should preferably be taken with food, and all 'didanosine preparations', (p.797), without food.

5. Ritonavir. Buffered didanosine 200 mg twice daily was given with ritonavir 600 mg twice daily to 13 HIV-positive subjects. Administration of the two drugs was separated by 2.5 hours, and treatment was given for 4 days. Treatment was staggered in this way since 'ritonavir', (p.818), should be given with food, and 'didanosine', (p.797) without food. There was little or no change in the pharmacokinetics of ritonavir, and the maximum serum levels and AUC of didanosine were reduced by 16% and 13%, respectively, which was not considered to be clinically significant. It was suggested that these changes may have been due to altered absorption in the presence of ritonavir.[18]

6. Saquinavir. In 8 healthy subjects a single 400-mg dose of didanosine decreased the AUC and maximum plasma concentration of saquinavir (as saquinavir/ritonavir 1600/100 mg soft capsules) by approximately 30% and 25%, respectively, but did not significantly affect the minimum plasma concentration of saquinavir. The manufacturer considers these changes are of doubtful clinical significance.[19] Note also that 'saquinavir', (p.818), should preferably be taken with food, and all 'didanosine preparations', (p.797) without.

7. Tipranavir with Ritonavir. Tipranavir plus low-dose ritonavir caused a 33% reduction in the AUC of didanosine in one of 3 studies,[8] but the clinical relevance of this has not been established.[7,8] Consequently, the manufacturer recommends that dosing of enteric-coated didanosine and tipranavir plus low-dose ritonavir should be separated by at least 2 hours to avoid formulation incompatibility.[7,8]

(c) Lamivudine

Lamivudine metabolism does not involve the cytochrome P450 isoenzyme CYP3A4. Therefore it is unlikely that it will interact with drugs, such as the protease inhibitors, which are metabolised by this system.[20] No pharmacokinetic interaction appears to occur between lamivudine and **amprenavir**,[3,4] **atazanavir**,[10,11] **indinavir**,[16] and **nelfinavir**.[21,22] The manufacturer of **lopinavir/ritonavir** notes that lamivudine did not alter the pharmacokinetics of **lopinavir**,[5,6] and **tipranavir** plus low-dose **ritonavir** did not cause a significant change in the AUC of lamivudine.[7,8]

(d) Stavudine

The manufacturer of **atazanavir**[10,11] notes that there was no pharmacokinetic interaction with stavudine.

The AUC of stavudine was increased by 25% when stavudine 40 mg twice daily was given with **indinavir** 800 mg every 8 hours for a week, which was not considered to be clinically significant. The serum levels of **indinavir** were unchanged.[23] Similarly, **indinavir/ritonavir** 800 mg/200 mg twice daily increased the AUC of stavudine by 24% in a study in 24 healthy subjects, but this change was not considered clinically relevant and does not require dosage modification.[24]

The manufacturer of **lopinavir/ritonavir** notes that stavudine did not alter the pharmacokinetics of **lopinavir**.[5,6]

In an early pilot study, combined **nelfinavir** and stavudine was well tolerated, and the adverse effects were similar to those seen when stavudine was given alone, although the incidence of diarrhoea did increase.[25] The manufacturer of **nelfinavir** notes that no clinically significant interactions have been observed with stavudine.[21,22]

In a study in HIV-positive children, **ritonavir** oral clearance was about 50% slower and the AUC about 2.5-fold higher in 6 children who received stavudine than in 7 who received zidovudine and lamivudine, although these differences did not reach statistical significance.[26]

Tipranavir plus low-dose **ritonavir** did not cause a significant change in the AUC of stavudine.[7,8]

(e) Zalcitabine

The manufacturer of zalcitabine noted that there is no pharmacokinetic interaction with **saquinavir**.[27,28] They stated that pharmacokinetic interactions with protease inhibitors would not be expected, since zalcitabine is mainly excreted unchanged in the urine.[27]

(f) Zidovudine

1. Amprenavir. The AUC and maximum levels of zidovudine were increased by 31% and 40%, respectively, when given with amprenavir. The pharmacokinetics of amprenavir were unchanged.[3,4] The UK manufacturer of amprenavir states that no dose adjustment of either drug is necessary when amprenavir and zidovudine are used together.[3]

2. Atazanavir. The manufacturer of atazanavir[10,11] notes that there was no clinically relevant pharmacokinetic interaction with zidovudine.

3. Indinavir. A study found that when zidovudine 200 mg every 8 hours and indinavir 1 g every 8 hours were given together for a week the AUC of zidovudine was increased by 17% and the AUC of indinavir was increased by 13%.[23] In another study, combined use of indinavir and zidovudine with lamivudine increased the zidovudine AUC by 39% but did not change indinavir pharmacokinetics.[16] These changes are not clinically relevant.

4. Lopinavir/Ritonavir. The manufacturer of lopinavir/ritonavir notes that it induces glucuronidation and therefore has the potential to reduce zidovudine levels. However this, and its clinical relevance, have yet to be studied.[5,6]

5. Nelfinavir. The manufacturer of nelfinavir notes that clinically significant interactions have not been observed with zidovudine, and no dose adjustments are needed.[21,22]

6. Ritonavir. A crossover study in 18 HIV-positive subjects found that the pharmacokinetics of ritonavir 300 mg every 6 hours were unchanged by zidovudine 200 mg every 8 hours. However, the maximum plasma levels and AUC of the zidovudine were both reduced by about 25%. The lack of change in the other pharmacokinetic parameters suggested that these changes were not due to altered metabolism.[29] Nevertheless, dose alternations are not considered necessary.[30]

7. Saquinavir. The UK manufacturer of saquinavir notes that there was no pharmacokinetic interaction with zidovudine.[19]

8. Tipranavir with Ritonavir. Tipranavir plus low-dose ritonavir decreased the AUC of zidovudine by approximately 35%, without affecting glucuronidated-zidovudine levels. The clinical relevance of this reduction has not been established,[7,8] but it may decrease the efficacy of zidovudine.[7] Therefore the UK manufacturer states that concurrent use of tipranavir plus low-dose ritonavir with zidovudine is not recommended unless there are no other available NRTIs suitable for patient management.[7]

1. Hoggard PG, Manion V, Barry MG, Back DJ. Effect of protease inhibitors on nucleoside analogue phosphorylation *in vitro*. *Br J Clin Pharmacol* (1998) 45, 164–7.
2. McDowell J, Sadler BM, Millard J, Nunnally P, Mustafa N. Evaluation of potential pharmacokinetic (PK) drug interaction between 141W94 and 1592U89 in HIV+ patients. *Intersci Conf Antimicrob Agents Chemother* (1997) 37, 13.
3. Agenerase (Amprenavir). GlaxoSmithKline UK. UK Summary of product characteristics, February 2007.
4. Agenerase (Amprenavir). GlaxoSmithKline. US Prescribing information, May 2005.
5. Kaletra Tablets (Lopinavir/ritonavir). Abbott Laboratories Ltd. UK Summary of product characteristics, March 2007.
6. Kaletra (Lopinavir/ritonavir). Abbott Laboratories. US Prescribing information, January 2007.
7. Aptivus (Tipranavir). Boehringer Ingelheim Ltd. UK Summary of product characteristics, March 2007.
8. Aptivus (Tipranavir). Boehringer Ingelheim. US Prescribing information, February 2007.
9. Shelton MJ, Giovanniello AA, Cloen D, Berenson CS, Keil K, DiFrancesco R, Hewitt RG. Effects of didanosine formulations on the pharmacokinetics of amprenavir. *Pharmacotherapy* (2003) 23, 835–42.
10. Reyataz (Atazanavir sulfate). Bristol-Myers Squibb Company. US Prescribing information, March 2007.
11. Reyataz (Atazanavir sulfate). Bristol-Myers Squibb Pharmaceuticals Ltd. UK Summary of product characteristics, April 2007.
12. Mummaneni V, Kaul S, Knupp CA. Single oral dose pharmacokinetic interaction study of didanosine and indinavir sulfate in healthy subjects (abstract 34). *J Clin Pharmacol* (1997) 37, 865.
13. Shelton MJ, Mei H, Hewitt RG, Defrancesco R. If taken 1 hour before indinavir (IDV), didanosine does not affect IDV exposure, despite persistent buffering effects. *Antimicrob Agents Chemother* (2001) 45, 298–300.
14. Damle BD, Mummaneni V, Kaul S, Knupp C. Lack of effect of simultaneously administered didanosine encapsulated enteric bead formulation (Videx EC) on oral absorption of indinavir, ketoconazole, or ciprofloxacin. *Antimicrob Agents Chemother* (2002) 46, 385–91.
15. Crixivan (Indinavir sulfate). Merck Sharp & Dohme Ltd. UK Summary of product characteristics, May 2007.
16. Crixivan (Indinavir sulfate). Merck & Co., Inc. US Prescribing information, November 2006.
17. Pedneault L, Elion R, Adler M, Anderson R, Kelleher T, Knupp C, Kaul S, Kerr B, Cross A, Dunkle L. Stavudine (d4T), didanosine (ddI), and nelfinavir combination therapy in HIV-infected subjects: antiviral effect and safety in an ongoing pilot study. 4th Conference on Retroviruses and Opportunistic Infections, Washington, 1997. Abstract 241.
18. Cato A, Qian J, Hsu A, Vomvouras S, Piergies AA, Leonard J, Granneman R. Pharmacokinetic interaction between ritonavir and didanosine when administered concurrently to HIV-infected patients. *J Acquir Immune Defic Syndr Hum Retrovirol* (1998) 18, 466–72.
19. Invirase Hard Capsules (Saquinavir mesilate). Roche Products Ltd. UK Summary of product characteristics, May 2007.
20. Epivir (Lamivudine). GlaxoSmithKline UK. UK Summary of product characteristics, March 2007.
21. Viracept (Nelfinavir mesilate). Roche Products Ltd. UK Summary of product characteristics, January 2007.
22. Viracept (Nelfinavir mesylate). Agouron Pharmaceuticals, Inc. US Prescribing information, January 2007.
23. The Indinavir (MK 639) Pharmacokinetic Study Group. Indinavir (MK 639) drug interaction studies. 11th International Conference on AIDS, Vancouver, 1996. Abstract Mo.B.174.
24. Kaul S, Agarwala S, Hess H, Nepal S, Gale J, O'Mara E, Stevens M. The effect of coadministration of indinavir (IDV) and ritonavir (RTV) on the pharmacokinetics of stavudine (d4T). *Intersci Conf Antimicrob Agents Chemother* (2002) 42, 26.
25. Gathe J, Burkhardt B, Hawley P, Conant M, Peterkin J, Chapman S. A randomized phase II study of Viracept™, a novel HIV protease inhibitor, used in combination with stavudine (D4T) vs. stavudine (D4T) alone. 11th International Conference on AIDS, Vancouver, 1996. Abstract Mo.B.413.
26. Fletcher CV, Yogev R, Nachman SA, Wiznia A, Pelton S, McIntosh K, Stanley K. Pharmacokinetic characteristics of ritonavir, zidovudine, lamivudine, and stavudine in children with human immunodeficiency virus infection. *Pharmacotherapy* (2004) 24, 453–9.
27. Hivid (Zalcitabine). Roche Products Ltd. UK Summary of product characteristics, November 2004.
28. Hivid (Zalcitabine). Roche Pharmaceuticals. US Prescribing information, September 2002.
29. Cato A, Qian J, Hsu A, Levy B, Leonard J, Granneman R. Multidose pharmacokinetics of ritonavir and zidovudine in human immunodeficiency virus-infected patients. *Antimicrob Agents Chemother* (1998) 42, 1788–93.
30. Norvir (Ritonavir). Abbott Laboratories Ltd. UK Summary of product characteristics, May 2007.

NRTIs + Ribavirin

The use of ribavirin with the NRTIs may result in increased toxicity (lactic acidosis, blood dyscrasias and hepatotoxicity), which may be more frequent with didanosine than other NRTIs. These effects may also be exacerbated by the additional use of interferon for hepatitis C. Early *in vitro* data suggested that ribavirin may reduce the antiretroviral effects of some NRTIs but this does not appear to have been demonstrated in practice.

Clinical evidence, mechanism, importance and management

In the UK, the manufacturers of **all NRTIs** state that patients co-infected with hepatitis C and treated with interferon alfa and ribavirin may be at increased risk of lactic acidosis. Patients at increased risk should be monitored closely.

(a) Didanosine

Ribavirin did not alter the pharmacokinetics of didanosine in HIV-positive adults or children.[1,2] However, *in vitro*, ribavirin increases the intracellular activation of didanosine, and the manufacturers note that this could result in increased adverse effects.[3-5] In one early study, no increase in adverse effects was seen when ribavirin 600 mg daily was given to 16 HIV-positive patients who had already been taking didanosine 125 to 200 mg twice daily for 4 weeks. Ribavirin was given 6 hours after the morning dose of didanosine. Over the 8 or 20 weeks of the study the combination was well tolerated.[1] Nevertheless, cases of mitochondrial toxicity (hepatotoxicity, pancreatitis, lactic acidaemia) have been reported when ribavirin was added to didanosine-containing antiretroviral regimens,[6-8] and fatalities have occurred.[6,9] In an analysis of data from the adverse event reporting system of the FDA in the US, 31 patients were identified who had adverse events suggestive of mitochondrial toxicity while taking ribavirin with an NRTI. Of these, nearly 90% had received didanosine, 71% stavudine, and 65% both didanosine and stavudine. Five patients died; all of who were taking didanosine, with stavudine in three of these cases. Use of ribavirin with didanosine was associated with an increased risk of mitochondrial toxicity (odds ratio 12.4) compared with patients receiving ribavirin in combination with other NRTIs (odds ratios: didanosine with stavudine, 8; stavudine, 3.3; abacavir, 1.1; lamivudine, 0.2; zidovudine, 0.06).[9] Some other studies have shown an increased risk of mitochondrial toxicity when ribavirin was given with didanosine.[10,11] As a result of these data, the manufacturers of ribavirin[4,12-14] and the US manufacturer of didanosine[5] say that concurrent use of ribavirin and didanosine is not recommended. Conversely, the UK manufacturer of didanosine[3] just advises that if these drugs need to be given together, caution is required, and that patients should be monitored closely. They advise that treatment with nucleoside analogues [such as didanosine] should be discontinued in the setting of symptomatic hyperlactataemia and metabolic/lactic acidosis, progressive hepatomegaly, or rapidly elevating aminotransferase levels. Similarly, others consider that didanosine should not be systematically replaced in patients requiring treatment for hepatitis C because the risk of lactic acidosis is only small.[15] Nevertheless, they suggest that if a modification of antiretroviral treatment is needed then it is best to avoid didanosine.[15]

(b) Lamivudine

In vitro, ribavirin reduced the intracellular activation and antiretroviral activity of lamivudine.[16] However, in a study in 22 HIV-positive patients with hepatitis C, ribavirin 800 mg daily had no statistically significant effect on the pharmacokinetics of lamivudine (a 27% increase in AUC), and no effect on the intracellular activation of lamivudine, when compared with 24 similar patients who received placebo.[17] As with all NRTIs, lamivudine has, rarely, been associated with lactic acidosis, and the UK manufacturers of all NRTIs state that patients co-infected with hepatitis C and treated with interferon alfa and ribavirin may be at increased risk of lactic acidosis. Patients at increased risk should be monitored closely.[18]

(c) Stavudine

In vitro, ribavirin reduced the intracellular activation and antiretroviral activity of stavudine.[4,19] However, in a study in 5 HIV-positive patients with hepatitis C, ribavirin 800 mg daily had no statistically significant effect on the pharmacokinetics of stavudine (a 45% increase in AUC), and no effect on intracellular activation of stavudine, when compared with similar patients who received placebo.[17] Similarly, no decrease in antiviral activity of stavudine (as assessed by plasma HIV-RNA levels) has been seen when ribavirin was given with interferon for hepatitis C infection in patients with HIV.[20,21] Nevertheless, the UK manufacturers of ribavirin continue to recommend that plasma HIV-RNA levels are closely monitored in patients taking ribavirin with stavudine to ensure continued efficacy.[4,13] In contrast, based on an analysis of data from the adverse event reporting system of the FDA in the US, (see *didanosine* above), the UK manufacturers of ribavirin consider that concurrent use of stavudine should be avoided to limit the risk of mitochondrial toxicity.[4,13] The UK manufacturer of stavudine notes that patients co-infected with hepatitis C and treated with interferon alfa and ribavirin may be at increased risk of NRTI-associated lactic acidosis. Patients at increased risk should be monitored closely.[22] Similarly, the US manufacturer of stavudine states that patients receiving interferon with or without ribavirin and stavudine should be closely monitored for treatment-associated toxicities, especially hepatic decompensation.[23]

(d) Zidovudine

In vitro, ribavirin reduced the intracellular activation and antiretroviral activity of zidovudine.[4,24] However, in a study in 7 HIV-positive patients with hepatitis C, ribavirin 800 mg daily had no statistically significant effect on the pharmacokinetics of zidovudine (a 22% decrease in AUC), and no effect on the intracellular activation of zidovudine, when compared with similar patients who received placebo.[17] Moreover, in a study in 8 patients taking zidovudine, there was no significant variation in HIV viral load or CD4 counts after 3 or 6 months of ribavirin treatment, compared with baseline values.[21] Nevertheless, the UK manufacturers of ribavirin continue to recommend that plasma HIV RNA levels are closely monitored in patients given ribavirin with zidovudine to ensure continued efficacy.[4,13] The US manufacturer of zidovudine states that nucleoside analogues that antagonise the antiretroviral activity of zidovudine, such as ribavirin, should be avoided.[25] However, they also state that patients receiving interferon alfa with or without ribavirin and zidovudine should be closely monitored for treatment-associated toxicities, especially hepatic decompensation, neutropenia, and anaemia.[25] In the UK, the manufacturers of all NRTIs state that patients co-infected with hepatitis C and treated with interferon alfa and ribavirin may be at increased risk of lactic acidosis. Patients at increased risk should be monitored closely. One US manufacturer of ribavirin includes details of a study in which patients treated with zidovudine, interferon alfa and ribavirin had a higher incidence of severe neutropenia (15% versus 9%) and severe anaemia (5% versus 1%) than other similar patients not receiving zidovudine.[12]

1. Japour AJ, Lertora JJ, Meehan PM, Erice A, Connor JD, Griffith BP, Clax PA, Holden-Wiltse J, Hussey S, Walesky M, Cooney E, Pollard R, Timpone J, McLaren C, Johanneson N, Wood K, Booth DK, Bassiakos Y, Crumpacker CS, for the AIDS Clinical Trials Group 231 Protocol Team. A phase-1 study of the safety, pharmacokinetics, and antiviral activity of combination didanosine and ribavirin in patients with HIV-1 disease. *J Acquir Immune Defic Syndr Hum Retrovirol* (1996) 13, 235–46.
2. Lertora JJL, Harrison M, Dreisbach AW, Van Dyke R. Lack of pharmacokinetic interaction between DDI and ribavirin in HIV infected children. *J Investig Med* (1999) 47, 106A.
3. Videx EC (Didanosine). Bristol-Myers Squibb Pharmaceuticals Ltd. UK Summary of product characteristics, December 2006.
4. Copegus (Ribavirin). Roche Products Ltd. UK Summary of product characteristics, October 2006.
5. Videx EC (Didanosine). Bristol-Myers Squibb Company. US Prescribing information, March 2007.
6. Butt AA. Fatal lactic acidosis and pancreatitis associated with ribavirin and didanosine therapy. *AIDS Read* (2003) 13, 344–8.
7. Lafeuillade A, Hittinger G, Chadapaud S. Increased mitochondrial toxicity with ribavirin in HIV/HCV coinfection. *Lancet* (2001) 357, 280–1.
8. Salmon-Céron D, Chauvelot-Moachon L, Abad S, Silbermann B, Sogni P. Mitochondrial toxic effects and ribavirin. *Lancet* (2001) 357, 1803–4.
9. Fleischer R, Boxwell D, Sherman KE. Nucleoside analogues and mitochondrial toxicity. *Clin Infect Dis* (2004) 38, e79–e80.
10. Moreno A, Quereda C, Moreno L, Perez-Elías MJ, Muriel A, Casado JL, Antela A, Dronda F, Navas E, Bárcena R, Moreno S. High rate of didanosine-related mitochondrial toxicity in HIV/HCV-coinfected patients receiving ribavirin. *Antivir Ther* (2004) 9, 133–8.
11. Laguno M, Milinkovic A, de Lazzari E, Murillas J, Martínez E, Blanco JL, Loncá M, Biglia A, Leon A, García M, Larrousse M, García F, Miró JM, Gatell JM, Mallolas J. Incidence and risk factors for mitochondrial toxicity in treated HIV/HCV-coinfected patients. *Antivir Ther* (2005) 10, 423–9.
12. Copegus (Ribavirin). Roche Pharmaceuticals. US Prescribing information, June 2007.
13. Rebetol (Ribavirin). Schering-Plough Ltd. UK Summary of product characteristics, January 2007.
14. Rebetol (Ribavirin). Schering Corporation. US Prescribing information, June 2004.
15. Anon. Hepatitis C and didanosine: risk of lactic acidosis. *Prescrire Int* (2005) 14, 222–3.
16. Huh A, Nam J, Chang K, Yeom J, Song Y, Kim S, Lee J, Kim J. Antagonistic effect of ribavirin on lamivudine against HIV-1 infection (abstract I-1939). *Intersci Conf Antimicrob Agents Chemother* (2001) 41, 348.
17. Rodriguez-Torres M, Torriani FJ, Soriano V, Borucki MJ, Lissen E, Sulkowski M, Dieterich D, Wang K, Gries J-M, Hoggard PG, Back D; APRICOT Study Group. Effect of ribavirin on intracellular and plasma pharmacokinetics of nucleoside reverse transcriptase inhibitors in patients with human immunodeficiency virus-hepatitis C virus coinfection: results of a randomized clinical study. *Antimicrob Agents Chemother* (2005) 49, 3997–4008.
18. Epivir (Lamivudine). GlaxoSmithKline UK. UK Summary of product characteristics, March 2007.
19. Hoggard PG, Kewn S, Barry MG, Khoo SH, Back DJ. Effects of drugs on 2',3'-dideoxy-2',3'-didehydrothymidine phosphorylation in vitro. *Antimicrob Agents Chemother* (1997) 41, 1231–6.
20. Salmon-Céron D, Lassalle R, Pruvost A, Benech H, Bouvier-Alias M, Payan C, Goujard C, Bonnet E, Zoulim F, Morlat P, Sogni P, Pérusat S, Tréluyer J-M, Chêne G, and the CORIST-ANRS HC1 Study Group. Interferon-ribavirin in association with stavudine has no impact on plasma human immunodeficiency virus (HIV) type 1 level in patients coinfected with HIV and hepatitis C virus: a CORIST-ANRS HC1 trial. *Clin Infect Dis* (2003) 36, 1295–1304.
21. Zylberberg H, Benhamou Y, Lagneaux JL, Landau A, Chaix M-L, Fontaine H, Bochet M, Poynard T, Katlama C, Pialoux G, Bréchot C, Pol S. Safety and efficacy of interferon-ribavirin combination therapy in HCV-HIV coinfected subjects: an early report. *Gut* (2000) 47, 694–7.
22. Zerit (Stavudine). Bristol-Myers Squibb Pharmaceuticals Ltd. UK Summary of product characteristics, January 2007.
23. Zerit (Stavudine). Bristol-Myers Squibb Company. US Prescribing information, August 2006.
24. Vogt MW, Hartshorn KL, Furman PA, Chou TC, Fyfe JA, Coleman LA, Crumpacker C, Schooley RT, Hirsch MS. Ribavirin antagonizes the effect of azidothymidine on HIV replication. *Science* (1987) 235, 1376–9.
25. Retrovir (Zidovudine). GlaxoSmithKline. US Prescribing information, November 2006.

NRTIs + Tenofovir

Tenofovir increases the levels of didanosine: an increased risk of pancreatitis and peripheral neuropathy has been reported, and a high level of treatment failure. There is no pharmacokinetic interaction between tenofovir and abacavir, emtricitabine, lamivudine or stavudine. However, the combination of tenofovir, lamivudine and abacavir was unexpectedly associated with a high level of treatment failure. Triple-NRTI regimens involving tenofovir are not recommended, with the possible exception of tenofovir, lamivudine and zidovudine.

Clinical evidence, mechanism, importance and management

Note that tenofovir is a nucleotide (nucleoside monophosphate) analogue and is often classed as an NRTI.

(a) Abacavir

There was no clinically relevant pharmacokinetic interaction between tenofovir and abacavir in 8 healthy subjects.[1,2] However, the combination of tenofovir, lamivudine and abacavir was unexpectedly associated with a high rate of treatment failure (early virological non-response) in clinical studies.[3] Consequently, in July 2003 the manufacturer and others recommended that this triple therapy should not be used alone, and if these three drugs are used with other antiretrovirals, virological response should be closely monitored.[3] US guidelines (October 2006) for treatment of HIV infections state that triple NRTI regimens like this should not be used routinely (with 2 specific exceptions) because of suboptimal virological activity or lack of data.[4] Similarly, UK guidelines (2006) state that nonthymidine-containing triple NRTI regimens such as tenofovir, abacavir and lamivudine should not be used because of unacceptably high rates of virological failure.[5]

(b) Didanosine

The AUC of buffered didanosine 250 or 400 mg was increased by 44% when it was given 1 hour before tenofovir.[1] Similarly the AUC of enteric-coated didanosine 400 mg was increased by 48% and 60% when didanosine was given 2 hours before and with tenofovir disoproxil fumarate 300 mg, respectively.[6] The pharmacokinetics of tenofovir were unchanged.[1,6] Another study found that the AUC of enteric-coated didanosine 250 mg (simultaneously or 2 hours apart, fasted or with food) was about equivalent to that seen with didanosine 400 mg alone when tenofovir was given.[6]

The main concern with raised didanosine levels is the increased risk of adverse effects, particularly pancreatitis and peripheral neuropathy. One retrospective analysis found that 5 of 185 patients receiving didanosine with tenofovir developed pancreatitis compared with one of 182 taking didanosine without tenofovir and none of 208 taking tenofovir without didanosine, suggesting an increased risk of pancreatitis with the combination. All 6 cases of pancreatitis were in women without renal impairment, who weighed less than 60 kg. Five had received a reduced dose of didanosine (250 mg) and one had received 400 mg. Pancreatitis developed after 12 to 24 weeks.[7] Similarly, another analysis found that use of tenofovir with didanosine (400 mg daily or 250 mg daily if weight less than 60 kg) was associated with a higher incidence of peripheral neuropathy (12% versus 4%) and pancreatitis (4% versus 0%) than use with lower doses of didanosine (100 to 250 mg daily).[8] However, another analysis failed to find an enhanced risk of toxicity with the combination of didanosine and tenofovir at full dose during the first 6 months of use.[9] Tenofovir is rarely associated with acute renal failure, and in one analysis it was suggested that since didanosine was one drug that appeared to be more commonly used in cases of tenofovir-associated renal failure, this might be due to an interaction,[10] although others contend that this does not necessarily infer an association.[11] Cases of pancreatitis[12,13] or lactic acidosis and renal failure[14-16] have been reported (the use of ritonavir may be a factor in at least one of these cases[16]).

Furthermore, a once daily combination of tenofovir disoproxil fumarate 300 mg, enteric-coated didanosine 250 mg and lamivudine 300 mg was unexpectedly associated with a high rate of treatment failure (early virological non-response) in a clinical study in treatment-naïve patients.[17] Similarly, other studies have shown a high rate of treatment failure with a once daily combination of tenofovir disoproxil fumarate 300 mg, enteric-coated didanosine 250 mg and either efavirenz or nevirapine in treatment-naïve patients with high baseline viral loads and low CD4 counts.[18] A poor immune response (lack of increase in CD4 cell counts) has also been seen with full-dose didanosine plus tenofovir regimens in treatment-experienced patients.[19]

The pharmacokinetic interaction is established, and raised didanosine levels would be expected when it is given with tenofovir. The US manufacturers recommend that the dose of didanosine should be reduced to 250 mg once daily when given with tenofovir in patients weighing more than 60 kg[1,20] and 200 mg once daily in patients weighing less than 60 kg.[20] Nevertheless, because of the high rates of treatment failure seen with didanosine in combination with tenofovir and an NNRTI or lamivudine, and the potential for tenofovir to potentiate didanosine-related toxicity, the EMEA,[21] the MHRA in the UK[22] and UK guidelines[5] now recommend that didanosine should not be used with tenofovir in any antiretroviral combination. Similarly, US guidelines (October 2006) also say that didanosine should not be used with tenofovir as part of initial therapy because of a high rate of early virological failure, rapid selection of resistant mutations, and the potential for immunological non-response/CD4 decline.[4] If the combination is considered necessary, the patient should be carefully monitored for didanosine-related adverse effects (e.g. pancreatitis, peripheral neuropathy) and for antiviral efficacy.

(c) Emtricitabine

There was no pharmacokinetic interaction between tenofovir disoproxil fumarate 300 mg daily and emtricitabine 200 mg daily in a study in healthy subjects.[1,23] UK and US guidelines (2006) for treatment of HIV infections recommend the combination of tenofovir and emtricitabine plus either an NNRTI or a protease inhibitor.[4,5] Tenofovir and emtricitabine are available in a fixed dose combination product.

(d) Lamivudine

The manufacturer briefly notes that there was no pharmacokinetic interaction between tenofovir and lamivudine.[24] UK guidelines (2006) for treatment of HIV infections recommend the combination of tenofovir and lamivudine plus either an NNRTI or a protease inhibitor.[5]

However, for studies showing a high rate of virological failure with the combination of tenofovir, lamivudine and one other NRTI, see *Abacavir*, and *Didanosine*, above. UK and US guidelines say to avoid sole use of all regimens of tenofovir plus two NRTIs (triple-NRTI regimens), with the possible exception of tenofovir plus lamivudine and zidovudine when a protease inhibitor or NNRTI-based regimen cannot be used.[4,5]

(e) Stavudine

There is information to suggest that tenofovir disoproxil fumarate 300 mg does not alter levels of stavudine 100 mg.[25]

1. Viread (Tenofovir disoproxil fumarate). Gilead Sciences, Inc. US Prescribing information, May 2007.
2. Kearney BP, Isaacson E, Sayre J, Ebrahimi R, Cheng AK. The pharmacokinetics of abacavir, a purine nucleoside analog, are not affected by tenofovir DF. *Intersci Conf Antimicrob Agents Chemother* (2003) 43, 36.
3. Manion DJ. Important drug warning. Re: early virologic non-response in patients with HIV infection treated with lamivudine, abacavir and tenofovir. GlaxoSmithKline, July 2003. Available at: http://www.fda.gov/medwatch/SAFETY/2003/ziagen_deardoc_07-25-03.pdf (accessed 21/08/07).
4. US Department of Health and Human Services; Panel on Antiretroviral Guidelines for Adults and Adolescents. Guidelines for the use of antiretroviral agents in HIV-1-infected adults and adolescents. October 10, 2006; 1–113. Available at: http://www.aidsinfo.nih.gov/contentfiles/AdultandAdolescentGL.pdf (accessed 21/08/07).
5. Gazzard B, Bernard EJ, Boffito M, Churchill D, Edwards S, Fisher M, Geretti AM, Johnson M, Leen C, Peters B, Pozniak A, Ross J, Walsh J, Wilkins E, Youle M. BHIVA Writing Committee, British HIV Association (BHIVA) guidelines for the treatment of HIV-infected adults with antiretroviral therapy (2006). *HIV Med* (2006) 7, 487–503. Available at: http://www.bhiva.org/files/file1001303.pdf (accessed 21/08/07).
6. Kearney BP, Sayre JR, Flaherty JF, Chen S-S, Kaul S, Cheng AK. Drug-drug and drug-food interactions between tenofovir disoproxil fumarate and didanosine. *J Clin Pharmacol* (2005) 45, 1360–7.
7. Martínez E, Milinkovic A, de Lazzari E, Ravasi G, Blanco JL, Larrousse M, Mallolas J, García F, Miró JM, Gatell JM. Pancreatic toxic effects associated with co-administration of didanosine and tenofovir in HIV-infected adults. *Lancet* (2004) 364, 65–7.
8. Young B, Weidle PJ, Baker RK, Armon C, Wood KC, Moorman AC, Holmberg SD; HIV Outpatient Study (HOPS) Investigators. Short-term safety and tolerability of didanosine combined with high- versus low-dose tenofovir disproxil fumarate in ambulatory HIV-1-infected persons. *AIDS Patient Care STDS* (2006) 20, 238–44.
9. Barrios A, Maida I, Perez-Saleme L, Negredo E, Clotet B, Vilaro J, Domingo P, Estrada V, Santos J, Asensi V, Labarga P, Terron J, Vergara A, Garcia-Benayas T, Martin-Carbonero L, Barreiro P, Gonzalez-Lahoz J, Soriano V. Safety and efficacy of combinations based on didanosine 400 mg od plus tenofovir 300 mg od. *Intersci Conf Antimicrob Agents Chemother* (2003) 43, 314.
10. Zimmermann AE, Pizzoferrato T, Bedford J, Morris A, Hoffman R, Braden G. Tenofovir-associated acute and chronic kidney disease: a case of multiple drug interactions. *Clin Infect Dis* (2006) 42, 283–90.
11. Winston JA, Shepp DH. The role of drug interactions and monitoring in the prevention of tenofovir-associated kidney disease. *Clin Infect Dis* (2006) 42, 1657–8; author reply ibid.,1658.
12. Blanchard JN, Wohlfeiler M, Canas A, King K, Lonergan JT. Pancreatitis with didanosine and tenofovir disoproxil fumarate. *Clin Infect Dis* (2003) 37, e57–e62. Correction. ibid. 995.
13. Kirian MA, Higginson RT, Pecora Fulco P. Acute onset of pancreatitis with concomitant use of tenofovir and didanosine. *Ann Pharmacother* (2004) 38, 1660–3.
14. Murphy MD, O'Hearn M, Chou S. Fatal lactic acidosis and acute renal failure after addition of tenofovir to an antiretroviral regimen containing didanosine. *Clin Infect Dis* (2003) 36, 1082–5.
15. Guo Y, Fung HB. Fatal lactic acidosis associated with coadministration of didanosine and tenofovir disoproxil fumarate. *Pharmacotherapy* (2004) 24, 1089–94.
16. Rollot F, Nazal E-M, Chauvelot-Moachon L, Kélaïdi C, Daniel N, Saba M, Abad S, Blanche P. Tenofovir-related Fanconi syndrome with nephrogenic diabetes insipidus in a patient with acquired immunodeficiency syndrome: the role of lopinavir-ritonavir-didanosine. *Clin Infect Dis* (2003) 37, e174–6.
17. EMEA Public Statement. High rate of virologic failure in patients with HIV infection treated with a once-daily triple nucleosides/nucleotide reverse transcriptase inhibitors combination containing didanosine, lamivudine and tenofovir. London, 22 October 2003. Available at: http://www.emea.eu.int/pdfs/human/press/pus/509403en.pdf (accessed 21/08/07).
18. Hodder SL. Re: Important new clinical data. Potential early virologic failure associated with the combination antiretroviral regimen of tenofovir disoproxil fumarate, didanosine, and either efavirenz or nevirapine in HIV treatment-naïve patients with high baseline viral loads. Bristol-Myers Squibb Company, November 2004. Available at: http://www.fda.gov/oashi/aids/listserv/bms.pdf (accessed 21/08/07).
19. Negredo E, Bonjoch A, Paredes R, Puig J, Clotet B. Compromised immunologic recovery in treatment-experienced patients with HIV infection receiving both tenofovir disoproxil fumarate and didanosine in the TORO studies. *Clin Infect Dis* (2005) 41, 901–5.
20. Videx EC (Didanosine). Bristol-Myers Squibb Company. US Prescribing information, March 2007.
21. EMEA Public Statement. Efficacy and safety concerns regarding the co-administration of tenofovir disoproxil fumarate (TDF, Viread) and didanosine (ddI, Videx). London, 3 March 2005. Available at: http://www.emea.europa.eu/pdfs/human/press/pus/6233105en.pdf (accessed 21/08/07).
22. CHM/MHRA. Tenofovir (Viread): interactions and renal adverse effects. *Current Problems* (2006) 31, 2. Available at: http://www.mhra.gov.uk/home/idcplg?IdcService=SS_GET_PAGE&useSecondary=true&ssDocName=CON2023859&ssTargetNodeId=368 (accessed 21/08/07).
23. Blum MR, Begley J, Zong J, Hill D, Adda N, Chittick G. Lack of a pharmacokinetic interaction between emtricitabine and tenofovir DF when coadministered to steady state in healthy volunteers. *Intersci Conf Antimicrob Agents Chemother* (2003) 43, 38.
24. Viread (Tenofovir disoproxil fumarate). Gilead Sciences International Ltd. UK Summary of product characteristics, May 2007.
25. Anon. E. Tenofovir drug interactions: ddI and d4T. *Treatmentupdate* (2003) 15 (Part 2), 7.

NRTIs; Didanosine + Allopurinol

Allopurinol markedly raises didanosine levels.

Clinical evidence, mechanism, importance and management

Buffered didanosine 400 mg was given to 14 healthy subjects, with and without allopurinol 300 mg daily for 7 days. The allopurinol significantly increased didanosine absorption, shown by a twofold increase in the AUC and a 69% rise in its maximum serum levels.[1] Similar findings were seen in HIV-positive subjects.[2] Moreover, the addition of allopurinol 300 mg daily allowed the dosage of didanosine to be halved from 400 mg to 200 mg daily in 4 patients taking buffered didanosine, hydroxycarbamide and chloroquine. Didanosine plasma levels and antiviral efficacy were unchanged.[3]

The manufacturer notes that allopurinol may increase the exposure to didanosine by inhibiting xanthine oxidase, an enzyme involved in didanosine metabolism.[4] This interaction has been studied for its therapeutic benefit.[3] However, if the dose of didanosine is not reduced, there is the potential for an increase in didanosine adverse effects.

The UK manufacturer recommends close monitoring for adverse effects if allopurinol is used with didanosine,[4] but the US manufacturer says that coadministration is not recommended.[5]

1. Liang D, Breaux K, Nornoo A Phadungpojna S, Rodriguez-Barradas M, Bates TR. Pharmacokinetic interaction between didanosine (ddI) and allopurinol in healthy volunteers. *Intersci Conf Antimicrob Agents Chemother* (1999) 39, 25.
2. Liang D, Breaux K, Rodriguez-Barradas M, Bates TR. Allopurinol increases didanosine absorption in HIV-infected patients. *Intersci Conf Antimicrob Agents Chemother* (2001) 41, 16.
3. Boelaert JR, Dom GM, Huitema ADR, Beijnen JH, Lange JMA. The boosting of didanosine by allopurinol permits a halving of the didanosine dosage. *AIDS* (2002) 16, 2221–3.
4. Videx EC (Didanosine). Bristol-Myers Squibb Pharmaceuticals Ltd. UK Summary of product characteristics, December 2006.
5. Videx EC (Didanosine). Bristol-Myers Squibb Company. US Prescribing information, March 2007.

NRTIs; Didanosine + Loperamide or Metoclopramide

Loperamide and metoclopramide do not appear to alter didanosine pharmacokinetics.

Clinical evidence, mechanism, importance and management

In 6 men and 6 women who were HIV-positive, the pharmacokinetics of oral buffered didanosine 300 mg were not altered to a clinically relevant extent by 4 mg of loperamide, given 19, 13, 7 and 1 hour before the didanosine. The rate of didanosine absorption was slightly decreased but the extent of absorption was unchanged. Similarly, the pharmacokinetics of oral buffered didanosine 300 mg were found to be unaffected by 10 mg of intravenous metoclopramide.[1] It appears that neither delaying nor accelerating gastrointestinal transit time appreciably alters the pharmacokinetics of didanosine, which is acid labile. On the basis of this study the authors conclude that neither the dose nor the frequency of didanosine administration need be altered if either loperamide or metoclopramide is given concurrently.[1]

1. Knupp CA, Milbrath RL, Barbhaiya RH. Effect of metoclopramide and loperamide on the pharmacokinetics of didanosine in HIV seropositive asymptomatic male and female patients. *Eur J Clin Pharmacol* (1993) 45, 409–13.

NRTIs; Stavudine + Doxorubicin

***In vitro* evidence suggests that doxorubicin may inhibit the activation of stavudine.**

Clinical evidence, mechanism, importance and management

Nucleoside reverse transcriptase inhibitors such as stavudine need to be phosphorylated within cells before they become effective. *In vitro* studies using mononucleated blood cells found that doxorubicin may interfere with stavudine phosphorylation at clinically relevant concentrations.[1] The clinical importance of this interaction awaits assessment. Until then, caution is required on concurrent use.

1. Hoggard PG, Kewn S, Barry MG, Khoo SH, Back DJ. Effects of drugs on 2',3'-dideoxy-2',3'-didehydrothymidine phosphorylation in vitro. *Antimicrob Agents Chemother* (1997) 41, 1231–6.

NRTIs; Zidovudine + Benzodiazepines

Oxazepam causes a modest increase in the bioavailability of zidovudine, and the combination can increase the incidence of headaches. Lorazepam possibly behaves similarly.

Clinical evidence, mechanism, importance and management

A pharmacokinetic study in 6 HIV-positive patients found that **oxazepam** did not significantly affect the bioavailability of zidovudine. All of the patients were sleepy and fatigued while taking **oxazepam** (as expected), but 5 of the 6 complained of headaches while taking both drugs, compared with only 1 of 6 while taking zidovudine alone and none while taking **oxazepam** alone. The authors of the report suggest that if headaches occur during concurrent use, the benzodiazepine should be stopped.[1] A previous *in vitro* study using human liver microsomes confirmed that **oxazepam** inhibits the metabolism of zidovudine to its glucuronide, and **lorazepam** behaves in the same way.[2] The same precautions suggested for **oxazepam** would therefore also appear to apply to **lorazepam**.

1. Mole L, Israelski D, Bubp J, O'Hanley P, Merigan T, Blaschke T. Pharmacokinetics of zidovudine alone and in combination with oxazepam in the HIV infected patient. *J Acquir Immune Defic Syndr* (1993) 6, 56–60.
2. Unadkat JD, Chien J. Lorazepam and oxazepam inhibit the metabolism of zidovudine (ZDV or azidothymidine) in an *in vitro* human liver microsomal system. *Pharm Res* (1988) 5 (Suppl), S177.

NRTIs; Zidovudine + Drugs that inhibit glucuronidation

***In vitro* evidence suggests that chloramphenicol, indometacin and naproxen inhibit the glucuronidation of zidovudine. However, neither indometacin nor naproxen altered zidovudine pharmacokinetics in subsequent clinical studies. Dipyridamole did not alter zidovudine pharmacokinetics.**

Clinical evidence and mechanism

(a) Aspirin or NSAIDs

A study of zidovudine use in 282 AIDS patients found that haematological abnormalities were not increased by aspirin in 47 patients.[1] An *in vitro* study using human liver microsomes found that **indometacin** and **naproxen** inhibited the glucuronidation of zidovudine by 50% or more, and aspirin also had some inhibitory effect.[2] This suggested that these drugs might possibly increase the effects and the toxicity of zidovudine. However, other *clinical* studies found no changes in the pharmacokinetics of zidovudine given with **indometacin** 25 mg twice daily for 3 days[3] or **naproxen** 500 mg to 1 g daily for 3 or 4 days.[3,4]

(b) Chloramphenicol

An *in vitro* study using human liver microsomes found that chloramphenicol inhibited the glucuronidation of zidovudine by 50% or more, suggesting that the effects and toxicity of zidovudine may be increased.[2] The effect of concurrent use in patients awaits assessment.

(c) Dipyridamole

Theoretically, dipyridamole and zidovudine might inhibit the metabolism of each other by competing for glucuronidation, the major clearance mechanism for both drugs. However, a study in 11 asymptomatic HIV-positive patients found that dipyridamole 75 to 100 mg every 4 hours for 5 days caused no significant changes in the pharmacokinetics of zidovudine 500 mg daily, but the dipyridamole adverse effects (headaches, nausea) when taking the higher dose were found to be intolerable.[5]

Importance and management

Many drugs that inhibit the glucuronidation of zidovudine *in vitro* appear to have only modest effects on zidovudine levels, which are unlikely to be clinically important in most patients. Consider also 'NRTIs + Atovaquone', p.793.

1. Richman DD, Fischl MA, Grieco MH, Gottlieb MS, Volberding PA, Laskin OL, Leedom JM, Groopman JE, Mildvan D, Hirsch MS, Jackson GG, Durack DT, Nusinoff-Lehrman S and the AZT Collaborative Working Group. The toxicity of azidothymidine (AZT) in the treatment of patients with AIDS and AIDS-related complex. A double-blind, placebo-controlled trial. *N Engl J Med* (1987) 317, 192–7.
2. Sim SM, Back DJ, Breckenridge AM. The effect of various drugs on the glucuronidation of zidovudine (azidothymidine; AZT) by human liver microsomes. *Br J Clin Pharmacol* (1991) 32, 17–21.
3. Barry M, Howe J, Back D, Breckenridge A, Brettle R, Mitchell R, Beeching NJ, Nye FJ. The effects of indomethacin and naproxen on zidovudine pharmacokinetics. *Br J Clin Pharmacol* (1993) 36, 82–5.
4. Sahai J, Gallicano K, Garber G, Pakuts A, Hawley-Foss N, Huang L, McGilveray I, Cameron DW. Evaluation of the in vivo effect of naproxen on zidovudine pharmacokinetics in patients infected with human immunodeficiency virus. *Clin Pharmacol Ther* (1992) 52, 464–70.
5. Hendrix CW, Flexner C, Szebeni J, Kuwahara S, Pennypacker S, Weinstein JN, Lietman PS. Effect of dipyridamole on zidovudine pharmacokinetics and short-term tolerance in asymptomatic human immunodeficiency virus-infected subjects. *Antimicrob Agents Chemother* (1994) 38, 1036–40.

NRTIs; Zidovudine + Lithium

Lithium can apparently oppose the neutropenic effects of zidovudine.

Clinical evidence, mechanism, importance and management

A study in 5 patients with AIDS found that serum lithium carbonate levels of 0.6 to 1.2 mmol/L increased their neutrophil counts sufficiently to allow the re-introduction of zidovudine, which had previously been withdrawn due to neutropenia. Withdrawal of the lithium resulted in a rapid fall in neutrophil levels in two patients.[1] Improvement in neutropenia occurred in another AIDS patient taking zidovudine 1.2 g daily when lithium carbonate 300 mg three times daily was also given.[2] Lithium has been found to induce granulopoiesis, and these reports suggest that no adverse reaction occurred in patients taking zidovudine and lithium, and that there may be some advantages to their use. However, lithium itself has a narrow therapeutic range and its toxic symptoms might be difficult to distinguish from neurological complications caused by the disease. The addition of lithium could also increase the risk of interactions with other drugs.[3,4] A study of 3 further patients found a lack of beneficial effect with lithium in 2 of the patients and only a short-term improvement in the neutrophil count in the third. In addition, one patient experienced severe diarrhoea necessitating discontinuation of the lithium.[5]

1. Roberts DE, Berman SM, Nakasato S, Wyle FA, Wishnow RM, Segal GP. Effect of lithium carbonate on zidovudine-associated neutropenia in the acquired immunodeficiency syndrome. *Am J Med* (1988) 85, 428–31.
2. Herbert V, Hirschman S, Jacobson J. Lithium for zidovudine-induced neutropenia in AIDS. *JAMA* (1988) 260, 3588.
3. Nathwani D, Green ST. Lithium for zidovudine-induced neutropenia in AIDS. *JAMA* (1989) 262, 775–6.
4. Klutman NE. Lithium carbonate therapy for zidovudine-associated neutropenia in patients with acquired immunodeficiency syndrome. *Am J Med* (1989) 87, 362–3.
5. Worthington M. Lack of effect of lithium carbonate on zidovudine-associated neutropenia in patients with AIDS. *J Infect Dis* (1990) 162, 777–8.

NRTIs; Zidovudine + Megestrol

Megestrol acetate does not affect the pharmacokinetics of zidovudine.

Clinical evidence, mechanism, importance and management

In 12 asymptomatic HIV-positive subjects megestrol acetate 800 mg daily for 13 days had no effect on the steady-state pharmacokinetics of zidovudine or its glucuronide metabolite.[1] Megestrol does not appear to affect the metabolism of zidovudine. No dose adjustments appear necessary.

1. Van Harken DR, Pei JC, Wagner J, Pike IM. Pharmacokinetic interaction of megestrol acetate with zidovudine in human immunodeficiency virus-infected patients. *Antimicrob Agents Chemother* (1997) 41, 2480–3.

NRTIs; Zidovudine + Myelosuppressive drugs

There have been reports of serious myelotoxicity when zidovudine was given with vancomycin or antineoplastics, and, on theoretical grounds, any drug causing bone marrow suppression might be additive with the effects of zidovudine. Moderate pharmacokinetic changes have been seen when zidovudine was given with chemotherapy regimens used for Kaposi's sarcoma, Hodgkin's disease, and non-Hodgkin's lymphoma.

Clinical evidence and mechanism

(a) Antineoplastics

In one preliminary report, the addition of **vinblastine** to zidovudine resulted in severe bone marrow depression.[1] Similarly, 9 of 21 patients could not tolerate zidovudine while receiving a chemotherapy regimen (**cyclophosphamide**, **doxorubicin**, **teniposide**, **prednisone**, **vincristine** and **bleomycin**) because of haematological toxicity.[2]

The pharmacokinetic interaction of chemotherapy with zidovudine was assessed in HIV-positive patients being treated for Kaposi's sarcoma, non-Hodgkin's lymphoma or Hodgkin's disease. The antineoplastics used were **bleomycin**, **cyclophosphamide**, **doxorubicin**, **epirubicin**, **etoposide**, **vinblastine**, **vincristine**, **vindesine** and **vinorelbine**. The zidovudine metabolism was unchanged, but a 43% decrease was noted in the maximum plasma levels of zidovudine and the time to peak level was prolonged by 51%, which was independent of the chemotherapy given.[3] The authors concluded that dose changes of zidovudine were not needed with the antineoplastics used, based on these pharmacokinetic changes alone, since the zidovudine AUC remained unchanged and maximum plasma levels have not been shown to clearly correlate with its activity.[3] Thus it appears that any interaction is likely to be attributable to additive myelosuppressive effects.

(b) Vancomycin

A report describes marked neutropenia in 4 HIV-positive patients receiving zidovudine when they were given vancomycin (which can also, rarely, have neutropenic effects).[4]

Importance and management

On theoretical grounds any drug causing bone marrow suppression might be additive with the effects of zidovudine. The UK manufacturer recommends that extra care be taken in monitoring haematological parameters if concurrent treatment with any myelosuppressive drug and zidovudine is required.[5] They specifically mention systemic **pentamidine**, **'dapsone'**, (p.796), **pyrimethamine**, **'co-trimoxazole'**, (p.795), **amphotericin** (myelotoxicity and nephrotoxicity seen in a study in *dogs*[6]), **flucytosine**, **'ganciclovir'**, (p.798), **'interferon'**, (p.795), **vinblastine**, and **doxorubicin**.[5] However, they also state[5] that limited clinical data do not indicate a significantly increased risk of adverse reactions to zidovudine if it is given with prophylactic doses of **co-trimoxazole**, aerosolised **pentamidine**, **pyrimethamine**, and **'aciclovir'**, (p.791).

1. Charakhanian S, De Sabb R, Vaseghi M, Cardon B, Rozenbaum W. Evaluation of the association of zidovudine and vinblastine in treatment of AIDS-related Kaposi's sarcoma. 5th International Conference on AIDS, Montreal, 1989. Abstract MBP368.
2. Tirelli U, Errante D, Oksenhendler E, Spina M, Vaccher E, Serraino D, Gastaldi R, Repetto L, Rizzardini G, Carbone A, et al. French-Italian Cooperative Study Group. Prospective study with combined low-dose chemotherapy and zidovudine in 37 patients with poor-prognosis AIDS-related non-Hodgkin's lymphoma. *Ann Oncol* (1992) 3, 843–7.
3. Toffoli G, Errante D, Corona G, Vaccher E, Bertola A, Robieux I, Aita P, Sorio R, Tirelli U, Boiocchi M. Interactions of antineoplastic chemotherapy with zidovudine pharmacokinetics in patients with HIV-related neoplasms. *Chemotherapy* (1999) 45, 418–28.
4. Kitchen LW, Clark RA, Hanna BJ, Pollock B, Valainis GT. Vancomycin and neutropenia in AZT-treated AIDS patients with staphylococcal infections. *J Acquir Immune Defic Syndr* (1990) 3, 925–6.
5. Retrovir (Zidovudine). GlaxoSmithKline UK. UK Summary of product characteristics, December 2006.
6. Abelcet (Amphotericin B lipid complex). Cephalon Ltd. UK Summary of product characteristics, November 2006.

Oseltamivir + Drugs that affect renal clearance

Probenecid inhibits the renal secretion of the active metabolite of oseltamivir and markedly raises its plasma levels, but this is not clinically relevant because of the wide safety margin of oseltamivir. There was no pharmacokinetic interaction between amoxicillin and oseltamivir, and cimetidine did not alter oseltamivir pharmacokinetics.

Clinical evidence

(a) Amoxicillin

In a study in healthy subjects, oseltamivir 75 mg twice daily for 4.5 days had no effect on the pharmacokinetics of a single 500-mg dose of amoxicillin given with the last dose of oseltamivir. Similarly, the amoxicillin had no effect on the pharmacokinetics of the active metabolite of oseltamivir.[1]

(b) Cimetidine

In a crossover study in 18 healthy subjects cimetidine 400 mg every 6 hours for 4 days had no effect on the pharmacokinetics of a single 150-mg dose of oseltamivir given on day 2.[1]

(c) Probenecid

In a crossover study in 18 healthy subjects probenecid 500 mg every 6 hours for 4 days approximately halved the renal clearance of the active metabolite of oseltamivir, and increased its AUC by about 2.5-fold when a single 150-mg dose of oseltamivir was given on day 2.[1]

Mechanism

Probenecid appears to completely inhibit the renal tubular secretion of the active metabolite of oseltamivir via the anionic renal transporter process. Oseltamivir does not alter amoxicillin pharmacokinetics, suggesting minimal potential to inhibit the renal anionic transport process.[1] Cimetidine, which inhibits the renal tubular secretion of drugs via the cationic secretion transport process, had no effect on oseltamivir.

Importance and management

Probenecid markedly increased the AUC of the active metabolite of oseltamivir, but because of the large safety margin of oseltamivir, this increase is not considered to be clinically relevant.[1-3] Oseltamivir did not alter amoxicillin pharmacokinetics, and is therefore unlikely to interact with other renally secreted organic acids. Other drugs that are involved in the active anionic tubular secretion mechanism are also unlikely to interact. Cimetidine does not interact with oseltamivir, and other drugs that are inhibitors of the renal cationic secretion transport process are unlikely to interact.[1]

Although the UK manufacturer does state that clinically important drug interactions involving competition for renal tubular secretion are unlikely, they recommend care should be taken when prescribing oseltamivir to patients taking other similarly excreted drugs with a narrow therapeutic margin, and they give **chlorpropamide**, **methotrexate**, and **phenylbutazone** as examples.[2]

1. Hill G, Cihlar T, Oo C, Ho ES, Prior K, Wiltshire H, Barrett J, Liu B, Ward P. The anti-influenza drug oseltamivir exhibits low potential to induce pharmacokinetic drug interactions via renal secretion–correlation of in vivo and in vitro studies. *Drug Metab Dispos* (2002) 30, 13–19.
2. Tamiflu (Oseltamivir phosphate). Roche Products Ltd. UK Summary of product characteristics, March 2007.
3. Tamiflu (Oseltamivir phosphate). Roche Pharmaceuticals. US Prescribing information, July 2007.

Oseltamivir or Zanamivir + Miscellaneous

Antacids do not affect the pharmacokinetics of oseltamivir, and there is no pharmacokinetic interaction between aspirin or paracetamol (acetaminophen) and oseltamivir. Aspirin and a variety of other drugs used for influenza management do not affect the antiviral activity of zanamivir *in vitro*.

Clinical evidence, mechanism, importance and management

(a) Oseltamivir

1. Antacids. In a single-dose study, the pharmacokinetics of oseltamivir 150 mg and its active carboxylate metabolite were not affected by antacids. The antacids used were an **aluminium/magnesium hydroxide** suspension *(Maalox)* and **calcium carbonate** tablet *(Titralac)*.[1]

2. Aspirin. In a study, 12 healthy subjects were given a single 900-mg dose of aspirin before, during and/or after oseltamivir 75 mg twice daily for 9 doses. There was no pharmacokinetic interaction between aspirin and oseltamivir.[2] A possible interaction was postulated since both drugs are hydrolysed by esterases and secreted by anionic tubular secretion.[2]

3. Paracetamol (Acetaminophen). The manufacturer notes that there is no pharmacokinetic interaction between paracetamol and oseltamivir.[3,4]

(b) Zanamivir

The *in vitro* antiviral potency of zanamivir was not affected by **aspirin**, **paracetamol**, **ibuprofen**, **phenylephrine**, **oxymetazoline**, **promethazine**, or **co-amoxiclav**.[5] Zanamivir is used as an inhalation, and has low systemic bioavailability, so interactions would not generally be expected.

1. Snell P, Oo C, Dorr A, Barrett J. Lack of pharmacokinetic interaction between the oral anti-influenza neuraminidase inhibitor prodrug oseltamivir and antacids. *Br J Clin Pharmacol* (2002) 54, 372–7.
2. Oo C, Barrett J, Dorr A, Liu B, Ward P. Lack of pharmacokinetic interaction between the oral anti-influenza prodrug oseltamivir and aspirin. *Antimicrob Agents Chemother* (2002) 46, 1993–5.
3. Tamiflu (Oseltamivir phosphate). Roche Products Ltd. UK Summary of product characteristics, March 2007.
4. Tamiflu (Oseltamivir phosphate). Roche Pharmaceuticals. US Prescribing information, July 2007.
5. Daniel MJ, Barnett JM, Pearson BA. The low potential for drug interactions with zanamivir. *Clin Pharmacokinet* (1999) 36 (Suppl 1), 41–50.

Protease inhibitors + Antiepileptics; Barbiturates

It is likely that phenobarbital and other barbiturates will increase the metabolism of the protease inhibitors, thereby reducing their levels and possibly resulting in failure of the antiretrovirals. However, one case suggested that this may not have occurred with primidone and ritonavir/saquinavir, although this should be viewed with caution.

Clinical evidence, mechanism, importance and management

The manufacturers of many of the protease inhibitors predict that their levels may be reduced by **phenobarbital**, due to induction of the cytochrome P450 isoenzyme CYP3A4 by which they are metabolised (see 'Table 21.2', (p.773)). There do not appear to be any controlled studies to demonstrate the extent of the pharmacokinetic interaction with different protease inhibitors. Data from one case report of carbamazepine toxicity with 'ritonavir/saquinavir', (p.810), provide indirect evidence to suggest the interaction with **primidone** is not clinically important. In this report, a patient taking an antiretroviral regimen including **ritonavir** and **saquinavir** had his antiepileptic medication changed from carbamazepine to **primidone** 500 mg daily. The authors noted that during follow-up (duration not stated), viral load was still undetectable and seizures remained under control.[1] **Primidone** is metabolised to **phenobarbital**, and might have been expected to cause antiretroviral therapy failure. Alternatively, the effect of **ritonavir**, which is a potent inhibitor of CYP3A4, may have been sufficient to offset the increased clearance associated with phenobarbital.

Another patient[2] taking phenobarbital, phenytoin and carbamazepine was found to have an unchanged phenobarbital level 2 days after switching from an antiretroviral regimen including indinavir to one containing ritonavir 300 mg twice daily and saquinavir. His plasma levels of 'carbamazepine', (p.810), had doubled, and there was a 32.7% drop in the levels of 'phenytoin', (p.812).

The combination of protease inhibitors and barbiturates should be used with caution, with increased monitoring of antiviral efficacy.

1. Berbel Garcia A, Latorre Ibarra A, Porta Etessam J, Martinez Salio A, Perez Martinez DA, Saiz Diaz R, Toledo Heras M. Protease inhibitor-induced carbamazepine toxicity. *Clin Neuropharmacol* (2000) 23, 216–18.
2. Mateu-de Antonio J, Grau S, Gimeno-Bayón J-L, Carmona A. Ritonavir-induced carbamazepine toxicity. *Ann Pharmacother* (2001) 35, 125–6.

Protease inhibitors + Antiepileptics; Carbamazepine

Case reports suggest that ritonavir markedly increases carbamazepine levels and toxicity. Cases have also been reported with lopinavir/ritonavir and nelfinavir. Carbamazepine reduces indinavir levels and efficacy, and would also be expected to decrease levels of other protease inhibitors.

Clinical evidence

(a) Indinavir

A report describes a 48-year-old man whose antiretrovirals (indinavir 800 mg every 8 hours, lamivudine 150 mg twice daily and zidovudine 200 mg three times daily) became ineffective after a 10-week course of carbamazepine for postherpetic neuralgia. Over this time indinavir levels were up to 16 times lower than those measured in the absence of carbamazepine.[1] In two further cases, patients taking carbamazepine had partial failure of indinavir-containing antiretroviral regimens, which prompted a change in their therapy to include ritonavir rather than indinavir.[2,3]

In 3 of the case reports described under *Ritonavir*, below, in which ritonavir increased carbamazepine levels,[2-4] patients had previously received indinavir (800 mg three times daily[2,4]) and carbamazepine (600 mg daily[2,3] or 400 mg three times daily[4]) without experiencing carbamazepine toxicity (therapeutic carbamazepine levels were reported in 2 of the cases[2,3]). This suggests that indinavir does not increase carbamazepine levels. However, in the case described above,[1] carbamazepine levels reached the therapeutic range for epilepsy even though the dosage of carbamazepine was only 200 mg daily, suggesting indinavir may increase carbamazepine levels.

(b) Lopinavir/Ritonavir

An HIV-positive patient who had a serum carbamazepine level of 10.3 mg/L while taking carbamazepine 400 mg three times daily reported feeling very drowsy within 9 days of starting to take tenofovir, lamivudine and lopinavir/ritonavir 400/100 mg twice daily. His carbamazepine serum level was found to have increased by 46%, to 15 mg/L. The carbamazepine dose was reduced to 400 mg twice daily, and 2 days later the carbamazepine level was 7.4 mg/L.[5]

(c) Nelfinavir

An HIV-positive patient who had a serum carbamazepine level of 9.8 mg/L while taking carbamazepine 400 mg three times daily started feeling more tired and unsteady on his feet 3 days after starting to take tenofovir, lamivudine and nelfinavir 1.25 g twice daily. His carbamazepine level was found to have increased by 53%, to 15 mg/L. The carbamazepine dose was reduced to 400 mg twice daily, and 2 days later the carbamazepine level was 9.3 mg/L.[5]

(d) Ritonavir

An 20-year-old HIV-positive man with epilepsy, who had his seizures controlled with carbamazepine 350 mg twice daily and zonisamide 140 mg twice daily, was admitted to hospital for review of his antiretrovirals. He started taking ritonavir 200 mg three times daily, but after the first dose of ritonavir his serum carbamazepine levels rose from 9.5 to 17.8 mg/L. This was accompanied by intractable vomiting and vertigo, so after 2 days the ritonavir was stopped. Symptoms resolved over the next few days. Subsequently ritonavir 200 mg daily was started, with the same effect, so the dose of carbamazepine dose was reduced to one-third, which resulted in carbamazepine levels of 6.2 micrograms/mL. Levels of ritonavir were not measured.[6] Three other cases also document two- to threefold rises in carbamazepine levels with associated toxicity caused by the addition of ritonavir 300 mg, 400 mg or 600 mg twice daily and **saquinavir** 400 mg twice daily.[2-4] In one case a carbamazepine dose reduction from 600 to 100 mg daily was needed to keep the levels within the therapeutic range before ritonavir was discontinued.[3]

Mechanism

Ritonavir is a potent inhibitor of the cytochrome P450 isoenzyme CYP3A4 and consequently markedly increases carbamazepine levels. Other protease inhibitors would be expected to interact similarly, although to a lesser degree (see also 'Antivirals', (p.772)). Moreover, carbamazepine is an inducer of CYP3A4 and therefore can increase the metabolism of the protease inhibitor causing the levels to become subtherapeutic. Use of ritonavir-boosted protease inhibitors could theoretically offset this effect, but it may lead to increased carbamazepine toxicity.

Importance and management

Although the evidence is limited, these interactions seem to be established. It would therefore appear that the use of carbamazepine with protease inhibitors should be avoided where possible (mainly because of the risk of antiviral treatment failure). If both must be used then extremely close monitoring of both antiviral efficacy and carbamazepine levels/toxicity is warranted. Symptoms of carbamazepine toxicity include nausea, vomiting, ataxia and drowsiness. The authors of one report suggest that amitriptyline or gabapentin would be possible alternatives for carbamazepine used for pain, or valproic acid or lamotrigine for carbamazepine used for seizures.[1]

1. Hugen PWH, Burger DM, Brinkman K, ter Hofstede HJM, Schuurman R, Koopmans PP, Hekster YA. Carbamazepine-indinavir interaction causes antiretroviral therapy failure. *Ann Pharmacother* (2000) 34, 465–70.
2. Berbel Garcia A, Latorre Ibarra A, Porta Etessam J, Martinez Salio A, Perez Martinez DA, Saiz Diaz R, Toledo Heras M. Protease inhibitor-induced carbamazepine toxicity. *Clin Neuropharmacol* (2000) 23, 216–18.
3. Burman W, Orr L. Carbamazepine toxicity after starting combination antiretroviral therapy including ritonavir and efavirenz. *AIDS* (2000) 14, 2793–4.
4. Mateu-de Antonio J, Grau S, Gimeno-Bayón J-L, Carmona A. Ritonavir-induced carbamazepine toxicity. *Ann Pharmacother* (2001) 35, 125–6.
5. Bates DE, Herman RJ. Carbamazepine toxicity induced by lopinavir/ritonavir and nelfinavir. *Ann Pharmacother* (2006) 40, 1190–5.
6. Kato Y, Fujii T, Mizoguchi N, Takata N, Ueda K, Feldman MD, Kayser SR. Potential interaction between ritonavir and carbamazepine. *Pharmacotherapy* (2000) 20, 851–4.

Protease inhibitors + Antiepileptics; Lamotrigine

Lopinavir/ritonavir halved lamotrigine plasma levels, whereas the protease inhibitor levels did not appear to be altered. Saquinavir/ritonavir had similar effects in another patient and therefore reduced lamotrigine levels should be anticipated with any ritonavir-boosted regimen.

Clinical evidence

In a study in 18 healthy subjects taking lamotrigine 100 mg twice daily, **lopinavir/ritonavir** 400/100 mg twice daily for 10 days decreased the steady-state minimum plasma level of lamotrigine by 55%, decreased the AUC of lamotrigine by 46%, and increased its clearance by 85%. Doubling the dose of lamotrigine to 200 mg twice daily increased the AUC to a similar level to that seen with the lower dose without **lopinavir/ritonavir**. Pharmacokinetic parameters for **lopinavir** and **ritonavir** were similar to those in historical controls.[1] The authors of a review describe a patient taking lamotrigine 25 mg twice daily who had a favourable decline in viral load 2 months after starting to take **lopinavir/ritonavir**, lamivudine and stavudine. There was no toxicity and no recurrence of seizures.[2]

A 30-year-old woman taking nevirapine, **saquinavir** 1.2 g daily, and **ritonavir** 600 mg daily with an undetectable viral load had her epilepsy medication changed from gabapentin and lorazepam to lamotrigine and phenytoin because of an increased frequency and severity of seizures. The lamotrigine dose was eventually increased to 1.8 g daily to achieve serum levels of 5 to 8 mg/L. The **ritonavir** dose was doubled and the **saquinavir** dose increased to 2 g daily to compensate for the enzyme-inducing effects of 'phenytoin', (p.812). The patient's viral load remained undetectable, and her seizures decreased over the next 6 months, but she died suddenly of unexplained causes following a tonic-clonic seizure (autopsy not performed).[3]

Mechanism

Lopinavir/ritonavir probably decreases lamotrigine levels by induction of glucuronidation (suggested by the increase in the AUC ratio of lamotrigine 2N-glucuronide to lamotrigine).

Importance and management

The pharmacokinetic interaction would appear to be established; however, since the relationship between lamotrigine levels and efficacy is not clear, the clinical relevance of the decrease is uncertain.[1] Lamotrigine efficacy should be monitored in patients taking lopinavir/ritonavir, and probably any ritonavir-boosted regimen. Anticipate the need to increase the lamotrigine dose.

1. van der Lee MJ, Dawood L, ter Hofstede HJM, de Graaff-Teulen MJA, van Ewijk-Beneken Kolmer EWJ, Caliskan-Yassen N, Koopmans PP, Burger DM. Lopinavir/ritonavir reduces lamotrigine plasma concentrations in healthy subjects. *Clin Pharmacol Ther* (2006) 80, 159–68.
2. Liedtke MD, Lockhart SM, Rathbun RC. Anticonvulsant and antiretroviral interactions. *Ann Pharmacother* (2004) 38, 482–9.
3. Leppik IE, Gapany S, Walczak T. An HIV-positive patient with epilepsy. *Epilepsy Behav* (2003) 4 (Suppl 1), S17–S19.

Protease inhibitors + Antiepileptics; Miscellaneous

Stiripentol did not alter single-dose saquinavir pharmacokinetics in a controlled study. In one case report, ritonavir did not alter zonisamide levels.

Clinical evidence, mechanism, importance and management

(a) Stiripentol

In a crossover study in 12 healthy subjects,[1] stiripentol 1 g twice daily for 8 days had no effect on the pharmacokinetics of a single 400-mg dose of **saquinavir** given on day 8.

(b) Zonisamide

A 20-year-old HIV-positive man with epilepsy, who had his seizures controlled with carbamazepine 350 mg twice daily and zonisamide 140 mg twice daily, was admitted to hospital for review of his antiretrovirals. He started taking **ritonavir**, and after the first 200-mg dose of ritonavir his zonisamide levels remained unchanged.[2] However, his levels of 'carbamazepine', (p.810), were almost doubled.

1. Cazali N, Tran A, Treluyer JM, Rey E, d'Athis P, Vincent J, Pons G. Inhibitory effect of stiripentol on carbamazepine and saquinavir metabolism in human. *Br J Clin Pharmacol* (2003) 56, 526–36.
2. Kato Y, Fujii T, Mizoguchi N, Takata N, Ueda K, Feldman MD, Kayser SR. Potential interaction between ritonavir and carbamazepine. *Pharmacotherapy* (2000) 20, 851–4.

Protease inhibitors + Antiepileptics; Phenytoin

Nelfinavir and lopinavir/ritonavir modestly reduced phenytoin levels in pharmacokinetic studies. In case reports, ritonavir has decreased, increased or not altered phenytoin levels. Phenytoin decreased lopinavir levels, and possibly also indinavir and ritonavir levels, but did not alter nelfinavir levels.

Clinical evidence

(a) Indinavir

A 39-year-old HIV-positive man, taking phenytoin 300 mg daily, started to take indinavir 800 mg three times daily. When the phenytoin dose was reduced to 200 mg daily, the viral load dropped by almost half and his CD4 count doubled.[1]

(b) Lopinavir/Ritonavir

The concurrent use of phenytoin 300 mg once daily and lopinavir/ritonavir 400/100 mg twice daily resulted in a 30% decrease in the AUC of lopinavir and a 23% decrease in the AUC of phenytoin in studies in healthy subjects.[2]

(c) Nelfinavir

An HIV-positive man taking phenytoin and phenobarbital for epilepsy had been taking nelfinavir 750 mg three times daily and stavudine 30 mg twice daily for nearly 3 months when he had a tonic-clonic seizure. After starting nelfinavir and stavudine, serum phenytoin levels were found to have dropped from around 10 mg/L to around 5 mg/L.[3] Similarly, nelfinavir 1.25 g twice daily for 7 days decreased the AUC of phenytoin by about 30% and the maximum serum level by 21%, in healthy subjects, whereas the nelfinavir levels were not altered.[4]

(d) Ritonavir

A case report describes the intentional use of ritonavir 600 mg twice daily to boost phenytoin levels in a 14-year-old boy who had been having seizures for 28 days, despite the use of several antiepileptics. Phenytoin at 20 mg/kg daily had originally failed to produce satisfactory plasma levels, although it did reduce the rate of seizures. After starting the ritonavir his seizures were controlled and the phenytoin level became therapeutic. Seizures started again after the ritonavir was stopped.[5] Conversely, an HIV-positive patient taking carbamazepine and phenytoin had little change in his phenytoin levels, which remained at around 15 mg/L, 2 months after switching from an antiretroviral regimen including indinavir to one containing ritonavir 600 mg twice daily and **saquinavir**.[6] This was despite a 2.8-fold increase in the levels of 'carbamazepine', (p.810). Another patient taking phenobarbital, phenytoin and carbamazepine had a 32.7% drop in his phenytoin level 2 days after switching from an antiretroviral regimen including indinavir to one containing ritonavir 300 mg twice daily and **saquinavir**. The level of 'carbamazepine', (p.810) had doubled, and the level of 'phenobarbital', (p.810) was unchanged.[7]

A 30-year-old woman taking nevirapine, **saquinavir** 1.2 g daily and ritonavir 600 mg daily with undetectable viral load had her epilepsy medication changed from gabapentin and lorazepam to lamotrigine and phenytoin because of increased frequency and severity of seizures. She required phenytoin 8 mg/kg daily to maintain therapeutic serum levels. The ritonavir dose was doubled and the saquinavir dose increased to 2 g daily to compensate for the enzyme-inducing effects of phenytoin. The patient's viral load remained undetectable, and her seizures decreased over the next 6 months but she died suddenly of unexplained causes following a tonic-clonic seizure (autopsy not performed).[8]

Mechanism

Phenytoin is an inducer of the cytochrome P450 isoenzyme CYP3A4, and would be expected to increase the metabolism of the protease inhibitors, although nelfinavir levels were not altered, possibly because it is a substrate for several other isoenzymes. Phenytoin is principally metabolised by CYP2C9 and CYP2C19, and would therefore, not be expected to be substantially affected by most protease inhibitors. However, both increases and modest decreases in phenytoin levels have been seen.

Importance and management

Although information is limited, some of these interactions are expected. Phenytoin may decrease plasma levels of indinavir, lopinavir and possibly ritonavir, and the manufacturers of **darunavir**[9,10] and **saquinavir**[11,12] also predict that their levels may be reduced by phenytoin, although they note that the effect on ritonavir-boosted saquinavir has not been assessed.[11,12] Phenytoin appears not to alter nelfinavir levels.

In addition, protease inhibitors appear to alter phenytoin levels. Therefore an alternative antiepileptic, such as sodium valproate, which does not affect cytochrome P450 isoenzymes, may be more appropriate in patients taking protease inhibitors. However, if there is no option but to use phenytoin, close monitoring of antiviral efficacy and phenytoin levels is essential.

1. Campagna KD, Torbert A, Bedsole GD, Ravis WR. Possible induction of indinavir metabolism by phenytoin. *Pharmacotherapy* (1997) 17, 182.
2. Lim ML, Min SS, Eron JJ, Bertz RJ, Robinson M, Gaedigk A, Kashuba ADM. Coadministration of lopinavir/ritonavir and phenytoin results in two-way drug interaction through cytochrome P-450 induction. *J Acquir Immune Defic Syndr* (2004) 36, 1034–40.
3. Honda M, Yasuoka A, Aoki M, Oka S. A generalized seizure following initiation of nelfinavir in a patient with human immunodeficiency virus type 1 infection, suspected due to interaction between nelfinavir and phenytoin. *Intern Med* (1999) 38, 302–3.
4. Shelton MJ, Cloen D, Becker M, Hsyu PH, Wilton JH, Hewitt RG. Evaluation of the pharmacokinetic interaction between phenytoin and nelfinavir in healthy volunteers at steady state. *Intersci Conf Antimicrob Agents Chemother* (2000) 40, 426.
5. Broderick A, Webb DW, McMenamin J, Butler K. A novel use of ritonavir. *AIDS* (1998) 12 (Suppl 4), S29.
6. Berbel Garcia A, Latorre Ibarra A, Porta Etessam J, Martinez Salio A, Perez Martinez DA, Saiz Diaz R, Toledo Heras M. Protease inhibitor-induced carbamazepine toxicity. *Clin Neuropharmacol* (2000) 23, 216–18.
7. Mateu-de Antonio J, Grau S, Gimeno-Bayón J-L, Carmona A. Ritonavir-induced carbamazepine toxicity. *Ann Pharmacother* (2001) 35, 125–6.
8. Leppik IE, Gapany S, Walczak T. An HIV-positive patient with epilepsy. *Epilepsy Behav* (2003) 4 (Suppl 1), S17–S19.
9. Prezista (Darunavir ethanolate). Janssen-Cilag Ltd. UK Summary of product characteristics, July 2007.
10. Prezista (Darunavir). Tibotec, Inc. US Prescribing information, June 2006.
11. Invirase Hard Capsules (Saquinavir mesilate). Roche Products Ltd. UK Summary of product characteristics, May 2007.
12. Invirase (Saquinavir mesylate). Roche Pharmaceuticals. US Prescribing information, July 2007.

Protease inhibitors + Antiepileptics; Valproate

Lopinavir levels appeared to be raised by valproic acid in one study in HIV-positive patients, whereas valproic acid levels were not significantly different to those in a control group not taking lopinavir with ritonavir. However, in one case, starting a lopinavir/ritonavir-based antiretroviral regimen caused a decrease of

about 50% in the valproic acid level, which resulted in an exacerbation of mania. A case of hepatotoxicity has occurred in a patient taking valproic acid with nevirapine and saquinavir/ritonavir.

Clinical evidence

In a study in 8 HIV-positive patients taking **lopinavir/ritonavir** 400/100 mg twice daily plus various NRTIs, the median AUC of **lopinavir** increased by 75% without any change in the estimated half-life after taking valproic acid 250 mg twice daily for 7 days. Although the maximum and minimum **lopinavir** levels were also higher, the difference was not statistically significant. **Ritonavir** levels were not assessed. Valproic acid levels achieved in the patients taking **lopinavir/ritonavir** were not significantly different from those in 11 HIV-positive control patients mainly taking NRTI antiretrovirals, even when the 3 patients taking a protease inhibitor or NNRTI (amprenavir, indinavir, or nelfinavir plus nevirapine) were excluded.[1]

However, there is one report of a possible decrease in valproate levels in a 30-year-old man after starting **lopinavir/ritonavir**.[2] This patient, who had been taking valproic acid 375 mg daily as divalproex sodium for 7 months after an episode of mania, had a subtherapeutic valproic acid level of 197 micromol/L, and the dose was increased to 250 mg three times daily. After 25 days his trough valproic acid level was 495 micromol/L, and an antiretroviral regimen of lamivudine, zidovudine, **lopinavir/ritonavir** was started, and paroxetine for depression. Four days later he was hypomanic and the paroxetine was replaced with sertraline, which the patient discontinued. Twenty-one days later he had become increasingly manic, and the valproic acid level was found to be 238 micromol/L, about 50% lower than the previous level. An increase in valproic acid dose to 1.5 g daily was eventually required to achieve a therapeutic level of 392 micromol/L.

A case of valproate-associated hepatotoxicity occurred in a 51-year-old man about 3 weeks after starting nevirapine 200 mg twice daily, **saquinavir** 400 mg twice daily, **ritonavir** 400 mg twice daily, and stavudine. Serum valproic acid levels remained therapeutic.[3]

Mechanism

Lopinavir/ritonavir might decrease the plasma levels of valproic acid by induction of glucuronidation. See also 'lamotrigine', (p.811), which is similarly affected.

Importance and management

It has been predicted that ritonavir might reduce valproate levels,[4,5] but the case report[2] appears to be the first clinical evidence of this occurring. Other evidence from the earlier study[1] suggested valproate levels were not affected by ritonavir to a statistically significant extent, although there was a downward trend in valproic acid levels. In addition, this study unexpectedly found that lopinavir levels appeared to be higher in patients taking valproic acid, although the increase is probably not clinically relevant.[1] If possible, monitor valproate levels when any antiretroviral regimen that includes ritonavir is used. Further study is needed. Note that there has been some concern about using valproate in HIV infection but there seems to be no established reason to avoid or specifically promote the use of valproate in HIV-infection *per se*.

1. DiCenzo R, Peterson D, Cruttenden K, Morse G, Riggs G, Gelbard H, Schifitto G. Effects of valproic acid coadministration on plasma efavirenz and lopinavir concentrations in human immunodeficiency virus-infected adults. *Antimicrob Agents Chemother* (2004) 48, 4328–31.
2. Sheehan NL, Brouillette M-J, Delisle M-S, Allan J. Possible interaction between lopinavir/ritonavir and valproic acid exacerbates bipolar disorder. *Ann Pharmacother* (2006) 40, 147–50.
3. Cozza KL, Swanton EJ, Humphreys CW. Hepatotoxicity with combination of valproic acid, ritonavir, and nevirapine: a case report. *Psychosomatics* (2000) 41, 452–3.
4. Norvir (Ritonavir). Abbott Laboratories Ltd. UK Summary of product characteristics, May 2007.
5. Norvir (Ritonavir). Abbott Laboratories. US Prescribing information, January 2006.

Protease inhibitors + Atovaquone

Atovaquone modestly reduces the minimum level of indinavir. Ritonavir alone and ritonavir-boosted protease inhibitors are predicted to decrease atovaquone levels.

Clinical evidence, mechanism, importance and management

(a) Indinavir

Preliminary results from a study in healthy subjects suggest that the concurrent use of atovaquone 750 mg twice daily and indinavir 800 mg three times daily results in a minor 5% decrease in the AUC of indinavir, and a 13% increase in the AUC of atovaquone.[1] The UK manufacturer of atovaquone notes that concurrent use decreased the minimum level and AUC of indinavir by 23% and 9%, respectively. They recommend that caution should be exercised on concurrent use because of the potential risk of failure of indinavir treatment.[2] However, note that the effect was small and that indinavir is often used with other antiretrovirals, which might modify the interaction by affecting indinavir levels.

(b) Ritonavir and ritonavir-boosted protease inhibitors

The manufacturer of ritonavir predicts that it will decrease the plasma levels of atovaquone,[3,4] by inducing atovaquone glucuronidation.[4] They say that the clinical significance of this prediction is unknown, but that an increase in the atovaquone dose might be needed.[3] Careful monitoring of serum levels and/or therapeutic effects is recommended when atovaquone is given with ritonavir as a pharmacokinetic enhancer or as an antiretroviral.[4] This predicted interaction would therefore apply to **lopinavir/ritonavir**[5] and any other boosted protease inhibitors. However, there does not appear to be any actual data to prove that the interaction occurs or is clinically relevant.

1. Emmanuel A, Gillotin C, Farinotti R, Sadler BM. Atovaquone suspension and indinavir have minimal pharmacokinetic interactions. *Int Conf AIDS* (1998) 12, 90.
2. Wellvone Oral Suspension (Atovaquone). GlaxoSmithKline UK. UK Summary of product characteristics, May 2006.
3. Norvir (Ritonavir). Abbott Laboratories. US Prescribing information, January 2006.
4. Norvir Soft Capsules (Ritonavir). Abbott Laboratories Ltd. UK Summary of product characteristics, May 2007
5. Kaletra (Lopinavir/ritonavir). Abbott Laboratories. US Prescribing information, January 2007.

Protease inhibitors + Azoles; Fluconazole

Fluconazole may modestly increase the levels of saquinavir and tipranavir, but does not significantly affect ritonavir, indinavir or nelfinavir levels.

Clinical evidence

Fluconazole 400 mg on day one, followed by 200 mg daily for 4 days did not alter any of the pharmacokinetic parameters of **ritonavir** 200 mg every 6 hours by more than 15%, when given to 8 healthy subjects.[1] Similarly, fluconazole had no effect on the pharmacokinetics of **ritonavir** in 3 HIV-positive subjects.[2]

The pharmacokinetics of both **indinavir** 1 g every 8 hours and fluconazole 400 mg daily were not significantly affected by concurrent use in 11 HIV-positive patients.[3] Another study also found no significant interaction between **indinavir** and fluconazole.[4]

A population pharmacokinetic analysis estimated that fluconazole decreased **nelfinavir** clearance by 26 to 30%, but this was not considered clinically significant.[5]

Fluconazole 400 mg on day 2, followed by 200 mg daily for 6 days increased the median AUC of **saquinavir** by 50%, and the maximum level by 56% in 5 HIV-positive subjects.[2]

Fluconazole increased the AUC of **tipranavir**, and its maximum and minimum levels by 50%, 32%, and 69%, respectively, when tipranavir/ritonavir 500/200 mg was given twice daily. Fluconazole levels were not affected.[6]

Mechanism

Fluconazole is a moderate inhibitor of CYP3A4 by which the protease inhibitors are metabolised.[1,3]

Importance and management

The small to modest changes in protease inhibitor pharmacokinetics seen with fluconazole are unlikely to be of clinical significance. Because fluconazole causes a more significant increase in tipranavir levels, the manufacturer of tipranavir states that fluconazole, in doses of greater than

200 mg daily, is not recommended. No dosage adjustments are recommended for lower doses of fluconazole.[6,7]

1. Cato A, Cao G, Hsu A, Cavanaugh J, Leonard J, Granneman R. Evaluation of the effect of fluconazole on the pharmacokinetics of ritonavir. *Drug Metab Dispos* (1997) 25, 1104–1106.
2. Koks CHW, Crommentuyn KML, Hoetelmans RMW, Burger DM, Koopmans PP, Mathôt RAA, Mulder JW, Meenhorst PL, Beijnen JH. The effect of fluconazole on ritonavir and saquinavir pharmacokinetics in HIV-1-infected individuals. *Br J Clin Pharmacol* (2001) 51, 631–5.
3. De Wit S, Debier M, De Smet M, McCrea J, Stone J, Carides A, Matthews C, Deutsch P, Clumeck N. Effect of fluconazole on indinavir pharmacokinetics in human immunodeficiency virus-infected patients. *Antimicrob Agents Chemother* (1998) 42, 223–7.
4. The indinavir (MK 639) pharmacokinetic study group. Indinavir (MK 639) drug interaction studies. 11th International Conference on AIDS, Vancouver, 1996. Abstract Mo.B.174.
5. Jackson KA, Rosenbaum SE, Kerr BM, Pithavala YK, Yuen G, Dudley MN. A population pharmacokinetic analysis of nelfinavir mesylate in human immunodeficiency virus-infected patients enrolled in a phase III clinical trial. *Antimicrob Agents Chemother* (2000) 44, 1832–7.
6. Aptivus (Tipranavir). Boehringer Ingelheim. US Prescribing information, February 2007.
7. Aptivus (Tipranavir). Boehringer Ingelheim Ltd. UK Summary of product characteristics, March 2007.

Protease inhibitors + Azoles; Itraconazole

Itraconazole increases the levels of amprenavir, indinavir, lopinavir/ritonavir, and saquinavir, and may theoretically increase the levels of other protease inhibitors.

Clinical evidence

Shortly after 2 patients taking **indinavir** and another taking **saquinavir/ritonavir** were given itraconazole they were noted to have eczematous eruptions and raised serum transaminases. These effects are seen with protease inhibitors alone, and were attributed to raised levels of both medications, arising from concurrent use. The patient taking **saquinavir/ritonavir** had a very prolonged itraconazole half-life.[1] In another patient, the itraconazole dose was halved when **lopinavir/ritonavir** was started, and after 5 weeks of concurrent use the itraconazole half-life had increased about tenfold, but no signs of itraconazole toxicity were observed.[2] In a study, itraconazole caused a median fivefold increase in the AUC of **saquinavir**, and it was considered that itraconazole may be an alternative to **ritonavir** for boosting **saquinavir** levels,[3] and another study has investigated this.[4] The UK manufacturer of **indinavir** says that giving **indinavir** 600 mg every 8 hours with itraconazole 200 mg twice daily produces an AUC similar to that achieved when **indinavir** 800 mg every 8 hours is given alone.[5] The manufacturer of **amprenavir** notes that it is possible that plasma levels of itraconazole may be raised by concurrent use.[6] The manufacturer of itraconazole[7,8] says that **ritonavir** and **indinavir** may increase the bioavailability of itraconazole, since they are potent inhibitors of CYP3A4.

Mechanism

Itraconazole is a known substrate and inhibitor of the cytochrome P450 isoenzyme CYP3A4, and the protease inhibitors also inhibit and share this pathway of metabolism. Thus enzyme inhibition, and competition for metabolism results in raised serum levels of both drugs.

Importance and management

The information about the interactions of protease inhibitors with itraconazole is limited. On the basis of the available data, it is possible that itraconazole has greater effects than 'ketoconazole', (below), on protease inhibitor levels. The manufacturers of indinavir advise modestly reducing the indinavir dose to 600 mg every 8 hours if it is to be given with itraconazole.[5,9] The UK manufacturer of saquinavir recommends monitoring for saquinavir toxicity if itraconazole is used.[10] Some protease inhibitors, especially ritonavir and possibly indinavir, may increase itraconazole levels and most manufacturers say that doses of itraconazole greater than 200 mg a day are not recommended. The US manufacturers of amprenavir recommend increased monitoring for adverse effects and state that the dose of itraconazole may need to be reduced if it is greater than 400 mg daily.[11]

1. MacKenzie-Wood AR, Whitfeld MJ, Ray JE. Itraconazole and HIV protease inhibitors: an important interaction. *Med J Aust* (1999) 170, 46–7.
2. Crommentuyn KML, Mulder JW, Sparidans RW, Huitema ADR, Schellens JHM, Beijnen JH. Drug-drug interaction between itraconazole and the antiretroviral drug lopinavir/ritonavir in an HIV-1-infected patient with disseminated histoplasmosis. *Clin Infect Dis* (2004) 38, e73–e75.
3. Koks CHW, Van Heeswijk RPG, Veldkamp AI, Meenhorst PL, Mulder J-W, van der Meer JTM, Beijnen JH, Hoetelmans RMW. Itraconazole as an alternative for ritonavir liquid formulation when combined with saquinavir. *AIDS* (2000) 14, 89–90.
4. Cardiello PG, Samor T, Burger D, Hoetelmans R, Mahanontharit A, Ruxrungtham K, Lange JM, Cooper DA, Phanuphak P. Pharmacokinetics of lower doses of saquinavir soft-gel caps (800 and 1200 mg twice daily) boosted with itraconazole in HIV-1-positive patients. *Antivir Ther* (2003) 8, 245–9.
5. Crixivan (Indinavir sulfate). Merck Sharp & Dohme Ltd. UK Summary of product characteristics, May 2007.
6. Agenerase (Amprenavir). GlaxoSmithKline UK. UK Summary of product characteristics, February 2007.
7. Sporanox Capsules (Itraconazole). Janssen-Cilag Ltd. UK Summary of product characteristics, March 2004.
8. Sporanox Capsules (Itraconazole). Janssen. US Prescribing information, June 2006.
9. Crixivan (Indinavir sulfate). Merck & Co., Inc. US Prescribing information, November 2006.
10. Invirase Hard Capsules (Saquinavir mesilate). Roche Products Ltd. UK Summary of product characteristics, May 2007.
11. Agenerase (Amprenavir). GlaxoSmithKline. US Prescribing information, May 2005.

Protease inhibitors + Azoles; Ketoconazole

Ketoconazole may increase the levels of protease inhibitors, but this is usually not clinically significant. The exception may be indinavir. Most protease inhibitors increase the levels of ketoconazole.

Clinical evidence

(a) Amprenavir or Fosamprenavir

The AUC of amprenavir was increased by 32% in one study,[1] but in another, the pharmacokinetics of amprenavir were not affected when ketoconazole was given with fosamprenavir/ritonavir.[2] In a single-dose study amprenavir 1.2 g caused a 44% rise in the AUC of ketoconazole 400 mg.[1] Similarly, the AUC of ketoconazole was increased by 2.7-fold by **fosamprenavir/ritonavir**.[2]

(b) Atazanavir

The pharmacokinetics of **atazanavir** 400 mg daily were not affected by the concurrent use of ketoconazole 200 mg daily for 7 days.[3]

(c) Darunavir

Pharmacokinetic changes have been seen with the concurrent use of ketoconazole and darunavir/ritonavir: the darunavir AUC was raised by 42% and the ketoconazole AUC was increased about threefold.[4]

(d) Indinavir

Ketoconazole raises the AUC of indinavir by 62%.[5]

(e) Lopinavir

A single 200-mg dose of ketoconazole had no effect on the pharmacokinetics of lopinavir.[6] However, ketoconazole 200 mg once daily for 14 days was associated with a 68% increase in trough lopinavir levels and a 33% increase in ritonavir levels in an HIV-positive patient.[7] The AUC of a single 200-mg dose of ketoconazole was increased threefold in patients taking lopinavir/ritonavir 400/100 mg twice daily.[6]

(f) Nelfinavir

Ketoconazole raises the AUC of nelfinavir by 35%.[8]

(g) Ritonavir

Ritonavir increased the AUC of ketoconazole 3.4-fold and the maximum plasma level 1.6-fold.[9]

(h) Saquinavir with Ritonavir

In one early clinical study, patients who received the combination of ketoconazole and saquinavir had a greater drop in viral load after 3 months than those not receiving ketoconazole.[10] However, in one pharmacokinetic study, ketoconazole 200 mg for 7 days then 400 mg daily for 7 days had no consistent effect on saquinavir peak and trough plasma levels in 7 HIV-positive patients, although inter-individual variability was great. Saquinavir [as hard gelatin capsules[11]] was given at the low dose of 600 mg three times daily.[12] Conversely, when saquinavir (soft gel capsule) 1.2 g three times daily was given to 12 healthy subjects with ketoconazole 400 mg daily for 7 days, the saquinavir AUC and maximum plasma levels were raised by 190% and 171%, respectively.[11] A similar study in 22 HIV-positive patients, using ketoconazole 200 mg daily, found that the saquinavir AUC and maximum plasma levels were raised by 69% and 36%, respectively.[11] In 12 HIV-positive patients, ketoconazole 200 or 400 mg increased the AUC of saquinavir and ritonavir in combination (both 400 mg twice daily) by 37% and 29%, respectively. The distribution of ritonavir was also affected, with disproportionate rises seen in CSF concentrations. All these changes appeared to be unrelated to the dose of ketoconazole used.[13]

The peak plasma level of ketoconazole 400 mg daily was similar to that usually seen with ketoconazole 800 mg alone when saquinavir/ritonavir were given.[13] Moreover, in this study, dose escalation to higher doses of ketoconazole was discontinued after the first patient given ketoconazole 600 mg daily stopped treatment early because of adverse gastrointestinal effects.[13] However, **saquinavir** alone did not affect ketoconazole pharmacokinetics.[11]

Mechanism

Ketoconazole is a known substrate and inhibitor of the cytochrome P450 isoenzyme CYP3A4, and the protease inhibitors also inhibit and share this pathway of metabolism.[1,11,13] Thus enzyme inhibition, and competition for metabolism results in raised serum levels of both drugs. Ketoconazole may also inhibit P-glycoprotein transport of saquinavir and ritonavir, causing a decrease in their clearance, and raising serum levels.[11,13] Inhibition of P-glycoprotein may reduce efflux of protease inhibitors from the CSF, so increasing CSF levels.[13]

Importance and management

The magnitude of the changes in protease inhibitor pharmacokinetics seen with **ketoconazole** are unlikely to warrant dose changes of the protease inhibitors or cause significant increase in their adverse effects. However, the US manufacturer of indinavir recommends that the dose of indinavir be reduced to 600 mg every 8 hours when used with ketoconazole.[14] Whether the ability of ketoconazole to boost CSF exposure to protease inhibitors has a role in improving therapeutic efficacy in the CNS remains to be seen.[13]

The data on the effect of protease inhibitors on ketoconazole are more limited. Amprenavir caused a modest increase in ketoconazole levels, and the UK manufacturer of amprenavir suggests that no ketoconazole dose adjustment is necessary with amprenavir alone,[15] although the US manufacturer recommends increased monitoring for adverse effects and states that a dose reduction may be needed in patients receiving ketoconazole in doses of more than 400 mg daily.[16] However, a marked effect was seen for ritonavir alone and for ritonavir combined with darunavir, fosamprenavir, lopinavir, saquinavir and theoretically **tipranavir**. This may increase the adverse effects of ketoconazole. Most protease inhibitor manufacturers say that doses greater than 200 mg a day of ketoconazole are not recommended. Similarly, the UK manufacturers of ketoconazole and ritonavir say that a dose reduction of ketoconazole should be considered when it is given with ritonavir.[9,17]

1. Polk RE, Crouch MA, Israel DS, Pastor A, Sadler BM, Chittick GE, Symonds WT, Gouldin W, Lou Y. Pharmacokinetic interaction between ketoconazole and amprenavir after single doses in healthy men. *Pharmacotherapy* (1999) 19, 1378–84.
2. Telzir (Fosamprenavir calcium). GlaxoSmithKline UK. UK Summary of product characteristics, February 2007.
3. O'Mara EM, Randall D, Mummaneni V, Uderman H, Knox L, Schuster A, Geraldes M, Raymond R. Steady-state pharmacokinetic interaction study between BMS-232632 and ketoconazole in healthy subjects. *Intersci Conf Antimicrob Agents Chemother* (2000) 40, 335.
4. Prezista (Darunavir). Tibotec, Inc. US Prescribing information, June 2006.
5. McCrea J, Woolf E, Sterrett A, Matthews C, Deutsch P, Yeh KC, Waldman S, Bjornsson T. Effects of ketoconazole and other P450 inhibitors on the pharmacokinetics of indinavir. *Pharm Res* (1996) 13 (Suppl 9), S465.
6. Bertz R, Hsu A, Lam W, Williams L, Renz C, Karol M, Dutta S, Carr R, Zhang Y, Wang Q, Schweitzer S, Foit C, Andre A, Bernstein B, Granneman GR, Sun E. Pharmacokinetic interactions between lopinavir/ritonavir (ABT-378r) and other non-HIV drugs (abstract P291). *AIDS* (2000) 14 (Suppl 4), S100.
7. Boffito M, Bonora S, Sales P, Dal Conte I, Sinicco A, Hoggard PG, Khoo S, Back DJ, Di Perri G. Ketoconazole and lopinavir/ritonavir coadministration: boosting beyond boosting. *AIDS Res Hum Retroviruses* (2003) 19, 941–2.
8. Kerr B, Lee C, Yuen G, Anderson R, Daniels R, Grettenberger H, Liang B-H, Quart B, Sandoval T, Shetty B, Wu E, Zhang K. Overview of *in-vitro* and *in-vivo* drug interaction studies of nelfinavir mesylate (NFV), a new HIV-1 protease inhibitor. 4th Conference on Retroviruses and Opportunistic Infections, Washington DC, 1997. Session 39, Slide 373.
9. Norvir (Ritonavir). Abbott Laboratories Ltd. UK Summary of product characteristics, May 2007.
10. Jordan WC. The effectiveness of combined saquinavir and ketoconazole treatment in reducing HIV viral load. *J Natl Med Assoc* (1998) 90, 622–4.
11. Grub S, Bryson H, Goggin T, Lüdin E, Jorga K. The interaction of saquinavir (soft gelatin capsule) with ketoconazole, erythromycin and rifampicin: comparison of the effect in healthy volunteers and in HIV-infected patients. *Eur J Clin Pharmacol* (2001) 57, 115–21.
12. Collazos J, Martínez E, Mayo J, Blanco M-S. Effect of ketoconazole on plasma concentrations of saquinavir. *J Antimicrob Chemother* (2000) 46, 151–2.
13. Khaliq Y, Gallicano K, Venance S, Kravcik S, Cameron DW. Effect of ketoconazole on ritonavir and saquinavir concentrations in plasma and cerebrospinal fluid from patients infected with human immunodeficiency virus. *Clin Pharmacol Ther* (2000) 68, 637–46.
14. Crixivan (Indinavir sulfate). Merck & Co., Inc. US Prescribing information, November 2006.
15. Agenerase (Amprenavir). GlaxoSmithKline UK. UK Summary of product characteristics, February 2007.
16. Agenerase (Amprenavir). GlaxoSmithKline. US Prescribing information, May 2005.
17. Nizoral Tablets (Ketoconazole). Janssen-Cilag Ltd. UK Summary of product characteristics, October 2006.

Protease inhibitors + Azoles; Posaconazole

The manufacturer of posaconazole predicts that it will increase plasma levels of protease inhibitors via inhibition of cytochrome P450 isoenzyme CYP3A4. They recommend patients should be carefully monitored for any occurrence of toxicity during concurrent use.[1]

1. Noxafil (Posaconazole). Schering-Plough Ltd. UK Summary of product characteristics, October 2006.

Protease inhibitors + Azoles; Voriconazole

The current use of protease inhibitors and voriconazole is predicted to interfere with the metabolism of both drugs. Studies suggest that ritonavir decreases voriconazole levels, but no interaction was seen between indinavir and voriconazole in one study.

Clinical evidence

In a study in 18 healthy subjects, the pharmacokinetics of both **indinavir** 800 mg three times daily and voriconazole 200 mg twice daily were unaffected by at least a week of concurrent use.[1] However, *in vitro* studies suggest that the metabolism of HIV-protease inhibitors may be inhibited by voriconazole, and the metabolism of voriconazole may be inhibited by HIV-protease inhibitors. The manufacturer therefore suggests that patients should be carefully monitored for evidence of drug toxicity and/or loss of efficacy during concurrent use of other HIV-protease inhibitors (**amprenavir**, **nelfinavir** and **saquinavir** are specifically mentioned).[2]

In healthy subjects **ritonavir** 400 mg twice daily for 9 days decreased the steady-state maximum levels and AUC of oral voriconazole (400 mg twice daily for 1 day, then 200 mg twice daily for 8 days) by 66% and 82%, respectively.[3] The pharmacokinetics of the **ritonavir** remained unchanged. Low-dose ritonavir (100 mg daily) decreased the AUC of voriconazole by 39% and the AUC of the ritonavir was decreased by 14%.[3]

Mechanism

Voriconazole is an inhibitor and a substrate of the cytochrome P450 isoenzyme CYP3A4: protease inhibitors are also metabolised by this route, and can, to varying degrees, also inhibit this isoenzyme.

Importance and management

The manufacturers of **voriconazole** say that the concurrent use of ritonavir (at doses of 400 mg and above twice daily) is contraindicated,[2,3] presumably because the efficacy of the voriconazole is expected to be markedly reduced. The manufacturer of ritonavir also recommends that when it is used as a pharmacokinetic enhancer (usually 100 mg twice daily) voriconazole should only be given if the benefits outweigh the risks.[4] Most protease inhibitors are given with ritonavir as a pharmacokinetic enhancer; however, caution is also warranted if they are given alone, as all the protease inhibitors can inhibit CYP3A4 to some extent and may therefore also increase voriconazole levels. Voriconazole may also affect protease inhibitor levels, but other than ritonavir and indinavir, which are not affected this does not appear to have been studied. Be aware that some increase in their levels is theoretically possible if voriconazole is given.

1. Purkins L, Wood N, Kleinermans D, Love ER. No clinically significant pharmacokinetic interactions between voriconazole and indinavir in healthy volunteers. *Br J Clin Pharmacol* (2003) 56 (Suppl 1), 62–8.
2. VFEND (Voriconazole). Pfizer Ltd. UK Summary of product characteristics, July 2007.
3. VFEND (Voriconazole). Pfizer Inc. US Prescribing information, November 2006.
4. Norvir (Ritonavir). Abbott Laboratories Ltd. UK Summary of product characteristics, May 2007.

Protease inhibitors + Cannabinoids

The short-term use of cannabis cigarettes or dronabinol did not appear to adversely affect indinavir or nelfinavir levels or viral loads in HIV-positive patients.

Clinical evidence

In 9 HIV-positive patients on a stable regimen containing **indinavir** (mostly 800 mg every 8 hours), smoking a **cannabis cigarette** (3.95% tetrahydrocannabinol) three times a day before meals for 14 days resulted in a median 14% decrease in AUC and maximum level and a 34% decrease in minimum indinavir level. However, only the change in maximum level was statistically significant.[1] Similarly, **dronabinol** 2.5 mg three times daily for 14 days had no significant effect on **indinavir** pharmacokinetics.[1]

In another 11 patients on a stable regimen containing **nelfinavir** 750 mg three times daily, there was a non-significant 10% decrease in AUC, 17% decrease in maximum level, and 12% decrease in minimum nelfinavir level after 14 days of **cannabis cigarettes.**[1] Similarly, **dronabinol** 2.5 mg three times daily for 14 days had no significant effect on **nelfinavir** pharmacokinetics.[1]

There was no adverse effect on viral load or CD4 count in the patients receiving cannabis cigarettes or dronabinol.[2]

Mechanism

Unknown.

Importance and management

Short-term use of cannabis cigarettes or dronabinol does not appear to have any important effect on levels of indinavir or nelfinavir, nor on markers of HIV infection.

1. Kosel BW, Aweeka FT, Benowitz NL, Shade SB, Hilton JF, Lizak PS, Abrams DI. The effects of cannabinoids on the pharmacokinetics of indinavir and nelfinavir. *AIDS* (2002) 16, 543–50.
2. Abrams DI, Hilton JF, Leiser RJ, Shade SB, Elbeik TA, Aweeka FT, Benowitz NL, Bredt BM, Kosel B, Aberg JA, Deeks SG, Mitchell TF, Mulligan K, Bacchetti P, McCune JM, Schambelan M. Short-term effects of cannabinoids in patients with HIV-1 infection: a randomized, placebo-controlled clinical trial. *Ann Intern Med* (2003) 139, 258–66.

Protease inhibitors + Co-trimoxazole

Minor pharmacokinetic changes have been seen when co-trimoxazole is given with the protease inhibitors, but these changes are not considered to be clinically significant.

Clinical evidence, mechanism, importance and management

A study in 12 healthy subjects given **indinavir** 400 mg every 6 hours with co-trimoxazole 960 mg every 12 hours found that there was no change in the AUC of **indinavir**, but a small 17% decrease in **indinavir** trough levels. In addition, there was an 18% increase in the AUC of **trimethoprim**, and a 5% increase in the AUC of **sulfamethoxazole**. None of these changes were considered to be clinically important.[1]

Ritonavir 500 mg twice daily caused a 20% increase in the AUC of **trimethoprim** and a 20% decrease in the AUC of **sulfamethoxazole** when a single 960-mg dose of co-trimoxazole was given to 15 healthy subjects. These changes were considered too small to be of clinical relevance.[2] The pharmacokinetics of **ritonavir** were not assessed.

The combination of **saquinavir** 600 mg three times daily and co-trimoxazole 960 mg three times weekly caused no changes in the pharmacokinetics of **saquinavir**.[3]

There would seem to be no reason for avoiding the use of co-trimoxazole with any of the protease inhibitors.

1. Sturgill MG, Seibold JR, Boruchoff SE, Yeh KC, Haddix H, Deutsch P. Trimethoprim/sulfamethoxazole does not affect the steady-state disposition of indinavir. *J Clin Pharmacol* (1999) 39, 1077–84.
2. Bertz RJ, Cao G, Cavanaugh JH, Hsu A, Granneman GR, Leonard JM. Effect of ritonavir on the pharmacokinetics of trimethoprim/sulfamethoxazole. 11th International Conference on AIDS, Vancouver, 1996. Abstract Mo.B.1197.
3. Maserati R, Villani P, Cocchi L, Regazzi MB. Co-trimoxazole administered for *Pneumocystis carinii* pneumonia prophylaxis does not interfere with saquinavir pharmacokinetics. *AIDS* (1998) 12, 815–6.

Protease inhibitors + Drugs that affect gastric pH

Proton pump inhibitors (marked effect) and H2-receptor antagonists (modest effect) reduce atazanavir levels. Other drugs that increase gastric pH are also predicted to reduce plasma levels of atazanavir. Fosamprenavir may be similarly affected (moderate effects seen with ranitidine), although antacids and esomeprazole had little effect in one study. Omeprazole decreases indinavir levels and an antacid modestly decreased tipranavir levels. Neither ranitidine nor omeprazole had any effect on darunavir/ritonavir or lopinavir/ritonavir levels. In contrast, cimetidine, ranitidine and omeprazole have been shown to increase saquinavir levels.

Clinical evidence

(a) Atazanavir

1. H_2-receptor antagonists. In a study in healthy subjects **famotidine** 40 mg twice daily reduced the atazanavir AUC, maximum, and minimum levels by 18%, 14%, and 28%, respectively, when given simultaneously with atazanavir/ritonavir 300/100 mg once daily.[1,2] A greater effect (41% reduction in AUC) was seen when the drugs were given again without ritonavir, but little effect was seen when the atazanavir was given 10 hours after and 2 hours before the **famotidine**.[2] In a randomised study in healthy subjects, **ranitidine** 150 mg one hour before breakfast reduced the atazanavir AUC, maximum, and minimum levels by 48%, 52%, and 43%, respectively, when atazanavir/ritonavir 300/100 mg once daily was taken 30 minutes after breakfast.[3]

2. Proton pump inhibitors. The AUC of atazanavir was reduced by 76% and the trough plasma level by 78% when atazanavir/ritonavir 300/100 mg was given with **omeprazole** 40 mg. Increasing the dose of atazanavir/ritonavir to 400/100 mg did not negate the effects of this interaction.[4,5] An even greater effect (94% reduction in AUC) was seen when atazanavir alone was given with omeprazole,[2] and the same effect was seen with **lansoprazole**.[6] Similar results were found in another study with **omeprazole**: ritonavir levels were not affected.[3]

Atazanavir trough levels were significantly lower in patients taking proton pump inhibitors than in those taking H_2-receptor antagonists in another study.[7] A 65-year-old HIV-positive man had a marked reduction in atazanavir trough levels and AUC in a 12-hour study while receiving **esomeprazole** and atazanavir/ritonavir.[8]

However, 9 of 12 subjects had a successful virological outcome while taking atazanavir with or without ritonavir together with a proton pump inhibitor (**esomeprazole**, **lansoprazole**, **omeprazole**, **pantoprazole**, **rabeprazole**) in a retrospective analysis of concurrent use.[9] Another retrospective analysis also found no difference in virological outcome in patients taking atazanavir/ritonavir with proton pump inhibitors (**rabeprazole**, **omeprazole**; 10 patients) and 66 patients not taking proton pump inhibitors.[10] Similarly, in one patient taking atazanavir/ritonavir 300/100 mg once daily, tenofovir and lamivudine, and **lansoprazole** 30 mg twice daily, the AUC, maximum, and minimum levels of atazanavir were higher than those seen historically with atazanavir/ritonavir plus tenofovir.[11] Another patient maintained virological suppression when **omeprazole** 20 mg daily was taken with ritonavir-boosted atazanavir 150 mg twice daily.[12]

(b) Darunavir with Ritonavir

In a crossover study in 16 healthy subjects, neither **omeprazole** 20 mg daily nor **ranitidine** 150 mg twice daily had a significant effect on the AUC or minimum level of darunavir after darunavir/ritonavir 400/100 mg was given twice daily for 5 days.[13]

(c) Fosamprenavir

In a crossover study in healthy subjects the AUC of amprenavir (derived from a single 1.4-g dose of fosamprenavir) was decreased by 18% and the maximum plasma level by 35%, but the minimum level was not significantly altered by the concurrent use of 30 mL of an **aluminium/magnesium hydroxide antacid** *(Maalox TC)*.[14]

In the same study, **ranitidine** 300 mg given one hour before fosamprenavir 1.4 g decreased the AUC of amprenavir by 30% and the maximum level by 51% without altering the minimum level.[14]

In contrast, **esomeprazole** 20 mg once daily had no effect on the steady-state pharmacokinetics of amprenavir after either fosamprenavir 1.4 g twice daily or fosamprenavir/ritonavir 700/100 mg twice daily in studies in healthy subjects. However, fosamprenavir 1.4 g twice daily increased the **esomeprazole** AUC by 55%. In this study, the daily dose of esomeprazole was given simultaneously with the first dose of protease inhibitor.[15] Similarly, no pharmacokinetic interaction was apparent in an 8-hour study in a 65-year-old HIV-positive who was given fosamprenavir/ritonavir with **esomeprazole**.[8]

(d) Indinavir

The manufacturer notes that **cimetidine** 600 mg twice daily for 6 days had no clinically significant effect on the pharmacokinetics of a single 400-mg dose of indinavir in a study in 12 healthy subjects.[16]

In a study in 8 healthy subjects given **omeprazole** 40 mg daily with a single 800-mg dose of indinavir, half of them had a clinically significant decrease in the plasma levels of indinavir; no significant pharmacokinetic changes occurred in the others.[17] In a review by the same authors, 4 of 9 patients taking **omeprazole** with indinavir had plasma levels of indinavir lower than expected. In two patients, increasing the indinavir dose from 800 mg to 1 g, three times daily, resulted in acceptable plasma levels.[18] In a later randomised controlled study, **omeprazole** 40 mg once daily for 7 days reduced the AUC of indinavir 800 mg by 47% in 14 subjects. However, the addition of ritonavir 200 mg to the indinavir negated the effect of the **omeprazole**.[19]

Note that 'buffered didanosine tablets', (p.804), has also been shown to reduce indinavir levels.

(e) Lopinavir/Ritonavir

In a randomised study in healthy subjects, **omeprazole** 40 mg once daily or **ranitidine** 150 mg one hour before breakfast had no effect on the relative bioavailability of either lopinavir or ritonavir when lopinavir/ritonavir 800/200 mg once daily was taken 30 minutes after breakfast, or when lopinavir/ritonavir 400/100 mg twice daily (30 minutes after a meal) was given 1.5 hours after the acid-reducing drug. The lopinavir/ritonavir was taken in a tablet form.[3]

In a clinical study of lopinavir/ritonavir once daily (8 study patients, 86 control patients) or twice daily (7 study patients, 45 control patients) in combination with tenofovir and emtricitabine, trough levels of lopinavir were assessed at 4, 8, 16, 24 and 48 weeks: patients taking acid-reducing drugs (**proton pump inhibitors** 67%, **H_2-receptor antagonists** or **antacids**) were then compared with control patients not using acid-reducing drugs. There was no significant difference in trough lopinavir levels between the patients taking acid-reducing drugs and the controls, except that at week 24 the trough level of lopinavir was 50% higher, and at week 48 it was 73% higher, in users of acid-reducing drugs taking lopinavir/ritonavir once daily. No difference was seen in the group taking lopinavir/ritonavir twice daily.[20]

(f) Saquinavir

When cimetidine was given with saquinavir the AUC of saquinavir 1.2 g *twice* daily was 120% greater when it was given with cimetidine 400 mg twice daily, when compared with saquinavir 1.2 g *three* times daily alone.[21] In a study in 12 healthy subjects, the AUC of saquinavir given with food was 67% higher when it was given after two 150-mg doses of **ranitidine** given 12 hours and 1 hour before the saquinavir.[22]

Omeprazole 40 mg daily increased the AUC of saquinavir by 82% when saquinavir/ritonavir 1000/100 mg was given twice daily to 18 healthy subjects.[23]

(g) Tipranavir

In a single-dose study in healthy subjects, 20 mL of an **aluminium/magnesium hydroxide** antacid *(Maalox Plus)* decreased the AUC, minimum and maximum levels of tipranavir by 25 to 29%, after simultaneous ingestion of tipranavir/ritonavir 500/200 mg.[24-26]

Mechanism

The UK manufacturer of indinavir states that a normal (acidic) gastric pH may be necessary for optimum absorption of indinavir.[27] Any drug that increases the gastric pH could therefore potentially reduce absorption. Altered gastric pH may also account for the interaction with atazanavir.[4] Cimetidine probably boosts saquinavir levels by inhibiting the first-pass metabolism of saquinavir.[21] It is not understood why ranitidine and omeprazole increase saquinavir levels.

Importance and management

The marked pharmacokinetic interaction of omeprazole with **atazanavir** (with or without ritonavir) is established, and lansoprazole appears to act similarly. Based on the available data, advice in Europe[4] and the USA[5] is that atazanavir or atazanavir/ritonavir should not be given with omeprazole or other proton pump inhibitors. Modest effects were seen with atazanavir and simultaneous famotidine, whereas ranitidine taken 1.5 hours before atazanavir/ritonavir had a more marked effect. The manufacturer says that no dosage adjustment of atazanavir/ritonavir is required when it is given with an H_2-receptor antagonist, all as a single daily dose with food. However, they caution that the magnitude of the interaction may be more pronounced in HIV-positive patients (as the intragastric pH may be higher in this population). To avoid any interaction they suggest that atazanavir/ritonavir should be given once daily with food, 2 hours before and at least 10 hours after the dose of the H_2-receptor antagonist. In addition, they recommend atazanavir should be given 2 hours before or 1 hour after buffered medicinal products.[1,2] This would include didanosine buffered tablets (see 'NRTIs + Protease inhibitors', p.804).

Based on the limited data with other protease inhibitors, the manufacturer of **amprenavir** also recommends it should not be given within 1 hour of antacids.[28,29] The decrease in amprenavir levels seen when **fosamprenavir** is given with an antacid are not considered clinically relevant, and no fosamprenavir dose adjustments are likely to be necessary. Greater decreases were seen with ranitidine, although the minimum levels were unchanged. The UK manufacturer[30] states that no fosamprenavir dose adjustment is needed with ranitidine or other H_2-receptor antagonists; however, the US manufacturer[31] says the combination should be used with caution because fosamprenavir may be less effective. However, no interaction occurred with esomeprazole, and this, or other proton pump inhibitors may be given at the same time as fosamprenavir.

The interaction between omeprazole and indinavir would appear to be established. Omeprazole should probably not be used with indinavir unless ritonavir is used to boost the indinavir levels.[19] This would likely apply to other proton pump inhibitors used with indinavir as well.

Antacids modestly decreased **tipranavir** levels, and administration should be separated by at least 2 hours.[26]

Cimetidine very markedly increases **saquinavir** levels, and further study is required to discover whether this is clinically useful.[21] Ranitidine and omeprazole cause a fairly marked increase in saquinavir levels, although this is probably not clinically relevant.

Omeprazole and ranitidine do not appear to alter the pharmacokinetics of **darunavir**/ritonavir or **lopinavir**/ritonavir.

1. Reyataz (Atazanavir sulfate). Bristol-Myers Squibb Pharmaceuticals Ltd. UK Summary of product characteristics, April 2007.
2. Reyataz (Atazanavir sulfate). Bristol-Myers Squibb Company. US Prescribing information, March 2007.
3. Klein CE, Chiu Y-L, Cai Y, Beck K, King KR, Causemaker SJ, Doan TT, Esslinger HU, Podsadecki TJ, Hanna GJ. Lack of effect of acid reducing agents on the pharmacokinetics of lopinavir/ritonavir tablet formulation. 13th Conference on Retroviruses and Opportunistic Infections, Denver, 5–8 Feb 2006. 578. Available at: http://www.retroconference.org/2006/PDFs/578.pdf (accessed 21/08/07).
4. EMEA public statement. Important new pharmacokinetic data demonstrating that REYATAZ (atazanavir sulfate) combined with NORVIR (ritonavir) and omeprazole should not be co-administered. London, 21 December 2004. Available at: http://www.emea.eu.int/pdfs/human/press/pus/20264904en.pdf (accessed 21/08/07).
5. Bristol-Myers Squibb Company. Re: Reyataz® (atazanavir sulfate) with or without Norvir® (ritonavir) and proton pump inhibitors should not be coadministered: important new pharmacokinetic data, December 2004. Available at: http://www.fda.gov/oashi/aids/listserv/2004/reyataz.pdf (accessed 21/08/07).
6. Tomilo DL, Smith PF, Ogundele AB, Difrancesco R, Berenson CS, Eberhardt E, Bednarczyk E, Morse GD. Inhibition of atazanavir oral absorption by lansoprazole gastric acid suppression in healthy volunteers. *Pharmacotherapy* (2006) 26, 341–6.
7. Khanlou H, Farthing C. Co-administration of atazanavir with proton-pump inhibitors and H_2 blockers. *J Acquir Immune Defic Syndr* (2005) 39, 503.
8. Kiser JJ, Lichtenstein KA, Anderson PL, Fletcher CV. Effects of esomeprazole on the pharmacokinetics of atazanavir and fosamprenavir in a patient with human immunodeficiency virus infection. *Pharmacotherapy* (2006) 26, 511–14.
9. Sahloff EG, Duggan JM. Clinical outcomes associated with concomitant use of atazanavir and proton pump inhibitors. *Ann Pharmacother* (2006) 40, 1731–6.
10. Furtek KJ, Crum NF, Olson PE, Wallace MR. Proton pump inhibitor therapy in atazanavir-treated patients: contraindicated? *J Acquir Immune Defic Syndr* (2006) 41, 394–6.
11. Kosel BW, Storey SS, Collier AC. Lack of interaction between atazanavir and lansoprazole. *AIDS* (2005) 19, 637–8.
12. Chan-Tack KM, Edozien A. Ritonavir-boosted atazanavir may be efficacious in HIV-infected patients concurrently receiving omeprazole. *Clin Infect Dis* (2006) 42, 1344.
13. Sekar VJ, Lefebvre E, De Paepe E, De Marez T, De Pauw M, Parys W, Hoetelmans RM. Pharmacokinetic interaction between darunavir boosted with ritonavir and omeprazole or ranitidine in human immunodeficiency virus-negative healthy volunteers. *Antimicrob Agents Chemother* (2007) 51, 958–61.
14. Ford SL, Wire MB, Lou Y, Baker KL, Stein DS. Effect of antacids and ranitidine on the single-dose pharmacokinetics of fosamprenavir. *Antimicrob Agents Chemother* (2005) 49, 467–9.
15. Shelton MJ, Ford SL, Borland J, Lou Y, Wire MB, Min SS, Xue ZG, Yuen G. Coadministration of esomeprazole with fosamprenavir has no impact on steady-state plasma amprenavir pharmacokinetics. *J Acquir Immune Defic Syndr* (2006) 42, 61–7.
16. Crixivan (Indinavir sulfate). Merck & Co., Inc. US Prescribing information, November 2006.

17. Hugen PWH, Burger DM, ter Hofstede HJM, Koopmans PP. Concomitant use of indinavir and omeprazole; risk of antiretroviral subtherapy. *AIDS* (1998) 12 (Suppl 4), S29.
18. Burger DM, Hugen PWH, Kroon FP, Groeneveld P, Brinkman K, Foudraine NA, Sprenger H, Koopmans PP, Hekster YA. Pharmacokinetic interaction between the proton pump inhibitor omeprazole and the HIV protease inhibitor indinavir. *AIDS* (1998) 12, 2080–2.
19. Rublein JC, Donovan BJ, Hollowell SB, Min SS, Theodore D, Raasch RH, Kashuba ADM. Effect of omeprazole on the plasma concentrations of indinavir in HIV-negative subjects. *Intersci Conf Antimicrob Agents Chemother* (2003) 43, 35.
20. Bertz RJ, Chiu Y-L, Naylor C, Luff K, Brun SC. Lack of effect of gastric acid reducing agents on lopinavir/ritonavir plasma concentrations in HIV-infected patients. 7th Int Cong Drug Therapy HIV, Glasgow, Nov 14–18 2004. P279.
21. Boffito M, Carriero P, Trentini L, Raiteri R, Bonora S, Sinicco A, Reynolds HE, Hoggard PG, Back DJ, Di Perri G. Pharmacokinetics of saquinavir co-administered with cimetidine. *J Antimicrob Chemother* (2002) 50, 1081–4.
22. Kakuda TN, Falcon RW. Effect of food and ranitidine on saquinavir pharmacokinetics and gastric pH in healthy volunteers. *Pharmacotherapy* (2006) 26, 1060–8.
23. Winston A, Back D, Fletcher C, Robinson L, Unsworth J, Tolowinska I, Schutz M, Pozniak AL, Gazzard B, Boffito M. Effect of omeprazole on the pharmacokinetics of saquinavir-500 mg formulation with ritonavir in healthy male and female volunteers. *AIDS* (2006) 20, 1401–6.
24. Boffito M, Maitland D, Pozniak A. Practical perspectives on the use of tipranavir in combination with other medications: lessons learned from pharmacokinetic studies. *J Clin Pharmacol* (2006) 46, 130–9.
25. Aptivus (Tipranavir). Boehringer Ingelheim. US Prescribing information, February 2007.
26. Aptivus (Tipranavir). Boehringer Ingelheim Ltd. UK Summary of product characteristics, March 2007.
27. Crixivan (Indinavir sulfate). Merck Sharp & Dohme Ltd. UK Summary of product characteristics, May 2007.
28. Agenerase (Amprenavir). GlaxoSmithKline UK. UK Summary of product characteristics, February 2007.
29. Agenerase (Amprenavir). GlaxoSmithKline. US Prescribing information, May 2005.
30. Telzir (Fosamprenavir calcium). GlaxoSmithKline UK. UK Summary of product characteristics, February 2007.
31. Lexiva (Fosamprenavir calcium). GlaxoSmithKline. US Prescribing information, June 2007.

Protease inhibitors + Food

Food increases the bioavailability of atazanavir, darunavir, lopinavir/ritonavir soft capsules and solution, nelfinavir, saquinavir (all formulations) and tipranavir, but decreases that of indinavir. Food only minimally affects the bioavailability of amprenavir, fosamprenavir, lopinavir/ritonavir tablets and ritonavir. Mixing ritonavir with enteral feeds does not affect the pharmacokinetics of ritonavir.

Clinical evidence, mechanism, importance and management

(a) Absorption decreased

A single 600-mg dose of **indinavir** was given to 7 HIV-positive subjects immediately after various types of meal. The **protein**, **carbohydrate**, **fat** and **high-viscosity meals** reduced the AUC of **indinavir** by 68%, 45%, 34% and 30%, respectively. The fat meal was associated with the largest inter-subject variation in bioavailability. The effect of the protein meal was attributed to the fact that it raised gastric pH and therefore impaired the absorption of **indinavir** (a weak base). The impairment of **indinavir** absorption caused by the other meals, which did not alter gastric pH, may have been due to delayed gastric emptying.[1] A similar study comparing a full breakfast with light breakfasts (toast or cereal) on indinavir absorption found that the full breakfast reduced the absorption of **indinavir** by 78% and reduced its maximum serum levels by 86%, while the light breakfasts had no significant effect.[2] The manufacturers advise that **indinavir** is given 1 hour before or 2 hours after meals, or with low-fat light meals only.[3,4] The US information gives examples of a light meal, such as dry toast with jam, juice, and coffee with skimmed milk and sugar; or corn flakes, skimmed milk and sugar.[4]

(b) Absorption increased

1. Atazanavir. The manufacturers of atazanavir note that administration with a light or high-fat meal decreased the wide variation in plasma levels. They recommend that atazanavir should be taken with food to enhance bioavailability and minimise variability.[5,6]

2. Darunavir with Ritonavir. The manufacturers of darunavir notes that the relative bioavailability of darunavir (with low-dose ritonavir) is 30% lower when it is given without food, compared with intake with food. Therefore, darunavir tablets should be taken with ritonavir and with food. They say that the type of food does not affect exposure to darunavir.[7,8]

3. Lopinavir/Ritonavir. A moderate-fat meal increased the AUC and maximum level of lopinavir capsules by 48% and 23%, respectively, and a high-fat meal by 96% and 43%, respectively. The corresponding increases for lopinavir solution were 80% and 54% for the moderate-fat meal, and 130% and 56% for the high-fat meal.[9] The manufacturers of lopinavir/ritonavir soft *capsules* and *oral solution* say that it should be taken with food.[9,10] No clinically significant difference was seen in the bioavailability of lopinavir/ritonavir *tablets* between fasting and fed subjects, therefore the manufacturers say that it can be taken with or without food.[10,11]

4. Nelfinavir. When nelfinavir 400 or 800 mg was given to 12 healthy subjects in the fasted state, the AUC was only 27% to 50% of that observed when nelfinavir was given with a meal.[12] Nelfinavir should be taken with food.[13,14]

5. Saquinavir. The manufacturer of saquinavir hard capsules and tablets notes that, in a crossover study in 22 HIV-positive patients taking saquinavir/ritonavir 1000/100 mg twice daily and receiving three consecutive doses under fasting conditions or after a high-fat, high-calorie meal, the AUC, maximum and minimum levels of saquinavir under fasting conditions were about 70% lower than with a high-fat meal. There were no clinically significant differences in the pharmacokinetic profile of ritonavir in fasting and fed conditions but the ritonavir minimum level was about 30% lower in the fasting state, when compared with its administration with a meal.[15,16] Saquinavir/ritonavir should be given with, or up to 2 hours after, a meal.[15-17]

6. Tipranavir. The US manufacturer states that the bioavailability of tipranavir is increased if it is taken with a high-fat meal.[18] In a study, tipranavir capsules were given with a high-fat meal or a light snack of toast and skimmed milk. A high-fat meal enhanced the AUC by 31%, but had minimal 16% effect on peak tipranavir levels. The UK manufacturer states that food improves the tolerability of tipranavir/ritonavir.[19] Both manufacturers recommend that tipranavir with ritonavir should be taken with food.[18,19]

(c) Absorption minimally affected

1. Amprenavir. Food resulted in a 25% reduction in the AUC of amprenavir, but no change in the steady-state trough level. Consequently, the manufacturers say it can be given with or without food,[20,21] but the US manufacturer says not with a high-fat meal.[21]

2. Fosamprenavir. The manufacturer states that taking the fosamprenavir tablet formulation with a high-fat meal did not alter plasma amprenavir pharmacokinetics (derived from fosamprenavir) when compared with taking this formulation in the fasted state. Fosamprenavir tablets may be taken without regard to food intake.[22,23]

3. Ritonavir. The US manufacturer notes that a meal increased the absorption of ritonavir capsules by 13%, when compared with the fasting state, whereas the absorption of the oral solution was decreased by 7%.[24] See also *Lopinavir* and *Saquinavir*, above. Although these changes are modest the manufacturers state that ritonavir capsules and solution are preferably taken with food.[24-26] There is also some evidence that mixing ritonavir with **enteral feeds** does not affect ritonavir pharmacokinetics. A 600-mg dose of **ritonavir** oral solution was mixed with 240 mL of **enteral feeds** (either *Advera* or *Ensure*), **chocolate milk** or water within 1 hour of dosing. When given up to 15 minutes after a low-fat meal, the pharmacokinetics of ritonavir in either of the **enteral feeds** or the **milk** were almost identical to those when ritonavir was given in water.[27]

1. Carver PL, Fleisher D, Zhou SY, Kaul D, Kazanjian P, Li C. Meal composition effects on the oral bioavailability of indinavir in HIV-infected patients. *Pharm Res* (1999) 16, 718–24.
2. Stone JA, Ju WD, Steritt A, Woolf EJ, Yeh KC, Deutsch P, Waldman S, Bjornsson TD. Effect of food on the pharmacokinetics of indinavir in man. *Pharm Res* (1996) 13 (Suppl 9), S414.
3. Crixivan (Indinavir sulfate). Merck Sharp & Dohme Ltd. UK Summary of product characteristics, May 2007.
4. Crixivan (Indinavir sulfate). Merck & Co., Inc. US Prescribing information, November 2006.
5. Reyataz (Atazanavir sulfate). Bristol-Myers Squibb Pharmaceuticals Ltd. UK Summary of product characteristics, April 2007.
6. Reyataz (Atazanavir sulfate). Bristol-Myers Squibb Company. US Prescribing information, March 2007.
7. Prezista (Darunavir ethanolate). Janssen-Cilag Ltd. UK Summary of product characteristics, July 2007.
8. Prezista (Darunavir). Tibotec, Inc. US Prescribing information, June 2006.
9. Kaletra Soft Capsules (Lopinavir/ritonavir). Abbott Laboratories Ltd. UK Summary of product characteristics, March 2007.
10. Kaletra (Lopinavir/ritonavir). Abbott Laboratories. US Prescribing information, January 2007.
11. Kaletra Tablets (Lopinavir/ritonavir). Abbott Laboratories Ltd. UK Summary of product characteristics, March 2007.
12. Quart BD, Chapman SK, Peterkin J, Webber S, Oliver S. Phase I safety, tolerance, pharmacokinetics and food effect studies of AG1343--a novel HIV protease inhibitor. The American Society for Microbiology in collaboration with NIH and CDC. 2nd National Conference Human Retroviruses and Related Infections, Washington DC, 1995. Abstract LB3.
13. Viracept (Nelfinavir mesilate). Roche Products Ltd. UK Summary of product characteristics, January 2007.
14. Viracept (Nelfinavir mesylate). Agouron Pharmaceuticals, Inc. US Prescribing information, January 2007.
15. Invirase Hard Capsules (Saquinavir mesilate). Roche Products Ltd. UK Summary of product characteristics, May 2007.
16. Invirase Tablets (Saquinavir mesilate). Roche Products Ltd. UK Summary of product characteristics, May 2007.

17. Invirase (Saquinavir mesylate). Roche Pharmaceuticals. US Prescribing information, July 2007.
18. Aptivus (Tipranavir). Boehringer Ingelheim. US Prescribing information, February 2007.
19. Aptivus (Tipranavir). Boehringer Ingelheim Ltd. UK Summary of product characteristics, March 2007.
20. Agenerase (Amprenavir). GlaxoSmithKline UK. UK Summary of product characteristics, February 2007.
21. Agenerase (Amprenavir). GlaxoSmithKline. US Prescribing information, May 2005.
22. Telzir (Fosamprenavir calcium). GlaxoSmithKline UK. UK Summary of product characteristics, February 2007.
23. Lexiva (Fosamprenavir calcium). GlaxoSmithKline. US Prescribing information, June 2007.
24. Norvir (Ritonavir). Abbott Laboratories. US Prescribing information, January 2006.
25. Norvir Oral Solution (Ritonavir). Abbott Laboratories Ltd. UK Summary of product characteristics, May 2007.
26. Norvir Soft Capsules (Ritonavir). Abbott Laboratories Ltd. UK Summary of product characteristics, May 2007.
27. Bertz R, Shi H, Cavanaugh J, Hsu A. Effect of three vehicles, Advera®, Ensure® and chocolate milk, on the bioavailability of an oral liquid formulation of Norvir (Ritonavir). *Intersci Conf Antimicrob Agents Chemother* (1996) 36, 5.

Protease inhibitors + Garlic

A garlic supplement reduced the plasma levels of saquinavir by 50% in one study, but had little effect in another. Another garlic supplement did not significantly affect the pharmacokinetics of a single dose of ritonavir.

Clinical evidence

In a study in 9 healthy subjects garlic reduced the AUC, and maximum and minimum plasma levels of **saquinavir** by about 50%. The garlic was taken in the form of a dietary supplement (*GarliPure, Maximum Allicin Formula* caplets) twice daily for 20 days. **Saquinavir** 1.2 g three times daily was given for 4-day periods before, during, and after the garlic supplement. Fourteen days after the garlic supplement was stopped the **saquinavir** pharmacokinetics had still not returned to baseline values. Of the 9 subjects, 6 had a substantial drop in the AUC of **saquinavir** while taking garlic, then a rise when garlic was stopped. The remaining 3 had no change in the AUC of **saquinavir** while taking garlic, but had a drop when garlic was stopped.[1] However, in another study, garlic extract (*Garlipure*) 1.2 g daily for 3 weeks had no significant effect on the pharmacokinetics of a single 1.2-g dose of **saquinavir** (a slight decrease in AUC in 7 subjects and a slight increase in 3).[2]

Gastrointestinal toxicity was noted in 2 patients taking garlic or garlic supplements when they started to take **ritonavir**-containing regimens.[3] However, in a study in 10 healthy subjects the use of a garlic extract (10 mg, equivalent to 1 g of fresh garlic) twice daily for 4 days did not significantly affect the pharmacokinetics of a single 400-mg dose of **ritonavir**. There was a non-significant 17% decrease in the AUC of **ritonavir**. The garlic was given in the form of capsules (*Natural Source Odourless Garlic Life Brand*).[4]

Mechanism

The mechanism of this interaction is uncertain, but it is thought that garlic reduced the bioavailability of saquinavir by increasing its metabolism in the intestine.[1] Why there was a disparity in the effect of garlic on saquinavir between patients is unclear.

Importance and management

Although information is limited, a reduction in saquinavir plasma levels of the magnitude seen in the first study could diminish its antiviral efficacy. All garlic supplements should probably be avoided in those taking saquinavir as the sole protease inhibitor (no longer generally recommended). While the pharmacokinetic effect on single-dose ritonavir was not clinically important, this requires confirmation in a multiple-dose study.

1. Piscitelli SC, Burstein AH, Welden N, Gallicano KD, Falloon J. The effect of garlic supplements on the pharmacokinetics of saquinavir. *Clin Infect Dis* (2002) 34, 234–8.
2. Jacek H, Rentsch KM, Steinert HC, Pauli-Magnus C, Meier PJ, Fattinger K. No effect of garlic extract on saquinavir kinetics and hepatic CYP3A4 function measured by the erythromycin breath test. *Clin Pharmacol Ther* (2004) 75, P80.
3. Laroche M, Choudhri S, Gallicano K, Foster B. Severe gastrointestinal toxicity with concomitant ingestion of ritonavir and garlic. *Can J Infect Dis* (1998) 9 (Suppl A), 76A.
4. Gallicano K, Foster B, Choudhri S. Effect of short-term administration of garlic supplements on single-dose ritonavir pharmacokinetics in healthy volunteers. *Br J Clin Pharmacol* (2003) 55, 199–202.

Protease inhibitors + Grapefruit and other fruit juices

Grapefruit juice does not have any clinically significant effects on the pharmacokinetics of either amprenavir or indinavir. Although the saquinavir AUC was doubled by grapefruit juice, these increases are not thought to be clinically relevant. Seville orange juice did not alter indinavir pharmacokinetics.

Clinical evidence, mechanism, importance and management

(a) Amprenavir and Fosamprenavir

The manufacturer of fosamprenavir notes that taking amprenavir with grapefruit juice was not associated with clinically significant changes in plasma amprenavir pharmacokinetics.[1] Note that fosamprenavir is metabolised to amprenavir in the gut.

(b) Indinavir

In a single-dose study in 10 healthy subjects grapefruit juice (8 oz, about 200 mL) reduced the AUC of indinavir 400 mg by 27%, although this was not considered clinically significant.[2] Conversely, in another study in 13 healthy subjects, grapefruit juice or Seville orange juice (both about 200 mL) had no effect on the pharmacokinetics of indinavir. In this study indinavir 800 mg was given every 8 hours for 4 doses; with water, grapefruit juice, or Seville orange juice given with the last 2 doses.[3] Similarly, in 15 HIV-positive subjects, grapefruit juice (about 150 mL of double strength) had no effect on the steady-state pharmacokinetics of indinavir (a non-significant 4.8% increase in AUC was seen).[4]

(c) Saquinavir

In a study of the effects of the concurrent use of grapefruit juice 400 mL and saquinavir (*Invirase;* hard capsules) 600 mg, grapefruit juice was found to increase the AUC of saquinavir by 50%, possibly by affecting the cytochrome P450 isoenzyme CYP3A4 in the intestine.[5] The manufacturer notes that the increase was 100% when double-strength grapefruit juice was used.[6] The manufacturer says that these increases are unlikely to be clinically relevant, and no dosage adjustment is necessary.[6] Various components of grapefruit juice have been shown to inhibit the metabolism of saquinavir *in vitro.*[7]

1. Telzir (Fosamprenavir calcium). GlaxoSmithKline UK. UK Summary of product characteristics, February 2007.
2. McCrea J, Woolf E, Sterrett A, Matthews C, Deutsch P, Yeh KC, Waldman S, Bjornsson T. Effects of ketoconazole and other P-450 inhibitors on the pharmacokinetics of indinavir. *Pharm Res* (1996) 13 (Suppl 9), S485.
3. Penzak SR, Acosta EP, Turner M, Edwards DJ, Hon YY, Desai HD, Jann MW. Effect of Seville orange juice and grapefruit juice on indinavir pharmacokinetics. *J Clin Pharmacol* (2002) 42, 1165–70.
4. Wynn H, Shelton MJ, Bartos L, Difrancesco R, Hewitt RG. Grapefruit juice (GJ) increases gastric pH, but does not affect indinavir (IDV) exposure, in HIV patients. *Intersci Conf Antimicrob Agents Chemother* (1999) 39, 25.
5. Kupferschmidt HHT, Fattinger KE, Ha HR, Follath F, Krähenbühl S. Grapefruit juice enhances the bioavailability of the HIV protease inhibitor saquinavir in man. *Br J Clin Pharmacol* (1998) 45, 355–9.
6. Invirase Hard Capsules (Saquinavir mesilate). Roche Products Ltd. UK Summary of product characteristics, May 2007.
7. Eagling VA, Profit L, Back DJ. Inhibition of the CYP3A4-mediated metabolism and P-glycoprotein-mediated transport of the HIV-1 protease inhibitor saquinavir by grapefruit juice components. *Br J Clin Pharmacol* (1999) 48, 543–52.

Protease inhibitors + Macrolides

Nelfinavir approximately doubles the serum levels of azithromycin, but the clinical significance of this is uncertain. Single doses of azithromycin have no effect on the levels of indinavir and nelfinavir. Ritonavir and atazanavir increase clarithromycin levels. Amprenavir, indinavir and saquinavir do not have a clinically significant effect on clarithromycin pharmacokinetics. Clarithromycin has no important effect on the pharmacokinetics of amprenavir, atazanavir, darunavir, indinavir or ritonavir, but it increases tipranavir levels. Although both clarithromycin and erythromycin markedly raise saquinavir levels, this is not considered clinically important for short courses of these antibacterials.

Clinical evidence

(a) Azithromycin

1. Indinavir. A single 1.2-g dose of azithromycin had no effect on the pharmacokinetics of indinavir in healthy subjects who had taken indinavir 800 mg three times daily for 5 days.[1]

2. Nelfinavir. A single 1.2-g dose of azithromycin was given to 12 healthy subjects who had taken nelfinavir 750 mg every 8 hours for 8 days. The pharmacokinetics of nelfinavir were minimally affected, but the AUC and maximum serum levels of azithromycin were about doubled.[2]

(b) Clarithromycin

1. Amprenavir. In a study in 12 healthy adults, amprenavir 1.2 g twice daily was given with clarithromycin 500 mg twice daily, for 4 days. The AUC and maximum serum levels of amprenavir were increased by 18% and 15%, respectively, whereas the pharmacokinetics of clarithromycin were not significantly altered. None of the changes were considered to be clinically significant.[3]

2. Atazanavir. The concurrent use of atazanavir 400 mg once daily and clarithromycin 500 mg twice daily for 4 days increased the AUC of clarithromycin by 94%, and reduced the AUC of the active metabolite 14-hydroxyclarithromycin by 70%. In addition, there was a minor 28% increase in the AUC of atazanavir.[4]

3. Darunavir. The manufacturer notes that the concurrent use of clarithromycin 500 mg twice daily and darunavir/ritonavir 400/100 mg twice daily increased the AUC of clarithromycin by 57% and increased its minimum level by 174%. The active metabolite 14-hydroxyclarithromycin was not detectable. Darunavir levels were not significantly changed.[5,6]

4. Indinavir. In 11 healthy subjects clarithromycin 500 mg every 12 hours, given with indinavir 800 mg every 8 hours caused no clinically important alterations in the pharmacokinetics of indinavir (the only significant change was a 52% increase in the trough level). The AUC of clarithromycin was increased by about 50%, and that of 14-hydroxyclarithromycin reduced by about 50%, but neither of these changes were considered clinically important because of the wide safety margin of clarithromycin.[7]

5. Ritonavir. When ritonavir 200 mg every 8 hours was given with clarithromycin 500 mg every 12 hours there were only minimal changes in ritonavir pharmacokinetics (12.5% increase in AUC and 15.3% increase in maximum plasma level). However, the AUC of clarithromycin increased by 77% with an almost total inhibition of 14-hydroxyclarithromycin formation (99.7% decrease in AUC).[8]

6. Saquinavir. In a study in healthy subjects the concurrent use of saquinavir soft capsules *(Fortovase)* [no longer available] 1.2 g three times daily and clarithromycin 500 mg twice daily increased the AUC and maximum serum levels of saquinavir by 177% and 187%, respectively. The AUC and maximum serum levels of clarithromycin were about 40% higher than when it was given alone.[9,10] The manufacturer notes that there are no data on the interaction using ritonavir-boosted saquinavir hard capsules or tablets (*Invirase*).[9,10]

7. Tipranavir. The manufacturer notes that tipranavir given with low-dose ritonavir increased the AUC and minimum levels of clarithromycin by 19% and 68%, respectively, and decreased the AUC of the 14-hydroxy active metabolite by over 95%. Clarithromycin more than doubled the minimum levels of tipranavir.[11,12]

(c) Erythromycin

The concurrent use of saquinavir soft capsules (*Fortovase*) [no longer available] 1.2 g three times daily and erythromycin 250 mg four times daily doubled the AUC and maximum serum levels of saquinavir in HIV-infected subjects.[13] The manufacturer notes that there are no data on the interaction using ritonavir-boosted saquinavir hard capsules or tablets (*Invirase*).[9]

Mechanism

Ritonavir is a potent inhibitor of the cytochrome P450 isoenzyme CYP3A4 and consequently markedly inhibits the 14-hydroxylation of clarithromycin by this isoenzyme. Other protease inhibitors would be expected to interact similarly, although to a lesser degree (see also 'Antivirals', (p.772)). Clarithromycin is a moderate to weak inhibitor of CYP3A4, and generally has only a small effect on the protease inhibitors, except for saquinavir. The effect of clarithromycin on saquinavir, and nelfinavir on azithromycin may involve inhibition of P-glycoprotein.[2,3]

Importance and management

The interaction of amprenavir or indinavir with **clarithromycin** does not appear to be clinically significant. Similarly, although large increases in saquinavir levels have been seen, the manufacturers say that for short courses no dosage adjustment is needed.[9,10] However, with ritonavir, because the hepatic metabolism of clarithromycin is so strongly inhibited it becomes more dependent on renal clearance, therefore the interaction may be significant in patients with renal failure.[8] The manufacturers of ritonavir and clarithromycin suggest that no dosage reductions should be needed in those with normal renal function, but they recommend a 50% reduction in the dose of clarithromycin for those with a creatinine clearance of 30 to 60 mL/minute and a 75% reduction for clearances of less than 30 mL/minute.[14-17] Some advise avoiding clarithromycin in dosages exceeding 1 g daily.[14,15] Similar clarithromycin dose reductions in renal impairment are recommended for ritonavir-boosted darunavir,[5,6]and ritonavir-boosted tipranavir.[11,12] Although there are no formal studies or specific dosage recommendations for other ritonavir-boosted protease inhibitors (fosamprenavir, lopinavir and saquinavir), similar precautions would seem prudent. Atazanavir also reduces the conversion of clarithromycin to its active metabolite, and is usually given with ritonavir. However, the UK manufacturer[18] cautions that reducing the dose of clarithromycin to avoid high levels of the parent drug may result in subtherapeutic levels of the active metabolite. The US manufacturer says that, other than for *Mycobacterium avium* complex infections, an alternative to clarithromycin should be considered.[19] If the combination is used they suggest a 50% dose reduction for the clarithromycin.

The increase in **azithromycin** levels with nelfinavir is likely to be of clinical significance,[2] and, although the outcome is presumed to be positive, this has yet to be assessed in practice. If concurrent use is necessary, monitor for azithromycin adverse effects. Single doses of azithromycin did not affect the pharmacokinetics of nelfinavir or indinavir, and the manufacturers of a combination product of lopinavir/ritonavir do not expect a clinically significant interaction with azithromycin.[20,21]

Despite the increases in saquinavir levels, the UK manufacturer says that no dose adjustment is needed when saquinavir is given with **erythromycin**.[9] The UK manufacturer of nelfinavir suggests that an interaction with erythromycin is unlikely, although it cannot be excluded.[22] The UK manufacturer of ritonavir suggests that because erythromycin levels may rise, due to inhibition of its metabolism by ritonavir, care should be taken if both drugs are given.[14] It would seem prudent to monitor for erythromycin adverse effects. A similar warning has been issued by the UK manufacturer of amprenavir about the use of erythromycin.[23]

Note that clarithromycin and erythromycin have been associated with QT prolongation, and rises in their levels may increase this risk. See 'Drugs that prolong the QT interval + Other drugs that prolong the QT interval', p.257.

1. Foulds G, LaBoy-Goral L, Wei GCG, Apseloff G. The effect of azithromycin on the pharmacokinetics of indinavir. *J Clin Pharmacol* (1999) 39, 842–6.
2. Amsden GW, Nafziger AN, Foulds G, Cabelus LJ. A study of the pharmacokinetics of azithromycin and nelfinavir when coadministered in healthy volunteers. *J Clin Pharmacol* (2000) 40, 1522–7.
3. Brophy DF, Israel DS, Pastor A, Gillotin C, Chittick GE, Symonds WT, Lou Y, Sadler BM, Polk RE. Pharmacokinetic interaction between amprenavir and clarithromycin in healthy male volunteers. *Antimicrob Agents Chemother* (2000) 44, 978–84.
4. Mummaneni V, Randall D, Chabuel D, Geraldes M, O'Mara E. Steady-state pharmacokinetic interaction study of atazanavir with clarithromycin in healthy subjects. *Intersci Conf Antimicrob Agents Chemother* (2002) 42, 275.
5. Prezista (Darunavir ethanolate). Janssen-Cilag Ltd. UK Summary of product characteristics, July 2007.
6. Prezista (Darunavir). Tibotec, Inc. US Prescribing information, June 2006.
7. Boruchoff SE, Sturgill MG, Grasing KW, Seibold JR, McCrea J, Winchell GA, Kusma SE, Deutsch PJ. The steady-state disposition of indinavir is not altered by the concomitant administration of clarithromycin. *Clin Pharmacol Ther* (2000) 67, 351–9.
8. Ouellet D, Hsu A, Granneman GR, Carlson G, Cavanaugh J, Guenther H, Leonard JM. Pharmacokinetic interaction between ritonavir and clarithromycin. *Clin Pharmacol Ther* (1998) 64, 355–62.
9. Invirase Hard Capsules (Saquinavir mesilate). Roche Products Ltd. UK Summary of product characteristics, May 2007.
10. Invirase (Saquinavir mesylate). Roche Pharmaceuticals. US Prescribing information, July 2007.
11. Aptivus (Tipranavir). Boehringer Ingelheim. US Prescribing information, February 2007.
12. Aptivus (Tipranavir). Boehringer Ingelheim Ltd. UK Summary of product characteristics, March 2007.
13. Grub S, Bryson H, Goggin T, Lüdin E, Jorga K. The interaction of saquinavir (soft gelatin capsule) with ketoconazole, erythromycin and rifampicin: comparison of the effect in healthy volunteers and in HIV-infected patients. *Eur J Clin Pharmacol* (2001) 57, 115–21.
14. Norvir (Ritonavir). Abbott Laboratories Ltd. UK Summary of product characteristics, May 2007.
15. Klaricid (Clarithromycin). Abbott Laboratories Ltd. UK Summary of product characteristics, September 2006.
16. Norvir (Ritonavir). Abbott Laboratories. US Prescribing information, January 2006.
17. Biaxin (Clarithromycin). Abbott Laboratories. US Prescribing information, March 2007.

18. Reyataz (Atazanavir sulfate). Bristol-Myers Squibb Pharmaceuticals Ltd. UK Summary of product characteristics, April 2007.
19. Reyataz (Atazanavir sulfate). Bristol-Myers Squibb Company. US Prescribing information, March 2007.
20. Kaletra Soft Capsules (Lopinavir/ritonavir). Abbott Laboratories Ltd. UK Summary of product characteristics, March 2007.
21. Kaletra (Lopinavir/ritonavir). Abbott Laboratories. US Prescribing information, January 2007.
22. Viracept (Nelfinavir mesilate). Roche Products Ltd. UK Summary of product characteristics, January 2007.
23. Agenerase (Amprenavir). GlaxoSmithKline UK. UK Summary of product characteristics, February 2007.

Protease inhibitors + Mefloquine

Data from individual patients suggest there is no pharmacokinetic interaction between mefloquine and indinavir or nelfinavir. In pharmacokinetic studies in healthy subjects, ritonavir did not alter mefloquine pharmacokinetics, but mefloquine modestly decreased steady-state ritonavir levels.

Clinical evidence

Two HIV-positive patients using HAART, one taking **indinavir** 800 mg three times daily, the other taking **nelfinavir** 1.25 g twice daily were given mefloquine 250 mg weekly, before a trip to Africa. Mefloquine achieved therapeutic levels, and its half-life was similar to that found in healthy subjects. In addition, no consistent changes in the plasma levels of the protease inhibitors were found.[1]

In 12 healthy subjects **ritonavir** 200 mg twice daily for one week had no significant effect on the pharmacokinetics of mefloquine.[2] Conversely, mefloquine (250 mg once daily for 3 days, then 250 mg weekly) significantly reduced the steady-state AUC, and maximum and minimum plasma levels of **ritonavir** 200 mg twice daily, by 31%, 36%, and 43%, respectively, but had no effect on the pharmacokinetics of single-dose **ritonavir**.[2]

Mechanism

Despite being inhibitors of the cytochrome P450 isoenzyme CYP3A4, the protease inhibitors do not appear to alter mefloquine pharmacokinetics.[1,2] It was suggested that the decrease in ritonavir levels was due to decreased absorption, perhaps due to mefloquine-induced inhibition of bile acid production or induction of P-glycoprotein.[2]

Importance and management

The limited evidence suggests that protease inhibitors do not affect mefloquine pharmacokinetics. The data on the effect of mefloquine on ritonavir are less clear. Until further evidence is available, it may be prudent to closely monitor ritonavir levels/efficacy if mefloquine is required.

1. Schippers EF, Hugen PWH, den Hartigh J, Burger DM, Hoetelmans RMW, Visser LG, Kroon FP. No drug-drug interaction between nelfinavir or indinavir and mefloquine in HIV-1 infected patients. *AIDS* (2000) 14, 2794–5.
2. Khaliq Y, Gallicano K, Tisdale C, Carignan G, Cooper C, McCarthy A. Pharmacokinetic interaction between mefloquine and ritonavir in healthy volunteers. *Br J Clin Pharmacol* (2001) 51, 591–600.

Protease inhibitors + Miscellaneous

Indinavir levels are raised by interleukin-2, but not affected by influenza vaccine or quinidine. Protease inhibitors are predicted to increase quinidine levels. Nelfinavir does not appear to interact with pancreatic enzyme supplements. In one case report, the combination of ritonavir/saquinavir and fusidic acid raised plasma levels of all three drugs.

Clinical evidence, mechanism, importance and management

(a) Fusidic acid

A 32-year-old HIV-positive man was admitted with suspected fusidic acid toxicity after taking fusidic acid 500 mg three times daily for one week, with his usual treatment of **ritonavir** 400 mg twice daily, **saquinavir** 400 mg twice daily and stavudine 40 mg twice daily. His plasma fusidic acid level was found to be twice the expected level, and his **ritonavir** and **saquinavir** levels were also elevated. He improved spontaneously, but 4 days later he returned with jaundice, nausea and vomiting. All medications were stopped, but after 6 days his fusidic acid level was still 1.3 times that expected, his **saquinavir** level was 16.3 micrograms/mL (expected range 1 to 4 micrograms/mL) and his **ritonavir** level was 43.4 micrograms/mL (expected range 4 to 12 micrograms/mL). He was later able to restart his antivirals without problem. It is possible that there was mutual inhibition of drug metabolism. The authors recommend avoiding this drug combination.[1] Further study is needed.

(b) Influenza vaccine

Influenza whole virus vaccine was given to 9 patients taking **indinavir** containing HAART. No significant changes were found in **indinavir** pharmacokinetics.[2]

(c) Interleukins

In a pharmacokinetic study in 9 HIV-positive patients, the subjects continued taking their usual antiretrovirals and were given a 4-week course of **indinavir** 800 mg three times daily followed by 3 to 12 million-unit infusions of interleukin-2 daily for 5 days. The AUC of **indinavir** increased in 8 of the 9 subjects (average increase 88%). During this time interleukin-6 was also elevated, so it was thought that the increased **indinavir** concentrations were due to the inhibitory effects of interleukin-6 on the cytochrome P450 isoenzyme CYP3A4. Increased **indinavir** trough levels were also seen in a further 8 patients not participating in the pharmacokinetic study.[3]

(d) Pancreatic enzymes

Combined use of pancreatic enzymes (pancrelipase 20,000 USP units, amylase 65,000 USP units and protease 65,000 USP units) and **nelfinavir** 1.25 g twice daily for 14 days resulted in no significant changes in the pharmacokinetics of **nelfinavir** in 9 HIV-positive subjects.[4]

(e) Quinidine

Quinidine sulphate 200 mg was given to 10 healthy subjects, followed 1 hour later by a single 400-mg dose of **indinavir**. Quinidine had no clinically significant effects on the pharmacokinetics of **indinavir**.[5] However, **indinavir** is predicted to increase quinidine levels, and the US manufacturer recommends caution and monitoring of quinidine levels.[6]

Lopinavir/ritonavir is also predicted to increase quinidine levels, and the combination should be monitored.[7,8] Similarly, **atazanavir/ritonavir**, **darunavir/ritonavir**, **amprenavir** and **fosamprenavir** are predicted to increase quinidine levels, and the UK manufacturers contraindicate the combinations[9-11] while the US manufacturers recommend monitoring quinidine concentrations.[12-14] Conversely, for **saquinavir/ritonavir**, the UK manufacturer recommends caution and monitoring quinidine levels,[15] and the US manufacturer contraindicates the combination.[16] Both the UK and US manufacturers contraindicate the use of quinidine with **nelfinavir**,[17,18] **ritonavir**[19,20] or **tipranavir/ritonavir**.[21,22]

1. Khaliq Y, Gallicano K, Leger R, Foster B, Badley A. A drug interaction between fusidic acid and a combination of ritonavir and saquinavir. *Br J Clin Pharmacol* (2000) 50, 82–3.
2. Maserati R, Villani P, Barasolo G, Mongiovetti M, Regazzi MB. Influenza immunization and indinavir pharmacokinetics. *Scand J Infect Dis* (2000) 32, 449–50.
3. Piscitelli SC, Vogel S, Figg WD, Raje S, Forrest A, Metcalf JA, Baseler M, Falloon J. Alteration in indinavir clearance during interleukin-2 infusions in patients infected with the human immunodeficiency virus. *Pharmacotherapy* (1998) 18, 1212–16.
4. Price J, Shalit P, Carlsen J, Becker MI, Frye J, Hsyu P. Pharmacokinetic interaction between Ultrase® MT-20 and nelfinavir in HIV-infected individuals. *Intersci Conf Antimicrob Agents Chemother* (1999) 39, 20.
5. McCrea J, Woolf E, Sterrett A, Matthews C, Deutsch P, Yeh KC, Waldman S, Bjornsson T. Effects of ketoconazole and other P-450 inhibitors on the pharmacokinetics of indinavir. *Pharm Res* (1996) 13 (9 Suppl), S485.
6. Crixivan (Indinavir sulfate). Merck & Co., Inc. US Prescribing information, November 2006.
7. Kaletra Tablets (Lopinavir/ritonavir). Abbott Laboratories Ltd. UK Summary of product characteristics, March 2007.
8. Kaletra (Lopinavir/ritonavir). Abbott Laboratories. US Prescribing information, January 2007.
9. Reyataz (Atazanavir sulfate). Bristol-Myers Squibb Pharmaceuticals Ltd. UK Summary of product characteristics, April 2007.
10. Prezista (Darunavir ethanolate). Janssen-Cilag Ltd. UK Summary of product characteristics, July 2007.
11. Telzir (Fosamprenavir calcium). GlaxoSmithKline UK. UK Summary of product characteristics, February 2007.
12. Reyataz (Atazanavir sulfate). Bristol-Myers Squibb Company. US Prescribing information, March 2007.
13. Prezista (Darunavir). Tibotec, Inc. US prescribing information, June 2006.
14. Lexiva (Fosamprenavir calcium). GlaxoSmithKline. US Prescribing information, June 2007.
15. Invirase Hard Capsules (Saquinavir mesilate). Roche Products Ltd. UK Summary of product characteristics, May 2007.
16. Invirase (Saquinavir mesylate). Roche Pharmaceuticals. US Prescribing information, July 2007.
17. Viracept (Nelfinavir mesilate). Roche Products Ltd. UK Summary of product characteristics, January 2007.
18. Viracept (Nelfinavir mesylate). Agouron Pharmaceuticals, Inc. US Prescribing information, January 2007
19. Norvir (Ritonavir). Abbott Laboratories. US Prescribing information, January 2006.

20. Norvir Soft Capsules (Ritonavir). Abbott Laboratories Ltd. UK Summary of product characteristics, May 2007.
21. Aptivus (Tipranavir). Boehringer Ingelheim. US Prescribing information, February 2007.
22. Aptivus (Tipranavir). Boehringer Ingelheim Ltd. UK Summary of product characteristics, March 2007.

Protease inhibitors + Protease inhibitors

Various dual combinations of protease inhibitors have been tried, or are used, to boost the levels and consequently the efficacy of one of the protease inhibitors. Ritonavir is the most potent at boosting levels of the other protease inhibitors, and current guidelines recommend the use of low-dose ritonavir in combination with atazanavir, darunavir, fosamprenavir, lopinavir, saquinavir, or tipranavir. Some protease inhibitor combinations may result in additive toxicity (indinavir and ritonavir or atazanavir). Although this monograph summarises the pharmacokinetic interactions and dosing recommendations current guidelines should be consulted when choosing protease inhibitor combinations.

Clinical evidence

A. Amprenavir or Fosamprenavir

(a) Indinavir

The steady-state AUC of amprenavir was 33% higher when amprenavir 750 or 800 mg three times daily was given with indinavir 800 mg three times daily. In this study, the AUC of indinavir was 38% lower than historical control data.[1] Similarly, in a model-based pharmacokinetic analysis of data from a clinical study, amprenavir intrinsic clearance was reduced by 54% by indinavir.[2] This agrees with *in vitro* data.[3] It was suggested[1] that the effect of amprenavir on indinavir was due to the lipid-like formulation of amprenavir reducing the absorption of indinavir (analogous to 'food', (p.818)). The changes in amprenavir levels were not considered to be clinically relevant.[1]

- No dose adjustment of amprenavir or indinavir needed.[4]
- The appropriate dose of fosamprenavir with indinavir is not established.[5]

(b) Lopinavir/Ritonavir

Preliminary data suggest that the combination of amprenavir 600 mg twice daily with lopinavir/ritonavir 400/100 mg twice daily resulted in amprenavir trough plasma levels that were lower than with the combination of amprenavir/ritonavir at the same doses. Similarly the lopinavir levels were lower than those without amprenavir.[6] Others have reported similar findings,[7] and increasing the dose of ritonavir did not prevent a decrease in amprenavir levels with lopinavir.[8] Similar findings were also reported for fosamprenavir with lopinavir/ritonavir,[9] and further study showed that separation of doses reduced the effect of amprenavir on lopinavir/ritonavir levels, but increased the effect on amprenavir levels.[10] However, the manufacturer notes that combining lopinavir/ritonavir 400/100 mg with fosamprenavir/ritonavir 700/100 mg, both twice daily, increased the AUC and minimum level of lopinavir by 37% and 52%, respectively, whereas the AUC and minimum level of amprenavir were decreased by 63% and 65%, respectively.[5,11] In addition, the US manufacturer says that the rate of adverse effects was higher with this combination.[5]

- An optimum dosage for concurrent use has not been established. A dose increase of lopinavir/ritonavir *oral solution* to 533/133 mg twice daily (dose rounded to 6.5 mL) or 600/150 mg twice daily may be needed if amprenavir is given. Avoid once daily regimens.[12]
- An optimum dosage for concurrent use has not been established.[5,12] A dose increase of lopinavir/ritonavir *tablets* to 600/150 mg twice daily may be needed if fosamprenavir is given.[12]

(c) Nelfinavir

The trough concentration of amprenavir 750 or 800 mg three times daily was increased by 189% by nelfinavir 750 mg three times daily, but the AUC and maximum level of amprenavir were not significantly altered. In this study, the pharmacokinetics of nelfinavir were not altered when compared with historical control data.[1] In a model-based pharmacokinetic analysis of data from a clinical study. amprenavir intrinsic clearance was reduced by about 40% by nelfinavir,[2] which agrees with *in vitro* data.[3] The increase in amprenavir trough concentration could result in improved antiviral efficacy, but further study is needed.[1]

- No dose adjustment of either drug is needed when amprenavir is given with nelfinavir (UK).[4,13]
- Appropriate dose of fosamprenavir with nelfinavir is not established.[5]

(d) Ritonavir

The AUC, minimum, and maximum levels of amprenavir 1.2 g twice daily were increased by 131%, 484%, and 33%, respectively, by ritonavir 200 mg twice daily.[4] This agrees with *in vitro* data.[3] The manufacturer recommends that doses of both protease inhibitors be reduced when they are used together.[4,14] Based on modelling of pharmacokinetic data, a dose of amprenavir 600 mg with ritonavir 100 mg, both twice daily, has been suggested.[15] This combination has shown good clinical efficacy in at least one study,[16] and resulted in satisfactory amprenavir levels when efavirenz was also used[17] (see also 'NNRTIs + Protease inhibitors', p.785). Amprenavir levels with fosamprenavir/ritonavir 700/100 mg twice daily were similar to those achieved with amprenavir/ritonavir 600/100 mg twice daily.[18]

- If ritonavir is given as a pharmacokinetic booster the recommended dose is amprenavir/ritonavir 600/100 mg twice daily.
- If ritonavir is given as a pharmacokinetic booster the recommended dose is fosamprenavir/ritonavir 700/100 mg twice daily.[5]

(e) Saquinavir

The steady-state AUC of amprenavir was reduced by 32% when amprenavir 750 or 800 mg three times daily was given with saquinavir (soft gel capsule) 800 mg three times daily, and the maximum plasma level was reduced by 37%. In this study, the pharmacokinetics of saquinavir were not changed when compared with historical control data.[1] In a model-based pharmacokinetic analysis of data from a clinical study, amprenavir intrinsic clearance was not altered by saquinavir,[2] which agrees with *in vitro* data.[3] It was suggested that, as amprenavir was given with 'food', (p.818), in the first study, this may have accounted for the reduced amprenavir levels.[1]

- No dose adjustment of amprenavir or saquinavir is needed when they are given together.[4]
- Appropriate dose of fosamprenavir with saquinavir not established.[5]

(f) Tipranavir with Ritonavir

In a clinical study of dual-boosted protease inhibitor combination therapy in multiple-treatment experienced HIV-positive adults there was a 55% reduction in minimum amprenavir levels when tipranavir/ritonavir 500/200 mg twice daily was added to amprenavir/ritonavir 600/100 mg twice daily.[19,20] Therefore the use of tipranavir/ritonavir with amprenavir/ritonavir is not recommended, as the clinical relevance of the reduction in amprenavir levels has not been established. If the combination is nevertheless considered necessary, a monitoring of the plasma levels of the protease inhibitors is strongly encouraged.[20]

- Combination not recommended.

B. Atazanavir

(a) Darunavir with Ritonavir

The manufacturer notes that combining atazanavir 300 mg once daily with darunavir/ritonavir 400/100 mg twice daily did not significantly alter the AUC and minimum level of darunavir. In addition, the AUC and minimum level of atazanavir were not significantly changed, when compared with atazanavir/ritonavir 300/100 mg once daily alone, although the minimum level was increased by 52%.[21,22]

- No dose change needed.[21,22]

(b) Indinavir

There are no pharmacokinetic data on the combination of atazanavir plus indinavir, but it is predicted that there may be an additive risk of hyperbilirubinaemia, so the combination is not recommended.[23-25]

- Combination not recommended.

(c) Ritonavir

The addition of ritonavir 100 mg to atazanavir 300 mg increased the AUC of atazanavir about twofold, and the trough plasma level sevenfold, in healthy subjects. The effect on the trough level was less marked in patients (about a threefold increase).[23] The manufacturer of atazanavir recommends that it is given with ritonavir when used in patients who have already received antiretroviral treatment.[23,24]

- Ritonavir is recommended as a pharmacokinetic booster with atazanavir.

(d) Saquinavir

The addition of atazanavir 400 mg once daily to saquinavir soft capsules 1.2 g once daily increased the AUC of saquinavir about 5.5-fold, and the trough plasma level sevenfold.[24] However, the manufacturer notes that a regimen including this combination did not provide adequate efficacy.[24]

- Not an effective combination

(e) Tipranavir with Ritonavir

The manufacturer notes that concurrent use of atazanavir 300 mg once daily with tipranavir/ritonavir 500/100 mg twice daily increased tipranavir exposure (minimum plasma level by 75%) and ritonavir exposure (AUC by 51%) while markedly reducing atazanavir exposure (AUC by 68%, and minimum level by 81%). Consequently, this combination is not recommended.[20]

- Combination not recommended.

C. Darunavir with Ritonavir

(a) Indinavir

The manufacturer notes that combining indinavir 800 mg twice daily with darunavir/ritonavir 400/100 mg twice daily increased the AUC and minimum level of darunavir by 24% and 44%, respectively. In addition, the AUC and minimum level of indinavir were increased by 23% and 125%, respectively, when compared with indinavir/ritonavir 800/100 mg twice daily alone.[21,22]

- No dose change is usually needed. Decreasing the dose of indinavir to 600 mg twice daily may be necessary if the combination is poorly tolerated.[21]

(b) Lopinavir/Ritonavir

The manufacturer notes that combining lopinavir/ritonavir 400/100 mg with darunavir/ritonavir 300/100 mg, both twice daily, increased the AUC and minimum level of lopinavir by 37% and 72%, respectively, whereas the AUC and minimum level of darunavir were decreased by 53% and 65%, respectively.[21,22]

- Combination not recommended.[21,22]

(c) Saquinavir

The manufacturer notes that combining saquinavir hard capsules 1 g twice daily with darunavir/ritonavir 400/100 mg twice daily decreased the AUC and minimum level of darunavir by 26% and 42%, respectively. The levels of saquinavir were not changed when compared with using saquinavir/ritonavir 1000/100 mg twice daily alone.[21,22]

- Combination not recommended.[21,22]

D. Indinavir

(a) Lopinavir/Ritonavir

Indinavir 600 mg twice daily in combination with lopinavir/ritonavir 400/100 mg twice daily produced a similar indinavir AUC, higher minimum level (by 3.5-fold) and 29% lower maximum level relative to indinavir 800 mg three times daily alone.[12,26] Based on historical comparisons, lopinavir levels were similar to those seen without indinavir.[26]

- Reduce the dose to indinavir 600 mg twice daily if lopinavir/ritonavir given.[12]

(b) Nelfinavir

The combination of indinavir 1.2 g every 12 hours with nelfinavir 1.25 g every 12 hours produced plasma levels that were equivalent to the standard dose of indinavir 800 mg every 8 hours in HIV-positive subjects. This suggests that nelfinavir only modestly inhibits indinavir metabolism. In this multiple-dose study, indinavir did not affect the pharmacokinetics of nelfinavir.[27] In contrast, a single 750-mg dose of nelfinavir, given after indinavir 800 mg every 8 hours for 7 days resulted in an 83% increase in the AUC of nelfinavir and a 22% increase its elimination half-life. In addition, administration of a single 800-mg dose of indinavir after nelfinavir 750 mg three times daily for 7 days resulted in a 51% increase in the indinavir plasma AUC, with a fivefold increase in trough concentrations measured at 8 hours, but no increase in peak concentrations.[13,28]

- Appropriate dose of indinavir with nelfinavir not established.[29]

(c) Ritonavir

The effects of a range of doses of ritonavir (200, 300, or 400 mg every 12 hours) on indinavir pharmacokinetics were assessed in 39 healthy subjects. The AUC of indinavir 400 or 600 mg was increased two- to fivefold by the ritonavir. It is suggested that the combination of indinavir 400 mg every 12 hours with ritonavir 400 mg every 12 hours will result in an AUC of indinavir roughly equivalent to that of indinavir 800 mg every 8 hours, without any effect on the pharmacokinetics of ritonavir.[30] In another similar study, when compared with historical data for indinavir 800 mg every 8 hours, the AUC of indinavir was at least 1.4-, 2.3-, and 3.3-fold higher when given indinavir/ritonavir in twice daily doses of 400/400 mg, 800/100 mg, and 800/200 mg, respectively. The regimens also produced markedly higher trough indinavir levels. The 800/100 mg regimen was the best tolerated.[31]

- If ritonavir is given as a pharmacokinetic booster the recommended dose is indinavir/ritonavir 800/100 or 200 mg twice daily.[31,32]
- Caution is needed when indinavir is used at a dose of 800 mg twice daily with ritonavir, because of the possibility of an increased risk of nephrolithiasis.[29,33] Appropriate hydration is strongly recommended.[33]
- The US guidelines say that the combination is not recommended as part of initial therapy because of the risk of nephrolithiasis.[25]

(d) Saquinavir

In a single-dose study, the concurrent use of indinavir and saquinavir 600 mg (hard capsule) or 800 mg or 1.2 g (soft capsule) increased the AUC of saquinavir by 500%, 620% and 360%, respectively.[33] This is supported by *in vitro* data.[34] However, in another *in vitro* study of antiviral activity, the combination of saquinavir and indinavir was antagonistic.[35] Further study is needed.

- Appropriate dose of indinavir with saquinavir not established.[29]

E. Lopinavir/Ritonavir

(a) Nelfinavir

The US manufacturer notes that the concurrent use of nelfinavir 1 g twice daily and lopinavir/ritonavir 400/100 mg twice daily resulted in similar nelfinavir pharmacokinetics to nelfinavir 1.25 g twice daily alone, but with markedly increased levels of the M8 metabolite of nelfinavir. Lopinavir levels were modestly reduced (27% decrease in AUC and 38% decrease in minimum level).[12]

- Dosage decrease of nelfinavir to 1 g twice daily recommended. Avoid once daily regimens. A dose increase of lopinavir/ritonavir *oral solution* to 533/133 mg twice daily or lopinavir/ritonavir *tablets* to 600/150 mg twice daily may be needed.[12]

(b) Ritonavir

Ritonavir is used to increase the plasma levels of lopinavir. The marketed dose combination is lopinavir/ritonavir 400/100 mg twice daily.[12,26] When an additional 100 mg of ritonavir twice daily was added to the marketed combination, the AUC of lopinavir increased by 33% and the trough concentration by 64%.[26]

- The use of lopinavir with ritonavir as a pharmacokinetic enhancer is established. The dose of additional ritonavir is not established.

(c) Saquinavir

Saquinavir 800 mg twice daily given with lopinavir/ritonavir produced a 9.6-fold increase in saquinavir AUC relative to saquinavir 1.2 g three times daily given alone. When compared with saquinavir/ritonavir 1000/100 mg twice daily, the increase in saquinavir AUC was about 30%, and was similar to that reported after saquinavir/ritonavir 400/400 mg twice daily. When saquinavir 1.2 g twice daily was combined with lopinavir/ritonavir, no further increase of concentrations was noted. Lopinavir levels did not appear to be affected by saquinavir, based on historical comparison with lopinavir/ritonavir alone.[26]

- In the US, the manufacturer recommends that saquinavir 1 g twice daily be used with lopinavir/ritonavir 400/100 mg twice daily.[12]

(d) Tipranavir with Ritonavir

In a clinical study of dual-boosted protease inhibitor combination therapy in multiple-treatment experienced HIV-positive adults there was a 70% reduction in minimum lopinavir levels when tipranavir/ritonavir 500/200 mg twice daily was added to lopinavir/ritonavir 400/100 mg twice daily.[19,20] The clinical relevance of the reduction in lopinavir levels has not been established.

- Combination not recommended, but if it is given monitoring the plasma levels of the protease inhibitors is strongly encouraged.[20]

E. Nelfinavir

(a) Ritonavir

Single-dose data indicate that ritonavir increases the AUC of nelfinavir by 1.8- to 2.5-fold, whereas the AUC of ritonavir is unchanged.[36] In a multiple-dose study in healthy subjects, ritonavir 100 or 200 mg twice daily increased the steady-state AUC of nelfinavir 1.25 g twice daily by 20% and 39%, after morning and evening doses, respectively. The AUC of the M8 metabolite of nelfinavir was increased by 74% and 86%, respectively. There was no difference in the effect of the two doses of ritonavir on nelfinavir AUC.[37]

- Appropriate dose of nelfinavir with ritonavir not established.[28]

(b) Saquinavir

A single 1.2-g dose of saquinavir (soft gel capsules), given after 3 days of nelfinavir 750 mg every 8 hours had no effect on the pharmacokinetics of nelfinavir, but the nelfinavir caused a fourfold increase in the AUC of saquinavir.[38] Similar two- to twelvefold increases have been found in other studies in HIV-positive subjects.[39-42] A study in which 157 patients received 12 weeks of combined saquinavir/nelfinavir treatment (doses unstated) found that the combination was well tolerated.[43] It appears that nelfinavir inhibits the hepatic clearance of saquinavir.[44]

- Appropriate dose of nelfinavir with saquinavir not established.[28]

F. Ritonavir

(a) Saquinavir

A study in 6 patients with advanced HIV disease found that while taking saquinavir 600 mg three times daily the addition of ritonavir 300 mg twice daily increased the maximum saquinavir plasma levels 33-fold, and increased the AUC 58-fold at steady state.[45] A pilot study in HIV-positive patients given both drugs together (saquinavir 800 mg daily, ritonavir 400 to 600 mg daily) found that the ritonavir serum levels were unaffected. However, the saquinavir levels were substantially higher than those achieved with saquinavir alone in daily doses of 3.6 to 7.2 g.[46] A study of a range of ritonavir and saquinavir *(Invirase)* doses (200 to 600 mg) in 57 healthy subjects found that saquinavir did not affect ritonavir pharmacokinetics, but ritonavir increased the AUC of saquinavir 50 to 132-fold. The authors suggested that giving both drugs in the dosage 400 mg every 12 hours might be optimal.[47] Subsequent study has revealed that the effect of ritonavir on saquinavir is not related to the ritonavir dose in the range of 100 to 400 mg twice daily,[48-50] and that the use of a combination with a higher dose of saquinavir and a lower dose of ritonavir may be preferable, as the lower doses of ritonavir are associated with fewer adverse effects.[50] A dose of saquinavir 1 g twice daily with ritonavir 100 mg twice daily is suggested by the manufacturer of saquinavir.[51,52] The UK manufacturer of ritonavir also says that doses of ritonavir higher than 100 mg twice daily should not be used in combination with saquinavir,[53] whereas the US manufacturer of ritonavir gives information solely on the saquinavir/ritonavir 400/400 or 600 mg twice daily regimen.[54] The UK manufacturer of ritonavir notes that higher doses of ritonavir have been associated with an increased incidence of adverse events. Concurrent use of saquinavir and ritonavir has led to severe adverse events, mainly diabetic ketoacidosis and liver disorders, especially in patients with pre-existing liver disease.[53]

- When ritonavir is given as a pharmacokinetic booster the recommended dose is saquinavir/ritonavir 1000/100 mg twice daily. Higher ritonavir doses are associated with increased adverse effects.[53]

G. Saquinavir with Ritonavir

(a) Tipranavir with Ritonavir

In a clinical study of dual-boosted protease inhibitor combination therapy in multiple-treatment experienced HIV-positive adults there was a marked, approximately 80%, reduction in minimum saquinavir levels when tipranavir/ritonavir 500/200 mg twice daily was added to saquinavir/ritonavir 600/100 mg twice daily.[19,20] The clinical relevance of the reduction in saquinavir levels has not been established.

- Combination is not recommended, but if it is given monitoring the plasma levels of the protease inhibitors is strongly encouraged.[20]

Mechanism

Protease inhibitors are inhibitors and substrates of the cytochrome P450 isoenzyme CYP3A4, with ritonavir being the most potent inhibitor and saquinavir the least (see 'Antivirals', (p.772)). They probably interact by inhibiting each other's gut (pre-absorption) and hepatic (post-absorption) metabolism, so resulting in increased absorption and decreased elimination.[44,47] A mechanism involving inhibition of P-glycoprotein may also be involved.[44]

Importance and management

Ritonavir inhibits the metabolism of amprenavir (and amprenavir derived from fosamprenavir), atazanavir, darunavir, indinavir, lopinavir, nelfinavir, tipranavir, and especially saquinavir. Ritonavir is therefore used in combination with other protease inhibitors to boost their levels, and allow a reduction in the protease inhibitor dose and the frequency of dosing. In US guidelines, the combination of atazanavir with ritonavir, fosamprenavir with ritonavir or lopinavir with ritonavir are currently the protease inhibitors preferred as alternative options to efavirenz for use with dual NRTIs for the treatment of HIV-infection in treatment naïve patients. Ritonavir-boosted saquinavir is considered inferior to the preferred options.[25] In UK guidelines, dual NRTIs plus a boosted protease inhibitor is a recommended alternative option to dual NRTIs plus efavirenz. The preferred boosted protease inhibitors are lopinavir with ritonavir and fosamprenavir with ritonavir, with saquinavir plus ritonavir as an alternative regimen, and atazanavir plus ritonavir recommended for specific groups.[55] The newer ritonavir-boosted protease inhibitors, darunavir and tipranavir are not currently recommended as initial therapy, and are used in extensively pre-treated patients with resistance to other protease inhibitors. The US guidelines state that ritonavir-boosted indinavir should be avoided because of a high incidence of nephrolithiasis, and that atazanavir plus indinavir should never be used because of potential additive hyperbilirubinaemia.[25] There appears to be no clinically important pharmacokinetic interactions between amprenavir with indinavir, nelfinavir, or saquinavir, between atazanavir with darunavir and ritonavir, and probably also indinavir with nelfinavir. Various dual ritonavir-boosted protease inhibitor combinations act to lower the levels of one of the protease inhibitors and should therefore probably be avoided. These include lopinavir/ritonavir with amprenavir or fosamprenavir, darunavir/ritonavir with lopinavir/ritonavir or saquinavir, and tipranavir/ritonavir with ritonavir-boosted amprenavir, lopinavir or saquinavir, or with atazanavir. When considering appropriate protease inhibitor combinations, in addition to pharmacokinetic interactions, cross resistance patterns and adverse effects should also be considered.

1. Sadler BM, Gillotin C, Lou Y, Eron JJ, Lang W, Haubrich R, Stein DS. Pharmacokinetic study of human immunodeficiency virus protease inhibitors used in combination with amprenavir. *Antimicrob Agents Chemother* (2001) 45, 3663–8.
2. Pfister M, Labbé L, Lu J-F, Hammer SM, Mellors J, Bennett KK, Rosenkranz S, Sheiner LB, and the AIDS Clinical Trial Group Protocol 398 Investigators. Effect of coadministration of nelfinavir, indinavir, and saquinavir on the pharmacokinetics of amprenavir. *Clin Pharmacol Ther* (2002) 72, 133–41.
3. Decker CJ, Laitinen LM, Bridson GW, Raybuck SA, Tung RD, Chaturvedi PR. Metabolism of amprenavir in liver microsomes: role of CYP3A4 inhibition for drug interactions. *J Pharm Sci* (1998) 87, 803–7.
4. Agenerase (Amprenavir). GlaxoSmithKline UK. UK Summary of product characteristics, February 2007.
5. Lexiva (Fosamprenavir calcium). GlaxoSmithKline. US Prescribing information, June 2007.
6. Mauss S, Schmutz G, Kuschak D. Unfavourable interaction of amprenavir and lopinavir in combination with ritonavir? *AIDS* (2002) 16, 296–7.
7. Khanlou H, Graham E, Brill M, Farthing C. Drug interaction between amprenavir and lopinavir/ritonavir in salvage therapy. *AIDS* (2002) 16, 797–8.
8. Mauss S, Scholten S, Wolf E, Berger F, Schmutz G, Jaeger H, Kurowski M, Rockstroh JK; Klinische Arbeitsgruppe AIDS Deutschland, Germany. A prospective, controlled study assessing the effect of lopinavir on amprenavir concentrations boosted by ritonavir. *HIV Med* (2004) 5, 15–17.
9. Kashuba ADM, Tierney C, Downey GF, Acosta EP, Vergis EN, Klingman K, Mellors JW, Eshleman SH, Scott TR, Collier AC. Combining fosamprenavir with lopinavir/ritonavir substantially reduces amprenavir and lopinavir exposure: ACTG protocol A5143 results. *AIDS* (2005) 19, 145–52.
10. Corbett AH, Patterson KB, Tien H-C, Kalvass LA, Eron JJ, Ngo LT, Lim ML, Kashuba ADM. Dose separation does not overcome the pharmacokinetic interaction between fosamprenavir and lopinavir/ritonavir. *Antimicrob Agents Chemother* (2006) 50, 2756–61.
11. Telzir (Fosamprenavir calcium). GlaxoSmithKline UK. UK Summary of product characteristics, February 2007.
12. Kaletra (Lopinavir/ritonavir). Abbott Laboratories. US Prescribing information, January 2007.
13. Viracept (Nelfinavir mesilate). Roche Products Ltd. UK Summary of product characteristics, January 2007.
14. Agenerase (Amprenavir). GlaxoSmithKline. US Prescribing information, May 2005.
15. Sale M, Sadler BM, Stein DS. Pharmacokinetic modeling and simulations of interaction of amprenavir and ritonavir. *Antimicrob Agents Chemother* (2002) 46, 746–54.
16. Duval X, Lamotte C, Race E, Descamps D, Damond F, Clavel F, Leport C, Peytavin G, Vilde J-L. Amprenavir inhibitory quotient and virological response in human immunodeficiency virus-infected patients on an amprenavir-containing salvage regimen without or with ritonavir. *Antimicrob Agents Chemother* (2002) 46, 570–4.

17. Goujard C, Vincent I, Meynard J-L, Choudet N, Bollens D, Rousseau C, Demarles D, Gillotin C, Bidault R, Taburet A-M. Steady-state pharmacokinetics of amprenavir coadministered with ritonavir in human immunodeficiency virus type 1-infected patients. *Antimicrob Agents Chemother* (2003) 47, 118–23.
18. Wire MB, Baker KL, Jones LS, Shelton MJ, Lou Y, Thomas GJ, Berrey MM. Ritonavir increases plasma amprenavir (APV) exposure to a similar extent when coadministered with either fosamprenavir or APV. *Antimicrob Agents Chemother* (2006) 50, 1578–80.
19. Aptivus (Tipranavir). Boehringer Ingelheim. US Prescribing information, February 2007.
20. Aptivus (Tipranavir). Boehringer Ingelheim Ltd. UK Summary of product characteristics, March 2007.
21. Prezista (Darunavir ethanolate). Janssen-Cilag Ltd. UK Summary of product characteristics, July 2007.
22. Prezista (Darunavir). Tibotec, Inc. US Prescribing information, June 2006.
23. Reyataz (Atazanavir sulfate). Bristol-Myers Squibb Pharmaceuticals Ltd. UK Summary of product characteristics, April 2007.
24. Reyataz (Atazanavir sulfate). Bristol-Myers Squibb Company. US Prescribing information, March 2007.
25. US Department of Health and Human Services; Panel on Antiretroviral Guidelines for Adults and Adolescents. Guidelines for the use of antiretroviral agents in HIV-1-infected adults and adolescents. October 10, 2006; 1–113. Available at: http://www.aidsinfo.nih.gov/contentfiles/AdultandAdolescentGL.pdf (accessed 21/08/07).
26. Kaletra Tablets (Lopinavir/ritonavir). Abbott Laboratories Ltd. UK Summary of product characteristics, March 2007.
27. Riddler SA, Havlir D, Squires KE, Kerr B, Lewis RH, Yeh K, Hawe Wynne L, Zhong L, Peng Y, Deutsch P, Saah A. Coadministration of indinavir and nelfinavir in human immunodeficiency virus type 1-infected adults: safety, pharmacokinetics, and antiretroviral activity. *Antimicrob Agents Chemother* (2002) 46, 3877–82.
28. Viracept (Nelfinavir mesylate). Agouron Pharmaceuticals, Inc. US Prescribing information, January 2007.
29. Crixivan (Indinavir sulfate). Merck & Co., Inc. US Prescribing information, November 2006.
30. Hsu A, Granneman GR, Cao G, Carothers L, Japour A, El-Shourbagy T, Dennis S, Berg J, Erdman K, Leonard JM, Sun E. Pharmacokinetic interaction between ritonavir and indinavir in healthy volunteers. *Antimicrob Agents Chemother* (1998) 42, 2784–91.
31. Saah AJ, Winchell GA, Nessly ML, Seniuk MA, Rhodes RR, Deutsch PJ. Pharmacokinetic profile and tolerability of indinavir-ritonavir combinations in healthy volunteers. *Antimicrob Agents Chemother* (2001) 45, 2710–15.
32. van Heeswijk RP, Veldkamp AI, Hoetelmans RM, Mulder JW, Schreij G, Hsu A, Lange JM, Beijnen JH, Meenhorst PL. The steady-state plasma pharmacokinetics of indinavir alone and in combination with a low dose of ritonavir in twice daily dosing regimens in HIV-1-infected individuals. *AIDS* (1999) 13, F95–F99.
33. Crixivan (Indinavir sulfate). Merck Sharp & Dohme Ltd. UK Summary of product characteristics, May 2007.
34. Fitzsimmons ME, Collins JM. Selective biotransformation of the human immunodeficiency virus protease inhibitor saquinavir by human small-intestinal cytochrome P4503A4: Potential contribution to high first-pass metabolism. *Drug Metab Dispos* (1997) 25, 256–66.
35. Merrill DP, Manion DJ, Chou T-C, Hirsch MS. Antagonism between human immunodeficiency virus type 1 protease inhibitors indinavir and saquinavir in vitro. *J Infect Dis* (1997) 176, 265–8.
36. Washington CB, Flexner C, Sheiner LB, Rosenkranz SL, Segal Y, Aberg JA, Blaschke TF, AIDS Clinical Trials Group Protocol (ACTG 378) study team. *Clin Pharmacol Ther* (2003) 73, 406–16.
37. Kurowski M, Kaeser B, Sawyer A, Popescu M, Mrozikiewicz A. Low-dose ritonavir moderately enhances nelfinavir exposure. *Clin Pharmacol Ther* (2002) 72, 123–32.
38. Kerr B, Yuep G, Daniels R, Quart B, Kravcik S, Sahai J, Anderson R. Strategic approach to nelfinavir mesylate (NFV) drug interactions involving CYP3A metabolism. 6th European Conference on Clinical Aspects and Treatment of HIV-infection, Hamburg, Germany, 1997.
39. Merry C, Ryan M, Mulchay F, Halifax K, Barry M, Back D. The effect of nelfinavir on plasma saquinavir levels. 6th European Conference on Clinical Aspects and Treatment of HIV-infection, Hamburg, Germany, 1997. Abstract 455.
40. Merry C, Barry MG, Mulcahy FM, Back DJ. Saquinavir pharmacokinetics alone and in combination with nelfinavir in HIV infected patients. 5th Conference on Retroviruses and Opportunistic Infections, Chicago, 1998. Abstract 352.
41. Gallicano K, Sahai J, Kravcik S, Seguin I, Bristow N, Cameron DW. Nelfinavir (NFV) increases plasma exposure of saquinavir in hard gel capsule (SQV-HGC) in HIV+ patients. 5th Conference on Retroviruses and Opportunistic Infections, Chicago, 1998. Abstract 353.
42. Hoetelmans RMW, Reijers MHE, Wit FW, ten Kate RW, Weige HM, Frissen PHJ, Bruisten SM, Beijnen JH, Lange JMA. Saquinavir (SQV) pharmacokinetics in combination with nelfinavir (NFV) in the ADAM study. 6th European Conference on Clinical Aspects and Treatment of HIV-infection, Hamburg, Germany, 1997. Abstract 255.
43. Posniak A and the SPICE study team. Study of protease inhibitors in combination in Europe (SPICE). 6th European Conference on Clinical Aspects and Treatment of HIV-infection, Hamburg, Germany, 1997. Abstract 209.
44. Lu J-F, Blaschke TF, Flexner C, Rosenkranz SL, Sheiner LB, and AIDS Clinical Trials Group protocol 378 investigators. Model-based analysis of the pharmacokinetic interactions between ritonavir, nelfinavir, and saquinavir after simultaneous and staggered oral administration. *Drug Metab Dispos* (2002) 30, 1455–61.
45. Merry C, Barry MG, Mulcahy F, Ryan M, Heavey J, Tjia JF, Gibbons SE, Breckenridge AM, Back DJ. Saquinavir pharmacokinetics alone and in combination with ritonavir in HIV-infected patients. *AIDS* (1997) 11, F29–F33.
46. Cameron DW, Hsu A, Granneman GR, Sun E, McMahon D, Farthing C, Poretz D, Markowitz M, Cohen C, Follansbee S, Mellors J, Ho D, Xu Y, Rode R, Salgo M, Leonard J. Pharmacokinetics of ritonavir-saquinavir combination therapy. *AIDS* (1996) 10 (Suppl 2), S16.
47. Hsu A, Granneman GR, Cao G, Carothers L, El-Shourbagy T, Baroldi P, Erdman K, Brown F, Sun E, Leonard JM. Pharmacokinetic interactions between two human immunodeficiency virus protease inhibitors, ritonavir and saquinavir. *Clin Pharmacol Ther* (1998) 63, 453–64.
48. Kilby JM, Hill A, Buss N. The effect of ritonavir on saquinavir plasma concentration is independent of ritonavir dosage: combined analysis of pharmacokinetic data from 97 subjects. *HIV Med* (2002) 3, 97–104.
49. Kurowski M, Arslan A, Moecklinghoff C, Sawyer W, Hill A. Effects of ritonavir on saquinavir plasma concentration: analysis of 271 patients in routine clinical practice (P261A). *AIDS* (2000) 14 (Suppl 4), 591.
50. Buss N, Snell P, Bock J, Hsu A, Jorga K. Saquinavir and ritonavir pharmacokinetics following combined ritonavir and saquinavir (soft gelatin capsules) administration. *Br J Clin Pharmacol* (2001) 52, 255–64.
51. Invirase Hard Capsules (Saquinavir mesilate). Roche Products Ltd. UK Summary of product characteristics, May 2007.
52. Invirase (Saquinavir mesylate). Roche Pharmaceuticals. US Prescribing information, July 2007.
53. Norvir (Ritonavir). Abbott Laboratories Ltd. UK Summary of product characteristics, May 2007.
54. Norvir (Ritonavir). Abbott Laboratories. US Prescribing information, January 2006.
55. Gazzard B, Bernard EJ, Boffito M, Churchill D, Edwards S, Fisher M, Geretti AM, Johnson M, Leen C, Peters B, Pozniak A, Ross J, Walsh J, Wilkins E, Youle M. BHIVA Writing Committee. British HIV Association (BHIVA) guidelines for the treatment of HIV-infected adults with antiretroviral therapy (2006). *HIV Med* (2006) 7, 487–503. Available at: http://www.bhiva.org/files/file1001303.pdf (accessed 21/08/07).

Protease inhibitors + Rifamycins

Rifabutin bioavailability is increased by amprenavir, atazanavir, fosamprenavir/ritonavir, indinavir, lopinavir/ritonavir, nelfinavir, tipranavir/ritonavir, and especially ritonavir, with an increased risk of toxicity. Rifabutin modestly decreases the bioavailability of indinavir, nelfinavir, and particularly saquinavir (with an increased risk of therapeutic failure), but has no effect on amprenavir, atazanavir, and ritonavir-boosted fosamprenavir. The combination of rifabutin with protease inhibitors may be used, but dosage adjustments of rifabutin or both drugs are often necessary.

Rifampicin (rifampin) bioavailability is increased by indinavir, but amprenavir has no effect. Rifampicin markedly reduces the bioavailability of amprenavir, atazanavir/ritonavir, indinavir, indinavir with ritonavir, lopinavir/ritonavir, nelfinavir and saquinavir, but only modestly reduces that of ritonavir. The effects of rifampicin on lopinavir/ritonavir and saquinavir/ritonavir can be overcome by increasing the protease inhibitor dose, but this appears to increase adverse effects (hepatotoxicity).

Clinical evidence

(a) Amprenavir or Fosamprenavir

1. Rifabutin. When amprenavir 1.2 g twice daily was given with rifabutin 300 mg daily to 11 healthy subjects for 10 days there was an almost threefold increase in the AUC of rifabutin, but the pharmacokinetics of amprenavir were not significantly altered. The combination was poorly tolerated, with 5 of 11 subjects stopping treatment between days 1 and 9 due to adverse events.[1] When reduced doses of rifabutin (150 mg every other day) were given with fosamprenavir/ritonavir 700/100 mg twice daily the rifabutin AUC was unchanged and the maximum level was decreased by 14%, when compared with rifabutin 300 mg once daily given alone. However, the 25-*O*-desacetylrifabutin AUC and maximum level were increased 11-fold and sixfold, respectively, which could potentially lead to an increase of rifabutin-related adverse events such as uveitis. Based on historical comparison, rifabutin did not appear to reduce amprenavir exposure from fosamprenavir/ritonavir.[2,3]

2. Rifampicin (Rifampin). When 11 healthy subjects were given amprenavir 1.2 g twice daily with rifampicin 600 mg daily to for 4 days the pharmacokinetics of rifampicin were not affected, but the AUC of amprenavir was reduced by 82%. The maximum plasma level of amprenavir was also reduced by 70%, from 9.2 to 2.78 micrograms/mL.[1]

It is expected that concurrent use of fosamprenavir or fosamprenavir/ritonavir with rifampicin will also result in large decreases in plasma concentrations of amprenavir.[2,3]

(b) Atazanavir

1. Rifabutin. The manufacturer notes that atazanavir 400 mg daily given with rifabutin 150 mg once daily for 14 days did not have any important effect on the AUC of atazanavir. However, the AUC of rifabutin 150 mg was 2.3-fold higher than historical data for a standard 300-mg dose.[4]

2. Rifampicin (Rifampin). When rifampicin 600 mg daily was given with atazanavir/ritonavir 300/100 mg once daily, the AUC and minimum levels of atazanavir were markedly reduced, by 72% and 98%, respectively.[5]

(c) Darunavir

Although there are no data, the manufacturer predicts that **rifabutin** will decrease ritonavir-boosted darunavir levels, and that darunavir/ritonavir will increase rifabutin levels. They also predict that **rifampicin** will markedly reduce ritonavir-boosted darunavir levels.[6,7]

(d) Indinavir

1. Rifabutin. When 10 healthy subjects were given rifabutin 300 mg once daily with indinavir 800 mg every 8 hours to for 10 days, the indinavir maximum serum levels and AUC were reduced by about one-third, whereas the rifabutin maximum serum levels and AUC were increased two- to threefold.[8] When the same dose of indinavir (800 mg every 8 hours) was given with half the dose of rifabutin (150 mg once daily), the AUC of indinavir was similarly reduced (by 32%), but the increase in the AUC of rifabutin was less (54% increase).[8] In a further study, the pharmacokinetics of indinavir 1 g every 8 hours (increased dose) and rifabutin 150 mg daily (reduced dose) were investigated in healthy and HIV-positive subjects. The indinavir AUC was the same with this increased dose as with indinavir 800 mg every 8 hours alone. However, despite halving the rifabutin dose, the AUC was still up to 70% higher than with the 300-mg dose alone.[9] When the combination was used in practice, there were no treatment failures in 25 patients being treated with rifabutin while receiving HAART (containing indinavir and/or nelfinavir). The rifabutin was given as 300 mg twice weekly and the indinavir dose was increased from 800 mg to 1.2 g every 8 hours to achieve satisfactory levels.[10]

2. Rifampicin (Rifampin). A study in 11 AIDS patients given indinavir 800 mg every 8 hours and rifampicin 600 mg daily for 14 days found that the AUC of rifampicin was increased by 73%.[11] In a similar study looking at the effects of the rifampicin on indinavir, the indinavir AUC and maximum serum levels were decreased by 92% and 86%, respectively.[12] In another study, giving rifampicin 300 mg daily for 4 days to 6 HIV-positive patients already receiving ritonavir-boosted indinavir (indinavir/ritonavir 800/100 mg twice daily) decreased the median indinavir plasma levels (measured 12 hours after the last dose) by 87% and the median ritonavir levels by 94%.[13]

(e) Lopinavir

1. Rifabutin. When healthy subjects were given lopinavir/ritonavir 400/100 mg twice daily with rifabutin 150 or 300 mg daily for 10 days the AUC of rifabutin was increased threefold and the AUC of lopinavir was increased by 17%.[14]

2. Rifampicin (Rifampin). Rifampicin 600 mg daily for 10 days decreased the AUC of lopinavir (given as lopinavir/ritonavir 400/100 mg twice daily) by 75% in a study in healthy subjects.[14] A dose titration of lopinavir/ritonavir was carried out in healthy subjects to try and overcome the interaction with rifampicin.[15] In 10 evaluable subjects, use of rifampicin 600 mg daily with lopinavir/ritonavir 800/200 mg twice daily decreased the minimum lopinavir level by 57% without affecting the maximum level, when compared with lopinavir/ritonavir 400/100 mg twice daily without rifampicin. In another 9 evaluable subjects, rifampicin 600 mg daily with lopinavir/ritonavir 400/400 mg twice daily did not alter the maximum or minimum level of lopinavir, but markedly increased ritonavir levels, when compared with lopinavir/ritonavir 400/100 mg twice daily without rifampicin. Of 29 subjects who received the adjusted doses of lopinavir/ritonavir with rifampicin, 9 subjects had grade 2 to 3 elevations in liver enzymes, and this was more common in the lopinavir/ritonavir 400/400 mg group than the lopinavir/ritonavir 800/200 mg group.[15]

(f) Nelfinavir

1. Rifabutin. When rifabutin 300 mg daily for 8 days was given with nelfinavir 750 mg every 8 hours for 7 to 8 days, the nelfinavir AUC was reduced by 32% and the rifabutin AUC was increased by 207%.[16] When nelfinavir 750 mg every 8 hours was given with half the dose of rifabutin (150 mg daily), the nelfinavir AUC was reduced by a similar amount (23%), whereas the rifabutin AUC was increased by a lower amount (83%).[17,18]

2. Rifampicin (Rifampin). Rifampicin 600 mg daily for 7 days decreased the AUC of nelfinavir 750 mg every 8 hours for 6 days by 82%.[16] A 7-month-old infant with HIV and tuberculosis was given a rifampicin-based antimycobacterial regimen with nelfinavir-based HAART. Nelfinavir plasma levels were found to be very low, so ritonavir was added. This improved nelfinavir levels, and also greatly increased those of the principal active metabolite of nelfinavir. The regimen was well tolerated and had a good clinical response.[19]

(g) Ritonavir

1. Rifabutin. In a study in 5 healthy subjects when ritonavir 500 mg twice daily was given with rifabutin 150 mg daily for 8 days, the maximum serum level of rifabutin was increased threefold and the AUC was increased fourfold (and the AUC of its active metabolite, 25-*O*-desacetylrifabutin, 35-fold). Seven subjects had to be withdrawn due to adverse events, primarily leucopenia.[20] Retrospective analysis of regimens containing ritonavir found that the concurrent use of rifabutin was associated with a higher incidence of rifabutin-related adverse effects including arthralgia, joint stiffness, uveitis and leucopenia.[21]

2. Rifampicin (Rifampin). When ritonavir 500 mg every 12 hours was given with rifampicin 300 or 600 mg daily for 10 days, the AUC of ritonavir was 35% lower and the maximum level 25% lower than in subjects receiving ritonavir alone.[22]

(h) Saquinavir

1. Rifabutin. The AUC of saquinavir 600 mg three times daily was reduced by about 40% by rifabutin 300 mg daily, in 12 HIV-positive subjects.[23] Similarly, the AUC of saquinavir (soft capsules) 1.2 g three times daily was decreased by 47% by rifabutin 300 mg once daily in 14 HIV-positive patients. In addition, the rifabutin AUC was increased by 44% by saquinavir.[24] However, combined use of ritonavir and saquinavir (hard capsules), both 400 mg twice daily, with intermittent rifabutin dosing (300 mg weekly or 150 mg every 3 days) for 8 weeks was reported to be safe and manageable. Rifabutin did not significantly alter the protease inhibitor levels, and the rifabutin pharmacokinetics were similar to those usually seen with rifabutin 300 mg daily alone.[25]

2. Rifampicin (Rifampin). Rifampicin 600 mg once daily decreased the AUC of saquinavir (soft capsules) 1.2 g three times daily by 70%.[26] It was suggested that the combination of ritonavir and saquinavir (both 400 mg twice daily) could cancel out the effects of rifampicin on saquinavir, so therapeutic levels of all three drugs could be achieved. This assumption has been confirmed in HIV-positive patients.[27,28] Five of 20 patients originally given the combination developed hepatotoxicity, 2 of whom had comorbidities.[28] However, in a further study in healthy subjects, severe hepatotoxicity with transaminase elevations of about 20 times the upper limit of normal occurred in 11 of 17 subjects after they took saquinavir/ritonavir 1000/100 mg twice daily with rifampicin 600 mg once daily for 1 to 5 days.[29,30]

(i) Tipranavir

The manufacturer notes that tipranavir/ritonavir 500/200 mg twice daily increased plasma rifabutin levels by up to threefold, and its active metabolite by up to 20-fold after a single 150-mg dose of rifabutin.[31,32]

Although there are no data, the manufacturer predicts that rifampicin will markedly reduce ritonavir-boosted tipranavir levels.[31,32]

Mechanism

Rifampicin is a potent inducer of the cytochrome P450 isoenzyme CYP3A4, by which the protease inhibitors are at least partially metabolised, and therefore it markedly reduces protease inhibitor levels. Rifabutin is a weak inducer of CYP3A4. The protease inhibitors are inhibitors of CYP3A4, with ritonavir being the most potent, and can therefore increase the levels of the rifamycins.

Importance and management

Established interactions of clinical importance. The protease inhibitors increase the levels of rifabutin, with a consequent increase in adverse effects unless the rifabutin dose is reduced. Ritonavir is the most potent protease inhibitor in this regard, and the combination has been considered contraindicated. However, the CDC in the US say that the combination may be used if the dose of rifabutin is markedly reduced.[33] In addition, rifabutin decreases the levels of some protease inhibitors, particularly saquinavir, increasing the risk of treatment failure. Rifabutin should not be used when saquinavir is the sole protease inhibitor (no longer recommended). However, there is some evidence that rifabutin can be used with ritonavir-boosted saquinavir. 'Table 21.5', (p.827) summarises the clinical recommendations for the concurrent use of protease inhibitors and rifabutin. Therapy should be well monitored. Note that, in one analysis, the use of rifabutin 150 mg twice weekly with low-dose ritonavir and a second protease inhibitor was associated with low rifabutin levels.[34] Recommended doses of rifabutin in patients taking ritonavir-boosted protease inhibitors are 150 mg every other day or three times per week.[33]

Rifampicin markedly reduces the levels of many of the protease inhibitors, and its use with unboosted protease inhibitors should be avoided, because of the risk of reduced antiviral efficacy and emergence of resistant viral strains. There are limited data to suggest that ritonavir as the sole protease inhibitor, or ritonavir used as a pharmacokinetic enhancer with other protease inhibitors such as saquinavir, can be used with rifampicin.[33] However, further study has shown a high incidence of hepatotoxicity with saquinavir/ritonavir 1000/100 mg twice daily and rifampicin, and the manufacturers of ritonavir and saquinavir advise that these drugs should not be given together with rifampicin.[22,29,30,35] Current UK guidelines state that, until more data are available, ritonavir-boosted protease inhibi-

Table 21.5 Summary of the manufacturers' dosage recommendations (unless stated otherwise) for combined use of protease inhibitors and rifamycins

Protease inhibitor	*Rifabutin*	*Rifampicin*	*Refs*
Protease inhibitors			
Amprenavir	Rifabutin dose at least halved (150 mg daily or every other day, or 300 mg three times per week). Amprenavir dose unchanged.	Not recommended (amprenavir levels markedly reduced).	1-3
Fosamprenavir	Rifabutin dose at least halved (150 mg daily or 300 mg three times per week). Fosamprenavir dose unchanged.	Not recommended (amprenavir levels expected to be markedly reduced).	3-5
Indinavir	Rifabutin dose halved (150 mg daily or 300 mg three times per week). Indinavir dose increased (1 to 1.2 g every 8 hours).	Not recommended (indinavir levels markedly reduced, rifampicin levels raised).	3, 6-8
Nelfinavir	Rifabutin dose at least halved (150 mg once daily or 300 mg three times per week). Nelfinavir dose unchanged (1.25 g twice daily preferred) or increase to 1 g every 8 hours.	Not recommended (nelfinavir levels markedly reduced).	3, 9, 10
Ritonavir alone	Rifabutin dose reduced by at least 75% (150 mg every other day or three times per week). Further dose reductions may be necessary.* Ritonavir dose unchanged.	May be used at usual doses, although limited data (ritonavir levels reduced). May lead to loss of virologic response.	3, 11
Saquinavir alone	Not recommended (saquinavir levels reduced).	Not recommended (saquinavir levels markedly reduced).	3
Ritonavir boosted protease inhibitors			
Atazanavir/ritonavir	Rifabutin dose reduced by up to 75% (150 mg every other day or three times per week). Atazanavir/ritonavir dose unchanged.	Not recommended (atazanavir levels markedly reduced).	3, 12, 13
Darunavir/ritonavir	Rifabutin dose reduced to 150 mg every other day.	Not recommended (darunavir levels predicted to be markedly reduced).	14, 15
Fosamprenavir/ritonavir	Rifabutin dose reduced by at least 75% (150 mg every other day or three times per week). Fosamprenavir/ritonavir dose unchanged.	Not recommended (amprenavir levels predicted to be markedly reduced).	3-5
Indinavir/ritonavir	Rifabutin dose reduced by at least 75% (150 mg every other day or three times per week). Indinavir/ritonavir dose unchanged.	Not recommended (indinavir levels markedly reduced).	3, 16
Lopinavir/ritonavir	Rifabutin dose reduced by at least 75% (150 mg every other day or three times per week). Lopinavir/ritonavir dose unchanged.	Not recommended (lopinavir levels markedly reduced). However, adjusted doses of lopinavir/ritonavir (800/200 mg or 400/400 mg twice daily) may overcome the pharmacokinetic interaction, but have a high incidence of elevated liver enzymes, and so if used, close monitoring is needed.	3, 17-19
Saquinavir/ritonavir	Rifabutin dose reduced by at least 75% (150 mg every other day or three times per week). Appropriate saquinavir/ritonavir dose not established. Consider usual dose (1000/100 mg twice daily).	Rifampicin dose unchanged. Saquinavir/ritonavir 400/400 mg twice daily. Note that a regimen of 1000/100 mg twice daily with rifampicin was associated with severe hepatotoxicity, and the combination is contraindicated.	3, 20, 21
Tipranavir/ritonavir	Rifabutin dose reduced by at least 75% (150 mg every other day or three times per week). Further dose reductions may be necessary. Tipranavir/ritonavir dose unchanged.	Not recommended (tipranavir levels predicted to be markedly reduced).	22, 23

*Formerly considered contraindicated (rifabutin levels markedly increased with risk of toxicity)

1. Agenerase (Amprenavir). GlaxoSmithKline UK. UK Summary of product characteristics, February 2007.
2. Agenerase (Amprenavir). GlaxoSmithKline. US Prescribing information, May 2005.
3. Centers for Disease Control and Prevention. Updated guidelines for the use of rifamycins for the treatment of tuberculosis among HIV-infected patients taking protease inhibitors or nonnucleoside reverse transcriptase inhibitors. January 20, 2004. Available at http://www.cdc.gov/tb/TB_HIV_Drugs/default.htm (accessed 22/08/07).
4. Telzir (Fosamprenavir). GlaxoSmithKline UK. UK Summary of product characteristics, February 2007.
5. Lexiva (Fosamprenavir). GlaxoSmithKline. US Prescribing information, February 2007.
6. Jaruratanasirikul S, Sriwiriyajan S. Pharmacokinetics of rifampicin administered alone and with indinavir. *J Antimicrob Chemother* (1999) 44 (Suppl A), 58.
7. Crixivan (Indinavir sulfate). Merck Sharp & Dohme Ltd. UK Summary of product characteristics, May 2007.
8. Crixivan (Indinavir sulfate). Merck & Co., Inc. US Prescribing information, November 2006.
9. Viracept (Nelfinavir mesilate). Roche Products Ltd. UK Summary of product characteristics, January 2007.
10. Viracept (Nelfinavir mesilate). Agouron Pharmaceuticals, Inc. US Prescribing information, January 2007.
11. Norvir Soft Capsules (Ritonavir). Abbott Laboratories. US Prescribing information, January 2006.
12. Reyataz (Atazanavir sulfate). Bristol-Myers Squibb Pharmaceuticals Ltd. UK Summary of product characteristics, April 2007.

Continued

Table 21.5 Summary of the manufacturers' dosage recommendations (unless stated otherwise) for combined use of protease inhibitors and rifamycins (continued)

13. Reyataz (Atazanavir sulfate). Bristol-Myers Squibb Company. US Prescribing information, March 2007.
14. Prezista (Darunavir). Janssen-Cilag Ltd. UK Summary of product characteristics, February 2007.
15. Prezista (Darunavir). Tibotec, Inc. US prescribing information, June 2006.
16. Justesen US, Andersen ÅB, Klitgaard NA, Brøsen K, Gerstoft J, Pedersen C. Pharmacokinetic interaction between rifampin and the combination of indinavir and low-dose ritonavir in HIV-infected patients. *Clin Infect Dis* (2004) 38, 426-9.
17. Kaletra (Lopinavir/ritonavir). Abbott Laboratories Ltd. UK Summary of product characteristics, March 2007.
18. Kaletra Tablets (Lopinavir/ritonavir). Abbott Laboratories. US Prescribing information, January 2007.
19. la Porte CJL, Colbers EPH, Bertz R, Voncken DS, Wikstrom K, Boeree MJ, Koopmans PP, Hekster YA, Burger DM. Pharmacokinetics of adjusted-dose lopinavir-ritonavir combined with rifampin in healthy volunteers. *Antimicrob Agents Chemother* (2004) 48, 1553–60.
20. Invirase (Saquinavir mesilate). Roche Products Ltd. UK Summary of product characteristics, May 2007.
21. Invirase (Saquinavir mesilate). Roche Pharmaceuticals. US Prescribing information, September 2005.
22. Aptivus (Tipranavir). Boehringer Ingelheim Ltd. UK Summary of product characteristics, March 2007.
23. Aptivus (Tipranavir). Boehringer Ingelheim. US Prescribing information, February 2007.

tors should not be used with rifampicin. They say that rifampicin should be switched to rifabutin for use with protease inhibitors, or the protease inhibitor should be changed to an alternative antiretroviral if this is possible.[36] Similarly, US guidelines say that rifampicin may only be used with full-dose ritonavir, and cannot be used safely with ritonavir-boosted regimens. They recommend the use of rifabutin.[37]

1. Polk RE, Brophy DF, Israel DS, Patron R, Sadler BM, Chittick GE, Symonds WT, Lou Y, Kristoff D, Stein DS. Pharmacokinetic interaction between amprenavir and rifabutin or rifampin in healthy males. *Antimicrob Agents Chemother* (2001) 45, 502–508.
2. Telzir (Fosamprenavir calcium). GlaxoSmithKline UK. UK Summary of product characteristics, February 2007.
3. Lexiva (Fosamprenavir calcium). GlaxoSmithKline. US Prescribing information, June 2007.
4. Reyataz (Atazanavir sulfate). Bristol-Myers Squibb Pharmaceuticals Ltd. UK Summary of product characteristics, April 2007.
5. Reyataz (Atazanavir sulfate). Bristol-Myers Squibb Company. US Prescribing information, March 2007.
6. Prezista (Darunavir ethanolate). Janssen-Cilag Ltd. UK Summary of product characteristics, July 2007.
7. Prezista (Darunavir). Tibotec, Inc. US Prescribing information, June 2006.
8. Kraft WK, McCrea JB, Winchell GA, Carides A, Lowry R, Woolf EJ, Kusma SE, Deutsch PJ, Greenberg HE, Waldman SA. Indinavir and rifabutin drug interactions in healthy volunteers. *J Clin Pharmacol* (2004) 44, 305–13.
9. Hamzeh FM, Benson C, Gerber J, Currier J, McCrea J, Deutsch P, Ruan P, Wu H, Lee J, Flexner C, for the AIDS Clinical Trials Group 365 Study Team. Steady-state pharmacokinetic interaction of modified-dose indinavir and rifabutin. *Clin Pharmacol Ther* (2003) 73, 159–69.
10. Narita M, Stambaugh JJ, Hollender ES, Jones D, Pitchenik AE, Ashkin D. Use of rifabutin with protease inhibitors for human immunodeficiency virus-infected patients with tuberculosis. *Clin Infect Dis* (2000) 30, 779–83. Correction. ibid. 992.
11. Jaruratanasirikul S, Sriwiriyajan S. Pharmacokinetics of rifampicin administered alone and with indinavir. *J Antimicrob Chemother* (1999) 44 (Suppl A), 58.
12. McCrea J, Wyss D, Stone J, Carides A, Kusma S, Kleinbloesem C, Al-Hamdan Y, Yeh K, Deutsch P. Pharmacokinetic interaction between indinavir and rifampin. *Clin Pharmacol Ther* (1997) 61, 152.
13. Justesen US, Andersen AB, Klitgaard NA, Brøsen K, Gerstoft J, Pedersen C. Pharmacokinetic interaction between rifampin and the combination of indinavir and low-dose ritonavir in HIV-infected patients. *Clin Infect Dis* (2004) 38, 426–9.
14. Bertz R, Hsu A, Lam W, Williams L, Renz C, Karol M, Dutta S, Carr R, Zhang Y, Wang Q, Schweitzer S, Foit C, Andre A, Bernstein B, Granneman GR, Sun E. Pharmacokinetic interactions between lopinavir/ritonavir (ABT-378r) and other non-HIV drugs (abstract P291). *AIDS* (2000) 14 (Suppl 4), S100.
15. la Porte CJL, Colbers EPH, Bertz R, Voncken DS, Wikstrom K, Boeree MJ, Koopmans PP, Hekster YA, Burger DM. Pharmacokinetics of adjusted-dose lopinavir-ritonavir combined with rifampin in healthy volunteers. *Antimicrob Agents Chemother* (2004) 48, 1553–60.
16. Kerr B, Yuep G, Daniels R, Quart B, Kravcik S, Sahai J, Anderson R. Strategic approach to nelfinavir mesylate (NFV) drug interactions involving CYP3A metabolism. 6th European Conference on Clinical Aspects and Treatment of HIV-infection, Hamburg, 1997. 256.
17. Viracept (Nelfinavir mesilate). Roche Products Ltd. UK Summary of product characteristics, January 2007.
18. Viracept (Nelfinavir mesylate). Agouron Pharmaceuticals, Inc. US Prescribing information, January 2007.
19. Bergshoeff AS, Wolfs TFW, Geelen SPM, Burger DM. Ritonavir-enhanced pharmacokinetics of nelfinavir/M8 during rifampin use. *Ann Pharmacother* (2003) 37, 521–5.
20. Cato A, Cavanaugh J, Shi H, Hsu A, Leonard J, Granneman R. The effect of multiple doses of ritonavir on the pharmacokinetics of rifabutin. *Clin Pharmacol Ther* (1998) 63, 414–21.
21. Sun E, Heath-Chiozzi M, Cameron DW, Hsu A, Granneman RG, Maurath CJ, Leonard JM. Concurrent ritonavir and rifabutin increases risk of rifabutin-associated adverse events. 11th International Conference on AIDS, Vancouver, 1996. Mo.B.171.
22. Norvir (Ritonavir). Abbott Laboratories. US Prescribing information, January 2006.
23. Sahai J, Stewart F, Swick L, Gallicano K, Garber G, Seguin I, Tucker A, Bristow N, Cameron W. Rifabutin (RBT) reduces saquinavir (SAQ) plasma levels in HIV-infected patients. *Intersci Conf Antimicrob Agents Chemother* (1996) 36, 6.
24. Moyle GJ, Buss NE, Goggin T, Snell P, Higgs C, Hawkins DA. Interaction between saquinavir soft-gel and rifabutin in patients infected with HIV. *Br J Clin Pharmacol* (2002) 54, 178–82.
25. Gallicano K, Khaliq Y, Carignan G, Tseng A, Walmsley S, Cameron DW. A pharmacokinetic study of intermittent rifabutin dosing with a combination of ritonavir and saquinavir in patients infected with human immunodeficiency virus. *Clin Pharmacol Ther* (2001) 70, 149–58.
26. Fortovase (Saquinavir). Roche Products Ltd. UK Summary of product characteristics, January 2005.
27. Veldkamp AI, Hoetelmans RMW, Beijnen JH, Mulder JW, Meenhorst PL. Ritonavir enables combined therapy with rifampicin and saquinavir. *Clin Infect Dis* (1999) 29, 1586.
28. Rolla VC, da Silva Vieira MA, Pereira Pinto D, Lourenço MC, de Jesus C da S, Gonçalves Morgado M, Ferreira Filho M, Werneck-Barroso E. Safety, efficacy and pharmacokinetics of ritonavir 400mg/saquinavir 400mg twice daily plus rifampicin combined therapy in HIV patients with tuberculosis. *Clin Drug Invest* (2006) 26, 469–79.
29. Invirase Hard Capsules (Saquinavir mesilate). Roche Products Ltd. UK Summary of product characteristics, May 2007.
30. Invirase (Saquinavir mesylate). Roche Pharmaceuticals. US Prescribing information, July 2007.
31. Aptivus (Tipranavir). Boehringer Ingelheim Ltd. UK Summary of product characteristics, March 2007.
32. Aptivus (Tipranavir). Boehringer Ingelheim. US Prescribing information, February 2007.
33. Centers for Disease Control and Prevention. Updated guidelines for the use of rifamycins for the treatment of tuberculosis among HIV-infected patients taking protease inhibitors or non-nucleoside reverse transcriptase inhibitors, January 20th 2004. Available at: http://www.cdc.gov/tb/TB_HIV_Drugs/default.htm (accessed 21/08/07).
34. Spradling P, Drociuk D, McLaughlin S, Lee LM, Peloquin CA, Gallicano K, Pozsik C, Onorato I, Castro KG, Ridzon R. Drug-drug interactions in inmates treated for human immunodeficiency virus and *Mycobacterium tuberculosis* infection or disease: an institutional tuberculosis outbreak. *Clin Infect Dis* (2002) 35, 1106–12.
35. Norvir Soft Capsules (Ritonavir). Abbott Laboratories Ltd. UK Summary of product characteristics, May 2007.
36. Pozniak AL, Miller RF, Lipman MCI, Freedman AR, Ormerod LP, Johnson MA, Collins S, Lucas SB, on behalf of the BHIVA guidelines writing committee. BHIVA treatment guidelines for TB/HIV infection, February 2005. Available at: http://www.bhiva.org/files/file1001577.pdf (accessed 21/08/07).
37. US Department of Health and Human Services; Panel on Antiretroviral Guidelines for Adults and Adolescents. Guidelines for the use of antiretroviral agents in HIV-infected adults and adolescents. October 10, 2006; 1–113. Available at: http://www.aidsinfo.nih.gov/contentfiles/AdultandAdolescentGL.pdf (accessed 21/08/07)

Protease inhibitors + St John's wort (*Hypericum perforatum*)

St John's wort causes a marked reduction in the serum levels of indinavir, which may result in HIV treatment failure. Other protease inhibitors, whether used alone or boosted by ritonavir, are predicted to interact similarly.

Clinical evidence

In a single-drug pharmacokinetic study, 8 healthy subjects were given three 800-mg doses of **indinavir** on day 1 of to achieve steady-state serum levels, and then an 800-mg dose on day 2. For the next 14 days they were given St John's wort extract 300 mg three times daily. Starting on day 16, the indinavir dosing was repeated. It was found that the St John's wort reduced the mean AUC of **indinavir** by 54% and decreased the 8-hour **indinavir** trough serum level by 81%.[1]

Mechanism

Not fully understood, but it seems highly likely that the St John's wort induces the activity of the cytochrome P450 isoenzyme CYP3A4, thereby increasing the metabolism of indinavir and therefore reducing its levels.

Importance and management

Direct information seems to be limited to this study, but the interaction would appear to be established. Such a large reduction in the serum levels of indinavir is likely to result in treatment failures and the development of viral resistance. Therefore St John's wort should be avoided. There seems to be no direct information about other protease inhibitors, but since they are also metabolised by CYP3A4 it is reasonable to expect that they will be similarly affected by St John's wort. The FDA in the US has suggested that concurrent use of St John's wort and protease inhibitors is not recommended.[2] Similarly, the CSM in the UK has advised that patients taking protease inhibitors should avoid St John's wort and that anyone already taking both should stop the St John's wort and have their HIV RNA viral load measured.[3] The manufacturers of indinavir give similar advice,[4,5] and also note that protease inhibitor levels may increase on stopping St John's wort, and the dose may need adjusting.[4] They note the inducing effect may persist for up to 2 weeks after stopping treatment with St John's wort.[4] US and UK manufacturers of all protease inhibitors (**amprenavir, atazanavir, darunavir, fosamprenavir, lopinavir/ritonavir, nelfinavir, ritonavir, saquinavir, tipranavir**) either contraindicate or advise against the use of St John's wort.

1. Piscitelli SC, Burstein AH, Chaitt D, Alfaro RM, Falloon J. Indinavir concentrations and St John's wort. *Lancet* (2000) 355, 547–8. Erratum *ibid.* (2001) 357, 1210.
2. Lumpkin MM, Alpert S; FDA Public Healthy Advisory. Risk of drug interactions with St John's wort and indinavir and other drugs, February 10, 2000. Available at: http://www.fda.gov/cder/drug/advisory/stjwort.htm (accessed 21/08/07).
3. Committee on Safety of Medicines. Message from Professor A Breckenridge (Chairman of CSM) and Fact Sheet for Health Care Professionals, 29th February 2000.
4. Crixivan (Indinavir sulfate). Merck Sharp & Dohme Ltd. UK Summary of product characteristics, May 2007.
5. Crixivan (Indinavir sulfate). Merck & Co., Inc. US Prescribing information, November 2006.

Protease inhibitors + Tenofovir

Atazanavir/ritonavir, darunavir/ritonavir and lopinavir/ritonavir modestly increased the levels of tenofovir, and there is at least one case report of nephrotoxicity with the combination of tenofovir, didanosine, and lopinavir/ritonavir. Saquinavir/ritonavir, tipranavir/ritonavir, and probably also fosamprenavir/ritonavir, have little effect on tenofovir levels. Tenofovir modestly decreased atazanavir levels, and this was minimised when ritonavir was also given. Tenofovir had no important effect on ritonavir-boosted darunavir, lopinavir, and tipranavir levels, and modestly increased those of ritonavir-boosted saquinavir in one of two studies. Indinavir and nelfinavir do not interact pharmacokinetically with tenofovir.

Clinical evidence

(a) Atazanavir

The AUC of atazanavir was decreased by 25%, and the trough level by 40% when atazanavir 400 mg daily was given with tenofovir disoproxil fumarate 300 mg daily, and the AUC of tenofovir was increased by 24%.[1-3] Similar results were seen when administration was separated by 12 hours.[3]

When atazanavir 300 mg once daily was given with ritonavir 100 mg once daily (as a pharmacokinetic booster), tenofovir disoproxil fumarate 300 mg once daily reduced the AUC of atazanavir by a similar amount (25%), but had less effect on the trough level (23% reduction), when compared with atazanavir/ritonavir alone.[4] Similarly, the pharmacokinetics of atazanavir/ritonavir did not differ significantly between patients taking tenofovir and those not.[5] Combined use increased the tenofovir AUC by 37% and the minimum level by 29%.[2,3]

(b) Darunavir with Ritonavir

The manufacturer notes that concurrent use of darunavir/ritonavir 300/100 mg twice daily with tenofovir disoproxil fumarate 300 mg once daily modestly increased the tenofovir AUC and minimum level by 22% and 37%, respectively. Darunavir levels were not significantly changed (minimum level increased by 24%).[6,7]

(c) Fosamprenavir with Ritonavir

The US manufacturer notes that, in a phase III clinical study plasma amprenavir trough levels (derived from fosamprenavir) were similar in subjects receiving tenofovir with fosamprenavir and ritonavir to those in subjects not receiving tenofovir.[8] Similarly, in a pharmacokinetic study in healthy subjects, tenofovir disoproxil fumarate 300 mg once daily had no significant effect on the pharmacokinetics of amprenavir after fosamprenavir/ritonavir 1400/100 mg once daily or fosamprenavir/ritonavir 1400/200 mg once daily.[9]

(d) Indinavir

The manufacturer of tenofovir notes that there was no pharmacokinetic interaction between tenofovir disoproxil fumarate 300 mg once daily and indinavir 800 mg three times daily in healthy subjects.[1,10]

(e) Lopinavir/Ritonavir

The concurrent use of lopinavir/ritonavir 400/100 mg twice daily and tenofovir resulted in a 30% increase in the AUC and a 50% increase in the trough level of tenofovir, but no change in the pharmacokinetics of lopinavir/ritonavir.[1,10] There is one case report of Fanconi syndrome with nephrogenic diabetes insipidus, which developed in a patient taking lopinavir/ritonavir 800/200 mg daily, tenofovir disoproxil fumarate 300 mg daily, didanosine and lamivudine (for an interaction between tenofovir and didanosine, see 'NRTIs', (p.806)). The tenofovir level was 3.7-fold higher than expected and the didanosine level was eightfold higher than it had been before tenofovir was started. Lopinavir levels were unchanged.[11]

(f) Nelfinavir

The manufacturer of tenofovir notes that there was no pharmacokinetic interaction between tenofovir disoproxil fumarate 300 mg once daily and nelfinavir 1.25 g twice daily in healthy subjects.[1,10]

(g) Saquinavir with Ritonavir

Tenofovir disoproxil fumarate 300 mg once daily modestly increased the saquinavir AUC and minimum level by 29% and 47%, respectively, after administration of saquinavir/ritonavir 1000/100 mg twice daily in healthy subjects. The only change in tenofovir pharmacokinetics was a slight 23% increase in minimum level.[10,12] In another study,[13] mentioned by the manufacturer of saquinavir,[14,15] in 18 HIV-positive patients treated with saquinavir/ritonavir 1000/100 mg twice daily and tenofovir disoproxil fumarate 300 mg once daily, saquinavir AUC and maximum values were just 1% and 7% lower, respectively, than those seen with saquinavir/ritonavir alone.

(h) Tipranavir with Ritonavir

Tipranavir/ritonavir 500/100 mg twice daily had no effect on the AUC and minimum level of a single 300-mg dose of tenofovir disoproxil fumarate, but it decreased the tenofovir maximum level by 23%. The tipranavir AUC and minimum level were decreased by 18% and 21%, respectively. With an increased dose of tipranavir/ritonavir 750/200 mg twice daily, the maximum level of tenofovir was reduced by 38% with no change in AUC or minimum level, and the decreases in tipranavir AUC and minimum levels were less (9% AUC and 12% minimum level).[16]

Mechanism

It has been suggested that ritonavir increases tenofovir levels via its effect on drug transporter proteins in the renal tubuli.[6,11]

Importance and management

The modest increase in tenofovir levels with ritonavir-boosted **atazanavir**, **darunavir** and **lopinavir** is of uncertain clinical relevance. However, it has been suggested that higher tenofovir levels could potentiate tenofovir-associated adverse events, including renal disorders.[2,3,17] For this reason, the UK manufacturer of darunavir says that monitoring of renal function may be indicated when ritonavir-boosted darunavir is given in combination with tenofovir, particularly in patients with underlying systemic or renal disease, or in patients taking nephrotoxic drugs.[6] The US manufacturer of lopinavir/ritonavir also recommends monitoring,[18] and this seems a prudent precaution.

The decrease in atazanavir levels with tenofovir is not of clinical importance if ritonavir is also used, and this combination has been used successfully as part of antiretroviral therapy in clinical studies.[1,2] Unboosted atazanavir should be used with caution[19] or not given[3] with tenofovir because of the potential for reduced efficacy and development of resistance. Ritonavir-boosted darunavir and lopinavir levels were not significantly affected by tenofovir, **amprenavir** levels were also unaffected following boosted fosamprenavir administration, and the increase in ritonavir-boosted **saquinavir** levels are not likely to be clinically relevant. The slight interaction between tenofovir and **tipranavir**/ritonavir is unlikely to be clinically relevant. There is no clinically relevant interaction between **nelfinavir** or **indinavir** and tenofovir.

Current UK guidelines give tenofovir as one of the preferred drugs as part of a dual NRTI regimen, to be used with either fosamprenavir/ritonavir or lopinavir/ritonavir, for the treatment of HIV infection in treatment naïve patients. They say that saquinavir/ritonavir is an alternative, and atazanavir/ritonavir may be used in specific groups.[20] US guidelines are similar.[21]

1. Viread (Tenofovir disoproxil fumarate). Gilead Sciences International Ltd. UK Summary of product characteristics, May 2007.
2. Reyataz (Atazanavir sulfate). Bristol-Myers Squibb Pharmaceuticals Ltd. UK Summary of product characteristics, April 2007.
3. Reyataz (Atazanavir sulfate). Bristol-Myers Squibb Company. US Prescribing information, March 2007.
4. Taburet A-M, Piketty C, Chazallon C, Vincent I, Gérard L, Calvez V, Clavel F, Aboulker J-P, Girard P-M, and the ANRS Protocol 107 Puzzle 2 Investigators. Interactions between atazanavir-ritonavir and tenofovir in heavily pretreated human immunodeficiency virus-infected patients. *Antimicrob Agents Chemother* (2004) 48, 2091–6.
5. Hentig NV, Haberl A, Lutz T, Klauke S, Kurowski M, Harder S, Staszewski S. Concomitant intake of tenofovir disoproxil fumarate (TDF) does not impair plasma exposure of ritonavir (RTV) boosted atazanavir (ATV) in HIV-1 infected adults. *Clin Pharmacol Ther* (2005) 77, P18.
6. Prezista (Darunavir ethanolate). Janssen-Cilag Ltd. UK Summary of product characteristics, July 2007.
7. Prezista (Darunavir). Tibotec, Inc. US Prescribing information, June 2006.
8. Lexiva (Fosamprenavir calcium). GlaxoSmithKline. US Prescribing information, June 2007.
9. Kurowski M, Walli R, Breske A, Kruse G, Stocker H, Banik N, Richter H, Mazur D. Coadministration of tenofovir 300 mg QD with fosamprenavir/ritonavir 1.400/100mg QD or 1.400/200mg QD does not affect amprenavir pharmacokinetics. 6th International Workshop on Clinical Pharmacology of HIV Therapy, Québec, 28 – 30 April, 2005. Abstract 10. Available at: http://www.hivpresentation.com/assets/85C4305C-E0C4-D510-02B06CE974717ADB.PDF (accessed 21/08/07).
10. Viread (Tenofovir disoproxil fumarate). Gilead Sciences, Inc. US Prescribing information, May 2007.
11. Rollot F, Nazal E-M, Chauvelot-Moachon L, Kélaïdi C, Daniel N, Saba M, Abad S, Blanche P. Tenofovir-related Fanconi syndrome with nephrogenic diabetes insipidus in a patient with acquired immunodeficiency syndrome: the role of lopinavir-ritonavir-didanosine. *Clin Infect Dis* (2003) 37, e174–e176.
12. Chittick GE, Zong J, Blum MR, Sorbel JJ, Begley JA, Adda N, Kearney BP. Pharmacokinetics of tenofovir disoproxil fumarate and ritonavir-boosted saquinavir mesylate administered alone or in combination at steady state. *Antimicrob Agents Chemother* (2006) 50, 1304–10.
13. Boffito M, Back D, Stainsby-Tron M, Hill A, Di Perri G, Moyle G, Nelson M, Tomkins J, Gazzard B, Pozniak A. Pharmacokinetics of saquinavir hard gel/ritonavir (1000/100 mg twice daily) when administered with tenofovir diproxil fumarate in HIV-1-infected subjects. *Br J Clin Pharmacol* (2005) 59, 38–42.
14. Invirase Tablets (Saquinavir mesilate). Roche Products Ltd. UK Summary of product characteristics, May 2007.
15. Invirase (Saquinavir mesylate). Roche Pharmaceuticals. US Prescribing information, July 2007.
16. Aptivus (Tipranavir). Boehringer Ingelheim. US Prescribing information, February 2007.
17. Kaletra Tablets (Lopinavir/ritonavir). Abbott Laboratories Ltd. UK Summary of product characteristics, March 2007.
18. Kaletra (Lopinavir/ritonavir). Abbott Laboratories. US Prescribing information, January 2007.
19. Hodder S, Bristol-Myers Squibb Company, Klein R, Struble K, FDA. Letter to health care providers. Re: Important new pharmacokinetic data for REYATAZ™ (atazanavir sulfate) in combination with Viread® (tenofovir disoproxil fumarate). August 8, 2003. Available at: http://www.fda.gov/oashi/aids/listserve/listserve2003.html (accessed 21/08/07).
20. Gazzard B on behalf of the writing committee, British HIV Association. British HIV Association (BHIVA) guidelines for the treatment of HIV-infected adults with antiretroviral therapy (2006). *HIV Med* (2006) 7, 487–503. Available at: http://www.bhiva.org/files/file1001303.pdf (accessed 21/08/07).
21. US Department of Health and Human Services; Panel on Antiretroviral Guidelines for Adult and Adolescents. Guidelines for the use of antiretroviral agents in HIV-1-infected adults and adolescents. October 10, 2006; 1–113. Available at: http://www.aidsinfo.nih.gov/contentfiles/AdultandAdolescentGL.pdf (accessed 21/08/07).

Protease inhibitors; Fosamprenavir + Miscellaneous

Fosamprenavir is a prodrug of amprenavir, and is rapidly and almost completely hydrolysed to amprenavir and inorganic phosphate primarily in the lining of the gut.[1,2] The interactions of fosamprenavir are therefore primarily those of amprenavir.

1. Telzir (Fosamprenavir calcium). GlaxoSmithKline UK. UK Summary of product characteristics, February 2007.
2. Lexiva (Fosamprenavir calcium). GlaxoSmithKline. US Prescribing information, June 2007.

Protease inhibitors; Indinavir + Ascorbic acid (Vitamin C)

Vitamin C 1 g daily caused a minor decrease in indinavir levels in healthy subjects.

Clinical evidence, mechanism, importance and management

In a study in healthy subjects high-dose vitamin C 1 g daily for 7 days caused a 14% reduction in the AUC of indinavir and a 20% reduction in its maximum plasma level: indinavir 800 mg was given every 8 hours for 4 doses beginning on day 6,.[1] However, whether this is a real effect needs further study as a similar reduction in plasma levels after a similar indinavir regimen was thought to be a time-dependent effect, see 'milk thistle', (p.830).

1. Slain D, Amsden JR, Khakoo RA, Fisher MA, Lalka D, Hobbs GR. Effect of high-dose vitamin C on the steady-state pharmacokinetics of the protease inhibitor indinavir in healthy volunteers. *Pharmacotherapy* (2005) 25, 165–70.

Protease inhibitors; Indinavir + Goldenseal (*Hydrastis*)

Goldenseal root had no effect on the pharmacokinetics of a single dose of indinavir in one study.

Clinical evidence

In a study in 10 healthy subjects, the peak plasma level and oral clearance of indinavir after a single 800-mg dose was not changed by goldenseal root (*Nature's Way*) 1.14 g twice daily for 2 weeks. In addition, there was no change in the indinavir half-life. Eight of the subjects had less than a 20% change in oral clearance, but one subject had a 46% increase and one a 46% decrease.[1]

Mechanism

Goldenseal (*Hydrastis canadensis*) was found to be an inhibitor of cytochrome P450 isoenzyme CYP3A4 *in vitro*.[2] This was confirmed in a clinical study using oral midazolam as a probe substrate for CYP3A4, which found a decrease of about 40% in the metabolism of midazolam to hydroxymidazolam.[3] Goldenseal root might therefore be expected to inhibit the metabolism of indinavir.

Importance and management

This study suggests that goldenseal root has no effect on indinavir levels, and may be taken without any undue concern in patients on this protease inhibitor, although confirmation may be required in the light of the midazolam probe study, and the two subjects who experienced greater effects. The contrasting results from the indinavir study and the midazolam study might be explained by indinavir having a relatively high oral bioavailability compared with midazolam.[3]

1. Sandhu RS, Prescilla RP, Simonelli TM, Edwards DJ. Influence of goldenseal root on the pharmacokinetics of indinavir. *J Clin Pharmacol* (2003) 43, 1283–8.
2. Budzinski JW, Foster BC, Vandenhoek S, Arnason JT. An in vitro evaluation of human cytochrome P450 3A4 inhibition by selected commercial herbal extracts and tinctures. *Phytomedicine* (2000) 7, 273–82.
3. Gurley BJ, Gardner SF, Hubbard MA, Williams DK, Gentry WB, Khan IA, Shah A. In vivo effects of goldenseal, kava kava, black cohosh, and valerian on human cytochrome P450 1A2, 2D6, 2E1, and 3A4/5 phenotypes. *Clin Pharmacol Ther* (2005) 77, 415–26.

Protease inhibitors; Indinavir + Milk thistle

Although some studies have found that milk thistle slightly lowers indinavir levels, it appears that this is a time-dependent effect rather than a drug interaction, since it also occurred in a control group in one study. The balance of evidence suggests that no important pharmacokinetic interaction occurs.

Clinical evidence

Milk thistle (*Silybum marianum*) 175 mg three times daily (*Thisilyn; Nature's Way,* standardised for silymarin content) for 3 weeks caused a 9% reduction in the AUC of indinavir and a 25% reduction its trough plasma level after four doses of indinavir 800 mg every 8 hours, but only the value for the trough level reached statistical significance.[1] The authors suggested that the effect on the trough level could represent a time-dependent effect of indinavir pharmacokinetics, since the plasma levels without milk thistle were found to be similarly lowered after a washout phase.[1] In another similar study, in 10 healthy subjects, milk thistle standardised for silymarin 160 mg (*General Nutrition Corp.*) three times daily for 13 days and then with indinavir 800 mg every 8 hours for 4 doses did not cause any statistically significant changes in the indinavir pharmacokinetics (6% reduction in AUC and 32% reduction in minimum level).[2] In yet another similar study, in 8 healthy subjects, milk thistle extract 456 mg, standardised for silymarins (*Kare and Hope Ltd*) three times daily for 28 days had no effect on the pharmacokinetics of indinavir 800 mg every 8 hours for four doses when compared with 6 subjects in a control group not receiving milk thistle extract. Both the control and indinavir group had a lower indinavir AUC after the second and third time of administration compared with the first, and this decline was greater in the control group.[3] A meta-analysis of these 3 studies showed no effect of milk thistle on indinavir levels.[3]

Mechanism

Based on *animal* data, milk thistle might be expected to increase indinavir levels by inhibiting its metabolism,[1] or to have effects via P-glycoprotein.[2]

Importance and management

The currently available data suggest that milk thistle extract does not have an effect on the pharmacokinetics of indinavir, although it is not totally conclusive. The reduction in indinavir levels appears to be just a time-dependent effect rather than an effect of the milk thistle, and further study is needed with longer exposure to indinavir than just four doses.

1. Piscitelli SC, Formentini E, Burstein AH, Alfaro R, Jagannatha S, Falloon J. Effect of milk thistle on the pharmacokinetics of indinavir in healthy volunteers. *Pharmacotherapy* (2002) 22, 551–6.
2. DiCenzo R, Shelton M, Jordan K, Koval C, Forrest A, Reichman R, Morse G. Coadministration of milk thistle and indinavir in healthy subjects. *Pharmacotherapy* (2003) 23, 866–70.
3. Mills E, Wilson K, Clarke M, Foster B, Walker S, Rachlis B, DeGroot N, Montori VM, Gold W, Phillips E, Myers S, Gallicano K. Milk thistle and indinavir: a randomized controlled pharmacokinetics study and meta-analysis. *Eur J Clin Pharmacol* (2005) 61, 1–7.

Protease inhibitors; Indinavir + Venlafaxine

In a single-dose study, venlafaxine lowered indinavir levels.

Clinical evidence, mechanism, importance and management

In a study, 9 healthy subjects were given a single dose of indinavir before and after 10 days of venlafaxine 150 mg daily in divided doses. Indinavir did not affect the pharmacokinetics of venlafaxine, but venlafaxine reduced the AUC and maximum plasma levels of indinavir by 28% and 36%, respectively. This is possibly enough to reduce the efficacy of indinavir.[1] Quite why this happens is not clear. More study is needed to establish the effects of multiple doses. Until more is known it would seem prudent to monitor closely to ensure that the antiviral effects of indinavir are not compromised.

1. Levin GM, Nelson LA, DeVane CL, Preston SL, Eisele G, Carson SW. A pharmacokinetic drug-drug interaction study of venlafaxine and indinavir. *Psychopharmacol Bull* (2001) 35, 62–71.

Protease inhibitors; Nelfinavir + Calcium

Calcium supplements do not affect the plasma levels of nelfinavir.

Clinical evidence, mechanism, importance and management

Calcium supplements had no effect on plasma levels of nelfinavir or its M8 metabolite in 15 patients receiving nelfinavir 1.25 g twice daily as part of a HAART regimen. Calcium was given as calcium carbonate 1350 mg twice daily to 9 patients, and calcium gluconate/calcium carbonate 2950/300 mg twice daily to 6 patients, both for 14 days. Plasma levels of nelfinavir were measured before a dose and 3 hours after a dose.[1] Similar results were reported in another study.[2] No nelfinavir dosage adjustments appear necessary if calcium supplements are given.

1. Jensen-Fangel S, Justesen US, Black FT, Pedersen C, Obel N. The use of calcium carbonate in nelfinavir-associated diarrhoea in HIV-1-infected patients. *HIV Med* (2003) 4, 48–52.
2. Kopp Hutzler B, Perez-Rodriguez E, Norton S, Hsyu PH. Pharmacokinetics (PK) interactions between nelfinavir (NFV) and calcium supplements (P277). *AIDS* (2000) 14 (Suppl 4), S96.

Ribavirin + Antacids

The manufacturers of ribavirin note that there was a minor 14% decrease in the AUC of ribavirin 600 mg when it was given with an antacid containing aluminium, magnesium, and simeticone,[1-3] but this is not considered clinically relevant.[1,2] No special precautions are needed.

1. Copegus (Ribavirin). Roche Products Ltd. UK Summary of product characteristics, October 2006.
2. Rebetol (Ribavirin). Schering-Plough Ltd. UK Summary of product characteristics, January 2007.
3. Rebetol (Ribavirin). Schering Corporation. US Prescribing information, June 2004.

Rimantadine + Aspirin or Paracetamol (Acetaminophen)

Both aspirin and paracetamol slightly reduce the levels of rimantadine, but this is unlikely to be clinically relevant.

Clinical evidence, mechanism, importance and management

(a) Aspirin

In a study in healthy subjects, rimantadine 100 mg twice daily was given for 13 days. On day 11, aspirin 650 mg four times daily was started and continued for 8 days. The peak plasma levels and AUC of rimantadine were reduced by about 10% in the presence of aspirin.[1] This reduction is unlikely to be clinically relevant.

(b) Paracetamol

In a study in healthy subjects, rimantadine 100 mg twice daily was given for 13 days. On day 11, paracetamol 650 mg four times daily was started and continued for 8 days. The peak plasma levels and AUC of rimantadine were reduced by about 11% in the presence of paracetamol.[1] This reduction is unlikely to be clinically relevant.

1. Flumadine (Rimantadine hydrochloride). Forest Pharmaceuticals, Inc. US Prescribing information, June 2006.

Rimantadine + Cimetidine

Cimetidine causes a small but probably clinically unimportant rise in the plasma levels of rimantadine.

Clinical evidence, mechanism, importance and management

In 23 healthy subjects the AUC of a single 100-mg dose of rimantadine was increased by 20% and the apparent total clearance reduced by 18% when it was taken one hour after the first dose of cimetidine 300 mg four times daily for 6 days. The authors of the study suggest that these changes are likely to have little, if any, clinical consequences.[1] The effects of multiple dose concurrent use are not known.

1. Holazo AA, Choma N, Brown SY, Lee LF, Wills RJ. Effect of cimetidine on the disposition of rimantadine in healthy subjects. *Antimicrob Agents Chemother* (1989) 33, 820–3.

Telbivudine + Miscellaneous

There appears to be no pharmacokinetic interaction between telbivudine and adefovir, ciclosporin or lamivudine. Peginterferon alfa 2a and food do not alter telbivudine pharmacokinetics. No interactions mediated by the cytochrome P450 isoenzymes are predicted for telbivudine.

Clinical evidence, mechanism, importance and management

(a) Adefovir

In a study in healthy subjects the concurrent use of telbivudine 600 mg daily and adefovir 10 mg daily for 7 days did not alter the pharmacokinetics of either drug, when compared to their use alone.[1] No dosage adjustments of either drug are anticipated to be needed if they are used together.

(b) Ciclosporin

The manufacturer notes that there was no pharmacokinetic interaction between ciclosporin and telbivudine.[2]

(c) Food

In a study in healthy subjects, when a single 600-mg dose of telbivudine was given immediately after a high-fat/high-calorie meal there was no effect on the pharmacokinetics of telbivudine, when compared with the fasting state.[3] Telbivudine may be taken with or without food.

(d) Interferons

The manufacturer notes that peginterferon-alfa 2a did not alter the pharmacokinetics of telbivudine. However, no conclusion could be made about the effect of telbivudine on peginterferon-alfa 2a because of high interindividual variability in its levels.[2]

(e) Lamivudine

In a study in healthy subjects, when telbivudine 200 mg daily and lamivudine 100 mg daily were given concurrently for 7 days the pharmacokinetics of both drugs were unchanged.[1] No dosage adjustments of either drug are anticipated to be needed if they are used together.

(f) Cytochrome P450-mediated interactions

The manufacturer notes that telbivudine is not metabolised and is principally excreted by the kidneys. It is therefore unlikely to be affected by drugs that induce or inhibit cytochrome P450 isoenzymes.[2]

Furthermore, *in vitro* studies suggest that telbivudine does not inhibit any of the cytochrome P450 isoenzymes commonly responsible for drug metabolism, and is therefore unlikely to interact with drugs that are substrates for these isoenzymes.[2]

1. Zhou X-J, Fielman BA, Lloyd DM, Chao GC, Brown NA. Pharmacokinetics of telbivudine in healthy subjects and absence of drug interaction with lamivudine or adefovir dipivoxil. *Antimicrob Agents Chemother* (2006) 50, 2309–15.
2. Tyzeka (Telbivudine). Idenix Pharmaceuticals, Inc. US Prescribing information, October 2006.
3. Zhou X-J, Lloyd DM, Chao GC, Brown NA. Absence of food effect on the pharmacokinetics of telbivudine following oral administration in healthy subjects. *J Clin Pharmacol* (2006) 46, 275–81.

Tenofovir + Miscellaneous

Tenofovir absorption is increased by high-fat food. Caution is recommended with drugs causing renal toxicity. Tenofovir did not alter the pharmacokinetics of ribavirin, and there was no clinically significant pharmacokinetic interaction with rifampicin (rifampin).

Clinical evidence, mechanism, importance and management

(a) Cidofovir

Tenofovir is actively secreted by human organic anion transporter 1 (hOAT1) in the kidneys. Therefore, the manufacturers suggest that if it is given with other drugs that are also secreted by this renal transporter, such as cidofovir, increased levels of tenofovir or the other drug could result. In the UK, they specifically recommend that tenofovir and cidofovir are not given together, unless clearly necessary, when renal function should be monitored weekly.[1]

(b) Food

Administration of tenofovir with a high-fat meal increased its AUC by about 40%, and its maximum level by about 14%, when compared with the fasted state, whereas administration with a light meal had no effect.[1,2] The UK manufacturer recommends that tenofovir is taken with food,[1] whereas the US manufacturer says that it can be taken without regard to food.[2]

(c) Other nephrotoxic drugs

Tenofovir has the potential to cause nephrotoxicity, and the manufacturer recommends monthly monitoring of renal function. Although the concurrent administration of other nephrotoxic drugs has not been studied, the manufacturer suggests that renal function should be monitored more frequently (weekly) if concurrent use is unavoidable. They specifically name **aminoglycosides**, **amphotericin B**, **cidofovir** (see above), **foscarnet**, **ganciclovir**, **interleukin-2**, **pentamidine** and **vancomycin**.[1]

(d) Ribavirin

Tenofovir disoproxil fumarate 300 mg daily did not alter the pharmacokinetics of a single 600-mg dose of ribavirin in 22 subjects, and the pharmacokinetics of tenofovir did not appear to be changed by ribavirin when compared with historical data.[3] Note that, there is evidence that HIV-positive patients co-infected with hepatitis C and treated with interferon alfa and ribavirin may be at increased risk of lactic acidosis and hepatic decompensation when receiving any 'NRTI', (p.805), including tenofovir, and increased monitoring is recommended.[1]

(e) Rifampicin (Rifampin)

In 23 subjects when rifampicin 600 mg once daily was given with tenofovir disoproxil fumarate 300 mg once daily the pharmacokinetics of both drugs were not significantly changed (tenofovir compared with historical data). One subject who was withdrawn from the study had raised liver enzyme values.[4]

1. Viread (Tenofovir disoproxil fumarate). Gilead Sciences International Ltd. UK Summary of product characteristics, May 2007.
2. Viread (Tenofovir disoproxil fumarate). Gilead Sciences, Inc. US Prescribing information, May 2007.
3. Ramanathan S, Cheng A, Mittan A, Ebrahimi R, Kearney BP. Absence of clinically relevant pharmacokinetic interaction between ribavirin and tenofovir in healthy subjects. *J Clin Pharmacol* (2006) 46, 559–66.
4. Droste JAH, Verweij-van Wissen CPWGM, Kearney BP, Buffels R, vanHorssen PJ, Hekster YA, Burger DM. Pharmacokinetic study of tenofovir disoproxil fumarate combined with rifampin in healthy volunteers. *Antimicrob Agents Chemother* (2005) 49, 680–4.

Vidarabine + Allopurinol

There is some evidence to suggest that if allopurinol and vidarabine (adenine arabinoside) are given together the toxicity of vidarabine may be increased.

Clinical evidence

Two patients with chronic lymphocytic leukaemia taking allopurinol 300 mg daily developed severe neurotoxicity (coarse rhythmic tremors of the extremities and facial muscles, and impaired mentation) 4 days after vidarabine was added for the treatment of viral infections.[1] A retrospective search to find other patients who had taken both drugs for 4 days revealed a total of 17 patients, 5 of whom had experienced adverse reactions including tremors, nausea, pain, itching and anaemia.[1] Another possible case of neurological toxicity has also been reported.[2]

Mechanism

Uncertain. One suggestion is that the allopurinol causes hypoxanthine arabinoside, the major metabolite of vidarabine, to accumulate by inhibiting xanthine oxidase. A study with *rat* liver cytosol found that allopurinol greatly increased the half-life of this metabolite.[3]

Importance and management

Information seems to be limited to these reports, and so the general clinical importance of this possible interaction is uncertain, but it would be prudent to exercise particular care if these drugs are used together.

1. Friedman HM, Grasela T. Adenine arabinoside and allopurinol – possible adverse drug interaction. *N Engl J Med* (1981) 304, 423.
2. Collignon PJ, Sorrell TC. Neurological toxicity associated with vidarabine (adenine arabinoside) therapy. *Aust N Z J Med* (1983) 13, 627–9.
3. Drach JC, Rentea RG, Cowen ME. The metabolic degradation of 9-β-D-arabinofuranosyladenine (ara-A) *in vitro*. *Fedn Proc* (1973) 32, 777.

22

Beta blockers

The adrenoceptors of the sympathetic nervous system are of two main types, namely alpha and beta. Drugs that block the beta adrenoceptors (better known as the beta blockers) are therapeutically exploited to reduce, for example, the normal sympathetic stimulation of the heart. The activity of the heart in response to stress and exercise is reduced, its consumption of oxygen is diminished, and in this way exercise-induced angina can be managed. Beta blockers given orally can also be used in the management of cardiac arrhythmias, hypertension, myocardial infarction, and heart failure. They may also be used for some symptoms of anxiety and for migraine prophylaxis. Some beta blockers are used in the form of eye drops for glaucoma and ocular hypertension.

Not all beta receptors are identical but can be further subdivided into two groups, $beta_1$ and $beta_2$. The former are found in the heart and the latter in the bronchi. Since one of the unwanted adverse effects of generalised beta blockade can be the loss of the normal noradrenaline-stimulated bronchodilation (leading to bronchospasm), cardioselective $beta_1$-blocking drugs (e.g. atenolol, metoprolol) were developed, which have less effect on $beta_2$ receptors. However, it should be emphasised that the selectivity is not absolute because bronchospasm can still occur with these drugs, particularly at high doses. 'Table 22.1', (below) includes an indication of the cardioselectivity of commonly used systemic beta blockers. Some beta blockers also have $alpha_1$-blocking activity, which causes vasodilatation, and this is also indicated in 'Table 22.1', (below). Some beta blockers, such as celiprolol and nebivolol, also have vasodilator activity but produce this by mechanisms other than blocking $alpha_1$ receptors. Other beta blockers also possess intrinsic sympathomimetic activity in that they can *activate* beta receptors and are therefore partial agonists. Sotalol has additional class III antiarrhythmic activity, and therefore it has a range of interactions not shared by most other beta blockers.

Beta blockers may be lipophilic drugs (such as metoprolol) or hydrophilic (such as atenolol). The lipophilic beta blockers are more likely to be involved in pharmacokinetic interactions than the hydrophilic drugs. Many of the lipophilic beta blockers are principally metabolised by the cytochrome P450 isoenzyme CYP2D6 (see 'Table 22.1', (below)), and drugs that are inhibitors or inducers of this isoenzyme (see 'Table 1.3', (p.6)) increase or decrease their levels. Propranolol is also metabolised in part by CYP1A2 (see 'Beta blockers + SSRIs', p.855).

Beta blockers may also be involved in pharmacodynamic interactions with other drugs that are based on enhancement or antagonism of pharmacological effects (such as additive blood pressure reduction).

This section is generally concerned with those drugs that affect the activity of the beta blockers. Where the beta blocker is the affecting drug, the interaction is dealt with elsewhere.

Table 22.1 The actions and metabolism of widely used systemic beta blockers

Drug	*$Beta_1$-receptor selectivity*	*Alpha-blocking activity?*	*ISA**	*Lipophilicity*	*Bioavailability*	*First pass metabolism*	*Metabolism*
Acebutolol	Selective	No	Yes (weak)	Hydrophilic	50 to 70%	30 to 50%	Rapidly metabolised to an active metabolite after which about 50% is excreted by the liver and 50% excreted in the urine.
Atenolol	Selective	No	No	Hydrophilic	40 to 50%	Less than 10%	Largely excreted unchanged in the urine.
Bisoprolol	Selective	No	No	Intermediate	88%	Less than 10%	50% hepatic metabolism and 50% excreted unchanged in the urine.
Carvedilol	Non-selective	Yes ($alpha_1$)	No	Lipophilic	25 to 35%	60 to 80%	Primarily metabolised by CYP2D6, although other isoenzymes do contribute.
Celiprolol	Selective	Yes (weak $alpha_2$)	Yes	Hydrophilic	30 to 70%	Little	Mostly excreted unchanged (only 1-3% metabolised) with 50% excreted in the bile and 50% excreted in the urine.
Esmolol	Selective	No	No	Relatively hydrophilic	N/A	Extensive	Rapidly hydrolysed in red blood cells (half-life 9 minutes).
Labetalol	Non-selective	Yes (postsynaptic $alpha_2$)	No	Moderately lipophilic	25 to 40%	Extensive	Conjugated in the liver.
Metoprolol	Selective	No	No	Lipophilic	50%	About 40 to 60%	Metabolised by CYP2D6.
Nadolol	Non-selective	No	No	Hydrophilic	20 to 40%	Little	Largely excreted unchanged in the urine.
Nebivolol	Selective	No	No		12 to 96%	Extensive	Metabolised by CYP2D6.
Oxprenolol	Non-selective	No	Yes	Lipophilic	19 to 74%	25 to 80%	Extensively metabolised by the liver.
Pindolol	Non-selective	No	Yes	Moderately lipophilic	90 to 100%	Little	30 to 40% excreted unchanged in the urine, rest excreted by liver and kidney as inactive metabolites.
Propranolol	Non-selective	No	No	Lipophilic	30 to 70%	Up to 95%	Mainly metabolised by CYP2D6 with some contribution by CYP1A2.
Sotalol	Non-selective	No	No	Hydrophilic	75 to 90%	None	Largely excreted unchanged in the urine.
Timolol	Non-selective	No	No	Lipophilic	61%	About 50 to 70%	Mostly metabolised by the liver, with some involvement from CYP2D6. 20% excreted unchanged. Timolol and metabolites renally excreted.

*Intrinsic sympathomimetic activity (partial agonists)

Beta blockers + Antacids or Antidiarrhoeals

Some antacids and antidiarrhoeals may cause a modest reduction in the absorption of atenolol, indenolol, propranolol, or sotalol, and possibly a slight increase in the absorption of metoprolol. However, the clinical importance of these interactions is probably minimal.

Clinical evidence

(a) Atenolol

Aluminium hydroxide 5.6 g given to 6 healthy subjects caused an insignificant 20% fall in the plasma levels of a single 100-mg dose of atenolol, which had no effect on the atenolol-induced reduction in exercising heart rate. Similarly, **aluminium hydroxide** had no significant effect on atenolol pharmacokinetics when both drugs were given together for 6 days.[1] Conversely, in 6 healthy subjects a single 500-mg dose of **calcium** (as the lactate, gluconate and carbonate) caused a 51% reduction in the peak plasma level of a single 100-mg dose of atenolol. **Calcium** also reduced the AUC of atenolol by 32%, and increased the elimination half-life from 6.2 to 11 hours. The effect of atenolol on heart rate was decreased by 12%. However, these changes were no longer significant after 6 days of concurrent use, except for a 21% reduction in peak plasma atenolol levels. In a further 6 hypertensive subjects, neither **calcium** 500 mg daily nor **aluminium hydroxide** 5.6 g daily had any influence on the blood pressure lowering effect of atenolol 100 mg daily for 4 weeks.[1]

Another study in 6 healthy subjects found that 30 mL of *Novalucol forte* (an **aluminium/magnesium-containing antacid**) reduced the peak plasma level and AUC of a single 100-mg dose of atenolol by 37% and 33%, respectively, which was considered to be of possible significance in some patients.[2]

(b) Indenolol

A study in *rats* found that when indenolol was given with either *Simeco* (**aluminium/magnesium hydroxide** with **simeticone**) or *Kaopectate* (**kaolin-pectin**), the AUC_{0-6} was reduced by 15% and 30%, respectively.[3]

(c) Metoprolol

In 6 healthy subjects, 30 mL of *Novalucol forte* (an **aluminium/magnesium-containing antacid**) increased the peak plasma level and AUC of a single 100-mg dose of metoprolol by 25% and 11%, respectively.[2]

(d) Propranolol

Aluminium hydroxide gel 30 mL did not affect the plasma level of a single 40-mg dose of propranolol in 6 healthy subjects: the reduction in exercise heart rate was also unaffected.[4] In contrast, a study in 5 healthy subjects found that 30 mL of an **aluminium hydroxide gel** reduced the levels and AUC of a single 80-mg dose of propranolol by almost 60%.[5] *In vitro* and *animal* data suggest that **bismuth subsalicylate, kaolin-pectin** and **magnesium trisilicate** can also reduce the absorption of propranolol.[6,7]

(e) Sotalol

A study in 5 healthy subjects found that single doses of **aluminium hydroxide** suspension (*Neutragel*) or **calcium carbonate** suspension, given after an overnight fast, had negligible effects on the pharmacokinetics of a single 160-mg dose of sotalol.[8] In contrast, a single dose of **magnesium hydroxide** slightly reduced the AUC of sotalol by 16%.[8] A further study in 6 healthy subjects found that when 20 mL of *Maalox* (**aluminium/magnesium hydroxide**) was given at the same time as 160 mg of sotalol, the maximum plasma level of the sotalol was reduced by 26% and its AUC was reduced by 21%. Changes in heart rates reflected these pharmacokinetic changes.[9] No interaction occurred when the *Maalox* was given 2 hours after the sotalol.[9]

Mechanism

Uncertain. The reduction in absorption could possibly be related to a delay in gastric emptying caused by the antacid, delayed dissolution due to an increase in gastric pH, or to the formation of a complex of the two drugs in the gut, which reduces absorption. However, one *in vitro* study indicated that sotalol was only subject to minor absorption or complexation interactions.[9] Another study found that 35 to 40% of sotalol was bound by magnesium hydroxide, but this may be reversible under physiological conditions and therefore unlikely to be relevant during long-term clinical use.[8]

Importance and management

The documentation is limited, in some instances somewhat contradictory, and largely confined to *animal* or single-dose studies, which may not be clinically relevant. Some changes in absorption may possibly occur but no study seems to have shown that there is a significant effect on the therapeutic effectiveness of the beta blockers. The one study using atenolol in patients found that the pharmacokinetic changes seen with single doses of **aluminium** or calcium-containing antacids were not clinically significant.[1] However, be alert for any changes during concurrent use. Separating the dosages by 2 hours was shown to avoid the interaction in one study,[9] and would seem a simple way of avoiding problems should they occur.

1. Kirch W, Schäfer-Korting M, Axthelm T, Köhler H, Mutschler E. Interaction of atenolol with furosemide and calcium and aluminium salts. *Clin Pharmacol Ther* (1981) 30, 429–35.
2. Regårdh CG, Lundborg P, Persson BA. The effect of antacid, metoclopramide and propantheline on the bioavailability of metoprolol and atenolol. *Biopharm Drug Dispos* (1981) 2, 79–87.
3. Tariq M, Babhair SA. Effect of antacid and antidiarrhoeal drugs on the bioavailability of indenolol. *IRCS Med Sci* (1984) 12, 87–8.
4. Hong CY, Hu SC, Lin SJ, Chiang BN. Lack of influence of aluminium hydroxide on the bioavailability and beta-adrenoceptor blocking activity of propranolol. *Int J Clin Pharmacol Ther Toxicol* (1985) 23, 244–6.
5. Dobbs JH, Skoutakis VA, Acchardio SR, Dobbs BR. Effects of aluminium hydroxide on the absorption of propranolol. *Curr Ther Res* (1977) 21, 887–92.
6. Moustafa MA, Gouda MW, Tariq M. Decreased bioavailability of propranolol due to interactions with adsorbent antacids and antidiarrhoeal mixtures. *Int J Pharmaceutics* (1986) 30, 225–8.
7. McElnay JC, D'Arcy PF, Leonard JK. The effect of activated dimethicone, other antacid constituents, and kaolin on the absorption of propranolol. *Experientia* (1982) 38, 605–7.
8. Kahela P, Anttila M, Sundqvist H. Antacids and sotalol absorption. *Acta Pharmacol Toxicol (Copenh)* (1981) 49, 181–3.
9. Läer S, Neumann J, Scholz H. Interaction between sotalol and an antacid preparation. *Br J Clin Pharmacol* (1997) 43, 269–72.

Beta blockers + Anticholinesterases

A small number of reports describe marked bradycardia and hypotension during the recovery period from anaesthesia and neuromuscular blockade, when patients taking beta blockers were given anticholinesterase drugs. However, normally no adverse reaction seems to occur. Myasthenic symptoms and myasthenia gravis have occurred when oral or topical beta blockers were given alone, and so beta blockers could oppose the efficacy of anticholinesterases in treating myasthenia gravis.

Clinical evidence

(a) Anticholinesterase effects

Three patients developed myasthenic symptoms when given beta blockers (two taking **propranolol** and one taking **oxprenolol**). Two of them were effectively treated with **pyridostigmine**.[1] Another patient developed fulminant myasthenia gravis within 2 weeks of starting to take **acebutolol**.[2] Similarly, in a patient with myasthenia gravis, the use of **timolol** eye drops was associated with a deterioration in muscle strength,[3] and in another patient, a serious deterioration in myasthenia.[4]

However, in a study in 10 myasthenic patients with mild to moderate symptoms, intravenous **propranolol** 100 micrograms/kg did not result in a worsening of neuromuscular transmission (assessed by muscle function tests and repetitive nerve stimulation), even though 8 of those with mild symptoms had reduced their **pyridostigmine** dose during the study to allow the effects of the additional drug to be more readily seen.[5]

(b) Bradycardia

A patient taking **nadolol** 40 mg daily, recovering from surgery during which suxamethonium (succinylcholine) and pancuronium had been given, developed prolonged bradycardia of 32 to 36 bpm and hypotension (systolic pressure 60 to 70 mmHg) when **neostigmine** and atropine were given to reverse the neuromuscular blockade. Isoprenaline and phenylephrine infusions were required to maintain a systolic blood pressure of 90 mmHg, and were gradually reduced over 3 days. **Propranolol** was substituted for **nadolol**, and about 10 weeks later the patient underwent general anaesthesia again (this time without a neuromuscular blocker/**neostigmine**) and she recovered uneventfully.[6] A patient taking **pro-**

pranolol 20 mg twice daily, recovering from surgery during which alcuronium had been used, received glycopyrronium and **neostigmine** without any change in heart rate. However, one hour later he developed severe bradycardia (a fall from 65 to 40 bpm) and hypotension (systolic blood pressure 70 mmHg) when given intravenous **physostigmine** 2 mg over 5 minutes, for extreme drowsiness attributed to the premedication. His symptoms responded to glycopyrronium.[7] Prolonged bradycardia and hypotension, requiring isoprenaline then adrenaline (epinephrine), were seen in an elderly woman taking **atenolol** 50 mg daily and nitrates when she was given **neostigmine** and atropine for the reversal of muscle relaxation at the end of general anaesthesia.[8] Another report similarly describes bradycardia in a patient taking **propranolol** when intravenous **neostigmine** was used to reverse pancuronium-induced blockade. This responded to atropine.[9]

However, a study in 8 hypertensive patients taking long-term **atenolol** or **propranolol** found no significant changes in heart rate and no serious adverse reactions when they were given low-dose oral **pyridostigmine** 30 mg three times daily for 2 days.[10]

Mechanism

It would appear that the bradycardic effects of the beta blockers and the acetylcholine-like effects of these anticholinesterase drugs can be additive. These were inadequately controlled by the use of atropine in some of the instances cited. The myasthenic symptoms may be due to beta blockers exerting a depressant effect on the neuromuscular junction.[2,3]

Importance and management

The information available indicates that marked adverse reactions between beta blockers and anticholinesterases after surgery are uncommon, but be aware of the possibility of an interaction if a patient becomes bradycardic or hypotensive shortly after surgery.

Limited information suggests that beta blockers given orally or topically could oppose the efficacy of anticholinesterases in the treatment of myasthenia gravis. However, one study suggests that, in cardiovascular emergencies, propranolol may be given to patients with myasthenia gravis, provided that resuscitation equipment and specific antidotes are available.[5] Strictly speaking this is a drug-disease rather than a drug-drug interaction.

1. Herishanu Y, Rosenberg P. Beta-blockers and myasthenia gravis. *Ann Intern Med* (1975) 83, 834–5.
2. Confavreux C, Charles N, Aimard G. Fulminant myasthenia gravis soon after initiation of acebutolol therapy. *Eur Neurol* (1990) 30, 279–81.
3. Verkijk A. Worsening of myasthenia gravis with timolol maleate eyedrops. *Ann Neurol* (1985) 17, 211–12.
4. Shaivitz SA. Timolol and myasthenia gravis. *JAMA* (1979) 242, 1611–12.
5. Jonkers I, Swerup C, Pirskanen R, Bjelak S, Matell G. Acute effects of intravenous injection of beta-adrenoreceptor- and calcium channel antagonists and agonists in myasthenia gravis. *Muscle Nerve* (1996) 19, 959–65.
6. Seidl DC, Martin DE. Prolonged bradycardia after neostigmine administration in a patient taking nadolol. *Anesth Analg* (1984) 63, 365–7.
7. Baraka A, Dajani A. Severe bradycardia following physostigmine in the presence of beta-adrenergic blockade. *Middle East J Anesthesiol* (1984) 7, 291–3.
8. Eldor J, Hoffman B, Davidson JT. Prolonged bradycardia and hypotension after neostigmine administration in a patient receiving atenolol. *Anaesthesia* (1987) 42, 1294–7.
9. Sprague DH. Severe bradycardia after neostigmine in a patient taking propranolol to control paroxysmal atrial tachycardia. *Anesthesiology* (1975) 42, 208–10.
10. Arad M, Roth A, Zelinger J, Zivner Z, Rabinowitz B, Atsmon J. Safety of pyridostigmine in hypertensive patients receiving beta blockers. *Am J Cardiol* (1992) 69, 518–22.

Beta blockers + Aspirin or NSAIDs

There is evidence that most NSAIDs can increase blood pressure in patients taking antihypertensives, although some studies have not found the increase to be clinically relevant. In various small studies, indometacin reduced the antihypertensive effects of the beta blockers. There is some evidence that piroxicam usually interacts similarly. Ibuprofen and naproxen have reduced the effect of beta blockers in some small studies but not others. Two isolated cases of hypertension have been reported with naproxen and ibuprofen in patients treated with propranolol and pindolol, respectively. Celecoxib, but not rofecoxib, inhibits the metabolism of metoprolol. Limited information suggests that normally diclofenac, imidazole salicylate, oxaprozin, tenoxicam and probably sulindac do not interact.

Multiple-dose aspirin, both in high and low dose, did not reduce the efficacy of antihypertensives including beta blockers in three studies, but one study using single, high doses showed antagonism of the effect of intravenous beta blockers. Another study suggested aspirin may attenuate the benefit of carvedilol in heart failure.

Clinical evidence

Various large epidemiological studies and meta-analyses of clinical studies have been conducted to assess the effect of NSAIDs on blood pressure in patients treated with **antihypertensives**, and the findings of these are summarised in 'Table 23.2', (p.862). In these studies, NSAIDs were not always associated with an increase in blood pressure, and the maximum increase was 6.2 mmHg. The effect has been shown for both COX-2 inhibitors and non-selective NSAIDs. In two meta-analyses,[1,2] the effects were evaluated by NSAID. The confidence intervals for all the NSAIDs overlapped, showing that there was no statistically significant difference between the NSAIDs, with the exception of the comparison between **indometacin** and **sulindac** in one analysis.[1] Nevertheless, an attempt was made at ranking the NSAIDs based on the means. In one analysis,[1] the effect was greatest for **piroxicam**, **indometacin**, and **ibuprofen**, intermediate for **naproxen**, and least for **sulindac** and **flurbiprofen**. In the other meta-analysis,[2] the effect was greatest for **indometacin** and **naproxen**, intermediate for **piroxicam**, and least for **ibuprofen** and **sulindac**. An attempt was also made to evaluate the effect by **antihypertensive** in one analysis.[1] The mean effect was greatest for beta blockers, intermediate for vasodilators (includes ACE inhibitors and calcium-channel blockers), and least for diuretics. However, the differences between the groups were not significant.

The findings of individual clinical and pharmacological studies that have studied the effects of aspirin or specific NSAIDs on beta blockers are outlined in the subsections below.

(a) Aspirin and other salicylates

A small study in patients taking various antihypertensives (including beta blockers and diuretics) found that aspirin, in both low doses (650 mg daily) and high doses (3.9 g daily) for 3 or 4 weeks, did not cause clinically significant increases in blood pressure.[3] Similarly, a study in 11 patients taking a number of antihypertensives (which included a few patients taking **propranolol** or **pindolol**) found that aspirin 650 mg three times daily for 7 days did not affect the control of blood pressure.[4] In contrast, another study found that 5 g of aspirin given over 24 hours prevented the antihypertensive effects of a single 1-mg intravenous dose of **pindolol**, and a single 1- to 1.5-g dose of aspirin reduced the antihypertensive effect of a single 5-mg intravenous dose of **propranolol**.[5] Aspirin was reported not to affect the control of hypertension by **metipranolol**.[6] A retrospective study of patients with heart failure taking **carvedilol** found that aspirin did not significantly affect systolic blood pressure or heart rate but did observe that left ventricular ejection fraction improved less in those patients taking aspirin in addition to **carvedilol** The effect appeared to be dose-related.[7]

A single-dose study in 6 healthy subjects found that aspirin 500 mg did not affect the pharmacokinetics of **atenolol**.[8] Another study in 6 healthy subjects found that aspirin did not affect the pharmacokinetics of **metoprolol**, but the maximum plasma levels of aspirin were increased by **metoprolol**, although this was not considered to be clinically relevant.[9]

Sodium salicylate did not affect either the pharmacokinetics of **alprenolol** or its effects on heart rate and blood pressure during exercise in a single-dose study in healthy subjects.[10] **Imidazole salicylate** did not affect the blood pressure control of patients treated with **atenolol**.[11]

(b) Celecoxib or Rofecoxib

In an open, randomised crossover study in 12 healthy subjects, celecoxib 200 mg twice daily for 7 days increased the AUC of a single 50-mg dose of **metoprolol** by 64%. In contrast, rofecoxib 25 mg daily for 7 days did not significantly affect the pharmacokinetics of **metoprolol**.

(c) Diclofenac

A study in 16 patients taking **atenolol**, **metoprolol**, **propranolol** or **pindolol** and/or a diuretic found that diclofenac 50 mg three times daily had no effect on the control of blood pressure.[12]

(d) Flurbiprofen

A study in 10 patients with hypertension found that flurbiprofen 100 mg daily for 7 days did not affect the pharmacokinetics of single-doses of either **propranolol** 80 mg or **atenolol** 100 mg. However, the hypotensive effects of **propranolol** but not **atenolol** were reduced by the flurbiprofen.[13]

(e) Ibuprofen

In a randomised study, ibuprofen 400 mg every 8 hours caused significant increases in blood pressure (mean increases of about 5 to 7 mmHg) in 6 hypertensive patients treated with thiazides and beta blockers.[14] The antihypertensive effect of **pindolol** was antagonised by ibuprofen in one patient.[15] However, ibuprofen 400 mg four times daily had no effect on the control of blood pressure in patients taking **propranolol** in one randomised controlled study.[16]

(f) Indometacin

A study found that when indometacin 25 mg three times daily was given to hypertensive patients taking thiazides with or without beta blockers, their blood pressure increased by 8 to 10 mmHg.[3] The diastolic blood pressures of 7 hypertensive patients treated with **pindolol** 15 mg daily or **propranolol** 80 to 160 mg daily rose from 82 to 96 mmHg when they were given indometacin 100 mg daily over a 10-day period. Changes in systolic pressures were not statistically significant.[17]

In another study, indometacin 50 mg twice daily raised the systolic/diastolic blood pressures of patients taking **propranolol** 60 to 320 mg daily by 14/5 mmHg when lying and 16/9 mmHg when standing.[18] This interaction has also been seen in other studies in patients taking **atenolol**,[11,19,20] **labetalol**,[21] **metipranolol**,[6] **oxprenolol**,[22,23] and **propranolol**.[4,24] Two women with pre-eclampsia taking **propranolol** or **pindolol** became markedly hypertensive (rises in blood pressure from 135/85 to 240/140 mmHg, and from 130/70 to 230/130 mmHg, respectively) within 4 to 5 days of being given indometacin to inhibit premature contractions.[25]

(g) Naproxen

A study in hypertensive patients taking **timolol** and hydrochlorothiazide with amiloride found that naproxen 250 mg twice daily caused a significant 4 mmHg rise in diastolic blood pressure, but did not significantly increase systolic blood pressure.[26] Similarly, in another study, naproxen 500 mg twice daily caused an average 4 mmHg rise in systolic blood pressure in patients taking **atenolol**, but did not significantly increase diastolic blood pressure.[27] In contrast, another study found that naproxen caused no changes in hypertension controlled with **propranolol**,[28] and a study in patients taking antihypertensives [drugs not specified] found that naproxen did not cause clinically significant increases in blood pressure.[3] A case report describes one patient taking **propranolol** who had a marked rise in blood pressure when given naproxen.[29]

(h) Oxaprozin

A study in 32 hypertensive arthritic patients found that oxaprozin 1.2 g daily for 4 weeks did not affect the antihypertensive effects of **metoprolol** 100 mg twice daily, although at 2 weeks there was a significant increase in systolic blood pressure.[30]

(i) Piroxicam

A double-blind study found that about one-quarter of the patients given piroxicam 20 mg daily and **propranolol** 80 to 160 mg daily developed diastolic pressure rises of 10 mmHg or more when lying or standing.[31,32] Increases in both systolic and diastolic pressures (8.1/5.2 mmHg lying and 8.5/8.9 mmHg standing) were seen in another study in 3 patients.[33] In contrast, patients taking **propranolol** and piroxicam 20 mg daily had blood pressure rises of 5.8/2.4 mmHg when lying and 3.5/0.5 mmHg when standing, after 2 weeks, but these increases were not statistically significant.[34] Blood pressure showed a trend towards higher levels in another study in 20 patients given **timolol** and piroxicam 20 mg daily.[26]

A study in 6 healthy subjects given **atenolol** 100 mg daily and piroxicam 20 mg daily for 7 days found no pharmacokinetic interaction. An associated study in another 6 healthy subjects given **metoprolol** 100 mg twice daily and piroxicam 20 mg daily for 7 days found that **metoprolol** levels were increased by piroxicam, but not to a statistically significant extent.[35]

(j) Sulindac

Sulindac 200 mg twice daily had little or no effect on the control of hypertension in patients taking hydrochlorothiazide with amiloride and **atenolol**, **metoprolol**, **propranolol** or **pindolol**.[12] In another study, diastolic blood pressure was slightly and significantly lower when sulindac was given with **timolol**.[26] No statistically significant rises in blood pressure occurred in other studies in patients taking **propranolol**[28,31-33] or **atenolol**[20,27] or unspecified antihypertensives[3] given sulindac 200 mg twice daily. In contrast, another study claimed that patients given **propranolol** with sulindac 200 mg twice daily had blood pressure rises of 10.3/4.8 mmHg when standing and 2.4/7.1 mmHg when lying, after 2 weeks, but only the increase in standing systolic blood pressure statistically significant.[34] Similarly, a crossover study in 26 hypertensive patients taking **labetalol** found that sulindac 200 mg twice daily for 7 days raised the mean systolic blood pressure by 6 mmHg when sitting, and by 9 to 14 mmHg when standing, which was considered potentially clinically significant. Diastolic pressures were not affected.[21]

(k) Tenoxicam

The control of hypertension in 16 patients taking **atenolol** was found not to be affected by tenoxicam 40 mg daily.[36]

Mechanism

Indometacin alone can raise blood pressure (13 hypertensive patients given indometacin 150 mg daily for 3 days had a mean systolic blood pressure rise from 118 to 131 mmHg).[37] One suggested reason is that indometacin inhibits the synthesis and release of two prostaglandins (PGA and PGE), which have a potent dilating effect on peripheral arterioles throughout the body. In their absence the blood pressure rises. Thus the hypotensive actions of the beta blockers are opposed by the hypertensive actions of indometacin. This mechanism has been questioned and it is possible that other physiological and pharmacological mechanisms have a part to play.[3,38,39] One study found that although indometacin caused increases in blood pressure in treated hypertensive patients, other inhibitors of prostaglandin synthesis (aspirin, naproxen and sulindac) did not.[3] Further, all four drugs caused similar reductions in plasma renin activity and aldosterone concentration, which suggests that the effect of indometacin on blood pressure may not be dependent on such changes.[3]

Celecoxib, but not rofecoxib, inhibits the metabolism of metoprolol by the cytochrome P450 isoenzyme CYP2D6.[40]

Importance and management

Overall, the evidence suggests that some patients treated with beta blockers can show a rise in blood pressure when given NSAIDs, but this may not always be clinically relevant. Some consider that the use of NSAIDs should be kept to a minimum in patients on antihypertensives.[41] The effects may be greater in the elderly and in those with blood pressures that are relatively high, as well as in those with high salt intake.[41] However, others consider that the clinical importance of an interaction between NSAIDs and antihypertensives is less than has previously been suggested.[42] While their findings do not rule out a 2/1 mmHg increase in blood pressure with NSAIDs in treated hypertensives, they suggest that if patients in primary care have inadequate control of blood pressure, other reasons may be more likely than any effect of concurrent NSAIDs.[42] There is insufficient data at present to clearly differentiate between NSAIDs, although there is some evidence that the effects of indometacin are greatest and sulindac least. Further study is needed.

For the effects of NSAIDs on other antihypertensive drug classes see 'ACE inhibitors', (p.28), 'calcium-channel blockers', (p.861) and 'thiazide diuretics', (p.956).

A few multiple-dose studies have not found aspirin to alter the antihypertensive effect of beta blockers, even in high doses, but one single-dose high-dose study reported an interaction. Another study suggested that aspirin might attenuate the benefit of carvedilol in heart failure, but the evidence is currently too slim to warrant a change in practice.

Although celecoxib increased levels of metoprolol, increases in plasma metoprolol levels of this size are unlikely to be clinically relevant.

1. Johnson AG, Nguyen TV, Day RO. Do nonsteroidal anti-inflammatory drugs affect blood pressure? A meta-analysis. *Ann Intern Med* (1994) 121, 289–300.
2. Pope JE, Anderson JJ, Felson DT. A meta-analysis of the effects of nonsteroidal anti-inflammatory drugs on blood pressure. *Arch Intern Med* (1993) 153, 477–84.
3. Chalmers JP, West MJ, Wing LMH, Bune AJC, Graham JR. Effects of indomethacin, sulindac, naproxen, aspirin, and paracetamol in treated hypertensive patients. *Clin Exp Hypertens A* (1984) 6, 1077–93.

4. Mills EH, Whitworth JA, Andrews J, Kincaid-Smith P. Non-steroidal anti-inflammatory drugs and blood pressure. *Aust N Z J Med* (1982) 12, 478–82.
5. Sziegoleit W, Rausch J, Polák G, György M, Dekov E, Békés M. Influence of acetylsalicylic acid on acute circulatory effects of the beta-blocking agents pindolol and propranolol in humans. *Int J Clin Pharmacol Ther Toxicol* (1982) 20, 423–30.
6. Macek K, Jurin I. Effects of indomethacine and aspirin on the antihypertensive action of metipranolol — a clinical study. *Eur J Pharmacol* (1990) 183, 839–40.
7. Lindenfeld J, Robertson AD, Lowes BD, Brisow MR. Aspirin impairs reverse myocardial remodelling in patients with heart failure treated with beta-blockers. *J Am Coll Cardiol* (2001) 38, 1950–6.
8. Schäfer-Korting M, Kirch W, Axthelm T, Köhler H, Mutschler E. Atenolol interaction with aspirin, allopurinol, and ampicillin. *Clin Pharmacol Ther* (1983) 33, 283–8.
9. Spahn H, Langguth P, Kirch W, Mutschler E, Ohnhaus EE. Pharmacokinetics of salicylates administered with metoprolol. *Arzneimittelforschung* (1986) 36, 1697–9.
10. Johnsson G, Regårdh CG, Sölvell L. Lack of biological interaction of alprenolol and salicylate in man. *Eur J Clin Pharmacol* (1973) 6, 9–14.
11. Abdel-Haq B, Magagna A, Favilla S, Salvetti A. The interference of indomethacin and of imidazole salicylate on blood pressure control of essential hypertensive patients treated with atenolol. *Int J Clin Pharmacol Ther Toxicol* (1987) 25, 598–600.
12. Stokes GS, Brooks PM, Johnston HJ, Monaghan JC, Okoro EO, Kelly D. The effects of sulindac and diclofenac in essential hypertension controlled by treatment with a beta blocker and/or diuretic. *Clin Exp Hypertens A* (1991) 13, 1169–78.
13. Webster J, Petrie JC, McLean I, Hawksworth GM. Flurbiprofen interaction with single doses of atenolol and propranolol. *Br J Clin Pharmacol* (1984) 18, 861–6.
14. Radack KL, Deck CC, Bloomfield SS. Ibuprofen interferes with the efficacy of antihypertensive drugs. A Randomized, double-blind, placebo-controlled trial of ibuprofen compared with acetaminophen. *Ann Intern Med* (1987) 107, 628–35.
15. Reid ALA. Antihypertensive effect of thiazides. *Med J Aust* (1981) 2, 109–10.
16. Davies JG, Rawlins DC, Busson M. Effect of ibuprofen on blood pressure control by propranolol and bendrofluazide. *J Int Med Res* (1988) 16, 173–81.
17. Durão V, Prata MM, Gonçalves LMP. Modification of antihypertensive effects of β-adrenoceptor blocking agents by inhibition of endogenous prostaglandin synthesis. *Lancet* (1977) ii, 1005–7.
18. Watkins J, Abbott EC, Hensby CN, Webster J, Dollery CT. Attenuation of hypotensive effects of propranolol and thiazide diuretics by indomethacin. *BMJ* (1980) 281, 702–5.
19. Ylitalo P, Pitkäjärvi T, Pyykönen M-L, Nurmi A-K, Seppälä E, Vapaatalo H. Inhibition of prostaglandin synthesis by indomethacin interacts with the antihypertensive effect of atenolol. *Clin Pharmacol Ther* (1985) 38, 443–9.
20. Salvetti A, Pedrinelli R, Alberici A, Magagna A and Abdel-Haq B. The influence of indomethacin and sulindac on some pharmacological actions of atenolol in hypertensive patients. *Br J Clin Pharmacol* (1984) 17, 108S–111S.
21. Abate MA, Neeley JL, Layne RD, D'Alessandri R. Interaction of indomethacin and sulindac with labetalol. *Br J Clin Pharmacol* (1991) 31, 363–6.
22. Salvetti A, Arzilli F, Pedrinelli R, Beggi P, Motolese M. Interaction between oxprenolol and indomethacin on blood pressure in essential hypertensive patients. *Eur J Clin Pharmacol* (1982) 22, 197–201.
23. Sörgel F, Hemmerlein M, Lang E. Wirkung von Pirprofen und Indometacin auf die Effekte von Oxprenolol und Furosemid. *Arzneimittelforschung* (1984) 34, 1330–2.
24. Lopez-Ovejero JA, Weber MA, Drayer JIM, Sealey JE, Laragh JH. Effects of indomethacin alone and during diuretic or beta-adrenoceptor blockade therapy on blood pressure and the renin system in essential hypertension. *Clin Sci Mol Med* (1978) 55, 203S–205S.
25. Schoenfeld A, Freedman S, Hod M, Ovadia Y. Antagonism of antihypertensive drug therapy in pregnancy by indomethacin? *Am J Obstet Gynecol* (1989) 161, 1204–5.
26. Wong DG, Spence JD, Lamki L, Freeman D, McDonald JWD. Effect of non-steroidal anti-inflammatory drugs on control of hypertension by beta-blockers and diuretics. *Lancet* (1986) i, 997–1001.
27. Abate MA, Layne RD, Neeley JL, D'Alessandri R. Effect of naproxen and sulindac on blood pressure response to atenolol. *DICP Ann Pharmacother* (1990) 24, 810–3.
28. Schuna AA, Vejraska BD, Hiatt JG, Kochar M, Day R, Goodfriend TL. Lack of interaction between sulindac or naproxen and propranolol in hypertensive patients. *J Clin Pharmacol* (1989) 29, 524–8.
29. Anon. Adverse Drug Reactions Advisory Committee. Seven case studies. *Med J Aust* (1982) 2, 190–1.
30. Halabi A, Linde M, Zeidler H, König J, Kirch W. Double-blind study on the interaction of oxaprozin with metoprolol in hypertensives. *Cardiovasc Drugs Ther* (1989) 3, 441–3.
31. Ebel DL, Rhymer AR, Stahl E. Effect of sulindac, piroxicam and placebo on the hypotensive effect of propranolol in patients with mild to moderate essential hypertension. *Adv Therapy* (1985) 2, 131–42.
32. Ebel DL, Rhymer AR, Stahl E, Tipping R. Effect of Clinoril (sulindac, MSD), piroxicam and placebo on the hypotensive effect of propranolol in patients with mild to moderate essential hypertension. *Scand J Rheumatol* (1986) (Suppl), 62, 41–49.
33. Pugliese F, Simonetti BM, Cinotti GA, Ciabattoni G, Catella F, Vastano S, Ghidini Ottonelli A, Pierucci A. Differential interaction of piroxicam and sulindac with the anti-hypertensive effect of propranolol. *Eur J Clin Invest* (1984) 14, 54.
34. Baez MA, Alvarez CR, Weidler DJ. Effects of the non-steroidal anti-inflammatory drugs, piroxicam or sulindac, on the antihypertensive actions of propranolol and verapamil. *J Hypertens* (1987) 5 (Suppl): S563–S566.
35. Spahn H, Langguth P, Krauss D, Kirch W, Mutschler E. Pharmacokinetics of atenolol and metoprolol administered together with piroxicam. *Arch Pharm (Wienheim)* (1987) 320, 103–7.
36. Hartmann D, Stief G, Lingenfelder M, Güzelhan C, Horsch AK. Study on the possible interaction between tenoxicam and atenolol in hypertensive patients. *Arzneimittelforschung* (1995) 45, 494–8.
37. Barrientos A, Alcazar V, Ruilope L, Jarillo D, Rodicio JL. Indomethacin and beta-blockers in hypertension. *Lancet* (1978) i, 277.
38. Frölich JC, Whorten AR, Walker L, Smigel M, Oates JA, France R, Hollifield JW, Data JL, Gerber JG, Nies AS, Williams W, Robertson GL. Renal prostaglandins: regional differences in synthesis and role in renin release and ADH action. 7th Int Congr Nephrol, Montreal, 1978. 107–114.
39. Walker LA, Frölich JC. Renal prostaglandins and leukotrienes. *Rev Physiol Biochem Pharmacol* (1987) 107, 1–72.
40. Werner U, Werner D, Rau T, Fromm MF, Hinz B, Brune K. Celecoxib inhibits metabolism of cytochrome P450 2D6 substrate metoprolol in humans. *Clin Pharmacol Ther* (2003) 74, 130–7.
41. Johnson AG. NSAIDs and blood pressure. Clinical importance for older patients. *Drugs Aging* (1998) 12, 17–27.
42. Sheridan R, Montgomery AA, Fahey T. NSAID use and BP in treated hypertensives: a retrospective controlled observational study. *J Hum Hypertens* (2005) 19, 445–50.

Beta blockers + Barbiturates

The plasma levels and the effects of beta blockers that are mainly metabolised by the liver (e.g. alprenolol, metoprolol, timolol) are reduced by the barbiturates. Alprenolol concentrations are halved, but the other beta blockers are possibly not affected as much. Beta blockers that are mainly excreted unchanged in the urine (e.g. atenolol, sotalol, nadolol) would not be expected to be affected by the barbiturates.

Clinical evidence

Pentobarbital 100 mg daily for 10 days at bedtime reduced the plasma levels of **alprenolol** 400 mg twice daily by 59% in 6 hypertensive patients. On day 11, the mean pulse rate at rest had risen from 70 to 74 bpm and blood pressure had risen from 134/89 to 145/97 mmHg. The changes were seen within 4 to 5 days of starting the barbiturate, and decreased within 8 to 9 days of stopping it.[1] These results confirm previous studies by the same research group using **pentobarbital** 100 mg daily in healthy subjects.[2,3] In one of these studies, **pentobarbital** was found to cause a 38% reduction in plasma **alprenolol** levels 90 minutes after a single 200-mg dose of **alprenolol** was given, and a 43% reduction in the **alprenolol** AUC, with no change in the elimination half-life. There was also a 20% reduction in the effects of the beta blocker on heart rate during exercise.[3] In the other study, the AUC of oral **alprenolol** was reduced by about 80%, but that of intravenous **alprenolol** was unaffected.[2]

Another study in 8 healthy subjects has shown that **pentobarbital** 100 mg daily for 10 days reduced the AUC of **metoprolol** 100 mg by 32% (range 2 to 46%).[4] **Phenobarbital** 100 mg daily for 7 days reduced the AUC of **timolol** by 24% in 12 healthy subjects, but this was not statistically significant.[5]

Mechanism

Barbiturates are potent liver enzyme inducers that can increase the metabolism and clearance of other drugs from the body. Beta blockers that are removed from the body principally by liver metabolism (e.g. alprenolol, metoprolol, timolol) can therefore possibly be cleared more quickly in the presence of a barbiturate.

Importance and management

The interaction between alprenolol and pentobarbital is well documented and likely to be of modest clinical importance when the beta blocker is being used to treat hypertension, and possibly angina. Monitor the effects of alprenolol and increase the dose as necessary. Where possible it may be preferable to replace the barbiturate with a non-interacting alternative, such as one of the 'benzodiazepines', (p.723), which only have minor effects on the beta blockers, or consider using an alternative non-interacting beta blocker.

A reduced response is possible with any of the beta blockers that are extensively metabolised (see 'Table 22.1', (p.833)), but the effects on the AUCs of metoprolol and timolol appear to be less than the effects on alprenolol. Detailed information about the clinical importance of this interaction is largely lacking, but seems likely to be minor. However, if a problem does occur consider the alternative measures suggested for alprenolol, above. Any possible interaction can almost certainly be avoided by using one of the beta blockers that are primarily excreted unchanged in the urine (see 'Table 22.1', (p.833)). Evidence is largely lacking, but all barbiturates would be expected to interact similarly, although the extent of the interaction may vary.

1. Seideman P, Borg K-O, Haglund K, von Bahr C. Decreased plasma concentrations and clinical effects of alprenolol during combined treatment with pentobarbitone in hypertension. *Br J Clin Pharmacol* (1987) 23, 267–71.
2. Alvan G, Piafsky K, Lind M, von Bahr C. Effect of pentobarbital on the disposition of alprenolol. *Clin Pharmacol Ther* (1977) 22, 316–21.
3. Collste P, Seideman P, Borg K-O, Haglund K, von Bahr C. Influence of pentobarbital on effects and plasma levels of alprenolol and 4-hydroxy-alprenolol. *Clin Pharmacol Ther* (1979) 25, 423–7.
4. Haglund K, Seideman P, Collste P, Borg K-O, von Bahr C. Influence of pentobarbital on metoprolol plasma levels. *Clin Pharmacol Ther* (1979) 26, 326–9.
5. Mäntylä R, Männistö P, Nykänen S, Koponen A, Lamminsivu U. Pharmacokinetic interactions of timolol with vasodilating drugs, food and phenobarbitone in healthy human volunteers. *Eur J Clin Pharmacol* (1983) 24, 227–30.

Beta blockers + Bile-acid binding resins

Although both colestyramine and colestipol can moderately reduce the absorption of propranolol, this does not seem to reduce its effects. Colesevelam does not appear to affect the absorption of metoprolol.

Clinical evidence

(a) Colesevelam

A single-dose study in 33 healthy subjects found that colesevelam 4.5 g did not cause a clinically relevant alteration in the plasma levels of sustained-release **metoprolol** 100 mg.[1]

(b) Colestipol

When 6 healthy subjects took a single 120-mg dose of **propranolol** with a 10-g dose of colestipol the peak plasma **propranolol** levels were *raised* by 30%. However, if an additional 10 g dose of colestipol was taken 12 hours before the **propranolol** the peak plasma levels were decreased by 36% and the AUC was reduced by about 30%. No changes in blood pressure or pulse rates were seen.[2]

(c) Colestyramine

When 6 healthy subjects took a single 120-mg dose of **propranolol** with an 8-g dose of colestyramine the peak **propranolol** plasma levels were reduced by almost 25% and the AUC was reduced by 13%. An additional dose of colestyramine 12 hours before the **propranolol** reduced the AUC by 43%. However, no changes in blood pressure or pulse rate were seen.[2] Preliminary results of another study found that colestyramine (single unstated dose) caused no significant changes in the blood levels of **propranolol** in 5 patients with type II hyperlipidaemia taking **propranolol** 40 mg four times daily.[3]

Mechanism

Uncertain. It seems probable that both colestyramine and colestipol can bind to propranolol in the gut, thereby reducing its absorption.

Importance and management

Information is limited. Even though both colestyramine and colestipol can apparently reduce the absorption of a single dose of propranolol, no changes in its effects were reported,[2] suggesting that the interaction is of minimal clinical importance. There is therefore no obvious reason for avoiding concurrent use. However, note that it is usually recommended that other drugs are given 1 hour before or 4 to 6 hours after colestyramine, and 1 hour before or 4 hours after colestipol.

1. Donovan JM, Stypinski D, Stiles MR, Olson TA, Burke SK. Drug interactions with colesevelam hydrochloride, a novel, potent lipid-lowering agent. *Cardiovasc Drugs Ther* (2000) 14, 681–90.
2. Hibbard DM, Peters JR, Hunninghake DB. Effects of cholestyramine and colestipol on the plasma concentrations of propranolol. *Br J Clin Pharmacol* (1984) 18, 337–42.
3. Schwartz DE, Schaeffer E, Brewer HB, Franciosa JA. Bioavailability of propranolol following administration of cholestyramine. *Clin Pharmacol Ther* (1982) 31, 268.

Beta blockers + Bupropion

A patient taking metoprolol developed bradycardia and hypotension when bupropion was also given.

Clinical evidence, mechanism, importance and management

A 50-year-old man taking **metoprolol** 75 mg twice daily and diltiazem 240 mg twice daily for hypertension developed fatigue 12 days after starting to take bupropion 150 mg twice daily. He was found to have a pulse rate of 43 bpm, a blood pressure of 102/65 mmHg, and signs of mild heart failure. He recovered within 24 hours of stopping all three drugs.[1] It was suggested that these effects had occurred as a result of raised **metoprolol** levels, which had occurred because bupropion inhibited the metabolism of **metoprolol** by the cytochrome P450 isoenzyme CYP2D6.

The manufacturers of bupropion have predicted this interaction and recommend that if **metoprolol** is added to treatment with bupropion, doses at the lower end of the range should be used. If bupropion is added to existing treatment, decreased dosages of **metoprolol** should be considered.[2,3]

It seems likely that this interaction could occur with any of the beta blockers metabolised by CYP2D6 (see 'Table 22.1', (p.833)).

1. McCollum DL, Greene JL, McGuire DK. Severe sinus bradycardia after initiation of bupropion therapy: a probable drug-drug interaction with metoprolol. *Cardiovasc Drugs Ther* (2004) 18, 329–30.
2. Zyban (Bupropion hydrochloride). GlaxoSmithKline UK. UK Summary of product characteristics, October 2006.
3. Zyban (Bupropion hydrochloride). GlaxoSmithKline. US Prescribing information, August 2007.

Beta blockers + Calcium-channel blockers; Dihydropyridines

The use of beta blockers with felodipine, isradipine, lacidipine, nicardipine, nimodipine and nisoldipine normally appears to be useful and safe. However, severe hypotension and heart failure have occurred rarely when a beta blocker was given with nifedipine or nisoldipine. Changes in the pharmacokinetics of the beta blockers and calcium-channel blockers may also occur on concurrent use, but they do not appear to be clinically important.

Clinical evidence

(a) Felodipine

A double-blind, crossover study in 8 healthy subjects found that over a 5-day period, **metoprolol** 100 mg twice daily did not affect the pharmacokinetics of felodipine 10 mg twice daily. On the other hand, the bioavailability and peak plasma levels of **metoprolol** were increased by 31% and 38%, respectively.[1] Another study in 10 healthy subjects given felodipine 10 mg with either **metoprolol** 100 mg, **pindolol** 5 mg, **propranolol** 80 mg, or **timolol** 10 mg found no changes in heart rate, PR interval or blood pressure that might be considered to be harmful to patients with hypertension or angina. However, 7 of the 10 subjects reported some increase in adverse effects.[2]

(b) Isradipine

A preliminary report of a study in 24 healthy subjects found that **propranolol** 40 mg twice daily given with isradipine 5 mg twice daily caused some modest changes in the pharmacokinetics of both drugs (peak **propranolol** plasma levels increased by 17%, peak isradipine plasma levels reduced by 18%), but the AUCs were not significantly altered.[3] However, an earlier preliminary report by the same research group in 17 subjects found an increase in the **propranolol** AUC of 28%, a reduction in the isradipine AUC of 22% and a 59% increase in the peak **propranolol** levels.[4]

(c) Lacidipine

Twelve patients with mild to moderate hypertension not satisfactorily controlled by **atenolol** alone were given lacidipine 4 mg once daily with or without **atenolol** 100 mg daily for 14 days. There was no evidence of a significant change in drug levels, but there was a significant additive reduction in blood pressure during concurrent use, when compared with the reductions observed with either drug alone.[5]

Single-dose studies in 24 healthy subjects found that **propranolol** 160 mg reduced the peak plasma levels and AUC of lacidipine 4 mg by 38% and 42%, respectively, while the peak plasma levels and AUC of the **propranolol** were increased by 35% and 26%, respectively. There was a modest additive reduction of 4 to 6 mmHg in blood pressure, and the combination reduced the heart rate, but not to an extent greater than **propranolol** alone. No significant adverse effects were seen.[6] However, a further preliminary report of a study by the same authors, in which 12 hypertensive patients were given **propranolol** 160 mg twice daily and lacidipine 4 mg daily for 2 weeks, found a non-significant 30% increase in systemic availability of lacidipine, and no change in **propranolol** pharmacokinetics. In addition, no clinically significant alterations in ECG recordings, blood pressure, or pulse rate were seen.[7]

(d) Lercanidipine

The manufacturer notes that when lercanidipine was given with **metoprolol**, the bioavailability of lercanidipine was reduced by 50% while the bioavailability of **metoprolol** was not changed. They suggest this may occur with any beta blocker, and that some adjustment of the lercanidipine dose may be needed.[8]

(e) Nicardipine

Nicardipine 30 mg did not affect the pharmacokinetics or pharmacodynamics of **atenolol** 100 mg in a single-dose study in healthy subjects.[9]

In another study, 14 healthy subjects were given nicardipine 50 mg every 12 hours and **metoprolol** 100 mg every 12 hours, both together and alone, for 11 doses. **Metoprolol** plasma levels were raised by 28% by the nicardipine in the 7 subjects who were of the extensive CYP2D6 metaboliser phenotype, but had no significant effect in the poor metabolisers. The extent of the beta-blockade was unchanged in all of them.[10]

Preliminary analysis of another study in healthy subjects found that the pharmacokinetics of both **propranolol** 80 mg twice daily and nicardipine 30 mg three times daily were unaffected when they were given together for 6 days.[11] However, this contrasts with two single-dose studies, which found that nicardipine 30 mg increased the AUC and peak plasma levels of a single 80-mg dose of **propranolol** by 47% and 80%, respectively,[12] and raised the AUC and peak plasma levels of an 80-mg dose of sustained-release **propranolol** to a lesser extent (17% and 22%, respectively).[13] A related single-dose study found that in elderly healthy subjects nicardipine 30 mg increased the maximum plasma levels and AUC of **propranolol** 40 mg by about 100% and 80%, respectively. Nicardipine caused a further decrease in blood pressure, and attenuated the reduction in heart rate seen with **propranolol** alone.[14]

A study in 8 healthy subjects found that the increase in heart rate during exercise associated with a single 40-mg dose of nicardipine was reduced by one drop of **timolol** 0.5% put into each eye. Systolic blood pressure was also reduced during concurrent use, but nicardipine did not cause any further reduction in the intraocular pressure reduction produced by **timolol**.[15]

(f) Nifedipine

Nifedipine 10 mg three times daily did not alter the pharmacokinetics of **atenolol** 100 mg daily,[16,17] **betaxolol**,[18] **metoprolol** 100 mg twice daily[16,17] or **propranolol** 80 mg twice daily.[16] A single-dose study also found no pharmacokinetic interaction between nifedipine and **atenolol**.[19] However, another study found that nifedipine 10 mg three times daily caused an increase in the peak plasma level and AUC of **propranolol** 80 mg twice daily of 56% and 23%, respectively.[18] Another study found that the absorption of a single-dose of **propranolol** appeared to be faster, leading to higher initial concentrations, when it was given after nifedipine.[20] Regardless of the pharmacokinetic changes, none of these studies in healthy subjects found any adverse haemodynamic effects from the combination of nifedipine and these beta blockers.[16,18,19]

Similarly, in studies in patients with normal left ventricular function there was no evidence of adverse haemodynamic effects when nifedipine (single-dose sublingual[21,22] or intravenously,[23] or daily dose orally[23]) was given with **atenolol**,[23] **celiprolol**[22] or **propranolol**.[21,24]

However, there are a few earlier isolated case reports of hypotension and heart failure with the combination. Two patients with angina taking **alprenolol** or **propranolol** developed heart failure when they were given nifedipine 10 mg three times daily. The signs of heart failure disappeared when the nifedipine was withdrawn.[25] One out of 15 patients with hypertension and exertional angina progressively developed hypotension (90/60 mmHg) when given nifedipine 10 mg twice daily in addition to treatment with **atenolol** 50 mg daily and a diuretic for one month.[26] A patient with angina taking **propranolol** 160 mg four times daily developed severe and prolonged hypotension (blood pressure initially not recordable, then 60 mmHg systolic) 18 days after nifedipine 10 mg three times daily was substituted for 'isosorbide', and this may have been a factor that led to fatal myocardial infarction.[27] Heart failure is also described in another patient with angina taking **atenolol** (and various other drugs) when nifedipine 20 mg three times daily was given.[28]

A patient developed hypotension and severe bradycardia on two occasions after being given her usual antihypertensive medication of **labetalol** and extended-release nifedipine crushed and given via a nasogastric tube. Crushing the nifedipine tablet altered its release characteristics so that the total dose was released quickly resulting in profound hypotension. The **labetalol** produced additional hypotensive effects and prevented a compensatory increase in heart rate.[29]

(g) Nimodipine

In a preliminary report of a study in 12 healthy subjects, nimodipine 30 mg three times daily for 4 days had no significant effect on the changes in heart rate, blood pressure or cardiac output seen with either **propranolol** 40 mg or **atenolol** 25 mg three times daily. The pharmacokinetics of the beta blockers were also unaltered.[30]

(h) Nisoldipine

A single 20-mg dose of nisoldipine increased the steady-state AUC and peak plasma level of **propranolol** 160 mg daily by 35% and 55%, respectively. After combined treatment for 7 days, the AUC of **propranolol** was increased by 60% and the peak plasma level was increased by 55%. The combination enhanced blood pressure reduction to a small extent, but nisoldipine did not significantly reduce the effect of **propranolol** on heart rate.[31] Similarly, another study found that a single 20-mg dose of nisoldipine increased the AUC and peak plasma level of a single 40-mg dose of **propranolol** by 43% and 68%, respectively, and that the AUC and peak plasma level of nisoldipine increased 30% and 57%, respectively. In this study, nisoldipine was reported to enhance beta-blockade.[32] However, the same research group later found that the steady-state pharmacokinetics of **propranolol** 80 mg twice daily and nisoldipine 10 mg twice daily were not affected by concurrent use for 7 days, but nisoldipine attenuated the decrease in forearm blood flow seen with propranolol.[33] The manufacturer of nisoldipine notes that severe hypotension can occur when it is given at the same time as beta blockers, and that, in isolated cases, signs of heart failure can also occur.[34]

Mechanism

Not understood. Where pharmacokinetic changes are seen, a possible reason is that the metabolism of the beta blockers is altered by changes in blood flow through the liver. The pharmacodynamic changes with nifedipine may be explained by the fact that nifedipine reduces the contractility of the heart muscle. This is counteracted by a sympathetic reflex increase in heart rate due to nifedipine-induced peripheral vasodilation, so that the ventricular output stays the same or is even improved. The presence of a beta blocker may oppose this to some extent by slowing the heart rate, which allows the negative inotropic effects of nifedipine to go unchecked.

Importance and management

The concurrent use of beta blockers and the dihydropyridine calcium-channel blockers is common, and normally valuable. However, isolated cases of severe hypotension and heart failure have been seen in a few patients taking beta blockers and nifedipine or nisoldipine. It has been suggested that those likely to be most at risk are patients with impaired left ventricular function[35] (which is a caution for the use of nifedipine anyway) and/or those taking beta blockers in high dosage. Bear this in mind. It should also be noted that the topical use of beta blockers (such as timolol eye drops) may reduce heart rate and blood pressure. Changes in the pharmacokinetics of the beta blockers and calcium-channel blockers may also occur, but these do not appear to be clinically important. It may also be worth noting that all but one of the cases of an adverse reaction with a beta blocker and nifedipine occurred with 'short-acting' formulations, which are now considered unsuitable for long-term management of angina or hypertension, since they are associated with larger variations in blood pressure and heart rate. The remaining case was associated with the incorrect use of an extended-release nifedipine preparation.

1. Smith SR, Wilkins MR, Jack DB, Kendall MJ, Laugher S. Pharmacokinetic interactions between felodipine and metoprolol. *Eur J Clin Pharmacol* (1987) 31, 575–8.
2. Carruthers SG, Bailey DG. Tolerance and cardiovascular effects of single dose felodipine/β-blocker combinations in healthy subjects. *J Cardiovasc Pharmacol* (1987) 10 (Suppl 1), S169–S176.
3. Schran HF, Shepherd AM, Choc MM, Gonasun LM, Brodie CL. The effect of concomitant administration of isradipine and propranolol on their steady-state bioavailability. *Pharmacologist* (1989) 31, 153.
4. Shepherd AMM, Brodie CL, Carrillo DW, Kwan CM. Pharmacokinetic interaction between isradipine and propranolol. *Clin Pharmacol Ther* (1988) 43,194.
5. Lyons D, Fowler G, Webster J, Hall ST, Petrie JC. An assessment of lacidipine and atenolol in mild to moderate hypertension. *Br J Clin Pharmacol* (1994) 37, 45–51.
6. Hall ST, Harding SM, Hassani H, Keene ON, Pellegatti M. The pharmacokinetic and pharmacodynamic interaction between lacidipine and propranolol in healthy volunteers. *J Cardiovasc Pharmacol* (1991) 18, (Suppl 11), S13–S17.

7. Hall ST, Saul P, Keene ON, Hassani H. Pharmacodynamic and pharmacokinetic interaction between lacidipine and propranolol. *Pharm Res* (1992) 9 (10 Suppl), S88.
8. Zanidip (Lercanidipine hydrochloride). Recordati Pharmaceuticals Ltd. UK Summary of product characteristics, October 2004.
9. Vercruysse I, Schoors DF, Musch G, Massart DL, Dupont AG. Nicardipine does not influence the pharmacokinetics and pharmacodynamics of atenolol. *Br J Clin Pharmacol* (1990) 30, 499–500.
10. Laurent-Kenesi M-A, Funck-Brentano C, Poirier J-M, Decolin D, Jaillon P. Influence of CYP2D6-dependent metabolism on the steady-state pharmacokinetics and pharmacodynamics of metoprolol and nicardipine, alone and in combination. *Br J Clin Pharmacol* (1993) 36, 531–8.
11. Macdonald FC, Dow RJ, Wilson RAG, Yee KF, Finlayson J. A study to determine potential interactions between nicardipine and propranolol in healthy volunteers. *Br J Clin Pharmacol* (1987), 23, 626P.
12. Schoors DF, Vercruysse I, Musch G, Massart DL, Dupont AG. Influence of nicardipine on the pharmacokinetics and pharmacodynamics of propranolol in healthy volunteers. *Br J Clin Pharmacol* (1990) 29, 497–501.
13. Vercruysse I, Massart DL, Dupont AG. Increase in plasma propranolol caused by nicardipine is dependent on the delivery rate of propranolol. *Eur J Clin Pharmacol* (1995) 49, 121–5.
14. Hartmann C, Vercruysse I, Metz T, Massart DL, Dupont AG. Influence of nicardipine on the pharmacokinetics of propranolol in the elderly. *Br J Clin Pharmacol* (1995) 39, 540P.
15. Yatsuka YI, Tsutsumi K, Kotegawa T, Nakamura K, Nakano S, Nakatsuka K. Interaction between timolol eyedrops and oral nicardipine or oral diltiazem in healthy Japanese subjects. *Eur J Clin Pharmacol* (1998) 54, 149–54.
16. Gangji D, Juvent M, Niset G, Wathieu M, Degreve M, Bellens R, Poortmans J, Degre S, Fitzsimons TJ, Herchuelz A. Study of the influence of nifedipine on the pharmacokinetics and pharmacodynamics of propranolol, metoprolol and atenolol. *Br J Clin Pharmacol* (1984) 17, 29S–35S.
17. Kendall MJ, Jack DB, Laugher SJ, Lobo J, Smith RS. Lack of a pharmacokinetic interaction between nifedipine and the β-adrenoceptor blockers metoprolol and atenolol. *Br J Clin Pharmacol* (1984) 18, 331–5.
18. Vinceneux Ph, Canal M, Domart Y, Roux A, Cascio B, Orofiamma B, Larribaud J, Flouvat B, Carbon C. Pharmacokinetic and pharmacodynamic interactions between nifedipine and propranolol or betaxolol. *Int J Clin Pharmacol Ther Toxicol* (1986) 24, 153–8.
19. Rosenkranz B, Ledermann H, Frölich JC. Interaction between nifedipine and atenolol: pharmacokinetics and pharmacodynamics in normotensive volunteers. *J Cardiovasc Pharmacol* (1986) 8, 943–9.
20. Bauer LA, Murray K, Horn JR, Opheim K, Olsen J. Influence of nifedipine therapy on indocyanine green and oral propranolol pharmacokinetics. *Eur J Clin Pharmacol* (1989) 37, 257–60.
21. Elkayam U, Roth A, Weber L, Kulick D, Kawanishi D, McKay C, Rahimtoola SH. Effects of nifedipine on hemodynamics and cardiac function in patients with normal left ventricular ejection fraction already treated with propranolol. *Am J Cardiol* (1986) 58, 536–40.
22. Silke B, Verma SP, Guy S. Hemodynamic interactions of a new beta blocker, celiprolol, with nifedipine in angina pectoris. *Cardiovasc Drugs Ther* (1991) 5, 681–8.
23. Rowland E, Razis P, Sugrue D, Krikler DM. Acute and chronic haemodynamic and electrophysiological effects of nifedipine in patients receiving atenolol. *Br Heart J* (1983) 50, 383–9.
24. Vetrovec GW, Parker VE. Nifedipine, beta blocker interaction: effect on left ventricular function. *Clin Res* (1984) 32, 833A.
25. Anastassiades CJ. Nifedipine and beta-blocker drugs. *BMJ* (1980) 281, 1251–2.
26. Opie LH, White DA. Adverse interaction between nifedipine and β-blockade. *BMJ* (1980) 281, 1462.
27. Staffurth JS, Emery P. Adverse interaction between nifedipine and beta-blockade. *BMJ* (1981) 282, 225.
28. Robson RH, Vishwanath MC. Nifedipine and beta-blockade as a cause of cardiac failure. *BMJ* (1982) 284, 104.
29. Schier JG, Howland MA, Hoffman RS, Nelson LS. Fatality from administration of labetalol and crushed extended-release nifedipine. *Ann Pharmacother* (2003) 37, 1420–3.
30. Horstmann R, Weber H, Wingender W, Rämsch K-D, Kuhlmann J. Does nimodipine interact with beta adrenergic blocking agents? *Eur J Clin Pharmacol* (1989) 36, A258.
31. Elliott HL, Meredith PA, McNally C, Reid JL. The interactions between nisoldipine and two β-adrenoceptor antagonists—atenolol and propranolol. *Br J Clin Pharmacol* (1991) 32, 379–85.
32. Levine MAH, Ogilvie RI, Leenen FHH. Pharmacokinetic and pharmacodynamic interactions between nisoldipine and propranolol. *Clin Pharmacol Ther* (1988) 43, 39–48.
33. Shaw-Stiffel TA, Walker SE, Ogilvie RI, Leenen FH. Pharmacokinetic and pharmacodynamic interactions during multiple-dose administration of nisoldipine and propranolol. *Clin Pharmacol Ther* (1994) 55, 661–9.
34. Syscor MR (Nisoldipine). Forest Laboratories UK Ltd. UK Summary of product characteristics, August 1998.
35. Brooks N, Cattell M, Pigeon J, Balcon R. Unpredictable response to nifedipine in severe cardiac failure. *BMJ* (1980) 281, 1324.

Beta blockers + Calcium-channel blockers; Diltiazem

The cardiac depressant effects of diltiazem and beta blockers are additive, and although concurrent use can be beneficial, close monitoring is recommended. A number of patients, (usually those with pre-existing ventricular failure or conduction abnormalities) have developed serious and potentially life-threatening bradycardia. Diltiazem increases the serum levels of propranolol and metoprolol, but not those of atenolol, but these changes are probably not clinically important.

Clinical evidence

(a) Cardiac depressant effects

Ten patients were admitted to an intensive coronary care unit during one year with severe bradycardia (heart rates of 24 to 44 bpm) after taking diltiazem 90 to 360 mg daily with **propranolol** 30 to 120 mg daily, **atenolol** 50 to 100 mg daily, or **pindolol** 90 mg daily. All were relatively elderly and presented with lethargy, dizziness, syncope, chest pain, and in one case pulmonary oedema. The ECG abnormalities were localised in the sinus node, the primary rhythm disorders being junctional escape rhythms, sinus bradycardia and sinus pause. These resolved within 24 hours of withdrawing the drugs, although a temporary pacemaker was needed in 4 patients.[1]

Symptomatic and severe bradyarrhythmias of this kind have been described in case reports in 16 other patients taking diltiazem with **atenolol**,[2] **carteolol**,[3] **metoprolol**,[2,4,5] **nadolol**,[6] **pindolol**,[7] **propranolol**,[2,4,6,8] or **sotalol**.[3,7] AV block with unusual ECG changes (T-wave inversion and ST-segment depression) was found in a 16-year-old girl following an overdose of diltiazem and **propranolol**.[9] In a later prospective study of hospital admissions due to cardiovascular adverse drug reactions, bradycardia, hypotension, syncope and worsening heart failure were noted in 21 patients taking beta blockers with diltiazem. The beta blockers involved were **propranolol** (13 patients), **atenolol** (5), **metoprolol** (2) and **oxprenolol** (1).[10] Similarly severe sinus bradycardia occurred in 8 of 59 patients in three early clinical studies of the combination of diltiazem and **propranolol**.[11-13] One patient developed congestive heart failure.[13] In contrast, four other similar clinical trials did not report any adverse effects,[14-17] and in a single-dose study, one drop of **timolol** 0.5% eye drops did not cause an additional reduction in heart rate when it was given to healthy subjects with a 60-mg dose of diltiazem.[18]

(b) Pharmacokinetics

In healthy subjects, diltiazem increased the AUC of **propranolol** and **metoprolol** by 48% and 33%, respectively, and increased the maximum serum levels by 45% and 71%, respectively, but **atenolol** was not significantly affected.[19] Another study found that diltiazem caused a 24% to 27% reduction in **propranolol** clearance.[20]

Mechanism

The bradycardic effects of the beta blockers can be additive with the delay in conduction through the atrioventricular node caused by diltiazem.[7] This advantageously increases the antianginal effects in most patients, but in a few these effects may exacerbate existing cardiac abnormalities. Diltiazem apparently also inhibits the metabolism of propranolol and metoprolol, but the exact mechanism for this is not clear.[19]

Importance and management

Concurrent use is unquestionably valuable and uneventful in many patients, but severe adverse effects can develop. This is well established. A not dissimilar adverse interaction can occur with 'verapamil', (p.841). On the basis of 6 reports, the incidence of symptomatic bradyarrhythmia was estimated to be about 10 to 15%.[1] It can occur with different beta blockers, even with very low doses, and at any time from within a few hours of starting treatment to 2 years of concurrent use.[1] The main risk factors seem to be ventricular dysfunction, or sinoatrial or AV nodal conduction abnormalities.[1] Note that these are usually contraindications to the use of diltiazem. Patients with normal ventricular function and no evidence of conduction abnormalities are usually not at risk. Concurrent use should be well monitored for evidence of adverse effects. Changes in the pharmacokinetics of the beta blockers may also occur, but these changes are probably not clinically important.

1. Sagie A, Strasberg B, Kusnieck J, Sclarovsky S. Symptomatic bradycardia induced by the combination of oral diltiazem and beta blockers. *Clin Cardiol* (1991) 14, 314–16.
2. Yust I, Hoffman M, Aronson RJ. Life-threatening bradycardic reactions due to beta blocker-diltiazem interactions. *Isr J Med Sci* (1992) 28, 292–4.
3. Lamaison D, Vacher D, Berenfeld A, Schandrin C, Lavarenne V. Association de diltiazem à libération prolongée et d'un bêta-bloquant dans l'hypertension artérielle. Deux cas de choc cardiogénique avec bradycardie extrême. *Therapie* (1990) 45, 411–13.
4. Lan Cheong Wah LSH, Robinet G, Guiavarc'h M, Garo B, Boles JM. États de choc au cours de l'association diltiazem-β-bloquant. *Rev Med Interne* (1992) 13, 80.
5. Kjeldsen SE, Syvertsen J-O, Hedner T. Cardiac conduction with diltiazem and beta-blockade combined. A review and report on cases. *Blood Pressure* (1996) 5, 260–3.
6. Hossack KF. Conduction abnormalities due to diltiazem. *N Engl J Med* (1982) 307, 953–4.
7. Hassell AB, Creamer JE. Profound bradycardia after the addition of diltiazem to a beta-blocker. *BMJ* (1989) 298, 675.
8. Ishikawa T, Imamura T, Koiwaya Y, Tanaka K. Atrioventricular dissociation and sinus arrest induced by oral diltiazem. *N Engl J Med* (1983) 309, 1124–5.
9. Satar S, Acikalin A, Akpinar O. Unusual electrocardiographic changes with propranolol and diltiazem overdosage: a case report. *Am J Ther* (2003) 10, 299–302.

10. Edoute Y, Nagachandran P, Svirski B, Ben-Ami H. Cardiovascular adverse drug reaction associated with combined β-adrenergic and calcium entry-blocking agents. *J Cardiovasc Pharmacol* (2000) 35, 556–9.
11. O'Hara MJ, Khurmi NS, Bowles MJ, Raftery EB. Diltiazem and propranolol combination for the treatment of chronic stable angina pectoris. *Clin Cardiol* (1987) 10, 115–23.
12. Hung J, Lamb IH, Connolly SJ, Jutzy KR, Goris ML, Schroeder JS. The effect of diltiazem and propranolol, alone and in combination, on exercise performance and left ventricular function in patients with stable effort angina: a double-blind, randomized, and placebo-controlled study. *Circulation* (1983) 68, 560–7.
13. Strauss WE, Parisi AF. Superiority of combined diltiazem and propranolol therapy for angina pectoris. *Circulation* (1985) 71, 951–7.
14. Tilmant PY, Lablanche JM, Thieuleux FA, Dupuis BA, Bertrand ME. Detrimental effect of propranolol in patients with coronary arterial spasm countered by combination with diltiazem. *Am J Cardiol* (1983) 52, 230–33.
15. Rocha P, Baron B, Delestrain A, Pathe M, Cazor J-L, Kahn J-C. Hemodynamic effects of intravenous diltiazem in patients treated chronically with propranolol. *Am Heart J* (1986) 111, 62–8.
16. Humen DP, O'Brien P, Purves P, Johnson D, Kostuk WJ. Effort angina with adequate beta-receptor blockade: comparison with diltiazem alone and in combination. *J Am Coll Cardiol* (1986) 7, 329–35.
17. Kenny J, Daly K, Bergman G, Kerkez S, Jewitt DE. Beneficial effects of diltiazem combined with beta blockade in angina pectoris. *Eur Heart J* (1985) 6, 418–23.
18. Yatsuka YI, Tsutsumi K, Kotegawa T, Nakamura K, Nakano S, Nakatsuka K. Interaction between timolol eyedrops and oral nicardipine or oral diltiazem in healthy Japanese subjects. *Eur J Clin Pharmacol* (1998) 54, 149–54.
19. Tateishi T, Nakashima H, Shitou T, Kumagai Y, Ohashi K, Hosoda S, Ebihara A. Effect of diltiazem on the pharmacokinetics of propranolol, metoprolol and atenolol. *Eur J Clin Pharmacol* (1989) 36, 67–70.
20. Hunt BA, Bottorff MB, Herring VL, Self TH, Lalonde RL. Effects of calcium channel blockers on the pharmacokinetics of propranolol stereoisomers. *Clin Pharmacol Ther* (1990) 47, 584–91.

Beta blockers + Calcium-channel blockers; Verapamil

The cardiac depressant effects of verapamil and beta blockers are additive, and although concurrent use can be beneficial, serious cardiodepression (bradycardia, asystole, sinus arrest) sometimes occurs. It has been suggested that the combination should only be given to those who can initially be closely supervised. An adverse interaction can also occur with beta blockers given as eye drops.

Clinical evidence

(a) Adverse interactions

1. Intravenous administration. Ventricular asystole developed in 2 cases when intravenous verapamil was given after the unsuccessful use of intravenous **practolol**, to treat supraventricular tachycardia in a 70-year-old man and a 6-month-old baby.[1] In a later study, the combination of intravenous verapamil and intravenous **practolol** produced a marked reduction in cardiac contractility, which was more evident when **practolol** was given first.[2]

2. Oral administration. In one series, 34 out of 42 patients taking beta blockers (daily dose: **atenolol** 100 mg (34 patients), **atenolol** 50 mg (2), **propranolol** 160 mg (4), **pindolol** 20 mg (1), or **metoprolol** 100 mg (1)) with verapamil 360 mg daily experienced a reduction in anginal episodes over a mean period of 6.5 months while taking both drugs. However, 12 patients needed a reduced dosage or withdrawal of one or both drugs. One had non-specific symptoms (drugs withdrawn), 2 had bradyarrhythmias (drugs withdrawn) and 6 experienced dyspnoea (3 withdrawals and 3 dosage reductions), presumed to be secondary to left ventricular failure. Other complications were tiredness (2 patients) and postural hypotension (1 patient), which were dealt with by reducing the dosage.[3] In another study in 15 patients with angina who were taking **atenolol** with verapamil, 4 experienced profound lethargy, one had left ventricular failure and 4 had bradyarrhythmias.[4]

Other case reports and studies describe heart failure,[5,6] dyspnoea,[5,7,8] sinus arrest,[9,10] heart block,[9,11-13] hypotension,[5,6,8,10,13-16] and bradycardia[4,5,8,10,11,14-18] in patients taking verapamil with **alprenolol**,[9] **atenolol**,[6,9,10,12] **metoprolol**,[5,11,13,15] **propranolol**[7,8,14,16-18] or **pindolol**.[5] In two further cases, bradycardia occurred in patients taking verapamil and using **timolol** eye drops.[19,20] Another case has been reported, but this was complicated by the presence of 'flecainide', (p.844). A number of reports noted that patients experiencing this interaction had reasonable left ventricular function.[5,10,12,19] Heart block and hypotension or cardiogenic shock has also been reported after verapamil was given with **atenolol**[21] or **propranolol**[22] in overdose.

(b) Pharmacokinetic interactions

The pharmacokinetics of **atenolol** were not altered by verapamil in one study in a single patient.[23] In a study in 15 patients the plasma levels of verapamil and **atenolol** varied greatly during individual and concurrent use but mean concentrations were not significantly changed.[4] In another study in 10 patients the mean AUC of **atenolol** was not significantly increased by verapamil, but individual patients had **atenolol** AUC increases of up to 112%.[24]

Verapamil raised the **metoprolol** AUC in 10 patients by 33% and the peak plasma levels by 41%. The minimum pulse rate and systolic blood pressure (1 to 3 hours post dose) were also lower in those taking the combination than with **metoprolol** alone.[15] Similarly, in a single-dose study in 9 healthy subjects, the AUC and maximum plasma level of **metoprolol** increased by 35% and 64%, respectively, and the AUC and half-life of verapamil increased by 57% and 29%, respectively, on concurrent use.[25]

In healthy subjects, verapamil reduced the clearance of **propranolol** by 26 to 32% and increased its AUC by 46 to 58% after 6 days of concurrent use.[26] Similarly, in 5 patients, verapamil increased the peak plasma levels of **propranolol** by 94%, and its AUC by 66%.[18] **Propranolol** did not affect the pharmacokinetics of verapamil.[18] However, in another study in healthy subjects no pharmacokinetic interaction was noted between **propranolol** and verapamil after they were taken together for 6 days.[27]

In a randomised, crossover study, a single 120-mg dose of *(R)*-verapamil reduced the bioavailability of a single 50-mg dose of **talinolol** by 25% in 9 healthy subjects.[28]

Mechanism

Both beta blockers and verapamil have negative inotropic effects on the heart, which can be additive.[27] Given together they can cause marked bradycardia and may even depress the contraction of the ventricle completely. Verapamil can also raise the serum levels of beta blockers that are extensively metabolised in the liver (e.g. metoprolol, propranolol), probably by inhibiting their metabolism,[29] although the exact mechanism for this is unclear. It is thought that verapamil affects talinolol bioavailability by modulating intestinal P-glycoprotein.[28,30]

Importance and management

Well documented and well established interactions. Although concurrent use can be uneventful and successful, the reports cited here amply demonstrate that it may not always be safe. The difficulty is identifying the patients most at risk. In the UK, the BNF says that oral concurrent use should only be considered if myocardial function is well preserved, and that verapamil should not be injected in patients recently given beta blockers because of the risk of hypotension and asystole. They also note that, although 30 minutes has been suggested as a sufficient interval before giving a beta blocker when a verapamil injection has been given first, the safety of this has not been established.[31] The manufacturers of verapamil contraindicate its intravenous use in those receiving intravenous beta blockers.[32]

It has been advised that the initiation of treatment should be restricted to hospital practice, where the dose of each drug can be carefully titrated and the patient closely supervised, particularly during the first few days when adverse effects are most likely to develop.[3,4,18] Some have suggested that beta blockers that are extensively metabolised (e.g. metoprolol, propranolol) may possibly carry some additional risk because verapamil raises their serum levels.[23] However, others contend that, since the interaction occurs with atenolol (which is largely excreted unchanged in the urine), the pharmacodynamic effects are more important than any pharmacokinetic changes.[4,10,18] Note that the latter argument is probably valid, as changes of this size, or even more, in the AUC of beta blockers have proved not to be clinically important.

1. Boothby CB, Garrard CS, Pickering D. Verapamil in cardiac arrhythmias. *BMJ* (1972) 2, 349.
2. Seabra-Gomes R, Rickards A, Sutton R. Hemodynamic effects of verapamil and practolol in man. *Eur J Cardiol* (1976) 4, 79–85.
3. McGourty JC, Silas JH, Solomon SA. Tolerability of combined treatment with verapamil and beta-blockers in angina resistant to monotherapy. *Postgrad Med J* (1985) 61, 229–32.
4. Findlay IN, MacLeod K, Gillen G, Elliott AT, Aitchison T, Dargie HJ. A double blind placebo controlled comparison of verapamil, atenolol, and their combination in patients with chronic stable angina pectoris. *Br Heart J* (1987) 57, 336–43.
5. Wayne VS, Harper RW, Laufer E, Federman J, Anderson ST, Pitt A. Adverse interaction between beta-adrenergic blocking drugs and verapamil-report of three cases. *Aust N Z J Med* (1982) 12, 285–9.
6. Sakurai H, Kei M, Matsubara K, Yokouchi K, Hattori K, Ichihashi R, Hirakawa Y, Tsukamoto H, Saburi Y. Cardiogenic shock triggered by verapamil and atenolol—a case report of therapeutic experience with intravenous calcium. *Jpn Circ J* (2000) 64, 893–6.

7. Balasubramian V, Bowles M, Davies AB, Raferty EB. Combined treatment with verapamil and propranolol in chronic stable angina. *Br Heart J* (1981) 45, 349–50.
8. Leon MB, Rosing DR, Bonow RO, Lipson LC, Epstein SE. Clinical efficacy of verapamil alone and combined with propranolol in treating patients with chronic stable angina pectoris. *Am J Cardiol* (1981) 48, 131–9.
9. McQueen EG. New Zealand Committee on Adverse Reactions: 14th Annual Report 1979. *N Z Med J* (1980) 91, 226–9.
10. Misra M, Thakur R, Bhandari K. Sinus arrest caused by atenolol-verapamil combination. *Clin Cardiol* (1987) 10, 365–7.
11. Eisenberg JNH, Oakley GDG. Probable adverse interaction between oral metoprolol and verapamil. *Postgrad Med J* (1984) 60, 705–6.
12. Hutchison SJ, Lorimer AR, Lakhdar A, McAlpine SG. β-blockers and verapamil: a cautionary tale. *BMJ* (1984) 289, 659–60.
13. Lee DW, Cohan B. Refractory cardiogenic shock and complete heart block after verapamil SR and metoprolol treatment. *Angiology* (1995) 46, 517–19.
14. Ljungström A, Åberg H. Interaktion mellan betareceptorblockerare och verapamil. *Lakartidningen* (1973) 70, 3548.
15. Keech AC, Harper RW, Harrison PM, Pitt A, McLean AJ. Pharmacokinetic interaction between oral metoprolol and verapamil for angina pectoris. *Am J Cardiol* (1986) 58, 551–2.
16. Zatuchni J. Bradycardia and hypotension after propranolol HCl and verapamil. *Heart Lung* (1985) 14, 94–5.
17. Rumboldt Z, Baković Z, Bagatin J. Opasna kardiodepresivna interakcija izmedu verapamila i propranolola. *Lijec Vjesn* (1979) 101, 430–2.
18. McCourty JC, Silas JH, Tucker GT, Lennard MS. The effect of combined therapy on the pharmacokinetics and pharmacodynamics of verapamil and propranolol in patients with angina pectoris. *Br J Clin Pharmacol* (1988) 25, 349–57.
19. Sinclair NI, Benzie JL. Timolol eye drops and verapamil — a dangerous combination. *Med J Aust* (1983) 1, 548.
20. Pringle SD, MacEwen CJ. Severe bradycardia due to interaction of timolol eye drops and verapamil. *BMJ* (1987) 294, 155–6.
21. Frierson J, Bailly D, Shultz T, Sund S, Dimas A. Refractory cardiogenic shock and complete heart block after unsuspected verapamil-SR and atenolol overdose. *Clin Cardiol* (1991) 14, 933–5.
22. Waxman AB, White KP, Trawick DR. Electromechanical dissociation following verapamil and propranolol ingestion: a physiologic profile. *Cardiology* (1997) 88, 478–81.
23. McLean AJ, Knight R, Harrison PM, Harper RW. Clearance-based oral drug interaction between verapamil and metoprolol and comparison with atenolol. *Am J Cardiol* (1985) 55, 1628–9.
24. Keech AC, Harper RW, Harrison PM, Pitt A, McLean AJ. Extent and pharmacokinetic mechanisms of oral atenolol-verapamil interaction in man. *Eur J Clin Pharmacol* (1988) 35, 363–6.
25. Bauer LA, Horn JR, Maxon MS, Easterling TR, Shen DD, Strandness DE. Effect of metoprolol and verapamil administered separately and concurrently after single doses on liver blood flow and drug disposition. *J Clin Pharmacol* (2000) 40, 533–43.
26. Hunt BA, Bottorff MB, Herring VL, Self TH, Lalonde RL. Effects of calcium channel blockers on the pharmacokinetics of propranolol stereoisomers. *Clin Pharmacol Ther* (1990) 47, 584–91.
27. Murdoch DL, Thomson GD, Thompson GG, Murray GD, Brodie MJ, McInnes GT. Evaluation of potential pharmacodynamic interactions between verapamil and propranolol in normal subjects. *Br J Clin Pharmacol* (1991) 31, 323–32.
28. Schwarz UI, Gramatté T, Krappweis J, Berndt A, Oertel R, von Richter O, Kirch W. Unexpected effect of verapamil on oral bioavailability of the β-blocker talinolol in humans. *Clin Pharmacol Ther* (1999) 65, 283–90.
29. Kim M, Shen DD, Eddy AC, Nelson WL. Inhibition of the enantioselective oxidative metabolism of metoprolol by verapamil in human liver microsomes. *Drug Metab Dispos* (1993) 21, 309–17.
30. Gramatté T, Oertel R. Intestinal secretion of intravenous talinolol is inhibited by luminal *R*-verapamil. *Clin Pharmacol Ther* (1999) 66, 239–45.
31. British National Formulary. 53rd ed. London: The British Medical Association and The Pharmaceutical Press; 2007. p. 115.
32. Securon IV (Verapamil hydrochloride). Abbott Laboratories Ltd. UK Summary of product characteristics, June 2003.

Beta blockers + Chloroquine or Hydroxychloroquine

Hydroxychloroquine and possibly chloroquine may increase the blood levels of metoprolol, but this is probably not clinically important.

Clinical evidence, mechanism, importance and management

Hydroxychloroquine 400 mg daily for 8 days increased the AUC and peak plasma levels of a single 100-mg dose of **metoprolol** by 65% and 72%, respectively, in 7 healthy subjects who were of the extensive CYP2D6 metaboliser phenotype,[1] see 'Genetic factors', (p.4). Hydroxychloroquine may inhibit the metabolism of **metoprolol** by the cytochrome P450 isoenzyme CYP2D6. The clinical significance of this interaction is unknown, but changes of this size in the AUC of beta blockers have proved not to be clinically important. Other beta blockers that are extensively metabolised (see 'Table 22.1', (p.833).) may behave like **metoprolol**, but those that are excreted unchanged in the urine would not be expected to interact. *In vitro* study suggests that **chloroquine** may interact with **metoprolol** in the same way as hydroxychloroquine.[2] More study is needed.

1. Somer M, Kallio J, Pesonen U, Pyykkö K, Huupponen R, Scheinin M. Influence of hydroxychloroquine on the bioavailability of oral metoprolol. *Br J Clin Pharmacol* (2000) 49, 549–54.
2. Lancaster DL, Adio RA, Tai KK, Simooya OO, Broadhead GD, Tucker GT, Lennard MS. Inhibition of metoprolol metabolism by chloroquine and other antimalarial drugs. *J Pharm Pharmacol* (1990) 42, 267–71.

Beta blockers + Dextropropoxyphene (Propoxyphene)

A single-dose study has shown that the bioavailability of metoprolol is markedly increased by dextropropoxyphene and a case report supports these findings. The bioavailability of propranolol is also increased, but to a lesser extent.

Clinical evidence

A 48-year-old man taking **metoprolol** 100 mg daily developed dizziness and sweating 3 hours after taking dextropropoxyphene 200 mg and paracetamol (acetaminophen) 1.3 g. He was found to have a heart rate of 30 to 40 bpm and a blood pressure of 98/65 mmHg, which returned to normal over the following 8 hours. Assessment of blood samples showed that his normal **metoprolol** level was 89 nanograms/mL, but that this had risen to 160 nanograms/mL in the presence of dextropropoxyphene.[1]

Preliminary results of a study suggest that after taking dextropropoxyphene [dose not stated] for a day the bioavailability of a single 100-mg oral dose of **metoprolol** was increased by almost 260% and the total body clearance was reduced by 18% in healthy subjects. The bioavailability of a single 40-mg oral dose of **propranolol** was increased by about 70%.[2]

Mechanism

Dextropropoxyphene inhibits the metabolism of metoprolol and propranolol by the cytochrome P450 isoenzyme CYP2D6, which results in increased levels and therefore increased effects. Propranolol is probably affected to a lesser extent as it is also metabolised by CYP1A2.

Importance and management

Evidence is limited, but an interaction seems established. It seems likely that this interaction could occur with any of the beta blockers metabolised by CYP2D6 (see 'Table 22.1', (p.833)). Therefore it would be prudent to be alert for evidence of an increased response but so far there seems to be very little evidence to suggest that concurrent use causes problems. No interaction would be expected with those beta blockers that are largely excreted unchanged in the urine (see 'Table 22.1', (p.833)).

1. Marraffa JM, Lang L, Ong G, Lehmann DF. Profound metoprolol-induced bradycardia precipitated by acetaminophen-propoxyphene. *Clin Pharmacol Ther* (2006) 79, 282–6.
2. Lundborg P, Regårdh CG. The effect of propoxyphene pretreatment on the disposition of metoprolol and propranolol. *Clin Pharmacol Ther* (1981) 29, 263–4.

Beta blockers + Diphenhydramine

Diphenhydramine inhibits the metabolism of metoprolol, but this is probably not clinically important.

Clinical evidence

In a placebo-controlled study, a single 100-mg dose of **metoprolol** was given to 16 healthy male subjects on day 3 of a 5-day course of diphenhydramine 50 mg three times daily. Diphenhydramine decreased the clearance of **metoprolol** by 46% and increased its AUC by 61% in the 10 subjects who were of the extensive CYP2D6 metaboliser phenotype, but had no significant effect in the 6 poor metabolisers. However, the **metoprolol** AUC in the extensive metabolisers taking diphenhydramine was still only about one-third of that in the poor metabolisers taking placebo. The effect of **metoprolol** on heart rate and systolic blood pressure during exercise was also increased by diphenhydramine in extensive metabolisers. However, as before, it was not as great as the effect of **metoprolol** alone in poor metabolisers.[1] The same group of researchers repeated this study in 20 healthy women and found broadly similar results.[2]

Mechanism

Diphenhydramine inhibits the cytochrome P450 isoenzyme CYP2D6, which is responsible, in part, for the metabolism of metoprolol and some other beta blockers. CYP2D6 shows polymorphism, with some individuals lacking significant CYP2D6 activity (poor metabolisers), in whom diphenhydramine would have little or no effect. See 'Genetic factors', (p.4), for more on polymorphism.

Importance and management

Information appears to be limited to these studies. Increases in plasma metoprolol levels of this size are unlikely to be clinically relevant. Indeed, despite the likely widespread use of 'extensively metabolised' beta blockers (see 'Table 22.1', (p.833)) and diphenhydramine, no problems seem to have been reported.

1. Hamelin BA, Bouayad A, Méthot J, Jobin J, Desgagnés P, Poirier P, Allaire J, Dumesnil J, Turgeon J. Significant interaction between the nonprescription antihistamine diphenhydramine and the CYP2D6 substrate metoprolol in healthy men with high or low CYP2D6 activity. *Clin Pharmacol Ther* (2000) 67, 466–77.

2. Sharma A, Pibarot P, Pilote S, Dumesnil JG, Arsenault M, Bélanger PM, Meibohn B, Hamelin BA. Modulation of metoprolol pharmacokinetics and hemodynamics by diphenhydramine coadministration during exercise testing in healthy premenopausal women. *J Pharmacol Exp Ther* (2005) 313, 1172–81.

Beta blockers + Dronedarone

Dronedarone increases the AUC of metoprolol in patients with a CYP2D6 extensive metaboliser phenotype. The increase in negative inotropic effects are modest at the recommended therapeutic dose of dronedarone.

Clinical evidence

In a study, 44 healthy subjects (39 extensive and 5 poor CYP2D6 metabolisers) were given **metoprolol** 200 mg daily for 13 days. Concurrent dronedarone 800 mg, 1.2 g or 1.6 g daily from day 5 increased the AUC of **metoprolol** in a dose-dependent manner in the 39 subjects who were extensive metabolisers by 1.63-, 2.08- and 2.53-fold, respectively. In addition, concurrent use resulted in an additive dose-dependent negative inotropic effect. In contrast, **metoprolol** plasma levels were not affected by dronedarone.[1]

Mechanism

Dronedarone is structurally related to amiodarone, which is known to inhibit the cytochrome P450 isoenzyme CYP2D6, by which metoprolol is metabolised (see 'Amiodarone + Beta blockers', p.246). This study also shows that dronedarone inhibits CYP2D6, effectively making extensive metabolisers into poor metabolisers. For more information on metaboliser status see 'Genetic factors', (p.4).

Importance and management

A pharmacokinetic interaction is established, but its clinical relevance is uncertain. The negative inotropic effect of metoprolol was almost doubled by the addition of dronedarone 1.6 g daily, but at the anticipated therapeutic dose of 800 mg the effects were modest. Other beta blockers that are metabolised by CYP2D6 (see 'Table 22.1', (p.833)) would be expected to interact similarly.

1. Damy T, Pousset F, Caplain H, Hulot J-S, Lechat P. Pharmacokinetic and pharmacodynamic interactions between metoprolol and dronedarone in extensive and poor CYP2D6 metabolizers healthy subjects. *Fundam Clin Pharmacol* (2004) 18, 113–23.

Beta blockers + Ergot derivatives

The use of beta blockers with ergot derivatives in the management of migraine is not uncommon, but concurrent use has resulted in three cases of severe peripheral vasoconstriction and one of hypertension.

Clinical evidence

A man with recurrent migraine headaches, reasonably well-controlled over a 6-year period with 2 daily suppositories of *Cafergot* (containing **ergotamine tartrate**) developed progressively painful and purple feet a short while after starting to take **propranolol** 30 mg daily. When he eventually resumed taking the *Cafergot* alone there was no further evidence of peripheral vasoconstriction.[1]

A similar case has been reported elsewhere, although an interaction is inconclusive in this patient, as neither the **ergotamine** nor the **propranolol** were taken alone.[2] Another similar case occurred in a woman taking **oxprenolol** and **ergotamine tartrate** [dosages unknown] for some considerable time. Arteriography showed severe spasm in a number of arteries, which responded eventually to an intra-arterial infusion of glyceryl trinitrate and heparin.[3] Severe pain in the legs and feet occurred in another man after he took **methysergide** 3 mg and **propranolol** 120 mg daily for 2 weeks. He did not respond to various therapies, and in 6 days it was necessary to amputate both his legs below the knee because of gangrene.[3] A woman taking **propranolol** for migraine prophylaxis became hypertensive (BP 180/120 mmHg) with a crushing substernal pain immediately after being given oxygen, prochlorperazine 5 mg and intravenous **dihydroergotamine** 750 micrograms for an acute migraine headache. She recovered uneventfully. She was later found to be hyperthyroid.[4]

These reports contrast with another stating that the use of **propranolol** with **ergotamine** was both effective and uneventful in 50 patients.[5]

Mechanism

Uncertain. One suggestion is that additive vasoconstriction occurs.[1,3] Ergot derivatives cause vasoconstriction, and the beta blockers do the same by blocking the normal (beta$_2$-stimulated) sympathetic vasodilatation. The beta blockers also reduce blood flow by reducing cardiac output.

Importance and management

Concurrent use is usually safe and effective, and there are only a handful of reports of adverse interactions. It was suggested that at least one of these could have been due to the ergotamine alone (i.e. ergotism).[5] However, it would clearly be prudent to be extra alert for any signs of an adverse response, particularly those suggestive of reduced peripheral circulation (coldness, numbness or tingling of the hands and feet).

1. Baumrucker JF. Drug interaction — propranolol and cafergot. *N Engl J Med* (1973) 288, 916–17.

2. Greenberg DJ, Hallett JW. Lower extremity ischemia due to combined drug therapy for migraine. *Postgrad Med* (1982) 72, 103–7.

3. Venter CP, Joubert PH, Buys AC. Severe peripheral ischaemia during concomitant use of beta blockers and ergot alkaloids. *BMJ* (1984) 289, 288–9.

4. Gandy W. Dihydroergotamine interaction with propranolol. *Ann Emerg Med* (1990) 19, 221.

5. Diamond S. Propranolol and ergotamine tartrate (cont.). *N Engl J Med* (1973) 289, 159.

Beta blockers + Finasteride

Finasteride 5 mg daily for 10 days caused no change in the pharmacokinetics or pharmacodynamics of a single 80-mg dose of propranolol in healthy subjects.[1] Further, the manufacturers say that finasteride was used with beta blockers in clinical studies without any evidence of an interaction.[2,3] Similarly, 'dutasteride', (p.1257) does not appear to interact with beta blockers.

1. Gregoire S, Williams R, Gormely G, Lin E. Effect of finasteride (Mk-906), a new potent 5 alpha reductase inhibitor on the disposition of D and L-propranolol. *J Clin Pharmacol* (1990) 30, 847.

2. Proscar (Finasteride). Merck Sharp & Dohme Ltd. UK Summary of product characteristics, February 2004.

3. Proscar (Finasteride). Merck and Co. Inc. US Prescribing information, March 2007.

Beta blockers + Fish oils

The hypotensive effect of propranolol may be enhanced by fish oil.

Clinical evidence, mechanism, importance and management

In a study 36 patients with mild hypertension were given either **propranolol** 80 mg daily or fish oil 9 g daily (as capsules and equivalent to **eicosapentaenoic acid** 1.8 g and **docosahexaenoic acid** 1.1 g daily) for 36 weeks followed by placebo for 4 weeks. A further group of 16 patients were given **propranolol** 80 mg daily for 12 weeks, **propranolol** plus fish oil 9 g daily for 12 weeks, **propranolol** plus fish oil placebo for 12 weeks, and finally **propranolol** placebo for 4 weeks. Fish oil alone decreased blood pressure to a similar extent to **propranolol**, and decreases in blood pressure with the combination were greater than with either **propranolol** or fish oil alone.[1] A further similar study in 14 patients taking a beta blocker found that when they were also given 4 capsules of *Omacor* (equivalent to **eicosapentaenoic acid** 1.9 g and **docosahexaenoic acid** 1.5 g) daily for 6 weeks their blood pressure decreased by a further 3.3/1.9 mmHg.[2]

The mechanism is uncertain, but as fish oil seems to have a hypotensive effect of its own, it may enhance the hypotensive effect of any beta blocker.

1. Singer P, Melzer S, Goschel M, Augustin S. Fish oil amplifies the effect of propranolol in mild essential hypertension. *Hypertension* (1990) 16, 682–91.
2. Lungershausen YK, Abbey M, Nestel PJ, Howe PRC. Reduction of blood pressure and plasma triglycerides by omega-3 fatty acids in treated hypertensives. *J Hypertens* (1994) 12, 1041–5.

Beta blockers + Flecainide

The combined use of flecainide and beta blockers may have additive cardiac depressant effects. An isolated case of bradycardia and fatal AV block has been reported during the use of flecainide with sotalol, and bradycardia has been reported in a patient taking flecainide who was given timolol eye drops.

Clinical evidence, mechanism, importance and management

A study on cardiac function and drug clearance in 10 healthy subjects found that when **propranolol** 80 mg three times daily was given with flecainide 200 mg twice daily for 4 days the AUCs of both drugs were increased by 20 to 30%, and they had some additive negative inotropic effects.[1] A report describes a patient taking flecainide 100 mg twice daily who developed bradycardia and fatal atrioventricular conduction block 3 hours after taking a second dose of **sotalol** 40 mg.[2] Another report describes a patient with chronic atrial fibrillation that had been stable for 5 years during treatment with flecainide and verapamil. Within 3 days of starting **timolol** 0.1% eye drops twice daily, she developed bradycardia with a heart rate of 35 to 40 bpm. The eye drops were stopped and 16 hours after the last dose, her heart rate had increased to 90 to 100 bpm.[3] Careful monitoring has therefore been recommended if beta blockers are added to flecainide. Note that serious cardiac depression has been seen following the use of flecainide with other drugs that have negative inotropic effects such as 'verapamil', (p.261).

1. Holtzman JL, Kvam DC, Berry DA, Mottonen L, Borrell G, Harrison LI, Conard GJ. The pharmacodynamic and pharmacokinetic interaction of flecainide acetate with propranolol: effects on cardiac function and drug clearance. *Eur J Clin Pharmacol* (1987) 33, 97–9.
2. Warren R, Vohra J, Hunt D, Hamer A. Serious interactions of sotalol with amiodarone and flecainide. *Med J Aust* (1990) 152, 277.
3. Minish T, Herd A. Symptomatic bradycardia secondary to interaction between timolol maleate, verapamil, and flecainide: a case report. *J Emerg Med* (2002) 22, 247–9.

Beta blockers + Food

Food can increase, decrease or not affect the bioavailability of beta blockers, but none of the changes has been shown to be of clinical importance.

Clinical evidence, mechanism, importance and management

Food increased the AUC of **propranolol** by 50 to 80%,[1-3] **metoprolol** by about 40%[1] and **labetalol** by about 40%,[4] probably by changing the extent of their first pass metabolism through the liver.[2-4] Food did not affect the extent of absorption of a sustained-release formulation of **propranolol**.[2] Food had very little effect on the absorption of **oxprenolol**[5,6] or **pindolol**,[7] whereas the AUC of **atenolol** was reduced by about 20%.[8] A later study suggested that **atenolol** (and possibly other hydrophilic beta blockers, see 'Table 22.1', (p.833)) become tightly associated with bile acid micelles, preventing their absorption.[9] None of these changes have been shown to be of clinical importance, nor is it clear whether it matters if patients take these drugs in a regular pattern in relation to meals. Beta blocker serum levels vary widely between patients (a 20-fold difference in propranolol AUC has been noted between individuals),[1] and individualising the dose is therefore more of an issue than food intake.

1. Melander A, Danielson K, Scherstén B, Wåhlin E. Enhancement of the bioavailability of propranolol and metoprolol by food. *Clin Pharmacol Ther* (1977) 22, 108–12.
2. Liedholm H, Melander A. Concomitant food intake can increase the bioavailability of propranolol by transient inhibition of its presystemic primary conjugation. *Clin Pharmacol Ther* (1986) 40, 29–36.
3. McLean AJ, Isbister C, Bobik A, Dudley F. Reduction of first-pass hepatic clearance of propranolol by food. *Clin Pharmacol Ther* (1981) 30, 31–4.
4. Daneshmend TK, Roberts CJC. The influence of food on the oral and intravenous pharmacokinetics of a high clearance drug: a study with labetalol. *Br J Clin Pharmacol* (1982) 14, 73–8.
5. Dawes CP, Kendall MJ, Welling PG. Bioavailability of conventional and slow-release oxprenolol in fasted and nonfasted individuals. *Br J Clin Pharmacol* (1979) 7, 299–302.
6. John VA, Smith SE. Influence of food intake on plasma oxprenolol concentrations following oral administration of conventional and Oros preparations. *Br J Clin Pharmacol* (1985) 19, 191S–195S.
7. Kiger JL, Lavene D, Guillaume MF, Guerret M, Longchampt J. The effect of food and clopamide on the absorption of pindolol in man. *Int J Clin Pharmacol Biopharm* (1976) 13, 228–32.
8. Melander A, Stenberg P, Liedholm H, Scherstén B, Wåhlin-Boll E. Food-induced reduction in bioavailability of atenolol. *Eur J Clin Pharmacol* (1979) 16, 327–30.
9. Barnwell SG, Laudanski T, Dwyer M, Story MJ, Guard P, Cole S, Attwood D. Reduced bioavailability of atenolol in man: the role of bile acids. *Int J Pharmaceutics* (1993) 89, 245–50.

Beta blockers + Grapefruit and other fruit juices

The bioavailability of celiprolol is markedly reduced by both grapefruit juice and orange juice, the bioavailability of atenolol is moderately reduced by orange juice, and the bioavailability of talinolol is reduced by grapefruit juice.

Clinical evidence, mechanism, importance and management

(a) Acebutolol

In a randomised, crossover study, 10 healthy subjects were given a 200-mL drink of normal-strength **grapefruit juice** three times a day for 4 days (total of 11 drinks), with a single 400-mg dose of acebutolol on the morning of day 3. **Grapefruit juice** decreased the maximum levels and AUC of acebutolol by a modest 19% and 6%, respectively. No significant changes in the heart rate or blood pressure were seen.[1]

(b) Atenolol

In a randomised crossover study 10 healthy subjects were given 200 mL of **orange juice** (from concentrate) three times daily with a single 50-mg dose of atenolol on the third day. **Orange juice** reduced the AUC and maximum serum levels of atenolol by 40% and 49%, respectively, and also attenuated the atenolol-induced reduction in heart rate. The effect of atenolol on blood pressure was unchanged.[2] This suggests that orange juice may make atenolol less effective when it is used for rate control, but the clinical significance of this effect is unclear.

(c) Celiprolol

In a study 12 healthy subjects were given **grapefruit juice** 200 mL three times daily for 2 days. On the third day celiprolol 100 mg was given with the second of four 200 mL volumes of **grapefruit juice**, and on day 4 two further 200 mL volumes of **grapefruit juice** were given. The AUC and peak plasma levels of celiprolol were reduced by about 87% and 95%, respectively. The half-life of celiprolol was slightly prolonged. However, **grapefruit juice** did not affect the changes in blood pressure or heart rate caused by celiprolol.[3] In a similar study in 10 healthy subjects, 200 mL of 'normal-strength' **orange juice**, given 2 to 4 times daily for 4 days, reduced the AUC and peak plasma levels of a single 100-mg dose of celiprolol given on day 3 by 83% and 89%, respectively. The half-life of celiprolol was prolonged from 4.6 to 10.8 hours and the renal excretion of celiprolol was reduced by 77%. However, **orange juice** did not alter the effects of celiprolol on blood pressure or heart rate.[4]

The mechanism of this effect is not known, but suggestions include an effect on intraduodenal pH and the lipid solubility of celiprolol, or the formation of a complex between celiprolol and an ingredient of **grapefruit** or **orange juice** that interfered with celiprolol absorption. Alternatively, inhibition of uptake transporter proteins in the intestine may have reduced absorption.[3,4]

Although the clinical relevance of these effects has not been fully assessed, the studies suggest that the effects of celiprolol on blood pressure and heart rate are not affected. Nevertheless the marked reduction in celiprolol bioavailability in the presence of **grapefruit** or **orange juice** suggests this interaction may be of clinical significance in some patients.[3,4]

(d) Talinolol

Grapefruit juice 300 mL decreased the AUC of a single 50-mg dose of talinolol by 44%, increased the maximum level by 42%, and increased the oral clearance by 62%. Similar results were seen after repeated administration of **grapefruit juice** over 6 days. However, the haemodynamic effects of talinolol were not altered by **grapefruit juice**.[5] Because P-glycoprotein levels did not appear to be affected by **grapefruit juice**, it was suggested that constituents in the juice might inhibit an uptake process other than P-glycoprotein. [Note that, in contrast, a study in *animals* found that the bioavailability of talinolol was increased by **grapefruit juice**.[6]] The decreases in talinolol levels are unlikely to be clinically relevant.

1. Lilja JJ, Raaska K, Neuvonen PJ. Effects of grapefruit juice on the pharmacokinetics of acebutolol. *Br J Clin Pharmacol* (2005) 60, 659–63.
2. Lilja JJ, Raaska K, Neuvonen PJ. Effects of orange juice on the pharmacokinetics of atenolol. *Eur J Clin Pharmacol* (2005) 61, 337–40.
3. Lilja JJ, Backman JT, Laitila J, Luurila H, Neuvonen PJ. Itraconazole increases but grapefruit juice greatly decreases plasma concentrations of celiprolol. *Clin Pharmacol Ther* (2003) 73, 192–8.
4. Lilja JJ, Juntti-Patinen L, Neuvonen PJ. Orange juice substantially reduces the bioavailability of the β-adrenergic-blocking agent celiprolol. *Clin Pharmacol Ther* (2004) 75, 184–90.
5. Schwarz UI, Seemann D, Oertel R, Miehlke S, Kuhlisch E, Fromm MF, Kim RB, Bailey DG, Kirch W. Grapefruit juice ingestion significantly reduces talinolol bioavailability. *Clin Pharmacol Ther* (2005) 77, 291–301.
6. Spahn-Langguth H, Langguth P. Grapefruit juice enhances intestinal absorption of the P-glycoprotein substrate talinolol. *Eur J Pharm Sci* (2001) 12, 361–7.

Beta blockers + H_2-receptor antagonists; Cimetidine

No clinically significant interaction appears to occur between the beta blockers and cimetidine, although the blood levels of some extensively metabolised beta blockers (e.g. metoprolol, propranolol) can be doubled. Isolated case reports describe bradycardia, an irregular heart beat, or hypotension in patients taking cimetidine with atenolol, metoprolol, or labetalol, respectively.

Clinical evidence

(a) Acebutolol

A study *in animals* found that the pharmacokinetics of acebutolol were not affected by cimetidine, which suggests that a clinical interaction is unlikely.[1]

(b) Atenolol

A report briefly mentions a patient taking a beta blocker for angina who developed profound sinus bradycardia (36 bpm) and hypotension when cimetidine was also given.[2] The beta blocker was not specified, but it was identified as atenolol elsewhere.[3] Three well controlled studies in healthy subjects and patients found that cimetidine did not significantly alter blood levels of atenolol, nor did it alter the affect of atenolol on heart rate.[4-9] Atenolol did not affect cimetidine pharmacokinetics.[6]

(c) Betaxolol

The blood levels and pharmacokinetics of betaxolol were unaffected by cimetidine in one study.[10]

(d) Bisoprolol

A study in 6 healthy subjects found that the maximum plasma level, AUC and clearance of bisoprolol were not significantly affected by cimetidine[11,12] although an analysis of the results by other authors suggested that cimetidine may cause a significant reduction in the renal clearance of bisoprolol.[13]

(e) Carvedilol

The blood levels and pharmacokinetics of carvedilol were unaffected by cimetidine in one study.[14]

(f) Labetalol

The AUC and bioavailability of a single 200-mg oral dose of labetalol was increased by 66% and 56%, respectively, in 6 healthy subjects who took cimetidine 400 mg four times daily for 4 days.[15] One subject developed postural hypotension (70/40 mmHg), felt light-headed and almost fainted on standing.[15] Conversely, the AUC of intravenous labetalol was unaffected by cimetidine.[15]

(g) Metoprolol

A study in 6 healthy subjects given metoprolol 100 mg twice daily for a week found that the cimetidine 1 g daily in divided doses increased the peak plasma levels of metoprolol by 70% and the AUC by 61%, but this did not increase the effect of metoprolol on the heart rate during exercise.[4-6] Metoprolol did not affect cimetidine pharmacokinetics.[6]

Three other studies confirmed that cimetidine increased metoprolol serum levels after single or multiple doses, but none of the studies found that this interaction resulted in an increase the effect of metoprolol on the heart rate during exercise.[16-19] An isolated case describes one patient who complained of a "very irregular heart beat" while taking both drugs, which was much less marked when he took the two drugs separated by as much time as possible.[20] In contrast, two other studies found that cimetidine did not affect the serum levels of a single 100-mg dose of metoprolol.[7,8]

(h) Nadolol

The blood levels and pharmacokinetics of nadolol were unaffected by cimetidine, and the effects of the beta blocker on heart rate and blood pressure were not changed.[21]

(i) Nebivolol

Cimetidine 400 mg twice daily increased the AUC and peak plasma levels of a single 5-mg dose of nebivolol by 48% and 23%, respectively, but did not alter the effect of nebivolol on blood pressure or heart rate.[22]

(j) Penbutolol

The blood levels and pharmacokinetics of penbutolol[9,23] were unaffected by cimetidine, and the effects of the beta blocker on heart rate and blood pressure were not changed.[23]

(k) Pindolol

Cimetidine 1 g daily in divided doses increased the AUC and peak plasma levels of pindolol 10 mg twice daily by 30% and 33%, respectively, although these changes were not statistically significant.[9] In another study, cimetidine 400 mg twice daily increased the AUC of the pindolol by about 40% and decreased the renal clearance by about 35%.[24]

(l) Propranolol

Cimetidine 300 mg four times daily for a week was given to 12 healthy subjects with propranolol 80 mg every 12 hours from day 3 onwards. The mean steady-state blood levels and the AUC of propranolol were raised by 47%, and the half-life was prolonged by 17%, but cimetidine did not alter the effect of propranolol on heart rate.[25] A number of other single-dose and steady-state studies confirmed that cimetidine caused rises of 35 to 136% in the blood levels, AUC and clearance of propranolol,[4-6,10,21,26-32] but this did not increase the effect of the beta blocker on blood pressure,[21,27,29] or on heart rate, either at rest or during exercise.[4,21,27-29] In contrast, one study did show a further reduction in heart rate when cimetidine was given with propranolol.[33] A letter describes one patient given cimetidine 1 g daily for 6 weeks who had an increase in the serum propranolol level of about threefold and an AUC increase of 340% when a single 80-mg dose of propranolol was given.[2] In one study, the increase in the steady-state AUC of propranolol tended to be higher when cimetidine was given simultaneously with propranolol than when they were given separated by 10 hours (41% versus 26%), but the difference was not significant.[34]

In one study propranolol did not affect cimetidine pharmacokinetics.[6]

(m) Timolol

A double-blind study in 12 healthy subjects found that cimetidine 400 mg twice daily for 3 days did not modify the effect of a single drop of timolol 0.5%, put into each eye on heart rate or intraocular pressure to either a statistically or clinically relevant extent.[35]

Mechanism

The blood levels of beta blockers extensively metabolised in the liver by the cytochrome P450 isoenzyme CYP2D6 (e.g. metoprolol, nebivolol and propranolol) are increased because cimetidine reduces their metabolism by inhibiting the activity of the liver enzymes. However, this does not seem to be a complete explanation as cimetidine does not affect carvedilol, which is metabolised by CYP2D6, but affects labetalol, a beta blocker that is not metabolised by CYP2D6.[15] Pindolol is partly excreted by an active renal tubular secretion mechanism, and cimetidine increases pindolol blood levels by inhibiting this mechanism.[24] Cimetidine may reduce the renal clearance of bisoprolol by a similar mechanism.[12] Those beta blockers that are largely excreted unchanged in the urine (e.g. atenolol, nadolol) are not affected by cimetidine.[8,21]

Importance and management

Well studied and established interactions but, despite the considerable rises in blood levels that can occur when some beta blockers are given with cimetidine, the effects normally appear to be clinically unimportant. Concurrent use is common, but only one isolated case of profound bradycardia (involving atenolol) appears to have been reported. Marked hypotension also seems to be rare. Combined use need not be avoided. However, it has been suggested that patients with impaired liver function who are given cimetidine with beta blockers that are extensively metabolised in the liver (see 'Table 22.1', (p.833)) might possibly develop grossly elevated blood levels, which could cause adverse effects. It would seem prudent to either monitor this type of patient (for effects such as hypotension) until more is known, or to use a non-interacting H_2-receptor antagonist such as 'ranitidine', (below).

1. Mostafavi SA, Foster RT. Influence of cimetidine co-administration on the pharmacokinetics of acebutolol enantiomers and its metabolite diacetolol in a rat model: the effect of gastric pH on double-peak phenomena. *Int J Pharm* (2003) 255, 81–6.
2. Donovan MA, Heagerty AM, Patel L, Castleden M, Pohl JEF. Cimetidine and bioavailability of propranolol. *Lancet* (1981) i, 164.
3. Rowley-Jones D, Flind AC. Drug interactions with cimetidine. *Pharm J* (1981) 283, 659.
4. Kirch W, Spahn H, Köhler H, Mutschler E. Accumulation and adverse effects of metoprolol and propranolol after concurrent administration of cimetidine. *Arch Toxicol* (1983) (Suppl 6), 379–83.
5. Kirch W, Spahn H, Köhler H, Mutschler E. Interaction of metoprolol, propranolol and atenolol with cimetidine. *Clin Sci* (1982) 63 (Suppl 8), 451S–453S.
6. Kirch W, Spahn H, Köhler H, Mutschler E. Influence of β-receptor antagonists on the pharmacokinetics of cimetidine. *Drugs* (1983) 25 (Suppl 2), 127–30.
7. Houtzagers JJR, Streurman O, Regårdh CG. The effect of pretreatment with cimetidine on the bioavailability and disposition of atenolol and metoprolol. *Br J Clin Pharmacol* (1982) 14, 67–72.
8. Ellis ME, Hussain M, Webb AK, Barker NP, Fitzsimons TJ. The effect of cimetidine on the relative cardioselectivity of atenolol and metoprolol in asthmatic patients. *Br J Clin Pharmacol* (1984) 17, 59S–64S.
9. Mutschler E, Spahn H, Kirch W. The interaction between H2-receptor antagonists and β-adrenoceptor blockers. *Br J Clin Pharmacol* (1984) 17, 51S–57S.
10. Rey E, Jammet P, d'Athis P, de Lauture D, Christoforov B, Weber S, Olive G. Effect of cimetidine on the pharmacokinetics of the new beta-blocker betaxolol. *Arzneimittelforschung* (1987) 37, 953–6.
11. Kirch W, Rose I, Klingmann I, Pabst J, Ohnhaus EE. Interaction of bisoprolol with cimetidine and rifampicin. *Eur J Clin Pharmacol* (1986) 31, 59–62.
12. Kirch W, Ohnhaus EE, Pabst J. Reply. *Eur J Clin Pharmacol* (1987) 33, 110.
13. Somogyi A, Muirhead M. Interaction of cimetidine with bisoprolol. *Eur J Clin Pharmacol* (1987) 33, 109–110.
14. Data on file, database on carvedilol, SmithKline Beecham, quoted by Ruffolo RR, Boyle DA, Venuti RP, Lukas MA. Carvedilol (Kredex®): a novel multiple action cardiovascular agent. *Drugs Today* (1991) 27, 465–92.
15. Daneshmend TK, Roberts CJC. The effects of enzyme induction and enzyme inhibition on labetalol pharmacokinetics. *Br J Clin Pharmacol* (1984) 18, 393–400.
16. Kendall MJ, Laugher SJ, Wilkins MR. Ranitidine, cimetidine and metoprolol: a pharmacokinetic interaction study. *Gastroenterology* (1986) 90, 1490.
17. Kirch W, Rämsch K, Janisch HD, Ohnhaus EE. The influence of two histamine H_2-receptor antagonists, cimetidine and ranitidine, on plasma levels and clinical effect of nifedipine and metoprolol. *Arch Toxicol* (1984) (Suppl 7), 256–9.
18. Chellingsworth MC, Laugher S, Akhlaghi S, Jack DB, Kendall MJ. The effects of ranitidine and cimetidine on the pharmacokinetics and pharmacodynamics of metoprolol. *Aliment Pharmacol Ther* (1988) 2, 521–7.
19. Toon S, Davidson EM, Garstang FM, Batra H, Bowes RJ, Rowland M. The racemic metoprolol H_2-antagonist interaction. *Clin Pharmacol Ther* (1988) 43, 283–9.
20. Anon. Adverse Drug Reactions Advisory Committee. Seven case studies. *Med J Aust* (1982) 2, 190–1.
21. Duchin KL, Stern MA, Willard DA, McKinstry DN. Comparison of kinetic interactions of nadolol and propranolol with cimetidine. *Am Heart J* (1984) 108, 1084–6.
22. Kamali F, Howes A, Thomas SHL, Ford GA, Snoeck E. A pharmacokinetic and pharmacodynamic interaction study between nebivolol and the H_2-receptor antagonists cimetidine and ranitidine. *Br J Clin Pharmacol* (1997) 43, 201–4.
23. Spahn H, Kirch W, Hajdu P, Mutschler E, Ohnhaus EE. Penbutolol pharmacokinetics: the influence of concomitant administration of cimetidine. *Eur J Clin Pharmacol* (1986) 29, 555–60.
24. Somogyi AA, Bochner F, Sallustio BC. Stereoselective inhibition of pindolol renal clearance by cimetidine in humans. *Clin Pharmacol Ther* (1992) 51, 379–87.
25. Donn KH, Powell JR, Rogers JF, Eshelman FN. The influence of H2-receptor antagonists on steady-state concentrations of propranolol and 4-hydroxypropranolol. *J Clin Pharmacol* (1984) 24, 500–8.
26. Kirch W, Köhler H, Spahn H, Mutschler E. Interaction of cimetidine with metoprolol, propranolol or atenolol. *Lancet* (1981) 2, 531–2.
27. Reimann IW, Klotz U, Frölich JC. Effects of cimetidine and ranitidine on steady-state propranolol kinetics and dynamics. *Clin Pharmacol Ther* (1982) 32, 749–57.
28. Reimann IW, Klotz U, Siems B, Frölich JC. Cimetidine increases steady-state plasma levels of propranolol. *Br J Clin Pharmacol* (1981) 12, 785–90.
29. Markiewicz A, Hartleb M, Lelek A, Boldys H, Nowak A. The effect of treatment with cimetidine and ranitidine on bioavailability of, and circulatory response to, propranolol. *Zbl Pharm* (1984) 123, 516–18.
30. Heagerty AM, Donovan MA, Castleden CM, Pohl JF, Patel L, Hedges A. Influence of cimetidine on pharmacokinetics of propranolol. *BMJ* (1981) 282, 1917–19.
31. Heagerty AM, Donovan MA, Casteleden CM, Pohl JEF, Patel L. The influence of histamine (H_2) antagonists on propranolol pharmacokinetics. *Int J Clin Pharmacol Res* (1982) 2, 203–5.
32. Reilly CS, Biollaz J, Koshakji RP, Wood AJJ. Enprostil, in contrast to cimetidine, does not inhibit propranolol metabolism. *Clin Pharmacol Ther* (1986) 40, 37–41.
33. Feely J, Wilkinson GR, Wood AJJ. Reduction in liver blood flow and propranolol metabolism by cimetidine. *N Engl J Med* (1981) 304, 692–5.
34. Asgharnejad M, Powell JR, Donn KH, Danis M. The effect of cimetidine dose timing on oral propranolol kinetics in adults. *J Clin Pharmacol* (1988) 28, 339–43.
35. Ishii Y, Nakamura K, Tsutsumi K, Kotegawa, Nakano S, Natasuka K. Drug interaction between cimetidine and timolol ophthalmic solution: effect on heart rate and intraocular pressure in healthy Japanese volunteers. *J Clin Pharmacol* (2000) 40, 193–9.

Beta blockers + H_2-receptor antagonists; Famotidine

Famotidine does not appear to interact with the beta blockers.

Clinical evidence, mechanism, importance and management

A survey of 15 patients taking beta blockers (**acebutolol**, **atenolol**, **betaxolol**, **nadolol**, **pindolol**, **propranolol** or **sotalol**) for 6 to 8 weeks found no evidence of changes in antihypertensive effects or bradycardia while they were taking famotidine 40 mg daily.[1] No interaction would be expected, and no special precautions would seem necessary if famotidine is taken with these or any other beta blocker.

1. Chichmanian RM, Mignot G, Spreux A, Jean-Girard C, Hofliger P. Tolérance de la famotidine. Étude due réseau médecins sentinelles en pharmacovigilance. *Therapie* (1992) 47, 239–43.

Beta blockers + H_2-receptor antagonists; Nizatidine

The bradycardic effects of atenolol are increased by nizatidine.

Clinical evidence, mechanism, importance and management

After taking **atenolol** 100 mg daily for 7 days the mean resting heart rate of 12 healthy subjects fell from about 64 to 53 bpm 3 hours after dosing. A further fall of 6 bpm occurred when they were also given nizatidine 300 mg daily for 7 days. Nizatidine alone caused a fall in heart rate of about 8 bpm.[1] Thus the effects of nizatidine and **atenolol** on heart rate appear to be additive. It seems likely that nizatidine would have the same effects in the presence of other beta blockers. The clinical significance of these effects is uncertain, but it might be important in elderly patients.[1] More study is needed.

1. Halabi A, Kirch W. Negative chronotropic effects of nizatidine. *Gut* (1991) 32, 630–4.

Beta blockers + H_2-receptor antagonists; Ranitidine

Ranitidine does not alter either the steady-state plasma levels or the therapeutic effects of atenolol, nebivolol, propranolol or tertatolol. Some studies have shown moderate rises in metoprolol levels in those also given ranitidine, but this is not clinically important.

Clinical evidence

The plasma levels of **metoprolol** 100 mg twice daily were unaffected by ranitidine 300 mg daily for 7 days in 12 healthy subjects.[1] Two other studies have confirmed that ranitidine did not significantly affect the plasma levels of **metoprolol**.[2-5] However, these studies found increases of up to 38% in the AUC of single intravenous or oral doses of **metoprolol**,[2-5] and another study found that ranitidine increased the AUC and plasma levels of **metoprolol** 100 mg twice daily by 55 and 34%, respectively.[6-8] All of these studies found that ranitidine did not alter the effect of **metoprolol** on heart rate during exercise.[1,2,5,6]

Ranitidine 300 mg daily for 6 days did not affect the steady-state plasma levels of **propranolol** 160 mg daily nor did it alter the effect of **propranolol** on heart rate or blood pressure in 5 healthy subjects.[9] Similarly no changes in plasma **propranolol** levels were seen in other multiple-dose[10] or single-dose studies.[11-14]

Similarly, in other studies, ranitidine 150 mg twice daily did not significantly alter the pharmacokinetic or pharmacodynamic effects of a single 5-mg dose of **nebivolol**,[15] a single 5-mg dose of **tertatolol**,[16] or **atenolol** 100 mg daily for 7 days.[6,8]

Mechanism

The rises in metoprolol serum levels caused by ranitidine in the two single-dose metoprolol studies are not understood, nor is it clear why one of four studies found an increase after multiple doses.

Importance and management

The possible effects of ranitidine on the plasma levels and effects of propranolol and metoprolol have been well studied. Although some studies have shown moderate rises in metoprolol levels, particularly after single-doses, these increases are of a magnitude that is unlikely to be clinically important. Less is known about atenolol, nebivolol and tertatolol, although no clinically relevant interactions have been seen. There is nothing to suggest that the concurrent use of ranitidine and any beta blocker should be avoided, nor that there is any need to take particular precautions.

1. Toon S, Davidson EM, Garstang FM, Batra H, Bowers RJ, Rowland M. The racemic metoprolol H_2-antagonist interaction. *Clin Pharmacol Ther* (1988) 43, 283–9.
2. Kelly JG, Salem SAM, Kinney CD, Shanks RG, McDevitt DG. Effects of ranitidine on the disposition of metoprolol. *Br J Clin Pharmacol* (1985) 19, 219–24.
3. Kelly JG, Shanks RG, McDevitt DG. Influence of ranitidine on plasma metoprolol concentrations. *BMJ* (1983) 287, 1218–19.
4. Kendall MJ, Laugher SJ, Wilkins MR. Ranitidine, cimetidine and metoprolol-a pharmacokinetic interaction study. *Gastroenterology* (1986) 90, 1490.
5. Chellingsworth MC, Laugher S, Akhlaghi S, Jack DB, Kendall MJ. The effects of ranitidine and cimetidine on the pharmacokinetics and pharmacodynamics of metoprolol. *Aliment Pharmacol Ther* (1988) 2, 521–7.
6. Spahn H, Mutschler E, Kirch W, Ohnhaus EE, Janisch HD. Influence of ranitidine on plasma metoprolol and atenolol concentrations. *BMJ* (1983) 286, 1546–7.
7. Kirch W, Rämsch K, Janisch HD, Ohnhaus EE. The influence of two histamine H_2-receptor antagonists, cimetidine and ranitidine, on the plasma levels and clinical effect of nifedipine and metoprolol. *Arch Toxicol* (1984) 7 (Suppl), 256–9.
8. Mutschler E, Spahn H, Kirch W. The interaction between H_2-receptor antagonists and beta-adrenoceptor blockers. *Br J Clin Pharmacol* (1984) 17, 51S–57S.
9. Reimann IW, Klotz U, Frölich JC. Effects of cimetidine and ranitidine on steady-state propranolol kinetics and dynamics. *Clin Pharmacol Ther* (1982) 32, 749–57.
10. Donn KH, Powell JR, Rogers JF, Eshelman FN. The influence of H_2-receptor antagonists on steady-state concentrations of propranolol and 4-hydroxypropranolol. *J Clin Pharmacol* (1984) 24, 500–8.
11. Markiewicz A, Hartleb M, Lelek H, Boldys H, Nowak A. The effect of treatment with cimetidine and ranitidine on bioavailability of, and circulatory response to, propranolol. *Zbl Pharm* (1984) 123, 516–18.
12. Heagerty AM, Castleden CM, Patel L. Failure of ranitidine to interact with propranolol. *BMJ* (1982) 284, 1304.
13. Heagerty AM, Donovan MA, Castleden CM, Pohl JEF, Patel L. The influence of histamine (H_2) antagonists on propranolol pharmacokinetics. *Int J Clin Pharmacol Res* (1982) 2, 203–5.
14. Patel L, Weerasuriya K. Effect of cimetidine and ranitidine on propranolol clearance. *Br J Clin Pharmacol* (1983) 15, 152P.
15. Kamali F, Howes A, Thomas SHL, Ford GA, Snoeck E. A pharmacokinetic and pharmacodynamic interaction study between nebivolol and the H_2-receptor antagonists cimetidine and ranitidine. *Br J Clin Pharmacol* (1997) 43, 201–4.
16. Kirch W, Milferstädt S, Halabi A, Rocher I, Efthymiopoulos C, Jung L. Interaction of tertatolol with rifampicin and ranitidine pharmacokinetics and antihypertensive activity. *Cardiovasc Drugs Ther* (1990) 4, 487–92.

Beta blockers + Haloperidol

An isolated case report describes severe hypotension and cardiopulmonary arrest in a woman shortly after she was given haloperidol and propranolol. Plasma levels of haloperidol in three patients were not significantly changed by propranolol. The concurrent use of sotalol and haloperidol should generally be avoided because of the possible increased risk of QT prolongation.

Clinical evidence, mechanism, importance and management

A middle-aged woman with schizophrenia and hypertension experienced three episodes of severe hypotension within 30 to 120 minutes of being given **propranolol** 40 to 80 mg and haloperidol 10 mg.[1] On two of the occasions she had a cardiopulmonary arrest. She fainted each time, became cyanotic, had no palpable pulses and had severe hypotension, but rapidly responded to cardiopulmonary resuscitation. She suffered no adverse consequences.[1] The reasons for the severe hypotension are not understood, although both drugs alone can cause hypotension.

A study found that the steady-state plasma levels of haloperidol 6 to 15 mg daily were not significantly changed in 3 patients by long-acting **propranolol**, in incremental doses up to 480 mg daily.[2]

There seems to be only one case of an interaction between haloperidol and **propranolol** on record. Bearing in mind the widespread use of these drugs, this interaction would appear to be rare. There would seem to be little reason for avoiding concurrent use.

Note that both haloperidol and **sotalol** can prolong the QT interval and should therefore not generally be used together, see 'Drugs that prolong the QT interval + Other drugs that prolong the QT interval', p.257.

1. Alexander HE, McCarty K, Giffen MB. Hypotension and cardiopulmonary arrest associated with concurrent haloperidol and propranolol therapy. *JAMA* (1984) 252, 87–8.
2. Greendyke RM, Kanter DR. Plasma propranolol levels and their effect on plasma thioridazine and haloperidol concentrations. *J Clin Psychopharmacol* (1987) 7, 178–82.

Beta blockers + Hormonal contraceptives

The blood levels of metoprolol are increased in women taking oral contraceptives, but the clinical importance of this is probably very small. Acebutolol, oxprenolol and propranolol pharmacokinetics are minimally affected by contraceptive use.

Clinical evidence

The peak plasma levels and the AUC of a single 100-mg dose of **metoprolol** were 36 and 70% higher, respectively, in 12 women taking low-dose combined oral contraceptives, when compared with a similar group not taking contraceptives. The elimination half-life of **metoprolol** was unaffected.[1] In a further study by the same research group, the AUC of **metoprolol** was 71% higher, the AUC of **oxprenolol** was 26% higher, the AUC of **propranolol** was 42% higher, and the AUC of **acebutolol** was marginally lower in women taking combined oral contraceptives, when compared to those not taking contraceptives, but only the **metoprolol** difference was statistically significant.[2] In another study, the total clearance of a single 80-mg dose of **propranolol** was increased (although not significantly) in 8 women given **ethinylestradiol** 50 micrograms daily, and an even smaller increase was seen when they were taking a combined oral contraceptive containing **ethinylestradiol** and **norethisterone**.[3]

Mechanism

The reason for the changes appears to be that ethinylestradiol alters the metabolism of these beta blockers. In the case of propranolol its conjugation and oxidation are increased by the ethinylestradiol.[3]

Importance and management

The changes seen with propranolol, oxprenolol and acebutolol are almost certainly too small to matter, but with metoprolol the changes are somewhat larger. Even so, changes of this size caused by the interactions of other drugs with beta blockers are not usually clinically relevant. No special precautions are generally necessary if any of these beta blockers are given to women taking combined oral contraceptives containing ethinylestradiol, or those taking ethinylestradiol alone, although note that the effects of a moderate rise may be more significant in those taking metoprolol for heart failure. Also be aware that some of the indications for beta blockers are cautions for, or preclude the use of, combined oral contraceptives.

1. Kendall MJ, Quarterman CP, Jack DB, Beeley L. Metoprolol pharmacokinetics and the oral contraceptive pill. *Br J Clin Pharmacol* (1982) 14, 120–2.
2. Kendall MJ, Jack DB, Quarterman CP, Smith SR, Zaman R. β-adrenoceptor blocker pharmacokinetics and the oral contraceptive pill. *Br J Clin Pharmacol* (1984) 17, 87S–89S.
3. Walle T, Fagan TC, Walle UK, Topmiller MJ. Stimulatory as well as inhibitory effects of ethinyloestradiol on the metabolic clearances of propranolol in young women. *Br J Clin Pharmacol* (1996) 41, 305–9.

Beta blockers + Hydralazine

The plasma levels of propranolol and other extensively metabolised beta blockers (such as metoprolol and oxprenolol) are

increased by hydralazine, but no increase in adverse effects seems to have been reported.

Clinical evidence

(a) Effect of hydralazine on beta blockers

Single 25- and 50-mg doses of hydralazine increased the AUC of a single 40-mg dose of **propranolol** by 60% and 110%, respectively, and raised the peak plasma levels by 144 and 240%, respectively, in 5 healthy subjects.[1] Similarly, in another single-dose study, hydralazine increased the AUC of **propranolol** by 62 to 77%.[2] However, a further single-dose study using sustained-release **propranolol** found that hydralazine had no effect on **propranolol** pharmacokinetics.[3]

In other studies hydralazine increased the AUC of sustained-release **oxprenolol** by 41% at steady-state;[4] and of **metoprolol** by 30% after a single dose,[5] and by 38% at steady-state.[6] In contrast, single-dose studies found that hydralazine did not affect the AUC of **acebutolol** or **nadolol**.[5]

(b) Effect of beta blockers on hydralazine

Oxprenolol was found not to have a significant effect on the pharmacokinetics of hydralazine.[4]

Mechanism

Uncertain. Hydralazine appears to increase the bioavailability only of those beta blockers that undergo high hepatic extraction and not those that are largely excreted unchanged in the urine. Hepatic extraction is discussed in more detail under 'Changes in first-pass metabolism', (p.4), and 'Table 22.1', (p.833), lists the metabolic routes of the commonly used systemic beta blockers. It has been suggested that hydralazine may alter hepatic blood flow or inhibit hepatic enzymes,[1,5,6] although other mechanisms may also be involved.[3,7,8]

Importance and management

Moderately well documented and established interactions, but the increased beta blocker serum levels appear to cause no adverse clinical effect. Concurrent use is usually valuable in the treatment of hypertension. No particular precautions seem to be necessary.

1. Schneck DW, Vary JE. Mechanism by which hydralazine increases propranolol bioavailability. *Clin Pharmacol Ther* (1984) 35, 447–53.
2. McLean AJ, Skews H, Bobik A, Dudley FJ. Interaction between oral propranolol and hydralazine. *Clin Pharmacol Ther* (1980) 27, 726–32.
3. Byrne AJ, McNeil JJ, Harrison PM, Louis W, Tonkin AM, McLean AJ. Stable oral availability of sustained release propranolol when co-administered with hydralazine or food: evidence implicating substrate delivery rate as a determinant of presystematic drug interactions. *Br J Clin Pharmacol* (1984) 17, 45S–50S.
4. Hawksworth GM, Dart AM, Chiang K, Parry K, Petrie JC. Effect of oxprenolol on the pharmacokinetics and pharmacodynamics of hydralazine. *Drugs* (1983) 25 (Suppl 2), 136–40.
5. Jack DB, Kendall MJ, Dean S, Laugher SJ, Zaman R, Tenneson ME. The effect of hydralazine on the pharmacokinetics of three different beta adrenoceptor antagonists: metoprolol, nadolol, and acebutolol. *Biopharm Drug Dispos* (1982) 3, 47–54.
6. Lindeberg S, Holm B, Lundborg P, Regårdh CG, Sandström B. The effect of hydralazine on steady-state plasma concentrations of metoprolol in pregnant hypertensive women. *Eur J Clin Pharmacol* (1988) 35, 131–5.
7. Svensson CK, Cumella JC, Tronolone M, Middleton E, Lalka D. Effects of hydralazine, nitroglycerin, and food on estimated hepatic blood flow. *Clin Pharmacol Ther* (1985) 37, 464–8.
8. Svensson CK, Knowlton PW, Ware JA. Effect of hydralazine on the elimination of antipyrine in the rat. *Pharm Res* (1987) 4, 515–18.

Beta blockers + Inotropes and Vasopressors

Effects on blood pressure and heart rate: The hypertensive effects of adrenaline (epinephrine) can be markedly increased in patients taking non-selective beta blockers such as propranolol. A severe and potentially life-threatening hypertensive reaction and/or marked bradycardia can develop. Cardioselective beta blockers such as atenolol and metoprolol interact minimally. An isolated report describes a fatal hypertensive reaction in a patient given propranolol and phenylephrine, but concurrent use normally seems to be uneventful. Paradoxically, marked hypotension occurred in one patient given low-dose carvedilol and dobutamine. Anaphylaxis: Some evidence suggests that anaphylactic shock in patients taking beta blockers may be resistant to treatment with adrenaline (epinephrine).

Clinical evidence

A. Effects on blood pressure and heart rate

(a) Adrenaline (Epinephrine)

An early study in 10 healthy subjects found that intravenous adrenaline (epinephrine) 5 micrograms/minute increased heart rates and caused minimal changes in blood pressure. However, after pretreatment with intravenous **propranolol** 10 mg, the same dose of adrenaline caused a *fall* in heart rate of 12 bpm and an increase in arterial pressure of 20/10 mmHg.[1] One case report describes 6 patients taking **propranolol** 20 to 80 mg daily, undergoing plastic surgery, who experienced marked hypertensive reactions (blood pressures in the range of 190/110 to 260/150 mmHg) and bradycardia when their eyelids and/or faces were infiltrated with 8 to 40 mL of local anaesthetic solutions of lidocaine containing 1:100 000 or 1:200 000 (10 or 5 micrograms/mL) of adrenaline. Cardiac arrest occurred in one patient.[2]

Similar marked increases in blood pressure, associated with marked bradycardia, have been described in other studies and case reports involving **propranolol**.[3-11] In contrast, only a small blood pressure rise was seen in a comparative study with **metoprolol**.[4] This was confirmed in another study in which patients given identical infusions of adrenaline developed a hypertensive/bradycardic reaction while taking **propranolol** but not while taking **metoprolol**.[5] After pretreatment with a single 5-mg dose of **pindolol**, only small reductions in blood pressure (4 mmHg) and heart rate (about 5 bpm) were seen with the intra-oral injection of 3.6 mL of 2% lidocaine containing 1:80 000 adrenaline (45 micrograms of adrenaline) in healthy subjects.[12] In 24 healthy subjects given either **nadolol**, **atenolol** or placebo for 1 week followed by an infusion of adrenaline, mean arterial pressure and calf vascular resistance rose markedly in the **nadolol**-treated group but not the **atenolol** group. Marked bradycardia also occurred in those given **nadolol** and adrenaline.[13]

In 6 healthy subjects, giving adrenaline after intravenous **labetalol** 1 mg/kg, resulted in a 13 to 21 mmHg increase in mean arterial pressure and a 23 to 29 bpm reduction in heart rate, compared with adrenaline alone.[14]

(b) Dobutamine

A 54-year-old man with severe heart failure was given **carvedilol** 3.125 to 6.25 mg twice daily. His symptoms worsened and he was admitted for treatment with intravenous dobutamine; the **carvedilol** was discontinued and other medications apart from furosemide were withheld short-term. Dobutamine was started at 1 microgram/kg per minute and gradually increased to 5 micrograms/kg per minute. However, with each 1 microgram/kg increment the systolic blood pressure *dropped* to about 70 mmHg for 5 to 10 minutes and then quickly returned to the baseline level of 80 to 84 mmHg. When the dose of dobutamine reached 5 micrograms/kg per minute, his systolic blood pressure dropped to 56 mmHg and the dobutamine was discontinued. The blood pressure returned to normal over the next 30 minutes. Two months later when the patient was no longer taking **carvedilol** he was again given intravenous dobutamine and his systolic blood pressure increased, as would be expected.[15]

(c) Phenylephrine

A woman taking **propranolol** 40 mg four times daily for hypertension was given one drop of a 10% phenylephrine hydrochloride solution in each eye during an ophthalmic examination. About 45 minutes later she complained of a sudden and sharp bi-temporal pain and shortly afterwards became unconscious. She later died of an intracerebral haemorrhage due to the rupture of a berry aneurysm. She had received a similar dose of phenylephrine on a previous occasion in the absence of **propranolol** without any problems.[16]

However, no change in blood pressure was seen in a study in both normotensive subjects and patients taking **metoprolol** who were given 0.5 to 4-mg doses of phenylephrine intranasally every hour, to a total of 7.5 to 15 mg (4 to 30 times the usual dose).[17] Similarly, in a placebo-controlled study in 12 hypertensive patients, neither **propranolol** nor **metoprolol** significantly altered the dose of intravenous phenylephrine required to cause a 25 mmHg increase in systolic blood pressure.[18]

B. Anaphylaxis: resistance to treatment

A patient taking **propranolol** who suffered an anaphylactic reaction after receiving an allergy injection for desensitisation did not respond to adrenaline (epinephrine) and required intubation.[19] Resistance to adrenaline treatment for anaphylaxis occurred in another patient using **timolol** eye drops.[20] It has also been proposed that the incidence and severity of anaphylactic reactions may be increased in those taking beta blockers,[21,22] one idea being that the adrenoceptors concerned with suppressing the release of the mediators of anaphylaxis may be blocked by either $beta_1$ or $beta_2$ antagonists.[21] However, one study failed to find any evidence to support an increased incidence of systemic reactions in patients taking beta blockers receiving allergen immunotherapy.[23] See also 'X-ray contrast media', (p.857), and 'penicillins', (p.850), for other anaphylactic reactions potentially exacerbated by beta blockers.

A beta-agonist bronchodilator (e.g. isoprenaline, salbutamol) may be effective in patients taking beta blockers with anaphylaxis resistant to adrenaline,[21] and glucagon was effective in treating a severe anaphylactoid reaction in one patient taking a beta blocker.[22] Severe hypertension, sometimes with bradycardia, has been described following the use of adrenaline to treat allergic reactions, including presumed anaphylaxis, in patients taking **propranolol**.[6-8] These are discussed under A. above.

Mechanism

Adrenaline (epinephrine) stimulates alpha- and beta-receptors of the cardiovascular system, the former results in vasoconstriction (mainly $alpha_1$) and the latter in both vasodilatation (mainly $beta_2$) and stimulation of the heart (mainly $beta_1$). The net result is usually a modest increase in heart rate and a small rise in blood pressure. However, if the beta-receptors are blocked by a non-selective beta blocker, such as propranolol or nadolol (see 'Table 22.1', (p.833) for a list), the unopposed alpha vasoconstriction causes a marked rise in blood pressure, followed by reflex bradycardia. Cardioselective beta blockers such as atenolol and metoprolol, which are more selective for $beta_1$ receptors, do not prevent the vasodilator action of adrenaline at $beta_2$ receptors to the same extent, and therefore the effect of any interaction is relatively small. Consequently, adrenaline has been used to assess the degree of beta blockade produced by propranolol and other beta blockers.[13,24] Phenylephrine is largely an alpha stimulator, therefore beta blockers should have a minimal effect on its action.

Dobutamine is a $beta_1$, $beta_2$ and $alpha_1$ adrenergic agonist and carvedilol is a non-selective beta blocker, but at low doses it is primarily a selective $beta_1$ adrenergic antagonist and it is also an $alpha_1$ antagonist. It was proposed that the drop in blood pressure was caused by vasodilation due to vascular $beta_2$ receptor activation, which was not blocked by low doses of carvedilol.[15]

Importance and management

The interaction between propranolol and adrenaline (epinephrine) is established. It may be serious and potentially life-threatening, depending on the dosage of adrenaline used. Marked and serious blood pressure rises and severe bradycardia have occurred in patients given 300 micrograms of adrenaline (0.3 mL of 1:1000) subcutaneously[6-8] or 40 to 400 micrograms by infiltration of the skin and eyelids during plastic surgery.[2] Adrenaline 15 micrograms given intravenously can cause an almost 40% fall in heart rate.[9] Patients taking non-selective beta blockers such as propranolol (see 'Table 22.1', (p.833) for a list) should only be given adrenaline in very reduced dosages because of the marked bradycardia and hypertension that can occur. A less marked effect is likely with the cardioselective beta blockers,[4] such as atenolol and metoprolol (see 'Table 22.1', (p.833) for a list). Local anaesthetics used in dental surgery usually contain very low concentrations of adrenaline (e.g. 5 to 20 micrograms/mL, i.e. 1:200 000 to 1:50 000) and only small volumes are usually given, so that an undesirable interaction is unlikely.

No interaction between phenylephrine and the beta blockers would be expected, and apart from the single unexplained case cited above, the literature appears to support this. Concurrent use normally appears to be clinically unimportant, particularly bearing in mind the widespread use of beta blockers and the ready availability of phenylephrine in the form of non-prescription cough-and-cold remedies and nasal decongestants.

Acute hypertensive episodes have been controlled with chlorpromazine or phentolamine (both of which are alpha blockers). Hydralazine,[2,10] nifedipine[7] and aminophylline[10] have also been used. Reflex bradycardia may be managed with atropine and the pre-emptive use of glycopyrrolate has also been suggested.[10]

The paradoxical case of hypotension with dobutamine and low-dose carvedilol suggests that this combination should be monitored carefully.

1. Harris WS, Schoenfeld CD, Brooks RH, Weissler AM. Effect of beta adrenergic blockade on the hemodynamic responses to epinephrine in man. *Am J Cardiol* (1966) 17, 484–92.
2. Foster CA, Aston SJ. Propranolol-epinephrine interaction: a potential disaster. *Plast Reconstr Surg* (1983) 72, 74–8.
3. Kram J, Bourne HR, Melmon KL, Maibach H. Propranolol. *Ann Intern Med* (1974) 80, 282–3.
4. van Herwaarden CLA, Binkhorst RA, Fennis JFM, van'T Laar A. Effects of adrenaline during treatment with propranolol and metoprolol. *BMJ* (1977) 2, 1029.
5. Houben H, Thien T, Laor VA. Effect of low-dose epinephrine infusion on hemodynamics after selective and non-selective beta-blockade in hypertension. *Clin Pharmacol Ther* (1982) 31, 685.
6. Hansbrough JF, Near A. Propranolol-epinephrine antagonism with hypertension and stroke. *Ann Intern Med* (1980) 92, 717.
7. Whelan TV. Propranolol, epinephrine and accelerated hypertension during hemodialysis. *Ann Intern Med* (1987) 106, 327.
8. Gandy W. Severe epinephrine-propranolol interaction. *Ann Emerg Med* (1989) 18, 98–9.
9. Mackie K, Lam A. Epinephrine-containing test dose during beta-blockade. *J Clin Monit* (1991) 7, 213–6.
10. Centeno RF, Yu YL. The propranolol-epinephrine interaction revisited: a serious and potentially catastrophic adverse drug interaction in facial plastic surgery. *Plast Reconstr Surg* (2003) 111, 944–5.
11. Lampman RM, Santinga JT, Bassett DR, Savage PJ. Cardiac arrhythmias during epinephrine-propranolol infusions for measurement on in vivo insulin resistance. *Diabetes* (1981) 30, 618–20.
12. Sugimura M, Hirota Y, Shibutani T, Niwa H, Hori T, Kim Y, Matsuura H. An echocardiographic study of interactions between pindolol and epinephrine contained in a local anesthetic solution. *Anesth Prog* (1995) 42, 29–35.
13. Hiatt WR, Wolfel EE, Stoll S, Nies AS, Zerbe GO, Brammell HL, Horwitz LD. Beta-2 Adrenergic blockade evaluated with epinephrine after placebo, atenolol, and nadolol. *Clin Pharmacol Ther* (1985) 37, 2–6.
14. Richards DA, Prichard BNC, Hernández R. Circulatory effects of noradrenaline and adrenaline before and after labetalol. *Br J Clin Pharmacol* (1979) 7, 371–8.
15. Lindenfield J, Lowes BD, Bristow MR. Hypotension with dobutamine: β-adrenergic antagonist selectivity at low doses of carvedilol. *Ann Pharmacother* (1999) 33, 1266–9.
16. Cass E, Kadar D, Stein HA. Hazards of phenylephrine topical medication in persons taking propranolol. *Can Med Assoc J* (1979) 120, 1261–2.
17. Myers MG, Iazzetta JJ. Intranasally administered phenylephrine and blood pressure. *Can Med Assoc J* (1982) 127, 365–8.
18. Myers MG. Beta adrenoceptor antagonism and pressor response to phenylephrine. *Clin Pharmacol Ther* (1984) 36, 57–63.
19. Newman BR, Schultz LK. Epinephrine-resistant anaphylaxis in a patient taking propranolol hydrochloride. *Ann Allergy* (1981) 47, 35–7.
20. Moneret-Vautrin DA, Kanny G, Faller JP, Levan D, Kohler C.Choc anaphylactique grave avec arrêt cardiaque au café et à la gomme arabique, potentialisé par un collyre bêta-bloquant. *Rev Med Interne* (1993) 14, 107–11.
21. Toogood JH. Beta-blocker therapy and the risk of anaphylaxis. *Can Med Assoc J* (1987) 136, 929–33.
22. Lang DM. Anaphylactoid and anaphylactic reactions. Hazards of beta-blockers. *Drug Safety* (1995) 12, 299–304.
23. Hepner MJ, Ownby DR, Anderson JA, Rowe MS, Sears-Ewald D, Brown EB. Risk of systemic reactions in patients taking beta-blocker drugs receiving allergen immunotherapy injections. *J Allergy Clin Immunol* (1990) 86, 407–11.
24. Varma DR, Sharma KK, Arora RC. Response to adrenaline and propranolol in hyperthyroidism. *Lancet* (1976), i, 260.

Beta blockers + Itraconazole

Itraconazole markedly increased the bioavailability of celiprolol and only slightly affected the pharmacokinetics of atenolol, without affecting heart rate or blood pressure These interactions are not expected to be clinically relevant.

Clinical evidence, mechanism, importance and management

(a) Atenolol

In a study in 10 healthy subjects itraconazole 200 mg twice daily for 5 doses had only minor effects on the pharmacokinetics of a single 50-mg dose of atenolol and no effects on heart rate or blood pressure were seen.[1]

(b) Celiprolol

In a study in 12 healthy subjects itraconazole 200 mg twice daily for 5 doses increased the AUC of a single 100-mg dose of celiprolol by 80%, without increasing the half-life. However, itraconazole did not increase the effect of celiprolol on heart rate or blood pressure.[2]

It was suggested that itraconazole probably increases the absorption of celiprolol by inhibiting P-glycoprotein in the intestinal wall.[2]

Although the increase in plasma levels was marked, it was suggested that it is unlikely to be clinically relevant because celiprolol has a wide therapeutic range.[2]

1. Lilja JJ, Backman JT, Neuvonen PJ. Effect of itraconazole on the pharmacokinetics of atenolol. *Basic Clin Pharmacol Toxicol* (2005) 97, 395–8.
2. Lilja JJ, Backman JT, Laitila J, Luurila H, Neuvonen PJ. Itraconazole increases but grapefruit juice greatly decreases plasma concentrations of celiprolol. *Clin Pharmacol Ther* (2003) 73, 192–8.

Beta blockers + Macrolides

The serum levels of talinolol and possibly nadolol are increased by erythromycin, but the clinical importance of this is uncertain. Telithromycin does not appear to adversely affect sotalol-induced QT prolongation. However, the combined use of sotalol and intravenous erythromycin should generally be avoided because of the possible additive effects on QT interval prolongation.

Clinical evidence, mechanism, importance and management

(a) Nadolol

A study, in which 7 healthy subjects were given a single 80-mg dose of nadolol after **erythromycin** 500 mg plus neomycin 500 mg every 6 hours for 2 days, suggested an increase in the rate of beta blocker absorption (reduced time to maximum plasma level, but no effect on AUC). A decrease in the elimination half-life was also seen.[1] More study is needed to determine the clinical significance of these findings.

(b) Sotalol

Sotalol prolongs the QT interval and should generally not be given with other drugs that do the same, such as intravenous **erythromycin**, because of the increased risk of torsade de pointes arrhythmia (see also 'Drugs that prolong the QT interval + Other drugs that prolong the QT interval', p.257). **Telithromycin** does not appear to be associated with QT prolongation and a study in 24 healthy women found that a single 800-mg dose of **telithromycin** had no adverse effect on the QT-prolongation induced by a 160-mg dose of sotalol. The **telithromycin** slightly reduced the AUC and maximum serum levels of sotalol, which was attributed to a decrease in its absorption,[2] but this is expected to be of little clinical significance.

(c) Talinolol

A single-dose study in 8 healthy subjects found that the AUC and serum levels of talinolol 50 mg were increased by 51% and 26%, respectively, by **erythromycin** 2 g. It was suggested that the increased bioavailability of talinolol was due to increased intestinal absorption caused by the inhibition of P-glycoprotein by **erythromycin**.[3]

1. du Souich P, Caillé G, Larochelle P. Enhancement of nadolol elimination by activated charcoal and antibiotics. *Clin Pharmacol Ther* (1983) 33, 585–90.
2. Démolis J-L, Strabach S, Vacheron F, Funck-Bretano C. Assessment of the effect of a single oral dose of telithromycin on sotalol-induced QT interval prolongation in healthy women. *Br J Clin Pharmacol* (2005) 60, 120–7.
3. Schwarz UI, Gramatté T, Krappweis J, Oertel R, Kirch W. P-glycoprotein inhibitor erythromycin increases oral bioavailability of talinolol in humans. *Int J Clin Pharmacol Ther* (2000) 38, 161–7.

Beta blockers + Metoclopramide

A patient with scleroderma suffered a fatal cardiac arrest after receiving postoperative intravenous labetalol and intravenous metoclopramide. Metoclopramide increased the rate of absorption of a conventional formulation of propranolol, but did not affect a sustained-release preparation.

Clinical evidence, mechanism, importance and management

(a) Labetalol

A 38-year-old patient with scleroderma, hypertension (for which she was taking lisinopril) and gangrene of her left index finger underwent minor hand surgery. While in postoperative care her blood pressure rose to 153/120 mmHg and she was given intravenous labetalol 10 mg. About 15 minutes later she experienced nausea and vomiting, which was treated with intravenous metoclopramide 10 mg. About 5 minutes later her heart rate decreased to 38 bpm and she became unresponsive with no palpable pulse: an ECG showed junctional bradycardia. She was initially resuscitated but died about 13 hours later after a further episode of bradycardia, despite full supportive treatment. It was noted that the bradycardia did not respond well to atropine, and there was persistent hypotension, despite escalating vasopressor use. Scleroderma and lisinopril may have contributed to the failure to resuscitate the patient. However, bradycardia or heart block and hypotension may occur with intravenous metoclopramide. In this patient the use of labetalol may have exacerbated the effects of metoclopramide by causing reductions in ventricular contractility due to its beta-adrenergic effects and limiting vasoconstrictive compensatory mechanisms due to alpha-adrenergic effects.[1] However, it has subsequently been suggested that this reaction may have been due to local anaesthetic toxicity rather than a drug interaction,[2] although this was disputed by the original authors.[3] A study in 11 untreated hypertensive patients found that intravenous metoclopramide (7.5 micrograms/kg per minute for 30 minutes) caused a slight decrease in the responsiveness to labetalol 400 to 600 mg daily. However, as metoclopramide only attenuated the systolic blood pressure response to labetalol by 3 mmHg this effect seems unlikely to be clinically significant in most patients.[4]

(b) Propranolol

Oral metoclopramide syrup 20 mg, given 30 minutes before sustained-release propranolol 160 mg, had no effect on the pharmacokinetics of propranolol in 12 healthy subjects.[5] In contrast, an earlier brief report found that the rate of absorption of a conventional formulation of propranolol 80 mg was increased by intravenous metoclopramide 10 mg in 4 healthy subjects. In the first 2 hours after dosing, propranolol levels were increased by 1.3 to 2.5-fold.[6] However, these changes are unlikely to be clinically relevant.

1. Tung A, Sweitzer B, Cutter T. Cardiac arrest after labetalol and metoclopramide administration in a patient with scleroderma. *Anesth Analg* (2002) 95, 1667–8.
2. Schwartz D, VadeBoncour T, Weinberg G. Was case report a case of unrecognized local anesthetic toxicity? *Anesth Analg* (2003) 96, 1844–5.
3. Tung A, Sweitzer BJ, Cutter TW. Was case report a case of unrecognized local anesthetic toxicity? In response. *Anesth Analg* (2003) 96, 1845.
4. Blanco M, Gomez J, Negrín C, Blanco G, Rodriguez M, Torres M, Vásquez M, Alcalá I, Vargas R, Velasco M. Metoclopramide enhances labetalol-induced antihypertensive effect during handgrip in hypertensive patients. *Am J Ther* (1998) 5, 221–4.
5. Charles BG, Renshaw PJ, Kay JJ, Ravenscroft PJ. Effect of metoclopramide on the bioavailability of long-acting propranolol. *Br J Clin Pharmacol* (1981) 517–18.
6. George CF, Castleden M. Propranolol absorption. *BMJ* (1977) 1, 47.

Beta blockers + Morphine

Morphine may moderately raise the serum levels of esmolol, but this is unlikely to be clinically important. The fatal doses of morphine and propranolol are markedly reduced by concurrent use in *animals*, but the clinical relevance of this in man is uncertain.

Clinical evidence, mechanism, importance and management

In a study in 10 healthy men a 3-mg injection of morphine sulfate increased the steady-state levels of a 300 microgram/kg per minute infusion of **esmolol**, given over 4 hours. However, the increases were only statistically significant in 2 of the subjects (increase of 46%), and were considered to be of no clinical importance. The pharmacokinetics of morphine were unchanged.[1]

Studies in *animals* have shown that the median fatal dose of **propranolol** was reduced two to sevenfold by morphine in *mice*[2] and the median lethal dose of morphine was reduced fifteen to sixteenfold by **propranolol** in *rats*.[3] The same interaction has also been seen in *dogs*.[3] There do not appear to be any published reports of synergistic toxicity involving morphine and **propranolol**, so the clinical relevance of this is uncertain.

1. Lowenthal DT, Porter RS, Saris SD, Bies CM, Slegowski MB, Staudacher A. Clinical pharmacology, pharmacodynamics and interactions with esmolol. *Am J Cardiol* (1985) 56, 14F–18F.
2. Murmann W, Almirante L, Saccani-Guelfi M. Effects of hexobarbitone, ether, morphine, and urethane upon the acute toxicity of propranolol and D-(-)-INPEA. *J Pharm Pharmacol* (1966) 18, 692–4.
3. Davis WM, Hatoum NS. Possible toxic interaction of propranolol and narcotic analgesics. *Drug Intell Clin Pharm* (1981) 15, 290–1.

Beta blockers + Penicillins

Plasma atenolol levels are halved by 1-g doses of ampicillin. The clinical importance of this is uncertain, but probably small. No important interaction occurs if atenolol is given with ampicillin

250 mg every 6 hours. One brief report suggests that anaphylactic reactions to penicillins may be more severe in patients taking beta blockers.

Clinical evidence

A single 1-g dose of **ampicillin** reduced the AUC of a single 100-mg dose of **atenolol** by 40%, and decreased its bioavailability from 60 to 36% in 6 healthy subjects. Similarly, when **atenolol** 100 mg was given with **ampicillin** 1 g daily for 6 days, the mean steady-state plasma atenolol level was reduced by 52% (from 199 to 95 nanograms/mL), and the AUC was reduced by 52%. The blood pressure lowering effect of **atenolol** at rest was not affected, but after exercise a small rise in systolic pressure of up to 17 mmHg occurred, whereas diastolic pressure was unchanged. The effects of **atenolol** on reducing heart rate during exercise were diminished from 24% to 11% at 12 hours.[1]

Another study showed that when a single 50-mg oral dose of **atenolol** was given with a single 1-g oral dose of **ampicillin** the AUC of **atenolol** was reduced by 51.5%, whereas when **ampicillin** 250 mg four times daily was given for 24 hours, the AUC was only reduced by 18.2%.[2]

A brief report describes 2 patients, one taking **nadolol** and one taking **propranolol**, who developed fatal anaphylactic shock after taking **phenoxymethylpenicillin**. The authors suggested that, as fatal reactions to penicillins are rare, the reaction had been exacerbated by the presence of a non-selective beta blocker.[3]

Mechanism

Uncertain. Ampicillin apparently affects the absorption of atenolol.

Importance and management

Information is limited, but the absorption interaction appears to be established. The clinical importance awaits full evaluation but the modest effects on blood pressure and heart rate[1] suggest that it is of limited importance. Information about other beta blockers and penicillins is lacking. Information on potentiation of anaphylaxis is too limited to make comment, but note that some evidence suggests that anaphylactic shock in patients taking beta blockers may be resistant to treatment with adrenaline (epinephrine), see 'Beta blockers + Inotropes and Vasopressors', p.848.

1. Schäfer-Korting M, Kirch W, Axthelm T, Köhler H, Mutschler E. Atenolol interaction with aspirin, allopurinol, and ampicillin. *Clin Pharmacol Ther* (1983) 33, 283–8.
2. McLean AJ, Tonkin A, McCarthy P, Harrison P. Dose-dependence of atenolol-ampicillin interaction. *Br J Clin Pharmacol* (1984) 18, 969–71.
3. Berkelman RL, Finton RJ, Elsea WR. Beta-adrenergic antagonists and fatal anaphylactic reactions to oral penicillins. *Ann Intern Med* (1986) 104, 134.

Beta blockers + Phenothiazines

The concurrent use of chlorpromazine with propranolol, or thioridazine with pindolol, can result in a marked rise in the plasma levels of both drugs. Propranolol markedly increases plasma thioridazine levels. Both beta blockers and phenothiazines can cause hypotension, and these effects could be additive: a handful of case reports suggest that this could occasionally be serious. The concurrent use of sotalol and phenothiazines that prolong the QT interval should generally be avoided.

Clinical evidence

(a) Chlorpromazine

In 4 healthy subjects and one hypertensive patient the mean steady-state levels of **propranolol** 80 mg every 8 hours were raised by 70% (from 41.5 to 70.2 nanograms/mL) when they were given chlorpromazine 50 mg every 8 hours.[1] The increase was considerable in some subjects but barely detectable in others. A sixth subject taking **propranolol** promptly fainted when getting out of bed after the first dose of chlorpromazine. He was found to have a pulse rate of 35 to 40 bpm and a blood pressure of 70/0 mmHg. He rapidly recovered, achieving a pulse rate of 85 bpm and a blood pressure of 120/70 mmHg when given atropine 3 mg. However, it is unclear whether the adverse effect was due to chlorpromazine alone, or to an interaction with **propranolol**.[1]

Propranolol (mean daily dose 8.1 mg/kg) increased the serum chlorpromazine levels of 7 schizophrenics by about 100 to 500%, and raised the plasma levels of the active metabolites of chlorpromazine by about 50 to 100%.[2] The same or similar work by the same authors is described elsewhere.[3] One of the patients was withdrawn from the study because he suffered a cardiovascular collapse while taking both drugs.[3] It has been suggested that the value of **propranolol** in the treatment of schizophrenia probably results from the rise in serum chlorpromazine levels.[3]

A report briefly mentions a diabetic girl who had an episode of minor hypotension with chlorpromazine that appeared to have been exacerbated by **sotalol**.[4] A schizophrenic patient taking chlorpromazine and **tiotixene** experienced delirium, grand mal seizures and skin photosensitivity, attributed to a rise in the serum levels of the antipsychotic drugs caused by increasing doses of **propranolol** (up to a total of 1200 mg daily).[5]

(b) Thioridazine

Serum **pindolol** levels were 2.5-fold higher in 7 patients taking thioridazine than in 17 patients taking haloperidol, phenytoin, and/or phenobarbital.[6] Furthermore, **pindolol** 40 mg daily increased serum thioridazine levels by about 50% in 8 patients.[6]

Two patients stable taking thioridazine 600 or 800 mg daily had three and fivefold rises in plasma levels, respectively, when given **propranolol**, in increasing doses up to a total of 800 mg daily, over 26 to 40 days. No signs or symptoms of thioridazine toxicity were seen even though plasma levels had risen into the toxic range.[7] Similarly, in another study thioridazine levels rose by about 55 to 370% in 5 patients taking **propranolol** 320 to 520 mg daily.[8]

Mechanism

Pharmacokinetic evidence[1] and *animal* studies[9] suggest that propranolol and chlorpromazine mutually inhibit the liver metabolism of the other drug so that both accumulate within the body. The mechanism of the interaction between propranolol and thioridazine is probably similar. Both beta blockers and phenothiazines can cause hypotension, and these effects could be additive.

Importance and management

The interaction between propranolol and chlorpromazine appears to be established although information is limited. Concurrent use should be well monitored and the dosages reduced if necessary. The same precautions apply with propranolol and thioridazine.[7] There seems to be no information about any interaction between other beta blockers and phenothiazines, but if the mechanism of interaction suggested above is true, it seems possible that other beta blockers that are mainly cleared from the body by liver metabolism might interact similarly with chlorpromazine, whereas those mainly cleared unchanged in the urine are less likely to have a pharmacokinetic interaction, although additive hypotensive effects would still be expected. See 'Table 22.1', (p.833), for information on the metabolism of the commonly used systemic beta blockers.

Note that **sotalol** and some phenothiazines, including chlorpromazine and thioridazine prolong the QT interval (see 'Table 9.2', (p.257) for a more extensive list). Combined use should therefore generally be avoided, because of the increased risk of torsade de pointes. See also 'Drugs that prolong the QT interval + Other drugs that prolong the QT interval', p.257.

1. Vestal RE, Kornhauser DM, Hollifield JW, Shand DG. Inhibition of propranolol metabolism by chlorpromazine. *Clin Pharmacol Ther* (1979) 25, 19–24.
2. Peet M, Middlemiss DN, Yates RA. Pharmacokinetic interaction between propranolol and chlorpromazine in schizophrenic patients. *Lancet* (1980) ii, 978.
3. Peet M, Middlemiss DN, Yates RA. Propranolol in schizophrenia II. Clinical and biochemical aspects of combining propranolol with chlorpromazine. *Br J Psychiatry* (1981) 138, 112–17.
4. Baker L, Barcai A, Kaye R, Haque N. Beta adrenergic blockade and juvenile diabetes: acute studies and long-term therapeutic trial. *J Pediatr* (1969) 75, 19–29.
5. Miller FA, Rampling D. Adverse effects of combined propranolol and chlorpromazine therapy. *Am J Psychiatry* (1982) 139, 1198–9.
6. Greendyke RM, Gulya A. Effect of pindolol administration on serum levels of thioridazine, haloperidol, phenytoin, and phenobarbital. *J Clin Psychiatry* (1988) 49, 105–7.
7. Silver JM, Yudofsky SC, Kogan M, Katz BL. Elevation of thioridazine plasma levels by propranolol. *Am J Psychiatry* (1986) 143, 1290–2.
8. Greendyke RM, Kanter DR. Plasma propranolol levels and their effect on plasma thioridazine and haloperidol concentrations. *J Clin Psychopharmacol* (1987) 7, 178–82.
9. Shand DG, Oates JA. Metabolism of propranolol by rat liver microsomes and its inhibition by phenothiazine and tricyclic antidepressant drugs. *Biochem Pharmacol* (1971) 20, 1720–3.

Beta blockers + Phenylpropanolamine

A small rise in blood pressure may occur in patients taking beta blockers who take single doses of phenylpropanolamine. A marked rise in blood pressure has been seen in one patient taking

oxprenolol with methyldopa when phenylpropanolamine was also taken. Propranolol attenuates the blood pressure rise seen with phenylpropanolamine.

Clinical evidence, mechanism, importance and management

(a) Effect on beta blockers

A study in 13 patients taking various antihypertensives including 5 taking unnamed beta blockers found that a single dose of *Dimetapp Extentabs* (phenylpropanolamine 75 mg with brompheniramine 12 mg) caused a blood pressure rise of 1.7/0.9 mmHg over a 4-hour period, which was not statistically or clinically significant.[1] These rises in blood pressure after single doses are small and relatively short-lived, and probably of little clinical importance. Another study in 7 stabilised hypertensive patients taking beta blockers (**atenolol** 5 patients, **metoprolol** 1, **propranolol** 1) found that a single 25-mg dose of rapid-release phenylpropanolamine (*Super Odrinex*) increased the mean peak blood pressures by about 8/5 mmHg over a 6-hour period.[2] A later multiple dose study in the same subjects (only 5 of whom completed the study), taking the same beta blockers, found that on day 1 phenylpropanolamine increased diastolic blood pressure by 9 to 16 mmHg, and on day 7 by 0 to 14 mmHg. The day 1 and day 7 results were not statistically different, which suggests that the increase in blood pressure is not enhanced by multiple dosing.[3] Note that a marked rise in blood pressure was seen in one patient taking methyldopa and **oxprenolol** when phenylpropanolamine was also given, see 'Methyldopa + Sympathomimetics; Indirectly-acting', p.898.

(b) Effect on phenylpropanolamine

In a placebo-controlled study in 6 healthy subjects, **propranolol** given either orally as a pretreatment or intravenously after phenylpropanolamine, was found to antagonise the rise in blood pressure induced by the phenylpropanolamine. Oral phenylpropanolamine 75 mg alone increased blood pressure from 116/63 to 148/83 mmHg; pretreatment with oral **propranolol** 80 mg every 6 hours reduced the baseline blood pressure to 107/62 mmHg and the increase with phenylpropanolamine was lower, reaching only 119/72 mmHg. Intravenous **propranolol** 0.3 mg/kg given after the phenylpropanolamine decreased blood pressure from 144/87 to 121/84 mmHg.[4]

1. Petrulis AS, Imperiale TF, Speroff T. The acute effect of phenylpropanolamine and brompheniramine on blood pressure in controlled hypertension. *J Gen Intern Med* (1991) 6, 503–6.
2. O'Connell MB, Gross CR. The effect of single-dose phenylpropanolamine on blood pressure in patients with hypertension controlled by β blockers. *Pharmacotherapy* (1990) 10, 85–91.
3. O'Connell MB, Gross CR. The effect of multiple doses of phenylpropanolamine on the blood pressure of patients whose hypertension was controlled with β blockers. *Pharmacotherapy* (1991) 11, 376–81.
4. Pentel PR, Asinger RW, Benowitz, NL. Propranolol antagonism of phenylpropanolamine-induced hypertension. *Clin Pharmacol Ther* (1985) 37, 488–94.

Beta blockers + Potassium-depleting drugs

The use of potassium-depleting diuretics can precipitate the development of potentially life-threatening torsade de pointes arrhythmias in patients taking sotalol unless potassium levels are maintained. This would also be expected with other potassium-depleting drugs such as corticosteroids, some laxatives, and intravenous amphotericin. Chlortalidone and hydrochlorothiazide may reduce the bioavailability of celiprolol, but the evidence for this is sparse.

Clinical evidence

(a) Pharmacokinetic effects

A study in 12 healthy subjects found that when **sotalol** 160 mg was given with **hydrochlorothiazide** 25 mg the pharmacokinetics of both drugs were unchanged.[1]

The manufacturers of **celiprolol** suggest that **chlortalidone** and **hydrochlorothiazide** reduce its bioavailability.[2] This appears to be based on an *in vitro* study,[3] which found that **chlortalidone** and **hydrochlorothiazide** blocked the active transport of **celiprolol** across the intestinal epithelium. The authors of this study also cite a single dose study that found that **chlortalidone** decreased the bioavailability of **celiprolol** but details are not given.

(b) QT-prolongation

A 4-year study in cardiac clinics in South Africa identified 13 patients who developed syncope and a prolonged QT interval while taking **sotalol** 80 to 480 mg daily. Twelve patients were taking a combined preparation (*Sotazide*) containing **sotalol** 160 mg and **hydrochlorothiazide** 25 mg. Eleven patients were being treated for hypertension, one for ventricular asystoles, and one for both. Polymorphous ventricular tachycardia was seen in 12 of the patients, and torsade de pointes were seen in 10 of these 12. Arrhythmias occurred within 72 hours of starting **sotalol** in 6 patients, and at varying intervals from 10 days to 3 years in the other 6 patients. Definite hypokalaemia (defined by the study as serum potassium of less than 3.5 mmol/L) was detected in 8 of the 13 patients. Four of the patients were also taking other drugs known to prolong the QT interval, namely disopyramide and tricyclic antidepressants. The problems resolved in all of the cases within 12 hours of stopping the **sotalol** and giving potassium supplements when indicated.[4] A further case has also been reported.[5]

Mechanism

Potassium-depleting drugs may cause hypokalaemia, which increases the potential for torsade de pointes arrhythmia with any drug that prolongs the QT interval, including sotalol.

Importance and management

The interaction between potassium-depleting diuretics such as hydrochlorothiazide and sotalol that results in QT prolongation is established, clinically important and potentially life threatening. Prolongation of the QT interval and the development of torsade de pointes in patients taking sotalol, particularly at high doses (said to be greater than 320 mg daily),[6] is a recognised adverse effect, but it can occur even with small doses of sotalol if potassium depletion is allowed to develop. It is clearly very important therefore to ensure that potassium levels are maintained if potassium-depleting drugs are given with sotalol. A list of potassium-depleting diuretics is given in 'Table 26.1', (p.944). Other drugs that may cause potassium depletion include **corticosteroids**, some **laxatives**, and intravenous **amphotericin**.

The interactions of chlortalidone and hydrochlorothiazide with celiprolol are poorly documented and their clinical significance is unclear, although it would be expected to be limited.

1. Sundquist H, Anttila M, Simon A, Reich JW. Comparative bioavailability and pharmacokinetics of sotalol administered alone and in combination with hydrochlorothiazide. *J Clin Pharmacol* (1979) 19, 557–64.
2. Celectol (Celiprolol hydrochloride). Winthrop Pharmaceuticals UK Ltd. UK Summary of product characteristics, September 2004.
3. Karlsson J, Kuo S-M, Zeiminak J, Artursson P. Transport of celiprolol across human intestinal epithelial (Caco-2) cells: mediation of secretion by multiple transporters including P-glycoprotein. *Br J Pharmacol* (1993) 110, 1009–1016.
4. McKibbin JK, Pocock WA, Barlow JB, Scott Millar RN, Obel IWP. Sotalol, hypokalaemia, syncope, and torsade de pointes. *Br Heart J* (1984) 51, 157–62.
5. Bennett JM, Gourassas J, Konstantinides S. Torsade de pointes induced by sotalol and hypokalaemia. *S Afr Med J* (1995) 68, 591–2.
6. Tan HH, Hsu LF, Kam RML, Chua T, Teo WS. A case series of sotalol-induced torsade de pointes in patients with atrial fibrillation a tale with a twist. *Ann Acad Med Singapore* (2003) 32, 403–7.

Beta blockers + Propafenone

Plasma metoprolol and propranolol levels can be markedly raised (two to fivefold) by propafenone. Toxicity may develop.

Clinical evidence

Four patients with ventricular arrhythmias taking **metoprolol** 150 to 200 mg daily had a two to fivefold rise in steady-state **metoprolol** serum levels when they were given propafenone 150 mg three times daily. One of them developed distressing nightmares, and another had acute left ventricular failure with pulmonary oedema and haemoptysis, which disappeared when the **metoprolol** dosage was reduced or stopped. In 4 other patients taking **metoprolol** 50 mg three times daily and propafenone 150 mg three times daily, it was found that stopping **metoprolol** did not affect propafenone plasma levels.[1] Single-dose studies in healthy subjects found a twofold decrease in the clearance of **metoprolol** and a further 20% reduction in exercise-induced tachycardia at 90 minutes when propafenone was also given.[1]

A patient developed neurotoxicity (including vivid nightmares, fatigue, headache) when given **metoprolol** 100 mg daily in divided doses, which worsened while it was being withdrawn and replaced by propafenone 300 mg daily. The symptoms disappeared when both drugs were stopped.[2]

Propafenone 225 mg every 8 hours more than doubled the steady-state levels of **propranolol** 50 mg every 8 hours in 12 healthy subjects. However, the beta-blocking effects were only modestly increased and the propafenone pharmacokinetics remained unchanged.[3]

Mechanism

It is suggested that propafenone reduces the metabolism of metoprolol and propranolol by the liver, thereby reducing their clearance and raising serum levels.[1,3]

Importance and management

Information is limited but the interaction would seem to be established. Concurrent use need not be avoided but anticipate the need to reduce the dosage of metoprolol and propranolol. Monitor closely because some patients may experience adverse effects. If the suggested mechanism of interaction is correct it is possible (but not confirmed) that other beta blockers that undergo liver metabolism will interact similarly but not those largely excreted unchanged in the urine. See 'Table 22.1', (p.833) for the metabolism of some commonly used beta blockers. Also note that propafenone and the beta blockers have negative inotropic effects, which could be additive and result in unwanted cardiodepression.

1. Wagner F, Kalusche D, Trenk D, Jähnchen E, Roskamm H. Drug interaction between propafenone and metoprolol. *Br J Clin Pharmacol* (1987) 24, 213–20.
2. Ahmad S. Metoprolol-induced delirium perpetuated by propafenone. *Am Fam Physician* (1991) 44, 1142–3.
3. Kowey PR, Kirsten EB, Fu C-HJ, Mason WD. Interaction between propranolol and propafenone in healthy volunteers. *J Clin Pharmacol* (1989) 29, 512–17.

Beta blockers + Proton pump inhibitors

Omeprazole does not interact with metoprolol or propranolol, and lansoprazole does not interact with propranolol.

Clinical evidence, mechanism, importance and management

Omeprazole 20 mg daily for 8 days had no effect on the steady-state plasma levels of **propranolol** 80 mg twice daily, and no effect on resting and exercised heart rates or blood pressure in 8 healthy subjects.[1] Another study found that **omeprazole** 40 mg daily for 8 days had no effect on the steady-state plasma levels of **metoprolol** 100 mg daily.[2]

A double-blind crossover study in 18 healthy subjects found that **lansoprazole** 60 mg daily for 7 days did not significantly affect the pharmacokinetics of a single 80-mg dose of **propranolol**.[3]

No special precautions would seem necessary if these proton pump inhibitors are used with **propranolol** or **metoprolol**.

1. Henry D, Brent P, Whyte I, Mihaly G, Devenish-Meares S. Propranolol steady-state pharmacokinetics are unaltered by omeprazole. *Eur J Clin Pharmacol* (1987) 33, 369–73.
2. Andersson T, Lundborg P, Regårdh CG. Lack of effect of omeprazole treatment on steady-state plasma levels of metoprolol. *Eur J Clin Pharmacol* (1991) 40, 61–5.
3. Karol MD, Locke CS, Cavanaugh JH. Lack of interaction between lansoprazole and propranolol, a pharmacokinetic and safety assessment. *J Clin Pharmacol* (2000) 40, 301–8.

Beta blockers + Quinidine

An isolated report describes a patient taking quinidine who developed marked bradycardia when using timolol eye drops. Other reports describe orthostatic hypotension when quinidine was given with atenolol or propranolol. Quinidine can raise plasma metoprolol, propranolol, and timolol levels, but the clinical relevance of this is uncertain.

Both sotalol and quinidine can prolong the QT interval, which may increase the risk of torsade de pointes arrhythmia if they are used together.

Clinical evidence

(a) Atenolol

Orthostatic hypotension occurred in a 56-year-old woman taking isosorbide dinitrate, diltiazem and quinidine sulfate 300 mg four times daily, 3 days after she started atenolol 50 mg daily. This resolved within 2 days of stopping the atenolol. Before starting the quinidine, she had previously taken atenolol and the other drugs without problems.[1]

(b) Metoprolol

A metabolic study in 5 healthy subjects who were extensive CYP2D6 metabolisers found that a single 50-mg dose of quinidine markedly inhibited the metabolism of a single 100-mg dose of metoprolol, which effectively made the subjects into poor metabolisers. The plasma levels of metoprolol were approximately tripled. Quinidine had no effect on metoprolol pharmacokinetics in 5 poor metabolisers.[2] Similar results have been found when quinidine 50 mg daily was given with metoprolol 100 mg twice daily for 7 days,[3] and when a 20-mg dose of metoprolol was given intravenously following either a single 50-mg dose of quinidine or quinidine slow-release tablets 250 mg twice daily for 3 days.[4] The effect on heart-rate reduction was small given the increase in metoprolol levels.[3]

(c) Propranolol

A single-dose pharmacokinetic study found that quinidine 200 mg doubled the AUC and the peak plasma levels of a 20-mg dose of propranolol. Maximum heart rates during exercise were suppressed by a further 45%.[5] A similar study by the same research group found that the AUC of propranolol was increased by about threefold by quinidine.[6] A further study found that quinidine doubled the AUC of propranolol and halved its clearance resulting in increased beta-blockade.[7]

After a single 200-mg dose of quinidine the peak plasma quinidine levels were over 50% higher and its clearance almost 40% lower in 7 patients taking propranolol 40 to 400 mg daily, when compared with 8 control patients, but the quinidine elimination half-life did not differ.[8] However, this interaction was not found in two other studies.[9,10]

A man taking propranolol 40 mg four times daily developed orthostatic hypotension, with symptoms of dizziness and faintness on standing, when he took quinidine 200 mg four times daily. This resolved when quinidine was withdrawn.[11] The same authors subsequently briefly reported another two cases of orthostatic hypotension when quinidine was given with unnamed beta blockers.[12]

(d) Sotalol

Although one study reports the safe concurrent use of sotalol and quinidine,[13] both drugs can prolong the QT interval, which may increase the risk of torsade de pointes arrhythmia if they are used together. See 'Drugs that prolong the QT interval + Other drugs that prolong the QT interval', p.257, for a general review of QT-prolongation and drug interactions.

(e) Timolol

An elderly man taking quinidine sulfate 500 mg three times daily for premature atrial beats was hospitalised with dizziness 12 weeks after starting to use timolol 0.5% eye drops for open-angle glaucoma. He was found to have a sinus bradycardia of 36 bpm. The symptoms abated when the drugs were withdrawn and normal sinus rhythm returned after 24 hours. The same symptoms developed within 30 hours of re-starting both drugs, but disappeared when the quinidine was withdrawn.[14] In a later study in healthy subjects, a single 50-mg oral dose of quinidine was given 30 minutes before 2 drops of timolol 0.5% ophthalmic solution, put into each *nostril*. In 13 extensive CYP2D6 metabolisers, quinidine caused a further decrease in heart rate and increase in plasma timolol levels compared with timolol alone. Giving quinidine with timolol in these extensive metabolisers gave results similar to giving timolol alone in 5 poor metabolisers.[15] In another study, quinidine augmented the plasma levels and cardiac effects of intravenous timolol.[16]

Mechanism

Quinidine appears to increase metoprolol, propranolol and timolol plasma levels by inhibiting the cytochrome P450 isoenzyme CYP2D6, thereby reducing their clearance.[2,7,15] As CYP2D6 shows polymorphism, these interactions would be most apparent in patients with high CYP2D6 activity (extensive metabolisers), effectively making them poor metabolisers. See 'Genetic factors', (p.4), for further information on polymorphism.

Importance and management

The pharmacokinetic interaction would seem to be established, but of uncertain clinical importance. Only one isolated case of possible excessive beta-blockade has been reported (with quinidine and timolol eye drops). Concurrent use need not be avoided (and may be beneficial in the treatment of atrial fibrillation), but some care is warranted as both quinidine and the beta blockers have negative inotropic effects, which could be additive and result in unwanted cardiodepression. The general relevance of the isolated reports of orthostatic hypotension with atenolol or propranolol and quinidine is uncertain.

The general consensus is that the combination of two drugs that prolong the QT interval such as quinidine and sotalol should usually be avoided, or only used with great caution. See also 'Drugs that prolong the QT interval + Other drugs that prolong the QT interval', p.257.

1. Manolis AS, Estes NA. Orthostatic hypotension due to quinidine and atenolol. *Am J Med* (1987) 82, 1083–4.
2. Leemann T, Dayer P, Meyer UA. Single-dose quinidine treatment inhibits metoprolol oxidation in extensive metabolizers. *Eur J Clin Pharmacol* (1986) 29, 739–41.
3. Schlanz KD, Yingling KW, Verme CN, Lalonde RL, Harrison DC, Bottorff MB. Loss of stereoselective metoprolol metabolism following quinidine inhibition of P450IID6. *Pharmacotherapy* (1991) 11, 272.
4. Leeman TD, Devi KP, Dayer P. Similar effect of oxidation deficiency (debrisoquine polymorphism) and quinidine on the apparent volume of distribution of (±)-metoprolol. *Eur J Clin Pharmacol* (1993) 45, 65–71.
5. Sakurai T, Kawai C, Yasuhara M, Okumura K, Hori R. Increased plasma concentration of propranolol by a pharmacokinetic interaction with quinidine. *Jpn Circ J* (1983) 47, 872–3.
6. Yasuhara M, Yatsuzuka A, Yamada K, Okumura K, Hori R, Sakurai T, Kawai C. Alteration of propranolol pharmacokinetics and pharmacodynamics by quinidine in man. *J Pharmacobiodyn* (1990) 13, 681–7.
7. Zhou H-H, Anthony LB, Roden DM, Wood AJJ. Quinidine reduces clearance of (+)-propranolol more than (–)-propranolol through marked reduction in 4-hydroxylation. *Clin Pharmacol Ther* (1990) 47, 686–93.
8. Kessler KM, Humphries WC, Black M, Spann JF. Quinidine pharmacokinetics in patients with cirrhosis or receiving propranolol. *Am Heart J* (1978) 96, 627–35.
9. Kates RE, Blanford MF. Disposition kinetics of oral quinidine when administered concurrently with propranolol. *J Clin Pharmacol* (1979) 19, 378–83.
10. Fenster P, Perrier D, Mayersohn M, Marcus FI. Kinetic evaluation of the propranolol-quinidine combination. *Clin Pharmacol Ther* (1980) 27, 450–3.
11. Loon NR, Wilcox CS, Folger W. Orthostatic hypotension due to quinidine and propranolol. *Am J Med* (1986) 81, 1101–4.
12. Loon NR, Wilcox CS. Orthostatic hypotension due to quinidine and propranolol. The reply. *Am J Med* (1987) 82, 1276–7.
13. Dorian P, Newman D, Berman N, Hardy J, Mitchell J. Sotalol and type IA drugs in combination prevent recurrence of sustained ventricular tachycardia. *J Am Coll Cardiol* (1993) 22, 106–13.
14. Dinai Y, Sharir M, Naveh N, Halkin H. Bradycardia induced by interaction between quinidine and ophthalmic timolol. *Ann Intern Med* (1985) 103, 890–1.
15. Edeki TI, He H, Wood AJJ. Pharmacogenetic explanation for excessive β-blockade following timolol eye drops. *JAMA* (1995) 274, 1611–13.
16. Kaila T, Huupponen R, Karhuvaara S, Havula P, Scheinin M, Iisalo E, Salminen L. Beta-blocking effects of timolol at low plasma concentrations. *Clin Pharmacol Ther* (1991) 49, 53–8.

Beta blockers + Quinolones

Ciprofloxacin reduces metoprolol clearance, but this is probably clinically unimportant. The concurrent use of sotalol and quinolones that prolong the QT interval should generally be avoided.

Clinical evidence, mechanism, importance and management

(a) Ciprofloxacin

Preliminary evidence from 7 healthy subjects given a single 100-mg dose of **metoprolol** suggested that pretreatment with 5 doses of ciprofloxacin 500 mg, given every 12 hours, increased the AUC of *(+)*-metoprolol by 54% and reduced its clearance by 38.5%. The AUC of *(–)*-metoprolol was increased by 29% and its clearance reduced by 12%.[1] It has been suggested that this interaction may occur because ciprofloxacin inhibits the activity of the cytochrome P450 isoenzymes concerned with the metabolism and clearance of **metoprolol**. However, this is questionable as **metoprolol** is metabolised, predominantly, by CYP2D6 while ciprofloxacin inhibits CYP1A2. Changes of this size, or even more, in the AUC of beta blockers have proved not to be clinically important with other enzyme-inhibiting drugs, and it seems probable that this will be the case with ciprofloxacin, but this needs confirmation.

(b) Quinolones that prolong the QT interval

In an analysis of cases of torsade de pointes associated with fluoroquinolones on the FDA Adverse Events Reporting System database, two cases of torsade de pointes were noted in patients taking a fluoroquinolone with **sotalol** (there were 37 cases identified, and 19 occurred in patients also taking other drugs known to prolong the QT interval).[2] **Sotalol** has class III antiarrhythmic effects and prolongs the QT interval, and this could be additive with the effects of quinolones that prolong the QT interval (e.g. **gatifloxacin**, **moxifloxacin**, **sparfloxacin**, see 'Table 9.2', (p.257)). The concurrent use of **sotalol** and these quinolones should generally be avoided (see 'Drugs that prolong the QT interval + Other drugs that prolong the QT interval', p.257).

1. Waite NM, Rutledge DR, Warbasse LH, Edwards DJ. Disposition of the (+) and (–) isomers of metoprolol following ciprofloxacin treatment. *Pharmacotherapy* (1990) 10, 236.
2. Frothingham R. Rates of torsades de pointes associated with ciprofloxacin, ofloxacin, levofloxacin, gatifloxacin, and moxifloxacin. *Pharmacotherapy* (2001) 21, 1468–72.

Beta blockers + Rifampicin (Rifampin)

Rifampicin increases the clearance of bisoprolol, carvedilol, celiprolol, metoprolol, propranolol, tertatolol and talinolol, and reduces their serum levels. The extent to which this reduces the effects of these beta blockers is uncertain, but it is probably small. Similar effects have been seen when atenolol is given with rifampicin, but a case report suggests that occasionally the effects may be of clinical relevance.

Clinical evidence

(a) Atenolol

A case report describes a man taking atenolol for angina whose exercise threshold before developing angina symptoms appreciably worsened when he was given rifampicin. Rifampicin was stopped, and after a week **rifabutin** was started. **Rifabutin** did not cause any change in his baseline exercise tolerance.[1] In a randomised, placebo-controlled, crossover study, 9 healthy subjects were given rifampicin 600 mg daily for 5 days, with a single 100-mg dose of atenolol on day 6. Although some pharmacokinetic changes were seen they were variable between subjects and in most cases slight. Heart rate and blood pressure were on average slightly higher in the presence of rifampicin (3.5 bpm and 4.3/3.9 mmHg, respectively), suggesting a modest reduction in the effects of atenolol, which was expected to be of only minor clinical relevance.[2]

(b) Bisoprolol

The AUC of bisoprolol 10 mg daily was reduced by 34% in healthy subjects given rifampicin 600 mg daily.[3]

(c) Carvedilol

Rifampicin 600 mg daily for 12 days caused a 60% decrease in the maximum serum levels and the AUC of carvedilol.[4]

(d) Celiprolol

In a study in healthy subjects, rifampicin 600 mg daily reduced the AUC of a single 200-mg dose of celiprolol by 55%.[5]

(e) Metoprolol

In a study in healthy subjects, rifampicin 600 mg daily reduced the AUC of a single 100-mg dose of **metoprolol** by 33%.[6]

(f) Propranolol

Rifampicin 600 mg daily for 3 weeks increased the oral clearance of propranolol in 6 healthy subjects by almost threefold. Increasing the rifampicin dosage to 900 or 1200 mg daily did not further increase the clearance. Four weeks after withdrawing the rifampicin the blood levels of propranolol had returned to normal.[7] In a similar study the oral clearance of propranolol was increased by about fourfold by rifampicin 600 mg daily for 3 weeks in both poor and extensive metabolisers of propranolol.[8]

(g) Talinolol

Rifampicin 600 mg daily decreased the AUC of a single-dose of talinolol 30 mg intravenously or 100 mg orally by 21 and 35%, respectively, in 8 healthy subjects.[9]

(h) Tertatolol

Rifampicin 600 mg daily for a week increased the clearance of tertatolol almost threefold and reduced the half-life from 9 to 3.4 hours. A slight reduction in the effects of tertatolol on blood pressure was seen and heart rates were raised from 68 to 74 bpm.[10]

Mechanism

Rifampicin is a potent liver-enzyme inducer that increases the metabolism and loss of extensively metabolised beta blockers such as propranolol and metoprolol. Rifampicin may also interact by mechanisms other than enzyme induction. Rifampicin increases duodenal P-glycoprotein expression, so increased clearance of talinolol (which is not metabolised) may be due to induction of P-glycoprotein excretion.[9] The effects on atenolol, which is not extensively metabolised, are also possibly due to induction of P-glycoprotein,[2] although this needs confirmation.

Importance and management

These interactions are established. Their clinical importance is uncertain but probably small.[10] Nevertheless, they cannot be completely dismissed as the case report with atenolol shows. Consider increasing the dosage of the beta blocker if there is any evidence that the therapeutic response is inadequate. Beta blockers that undergo extensive liver metabolism would be expected to be affected by the enzyme-inducing effects of rifampicin (see 'Table 22.1', (p.833)). Those beta blockers mainly lost unchanged in the urine would not be expected to be affected, but it appears that a reaction may occur with non-metabolised drugs, such as talinolol, that are substrates for P-glycoprotein. More study is required.

1. Goldberg SV, Hanson D, Peloquin CA. Rifamycin treatment of tuberculosis in a patient receiving atenolol: less interaction with rifabutin than with rifampin. *Clin Infect Dis* (2003), 37, 607–8.
2. Lilja JJ, Juntti-Patinen L, Neuvonen PJ. Effect of rifampicin on the pharmacokinetics of atenolol. *Basic Clin Pharmacol Toxicol* (2006) 98, 555–8.
3. Kirch W, Rose I, Klingmann I, Pabst J, Ohnhaus EE. Interaction of bisoprolol with cimetidine and rifampicin. *Eur J Clin Pharmacol* (1986) 31, 59–62.
4. Data on file, database on carvedilol, SmithKline Beecham, quoted by Ruffolo RR, Boyle DA, Venuti RP, Lukas MA. Carvedilol (Kredex®): a novel multiple action cardiovascular agent. *Drugs Today* (1991) 27, 465–92.
5. Lilja JJ, Niemi M, Neuvonen PJ. Rifampicin reduces plasma concentrations of celiprolol. *Eur J Clin Pharmacol* (2004) 59, 819–24.
6. Bennett PN, John VA, Whitmarsh VB. Effect of rifampicin on metoprolol and antipyrine kinetics. *Br J Clin Pharmacol* (1982) 13, 387–91.
7. Herman RJ, Nakamura K, Wilkinson GR, Wood AJJ. Induction of propranolol metabolism by rifampicin. *Br J Clin Pharmacol* (1983) 16, 565–9.
8. Shaheen O, Biollaz J, Koshakji RP, Wilkinson GR, Wood AJJ. Influence of debrisoquin phenotype on the inducibility of propranolol metabolism. *Clin Pharmacol Ther* (1989) 45, 439–43.
9. Westphal K, Weinbrenner A, Zschiesche M, Franke G, Knoke M, Oertel R, Fritz P, von Richter O, Warzok R, Hachenberg T, Kauffmann H-M, Schrenk D, Terhaag B, Kroemer HK, Siegmund W. Induction of P-glycoprotein by rifampin increases intestinal secretion of talinolol in human beings: a new type of drug/drug interaction. *Clin Pharmacol Ther* (2000) 68, 345–55.
10. Kirch W, Milferstädt S, Halabi A, Rocher I, Efthymiopoulos C, Jung L. Interaction of tertatolol with rifampicin and ranitidine pharmacokinetics and antihypertensive activity. *Cardiovasc Drugs Ther* (1990) 4, 487–92.

Beta blockers + Sevelamer

The concurrent use of a single 2.418-g dose of sevelamer did not alter the AUC of a single 100-mg dose of metoprolol in 31 healthy subjects.[1]

1. Burke SK, Amin NS, Incerti C, Plone MA, Lee JW. Sevelamer hydrochloride (Renagel®), a phosphate-binding polymer, does not alter the pharmacokinetics of two commonly used antihypertensives in healthy volunteers. *J Clin Pharmacol* (2001) 41, 199–205.

Beta blockers + SSRIs

Fluoxetine can increase serum pindolol and carvedilol levels, but the clinical effects of this are minimal. Isolated reports describe lethargy and bradycardia in patients taking metoprolol with fluoxetine and propranolol with fluoxetine or fluvoxamine. Fluvoxamine may increase the levels of propranolol, but not atenolol. Paroxetine may increase levels of metoprolol resulting in increased beta-blocking effects. Citalopram and escitalopram may interact similarly. Sertraline does not interact with atenolol.

Clinical evidence

(a) Citalopram

The UK manufacturers of citalopram say that no pharmacodynamic interactions have been noted in clinical studies in which citalopram was given with beta blockers.[1] However the US manufacturers say that although the concurrent use of **metoprolol** and citalopram has no clinically significant effect on heart rate and blood pressure, the plasma levels of **metoprolol** are increased twofold, which may decrease its cardioselectivity.[2]

(b) Escitalopram

The manufacturers say that escitalopram causes a 50% increase in the plasma levels of **metoprolol** and an 82% increase in its AUC. They note that although the concurrent use of **metoprolol** and escitalopram has no clinically significant effect on heart rate and blood pressure, this increase in plasma levels may decrease the cardioselectivity of **metoprolol**.[3]

(c) Fluoxetine

Metoprolol 100 mg daily improved the angina of a man who had undergone a coronary artery bypass 4 years earlier. A month later he was given fluoxetine 20 mg daily for depression. Within 2 days he complained of profound lethargy, and his resting heart rate was found to have fallen from 64 to 36 bpm. The fluoxetine was withdrawn, and within 5 days his heart rate returned to 64 bpm. The **metoprolol** was replaced by **sotalol** 80 mg twice daily and fluoxetine reintroduced without problems.[4]

A patient taking **propranolol** 40 mg twice daily developed bradycardia of 30 bpm, heart block and syncope 2 weeks after starting fluoxetine 20 mg daily. This patient possibly also had some pre-existing conduction disease contributing to the effect.[5]

When 9 healthy subjects were given **pindolol** 5 mg every 6 hours with fluoxetine 20 mg daily for 3 days and then 60 mg daily for another 7 days, the **pindolol** AUC rose by about 75% and its clearance fell by about 45%, when compared with a single 5-mg dose of **pindolol**. Only mild to moderate alterations in pulse rate and blood pressure were seen.[6] Some studies including a high proportion of patients with first-episode depression have suggested that the antidepressant response to fluoxetine is accelerated by **pindolol**[7] while other studies in patients with predominantly chronic or recurrent depression did not find an enhanced response.[8] A double-blind crossover study in 10 patients with heart failure, taking **carvedilol** 25 to 50 mg twice daily, found that the addition of fluoxetine 20 mg daily for 28 days increased the AUC of ***(R)*-carvedilol** by 77%, and decreased the clearance of both enantiomers by 44 to 56%. However, these pharmacokinetic changes were of little clinical significance, since there were no changes in blood pressure, heart rate, and heart rate variability.[9]

(d) Fluvoxamine

A 79-year-old man who had taken **propranolol** for prophylaxis of migraine for several years developed fatigue and lightheadedness within a few days of starting fluvoxamine. He was admitted to hospital with syncope and bradycardia of 38 bpm but recovered after both drugs were discontinued.[10] Fluvoxamine 100 mg daily raised the plasma levels of **propranolol** 160 mg daily fivefold in healthy subjects, but the bradycardic effects were only slightly increased (by 3 bpm). The diastolic pressure following exercise was only slightly reduced but the general hypotensive effects remained unaltered.[11] Fluvoxamine did not change the plasma levels of **atenolol** 100 mg daily, but the heart-slowing effects were slightly increased and the hypotensive effects were slightly decreased.[11]

(e) Paroxetine

A study in 8 healthy subjects found that paroxetine 20 mg daily for 6 days increased the AUCs of ***(R)*-** and ***(S)*-metoprolol** by eightfold and fivefold, respectively, after a single 100-mg dose of **metoprolol**. The maximum plasma concentration and elimination half-life were increased about twofold. The beta-blocking effects of **metoprolol** were more sustained and the reduction in exercise systolic pressure was more pronounced when paroxetine was also taken, when compared with **metoprolol** alone.[12]

(f) Sertraline

No changes in the beta-blocking effects of **atenolol** were found in a single-dose study in 10 healthy subjects given sertraline 100 mg five hours before **atenolol** 50 mg.[13,14]

Mechanism

Fluoxetine and paroxetine inhibit the cytochrome P450 isoenzyme CYP2D6 thus inhibiting the metabolism of some beta blockers (e.g. propranolol, metoprolol, carvedilol) so that they accumulate, the result being that their effects, such as bradycardia, may be increased.[4] Citalopram and escitalopram may also inhibit CYP2D6. *In vitro* studies with human liver microsomes found that fluoxetine and paroxetine are potent inhibitors of metoprolol metabolism and fluvoxamine, sertraline and citalopram less potent.[15] However, fluvoxamine also potently inhibits the metabolism of propranolol by CYP1A2.[10,16] Beta blockers that are not extensively metabolised, such as atenolol and sotalol, would not be expected to be affected.

Pindolol may augment the antidepressant effect of fluoxetine by its antagonistic effects at 5-HT_{1A} receptors.[7,8,17]

Importance and management

Pharmacokinetic interactions have been found between fluoxetine, fluvoxamine or paroxetine and some beta blockers, but despite marked pharmacokinetic changes, the clinical effects are not generally significant. However, be aware that there are a few isolated reports of severe bradycardia with beta blockers and fluoxetine or fluvoxamine. If problems arise, the interaction can apparently be avoided by giving a beta blocker (such as atenolol), which is not extensively metabolised. Alternatively, sertraline and citalopram seem to be less likely than the other SSRIs to interact with extensively-metabolised beta blockers.[15] However, because metoprolol is considered to have a narrow therapeutic index in the treatment of heart failure, the UK manufacturers of escitalopram say that caution and possible dosage adjustments are warranted on concurrent use.[18] Similarly the manufacturers of paroxetine suggest that concurrent use should be avoided if metoprolol is being used for heart failure.[19] Remember that fluoxetine and particularly its metabolite have long half-lives so that this interaction may possibly still occur for some days after the fluoxetine has been stopped. Also note that bradycardia occurs rarely with fluoxetine alone and in some cases an interaction may be pharmacodynamic rather than pharmacokinetic, and so swapping the beta blocker could, rarely, be ineffective.

The combination of pindolol with fluoxetine may be advantageous in the treatment of depression in some patients.[7,8]

1. Cipramil (Citalopram hydrobromide). Lundbeck Ltd. UK Summary of product characteristics, January 2007.
2. Celexa (Citalopram hydrobromide). Forest Pharmaceuticals, Inc. US Prescribing information, May 2007.
3. Lexapro (Escitalopram oxalate). Forest Pharmaceuticals Inc. US Prescribing information, May 2007.
4. Walley T, Pirmohamed M, Proudlove C, Maxwell D. Interaction of metoprolol and fluoxetine. *Lancet* (1993) 341, 967–8.
5. Drake WM, Gordon GD. Heart block in a patient on propranolol and fluoxetine. *Lancet* (1994) 343, 425–6.
6. Goldberg MJ, Bergstrom RF, Cerimele BJ, Thomassom HR, Hatcher BL, Simcox EA. Fluoxetine effects on pindolol pharmacokinetics. *Clin Pharmacol Ther* (1997) 61, 178.
7. Pérez V, Gilaberte I, Faries D, Alvarez E, Artigas F. Randomised, double-blind, placebo-controlled trial of pindolol in combination with fluoxetine antidepressant treatment. *Lancet* (1997) 349, 1594–7.
8. Berman RM, Anand A, Cappiello A, Miller HL, Hu XS, Oren DA, Charney DS. The use of pindolol with fluoxetine in the treatment of major depression: final results from a double-blind, placebo-controlled trial. *Biol Psychiatry* (1999) 45, 1170–7.
9. Graff DW, Williamson KM, Pieper JA, Carson SW, Adams KF, Cascio WE, Patterson JH. Effect of fluoxetine on carvedilol pharmacokinetics, CYP2D6 activity, and autonomic balance in heart failure patients. *J Clin Pharmacol* (2001) 41, 97–106.
10. Morocco AP, Hendrickson RG. Propranolol-induced symptomatic bradycardia after initiation of fluvoxamine therapy. *J Toxicol Clin Toxicol* (2001) 39, 490–1.
11. Data on file (Duphar), quoted by Benfield P, Ward A. Fluvoxamine, a review of its pharmacodynamic and pharmacokinetic properties and therapeutic efficacy in depressive illness. *Drugs* (1986) 32, 313–34.
12. Hemeryck A, Lefebvre RA, De Vriendt C, Belpaire FM. Paroxetine affects metoprolol pharmacokinetics and pharmacodynamics in healthy volunteers. *Clin Pharmacol Ther* (2000) 67, 283–9.
13. Warrington SJ. Clinical implications of the pharmacology of sertraline. *Int Clin Psychopharmacol* (1991) 6 (Suppl 2), 11–21.
14. Ziegler MG, Wilner KD. Sertraline does not alter the β-adrenergic blocking activity of atenolol in healthy male volunteers. *J Clin Psychiatry* (1996) 57, (Suppl 1), 12–15.
15. Belpaire FM, Wijnant P, Temmerman A, Rasmussen BB, Brøsen K. The oxidative metabolism of metoprolol in human liver microsomes: inhibition by the selective serotonin reuptake inhibitors. *Eur J Clin Pharmacol* (1998) 54, 261–4.
16. Brøsen K, Skelbo E, Rasmussen BB, Poulsen HE, Loft S. Fluvoxamine is a potent inhibitor of cytochrome P4501A2. *Biochem Pharmacol* (1993) 45, 1211–14.
17. Dawson LA, Nguyen HQ, Smith DI, Schechter LE. Effects of chronic fluoxetine treatment in the presence and absence of (+/-)pindolol: a microdialysis study. *Br J Pharmacol* (2000) 130, 797–804.
18. Cipralex (Escitalopram oxalate). Lundbeck Ltd. UK Summary of product characteristics, December 2005.
19. Seroxat (Paroxetine hydrochloride hemihydrate). GlaxoSmithKline UK. UK Summary of product characteristics, April 2007.

Beta blockers + Sulfinpyrazone

The antihypertensive effects of oxprenolol can be reduced or abolished by sulfinpyrazone. The pharmacokinetics of metoprolol are not affected by sulfinpyrazone.

Clinical evidence

Oxprenolol 80 mg twice daily was given to 10 hypertensive subjects for 15 days, which reduced their mean supine blood pressure from 161/101 to 149/96 mmHg, and their heart rate from 72 to 66 bpm. When they were additionally given sulfinpyrazone 400 mg twice daily for 15 days, their mean blood pressure rose to about the former level. The reduction in mean heart rate remained unaffected. Sulfinpyrazone attenuated the reduction in cardiac workload seen with **oxprenolol** alone by about half.[1]

A study in 9 healthy subjects found that sulfinpyrazone 400 mg twice daily did not affect the pharmacokinetics of **metoprolol** 100 mg twice daily. No adverse effects were noted in healthy subjects during concurrent use.[2]

Mechanism

Not understood. One idea is that the sulfinpyrazone inhibits the production of vasodilatory (antihypertensive) prostaglandins by the kidney. This would oppose the actions of the oxprenolol.

Importance and management

Information seems to be limited. If sulfinpyrazone is given to patients taking oxprenolol for hypertension, the effects should be monitored. It seems likely that this interaction could be accommodated by raising the dosage of the oxprenolol but this needs confirmation. The effect of this interaction on cardiac workload appears to be less important, but it would still be prudent to monitor concurrent use if oxprenolol is used for angina. Metoprolol may be a suitable alternative to oxprenolol as it does not appear to interact with sulfinpyrazone.

1. Ferrara LA, Mancini M, Marotta T, Pasanisi F, Fasano ML. Interference by sulphinpyrazone with the antihypertensive effects of oxprenolol. *Eur J Clin Pharmacol* (1986) 29, 717–19.
2. Cortellaro M, Boschetti C, Antoniazzi V, Polli EE, de Gaetano G, De Blasi A, Gerna M, Pezzi L, Garattini S. A pharmacokinetic and platelet function study of the combined administration of metoprolol and sulfinpyrazone to healthy volunteers. *Thromb Res* (1984) 34, 65–74.

Beta blockers + Tobacco ± Coffee and Tea

Tobacco smoking can reduce the beneficial effects of beta blockers on heart rate and blood pressure. Some increase in the dosage of the beta blocker may be necessary. Drinking tea or coffee may have a similar but smaller effect.

Clinical evidence

(a) Caffeine

Two 150-mL cups of coffee (made from 24 g of coffee) increased the mean blood pressure of 12 healthy subjects taking **propranolol** 240 mg, **metoprolol** 300 mg or a placebo. Mean blood pressure rises were 7%/22% with **propranolol**, 7%/19% with **metoprolol** and 4%/16% mmHg with placebo. The beta blockers and placebo were given in divided doses over 15 hours before the test.[1]

(b) Tobacco smoking

A double-blind study in 10 smokers with angina pectoris, taking daily doses of either **propranolol** 240 mg, **atenolol** 100 mg or a placebo, found that smoking reduced their plasma **propranolol** levels by 25% when compared with a non-smoking phase. Plasma **atenolol** levels were not significantly altered. Both of the beta blockers reduced heart rate at rest and during exercise, but the reductions were less when subjects smoked (effects attenuated by 8 to 14%).[2]

Other studies found that serum **propranolol** levels in smokers were about half those in non-smokers.[3,4] Smoking caused an increase in blood pressure and heart rate in patients with angina and these effects were still evident, to a reduced extent, during **propranolol** treatment. In addition smoking abolished the beneficial effects of **propranolol** on ST-segment depression.[5]

(c) Tobacco smoking and caffeine

Eight patients with mild hypertension taking **propranolol** 80 mg twice daily, **oxprenolol** 80 mg twice daily or **atenolol** 100 mg daily over a 6-week period had their blood pressure monitored after smoking 2 tipped cigarettes and drinking coffee, containing 200 mg of caffeine.

Their mean blood pressure rises over the following 2 hours were 8.5/8 mmHg in those taking **propranolol**, 12.1/9.1 mmHg in those taking **oxprenolol** and 5.2/4.4 mmHg in those taking **atenolol**.[6]

Mechanism

Smoking tobacco increases heart rate, blood pressure and the severity of myocardial ischaemia, probably as a direct effect of the nicotine and due to the reduced oxygen-carrying capacity of the blood.[2,5] These actions oppose and may even totally abolish the beneficial actions of the beta blockers. In addition, smoking stimulates the liver enzymes concerned with the metabolism of some beta blockers (e.g. propranolol) so that their serum levels are reduced.

Caffeine causes the release of catecholamines, such as adrenaline, into the blood, which could account for the increases in heart rate and blood pressure that are seen.[6] The blood pressure rise may be exaggerated in the presence of non-selective beta blockers, which block vasodilatation leaving the alpha (vasoconstrictor) effects of adrenaline unopposed. This will also oppose the actions of the beta blockers.

Importance and management

Established interactions. Smoking tobacco and (to a very much lesser extent) drinking tea or coffee oppose the effects of the beta blockers in the treatment of angina or hypertension. Patients should be encouraged to stop smoking because, quite apart from its other toxic effects, it aggravates myocardial ischaemia, increases heart rate and can impair blood pressure control. If patients continue to smoke, it may be necessary to raise the dosages of the beta blockers. The effects of the caffeine in tea, coffee, cola drinks, etc. are quite small and there seems to be no strong reason to forbid them, but the excessive consumption of large amounts may not be a good idea, particularly in those who also smoke.

1. Smits P, Hoffmann H, Thien T, Houben H, van't Laar A. Hemodynamic and humoral effects of coffee after β_1-selective and nonselective β-blockade. *Clin Pharmacol Ther* (1983) 34, 153–8.
2. Fox K, Deanfield J, Krikler S, Ribeiro P, Wright C. The interaction of cigarette smoking and β-adrenoceptor blockade. *Br J Clin Pharmacol* (1984) 17, 92S–93S.
3. Vestal RE, Wood AJJ, Branch RA, Shand DG, Wilkinson GR. Effects of age and cigarette smoking on propranolol disposition. *Clin Pharmacol Ther* (1979) 26, 8–15.
4. Gardner SK, Cady WJ, Ong YS. Effect of smoking on the elimination of propranolol hydrochloride. *Int J Clin Pharmacol Ther Toxicol* (1980) 18, 421–4.
5. Fox K, Jonathan A, Williams H, Selwyn A. Interaction between cigarettes and propranolol in treatment of angina pectoris. *BMJ* (1980) 281, 191–3.
6. Freestone S, Ramsey LE. Effect of β-blockade on the pressor response to coffee plus smoking in patients with mild hypertension. *Drugs* (1983) 25 (Suppl 2), 141–5.

Beta blockers + X-ray contrast media

There is some evidence that use of beta blockers is a risk factor for anaphylactoid reactions to X-ray contrast media. Severe hypotension has been seen in two patients taking beta blockers who were given sodium meglumine amidotrizoate and in a further patient taking atenolol who was given iohexol.

Clinical evidence

A case-control study of anaphylactoid reactions to X-ray contrast media found that the risk of bronchospasm during intravenous contrast media procedures was associated with beta blocker use and also with asthma, while the risk of major and life-threatening anaphylactoid reactions were associated with cardiovascular disorders. Use of beta blockers also increased the risk of hospitalisation in those patients who had a severe anaphylactoid reaction.[1]

Two patients, one taking **nadolol** and the other **propranolol**, developed severe hypotensive reactions when given **sodium meglumine amidotrizoate** as a contrast agent for X-ray urography. Both patients developed slowly progressive erythema on the face and arms followed by tachycardia and a weak pulse. Each was successfully treated with subcutaneous adrenaline (epinephrine) and hydrocortisone.[2]

Another patient who had developed a transient rash during cardiac catheterisation 6 years earlier and who was subsequently given **atenolol** developed generalised urticaria and severe hypotension immediately after an injection of **iohexol** for coronary angiography. The hypotension was refractory to aggressive standard treatment with adrenaline, atropine, and dopamine and the patient remained in shock (BP 60/34 mmHg). Noradrenaline (norepinephrine) infusion produced a modest improvement (BP 80/40 mmHg), but significant improvement in blood pressure occurred only after intravenous injections of glucagon 1 mg.[3]

See also, Anaphylaxis under 'Beta blockers + Inotropes and Vasopressors', p.848.

Mechanism

Iodinated contrast media are associated with hypersensitivity reactions due to the release of histamine. It is suggested that beta blockers compromise the ability of the body to cope with the effects of histamine release.[2]

Importance and management

Limited documentation. Withdrawal of the beta blocker 2 to 3 days before use of contrast media has been suggested,[2] but because of the potential for beta blocker withdrawal syndromes this must be considered on an individual risk/benefit basis.[1] Pretreatment with an antihistamine such as diphenhydramine and a corticosteroid such as prednisone may reduce the risk of reactions.[3-5] Ephedrine and cimetidine have also been tried, but their use is controversial.[5] Use of low osmolality, non-ionic contrast media may reduce the risk of adverse reactions, including anaphylaxis.[1,5,6] However, even mild reactions to contrast media may sensitise the patient and a serious anaphylactoid reaction may occur on further exposure despite pretreatment and the use of low osmolality contrast media.[3] Pre-testing with a small amount of the contrast media has been shown to be a poor predictor of a reaction.[5]

When anaphylactic reactions do occur in patients taking beta blockers, it may be preferable to use a beta-agonist bronchodilator such as isoprenaline rather than adrenaline (epinephrine).[2] Glucagon, which has inotropic and chronotropic actions that are only minimally antagonised by beta blockers, may also be effective in reversing anaphylactoid shock in patients taking beta blockers.[3]

1. Lang DM, Alpern MB, Visintainer PF, Smith ST. Elevated risk of anaphylactoid reaction from radiographic contrast media is associated with both β-blocker exposure and cardiovascular disorders. *Arch Intern Med* (1993) 153, 2033–40.
2. Hamilton G. Severe adverse reactions to urography in patients taking beta-adrenergic blocking agents. *Can Med Assoc J* (1985) 133, 122.
3. Javeed N, Javeed H, Javeed S, Moussa G, Wong P, Rezai F. Refractory anaphylactoid shock potentiated by beta-blockers. *Cathet Cardiovasc Diagn* (1996) 39, 383–4.
4. Greenberger PA, Patterson R, Tapio CM. Prophylaxis against repeated radiocontrast media reactions in 857 cases. *Arch Intern Med* (1985) 145, 2197–2200.
5. Wittbrodt ET, Spinler SA. Prevention of anaphylactoid reactions in high-risk patients receiving radiographic contrast media. *Ann Pharmacother* (1994) 28, 236–41.
6. Greenberger PA, Patterson R. The prevention of immediate generalized reactions to radiocontrast media in high-risk patients. *J Allergy Clin Immunol* (1991) 87, 867–72.

Atenolol + Allopurinol

Allopurinol 300 mg daily for 6 days did not affect the steady-state pharmacokinetics of atenolol 100 mg daily in 6 healthy subjects.[1] No special precautions would therefore appear to be necessary on concurrent use.

1. Schäfer-Korting M, Kirch W, Axthelm T, Köhler H, Mutschler E. Atenolol interaction with aspirin, allopurinol, and ampicillin. *Clin Pharmacol Ther* (1983) 33, 283–8.

Metoprolol + Acetylcholine

An isolated case describes bronchospasm, which developed in a patient taking metoprolol when intra-ocular acetylcholine was given.

Clinical evidence, mechanism, importance and management

An elderly patient with a history of hypertension, obstructive pulmonary disease and stable angina, taking several drugs including metoprolol, experienced severe bronchospasm and pulmonary oedema immediately following the intra-ocular injection of acetylcholine chloride during cataract surgery. Her blood pressure rapidly increased, and she became tachycardic. She had also received phenylephrine eye drops before surgery. The patient may have been more sensitive to the pulmonary effects of acetylcholine, such as bronchospasm, because of pre-existing disease and the presence of metoprolol. Phenylephrine may also have been involved,[1] (see also 'Beta blockers + Inotropes and Vasopressors', p.848). The general clinical relevance of this single case is uncertain but it seems likely to be small.

1. Rasch D, Holt J, Wilson M, Smith RB. Bronchospasm following intraocular injection of acetylcholine in a patient taking metoprolol. *Anesthesiology* (1983) 59, 583–5.

Propranolol + Ascorbic acid (Vitamin C)

Vitamin C reduces the bioavailability of propranolol but the extent is too small to be of clinical significance.

Clinical evidence, mechanism, importance and management

A study in 5 healthy subjects given a single 80-mg dose of propranolol found that a single 2-g dose of vitamin C reduced the maximum plasma levels of propranolol by 28%, reduced the AUC by 37% and reduced its recovery in the urine by 66%. The fall in heart rate was also slightly reduced. The reason for this interaction appears to be that vitamin C reduces both the absorption and the metabolic conjugation of propranolol.[1] However, none of the changes seen would appear to be of clinical relevance.

1. Gonzalez JP, Valdivieso A, Calvo R, Rodríguez-Sasiaín JM, Jimenez R, Aguirre C, du Souich P. Influence of vitamin C on the absorption and first pass metabolism of propranolol. *Eur J Clin Pharmacol* (1995) 48, 295–7.

Propranolol + Dextromoramide

An isolated report describes two patients who developed marked bradycardia and severe hypotension when they were given propranolol and dextromoramide following the induction of anaesthesia.

Clinical evidence, mechanism, importance and management

Two women about to undergo a partial thyroidectomy were given propranolol 30 mg and dextromoramide 1.25 or 4 mg by injection during the pre-operative period, after which anaesthesia was induced with a barbiturate. Each woman developed marked bradycardia and severe hypotension, which responded rapidly to intravenous atropine.[1] The reasons for this response are not understood and the general significance of this interaction is unclear.

1. Cabanne F, Wilkening M, Caillard B, Foissac JC, Aupecle P. Interférences médicamenteuses induites par l'association propranolol-dextromoramide. *Anesth Analg Reanim* (1973) 30, 369–75.

Propranolol + Miscellaneous

The manufacturers predict that propranolol levels will be raised by a number of drugs, but only the possible interaction with ritonavir appears to be of much concern.

Clinical evidence, mechanism, importance and management

(a) CYP2D6 inhibitors

As propranolol is metabolised by CYP2D6 the US manufacturers[1] suggest that inhibitors of this isoenzyme may inhibit propranolol metabolism. Some CYP2D6 inhibitors have been seen to interact (such as 'quinidine', (p.853)), but the pharmacokinetic effects seem modest in many cases, probably because propranolol is also metabolised by CYP1A2. An interaction with **ritonavir** (as predicted by the manufacturers) therefore seems possible, and the effects may be greater than those seen with other CYP2D6 inhibitors (see (b) below).

(b) CYP1A2 substrates or inhibitors

As propranolol is partly metabolised by CYP1A2 the US manufacturers[1] predict that its levels may be raised by substrates or inhibitors of this isoenzyme.

However, data for 'imipramine', (p.1246), 'isoniazid', (p.310), and 'theophylline', (p.1175), (substrates of CYP1A2) suggest that in fact propranolol raises the levels of these drugs.

Inhibitors of CYP1A2 raise propranolol levels (as seen with 'fluvoxamine', (p.855)) and therefore an interaction with **ciprofloxacin** (as predicted by the manufacturers) seems possible. However, note that propranolol levels fluctuate greatly between individuals, and propranolol is not exclusively metabolised by CYP1A2, and so any interaction seems likely only to produce moderate clinical effects. Note that the manufacturers of propranolol also list **ritonavir** as an inhibitor of CYP1A2, and this possible interaction may be of greater clinical significance as **ritonavir** can also inhibit CYP2D6, the other main route of propranolol metabolism (see (a) above). A large rise in propranolol levels may therefore occur. It would therefore seem prudent to be cautious if **ritonavir** is given with propranolol.

(c) CYP2C19 substrates or inhibitors

The US manufacturers[1] suggest that raised propranolol levels may occur with **fluconazole** or **tolbutamide**, which are inhibitors of CYP2C19 and a substrate for CYP2C19, respectively. However, CYP2C19 only plays a small part in propranolol metabolism. Further, the manufacturers also note that **omeprazole** and **lansoprazole** (inhibitors and substrates for CYP2C19) do not interact, and so a clinically significant interaction involving CYP2C19 seems unlikely.

1. Inderal (Propranolol hydrochloride). Wyeth Pharmaceuticals Inc. US Prescribing information, January 2007.

Propranolol + Misoprostol

Misoprostol does not significantly alter the pharmacokinetics of propranolol.

Clinical evidence, mechanism, importance and management

In 12 healthy subjects misoprostol 400 micrograms twice daily raised the AUC of propranolol 80 mg twice daily by about 20 to 40%, and this remained raised 7 days after misoprostol was discontinued.[1] However, as these findings were unexpected, the authors conducted a randomised, crossover, placebo-controlled study and ensured that propranolol was at steady state before assessing the effect of misoprostol. No significant effects on the pharmacokinetics of propranolol were found.[2] No special precautions would therefore seem necessary during concurrent use.

1. Bennett PN, Fenn GC, Notarianni LJ. Potential drug interactions with misoprostol: effects on the pharmacokinetics of antipyrine and propranolol. *Postgrad Med J* (1988) 64 (Suppl 1), 21–4.
2. Bennett PN, Fenn GC, Notarianni LJ, Lee CE. Misoprostol does not alter the pharmacokinetics of propranolol. *Postgrad Med J* (1991) 67, 455–7.

Propranolol + Nefazodone

Nefazodone does not significantly affect the pharmacokinetics of propranolol.

Clinical evidence, mechanism, importance and management

A study in 18 healthy subjects found that nefazodone 200 mg every 12 hours reduced the AUC of propranolol 40 mg every 12 hours by 14% and decreased the maximum plasma levels by 29%, but no clinically significant changes in the response to propranolol or relevant adverse responses were seen. The pharmacokinetics of the nefazodone were largely unchanged.[1] No special precautions would therefore seem to be necessary if both drugs are used.

1. Salazar DE, Marathe PH, Fulmor IE, Lee JS, Raymond RH, Uderman HD. Pharmacokinetic and pharmacodynamic evaluation during coadministration of nefazodone and propranolol in healthy men. *J Clin Pharmacol* (1995) 35, 1109–18.

Propranolol + Sucrose polyesters

There is evidence that sucrose polyesters (e.g. *Olestra*) do not interact with propranolol.

Clinical evidence, mechanism, importance and management

Eight healthy subjects were given sucrose polyester 18 g and a single unstated dose of propranolol. Sucrose polyester had no effect on the pharmacokinetics of propranolol.[1] Sucrose polyesters, are non-absorbable, non-calorific fat replacements. It has been concluded that sucrose polyesters are unlikely to reduce the absorption of oral drugs in general.[2]

1. Roberts RJ, Leff RD. Influence of absorbable and nonabsorbable lipids and lipidlike substances on drug bioavailability. *Clin Pharmacol Ther* (1989) 45, 299–304.
2. Goldman P. Olestra: assessing its potential to interact with drugs in the gastrointestinal tract. *Clin Pharmacol Ther* (1997) 61, 613–18.

Sotalol + Terfenadine

Episodes of torsade de pointes arrhythmia developed in a woman taking sotalol when terfenadine was added.

Clinical evidence, mechanism, importance and management

A 71-year-old woman with a history of atrial fibrillation was successfully treated with sotalol 80 mg twice daily. She started to take terfenadine 60 mg twice daily, and 8 days later she developed repeated self-limiting episodes of torsade de pointes arrhythmia. On one occasion she required resuscitation. Both drugs were stopped and no further episodes of arrhythmia occurred 72 hours after temporary pacing was discontinued.[1] It seems likely that what happened resulted from the additive effects of both drugs on the QT interval, which can lead to the development of torsade de pointes. This case confirms a previous mention of the possibility of this interaction.[2]

Although this seems to be the first report of this interaction, it is consistent with the known pharmacology of both drugs. Torsade de pointes is potentially life threatening, so the concurrent use of these two drugs should generally be avoided. See also 'Drugs that prolong the QT interval + Other drugs that prolong the QT interval', p.257.

1. Feroze H, Suri R, Silverman DI. Torsades de pointes from terfenadine and sotalol given in combination. *Pacing Clin Electrophysiol* (1996) 19, 1519–21.
2. Woosley RL, Chen Y, Freiman JP, Gillis RA. Mechanism of the cardiotoxic actions of terfenadine. *JAMA* (1993) 269, 1532–6.

Talinolol + Sulfasalazine

Sulfasalazine markedly reduces the absorption of talinolol.

Clinical evidence

The AUC of talinolol 50 mg was reduced by 91% (from 958 to 84 nanograms/mL per hour) in 8 healthy subjects given sulfasalazine 4 g. The maximum serum levels were also markedly reduced, from 112 to 23 nanograms/mL in 3 subjects, and to undetectable levels in the other 5 subjects.[1]

Mechanism

Not known. It is suggested that talinolol is adsorbed onto the sulfasalazine, thereby preventing its absorption.[1]

Importance and management

Information is limited to this study, but it would appear to be an established and probably clinically important interaction. The efficacy of the talinolol would be expected to be markedly reduced, but this does not appear to have been studied. If the mechanism suggested by the authors is true, their advice to separate the dosages by 2 to 3 hours should minimise this interaction.[1] More study is needed to confirm how effective this action is, and whether other beta blockers behave similarly.

1. Terhaag B, Palm U, Sahre H, Richter K, Oertel R. Interaction of talinolol and sulfasalazine in the human gastrointestinal tract. *Eur J Clin Pharmacol* (1992) 42, 461–2.

23

Calcium-channel blockers

Calcium-channel blockers in current clinical usage affect the slow L-type channel. They are usually classified by their chemical structure, which determines their selectivity for vascular smooth muscle over myocardium, and hence their potential to slow the heart rate (negative inotropic activity) see 'Table 23.1', (below). Interactions due to additive inotropic effects will therefore apply only to the benzothiazepine (diltiazem) and phenylalkylamine-type (verapamil) calcium-channel blockers, and usually not to the dihydropyridine-type (e.g. nifedipine) calcium-channel blockers. All three types of calcium-channel blocker will have additive hypotensive effects with other drugs with blood-pressure lowering activity.

Calcium-channel blockers also undergo interactions due to altered metabolism. Both verapamil and diltiazem are principally metabolised by the cytochrome P450 isoenzyme CYP3A4, and also inhibit this enzyme (see 'Table 1.4', (p.6)). They are therefore affected by drugs that induce or inhibit CYP3A4, and also themselves interact with drugs metabolised by CYP3A4.

Many of the dihydropyridine-type calcium-channel blockers are also metabolised by CYP3A4, and are affected by inducers or inhibitors of this isoenzyme. However, they do not generally inhibit CYP3A4, or other isoenzymes to a clinically relevant extent. The exception is perhaps nicardipine, which may cause a clinically relevant inhibition of CYP3A4 (see 'Table 1.4', (p.6)).

This section is primarily concerned with those interactions where the activity of the calcium-channel blockers is changed by the presence of another drug. Where the calcium-channel blocker is the affecting agent, the relevant monograph is usually categorised under the heading of the affected drug.

Mibefradil is a calcium-channel blocker that acts on the fast T-type calcium channel. It was withdrawn soon after it was launched because of identification of an increasing number of serious drug interactions caused by its inhibitory effects on CYP3A4 and 2D6. It was thought that the practical problems of implementing all the warnings relating to these interactions were too difficult and risky.

Table 23.1 Classification of calcium-channel blockers that act on slow L-type channels

Class	*Rate limiting?*	*Effect on AV or SA node*	*Examples*
Dihydropyridine	No	Little or none	Amlodipine, Barnidipine, Benidipine, Felodipine, Isradipine, Lacidipine, Lercanidipine, Manidipine, Nicardipine, Nifedipine, Nilvadipine, Nimodipine,† Nisoldipine, Nitrendipine
Benzothiazepine	Yes	Depression (negative inotropic activity)	Diltiazem
Phenylalkylamine	Yes	Depression (negative inotropic activity)	Gallopamil, Verapamil

†Nimodipine crosses the blood-brain barrier and therefore affects cerebral blood vessels, and is used for cerebral ischaemia.

Calcium-channel blockers + Antihistamines

An isolated report describes increased adverse effects in two patients when terfenadine was given to patients taking nifedipine or verapamil. Verapamil markedly increased the AUC of a single dose of fexofenadine in one study, but another study found a much more modest effect. However, even a marked increase may not be clinically important.

No pharmacodynamic interaction appears to occur between diltiazem and mizolastine, and mizolastine did not alter diltiazem pharmacokinetics. Nifedipine is predicted to increase the levels of mizolastine.

Clinical evidence, mechanism, importance and management

(a) Fexofenadine

In a study in 12 healthy subjects **verapamil** 240 mg daily for 6 days increased the AUC of a single 120-mg dose of fexofenadine 2.5-fold and increased the maximum level 2.9-fold with marked interindividual variation. Fexofenadine is not metabolised by the cytochrome P450 system, and it was suggested that **verapamil** may have increased fexofenadine bioavailability by inhibiting the drug transporters, P-glycoprotein or OATPs.[1] Another study showed a smaller 30% increase in maximum level of fexofenadine when a single 60-mg dose was given to subjects who had taken **verapamil** 240 mg daily for 10 days. Moreover, after 38 days of **verapamil**, the maximum level and clearance of fexofenadine was not significantly changed.[2]

Note that marked increases in fexofenadine levels with 'erythromycin', (p.589) and 'ketoconazole', (p.584) did not increase adverse effects and were not associated with any prolongation of the QT interval. This suggests that a clinically relevant interaction between **verapamil** and fexofenadine is not expected, but some caution may be warranted until further experience is gained.

(b) Mizolastine

A double-blind crossover study in 12 healthy subjects taking **diltiazem** 60 mg three times daily found that the concurrent use of mizolastine 10 mg daily for 5 days did not alter ECGs or blood pressures. No significant increases in adverse effects were seen and the pharmacokinetics of the **diltiazem** remained unchanged. However, mizolastine pharmacokinetics were not assessed.[3] Some manufacturers of **nifedipine**[4] and those of mizolastine[5] suggest that concurrent use may raise mizolastine levels by inhibition of the cytochrome P450 isoenzyme CYP3A4, and caution is therefore advised,[5] presumably because mizolastine has a weak potential to prolong the QT interval. If caution is required with **nifedipine**, then this should be extended to both **diltiazem** and **verapamil**, since these are both more potent inhibitors of CYP3A4 than **nifedipine**. Further study is needed.

(c) Terfenadine

An isolated report describes severe angina in a patient stabilised on **nifedipine** 10 mg three times daily when she took terfenadine 60 mg for seasonal allergy. A second patient taking **verapamil** 80 mg three times daily also experienced adverse effects (including severe headache and confusion) when a single 60-mg dose of terfenadine was taken.[6] **Verapamil**, **diltiazem**, and to a lesser extent some dihydropyridine calcium-channel blockers (e.g. **nicardipine**) are inhibitors of CYP3A4, but there appear to be no other reports of interactions with either terfenadine or **astemizole** (substrates of CYP3A4). Of all the calcium-channel blockers, only the manufacturers of **lercanidipine** advise caution during the concurrent use of terfenadine and **astemizole**.[7]

1. Yasui-Furukori N, Uno T, Sugawara K, Tateishi T. Different effects of three transporting inhibitors, verapamil, cimetidine, and probenecid, on fexofenadine pharmacokinetics. *Clin Pharmacol Ther* (2005) 77, 17–23.
2. Lemma GL, Hamman MA, Hall SD, Wang Z. The effect of verapamil administration on the pharmacokinetics of fexofenadine. *Clin Pharmacol Ther* (2003), 73, P16.
3. Miget N, Herrmann WM, Bergougnan L, Dubruc C, Weber F, Rosenzweig P. Lack of interaction between mizolastine and diltiazem in healthy volunteers. *Methods Find Exp Clin Pharmacol* (1996) 18 (Suppl B), 204.
4. Coracten SR (Nifedipine). UCB Pharma Ltd. UK Summary of product characteristics, June 2005.
5. Mizollen (Mizolastine). Schwarz Pharma Ltd. UK Summary of product characteristics, May 2006.
6. Falkenberg HM. Possible interaction report. *Can Pharm J* (1988) 121, 294.
7. Zanidip (Lercanidipine hydrochloride). Recordati Pharmaceuticals Ltd. UK Summary of product characteristics, October 2004.

Calcium-channel blockers + Antineoplastics

The absorption of verapamil can be modestly reduced by antineoplastic regimens containing cyclophosphamide, vincristine, and procarbazine, or vindesine, doxorubicin, cisplatin.

Clinical evidence, mechanism, importance and management

A study in 9 patients with a variety of malignant diseases found that treatment with antineoplastics reduced the absorption of a single 160-mg oral dose of **verapamil**. The **verapamil** AUC in 8 patients was reduced by 40% (range 7 to 58%), and one patient conversely had a 26% increase. Five patients received a modified **COPP** regimen (**cyclophosphamide**, **vincristine**, **procarbazine**, prednisone) and four received **VAC** (**vindesine**, **doxorubicin**, **cisplatin**).[1] It is believed that these antineoplastics damage the lining of the upper part of the small intestine, which impairs the absorption of **verapamil**. The clinical relevance of this reduction does not appear to have been studied. Note that **verapamil** may affect levels of 'anthracyclines', (p.611), 'etoposide', (p.631), and possibly 'docetaxel', (p.662). In addition, **nifedipine** may affect the levels of 'vincristine', (p.671).

1. Kuhlmann J, Woodcock B, Wilke J, Rietbrock N. Verapamil plasma concentrations during treatment with cytostatic drugs. *J Cardiovasc Pharmacol* (1985) 7, 1003–6.

Calcium-channel blockers + Aprepitant

The concurrent use of aprepitant and diltiazem markedly increases the levels of both drugs.

Clinical evidence, mechanism, importance and management

The US manufacturer notes that the use of aprepitant 230 mg daily with **diltiazem** 120 mg three times daily for 5 days increased the AUC of aprepitant twofold and increased the **diltiazem** AUC 1.7-fold in patients with hypertension. Nevertheless, aprepitant did not alter the effects of **diltiazem** on heart rate or blood pressure.[1]

Both aprepitant and **diltiazem** are substrates and inhibitors of the cytochrome P450 isoenzyme CYP3A4, therefore they each inhibit the other drugs metabolism. The clinical relevance of this interaction is uncertain, but the manufacturers recommend caution with **diltiazem** and other moderate inhibitors of CYP3A4.[1]

1. Emend (Aprepitant). Merck & Co., Inc. US Prescribing information, June 2006.

Calcium-channel blockers + Aspirin or NSAIDs

There is evidence that most NSAIDs can increase blood pressure in patients treated with antihypertensives, although some studies have not found the increase to be clinically relevant. In various small studies, indometacin appeared not to reduce the hypotensive effects of amlodipine, felodipine, nicardipine, nimodipine or verapamil, but it did in one of two studies with nifedipine, and one study with nitrendipine. Similarly, ibuprofen caused a small reduction in the antihypertensive effects of amlodipine. Diclofenac and sulindac appear not to interact with nifedipine, nor ibuprofen, naproxen, piroxicam or sulindac with verapamil, nor naproxen with nicardipine. Low-dose aspirin did not alter the antihypertensive effect of felodipine or nifedipine in one study, and long-term aspirin did not alter the cardiovascular benefits of nitrendipine in another. Diclofenac reduces verapamil serum levels and raises those of isradipine, but these changes are probably unimportant.

Two reports describe abnormal bruising and prolonged bleeding times in two patients and one healthy subject taking verapamil with aspirin. There are conflicting reports as to whether or not gastrointestinal bleeding is increased by giving NSAIDs with calcium-channel blockers.

Clinical evidence

A. Antagonism of antihypertensive effects

Various large epidemiological studies and meta-analyses of clinical trials have been conducted to assess the effect of NSAIDs on blood pressure in patients treated with **antihypertensives**, and the findings of these are summarised in 'Table 23.2', (below). In these studies, NSAIDs were not always associated with an increase in blood pressure, and the maximum increase was 6.2 mmHg. The effect has been shown for both COX-2 inhibitors and non-selective NSAIDs. In two meta-analyses,[1,2] the effects were evaluated by NSAID. The confidence intervals for all the NSAIDs overlapped, showing that there was no statistically significant difference between the NSAIDs, with the exception of the comparison between **indometacin** and **sulindac** in one analysis.[2] Nevertheless, an attempt was made at ranking the NSAIDs based on the means. In one analysis,[1] the effect was greatest for **piroxicam**, **indometacin**, and **ibuprofen**, intermediate for **naproxen**, and least for **sulindac** and **flurbiprofen**. In the other meta-analysis,[2] the effect was greatest for **indometacin** and **naproxen**, intermediate for **piroxicam**, and least for **ibuprofen** and **sulindac**. An attempt was also made to evaluate the effect by **antihypertensive** in one analysis.[1] The mean effect was greatest for beta blockers, intermediate for vasodilators (includes ACE inhibitors and calcium-channel blockers), and least for diuretics. However, the differences between the groups were not significant.

The findings of individual clinical and pharmacological studies that have studied the effects of aspirin or specific NSAIDs on specific calcium-channel blockers are outlined in the subsections below.

(a) Aspirin

1. Felodipine. In the Hypertension Optimal Treatment (HOT) study, 18 790 treated hypertensive patients, about 82% of whom received a calcium-channel blocker, usually felodipine alone or in combination, were also given either aspirin 75 mg daily or placebo for an average of 3.8 years. It was found that long-term low-dose aspirin does not interfere with the blood pressure-lowering effects of the antihypertensive drugs studied.[3]

2. Nifedipine. In a small study in 18 patients, low-dose aspirin 100 mg daily for 2 weeks did not alter the blood pressure lowering effect of nifedipine 30 to 60 mg daily, given as a modified-release preparation.[4]

3. Nitrendipine. A post-hoc analysis of the Syst-Eur trial of nitrendipine-based antihypertensive treatment found no difference in cardiovascular outcome between 861 patients who were also using long-term aspirin (700 patients) and/or other NSAIDs (161) and 2882 patients who had never taken aspirin or NSAIDs. Patients in this trial were randomised to receive nitrendipine, which could be combined or replaced by enalapril, hydrochlorothiazide, or both.[5]

4. Unnamed calcium-channel blockers. In a randomised study, the use of low-dose aspirin 100 mg daily for 3 months did not alter blood pressure control in patients taking calcium-channel blockers or ACE inhibitors, when compared with placebo.[6]

(b) Diclofenac

Hypertensive subjects taking slow-release **verapamil** 240 mg daily had a 26% reduction in the AUC of **verapamil** when they took diclofenac 75 mg twice daily.[7] The AUC of **isradipine** 5 mg twice daily for a week was unaffected in 18 healthy subjects by a single 50-mg dose of diclofenac but the maximum serum levels were raised by about 20%. Platelet aggregation

Table 23.2 Summary of epidemiological studies and meta-analyses of the effect of NSAIDs on blood pressure in patients taking antihypertensive drugs

Study type	*Patients*	*Antihypertensives*	*NSAIDs*	*Findings*	*Refs*
Case-control (2005)	184 cases 762 controls (UK primary care)	Not stated. Median of 2 different drugs.	Ibuprofen (78 cases) Diclofenac (60) Other (25)	BP control in treated hypertensives was not affected by use of NSAIDs. No evidence that either SBP or DBP differed according to type of NSAID.	1
Retrospective analysis (2004)	8538 patients with rheumatic disease and hypertension	Not stated	NSAID (1164 patients) Celecoxib (654) Rofecoxib (417)	Other NSAID or celecoxib therapy not associated with difficulty in controlling blood pressure, but rofecoxib was (odds ratio 1.38).	2
Meta-analysis (1994)	50 randomised controlled trials in 771 patients or healthy subjects	Beta blockers (15) Vasodilators (18) Diuretics (12)	Indometacin (33 trials) Sulindac (7) Ibuprofen (5) Piroxicam (4) Flurbiprofen (4)	NSAIDs elevated mean supine BP by 5 mmHg. NSAIDs antagonised all antihypertensives, but only beta blockers was statistically significant (6.2 mmHg). Among the NSAIDs, only the effect of piroxicam was statistically significant, with piroxicam, indometacin and ibuprofen causing the greatest increase, and sulindac and flurbiprofen the least.	3
Case-control (1993)	133 cases 133 controls	Hydrochlorothiazide, furosemide, methyldopa, propranolol	Ibuprofen (30% of cases) Indometacin (22%) Naproxen (18%) Sulindac (13%)	SBP was about 5 mmHg higher (not statistically significant) in those on NSAIDs, but DBP did not differ. Findings the same if indometacin users removed.	4
Cross-sectional cohort (1993)	2800 elderly (12% on both an NSAID and antihypertensives)	Not stated	Not stated	NSAID use was associated with a 29% increased risk of hypertension in those on antihypertensives, but not in those not on antihypertensives.	5
Meta-analysis (1993)	54 studies with 108 NSAID treatment arms in 1213 hypertensive patients	Not stated	Indometacin (600 patients) Naproxen (72) Piroxicam (51) Ibuprofen (55) Sulindac (277)	Increase in mean arterial pressure with indometacin 3.6 mmHg, naproxen 3.7, piroxicam 0.5, decrease in mean arterial pressure with ibuprofen 0.8, sulindac 0.16. The difference between indometacin and sulindac was statistically significant.	6

1. Sheridan R, Montgomery AA, Fahey T. NSAID use and BP in treated hypertensives: a retrospective controlled observational study. *J Hum Hypertens* (2005) 19, 445–50.
2. Wolfe F, Zhao S, Pettitt D. Blood pressure destabilization and edema among 8538 users of celecoxib, rofecoxib, and nonselective nonsteroidal antiinflammatory drugs (NSAID) and nonusers of NSAID receiving ordinary clinical care. *J Rheumatol* (2004) 31, 1143–51.
3. Johnson AG, Nguyen TV, Day RO. Do nonsteroidal anti-inflammatory drugs affect blood pressure? A meta-analysis. *Ann Intern Med* (1994) 121, 289–300.
4. Chrischilles EA, Wallace RB. Nonsteroidal anti-inflammatory drugs and blood pressure in an elderly population. *J Gerontol* (1993) 48, M91–M96.
5. Johnson AG, Simons LA, Simons J, Friedlander Y, McCallum J. Non-steroidal anti-inflammatory drugs and hypertension in the elderly: a community-based cross-sectional study. *Br J Clin Pharmacol* (1993) 35, 455–9.
6. Pope JE, Anderson JJ, Felson DT. A meta-analysis of the effects of nonsteroidal anti-inflammatory drugs on blood pressure. *Arch Intern Med* (1993) 153, 477–84.

was unaffected and the pharmacokinetics of the diclofenac were unchanged.[8]

A study in elderly women with hypertension found that diclofenac sodium 25 mg three times daily for one week had no effect on the control of their blood pressure with **nifedipine**.[9]

(c) Ibuprofen

Fifty-three hypertensive patients had no changes in their blood pressure control with **verapamil** 240 or 480 mg daily when they also took ibuprofen 400 mg three times daily for 3 weeks.[10] However, another study in 12 patients with mild or moderate essential hypertension controlled with **amlodipine** 10 mg daily, found that ibuprofen 400 mg three times daily for 3 days increased the mean blood pressure by 7.8/3.9 mmHg.[11]

(d) Indometacin

Indometacin 100 mg daily for a week did not significantly affect the hypotensive effects of **nifedipine** 20 mg twice daily in 10 patients with mild to moderate essential hypertension.[12] In contrast, in another study, indometacin 100 mg in divided doses over 24 hours was found to raise the mean arterial pressure by 17 to 20 mmHg in 5 out of 8 hypertensive patients taking **nifedipine** 15 to 40 mg daily.[13]

Five other studies, two in healthy subjects[14,15] and 3 in patients with hypertension[16-18] found that indometacin did not alter the blood pressure-lowering effects of **amlodipine**,[18] **felodipine**,[14,16] **nicardipine**[15] or **verapamil**.[17] Similarly, the haemodynamic effects of **nimodipine** 30 mg three times daily were not affected to a clinically relevant extent by indometacin 25 mg twice daily in 24 healthy elderly subjects, although the AUC of **nimodipine** and its maximum plasma levels were slightly increased.[19] However, indometacin 25 mg three times daily raised systolic and diastolic blood pressure by a mean of 4 mmHg in 15 patients taking **nitrendipine** 5 to 20 mg twice daily.[20]

(e) Naproxen

Naproxen 375 mg twice daily had no effect on the pharmacokinetics of **verapamil** in hypertensive subjects.[7] Fifty-five hypertensive patients had no changes in their blood pressure control with **verapamil** 240 to 480 mg daily when they were given naproxen 250 mg twice daily for 3 weeks.[10]

A placebo-controlled study in 100 patients taking **nicardipine** 30 mg three times daily found that naproxen 375 mg twice daily caused no clinically relevant changes in the control of their blood pressure.[21]

(f) Piroxicam

A study in hypertensive patients given up to 440 mg of **verapamil** daily found that piroxicam 20 mg once daily for 4 weeks did not significantly alter the antihypertensive effects of **verapamil**.[22]

(g) Sulindac

A study in elderly women with hypertension found that sulindac 100 mg three times daily for one week had no effect on the control of their blood pressure with **nifedipine**.[9]

A study in hypertensive patients given up to 440 mg of **verapamil** daily found that sulindac 200 mg twice daily for 4 weeks did not significantly alter the antihypertensive effects of **verapamil**.[22]

B. Antiplatelet effects and gastrointestinal bleeding

Abnormal bruising and prolonged bleeding times occurred in a woman taking **verapamil** 80 mg three times daily when she took **aspirin** 650 mg several times a week for headaches. The bruising ceased when the **verapamil** was stopped. Her normal bleeding time of 1 minute rose to 4.5 minutes while she was taking **verapamil**, and to 9 minutes while she was taking **verapamil** and **aspirin**. A healthy subject taking the same dose of **verapamil** and **aspirin** observed the appearance of new petechiae and her bleeding time rose from a normal 4.5 minutes to more than 15 minutes in the presence of both drugs.[23] An 85-year-old man taking enteric-coated **aspirin** 325 mg daily developed widespread and serious ecchymoses of his arms and legs and a retroperitoneal bleed about 3 weeks after starting **verapamil** 240 mg daily.[24]

A prospective cohort study[25] in 1636 elderly hypertensive patients and a case-control study[26] found that calcium-channel blockers were associated with an increased risk of gastrointestinal bleeding compared with beta blockers; in one of the studies, **verapamil** had the highest rate of bleeding, followed by **diltiazem** and **nifedipine**.[25] Two studies indicated that gastrointestinal bleeding was not increased by calcium-channel blockers.[27,28] A post-hoc analysis of the Syst-Eur data found that there was no interaction between chronic NSAID intake (81% **aspirin**) and antihypertensive therapy based on **nitrendipine** in terms of incidence of gastrointestinal bleeding. Further, the results suggested that chronic NSAID therapy tended to be associated with a lower incidence of bleeding in patients taking **nitrendipine**-based therapy than those on placebo.[5]

Mechanism

A. Antagonism of antihypertensive effects

There is some evidence that NSAIDs may increase blood pressure in patients treated with antihypertensives. Possible explanations for this include inhibition of vasodilator and natriuretic prostaglandins in the kidney and/or a decrease in vascular or endothelial prostaglandin synthesis resulting in salt retention and vasoconstriction.[29] In contrast, low-dose aspirin appears not to affect the blood pressure-lowering effects of calcium-channel blocker-based antihypertensive therapy.[3]

B. Antiplatelet effects and gastrointestinal bleeding

The prolonged bleeding times noted with verapamil[23] are probably a result of inhibition of platelet aggregation, because calcium-channel blockers interfere with the movement of calcium ions through cell membranes, which can affect platelet function. This appears to be additive with the effects of other antiplatelet drugs. It was suggested that vasodilation produced by calcium-channel blockers in conjunction with inhibition of platelet aggregation may increase the risk of bleeding, or at least prevent the normal vasoconstrictive response to bleeding,[25] although a protective effect of beta blockers rather than an adverse effect of calcium-channel blockers may also be the reason.[27]

Importance and management

Although several studies exist, the evidence for an interaction between the calcium-channel blockers and NSAIDs or aspirin is still somewhat inconclusive. Some consider that the use of NSAIDs should be kept to a minimum in patients on antihypertensives. The effects may be greater in the elderly and in those with blood pressures that are relatively high, as well as in those with high salt intake.[30] However, others consider that the clinical importance of an interaction between NSAIDs and antihypertensives is less than has previously been suggested.[31] While their findings do not rule out a 2/1 mmHg increase in blood pressure with NSAIDs in treated hypertensives, they suggest that if patients in primary care have inadequate control of blood pressure, other reasons may be more likely than any effect of concurrent NSAIDs.[31] There is insufficient data at present to clearly differentiate between NSAIDs. Further study is needed.

There is some limited evidence that the interaction of NSAIDs with calcium-channel blockers is less than with ACE inhibitors.[4,16,18]

For the effects of NSAIDs on other antihypertensive drug classes see 'ACE inhibitors', (p.28), 'beta blockers', (p.835) and 'thiazide diuretics', (p.956).

Clinically significant interactions between NSAIDs and calcium-channel blockers that result in bleeding appear rare.

1. Johnson AG, Nguyen TV, Day RO. Do nonsteroidal anti-inflammatory drugs affect blood pressure? A meta-analysis. *Ann Intern Med* (1994) 121, 289–300.
2. Pope JE, Anderson JJ, Felson DT. A meta-analysis of the effects of nonsteroidal anti-inflammatory drugs on blood pressure. *Arch Intern Med* (1993) 153, 477–84.
3. Zanchetti A, Hansson L, Leonetti G, Rahn K-H, Ruilope L, Warnold I, Wedel H. Low-dose aspirin does not interfere with the blood pressure-lowering effects of antihypertensive therapy. *J Hypertens* (2002) 20, 1015–22.
4. Polónia J, Boaventura I, Gama G, Camões I, Bernardo F, Andrade P, Nunes JP, Brandão F, Cerqueira-Gomes M. Influence of non-steroidal anti-inflammatory drugs on renal function and 24 h ambulatory blood pressure-reducing effects of enalapril and nifedipine gastrointestinal therapeutic system in hypertensive patients. *J Hypertens* (1995) 13, 925–31.
5. Celis H, Thijs L, Staessen JA, Birkenhäger WH, Bulpitt CJ, de Leeuw PW, Leonetti G, Nachev C, Tuomilehto J, Fagard RH for the Syst-Eur investigators. Interaction between nonsteroidal anti-inflammatory drug intake and calcium-channel blocker-based antihypertensive treatment in the Syst-Eur trial. *J Hum Hypertens* (2001) 15, 613–18.
6. Avanzini F, Palumbo G, Alli C, Roncaglioni MC, Ronchi E, Cristofari M, Capra A, Rossi S, Nosotti L, Costantini C, Pietrofeso R. Collaborative Group of the Primary Prevention Progect (PPP)–Hypertension study. Effects of low-dose aspirin on clinic and ambulatory blood pressure in treated hypertensive patients. *Am J Hypertens* (2000) 13, 611–16.
7. Peterson C, Basch C, Cohen A. Differential effects of naproxen and diclofenac on verapamil pharmacokinetics. *Clin Pharmacol Ther* (1990) 49, 129.
8. Sommers DK, Kovarik JM, Meyer EC, van Wyk M, Snyman JR, Blom M, Ott S, Grass P, Kutz K. Effects of diclofenac on isradipine pharmacokinetics and platelet aggregation in volunteers. *Eur J Clin Pharmacol* (1993) 44, 391–3.
9. Takeuchi K, Abe K, Yasujima M, Sato M, Tanno M, Sato K, Yoshinaga K. No adverse effect of non-steroidal anti-inflammatory drugs, sulindac and diclofenac sodium, on blood pressure control with a calcium antagonist, nifedipine, in elderly hypertensive patients. *Tohoku J Exp Med* (1991) 165, 201–8.
10. Houston MC, Weir M, Gray J, Ginsberg D, Szeto C, Kaihlenen PM, Sugimoto D, Runde M, Lefkowitz M. The effects of nonsteroidal anti-inflammatory drugs on blood pressures of patients with hypertension controlled by verapamil. *Arch Intern Med* (1995) 155, 1049–54.
11. Minuz P, Pancera P, Ribul M, Priante F, Degan M, Campedelli A, Arosio E, Lechi A. Amlodipine and haemodynamic effects of cyclo-oxygenase inhibition. *Br J Clin Pharmacol* (1995) 39, 45–50.
12. Salvetti A, Pedrinelli R, Magagna A, Stornello M, Scapellato L. Calcium antagonists: interactions in hypertension. *Am J Nephrol* (1986) 6 (Suppl 1), 95–99.

13. Thatte UM, Shah SJ, Dalvi SS, Suraokar S, Temulkar P, Anklesaria P, Kshirsagar NA. Acute drug interaction between indomethacin and nifedipine in hypertensive patients. *J Assoc Physicians India* (1988) 36, 695–8.
14. Hardy BG, Bartle WR, Myers M, Bailey DG, Edgar B. Effect of indomethacin on the pharmacokinetics and pharmacodynamics of felodipine. *Br J Clin Pharmacol* (1988) 26, 557–62.
15. Debbas NMG, Raoof NT, Al Qassab HK, Jackson SHD, Turner P. Does indomethacin antagonise the effects of nicardipine? *Acta Pharmacol Toxicol (Copenh)* (1986) 59 (Suppl V), 181.
16. Morgan T, Anderson A. Interaction of indomethacin with felodipine and enalapril. *J Hypertens* (1993) 11 (Suppl 5), S338–S339.
17. Perreault MM, Foster RT, Lebel M, Du Souich P, Larochelle P, Cusson JR. Pharmacodynamic effects of indomethacin in essential hypertensive patients treated with verapamil. *Clin Invest Med* (1993) 16 (Suppl 4), B17.
18. Morgan TO, Anderson A, Bertram D. Effect of indomethacin on blood pressure in elderly people with essential hypertension well controlled on amlodipine or enalapril. *Am J Hypertens* (2000), 13, 1161–7.
19. Mück W, Heine PR, Schmage N, Niklaus H, Horkulak J, Breuel H-P. Steady-state pharmacokinetics of nimodipine during chronic administration of indometacin in elderly healthy volunteers. *Arzneimittelforschung* (1995) 45, 460–2.
20. Harvey PJ, Wing LM, Beilby J, Ramsay A, Tonkin AL, Goh SH, Russell AE, Bune AJ, Chalmers JP. Effect of indomethacin on blood pressure control during treatment with nitrendipine. *Blood Pressure* (1995) 4, 307–12.
21. Klassen DK, Jane LH, Young DY, Peterson CA. Assessment of blood pressure during naproxen therapy in hypertensive patients treated with nicardipine. *Am J Hypertens* (1995) 8, 146–53.
22. Baez MA, Alvarez CR, Weidler DJ. Effects of the non-steroidal anti-inflammatory drugs, piroxicam or sulindac, on the antihypertensive actions of propranolol and verapamil. *J Hypertens* (1987) 5 (Suppl 5) S563–S566.
23. Ring ME, Martin GV, Fenster PE. Clinically significant antiplatelet effects of calcium-channel blockers. *J Clin Pharmacol* (1986) 26, 719–20.
24. Verzino E, Kaplan B, Ashley JV, Burdette M. Verapamil–aspirin interaction. *Ann Pharmacother* (1994) 28, 536–7.
25. Pahor M, Guralnik JM, Furberg CD, Carbonin P, Havlik RJ. Risk of gastrointestinal haemorrhage with calcium antagonists in hypertensive persons over 67 years old. *Lancet* (1996) 347, 1061–5.
26. Kaplan RC, Heckbert SR, Koepsell TD, Rosendaal FR, Psaty BM. Use of calcium channel blockers and risk of hospitalized gastrointestinal tract bleeding. *Arch Intern Med* (2000) 160, 1849–55.
27. Suissa S, Bourgault C, Barkun A, Sheehy O, Ernst P. Antihypertensive drugs and the risk of gastrointestinal bleeding. *Am J Med* (1998) 105, 230–5.
28. Kelly JP, Laszlo A, Kaufman DW, Sundstrom A, Shapiro S. Major upper gastrointestinal bleeding and the use of calcium channel blockers. *Lancet* (1999) 353, 559.
29. Beilin LJ. Non-steroidal anti-inflammatory drugs and antihypertensive drug therapy. *J Hypertens* (2002) 20, 849–50.
30. Johnson AG. NSAIDs and blood pressure. Clinical importance for older patients. *Drugs Aging* (1998) 12, 17–27.
31. Sheridan R, Montgomery AA, Fahey T. NSAID use and BP in treated hypertensives: a retrospective controlled observational study. *J Hum Hypertens* (2005) 19, 445–50.

Calcium-channel blockers + Azoles

Itraconazole can markedly raise the serum levels of felodipine, which increases its adverse effects, in particular ankle and leg oedema. A few case reports suggest that isradipine and nifedipine can interact similarly with itraconazole, and that fluconazole can also interact with nifedipine. Ketoconazole can markedly raise the plasma levels of lercanidipine and nisoldipine. Caution is warranted with all calcium-channel blockers when azole antifungals, particularly itraconazole and ketoconazole, are used.

Clinical evidence

(a) Felodipine

When **itraconazole** 200 mg daily or a placebo was given to 9 healthy subjects for 4 days, followed by a single 5-mg dose of felodipine, it was found that the felodipine AUC was increased sixfold and the maximum plasma levels were increased eightfold. The effects of the felodipine on blood pressure and heart rate were also increased.[1]

A 52-year-old woman taking felodipine 10 mg daily for hypertension for a year, without problems, developed ankle and leg swelling within 7 days of starting **itraconazole** 100 mg daily for tinea pedis. The oedema disappeared within 2 to 4 days of stopping the **itraconazole**.[2] Virtually the same reaction occurred in another woman taking both drugs. Later tests found that her AUC_{0-6} of a single 5-mg dose of felodipine was increased at least fourfold (possibly up to tenfold) while taking **itraconazole**, and ankle swelling was noted.[2]

(b) Isradipine

Ankle swelling was noted in a patient taking isradipine 5 mg daily when **itraconazole** 200 mg twice daily was also taken.[2]

(c) Lercanidipine

The manufacturer notes that an interaction study found that **ketoconazole** increased the *S*-lercanidipine AUC and peak plasma levels 15-fold and eightfold, respectively.[3]

(d) Nifedipine

A report describes massive pitting oedema in the legs and ankles of a patient taking nifedipine when **itraconazole** 100 mg twice daily was also taken.[4] Another patient similarly had ankle oedema and markedly raised serum nifedipine levels (trough levels raised almost fivefold) while taking **itraconazole**.[5] A patient with malignant phaeochromocytoma whose persistent hypertension was controlled with nifedipine had a rise in blood pressure when **fluconazole** 200 mg daily was *stopped*. His blood pressure fell again when the **fluconazole** was restarted. A later study found that his maximum nifedipine plasma levels and AUC_{0-5} were raised about three-fold by **fluconazole**.[6]

(e) Nisoldipine

A study in 7 healthy subjects found that **ketoconazole** 200 mg daily for 5 days increased the AUC and peak plasma levels of a single 5-mg dose of nisoldipine by 24-fold and 11-fold, respectively. The levels of nisoldipine metabolite were similarly increased.[7]

Mechanism

Ankle swelling due to precapillary vasodilatation is a relatively common adverse effect of the dihydropyridine calcium-channel blockers, and this effect appears to be dose-related. Calcium-channel blockers are metabolised in the gut wall and liver by the cytochrome P450 CYP3A subfamily of isoenzymes, which are inhibited by itraconazole, ketoconazole and to a lesser extent by fluconazole, so that in the presence of these antifungals the levels of the calcium-channel blockers are raised and the adverse effects increased.

Importance and management

The interaction between felodipine and itraconazole would appear to be established and clinically important. It also seems that isradipine, lercanidipine, nifedipine and nisoldipine can interact similarly with fluconazole, itraconazole or ketoconazole and, because they are metabolised by CYP3A4, it is likely that other calcium-channel blockers will behave in the same way. If itraconazole, ketoconazole, or fluconazole is given to a patient on established treatment with any calcium-channel blocker be alert for the need to lower the dosage of the calcium-channel blocker. However, some manufacturers (e.g. felodipine,[8] lercanidipine[3]) actually contraindicate concurrent use of itraconazole or ketoconazole, and others (e.g. nisoldipine[9]) additionally contraindicate fluconazole. In the US the guidance differs slightly and only caution is considered necessary with felodipine.[10] The manufacturers of nimodipine predict that fluconazole, itraconazole and ketoconazole will substantially raise nimodipine levels. They say that concurrent use should be avoided, but, if this is not possible then the patient's blood pressure should be carefully monitored.[11]

1. Jalava K-M, Olkkola KT, Neuvonen PJ. Itraconazole greatly increases plasma concentrations and effects of felodipine. *Clin Pharmacol Ther* (1997) 61, 410–15.
2. Neuvonen PJ, Suhonen R. Itraconazole interacts with felodipine. *J Am Acad Dermatol* (1995) 33, 134–5.
3. Zanidip (Lercanidipine hydrochloride). Recordati Pharmaceuticals Ltd. UK Summary of product characteristics, October 2004.
4. Rosen T. Debilitating edema associated with itraconazole therapy. *Arch Dermatol* (1994) 130, 260–1.
5. Tailor SAN, Gupta AK, Walker SE, Shear NH. Peripheral edema due to nifedipine-itraconazole interaction: a case report. *Arch Dermatol* (1996) 132, 350–2.
6. Kremens B, Brendel E, Bald M, Czyborra P, Michel MC. Loss of blood pressure control on withdrawal of fluconazole during nifedipine therapy. *Br J Clin Pharmacol* (1999) 47, 707–8.
7. Heinig R, Adelmann HG, Ahr G. The effect of ketoconazole on the pharmacokinetics, pharmacodynamics and safety of nisoldipine. *Eur J Clin Pharmacol* (1999) 55, 57–60.
8. Plendil (Felodipine). AstraZeneca UK Ltd. UK Summary of product characteristics, March 2006.
9. Syscor MR (Nisoldipine). Forest Laboratories UK Ltd. UK Summary of product characteristics, August 1998.
10. Plendil (Felodipine). AstraZeneca. US Prescribing information, November 2003.
11. Nimotop (Nimodipine). Bayer plc. UK Summary of product characteristics, August 2005.

Calcium-channel blockers + Bile-acid binding resins

Colesevelam slightly reduces the bioavailability of verapamil and colestipol slightly reduces the bioavailability of diltiazem. These interactions are unlikely to be clinically important.

Clinical evidence, mechanism, importance and management

(a) Colesevelam

A study in 31 healthy subjects found that a single 4.5-g dose of colesevelam reduced the peak plasma levels and AUC of a single 240-mg dose of **verapamil** by about 33% and about 15%, respectively. These changes were not considered to be clinically significant.[1]

(b) Colestipol

A study in 12 healthy subjects found that colestipol reduced the AUC and peak plasma levels of a single 120-mg dose of sustained-release **diltiazem** by 22% and 36%, respectively, and those of a single 120-mg dose of immediate-release **diltiazem** by 27% and 33%, respectively. In a further study sustained-release **diltiazem** 120 mg was given alone, or 1 hour before or 4 hours after multiple doses of colestipol. The AUC of **diltiazem** was decreased by 17% when it was taken 1 hour before colestipol and by 22% when taken 4 hours after colestipol. This suggests that the effects of colestipol on **diltiazem** bioavailability are not reduced by separating their administration. However, these small reductions in levels are unlikely to result in reduced **diltiazem** efficacy, but the authors advise caution if these drugs are used concurrently.[2]

1. Donovan JM, Stypinski D, Stiles MR, Olson TA, Burke SK. Drug interactions with colesevelam hydrochloride, a novel, potent lipid-lowering agent. *Cardiovasc Drugs Ther* (2000) 14, 681–90.
2. Turner SW, Jungbluth GL, Knuth DW. Effect of concomitant colestipol hydrochloride administration on the bioavailability of diltiazem from immediate- and sustained-release formulations. *Biopharm Drug Dispos* (2002) 23, 369–77.

Calcium-channel blockers + Bile acids

Chenodeoxycholic acid and ursodeoxycholic acid reduce the bioavailability of nitrendipine.

Clinical evidence, mechanism, importance and management

In a single-dose study, 6 healthy subjects were given **nitrendipine** 10 mg with or without either **chenodeoxycholic acid** 200 mg or 600 mg, or **ursodeoxycholic acid** 50 mg. **Ursodeoxycholic acid** reduced the peak plasma level and AUC of **nitrendipine** by 54% and 75%, respectively. **Chenodeoxycholic acid** 200 mg decreased the peak plasma level and AUC of **nitrendipine** by about 20%, but the 600-mg dose reduced the peak plasma level and AUC of **nitrendipine** by 54% and 68%, respectively. The reduction in bioavailability of **nitrendipine** was possibly due to the effects of the bile acids on tablet disintegration or more probably on drug solubilisation. The clinical importance of the interaction is not known.[1]

1. Sasaki M, Maeda A, Sakamoto K-I, Fujimura A. Effect of bile acids on absorption of nitrendipine in healthy subjects. *Br J Clin Pharmacol* (2001) 52, 699–701.

Calcium-channel blockers + Calcium-channel blockers

Plasma levels of both nifedipine and diltiazem are increased by concurrent use and blood pressure is reduced accordingly. Verapamil is predicted to interact similarly. There are isolated reports of intestinal occlusion attributed to the concurrent use of nifedipine and diltiazem. Note that if nimodipine is used with another calcium-channel blocker, monitoring, with possible dose reduction or discontinuation of the other calcium-channel blocker is recommended.

Clinical evidence

Pretreatment of 6 healthy subjects with **diltiazem** 30 or 90 mg three times daily for 3 days was found to increase the AUC of a single 20-mg dose of **nifedipine** two- and threefold, respectively.[1] Similar and related results are reported elsewhere.[2] In another study it was found that **nifedipine** 10 mg three times daily for 3 days increased the maximum plasma levels of a single 60-mg dose of **diltiazem** by 54% and increased its AUC by 49%.[3]

A patient taking **nifedipine** 20 mg twice daily developed abdominal distension and vomiting 2 days after also being given **diltiazem** 100 mg twice daily. Both calcium-channel blockers were stopped and abdominal X-ray suggested paralytic ileus, which resolved but then recurred when the drugs were restarted. The excessive relaxation of the intestine was attributed to elevated **nifedipine** plasma levels, which were said to be caused by **diltiazem**.[4] Another report describes complete or partial intestinal occlusion in a patient taking **diltiazem** on three occasions, each time when **nifedipine** was added.[5]

Mechanism

A reduction in the metabolism of both the nifedipine and diltiazem in the liver seems to be the explanation for the increase in drug levels.[3] An increased relaxant effect on smooth muscle is suggested for the cases of intestinal occlusion.[5]

Importance and management

Established interactions but of uncertain clinical importance. The manufacturers of nifedipine advise caution when it is used with diltiazem[6,7] because of possible increases in nifedipine levels. They say a reduction in the dose of nifedipine should be considered.[7] **Verapamil** is predicted to interact similarly.[7] Information about the use of combinations of other calcium-channel blockers appears to be lacking. However, the UK manufacturers of **nimodipine**[8] advise that if it is used with other antihypertensive drugs, including other calcium-channel blockers such as nifedipine, diltiazem, or **verapamil**, blood pressure monitoring and careful dose titration of **nimodipine** should be carried out with possible reduction or discontinuation of the other calcium-channel blocker.

1. Tateishi T, Ohashi K, Sudo T, Sakamoto K, Toyosaki N, Hosoda S, Toyo-oka T, Kumagai Y, Sugimoto K, Fujimura A, Ebihara A. Dose dependent effect of diltiazem on the pharmacokinetics of nifedipine. *J Clin Pharmacol* (1989) 29, 994–7.
2. Ohashi K, Tateishi T, Sudo T, Sakamoto K, Toyosaki N, Hosoda S, Toyo-oka T, Sugimoto K, Kumagai Y, Ebihara A. Effects of diltiazem on the pharmacokinetics of nifedipine. *J Cardiovasc Pharmacol* (1990) 15, 96–101.
3. Tateishi T, Ohashi K, Sudo T, Sakamoto K, Fujimura A, Ebihara A. The effect of nifedipine on the pharmacokinetics and dynamics of diltiazem: the preliminary study in normal volunteers. *J Clin Pharmacol* (1993) 33, 738–40.
4. Harada T, Ohtaki E, Sumiyoshi T, Hosoda S. Paralytic ileus induced by the combined use of nifedipine and diltiazem in the treatment of vasospastic angina. *Cardiology* (2002) 97, 113–14.
5. Lamaison D, Abrieu V, Fialip J, Dumas R, Andronikoff M, Lavarenne J. Occlusion intestinale aiguë et antagonistes calciques. *Therapie* (1989) 44, 201–2.
6. Adalat LA (Nifedipine). Bayer plc. UK Summary of product characteristics, September 2006.
7. Adalat CC (Nifedipine). Bayer HealthCare. US Prescribing information, August 2005.
8. Nimotop (Nimodipine). Bayer plc. UK Summary of product characteristics, August 2005.

Calcium-channel blockers + Calcium compounds

An isolated report describes antagonism of the antiarrhythmic effects of oral verapamil due to the use of oral calcium and calciferol. Note that intravenous calcium compounds may be used prior to intravenous verapamil where the hypotensive effects of verapamil would be detrimental.

Clinical evidence, mechanism, importance and management

An elderly woman with atrial fibrillation, successfully treated for over a year with **verapamil**, developed atrial fibrillation within a week of starting to take an oral calcium compound 1.2 g with calciferol (vitamin D) 3000 units daily for diffuse osteoporosis. Her serum calcium levels had risen from 2.45 to 2.7 mmol/L. Normal sinus rhythm was restored by giving 500 mL of saline and repeated doses of furosemide 20 mg and **verapamil** 5 mg by intravenous injection.[1]

Verapamil acts by inhibiting the passage of calcium ions into cardiac muscle cells and it would appear that in this case the increased concentration of calcium ions outside the cells opposed the effects of the **verapamil**.

The general importance of this isolated case is uncertain, but bear it in mind in the event of an unexpected reduction in **verapamil** effects.

Note that intravenous calcium compounds are sometimes given prior to intravenous verapamil for the treatment of ventricular arrhythmias to prevent verapamil-induced hypotension in situations where a reduction in blood pressure could be detrimental. This use does not affect the antiarrhythmic efficacy.[2] Calcium, usually in the form of intravenous calcium gluconate, is used as an antidote in cases of overdose of calcium-channel blockers.

1. Bar-Or D, Yoel G. Calcium and calciferol antagonise effect of verapamil in atrial fibrillation. *BMJ* (1981) 282, 1585–6.
2. Moser LR, Smythe MA, Tisdale JE. The use of calcium salts in the prevention and management of verapamil-induced hypotension. *Ann Pharmacother* (2000) 34, 622–9.

Calcium-channel blockers + Ceftriaxone and Clindamycin

An isolated report describes the development of complete heart block in a man taking verapamil, which was attributed to the use of intravenous ceftriaxone and clindamycin. The validity of this interaction has been questioned.

Clinical evidence, mechanism, importance and management

A 59-year-old man who had been taking sustained-release **verapamil** 240 mg twice daily for 2 years and phenytoin 300 mg daily for several years, developed complete heart block an hour after being given intravenous ceftriaxone 1 g and clindamycin 900 mg for bilateral pneumonia. He needed cardiopulmonary resuscitation and the insertion of a temporary pacemaker, but spontaneously recovered normal sinus rhythm after 16 hours. He made a full recovery. The reasons for this serious reaction are not known, but the authors of the report postulate that these two antibacterials precipitated acute **verapamil** toxicity, possibly by displacing it from its plasma protein binding sites. Although both antibacterials are highly protein-bound (93% or more),[1] they are acidic and do not bind to the same sites as the **verapamil** (a base), so that this mechanism of interaction seems very unlikely. This seems to be the first and only report of this reaction, and the suggestion by the authors that it was due to a drug interaction has been seriously questioned.[2] There seems to be no other evidence that either of these antibacterials interact with **verapamil**, either given orally or intravenously.

1. Kishore K, Raina A, Misra V, Jonas E. Acute verapamil toxicity in a patient with chronic toxicity: possible interaction with ceftriaxone and clindamycin. *Ann Pharmacother* (1993) 27, 877–80.
2. Horn JR, Hansten PD. Comment: pitfalls in reporting drug interactions. *Ann Pharmacother* (1993) 27, 1545–6.

Calcium-channel blockers + Chlorpromazine

A patient taking chlorpromazine who was given nifedipine [dosage not stated] for 2 days before surgery, developed marked hypotension during surgery, which was eventually controlled with noradrenaline (norepinephrine).[1] Other phenothiazines and calcium-channel blockers may interact similarly, see 'Antihypertensives + Other drugs that affect blood pressure', p.880.

1. Stuart-Taylor ME, Crosse MM. A plea for noradrenaline. *Anaesthesia* (1989) 44, 916–7.

Calcium-channel blockers + Clonidine

Two hypertensive patients taking verapamil developed complete heart block when clonidine was added. The hypotensive effects of nifedipine and clonidine were additive in hypertensive patients. Transdermal clonidine has been successfully used with nifedipine or diltiazem in small studies.

Clinical evidence

(a) Diltiazem

In a clinical trial, transdermal clonidine decreased blood pressure in 58 of 60 patients with hypertension inadequately controlled by sustained-release diltiazem 90 mg twice daily. The addition of clonidine did not cause a significant decrease in heart rate.[1]

(b) Nifedipine

Sustained-release clonidine 250 micrograms daily for 2 weeks increased the hypotensive effects of nifedipine 20 mg twice daily by about 5 mmHg (mean blood pressure reduction) in 12 patients. Clonidine did not alter the slight heart rate increase seen with nifedipine.[2] In a clinical trial in 39 patients with hypertension inadequately controlled by nifedipine GITS 30 to 60 mg daily, transdermal clonidine successfully decreased blood pressure in all 35 patients who completed a one-week titration phase then an 8-week maintenance phase.[3]

(c) Verapamil

A 54-year-old woman with refractory hypertension (240/140 mmHg) and hyperaldosteronism, took verapamil 160 mg three times daily and spironolactone 100 mg daily for 10 days, and had a reduction in her blood pressure to 180/100 mmHg. She was additionally given clonidine 150 micrograms twice daily, and after the second dose she became confused and her blood pressure was found to have fallen to 90/70 mmHg, with a heart rate of 50 bpm. She had developed complete AV block, which resolved when all the drugs were stopped. A 65-year-old woman with persistent hypertension did not have a satisfactory reduction in blood pressure with extended-release verapamil 240 mg daily (blood pressure 165/100 mmHg). Clonidine 150 micrograms twice daily was then added, and the next day a routine ECG showed that she had a nodal rhythm of 80 bpm, which developed into complete AV block. Her blood pressure had fallen to 130/80 mmHg.[4]

Mechanism

Not fully understood. Verapamil very occasionally causes AV node disturbances, but both of these patients had normal sinus rhythm before the clonidine was added. Clonidine alone has been associated with AV node dysfunction in hypertensive patients. It would seem therefore that these effects were additive in these two patients.[4]

Importance and management

Information about the interaction between verapamil and clonidine seems to be limited to this report.[4] Its authors say that a review of the literature from 1966 to 1992 revealed no reports of any adverse interactions between these drugs. Nonetheless, they suggest that it would now be prudent to give these two drugs together with caution and good monitoring in any patient, even in those without sinus or AV node dysfunction. There was no adverse effect on heart rate in one trial in patients taking diltiazem and using transdermal clonidine. There seems to be no particular need for additional caution when nifedipine is given with clonidine.

1. Lueg MC, Herron J, Zellner S. Transdermal clonidine as an adjunct to sustained-release diltiazem in the treatment of mild-to-moderate hypertension. *Clin Ther* (1991) 13, 471–81.
2. Salvetti A, Pedrinelli R, Magagna A, Stornello M, Scapellato L. Calcium antagonists: interactions in hypertension. *Am J Nephrol* (1986) 6 (Suppl 1), 95–9.
3. Houston MC, Hays L. Transdermal clonidine as an adjunct to nifedipine-GITS therapy in patients with mild-to-moderate hypertension. *Am Heart J* (1993) 126, 918–23.
4. Jaffe R, Livshits T, Bursztyn M. Adverse interaction between clonidine and verapamil. *Ann Pharmacother* (1994) 28, 881–3.

Calcium-channel blockers + Co-trimoxazole

Adverse effects (leg cramps, facial flushing) have been reported in one patient taking nifedipine when co-trimoxazole was also taken. One study found that co-trimoxazole had no effect on the pharmacokinetics and hypotensive action of a single dose of nifedipine.

Clinical evidence, mechanism, importance and management

The observation of a patient taking **nifedipine** who developed leg cramps and facial flushing (possibly as a result of raised plasma **nifedipine** levels) when given co-trimoxazole, prompted further study of this possible interaction in 9 healthy subjects. After taking co-trimoxazole 960 mg twice daily for 3 days the pharmacokinetics and hypotensive effects of a single 20-mg dose of **nifedipine** were found to be unchanged.[1] No special precautions would therefore normally seem to be necessary on concurrent use.

1. Edwards C, Monkman S, Cholerton S, Rawlins MD, Idle JR, Ferner RE. Lack of effect of co-trimoxazole on the pharmacokinetics and pharmacodynamics of nifedipine. *Br J Clin Pharmacol* (1990) 30, 889–91.

Calcium-channel blockers + Dantrolene

An isolated report describes acute hyperkalaemia and cardiovascular collapse when dantrolene was given to a patient taking verapamil, but not when he was subsequently given nifedipine. *Animal* studies have found similar effects with the combination of dantrolene and verapamil or diltiazem, but not with nifedipine or amlodipine.

Clinical evidence, mechanism, importance and management

A case report describes a 60-year-old man with insulin-dependent diabetes undergoing a right hemicolectomy. Due to inoperable coronary artery disease, which was causing angina pain he was taking **verapamil** 80 mg three times daily. On the morning of surgery he was given **verapamil** 80 mg with his pre-operative sedation and then, 2 hours later at the start of surgery, he was given intravenous dantrolene 220 mg over 30 minutes, because he was known to have previously had malignant hypertension. After surgery, when he was on ITU, it was found that his potassium had risen from 4.6 mmol/L before surgery to 6.1 mmol/L at the end of surgery (about 90 minutes after the dantrolene infusion). He was given 10 units of insulin, but an hour later his potassium was 7.1 mmol/L. He was given more insulin, but then developed metabolic acidosis and some cardiac depression, which resolved when he was given bicarbonate and hetastarch 5%. He received three further doses of dantrolene without incident.[1]

The authors of the report attributed the effects seen to an interaction between **verapamil** and dantrolene. They note that hyperkalaemia has been seen following dantrolene infusions, but the case they cite was in response to suxamethonium, and the UK and US manufacturers of dantrolene do not include hyperkalaemia as an adverse effect.[2,3] Nevertheless, the overall picture is that hyperkalaemia, of whatever cause, can apparently increase the myocardial depression caused by **verapamil**.[4,5] This case seems to be the only report of an interaction between **verapamil**, and several factors do not make this a clear-cut case of an interaction. However, hyperkalaemia and cardiovascular collapse have been seen in *pigs* and *dogs* given dantrolene and **verapamil**,[6-8] and so an interaction cannot be completely ruled out. The manufacturers of dantrolene contraindicate its use in patients taking **verapamil**.[2,3] One animal study suggests that **diltiazem** may interact similarly,[9] and the combination of **diltiazem** and dantrolene may also cause ventricular arrhythmias.[10] The manufacturers of **diltiazem** similarly contraindicate concurrent use.[10] Studies suggest that **amlodipine**[4] and **nifedipine**[9] do not interact and they may therefore be safer alternatives. In the case above[1] the patient later underwent further surgery while taking **nifedipine**, without any significant adverse effect (although the potassium was moderately raised to 5.4 mmol/L).

1. Rubin AS, Zablocki AD. Hyperkalemia, verapamil, and dantrolene. *Anesthesiology* (1987) 66, 246–9.
2. Dantrium Intravenous (Dantrolene sodium). Procter & Gamble Pharmaceuticals UK Ltd. UK Summary of product characteristics, April 2005.
3. Dantrium Intravenous (Dantrolene sodium). Procter & Gamble Pharmaceuticals. US Prescribing information, May 2001.
4. Freysz M, Timour Q, Bernaud C, Bertrix L, Faucon G. Cardiac implications of amlodipine-dantrolene combinations. *Can J Anaesth* (1996) 43, 50–5.
5. Jolly SR, Keaton N, Movahed A, Rose GC, Reeves WC. Effect of hyperkalemia on experimental myocardial depression by verapamil. *Am Heart J* (1991) 121, 517–23.
6. Lynch C, Durbin CG, Fisher NA, Veselis RA, Althaus JS. Effects of dantrolene and verapamil on atrioventricular conduction and cardiovascular performance in dogs. *Anesth Analg* (1986) 65, 252–8.3954091
7. San Juan AC, Port JD, Wong KC. Hyperkalemia after dantrolene administration in dogs. *Anesth Analg* (1986) 65, S131.
8. Saltzman LS, Kates RA, Corke BC, Norfleet EA, Heath KR. Hyperkalemia and cardiovascular collapse after verapamil and dantrolene administration in swine. *Anesth Analg* (1984) 63, 473–8.
9. Saltzman LS, Kates RA, Norfleet EA, Corke BC, Heath KS. Hemodynamic interactions of diltiazem-dantrolene and nifedipine and nifedipine-dantrolene. *Anesthesiology* (1984) 61, A11.
10. Tildiem Retard (Diltiazem hydrochloride). Sanofi-Aventis. UK Summary of product characteristics, April 2004.

Calcium-channel blockers + Diuretics

No pharmacokinetic interaction appears to occur between hydrochlorothiazide and diltiazem or isradipine. Similarly, hydrochlorothiazide and triamterene did not alter nifedipine pharmacokinetics, and spironolactone does not alter felodipine pharmacokinetics. Combinations of diuretics and calcium-channel blockers are used clinically for their additive antihypertensive effects.

Clinical evidence, mechanism, importance and management

(a) Diltiazem

A study in 21 healthy subjects given **diltiazem** 60 mg 4 times daily (for 21 doses) and **hydrochlorothiazide** 25 mg twice daily (for 11 doses) either alone or in combination found that at steady-state there was no clinically significant pharmacokinetic interaction between the two drugs.[1]

(b) Dihydropyridine-type calcium-channel blockers

The pharmacokinetics of **isradipine** and **hydrochlorothiazide** are not affected by concurrent use,[2] and the pharmacokinetics of **nifedipine** are not affected by either **hydrochlorothiazide** or **triamterene**.[3] **Spironolactone** 50 mg was found not to affect either the pharmacokinetics or the clinical effects of **felodipine**.[4]

The manufacturers say that **amlodipine** has been safely given with **thiazide diuretics** and no dosage adjustment of **amlodipine** is required.[5]

Additive antihypertensive effects are expected when diuretics such as **hydrochlorothiazide** are used in combination with calcium-channel blockers, and such combinations are used clinically.

1. Weir SJ, Dimmitt DC, Lanman RC, Morrill MB, Geising DH. Steady-state pharmacokinetics of diltiazem and hydrochlorothiazide administered alone and in combination. *Biopharm Drug Dispos* (1998) 19, 365–71.
2. Prescal (Isradipine). Novartis Pharmaceuticals UK Ltd. UK Summary of product characteristics, February 2002.
3. Adalat Retard (Nifedipine). Bayer plc. UK Summary of product characteristics, September 2006.
4. Janzon K, Edgar B, Lundborg P, Regardh CG. The influence of cimetidine and spironolactone on the pharmacokinetics and haemodynamic effects of felodipine in healthy subjects. *Acta Pharmacol Toxicol (Copenh)* (1986) 59 (Suppl 4), 98.
5. Istin (Amlodipine besilate). Pfizer Ltd. UK Summary of product characteristics, July 2007.

Calcium-channel blockers + Fluoxetine

Two patients taking verapamil and two taking nifedipine developed increased adverse effects (oedema, headaches, nausea, flushing, orthostatic hypotension) due to the concurrent use of fluoxetine. Fluoxetine appears to increase nimodipine levels, whereas nimodipine may decrease fluoxetine levels. Fluoxetine does not appear to alter lercanidipine pharmacokinetics.

Clinical evidence

(a) Lercanidipine

The manufacturer notes that a study in elderly subjects found that fluoxetine had no clinically relevant effects on the pharmacokinetics of lercanidipine. No other details were given.[1]

(b) Nifedipine

A patient taking nifedipine 60 mg daily developed nausea and flushing after also starting to take fluoxetine 20 mg every other day. The adverse effects gradually disappeared over the next 2 to 3 weeks when the nifedipine dosage was halved.[2] An 80-year-old woman taking nifedipine developed tachycardia, hypotension and profound weakness 10 days after starting fluoxetine 20 mg daily. On admission to hospital 8 days later she was unable to stand, her standing blood pressure was 90/50 mmHg and her heart rate was 120 bpm. She fully recovered within a week of stopping the fluoxetine.[3]

(c) Nimodipine

The manufacturer notes that, in elderly patients, nimodipine 30 mg twice daily given with fluoxetine 20 mg daily resulted in an increase in plasma levels of nimodipine, a reduction in plasma levels of fluoxetine, and a trend towards increased levels of the metabolite norfluoxetine,[4] but no specific values were given.

(d) Verapamil

A woman taking verapamil 240 mg daily developed oedema of the feet and ankles, and neck vein distension within 6 weeks of starting fluoxetine 20 mg every other day. The oedema resolved within 2 to 3 weeks of reducing the verapamil dosage to 120 mg daily.[2] Another patient taking verapamil 240 mg daily for the prophylaxis of migraine developed morning headaches (believed by the patient not to be migraine) about one week after increasing his fluoxetine dosage from 20 to 40 mg daily. The headaches stopped when the verapamil dosage was reduced and then stopped.[2]

Mechanism

The calcium-channel blockers are metabolised by the cytochrome P450 isoenzyme CYP3A4, which can be inhibited by fluoxetine. This results in a marked reduction in the metabolism and clearance of the calcium-channel blockers. The reactions reported appear to be the exaggeration of the adverse effects of these calcium-channel blockers, possibly due to an increase in their levels.

Importance and management

Although a pharmacokinetic interaction might be predicted, information on an important clinical interaction appears to be limited to these reports.[2,3] This suggests that the incidence is very rare. Bear the possibility of a pharmacokinetic interaction in mind if a patient shows an exaggerated response to a calcium-channel blocker after starting fluoxetine, being alert for the need to reduce the drug dosages. The clinical significance of the interaction between nimodipine and fluoxetine is not known.[4] Information about other calcium-channel blockers with fluoxetine or other SSRIs appears to be lacking.

1. Zanidip (Lercanidipine hydrochloride). Recordati Pharmaceuticals Ltd. UK Summary of product characteristics, October 2004.
2. Sternbach H. Fluoxetine-associated potentiation of calcium-channel blockers. *J Clin Psychopharmacol* (1991) 11, 390–1.
3. Azaz-Livshits TLT, Danenberg HD. Tachycardia, orthostatic hypotension and profound weakness due to concomitant use of fluoxetine and nifedipine. *Pharmacopsychiatry* (1997) 30, 274–5.
4. Nimotop (Nimodipine). Bayer plc. UK Summary of product characteristics, August 2005.

Calcium-channel blockers + Food

Some modified-release preparations of felodipine, nifedipine, and nisoldipine show markedly increased levels when given with food, particularly when high in fat. The bioavailability of lercanidipine is markedly increased by food, and it should therefore be given on an empty stomach. Manidipine should be given with food, as this improves its absorption. Food modestly decreases the rate and extent of absorption of nimodipine capsules. Food had no effect on the absorption of amlodipine, bepridil, diltiazem, isradipine, or verapamil in the studies cited.

Clinical evidence

(a) Amlodipine

There was no difference in rate or extent of absorption of amlodipine capsules between the fed and fasted state in a study in healthy subjects.[1]

(b) Diltiazem

The rate and extent of absorption of both a slow-release and a conventional tablet of diltiazem were unaffected by food in healthy subjects.[2] Similarly, the pharmacokinetic parameters of another sustained-release formulation of diltiazem (*Mono-Tildiem LP)* showed only minor changes when given with food in a study in healthy subjects.[3]

(c) Felodipine

The manufacturer of one prolonged-release tablet of felodipine *(Vascalpha)* notes that taking it with a high-fat meal markedly increased the maximum level (2 to 2.5-fold) without altering the extent of absorption.[4]

(d) Isradipine

The pharmacokinetic parameters of isradipine differed by less than 20% when modified-release and nonretard formulations of isradipine were given with a light meal compared with the fasted state.[5]

(e) Lercanidipine

The manufacturer notes that the oral bioavailability of lercanidipine is increased up to fourfold when it is taken up to 2 hours after a high-fat meal.[6]

(f) Manidipine

The bioavailability of single 20-mg doses of manidipine was increased by 42% when given to 12 healthy subjects after a standard breakfast rather than in the fasting state. Peak plasma levels were increased by about 25% by food (not significant), and the rate of absorption was unaffected.[7]

(g) Nifedipine

Some single-dose studies suggested that food might delay the absorption of nifedipine[8] and reduce its peak levels,[9,10] but a multiple dose study found that food did not have an important effect on the steady-state levels of nifedipine in a 'biphasic' formulation.[11] A further single-dose study in healthy subjects found that the bioavailability of two modified-release preparations of nifedipine *(Adalat OROS* or *Nifedicron)* were not significantly different when they were given in the fasting state, although the maximum plasma levels were 31 and 53 micrograms/L respectively. The bioavailability and maximum plasma level (38 micrograms/L) of *Adalat OROS* were similar after a high-fat breakfast to those in the fasting state. However, the maximum plasma level of *Nifedicron* increased 2.4-fold to 128 micrograms/L after a high-fat breakfast. Although the bioavailability of *Nifedicron* was only modestly increased by food, the increase in plasma levels indicates a loss of modified-release characteristics and suggests that the effect of food on nifedipine may depend on the product formulation.[12] The manufacturer of another modified-release preparation of nifedipine (*Adalat CC*) also notes that administration immediately after a high-fat meal increased the peak plasma level by 60% without altering the AUC.[13]

(h) Nimodipine

The US manufacturer notes that taking nimodipine capsules after a standard breakfast reduced the AUC by 38% and the peak level by 68% when compared with the fasted state in healthy subjects.[14]

(i) Nisoldipine

The manufacturer of an extended-release nisoldipine preparation *(Sular)* notes that food with a high fat content markedly increases the maximum plasma level (by up to 300%), but decreases total exposure by 25%. They note that this appears to be specific to the controlled-release preparation, as food had a lesser effect on the immediate-release tablet.[15] A similar food interaction has been noted with *Syscor MR*, another extended-release nisoldipine preparation.[16]

(j) Verapamil

The absorption of verapamil from a multiparticulate sustained-release preparation was not affected when it was given with food.[17]

Mechanism

The increase in bioavailability of manidipine in the presence of food may be because it is lipophilic and solubilised by food and bile secretions. Other lipophilic dihydropyridine calcium-channel blockers include felodipine and nisoldipine.[7] Food may alter the release characteristics of modified-release preparations of drugs, increasing the rate of absorption of the drug, and thereby potentially increasing effects.

Importance and management

Some modified-release preparations of felodipine, nifedipine and nisoldipine have shown markedly increased peak levels when given with meals, particularly if they are high in fat content. Because of this increase, the manufacturers of *Vascalpha* (felodipine),[4] *Adalat CC* (nifedipine)[13] and *Sular* or *Syscor MR* (nisoldipine)[15,16] recommend that they are given on an empty stomach[4,13] before breakfast,[16] or with a light meal,[4] avoiding high fat meals.[4,15] Note that these precautions do not apply to all preparations of these calcium-channel blockers (e.g. *Plendil* (felodipine) can be taken irrespective of meals), so the manufacturers literature needs to be consulted. Food markedly increases the extent of absorption of lercanidipine, and this should therefore be taken at least 15 minutes before food.[6] Because food modestly increases the extent of absorption of manidipine, it has been recommended that manidipine should be given with food.[7]

In contrast, food modestly decreases the rate and extent of absorption of nimodipine *capsules,* and the US manufacturer says they should preferably be taken not less than one hour before, or two hours after, a meal.[14] Food also modestly decreases the peak level of nicardipine, but the clinical relevance of this is uncertain.

Food had no effect on the absorption of amlodipine, diltiazem, isradipine, or verapamil from the preparations studied (see *Clinical evidence*, above).

1. Faulkner JK, Hayden ML, Chasseaud LF, Taylor T. Absorption of amlodipine unaffected by food. Solid dose equivalent to solution dose. *Arzneimittelforschung* (1989) 39, 799–801.
2. Du Souich P, Lery N, Lery L, Varin F, Boucher S, Vezina M, Pilon D, Spenard J, Caillé G. Influence of food on the bioavailability of diltiazem and two of its metabolites following the administration of conventional tablets and slow-release capsules. *Biopharm Drug Dispos* (1990) 11, 137–47.
3. Bianchetti G, Bagheri H, Houin G, Dubruc C, Thénot JP. Pharmacokinetic and bioavailability of diltiazem sustained-release: influence of food and time of administration. *Fundam Clin Pharmacol* (1995) 9, 197–201.
4. Vascalpha (Felodipine). Actavis UK Ltd. UK Summary of product characteristics, September 2006.
5. Holmes DG, Kutz K. Bioequivalence of a slow-release and a non-retard formulation of isradipine. *Am J Hypertens* (1993) 6 (3 Pt 2), 70S–73S.
6. Zanidip (Lercanidipine hydrochloride). Recordati Pharmaceuticals Ltd. UK Summary of product characteristics, October 2004.
7. Rosillon D, Stockis A, Poli G, Acerbi D, Lins R, Jeanbaptiste B. Food effect on the oral bioavailability of manidipine: single dose, randomized, crossover study in healthy male subjects. *Eur J Drug Metab Pharmacokinet* (1998) 23, 197–202.
8. Ochs HR, Rämsch K-D, Verburg-Ochs B, Greenblatt DJ, Gerloff J. Nifedipine: kinetics and dynamics after single oral doses. *Klin Wochenschr* (1984) 62, 427–9.
9. Reitberg DP, Love SJ, Quercia GT, Zinny MA. Effect of food on nifedipine pharmacokinetics. *Clin Pharmacol Ther* (1987) 42, 72–5.
10. Challenor VF, Waller DG, Gruchy BS, Renwick AG, George CF. Food and nifedipine pharmacokinetics. *Br J Clin Pharmacol* (1987) 23, 248–9.

11. Rimoy GH, Idle JR, Bhaskar NK, Rubin PC. The influence of food on the pharmacokinetics of 'biphasic' nifedipine at steady state in normal subjects. *Br J Clin Pharmacol* (1989) 28, 612–15.
12. Schug BS, Brendel E, Wonnemann M, Wolf D, Wargenau M, Dingler A, Blume HH. Dosage form-related food interaction observed in a marketed once-daily nifedipine formulation after a high-fat American breakfast. *Eur J Clin Pharmacol* (2002) 58, 119–25.
13. Adalat CC (Nifedipine). Bayer HealthCare. US Prescribing information, August 2005.
14. Nimotop Capsules (Nimodipine). Bayer Pharmaceuticals Corp. US Prescribing information, December 2005.
15. Sular (Nisoldipine). First Horizon Pharmaceutical Corporation. US Prescribing information, March 2004.
16. Syscor MR (Nisoldipine). Forest Laboratories UK Ltd. UK Summary of product characteristics, August 1998.
17. Devane JG, Kelly JG. Effect of food on the bioavailability of a multiparticulate sustained-release verapamil formulation. *Adv Therapy* (1991) 8, 48–53.

Calcium-channel blockers + Grapefruit juice

Grapefruit juice very markedly increases the bioavailability of felodipine and nisoldipine and alters their haemodynamic effects. The bioavailability of nicardipine, nifedipine, nimodipine or nitrendipine is increased without significantly altering haemodynamic effects, whereas the bioavailability of amlodipine, diltiazem and verapamil is only minimally affected. An isolated report describes peripheral oedema and weight gain in a black man taking nifedipine when also drinking grapefruit juice.

Clinical evidence

(a) Dihydropyridine calcium-channel blockers

1. Grapefruit juice. Drinking 200 to 250 mL of grapefruit juice can increase the bioavailability of **felodipine** two to threefold in healthy subjects and patients with hypertension.[1-11] Its effects are proportionately increased. One study found that diastolic pressures were reduced by 20% (11% with water) and heart rates increased by 22% (9% with water) when blood **felodipine** levels were at their highest after a drink of grapefruit juice.[1] Adverse effects such as headaches, facial flushing and lightheadedness were also increased.[1] The interaction develops after taking the first glass of grapefruit juice and persists for about 24 hours.[7,12]
The bioavailabilities of **nicardipine**,[13] **nifedipine**,[1,14-17] **nimodipine**[18,19] and **nitrendipine**[20] have also been found to be increased, even about doubled in some instances, but usually only minor changes in haemodynamic effects (blood pressure and heart rate) were reported in healthy subjects.[17,19-21] However, the effect may be more pronounced in some hypertensive patients.[17] An isolated report describes a 54-year-old black African man taking **nifedipine** retard 60 mg daily, lisinopril 5 mg daily and aspirin 75 mg who presented with peripheral oedema, weight gain, and apparently improved blood pressure control of about 6 months' duration. Over this time he had been drinking about 400 mL of freshly squeezed grapefruit juice every morning as part of a diet regimen. He was advised to stop drinking grapefruit juice, and 2 weeks later the oedema had disappeared, he had lost 2 kg in weight, and his blood pressure was slightly higher (140/85 mmHg) than when he presented (130/80 mmHg).[22]
One study in 8 healthy subjects found that when **nisoldipine** was given with grapefruit juice it produced significantly larger decreases in blood pressure for 8 hours compared to **nisoldipine** alone. The effect of grapefruit juice decreased with time but lasted for at least 3 days.[23] However, in a further study in healthy subjects, grapefruit juice increased the maximum **nisoldipine** plasma levels fivefold, but only minor effects on blood pressure and heart rate were found.[21]
Other studies found that the bioavailability of **amlodipine** was at most only slightly increased by grapefruit juice.[24-26]

2. Whole Grapefruit. Some studies have found that grapefruit pulp, segments, or extract may increase the AUCs of **nifedipine**, **nisoldipine** and **felodipine** by 1.3-fold, 1.3-fold and threefold respectively.[27,28]

(b) Diltiazem

In one study grapefruit juice had no significant effect on the bioavailability of diltiazem,[29] and in another it increased the AUC of diltiazem by about 20% but differences in blood pressure and heart rate were not significant.[30]

(c) Verapamil

A study in 10 hypertensive patients found that a single drink of grapefruit juice had no significant effects on the pharmacokinetics of verapamil.[31] However, studies in healthy subjects[32,33] found that grapefruit juice given 2 to 4 times daily for 3 to 5 days increased the AUC of verapamil by about 40%. Pharmacodynamic parameters (blood pressure heart rate and PR interval) were not significantly altered by grapefruit juice in one study,[32] but prolongation of PR intervals occurred in the other[33] and were of borderline significance, with increases to above 350 milliseconds in 2 subjects (maximal PR intervals of 200 to 260 milliseconds were usually observed).

Mechanism

Uncertain. It has been suggested that the increases in bioavailability are due to components of the fruit juice including flavonoids such as naringin,[1,5,21] (but not quercetin[14]), sesquiterpenoids,[34] or furanocoumarins including bergamottin (also found in Seville oranges and lime juice) and 6',7'-dihydroxybergamottin.[9,23,35,36] These components inhibit the activity of the cytochrome P450 isoenzymes CYP3A subfamily in the intestinal wall so that the first-pass metabolism of these calcium-channel blockers is reduced, thereby increasing their bioavailability and therefore their effects. Grapefruit juice has little effect on hepatic CYP3A4 and this is borne out by the fact that it interacts with oral but not intravenous preparations. See also 'Grapefruit juice', (p.11).
Therefore, the sensitivity of the interaction with grapefruit juice may be related to the oral bioavailability of the calcium-channel blocker.[30] Thus, amlodipine and diltiazem with high bioavailability are least affected, nifedipine is intermediate, and felodipine,[30] which has a lower bioavailability, is most sensitive to the activity of grapefruit juice. The exception is verapamil, which has low bioavailability and appears to be only slightly affected by grapefruit juice, but this is possibly because cytochrome P450 isoenzymes other than CYP3A4 are involved in its metabolism.[30] In the reported case, it was suggested that black Africans may be more susceptible to any interaction, as they already show reduced systemic clearance of nifedipine when compared with caucasians.[22]
Furanocoumarins and possibly other components of grapefruit juice may also increase the levels of calcium-channel blockers by inhibition of intestinal P-glycoprotein efflux transport.[9,23,30]

Importance and management

These are established interactions and the manufacturers of felodipine[37,38] say that it should not be taken with grapefruit juice. It has been suggested that **whole grapefruit** or products made from **grapefruit peel** such as marmalade should also be avoided in patients on felodipine.[28] The manufacturers of **lercanidipine**,[39] and verapamil[40,41] also contraindicate grapefruit juice, although this interaction is normally of little clinical relevance in the majority of patients. The manufacturers of nifedipine,[42,43] and nisoldipine[44] say that grapefruit juice should not be taken concurrently, whereas the manufacturers of nimodipine[45] advise against concurrent use. It is noteworthy that only one probable case report of the interaction appears to have been published. Generally speaking the concurrent use of grapefruit juice and most calcium channel-blockers other than felodipine, and possibly nisoldipine or verapamil, need not be avoided. However, it would be worth checking the diet of any patient who complains of increased adverse effects with any of the calcium-channel blockers that are known to interact with grapefruit juice. Any problems can be solved either by avoiding grapefruit juice, or possibly by swapping the calcium-channel blocker for a non-interacting one (amlodipine appears not to interact).

1. Bailey DG, Spence JD, Munoz C, Arnold JMO. Interaction of citrus juices with felodipine and nifedipine. *Lancet* (1991) 337, 268–9.
2. Edgar B, Bailey DG, Bergstrand R, Johnsson G, Lurje L. Formulation dependent interaction between felodipine and grapefruit juice. *Clin Pharmacol Ther* (1990) 47, 181.
3. Bailey DG, Spence JD, Edgar B, Bayliff CD, Arnold JMO. Ethanol enhances the hemodynamic effects of felodipine. *Clin Invest Med* (1989) 12, 357–62.
4. Edgar B, Bailey D, Bergstrand R, Johnsson G, Regårdh CG. Acute effects of drinking grapefruit juice on the pharmacokinetics and dynamics on felodipine – and its potential clinical relevance. *Eur J Clin Pharmacol* (1992) 42, 313–17.
5. Bailey DG, Arnold JMO, Munoz C, Spence JD. Grapefruit juice–felodipine interaction: mechanism, predictability, and effect of naringin. *Clin Pharmacol Ther* (1993) 53, 637–42.
6. Bailey DG, Bend JR, Arnold JMO, Tran LT, Spence JD. Erythromycin-felodipine interaction: magnitude, mechanism, and comparison with grapefruit juice. *Clin Pharmacol Ther* (1996) 60, 25–33.
7. Lundahl JUE, Regårdh CG, Edgar B, Johnsson G. The interaction effect of grapefruit juice is maximal after the first glass. *Eur J Clin Pharmacol* (1998) 54, 75–81.
8. Lundahl J, Regårdh CG, Edgar B, Johnsson G. Effects of grapefruit juice ingestion – pharmacokinetics and haemodynamics of intravenously and orally administered felodipine in healthy men. *Eur J Clin Pharmacol* (1997) 52, 139–45.
9. Malhotra S, Bailey DG, Paine MF, Watkins PB. Seville orange juice-felodipine interaction: comparison with dilute grapefruit juice and involvement of furocoumarins. *Clin Pharmacol Ther* (2001) 69, 14–23.
10. Dresser GK, Bailey DG, Carruthers SG. Grapefruit juice—felodipine interaction in the elderly. *Clin Pharmacol Ther* (2000) 68, 28–34.
11. Bailey DG, Arnold JMO, Bend JR, Tran LT, Spence JD. Grapefruit juice-felodipine interaction: reproducibility and characterization with the extended release drug formulation. *Br J Clin Pharmacol* (1995) 40, 135–40.

12. Lundahl J, Regårdh CG, Edgar B, Johnsson G. Relationship between time of intake of grapefruit juice and its effect on pharmacokinetics and pharmacodynamics of felodipine in healthy subjects. *Eur J Clin Pharmacol* (1995) 49, 61–7.
13. Uno T, Ohkubo T, Sugawara K, Higashiyama A, Motomura S, Ishizaki T. Effects of grapefruit juice on the stereoselective disposition of nicardipine in humans: evidence for dominant presystemic elimination at the gut site. *Eur J Clin Pharmacol* (2000) 56, 643–9.
14. Rashid J, McKinstry C, Renwick AG, Dirnhuber M, Waller DG, George CF. Quercetin, an *in vitro* inhibitor of CYP3A, does not contribute to the interaction between nifedipine and grapefruit juice. *Br J Clin Pharmacol* (1993) 36, 460–3.
15. Sigusch H, Hippius M, Henschel L, Kaufmann K, Hoffmann A. Influence of grapefruit juice on the pharmacokinetics of a slow release nifedipine formulation. *Pharmazie* (1994) 49, 522–4.
16. Rashid TJ, Martin U, Clarke H, Waller DG, Renwick AG, George CF. Factors affecting the absolute bioavailability of nifedipine. *Br J Clin Pharmacol* (1995) 40, 51–8.
17. Pisaŕik P. Blood pressure-lowering effect of adding grapefruit juice to nifedipine and terazosin in a patient with severe renovascular hypertension. *Arch Fam Med* (1996) 5, 413–6.
18. Fuhr U, Maier A, Blume H, Mück W, Unger S, Staib AH. Grapefruit juice increases oral nimodipine bioavailability. *Eur J Clin Pharmacol* (1994) 47, A100.
19. Fuhr U, Maier-Brüggemann A, Blume H, Mück W, Unger S, Kuhlmann J, Huschka C, Zaigler M, Rietbrock S, Staib AH. Grapefruit juice increases oral nimodipine bioavailability. *Int J Clin Pharmacol Ther* (1998) 36, 126–32.
20. Soons PA, Vogels BAPM, Roosemalen MCM, Schoemaker HC, Uchida E, Edgar B, Lundahl J, Cohen AF, Breimer DD. Grapefruit juice and cimetidine inhibit stereoselective metabolism of nitrendipine in humans. *Clin Pharmacol Ther* (1991) 50, 394–403.
21. Bailey DG, Arnold JMO, Strong HA, Munoz C, Spence JD. Effect of grapefruit juice and naringin on nisoldipine pharmacokinetics. *Clin Pharmacol Ther* (1993) 54, 589–94.
22. Adigun AQ, Mudasiru Z. Clinical effects of grapefruit juice-nifedipine interaction in a 54-year-old Nigerian: a case report. *J Natl Med Assoc* (2002) 94, 276–8.
23. Takanaga H, Ohnishi A, Murakami H, Matsuo H, Higuchi S, Urae A, Irie S, Furuie H, Matsukuma K, Kimura M, Kawano K, Orii Y, Tanaka T, Sawada Y. Relationship between time after intake of grapefruit juice and the effect on pharmacokinetics and pharmacodynamics of nisoldipine in healthy subjects. *Clin Pharmacol Ther* (2000) 67, 201–14.
24. Josefsson M, Zackrisson A-L, Ahlner J. Effect of grapefruit juice on the pharmacokinetics of amlodipine in healthy volunteers. *Eur J Clin Pharmacol* (1996) 51, 189–93.
25. Vincent J, Harris SI, Foulds G, Dogolo LC, Willavize S, Friedman HL. Lack of effect of grapefruit juice on the pharmacokinetics and pharmacodynamics of amlodipine. *Br J Clin Pharmacol* (2000) 50, 455–63.
26. Josefsson M, Ahlner J. Amlodipine and grapefruit juice. *Br J Clin Pharmacol* (2002) 53, 405.
27. Ohtani M, Kawabata S, Kariya S, Uchino K, Itou K, Kotaki H, Kasuyama K, Morikawa A, Seo I, Nishida N. Effect of grapefruit pulp on the pharmacokinetics of the dihydropyridine calcium antagonists nifedipine and nisoldipine. *Yakugaku Zasshi* (2002) 122, 323–9.
28. Bailey DG, Dresser GK, Kreeft JH, Munoz C, Freeman DJ, Bend JR. Grapefruit-felodipine interaction: effect of unprocessed fruit and probable active ingredients. *Clin Pharmacol Ther* (2000) 68, 468–77.
29. Sigusch H, Henschel L, Kraul H, Merkel U, Hoffman A. Lack of effect of grapefruit juice on diltiazem bioavailability in normal subjects. *Pharmazie* (1994) 49, 675–9.
30. Christensen H, Åsberg A, Holmboe A-B, Berg KJ. Coadministration of grapefruit juice increases systemic exposure of diltiazem in healthy volunteers. *Eur J Clin Pharmacol* (2002) 58, 515–20.
31. Zaidenstein R, Dishi V, Gips M, Soback S, Cohen N, Weissgarten J, Blatt A, Golik A. The effect of grapefruit juice on the pharmacokinetics of orally administered verapamil. *Eur J Clin Pharmacol* (1998) 54, 337–40.
32. Ho P-C, Ghose K, Saville D, Wanwimolruk S. Effect of grapefruit juice on pharmacokinetics and pharmacodynamics of verapamil enantiomers in healthy volunteers. *Eur J Clin Pharmacol* (2000) 56, 693–8.
33. Fuhr U, Müller-Peltzer H, Kern R, Lopez-Rojas P, Jünemann M, Harder S, Staib AH. Effects of grapefruit juice and smoking on verapamil concentrations in steady state. *Eur J Clin Pharmacol* (2002) 58, 45–53.
34. Chayen R, Rosenthal T. Interaction of citrus juices with felodipine and nifedipine. *Lancet* (1991) 337, 854.
35. Bailey DG, Dresser GK, Bend JR. Bergamottin, lime juice, and red wine as inhibitors of cytochrome P450 3A4 activity: comparison with grapefruit juice. *Clin Pharmacol Ther* (2003) 73, 529–37.
36. Goosen TC, Cillié D, Bailey DG, Yu C, He K, Hollenberg PF, Woster PM, Cohen L, Williams JA, Rheeders M, Dijkstra HP. Bergamottin contribution to the grapefruit juice—felodipine interaction and disposition in humans. *Clin Pharmacol Ther* (2004) 76, 607–17.
37. Plendil (Felodipine). AstraZeneca UK Ltd. UK Summary of product characteristics, March 2006.
38. Vascalpha (Felodipine). Actavis UK Ltd. UK Summary of product characteristics, September 2006.
39. Zanidip (Lercanidipine hydrochloride). Recordati Pharmaceuticals Ltd. UK Summary of product characteristics, October 2004.
40. Securon (Verapamil hydrochloride). Abbott Laboratories Ltd. UK Summary of product characteristics, August 2003.
41. Univer (Verapamil hydrochloride). Cephalon Ltd. UK Summary of product characteristics, April 2007.
42. Adalat Retard (Nifedipine). Bayer plc. UK Summary of product characteristics, September 2006.
43. Coracten SR (Nifedipine). UCB Pharma Ltd. UK Summary of product characteristics, June 2005.
44. Syscor MR (Nisoldipine). Forest Laboratories UK Ltd. UK Summary of product characteristics, August 1998.
45. Nimotop (Nimodipine). Bayer plc. UK Summary of product characteristics, August 2005.

Calcium-channel blockers + H_2-receptor antagonists

The plasma levels of diltiazem, isradipine and nifedipine are increased by cimetidine and it may possibly be necessary to reduce the dosages of these calcium-channel blockers. High doses of cimetidine may increase the bioavailability of lercanidipine. Although studies suggest no important interactions occur between nicardipine or nisoldipine and cimetidine, the manufacturers advise caution. Plasma felodipine, lacidipine, nimodipine, and nitrendipine levels are also increased by cimetidine, but this seems to be clinically unimportant. Cimetidine does not interact with amlodipine. It is uncertain whether cimetidine interacts significantly with verapamil. Ranitidine appears to interact only minimally with calcium-channel blockers, if at all. Famotidine does not interact pharmacokinetically with nifedipine.

Clinical evidence

(a) Amlodipine

A crossover study in 12 healthy subjects found that **cimetidine** 400 mg twice daily for 14 days had no effect on the pharmacokinetics of amlodipine 10 mg.[1]

(b) Diltiazem

Cimetidine 300 mg before meals and at bedtime for a week increased the AUC of a single 60-mg oral dose of diltiazem by 50% in 6 healthy subjects and increased peak plasma levels by 57%. **Ranitidine** 150 mg twice daily for a week increased the AUC of diltiazem by 15%, but this was not statistically significant.[2] Increases in the serum levels and AUC of diltiazem of 40% and 25 to 50%, respectively, were seen in another study using **cimetidine**.[3]

(c) Felodipine

Cimetidine 1 g daily increased the AUC of felodipine 10 mg by 56%, and raised the peak serum level by 54% in 12 subjects. There was a short lasting effect on their heart rates but the clinical effects were minimal.[4]

(d) Isradipine

The manufacturer of isradipine[5] notes that **cimetidine** increases the bioavailability of isradipine by about 50%.

(e) Lacidipine

A single 800-mg dose of **cimetidine** increased the maximum plasma level of a single 4-mg dose of lacidipine by 59% and increased the AUC by 74% in one study in healthy subjects. Pulse rates and blood pressures were unaffected.[6]

(f) Lercanidipine

Cimetidine 800 mg daily causes no significant alteration in plasma levels of lercanidipine but the manufacturer says that the bioavailability of lercanidipine and its hypotensive effects may be increased by higher doses of **cimetidine**.[7]

(g) Nicardipine

No adverse interaction was seen in 22 patients given calcium-channel blockers, including nicardipine, with oral **famotidine** for 6 to 8 weeks.[8] No changes in the pharmacokinetics or pharmacodynamics of a 12-hour intravenous infusion of nicardipine 24 mg were seen in 12 healthy subjects given intravenous **cimetidine** 300 mg every 6 hours for 48 hours.[9]

(h) Nifedipine

Cimetidine 1 g daily for a week increased the AUC of nifedipine 40 mg daily by about 60% and increased the maximum plasma levels by about 90%. **Ranitidine** 150 mg twice daily for a week caused an insignificant rise of about 25% in maximum nifedipine plasma levels and AUC.[10] Seven hypertensive patients had a fall in mean blood pressure from 127 to 109 mmHg after taking nifedipine 40 mg daily for 4 weeks, and a further fall to 95 mmHg after they also took **cimetidine** 1 g daily for 3 weeks. When they took **ranitidine** 300 mg instead of cimetidine, there was an insignificant fall in blood pressure.[10,11]

Other studies clearly confirm that **cimetidine** causes a very significant rise in plasma nifedipine levels and an increase in its effects, whereas **ranitidine** interacts only minimally.[12-18]

A study found no pharmacokinetic interaction between nifedipine and **famotidine**, but the **famotidine** reversed the effects of nifedipine on systolic time intervals and significantly reduced the stroke volume and cardiac output.[19,20] No adverse interaction was seen in 22 patients given calcium-channel blockers, including nifedipine, with **famotidine** for 6 to 8 weeks.[8]

(i) Nimodipine

Cimetidine 1 g daily for 7 days increased the bioavailability of nimodipine 30 mg three times daily in 8 healthy subjects by 75%, but the haemodynamic effects were unchanged. **Ranitidine** did not interact.[21]

(j) Nisoldipine

A study in 8 healthy subjects found that taking **cimetidine** 1 g in divided doses on the day before the study and then three 200 mg doses every 4 hours on the study day, increased the bioavailability of a single 10-mg dose of nisoldipine by about 50%, but the haemodynamic effects of the nisoldipine were unaltered.[22] **Ranitidine** does not interact with nisoldipine.[23]

(k) Nitrendipine

Cimetidine 800 mg given before, and 400 mg in divided doses given after, a single 20-mg dose of nitrendipine was found to increase its bioavailability by 154% but the haemodynamic effects were unchanged.[24] Another study found that **ranitidine** increased the AUC of oral nitrendipine 20 mg daily for 1 week by about 50% and decreased its clearance, but there were no changes in the haemodynamic measurements (systolic time intervals, impedance cardiography).[25,26] A further study found that **ranitidine** increases the AUC of nitrendipine by 89%, but this does not appear to be clinically significant.[27]

(l) Verapamil

A study in 8 healthy subjects found that **cimetidine** 300 mg every 6 hours for 8 days did not affect the pharmacokinetics of a single 10-mg intravenous dose of verapamil, but the bioavailability of a 120-mg oral dose of verapamil was increased from 26 to 49%. A small insignificant change in clearance occurred but no change in AUC. The changes in the PR interval caused by the verapamil were unaltered in the presence of **cimetidine**.[28]

Another study found that **cimetidine** 300 mg four times daily for 5 days reduced the clearance of a single intravenous dose of verapamil by 21% and increased its elimination half-life by 50%.[29] **Cimetidine** 400 mg twice daily for a week increased the bioavailability of verapamil from 35 to 42% and its clearance was reduced by almost 30% in another study.[30] A further study found a small increase in the bioavailability of both enantiomers of verapamil.[31] In contrast, other studies have found that the pharmacokinetics of verapamil were unaffected by **cimetidine**.[32,33]

Mechanism

It is believed that cimetidine increases nifedipine levels by inhibiting its oxidative metabolism by the liver. Like ranitidine, it may also increase the bioavailability of nifedipine by lowering gastric acidity.[14] The mechanisms of the other interactions are probably similar.

Importance and management

The interactions of cimetidine with diltiazem and nifedipine are established. Concurrent use need not be avoided but the increase in the calcium-channel blocker effects should be taken into account. It has been suggested that the dosage of diltiazem should be reduced by 30 to 50%[34,35] and that of nifedipine by 40 to 50%.[34,35] The interaction between verapamil and cimetidine is not well established, but monitor the effects until more is known. It has been suggested that the verapamil dose may need to be reduced by 50%.[35] Monitoring is advised if isradipine is given with cimetidine and a reduction in isradipine dose may be required.[5]

Similarly, high doses of cimetidine may increase the hypotensive effects of lercanidipine and caution is advised.[7] The evidence available suggests that, although cimetidine increases the serum levels of felodipine, lacidipine, nimodipine, and nitrendipine, the haemodynamic changes are unimportant. However, this needs confirmation. The manufacturer of nisoldipine warns that the antihypertensive effect may be potentiated by cimetidine,[23] but the study available suggests that this is not significant, Although some studies indicate no interaction between nicardipine and cimetidine, the manufacturer notes that cimetidine increases nicardipine plasma levels and monitoring is recommended.[36] Amlodipine and cimetidine do not interact.

Ranitidine does not interact significantly with diltiazem, nimodipine, nisoldipine or nifedipine, and is possibly a non-interacting alternative for cimetidine with other calcium-channel blockers. Note that the nitrendipine AUC was increased by 50% and 89% by ranitidine, although this was not considered clinically relevant.

Famotidine does not have a pharmacokinetic interaction with nifedipine.

1. Quoted as unpublished data, Pfizer Central Research by Abernethy DR. Amlodipine: pharmacokinetic profile of a low-clearance calcium antagonist. *J Cardiovasc Pharmacol* (1991) 17 (Suppl 1), S4–S7.
2. Winship LC, McKenney JM, Wright JT, Wood JH, Goodman RP. The effect of ranitidine and cimetidine on single-dose diltiazem pharmacokinetics. *Pharmacotherapy* (1985) 5, 16–19.
3. Mazhar M, Popat KD, Sanders C. Effect of cimetidine on diltiazem blood levels. *Clin Res* (1984) 32, 741A.
4. Janzon K, Edgar B, Lundborg P, Regårdh CG. The influence of cimetidine and spironolactone on the pharmacokinetics and haemodynamic effects of felodipine in healthy subjects. *Acta Pharmacol Toxicol (Copenh)* (1986) 59 (Suppl 4), 98.
5. Prescal (Isradipine). Novartis Pharmaceuticals UK Ltd. UK Summary of product characteristics, February 2002.
6. Dewland PM. A study to assess the effect of food and a single 800 mg oral dose of cimetidine on the pharmacokinetics of a single 4 mg oral dose of calcium-channel inhibitor, GR43659X (lacidipine). Boehringer Ingelheim report GMH/88/030.
7. Zanidip (Lercanidipine hydrochloride). Recordati Pharmaceuticals Ltd. UK Summary of product characteristics, October 2004.
8. Chichmanian RM, Mignot G, Spreux A, Jean-Girard C, Hofliger P. Tolérance de la famotidine. Étude du réseau médecins sentinelles en pharmacovigilance. *Therapie* (1992) 47, 239–43.
9. Lai C-M, McEntegart CM, Maher KE, Bell VA, Turlapaty P, Quon CY. The effects of iv cimetidine on the pharmacokinetics (PK) and pharmacodynamics (PD) of iv nicardipine in man. *Pharm Res* (1994) 11 (Suppl 10), S386.
10. Kirch W, Janisch HD, Heidemann H, Rämsch K, Ohnhaus EE. Einfluss von Cimetidin und Ranitidin auf Pharmakokinetik und antihypertensiven Effekt von Nifedipin. *Dtsch Med Wochenschr* (1983) 108, 1757–61.
11. Kirch W, Rämsch K, Janisch HD, Ohnhaus EE. The influence of two histamine H_2-receptor antagonists, cimetidine and ranitidine, on the plasma levels and clinical effect of nifedipine and metoprolol. *Arch Toxicol* (1984) (Suppl 7), 256–9.
12. Kirch W, Hoensch H, Ohnhaus EE, Janisch HD. Ranitidin-Nifedipin-Interaktion. *Dtsch Med Wochenschr* (1984) 109, 1223.
13. Smith SR, Kendall MJ, Lobo J, Beerahee A, Jack DB, Wilkins MR. Ranitidine and cimetidine: drug interactions with single dose and steady-state nifedipine administration. *Br J Clin Pharmacol* (1987) 23, 311–15.
14. Adams LJ, Antonow DR, McClain CJ, McAllister R. Effect of ranitidine on bioavailability of nifedipine. *Gastroenterology* (1986) 90, 1320.
15. Kirch W, Ohnhaus EE, Hoensch H, Janisch HD. Ranitidine increases bioavailability of nifedipine. *Clin Pharmacol Ther* (1985) 37, 204.
16. Schwartz JB, Upton RA, Lin ET, Williams RL, Benet LZ. Effect of cimetidine or ranitidine administration on nifedipine pharmacokinetics and pharmacodynamics. *Clin Pharmacol Ther* (1988) 43, 673–80.
17. Renwick AG, Le Vie J, Challenor VF, Waller DG, Gruchy B, George CF. Factors affecting the pharmacokinetics of nifedipine. *Eur J Clin Pharmacol* (1987) 32, 351–5.
18. Khan A, Langley SJ, Mullins FGP, Dixon JS, Toon S. The pharmacokinetics and pharmacodynamics of nifedipine at steady state during concomitant administration of cimetidine or high dose ranitidine. *Br J Clin Pharmacol* (1991) 32, 519–22.
19. Kirch W, Halabi A, Linde M, Ohnhaus EE. Negativ-inotrope Wirkung von Famotidin. *Schweiz Med Wochenschr* (1988) 118, 1912–14.
20. Kirch W, Halabi A, Linde M, Santos SR, Ohnhaus EE. Negative effects of famotidine on cardiac performance assessed by noninvasive hemodynamic measurements. *Gastroenterology* (1989) 96, 1388–92.
21. Mück W, Wingender W, Seiberling M, Woelke E, Rämsch K-D, Kuhlmann J. Influence of the H2-receptor antagonists cimetidine and ranitidine on the pharmacokinetics of nimodipine in healthy volunteers. *Eur J Clin Pharmacol* (1992) 42, 325–8.
22. Van Harten J, van Brummelen P, Lodewijks MTM, Danhof M, Breimer DD. Pharmacokinetics and hemodynamic effects of nisoldipine and its interaction with cimetidine. *Clin Pharmacol Ther* (1988) 43, 332–41.
23. Syscor MR (Nisoldipine). Forest Laboratories UK Ltd. UK Summary of product characteristics, August 1998.
24. Soons PA, Vogels BAPM, Roosemalen MCM, Schoemaker HC, Uchida E, Edgar B, Lundahl J, Cohen AF, Breimer DD. Grapefruit juice and cimetidine inhibit stereoselective metabolism of nitrendipine in humans. *Clin Pharmacol Ther* (1991) 50, 394–403.
25. Kirch W, Nahoui R, Ohnhaus EE. Ranitidine/nitrendipine interaction. *Clin Pharmacol Ther* (1988) 43, 149.
26. Halabi A, Nahoui R, Kirch W. Influence of ranitidine on kinetics of nitrendipine and on noninvasive hemodynamic parameters. *Ther Drug Monit* (1990) 12, 303–4.
27. Santos SR, Storpirtis S, Moreira-Filho L, Donzella H, Kirch W. Ranitidine increases the bioavailability of nitrendipine in patients with arterial hypertension. *Braz J Med Biol Res* (1992) 25, 337–47.
28. Smith MS, Benyunes MC, Bjornsson TD, Shand DG, Pritchett ELC. Influence of cimetidine on verapamil kinetics and dynamics. *Clin Pharmacol Ther* (1984) 36, 551–4.
29. Loi C-M, Rollins DE, Dukes GE, Peat MA. Effect of cimetidine on verapamil disposition. *Clin Pharmacol Ther* (1985) 37, 654–7.
30. Mikus G, Stuber H. Influence of cimetidine treatment on the physiological disposition of verapamil. *Naunyn Schmiedebergs Arch Pharmacol* (1987) 335 (Suppl), R106.
31. Mikus G, Eichelbaum M, Fischer C, Gumulka S, Klotz U, Kroemer HK. Interaction of verapamil and cimetidine: stereochemical aspects of drug metabolism, drug disposition and drug action. *J Pharmacol Exp Ther* (1990) 253, 1042–8.
32. Abernethy DR, Schwartz JB, Todd EL. Lack of interaction between verapamil and cimetidine. *Clin Pharmacol Ther* (1985) 38, 342–9.
33. Wing LMH, Miners JO, Lillywhite KJ. Verapamil disposition—effects of sulphinpyrazone and cimetidine. *Br J Clin Pharmacol* (1985) 19, 385–91.
34. Piepho RW, Culbertson VL, Rhodes RS. Drug interactions with the calcium-entry blockers. *Circulation* (1987) 75 (Suppl V), V181–V194.
35. Piepho RW. Individualization of calcium entry–blocker dosage for systemic hypertension. *Am J Cardiol* (1985) 56, 105H–111H.
36. Cardene SR (Nicardipine hydrochloride). Yamanouchi Pharma Ltd. UK Summary of product characteristics, June 2006.

Calcium-channel blockers + Macrolides

Erythromycin markedly increases the bioavailability of felodipine. Isolated reports describe increased felodipine, nifedipine or verapamil effects and toxicity in patients also given erythromycin. There are also a few reports of verapamil toxicity with clarithromycin, and one with telithromycin.

A prolonged QT interval in one patient may have been due to increased levels of erythromycin in the presence of verapamil. A retrospective analysis revealed 3 cases of sudden cardiac death in patients taking erythromycin with diltiazem or verapamil, which represented about a fivefold increase in risk. No increased risk was seen with nifedipine and erythromycin.

Clinical evidence

(a) Diltiazem

A patient who had marked hypotension and bradycardia when **erythromycin** was added to verapamil and propranolol (see under verapamil, below) had previously taken **erythromycin** with diltiazem and a beta blocker without any reported adverse effects.[1]

In a retrospective cohort study, there was one sudden cardiac death in 106 person-years among patients taking diltiazem with **erythromycin**. When combined with the two deaths with concurrent verapamil and **erythromycin**, this represented about a fivefold increase in risk of sudden death when compared with those who used neither CYP3A4 inhibitors (defined as ketoconazole, itraconazole, fluconazole, diltiazem, verapamil or troleandomycin) nor **erythromycin**.[2]

(b) Felodipine

Twelve healthy subjects were given felodipine 10 mg before and after taking **erythromycin** 250 mg four times daily for a day.[3] The felodipine AUC was increased almost threefold by the **erythromycin**, the maximum plasma levels were more than doubled and the half-life prolonged from 6.9 to 11.1 hours.[3]

A hypertensive woman taking felodipine 10 mg daily developed tachycardia, flushing and massive ankle oedema within 2 to 3 days of starting to take **erythromycin** 250 mg twice daily. Her blood pressure had fallen from 120/90 to 110/70 mmHg. She fully recovered within a few days of stopping the **erythromycin**.[4]

(c) Nifedipine

1. Clarithromycin. A 77-year-old man taking sustained-release nifedipine 60 mg twice daily, captopril and doxazosin, and with slight renal impairment, had persistent systolic hypertension (170 to 180 mmHg). Two days after starting clarithromycin 500 mg twice daily for breathing difficulty and cough, his blood pressure was 140/70 mmHg at a routine appointment, and the doxazosin dose was halved and valsartan substituted for captopril. Later that day, he was admitted with hypotension (80/40 mmHg) and bradycardia (40 bpm). Clarithromycin was replaced with erythromycin and the antihypertensives stopped. After 3 days his blood pressure was stabilised with nifedipine 60 mg daily and furosemide, and the clarithromycin was restarted. Septic shock was ruled out as a cause of the hypotension.[5]

2. Erythromycin. In a retrospective cohort study, there were no sudden deaths from cardiac causes in 114 person-years of the use of oral erythromycin with calcium-channel blockers that do not inhibit CYP3A4 to a clinically relevant extent (stated as nearly all nifedipine).[2] This was in contrast to the increased risk of sudden death with erythromycin and diltiazem (see above) or verapamil (see below).

(d) Verapamil

1. Clarithromycin. A 53-year-old woman on haemodialysis 3 times a week, and a range of medicines including digoxin, was given clarithromycin 250 mg and verapamil 120 mg both twice daily because of an acute exacerbation of chronic obstructive pulmonary disease and a recurrence of atrial fibrillation. After 24 hours she experienced dizziness and episodes of fainting. A day later her supine blood pressure was 89/39 mmHg and her pulse rate 50 bpm. Verapamil was stopped and she recovered within 2 days, after which verapamil was re-started at a dose of 40 mg before each dialysis session.[6] Another report[1] describes a 77-year-old woman with hypertension, taking propranolol and verapamil, who developed marked bradycardia (37 to 50 bpm), within 4 days of starting a course of clarithromycin 500 mg twice daily. The problem was solved by temporarily reducing the dose of the verapamil from 80 mg to 40 mg twice daily and the propranolol to a half until the clarithromycin course was over. Essentially the same thing happened 2 years later while taking the same drugs when erythromycin was added (see below).

2. Erythromycin. A 79-year-old woman taking verapamil 240 mg twice daily and ramipril was admitted to hospital with extreme fatigue and dizziness one week after starting a course of erythromycin 2 g daily for a respiratory-tract infection. Her blood pressure was 80/60 mmHg and her respiratory rate was 18 breaths per minute. ECG showed complete AV block, escape rhythm of 50 bpm, pattern of left bundle-branch block and QTc interval prolongation (583 milliseconds compared with 436 milliseconds 20 days before admission). Verapamil and erythromycin were stopped and intravenous fluids, dopamine and calcium were given. Her blood pressure increased to 110/70 mmHg and after 4 days the QTc interval prolongation had resolved and her heart rate was 76 bpm.[7] Another patient taking verapamil and propranolol developed marked bradycardia and hypotension 2 days after starting to take erythromycin 333 mg three times daily.[1] Two years previously she had experienced a similar interaction with clarithromycin and verapamil, but not with erythromycin and diltiazem (see above).

In a retrospective cohort study, there were two sudden cardiac deaths in 78 person-years among patients taking verapamil with erythromycin. When combined with the one death with current diltiazem and erythromycin, this represented about a fivefold increase in risk of sudden death when compared with those who used neither CYP3A4 inhibitors (defined as ketoconazole, itraconazole, fluconazole, diltiazem, verapamil or troleandomycin) nor erythromycin.[2]

3. Telithromycin. A 76-year-old woman taking verapamil 180 mg daily experienced shortness of breath and weakness 2 days after starting telithromycin 800 mg daily for a sinus infection. She was found to have marked hypotension (systolic BP 50 to 60 mmHg) and bradycardia (30 bpm). She required a transvenous pacemaker for 3 days and pressor drugs.[8]

Mechanism

Calcium-channel blockers are metabolised in the gut wall and liver by the cytochrome P450 CYP3A subfamily of isoenzymes, which are inhibited by erythromycin, clarithromycin, and telithromycin, so that in their presence a normal oral dose becomes in effect an overdose with its attendant adverse effects.[1,3,4,8] Verapamil, erythromycin[7] and possibly clarithromycin are also P-glycoprotein inhibitors, which may contribute to the pharmacokinetic interaction by reducing the elimination of the calcium-channel blocker,[6] or by increasing macrolide absorption.[7]

Erythromycin has been associated with prolongation of the QT interval; an effect that is likely to be increased by drugs that increase erythromycin levels such as diltiazem and verapamil.[2]

Importance and management

Information seems to be limited but the interaction would appear to be established and clinically important, although its incidence is probably low. Anticipate the need to reduce the felodipine or verapamil dosage if erythromycin or clarithromycin, or possibly also telithromycin, is added. Nifedipine may also interact. Other reports suggests that the cardiac toxicity of erythromycin may be increased by verapamil,[2,7] and diltiazem,[2] and the authors of one of these reports consider that erythromycin should not be used with CYP3A4 inhibitors (that is diltiazem and verapamil).[2] There seem to be no reports of interactions between any of the other calcium-channel blockers and macrolides. However, because of the theoretical possibility of an interaction, many of the manufacturers of calcium-channel blockers warn of the possibility of increased plasma levels and the need to either avoid use with macrolides such as erythromycin, or **troleandomycin**, or to monitor and reduce doses where necessary.

1. Steenbergen JA, Stauffer VL. Potential macrolide interaction with verapamil. *Ann Pharmacother* (1998) 32, 387–8.
2. Ray WA, Murray KT, Meredith S, Narasimhulu SS, Hall K, Stein CM. Oral erythromycin and the risk of sudden death from cardiac causes. *N Engl J Med* (2004) 351, 1089–96.
3. Bailey DG, Bend JR, Arnold JMO, Tran LT, Spence JD. Erythromycin-felodipine interaction: magnitude, mechanism, and comparison with grapefruit juice. *Clin Pharmacol Ther* (1996) 60, 25–33.
4. Liedholm H, Nordin G. Erythromycin–felodipine interaction. *DICP Ann Pharmacother* (1991) 25, 1007–8.
5. Gerónimo-Pardo M, Cuartero-del-Pozo AB, Jiménez-Vizuete JM, Cortiñas-Sáez M, Peyró-García R. Clarithromycin-nifedipine interaction as possible cause of vasodilatory shock. *Ann Pharmacother* (2005) 39, 538–42.
6. Kaeser YA, Brunner F, Drewe J, Haefeli WE. Severe hypotension and bradycardia associated with verapamil and clarithromycin. *Am J Health-Syst Pharm* (1998) 55, 2417–18.
7. Goldschmidt N, Azaz-Livshits T, Gotsman I, Nir-Paz R, Ben-Yehuda A, Muszkat M. Compound cardiac toxicity of oral erythromycin and verapamil. *Ann Pharmacother* (2001) 35, 1396–9.
8. Reed M, Wall GC, Shah NP, Heun JM, Hicklin GA. Verapamil toxicity resulting from a probable interaction with telithromycin. *Ann Pharmacother* (2005) 39, 357–60.

Calcium-channel blockers + Magnesium compounds

Two pregnant women developed bilateral hand contractures after receiving magnesium sulfate either alone or with nifedipine. Two other pregnant women developed muscular weakness and then paralysis when they were given both nifedipine and intravenous magnesium sulfate. Profound hypotension occurred in two women when nifedipine was added to magnesium sulfate and

methyldopa. However, a retrospective study found no significant increase in neuromuscular weakness in women treated with both magnesium sulfate and nifedipine compared with magnesium sulfate and no antihypertensive, and the incidence of hypotension was actually lower.

Clinical evidence

(a) Hypotension

Two women with pre-eclampsia, unsuccessfully treated with methyldopa and magnesium sulfate, experienced severe hypotension when a single 10-mg oral dose of **nifedipine** was added.[1] In contrast, a study in 10 women with severe pre-eclampsia receiving magnesium sulfate found that oral **nifedipine** 10 mg followed by 20 mg every 20 minutes, caused a steady decrease in mean arterial pressure and severe hypotension was not observed.[2] Moreover, in a retrospective study, the incidence of hypotension in 162 women given **nifedipine** and magnesium sulfate was lower than in 183 receiving magnesium sulfate and no antihypertensive (41.4% versus 53%).[3] For further details of this study, see (b) below.

(b) Neuromuscular blockade and hypocalcaemia

A report describes symptomatic hypocalcaemia (serum calcium levels 5.4 mg/dL) in a woman at 33 weeks gestation after she received magnesium sulfate plus **nifedipine**.[4] However, this report also describes this effect in a patient taking magnesium sulfate alone. Both women experienced bilateral hand contractures and were successfully treated with calcium gluconate.[4]

A pregnant woman at 32 weeks gestation was effectively treated for premature uterine contractions with **nifedipine**, 60 mg orally over 3 hours, and later 20 mg every 8 hours. When contractions began again 12 hours later she was given magnesium sulfate 500 mg intravenously. She developed jerky movements of the extremities, complained of difficulty in swallowing, paradoxical respirations and an inability to lift her head from the pillow. The magnesium was stopped and the muscle weakness disappeared over the next 25 minutes.[5]

A woman at 28 weeks gestation with mild pre-eclampsia was started on an infusion of magnesium sulfate 2 g/hour. Her plasma magnesium levels were found to be 2.75 mmol/L. No untoward reactions developed when she took a 20-mg dose of **nifedipine**, but 30 minutes after taking a second dose [by implication 3 to 4 hours later] she complained of flushing and sweating and had difficulty in lifting her head and limbs. Shortly afterwards almost complete muscular paralysis developed. The magnesium sulfate was stopped and a dramatic improvement followed within 15 minutes of a 1-g intravenous injection of calcium gluconate.[6]

In contrast, a retrospective analysis found no increased risk of serious magnesium-related maternal adverse effects in 162 women with pre-eclampsia who were also treated with **nifedipine** compared with 32 women receiving another antihypertensive or 183 who received no antihypertensive. The women receiving **nifedipine** had more severe pre-eclampsia and a longer magnesium sulfate infusion. However, the incidence of neuromuscular weakness was 53.1% in these women compared with 53.1% in those receiving another antihypertensive and 44.8% in those receiving no antihypertensive. These differences were not statistically significant. Moreover, the incidence of maternal hypotension was lower in those receiving **nifedipine** than in those receiving no antihypertensive (see (a) above).[3]

Mechanism

The probable reason for neuromuscular effects is that both drugs can seriously reduce the amount of calcium ions needed for normal muscular contraction. Nifedipine inhibits the inflow of extracellular calcium across cell membranes. Magnesium probably acts in the same way, and also reduces intracellular calcium by activating adenyl cyclase and increasing cAMP. In addition magnesium stimulates calcium-dependent ATPase which promotes calcium uptake by the sarcoplasmic reticulum. The result is muscular paralysis, which is reversed by giving large amounts of calcium. Magnesium sulfate is also known to have neuromuscular blocking activity. Both drugs can also cause hypotension, which could be additive.

Importance and management

Direct information on the neuromuscular effects and hypotensive effects of the combination of nifedipine and magnesium seems to be limited. Although a few cases of possible additive effects have been reported, one large retrospective study did not find an increase in risk of neuromuscular effects or of hypotension with combined use. Nevertheless, at least one manufacturer of nifedipine advises particular caution when it is used in combination with intravenous magnesium sulfate in pregnant women.[7] The same interaction would be expected to occur with other calcium-channel blockers.

1. Waisman GD, Mayorga LM, Cámera MI, Vignolo CA, Martinotti A. Magnesium plus nifedipine: potentiation of hypotensive effect in preeclampsia? *Am J Obstet Gynecol* (1988) 159, 308–9.
2. Scardo JA, Vermillion ST, Hogg BB, Newman RB. Hemodynamic effects of oral nifedipine in preeclamptic hypertensive emergencies. *Am J Obstet Gynecol* (1996) 175, 336–8.
3. Magee LA, Miremadi S, Li J, Cheng C, Ensom MHH, Carleton B, Coté A-M, von Dadelszen P. Therapy with both magnesium sulfate and nifedipine does not increase the risk of serious magnesium-related maternal side effects in women with preeclampsia. *Am J Obstet Gynecol* (2005) 193, 153–63.
4. Koontz SL, Friedman SA, Schwartz ML. Symptomatic hypocalcemia after tocolytic therapy with magnesium sulfate and nifedipine. *Am J Obstet Gynecol* (2004) 190, 1773–6.
5. Snyder SW, Cardwell MS. Neuromuscular blockade with magnesium sulfate and nifedipine. *Am J Obstet Gynecol* (1989) 161, 35–6.
6. Ben-Ami M, Giladi Y, Shalev E. The combination of magnesium sulphate and nifedipine: a cause of neuromuscular blockade. *Br J Obstet Gynaecol* (1994) 101, 262–3.
7. Adalat Retard (Nifedipine). Bayer plc. UK Summary of product characteristics, September 2006.

Calcium-channel blockers + Nitrates

Enhanced hypotensive effects may occur when calcium-channel blockers are given with nitrates. The manufacturers of amlodipine say that long-acting nitrates and sublingual glyceryl trinitrate have been given safely with amlodipine.[1] Increased hypotensive effects and faintness due to additive vasodilating effects have been noted when diltiazem has been given with nitrate derivatives. In patients treated with calcium-channel blockers, the dosage of concurrent nitrate derivatives should be increased gradually.[2]

1. Istin (Amlodipine besilate). Pfizer Ltd. UK Summary of product characteristics, July 2007.
2. Tildiem Retard (Diltiazem hydrochloride). Sanofi-Aventis. UK Summary of product characteristics, April 2004.

Calcium-channel blockers + Phenobarbital

Limited evidence suggests that phenobarbital greatly reduces the levels and/or increases the clearance of felodipine, nifedipine, nimodipine, and verapamil. Other calcium-channel blockers are expected to be similarly affected.

Clinical evidence

(a) Felodipine

After taking felodipine 10 mg daily for 4 days, 10 epileptics (including one who was taking phenobarbital) had markedly reduced plasma felodipine levels (peak levels of 1.6 nanomol/L compared with 8.9 nanomol/L in 12 control subjects). The felodipine bioavailability was reduced to 6.6%.[1]

(b) Nifedipine

After taking phenobarbital 100 mg daily for 2 weeks the clearance of a single 20-mg dose of nifedipine in a 'cocktail' also containing sparteine, mephenytoin and antipyrine was increased almost threefold in 15 healthy subjects. The nifedipine AUC was reduced by about 60%.[2]

(c) Nimodipine

A study in 8 epileptic patients receiving long-term antiepileptic treatment (including 4 who were taking phenobarbital and 2 who were taking phenobarbital with carbamazepine) found that the AUC of a single 60-mg oral dose of nimodipine was only about 15% of that obtained from a group of healthy subjects.[3]

(d) Verapamil

A study in 7 healthy subjects found phenobarbital 100 mg daily for 3 weeks increased the clearance of verapamil 80 mg every 6 hours four-fold and reduced the bioavailability fivefold.[4]

Mechanism

Phenobarbital is an enzyme inducer which can increase the metabolism of the calcium-channel blockers by the cytochrome P450 isoenzyme CYP3A4 in the liver, resulting in lower serum levels.

Importance and management

Phenobarbital markedly reduces felodipine, nifedipine and verapamil levels. A considerable increase in the dosage of these calcium-channel blockers will probably be needed in patients taking phenobarbital. Nimodipine effects are also markedly reduced by phenobarbital and the manufacturer contraindicates concurrent use.[5] There is no direct information of interactions with other calcium-channel blockers, but as they are largely metabolised in the same way (see 'calcium-channel blockers', (p.860)) they would all be expected to interact similarly.

1. Capewell S, Freestone S, Critchley JAJH, Pottage A, Prescott LF. Reduced felodipine bioavailability in patients taking anticonvulsants. *Lancet* (1988) ii, 480–2.
2. Schellens JHM, van der Wart JHF, Brugman M, Breimer DD. Influence of enzyme induction and inhibition on the oxidation of nifedipine, sparteine, mephenytoin and antipyrine in humans assessed by a "cocktail" study design. *J Pharmacol Exp Ther* (1989) 249, 638–45.
3. Tartara A, Galimberti CA, Manni R, Parietti L, Zucca C, Baasch H, Caresia L, Mück W, Barzaghi N, Gatti G, Perucca E. Differential effects of valproic acid and enzyme-inducing anticonvulsants on nimodipine pharmacokinetics in epileptic patients. *Br J Clin Pharmacol* (1991) 32, 335–40.
4. Rutledge DR, Pieper JA, Sirmans SM, Mirvis DM. Verapamil disposition after phenobarbital treatment. *Clin Pharmacol Ther* (1987) 41, 245.
5. Nimotop (Nimodipine). Bayer plc. UK Summary of product characteristics, August 2005.

Calcium-channel blockers + Protease inhibitors

Symptomatic orthostasis occurred in a patient taking nelfinavir or ritonavir/indinavir and nifedipine. Another patient had similar symptoms when nelfinavir was added to felodipine therapy. Atazanavir markedly increased diltiazem bioavailability with an increase in cardiac effects in healthy subjects. Similarly, ritonavir/indinavir caused a modest to marked increase in diltiazem levels, and a 1.9-fold increase in amlodipine levels. Based on this evidence, raised calcium-channel blocker levels are predicted when any calcium-channel blocker is given with a protease inhibitor, especially ritonavir. Caution is required.

Clinical evidence

(a) Amlodipine

Ritonavir/indinavir 100/800 mg twice daily given with amlodipine 5 mg daily for 7 days increased the median AUC of amlodipine by 1.9-fold in 13 healthy subjects. Amlodipine had no effect on the steady-state AUCs of the protease inhibitors.[1]

(b) Diltiazem

1. Atazanavir. A study in healthy subjects found that atazanavir 400 mg once daily given with diltiazem 180 mg once daily resulted in a two- to threefold increase in the bioavailability of diltiazem and its metabolite desacetyl-diltiazem. The pharmacokinetics of atazanavir were not affected by diltiazem. There was an increase in the maximum PR interval with combined use compared to that found with atazanavir alone.[2,3]

2. Ritonavir with Indinavir. Ritonavir/indinavir 100/800 mg twice daily given with diltiazem 120 mg daily for 7 days modestly increased the median AUC of diltiazem by 27% (not statistically significant) in 13 healthy subjects. However, two of the subjects had a fourfold increase in the AUC of diltiazem, and the desacetyl-diltiazem AUC increased by 102%. Diltiazem had no effect on the steady-state AUCs of the protease inhibitors.[1]

(c) Felodipine

A woman taking metoprolol 50 mg daily and felodipine 5 mg daily for hypertension developed bilateral leg oedema, orthostatic hypotension, and other symptoms including dizziness and fatigue, 3 days after starting HAART following a needle-stick injury. The antiretroviral therapy included zidovudine, lamivudine, and **nelfinavir** 2 g daily. Antihypertensive treatment was stopped and the adverse effects abated within 3 days. The patient was then successfully switched to a diuretic-based regimen without recurrence of oedema.[4]

(d) Nifedipine

A 51-year-old HIV positive man with coronary artery disease, hypertension and osteoarthritis, and taking atenolol, was started on extended-release nifedipine 60 mg daily. When his blood pressure control improved he was started on zidovudine 300 mg, lamivudine 150 mg, and **nelfinavir** 1.25 g all twice daily. Within 3 days of starting the antiretroviral therapy he experienced dizziness, weakness and hypotension and developed complete heart block with a junctional escape rhythm. His ECG returned to normal within 24 hours of stopping the antiretroviral therapy, but he developed orthostatic symptoms within 2 days of restarting **nelfinavir**. He later tolerated a regimen consisting of stavudine, didanosine and efavirenz without any episodes of dizziness, hypotension or bradycardia. However, when he was given zidovudine, abacavir, **ritonavir**, and **indinavir**, he experienced hypotension, decreased heart rate, weakness and fatigue. His symptoms were controlled by modifying his antihypertensive therapy, including discontinuation of atenolol and reduction of the dose of nifedipine to 30 mg daily.[5]

Mechanism

Protease inhibitors, particularly ritonavir (see 'Antivirals', (p.772)), are potent inhibitors of cytochrome P450 isoenzyme CYP3A4, by which all the calcium-channel blockers are extensively metabolised. It appears that some protease inhibitors can cause a clinically relevant increase in calcium-channel blocker levels. In addition, verapamil, diltiazem and nicardipine can also inhibit CYP3A4, and might therefore theoretically reduce the metabolism of the protease inhibitors. However, the effect might depend on which is the more potent inhibitor, since, in the studies above, diltiazem did not affect atazanavir, indinavir or ritonavir levels.

Importance and management

Although information is limited, these pharmacokinetic interactions are predictable, and potentially serious. To date, clinically relevant increases in calcium-channel blocker levels or effects have been shown for nelfinavir with nifedipine or felodipine, indinavir/ritonavir with amlodipine, diltiazem or nifedipine, and atazanavir with diltiazem. Caution would be required with any of these combinations, anticipating the need to use lower doses of the calcium-channel blocker. The manufacturers specifically recommend that if diltiazem is given with **atazanavir** the initial dose of diltiazem should be reduced by 50% with subsequent dose titration and ECG monitoring.[2,3] They also note that **verapamil** levels may be raised and therefore advise caution.[2,3] Similarly, the manufacturers of nifedipine say that blood pressure monitoring is required and a reduction in nifedipine dose may be necessary if it is given with HIV-protease inhibitors.[6,7] However, some UK manufacturers (e.g. felodipine,[8] **lercanidipine**,[9] **nimodipine**[10]) recommend avoiding the concurrent use of ritonavir and other protease inhibitors if possible.

Until more is known, caution is warranted with any combination of a calcium-channel blocker and a protease inhibitor.

1. Glesby MJ, Aberg JA, Kendall MA, Fichtenbaum CJ, Hafner R, Hall S, Grosskopf N, Zolopa AR, Gerber JG. Pharmacokinetic interactions between indinavir plus ritonavir and calcium channel blockers. *Clin Pharmacol Ther* (2005) 78, 143–53.
2. Reyataz (Atazanavir sulfate). Bristol-Myers Squibb Pharmaceuticals Ltd. UK Summary of product characteristics, April 2007.
3. Reyataz (Atazanavir sulfate). Bristol-Myers Squibb Company. US Prescribing information, March 2007.
4. Izzedine H, Launay-Vacher V, Deray G, Hulot J-S. Nelfinavir and felodipine: A cytochrome P450 3A4-mediated drug interaction. *Clin Pharmacol Ther* (2004) 75, 362–3.
5. Rossi DR, Rathbun RC, Slater LN. Symptomatic orthostasis with extended-release nifedipine and protease inhibitors. *Pharmacotherapy* (2002) 22, 1312–16.
6. Adalat Retard (Nifedipine). Bayer plc. UK Summary of product characteristics, September 2006.
7. Adalat CC (Nifedipine). Bayer HealthCare. US Prescribing information, August 2005.
8. Vascalpha (Felodipine). Actavis UK Ltd. UK Summary of product characteristics, September 2006.
9. Zanidip (Lercanidipine hydrochloride). Recordati Pharmaceuticals Ltd. UK Summary of product characteristics, October 2004.
10. Nimotop (Nimodipine). Bayer plc. UK Summary of product characteristics, August 2005.

Calcium-channel blockers + Proton pump inhibitors

The clearance of both nifedipine and omeprazole is modestly reduced by their concurrent use, but these changes seem unlikely to be of clinical importance. Pantoprazole does not affect the pharmacokinetics of nifedipine.

Clinical evidence, mechanism, importance and management

(a) Omeprazole

After taking omeprazole 20 mg daily for 7 days the clearance of **nifedipine** was reduced 21% in 10 healthy subjects. The same subjects had a

14% reduction in the clearance of a 40-mg intravenous dose of omeprazole after 5 days of treatment with **nifedipine** 10 mg three times daily.[1] In a related study, the same group of workers found that omeprazole 20 mg daily for 8 days increased the AUC of a single 10-mg dose of **nifedipine** by 26%, but no changes in blood pressures or heart rates were seen.[2] None of these changes is large and they seem not to be of clinical importance.

(b) Pantoprazole

In an open, randomised, crossover study, 24 healthy subjects were given pantoprazole 40 mg daily for 10 days, with sustained-release **nifedipine** 20 mg twice daily from day 6 to 10. The pharmacokinetics of the **nifedipine** were unchanged by the pantoprazole.[3] No special precautions would seem to be necessary if pantoprazole and **nifedipine** are given concurrently.

1. Danhof M, Soons PA, van den Berg G, Van Brummelen P, Jansen JBMJ. Interactions between nifedipine and omeprazole. *Eur J Clin Pharmacol* (1989) 36 (Suppl), A258.
2. Soons PA, van den Berg G, Danhof M, van Brummelen P, Jansen JBMJ, Lamers CBHW, Breimer DD. Influence of single- and multiple-dose omeprazole treatment on nifedipine pharmacokinetics and effects in healthy subjects. *Eur J Clin Pharmacol* (1992) 42, 319–24.
3. Bliesath H, Huber R, Steinijans VW, Koch HJ, Kunz K, Wurst W. Pantoprazole does not interact with nifedipine in man under steady-state conditions. *Int J Clin Pharmacol Ther* (1996) 34, 51–5.

Calcium-channel blockers + Quinupristin/Dalfopristin

Quinupristin/dalfopristin modestly increased the AUC of nifedipine. Other calcium-channel blockers are predicted to be similarly affected.

Clinical evidence, mechanism, importance and management

The manufacturers note that the AUC of repeated-dose **nifedipine** was increased 1.4-fold by quinupristin/dalfopristin, and the maximum level was increased by 1.18-fold.[1] This is probably because quinupristin/dalfopristin inhibits the cytochrome P450 isoenzyme CYP3A4-mediated metabolism of **nifedipine**.[2] Although the clinical relevance of these increases have not been assessed, the manufacturers advise blood pressure monitoring and, if necessary, a reduction of **nifedipine** dosage during concurrent use.[1,3] It is predicted that other calcium-channel blockers (e.g. **verapamil**, **diltiazem**) will also have their levels raised by quinupristin/dalfopristin.[2]

1. Adalat CC (Nifedipine). Bayer HealthCare. US Prescribing information, August 2005.
2. Rubinstein E, Prokocimer P, Talbot GH. Safety and tolerability of quinupristin/dalfopristin: administration guidelines. *J Antimicrob Chemother* (1999) 44 (Suppl A) 37–46.
3. Adalat Retard (Nifedipine). Bayer plc. UK Summary of product characteristics, September 2006.

Calcium-channel blockers + Rifampicin (Rifampin)

Rifampicin markedly reduces the plasma levels of diltiazem, nifedipine, nilvadipine, verapamil and possibly reduces those of barnidipine, isradipine, lercanidipine, manidipine, nicardipine, nimodipine, and nisoldipine. They may become therapeutically ineffective unless the dose of the calcium-channel blocker is raised. Rifapentine and rifabutin would also be expected to reduce the levels of the calcium-channel blockers.

Clinical evidence

(a) Barnidipine and Manidipine

A brief report states that elderly patients with hypertension well-controlled with calcium-channel blockers including barnidipine or manidipine had blood pressure rises when rifampicin was added. Increased dosages or additional antihypertensives were needed to control the blood pressures, and reduced doses were required when the rifampicin was withdrawn.[1]

(b) Diltiazem

A study in 12 subjects found that the peak serum level following a single 120-mg oral dose of diltiazem alone was 186 nanograms/mL, but after taking rifampicin 600 mg daily for 8 days maximum serum diltiazem levels were less than 8 nanograms/mL.[2] One patient with angina controlled with diltiazem 120 mg daily began to feel chest pain at rest one month after starting rifampicin and isoniazid. Nifedipine was also not effective in this man while he was taking rifampicin.[3]

(c) Nifedipine

A woman with hypertension well controlled with nifedipine 40 mg twice daily, had a blood pressure rise from under 160/90 mmHg to 200/110 mmHg within 2 weeks of starting to take antitubercular treatment, which included rifampicin 450 mg daily. When the rifampicin was stopped and then restarted, the blood pressure fell and then rose again. The peak nifedipine plasma levels and the AUC fell by about 60% in the presence of rifampicin.[4] Another patient had anginal attacks refractory to both diltiazem and nifedipine while taking rifampicin, but which were controlled by nifedipine when the rifampicin was stopped. Restarting rifampicin reduced nifedipine levels (peak plasma levels and AUCs roughly halved) and increased the number of anginal attacks.[3] Yet another patient taking nifedipine had a loss of blood pressure control when given rifampicin.[5]

Six healthy subjects were given nifedipine 20 micrograms/kg intravenously and nifedipine 20 mg orally on separate days before and after taking rifampicin 600 mg daily for 7 days. The pharmacokinetics of the intravenous nifedipine were not significantly changed by the rifampicin, but the oral clearance increased from 1.5 to 20.9 L/minute and the bioavailability fell from 41.2 to 5.3%.[6] A pharmacokinetic study in 6 healthy subjects found that when a single 10-mg oral dose of nifedipine was taken 8 hours after a single 1.2-g dose of rifampicin its bioavailability was reduced to 36%, its half-life was more than halved and its clearance increased threefold.[7]

(d) Nilvadipine

A study in 5 healthy normotensive subjects found that rifampicin 450 mg daily for 6 days reduced the peak plasma level and AUC of a single 4-mg dose of nilvadipine by about 20-fold and 30-fold, respectively. The hypotensive effect and reflex tachycardia associated with nilvadipine alone in these subjects was also abolished by rifampicin.[8]

(e) Nisoldipine

There is some evidence that nisoldipine is ineffective in reducing blood pressure in the presence of rifampicin.[1,4]

(f) Verapamil

The observation that a patient whose raised blood pressure was not reduced by verapamil while on antitubercular drugs, prompted a study in 4 other patients.[9] No verapamil could be detected in the plasma of 3 patients who took a single 40-mg dose of verapamil with rifampicin 450 to 600 mg daily, isoniazid 5 mg/kg daily, and ethambutol 15 mg/kg daily. A maximum verapamil level of 20 nanograms/mL was found in the fourth patient. Six other subjects not taking antitubercular drugs had a maximum verapamil plasma concentration of 35 nanograms/mL.[9] Similar results have been reported by the same authors in another study.[10]

Supraventricular tachycardia was inadequately controlled in a patient taking rifampicin 600 mg daily and isoniazid 300 mg daily, despite a verapamil dose of 480 mg every 6 hours. Substitution of the rifampicin by ethambutol resulted in a fourfold rise in serum verapamil levels.[11] A later study in 6 healthy subjects found that after taking rifampicin 600 mg daily for 2 weeks the oral bioavailability of verapamil was reduced from 26 to 2%, and the effects of verapamil on the ECG were abolished.[12] Yet another study in elderly patients similarly found that rifampicin 600 mg daily markedly increased the clearance of verapamil 120 mg twice daily. The effects of verapamil on AV conduction were almost abolished.[13]

Mechanism

Rifampicin reduces the effectiveness of nifedipine and verapamil to a greater extent after oral than after intravenous use. The evidence suggests that rifampicin increases the cytochrome P450 isoenzyme CYP3A4-mediated metabolism of calcium-channel blockers in the gastrointestinal wall,[6,13,14] thereby reducing their oral bioavailability. Rifabutin and rifapentine are also inducers of CYP3A4, although to a lesser extent than rifampicin, and would therefore also be expected to reduce the levels of the calcium-channel blockers.

Importance and management

The interactions between diltiazem, nifedipine, or verapamil and rifampicin are established and of clinical importance. There is some evidence that barnidipine, manidipine, nilvadipine, and nisoldipine interact with rifampicin and the manufacturers of a number of other calcium-channel blockers warn of similar interactions. Monitor the effects closely if rifampicin is given with any calcium-channel blocker, being alert for the need to make a marked increase in their dosage. However, note that some manufacturers of nifedipine,[15] and nisoldipine[16] contraindicate their use with rifampicin. Although the manufacturers of **nimodipine**[17] do not strictly contraindicate concurrent use they say that both drugs should not be given together. **Rifabutin** and **rifapentine** would also be expected to reduce levels of calcium-channel blockers, although perhaps to a lesser extent than rifampicin. However, there does not appear to be any data to prove this.

1. Yoshimoto H, Takahashi M, Saima S. Influence of rifampicin on antihypertensive effects of dihydropiridine calcium-channel blockers in four elderly patients. *Nippon Ronen Igakkai Zasshi* (1996) 33, 692–6.
2. Drda KD, Bastian TL, Self TH, Lawson J, Lanman RC, Burlew BS, Lalonde RL. Effects of debrisoquine hydroxylation phenotype and enzyme induction with rifampin on diltiazem pharmacokinetics and pharmacodynamics. *Pharmacotherapy* (1991) 11, 278.
3. Tsuchihashi K, Fukami K, Kishimoto H, Sumiyoshi T, Haze K, Saito M, Hiramori K. A case of variant angina exacerbated by administration of rifampicin. *Heart Vessels* (1987) 3, 214–17.
4. Tada Y, Tsuda Y, Otsuka T, Nagasawa K, Kimura H, Kusaba T, Sakata T. Case report: nifedipine-rifampicin interaction attenuates the effect on blood pressure in a patient with essential hypertension. *Am J Med Sci* (1992) 303, 25–7.
5. Takasugi T. A case of hypertension suggesting nifedipine and rifampicin drug interaction. *Igaku To Yakugaku* (1989) 22, 132–5.
6. Holtbecker N, Fromm MF, Kroemer HK, Ohnhaus EE, Heidemann H. The nifedipine-rifampin interaction: Evidence for induction of gut wall metabolism. *Drug Metab Dispos* (1996) 24, 1121–3.
7. Ndanusa BU, Mustapha A, Abdu-Aguye I. The effect of single dose of rifampicin on the pharmacokinetics of oral nifedipine. *J Pharm Biomed Anal* (1997) 15, 1571–5.
8. Saima S, Furuie K, Yoshimoto H, Fukuda J, Hayashi T, Echizen H. The effects of rifampicin on the pharmacokinetics and pharmacodynamics of orally administered nilvadipine to healthy subjects. *Br J Clin Pharmacol* (2002) 53, 203–6.
9. Rahn KH, Mooy J, Böhm R, vd Vet, A. Reduction of bioavailability of verapamil by rifampin. *N Engl J Med* (1985) 312, 920–1.
10. Mooy J, Böhm R, van Baak M, van Kemenade J, vd Vet A, Rahn KH. The influence of antituberculosis drugs on the plasma level of verapamil. *Eur J Clin Pharmacol* (1987) 32, 107–9.
11. Barbarash RA. Verapamil-rifampin interaction. *Drug Intell Clin Pharm* (1985) 19, 559–60.
12. Barbarash RA, Bauman JL, Fischer JH, Kondos GT, Batenhorst RL. Near-total reduction in verapamil bioavailability by rifampin: electrocardiographic correlates. *Chest* (1988) 94, 954–9.
13. Fromm MF, Dilger K, Busse D, Kroemer HK, Eichelbaum M, Klotz U. Gut wall metabolism of verapamil in older people: effects of rifampicin-mediated enzyme induction. *Br J Clin Pharmacol* (1998) 45, 247–55.
14. Fromm MF, Busse D, Kroemer HK, Eichelbaum M. Differential induction of prehepatic and hepatic metabolism of verapamil by rifampin. *Hepatology* (1996) 24, 796–801.
15. Adalat Retard (Nifedipine). Bayer plc. UK Summary of product characteristics, September 2006.
16. Syscor MR (Nisoldipine). Forest Laboratories UK Ltd. UK Summary of product characteristics, August 1998.
17. Nimotop (Nimodipine). Bayer plc. UK Summary of product characteristics, August 2005.

Calcium-channel blockers + St John's wort (*Hypericum perforatum*)

St John's wort significantly reduces the bioavailability of verapamil.

Clinical evidence, mechanism, importance and management

In a study, racemic **verapamil** 24 mg was given as a jejunal perfusion over 100 minutes to 8 healthy subjects both before and after treatment with St John's wort tablets *(Movina;* containing 3 to 6% hyperforin) 300 mg three times daily for 14 days. St John's wort did not affect jejunal permeability or the absorption of either ***R***- or ***S*-verapamil**. The AUCs of ***R***- and ***S*-verapamil** were decreased by 78% and 80%, respectively, and the peak plasma levels were decreased by 76% and 78%, respectively. The terminal half-life was not changed significantly. The AUC for ***R*-verapamil** was sixfold higher than that of ***S*-verapamil** and St John's wort did not change this ratio.[1]

It appears that St John's wort decreased the bioavailability of both ***R***- and ***S*-verapamil** by inducing their metabolism by the cytochrome P450 isoenzyme CYP3A4 in the gut. An effect on P-glycoprotein-mediated transport is not likely, as intestinal permeability was not significantly altered.[1] The clinical importance of this interaction is not known but it may be prudent to avoid concurrent use. There appears to be no information about other calcium-channel blockers, but as they are also affected by other CYP3A4 enzyme inducers, it would seem prudent to monitor concurrent use carefully. More study is required.

1. Tannergren C, Engman H, Knutson L, Hedeland M, Bondesson U, Lennernäs H. St John's wort decreases the bioavailability of *R*- and *S*-verapamil through induction of first-pass metabolism. *Clin Pharmacol Ther* (2004) 75, 298–309.

Calcium-channel blockers + Sulfinpyrazone

The clearance of verapamil is markedly increased by sulfinpyrazone.

Clinical evidence, mechanism, importance and management

A study in 8 healthy subjects found that sulfinpyrazone 800 mg daily for a week, increased the clearance of a single oral dose of **verapamil** by about threefold, possibly due to an increase in its liver metabolism.[1] The clinical importance of this is uncertain, but be alert for reduced **verapamil** effects. It seems probable that the dosage may need to be increased.

1. Wing LMH, Miners JO, Lillywhite KJ. Verapamil disposition—effects of sulphinpyrazone and cimetidine. *Br J Clin Pharmacol* (1985) 19, 385–91.

Calcium-channel blockers + Terbinafine

A study in 12 healthy subjects found that terbinafine 250 mg did not alter the pharmacokinetics of nifedipine 30 mg (as *Procardia XL*).[1]

1. Cramer JA, Robbins B, Barbeito R, Bedman TC, Dreisbach A, Meligeni JA. Lamisil®: interaction study with a sustained release nifedipine formulation. *Pharm Res* (1996) 13 (9 Suppl), S436.

Calcium-channel blockers + Valproate

Nimodipine and possibly nifedipine levels are raised by valproate.

Clinical evidence, mechanism, importance and management

Eight epileptic patients who had been taking valproate alone for at least 4 months were given a single 60-mg dose of **nimodipine**. The AUC of nimodipine was about 50% higher than in the control group.[1] The **nimodipine** dosage may need to be reduced if it is given with valproate.

One of the UK manufacturers of **nifedipine** notes that there is a theoretical possibility that levels of **nifedipine** may be increased in the presence of valproate.[2] The US manufacturer recommends blood pressure monitoring during concurrent use and also suggests that a reduction in the dose of **nifedipine** should be considered.[3]

1. Tartara A, Galimberti CA, Manni R, Parietti L, Zucca C, Baasch H, Caresia L, Mück W, Barzaghi N, Gatti G, Perucca E. Differential effects of valproic acid and enzyme-inducing anticonvulsants on nimodipine pharmacokinetics in epileptic patients. *Br J Clin Pharmacol* (1991) 32, 335–40.
2. Adalat Retard (Nifedipine). Bayer plc. UK Summary of product characteristics, September 2006.
3. Adalat CC (Nifedipine). Bayer HealthCare. US Prescribing information, August 2005.

Calcium-channel blockers + Vancomycin

An isolated case report suggests that the hypotensive effects of the rapid infusion of vancomycin may occur more readily in those who are already vasodilated with nifedipine, but it seems likely that the effects seen were due to the rapid infusion alone.

Clinical evidence, mechanism, importance and management

A man with severe systemic sclerosis was hospitalised for Raynaud's phenomenon and dental extraction. After being started on **nifedipine** 40 mg daily, he was given intravenous vancomycin 1 g in 200 mL of dextrose 5% over 30 minutes. After 20 minutes he experienced a severe headache and was found to have a marked macular erythema on the upper trunk, head, neck and arms. His blood pressure fell to 100/60 mmHg and his pulse rate was 90 bpm. He recovered spontaneously.[1] The authors of the report acknowledge the possibility of 'red-man syndrome' caused by the vancomycin, and suggest that it may occur more readily in those already vasodilated with **nifedipine**. However, given that this is an isolated report, and the vancomycin was given over 3 times faster than the recommended rate, it seems likely that this is purely an adverse effect of vancomycin.

1. Daly BM, Sharkey I. Nifedipine and vancomycin-associated red man syndrome. *Drug Intell Clin Pharm* (1986) 20, 986.

Calcium-channel blockers + X-ray contrast media

The hypotensive effects of an intravenous bolus of an ionic X-ray contrast medium can be increased by the presence of calcium-channel blockers. No interaction or only a small interaction appears to occur with non-ionic contrast media.

Clinical evidence, mechanism, importance and management

It is well recognised that ionic X-ray contrast media used for ventriculography reduce the systemic blood pressure due to peripheral vasodilation. They also have a direct depressant effect on the heart muscle. A comparative study of the haemodynamic response of 65 patients found that the hypotensive effect of a bolus dose of an ionic agent (0.5 mL/kg of **meglumine amidotrizoate** and **sodium amidotrizoate** with edetate sodium or disodium) was increased by the concurrent use of **nifedipine** or **diltiazem**. Haemodynamic effects occurred earlier (3.1 seconds instead of 12.9 seconds), were more profound (a fall in systolic pressure of 48.4 instead of 36.9 mmHg) and more prolonged (62 seconds instead of 36 seconds).[1] A similar interaction was seen in *dogs* given **verapamil**.[2] No interaction or only a minimal interaction was seen in the patients and *dogs* when non-ionic contrast media (**iopamidol** or **iohexol**) were used instead.[1,2] The clinical relevance of these findings is uncertain. Note that calcium-channel blockers have been tried to prevent the nephrotoxicity of contrast media.

1. Morris DL, Wisneski JA, Gertz EW, Wexman M, Axelrod R, Langberg JJ. Potentiation by nifedipine and diltiazem of the hypotensive response after contrast angiography. *J Am Coll Cardiol* (1985) 6, 785–91.
2. Higgins CB, Kuber M, Slutsky RA. Interaction between verapamil and contrast media in coronary arteriography: comparison of standard ionic and new nonionic media. *Circulation* (1983) 68, 628–35.

Calcium-channel blockers + Zidovudine

***Animal* studies suggest that nimodipine may increase the bioavailability of zidovudine.**

Clinical evidence, mechanism, importance and management

Studies in *animals* have shown that the AUC of zidovudine is increased and its volume of distribution and clearance rate decreased when it is given with **nimodipine**.[1] The clinical relevance of the interaction is not known, but as the adverse effects of zidovudine are dose related, the manufacturer of **nimodipine** suggests that the possibility of this interaction should be borne in mind in patients given both drugs.[2]

1. Gallo JM, Swagler AR, Mehta M, Qian M. Pharmacokinetic evaluation of drug interactions with anti-human immunodeficiency virus drugs. VI. Effect of the calcium channel blocker nimodipine on zidovudine kinetics in monkeys. *J Pharmacol Exp Ther* (1993) 264, 315–20.
2. Nimotop (Nimodipine). Bayer plc. UK Summary of product characteristics, August 2005.

24

Cardiovascular drugs, miscellaneous

The drugs dealt with in this section include the centrally acting drugs (clonidine, methyldopa), inotropes and vasopressors (adrenaline, phenylephrine), adrenergic neurone blockers (guanethidine), some vasodilator antihypertensives (hydralazine, diazoxide), nitrates (glyceryl trinitrate), potassium channel activators (nicorandil), peripheral vasodilators (pentoxifylline), calcium sensitisers (levosimendan), endothelin antagonists (bosentan) and newer drugs used in the management of angina (ivabradine and ranolazine).

(a) Miscellaneous antihypertensives

The combination of two antihypertensive drugs often results in an increased antihypertensive action, likewise the combination of drugs which may have hypotension as an adverse effect, can lead to an unexpected increase in hypotension. Examples of this type of interaction are discussed in the monograph 'Antihypertensives + Other drugs that affect blood pressure', p.880. Some drugs are known to antagonise the effect of antihypertensives, and these are also generally discussed in this monograph.

(b) Sympathomimetics

Many of the inotropes and vasopressors have actions on the sympathetic nervous system. Noradrenaline (norepinephrine) is the principal neurotransmitter involved in the final link between nerve endings of the sympathetic nervous system and the adrenergic receptors of the organs or tissues innervated. The effects of stimulating this system can be reproduced or mimicked by exogenous noradrenaline and by a number of other drugs that also stimulate these receptors. The drugs that behave in this way are described as 'sympathomimetics' and act either directly, like noradrenaline, on the adrenergic receptors, or indirectly by releasing stored noradrenaline from the nerve endings. Some drugs do both. This is very simply illustrated in 'Figure 24.1', (below).

The adrenergic receptors of the sympathetic system are not identical but can be subdivided into two main types, namely alpha and beta receptors, which can then be further subdivided. The sympathomimetics are categorised in 'Table 24.1', (p.879), and a brief summary of the principal effects of stimulation of these receptors is listed below:

- $Alpha_1$ (vasoconstriction, increased blood pressure and sometimes reflex bradycardia; contraction of smooth muscle; mydriasis in the eye)
- $Alpha_2$ (role in feedback inhibition of neurotransmitter release; inhibition of insulin release)
- $Beta_1$ (increased rate and force of contraction or the heart)
- $Beta_2$ (vasodilatation and bronchodilation; uterine relaxation and decreased gastrointestinal motility; release of insulin)

A third distinct group of receptors, which occur primarily within the CNS and may be affected by some sympathomimetics, are the dopamine receptors.

It is therefore possible to broadly categorise the sympathomimetics into groups according to their activity.

Given these wide ranging actions on a number of different receptors the group 'sympathomimetics' is clearly a very diverse collection of drugs with a wide range of uses. One should not, therefore, extrapolate the interactions seen with one drug to any other without fully taking into account their differences. For this reason, where possible, this term has been avoided and drugs have been grouped by therapeutic use. This section is generally concerned with the interactions of sympathomimetics that have predominately cardiovascular actions (mainly through stimulation of $alpha_1$ and/or $beta_1$ receptors). Those used as decongestants (through stimulation of alpha receptors with or without beta activity) are mainly discussed in the Miscellaneous drugs section but some of these drugs are also given intravenously for their pressor actions, in which case their interactions are discussed here. Interactions involving beta agonists, such as salbutamol, which selectively stimulate the $beta_2$ receptors in bronchi causing bronchodilation, are mainly covered in 'Respiratory drugs', (p.1158) and interactions involving dopaminergics, such as levodopa, are dealt with in 'Antiparkinsonian and related drugs', (p.672).

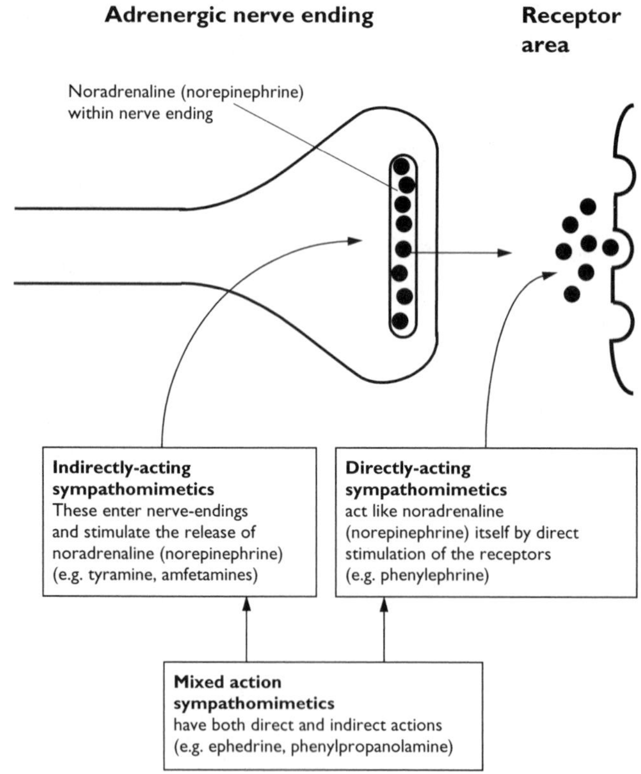
Adrenergic nerve ending
Receptor area
Noradrenaline (norepinephrine) within nerve ending
Indirectly-acting sympathomimetics
These enter nerve-endings and stimulate the release of noradrenaline (norepinephrine) (e.g. tyramine, amfetamines)
Directly-acting sympathomimetics
act like noradrenaline (norepinephrine) itself by direct stimulation of the receptors (e.g. phenylephrine)
Mixed action sympathomimetics
have both direct and indirect actions (e.g. ephedrine, phenylpropanolamine)

Fig. 24.1 A very simple illustration of the modes of action of indirectly-acting, directly-acting and mixed action sympathomimetics at adrenergic neurones.

Table 24.1 A categorisation of some sympathomimetic drugs

Drug	*Receptors stimulated*
Direct stimulators of alpha and beta receptors	
Adrenaline (Epinephrine)	Beta more marked than alpha
Mainly direct stimulators of alpha receptors	
Phenylephrine	Predominantly alpha
Metaraminol	Predominantly alpha
Methoxamine	Predominantly alpha
Noradrenaline (Norepinephrine)	Predominantly alpha
Mainly direct stimulators of beta-1 receptors	
Dobutamine	Predominantly beta-1, some beta-2 and alpha
Dopamine	Predominantly beta-1, some alpha
Direct stimulators of beta-1 and beta-2 receptors (beta-agonist bronchodilators)	
Bambuterol	Predominantly beta-2
Fenoterol	Predominantly beta-2
Formoterol	Predominantly beta-2
Isoetharine	Predominantly beta-2
Isoprenaline (Isoproterenol)	Beta-1 and beta-2
Orciprenaline	Predominantly beta-2
Pirbuterol	Predominantly beta-2
Reproterol	Predominantly beta-2
Rimiterol	Predominantly beta-2
Ritodrine	Predominantly beta-2
Salbutamol (Albuterol)	Predominantly beta-2
Salmeterol	Predominantly beta-2
Terbutaline	Predominantly beta-2
Tulobuterol	Predominantly beta-2
Direct and indirect stimulators of alpha and beta receptors	
Ephedrine	Alpha and beta
Etefedrine	Alpha and beta
Phenylpropanolamine	Alpha and beta
Pseudoephedrine	Alpha and beta
Mainly indirect stimulators of alpha and beta receptors	
Amfetamine (Amphetamine)	Alpha and beta – also central stimulant
Mephentermine	Alpha and beta – also central stimulant
Methylphenidate	Alpha and beta – also central stimulant
Tyramine	Alpha and beta

Antihypertensives + Hormonal contraceptives

Combined oral contraceptives are associated with increased blood pressure and may antagonise the efficacy of antihypertensive drugs. However, the effects are far greater with the high-dose contraceptives that were used historically, and the risks appear to be smaller with the newer low-dose contraceptives.

Clinical evidence, mechanism, importance and management

Early after the introduction of **combined oral contraceptives** it was realised that they can cause increases in blood pressure and clinical hypertension.[1,2] One study,[3] from the 1970s, in 83 women found that the average rise in blood pressure was 9.2/5 mmHg, and that it was about twice as likely to occur as in those not on the pill. Additionally, cases were noted where antihypertensives (at that time, commonly **guanethidine** and/or **methyldopa**) were not that effective in women with hypertension on combined oral contraceptives.[2,4] Although modern combined oral contraceptives are lower dose, they are still associated with a small increased risk of elevated blood pressure.[5] A UK study found that **combined oral contraceptives** were associated with a 2.6/1.8 mmHg rise in blood pressure, whereas **progestogen-only oral contraceptives** did not affect blood pressure.[5] Furthermore, in a study in 24 postmenopausal women with hypertension taking **enalapril** 10 mg twice daily the use of enalapril with **drospirenone/estradiol** 3/1 mg (12 women) produced a significant *decrease* in blood pressure of 9/5 mmHg after 14 days of treatment, when compared with the placebo group (12 patients). No serious adverse effects were reported.[6] Note that drospirenone is an analogue of spironolactone, and shares some of its effects, including its blood pressure-lowering effects.

This is only a very brief review of this subject, but the risks of hypertension with combined hormonal contraceptives appear to be modest. Nevertheless, they need to be considered in the context of other possible cardiovascular risk factors. Where possible, blood pressure should be monitored before and during contraceptive use.

1. Wallace MR. Oral contraceptives and severe hypertension. *Aust N Z J Med* (1971) 1, 49–52.
2. Woods JW. Oral contraceptives and hypertension. *Lancet* (1967) iii, 653–4.
3. Weir RJ, Briggs E, Mack A, Naismith L, Taylor L, Wilson E. Blood pressure in women taking oral contraceptives. *BMJ* (1974) 1, 533.
4. Clezy TM. Oral contraceptives and hypertension: the effect of guanethidine. *Med J Aust* (1970) 1, 638–40.
5. Dong W, Colhoun HM, Poulter NR. Blood pressure in women using oral contraceptives: results from the Health Survey for England 1994. *J Hypertens* (1997) 15, 1063–8.
6. Preston RA, Alonso A, Panzitta D, Zhang P, Karara AH. Additive effect of drospirenone/17-ß-estradiol in hypertensive postmenopausal women receiving enalapril. *Am J Hypertens* (2002) 15, 816–22.

Antihypertensives + Other drugs that affect blood pressure

The hypotensive effect of antihypertensives can be enhanced by other antihypertensives, as would be expected. Although 'first-dose hypotension' (dizziness, lightheadedness, fainting) can occur with some combinations, the additive effects are usually clinically useful. Perhaps of more concern is the use of antihypertensives with drugs that have hypotension as an adverse effect, where the effects may not be anticipated. Some drugs antagonise the blood pressure-lowering effects of the antihypertensives and should therefore be used with caution.

Clinical evidence, mechanism, importance and management

(a) Antihypertensive drugs

Enhanced hypotensive effects should be expected when using two antihypertensives together and it is now widely acknowledged that most people require more than one antihypertensive to control blood pressure.[1] In the US, more than two-thirds of patients receive two or more antihypertensives in order to reach the desired target blood pressure. Not only does this improve blood pressure control, but adverse effects can also be reduced as lower doses of each drug can be used.[2]

Therefore many antihypertensive combinations produce additive effects that are exploited clinically. 'Calcium-channel blockers and diuretics', (p.867) are often used together for additional blood pressure lowering in patients with hypertension. Although there are only a few reports describing these additive interactions, they are highly probable, and caution is advised when using two antihypertensives together. The most common symptoms seen in hypotensive patients are dizziness, fatigue, headache, nausea, confusion, general weakness, lightheadedness, faintness and possible loss of consciousness.

However, in some cases combining two or more antihypertensives has led to severe, first-dose hypotension, see 'Alpha blockers + ACE inhibitors', p.84. Further, life-threatening bradycardia, asystole and sinus arrest can occur when antihypertensives that cause cardiodepression are given together (see 'beta blockers and diltiazem', (p.840)).

In contrast, a sharp and serious rise in blood pressure (rebound hypertension) can occur following the sudden withdrawal of clonidine, and this can be exacerbated in the presence of a beta blocker (see 'clonidine', (p.882)). In some cases fatalities have occurred. 'Table 24.2', (p.881) lists antihypertensive combinations that have been implicated in adverse events.

(b) Drugs with significant hypotensive adverse effects

Caution must also be used when combining two or more drugs that, although not primarily indicated for hypertension, may have hypotensive adverse effects. In fact, it is these drugs, rather than drugs commonly given for their hypotensive effects that may cause more of a problem, as the effects are less likely to be deliberately sought. These drugs are listed in 'Table 24.3', (p.881) with cross-references to the individual monographs that discuss the reports of adverse effects from these combinations.

(c) Drugs that antagonise hypotensive effects

When using antihypertensive drugs it is important to consider the implications of using drugs that antagonise their effects. The NSAIDs are the prime example of this. Drugs that are thought to antagonise the effects of antihypertensives are listed in 'Table 24.4', (p.881), with cross-references to the individual monographs that discuss the reports of adverse effects from these combinations.

1. Williams B, Poulter NR, Brown MJ, Davis M, McInnes GT, Potter JF, Sever PS, McG Thom S. British Hypertension Society. Guidelines for management of hypertension: report of the fourth working party of the British Hypertension Society, 2004-BHS IV. *J Hum Hypertens* (2004) 18, 139–185.
2. Chobanian AV, Bakris GL, Black HR, Cushman WC, Green LA, Izzo JL, Jones DW, Materson BJ, Oparil S, Wright JT, Roccella EJ and the National High Blood Pressure Education Program Co-ordinating Committee. Seventh report of the Joint National Committee on Prevention, Detection, Evaluation, and Treatment of Blood Pressure. *Hypertension* (2003) 42, 1206–52.

Antihypertensives + Phenylpropanolamine

A single dose of a sustained-release preparation of phenylpropanolamine and brompheniramine was found to cause a minor and clinically insignificant rise in the blood pressures of patients on various antihypertensives.

Clinical evidence, mechanism, importance and management

A randomised, double-blind, crossover study in 13 patients with hypertension controlled with **unnamed diuretics** (7), **ACE inhibitors** (6), **beta blockers** (5), **calcium-channel blockers** (1) and a **centrally acting alpha-agonist** (1) found that a single dose of *Dimetapp Extentabs* (phenylpropanolamine 75 mg with brompheniramine 12 mg) caused only a minor rise in blood pressure of 1.7/0.9 mmHg over 4 hours.[1] This sustained-release preparation in this dosage has therefore no clinically important effect on blood pressure, but (as the authors point out), these results do not necessarily apply to different doses and immediate-release preparations. A marked rise in blood pressure was seen in one patient taking **methyldopa** and **oxprenolol** when given phenylpropanolamine, see 'Methyldopa + Sympathomimetics; Indirectly-acting', p.898. Consider also 'Beta blockers + Phenylpropanolamine', p.851.

1. Petrulis AS, Imperiale TF, Speroff T. The acute effect of phenylpropanolamine and brompheniramine on blood pressure in controlled hypertension. *J Gen Intern Med* (1991) 6, 503–6.

Table 24.2 Antihypertensive + Antihypertensive drug interactions

Drugs	*Additive antihypertensive interactions*
ACE inhibitors	Alpha blockers Beta blockers Calcium-channel blockers Clonidine Diuretics
Adrenergic neurone blockers (e.g. guanethidine)	Minoxidil + Guanethidine
Alpha blockers	ACE inhibitors Beta blockers Calcium-channel blockers Diuretics
Angiotensin II receptor antagonists	Beta blockers Calcium-channel blockers Diuretics
Beta blockers	ACE inhibitors Alpha blockers Angiotensin II receptor antagonists Calcium-channel blockers; Dihydropyridines Calcium-channel blockers; Diltiazem Calcium-channel blockers; Verapamil Clonidine Ketanserin Vasodilators
Calcium-channel blockers	ACE inhibitors Alpha blockers Angiotensin II receptor antagonists Beta blockers + Dihydropyridines Beta blockers + Diltiazem Beta blockers + Verapamil Calcium-channel blockers Diuretics Glyceryl trinitrate (Nitroglycerin) Nitrates
Centrally acting antihypertensives (e.g. clonidine, moxonidine)	ACE inhibitors + Clonidine Clonidine + Beta blockers Moxonidine + Miscellaneous
Diazoxide	Vasodilators
Diuretics	ACE inhibitors Alpha blockers Angiotensin II receptor antagonists Calcium-channel blockers
Nicorandil	Vasodilators
Nitrates	Calcium-channel blockers Calcium-channel blockers; Nifedipine Sodium nitroprusside + Miscellaneous
Rauwolfia alkaloids	—
Vasodilators (e.g. hydralazine)	Beta blockers + Hydralazine Diazoxide + Hydralazine Guanethidine + Minoxidil Nicorandil + Vasodilators

Table 24.3 Antihypertensive drug interactions involving drugs with significant hypotensive properties or adverse effects

Drugs	*Additive antihypertensive interactions*
Alcohol	Alcohol + Antihypertensives
Anaesthetics	General anaesthetics + Antihypertensives Local anaesthetics + Antihypertensives MAOIs Timolol
Antipsychotics	ACE inhibitors Beta blockers Clonidine Clozapine + Antihypertensives Guanethidine + Antipsychotics Methyldopa
Dopamine agonists (e.g. apomorphine, bromocriptine etc.)	Apomorphine + Miscellaneous Pergolide + ACE inhibitors
Levodopa	Guanethidine Methyldopa
Moxisylyte	Moxisylyte + Miscellaneous
Phosphodiesterase type-5 inhibitors	Alpha blockers Antihypertensives Nitrates
Procarbazine	Procarbazine + Miscellaneous
Tizanidine	Tizanidine + Antihypertensives
Other drugs suggested to cause hypotension but where no reports of adverse interaction found	Aldesleukin Alprostadil MAOIs

Table 24.4 Antihypertensive drugs and drugs antagonising their effect

Drugs	*Antagonising antihypertensive interactions*
Amfetamines	Guanethidine + Amfetamines and related drugs
High-dose aspirin	ACE inhibitors + Aspirin
Carbenoxolone	Carbenoxolone + Antihypertensives
Hormonal contraceptives	Antihypertensives + Hormonal contraceptives
Epoetin	ACE inhibitors or Angiotensin II receptor antagonists + Epoetin
NSAIDs	ACE inhibitors + NSAIDs Alpha blockers + NSAIDs Angiotensin II receptor antagonists + Aspirin or NSAIDs Beta blockers + Aspirin or NSAIDs Calcium-channel blockers + Aspirin or NSAIDs Guanethidine + NSAIDs Hydralazine + NSAIDs Thiazide and related diuretics + NSAIDs
Phenylpropanolamine	Antihypertensives + Phenylpropanolamine Beta blockers + Phenylpropanolamine
Other drugs suggested to antagonise the effects of antihypertensives	Corticosteroids

Bosentan + Azoles

Ketoconazole increases bosentan levels by twofold: fluconazole is predicted to have a greater effect.

Clinical evidence, mechanism, importance and management

In a randomised crossover study, 10 healthy subjects were given bosentan 62.5 mg twice daily for 11 doses, either alone, or with **ketoconazole** 200 mg daily. The maximum plasma level of bosentan was increased 2.1-fold, and the AUC was increased 2.3-fold (range 1.4- to 4-fold) by **ketoconazole**. This interaction probably occurs because bosentan is metabolised by the cytochrome P450 isoenzyme CYP3A4, of which ketoconazole is a known, potent inhibitor.[1]

Other potent CYP3A4 inhibitors (e.g. **itraconazole**) are expected to interact similarly to **ketoconazole**.[2] However, because **fluconazole** (a moderate inhibitor of CYP3A4) also inhibits CYP2C9, another enzyme involved in the metabolism of bosentan, it is anticipated that it could cause even larger increases in bosentan levels.

The clinical significance of raised the bosentan levels is unclear. Bosentan has been tolerated in single-doses of up to 2.4 g in healthy subjects, although elevations in liver transaminases have been seen during long-term, high-dose treatment.[1] Even so, the manufacturers do not recommend the combination of **fluconazole** with bosentan because of the risk of liver toxicity.[2] Similarly using **ketoconazole** or **itraconazole** in combination with a CYP2C9 inhibitor (the manufacturers name **voriconazole**) and bosentan is also not recommended.[2] Other drugs that inhibit CYP2C9 are listed in 'Table 1.3', (p.6).

Until more is known, it may be prudent to carefully monitor liver function when the combination is used. The manufacturers suggest that no dosage adjustment is likely to be required when **ketoconazole** is used with bosentan.[2]

1. van Giersbergen PLM, Halabi A, Dingemanse J. Single- and multiple-dose pharmacokinetics of bosentan and its interaction with ketoconazole. *Br J Clin Pharmacol* (2002) 53, 589–95.
2. Tracleer (Bosentan monohydrate). Actelion Pharmaceuticals UK. UK Summary of product characteristics, October 2006.

Bosentan + Food

In a study in 16 healthy subjects the pharmacokinetics of bosentan were not significantly changed by the presence of food. Bosentan may therefore be given without regard to meal times.[1]

1. Dingemanse J, Bodin F, Weidekamm E, Kutz K, van Giersbergen P. Influence of food intake and formulation on the pharmacokinetics and metabolism of bosentan, a dual endothelin receptor antagonist. *J Clin Pharmacol* (2002) 42, 283–9.

Bosentan + Miscellaneous

The pharmacokinetics of bosentan were not significantly altered when it was taken with losartan or nimodipine.

Clinical evidence, mechanism, importance and management

(a) Losartan

A study in healthy subjects found that the pharmacokinetics of bosentan 125 mg twice daily were unaffected by the concurrent use of losartan 100 mg once daily for 9 doses.[1]

(b) Nimodipine

In a study of 6 patients with subarachnoid haemorrhage, the pharmacokinetics of a single 500-mg intravenous dose of bosentan were not affected by the concurrent use of nimodipine (dose not specified).[2]

1. van Giersbergen PLM, Clozel M, Bodin F. A drug interaction study between bosentan and ketoconazole and losartan. *Clin Pharmacol Ther* (2001) 69, P67
2. Dingemanse J, van Giersbergen PLM. Clinical pharmacology of bosentan, a dual endothelin receptor antagonist. *Clin Pharmacokinet* (2004) 43, 1089–1115.

Clonidine + Antipsychotics

The hypotensive adverse effects of the phenothiazines, and possibly haloperidol may be additive with the antihypertensive effects of clonidine. Patients may feel faint and dizzy if they stand up quickly.

Clinical evidence

One report describes a patient who experienced dizziness and hypotension (systolic blood pressure 76 mmHg) about an hour after being given **chlorpromazine** 100 mg, clonidine 100 micrograms and **furosemide** 40 mg. Another patient also experienced hypotension 2 hours after being given clonidine 100 micrograms and a 1-mg intramuscular dose of **haloperidol**.[1]

There is also an isolated and unexplained case of a psychotic patient taking **fluphenazine decanoate** who began to exhibit delirium, agitation, disorientation, short-term memory loss, confusion and clouded consciousness within 10 days of starting to take clonidine 200 micrograms daily. These symptoms disappeared when the clonidine was stopped and returned when it was re-started. He had previously uneventfully taken **haloperidol** with clonidine.[2]

Mechanism

Simple addition of the hypotensive effects of both drugs seems to be the explanation for the increased hypotension and orthostasis. However, note that in contrast to the case report above, *animal* studies have shown that chlorpromazine *reduces* the antihypertensive effect of clonidine.[3]

Importance and management

The increased hypotension and orthostasis that can occur if phenothiazines are used with antihypertensive drugs such as clonidine is established. Note that, of the phenothiazines, **levomepromazine** is particularly associated with postural hypotension. One report suggests that haloperidol may interact similarly. Monitor, particularly during the initial stages of concurrent use, and warn patients that if they feel faint and dizzy they should lie down, and that they should remain lying down until symptoms abate completely. Dosage adjustment may be necessary.

The manufacturers of clonidine note that a reduced antihypertensive effect may occur with antipsychotics with alpha-blocking properties (e.g. chlorpromazine), as well as mentioning the risk of orthostatic hypotension.[4] Consider also 'Clonidine + Tricyclic and related antidepressants', p.884. Although antagonism of the antihypertensive effect of clonidine has been seen in *animals* given chlorpromazine, there appear to be no clinical reports.

1. Fruncillo RJ, Gibbons WJ, Vlasses PH, Ferguson RK. Severe hypotension associated with concurrent clonidine and antipsychotic medication. *Am J Psychiatry* (1985) 142, 274.
2. Allen RM, Flemenbaum A. Delirium associated with combined fluphenazine-clonidine therapy. *J Clin Psychiatry* (1979) 40, 236–7.
3. van Zwieten PA. The interaction between clonidine and various neuroleptic agents and some benzodiazepine tranquillizers. *J Pharm Pharmacol* (1977) 29, 229–34.
4. Catapres Tablets (Clonidine hydrochloride). Boehringer Ingelheim Ltd. UK Summary of product characteristics, May 2006.

Clonidine + Beta blockers

The use of clonidine with beta blockers can be therapeutically valuable, but a sharp and serious rise in blood pressure ('rebound hypertension') can follow the sudden withdrawal of clonidine, which may be worsened by the presence of a beta blocker. Isolated cases of marked bradycardia and hypotension have been seen in patients given clonidine with esmolol. There are also two reports describing paradoxical hypertension with the combination of clonidine and beta blockers.

Clinical evidence

(a) Exacerbation of the clonidine-withdrawal hypertensive rebound

A woman with a blood pressure of 180/140 mmHg was taking clonidine and **timolol**. When the clonidine was stopped in error, she developed a violent throbbing headache and became progressively confused, ataxic and semicomatose, and had a grand mal convulsion. Her blood pressure was found to have risen to over 300/185 mmHg.[1]

A number of other reports describe similar cases of hypertensive rebound (a sudden and serious rise in blood pressure) within 24 to 72 hours of stopping the clonidine, apparently worsened by the presence of **propranolol**.[2-6] The symptoms resemble those of phaeochromocytoma, and include tremor, apprehension, flushing, nausea, vomiting, severe headache, and a serious rise in blood pressure. One patient died from a cerebellar haemorrhage.[5]

(b) Bradycardia and hypotension

A man anaesthetised with thiopental and diamorphine, with oxygen, nitrous oxide, enflurane and atracurium, was given clonidine 50 micrograms to control hypertension. After 15 minutes he became tachycardic with a heart rate of up to 170 bpm. **Esmolol** 75 mg was given by slow infusion, whereupon his heart rate fell to 20 bpm. He responded to atropine 1.2 mg, adrenaline (epinephrine) 1 mg and calcium chloride 10 mL with a stable heart rate of 110 bpm.[7] Of 32 patients receiving **esmolol** during surgery in a clinical study, one patient developed marked hypotension and bradycardia, which responded to ephedrine 10 mg. It was noted that this patient had been receiving clonidine.[8] A subset of 5 patients involved in a study investigating the use of clonidine with **propranolol** and minoxidil had a reduction in blood pressure when clonidine (0.2 to 0.4 mg daily) was added. After the discontinuation of **propranolol**, blood pressure returned to that seen before clonidine was added, indicating that **propranolol** and clonidine have additive hypotensive actions.[9] Similarly, **atenolol** and clonidine have been shown to have additive hypotensive effects.[10,11]

(c) Antagonism of the hypotensive effects

The combination of **sotalol** 160 mg daily and clonidine 450 micrograms daily caused a marked rise in blood pressure in 6 of 10 patients, compared with either clonidine alone (3 patients) or **sotalol** alone (3 patients). Two of the 10 had blood pressures that were lower than with either drug alone, and the remaining 2 patients had no appreciable change in blood pressure.[12] Two cases of hypertension involving clonidine with **propranolol** have also been described,[13] and in some studies the combination of clonidine and **nadolol**[11] or **propranolol**[10] has been no more effective than either drug alone.

(d) Peripheral vascular disorders

The manufacturer of clonidine notes that the concurrent use of a beta blocker may possibly potentiate peripheral vascular disorders.[14] This is based on the known pharmacology of the drugs,[15] and no specific cases appear to have been reported.

Mechanism

The normal additive hypotensive effects of these drugs result from the two acting in concert at different but complementary sites in the cardiovascular system. Just why antagonism sometimes occurs is unexplained. The hypertensive rebound following clonidine withdrawal is thought to be due to an increase in the levels of circulating catecholamines. With the beta (vasodilator) effects blocked by a beta blocker, the alpha (vasoconstrictor) effects of the catecholamines are unopposed and the hypertension is further exaggerated.

Importance and management

It is well-known that beta blockers seriously worsen the rebound hypertension following clonidine withdrawal. Control this adverse effect by stopping the beta blocker several days before starting a gradual withdrawal of clonidine.[16] A successful alternative is to replace the clonidine and the beta blocker with labetalol,[17] which is both an alpha and a beta blocker: The blood catecholamine levels still rise markedly (20-fold) and the patient may experience tremor, nausea, apprehension and palpitations, but no serious blood pressure rise or headaches appear to occur.[17] The dosage of labetalol will need to be titrated to effect, with regular checks on the blood pressure over 2 to 3 days. If a hypertensive episode develops, control it with an alpha-blocking drug such as phentolamine.[2] Diazoxide is also said to be effective.[1,5] Re-introduction of oral or intravenous clonidine should also stabilise the situation. It is clearly important to emphasise to patients taking clonidine and beta blockers that they should not stop taking these drugs without seeking medical advice.

Clonidine and atenolol (a cardio-selective beta blocker) have additive hypotensive effects and smaller doses of clonidine can be given, which decreases its troublesome adverse effects (sedation and dry mouth). In contrast, limited evidence suggests that propranolol or nadolol (non-selective beta blockers) the blood pressure reductions were the same as with either drug alone, although this has not been confirmed in other studies. The weight of evidence suggests that paradoxical hypertension is rare.[12,13]

1. Bailey RR, Neale TJ. Rapid clonidine withdrawal with blood pressure overshoot exaggerated by beta-blockade. *BMJ* (1976) i, 942–3.
2. Bruce DL, Croley TF, Lee JS. Preoperative clonidine withdrawal syndrome. *Anesthesiology* (1979) 51, 90–2.
3. Cairns SA, Marshall AJ. Clonidine withdrawal. *Lancet* (1976) i, 368.
4. Strauss FG, Franklin SS, Lewin AJ, Maxwell MH. Withdrawal of antihypertensive therapy. Hypertensive crisis in renovascular hypertension. *JAMA* (1977) 238, 1734–6.
5. Vernon C, Sakula A. Fatal rebound hypertension after abrupt withdrawal of clonidine and propranolol. *Br J Clin Pract* (1979) 33, 112,121.
6. Reid JL, Wing LMH, Dargie HJ, Hamilton CA, Davies DS, Dollery CT. Clonidine withdrawal in hypertension. Changes in blood pressure and plasma and urinary noradrenaline. *Lancet* (1977) i, 1171–4.
7. Perks D, Fisher GC. Esmolol and clonidine — a possible interaction. *Anaesthesia* (1992) 47, 533–4.
8. Kanitz DD, Ebert TJ, Kampine JP. Intraoperative use of bolus doses of esmolol to treat tachycardia. *J Clin Anesth* (1990) 2, 238–42.
9. Pettinger WA, Mitchell HC, Güllner H-G. Clonidine and the vasodilating beta blocker antihypertensive drug interaction. *Clin Pharmacol Ther* (1977) 22, 164–71.
10. Lilja M, Jounela AJ, Juustila H, Mattila MJ. Interaction of clonidine and β-blockers. *Acta Med Scand* (1980) 207, 173–6.
11. Fogari R, Corradi L. Interaction of clonidine and beta blocking agents in the treatment of essential hypertension. In 'Low dose oral and transdermal therapy of hypertension' (Proceedings of Conference 1984), edited by Weber MA, Drayer JIM, Kolloch R. Springer-Verlag, 1985, pp. 118–21.
12. Saarimaa H. Combination of clonidine and sotalol in hypertension. *BMJ* (1976) i, 810.
13. Warren SE, Ebert E, Swerdlin A-H, Steinberg SM, Stone R. Clonidine and propranolol paradoxical hypertension. *Arch Intern Med* (1979) 139, 253.
14. Catapres Tablets (Clonidine hydrochloride). Boehringer Ingelheim Ltd. UK Summary of product characteristics, May 2006.
15. Boehringer Ingelheim. Personal communication, 29 March 2005.
16. Harris AL. Clonidine withdrawal and blockade. *Lancet* (1976) i, 596.
17. Rosenthal T, Rabinowitz B, Boichis H, Elazar E, Brauner A, Neufeld HN. Use of labetalol in hypertensive patients during discontinuation of clonidine therapy. *Eur J Clin Pharmacol* (1981) 20, 237–40.

Clonidine + Bupropion

Bupropion 100 mg three times daily for 9 days did not reduce the hypotensive effect of a single 300-microgram dose of oral clonidine in 8 healthy subjects.[1]

1. Cubeddu LX, Cloutier G, Gross K, Grippo R, Tanner L, Lerea L, Shakarjian M, Knowlton G, Harden TK, Arendshorst W and Rogers JF. Bupropion does not antagonize cardiovascular actions of clonidine in normal subjects and spontaneously hypertensive rats. *Clin Pharmacol Ther* (1984) 35, 576–84.

Clonidine and related drugs + CNS depressants

Increased sedation may occur if alcohol or other CNS depressants are taken with clonidine, guanfacine or guanabenz.

Clinical evidence, mechanism, importance and management

Sedation is a common adverse effect of clonidine and other central alpha-adrenoceptor agonists such as **guanfacine** and **guanabenz**, particularly during the initial stages of treatment.[1-3] Patients starting treatment with these drugs should be warned that their tolerance to **alcohol** and other CNS depressant drugs may be diminished. Patients who are affected should not drive or operate machinery. Consider also 'Moxonidine + Miscellaneous', p.899.

1. Catapres Tablets (Clonidine hydrochloride). Boehringer Ingelheim Ltd. UK Summary of product characteristics, May 2006.
2. Guanfacine hydrochloride. Watson Laboratories, Inc. US Prescribing information, April 2003.
3. Catapres Tablets (Clonidine hydrochloride). Boehringer Ingelheim Pharmaceuticals, Inc. US Prescribing information, January 2007.

Clonidine + Hormonal contraceptives

The sedative effects of intravenous clonidine have been increased by a combined oral contraceptive.

Clinical evidence, mechanism, importance and management

A study[1] in a group of 10 women found that the sedative effects of a single 1.3-microgram/kg dose of intravenous clonidine were increased by a combined oral contraceptive (**ethinylestradiol/levonorgestrel** 30 micrograms/150 or 250 micrograms). The clinical importance of this is uncertain. Consider also 'Antihypertensives + Hormonal contraceptives', p.880.

1. Chalmers JS, Fulli-Lemaire I, Cowen PJ. Effects of the contraceptive pill on sedative responses to clonidine and apomorphine in normal women. *Psychol Med* (1985) 15, 363–7.

Clonidine + Naloxone

A study in *animals* suggesting naloxone blocked the antihypertensive effects of clonidine prompted a placebo-controlled study in 6 patients with hypertension. Each patient received a single oral dose of clonidine 300 micrograms during an infusion of either naloxone 6 micrograms/kg per hour for 8 hours. Supine and standing blood pressure and heart rate were monitored. Naloxone was not found to affect the hypotensive or bradycardic effect of clonidine.[1]

1. Rogers JF, Cubeddu LX. Naloxone does not antagonize the antihypertensive effect of clonidine in essential hypertension. *Clin Pharmacol Ther* (1983) 34, 68–73.

Clonidine + Prazosin

There is some evidence to suggest that prazosin can reduce the antihypertensive effects of clonidine, whereas some other evidence suggests that this does not occur.

Clinical evidence, mechanism, importance and management

The hypotensive effect of a 150-microgram intravenous dose of clonidine was reduced by 47% in 18 patients with essential hypertension after they took prazosin (mean dose 11 mg three times daily for 4 days).[1] A later crossover study by the same research group in 17 patients with essential hypertension (mean blood pressures 170/103 mmHg) found that clonidine 300 micrograms daily for 4 days reduced the mean blood pressure by 38/18 mmHg and prazosin 6 mg daily for 3 days reduced the mean blood pressure by 10/4 mmHg. However, when prazosin and clonidine were given together the mean blood pressure was only reduced to a similar extent as prazosin alone (12/6 mmHg).[2] Similarly, some earlier studies had suggested that the combination of clonidine and prazosin produced only a modest,[3] or no additive antihypertensive effect.[4] Conversely, other studies using the combination have not reported a reduced antihypertensive effect.[5,6] In the presence of prazosin the rebound hypertension following clonidine withdrawal was said to be moderate (a rise from 145/85 to 169/104 mmHg).[6]

Clonidine is an $alpha_2$ agonist, whereas prazosin is an $alpha_1$ blocker. Consequently, it has been postulated that the drugs may be partially antagonistic when given together, and the authors of the first study cite a number of *animal* studies to support this.[1] Although not conclusive, it seems possible that concurrent use may not always be favourable. Monitor the effects.

1. Kapocsi J, Farsang C, Vizi ES. Prazosin partly blocks clonidine-induced hypotension in patients with essential hypertension. *Eur J Clin Pharmacol* (1987) 32, 331–4.
2. Farsang C, Varga K, Kapocsi J. Prazosin-clonidine and prazosin-guanfacine interactions in hypertension. *Pharmacol Res Commun* (1988) 20 (Suppl 1), 85–6.
3. Kuokkanen K, Mattila MJ. Antihypertensive effects of prazosin in combination with methyldopa, clonidine or propranolol. *Ann Clin Res* (1979) 11, 18–24.
4. Hubbell FA, Weber MA, Drayer JIM, Rose DE. Combined central and peripheral sympathetic blockade: absence of additive antihypertensive effects. *Am J Med Sci* (1983) 285: 18–26.
5. Stokes GS, Gain JM, Mahoney JE, Raaftos J, Steward JH. Long term use of prazosin in combination or alone for treating hypertension. *Med J Aust* (1977) 2 (Suppl), 13–16.
6. Andréjak M, Fievet P, Makdassi R, Comoy E, de Fremont JF, Coevoet B, Fournier A. Lack of antagonism in the antihypertensive effects of clonidine and prazosin in man. *Clin Sci* (1981) 61, 453s–455s.

Clonidine + Rifampicin (Rifampin)

Rifampicin does not interact with clonidine.

Clinical evidence, mechanism, importance and management

In 6 subjects taking clonidine 200 micrograms twice daily the use of rifampicin 600 mg twice daily for 7 days did not affect the elimination kinetics of clonidine, or its effects on pulse rate or blood pressure.[1] No special precautions would seem necessary on concurrent use.

1. Affrime MB, Lowenthal DT, Rufo M. Failure of rifampin to induce the metabolism of clonidine in normal volunteers. *Drug Intell Clin Pharm* (1981) 15, 964–6.

Clonidine + Tricyclic and related antidepressants

The tricyclic antidepressants, clomipramine, desipramine and imipramine, reduce or abolish the antihypertensive effects of clonidine. Other tricyclics are expected to behave similarly. A hypertensive crisis developed in a woman taking clonidine who was also given imipramine, and severe pain occurred in a man taking amitriptyline and diamorphine when he was given intrathecal clonidine. Conversely, the tetracyclics, maprotiline and mianserin do not appear to alter the antihypertensive effects of clonidine. An isolated case report describes a hypertensive crisis in a patient taking mirtazapine and clonidine. Hypotension occurred in a boy taking clonidine and trazodone.

Clinical evidence

(a) Tetracyclic and related antidepressants

Maprotiline 100 mg in 4 divided doses over 22 hours did not alter the effect of a single dose of clonidine on blood pressure or heart rate in 8 healthy subjects.[1] **Mianserin** 20 mg three times daily for 2 weeks had no effect on the control of blood pressure in 5 patients receiving clonidine.[2,3] Similarly, **mianserin** pretreatment did not significantly alter the hypotensive action of a single dose of clonidine in healthy subjects.[2,4] In contrast, an isolated report describes hypertensive urgency in a man with end-stage renal disease taking clonidine, metoprolol and losartan when **mirtazapine** (a **mianserin** analogue) was added for depression.[5]

(b) Trazodone

A 12-year-old boy taking clonidine 100 micrograms three times daily and dexamfetamine 15 mg twice daily was prescribed trazodone 50 mg at bedtime. After a few weeks his trazodone dosage was increased to 100 mg at bedtime. Within 45 minutes of taking his first increased dose he had a hypotensive episode with bradycardia and sedation. The trazodone dose was reduced back to 50 mg, but the drug was discontinued 2 weeks later because of low blood pressure.[6]

(c) Tricyclic antidepressants

Desipramine 75 mg daily for 2 weeks caused the lying and standing blood pressures of 4 out of 5 hypertensive patients taking clonidine 600 to 1800 micrograms daily (with chlortalidone or hydrochlorothiazide) to rise by 22/15 mmHg and 12/10 mmHg respectively.[7]

This interaction has been seen in other patients taking **clomipramine**, **desipramine** and **imipramine**.[8-11] In one study, the antihypertensive effects of a single intravenous dose of clonidine were reduced by about 50% in 6 patients given **desipramine** for 3 weeks.[12] Similarly the blood pressure lowering effect of a single 300-microgram dose of clonidine was reduced by 40 to 50% in 8 healthy subjects when it was given on day 9 of treatment with **imipramine** 25 mg three times daily.[13] An elderly woman taking clonidine 200 micrograms daily developed severe frontal headache, dizziness, chest and neck pain and tachycardia of 120 bpm with hypertension (230/124–130 mmHg) on the second day of taking **imipramine** 50 mg for incontinence.[14]

Rebound hypertension and tachycardia seen on the withdrawal of clonidine, may have been made worse by the presence of **amitriptyline** in a 73-year-old woman.[15]

A man with severe pain, well controlled with **amitriptyline**, sodium valproate and intrathecal boluses of diamorphine, experienced severe pain within 5 minutes of an intrathecal test dose of clonidine 75 micrograms.[16]

Mechanism

Not understood. One idea is that the tricyclics desensitise or block central $alpha_2$-receptors.[17] This would explain the interaction with mirtazapine (a mianserin analogue), which also has alpha-blocking properties.[5] However, mianserin (also an alpha-blocker) did not interact.[2] Another idea is that tricyclics block noradrenaline uptake. However, maprotiline, which also blocks noradrenaline uptake, did not interact.[1] Trazodone, which also has alpha-blocking properties was predicted to inhibit the effect of clonidine based on a study in *animals* where it antagonised the hypotensive effect of clonidine when given centrally (note this effect was not seen when it was administered intravenously).[18] The case of hypotension described could be explained by the hypotensive effect of trazodone alone, but may have been compounded by the hypotensive effect of clonidine.

Importance and management

The interaction between clonidine and the tricyclics is established and clinically important. The incidence is uncertain but it is not seen in all patients.[7] Avoid concurrent use unless the effects can be monitored. Increasing the dosage of clonidine may possibly be effective. The clonidine dosage was apparently successfully titrated in 10 out of 11 hypertensive patients already on amitriptyline or imipramine.[19] Only clomipramine, desipramine and imipramine have been implicated so far, but other tricyclics would be expected to behave similarly (amitriptyline, **nortriptyline** and **protriptyline** have been shown to interact in *animals*[20]). The tetracyclic antidepressants maprotiline and mianserin do not generally appear to interact with clonidine. The isolated case of hypotension with trazodone is of unknown general importance.

1. Gundert-Remy U, Amann E, Hildebrandt R, Weber E. Lack of interaction between the tetracyclic antidepressant maprotiline and the centrally acting antihypertensive drug clonidine. *Eur J Clin Pharmacol* (1983) 25, 595–9.
2. Elliott HL, Whiting B, Reid JL. Assessment of the interaction between mianserin and centrally-acting antihypertensive drugs. *Br J Clin Pharmacol* (1983) 15, 323S–328S.
3. Elliott HL, McLean K, Sumner DJ, Reid JL. Absence of an effect of mianserin on the actions of clonidine or methyldopa in hypertensive patients. *Eur J Clin Pharmacol* (1983) 24, 15–19.
4. Elliott HL, McLean K, Sumner DJ, Reid JL. Pharmacodynamic studies on mianserin and its interaction with clonidine. *Eur J Clin Pharmacol* (1981) 21, 97–102.
5. Abo-Zena RA, Bobek MB, Dweik RA. Hypertensive urgency induced by an interaction of mirtazapine and clonidine. *Pharmacotherapy* (2000) 20, 476–8.
6. Bhatara VS, Kallepalli BR, Misra LK, Awadallah S. A possible clonidine-trazodone-dextroamphetamine interaction in a 12-year-old boy. *J Child Adolesc Psychopharmacol* (1996) 6, 203–9.
7. Briant RH, Reid JL, Dollery CT. Interaction between clonidine and desipramine in man. *BMJ* (1973) i, 522–3.
8. Coffler DE. Antipsychotic drug interaction. *Drug Intell Clin Pharm* (1976) 10, 114–15.
9. Andrejak M, Fournier A, Hardin J-M, Coevoet B, Lambrey G, De Fremont J-F, Quichaud J. Suppression de l'effet antihypertenseur de la clonidine par la prise simultanée d'un antidépresseur tricyclique. *Nouv Presse Med* (1977) 6, 2603.
10. Lacomblez L, Warot D, Bouche P, Derouesné C. Suppression de l'effet antihypertenseur de la clonidine par la clomipramine. *Rev Med Interne* (1988) 9, 291–3.
11. Manchon ND, Bercoff E, Lemarchand P, Chassagne P, Senant J, Bourreille J. Fréquence et gravité des interactions médicamenteuses dans une population âgée: étude prospective concernant 639 malades. *Rev Med Interne* (1989) 10, 521–5.
12. Checkley SA, Slade AP, Shur E, Dawling S. A pilot study of the mechanism of action of desipramine. *Br J Psychiatry* (1981) 138, 248–51.
13. Cubeddu LX, Cloutier G, Gross K, Grippo PA-CR, Tanner L, Lerea L, Shakarjian M, Knowlton G, Harden TK, Arendshorst W, Rogers JF. Bupropion does not antagonize cardiovascular actions of clonidine in normal subjects and spontaneously hypertensive rats. *Clin Pharmacol Ther* (1984) 35, 576–84.
14. Hui KK. Hypertensive crisis induced by interaction of clonidine with imipramine. *J Am Geriatr Soc* (1983) 31, 164–5.
15. Stiff JL, Harris DB. Clonidine withdrawal complicated by amitriptyline therapy. *Anesthesiology* (1983) 59, 73–4.
16. Hardy PAJ, Wells JCD. Pain after spinal intrathecal clonidine. An adverse interaction with tricyclic antidepressants? *Anaesthesia* (1988) 43, 1026–7.
17. van Spanning HW, van Zwieten PA. The interference of tricyclic antidepressants with the central hypotensive effect of clonidine. *Eur J Pharmacol* (1973) 24, 402–4.
18. van Zwieten PA. Inhibition of the central hypotensive effect of clonidine by trazodone, a novel antidepressant. *Pharmacology* (1977) 15, 331–6.
19. Raftos J, Bauer GE, Lewis RG, Stokes GS, Mitchell AS, Young AA, Maclachlan I. Clonidine in the treatment of severe hypertension. *Med J Aust* (1973) 1, 786–93.
20. van Zwieten PA. Interaction between centrally active hypotensive drugs and tricyclic antidepressants. *Arch Int Pharmacodyn Ther* (1975) 214, 12–30.

Diazoxide + Hydralazine

Severe hypotension, in some cases fatal, has followed the use of high doses of intravenous diazoxide, given before or after hydralazine.

Clinical evidence

A previously normotensive 25-year-old woman had a blood pressure of 250/150 mmHg during the 34th week of pregnancy, which failed to respond to intravenous magnesium sulfate 4 g. Her blood pressure fell transiently to 170/120 mmHg when she was given hydralazine 15 mg intravenously. One hour later intravenous diazoxide 5 mg/kg resulted in a blood pressure fall to 60/0 mmHg. Despite large doses of noradrenaline (norepinephrine), the hypotension persisted and the woman died.[1]

Other cases of severe hypotension in patients given high doses of intravenous diazoxide and intravenous or oral hydralazine are described in this[1] and other studies and reports.[2-4] In some instances the patients had also received other antihypertensives such as methyldopa[1] or reserpine.[1,4] At least three of the cases had a fatal outcome.[4]

Mechanism

Not fully understood. The (vasodilatory) hypotensive effects of the two drugs are additive, and it would seem that in some instances the normal compensatory responses of the cardiovascular system to maintain an adequate blood pressure reach their limit. This can occur with intravenous diazoxide alone.[2]

Importance and management

The concurrent use of intravenous diazoxide and hydralazine should be undertaken extremely cautiously with thorough monitoring. Note that the doses of diazoxide used in the above reports were frequently higher than those currently recommended for hypertensive crises.[5] In addition, there are now many more options available for the treatment of very severe hypertension, and the BNF in the UK considers intravenous diazoxide to be one of the less suitable choices.[5] Moreover, diazoxide was frequently associated with clinically important hypotension when used in pregnancy, and is not considered a good choice in this situation.[6]

1. Henrich WL, Cronin R, Miller PD, Anderson RJ. Hypotensive sequelae of diazoxide and hydralazine therapy. *JAMA* (1977) 237, 264–5.
2. Kumar GK, Dastoor FC, Robayo JR, Razzaque MA. Side effects of diazoxide. *JAMA* (1976) 235, 275–6.
3. Tansey WA, Williams EG, Landesman RH and Schwarz MJ. Diazoxide. *JAMA* (1973) 225, 749.
4. Davey M, Moodley J, Soutter P. Adverse effects of a combination of diazoxide and hydrallazine therapy. *S Afr Med J* (1981) 59, 496–7.
5. British National Formulary. 53rd ed. London: The British Medical Association and The Pharmaceutical Press; 2007. p. 93.
6. Duley L, Henderson-Smart DJ, Meher S. Drugs for treatment of very high blood pressure during pregnancy. Available in the Cochrane Database of Systematic Reviews; Issue 3. Chichester: John Wiley; 2006 (accessed 12/09/06).

Diazoxide + Other drugs with hyperglycaemic activity

The risk of hyperglycaemia is increased if diazoxide is given with other drugs with hyperglycaemic activity (e.g. the thiazides, chlorpromazine, corticosteroids, combined oral contraceptives).

Clinical evidence, mechanism, importance and management

An isolated report[1] describes a child receiving long-term treatment for hypoglycaemia with diazoxide 8 mg/kg daily in divided doses and **bendroflumethiazide** 1.25 mg daily, who developed a diabetic pre-coma and severe hyperglycaemia after taking a single 30-mg dose of **chlorpromazine.** The reason for this reaction is not understood but one idea is that all three drugs had additive hyperglycaemic effects. Enhanced hyperglycaemia has been seen in other patients given diazoxide with **trichlormethiazide.**[2] Caution is clearly needed to ensure that the hyperglycaemic effects do not become excessive. The manufacturers of diazoxide also mention that the risk of hyperglycaemia may be increased by **corticosteroids** or oestrogen-progestogen combinations (e.g. **combined oral contraceptives**).[3]

1. Aynsley-Green A, Illig R. Enhancement by chlorpromazine of hyperglycaemic action of diazoxide. *Lancet* (1975) ii, 658–9.
2. Seltzer HS, Allen EW. Hyperglycemia and inhibition of insulin secretion during administration of diazoxide and trichlormethiazide in man. *Diabetes* (1969) 18, 19–28.
3. Eudemine Tablets (Diazoxide). UCB Pharma Ltd. UK Summary of product characteristics, June 2005.

Glyceryl trinitrate (Nitroglycerin) + Antimuscarinics

Drugs with antimuscarinic effects, such as the tricyclic antidepressants and disopyramide, depress salivation and many patients complain of having a dry mouth. In theory sublingual glyceryl trinitrate tablets will dissolve less readily under the tongue in these patients, thereby reducing their absorption and

effects. However, no formal studies seem to have been done to confirm that this actually happens. 'Table 18.1', (p.672), and 'Table 18.2', (p.674) list drugs that have antimuscarinic effects. A possible alternative is to use a glyceryl trinitrate spray in patients who suffer from dry mouth.

3. Levin RI, Feit F. The effect of aspirin on the hemodynamic response to nitroglycerin. *Am Heart J* (1988) 116, 77–84.
4. Key BJ, Keen M, Wilkes MP. Reduced responsiveness to nitro-vasodilators following prolonged low dose aspirin administration in man. *Br J Clin Pharmacol* (1992) 34, 453P–454P.
5. Karlberg K-E, Ahlner J, Henriksson P, Torfgård K, Sylvén C. Effects of nitroglycerin on platelet aggregation beyond the effects of acetylsalicylic acid in healthy subjects. *Am J Cardiol* (1993) 71, 361–4.

Glyceryl trinitrate (Nitroglycerin) + Aspirin

Some limited evidence suggests that analgesic doses of aspirin can increase the serum levels of glyceryl trinitrate given sublingually, possibly resulting in an increase in its adverse effects such as hypotension and headache. Paradoxically, long-term aspirin use appears to reduce the effects of intravenous glyceryl trinitrate used for vasodilatation in patients following coronary artery bypass surgery.

Clinical evidence

(a) Glyceryl trinitrate (sublingual) effects increased

When aspirin 1 g was given to 7 healthy subjects followed one hour later by 800 micrograms of glyceryl trinitrate sublingual spray, the mean plasma glyceryl trinitrate levels 30 minutes after administration were increased by 54% (from 0.24 to 0.37 nanograms/mL). The haemodynamic effects of the glyceryl trinitrate (including heart rate and reduced diastolic blood pressure) were enhanced. Some changes were seen when aspirin 500 mg was given every 2 days (described as an anti-aggregant dose) but the effects were not statistically significant.[1,2]

(b) Glyceryl trinitrate (sublingual) effects unchanged

A study in 40 healthy subjects who were given 650 mg aspirin or placebo, followed after 1 to 2 hours by sublingual glyceryl trinitrate 432 micrograms found no significant alterations in the peak haemodynamic response, nor the area under the time-pressure and time-pulse curves. There was a transient pressor response, which occurred 1 minute after glyceryl trinitrate was given: this was blunted by aspirin. Taken alone, this change was significant, but when the overall pattern of changes during the 30 minute study was considered, the differences were not significant.[3]

(c) Glyceryl trinitrate (intravenous) effects reduced

A study in patients following coronary artery bypass surgery found that those who had been taking aspirin 150 or 300 mg daily (33 patients) for at least 3 months, needed more glyceryl trinitrate to control blood pressure during the recovery period than those who had not taken aspirin (33 patients). To achieve the blood pressure criteria required, the aspirin-group needed an 8.2 microgram/minute infusion of glyceryl trinitrate. The dose remained relatively high at 3.3 micrograms/minute even after 8 hours, whereas the non-aspirin group needed only 5.5 micrograms/minute, which was reduced to 1.9 micrograms/minute after 8 hours.[4]

Mechanism

Not understood. Prostaglandin-synthetase inhibitors such as aspirin can, to some extent, suppress the vasodilator effects of glyceryl trinitrate by blocking prostaglandin release. However, it seems that a much greater pharmacodynamic interaction also occurs, in which aspirin reduces the flow of blood through the liver, so that the metabolism of the glyceryl trinitrate is reduced, thus increasing its levels, and therefore its effects.

Importance and management

A confusing and unexplained situation. It seems possible that patients taking sublingual glyceryl trinitrate may experience an exaggeration of its adverse effects such as hypotension and headaches if they are taking analgesic doses of aspirin. Also be aware that long-term aspirin use may reduce the vasodilatory effects of intravenous glyceryl trinitrate. The antiplatelet effects of aspirin and glyceryl trinitrate appear to be additive.[5]

1. Weber S, Rey E, Pipeau C, Lutfalla G, Richard M-O, Daoud-El-Assaf H, Olive G, Degeorges M. Influence of aspirin on the hemodynamic effects of sublingual nitroglycerin. *J Cardiovasc Pharmacol* (1983) 5, 874–7.
2. Rey E, El-Assaf HD, Richard MO, Weber S, Bourdon A, Picard G, Olive G. Pharmacological interaction between nitroglycerin and aspirin after acute and chronic aspirin treatment of healthy subjects. *Eur J Clin Pharmacol* (1983) 25, 779–82.

Glyceryl trinitrate (Nitroglycerin) + Nifedipine

The effect of sublingual glyceryl trinitrate was not altered by pretreatment with nifedipine in two studies. Nifedipine and intravenous glyceryl trinitrate had additive vasodilator effects in one study, but the preliminary results of another study found that patients undergoing coronary artery bypass surgery and taking nifedipine 20 mg twice daily required more intravenous glyceryl trinitrate than those taking nifedipine 10 mg twice daily or those not taking nifedipine.

Clinical evidence, mechanism, importance and management

(a) Sublingual glyceryl trinitrate

In 9 patients with stable chronic angina, there was no significant haemodynamic interaction between sublingual glyceryl trinitrate and a single-dose of nifedipine, or nifedipine three times daily for 5 days.[1] In another study in healthy subjects, the venodilatory effect of sublingual glyceryl trinitrate was not altered by pretreatment with nifedipine 10 mg.[2] No special precautions are required during concurrent use.

(b) Intravenous glyceryl trinitrate

In 7 patients with severe congestive heart failure, a single-dose of oral nifedipine increased stroke volume, with a peak effect at 30 minutes. The addition of intravenous glyceryl trinitrate at 2 hours further increased stroke volume and increased the cardiac index.[3] Therefore the addition of glyceryl trinitrate enhanced the vasodilator action of nifedipine. Conversely, in the preliminary findings of a comparative study of 3 groups of patients undergoing coronary bypass graft surgery, those taking nifedipine 20 mg twice daily needed initial doses of intravenous glyceryl trinitrate (to reduce cardiac workload, maintain graft patency and control blood pressure) that were about 40% higher than those in the other 2 groups; one taking nifedipine 10 mg twice daily for hypertension, and the other a control group of normotensive patients. Moreover, these higher doses had little effect on the initial mean systolic blood pressure of half of the group taking nifedipine 20 mg twice daily, and they needed an additional infusion of nitroprusside.[4] It was suggested that since glyceryl trinitrate is converted to nitric oxide to elicit its vasodilator effect, it is possible that the nifedipine inhibits the enzymic production of the nitrous oxide. This appears to be the only study to suggest a negative interaction, and the clinical relevance of its findings is unclear. Note that this study was non-randomised, and there may have been other important differences between the patients in each group that would account for the effects seen.

1. Boje KM, Fung H-L, Yoshitomi K, Parker JO. Haemodynamic effects of combined oral nifedipine and sublingual nitroglycerin in patients with chronic stable angina. *Eur J Clin Pharmacol* (1987) 33, 349–54.
2. Gascho JA, Apollo WP. Effects of nifedipine on the venodilatory response to nitroglycerin. *Am J Cardiol* (1990) 65, 99–102.
3. Kubo SH, Fox SC, Prida XE, Cody RJ. Combined hemodynamic effects of nifedipine and nitroglycerin in congestive heart failure. *Am Heart J* (1985) 110, 1032–4.
4. Key BJ, Wilkes MP, Keen M. Reduced responsiveness to glyceryl trinitrate following antihypertensive treatment with nifedipine in man. *Br J Clin Pharmacol* (1993) 36, 499P.

Guanethidine + Amfetamines and related drugs

The antihypertensive effects of guanethidine can be reduced or abolished by drugs including dexamfetamine, ephedrine, metamfetamine and methylphenidate. The blood pressure may even rise higher than before treatment with the antihypertensive.

Clinical evidence

When 16 hypertensive patients taking guanethidine 25 to 35 mg daily were given single-doses of **dexamfetamine** 10 mg orally, **ephedrine** 90 mg orally, **metamfetamine** 30 mg intramuscularly or **methylphenidate** 20 mg orally, the hypotensive effects of the guanethidine were completely abolished, and in some instances the blood pressures rose higher than before treatment with the guanethidine.[1] Another report describes the same interaction between guanethidine and **dexamfetamine**.[2]

Mechanism

These drugs are all indirectly-acting sympathomimetic amines, which not only prevent guanethidine-like drugs from entering the adrenergic neurones of the sympathetic nervous system, but also displace the antihypertensive drug already there.[3] As a result the blood pressure lowering effects are lost. In addition these amines release noradrenaline (norepinephrine) from the neurones, which raises the blood pressure. Thus the antihypertensive effects are not only opposed, but the pressure may even be raised higher than before treatment.[3-8]

Importance and management

Well documented, well established, and clinically important interactions. Other drugs, such as **phenylpropanolamine**, which is also an indirectly-acting sympathomimetic, are likely to interact similarly. Patients taking guanethidine should avoid indirectly-acting sympathomimetics, see 'Table 24.1', (p.879) for a list. Warn them against the temptation to use proprietary non-prescription nasal decongestants containing any of these amines to relieve the nasal stuffiness commonly associated with the use of guanethidine and related drugs. The same precautions apply to the sympathomimetics used as appetite suppressants. However, one brief report stated that **diethylpropion** has been used with guanethidine without any adverse events.[9] Note that guanethidine increases the hypertensive effects of 'directly-acting sympathomimetics', (p.891).

1. Gulati OD, Dave BT, Gokhale SD, Shah KM. Antagonism of adrenergic neuron blockade in hypertensive subjects. *Clin Pharmacol Ther* (1966) 7, 510–4.
2. Ober KF, Wang RIH. Drug interactions with guanethidine. *Clin Pharmacol Ther* (1973) 14, 190–5.
3. Flegin OT, Morgan DH, Oates JA, Shand DG. The mechanism of the reversal of the effect of guanethidine by amphetamines in cat and man. *Br J Pharmacol* (1970) 39, 253P–254P.
4. Day MD, Rand MJ. Antagonism of guanethidine and bretylium by various agents. *Lancet* (1962) 2, 1282–3.
5. Day MD, Rand MJ. Evidence for a competitive antagonism of guanethidine by dexamphetamine. *Br J Pharmacol* (1963) 20, 17–28.
6. Day MD. Effect of sympathomimetic amines on the blocking action of guanethidine, bretylium and xylocholine. *Br J Pharmacol* (1962) 18, 421–39.
7. Starke K. Interactions of guanethidine and indirectly-acting sympathomimetic amines. *Arch Int Pharmacodyn Ther* (1972) 195, 309–14.
8. Boura ALA, Green AF. Comparison of bretylium and guanethidine: tolerance and effects on adrenergic nerve function and responses to sympathomimetic amines. *Br J Pharmacol* (1962) 19, 13–41.
9. Seedat YK, Reddy J. Diethylpropion hydrochloride (Tenuate Dospan) in the treatment of obese hypertensive patients. *S Afr Med J* (1974) 48, 569.

Guanethidine + Antipsychotics

Large doses of chlorpromazine may reduce or even abolish the antihypertensive effects of guanethidine, although in some patients the inherent hypotensive effects of the chlorpromazine may possibly predominate. Case reports suggest that haloperidol and tiotixene may interact similarly. Molindone is reported not to interact with guanethidine, and a single-dose of prochlorperazine also did not interact with guanethidine.

Clinical evidence

Two severely hypertensive patients, with stable blood pressure while taking guanethidine 80 mg daily, were given **chlorpromazine** 200 to 300 mg daily. The diastolic blood pressure of one rose over 10 days from 94 to 112 mmHg and continued to rise to 116 mmHg, even when the **chlorpromazine** was withdrawn. The diastolic pressure of the other rose from 105 to 127 mmHg, and then to 150 mmHg, again, even after the **chlorpromazine** had been withdrawn.[1] Other reports similarly describe marked rises in blood pressure in patients taking guanethidine with **chlorpromazine** 100 to 400 mg daily.[2-4]

Three hypertensive patients taking guanethidine 60 to 150 mg daily had increases in their blood pressure when **haloperidol** 6 to 9 mg daily was added. The blood pressure rose from 132/95 to 149/99 mmHg in the first patient; from 125/84 to 148/100 mmHg in the second patient; and from 138/91 to 154/100 mmHg in the third patient. **Tiotixene** 60 mg daily was later given to one of the patients and the blood pressure rose from 126/87 to 156/110 mmHg.[2] These results have been reported elsewhere.[3,4]

However, a single 25-mg dose of **prochlorperazine** did not significantly antagonise the effect of guanethidine 15 to 20 mg daily in 5 patients.[5] In another study in 7 patients taking guanethidine 50 to 95 mg daily, the addition of **molindone** 30 to 120 mg daily had no effect on blood pressure.[6]

Mechanism

Chlorpromazine prevents the entry of guanethidine into the adrenergic neurones of the sympathetic nervous system resulting in a loss of its blood pressure-lowering effects. The other interacting antipsychotics probably have similar effects. This is essentially the same mechanism of interaction as that seen with the 'tricyclic antidepressants', (p.888).

Importance and management

Direct information is limited but the interaction between guanethidine and chlorpromazine is established and can be clinically important. It may take several days to develop. Not all patients may react to the same extent.[2,7] Monitor concurrent use and raise the guanethidine dosage if necessary. It is uncertain how much chlorpromazine is needed before a significant effect occurs, but the smallest dose of chlorpromazine used in the studies was 100 mg with 90 mg guanethidine, which raised the blood pressure by 40/23 mmHg.[2] The inherent hypotensive effects of the chlorpromazine may possibly reduce the effects of this interaction. Other antipsychotics (particularly the phenothiazines) might be expected to interact similarly and this has been seen with tiotixene an haloperidol. The effects should be monitored. However, molindone is reported not to interact, and a single-dose of prochlorperazine did not interact.

1. Fann WE, Janowsky DS, Davis JM, Oates JA. Chlorpromazine reversal of the antihypertensive action of guanethidine. *Lancet* (1971) ii, 436–7.
2. Janowsky DS, El-Yousef MK, Davis JM, Fann WE, Oates JA. Guanethidine antagonism by antipsychotic drugs. *J Tenn Med Assoc* (1972) 65, 620–2.
3. Janowsky DS, El-Yousef MK, Davis JM, Fann WE. Antagonism of guanethidine by chlorpromazine. *Am J Psychiatry* (1973) 130, 808–12.
4. Davis JM. Psychopharmacology in the aged. Use of psychotropic drugs in geriatric patients. *J Geriatr Psychiatry* (1974) 7, 145–59.
5. Ober KF, Wang RIH. Drug interactions with guanethidine. *Clin Pharmacol Ther* (1973) 14, 190–5.
6. Simpson LL. Combined use of molindone and guanethidine in patients with schizophrenia and hypertension. *Am J Psychiatry* (1979) 136, 1410–14.
7. Tuck D, Hamberger B and Sjoqvist F. Drug interactions: effect of chlorpromazine on the uptake of monoamines into adrenergic neurones in man. *Lancet* (1972) ii, 492.

Guanethidine + Levodopa

When two patients taking guanethidine were given levodopa it was possible to reduce the guanethidine dosage in one and to stop adjunctive diuretics in the other.

Clinical evidence, mechanism, importance and management

A brief report describes a patient taking guanethidine and a diuretic who, when given levodopa (dose not stated), required a reduction in his daily dose of guanethidine, from 60 to 20 mg. Another patient similarly treated was able to discontinue the diuretic.[1] The suggested reason is that the hypotensive adverse effects of the levodopa are additive with the effects of the guanethidine. Direct information seems to be limited to this report but it would be wise to confirm that excessive hypotension does not develop if levodopa is added to treatment with guanethidine.

1. Hunter KR, Stern GM, Laurence DR. Use of levodopa with other drugs. *Lancet* (1970) ii, 1283–5.

Guanethidine + MAOIs

The antihypertensive effects of guanethidine can be reduced by nialamide, and probably therefore other similar MAOIs.

Clinical evidence, mechanism, importance and management

Four out of 5 hypertensive patients taking guanethidine 25 to 35 mg daily had a rise in blood pressure from 140/85 to 165/100 mmHg six hours after being given a single 50-mg dose of **nialamide**.[1] The reason is not understood but one idea is that MAOIs possibly oppose the guanethidine-induced loss of noradrenaline from sympathetic neurones. In *animal* studies, effective antagonism of guanethidine was shown by those MAOIs that also possess sympathomimetic effects (**phenelzine** and **tranylcy-**

promine), but not by **iproniazid** or **nialamide**,[2] and the antagonism was weaker than that seen with some other sympathomimetics.[3]

Direct clinical information seems to be limited to the single dose study,[1] but it would be prudent to monitor the effects if any MAOI is given to patients taking any guanethidine-like drug. The manufacturers of guanethidine actually contraindicate the use of MAOIs because of the possibility of the release of large quantities of catecholamines and the risk of hypertensive crisis. They recommend that at least 14 days should elapse between stopping an MAOI and starting guanethidine.[4]

1. Gulati OD, Dave BT, Gokhale SD, Shah KM. Antagonism of adrenergic neuron blockade in hypertensive subjects. *Clin Pharmacol Ther* (1966) 7, 510–4.
2. Day MD. Effect of sympathomimetic amines on the blocking action of guanethidine, bretylium and xylocholine. *Br J Pharmacol* (1962) 18, 421–39.
3. Day MD, Rand MJ. Antagonism of guanethidine and bretylium by various agents. *Lancet* (1962) 2, 1282–3.
4. Ismelin Ampoules (Guanethidine monosulphate). Amdipharm. UK Summary of product characteristics, April 2005.

Guanethidine + NSAIDs

Phenylbutazone and kebuzone reduce the antihypertensive effects of guanethidine.

Clinical evidence, mechanism, importance and management

When 20 patients taking guanethidine 75 mg daily were given **phenylbutazone** or **kebuzone** 750 mg daily the mean systolic blood pressure rose by 20 mmHg (from 169 to 189 mmHg).[1] This rise represents about a 35% reduction in the antihypertensive effect of guanethidine. The mechanism of this interaction is uncertain but it is probably due to salt and water retention caused by these pyrazolone compounds. Direct evidence seems to be limited to this report. Patients taking guanethidine should be monitored if **phenylbutazone** or **kebuzone** is given concurrently. There does not appear to be any information on guanethidine and other NSAIDs, but indometacin in particular is well known to reduce the efficacy of other classes of antihypertensives, see for example 'ACE inhibitors + NSAIDs', p.28.

1. Polak F. Die hemmende Wirkung von Phenylbutazon auf die durch einige Antihypertonika hervorgerufene Blutdrucksenkung bei Hypertonikern. *Z Gesamte Inn Med* (1967) 22, 375–6.

Guanethidine + Tricyclic and related antidepressants

The antihypertensive effects of guanethidine are reduced or abolished by amitriptyline, desipramine, imipramine, nortriptyline and protriptyline. Doxepin in doses of 300 mg or more daily interacts similarly, but in smaller doses appears not to do so, although one case is reported with doxepin 100 mg daily. A few case reports suggest that maprotiline and mianserin do not interact with guanethidine.

Clinical evidence

(a) Tricyclic antidepressants

Five hypertensive patients taking guanethidine sulfate 50 to 150 mg daily had a mean arterial blood pressure rise of 27 mmHg when they were also given **desipramine** 50 or 75 mg or **protriptyline** 20 mg daily for 1 to 9 days. The full antihypertensive effects of the guanethidine were not re-established until 5 days after the antidepressants were withdrawn.[1]

The same interaction has been described in other reports, with guanethidine and **desipramine**,[2,3] **imipramine**,[4] **amitriptyline**,[5-7] **protriptyline**[3] or **nortriptyline**.[8] The interaction may take several days to develop fully and can last an average of 5 days after discontinuation of the tricyclic.[2] Some studies, and clinical experience suggests that **doxepin** does not begin to interact until doses of about 200 to 250 mg daily are used, then at 300 mg or more daily it interacts to the same extent as other tricyclics.[9-13] However, in one case excessive hypertension occurred in a man taking guanethidine and **doxepin** 100 mg daily.[14]

(b) Tetracyclic antidepressants

Maprotiline 25 mg three times daily caused no appreciable change in blood pressure in two patients taking guanethidine.[7] Similarly, in a study in two patients, **mianserin** 20 mg three times daily for 2 days did not alter the antihypertensive efficacy of guanethidine.[15]

Mechanism

The guanethidine-like drugs exert their hypotensive actions by entering the adrenergic nerve endings associated with blood vessels using the noradrenaline uptake mechanism. The tricyclics successfully compete for the same mechanism so that the antihypertensives fail to reach their site of action, and as a result, the blood pressure rises once again.[16] The differences in the rate of development, duration and extent of the interactions reflect the pharmacokinetic differences between the various tricyclics, as well as individual differences between patients.

Importance and management

A very well documented and well established interaction of clinical importance. Not every combination of guanethidine and tricyclic antidepressant has been studied but all are expected to interact similarly. Concurrent use should be avoided unless the effects are very closely monitored and the interaction balanced by raising the dosage of the antihypertensive. Note that the use of guanethidine and related adrenergic neurone blockers has largely been superseded by other antihypertensive drug classes.

1. Mitchell JR, Arias L, Oates JA. Antagonism of the antihypertensive actions of guanethidine sulfate by desipramine hydrochloride. *JAMA* (1967) 202, 973–6.
2. Oates JA, Mitchell JR, Feagin OT, Kaufmann JS, Shand DG. Distribution of guanidinium antihypertensives-mechanism of their selective action. *Ann N Y Acad Sci* (1971) 179, 302–9.
3. Mitchell JR, Cavanaugh JH, Arias L, Oates JA. Guanethidine and related agents. III. Antagonism by drugs which inhibit the norepinephrine pump in man. *J Clin Invest* (1970) 49, 1596–1604.
4. Leishman AWD, Matthews HL, Smith AJ. Antagonism of guanethidine by imipramine. *Lancet* (1963) i, 112.
5. Meyer JF, McAllister CK, Goldberg LI. Insidious and prolonged antagonism of guanethidine by amitriptyline. *JAMA* (1970) 213, 1487–8.
6. Ober KF, Wang RIH. Drug interactions with guanethidine. *Clin Pharmacol Ther* (1973) 14, 190–5.
7. Smith AJ, Bant WP. Interactions between post-ganglionic sympathetic blocking drugs and anti-depressants. *J Int Med Res* (1975) 3 (Suppl 2), 55–60.
8. McQueen EG. New Zealand Committee on Adverse Reactions: Ninth Annual Report 1974. *N Z Med J* (1974) 80, 305–11.
9. Oates JA, Fann WE, Cavanaugh JH. Effect of doxepin on the norepinephrine pump. A preliminary report. *Psychosomatics* (1969) 10 (Suppl), 12–13.
10. Fann WE, Cavanaugh JH, Kaufmann JS, Griffith JD, Davis JM, Janowsky DS, Oates JA. Doxepin: effects on transport of biogenic amines in man. *Psychopharmacologia* (1971) 22, 111–25.
11. Gerson IM, Friedman R, Unterberger H. Non-antagonism of antiadrenergic agents by dibenzoxepine (preliminary report). *Dis Nerv Syst* (1970) 31, 780–2.
12. Ayd FJ. Long-term administration of doxepin (Sinequan). *Dis Nerv Syst* (1971) 32, 617–22.
13. Ayd FJ. Doxepin with other drugs. *South Med J* (1973) 66, 465–71.
14. Poe TE, Edwards JL, Taylor RB. Hypertensive crisis possibly due to drug interaction. *Postgrad Med* (1979) 66, 235–7.
15. Burgess CD, Turner P, Wadsworth J. Cardiovascular responses to mianserin hydrochloride: a comparison with tricyclic antidepressant drugs. *Br J Clin Pharmacol* (1978) 5, 21S–28S.
16. Cairncross KD. On the peripheral pharmacology of amitriptyline. *Arch Int Pharmacodyn Ther* (1965) 154, 438–48.

Guanfacine + Phenobarbital or Phenytoin

In two patients, the concurrent use of phenobarbital or phenytoin increased the metabolism of guanfacine.

Clinical evidence, mechanism, importance and management

When a hypertensive patient with chronic renal failure who was taking guanfacine 4 mg daily, was given phenobarbital 10 mg daily the antihypertensive effects of guanfacine were noted to be reduced and its dose was progressively raised over about 18 months to 12 mg daily. Phenobarbital was eventually stopped. Single measurements of the pharmacokinetics of guanfacine, both when the patient was taking phenobarbital, and 2 months after cessation of phenobarbital, showed that the half-life of guanfacine increased fourfold when the phenobarbital was stopped.[1] The manufacturer also reports a similar case with phenytoin and guanfacine.[2] Phenobarbital and phenytoin probably induce the metabolism of guanfacine. Patients taking these drugs are likely to need more frequent doses of guanfacine.

1. Kiechel JR, Lavene D, Guerret M, Comoy E, Godin M, Fillastre JP. Pharmacokinetic aspects of guanfacine withdrawal syndrome in a hypertensive patient with chronic renal failure. *Eur J Clin Pharmacol* (1983) 25, 463–6.
2. Guanfacine hydrochloride. Watson Laboratories Inc. US Prescribing information, April 2003.

Guanfacine + Tricyclic antidepressants

A single report describes a reduced antihypertensive response to guanfacine in a patient given amitriptyline and later imipramine. The sedative effects of guanfacine and tricyclics are predicted to be additive.

Clinical evidence

A 38-year-old woman with stable hypertension, taking guanfacine 2 mg daily, had a rise in her mean blood pressure from 138/89 mmHg to 150/100 mmHg while taking **amitriptyline** 75 mg daily for 14 days. The pressure fell again when the **amitriptyline** was stopped. A month later her blood pressure rose to 142/98 mmHg after she had taken **imipramine** 50 mg daily for two days, and fell again when it was stopped.[1]

Mechanism

Uncertain. A possible reason is that, like clonidine (another alpha-2 agonist), the uptake of guanfacine into neurones within the brain is blocked by tricyclic antidepressants, thereby reducing its effects.

Importance and management

Direct information is limited to this report, but it is supported by *animal* studies[2] and consistent with the way another alpha-2 agonist interacts with tricyclic antidepressants (see 'Clonidine + Tricyclic and related antidepressants', p.884). Be alert for this interaction in any patient given guanfacine and any tricyclic antidepressant. **Guanabenz** is another alpha-2 agonist that might interact similarly, but as yet there is no direct clinical evidence that it does so. Note that the sedative effects of guanfacine or **guanabenz** and tricyclics would be predicted to be additive.

1. Buckley M, Feeley J. Antagonism of antihypertensive effect of guanfacine by tricyclic antidepressants. *Lancet* (1991) 337, 1173–4.
2. Ohkubo K, Suzuki K, Oguma T, Otorii T. Central hypotensive effects of guanfacine in anaesthetised rabbits. *Nippon Yakurigaku Zasshi* (1982) 79, 263–74.

Hydralazine + Adrenaline (Epinephrine)

The manufacturers note that patients taking hydralazine who develop hypotension while undergoing surgery should *not* be treated with adrenaline (epinephrine).[1] This is because hydralazine frequently causes tachycardia,[2] and adrenaline would enhance this.[1]

1. Apresoline (Hydralazine hydrochloride). Amdipharm. UK Summary of product characteristics, March 2005.
2. Lin M-S, McNay JL, Shepherd AMM, Musgrave GE, Keeton TK. Increased plasma norepinephrine accompanies persistent tachycardia after hydralazine. *Hypertension* (1983) 5, 257–63.

Hydralazine + Food

The effect of food on hydralazine absorption is uncertain: food increased the AUC of hydralazine in two studies, had no effect in one study, and decreased it in three others. In other studies, a bolus dose of enteral feed decreased the AUC of hydralazine, but an enteral feed infusion had no effect.

Clinical evidence, mechanism, importance and management

Food *enhanced* the bioavailability of a single 50-mg dose of hydralazine in healthy subjects by two to threefold in one study.[1] Similar findings were reported by the same research group with conventional hydralazine tablets, but not slow-release tablets.[2] In contrast, others found that food had no effect on the AUC of hydralazine in healthy subjects.[3] Furthermore, other studies have found that food decreases the AUC of hydralazine by 46% when it is given as oral solution,[4] by 44% after conventional tablets,[5] and by 29% (not significant) after a slow-release preparation.[5] A reduction in the antihypertensive effect of hydralazine was noted in the first of these studies,[4] but no significant alteration in antihypertensive effect was seen in the second.[5] Similarly, another study reported a decrease in the AUC of hydralazine of 55% when it was given with a meal, and 62% when it was given with a bolus dose of **enteral feed**, but no significant change when it was given during an **enteral feed infusion**.[6]

The widely different findings of these studies may be related to the problems in analysing hydralazine and its metabolites, all of which are unstable. All these studies were single-dose, and no studies have adequately assessed the possible clinical importance of any pharmacokinetic changes in long-term clinical use. Note that the bioavailability of hydralazine varies widely between individuals depending on their acetylator status. No recommendations can be made as to whether or not hydralazine should be taken at a set time in relation to meals.

1. Melander A, Danielson K, Hanson A, Rudell B, Schersten B, Thulin T, Wåhlin E. Enhancement of hydralazine bioavailability by food. *Clin Pharmacol Ther* (1977) 22, 104–7.
2. Liedholm H, Wåhlin-Boll E, Hanson A, Melander A. Influence of food on the bioavailability of 'real' and 'apparent' hydralazine from conventional and slow-release preparations. *Drug Nutr Interact* (1982) 1, 293–302.
3. Walden RJ, Hernadez R, Witts D, Graham BR, Prichard BN. Effect of food on the absorption of hydralazine in man. *Eur J Clin Pharmacol* (1981) 20, 53–8.
4. Shepherd AM, Irvine NA, Ludden TM. Effect of food on blood hydralazine levels and response in hypertension. *Clin Pharmacol Ther* (1984) 36, 14–18.
5. Jackson SHD, Shepherd AMM, Ludden TM, Jamieson MJ, Woodworth J, Rogers D, Ludden LK, Muir KT. Effect of food on oral bioavailability of apresoline and controlled release hydralazine in hypertensive patients. *J Cardiovasc Pharmacol* (1990) 16, 624–8.
6. Semple HA, Koo W, Tam YK, Ngo LY, Coutts RT. Interactions between hydralazine and oral nutrients in humans. *Ther Drug Monit* (1991) 13, 304–8.

Hydralazine + NSAIDs

Oral indometacin abolished the hypotensive effects of intravenous hydralazine in one study, but no effect was found in another. In patients with pulmonary hypertension, intravenous indometacin reduced the effects of intravenous hydralazine, and in patients with hypertension, intravenous diclofenac reduced the effects of intravenous dihydralazine.

Clinical evidence, mechanism, importance and management

In 9 healthy subjects, oral **indometacin** 50 mg every 6 hours for 4 doses abolished the hypotensive response to intravenous hydralazine 150 micrograms/kg, and the subjects only responded when given another dose of hydralazine 30 minutes later.[1] A study in 7 patients with pulmonary hypertension given **indometacin** 50 mg and hydralazine 350 micrograms/kg, both intravenously, either alone, or concurrently, also found that the effects of hydralazine (reduction in systemic arterial pressure, heart rate, cardiac index) were reduced by **indometacin**.[2] In contrast, another study in 9 healthy subjects[3] found that oral **indometacin** 25 mg four times daily for 2.5 days did not affect the hypotensive response to a single 200-microgram/kg intravenous dose of hydralazine.

Thus it is not clear if **indometacin** interacts with intravenous hydralazine, and it is uncertain if an interaction occurs when hydralazine is given orally.

On the other hand, a single-dose study in 4 hypertensive subjects found that the actions of intravenous **dihydralazine** (effects on blood pressure, urinary excretion, heart rate and sodium clearance) were reduced by intravenous **diclofenac**.[4]

NSAIDs can cause increases in blood pressure due to their effects on sodium and water retention. Various NSAIDs have been reported to reduce the efficacy of other antihypertensive drug classes, for example see 'ACE inhibitors + NSAIDs', p.28. It would therefore be prudent to monitor concurrent use of hydralazine and NSAIDs.

1. Cinquegrani MP, Liang C-S. Indomethacin attenuates the hypotensive action of hydralazine. *Clin Pharmacol Ther* (1986) 39, 564–70.
2. Adnot S, Defouilloy C, Brun-Buisson C, Piquet J, De Cremoux H, Lemaire F. Effects of indomethacin on pulmonary hemodynamics and gas exchange in patients with pulmonary artery hypertension, interference with hydralazine. *Am Rev Respir Dis* (1987) 136, 1343–9.
3. Jackson SHD, Pickles H. Indomethacin does not attenuate the effects of hydralazine in normal subjects. *Eur J Clin Pharmacol* (1983) 25, 303–5.
4. Reimann IW, Ratge D, Wisser H, Fröhlich JC. Are prostaglandins involved in the antihypertensive effect of dihydralazine? *Clin Sci* (1981) 61, 319S–321S.

Inotropes and Vasopressors + Antimuscarinics

The hypertensive and other serious adverse effects of intravenous phenylephrine and phenylephrine absorbed from *eye drops* can be markedly increased by intravenous or intramuscular atropine.

Clinical evidence

A brief report describes 7 cases of pseudo-phaeochromocytoma, with severe rises in blood pressure and tachycardia, which occurred in young adults and children when they underwent eye operations and were given phenylephrine 10% eye drops and atropine. Only two of them had any pre-existing cardiovascular illness (moderate hypertension). All were under general anaesthesia with propofol, phenoperidine and vecuronium, and premedicated with intramuscular **atropine**, and some were later given more intravenous **atropine** to control the bradycardia, which occurred as a result of stretching the oculomotor muscles. The total atropine doses were less than 10 micrograms/kg in adults and 20 micrograms/kg in children. At least 0.4 mL of phenylephrine 10% was used. In three cases left ventricular failure and pulmonary oedema occurred, which needed monitoring in intensive care. The authors say that no further cardiovascular adverse events were observed during similar procedures when steps were taken to reduce the amount of phenylephrine used and absorbed (see Importance and Management, below).[1] Prior to this case report, a number of cases of cardiovascular adverse effects (severe hypertension, cardiac arrhythmias, myocardial infarction) had been reported for phenylephrine eye drops (usually 10%), or as a subconjunctival injection, and many of these patients had also received antimuscarinics (**atropine**, **cyclopentolate**, **homatropine**, **hyoscine**, **tropicamide**),[2-6] although the contribution, if any, of these antimuscarinics to the adverse effects is unknown.

In a study, 6 healthy subjects were given an intravenous phenylephrine infusion at incremental rates before and after being given three intravenous doses of **atropine** (20, 10, and 10 micrograms/kg) at 90, 120 and 150 minutes. It was found that phenylephrine 420 nanograms/kg per minute raised the diastolic and systolic blood pressures by 4 mmHg before using atropine, and 17 mmHg after atropine was given. For safety reasons the increases in blood pressure were limited to 30 mmHg above the baseline.[7]

Mechanism

Phenylephrine causes vasoconstriction, which can raise the blood pressure. Normally this would be limited by a baroreflex mediated by the vagus nerve, but if this cholinergic mechanism is blocked by atropine or other antimuscarinics, the rise in blood pressure is largely uncontrolled. Severe hypertension may occur, and other adverse cardiac events such as acute cardiac failure may follow.

Importance and management

A surprisingly large amount of phenylephrine can be absorbed from eye drops, and the potential cardiovascular adverse effects of this are well documented. The reports cited here suggest that these risks are clearly increased by the systemic use of atropine. The authors of one of the reports[1] found that the systemic absorption of phenylephrine can be reduced by using lower concentrations of phenylephrine, swabbing to minimise the amount that drains into the nasolachrymal duct to the nasal mucosa where rapid absorption occurs, and reducing the drop size by using a thin-walled cannula. Others have demonstrated that a cannula reduced the dose of phenylephrine given by two-thirds without loss of efficacy.[8] Other suggestions for reducing systemic absorption of phenylephrine are punctal plugging, nasolachrymal duct compression, and lid closure after instillation of the eye drop.[8] Note that phenylephrine eye drops are contraindicated in those with cardiovascular disease.[9] Note also that topical phenylephrine is commonly used with a topical antimuscarinic to enhance mydriasis.

1. Daelman F, Andréjak M, Rajaonarivony D, Bryselbout E, Jezraoui P, Ossart M. Phenylephrine eyedrops, systemic atropine and cardiovascular adverse events. *Therapie* (1994) 49, 467.
2. Fraunfelder FT, Scafidi AF. Possible adverse effects from topical ocular 10% phenylephrine. *Am J Ophthalmol* (1978) 85, 447–53.
3. Van der Spek AFL, Hantler CB. Phenylephrine eyedrops and anesthesia. *Anesthesiology* (1986) 64, 812–14.
4. Lai Y-K. Adverse effect of intraoperative phenylephrine 10%: case report. *Br J Ophthalmol* (1989) 73, 468–9.
5. Miller SA, Mieler WF. Systemic reaction to subconjunctival phenylephrine. *Can J Ophthalmol* (1978) 13, 291–3.
6. Benatar-Haserfaty J, Tercero-López JQ. Crisis hipertensiva y coma tras la administración de colirio de escopolamina, atropine y fenilefrina durante dos casos de ciugía vitrorretiniana. *Rev Esp Anestesiol Reanim* (2002) 49, 440–1.
7. Levine MAH, Leenen FHH. Role of vagal activity in the cardiovascular responses to phenylephrine in man. *Br J Clin Pharmacol* (1992) 33, 333–6.
8. Craig EW, Griffiths PG. Effect on mydriasis of modifying the volume of phenylephrine drops. *Br J Ophthalmol* (1991) 75, 222–3.
9. Minims phenylephrine hydrochloride. Chauvin Pharmaceuticals Ltd. UK Summary of product characteristics, November 2002.

Inotropes and Vasopressors + Calcium compounds

Calcium chloride infusions reduce the cardiotonic effects of adrenaline (epinephrine) and dobutamine, but not those of amrinone.

Clinical evidence, mechanism, importance and management

In a double-blind, randomised, crossover study in 12 patients following coronary artery bypass grafting, calcium chloride (10 mg/kg bolus followed by 2 mg/kg per hour infusion) was found to attenuate the effects of **adrenaline (epinephrine)** 10 and 30 nanograms/kg per minute, given for 8 minutes each. **Adrenaline** alone produced a significant increase in the cardiac index, but following the calcium infusion **adrenaline** had no significant effect and the maximal **adrenaline**-induced increase in cardiac index was reduced by 70%. **Adrenaline** 30 nanograms/kg per minute alone increased mean arterial blood pressure from 87 to 95 mmHg; calcium chloride also raised blood pressure from 85 to 93 mmHg. After calcium was given, **adrenaline** had no further significant effect on blood pressure.[1]

Some of these workers also studied the mode of action of **dobutamine** in 22 patients recovering from coronary artery bypass surgery.[2] It was found that an infusion of calcium chloride (1 mg/kg per minute initially, then 0.25 mg/kg per minute) reduced the increase in cardiac output produced by an infusion of **dobutamine** 2.5 to 5 micrograms/kg per minute by 30%. In a group of 24 similar patients the cardiotonic actions of **amrinone** (a phosphodiesterase inhibitor) were unaffected by the calcium infusion.[2]

Just how the calcium alters the effects of **adrenaline** and **dobutamine** is not known, but since they are both beta-receptor agonists a reasonable suggestion is that calcium interferes with the signal transduction through the beta-adrenergic receptor complex. The clinical importance of these findings is uncertain.

1. Zaloga GP, Strickland RA, Butterworth JF, Mark LJ, Mills SA, Lake CR. Calcium attenuates epinephrine's ß-adrenergic effects in postoperative heart surgery patients. *Circulation* (1990) 81, 196–200.
2. Butterworth JF, Zaloga GP, Prielipp RC, Tucker WY, Royster RL. Calcium inhibits the cardiac stimulating properties of dobutamine but not of amrinone. *Chest* (1992) 101, 174–80.

Inotropes and Vasopressors + Cimetidine

An exaggerated hypertensive response to dobutamine occurred during anaesthetic induction in a patient taking cimetidine. Another case report describes supraventricular tachycardia, which occurred when a patient receiving dobutamine and dopamine was given cimetidine.

Clinical evidence, mechanism, importance and management

A patient about to undergo coronary artery bypass grafting was anaesthetised with midazolam, fentanyl, vecuronium and oxygen. When a 5 microgram/kg per minute infusion of dobutamine was given the patient developed unexpectedly marked hypertension of 210/100 mmHg. The infusion was stopped and over the next 15 minutes the blood pressure fell to 90/50 mmHg. A new infusion had the same hypertensive effect, and the patient's blood pressure was subsequently controlled at 120/80 mmHg with dobutamine 1 microgram/kg per minute.[1] The authors of the report suggest that this exaggerated response to dobutamine may have been due to cimetidine 1 g daily, which the patient was also taking. They postulate that the cimetidine may possibly have inhibited the metabolism and clearance of the dobutamine by the liver, thereby increasing its effects.[1]

A post-operative patient receiving dopamine and dobutamine infusions developed a supraventricular tachycardia 30 seconds after an intravenous injection of cimetidine. Similar episodes of tachycardia occurred on rechallenge with both drugs, but not when each drug was given separately.[2]

These are isolated cases and the general importance is not known but it seems likely to be small.

1. Baraka A, Nauphal M, Arab W. Cimetidine–dobutamine interaction? *Anaesthesia* (1992) 47, 965–6.
2. Grozel JM, Mignotte H, Descotes J. Une nouvelle interaction médicamenteuse: dopamine-cimétidine? *Nouv Presse Med* (1980) 9, 3548.

Inotropes and Vasopressors + Clonidine

Experimental studies in patients show that pretreatment with clonidine decreases the blood pressure response to small doses of dopamine; does not affect the blood pressure response to noradrenaline (norepinephrine); and can increase the blood pressure responses to dobutamine, ephedrine, isoprenaline (isoproterenol) and phenylephrine.

Clinical evidence

In a study in 70 patients undergoing elective surgery, 35 patients were given clonidine 5 micrograms/kg 90 minutes before the induction of anaesthesia and 35 patients were used as a control group. While under anaesthesia, and when haemodynamically stable for at least 10 minutes, all patients were given a 10-minute infusion of **dopamine** 3 or 5 micrograms/kg per minute or **dobutamine** 0.5, 1, or 3 micrograms/kg per minute.[1] Clonidine attenuated the response to the 5 micrograms/kg per minute dose of **dopamine** (blood pressure rise 19/10 mmHg in the control group but only 4/0 mmHg in the clonidine group). However, **dopamine** 3 micrograms/kg per minute did not significantly affect blood pressure in either the control group or the clonidine group. Conversely, clonidine enhanced the response to **dobutamine** at all 3 doses. The study had to be stopped after 2 minutes in the clonidine group receiving the highest dose of **dobutamine** as the rise in blood pressure exceed the study limits (rise 45/24 mmHg compared with 16/7 mmHg in the control group).[1] In a study of the same design, 20 clonidine-treated patients and 20 controls were given a bolus infusion of **phenylephrine** 3 micrograms/kg or **isoprenaline (isoproterenol)** 0.02 micrograms/kg. Those who received clonidine had a greater and more prolonged increase in arterial pressure and heart rate with **phenylephrine** (10 minutes compared with 2 to 3 minutes) and increase in heart rate (but not arterial pressure) with **isoprenaline (isoproterenol)**.[2]

In another similar study, 77 patients (38 premedicated with clonidine 5 micrograms/kg and famotidine 20 mg, 90 minutes before anaesthetic induction, and a control group of 39 given only famotidine) were given **noradrenaline (norepinephrine)** 0.5 micrograms/kg or **phenylephrine** 2 micrograms/kg. It was found that the overall response to **noradrenaline (norepinephrine)** was not significantly affected by clonidine, although 2 to 4 minutes after administration the mean arterial blood pressure was raised in the clonidine group. The blood pressure rise in response to **phenylephrine** was found to be augmented. There were no significant differences between the groups in terms of the incidence of hypertension, arrhythmias or bradycardia.[3] Similar results have been reported with phenylephrine in other studies (see below). The same group of workers repeated this study using two doses of **ephedrine** 100 micrograms/kg as the vasopressor. Clonidine prolonged the response to **ephedrine** by 2 minutes and increased the rise in blood pressure (rise in mean blood pressure in response to **ephedrine** at 3 minutes of 12.7 mmHg with clonidine, compared with 6.6 mmHg without clonidine). The rise in blood pressure was greater in both groups after a second dose of **ephedrine** was given but the effect in the clonidine group was still greater (rise in mean blood pressure in response to **ephedrine** at 4 minutes of 15 mmHg with clonidine compared with 9.4 mmHg without clonidine).[4]

Further study by these same workers, using enflurane and nitrous oxide/oxygen for anaesthesia, found that the mean maximum blood pressure increases in a group of patients premedicated with clonidine and given intravenous **phenylephrine** 2 micrograms/kg were 26% and 32%, for awake and anaesthetised subjects, respectively. This was greater than the blood pressure rises seen in a group not given clonidine, which were 13% and 18%, for awake and anaesthetised subjects, respectively.[5]

Similar additional effects on blood pressure were found in patients given intravenous **ephedrine** 100 micrograms/kg after pretreatment with clonidine.[6]

Mechanism

Not understood, although clonidine is an alpha$_2$ agonist, which blocks the release of noradrenaline (norepinephrine) from the nerve endings, and most suggested mechanisms consider noradrenaline release to be involved in some way.

Importance and management

An interaction is established, although the exact outcome of the concurrent use of clonidine and these sympathomimetic vasopressors is not clear. It has been suggested that the effects may be different at different doses of dopamine.[5] The authors of the one report,[3] studying phenylephrine and noradrenaline (norepinephrine) with clonidine, suggested that the increase in pressor response was unlikely to be clinically significant.

Be aware that dobutamine, ephedrine, and phenylephrine may have a greater than expected effect if clonidine has been taken. Some of these drugs may also be used as nasal decongestants (e.g. ephedrine, and phenylephrine). The outcome of the concurrent use of clonidine in these circumstances is unclear, but a rise in blood pressure seems possible. However, note that these products are usually cautioned in patients with hypertension.

1. Ohata H, Iida H, Watanabe Y, Dohi S. Hemodynamic responses induced by dopamine and dobutamine in anesthetized patients premedicated with clonidine. *Anesth Analg* (1999) 89, 843–8.
2. Watanabe Y, Iida H, Tanabe K, Ohata H, Dohi S. Clonidine premedication modifies responses to adrenoceptor agonists and baroreflex sensitivity. *Can J Anaesth* (1998) 45, 1084–1090.
3. Tanaka M, Nishikawa T. Effects of clonidine premedication on the pressor response to α-adrenergic agonists. *Br J Anaesth* (1995) 75, 593–7.
4. Tanaka M, Nishikawa T. Enhancement of pressor response to ephedrine following clonidine medication. *Anaesthesia* (1996) 51, 123–7.
5. Inomata S, Nishikawa T, Kihara S, Akiyoshi Y. Enhancement of pressor response to intravenous phenylephrine following oral clonidine medication in awake and anaesthetized patients. *Can J Anaesth* (1995) 42, 119–25.
6. Nishikawa T, Kimura T, Taguchi N, Dohi S. Oral clonidine preanesthetic medication augments the pressor responses to intravenous ephedrine in awake or anesthetized patients. *Anesthesiology* (1991) 74, 705–10.

Inotropes and Vasopressors + Ergometrine (Ergonovine)

An isolated report attributes the development of gangrene and subsequently fatal septicaemia to the use of dopamine following the use of ergometrine. A similar case has been reported with ergometrine and noradrenaline (norepinephrine).

Clinical evidence, mechanism, importance and management

One patient developed gangrene of the hands and feet after being given an infusion of **dopamine** (10 micrograms/kg per minute, later doubled) started approximately 2 hours after the use of ergometrine (two 400 microgram doses).[1] This would seem to have resulted from the additive peripheral vasoconstrictor effects of both drugs, which reduced the circulation to such an extent that gangrene and then fatal septicaemia developed. Note that gangrene has been reported with the use of both drugs alone, and it is recommended that peripheral tissue perfusion should be monitored in elderly patients or patients with a history of peripheral vascular disease receiving **dopamine**.[2] This would also seem to be a prudent precaution in those who have previously received ergometrine.

A similar case report describes a pregnant woman (24-week gestation) with severe burns who received ergometrine to treat post-partum bleeding after spontaneous abortion and **noradrenaline (norepinephrine)** to treat hypotensive septic shock. The combination of these two vasoconstrictors is thought to have contributed to ischaemia of the fingers, resulting in loss of some digits.[3] In the rare circumstances when it may be necessary to use both of these drugs, close attention should be paid to peripheral tissue perfusion.

1. Buchanan N, Cane RD, Miller M. Symmetrical gangrene of the extremities associated with the use of dopamine subsequent to ergometrine administration. *Intensive Care Med* (1977) 3, 55–6.
2. Dopamine Sterile Concentrate (Dopamine hydrochloride). Mayne Pharma plc. UK Summary of product characteristics, April 2003.
3. Chuang S-S. Finger ischemia secondary to the synergistic agonist effect of norepinephrine and ergonovine and in a burn patient. *Burns* (2003) 29, 92–4.

Inotropes and Vasopressors + Guanethidine

The pressor effects of noradrenaline (norepinephrine), phenylephrine, and metaraminol can be increased in the presence of guanethidine. These drugs can also be used as eye drops, and in this situation their mydriatic effects are similarly enhanced and prolonged by guanethidine.

Clinical evidence

(a) Blood pressure response

A study in 6 normotensive subjects given guanethidine 200 mg on the first day of the study and 100 mg daily for the next 2 days, found that their mean arterial blood pressure in response to a range of doses of **noradrenaline (norepinephrine)**, was increased by 6 to 18% (a 6 to 20 mmHg increase). Moreover, cardiac arrhythmias appeared at lower doses of **noradrenaline** and with greater frequency than in the absence of guanethidine, and were more serious in nature.[1]

In another report, a patient taking guanethidine 20 mg daily was given intramuscular **metaraminol** 10 mg, which rapidly caused the blood pressure to rise to 220/130 mmHg accompanied by severe headache and extreme angina.[2] An increase in blood pressure from 165/90 to 170/110 mmHg was also seen in a patient taking guanethidine who, prior to surgery, was given **phenylephrine** eye drops.[3]

(b) Mydriatic response

The mydriasis due to **phenylephrine** given as a 10% eye drop solution was prolonged for up to 10 hours in a patient taking guanethidine for hypertension.[4] This enhanced mydriatic response has been described in another study using guanethidine eye drops with **adrenaline (epinephrine)**, **phenylephrine** or **methoxamine** eye drops.[5]

Mechanism

By preventing the release of noradrenaline from adrenergic neurones, guanethidine and other adrenergic neurone blockers cause a temporary 'drug-induced sympathectomy', which is also accompanied by hypersensitivity of the receptors. This results in the increased response to the stimulation of the receptors by directly-acting sympathomimetics such as noradrenaline and phenylephrine.

Importance and management

An established, well-documented and potentially serious interaction. Since the pressor effects can be grossly exaggerated, dosages of directly-acting sympathomimetics (alpha-agonists) should be reduced appropriately. In addition it should be remembered that the incidence and severity of cardiac arrhythmias is increased.[1] Considerable care is required. Direct evidence seems to be limited to noradrenaline (norepinephrine), phenylephrine, metaraminol, and methoxamine. **Dopamine** also possess direct sympathomimetic activity and may be expected to interact similarly. If as a result of this interaction the blood pressure becomes grossly elevated, it can be controlled by giving an alpha-adrenergic blocker such as phentolamine.[6] Phenylephrine is contained in a number of non-prescription cough and cold preparations, which may contain 12 mg in a dose. A single dose of this size is only likely to cause a moderate blood pressure rise. However, this requires confirmation, particularly since the non-prescription products may be taken up to 4 times daily for up to 7 days, and higher doses may be available in some countries.

An exaggerated pressor response is clearly much more potentially serious than enhanced and prolonged mydriasis, but the latter is also possible and undesirable. The same precautions apply about using smaller amounts of the sympathomimetic drugs. Note that many indirectly-acting sympathomimetics can antagonise the blood pressure lowering effect of guanethidine, see 'Guanethidine + Amfetamines and related drugs', p.886. The sympathomimetics are classified in 'Table 24.1', (p.879).

1. Mulheims GH, Entrup RW, Paiewonsky D, Mierzwiak DS. Increased sensitivity of the heart to catecholamine-induced arrhythmias following guanethidine. *Clin Pharmacol Ther* (1965) 6, 757–62.
2. Stevens FRT. A danger of sympathomimetic drugs. *Med J Aust* (1966) 2, 576.
3. Kim JM, Stevenson CE, Mathewson HS. Hypertensive reactions to phenylephrine eyedrops in patients with sympathetic denervation. *Am J Ophthalmol* (1978) 85, 862–8.
4. Cooper B. Neo-synephrine (10%) eye drops. *Med J Aust* (1968) 55, 420.
5. Sneddon JM, Turner P. The interactions of local guanethidine and sympathomimetic amines in the human eye. *Arch Ophthalmol* (1969) 81,622–7.
6. Allum W, Aminu J, Bloomfield TH, Davies C, Scales AH, Vere DW. Interaction between debrisoquine and phenylephrine in man. *Br J Clin Pharmacol* (1974) 1, 51–7.

Inotropes and Vasopressors + Lithium

The pressor effects of noradrenaline (norepinephrine) and phenylephrine are slightly reduced by lithium carbonate.

Clinical evidence, mechanism, importance and management

A study in 8 patients with 'manic depression' found that after taking lithium carbonate for 7 to 10 days (serum level range 0.72 to 1.62 mmol/L) the dosage of a **noradrenaline (norepinephrine)** infusion had to be increased by 1.8 micrograms in 7 patients to maintain a blood pressure increase of 25 mmHg. This equated to a 22% reduction in the pressor effect of **noradrenaline (norepinephrine)**.[1] Another study in 17 depressed patients with serum lithium levels in the range 0.8 to 1.2 mmol/L found that 12% more **noradrenaline (norepinephrine)** and 31% more **phenylephrine** was needed to raise the blood pressure by 30 mmHg.[2] The reasons for this interaction are not known.

These decreases in the pressor response to **noradrenaline (norepinephrine)** and to **phenylephrine** in the presence of lithium carbonate are both relatively small and it seems unlikely that they will present any problems in practice.

1. Fann WE, Davis JM, Janowsky DS, Cavanaugh JH, Kaufmann JS, Griffith JD, Oates JA. Effects of lithium on adrenergic function in man. *Clin Pharmacol Ther* (1972) 13, 71–7.
2. Ghose K. Assessment of peripheral adrenergic activity and its interactions with drugs in man. *Eur J Clin Pharmacol* (1980) 17, 233–8.

Inotropes and Vasopressors + Reserpine

The effects of adrenaline (epinephrine), noradrenaline (norepinephrine) and other directly-acting sympathomimetics are slightly increased in the presence of reserpine.

Clinical evidence

Pretreatment with **phenylephrine** 10% eye drops caused a blood pressure increase of 30/12 mmHg in 11 patients taking reserpine, whereas no significant increase in blood pressure occurred in 176 patients who were given **phenylephrine** eye drops and who were not taking reserpine.[1] After 7 healthy subjects took reserpine 0.25 to 1 mg daily for 2 weeks the increase in the blood pressure response to **noradrenaline (norepinephrine)** was increased by 20 to 40%.[2] A man taking reserpine who became hypotensive while undergoing surgery failed to respond to an intravenous injection of ephedrine, but did so after 30 minutes treatment with **noradrenaline**, presumably because the stores of **noradrenaline** at adrenergic neurones had become replenished.[3] The mydriatic effects of **ephedrine** have also been shown to be antagonised by pretreatment with reserpine.[4] However, in contrast, one report claimed that ephedrine 25 mg given orally or intramuscularly, once or twice daily, proved to be an effective treatment for reserpine-induced hypotension and bradycardia in schizophrenic patients.[5]

Studies in dogs have demonstrated that **adrenaline (epinephrine)**, **noradrenaline (norepinephrine)** and **phenylephrine** (all sympathomimetics with direct actions) remain effective vasopressors after treatment with reserpine, and their actions are enhanced to some extent.[6-8] **Metaraminol** has also been successfully used to raise blood pressure in reserpine-treated patients.[9]

Mechanism

The rauwolfia alkaloids (e.g. reserpine) cause adrenergic neurones to lose their stores of noradrenaline (norepinephrine), so that they can no longer stimulate adrenergic receptors and transmission ceases. Indirectly-acting sympathomimetics, which work by stimulating the release of stored noradrenaline, may therefore be expected to become ineffective. In contrast, the effects of directly-acting sympathomimetics should remain unchanged. However, their effects may be enhanced (as described above) because when the receptors are deprived of stimulation by noradrenaline for any length of time they can become supersensitive. Drugs with mixed direct and indirect actions, such as ephedrine, should fall somewhere between the two, although the reports cited seem to indicate that ephedrine has predominantly indirect activity.[3,4]

Importance and management

These are established interactions, but the paucity of clinical information suggests that in practice they do not present many problems, perhaps because the effects of these vasopressors are so closely monitored, and titrated to effect. If a pressor drug is required, a directly-acting drug such as noradrenaline (norepinephrine) or phenylephrine may be expected to be effective. The receptors may show some supersensitivity so that a dosage reduction may be required. 'Table 24.1', (p.879) gives a classification of the sympathomimetics.

1. Kim JM, Stevenson CE, Mathewson HS. Hypertensive reactions to phenylephrine eyedrops in patients with sympathetic denervation. *Am J Ophthalmol* (1978) 85, 862–8.
2. Abboud FM, Eckstein JW. Effects of small oral doses of reserpine on vascular responses to tyramine and norepinephrine in man. *Circulation* (1964) 29, 219–23.
3. Ziegler CH, Lovette JB. Operative complications after therapy with reserpine and reserpine compounds. *JAMA* (1961) 176, 916–19.
4. Sneddon JM, Turner P. Ephedrine mydriasis in hypertension and the response to treatment. *Clin Pharmacol Ther* (1969) 10, 64–71.
5. Noce RH, Williams DB, Rapaport W. Reserpine (Serpasil) in the management of the mentally ill. *JAMA* (1955) 158, 11–15.
6. Stone CA, Ross CA, Wenger HC, Ludden CT, Blessing JA, Totaro JA, Porter CC. Effect of α-methyl-3,4-dihydroxyphenylalanine (methyldopa), reserpine and related agents on some vascular responses in the dog. *J Pharmacol Exp Ther* (1962) 136, 80–8.
7. Eger EI, Hamilton WK. The effect of reserpine on the action of various vasopressors. *Anesthesiology* (1959) 20, 641–5.
8. Moore JI, Moran NC. Cardiac contractile force responses to ephedrine and other sympathomimetic amines in dogs after pretreatment with reserpine. *J Pharmacol Exp Ther* (1962) 136, 89–96.
9. Smessaert AA, Hicks RG. Problems caused by rauwolfia drugs during anesthesia and surgery. *N Y State J Med* (1961) 61, 2399–2403.

Inotropes and Vasopressors; Dobutamine + Dipyridamole

The addition of dipyridamole to dobutamine for echocardiography can cause potentially hazardous hypotension.

Clinical evidence, mechanism, importance and management

Ten patients with a low probability of coronary artery disease underwent dobutamine echocardiography. Five were given dobutamine alone, while the other 5 were given a low intravenous dose of dipyridamole with the maximal dose of dobutamine, to see whether the sensitivity of the test could be improved. Four of the patients given both drugs experienced severe hypotension while no hypotension was seen in the control group. The conclusion was reached that this combination of drugs can be hazardous and should not be used in patients suspected of coronary heart disease.[1] Note that, although both of these drugs are commonly used in stress echocardiography, they are not given together.

1. Shaheen J, Rosenmann D, Tzivoni D. Severe hypotension induced by combination of dobutamine and dipyridamole. *Isr J Med Sci* (1996) 32, 1105–7.

Inotropes and Vasopressors; Dopamine + Phenytoin

Some limited evidence suggests that patients needing dopamine to support their blood pressure can become severely hypotensive if they are also given intravenous phenytoin.

Clinical evidence, mechanism, importance and management

Five critically ill patients treated with a number of different drugs, were given dopamine to maintain an adequate blood pressure. When seizures developed they were given intravenous phenytoin at an infusion rate of 5 to 25 mg/minute. Their previously stable blood pressures then fell rapidly, one patient became bradycardic, and two patients died from cardiac arrest. A similar reaction was found in *dogs* made hypovolaemic and hypotensive by bleeding, and then given dopamine followed by a phenytoin infusion.[1] However, another study in *dogs* was unable to find evidence of this serious adverse interaction,[2] and no evidence of marked hypotension occurred when a patient with cardiogenic shock was given a phenytoin infusion while receiving dopamine and dobutamine.[3]

The documentation of this adverse interaction therefore appears to be limited to this single report. However, intravenous phenytoin is known to cause hypotension if it is given rapidly, particularly in gravely ill patients. Blood pressure is doubtless being monitored in patients receiving dopamine, and should be measured when phenytoin is given intravenously. However, more frequent monitoring may be necessary initially, as this interaction develops rapidly.

1. Bivins BA, Rapp RP, Griffen WO, Blouin R, Bustrack J. Dopamine-phenytoin interaction. A cause of hypotension in the critically ill. *Arch Surg* (1978) 113, 245–9.
2. Smith RD, Lomas TE. Modification of cardiovascular responses to intravenous phenytoin by dopamine in dogs: evidence against an adverse interaction. *Toxicol Appl Pharmacol* (1978) 45, 665–73.
3. Torres E, Garcia B, Sosa P, Alba D. No interaction between dopamine and phenytoin. *Ann Pharmacother* (1995) 29, 1300–1.

Inotropes and Vasopressors; Dopamine + Selegiline

A case report describes a hypertensive reaction attributed to the concurrent use of dopamine and selegiline.

Clinical evidence, mechanism, importance and management

A 75-year-old man, who was taking selegiline 5 mg twice daily for Parkinson's disease, was given intravenous dopamine 3.5 micrograms/kg per minute because of a decline in blood pressure and urine output following a serious road traffic accident. Twenty minutes after the infusion was started his blood pressure had hardly changed, but 30 minutes later it had risen from 108/33 to 228/50 mmHg. The dopamine infusion was discontinued and the blood pressure decreased to 121/40 mmHg over the next 30 minutes. The dopamine infusion was reinstituted twice more at lower doses (1.03 and 0.9 micrograms/kg per minute), but each time similar reactions occurred. The exaggerated vasopressor response was thought to be due to inhibition of dopamine metabolism by selegiline.[1]

The authors of the report[1] and the manufacturers of selegiline recommend that dopamine should be used cautiously,[2] and only after careful risk-benefit assessment,[3] in patients who are currently taking selegiline or who have taken selegiline in the 2 weeks prior to dopamine therapy. In addition, the manufacturers of dopamine warn that in patients who have received **MAOIs** within the previous 2 to 3 weeks, the initial dose of dopamine should be no greater than 10% of the usual dose.[4]

1. Rose LM, Ohlinger MJ, Mauro VF. A hypertensive reaction induced by concurrent use of selegiline and dopamine. *Ann Pharmacother* (2000) 34, 1020–4.
2. Eldepryl (Selegiline hydrochloride). Orion Pharma (UK) Ltd. UK Summary of product characteristics, July 2006.
3. Zelapar (Selegiline hydrochloride). Cephalon Ltd. UK Summary of product characteristics, November 2006.
4. Dopamine Sterile Concentrate (Dopamine hydrochloride). Mayne Pharma plc. UK Summary of product characteristics, April 2003.

Inotropes and Vasopressors; Dopamine + Tolazoline

Acute and eventually fatal hypotension occurred in a patient given dopamine and tolazoline.

Clinical evidence

A patient receiving ventilatory support following surgery was given dopamine on the third postoperative day. Pulmonary arterial pressure had been steadily rising since the surgery, so on day 4 he was given a slow 2-mg/kg bolus injection of tolazoline. Systemic arterial pressure immediately fell to 50/30 mmHg so the dopamine infusion was increased but, contrary to the expected effect, the arterial pressure then fell even further to 38/15 mmHg. The dopamine was stopped and ephedrine, methoxamine and fresh frozen plasma were given. Two hours later his blood pressure was 70/40 mmHg. Two further attempts were made to give dopamine, but the arterial pressure fell to 40/15 mmHg on the first occasion, and to 38/20 mmHg on the second, which resulted in a fatal cardiac arrest.[1]

Mechanism

Not fully understood. Dopamine has both alpha (vasoconstrictor) and beta (vasodilator) activity. With the alpha effects on the systemic circulation competitively blocked by the tolazoline, its vasodilatory actions would predominate, resulting in paradoxical hypotension.

Importance and management

Information is limited but this interaction would appear to be established. The authors of this report warn that an infusion of dopamine should not be considered for several hours after even a small single dose of tolazoline has been given. They point out that impaired renal function often accompanies severe respiratory failure, which may significantly prolong the effects of tolazoline.

1. Carlon GC. Fatal association of tolazoline and dopamine. *Chest* (1979) 76, 336.

Ivabradine + CYP3A4 inducers

The metabolism of ivabradine may be increased by CYP3A4 inducers including barbiturates, phenytoin, rifampicin, and St John's wort.

Clinical evidence, mechanism, importance and management

St John's wort (*Hypericum perforatum*) reduced the AUC of ivabradine 10 mg twice daily by half.[1] St John's wort is a known inducer of the cytochrome P450 isoenzyme CYP3A4, by which ivabradine is metabolised. Concurrent use therefore decreases ivabradine levels, and as a result probably reduces its effects (although this does not appear to have been studied) increase the metabolism of ivabradine, which results in a reduction in its plasma levels.[1] The manufacturers suggest that the use of St John's wort should be restricted in patients taking ivabradine. They also advise that patients taking other CYP3A4 inducers (they specifically name **barbiturates**, **phenytoin**, and **rifampicin**) may need dosage increases of ivabradine.[1] Monitor concurrent use for ivabradine efficacy and adjust the dose as necessary. Remember to re-adjust the dose of ivabradine if concurrent use of these drugs is stopped.

1. Procoralan (Ivabradine hydrochloride) Servier Laboratories Ltd. UK Summary of product characteristics, March 2007.

Ivabradine + CYP3A4 inhibitors

Ivabradine is metabolised by CYP3A4 and its levels may therefore be increased significantly in the presence of inhibitors of this isoenzyme, such as some azoles, diltiazem, some macrolides, nefazodone, protease inhibitors, or verapamil.

Clinical evidence

A study found that ketoconazole 200 mg daily or josamycin 1 g twice daily increased ivabradine plasma levels by seven to eightfold. Studies in healthy subjects given diltiazem or verapamil have resulted in an increase in the AUC of ivabradine of two to threefold, and an additional heart rate reduction of 5 bpm.[1]

Mechanism

Ivabradine is a substrate of the cytochrome P450 isoenzyme CYP3A4, and its metabolism is reduced by inhibitors of CYP3A4, resulting in increased plasma levels and increased therapeutic effects.[1]

Importance and management

The manufacturers contraindicate the use of potent inhibitors of CYP3A4 with ivabradine, (they specifically mention **clarithromycin**, **oral erythromycin**, **itraconazole**, josamycin, ketoconazole, **nefazodone**, **nelfinavir**, **ritonavir**, and **telithromycin**).The manufacturers suggest that if moderate inhibitors of CYP3A4 are given (they name **fluconazole**) ivabradine may be used, but at a lower starting dose of 2.5 mg, with consideration of heart rate monitoring.[1] Diltiazem and verapamil are also moderate inhibitors of CYP3A4, but their use is not recommended because of their effects on heart rate. Note that clinically relevant inhibitors of CYP3A4 are listed in 'Table 1.4', (p.6).

1. Procoralan (Ivabradine hydrochloride) Servier Laboratories Ltd. UK Summary of product characteristics, March 2007.

Ivabradine + Drugs that prolong the QT interval

The manufacturers advise that ivabradine should not be taken with drugs that prolong the QT interval. Bradycardia is a pharmacological effect of ivabradine, and QT prolongation may be exacerbated by heart rate reductions.[1] For a list of drugs known to affect the QT interval see 'Table 9.2', (p.257).

1. Procoralan (Ivabradine hydrochloride). Servier Laboratories Ltd. UK Summary of product characteristics, March 2007.

Ivabradine + Grapefruit juice

Grapefruit juice inhibits the metabolism of ivabradine.

Clinical evidence, mechanism, importance and management

Grapefruit juice increases the exposure to ivabradine exposure twofold. This interaction probably occur because grapefruit inhibits the cytochrome P450 isoenzyme CYP3A4 in the intestine, by which ivabradine is metabolised. This leads to increased levels, which increases the risks of adverse effects such as profound bradycardia The manufacturers recommend that the intake of grapefruit juice by patients also taking ivabradine is restricted.[1] However, note that they contraindicate the use of other drugs that increase ivabradine levels by a similar amount, and so it would seem that concurrent use is best avoided.

1. Procoralan (Ivabradine hydrochloride) Servier Laboratories Ltd. UK Summary of product characteristics, March 2007.

Ivabradine + Miscellaneous

The manufacturers say that in specific drug-drug interaction studies, ivabradine was not found to interact with proton pump inhibitors (omeprazole, lansoprazole), sildenafil, statins (simvastatin), dihydropyridine calcium-channel blockers (amlodipine, lacidipine), digoxin and warfarin. During clinical studies, ivabradine was taken with ACE inhibitors, angiotensin II receptor antagonists, diuretics, short and long acting nitrates, statins, fibrates, proton pump inhibitors, oral antidiabetics, aspirin and other antiplatelet drugs, and there was no evidence of safety concerns.[1]

1. Procoralan (Ivabradine hydrochloride) Servier Laboratories Ltd. UK Summary of product characteristics, March 2007.

Ketanserin + Beta blockers

There is no pharmacokinetic interaction between ketanserin and propranolol, but additive hypotensive effects may occur. Very marked acute hypotension has been seen in two patients taking atenolol when they were first given ketanserin.

Clinical evidence, mechanism, importance and management

A study in 6 patients and 2 healthy subjects given ketanserin 40 mg twice daily for 3 weeks found that **propranolol** 80 mg twice daily for 6 days did not significantly alter the steady-state plasma levels of ketanserin.[1] Another study in healthy subjects, using single doses of both drugs, found that neither drug affected the pharmacokinetics of the other.[2] In a third study, **propranolol** 80 mg twice daily had no effect on the pharmacokinetics of a single 10-mg intravenous dose of ketanserin. However, ketanserin 40 mg twice daily modestly decreased the clearance of a single 160-mg dose of **propranolol** by 29% and increased its maximum serum level by 38%, although neither of these changes were statistically significant.[3] The hypotensive effects of ketanserin were slightly increased by **propranolol** in the first study,[1] and additive hypotensive effects were seen in another study in patients with essential hypertension.[4]

Acute hypotension is reported to have occurred in two patients taking **atenolol** within an hour of taking a 40-mg oral dose of ketanserin. One of them briefly lost consciousness.[5]

The concurrent use of ketanserin and beta blockers can be valuable and uneventful, but a few patients may experience marked hypotensive effects when first given ketanserin. Patients should be warned.

1. Trenk D, Lühr A, Radkow N, Jähnchen E. Lack of effect of propranolol on the steady-state plasma levels of ketanserin. *Arzneimittelforschung* (1985) 35, 1286–8.
2. Williams FM, Leeser JE, Rawlins MD. Pharmacodynamics and pharmacokinetics of single doses of ketanserin and propranolol alone and in combination in healthy volunteers. *Br J Clin Pharmacol* (1986) 22, 301–8.
3. Ochs HR, Greenblatt DJ, Höller M, Labedzky L. The interactions of propranolol and ketanserin. *Clin Pharmacol Ther* (1987) 41, 55–60.
4. Hedner T, Persson B. Antihypertensive properties of ketanserin in combination with β-adrenergic blocking agents. *J Cardiovasc Pharmacol* (1985) 7 (Suppl 7), S161–S163.
5. Waller PC, Cameron HA, Ramsey LE. Profound hypotension after the first dose of ketanserin. *Postgrad Med J* (1987) 63, 305–7.

Ketanserin + Diuretics

Sudden deaths, probably from cardiac arrhythmias, were markedly increased in patients taking potassium-depleting diuretics and high doses of ketanserin. No interaction occurred with low doses of ketanserin in those with normal potassium levels. Potassium-sparing diuretics do not interact in this way.

Clinical evidence

A large multi-national study[1] in 3899 patients found that a harmful and potentially fatal interaction could occur in those given ketanserin 40 mg three times daily and **potassium-depleting diuretics**. Of 249 patients taking both drugs, 35 died (16 suddenly) compared with only 15 (5 suddenly) of 260 patients taking a placebo and **potassium-depleting diuretics**. No significant increase in the number of deaths occurred in those taking ketanserin and **potassium-sparing diuretics**.

It was found that the corrected QT interval was prolonged as follows: ketanserin alone 18 milliseconds, ketanserin with **potassium-sparing diuretics** 24 milliseconds, ketanserin with **potassium-depleting diuretics** 30 milliseconds. Preliminary results of a later study in 33 patients using a smaller dose of ketanserin (20 mg twice daily) with **potassium-depleting diuretics** (**furosemide**, **thiazides**) found no evidence of a prolonged QTc interval in patients with normal potassium levels.[2] The pharmacokinetics of a single 20-mg dose of ketanserin were not altered by single 25-mg doses of **hydrochlorothiazide**.[3]

Mechanism

Potassium-depleting diuretics may cause hypokalaemia, which increases the risk of QT-prolongation and torsade de pointes arrhythmia, which can result in sudden death. Ketanserin also prolongs the QT interval in a dose-related way, and its effects would be expected to be additive with that of diuretic-induced hypokalaemia. See also 'Drugs that prolong the QT interval + Other drugs that prolong the QT interval', p.257.

Importance and management

The use of potassium-depleting diuretics (see 'Table 26.1', (p.944)) with ketanserin 40 mg three times daily should be avoided. Lower doses of ketanserin (20 mg twice daily) have less effect on the QT interval, and can probably be used cautiously with potassium-depleting diuretics, as long as serum potassium levels are maintained. Potassium-sparing diuretics do not interact.

1. Prevention of Atherosclerotic Complications with Ketanserin Trial Group. Prevention of atherosclerotic complications: controlled trial of ketanserin. *BMJ* (1989) 298, 424–30.
2. Van Gool R, Symoens J. Ketanserin in combination with diuretics: effect on QTc-interval. *Eur Heart J* (1990) 11 (Suppl), 57.
3. Botha JH, McFadyen ML, Leary WPP, Janssens M. No effect of single-dose hydrochlorothiazide on the pharmacokinetics of single-dose ketanserin. *Curr Ther Res* (1991) 49, 225–30.

Ketanserin + Miscellaneous

Ketanserin should not be given with certain antiarrhythmics, naftidrofuryl, or tricyclic antidepressants because of the risk of potentially fatal cardiac arrhythmias. Drowsiness and dizziness are common adverse effects, which may possibly be additive with the effects of other CNS depressants.

Clinical evidence, mechanism, importance and management

Ketanserin has weak class III antiarrhythmic activity and can prolong the QTc interval. For safety reasons it has therefore been advised that it should be avoided in patients with existing QTc prolongation, atrioventricular or sinoauricular block of higher degree, or severe bradycardia of less than 50 bpm.[1] For the same reason the concurrent use of drugs that affect repolarisation (**class Ia**, **Ic** and **III arrhythmics**) or those that cause conduction disturbances (**naftidrofuryl**, **tricyclic antidepressants**) should be avoided.[1] See also 'Drugs that prolong the QT interval + Other drugs that prolong the QT interval', p.257, and 'Ketanserin + Diuretics', above.

Dizziness and drowsiness are common adverse effects of ketanserin and therefore it seems likely that these will be additive with other **CNS depressants** and **alcohol**, which may possibly make driving more hazardous, but this needs confirmation.

1. Distler A. Clinical aspects during therapy with the serotonin antagonist ketanserin. *Clin Physiol Biochem* (1990) 8 (Suppl 3), 64–80.

Ketanserin + Nifedipine

Two patients experienced an increase in cardiac arrhythmias when they were given ketanserin with nifedipine.

Clinical evidence, mechanism, importance and management

A study in 20 subjects aged 60 years or more, with normal or slightly raised blood pressures, found that the concurrent use of ketanserin and nifedipine for a week did not, on average, affect their blood pressures, heart rates, or QT intervals, but two of the subjects monitored over 24 hours showed a marked increase in the frequency of ectopic beats, couplets and ventricular tachycardia.[1] The reasons are not understood. The authors of this study say that their findings do not exclude the possibility that the concurrent use of these two drugs might therefore increase arrhythmia in some elderly patients.[1] Concurrent use should be monitored.

1. Alberio L, Beretta-Piccoli C, Tanzi F, Koch P, Zehender M. Kardiale Interaktionen zwischen Ketanserin und dem Calcium-Antagonisten Nifedipin. *Schweiz Med Wochenschr* (1992) 122, 1723–7.

Levosimendan + Miscellaneous

Orthostatic hypotension occurred when levosimendan was given with isosorbide mononitrate. The haemodynamic effects of levosimendan were not significantly altered by captopril, carvedilol or other unnamed beta blockers, or felodipine. Levosimendan does not alter the effects of warfarin. Itraconazole does not alter the pharmacokinetics of levosimendan. Levosimendan appears not to interact adversely with alcohol.

Clinical evidence, mechanism, importance and management

(a) Alcohol

A double-blind, randomised, crossover study in 12 healthy subjects given oral alcohol 0.8 g/kg with intravenous levosimendan 1 mg found no clinically significant pharmacokinetic or pharmacodynamic interactions.[1]

(b) Beta blockers

In 12 healthy subjects carvedilol 25 mg twice daily for 7 to 9 days did not alter the effects of a single 2-mg intravenous dose of levosimendan on cardiac contractility. In addition, the heart rate and diastolic blood pressure responses were not altered, but the systolic blood pressure response was blunted.[2] In a study to compare levosimendan with dobutamine in patients with severe, low-output heart failure, 33 of the 102 patients receiving levosimendan were also given unnamed beta blockers. The use of a beta blocker was shown not to reduce the haemodynamic effects of levosimendan. The authors say this suggests that there may be a place for levosimendan in the management of exacerbations of heart failure not controlled by beta blockers.[3]

(c) Captopril

Captopril, in doses of up to 50 mg twice daily, did not change the haemodynamic effects of a single 1- or 2-mg intravenous dose of levosimendan in 24 patients with heart failure. No additional decrease in blood pressure was observed.[4] No special precautions appear to be required if levosimendan is given to patients taking captopril.

(d) Felodipine

A study of the use of oral levosimendan 500 micrograms four times daily and felodipine 5 mg once daily in 24 men with coronary heart disease found that concurrent use was well tolerated. The felodipine did not antagonise the positive inotropic effects of the levosimendan and had no effect on exercise capacity. Both drugs increased the heart rate during exercise, and there was a slight additional effect with the combination (5 to 8 bpm for levosimendan alone versus 6 to 10 bpm for the combination).[5] There would appear to be no reason for avoiding concurrent use.

(e) Isosorbide mononitrate

In 12 healthy subjects at rest giving an infusion of levosimendan (12 micrograms/kg over 10 minutes, then 0.2 micrograms/kg/minute for 110 minutes) with a single 20-mg oral dose of isosorbide mononitrate had no additional effects on haemodynamic parameters (heart rate, blood pressure, leg blood flow, cardiac output). However, during an orthostatic test, the circulatory response of the combination was significantly potentiated, and three subjects were unable to remain standing for the stipulated time.[6] Care is therefore required when levosimendan and isosorbide mononitrate, or similar drugs, are used concurrently.

(f) Itraconazole

A study in 12 healthy subjects found that the pharmacokinetics of a single 2-mg oral dose of levosimendan were unchanged by itraconazole 200 mg daily for 5 days, and there was no change in heart rates or ECGs (including the QTc interval). It was concluded that because itraconazole, a potent inhibitor of the cytochrome P450 isoenzyme CYP3A4, does not interact significantly with levosimendan, interactions with other CYP3A4 inhibitors are unlikely.[7]

(g) Warfarin

In an open, randomised, crossover study, 10 healthy subjects were given a single 25-mg oral dose of warfarin both before and on day 4 of a 9-day course of oral levosimendan 500 micrograms four times daily. No clinically relevant changes in the anticoagulant effects of the warfarin were seen, and levosimendan alone had no effect on blood coagulation. In addition, there was no important pharmacokinetic interaction between warfarin and levosimendan. No interactions would therefore be expected if both drugs are used concurrently.[8]

1. Antila S, Järvinen A, Akkila J, Honkanen T, Karlsson M, Lehtonen L. Studies on psychomotoric effects and pharmacokinetic interactions of the new calcium sensitizing drug levosimendan and ethanol. *Arzneimittelforschung* (1997) 47, 816–20.
2. Lehtonen L, Sundberg S. The contractility enhancing effect of the calcium sensitiser levosimendan is not attenuated by carvedilol in healthy subjects. *Eur J Clin Pharmacol* (2002) 58, 449–52.
3. Follath F, Cleland JGF, Just H, Papp JGY, Scholz H, Peuhkurinen K, Harjola VP, MItrovic V, Abdalla M, Sandell E-P, Lehtonen L, for the Steering Committee and Investigators of the Levosimendan Infusion versus Dobutamine (LIDO) Study. Efficacy and safety of intravenous levosimendan compared with dobutamine in severe low-output heart failure (the LIDO study): a randomised double-blind trial. *Lancet* (2002) 360, 196–202.
4. Antila S, Eha J, Heinpalu M, Lehtonen L, Loogna I, Mesikepp A, Planken U, Sandell E-P. Haemodynamic interactions of a new calcium sensitizing drug levosimendan and captopril. *Eur J Clin Pharmacol* (1996) 49, 451–8.
5. Põder P, Eha J, Antila S, Heinpalu M, Planken Ü, Loogna I, Mesikepp A, Akkila J, Lehtonen L. Pharmacodynamic interactions of levosimendan and felodipine in patients with coronary heart disease. *Cardiovasc Drugs Ther* (2003) 17, 451–8.
6. Sundberg S, Lehtonen L. Haemodynamic interactions between the novel calcium sensitiser levosimendan and isosorbide-5-mononitrate in healthy subjects. *Eur J Clin Pharmacol* (2000) 55, 793–9.
7. Antila S, Honkanen T, Lehtonen L, Neuvonen PJ. The CYP3A4 inhibitor itraconazole does not affect the pharmacokinetics of a new calcium-sensitizing drug levosimendan. *Int J Clin Pharmacol Ther* (1998) 36, 446–9.
8. Antila S, Jarvinen A, Honkanen T, Lehtonen L. Pharmacokinetic and pharmacodynamic interactions between the new calcium sensitiser levosimendan and warfarin. *Eur J Clin Pharmacol* (2000) 56, 705–10.

Methyldopa + Barbiturates

Methyldopa plasma levels are not altered by the use of phenobarbital.

Clinical evidence, mechanism, importance and management

Indirect evidence from one study in hypertensive subjects suggested that phenobarbital could reduce methyldopa levels,[1] but later work, which directly measured the plasma levels of methyldopa, did not find any evidence of a pharmacokinetic interaction.[2,3]

1. Káldor A, Juvancz P, Demeczky M, Sebestyen, Palotas J. Enhancement of methyldopa metabolism with barbiturate. *BMJ* (1971) 3, 518–19.
2. Kristensen M, Jørgensen M, Hansen T. Plasma concentration of alfamethyldopa and its main metabolite, methyldopa-O-sulphate, during long term treatment with alfamethyldopa with special reference to possible interaction with other drugs given simultaneously. *Clin Pharmacol Ther* (1973) 14, 139–40.
3. Kristensen M, Jørgensen M, Hansen T. Barbiturates and methyldopa metabolism. *BMJ* (1973) 1, 49.

Methyldopa + Bile-acid binding resins

Colestyramine and colestipol are reported to have no important effect on the absorption of methyldopa.[1]

1. Hunninghake DB, King S. Effect of cholestyramine and colestipol on the absorption of methyldopa and hydrochlorothiazide. *Pharmacologist* (1978) 20, 220.

Methyldopa + Cephalosporins

Pustular eruptions developed in two women taking methyldopa and cefradine or cefazolin. The use of methyldopa may have been coincidental.

Clinical evidence, mechanism, importance and management

A 74-year-old black woman taking methyldopa and insulin developed pruritus on her arms and legs within 2 hours of starting to take **cefradine** 250 mg every 6 hours. **Cefradine** was stopped after 7 doses. Over the next 2 days, fever and a widespread pustular eruption developed.[1] Another 65-year-old black woman taking methyldopa and furosemide experienced severe pruritus within 8 hours of starting to receive intravenous **cefazolin sodium** 1 g every 12 hours. Over the next 2 days superficial and coalescing pustules appeared on her trunk, arms and legs.[2] The authors of the first report attributed the reaction to **cefradine**.[1] The authors of the second report note that the concurrent use of methyldopa may or may not have been a contributing factor in both reports.[2] There seem to be no other reports of this reaction.

1. Kalb RE, Grossman ME. Pustular eruption following administration of cephradine. *Cutis* (1986) 38, 58–60.
2. Stough D, Guin JD, Baker GF, Haynie L. Pustular eruptions following administration of cefazolin: a possible interaction with methyldopa. *J Am Acad Dermatol* (1987) 16, 1051–2.

Methyldopa + Disulfiram

An isolated report describes a patient with hypertension, which was unresponsive to methyldopa in the presence of disulfiram.

Clinical evidence, mechanism, importance and management

An alcoholic patient taking disulfiram did not respond to moderate to high doses of intravenous methyldopa, given to control his hypertension, but responded to oral low-dose clonidine. The suggested reason for this lack of response to methyldopa is that disulfiram blocks the activity of dopamine beta-hydroxylase, the enzyme responsible for the conversion of the methyldopa to its active form.[1] The general importance of this apparent interaction is uncertain.

1. McCord RW, LaCorte WS. Hypertension refractory to methyldopa in a disulfiram-treated patient. *Clin Res* (1984) 32, 923A.

Methyldopa + Haloperidol

Two cases of marked CNS adverse effects have been attributed to the use of methyldopa and haloperidol. Another patient became irritable and aggressive. In a small pilot study, the combination of methyldopa and haloperidol lowered blood pressure, and symptomatic hypotension occurred in one patient. The combination also caused marked sedation.

Clinical evidence

Two patients who had been taking methyldopa 1 to 1.5 g daily for hypertension, without problems, developed a dementia syndrome (cognitive disabilities, loss of memory, disorientation, etc.) within 3 days of starting to take haloperidol 6 to 8 mg daily for anxiety. The symptoms totally cleared within 72 hours of stopping the haloperidol.[1] Another patient treated with haloperidol for schizophrenia, and methyldopa for hypertension, became very irritable and aggressive. When the methyldopa was replaced with hydrochlorothiazide, the patient's behaviour improved dramatically.[2]

In a pilot study of the therapeutic potential of using haloperidol 10 mg daily with methyldopa 500 mg daily for 4 weeks, in the treatment of schizophrenia, the supine diastolic blood pressure decreased significantly from 65 to 59.5 mmHg. Six of the 10 patients complained of dizziness, and one patient needed a reduction in the drug doses because of transient hypotension. Somnolence occurred in 8 of the 10 patients.[3]

Mechanism

The hypotensive effects of methyldopa and haloperidol might be expected to be additive. The CNS effects are not understood, although methyldopa can cause sedation, depression and dementia, and haloperidol can cause drowsiness, dizziness and depression.

Importance and management

Concurrent use need not be avoided, but it would be prudent to be on the alert for excessive sedation, excessive reductions in blood pressure or the development of other unexpected CNS adverse effects, particularly in the initial stages of concurrent use.

1. Thornton WE. Dementia induced by methyldopa with haloperidol. *N Engl J Med* (1976) 294, 1222.
2. Nadel I, Wallach M. Drug interaction between haloperidol and methyldopa. *Br J Psychiatry* (1979) 135, 484.
3. Chouinard G, Pinard G, Serrano M, Tetreault L. Potentiation of haloperidol by α-methyldopa in the treatment of schizophrenic patients. *Curr Ther Res* (1973) 15, 473–83.

Methyldopa + Iron compounds

The antihypertensive effects of methyldopa can be reduced by ferrous sulfate. Ferrous gluconate appears to interact similarly.

Clinical evidence

Ferrous sulfate 325 mg three times daily was given to 5 hypertensive patients who had been taking methyldopa 250 mg to 1.5 g daily for more than a year. After 2 weeks the blood pressures of all of them had risen, and the systolic pressures of 3 of them had risen by more than 15 mmHg. Four had diastolic blood pressure rises, two of them exceeding 10 mmHg.[1] The renal excretion of unmetabolised methyldopa was reduced by 88% and 79% when methyldopa was given with **ferrous sulfate** and **ferrous gluconate**, respectively.[1] A further study found that if the **ferrous sulfate** was given 2 hours before, 1 hour before or with the methyldopa, its bioavailability was reduced by 42%, 55%, and 83%, respectively.[2]

Mechanism

It appears that methyldopa chelates or complexes with the iron in the gut, reducing its absorption by about 50%.[1,3,4] The increase in the metabolic sulfonation of the methyldopa also seems to have a part to play.

Importance and management

Information is limited, but this interaction appears to be established and clinically important. Monitor the effects of concurrent use and increase the methyldopa dosage as necessary. Separating the dosages by up to 2 hours apparently only partially reduces the effects of this interaction. Ferrous gluconate appears to interact like ferrous sulfate, and all iron compounds would be expected to interact similarly.

1. Campbell N, Paddock V, Sundaram R. Alteration of methyldopa absorption, metabolism, and blood pressure control caused by ferrous sulfate and ferrous gluconate. *Clin Pharmacol Ther* (1988) 43, 381–6.
2. Campbell NRC, Hasinoff BB. Iron supplements: a common cause of drug interactions. *Br J Clin Pharmacol* (1991) 31, 251–55.
3. Campbell NRC, Campbell RRA, Hasinoff BB. Ferrous sulfate reduces methyldopa absorption: methyldopa: iron complex formation as a likely mechanism. *Clin Invest Med* (1990) 13, 329–32.
4. Greene RJ, Hall AD, Hider RC. The interaction of orally administered iron with levodopa and methyldopa therapy. *J Pharm Pharmacol* (1990) 42, 502–4.

Methyldopa + Oxazepam

A single, unsubstantiated case report suggests that blood pressure control with methyldopa may possibly be made more difficult in the presence of oxazepam.

Clinical evidence, mechanism, importance and management

A 54-year-old woman with insomnia and essential hypertension had unexplained variability in blood pressure while taking methyldopa 750 mg three times daily and a thiazide diuretic. Within a week of stopping oxazepam 60 mg at night, she developed grand mal convulsions and hypertension (190/90 mmHg standing, 240/140 mmHg lying). Her hypertension was then successfully controlled by switching to atenolol and prazosin. The authors of this report suggest that short-acting benzodiazepines such as oxazepam can cause transient hypotension after a dose, but that *hyper*tension may occur on withdrawal. These effects may complicate the management of hypertension.[1] The general importance of this possible interaction is not established, but it seems likely to be limited.

1. Stokes GS. Can short-acting benzodiazepines exacerbate essential hypertension? *Cardiovasc Rev Rep* (1989) 10, 60–1.

Methyldopa + Phenothiazines

The hypotensive adverse effects of chlorpromazine and other phenothiazines may be additive with the antihypertensive effects of methyldopa. Patients may feel faint and dizzy if they stand up quickly. An isolated report describes paradoxical hypertension in a patient given methyldopa and trifluoperazine.

Clinical evidence

In one study, 8 normotensive patients given methyldopa 500 mg to 1 g daily with **chlorpromazine** 200 to 400 mg daily for schizophrenia experienced orthostatic dizziness and had reductions in their standing systolic blood pressure.[1] In contrast, an isolated report describes a paradoxical *rise* in blood pressure in a patient with systemic lupus erythematosus and renal failure when methyldopa and **trifluoperazine** were given. When the **trifluoperazine** was stopped, the blood pressure fell.[2]

Mechanism

Simple addition of the hypotensive effects of both drugs seems to be the explanation for the increased hypotension and orthostasis. The suggested explanation for the hypertensive interaction with methyldopa and trifluoperazine is that the phenothiazine blocked the reuptake of the 'false transmitter' (alpha-methyl noradrenaline) that is produced during when methyldopa is given.[2]

Importance and management

The increased hypotension and orthostasis that can occur if chlorpromazine or other phenothiazines are used with antihypertensive drugs such as methyldopa is established. Note that, of the phenothiazines, **levomepromazine** is particularly associated with postural hypotension. Warn patients that they may feel faint and dizzy particularly during the initial stages of concurrent use, and that if this occurs they should lie down, and that they should remain lying down until symptoms abate completely. Dosage adjustments may be necessary.

The manufacturers of methyldopa note that a reduced antihypertensive effect may occur with phenothiazines, as well as mentioning the risk of additive hypotensive effects[3]

1. Chouinard G, Pinard G, Prenoveau Y, Tetreault L. Alpha methyldopa-chlorpromazine interaction in schizophrenic patients. *Curr Ther Res* (1973) 15, 60–72.
2. Westhervelt FB, Atuk NO. Methyldopa-induced hypertension. *JAMA* (1974) 227, 557.
3. Aldomet (Methyldopa). Merck Sharp & Dohme Ltd. UK Summary of product characteristics, August 2001.

Methyldopa + Phenoxybenzamine

An isolated case report describes a patient who had undergone bilateral lumbar sympathectomy who developed total urinary incontinence when taking methyldopa and phenoxybenzamine.

Clinical evidence, mechanism, importance and management

A woman who had previously had bilateral lumbar sympathectomy for Raynaud's disease developed total urinary incontinence when given methyldopa 500 mg to 1.5 g with phenoxybenzamine 12.5 mg daily, but not when she was taking either drug alone. This would seem to be the outcome of the additive effects of the sympathectomy and the two drugs on the sympathetic control of the bladder sphincters.[1] Stress incontinence has previously been described with these drugs. The general importance of this interaction is probably small.

1. Fernandez PG, Sahni S, Galway BA, Granter S, McDonald J. Urinary incontinence due to interaction of phenoxybenzamine and α-methyldopa. *Can Med Assoc J* (1981) 124, 174.

Methyldopa + Sympathomimetics; Indirectly-acting

Indirectly-acting sympathomimetics might be expected to cause a blood pressure rise in patients taking methyldopa, and an isolated case report describes such a reaction in a patient who took phenylpropanolamine, but in practice this interaction normally seems to be of little or no general practical importance. The mydriatic effects of ephedrine are reported to be reduced by methyldopa.

Clinical evidence, mechanism, importance and management

In a study in 5 hypertensive subjects taking methyldopa 2 to 3 g daily, the pressor (rise in blood pressure) effects of **tyramine** were doubled.[1] In another study the pressor effect of **tyramine** was 50/16 mmHg, compared with 18/10 mmHg before methyldopa treatment.[2]

A man with renal hypertension, whose blood pressure was well controlled with methyldopa 250 mg twice daily and oxprenolol 160 mg three times daily, had a rise in blood pressure from under 140/80 mmHg to 200/150 mmHg within 2 days of starting to take two tablets of *Triogesic* (**phenylpropanolamine** 12.5 mg and paracetamol 500 mg) three times daily. His blood pressure fell when the *Triogesic* was withdrawn.[3]

The reason for this is uncertain. One suggestion is that the methyldopa causes the replacement of noradrenaline at adrenergic nerve endings by methylnoradrenaline, which has weaker pressor (alpha) activity but greater vasodilator (beta) activity. With the vasodilator activity blocked by the oxprenolol, the vasoconstrictor (pressor) activity of the **phenylpropanolamine** would be unopposed and exaggerated. Alternatively it could have been that he was unusually sensitive to the pressor effects of **phenylpropanolamine**.

Despite the information derived from the studies outlined above[1,2] and the single report cited, there seems to be nothing else in the literature to suggest that indirectly-acting sympathomimetics normally cause an adverse reaction with methyldopa. One report briefly mentions that the antihypertensive effects of various drugs, including methyldopa, were not affected by **diethylpropion**.[4]

In 9 patients with untreated hypertension, the normal mydriatic effects of **ephedrine** were reduced by 54% after they started treatment with methyldopa 500 mg to 1.5 g daily.[5]

1. Pettinger W, Horwitz D, Spector S, Sjoerdsma A. Enhancement by methyldopa of tyramine sensitivity in man. *Nature* (1963) 200, 1107–8.

2. Dollery CT, Harington M, Hodge JV. Haemodynamic studies with methyldopa: effect on cardiac output and response to pressor amines. *Br Heart J* (1963) 25, 670–6.

3. McLaren EH. Severe hypertension produced by interaction of phenylpropanolamine with methyldopa and oxprenolol. *BMJ* (1976) 3, 283–4.

4. Seedat YK, Reddy J. Diethylpropion hydrochloride (Tenuate, Dospan) in the treatment of obese hypertensive patients. *S Afr Med J* (1974) 48, 569.

5. Sneddon JM, Turner P. Ephedrine mydriasis in hypertension and the response to treatment. *Clin Pharmacol Ther* (1969) 10, 64–71.

Methyldopa + Tricyclic and related antidepressants

The antihypertensive effects of methyldopa are not normally adversely affected by desipramine, but an isolated report describes hypertension, tachycardia, tremor and agitation in a man taking methyldopa and amitriptyline. The tetracyclic mianserin does not appear not to interact significantly.

Clinical evidence

A man with hypertension, taking methyldopa 250 mg three times daily and a thiazide diuretic, experienced tremor, agitation, tachycardia (148 bpm) and hypertension (a rise from under 150/90 mmHg to 170/110 mmHg) within 10 days of starting to take **amitriptyline** 25 mg three times daily. A week after stopping all treatment his pulse rate was 100 bpm and his blood pressure 160/90 mmHg.[1] In contrast, a double-blind, crossover study in 5 subjects (one with mild hypertension) found that **desipramine** 25 mg three times daily for 3 days had no significant effect on the hypotensive effects of a single 750-mg dose of methyldopa.[2] Another study in 3 hypertensive patients taking methyldopa 2.5 to 3 g daily found that **desipramine** 75 mg daily for 5 to 6 days did not antagonise the action of methyldopa. In fact, the blood pressure fell slightly.[3] **Mianserin** 20 mg three times daily for 2 weeks had no effect on the control of blood pressure in 6 patients receiving methyldopa, although 2 patients developed symptomatic hypotension after the first dose of **mianserin**.[4,5]

Mechanism

Not understood. Antagonism of the antihypertensive actions of methyldopa by tricyclic antidepressants is seen in *animals* and it seems to occur within the brain.[6,7]

Importance and management

Normally no adverse interaction occurs, nevertheless it would seem prudent to monitor the effects of concurrent use if amitriptyline or any other tricyclic antidepressant is given to patients taking methyldopa. Note that methyldopa sometimes induces depression, and so it is generally considered contraindicated in depressed patients.

1. White AG. Methyldopa and amitriptyline. *Lancet* (1965) ii, 441.
2. Reid JL, Porsius AJ, Zamboulis C, Polak G, Hamilton CA, Dean CR. The effects of desmethylimipramine on the pharmacological actions of alpha methyldopa in man. *Eur J Clin Pharmacol* (1979) 16, 75–80.
3. Mitchell JR, Cavanaugh JH, Arias L, Oates JA. Guanethidine and related agents. III. Antagonism by drugs which inhibit the norepinephrine pump in man. *J Clin Invest* (1970) 49, 1596–1604.
4. Elliott HL, Whiting B, Reid JL. Assessment of the interaction between mianserin and centrally-acting antihypertensive drugs. *Br J Clin Pharmacol* (1983) 15, 323S–328S.
5. Elliott HL, McLean K, Sumner DJ, Reid JL. Absence of an effect of mianserin on the actions of clonidine or methyldopa in hypertensive patients. *Eur J Clin Pharmacol* (1983) 24, 15–19.
6. van Spanning HW, van Zwieten PA. The interaction between alpha-methyl-dopa and tricyclic antidepressants. *Int J Clin Pharmacol Biopharm* (1975) 11, 65–7.
7. van Zwieten PA. Interaction between centrally acting hypotensive drugs and tricyclic antidepressants. *Arch Int Pharmacodyn Ther* (1975) 214, 12–30.

Minoxidil + Glibenclamide (Glyburide)

There is some evidence that a 5-mg dose of glibenclamide, but not a 2.5-mg dose, may reduce the hypotensive effect of minoxidil.

Clinical evidence, mechanism, importance and management

A single-dose study in 9 healthy subjects found that glibenclamide 2.5 mg did not alter the hypotensive effect of oral minoxidil 5 mg. However, in a further 4 subjects a 5-mg dose of glibenclamide appeared to cause some loss in the hypotensive effect of minoxidil, but this was not statistically significant. The authors therefore suggested that this interaction may be dose-related. The suggested reason for these effects is that these two drugs have opposing effects on the potassium channels of the smooth muscle of blood vessels.[1] In this study, subjects were pre-treated with propranolol to prevent reflex tachycardia when given minoxidil, which is how minoxidil is used clinically.[1] What is not yet clear is whether any interaction occurs between minoxidil and glibenclamide in a clinical setting.

1. Stein CM, Brown N, Carlson MG, Campbell P, Wood AJJ. Coadministration of glyburide and minoxidil, drugs with opposing effects on potassium channels. *Clin Pharmacol Ther* (1997) 61, 662–8.

Minoxidil + Miscellaneous

The manufacturer notes that excessive blood pressure reductions may occur if minoxidil is used in patients taking guanethidine, because of the adrenergic blocking effects of guanethidine.[1,2] If ex-

cessive hypotension occurs with minoxidil, this should *not* be treated with adrenaline (epinephrine) or noradrenaline (norepinephrine), because this may result in excessive tachycardia.[1]

1. Loniten Tablets (Minoxidil). Pharmacia Ltd. UK Summary of product characteristics, July 2007.
2. Minoxidil. Watson Pharmaceuticals, Inc. US Prescribing information, October 2002.

Minoxidil; Topical + Miscellaneous

A study in 19 healthy subjects found that the absorption of topical minoxidil was increased by almost threefold by the use of topical tretinoin 0.05% applied 1 hour before the minoxidil.[1] The manufacturers note that topical drugs that alter the stratum corneum barrier, such as tretinoin or dithranol, could result in increased absorption of minoxidil if applied concurrently. They suggest that, theoretically, one possible effect of minoxidil absorption would be potentiation of orthostatic hypotension caused by vasodilator drugs.[2] The exact drugs are not stated but this caution would be expected to cover drugs such as the nitrates and hydralazine.

1. Ferry JJ, Forbes KK, VanderLugt JT, Szpunar GJ. Influence of tretinoin on the percutaneous absorption of minoxidil from an aqueous topical solution. *Clin Pharmacol Ther* (1990) 47, 439–46.
2. Regaine for Men Gel (Minoxidil). Pfizer Consumer Healthcare. UK Summary of product characteristics, August 2005.

Moxonidine + Miscellaneous

On theoretical grounds the manufacturers of moxonidine advise withdrawing beta blockers before withdrawing moxonidine. They also advise avoiding alcohol and tricyclic antidepressants during the use of moxonidine. Moxonidine alone can cause sedation, and increases the sedative effects of lorazepam, therefore care is needed with other benzodiazepines, hypnotics and sedatives. No clinically significant pharmacokinetic interactions occur with moxonidine and digoxin, glibenclamide (glyburide), hydrochlorothiazide, moclobemide, or quinidine.

Clinical evidence, mechanism, importance and management

(a) Benzodiazepines and other sedatives and hypnotics

The cognitive function of 24 healthy subjects was not impaired by moxonidine 400 micrograms daily, but the presence of moxonidine was found to increase the cognitive impairment caused by **lorazepam** 1 mg daily.[1] For this reason the manufacturers warn that the sedative effects of the benzodiazepines may possibly be enhanced by moxonidine.[2] Sedation and dizziness may occur with moxonidine, which the manufacturers suggest may be additive with the effects of sedatives and hypnotics.[2] They also advise the avoidance of **alcohol**.[2]

(b) Beta blockers

The presence of a beta blocker can exacerbate the rebound hypertension that follows the withdrawal of clonidine (see 'Clonidine + Beta blockers', p.882). Moxonidine is reported to have less affinity for central alpha-receptors than clonidine, and no such rebound hypertension has actually been seen when moxonidine is withdrawn. However, to be on the safe side the manufacturers advise that any beta blocker should be stopped first, followed by the moxonidine a few days later.[2,3]

(c) Digoxin

No clinically relevant pharmacokinetic interaction was seen at steady state between moxonidine 200 micrograms twice daily and digoxin 200 micrograms daily in 15 healthy subjects.[4]

(d) Glibenclamide (Glyburide)

Glibenclamide 2.5 mg daily had no effect on the steady-state pharmacokinetics of moxonidine 200 micrograms twice daily in 18 healthy subjects. There was a minor 12% decrease in the AUC of glibenclamide, and a 14% increase in clearance, but these changes are unlikely to be of any clinical relevance.[5]

(e) Hydrochlorothiazide

No clinically relevant pharmacokinetic interaction was seen at steady state between moxonidine 200 micrograms twice daily and hydrochlorothiazide 25 mg twice daily.[6] A double-blind, placebo-controlled study showed that when moxonidine 400 micrograms daily was given with hydrochlorothiazide 25 mg daily an increased blood pressure lowering effect was seen, compared to either drug alone. A mean reduction of 27/16 mmHg was noted with the combination, compared to 13/9, 20/12, and 22/13 mmHg for placebo, moxonidine and hydrochlorothiazide, respectively.[7]

(f) Moclobemide

A study found no pharmacokinetic interaction occurred when healthy subjects were given moxonidine 400 micrograms daily and a single 300-mg dose of moclobemide. Moxonidine alone or with moclobemide did not significantly affect cognitive function.[1]

(g) Quinidine

In a single-dose study in 6 healthy subjects, quinidine sulfate 400 mg, given one hour before moxonidine 200 micrograms, caused a minor 11% increase in the AUC of moxonidine and decreased its clearance by 10%. These small changes are unlikely to be of any clinical relevance.[8]

(h) Tricyclic antidepressants

The manufacturers of moxonidine advise avoiding tricyclic antidepressants, because of the lack of clinical experience of combined use.[2] Presumably, this is because moxonidine is related to clonidine, and tricyclics may antagonise the blood pressure-lowering effects of clonidine, see 'Clonidine + Tricyclic and related antidepressants', p.884. Tricyclics can also cause postural hypotension and sedation, both of which could potentially be additive with the effects of moxonidine. If the combination is used, it would be prudent to carefully monitor blood pressure and sedation.

1. Wesnes K, Simpson PM, Jansson B, Grahnén A, Wemann H-J, Küppers H. Moxonidine and cognitive function: interactions with moclobemide and lorazepam. *Eur J Clin Pharmacol* (1997) 52, 351–8.
2. Physiotens (Moxonidine). Solvay Healthcare Ltd. UK Summary of product characteristics, March 2002.
3. Solvay Healthcare. Personal communication, September 1996.
4. Pabst G, Weimann H-J, Weber W. Lack of pharmacokinetic interactions between moxonidine and digoxin. *Clin Pharmacokinet* (1992) 23, 477–81.
5. Müller M, Weimann H-J, Eden G, Weber W, Michaelis K, Dilger C, Achtert G. Steady state investigation of possible pharmacokinetic interactions of moxonidine and glibenclamide. *Eur J Drug Metab Pharmacokinet* (1993) 18, 277–83.
6. Weimann H-J, Rudolph M. Clinical pharmacokinetics of moxonidine. *J Cardiovasc Pharmacol* (1992) 20 (Suppl 4), S37–S41.
7. Frei M, Küster L, Gardosch von Krosigk PP, Koch HF, Küppers H. Moxonidine and hydrochlorothiazide in combination: a synergistic antihypertensive effect. *J Cardiovasc Pharmacol* (1994) 24, (Suppl 1), S25–S28.
8. Wise SD, Chan C, Schaefer HG, He MM, Pouliquen IJ, Mitchell MI. Quinidine does not affect the renal clearance of moxonidine. *Br J Clin Pharmacol* (2002) 54, 251–4.

Nicorandil + Miscellaneous

Neither cimetidine nor rifampicin had any clinically relevant effect on the pharmacokinetics of nicorandil. Nicorandil did not alter the anticoagulant effects of acenocoumarol. Although *animal* studies suggest antagonism of effects, a study in patients found no pharmacodynamic interaction between nicorandil and glibenclamide. Nicorandil may potentiate the hypotensive effects of other vasodilators, tricyclic antidepressants and alcohol.

Clinical evidence, mechanism, importance and management

(a) Acenocoumarol

Nicorandil 10 mg twice daily for 4 days then 20 mg twice daily for 7 days did not alter the INR in 11 patients stabilised on acenocoumarol.[1]

(b) Cimetidine

Cimetidine 400 mg twice daily for 7 days had no effect on the pharmacokinetics of nicorandil 20 mg twice daily for 7 days, except that the nicorandil AUC showed a minor 10% increase, which is not clinically important.[1]

(c) Glibenclamide

Studies in *animals* have indicated that there may be antagonism between nicorandil and glibenclamide. However, in a study, 8 patients with diabetes and angina (taking glibenclamide), and 11 similar patients not receiving glibenclamide, were given nicorandil 15 mg daily for more than 8 weeks. In contrast to the findings in the *animal* studies, glibenclamide did not cause inhibition of the anti-anginal effects of nicorandil, nor was there any disturbance of diabetic control.[2]

(d) Miscellaneous drugs

Combined data from clinical studies in 1152 patients using nicorandil found no evidence of increased adverse effects or an increased number of withdrawals in patients taking unnamed **beta blockers** (210 patients), **calcium-channel blockers** (117), **long-acting nitrates** (130), **bepridil** (18), **diltiazem** (91), **verapamil** (9), **amiodarone** (23) or **molsidomine** (30). It has also been reported that unnamed **antihypertensives**, **antidiabetic** or **lipid-regulating drugs** do not appear to interact adversely with nicorandil.[3] No adverse ECG effects have been seen (including QT or ST segment modifications) with nicorandil.[3] However, the manufacturers suggest that nicorandil may possibly potentiate the blood pressure-lowering effects of other **vasodilators**, **tricyclic antidepressants** or **alcohol**.[4] For mention that phosphodiesterase inhibitors (e.g. **sildenafil**, **tadalafil**, **vardenafil**) should not be used with nicorandil, see 'Phosphodiesterase type-5 inhibitors + Nitrates', p.1272.

(e) Rifampicin

Rifampicin 600 mg daily for 5 days had no effect on the pharmacokinetics of nicorandil 20 mg twice daily for 5 days, except that the elimination half-life showed a minor 17% decrease, which is not clinically important.[1]

1. Frydman A. Pharmacokinetic profile of nicorandil in humans: an overview. *J Cardiovasc Pharmacol* (1992) 20 (Suppl 3), S34–S44.
2. Hata N, Takano M, Kunimi T, Kishida H, Takano T. Lack of antagonism between nicorandil and sulfonylurea in stable angina pectoris. *Int J Clin Pharmacol Res* (2001) 21, 59–63.
3. Witchitz S, Darmon J-Y. Nicorandil safety in the long-term treatment of coronary heart disease. *Cardiovasc Drugs Ther* (1995) 9, 237–43.
4. Ikorel (Nicorandil). Sanofi-Aventis. UK Summary of product characteristics, June 2004.

Pentoxifylline + Cimetidine

Cimetidine increases plasma pentoxifylline levels to a moderate extent, which may increase the incidence of adverse effects.

Clinical evidence, mechanism, importance and management

A study in 10 healthy subjects found that the mean steady-state plasma levels of controlled-release pentoxifylline 400 mg every 8 hours were raised by about 27% when cimetidine 300 mg four times daily for 7 days was added.[1] Adverse effects such as headache, nausea, and vomiting were said to be more common and bothersome while taking the cimetidine.[1]

The reason for this interaction is not known. However, cimetidine is known to inhibit the metabolism of 'theophylline', (p.1181), to which pentoxifylline is structurally related.

The findings of this study suggest that this interaction may be clinically relevant. If cimetidine is required in a patient taking pentoxifylline, monitor for adverse effects, and decrease the pentoxifylline dose if problems occur.

1. Mauro VF, Mauro LS, Hageman JH. Alteration of pentoxifylline pharmacokinetics by cimetidine. *J Clin Pharmacol* (1988) 28, 649–54.

Pentoxifylline + Ciprofloxacin

Evidence from one study suggests that ciprofloxacin increases the serum levels of pentoxifylline, and may increase the incidence of adverse effects. In some clinical studies ciprofloxacin has been used to boost the levels of pentoxifylline.

Clinical evidence

Because patients taking pentoxifylline and ciprofloxacin often complained of headache, the possibility of a pharmacokinetic interaction was studied in 6 healthy subjects. The study showed that ciprofloxacin 500 mg daily for 3 days increased the peak serum levels of a single 400-mg dose of pentoxifylline by almost 60% (from 114.5 to 179.5 nanograms/mL), and increased the AUC by 15%. All 6 subjects complained of a frontal headache.[1]

Mechanism

The evidence suggests that ciprofloxacin inhibits the metabolism of the pentoxifylline (a xanthine derivative) by the liver. Compare 'Theophylline + Quinolones', p.1192.

Importance and management

Information on this interaction and its clinical relevance is limited. The author of the pharmacokinetic study suggests that, if the drugs need to be used together, the dosage of pentoxifylline should be halved.[1] In the absence of other information, if a short-course of ciprofloxacin is required in a patient taking pentoxifylline, this may be a sensible precaution. Alternatively, because the increase in AUC was minor, it may be sufficient to recommend a reduction in pentoxifylline dose only in those who experience adverse effects (e.g. nausea, headache). Note that ciprofloxacin has been used to boost pentoxifylline levels in studies investigating the possible therapeutic value of pentoxifylline's ability to inhibit various cytokines. For example, ciprofloxacin 500 mg twice daily was used with pentoxifylline 800 mg three times daily for up to one year in patients with myelodysplastic syndrome.[2]

1. Cleary JD. Ciprofloxacin (CIPRO) and pentoxifylline (PTF): a clinically significant drug interaction. *Pharmacotherapy* (1992) 12, 259–60.
2. Raza A, Qawi H, Lisak L, Andric T, Dar S, Andrews C, Venugopal P, Gezer S, Gregory S, Loew J, Robin E, Rifkin S, Hsu W-T, Huang R-W. Patients with myelodysplastic syndromes benefit from palliative therapy with amifostine, pentoxifylline, and ciprofloxacin with or without dexamethasone. *Blood* (2000) 95, 1580–87.

Perhexiline + SSRIs

Case reports describe an increase in perhexiline serum levels resulting in toxicity when citalopram, fluoxetine or paroxetine were given.

Clinical evidence, mechanism, importance and management

An 86-year-old woman taking perhexiline was admitted to hospital because of ataxia, falls, lethargy, nausea, and an inability to cope at home. She had started to take **paroxetine** 20 mg daily 5 weeks earlier. Her serum perhexiline levels were 2.02 mg/L, compared with the normal range of 0.15 to 0.6 mg/L.[1] Perhexiline toxicity was also seen in two other elderly women, following the use of **paroxetine** in one case, and **fluoxetine** in the other. The perhexiline serum levels fell when both drugs were stopped, but in one case the fall was very slow.[2] Another case report describes toxicity and raised perhexiline levels in an elderly man shortly after he started taking **citalopram**.[3]

The reason for the rise in perhexiline levels is not known, but it seems likely that these SSRIs can inhibit its metabolism, probably via the cytochrome P450 isoenzyme CYP2D6. The general importance of these interactions is also not known, but it would now be prudent to monitor the outcome of concurrent use for perhexiline toxicity and consider monitoring perhexiline serum levels where possible. The perhexiline dosage may need to be reduced. More study is needed.

1. Alderman CP. Perhexiline-paroxetine interaction. *Aust J Hosp Pharm* (1998) 28, 254–5.
2. Alderman CP, Hundertmark JD, Soetratma TW. Interaction of serotonin re-uptake inhibitors with perhexiline. *Aust N Z J Psychiatry* (1997) 31, 601–3.
3. Nyfort-Hansen K. Perhexiline toxicity related to citalopram use. *Med J Aust* (2002) 176, 560–61.

Ranolazine + Miscellaneous

The concurrent use of ranolazine and moderate or potent inhibitors of CYP3A4, such as some azoles, diltiazem, grapefruit juice, macrolides, protease inhibitors, or verapamil will result in increased levels of ranolazine, and can predispose the patient to adverse effects including QT interval prolongation. Cimetidine and paroxetine do not interact to a clinically significant extent. Ranolazine may increase levels of ciclosporin, digoxin or simvastatin.

Clinical evidence, mechanism, importance and management

(a) CYP3A4 inhibitors

Moderate inhibitors of CYP3A4 (e.g. diltiazem and verapamil) cause a two- to threefold rise in ranolazine levels, and ketoconazole, a potent inhibitor of CYP3A4 causes an ever greater rise (see below). Raised ranolazine levels can cause clinically significant QT prolongation. The manufacturer of ranolazine therefore contraindicates its use with these and other potent or moderately potent CYP3A4 inhibitors. They specifically name **grapefruit juice** and **grapefruit-containing products**, **macrolides** and **protease inhibitors**.[1]

A list of clinically relevant CYP3A4 inhibitors is given in 'Table 1.4', (p.6).

1. Diltiazem. In a placebo-controlled study in 12 healthy subjects diltiazem 60 mg three times daily was given to 12 healthy subjects for 7 days, with ranolazine 240 mg three times daily on days 4 to 7. Ranolazine did not alter the pharmacokinetics of diltiazem, but diltiazem increased the AUC and maximum plasma level of ranolazine by 85% and twofold, respectively. A further study using modified-release diltiazem 180 mg, 240 mg, and 360 mg once daily, and a slow-release preparation of ranolazine 1 g twice daily, resulted in increases in the AUC of ranolazine of 52%, 93%, and 139%, respectively.[2]

2. Ketoconazole. In a double-blind, randomised study, healthy subjects were given slow-release ranolazine 375 mg twice daily for 9 days, with ketoconazole 200 mg twice daily on days 5 to 9. The same study was repeated with ranolazine 1 g twice daily. It was found that ketoconazole increased the AUC, levels (mean, peak and trough) and half-life of ranolazine by 2.5- to 4.5-fold. The most common adverse events were headaches, dizziness and nausea. In some patients the higher dose of ranolazine with ketoconazole resulted in intolerable adverse events.[2]

3. Verapamil. Plasma levels of ranolazine 750 mg twice daily are reported to be increased twofold by concurrent verapamil 120 mg three times daily.[1]

(b) Ciclosporin

Ranolazine inhibits P-glycoprotein. and has been shown to raise digoxin levels (see below), presumably by this mechanism. However, it is also a substrate of P-glycoprotein. The manufacturers of ranolazine therefore advise caution if it is given to patients taking ciclosporin, which is also a P-glycoprotein inhibitor [and substrate].[1] Until more is known it would seem prudent to increase the frequency of ciclosporin and ranolazine monitoring if both drugs are given.

(c) CYP3A4 substrates

In an open-label study, simvastatin 80 mg daily was given with ranolazine 1 g twice daily for 4 days. Simvastatin had no effect on the pharmacokinetics of ranolazine, but ranolazine increased the maximum plasma levels of simvastatin and its active metabolites by about twofold and increased its AUC by 40 to 60%.[2]

These changes may be clinically significant in some patients. If simvastatin is given to a patient taking ranolazine, it would seem prudent to start at the lowest dose and titrate cautiously. If ranolazine is given to patients already taking simvastatin consider reducing the dose of simvastatin (particularly with high simvastatin doses). All patients taking statins should be warned about the symptoms of myopathy and told to report muscle pain or weakness. It would be prudent to reinforce this advice if they are given ranolazine.

(d) Digoxin

A study in healthy subjects given ranolazine 1 g twice daily and digoxin 125 micrograms found that ranolazine increased the plasma levels of digoxin by about 1.5-fold. Plasma levels of ranolazine were not significantly affected by concurrent digoxin.[1] Ranolazine probably raises digoxin levels by inhibiting P-glycoprotein. It would seem prudent to monitor digoxin levels if ranolazine is started, anticipating the need to reduce the digoxin dose.

(e) Paroxetine

Paroxetine has been reported to increase the average steady state plasma concentrations of ranolazine 1.2-fold.[1] Ranolazine is metabolised by the cytochrome P450 isoenzymes CYP2D6, which paroxetine inhibits. However, as CYP2D6 is not the main route of metabolism, only very modest effects are seen, and no dosage adjustment is necessary.[1]

(f) Ritonavir

Ranolazine and ritonavir are both substrates for and inhibitors of P-glycoprotein. The manufacturers of ranolazine advise caution if ranolazine is given to patients taking ritonavir.[1]

1. Ranexa (Ranolazine). CV Therapeutics, Inc. US Prescribing Information, February 2006
2. Jerling M, Huan B-L, Leung K, Chu N, Abdallah H, Hussein Z. Studies to investigate the pharmacokinetic interactions between ranolazine and ketoconazole, diltiazem or simvastatin during combined administration in healthy subjects. J Clin Pharmacol. (2005) 45, 422–33.

Sodium nitroprusside + Miscellaneous

Smaller doses of sodium nitroprusside might be required in patients receiving antihypertensive drugs. There is a risk of severe hypotension if phosphodiesterase inhibitors (e.g. sildenafil, tadalafil and vardenafil) are used with sodium nitroprusside.

Clinical evidence, mechanism, importance and management

(a) Antihypertensives

The manufacturer notes that smaller doses of sodium nitroprusside might be required in patients receiving antihypertensive drugs. In any event the required dose varies considerably between patients and so should be titrated to effect. When used for controlled hypotension during anaesthesia, the hypotensive effect of other drugs, particularly anaesthetics, should be remembered.[1] They name **halothane** and **enflurane**.

(b) Phosphodiesterase inhibitors

The use of phosphodiesterase inhibitors (e.g. **sildenafil**, **tadalafil** and **vardenafil**) with sodium nitroprusside is contraindicated by the manufacturers, due to the risk of severe hypotension. See also 'Phosphodiesterase type-5 inhibitors + Nitrates', p.1272. A case report describes the therapeutic use of **sildenafil** to enhance the hypotensive effect of sodium nitroprusside and other antihypertensives in a patient with a hypertensive crisis.[2]

1. Sodium Nitroprusside. Mayne Pharma plc. UK Summary of product characteristics, May 2005.
2. Bahadur MM, Aggarwal VD, Mali M, Thamba A. Novel therapeutic option in hypertensive crisis: sildenafil augments nitroprusside-induced hypotension. *Nephrol Dial Transplant* (2005) 20, 1254–6.

Tirilazad mesilate + Miscellaneous

Phenobarbital and phenytoin reduce the serum levels of tirilazad mesilate whereas ketoconazole increases them. Finasteride inhibits the metabolism of tirilazad to its active metabolite. No pharmacokinetic interaction appears to occur between cimetidine or nimodipine and tirilazad.

Clinical evidence, mechanism, importance and management

(a) Cimetidine

A study in 16 healthy men found that cimetidine 300 mg every 6 hours for 4 days had no effect on the pharmacokinetics of a single 2-mg/kg dose of tirilazad mesilate, given by infusion over 10 minutes on day 2, nor on U-89678, its active metabolite.[1] No special precautions would seem necessary if cimetidine is given with tirilazad mesilate.

(b) Finasteride

In a study, 8 healthy men were given finasteride 5 mg daily for 10 days, with tirilazad mesilate 10 mg/kg orally or 2 mg/kg intravenously on day 7. Finasteride increased the AUCs of intravenous and oral tirilazad by 21% and 29%, respectively. Oral finasteride reduced the AUCs of the active metabolite (U-89678) by 92% when tirilazad was given intravenously and by 75% when tirilazad was given orally. Although the metabolism of tirilazad to U-89678 was inhibited there was only a moderate effect on the overall clearance of tirilazad and the interaction was considered unlikely to be of clinical significance.[2]

(c) Ketoconazole

Tirilazad mesilate, 10 mg/kg orally or 2 mg/kg intravenously, was given to 12 healthy men and women, either alone or on day 4 of a 7-day regimen of ketoconazole 200 mg daily. The ketoconazole more than doubled the absolute bioavailability of the oral tirilazad mesilate (from 8.7% to 20.9%), apparently because its metabolism by the cytochrome P450 isoenzyme CYP3A in the gut wall and during the first pass through the liver was inhibited.[3] The clinical importance of this interaction awaits assessment.

(d) Nimodipine

In a single-dose study in 12 healthy men, there was no pharmacokinetic or pharmacodynamic interaction between intravenous tirilazad mesilate 2 mg/kg and oral nimodipine 60 mg.[4] No special precautions would seem necessary if nimodipine is given with tirilazad mesilate

(e) Phenobarbital

The pharmacokinetics of tirilazad mesilate (1.5 mg/kg as 10 minute intravenous infusions every 6 hours for 29 doses) were studied in 15 healthy subjects before and after they took phenobarbital 100 mg daily for 8 days. The phenobarbital increased the clearance of the tirilazad by 25% in the male subjects and 29% in the female, and the AUC of the active metabolite of tirilazad (U-89678) was reduced by 51% in the males and 69% in the females. The reason is thought to be that the phenobarbital acts as an enzyme inducer, which increases the metabolism of the tirilazad.[5] The clinical importance of these reductions awaits assessment, but be alert for evidence of reduced effects if both drugs are given. It is doubtful if the full enzyme-inducing effects of the phenobarbital would have been reached in this study after only one week, so anticipate a greater effect if it is given for a longer period.

(f) Phenytoin

After taking phenytoin 200 mg every 8 hours for 11 doses then 100 mg every 8 hours for 5 doses, the AUC_{0-6} of tirilazad mesilate was reduced by 35% in 12 healthy subjects. The AUC of the active metabolite, U-89678, was reduced by 87%.[6] Another report by the same group of workers[7] found that phenytoin every 8 hours for 7 days (9 doses of 200 mg followed by 13 doses of 100 mg) reduced the clearance of tirilazad by 92% and of U-89678 by 93%. In another report the authors noted that phenytoin increased the metabolism of tirilazad and its metabolite in men and women to similar extents.[8] The clinical importance of these reductions is still to be assessed, but be alert for any evidence of reduced tirilazad effects if both drugs are given.

1. Fleishaker JC, Hulst LK, Peters GR. Lack of pharmacokinetic interaction between cimetidine and tirilazad mesylate. *Pharm Res* (1994) 11, 341–4.
2. Fleishaker JC, Pearson PG, Wienkers LC, Pearson LK, Moore TA, Peters GR. Biotransformation of tirilazad in human: 4. effect of finasteride on tirilazad clearance and reduced metabolite formation. J Pharmacol Exp Ther. (1998) 287, 591–7.
3. Fleishaker JC, Pearson PG, Wienkers LC, Pearson LK, Peters GR. Biotransformation of tirilazad in humans: 2. Effect of ketoconazole on tirilazad clearance and oral bioavailability. *J Pharmacol Exp Ther* (1996) 277, 991–8.
4. Fleishaker JC, Hulst LK, Peters GR. Lack of a pharmacokinetic/pharmacodynamic interaction between nimodipine and tirilazad mesylate in healthy volunteers. *J Clin Pharmacol* (1994) 34, 837–41.
5. Fleishaker JC, Pearson LK, Peters GR. Gender does not affect the degree of induction of tirilazad clearance by phenobarbital. *Eur J Clin Pharmacol* (1996) 50, 139–45.
6. Fleishaker JC, Hulst LK, Peters GR. The effect of phenytoin on the pharmacokinetics of tirilazad mesylate in healthy male volunteers. *Clin Pharmacol Ther* (1994) 56, 389–97.
7. Fleishaker JC, Pearson LK, Peters GR. Induction of tirilazad clearance by phenytoin. *Biopharm Drug Dispos* (1998) 19, 91–6.
8. Fleishaker JC, Pearson LK, Peters GR. Effect of gender on the degree of induction of tirilazad clearance by phenytoin. *Clin Pharmacol Ther* (1996) 59, 168.

Tolazoline + H_2-receptor antagonists

Cimetidine and ranitidine can reduce or abolish the effects of tolazoline used as a pulmonary vasodilator in children.

Clinical evidence

A newborn infant with persistent foetal circulation was given a continuous infusion of tolazoline to reduce pulmonary hypertension. The oxygenation improved but gastrointestinal bleeding occurred. When **cimetidine** was given, the condition of the child deteriorated with a decrease in oxygen saturation and arterial pO_2 values.[1] A second case report describes a similar outcome in a 2-day-old neonate, who had an initial improvement with tolazoline alone, but then developed worsening hypoxaemia when cimetidine was given.[2]

These reports are similar to another, in which the tolazoline-induced reduction in pulmonary arterial pressure in a child was reversed when **cimetidine** was given, for acute gastrointestinal haemorrhage.[3] Another study in 12 children found that intravenous **ranitidine** 3 mg/kg abolished the tolazoline-induced reduction in pulmonary and systemic vascular.[4]

Mechanism

Tolazoline dilates the pulmonary vascular system by stimulating both H_1- and H_2-receptors. Cimetidine and ranitidine block H_2-receptors so that at least part of the effects of tolazoline are abolished. It has been suggested that this interaction is confined to children.[3]

Importance and management

An established interaction. Cimetidine and ranitidine are not suitable drugs for prophylaxis of the gastrointestinal adverse effects of tolazoline in children. Other H_2-receptor antagonists would be expected to behave similarly.

1. Roll C, Hanssler L. Interaktion von Tolazolin und Cimetidin bei persistierender fetaler Zirkulation des Neugeborenen. *Monatsschr Kinderheilkd* (1993) 141, 297–9.
2. Huang C-B, Huang S-C. Caution with use of cimetidine in tolazoline induced upper gastrointestinal bleeding. Changgeng Yi Xue Za Zhi. (1996) 19, 268–71.
3. Jones ODH, Shore DF, Rigby ML. The use of tolazoline hydrochloride as a pulmonary vasodilator in potentially fatal episodes of pulmonary vasoconstriction after cardiac surgery in children. *Circulation* (1981) 64 (Suppl II), 134–9.
4. Bush A, Busst CM, Knight WB, Shinebourne EA. Cardiovascular effects of tolazoline and ranitidine. *Arch Dis Child* (1987) 62, 241–6.

25

Digitalis glycosides

Plant extracts containing cardiac glycosides have been in use for thousands of years. The ancient Egyptians were familiar with squill (a source of **proscillaridin**), as were the Romans who used it as a heart tonic and diuretic. The foxglove was mentioned in the writings of Welsh physicians in the thirteenth century and features in 'An Account of the Foxglove and some of its Medical Uses', published by William Withering in 1785, in which he described its application in the treatment of 'dropsy' or the oedema that results from heart failure.

The most commonly used cardiac glycosides are those obtained from the members of the foxglove family, *Digitalis purpurea* and *Digitalis lanata*. The leaves of *D. lanata* are the source of a number of purified glycosides including **digoxin**, **digitoxin**, **acetyldigoxin**, **acetyldigitoxin**, **lanatoside C**, **deslanoside**, of gitalin (an amorphous mixture largely composed of digitoxin and digoxin), and of powdered whole leaf **digitalis lanata leaf**. *D. purpurea* is the source of **digitoxin**, **digitalis leaf**, and the standardised preparation **digitalin**. **Metildigoxin** is a semi-synthetic digitalis glycoside. Occasionally ouabain or strophanthin-K (also of plant origin) are used for particular situations, while for a number of years the Russians have exploited cardiac glycosides from lily of the valley (**convallaria**). Bufalin is a related cardioactive compound obtained from toads, and is found in a number of Chinese medicines.

Digitalisation

The cardiac glycosides have two main actions and two main applications. They reduce conductivity within the atrioventricular (AV) node, hence are used for treating supraventricular tachycardias (especially atrial fibrillation), and they have a positive inotropic effect (i.e. increase the force of contraction), hence are used for congestive heart failure, although this use has declined.

Because the most commonly used glycosides are derived from digitalis, the achievement of the desired therapeutic serum concentration of any cardiac glycoside is usually referred to as digitalisation. Treatment may be started with a large loading dose so that the therapeutic concentrations are achieved reasonably quickly, but once these have been reached the amount is reduced to a maintenance dose. This has to be done carefully because there is a relatively narrow gap between therapeutic and toxic serum concentrations. Normal therapeutic levels are about one-third of those that are fatal, and serious toxic arrhythmias begin at about two-thirds of the fatal levels. The normal range for digoxin levels is 0.8 to 2 nanograms/mL (or 1.02 to 2.56 nanomol/L). To convert nanograms/mL to nanomol/L multiply by 1.28, or to convert nanomol/L to nanograms/mL multiply by 0.781. Note that micrograms/L is the same as nanograms/mL.

If a patient is over-digitalised, signs of toxicity will occur, which may include loss of appetite, nausea and vomiting, and bradycardia. These symptoms are often used as clinical indicators of toxicity, and a pulse rate of less than 60 bpm is usually considered to be an indication of over-treatment. Note that paroxysmal atrial tachycardia with AV block and junctional tachycardia can also occur as a result of digitalis toxicity. Other symptoms include visual disturbances, headache, drowsiness and occasionally diarrhoea. Death may result from cardiac arrhythmias. Patients treated for cardiac arrhythmias can therefore demonstrate arrhythmias when they are both under- as well as over-digitalised.

Interactions of the cardiac glycosides

The pharmacological actions of these glycosides are very similar, but their rates and degree of absorption, metabolism and clearance are different. For example, digoxin is mainly renally cleared whereas digitoxin undergoes a degree of metabolism by the liver. It is therefore most important not to extrapolate an interaction seen with one glycoside and apply it uncritically to any other. Because the therapeutic ratio of the cardiac glycosides is low, a quite small change in serum levels may lead to inadequate digitalisation or to toxicity. For this reason interactions that have a relatively modest effect on serum levels may sometimes have serious consequences.

Many interactions between digoxin and other drugs are mediated by P-glycoprotein. Drugs that inhibit the activity of P-glycoprotein in the renal tubules may reduce the elimination of digoxin in the urine and this may result in toxic serum levels. Further, the induction or inhibition of P-glycoprotein in the gut may affect the oral absorption of digoxin. See also 'Drug transporter proteins', (p.8).

Digitalis glycosides + ACE inhibitors

Most ACE inhibitors do not interact with digoxin to a clinically relevant extent. Some studies have found that serum digoxin levels rise by about 20% or more if captopril is used, but others have found no significant changes. It has been suggested that any interaction is likely to occur only in those patients who have pre-existing renal impairment. Digitoxin and captopril appear not to interact.

Clinical evidence

(a) Digitoxin and Captopril

A study in 12 healthy subjects given digitoxin 70 micrograms daily for up to 58 days found no evidence that the addition of captopril 25 mg daily had a relevant effect on the pharmacokinetics of digitoxin, or its effects on the heart.[1]

(b) Digoxin and Captopril

The serum digoxin levels of 16 patients with severe chronic congestive heart failure rose by 21%, from 1.1 to 1.3 nanograms/mL, while taking captopril (average dose 93.7 mg daily). Serum digoxin levels were above the therapeutic range at 2 nanograms/mL on 3 out of 63 occasions, but no toxicity was seen. All patients had impaired renal function and were being treated with diuretics.[2,3] Another study[4] found an approximate 30% rise in serum digoxin levels in patients with congestive heart failure class II and a further study[5] found an approximate 60% rise in peak serum digoxin levels in patients with congestive heart failure class IV. Conversely, another study in 31 patients with stable congestive heart failure, given captopril 25 mg three times daily, found no significant changes in serum digoxin levels over a 6-month period.[6] Two other studies in healthy subjects[7] and patients with congestive heart failure[8] also found no evidence of an interaction.

(c) Digoxin and Other ACE inhibitors

In general no significant interactions have been seen between ACE inhibitors and digoxin.

- **Cilazapril** 5 mg for 14 days did not alter the trough plasma digoxin levels in healthy subjects.[9]
- **Enalapril** 20 mg daily for 30 days had no significant effect on the pharmacokinetics of digoxin 250 micrograms daily in 7 patients with congestive heart failure.[10]
- **Imidapril** 10 mg daily had no effect on the serum digoxin levels of 12 healthy subjects, but slight reductions in levels of the active form imidaprilat and in ACE inhibition of about 15% were seen, which were of uncertain clinical relevance.[11]
- **Lisinopril** 5 mg daily for 4 weeks had no significant effect on the serum digoxin levels of 9 patients.[12] This confirms the findings of a single-dose study.[13]
- **Moexipril** has been reported, by the manufacturer, to have had no important pharmacokinetic interaction with digoxin in healthy subjects.[14] They also have clinical studies that show no evidence of clinically important adverse interactions when moexipril was used with digoxin.[15]
- **Perindopril** 2 to 4 mg daily for a month had no effect on the steady-state serum digoxin levels of 10 patients with mild chronic heart failure.[16]
- **Quinapril** is also reported not to alter the steady-state levels of digoxin in healthy subjects,[17] and patients with congestive heart failure.[18]
- **Ramipril** 5 mg daily for 14 days had no effect on the serum digoxin levels of 12 healthy subjects.[19]
- **Spirapril** 12 to 48 mg daily did not significantly affect the pharmacokinetics nor the steady-state serum levels of digoxin in 15 healthy subjects taking digoxin 250 micrograms twice daily.[20]
- **Trandolapril** has been shown to have no significant pharmacokinetic interaction with digoxin in healthy subjects.[21] The manufacturers also note that, in patients with left ventricular dysfunction after myocardial infarction, no clinical interactions have been found between trandolapril and digoxin.[22,23]

Mechanism

Not fully understood. It has been suggested that an interaction is only likely to occur in those who have renal impairment because the glomerular filtration rate of these patients may be maintained by the vasoconstrictor action of angiotensin II on the post-glomerular blood vessels, which would be impaired by ACE inhibition. As a result some of the loss of digoxin through the tubules is reduced.[7]

Importance and management

The overall picture is that no clinically important adverse interaction occurs between digoxin and ACE inhibitors in patients with normal renal function, and that serum digoxin monitoring is only needed in those who have a high risk of reversible ACE inhibitor induced renal failure (e.g. patients with congestive heart failure during chronic diuretic treatment, with bilateral renal artery stenosis or unilateral renal artery stenosis in a solitary kidney);[7] however, note these latter two conditions are contraindications to the use of ACE inhibitors. The critical factor does not seem to be the particular ACE inhibitor used but the existence of abnormal renal function or conditions that increase the risk of renal impairment. This needs confirmation.

No interaction apparently occurs between digitoxin and captopril in healthy subjects, but this needs confirmation in patients.

1. de Mey C, Elich D, Schroeter V, Butzer R, Belz GG. Captopril does not interact with the pharmacodynamics and pharmacokinetics of digitoxin in healthy man. *Eur J Clin Pharmacol* (1992) 43, 445–7.
2. Cleland JGF, Dargie HJ, Hodsman GP, Robertson JIS, Ball SG. Interaction of digoxin and captopril. *Br J Clin Pharmacol* (1984) 17, 214P.
3. Cleland JGF, Dargie HJ, Pettigrew A, Gillen C, Robertson JIS. The effects of captopril on serum digoxin and urinary urea and digoxin clearances in patients with congestive heart failure. *Am Heart J* (1986) 112, 130–5.
4. Mazurek W, Haczyński J, Interakcja kaptoprilu i digoksyny. *Pol Tyg Lek* (1993) 48, 834–5.
5. Kirimli O, Kalkan S, Guneri S, Tuncok Y, Akdeniz B, Ozdamar M, Guven H. The effects of captopril on serum digoxin levels in patients with severe congestive heart failure. *Int J Clin Pharmacol Ther* (2001) 39, 311–14.
6. Magelli C, Bassein L, Ribani MA, Liberatore S, Ambrosioni E, Magnani B. Lack of effect of captopril on serum digoxin in congestive heart failure. *Eur J Clin Pharmacol* (1989) 36, 99–100.
7. Rossi GP, Semplicini A, Bongiovi S, Mozzato MG, Paleari CD, Pessina AC. Effect of acute captopril administration on digoxin pharmacokinetics in normal subjects. *Curr Ther Res* (1989) 46, 439–44.
8. Miyakawa T, Shionoiri H, Takasaki I, Kobayashi K, Ishii M. The effect of captopril on pharmacokinetics of digoxin in patients with mild congestive heart failure. *J Cardiovasc Pharmacol* (1991) 17, 576–80.
9. Kleinbloesem CH, van Brummelen P, Francis RJ, Wiegand U-W. Clinical pharmacology of cilazapril. *Drugs* (1991) 41 (Suppl 1), 3–10.
10. Douste-Blazy Ph, Blanc M, Montastruc JL, Conte D, Cotonat J, Galinier F. Is there any interaction between digoxin and enalapril? *Br J Clin Pharmacol* (1986) 22, 752–3.
11. Harder S, Thürmann PA. Pharmacokinetic and pharmacodynamic interaction trial after repeated oral doses of imidapril and digoxin in healthy volunteers. *Br J Clin Pharmacol* (1997) 43, 475–80.
12. Vandenburg MJ, Kelly JG, Wiseman HT, Mannering D, Long C, Glover DR. The effect of lisinopril on digoxin pharmacokinetics in patients with congestive heart failure. *Br J Clin Pharmacol* (1988) 21, 656P–657P.
13. Vandenburg MJ, Morris F, Marks C, Kelly JG, Dews IM, Stephens JD. A study of the potential pharmacokinetic interaction of lisinopril and digoxin in normal volunteers. *Xenobiotica* (1988) 18, 1179–84.
14. Perdix (Moexipril hydrochloride). Schwarz Pharma Ltd. UK Summary of product characteristics, July 2006.
15. Perdix (Moexipril). Schwarz Pharma. Product Monograph. Data on file, September 1995.
16. Vandenburg MJ, Stephens JD, Resplandy G, Dews IM, Robinson J, Desche P. Digoxin pharmacokinetics and perindopril in heart failure patients. *J Clin Pharmacol* (1993) 33, 146–9.
17. Ferry JJ, Sedman AJ, Hengy H, Vollmer KO, Dunkey A, Klotz U, Colburn WA. Concomitant multiple dose quinapril administration does not alter steady-state pharmacokinetics of digoxin. *Pharm Res* (1987) 4, S98.
18. Kromer EP, Elsner D, Riegger GAJ. Digoxin, converting-enzyme inhibition (quinapril) and the combination in patients with congestive heart failure functional class II and sinus rhythm. *J Cardiovasc Pharmacol* (1990) 16, 9–14.
19. Doering W, Maass L, Irmisch R and König E. Pharmacokinetic interaction study with ramipril and digoxin in healthy volunteers. *Am J Cardiol* (1987) 59, 60D–64D.
20. Johnson BF, Wilson J, Johnson J, Flemming J. Digoxin pharmacokinetics and spirapril, a new ACE inhibitor. *J Clin Pharmacol* (1991) 31, 527–30.
21. New horizons in antihypertensive therapy. Gopten® Trandolapril. Knoll AG, 1992.
22. Gopten (Trandolapril). Abbott Laboratories Ltd. UK Summary of product characteristics, May 2007.
23. Mavik (Trandolapril). Abbott Laboratories. US Prescribing information, July 2003.

Digitalis glycosides + Acipimox

One study suggests that acipimox does not interact with digoxin.

Clinical evidence, mechanism, importance and management

In 6 elderly patients acipimox 250 mg three times daily for a week was found to have no significant effect on plasma **digoxin** levels, clinical condition, ECGs, plasma urea or electrolyte levels.[1] No special precautions during concurrent use would seem necessary.

1. Chijioke PC, Pearson RM, Benedetti S. Lack of acipimox-digoxin interaction in patient volunteers. *Hum Exp Toxicol* (1992) 11, 357–9.

Digitalis glycosides + Allopurinol

Allopurinol does not appear to affect serum digoxin levels.

Clinical evidence, mechanism, importance and management

No significant changes in the serum **digoxin** levels of 5 healthy subjects occurred over a 7-day period while they were taking allopurinol 300 mg daily.[1] No additional precautions would appear to be necessary on concurrent use.

1. Havelund T, Abildtrup N, Birkebaek N, Breddam E, Rosager AM. Allopurinols effekt på koncentrationen af digoksin i serum. *Ugeskr Laeger* (1984) 146, 1209–11.

Digitalis glycosides + Alpha blockers

A rapid and marked rise in serum digoxin levels occurred in one study when prazosin was also given. Alfuzosin, doxazosin, tamsulosin and terazosin appear not to interact with digoxin.

Clinical evidence, mechanism, importance and management

(a) Alfuzosin

The manufacturers of alfuzosin report that no pharmacodynamic or pharmacokinetic interaction was observed in healthy subjects given alfuzosin 10 mg [daily] with **digoxin** 250 micrograms daily for 7 days.[1,2]

(b) Doxazosin

Doxazosin is highly bound to plasma proteins (98%), but the manufacturer notes that *in vitro* data in human plasma indicated that doxazosin did not affect the protein binding of **digoxin**.[3,4] Although there appears to be no clinical evidence of an interaction between **digoxin** and doxazosin, an *in vitro* study found that doxazosin inhibited the P-glycoprotein-mediated transcellular transport of **digoxin**, suggesting that an interaction is possible, as **digoxin** renal transport may be inhibited.[5] More study is needed.

(c) Prazosin

In 20 patients prazosin 2.5 mg twice daily increased the mean steady-state plasma **digoxin** level by 43% from 0.94 to 1.34 nanograms/mL after one day, and by 60% from 0.94 to 1.51 nanograms/mL after 3 days, although the individual response varied from an increase to a decrease, or no effect. Three days after the prazosin was stopped, by which time it would be totally cleared from the body, the serum **digoxin** concentrations had fallen to their previous levels.[6] The reason for this response is not understood. There do not appear to be any other reports in the literature, and the manufacturer notes that, in clinical experience, prazosin has been given with **digoxin** (and 'digitalis') without any adverse drug interaction.[7] However, bear this interaction in mind in case of an unexpected response to treatment.

(d) Tamsulosin

A placebo-controlled study in 10 healthy subjects found that tamsulosin 800 micrograms daily had no effect on the pharmacokinetics of a single 500-microgram intravenous dose of **digoxin**. The most frequently reported adverse effect was dizziness and the safety profile was considered acceptable.[8] The manufacturers note that dosage adjustments are not necessary when tamsulosin is given with **digoxin**.[9]

(e) Terazosin

The manufacturer of terazosin states that terazosin has been given with cardiac glycosides without evidence of an interaction.[10]

1. Xatral (Alfuzosin hydrochloride). Sanofi-Aventis. UK Summary of product characteristics, April 2005.
2. Uroxatral (Alfuzosin hydrochloride extended-release tablets). Sanofi-Aventis US LLC. US Prescribing information, March 2007.
3. Cardura (Doxazosin mesilate). Pfizer Ltd. UK Summary of product characteristics, February 2007.
4. Cardura (Doxazosin mesylate). Pfizer Inc. US Prescribing information, April 2002.
5. Takara K, Kakumoto M, Tanigawara Y, Funakoshi J, Sakaeda T, Okumura K. Interaction of digoxin with antihypertensive drugs *via* MDR1. *Life Sci* (2002) 70, 1491–1500.
6. Çopur S, Tokgözoğlu L, Oto A, Oram E, Uğurlu Ş. Effects of oral prazosin on total plasma digoxin levels. *Fundam Clin Pharmacol* (1988) 2, 13–17.
7. Hypovase (Prazosin hydrochloride). Pfizer Ltd. UK Summary of product characteristics, May 2007.
8. Miyazawa Y, Starkey LP, Forrest A, Schentag JJ, Kamimura H, Swarz H, Ito Y. Effects of the concomitant administration of tamsulosin (0.8 mg) on the pharmacokinetic and safety profile of intravenous digoxin (Lanoxin®) in normal healthy subjects: a placebo-controlled evaluation. *J Clin Pharm Ther* (2002) 27, 13–19.
9. Flomax (Tamsulosin hydrochloride). Boehringer Ingelheim Pharmaceuticals Inc. US Prescribing information, February 2007.
10. Hytrin (Terazosin). Abbott Laboratories Ltd. UK Summary of product characteristics, January 2006.

Digitalis glycosides + Alpha-glucosidase inhibitors

Some but not all studies have found that digoxin plasma levels can be markedly reduced by acarbose. Miglitol modestly reduced digoxin levels in healthy subjects, but no change was seen in diabetic patients. Voglibose does not appear to interact adversely with digoxin.

Clinical evidence, mechanism, importance and management

(a) Acarbose

A woman taking **digoxin** 250 micrograms daily, insulin, nifedipine, isosorbide dinitrate, clorazepate and nabumetone had subtherapeutic plasma **digoxin** levels of 0.48 to 0.64 nanograms/mL while taking acarbose, even when her **digoxin** dosage was raised by adding 125 micrograms on two days of the week. Later, in the absence of acarbose and with the original **digoxin** dosage, her plasma levels were 1.9 nanograms/mL.[1,2] Two other patients similarly had markedly reduced plasma **digoxin** levels while taking acarbose. When the acarbose was stopped, the plasma **digoxin** levels rose from 0.23 to 1.6 nanograms/mL and from 0.56 to 1.9 nanograms/mL, respectively.[3] Another patient with heart failure and type 2 diabetes taking **digoxin** and voglibose, was found to have subtherapeutic levels of **digoxin** when his treatment was changed from voglibose (see below) to acarbose. The serum levels unexpectedly remained subtherapeutic for at least a month when treatment was switched back to voglibose.[4]

A pharmacokinetic study in 7 healthy subjects, using either a 200-mg dose of acarbose or pretreatment with acarbose 100 mg doses three times daily, similarly found that the serum levels and AUC of a single 500-microgram dose of **digoxin** were reduced. Maximum **digoxin** serum levels were reduced by about 30 to 40% and the AUC was reduced by about 40%.[5] The reasons for this interaction are not understood but a reduction in the absorption of the **digoxin** from the gut has been suggested.[5] These reports contrast with other studies that found no significant interaction between single-dose **digoxin** and acarbose at therapeutic doses in healthy subjects.[6,7] Just why there is an inconsistency between these reports is not understood but it would clearly be prudent to consider monitoring **digoxin** levels if both drugs are used, being alert for any evidence of reduced levels.

(b) Miglitol

The manufacturer notes that in a study in healthy subjects, miglitol 50 mg or 100 mg three times daily reduced the average plasma concentrations of **digoxin** by 19% and 28%, respectively. However, in diabetic patients receiving treatment with **digoxin**, plasma **digoxin** levels were not altered by the concurrent use of miglitol 100 mg three times daily for 14 days.[8] It would seem prudent to monitor digoxin levels if both drugs are used together.

(c) Voglibose

A randomised, crossover study in 8 healthy subjects taking **digoxin** 250 micrograms daily after breakfast for 8 days found that voglibose 200 micrograms three times daily had no effect on the pharmacokinetics of the **digoxin**.[9] For mention of a patient whose **digoxin** levels became subtherapeutic when acarbose was substituted for voglibose, see above. There would therefore appear to be no reason for avoiding concurrent use. No special precautions are needed.

1. Serrano JS, Jiménez CM, Serrano MI, Balboa B. A possible interaction of potential clinical interest between digoxin and acarbose. *Clin Pharmacol Ther* (1996) 60, 589–92.

2. Menchén del Cerro E. Acarbosa y digoxina. *Aten Primaria* (1995) 16, 508.
3. Ben-Ami H, Krivoy N, Nagachandran P, Roguin A, Edoute Y. An interaction between digoxin and acarbose. *Diabetes Care* (1999) 22, 860–1.
4. Nagai Y, Hayakawa T, Abe T, Nomura G. Are there different effects of acarbose and voglibose on serum levels of digoxin in a diabetic patient with congestive heart failure? *Diabetes Care* (2000) 23, 1703.
5. Miura T, Ueno K, Tanaka K, Sugiura Y, Mizutani M, Takatsu F, Takano Y, Shibakawa M. Impairment of absorption of digoxin by acarbose. *J Clin Pharmacol* (1998) 38, 654–7.
6. Cohen E, Almog S, Staruvin D, Garty M. Do therapeutic doses of acarbose alter the pharmacokinetics of digoxin? *Isr Med Assoc J* (2002) 4, 772–5.
7. Hillebrand I, Graefe KH, Bischoff H, Frank G, Raemsch KD, Berchtold P. Serum digoxin and propranolol levels during acarbose treatment. *Int Congr Ser* (1982) 594, 244–6.
8. Glyset (Miglitol). Pfizer Inc. US prescribing information, October 2004
9. Kusumoto M, Ueno K, Fujimura Y, Kameda T, Mashimo K, Takeda K, Tatami R, Shibakawa M. Lack of kinetic interaction between digoxin and voglibose. *Eur J Clin Pharmacol* (1999) 55, 79–80.

Digitalis glycosides + Aminoglutethimide

The clearance of digitoxin is markedly increased by aminoglutethimide and a reduction in its effects would be expected.

Clinical evidence, mechanism, importance and management

The clearance of **digitoxin** was increased by a mean of 109% in 5 patients who took aminoglutethimide (250 mg four times a day in four, and 125 mg twice daily in one).[1,2] The likely reason is that aminoglutethimide increases the metabolism of the **digitoxin** by the liver.

This increase in clearance would be expected to be clinically important, but this does not appear to have been assessed. Check that patients do not become under-digitalised during concurrent treatment. No interaction would be expected with **digoxin** because it is largely excreted unchanged in the urine and therefore metabolism by the liver has little part to play in its clearance.

1. Lønning PE, Kvinnsland S and Bakke OM. Effect of aminoglutethimide on antipyrine, theophylline and digitoxin disposition in breast cancer. *Clin Pharmacol Ther* (1984) 36, 796–802.
2. Lønning PE. Aminoglutethimide enzyme induction: pharmacological and endocrinological implications. *Cancer Chemother Pharmacol* (1990) 26, 241–4.

Digitalis glycosides + Aminoglycosides

Serum levels of digoxin can be reduced by the concurrent use of oral neomycin and increased by intramuscular gentamicin.

Clinical evidence

(a) Gentamicin

In a study in 12 patients with congestive heart failure taking **digoxin** 250 micrograms daily, the addition of gentamicin 80 mg intramuscularly twice daily for 7 days was found to increase serum **digoxin** levels by 129%. In a further 12 patients with congestive heart failure and diabetes, the same dosage of gentamicin increased **digoxin** levels more than two-fold to 2 nanograms/mL. However, no symptoms of **digoxin** toxicity were seen. It should be noted that serum creatinine levels were higher in both groups than those in healthy controls even before receiving gentamicin, and were further increased after gentamicin.[1]

An earlier study similarly found that gentamicin prolonged the half-life of **digoxin** and increased serum levels from 1.9 to 2.8 nanograms/mL.[2]

(b) Neomycin

Neomycin 1 to 3 g orally was found to reduce and delay the absorption of a single 500-microgram dose of **digoxin** in healthy subjects.[3] The AUC was reduced by 41 to 51%. Absorption was affected even when the neomycin was given 3 to 6 hours before the **digoxin**. In a steady-state study, neomycin 2 g given with **digoxin** 250 to 500 micrograms daily reduced the serum level of **digoxin** by 8 to 49% (mean 28.2%).[3]

Mechanism

Gentamicin impairs renal function, so decreasing digoxin clearance.[2] Higher digoxin levels and serum creatinine levels in diabetic compared with non-diabetic patients may be due to differences in renal function,[1] with concurrent gentamicin causing further renal function impairment and even higher digoxin levels. The reduction in digoxin toxicity is not fully understood but changes in ionic transport may be involved. The inhibition by gentamicin of Na^+/K^+ ATPase, which acts as a specific receptor for digoxin, may also be a factor.[1]

Neomycin can cause a general but reversible malabsorption syndrome, which affects the absorption of several drugs. The extent of this is probably offset in some patients, because the neomycin also reduces the breakdown of digoxin by the bacteria in the gut.[4]

Importance and management

Information is limited, but patients should be monitored for increased digoxin effects if gentamicin is given, especially those with diabetes or any other patient with impaired renal function. Initially, checking pulse rate is probably adequate. There seems to be no information about other parenteral aminoglycosides.

Patients should be monitored for reduced digoxin effects if neomycin is given and suitable dosage adjustments made if necessary. Separating the dosages of the two drugs does not prevent this interaction. Other aminoglycosides that can be given orally such as **kanamycin** and **paromomycin** might possibly interact similarly to neomycin, but this requires confirmation.

1. Alkadi HO, Nooman MA, Raja'a YA. Effect of gentamicin on serum digoxin level in patients with congestive heart failure. *Pharm World Sci* (2004) 26, 107–9.
2. Halawa B. Interakcje digoksyny z cefradina (Sefril), tetracyklina (Tetracyclinum), gentamycyna (Gentamycin) i wankomycyna (Vancocin). *Pol Tyg Lek* (1984) 39, 1717–20.
3. Lindenbaum J, Maulitz RM, Butler VP. Inhibition of digoxin absorption by neomycin. *Gastroenterology* (1976) 71, 399–404.
4. Lindenbaum J, Tse-Eng D, Butler VP, Rund DG. Urinary excretion of reduced metabolites of digoxin. *Am J Med* (1981) 71, 67–74.

Digitalis glycosides + 5-Aminosalicylates

Serum digoxin levels can be reduced by sulfasalazine. The manufacturers of balsalazide suggest that it may interact similarly.

Clinical evidence, mechanism, importance and management

The observation that a patient taking **sulfasalazine** 8 g daily had low serum **digoxin** levels, prompted a crossover study in 10 healthy subjects. In this study a single 500-microgram dose of **digoxin** syrup was given alone, and after 6 days of treatment with **sulfasalazine** 2 to 6 g daily. **Digoxin** absorption was reduced, ranging from 0 to 50% depending on the dosage of **sulfasalazine** used.[1] Serum **digoxin** levels were reduced accordingly.[1] The reasons for this effect are not understood. This seems to be the only report of this interaction. Concurrent use need not be avoided, but it would be prudent to check for under-digitalisation, initially by checking symptoms and pulse rate, and then taking **digoxin** levels if an interaction is suspected. In the one patient examined, separating the dosages appeared not to prevent this interaction.[1]

Although no interaction involving **digoxin** and **balsalazide** has been reported, based on the information with sulfasalazine, the manufacturers of **balsalazide** recommend that plasma levels of **digoxin** should be monitored in digitalised patients starting **balsalazide**.[2]

1. Juhl RP, Summers RW, Guillory JK, Blaug SM, Cheng FH, Brown DD. Effect of sulfasalazine on digoxin bioavailability. *Clin Pharmacol Ther* (1976) 20, 387–94.
2. Colazide (Balsalazide). Shire Pharmaceuticals Ltd. UK Summary of product characteristics, September 2005.

Digitalis glycosides + Aminosalicylic acid

Aminosalicylic acid causes a small reduction in digoxin levels in healthy subjects but the importance of this in patients is uncertain.

Clinical evidence, mechanism, importance and management

In one study in 10 healthy subjects, the bioavailability of a single 750-microgram dose of **digoxin**, using urinary excretion as a measure, was reduced by 20% by aminosalicylic acid 2 g four times daily for 2 weeks.[1] This seems to be just another aspect of the general malabsorption caused by aminosalicylic acid. The importance of this interaction in patients is not known (it is probably small) but it would be prudent to monitor concurrent use.

1. Brown DD, Juhl RP, Warner SL. Decreased bioavailability of digoxin due to hypocholesterolemic interventions. *Circulation* (1978) 58, 164–72.

Digitalis glycosides + Amiodarone

Digoxin levels can be approximately doubled by amiodarone. Some individuals may show even greater increases. The same interaction also appears to occur with digitoxin.

Clinical evidence

(a) Acetyldigoxin

Torsade de pointes developed in one patient 3 days after the amiodarone dose was increased to 600 mg daily, and beta-acetyldigoxin 100 micrograms and bisoprolol 1.25 mg daily were added, for persistent atrial fibrillation. Serum levels of digoxin and amiodarone were normal. Withdrawal of all medications and treatment with intravenous magnesium resolved the arrhythmias. It has been suggested that the bradycardia caused by treatment with these three drugs may have placed the patient at risk of such arrhythmias.[1] Cases of proarrhythmic effects of amiodarone with digoxin have also been reported, see *Digoxin*, below.

(b) Digitoxin

Two elderly patients (aged 77 and 78) taking digitoxin 100 micrograms daily were given loading doses of amiodarone followed by maintenance doses of 200 to 400 mg daily. Within 2 months in one case, and 4 months in the other, they were hospitalised because of bradycardia, dyspnoea, nausea and malaise. One of them had total AV block (38 bpm). The serum digitoxin levels of both of them were found to be elevated (54 and 45 nanograms/mL, respectively) well above the therapeutic range of 9 to 30 nanograms/mL. Serum amiodarone and desethylamiodarone levels were normal. Both patients recovered when the digitoxin was stopped.[2]

(c) Digoxin

The observation that patients taking digoxin developed digoxin toxicity when given amiodarone[3] prompted a study of this interaction. Seven patients receiving maintenance digoxin had a mean rise in their plasma digoxin levels of 69%, from 1.17 to 1.98 nanograms/mL, when they were given amiodarone 200 mg three times daily. Two other patients similarly treated also showed this interaction.[3]

Numerous studies in patients have confirmed this interaction with reported increases in serum digoxin levels of 75%,[4] 90%,[5] 95%[6] and 104%.[7] The occasional patient may show three- to fourfold increases, whereas others may show little or no change.[5,8] Children seem particularly sensitive, with threefold, and even as much as ninefold rises.[9] Other reports confirm that the digoxin levels are markedly increased or roughly doubled, and toxicity can occur.[8,10-19] In contrast, one group of workers state that they observed no change in serum digoxin levels in 5 patients given amiodarone.[20,21]

There is also some evidence that, in the treatment of resistant atrial tachyarrhythmias, the risk of arrhythmias may be increased by the concurrent use of digoxin and amiodarone,[18,22] and another study found that combined use had an unfavourable effect on survival in patients with atrial fibrillation and sinus rhythm.[23]

A review of prescribing in an Australian hospital revealed 42 patients who had received amiodarone with digoxin (both long-term (16), either drug recently started (21), or both drugs recently started (5)). Of 31 patients who had digoxin levels monitored, 12 required a change in dose of the digoxin, and in 3, digoxin was stopped.[24] It is unclear whether this was purely on the basis of serum levels, or whether patients experienced adverse effects.

Mechanism

Not fully understood. Amiodarone reduces both the renal and non-renal excretion of digoxin.[25] *In vitro* studies have found that amiodarone (and possibly desethylamiodarone) inhibit P-glycoprotein-mediated transcellular transport of digoxin. This suggests that any interaction may occur, at least in part, by inhibiting digoxin renal tubular secretion.[26,27] Other possible mechanisms that have been suggested include changes in thyroid function,[28] protein-binding displacement[29,30] or increased absorption.[31]

It is thought that amiodarone can also inhibit the metabolism of digitoxin by the liver, which would explain why its serum levels are increased.[2]

Importance and management

The pharmacokinetic interaction between digoxin and amiodarone is well documented, well established and of considerable clinical importance. It occurs in most patients. It is clearly evident after a few days and develops over the course of 1 to 4 weeks.[6] If no account is taken of this interaction the patient may develop digitalis toxicity. Reduce the digoxin dosage by between one-third to one-half when amiodarone is added,[3,4,13,31] with further adjustment of the dosage after a week or two, and possibly a month or more,[13] depending on digoxin levels. Particular care is needed in children, who may show much larger rises in digoxin levels than adults. Amiodarone has a long half-life so that the effects of this interaction will persist for several weeks after its withdrawal.[17] A synergistic effect on heart rate and atrioventricular conduction is also possible, which may result in the development of new arrhythmias. Also note that some authors suggest that concurrent use may possibly worsen the prognosis in some patients.[22,23]

Far less is known about the interaction between digitoxin and amiodarone but the limited evidence available suggests that all of the precautions appropriate for digoxin should be used for digitoxin as well. Note that the interaction may possibly take months to develop.

1. Schrickel J, Bielik H, Yang A, Schwab JO, Shlevkov N, Schimpf R, Lüderitz B, Lewalter T. Amiodarone-associated 'torsade de pointes'. *Z Kardiol* (2003) 92, 889–92.
2. Läer S, Scholz H, Buschmann I, Thoenes M, Meinertz T. Digitoxin intoxication during concomitant use of amiodarone. *Eur J Clin Pharmacol* (1998) 54, 95–6.
3. Moysey JO, Jaggarao NSV, Grundy EN, Chamberlain DA. Amiodarone increases plasma digoxin concentrations. *BMJ* (1981) 282, 272.
4. Fornaro G, Rossi P, Padrini R, Piovan D, Ferrari M, Fortina A, Tomassini G, Aquili C. Ricerca farmacologico-clinica sull'interazione digitale-amiodarone in pazienti cardiopatici con insufficiencza cardiaca di vario grado. *G Ital Cardiol* (1984) 14, 990–8.
5. Oetgen WJ, Sobol SM, Tri TB, Heydorn WH, Rakita L. Amiodarone-digoxin interaction. Clinical and experimental observations. *Chest* (1984) 86, 75–9.
6. Vitale P, Jacono A, Gonzales y Reyero E, Zeuli L. Effect of amiodarone on serum digoxin levels in patients with atrial fibrillation. *Clin Trials J* (1984) 21, 199–206.
7. Nademanee K, Kannan R, Hendrickson J, Ookhtens M, Kay I, Singh BN. Amiodarone-digoxin interaction: clinical significance, time course of development, potential pharmacokinetic mechanisms and therapeutic implications. *J Am Coll Cardiol* (1984) 4, 111–16.
8. Nager G, Nager F. Interaktion zwischen Amiodaron und Digoxin. *Schweiz Med Wochenschr* (1983) 113, 1727–30.
9. Koren G, Hesslein PS, MacLeod SM. Digoxin toxicity associated with amiodarone therapy in children. *J Pediatr* (1984) 104, 467–70.
10. Nademanee K, Kannan R, Hendrickson JA, Burnam M, Kay I, Singh B. Amiodarone-digoxin interaction during treatment of resistant cardiac arrhythmias. *Am J Cardiol* (1982) 49, 1026.
11. McQueen EG. New Zealand Committee on Adverse Drug Reactions. 17th Annual Report 1982. *N Z Med J* (1983) 96, 95–9.
12. McGovern B, Garan H, Kelly E, Ruskin JN. Adverse reactions during treatment with amiodarone hydrochloride. *BMJ* (1983) 287, 175–80.
13. Marcus FI, Fenster PE. Drug therapy. Digoxin interactions with other cardiac drugs. *J Cardiovasc Med* (1983) 8, 25–8.
14. Strocchi E, Malini PL, Graziani A, Ambrosioni E, Magnani B. L'interazione tra digossina ed amiodarone. *G Ital Cardiol* (1984) 14, 12–15.
15. Robinson KC, Walker S, Johnston A, Mulrow JP, McKenna WJ, Holt DW. The digoxin-amiodarone interaction. *Circulation* (1986) 74, II-225.
16. Johnston A, Walker S, Robinson KC, McKenna WJ and Holt DW. The digoxin-amiodarone interaction. *Br J Clin Pharmacol* (1987) 24, 253P.
17. Robinson K, Johnston A, Walker S, Mulrow JP, McKenna WJ, Holt DW. The digoxin-amiodarone interaction. *Cardiovasc Drugs Ther* (1989) 3, 25–28.
18. Lien W-C, Huang C-H, Chen W-J. Bidirectional ventricular tachycardia resulting from digoxin and amiodarone treatment of rapid atrial fibrillation. *Am J Emerg Med* (2004) 22, 235–6.
19. Giordano G, Franciosini MF, Zuanetti G, Latini R. Intossicazione digitalica in presenza di epatite acuta da amiodarone. *G Ital Cardiol* (1988) 18, 862–4
20. Achilli A, Serra N. Amiodarone increases plasma digoxin concentrations. *BMJ* (1981) 282, 1630.
21. Achilli A, Giacci M, Capezzuto A, de Luca F, Guerra R, Serra N. Interazione digossina-chinidina e digossina-amiodarone. *G Ital Cardiol* (1981) 11, 918–25.
22. Bajaj BP, Baig MW, Perrins EJ. Amiodarone-induced torsades de pointes: the possible facilitatory role of digoxin. *Int J Cardiol* (1991) 33, 335–8.
23. Mortara A, Cioffi G, Opasich C, Pozzoli M, Febo O, Riccardi G, Cobelli F, Tavazzi L. Combination of amiodarone plus digoxin in chronic heart failure: an adverse effect on survival independently of the presence of sinus rhythm or atrial fibrillation. *Circulation* (1996) 94 (8 Suppl), I-21.
24. Freitag D, Bebee R, Sunderland B. Digoxin–quinidine and digoxin–amiodarone interactions: frequency of occurrence and monitoring in Australian repatriation hospitals. *J Clin Pharm Ther* (1995) 20, 179–83.
25. Fenster PE, White NW, Hanson CD. Pharmacokinetic evaluation of the digoxin-amiodarone interaction. *J Am Coll Cardiol* (1985) 5, 108–12.
26. Kakumoto M, Takara K, Sakaeda T, Tanigawara Y, Kita T, Okumura K. MDR1-mediated interaction of digoxin with antiarrhythmic or antianginal drugs. *Biol Pharm Bull* (2002) 25, 1604–7.
27. Kodawara T, Masuda S, Wakasugi H, Uwai Y, Futami T, Saito H, Abe T, Inui K-i. Organic anion transporter oatp2-mediated interaction between digoxin and amiodarone in the rat liver. *Pharm Res* (2002) 19, 738–43.
28. Ben-Chetrit E, Ackerman Z, Eliakim M. Case-report: Amiodarone-associated hypothyroidism — a possible cause of digoxin intoxication. *Am J Med Sci* (1985) 289, 114–16.
29. Douste-Blazy P, Montastruc JL, Bonnet B, Auriol P, Conte D, Bernadet P. Influence of amiodarone on plasma and urine digoxin concentrations. *Lancet* (1984) i, 905.
30. Mingardi G. Amiodarone and plasma digoxin levels. *Lancet* (1984) i, 1238.
31. Santostasi G, Fantin M, Maragno I, Gaion RM, Basadonna O, Dalla-Volta S. Effects of amiodarone on oral and intravenous digoxin kinetics in healthy subjects. *J Cardiovasc Pharmacol* (1987) 9, 385–90.

Digitalis glycosides + Angiotensin II receptor antagonists

Candesartan, eprosartan, irbesartan, losartan, and valsartan do not appear to affect the pharmacokinetics of digoxin, but telmisartan may cause a rise in serum digoxin levels.

Clinical evidence

(a) Candesartan

There was no pharmacokinetic interaction between candesartan 16 mg daily and **digoxin** given as a loading dose of 750 micrograms then 250 micrograms daily in 12 healthy subjects.[1]

(b) Eprosartan

A study in 12 healthy men given a single 600-microgram dose of **digoxin** found that eprosartan 200 mg every 12 hours for 4 days had no significant effect on the pharmacokinetics of **digoxin**.[2]

(c) Irbesartan

A study in 10 healthy subjects taking **digoxin** for 2 weeks found no changes in the AUC or maximum serum levels of **digoxin**, when, during the second week, they also took irbesartan 150 mg daily.[3]

(d) Losartan

In 13 healthy subjects the pharmacokinetics of a single 500-microgram oral or intravenous dose of **digoxin** were not affected by losartan 50 mg daily for a week.[4]

(e) Telmisartan

A study in 12 healthy subjects given a 500-microgram loading dose of **digoxin** followed by 250 micrograms daily found that the maximum serum concentration, the trough serum concentration and the AUC were increased by 50%, 13%, and 22%, respectively, when telmisartan 120 mg daily was given for 7 days.[5] No clinically relevant changes in vital signs or ECGs were noted.

(f) Valsartan

There was no adverse interaction between a single 160-mg dose of valsartan and **digoxin** 250 micrograms in a study in 12 healthy subjects.[6]

Mechanism

It has been suggested that telmisartan may have caused digoxin to be more rapidly absorbed.[5] An *in vitro* study found that candesartan and losartan do not appear to inhibit P-glycoprotein-mediated transcellular transport. Therefore interactions resulting in reduced digoxin renal excretion are unlikely.[7]

Importance and management

No special precautions seem to be necessary when digoxin is used with candesartan, eprosartan, irbesartan, losartan, or valsartan. However, note that information for eprosartan, losartan, and valsartan is from single-dose studies, although the authors of the eprosartan study consider that a clinically relevant interaction with multiple doses of digoxin is unlikely.[2] The small increase in trough serum digoxin level with telmisartan suggests that the dose of digoxin need not automatically be reduced when telmisartan is started, but consideration should be given to monitoring digoxin effects (e.g. monitor for bradycardia) and take digoxin levels if necessary.

1. Jonkman JH, van Lier JJ, van Heiningen PN, Lins R, Sennewald R, Hogemann A. Pharmacokinetic drug interaction studies with candesartan cilexetil. *J Hum Hypertens* (1997) 11 (Suppl 2), S31–S35.
2. Martin DE, Tompson D, Boike SC, Tenero D, Ilson B, Citerone D, Jorkasky DK. Lack of effect of eprosartan on the single dose pharmacokinetics of orally administered digoxin in healthy male volunteers. *Br J Clin Pharmacol* (1997) 43, 661–4.
3. Marino MR, Vachharajani NN. Drug interactions with irbesartan. *Clin Pharmacokinet* (2001) 40, 605–14.
4. De Smet M, Schoors DF, De Meyer G, Verbesselt R, Goldberg MR, Fitzpatrick V, Somers G. Effect of multiple doses of losartan on the pharmacokinetics of single doses of digoxin in healthy volunteers. *Br J Clin Pharmacol* (1995) 40, 571–5.
5. Stangier J, Su C-APF, Hendricks MGC, van Lier JJ, Sollie FAE, Oosterhuis B, Jonkman JHG. The effect of telmisartan on the steady-state pharmacokinetics of digoxin in healthy male volunteers. *J Clin Pharmacol* (2000) 40, 1373–9.
6. Ciba Laboratories. Data on file, Protocols 07, 36–40, 42, 43, 52.
7. Takara K, Kakumoto M, Tanigawara Y, Funakoshi J, Sakaeda T, Okumura K. Interaction of digoxin with antihypertensive drugs *via* MDR1. *Life Sci* (2002) 70, 1491–1500.

Digitalis glycosides + Antacids

Although some studies suggest that antacids can reduce the bioavailability of digoxin and digitoxin, there is other evidence suggesting that no clinically relevant interactions occur.

Clinical evidence

(a) Digoxin

1. Evidence of an interaction. A study in 10 healthy subjects given digoxin 750 micrograms with 60 mL of either 4% **aluminium hydroxide gel**, 8% **magnesium hydroxide gel** or **magnesium trisilicate** found that the cumulative 6-day urinary excretion, expressed as a percentage of the original dose, was 40% for control; 31% for **aluminium hydroxide**; 27% for **magnesium hydroxide**; and 29% for **magnesium trisilicate**.[1]
Other studies describe reductions in digoxin absorption of 11% with **aluminium hydroxide**, 15% with **bismuth carbonate** and **light magnesium carbonate**, and 99.5% with **magnesium trisilicate**.[2]
When digoxin was given with 30 mL of an **aluminium/magnesium hydroxide** antacid and mexiletine, the digoxin AUC was approximately halved. As 'mexiletine', (p.931) does not appear to interact with digoxin the interaction was attributed to the antacid.[3]

2. Evidence of no interaction. A study in 4 patients chronically treated with digoxin 250 to 500 micrograms daily, found that the concurrent use of either 10 mL of **aluminium hydroxide mixture BP** or **magnesium trisilicate mixture BP**, three times daily, did not reduce the bioavailability of the digoxin and none of the patients showed any reduction in the control of their symptoms.[4]
Other bioavailability studies have not found a significant interaction between digoxin capsules and **aluminium/magnesium hydroxide**.[5]

(b) Other cardiac glycosides

In vitro studies with **digitoxin** suggest that it might possibly interact like digoxin, and be absorbed by various antacids,[6] but **lanatoside C** probably does not interact.[7] Bioavailability studies have not found a significant interaction between **beta-acetyldigoxin** and **aluminium/magnesium hydroxide**.[8]

A study in 10 patients with heart failure showed that their steady-state serum **digitoxin** levels were slightly, but not significantly raised (from 13.6 to 15.1 nanograms/mL) while taking 20 mL of **aluminium/magnesium hydroxide** gel three or four times daily, separated from the **digitoxin** dosage by at least 1 to 2 hours.[9]

Mechanism

Not established. One suggestion is that the digoxin can become adsorbed onto the antacids and therefore unavailable for absorption.[1,6] This is probably also true for digitoxin. However, some results are not consistent with this idea.

Importance and management

The interactions between digoxin or digitoxin and antacids are only moderately well documented, and the evidence is inconsistent. No clearly clinically relevant interactions have been reported. Separating the dosages by 1 to 2 hours to minimise admixture is effective with many other drugs that interact in the gut, and seems to work with digitoxin. However, unless further information becomes available it seems unlikely that separating administration is necessary, although it may be worth bearing in mind if, on rare occasions, a patient experiences an interaction.

1. Brown DD, Juhl RP, Lewis K, Schrott M, Bartels B. Decreased bioavailability of digoxin due to antacids and kaolin-pectin. *N Engl J Med* (1976) 295, 1034–7.
2. McElnay JC, Harron DWG, D'Arcy PF, Eagle MRG. Interaction of digoxin with antacid constituents. *BMJ* (1978) i, 1554.
3. Saris SD, Lowenthal DT, Affrime MB. Steady-state digoxin concentration during oral mexiletine administration. *Curr Ther Res* (1983) 34, 662–66.
4. Cooke J, Smith JA. Absence of interaction of digoxin with antacids under clinical conditions. *BMJ* (1978) 2, 1166.
5. Allen MD, Greenblatt DJ, Harmatz JS, Smith TW. Effect of magnesium-aluminum hydroxide and kaolin-pectin on the absorption of digoxin from tablets and capsules. *J Clin Pharmacol* (1981) 21, 26–30.
6. Khalil SAH. The uptake of digoxin and digitoxin by some antacids. *J Pharm Pharmacol* (1974) 26, 961–7.
7. Aldous S, Thomas R. Absorption and metabolism of lanatoside C. *Clin Pharmacol Ther* (1977) 21, 647–58.

8. Bonelli J, Hruby K, Magometschnigg D, Hitzenberger G, Kaik G. The bioavailability of β-acetyldigoxine alone and combined with aluminium hydroxide and magnesium hydroxide (Alucol®). *Int J Clin Pharmacol* (1977) 15, 337–9.
9. Kuhlmann J. Plasmaspiegel und renale Elimination von Digitoxin bei Langzeittherapie mit Aluminium-Magnesium-Hydroxid-Gel. *Dtsch Med Wochenschr* (1984) 109, 59–61.

Digitalis glycosides + Anticholinesterases; Centrally acting

There is no pharmacokinetic interaction between digoxin and tacrine or donepezil. The bradycardic effects of anticholinesterases and digoxin may possibly be additive.

Clinical evidence, mechanism, importance and management

A single-dose study in 12 healthy subjects found that the pharmacokinetics of **donepezil** 5 mg and **digoxin** 250 micrograms were not affected by concurrent use and no clinically relevant changes in cardiac conduction parameters occurred.[1]

In one study in healthy subjects given a single 500-microgram dose of **digoxin**, the pharmacokinetics of the **digoxin** were unchanged by **tacrine** 20 mg every 6 hours.[2] Although no special precautions would seem necessary on a pharmacokinetic basis, check to see that the combined bradycardic effects of **digoxin** and **tacrine** do not become excessive.

Similarly, the manufacturers of **galantamine**[3] say that no pharmacokinetic interactions have been seen with **digoxin**, but caution about the possibility of a pharmacodynamic interaction that may result in bradycardia. The manufacturers of **rivastigmine**[4] say that the combination has no pharmacokinetic interaction, nor does it interfere with cardiac conduction. It would however seem prudent to monitor heart rate if any of these combinations are used.

1. Tiseo PJ, Perdomo CA, Friedhoff LT. Concurrent administration of donepezil HCl and digoxin: assessment of pharmacokinetic changes. *Br J Clin Pharmacol* (1998) 46 (Suppl 1), 40–4.
2. deVries TM, Siedlik P, Smithers JA, Brown RR, Reece PA, Posvar EL, Sedman AJ, Koup JR, Forgue ST. Effect of multiple-dose tacrine administration on single-dose pharmacokinetics of digoxin, diazepam, and theophylline. *Pharm Res* (1993) 10 (10 Suppl), S-333.
3. Reminyl (Galantamine hydrobromide). Shire Pharmaceuticals Ltd. UK Summary of product characteristics, July 2005.
4. Exelon (Rivastigmine hydrogen tartrate). Novartis Pharmaceuticals UK Ltd. UK Summary of product characteristics, October 2006.

Digitalis glycosides + Antiepileptics; Miscellaneous

There is little evidence to suggest that carbamazepine interacts with digoxin, and topiramate causes only a small reduction in digoxin serum levels. Levetiracetam and tiagabine do not appear to interact with digoxin.

Clinical evidence, mechanism, importance and management

(a) Carbamazepine

In an early clinical study, bradycardia seen in 3 patients taking **digitalis** and carbamazepine was tentatively attributed to their concurrent use.[1]There appear to be no other reports to confirm or refute this.

(b) Levetiracetam

In a placebo-controlled study, 11 healthy subjects were given an initial loading dose of **digoxin** 500 micrograms followed by 250 micrograms daily with levetiracetam 1 g twice daily for one week. Levetiracetam did not significantly affect the pharmacokinetics or pharmacodynamics of **digoxin**, and the pharmacokinetics of levetiracetam were not significantly altered by **digoxin**.[2] No additional precautions seem necessary on concurrent use.

(c) Tiagabine

In a crossover study, 13 healthy subjects were given a loading dose of **digoxin** 500 micrograms twice daily for one day then 250 micrograms daily for 8 days, either alone or with tiagabine 4 mg three times daily for 9 days. It was found that the pharmacokinetics of **digoxin** were not significantly altered by tiagabine.[3]

(d) Topiramate

Topiramate 100 mg twice daily for 9 days caused a small reduction in the serum **digoxin** levels of 12 healthy subjects. The maximum serum levels and the AUC were reduced by 15.8% and 12%, respectively, and the oral **digoxin** clearance was increased by 13%.[4-6] The manufacturers suggest good monitoring of **digoxin** if topiramate is added or withdrawn,[5] but changes in the pharmacokinetics of **digoxin** of this magnitude seem unlikely to be clinically relevant in most patients.

1. Killian JM, Fromm GH. Carbamazepine in the treatment of neuralgia. Use and side effects. *Arch Neurol* (1968) 19, 129–36.
2. Levy RH, Ragueneau-Majlessi I, Baltes E. Repeated administration of the novel antiepileptic agent levetiracetam does not alter digoxin pharmacokinetics and pharmacodynamics in healthy volunteers. *Epilepsy Res* (2001) 46, 93–9.
3. Snel S, Jansen JA, Pedersen PC, Jonkman JHG, van Heiningen PNM. Tiagabine, a novel antiepileptic agent: lack of pharmacokinetic interaction with digoxin. *Eur J Clin Pharmacol* (1998) 54, 355–7.
4. Liao S, Palmer M. Digoxin and topiramate drug interaction study in male volunteers. *Pharm Res* (1993) 10 (10 Suppl), S405.
5. Topamax (Topiramate). Janssen-Cilag Ltd. UK Summary of product characteristics, November 2006.
6. Topamax (Topiramate) Ortho-McNeil Neurologics, Inc. US Prescribing information, March 2007.

Digitalis glycosides + Antiepileptics; Phenytoin

Phenytoin reduces the serum levels of digoxin and digitoxin. Cases of bradycardia have been seen in digitalised patients given phenytoin. Phenytoin was formerly used for the treatment of digitalis-induced cardiac arrhythmias, but sudden cardiac arrest has been reported.

Clinical evidence

(a) Bradycardia and cardiac arrest

A patient with suspected digitalis-induced cardiac arrhythmias developed bradycardia, then became asystolic and died, following an intravenous injection of phenytoin.[1] The discussion of this case briefly mentions a further 6 fatalities in patients similarly treated.[1] A patient with Down's syndrome and mitral valve insufficiency taking **digoxin** 250 micrograms daily developed bradycardia of 34 bpm and complete heart block when his phenytoin dose was increased from 200 to 300 mg daily.[2]

(b) Reduced digoxin levels

A study in 6 healthy subjects given **beta-acetyldigoxin** 400 micrograms daily found that the half-life of digoxin was reduced by 30% (from 33.9 to 23.7 hours) and the AUC was reduced by 23% after they took phenytoin 200 mg twice daily for a week. Total digoxin clearance increased by 27% (from 258.6 to 328.3 mL/minute).[3]

(c) Reduced digitoxin levels

The plasma digitoxin levels of a man were reduced on three occasions when he was given phenytoin. On the third occasion, while taking digitoxin 200 micrograms daily, the addition of phenytoin 900 mg daily caused a 60% fall in digitoxin levels (from 25 to 10 nanograms/mL) over a 7 to 10 day period.[4]

Mechanism

Phenytoin has a stabilising effect on the myocardial cells so that the toxic threshold of digoxin at which arrhythmias occur is raised. However, the bradycardic effects of the digitalis glycoside are not opposed and the lethal dose is unaltered, so that the cardiac arrest reported would appear to be the result of excessive bradycardia. It seems possible that the fall in plasma digitoxin levels may be due to a phenytoin-induced increase in the metabolism of the digitoxin by the liver.[5]

Importance and management

Phenytoin was formerly used for treating digitalis-induced arrhythmias, but this use now appears to be obsolete. Intravenous phenytoin should not be used in patients with a high degree of heart block or marked bradycardia because of the risk that cardiac arrest may occur. Information about the effects of phenytoin on digitalis glycoside levels seems to be confined to these single reports, but it may be prudent to check that patients who are taking digitoxin (and possibly digoxin), and are subsequently given phenytoin, do not become under-digitalised.

1. Zoneraich S, Zoneraich O, Siegel J. Sudden death following intravenous sodium diphenylhydantoin. *Am Heart J* (1976) 91, 375–7.
2. Viukari NMA, Aho K. Digoxin-phenytoin interaction. *BMJ* (1970) 2, 51.
3. Rameis H. On the interaction between phenytoin and digoxin. *Eur J Clin Pharmacol* (1985) 29, 49–53.

4. Solomon HM, Reich S, Spirt N, Abrams WB. Interactions between digitoxin and other drugs *in vitro* and *in vivo*. *Ann N Y Acad Sci* (1971) 179, 362–9.
5. Rameis H. The importance of prospective planning of pharmacokinetic trials. Considerations of studies on the phenytoin-digoxin-(P-D) and phenytoin-digitoxin-(P-DT) interaction. *Int J Clin Pharmacol Ther Toxicol* (1992) 30, 528–9.

Digitalis glycosides + Antineoplastics

Treatment with radiation and/or antineoplastic cytotoxics can damage the lining of the intestine so that digoxin (given as tablets) is much less readily absorbed. This appears to be resolved by giving the digoxin in liquid or liquid-in-capsule form, or by substituting digitoxin.

Clinical evidence

A study in 13 patients with various forms of neoplastic disease showed that radiation therapy and/or various high-dose cytotoxic regimens (including **carmustine**, **cyclophosphamide**, **melphalan**, **cytarabine** and **methotrexate**) reduced the absorption of **digoxin** from tablets (*Lanoxin*) by almost 46%, but the reduction was not significant (15%) when the **digoxin** was given as capsules (*Lanoxicaps*).[1]

Other studies confirm that a 50% reduction in serum **digoxin** levels (using **beta-acetyldigoxin**) occurred in patients given **cyclophosphamide**, **vincristine**, **procarbazine** and prednisone (COPP); **cyclophosphamide**, **vincristine** and prednisone (COP); **cyclophosphamide**, **vincristine**, **cytarabine** and prednisone (COAP); and **doxorubicin**, **bleomycin** and prednisone (ABP). These effects disappeared about a week after cytotoxic therapy finished.[2] Radiation has a smaller effect.[3] **Digitoxin** absorption does not seem to be affected by antineoplastics.[4]

Mechanism

The reduced absorption is thought to result from damage to the intestinal epithelium caused by the antineoplastic cytotoxics.[5]

Importance and management

The interaction appears to be established. Patients taking digoxin and receiving treatment with antineoplastic cytotoxics should be monitored for signs of under-digitalisation. The problem can be overcome by replacing digoxin tablets with digoxin in liquid form or in solution inside a capsule. The effects of the interaction are short-lived so that a downward readjustment may be necessary about a week after treatment is withdrawn. An alternative is to use digitoxin, which does not appear to be affected.

1. Bjornsson TD, Huang AT, Roth P, Jacob DS, Christenson R. Effects of high-dose cancer chemotherapy on the absorption of digoxin in two different formulations. *Clin Pharmacol Ther* (1986) 39, 25–8.
2. Kuhlmann J, Zilly W, Wilke J. Effects of cytostatic drugs on plasma levels and renal excretion of β-acetyldigoxin. *Clin Pharmacol Ther* (1981) 30, 518–27.
3. Sokol GH, Greenblatt DJ, Lloyd BL, Georgotas A, Allen MD, Harmatz JS, Smith TW, Shader RI. Effect of abdominal radiation therapy on drug absorption in humans. *J Clin Pharmacol* (1978) 18, 388–96.
4. Kuhlmann J, Wilke J, Rietbrock N. Cytostatic drugs are without significant effect on digitoxin plasma level and renal excretion. *Clin Pharmacol Ther* (1982) 32, 646–51.
5. Jusko WB, Conti DR, Molson A, Kuritzky P, Giller J, Schultz R. Digoxin absorption from tablets and elixir: the effect of radiation-induced malabsorption. *JAMA* (1974) 230, 1554–5.

Digitalis glycosides + Aprepitant

Aprepitant does not affect the pharmacokinetics of digoxin.

Clinical evidence, mechanism, importance and management

A placebo-controlled, randomised, study in 11 healthy subjects found that the pharmacokinetics of **digoxin** 250 micrograms daily were not affected by aprepitant (125 mg given on day 7 and 80 mg given daily on days 8 to 11). *In vitro* evidence indicates that aprepitant is a substrate and weak inhibitor of P-glycoprotein. However, at the doses used for the prevention of chemotherapy-induced nausea and vomiting, it appears unlikely to interact with P-glycoprotein substrates such as **digoxin**.[1]

1. Feuring M, Lee Y, Orlowski LH, Michiels N, De Smet M, Majumdar AK, Petty KJ, Goldberg MR, Murphy MG, Gottesdiener KM, Hesney M, Brackett LE, Wehling M. Lack of effect of aprepitant on digoxin pharmacokinetics in healthy subjects. *J Clin Pharmacol* (2003) 43, 912–17.

Digitalis glycosides + Argatroban

No significant pharmacokinetic interaction occurs between digoxin and argatroban.

Clinical evidence, mechanism, importance and management

A placebo-controlled, crossover study in 12 healthy subjects found that the pharmacokinetics of steady-state **digoxin** 375 micrograms daily were not affected by an infusion of argatroban 2 micrograms/kg per minute for 120 hours. Steady-state argatroban levels were obtained within 3 hours and maintained throughout the infusion. Dosage adjustments should not be necessary during concurrent use.[1]

1. Inglis AML, Sheth SB, Hursting MJ, Tenero DM, Graham AM, DiCicco RA. Investigation of the interaction between argatroban and acetaminophen, lidocaine, or digoxin. *Am J Health-Syst Pharm* (2002) 59, 1258–66.

Digitalis glycosides + Aspirin

Aspirin may cause a moderate rise in serum digoxin levels, but no interaction of clinical relevance seems to occur.

Clinical evidence, mechanism, importance and management

Although aspirin can double the serum concentrations of **digoxin** in *dogs*, a study in 8 healthy subjects found no interaction, even when high doses of aspirin (975 mg three times daily) were given.[1] However, in another study in 9 healthy subjects given aspirin 1.5 g daily for 10 days, the serum **digoxin** levels were increased by 31%.[2] A further study found a 49% increase in **digoxin** levels when it was given with aspirin 1.5 g daily.[3] Bearing in mind that both drugs have been in use for a very considerable number of years, the lack of reports in the literature describing problems suggests that no clinically important interaction normally occurs.

1. Fenster PE, Comess KA, Hanson CD and Finley PR. Kinetics of digoxin-aspirin combination. *Clin Pharmacol Ther* (1982) 32, 428–30.
2. Isbary J, Doering W, König E.Der Einfluβ von Tiaprofensäure auf die Digoxinkonzentration im Serum (DKS) im Vergleich zu anderen Antirheumatika (AR). *Z Rheumatol* (1982) 41, 164.
3. Halawa B, Mazurek W. Interakcja digoksyny i niektórych niesteroidowych leków przeciwzapalnych, kwasu acetylosalicylowego i nifedipiny. *Pol Tyg Lek* (1982) 37, 1475–6.

Digitalis glycosides + Azoles; Itraconazole

Itraconazole causes a marked increase in serum digoxin levels. Toxicity may occur unless the digoxin dosage is suitably reduced. Theoretically, itraconazole might also oppose the positive inotropic effects of digoxin.

Clinical evidence

In a placebo-controlled, crossover study, 10 healthy subjects taking **digoxin** 250 micrograms daily were given itraconazole 200 mg daily for 10 days. The serum **digoxin** levels increased by about 80% (from 1 to 1.8 nanograms/mL). New steady-state **digoxin** levels were not fully achieved during the 10-day period with itraconazole, so greater rises might occur on longer use.[1] A study in 3 patients with congestive heart failure taking **digoxin** found that itraconazole decreased **digoxin** clearance by 50% and increased **digoxin** levels, and ECG changes (premature ventricular contractions, AV block and ST depression) occurred.[2]

A 68-year-old man taking **digoxin** 250 micrograms twice daily and ibuprofen developed nausea and fatigue (interpreted later as **digoxin** toxicity) after starting itraconazole 400 mg daily for an infected elbow. The symptoms disappeared when both the itraconazole and ibuprofen were stopped, but returned when the itraconazole was restarted. After 7 days his heart rate had fallen, from 60 to 40 bpm, and his **digoxin** level had doubled, from 1.6 to 3.2 nanograms/mL. He was later satisfactorily restabilised on a quarter of the **digoxin** dosage while taking the same dose of itraconazole.[3] Several other patients developed **digoxin** toxicity (a sixfold increase in one case) within 3 to 13 days of starting to take itraconazole,[4-10] and after 4 weeks in one case.[11] A possible case of **digoxin** toxicity has also occurred with itraconazole pulse therapy.[12] Two cases of **digoxin** toxicity have been reported when itraconazole was given to renal transplant patients, but other factors may have contributed to the high levels of **digoxin** in these 2 patients.[13]

Mechanism

Itraconazole inhibits P-glycoprotein, which transports digoxin out of kidney tubule cells into the urine,[14-17] and therefore digoxin urinary clearance is reduced and serum levels are increased.[5,10]

Importance and management

An established and clinically important pharmacokinetic interaction. Monitor the effects of digoxin (e.g. bradycardia, nausea, vomiting) if itraconazole is started, anticipating the need to reduce the digoxin dosage. Halving the dose was suggested in one study.[2] Two of the patients cited above were restabilised with a quarter of the digoxin dosage[3,4] and another with about one-third of the original digoxin dose[5] while taking itraconazole. More recent findings suggest that itraconazole may possess significant negative inotropic properties, and the CSM in the UK suggest that it should be used with caution in patients at risk of heart failure.[18] This suggests that itraconazole might oppose the pharmacological effects of digoxin.

1. Partanen J, Jalava K-M, Neuvonen PJ. Itraconazole increases serum digoxin concentration. *Pharmacol Toxicol* (1996) 79, 274–6.
2. Wagasugi H, Isizuka R, Koreeda N, Yano I, Futami T, Nohara R, Sasayoma S, Inui K. Effect of itraconazole on digoxin clearance in patients with congestive heart failure. *Yakugaku Zasshi* (2000) 120, 807–11.
3. Rex J. Itraconazole-digoxin interaction. *Ann Intern Med* (1992) 116, 525.
4. Kauffman CA, Bagnasco FA. Digoxin toxicity associated with itraconazole therapy. *Clin Infect Dis* (1992) 15, 886–7.
5. Sachs MK, Blanchard LM, Green PJ. Interaction of itraconazole and digoxin. *Clin Infect Dis* (1993) 16, 400–3.
6. Alderman CP, Jersmann HPA. Digoxin-itraconazole interaction. *Med J Aust* (1993) 159, 838–9.
7. McClean KL, Sheehan GJ. Interaction between itraconazole and digoxin. *Clin Infect Dis* (1994) 18, 259–60.
8. Meyboom RH, de Jonge K, Veentjer H, Dekens-Konter JA, de Koning GH. Potentiering van digoxine door itraconazol. *Ned Tijdschr Geneeskd* (1994) 138, 2353–6.
9. Cone LA, Himelman RB, Hirschberg JN, Hutcheson JW. Itraconazole-related amaurosis and vomiting due to digoxin toxicity. *West J Med* (1996) 165, 322.
10. Alderman CP, Allcroft PD. Digoxin-itraconazole interaction: possible mechanisms. *Ann Pharmacother* (1997) 31, 438–40.
11. Lopez F, Hancock EW. Nausea and malaise during treatment of coccidioidomycosis. *Hosp Pract* (1997) 32, 21–2.
12. Brodell RT, Elewski B. Antifungal drug Interactions. Avoidance requires more than memorization. *Postgrad Med* (2000) 107, 41–3.
13. Mathis AS, Friedman GS. Coadministration of digoxin with itraconazole in renal transplant recipients. *Am J Kidney Dis* (2001) 37, 1–8.
14. Ito S, Koren G. Comment: possible mechanism of digoxin-itraconazole interaction. *Ann Pharmacother* (1997) 31, 1091–2.
15. Woodland C, Ito S, Koren G. A model for the prediction of digoxin–drug interactions at the renal tubular cell level. *Ther Drug Monit* (1998) 20, 134–8.
16. Angirasa AK, Koch AZ. P-glycoprotein as the mediator of itraconazole–digoxin interaction. *J Am Podiatr Med Assoc* (2002) 92, 471–2.
17. Jalava K-M, Partanen J, Neuvonen PJ. Itraconazole decreases renal clearance of digoxin. *Ther Drug Monit* (1997) 19, 609–13.
18. Committee on Safety of Medicines/Medicines Control Agency. Cardiodepressant effects of itraconazole. *Current Problems* (2001) 27, 11.

Digitalis glycosides + Azoles; Posaconazole

The UK manufacturer of posaconazole advises that digoxin levels should be monitored when initiating or discontinuing treatment with posaconazole, in the light of the rise in digoxin levels when given with other azoles.[1] See 'itraconazole', (p.910).

1. Noxafil (Posaconazole). Schering-Plough Ltd. UK Summary of product characteristics, October 2006.

Digitalis glycosides + Azoles; Voriconazole

Voriconazole did not affect the steady-state pharmacokinetics of digoxin in a study in healthy patients. One study briefly mentions increased digoxin levels in two patients receiving voriconazole.

Clinical evidence, mechanism, importance and management

A placebo-controlled study in healthy subjects given a **digoxin** loading dose over 2 days, then **digoxin** 250 micrograms daily for 20 days, found that voriconazole 200 mg twice daily for the last 12 days had no significant effect on the steady-state pharmacokinetics of **digoxin**.[1] Unlike 'itraconazole', (p.910), voriconazole appears not to alter the P-glycoprotein-mediated transport of **digoxin**.

However, a clinical study in severely ill patients with invasive mycosis briefly mentions that two patients receiving voriconazole developed high trough **digoxin** levels, which required the **digoxin** to be withdrawn. One patient was symptomatic with an arrhythmia and ECG changes.[2]

1. Purkins L, Wood N, Kleinermans D, Nichols D. Voriconazole does not affect the steady-state pharmacokinetics of digoxin. *Br J Clin Pharmacol* (2003) 56, 45–50.
2. Cesaro S, Toffolutti T, Messina C, Calore E, Alaggio R, Cusinato R, Pillon M, Zanesco L. Safety and efficacy of caspofungin and liposomal amphotericin B, followed by voriconazole in young patients affected by refractory invasive mycosis. *Eur J Haematol* (2004) 73, 50–5.

Digitalis glycosides + Barbiturates

Blood levels of digitoxin can be halved by phenobarbital and its effects may be expected to be reduced accordingly. However, another study found that phenobarbital did not affect digitoxin, digoxin or acetyldigitoxin pharmacokinetics.

Clinical evidence

Phenobarbital 60 mg three times daily for 12 weeks, halved the steady-state plasma levels of **digitoxin** 100 micrograms daily.[1] In associated studies the half-life of **digitoxin** decreased from 7.8 to 4.5 days during **phenobarbital** treatment.[1] In another study[2] the rate of conversion of **digitoxin** to digoxin increased from 4% to 27% in one patient who took **phenobarbital** 96 mg daily for 13 days.

In contrast, a study in groups of 10 healthy subjects given either **digitoxin** 400 micrograms, **digoxin** 1 mg or **acetyldigitoxin** 800 micrograms daily did not find any changes in the serum concentrations of any of these digitalis glycosides when **phenobarbital** 100 mg was given three times daily for 7 to 9 days.[3]

Mechanism

Phenobarbital and other barbiturates are well-known potent liver enzyme inducers which, it would seem, can increase the metabolism and conversion of digitoxin to digoxin.[1,2] The lack of interaction in one study may possibly have been because the barbiturate was taken for a relatively short time.[3]

Importance and management

An established interaction, although its clinical importance is somewhat uncertain because there seem to be few reports of the effects of using digitoxin with phenobarbital, or of problems in practice. Nevertheless, patients taking both drugs should be monitored for possible under-digitalisation and the dosage of digitoxin increased if necessary. It seems likely that digoxin will not be affected by the barbiturates because it is largely excreted unchanged in the urine. Other barbiturates would be expected to behave like phenobarbital.

1. Solomon HM, Abrams WB. Interactions between digitoxin and other drugs in man. *Am Heart J* (1972) 83, 277–80.
2. Jelliffe RW, Blankenhorn DH. Effect of phenobarbital on digitoxin metabolism. *Clin Res* (1966) 14, 160.
3. Káldor A, Somogyi G, Debreczeni LA, Gachályi B. Interaction of heart glycosides and phenobarbital. *Int J Clin Pharmacol* (1975) 12, 403–7.

Digitalis glycosides + Benzodiazepines and related drugs

Digoxin toxicity occurred in two elderly patients and rises in serum digoxin levels have been seen in others when they were given alprazolam. A reduction in the urinary clearance of digoxin has been described during the use of diazepam. No pharmacokinetic interaction seems to occur with digoxin and eszopiclone, zaleplon, or zolpidem.

Clinical evidence

(a) Benzodiazepines

1. Alprazolam. An elderly woman taking **digoxin**, maprotiline, isosorbide dinitrate, furosemide and potassium chloride showed signs of **digoxin** toxicity during the second week of taking alprazolam 1 mg daily. Her serum **digoxin** levels were later found to have risen almost 300%, from 1.6 to 4.3 nanograms/mL, and her apparent **digoxin** clearance had fallen from 126.3 to 49.8 L/day.[1] A later study in 12 patients confirmed that **digoxin** levels can be significantly raised by alprazolam, particularly in those over 65 years old. One elderly man developed clinical **digoxin** toxicity.[2] In contrast, a study in 8 healthy subjects found no changes in the clearance of **digoxin** after they took alprazolam 1.5 mg daily.[3]

2. Diazepam. The observation that 3 patients developed raised **digoxin** levels while also taking diazepam prompted a further study in 7 healthy subjects.[4] After taking diazepam 5 mg with a single 500-microgram dose of **digoxin**, and diazepam 5 mg every 12 hours thereafter, all of them had a substantial reduction in the urinary excretion of **digoxin** and 5 of them had a moderate increase in the **digoxin** half-life. No further details were given.[4]

3. Metaclazepam. No statistically significant interaction was seen in 9 patients taking **beta-acetyldigoxin** when they were given metaclazepam.[5]

(b) Non-benzodiazepine hypnotics

1. Eszopiclone. In a study in 12 healthy subjects, a 3-mg single dose of eszopiclone did not alter the pharmacokinetics of **digoxin**, given for 7 days.[6]

2. Zaleplon. Zaleplon 10 mg daily given to 20 healthy subjects for 5 days had no significant effects on the steady-state pharmacokinetics of **digoxin** 375 micrograms daily. There were no significant differences in QTc or PR intervals.[7]

3. Zolpidem. No significant pharmacokinetic interaction occurs between zolpidem and **digoxin**.[8]

Mechanism

Uncertain. The suggestion is that diazepam may possibly alter the extent of the protein binding of digoxin within the plasma, which may have some influence on the renal tubular excretion,[4] but see comments on protein binding interactions in 'Drug distribution interactions', (p.3). The reason for the interaction between digoxin and alprazolam is not understood.

Importance and management

The interaction between digoxin and alprazolam is established and clinically important. Monitor the effects of digoxin (e.g. bradycardia) in any patient if alprazolam is added, and reduce the digoxin dosage as necessary. What is known suggests that toxicity is more likely in the elderly. Other benzodiazepines and digoxin have been used for a considerable time but there seem to be no other reports of adverse interactions. The newer non-benzodiazepine hypnotics, eszopiclone, zaleplon and zolpidem do not appear to affect the pharmacokinetics of digoxin.

1. Tollefson G, Lesar T, Grothe D, Garvey M. Alprazolam-related digoxin toxicity. *Am J Psychiatry* (1984) 141, 1612–14.
2. Guven H, Tuncok Y, Guneri S, Cavdar C, Fowler J. Age-related digoxin-alprazolam interaction. *Clin Pharmacol Ther* (1993) 54, 42–4.
3. Ochs HR, Greenblatt DJ, Verburg-Ochs B. Effect of alprazolam on digoxin kinetics and creatinine clearance. *Clin Pharmacol Ther* (1985) 38, 595–8.
4. Castillo-Ferrando JR, Garcia M, Carmona J. Digoxin levels and diazepam. *Lancet* (1980) ii, 368.
5. Völker D, Müller R, Günther C, Bode R. Digoxin-Plasmaspiegel während der Behandlung mit Metaclazepam. *Arzneimittelforschung* (1988) 38, 923–5.
6. Caron J, Wessel T, Maier G. Evaluation of a pharmacokinetic interaction between eszopiclone and digoxin. *Sleep* (2004) 27, A55.
7. Sanchez Garcia P, Paty I, Leister CA, Guerra P, Frías J, García Pérez LE, Darwish M. Effect of zaleplon on digoxin pharmacokinetics and pharmacodynamics. *Am J Health-Syst Pharm* (2000) 57, 2267–70.
8. Salvà P, Costa J. Clinical pharmacokinetics and pharmacodynamics of zolpidem: therapeutic implications. *Clin Pharmacokinet* (1995) 29, 142–53.

Digitalis glycosides + Beta-agonist bronchodilators

Oral salbutamol (albuterol) causes a small reduction in serum digoxin levels. Beta agonists can cause hypokalaemia, which could lead to the development of digitalis toxicity.

Clinical evidence, mechanism, importance and management

A study in 10 healthy subjects who had taken **digoxin** 500 micrograms daily for 10 days[1] found that, 3 hours after taking oral **salbutamol** (albuterol) 3 to 4 mg, their serum **digoxin** levels had fallen by 0.23 nanograms/mL and their serum potassium levels had fallen by 0.58 mmol/L. A follow-up study suggested that the **digoxin** distribution to skeletal muscle may have been increased.[2]

Note that all $beta_2$ agonists can cause a fall in serum potassium, which could possibly affect the response of patients to **digoxin**. The clinical importance of these changes is uncertain but concurrent use should be monitored. Consider monitoring potassium levels if the effects of **digoxin** seem excessive.

1. Edner M, Jogestrand T. Oral salbutamol decreases serum digoxin concentration. *Eur J Clin Pharmacol* (1990) 38, 195–7.
2. Edner M, Jogestrand T, Dahlqvist R. Effect of salbutamol on digoxin pharmacokinetics. *Eur J Clin Pharmacol* (1992) 42, 197–201.

Digitalis glycosides + Beta blockers

In general there appears to be no pharmacokinetic interaction between digoxin and beta blockers, although talinolol and carvedilol appear to increase the bioavailability of digoxin. Pharmacodynamic interactions, resulting in additive bradycardia, are possible. A few cases of excessive bradycardia have been reported when propranolol was used to control digitalis-induced arrhythmias.

Clinical evidence

(a) Pharmacokinetic interactions

1. Carvedilol. A 12-year-old boy with dilated cardiomyopathy taking **digoxin** 250 micrograms in the morning and 125 micrograms in the evening was subsequently given carvedilol 70 micrograms/kg twice daily. Several days later he became anorexic and started vomiting and his **digoxin** serum level was found to have increased from 1.6 to 2.3 nanograms/mL up to 4.2 nanograms/mL. **Digoxin** was stopped and subsequently restarted at half the original dose.[1] In one study, 8 children aged 2 weeks to 8 years were given **digoxin** for ventricular failure secondary to congenital heart disease. When they were also given carvedilol 0.06 to 1.06 mg/kg daily the clearance of **digoxin** was approximately halved and 2 children experienced **digoxin** toxicity.[1]

A single-dose study in healthy adults given carvedilol 25 mg found that maximum plasma levels of a 500-microgram dose of **digoxin** were increased by 0.97 nanograms/mL (60%) and the AUC was increased by about 20%, but the clinical effects of these changes were considered likely to be small.[2] No significant pharmacokinetic interaction was found in other single-dose studies in adults given carvedilol and **digitoxin**,[3] or carvedilol and intravenous **digoxin**.[2]

In a multiple-dose study in adult patients with hypertension, carvedilol raised the maximum serum levels and AUC of **digoxin** 250 micrograms daily by 32% and 14%, respectively, after 2 weeks of treatment. Again, these changes were considered unlikely to be clinically significant.[4] In another study in 12 male and 12 female patients taking **digoxin** 62.5 to 250 micrograms daily for heart failure, the addition of carvedilol 6.25 mg twice daily for 7 days increased the maximum concentration and the AUC_{0-16} of **digoxin** by 37% and 56%, respectively, in the men, but no significant changes to the pharmacokinetics of **digoxin** were noted in the women.[5]

2. Talinolol. In healthy subjects talinolol 100 mg orally substantially increased the bioavailability of a single 500-microgram dose of **digoxin**. The AUC_{0-72} and the maximum serum levels of **digoxin** were increased by 23% and 45%, respectively.[6] Conversely, intravenous talinolol 30 mg had no effect on **digoxin** pharmacokinetics.[6]

3. Miscellaneous. A single dose of intravenous **esmolol** did not affect the pharmacokinetics of multiple-dose **digoxin**, except that a small increase was seen in the AUC_{0-6} of **digoxin**.[7] The pharmacokinetics of multiple-dose **digoxin** have been shown to be unaffected by **acebutolol**,[8] **bevantolol** 200 mg daily,[9] **bisoprolol** 10 mg daily,[10] **nebivolol** 10 mg daily,[11] or **sotalol** 80 to 320 mg daily.[12]

(b) Pharmacodynamic interactions

Increased bradycardia is expected to occur with combinations of **digoxin** and beta blockers, but reports of this becoming a problem seem rare. One report notes marked bradycardia of 35 to 50 bpm in a 91-year-old patient taking **digoxin** and using **timolol** 0.25% eye drops.[13] Bradycardia persisted on withdrawal of **digoxin**, and improved only after discontinuation of the timolol as well. Two cases, where **propranolol** 10 mg orally was used to treat arrhythmias associated with **digoxin** toxicity, are reported.[14] The first patient (who had heart failure) became bradycardic, asystolic and then died, while the second patient became bradycardic (30 bpm) but recovered after being given atropine. A further fatality was reported when intravenous **propranolol** was used.[15] In a placebo-controlled study of the use of **sotalol** in digitalised patients with chronic atrial fibrillation, 2 of 24 **sotalol** recipients were withdrawn due to bradycardia compared with none of 10 given placebo. However, the combination was still considered valuable.[12] In a prospective analysis of adverse drug reactions leading to hospital admission over a 4-year period, 83 patients were identified who had been admitted with bradycardia. Of these, 62 were taking **digitalis glycosides**, and 14 were also taking a beta blocker.[16]

In healthy subjects, the pharmacodynamics of **digoxin** were unaffected by **bevantolol**,[9] and **esmolol**,[7] with no significant changes in heart rate or blood pressure occurring.

Mechanism

In most cases where the situation has had an adverse outcome the interaction seems to be due to the additive effects on the slowing of the heart.

It has been suggested that the pharmacokinetic interaction with talinolol is due to competition with digoxin for *intestinal* P-glycoprotein, although this needs confirmation.[6] It would seem possible that this mechanism also accounts for the interaction between digoxin and carvedilol, and an *in vitro* study found that carvedilol (but not atenolol or metoprolol) inhibits P-glycoprotein-mediated transcellular transport of digoxin,[17] which may mean *renal* tubular secretion of digoxin is inhibited. It is conceivable that P-glycoprotein inhibition by carvedilol enhances the intestinal absorption of digoxin and also decreases its renal excretion. This may explain why the interaction is possibly more significant in children, as they have a higher renal clearance rate of digoxin than adults.[1] Women have lower P-glycoprotein activity in the gut than men, which may account for the gender differences seen with the interaction of carvedilol and digoxin.[5]

It has also been suggested that the interaction between digoxin and talinolol may be dosage form dependent. More study is needed.

Importance and management

Concurrent use appears, on the whole, beneficial, but the potential for additive bradycardia should be borne in mind. Use of beta blockers in cases of digoxin toxicity should be undertaken with great care. In addition, it may be prudent to monitor digoxin levels with talinolol, and also with carvedilol, particularly in children. It has been suggested that the dose of digoxin should be reduced by at least 25% in children given carvedilol, with further adjustments as required.[1]

1. Ratnapalan S, Griffiths K, Costei AM, Benson L, Koren G. Digoxin-carvedilol interactions in children. *J Pediatr* (2003) 142, 572–4.
2. De Mey C, Brendel E, Enterling D. Carvedilol increases the systemic bioavailability of oral digoxin. *Br J Clin Pharmacol* (1990) 29, 486–90.
3. Harder S, Brei R, Caspary S, Merz PG. Lack of a pharmacokinetic interaction between carvedilol and digitoxin or phenprocoumon. *Eur J Clin Pharmacol* (1993) 44, 583–6.
4. Wermeling DP, Feild CJ, Smith DA, Chandler MHH, Clifton GD, Boyle DA. Effects of long-term oral carvedilol on the steady-state pharmacokinetics of oral digoxin in patients with mild to moderate hypertension. *Pharmacotherapy* (1994) 14, 600–6.
5. Baris N, Kalkan S, Güneri S, Bozdemir V, Guven H. Influence of carvedilol on serum digoxin levels in heart failure: is there any gender difference? *Eur J Clin Pharmacol* (2006) 62, 535–38.
6. Westphal K, Weinbrenner A, Giessmann T, Stuhr M, Gerd F, Zschiesche M, Oertel R, Terhaag B, Kroemer HK, Siegmund W. Oral bioavailability of digoxin is enhanced by talinolol: Evidence for involvement of P-glycoprotein. *Clin Pharmacol Ther* (2000) 68, 6–12.
7. Lowenthal DT, Porter RS, Achari R, Turlapaty P, Laddu AR and Matier WL. Esmolol-digoxin drug interaction. *J Clin Pharmacol* (1987) 27, 561–6.
8. Ryan JR. Clinical pharmacology of acebutolol. *Am Heart J* (1985) 109, 1131–6.
9. Frishman WH, Goldberg RJ, Benfield P. Bevantolol. A preliminary review of its pharmacodynamic and pharmacokinetic properties, and therapeutic efficacy in hypertension and angina pectoris. *Drugs* (1988) 35, 1–21.
10. Vechlekar DL, Cheung WK, Pearse S, Greene DS, Dukart G, Unczowsky R, Weiss AI, Silber BM, Faulkner RD. Bisoprolol does not alter the pharmacokinetics of digoxin. *Pharm Res* (1988) 5 (Suppl), S176.
11. Lawrence TE, Liu S, Fischer JW, Vukic-Bugarski T, Donnelly CM, Huang MY, Rackley RJ. No interaction between nebivolol and digoxin in healthy volunteers. *Clin Pharmacol Ther* (2005) 77, P76.
12. Singh S, Saini RK, DiMarco J, Kluger J, Gold R, Chen Y. Efficacy and safety of sotalol in digitalized patients with chronic atrial fibrillation. *Am J Cardiol* (1991) 68, 1227–30.
13. Rynne MV. Timolol toxicity: ophthalmic medication complicating systemic disease. *J Maine Med Assoc* (1980) 71, 82.
14. Watt DAL. Sensitivity to propranolol after digoxin intoxication. *BMJ* (1968) 3, 413–14.
15. Schamroth L. The immediate effects of intravenous propranolol in various cardiac arrhythmias. *Am J Cardiol* (1966) 18, 438.
16. Haase G, Pietzsch M, Fähnrich A, Voss W, Riethling A-K. Results of a systematic adverse drug reaction (ADR)-screening concerning bradycardia caused by drug interactions in departments of internal medicine in Rostock. *Int J Clin Pharmacol Ther* (2002) 40,116–19.
17. Takara K, Kakumoto M, Tanigawara Y, Funakoshi J, Sakaeda T, Okumura K. Interaction of digoxin with antihypertensive drugs *via* MDR1. *Life Sci* (2002) 70, 1491–1500.

Digitalis glycosides + Beta-lactam antibacterials

No interaction normally occurs between digoxin and amoxicillin, cefazolin, cefuroxime, flucloxacillin, phenoxymethylpenicillin or ticarcillin/clavulanic acid. No pharmacokinetic interaction occurs between ampicillin and digitoxin. In contrast, one early study found that cefradine increased serum levels of digoxin.

Clinical evidence

Ampicillin 500 mg four times daily for 5 days had no significant effect on the pharmacokinetics of a single 1-mg dose of **digitoxin** in 6 healthy subjects.[1] No significant changes in **digoxin** serum concentrations were found in 16 elderly patients given **amoxicillin** (2 patients also took erythromycin and one **flucloxacillin**), and 2 patients who took **flucloxacillin** and **phenoxymethylpenicillin**. However, a few patients complained of some 'toxic' symptoms (nausea, vomiting, anorexia, headache, fatigue, blurred vision, confusion), which the authors of the report attributed to the underlying illness or the antibacterials rather than to an interaction.[2] There was no significant change in digoxin pharmacokinetics in 15 patients given **ticarcillin/clavulanic acid** 1 g/200 mg intramuscularly every 12 hours for one week.[3] There was no reduction in the excretion of **digoxin** metabolites from the gut (see Mechanism) in 3 patients taking **cefazolin**, and a reduction occurred in only 1 of 10 patients taking penicillins (**ampicillin** 6, **oxacillin** 3, **penicillin** 1).[4]

A case-control study using data from healthcare databases in Ontario from 1994 to 2000 identified 1051 patients who had been admitted to hospital with **digoxin** toxicity. Of these, 5 patients (0.5%) had been exposed to **cefuroxime** in the preceding 3 weeks when compared with 0.3% of controls, suggesting that digoxin toxicity was not significantly related to **cefuroxime** exposure.[5]

In an early study, **cefradine** prolonged the half-life of **digoxin** and increased serum levels from 1.8 to 2.6 nanograms/mL. This effect was considered to occur as a result of reduced renal clearance.[6]

Mechanism

Up to 10% of patients receiving oral digoxin excrete it in substantial amounts in the faeces and urine as inactive metabolites (digoxin reduction products or DRPs). This metabolism seems to be due to gut flora,[7] in particular *Eubacterium lentum*, which is anaerobic and Gram positive. It was suggested that inhibition of digoxin metabolism by gut flora was responsible for any interaction, but doubt has been thrown on this theory, see *Mechanism* in 'Digitalis glycosides + Macrolides', (p.929).

Importance and management

The silence of the literature on adverse interactions between digoxin and beta-lactam antibacterials, and the limited evidence for a plausible mechanism suggest that interactions are unlikely.

1. Lucena MI, Moreno A, Fernandez MC, Garcia-Morillas M, Andrade R. Digitoxin elimination in healthy subjects taking ampicillin. *Int J Clin Pharmacol Res* (1987) VII, 33–7.
2. Rhodes KM, Brown SN. Do the penicillin antibiotics interact with digoxin? *Eur J Clin Pharmacol* (1994) 46, 479–80.
3. Cazzola M, Matera MG, Santangelo G, Angrisani M, Loffreda A, de Prisco F, Paizis G, Rossi F. Serum digoxin levels after concomitant ticarcillin and clavulanic acid administration. *Ther Drug Monit* (1994) 16, 46–8.
4. Dobkin JF, Saha JR, Butler VP, Lindenbaum J. Effects of antibiotic therapy on digoxin metabolism. *Clin Res* (1982) 30, 517A.
5. Juurlink DN, Mamdani M, Kopp A, Laupacis A, Redelmeier DA. Drug-drug interactions among elderly patients hospitalized for drug toxicity. *JAMA* (2003) 289, 1652–8.
6. Halawa B. Interakcje digoksyny z cefradina (Sefril), tetracyklina (Tetracyclinum), gentamycyna (Gentamycin) i wankomycyna (Vancocin). *Pol Tyg Lek* (1984) 39, 1717–20.
7. Lindenbaum J, Rund DG, Butler VP, Tse-Eng D, Saha JR. Inactivation of digoxin by the gut flora: reversal by antibiotic therapy. *N Engl J Med* (1981) 305, 789–94.

Digitalis glycosides + Bosentan

Bosentan does not appear to affect the pharmacokinetics of digoxin.

Clinical evidence, mechanism, importance and management

In 18 healthy subjects bosentan 500 mg twice daily for a week did not significantly affect the steady-state peak or trough levels of **digoxin** 375 micrograms daily. There was a small reduction of about 12% in the AUC of **digoxin**, although this was not considered to be clinically relevant. There were no changes in ECG recordings and vital signs.[1]

The results suggest that bosentan does not interact with **digoxin**, and that concurrent use need not be avoided. However, the authors note that further studies over the longer term, and in patients with renal impairment may be necessary to confirm this.

1. Weber C, Banken L, Birnboeck H, Nave S, Schulz R. The effect of bosentan on the pharmacokinetics of digoxin in healthy male subjects. *Br J Clin Pharmacol* (1999) 47, 701–6.

Digitalis glycosides + Calcium-channel blockers

Concurrent use can be valuable. Felodipine, gallopamil, lacidipine, nicardipine and nisoldipine cause small but normally clinically unimportant increases in digoxin levels, while amlodipine, isradipine and nimodipine appear not to interact. The situation with nitrendipine is uncertain but it possibly causes only a small rise in digoxin levels.

Clinical evidence

(a) Amlodipine

Amlodipine 5 mg daily had no significant effect on the serum levels or renal clearance of **digoxin** 375 micrograms daily given to 21 healthy subjects.[1]

(b) Bepridil

In 12 healthy subjects bepridil 300 mg daily for a week raised the serum levels of **digoxin** 375 micrograms daily by 34% (from 0.93 to 1.25 nanograms/mL).[2] Five of them had mild to moderate headache, nausea and dizziness for 1 to 3 days shortly after concurrent use was started. The bradycardic effects of the two drugs were found to be additive, while the negative inotropic effects of the bepridil and the positive inotropism of the increased serum **digoxin** levels were almost balanced.[2]

In another study in 23 subjects given **digoxin** 250 micrograms and bepridil 300 mg daily for 14 days, peak plasma **digoxin** levels rose by 48% (from 1.49 to 2.2 nanograms/mL) and the AUC rose by 21%.[3]

(c) Felodipine

Felodipine 10 mg twice daily for 8 weeks raised the serum **digoxin** levels in 11 patients by 15%, which was not clinically significant.[4] In another study, 14 patients were given felodipine 10 mg daily for a week. Plain tablets raised the steady-state **digoxin** serum levels by 11%, but extended-release tablets had no significant effect.[5] A third study found that, when taking felodipine, peak plasma **digoxin** levels were transiently raised by about 40% one hour after intake, but that **digoxin** AUCs were not significantly increased.[6]

(d) Gallopamil

Gallopamil 50 mg three times daily for 2 weeks raised the serum levels of **digoxin** 375 micrograms daily by 16% (from 0.58 to 0.67 nanograms/mL) in 12 healthy subjects.[7]

(e) Isradipine

Isradipine (given as 2.5 mg every 12 hours for 2 days, 5 mg every 12 hours for 2 days and then 5 mg three times daily for 10 days) did not interact significantly with a single 1-mg intravenous dose of **digoxin** given to 24 healthy subjects.[8] A similar study by the same group found that the same dosage regimen of isradipine given with oral **digoxin** 250 micrograms twice daily caused a small increase in peak serum **digoxin** levels but no changes in its steady-state levels or AUC.[9]

(f) Lacidipine

In 12 healthy subjects, a single 4-mg oral dose of lacidipine did not affect the AUC or minimum serum levels of **digoxin** 250 micrograms daily for 7 days, but the maximum serum levels of **digoxin** were increased by 34%. These changes were not considered to be clinically significant.[10]

(g) Lercanidipine

The maximum serum levels of **digoxin** rose by 33% in healthy subjects also given lercanidipine. However, there was no evidence of a pharmacokinetic interaction in patients given **metildigoxin** with lercanidipine.[11]

(h) Nicardipine

In 10 patients given nicardipine 20 mg three times daily for 14 days the plasma levels of **digoxin** 130 to 250 micrograms daily were increased by 15%, but this was not statistically significant.[12] Another 20 patients with congestive heart failure also had no significant changes in steady-state serum **digoxin** levels while taking nicardipine 30 mg three times daily for 5 days.[13] Yet another study in 9 patients confirmed the absence of an interaction.[14]

(i) Nimodipine

Nimodipine 30 mg twice daily caused no change in the pharmacokinetics or haemodynamic effects of **beta-acetyldigoxin** in 12 healthy subjects.[15]

(j) Nisoldipine

In 10 patients with heart failure nisoldipine 20 mg daily increased the plasma trough **digoxin** levels by about 15%.[16,17] Nisoldipine 10 mg twice daily caused no changes in the pharmacokinetics or haemodynamic effects of **digoxin** in 8 healthy subjects.[15]

(k) Nitrendipine

A study in 8 healthy subjects who had been taking **digoxin** 250 micrograms twice daily for 2 weeks, showed that nitrendipine 10 mg daily caused a slight but insignificant rise in plasma **digoxin** levels. Nitrendipine 20 mg daily increased the AUC of **digoxin** by 15%, its maximum plasma levels rose from 1.34 to 2.1 nanograms/mL, and its clearance fell by 13%. One subject dropped out of the study because of dizziness, nausea and vomiting, palpitations, insomnia and nervousness.[18,19]

Another study found that plasma **digoxin** levels were approximately doubled when nitrendipine was given,[20] but other studies in healthy subjects and patients found that nitrendipine 20 mg twice daily caused no changes in the pharmacokinetics or haemodynamic effects of **digoxin**,[15,21] or **beta-acetyldigoxin**.[22]

Mechanism

Where an interaction occurs it is probably due to changes in the renal excretion of the digoxin. An *in vitro* study found that several calcium-channel blockers including bepridil, nicardipine, and to a lesser extent nisoldipine (as well as barnidipine, benidipine, efonidipine, manidipine, nilvadipine, and verapamil) inhibited P-glycoprotein-mediated transcellular transport of digoxin. This suggests that any interaction may occur, at least in part, by affecting digoxin renal tubular excretion. Nitrendipine (and also diltiazem and nifedipine) only weakly inhibited the transcellular transport of digoxin.[23]

Importance and management

The extent of the information varies from drug to drug, but the concurrent use of digoxin and calcium-channel blockers can be therapeutically valuable. Monitor the effects of digoxin (e.g. bradycardia) in patients given digoxin and bepridil or lercanidipine, and consider measuring levels if the effects of digoxin seem excessive. Reduce the digoxin dosage as necessary. The other calcium-channel blockers listed here either cause only minimal increases in digoxin levels, which are unlikely to be clinically important in most patients, or do not interact at all. The situation with nitrendipine needs clarification. For the interactions of digoxin with other calcium-channel blockers see 'diltiazem', (p.915), 'nifedipine', (p.915), and 'verapamil', (p.916).

1. Schwartz JB. Effects of amlodipine on steady-state digoxin concentrations and renal digoxin clearance. *J Cardiovasc Pharmacol* (1988) 12, 1–5.
2. Belz GG, Wistuba S, Matthews JH. Digoxin and bepridil: pharmacokinetic and pharmacodynamic interactions. *Clin Pharmacol Ther* (1986) 39, 65–71.
3. Doose DR, Wallen S, Nayak RK, Minn FL. Pharmacokinetic interaction of bepridil and digoxin at steady-state. *Clin Pharmacol Ther* (1987) 41, 204.
4. Dunselman PHJM, Scaf AHJ, Kuntze CEE, Lie KI, Wesseling H. Digoxin-felodipine interaction in patients with congestive heart failure. *Eur J Clin Pharmacol* (1988) 35, 461–5.
5. Kirch W, Laskowski M, Ohnhaus EE, Åberg J. Effects of felodipine on plasma digoxin levels and haemodynamics in patients with heart failure. *J Intern Med* (1989) 225, 237–39.

6. Rehnqvist N, Billing E, Moberg L, Lundman T, Olsson G. Pharmacokinetics of felodipine and effect on digoxin plasma levels in patients with heart failure. *Drugs* (1987) 34 (Suppl 3), 33–42.
7. Belz GG, Doering W, Munkes R, Matthews J. Interaction between digoxin and calcium antagonists and antiarrhythmic drugs. *Clin Pharmacol Ther* (1983) 33, 410–17.
8. Johnson BF, Wilson J, Marwaha R, Hoch K, Johnson J. The comparative effects of verapamil and a new dihydropyridine calcium channel blocker on digoxin pharmacokinetics. *Clin Pharmacol Ther* (1987) 42, 66–71.
9. Rodin SM, Johnson BF, Wilson J, Ritchie P, Johnson J. Comparative effects of verapamil and isradipine on steady-state digoxin kinetics. *Clin Pharmacol Ther* (1988) 43, 668–72.
10. Hall ST, Harding SM, Anderson DM, Ward C, Stevens LA. The effect of single 4 mg oral dose of calcium antagonist lacidipine on the pharmacokinetics of digoxin. In: Carpi C, Zanchetti A, eds. IVth Int Symp Calcium Antagonists: Pharmacology and Clinical Research. Florence, May 1989: 161.
11. Zanidip (Lercanidipine hydrochloride). Recordati Pharmaceuticals Ltd. UK Summary of product characteristics, October 2004.
12. Lessem J, Bellinetto A. Interaction between digoxin and the calcium antagonists nicardipine and tiapamil. *Clin Ther* (1983) 5, 595–602.
13. Debruyne D, Commeau Ph, Grollier G, Huret B, Scanu P, Moulin M. Nicardipine does not significantly affect serum digoxin concentrations at the steady state of patients with congestive heart failure. *Int J Clin Pharmacol Res* (1989) IX, 15–19.
14. Scanu P, Commeau P, Huret B, Gérard JL, Debruyne D, Moore N, Lamy E, Dorey H, Grolier G, Potier JC. Pharmacocinétique et effets pharmacodynamiques de la digoxine dans les myocardiopathies dilatées. Influence de la nicardipine. *Arch Mal Coeur Vaiss* (1987) 80, 1773–83.
15. Ziegler R, Horstmann R, Wingender W, Kuhlmann J. Do dihydropyridines influence pharmacokinetic and hemodynamic parameters of digoxin? *J Clin Pharmacol* (1987) 27, 712.
16. Kirch W, Stenzel J, Dylewicz P, Hutt HJ, Santos SR, Ohnhaus EE. Influence of nisoldipine on haemodynamic effects and plasma levels of digoxin. *Br J Clin Pharmacol* (1986) 22, 155–9.
17. Kirch W, Stenzel J, Santos SR, Ohnhaus EE. Nisoldipine, a new calcium channel antagonist, elevates plasma levels of digoxin. *Arch Toxicol* (1987) (Suppl 11), 310–12.
18. Kirch W, Logemann C, Heidemann H, Santos SR, Ohnhaus EE. Effect of two different doses of nitrendipine on steady-state plasma digoxin levels and systolic time intervals. *Eur J Clin Pharmacol* (1986) 31, 391–5.
19. Kirch W, Logemann C, Heidemann H, Santos SR, Ohnhaus EE. Nitrendipine/digoxin interaction. *J Cardiovasc Pharmacol* (1987) 10 (Suppl 10), S74–S75.
20. Kirch W, Hutt HJ, Heidemann H, Rämsch K, Janisch HD, Ohnhaus EE. Drug interactions with nitrendipine. *J Cardiovasc Pharmacol* (1984) 6 (Suppl 7), S982–S985.
21. Debbas NMG, Johnston A, Jackson SHD, Banim SO, Camm AJ, Turner P. The effect of nitrendipine on predose digoxin serum concentration. *Br J Clin Pharmacol* (1988) 25, 151P.
22. Ziegler R, Wingender W, Boehme K, Raemsch K, Kuhlmann J. Study of pharmacokinetic and pharmacodynamic interaction between nitrendipine and digoxin. *J Cardiovasc Pharmacol* (1987) 9 (Suppl 4), S101–S106.
23. Takara K, Kakumoto M, Tanigawara Y, Funakoshi J, Sakaeda T, Okumura K. Interaction of digoxin with antihypertensive drugs *via* MDR1. *Life Sci* (2002) 70, 1491–1500.

Digitalis glycosides + Calcium-channel blockers; Diltiazem

Serum digoxin levels are reported to be unchanged by diltiazem in a number of studies but others describe increases ranging from 20 to 85%. Serum digitoxin levels have also been reported to rise in some patients, but only by about 20%. There is a risk of additive bradycardia when cardiac glycosides are given with diltiazem.

Clinical evidence

(a) Digitoxin

Five out of 10 patients taking digitoxin had a 6 to 31% (mean 21%) rise in plasma digitoxin levels while taking diltiazem 180 mg daily for 4 to 6 weeks.[1]

(b) Digoxin

1. Evidence of no interaction. Diltiazem 30 or 60 mg four times daily had no significant effect on the serum levels of digoxin 250 micrograms daily in 9 patients with cardiac diseases.[2] Two similar studies in 12 patients[3] and 8 healthy subjects,[4] taking digoxin with diltiazem 120 to 360 mg daily confirmed the absence of an interaction. Two further studies in healthy subjects,[5,6] found that diltiazem 120 mg daily did not affect the pharmacokinetics of a single 1-mg intravenous dose of digoxin.

2. Evidence of an interaction. A study in 17 Japanese patients (some with rheumatic valvular disease) taking either digoxin or **metildigoxin** found that diltiazem 60 mg three times daily for 2 weeks increased their serum digoxin levels measured at 24 hours by 36% and 51%, respectively.[7] Another study in 8 patients with chronic heart failure secondary to ischaemic disease, taking digoxin 250 micrograms daily, found that diltiazem 60 mg three times daily increased the digoxin AUC and mean steady-state serum levels by about 50%, its peak serum level by 37% and elimination half-life by 29%. Diltiazem had no significant effects on haemodynamic parameters.[8]

Other studies in Western patients[9,10] and healthy subjects[11-14] have shown rises of 20 to 85% in plasma digoxin levels during diltiazem use. In one case report a 143% increase was seen.[15] The authors of two of these studies noted that the effect was highly individual with some subjects showing no increase and some a large increase.[10,12] There is also a case report of raised serum **digoxin** levels and toxicity in a man taking digoxin when given diltiazem with or without nifedipine.[16]

Mechanism

Not understood. In those individuals showing a pharmacokinetic interaction, falls in total digoxin clearance of about 25% have been described.[8,10,11,17,18] Although several calcium-channel blockers may inhibit the P-glycoprotein-mediated renal clearance of digoxin, the results of an *in vitro* study[19] suggest that this may not occur with diltiazem.

A synergistic effect on heart rate and atrioventricular conduction is also possible.

Importance and management

A thoroughly investigated and well documented pharmacokinetic interaction but there is no clear explanation for the inconsistent results. All patients taking digoxin given diltiazem should be well monitored for signs of over-digitalisation (e.g. bradycardia) with digoxin levels measured as necessary. Dosage reductions may be necessary. Those most at risk are patients with digoxin levels near the top end of the range. Similar precautions would appear to be necessary with digitoxin, although the documentation of this interaction is very limited and the expected rise in levels only small. The potential for additive bradycardia and heart block should be borne in mind when using diltiazem with any digitalis glycoside.

1. Kuhlmann J. Effects of verapamil, diltiazem, and nifedipine on plasma levels and renal excretion of digitoxin. *Clin Pharmacol Ther* (1985) 38, 667–73.
2. Elkayam U, Parikh K, Torkan B, Weber L, Cohen JL, Rahimtoola SH. Effect of diltiazem on renal clearance and serum concentration of digoxin in patients with cardiac disease. *Am J Cardiol* (1985) 55, 1393–5.
3. Schrager BR, Pina I, Frangi M, Applewhite S, Sequeira R, Chahine RA. Diltiazem, digoxin interaction? *Circulation* (1983) 68 (Suppl), III-368.
4. Boden WE, More G, Sharma S, Bough EW, Korr KS, Young PM, Shulman RS. No increase in serum digoxin concentrations with high dose diltiazem. *Am J Med* (1986) 81, 425–8.
5. Beltrami TR, May JJ, Bertino JS. Lack of effects of diltiazem on digoxin pharmacokinetics. *J Clin Pharmacol* (1985) 25, 390–392.
6. Jones WN, Kern KB, Rindone JP, Mayersohn M, Bliss M, Goldman S. Digoxin-diltiazem interaction: a pharmacokinetic evaluation. *Eur J Clin Pharmacol* (1986) 31, 351–3.
7. Oyama Y, Fujii S, Kanda K, Akino E, Kawasaki H, Nagata M, Goto K. Digoxin-diltiazem interaction. *Am J Cardiol* (1984) 53, 1480–1.
8. Mahgoub AA, El-Medany AH, Abdulatif AS. A comparison between the effects of diltiazem and isosorbide dinitrate on digoxin pharmacodynamics and kinetics in the treatment of patients with chronic ischemic heart failure. *Saudi Med J* (2002) 23, 725–31.
9. Andrejak M, Hary L, Andrjak M-Th, Lesbre J Ph. Diltiazem increases steady state digoxin serum levels in patients with cardiac disease. *J Clin Pharmacol* (1987) 27, 967–70.
10. Kuhlmann J. Effects of nifedipine and diltiazem on plasma levels and renal excretion of beta-acetyldigoxin. *Clin Pharmacol Ther* (1985) 37, 150–6.
11. Rameis H, Magometschnigg D, Ganzinger U. The diltiazem-digoxin interaction. *Clin Pharmacol Ther* (1984) 36, 183–9.
12. North DS, Mattern AL, Hiser WW. The influence of diltiazem hydrochloride on trough serum digoxin levels. *Drug Intell Clin Pharm* (1986) 20, 500–503.
13. Gallet M, Aupetit JF, Lopez M, Manchon J, Lestaevel M, Lefrancois JJ. Interaction diltiazem-digoxine. Évolution de la digoxinémie et des paramtres électrocardiographiques chez le sujet sain. *Arch Mal Coeur* (1986) 79, 1216–20.
14. Larman RC. A pharmacokinetic evaluation of the digoxin-diltiazem interaction. *J Pharm Sci* (1987) 76, S79.
15. King T, Mallet L. Diltiazem-digoxin interaction in an elderly woman: a case report. *J Geriatr Drug Ther* (1991) 5, 79–83.
16. Kasmer RJ, Jones EM. Diltiazem-nifedipine-digoxin interaction. *Drug Intell Clin Pharm* (1986) 20, 985–6.
17. Yoshida A, Fujita M, Kurosawa N, Nioka M, Shichinohe T, Arakawa M, Fukuda R, Owada E, Ito K. Effects of diltiazem on plasma level and urinary excretion of digoxin in healthy subjects. *Clin Pharmacol Ther* (1984) 35, 681–5.
18. Suematsu F, Yukawa E, Yukawa M, Minemoto M, Ohdo S, Higuchi S, Goto Y. Pharmacoepidemiologic detection of calcium channel blocker-induced change on digoxin clearance using multiple trough screen analysis. *Biopharm Drug Dispos* (2002) 23, 173–81.
19. Takara K, Kakumoto M, Tanigawara Y, Funakoshi J, Sakaeda T, Okumura K. Interaction of digoxin with antihypertensive drugs *via* MDR1. *Life Sci* (2002) 70, 1491–1500.

Digitalis glycosides + Calcium-channel blockers; Nifedipine

Serum digoxin levels are normally unchanged or increased only to a small extent by nifedipine. However, one unexplained and conflicting study indicated that a 45% rise could occur. Digitoxin appears not to interact.

Clinical evidence

(a) Digitoxin

A study in 18 subjects showed that nifedipine 40 to 60 mg daily had no significant effect on their steady-state plasma digitoxin levels over a 6-week period.[1] This study has also been published elsewhere.[2]

(b) Digoxin

1. Serum digoxin levels unchanged. Studies in 25 patients[3-5] and 28 healthy subjects[6-8] showed that serum digoxin levels were not significantly altered by nifedipine 30 to 60 mg daily. Similarly no significant changes in the pharmacokinetics of a single intravenous dose of digoxin were found in 6 patients[9] or 16 healthy subjects[10,11] taking nifedipine 40 to 90 mg daily. Furthermore, no changes in the pharmacokinetics of nifedipine were seen.[10]

2. Serum digoxin levels increased. in 12 healthy subjects nifedipine 30 mg increased the plasma levels of digoxin 375 micrograms daily by 45% (from 0.505 to 0.734 nanograms/mL) over 14 days.[12] In a study in 7 healthy subjects, nifedipine 15 to 60 mg daily increased the levels of digoxin 250 micrograms twice daily by a modest 15%.[13] These studies have been reported elsewhere.[14,15]

Nifedipine 20 mg twice daily increased the steady-state serum digoxin levels of 9 patients by 15% (from 0.87 to 1.04 nanograms/mL).[16] A 61% increase in serum digoxin levels was found in a study involving nifedipine in daily doses of 30 mg.[17]

Mechanism

Not understood. Changes and lack of changes in both the renal and non-renal excretion of digoxin have been reported. A retrospective analysis of pharmacokinetic data suggests that clearance of digoxin may be reduced by 10% in patients also taking nifedipine.[18] Although several calcium-channel blockers may inhibit the P-glycoprotein mediated renal clearance of digoxin, the results of an *in vitro* study[19] suggest that this may not occur with nifedipine.

Importance and management

The pharmacokinetic interaction of digoxin and nifedipine is well documented but the findings are inconsistent. The weight of evidence appears to be that serum digoxin levels are normally unchanged or only modestly increased by nifedipine. Concurrent use appears normally to be safe and effective.[20] One report suggests that nifedipine has some attenuating effect on the digoxin-induced inotropism.[21] Another points out that under some circumstances (renal impairment or pre-existing digoxin overdosage) some risk of an undesirable interaction still exists.[13] If undesirable bradycardia occurs in a patient taking digoxin and nifedipine consider measuring digoxin levels, and adjust the dose accordingly. Nifedipine appears not to interact with digitoxin to a clinically significantly extent.

1. Kuhlmann J. Effects of quinidine, verapamil and nifedipine on the pharmacokinetics and pharmacodynamics of digitoxin during steady-state conditions. *Arzneimittelforschung* (1987) 37, 545–8.
2. Kuhlmann J. Effects of verapamil, diltiazem, and nifedipine on plasma levels and renal excretion of digitoxin. *Clin Pharmacol Ther* (1985) 38, 667–73.
3. Schwartz JB, Raizner A, Akers S. The effect of nifedipine on serum digoxin concentrations in patients. *Am Heart J* (1984) 107, 669–73.
4. Kuhlmann J, Marcin S, Frank KH. Effects of nifedipine and diltiazem on the pharmacokinetics of digoxin. *Naunyn Schmiedebergs Arch Pharmacol* (1983) 324 (Suppl), R81.
5. Kuhlmann J. Effects of nifedipine and diltiazem on plasma levels and renal excretion of beta-acetyldigoxin. *Clin Pharmacol Ther* (1985) 37, 150–6.
6. Schwartz JB, Migliore PJ. Nifedipine does not alter digoxin level or clearance. *J Am Coll Cardiol* (1984) 3, 478.
7. Schwartz JB, Migliore PJ. Effect of nifedipine on serum digoxin concentration and renal clearance. *Clin Pharmacol Ther* (1984) 36, 19–24.
8. Pedersen KE, Madsen JL, Klitgaard NA, Kjoer K, Hvidt S. Non-interaction between nifedipine and digoxin. *Dan Med Bull* (1986) 33, 109–10.
9. Garty M, Shamir E, Ilfeld D, Pitlik S, Rosenfeld JB. Non interaction of digoxin and nifedipine in cardiac patients. *J Clin Pharmacol* (1986) 26, 304–5.
10. Koren G, Zylber-Katz E, Granit L, Levy M. Pharmacokinetic studies of nifedipine and digoxin co-administration. *Int J Clin Pharmacol Ther Toxicol* (1986) 24, 39–42.
11. Pedersen KE, Dorph-Pedersen A, Hvidt S, Klitgaard NA, Kjaer K, Nielsen-Kudsk F. Effect of nifedipine on digoxin kinetics in healthy subjects. *Clin Pharmacol Ther* (1982) 32, 562–5.
12. Belz GG, Doering W, Munkes R, Matthews J. Interaction between digoxin and calcium antagonists and antiarrhythmic drugs. *Clin Pharmacol Ther* (1983) 33, 410–17.
13. Kirch W, Hutt HJ, Dylewicz P, Gräf KJ, Ohnhaus EE. Dose-dependence of the nifedipine-digoxin interaction? *Clin Pharmacol Ther* (1986) 39, 35–9.
14. Belz GG, Aust PE, Munkes R. Digoxin plasma concentrations and nifedipine. *Lancet* (1981) i, 844–5.
15. Hutt HJ, Kirch W, Dylewicz P, Ohnhaus EE. Dose-dependence of the nifedipine/digoxin interaction? *Arch Toxicol* (1986) (Suppl 9), 209–12.
16. Kleinbloesem CH, van Brummelen P, Hillers J, Moolenaar AJ, Breimer DD. Interaction between digoxin and nifedipine at steady state in patients with atrial fibrillation. *Ther Drug Monit* (1985) 7, 372–6.
17. Halawa B, Mazurek W. Interakcja digoksyny i niektórych niesteroidowych leków przeciwzapalnych, kwasu acetylosalicylowego i nifedipiny. *Pol Tyg Lek* (1982) 37, 1475–6.
18. Suematsu F, Yukawa E, Yukawa M, Minemoto M, Ohdo S, Higuchi S, Goto Y. Pharmacoepidemiologic detection of calcium channel blocker-induced change on digoxin clearance using multiple trough screen analysis. *Biopharm Drug Dispos* (2002) 23, 173–81.
19. Takara K, Kakumoto M, Tanigawara Y, Funakoshi J, Sakaeda T, Okumura K. Interaction of digoxin with antihypertensive drugs *via* MDR1. *Life Sci* (2002) 70, 1491–1500.
20. Cantelli I, Pavesi PC, Parchi C, Naccarella F, Bracchetti D. Acute hemodynamic effects of combined therapy with digoxin and nifedipine in patients with chronic heart failure. *Am Heart J* (1983) 106, 308–15.
21. Hansen PB, Buch J, Rasmussen OØ, Waldorff S, Steiness E. Influence of atenolol and nifedipine on digoxin-induced inotropism in humans. *Br J Clin Pharmacol* (1984) 18, 817–22.

Digitalis glycosides + Calcium-channel blockers; Verapamil

Serum digoxin levels are increased by about 40% by verapamil 160 mg daily, and by about 70% by verapamil 240 mg daily. Digoxin toxicity may develop if the dosage is not reduced. Deaths have occurred. Verapamil causes a rise of about 35% in digitoxin levels. There is a risk of additive bradycardia and conduction disturbances when cardiac glycosides are given with verapamil.

Clinical evidence

(a) Digitoxin

Eight out of 10 patients had a mean 35% rise (range 14 to 97%) in plasma digitoxin levels over a 4 to 6 week period while taking verapamil 240 mg daily, in three divided doses. In 2 patients (and 3 other healthy subjects given a single dose of digitoxin) the pharmacokinetics of digitoxin were not affected by verapamil.[1,2]

(b) Digoxin

After 2 weeks of treatment with verapamil 240 mg daily, in three divided doses, the mean serum digoxin levels of 49 patients with chronic atrial fibrillation had risen by 72%. The rise was seen in most patients, and it occurred largely within the first 7 days. A rise of about 40% has been seen with verapamil 160 mg daily.[3,4]

Reports in a total of 21 healthy subjects,[5,6] and 54 patients[7-9] describe rises in serum digoxin levels of 22 to 147% when verapamil 240 to 360 mg daily was added to digoxin. Similar rises are reported elsewhere.[4,10-12]

A rise in digoxin levels of about 50% was seen in chronic haemodialysis patients given verapamil 120 to 240 mg daily.[13] Nine healthy subjects had a 53% rise in their digoxin levels while taking verapamil 240 mg three times daily for two weeks.[5] Toxicity[14] and a fatality[15] occurred in patients whose digoxin levels became markedly increased by verapamil. Both asystole and sinus arrest have been described.[16,17] A single-dose study indicated that cirrhosis magnifies the extent of this interaction.[18]

Mechanism

The rise in serum digoxin levels is due to reductions in renal and especially extra-renal (biliary) clearance; a diminution in the volume of distribution also takes place.[4,9,10,19] It has been suggested that P-glycoprotein may be involved.[20] An *in vitro* study found that verapamil can inhibit the P-glycoprotein-mediated transcellular transport of digoxin,[21] which suggests that any interaction may occur, at least in part, by inhibiting the renal tubular excretion of digoxin. Impaired extra-renal excretion is suggested as the reason for the rise in serum digitoxin levels.[1]

The increased plasma levels of digoxin caused by verapamil are reported to increase both inotropism[22] and toxic effects.[23] Verapamil may enhance the digoxin-induced elevation of intracellular sodium, which may increase the risk of arrhythmias.[23,24] A synergistic effect on heart rate and atrioventricular conduction is also possible.

Importance and management

The pharmacokinetic interaction between digoxin and verapamil is well documented, well established and it occurs in most patients.[10,25] Serum digoxin levels should be well monitored and downward dosage adjustments made to avoid digoxin toxicity (deaths have occurred[15]). An initial 33 to 50% dosage reduction has been recommended.[26,27] The interaction develops within 2 to 7 days, approaching or reaching a maximum within 14 days or so.[3,8] The magnitude of the rise in serum digoxin is dose-dependent[28] with a significant increase if the verapamil dosage is increased from 160 to 240 mg daily,[3] but with no further significant increase if the dose is raised any higher.[6] The mean rise with verapamil 160 mg daily is about 40%, and with 240 mg or more is about 60 to 80%, but the response is variable. Some patients may show rises of up to 150% while others show only a modest increase. One study found that although the rise in serum digoxin levels was 60% within a week, this had lessened to about 30% five weeks later.[10] Regular monitoring and dosage adjustments would seem to be necessary. Note that the potential for additive bradycardia and heart block should also be borne in mind.

The documentation of the digitoxin and verapamil interaction is limited, but the interaction appears to be established. Downward dosage adjustment may be necessary, particularly in some patients.[1]

1. Kuhlmann J, Marcin S. Effects of verapamil on pharmacokinetics and pharmacodynamics of digitoxin in patients. *Am Heart J* (1985) 110, 1245–50.
2. Kuhlmann J. Effects of verapamil, diltiazem, and nifedipine on plasma levels and renal excretion of digitoxin. *Clin Pharmacol Ther* (1985) 38, 667–73.
3. Klein HO, Lang R, Weiss E, Di Segni E, Libhaber C, Guerrero J, Kaplinsky E. The influence of verapamil on serum digoxin concentration. *Circulation* (1982) 65, 998–1003.
4. Lang R, Klein HO, Weiss E, Libhaber C, Kaplinsky E. Effect of verapamil on digoxin blood level and clearance. *Chest* (1980) 78, 525.
5. Doering W. Effect of coadministration of verapamil and quinidine on serum digoxin concentration. *Eur J Clin Pharmacol* (1983) 25, 517–21.
6. Belz GG, Doering W, Munkes R, Matthews J. Interaction between digoxin and calcium antagonists and antiarrhythmic drugs. *Clin Pharmacol Ther* (1983) 33, 410–17.
7. Klein HO, Lang R, Di Segni E, Kaplinsky E. Verapamil-digoxin interaction. *N Engl J Med* (1980) 303, 160.
8. Merola P, Badin A, Paleari DC, De Petris A, Maragno I. Influenza del verapamile sui livelli plasmatici di digossina nell'uomo. *Cardiologia* (1982) 27, 683–7.
9. Hedman A, Angelin B, Arvidsson A, Beck O, Dahlqvist R, Nilsson B, Olsson M, Schenck-Gustafsson K. Digoxin-verapamil interaction: reduction of biliary but not renal digoxin clearance. *Clin Pharmacol Ther* (1991) 49, 256–62.
10. Pedersen KE, Dorph-Pedersen A, Hvidt S, Klitgaard NA, Pedersen KK. The long-term effect of verapamil on plasma digoxin concentration and renal digoxin clearance in healthy subjects. *Eur J Clin Pharmacol* (1982) 22, 123–7.
11. Klein HO, Lang R, Di Segni E, Sareli P, David D, Kaplinsky E. Oral verapamil versus digoxin in the management of chronic atrial fibrillation. *Chest* (1980) 78, 524.
12. Schwartz JB, Keefe D, Kates RE, Harrison DC. Verapamil and digoxin. Another drug-drug interaction. *Clin Res* (1981) 29, 501A.
13. Rendtorff C, Johannessen AC, Halck S, Klitgaard NA. Verapamil-digoxin interaction in chronic hemodialysis patients. *Scand J Urol Nephrol* (1990) 24, 137–9.
14. Gordon M, Goldenberg LMC. Clinical digoxin toxicity in the aged in association with co-administered verapamil. A report of two cases and a review of the literature. *J Am Geriatr Soc* (1986) 34, 659–62.
15. Zatuchni J. Verapamil-digoxin interaction. *Am Heart J* (1984) 108, 412–3.
16. Kounis NG. Asystole after verapamil and digoxin. *Br J Clin Pract* (1980) 34, 57–8.
17. Kounis NG, Mallioris C. Interactions with cardioactive drugs. *Br J Clin Pract* (1986) 40, 537–8.
18. Maragno I, Gianotti C, Tropeano PF, Rodighiero V, Gaion RM, Paleari C, Prandoni R, Menozzi L. Verapamil-induced changes in digoxin kinetics in cirrhosis. *Eur J Clin Pharmacol* (1987) 32, 309–11.
19. Pedersen KE, Dorph-Pedersen A, Hvidt S, Klitgaard NA, Nielsen-Kudsk F. Digoxin-verapamil interaction. *Clin Pharmacol Ther* (1981) 30, 311–16.
20. Verschraagen M, Koks CHW, Schellens JHM, Beijnen JH. P-glycoprotein system as a determinant of drug interactions: the case of digoxin-verapamil. *Pharmacol Res* (1999) 40, 301–6.
21. Takara K, Kakumoto M, Tanigawara Y, Funakoshi J, Sakaeda T, Okumura K. Interaction of digoxin with antihypertensive drugs *via* MDR1. *Life Sci* (2002) 70, 1491–1500.
22. Pedersen KE, Thayssen P, Klitgaard NA, Christiansen BD, Nielsen-Kudsk F. Influence of verapamil on the inotropism and pharmacokinetics of digoxin. *Eur J Clin Pharmacol* (1983) 25, 199–206.
23. Pedersen KE. The influence of calcium antagonists on plasma digoxin concentration. *Acta Med Scand* (1984) (Suppl 681), 31–6.
24. Pedersen KE, Christiansen BD, Kjaer K, Klitgaard NA, Nielsen-Kudsk F. Verapamil-induced changes in digoxin kinetics and intraerythrocytic sodium concentration. *Clin Pharmacol Ther* (1983) 34, 8–13.
25. Belz GG, Aust PE, Munkes R. Digoxin plasma concentrations and nifedipine. *Lancet* (1981) i, 844–5.
26. Marcus FI. Pharmacokinetic interactions between digoxin and other drugs. *J Am Coll Cardiol* (1985) 5, 82A–90A.
27. Klein HO, Kaplinsky E. Verapamil and digoxin: their respective effects on atrial fibrillation and their interaction. *Am J Cardiol* (1982) 50, 894–902.
28. Schwartz JB, Keefe D, Kates RE, Kirsten E, Harrison DC. Acute and chronic pharmacodynamic interaction of verapamil and digoxin in atrial fibrillation. *Circulation* (1982) 65, 1163–70.

Digitalis glycosides + Chinese herbal medicines

Bufalin can interfere with the assay of cardiac glycosides. Danshen appears not to interact with digoxin, but it can falsify the results of serum immunoassay methods. Digoxin toxicity in an elderly man was attributed to the use of a herbal laxative containing kanzo (liquorice).

Clinical evidence, mechanism, importance and management

(a) Bufalin (Chan Su, Kyushin, and Lu-Shen-Wan)

Bufalin, a cardioactive substance of amphibian origin and Chinese medicines such as Chan Su, Lu-Shen-Wan and Kyushin that contain bufalin can interfere with some immunoassay methods of **digitoxin** and **digoxin**, particularly the fluorescence polarisation immunoassay.[1-3] The digoxin-like immunoreactivity of Kyushin was found to be equivalent to varying amounts of **digoxin** because of differences in the cross-reactivity of the antibody used in different immunoassays.[3] A chemiluminescent assay for **digitoxin**[2,4] and **digoxin**[2] did not cross-react with bufalin.

Bufalin and an extract of Chan Su displaced **digitoxin** from protein-binding sites *in vitro*.[4] Whether this would result in elevated free **digitoxin** levels and toxicity *in vivo* is not known. However, this is probably unlikely, since *in vivo* the free drug would be available for metabolism (see 'protein-binding interactions', (p.3)).

Another possibility, given the similarities between bufalin and cardiac glycosides, is that toxicity could result from additive cardiac effects. Cases of cardiotoxicity following the ingestion of bufalin (or toads) alone have been reported. In one case, the symptoms seen were very similar to those of **digoxin** toxicity, with nausea, vomiting, blurred vision, mental confusion, cardiopulmonary arrest and severe bradyarrhythmia. Assay for digoxin was positive (2.1 nanograms/mL) when measured by the fluorescence energy transfer immunoassay. The patient had ingested a bowl of toad soup (Bufo melanosticus Schneider) shortly before his symptoms developed.[5]

(b) Danshen

Danshen appears not to have been reported to affect serum **digoxin** levels, but it can falsify laboratory measurements. A study found that a fluorescent polarization immunoassay method (Abbott Laboratories) for **digoxin** gave falsely high readings in the presence of danshen, whereas a microparticle enzyme immunoassay (Abbott Laboratories) gave falsely low readings. These false readings could be eliminated by monitoring the free (i.e. unbound) **digoxin** concentrations[6] or by choosing assay systems that are unaffected by the presence of danshen (said to be the Roche and Beckman systems[1] or an enzyme linked chemiluminescent immunisorbent digoxin assay by Bayer HealthCare[7]).

(c) Kanzo (Liquorice)

An 84-year-old man taking **digoxin** 125 micrograms daily and furosemide complained of loss of appetite, fatigue and oedema of the lower extremities 5 days after starting to take a Chinese herbal laxative containing liquorice (kanzo) 400 mg and rhubarb (daio) 1.6 g three times daily. It was suggested that heart failure occurred because of **digoxin** toxicity induced by liquorice-associated electrolyte imbalance, which may also have been exacerbated by the age of the patient, the diuretic and his existing cardiovascular disease.[8]

1. Chow L, Johnson M, Wells A, Dasgupta A. Effect of the traditional Chinese medicines Chan Su, Lu-Shen-Wan, Dan Shen, and Asian ginseng on serum digoxin measurement by Tina-quant (Roche) and Synchron LX System (Beckman) digoxin immunoassays. *J Clin Lab Anal* (2003) 17, 22–7.
2. Dasgupta A, Datta P. Rapid detection of cardioactive bufalin toxicity using fluorescence polarization immunoassay for digitoxin. *Ther Drug Monit* (1998) 20, 104–8.
3. Fushimi R, Koh T, Iyama S, Yasuhara M, Tachi J, Kohda K, Amino N, Miyai K. Digoxin-like immunoreactivity in Chinese medicine. *Ther Drug Monit* (1990) 12, 242–5.
4. Datta P, Dasgupta A. Interactions between drugs and Asian medicine: displacement of digitoxin from protein binding site by bufalin, the constituent of Chinese medicines Chan Su and Lu-Shen-Wan. *Ther Drug Monit* (2000) 22, 155–9.
5. Chern M-S. Ray C-Y, Wu D. Biologic intoxication due to digitalis-like substance after ingestion of cooked toad soup. *Am J Cardiol* (1991) 67, 443–4.
6. Wahed A, Dasgupta A. Positive and negative in vitro interference of Chinese medicine dan shen in serum digoxin measurement. Elimination of interference by monitoring free digoxin concentration. *Am J Clin Pathol* (2001) 116, 403–8.
7. Dasgupta A, Kang E, Olsen M, Actor JK, Datta P. New enzyme-linked chemiluminescent immunosorbent digoxin assay is free from interference of Chinese medicine DanShen. *Ther Drug Monit* (2006) 28, 775–8.
8. Harada T, Ohtaki E, Misu K, Sumiyoshi T, Hosoda S. Congestive heart failure caused by digitalis toxicity in an elderly man taking a licorice-containing Chinese herbal laxative. *Cardiology* (2002) 98, 218.

Digitalis glycosides + Chloroquine or Hydroxychloroquine

The levels of digoxin were found to be increased by over 70% in two elderly patients when they were given hydroxychloroquine. A similar increase has been seen with chloroquine in *dogs*.

Clinical evidence, mechanism, importance and management

Two women aged 65 and 68 who had been taking **digoxin** 250 micrograms daily for 2 to 3 years for arrhythmias were given hydroxychloroquine 250 mg twice daily for rheumatoid arthritis. When the hydroxychloroquine was withdrawn the plasma **digoxin** levels of both women fell by 70 to 75% (from 2.3 to 0.5 nanograms/mL and from 2.4 to 0.7 nanograms/mL, respectively). Neither showed any evidence of toxicity during concurrent use, and one of them claimed that the regularity of her heart rhythm had been improved.[1] The reason for this apparent interaction is not understood and its general significance is uncertain.

No interaction between digoxin and chloroquine has been described clinically, but increases in peak serum **digoxin** levels of about 77% have been seen in *dogs*.[2]

1. Leden I. Digoxin-hydroxychloroquine interaction? *Acta Med Scand* (1982) 211, 411–12.
2. McElnay JC, Sidahmed AM, D'Arcy PF and McQuade RD. Chloroquine-digoxin interaction. *Int J Pharmaceutics* (1985) 26, 267–74.

Digitalis glycosides + Cibenzoline (Cifenline)

Cibenzoline did not affect plasma digoxin levels.

Clinical evidence, mechanism, importance and management

A study in 12 healthy subjects taking **digoxin** 250 to 375 micrograms daily showed that cibenzoline 160 mg twice daily for 7 days had no effect on the pharmacokinetics of **digoxin**.[1] An *in vitro* study found that cibenzoline only slightly inhibited the P-glycoprotein-mediated transcellular transport of **digoxin** and therefore inhibition of the renal tubular secretion of **digoxin** is unlikely.[2]

1. Khoo K-C, Givens SV, Parsonnet M, Massarella JW. Effect of oral cibenzoline on steady-state digoxin concentrations in healthy volunteers. *J Clin Pharmacol* (1988) 28, 29–35.
2. Kakumoto M, Takara K, Sakaeda T, Tanigawara Y, Kita T, Okumura K. MDR1-mediated interaction of digoxin with antiarrhythmic or antianginal drugs. *Biol Pharm Bull* (2002), 25, 1604–7.

Digitalis glycosides + Ciclosporin

Ciclosporin causes a marked rise in serum digoxin levels in some patients.

Clinical evidence

Digoxin toxicity developed in 4 patients when they were given ciclosporin before cardiac transplantation. In the two cases described in detail, ciclosporin 10 mg/kg daily was added to **digoxin** 375 micrograms daily. Fourfold rises in **digoxin** levels, from 1.2 to 4.5 nanograms/mL and from 2 to 8.3 nanograms/mL, were seen within 2 to 3 days. This was accompanied by rises in serum creatinine levels from 110 to 120 micromol/L and from 84 to 181 micromol/L respectively, which were considered insufficient to explain the rise in **digoxin** levels. As a consequence of these findings, the same authors conducted a study in 4 patients given ciclosporin and **digoxin**. Two patients developed acute renal failure. In the other 2 patients, the volume of distribution of **digoxin** was decreased by 69% and 72%, while the clearance was reduced by 47% and 58%.[1] In a further 7 patients, **digoxin** pharmacokinetics were assessed before cardiac transplantation, then after transplantation during maintenance ciclosporin therapy.[2] The total body clearance of **digoxin** remained unchanged, which appeared to be at odds with the earlier results.[1] It was suggested that haemodynamic improvements brought about by successful cardiac transplantation may have counterbalanced any inhibitory effect ciclosporin had on renal clearance.[2]

Mechanism

Not fully understood. The authors of the studies concluded that ciclosporin has no specific inhibitory effect on the renal elimination of digoxin, but that it causes a non-specific reduction in renal function after acute administration, which reduces digoxin elimination.[2] Conversely, another study in *animals* suggested that ciclosporin can reduce the secretion of digoxin by the kidney tubular cells by inhibiting P-glycoprotein.[3]

Importance and management

Information seems limited to the studies cited. Nevertheless, the effects of concurrent use should be monitored very closely, and the digoxin dosage should be adjusted as necessary.

1. Dorian P, Cardella C, Strauss M, David T, East S, Ogilvie R. Cyclosporine nephrotoxicity and cyclosporine-digoxin interaction prior to heart transplantation. *Transplant Proc* (1987) 19, 1825–7.
2. Robieux I, Dorian P, Klein J, Chung D, Zborowska-Sluis D, Ogilvie R, Koren G. The effects of cardiac transplantation and cyclosporine therapy on digoxin pharmacokinetics. *J Clin Pharmacol* (1992) 32, 338–43.
3. Okamura N, Hirai M, Tanigawara Y, Tanaka K, Yasuhura M, Ueda K, Komano T, Hori R. Digoxin-cyclosporin A interaction: modulation of the multidrug transporter P-glycoprotein in the kidney. *J Pharmacol Exp Ther* (1993) 266, 1614–9.

Digitalis glycosides + Colesevelam

The absorption of a single dose of digoxin is not affected by colesevelam.

Clinical evidence, mechanism, importance and management

A single-dose study in which 26 healthy subjects were given **digoxin** 250 micrograms with or without **colesevelam** 4.5 g, followed by a standard meal, found that **colesevelam** did not significantly affect the absorption of **digoxin**.[1] Because the bile-acid binding resins 'colestyramine', (p.919) and 'colestipol', (below) may interact with digoxin it was suggested that **colesevelam** could also interact, although this appears not to be the case.

1. Donovan JM, Stypinski D, Stiles MR, Olson TA, Burke SK. Drug interactions with colesevelam hydrochloride, a novel, potent lipid-lowering agent. *Cardiovasc Drugs Ther* (2000) 14, 681–90.

Digitalis glycosides + Colestipol

Colestipol appears not to interfere with the absorption of either digoxin or digitoxin if it is given at least 1.5 hours after the digitalis glycoside.

Clinical evidence

(a) Digitalis glycoside levels reduced

Four patients with **digitoxin** toxicity were given colestipol 10 g at once and 5 g every 6 to 8 hours thereafter to reduce their **digitoxin** serum levels. The average **digitoxin** half-life fell to 2.75 days compared with an untreated control patient in whom the **digitoxin** half-life was 9.3 days. In another patient with **digoxin** toxicity who was similarly treated, the **digoxin** half-life was 16 hours compared with 1.8 to 2 days in two other control patients.[1]

(b) Digitalis glycoside levels unaffected

Ten patients receiving long-term treatment with either **digoxin** 125 to 250 micrograms daily or **digitoxin** 100 to 200 micrograms daily were given colestipol 15 g daily or a placebo, taken 1.5 hour after the digitalis. Their serum digitalis levels were not significantly altered over a 1-year period by the colestipol.[2]

A comparative study in 11 patients with plasma **digitoxin** levels greater than 40 nanograms/mL found that when the **digitoxin** was stopped and colestipol 5 g four times daily was given before meals, the **digitoxin** half-life (6.3 days) was unaffected, when compared with 11 other patients not given colestipol (6.8 days).[3]

Mechanism

Colestipol is an ion-exchange resin, which can bind to digitalis glycosides.[1] In cases of toxicity colestipol may possibly reduce serum digitalis levels because under these circumstances the excretion of digitalis in the bile increases and more becomes available for binding in the gut.[2]

Importance and management

This interaction is not well established. Giving either digoxin or digitoxin 1.5 hours before colestipol appears to avoid any possible interaction in the gut.[2] It is usually recommended that other drugs are given 1 hour before or 4 hours after colestipol.

1. Bazzano G, Bazzano GS. Digitalis intoxication. Treatment with a new steroid-binding resin. *JAMA* (1972) 220, 828–30.
2. Bazzano G, Bazzano GS. Effect of digitalis-binding resins on cardiac glycosides plasma levels. *Clin Res* (1972) 20, 24.
3. van Bever RJ, Duchateau AMJA, Pluym BFM, Merkus FWHM. The effect of colestipol on digitoxin plasma levels. *Arzneimittelforschung* (1976) 26, 1891–3.

Digitalis glycosides + Colestyramine

The levels of both digoxin and digitoxin can be reduced by colestyramine, but the clinical importance of this is uncertain. Minimise the possible effects of this interaction by separating administration.

Clinical evidence

(a) Digitalis glycoside levels reduced

A study in 12 healthy subjects given **digoxin** 750 micrograms showed that the cumulative 6-day recovery of **digoxin** from the urine was reduced by almost 20% (from 40.5 to 33.1%) when colestyramine 4 g was given.[1] Two patients with congestive heart failure and toxic serum levels of **digoxin** of 3 and 4 nanograms/mL were given colestyramine 4 g every 4 hours for 4 doses. The levels of **digoxin** fell to therapeutic levels within 13 to 24 hours.[2]

Other reports describe a fall in serum **digoxin** levels during the concurrent use of colestyramine[3-5] and an increase in the loss of **digoxin** and its metabolites in the faeces during long-term use.[6] Another study showed that giving **digoxin** as a solution in a capsule reduced the effects of this interaction.[5] Other studies have found that colestyramine reduces the half-life of **digitoxin** by 35 to 40%.[7,8]

(b) Digitalis glycoside levels unaffected

Ten patients receiving long-term treatment with either **digoxin** 125 to 250 micrograms daily or **digitoxin** 100 to 200 micrograms daily were given colestyramine 12 g daily or a placebo taken 1.5 hour after the digitalis. Their plasma digitalis levels were not significantly altered by the colestyramine over a 1-year period.[9] The half-life of **digitoxin** is reported to have remained unchanged when colestyramine was given.[10] One study suggested that **metildigoxin** may be minimally affected by colestyramine.[11]

Mechanism

Not totally understood. Colestyramine appears to bind with digitoxin in the gut, thereby reducing its bioavailability and interfering with enterohepatic recirculation so that its half-life is shortened. Digoxin may interact similarly.[2]

Importance and management

The overall picture is far from clear. Some interaction seems possible but the extent to which it impairs the treatment of patients receiving these glycosides is uncertain. Be alert for any evidence of under-digitalisation if digoxin or, more particularly, digitoxin is given with colestyramine. The studies suggest that colestyramine should not be given less than 1.5 to 2 hours after the digitalis to minimise the possibility of an interaction.[9] Note that the standard recommendation is to give other drugs 1 hour before or 4 to 6 hours after colestyramine.

1. Brown DD, Juhl RP, Warner SL. Decreased bioavailability of digoxin produced by dietary fiber and cholestyramine. *Am J Cardiol* (1977) 39, 297.
2. Roberge RJ, Sorensen T. Congestive heart failure and toxic digoxin levels: role of cholestyramine. *Vet Hum Toxicol* (2000) 42, 172–3.
3. Smith TW. New approaches to the management of digitalis intoxication, In 'Symposium on Digitalis'. *Gyldenkal Norsk Forlag* (1977) 39, 312.
4. Brown DD, Juhl RP, Warner SL. Decreased bioavailability of digoxin due to hypocholesterolemic interventions. *Circulation* (1978) 58, 164–72.
5. Brown DD, Schmid J, Long RA, Hull JH. A steady-state evaluation of the effects of propantheline bromide and cholestyramine on the bioavailability of digoxin when administered as tablets or capsules. *J Clin Pharmacol* (1985) 25, 360–4.
6. Hall WH, Shappell SD, Doherty JE. Effect of cholestyramine on digoxin absorption and excretion in man. *Am J Cardiol* (1977) 39, 213–16.
7. Caldwell JH, Bush CA, Greenberger NJ. Interruption of the enterohepatic circulation of digitoxin by cholestyramine. *J Clin Invest* (1971) 50, 2638–44.
8. Carruthers SG, Dujovne CA. Cholestyramine and spironolactone and their combination in digitoxin elimination. *Clin Pharmacol Ther* (1980) 27, 184–7.
9. Bazzano G, Bazzano GS. Effects of digitalis binding resins on cardiac glycoside plasma levels. *Clin Res* (1972) 20, 24.
10. Pabst J, Leopold G, Schad W, Meub R. Bioavailability of digitoxin during chronic administration and influence of food and cholestyramine on the bioavailability after a single dose. *Naunyn Schmiedebergs Arch Pharmacol* (1979) 307, R70.
11. Blondheim SH, Alkan WJ, Brunner D. Frontiers of Internal Medicine. Basel: Karger; 1975 p. 409–11.

Digitalis glycosides + Co-trimoxazole or Trimethoprim

Serum digoxin levels can be modestly increased by about 22% by trimethoprim, although some individuals may show a much greater rise.

Clinical evidence

(a) Elderly patients

After taking trimethoprim 200 mg twice daily for 14 days the mean serum **digoxin** levels in 9 elderly patients (aged 62 to 92) had risen by an average of 22%, from 0.9 to 1.2 nanograms/mL. One patient had a 75% rise. A 34% increase in mean serum creatinine was also seen. When the trimethoprim was withdrawn, the serum **digoxin** levels returned to their previous value.[1,2]

(b) Young healthy adult subjects

Trimethoprim 200 mg twice daily for 10 days did not affect the total body clearance of a single 1-mg intravenous dose of **digoxin** in 6 young healthy subjects (aged 24 to 31). Renal clearance was reduced, but this was compensated for by an increase in extra-renal clearance.[2]

Mechanism

It is suggested that trimethoprim reduces the renal excretion of digoxin.[1,2] The paradoxical finding between the elderly patients and the young healthy subjects may be the age difference, probably as the elderly patients may not be able to accommodate an increase in extra-renal digoxin clearance.

Importance and management

Information seems to be limited to the information cited. Although the serum digoxin rise in the elderly was modest, it would seem prudent to monitor the effects because some individuals can apparently experience a marked rise. Reduce the digoxin dosage if necessary. Trimethoprim is contained in co-trimoxazole but it is not known whether prophylactic doses of co-trimoxazole (160 mg trimethoprim a day, from 960 mg co-trimoxazole) will interact to a clinically significant degree. An interaction would seem likely with high-dose co-trimoxazole regimens and care with any co-trimoxazole regimen is needed in the elderly.

1. Kastrup J, Bartram R, Petersen P, Hansen JM. Trimetoprims indvirkning på serum-digoksin og serum-kreatinin. *Ugeskr Laeger* (1983) 145, 2286–8.
2. Petersen P, Kastrup J, Bartram R, Hansen JM. Digoxin-trimethoprim interaction. *Acta Med Scand* (1985) 217, 423–7.

Digitalis glycosides + Danaparoid

No clinically significant interaction appears to occur between digoxin and danaparoid.

Clinical evidence, mechanism, importance and management

In a study, 6 healthy subjects were given digoxin 250 micrograms daily for 8 days, with a single 3250 anti-Xa-unit-bolus dose of danaparoid during day 7. The AUC of digoxin was slightly decreased, although this did not appear to be clinically significant. Digoxin did not alter the effects of danaparoid on clotting tests (including aPTT).[1]

1. de Boer A, Stiekema JCJ, Danhof M, Moolenaar AJ, Breimer DD. Interaction of ORG 10172, a low molecular weight heparinoid, and digoxin in healthy volunteers. *Eur J Clin Pharmacol* (1991) 41, 245–50.

Digitalis glycosides + Darifenacin or Solifenacin

Darifenacin increased digoxin exposure by a modest 16%, which would usually not be clinically important. Solifenacin did not alter the pharmacokinetics of digoxin.

Clinical evidence, mechanism, importance and management

(a) Darifenacin

The manufacturer notes that the concurrent use of **digoxin** 250 micrograms and darifenacin 30 mg daily increased **digoxin** exposure at steady state by a modest 16%. This small increase would generally not be clinically relevant.[1]

(b) Solifenacin

In a crossover study in 24 healthy subjects, solifenacin 10 mg daily for 10 days had no effect on the pharmacokinetics of **digoxin** 125 micrograms daily.[2]

This study suggests that no pharmacokinetic interaction occurs, and that no **digoxin** dose adjustment would be expected to be needed on concurrent use.

1. Enablex (Darifenacin hydrobromide). Novartis. US Prescribing information, February 2007.
2. Smulders RA, Kuipers ME, Krauwinkel WJJ. Multiple doses of the antimuscarinic agent solifenacin do not affect the pharmacodynamics or pharmacokinetics of warfarin or the steady-state pharmacokinetics of digoxin in healthy subjects. *Br J Clin Pharmacol* (2006) 62, 210–17.

Digitalis glycosides + Dexmedetomidine

An isolated report describes bradycardia when an infant receiving digoxin was given dexmedetomidine.

Clinical evidence, mechanism, importance and management

A 5-week-old infant with an atrioventricular septal defect, taking **digoxin** 10 micrograms twice daily and furosemide for mild congestive heart failure, developed respiratory failure requiring intubation and mechanical ventilation. She was given dexmedetomidine for sedation and received a loading dose of 0.5 micrograms/kg over 15 minutes, followed by an infusion of 0.44 micrograms/kg per hour. During the loading dose period her heart rate decreased from 133 to 116 bpm. Throughout the next 13 hours the rate continued to decrease to about 90 bpm, with episodes of sinus bradycardia (heart rate around 50 bpm). Within 1 hour of discontinuing dexmedetomidine, the heart rate increased to its baseline value and no further episodes of bradycardia were observed. The reasons for the interaction are not known, but caution is advised if dexmedetomidine is used for sedation in patients receiving **digoxin**.[1]

1. Berkenbosch JW, Tobias JD. Development of bradycardia during sedation with dexmedetomidine in an infant concurrently receiving digoxin. *Pediatr Crit Care Med* (2003) 4, 203–5.

Digitalis glycosides + Dietary fibre and Laxatives

Bisacodyl reduces serum digoxin levels to a small extent. Large amounts of dietary fibre, guar gum and bulk-forming laxatives containing ispaghula or psyllium appear to have no significant effect on the absorption of digoxin. Single-dose studies show that macrogol 4000, a laxative polymer, reduces the serum levels of digoxin.

Clinical evidence

(a) Bisacodyl

Bisacodyl reduced the mean serum **digoxin** levels of 11 healthy subjects by about 12%. When the bisacodyl was taken 2 hours before the **digoxin**, serum **digoxin** levels were slightly raised, but not to a statistically significant extent.[1]

(b) Fibre

The serum **digoxin** levels of 12 patients taking **digoxin** 125 to 250 micrograms daily 15 to 30 minutes before breakfast were unchanged over a 10-day period when they were given a diet supplemented each day with 22 g of dietary fibre. The fibre was given in this way to simulate the conditions that might be encountered clinically (for example to reduce the symptoms of diverticular disease).[2]

Wheat bran 7.5 g twice daily caused a small 10% reduction in the plasma **digoxin** levels of 14 geriatric patients after 2 weeks, but there was no significant change after 4 weeks.[3] Bran fibre 11 g caused a 6 to 7% reduction in the absorption and the steady-state serum levels of **digoxin** in 16 healthy subjects.[4] The cumulative urinary recovery of a single oral dose of **digoxin** in healthy subjects was reduced almost 20% by 5 g of fibre, whereas 0.75 g of fibre had no effect.[5]

(c) Guar gum

In 10 healthy subjects *Guarem* (95% guar gum) 5 g reduced the peak serum levels of a single 500-microgram oral dose of **digoxin** by 21% and the AUC_{0-6} was reduced by 16%, but the amount excreted in the urine over 24 hours was only minimally reduced.[6] Guar gum 18 g with a test meal did not affect steady-state plasma **digoxin** levels in 11 healthy subjects given **digoxin** 1 mg on day 1, then 750 micrograms on day 2, then 500 micrograms daily for 3 days.[7]

(d) Ispaghula or psyllium

An ispaghula preparation (*Vi-Siblin S*) was found to have no significant effect on serum **digoxin** levels of 16 geriatric patients.[3] The same lack of effect was seen in another study in 15 patients given 3.6 g of a psyllium preparation (*Metamucil*) three times a day.[8]

(e) Macrogol 4000

A randomised, crossover study in 18 healthy subjects found that 20 g of macrogol 4000 daily over an 8-day period reduced the maximum serum levels of a single 500-microgram dose of **digoxin** by 40%, and reduced the AUC by 30%. Heart rate and the PR interval were unchanged.[9] More study is needed to assess the effects of this interaction on steady-state **digoxin** levels.

Mechanism

Not established. Digoxin can bind to some extent to fibre within the gut.[10] However, *in vitro* studies (with bran, carrageenan, pectin, sodium pectinate, xylan and carboxymethylcellulose) have shown that most of the binding is reversible.[11]

Importance and management

Information seems to be limited to these reports. The reduction in serum digoxin levels caused by bisacodyl is small, and not expected to be of clinical importance, and apparently preventable by giving the bisacodyl 2 hours before the digoxin. Neither dietary fibre (bran), guar gum nor the two bulk-forming laxatives (*Vi-Siblin* and *Metamucil*) have a clinically important effect on serum digoxin levels. No special precautions would appear to be necessary. The importance of the interaction between digoxin and macrogol 4000 awaits further assessment, but on the available evidence it would be prudent to be alert for the need to increase the digoxin dosage.

1. Wang D-J, Chu K-M, Chen J-D. Drug interaction between digoxin and bisacodyl. *J Formos Med Assoc* (1990) 89, 913, 915–9.
2. Woods MN, Ingelfinger JA. Lack of effect of bran on digoxin absorption. *Clin Pharmacol Ther* (1979) 26, 21–3.
3. Nordström M, Melander A, Robertsson E, Steen B. Influence of wheat bran and of a bulk-forming ispaghula cathartic on the bioavailability of digoxin in geriatric in-patients. *Drug Nutr Interact* (1987) 5, 67–9.
4. Johnson BF, Rodin SM, Hoch K, Shekar V. The effect of dietary fiber on the bioavailability of digoxin in capsules. *J Clin Pharmacol* (1987) 27, 487–90.
5. Brown DD, Juhl RP, Warner SL. Decreased bioavailability of digoxin due to hypocholesterolemic interventions. *Circulation* (1978) 58, 164–72.
6. Huupponen R, Seppälä P, Iisalo E. Effect of guar gum, a fibre preparation, on digoxin and penicillin absorption in man. *Eur J Clin Pharmacol* (1984) 26, 279–81.
7. Lembcke B, Häsler K, Kramer P, Caspary WF, Creuzfeldt W. Plasma digoxin concentrations during administration of dietary fibre (guar gum) in man. *Z Gastroenterol* (1982) 20, 164–7.
8. Walan A, Bergdahl B, Skoog M-L. Study of digoxin bioavailability during treatment with a bulk forming laxative (*Metamucil*). *Scand J Gastroenterol* (1977) 12 (Suppl 45), 111.
9. Ragueneau I, Poirier J-M, Radembino N, Sao AB, Funck-Brentano C, Jaillon P. Pharmacokinetic and pharmacodynamic drug interactions between digoxin and macrogol 4000, a laxative polymer, in healthy volunteers. *Br J Clin Pharmacol* (1999) 48, 453–6.
10. Floyd RA. Digoxin interaction with bran and high fiber foods. *Am J Hosp Pharm* (1978) 35, 660.
11. Hamamura J, Burros BC, Clemens RA, Smith CH. Dietary fiber and digoxin. *Fedn Proc* (1985) 44, 759.

Digitalis glycosides + Dihydroergocryptine

Dihydroergocryptine appears not to interact with digoxin.

Clinical evidence, mechanism, importance and management

In a randomised study in 12 healthy subjects dihydroergocryptine 20 mg did not affect the pharmacokinetics of a single 500-microgram dose of **digoxin**. No clinically significant changes were seen in the ability of the heart to initiate and conduct impulses, or repolarise. The slight drop in blood pressure during the first 2 to 4 hours after **digoxin** was more pronounced in the presence of dihydroergocryptine, but there was no evidence of impaired orthostatic blood pressure control.[1] No special precautions would seem necessary during concurrent use.

1. Retzow A, Althaus M, de Mey C, Mazur D, Vens-Cappell B. Study on the interaction of the dopamine agonist α-dihydroergocryptine with the pharmacokinetics of digoxin. *Arzneimittelforschung* (2000) 50, 591–6.

Digitalis glycosides + Dipyridamole

Dipyridamole may cause a minor increase in the absorption of digoxin.

Clinical evidence, mechanism, importance and management

A study in 12 healthy subjects found that dipyridamole 150 mg twice daily for 5 doses increased the AUC_{0-4} and the AUC_{0-24} of a single 500-microgram oral dose of **digoxin** by 20% and 13%, respectively. This was attributed to an increase in **digoxin** absorption possibly mediated by intestinal P-glycoprotein inhibition.[1] *In vitro* studies[1,2] found that dipyridamole inhibits P-glycoprotein-mediated transport of **digoxin**, but in one study this was only at higher levels than those achieved clinically.[2] Therefore these minor changes are not fully explained. The changes in **digoxin** pharmacokinetics in the presence of dipyridamole are probably not clinically significant.

1. Verstuyft C, Strabach S, El Morabet H, Kerb R, Brinkmann U, Dubert L, Jaillon P, Funck-Brentano C, Trugnan G, Becquemont L. Dipyridamole enhances digoxin bioavailability via P-glycoprotein inhibition. *Clin Pharmacol Ther* (2003) 73, 51–60.
2. Kakumoto M, Takara K, Sakaeda T, Tanigawara Y, Kita T, Okumura K. MDR1-mediated interaction of digoxin with antiarrhythmic or antianginal drugs. *Biol Pharm Bull* (2002) 25, 1604–7.

Digitalis glycosides + Disopyramide or Procainamide

Neither disopyramide nor procainamide normally cause a significant change in serum digoxin levels. A single report describes toxicity in a patient taking digitoxin and disopyramide.

Clinical evidence, mechanism, importance and management

(a) Disopyramide

A number of studies have clearly shown that disopyramide causes only a very small increase or no increase at all in the serum levels of **digoxin**.[1-6] A small but insignificant reduction in heart rate has been seen[7] but the weight of evidence suggests that no adverse interaction occurs if **digoxin** and disopyramide are used together. However, a very brief report describes toxicity and serious arrhythmia in one patient given **digitoxin** and disopyramide.[8]

(b) Procainamide

A study in patients who had been taking **digoxin** for at least 7 days showed that procainamide did not affect their serum **digoxin** levels.[2] However, it should be noted that the manufacturers of procainamide say that, in digitalis toxicity, procainamide may further depress conduction, which may result in ventricular asystole or fibrillation.[9]

1. Doering W. Quinidine-digoxin interaction. *N Engl J Med* (1979) 301, 400–4.
2. Leahey EB, Reiffel JA, Giardina E-GV, Bigger JT. The effect of quinidine and other oral antiarrhythmic drugs on serum digoxin: a prospective study. *Ann Intern Med* (1980) 92, 605–8.
3. Manolas EG, Hunt D, Sloman G. Effects of quinidine and disopyramide on serum digoxin concentrations. *Aust N Z J Med* (1980) 10, 426–9.
4. Wellens HJ, Gorgels AP, Braat SJ, Bär FW, Vanagt EJ, Phaf B. Effect of oral disopyramide on serum digoxin levels. A prospective study. *Am Heart J* (1980) 100, 934–5.
5. Risler T, Burk M, Peters U, Grabensee B, Seipel L. On the interaction between digoxin and disopyramide. *Clin Pharmacol Ther* (1983) 34, 176–80.
6. García-Barreto D, Groning E, González-Gómez A, Pérez A, Hernández-Cañero A, Toruncha A. Enhancement of the antiarrhythmic action of disopyramide by digoxin. *J Cardiovasc Pharmacol* (1981) 3, 1236–42.
7. Elliott HL, Kelman AW, Sumner DJ, Bryson SM, Campbell BC, Hillis WS, Whiting B. Pharmacodynamic and pharmacokinetic evaluation of the interaction between digoxin and disopyramide. *Br J Clin Pharmacol* (1982) 14, 141P.
8. Manchon ND, Bercoff E, Lemarchand P, Chassagne P, Senant J, Bourreille J. Fréquence et gravité des interactions médicamenteuses dans une population âgée: étude prospective concernant 63 malades. *Rev Med Interne* (1989) 10, 521–5.
9. Pronestyl (Procainamide hydrochloride).E.R. Squibb & Sons Ltd. UK Summary of product characteristics, June 2005.

Digitalis glycosides + Diuretics; Potassium-depleting

The potassium loss caused by potassium-depleting diuretics increases the toxicity of the digitalis glycosides.

Clinical evidence

(a) Evidence suggesting an interaction

A comparative study[1] of the medical records of 418 patients taking digitalis over the period 1950 to 1952, and of 679 patients over the period 1964 to 1966, showed that the incidence of digitalis toxicity had more than doubled. Of the earlier group 8.6% developed toxicity (58% taking diuretics, mainly of the **organomercurial type**) compared with 17.2% of the latter group (81% taking diuretics, mainly **chlorothiazides**, **furosemide**, **etacrynic acid**, **chlortalidone**). It was concluded that the increased toxicity was related to the increased usage of potassium-depleting diuretics.

A retrospective study of over 400 patients taking **digoxin** showed that almost one in five had some toxic reactions attributable to the use of the glycoside. Of these, 16% had demonstrable hypokalaemia (defined as serum potassium less than 3.5 mmol/L). Almost half of the patients who showed toxicity were taking potassium-depleting diuretics, notably **hydrochlorothiazide** or **furosemide**.[2] Similar results were found in other studies[3-9] in a considerable number of patients. There are other reports not listed here. In addition there is also some evidence that **furosemide** may raise serum **digoxin** levels,[10] although two other studies found no evidence that **furosemide** affects the urinary excretion of **digoxin**.[11,12]

(b) Evidence suggesting no interaction

A retrospective study of patients who developed digitalis toxicity showed that the likelihood of its development in those with potassium levels below 3.5 mmol/L was no greater than those with normal potassium levels.[13]

Two other studies in a total of almost 200 patients failed to detect any association between the development of digitalis toxicity and the use of diuretics or changes in potassium levels.[14,15]

A pharmacokinetic study in 6 patients found that single 50-mg and 100-mg doses of cicletanine had no effect on the plasma levels of **digoxin** 125 to 250 micrograms daily.[16]

Mechanism

Not fully understood. The cardiac glycosides inhibit sodium-potassium ATP-ase, which is concerned with the transport of sodium and potassium ions across the membranes of the myocardial cells. This is associated with an increase in the availability of calcium ions concerned with the contraction of the cells. Potassium loss caused by these diuretics exacerbates the potassium loss from the myocardial cells, thereby increasing the activity and the toxicity of the digitalis. Some loss of magnesium may also have a part to play. The mechanism of this interaction is still being debated.

Importance and management

A direct link between the use of these potassium-depleting diuretics and the development of digitalis toxicity is not established beyond doubt, but concurrent use can result in digitalis toxicity. It is therefore important that potassium levels remain within the accepted normal range during digitalis treatment. Potassium levels should be routinely monitored when diuretics are given and it may be prudent to recheck levels if patients develop symptoms of digitalis toxicity. See 'Table 26.1', (p.944) for a list of potassium-depleting diuretics.

1. Jørgenson AW, Sørensen OH. Digitalis intoxication. A comparative study on the incidence of digitalis intoxication during the periods 1950–52 and 1964–66. *Acta Med Scand* (1970) 188, 179–83.
2. Shapiro S, Slone D, Lewis GP, Jick H. The epidemiology of digoxin. A study in three Boston Hospitals. *J Chron Dis* (1969) 22, 361–71.
3. Tawakkol AA, Nutter DO, Massumi RA. A prospective study of digitalis toxicity in a large city hospital. *Med Ann Dist Columbia* (1967) 36, 402–9.
4. Soffer A. The changing clinical picture of digitalis intoxication. *Arch Intern Med* (1961) 107, 681–8.
5. Rodensky PL, Wasserman F. Observations on digitalis intoxication. *Arch Intern Med* (1961) 108, 171–88.
6. Steiness E, Olesen KH. Cardiac arrhythmias induced by hypokalaemia and potassium loss during maintenance digoxin therapy. *Br Heart J* (1976) 38, 167–72.
7. Binnion PF. Hypokalaemia and digoxin-induced arrhythmias. *Lancet* (1975) i, 343–4.
8. Poole-Wilson PA, Hall R, Cameron IR. Hypokalaemia, digitalis, and arrhythmias. *Lancet* (1975) i, 575–6.
9. Shapiro W, Taubert K. Hypokalaemia and digoxin-induced arrhythmias. *Lancet* (1975) ii, 604–5.

10. Tsutsumi E, Fujiki H, Takeda H, Fukushima H. Effect of furosemide on serum clearance and renal excretion of digoxin. *J Clin Pharmacol* (1979) 19, 200–204.
11. Malcolm AD, Leung FY, Fuchs JCA, Duarte JE. Digoxin kinetics during furosemide administration. *Clin Pharmacol Ther* (1977) 21, 567–574.
12. Brown DD, Dormois JC, Abraham GN, Lewis K, Dixon K. Effect of furosemide on the renal excretion of digoxin. *Clin Pharmacol Ther* (1976) 20, 395–400.
13. Ogilvie RI, Ruedy J. An educational program in digitalis therapy. *JAMA* (1972) 222, 50–55.
14. Smith TW, Haber E. Digoxin intoxication: the relationship of clinical presentation to serum digoxin concentration. *J Clin Invest* (1970) 49, 2377–86.
15. Beller GA, Smith TW, Abelmann WH, Haber E, Hood WB. Digitalis intoxication. A prospective clinical study with serum level correlations. *N Engl J Med* (1971) 284, 989–97.
16. Clement DL, Teirlynck O, Belpaire F. Lack of effect of cicletanine on plasma digoxin levels. *Int J Clin Pharmacol Res* (1988) 8, 9–11.

Digitalis glycosides + Diuretics; Potassium-sparing

Serum digoxin levels may be increased by 25% by spironolactone, but because spironolactone or its metabolite, canrenone, can interfere with some digoxin assay methods, the evaluation of this interaction is difficult. Eplerenone may also cause a minor increase in digoxin levels. Amiloride has little effect on digoxin levels in healthy subjects, but it may reduce its inotropic effects. In patients with renal impairment it possibly raises plasma digoxin levels. The effects of digitoxin are reported to be both increased and decreased by spironolactone.

Clinical evidence

(a) Digitoxin

A study in 6 healthy subjects who had been taking digitoxin 100 or 150 micrograms daily for 30 days showed that **spironolactone** 300 mg daily increased the digitoxin half-life by one-third (from 142 to 192 hours).[1]

In contrast, other studies have found that the digitoxin half-life was reduced (from 256 to 205 hours) by **spironolactone**.[2]

(b) Digoxin

1. Amiloride. In 6 healthy subjects amiloride 5 mg twice daily for 8 days almost doubled the renal clearance of digoxin from 1.3 to 2.4 mL/kg per minute, but reduced the extra-renal clearance from 2.1 to 0.1 mL/kg per minute. The balance of the two effects was to cause a small fall in total clearance and a small rise in plasma digoxin levels.[3] The positive inotropic effects of digoxin were reduced, but whether this is clinically important is uncertain. In contrast, a later study in 8 healthy subjects found that a single 75-mg [sic] oral dose of amiloride given 3 hours before an infusion of digoxin did not reduce the inotropic effects of digoxin.[4]

2. Eplerenone. The UK manufacturer of eplerenone states that the AUC of digoxin increased by 16% (90% confidence interval: 4% to 30%) when it was given with eplerenone.[5]

3. Spironolactone. The plasma digoxin levels of 9 patients were increased by about 20% (from 0.8 to 1 nanograms/mL) when they were given spironolactone 100 mg daily. One patient had a three to fourfold rise in digoxin levels.[6]
The clearance of a single 750-microgram intravenous dose of digoxin was reduced by about 25% in 4 patients and 4 healthy subjects following 5 days of treatment with spironolactone 100 mg twice daily.[7] A marked fall in serum digoxin levels occurred in an elderly patient when spironolactone was withdrawn,[8] but the accuracy of the assay method used is uncertain (see *Importance and management* below). One study found that no clinically important reduction in digoxin clearance occurred when *Aldactazide* (spironolactone-hydrochlorothiazide) was also given.[9]

Mechanism

Not fully understood. Spironolactone inhibits the excretion of digoxin by the kidney (by 13%) but does not affect its biliary clearance.[10] *Animal* studies have suggested that spironolactone may induce P-glycoprotein expression, resulting in reduced intestinal absorption of substrates such as digoxin.[11] Spironolactone probably also causes a reduction in the volume of distribution of digoxin.

It has been suggested that amiloride may have increased the production of aldosterone, which suppressed the positive inotropic effects of digoxin.[3] Studies in patients with congestive heart failure are needed.

Importance and management

The pharmacokinetic interaction between digoxin and spironolactone appears to be established. What is known suggests that a rise in digoxin levels of up to 25% is likely to occur, although much greater increases can apparently occur in some patients.[6] Monitor concurrent use carefully for signs of over-digitalisation. Note that spironolactone or its metabolite, canrenone, can interfere with some digoxin assay methods.[12] In one report, radioimmunoassay (RIA) and affinity-column-mediated immunoassay (ACMIA) were particularly affected by spironolactone and its metabolites.[13] Conversely, falsely low digoxin readings with the AxSym MEIA assay method led to digoxin overdose and toxicity in one patient.[14] This means that monitoring is difficult unless the digoxin assay method is known to be reliable. Measurement of free digoxin levels or use of a chemiluminescent assay (CLIA) or turbidometric immunoassay for digoxin has been reported to mostly eliminate interference from spironolactone, potassium canrenoate and canrenone.[15,16]

Eplerenone also appears to cause a small increase in digoxin levels. The UK manufacturers recommend that caution is warranted when digoxin is dosed near the upper limit of therapeutic range.[5] However, the US manufacturer states that the pharmacokinetic interaction is not clinically significant.[17]

The situation with digitoxin and spironolactone is confusing because the reports are contradictory and the outcome uncertain. Concurrent use should be well monitored.

Patients with poor renal function would be expected to have a rise in digoxin levels when given amiloride (due to the increased reliance on renal clearance) but the clinical importance of this awaits confirmation.

1. Carruthers SG, Dujovne CA. Cholestyramine and spironolactone and their combination in digitoxin elimination. *Clin Pharmacol Ther* (1980) 27, 184–7.
2. Wirth KE, Frölich JC, Hollifield JW, Falkner FC, Sweetman BS, Oates JA. Metabolism of digitoxin in man and its modification by spironolactone. *Eur J Clin Pharmacol* (1976) 9, 345–54.
3. Waldorff S, Hansen PB, Kjærgård H, Buch J, Egeblad H, Steiness E. Amiloride-induced changes in digoxin dynamics and kinetics: abolition of digoxin-induced inotropism with amiloride. *Clin Pharmacol Ther* (1981) 30, 172–6.
4. Richter JP, Sommers De K, Snyman JR, Millard SM. The acute effects of amiloride and potassium canrenoate on digoxin-induced positive inotropism in healthy volunteers. *Eur J Clin Pharmacol* (1993) 45, 195–6.
5. Inspra (Eplerenone). Pfizer Ltd. UK Summary of product characteristics, May 2006.
6. Steiness E. Renal tubular secretion of digoxin. *Circulation* (1974) 50. 103–7.
7. Waldorff S, Andersen JD, Heebøll-Nielsen N, Nielsen OG, Moltke E, Sørensen U, Steiness E. Spironolactone-induced changes in digoxin kinetics. *Clin Pharmacol Ther* (1978) 24, 162–7.
8. Paladino JA, Davidson KH, McCall BB. Influence of spironolactone on serum digoxin concentration. *JAMA* (1984) 251, 470–1.
9. Finnegan TP, Spence JD, Cape R. Potassium-sparing diuretics: interaction with digoxin in elderly men. *J Am Geriatr Soc* (1984) 32, 129–31.
10. Hedman A, Angelin B, Arvidsson A, Dahlqvist R. Digoxin-interactions in man: spironolactone reduces renal but not biliary digoxin clearance. *Eur J Clin Pharmacol* (1992) 42, 481–5.
11. Ghanem CI, Gómez PC, Arana MC, Perassolo M, Delli Carpini G, Luquita MG, Veggi LM, Catania VA, Bengochea LA, Mottino AD. Induction of rat intestinal P-glycoprotein by spironolactone and its effect on absorption of orally administered digoxin. *J Pharmacol Exp Ther* (2006) 318, 1146–52.
12. Steimer W, Müller C, Eber B. Digoxin assays: frequent, substantial, and potentially dangerous interference by spironolactone, canrenone, and other steroids. *Clin Chem* (2002) 48, 507–16.
13. Pleasants RA, Williams DM, Porter RS, Gadsden RH. Reassessment of cross-reactivity of spironolactone metabolites with four digoxin immunoassays. *Ther Drug Monit* (1989) 11, 200–4.
14. Steimer W, Müller C, Eber B, Emmanuilidis K. Intoxication due to negative canrenone interference in digoxin drug monitoring. *Lancet* (1999) 354, 1176–7.
15. Dasgupta A, Saffer H, Wells A, Datta P. Bidirectional (positive/negative) interference of spironolactone, canrenone, and potassium canrenoate on serum digoxin measurement: elimination of interference by measuring free digoxin or using a chemiluminescent assay for digoxin. *J Clin Lab Anal* (2002) 16, 172–7.
16. Datta P, Dasgupta A. A new turbidometric digoxin immunoassay on the ADVIA 1650 analyzer is free from interference by spironolactone, potassium canrenoate, and their common metabolite canrenone. *Ther Drug Monit* (2003) 25, 478–82.
17. Inspra (Eplerenone). Pfizer Inc. US Prescribing information, May 2005.

Digitalis glycosides + Dofetilide

Dofetilide does not affect the pharmacokinetics of digoxin.

Clinical evidence, mechanism, importance and management

In a placebo-controlled study in 13 subjects, dofetilide 250 micrograms twice daily for 5 days had no effect on the steady-state pharmacokinetics of **digoxin**, given at a dose of 250 micrograms daily after a loading dose.[1]

1. Kleinermans D, Nichols DJ, Dalrymple I. Effect of dofetilide on the pharmacokinetics of digoxin. *Am J Cardiol* (2001) 87, 248–50.

Digitalis glycosides + Drugs that affect calcium

The effects of digitalis glycosides might be increased by rises in blood calcium levels, and the use of intravenous calcium may result in the development of potentially life-threatening digitalis-induced cardiac arrhythmias. Teriparatide appears not to affect the calcium-mediated pharmacodynamics of digoxin.

Clinical evidence

(a) Calcium

Two patients developed cardiac arrhythmias and died after being given **digitalis** intramuscularly and either **calcium chloride** or **calcium gluconate** intravenously. No absolutely certain causative relationship was established.[1]

There is some evidence that increases or decreases in blood **calcium** levels can increase or decrease, respectively, the effects of **digitalis**. A patient with congestive heart failure and atrial fibrillation was resistant to the actions of **digoxin** serum levels of 1.5 to 3 nanograms/mL until his serum **calcium** levels were raised from 1.68 to about 2.13 mmol/L by oral **calcium and vitamin D**.[2]

(b) Other drugs affecting calcium

1. Disodium edetate. Disodium edetate,[3-5] which lowers blood calcium levels, has been used successfully in the treatment of digitalis toxicity, although less toxic drugs are generally preferred.

2. Teriparatide. A placebo-controlled study in 15 healthy subjects given **digoxin** 500 micrograms daily, adjusted to maintain steady-state serum levels in the range 1 to 2 nanograms/mL, found that a single 20-microgram subcutaneous dose of teriparatide on day 15 or 16 did not alter the calcium-mediated effects of **digoxin** (systolic time interval), or heart rate. Serum calcium increased slightly, with a maximum increase of 0.05 mmol/L.[6]

Mechanism

The actions of the cardiac glycosides (even now not fully understood) are closely tied up with movement of calcium ions into heart muscle cells. Increased concentrations of calcium outside these cells increase the inflow of calcium and this enhances the activity of the glycosides. This can lead to effective over-digitalisation and even potentially life-threatening arrhythmias. Conversely, a drop in calcium levels can attenuate the activity of the glycosides. However, the clinical relevance of these changes in calcium is not fully established.

Importance and management

The report of deaths associated with digitalis and calcium compounds (published in 1936) seems to be the only direct clinical evidence of a serious adverse interaction, although there is plenty of less direct evidence that an interaction is possible. Intravenous calcium should be avoided in patients receiving cardiac glycosides. If that is not possible, it has been suggested[7] that it should be given slowly or only in small amounts in order to avoid transient serum calcium levels higher than 7.5 mmol/L, but it seems likely that very large doses of calcium would be required to reach this level, even transiently.

The very slight increases in calcium observed with teriparatide were considered insufficient to increase cardiac sensitivity to **digoxin** at therapeutic dosage.[6] Nevertheless, the manufacturer of **teriparatide** still advises caution in patients taking digitalis, because of the possibility for transiently raised calcium levels.[8,9]

1. Bower JO, Mengle HAK. The additive effects of calcium and digitalis. A warning with a report of two deaths. *JAMA* (1936) 106, 1151.
2. Chopra D, Janson P, Sawin CT. Insensitivity to digoxin associated with hypocalcaemia. *N Engl J Med* (1977) 296, 917–8.
3. Jick S, Karsh R. The effect of calcium chelation on cardiac arrhythmias and conduction disturbances. *Am J Cardiol* (1959) 4, 287–93.
4. Szekely P, Wynne NA. Effects of calcium chelation on digitalis-induced cardiac arrhythmias. *Br Heart J* (1963) 25, 589–94.
5. Rosenbaum JL, Mason D, Seven MJ. The effect of disodium EDTA on digitalis intoxication. *Am J Med Sci* (1960) 240, 111–18.
6. Benson CT, Voelker JR. Teriparatide has no effect on the calcium-mediated pharmacodynamics of digoxin. *Clin Pharmacol Ther* (2003) 73, 87–94.
7. Nola GT, Pope S, Harrison DC. Assessment of the synergistic relationship between serum calcium and digitalis. *Am Heart J* (1970) 79, 499–507.
8. Forsteo (Teriparatide). Eli Lilly and Company Ltd. UK Summary of product characteristics, June 2007.
9. Forteo (Teriparatide). Eli Lilly and Company. US Prescribing information, September 2004.

Digitalis glycosides + Drugs that reduce potassium levels

A number of drugs, including amphotericin B, carbenoxolone, and corticosteroids, cause potassium loss, which could lead to the development of digitalis toxicity.

Clinical evidence, mechanism, importance and management

Among the well-recognised adverse effects of **amphotericin B** is hypokalaemia, which can be severe. Although there seem to be no reports of adverse interactions, it would be logical to expect that digitalis toxicity could develop in patients given both drugs if the potassium levels fall. Amiloride has been successfully used to counteract the potassium loss caused by **amphotericin B**.[1]

The adverse effects of **carbenoxolone** include an increase in blood pressure (both systolic and diastolic), fluid retention and reduced serum potassium levels. The incidence of these adverse effects is said in some reports to be as high as 50%; others quote lower figures. Hypertension and fluid retention occur early in **carbenoxolone** treatment, whereas the hypokalaemia develops later and may occur in the absence of the other two adverse effects.[2-5] **Carbenoxolone** is therefore unsuitable for patients with congestive heart failure, or those taking digitalis glycosides, unless measures to avoid hypokalaemia are taken.

Systemic corticosteroids can increase the loss of potassium, particularly those that are naturally occurring (**cortisone**, **deoxycortone**, **hydrocortisone**) whereas the synthetic derivatives (**betamethasone**, **dexamethasone, methylprednisolone**, **prednisolone**, **prednisone**, **triamcinolone**) have much less mineralocorticoid activity. There is therefore the possibility of potassium depletion, particularly when corticosteroids are used long-term, which may increase the risk of digitalis toxicity. These corticosteroids also cause sodium and water retention, resulting in oedema and hypertension, which can lead to cardiac failure in some individuals.

It is therefore important to monitor the use of **digoxin** and any of these drugs well. Potassium levels should be routinely monitored in any patient taking **amphotericin B**, but it is particularly important in those taking **digoxin**. With other drugs where potassium monitoring is not routine, it would seem prudent to watch for signs of **digoxin** toxicity (e.g. bradycardia) and consider measuring potassium levels. No problems of this kind would be expected with corticosteroids used topically or by inhalation, because the amounts absorbed are likely to be relatively small.

1. Smith SR, Galloway MJ, Reilly JT, Davies JM. Amiloride prevents amphotericin B related hypokalaemia in neutropenic patients. *J Clin Pathol* (1988) 41, 494–7.
2. Geismar P, Mosbech J, Myren J. A double-blind study of the effect of carbenoxolone sodium in the treatment of gastric ulcer. *Scand J Gastroenterol* (1973) 8, 251–6.
3. Turpie AGG, Thomson TJ. Carbenoxolone sodium in the treatment of gastric ulcer with special reference to side-effects. *Gut* (1965) 6, 591–4.
4. Langman MJS, Knapp DR, Wakley EJ. Treatment of chronic gastric ulcer with carbenoxolone and gefarnate: a comparative trial. *BMJ* (1973) 3, 84–6.
5. Davies GJ, Rhodes J, Calcraft BJ. Complications of carbenoxolone therapy. *BMJ* (1974) 3, 400–402.

Digitalis glycosides + Edrophonium

Excessive bradycardia and AV-block may occur if patients taking digitalis glycosides are given edrophonium.

Clinical evidence, mechanism, importance and management

The rapid intravenous injection of edrophonium 10 mg has been used in the differentiation of cardiac arrhythmias, but in one study, 4 of 10 digitalised patients given edrophonium developed atrial tachycardia with AV block. The effect was transient; recovery of baseline ECGs occurred 15 to 20 minutes after administration.[1] Nevertheless, the authors recommended that edrophonium should not be given to patients with atrial flutter or tachycardia who are taking digitalis glycosides. This recommendation is reinforced by the case of an elderly woman[2] who developed bradycardia, AV block and asystole following concurrent use. She recovered after being given atropine 1 mg.

1. Reddy RCV, Gould L, Gomprecht RF. Use of edrophonium (Tensilon) in the evaluation of cardiac arrhythmias. *Am Heart J* (1971) 82, 742–9.
2. Gould L, Zahir M, Gomprecht RF. Cardiac arrest during edrophonium administration. *Am Heart J* (1971) 81, 437–8.

Digitalis glycosides + Enoximone

Studies in patients receiving long-term treatment with digitalis glycosides (digoxin or digitoxin) showed that *oral* enoximone 100 mg three times daily for a week had no significant effect on the plasma levels of either of these digitalis glycosides.[1,2] Cardiac function was improved.

1. Glauner T, Hertrich F, Winkelmann B, Dieterich HA, Trenk D, Jähnchen E. Lack of effect of enoximone on steady-state plasma concentrations of digoxin and digitoxin. *Eur Heart J* (1988) 9 (Suppl 1), 151.
2. Trenk D, Hertrich F, Winkelmann B, Glauner T, Dieterich HA, Jähnchen E. Lack of effect of enoximone on the pharmacokinetics of digoxin in patients with congestive heart failure. *J Clin Pharmacol* (1990) 30, 235–40.

Digitalis glycosides + Etanercept

No clinically significant interaction appears to occur between digoxin and etanercept.

Clinical evidence, mechanism, importance and management

A study in 12 healthy subjects given an oral loading dose of **digoxin** 500 micrograms twice daily on day one followed by 250 micrograms daily found that subcutaneous etanercept 25 mg twice weekly did not significantly affect the pharmacokinetics of **digoxin**. The maximum serum levels and AUC of etanercept were 4.2% and 12.5% lower, respectively, during concurrent use but this was not considered to be clinically significant. The combination was well tolerated and there were no changes in ECG parameters.[1] No special precautions therefore seem necessary if both drugs are given.

1. Zhou H, Parks V, Patat A, Le Coz F, Simcoe D, Korth-Bradley J. Absence of a clinically relevant interaction between etanercept and digoxin. *J Clin Pharmacol* (2004) 44, 1244–51.

Digitalis glycosides + Exenatide

Exenatide delayed the time to peak plasma digoxin levels, but this change is not expected to be clinically relevant.

Clinical evidence, mechanism, importance and management

To determine the effects of exenatide on the pharmacokinetics of **digoxin**, 21 healthy subjects were given a loading dose of **digoxin** 500 micrograms twice daily on day one, then 250 micrograms daily for 11 days, with subcutaneous exenatide 10 micrograms twice daily on days 8 to 12. The median time to maximum concentration of **digoxin** was increased from 1.5 hours to 4 hours, and there was a reduction of 17% in its maximum plasma levels. There was no change in AUC and trough **digoxin** levels, and the renal clearance of **digoxin** was not altered. It is thought that the changes in **digoxin** pharmacokinetics occurred as a result of altered gastric emptying caused by exenatide.[1]

Nevertheless, the changes in **digoxin** pharmacokinetics are unlikely to be clinically relevant, and no **digoxin** dose adjustment is likely to be required on concurrent use.

1. Kothare AP, Soon DKW, Linnebjerg H, Park S, Chan C, Yeo A, Lim M, Mace KF, Wise SD. Effect of Exenatide on the steady-state pharmacokinetics of digoxin. *J Clin Pharmacol* (2005) 45, 1032–7.

Digitalis glycosides + Ezetimibe

In a study in 12 healthy subjects ezetimibe 10 mg daily for 7 days did not alter the pharmacokinetics of a single 500-microgram dose of digoxin. In addition, ezetimibe did not alter the ECG effects of digoxin.[1]

1. Kosoglou T, Statkevick P, Johnson-Levonas AO, Paolini JF, Bergman AJ, Alton KB. Ezetimibe. A review of its metabolism, pharmacokinetics and drug interactions. *Clin Pharmacokinet* (2005) 44, 467–94.

Digitalis glycosides + Fenoldopam

Oral fenoldopam appears to cause a small and clinically unimportant reduction in serum digoxin levels in most patients, but more marked changes may occur in a few individuals.

Clinical evidence, mechanism, importance and management

Ten patients with congestive heart failure receiving **digoxin** long-term (doses not stated) were additionally given *oral* fenoldopam 100 mg three times daily for 9 days. The mean AUC and steady-state **digoxin** levels were reduced by about 20%. In two patients, the steady-state serum levels of **digoxin** fell by 48%, from 1.36 to 0.71 nanograms/mL, and 68%, from 1.93 to 0.61 nanograms/mL, respectively, and in a further patient, rose by 45% (from 1.03 to 1.49 nanograms/mL).[1] Most patients appear therefore not to show marked changes in serum **digoxin** levels, but a few individuals may possibly need some dosage adjustment. Monitor the effects of concurrent use.

1. Strocchi E, Tartagni F, Malini PL, Valtancoli G, Ambrosioni E, Pasinelli F, Riva E, Fuccella LM. Interaction study of fenoldopam-digoxin in congestive heart failure. *Eur J Clin Pharmacol* (1989) 37, 395–7.

Digitalis glycosides + Finasteride

Finasteride does not appear to affect the pharmacokinetics of digoxin.

Clinical evidence, mechanism, importance and management

In a randomised study, 17 healthy subjects were given a single 400-microgram dose of **digoxin** while taking finasteride 5 mg daily for 10 days. Finasteride had no significant effect on the pharmacokinetics of **digoxin**.[1] No adverse effects are expected on concurrent use.

1. Gregoire S, Williams R, Gormely G, Lin E. Effect of finasteride (MK-906) on the disposition of digoxin. *J Clin Pharmacol* (1990) 30, 847.

Digitalis glycosides + Flecainide

Plasma digoxin levels are unaltered or only modestly increased by the use of flecainide, but this is not likely to be important in most patients.

Clinical evidence

The plasma **digoxin** levels of 10 patients with congestive heart failure were unchanged when they took flecainide 100 to 200 mg twice daily for 7 days. A similar lack of interaction was also seen in 4 patients who took both drugs over a 4-week period.[1]

In contrast, a study in 15 healthy subjects found that flecainide 200 mg twice daily increased the trough and peak plasma levels of **digoxin** 250 micrograms by 24% and 13%, respectively.[2] The changes observed in vital signs were not clinically significant. Based on the results of a single-dose study the steady-state **digoxin** levels were predicted to rise by about 15% during the use of flecainide 200 mg twice daily.[3]

Mechanism

Uncertain. It is suggested that any changes may be due to alterations in the volume of distribution.[3]

Importance and management

Documentation is limited but what is known suggests that either no interaction occurs, or any changes are small and unlikely to be clinically relevant in most patients. However, the UK manufacturers of flecainide recommend that digoxin plasma levels should be measured not less than 6 hours after any digoxin dose, before or after the administration of flecainide.[4] The US manufacturers do not advise any additional monitoring.[5] The authors of one of the reports[2] suggest that patients with high drug levels, atrioventricular nodal dysfunction, or both, should be monitored during concurrent treatment.

1. McQuinn RL, Kvam DC, Parrish SL, Fox TL, Miller AM, Franciosa JA. Digoxin levels in patients with congestive heart failure are not altered by flecainide. *Clin Pharmacol Ther* (1988) 43, 150.
2. Weeks CE, Conard GJ, Kvam DC, Fox JM, Chang SF, Paone RP, Lewis GP. The effect of flecainide acetate, a new antiarrhythmic, on plasma digoxin levels. *J Clin Pharmacol* (1986) 26, 27–31.
3. Tjandramaga TB, Verbesselt R, Van Hecken A, Mullie A, De Schepper PJ. Oral digoxin pharmacokinetics during multiple-dose flecainide treatment. *Arch Int Pharmacodyn Ther* (1982) 260, 302–3.
4. Tambocor (Flecainide acetate). 3M Health Care Ltd. UK Summary of product characteristics, May 2006.
5. Tambocor (Flecainide acetate). 3M Pharmaceuticals. US Prescribing information, June 1998.

Digitalis glycosides + Fondaparinux

No significant interaction appears to occur between digoxin and fondaparinux.

Clinical evidence, mechanism, importance and management

A phase I randomised study in 24 healthy subjects found that the pharmacokinetics of oral **digoxin** 250 micrograms twice daily for one day then 250 micrograms daily for 6 days was unaffected by subcutaneous fondaparinux 10 mg daily. The pharmacokinetics of fondaparinux were not affected by **digoxin**. The combination was well tolerated and no clinically significant changes in vital signs and ECGs were observed.[1] No additional precautions therefore seem necessary on concurrent use.

1. Mant T, Fournié P, Ollier C, Donat F, Necciari J. Absence of interaction of fondaparinux sodium with digoxin in healthy volunteers. *Clin Pharmacokinet* (2002), 41 (Suppl 2), 39–45.

Digitalis glycosides + Grapefruit juice

Plasma digoxin levels are generally unaltered or only modestly increased by grapefruit juice, but in some individuals significant changes may occur.

Clinical evidence

A crossover study in 12 healthy subjects found that when they were given either grapefruit juice 220 mL or water, 30 minutes before and 3.5, 7.5, and 11.5 hours after a single 500-microgram dose of **digoxin** (taken with 50 mL of grapefruit juice or water respectively), the 0 to 4-hour and 0 to 24-hour **digoxin** AUCs were increased by about 10%. The maximum plasma levels and renal clearance of **digoxin** were not significantly affected. However, in 2 subjects taking grapefruit juice, the ECGs taken 90 minutes after **digoxin** ingestion revealed an asymptomatic first-degree atrioventricular block. Plasma levels in these subjects had increased by 50% to 2.4 and 2.8 nanograms/mL, respectively.[1] Another study found that grapefruit juice decreased the rate but not the extent of absorption of **digoxin** and had no effect on AUC or renal clearance, but there was significant inter-individual variability.[2]

Mechanism

The modest increases in digoxin levels may be due to increased intestinal absorption of digoxin, possibly due to inhibition of P-glycoprotein-mediated digoxin transport by grapefruit juice, although this mechanism has been questioned.[1] *In vitro*, pomelo (*Citrus grandis*) and grapefruit juices inhibited P-glycoprotein transport of digoxin.[3]

Importance and management

Although grapefruit juice appears to have little effect on digoxin bioavailability, it is possible that in some individuals the interaction could be of clinical significance.[2] Bear this interaction in mind in the case of an unexpected response to digoxin. More study is needed.

1. Becquemont L, Verstuyft C, Kerb R, Brinkmann U, Lebot M, Jaillon P, Funck-Brentano C. Effect of grapefruit juice on digoxin pharmacokinetics in humans. *Clin Pharmacol Ther* (2001) 70, 311–6.
2. Parker RB, Yates CR, Soberman JE, Laizure SC. Effects of grapefruit juice on intestinal P-glycoprotein: evaluation using digoxin in humans. *Pharmacotherapy* (2003) 23, 979–87.
3. Xu J, Go ML, Lim L-Y. Modulation of digoxin transport across Caco-2 cell monolayers by citrus fruit juices: lime, lemon, grapefruit and pummelo. *Pharm Res* (2003) 20, 169–76.

Digitalis glycosides + Guanadrel

Guanadrel did not affect the pharmacokinetics of a single dose of digoxin.

Clinical evidence, mechanism, importance and management

In 13 healthy subjects guanadrel 10 mg orally every 12 hours for 8 days did not affect the pharmacokinetics of a single intravenous dose of **digoxin** given on day 5. One subject experienced a 10-minute episode of asymptomatic second-degree heart block (Wenckebach) 3 hours after the dose of **digoxin**, but the reason for this effect was not clear.[1] There seem to be no reports of adverse interactions between the digitalis glycosides and any of the guanethidine-like antihypertensive drugs.

1. Wright CE, Andreadis NA. Digoxin pharmacokinetics when administered concurrently with guanadrel sulfate. *Drug Intell Clin Pharm* (1986) 20, 465.

Digitalis glycosides + H_2-receptor antagonists

Small changes in serum digoxin levels, both rises and falls, have been seen in patients also given cimetidine, but these do not appear to be of clinical importance. Ranitidine does not appear to interact with metildigoxin.

Clinical evidence, mechanism, importance and management

While taking **cimetidine** 300 mg every 6 or 12 hours the steady-state serum **digoxin** levels of 11 patients with congestive heart failure fell, on average, by 25% (from 2 to 1.5 nanograms/mL), but none of them showed any ECG changes or signs that their condition had worsened.[1] Four other patients with stable congestive heart failure had no significant changes in the pharmacokinetics of **digoxin** 125 to 250 micrograms daily when they were given **cimetidine** 300 mg every 6 hours.[2] Three single-dose studies in a total of 19 healthy subjects, and 6 patients with duodenal ulcers[3] found that **cimetidine** 600 mg to 1.2 g daily had no significant effect on the absorption[4] or the pharmacokinetics[3,5] of **digoxin**. Another study found a small increase in **digoxin** levels in healthy subjects, but only a small statistically insignificant rise in the steady-state levels of 11 patients given **cimetidine** 400 mg four times daily.[6] Six patients with chronic congestive heart failure given **metildigoxin** had no changes in their serum **digoxin** levels when they were given **ranitidine** 150 mg twice daily for a week.[7]

No interaction of clinical importance with either of these H_2-receptor antagonists has been established and no special precautions would seem to be necessary.

1. Fraley DS, Britton HL, Schwinghammer TL, Kalla R. Effect of cimetidine on steady-state serum digoxin concentrations. *Clin Pharm* (1983) 2, 163–5.
2. Mouser B, Nykamp D, Murphy JE, Krissman PH. Effect of cimetidine on oral digoxin absorption. *DICP Ann Pharmacother* (1990) 24, 286–8.
3. Garty M, Perry G, Shmueli H, Ilfeld D, Boner G, Pitlik S, Rosenfeld J. Effect of cimetidine on digoxin disposition in peptic ulcer patients. *Eur J Clin Pharmacol* (1986) 30, 489–91.
4. Jordaens L, Hoegaerts J, Belpaire F. Non-interaction of cimetidine with digoxin absorption. *Acta Clin Belg* (1981) 36, 109–10.
5. Ochs HR, Gugler R, Guthoff T, Greenblatt DJ. Effect of cimetidine on digoxin kinetics and creatinine clearance. *Am Heart J* (1984) 107, 170–2.
6. Crome P, Curl B, Holt D, Volans GN, Bennett PN, Cole DS. Digoxin and cimetidine: investigation of the potential for a drug interaction. *Hum Toxicol* (1985) 4, 391–9.
7. Enomoto N, Kurasawa T, Ichikawa M, Shimuzu T, Matsuyama T, Sakai K, Shimamura K, Oda M. Lack of interaction of β-methyldigoxin with ranitidine in patients with chronic congestive heart failure. *Eur J Clin Pharmacol* (1992) 43, 205–6.

Digitalis glycosides + Herbal medicines; Cimicifuga

A standardised black cohosh extract (Cimicifuga) did not alter the pharmacokinetics of digoxin.

Clinical evidence, mechanism, importance and management

A study in 16 healthy subjects who were given a single 400-microgram dose of **digoxin** before and on the last day of a 14-day course of a standardised black cohosh (*Cimicifuga racemosa*) extract 20 mg twice daily, found no statistically significant changes in the pharmacokinetics of **digoxin**. The product used was standardised to 2.5% triterpene glycosides.[1]

Digoxin is a substrate of P-glycoprotein, and this study was conducted to see if black cohosh had any clinically relevant effect on P-glycoprotein.[1] The findings indicated that black cohosh does not cause clinically relevant changes in digoxin pharmacokinetics, and no alteration in **digoxin** levels would therefore be expected on concurrent use. For mention of a case of digoxin-like toxicity attributed to a herbal preparation, containing amongst other ingredients, black cohosh, see 'Digitalis glycosides + Herbal medicines; Digoxin-like', below.

1. Gurley BJ, Barone GW, Williams DK, Carrier J, Breen P, Yates CR, Song P-f, Hubbard MA, Tong Y, Cheboyina S. Effect of milk thistle (*Silybum marianum*) and black cohosh (*Cimicifuga racemosa*) supplementation on digoxin pharmacokinetics in humans. *Drug Metab Dispos* (2006) 34, 69–74.

Digitalis glycosides + Herbal medicines; Digoxin-like

Many herbal remedies contain cardiac glycosides, which could in theory have additive effects with digoxin or digitoxin, or interfere with their assays. However, there appear to be few such interactions reported.

Clinical evidence, mechanism, importance and management

(a) Additive effects possible

A 26-year-old woman developed severe and unexplained chest pain, and was later noted to have a heart rate of 39 bpm and a blood pressure of 59/36 mmHg, but these rose to normal with conservative management. She was found to have a **digoxin** level of 0.9 nanograms/mL and was diagnosed as having **digoxin** toxicity, despite not taking any prescribed **digoxin**. The digoxin-like cardiac glycosides were thought to have come from an unnamed herbal remedy for stress, which contained **black cohosh root** (*Cimicifuga racemosa*), **cayenne pepper fruit** (*Capsicum annuum*), **hops flowers** (*Humulus lupulus*), **skullcap herb** (*Scutellaria lateriflora*), **valerian root** (*Valeriana officinalis*) and **wood betony herb** (*Pedicularis canadensis*).[1] All of these had previously been shown to contain small amounts of digoxin-like compounds, which were only partially detected by **digoxin** antibody immunoassays.[1,2] In this previous *in vitro* study, 46 commercially packaged herb teas and 78 teas prepared from herbs were assayed for digoxin-like factors by their cross-reactivity with **digoxin** antibody or inhibition of ouabain binding, and these values were used to give approximate equivalent daily doses of **digoxin**. Three packaged teas (***Breathe Easy***, **blackcurrant**, and **jasmine**) and 3 herbs (**pleurisy root**, **chaparral**, **peppermint**) were found to contain greater than 30 micrograms of **digoxin** equivalents per cup and were postulated to provide a therapeutic daily dose of **digoxin** if 5 cups a day were drunk.[2] However, note that some common teas sampled in this study (e.g. English Breakfast, Earl Grey) contained over 20 micrograms of **digoxin** equivalents per cup, and tea drinking has not been associated with adverse cardiovascular risk.[3] Therefore the interpretation of the findings of this study is unclear.

Theoretical interactions with herbal remedies are not always translated into practice, and there do not appear to be any cases of herbals interacting with **digoxin** because of their cardiac glycoside content. See also 'Digitalis glycosides + Chinese herbal medicines', p.917.

(b) Effects on digoxin assays

A 68-year-old woman who was given a loading dose of **digitoxin** 750 micrograms then 100 micrograms on the second day was found to have markedly elevated levels of **digitoxin** (greater than 100 nanograms/mL), but no clinical signs of toxicity. Two days before admission she had ingested 90 drops of **Uzara**, a preparation from *Xysmalobium undulatum,* which contains weak cardiac glycosides. Later investigations in 4 healthy subjects given 30 drops of **Uzara** confirmed that assays for **digitoxin** (CEDIA digitoxin test, Roche Diagnostics, Germany) and **digoxin** (Tina-quant digoxin test, Roche Diagnostics, Germany) were markedly elevated by **Uzara** to levels well above usual therapeutic concentrations, but that there were no clinically relevant changes in heart rate and blood pressure.[4]

In an *in vitro* study, **plantain** (*Plantago major*) extract from capsules, liquid extract, or dry leaf did not affect the results of **digoxin** assays when using fluorescence polarization immunoassay or microparticle enzyme immunoassay.[5] Note that contamination of plantain with *Digitalis lanata* has been reported.[6]

See also 'Digitalis glycosides + Chinese herbal medicines', p.917 and 'Digitalis glycosides + Herbal medicines; Ginseng', below for other herbals that can affect the results of **digoxin** assays.

1. Scheinhost ME. Digoxin toxicity in a 26-year-old woman taking a herbal dietary supplement. *J Am Osteopath Assoc* (2001), 101, 444–6.
2. Longerich L, Johnson E, Gault MH. Digoxin-like factors in herbal teas. *Clin Invest Med* (1993) 16, 210–8.
3. Sweetman SC, ed. Martindale: The complete drug reference. 35th ed. London: Pharmaceutical Press; 2007. p. 2188.
4. Thürmann PA, Neff A, Fleisch J. Interference of uzara glycosides in assays of digitalis glycosides. *Int J Clin Pharmacol Ther* (2004) 42, 281–4.
5. Dasgupta A, Davis B, Wells A. Effect of plantain on therapeutic drug monitoring of digoxin and thirteen other common drugs. *Ann Clin Biochem* (2006) 43, 223–5.
6. Slifman NR, Obermeyer WR, Aloi BK, Musser SM, Correll WA, Cichowicz SM, Betz JM, Love LA. Contamination of botanical dietary supplements by Digitalis lanata. *N Engl J Med* (1998) 339, 806–11.

Digitalis glycosides + Herbal medicines; *Ginkgo biloba*

A study in 8 healthy subjects found that ginkgo biloba leaf extract 80 mg three times daily had no significant effects on the pharmacokinetics of a single 500-microgram dose of digoxin.[1]

1. Mauro VF, Mauro LS, Kleshinski JF, Khuder SA, Wang Y, Erhardt PW. Impact of Ginkgo biloba on the pharmacokinetics of digoxin. *Am J Ther* (2003) 10, 247–51.

Digitalis glycosides + Herbal medicines; Ginseng

A man taking digoxin developed grossly elevated serum digoxin levels, without symptoms of toxicity, while taking Siberian ginseng. This was eventually attributed to an effect of ginseng on the digoxin assay. Both Chinese and Siberian ginseng may interfere with some digoxin assays.

Clinical evidence, mechanism, importance and management

A 74-year-old man who had been taking **digoxin** for many years (serum levels normally in the range 0.9 to 2.2 nanograms/mL) was found, during a routine check, to have **digoxin** levels of 5.2 nanograms/mL, but without evidence of toxicity or bradycardia or any other ECG changes.[1] The levels remained high even when the **digoxin** was stopped. It turned out he had also been taking **Siberian ginseng** capsules. When the ginseng was stopped, the **digoxin** levels returned to the usual range, and **digoxin** was resumed. Later rechallenge with the ginseng caused a rise in his serum **digoxin** levels. No digoxin or digitoxin contamination was found in the capsules, and the authors of the report also rejected the idea that the eleutherosides (chemically related to cardiac glycosides) in ginseng might have been converted *in vivo* into **digoxin**, or that the renal elimination of **digoxin** might have been impaired, since the patient showed no signs of toxicity. One possible explanation is that the ginseng affected the accuracy of the **digoxin** assay so that it gave false results.[1]

Asian or **Chinese ginseng** *(Panax ginseng)* and **Siberian ginseng** *(Eleutherococcus senticosus)* have both been found to interfere with some **digoxin** assays including fluorescence polarisation immunoassay (FPIA) and microparticle enzyme immunoassay (MEIA).[2]

Whether serum digoxin levels are actually affected is uncertain. Nevertheless is may be sensible to ask about ginseng use when interpreting **digoxin** levels.

1. McRae S. Elevated serum digoxin levels in a patient taking digoxin and Siberian ginseng. *Can Med Assoc J* (1996) 155, 293–5.
2. Dasgupta A, Wu S, Actor J, Olsen M, Wells A, Datta P. Effect of Asian and Siberian ginseng on serum digoxin measurement by five digoxin immunoassays. Significant variation in digoxin-like immunoreactivity among commercial ginsengs. *Am J Clin Pathol* (2003) 119, 298–303.

Digitalis glycosides + Herbal medicines; Goldenseal (*Hydrastis*)

A standardised goldenseal root extract did not alter the pharmacokinetics of digoxin.

Clinical evidence, mechanism, importance and management

A study in 20 healthy subjects given a single 500-microgram dose of **digoxin** before and on the last day of treatment with standardised **goldenseal root extract** (*Hydrastis canadensis*) 1070 mg three times daily for 14 days, found a 14% increase in the maximum **digoxin** plasma levels, but no other changes in the pharmacokinetics of **digoxin**. The product was standardised for isoquinoline alkaloid content.[1]

It was suggested that constituents of goldenseal may alter **digoxin** pharmacokinetics by affecting P-glycoprotein, since goldenseal alkaloids are modulators of P-glycoprotein *in vitro*. However, the clinical study showed that goldenseal does not cause clinically relevant changes in **digoxin** pharmacokinetics. Therefore no changes in **digoxin** levels would be anticipated on concurrent use, the caveat being that, as with all herbals, these results may not be applicable to all goldenseal products.[1]

1. Gurley BJ, Swain A, Barone GW, Williams DK, Breen P, Yates CR, Stuart LB, Hubbard MA, Tong Y, Cheboyina S. Effect of goldenseal (*Hydrastis canadensis*) and kava kava (*Piper methysticum*) supplementation on digoxin pharmacokinetics in humans. *Drug Metab Dispos* (2007) 35, 240–5.

Digitalis glycosides + Herbal medicines; Hawthorn (Crataegus)

A standardised extract of hawthorn (Crataegus) did not have any clinically relevant effect on digoxin levels.

Clinical evidence, mechanism, importance and management

In a crossover study in 8 healthy subjects, a standardised extract of hawthorn leaves and flowers (*Crataegus oxyacantha*) 450 mg twice daily for 21 days had no effect on the steady-state pharmacokinetics of **digoxin**. The biggest difference was a non-significant 23% reduction in the **digoxin** trough level. There were no changes in ECG or blood pressure from baseline values for either **digoxin** alone or combined with hawthorn.[1]

It was suggested that flavonol constituents of hawthorn might induce P-glycoprotein and therefore decrease **digoxin** levels,[1] similar to 'St John's wort', (below).

This study suggests that, at the most, hawthorn might cause a minor decrease in **digoxin** levels, and no adjustment of the **digoxin** dose is therefore likely to be needed on concurrent use. Although no pharmacodynamic effects were seen, the possibility that hawthorn's cardioactive constituents might increase the effect of **digoxin** on cardiac contractility cannot be ruled out.[1]

1. Tankanow R, Tamer HR, Streetman DS, Smith SG, Welton JL, Annesley T, Aaronson KD, Bleske BE. Interaction study between digoxin and a preparation of hawthorn (*Crataegus oxyacantha*). *J Clin Pharmacol* (2003) 43, 637–42.

Digitalis glycosides + Herbal medicines; Kava

A standardised kava extract did not alter the pharmacokinetics of digoxin.

Clinical evidence, mechanism, importance and management

A study in 20 healthy subjects given a single 500-microgram dose of **digoxin** before and on the last day of treatment with a standardised kava rhizome (*Piper methysticum*) extract 1227 mg three times daily for 14 days, found no changes in the pharmacokinetics of **digoxin**. The product used was standardised for kavalactone content.[1]

It was suggested that kava may alter **digoxin** pharmacokinetics by affecting P-glycoprotein, since kavalactones are modulators of P-glycoprotein *in vitro*. However, the clinical study showed that kava does not cause clinically relevant changes in **digoxin** pharmacokinetics. Therefore no changes in **digoxin** levels would be anticipated on concurrent use, the caveat being that, as with all herbals, these results may not be applicable to all kava products.[1]

1. Gurley BJ, Swain A, Barone GW, Williams DK, Breen P, Yates CR, Stuart LB, Hubbard MA, Tong Y, Cheboyina S. Effect of goldenseal (*Hydrastis canadensis*) and kava kava (*Piper methysticum*) supplementation on digoxin pharmacokinetics in humans. *Drug Metab Dispos* (2007) 35, 240–5.

Digitalis glycosides + Herbal medicines; Milk thistle

A standardised milk thistle extract did not alter the pharmacokinetics of digoxin.

Clinical evidence, mechanism, importance and management

A study in 16 healthy subjects who were given a single 400-microgram dose of **digoxin** before and on the last day of a 14-day course of a standardised milk thistle (*Silybum marianum*) extract 300 mg three times daily, found no statistically significant changes in the pharmacokinetics of **digoxin**. There was a trend towards a minor 10% reduction in the AUC of **digoxin**, but this did not reach statistical significance. The extract used was standardised to contain 80% silymarin.[1]

It was suggested that milk thistle may alter **digoxin** pharmacokinetics by affecting P-glycoprotein, since silymarin is a modulator of P-glycoprotein *in vitro*. However, the clinical study showed that milk thistle does not cause clinically relevant changes in **digoxin** pharmacokinetics. Therefore no changes in **digoxin** levels would be anticipated on concurrent use, the caveat being that, as with all herbals, these results may not be applicable to all milk thistle products.[1]

1. Gurley BJ, Barone GW, Williams DK, Carrier J, Breen P, Yates CR, Song P-f, Hubbard MA, Tong Y, Cheboyina S. Effect of milk thistle (*Silybum marianum*) and black cohosh (*Cimicifuga racemosa*) supplementation on digoxin pharmacokinetics in humans. *Drug Metab Dispos* (2006) 34, 69–74.

Digitalis glycosides + Herbal medicines; St John's wort (*Hypericum perforatum*)

Digoxin toxicity occurred in a patient taking digoxin when he stopped taking St John's wort. There is good evidence that some preparations of St John's wort can reduce the levels of digoxin by about one-quarter to one-third.

Clinical evidence

An 80-year-old man taking long-term **digoxin** and St John's wort herbal tea (2 litres daily) developed symptoms of **digoxin** toxicity (nodal bradycardia of 36 bpm and bigeminy) when he stopped taking the herbal tea.[1]

In a study 13 healthy subjects were given **digoxin** for 5 days until steady-state had been achieved, and then St John's wort extract (LI 160, Lichtwer Pharma) 300 mg three times daily for a further 10 days. The AUC and trough level of **digoxin** decreased by 28% and 37%, respectively. When compared with a parallel group of 12 subjects taking digoxin and placebo, the St John's wort group had 26.3% lower maximum plasma **digoxin** levels, 33.3% lower trough **digoxin** levels and a 25% lower AUC.[2]

In a further randomised placebo-controlled study, 93 healthy subjects were given **digoxin** alone for 7 days and then with one of ten St John's wort preparations for 14 days. The extract used in the earlier study (LI 160, *Jarsin 300*, Lichtwer Pharma) 300 mg three time daily similarly reduced the **digoxin** AUC, peak and trough plasma levels by 25%, 37%, and 19%, respectively. Comparable results were found with hypericum powder containing similar amounts of hyperforin (about 21 mg daily), while hypericum powder with half the hyperforin content (about 10 mg daily) reduced the AUC, peak and trough plasma levels by about 18%, 21%, and 13%, respectively. Some St John's wort products, including tea, juice, oil extract, and powder with low-dose hyperforin (all 5 mg daily or less), did not significantly affect the pharmacokinetics of **digoxin**.[3] Similarly, a further study in 28 healthy subjects found no statistically significant change in **digoxin** pharmacokinetics when another low-hyperforin (about 3.5 mg daily) St John's wort extract (***Esbericum***) 120 mg was given twice daily for 11 days to patients who had received a digoxin loading dose of 750 micrograms daily for 2 days before starting St John's wort, and then received digoxin 250 micrograms daily each day during the study.[4]

Mechanism

St John's wort has been shown to increase the activity of the P-glycoprotein drug transporter protein in the intestines, which reduces the absorption of digoxin.[2,5]

Importance and management

Information seems to be limited to these reports, but the interaction would appear to be established. The extent of the interaction may depend on the St John's wort preparation involved and dose used and seems to be correlated with the dose of hyperforin.[3,4] See also 'Drug-herb interactions', (p.10). Reductions in serum digoxin levels of the size seen with LI 160 could diminish the control of arrhythmias or heart failure. Digoxin serum levels should therefore be well monitored if St John's wort is either started or stopped and appropriate dosage adjustments made if necessary. The recommendation of the CSM in the UK is that St John's wort should not be used by patients taking digoxin.[6]

1. Anđelić S. Bigeminija – rezultat interakcije digoksina i kantariona. *Vojnosanit Pregl* (2003) 60, 361–4.
2. Johne A, Brockmöller J, Bauer S, Maurer A, Langheinrich M, Roots I. Pharmacokinetic interaction of digoxin with an herbal extract from St John's wort (*Hypericum perforatum*). *Clin Pharmacol Ther* (1999) 66, 338–45.
3. Mueller SC, Uehleke B, Woehling H, Petzsch M, Majcher-Peszynska J, Hehl E-M, Sievers H, Frank B, Riethling A-K, Drewelow B. Effect of St John's wort dose and preparations on the pharmacokinetics of digoxin. *Clin Pharmacol Ther* (2004) 75, 546–57.
4. Arold G, Donath F, Maurer A, Diefenbach K, Bauer S, Henneicke-von Zepelin HH, Friede M, Roots I. No relevant interaction with alprazolam, caffeine, tolbutamide and digoxin by treatment with a low-hyperforin St John's wort extract. *Planta Med* (2005) 71, 331–337.
5. Dürr D, Stieger B, Kullak-Ublick GA, Rentsch KM, Steinert HC, Meier PJ, Fattinger K. St John's wort induces intestinal P-glycoprotein/MDR1 and intestinal and hepatic CYP3A4. *Clin Pharmacol Ther* (2000) 68, 598–604.
6. Committee on the Safety of Medicines (UK). Message from Professor A Breckenridge (Chairman of CSM) and Fact Sheet for Health Care Professionals, 29th February 2000.

Digitalis glycosides + HRT

Post hoc analysis of one study found an increased rate of cardiovascular adverse events in women using digitalis and also taking HRT.

Clinical evidence, mechanism, importance and management

Retrospective analysis of data from a large randomised, placebo-controlled study of HRT (conjugated estrogens/medroxyprogesterone 0.625/2.5 mg daily) in women with coronary heart disease was conducted to see if there were any subgroups of patients who responded differently. Use of digitalis was associated with a fivefold excess rate of cardiovascular events in the first year in women receiving HRT, when compared with the control group. A lower 1.5-fold excess rate was seen over the whole duration of the study (average 4.1 years). Possible mechanisms could be a drug-drug interaction or a drug-disease (HRT with congestive heart failure) interaction.[1]

However, it is impossible to say whether this represents a true effect, because the number of positive sub-group analyses in this study was the same as the number predicted by chance alone. Confirmatory evidence is required.[1]

1. Furberg CD, Vittinghoff E, Davidson M, Herrington DM, Simon JA, Wenger NK, Hulley S. Subgroup interactions in the Heart and Estrogen/Progestin replacement study. Lessons learned. *Circulation* (2002) 105, 917–22.

Digitalis glycosides + Kaolin-pectin

Plasma digoxin levels can be reduced by kaolin-pectin, but the reduction is small and probably of minimal clinical importance.

Clinical evidence

The concurrent use of kaolin-pectin suspension and **digoxin** reduced the peak plasma **digoxin** levels of 7 patients by 36%, while the AUC_{0-24} was reduced by 15%. Conversely, when two doses of kaolin-pectin were taken, the first 2 hours before and the other 2 hours after the **digoxin**, no significant changes were seen.[1]

Two single-dose studies have found 42% and 62% reductions in the bioavailability of **digoxin** caused by kaolin-pectin.[2,3] Another study found an interaction with **digoxin** tablets but not with **digoxin** capsules.[4]

Mechanism

Not understood. The digoxin may possibly become adsorbed onto the kaolin so that less is available for absorption. Another possibility is that the kaolin reduces the motility of the gut, which normally increases mixing and brings the digoxin into contact with the absorbing surface.

Importance and management

Steady-state studies reflect the every-day situation much more closely than single-dose studies, and the one cited above[1] indicates that the total reduction in digoxin absorption is small (15%). This is unlikely to be of clinical importance. However, if an interaction does occur the effects can seemingly be minimised by separating the dosages by 2 hours.

1. Albert KS, Elliott WJ, Abbott RD, Gilbertson TJ, Data JL. Influence of kaolin-pectin suspension on steady-state plasma digoxin levels. *J Clin Pharmacol* (1981) 21, 449–55.
2. Brown DD, Juhl RP, Lewis K, Schrott M, Bartels B. Decreased bioavailability of digoxin due to antacids and kaolin-pectin. *N Engl J Med* (1976) 295, 1034–7.
3. Albert KS, Ayres JW, Disanto AR, Weidler DJ, Sakmar E, Hallmark MR, Stoll RG, DeSante KA, Wagner JG. Influence of kaolin-pectin suspension on digoxin bioavailability. *J Pharm Sci* (1978) 67, 1582–6.
4. Allen MD, Greenblatt DJ, Harmatz JS, Smith TW. Effect of magnesium aluminum hydroxide and kaolin-pectin on absorption of digoxin from tablets and capsules. *J Clin Pharmacol* (1981) 21, 26–30.

Digitalis glycosides + Ketanserin

Ketanserin does not appear to affect the pharmacokinetics of either digoxin or digitoxin.

Clinical evidence, mechanism, importance and management

Ketanserin 40 mg twice daily did not cause any significant changes in the pharmacokinetics of single doses of either **digoxin** 1.25 mg or **digitoxin** 1 mg in healthy subjects, and it was concluded that ketanserin is unlikely to alter serum concentrations of either digitalis glycoside during clinical use.[1]

1. Ochs HR, Verburg-Ochs B, Höller M, Greenblatt DJ. Effect of ketanserin on the kinetics of digoxin and digitoxin. *J Cardiovasc Pharmacol* (1985) 7, 205–7.

Digitalis glycosides + Lanthanum

Lanthanum did not significantly affect the pharmacokinetics of digoxin in a single-dose study.

Clinical evidence, mechanism, importance and management

In a crossover study, 14 healthy subjects were given lanthanum 1 g for 3 doses on one day, followed by a fourth dose the next day. A single 500-microgram dose of **digoxin** was given 30 minutes after the fourth dose of lanthanum. The **digoxin** half-life was increased during concurrent treatment from 11.4 to 14.8 hours but this was not considered to be clinically significant. Other pharmacokinetic parameters were not significantly affected.[1] Further multiple dose studies are needed to confirm this lack of interaction in patients.

1. Fiddler G. Fosrenol™ (lanthanum carbonate) does not affect the pharmacokinetics of concomitant treatment with digoxin. *J Am Soc Nephrol* (2002) 13, 749A.

Digitalis glycosides + Lithium

No pharmacokinetic interaction occurs between digoxin and lithium but the addition of digoxin to lithium possibly has a detrimental short-term effect on the control of mania. An isolated report describes severe bradycardia in one patient given both drugs.

Clinical evidence, mechanism, importance and management

A study in 6 healthy subjects taking lithium carbonate sufficient to achieve mean steady-state serum levels of 0.76 mmol/L (range 0.4 to 1 mmol/L) showed that the pharmacokinetics of a 750-microgram intravenous dose of **digoxin** were unchanged by lithium, and that there were no significant effects on sodium pump activity or electrolyte concentrations.[1] However an experimental 7-day study in patients with manic-depressive psychoses found that there was a greater improvement in those given lithium with placebo than those given lithium with **digoxin**. This may be a reflection of changes in Na-K ATP-ase.[2] An isolated report describes tremor, confusion and severe nodal bradycardia in a patient given both drugs. The bradycardia worsened (30 bpm) even after both drugs were stopped.[3] The clinical significance of all of these findings is uncertain. Note that one UK manufacturer of **digoxin**[4] lists lithium as a drug that may increase sensitivity to **digoxin** because it may cause hypokalaemia or intracellular potassium deficiency, consider also 'drugs that lower potassium', (p.923).

1. Cooper SJ, Kelly JG, Johnston GD, Copeland S, King DJ, McDevitt DG. Pharmacodynamics and pharmacokinetics of digoxin in the presence of lithium. *Br J Clin Pharmacol* (1984) 18, 21–5.
2. Chambers CA, Smith AHW, Naylor GJ. The effect of digoxin on the response to lithium therapy in mania. *Psychol Med* (1982) 12, 57–60.
3. Winters WD, Ralph DD. Digoxin-lithium drug interaction. *Clin Toxicol* (1977) 10, 487–8.
4. Lanoxin (Digoxin). GlaxoSmithKline UK. UK Summary of product characteristics, May 2003.

Digitalis glycosides + Macrolides

Clarithromycin markedly increases digoxin levels, and numerous cases of digoxin toxicity have been reported. Increases in serum digoxin levels also occur with telithromycin. Cases of rapid and marked two to fourfold increase in serum digoxin levels have also been reported for azithromycin, erythromycin, josamycin and roxithromycin. A similar case has been seen with digitoxin and azithromycin.

Clinical evidence

A. Digitoxin

A man with congestive heart failure taking digitoxin 70 micrograms daily for 5 days of each week, with enalapril and furosemide, was admitted to hospital with nausea and bradycardia of 26 bpm 4 days after starting a 3-day course of **azithromycin** (dosage not stated). His serum digitoxin levels were found to be raised from his usual baseline range of 9.9 to 19 nanograms/mL up to 34 nanograms/mL. His renal function was normal. Another patient treated with intravenous digitoxin 250 micrograms once daily had a marked rise from his steady-state digitoxin range of 11 to 15 nanograms/mL after being given **azithromycin** 500 mg daily for 3 days. The digitoxin was withdrawn one day later, but even so the levels climbed to a peak of 32 nanograms/mL after a further 3 days, and remained in the toxic range for yet another 3 days.[1]

B. Digoxin

(a) Azithromycin

A 31-month-old boy with Down's syndrome and tetralogy of Fallot (a congenital heart defect resulting in reduced blood flow to the lungs) was discharged from hospital after repair of his heart defect. He was taking digoxin 60 micrograms twice daily, furosemide, and potassium chloride. Eight days later, when readmitted with symptoms of heart failure, intermittent fever and wheezing, he was given azithromycin (10 mg/kg on day 1, then 5 mg/kg daily for 4 days). Three days later his steady-state serum digoxin levels had risen from 1.79 to 2.37 nanograms/mL and he experienced anorexia, nausea, and second degree atrioventricular block. All the symptoms resolved when the digoxin was withdrawn. Digoxin was restarted at 50 micrograms twice daily after the azithromycin course was completed and steady-state digoxin levels of 1.42 nanograms/mL were noted.[2]

The manufacturers of azithromycin said that, as of October 2000, there were 230 cases of the concurrent use of azithromycin and digoxin on their database. Of these, 78 cases had adverse events indicating possible digoxin toxicity. However on review, 21 cases were clearly excluded. Of the remaining cases, only 13 provided digoxin levels, and of these, high serum digoxin concentrations were reported in 6, but generally insufficient data made interpretation difficult.[3] The manufacturers concluded that the possibility that a patient may experience an increase in digoxin levels while taking azithromycin cannot be entirely excluded.[3]

(b) Clarithromycin

A woman receiving treatment with warfarin, heparin, carbamazepine and digoxin was admitted to hospital with syncope, vomiting and an irregular heart rhythm shortly after starting clarithromycin 1 g daily. Her serum digoxin levels were found to be raised. The clarithromycin was decreased, the carbamazepine and digoxin stopped, and she was treated with digoxin-specific antibody fragments (*Digibind*) and intravenous fluids. Her serum digoxin levels fell again and the digitalis toxicity disappeared.[4]

In 1995, the manufacturers of clarithromycin had a few other cases on their records of raised digoxin levels in patients following treatment with clarithromycin[4] and there are many other case reports of this interaction in the literature,[5-19] including a case series of 6 patients with end stage renal disease.[20]

A subsequent randomised, placebo-controlled study in 12 healthy subjects confirmed that clarithromycin 250 mg twice daily for 3 days increased the AUC of a single 750-microgram oral dose of digoxin by 70%. The non-glomerular renal clearance of digoxin was reduced by 40%.[21] Intravenous digoxin was much less affected.[21,22] In two further studies in which clarithromycin (500 mg twice daily for 7 days) was used as a positive control, a 57% and 35% increase in the AUC of digoxin was seen.[23,24]

Two studies that prospectively measured digoxin levels in patients before and during clarithromycin therapy found an important increase in all patients of 70%,[25] and from a range of 1 to 1.6 nanograms/mL up to 2.3 to greater than 4 nanograms/mL.[26] In one of these studies, there was a significant correlation between the dose of clarithromycin and the increase in digoxin serum levels.[25]

A case-control study using data from healthcare databases in Ontario from 1994 to 2000 identified 1051 patients who had been admitted to hospital with digoxin toxicity. Of these, 55 patients (5.2%) had been exposed to clarithromycin in the preceding 3 weeks, when compared with just 0.5% of controls, showing about a tenfold increase in risk.[27]

(c) Erythromycin

An elderly woman with a prosthetic heart valve being treated for left ventricular dysfunction with warfarin, furosemide, hydralazine, isosorbide dinitrate and digoxin, was given erythromycin. She took only four 250-mg doses. Four days later her serum digoxin levels were found to have risen to 2.6 nanograms/mL from a normal steady-state range of 1.4 to 1.7 nanograms/mL, and she showed evidence of digitalis toxicity.[28] Another four similar cases have also been reported.[29-31]

A study in a man who was resistant to digoxin found that erythromycin 1 g daily increased the AUC of digoxin by 300%.[32] A neonate given oral digoxin 5 micrograms/kg daily developed digoxin toxicity two days after erythromycin (10 mg three times daily, then 17 mg three times daily) was given. Digoxin levels rose from 1.8 to 16 nanograms/mL.[33]

(d) Josamycin

A case report describes a premature neonate receiving digoxin who had a 50% increase in digoxin levels from 2 to 2.95 nanograms/mL, resulting in bradycardia, and sinoatrial block after being given josamycin for 4 days. This was treated with antidigitalis Fab fragments.[34]

(e) Rokitamycin

Rokitamycin did not affect serum digoxin levels in a study in 10 subjects.[35]

(f) Roxithromycin

A 76-year-old woman taking digoxin and a number of other drugs (enalapril, isosorbide mononitrate, furosemide, diltiazem, glyceryl trinitrate, slow-release potassium, prednisolone, omeprazole, calcitriol) developed signs of digoxin toxicity (nausea, vomiting, first degree heart block) within 4 days of starting to take roxithromycin 150 mg twice daily. Her serum digoxin levels were raised by about fourfold.[36]

(g) Telithromycin

A study in 26 healthy subjects given digoxin 500 micrograms twice daily on the first day followed by 250 micrograms twice daily found that telithromycin 800 mg daily increased the digoxin AUC by 37% and the maximum blood levels by 74%. Trough plasma levels were increased by 21% and remained within the therapeutic range. No signs of digoxin toxicity were observed on ECGs.[37]

A 58-year-old woman taking digoxin 250 micrograms daily developed syncope and malaise after a 5-day course of telithromycin 800 mg daily. Her digoxin levels were 55% higher than her normal baseline level, and there were ECG changes.[38]

Mechanism

It was originally thought that this interaction was due to the effect of the antibacterials on gut flora. Up to 10% of patients receiving oral digoxin excrete it in substantial amounts in the faeces and urine as inactive metabolites (digoxin reduction products or DRPs). This metabolism seems to be the responsibility of the gut flora,[29] in particular *Eubacterium lentum*, which is anaerobic and Gram positive.[31,39] In the presence of antibacterials that inhibit this organism, much more digoxin becomes available for absorption, which results in a marked rise in serum levels. At the same time the inactive metabolites derived from the gut disappear.[29,40] However, it is worth noting that most classes of antibacterials do not appear to interact with digoxin despite inhibiting *E. lentum in vitro*.[39] See 'Digitalis glycosides + Beta-lactam antibacterials', p.913. In addition, more recent data showing that digoxin levels are affected by clarithromycin in all, or the majority, of patients or subjects throw doubt on this theory.

A more plausible explanation for the interaction between digoxin and clarithromycin, and probably also erythromycin, is that the antibacterials inhibit the intestinal[22,41] or renal[14,25] P-glycoprotein transport of digoxin, which would increase the oral bioavailability and reduce the nonglomerular renal clearance respectively. Both mechanisms may be important.[21]

Further, the increased gastric emptying due to erythromycin may also increase the bioavailability of digoxin[42] or digitoxin.[39]

Importance and management

The pharmacokinetic interaction between oral digoxin and clarithromycin is established, and likely to occur in the majority of patients. Digoxin toxicity has been commonly reported. Monitor all patients well for signs of increased digoxin effects when clarithromycin is first given, reducing the digoxin dosage as necessary. Intravenous digoxin is unlikely to be affected to a clinically relevant extent. Telithromycin appears to interact similarly to clarithromycin, and similar advice applies.

Information about azithromycin and erythromycin is limited to a relatively small number of patients, and there is only one report of an interaction between digoxin and josamycin or digoxin and roxithromycin. Until more is known, it would be prudent to monitor all patients well for signs of increased digoxin effects when any of these macrolide antibacterials is first given, reducing the digoxin dosage as necessary. In addition, remember that azithromycin has a long serum half-life (60 hours), which means that it can continue to interact for several days after it has been withdrawn. Rokitamycin appears not to interact.

1. Thalhammer F, Hollenstein UM, Locker GJ, Janata K, Sunder-Plassmann G, Frass M, Burgmann H. Azithromycin-related toxic effects of digitoxin. *Br J Clin Pharmacol* (1998) 45, 91–2.
2. Ten Eick AP, Sallee D, Preminger T, Weiss A, Reed DM. Possible drug interaction between digoxin and azithromycin in a young child. *Clin Drug Invest* (2000) 20, 61–4.
3. Pfizer Ltd. Personal Communication, February 2001.
4. Abbott Labs, Personal communication 1995.
5. Midoneck SR, Etingin OR. Clarithromycin-related toxic effects of digoxin. *N Engl J Med* (1995) 333, 1505.
6. Taylor JW, Gammenthaler SA, Rape JM. Clarithromycin (Biaxin) induced digoxin toxicity. Presented at the American Society of Healthcare Pharmacists Midyear Clinical Meeting, Miami, December 1994.
7. Ford A, Crocker Smith L, Baltch AL, Smith RP. Clarithromycin-induced digoxin toxicity in a patient with AIDS. *Clin Infect Dis* (1995) 21, 1051–2.
8. Brown BA, Wallace RJ, Griffith DE, Warden R. Clarithromycin-associated digoxin toxicity in the elderly. *Clin Infect Dis* (1997) 24, 92–3.
9. Guillemet C, Alt M, Arpin-Bott MP, Imler M. Clarithromycine-digoxine: une interaction méconnue chez certains patients? *Presse Med* (1997) 26, 512.
10. Nordt S, Williams S, Manoguerra A, Clark R. Clarithromycin-induced digoxin poisoning. *J Toxicol Clin Toxicol* (1997) 35, 501–2.
11. Guerriero SE, Ehrenpreis E, Gallagher KL. Two cases of clarithromycin-induced digoxin toxicity. *Pharmacotherapy* (1997) 17, 1035–7.
12. Laberge P, Martineau P. Clarithromycin-induced digoxin intoxication. *Ann Pharmacother* (1997) 31, 999–1001.
13. Trivedi S, Hyman J, Lichstein E. Clarithromycin and digoxin toxicity. *Ann Intern Med* (1998) 128, 604.
14. Wakasugi H, Yano I, Ito T, Hashida T, Futami T, Nohara R, Sasayama S, Inui K-I. Effect of clarithromycin on renal excretion of digoxin: interaction with P-glycoprotein. *Clin Pharmacol Ther* (1998) 64, 123–8.
15. Nawarskas JJ, McCarthy DM, Spinler SA. Digoxin toxicity secondary to clarithromycin therapy. *Ann Pharmacother* (1997) 31, 864–6.
16. Nordt SP, Williams SR, Manoguerra AS, Clark RF. Clarithromycin induced digoxin toxicity. *J Accid Emerg Med* (1998) 15, 194–5.
17. Juurlink DN, Ito S. Comment: clarithromycin-digoxin interaction. *Ann Pharmacother* (1999) 33, 1375–6.
18. Kiran N, Azam S, Dhakam S. Clarithromycin induced digoxin toxicity: Case report and review. *J Pakistan Med Assoc* (2004) 54, 440–41.
19. Gooderham MJ, Bolli P, Fernandez PG. Concomitant digoxin toxicity and warfarin interaction in a patient receiving clarithromycin. *Ann Pharmacother* (1999) 33, 796–9.
20. Hirata S, Izumi S, Furukubo T, Ota M, Fujita M, Yamakawa T, Hasegawa I, Ohtani H, Sawada Y. Interactions between clarithromycin and digoxin in patients with end-stage renal disease. *Int J Clin Pharmacol Ther* (2005) 43, 30–36.
21. Rengelshausen J, Göggelmann C, Burhenne J, Riedel K-D, Ludwig J, Weiss J, Mikus G, Walter-Sack I, Haefeli WE. Contribution of increased oral bioavailability and reduced nonglomerular renal clearance of digoxin to the digoxin–clarithromycin interaction. *Br J Clin Pharmacol* (2003) 56, 32–8.
22. Tsutsumi K, Kotegawa T, Kuranari M, Otani Y, Morimoto T, Matsuki S, Nakano S. The effect of erythromycin and clarithromycin on the pharmacokinetics of intravenous digoxin in healthy volunteers. *J Clin Pharmacol* (2002) 42, 1159–64.
23. Gurley BJ, Swain A, Barone GW, Williams DK, Breen P, Yates CR, Stuart LB, Hubbard MA, Tong Y, Cheboyina S. Effect of goldenseal (*Hydrastis canadensis*) and kava kava (*Piper methysticum*) supplementation on digoxin pharmacokinetics in humans. *Drug Metab Dispos* (2007) 35, 240–5.
24. Gurley BJ, Barone GW, Williams DK, Carrier J, Breen P, Yates CR, Song P-f, Hubbard MA, Tong Y, Cheboyina S. Effect of milk thistle (*Silybum marianum*) and black cohosh (*Cimicifuga racemosa*) supplementation on digoxin pharmacokinetics in humans. *Drug Metab Dispos* (2006) 34, 69–74.
25. Tanaka H, Matsumoto K, Ueno K, Kodama M, Yoneda K, Katayama Y, Miyatake K. Effect of clarithromycin on steady-state digoxin concentrations. *Ann Pharmacother* (2003) 37, 178–81.
26. Zapater P, Reus S, Tello A, Torrús D, Pérez-Mateo M, Horga JF. A prospective study of the clarithromycin–digoxin interaction in elderly patients. *J Antimicrob Chemother* (2002) 50, 601–6.
27. Juurlink DN, Mamdani M, Kopp A, Laupacis A, Redelmeier DA. Drug-drug interactions among elderly patients hospitalized for drug toxicity. *JAMA* (2003) 289, 1652–8.
28. Friedman HS, Bonventre MV. Erythromycin-induced digoxin toxicity. *Chest* (1982) 82, 202.
29. Lindenbaum J, Rund DG, Butler VP, Tse-Eng D, Saha JR. Inactivation of digoxin by the gut flora: reversal by antibiotic therapy. *N Engl J Med* (1981) 305, 789–94.
30. Maxwell DL, Gilmour-White SK, Hall MR. Digoxin toxicity due to interaction of digoxin with erythromycin. *BMJ* (1989) 298, 572.
31. Morton MR, Cooper JW. Erythromycin-induced digoxin toxicity. *DICP Ann Pharmacother* (1989) 23, 668–70.
32. Nørregaard-Hansen K, Klitgaard NA, Pedersen KE. The significance of the enterohepatic circulation on the metabolism of digoxin in patients with the ability of intestinal conversion of the drug. *Acta Med Scand* (1986) 220, 89–92.
33. Coudray S, Janoly A, Belkacem-Kahlouli A, Bourhis Y, Bleyzac N, Bourgeois J, Putet G, Aulagner G. L'érythromycine responsable d'une intoxication sévère par la digoxine dans un service de réanimation néonatale. *J Pharm Clin* (2001) 20, 129–31.
34. Cambonie G, Sabatier E, Guillaumont S, Masson F, Charbit J, Pidoux O, Hillaire-Buys D, Picaud JC. Digoxin-Josamycin: a dangerous drug interaction in children. *Arch Pediatr* (2006) 13, 1118–20.
35. Ishioka T. Effect of a new macrolide antibiotic 3″-O-propionyl-leucomycin A_5 (Rokitamycin) on serum concentrations of theophylline and digoxin in the elderly. *Acta Ther* (1987) 13, 17–23.
36. Corallo CE, Rogers IR. Roxithromycin-induced digoxin toxicity. *Med J Aust* (1996) 165, 433–4.
37. Montay G, Shi J, Leroy B, Bhargava V. Effects of telithromycin on the pharmacokinetics of digoxin in healthy men. *Intersci Conf Antimicrob Agents Chemother* (2002) 42, 28.
38. Nenciu LM, Laberge P, Thirion DJG. Telithromycin-induced digoxin toxicity and electrocardiographic changes. *Pharmacotherapy* (2006) 26, 872–6.
39. Ten Eick AP, Reed MD. Hidden dangers of coadministration of antibiotics and digoxin in children: focus on azithromycin. *Curr Ther Res* (2000) 61, 148–60.
40. Lindenbaum J, Tse-Eng D, Butler VP, Rund DG. Urinary excretion of reduced metabolites of digoxin. *Am J Med* (1981) 71, 67–74.
41. Berndt A, Gramatté T, Kirch W. Digoxin-erythromycin interaction: in vitro evidence for competition for intestinal P-glycoprotein. *Eur J Clin Pharmacol* (1996) 50, 538.
42. Sutton A, Pilot M-A. Digoxin toxicity and erythromycin. *BMJ* (1989) 298, 1101.

Digitalis glycosides + Medroxyprogesterone acetate or Megestrol

Doses of medroxyprogesterone acetate or megestrol used for malignant disease do not appear to interact with digitoxin to a clinically relevant extent.

Clinical evidence, mechanism, importance and management

Steady-state **digitoxin** levels were monitored in 3 patients before and after 5 weeks of treatment with oral medroxyprogesterone acetate 500 mg twice daily or megestrol 160 mg daily. Only small and clinically irrelevant changes in **digitoxin** levels and clearance were seen.[1] For the possible effect of HRT including medroxyprogesterone on digitalis, see 'Digitalis glycosides + HRT', p.928.

1. Lundgren S, Kvinnsland S, Utaaker E, Bakke O, Ueland PM. Effect of oral high-dose progestins on the disposition of antipyrine, digitoxin, and warfarin in patients with advanced breast cancer. *Cancer Chemother Pharmacol* (1986) 18, 270–5.

Digitalis glycosides + Methyldopa

Methyldopa does not appear to affect serum digoxin levels, but marked bradycardia has been seen in two elderly women given both drugs.

Clinical evidence

Methyldopa 250 mg daily had no effect on the steady-state serum levels of **digoxin** 250 micrograms daily in 8 healthy subjects.[1]

However, two elderly women with hypertension and left ventricular failure developed marked bradycardia when they were given **digoxin** with methyldopa 750 mg or 3.75 g daily but not when they were given **digoxin** alone. Average heart rates were 50 and 48 bpm while minimum heart rates were 32 and 38 bpm, respectively. They were subsequently discharged taking **digoxin** and hydralazine with heart rates within the normal range.[2]

Mechanism

Uncertain. Both digoxin and methyldopa[3] can cause some bradycardia, but these effects seem to have been more than simply the sum of the individual drug effects on the autonomic nervous system.[2]

Importance and management

Information is limited but it would seem that concurrent use need not be avoided, but be aware that on rare occasions undesirable bradycardia has occurred.

1. May CA, Vlasses PH, Rocci ML, Rotmensch HH, Swanson BN, Tannenbaum RP, Ferguson RK, Abrams WB. Methyldopa does not alter the disposition of digoxin. *J Clin Pharmacol* (1984) 24, 386–9.
2. Davis JC, Reiffel JA, Bigger JT. Sinus node dysfunction caused by methyldopa and digoxin. *JAMA* (1981) 245, 1241–3.
3. Lund-Johansen P. Hemodynamic changes in long term α-methyldopa therapy of essential hypertension. *Acta Med Scand* (1972) 192, 221–6.

Digitalis glycosides + Metoclopramide

The serum levels of digoxin may be reduced by about one-third if metoclopramide is given with slowly dissolving forms of digoxin. No interaction is likely with digoxin in liquid form or in fast-dissolving preparations.

Clinical evidence

A study in 11 patients taking slowly dissolving **digoxin** tablets (*Orion*) found that metoclopramide 10 mg three times a day for 10 days reduced the serum **digoxin** levels by 36%, from 0.72 to 0.46 nanograms/mL.[1] The **digoxin** concentrations rose to their former levels when the metoclopramide was withdrawn.

Another study in healthy subjects found metoclopramide 10 mg three times daily caused a 19% reduction in the AUC of **digoxin** and a 27% reduction in peak serum **digoxin** levels (**digoxin** formulation not stated).[2] Yet another study in healthy subjects clearly showed that metoclopramide decreased the absorption of **digoxin** from tablets (*Lanoxin*) but not capsules (*Lanoxicaps*).[3]

Mechanism

It would seem[4-6] that the metoclopramide increases the motility of the gut to such an extent that full dissolution and absorption of some digoxin formulations does not occur.

Importance and management

Information is very limited, but the interaction seems to be established. It is not likely to occur with solid form, fast-dissolving digoxin preparations (e.g. liquid-filled capsules) or digoxin in liquid form, but only with those preparations which are slowly dissolving (i.e. some tablet formulations). A reduction in digoxin levels of one-third could result in under-digitalisation. There seems to be no information about **digitoxin**.

1. Manninen V, Apajalahti A, Melin J, Karesoja M. Altered absorption of digoxin in patients given propantheline and metoclopramide. *Lancet* (1973) i, 398–400.
2. Kirch W, Janisch HD, Santos SR, Duhrsen U, Dylewicz P, Ohnhaus EE. Effect of cisapride and metoclopramide on digoxin bioavailability. *Eur J Drug Metab Pharmacokinet* (1986) 11, 249–50.
3. Johnson BF, Bustrack JA, Urbach DR, Hull JH, Marwaha R. Effect of metoclopramide on digoxin absorption from tablets and capsules. *Clin Pharmacol Ther* (1984) 36, 724–30.
4. Manninen V, Apajalahti A, Simonen H, Reissell P. Effect of propantheline and metoclopramide on the absorption of digoxin. *Lancet* (1973) i, 1118–9.
5. Medin S, Nyberg L. Effect of propantheline and metoclopramide on the absorption of digoxin. *Lancet* (1973) i, 1393.
6. Fraser EJ, Leach RH, Poston JW, Bold AM, Culank LS, Lipede AB. Dissolution-rates and bioavailability of digoxin tablets. *Lancet* (1973) i, 1393.

Digitalis glycosides + Mexiletine

Serum digoxin levels are not significantly altered by mexiletine.

Clinical evidence, mechanism, importance and management

Mexiletine 200 mg every 8 hours for 4 days slightly reduced the serum levels of **digoxin** 250 micrograms daily from 0.32 to 0.27 nanograms/mL in 10 healthy subjects.[1] Two other studies in a total of 17 patients[2,3] confirmed that mexiletine does not significantly affect serum **digoxin** levels.

1. Saris SD, Lowenthal DT, Affrime MB. Steady-state digoxin concentration during oral mexiletine administration. *Curr Ther Res* (1983) 34, 662–66.
2. Leahey EB, Reiffel JA, Giardina E-GV, Bigger T. The effect of quinidine and other oral antiarrhythmic drugs on serum digoxin. *Ann Intern Med* (1980) 92, 605–8.
3. Day T, Hunt D. Interaction between mexiletine and digoxin. *Med J Aust* (1983) 2, 630.

Digitalis glycosides + Mizolastine

Mizolastine can cause a small but clinically irrelevant rise in serum digoxin levels.

Clinical evidence, mechanism, importance and management

A placebo-controlled, crossover study in 12 healthy subjects found that mizolastine 10 mg daily for a week caused a 17% increase in the maximum serum levels of **digoxin** 250 micrograms daily. The **digoxin** AUC and half-life were unchanged and the haemodynamic parameters measured (blood pressure, ECG) were unaltered.[1] No special precautions would seem necessary during concurrent use.

1. Chaufour S, Le Coz F, Denolle T, Dubruc C, Cimarosti I, Deschamps C, Ulliac N, Delhotal-Landes B, Rosenweig P. Lack of effect of mizolastine on the safety and pharmacokinetics of digoxin administered orally in repeated doses to healthy volunteers. *Int J Clin Pharmacol Ther* (1998) 36, 286–91.

Digitalis glycosides + Moclobemide

Moclobemide had no clinically relevant effect on the pharmacokinetics of beta-acetyldigoxin.

Clinical evidence, mechanism, importance and management

A study in 14 patients with decompensated heart failure given an individualised dose of **beta-acetyldigoxin** for 2 weeks found that moclobemide 100 mg three times daily given for 8 days caused a non-significant 14% reduction (from 0.99 to 0.85 nanograms/mL) in plasma **beta-acetyldigoxin** levels. No adverse effects attributable to an interaction were seen.[1] No special precautions appear to be required during concurrent use of acetyldigoxin and moclobemide.

1. Amrein R, Güntert TW, Dingemanse J, Lorscheid T, Stabl M, Schmid-Burgk W. Interactions of moclobemide with concomitantly administered medication: evidence from pharmacological and clinical studies. *Psychopharmacology (Berl)* (1992) 106, S24–S31.

Digitalis glycosides + Montelukast

Montelukast does not affect the pharmacokinetics of digoxin.

Clinical evidence, mechanism, importance and management

In a randomised study in 11 healthy subjects montelukast 10 mg was given for 12 days with a single 500-microgram dose of digoxin on day 7. It was found that the pharmacokinetic profile of the digoxin was unchanged by the montelukast.[1] No special precautions are needed if both drugs are used concurrently.

1. Depre M, Van Hecken A, Verbesselt R, Wynants K, De Lelepeire I, Freeman A, Holland S, Shahane A, Gertz B, De Schepper PJ. Effect of multiple doses of montelukast, a CysLT1 receptor agonist, on digoxin pharmacokinetics in healthy volunteers. *J Clin Pharmacol* (1999) 39, 941–4.

Digitalis glycosides + Moracizine

Moracizine does not significantly increase serum digoxin levels in patients with normal renal function. However, some adverse conduction effects have been seen.

Clinical evidence

Thirteen patients taking **digoxin** 125 to 250 micrograms daily showed a non-significant rise in their serum **digoxin** levels of 10 to 15% when they were given moracizine 10 mg/kg daily in three divided doses for 2 weeks. Nine patients taking **digoxin** and moracizine for 1 to 6 months had no significant changes in their serum **digoxin** levels.[1]

No changes in the pharmacokinetics of **digoxin** were seen in a single-dose study of intravenous **digoxin** and moracizine in 9 healthy subjects[2] or in a study in patients receiving maintenance treatment with **digoxin** over a 13-day period. However, cardiac arrhythmias (AV junctional rhythm and heart block) were seen, which resolved when the moracizine was stopped.[3]

Mechanism

Not established. There does not appear to be a pharmacokinetic interaction between moracizine and digoxin. Concurrent use can cause a significant increase in the PR interval and QRS duration, which can result in AV block.[4]

Importance and management

Although no clinically important changes in serum digoxin levels appear to occur during concurrent use, the occurrence of arrhythmias in a few patients indicates that good monitoring is advisable. It has been pointed out that the additive effects of both drugs on intranodal and intraventricular conduction may be excessive in some patients with heart disease.[4] More study is needed.

1. Kennedy HL, Sprague MK, Redd RM, Wiens RD, Blum RI, Buckingham TA. Serum digoxin concentrations during ethmozine antiarrhythmic therapy. *Am Heart J* (1986) 111, 667–72.
2. MacFarland RT, Moeller VR, Pieniaszek HJ, Whitney CC, Marcus FI. Assessment of the potential pharmacokinetic interaction between digoxin and ethmozine. *J Clin Pharmacol* (1985) 25, 138–43.
3. Antman EM, Arnold JMO, Friedman PL, White H, Bosak M, Smith TW. Drug interactions with cardiac glycosides: evaluation of a possible digoxin-ethmozine pharmacokinetic interaction. *J Cardiovasc Pharmacol* (1987) 9, 622–7.
4. Siddoway LA, Schwartz SL, Barbey JT, Woosley RL. Clinical pharmacokinetics of moricizine. *Am J Cardiol* (1990) 65, 21D–25D.

Digitalis glycosides + Nateglinide or Repaglinide

The pharmacokinetics of nateglinide and digoxin are not altered when they are given together. Repaglinide does not affect the pharmacokinetics of digoxin.

Clinical evidence, mechanism, importance and management

(a) Nateglinide

A crossover study in 12 healthy subjects found that when a single 1-mg dose of **digoxin** was given with the first dose of nateglinide 120 mg three times daily for 2 days, there were no changes in the pharmacokinetics of **digoxin**, nor were the pharmacokinetics of nateglinide altered by the **digoxin**.[1]

(b) Repaglinide

A crossover, multiple-dose study in 14 healthy subjects found that repaglinide 2 mg three times daily before meals had no effect on the pharmacokinetics of **digoxin** 250 micrograms daily. Concurrent use was well tolerated.[2]

1. Zhou H, Walter YH, Smith H, Devineni D, McLeod JF. Nateglinide, a new mealtime glucose regulator. Lack of pharmacokinetic interaction with digoxin in healthy volunteers. *Clin Drug Invest* (2000) 19, 465–71.
2. Hatorp V, Thomsen MS. Drug interaction studies with repaglinide: repaglinide on digoxin or theophylline pharmacokinetics and cimetidine on repaglinide pharmacokinetics. *J Clin Pharmacol* (2000) 40, 184–92.

Digitalis glycosides + Nefazodone

Nefazodone causes a moderate increase in serum digoxin levels but this is of uncertain clinical importance. Digoxin does not appear to affect the pharmacokinetics of nefazodone.

Clinical evidence

Eighteen healthy subjects were given **digoxin** 200 micrograms daily for 8 days, then nefazodone 200 mg twice daily for 8 days, and then both drugs together for 8 days. Nefazodone increased the AUC of **digoxin** by 15%, and increased the peak and trough serum levels of **digoxin** by 29% and 27%, respectively. However, no clinically significant changes in ECG measurements occurred (PR, QRS and QT intervals), nor was the heart rate nor any other vital sign altered. The pharmacokinetics of the nefazodone were unchanged.[1]

Mechanism

Not understood.

Importance and management

This interaction appears to be established, but its clinical importance is uncertain. The increase in the AUC of digoxin is modest, and would not generally be expected to be clinically significant, although some effect may be seen in patients with digoxin levels at the higher end of the therapeutic range. It may be prudent to monitor for symptoms of digoxin excess (e.g. bradycardia) and take digoxin levels if necessary.

1. Dockens RC, Greene DS, Barbhaiya RH. Assessment of pharmacokinetic and pharmacodynamic drug interactions between nefazodone and digoxin in healthy male volunteers. *J Clin Pharmacol* (1996) 36, 160–7.

Digitalis glycosides + Neuromuscular blockers

Serious cardiac arrhythmias can develop in patients receiving digitalis glycosides who are given suxamethonium (succinylcholine) or pancuronium.

Clinical evidence

Eight out of 17 digitalised patients (anaesthetised with thiamylal and then maintained with nitrous oxide and oxygen) developed serious ventricular arrhythmias following the intravenous injection of **suxamethonium (succinylcholine)** 40 to 100 mg. Four out of the 8 patients reverted to their previous rhythm when they were given tubocurarine 15 to 30 mg, with one patient returning to a regular nodal rhythm from ventricular tachycardia.[1]

Of the other 9 patients, 3 had immediate and definite ST-T wave changes, and the remaining 6 had no demonstrable changes.[1] There are other reports of this interaction,[2-4] including one that describes sinus tachycardia and atrial flutter in 6 out of 18 patients taking **digoxin** after they were given **pancuronium**.[4]

Mechanism

Not understood. One possibility is that the suxamethonium may cause the rapid removal of potassium from the myocardial cells. Another idea is that it affects catecholamine-releasing cholinergic receptors.

Importance and management

Information is limited but the interaction appears to be established. Suxamethonium should be used with great caution in patients taking digitalis glycosides. Similarly, caution would seem appropriate with pancuronium.

1. Dowdy EG, Fabian LW. Ventricular arrhythmias induced by succinylcholine in digitalized patients: A preliminary report. *Anesth Analg* (1963) 42, 501–13.
2. Pérez HR. Cardiac arrhythmia after succinylcholine. *Anesth Analg* (1970) 49, 33–8.
3. Smith RB, Petrusack J. Succinylcholine, digitalis, and hypercalcaemia: a case report. *Anesth Analg* (1972) 51, 202–5.
4. Bartolone RS, Rao TLK. Dysrhythmias following muscle relaxant administration in patients receiving digitalis. *Anesthesiology* (1983) 58, 567–9.

Digitalis glycosides + NSAIDs

Diclofenac and indometacin can cause potentially toxic rises in digitalis glycoside levels, while azapropazone, fenbufen and tiaprofenic acid raise levels to a lesser degree. Two studies found that ibuprofen raised serum digoxin levels, whereas another found no evidence of an interaction. Isoxicam, ketoprofen, lornoxicam, meloxicam, nimesulide, piroxicam, and rofecoxib do not appear to interact significantly with digoxin. In contrast, phenylbutazone appears to lower plasma digitalis glycoside levels. NSAIDs can cause a deterioration in renal function, which could result in digoxin toxicity.

Clinical evidence

(a) Azapropazone

In 8 arthritic patients azapropazone 900 mg daily did not significantly alter the AUC of a single 500-microgram intravenous dose of **digitoxin**, but its mean half-life was increased by about 10%. Two of the patients showed individual half-life increases of almost one-third.[1]

(b) Diclofenac

A study in 7 healthy subjects found that diclofenac 100 mg daily for 10 days increased the serum levels of **digoxin** by 29%.[2] Another study in 6 healthy subjects similarly found that diclofenac 50 mg three times daily raised the serum **digoxin** levels by about one-third.[3] **Digitoxin** 100 micrograms had no effect on the plasma levels of diclofenac 50 mg twice daily in 8 subjects; **digitoxin** levels were not reported.[4]

(c) Etoricoxib

A study in healthy subjects given **digoxin** found that the addition of etoricoxib 120 mg daily for 10 days did not alter the steady-state AUC of **digoxin** or its renal elimination, but the maximum serum **digoxin** levels were increased by about 33%.[5] This change is unlikely to be clinically relevant in most patients but it might possibly affect a very small number whose **digoxin** levels are already high.

(d) Fenbufen

Fenbufen 900 mg daily was found to cause an insignificant rise in the serum levels of **digoxin**.[6]

(e) Ibuprofen

The serum **digoxin** levels of 12 patients were reported to have risen by about 60% after they were given at least 1.6 g of ibuprofen daily for a week. However, after a month the **digoxin** levels had returned to their former amount.[7] These findings may be unreliable because half of the patients were not satisfactorily compliant with treatment. Another study found that ibuprofen 1.2 g daily for 10 days raised the serum **digoxin** levels of 9 healthy subjects by 25%.[2] Yet another study found that ibuprofen 600 mg three times daily for 10 days had no effect on steady-state serum **digoxin** levels of 8 patients.[8]

(f) Indometacin

1. Neonates. A study in 11 premature neonates (gestational age 25 to 33 weeks) given **digoxin** showed that when they were given indometacin (mean total dose of 320 micrograms/kg over 12 to 24 hours) for patent ductus arteriosus, their mean serum **digoxin** levels rose on average by 40%. The **digoxin** was stopped in 5 of them because serum levels were potentially toxic.[9] This confirms the observation of digitalis toxicity in 3 similarly treated premature neonates,[10] and of toxic serum **digoxin** levels in another neonate.[11] A further report describes very high **digoxin** levels (8.2 nanograms/mL) without symptoms of toxicity in a full-term neonate given indometacin.[12]

2. Adults. Indometacin 50 mg three times daily for 10 days increased steady-state **digoxin** levels of 10 patients by about 40% (from 0.57 to 0.8 nanograms/mL), with a range of 0 to 100%.[8] Indometacin 150 mg daily for 10 days increased the serum **digoxin** levels of 9 healthy subjects by 25%.[2] In yet another study, a 60% increase in digoxin levels was seen with indometacin 150 mg daily.[13] This contrasts with the results of single-dose studies in 2 groups of 6 healthy adult subjects[14,15] who were given a 4-hour infusion of **digoxin**. Both studies suggested that no interaction occurs with indometacin.

(g) Isoxicam

Isoxicam 200 mg daily did not affect the steady-state plasma levels of 12 healthy subjects taking **beta-acetyldigoxin**.[16] This confirms the findings of a previous study.[17]

(h) Ketoprofen

Ketoprofen 50 mg four times daily for 4 days had no effect on the serum **digoxin** levels of 12 patients.[18]

(i) Lornoxicam

In 12 healthy subjects the concurrent use of lornoxicam 4 mg twice daily for 14 days and **digoxin** 250 micrograms daily had only a small effect on the pharmacokinetics of each drug. The apparent clearance of the **digoxin** was decreased by 14% while the maximum serum level of the lornoxicam was decreased by 21% and its elimination half-life increased by 36%.[19]

(j) Meloxicam

Meloxicam 15 mg daily for 8 days had no effect on the pharmacokinetics of **digoxin** (given as **beta-acetyldigoxin**) in 12 healthy subjects.[20]

(k) Nimesulide

Nimesulide 100 mg twice daily for 7 days had little effect on the pharmacokinetics of **digoxin** 250 micrograms daily in 9 patients with mild heart failure. No major change in their clinical condition occurred.[21]

(l) Phenylbutazone

Phenylbutazone 200 or 400 mg daily halved the plasma levels of **digitoxin** 100 micrograms daily in 6 patients, on two separate occasions. **Digitoxin** levels returned to their former values within roughly the same period of time after phenylbutazone was withdrawn.[22] A similar response has been described elsewhere in one patient.[23] Six healthy subjects showed an a decrease of about 20% in their serum **digoxin** levels while taking phenylbutazone 200 mg three times daily for 4 days.[3] In contrast, one study found no alteration in the levels of **digoxin** when it was given with phenylbutazone 600 mg daily.[13]

(m) Piroxicam

In 10 patients taking **digoxin** for mild heart failure, piroxicam 10 or 20 mg daily for 15 days had no effect on the steady-state **digoxin** levels, nor were consistent effects seen on the pharmacokinetics of **digoxin**.[24] Piroxicam 20 mg daily for 10 days was found to have no effect on serum **digoxin** levels in 6 healthy subjects.[2]

(n) Rofecoxib

Rofecoxib 75 mg once daily did not cause significant changes in the plasma pharmacokinetics or renal elimination of single 500-microgram doses of **digoxin** elixir.[25]

(o) Tiaprofenic acid

Tiaprofenic acid 200 mg three times daily for 10 days caused a non-significant 15% rise, from 0.97 to 1.12 nanograms/mL, in the serum **digoxin** levels of 12 healthy subjects.[26]

Mechanism

The reasons for the altered digoxin pharmacokinetics in some of the studies are not clear. However, in the studies in neonates, the elevated digoxin levels were clearly related to an indometacin-induced deterioration in renal function.[9,11,12] It should be noted that all NSAIDs have the potential to cause renal impairment.

It is suggested that phenylbutazone lowers digitoxin levels by increasing its rate of metabolism by the liver.[22]

Importance and management

The interaction between digoxin and **indometacin** seems established in neonates, but documentation is limited. It has been suggested that the digoxin dosage should be halved if indometacin is given to premature or full-term infants and the serum digoxin levels and urinary output monitored. Also be alert for moderate increases in serum digoxin levels in adults if indometacin is given. In adults it may be sufficient to monitor pulse rate (for bradycardia) and take digoxin levels if an interaction is suspected. The interaction between digoxin and **diclofenac** is less well established and its clinical importance is somewhat uncertain as the rises in digoxin levels were mostly modest. It would be prudent to monitor concurrent use (e.g. for bradycardia) and monitor digoxin levels as necessary. Adjust the digoxin dosage accordingly.

The importance of the interaction with azapropazone, etoricoxib, fenbufen and tiaprofenic acid is not known. In most cases changes to doses are unlikely to be necessary, but remain aware of the potential for an interaction. No special precautions would appear to be necessary with isoxicam, ketoprofen, meloxicam, piroxicam, and rofecoxib. More study is needed in most cases, but especially with ibuprofen, where the evidence is conflicting (although note that the one study reporting a significant interaction was poor).

The interaction with phenylbutazone appears to be in direct contrast to that with the other NSAIDs, but documentation is limited. The dosage of digoxin and digitoxin may possibly need to be increased to avoid under-digitalisation if phenylbutazone is added to established treatment. Monitor concurrent use well.

1. Faust-Tinnefeldt G, Gilfrich HJ. Digitoxin-Kinetik unter antirheumatischer Therapie mit Azapropazon. *Arzneimittelforschung* (1977) 27, 2009–11.
2. Isbary J, Doering W, König E. Der Einfluβ von Tiaprofensäure auf die Digoxinkonzentration im Serum (DKS) im Vergleich zu anderen Antirheumatika (AR). *Z Rheumatol* (1982) 41, 164.
3. Rau R, Georgiopoulos G, Neumann P, Gross D. Die Beeinflussung des Digoxinblutspiegels durch Antirheumatika. *Akt Rheum* (1980) 5, 349–58.
4. Schumacher A, Faust-Tinnefeldt G, Geissler HE, Gilfrich HJ, Mutschler E. Untersuchungen potentieller Interaktionen von Diclofenac-Natrium (Voltaren) mit einem Antazidum und mit Digitoxin. *Therapiewoche* (1983) 33, 2619–25.
5. Arcoxia (Etoricoxib). Merck Sharp & Dohme Ltd. UK Summary of product characteristics, January 2007.
6. Dunky A, Eberi R. Anti-inflammatory effects of a new anti-rheumatic drug fenbufen in rheumatoid arthritis. XIV Int Congr Rheumatology, San Francisco, 1977. Abstract No 379.

7. Quattrocchi FP, Robinson JD, Curry RW, Grieco ML, Schulman SG. The effect of ibuprofen on serum digoxin concentrations. *Drug Intell Clin Pharm* (1983) 17, 286–8.
8. Jørgensen HS, Christensen HR, Kampmann JP. Interaction between digoxin and indomethacin or ibuprofen. *Br J Clin Pharmacol* (1991) 31, 108–110.
9. Koren G, Zarfin Y, Perlman M, MacLeod SM. Effects of indomethacin on digoxin pharmacokinetics in preterm infants. *Pediatr Pharmacol* (1984) 4, 25–30.
10. Mayes LC, Boerth RC. Digoxin-indomethacin interaction. *Pediatr Res* (1980) 14, 469.
11. Schimmel MS, Inwood RL, Eidelman AI, Eylath U. Toxic digitalis levels associated with indomethacin therapy in a neonate. *Clin Pediatr (Phila)* (1980) 19, 768–9.
12. Haig GM, Brookfield EG. Increase in serum digoxin concentrations after indomethacin therapy in a full-term neonate. *Pharmacotherapy* (1992) 12, 334–6.
13. Halawa B, Mazurek W. Interakcja digoksyny i niektórych niesteroidowych leków przeciwzapalnych, kwasu acetylosalicylowego i nifedipiny. *Pol Tyg Lek* (1982) 37, 1475–6.
14. Finch MB, Johnston GD, Kelly JG, McDevitt DG. Pharmacokinetics of digoxin alone and in the presence of indomethacin therapy. *Br J Clin Pharmacol* (1984) 17, 353–5.
15. Sziegoleit W, Weiss M, Fahr A, Förster W. Are serum levels and cardiac effects of digoxin influenced by indometacin? *Pharmazie* (1986) 41, 340–2.
16. Zöller B, Engel HJ, Faust-Tinnefeldt G, Gilfrich HJ, Zimmer M. Untersuchungen zur Wechselwirkung von Isoxicam und Digoxin. *Z Rheumatol* (1984) 43, 182–4.
17. Chlud K. Zur Frage der Interaktionen in der Rheumatherapie: Untersuchungen von Isoxicam und Glibenclamid bei Diabetien mit rheumatischen Enkrankungen. *Tempo Med* (1983) 12A, 15–18.
18. Lewis GR, Jacobs SG, Vavra I. Effect of ketoprofen on serum digoxin concentrations. *Curr Ther Res* (1985) 38, 494–9.
19. Ravic M, Johnston A, Turner P. Clinical pharmacological studies of some possible interactions of lornoxicam with other drugs. *Postgrad Med J* (1990) 66 (Suppl 4), S30–S34.
20. Degner FL, Heinzel G, Narjes H, Türck D. The effect of meloxicam on the pharmacokinetics of β-acetyl-digoxin. *Br J Clin Pharmacol* (1995) 40, 486–8.
21. Baggio E, Maraffi F, Montalto C, Nava ML, Torti L, Casciarri I. A clinical assessment of the potential for pharmacological interaction between nimesulide and digoxin in patients with heart failure. *Drugs* (1993) 46 (Suppl 1), 91–4.
22. Wirth KE. Arzneimittelinteraktionen bei der Anwendung herzwirksamer Glykoside. *Med Welt* (1981) 32, 234–8.
23. Solomon HM, Reich S, Spirt N, Abrams WB. Interactions between digitoxin and other drugs *in vitro* and *in vivo*. *Ann N Y Acad Sci* (1971) 179, 362–9.
24. Rau R. Interaction study of piroxicam with digoxin. In 'Piroxicam: A New Non-steroidal Anti-inflammatory Agent.' Proc IXth Eur Cong Rheumatol, Wiesbaden, September 1979, pp 41–6. Academy Professional Information Services, NY.
25. Schwartz JI, De Smet M, Larson PJ, Verbesselt R, Ebel DL, Lins R, Lens S, Porras AG, Gertz BJ. Effect of rofecoxib on the pharmacokinetics of digoxin in healthy volunteers. *J Clin Pharmacol* (2001) 41, 107–112.
26. Doering W, Isbary J. Der Einfluß von Tiaprofensäure auf die Digoxin-konzentration im Serum. *Arzneimittelforschung* (1983) 33, 167–8.

Digitalis glycosides + Orlistat

Orlistat appears not to interact with digoxin.

Clinical evidence, mechanism, importance and management

Orlistat 120 mg three times daily for 6 days was found to have no effect on the pharmacokinetics of a single 400-microgram oral dose of **digoxin** (in soft gelatin capsules) in 12 healthy subjects.[1] This suggests that an approximate 30% reduction in dietary fat absorption induced by orlistat should not change the efficacy of **digoxin** and that no special precautions will be needed in patients who are given both drugs.

1. Melia AT, Zhi J, Koss-Twardy SG, Min BH, Smith BL, Freundlich NL, Arora S, Passe SM. The influence of reduced dietary fat absorption induced by orlistat on the pharmacokinetics of digoxin in healthy volunteers. *J Clin Pharmacol* (1995) 35, 840–3.

Digitalis glycosides + Penicillamine

Serum digoxin levels can be reduced by penicillamine.

Clinical evidence

In 10 patients, penicillamine 1 g daily taken 2 hours after an oral dose of **digoxin**, reduced the serum **digoxin** levels measured 2, 4 and 6 hours later, by 13%, 20% and 39%, respectively. In 10 other patients similarly treated but given **digoxin** intravenously, the serum **digoxin** levels measured 4 and 6 hours later were reduced by 23% and 64%, respectively.[1] The same authors have also reported this interaction in children.[2]

Mechanism

Unknown.

Importance and management

Information seems to be limited to the reports cited. Patients taking digoxin should be checked for signs of under-digitalisation if penicillamine is added. Information about digitoxin appears to be lacking.

1. Moezzi B, Fatourechi V, Khozain R, Eslami B. The effect of penicillamine on serum digoxin levels. *Jpn Heart J* (1978) 19, 366–70.
2. Moezzi B, Khozein R, Pooymehr F, Shakibi JG. Reversal of digoxin-induced changes in erythrocyte electrolyte concentrations by penicillamine in children. *Jpn Heart J* (1980) 21, 335–9.

Digitalis glycosides + Pinaverium

Plasma digoxin levels are not affected by pinaverium in patients taking either beta-acetyldigoxin or metildigoxin.

Clinical evidence, mechanism, importance and management

A study in 25 patients, taking either **beta-acetyldigoxin** or **metildigoxin** for congestive heart failure, found that pinaverium 50 mg three times daily for 12 days had no significant effect on their plasma digoxin levels.[1] No special precautions seem necessary on concurrent use.

1. Weitzel O, Seidel G, Engelbert S, Berksoy M, Eberhardt G, Bode R. Investigation of possible interaction between pinaverium bromide and digoxin. *Curr Med Res Opin* (1983) 8, 600–2.

Digitalis glycosides + Pioglitazone or Rosiglitazone

Pioglitazone and rosiglitazone do not affect the pharmacokinetics of digoxin, but they may adversely affect cardiac function in patients with cardiac failure.

Clinical evidence

(a) Pioglitazone

In healthy subjects, pioglitazone did not alter the steady-state pharmacokinetics of **digoxin** 250 micrograms daily.[1,2]

(b) Rosiglitazone

A study in healthy subjects found that rosiglitazone 8 mg once daily for 14 days had no effect on the steady-state pharmacokinetics of **digoxin** 375 micrograms daily. Concurrent use was safe and well tolerated (aside from one patient who withdrew because of a rash).[3]

Mechanism

Pioglitazone and rosiglitazone can cause fluid retention, which may cause or exacerbate heart failure.

Importance and management

No pharmacokinetic interaction occurs. However, the US manufacturers advise caution with the use of pioglitazone or rosiglitazone in those with a history of heart failure because it may cause fluid retention which could lead to a deterioration in cardiac function.[1,4] For the same reason the UK manufacturers contraindicate use in heart failure.[5,6] If **digoxin** or any other **digitalis glycoside** is being used to treat cardiac failure, the use of pioglitazone or rosiglitazone would not therefore be recommended. This is not a drug-drug interaction but a drug-disease interaction.

1. Actos (Pioglitazone hydrochloride). Takeda Pharmaceutical Company Ltd. US Prescribing information, February 2007.
2. Kortboyer JM, Eckland DJA. Pioglitazone has low potential for drug interactions. *Diabetologia* (1999) 42 (Suppl 1), A228.
3. Di Cicco RA, Miller AK, Patterson S, Freed MI. Rosiglitazone does not affect the steady-state pharmacokinetics of digoxin. *J Clin Pharmacol* (2000) 40, 1516–21.
4. Avandia (Rosiglitazone maleate). GlaxoSmithKline. US Prescribing information, June 2007.
5. Actos (Pioglitazone hydrochloride). Takeda UK Ltd. UK Summary of product characteristics, January 2007.
6. Avandia (Rosiglitazone maleate). GlaxoSmithKline UK. UK Summary of product characteristics, May 2007.

Digitalis glycosides + Probenecid

Probenecid has no clinically significant effect on plasma digoxin levels.

Clinical evidence, mechanism, importance and management

A study in 2 healthy subjects taking **digoxin** 250 micrograms daily showed that after taking *ColBenemid* (probenecid 500 mg with colchicine

500 micrograms) twice daily for 3 days, their plasma **digoxin** levels were slightly but not significantly raised (from 0.67 to 0.7 nanograms/mL, and from 0.6 to 0.67 nanograms/mL, respectively).[1] Another study in 6 healthy subjects found that probenecid 2 g daily for 8 days had no significant effect on the pharmacokinetics of **digoxin**.[2] No special precautions would seem necessary during concurrent use.

1. Jaillon P, Weissenburger J, Cheymol G, Graves P, Marcus F. Les effets du probénécide sur la concentration plasmatique à l'équilibre de digoxine. *Therapie* (1980) 35, 655–6.
2. Hedman A, Angelin B, Arvidsson A, Dahlqvist R. No effect of probenecid on the renal and biliary clearances of digoxin in man. *Br J Clin Pharmacol* (1991) 32, 63–7.

Digitalis glycosides + Propafenone

Propafenone can increase serum digoxin levels by 30 to 90% or even more in children.

Clinical evidence

Propafenone (increasing over 6 days to 300 mg every 8 hours) increased the mean steady-state serum levels of **digoxin** 125 to 250 micrograms daily by 83% in 5 patients. Three patients continued to take both drugs for 6 months, at which point the **digoxin** levels were 63% higher. No digitalis toxicity was seen.[1] In another study, propafenone 600 mg daily in divided doses increased the steady-state serum **digoxin** levels of 10 patients by 90% (from 0.97 to 1.54 nanograms/mL), and two of them developed symptoms of toxicity (nausea, vomiting).[2] An even greater increase was seen in 3 children who showed rises in serum **digoxin** levels of 112 to 254% over 3 to 24 days when given propafenone 250 to 500 mg/m^2 daily.[3] The mean AUC of **digoxin** increased by 13.8% in 27 patients receiving propafenone 10 mg/kg daily in divided doses. However, there was great inter-individual variability, with 22 patients showing an increase in AUC, and 5 a decrease. One patient experienced **digoxin** toxicity resulting in fatal ventricular fibrillation.[4]

Propafenone 450 mg daily increased the mean steady-state serum **digoxin** levels of 12 healthy subjects by about 35% (from 0.58 to 0.78 nanograms/mL), and the cardiac effects were increased accordingly.[5] In a study in 6 subjects[6] given a single 1-mg intravenous dose of **digoxin**, propafenone 150 or 300 mg every 8 hours increased the AUC of **digoxin** by 28% and decreased the total clearance of **digoxin** by 21.9%. A similar study with oral **digoxin** found a 25% increase in the AUC of **digoxin** when healthy subjects were given propafenone.[7]

Mechanism

Not understood. One suggestion is that propafenone increases the bioavailability of the digoxin.[7] Another is that the volume of distribution and non-renal clearance of digoxin are changed by the propafenone.[6] Conversely, others reported that propafenone decreased the renal clearance of digoxin.[2,5] There is certainly some *in vitro* evidence that propafenone and its metabolite inhibit the P-glycoprotein transporter, which is concerned with digoxin secretion by the renal tubular cells.[8,9]

Importance and management

A very well established interaction of clinical importance. Monitor the effects of concurrent use and reduce the digoxin dosage appropriately in order to avoid toxicity. Most patients appear to be affected and dosage reductions in the range 15 to 70% were found necessary in one of the studies cited.[2] The data available suggest that the extent of the rise may possibly depend on the propafenone serum concentration rather than on its dose.[6,10]

1. Salerno DM, Granrud G, Sharkey P, Asinger R, Hodges M. A controlled trial of propafenone for treatment of frequent and repetitive ventricular premature complexes. *Am J Cardiol* (1984) 53, 77–83.
2. Calvo MV, Martin-Suarez A, Luengo CM, Avila C, Cascon M, Hurlé AD-G. Interaction between digoxin and propafenone. *Ther Drug Monit* (1989) 11, 10–15.
3. Zalzstein E, Koren G, Bryson SM, Freedom RM. Interaction between digoxin and propafenone in children. *J Pediatr* (1990) 116, 310–2.
4. Palumbo E, Svetoni N, Casini M, Spargi T, Biagi G, Martelli F, Lanzetta T. Interazione digoxina-propafenone: valori e limiti del dosaggio plasmatico dis due farmaci. *G Ital Cardiol* (1986) 16, 855–62.
5. Belz GG, Doering W, Munkes R, Matthews J. Interaction between digoxin and calcium antagonists and antiarrhythmic drugs. *Clin Pharmacol Ther* (1983) 33, 410–17.
6. Nolan PE, Marcus FI, Erstad BL, Hoyer GK, Furman C, Kirsten EB. Effects of coadministration of propafenone on the pharmacokinetics of digoxin in healthy volunteer subjects. *J Clin Pharmacol* (1989) 29, 46–52.
7. Cardaioli P, Compostella L, De Domenico R, Papalia D, Zeppellini R, Libardoni M, Pulido E, Cucchini F. Influenza del propafenone sulla farmacocinetica della digossina somministrata per via orale: studio su volontari sani. *G Ital Cardiol* (1986) 16, 237–40.
8. Woodland C, Verjee Z, Giesbrecht E, Koren G, Ito S. The digoxin-propafenone interaction: characterization of a mechanism using renal tubular cell monolayers. *J Pharmacol Exp Ther* (1997) 283, 39–45.
9. Bachmakov I, Rekersbrink S, Hofmann U, Eichelbaum M, Fromm MF. Characterisation of (*R/S*)-propafenone and its metabolites as substrates and inhibitors of P-glycoprotein. *Naunyn Schmiedebergs Arch Pharmacol* (2005) 371, 195–201.
10. Bigot M-C, Debruyne D, Bonnefoy L, Grollier G, Moulin M, Potier J-C. Serum digoxin levels related to plasma propafenone levels during concomitant treatment. *J Clin Pharmacol* (1991) 31, 521–6.

Digitalis glycosides + Propantheline

Serum digoxin levels may be increased by at least one-third if propantheline is given with slow-dissolving forms of digoxin tablets. No clinically significant interaction is likely with digoxin given as a liquid or in soft-gelatin capsules or in the form of fast-dissolving tablets.

Clinical evidence

The serum **digoxin** levels of 9 out of 13 patients rose by 30%, from 1.02 to 1.33 nanograms/mL when they took a slow-dissolving formulation of **digoxin** tablets (*Orion*) with propantheline 15 mg three times daily for 10 days. The serum levels stayed the same in 3 patients and fell slightly in one. An associated study in 4 healthy subjects given **digoxin** in liquid form found that serum **digoxin** levels were unaffected by propantheline.[1]

Another study by the same workers showed that propantheline increased the **digoxin** serum levels of a slow-dissolving tablet formulation (*Orion*) by 40%, but had no effect on serum **digoxin** levels with a fast-dissolving tablet formulation (*Lanoxin*).[2] In a further study, propantheline increased the AUC of **digoxin** from *Lanoxin* tablets by 24%, compared with a non-significant increase of 13% with digoxin in the form of a solution in a capsule (*Lanoxicaps*).[3]

Mechanism

Propantheline is an antimuscarinic, which reduces gut motility. This allows the slow-dissolving formulations of digoxin more time to pass into solution so that more is available for absorption.

Importance and management

An established interaction, but only of importance if slow-dissolving digoxin formulations are used. No interaction is likely with liquid or liquid-filled capsule forms of digoxin. With slow-dissolving forms of digoxin tablets it may be necessary to reduce the digoxin dosage. No interaction seems likely with **digitoxin** because it is better absorbed from the gut than digoxin, but this requires confirmation.

1. Manninen V, Apajalahti A, Melin J, Karesoja M. Altered absorption of digoxin in patients given propantheline and metoclopramide. *Lancet* (1973) i, 398–400.
2. Manninen V, Apajalahti A, Simonen H, Reissell P. Effect of propantheline and metoclopramide on absorption of digoxin. *Lancet* (1973) i, 1118–19.
3. Brown DD, Schmid J, Long RA, Hull JH. A steady-state evaluation of the effects of propantheline bromide and cholestyramine on the bioavailability of digoxin when administered as tablets or capsules. *J Clin Pharmacol* (1985) 25, 360–4.

Digitalis glycosides + Prostaglandins

Iloprost does not significantly alter digoxin pharmacokinetics. Epoprostenol caused a small decrease in digoxin clearance in the short-term, which is of uncertain clinical importance.

Clinical evidence, mechanism, importance and management

A 6-hour intravenous infusion of **iloprost** 2 nanograms/kg per minute was given to 12 patients taking **digoxin** 250 micrograms daily over a period of 20 days. The mean time to maximum serum **digoxin** levels was delayed by an hour, but overall the pharmacokinetics of the **digoxin** were unchanged.[1,2] No special precautions would seem to be necessary on concurrent use.

The **digoxin** clearance of 14 patients with congestive heart failure was reduced by an estimated 15% by **epoprostenol** given for 3 days, but this effect was no longer apparent by the end of 12 weeks concurrent use. The clinical relevance of this awaits evaluation but it seems unlikely to be important. However, the authors of the report suggest that the possible short-term changes in patients with high trough-serum **digoxin** levels and those prone to **digoxin** toxicity should be borne in mind when using the combination.[3]

1. Cabane J, Penin I, Bouslama K, Benchouieb A, Giral Ph, Picard O, Wattiaux MJ, Cheymol G, Souvignet G, Imbert JC. Traitement par iloprost des ischémies critiques des membres inférieurs associées à une insuffisance cardiaque. *Therapie* (1991) 46, 235–40.
2. Penin E, Cheymol G, Bouslama K, Benchouieb A, Cabane J, Souvignet G. No pharmacokinetic interaction between iloprost and digoxin. *Eur J Clin Pharmacol* (1991) 41, 505–6.
3. Carlton LD, Patterson JH, Mattson CN, Schmith VD. The effects of epoprostenol on drug disposition I. A pilot study of the pharmacokinetics of digoxin with and without epoprostenol in patients with congestive heart failure. *J Clin Pharmacol* (1996) 36, 247–56.

Digitalis glycosides + Proton pump inhibitors

A small rise in serum digoxin levels may occur with omeprazole, pantoprazole or rabeprazole, but this is not thought to be clinically significant. One case of digoxin toxicity has been reported with omeprazole.

Clinical evidence

(a) Lansoprazole

A study in 47 patients regularly taking **digoxin** and either lansoprazole or omeprazole found that changing the proton pump inhibitor to an equivalent dose of rabeprazole did not significantly change the mean serum **digoxin** level, although 12 of the patients had increases of more than 15%.[1]

(b) Omeprazole

In a study in healthy subjects, omeprazole 20 mg daily for 11 days caused only minor changes in the disposition of a single 1-mg oral dose of **digoxin**. On average the AUC was increased by 10%.[2] See also *Lansoprazole*, above. However, a 65-year-old woman showed signs of digoxin toxicity 3 months after starting to take omeprazole 20 mg daily. She was found to have a **digoxin** level of 3.9 nanograms/mL (previous level 1.1 nanograms/mL) and ECG changes, which resolved after the administration of **digoxin** immune fab. No changes in renal function were noted in this patient.[3]

(c) Pantoprazole

Beta-acetyldigoxin 200 micrograms twice daily was given to 18 healthy subjects, with and without pantoprazole 40 mg daily, for 5 days. The pantoprazole caused a 10% rise in the **digoxin** AUC and a 9% rise in the maximum **digoxin** serum levels, but both were considered to be clinically irrelevant. No changes in the **digoxin**-induced height reduction in the T-wave occurred.[4]

(d) Rabeprazole

A preliminary report, giving few details, states that rabeprazole increased the minimum **digoxin** levels by about 20%, and increased the AUC and maximum level.[5] The US manufacturer states that rabeprazole increased the AUC and maximum level of **digoxin** by 19%, and 29%, respectively.[6] However, these changes are thought to be within the normal variations of **digoxin** levels and so are not considered clinically significant.[7] See also *Lansoprazole*, above.

Mechanism

The increase in digoxin levels with omeprazole may be the result of higher gastric pH which results in less digoxin hydrolysis and an increase in digoxin absorption.[8] Non-selective digoxin assay methods may fail to detect an interaction, whereas selective HPLC assay methods and ECG studies provide evidence that the bioavailability of digoxin may be increased by omeprazole.[8] An *in vitro* study found that omeprazole, pantoprazole and lansoprazole inhibit P-glycoprotein-mediated intestinal transport of digoxin.[9]

Importance and management

Although some studies suggest small changes in digoxin pharmacokinetics may occur these changes are usually small and unlikely to be clinically significant. No special precautions would therefore seem to be necessary if proton pump inhibitors and digoxin are given concurrently.

1. Le GH, Schaefer MG, Plowman BK, Morreale AP, Delattre M, Okino L, Felicio L. Assessment of potential digoxin-rabeprazole interaction after formulary conversion of proton-pump inhibitors. *Am J Health-Syst Pharm* (2003) 60, 1343–5.
2. Oosterhuis B, Jonkman JHG, Andersson T, Zuiderwijk PBM, Jedema JN. Minor effect of multiple dose omeprazole on the pharmacokinetics of digoxin after a single oral dose. *Br J Clin Pharmacol* (1991) 32, 569–72.
3. Kiley CA, Cragin DJ, Roth BJ. Omeprazole-associated digoxin toxicity. *South Med J* (2007) 100, 400–2.
4. Hartmann M, Huber R, Bliesath H, Steinijans VW, Koch HJ, Wurst W, Kunz K. Lack of interaction between pantoprazole and digoxin at therapeutic doses in man. *Int J Clin Pharmacol Ther* (1995) 33, 481–5.
5. Humphries TJ, Nardi RV, Lazar JD, Spanyers SA. Drug-drug interaction evaluation of rabeprazole sodium: a clean/expected slate? *Gut* (1996) 39 (Suppl 3), A47.
6. AcipHex (Rabeprazole sodium). Eisai Inc. US Prescribing information, February 2007.
7. Anon. Notice board. *Pharm J* (2003) 271, 541.
8. Cohen AF, Kroon R, Schoemaker HC, Hoogkamer JFW, van Vliet-Verbeek A. Effects of gastric acidity on the bioavailability of digoxin. Evidence for a new mechanism for interactions with omeprazole. *Br J Clin Pharmacol* (1991) 31, 565P.
9. Pauli-Magnus C, Rekersbrink S, Klotz U, Fromm MF. Interaction of omeprazole, lansoprazole and pantoprazole with P-glycoprotein. *Naunyn Schmiedebergs Arch Pharmacol* (2001) 364, 551–7.

Digitalis glycosides + Quinidine

In most patients, on average, the serum levels of digoxin doubled within five days of starting quinidine. The digoxin dosage usually needs to be halved if toxicity is to be avoided. Digitoxin levels are also increased but to a lesser extent and takes a longer period of time to develop.

Clinical evidence

(a) Digitoxin

Quinidine 750 mg daily increased the steady-state serum digitoxin levels of 8 healthy subjects by 45%, from 13.6 to 19.7 nanograms/mL, over 32 days.[1] Another study found a 31% increase in serum digitoxin levels over 10 days,[2] whereas yet another found a 115% increase after 70 days of treatment with 360 mg quinidine three times daily.[3] A study in 5 healthy subjects found that quinidine reduced the total body clearance of digitoxin by 63%, resulting in raised serum digitoxin levels.[4]

(b) Digoxin

The observation that quinidine appeared to increase serum digoxin levels prompted a retrospective study of patient records, which revealed that 25 out of 27 patients taking digoxin had shown a significant rise in serum digoxin levels from 1.4 to 3.2 nanograms/mL when given quinidine. Of the patients who showed a rise,16 showed typical signs of digoxin toxicity (nausea, vomiting, anorexia), which resolved in 10 of them when the digoxin dosage was reduced or withdrawn, and in 5 when the quinidine was withdrawn.[5]

This is one of the first reports published in 1978 (two other groups independently reported it at a similar time[6,7]) that clearly describes this interaction, although hints of its existence can be found in papers published over the previous 50 years. Since then large numbers of research reports, both retrospective and prospective, and case studies have confirmed and established the incidence and magnitude of this interaction. It occurs in over 90% of patients and, on average, there is a 100% increase in serum digoxin levels, although there are pronounced inter-individual differences, and the increase is somewhat dependent on the quinidine dose. There are numerous reports and reviews of this interaction, only a selection of which are listed here. Two reviews published in 1982 and 1983 contain valuable bibliographies.[8,9]

Mechanism

Quinidine reduces the renal excretion of digoxin by 40 to 50%, and it also appears to have some effects on non-renal clearance, which includes a reduction in digoxin excretion in the bile.[10] There is also evidence that increases in the rate and extent of absorption of digoxin from the gut occur.[11] More recent studies show that the mechanism behind these effects on absorption and renal excretion is likely to be P-glycoprotein inhibition by quinidine.[12-14] Digoxin also appears to cause a small reduction in the renal clearance of quinidine.[15] Quinidine appears to increase digitoxin serum levels by reducing its non-renal clearance.

Importance and management

The interaction between digoxin and quinidine is very well-documented, well-established and of definite clinical importance. Since serum digoxin levels are usually roughly doubled (up to fivefold increases have been seen[8]) and over 90% of patients are affected, digitalis toxicity will develop unless the dosage of digoxin is reduced (approximately halved).[5,8,16,17] A suggested rule-of-thumb is that if serum digoxin levels are no greater than 0.9 nanograms/mL the addition of quinidine is unlikely to cause toxic digoxin levels (if serum potassium levels are normal) whereas with levels of 1 nanogram/mL or more, toxic concentrations may develop.[18] Monitor the effects and readjust the dosage as necessary. Significant effects occur within a day of taking the quinidine and reach a maximum after about 3 to 6 days (quicker or slower in some patients), but digoxin levels will only stabilise when the quinidine has reached steady-state and that depends on whether a loading dose of quinidine is given. The effects are to some extent dose-related but the correlation is not good: less than 400 to 500 mg of quinidine daily has minimal effects, and increasing doses up to 1.2 g has greater effects.[16,19] About 5 days are needed after withdrawing the quinidine before serum digoxin levels fall to their former levels. It has been recommended that patients with chronic renal failure should have their digoxin dosage reduced by as much as two-thirds.[20-22] An appropriate upward readjustment will be necessary if the quinidine is subsequently withdrawn.

Far less is known about the interaction between digitoxin and quinidine but similar precautions should be taken. It develops much more slowly.

1. Kuhlmann J, Dohrmann M, Marcin S. Effects of quinidine on pharmacokinetics and pharmacodynamics of digitoxin achieving steady-state conditions. *Clin Pharmacol Ther* (1986) 39, 288–94.
2. Peters U, Risler T, Grabensee B, Falkenstein U, Kroukou J. Interaktion von Chinidin und Digitoxin beim Menschen. *Dtsch Med Wochenschr* (1980) 105, 438–42.
3. Kreutz G, Keller F, Gast D and Prokein E. Digitoxin-quinidine interaction achieving steady-state conditions for both drugs. *Naunyn Schmiedebergs Arch Pharmacol* (1982) 319, R82.
4. Garty M, Sood P, Rollins DE. Digitoxin elimination reduced during quinidine therapy. *Ann Intern Med* (1981) 94, 35–7.
5. Leahey EB, Reiffel JA, Drusin RE, Heisenbuttel RH, Lovejoy WP, Bigger JT. Interaction between quinidine and digoxin. *JAMA* (1978) 240, 533–4.
6. Ejvinsson G. Effect of quinidine on plasma concentrations of digoxin. *BMJ* (1978) i, 279–80.
7. Reid PR, Meek AG. Digoxin-quinidine interaction. *Johns Hopkins Med J* (1979) 145, 227–9.
8. Bigger JT, Leahey EB. Quinidine and digoxin. An important interaction. *Drugs* (1982) 24, 229–39.
9. Fichtl B, Doering W. The quinidine-digoxin interaction in perspective. *Clin Pharmacokinet* (1983) 8, 137–54.
10. Schenck-Gustafsson K, Angelin B, Hedman A, Arvidsson A, Dahlqvist R. Quinidine-induced reduction of the biliar excretion of digoxin in patients. *Circulation* (1985) 72 (Suppl), III-19.
11. Pedersen KE, Christiansen BD, Klitgaard NA, Nielsen-Kudsk F. Effect of quinidine on digoxin bioavailability. *Eur J Clin Pharmacol* (1983) 24, 41–7.
12. Su S-F, Huang J-D. Inhibition of the intestinal digoxin absorption and exsorption by quinidine. *Drug Metab Dispos* (1996) 24, 142–7.
13. Fromm MF, Kim RB, Stein CM, Wilkinson GR, Roden DM. Inhibition of P-glycoprotein–mediated drug transport. A unifying mechanism to explain the interaction between digoxin and quinidine. *Circulation* (1999) 99, 552–7.
14. Drescher S, Glaeser H, Mürdter T, Hitzl M, Eichelbaum M, Fromm MF. P-glycoprotein–mediated intestinal and biliary digoxin transport in humans. *Clin Pharmacol Ther* (2003) 73, 223–31.
15. Rameis H. Quinidine-digoxin interaction: are the pharmacokinetics of both drugs altered? *Int J Clin Pharmacol Ther Toxicol* (1985) 23, 145–53.
16. Doering W. Quinidine-digoxin interaction: pharmacokinetics, underlying mechanism and clinical implications. *N Engl J Med* (1979) 301, 400–4.
17. Leahey EB, Reiffel JA, Heissenbuttel RH, Drusin RE, Lovejoy WP, Bigger JT. Enhanced cardiac effect of digoxin during quinidine treatment. *Arch Intern Med* (1979) 139, 519–21.
18. Friedman HS, Chen T-S. Use of control steady-state serum digoxin levels for predicting serum digoxin concentration after quinidine administration. *Am Heart J* (1982) 104, 72–6.
19. Fenster PE, Powell JR, Hager WD, Graves PE, Conrad K, Goldman S. Onset and dose dependence of digoxin-quinidine interaction. *Am J Cardiol* (1980) 45, 413.
20. Fichtl B, Doering W, Seidel H. The quinidine-digoxin interaction in patients with impaired renal function. *Int J Clin Pharmacol Ther Toxicol* (1983) 21, 229–33.
21. Fenster PE, Hager WD, Perrier D, Powell JR, Graves PE, Michael UF. Digoxin-quinidine interaction in patients with chronic renal failure. *Circulation* (1982) 66, 1277–80.
22. Woodcock BG, Rietbrock N. Digitalis-quinidine interactions. *Trends Pharmacol Sci* (1982) 3, 118–22.

Digitalis glycosides + Quinine

The digoxin levels of some but not all patients may rise by more than 60% if they are given quinine.

Clinical evidence

After taking quinine 300 mg four times daily for a day the steady-state **digoxin** levels of 4 subjects taking **digoxin** 250 micrograms daily rose by 63%, from 0.49 to 0.8 nanograms/mL. After taking the quinine for a further 3 days the **digoxin** levels rose a further 11% (to 0.86 nanograms/mL). **Digoxin** renal clearance fell by 20%.[1]

Quinine sulfate 250 mg daily for 7 days increased the mean serum **digoxin** levels of 7 healthy subjects by 25%, from 0.64 to 0.8 nanograms/mL. When quinine sulfate 250 mg was given three times daily there was a further 8% rise. Considerable individual differences were seen; one subject had a 92% rise.[2] In contrast, 17 patients given quinine 750 mg daily had only a small and statistically insignificant rise in mean serum **digoxin** levels, from 0.8 to 0.91 nanograms/mL. Serum levels were virtually unaltered in 11 patients, decreased in two and markedly increased (amount not stated) in four.[3] Another study found that **quinine** reduced the total clearance of **digoxin** by 26%.[4]

Mechanism

Not fully understood. A reduction in non-renal clearance is apparently largely responsible for the rise in serum digoxin levels with quinine.[2,4,5] This is possibly due to changes in digoxin metabolism or in its biliary excretion.[4,5]

Importance and management

An established interaction of clinical importance but only moderately documented. Monitor the effects of concurrent use (e.g. for bradycardia) and reduce the digoxin dosage where necessary. Some patients may have a substantial increase in serum digoxin levels whereas others will have only a small or moderate rise. There appear to be no case reports of digoxin toxicity arising from this interaction.

1. Aronson JK, Carver JG. Interaction of digoxin with quinine. *Lancet* (1981) i, 1418.
2. Pedersen KE, Madsen JL, Klitgaard NA, Kjær K, Hvidt S. Effect of quinine on plasma digoxin concentration and renal digoxin clearance. *Acta Med Scand* (1985) 218, 229–32.
3. Doering W. Is there a clinically relevant interaction between quinine and digoxin in human beings? *Am J Cardiol* (1981) 48, 975–6.
4. Wandell M, Powell JR, Hager WD, Fenster PE, Graves PE, Conrad KA, Goldman S. Effect of quinine on digoxin kinetics. *Clin Pharmacol Ther* (1980) 28, 425–30.
5. Hedman A, Angelin B, Arvidsson A, Dahlqvist R, Nilsson B. Interactions in the renal and biliary elimination of digoxin: stereoselective difference between quinine and quinidine. *Clin Pharmacol Ther* (1990) 47, 20–6.

Digitalis glycosides + Quinolones

Levofloxacin, gemifloxacin, moxifloxacin and sparfloxacin do not affect the pharmacokinetics of digoxin. Similarly moxifloxacin does not interact with beta-acetyldigoxin. Gatifloxacin may cause small increases in digoxin levels, which are probably not clinically significant. The effects of garenoxacin are unclear.

Clinical evidence

(a) Garenoxacin

In a study designed to look at the effects of garenoxacin on gut flora, 16 healthy subjects were given **digoxin** 250 micrograms every 6 hours on day 1, then 250 micrograms daily to day 14, with garenoxacin 600 mg daily on days 8 to 14. Garenoxacin did not decrease (but may actually increase) the numbers of *E. lentum* in faeces (see 'Digitalis glycosides + Macrolides', p.929, for an explanation of the possible significance of these findings). Thus an interaction due to the effect of garenoxacin on intestinal microflora is unlikely.[1]

(b) Gatifloxacin

The vital signs of 12 healthy subjects given gatifloxacin 400 mg daily for 7 days while taking **digoxin** 250 micrograms daily were not altered. The AUC and steady-state levels of **digoxin** were increased by 19% and 12% respectively. Dosage adjustments were not considered necessary.[2]

(c) Gemifloxacin

No clinically relevant pharmacokinetic changes were seen in a study in 14 healthy elderly subjects given gemifloxacin 320 mg daily for 7 days while taking **digoxin** (*Lenoxin*) 250 micrograms daily. No clinically important changes in vital signs or ECGs were found.[3]

(d) Levofloxacin

The pharmacokinetics of a single 400-microgram dose of **digoxin** (*Lanoxicaps*) were unchanged when 12 healthy subjects were given levofloxacin 500 mg twice daily for 6 days.[4]

(e) Moxifloxacin

In 14 healthy subjects, moxifloxacin 400 mg daily for 14 days did not cause any clinically relevant changes in the steady-state pharmacokinetics of **digoxin** 250 micrograms daily.[5] No pharmacokinetic changes were seen in another study in 12 healthy subjects given a single 600-microgram dose of **beta-acetyldigoxin** with moxifloxacin 400 mg daily for 2 days.[6]

(f) Sparfloxacin

Sparfloxacin, 400 mg as a loading dose, followed by 200 mg daily for 9 days did not affect the pharmacokinetics of **digoxin** (*Lanoxicaps*) 300 micrograms daily in 24 healthy subjects.[7]

Mechanism, importance and management

Information about other digitalis glycosides and quinolones seems to be lacking, but bearing in mind their extensive use, this silence in the literature would suggest that no problems normally arise. Despite *in vitro* susceptibility of *E. lentum* to a range of antibacterials including some quinolones there is currently no information to suggest such an interaction occurs between the quinolones and digoxin.[8] See 'Digitalis glycosides + Macrolides', p.929, for an explanation of the possible significance of *E. lentum*.

1. Nord CE, Meurling L, Russo RL, Bello A, Grasela DM, Gajjar DA. Effect of garenoxacin on Eubacteria in the normal intestinal microflora when administered concomitantly with digoxin. *J Chemother* (2003) 15, 244–7.
2. Olsen SJ, Uderman HD, Kaul S, Kollia GD, Birkhoffer MJ, Grasela DM. Pharmacokinetics of concomitantly administered gatifloxacin and digoxin. *Intersci Conf Antimicrob Agents Chemother* (1999) 39, 12.
3. Vousden M, Allen A, Lewis A, Ehren N. Lack of pharmacokinetic interaction between gemifloxacin and digoxin in healthy elderly volunteers. *Chemotherapy* (1999) 45, 485–90.
4. Chien S-C, Rogge MC, Williams RR, Natarajan J, Wong F, Chow AT. Absence of a pharmacokinetic interaction between digoxin and levofloxacin. *J Clin Pharm Ther* (2002) 27, 7–12.
5. Staß H, Frey R, Kubitza D, Möller J-G, Zühlsdorf M. Influence of orally administered moxifloxacin (MOX) on the steady state pharmacokinetics (PK) of digoxin (D) in healthy male volunteers. *J Antimicrob Chemother* (1999) 44 (Suppl A), 134–5.
6. Horstmann R, Delesen H, Dietrich H, Ochmann K, Sachse R, Staß H, Zuehlsdorf M, Kuhlmann J. No drug-drug interaction between moxifloxacin and β-acetyldigoxin. *Clin Invest Med* (1998) (Suppl), S20.
7. Johnson RD, Dorr MB, Hunt TL, Conway S, Talbot GH. Pharmacokinetic interaction of sparfloxacin and digoxin. *Clin Ther* (1999) 21, 368–79.
8. Ten Eick AP, Reed MD. Hidden dangers of coadministration of antibiotics and digoxin in children: focus on azithromycin. *Curr Ther Res* (2000) 61, 148–60.

Digitalis glycosides + Rauwolfia alkaloids

Concurrent use of digitalis glycosides and rauwolfia alkaloids is usually uneventful, but the incidence of arrhythmias appears to be increased, particularly in those with atrial fibrillation. Excessive bradycardia and syncope have also been described.

Clinical evidence

Three patients taking **digoxin** and either **reserpine** or whole root ***Rauwolfia serpentina*** developed arrhythmias, namely atrial tachycardia with 4:1 Wenckebach irregular block, ventricular bigeminy and tachycardia, and atrial fibrillation. A large number of other patients received both drugs without problems.[1]

The incidence of premature ventricular systoles was roughly doubled in patients taking **digoxin** and **rauwolfia** compared with a similar group taking **rauwolfia** alone.[2] **Reserpine** reduced the tolerated dose of **acetyl strophanthidin** in 15 patients with congestive heart failure; 8 out of 9 patients with atrial fibrillation developed ECG abnormalities, including complete heart block and ventricular ectopics, during acute digitalisation following **reserpine** use, compared with only one of 9 patients not taking **reserpine**.[3]

A man taking **digoxin** 250 and 375 micrograms on alternate days and **reserpine** 25 micrograms daily developed sinus bradycardia and carotid sinus supersensitivity. He was hospitalised because of syncope, which resolved when the **reserpine** was withdrawn.[4]

Mechanism

Not understood. A possible explanation is that because the rauwolfia alkaloids deplete the neurotransmitter from the sympathetic nerve supply to the heart, the parasympathetic vagal supply (i.e. heart slowing) has full rein. Digitalis also causes bradycardia which in the presence of the rauwolfia becomes excessive. In this situation the rate could become so slow that ectopic foci, which would normally be swamped by a faster, more normal beat, begin to fire, leading to the development of arrhythmias. Syncope could also result from the combination of bradycardia and the hypotensive effects of reserpine.

Importance and management

Some caution is advisable. One group of authors, despite having described the adverse reactions cited above,[1] conclude that time has proven the safety of the combination. However, they warn that arrhythmias must be anticipated. Particular risk of arrhythmias seems to occur in patients with atrial fibrillation, and in digitalised patients given reserpine parenterally, because of the sudden release of catecholamines that takes place.[4]

1. Dick HLH, McCawley EL, Fisher WA. Reserpine-digitalis toxicity. *Arch Intern Med* (1962) 109, 503–6.
2. Schreader CJ, Etzl MM. Premature ventricular contractions due to rauwolfia therapy. *JAMA* (1956) 162, 1256.
3. Lown B, Ehrlich L, Lipschultz B, Blake J. Effect of digitalis in patients receiving reserpine. *Circulation* (1961) 24, 1185–91.
4. Bigger JT, Strauss HC. Digitalis toxicity: drug interactions promoting toxicity and the management of toxicity. *Semin Drug Treat* (1972) 2, 147–77.

Digitalis glycosides + Rifamycins

The serum levels of digitoxin can be halved by rifampicin (rifampin). Digoxin serum levels are modestly reduced by rifampicin.

Clinical evidence

(a) Digitoxin

A comparative study in 21 patients with tuberculosis and 19 healthy subjects taking digitoxin 100 micrograms daily found that the serum digitoxin levels of the patients taking **rifampicin (rifampin)** were about half of the levels in healthy subjects not taking **rifampicin** (18.4 nanograms/mL compared with 39.1 nanograms/mL).[1] The half-life of digitoxin was reduced from 8.2 to 4.5 days by the **rifampicin**. There are case reports confirming that **rifampicin** can markedly reduce serum digitoxin levels.[2,3]

(b) Digoxin

A woman, hospitalised for endocarditis, taking digoxin 250 to 375 micrograms daily, furosemide, aspirin, isosorbide dinitrate and potassium chloride, had a marked fall of about 80% in her serum digoxin level when she was given **rifampicin** 600 mg daily. The serum digoxin returned to its former level over the 2 weeks following **rifampicin** withdrawal.[4] She had only moderate renal impairment (serum creatinine 221 micromol/L).

Another report describes 2 patients undergoing renal dialysis whose digoxin dosage needed to be doubled while they were taking **rifampicin**, and similarly reduced when the **rifampicin** was withdrawn.[5] This confirms an earlier report.[6]

A study in 8 healthy subjects found that the AUC and maximum plasma levels of a single 1-mg oral dose of digoxin were reduced by 30% and 52%, respectively, by **rifampicin** 600 mg daily for 10 days.[7] In two further studies in which **rifampicin** 300 mg twice daily for 7 days was used as a positive control, the AUC of a single oral dose of digoxin was reduced by 16%, and the maximum levels were reduced by about 25%.[8,9]

A 15% reduction in the AUC and maximum plasma levels of digoxin was seen when a single 1-mg intravenous dose of digoxin was given after pre-treatment with **rifampicin** 600 mg daily for 10 days.[7] Similarly, a study in 8 healthy subjects who were given a single 1-mg intravenous dose of digoxin after 14 days of treatment with **rifampicin** 600 mg daily found an increased excretion of digoxin into the bile, and a 27% reduction in the AUC of digoxin.[10]

Mechanism

The interaction between digitoxin and rifampicin is almost certainly due to the increase in digitoxin metabolism caused by rifampicin, which is a potent enzyme inducer.[1] Digoxin is largely excreted unchanged in the urine and the interaction with rifampicin appears to be mainly due to induction of P-glycoprotein, resulting in reduced digoxin absorption from the intestine,[7,10] and increased biliary excretion.[10]

Importance and management

The interaction between digitoxin and rifampicin is established and clinically important. Under-digitalisation may occur unless the digitoxin dosage is increased appropriately. Good monitoring is obviously advisable.

The pharmacokinetic interaction with digoxin is also established, but rifampicin causes only a minor to modest reduction in digoxin levels, and the few case reports suggest that these changes are generally not clinically relevant. However, it would be prudent to monitor the concurrent use of these drugs, being alert for the need to increase the digoxin dosage. It may be that renal impairment increases the extent of this interaction, as several of the cases cited involved patients with some degree of renal impairment.

There does not seem to be any information regarding the other rifamycins, **rifabutin** (a weak enzyme inducer) and **rifapentine** (a moderate enzyme inducer). However, the UK manufacturers and the CSM in the UK warn that rifabutin may possibly reduce the effects of a number of drugs, including digitalis (but not digoxin).[11,12]

1. Peters U, Hausamen T-U, Grosse-Brockhoff F. Einfluβ von Tuberkulostatika auf die Pharmakokinetik des Digitoxins. *Dtsch Med Wochenschr* (1974) 99, 2381–6.
2. Boman G, Eliasson K, Odarcederlöf I. Acute cardiac failure during treatment with digitoxin - an interaction with rifampicin. *Br J Clin Pharmacol* (1980) 10, 89–90.
3. Poor DM, Self TH, Davis HL. Interaction of rifampin and digitoxin. *Arch Intern Med* (1983) 143, 599.
4. Bussey HI, Merritt GJ, Hill EG. The influence of rifampin on quinidine and digoxin. *Arch Intern Med* (1984) 144, 1021–3.
5. Gault H, Longerich L, Dawe M, Fine A. Digoxin-rifampin interaction. *Clin Pharmacol Ther* (1984) 35, 750–4.
6. Novi C, Bissoli F, Simonati V, Volpini T, Baroli A, Vignati G. Rifampin and digoxin: possible drug interaction in a dialysis patient. *JAMA* (1980) 244, 2521–2.
7. Greiner B, Eichelbaum M, Fritz P, Kreichgauer H-P, von Richter O, Zundler J, Kroemer HK. The role of intestinal P-glycoprotein in the interaction of digoxin and rifampin. *J Clin Invest* (1999) 104, 147–53. Correction. ibid. (2002) 110, 571.
8. Gurley BJ, Swain A, Barone GW, Williams DK, Breen P, Yates CR, Stuart LB, Hubbard MA, Tong Y, Cheboyina S. Effect of goldenseal (*Hydrastis canadensis*) and kava kava (*Piper methysticum*) supplementation on digoxin pharmacokinetics in humans. *Drug Metab Dispos* (2007) 35, 240–5.
9. Gurley BJ, Barone GW, Williams DK, Carrier J, Breen P, Yates CR, Song P-f, Hubbard MA, Tong Y, Cheboyina S. Effect of milk thistle (*Silybum marianum*) and black cohosh (*Cimicifuga racemosa*) supplementation on digoxin pharmacokinetics in humans. *Drug Metab Dispos* (2006) 34, 69–74.
10. Drescher S, Glaeser H, Mürdter T, Hitzl M, Eichelbaum M, Fromm MF. P-glycoprotein-mediated intestinal and biliary digoxin transport in humans. *Clin Pharmacol Ther* (2003) 73, 223–31.
11. Mycobutin (Rifabutin). Pharmacia Ltd. UK Summary of product characteristics, October 2006.
12. Committee on the Safety of Medicines/Medicines Control Agency. Revised indication and drug interactions of rifabutin. *Current Problems* (1997) 23, 14.

Digitalis glycosides + Ritonavir

A woman had elevated serum digoxin levels and signs of toxicity after she was given ritonavir. Pharmacokinetic studies have shown that ritonavir causes modest to marked increases in single-dose digoxin levels.

Clinical evidence

A 61-year-old HIV-positive woman taking lamivudine, indinavir, stavudine, pentamidine, warfarin with **digoxin** 250 micrograms daily for atrial fibrillation, presented with increasing nausea and vomiting 3 days after starting to take ritonavir 200 mg twice daily. **Digoxin** levels about 5 and 27 hours after her last dose were 5.6 nanograms/mL and 2.1 nanograms/mL, respectively.[1]

A study in 12 healthy subjects found that ritonavir 300 mg twice daily for 11 days significantly increased the AUC and volume of distribution of a single 500-microgram intravenous dose of **digoxin** by 86% and 77%, respectively. Non-renal and renal **digoxin** clearance were decreased by 48% and 35%, respectively, and its half-life increased by 156%.[2] Another study found that ritonavir 200 mg twice daily for 15 days increased the AUC of a single 400-microgram oral dose of **digoxin** by 22%, with 9 of 12 subjects having an increase. Non-renal but not renal clearance was reduced.[3]

Mechanism

Raised digoxin levels are possibly due to inhibition of the P-glycoprotein-mediated renal transport of digoxin by ritonavir.[1-3]

Importance and management

A pharmacokinetic interaction between ritonavir and digoxin would appear to be established, although its extent is uncertain. The study with intravenous digoxin showed a marked effect, whereas the study with oral digoxin showed a much smaller effect. Nevertheless, given the case report, it would seem prudent to closely monitor patients taking digoxin when ritonavir is started or stopped. There do not appear to be any reports or studies of the interaction of digoxin with other protease inhibitors.

1. Phillips EJ, Rachlis AR, Ito S. Digoxin toxicity and ritonavir: a drug interaction mediated through p-glycoprotein? *AIDS* (2003) 17, 1577–8.
2. Ding R, Tayrouz Y, Riedel K-D, Burhenne J, Weiss J, Mikus G, Haefeli WE. Substantial pharmacokinetic interaction between digoxin and ritonavir in healthy volunteers. *Clin Pharmacol Ther* (2004) 76, 73–84.
3. Penzak SR, Shen JM, Alfaro RM, Remaley AT, Natarajan V, Falloon J. Ritonavir decreases the nonrenal clearance of digoxin in healthy volunteers with known MDR1 genotypes. *Ther Drug Monit* (2004) 26, 322–30.

Digitalis glycosides + Ropinirole

Ropinirole does not significantly affect the pharmacokinetics of digoxin.

Clinical evidence, mechanism, importance and management

In a placebo-controlled study, 10 patients with Parkinson's disease were given ropinirole (initially 250 micrograms increasing to 2 mg three times daily) in addition to their usual treatment with **digoxin** 125 or 250 micrograms daily. Although ropinirole decreased the **digoxin** AUC by 10%, and the maximum plasma concentration by 25%, the **digoxin** minimum plasma concentration was not significantly altered. The authors therefore concluded that no dosage adjustment would be needed on concurrent use.[1]

1. Taylor A, Beerahee A, Citerone D, Davy M, Fitzpatrick K, Lopez-Gil A, Stocchi F. The effect of steady-state ropinirole on plasma concentrations of digoxin in patients with Parkinson's disease. *Br J Clin Pharmacol* (1999) 47, 219–22.

Digitalis glycosides + Sevelamer

The pharmacokinetics of single doses of digoxin are not affected by sevelamer.

Clinical evidence, mechanism, importance and management

In a randomised study a single 1-mg oral dose of **digoxin** was given with or without sevelamer 2.4 g followed by a standard breakfast. Five further doses of sevelamer were given immediately before subsequent meals over the following 2 days. During this time, the pharmacokinetic profile of **digoxin** was not altered.[1]

Sevelamer is a non-absorbed phosphate-binding polymer with bile-acid binding properties. Because the bile-acid binding resins 'colestyramine', (p.919) and 'colestipol', (p.918) may interact with **digoxin**, it was suggested that sevelamer could also interact, although this does not appear to be the case. This finding requires confirmation in long-term studies.

1. Burke S, Amin N, Incerti C, Plone M, Watson N. Sevelamer hydrochloride (Renagel®), a non-absorbed phosphate-binding polymer, does not interfere with digoxin or warfarin pharmacokinetics. *J Clin Pharmacol* (2001) 41, 193–8.

Digitalis glycosides + SSRIs

Citalopram, fluvoxamine, paroxetine, and sertraline appear not to affect the pharmacokinetics of digoxin. However, one case-control study found a small increased risk of digoxin toxicity after starting sertraline, paroxetine, fluoxetine or fluvoxamine, and two isolated reports describe increased serum digoxin levels attributed to the use of fluoxetine or paroxetine.

Clinical evidence

A study in 11 healthy subjects found that **citalopram** 40 mg once daily for 28 days did not have any significant effect on the pharmacokinetics of a single 1-mg dose of **digoxin** taken on day 21. No clinically significant ECG changes were observed.[1]

After taking **fluvoxamine** 100 mg daily for 15 days, the pharmacokinetics of a single 1.25-mg intravenous dose of **digoxin** were unchanged in 8 healthy subjects.[2]

A study in healthy subjects found that **paroxetine** 30 mg daily had no effect on the pharmacokinetics of **digoxin** 250 micrograms daily. The pharmacokinetics of **paroxetine** were unaffected by **digoxin**.[3]

A placebo-controlled study in 19 healthy subjects found that **sertraline**, in an initial dose of 50 mg daily titrated to 200 mg daily, had no effect on the steady-state pharmacokinetics of **digoxin**, except for a decrease in time to maximum plasma levels.[4]

However, in a case-control study in 3144 patients who had been admitted to hospital with **digoxin** toxicity, these patients were significantly more likely than controls to have received a new prescription for **sertraline**, **fluoxetine**, **fluvoxamine**, or **paroxetine** in the 30 days prior to admission (adjusted odds ratios, 3, 2.9, 3 and 2.8, for the SSRIs, respectively). This was after adjusting for renal disease and other interacting drugs. Nevertheless, this increased risk was not statistically significantly different to that in patients taking tricyclics (1.5) or benzodiazepines (2.1), which the authors considered have no known basis for an interaction (see 'Digitalis glycosides + Benzodiazepines and related drugs', p.911). In addition, it was small compared with the 12-fold increased risk found by the same authors in a similar study[5] of 'clarithromycin', (p.929).

An isolated report describes a 93-year-old woman with congestive heart failure who developed increased serum **digoxin** levels on two occasions when **fluoxetine** was added.[6] Another case report describes **digoxin** toxicity in a 68-year-old woman with atrial fibrillation and depression, which was attributed to the addition of **paroxetine** 20 mg daily. Her **digoxin** levels reached 5.2 nanograms/mL.[7]

Mechanism

It has been suggested that paroxetine might inhibit P-glycoprotein leading to reduced renal excretion of digoxin.[7] This suggestion has been criticised by other authors who propose that the increase in levels seen in the case with paroxetine may be due to hospital-induced compliance or renal impairment.[8,9] Moreover, the case-control study found no evidence of a significantly different risk of digoxin toxicity between those SSRIs with greater P-glycoprotein inhibitory activity (sertraline and paroxetine) than those with less (fluoxetine, fluvoxamine).[5]

Importance and management

The pharmacokinetic studies show that it is unlikely that, in general, SSRIs will affect the steady-state serum levels of digoxin. The excess risk seen in the case-control study was considered to be small and related to detection bias or confounding by indication,[5] although the findings do introduce a note of caution. Nevertheless, the fact that there are only isolated case reports of possible interactions with digoxin for such a widely used class of drugs suggests that problems are rarely encountered. No special precautions would seem to be necessary.

1. Larsen F, Priskorn M, Overø KF. Lack of citalopram effect on oral digoxin pharmacokinetics. *J Clin Pharmacol* (2001) 41, 340–6.
2. Ochs HR, Greenblatt DJ, Verburg-Ochs B, Labedski L. Chronic treatment with fluvoxamine, clovoxamine and placebo: interaction with digoxin and effects on sleep and alertness. *J Clin Pharmacol* (1989) 29, 91–95.
3. Bannister SJ, Houser VP, Hulse JD, Kisicki JC, Rasmussen JGC. Evaluation of the potential for interactions of paroxetine with diazepam, cimetidine, warfarin, and digoxin. *Acta Psychiatr Scand* (1989) 80 (Suppl 350), 102–6.
4. Rapeport WG, Coates PE, Dewland PM, Forster PL. Absence of a sertraline-mediated effect on digoxin pharmacokinetics and electrocardiographic findings. *J Clin Psychiatry* (1996) 57 (Suppl 1), 16–19.
5. Juurlink DN, Mamdani MM, Kopp A, Herrmann N, Laupacis A. A population-based assessment of the potential interaction between serotonin-specific reuptake inhibitors and digoxin. *Br J Clin Pharmacol* (2005) 59, 102–7.
6. Leibovitz A, Bilchinsky T, Gil I, Habot B. Elevated serum digoxin level associated with coadministered fluoxetine. *Arch Intern Med* (1998) 158, 1152–3.
7. Yasui-Furukori N, Kaneko S. Digitalis intoxication induced by paroxetine co-administration. *Lancet* (2006) 367, 788.
8. Bateman DN, Thanacoody HKR, Waring WS. Digitalis intoxication induced by paroxetine co-administration. *Lancet* (2006) 368, 1962–3.
9. Hallberg P, Melhus H. Digitalis intoxication induced by paroxetine co-administration. *Lancet* (2006) 368, 1963.

Digitalis glycosides + Statins

Atorvastatin, fluvastatin and simvastatin cause small but probably clinically unimportant increases in the serum levels of digoxin. Pravastatin and rosuvastatin appear to have no effect on digoxin pharmacokinetics.

Clinical evidence

(a) Atorvastatin

Digoxin 250 micrograms daily was given to 24 healthy subjects for 10 days, with atorvastatin 10 or 80 mg daily for a further 10 days. The mean steady-state **digoxin** levels were unaffected by atorvastatin 10 mg, but atorvastatin 80 mg caused a 20% rise in maximum **digoxin** levels and a 15% rise in its AUC.[1]

(b) Fluvastatin

In a crossover study in 18 patients, fluvastatin 40 mg caused no significant changes in the pharmacokinetics of **digoxin** 100 to 375 micrograms daily.[2] Another similar study in patients found changes of up to 15% in maximum plasma **digoxin** levels and clearance, but these were not considered to be clinically relevant.[3]

(c) Pravastatin

Pravastatin 20 mg daily for 9 days had no significant effect on the steady-state levels of **digoxin** 200 micrograms daily in 18 healthy subjects.[4]

(d) Rosuvastatin

In a randomised study, 18 healthy subjects were given rosuvastatin 40 mg daily or placebo for 12 days, with a single 500-microgram dose of **digoxin** on day 8. The absorption, renal excretion, AUC and maximum serum levels of **digoxin** were unaffected by rosuvastatin.[5]

(e) Simvastatin

Plasma **digoxin** levels can be slightly raised, by about 0.3 nanograms/mL, by simvastatin but this appears to be of little or no clinical importance.[6]

Mechanism

The small changes seen in digoxin levels are probably due to the inhibitory effects of these statins on P-glycoprotein. Pravastatin does not appear to inhibit P-glycoprotein.[7]

Importance and management

The small changes seen in the digoxin levels with statins seem unlikely to be clinically relevant in most patients.

1. Boyd RA, Stern RH, Stewart BH, Wu X, Reyner EL, Zegarac EA, Randinitis EJ, Whitfield L. Atorvastatin coadministration may increase digoxin concentrations by inhibition of intestinal P-glycoprotein-mediated secretion. *J Clin Pharmacol* (2000) 40, 91–8.
2. Smith HT, Jokubaitis LA, Troendle AJ, Hwang DS, Robinson WT. Pharmacokinetics of fluvastatin and specific drug interactions. *Am J Hypertens* (1993) 6 (Suppl), 375S–382S.
3. Garnett WR, Venitz J, Wilkens RC, Dimenna G. Pharmacokinetic effects of fluvastatin in patients chronically receiving digoxin. *Am J Med* (1994) 96 (Suppl 6A), 84S–86S.
4. Triscari J, Swanson BN, Willard DA, Cohen AI, Devault A, Pan HY. Steady state serum concentrations of pravastatin and digoxin when given in combination. *Br J Clin Pharmacol* (1993) 36, 263–5.
5. Martin PD, Kemp J, Dane AL, Warwick MJ, Schneck DW. No effect of rosuvastatin on the pharmacokinetics of digoxin in healthy volunteers. *J Clin Pharmacol* (2002) 42, 1352–7.
6. Garnett WR. Interactions with hydroxymethylglutaryl-coenzyme A reductase inhibitors. *Am J Health-Syst Pharm* (1995) 52, 1639–45.
7. Sakaeda T, Takara K, Kakumoto M, Ohmoto N, Nakamura T, Iwaki K, Tanigawara Y, Okumura K. Simvastatin and lovastatin, but not pravastatin, interact with MDR1. *J Pharm Pharmacol* (2002) 54, 419–23.

Digitalis glycosides + Sucralfate

Sucralfate caused only a small reduction in the absorption of digoxin in one study, but an isolated report describes a marked reduction in one patient.

Clinical evidence

Sucralfate 1 g four times daily given to 12 healthy subjects for 2 days had no effect on most of the pharmacokinetics of a single 750-microgram dose of **digoxin**; however, the AUC was reduced by 19% and the amount of **digoxin** eliminated in the urine was reduced by 12%. **Digoxin** was also absorbed faster.[1] No interaction occurred when the **digoxin** was given 2 hours before the sucralfate.[1] One elderly patient is reported to have had subtherapeutic serum **digoxin** levels while taking sucralfate, even though the dosages were separated by 2 hours.[2]

Mechanism

Uncertain. One possibility is that the digoxin and sucralfate bind together in the gut, which reduces the digoxin absorption.

Importance and management

Information appears to be limited to the reports cited. The reduction in digoxin levels reported in the study is small and therefore normally unlikely to be clinically relevant, but the unexplained and isolated case suggests that clinicians should at least be aware of the possibility of an interaction.

1. Giesing DH, Lanman RC, Dimmitt DC, Runser DJ. Lack of effect of sucralfate on digoxin pharmacokinetics. *Gastroenterology* (1983) 84,1165.
2. Rey AM, Gums JG. Altered absorption of digoxin, sustained-release quinidine, and warfarin with sucralfate administration. *Ann Pharmacother* (1991) 25, 745–6.

Digitalis glycosides + Surfactant excipients

Non-ionic surfactants used as pharmaceutical excipients such as polyoxyl castor oil (Cremophor) may slightly enhance the absorption of digoxin.

Clinical evidence, mechanism, importance and management

A placebo-controlled study in 12 healthy subjects found that **polyoxyl castor oil** (***Cremophor RH40***) 600 mg three times daily increased the AUC_{0-5} and peak plasma levels of a single 500-microgram oral dose of **digoxin** by about 22%. The absorption of **digoxin** was delayed. The pharmacodynamic effects of **digoxin** were not affected by ***Cremophor***.

It was suggested that ***Cremophor*** increases **digoxin** plasma levels by inhibiting intestinal P-glycoprotein, or that the ***Cremophor*** prolongs the dissolution of **digoxin** tablets resulting in delayed absorption from the intestines.[1]

Other surfactants inhibit P-glycoprotein mediated intestinal transport and an *in vitro* study found that the order of effectiveness for enhanced intestinal uptake of **digoxin** (starting with the most effective) was ***Labrasol***, ***Imwitor 742***, ***Acconon E***, ***Softigen 767***, ***Cremophor EL***, ***Miglyol***, ***Solutol HS 15***, **Sucrose monolaurate**, **Polysorbate 20**, ***TPGS***, **Polysorbate 80**.[2] See also 'Digitalis glycosides + Vitamin E substances', p.943.

1. Tayrouz Y, Ding R, Burhenne J, Riedel K-D, Weiss J, Hoppe-Tichy T, Haefeli WE, Mikus G. Pharmacokinetic and pharmaceutic interaction between digoxin and Cremophor RH40. *Clin Pharmacol Ther* (2003) 73, 397–405.
2. Cornaire G, Woodley J, Hermann P, Cloarec A, Arellano C, Houin G. Impact of excipients on the absorption of P-glycoprotein substrates in vitro and in vivo. *Int J Pharm* (2004) 278, 119–31.

Digitalis glycosides + Tegaserod

Tegaserod slightly reduces the AUC of digoxin, but this is unlikely to be clinically relevant.

Clinical evidence, mechanism, importance and management

A study in 12 healthy subjects given tegaserod 6 mg twice daily for 5 days found that the time to peak levels of a single 1-mg dose of **digoxin** on day 4 was reduced by 30 minutes, and the mean AUC and maximum plasma concentrations were slightly reduced by 11.9% and 15%, respectively.[1] These small changes are unlikely to be clinically relevant. Note that the manufacturer has discontinued marketing of tegaserod in the US because of a finding of an excess risk of serious cardiovascular ischaemic events.[2]

1. Zhou H, Horowitz A, Ledford PC, Hubert M, Appel-Dingemanse S, Osborne S, McLeod JF. The effects of tegaserod (HTF 919) on the pharmacokinetics and pharmacodynamics of digoxin in healthy subjects. *J Clin Pharmacol* (2001) 41, 1131–9.
2. Dear Dr Letter. Novartis Pharmaceuticals Corp. March 30, 2007. Available at: http://www.zelnorm.com/Dr_Doctor_Letter.pdf (accessed 22/08/07).

Digitalis glycosides + Tetracycline

Limited early evidence suggested that tetracycline may cause a rise in serum digoxin levels.

Clinical evidence

A patient taking **digoxin** tablets 500 micrograms daily was given tetracycline 500 mg every 6 hours for 5 days. His urinary excretion of **digoxin** metabolites (see *Mechanism*, below) fell sharply within 2 days, and his steady-state serum **digoxin** levels rose by 43%.[1] Another subject had a marked fall in the excretion of **digoxin** metabolites from the gut after taking tetracycline.[2]

In one study, tetracycline prolonged the half-life of **digoxin** and increased serum levels from 1.7 to 2.9 nanograms/mL.[3]

Mechanism

Uncertain. Up to 10% of patients taking oral digoxin excrete it in substantial amounts in the faeces and urine as inactive metabolites (digoxin reduction products or DRPs). This metabolism seems to be performed by the gut flora,[1] in particular *Eubacterium lentum*, which is anaerobic and Gram positive.[2,4] In the presence of some antibacterials, such as tetracycline, which can inhibit this organism, more digoxin becomes available for absorption, which results in a rise in serum levels. At the same time the inactive metabolites derived from the gut disappear.[2] However, this is not necessarily the full explanation, see also 'Digitalis glycosides + Macrolides', p.929.

Importance and management

The interaction between digoxin and tetracycline is not well established, the evidence is very limited, and its general clinical importance is uncertain. Bear this interaction in mind in case of an unexpected response to digoxin.

1. Lindenbaum J, Rund DG, Butler VP, Tse-Eng D, Saha JR. Inactivation of digoxin by the gut flora: reversal by antibiotic therapy. *N Engl J Med* (1981) 305, 789–94.
2. Dobkin JF, Saha JR, Butler VP, Lindenbaum J. Effects of antibiotic therapy on digoxin metabolism. *Clin Res* (1982) 30, 517A.
3. Halawa B. Interakcje digoksyny z cefradina (Sefril), tetracyklina (Tetracyclinum), gentamycyna (Gentamycin) i wankomycyna (Vancocin). *Pol Tyg Lek* (1984) 39, 1717–20.
4. Ten Eick AP, Reed MD. Hidden dangers of coadministration of antibiotics and digoxin in children: focus on azithromycin. *Curr Ther Res* (2000) 61, 148–60.

Digitalis glycosides + Thyroid hormones and Antithyroid drugs

Thyrotoxic patients are relatively resistant to the effects of digitalis glycosides and may need reduced doses as treatment with antithyroid drugs (carbimazole, thiamazole) progresses, whereas patients with hypothyroidism may need increased doses of digitalis glycosides as treatment with thyroid hormones progresses. Carbimazole has been shown to reduce serum digoxin in healthy subjects.

Clinical evidence

(a) Carbimazole

The observation of relatively low plasma **digoxin** levels in a patient taking carbimazole prompted a further study in 10 healthy subjects. In 9 out of the 10, steady-state peak serum **digoxin** levels were reduced by 23% (from 1.72 to 1.33 nanograms/mL) by a single 60-mg dose of carbimazole, but in the other subject the serum **digoxin** levels were increased. Other pharmacokinetic parameters were unaffected.

Carbimazole abolished the systolic blood pressure decrease seen in the first 3 hours with **digoxin**, and also reduced the duration of the **digoxin**-induced diastolic blood pressure fall from 12 to 6 hours. The changes in heart rates, cardiac output and stroke volumes were not statistically significant, but inter-individual differences were large.[1-3]

(b) Thiamazole

A study in 12 patients with hyperthyroidism found that normalisation of serum T3 and T4 by thiamazole treatment did not produce significant changes in the pharmacokinetics of **digoxin**.[4]

Mechanism

One explanation for the changed response to digitalis with carbimazole is that there is a direct and altered response of the heart due to the raised or lowered thyroid hormone levels. Another is that changes in glomerular filtration rate associated with hypo- or hyperthyroidism result in increased or decreased serum digoxin, respectively.[5] Why carbimazole *reduced* serum digoxin in healthy subjects (normal thyroid status) is not known.

Importance and management

As thyroid status is returned to normal by the use of drugs (antithyroid drugs or thyroid hormones), the dosage of the digitalis glycosides may need to be adjusted appropriately. Hyperthyroid patients may need to have their digitalis dosage gradually reduced as treatment proceeds (because initially they are relatively resistant to the effects of digitalis and start off needing higher doses). They are also relatively insensitive to the chronotropic effects of digitalis.[6,7] Hypothyroid patients on the other hand may need a gradually increasing dosage (because initially they are relatively sensitive to digitalis).[5,6] In either of these situations it would be prudent to monitor serum digoxin levels and glomerular filtration rate as treatment continues. The reduction of serum digoxin by carbimazole in healthy subjects does not fit with the need to decrease digoxin doses when antithyroid drugs are used in patients. Further study is needed.

1. Petereit G, Ramesh Rao B, Siepmann M, Kirch W. Influence of carbimazole on the steady state serum levels and haemodynamic effects of digoxin in healthy subjects. *Eur J Clin Pharmacol* (1995) 49, A159.
2. Rao BR, Petereit G, Ebert U, Siepmann M, Kirch W. Influence of carbimazole on the steady state serum levels and haemodynamic effects of digoxin in healthy subjects. *Therapie* (1995) 50 (Suppl), 406.
3. Rao R, Petereit G, Ebert U, Kirch W. Influence of carbimazole on serum levels and haemodynamic effects of digoxin. *Clin Drug Invest* (1997) 13, 350–4.
4. Gasińska T, Izbicka M, Dec R. Digoxin pharmacokinetics in hyperthyroid patients treated with methimazole. *J Endocrinol* (1997) 152 (Suppl), P285.
5. Croxson MS, Ibbertson HK. Serum digoxin in patients with thyroid disease. *BMJ* (1975) 3, 566–8.
6. Lawrence JR, Sumner DJ, Kalk WJ, Ratcliffe WA, Whiting B, Gray K, Lindsay M. Digoxin kinetics in patients with thyroid dysfunction. *Clin Pharmacol Ther* (1977) 22, 7–13.
7. Huffman DH, Klaassen CD, Hartman CR. Digoxin in hyperthyroidism. *Clin Pharmacol Ther* (1977) 22, 533–8.

Digitalis glycosides + Ticlopidine

In 15 subjects ticlopidine 250 mg twice daily for 10 days reduced the peak serum levels and AUC of digoxin by about 10%.[1] This reduction is small and unlikely to be of clinical importance.

1. Vargas R, Reitman M, Teitelbaum P, Ryan JR, McMahon FG, Jain AK, Ryan M, Regel G. Study of the effect of ticlopidine on digoxin blood levels. *Clin Pharmacol Ther* (1988) 43, 176.

Digitalis glycosides + Tiludronate

Tiludronate does not appear to affect the pharmacokinetics of digoxin.

Clinical evidence, mechanism, importance and management

A study in 12 healthy subjects found that **tiludronate**, 600 mg daily for 2 days then 400 mg daily for the next 10 days, caused no significant changes in the pharmacokinetics of **digoxin** 250 micrograms daily.[1] No special precautions appear to be needed.

1. Sanofi Winthrop. Data on file, June 1996.

Digitalis glycosides + Trapidil

Trapidil does not alter serum digoxin levels.

Clinical evidence, mechanism, importance and management

Trapidil 400 mg daily for 8 days had no effect on the steady-state serum levels of **digoxin** 375 micrograms daily in 10 healthy subjects. It was noted that the positive chronotropic effect of trapidil opposed the negative chronotropic effect of **digoxin**, which should be remembered when using both drugs, but overall no adverse effects that would prevent concurrent use were noted.[1]

1. Sziegoleit W, Weiss M, Fahr A, Scharfe S. Trapidil does not affect serum levels and cardiotonic action of digoxin in healthy humans. *Jpn Circ J* (1987) 51, 1305–9.

Digitalis glycosides + Trazodone

A rise in serum digoxin levels, accompanied by toxicity in one instance, has been seen when two patients taking digoxin were given trazodone.

Clinical evidence, mechanism, importance and management

An elderly woman taking **digoxin** 125 micrograms daily (and also taking quinidine, clonidine and a triamterene/hydrochlorothiazide diuretic) complained of nausea and vomiting within about 2 weeks of starting to take trazodone (initially 50 mg, increasing to 300 mg daily over 11 days). Her serum **digoxin** levels had risen more than threefold, from 0.8 to 2.8 nanograms/mL. The **digoxin** was stopped and then restarted at half the original dosage, which maintained therapeutic levels.[1] The patient had poor renal function, but this did not change significantly during this incident. Another case of raised **digoxin** levels, apparently caused by trazodone, has been reported.[2]

Direct information seems to be limited to these two reports, which is insufficient evidence to make any general recommendations; however, bear this interaction in mind in case of an unexpected response to **digoxin**.

1. Rauch PK, Jenike MA. Digoxin toxicity possibly precipitated by trazodone. *Psychosomatics* (1984) 25, 334–5.
2. Knapp JE. Mead Johnson Pharmaceutical Newsletter, 1983.

Digitalis glycosides + Trimetazidine

Trimetazidine does not appear to affect the pharmacokinetics of digoxin.

Clinical evidence, mechanism, importance and management

After taking trimetazidine 20 mg twice daily for at least 14 days the pharmacokinetics of a single 500-microgram dose of **digoxin** remained unchanged in 13 healthy subjects.[1] These results suggest that treatment with **digoxin** is unlikely to be altered in patients concurrently treated with trimetazidine.

1. Edeki TI, Johnston A, Campbell DB, Ings RMJ, Brownsill R, Genissel P, Turner P. An examination of the possible pharmacokinetic interaction of trimetazidine with theophylline, digoxin and antipyrine. *Br J Clin Pharmacol* (1989) 26, 657P.

Digitalis glycosides + Trospium

In a study in 40 healthy subjects trospium 20 mg twice daily for 12 days did not affect the pharmacokinetics of a single 500-microgram dose of digoxin elixir given on day 7.[1]

1. Sandage B, Sabounjian L, Shipley J, Profy A, Lasseter K, Fox L, Harnett M. Predictive power of an in vitro system to assess drug interactions of an antimuscarinic medication: a comparison of in vitro and in vivo drug-drug interaction studies of trospium chloride with digoxin. *J Clin Pharmacol* (2006) 46, 776–84.

Digitalis glycosides + Urapidil

Urapidil does not appear to affect the pharmacokinetics of digoxin.

Clinical evidence, mechanism, importance and management

In 12 healthy subjects urapidil 60 mg twice daily on days 5 to 8 had no significant effects on the serum levels of **digoxin** 250 micrograms twice daily on day one, then 250 micrograms daily on days 2 to 8. Blood pressures and pulse rates were not significantly changed.[1] No special precautions seem necessary if both drugs are given.

1. Solleder P, Haerlin R, Wurst W, Klingmann I, Mosberg H. Effect of urapidil on steady-state serum digoxin concentration in healthy subjects. *Eur J Clin Pharmacol* (1989) 37, 193–4.

Digitalis glycosides + Valaciclovir

Valaciclovir appears not to interact with digoxin.

Clinical evidence, mechanism, importance and management

In a randomised study, 12 healthy subjects were given 1 g of oral valaciclovir alone, two 750-microgram doses of **digoxin** alone, valaciclovir 1 g after the second of two 750-microgram doses of **digoxin** given 12 hours apart, and finally valaciclovir 1 g three times daily for 8 days starting 12 hours before the first **digoxin** dose.[1]

It was found that no clinically significant changes occurred in the pharmacokinetics of either drug and no ECG changes were seen and it was therefore concluded that no dosage adjustments of either drug are needed if they are given concurrently.[1] Since valaciclovir is a prodrug of **aciclovir**, it also seems unlikely that an interaction will occur between **aciclovir** and **digoxin**. Information about **digitoxin** and other analogues of aciclovir seems to be lacking.

1. Soul-Lawton JH, Weatherley BC, Posner J, Layton G, Peck RW. Lack of interaction between valaciclovir, the L-valyl ester of aciclovir and digoxin. *Br J Clin Pharmacol* (1998) 45, 87–9.

Digitalis glycosides + Valspodar

Valspodar increases the AUC of digoxin two to threefold.

Clinical evidence, mechanism, importance and management

Twelve healthy subjects were given **digoxin** 1 mg on day 1, followed by 125 micrograms daily for the next 10 days. Starting on day 7 they were also given a single 400-mg dose of valspodar, followed by valspodar 200 mg twice daily for the following 4 days. The steady-state **digoxin** AUC was increased by 76% after the first valspodar dose, and by the end of valspodar dosing it had increased by 211%. This was apparently due to a 73% reduction in **digoxin** renal clearance and a 58% reduction in non-renal clearance, probably because of reduced tubular secretion, reduced biliary elimination, and increased intestinal absorption caused by P-glycoprotein inhibition. No symptoms of digitalis toxicity were seen and there were no changes in vital signs or ECG parameters.[1]

Information seems to be limited to this study in healthy subjects but it suggests that the **digoxin** dosage should be reduced if valspodar is given. An initial 50% reduction has been suggested.

1. Kovarik JM, Rigaudy L, Guerret M, Gerbeau C, Rost K-L. Longitudinal assessment of a P-glycoprotein-mediated drug interaction of valspodar on digoxin. *Clin Pharmacol Ther* (1999) 66, 391–400.

Digitalis glycosides + Vancomycin

In one early study, vancomycin prolonged the half-life of digoxin and increased its serum levels from 1.6 to 3 nanograms/mL. It was suggested that this effect might be as a result of reduced renal clearance.[1] This appears to be the only evidence of a possible interaction.

1. Halawa B. Interakcje digoksyny z cefradina (Sefril), tetracylina (Tetracyclinum), gentamycyna (Gentamycin) i wankomycyna (Vancocin). *Pol Tyg Lek* (1984) 39, 1717–20.

Digitalis glycosides + Vardenafil

Vardenafil does not appear to interact with digoxin.

Clinical evidence, mechanism, importance and management

In a placebo-controlled study, 19 healthy subjects were given **digoxin** 375 micrograms daily for 28 days, with vardenafil 20 mg once daily on alternate days from day 16 to day 28. The pharmacokinetics of **digoxin** were not significantly changed by vardenafil, and there was no alteration in vital signs, ECG readings and laboratory parameters (not stated). The incidence of mild to moderate headache rose slightly from 7 out of 19 with placebo to 13 out of 19 with **digoxin**.[1] There would appear to be no reason to monitor **digoxin** levels in patients given vardenafil.

1. Rohde G, Bauer R-J, Unger S, Ahr G, Wensing G. Vardenafil, a new selective PDE5 inhibitor, produces no interaction with digoxin. *Pharmacotherapy* (2001) 21, 1254.

Digitalis glycosides + Vasodilators

Sodium nitroprusside or hydralazine infusions can reduce serum digoxin levels, but the importance of this is uncertain. Isosorbide dinitrate did not alter digoxin pharmacokinetics in one study.

Clinical evidence, mechanism, importance and management

(a) Hydralazine or Sodium nitroprusside

An experimental study in 8 patients with congestive heart failure found that when they were given either **sodium nitroprusside** by infusion (7 to 425 micrograms/minute) or **hydralazine** by intravenous injection (5 mg every 10 to 20 minutes to a total dose of 10 to 60 mg) the total renal **digoxin** clearance was increased by about 50% by both drugs and the serum **digoxin** levels were decreased by 20% by the **nitroprusside** and 11% by the **hydralazine**.[1]

It is not known whether these changes would be sustained during chronic concurrent use, or the extent to which the **digoxin** dosage might need to be increased. More study is needed to find out if this interaction is of practical importance.

(b) Isosorbide dinitrate

In a crossover study in 8 patients with chronic heart failure given **digoxin** 250 micrograms daily for 20 days with isosorbide dinitrate 10 mg three times daily for the last 10 days, there was no change in the mean steady-state concentration, AUC or half-life of digoxin.[2]

1. Cogan JJ, Humphreys MH, Carlson CJ, Benowitz NL, Rapaport E. Acute vasodilator therapy increases renal clearance of digoxin in patients with congestive heart failure. *Circulation* (1981) 64, 973–6.
2. Mahgoub AA, El-Medany AH, Abdulatif AS. A comparison between the effects of diltiazem and isosorbide dinitrate on digoxin pharmacodynamics and kinetics in the treatment of patients with chronic ischemic heart failure. *Saudi Med J* (2002) 23, 725–31.

Digitalis glycosides + Vitamin E substances

Alpha tocoferil acetate had no effect on digoxin pharmacokinetics, but vitamin E formulations with polyethylene glycol might.

Clinical evidence, mechanism, importance and management

In a study in healthy subjects, **alpha tocoferil acetate** 400 units twice daily for 15 days did not affect the pharmacokinetics of a single 500-microgram dose of **digoxin** given on day 15. This was in contrast to a formulation of vitamin E containing polyethylene glycol (**alpha tocoferil acid succinate**), which altered **digoxin** pharmacokinetics (amount not stated) without altering its ECG effects.

It was suggested that the effect of polyethylene glycol on **digoxin** was via P-glycoprotein inhibition,[1] see also 'Digitalis glycosides + Surfactant excipients', p.941.

1. Chan L, Humma LM, Schriever CA, Fahsingbauer BS, Dominguez CP, Baum CL. Vitamin E formulation affects digoxin absorption by inhibiting P-glycoprotein (P-GP) in humans. *Clin Pharmacol Ther* (2004) 75, P95.

Digitalis glycosides + Zileuton

Zileuton appears not to interact with digoxin.

Clinical evidence, mechanism, importance and management

In a placebo-controlled study, 12 healthy subjects were given zileuton 600 mg every 6 hours for 13 days, with **digoxin** 250 micrograms daily from days 1 to 11. The zileuton had no effect on the steady-state **digoxin** pharmacokinetics, although the time to reach maximum plasma levels was reduced from 1.43 to 0.95 hours. Concurrent use was well tolerated.[1] This evidence suggests that no special precautions are needed if these two drugs are used together.

1. Awni WM, Hussein Z, Cavanaugh JH, Granneman GR, Dube LM. Assessment of the pharmacokinetic interaction between zileuton and digoxin in humans. *Clin Pharmacokinet* (1995) 29 (Suppl 2), 92–7.

26

Diuretics

The majority of the interactions of the diuretics appear to be pharmacodynamic in nature, that is, they appear to be due to the combined effects of the diuretic and the other interacting drug. Obvious examples of this would be hypotension caused by the use of a loop diuretic and a beta blocker, or hyperkalaemia caused by an ACE inhibitor and a potassium-sparing diuretic. Some commonly accepted interactions appear to be sparsely documented, most probably because they are perceived to be a predictable effect of using two drugs with similar actions together. 'Table 26.1', (below) lists the major diuretic drug groups classified by their effect on potassium. Carbonic anhydrase inhibitors are included under potassium-depleting diuretics, but note that hypokalaemia caused by this type of drug is said to be transient and rarely clinically significant.

Eplerenone, a selective aldosterone antagonist similar to spironolactone, is metabolised by the cytochrome P450 isoenzyme CYP3A4 and is therefore affected by other drugs that are inhibitors or inducers of this enzyme.

The interactions covered in this section are mainly those in which the diuretic is affected. There are many other interactions throughout the publication where diuretics affect the actions of other drugs.

Table 26.1 Diuretics

Group	*Drugs*
Potassium-depleting diuretics	
Carbonic anhydrase inhibitors*	Acetazolamide, Diclofenamide (Dichlorphenamide), Methazolamide
Loop diuretics	Bumetanide, Etacrynic acid, Furosemide, Piretanide, Torasemide
Thiazides and related diuretics	Altizide, Bemetizide, Bendroflumethiazide, Benzthiazide, Butizide, Chlorothiazide, Chlortalidone, Clopamide, Cyclopenthiazide, Cyclothiazide, Epitizide, Hydrochlorothiazide, Hydroflumethiazide, Indapamide, Mefruside, Methyclothiazide, Metolazone, Polythiazide, Teclothiazide, Trichlormethiazide, Xipamide
Potassium-sparing diuretics	
Aldosterone inhibitors	Eplerenone, Potassium canrenoate, Spironolactone
Other	Amiloride, Triamterene

*Note that hypokalaemia caused by this type of drug is said to be transient and rarely clinically significant

Acetazolamide + NSAIDs

A case of acute renal failure has been reported in a woman who underwent retinal surgery, which occurred after the postoperative use of a total of 2 g of acetazolamide, 80 g of mannitol and 700 mg of ketoprofen.[1] There appear to be no other similar case reports, but note that 'loop diuretics', (p.949) are known to increase the risk of NSAID-induced acute renal failure.

1. Truc C, Rigal E, Pernot A, Vaudelin G, Boulétreau P. Anti-inflammatoires non stéroïdiens et diurétiques: une association à risqué néphrotoxique. *Ann Fr Anesth Reanim* (2000) 19, 675–7.

Acetazolamide + Sodium bicarbonate

Acetazolamide is associated with development of renal calculi and it is claimed that sodium bicarbonate, even on alternate days, potentiates the risk of calculus formation.[1]

1. Rubenstein MA, Bucy JG. Acetazolamide-induced renal calculi. *J Urol (Baltimore)* (1975) 114, 610–12.

Acetazolamide + Timolol

The use of acetazolamide tablets with timolol eye drops resulted in severe mixed acidosis in a patient with chronic obstructive pulmonary disease.

Clinical evidence, mechanism, importance and management

An elderly man with severe chronic obstructive pulmonary disease was given oral acetazolamide 750 mg daily and timolol maleate 0.5% eye drops, one drop in each eye twice daily, as premedication to reduce ocular hypertension before surgery for glaucoma. Five days later he developed progressively worsening dyspnoea and he was found to have a severe, mixed acidosis.[1] This seems to have been caused by the additive effects of acetazolamide, which blocked the excretion of hydrogen ions in the kidney, and the bronchoconstrictor effects of the timolol, which was absorbed in sufficient amounts to exacerbate the airway obstruction in this patient, and thereby reduced the respiration. This isolated case emphasises the potential risks of using beta blockers, even as non-systemic preparations such as eye drops, in patients with obstructive pulmonary disease. The manufacturers of acetazolamide note that it should be used with caution in those with pulmonary obstruction or emphysema because of the increased risk of acidosis.[2] This is, in part, a drug-disease interaction.

1. Boada JE, Estopa R, Izquierdo J, Dorca J, Manresa F. Severe mixed acidosis by combined therapy with acetazolamide and timolol eyedrops. *Eur J Respir Dis* (1986) 68, 226–8.
2. Diamox (Acetazolamide). Wyeth Pharmaceuticals. UK Summary of product characteristics, February 2004.

Cyclothiazide/triamterene + Pravastatin

Reversible diabetes mellitus developed in a woman taking cyclothiazide/triamterene when she was also given pravastatin.

Clinical evidence, mechanism, importance and management

A 63-year-old woman who had been taking cyclothiazide/triamterene and acebutolol for 4 years, developed polyuria and polydipsia within 3 weeks of starting to take pravastatin 20 mg daily, which gradually worsened. After another 4 months she was hospitalised for hyperglycaemia, which was treated with insulin and later glibenclamide (glyburide). The cyclothiazide/triamterene and pravastatin were stopped and gradually the diabetic symptoms began to abate. Five weeks after admission she was discharged without the need for any antidiabetic treatment with the diabetes fully resolved.[1] The detailed reasons for this reaction are not understood, but it would seem that the pravastatin increased the hyperglycaemic potential of the thiazide diuretic to the point where frank diabetes developed. This is an isolated case and there would seem to be little reason normally to avoid the concurrent use of these drugs.

1. Jonville-Bera A-P, Zakian A, Bera FJ, Carré P, Autret E. Possible pravastatin and diuretics-induced diabetes mellitus. *Ann Pharmacother* (1994) 28, 964–5.

Eplerenone + CYP3A4 inducers

St John's wort slightly decreased the AUC of eplerenone. The manufacturer recommends the avoidance of St John's wort and other stronger inducers of CYP3A4 such as rifampicin because of the possible risk of decreased eplerenone efficacy.

Clinical evidence, mechanism, importance and management

St John's wort (*Hypericum perforatum*) caused a slight 30% decrease in the AUC of a single 100-mg dose of eplerenone.[1,2] Eplerenone is metabolised by the cytochrome P450 isoenzyme CYP3A4, and therefore inducers of this isoenzyme, such as **St John's wort**, would be expected to decrease its levels. In the UK, the manufacturer predicts that a more pronounced decrease in the AUC of eplerenone might occur with stronger CYP3A4 inducers, such as **rifampicin (rifampin)**.[1] Because of the possibility of decreased efficacy, they do not recommend the concurrent use of potent CYP3A4 inducers with eplerenone, and they specifically name **carbamazepine**, **phenytoin**, **phenobarbital**, **rifampicin**, and **St John's wort**.[1] However, it is unlikely that the decrease seen with **St John's wort** is clinically relevant. Further study is needed of the other potential interactions to demonstrate their clinical significance.

1. Inspra (Eplerenone). Pfizer Ltd. UK Summary of product characteristics, May 2006.
2. Inspra (Eplerenone). Pfizer Inc. US Prescribing information, May 2005.

Eplerenone + CYP3A4 inhibitors

Ketoconazole markedly raises the AUC of eplerenone, and the manufacturer contraindicates concurrent use. Similarly, the concurrent use of other potent inhibitors of CYP3A4 should be avoided. Mild to moderate inhibitors of CYP3A4 (including diltiazem, fluconazole, saquinavir and verapamil) increase the AUC of eplerenone by up to almost threefold. Grapefruit juice had a small but unimportant effect.

Clinical evidence

(a) Azoles

Ketoconazole 200 mg twice daily for 7 days increased the AUC of a single 100-mg dose of eplerenone 5.4-fold in 18 healthy subjects,[1,2] and **fluconazole** 200 mg daily for 7 days increased the AUC of eplerenone 2.2-fold in 18 healthy subjects.[2] The manufacturer predicts that **itraconazole** will have a similar effect to **ketoconazole**.[3]

(b) Calcium-channel blockers

In 24 healthy subjects the steady-state AUC of eplerenone 100 mg daily was increased by about twofold by **verapamil** 240 mg daily for 7 days.[2] **Diltiazem** has caused similar increases.[3]

(c) Grapefruit juice

Grapefruit juice caused only a small 25% increase in the AUC of eplerenone 100 mg.[1]

(d) Macrolides

In 24 healthy subjects **erythromycin** 500 mg twice daily increased the steady-state AUC of eplerenone 100 mg daily by 2.9-fold.[2] The manufacturer predicts that **clarithromycin**,[1,3] **telithromycin**,[3] and **troleandomycin**[1] will have a greater effect. Eplerenone reduced the AUC of **erythromycin** by 14%, which was not considered clinically relevant.[2]

(e) Protease inhibitors

in 24 healthy subjects **saquinavir** 1.2 g three times daily increased the steady-state AUC of eplerenone 100 mg daily by 2.1-fold.[2] The manufacturer predicts that **ritonavir** and **nelfinavir** will have a greater effect.[3]

Eplerenone reduced the maximum level of **saquinavir** by 30%, and the AUC by 21%,[2] but the clinical relevance of this has not been assessed.

Mechanism

Eplerenone is metabolised by the cytochrome P450 isoenzyme CYP3A4, and therefore inhibitors of this isoenzyme will raise its levels.

Importance and management

These pharmacokinetic interactions are established. Although the clinical relevance has not been assessed, it is known that the risk of hyperkalaemia with eplerenone is related to its dose.[3] Because the increase in the AUC of eplerenone with ketoconazole is so great, the manufacturers contraindicate this combination.[1,3] They also contraindicate the concurrent use of other potent inhibitors of CYP3A4, and they list clarithromycin, itraconazole, **nefazodone**, nelfinavir, ritonavir,[1,3] telithromycin[3] and troleandomycin.[1]

In the UK, the manufacturers recommend that the dose of eplerenone should not exceed 25 mg daily in patients taking mild to moderate CYP3A4 inhibitors such as **amiodarone**, diltiazem, erythromycin, fluconazole, saquinavir and verapamil.[3] In the US, the manufacturer recommends that the starting dose for hypertension should be reduced to 25 mg daily for patients taking these drugs.[1] This seems a sensible precaution. However, note that in many cases erythromycin appears to be a more potent inhibitor of CYP3A4 than clarithromycin (and certainly the other moderate CYP3A4 inhibitors listed above), and so extra caution is probably warranted with this combination.

1. Inspra (Eplerenone). Pfizer Inc. US Prescribing information, May 2005.
2. Cook CS, Berry LM, Burton E. Prediction of *in vivo* drug interactions with eplerenone in man from *in vitro* metabolic inhibition data. *Xenobiotica* (2004) 34, 215–28.
3. Inspra (Eplerenone). Pfizer Ltd. UK Summary of product characteristics, May 2006.

Eplerenone + Miscellaneous

Caution is recommended when eplerenone is used with alpha blockers, antipsychotics, amifostine, baclofen, corticosteroids, tetracosactide and tricyclic antidepressants. Lithium, ciclosporin, and tacrolimus should generally not be used with eplerenone. Antacids, cisapride, midazolam and simvastatin had no effect on eplerenone pharmacokinetics. Eplerenone had no important effect on cisapride, midazolam, warfarin or contraceptive steroid pharmacokinetics, but caused a slight increase in digoxin levels.

Clinical evidence, mechanism, importance and management

(a) Antacids

The manufacturer notes that **aluminium/magnesium**-containing antacids had no effect on the pharmacokinetics of eplerenone.[1]

(b) Ciclosporin and Tacrolimus

No clinically significant pharmacokinetic interaction was noted when eplerenone was given with ciclosporin.[1,2] Nevertheless, in the UK, the manufacturers state that ciclosporin and tacrolimus may impair renal function and increase the risk of hyperkalaemia. Therefore, they recommend that the concurrent use of either ciclosporin or tacrolimus with eplerenone should be avoided, or renal function and serum potassium should be closely monitored.[3] See also 'Ciclosporin + Diuretics', p.1032 and 'Tacrolimus + Miscellaneous', p.1080.

(c) Cisapride

A pharmacokinetic study found no interaction between cisapride (a cytochrome P450 isoenzyme CYP3A4 substrate) and eplerenone.[1,3]

(d) Combined hormonal contraceptives

Eplerenone 100 mg daily was given to 24 healthy subjects on days 1 to 11 of a 28-day cycle of a combined hormonal contraceptive (**ethinylestradiol/norethisterone** 35 micrograms/1 mg). There was no change in the **ethinylestradiol** AUC, but there was a small 17% increase in the **norethisterone** AUC, which is unlikely to be clinically relevant.[1,2]

(e) Corticosteroids

The concurrent use of corticosteroids may reduce the antihypertensive effect of eplerenone as they may cause fluid and sodium retention.[3]

(f) Digoxin

The steady-state AUC of digoxin 200 micrograms daily increased by 16% when it was given to healthy subjects with eplerenone 100 mg daily.[2,3] The UK manufacturers warn that caution may be warranted in patients with digoxin levels near the upper end of the therapeutic range.[3] Note that changes of this size are within the usual expected variation in the AUC of digoxin.

(g) Drugs that may cause postural hypotension

The manufacturer suggests that there is a risk of increased hypotensive effects and/or postural hypotension if eplerenone is given with **alpha blockers** (e.g. prazosin), **tricyclic antidepressants**, **antipsychotics**, **amifostine** and **baclofen**. They suggest increased monitoring.[3]

(h) Lithium

No interaction study has been done with lithium and eplerenone.[1,3] Serum lithium should be monitored frequently if eplerenone is given with lithium,[1,3] although, in the UK, the manufacturers advise avoidance of the combination.[3] This is because lithium toxicity has occurred with lithium and 'ACE inhibitors', (p.1112) or 'diuretics', (p.1122).

(i) Midazolam

A pharmacokinetic study has shown no pharmacokinetic interaction between midazolam (a cytochrome P450 isoenzyme CYP3A4 substrate) and eplerenone.[1,3]

(j) Simvastatin

In 18 healthy subjects simvastatin 40 mg once daily had no effect on the pharmacokinetics of eplerenone 100 mg once daily. The maximum level of simvastatin was modestly decreased by 32%, and the AUC by 14%, but this was not considered to be clinically relevant.[1,2]

(k) Tetracosactide

Tetracosactide can cause fluid and sodium retention and this may reduce the antihypertensive effect of eplerenone.[3]

(l) Warfarin

Eplerenone did not alter the pharmacokinetics of warfarin to a clinically significant extent.[1,3] However, in the UK the manufacturer still recommends caution when the warfarin dose is near the upper limit of the therapeutic range.[3]

1. Inspra (Eplerenone). Pfizer Inc. US Prescribing information, May 2005.
2. Cook CS, Berry LM, Burton E. Prediction of *in vivo* drug interactions with eplerenone in man from *in vitro* metabolic inhibition data. *Xenobiotica* (2004) 34, 215–28.
3. Inspra (Eplerenone). Pfizer Ltd. UK Summary of product characteristics, May 2006.

Furosemide + Bile-acid binding resins

Colestyramine and colestipol markedly reduce the absorption and diuretic effects of furosemide.

Clinical evidence

In 6 healthy subjects **colestyramine** 8 g reduced the absorption of a single 40-mg dose of furosemide by 95%. The 4-hour diuretic response was reduced by 77% (urinary output reduced from 1510 to 350 mL). **Colestipol** 10 g reduced the furosemide absorption by 80% and the 4-hour diuretic response by 58% (urinary output reduced from 1510 to 630 mL).[1]

Mechanism

Both colestyramine and colestipol are anionic exchange resins, which can bind with furosemide within the gut, thereby reducing its absorption and its effects.

Importance and management

An established interaction, although direct evidence seems to be limited to this study. The absorption of furosemide is relatively rapid so that giving it 2 to 3 hours before either the colestyramine or colestipol should be an effective way of overcoming this interaction. This needs confirmation. Note that it is normally recommended that other drugs are given 1 hour before or 4 to 6 hours after colestyramine and 1 hour before or 4 hours after colestipol.

1. Neuvonen PJ, Kivistö K, Hirvisalo EL. Effects of resins and activated charcoal on the absorption of digoxin, carbamazepine and frusemide. *Br J Clin Pharmacol* (1988) 25, 229–33.

Furosemide + Cloral hydrate

Intravenous injection of furosemide after treatment with cloral hydrate occasionally causes sweating, hot flushes, a variable blood pressure and tachycardia.

Clinical evidence

Six patients in a coronary care unit given an intravenous bolus of 40 to 120 mg of furosemide and who had received cloral hydrate during the previous 24 hours developed sweating, hot flushes, variable blood pressure, and tachycardia. The reaction was immediate and lasted for about 15 minutes. No special treatment was given. Furosemide had caused no problems when given before the cloral hydrate was started.[1]

A retrospective study of hospital records revealed that, out of 43 patients who had received both cloral hydrate and furosemide, one patient developed this reaction and 2 others may have done so.[2] The interaction has also been described in an 8-year-old boy.[3]

Mechanism

Not understood. One suggestion is that furosemide displaces trichloroacetic acid (the metabolite of cloral hydrate) from its protein binding sites, which in its turn displaces levothyroxine or alters the serum pH so that the levels of free levothyroxine rise leading to a hypermetabolic state.[1]

Importance and management

An established interaction, but information is limited to three reports. The incidence is uncertain but probably low. Concurrent use need not be avoided, but it would be prudent to give intravenous furosemide cautiously if cloral hydrate has been given recently. It seems possible that derivatives of cloral hydrate that break down in the body to release cloral hydrate (e.g. **dichloralphenazone**, **cloral betaine**) might interact similarly. There is no evidence that furosemide given orally or cloral hydrate given to patients already taking furosemide causes this reaction.[2]

1. Malach M, Berman N. Furosemide and chloral hydrate. Adverse drug interaction. *JAMA* (1975) 232, 638–9.
2. Pevonka MP, Yost RL, Marks RG, Howell WS, Stewart RB. Interaction of chloral hydrate and furosemide. A controlled retrospective study. *Drug Intell Clin Pharm* (1977) 11, 332–5.
3. Dean RP, Rudinsky BF, Kelleher MD. Interaction of chloral hydrate and intravenous furosemide in a child. *Clin Pharm* (1991) 10, 385–7.

Furosemide + Epoprostenol

An epoprostenol infusion did not significantly alter the pharmacokinetics of furosemide in a study modelling data from 23 patients with heart failure.[1] Note that the combination of loop diuretics with epoprostenol may lead to an enhanced hypotensive effect.

1. Carlton LD, Patterson JH, Mattson CN, Schmith VD. The effects of epoprostenol on drug disposition II: a pilot study of the pharmacokinetics of furosemide with and without epoprostenol in patients with congestive heart failure. *J Clin Pharmacol* (1996) 36, 257–64.

Furosemide + Germanium

An isolated case report describes a man who became resistant to furosemide after he took germanium.

Clinical evidence, mechanism, importance and management

A 63-year-old man was hospitalised for hypertension and oedema 10 days after adding ginseng containing germanium to his usual treatment with cyclophosphamide and furosemide. He gained almost 13 kg in weight. After treatment with intravenous furosemide he was discharged and again took ginseng with germanium. This time he gained 12 kg in weight over 14 days, despite an increase in the dose of furosemide from 80 to 240 mg twice daily. The weight gain and oedema again resolved when the ginseng and germanium was withdrawn and he was given intravenous furosemide. The authors suggest that germanium was responsible for this interaction.[1]

This is an isolated report, and its general significance is unclear. However, note that it has been said that the use of germanium should be discouraged due to its potential to cause renal toxicity.[2]

1. Becker BN, Greene J, Evanson J, Chidsey J, Stone WJ. Ginseng-induced diuretic resistance. *JAMA* (1996) 276, 606–7.
2. Sweetman SC, ed. Martindale: The complete drug reference. 35th ed. London: Pharmaceutical Press; 2007. p. 2097.

Furosemide + Paracetamol (Acetaminophen)

In 10 healthy women paracetamol 1 g four times daily for 2 days was found to have no effect on the diuresis or natriuresis in response to intravenous furosemide 20 mg.[1]

1. Martin U, Prescott LF. The interaction of paracetamol with frusemide. *Br J Clin Pharmacol* (1994) 37, 464–7.

Furosemide + Phenytoin

The diuretic effects of furosemide can be reduced as much as 50% if phenytoin is also given.

Clinical evidence

The observation that dependent oedema in a group of epileptics was higher than expected, and that the response to diuretic treatment seemed to be reduced, prompted further study. In 30 patients taking **phenytoin** 200 to 400 mg daily with phenobarbital 60 to 180 mg daily the maximal diuresis in response to furosemide 20 or 40 mg occurred after 3 to 4 hours instead of the usual 2 hours, and the total diuresis was reduced by 32% for the 20-mg dose and 49% for the 40-mg dose. When intravenous furosemide 20 mg was given, the total diuresis was reduced by 50%. Some of the patients were also taking carbamazepine, pheneturide, ethosuximide, diazepam or chlordiazepoxide.[1]

Another study in 5 healthy subjects given **phenytoin** 100 mg three times daily for 10 days found that the maximum serum levels of furosemide 20 mg, given orally or intravenously, were reduced by 50%.[2]

Mechanism

Not fully understood. One suggestion is that the phenytoin causes changes in the jejunal sodium pump activity, which reduces the absorption of the furosemide,[2] but this is not the whole story because an interaction also occurs when furosemide is given intravenously.[1] Another suggestion, based on *in vitro* evidence, is that the phenytoin generates a 'liquid membrane,' which blocks the transport of the furosemide to its active site.[3]

Importance and management

Information is limited but the interaction is established. A reduced diuretic response should be expected in the presence of phenytoin. A dosage increase may be needed.

1. Ahmad S. Renal insensitivity to frusemide caused by chronic anticonvulsant therapy. *BMJ* (1974) 3, 657–9.
2. Fine A, Henderson JS, Morgan DR, Tilstone WJ. Malabsorption of frusemide caused by phenytoin. *BMJ* (1977) 2, 1061–2.
3. Srivastava RC, Bhise SB, Sood R, Rao MNA. On the reduced furosemide response in the presence of diphenylhydantoin. *Colloids and Surfaces* (1986) 19, 83–8.

Furosemide + Sevelamer

Sevelamer abolished the diuretic effect of furosemide in a haemodialysis patient.

Clinical evidence, mechanism, importance and management

A haemodialysis patient taking furosemide 250 mg twice daily found that her urine output reduced from 950 mL/day to zero when she started taking sevelamer 800 mg at breakfast and lunchtime, and 1.6 g with dinner. Urine output returned to the previous level within 24 hours of stopping the sevelamer. This effect also occurred on rechallenge. The dose times were adjusted so that she took furosemide 500 mg in the morning and sevelamer 1.6 g at lunch and dinner, and her urine output was unaffected and remained stable.[1]

The authors suggest that furosemide became bound to sevelamer in the gut, and this prevented its absorption.

This appears to be the only case report of an interaction between these drugs so far; however, it is worth bearing this case in mind should a similar situation arise in other patients. Note that the manufacturers of sevelamer[2,3] suggest that when giving any other oral drug for which a reduction in the bioavailability could have a clinically significant effect on safety or efficacy, the drug should be given at least 1 hour before or 3 hours after sevelamer.

1. Fleuren HWHA, Kho Y, Schuurmans MMJ, Vollaard EJ. Drug interaction between sevelamer and furosemide. *Nephrol Dial Transplant* (2005) 20, 2288–9.
2. Renagel (Sevelamer). Genzyme Therapeutics. UK Summary of product characteristics, June 2007.
3. Renagel Capsules (Sevelamer hydrochloride). Genzyme. US Prescribing information, April 2007.

Loop diuretics + Aspirin

Aspirin may reduce the diuretic effect of bumetanide or furosemide, and the venodilation produced by furosemide.

Clinical evidence

(a) Bumetanide

In 8 healthy subjects aspirin 640 mg four times daily reduced the 24-hour urinary output in response to bumetanide 1 mg by 18%.[1]

(b) Furosemide

A study in 11 patients with chronic heart failure found that both aspirin 75 mg daily and aspirin 300 mg daily for 14 days reduced the venodilatory effects produced by a single 20-mg intravenous dose of furosemide (as measured by the forearm venous capacitance).[2] Six patients with cirrhosis and ascites had a reduced diuretic response to intravenous furosemide 40 mg when a single 450-mg dose of **lysine aspirin** was given before the injection.[3]

Mechanism

See 'Loop diuretics + NSAIDs', p.949.

Importance and management

The clinical significance of these interactions is unclear. Note that the European Society of Cardiology (ESC) and American College of Cardiology/American Heart Association (ACC/AHA) heart failure guidelines say that the prophylactic use of aspirin in patients with heart failure has not been proven unless the patient has underlying ischaemic heart disease[4,5] and should be avoided in patients with recurrent hospital admissions for worsening heart failure.[5]

1. Kaufman J, Hamburger R, Matheson J, Flamenbaum W. Bumetanide-induced diuresis and natriuresis: effect of prostaglandin synthetase inhibition. *J Clin Pharmacol* (1981) 21, 663–7.
2. Jhund PS, Davie AP, McMurray JJV. Aspirin inhibits the acute venodilator response to furosemide in patients with chronic heart failure. *J Am Coll Cardiol* (2001) 37, 1234–8.
3. Planas R, Arroyo V, Rimola A, Pérez-Ayuso RM, Rodés J. Acetylsalicylic acid suppresses the renal hemodynamic effect and reduces the diuretic action of furosemide in cirrhosis with ascites. *Gastroenterology* (1983) 84, 247–52.
4. Hunt SA. ACC/AHA 2005 guideline update for the diagnosis and management of chronic heart failure in the adult. A report of the American College of Cardiology/American Heart Association Task Force on Practice Guidelines (Writing Committee to Update the 2001 Guidelines for the Evaluation and Management of Heart Failure). *J Am Coll Cardiol* (2005) 46, e1–e82. Available at: http://content.onlinejacc.org/cgi/reprint/46/6/e1.pdf (accessed 22/08/2007).
5. Swedberg K, Cleland J, Dargie H, Drexler H, Follath F, Komajda M, Tavazzi L, Smiseth OA, Gavazzi A, Haverich A, Hoes A, Jaarsma T, Korewicki J, Lévy S, Linde C, Lopez-Sendon J-L, Nieminen MS, Piérard L, Remme WJ; The Task Force for the Diagnosis and Treatment of Chronic Heart Failure of the European Society of Cardiology. Guidelines for the diagnosis and treatment of chronic heart failure (update 2005). *Eur Heart J* (2005) 26, 1115–40. Available at: http://www.escardio.org/NR/rdonlyres/8A2848B4-5DEB-41B9-9A0A-5B5A90494B64/0/guidelines_CHF_FT_2005.pdf (accessed 22/08/2007).

Loop diuretics + Food

Some studies suggest that food modestly reduces the bioavailability and diuretic effects of furosemide. However, other studies have found that the bioavailability of furosemide and its diuretic effect is not affected by food. Food does not appear to affect bumetanide bioavailability.

Clinical evidence

(a) Solutions or standard tablets

Ten healthy subjects were given **furosemide** 40 mg with and without a standard breakfast. The food reduced the peak plasma levels of **furosemide** by 55% and the bioavailability by about 30%.[1] The results were almost identical when 5 of the subjects were given a heavy meal.[1] The diuresis over 10 hours was reduced by 21% (from 2072 to 1640 mL) and over 24 hours by 15% (from 2668 to 2270 mL) by **furosemide** taken with breakfast.[1] A comparative study in healthy subjects found that the absorption of both **bumetanide** 2 mg (9 subjects) and **furosemide** 40 mg (8 subjects), given as *solutions*, was delayed, and peak plasma levels were reduced, by a standard breakfast.[2] However, although food reduced the oral bioavailability of **furosemide** by about one-third, from 76% to 43%, the bioavailability of **bumetanide** was not significantly reduced (75% with food and 84% fasting). Food delayed the absorption but did not significantly alter the bioavailability of **furosemide** as tablets or solutions in two other studies.[3,4] In one of these studies, there was no difference in diuresis between fed and fasting subjects.[4]

(b) Sustained-release tablets

In a single-dose, crossover study in 28 subjects given two different controlled-release formulations of furosemide 60 mg, the absorption of one preparation (*Furix Retard*) was reduced by about 32% when it was given with breakfast, but the extent of absorption of the other formulation (*Lasix Retard*) was *increased* by about 18%. In the fasting phase of the study, the first formulation had a higher extent and rate of absorption than the second formulation. However, the differences in diuresis and total natriuresis between the formulations, and between the fed and fasted state, were minor.[5]

Mechanism

Not understood.

Importance and management

Information about the effect of food on **furosemide** absorption is somewhat contradictory. Of the four studies using solutions or standard tablets, just two found that the bioavailability of furosemide was modestly reduced by food (by about 30%) and the others found no effect. Moreover, the modest reduction in the AUC of furosemide did not result in a clinically relevant decrease in diuresis in the one study that assessed this. It would also seem that the absorption of controlled-release formulations of furosemide may be modestly affected by food, but this may lead to increased absorption depending on the preparation.[5] The authors of this study noted that the amount of furosemide absorbed did not correlate with the extent of diuresis, and concluded that the urinary excretion profile of furosemide may be more important for producing diuresis than the amount of furosemide absorbed. It would seem that furosemide and **bumetanide** can be given to most patients without regard to meal times. Food does not affect the bioavailability of bumetanide given as solution.

1. Beermann B, Midskov C. Reduced bioavailability and effect of furosemide given with food. *Eur J Clin Pharmacol* (1986) 29, 725–7.
2. McCrindle JL, Li Kam Wa TC, Barron W, Prescott LF. Effect of food on the absorption of frusemide and bumetanide in man. *Br J Clin Pharmacol* (1996) 42, 743–6.
3. Hammarlund MM, Paalzow LK, Odlind B. Pharmacokinetics of furosemide in man after intravenous and oral administration. Application of moment analysis. *Eur J Clin Pharmacol* (1984) 26, 197–207.
4. Kelly MR, Cutler RE, Forrey AW, Kimpel BM. Pharmacokinetics of orally administered furosemide. *Clin Pharmacol Ther* (1974) 15, 178–86.
5. Paintaud G, Alván G, Eckernäs SÅ, Wakelkamp M, Grahnén A. The influence of food intake on the effect of two controlled release formulations of furosemide. *Biopharm Drug Dispos* (1995) 16, 221–32.

Loop diuretics + H_2-receptor antagonists

Ranitidine and cimetidine may cause a moderate increase in the bioavailability of furosemide, but with no associated increase in diuretic effect. Cimetidine appears not to interact with torasemide.

Clinical evidence, mechanism, importance and management

(a) Furosemide

In a study in 6 healthy subjects, a single 400-mg dose of **cimetidine** increased the mean AUC of furosemide by one-third, although there was wide inter-patient variation. However, there were no changes in the diuretic effects of furosemide or in the pharmacokinetics of cimetidine, and an associated study using multiple doses of **cimetidine** over 5 days found no pharmacokinetic or pharmacodynamic interaction.[1] A similar study in patients with hepatic cirrhosis also found that **cimetidine** does not interact with furosemide.[2]

Eighteen healthy subjects were given oral furosemide 40 mg one hour after intravenous **ranitidine** 50 mg or saline. The **ranitidine** increased the AUC of furosemide by 28% and increased the maximum serum levels by 37%.[3] The effects of furosemide could possibly be slightly increased by **ranitidine**, but the clinical importance of this is probably small. No special precautions seem necessary.

(b) Torasemide

In 11 healthy subjects **cimetidine** 300 mg four times daily for 3 days was found to have no effect on the pharmacokinetics of a single 10-mg oral dose of torasemide, nor were there any changes in the volume of urine or the excretion of sodium, potassium or chloride.[4]

1. Rogers HJ, Morrison P, House FR, Bradbrook ID. Effect of cimetidine on the absorption and efficacy of orally administered furosemide. *Int J Clin Pharmacol Ther Toxicol* (1982) 20, 8–11.
2. Sanchis Closa A, Lambert C, du Souich P. Lack of effect of cimetidine on furosemide kinetics and dynamics in patients with hepatic cirrhosis. *Int J Clin Pharmacol Ther Toxicol* (1993) 31, 461–6.
3. Müller FO, De Vaal AC, Hundt KL, Luus HG. Intravenous ranitidine enhances furosemide bioavailability. *Klin Pharmakol Akt* (1993) 4, 26.
4. Kramer WG. Lack of effect of cimetidine on torasemide pharmacokinetics and pharmacodynamics in healthy subjects. *Int Congr Ser* (1993), 361–4.

Loop diuretics + NSAIDs

The antihypertensive and diuretic effects of the loop diuretics appear to be reduced by NSAIDs, including coxibs, although the extent of this interaction largely depends on individual NSAIDs. Diuretics increase the risk of NSAID-induced acute renal failure. The concurrent use of NSAIDs with loop diuretics may exacerbate congestive heart failure and increase the risk of hospitalisation.

Clinical evidence

A. Bumetanide

(a) Celecoxib and other Coxibs

A patient taking celecoxib with bumetanide developed a moderately raised serum creatinine. Another patient taking an ACE inhibitor, spironolactone and bumetanide developed severely raised serum creatinine, hyperkalaemia, and worsening of congestive heart failure shortly after starting celecoxib.[1] A similar case occurred in another patient taking bumetanide about 8 days after starting **rofecoxib**.[1]

(b) Indometacin

In two studies, a single 100-mg dose of indometacin was found to reduce the bumetanide-induced output of urine, sodium and chloride (but not potassium) by about 25%.[2-4] Diuresis was reduced by 42% and weight gain was noted.[2] There are other reports confirming this interaction between bumetanide and indometacin, including a clinical study,[5] and a report of a patient who developed heart failure as a result of this interaction.[6]

(c) Sulindac

A study in 8 healthy subjects found that a single 300-mg dose of sulindac did not significantly reduce the diuretic response (measured by urinary volume, sodium, potassium and chloride) to a single 1-mg dose of bumetanide.[7] However, another study in 9 healthy subjects found that pre-treatment with sulindac 200 mg twice daily for 5 days reduced the diuretic effect of a single 1-mg dose of bumetanide (mean urine flow rate after 2 hours reduced by 21% and cumulative sodium excretion at 3 hours reduced by 22%).[8]

(d) Tolfenamic acid

A study in 8 healthy subjects found that tolfenamic acid 300 mg reduced the diuretic response to a single 1-mg dose of bumetanide by 34% at 2 hours (measured by urinary volume, sodium, potassium and chloride).[7]

B. Furosemide

(a) Azapropazone

Ten healthy subjects had no change in their urinary excretion in response to furosemide 40 mg daily when they were also given azapropazone 600 mg twice daily. The furosemide did not antagonise the uricosuric effects of the azapropazone.[9]

(b) Celecoxib and other Coxibs

In a placebo-controlled study, 7 patients with cirrhosis and ascites were given a single 40-mg intravenous dose of furosemide before and after receiving celecoxib 200 mg twice daily for 5 doses. It was found that this short-term use of celecoxib did not reduce the natriuretic or diuretic effects of furosemide.[10]

Two patients with a history of chronic heart failure, taking furosemide 40 or 80 mg daily, developed acute renal failure when they started to take celecoxib 100 or 200 mg twice daily. Neither patient showed any sign of decompensated heart failure on admission (which can in itself cause renal failure) and both recovered on stopping the celecoxib and furosemide combination. One patient was also taking enalapril, and the combination of the enalapril with furosemide was restarted without any changes in renal function.[11] The same authors also described two other patients taking furosemide who developed renal failure when they started to take **rofecoxib**.[11] Other cases have occurred in patients taking furosemide, often with ACE inhibitors, after they started **rofecoxib**.[1]

(c) Diclofenac

A study in patients with heart failure and cirrhosis found that diclofenac 150 mg daily reduced the furosemide-induced excretion of sodium by 38%, but the excretion of potassium was unaltered.[12]

(d) Diflunisal

A study in 12 healthy subjects found that diflunisal 500 mg twice daily reduced sodium excretion in response to furosemide by 59%, but potassium excretion remained unchanged.[13] In patients with heart failure and cirrhosis taking furosemide, diflunisal 500 to 700 mg daily decreased the sodium excretion by 36% and the potassium excretion by 47%.[12] However, another study found no interaction between diflunisal and furosemide.[14]

(e) Flupirtine

A study in healthy subjects found that a single 200-mg dose of flupirtine did not affect the overall furosemide diuresis, but the diuretic effect was slightly delayed.[15]

(f) Flurbiprofen

A study in 7 healthy subjects found that the increase in renal osmolal clearance of a standard water load in response to furosemide 40 mg orally or 20 mg intravenously fell from 105% to 19% and from 140% to 70%, respectively, after flurbiprofen 100 mg was given.[16] A single-dose study in 10 healthy subjects found that flurbiprofen 100 mg reduced the urinary volume, urinary sodium and urinary potassium, in response to oral furosemide 80 mg by 10%, 9%, and 12%, respectively.[17,18]

(g) Ibuprofen

An elderly man with heart failure taking digoxin, isosorbide dinitrate and furosemide 80 mg daily, developed symptomatic congestive heart failure with ascites when given ibuprofen 400 mg three times daily. His serum urea and creatinine levels rose and no diuresis occurred, even when the furosemide dosage was doubled. Two days after withdrawing the ibuprofen, brisk diuresis took place, renal function returned to normal, and his condition improved steadily.[19] Another elderly patient similarly had a poor response to furosemide (and later to metolazone as well) until he stopped taking ibuprofen 600 mg four times daily and at least two **aspirin** daily (for headache).[20] This was due to hyponatraemic hypovolaemia brought on by the drug combination.

In a small, placebo-controlled, crossover study in 8 healthy subjects, ibuprofen 400 mg and 800 mg three times daily for 3 days significantly reduced the glomerular filtration rate and the diuresis produced by a single 20-mg intravenous dose of furosemide, but did not alter sodium excretion.[21]

(h) Indometacin

A study in 4 healthy subjects and 6 patients with essential hypertension found that furosemide 80 mg three times daily reduced the mean blood pressure by 13 mmHg, but when indometacin 50 mg four times daily was also given the blood pressures returned to virtually pre-treatment levels. Moreover, the normal urinary sodium loss induced by the furosemide was significantly reduced.[22]

A study in healthy subjects and patients with congestive heart failure given furosemide found that indometacin 100 mg reduced the urinary output by 53% and also reduced the excretion of sodium, potassium, and chloride by 64%, 49%, and 62%, respectively.[23] A study in 14 patients with ascites secondary to liver cirrhosis found that indometacin 50 mg every 6 hours for 2 doses significantly reduced the urinary volume and the natriuretic response to furosemide, by 82% and 69%, respectively, but produced only a small, non-significant reduction in creatinine clearance.[24] Another study found that indometacin reduced the urinary output in response to furosemide by 20 to 30%.[25] There are other case reports and studies confirming the interaction between furosemide and indometacin.[21,26-31]

(i) Ketoprofen

A study in 12 healthy subjects given furosemide 40 mg daily found that ketoprofen 100 mg twice daily reduced the 6-hour urine output by 67 mL, and the 24-hour urine output by 651 mL on the first day of treatment. However no significant differences were seen after 5 days of treatment.[32]

(j) Ketorolac

Twelve healthy subjects were given oral ketorolac 30 mg four times daily, and then a single 30-mg intramuscular dose of ketorolac 30 minutes before a 40-mg intravenous dose of furosemide. No precise figures are given, but the maximum serum level of the furosemide, its diuretic effect, and the electrolyte loss were said to be significantly reduced by the ketorolac.[33] Another study in healthy elderly subjects found that when they were given oral ketorolac 120 mg, then, on the following day, intramuscular ketorolac 30 mg, followed 30 minutes later by furosemide 40 mg, the urinary output fell by 16% and the sodium output fell by 26% over the next 8 hours, when compared with furosemide alone.[34]

(k) Lornoxicam

A study in 12 healthy subjects found that lornoxicam 4 mg significantly antagonised the diuretic and natriuretic effects of furosemide, but this was not quantified.[35]

(l) Meloxicam

Meloxicam 15 mg daily for 3 days had no significant effect on the pharmacokinetics of furosemide 40 mg in 12 healthy subjects. The furosemide-induced diuresis was unchanged, and although the cumulative urinary electrolyte excretion was somewhat lower, but this was not considered to be clinically significant.[36] A similar study in patients with heart failure taking an ACE inhibitor also found no clinically significant pharmacokinetic or pharmacodynamic interaction between furosemide and meloxicam.[37]

(m) Metamizole sodium (Dipyrone)

A study in 9 healthy subjects found that metamizole sodium 3 g daily for 3 days, reduced the clearance of intravenous furosemide 20 mg from 175 to 141 mL/minute but the diuretic effects of the furosemide were unchanged.[38]

(n) Mofebutazone

A study in 10 healthy subjects found that mofebutazone 600 mg had no effect on the diuretic effects of furosemide 40 mg. The urinary volume and excretion of sodium, potassium and chloride were unchanged.[39]

(o) Naproxen

Two elderly women with congestive heart failure did not respond to treatment with furosemide and digoxin until the naproxen they were taking was withdrawn.[19] A single-dose study in patients with heart failure found that the volume of urine excreted in response to furosemide was reduced about 50% by naproxen.[25] In a placebo-controlled study, 6 patients with cirrhosis and ascites were given a single 40-mg intravenous dose of furosemide before and after naproxen 500 mg twice daily for 5 doses. It was found that this short-term use of naproxen reduced the glomerular filtration rate and the natriuretic and diuretic effects of furosemide.[10]

(p) Nimesulide

A study in 8 healthy subjects found that nimesulide 200 mg twice daily attenuated the effects of furosemide 40 mg twice daily. Subjects who had initially lost weight when taking furosemide regained weight, diuresis was slightly reduced, and the glomerular filtration rate was reduced.[40]

(q) Piroxicam

A 96-year-old woman with congestive heart failure did not adequately respond to furosemide until the dosage of piroxicam she was taking was reduced from 20 to 10 mg daily.[41]

In one study in 9 hypertensive patients with a creatinine clearance of less than 60 mL/minute, who were taking furosemide, piroxicam 20 mg daily for 3 days produced a significant reduction in the natriuretic and kaliuretic effects of an additional single 40-mg dose of furosemide. However, in 13 other patients, with a creatinine clearance of greater than 60 mL/minute, who were taking a thiazide diuretic, piroxicam did not alter the effects of a single 40-mg dose of furosemide. In a third group of 8 healthy subjects, the same dose of piroxicam reduced the natriuretic effects, but not the kaliuretic effects, of a single 40-mg dose of furosemide.[42]

(r) Sulindac

A study in 5 healthy subjects found that pre-treatment with two 150-mg doses of sulindac reduced the urinary volume and urinary sodium following an intravenous furosemide 80 mg by 25% and 37.5%, respectively. In patients with cirrhosis and ascites, sulindac 150 mg reduced the urinary volume, urinary sodium, and urinary potassium following an 80-mg intravenous dose of furosemide by 38%, 52%, and 8%, respectively.[43] In another placebo-controlled study in 15 healthy women, sulindac 200 mg twice daily for 5 days produced a similar but slightly smaller reduction in the natriuretic effect of a single 40-mg intravenous dose of furosemide, when compared with indometacin.[31]

(s) Tenoxicam

A study in 12 patients found that tenoxicam 20 to 40 mg daily had no significant effect on the urinary excretion of sodium or chloride due to furosemide 40 mg daily, and blood pressure, heart rate and body-weight also were not affected.[44]

C. Piretanide

(a) Indometacin

A comparative study[45] into the pharmacological mechanisms underlying the way drugs interfere with the actions of loop diuretics found that indometacin 50 mg three times daily for 2 days reduced the peak fractional excretion of sodium in response to a single 6-mg dose of piretanide. The clinical importance of this change was not studied.

(b) Piroxicam

A comparative study into the pharmacological mechanisms underlying the way drugs interfere with the actions of loop diuretics found that piroxicam 20 mg twice daily for 2 days did not significantly affect the peak fractional excretion of sodium in response to a single 6-mg dose of piretanide.[45]

D. Torasemide

A study in healthy subjects suggested that indometacin did not affect the natriuretic effects of torasemide,[46] but on the basis of later study the same workers suggest that pathological factors in patients may allow an interaction similar to that with furosemide and indometacin to occur.[47]

Mechanism

Uncertain and complex. It is likely that a number of different mechanisms come into play. One probable mechanism involves the synthesis of renal prostaglandins, which occurs when the loop diuretics cause sodium excretion. If this synthesis is blocked by drugs such as the NSAIDs, then renal blood flow and diuresis will be altered.[48] NSAIDs cause fluid and salt retention, which would antagonise the effects produced by diuretics.

Importance and management

NSAIDs can cause renal impairment, particularly in patients in whom prostaglandins are playing an important role in maintaining renal function. Such patients include those taking diuretics, the elderly and those with concurrent conditions such as congestive heart failure and ascites. Hence the combination of diuretics and NSAIDs may increase the nephrotoxicity of NSAIDs.[30,49-51]

The antihypertensive and diuretic effects of the loop diuretics are reduced by NSAIDs. This interaction is very well documented between furosemide and indometacin, and of clinical importance, whereas less is known about the interactions with other NSAIDs, although the interaction should be anticipated with all of them. Use of an alternative non-NSAID analgesic should always be considered if possible. However, in cases where concurrent use cannot be avoided, the loop diuretic dosage may need to be raised (according to clinical response), but the effects on renal function and electrolytes, as well as efficacy, should be closely monitored. Patients at greatest risk of an adverse interaction include the elderly and patients with cirrhosis, cardiac failure and/or renal impairment, and NSAIDs should usually be used with caution in these patient groups regardless of concurrent use of diuretics. Note that a retrospective analysis of records of patients taking diuretics (thiazides, loop and/or potassium-sparing) with NSAIDs found a twofold increase in the risk of hospitalisation for congestive heart failure on concurrent use. The most common

NSAIDs taken by this cohort of patients were diclofenac, ibuprofen, indometacin and naproxen.[52]

Much less is known about the interactions of NSAIDs with **bumetanide**, and even less about **piretanide** and **torasemide**, but the evidence suggests that they probably interact in the same way as furosemide and indometacin. It would therefore seem prudent to be alert for interactions with any of the NSAIDs with which furosemide interacts. See also 'Loop diuretics + Aspirin', p.948, for a discussion of the interactions between aspirin and bumetanide or furosemide.

Various large epidemiological studies and meta-analyses of clinical studies have been conducted to assess the effect of NSAIDs on blood pressure in patients treated with **antihypertensives**, including diuretics, and the findings of these are summarised in 'Table 23.2', (p.862).

1. Verrico MM, Weber RJ, McKaveney TP, Ansani NT, Towers AL. Adverse drug events involving COX-2 inhibitors. *Ann Pharmacother* (2003) 37, 1203–13.
2. Aggernæs KH. Indometacinhæmning af bumetaniddiurese. *Ugeskr Laeger* (1980) 142, 691–3.
3. Brater C, Chennavasin P. Indomethacin and the response to bumetanide. *Clin Pharmacol Ther* (1980) 27, 421–5.
4. Brater DC, Fox WR, Chennavasin P. Interaction studies with bumetanide and furosemide. Effects of probenecid and of indomethacin on response to bumetanide in man. *J Clin Pharmacol* (1981) 21, 647–53.
5. Kaufman J, Hamburger R, Matheson J, Flamenbaum W. Bumetanide-induced diuresis and natriuresis: effect of prostaglandin synthetase inhibition. *J Clin Pharmacol* (1981) 21, 663–7.
6. Ahmad S. Indomethacin-bumetanide interaction: an alert. *Am J Cardiol* (1984) 54, 246–7.
7. Pentikäinen PJ, Tokola O, Vapaatalo H. Non-steroidal anti-inflammatory drugs and bumetanide response in man. Comparison of tolfenamic acid and sulindac. *Clin Pharmacol Ther* (1986) 39, 219.
8. Skinner MH, Mutterperl R, Zeitz HJ. Sulindac inhibits bumetanide-induced sodium and water excretion. *Clin Pharmacol Ther* (1987) 42, 542–6.
9. Williamson PJ, Ene MD, Roberts CJC. A study of the potential interactions between azapropazone and frusemide in man. *Br J Clin Pharmacol* (1984) 18, 619–23.
10. Clària J, Kent JD, López-Parra M, Escolar G, Ruiz-del-Arbol L, Ginès P, Jiménez W, Vucelic B, Arroyo V. Effects of celecoxib and naproxen on renal function in nonazotemic patients with cirrhosis and ascites. *Hepatology* (2005) 41, 579–87.
11. Braden GL, O'Shea MH, Mulhern JG, Germain MJ. Acute renal failure and hyperkalaemia associated with cyclooxygenase-2 inhibitors. *Nephrol Dial Transplant* (2004) 19, 1149–53.
12. Jean G, Meregalli G, Vasilicò M, Silvani A, Scapaticci R, Della Ventura GF, Baiocchi C, Thiella G. Interazioni tra terapia diuretica e farmaci antiinfiammatori non steroidei. *Clin Ter* (1983) 105, 471–5.
13. Favre L, Glasson PH, Riondel A, Vallotton MB. Interaction of diuretics and non-steroidal anti-inflammatory drugs in man. *Clin Sci* (1983) 64, 407–15.
14. Tobert JA, Ostaszewski T, Reger B, Mesinger MAP, Cook TJ. Diflunisal-furosemide interaction. *Clin Pharmacol Ther* (1980) 27, 289–90.
15. Johnston A, Warrington SJ, Turner P, Riethmuller-Winzen H. Comparison of flupirtine and indomethacin on frusemide-induced diuresis. *Postgrad Med J* (1987) 63, 959–61.
16. Rawles JM. Antagonism between non-steroidal anti-inflammatory drugs and diuretics. *Scott Med J* (1982) 27, 37–40.
17. Symmons D, Kendall MJ. Non-steroidal anti-inflammatory drugs and frusemide-induced diuresis. *BMJ* (1981) 283, 988–9.
18. Symmons DPM, Kendall MJ, Rees JA, Hind ID. The effect of flurbiprofen on the responses to frusemide in healthy volunteers. *Int J Clin Pharmacol Ther Toxicol* (1983) 21, 350–4.
19. Laiwah ACY, Mactier RA. Antagonistic effect of non-steroidal anti-inflammatory drugs on frusemide-induced diuresis in cardiac failure. *BMJ* (1981) 283, 714.
20. Goodenough GK, Lutz LJ. Hyponatremic hypervolemia caused by a drug-drug interaction mistaken for syndrome of inappropriate ADH. *J Am Geriatr Soc* (1988) 36, 285–6.
21. Passmore AP, Copeland S, Johnston GD. A comparison of the effects of ibuprofen and indomethacin upon renal haemodynamics and electrolyte excretion in the presence and absence of furosemide. *Br J Clin Pharmacol* (1989) 27, 483–90.
22. Patak RV, Mookerjee BK, Bentzel CJ, Hysert PE, Babej M, Lee JB. Antagonism of the effects of furosemide by indomethacin in normal and hypertensive man. *Prostaglandins* (1975) 10, 649–59.
23. Sörgel F, Koob R, Gluth WP, Krüger B, Lang E. The interaction of indomethacin and furosemide in patients with congestive heart failure. *Clin Pharmacol Ther* (1985) 37, 231.
24. Mirouze D, Zipser RD, Reynolds TB. Effect of inhibitors of prostaglandin synthesis on induced diuresis in cirrhosis. *Hepatology* (1983) 3, 50–5.
25. Faunch R. Non-steroidal anti-inflammatory drugs and frusemide-induced diuresis. *BMJ* (1981) 283, 989.
26. Allan SG, Knox J, Kerr F. Interaction between diuretics and indomethacin. *BMJ* (1981) 283, 1611.
27. Poe TE, Scott RB, Keith JF. Interaction of indomethacin with furosemide. *J Fam Pract* (1983) 16, 610–16.
28. Ritland S. Alvorlig interaksjon mellom indometacin og furosemid. *Tidsskr Nor Laegeforen* (1983) 103, 2003.
29. Nordrehaug JE. Alvorlig interaksjon mellom indometacin og furosemid. *Tidsskr Nor Laegeforen* (1983) 103, 1680–1.
30. Thomas MC. Diuretics, ACE inhibitors and NSAIDs—the triple whammy. *Med J Aust* (2000) 172, 184–5.
31. Roberts DG, Gerber JG, Barnes JS, Zerbe GO, Nies AS. Sulindac is not renal sparing in man. *Clin Pharmacol Ther* (1985) 38, 258–65.
32. Wa TC, Lawson M, Jackson SHD, Hitoglou-Makedou A, Turner P. Interaction of ketoprofen and frusemide in man. *Postgrad Med J* (1991) 67, 655–8.
33. Shah J, Bullingham R, Jonkman J, Curd J, Taylor R, Fratis A. PK-PD interaction of ketorolac and furosemide in healthy volunteers in a normovolemic state. *Clin Pharmacol Ther* (1994) 55, 198.
34. Jones RW, Notarianni LJ, Parker G. The effect of ketorolac tromethamine on the diuretic response of frusemide in healthy elderly people. *Therapie* (1995) 50 (Suppl), Abstract 98.
35. Ravic M, Johnston A, Turner P. Clinical pharmacological studies of some possible interactions of lornoxicam with other drugs. *Postgrad Med J* (1990) 66 (Suppl 4), S30–S34.
36. Müller FO, Schall R, de Vaal AC, Groenewoud G, Hundt HKL, Middle MV. Influence of meloxicam on furosemide pharmacokinetics and pharmacodynamics in healthy volunteers. *Eur J Clin Pharmacol* (1995) 48, 247–51.
37. Müller FO, Middle MV, Schall R, Terblanché J, Hundt HKL Groenewoud G. An evaluation of the interaction of meloxicam with furosemide in patients with compensated chronic cardiac failure. *Br J Clin Pharmacol* (1997) 44, 393–8.
38. Rosenkranz B, Lehr K-H, Mackert G, Seyberth HW. Metamizole-furosemide interaction study in healthy volunteers. *Eur J Clin Pharmacol* (1992) 42, 593–8.
39. Matthei U, Grabensee B, Loew D. The interaction of mofebutazone with furosemide. *Curr Med Res Opin* (1987) 10, 638–44.
40. Steinhäuslin F, Munafo A, Buclin T, Macciocchi A. Renal effects of nimesulide in furosemide-treated subjects. *Drugs* (1993) 46 (Suppl 1), 257–62.
41. Baker DE. Piroxicam-furosemide drug interaction. *Drug Intell Clin Pharm* (1988) 22, 505–6.
42. Lin MS. Effects of piroxicam on natriuresis and kaliuresis in hypertensives and healthy subjects. *Scand J Rheumatol* (1990) 19, 145–9.
43. Daskalopoulos G, Kronborg I, Katkov W, Gonzalez M, Laffi G, Zipser RD. Sulindac and indomethacin suppress the diuretic action of furosemide in patients with cirrhosis and ascites: evidence that sulindac affects renal prostaglandins. *Am J Kidney Dis* (1985) 6, 217–21.
44. Hartmann D, Kleinbloesem CH, Lücker PW, Vetter G. Study on the possible interaction between tenoxicam and furosemide. *Arzneimittelforschung* (1987) 37, 1072–6.
45. Dixey JJ, Noormohamed FH, Pawa JS, Lant AF, Brewerton DA. The influence of nonsteroidal anti-inflammatory drugs and probenecid on the renal response to and kinetics of piretanide in man. *Clin Pharmacol Ther* (1988) 44, 531–9.
46. van Ganse E, Douchamps J, Deger F, Staroukine M, Verniory A, Herchuelz A. Failure of indomethacin to impair the diuretic and natriuretic effects of the loop diuretic torasemide in healthy volunteers. *Eur J Clin Pharmacol* (1986) 31 (Suppl), 43–7.
47. Herchuelz A, Derenne F, Deger F, Juvent M, van Ganse E, Staroutkine M, Verniory A, Boeynaems JM, Douchamps J. Interaction between nonsteroidal anti-inflammatory drugs and loop diuretics: modulation by sodium balance. *J Pharmacol Exp Ther* (1989) 248, 1175–81.
48. Passmore AP, Copeland CS, Johnston GD. The effects of ibuprofen and indomethacin on renal function in the presence and absence of frusemide in healthy volunteers on a restricted sodium diet. *Br J Clin Pharmacol* (1990) 29, 311–19.
49. Murray MD, Brater DC, Tierney WM, Hui SL, McDonald CJ. Ibuprofen-associated renal impairment in a large general internal medicine practice. *Am J Med Sci* (1990) 299, 222–9.
50. Blackshear JL, Davidman M, Stillman MT. Identification of risk for renal insufficiency from nonsteroidal anti-inflammatory drugs. *Arch Intern Med* (1983) 143, 1130–4.
51. Menkes CJ. Renal and hepatic effects of NSAIDs in the elderly. *Scand J Rheumatol* (1989) 83 (Suppl), 11–13.
52. Heerdink ER, Leufkens HG, Herings RMC, Ottervanger JP, Stricker BHC, Bakker A. NSAIDs associated with increased risk of congestive heart failure in elderly patients taking diuretics. *Arch Intern Med* (1998) 158, 1108–12.

Loop diuretics + Probenecid

Probenecid decreases the renal clearance of furosemide, but it appears not to alter its overall diuretic effect. Probenecid reduces the natriuretic effects of piretanide, but the clinical relevance of this is not known. Probenecid does not appear to significantly affect bumetanide diuresis.

Clinical evidence, mechanism, importance and management

(a) Bumetanide

Probenecid 1 g did not affect the response of 8 healthy subjects to 500 micrograms or 1 mg of intravenous bumetanide.[1] Another study reported a fall in natriuresis and in the clearance of bumetanide, but this was of minimal clinical importance.[2]

(b) Furosemide

The concurrent use of furosemide and probenecid has been closely studied to determine the renal pharmacological mechanisms of loop diuretics. One study in patients given furosemide 40 mg daily found that the addition of probenecid 500 mg twice daily for 3 days reduced their urinary excretion of sodium by about 36% (from 56.3 to 35.9 mmol daily).[3] Other studies have also found some changes in overall diuresis (a fall,[4] a rise,[5] and no change[6,7] in some studies), and a reduction of 35 to 80% in the renal clearance of furosemide.[4,6-9] One study found that probenecid 1 g increased the half-life of furosemide by 70% and decreased its oral clearance by 65%.[8] Similar results were found in another study.[10] The clinical importance of these changes is uncertain, but probably small.

(c) Piretanide

A comparative study[11] into the pharmacological mechanisms underlying the way drugs interfere with the actions of loop diuretics found that probenecid 1 g reduced the peak fractional excretion of sodium produced by a 6-mg dose of oral piretanide by 65%. Another study confirmed that probenecid reduces the natriuretic effects of piretanide.[12] The clinical importance of these changes was not studied.

1. Brater DC, Chennavasin P. Effect of probenecid on response to bumetanide in man. *J Clin Pharmacol* (1981) 21, 311–15.
2. Lant AF. Effects of bumetanide on cation and anion transport. *Postgrad Med J* (1975) 51 (Suppl 6), 35–42.
3. Hsieh Y-Y, Hsieh B-S, Lien W-P, Wu T-L. Probenecid interferes with the natriuretic action of furosemide. *J Cardiovasc Pharmacol* (1987) 10, 530–4.
4. Honari J, Blair AD, Cutler RE. Effects of probenecid on furosemide kinetics and natriuresis in man. *Clin Pharmacol Ther* (1977) 22, 395–401.
5. Brater DC. Effects of probenecid on furosemide response. *Clin Pharmacol Ther* (1978) 24, 548–54.
6. Homeida M, Roberts C, Branch RA. Influence of probenecid and spironolactone on furosemide kinetics and dynamics in man. *Clin Pharmacol Ther* (1977) 22, 402–9.

7. Smith DE, Gee WL, Brater DC, Lin ET, Benet LZ. Preliminary evaluation of furosemide-probenecid interaction in humans. *J Pharm Sci* (1980) 69, 571–5.
8. Vree TB, van den Biggelaar-Martea M, Verwey-van Wissen CPWGM. Probenecid inhibits the renal clearance of frusemide and its acyl glucuronide. *Br J Clin Pharmacol* (1995) 39, 692–5.
9. Sommers DK, Meyer EC, Moncrieff J. The influence of co-administered organic acids on the kinetics and dynamics of frusemide. *Br J Clin Pharmacol* (1991) 32, 489–93.
10. Chennavasin P, Seiwell R, Brater DC, Liang WMM. Pharmacodynamic analysis of the furosemide-probenecid interaction in man. *Kidney Int* (1979) 16, 187–95.
11. Dixey JJ, Noormohamed FH, Pawa JS, Lant AF, Brewerton DA. The influence of nonsteroidal anti-inflammatory drugs and probenecid on the renal response to and kinetics of piretanide in man. *Clin Pharmacol Ther* (1988) 44, 531–9.
12. Noormohamed FH, Lant AF. Analysis of the natriuretic action of a loop diuretic, piretanide, in man. *Br J Clin Pharmacol* (1991) 31, 463–9.

Potassium-sparing diuretics + H_2-receptor antagonists

Although minor interactions occasionally occur between potassium-sparing diuretics and the H_2-receptor antagonists, none of these have been shown to be of clinical significance. The combinations that have been studied are; amiloride or triamterene with cimetidine, and triamterene with ranitidine.

Clinical evidence, mechanism, importance and management

(a) Amiloride

A study in 8 healthy subjects given amiloride 5 mg daily found that **cimetidine** 400 mg twice daily for 12 days reduced the renal clearance of amiloride by 17% and reduced its urinary excretion from 65% to 53%. Amiloride also reduced the excretion of **cimetidine** from 43% to 32%, and the AUC was reduced by 14%.[1] No changes in the diuretic effects (urinary volume, sodium or potassium excretion) occurred. It seems that each drug reduces the gastrointestinal absorption of the other drug by as yet unidentified mechanisms. The overall plasma levels of the amiloride remain unchanged because the reduced absorption is offset by a reduction in its renal excretion. These mutual interactions do not seem to be clinically significant.

(b) Triamterene

A study in 6 healthy subjects given triamterene 100 mg daily for 4 days found that **cimetidine** 400 mg twice daily increased the AUC of triamterene by 22%, reduced its metabolism (hydroxylation) by 32%, and reduced its renal clearance by 28%. There also appeared to be a reduction in the absorption of triamterene. However, the loss of sodium in the urine was not significantly changed, and the potassium-sparing effects of triamterene were not altered.[2] Because the diuretic effects of triamterene are minimally changed, this interaction is unlikely to be clinically important.[2]

In 8 healthy subjects **ranitidine** 150 mg twice daily for 4 days roughly halved the absorption (as measured by renal clearance) of triamterene 100 mg daily. Its metabolism was also reduced, with the total effect being a 21% reduction in the AUC. As a result of the reduced plasma triamterene levels, the urinary sodium loss was reduced to some extent but potassium excretion remained unchanged.[3] Overall the diuretic effects of triamterene were only mildly affected. Another study found that a 22% reduction in the AUC of triamterene is unlikely to result in a significant change in its diuretic effects.[2] No clinically significant interaction is anticipated.

1. Somogyi AA, Hovens CM, Muirhead MR, Bochner F. Renal tubular secretion of amiloride and its inhibition by cimetidine in humans and in an animal model. *Drug Metab Dispos* (1989) 17, 190–6.
2. Muirhead MR, Somogyi AA, Rolan PE, Bochner F. Effect of cimetidine on renal and hepatic drugs elimination: studies with triamterene. *Clin Pharmacol Ther* (1986) 40, 400–7.
3. Muirhead M, Bochner F, Somogyi A. Pharmacokinetic drug interactions between triamterene and ranitidine in humans: alterations in renal and hepatic clearances and gastrointestinal absorption. *J Pharmacol Exp Ther* (1988) 244, 734–9.

Potassium-sparing diuretics + NSAIDs

The concurrent use of triamterene and indometacin has, in several cases, rapidly lead to acute renal failure. An isolated case of renal impairment with diclofenac has been reported in a patient taking triamterene plus a thiazide. A case of exercise-induced acute renal failure has also been reported in a patient taking ibuprofen with triamterene plus a thiazide. Indometacin reduced the diuretic effect of spironolactone.

Clinical evidence

(a) Spironolactone with Indometacin

A study in healthy subjects found that indometacin 150 mg daily reduced the natriuretic effect of spironolactone 300 mg daily by 54%.[1]

(b) Triamterene with Diclofenac

A patient receiving triamterene 100 mg plus trichlormethiazide 2 mg daily was given intramuscular diclofenac 75 mg before admission to hospital with breast pain. On admission serum creatinine was 91 micromol/L and after 2 days it had increased to 248 micromol/L, but it returned to normal over 2 weeks. Subsequent oral diclofenac produced no adverse effects. The observed deterioration in renal function was attributed to an interaction between triamterene and diclofenac.[2]

(c) Triamterene with Diflunisal

Diflunisal had no effects on the pharmacokinetics of triamterene in healthy subjects, but the plasma AUC of an active metabolite, *p*-hydroxytriamterene was increased by more than fourfold.[3]

(d) Triamterene with Ibuprofen

A 37-year-old patient developed acute renal failure after strenuous exercise while taking hydrochlorothiazide/triamterene 50/75 mg daily and ibuprofen (800 mg 12 hours and 2 hours before the exercise, and 800 mg 24 hours after). A renal biopsy showed acute tubular necrosis.[4]

(e) Triamterene with Indometacin

A study in 4 healthy subjects found that indometacin 150 mg daily given with triamterene 200 mg daily over a 3-day period reduced the creatinine clearance in 2 subjects by 62% and 72%, respectively. Renal function returned to normal after a month. Indometacin alone caused an average 10% fall in creatinine clearance, but triamterene alone caused no consistent change in renal function. No adverse reactions were seen in 18 other subjects treated in the same way with indometacin and furosemide, hydrochlorothiazide or spironolactone.[5,6] Five patients are reported to have rapidly developed acute renal failure after receiving indometacin and triamterene, either concurrently or sequentially.[7-10]

Mechanism

Uncertain. One suggestion is that triamterene causes renal ischaemia, for which the kidney compensates by increasing prostaglandin (PGE_2) production, thereby preserving renal blood flow. Indometacin opposes this by inhibiting prostaglandin synthesis, so that the damaging effects of triamterene on the kidney continue unchecked. Increases in pharmacologically active metabolites of triamterene may occur due to competition for renal excretory pathways but the clinical significance is uncertain.

As prostaglandins may contribute to the natriuretic effects of spironolactone, the NSAIDs may exert their effects by blocking prostaglandin synthesis. See also 'Loop diuretics + NSAIDs', p.949.

Importance and management

Information is limited to these reports, but the interaction with **indometacin** is established. The incidence is uncertain. Since acute renal failure can apparently develop unpredictably and very rapidly it would seem prudent to use triamterene and indometacin cautiously, or avoid it altogether. The authors of the report with **diclofenac** suggest caution with the use of any NSAID with triamterene.[2] Strenuous exercise can reduce renal blood flow, and the author of the case report with **ibuprofen** notes that although renal failure secondary to this is rare, patients taking medication that also reduces renal blood flow are more at risk of this complication.[4] A retrospective analysis of records of patients taking diuretics (thiazides, loop and/or potassium-sparing) and NSAIDs found a twofold increase in the risk of hospitalisation for congestive heart failure on concurrent use, although the relative risk (1.4) with potassium-sparing diuretics was less than that when combined with a thiazide (2.9). The most common NSAIDs taken by this cohort of patients were diclofenac, ibuprofen, indometacin and naproxen.[11] The European Society of Cardiology (ESC) Task Force and the joint American College of Cardiology/American Heart Association guidelines on the management of chronic heart failure both recommend that NSAIDs, including coxibs, should be avoided, if possible, with aldosterone antagonists (such as **eplerenone** or **spironolactone**), as this increases the risk of developing hyperkalaemia and renal failure.[12,13] For a discussion of the interaction of spironolactone with aspirin, see 'Spironolactone + Aspirin', p.954.

Various large epidemiological studies and meta-analyses of clinical studies have been conducted to assess the effect of NSAIDs on blood pressure in patients treated with antihypertensives, including diuretics, and the findings of these are summarised in 'Table 23.2', (p.862).

1. Hofmann LM, Garcia HA. Interaction of spironolactone and indomethacin at the renal level. *Proc Soc Exp Biol Med* (1972) 141, 353–5.
2. Härkönen M, Ekblom-Kullberg S. Reversible deterioration of renal function after diclofenac in patient receiving triamterene. *BMJ* (1986) 293, 698–9.
3. Jacob SS, Franklin ME, Dickinson RG, Hooper WD. The effect of diflunisal on the elimination of triamterene in human volunteers. *Drug Metabol Drug Interact* (2000) 16, 159–71.
4. Sanders LR. Exercise-induced acute renal failure associated with ibuprofen, hydrochlorothiazide, and triamterene. *J Am Soc Nephrol* (1995) 5, 2020–3.
5. Favre L, Glasson P, Vallotton MB. Reversible acute renal failure from combined triamterene and indomethacin. A study in healthy subjects. *Ann Intern Med* (1982) 96, 317–20.
6. Favre L, Glasson PH, Riondel A, Vallotton MB. Interaction of diuretics and non-steroidal anti-inflammatory drugs in man. *Clin Sci* (1983) 64, 407–15.
7. McCarthy JT, Torres VE, Romero JC, Wochos DN, Velosa JA. Acute intrinsic renal failure induced by indomethacin: role of prostaglandin synthetase inhibition. *Mayo Clin Proc* (1982) 57, 289–96.
8. McCarthy JT. Drug-induced renal failure. *Mayo Clin Proc* (1982) 57, 463.
9. Weinberg MS, Quigg RJ, Salant DJ, Bernard DB. Anuric renal failure precipitated by indomethacin and triamterene. *Nephron* (1985) 40, 216–18.
10. Mathews A, Baillie GR. Acute renal failure and hyperkalemia associated with triamterene and indomethacin. *Vet Hum Toxicol* (1986) 28, 224–5.
11. Heerdink ER, Leufkens HG, Herings RMC, Ottervanger JP, Stricker BHC, Bakker A. NSAIDs associated with increased risk of congestive heart failure in elderly patients taking diuretics. *Arch Intern Med* (1998) 158, 1108–12.
12. Hunt SA. ACC/AHA 2005 guideline update for the diagnosis and management of chronic heart failure in the adult. A report of the American College of Cardiology; American Heart Association Task Force on Practice Guidelines (Writing Committee to Update the 2001 Guidelines for the Evaluation and Management of Heart Failure). *J Am Coll Cardiol* (2005) 46, e1–e82. Available at: http://content.onlinejacc.org/cgi/reprint/46/6/e1.pdf (accessed 22/08/2007).
13. Swedberg K, Cleland J, Dargie H, Drexler H, Follath F, Komajda M, Tavazzi L, Smiseth OA, Gavazzi A, Haverich A, Hoes A, Jaarsma T, Korewicki J, Lévy S, Linde C, Lopez-Sendon JL, Nieminen MS, Piérard L, Remme WJ; The Task Force for the Diagnosis and Treatment of Chronic Heart Failure of the European Society of Cardiology. Guidelines for the diagnosis and treatment of chronic heart failure (update 2005). *Eur Heart J* (2005) 26, 1115–40. Available at: http://www.escardio.org/NR/rdonlyres/8A2848B4-5DEB-41B9-9A0A-5B5A90494B64/0/guidelines_CHF_FT_2005.pdf (accessed 22/08/2007).

Potassium-sparing diuretics + Potassium compounds

The concurrent use of spironolactone or triamterene and potassium supplements can result in severe and even life-threatening hyperkalaemia. Amiloride and eplerenone are expected to interact similarly. Potassium-containing salt substitutes can be as hazardous as potassium supplements.

Clinical evidence

In a retrospective analysis of hospitalised patients who had received **spironolactone**, hyperkalaemia had developed in 5.7% of patients taking **spironolactone** alone and in 15.4% of those also taking a **potassium chloride** supplement. The incidence was 42% in those with severe azotaemia given **spironolactone** and **potassium chloride**.[1] A retrospective survey of another group of 25 patients taking **spironolactone** and oral **potassium chloride** supplements found that half of them had developed hyperkalaemia.[2] Another patient developed severe hyperkalaemia and cardiotoxicity as a result of treatment with **spironolactone** and a **potassium supplement**.[3] Three patients taking furosemide and **spironolactone** became hyperkalaemic[4,5] because they took **potassium-containing salt substitutes** (*No Salt* in one case[4]). Two developed cardiac arrhythmias.[5]

The pacemaker of a patient failed because of hyperkalaemia caused by the concurrent use of **triamterene**/hydrochlorothiazide (*Dyazide*) and **potassium chloride** (*Slow-K*).[6]

Mechanism

The effects of these potassium-sparing diuretics and potassium compounds are additive, which can result in hyperkalaemia.

Importance and management

The interaction with spironolactone is established and of clinical importance. A case has also been reported with triamterene; amiloride and eplerenone would be expected to behave similarly. Avoid potassium compounds in patients taking potassium-sparing diuretics except in cases of marked potassium depletion and where the effects can be closely monitored. Warn patients about the risks of salt substitutes containing potassium, which may increase the potassium intake by 50 to 60 mmol daily.[5] The signs and symptoms of hyperkalaemia include muscular weakness, fatigue, paraesthesia, flaccid paralysis of the extremities, bradycardia, shock and ECG abnormalities, which may develop slowly and insidiously.

1. Greenblatt DJ, Koch-Weser J. Adverse reactions to spironolactone. A report from the Boston Collaborative Drug Surveillance Program. *Clin Pharmacol Ther* (1973) 14, 136–7.
2. Simborg DN. Medication prescribing on a university medical service — the incidence of drug combinations with potential adverse interactions. *Johns Hopkins Med J* (1976) 139, 23–6.
3. Kalbian VV. Iatrogenic hyperkalemic paralysis with electrocardiographic changes. *South Med J* (1974) 67, 342–5.
4. McCaughan D. Hazards of non-prescription potassium supplements. *Lancet* (1984) i, 513–14.
5. Yap V, Patel A, Thomsen J. Hyperkalemia with cardiac arrhythmia. Induction by salt substitutes, spironolactone, and azotemia. *JAMA* (1976) 236, 2775–6.
6. O'Reilly MV, Murnaghan DP, Williams MB. Transvenous pacemaker failure induced by hyperkalemia. *JAMA* (1974) 228, 336–7.

Potassium-sparing diuretics + Total parenteral nutrition

Metabolic acidosis occurred in two patients receiving total parenteral nutrition, which was attributed to the use of triamterene or amiloride.

Clinical evidence, mechanism, importance and management

Metabolic acidosis developed in two patients receiving total parenteral nutrition associated with the concurrent use of **triamterene** or **amiloride**. The cases were complicated by a number of pathological and other factors, but it was suggested that the major reason for the acidosis was because the diuretics prevented the kidneys from responding normally to the acid load. Caution is advised during concurrent use.[1]

1. Kushner RF, Sitrin MD. Metabolic acidosis. Development in two patients receiving a potassium-sparing diuretic and total parenteral nutrition. *Arch Intern Med* (1986) 146, 343–5.

Potassium-sparing/Thiazide diuretics + Trimethoprim

Excessively low sodium levels have been seen in a few patients taking hydrochlorothiazide with amiloride or triamterene when they were given trimethoprim or co-trimoxazole. Trimethoprim may cause hyperkalaemia and this may be additive with potassium-sparing diuretics, including the aldosterone antagonists.

Clinical evidence

A 75-year-old woman with multiple medical conditions taking methyldopa, levothyroxine and **co-amilozide** (**hydrochlorothiazide** with **amiloride**) developed nausea and anorexia, and was found to have hyponatraemia (plasma sodium 107 mmol/L), within 4 days of starting to take trimethoprim 200 mg twice daily. The problem resolved when the diuretics and trimethoprim were stopped. When re-challenged 4 months later with trimethoprim, hyponatraemia did not occur, but it developed rapidly when **co-amilozide** was also restarted.[1] The authors of this report say that they have seen several other patients who developed hyponatraemia within 4 to 12 days of starting trimethoprim or co-trimoxazole, all of whom were elderly and all but one of whom were taking a diuretic [unnamed].[1]

Another report describes hyponatraemia in two other patients after co-trimoxazole was added to treatment with **co-amilozide** or **co-triamterzide** (**hydrochlorothiazide** with **triamterene**).[2]

Mechanism

Not established. Thiazide diuretics combined with potassium-sparing diuretics are said to be particularly liable to cause hyponatraemia.[3] Trimethoprim can also cause hyperkalaemia[4], by blocking amiloride-sensitive sodium channels in the collecting duct (this produces a similar effect to that of a potassium-sparing diuretic). It seems likely that these adverse effects can be additive with the effects of other drugs.

Importance and management

Information is very limited but it would seem prudent to be on the alert for any signs of hyponatraemia (nausea, anorexia, etc.) in any patient taking potassium-sparing diuretics with thiazides and trimethoprim. Although there appears to have been no specific case reports of hyperkalaemia in patients taking trimethoprim with potassium-sparing diuretics (including the **aldosterone antagonists**), in theory the risk of hyperkalaemia would be increased by concurrent use. It may therefore be prudent to also monitor potassium levels. The UK manufacturers of eplerenone note that the concurrent use of trimethoprim increases the risk of hyperkalaemia and patients should be closely monitored.[5]

1. Eastell R, Edmonds CJ. Hyponatraemia associated with trimethoprim and a diuretic. *BMJ* (1984) 289, 1658–9.
2. Hart TL, Johnston LJ, Edmonds MW, Brownscombe L. Hyponatremia secondary to thiazide-trimethoprim interaction. *Can J Hosp Pharm* (1989) 42, 243–6.
3. Hornick P. Severe hyponatraemia in elderly patients: cause for concern. *Ann R Coll Surg Engl* (1996) 78, 230–1.
4. Perazella MA. Trimethoprim-induced hyperkalaemia. Clinical data, mechanism, prevention and management. *Drug Safety* (2000) 22, 227–36.
5. Inspra (Eplerenone). Pfizer Ltd. UK Summary of product characteristics, May 2006.

Spironolactone + Aspirin

The antihypertensive effects of spironolactone in patients with hypertension were unaffected by anti-inflammatory doses of aspirin in one small study, although there is evidence that these doses of aspirin reduce the spironolactone-induced loss of sodium in the urine.

Clinical evidence

(a) Effects on blood pressure

Five patients with low-renin essential hypertension, well-controlled for 4 months or more with spironolactone 100 to 300 mg daily, took part in a crossover study. Aspirin 2.4 to 4.8 g daily given over 6-week periods had no effect on blood pressure, serum electrolytes, body-weight, blood-urea-nitrogen or plasma renin activity.[1]

(b) Effects on natriuresis

A study in 10 healthy subjects given single 25-, 50- and 100-mg doses of spironolactone, found that a single 600-mg dose of aspirin reduced the urinary excretion of sodium in response to spironolactone.[2] In a further study in 7 of these subjects, the effectiveness of the spironolactone was reduced by 70%, and the overnight sodium excretion was reduced by one-third when they were given spironolactone 25 mg four times daily for one week followed by a single 600-mg dose of aspirin.[2] Reductions in sodium excretion are described in other studies of this interaction.[3,4] In one of these the sodium excretion brought about by spironolactone was completely abolished when aspirin was given 90 minutes after the spironolactone, but when the drugs were given in the reverse order the inhibition of sodium excretion, which was caused by aspirin, was not completely reversed by spironolactone.[4]

In another study in 7 patients with ascites due to liver cirrhosis, pre-treatment with two doses of aspirin 900 mg reduced the natriuretic effect of spironolactone 300 mg daily by 33%. However, there was no significant change in urinary output.[5]

Mechanism

Uncertain. There is evidence that the active secretion of canrenone (the active metabolite of spironolactone) is blocked by aspirin, but the significance of this is not entirely clear.[3]

Importance and management

An adequately but not extensively documented interaction. Despite the results of the studies showing a reduced natriuretic effect, the small study in hypertensive patients shows that the blood pressure-lowering effects of spironolactone might not be affected by anti-inflammatory doses of aspirin. In general, concurrent use need not be avoided, but if the diuretic response to spironolactone is less than expected consider this interaction as a cause.

None of these studies looked at the effects of low-dose aspirin on spironolactone. Nevertheless, it is likely that the proven protective cardiovascular benefits of low-dose aspirin in patients with hypertension and/or coronary artery disease would usually outweigh the possible reduction in the efficacy of spironolactone. However, note that, when spironolactone is being used for congestive heart failure, the European Society of Cardiology (ESC) and American College of Cardiology/American Heart Association (ACC/AHA) heart failure guidelines say that the prophylactic use of aspirin in patients with heart failure has not been proven unless the patient has underlying ischaemic heart disease[6,7] and should be avoided in patients with recurrent hospital admissions for worsening heart failure.[7] See also 'Potassium-sparing diuretics + NSAIDs', p.952, for a discussion of the interactions of spironolactone with NSAIDs.

1. Hollifield JW. Failure of aspirin to antagonize the antihypertensive effect of spironolactone in low-renin hypertension. *South Med J* (1976) 69, 1034–6.
2. Tweeddale MG, Ogilvie RI. Antagonism of spironolactone-induced natriuresis by aspirin in man. *N Engl J Med* (1973) 289, 198.
3. Ramsay LE, Harrison IR, Shelton JR, Vose CW. Influence of acetylsalicylic acid on the renal handling of a spironolactone metabolite in healthy subjects. *Eur J Clin Pharmacol* (1976) 10, 43–8.
4. Elliott HC. Reduced adrenocortical steroid excretion rates in man following aspirin administration. *Metabolism* (1962) 11, 1015–18.
5. Mirouze D, Zipser RD, Reynolds TB. Effect of inhibitors of prostaglandin synthesis on induced diuresis in cirrhosis. *Hepatology* (1983) 3, 50–5.
6. Hunt SA. ACC/AHA 2005 guideline update for the diagnosis and management of chronic heart failure in the adult. A report of the American College of Cardiology/ American Heart Association Task Force on Practice Guidelines (Writing Committee to Update the 2001 Guidelines for the Evaluation and Management of Heart Failure). *J Am Coll Cardiol* (2005) 46, e1–e82. Available at: http://content.onlinejacc.org/cgi/reprint/46/6/e1.pdf (accessed 22/08/2007).
7. Swedberg K, Cleland J, Dargie H, Drexler H, Follath F, Komajda M, Tavazzi L, Smiseth OA, Gavazzi A, Haverich A, Hoes A, Jaarsma T, Korewicki J, Lévy S, Linde C, Lopez-Sendon JL, Nieminen MS, Piérard L, Remme WJ; Task Force for the Diagnosis and Treatment of Chronic Heart Failure of the European Society of Cardiology. Guidelines for the diagnosis and treatment of chronic heart failure (update 2005). *Eur Heart J* (2005) 26, 1115–40. Available at: http://www.escardio.org/NR/rdonlyres/8A2848B4-5DEB-41B9-9A0A-5B5A90494B64/0/guidelines_CHF_FT_2005.pdf (accessed 22/08/2007).

Spironolactone + Colestyramine

A few case reports have described hyperchloraemic metabolic acidosis, which was associated with the use of colestyramine and spironolactone.

Clinical evidence

Four case reports describe the development of hyperchloraemic metabolic acidosis in patients with liver cirrhosis taking colestyramine (up to about 25 g daily), who were also taking spironolactone 75 mg or 100 mg daily.[1-4] One patient developed significant hyperkalaemia (potassium 8 mmol/L),[4] and 2 patients developed mild renal impairment.[1,3] One patient had recently recovered from a respiratory tract infection, which the authors suggested may have contributed to the acidosis.[1] Acidosis resolved when the colestyramine was stopped.

Mechanism

Bicarbonate has been shown to compete *in vitro* with bile acids for binding sites on the colestyramine resin.[1,3] The chloride ions in the colestyramine resin may cause an anion exchange of not only the bile salts, as is the intention, but also bicarbonate in the small bowel. This removal of bicarbonate from the body can predispose to the development of a hyperchloraemic metabolic acidosis and hyperkalaemia. This might be exacerbated by the bicarbonate-losing and hyperkalaemic effects of spironolactone.[1-4]

Importance and management

In healthy subjects with normal renal function, acidosis does not usually occur, as the kidneys correct it by increasing the excretion of chloride and production of bicarbonate.[1-4] However, in patients with renal impairment, volume depletion (e.g. secondary to diuretics) or concurrent conditions that predispose to acidosis, this interaction may be significant. It has been suggested that electrolytes should be closely monitored when patients who are at risk of an interaction are taking colestyramine and spironolactone,[1] although note that the interaction appears to be rare.

1. Eaves ER, Korman MG. Cholestyramine induced hyperchloremic metabolic acidosis. *Aust N Z J Med* (1984) 14, 670–2.
2. Clouston WM, Lloyd HM. Cholestyramine induced hyperchloremic metabolic acidosis. *Aust N Z J Med* (1985) 15, 271.
3. Scheel PJ, Whelton A, Rossiter K, Watson A. Cholestyramine-induced hyperchloremic metabolic acidosis. *J Clin Pharmacol* (1992) 32, 536–8.
4. Zapater P, Alba D. Acidosis and extreme hyperkalemia associated with cholestyramine and spironolactone. *Ann Pharmacother* (1995) 29, 199–200.

Spironolactone + Dextropropoxyphene (Propoxyphene)

A single case report describes the development of gynaecomastia and a rash when a man taking spironolactone was given dextropropoxyphene.

Clinical evidence, mechanism, importance and management

A patient who had been taking spironolactone uneventfully for 4 years developed swollen, tender breasts and a rash on his chest and neck a fortnight after starting to take *Darvon Compound* (dextropropoxyphene, **aspirin**, **phenacetin** and **caffeine**). The problem disappeared when both drugs were withdrawn but the rash reappeared when the *Darvon Compound* alone was given and disappeared when it was withdrawn. No problems occurred when the spironolactone was given alone, but both the rash and the gynaecomastia recurred when the *Darvon Compound* was again added.[1] The reasons for this reaction are not understood. Gynaecomastia is a known adverse effect of spironolactone (incidence 1.2%), but the authors considered it unlikely that it should spontaneously develop after so many years of treatment. Consequently they attribute the reaction to an interaction with *Darvon Compound*, but say they cannot be sure which of the components is responsible. This is an isolated case, and would therefore not be expected to be of general relevance.

1. Licata AA, Bartter FC. Spironolactone-induced gynaecomastia related to allergic reaction to 'Darvon Compound'. *Lancet* (1976) ii, 905.

Spironolactone + Food

Food may increase the plasma levels of spironolactone, but this did not alter antihypertensive efficacy in one long-term study.

Clinical evidence, mechanism, importance and management

In a study in healthy subjects food increased the AUC of canrenone (the major active metabolite of spironolactone) by about 30% after a single 100-mg dose of spironolactone, when compared to the fasted state.[1] However, the same research group later found that the steady-state canrenone levels did not differ when spironolactone 100 mg daily was taken at least 30 minutes before eating for 60 days, compared with immediately after eating for 60 days. Furthermore, in a crossover study in 10 hypertensive patients, the antihypertensive efficacy of spironolactone was not altered by food. They suggest that the difference is due to a more specific drug assay in the second study.[2] Other authors have also found that, in healthy subjects, food increased the AUC of a single dose of spironolactone by 71%, and also increased the AUC of three of its metabolites (including canrenone) by 32%, but they did not assess whether this altered the hypotensive effect.[3] It appears from the long-term study, that food does not alter the antihypertensive efficacy of spironolactone. It has been recommended that spironolactone be taken with food to try and reduce the gastric irritant effects of the drug.[2]

1. Melander A, Danielson K, Schersten B, Thulin T, Wåhlin E. Enhancement by food of canrenone bioavailability from spironolactone. *Clin Pharmacol Ther* (1977) 22, 100–3.
2. Thulin T, Wåhlin-Boll E, Liedholm H, Lindholm L, Melander A. Influence of food intake on antihypertensive drugs: spironolactone. *Drug Nutr Interact* (1983) 2, 169–73.
3. Overdiek HW, Merkus FW. Influence of food on the bioavailability of spironolactone. *Clin Pharmacol Ther* (1986) 40, 531–6.

Thiazide diuretics + Bile-acid binding resins

The absorption of hydrochlorothiazide (and probably chlorothiazide) can be reduced by more than one-third if colestipol is given concurrently. Colestyramine also reduces the absorption of hydrochlorothiazide by more than two-thirds.

Clinical evidence

In 6 healthy subjects the plasma levels of **hydrochlorothiazide** were reduced by about two-thirds by **colestyramine** 8 g, taken 2 minutes before and 6 and 12 hours after a single 75-mg oral dose of **hydrochlorothiazide**. Total urinary excretion of **hydrochlorothiazide** fell by 83%. In a parallel study with **colestipol** 10 g, the blood levels of **hydrochlorothiazide** fell by about 14% and the total urinary excretion fell by 31%.[1] A further study found that giving the **colestyramine** 4 hours after the **hydrochlorothiazide** reduced the effects of the interaction but the absorption was still reduced by one-third.[2] In another study **colestipol**, given simultaneously or one hour after **chlorothiazide**, reduced the urinary excretion of **chlorothiazide** by 58% and 54%, respectively.[3]

Mechanism

Hydrochlorothiazide becomes bound to these non-absorbable anionic exchange resins within the gut, and less is available for absorption.

Importance and management

Established interactions of clinical importance. The best dosing schedule would appear to be to give hydrochlorothiazide 4 hours before colestyramine to minimise mixing in the gut. Even so, a one-third reduction in thiazide absorption occurs[2] and the possibility of this interaction should be considered in patients taking colestyramine or colestipol who have a reduced response to a thiazide diuretic. The optimum time-interval with colestipol has not been investigated but it would be reasonable to take similar precautions. Information about other thiazides is lacking although it seems likely that they will interact similarly. Note that it is normally recommended that other drugs are given 1 hour before or 4 to 6 hours after colestyramine and 1 hour before or 4 hours after colestipol.

1. Hunninghake DB, King S, La Croix K. The effect of cholestyramine and colestipol on the absorption of hydrochlorothiazide. *Int J Clin Pharmacol Ther Toxicol* (1982) 20, 151–4.
2. Hunninghake DB, Hibbard DM. Influence of time intervals for cholestyramine dosing on the absorption of hydrochlorothiazide. *Clin Pharmacol Ther* (1986) 39, 329–34.
3. Kauffmann RE, Azarnoff DL. Effect of colestipol on gastrointestinal absorption of chlorothiazide in man. *Clin Pharmacol Ther* (1973) 14, 886.

Thiazide diuretics + Calcium and/or Vitamin D

Hypercalcaemia and possibly metabolic alkalosis can develop in patients who are given high doses of vitamin D and/or large amounts of calcium if they are also given diuretics such as the thiazides, which can reduce the urinary excretion of calcium. One case of hypercalcaemia has been reported in a patient using a high-strength topical tacalcitol with a thiazide diuretic.

Clinical evidence

(a) Calcium and vitamin D

An elderly woman taking **hydrochlorothiazide** 25 mg and **triamterene** 50 mg daily became confused, disorientated and dehydrated 6 months after starting to take vitamin D_2 50 000 units and calcium 1.5 g daily (as calcium carbonate) for osteoporosis. Her serum calcium level had risen to about 3.5 mmol/L (normal range about 2 to 2.6 mmol/L).[1]

A young woman with osteoporosis taking 3 mg of vitamin D_2 and calcium 2 g daily (as lactate) became hypercalcaemic 3 days after starting to take **chlorothiazide** 500 mg every 6 hours.[2]

(b) Calcium carbonate

A 47-year-old man was admitted to hospital complaining of dizziness and general weakness, which had begun 2 months previously. He was taking **chlorothiazide** 500 mg daily for hypertension, 'thyroid' 120 mg daily for hypothyroidism and calcium carbonate 7.5 to 10 g daily for heartburn. On examination he was found to have metabolic alkalosis with respiratory compensation, a total serum calcium concentration of 3.4 mmol/L (range given as 2.15 to 2.6 mmol/L) and an abnormal ECG. He was diagnosed as having the milk-alkali syndrome. Recovery was rapid when the thiazide and calcium carbonate were withdrawn and a sodium chloride infusion, furosemide and oral phosphates were given.[3]

An elderly woman with normal renal function taking **hydrochlorothiazide** 50 mg daily developed hypercalcaemia about 3 weeks after increasing her dose of calcium carbonate from 2.5 g daily to 7.5 g daily.[4]

In both cases the thiazide diuretic was thought to be implicated as the levels of calcium ingestion were in the region of the normally recommended doses.

(c) Oral vitamin D

In a group of 12 patients treated for hypoparathyroidism with vitamin D (**dihydrotachysterol** or **ergocalciferol**), 5 patients became hypercalcaemic when they took **bendroflumethiazide** or **methyclothiazide**.[5] A significant rise in plasma calcium levels occurred in 7 patients given vitamin D and **methyclothiazide** or **chlorothiazide**, and hypercalcaemia developed in 3 of them.[6] A study in 12 children taking **calcitriol** (31 nanograms/kg daily) found that the addition of **hydrochlorothiazide** (1 to 2 micrograms/kg daily) reduced the urinary excretion of calcium caused by the calcitriol.[7] Another study in 7 patients with vitamin D-induced calciuria found that the addition of **hydrochlorothiazide** and **amiloride** reduced the urinary excretion of calcium due to the **calcitriol** to a greater extent than **hydrochlorothiazide** alone. Moreover, the addition of amiloride helped to prevent adverse effects associated with the use of **hydrochlorothiazide**, such as hypokalaemia and alkalosis.[8]

(d) Topical vitamin D analogues

A case of asymptomatic hypercalcaemia has been reported in a patient taking **trichlormethiazide** 6 mg daily and using 10 g of a high-strength topical **tacalcitol** ointment (20 micrograms/g) daily for psoriasis as part of a clinical study. His calcium level reached a peak of 3.55 mmol/L 28 days after starting the tacalcitol ointment and it fell back to within the normal range within 7 days of stopping the ointment.[9]

Mechanism

The thiazide diuretics (and triamterene) can cause calcium retention by reducing its urinary excretion. This, added to the increased intake of calcium, resulted in excessive calcium levels. Alkalosis (the milk-alkali syndrome, associated with hypercalcaemia, alkalosis, and renal impairment) may also occur in some individuals because the thiazide limits the excretion of bicarbonate.

Importance and management

An established interaction. The incidence is unknown but the reports cited[5,6] suggest that it can be considerable if the intake of vitamin D and calcium are high. Concurrent use need not be avoided; thiazides have been used clinically to reduce vitamin-D induced hypercalciuria,[7,8] but the serum calcium levels should be regularly monitored to ensure that they do not become excessive. Patients should be warned about the ingestion of very large amounts of calcium carbonate (readily available without prescription) if they are taking thiazide diuretics.

The case of hypercalcaemia with the use of a topical vitamin D analogue is rare and the strength of the preparation of tacalcitol used was fivefold higher than the current licensed preparation of 4 micrograms/g (*Curatoderm*). However, bear this case in mind should a patient taking thiazides with a topical vitamin D analogue develop hypercalcaemia.

1. Drinka PJ, Nolten WE. Hazards of treating osteoporosis and hypertension concurrently with calcium, vitamin D, and distal diuretics. *J Am Geriatr Soc* (1984) 32, 405–7.
2. Parfitt AM. Chlorothiazide-induced hypercalcaemia in juvenile osteoporosis and hyperparathyroidism. *N Engl J Med* (1969) 281, 55–9.
3. Gora ML, Seth SK, Bay WH, Visconti JA. Milk-alkali syndrome associated with use of chlorothiazide and calcium carbonate. *Clin Pharm* (1989) 8, 227–9.
4. Hakim R, Tolis G, Goltzman D, Meltzer S, Friedman R. Severe hypercalcemia associated with hydrochlorothiazide and calcium carbonate therapy. *Can Med Assoc J* (1979) 121, 591–4.
5. Parfitt AM. Thiazide-induced hypercalcaemia in vitamin D-treated hypoparathyroidism. *Ann Intern Med* (1972) 77, 557–63.
6. Parfitt AM. Interactions of thiazide diuretics with parathyroid hormone and vitamin D. Studies in patients with hypoparathyroidism. *J Clin Invest* (1972) 51, 1879–88.
7. Santos F, Smith MJ, Chan JCM. Hypercalciuria associated with long-term administration of calcitriol (1,25-dihydroxyvitamin D_3). Action of hydrochlorothiazide. *Am J Dis Child* (1986) 140, 139–42.
8. Alon U, Costanzo LS, Chan JCM. Additive hypocalciuric effects of amiloride and hydrochlorothiazide in patients treated with calcitriol. *Miner Electrolyte Metab* (1984) 10, 379–86.
9. Kawaguchi M, Mitsuhashi Y, Kondo S. Iatrogenic hypercalcemia due to vitamin D_3 ointment (1,24$(OH)_2D_3$) combined with thiazide diuretics in a case of psoriasis. *J Dermatol* (2003) 30, 801–4.

Thiazide and related diuretics + NSAIDs

There is evidence that most NSAIDs can increase blood pressure in patients taking antihypertensives, including diuretics, although some studies have not found the increase to be clinically relevant. The concurrent use of NSAIDs with thiazide diuretics may exacerbate congestive heart failure and increase the risk of hospitalisation.

Clinical evidence

Various large epidemiological studies and meta-analyses of clinical studies have been conducted to assess the effect of NSAIDs on blood pressure in patients treated with **antihypertensives**, and the findings of these are summarised in 'Table 23.2', (p.862). In these studies, NSAIDs were not always associated with an increase in blood pressure, and the maximum increase was 6.2 mmHg. The effect has been shown for both coxibs and non-selective NSAIDs. In two meta-analyses,[1,2] the effects were evaluated by NSAID. The confidence intervals for all the NSAIDs overlapped, showing that there was no statistically significant difference between the NSAIDs, with the exception of the comparison between **indometacin** and **sulindac** in one analysis.[2] Nevertheless, an attempt was made at ranking the NSAIDs based on the means. In one analysis,[1] the effect was greatest for **piroxicam**, **indometacin**, and **ibuprofen**, intermediate for **naproxen**, and least for **sulindac** and **flurbiprofen**. In the other meta-analysis,[2] the effect was greatest for **indometacin** and **naproxen**, intermediate for **piroxicam**, and least for **ibuprofen** and **sulindac**. An attempt was also made to evaluate the effect by **antihypertensive** in one analysis.[1] The mean effect was greatest for beta blockers, intermediate for vasodilators (includes ACE inhibitors and calcium-channel blockers), and least for **diuretics**. However, the differences between the groups were not significant.

The findings of individual clinical and pharmacological studies that have studied the effects of specific NSAIDs on diuretics are outlined in the subsections below and in 'Table 26.2', (p.957).

A. Bemetizide

Indometacin 100 mg was found to reduce the urinary excretion of sodium and chloride caused by bemetizide by 47% and 44%, respectively, in healthy subjects.[3]

B. Bendroflumethiazide

(a) Ibuprofen

In a randomised, placebo-controlled study, 7 hypertensive patients taking bendroflumethiazide 5 to 10 mg daily were also given ibuprofen 400 mg four times daily for 2 weeks. Although some small increases in blood pressure occurred, the diastolic blood pressure of all patients remained below 90 mmHg throughout the ibuprofen phase. Overall no statistically significant weight gain was noted, although 2 patients gained more than 2 kg.[4]

(b) Indometacin

A controlled study in 7 hypertensive patients taking bendroflumethiazide 5 to 10 mg daily found that indometacin 100 mg daily for 3 weeks raised their blood pressure by 13/9 mmHg when lying and by 16/9 mmHg when standing. Body-weight increased by 1.1 kg.[5] Indometacin also attenuated the hypotensive effect of bendroflumethiazide in another study.[6]

(c) Sulindac

A brief report suggested that sulindac *enhanced* the hypotensive effects of bendroflumethiazide in 5 hypertensive patients.[6]

C. Hydrochlorothiazide

(a) Diclofenac

Diclofenac 25 mg three times daily was given to 8 patients with essential hypertension who were taking hydrochlorothiazide. Blood pressure was not significantly altered after the addition of diclofenac, but a weight gain of about 1 to 2 kg was noted, which was thought to have been caused by the sodium retaining effects of diclofenac.[7] In another study, diclofenac 75 mg twice daily for one month did not alter the antihypertensive effect of the combination of hydrochlorothiazide 25 mg daily and lisinopril 10 to 40 mg daily.[8]

(b) Diflunisal

Diflunisal 375 mg twice daily caused the plasma levels of hydrochlorothiazide to rise by 25 to 30%, but this does not appear to be clinically significant.[9,10] Diflunisal also has uricosuric activity, which counteracts the uric acid retention that occurs with hydrochlorothiazide.

(c) Ibuprofen

In two studies in patients taking hydrochlorothiazide, ibuprofen 400 or 600 mg three times daily for 4 weeks caused a small rise in systolic but not in diastolic blood pressure.[7,11] However, a weight gain of about 1 to 2 kg was noted in one of the studies.[7] Another study found that ibuprofen 400 mg three times daily had no effect on blood pressure controlled by triamterene with hydrochlorothiazide, although one patient had a marked fall in renal function.[12] Ibuprofen 800 mg four times daily for a week had little effect on blood pressure controlled with hydrochlorothiazide in yet another study.[13] In two further studies, ibuprofen 800 mg three times daily for

Table 26.2 Interactions of diuretics and NSAIDs

	Bumetanide	*Furosemide*	*Piretanide*	*Torasemide*	*Bemetizide*	*Bendroflume-thiazide*	*Hydrochloro-thiazide*	*Hydrochloro-thiazide and amiloride*	*Hydrochloro-thiazide and triamterene*	*Metolazone*	*Spironolactone*	*Triamterene*
Azapropazone		N/S										
Celecoxib		ARF										
Diclofenac		Excretion of Na^+ ↓ 38%					N/S Weight gain	N/S				ARF
Diflunisal		Excretion of Na^+ ↓ 36 to 59%, Excretion of K^+ ↓ 47%					N/S					
Flupirtine		Delayed diuresis										
Flurbiprofen		Urinary volume ↓ 10%										
Ibuprofen		CHF, ↓ GFR & diuresis				N/S Weight gain	↑ BP		ARF			
Indometacin	Excretion of Na^+ ↓ 25% & ↓ diuresis. Case of heart failure	Mean BP ↑ by 13 mmHg; Urinary output ↓ 53%; Na^+ ↓ 64%	Excretion of Na^+ ↓ 35%	Possibly as furosemide	Excretion of Na^+ ↓ 47%	↑ BP by 13/9 mmHg; Weight gain	↑ BP by 6/3 mmHg	↑ BP by 16/9 mmHg		Excretion of Na^+ ↓ and K^+ ↓	Excretion of Na^+ ↓	ARF
Kebuzone							↑ systolic BP by 18 mmHg					
Ketoprofen		24-h Urinary output ↓ 651 mL										
Ketorolac		Diuretic effect ↓ 20%										
Lornoxicam		Diuretic effect ↓										
Meloxicam		N/S										
Metamizole (Dipyrone)		↓ furosemide clearance										
Mofebutazone		N/S										
Naproxen		Urinary volume ↓ 50%, ↓ GFR & diuresis					↑ BP					
Nimesulide		↓ GFR & diuresis										
Phenylbutazone							↑ systolic BP by 18 mmHg					
Piroxicam		Diuretic effect ↓, excretion of Na^+ ↓	N/S				↑ BP					
Sulindac	Na^+ ↓ 22%; urine flow rate ↓ 21%	Diuretic effect ↓ 76%				Enhanced hypotensive effects	N/S	N/S		Excretion of Na^+ & K^+ ↓		
Tenoxicam		N/S										
Tolfenamic acid	Diuretic effect ↓ 34%											

Abbreviations: ARF = acute renal failure; CHF = congestive heart failure; GFR; glomerular filtration rate; N/S = non-significant one month did not alter the antihypertensive effect of the combinations of hydrochlorothiazide 25 mg daily with fosinopril 10 to 40 mg daily[14] or lisinopril 10 to 40 mg daily.[8]

(d) Indometacin

A controlled study in 7 patients with hypertension taking amiloride 5 to 10 mg with hydrochlorothiazide 50 to 100 mg, found that indometacin 100 mg daily for 3 weeks raised their blood pressure by 13/9 mmHg when lying and by 16/9 mmHg when standing. Body-weight increased by 1.1 kg.[5] A later study in patients taking hydrochlorothiazide found a 6/3 mmHg blood pressure rise after they took indometacin for 2 weeks, but this had gone after 4 weeks.[15] A blood pressure rise of only 5/1 mmHg was seen in another study in hypertensive patients taking hydrochlorothiazide with indometacin 100 mg daily.[16] Indometacin also attenuated the hypotensive effect of hydrochlorothiazide (given with amiloride) in another study.[6]

In other studies indometacin had no effect on blood pressure in healthy subjects,[17] no effect on the sodium excretion caused by hydrochlorothiazide,[18] and did not affect the pharmacokinetics of hydrochlorothiazide.[17,18]

(e) Kebuzone

A mean systolic blood pressure rise of 18 mmHg (from 171 to 189 mmHg) occurred in 15 patients taking hydrochlorothiazide 50 mg daily, when they were given kebuzone 750 mg daily. This rise represents about a 35% reduction in the antihypertensive effect of hydrochlorothiazide.[19]

(f) Naproxen

One study found that naproxen had no clinically relevant interaction with hydrochlorothiazide alone,[15] while another found that naproxen attenuated the antihypertensive efficacy of hydrochlorothiazide taken with timolol, but how much of the attenuation is due to an interaction with the diuretic is unclear.[20]

(g) Phenylbutazone

A mean systolic blood pressure rise of 18 mmHg (from 171 to 189 mmHg) occurred in 15 patients taking hydrochlorothiazide 50 mg daily, when they were given phenylbutazone 750 mg daily. This rise represents about a 35% reduction in the antihypertensive effect of hydrochlorothiazide.[19]

(h) Piroxicam

One study found that piroxicam attenuated the antihypertensive efficacy of hydrochlorothiazide taken with timolol, but how much of the attenuation is due to an interaction with the diuretic is unclear.[20]

(i) Sulindac

Sulindac does not appear to reduce either the hypotensive or diuretic effects of hydrochlorothiazide, and may even slightly *enhance* the antihypertensive effects.[6,7,15,16,20,21] Another study found that sulindac did not alter the antihypertensive efficacy of hydrochlorothiazide/amiloride given with beta blockers.[22] Similarly, sulindac 200 mg twice daily for one month did not alter the antihypertensive effect of the combinations of hydrochlorothiazide 25 mg daily with fosinopril 10 to 40 mg daily,[14] or lisinopril 10 to 40 mg daily.[8]

D. Metolazone

(a) Indometacin

Indometacin was found to reduce the urinary sodium excretion due to metolazone by 34% in 6 healthy subjects.[23] The excretion of total potassium fell by 30%.

(b) Sulindac

Sulindac was found to reduce the urinary sodium excretion due to metolazone by 19% in 6 healthy subjects.[23] The excretion of total potassium fell by 16%.

E. Unspecified

In a randomised study, **ibuprofen** 400 mg every 8 hours caused a significant increase in blood pressure (mean increase of about 5 to 7 mmHg) in 12 hypertensive patients taking thiazides with beta blockers or centrally acting antihypertensives.[24]

Mechanism

Not understood. NSAIDs can cause salt and water retention, which antagonises the effects of diuretics. Prostaglandins have a role to play in renal function and drugs such as the NSAIDs, which inhibit prostaglandin synthesis, would therefore be expected to have some effect on the actions of diuretics, whose venodilatory effects also depend on the activity of the prostaglandins. A study in *rats* suggested that indometacin may oppose the effects of the thiazides by reducing chloride delivery to the site of thiazide action in the distal tubule.[25]

Importance and management

Overall, the evidence suggests that some patients taking thiazide diuretics can have a rise in blood pressure when given NSAIDs, but this may not always be clinically relevant. Some consider that the use of NSAIDs should be kept to a minimum in patients taking antihypertensives.[26] The effects may be greater in the elderly and in those with blood pressures that are relatively high, as well as in those with high salt intake.[26] However, others consider that the clinical importance of an interaction between NSAIDs and antihypertensives is less than has previously been suggested.[27] While their findings do not rule out a 2/1 mmHg increase in blood pressure with NSAIDs in treated hypertensives, they suggest that if patients in primary care have inadequate control of blood pressure, other reasons may be more likely than any effect of concurrent NSAIDs.[27] There is insufficient data at present to clearly differentiate between NSAIDs, although there is some evidence that the effects of indometacin are greatest and sulindac least. Further study is needed. A retrospective analysis of records of patients taking diuretics (thiazides, loop and/or potassium-sparing) with NSAIDs found a twofold increase in the risk of hospitalisation for congestive heart failure on concurrent use. The most common NSAIDs taken by this cohort of patients were diclofenac, ibuprofen, indometacin and naproxen.[28] The European Society of Cardiology (ESC) Task Force and the joint American College of Cardiology/American Heart Association both recommend avoiding NSAID use, if possible, in patients with congestive heart failure.[29,30]

For the effects of NSAIDs on other antihypertensive drug classes see 'ACE inhibitors', (p.28), 'beta blockers', (p.835) and 'calcium-channel blockers', (p.861).

1. Johnson AG, Nguyen TV, Day RO. Do nonsteroidal anti-inflammatory drugs affect blood pressure? A meta-analysis. *Ann Intern Med* (1994) 121, 289–300.
2. Pope JE, Anderson JJ, Felson DT. A meta-analysis of the effects of nonsteroidal anti-inflammatory drugs on blood pressure. *Arch Intern Med* (1993) 153, 477–84.
3. Düsing R, Nicolas V, Glatte B, Glänzer K, Kipnowski J, Kramer HJ. Interaction of bemetizide and indomethacin in the kidney. *Br J Clin Pharmacol* (1983) 16, 377–84.
4. Davies JG, Rawlins DC, Busson M. Effect of ibuprofen on blood pressure control by propranolol and bendrofluazide. *J Int Med Res* (1988) 16, 173–81.
5. Watkins J, Abbott EC, Hensby CN, Webster J, Dollery CT. Attenuation of hypotensive effect of propranolol and thiazide diuretics by indomethacin. *BMJ* (1980) 281, 702–5.
6. Steiness E, Waldorff S. Different interactions of indomethacin and sulindac with thiazides in hypertension. *BMJ* (1982) 285, 1702–3.
7. Koopmans PP, Thien Th, Gribnau FWJ. The influence of ibuprofen, diclofenac and sulindac on the blood pressure lowering effect of hydrochlorothiazide. *Eur J Clin Pharmacol* (1987) 31, 553–7.
8. Bhagat K. Effects of non-steroidal anti-inflammatory drugs on hypertension control using angiotensin converting enzyme inhibitors and thiazide diuretics. *East Afr Med J* (2001) 78, 507–9.
9. Tempero KF, Cirillo VJ, Steelman SL. Diflunisal: a review of the pharmacokinetic and pharmacodynamic properties, drug interactions and special tolerability studies in humans. *Br J Clin Pharmacol* (1977) 4, 31S–36S.
10. Tempero KF, Cirillo VJ, Steelman SL, Besselaar GH, Smit Sibinga CTh, De Schepper P, Tjandramaga TB, Dresse A, Gribnau FWJ. Special studies on diflunisal, a novel salicylate. *Clin Res* (1975) 23, 224A.
11. Gurwitz JH, Everitt DE, Monane M, Glynn RJ, Choodnovskiy I, Beaudet MP, Avorn J. The impact of ibuprofen on the efficacy of antihypertensive treatment with hydrochlorothiazide in elderly persons. *J Gerontol* (1996) 51A, M74–M79.
12. Gehr TWB, Sica DA, Steiger BW, Marshall C. Interaction of triamterene-hydrochlorothiazide and ibuprofen. *Clin Pharmacol Ther* (1990) 47, 200.
13. Wright JT, McKenney JM, Lehany AM, Bryan DL, Cooper LW, Lambert CM. The effect of high-dose short-term ibuprofen on antihypertensive control with hydrochlorothiazide. *Clin Pharmacol Ther* (1989) 46, 440–4.
14. Thakur V, Cook ME, Wallin JD. Antihypertensive effect of the combination of fosinopril and HCTZ is resistant to interference by nonsteroidal antiinflammatory drugs. *Am J Hypertens* (1999) 12, 925–8.
15. Koopmans PP, Thien Th, Gribnau FWJ. Influence of non-steroidal anti-inflammatory drugs on diuretic treatment of mild to moderate essential hypertension. *BMJ* (1984) 289, 1492–4.
16. Koopmans PP, Thien Th, Thomas CMG, van den Berg RJ, Gribnau FWJ. The effects of sulindac and indomethacin on the antihypertensive and diuretic action of hydrochlorothiazide in patients with mild to moderate essential hypertension. *Br J Clin Pharmacol* (1986) 21, 417–23.
17. Koopmans PP, Kateman WGPM, Tan Y, van Ginneken CAM, Gribnau FWJ. Effects of indomethacin and sulindac on hydrochlorothiazide kinetics. *Clin Pharmacol Ther* (1985) 37, 625–8.
18. Williams RL, Davies RO, Berman RS, Holmes GI, Huber P, Gee WL, Lin ET, Benet LZ. Hydrochlorothiazide pharmacokinetics and pharmacologic effect: the influence of indomethacin. *J Clin Pharmacol* (1982) 22, 32–41.
19. Polak F. Die hemmende Wirkung von Phenylbutazon auf die durch einige Antihypertonika hervorgerufene Blutdrucksenkung bei Hypertonikern. *Z Gesamte Inn Med* (1976) 22, 375–6.

20. Wong DG, Spence JD, Lamki L, Freeman D, McDonald JWD. Effect of non-steroidal anti-inflammatory drugs on control of hypertension by beta-blockers and diuretics. *Lancet* (1986) 3, 997–1001.
21. Steiness E, Waldorff S. Different interactions of indomethacin and sulindac with thiazides in hypertension. *BMJ* (1982) 285, 1702–3.
22. Stokes GS, Brooks PM, Johnson HJ, Monaghan JC, Okoro EO, Kelly D. The effects of sulindac and diclofenac in essential hypertension controlled by treatment with a beta-blocker and/or diuretic. *Clin Exp Hypertens A* (1991) 13, 1169–78.
23. Ripley EBD, Gehr TWB, Wallace H, Wade J, Kish C, Sica DA. The effect of nonsteroidal agents (NSAIDs) on the pharmacokinetics and pharmacodynamics of metolazone. *Int J Clin Pharmacol Ther* (1994) 32, 12–18.
24. Radack KL, Deck CC, Bloomfield SS. Ibuprofen interferes with the efficacy of antihypertensive drugs. A Randomized, double-blind, placebo-controlled trial of ibuprofen compared with acetaminophen. *Ann Intern Med* (1987) 107, 628–35.
25. Kirchner KA, Brandon S, Mueller RA, Smith MJ, Bower JD. Mechanism of attenuated hydrochlorothiazide response during indomethacin administration. *Kidney Int* (1987) 31, 1097–1103.
26. Johnson AG. NSAIDs and blood pressure. Clinical importance for older patients. *Drugs Aging* (1998) 12, 17–27.
27. Sheridan R, Montgomery AA, Fahey T. NSAID use and BP in treated hypertensives: a retrospective controlled observational study. *J Hum Hypertens* (2005) 19, 445–50.
28. Heerdink ER, Leufkens HG, Herings RMC, Ottervanger JP, Stricker BHC, Bakker A. NSAIDs associated with increased risk of congestive heart failure in elderly patients taking diuretics. *Arch Intern Med* (1998) 158, 1108–12.
29. Hunt SA. ACC/AHA 2005 guideline update for the diagnosis and management of chronic heart failure in the adult. A report of the American College of Cardiology/American Heart Association Task Force on Practice Guidelines (Writing Committee to Update the 2001 Guidelines for the Evaluation and Management of Heart Failure). *J Am Coll Cardiol* (2005) 46, e1–e82. Available at: http://content.onlinejacc.org/cgi/reprint/46/6/e1.pdf (accessed 22/08/2007).
30. Swedberg K, Cleland J, Dargie H, Drexler H, Follath F, Komajda M, Tavazzi L, Smiseth OA, Gavazzi A, Haverich A, Hoes A, Jaarsma T, Korewicki J, Lévy S, Linde C, Lopez-Sendon J-L, Nieminen MS, Piérard L, Remme WJ; The Task Force for the Diagnosis and Treatment of Chronic Heart Failure of the European Society of Cardiology. Guidelines for the diagnosis and treatment of chronic heart failure (update 2005). *Eur Heart J* (2005) 26, 1115–40. Available at: http://www.escardio.org/NR/rdonlyres/8A2848B4-5DEB-41B9-9A0A-5B5A90494B64/0/guidelines_CHF_FT_2005.pdf (accessed 22/08/2007).

Thiazide diuretics + Propantheline

Propantheline can slightly increase the absorption of hydrochlorothiazide.

Clinical evidence, mechanism, importance and management

In 6 healthy fasting subjects the absorption of hydrochlorothiazide 75 mg was delayed and increased (AUC increased by 23% and urinary recovery increased by 36%) by propantheline 60 mg. It is suggested that this occurs because propantheline causes a slower delivery of the hydrochlorothiazide to its areas of absorption.[1] This small increase is unlikely to be clinically important.

1. Beermann B, Groschinsky-Grind M. Enhancement of the gastrointestinal absorption of hydrochlorothiazide by propantheline. *Eur J Clin Pharmacol* (1978) 13, 385–7.

27

Gastrointestinal drugs

The various gastrointestinal drug groups covered in this section are listed in 'Table 27.1', (see below). 'Drug absorption interactions', (p.3) discusses how absorption interactions occur and contains more detailed information on some of the mechanisms of interaction covered in this section.

Metabolism of proton pump inhibitors

The main metabolic pathway for esomeprazole, lansoprazole, omeprazole, pantoprazole, and to a lesser extent rabeprazole, is through the cytochrome P450 isoenzyme CYP2C19. This isoenzyme is subject to genetic polymorphism,[1] (see 'Genetic factors', (p.4), for a further explanation of polymorphism). The poor metaboliser phenotype for CYP2C19 is found in approximately 1 to 6% of Caucasians, 1 to 7.5% of Blacks and 12 to 23% of Oriental and Indian Asians.[2]

Therefore most patients will be extensive CYP2C19 metabolisers, and their major route for the metabolism of these PPIs will be through this isoenzyme. As a consequence, the levels of PPIs in these patients are likely to be affected by drugs that inhibit or induce CYP2C19, such as 'fluvoxamine', (p.973).[2] Patients of the extensive metaboliser phenotype have also been shown in some studies to have a poorer clinical outcome, when compared with poor metabolisers e.g. in the eradication of *H. pylori,* as they tend to have lower therapeutic levels of PPIs.[2-4]

Poor metabolisers, who lack CYP2C19 metabolising capacity, use alternative pathways to metabolise PPIs, and this is mainly CYP3A4. Because poor metabolisers are more dependent on CYP3A4 for metabolism of the PPIs the levels of PPIs may be raised in these patients when they are given CYP3A4 inhibitors, such as 'clarithromycin' , (p.971), and 'ketoconazole', (p.218).

Omeprazole and esomeprazole are also inhibitors of CYP2C19, and therefore they may increase the levels of drugs that are metabolised by CYP2C19, such as diazepam. Other CYP2C19 substrates are listed in 'Table 1.3', (p.6).[1,2] Particular care may be required when giving drugs that are CYP2C19 inhibitors to patients in those ethnic groups who have a higher percentage of poor CYP2C19 metabolisers, such as Indian Asians.[1,2]

1. Robinson M, Horn J. Clinical pharmacology of proton pump inhibitors. What the practising physician needs to know. *Drugs* (2003) 63, 2739–54.
2. Desta Z, Zhao X, Shin JG, Flockhart DA. Clinical significance of the cytochrome P450 2C19 genetic polymorphism. *Clin Pharmacokinet* (2002) 41, 913–58.
3. Furuta T, Shirai N, Sugimoto M, Nakamura A, Hishida A, Ishizaki T. Influence of CYP2C19 pharmacogenetic polymorphism on proton pump inhibitor-based therapies. *Drug Metab Pharmacokinet* (2005) 20, 153–67.
4. Klotz U. Pharmacokinetic considerations in the eradication of *Helicobacter pylori. Clin Pharmacokinet* (2000) 38, 243–70.

Table 27.1 Gastrointestinal drugs covered in this section

Group	*Drugs*
5-aminosalicylates	Balsalazide, Mesalazine, Olsalazine, Sulfasalazine
Antidiarrhoeals	Loperamide
Antimuscarinics	Pirenzepine
Bismuth compounds	Bismuth biskalcitrate, Bismuth salicylate, Bismuth subnitrate, Tripotassium dicitratobismuthate
H_2-receptor antagonists	Cimetidine, Famotidine, Nizatidine, Ranitidine, Roxatidine
Mucosal protectants	Carbenoxolone, Liquorice, Sucralfate
Prokinetic drugs	Cisapride
Proton pump inhibitors	Esomeprazole, Lansoprazole, Omeprazole, Pantoprazole, Rabeprazole

Antacids + Milk

Hypercalcaemia, alkalosis and renal insufficiency (milk-alkali syndrome) can develop in patients taking antacids with calcium-containing substances, including dairy products.

Clinical evidence

A man presented with nausea, vomiting, constipation, polyuria and polydipsia, which was diagnosed as milk-alkali syndrome, due to daily treatment with 6 tablets of ***Caved-S*** and 3.5 pints of milk, for dyspepsia related to a peptic ulcer.[1] This dose of ***Caved-S*** meant he was taking 600 mg of **aluminium hydroxide**, 1200 mg of **magnesium carbonate**, 600 mg of **sodium bicarbonate** and 2280 mg of **deglycyrrhizinised liquorice** daily.[1] Another case report describes a 42-year-old man who presented with confusion, agitation, involuntary movements of his limbs, severe dehydration, and metabolic and respiratory alkalosis. He had taken large amounts of a **calcium/magnesium carbonate**-containing antacid preparation (*Rennies)* and had also consumed at least 3 litres of diary products a day for upper abdominal complaints. Milk-alkali syndrome was diagnosed and he was successfully treated with isotonic saline and potassium.[2] A pregnant woman developed vomiting, drowsiness, abdominal pain and acute pancreatitis after excessive antacid use. She had been taking up to 10 tablets of *Rennies* antacid (**calcium/magnesium carbonate**), containing about 3 g of elemental calcium with up to 3 glasses of milk a day.[3] In a study in 125 patients with non end-stage renal disease, milk-alkali syndrome was found to be the cause of hypercalcaemia in 11 (8.8%) of the patients, 9 of who had severe hypercalcaemia (serum calcium greater than 3.5 mmol/L).[4] Several other cases have been reported in recent years involving excessive use of non-prescription **calcium carbonate**,[5-7] one of which was in a pregnant woman.[6]

Mechanism

High intake and absorption of calcium can suppress the parathyroid hormone, which leads to bicarbonate retention by the kidneys, leading to metabolic and respiratory alkalosis. The alkalosis also causes reduced excretion of calcium by the kidneys. Hypermagnesaemia may also have a part to play.

Importance and management

The milk-alkali syndrome was a common adverse effect of antacid use when it was the primary treatment of peptic ulcer disease, but has become very uncommon with the advent of H_2-blockers and proton pump inhibitors. However, the above cases illustrate that while taking antacids, even well within the recommended dosage range, as in the first case, it is still possible to develop a serious and potentially life-threatening reaction if the intake of calcium is high. This should be borne in mind in patients who take both prescribed or non-prescription medications containing calcium, such as antacids or supplements for the prophylaxis of osteoporosis, and also consume large quantities of dairy products in their diet. Chronic milk-alkali syndrome can lead to the formation of calcification and kidney damage, which may be irreversible. The quantity of calcium ingested does not appear to be directly correlated to either the development or severity of milk-alkali syndrome, which has been reported with an intake of between 4 g to 60 g of calcium carbonate.[3] However, a safe maximum calcium intake of 1.2 to 1.5 g of elemental calcium (3 to 3.75 g of calcium carbonate) has been suggested.[3]

1. Gibbs CJ, Lee HA. Milk-alkali syndrome due to Caved-S. *J R Soc Med* (1992) 85, 498–9.
2. Verburg FA, van Zanten RAA, Brouwer RML, Woittiez AJJ, Veneman TF. Een man met een ernstig klassiek melk-alkalisyndroom en een maagcarcinoom. *Ned Tijdschr Geneeskd* (2006) 150, 1624–7.
3. Gordon MV, Hamblin PS, McMahon LP. Life-threatening milk-alkali syndrome resulting from antacid ingestion during pregnancy. *Med J Aust* (2005) 182, 350–351
4. Picolos MK, Lavis VR, Orlander PR. Milk–alkali syndrome is a major cause of hypercalcaemia among non-end-stage renal disease (non-ESRD) inpatients. *Clin Endocrinol (Oxf)* (2005) 63, 566–76.
5. McGuinness B, Logan JI. Milk alkali syndrome. *Ulster Med J* (2002) 71, 132–5.
6. Ennen CS, Magann EF. Milk-alkali syndrome presenting as acute renal insufficiency during pregnancy. *Obstet Gynecol* (2006) 108, 785–6.
7. George S, Clark JDA. Milk alkali syndrome – an unusual syndrome causing an unusual complication. *Postgrad Med J* (2000) 76, 422–4.

Bismuth compounds + H_2-receptor antagonists

Ranitidine possibly causes an increase in the absorption of bismuth from tripotassium dicitratobismuthate, but not bismuth salicylate or bismuth subnitrate. Any increase is considered unlikely to be clinically relevant with recommended short courses for *H. pylori* eradication. Other H_2-receptor antagonists would be expected to interact similarly.

Clinical evidence, mechanism, importance and management

The AUC of a single 240-mg dose of **tripotassium dicitratobismuthate (TDB**, *De Noltabs*), was increased fourfold in 12 healthy subjects given two 300-mg doses of ranitidine (one the night before and one 2 hours before the bismuth compound). The maximum serum levels were approximately doubled. The same regimen of ranitidine had no significant effect on the absorption of bismuth from **bismuth salicylate** (*Pepto-Bismol)* or **bismuth subnitrate** (*Roter tablets*).[1]

The authors suggest that the reduction in gastric acidity maintains **TDB** in its colloidal form, which is more likely to be absorbed, and that this may result in increased bismuth toxicity.[1] Other H_2-receptor antagonists, and other drugs that reduce gastric acidity would be expected to interact similarly (see also 'Bismuth compounds + Proton pump inhibitors', p.961).

However, the manufacturers of **TDB** say that the toxic range of bismuth is arbitrary and a small increase in absorption is not clinically relevant, except perhaps in patients with renal failure, in whom this bismuth compound should be avoided in any case.[2] Note that a complex of ranitidine with bismuth and citrate (**ranitidine bismuth citrate**) is available in many countries and is a recommended constituent in one of the triple therapy regimens for *H. pylori* eradication. As with all bismuth compounds, it is recommended that this is used only for limited periods: a maximum of 16 weeks (two 8-week courses or four 4-week courses) in a 12-month period.[3]

1. Nwokolo CU, Prewett EJ, Sawyerr AM, Hudson M, Pounder RE. The effect of histamine H_2-receptor blockade on bismuth absorption from three ulcer-healing compounds. *Gastroenterology* (1991) 101, 889–94.
2. Yamanouchi Pharma Ltd. Personal communication, November 1994.
3. Pylorid Tablets (Ranitidine bismuth citrate). GlaxoSmithKline UK. UK Summary of product characteristics, December 2005.

Bismuth compounds + Proton pump inhibitors

Omeprazole markedly increases the absorption and bioavailability of bismuth from tripotassium dicitratobismuthate and bismuth biskalcitrate. Other proton pump inhibitors are expected to interact similarly. However, this is probably unlikely to be clinically relevant.

Clinical evidence

Thirty-four healthy subjects were randomised to receive a triple therapy capsule *Helizide* (containing **bismuth biskalcitrate** 140 mg, metronidazole 125 mg, and tetracycline 125 mg) at a dose of three capsules four times daily with or without omeprazole 20 mg twice daily for 6 days. Omeprazole increased the maximum serum levels and AUC of bismuth by about threefold. However, the maximum serum level achieved was 25.5 micrograms/L, which was still well below 50 micrograms/L, a level reported to be highly unlikely to cause toxicity.[1] The authors also state that in clinical trials of *Helizide* with omeprazole for 10 days in several hundred patients,[2] no patient showed signs of encephalopathy, a notable toxic adverse effect of bismuth.[1]

In an earlier single-dose study in 6 healthy subjects, a single 240-mg dose of **tripotassium dicitratobismuthate** was taken 1 hour after the last dose of a 1-week course of omeprazole 40 mg daily. Omeprazole increased the AUC of bismuth fourfold, and increased the maximum serum levels from 36.7 to 86.7 micrograms/L, which the authors pointed out approaches the considered "toxic range" for bismuth (100 micrograms/L and above).

Mechanism

The solubility and absorption of some bismuth compounds are known to be increased by decreased acidity of the stomach,[1] see also 'Bismuth compounds + H_2-receptor antagonists', p.961).

Importance and management

The authors of the single-dose study recommended that the dosage of tripotassium dicitratobismuthate should be halved when given with omeprazole because of the possibility of systemic bismuth toxicity.[3] However, an increased risk of toxicity has not been seen in subsequent studies using bismuth biskalcitrate for up to 10 days.[1,2] The manufacturers of tripotassium dicitratobismuthate say that the toxic range of bismuth is arbitrary and the small increase in absorption is not clinically relevant, except perhaps in patients with renal failure, in whom this bismuth compound should be avoided in any case.[4] No clinically significant effect would be expected if combined treatment is limited to the recommended 2-week regimen for resistant *Helicobacter pylori* infection. As this interaction is due to changes in gastric pH other **proton pump inhibitors** would be expected to interact similarly.

1. Spénard J, Aumais C, Massicotte J, Tremblay C, Lefebvre M. Influence of omeprazole on bioavailability of bismuth following administration of a triple capsule of bismuth biskalcitrate, metronidazole, and tetracycline. *J Clin Pharmacol* (2004) 44, 640–5.
2. O'Morain C, Borody T, Farley A, De Boer WA, Dallaire C, Schuman R, Piotrowski J, Fallone CA, Tytgat G, Mégraud F, Spénard J. Efficacy and safety of single-triple capsules of bismuth biskalcitrate, metronidazole and tetracycline, given with omeprazole, for the eradication of Helicobacter pylori: an international multicentre study. *Aliment Pharmacol Ther* (2003) 17, 415–20.
3. Treiber G, Walker S, Klotz U. Omeprazole-induced increase in the absorption of bismuth from tripotassium dicitrato bismuthate. *Clin Pharmacol Ther* (1994) 55, 486–91.
4. Yamanouchi Pharma Ltd. Personal communication, November 1994.

Carbenoxolone + Antacids

There is some evidence that antacids may possibly reduce the bioavailability of carbenoxolone liquid.

Clinical evidence, mechanism, importance and management

The bioavailability of carbenoxolone, in a liquid formulation, when given with **aluminium/magnesium hydroxide** antacids, was found to be approximately half that of carbenoxolone in granular and capsule formulations.[1] The extent to which antacids might reduce the ulcer-healing effects of carbenoxolone liquid seems not to have been assessed, but the possibility of a reduction should be borne in mind.

1. Crema F, Parini J, Visconti M, Perucca E. Effetto degli antiacidi sulla biodisponibilità del carbenoxolone. *Farmaco (Prat)* (1987) 42, 357–64.

Carbenoxolone + Antihypertensives

Carbenoxolone causes fluid retention and raises blood pressure in some patients. This may be expected to oppose the effects of antihypertensive drugs. The potassium-depleting effects of carbenoxolone and diuretics such as the thiazides or loop diuretics can be additive. Spironolactone or amiloride can oppose the ulcer-healing effects of carbenoxolone.

Clinical evidence, mechanism, importance and management

(a) Antihypertensives (unnamed)

Carbenoxolone can raise blood pressure. Five out of 10 patients taking carbenoxolone 300 mg daily, and 2 out of 10 patients taking carbenoxolone 150 mg daily, had a rise in diastolic blood pressure of 20 mmHg or more.[1] Other reports[2-8] confirm that fluid retention and hypertension occur in those taking carbenoxolone, with the reported incidence of hypertension varying from as low as 4%[8] to as high as 50%,[7] and fluid retention occurring in 0%[2] to 46% of patients.[7] The reason for the blood pressure rise is that carbenoxolone has mineralocorticoid-like activity and therefore causes sodium and water retention. There appear to be few direct reports of adverse interactions between antihypertensives and carbenoxolone. Patients taking carbenoxolone should have regular checks on their weight and blood pressure, and carbenoxolone should be used with caution, if at all, in those with cardiac disease such as hypertension or congestive heart failure (see also Diuretics, below).

(b) Diuretics

Thiazide diuretics have been used to control the oedema and hypertension caused by carbenoxolone, but **spironolactone**[3] (an aldosterone antagonist) and **amiloride**[9] are best avoided because they oppose its ulcer-healing effects. If **thiazides** or other potassium-depleting diuretics (see 'Table 26.1', (p.944)) are used it should be remembered that the potassium-losing effects of the carbenoxolone and the diuretic will be additive, so that a potassium supplement may be needed to prevent hypokalaemia. For example, rhabdomyolysis and acute tubular necrosis associated with severe hypokalaemia occurred in a patient given carbenoxolone and **chlortalidone**, without a potassium supplement.[10] Laryngospasm and stridor have been reported in a patient secondary to hypokalaemia and alkalosis caused by long-term use of **furosemide** and a carbenoxolone-containing antacid (*Pyrogastrone*).[11] Possible alternatives to carbenoxolone are the **H_2-receptor antagonists**, or the **proton pump inhibitors**, which do not appear to interact with antihypertensives.

1. Turpie AGG, Thomson TJ. Carbenoxolone sodium in the treatment of gastric ulcer with special reference to side-effects. *Gut* (1965) 6, 591.
2. Baron A, Sullivan S, eds. Carbenoxolone Sodium: Maintenance carbenoxolone sodium in the prevention of gastric ulcer recurrence. London: Butterworths; 1970 p. 103–16.
3. Doll R, Langman MJS, Shawdon HH. Treatment of gastric ulcer with carbenoxolone: antagonistic effect of spironolactone. *Gut* (1968) 9, 42–5.
4. Montgomery RD, Cookson JB. Comparative trial of carbenoxolone and a deglycyrrhizinated liquorice preparation (Caved-S). *Clin Trials J* (1972) 9, 33–5.
5. Langman MJS, Knapp DR, Wakley EJ. Treatment of chronic gastric ulcer with carbenoxolone and gefarnate: a comparative trial. *BMJ* (1973) 3, 84–6.
6. Horwich L, Galloway R. Treatment of gastric ulceration with carbenoxolone sodium: clinical and radiological evaluation. *BMJ* (1965) 2, 1274–7.
7. Fraser PM, Doll R, Langman MJS, Misiewicz JJ, Shawdon HH. Clinical trial of a new carbenoxolone analogue (BX-24), zinc sulphate, and vitamin A in the treatment of gastric ulcer. *Gut* (1972) 13, 459–63.
8. Montgomery RD. Side effects of carbenoxolone sodium: a study of ambulant therapy of gastric ulcer. *Gut* (1967) 8, 148–50.
9. Reed PI, Lewis SI, Vincent-Brown A, Holdstock DJ, Gribble RJN, Murgatroyd RE, Baron JH. The influence of amiloride on the therapeutic and metabolic effects of carbenoxolone in patients with gastric ulcer. *Scand J Gastroenterol* (1980) 15 (Suppl 65), 51–5.
10. Descamps C, Vandenbroucke JM, van Ypersele de Strihou C. Rhabdomyolysis and acute tubular necrosis associated with carbenoxolone and diuretic treatment. *BMJ* (1977) 1, 272.
11. Sarkar SK. Stridor due to drug-induced hypokalaemic alkalosis. *J Laryngol Otol* (1987) 101, 197–8.

Carbenoxolone + Phenytoin

A single 100-mg dose of phenytoin had no significant effect on the half-life of a single 100-mg dose of carbenoxolone in 4 healthy subjects.[1] This limited evidence would seem to suggest that there is no reason for avoiding concurrent use.

1. Thornton PC, Papouchado M, Reed PI. Carbenoxolone interactions in man - preliminary report. *Scand J Gastroenterol* (1980) 15 (Suppl 65), 35–9.

Carbenoxolone + Sulphonylureas

Chlorpropamide appears to reduce the serum levels of carbenoxolone. Tolbutamide does not appear to have any significant effect on the pharmacokinetics of carbenoxolone.

Clinical evidence, mechanism, importance and management

A single 500-mg dose of **tolbutamide** had no significant effect on the half-life of a single 100-mg dose of carbenoxolone in 4 healthy subjects, whereas a single 250-mg dose of **chlorpropamide** delayed the absorption of carbenoxolone and reduced its plasma levels in 6 patients taking carbenoxolone 100 mg three times daily.[1] The clinical importance of this latter interaction is uncertain.

1. Thornton PC, Papouchado M, Reed PI. Carbenoxolone interactions in man - preliminary report. *Scand J Gastroenterol* (1980) 15 (Suppl 65), 35–9.

Cimetidine + Dimeticone

The pharmacokinetics of a 200-mg dose of cimetidine were not significantly changed by dimeticone 2.25 g in 11 healthy subjects.[1] For the effect of antacids containing dimeticone, see 'H_2-receptor antagonists + Antacids', p.966.

1. Boismare F, Flipo JL, Moore N, Chanteclair G. Etude de l'effet du diméticone sur la biodisponibilité de la cimétidine. *Therapie* (1987) 42, 9–11.

Cimetidine + Phenobarbital

Phenobarbital modestly reduces the AUC of cimetidine, although this is probably not clinically relevant.

Clinical evidence, mechanism, importance and management

Phenobarbital 100 mg daily for 3 weeks reduced the AUC of a single 400-mg oral dose of cimetidine in 8 healthy subjects by 15%, and the time during which the plasma concentrations of the cimetidine exceeded 0.5 micrograms/mL (regarded as therapeutically desirable) was reduced by 11%.[1]

Phenobarbital apparently stimulates the enzymes in the gut wall so that the metabolism of the cimetidine is increased. Thus the amount of cimetidine absorbed and released into the circulation is reduced.

Direct information is very limited, but the effect of phenobarbital on cimetidine is small and unlikely to be clinically important. No special precautions seem to be necessary.

1. Somogyi A, Thielscher S, Gugler R. Influence of phenobarbital treatment on cimetidine kinetics. *Eur J Clin Pharmacol* (1981) 19, 343–7.

Cimetidine + Rifampicin (Rifampin)

Antituberculous treatment with rifampicin, isoniazid and ethambutol has been shown to increase the non-renal clearance of cimetidine by about 50%. This is probably due to enzyme induction caused by rifampicin. However, the total clearance is unchanged and so this interaction would appear to be of little clinical importance.[1]

1. Keller E, Schollmeyer P, Brandenstein U, Hoppe-Seyler G. Increased nonrenal clearance of cimetidine during antituberculous therapy. *Int J Clin Pharmacol Ther Toxicol* (1984) 22, 307–11.

Cisapride + Miscellaneous

Ketoconazole, erythromycin, and clarithromycin can cause a marked rise in serum cisapride levels, increasing the risk of serious and life-threatening ventricular arrhythmias including torsade de pointes. Nefazodone and protease inhibitors are also predicted to have this effect. Although there do not appear to be any specific reports, cisapride should not be used with other drugs that prolong the QT interval (see also 'Drugs that prolong the QT interval + Other drugs that prolong the QT interval', p.257). No clinically relevant interactions with cisapride are apparent when it is given with antacids, cimetidine, esomeprazole, fluoxetine or pantoprazole, but two isolated reports attribute cardiotoxicity to the concurrent use of cisapride and ranitidine or diltiazem. Cisapride increases the rate of absorption of bromperidol, ciclosporin, diazepam, disopyramide, and nifedipine, but appears to have no important effect on digoxin, morphine, paracetamol (acetaminophen) or propranolol. The effects of anticoagulants may be altered by cisapride.

Clinical evidence, mechanism, importance and management

In many countries cisapride has been withdrawn from the market, or is only available for restricted use because of its potential to cause torsade de pointes arrhythmias, especially when cisapride serum levels are elevated.[1] This can lead to cardiac arrest and sudden death. The interactions of cisapride and their importance and management are summarised in 'Table 27.2', (p.964).

Enteral feeds + Aluminium compounds and/or Sucralfate

Aluminium-containing antacids and sucralfate can interact with high-protein liquid enteral feeds to produce an obstructive plug.

Clinical evidence

(a) Aluminium-containing antacids

Three patients, who were being fed with a liquid high-protein nutrient (***Fresubin liquid***) through an enteral tube, developed an obstructing protein-aluminium-complex oesophageal plug when intermittently given an aluminium/magnesium hydroxide antacid (*Alucol-Gel*).[1] Another report also describes blockage of a nasogastric tube in a patient treated with aluminium hydroxide (*Aludrox*) and ***Nutrison***.[2]

(b) Sucralfate alone or with aluminium-containing antacids

A number of reports describe the development of hard putty-like or creamy precipitations and encrustations that have blocked the oesophagus or stomach of patients given **sucralfate** with enteral feeds (***Ensure Plus***,[3] ***Fresubin plus F***[4] or ***Osmolite***[5]). Another patient developed this precipitate when treated with ***Isocal*** and **sucralfate** with aluminium/magnesium hydroxide.[6] Similarly, a patient receiving ***Pulmocare*** nasogastric feed, sucralfate and aluminium hydroxide gel also developed an oesophageal bezoar, which was analysed and found to contain components of both the drugs and the enteral feed.[7]

Data from the French Pharmacovigilance system database found 16 adults and 5 newborn babies who developed bezoars while taking sucralfate, and identified nasogastric feeding as a risk factor.[8]

Mechanism

It seems that a bezoar (a relatively insoluble complex) forms between the protein in the enteral feeds, and the aluminium from the antacids or sucralfate (sucralfate is about 18% aluminium). It thickens when the pH falls.[3]

Importance and management

An established and clinically important interaction that can result in the blockage of enteral or nasogastric tubes. The authors of one report say that high molecular protein solutions should not be mixed with antacids or followed by antacids, and if an antacid is needed, it should be given some time after the nutrients and the tube should be vigorously flushed beforehand.[1] The authors of another report say that they feed for 18 hours daily and then give the sucralfate overnight without problems.[2] The manufacturers recommend separating the administration of sucralfate suspension and enteral feeds given by nasogastric tube by one hour.[9]

1. Valli C, Schulthess H-K, Asper R, Escher F, Häcki WH. Interaction of nutrients with antacids: a complication during enteral tube feeding. *Lancet* (1986) i, 747–8.
2. Tomlin ME, Dixon S. Aluminium and nasogastric feeds. *Pharm J* (1996) 256, 40.
3. Rowbottom SJ, Wilson J, Samuel L, Grant IS. Total oesophageal obstruction in association with combined enteral feed and sucralfate therapy. *Anaesth Intensive Care* (1993) 21, 372–4.
4. Vohra SB, Strang TI. Sucralfate therapy - a caution. *Br J Intensive Care* (1994) 4, 114.
5. Anderson W. Esophageal medication bezoar in a patient receiving enteral feedings and sucralfate. *Am J Gastroenterol* (1989) 84, 205–6.
6. Algozzine GJ, Hill G, Scoggins WG, Marr MA. Sucralfate bezoar. *N Engl J Med* (1983) 309, 1387.
7. Krupp KB, Johns P, Troncoso V. Esophageal bezoar formation in a tude-fed patient receiving sucralfate and antacid therapy: a case report. *Gastroenterol Nurs* (1995) 18, 46–8.
8. Guy C, Ollagnier M. Sucralfate et bézoard: bilan de l'enquête officielle de pharmacovigilance et revue de la littérature. *Therapie* (1999) 54, 55–8.
9. Antepsin Suspension (Sucralfate). Chugai Pharma Ltd. UK Summary of product characteristics, November 2006.

Table 27.2 Summary of the interactions of cisapride

Interacting drugs	*Reported effects*	*Action*	*Refs*
Alcohol	Cisapride increases gastric emptying and can modestly increase serum alcohol levels. A modest 22% increase in the AUC of cisapride seen in one study.	Unlikely to be significant, however the sedative effects might be accelerated. Unknown significance; monitor patient for sedation.	1-5
Antacids **Aluminium oxide and magnesium hydroxide**	No effect on cisapride absorption seen.	None.	6
Antiepileptics **e.g. Phenytoin**	Increase in gastrointestinal motility caused by cisapride may affect the rate and/or extent of absorption, which may be important for some drugs with a narrow therapeutic index, such as some antiepileptics. However, no available case reports to suggest this is a problem, and one case reporting no interaction.	Uncertain. Monitor antiepileptic drug levels as usual practice. Advise the patient to report any increase in adverse effects.	1, 7
Antimuscarinics **e.g. Disopyramide**	Cisapride increases gastric emptying but anticholinergics slow gastric emptying. **Disopyramide** absorption and serum levels were increased in one study.	The clinical outcome is uncertain but caution is warranted if increased levels of the other drug likely to be significant e.g. **Disopyramide** is contraindicated as it can prolong the QT interval.	8
Bromperidol	Increased psychotic symptoms and bromperidol levels occurred in one case report.	Significance uncertain, but probably small.	9
Ciclosporin	An increase in AUC and serum levels of ciclosporin has been reported.	Monitor ciclosporin levels more frequently.	10
CYP3A4 inhibitors: ***Macrolides* e.g.** **Clarithromycin,** **Erythromycin** ***Azole antifungals* e.g.** **Ketoconazole** ***Protease inhibitors*** **Nefazodone** **Diltiazem** **Cimetidine** **See also Table 1.4, p. 6**	Increased levels of cisapride result in an increase in the risk of QT prolongation and life-threatening ventricular arrhythmias e.g. *torsade de pointes*.	Avoid.	1, 11-20
Diazepam	Accelerated absorption of diazepam reported. Transient increase in sedation possible.	Monitor the patient and advise that sedation may occur more quickly.	1, 21
Digoxin	Small reduction in the AUC and serum levels of digoxin seen in one study.	Unlikely to be clinically significant.	22
Diltiazem	A case of syncope and prolonged QT interval reported – see also CYP3A4 inhibitors above.	See CYP3A4 inhibitors above.	23
Drugs that prolong the QT interval	Increased risk of QT prolongation and life-threatening ventricular arrythmias.	Avoid. Should not be used with other drugs that prolong the QT interval.	1, 15
Esomeprazole	An increase in AUC and elimination half-life of cisapride reported, but no increase in serum levels. No QT-prolonging effects seen.	Unlikely to be clinically significant.	1, 24
Fluoxetine	No effect on the QT interval seen.	None.	25
Grapefruit juice	Significant increases in cisapride levels seen but high inter-subject variability occurred. No QT interval changes were seen.	May be of more significance in patients taking higher doses of cisapride or also taking other interacting drugs. Avoid concurrent use if possible.	26-28
H_2-receptor antagonists: **Cimetidine, ranitidine**	Increase in cisapride levels and reduction in cimetidine and ranitidine bioavailability seen.	Unlikely to be clinically significant. For cimetidine, see also CYP3A4 inhibitors, above.	1, 29-32
Morphine	An increase in peak morphine serum levels was seen but with no increase in the adverse effects of morphine.	Uncertain but be aware in case of increased morphine adverse effects.	33
Nifedipine	An increase in nifedipine levels with increased nifedipine effects seen, probably due to increased absorption.	Monitor patient and adjust the nifedipine dose accordingly.	34
Pantoprazole	Small reduction in cisapride levels and no QT interval effects seen.	None.	35
Paracetamol	No significant effect on the pharmacokinetics of paracetamol was found in one study but another small study found that the metabolism of paracetamol was reduced.	Unlikely to be clinically significant.	36, 37
Propranolol	No change in levels or effect of propranolol.	None.	38

Continued

Table 27.2 Summary of the interactions of cisapride (continued)

Interacting drugs	*Reported effects*	*Action*	*Refs*
Red wine	Minor changes in cisapride levels seen in one single-dose study.	Significance is unclear.	28
Simvastatin	Slightly increased cisapride levels and reduced simvastatin levels.	Unlikely to be generally significant although it may be prudent to check that simvastatin remains effective.	39
Warfarin and related anticoagulants	**Warfarin**: A small but insignificant increase in INR was seen in healthy subjects, but one case report describes large rise in INR. **Acenocoumarol**: Increased anticoagulant effect reported, which resolved when cisapride stopped. **Phenoprocoumon**: No significant change in anticoagulant effects.	It seems prudent to monitor patients taking anticoagulants who are given cisapride until their INR is stable.	1, 40-43

1. Prepulsid (Cisapride). Janssen Pharmaceuticals. ABPI Compendium of Datasheets and Summaries of Product Characteristics 1999–2000, p 655–6.
2. Janssen Pharmaceuticals. An evaluation of possible interactions between ethanol and cisapride. Data on file (Unpublished report, N 49087), 1986.
3. Roine R, Heikkonen E, Salaspuro M. Cisapride enhances alcohol absorption and leads to high blood alcohol levels. *Gastroenterology* (1992) 102, A507.
4. Dziekan G, Contesse J, Werth B, Schwarzer G, Reinhardt WH. Cisapride increases peak plasma and saliva ethanol levels under fasting conditions. *J Intern Med* (1997) 242, 479–82.
5. Kechagias S, Jönsson K-Å, Jones AW. Impact of gastric emptying on the pharmacokinetics of ethanol as influenced by cisapride. *Br J Clin Pharmacol* (1999) 48, 728–32.
6. Janssen Pharmaceuticals. Unaltered oral absorption of cisapride on coadministration of antacids. Data on file (Study R 51 619/69), 1986.
7. Roberts GW, Kowalski SR, Calabretto JP. Lack of effect of cisapride on phenytoin free fraction. *Ann Pharmacother* (1992) 26, 1016–17.
8. Kuroda T, Yoshihara Y, Nakamura H, Azumi T, Inatome T, Fukuzaki H, Takanashi H, Yogo K, Akima M. Effects of cisapride on gastrointestinal motor activity and gastric emptying of disopyramide. *J Pharmacobiodyn* (1992) 15, 395–402.
9. Ishida M, Iotani K, Yasui N, Inoue Y, Kaneko S. Possible interaction between cisapride and bromperidol. *Prog Neuropsychopharmacol Biol Psychiatry* (1997) 21, 235–8.
10. Finet L, Westeel PF, Hary G, Maurel M, Andrejak M, Dupas JL. Effects of cisapride on the intestinal absorption of cyclosporine in renal transplant recipients. *Gastroenterology* (1991) 100, A209.
11. Ahmad SR, Wolfe SM. Cisapride and torsades de pointes. *Lancet* (1995) 345, 508.
12. van Haarst AD, van't Klooster GEA, van Gerven JMA, Schoemaker RC, van Oene JC, Burggraaf J, Coene M-C, Cohen AF. The influence of cisapride and clarithromycin on QT intervals in healthy volunteers. *Clin Pharmacol Ther* (1998) 64, 542–6.
13. Sekkarie MA. Torsades de pointes in two chronic renal failure patients treated with cisapride and clarithromycin. *Am J Kidney Dis* (1997) 30, 437–9.
14. Gray VS. Syncopal episodes associated with cisapride and concurrent drugs. *Ann Pharmacother* (1998) 32, 648–51.
15. Janssen-Cilag Ltd. Dear Doctor letter, November 1995.
16. Janssen-Cilag UK Ltd. Confidential Report from Medical Information Department and Drug Safety Unit, December 18th 1995.
17. Jenkins IR, Gibson J. Cisapride, erythromycin and arrhythmia. *Anaesth Intensive Care* (1996) 24, 728.
18. Wysowski DK, Bacsanyi J. Cisapride and fatal arrhythmia. *N Engl J Med* (1996) 335, 290–1.
19. Janssen-Cilag Ltd. Personal communication, April 1995.
20. Committee on Safety of Medicines/Medicines Control Agency. Cisapride (Prepulsid): Risk of arrhythmias. Current Problems (1998) 24, 11.
21. Bateman DN. The action of cisapride on gastric emptying and the pharmacodynamics and pharmacokinetics of oral diazepam. *Eur J Clin Pharmacol* (1986) 30, 205–8.
22. Kirch W, Janisch HD, Santos SR, Duhrsen U, Dylewicz P, Ohnhaus EE. Effect of cisapride and metoclopramide on digoxin bioavailability. *Eur J Drug Metab Pharmacokinet* (1986) 11, 249–50.
23. Thomas AR, Chan L-N, Bauman JL, Olopade CO. Prolongation of the QT interval related to cisapride-diltiazem interaction. *Pharmacotherapy* (1998) 18, 381–5.
24. Nexium (Esomeprazole). AstraZeneca UK Ltd. UK Summary of product characteristics, October 2004.
25. Zhao Q, Wojcik MA, Parier J-L, Pesco-Koplowitz L. Influence of coadministration of fluoxetine on cisapride pharmacokinetics and QTc intervals in healthy volunteers. *Pharmacotherapy* (2001) 21, 149–57.
26. Gross AS, Goh YD, Addison RS, Shenfield GM. Influence of grapefruit juice on cisapride pharmacokinetics. *Clin Pharmacol Ther* (1999) 65, 395–401.
27. Kivistö KT, Lilja JJ, Backman JT, Neuvonen PJ. Repeated consumption of grapefruit juice considerably increases plasma concentrations of cisapride. *Clin Pharmacol Ther* (1999) 66, 448–53.
28. Offman EM, Freeman DJ, Dresser GK, Munoz C, Bend JR, Bailey DG. Red wine–cisapride interaction: comparison with grapefruit juice. *Clin Pharmacol Ther* (2001) 70, 17–23.
29. Kirch W, Janisch HD, Ohnhaus EE, van Peer A. Cisapride-cimetidine interaction: enhanced cisapride bioavailability and accelerated cimetidine absorption. *Ther Drug Monit* (1989) 11, 411–14.
30. Milligan KA, McHugh P, Rowbotham DJ. Effects of concomitant administration of cisapride and ranitidine on plasma concentrations in volunteers. *Br J Anaesth* (1989) 63, 628P.
31. Janssen Pharmaceuticals. Cisapride-ranitidine interaction. Data on file (Study R 51 619/74), 1986.
32. Valdes L, Champel V, Olivier C, Jonville-Bera AP, Autret E. Malaise avec allongement de l'espace QT chez un nourrisson de 39 jours traité par cisapride. *Arch Pediatr* (1997) 4, 535–7.
33. Rowbotham DJ, Milligan K, McHugh P. Effect of cisapride on morphine absorption after oral administration of sustained-release morphine. *Br J Anaesth* (1991) 67, 421–5.
34. Satoh C, Sakai T, Kashiwagi H, Hongo K, Aizawa O, Watanabe H, Mochizuki S, Okamura T. Influence of cisapride on the pharmacokinetics and antihypertensive effect of sustained-release nifedipine. *Int Med* (1996) 35, 941–5.
35. Ferron GM, Paul JC, Fruncillo RJ, Martin PT, Yacoub L, Mayer PR. Lack of pharmacokinetic interaction between oral pantoprazole and cisapride in healthy adults. *J Clin Pharmacol* (1999) 39, 945–50.
36. Rowbotham DJ, Parnacott S, Nimmo WS. No effect of cisapride on paracetamol absorption after oral simultaneous administration. *Eur J Clin Pharmacol* (1992) 42, 235–6.
37. Itoh H, Nagano T, Takeyama M. Cisapride raises the bioavailability of paracetamol by inhibiting its glucuronidation in man. *J Pharm Pharmacol* (2001) 53, 1041-45.
38. Janssen Pharmaceuticals. Effect of cisapride on the plasma concentrations of a delayed formulation of propranolol and on its clinical effects on blood pressure in mildly hypertensive patients. Data on file (Study R 51619/23-NL), 1986.
39. Simard C, O'Hara GE, Prévost J, Guilbaud R, Massé R, Turgeon J. Study of the drug-drug interaction between simvastatin and cisapride in man. *Eur J Clin Pharmacol* (2001) 57, 229–34.
40. Janssen Pharmaceutica (Jonker JJC). Effect of cisapride on anticoagulant treatment with acenocoumarol. Data on file (Clinical Research Report, R 51619-NL), August 1985.

Continued

Table 27.2 Summary of the interactions of cisapride (continued)

41. Wesemeyer D, Mönig H, Gaska T, Masuch S, Seiler KU, Huss H, Bruhn HD. Der Einfluß von Cisaprid und Metoclopramid auf die Bioverfügbarkeit von Phenprocoumon. *Hamostaseologie* (1991) 11, 95–102.
42. Daneshmend TK, Mahida YR, Bhaskar NK, Hawkey CJ. Does cisapride alter the anticoagulant effect of warfarin? A pharmacodynamic assessment. British Society of Gastroenterology Spring Meeting, 12–14 April 1989.
43. Darlington MR. Hypoprothrombinemia induced by warfarin sodium and cisapride. *Am J Health-Syst Pharm* (1997) 54, 320–1.

H_2-receptor antagonists + Antacids

The absorption of cimetidine, famotidine, nizatidine, and ranitidine may possibly be reduced to some extent by antacids, but it seems doubtful if this significantly reduces their effects. Separating the dosages by 1 to 2 hours minimises any interaction. Roxatidine absorption appears not to be affected by antacids. Cimetidine appears not to interfere with the effectiveness of *Gaviscon* (sodium alginate compound).

Clinical evidence

(a) Cimetidine

When 12 healthy subjects were given oral cimetidine 300 mg four times daily for 5 doses, with and without 30 mL of *Mylanta II* (**aluminium/magnesium hydroxide** mixture), the absorption of cimetidine was unaffected.[1] No interaction was found in other single-dose studies using **aluminium phosphate**[2,3] or **aluminium/magnesium hydroxide**[4,5] antacids.

In contrast, a number of other single-dose studies indicated that antacids reduce the absorption of cimetidine. The AUCs of 200- to 800-mg doses of cimetidine were reduced by an average of 19 to 34% by 10 to 45 mL doses of a variety of **aluminium/magnesium**-containing antacids.[6-10] When the antacids were given 1 to 3 hours after cimetidine 'marginal' or insignificant reductions occurred in the AUCs.[7,11,12]

Gaviscon (**sodium alginate/antacid**) is an anti-reflux preparation that needs a small amount of gastric acid to be present in order for the alginic acid 'raft' to form. A study in 12 healthy subjects designed to find out if an H_2-receptor antagonist would alter the effectiveness of *Liquid Gaviscon* found that cimetidine 400 mg four times daily for 7 days caused some slight changes in gastric emptying, but the distribution of the *Gaviscon* in the fundus of the stomach was not altered.[13]

(b) Famotidine

Mylanta II (**aluminium/magnesium hydroxide** mixture) 30 mL reduced the AUC and peak serum levels of famotidine by about a third when taken simultaneously, but no significant interaction occurred when the antacid was taken 2 hours after famotidine.[14] Another study found that the peak serum levels of famotidine were reduced by about 25% by *Mylanta II* in 17 healthy subjects.[15]

In contrast, *Mylanta Double Strength* (**aluminium/magnesium hydroxide** with **simeticone**) was found to reduce the absorption of famotidine by 19%, a difference that was considered unimportant.[10] Two chewable tablets of *Mylanta II* were found to have no effect on the pharmacokinetics or pharmacodynamics of famotidine 10 or 20 mg in 18 healthy subjects.[16]

(c) Nizatidine

Mylanta Double Strength (**aluminium/magnesium hydroxide** with **simeticone**) reduced the absorption of nizatidine by 12%, which was considered clinically insignificant.[10] In a study in 11 healthy subjects a single 30-mL dose of *Gelusil* (**aluminium/magnesium hydroxide** with **simeticone**) reduced the mean AUC and maximum serum levels of nizatidine (given simultaneously) by 13 and 17%, respectively.[17] Another study found that the pharmacokinetics of nizatidine were not affected by an **aluminium/magnesium hydroxide** antacid (*Maalox)* although a non-significant reduction in the AUC of 8% and an increase in the time to peak effect of nizatidine were seen.[18]

(d) Ranitidine

Mylanta II (**aluminium/magnesium hydroxide** mixture) 30 mL reduced the ranitidine peak serum levels and AUC after a single 150-mg dose by about one-third in 6 healthy subjects.[19] *Mylanta Double Strength* (**aluminium/magnesium hydroxide** with **simeticone**) reduced the absorption of ranitidine by 26%, which was not thought to be clinically significant.[10] Reductions of up to 59% were found in another study.[9] Yet another study showed that **aluminium phosphate** reduced the bioavailability of ranitidine by 30%.[20] In contrast, another study found no significant changes in the pharmacokinetics of ranitidine given with an **aluminium/magnesium hydroxide** antacid (*Maalox).*[18]

(e) Roxatidine

In an open-label crossover study, 24 healthy subjects were given roxatidine 150 mg with 10 mL of *Maalox* (**aluminium/magnesium hydroxide**) four times daily. The pharmacokinetics of roxatidine were unchanged, apart from a clinically insignificant lengthening of the half-life.[21]

Mechanism

Not fully understood. Changes in gastric pH caused by the antacid, and retarded gastric motility have been suggested as potential mechanisms. An *in vitro* study showed no absorption interaction occurred between cimetidine and antacids.[5]

Importance and management

A modest reduction in the bioavailability of cimetidine, famotidine, nizatidine and ranitidine can occur with some antacids although this appears to be more likely when larger doses of antacids are used. None of these interactions are well established and evidence that the effects of the H_2-receptor antagonists are reduced seems to be lacking. If the antacids are given 1 to 2 hours before or after the H_2-receptor antagonist (if fasting), or 1 hour after (if the H_2-receptor antagonist is taken with food), no reduction in absorption should occur.[7,14,15,22] Preliminary evidence suggests that roxatidine is unaffected. Given the evidence available it seems unlikely that a clinically significant interaction will occur between any H_2-receptor antagonist and standard doses of an antacid. The action of *Gaviscon* (sodium alginate) does not appear to be compromised by cimetidine.[13]

1. Shelly DW, Doering PL, Russell WL, Guild RT, Lopez LM, Perrin J. Effect of concomitant antacid administration on plasma cimetidine concentrations during repetitive dosing. *Drug Intell Clin Pharm* (1986) 20, 792–5.
2. Albin H, Vinçon G, Pehoucq F, Dangoumau J. Influence d'un antacide sur la biodisponibilité de la cimétidine. *Therapie* (1982) 37, 563–6.
3. Albin H, Vinçon G, Demotes-Mainard F, Begaud B, Bedjaoui A. Effect of aluminium phosphate on the bioavailability of cimetidine and prednisolone. *Eur J Clin Pharmacol* (1984) 26, 271–3.
4. Burland WL, Darkin DW, Mills MW. Effect of antacids on absorption of cimetidine. *Lancet* (1976) ii, 965.
5. Allgayer H, Röllinghoff W, Paumgartner G. Absence of in vivo and in vitro interactions of an aluminium hydroxide, magnesium hydroxide containing antacid with cimetidine in patients with peptic ulcer. *Z Gastroenterol* (1983) 21, 351–4.
6. Bodemar G, Norlander B, Walan A. Diminished absorption of cimetidine caused by antacids. *Lancet* (1979) i, 444–5.
7. Steinberg WM, Lewis JH, Katz DM. Antacids inhibit absorption of cimetidine. *N Engl J Med* (1982) 307, 400–4.
8. Gugler R, Brand M, Somogyi A. Impaired cimetidine absorption due to antacids and metoclopramide. *Eur J Clin Pharmacol* (1981) 20, 225–8.
9. Desmond PV, Harman PJ, Gannoulis N, Kamm M, Mashford ML. The effect of an antacid and food on the absorption of cimetidine and ranitidine. *J Pharm Pharmacol* (1990) 42, 352–4.
10. Sullivan TJ, Reese JH, Jauregui L, Miller K, Levine L, Bachmann KA. Short report: a comparative study of the interaction between antacid and H_2-receptor antagonists. *Aliment Pharmacol Ther* (1994) 8, 123–6.
11. Russell WL, Lopez LM, Normann SA, Doering PL, Guild RT. Effect of antacids on predicted steady-state cimetidine concentrations. *Dig Dis Sci* (1984) 29, 385–9.
12. Barzaghi N, Crema F, Mescoli G, Perucca E. Effects on cimetidine bioavailability of metoclopramide and antacids given two hours apart. *Eur J Clin Pharmacol* (1989) 37, 409–10.
13. Washington N, Wilson CG, Williams DL, Robertson C. An investigation into the effect of cimetidine pre-treatment on raft formation of an anti-reflux agent. *Aliment Pharmacol Ther* (1993) 7, 553–9.
14. Barzaghi N, Gatti G, Crema F, Perucca E. Impaired bioavailability of famotidine given concurrently with a potent antacid. *J Clin Pharmacol* (1989) 29, 670–2.
15. Tupy-Visich MA, Tarzian SK, Schwartz S, Lin JH, Hessey GA, Kanovsky SM, Chremos AN. Bioavailability of oral famotidine when administered with antacid or food. *J Clin Pharmacol* (1986) 26, 555.
16. Schwartz JI, Yeh KC, Bolognese J, Laskin OL, Patterson PM, Shamblen EC, Han R, Lasseter KC. Lack of effect of chewable antacid on famotidine pharmacodynamics and pharmacokinetics. *Pharmacotherapy* (1994) 14, 375.
17. Knadler MP, Bergstrom RF, Callaghan JT, Obermeyer BD, Rubin A. Absorption studies of the H_2-blocker nizatidine. *Clin Pharmacol Ther* (1987) 42, 514–20.
18. Desager JP, Harvengt C. Oral bioavailability of nizatidine and ranitidine concurrently administered with antacid. *J Int Med Res* (1989) 17, 62–7.

19. Mihaly GW, Marino AT, Webster LK, Jones DB, Louis WJ, Smallwood RA. High dose of antacid (Mylanta II) reduces the bioavailability of ranitidine. *BMJ* (1982) 285, 998–9.
20. Albin H, Vinçon G, Begaud B, Bistue C, Perez P. Effect of aluminum phosphate on the bioavailability of ranitidine. *Eur J Clin Pharmacol* (1987) 32, 97–99.
21. Labs RA. Interaction of roxatidine acetate with antacids, food and other drugs. *Drugs* (1988) 35 (Suppl 3), 82–9.
22. Frislid K, Berstad A. High dose of antacid reduces bioavailability of ranitidine. *BMJ* (1983) 286, 1358.

H_2-receptor antagonists + Probenecid

Probenecid markedly decreases the renal clearance of famotidine and modestly reduces the renal clearance of cimetidine. However, these effects are not expected to result in adverse clinical effects.

Clinical evidence, mechanism, importance and management

In a randomised, crossover study 6 healthy subjects were given probenecid 500 mg every 6 hours for 13 doses, with a single 300-mg intravenous dose of **cimetidine** 3 hours after the last probenecid dose. Probenecid reduced the renal clearance of **cimetidine** by 22%, without affecting overall clearance.[1] Probenecid 1.5 g increased the AUC of a single 20-mg dose of **famotidine** in 8 healthy subjects by 81%, and reduced the renal tubular clearance by 89%.[2] It has been suggested that probenecid inhibits the renal secretion of cimetidine and famotidine, thereby reducing their loss from the body. This is consistent with the way that probenecid affects some other drugs. The effects of famotidine would be expected to be increased, but dose-related toxicity arising from this interaction seems unlikely. The effects of cimetidine are unlikely to be significantly altered. There would therefore seem to be no reason for avoiding concurrent use. Other H_2-receptor antagonists are also renally excreted and therefore they may behave similarly.

1. Gisclon LG, Boyd RA, Williams RL, Giacomini KM. The effect of probenecid on the renal elimination of cimetidine. *Clin Pharmacol Ther* (1989) 45, 444–52.
2. Inotsume N, Nishimura M, Nakano M, Fujiyama S, Sato T. The inhibitory effect of probenecid on renal excretion of famotidine in young, healthy volunteers. *J Clin Pharmacol* (1990) 30, 50–56.

H_2-receptor antagonists + Sucralfate

Most *in vitro* and human studies have found that sucralfate does not affect the absorption of either cimetidine,[1-3] ranitidine,[4] or roxatidine,[5] but two studies found 22 to 29% reductions in ranitidine bioavailability due to concurrent use of sucralfate.[6,7] There is no clear reason for avoiding concurrent use.

1. Albin H, Vincon G, Lalague MC, Couzigou P, Amouretti M. Effect of sucralfate on the bioavailability of cimetidine. *Eur J Clin Pharmacol* (1986) 30, 493–4.
2. D'Angio R, Mayersohn M, Conrad KA, Bliss M. Cimetidine absorption in humans during sucralfate coadministration. *Br J Clin Pharmacol* (1986) 21, 515–20.
3. Beck CL, Dietz AJ, Carlson JD, Letendre PW. Evaluation of potential cimetidine sucralfate interaction. *Clin Pharmacol Ther* (1987) 41, 168.
4. Mullersman G, Gotz VP, Russell WL, Derendorf H. Lack of clinically significant in vitro and in vivo interactions between ranitidine and sucralfate. *J Pharm Sci* (1986) 75, 995–8.
5. Seibert-Grafe M, Pidgen A. Lack of effect of multiple dose sucralfate on the pharmacokinetics of roxatidine acetate. *Eur J Clin Pharmacol* (1991) 40, 637–8.
6. Maconochie JG, Thomas M, Michael MF, Jenner WR, Tanner RJN. Ranitidine sucralfate interaction study. *Clin Pharmacol Ther* (1987) 41, 205.
7. Kimura K, Sakai H, Yoshida Y, Kasano T, Hirose M. Effects of concomitant drugs on the blood concentration of a histamine H_2 antagonist (the 2nd report) - concomitant or time lag administration of ranitidine and sucralfate. *Nippon Shokakibyo Gakkai Zasshi* (1986) 83, 603–7.

H_2-receptor antagonists + Tobacco or Nicotine

Smoking may reduce the plasma levels of cimetidine and ranitidine, but does not appear to affect famotidine. Cimetidine, and to a lesser extent ranitidine, reduce the clearance of nicotine from the body in non-smokers, but there is some evidence to suggest that cimetidine has no effect on nicotine clearance in smokers.

Clinical evidence

(a) Nicotine

Cimetidine 600 mg twice daily for one day, given before intravenous nicotine (1 microgram/kg per minute given intravenously for 30 minutes), reduced the nicotine clearance in 6 healthy non-smokers by 27 to 30%. **Ranitidine** (300 mg twice daily taken for one day) reduced the clearance of nicotine by about 7 to 10%.[1] See also tobacco smoking, below.

(b) Tobacco

In one study, tobacco smokers were given single oral doses of either **ranitidine** 150 mg or **cimetidine** 200 mg on two separate days. On one of the days they were allowed to smoke as normal and on the other they were not allowed to smoke. Peak levels for both drugs occurred sooner and were higher on the smoking day than on the non-smoking day. However, the plasma levels of the H_2-receptor antagonists after peak levels were achieved were lower. No effect was seen when intravenous **cimetidine** or **ranitidine** were given.[2]

A study in heavy smokers (more than 20 cigarettes per day for at least 1 year) given cimetidine 400 mg three times daily for 2 weeks found no reduction in the clearance of **nicotine** or in the number of cigarettes smoked, when compared with placebo.[3]

There was no difference in the pharmacokinetics and gastric acid-lowering effect of **famotidine** between 12 healthy smokers and 8 non-smokers.[4]

Mechanism, importance and management

The authors of one of the above studies[3] noted that tobacco smoking induces nicotine metabolism and that this may have been a factor in the lack of effect of cimetidine on nicotine clearance compared with their previous study in non-smokers.[1] On balance cimetidine and other H_2-receptor antagonists probably have little effect on nicotine replacement therapy or tobacco smoking.

The healing of duodenal ulcers in patients taking H_2-receptor antagonists such as **cimetidine**,[5,6] **famotidine**,[7] **nizatidine**[8] and **ranitidine**[6,7] is slower and ulcer recurrence is more common in smokers than in non-smokers. It is quite possible that this is due to smoking being a risk factor for the occurrence of duodenal ulcers[5,7-9] rather than a significant interaction between smoking and H_2-receptor antagonists.

1. Bendayan R, Sullivan JT, Shaw C, Frecker RC, Sellers EM. Effect of cimetidine and ranitidine on the hepatic and renal elimination of nicotine in humans. *Eur J Clin Pharmacol* (1990) 38, 165–9.
2. Boyd EJS, Johnston DA, Wormsley KG, Jenner WN, Salanson X. The effects of cigarette smoking on plasma concentrations of gastric antisecretory drugs. *Aliment Pharmacol Ther* (1987) 1, 57–65.
3. Bendayan R, Kennedy G, Frecker RC, Sellers EM. Lack of effect of cimetidine on cigarette smoking. *Eur J Clin Pharmacol* (1993) 44, 51–55.
4. Baak LC, Ganesh S, Jansen JBMJ, Lamers CBHW. Does smoking influence the pharmacokinetics and pharmacodynamics of the H_2-receptor antagonist famotidine. *Br J Clin Pharmacol* (1992) 33, 193–6.
5. Hetzel DJ, Korman MG, Hansky J, Shearman DJ, Eaves ER, Schmidt GT, Hecker R, Fitch RJ. The influence of smoking on the healing of duodenal ulcer treated with oxmetidine or cimetidine. *Aust N Z J Med* (1983) 13, 587–90.
6. Korman MG, Hansky J, Merrett AC, Schmidt GT. Ranitidine in duodenal ulcer: incidence of healing and effect of smoking. *Dig Dis Sci* (1982) 27, 712–15.
7. Reynolds JC, Schoen RE, Maislin G, Zangari GG. Risk factors for delayed healing of duodenal ulcers treated with famotidine and ranitidine. *Am J Gastroenterol* (1994) 89, 571–80.
8. Battaglia G. Risk factors of relapse in gastric ulcer: a one-year, double-blind comparative study of nizatidine versus placebo. *Ital J Gastroenterol* (1994) 26 (1 Suppl 1), 19–22.
9. Boyd EJS, Wilson JA, Wormsley KG. Smoking impairs therapeutic gastric inhibition. *Lancet* (1983) i, 95–7.

Loperamide + Colestyramine

An isolated report, supported by an *in vitro* study, indicates that the effects of loperamide can be reduced by colestyramine.

Clinical evidence, mechanism, importance and management

A man who had undergone extensive surgery to the gut, with the creation of an ileostomy, needed treatment for excessive fluid loss. His fluid loss was observed to be "substantially less" when he took loperamide 2 mg every 6 hours alone, than when he took loperamide in combination with colestyramine 2 g every 4 hours.[1] The probable reason is that the colestyramine binds to the loperamide in the gut, thereby reducing its activity. An *in vitro* study using 50 mL of simulated gastric fluid found that 64% of a 5.5-mg dose of loperamide was bound by 4 g of colestyramine.[1] Direct information is limited to this report, but what occurred is consistent with the way colestyramine interacts with other drugs. It has been suggested that the two drugs should be separated as much as possible to prevent mixing in the gut, or that the loperamide dosage should be increased.[1] It is a standard recommendation that other drugs should be given 1 hour before or 4 to 6 hours after colestyramine.

1. Ti TY, Giles HG, Sellers EM. Probable interaction of loperamide and cholestyramine. *Can Med Assoc J* (1978) 119, 607–8.

Loperamide + Co-trimoxazole

Co-trimoxazole increases the plasma levels of loperamide.

Clinical evidence, mechanism, importance and management

Co-trimoxazole 960 mg twice daily was given to healthy subjects for 24 hours before and then 48 hours after they took a single 4-mg dose of loperamide (12 subjects) or loperamide oxide (a prodrug of loperamide, 10 subjects). The co-trimoxazole increased the loperamide AUC by 89% and doubled its maximum plasma levels. The loperamide oxide AUC was raised by 54% and its maximum plasma levels were raised by 41%. It is thought that co-trimoxazole inhibits the metabolism of loperamide, possibly by reducing its first pass metabolism.[1] However, despite these rises, because loperamide has a very wide margin of safety, it is thought unlikely that any dosage changes are needed.

1. Kamali F, Huang ML. Increased systemic availability of loperamide after oral administration of loperamide and loperamide oxide with cotrimoxazole. *Br J Clin Pharmacol* (1996) 41, 125–8.

Loperamide + Protease inhibitors

Ritonavir increases the plasma levels of loperamide. Tipranavir, alone and combined with ritonavir, reduces the bioavailability and plasma levels of loperamide and its metabolites. No central opioid adverse effects are seen when loperamide is given with ritonavir alone, tipranavir alone, or tipranavir/ritonavir.

Clinical evidence

In a double-blind, placebo-controlled study, 12 healthy subjects were given a single 600-mg dose of **ritonavir** with either loperamide 16 mg or placebo. The loperamide AUC and maximum plasma level were increased threefold and 17%, respectively, by ritonavir, but no additional CNS adverse effects were seen.[1] Another study in 20 healthy subjects looked at the pharmacokinetics and pharmacodynamics of a single 16-mg dose of loperamide taken with either **tipranavir** 750 mg twice daily, **ritonavir** 200 mg twice daily or both drugs together. (Note that this dose of tipranavir is higher than the usual ritonavir-boosted dose of 500 mg twice daily.) **Tipranavir** alone *reduced* the maximum concentration and AUC of loperamide by 58% and 63%, respectively, whereas **ritonavir** *increased* these parameters by 83% and 121%, respectively. The combination of **tipranavir/ritonavir**, as is usual clinical practice, resulted in a net reduction in the maximum concentration and AUC of loperamide by 61% and 51%, respectively, similar to the effect seen with **tipranavir** alone. The maximum concentration and AUC of the metabolites of loperamide were also reduced. There were no clinically significant loperamide adverse effects on respiration or pupil contractility with either ritonavir alone, tipranavir alone, or the combination.[2]

Mechanism

Loperamide is primarily metabolised by cytochrome P450 isoenzyme CYP3A4, and is thought to lack CNS effects because it is a substrate for P-glycoprotein, which transports drugs out of the cells at the blood-brain barrier, thereby restricting CNS penetration.[2] The increase in loperamide levels with ritonavir alone is thought to be due to ritonavir inhibiting CYP3A4. The lack of an increase in loperamide CNS effects suggests that ritonavir alone does not inhibit P-glycoprotein.[1,2] The reduction in loperamide levels with tipranavir alone or tipranavir/ritonavir is not thought to be via effects on CYP3A4, but is due to induction of gastrointestinal P-glycoprotein by tipranavir, resulting in decreased systemic bioavailability of loperamide.[2]

Importance and management

Despite the increases seen in loperamide plasma levels seen in both studies with ritonavir alone, a lack of central opioid effects with loperamide (such as pupillary constriction, respiratory depression and also analgesic effects) was demonstrated. This suggests that the combination of loperamide with ritonavir is potentially safe to use as an antidiarrhoeal for protease inhibitor-induced diarrhoea.[1]

The clinical relevance of the decrease in loperamide bioavailability with tipranavir alone or tipranavir/ritonavir is unknown.

1. Tayrouz Y, Ganssmann B, Ding R, Klingmann A, Aderjan R, Burhenne J, Haefeli WE, Mikus G. Ritonavir increases loperamide plasma concentrations without evidence for P-glycoprotein involvement. *Clin Pharmacol Ther* (2001) 70, 405–14.
2. Mukwaya G, MacGregor T, Hoelscher D, Heming T, Legg D, Kavanaugh K, Johnson P, Sabo JP, McCallister S. Interaction of ritonavir-boosted tipranavir with loperamide does not result in loperamide-associated neurologic side effects in healthy volunteers. *Antimicrob Agents Chemother* (2005) 49, 4903–10.

Mesalazine (Mesalamine) + Ispaghula, Lactitol, or Lactulose

On theoretical grounds, formulations designed to release mesalazine in response to the higher pH in the colon should not be given with lactulose, lactitol or other preparations that lower the colonic pH. However, neither ispaghula or lactulose appear to affect the bioavailability of mesalazine.

Clinical evidence, mechanism, importance and management

Asacol is a preparation of mesalazine coated with an acrylic based resin (*Eudragit S*) that disintegrates above pH 7 and thereby releases the mesalazine into the terminal ileum and colon. Since the disintegration depends upon this alkaline pH, the UK manufacturers of ***Asacol*** say that the concurrent use of preparations that lower the pH in the lower part of the gut should be avoided.[1] ***Salofalk*** is another preparation of mesalazine with a pH-dependent enteric coating.

The pH in the colon can be lowered by lactulose and lactitol, which are metabolised by gut bacteria to a number of acids (e.g. acetic, butyric, propionic, and lactic acid).[2] In healthy subjects, lactulose 30 to 80 g daily has been found to cause slight falls in colonic pH;[2,3] from about 6 to 5 in the right colon and from 7 to 6.7 in the left colon. Lactitol 40 to 180 g daily can cause similar falls in pH.[2] Ispaghula can also lower colonic pH (from 6.5 to 5.8 in the right colon, and from 7.3 to 6.6 in the left colon).[4] However, a study in patients given mesalazine found that despite this colonic acidification by ispaghula husk (*Fybogel*), the release of mesalazine appeared not to be affected, as 24-hour faecal and urinary excretion of mesalazine metabolites were unchanged.[5] Similarly, another study in 14 healthy subjects given delayed-release mesalazine (*Asacol*) 400 mg three times daily found that lactulose (15 mL increased to 30 mL twice daily) did not affect urinary or faecal excretion of mesalazine and its metabolites.[6]

Thus, although on theoretical grounds ispaghula husk and lactulose might be expected to reduce the effects of mesalazine, no interaction of clinical importance seems to occur, and there have been no reports as yet that a clinically important interaction occurs with either ispaghula husk, lactulose or lactitol. Also note that this interaction is not mentioned by the US manufacturers of *Asacol*.[7]

1. Asacol Tablets (Mesalazine). Procter & Gamble Pharmaceuticals UK Ltd. UK Summary of product characteristics, April 2003.
2. Patil DH, Westaby D, Mahida YR, Palmer KR, Rees R, Clark ML, Dawson AM, Silk DBA. Comparative modes of action of lactitol and lactulose in the treatment of hepatic encephalopathy. *Gut* (1987) 28, 255–9.
3. Brown RL, Gibson JA, Sladen GE, Hicks B, Dawson AM. Effects of lactulose and other laxatives on ileal and colonic pH as measured by a radiotelemetry device. *Gut* (1974) 15, 999–1004.
4. Evans DF, Crompton J, Pye G, Hardcastle JD. The role of dietary fibre on acidification of the colon in man. *Gastroenterology* (1988) 94, A118.
5. Riley SA, Tavares IA, Bishai PM, Bennett A, Mani V. Mesalazine release from coated tablets: effect of dietary fibre. *Br J Clin Pharmacol* (1991) 32, 248–50.
6. Hussain FN, Ajjan RA, Moustafa M, Weir NW, Riley SA. Mesalazine release from a pH dependent formulation: effects of omeprazole and lactulose co-administration. *Br J Clin Pharmacol* (1998) 46, 173–5.
7. Asacol (Mesalamine). Procter & Gamble Pharmaceuticals. US Prescribing information, September 2006.

Mesalazine (Mesalamine) + Proton pump inhibitors

Omeprazole does not affect the release of mesalazine from a delayed-release preparation (*Asacol*).

Clinical evidence, mechanism, importance and management

Asacol is a preparation of mesalazine coated with an acrylic based resin (*Eudragit S*) that disintegrates above pH 7 and thereby releases the mesalazine into the terminal ileum and colon. The release is rapid at pH values of 7 and above, but it can also occur between pH 6 and 7. Since the proton pump inhibitors can raise the pH in the stomach to 6 and above, the potential exists for the premature release of mesalazine from *Asacol*. However, a study in 6 healthy subjects given *Asacol* 400 mg three times daily for 3 weeks found that when they were also given omeprazole 20 mg daily during the second week, and omeprazole 40 mg daily during the third week, the steady-state pharmacokinetics of the mesalazine remained unchanged.[1] Had mesalazine been released earlier, the absorption characteristics would have changed. There would therefore appear to be no reason for avoiding the concurrent use of *Asacol* and omeprazole in doses of up to 40 mg daily. On the basis of this study, it seems likely that other proton pump inhibitors will behave similarly at equivalent doses.

1. Hussain FN, Ajjan RA, Moustafa M, Weir NW, Riley SA. Mesalazine release from a pH dependent formulation: effects of omeprazole and lactulose co-administration. *Br J Clin Pharmacol* (1998) 46, 173–5.

Omeprazole + Artemisinin

Artemisinin modestly increases the metabolism of omeprazole, but the clinical significance of this is unclear.

Clinical evidence, mechanism, importance and management

A study in 9 healthy subjects found that the AUC of a single 20-mg dose of omeprazole was reduced by 35% by artemisinin 250 mg twice daily for 7 days. The pharmacokinetics of the omeprazole metabolites were unchanged, but the ratio of hydroxyomeprazole/omeprazole increased 2.2-fold in those of an extensive CYP2C19 metabolisers phenotype (see 'metabolism of proton pump inhibitors', (p.960)). This suggests that artemisinin affects the pharmacokinetics of omeprazole by inducing the cytochrome P450 isoenzyme CYP2C19, an enzyme involved in its metabolism, although other isoenzymes may also be involved. A single 250-mg dose of artemisinin had no effect on the pharmacokinetics of omeprazole, which supports the proposed mechanism of enzyme induction.[1] A subsequent study in 8 healthy subjects who were of the extensive CYP2C19 metaboliser phenotype similarly found that artemisinin 500 mg daily for 7 days decreased the AUC of both the *S* and *R*-enantiomers of a single 20-mg dose of omeprazole to the same extent, and increased the oral clearance of both enantiomers by about threefold.[2] The clinical significance of this interaction is unclear.

1. Svensson USH, Ashton M, Hai TN, Bertilsson L, Huong DX, Huong NV, Niêu NT, Sy ND, Lykkesfeldt J, Công LD. Artemisinin induces omeprazole metabolism in human beings. *Clin Pharmacol Ther* (1998) 64, 160–67.

2. Mihara K, Svensson USH, Tybring G, Hai TN, Bertilsson L, Ashton M. Stereospecific analysis of omeprazole supports artemisinin as a potent inducer of CYP2C19. *Fundam Clin Pharmacol* (1999) 13, 671–5.

Omeprazole + Disulfiram

An isolated case describes a catatonic reaction in a patient given omeprazole and disulfiram.

Clinical evidence, mechanism, importance and management

A patient who had been taking omeprazole 40 mg daily for 7 months was also given disulfiram 500 mg daily. Six days later he gradually developed confusion, which progressed to a catatonic state with muscle rigidity and trismus (spasm of the muscles used to chew food) after 15 days. Both drugs were withdrawn and he gradually recovered. Some months later while taking disulfiram 250 mg daily, he again developed confusion, disorientation and nightmares within 72 hours of starting to take omeprazole 40 mg each morning. Again he recovered when both drugs were stopped.[1] The reason for this reaction is not understood, but the authors of the report suggest that the omeprazole may have allowed the accumulation of one of the metabolites of disulfiram, carbon disulphide, which could have been responsible for the toxic effects.[1]

This is the first and only report of a possible interaction between omeprazole and disulfiram. Other patients given both drugs are said not to have shown adverse effects.[2] The general importance of this adverse interaction is therefore uncertain, but it seems likely to be small.

1. Hajela R, Cunningham G M, Kapur B M, Peachey J E, Devenyi P. Catatonic reaction to omeprazole and disulfiram in a patient with alcohol dependence. *Can Med Assoc J* (1990) 143, 1207–8.
2. Astra Pharmaceuticals. Personal communication, 1991.

Pirenzepine + Antacids

***Mylanta* reduces the bioavailability of pirenzepine by about 30%. Another antacid, *Trigastril*, modestly *increases* the bioavailability of pirenzepine, but these changes are probably of little clinical importance.**

Clinical evidence, mechanism, importance and management

The AUC of a single 50-mg dose of pirenzepine was reduced by about 30% in 20 healthy subjects by 30 mL of *Mylanta* (**aluminium/magnesium hydroxide** and **simeticone**). The **antacid** reduced the peak plasma levels of pirenzepine by about 45%.[1] Another study in 10 healthy subjects found that the AUC of a single 50-mg dose of pirenzepine was increased by almost 25% by 10 mL of an **antacid** (*Trigastril*, **aluminium/magnesium hydroxide, calcium carbonate**).[2] In practical terms these modest changes in bioavailability are probably too small to matter.

1. Matzek KM, MacGregor TR, Keirns JJ, Vinocur M. Effect of food and antacids on the oral absorption of pirenzepine in man. *Int J Pharmaceutics* (1986) 28, 151–5.
2. Vergin H, Herrlinger C, Gugler R. Effect of an aluminium-hydroxide containing antacid on the oral bioavailability of pirenzepine. *Arzneimittelforschung* (1989) 39, 520–3.

Pirenzepine + Cimetidine

The pharmacokinetics of pirenzepine and cimetidine are not affected by the presence of the other drug, but pirenzepine increases the cimetidine-induced reduction in gastric acid secretion, which is an apparently advantageous interaction.[1]

1. Jamali F, Mahachai V, Reilly PA, Thomson ABR. Lack of pharmacokinetic interaction between cimetidine and pirenzepine. *Clin Pharmacol Ther* (1985) 38, 325–30.

Pirenzepine + Food

Food reduces the bioavailability of pirenzepine by about 30%, but this is probably of little clinical importance.

Clinical evidence, mechanism, importance and management

The AUC of a single 50-mg dose of pirenzepine was reduced by about 30% in 20 healthy subjects when pirenzepine was taken half-an-hour before food, or with food. Peak plasma levels were reduced by about 30% and 45%, respectively. The time to achieve peak levels was also reduced.[1] In practical terms this modest change in bioavailability is probably too small to matter. The authors of this report suggest taking it with food because compliance is better if associated with a convenient daily ritual.[1]

1. Matzek KM, MacGregor TR, Keirns JJ, Vinocur M. Effect of food and antacids on the oral absorption of pirenzepine in man. *Int J Pharmaceutics* (1986) 28, 151–5.

Proton pump inhibitors + Antacids

***Maalox* does not appear to alter the pharmacokinetics of omeprazole, pantoprazole or rabeprazole. Antacids may cause a slight reduction in the bioavailability of lansoprazole. This is probably not clinically relevant but can be accommodated by separating their administration by one hour. There is no interaction between sodium alginate and omeprazole.**

Clinical evidence, mechanism, importance and management

(a) Lansoprazole

In a study in 12 healthy subjects a single 30-mL dose of *Maalox* (**aluminium/magnesium hydroxide**) slightly reduced the AUC of a 30-mg dose of lansoprazole by 13% (not statistically significant), and reduced the maximum plasma level by 27%. However, no changes were seen when the lansoprazole was given 1 hour after the antacid.[1] Note that in this study, the bioavailability of lansoprazole was highly variable between subjects (the AUC varied by a factor of 6), and the effect of 'food', (below), was greater than the effect of the antacid. In another study, **magaldrate** had no effect on the AUC of lansoprazole, and slightly reduced the maximum level (by 28%), but this change was not considered clinically relevant.[2] Nevertheless, the manufacturer recommends that antacids should not be taken within one hour of lansoprazole,[3] but this seems to be an overcautious recommendation.

(b) Omeprazole

Two single-dose studies have shown that *Maalox* suspension (**aluminium/magnesium hydroxide**) did not affect the absorption or disposition of omeprazole from an enteric-coated formulation.[4,5] Similar findings were reported for *Maalox* suspension in another single-dose study. In contrast, this study found that *Maalox granules* modestly reduced the AUC of omeprazole enteric-coated tablets by 26% and reduced its plasma levels.[6]

A randomised, crossover study in healthy subjects given omeprazole capsules 20 mg daily for 3 days, with two *Gaviscon* tablets (aluminium hydroxide, **magnesium trisilicate** and **sodium alginate**) on day 3, found that omeprazole did not significantly affect the alginate raft formation or the length of time the raft stayed in the stomach.[7] In another study in healthy subjects, concurrent use of *Gaviscon Advance* (**sodium alginate**) 10 mL four times daily and omeprazole (*Losec MUPS)* 20 mg daily for 3 days did not affect the pharmacokinetics of omeprazole, although it was noted that *Gaviscon Advance,* unlike *Gaviscon,* does not contain any antacid.[8] No special precautions appear to be necessary if omeprazole is given with these antacids.

(c) Pantoprazole

Pantoprazole 40 mg daily was given to 24 healthy subjects with and without 10 mL of *Maalox* (**aluminium/magnesium hydroxide**). The AUC, maximum serum levels, and the half-life of the pantoprazole were unchanged by the antacid.[9] No special precautions would seem to be necessary if pantoprazole is given with *Maalox.*

(d) Rabeprazole

In a single-dose study, 12 healthy subjects were, on separate occasions, given 20 mg of rabeprazole with, without, and 1-hour after a dose of **aluminium/magnesium hydroxide** antacid (*Maalox*).[10] The antacid had no effect on the pharmacokinetics of rabeprazole, so no special precautions would seem necessary on concurrent use.

1. Delhotal-Landes B, Cournot A, Vermerie N, Dellatolas F, Benoit M, Flouvat B. The effect of food and antacids on lansoprazole absorption and disposition. *Eur J Drug Metab Pharmacokinet* (1991), Spec No 3, 315–20.
2. Gerloff J, Barth H, Mignot A, Fuchs W, Heintze K. Does the proton pump inhibitor lansoprazole interact with antacids? *Naunyn Schmiedebergs Arch Pharmacol* (1993) 347, R31.
3. Zoton FasTab (Lansoprazole). Wyeth Pharmaceuticals. UK Summary of product characteristics, May 2007.
4. Tuynman HARE, Festern HPM, Röhss K, Meuwissen SGM. Lack of effect of antacids on plasma concentrations of omeprazole given as enteric-coated granules. *Br J Clin Pharmacol* (1987) 24, 833–5.
5. Howden CW, Reid JL. The effect of antacids and metoclopramide on omeprazole absorption and disposition. *Br J Clin Pharmacol* (1988) 25, 779–80.
6. Iwao K, Saitoh H, Takeda K, Azuumi Y, Takada M. Decreased plasma levels of omeprazole after coadministration with magnesium-aluminium hydroxide dry suspension granules. *Yakugaku Zasshi* (1999) 119, 221–8.
7. Dettmar PW, Little SL, Baxter T. The effect of omeprazole pre-treatment on rafts formed by reflux suppressant tablets containing alginate. *J Int Med Res* (2005) 33, 301–8.
8. Dettmar PW, Hampson FC, Jain A, Choubey S, Little SL, Baxter T. Administration of an alginate based gastric reflux suppressant on the bioavailability of omeprazole. *Indian J Med Res* (2006) 123, 517–24.
9. Hartmann M, Bliesath H, Huber R, Koch H, Steinijans VW, Wurst W. Lack of influence of antacids on the pharmacokinetics of the new gastric H^+/K^+-ATPase inhibitor pantoprazole. *Gastroenterology* (1994) 106 (Suppl), A91.
10. Yasuda S, Higashi S, Murakami M, Tomono Y, Kawaguchi M. Antacids have no influence on the pharmacokinetics of rabeprazole, a new proton pump inhibitor, in healthy volunteers. *Int J Clin Pharmacol Ther* (1999) 37, 249–53.

Proton pump inhibitors + Food or Drinks

Food modestly reduces the bioavailability of lansoprazole and esomeprazole, but not omeprazole, pantoprazole, or rabeprazole. Foods such as apple sauce, apple or orange juice, and yoghurt do not seem to significantly affect the bioavailability of the contents of lansoprazole or omeprazole capsules, and apple sauce did not alter the bioavailability of the contents of esomeprazole capsules.

Clinical evidence, mechanism, importance and management

(a) Esomeprazole

In a crossover study in fasting healthy subjects, the bioavailability of the contents of an esomeprazole capsule mixed with one tablespoonful of **apple sauce** were similar to those of an intact esomeprazole capsule taken with water. Apple sauce was chosen because it is acidic and would therefore be unlikely to affect the enteric coat of the esomeprazole granules from the capsule.[1] An *in vitro* study found that esomeprazole enteric-coated granules from an opened capsule were stable when mixed with 100 mL tap water, yogurt, orange juice or apple juice.[2] The authors suggest that it is likely that esomeprazole could be mixed with these **juices** or other **soft acidic foods** in patients who cannot swallow a capsule.[1,2] Nevertheless, for patients unable to swallow, the UK manufacturers recommend dispersing esomeprazole *tablets* in non-carbonated water only to avoid dissolving the enteric coating. They also note that food delays and decreases the absorption of esomeprazole *tablets,* but that this has little effect on the efficacy to reduce gastric acidity.[3] The US manufacturers say that because the AUC of esomeprazole can be reduced by 43 to 54% by food, esomeprazole *capsules* and *oral suspension* should be taken at least one hour before meals.[4]

(b) Lansoprazole

A study found that food (a **standard meal**) reduced lansoprazole bioavailability by 27%.[5] Another study found a 50% reduction in lansoprazole bioavailability with food (a **standard breakfast**).[6] The authors of both these studies therefore recommended that lansoprazole should not be given with food.[5,6] The maximum serum levels and AUC of lansoprazole are reduced by 50 to 70% when it is given 30 minutes after food. No significant effect was found when lansoprazole was given before meals.[7] The manufacturers recommend that, to achieve optimal efficacy, lansoprazole should be given in the morning at least 30 minutes before food.[7,8] However, in a crossover study in fasting healthy patients the bioavailability of the contents of a lansoprazole 30 mg capsule mixed with either **orange juice**, **tomato juice**, or one tablespoonful of **strained pear** was comparable to that of an intact capsule given with water.[9] This study suggests that, for patients who are unable to swallow or who have difficulty swallowing, mixing the capsule contents with these specific juices or soft foods is acceptable. The US manufacturers also say that the intact contents of the *delayed-release capsules* may be mixed in with a small volume (60 mL) of **apple sauce**, ***Ensure* pudding**, **cottage cheese**, or **yoghurt**. However, the *soluble tablets* may only be dispersed in **water**, and, if given via a nasogastric tube, the tube should be flushed with water before and after administration. The *suspension* may only be mixed with **water** and must not be given through a nasogastric tube.[7]

(c) Omeprazole

In a study in healthy subjects, giving omeprazole with **breakfast** delayed its absorption, but did not affect the total amount absorbed.[10] Similarly, in another study in healthy subjects, a **standardised breakfast** did not affect the bioavailability or maximum concentration of omeprazole enteric-coated tablets, when compared to the fasting state, or when taken immediately before a meal, although an increase in time to maximum concentration was seen.[11] Omeprazole may therefore be taken without regard to the timing of meals. For patients unable to swallow, the manufacturers recommend mixing the intact contents of the opened capsule with **non-carbonated water**, **apple**, **orange** or **pineapple juice**, **yoghurt**[12] or **apple sauce**.[12,13]

(d) Pantoprazole

The manufacturers state that food has no effect on the bioavailability of pantoprazole. The US manufacturers recommend that the tablet is swallowed whole with water with or without food,[14] whereas the UK manufacturers recommend taking it before a meal.[15]

(e) Rabeprazole

A high-fat meal may delay the absorption of rabeprazole but does not alter the AUC and maximum serum levels[16] and so rabeprazole may be taken with or without food.[16,17] The UK manufacturers note that, although food has no effect on the activity of rabeprazole, for once daily regimens they recommend taking it in the morning, before breakfast, to aid compliance.[17]

1. Andersson T, Magner D, Patel J, Rogers P, Levine JG. Esomeprazole 40 mg capsules are bioequivalent when administered intact or as the contents mixed with applesauce. *Clin Drug Invest* (2001) 21, 67–71.
2. Johnson DA, Roach AC, Carlsson AS, Karlsson AAS, Behr DE. Stability of esomeprazole capsule contents after in vitro suspension in common soft foods and beverages. *Pharmacotherapy* (2003) 23, 731–4.
3. Nexium Tablets (Esomeprazole magnesium trihydrate). AstraZeneca UK Ltd. UK Summary of product characteristics, May 2007.
4. Nexium (Esomeprazole magnesium). AstraZeneca. US Prescribing information, April 2007.
5. Delhotal-Landes B, Cournot A, Vermerie N, Dellatolas F, Benoit M, Flouvat B. The effect of food and antacids on lansoprazole absorption and disposition. *Eur J Drug Metab Pharmacokinet* (1991), Spec No 3, 315–20.
6. Bergstrand R, Grind M, Nyberg G, Olofsson B. Decreased oral bioavailability of lansoprazole in healthy volunteers when given with a standardised breakfast. *Clin Drug Invest* (1995) 9, 67–71.
7. Prevacid (Lansoprazole delayed-release). Tap Pharmaceutical Inc. US Prescribing information, June 2007.
8. Zoton FasTab (Lansoprazole). Wyeth Pharmaceuticals. UK Summary of product characteristics, May 2007.
9. Chun AHC, Erdman K, Chiu YL, Pilmer BL, Achari R, Cavanaugh JH. Bioavailability of lansoprazole granules administered in juice or soft food compared to the intact capsule formulation. *Clin Ther* (2002) 24, 1322–31.
10. Rohss K, Andren K, Heggelund A, Lagerstrom P-O, Lundborg P. Bioavailability of omeprazole given in conjunction with food. III World Conf Clin Pharmacol Ther, Stockholm July-Aug 1986. *Acta Pharmacol Toxicol (Copenh)* (1986) 85 (Suppl 5), Abstract 207.
11. Thomson ABR, Sinclair P, Matisko A, Rosen E, Andersson T, Olofsson B. Influence of food on the bioavailability of an enteric-coated tablet formulation of omeprazole under repeated dose conditions. *Can J Gastroenterol* (1997) 11, 663–7.
12. Losec Capsules (Omeprazole). AstraZeneca UK Limited. UK Summary of product characteristics, July 2006.
13. Prilosec (Omeprazole delayed-release). AstraZeneca. US Prescribing information, April 2007.
14. Protonix (Pantoprazole sodium). Wyeth Pharmaceuticals Inc. US Prescribing information, June 2007.
15. Protium Tablets (Pantoprazole sodium sesquihydrate). Altana Pharma Ltd. UK Summary of product characteristics, December 2005.
16. AcipHex Tablets (Rabeprazole sodium). Eisai Inc. US Prescribing information, February 2007.
17. Pariet (Rabeprazole sodium). Eisai Ltd. UK Summary of product characteristics, September 2004.

Proton pump inhibitors + Grapefruit juice

Grapefruit juice has little effect on the AUC of lansoprazole or omeprazole, but modestly reduces the formation of the sulphone metabolites, which is unlikely to be clinically relevant.

Clinical evidence

(a) Lansoprazole

In a randomised, crossover study 21 subjects were given a single 60-mg dose of lansoprazole with either 200 mL of water or freshly-squeezed grapefruit juice. The AUC of lansoprazole was slightly increased by 18%, and the formation of the sulphone metabolite was reduced by the grapefruit juice. Metabolism to the hydroxyl metabolite was not significantly affected.[1]

(b) Omeprazole

In a single-dose study in 12 healthy subjects, grapefruit juice 300 mL had no significant effect on the AUC or half-life of omeprazole 20 mg: the results were similar in both CYP2C19 metaboliser phenotypes, as indicated by plasma levels of hydroxyomeprazole. However, there was a 20% reduction in AUC of omeprazole sulphone..[2]

Mechanism

From the studies above[1,2] it appears that grapefruit juice may have a minor inhibitory effect on the metabolism of omeprazole and lansoprazole by the cytochrome P450 isoenzyme CYP3A4 (which results in the sulphone metabolites). This was suggested to be due to intestinal inhibition of CYP3A4. , Grapefruit juice does not affect the metabolism (hydroxylation) of the proton pump inhibitors by CYP2C19.

Importance and management

The small changes in lansoprazole and omeprazole pharmacokinetics are not clinically relevant, so it appears that they may be taken with grapefruit juice. See also 'Proton pump inhibitors + Food or Drinks', p.970, for the finding that other fruit juices had no effect on lansoprazole or omeprazole bioavailability.

1. Uno T, Yasui-Furukori N, Takahata T, Sugawara K, Tateishi T. Lack of significant effect of grapefruit juice on the pharmacokinetics of lansoprazole and its metabolites in subjects with different CYP2C19 genotypes. *J Clin Pharmacol* (2005) 45, 690–4.
2. Tassaneeyakul W, Tassaneeyakul W, Vannaprasaht S, Yamazoe Y. Formation of omeprazole sulphone but not 5-hydroxyomeprazole is inhibited by grapefruit juice. *Br J Clin Pharmacol* (2000) 49, 139–44.

Proton pump inhibitors + Herbal medicines

Both *Gingko biloba* and St John's wort induce the metabolism of omeprazole, and this might result in reduced efficacy. Other proton pump inhibitors are likely to be similarly affected.

Clinical evidence and mechanism

(a) Gingko biloba

In one study, 18 healthy Chinese subjects were given a single 40-mg dose of omeprazole before and after a 12-day course of a standardised extract of *Gingko biloba* 140 mg twice daily. The subjects were divided into three groups: homozygous extensive CYP2C19 metabolisers (6 subjects), heterozygous extensive CYP2C19 metabolisers (5) and poor CYP2C19 metabolisers (7). The AUC of omeprazole was modestly decreased by 42%, 27% and 40%, respectively, and levels of the inactive metabolite, hydroxyomeprazole, were increased by 38%, 100%, and 232%, in the three groups, respectively. Renal clearance of hydroxyomeprazole was also reduced by *Gingko biloba.* It was concluded that Gingko biloba increases the metabolism (hydroxylation) of omeprazole by inducing the cytochrome P450 isoenzyme CYP2C19.[1]

(b) St John's wort (Hypericum perforatum)

In a crossover study 12 healthy subjects (6 of the extensive CYP2C19 metaboliser phenotype and 6 of the poor CYP2C19 metaboliser phenotype) were given St John's wort 300 mg three times daily or placebo for 14 days, followed by a single 20-mg dose of omeprazole on day 15. St John's wort modestly decreased the AUC of omeprazole in all subjects (by 49% in extensive metabolisers and 41% in poor metabolisers), and also increased the levels of hydroxyomeprazole by 35% in those who were extensive metabolisers. It also markedly increased the levels of the inactive CYP3A4 sulfone metabolite of omeprazole in both extensive and poor metabolisers (by 148% and 132%, respectively).[2] It was concluded that St John's wort increases the metabolism of omeprazole by inducing both CYP2C19 and CYP3A4.

Importance and management

These appear to be the only studies examining the effects of *Gingko biloba* and St John's wort on proton pump inhibitors. However, the reduction in the AUCs of omeprazole seen (about 40%) suggest that there is a possibility that omeprazole will be less effective in patients taking these herbal medicines. As all PPIs are metabolised by CYP2C19 to varying extents, it is likely that the effects of *Gingko biloba* and St John's wort seen in these studies will be similar with other PPIs. There is insufficient evidence to suggest that these herbs should be avoided in patients taking PPIs. However, the potential reduction in the efficacy of the PPI should be borne in mind, particular where the consequences may be serious, such as in patients with healing ulcers.

1. Yin OQP, Tomlinson B, Waye MMY, Chow AHL, Chow MSS. Pharmacogenetics and herb–drug interactions: experience with Gingko biloba and omeprazole. *Pharmacogenetics* (2004) 14, 841–50.
2. Wang LS, Zhou G, Zhu B, Wu J, Wang JG, Abd El-Aty AM, Li T, Liu J, Yang TL, Wang D, Zhong XY, Zhou HH. St John's wort induces both cytochrome P450 3A4–catalyzed sulfoxidation and 2C19–dependent hydroxylation of omeprazole. *Clin Pharmacol Ther* (2004) 75, 191–7.

Proton pump inhibitors + Macrolides

Clarithromycin approximately doubles the serum levels of esomeprazole, lansoprazole and omeprazole, but has no effect on pantoprazole. A small rise in the serum levels of clarithromycin might also occur, which may be therapeutically useful. Some very limited evidence indicates that erythromycin raises serum omeprazole

levels, without significantly altering its effects. Lansoprazole and omeprazole do not appear to affect the pharmacokinetics of roxithromycin.

Clinical evidence

(a) Clarithromycin

When 11 healthy subjects taking **omeprazole** 40 mg daily were also given clarithromycin 500 mg every 8 hours for 5 days, the maximum serum levels of **omeprazole** rose by 30% and its AUC_{0-24} rose by 89%, but the effect of **omeprazole** on gastric pH was unchanged. The maximum serum clarithromycin levels rose by 11% and the AUC_{0-8} was increased by 15%.[1] In a similar study, approximately twofold increases in the AUC of **omeprazole** were reported.[2] In another study in 8 subjects (all extensive metabolisers of CYP2C19), clarithromycin 500 mg twice daily for 7 days caused a similar twofold increase in the AUC of **omeprazole** 20 mg twice daily but did not affect the AUC of **pantoprazole** 40 mg twice daily. The levels of clarithromycin itself were not affected.[3]

The AUC of a single 60-mg dose of **lansoprazole** was raised 1.55-fold to 1.8-fold by clarithromycin 500 mg twice daily for 6 days in both extensive and poor metabolisers of CYP2C19.[4] In another study in healthy subjects, the AUC of lansoprazole 30 mg twice daily was increased by just 25% by clarithromycin 500 mg twice daily and amoxicillin 1 g twice daily for 4 days. The AUC of the hydroxyl metabolite of clarithromycin was also increased by about 25%.[5]

In a study in 18 healthy subjects the AUC, maximum serum levels and half-life of **esomeprazole** 40 mg once daily were increased by 70%, 18% and 35%, respectively, when taken with clarithromycin 500 mg twice daily and amoxicillin 1 g twice daily for 7 days. When the study was repeated in 19 healthy subjects with esomeprazole 20 mg the AUC, maximum serum levels and half-life of **esomeprazole** were increased by 127%, 39% and 50%, respectively. All subjects were of the CYP2C19 extensive metaboliser phenotype. Similar increases in **esomeprazole** levels (e.g. AUC doubled) were seen in a further 6 subjects who were of the CYP2C19 poor metaboliser phenotype. In these studies, **esomeprazole** did not alter clarithromycin levels.[6]

See also 'Proton pump inhibitors + Penicillins', below, for information on case reports of glossitis, stomatitis and a black tongue with lansoprazole and antibacterial regimens including clarithromycin.

(b) Erythromycin

A study was undertaken in a patient to confirm the *in vitro* findings that erythromycin inhibits the metabolism of **omeprazole**. After taking 500 mg of erythromycin base and 20 mg of **omeprazole** daily for 8 weeks, it was found that the AUC of **omeprazole** was increased almost fourfold, and the metabolite of **omeprazole** was undetectable. These raised **omeprazole** levels might have been expected to increase its effectiveness, but in this patient the time during which gastric pH was less than 4 *decreased* by 22%.[7]

(c) Roxithromycin

A study of roxithromycin 300 mg twice daily with **omeprazole** 20 mg twice daily or with **lansoprazole** 30 mg twice daily, for 6 days found that neither PPI significantly affected the pharmacokinetics of roxithromycin.[8]

Mechanism

Clarithromycin appears to inhibit the metabolism of esomeprazole, lansoprazole[4] and omeprazole[1,2] by the cytochrome P450 isoenzyme CYP3A4, one of the enzymes involved in their metabolism. Pantoprazole is metabolised by CYP2C19 only and was therefore not affected by the inhibition of CYP3A4. See 'Gastrointestinal drugs', (p.960) for an overview of the metabolism of PPIs and the role of CYP2C19 polymorphism. Erythromycin interacts similarly, whereas roxithromycin has only weak effects on CYP3A4.

Importance and management

The pharmacokinetic interactions between clarithromycin and **omeprazole**, **esomeprazole** and **lansoprazole** are established. However, none of the changes reported represents an adverse interaction, but they may help to explain why concurrent use is valuable in the eradication of *Helicobacter pylori*. Erythromycin is likely to interact similarly, whereas roxithromycin does not. Pantoprazole is not affected by macrolides.

1. Gustavson LE, Kaiser JF, Edmonds AL, Locke CS, DeBartolo ML, Schneck DW. Effect of omeprazole on concentrations of clarithromycin in plasma and gastric tissue at steady state. *Antimicrob Agents Chemother* (1995) 39, 2078–83.
2. Furuta T, Ohashi K, Kobayashi K, Iida I, Yoshida H, Shirai N, Takashima M, Kosuge K, Hanai H, Chiba K, Ishizaki T, Kaneko E. Effects of clarithromycin on the metabolism of omeprazole in relation to CYP2C19 genotype status in humans. *Clin Pharmacol Ther* (1999) 66, 265–74.
3. Calabresi L, Pazzucconi F, Ferrara S, di Paolo A, Del Tacca M, Sirtori C. Pharmacokinetic interactions between omeprazole/pantoprazole and clarithromycin in healthy volunteers. *Pharmacol Res* (2004) 49, 493–9.
4. Saito M, Yasui-Furukori N, Uno T, Takahata T, Sugawara K, Munakata A, Tateishi T. Effects of clarithromycin on lansoprazole pharmacokinetics between CYP2C19 genotypes. *Br J Clin Pharmacol* (2005) 59, 302–9.
5. Mainz D, Borner K, Koeppe P, Kotwas J, Lode H. Pharmacokinetics of lansoprazole, amoxicillin and clarithromycin after simultaneous and single administration. *J Antimicrob Chemother* (2002) 50, 699–706.
6. Hassan-Alin M, Andersson T, Niazi M, Liljeblad M, Persson BA, Röhss K. Studies on drug interactions between esomeprazole, amoxicillin and clarithromycin in healthy subjects. *Int J Clin Pharmacol Ther* (2006) 44, 119–27.
7. Salcedo JA, Benjamin SB, Maher KA, Sukhova N. Erythromycin inhibits the metabolism of omeprazole. *Gastroenterology* (1997) 112 (4 Suppl), A277.
8. Kees F, Holstege A, Ittner KP, Zimmermann M, Lock G, Schölmerich J, Grobecker H. Pharmacokinetic interaction between proton pump inhibitors and roxithromycin in volunteers. *Aliment Pharmacol Ther* (2000) 14, 407–12.

Proton pump inhibitors + Metronidazole

Omeprazole has no clinically significant effect on the pharmacokinetics of oral or intravenous metronidazole.

Clinical evidence, mechanism, importance and management

The plasma pharmacokinetics of a single oral dose of metronidazole were unaffected by 5 days pre-treatment with **omeprazole** 20 mg twice daily in 14 healthy subjects.[1] Similar results were found in another study with oral and intravenous metronidazole, but when the gastric juice was further studied it was found that the transfer of metronidazole into the gastric juice following an intravenous dose dropped from 15.5 to 2.6% in the presence of **omeprazole**.[2] The significance of these findings is unclear, but the clinical relevance seems small.

See also 'Proton pump inhibitors + Penicillins', below, for case reports of glossitis, stomatitis and a black tongue with lansoprazole and antibacterial regimens including metronidazole.

1. David FL, Da Silva CMF, Mendes FD, Ferraz JGP, Muscara MN, Moreno H, De Nucci G, Pedrazzoli J. Acid suppression by omeprazole does not affect orally administered metronidazole bioavailability and metabolism in healthy male volunteers. *Aliment Pharmacol Ther* (1998) 12, 349–54.
2. Jessa MJ, Goddard AF, Barrett DA, Shaw PN, Spiller RC. The effect of omeprazole on the pharmacokinetics of metronidazole and hydroxymetronidazole in human plasma, saliva and gastric juice. *Br J Clin Pharmacol* (1997) 44, 245–53.

Proton pump inhibitors + Penicillins

Esomeprazole, lansoprazole and omeprazole do not alter the pharmacokinetics of amoxicillin, and omeprazole does not alter bacampicillin bioavailability. Isolated reports describe glossitis, stomatitis and/or black tongue in a small number of patients when treated with lansoprazole and antibacterials, which included amoxicillin, clarithromycin and metronidazole.

Clinical evidence and mechanism

(a) Pharmacokinetic interactions

A study in 12 healthy subjects found no significant changes in the pharmacokinetics of **amoxicillin** 1 g twice daily when it was given with **lansoprazole** 30 mg twice daily and clarithromycin 500 mg twice daily for 4 days.[1] Other randomised, crossover studies in a total of 36 healthy subjects also found no changes in the bioavailability or half-life of **amoxicillin** 1 g twice daily when it was given with clarithromycin 500 mg twice daily and either **esomeprazole** 20 mg twice daily or 40 mg once daily for 7 days.[2]

In other studies **omeprazole** caused a few small changes in the pharmacokinetics of **bacampicillin** and **amoxicillin**, but their bioavailabilities were not reduced,[3-5] and the use of **amoxicillin** with **omeprazole** had a synergistic effect on *Helicobacter pylori* eradication.[4] Similarly, in another study, **omeprazole** 40 mg twice daily for 5 days did not affect the pharmacokinetics of amoxicillin 750 mg twice daily for 5 days, although the mean serum concentration of omeprazole was 12% lower and intragastric pH was slightly lower with the combination than with omeprazole alone. This was felt to be partly due to suppression of *H. pylori*.[6]

(b) Stomatitis and similar adverse effects

Six cases of glossitis, stomatitis and/or black tongue were reported to the Sicilian Regional Pharmacovigilance Centre in patients on **lansoprazole**, when combined with antibacterials used to treat *H. pylori* infections. All 6 patients had been given daily doses of **lansoprazole** 60 mg with clarithromycin 1 g and either metronidazole 1 g (3 patients) or **amoxicillin** 2 g (3 patients) for one week, after which the antibacterials were stopped. The **lansoprazole** continued at 30 mg for periods of up to 3 weeks. The glossitis (1 patient), black tongue (3 patients) and stomatitis (2 patients) developed between days 2 and 19 of the courses of treatment.[7] In one small randomised study, nine cases of glossitis occurred when **lansoprazole** was given with **amoxicillin** but none occurred with **lansoprazole** alone.[8]

Importance and management

The incidence of glossitis, stomatitis and black tongue reported with lansoprazole and antibacterials appears to be rare and no new cases appear to have been published since these reports, whereas these drug combinations are commonly used for the eradication of *H. pylori*. Just why these drugs cause these adverse effects, and whether they are due to just one drug or to an interaction is not understood. Note that the CSM in the UK have received reports of stomatitis, glossitis and a black, hairy tongue or discolouration with each of the reported drugs individually. The CSM in the UK have received reports of 4 cases of stomatitis, one case of glossitis and one case of a black hairy tongue with sole use of lansoprazole, but these are rare effects.[9]

The pharmacokinetics of amoxicillin do not appear to be affected by concurrent use of esomeprazole, lansoprazole and omeprazole, and omeprazole was not affected by amoxicillin.

1. Mainz D, Borner K, Koeppe P, Kotwas J, Lode H. Pharmacokinetics of lansoprazole, amoxicillin and clarithromycin after simultaneous and single administration. *J Antimicrob Chemother* (2002) 50, 699–706.
2. Hassan-Alin M, Andersson T, Niazi M, Liljeblad M, Persson BA, Röhss K. Studies on drug interactions between esomeprazole, amoxicillin and clarithromycin in healthy subjects. *Int J Clin Pharmacol Ther* (2006) 44, 119–27.
3. Paulsen O, Högland P, Walder M. No effect of omeprazole-induced hypoacidity on the bioavailability of amoxycillin and bacampicillin. *Scand J Infect Dis* (1989) 21, 219–23.
4. Cardaci G, Lambert JR, Aranda-Michel J, Underwood B. Omeprazole has no effect on the gastric mucosal bioavailability of amoxycillin. *Gut* (1995) 37 (Suppl 1), A90.
5. Goddard AF, Jessa MJ, Barrett DA, Shaw PN, Idström J-P, Wason C, Wrangstadh M, Spiller RC. Effect of omeprazole on the distribution of antibiotics in gastric juice. *Gastroenterology* (1995) 108 (Suppl), A102.
6. Pommerien W, Braun M, Idström JP, Wrangstadh M, Londong W. Pharmacokinetic and pharmacodynamic interactions between omeprazole and amoxycillin in Helicobacter pylori-positive healthy subjects. *Aliment Pharmacol Ther* (1996) 10, 295–301.
7. Greco S, Mazzaglia G, Caputi AP, Pagliaro L. Glossitis, stomatitis and black tongue with lansoprazole plus clarithromycin and other antibiotics. *Ann Pharmacother* (1997) 31, 1548.
8. Hatlebakk JG, Nesje LB, Hausken T, Bang CJ, Berstad A. Lansoprazole capsules and amoxicillin oral suspension in the treatment of peptic ulcer disease. *Scand J Gastroenterol* (1995) 30, 1053–7.
9. Drug analysis prints (Amoxicillin, clarithromycin, lansoprazole and metronidazole). Medicines and Healthcare Regulatory Agency, UK. Available at: http://www.mhra.gov.uk/home/idcplg?IdcService=SS_GET_PAGE&nodeId=742 (accessed 24/08/07).

Proton pump inhibitors + SSRIs

Fluvoxamine markedly inhibits the metabolism of the proton pump inhibitors lansoprazole, omeprazole and rabeprazole in those of the CYP2C19 extensive metaboliser phenotype, producing levels comparable to those in poor metabolisers. However, these increases are probably of little clinical relevance. Theoretically escitalopram may have the same effect. Omeprazole may increase escitalopram levels.

Clinical evidence

(a) Escitalopram

Omeprazole 30 mg daily caused a 50% increase in the plasma levels of escitalopram. This is only a moderate increase, but the manufacturer suggests that caution is warranted and a dose adjustment of the escitalopram may be needed.[1]

(b) Fluvoxamine

Several studies in healthy subjects have investigated the effects of fluvoxamine (a CYP2C19 inhibitor) on the metabolism of PPIs. In these studies, fluvoxamine 25 mg twice daily for 6 days had significant effects on the pharmacokinetics of three different PPIs in patients who were of the extensive CYP2C19 metaboliser phenotype (the most common phenotype) as follows:

- **Lansoprazole**: Fluvoxamine increased the AUC and elimination half-life of a single 40-mg dose of lansoprazole by 3.8-fold and 3-fold, respectively.[2]
- **Omeprazole**: Fluvoxamine increased the AUC, half-life and maximum plasma concentration of a single 40-mg dose of omeprazole by 6-fold, 2.6-fold and 3.7-fold, respectively.[3]
- **Rabeprazole**: Fluvoxamine increased the AUC, elimination half-life and maximum plasma concentration of a single 20-mg dose of rabeprazole by 2.8-fold, 2.4-fold and 2-fold, respectively.[4]

However, these pharmacokinetic changes essentially had the effect of turning the extensive metabolisers into poor metabolisers.[2-4] In contrast, in patients who were of the CYP2C19 poor metabolisers phenotype, fluvoxamine did not have any significant effect on the pharmacokinetics of either of these three PPIs.[2-4]

In an earlier study in 12 healthy subjects (7 extensive metabolisers and 5 poor metabolisers of CYP2C19) given fluvoxamine 10 to 50 mg daily for 7 days, with a single 20-mg dose of omeprazole on day 7, the AUC of omeprazole was increased by nearly threefold by fluvoxamine 10 to 20 mg and by over fourfold by fluvoxamine 25 to 50 mg (all subjects combined).[5]

Mechanism

All proton pump inhibitors are primarily metabolised by the cytochrome P450 isoenzyme CYP2C19, which is subject to genetic polymorphism, see 'Gastrointestinal drugs', (p.960). As fluvoxamine inhibits CYP2C19, it can increase the levels of PPIs in patients who are extensive CYP2C19 metabolisers, but does not significantly affect the metabolism of PPIs in patients who are poor metabolisers.

Importance and management

An established interaction. The increased levels of these PPIs seen in extensive metabolisers taking fluvoxamine are similar to those seen in poor metabolisers not taking fluvoxamine, and are unlikely to lead to an increase in adverse effects because of the wide therapeutic margin of PPIs.

Some studies have shown that CYP2C19 genotype is a factor in the success of PPI-based eradication regimens, as poor metabolisers of CYP2C19 appear to have higher *H. pylori* eradication rates with these regimens than extensive metabolisers.[6,7] Therefore, treatment of *H. pylori* is likely to be more successful in patients who are extensive metabolisers and are also taking an inhibitor of CYP2C19 such as fluvoxamine (see 'Table 1.3', (p.6)). However, the addition of fluvoxamine to improve PPI-based eradication regimens is not clinically appropriate because of the risk of fluvoxamine adverse effects.

1. Cipralex (Escitalopram oxalate). Lundbeck Ltd. UK Summary of product characteristics, December 2005.
2. Yasui-Furukori N, Saito M, Uno T, Takahata T, Sugawara K, Tateishi T. Effects of fluvoxamine on lansoprazole pharmacokinetics in relation to CYP2C19 genotypes. *J Clin Pharmacol* (2004) 44, 1223–9.
3. Yasui-Furukori N, Takahata T, Nakagami T, Yoshiya G, Inoue Y, Kaneko S, Tateishi T. Different inhibitory effect of fluvoxamine on omeprazole metabolism between CYP2C19 genotypes. *Br J Clin Pharmacol* (2004) 57, 487–94.
4. Uno T, Shimizu M, Yasui-Furukori N, Sugawara K, Tateishi T. Different effects of fluvoxamine on rabeprazole pharmacokinetics in relation to CYP2C19 genotype status. *Br J Clin Pharmacol* (2006) 61, 309–14.
5. Christensen M, Tybring G, Mihara K, Yasui-Furokori N, Carrillo JA, Ramos SI, Andersson K, Dahl M-L, Bertilsson L. Low daily 10-mg and 20-mg doses of fluvoxamine inhibit the metabolism of both caffeine (cytochrome P4501A2) and omeprazole (cytochrome P4502C19). *Clin Pharmacol Ther* (2002) 71, 141–52.
6. Furuta T, Shirai N, Takashima M, Xiao F, Hanai H, Sugimura H, Ohashi K, Ishizaki T, Kaneko E. Effect of genotypic differences in CYP2C19 on cure rates of *Helicobacter pylori* infection by triple therapy with a proton pump inhibitor, amoxicillin, and clarithromycin. *Clin Pharmacol Ther* (2001) 69, 158–68.
7. Furuta T, Ohashi K, Kamata T, Takashima M, Kosuge K, Kawasaki T, Hanai H, Kubota T, Ishizaki T, Kaneko E. Effect of genetic differences in omeprazole metabolism on cure rates for *Helicobacter pylori* infection and peptic ulcer. *Ann Intern Med* (1998) 129, 1027–30.

Sulfasalazine + Antibacterials

Ampicillin and rifampicin markedly reduce the colonic release of 5-aminosalicylate (the active drug) from sulfasalazine. Metronidazole appears not to interact adversely with sulfasalazine.

Clinical evidence

(a) Ampicillin

In a study in 5 healthy subjects the conversion and release of the active metabolite of sulfasalazine, 5-aminosalicylic acid was reduced by one third when a single 2-g dose of sulfasalazine was given after a 5-day course of ampicillin 250 mg four times daily.[1]

(b) Metronidazole

A study in 10 patients (7 with Crohn's disease and 5 with ulcerative colitis) taking long-term sulfasalazine 2 to 4 g daily found that no statistically significant changes in serum sulfapyridine levels occurred while they were also taking metronidazole 400 mg twice daily for 8 to 14 days.[2]

(c) Rifampicin (Rifampin)

A crossover trial in 11 patients with Crohn's disease receiving long-term treatment with sulfasalazine found that rifampicin 10 mg/kg daily and ethambutol 15 mg/kg daily reduced the plasma levels of both 5-aminosalicylic acid and sulphapyridine by about 60%.[3] A similar study in patients taking sulfasalazine 1.5 g to 4 g daily found that the plasma sulfapyridine levels were reduced by 57% when patients were taking rifampicin 10 mg/kg and ethambutol 15 mg/kg daily, when compared with placebo. They also noted an increase in the erythrocyte sedimentation rate (ESR) during antibacterial treatment.[4]

Mechanism

The azo link of sulfasalazine is split by anaerobic bacteria in the colon to release sulphapyridine and 5-aminosalicylic acid, the latter being the active metabolite that acts locally in the treatment of inflammatory bowel disease. Antibacterials that decimate the gut flora can apparently reduce this conversion and this is reflected in lower plasma levels. Rifampicin also possibly increases the metabolism of the sulphapyridine.

Importance and management

Information is limited, but the interaction appears to be established. However, the extent to which these antibacterials actually reduce the effectiveness of sulfasalazine in the treatment of Crohn's disease or ulcerative colitis seems not to have been assessed, but be alert for evidence of a reduced effect if ampicillin, rifampicin or any other oral antibacterial is given. **Neomycin**, which also affects the activity of the gut microflora, has been seen to interact similarly in *animal* studies,[5] but limited evidence suggests metronidazole does not interact.

1. Houston JB, Day J, Walker J. Azo reduction of sulphasalazine in healthy volunteers. *Br J Clin Pharmacol* (1982) 14, 395–8.
2. Shaffer JL, Kershaw A, Houston JB. Disposition of metronidazole and its effects on sulphasalazine metabolism in patients with inflammatory bowel disease. *Br J Clin Pharmacol* (1986) 21, 431–5.
3. Shaffer JL, Houston JB. The effect of rifampicin on sulphapyridine plasma concentrations following sulphasalazine administration. *Br J Clin Pharmacol* (1985) 19, 526–8.
4. Shaffer JL, Hughes S, Linaker BD, Baker RD, Turnberg LA. Controlled trial of rifampicin and ethambutol in Crohn's disease. *Gut* (1984) 25, 203–5.
5. Peppercorn MA, Goldman P. The role of intestinal bacteria in the metabolism of salicylazosulfapyridine. *J Pharmacol Exp Ther* (1972) 181, 555–62.

Sulfasalazine + Cimetidine

Cimetidine does not interact with sulfasalazine.

Clinical evidence, mechanism, importance and management

In a study, 5 patients with rheumatoid arthritis were given sulfasalazine alone, and another 9 patients were given cimetidine 400 mg three times daily for 18 weeks as well as their usual sulfasalazine. On comparing the two groups, it was found that cimetidine did not affect the plasma or urinary levels of sulfasalazine and there were no changes in blood cell counts or haemoglobin levels. It was concluded that no clinically important interaction occurs between these two drugs.[1]

1. Pirmohamed M, Coleman MD, Galvani D, Bucknall RC, Breckenridge AM, Park BK. Lack of interaction between sulphasalazine and cimetidine in patients with rheumatoid arthritis. *Br J Rheumatol* (1993) 32, 222–6.

Sulfasalazine + Colestyramine

***Animal* studies show that colestyramine can bind with sulfasalazine in the gut, thereby reducing its activity, but it is not known if this also occurs in clinical use.**

Clinical evidence, mechanism, importance and management

A study in *rats* found that colestyramine binds with sulfasalazine so that the azo-bond is protected against attack by the bacteria within the gut. As a result the active 5-aminosalicylic acid is not released and the faecal excretion of intact sulfasalazine increases 30-fold.[1] It seems possible that this interaction could also occur in humans, but confirmation of this is lacking. Separating the drug dosages to prevent their admixture in the gut has proved effective with other drugs that bind with colestyramine. Standard advice is to avoid other drugs for one hour before, and 4 to 6 hours after colestyramine.

1. Pieniaszek HJ, Bates TR. Cholestyramine-induced inhibition of salicylazosulfapyridine (sulfasalazine) metabolism by rat intestinal microflora. *J Pharmacol Exp Ther* (1976) 198, 240–5.

Sulfasalazine + Iron compounds

Sulfasalazine and iron appear to bind together in the gut, but whether this reduces the therapeutic response to either drug is uncertain.

Clinical evidence, mechanism, importance and management

Ferrous iron 400 mg reduced the peak serum levels of a single 50-mg/kg dose of sulfasalazine by 40% in 5 healthy subjects. The reasons are not known, but it seems likely that the sulfasalazine chelates with the **iron** in the gut and thereby interferes with its absorption.[1] The extent to which this suggested chelation affects the ability of the intestinal bacteria to split the sulfasalazine and release its locally active metabolite 5-aminosalicylic acid seems not to have been studied. Therefore the effect of this interaction on the clinical response to sulfasalazine is unclear.

1. Das KM, Eastwood MA. Effect of iron and calcium on salicylazosulphapyridine metabolism. *Scott Med J* (1973) 18, 45–50.

Sulfasalazine + Zileuton

No pharmacokinetic interaction appears to occur between sulfasalazine and zileuton.

Clinical evidence, mechanism, importance and management

In a randomised, double-blind, placebo-controlled study, 14 healthy subjects were given sulfasalazine 1 g every 12 hours for 8 days, with zileuton 800 mg or a placebo every 12 hours on days 3 to 8. It was found that the pharmacokinetics of the sulfasalazine and its metabolites (sulphapyridine and *N*-acetyl sulphapyridine) were not significantly changed. The study did not directly look at the pharmacokinetics of the zileuton but the parameters measured were similar to those seen in a previous study.[1] There would seem to be no reason for special precautions if both drugs are used.

1. Awni WM, Braeckman RA, Locke CS, Dubé LM, Granneman GR. The influence of multiple oral doses of zileuton on the steady-state pharmacokinetics of sulfasalazine and its metabolites, sulfapyridine and N-acetylsulfapyridine. *Clin Pharmacokinet* (1995) 29 (Suppl 2), 98–104.

28

Hormonal contraceptives and Sex hormones

The oral contraceptives are of two main types: the **combined hormonal contraceptives** containing both an oestrogen and a progestogen (monophasic, biphasic, triphasic, or sequential), available as tablets or a patch, and the **progestogen-only contraceptives**, which are available as tablets (sometimes called 'mini' pills), parenteral preparations (implants, depot injections) and intrauterine devices.

The oestrogen most commonly used in combined hormonal contraceptives is ethinylestradiol, in a usual daily dose of 20 to 50 micrograms, although higher doses of ethinylestradiol may be used with liver enzyme-inducing drugs such as rifampicin. Mestranol (a pro-drug of ethinylestradiol) is used only rarely (daily dose 50 micrograms). The progestogens used in both combined and progestogen-only oral contraceptives are commonly those derived from 19-nortestosterone and can be subdivided into first generation (e.g. etynodiol diacetate, lynestrenol, norethisterone), second generation (levonorgestrel, norgestrel) and third generation (e.g. desogestrel, drospirenone, gestodene, norgestimate). Note that drospirenone is an analogue of spironolactone and has antiandrogenic and antimineralocorticoid effects. A patch containing ethinylestradiol and norelgestromin is also available. The progestogens used in parenteral progestogen-only contraceptives are either 19-nortestosterone derivatives (e.g. etonogestrel, norethisterone) or derived from progesterone (e.g. medroxyprogesterone acetate). Those in intra-uterine devices are 19-nortestosterone derivatives (e.g. levonorgestrel).

Combined oral preparations are most usually taken for 21 days, followed by a period of 7 days during which withdrawal bleeding occurs. Some of them include 7 inert tablets to be taken at this time so that the daily routine of taking a tablet is not broken. The combined patch is applied weekly for 3 weeks followed by a patch-free week. The oestrogenic and progestogenic components of these contraceptives act together to consistently suppress ovulation.

The progestogen-only oral contraceptives are taken continuously; the implants, injections or intra-uterine devices slowly release the progestogen over an extended period of time. They do not inhibit ovulation reliably in all cycles and probably act mainly by increasing the viscosity of the cervical mucus so that the movement of the sperm is retarded. They may also cause changes in the endometrium, which inhibit successful implantation.

Interactions

(a) Combined hormonal contraceptives

Almost all of the interactions of the hormonal contraceptives described in this publication involve the combined hormonal contraceptives. Most of the clinically important interactions with the combined hormonal contraceptives involve increased metabolism. The major route for hepatic metabolism of ethinylestradiol is hydroxylation by the cytochrome P450 isoenzyme CYP3A4, and progestogens are also substrates for this enzyme. Thus, inducers of this enzyme can increase the clearance of the contraceptive steroids and possibly increase breakthrough bleeding and decrease contraceptive efficacy (see 'Hormonal contraceptives + Antiepileptics; Barbiturates or Phenytoin', p.985). The drugs that have been shown to induce the metabolism of hormonal contraceptives are listed in 'Table 28.1', (see below). Conversely, inhibitors of CYP3A4 may increase the incidence of adverse effects such as nausea, breast tenderness, headaches, and potentially more serious complications such as thromboembolic events, although the latter has yet to be demonstrated.

Some of the conjugated metabolites of ethinylestradiol undergo enterohepatic recirculation, and certain antibacterials are postulated to reduce this by inhibiting gut flora, thereby possibly decreasing contraceptive efficacy, although this is unproven (see 'Hormonal contraceptives + Antibacterials; Penicillins', p.981). Low-dose combined oral contraceptives may be more susceptible to drug interactions than standard-dose or high-dose preparations, but evidence to support this is scant. When considering any pharmacokinetic interactions, it should be noted that there is a large interindividual variation in plasma levels of ethinylestradiol and progestogens.

Table 28.1 Enzyme-inducing drugs shown to reduce the efficacy and/or increase the metabolism of hormonal contraceptives

Group	*Drugs*
Antibacterials	Rifabutin, Rifampicin (Rifampin)
Antiepileptics	Barbiturates (e.g. phenobarbital, primidone), Carbamazepine, Phenytoin, Topiramate
Antifungals	Griseofulvin
Antivirals	Nevirapine, Protease inhibitors (e.g. nelfinavir, ritonavir)
Other drugs	Aprepitant, Modafinil, St John's wort (*Hypericum perforatum*)

(b) Progestogen-only contraceptives

There is very little direct information about interactions with the progestogen-only contraceptives (oral, parenteral, and intrauterine). It is unwise to uncritically assume that interactions known to occur with the combined oral contraceptives also occur with these. However, it seems probable that an increased risk of failure with the oral and parenteral progestogen-only contraceptives is likely with drugs that cause enzyme induction (listed in 'Table 28.1', (see above)), which results in an increased clearance of the progestogen, with an accompanying loss of efficacy. The progestogen-releasing intrauterine system is thought to have a primarily local effect, and may not be affected by enzyme-inducers (see 'Progestogen-only contraceptives + Enzyme inducers', p.1007). However, much more study is needed to clarify the situation.

(c) Emergency hormonal contraceptives

It is not known whether interacting drugs are likely to affect the emergency hormonal contraceptives, although it is common practice that women taking enzyme-inducing drugs (see 'Table 28.1', (see above)) are given an increased dosage to accommodate the increased rate of metabolism by the liver (see 'Emergency hormonal contraceptives + Enzyme inducers', p.977). The efficacy of progestogen-only emergency hormonal contraceptives is not affected by antibacterials that do not induce liver enzymes (see 'Emergency hormonal contraceptives + Antibacterials', p.977).

(d) Hormone replacement therapy (HRT)

The preparations used for HRT contain oestrogens, either alone or combined with progestogens. They differ from the hormonal contraceptives as the most commonly used oestrogens in HRT are natural oestrogens such as estradiol and conjugated oestrogens, and their dosages are generally lower than equivalent doses of ethinylestradiol used in combined hormonal contraceptives. There are only a few reports of interactions with HRT preparations, but generally they are expected to behave very much like the combined oral contraceptives.

(e) Other preparations

Cyproterone acetate combined with ethinylestradiol (co-cyprindiol) is intended for use in women with androgen-dependent skin conditions, but it also acts as an oral contraceptive and is therefore predicted to interact like conventional oestrogen-containing oral contraceptives (see 'Co-cyprindiol (Cyproterone/Ethinylestradiol) + Miscellaneous', p.977).

General references

1. Back DJ, Breckenridge AM, Crawford FE, MacIver M, Orme ML'E, Rowe PH. Interindividual variation and drug interactions with hormonal steroid contraceptives. *Drugs* (1981) 21, 46–61.
2. Shader RI, Oesterheld JR. Contraceptive effectiveness: cytochromes and induction. *J Clin Psychopharmacol* (2000) 20, 119–121.
3. Shader RI, Greenblatt DJ. More on oral contraceptives, drug interactions, herbal medicines, and hormone replacement therapy. *J Clin Psychopharmacol* (2000) 20, 397–8.
4. Elliman A. Interactions with hormonal contraception. *Br J Fam Plann* (2000) 26, 109–11.

Co-cyprindiol (Cyproterone/Ethinylestradiol) + Miscellaneous

Co-cyprindiol is expected to interact with enzyme inducers in a similar manner to the combined oral contraceptives, and therefore the risk of contraceptive failure is increased. Like combined oral contraceptives, there may be rare cases of contraceptive failure with broad-spectrum antibacterials. There is some evidence that co-cyprindiol also interacts with minocycline to increase facial pigmentation.

Clinical evidence, mechanism, importance and management

Co-cyprindiol is a mixture of the anti-androgenic progestogen, cyproterone acetate 2 mg, with ethinylestradiol 35 micrograms. It is used for the treatment of acne and moderately severe hirsutism in women who may also wish to use it as an oral contraceptive, and its contraceptive efficacy is expected to be reduced by the same hepatic enzyme inducers (see 'Table 28.1', (p.975)) that interact with conventional combined oral contraceptives.[1] The precautions described in this section for the combined hormonal contraceptives with the various drugs listed in 'Table 28.1', (p.975), should therefore be followed, see 'Hormonal contraceptives + Antiepileptics; Barbiturates or Phenytoin', p.985.

Similarly, it is anticipated that the use of broad-spectrum antibacterials that do not induce liver enzymes may rarely reduce the contraceptive efficacy of co-cyprindiol and the Faculty of Family Planning and Reproductive Health Care (FFPRHC) guidance under 'Hormonal contraceptives + Antibacterials; Penicillins', p.981, should be followed. Usually these precautions (additional barrier methods) are considered unnecessary after 3 weeks of concurrent use. However, the manufacturer of co-cyprindiol says that when **tetracyclines** are being taken it is advisable to use additional non-hormonal methods of contraception (except the rhythm or temperature methods) since an extremely high degree of contraceptive protection must be provided with co-cyprindiol due to the theoretical risk of cyproterone causing feminization of a male foetus. However, they do also note that oral **tetracyclines** have not actually been shown to reduce the contraceptive efficacy of co-cyprindiol. In addition co-cyprindiol may also possibly interact with **minocycline** to accentuate facial pigmentation (see 'Tetracyclines; Minocycline + Ethinylestradiol', p.350).

The manufacturer also points out that **combined oral contraceptives** (and presumably the combined hormonal contraceptive patch) must not be taken with co-cyprindiol.[1] To do this would be analogous to doubling the ethinylestradiol dose with consequent increased risk of adverse effects. In addition, some of the progestogens in combined oral contraceptives have weak androgenic effects, which could oppose the benefits of cyproterone.

1. Dianette (Cyproterone/ethinylestradiol). Schering Health Care Ltd. UK Summary of product characteristics, June 2007.

Drospirenone + Potassium-sparing drugs

Drospirenone has the potential to cause hyperkalaemia and may have additive effects with other potassium-sparing drugs.

Clinical evidence, mechanism, importance and management

Drospirenone is an analogue of spironolactone and has antimineralocorticoid and potassium-sparing effects, and therefore may increase the risk of hyperkalaemia if it is given to patients with conditions that predispose to hyperkalaemia (e.g. renal failure), and/or with potassium supplements or other drugs that may increase potassium levels such as ACE inhibitors, angiotensin II receptor antagonists, ciclosporin, heparin, NSAIDs (uncommon), potassium-sparing diuretics (such as amiloride, triamterene) and other aldosterone antagonists (such as spironolactone and eplerenone).[1-3] Note that the US manufacturer[3] notes that hyperkalaemia did not occur in a study in which drospirenone was given to patients with mild to moderate renal impairment, or when drospirenone was given with potassium-sparing diuretics (although in 5 patients in the potassium-sparing diuretic group had a rise in potassium level of 0.33 mmol/L). Furthermore, in a study where drospirenone was given with enalapril 10 mg twice daily, no subject developed hyperkalaemia (defined as serum potassium greater than 5.5 mmol/L). It is generally recommended that serum potassium is measured during the first cycle of treatment with drospirenone.

1. Yasmin (Drospirenone/Ethinylestradiol). Schering Health Care Ltd. UK Summary of product characteristics, August 2006.
2. Angeliq (Drospirenone/Estradiol). Schering Health Care Ltd. UK Summary of product characteristics, December 2006.
3. Yaz (Drospirenone/Ethinylestradiol). Bayer HealthCare Pharmaceuticals, Inc. US Prescribing information, February 2007.

Emergency hormonal contraceptives + Antibacterials

There is a theoretical possibility that the emergency contraceptive efficacy of norgestrel/ethinylestradiol could be affected by antibacterials that do not induce liver enzymes, such as the penicillins and tetracyclines. The efficacy of levonorgestrel given for emergency contraception is not likely to be affected by these antibacterials.

Clinical evidence, mechanism, importance and management

(a) Combined oestrogen/progestogen

The manufacturer has stated that the efficacy of **norgestrel** with **ethinylestradiol** (***Schering PC4***) may be reduced by **ampicillin** and other antibacterials.[1] This is presumably an extrapolation from the rare cases of combined oral contraceptive failure seen with various other antibacterials that do not induce liver enzymes, which, it has been suggested, are due to reduced enterohepatic recycling of **ethinylestradiol** (see 'Hormonal contraceptives + Antibacterials; Penicillins', p.981). However, it has been suggested that it is likely that sufficient hormone is absorbed initially for the emergency contraceptive to be effective[2] (it is taken as 2 doses within 12 hours of each other). Note that **rifampicin** and **rifabutin** are likely to reduce the efficacy of all forms of combined hormonal contraceptives, as they induce the metabolism of oestrogens and progestogens, see 'Hormonal contraceptives + Rifamycins', p.1001. The use of combined oestrogen/progestogen as an emergency contraceptive has been superseded by a progestogen-only preparation, as the latter is associated with a higher efficacy and less oestrogen-related adverse effects.

(b) Progestogen only

Levonorgestrel is metabolised to inactive substances before it is conjugated,[3] and does not therefore undergo enterohepatic recycling of the active moiety.[4] There is no reason to expect that its efficacy as an emergency contraceptive would be affected by antibacterials that alter gut flora and do not induce liver enzymes.[4] No special precautions are necessary with these antibacterials. However, **rifampicin** and **rifabutin** are likely to reduce the efficacy of most forms of hormonal contraceptives, as they induce the metabolism of oestrogens and progestogens, see 'Hormonal contraceptives + Rifamycins', p.1001.

1. Schering PC4 (Norgestrel/ethinylestradiol). Schering Health Care Ltd. UK Summary of product characteristics, July 1995.
2. Elliman A. Interactions with hormonal contraception. *Br J Fam Plann* (2000) 26, 109–11.
3. Levonelle One Step (Levonorgestrel). Schering Health Care Ltd. UK Summary of product characteristics, June 2004.
4. Faculty of Family Planning and Reproductive Health Care Clinical Effectiveness Unit. FFPRHC Guidance: Drug interactions with hormonal contraception. April 2005. Available at: http://www.ffprhc.org.uk/admin/uploads/DrugInteractionsFinal.pdf (accessed 23/08/07).

Emergency hormonal contraceptives + Enzyme inducers

The efficacy of both the progestogen-only and combined emergency hormonal contraceptive is likely to be reduced by enzyme inducers such as rifampicin and some antiepileptics.

Clinical evidence, mechanism, importance and management

The manufacturer has stated that some enzyme inducers (see 'Table 28.1', (p.975)) might reduce the efficacy of **norgestrel/ethinylestradiol** *(Schering PC4)*[1] [withdrawn from the UK market in 2001] and **levonorgestrel** *(Levonelle One Step)*[2] used as emergency contraceptives. Cases of failure of emergency contraceptives have been reported with **'St John's wort'**, (p.1002). Various enzyme inducers have specifically been shown to decrease the levels of contraceptive steroids when used as components of combined oral contraceptives (see individual monographs). This would also be expected when they are used as postcoital emergency contraceptives. However, it is difficult to envisage a study design that would show whether this reduced metabolism results in reduced efficacy of emergency contraception (e.g. indicators of ovulation do not necessarily indicate likely reduced efficacy).

The Faculty of Family Planning and Reproductive Health Care (FFPRHC) Clinical Effectiveness Unit notes that there appears to be no good evidence on how to manage this interaction, but current clinical practice is to increase the contraceptive dose by approximately 50%.[3] The British National Formulary recommends giving a dose of levonorgestrel 1.5 mg immediately followed by another 1.5-mg dose 12 hours later, although this is unlicensed.[4] A copper IUD may also be used as an effective alternative.[3] In the UK it is possible to buy emergency hormonal contraception without a prescription; however, it has been advised that patients taking enzyme inducers should not be supplied the emergency hormonal contraceptive but should be referred to a doctor or family planning service.[3,5] Given the potential consequences of an unwanted pregnancy, these seem sensible precautions.

1. Schering PC4 (Norgestrel/ethinylestradiol). Schering Health Care Ltd. UK Summary of product characteristics, July 1995.
2. Levonelle One Step (Levonorgestrel). Schering Health Care Ltd. UK Summary of product characteristics, June 2004.
3. Faculty of Family Planning and Reproductive Health Care Clinical Effectiveness Unit. FFPRHC Guidance: Drug interactions with hormonal contraception. April 2005. Available at: http://www.ffprhc.org.uk/admin/uploads/DrugInteractionsFinal.pdf (accessed 23/08/07).
4. British National Formulary. 53rd ed. London: The British Medical Association and The Pharmaceutical Press; 2007. p. 425.
5. Royal Pharmaceutical Society of Great Britain. Practice guidance on the supply of emergency hormonal contraception as a pharmacy medicine. September 2004. Available at: http://www.rpsgb.org/pdfs/ehcguid.pdf (accessed 23/08/07).

Gestrinone + Enzyme inducers

The manufacturer says that rifampicin and antiepileptics may reduce the effects of gestrinone.

Clinical evidence, mechanism, importance and management

The manufacturer suggests that **rifampicin** and **antiepileptics** (not named, but by implication those that are enzyme-inducers, see 'Table 28.1', (p.975)) can accelerate the metabolism of gestrinone thereby reducing its effects.[1] However, there appear to be no reports that this actually occurs.[2] Good monitoring is advisable if any of these drugs are given concurrently, with dosage adjustments if necessary.

1. Dimetriose (Gestrinone). Sanofi-Aventis. UK Summary of product characteristics, October 2003.
2. Roberts G (Roussel Labs). Personal Communication 1992.

Hormonal contraceptives + Antacids

Despite *in vitro* evidence that some antacids might reduce the availability of norethisterone acetate, evidence from healthy women indicates that no interaction occurs. This also appears to be true for ethinylestradiol and levonorgestrel.

Clinical evidence, mechanism, importance and management

An *in vitro* study found that a 1% suspension of **magnesium trisilicate** in water adsorbed about 80% of **mestranol** and 50% of **norethisterone**, but minimal amounts of **ethinylestradiol**.[1,2] Similarly, another *in vitro* study reported reduced dissolution of **norethisterone acetate** from combined oral contraceptive tablets in the presence of **magnesium trisilicate, kaolin mixture**, and **aluminium hydroxide**.[3] In contrast, a single dose study in 12 healthy women given a combined oral contraceptive (**ethinylestradiol** 30 micrograms and either **norethisterone acetate** 1 mg or **levonorgestrel** 150 micrograms) with **magnesium trisilicate** 500 mg and **aluminium hydroxide** 250 mg, showed that the AUC and peak levels of all three steroids were unchanged.[4] This is in line with common experience. There do not appear to be any reports of contraceptive failure with antacids and **norethisterone acetate** or **mestranol**-containing combined oral contraceptives. No special precautions seem to be necessary.

1. Khalil SAH, Iwuagwu M. The in vitro uptake of some oral contraceptive steroids by magnesium trisilicate. *J Pharm Pharmacol* (1976) 28 (Suppl), 47P.
2. Khalil SAH, Iwuagwu M. *In vitro* uptake of oral contraceptive steroids by magnesium trisilicate. *J Pharm Sci* (1978) 67, 287–9.
3. Fadel H, Abd Elbary A, Nour El-Din E, Kassem AA. Availability of norethisterone acetate from combined oral contraceptive tablets. *Pharmazie* (1979) 34, 49–50.
4. Joshi JV, Sankolli GM, Shah RS, Joshi UM. Antacid does not reduce the bioavailability of oral contraceptive steroids in women. *Int J Clin Pharmacol Ther Toxicol* (1986) 24, 192–5.

Hormonal contraceptives + Anthelmintics

The use of praziquantel or metrifonate does not appear to alter the pharmacokinetics of combined oral contraceptives. The manufacturer of albendazole recommends that women should use effective methods of contraception because of a possible teratogenic risk.

Clinical evidence, mechanism, importance and management

(a) Albendazole

The manufacturer recommends that women taking albendazole should use effective methods of contraception during and for one month after stopping the drug.[1] This is because albendazole is teratogenic in some *animal* species.[1,2]

(b) Metrifonate and Praziquantel

A study in 25 women with early active schistosomiasis (*S. haematobium* or *S. mansoni*) without signs of liver disease and 6 healthy women showed that neither the disease itself nor the concurrent use of antischistosomal drugs (a single 40-mg/kg dose of praziquantel, or metrifonate in three doses of 10 mg/kg at fortnightly intervals) had any effect on the plasma levels of steroids from a combined oral contraceptive (**ethinylestradiol/levonorgestrel** 50/500 micrograms).[3] Moreover, in another study there was no evidence that women with early active schistosomiasis without signs of liver disease were at any greater risk of hepatic impairment while using combined oral contraceptives.[4] No special precautions would therefore appear necessary in women with early active schistosomiasis taking oral contraceptives and praziquantel or metrifonate. Note that oral contraceptives are considered contraindicated in schistosomiasis with liver involvement.

1. Eskazole (Albendazole). GlaxoSmithKline Australia Pty Ltd. Australian product information, November 2004.
2. Albenza (Albendazole). GlaxoSmithKline. US Prescribing information, February 2007.
3. El-Raghy I, Back DJ, Osman F, Orme ML'E, Fathalla M. Contraceptive steroid concentrations in women with early active schistosomiasis: lack of effect of antischistosomal drugs. *Contraception* (1986) 33, 373–7.
4. Shaaban MM, Hammad WA, Fathalla MF, Ghaneimah SA, El-Sharkawy MM, Salim TH, Liao WC, Smith SC. Effects of oral contraception on liver function tests and serum proteins in women with active schistosomiasis. *Contraception* (1982) 26, 75–82.

Hormonal contraceptives + Antibacterials; Cephalosporins

A few anecdotal cases of combined oral contraceptive failure have been reported with cefalexin, cefalexin with clindamycin, and unspecified cephalosporins. The interaction (if such it is) appears to be very rare indeed.

Clinical evidence

Two pregnancies were attributed to the use of cephalosporins (unspecified) and an oral contraceptive (unspecified) in the adverse reactions register of the CSM in the UK for the years 1968 to 1984 (61 cases were attributed to other antibacterials).[1] One case of contraceptive failure has been attributed to **cefalexin**,[2] and one to **cefalexin** used with clindamycin.[3] In a case-control study, 356 women were who had received oral contraceptives and antibacterials (said to be cephalosporins, penicillins, tetracyclines) were identified over a 5-year period in 3 dermatological practices. The contraceptive failure rate in these women (1.6% per year; 2 pregnancies occurred in women taking a cephalosporin and 3 in women taking minocycline) was indistinguishable from the failure rate seen in control patients taking oral contraceptives and no antibacterials (1% per year).[4]

Mechanism

Suppression of intestinal bacteria, which results in reduced enterohepatic recirculation of ethinylestradiol and a fall in serum levels, is the suggested explanation for any interaction (see 'Hormonal contraceptives and sex hormones', (p.975)). Note that broad-spectrum antibacterials do not affect progestogens, as their metabolites are inactive.[5]

Importance and management

The interaction between the combined hormonal contraceptives and cephalosporins that are summarised here are all that have been identified in the literature. These interactions are not adequately established and the whole issue remains very controversial.[5] Bearing in mind the extremely wide use of both groups of drugs, any increased incidence of contraceptive failure above that normally seen is clearly very low indeed. On the other hand, the personal and ethical consequences of an unwanted pregnancy can be very serious. For this reason, the Faculty of Family Planning and Reproductive Health Care (FFPRHC) Clinical Effectiveness Unit recommends that patients taking antibacterials that do not induce liver enzymes should use a second form of non-hormonal contraception, such as condoms, while taking a short course of less than 3 weeks of a cephalosporin, and also for 7 days after the antibiotic has been stopped. This advice applies to both the oral and patch form of the combined contraceptive.[5] For further comment and advice see also 'Hormonal contraceptives + Antibacterials; Penicillins', p.981.

Note that antibacterials that do not induce liver enzymes do not affect the reliability of the **progestogen-only contraceptives**, see 'Progestogen-only contraceptives + Antibacterials, p.1007, or the progestogen-only **emergency hormonal contraceptive**, see 'Emergency hormonal contraceptives + Antibacterials', p.977.

1. Back DJ, Grimmer SFM, Orme ML'E, Proudlove C, Mann RD, Breckenridge AM. Evaluation of Committee on Safety of Medicines yellow card reports on oral contraceptive-drug interactions with anticonvulsants and antibiotics. *Br J Clin Pharmacol* (1988) 25, 527–32.
2. DeSano EA, Hurley SC. Possible interactions of antihistamines and antibiotics with oral contraceptive effectiveness. *Fertil Steril* (1982) 37, 853–4.
3. Back DJ, Breckenridge AM, Crawford FE, MacIver M, Orme L'E, Rowe PH. Interindividual variation and drug interactions with hormonal steroids. *Drugs* (1981) 21, 46.
4. Helms SE, Bredle DL, Zajic J, Jarjoura D, Brodell RT, Krishnarao I. Oral contraceptive failure rates and oral antibiotics. *J Am Acad Dermatol* (1997) 36, 705–10.
5. Faculty of Family Planning and Reproductive Health Care Clinical Effectiveness Unit. FFPRHC Guidance: Drug interactions with hormonal contraception. April 2005. Available at: http://www.ffprhc.org.uk/admin/uploads/DrugInteractionsFinal.pdf (accessed 23/08/07).

Hormonal contraceptives + Antibacterials; Macrolides

The macrolides clarithromycin, dirithromycin, roxithromycin and telithromycin appear unlikely to cause combined hormonal contraceptive failure. Erythromycin is also not considered to cause failure of combined hormonal contraceptives, but isolated anecdotal cases have been reported. An isolated case has also been reported with spiramycin.

Clinical evidence

(a) Clarithromycin

Ten women taking a combined oral contraceptive (**ethinylestradiol** with **levonorgestrel** or **desogestrel**) showed a very slight but not statistically significant rise in serum **ethinylestradiol** levels while taking clarithromycin 250 mg twice daily for 7 days. No changes in **levonorgestrel** levels occurred, but levels of the active metabolite of desogestrel were increased. Ovulation did not occur (progesterone levels remained suppressed, and FSH and LH levels were reduced). These hormonal changes suggest that clarithromycin may even *increase* the efficacy of combined oral contraceptives.[1]

(b) Dirithromycin

Fifteen women taking a triphasic combined oral contraceptive (**ethinylestradiol/norethisterone**) were given dirithromycin 500 mg daily for 14 days starting on day 21 of the cycle. A small but statistically significant decrease of 7.6% occurred in the mean **ethinylestradiol** AUC, but no woman ovulated (as assessed by ultrasound and ovarian hormone levels).[2]

(c) Erythromycin

Isolated cases of contraceptive failure have been attributed to erythromycin, and two pregnancies were attributed to the use of erythromycin and an oral contraceptive (unspecified) in the adverse reactions register of the CSM in the UK for the years 1968 to 1984 (61 cases were attributed to other antibacterials).[3] Another survey of oral contraceptive failure identified 1 failure due to erythromycin (48 of 209 pill failures were attributed to antibacterials),[4] and break-through bleeding due to erythromycin has also been described in 2 cases.[5] Conversely, in 2 studies of contraceptive failures in dermatology patients, no pregnancies were identified in a total of 74 women taking erythromycin and an oral contraceptive.[6,7]

(d) Roxithromycin

While taking roxithromycin 150 mg twice daily, the anti-ovulatory effects of a triphasic combined oral contraceptive (**ethinylestradiol/levonorgestrel**) remained unchanged during one cycle in 21 healthy women. Efficacy was measured by monitoring ovulation, which was assessed by ultrasound and progesterone levels.[8]

(e) Spiramycin

One case of contraceptive failure has been attributed to concurrent treatment with spiramycin.[9]

(f) Telithromycin

Telithromycin 800 mg once daily for 10 days had no effect on the pharmacokinetics of **ethinylestradiol**, but increased the plasma levels of **levonorgestrel** in 38 healthy women taking a triphasic combined oral contraceptive. None of the women ovulated, as assessed by progesterone levels.[10]

Mechanism

The macrolides such as erythromycin might possibly be expected to suppress the bacteria responsible for the enterohepatic recycling of ethinylestradiol, but good evidence that this is clinically important is scant (see 'Hormonal contraceptives + Antibacterials; Penicillins', p.981). Erythromycin, and to a lesser extent the other macrolides discussed here, also inhibit the cytochrome P450 isoenzyme CYP3A4, which is responsible for the metabolism of the contraceptive steroids. Therefore they might be expected to increase rather than reduce contraceptive efficacy. This would be expected to offset any possible reduced enterohepatic recycling.

Importance and management

Information about erythromycin is very limited, but the fact that there are only isolated reports of pregnancies with this drug, coupled with its known enzyme-inhibiting properties, suggest that it is unlikely to cause contraceptive failure. The UK Family Planning Association considered that it was almost certain that erythromycin did not interact with combined oral contraceptives.[11] Information on the other macrolides seems to be limited to the studies cited, on the basis of which no interaction appears to be likely with clarithromycin, roxithromycin and telithromycin. Dirithromycin also appears unlikely to cause oral contraceptive failure. No cases of contraceptive failure with these newer macrolides appear to have been reported. If one accepts the theory that there are an as yet unidentifiable tiny group of women for whom enterohepatic recirculation of ethinylestradiol is important, then additional contraceptive precautions should be taken. However, if one tends to the theory that the anecdotal cases of contraceptive failure with broad-spectrum antibacterials are indistinguishable from the normal accepted failure rate, no special precautions are necessary. The Faculty of Family Planning and Reproductive Health Care (FFPRHC) Clinical Effectiveness Unit has issued guidance on the use of antibacterials with hormonal contraceptives. Although they recognise that there is poor evidence for contraceptive failure with the macrolides, they recommend that additional contraceptives, such as condoms, should be used for short courses of antibacterials, see 'Hormonal contraceptives + Antibacterials; Penicillins', p.981, for more detailed information. This advice has usually been applied to only broad-spectrum antibacterials that do not induce liver enzymes, but the FFPRHC notes that some confusion has occurred over which antibacterials are considered to be 'broad-spectrum', and thus they recommend that this advice is applied to all antibacterials that do not induce liver enzymes, which would include the macrolides.[12] This applies to both the oral and the patch form of the combined hormonal contraceptive. Note that antibacterials that do not induce liver enzymes do not affect the reliability of the **progestogen-only contraceptives**, see 'Progestogen-only contraceptives + Antibacterials, p.1007), or the **emergency hormonal contraceptive**, see 'Emergency hormonal contraceptives + Antibacterials', p.977.

For a discussion of the adverse hepatic interaction between oral contraceptives and the macrolide troleandomycin, see 'Hormonal contraceptives or HRT + Antibacterials; Troleandomycin', p.984.

1. Back DJ, Tjia J, Martin C, Millar E, Salmon P, Orme M. The interaction between clarithromycin and combined oral-contraceptive steroids. *J Pharm Med* (1991) 2, 81–7.
2. Wermeling DP, Chandler MHH, Sides GD, Collins D, Muse KN. Dirithromycin increases ethinyl estradiol clearance without allowing ovulation. *Obstet Gynecol* (1995) 86, 78–84.
3. Back DJ, Grimmer SFM, Orme ML'E, Proudlove C, Mann RD, Breckenridge AM. Evaluation of Committee on Safety of Medicines yellow card reports on oral contraceptive-drug interactions with anticonvulsants and antibiotics. *Br J Clin Pharmacol* (1988) 25, 527–32.
4. Kovacs GT, Riddoch G, Duncombe P, Welberry L, Chick P, Weisberg E, Leavesley GM, Baker HWG. Inadvertent pregnancies in oral contraceptive users. *Med J Aust* (1989) 150, 549–51.
5. Hetényi G. Possible interactions between antibiotics and oral contraceptives. *Ther Hung* (1989) 37, 86–9.
6. Hughes BR, Cunliffe WJ. Interactions between the oral contraceptive pill and antibiotics. *Br J Dermatol* (1990) 122, 717–18.
7. London BM, Lookingbill DP. Frequency of pregnancy in acne patients taking oral antibiotics and oral contraceptives. *Arch Dermatol* (1994) 130, 392–3.
8. Meyer BH, Müller FO, Wessels P, Maree J. A model to detect interactions between roxithromycin and oral contraceptives. *Clin Pharmacol Ther* (1990) 47, 671–4.
9. Pedretti E, Brunenghi GM, Morali GC. Interazione tra antibiotici e contraccettivi orali: la spiramicina. *Quad Clin Ostet Ginecol* (1991) 46, 153–4.
10. Scholtz HE, Sultan E, Wessels D, Hundt AF, Passot V, Renouz A, van Neikerk N. HMR 3647, a new ketolide antimicrobial, does not affect the reliability of low-dose, triphasic oral contraceptives. *Intersci Conf Antimicrob Agents Chemother* (1999) 39, 3.
11. Belfield T, ed. FPA Contraceptive Handbook: a guide for family planning and other health professionals. 3rd ed. London: Family Planning Association, 1999.
12. Faculty of Family Planning and Reproductive Health Care Clinical Effectiveness Unit. FFPRHC Guidance: Drug interactions with hormonal contraception. April 2005. Available at: http://www.ffprhc.org.uk/admin/uploads/DrugInteractionsFinal.pdf (accessed 23/08/07).

Hormonal contraceptives + Antibacterials; Metronidazole

Isolated cases of combined oral contraceptive failure have been reported with metronidazole. The interaction (if such it is) appears to be very rare indeed. In a controlled study, metronidazole did not affect contraceptive steroid levels.

Clinical evidence, mechanism, importance and management

In 10 women taking a combined oral contraceptive metronidazole 400 mg three times daily for 6 to 8 days had no effect on the AUC of **ethinylestradiol** and **norethisterone**. However, 2 of the 10 women had a rise in plasma progesterone levels suggesting that ovulation may have occurred. One of a further 15 women taking metronidazole and a combined oral contraceptive also appeared to ovulate. Of the 3 women who ovulated one also ovulated during a cycle while not taking metronidazole.[1] Another similar study in 10 women found that none ovulated while taking metronidazole and a combined oral contraceptive (**ethinylestradiol/norethisterone**).[2]

Only 3 reports of pregnancies were identified in women who took metronidazole and an oral contraceptive (unspecified) in the adverse reactions register of the CSM in the UK for the years 1968 to 1984.[3] A survey of oral contraceptive failure identified one failure due to metronidazole (48 of a total of 209 cases were attributed to antibacterials),[4] and a follow-up study identified one further case.[5] Another survey[6] found one contraceptive failure in a woman taking metronidazole, but she was also taking **doxycycline** (see 'Hormonal contraceptives + Antibacterials; Tetracyclines', p.983). It is possible that these cases represent chance associations.

The interaction between metronidazole and combined oral contraceptives is not established, and the whole issue of any interaction with broad-spectrum antibacterials remains very controversial. Bearing in mind the extremely wide use of both metronidazole and combined oral contraceptives, any increased incidence of contraceptive failure above that seen in general usage is clearly very low indeed. The Faculty of Family Planning and Reproductive Health Care (FFPRHC) Clinical Effectiveness Unit has issued guidance on the use of antibacterials with combined hormonal contraceptives. Although they recognise that there is poor evidence for contraceptive failure, they recommend that additional form of contraception, such as condoms, should be used for short courses of antibacterials, see 'Hormonal contraceptives + Antibacterials; Penicillins', p.981, for more detailed information. This applies to both the oral and the patch form of the combined contraceptive. This advice has usually been applied to only broad-spectrum antibacterials that do not induce liver enzymes but the FFPRHC notes that some confusion has occurred over which antibacterials are considered to be 'broad-spectrum', and thus they recommend that this advice is applied to all antibacterials that do not induce liver enzymes, which would include metronidazole.[7]

Note that antibacterials that do not induce liver enzymes do not affect the reliability of the **progestogen-only contraceptives**, see 'Progestogen-only contraceptives + Antibacterials, p.1007, or the progestogen-only **emergency hormonal contraceptive**, see 'Emergency hormonal contraceptives + Antibacterials', p.977.

1. Joshi JV, Joshi UM, Sankholi GM, Krishna U, Mandlekar A, Chowdhury V, Hazari K, Gupta K, Sheth UK, Saxena BN. A study of interaction of low-dose combination oral contraceptive with ampicillin and metronidazole. *Contraception* (1980) 22, 643–52.
2. Viswanathan MK, Govindarajulu P. Metronidazole therapy on the efficacy of oral contraceptive steroid pills. *J Reprod Biol Comp Endocrinol* (1985) 5, 69–72.
3. Back DJ, Grimmer SFM, Orme ML'E, Proudlove C, Mann RD, Breckenridge AM. Evaluation of Committee on Safety of Medicines yellow card reports on oral contraceptive-drug interactions with anticonvulsants and antibiotics. *Br J Clin Pharmacol* (1988) 25, 527–32.
4. Kovacs GT, Riddoch G, Duncombe P, Welberry L, Chick P, Weisberg E, Leavesley GM, Baker HWG. Inadvertent pregnancies in oral contraceptive users. *Med J Aust* (1989) 150, 549–51.
5. Kakouris H, Kovacs GT. Pill failure and non-use of secondary precautions. *Br J Fam Plann* (1992) 18, 41–4.
6. Sparrow MJ. Pill method failures. *N Z Med J* (1987) 100, 102–5.
7. Faculty of Family Planning and Reproductive Health Care Clinical Effectiveness Unit. FFPRHC Guidance: Drug interactions with hormonal contraception. April 2005. Available at: http://www.ffprhc.org.uk/admin/uploads/DrugInteractionsFinal.pdf (accessed 23/08/07).

Hormonal contraceptives + Antibacterials; Miscellaneous

One or two cases of combined oral contraceptive failure have been reported in patients given chloramphenicol, clindamycin (used with cefalexin), dapsone, fusidic acid, isoniazid, nifurtoinol and nitrofurantoin. These isolated cases are anecdotal and unconfirmed, and the interaction (if such it is) appears to be very rare indeed. The combination of aminosalicylic acid, isoniazid and streptomycin does not appear to affect contraceptive efficacy.

Clinical evidence, mechanism, importance and management

One woman taking a combined oral contraceptive was briefly reported to have developed breakthrough bleeding and to have become pregnant while taking **chloramphenicol**.[1,2] One or two cases of contraceptive failure have been briefly attributed to **clindamycin** (used with cefalexin),[3] **dapsone**,[3] **fusidic acid**,[4] **isoniazid**,[3,5] **nifurtoinol**[6] and **nitrofurantoin**.[3,6] Breakthrough bleeding, due to **clindamycin** in one case and **chloramphenicol** in another case, have also been reported.[7] Conversely, no evidence of ovulation or of changes in plasma **ethinylestradiol** and **norethisterone** levels were seen in a study of 8 women taking a combined oral contraceptive with **aminosalicylic acid**, **isoniazid** and **streptomycin**.[8]

The interactions between the oral contraceptives and antibacterials summarised here are all that have been identified in the literature involving the drugs cited. These interactions are not established, and given the few anecdotal cases with each drug, could just be coincidental. With **isoniazid** in particular, there is evidence that the drug does not cause contraceptive failure when used in combination antitubercular therapy (without rifampicin). On the other hand, the personal and ethical consequences of an unwanted pregnancy can be very serious. For this reason, the Faculty of Family Planning and Reproductive Health Care (FFPRHC) Clinical Effectiveness Unit recommends that women taking combined hormonal contraceptives should routinely use an additional form of contraception, such as condoms, while taking a short course of antibacterials that do not induce liver enzymes, and for 7 days after the antibiotic has been stopped.[9] This advice applies to both the oral and patch form of the combined hormonal contraceptives. For further details of this advice see 'Hormonal contraceptives + Antibacterials; Penicillins', p.981. Although this advice has previously been applied to only broad-spectrum antibacterials that do not induce liver enzymes, the FFPRHC notes that some confusion has occurred over which antibacterials are considered to be 'broad-spectrum', and thus they recommend that this advice is applied to all antibacterials that do not induce liver enzymes.[9]

Note that antibacterials that do not induce liver enzymes do not affect the reliability of the **progestogen-only contraceptives**, see 'Progestogen-only contraceptives + Antibacterials, p.1007, or the progestogen-only **emergency hormonal contraceptive**, see 'Emergency hormonal contraceptives + Antibacterials', p.977.

1. Hempel E, Böhm W, Carol W, Klinger G. Medikamentöse enzyminduktion und hormonale kontrazeption. *Zentralbl Gynakol* (1973) 95, 1451–7.
2. Hempel E. Personal communication, 1975.

3. Back DJ, Breckenridge AM, Crawford FE, MacIver M, Orme ML'E, Rowe PH. Interindividual variation and drug interactions with hormonal steroid contraceptives. *Drugs* (1981) 21, 46–61.
4. Back DJ, Grimmer SFM, Orme ML'E, Proudlove C, Mann RD, Breckenridge AM. Evaluation of Committee on Safety of Medicines yellow card reports on oral contraceptive-drug interactions with anticonvulsants and antibiotics. *Br J Clin Pharmacol* (1988) 25, 527–32.
5. Kovacs GT, Riddoch G, Duncombe P, Welberry L, Chick P, Weisberg E, Leavesley GM, Baker HWG. Inadvertent pregnancies in oral contraceptive users. *Med J Aust* (1989) 150, 549–51.
6. De Groot AC, Eshuis H, Stricker BHC. Ineffectiviteit van orale anticonceptie tijdens gebruik van minocycline. *Ned Tijdschr Geneeskd* (1990) 134, 1227–9.
7. Hetényi G. Possible interactions between antibiotics and oral contraceptives. *Ther Hung* (1989) 37, 86–9.
8. Joshi JV, Joshi UM, Sankolli GM, Gupta K, Rao AP, Hazari K, Sheth UK, Saxena BN. A study of interaction of low-dose combination oral contraceptive with anti-tubercular drugs. *Contraception* (1980) 21, 617–29.
9. Faculty of Family Planning and Reproductive Health Care Clinical Effectiveness Unit. FFPRHC Guidance (April 2005): Drug interactions with hormonal contraception. April 2005. Available at: http://www.ffprhc.org.uk/admin/uploads/DrugInteractionsFinal.pdf (accessed 23/08/07).

Hormonal contraceptives + Antibacterials; Penicillins

Combined oral contraceptive failure has been attributed to ampicillin, amoxicillin, flucloxacillin, oxacillin, phenoxymethylpenicillin, pivampicillin and talampicillin. However, the interaction (if such it is), appears to be very rare. Controlled studies have not shown any effect of ampicillin on contraceptive steroid levels and ovarian suppression.

Clinical evidence

A case report describes 3 women taking an oral contraceptive who became pregnant when given **ampicillin**.[1] One woman had two unwanted pregnancies while taking a combined oral contraceptive (**ethinylestradiol/norethisterone**). On both occasions conception occurred when she was being treated with **ampicillin** for tonsillitis.[2] Another woman taking **ethinylestradiol/norethisterone** for 5 years with no history of breakthrough bleeding, lost a quantity of blood similar to a normal period loss within a day of starting to take **ampicillin** (exact dose unknown). There was no evidence of diarrhoea or vomiting in either case.[2] Two other case reports attributed contraceptive failure to oxacillin,[3] and to an intramuscular injection of **benethamine penicillin**, **procaine penicillin** and **benzylpenicillin**.[4]

The use of a penicillin (unspecified) was implicated in 32 pregnancies in women taking an oral contraceptive (unspecified) in the adverse reactions register of the CSM in the UK for the years 1968 to 1984 (a further 31 cases were attributed to other antibacterials).[5] In an earlier review, the penicillins in 15 cases of contraceptive failure were named as **ampicillin** (alone or with fusidic acid, tetracycline or **flucloxacillin**), **amoxicillin**, **talampicillin**, **phenoxymethylpenicillin** (one also with **oxytetracycline**) and 'penicillin'.[6] A survey of contraceptive failure described failures due to **amoxicillin** (16 cases), **flucloxacillin**, **phenoxymethylpenicillin**, **pivampicillin** (5 cases) and **amoxicillin** with **phenoxymethylpenicillin** (1 case),[7] and a follow-up survey identified 9 further cases involving **amoxicillin** and one with 'penicillin'.[8] Another similar survey described a total of 17 cases with **amoxicillin** and 5 cases with 'penicillin',[9] and a follow-up survey identified 8 further cases with **amoxicillin** and 1 case with 'penicillin'.[10]

In contrast, 3 controlled studies have provided evidence that **ampicillin** does not alter the plasma levels of contraceptive steroids nor reduce their anti-ovulatory effects.[11-13] In the first study, **ampicillin** 250 mg four times daily for 16 days was given to women taking **ethinylestradiol/etynodiol**. No women ovulated, as assessed by FSH, LH and progesterone levels. Two women had breakthrough bleeding while receiving **ampicillin**, and one had spotting while receiving placebo.[11] In another study in 7 patients and 6 healthy women, **ampicillin** 500 mg three times daily for 8 days had no significant effect on the plasma levels of **ethinylestradiol** and **levonorgestrel**. However, one woman had a large fall in **ethinylestradiol** levels. Despite this, none of the women ovulated, as assessed by progesterone levels.[12] The third study in 6 women found that **ampicillin** 1 g twice daily had no effect on the plasma levels of **ethinylestradiol** and **norethisterone**, and ovulation did not occur.[13] A crossover study involving 16 healthy women also found that a 10-day course of **amoxicillin** 875 mg twice daily did not affect **etonogestrel** or **ethinylestradiol** released from the *NuvaRing* vaginal contraceptive ring.[14]

Mechanism

Not understood. The oestrogen component of the contraceptive undergoes enterohepatic recirculation (i.e. it is repeatedly secreted in the bile as sulfate and glucuronide conjugates, which are hydrolysed by the gut bacteria before reabsorption). One idea is that if these bacteria are suppressed by the use of an antibacterial, the steroid conjugates are not hydrolysed and are therefore only poorly reabsorbed, resulting in lower than normal concentrations of circulating oestrogen in some women. This may result in inadequate suppression of ovulation.[6] However, although the penicillins reduce *urinary* oestriol secretion in pregnant women,[15-19] no marked changes in *serum* ethinylestradiol levels have been found in controlled studies in women taking an oral contraceptive with ampicillin or any other broad-spectrum antibacterial (see 'tetracyclines', (p.983), 'macrolides', (p.979), 'quinolones', (p.982)). It may be that the enterohepatic recirculation of ethinylestradiol is not clinically important: note that women with an ileostomy have normal serum contraceptive steroid levels.[20] Alternatively, it may be that the proportion of women for whom enterohepatic recirculation is important is extremely small.[20] The progestogens do not take part in enterohepatic recirculation in their active forms.

Importance and management

The interaction between combined hormonal contraceptives and penicillins is inadequately established and controversial. Almost all of the evidence is anecdotal with no controls. The total number of failures is extremely small when viewed against the number of women worldwide using combined hormonal contraceptives (estimated at 70 million in 1996 by WHO[21]), so most women are apparently not at risk.

On the other hand, the personal and ethical consequences of an unwanted pregnancy can be very serious. For this reason, the Faculty of Family Planning and Reproductive Health Care (FFPRHC) Clinical Effectiveness Unit recommends that women taking combined hormonal contraceptives should routinely use a second form of contraception, such as condoms, while taking a short course of less than 3 weeks of an antibacterial,[22] and for 7 days after the antibacterial has been stopped.[22] In addition, the FFPRHC recommends that if fewer than 7 active pills are left in the pack after the antibacterial has been stopped, the new packet should be started without a pill-free break, omitting any of the inactive tablets. For patients using the combined contraceptive patch, if the 7 days after the antibacterial has been stopped runs into the usual 7 day patch-free period, a new patch should be applied when it is due to be changed and the patch-free week delayed by 7 days.[22]

Although this advice has previously only been applied to broad-spectrum antibacterials that do not induce liver enzymes the FFPRHC notes that some confusion has occurred over which antibacterials are considered to be 'broad-spectrum', and thus they recommend that this advice is applied to all antibacterials that do not induce liver enzymes, which would include penicillins.[22] However, others contend that these instructions may confuse patients, and complicate pill taking, and could have the opposite effect of increasing the failure rate of oral contraceptives.[23]

The FFPRHC also says that after 3 weeks of treatment the gut flora becomes resistant to the antibacterial. Therefore women taking a long-term antibacterial that does not induce liver enzymes (for example, for acne) no longer need additional contraceptive protection after the initial 3 weeks of concurrent use. However, if the antibacterial is changed or another antibacterial is started, additional contraceptive cover is required. Women who have already been taking long-term antibacterials that do not induce liver enzymes, who start a combined hormonal contraceptive, do not require additional contraception, unless the antibacterial is changed.[22]

Note that antibacterials that do not induce liver enzymes do not affect the reliability of the **progestogen-only contraceptives**, see 'Progestogen-only contraceptives + Antibacterials', p.1007, or the progestogen-only **emergency hormonal contraceptive**, see 'Emergency hormonal contraceptives + Antibacterials', p.977.

1. Dossetor J. Drug interactions with oral contraceptives. *BMJ* (1975) 4, 467–8.
2. Dossetor J. Personal communication, 1975.
3. Silber TJ. Apparent oral contraceptive failure associated with antibiotic administration. *J Adolesc Health Care* (1983) 4, 287–9.
4. Bainton R. Interaction between antibiotic therapy and contraceptive medication. *Oral Surg Oral Med Oral Pathol* (1986) 61, 453–5.
5. Back DJ, Grimmer SFM, Orme ML'E, Proudlove C, Mann RD, Breckenridge AM. Evaluation of Committee on Safety of Medicines yellow card reports on oral contraceptive-drug interactions with anticonvulsants and antibiotics. *Br J Clin Pharmacol* (1988) 25, 527–32.
6. Back DJ, Breckenridge AM, Crawford FE, MacIver M, Orme ML'E, Rowe PH. Interindividual variation and drug interactions with hormonal steroid contraceptives. *Drugs* (1981) 21, 46–61.
7. Sparrow MJ. Pill method failures. *N Z Med J* (1987) 100, 102–5.
8. Sparrow MJ. Pregnancies in reliable pill takers. *N Z Med J* (1989) 102, 575–7.

9. Kovacs GT, Riddoch G, Duncombe P, Welberry L, Chick P, Weisberg E, Leavesley GM, Baker HWG. Inadvertent pregnancies in oral contraceptive users. *Med J Aust* (1989) 150, 549–51.
10. Kakouris H, Kovacs GT. Pill failure and non-use of secondary precautions. *Br J Fam Plann* (1992) 18, 41–4.
11. Friedman CI, Huneke AL, Kim MH, Powell J. The effect of ampicillin on oral contraceptive effectiveness. *Obstet Gynecol* (1980) 55, 33–7.
12. Back DJ, Breckenridge AM, MacIver M, Orme M, Rowe PH, Staiger Ch, Thomas E, Tjia J. The effects of ampicillin on oral contraceptive steroids in women. *Br J Clin Pharmacol* (1982) 14, 43–8.
13. Joshi JV, Joshi UM, Sankholi GM, Krishna U, Mandlekar A, Chowdhury V, Hazari K, Gupta K, Sheth UK, Saxena BN. A study of interaction of low-dose combination oral contraceptive with ampicillin and metronidazole. *Contraception* (1980) 22, 643–52.
14. Dogterom P, van den Heuvel MW, Thomsen T. Absence of pharmacokinetic interactions of the combined contraceptive vaginal ring NuvaRing® with oral amoxicillin or doxycycline in two randomised trials. *Clin Pharmacokinet* (2005) 44, 429–38.
15. Willman K, Pulkkinen MO. Reduced maternal plasma and urinary estriol during ampicillin treatment. *Am J Obstet Gynecol* (1971) 109, 893–6.
16. Tikkanen MJ, Aldercreutz H, Pulkkinen MO. Effect of antibiotics on oestrogen metabolism. *BMJ* (1973) 1, 369.
17. Pulkkinen MO, Willman K. Maternal oestrogen levels during penicillin treatment. *BMJ* (1971) 4, 48.
18. Sybulski S, Maughan GB. Effect of ampicillin administration on estradiol, estriol, and cortisol levels in maternal plasma and on estriol levels in urine. *Am J Obstet Gynecol* (1976) 124, 379–81.
19. Trybuchowski H. Effect of ampicillin on the urinary output of steroidal hormones in pregnant and non-pregnant women. *Clin Chim Acta* (1973) 45, 9–18.
20. Orme M, Back DJ. Oral contraceptive steroids – pharmacological issues of interest to the prescribing physician. *Adv Contracept* (1991) 7, 325–31.
21. WHO. New program research on the safety of oral contraceptive pills. Available at: http://www.who.int/reproductive-health/hrp/progress/39/prog39.pdf (accessed 23/08/07).
22. Faculty of Family Planning and Reproductive Health Care Clinical Effectiveness Unit. FFPRHC Guidance: Drug interactions with hormonal contraception. April 2005. Available at: http://www.ffprhc.org.uk/admin/uploads/DrugInteractionsFinal.pdf (accessed 23/08/07).
23. Weaver K, Glasier A. Interaction between broad-spectrum antibiotics and the combined oral contraceptive pill. *Contraception* (1999) 59, 71–8.

Hormonal contraceptives + Antibacterials; Quinolones

Ciprofloxacin, moxifloxacin and ofloxacin have been shown not to affect the pharmacokinetics of combined oral contraceptives in controlled studies. No cases of contraceptive failure appear to have been reported, and ovarian suppression is not affected. The plasma levels of moxifloxacin may be modestly reduced by combined oral contraceptives.

Clinical evidence

(a) Ciprofloxacin

No ovulation occurred (as assessed by LH, FSH and estradiol levels) in 10 healthy women taking a combined oral contraceptive (**ethinylestradiol** plus **desogestrel**, **gestodene** or **levonorgestrel**) with ciprofloxacin 500 mg twice daily for 7 days (started on the first day of contraceptive intake). No breakthrough bleeding occurred.[1] Another study in 24 healthy women taking a combined oral contraceptive (**ethinylestradiol/desogestrel**) found that ciprofloxacin 500 mg twice daily for 10 days had no effect on the pharmacokinetics of **ethinylestradiol**. In addition, no subject ovulated, as assessed by progesterone and estradiol levels. However, 2 of the subjects were potentially ovulatory while taking a placebo instead of ciprofloxacin, as detected by an ultrasound of ovarian activity. A further 4 subjects taking ciprofloxacin and 2 taking placebo had lesser indications of ovarian activity.[2]

(b) Moxifloxacin

A placebo-controlled, crossover study in 29 young healthy women taking a combined oral contraceptive (**ethinylestradiol/levonorgestrel**) found that moxifloxacin 400 mg daily on cycle days 1 to 7 had no clinically relevant effect on the pharmacokinetics of either contraceptive steroid. The hormonal parameters measured (estradiol, progesterone, LH, FSH) were also unchanged by the presence of the quinolone, indicating that ovulation continued to be suppressed.[3] Another study looking at the effects of combined oral contraceptives (unspecified) on the pharmacokinetics of a single 400-mg dose of moxifloxacin found that the total oral clearance of moxifloxacin was increased by 20% and its AUC and maximum plasma concentrations were reduced by approximately 15%. This was not considered to be clinically significant except in cases of borderline sensitivity of the bacteria to the drug.[4]

(c) Ofloxacin

Ofloxacin had no effect on the suppression of ovulation in 19 women taking a combined oral contraceptive (**ethinylestradiol/levonorgestrel**). In this placebo-controlled, crossover study, two courses of ofloxacin 200 mg twice daily for 7 days were given on days 1 to 7 of two consecutive contraceptive cycles. Ovulation was assessed by ultrasound of the ovaries, and by measuring FSH, estradiol and progesterone levels. Four of the women showed signs of ovarian activity in both the placebo and ofloxacin cycles.[5]

Mechanism

The fluoroquinolones are broad-spectrum antibacterials, and so might be expected to interrupt the enterohepatic recirculation of ethinylestradiol,[1,6] but the evidence that this is clinically important is scant (for a more detailed discussion of this mechanism see 'Hormonal contraceptives + Antibacterials; Penicillins', p.981).

Importance and management

The pharmacokinetic and pharmacodynamic data indicate a likely absence of interactions between combined oral contraceptives and these quinolones. In addition, reports of cases of contraceptive failure with these or any other quinolone antibacterial seem to be lacking. No special extra contraceptive precautions would therefore seem to be necessary during concurrent use. However, if one accepts the theory that there are an as yet unidentifiable tiny group of women for whom enterohepatic recirculation of ethinylestradiol is important, then it could be argued that insufficient patients were assessed in the above studies to include anyone from this group, and that the general precautions should be applied. However, if one tends to the theory that the anecdotal cases of contraceptive failure with broad-spectrum antibacterials are indistinguishable from the normal accepted failure rate, no special precautions are necessary with these quinolones, or indeed, any other antibacterials that do not induce liver enzymes. The Faculty of Family Planning and Reproductive Health Care (FFPRHC) Clinical Effectiveness Unit has issued guidance on the use of antibacterials with hormonal contraceptives. Although they recognise that there is poor evidence for contraceptive failure, they recommend that additional contraceptives, such as condoms, should be used for short courses of antibacterials, see 'Hormonal contraceptives + Antibacterials; Penicillins', p.981, for more detailed information. This applies to both the oral and the patch form of the combined contraceptive. This advice has usually been applied to only broad-spectrum non-liver enzyme-inducing antibacterials but the FFPRHC notes that some confusion has occurred over which antibacterials are considered to be 'broad-spectrum', and thus they recommend that this advice is applied to all antibacterials that do not induce liver enzymes, which would include the quinolones.[7]

Note that antibacterials that do not induce liver enzymes do not affect the reliability of the **progestogen-only contraceptives**, see 'Progestogen-only contraceptives + Antibacterials, p.1007, or the progestogen-only **emergency hormonal contraceptive**, see 'Emergency hormonal contraceptives + Antibacterials', p.977.

1. Maggiolo F, Puricelli G, Dottorini M, Caprioli S, Bianchi W, Suter F. The effect of ciprofloxacin on oral contraceptive steroid treatments. *Drugs Exp Clin Res* (1991) 17, 451–4.
2. Scholten PC, Droppert RM, Zwinkels MGJ, Moesker HL, Nauta JJP, Hoepelman IM. No interaction between ciprofloxacin and an oral contraceptive. *Antimicrob Agents Chemother* (1998) 42, 3266–8.
3. Staß H, Sachse R, Heinig R, Zühlsdorf M, Horstmann R. Pharmacokinetics (PK) of steroid hormones in oral contraceptives (OC) are not altered by oral moxifloxacin (MOX). *J Antimicrob Chemother* (1999) 44 (Suppl A) 138–9.
4. Shain CS, Whitaker A-M, Amsden GW. Effects of oral contraceptives on the pharmacokinetics of moxifloxacin in premenopausal women. *Clin Drug Invest* (2002) 22, 429–34.
5. Csemiczky G, Alvendal C, Landgren B-M. Risk for ovulation in women taking a low-dose oral contraceptive (Microgynon) when receiving antibacterial treatment with a fluoroquinolone (ofloxacin). *Adv Contracept* (1996) 12, 101–9.
6. Back DJ, Tija J, Martin C, Millar E, Mant T, Morrison P, Orme M. The lack of interaction between temafloxacin and combined oral contraceptive steroids. *Contraception* (1991) 43, 317–23.
7. Faculty of Family Planning and Reproductive Health Care Clinical Effectiveness Unit. FFPRHC Guidance: Drug interactions with hormonal contraception. April 2005. Available at: http://www.ffprhc.org.uk/admin/uploads/DrugInteractionsFinal.pdf (accessed 23/08/07).

Hormonal contraceptives + Antibacterials; Sulfonamides and/or Trimethoprim

Co-trimoxazole (sulfamethoxazole/trimethoprim) *increases* ethinylestradiol levels. However, there are about 15 anecdotal cases on record of contraceptive failure attributed to co-trimoxazole. There are also isolated cases of contraceptive failure attributed to various sulfonamides and trimethoprim.

Clinical evidence

(a) Co-trimoxazole

In a study in 9 women taking a triphasic combined oral contraceptive (**ethinylestradiol/levonorgestrel**) the use of co-trimoxazole (trimethoprim/sulfamethoxazole) 960 mg twice daily for 7 days starting on day 10 of the cycle increased **ethinylestradiol** plasma levels by 30 to 50%. **Levonorgestrel** plasma levels remained unaltered. No subjects ovulated, as assessed by progesterone and FSH levels: FSH levels actually decreased, indicating increased suppression of ovulation.[1]

In contrast, 5 cases of oral contraceptive failure attributed to the use of co-trimoxazole were identified in the adverse reactions register of the CSM in the UK for the years 1968 to 1984 (58 cases were attributed to other antibacterials).[2,3] Contraceptive failure has been reported in another 10 patients taking co-trimoxazole,[4-8] and 3 further cases of contraceptive failure are attributed to the use of co-trimoxazole or trimethoprim.[9]

(b) Sulphonamides

One woman taking a combined oral contraceptive is briefly reported to have shown breakthrough bleeding and to have become pregnant while taking **sulfamethoxypyridazine**.[10,11] One case of a pregnancy, in a woman who had taken a sulphonamide (unspecified) and an oral contraceptive (unspecified), was identified in the adverse reactions register of the CSM in the UK for the years 1968 to 1984 (a total of 62 cases were attributed to other antibacterials).[3] Three further cases of failure have been attributed to the use of **sulfafurazole** (**sulfisoxazole**) and a sulphonamide (unspecified).[12]

(c) Trimethoprim

Two pregnancies were attributed to the use of trimethoprim with an oral contraceptive (unspecified) in the adverse reactions register of the CSM in the UK for the years 1968 to 1984 (a total of 61 cases were attributed to other antibacterials).[3] Another survey of oral contraceptive failure identified one pregnancy due to trimethoprim (23 of a total of 137 cases were attributed to antibacterials),[6] while an earlier survey attributed 3 cases of contraceptive failure to either **co-trimoxazole** or trimethoprim.[9] One case with trimethoprim and one with trimethoprim plus nitrofurantoin are briefly mentioned in another report.[7]

Mechanism

A possible explanation for the rise in ethinylestradiol levels is that co-trimoxazole inhibits the liver enzymes concerned with the metabolism of this oestrogen. Broad-spectrum antibacterials might be expected to interrupt the enterohepatic recirculation of ethinylestradiol leading to contraceptive failure, but the evidence that this is clinically important is scant (see also 'Hormonal contraceptives + Antibacterials; Penicillins', p.981).

Importance and management

Not established. The pharmacokinetic and pharmacodynamic evidence indicates that co-trimoxazole is not likely to reduce the effectiveness of combined oral contraceptives. Although there are a number of reports of contraceptive failure attributed to co-trimoxazole, these are anecdotal and unconfirmed, whereas the studies suggest *increased* contraceptive efficacy (but see below). It is possible that the cases are coincidental, and fit within the normal failure rate of combined oral contraceptives. The UK Family Planning Authority considered that it was almost certain that co-trimoxazole and sulphonamides did not interact with combined oral contraceptives.[13] However, the Faculty of Family Planning and Reproductive Health Care (FFPRHC) Clinical Effectiveness Unit has issued guidance on the use of antibacterials with hormonal contraceptives. Although they recognise that there is poor evidence for contraceptive failure, they recommend that additional contraceptives, such as condoms, should be used for short courses of antibacterials, see 'Hormonal contraceptives + Antibacterials; Penicillins', p.981, for more detailed information. This applies to both the oral and the patch form of the combined contraceptive. This advice has usually been applied to only broad-spectrum antibacterials that do not induce liver enzymes but the FFPRHC notes that some confusion has occurred over which antibacterials are considered to be 'broad-spectrum', and thus they recommend that this advice is applied to all antibacterials that do not induce liver enzymes, which would include co-trimoxazole, sulfonamides and trimethoprim.[14]

Note that antibacterials that do not induce liver enzymes do not affect the reliability of the **progestogen-only contraceptives**, see 'Progestogen-only contraceptives + Antibacterials, p.1007, or the progestogen-only **emergency hormonal contraceptive**, see 'Emergency hormonal contraceptives + Antibacterials', p.977.

Aside from contraceptive failure the other aspect of using this drug combination is the potential for increased ethinylestradiol levels. The main concern is whether this would increase the risk of adverse effects of the oestrogen, but there are no data on the clinical significance of these modest (30 to 50%) increases on various adverse effects. It could be argued that a 40% increase would turn a standard-strength contraceptive (35 micrograms) into a high-dose contraceptive (50 micrograms). However, early studies showed that the interindividual variation in ethinylestradiol pharmacokinetics was greater than this anyway.[2] Further study is needed on this issue.

1. Grimmer SFM, Allen WL, Back DJ, Breckenridge AM, Orme M, Tjia J. The effect of cotrimoxazole on oral contraceptive steroids in women. *Contraception* (1983) 28, 53–9.
2. Back DJ, Breckenridge AM, Crawford FE, MacIver M, Orme ML'E, Rowe PH. Interindividual variation and drug interactions with hormonal steroid contraceptives. *Drugs* (1981) 21, 46–61.
3. Back DJ, Grimmer SFM, Orme ML'E, Proudlove C, Mann RD, Breckenridge AM. Evaluation of Committee on Safety of Medicines yellow card reports on oral contraceptive-drug interactions with anticonvulsants and antibiotics. *Br J Clin Pharmacol* (1988) 25, 527–32.
4. Beeley L, Magee P, Hickey FM. *Bulletin of the West Midlands Centre for Adverse Drug Reaction Reporting* (1989) 28, 32.
5. Kovacs GT, Riddoch G, Duncombe P, Welberry L, Chick P, Weisberg E, Leavesley GM, Baker HWG. Inadvertent pregnancies in oral contraceptive users. *Med J Aust* (1989) 150, 549–51.
6. Sparrow MJ. Pregnancies in reliable pill takers. *N Z Med J* (1989) 102, 575–7.
7. De Groot AC, Eshuis H, Stricker BHC. Ineffectiviteit van orale anticonceptie tijdens gebruik van minocycline. *Ned Tijdschr Geneeskd* (1990) 134, 1227–9.
8. Kakouris H, Kovacs GT. Pill failure and non-use of secondary precautions. *Br J Fam Plann* (1992) 18, 41–4.
9. Sparrow MJ. Pill method failures. *N Z Med J* (1987) 100, 102–5.
10. Hempel E, Böhm W, Carol W, Klinger G. Medikamentöse enzyminduktion und hormonale kontrazeption. *Zentralbl Gynakol* (1973) 95, 1451–7.
11. Hempel E. Personal communication, 1975.
12. DeSano EA, Hurley SC. Possible interactions of antihistamines and antibiotics with oral contraceptive effectiveness. *Fertil Steril* (1982) 37, 853–4.
13. Belfield T, ed. FPA Contraceptive Handbook: a guide for family planning and other health professionals. 3rd ed. London: Family Planning Association, 1999.
14. Faculty of Family Planning and Reproductive Health Care Clinical Effectiveness Unit. FFPRHC Guidance: Drug interactions with hormonal contraception. April 2005. Available at: http://www.ffprhc.org.uk/admin/uploads/DrugInteractionsFinal.pdf (accessed 23/08/07).

Hormonal contraceptives + Antibacterials; Tetracyclines

Contraceptive failure has been attributed to doxycycline, lymecycline, minocycline, oxytetracycline and tetracycline in about 40 reported cases, 7 of which specified long-term antibacterial use, but the interaction (if such it is) appears to be rare. Controlled studies have not shown any effect of tetracycline or doxycycline on contraceptive steroid levels.

Clinical evidence

A woman taking a combined oral contraceptive (**ethinylestradiol** with **levonorgestrel**) became pregnant, the evidence indicating that she had conceived during or in the week after taking **tetracycline** 500 mg every 6 hours for 3 days and then 250 mg every 6 hours for 2 days. There was no evidence of either nausea or vomiting, which might have been an alternative explanation for the contraceptive failure.[1] A case of breakthrough bleeding attributed to **tetracycline** was also mentioned in this report.[1] Two other case reports describe pregnancies in women taking a combined oral contraceptive and long-term **tetracycline** 500 mg daily[2] or long-term **minocycline** 100 mg daily.[3] The latter also briefly mentions 2 cases of contraceptive failure with **doxycycline**.[3]

Twelve reports of pregnancies were attributed to the use of tetracyclines (unspecified) and an oral contraceptive (unspecified) in the adverse reactions register of the CSM in the UK for the years 1968 to 1984 (51 cases were attributed to other antibacterials).[4] In an earlier report, the tetracyclines in 6 cases were named as **tetracycline** and **oxytetracycline**.[5] A survey of oral contraceptive failure identified 7 failures due to **doxycycline**, **lymecycline** or **minocycline** (37 of a total of 163 cases were attributed to antibacterials),[6] and a follow-up survey identified 3 further cases involving short courses of **tetracycline**.[7] Similar surveys identified 5 contraceptive failures with **tetracycline**,[8-10] and 2 failures with **doxycycline**.[9] Breakthrough bleeding was attributed to **doxycycline** or **oxytetracycline** in 3 other cases.[11]

In a dermatological practice, of 124 women taking an oral contraceptive and antibacterials (mostly tetracyclines or erythromycin), 2 became pregnant, with a calculated failure rate of 1.2%. One patient was taking long-term **minocycline** and **ethinylestradiol/norethisterone**, and one had taken a 5-day course of **oxytetracycline** while taking **ethinylestradiol/levonorgestrel**. This failure rate was reported to be sixfold higher than a normal failure rate of 0.2%.[12] However, a rate of 0.2% represents perfect rather than typical use of combined oral contraceptives. In a similar analysis,[13] one of 34 women became pregnant after taking long-term **tetracycline** and **ethinylestradiol/norethisterone**. This failure rate of 1.4% was not considered to be significantly different from a normal failure rate of 0.27%. In a larger, better-designed, case-control study, 356 women were identified who had received oral contraceptives and antibacterials (cephalosporins, penicillins, tetracyclines) over a 5-year period in 3 dermatological practices. The failure rate in these women (1.6% per year, 3 pregnancies occurred in women taking long-term **minocycline** and 2 taking a cephalosporin) was indistinguishable from the failure rate seen in control patients taking oral contraceptives and no antibacterials (1% per year).[14]

Moreover, two controlled studies have shown that tetracyclines do not affect the pharmacokinetics of contraceptive steroids.[15,16] In the first, in 7 healthy women taking a combined oral contraceptive, **tetracycline** 500 mg every 6 hours for 10 days had no effect on the AUC of **ethinylestradiol** and **norethisterone** (measured on days 1, 5 and 10).[15] Similarly, in 23 healthy women taking a combined oral contraceptive, **doxycycline** 100 mg twice daily for 7 days had no effect on the serum levels of **ethinylestradiol** and **norethisterone** (measured on days 5 to 7). In addition, ovulation did not occur, as assessed by progesterone levels, but 2 women did experience breakthrough bleeding.[16] A further study has found no pharmacokinetic interaction between a combined contraceptive patch and **tetracycline**.[17] A crossover study involving 16 healthy women also found that a 10-day course of **doxycycline** did not affect **etonogestrel** or **ethinylestradiol** released from the *NuvaRing* vaginal contraceptive ring.[18]

The pharmacokinetics of **tetracycline** (4-hour AUC and peak level) were not significantly different between 7 healthy women taking a combined oral contraceptive (**ethinylestradiol/norethisterone**) and 4 healthy women not taking any medication.[15] For reports of facial pigmentation due to **minocycline** and **ethinylestradiol**, see 'Tetracyclines; Minocycline + Ethinylestradiol', p.350.

Mechanism

Not understood. If an interaction occurs, suppression of intestinal bacteria resulting in a fall in enterohepatic recirculation of ethinylestradiol is the usual suggested explanation, but there is no evidence that this is clinically important. For a full discussion of this mechanism, see 'Hormonal contraceptives + Antibacterials; Penicillins', p.981.

Importance and management

The interactions between the oral contraceptives and tetracyclines summarised here are all that have been identified in the literature. Much of the evidence is anecdotal with insufficient controls (if any). These interactions are not adequately established and the whole issue remains controversial. Bearing in mind the extremely wide use of both drugs, any increase in the incidence of contraceptive failure above the accepted failure rate is clearly very low indeed. On the other hand, the personal and ethical consequences of an unwanted pregnancy can be very serious. For this reason, the Faculty of Family Planning and Reproductive Health Care (FFPRHC) Clinical Effectiveness Unit recommends that an additional form of contraception, such as condoms, should be used while taking a short course of antibacterials that do not induce liver enzymes, and for 7 days after the antibacterial has been stopped.[19] See 'Hormonal contraceptives + Antibacterials; Penicillins', p.981, for more detailed information on how to manage this interaction.

In the case of long-term use of tetracyclines for acne, at least 7 cases of contraceptive failure have been reported. Nevertheless, in statistical terms the only well-designed case-controlled study in dermatological practice indicated that the incidence of contraceptive failure due to this interaction could not be distinguished from the general and recognised failure rate of oral contraceptives.[14]

The FFPRHC advise that additional contraceptive protection is not required in established users of the combined hormonal contraceptive patch taking tetracycline.[19] This is in line with the findings of the study cited above.

Note that antibacterials that do not induce liver enzymes do not affect the reliability of the **progestogen-only contraceptives**, see 'Progestogen-only contraceptives + Antibacterials, p.1007, or the progestogen-only **emergency hormonal contraceptive**, see 'Emergency hormonal contraceptives + Antibacterials', p.977.

1. Bacon JF, Shenfield GM. Pregnancy attributable to interaction between tetracycline and oral contraceptives. *BMJ* (1980) 1, 293.
2. Lequeux A. Grossesse sous contraceptif oral après prise de tétracycline. *Louvain Med* (1980) 99, 413–14.
3. de Groot AC, Eshuis H, Stricker BHC. Ineffectiviteit van orale anticonceptie tijdens gebruik van minocycline. *Ned Tijdschr Geneeskd* (1990) 134, 1227–9.
4. Back DJ, Grimmer SFM, Orme ML'E, Proudlove C, Mann RD, Breckenridge AM. Evaluation of Committee on Safety of Medicines yellow card reports on oral contraceptive-drug interactions with anticonvulsants and antibiotics. *Br J Clin Pharmacol* (1988) 25, 527–32.
5. Back DJ, Breckenridge AM, Crawford FE, MacIver M, Orme ML'E, Rowe PH. Interindividual variation and drug interactions with hormonal steroid contraceptives. *Drugs* (1981) 21, 46–61.
6. Sparrow MJ. Pill method failures. *N Z Med J* (1987) 100, 102–5.
7. Sparrow MJ. Pregnancies in reliable pill takers. *N Z Med J* (1989) 102, 575–7.
8. Kovacs GT, Riddoch G, Duncombe P, Welberry L, Chick P, Weisberg E, Leavesley GM, Baker HWG. Inadvertent pregnancies in oral contraceptive users. *Med J Aust* (1989) 150, 549–51.
9. Kakouris H, Kovacs GT. Pill failure and non-use of secondary precautions. *Br J Fam Plann* (1992) 18, 41–4.
10. DeSano EA, Hurley SC. Possible interactions of antihistamines and antibiotics with oral contraceptive effectiveness. *Fertil Steril* (1982) 37, 853–4.
11. Hetényi G. Possible interactions between antibiotics and oral contraceptives. *Ther Hung* (1989) 37, 86–9.
12. Hughes BR, Cunliffe WJ. Interactions between the oral contraceptive pill and antibiotics. *Br J Dermatol* (1990) 122, 717.
13. London BM, Lookingbill DP. Frequency of pregnancy in acne patients taking oral antibiotics and oral contraceptives. *Arch Dermatol* (1994) 130, 392–3.
14. Helms SE, Bredle DL, Zajic J, Jarjoura D, Brodell RT, Krishnarao I. Oral contraceptive failure rates and oral antibiotics. *J Am Acad Dermatol* (1997) 36, 705–10.
15. Murphy AA, Zacur HA, Charache P, Burkman RT. The effect of tetracycline on levels of oral contraceptives. *Am J Obstet Gynecol* (1991) 164, 28–33.
16. Neely JL, Abate M, Swinker M, D'Angio R. The effect of doxycycline on serum levels of ethinyl estradiol, norethindrone, and endogenous progesterone. *Obstet Gynecol* (1991) 77, 416–20.
17. Abrams LS, Skee D, Natarajan J, Hutman W, Wong F. Tetracycline HCl does not affect the pharmacokinetics of a contraceptive patch. *Int J Gynaecol Obstet* (2000) 70, 57–8.
18. Dogterom P, van den Heuvel MW, Thomsen T. Absence of pharmacokinetic interactions of the combined contraceptive vaginal ring NuvaRing® with oral amoxicillin or doxycycline in two randomised trials. *Clin Pharmacokinet* (2005) 44, 429–438.
19. Faculty of Family Planning and Reproductive Health Care Clinical Effectiveness Unit. FFPRHC Guidance: Drug interactions with hormonal contraception. April 2005. Available at: http://www.ffprhc.org.uk/admin/uploads/DrugInteractionsFinal.pdf (accessed 23/08/07).

Hormonal contraceptives or HRT + Antibacterials; Troleandomycin

Severe pruritus and jaundice have been observed in women taking oral contraceptives shortly after starting treatment with troleandomycin. One case has also been reported with oestrogens for HRT.

Clinical evidence

A report describes 10 cases of cholestatic jaundice and pruritus in women taking oral contraceptives and troleandomycin. All had been using the contraceptive for 7 to 48 months and were given the antibacterial in daily doses of 1 to 3 g. The pruritus was intense, and started within 2 to 24 days of the first dose of troleandomycin, and preceding the jaundice. In 8 of the patients the pruritus and jaundice persisted for over a month.[1] A later report and letter by the same authors describes a total of 24 cases of this reaction.[2,3]

There are numerous other reports of this adverse reaction in a total of over 40 other women.[4-12] The adverse reactions (fatigue, anorexia, severe itching, jaundice) can begin very rapidly, sometimes even within 2 days of starting the troleandomycin, and may last up to 14 weeks or more.[3,4,12] One report also describes a similar reaction in a 48-year-old woman taking **oestrogens** for HRT.[4]

Mechanism

Uncertain. Hepatotoxicity has been associated with the use of both types of drug, but it is not common. The reaction suggests that their damaging effects on the liver may be additive or synergistic.[10,11] Troleandomycin may cause an increase in levels of contraceptive steroids, since it is an liver enzyme inhibitor.[12,13]

Importance and management

A well established, well documented and clinically important interaction. The incidence is unknown. Concurrent use should be avoided. Other macrolides may be suitable alternatives, but see 'Hormonal contraceptives + Antibacterials; Macrolides', p.979.

1. Miguet JP, Monange C, Vuitton D, Allemand H, Hirsch JP, Carayon P, Gisselbrecht H. Ictère cholestatique survenu après administration de triacétyloléandomycine: interférence avec les contraceptifs oraux? Dix observations. *Nouv Presse Med* (1978) 7, 4304.
2. Miguet J-P, Vuitton D, Pessayre D, Allemand H, Metreau J-M, Poupon R, Capron J-P, Blanc F. Jaundice from troleandomycin and oral contraceptives. *Ann Intern Med* (1980) 92, 434.
3. Miguet J-P, Vuitton D, Allemand H, Pessayre D, Monange C, Hirsch J-P, Metreau J-M, Poupon R, Capron J-P, Blanc F. Une épidémie d'ictères due a l'association troléandomycine – contraceptifs oraux. *Gastroenterol Clin Biol* (1980) 4, 420–4.
4. Perol R, Hincky J, Desnos M. Hépatites cholestatiques lors de la prise de troléandomycine chez deux femmes prenant des estrogènes. *Nouv Presse Med* (1978) 7, 4302.
5. Goldfain D, Chauveinc L, Guillan J, Verduron J. Ictère cholestatique chez des femmes prenant simultanément de la triacétyloléandomycine et des contraceptifs oraux. *Nouv Presse Med* (1979) 8, 1099.
6. Rollux R, Plottin F, Mingat J, Bessard G. Ictère apres association estroprogestatif-troléandomycine. Trois observations. *Nouv Presse Med* (1979) 8, 1694.
7. Haber I, Hubens H. Cholestatic jaundice after triacetyloleandomycin and oral contraceptives. *Acta Gastroenterol Belg* (1980) 43, 475–82.
8. Descotes J, Evreux JC, Foyatier N, Gaumer R, Girard D, Savoye B. Trois nouvelles observations d'ictère après estroprogestatifs et troléandomycine. *Nouv Presse Med* (1979) 8, 1182–3.
9. Belgian Centre for Drug Supervison. Levertoxiciteit van troleandomycine en oestrogen. *Folia Pharmaceutica (Brussels)* (1979) 6, 64.
10. Dellas JA, Hugues FC, Roussel G, Marche J. Contraception orale et troléandomycine. Un nouveau cas d'ictère. *Therapie* (1982) 37, 443–6.
11. Girard D, Pillon M, Bel A, Petigny A, Savoye B. Hepatite au decours d'un traitment a la triacetyloleandomycine chez les jeunes femmes sous estro-progestatifs. *Lyon Mediterr Med Med Sud Est* (1980) 16, 2335–44.
12. Fevery J, Van Steenbergen W, Desmet V, Deruyttere M, De Groote J. Severe intrahepatic cholestasis due to the combined intake of oral contraceptives and triacetyloleandomycin. *Acta Clin Belg* (1983) 38, 242–5.
13. Claudel S, Euvrard P, Bory R, Chavaillon A, Paliard P. Cholestase intra-hépatique après association triacétyloléandomycine-estroprogestatif. *Nouv Presse Med* (1979) 8, 1182.

Hormonal contraceptives + Antiepileptics; Barbiturates or Phenytoin

Hormonal contraceptives are less reliable during the use of phenytoin and barbiturates such as phenobarbital and primidone. Intermenstrual breakthrough bleeding and spotting can take place, and pregnancies have occurred. Controlled studies have shown that phenytoin and phenobarbital can reduce contraceptive steroid levels.

Clinical evidence

An epileptic woman taking phenytoin 200 mg and sultiame 50 mg daily (with ferrous gluconate and folic acid) became pregnant despite the regular use of a combined oral contraceptive (**ethinylestradiol/norethisterone** 50 micrograms/3 mg).[1] Since this first report in 1972, at least 33 pregnancies have been reported in the literature in women taking a range of oral contraceptives (mostly combined) and a barbiturate (such as **phenobarbital** or **primidone**) and/or phenytoin (see 'Table 28.2', (p.986)). Note that most of these cases were with a combined oral contraceptive containing at least 50 micrograms of **ethinylestradiol**. In addition, between the years 1968 to 1984, a further 25 pregnancies in women who took phenytoin and an oral contraceptive, and 20 pregnancies in women who took **phenobarbital** and an oral contraceptive were reported to in the CSM in the UK. However, it is unclear how many of these patients were receiving just the antiepileptic mentioned, since the authors note that some women were taking multiple antiepileptics (combinations not stated).[2] Even so, the total number of unwanted pregnancies due to this interaction is fairly large. In this report, over half the cases of contraceptive failure with antiepileptics related to high-dose combined oral contraceptives (50 micrograms of oestrogen). Three were in women taking **progestogen-only oral contraceptives**.[2]

In one study, breakthrough bleeding (which was regarded as loss of reliability of the contraceptive) occurred in 30 of 51 women taking a combined oral contraceptive (**ethinylestradiol/norethisterone** or **mestranol/chlormadinone**) given **phenobarbital**.[3] In another study, 7 out of 11 patients taking **phenobarbital** and 1 of 2 patients taking phenytoin had breakthrough bleeding.[4] The incidence of breakthrough bleeding was 90% with preparations containing **ethinylestradiol** 30 micrograms and 29% with preparations containing 75 micrograms of ethinylestradiol. Similarly, with preparations containing **ethinylestradiol** 50 micrograms, decreasing the dose of **norgestrel** from 500 to 125 micrograms increased breakthrough bleeding from 50% to 62%.[4]

A pharmacokinetic study in 6 women taking a combined oral contraceptive found that the AUCs of **ethinylestradiol** 50 micrograms and **levonorgestrel** 250 micrograms were lowered by 49% and 42%, respectively, by phenytoin 200 to 300 mg daily for 8 to 12 weeks.[5] In another study, **phenobarbital** 30 mg twice daily did not significantly alter the plasma levels of contraceptive steroids in 4 women taking combined oral contraceptives (**ethinylestradiol** with **norethisterone** or **norgestrel**), but 2 of the women did have 54% and 60% falls, respectively, in their **ethinylestradiol** levels. These 2 women had breakthrough bleeding, but ovulation suppression was maintained.[6]

Mechanism

The likeliest explanation for the unreliability and failure of oral contraceptives is that phenytoin and the barbiturates (known potent liver enzyme inducers) increase the metabolism and clearance of the contraceptive steroids from the body, thereby reducing their effects, and in some instances, allowing ovulation to occur.

Importance and management

The interactions between combined oral contraceptives and phenobarbital and phenytoin are clinically important and well documented. As primidone is metabolised to phenobarbital it would be prudent to assume that it will interact similarly. The risk of breakthrough bleeding and spotting is high (bleeding disturbances are usually regarded as an indication of reduced efficacy if cycles were previously regular[7]). However, the actual incidence of contraceptive failure when combined oral contraceptives are given with these drugs is unknown. It appears that the incidence of unintended pregnancies is quite small: in one series, a failure rate of 3.1 per 100 woman years was calculated, compared with an expected 0.7 per 100 woman years.[8] Note that this failure rate is still less than that seen with barrier methods such as condoms.

Reliable contraception in most patients is said to be achievable with ethinylestradiol 80 to 100 micrograms daily.[4,9,10] If these larger doses are required for good cycle control, there should be no increase in adverse effects because the enzyme-inducing effects of the antiepileptics reduce the blood levels of the steroids. However, note that many of the cases of unintended pregnancies were with products containing 50 micrograms of ethinylestradiol or more, and one review of contraceptive interactions suggested that women taking low-dose oestrogen contraceptives may not be at a greater risk of an interaction.[11]

Nevertheless, since the personal and ethical consequences of an unplanned pregnancy can be very serious, it is important to take the necessary practical steps to reduce this increased risk. Moreover, pregnancy in women with epilepsy should ideally be planned so that therapy can be reviewed to minimise the risks of foetal malformation.[9] In this regard, it is of concern that some surveys have shown a lack of knowledge of these interactions and their management among prescribers,[12] and the frequent use of enzyme-inducing antiepileptics with hormonal contraceptives containing less than 50 micrograms of ethinylestradiol.[13] Almost all of the evidence cited here originates from studies with combined oral contraceptives, but the enzyme-inducing antiepileptics can also increase the metabolism of progestogens thereby reducing their efficacy, so that there is also a risk of contraceptive failure with **progestogen-only oral contraceptives**.[14] This is of particular concern since progestogen-only oral contraceptives are not as effective as combined oral contraceptives. Some have suggested at least doubling the dose of the progestogen-only oral contraceptive.[9] However, others consider that this is not an option as it tends to increase the rate of irregular bleeding (a common adverse effect of these contraceptives). They consider that progestogen-only oral contraceptives are not suitable for use in women taking enzyme-inducing antiepileptics.[14,15] The use of an alternative, non-interacting antiepileptic drug should be considered in patients taking hormonal contraceptives. Note that 'ethosuximide', (p.987), 'gabapentin', (p.988), 'lamotrigine', (p.988), 'levetiracetam', (p.989), 'sodium valproate', (p.990), 'tiagabine', (p.990), and 'vigabatrin', (p.991) do not appear to interact with the hormonal contraceptives.

The Faculty of Family Planning and Reproductive Health Care (FFPRHC) Clinical Effectiveness Unit have issued guidance on the use of drugs that induce liver enzyme with hormonal contraceptives:[15]

- Women taking **combined oral contraceptives** should use an ethinylestradiol dose of at least 50 micrograms daily. The dose may be increased further above 50 micrograms if breakthrough bleeding occurs. Omitting or reducing the pill-free interval has not been shown to reduce the risk of ovulation with liver enzyme inducers. Additional non-hormonal methods of contraception, such as condoms, should also be used by patients using combined hormonal contraceptives, both when taking the

Table 28.2 Case reports of pregnancies in women taking hormonal contraceptives with barbiturates and/or phenytoin

Antiepileptic	*Oestrogen*	*Progestogen*	*Number of cases*	*Refs*
Phenytoin + Sultiame	Ethinylestradiol 50 micrograms	Norethisterone 3 mg	1	1
Phenytoin + Primidone, Phenobarbital or Methylphenobarbital	Not stated	Not stated	7	2, 3
Primidone	Ethinylestradiol 50 or 100 micrograms	Norgestrel 0.5 mg or Megestrol 1 mg	2	4, 5
Phenytoin + Primidone or Phenobarbital	Ethinylestradiol 50 micrograms	Norgestrel 0.25 or 0.5 mg or Norethisterone 1 mg	3	4, 5
Phenytoin + Primidone or Phenobarbital + Other	Ethinylestradiol 50 micrograms	Norgestrel 0.5 mg	2	4, 5
Phenytoin + Carbamazepine	Ethinylestradiol 50 micrograms	Norgestrel 0.25 mg	1	4, 5
Primidone or Phenobarbital	Ethinylestradiol	Norgestrel	3	6
Phenobarbital or Butobarbital	Ethinylestradiol or Mestranol	Norethisterone	3	7
Phenytoin	Ethinylestradiol 100 micrograms	Dimethisterone 25 mg	1	8
Phenobarbital or Methylphenobarbital	Ethinylestradiol 50 micrograms or Mestranol 80 micrograms	Etynodiol 1 mg or Chlormadinone 2 mg	2	8
Phenytoin + Phenobarbital	Mestranol 100 micrograms	Noretynodrel 2.5 mg	1	8
Phenobarbital	Ethinylestradiol 50 micrograms	Desogestrel 75 mg	1	9
Phenytoin + Phenobarbital	Ethinylestradiol	Levonorgestrel	1	10
Phenytoin then Carbamazepine	Ethinylestradiol	Lynestrol	1	10
Phenytoin with or without other antiepileptics	Ethinylestradiol 30 or 50 micrograms or Mestranol 50 micrograms	Megestrol, Norethisterone, Etynodiol, Norgestrel or Levonorgestrel	25	11
Phenobarbital with or without other antiepileptics		Progestogen-only pill	20	11
Phenytoin	Ethinylestradiol 50 micrograms	Not stated	1	12
Phenytoin	Ethinylestradiol less than 50 micrograms	Not stated	2	13
Phenobarbital	Ethinylestradiol 35 micrograms ('back up' contraception also used)	Norgestimate 0.18 to 0.25 mg	1	14

1. Kenyon IE. Unplanned pregnancy in an epileptic. *BMJ* (1972) 1, 686–7.
2. Hempel E, Böhm W, Carol W, Klinger G. Medikamentöse Enzyminduktion und hormonale Kontrazeption. *Zentralbl Gynakol* (1973) 95, 1451–7.
3. Hempel E, Klinger W. Drug stimulated biotransformation of hormonal steroid contraceptives: clinical implications. *Drugs* (1976) 12, 442–8.
4. Janz D, Schmidt D. Anti-epileptic drugs and failure of oral contraceptives. *Lancet* (1974) i, 1113.
5. Janz D, Schmidt D. Antiepileptika und die Sicherheit oraler Kontrazeptiva. *Bibl Psychiatr* (1975) 151, 82–5.
6. Belaisch J, Driguez P, Janaud A. Influence de certains médicaments sur l'action des pilules contraceptives. *Nouv Presse Med* (1976) 5, 1645–6.
7. Gagnaire JC, Tchertchian J, Revol A, Rochet Y. Grossesses sous contraceptifs oraux chez les patientes recevant des barbituriques. *Nouv Presse Med* (1975) 4, 3008.
8. Coulam CB, Annegers JF. Do anticonvulsants reduce the efficacy of oral contraceptives? *Epilepsia* (1979) 20, 519–26.
9. Fanøe E. P-pillesvigt – antagelig på grund af interaktion med fenemal. *Ugeskr Laeger* (1977) 139, 1485.
10. Sparrow MJ. Pill method failures. *N Z Med J* (1987) 100, 102–5.
11. Back DJ, Grimmer FM, Orme ML'E, Proudlove C, Mann RD, Breckenridge AM. Evaluation of Committee on Safety of Medicines yellow card reports on oral contraceptive-drug interactions with anticonvulsants and antibiotics. *Br J Clin Pharmacol* (1988) 25, 527–32.
12. Kovacs GT, Riddoch G, Duncombe P, Welberry L, Chick P, Weisberg E, Leavesley GM, Baker HWG. Inadvertent pregnancies in oral contraceptive users. *Med J Aust* (1989) 150, 549–51.
13. van der Graaf WT, van Loon AJ, Postmus PE, Sleijfer DT. Twee patiënten met hersenmetastasen die zwanger werden tijdens fenytoïnegebruik. *Ned Tijdschr Geneeskd* (1992) 136, 2236–8.
14. Shane-McWhorter L, Cerveny JD, MacFarlane LL, Osborn C. Enhanced metabolism of levonorgestrel during phenobarbital treatment and resultant pregnancy. *Pharmacotherapy* (1998) 18, 1360–4.

liver enzyme inducers and for at least 4 weeks after stopping the drug. Alternatives to all forms of combined hormonal contraceptives should be considered with long-term use of liver enzyme inducers.

- The **combined contraceptive patch** may be continued in the usual manner. Using more than one patch is not recommended. Additional, non-hormonal methods of contraception, such as condoms, should also be used by patients using the combined contraceptive patch, both when taking the liver enzyme inducers and for at least 4 weeks after stopping the drug.
- The **progestogen-only implant** may be continued with *short* courses of enzyme inducers. Additional non-hormonal methods of contraception, such as condoms, should also be used by patients using the progestogen-only implant, both when taking the liver enzyme inducers and for at least 4 weeks after stopping the drug. Alternatives to the progestogen-only implant should be considered with long-term use of liver enzyme inducers.
- The **progestogen-only pill** is not recommended for use with liver enzyme inducers and alternative methods of contraception are advised.
- The effectiveness of the **progestogen-only *emergency* hormonal contraceptive** will be reduced in women taking liver enzyme inducers, see 'Emergency hormonal contraceptives + Enzyme inducers', p.977, for further guidance.
- **Copper** or **levonorgestrel-releasing intrauterine devices** (IUD) and **depot progestogen-only injections** may be used as alternative contraceptive methods, particularly for women requiring hormonal contracep-

tion who are likely to be taking the enzyme inducer in the long-term, as these are unaffected by liver enzyme inducers.

1. Kenyon IE. Unplanned pregnancy in an epileptic. *BMJ* (1972) 1, 686–7.
2. Back DJ, Grimmer FM, Orme ML'E, Proudlove C, Mann RD, Breckenridge AM. Evaluation of Committee on Safety of Medicines yellow card reports on oral contraceptive-drug interactions with anticonvulsants and antibiotics. *Br J Clin Pharmacol* (1988) 25, 527–32.
3. Hempel E, Böhm W, Carol W, Klinger G. Medikamentöse Enzyminduktion und hormonale Kontrazeption. *Zentralbl Gynakol* (1973) 95, 1451–7.
4. Akimoto H, Kazamatsuri H, Seino M, Ward A, Eds. Advances in Epileptology: Sodium valproate and the pill. New York: Raven Press, 1982 429–32.
5. Crawford P, Chadwick DJ, Martin C, Tjia J, Back DJ, Orme M. The interaction of phenytoin and carbamazepine with combined oral contraceptive steroids. *Br J Clin Pharmacol* (1990) 30, 892–6.
6. Back DJ, Bates M, Bowden A, Breckenridge AM, Hall MJ, Jones H, MacIver M, Orme M, Perucca E, Richens A, Rowe PH, Smith E. The interaction of phenobarbital and other anticonvulsants with oral contraceptive steroid therapy. *Contraception* (1980) 22, 495–503.
7. Hempel E, Klinger W. Drug stimulated biotransformation of hormonal steroid contraceptives: clinical implications. *Drugs* (1976) 12, 442–8.
8. Coulam CB, Annegers JF. Do anticonvulsants reduce the efficacy of oral contraceptives? *Epilepsia* (1979) 20, 519–26.
9. O'Brien MD, Gilmour-White S. Epilepsy and pregnancy. *BMJ* (1993) 307, 492–5.
10. Orme M, Back DJ. Oral contraceptive steroids – pharmacological issues of interest to the prescribing physician. *Adv Contracept* (1991) 7, 325–31.
11. Szoka PR, Edgren RA. Drug interactions with oral contraceptives: compilation and analysis of an adverse experience report database. *Fertil Steril* (1988) 49 (Suppl), S31–S38.
12. Krauss GL, Brandt J, Campbell M, Plate C, Summerfield M. Antiepileptic medication and oral contraceptive interactions: a national survey of neurologists and obstetricians. *Neurology* (1996) 46, 1534–9.
13. Shorvon SD, Tallis RC, Wallace HK. Antiepileptic drugs: coprescription of proconvulsant drugs and oral contraceptives: a national study of antiepileptic drug prescribing practice. *J Neurol Neurosurg Psychiatry* (2002) 72, 114–15.
14. McCann MF, Potter LS. Progestin-only contraception: a comprehensive review. *Contraception* (1994) 50 (Suppl 1), S1–S198.
15. Faculty of Family Planning and Reproductive Health Care Clinical Effectiveness Unit. FFPRHC Guidance: Drug interactions with hormonal contraception. April 2005. Available at: http://www.ffprhc.org.uk/admin/uploads/DrugInteractionsFinal.pdf (accessed 23/08/07).

Hormonal contraceptives + Antiepileptics; Carbamazepine or Oxcarbazepine

Hormonal contraceptives are less reliable during treatment with carbamazepine and oxcarbazepine. Breakthrough bleeding and spotting can take place, and unintended pregnancies have occurred with carbamazepine. Controlled studies have shown that carbamazepine and oxcarbazepine can reduce contraceptive steroid levels.

Clinical evidence

(a) Carbamazepine

In a pharmacokinetic study, carbamazepine 300 to 600 mg daily reduced the AUC of **ethinylestradiol** by 42% and **levonorgestrel** by 40% in 4 women given a single dose of a combined oral contraceptive (**ethinylestradiol/levonorgestrel** 50/250 micrograms) before and after 8 to 12 weeks of carbamazepine use.[1] Another study compared the effects of topiramate or carbamazepine on a combined oral contraceptive containing **norethisterone/ethinylestradiol** 1 mg/35 micrograms (*Ortho-Novum*). In the 10 patients who received carbamazepine 600 mg daily, the AUC of norethisterone and ethinylestradiol were reduced by 58% and 42%, respectively.[2]

In an early study, 6 of 12 women taking a combined oral contraceptive (**ethinylestradiol/norethisterone**) developed spotting or breakthrough bleeding while taking carbamazepine (this is regarded as a possible loss of reliability of the contraceptive).[3] A similar study reported breakthrough bleeding in 4 of 6 patients taking carbamazepine and a combined oral contraceptive,[4] and the same author later briefly reported 37 out of 59 patients had breakthrough bleeding while taking this combination.[5]

One woman taking a low-dose combined oral contraceptive (not specified) conceived 6 weeks after starting carbamazepine, initially 200 mg daily then 600 mg daily.[6] In two other cases the failure of a combined oral contraceptive containing **ethinylestradiol** 30 micrograms has been attributed to carbamazepine.[7,8] Six pregnancies were identified in women who took carbamazepine and an oral contraceptive (unspecified) in the adverse reactions register of the CSM in the UK for the years 1968 to 1984. However, it is unclear how many of these 6 women were taking carbamazepine alone, as the authors note that some women were taking multiple antiepileptics.[9] Two further pregnancies have been reported in women taking combined oral contraceptives and antiepileptics including carbamazepine and phenytoin,[10] and one in a woman who was switched from phenytoin to carbamazepine.[11]

(b) Oxcarbazepine

Preliminary observations revealed that 4 of 6 women receiving oxcarbazepine had breakthrough bleeding when they were given a combined oral contraceptive containing **ethinylestradiol** 30 micrograms. This resolved in two women when they took double the dose of **ethinylestradiol**.[5] In a pharmacokinetic study in 10 healthy women taking a triphasic combined oral contraceptive, oxcarbazepine 300 mg three times daily for 4 weeks reduced the AUCs of **ethinylestradiol** and **levonorgestrel** by 47% and 36%, respectively. Three women had menstrual bleeding disturbances.[12] Similar results were reported in a later study with oxcarbazepine 1.2 g daily and a combined oral contraceptive (**ethinylestradiol/levonorgestrel** 50/250 micrograms).[13] So far, no cases of unintended pregnancy have been reported.

Mechanism

The most likely explanation for these interactions is that both carbamazepine and oxcarbazepine reduce the levels of the contraceptive steroids, presumably by inducing their metabolism. This may result in loss of contraceptive efficacy.

Importance and management

The reduction in contraceptive steroid levels caused by carbamazepine and oxcarbazepine is well established. However, the actual incidence of contraceptive failure when oral contraceptives are given with these drugs is unknown. Given the few published reports, it appears that unintended pregnancies with carbamazepine are rare, and still less frequent than that seen with barrier methods such as condoms. No pregnancies have been reported in patients taking an oral contraceptive and oxcarbazepine. Nevertheless, given the personal and ethical consequences of an unwanted pregnancy, any reduction in contraceptive efficacy is of concern. The Faculty of Family Planning and Reproductive Health Care (FFPRHC) Clinical Effectiveness Unit has issued guidelines on the management of patients taking liver enzyme inducers with hormonal contraceptives. These are discussed in further detail under 'Hormonal contraceptives + Antiepileptics; Barbiturates or Phenytoin', p.985.

1. Crawford P, Chadwick DJ, Martin C, Tjia J, Back DJ, Orme M. The interaction of phenytoin and carbamazepine with combined oral contraceptive steroids. *Br J Clin Pharmacol* (1990) 30, 892–6.
2. Doose DR, Wang S-S, Padmanabhan M, Schwabe S, Jacobs D, Bialer M. Effect of topiramate or carbamazepine on the pharmacokinetics of an oral contraceptive containing norethindrone and ethinyl estradiol in healthy obese and nonobese female subjects. *Epilepsia* (2003) 44, 540–9.
3. Hempel E, Klinger W. Drug stimulated biotransformation of hormonal steroid contraceptives: clinical implications. *Drugs* (1976) 12, 442–8.
4. Akimoto H, Kazamatsuri H, Seino M, Ward A, Eds. Advances in Epileptology. New York: Raven Press, 1982 429–32.
5. Sonnen AEH. Oxcarbazepine and oral contraceptives. *Acta Neurol Scand* (1990) 82 (Suppl 133) 37.
6. Rapport DJ, Calabrese JR. Interactions between carbamazepine and birth control pills. *Psychosomatics* (1989) 30, 462–4.
7. Beeley L, Magee P, Hickey FM. *Bulletin of the West Midlands Centre for Adverse Drug Reaction Reporting* (1989) 28, 21.
8. Kovacs GT, Riddoch G, Duncombe P, Welberry L, Chick P, Weisberg E, Leavesley GM, Baker HWG. Inadvertent pregnancies in oral contraceptive users. *Med J Aust* (1989) 150, 549–51.
9. Back DJ, Grimmer FM, Orme ML'E, Proudlove C, Mann RD, Breckenridge AM. Evaluation of Committee on Safety of Medicines yellow card reports on oral contraceptive-drug interactions with anticonvulsants and antibiotics. *Br J Clin Pharmacol* (1988) 25, 527–32.
10. Janz D, Schmidt D. Antiepileptika und die Sicherheit oraler Kontrazeptiva. *Bibl Psychiatr* (1975) 151, 82–5.
11. Sparrow MJ. Pill method failures. *N Z Med J* (1987) 100, 102–5.
12. Klosterskov Jensen P, Saano V, Haring P, Svenstrup B, Menge GP. Possible interaction between oxcarbazepine and an oral contraceptive. *Epilepsia* (1992) 33, 1149–52.
13. Fattore C, Cipolla G, Gatti G, Limido GL, Sturm Y, Bernasconi C, Perucca E. Induction of ethinylestradiol and levonorgestrel metabolism by oxcarbazepine in healthy women. *Epilepsia* (1999) 40, 783–7.

Hormonal contraceptives + Antiepileptics; Ethosuximide

Ethosuximide appears not to alter the efficacy of combined oral contraceptives.

Clinical evidence, mechanism, importance and management

Four pregnancies were identified in women who took ethosuximide and an oral contraceptive (unspecified) in the adverse reactions register of the CSM in the UK for the years 1968 to 1984. However, the authors note that in only one of the cases reported was ethosuximide the sole antiepileptic prescribed.[1] Since ethosuximide is not an inducer of hepatic enzymes, it is likely that this one case is a chance association. Another case describes pregnancy in a woman who had been taking ethosuximide, phenytoin, and phenobarbital, with a combined oral contraceptive for 6 years.[2] If indeed this case does represent an interaction, the known enzyme-inducers phenytoin and phenobarbital are more likely to be implicated than ethosuximide (see 'Hormonal contraceptives + Antiepileptics; Barbiturates or Phenytoin', p.985). There do not appear to have been any pharmacokinetic or pharmacodynamic studies of the use of ethosuximide with oral contraceptives and no further case reports have been published. The Faculty of Family Planning and Reproductive Health Care (FFPRHC) Clinical Effectiveness Unit guidelines on the management of hormonal contraceptives and drug interactions state that ethosuximide does not induce liver enzymes and causes no reduction in ethinylestradiol or progestogens.[3] No special contraceptive precautions appear to be necessary on concurrent use.

1. Back DJ, Grimmer FM, Orme ML'E, Proudlove C, Mann RD, Breckenridge AM. Evaluation of Committee on Safety of Medicines yellow card reports on oral contraceptive-drug interactions with anticonvulsants and antibiotics. *Br J Clin Pharmacol* (1988) 25, 527–32.
2. Janz D, Schmidt D. Anti-epileptic drugs and failure of oral contraceptives. *Lancet* (1974) i, 1113.
3. Faculty of Family Planning and Reproductive Health Care Clinical Effectiveness Unit. FFPRHC Guidance: Drug interactions with hormonal contraception. April 2005. Available at: http://www.ffprhc.org.uk/admin/uploads/DrugInteractionsFinal.pdf (accessed 23/08/07).

Hormonal contraceptives + Antiepileptics; Felbamate

Felbamate increases the clearance of gestodene from a combined oral contraceptive but it is not known if this reduces contraceptive efficacy.

Clinical evidence, mechanism, importance and management

In a randomised, placebo-controlled study 23 healthy women were given a combined oral contraceptive (**ethinylestradiol/gestodene** 30/75 micrograms) for 3 months or more. During months 1 and 2 they were also given either felbamate in a dose of up to 2.4 g daily, or a placebo, from day 15 of month 1 to day 14 of month 2. None of the women showed any evidence of ovulation during the entire 3 months, although one had intermenstrual spotting. However, felbamate reduced the **gestodene** AUC by 42% and the **ethinylestradiol** AUC by 13%.[1] The reasons for this effect are not understood. What this change means in terms of the reliability of the oral contraceptive is not known, but some reduction in its efficacy might be expected. More study is needed to assess the clinical relevance and to see whether other progestogens are similarly affected.

1. Saano V, Glue P, Banfield CR, Reidenberg P, Colucci RD, Meehan JW, Haring P, Radwanski E, Nomeir A, Lin C-C, Jensen PK, Affrime MB. Effects of felbamate on the pharmacokinetics of a low-dose combination oral contraceptive. *Clin Pharmacol Ther* (1995) 58, 523–31.

Hormonal contraceptives + Antiepileptics; Gabapentin

In a controlled study, gabapentin did not alter the levels of ethinylestradiol or norethisterone.

Clinical evidence, mechanism, importance and management

Gabapentin 400 mg every 8 hours for 7 days had no effect on the AUC of **ethinylestradiol** or **norethisterone** in 13 healthy women taking a combined oral contraceptive (**ethinylestradiol/norethisterone** 50 micrograms/2.5 mg). Ovulation suppression was not assessed.[1] The Faculty of Family Planning and Reproductive Health Care (FFPRHC) Clinical Effectiveness Unit guidelines on the management of hormonal contraceptives and drug interactions state that gabapentin does not induce liver enzymes responsible for the metabolism of contraceptive steroids and causes no reduction in ethinylestradiol or progestogens.[2] Thus, no special contraceptive precautions appear to be required during concurrent use.

1. Eldon MA, Underwood BA, Randinitis EJ, Sedman AJ. Gabapentin does not interact with a contraceptive regimen of norethindrone acetate and ethinyl estradiol. *Neurology* (1998) 50, 1146–8.
2. Faculty of Family Planning and Reproductive Health Care Clinical Effectiveness Unit. FFPRHC Guidance: Drug interactions with hormonal contraception. April 2005. Available at: http://www.ffprhc.org.uk/admin/uploads/DrugInteractionsFinal.pdf (accessed 23/08/07).

Hormonal contraceptives + Antiepileptics; Lamotrigine

One study suggests that lamotrigine does not alter the contraceptive efficacy or plasma levels of combined oral contraceptives. Another study found a slight reduction in levonorgestrel levels but no evidence of ovulation, however, based on this, the manufacturer says that the possibility of reduced contraceptive efficacy cannot be ruled out.
Hormonal contraceptives may reduce the levels of lamotrigine, which can lead to a decrease in seizure control.

Clinical evidence and mechanism

(a) Contraceptive efficacy

Preliminary results of a study showed that lamotrigine 150 mg daily for 10 to 14 days had no significant effect on the mean plasma levels of **ethinylestradiol** and **levonorgestrel** in women taking a combined oral contraceptive (**ethinylestradiol/levonorgestrel** 30/150 micrograms). No ovulation occurred (assessed by progesterone levels) and no changes in menstrual pattern were observed. Furthermore, lamotrigine did not induce hepatic enzymes (assessed by 6-β-hydroxycortisol excretion).[1] A study by the manufacturer in 16 healthy women taking the combined oral contraceptive *Microgynon 30* (**ethinylestradiol/levonorgestrel** 30/150 micrograms) and given lamotrigine (titrated to 300 mg daily) found a slight but non-significant reduction in the AUC and the maximum serum concentration of **levonorgestrel** of 19% and 12%, respectively, compared with hormone levels before starting lamotrigine. **Ethinylestradiol** levels were not affected. Significant increases in FSH and LH were also seen, although there was no increase in the levels of progesterone, indicating that ovulation probably did not occur. Intermenstrual bleeding was reported in 32% of subjects when receiving lamotrigine.[2]

(b) Lamotrigine efficacy

A case report describes 7 women in whom lamotrigine plasma levels were decreased by 41 to 64% by combined oral contraceptives (**ethinylestradiol** with **desogestrel** or **norethisterone**). Five had increased seizure frequency or recurrence of seizures after starting an oral contraceptive, and two had lamotrigine adverse effects on stopping the oral contraceptive. It was suggested that hormonal contraceptives can increase the glucuronidation of lamotrigine, thereby increasing its clearance.[3] A subsequent study found a more than 50% reduction in lamotrigine levels in women taking the combined oral contraceptive.[4] A study by the manufacturer in 16 healthy women taking the combined oral contraceptive *Microgynon 30* (**ethinylestradiol/levonorgestrel** 30/150 micrograms) and lamotrigine (titrated to 300 mg daily) found that the maximum serum concentration and AUC of lamotrigine were decreased by approximately 39% and 52%, respectively, when compared with lamotrigine alone.[2] A further study in 8 epileptic women found that lamotrigine plasma concentrations varied with hormonal contraceptive monthly cycles. The median lamotrigine plasma concentration was 15% higher during the hormonal contraceptive washout week than during the phase of hormonal contraceptive intake, although there was a wide interpatient variability.[5]

Another study in 45 women found that a reduction in lamotrigine levels occurred with **ethinylestradiol** (given as a combined hormonal contraceptive in 11 subjects and a vaginal ring also containing etonogestrel in one subject) compared with 18 women using no hormonal contraception. However, lamotrigine serum concentrations were not affected in 16 women using a progestogen-only contraceptive (4 using oral **desogestrel** or **norethisterone**, 8 using subdermal **etonogestrel** or **levonorgestrel**, 1 using depot **medroxyprogesterone,** and 3 using intrauterine **levonorgestrel**).[6]

Importance and management

Based on the small reduction in levonorgestrel levels the manufacturer of lamotrigine suggests that the possibility of decreased contraceptive efficacy cannot be ruled out, and advises that the use of non-hormonal contraceptives is preferable. If a hormonal contraceptive is used as the only form of contraception, they advise that women should be alert for signs of breakthrough bleeding, which may be a sign of reduced contraceptive efficacy.[7] Note that the Faculty of Family Planning and Reproductive Health Care (FFPRHC) Clinical Effectiveness Unit has issued guidance on the use of lamotrigine in patients taking hormonal contraceptives in response to the manufacturer's guidance. They found no evidence of reduced contraceptive effectiveness in patients taking combined oral contraceptives (tablets, patch or vaginal ring) or progestogen-only contraceptives (tablets, implant, injectable or intrauterine system) with lamotrigine. They concluded that there is no good evidence that non-hormonal methods of contraception are preferable in patients taking lamotrigine.[8]

Lamotrigine can be started as normal in patients already taking hormonal contraceptives.[7] In those already taking lamotrigine with inducers of lamotrigine glucuronidation, such as phenytoin and carbamazepine, changes in the dose of lamotrigine are unlikely to be necessary when starting hormonal contraceptives. However, for women already taking lamotrigine and *not* taking inducers of lamotrigine glucuronidation, the maintenance dose of lamotrigine may need to be increased by as much as twofold, according to clinical response when hormonal contraceptives are started. If this group of patients stop taking an oral contraceptive, the lamotrigine dose should be reviewed (and may need to be decreased by as much as 50%) to reduce the risk of adverse effects occurring.[7,8] Note that apart from interindividual variations, lamotrigine plasma concentrations may vary with the hormonal contraceptive monthly cycles.[5] Patients should also be advised that an increase in seizure frequency may occur when the combined oral contraceptive is started.[8]

1. Holdich T, Whiteman P, Orme M, Back D, Ward S. Effect of lamotrigine on the pharmacology of the combined oral contraceptive pill. *Epilepsia* (1991) 32 (Suppl 1), 96.
2. Sidhu J, Job S, Singh S, Philipson R. The pharmacokinetic and pharmacodynamic consequences of the co-administration of lamotrigine and a combined oral contraceptive in healthy female subjects. *Br J Clin Pharmacol* (2006) 61, 191–9.
3. Sabers A, Buchholt JM, Uldall P, Hansen EL. Lamotrigine plasma levels reduced by oral contraceptives. *Epilepsy Res* (2001) 47, 151–4.
4. Sabers A, Öhman I, Christensen J, Tomson T. Oral contraceptives reduce lamotrigine plasma levels. *Neurology* (2003) 61, 570–1.
5. Contin M, Albani F. Ambrosetto G, Avoni P, Bisulli F, Riva R, Tinuper P, Baruzzi A. Variation in lamotrigine plasma concentrations with hormonal contraceptive monthly cycles in patients with epilepsy. *Epilepsia* (2006) 47, 1573–5.
6. Reimers A, Helde G, Brodtkorb E. Ethinyl estradiol, not progestogens, reduces lamotrigine serum concentrations. *Epilepsia* (2005) 46, 1414–17.
7. Lamictal (Lamotrigine). GlaxoSmithKline UK. UK Summary of product characteristics, March 2007.
8. Faculty of Family Planning and Reproductive Health Care Clinical Effectiveness Unit. Faculty statement from the CEU on changes to prescribing information for lamotrigine. August 2005. Available at: http://www.ffprhc.org.uk/admin/uploads/831_lamotrigine.pdf (accessed 23/08/07).

Hormonal contraceptives + Antiepileptics; Levetiracetam

Levetiracetam appears not to alter the contraceptive efficacy and plasma levels of ethinylestradiol and levonorgestrel given as a combined oral contraceptive.

Clinical evidence, mechanism, importance and management

The pharmacokinetics of a combined oral contraceptive (**ethinylestradiol/levonorgestrel**) were found not to be affected by levetiracetam 500 mg twice daily, nor was ovulation suppression altered (there were no changes in LH or progesterone levels). The pharmacokinetics of levetiracetam also remained unaffected.[1] A placebo-controlled study in 18 subjects taking a combined oral contraceptive containing **ethinylestradiol** 30 micrograms and **levonorgestrel** 150 micrograms with levetiracetam 500 mg twice daily found that levetiracetam did not affect the serum levels of either steroid or alter the contraceptive efficacy of these drugs, as measured by progesterone and LH levels.[2] The Faculty of Family Planning and Reproductive Health Care (FFPRHC) Clinical Effectiveness Unit guidelines on the management of drug interactions with hormonal contraceptives state that levetiracetam does not induce liver enzymes and causes no reduction in ethinylestradiol or progestogens.[3] These findings indicate that no special or additional precautions are needed if oral contraceptives and levetiracetam are used concurrently.

1. Giuliano RA, Hiersemenzel R, Baltes E, Johnscher G, Janik F, Weber W. Influence of a new antiepileptic drug (Levetiracetam, ucb L059) on the pharmacokinetics and pharmacodynamics of oral contraceptives. *Epilepsia* (1996) 37, 90.
2. Ragueneau-Majlessi I, Levy RH, Janik F. Levetiracetam does not alter the pharmacokinetics of an oral contraceptive in healthy women. *Epilepsia* (2002) 43, 697–702.
3. Faculty of Family Planning and Reproductive Health Care Clinical Effectiveness Unit. FFPRHC Guidance: Drug interactions with hormonal contraception. April 2005. Available at: http://www.ffprhc.org.uk/admin/uploads/DrugInteractionsFinal.pdf (accessed 23/08/07).

Hormonal contraceptives + Antiepileptics; Pregabalin

Pregabalin does not appear to affect the pharmacokinetics or contraceptive efficacy of ethinylestradiol or norethisterone. In addition, the pharmacokinetics of pregabalin were not affected by the contraceptive steroids.

Clinical evidence, mechanism, importance and management

A study in 16 subjects found that pregabalin 200 mg every 8 hours had no effect on the pharmacokinetics of **ethinylestradiol** or **norethisterone** taken as a combined oral contraceptive *(Orthonovum)* and did not reduce the contraceptive effect as measured by progesterone levels. Neither contraceptive steroid had an effect on the pharmacokinetics of pregabalin.[1] No special contraceptive precautions therefore appear to be required during concurrent use.

1. Bockbrader HN, Posvar EL, Hunt T, Randinitis EJ. Pharmacokinetics of pregabalin and a concomitantly administered oral contraceptive show no-drug drug interaction. *Epilepsia* (2004) 45 (Suppl 3), 153.

Hormonal contraceptives + Antiepileptics; Remacemide

Remacemide appears not to interact with combined oral contraceptives.

Clinical evidence, mechanism, importance and management

Preliminary results of a study show that remacemide 200 mg twice daily for 14 days had no effect on the pharmacokinetics of **ethinylestradiol, desogestrel**, or **levonorgestrel**, when compared with placebo, in women taking a combined oral contraceptive (**ethinylestradiol/levonorgestrel** 30/150 micrograms or **ethinylestradiol/desogestrel** 30/150 micrograms). Inhibition of ovulation was maintained (assessed by measurement of progesterone, FSH, and LH levels).[1] It appears that no special contraceptive precautions are needed during concurrent use.

1. Blakey GE, Lockton JA, Corfield J, Oliver SD, Back D. Absence of interaction of remacemide with oral contraceptives. *Epilepsia* (1999) 40 (Suppl 2), 95.

Hormonal contraceptives + Antiepileptics; Retigabine

Retigabine did not alter the plasma levels of ethinylestradiol or norgestrel given as a combined oral contraceptive.

Clinical evidence, mechanism, importance and management

Preliminary results of a study show that retigabine 150 mg three times daily had no effect on the pharmacokinetics of **ethinylestradiol** or **norgestrel** in women taking a combined oral contraceptive (**ethinylestradiol/norgestrel** 30/300 micrograms).[1] This suggests that no special contraceptive precautions are needed during concurrent use.

1. Paul J, Ferron GM, Richards L, Getsy J, Troy SM. Retigabine does not alter the pharmacokinetics of a low-dose oral contraceptive in women. *Neurology* (2001) 56 (Suppl 3), A335.

Hormonal contraceptives + Antiepileptics; Rufinamide

Rufinamide caused a modest decrease in the plasma levels of ethinyloestradiol and norethisterone given as a combined oral contraceptive.

Clinical evidence, mechanism, importance and management

Preliminary results of a study show that rufinamide 800 mg twice daily for 14 days decreased the AUC of **ethinylestradiol** 35 micrograms by 22% and of **norethisterone** 1 mg by 14% in healthy women taking a combined oral contraceptive. Inhibition of ovulation was not assessed.[1] These reductions in plasma levels of the contraceptive hormones are similar to those seen with topiramate (see 'Hormonal contraceptives + Antiepileptics; Topiramate', below), and their clinical relevance is unknown. However, given these findings, low-dose contraceptives (**ethinylestradiol** 20 micrograms) may be considered unsuitable for use with rufinamide. Further study is needed.

1. Svendsen KD, Choi L, Chen B-L, Karolchyk MA. Single-center, open-label, multiple-dose pharmacokinetic trial investigating the effect of rufinamide administration on Ortho-Novum 1/35 in healthy women. *Epilepsia* (1998) 39 (Suppl 6), 59.

Hormonal contraceptives + Antiepileptics; Tiagabine

Tiagabine appears not to alter the contraceptive efficacy and plasma levels of combined oral contraceptives.

Clinical evidence, mechanism, importance and management

A study in 10 healthy women found that tiagabine 2 mg, four times daily from day 24 to day 7 of the next cycle, had no effect on the mean plasma levels of any of steroids in two combined oral contraceptives (**ethinylestradiol/levonorgestrel** or **ethinylestradiol/desogestrel**, both 30/150 micrograms). There was no evidence that the suppression of ovulation was altered in any way (no significant changes in the plasma concentrations of progesterone, FSH, or LH were seen between the first and second cycles, and progesterone levels remained in the non-ovulatory range). Tiagabine did not induce hepatic enzymes, as assessed by 6β-hydroxycortisol excretion. Two women did develop breakthrough bleeding, but given the above findings, this was not thought to represent reduced efficacy of the contraceptive.[1] There would appear to be no reason for any special contraceptive precautions during concurrent use.

1. Mengel HB, Houston A, Back DJ. An evaluation of the interaction between tiagabine and oral contraceptives in female volunteers. *J Pharm Med* (1994) 4, 141–50.

Hormonal contraceptives + Antiepileptics; Topiramate

The serum levels of ethinylestradiol may be reduced by topiramate, increasing the risk of breakthrough bleeding in women taking combined oral contraceptives. It is suggested that oral contraceptives with a higher dosage of oestrogen should be used.

Clinical evidence

Eleven epileptic women taking sodium valproate and a combined oral contraceptive (**ethinylestradiol/norethisterone** 35 micrograms/1 mg) were also given three escalating doses of topiramate 100, 200 and 400 mg twice daily for 28-day periods.[1] The mean AUC of the **ethinylestradiol** fell by 18%, 21%, and 30%, with the three doses respectively. Although no significant changes were found in the **norethisterone** AUC, the authors considered that the study was not sufficiently powered to detect small changes. No ovulation occurred, as assessed by progestogen levels, but one patient had breakthrough bleeding.[2] A follow-up study evaluated the effect of lower doses of topiramate on the pharmacokinetics of a combined oral contraceptive containing **ethinylestradiol/norethisterone** 35 micrograms/1 mg (*Ortho-Novum*). Subjects were randomised to take daily doses of topiramate of 50 mg (11 subjects), 100 mg (10 subjects) or 200 mg (2 groups of 12 subjects). This study found a minor, non-significant change in the pharmacokinetics of both **ethinylestradiol** and **norethisterone**; this change was further reduced when the data from 2 subjects were excluded due to compliance issues. The authors noted that the difference between this study and the study cited above[2] was due to the difference in the doses of topiramate used, as topiramate is a weak liver enzyme-inducer, and this effect is dose-related.[3]

Mechanism

Not understood. It is suggested that topiramate weakly induces enzymes in the liver, which increases the metabolism of the ethinylestradiol.[2,3]

Importance and management

An established interaction but supported by limited evidence. The modest changes in pharmacokinetics of the combined oral contraceptive seen here are lower than those seen with other enzyme-inducing antiepileptics (see 'Hormonal contraceptives + Antiepileptics; Carbamazepine or Oxcarbazepine', p.987, and 'Hormonal contraceptives + Antiepileptics; Barbiturates or Phenytoin', p.985) and may be dose-dependent. However, it is possible that they would be sufficient to cause failure of combined oral contraceptives in rare cases, particularly at high therapeutic doses of topiramate. As there is a risk of failure of contraception with the concurrent use of topiramate, and possibly more importantly, because topiramate is teratogenic, the manufacturer of topiramate advises the use of a non-hormonal contraceptive or a high-dose combined oral contraceptive (at least 50 micrograms of oestrogen), and also that patients should be told to report any changes in their bleeding patterns.[1] The Faculty of Family Planning and Reproductive Health Care (FFPRHC) Clinical Effectiveness Unit has issued guidance on the use of liver enzyme inducers, including topiramate, with hormonal contraceptives, see 'Hormonal contraceptives + Antiepileptics; Barbiturates or Phenytoin', p.985, for details of this guidance.

1. Topamax (Topiramate). Janssen-Cilag Ltd. UK Summary of product characteristics, November 2006.
2. Rosenfeld WE, Doose DR, Walker SA, Nayak RK. Effect of topiramate on the pharmacokinetics of an oral contraceptive containing norethindrone and ethinyl estradiol in patients with epilepsy. *Epilepsia* (1997) 38, 317–23.
3. Doose DR, Wang S-S, Padmanabhan M, Schwabe S, Jacobs D, Bialer M. Effect of topiramate or carbamazepine on the pharmacokinetics of an oral contraceptive containing norethindrone and ethinyl estradiol in healthy obese and nonobese female subjects. *Epilepsia* (2003) 44, 540–9.

Hormonal contraceptives + Antiepileptics; Valproate

Sodium valproate and valproate semisodium do not appear to alter the efficacy of combined oral contraceptives. In one study, sodium valproate increased ethinylestradiol levels. Ethinylestradiol may reduce valproate levels but there appears to be only one case where this resulted in a loss of seizure control.

Clinical evidence and mechanism

(a) Contraceptive efficacy

In a series of 32 patients taking an oral contraceptive, none of 7 taking sodium valproate 600 mg to 1.8 g daily had breakthrough bleeding, whereas about two-thirds of those taking carbamazepine or phenobarbital had breakthrough bleeding (a sign of possible reduced contraceptive efficacy). Most of the 7 patients taking valproate were taking combined oral contraceptives containing 50 micrograms of **ethinylestradiol**; one was taking less than 50 micrograms, and one was using a **progestogen-only oral contraceptive**. One of the 7 patients had previously experienced breakthrough bleeding while taking phenobarbital, but this stopped when it was replaced with sodium valproate. Two further patients did not have breakthrough bleeding while taking sodium valproate and benzodiazepines, but breakthrough bleeding started when phenytoin was also given.[1]

In a pharmacokinetic study, sodium valproate 200 mg twice daily had no effect on the AUC of a single dose of a combined oral contraceptive (**ethinylestradiol/levonorgestrel** 50/250 micrograms) given to women with epilepsy 8 to 16 weeks after they started sodium valproate. However, a 50% *increase* in the peak plasma levels of **ethinylestradiol** was noted.[2]

Conversely, one pregnancy was identified in a woman who took sodium valproate and an oral contraceptive (unspecified) in the adverse reactions register of the CSM in the UK for the years 1968 to 1984. However, the authors consider this one case to be a chance association.[3]

(b) Valproate efficacy

A study in 9 women with epilepsy taking valproic acid found an increase in the apparent oral clearance of both total and unbound valproic acid during oral contraceptive intake compared with the pill-free period. The authors report that this may be due to induction of glucuronosyltransferase by ethinylestradiol and that the magnitude of this effect can differ between individuals.[4] Reduced valproate levels and an increase in seizure frequency have been reported to occur in one patient taking a combined oral contraceptive during the active pill phase, when compared with the inactive 7-day period.[5] No further cases appear to have been published.

Importance and management

The Faculty of Family Planning and Reproductive Health Care (FFPRHC) Clinical Effectiveness Unit guidelines on the management of hormonal contraceptives and drug interactions state that valproate does not induce liver enzymes and causes no reduction in ethinylestradiol or progestogens.[6] The manufacturers of sodium valproate and valproate semisodium state that valproate does not affect the efficacy of hormonal contraceptives.[7,8] No special contraceptive precautions are required during concurrent use.

The significance of the reduction in valproate levels and the case report above is unclear.

1. Akimoto H, Kazamatsuri H, Seino M, Ward A, Eds. Advances in Epileptology: Sodium valproate and the pill. New York: Raven Press, 1982 429–32.
2. Crawford P, Chadwick D, Cleland P, Tjia J, Cowie A, Back DJ, Orme ML'E. The lack of effect of sodium valproate on the pharmacokinetics of oral contraceptive steroids. *Contraception* (1986) 33, 23–9.
3. Back DJ, Grimmer FM, Orme L'E, Proudlove C, Mann RD, Breckenridge AM. Evaluation of Committee on Safety of Medicines yellow card reports on oral contraceptive-drug interactions with anticonvulsants and antibiotics. *Br J Clin Pharmacol* (1988) 25, 527–32.
4. Galimberti CA, Mazzucchelli I, Arbasino C, Canevini MP, Fattore C, Perucca E. Increased apparent oral clearance of valproic acid during intake of combined contraceptive steroids in women with epilepsy. *Epilepsia* (2006) 47, 1569–72.
5. Herzog AG, Farina EL, Blum AS. Serum valproate levels with oral contraceptive use. *Epilepsia* (2005) 46, 970–1.
6. Faculty of Family Planning and Reproductive Health Care Clinical Effectiveness Unit. FFPRHC Guidance: Drug interactions with hormonal contraception. April 2005. Available at: http://www.ffprhc.org.uk/admin/uploads/DrugInteractionsFinal.pdf (accessed 23/08/07).
7. Depakote (Valproate semisodium). Sanofi-Aventis. UK Summary of product characteristics, September 2005.
8. Epilim (Sodium valproate). Sanofi-Aventis. UK Summary of product characteristics, October 2005.

Hormonal contraceptives + Antiepileptics; Vigabatrin

Vigabatrin appears not to alter the pharmacokinetics of ethinyloestradiol or levonorgestrel given as a combined oral contraceptive.

Clinical evidence, mechanism, importance and management

Vigabatrin 3 g daily had no statistically significant effect on the pharmacokinetics of **ethinylestradiol** and **levonorgestrel** in 13 healthy women given a single dose of a combined oral contraceptive (**ethinylestradiol/levonorgestrel** 30/150 micrograms); although 2 of the women had a 39% and a 50% fall in the AUC of **ethinylestradiol**. Vigabatrin did not induce hepatic enzymes as assessed by antipyrine clearance and 6β-hydroxycortisol excretion.[1]

This study would seem to confirm the lack of reports of an interaction between oral contraceptives and vigabatrin, but the authors of the report introduce a small note of caution because it is not clear whether the reduced **ethinylestradiol** AUCs seen in two of the women resulted from an interaction or were simply normal individual variations.[1] The Faculty of Family Planning and Reproductive Health Care (FFPRHC) Clinical Effectiveness Unit guidelines on the management of hormonal contraceptives and drug interactions state that vigabatrin does not induce liver enzymes and causes no reduction in ethinylestradiol or progestogens.[2] No special precautions are recommended.

1. Bartoli A, Gatti G, Cipolla G, Barzaghi N, Veliz G, Fattore C, Mumford J, Perucca E. A double-blind, placebo-controlled study on the effect of vigabatrin on in vivo parameters of hepatic microsomal enzyme induction and on the kinetics of steroid oral contraceptives in healthy female volunteers. *Epilepsia* (1997) 38, 702–7.
2. Faculty of Family Planning and Reproductive Health Care Clinical Effectiveness Unit. FFPRHC Guidance: Drug interactions with hormonal contraception. April 2005. Available at: http://www.ffprhc.org.uk/admin/uploads/DrugInteractionsFinal.pdf (accessed 23/08/07).

Hormonal contraceptives + Antiepileptics; Zonisamide

A study in healthy women taking a combined oral contraceptive found that steady-state zonisamide 100 to 400 mg daily did not affect the levels of ethinylestradiol or norethisterone. Contraceptive efficacy was not reduced.[1]

1. Griffith SG, Dai Y. Effect of zonisamide on the pharmacokinetics and pharmacodynamics of a combination ethinyl estradiol-norethindrone oral contraceptive in healthy women. *Clin Ther* (2004) 26, 2056–65.

Hormonal contraceptives + Antihistamines

The pharmacokinetics of single doses of doxylamine and diphenhydramine do not appear to be altered by combined oral contraceptives.

Clinical evidence, mechanism, importance and management

The pharmacokinetics of a single 25-mg dose of **doxylamine** in 13 subjects and the pharmacokinetics of a single 50-mg dose of **diphenhydramine** in 10 subjects were not significantly altered by the use of low-dose combined oral contraceptives.[1] Cases of oral contraceptive failure have been attributed to the use of **doxylamine**, **chlorpheniramine**, and an unnamed antihistamine,[2] but these antihistamines were all used in conjunction with penicillins, which would seem to be a more likely cause of contraceptive failure (see 'Hormonal contraceptives + Antibacterials; Penicillins', p.981). The effect of the antihistamines on the pharmacokinetics and pharmacodynamics of contraceptive steroids appear not to have been studied. No particular precautions would seem necessary during concurrent use.

1. Luna BG, Scavone JM, Greenblatt DJ. Doxylamine and diphenhydramine pharmacokinetics in women on low-dose estrogen oral contraceptives. *J Clin Pharmacol* (1989) 29, 257–60.
2. DeSano EA, Hurley SC. Possible interactions of antihistamines and antibiotics with oral contraceptive effectiveness. *Fertil Steril* (1982) 37, 853–4.

Hormonal contraceptives + Antimalarials

No clinically significant interaction appears to occur between combined oral contraceptives and chloroquine or primaquine, or between oral contraceptives and mefloquine or quinine. There is some evidence to suggest that a combined oral contraceptive reduced the conversion of proguanil to its active metabolite, cycloguanil.

Clinical evidence and mechanism

(a) Chloroquine

A pharmacokinetic study in 12 healthy women taking a combined oral contraceptive (**ethinylestradiol/norethisterone** 30 micrograms/1 mg) found that the prophylactic use of chloroquine phosphate 500 mg once a week for 4 weeks caused a small 15% increase in the AUC of **ethinylestradiol**, and no change in the levels of **norethisterone**. Chloroquine use did not alter ovulation inhibition, as assessed by mid-luteal progesterone levels and the lack of breakthrough spotting and bleeding. In a further group of 7 women, the same combined oral contraceptive did not alter the pharmacokinetics of a single 500-mg dose of chloroquine phosphate.[1] Another study in 6 healthy women given a single dose of a combined oral contraceptive (**ethinylestradiol/levonorgestrel** 30 micrograms/150 micrograms) confirmed that a single 300-mg dose of chloroquine had no significant effect on the pharmacokinetics of either the oestrogen or the progestogen.[2] Furthermore studies in *rhesus monkeys* infected with malaria, suggest that the curative efficacy of chloroquine is not altered by the use of combined oral contraceptives (**ethinylestradiol/norethisterone** or **ethinylestradiol/norgestrel**).[3]

(b) Mefloquine

A study in 12 Thai women with falciparum malaria, 6 of whom were taking unnamed oral contraceptives, found that their response to mefloquine (parasite and fever clearance) was not affected by oral contraceptives.

Similarly, the pharmacokinetics of mefloquine were not affected by oral contraceptives in patients with malaria.[4]

(c) Primaquine

A study in 6 healthy women given a single dose of a combined oral contraceptive (**ethinylestradiol/levonorgestrel** 30 micrograms/150 micrograms) confirmed that a single 45-mg dose of primaquine had no significant effect on the pharmacokinetics of either the oestrogen or the progestogen.[2]

(d) Proguanil

In women who were CYP2C19 extensive metabolisers the use of a combined oral contraceptive (**ethinylestradiol/levonorgestrel**) reduced the levels of cycloguanil (the active metabolite of proguanil) by 34% after 3 weeks, when compared with the cycloguanil levels before starting the contraceptive.[5] It was suggested that the oestrogen might have inhibited the metabolism of proguanil by the cytochrome P450 isoenzyme CYP2C19. However, inhibition of CYP2C19 makes extensive metabolisers into poor metabolisers, and there is some evidence that CYP2C19 poor metaboliser status does not reduce the efficacy of proguanil for prophylaxis[6] or treatment[7] of malaria (see also 'Proguanil + Fluvoxamine', p.238).

(e) Quinine

A controlled study in Thai women showed that the pharmacokinetics of a single 600-mg dose of quinine sulfate in 7 women taking oral contraceptives were not significantly different from those in 7 other women not taking contraceptives. The contraceptives being used were combined oral contraceptives (**ethinylestradiol/levonorgestrel** or **ethinylestradiol/norgestrel**) and a progestogen-only oral contraceptive (**norethisterone**).[8] There seem to be no reports that quinine affects the reliability of the oral contraceptives.

Importance and management

No clinically significant interaction appears to occur between the combined oral contraceptives and chloroquine, primaquine or quinine, between oral contraceptives and mefloquine, or between a progestogen-only oral contraceptive and quinine. There would seem to be no reason for avoiding concurrent use.

The decrease in the active metabolite of proguanil caused by a combined oral contraceptive has not been fully assessed, although the authors recommended that the dose of proguanil should be increased by 50% in women taking oral contraceptives.[5] However, there is limited evidence that this pharmacokinetic interaction may not be clinically relevant. More study is needed.

The Faculty of Family Planning and Reproductive Health Care (FFPRHC) Clinical Effectiveness Unit has issued guidance (adapted from the World Health Organization Medical Eligibility Criteria (WHOMEC) guidance on contraceptive use) stating that malaria as a condition does not restrict the choice of various contraceptive methods including combined and progesterone-only oral contraceptives.[9]

Note that **doxycycline** is increasingly used in the treatment of malaria. See 'Hormonal contraceptives + Antibacterials; Tetracyclines', p.983, for further information on possible combined hormonal contraceptive failure with tetracyclines.

1. Gupta KC, Joshi JV, Desai NK, Sankolli GM, Chowdhary VN, Joshi UM, Chitalange S, Satoskar RS. Kinetics of chloroquine and contraceptive steroids in oral contraceptive users during concurrent chloroquine prophylaxis. *Indian J Med Res* (1984) 80, 658–62.
2. Back DJ, Breckenridge AM, Grimmer SFM, Orme ML'E, Purba HS. Pharmacokinetics of oral contraceptive steroids following the administration of the antimalarial drugs primaquine and chloroquine. *Contraception* (1984) 30, 289–95.
3. Dutta GP, Puri SK, Kamboj KK, Srivastava SK, Kamboj VP. Interactions between oral contraceptives and malaria infections in rhesus monkeys. *Bull WHO* (1984) 62, 931–9.
4. Karbwang J, Looareesuwan S, Back DJ, Migasana S, Bunnag D, Breckenridge AM. Effect of oral contraceptive steroids on the clinical course of malaria infection and on the pharmacokinetics of mefloquine in Thai women. *Bull WHO* (1988) 66, 763–7.
5. McGready R, Stepniewska K, Seaton E, Cho T, Cho D, Ginsberg A, Edstein MD, Ashley E, Looareesuman S, White NJ, Nosten F. Pregnancy and use of oral contraceptives reduces the biotransformation of proguanil to cycloguanil. *Eur J Clin Pharmacol* (2003) 59, 553–7.
6. Mberu EK, Wansor T, Sato H, Nishikawa Y, Watkins WM. Japanese poor metabolizers of proguanil do not have an increased risk of malaria chemoprophylaxis breakthrough. *Trans R Soc Trop Med Hyg* (1995) 89, 658–9.
7. Kaneko A, Bergqvist Y, Takechi M, Kalkoa M, Kaneko O, Kobayakawa T, Ishizaki T, Bjorkman A. Intrinsic efficacy of proguanil against falciparum and vivax malaria independent of the metabolite cycloguanil. *J Infect Dis* (1999) 179; 974–9.
8. Wanwimolruk S, Kaewvichit S, Tanthayaphinant O, Suwannarach C, Oranratnachai A. Lack of effect of oral contraceptive use on the pharmacokinetics of quinine. *Br J Clin Pharmacol* (1991) 31,179–81.
9. Faculty of Family Planning and Reproductive Health Care (FFPRHC). UK Medical eligibility criteria for contraceptive use (UKMEC 2005/2006), July 2006. Available at: http://www.ffprhc.org.uk/admin/uploads/298_UKMEC_200506.pdf (accessed 23/08/07).

Hormonal contraceptives + Aprepitant

Aprepitant reduced the levels of ethinylestradiol and norethisterone given as an oral contraceptive.

Clinical evidence

The manufacturers[1,2] note that aprepitant 100 mg daily for 14 days given with a combined oral contraceptive (**ethinylestradiol/norethisterone** 35 micrograms/1 mg) decreased the AUC of **ethinylestradiol** and **norethisterone** by 43% and 8%, respectively. Reduced contraceptive steroid levels were reported in another study using a recommended antiemetic regimen including aprepitant (125 mg on the first day, then 80 mg daily for 2 days with dexamethasone 12 mg on the first day, then 8 mg daily for 3 days and ondansetron 32 mg on the first day), which was started on day 8 of a 21-day cycle of a combined oral contraceptive (**ethinylestradiol/norethisterone**).[1,2] Within 2 days of starting the antiemetics (day 10) the **ethinylestradiol** AUC was reduced by 19% and the **norethisterone** level was unchanged.[2] However, the trough level of **ethinylestradiol** was reduced by as much as 64% and that of **norethisterone** by 60% during days 9 to 21.[1,2]

Mechanism

During the first few days of use aprepitant is an inhibitor of the cytochrome P450 isoenzyme CYP3A4 and therefore it would be expected to *increase* the levels of the contraceptive steroids. However, aprepitant then becomes an inducer of CYP3A4 (which is usually after the end of a standard 3-day course), reaching a maximal induction effect within 3 to 5 days of stopping aprepitant. This effect lasts only a few days and then reduces to become clinically insignificant within 2 weeks of stopping aprepitant,[1] and hence reduces the levels of the contraceptive steroids.

Importance and management

Although the effects of these reduced contraceptive steroids levels on ovulation were not assessed, it is likely that they could result in reduced efficacy. The manufacturer therefore recommends that alternative or additional contraceptive methods should be used during, and for 2 months (UK advice)[1] or one month (US advice)[2] after, aprepitant use. This seems a sensible precaution. No studies have been done on the effect of a single 40-mg dose of aprepitant 40 mg, as licensed in the US for postoperative nausea and vomiting. However, the US manufacturer states that the timing of the dose may cause contraceptive failure and the same guidance, as stated above, should be used.[2]

1. Emend (Aprepitant). Merck Sharp & Dohme Ltd. UK Summary of product characteristics, February 2007.
2. Emend (Aprepitant). Merck & Co., Inc. US prescribing information, June 2006.

Hormonal contraceptives or HRT + Ascorbic acid (Vitamin C)

Ascorbic acid does not appear to cause a clinically important alteration in the levels of ethinylestradiol or levonorgestrel, but there are a few unconfirmed anecdotal reports of contraceptive failure associated with ascorbic acid. There is some evidence that ascorbic acid may modestly increase estradiol levels in women receiving HRT.

Clinical evidence

(a) Combined oral contraceptives

One study found that ascorbic acid 1 g raised serum **ethinylestradiol** levels by 16% at 6 hours post-dose and 48% at 24 hours post-dose in 5 women taking combined oral contraceptives.[1] However, a later well-controlled study found that ascorbic acid 1 g daily caused no significant changes in **ethinylestradiol** serum levels in 37 women taking a combined oral contraceptive (**ethinylestradiol/levonorgestrel** 30/150 micrograms).[2] A similar study by the same workers found that ascorbic acid 1 g did not affect the pharmacokinetics of **levonorgestrel**.[3]

A single case report describes a woman taking a combined oral contraceptive (**ethinylestradiol/levonorgestrel**) who experienced heavy breakthrough bleeding in 3 cycles within 2 to 3 days of stopping ascorbic acid 1 g daily. This did not occur in 3 other cycles when no ascorbic acid was taken. This was postulated to be due to a fall in **ethinylestradiol** levels when the vitamin C was stopped, which could increase the risk of contraceptive failure.[4] One report attributed contraceptive failure in one case to ascorbic acid and **multivitamins**.[5] Another two studies of pregnancies in oral contraceptive users found that vitamin C had been taken in 44 of 209 cases[6] and 15 of 137 cases,[7] although other drugs and/or factors may possibly have been involved in some of these cases.

(b) Hormone replacement therapy

Ascorbic acid 500 mg twice daily for one month caused a non-significant 21% increase in plasma estradiol levels in 25 postmenopausal women receiving **transdermal estradiol** HRT. However, in the 9 women with initially low estradiol levels, ascorbic acid doubled the levels, and this reached significance.[8]

Mechanism

Both ascorbic acid and ethinylestradiol undergo sulfate conjugation. It was suggested that large doses of ascorbic acid might compete for the metabolism of ethinylestradiol, and therefore increase its levels.[1] This would be expected to increase the efficacy of the oral contraceptive. However, some have postulated that enhanced levels could be followed by rebound ovulation,[4] but there is no evidence to support this. Ascorbic acid may reverse the oxidation of oestrogens.[8]

Importance and management

Documentation about an interaction with contraceptives is limited. From the point of view of reliability, there seems to be little reason for avoiding the use of oral contraceptives and ascorbic acid. No special precautions are required.

The authors of the report on ascorbic acid and HRT say that their findings do not support the general use of ascorbic acid as an adjuvant to HRT, but that further study is needed. No special precautions are required.

1. Back DJ, Breckenridge AM, MacIver M, Orme ML'E, Purba H, Rowe PH. Interaction of ethinyloestradiol with ascorbic acid in man. *BMJ* (1981) 282, 1516.
2. Zamah NM, Hümpel M, Kuhnz W, Louton T, Rafferty J, Back DJ. Absence of an effect of high vitamin C dosage on the systemic availability of ethinyl estradiol in women using a combination oral contraceptive. *Contraception* (1993) 48, 377–91.
3. Kuhnz W, Louton T, Hümpel M, Back DJ, Zamah NM. Influence of high doses of vitamin C on the bioavailability and the serum protein binding of levonorgestrel in women using a combination oral contraceptive. *Contraception* (1995) 51, 111–16.
4. Morris JC, Beeley L, Ballantine N. Interaction of ethinyloestradiol with ascorbic acid in man. *BMJ* (1981) 283, 503.
5. DeSano EA, Hurley SC. Possible interactions of antihistamines and antibiotics with oral contraceptive effectiveness. *Fertil Steril* (1982) 37, 853–4.
6. Kovacs GT, Riddoch G, Duncombe P, Welberry L, Chick P, Weisberg E, Leavesley GM, Baker HWG. Inadvertent pregnancies in oral contraceptive users. *Med J Aust* (1989) 150, 549–51.
7. Sparrow MJ. Pregnancies in reliable pill takers. *N Z Med J* (1989) 102, 575–7.
8. Vihtamäki T, Parantainen J, Koivisto A-M, Metsä-Ketelä T, Tuimala R. Oral ascorbic acid increases plasma oestradiol during postmenopausal hormone replacement therapy. *Maturitas* (2002) 42, 129–35.

Hormonal contraceptives or HRT + Azoles

There are isolated reports of breakthrough bleeding and failure of combined oral contraceptives with fluconazole (including single 150 mg doses), itraconazole and ketoconazole. Conversely, fluconazole, itraconazole and voriconazole have been shown to modestly *increase* the serum levels of the contraceptive steroids. Ketoconazole slightly increases the levels of estrone following oestrogen administration. Miconazole slightly increases the serum levels of ethinylestradiol and etonogestrel released from an intravaginal contraceptive ring.

Clinical evidence

(a) Fluconazole

Up to 1990 the UK manufacturer of fluconazole had received 11 reports of menstrual disorders possibly associated with single-dose fluconazole 150 mg. Eight of these were in women taking an oral contraceptive who developed breakthrough bleeding (5 cases), no withdrawal bleeding (1 case), unintended pregnancies (2 cases).[1] Three other cases of unintended pregnancy have been very briefly mentioned elsewhere.[2]

However, one study found that a single 150-mg dose of fluconazole *increased* the AUC of **ethinylestradiol** by 29% in women taking a combined oral contraceptive (**ethinylestradiol** and **norethisterone** or **levonorgestrel**).[3] Similarly, fluconazole 300 mg once weekly for 4 weeks caused a 24% increase in the AUC of **ethinylestradiol** and a 13% increase in the AUC of **norethisterone**.[4] Moreover, the manufacturer has data on file showing that multiple doses of fluconazole 200 mg daily raised the levels of **ethinylestradiol** by 40% and of **levonorgestrel** by 24%,[5] whereas a lower dose of fluconazole (a single 50-mg dose or 50 mg of fluconazole daily for 10 days) had no significant effect on the pharmacokinetics of **ethinylestradiol** and **norgestrel**.[6] One other study in 10 women taking combined oral contraceptives found no changes in progesterone levels (suggesting no ovulation occurred) and no menstrual disorders while they were taking fluconazole 50 mg daily.[7] Furthermore, during clinical studies in which single 150-mg doses of fluconazole were used by over 700 women taking oral contraceptives, no evidence of an interaction was seen.[8]

(b) Itraconazole

A 25-year-old woman who had been taking a combined oral contraceptive (**ethinylestradiol/levonorgestrel** 30/150 micrograms) for a year, without problems, became pregnant when she was given itraconazole 200 mg daily for 3 months for a fungal infection. The patient was said to be compliant, had suffered no gastrointestinal upset, and was not taking any other drugs that might have accounted for the failure of the pill.[2]

The Netherlands Pharmacovigilance Foundation (LAREB) have 9 cases of menstrual changes on their records in women taking an oral contraceptive during or after taking itraconazole 100 to 400 mg daily for 1 to 4 weeks. Seven women reported delayed withdrawal bleeding (2 to 5 days). In 2 of them the menstrual flow was decreased and one transiently had a positive pregnancy test after having previously experienced an intermenstrual blood loss. The remaining two reports were of amenorrhoea during one cycle, and breakthrough bleeding. The women were taking **ethinylestradiol** plus either **desogestrel** or **levonorgestrel**.[9] A later extension of this report from LAREB, covering the period 1991 to 1997, describes 12 women taking contraceptives containing **ethinylestradiol** with **desogestrel**, whose withdrawal bleeding was either delayed or did not occur at all while taking itraconazole. Three other women taking **ethinylestradiol** with **levonorgestrel** had breakthrough bleeding, and yet another taking **ethinylestradiol** with **cyproterone** became pregnant while taking itraconazole.[10]

However, the manufacturer has data on file of a study showing that itraconazole 200 mg daily for 15 days had no effect on the pharmacokinetics of **ethinylestradiol**, and *increased* the bioavailability of **norethisterone** by about 40%. In this study, a single dose of **ethinylestradiol/norethisterone** was given before the first dose and with the last dose of itraconazole.[11]

(c) Ketoconazole

An early report described 7 out of 147 women taking combined oral contraceptives (**ethinylestradiol/norgestrel**) who experienced breakthrough bleeding or spotting within 2 to 5 days of starting a 5-day course of ketoconazole 400 mg daily. No pregnancies occurred.[12] One unintended pregnancy attributed to contraceptive failure due to ketoconazole has been very briefly mentioned elsewhere.[2] A study in 6 postmenopausal women given a single 2-mg dose of **estradiol** found that ketoconazole 100 mg twice daily for 4 days increased the AUC and maximum plasma levels of estrone (a metabolite of estradiol) by 16% and 30%, respectively. The small increases were not thought to be clinically significant.[13]

(d) Miconazole

A study found that both single and multiple-dose intravaginal regimens of miconazole pessaries and cream slightly increased the serum levels of **ethinylestradiol** and **etonogestrel** released from an intravaginal ring *(NuvaRing)*.[14]

(e) Voriconazole

The maximum levels and AUC of **ethinylestradiol** 35 micrograms (given as a combined oral contraceptive) were increased by 36% and 61%, respectively, by concurrent use of voriconazole. Similarly, the maximum levels and AUC of **norethisterone** 1 mg were also increased by 15% and 53%, respectively, by voriconazole. The maximum levels and AUC of voriconazole were increased by 14% and 46%, respectively, by these contraceptive steroids.[15]

Mechanism

The azole antifungals are, to varying degrees, inhibitors of the cytochrome P450 isoenzyme CYP3A4. They would therefore be expected to increase the levels of the contraceptive steroids, as has been shown for fluconazole, itraconazole and voriconazole. Similarly, ketoconazole and miconazole have been seen to raise the levels of some oestrogens. Therefore the azoles would *not* be expected to increase the incidence of breakthrough bleeding or contraceptive failure when used with combined oral contraceptives. It should be noted that the manufacturers list menstrual irregularities as adverse effects of itraconazole, ketoconazole and **posaconazole** irrespective of the use of combined oral contraceptives,[16-18] and menstrual disorders have also been reported with fluconazole alone.[1]

Importance and management

The picture presented by these reports is somewhat confusing and contradictory. The anecdotal reports of contraceptive failure and the cases of breakthrough bleeding would suggest that these antifungals can, rarely, make oral contraception less reliable in some individuals. However, the problem with this interpretation is that the pharmacokinetic data suggest that, if anything, an *enhanced* effect of the combined oral contraceptives is likely. Note that, of all the drugs proven to decrease the efficacy of combined oral contraceptives, all have also been shown to decrease the steroid levels. Menstrual disorders have occurred with the azole antifungals alone, and may not be indicative of reduced contraceptive efficacy. Since there are so few reports of pregnancy, it could just be that they fall within the accepted failure rate of combined oral contraceptives, and it was just coincidental they occurred when the antifungal was being taken. Note that the manufacturers do not advise any special precautions when taking oral contraceptives and these azole antifungals.[5,15,16] However, some consider that the data warrant consideration being given to the use of additional contraceptive measures.[10] The theoretical teratogenic risk[5,15-18] from these azole antifungals may have a bearing on this, and the UK manufacturers of a number of the azoles recommend using effective contraception during azole treatment to reduce this risk.[5,15,16,18] More study is clearly needed.

The main concern regarding the increased levels of ethinylestradiol or progestogens is whether this would increase the risk of adverse effects of the steroid. There are no data on the effect of these modest 25 to 40% increases in steroid levels on adverse effects. It could be argued that a 40% increase would turn a standard-strength contraceptive (35 micrograms) into a high-dose contraceptive (50 micrograms). However, early studies showed that the interindividual variation in ethinylestradiol pharmacokinetics was greater than this anyway.[19] Further study is needed.

1. Pfizer Ltd. Summary of unpublished reports: female reproductive disorders possibly associated with Diflucan. Data on file (Ref DIFLU:diflu41.1), 1990.
2. Pillans PI, Sparrow MJ. Pregnancy associated with a combined oral contraceptive and itraconazole. *N Z Med J* (1993) 106, 436.
3. Sinofsky FE, Pasquale SA. The effect of fluconazole on circulating ethinyl estradiol levels in women taking oral contraceptives. *Am J Obstet Gynecol* (1998) 178, 300–4.
4. Hilbert J, Messig M, Kuye O, Friedman H. Evaluation of interaction between fluconazole and an oral contraceptive in healthy women. *Obstet Gynecol* (2001) 98, 218–23.
5. Diflucan (Fluconazole). Pfizer Ltd. UK Summary of product characteristics, April 2007.
6. Lazar JD, Wilner KD. Drug interactions with fluconazole. *Rev Infect Dis* (1990) 12, Suppl 3, S327–S333.
7. Devenport MH, Crook D, Wynn V, Lees LJ. Metabolic effects of low-dose fluconazole in healthy female users and non-users of oral contraceptives. *Br J Clin Pharmacol* (1989) 27, 851–9.
8. Dodd GK (Pfizer Ltd). Personal communication, 1990.
9. Meyboom RHB, van Puijenbroek EP, Vinks MHAM, Lastdrager CJ. Disturbance of withdrawal bleeding during concomitant use of itraconazole and oral contraceptives. *N Z Med J* (1997) 110, 300.
10. van Puijenbroek EP, Feenstra J, Meyboom RHB. Verstoring van de pilcyclus tijdens het gelijktijdig gebruik van itraconazol en orale anticonceptiva. *Ned Tijdschr Geneeskd* (1998) 142, 146–9.
11. Jones AR (Janssen). Personal communication, 1994.
12. Kovács I, Somos P, Hámori M. Examination of the potential interaction between ketoconazole (Nizoral) and oral contraceptives with special regard to products of low hormone content (Rigevidon, Anteovin). *Ther Hung* (1986) 34, 167–70.
13. Annas A, Carlström K, Alván G, AL-Shurbaji A. The effect of ketoconazole and diltiazem on oestrogen metabolism in postmenopausal women after single dose oestradiol treatment. *Br J Clin Pharmacol* (2003) 56, 334–6.
14. Verhoeven CHJ, van den Heuvel MW, Mulders TMT, Dieben TOM. The contraceptive vaginal ring, NuvaRing®, and antimycotic co-medication. *Contraception* (2004) 69, 129–32.
15. VFEND (Voriconazole). Pfizer Ltd. UK Summary of product characteristics, July 2007.
16. Sporanox Capsules (Itraconazole). Janssen-Cilag Ltd. UK Summary of product characteristics, March 2004.
17. Nizoral Tablets (Ketoconazole). Janssen-Cilag Ltd. UK Summary of product characteristics, October 2006.
18. Noxafil (Posaconazole). Schering-Plough Ltd. UK Summary of product characteristics, October 2006.
19. Back DJ, Breckenridge AM, Crawford FE, MacIver M, Orme ML'E, Rowe PH. Interindividual variation and drug interactions with hormonal steroids. *Drugs* (1981) 21, 46–61.

Hormonal contraceptives + Bosentan

Bosentan reduces the levels of ethinylestradiol and norethisterone given as a combined oral contraceptive.

Clinical evidence, mechanism, importance and management

In randomised, crossover study in 19 healthy subjects a single dose of a combined oral contraceptive containing **norethisterone** 1 mg and **ethinylestradiol** 35 micrograms (*Ortho-Novum*) was given with bosentan 125 mg twice daily for one week. Bosentan reduced the mean AUC of norethisterone by 14% (maximum reduction 56%) and the mean AUC of ethinylestradiol by 31% (maximum reduction 66%). Note that there was marked inter-individual variability. The maximum concentration and half-life of both contraceptive steroids were not significantly affected. The contraceptive steroids are metabolised by the cytochrome P450 isoenzyme CYP3A4, and it was thought that the changes in their pharmacokinetics may have been caused by induction of CYP3A4 by bosentan. However other mechanisms could not be excluded. The link between these results and actual contraceptive failure is unclear.[1]

The Pulmonary Hypertension Association has suggested that there is the potential for bosentan to reduce the effectiveness of hormonal contraceptives by any route. They also state that bosentan may have teratogenic effects and therefore it should not be used as the only method of contraception in patients taking bosentan.[2] Similarly, the manufacturer contraindicates the use of bosentan in women who are not using reliable methods of contraception and recommends that additional or alternative methods to hormonal contraceptives are used. This must be continued for at least 3 months after treatment is stopped.[3]

1. Van Giersbergen PLM, Halabi A, Dingemanse J. Pharmacokinetic interaction between bosentan and the oral contraceptives norethisterone and ethinyl estradiol. *Int J Clin Pharmacol Ther* (2006) 44, 113–18.
2. Pulmonary Hypertension Association. Treatments: Bosentan (Tracleer®). Available at: http://www.phassociation.org/Learn/treatment/bosentan.asp (accessed on 23/08/2007).
3. Tracleer (Bosentan monohydrate). Actelion Pharmaceuticals UK. UK Summary of product characteristics, October 2006.

Hormonal contraceptives + Candesartan

Candesartan cilexetil 8 mg daily had no effect on the pharmacokinetics of ethinylestradiol and levonorgestrel in a combined oral contraceptive, and no ovulation occurred during concurrent treatment.[1] No special precautions would therefore appear to be needed. Consider also 'Drospirenone + Potassium-sparing drugs', p.977, for a possible interaction between angiotensin II receptor antagonists and drospirenone, and 'Antihypertensives + Hormonal contraceptives', p.880.

1. Jonkman JHG, van Lier JJ, van Heiningen PNM, Lins R, Sennewald R, Högemann A. Pharmacokinetic drug interaction studies with candesartan cilexetil. *J Hum Hypertens* (1997) 11 (Suppl 2), S31–S35.

Hormonal contraceptives or HRT + Coxibs

Rofecoxib increases contraceptive steroid levels to a small extent, and would not therefore be expected to reduce contraceptive efficacy. Etoricoxib raises ethinylestradiol levels by 50 to 60%, and also appears to raise the levels of conjugated oestrogens in HRT. Celecoxib appears to have no effect on combined oral contraceptive levels. One case of pulmonary embolism has been reported in a patient taking valdecoxib with a combined oral contraceptive.

Clinical evidence, mechanism, importance and management

(a) Celecoxib

Celecoxib had no clinically significant effects on the pharmacokinetics of a combined oral contraceptive containing **norethisterone** 1 mg and **ethinylestradiol** 35 micrograms.[1] No precautions seem necessary.

(b) Etoricoxib

A study in women taking a combined oral contraceptive (**ethinylestradiol/norethisterone** 35 micrograms/0.5 to 1 mg) for 21 days found that the addition of etoricoxib 120 mg with or 12 hours after the oral contraceptive increased the 24-hour steady-state levels of **ethinylestradiol** by 50 to 60%. It is thought that etoricoxib increases **ethinylestradiol** levels because it inhibits human sulfotransferase activity. The manufacturer suggests that this increase in **ethinylestradiol** levels should be considered when choosing the oral contraceptive because of the possible increased risk of adverse events.[2] It may therefore be appropriate to use a contraceptive with a lower dose of **ethinylestradiol**.

Etoricoxib 120 mg taken with HRT containing 0.625 mg of conjugated oestrogens (*Premarin*) increased the $AUC_{0\text{-}24}$ of unconjugated estrone, equilin and 17-ß estradiol by 41%, 76%, and 22%, respectively; however, the AUCs of these metabolites were less than those seen with 1.25 mg of conjugated oestrogens. The effects of lower doses of etoricoxib have not been studied. The manufacturers say that these increases should be taken into account when selecting HRT in patients taking etoricoxib.[2]

(c) Rofecoxib

In a placebo-controlled, crossover study in 18 healthy women taking a combined oral contraceptive (**ethinylestradiol/norethisterone** 35 micrograms/1 mg), rofecoxib 175 mg daily for 2 weeks raised the AUCs of **ethinylestradiol** and **norethisterone** by 13% and 18%, respectively. These small changes, although statistically significant, are within the accepted criteria for bioequivalence, and are unlikely to be clinically important. No abnormal menstrual bleeding was reported.[3] No special precautions are required during concurrent use.

(d) Valdecoxib

A single case of pulmonary embolism has been reported with the concurrent use of a combined oral contraceptive containing **norgestimate/ethinylestradiol** (*Ortho Tri-Cyclen)* and valdecoxib. The patient had been taking the same combined oral contraceptive (containing ethinylestradiol doses of 35 and then 25 micrograms) for 3 years prior to taking valdecoxib with no adverse effects. The authors note that multiple factors may have contributed to this case, as prolonged stasis (a 6-hour car journey) and oral contraceptives themselves can cause venous thromboembolism.[4] There appear to be no further similar published reports and the clinical significance of this case is unclear. Note that valdecoxib has been withdrawn.

1. Celebrex (Celecoxib). Pharmacia Ltd. UK Summary of product characteristics, February 2007.
2. Arcoxia (Etoricoxib). Merck Sharp & Dohme Ltd. UK Summary of product characteristics, January 2007.
3. Schwartz JI, Wong PH, Porras AG, Ebel DL, Hunt TR, Gertz BJ. Effect of rofecoxib on the pharmacokinetics of chronically administered oral contraceptives in healthy female volunteers. *J Clin Pharmacol* (2002) 42, 215–21.
4. Westgate EJ, Fitzgerald GA. Pulmonary embolism in a woman taking oral contraceptives and valdecoxib. *PLoS Med* (2005) 2, e197.

Hormonal contraceptives + Danazol or Gestrinone

There is a theoretical risk that the effects of danazol or gestrinone and hormonal contraceptives might be altered or reduced by concurrent use.

Clinical evidence, mechanism, importance and management

(a) Danazol

Danazol inhibits ovulation, but it is not considered reliable enough to be used as a hormonal contraceptive.[1-3] Danazol should not be used during pregnancy, because it can cause virilisation of a female foetus. The manufacturer advises the use of reliable non-hormonal contraceptive methods while taking danazol,[4] and by inference the avoidance of hormonal contraceptives. They say that there is a theoretical risk that danazol and exogenously administered oestrogens and/or progestogens, including oral contraceptives, might possibly compete for the same oestrogen, progestogen, and androgen receptors, thereby altering the effects of both drugs.[3] This would also apply to other hormonal contraceptives such as **etonogestrel** implants and depot preparations of **medroxyprogesterone** and **norethisterone**. However, as yet there appears to be no direct evidence that any interaction actually occurs.

(b) Gestrinone

Although gestrinone, at the dose used for endometriosis, can inhibit ovulation, it is not sufficiently reliable to be used as a contraceptive. The manufacturer strongly emphasises the importance of using a barrier method of contraception while taking gestrinone because they say that not only are the effects of gestrinone possibly modified by oral contraceptives, but its use in pregnancy is totally contraindicated (high doses have been shown to be embryotoxic in some *animal* species).[5]

1. Greenblatt RB, Oettinger M, Borenstein R, Bohler CS-S. Influence of danazol (100 mg) on conception and contraception. *J Reprod Med* (1974) 13, 201–3.
2. Colle ML, Greenblatt RB. Contraceptive properties of danazol. *J Reprod Med* (1976) 17, 98–102.
3. Sterling-Winthrop, Personal communication 1990.
4. Danol (Danazol). Sanofi-Aventis. UK Summary of product characteristics, April 2006.
5. Dimetriose (Gestrinone). Sanofi-Aventis. UK Summary of product characteristics, October 2003.

Hormonal contraceptives + Ezetimibe

No significant pharmacokinetic interaction appears to occur between ezetimibe and an ethinylestradiol/norgestrel-containing oral contraceptive.

Clinical evidence, mechanism, importance and management

In a randomised, crossover study, 18 healthy women who had been taking a triphasic oral contraceptive (containing **ethinylestradiol/norgestrel**) were also given ezetimibe 10 mg daily or placebo on days 8 to 14 of two consecutive contraceptive cycles. Ezetimibe did not significantly affect the pharmacokinetics of ethinylestradiol or norgestrel.[1] The manufacturers note that ezetimibe had no effect on the pharmacokinetics of **ethinylestradiol/*levo*norgestrel**-containing contraceptives, therefore no additional precautions seem necessary if ezetimibe is given to women taking these contraceptives.[2]

1. Keung ACF, Kosoglou T, Statkevich P, Anderson L, Boutros T, Cutler DL, Batra V, Sellers EM. Ezetimibe does not affect the pharmacokinetics of oral contraceptives. *Clin Pharmacol Ther* (2001) 69, P55.
2. Ezetrol (Ezetimibe). MSD-SP Ltd. UK Summary of product characteristics, December 2006.

Hormonal contraceptives + Griseofulvin

The effects of the oral contraceptives may possibly be disturbed (either intermenstrual bleeding or amenorrhoea) if griseofulvin is taken concurrently. Reports describe women taking oral contraceptives who became pregnant while taking griseofulvin.

Clinical evidence

In 1984, regulatory authorities in the UK and the Netherlands noted that they had received a total of 22 reports of possible interactions between oral contraceptives and griseofulvin. These included 15 reports of transient intermenstrual bleeding and 5 of amenorrhoea, occurring during the first or second cycle, after griseofulvin 500 mg to 1 g daily was started. Four of these patients were rechallenged with griseofulvin (2 with intermenstrual bleeding and 2 with amenorrhoea) and all developed their original reactions. The other two women were reported to have become pregnant while taking griseofulvin and a sulphonamide ('co-trimoxazole', (p.982) in one instance and an unknown sulphonamide in the other).[1] One other case of contraceptive failure has been reported from an analysis of the database of the CSM in the UK from 1968 to 1984,[2] but note this case may be included in the two already reported.[1] One other case report describes a woman taking a triphasic combined oral contraceptive who became pregnant about 2 months after she started to take griseofulvin 330 mg twice daily,[3] and another report describes a woman taking an oral contraceptive who became pregnant 6 weeks after starting to take griseofulvin 500 mg daily for 3 months and a 7-day course of 'erythromycin', (p.979).[4] Irregular menses and reduced menstrual flow have been described in another woman taking a combined oral contraceptive (**ethinylestradiol** 35 micrograms/**norethisterone** 0.5 to 1 mg) with griseofulvin 250 to 500 mg daily. When the oral contraceptive was substituted with another with more oestrogen (**ethinylestradiol/norgestrel** 50/500 micrograms), the menstrual cycle became normal again.[5] Breakthrough bleeding has also been seen in one other woman taking an oral contraceptive with griseofulvin.[6]

Mechanism

Not understood. Griseofulvin may possibly stimulate the activity of the liver enzymes concerned with the metabolism of the contraceptive steroids, thereby reducing their effects (see 'Hormonal contraceptives and sex hormones', (p.975)).

Importance and management

Information about this interaction is very limited. The risk of contraceptive failure is uncertain but probably very small. However, it would be prudent for prescribers to warn women taking a **combined oral contraceptive** who are given griseofulvin that menstrual disturbances may possibly be signs of contraceptive unreliability, and that additional contraceptive precautions should be taken. The CSM in the UK has pointed out the importance of ensuring adequate contraception during and for one month after taking griseofulvin because it can induce aneuploidy (abnormal segregation of chromosomes during cell division), which carries the potential risk of teratogenicity.[7] For maximal contraceptive protection additional contraceptive measures (such as a barrier method) should be used routinely while taking griseofulvin and for one month afterwards.

The situation with **progestogen-only contraceptives** is not clear, but it has been suggested that they are not the contraceptive of choice in those taking griseofulvin, not because of reduced efficacy but because of increased menstrual irregularities.[8] The Faculty of Family Planning and Reproductive Health Care (FFPRHC) Clinical Effectiveness Unit states that griseofulvin may reduce the efficacy of hormonal contraceptives as it is a liver enzyme inducer and additional contraceptive protection is advised with concurrent use.[9] They have issued guidance on the use of contraceptives with liver enzyme inducers, see 'Hormonal contraceptives + Antiepileptics; Barbiturates or Phenytoin', p.985.

1. van Dijke CPH, Weber JCP. Interaction between oral contraceptives and griseofulvin. *BMJ* (1984) 288, 1125–6.
2. Back DJ, Grimmer SFM, Orme ML'E, Proudlove C, Mann RD, Breckenridge AM. Evaluation of Committee on Safety of Medicines yellow card reports on oral contraceptive-drug interactions with anticonvulsants and antibiotics. *Br J Clin Pharmacol* (1988) 25, 527–32.
3. Côté J. Interaction of griseofulvin and oral contraceptives. *J Am Acad Dermatol* (1990) 22, 124–5.
4. Bollen M. Use of antibiotics when taking the oral contraceptive pill. *Aust Fam Physician* (1995) 24, 928–9.
5. McDaniel PA, Caldroney RD. Oral contraceptives and griseofulvin interaction. *Drug Intell Clin Pharm* (1986) 20, 384.
6. Beeley L, Stewart P. *Bulletin of the West Midlands Centre for Adverse Drug Reaction Reporting* (1987) 25, 23.
7. Committee on Safety of Medicines/Medicines Control Agency. Griseofulvin (Fulcin, Grisovin): contraceptive precautions. *Current Problems* (1996) 22, 8.
8. McCann MF, Potter LS. Progestin-only contraception: a comprehensive review. *Contraception* (1994) 50 (Suppl 1), S1–S198.
9. Faculty of Family Planning and Reproductive Health Care Clinical Effectiveness Unit. FFPRHC Guidance: Drug interactions with hormonal contraception. April 2005. Available at: http://www.ffprhc.org.uk/admin/uploads/DrugInteractionsFinal.pdf (accessed 23/08/07).

Hormonal contraceptives + Immunosuppressants

No clinically relevant interactions have been seen between leflunomide, mycophenolate or sirolimus and combined oral contraceptives, but the manufacturer of sirolimus suggests some caution. Mycophenolate has been shown to be teratogenic in *animals* and so the manufacturer suggests contraceptive precautions in addition to the use of hormonal contraceptives. Tacrolimus may increase the plasma levels of hormonal contraceptives.

Clinical evidence, mechanism, importance and management

(a) Ciclosporin

For the interactions of ciclosporin with hormonal contraceptives see, 'Ciclosporin + Hormonal contraceptives and Progestogens', p.1038.

(b) Leflunomide

Leflunomide was given to healthy women taking a triphasic oral contraceptive containing 30 micrograms of **ethinylestradiol**. During the study it was found that the leflunomide had no effect on the activity of the oral contraceptive and the pharmacokinetics of the active metabolite of leflunomide (A771726) were not changed to a clinically relevant extent.[1] No special precautions would therefore appear to be needed on concurrent use.

(c) Mycophenolate

The manufacturer says that no pharmacokinetic interaction was seen in a single-dose study in 15 healthy women taking mycophenolate and *Orthonovum* (**norethisterone/ethinylestradiol** 1 mg/35 micrograms).[2] A study of mycophenolate 1 g twice daily given with a combined oral contraceptive (containing **ethinylestradiol** 20 to 40 micrograms and **levonorgestrel** 50 to 150 micrograms, **desogestrel** 150 micrograms or **gestodene** 50 to 100 micrograms) over 3 consecutive menstrual cycles in 18 women not previously taking immunosuppressants found no clinically relevant influence of mycophenolate on the suppression of ovulation by the oral contraceptives.[3,4] Large interpatient variability was seen especially for **ethinylestradiol**. However, the mean **levonorgestrel** AUC was decreased by about 15%.[4] In addition, mycophenolate has been shown to be teratogenic in *animal* studies at doses lower than those causing maternal toxicity. The manufacturers say that effective contraception must be used before mycophenolate, during, and for 6 weeks after mycophenolate has been stopped.[3,4] The US manufacturer also advises that oral contraceptives should be used with caution, and additional birth control methods used.[4]

(d) Sirolimus

A single-dose study found that the pharmacokinetics of an oral contraceptive (**ethinylestradiol/norgestrel** 30/300 micrograms) were unaffected by sirolimus. This suggests that the efficacy of the contraceptive is likely to be unchanged, but the UK manufacturer cautiously points out that the effects of long-term sirolimus on oral contraception are unknown.[5] They advise that contraception should be continued for 12 weeks after sirolimus is stopped.

(e) Tacrolimus

The UK manufacturer of tacrolimus says that during clinical use **ethinylestradiol** has been shown to be a weak inhibitor of tacrolimus metabolism and may increase tacrolimus levels, presumably because it inhibits the cytochrome P450 isoenzyme CYP3A4. *In vitro* data suggest that **gestodene** and **norethisterone** may do the same. In addition, tacrolimus may reduce the clearance of steroid-based contraceptives, leading to increased hormone exposure, and therefore the manufacturers suggest that care should be taken when deciding upon contraceptive measures.[6]

1. Arava (Leflunomide). Sanofi-Aventis. UK Summary of product characteristics, January 2006.
2. Syntex. Data on file. A single-dose pharmacokinetic drug interaction study of oral mycophenolate mofetil and an oral contraceptive in normal subjects. (Study No. MYCS2308) 1994.
3. CellCept (Mycophenolate mofetil). Roche Products Ltd. UK Summary of product characteristics, March 2006.
4. CellCept (Mycophenolate mofetil). Roche Laboratories Inc. US Prescribing information, October 2005.
5. Rapamune (Sirolimus). Wyeth Pharmaceuticals. UK Summary of product characteristics, March 2007.
6. Prograf (Tacrolimus monohydrate). Astellas Pharma Ltd. UK Summary of product characteristics, May 2007.

Hormonal contraceptives + Leukotriene antagonists

Montelukast and zafirlukast do not alter the contraceptive efficacy of oral contraceptives.

Clinical evidence, mechanism, importance and management

(a) Montelukast

The manufacturers of montelukast say that it does not affect the pharmacokinetics of an oral contraceptive (**ethinylestradiol/norethisterone** 35 micrograms/1 mg).[1,2] No special precautions are therefore needed if both drugs are given together.

(b) Zafirlukast

A single-blind, parallel-group study in 39 healthy women taking unnamed oral contraceptives found that zafirlukast 40 mg twice daily had no effect on the serum levels of **ethinylestradiol** nor on its contraceptive efficacy.[3] This study suggests that concurrent use need not be avoided.

1. Singulair (Montelukast sodium). Merck Sharp & Dohme Ltd. UK Summary of product characteristics, November 2006.
2. Singulair (Montelukast sodium). Merck & Co., Inc. US Prescribing information, April 2007.
3. Accolate (Zafirlukast). AstraZeneca Pharmaceuticals LP. US Prescribing information, July 2004.

Hormonal contraceptives + Moclobemide

Moclobemide did not alter the efficacy of combined oral contraceptives, as assessed by measures of ovulation suppression.

Clinical evidence, mechanism, importance and management

A study in 7 women taking combined oral contraceptives found no evidence of any significant alterations in estradiol, progesterone, FSH, or LH levels when they took moclobemide 200 mg three times daily for one cycle. This suggests that ovulation did not occur. No serious adverse reactions occurred. It was considered that the efficacy of the oral contraceptives is likely to be maintained during concurrent use.[1]

1. Amrein R, Güntert TW, Dingemanse J, Lorscheid T, Stabl M, Schmid-Burgk W. Interactions of moclobemide with concomitantly administered medication: evidence from pharmacological and clinical studies. *Psychopharmacology (Berl)* (1992) 106, S24–S31.

Hormonal contraceptives + Modafinil

Modafinil slightly reduces the levels of ethinylestradiol given as part of a combined oral contraceptive.

Clinical evidence, mechanism, importance and management

In 16 healthy women taking a combined oral contraceptive (**ethinylestradiol/norgestimate**), modafinil 200 mg daily for 7 days followed by 400 mg daily for 21 days decreased the AUC and the maximum plasma levels of **ethinylestradiol** by 18% and 11%, respectively. Increases in plasma FSH and LH were not significant.[1] Modafinil is an inducer of the cytochrome P450 isoenzyme CYP3A4, which is partially responsible for the metabolism of **ethinylestradiol**. These small changes are lower than those seen with other enzyme inducers known to reduce the reliability of combined oral contraceptives (e.g. see 'phenytoin', (p.985)). However, it cannot be ruled out that they would be sufficient to cause failure of combined oral contraceptives in very rare cases. The UK manufacturer recommends that additional or alternative methods of contraception should be used during and for up to 2 cycles after stopping modafinil.[2] The US manufacturer gives similar guidance but advises that additional or alternative contraceptive methods need only be continued for one month after stopping modafinil.[3] Note that this advice applies to other forms of hormonal contraception including implants and patches.[3,4] The Faculty of Family Planning and Reproductive Health Care (FFPRHC) Clinical Effectiveness Unit has issued guidance on the use of liver enzyme inducers with hormonal contraceptives,[4] see 'Hormonal contraceptives + Antiepileptics; Barbiturates or Phenytoin', p.985, for further information.

1. Robertson P, Hellriegel ET, Arora S, Nelson M. Effect of modafinil on the pharmacokinetics of ethinyl estradiol and triazolam in healthy volunteers. *Clin Pharmacol Ther* (2002) 71, 46–56.

2. Provigil (Modafinil). Cephalon Ltd. UK Summary of product characteristics, July 2007.

3. Provigil (Modafinil). Cephalon, Inc. US Prescribing information, December 2004.

4. Faculty of Family Planning and Reproductive Health Care Clinical Effectiveness Unit. FFPRHC Guidance: Drug interactions with hormonal contraception. April 2005. Available at: http://www.ffprhc.org.uk/admin/uploads/DrugInteractionsFinal.pdf (accessed 23/08/07).

Hormonal contraceptives + Nefazodone

A woman experienced increased combined oral contraceptive adverse effects while taking nefazodone.

Clinical evidence, mechanism, importance and management

Within a week of starting to take nefazodone 50 mg twice daily, a woman taking a low-dose combined oral contraceptive (**ethinylestradiol** 20 micrograms/**desogestrel**) reported breast tenderness, bloating, weight gain, and increased premenstrual irritability. She had previously experienced identical symptoms while taking a combined oral contraceptive with a higher dose of oestrogen. Nefazodone was discontinued after 6 weeks, and within 24 hours the adverse effects resolved.[1] Nefazodone is a known inhibitor of the cytochrome P450 isoenzyme CYP3A4, by which **ethinylestradiol** is metabolised, and might therefore be expected to increase **ethinylestradiol** levels. However, the general importance of this isolated case is unknown.

1. Adson DE, Kotlyar M. A probable interaction between a very low-dose oral contraceptive and the antidepressant nefazodone: a case report. *J Clin Psychopharmacol* (2001) 21, 618–19.

Hormonal contraceptives + NNRTIs

Nevirapine modestly reduces ethinylestradiol and norethisterone levels. Efavirenz and delavirdine increased the levels of ethinylestradiol, while ethinylestradiol had no effect on efavirenz levels. Potential contraceptive failures have been reported in two women taking efavirenz.
Note that whatever other methods of contraception are being used, barrier methods are also advisable to reduce the risk of HIV transmission.

Clinical evidence, mechanism, importance and management

(a) Delavirdine

The manufacturer of delavirdine notes that it may increase the levels of **ethinylestradiol**, but the clinical relevance of this is unknown.[1]

(b) Efavirenz

The manufacturer notes that efavirenz *increased* the AUC of a single dose of **ethinylestradiol** by 37% while the maximum plasma levels remained unchanged. **Ethinylestradiol** had no effect on the AUC of maximum plasma levels of efavirenz.[2,3] These findings suggest that efavirenz does not adversely alter the efficacy of combined oral contraceptives. Nevertheless, the manufacturer notes that because the interaction has not been fully characterised, a reliable method of barrier contraception must be used in addition to other methods of contraception such as hormonal contraceptives.[2,3] Furthermore, a retrospective review identified 22 women who were prescribed oral contraceptives and also received an NNRTI. Two of the 16 women taking efavirenz experienced contraceptive failure. However, medication adherence could not be confirmed.[4] The Faculty of Family Planning and Reproductive Health Care (FFPRHC) Clinical Effectiveness Unit states that efavirenz can induce liver enzymes and may *reduce* ethinylestradiol and progestogens. They therefore recommend that their guidance on hormonal contraceptives and liver enzyme inducers is followed,[5] see 'Hormonal contraceptives + Antiepileptics; Barbiturates or Phenytoin', p.985 for further detail. Note that, a barrier method of contraception would usually be considered advisable to reduce the risk of HIV transmission.

(c) Nevirapine

A study in 10 HIV-positive women found that nevirapine 200 mg once daily for 2 weeks then twice daily for a further 2 weeks decreased the median AUC and elimination half-life of **ethinylestradiol** by 29% and 31%, respectively, and decreased the median AUC of **norethisterone** by 19%. The women received two single doses of a combined oral contraceptive (**ethinylestradiol/norethisterone** 35 micrograms/1 mg); 2 days before the nevirapine and on the last day of the nevirapine. Nevirapine was added to established antiretroviral therapy (commonly 3 drugs), which had been unchanged for at least 4 weeks.[6] A retrospective study identified 22 women who were prescribed oral contraceptives and also received an NNRTI. None of the 6 women taking nevirapine experienced contraceptive failure. However, medication adherence could not be confirmed.[4]

It is likely that nevirapine induces the metabolism of the components of the oral contraceptive by cytochrome P450 isoenzymes.[6] Although it is not known whether these modest reductions in levels would reduce the anti-ovulatory efficacy of the combined oral contraceptive, it would be prudent to assume they could. The manufacturers recommend that combined oral contraceptives and other hormonal methods of birth control should not be used as the sole method of contraception in women taking nevirapine. They suggest that a barrier method (e.g. condoms) should also be used, and note that this is also advisable to reduce the risk of HIV transmission.[6,7] The Faculty of Family Planning and Reproductive Health Care (FFPRHC) Clinical Effectiveness Unit notes that nevirapine can induce liver enzymes and may reduce the levels of ethinylestradiol and progestogens. They therefore recommend that their guidance on hormonal contraceptives and liver enzyme inducers is followed,[5] see 'Hormonal contraceptives + Antiepileptics; Barbiturates or Phenytoin', p.985 for further detail.

The manufacturer also suggests that if combined oral contraceptives are used for reasons other than contraception (e.g. endometriosis), that the therapeutic effect should be monitored and the dose increased if necessary.[6,7] These precautions seem prudent.

1. Rescriptor (Delavirdine mesylate). Pfizer Inc. US Prescribing information, June 2006.

2. Sustiva (Efavirenz). Bristol-Myers Squibb Pharmaceuticals Ltd. UK Summary of product characteristics, May 2007.
3. Sustiva (Efavirenz). Bristol-Myers Squibb Company. US Prescribing information, January 2007.
4. Clark RA, Theall K. Population-based study evaluating association between selected antiretroviral therapies and potential oral contraceptive failure. *J Acquir Immune Defic Syndr* (2004) 37, 1219–20.
5. Faculty of Family Planning and Reproductive Health Care Clinical Effectiveness Unit. FFPRHC Guidance: Drug interactions with hormonal contraception. April 2005. Available at: http://www.ffprhc.org.uk/admin/uploads/DrugInteractionsFinal.pdf (accessed 23/08/07).
6. Mildvan D, Yarrish R, Marshak A, Hutman HW, McDonough M, Lamson M, Robinson P. Pharmacokinetic interaction between nevirapine and ethinyl estradiol/norethindrone when administered concurrently to HIV-infected women. *J Acquir Immune Defic Syndr* (2002) 29, 471–7.
7. Viramune (Nevirapine anhydrate). Boehringer Ingelheim Ltd. UK Summary of product characteristics, January 2007.

Hormonal contraceptives + NRTIs

There do not appear to have been any reports of hormonal contraceptive or NRTI failure during concurrent use. Tenofovir does not appear to affect the pharmacokinetics of ethinylestradiol or norgestimate. *In-vitro* evidence suggests that ethinylestradiol might possibly reduce the metabolism of zidovudine but the significance of this is unclear.

Note that whatever other methods of contraception are being used, barrier methods are also advisable to reduce the risk of HIV transmission.

Clinical evidence and mechanism

(a) Tenofovir

In a study in 20 women taking a combined oral contraceptive containing **ethinylestradiol** and **norgestimate** *(Ortho Tri-Cyclen),* tenofovir 300 mg daily for 7 days had no effect on the pharmacokinetics of ethinylestradiol or norgestimate. The pharmacokinetics of tenofovir were also not affected when compared with historical data.[1]

(b) Zidovudine

An *in vitro* study using human liver microsomes found that **ethinylestradiol** inhibited the glucuronidation of **zidovudine** by 50% or more, suggesting that **ethinyloestradiol** may increase the effects and toxicity of **zidovudine**.[2] However, note that other drugs that had a similar effect *in vitro* did not alter zidovudine pharmacokinetics in subsequent clinical studies, see 'NRTIs; Zidovudine + Drugs that inhibit glucuronidation', p.808. Further study is needed.

Importance and management

There appears to be no published evidence at present of a clinically significant interaction between the NRTIs (**abacavir**, **didanosine**, **emtricitabine**, **lamivudine**, **stavudine**, **tenofovir**, **zalcitabine** and **zidovudine**) and hormonal contraceptives. The Faculty of Family Planning and Reproductive Health Care (FFPRHC) Clinical Effectiveness Unit guidance on drug interactions with hormonal contraception also notes this.[3] A study[4] found no evidence to suggest that hormonal contraceptives affect the efficacy of HAART. The specific HAART drugs were not named, however most patients were noted to be on a regimen containing an NRTI and a protease inhibitor, but no NNRTI

Note that whatever other methods of contraception are being used, barrier methods are also advisable to reduce the risk of HIV transmission.

1. Kearney BP, Isaacson E, Sayre J, Cheng AK. Tenofovir DF and oral contraceptives: Lack of a pharmacokinetic drug interaction. *Intersci Conf Antimicrob Agents Chemother* (2003) 43, 37.
2. Sim SM, Back DJ, Breckenridge AM. The effect of various drugs on the glucuronidation of zidovudine (azidothymidine, AZT) by human liver microsomes. *Br J Clin Pharmacol* (1991) 32, 17–21.
3. Faculty of Family Planning and Reproductive Health Care Clinical Effectiveness Unit. FFPRHC Guidance: Drug interactions with hormonal contraception. April 2005. Available at: http://www.ffprhc.org.uk/admin/uploads/DrugInteractionsFinal.pdf (accessed 23/08/07).
4. Chu JH, Gange SJ, Anastos K, Minkoff H, Cejtin H, Bacon M, Levine A, Greenblatt RM. Hormonal contraceptive use and the effectiveness of highly active antiretroviral therapy. *Am J Epidemiol* (2005) 161, 881–90.

Hormonal contraceptives + Orlistat

Studies suggest that orlistat does not interact with combined oral contraceptives. However, the manufacturers say that pregnancies have occurred.

Clinical evidence, mechanism, importance and management

Two groups of 10 healthy women taking a combined oral contraceptive were given **orlistat** 120 mg three times daily or a placebo on days 1 to 23 of two menstrual cycles.[1] Orlistat had no effect on ovulation (measured by luteinising hormone and progesterone levels). The contraceptives used all contained **ethinylestradiol**, but the progestogens differed: 10 contained **desogestrel**, 4 **levonorgestrel**, 3 **gestodene**, 2 **cyproterone acetate** and 1 **lynestrenol**. However, the manufacturer has received reports of unexpected pregnancies in patients taking orlistat and hormonal contraceptives. They state that orlistat may indirectly reduce the bioavailability of oral contraceptives as it can cause severe diarrhoea. Therefore, as is standard practice, they recommend using additional contraceptives in patients who develop severe diarrhoea.[2] Note that the contraceptive effect of the combined hormonal patch is said not to be affected by diarrhoea.

1. Hartmann D, Güzelhan C, Zuiderwijk PBM, Odink J. Lack of interaction between orlistat and oral contraceptives. *Eur J Clin Pharmacol* (1996) 50, 421–4.
2. Xenical (Orlistat). Roche Products Ltd. UK Summary of product characteristics, May 2006.

Hormonal contraceptives or HRT + Protease inhibitors

Amprenavir and atazanavir, given alone increase the levels of ethinylestradiol and norethisterone. Ritonavir and nelfinavir, in contrast to the effect that would normally be expected *decrease* the levels of ethinylestradiol. *Reduced* ethinylestradiol and norethisterone levels occur with fosamprenavir, lopinavir and tipranavir given with ritonavir. Indinavir does not appear to interact.

A combined oral contraceptive modestly reduced amprenavir levels, but did not affect the levels of amprenavir derived from fosamprenavir, nor saquinavir levels.

Note that whatever other methods of contraception are being used, barrier methods are also advisable to reduce the risk of HIV transmission.

Clinical evidence

(a) Amprenavir

The UK manufacturer briefly notes that amprenavir *increased* the minimum plasma concentrations of **ethinylestradiol** and **norethisterone**, given as a combined oral contraceptive, by 32% and 45%, respectively. Conversely, the amprenavir minimum concentration and AUC were *decreased* by 20% and 22%, respectively.[1]

(b) Atazanavir

Atazanavir 400 mg once daily alone *increased* the concentration of **ethinylestradiol** 35 micrograms (when given as a combined oral contraceptive with norethisterone) to a level between the mean concentrations produced by a 35-microgram and a 50-microgram ethinylestradiol dose. The AUC of **norethisterone** was *increased* about twofold.[2]

(c) Fosamprenavir

When fosamprenavir 700 mg twice daily with **ritonavir** 100 mg twice daily was given with an oral contraceptive containing **ethinylestradiol/norethisterone** 35/500 micrograms the AUC and maximum plasma concentration of ethinylestradiol were *decreased* by 37% and 28%, respectively, and the AUC and maximum concentration of norethisterone were *decreased* by 34% and 38%, respectively. The pharmacokinetics of amprenavir (derived from fosamprenavir) were not significantly affected.[3] However, the AUC and maximum concentration of **ritonavir** were 45% and 63% higher, respectively, compared with historical data in female subjects taking fosamprenavir and ritonavir alone.[3] Coadministration of fosamprenavir with ritonavir and a combined oral contraceptive containing ethinylestradiol and norethisterone also resulted in clinically significant increases in liver transaminases in some healthy subjects.[3] The clinical relevance of this is not known.

(d) Indinavir

The manufacturer briefly notes that no clinically significant interaction was seen between indinavir and a combined oral contraceptive containing **ethinylestradiol** and **norethisterone**.[4] In a retrospective study there were no reports of contraceptive failure in 9 patients taking indinavir (overall there were 8 contraceptive failures out of 33 women taking protease inhibitors). However, medication adherence could not be confirmed.[5]

(e) Lopinavir

A study in 12 healthy subjects found that lopinavir/**ritonavir** 400/100 mg twice daily for 14 days *decreased* the AUC of **ethinylestradiol** and **norethisterone** (given as a combined oral contraceptive for 21 days) by 42% and 17%, respectively.[6]

(f) Nelfinavir

The manufacturer briefly notes that in women taking a combined oral contraceptive (ethinylestradiol/norethisterone 35/400 micrograms) nelfinavir 750 mg three times daily for one week *decreased* the AUCs of **ethinylestradiol** and **norethisterone** by 47% and 18%, respectively.[7] In a retrospective study 7 of 21 women taking nelfinavir experienced contraceptive failure (overall there were 8 contraceptive failures out of 33 women taking protease inhibitors). However, medication adherence could not be confirmed.[5]

(g) Ritonavir

In a study in 23 healthy women ritonavir 500 mg every 12 hours for 16 days *decreased* the AUC of **ethinylestradiol** by 41% and decreased its elimination half-life from 17 to 13 hours. The women received a single dose of a combined oral contraceptive (**ethinylestradiol/ethynodiol** 50 micrograms/ 1 mg), 14 days before the ritonavir and on day 15 of ritonavir.[8] In a retrospective study there were no reports of contraceptive failure in 6 women taking ritonavir (overall there were 8 contraceptive failures out of 33 women taking protease inhibitors). However, medication adherence could not be confirmed.[5].

(h) Saquinavir

A study in 8 healthy women found that the pharmacokinetics of a single 600-mg dose of saquinavir were not affected by a combined oral contraceptive containing **ethinylestradiol/gestodene** 30/75 micrograms (*Minulet*) taken for 21 days.[9] In a retrospective study there was one report of contraceptive failure out of 5 women taking saquinavir (overall there were 8 contraceptive failures out of 33 women taking protease inhibitors). However, medication adherence could not be confirmed.[5].

(i) Tipranavir

Tipranavir given with low-dose **ritonavir** *decreased* the AUC and maximum concentration of **ethinylestradiol** by 50%, but did not significantly alter the pharmacokinetics of **norethisterone**.[10,11]

Mechanism

Ritonavir more commonly *inhibits* the cytochrome P450 isoenzyme CYP3A4 and the results for ritonavir are the opposite of those originally predicted based on *in vitro* data showing *inhibition* of ethinylestradiol metabolism (cytochrome P450 isoenzyme CYP3A mediated 2-hydroxylation).[12] It is possible that ritonavir induces the metabolism of hormonal contraceptives rather than inhibits CYP3A after chronic use. It is also likely that ritonavir induces ethinylestradiol glucuronosyl transferase activity.[8] Nelfinavir probably interacts similarly. Amprenavir, atazanavir, fosamprenavir, indinavir and tipranavir (when combined with ritonavir) may inhibit CYP3A4. However, note that, although indinavir is a relatively potent inhibitor of CYP3A4, it does not appear to interact.

Importance and management

Although information is limited, the pharmacokinetic interaction between the ethinylestradiol component of **combined hormonal contraceptives** and nelfinavir or ritonavir appears to be established and is likely to be clinically important. Similar *decreases* in plasma levels of ethinylestradiol caused by other drugs have resulted in reduced efficacy and reliability of combined oral contraceptives, and one retrospective report suggests that this has occurred with nelfinavir.[5] It seem likely that the reduced contraceptive levels seen with fosamprenavir, lopinavir and tipranavir were due to the concurrent use of ritonavir (as would be common in practice). Similarly, although no interaction was reported with saquinavir, and *raised* contraceptive steroid levels were reported with amprenavir and atazanavir, in practice these drugs would be given with ritonavir (as a pharmacokinetic enhancer), and so the levels of combined hormonal contraceptives can reasonably be expected to be reduced. The Faculty of Family Planning and Reproductive Health Care (FFPRHC) Clinical Effectiveness Unit has given general guidance on how to manage the interaction of combined hormonal contraceptives with liver enzyme inducers. See 'Hormonal contraceptives + Antiepileptics; Barbiturates or Phenytoin', p.985. Note that there appears to be no clinically significant interaction between indinavir and combined oral contraceptives.

There is no direct information about **progestogen-only contraceptives** but since lopinavir/ritonavir and nelfinavir cause small *reductions* in the levels of norethisterone (when given as part of a combined oral contraceptive) it is possible that these protease inhibitors could reduce the contraceptive efficacy of progestogen-only contraceptives containing norethisterone. The progestogen-only oral contraceptives have a higher failure rate than the combined oral contraceptives, so it would seem prudent to use additional or alternative contraceptive measures in this situation as well. Whether this applies to other progestogens used in progestogen-only contraceptives does not appear to have been specifically studied. See 'Hormonal contraceptives + Antiepileptics; Barbiturates or Phenytoin', p.985, for the Faculty of Family Planning and Reproductive Health Care (FFPRHC) Clinical Effectiveness Unit general guidance on how to manage the interaction between liver enzyme inducers and hormonal contraceptives in women using the progestogen-only pill or implant. The progestogen-only depot injection and progestogen-releasing intrauterine system are not affected by liver enzyme inducers.[13]

However, note that whatever other methods of contraception are being used, barrier methods are always advisable to reduce the risk of HIV transmission.

The effects of the protease inhibitors on **HRT** does not appear to have been studied, although it would be prudent to anticipate some reduction in their effects. The manufacturers of tipranavir specifically note that patients using oestrogens as HRT together with tipranavir and ritonavir should be monitored for signs of oestrogen deficiency. They also note that women using oestrogens with tipranavir may also have an increased risk of non-serious rash.[10,11]

Amprenavir levels are decreased by combined hormonal contraceptives, but the effects are modest. There appears to be no evidence to suggest that combined hormonal contraceptives decrease the antiretroviral efficacy of HAART.[14] but evidence is preliminary and more study is needed.

1. Agenerase (Amprenavir). GlaxoSmithKline UK. UK Summary of product characteristics, February 2007.
2. Reyataz (Atazanavir). Bristol-Myers Squibb Pharmaceuticals Ltd. UK Summary of product characteristics, April 2007.
3. Telzir (Fosamprenavir calcium). GlaxoSmithKline UK. UK Summary of product characteristics, February 2007.
4. Crixivan (Indinavir sulfate). Merck Sharp & Dohme Ltd. UK Summary of product characteristics, May 2007.
5. Clark RA, Theall K. Population-based study evaluating association between selected antiretroviral therapies and potential oral contraceptive failure. *J Acquir Immune Defic Syndr* (2004) 37, 1219–20.
6. Bertz R, Hsu A, Lam W, Williams L, Renz C, Karol M, Dutta S, Carr R, Zhang Y, Wang Q, Schweitzer S, Foit C, Andre A, Bernstein B, Granneman GR, Sun E. Pharmacokinetic interaction between lopinavir/ritonavir (ABT-378r) and other non-HIV drugs (P291). *AIDS* (2000) 14 (Suppl 4), S100.
7. Viracept (Nelfinavir mesilate). Roche Products Ltd. UK Summary of product characteristics, January 2007.
8. Ouellet D, Hsu A, Qian J, Locke CS, Eason CJ, Cavanaugh JH, Leonard JM, Granneman GR. Effect of ritonavir on the pharmacokinetics of ethinyl oestradiol in healthy female volunteers. *Br J Clin Pharmacol* (1998) 46, 111–16.
9. Fröhlich M, Burhenne J, Martin-Facklam M, Weiss J, von Wolff M, Strowitzki T, Walter-Sack I, Haefeli WE. Oral contraception does not alter single dose saquinavir pharmacokinetics in women. *Br J Clin Pharmacol* (2004) 57, 244–52.
10. Aptivus (Tipranavir). Boehringer Ingelheim Ltd. UK Summary of product characteristics, March 2007.
11. Aptivus (Tipranavir). Boehringer Ingelheim. US Prescribing information, February 2007.
12. Kumar GN, Rodrigues AD, Buko AM, Denissen JF. Cytochrome P450-mediated metabolism of the HIV-1 protease inhibitor ritonavir (ABT-538) in human liver microsomes. *J Pharmacol Exp Ther* (1996) 277, 423–31.
13. Faculty of Family Planning and Reproductive Health Care Clinical Effectiveness Unit. FFPRHC Guidance: Drug interactions with hormonal contraception. April 2005. Available at: http://www.ffprhc.org.uk/admin/uploads/DrugInteractionsFinal.pdf (accessed 23/08/07).
14. Chu JH, Gange SJ, Anastos K, Minkoff H, Cejtin H, Bacon M, Levine A, Greenblatt RM. Hormonal contraceptive use and the effectiveness of highly active antiretroviral therapy. *Am J Epidemiol* (2005) 161, 881–90.

Hormonal contraceptives or HRT + Proton pump inhibitors

Lansoprazole and pantoprazole appear not to interact with combined oral contraceptives. Ethinylestradiol may inhibit the me-

tabolism of omeprazole, but levonorgestrel appears to have no effect. Omeprazole does not appear to interact with estradiol.

Clinical evidence, mechanism, importance and management

(a) Lansoprazole

In a placebo-controlled, crossover study, 24 healthy women were given a combined oral contraceptive (**ethinylestradiol/levonorgestrel** 30/150 micrograms) for two monthly cycles, with and without lansoprazole 60 mg daily. The levels of the oral contraceptive steroids were not significantly altered by lansoprazole, nor were endogenous progesterone levels raised, suggesting that ovulation did not occur.[1] The manufacturer has information about 3 other unpublished studies in a total of 59 women, which have also found no evidence to suggest that lansoprazole interacts with oral contraceptives in any way which would affect their reliability.[2] No special precautions are necessary on concurrent use.

(b) Omeprazole

A study in 10 subjects taking a combined oral contraceptive containing **ethinylestradiol/levonorgestrel** 40/75 micrograms (*Trikvilar*) for 10 days found that the combined contraceptive increased the AUC of a single 40-mg dose of omeprazole (*Losec MUPS*) by 38%. This increase was not seen when patients were given **levonorgestrel** alone. Changes in hormonal steroid levels were not studied.[3] No cases of contraceptive failure appear to have been reported with omeprazole. No special precautions appear to be necessary on concurrent use. Note that the UK manufacturer of omeprazole says that there is no evidence of an interaction with **estradiol**.[4]

(c) Pantoprazole

A study over four menstrual cycles was completed by 64 pre-menopausal women. The women were confirmed to be ovulating before taking a low-dose triphasic oral contraceptive (**ethinylestradiol/levonorgestrel**), and not ovulating during contraceptive use. They continued not ovulating when pantoprazole 40 mg daily was given, so it was concluded that pantoprazole does not affect the efficacy of oral contraception.[5]

1. Fuchs W, Sennewald R, Klotz U. Lansoprazole does not affect the bioavailability of oral contraceptives. *Br J Clin Pharmacol* (1994) 38, 376–80.
2. Wyeth, Personal communication, February 1998.
3. Palovaara S, Tybring G, Laine K. The effect of ethinyloestradiol and levonorgestrel on the CYP2C19-mediated metabolism of omeprazole in healthy female subjects. *Br J Clin Pharmacol* (2003) 56, 232–7.
4. Losec MUPS (Omeprazole magnesium). AstraZeneca UK Ltd. UK Summary of product characteristics, July 2006.
5. Middle MV, Müller FO, Schall R, Hundt HKL, Mogilnicka EM, Beneke PC. Effect of pantoprazole on ovulation suppression by a low-dose hormonal contraceptive. *Clin Drug Invest* (1995) 9, 54–6.

Hormonal contraceptives + Retinoids

There seems to be no evidence that the reliability of the combined oral contraceptives is affected by acitretin, etretinate or isotretinoin, and they are the contraceptive method of choice with these teratogenic drugs. It is unclear whether the effects of the progestogen-only oral contraceptives are altered by acitretin, but, in any case, progestogen-only oral contraceptives are not generally considered reliable enough for use with these teratogenic drugs. The adverse effects of isotretinoin on lipids may be additive with those of oral contraceptives.

Clinical evidence

(a) Combined oral contraceptives

1. Acitretin. Eight women taking a combined oral contraceptive (**ethinylestradiol/levonorgestrel**) were given acitretin 25 to 40 mg daily for at least two cycles. Suppression of ovulation was not affected by acitretin, as assessed by plasma progesterone levels.[1]

2. Etretinate. In a study in 12 women taking a combined oral contraceptive (**ethinylestradiol** plus **levonorgestrel**, **norethisterone**, **norgestrel**, or **cyproterone**) the use of **etretinate** 0.7 to 1 mg/kg did not affect the suppression of ovulation.[2]

3. Isotretinoin. A pharmacokinetic study in 9 women taking a combined oral contraceptive found that the plasma levels of **ethinylestradiol** and **levonorgestrel** were not significantly changed by the use of isotretinoin 500 micrograms/kg. Suppression of ovulation was maintained.[3] Another study in 26 women taking a combined oral contraceptive containing **ethinylestradiol** 35 micrograms and **norethisterone** 0.5/0.75/1 mg (*Ortho Novum 7/7/7*) found a small reduction in the levels of ethinylestradiol and norethisterone when isotretinoin 1 mg/kg daily was also given. These changes were not associated with significant changes in the levels of FSH, LH or progesterone. However large inter-patient variability in the results was noted and two patients showed increases in progesterone levels, possibly indicating that ovulation had occurred. One of these patients was noted to be non-compliant.[4]
The adverse effects of isotretinoin and combined oral contraceptives on plasma lipids may be additive. A case-control study found that women who had hypertriglyceridaemia and/or hypercholesterolaemia while taking isotretinoin were 2 to 12 times as likely to be also taking an oral contraceptive.[5]

(b) Progestogen-only oral contraceptives

One woman taking a progestogen-only contraceptive (**levonorgestrel** 30 micrograms) had a significant increase in her progesterone levels after 3 cycles while taking **acitretin** 400 micrograms/kg daily. Plasma progesterone levels rose from 2.15 nanograms/mL before taking the **acitretin** to 3.87 to 13.46 nanograms/mL with **acitretin**. This rise in progesterone levels was taken as evidence that ovulation had occurred.[1]

Mechanism, importance and management

Information is limited, but it appears that these retinoids do not usually alter the efficacy of combined oral contraceptives. The one available case suggests that acitretin reduces the efficacy of progestogen-only oral contraceptives. However, note that **progestogen-only oral contraceptives** do not reliably suppress ovulation in all cycles, and that this is not considered their primary mechanism of action (see 'Hormonal contraceptives and Sex hormones', (p.975)). The single report cannot therefore be taken as evidence that acitretin reduces the efficacy of progestogen-only contraceptives.

Also note that because the retinoids are established human teratogens, it is very important that women taking them do not become pregnant. For this reason, progestogen-only oral contraceptives are generally not considered suitable for use with retinoids.[6] Unless contraindicated, combined oral contraceptives are the method of choice.[6-8] The combined oral contraceptive should be started one month before the retinoids and continued for one month after stopping isotretinoin,[7,8] and for 2 years after stopping etretinate or acitretin.[6] In the US, it is standard practice to recommend that a second form of contraception, such as a barrier method, should also be used.[9] This is also recommended by the UK manufacturer of isotretinoin.[10] This is because, even though hormonal methods of contraception are highly effective, they do, on rare occasions, fail.[7] The general significance of the reduction in steroid levels seen in one study with isotretinoin is unclear and the results were subject to wide inter-patient variability, however the authors state that their results reinforce the advice of using two forms of contraception,[4] one of which should usually be a barrier method, such as condoms.[9] Note that an oral contraceptive containing a non-androgenic (third generation) progestogen (e.g. desogestrel, gestodene, norgestimate) is preferred, since these have less detrimental effects on lipids,[6] and some favour the use of the anti-androgen cyproterone.[8]

1. Berbis Ph, Bun H, Geiger JM, Rognin C, Durand A, Serradimigni A, Hartmann D, Privat Y. Acitretin (RO10-1670) and oral contraceptives: interaction study. *Arch Dermatol Res* (1988) 280, 388–9.
2. Berbis P, Bounameaux Y, Rognin C, Hartmann D, Privat Y. Study on the influence of etretinate on biologic activity of oral contraceptives. *J Am Acad Dermatol* (1987) 17, 302–3.
3. Orme M, Back DJ, Shaw MA, Allen WL, Tjia J, Cunliffe WJ, Jones DH. Isotretinoin and contraception. *Lancet* (1984) ii, 752–3.
4. Hendrix CW, Jackson KA, Whitmore E, Guidos A, Kretzer R, Liss CM, Shah LP, Khoo K-C, McLane J, Trapnell CB. The effect of isotretinoin on the pharmacokinetics and pharmacodynamics of ethinyl estradiol and norethindrone. *Clin Pharmacol Ther* (2004) 75, 464–75.
5. Chen Y, Xue S, Dai W, LaBraico J. Evaluation of serum triglyceride and cholesterol levels from isotretinoin therapy with concomitant oral contraceptives. *Pharmacoepidemiol Drug Safety* (1995) 4, 91–6.
6. Ceyrac DL, Serfaty D, Lefrancq H. Retinoids and contraception. *Dermatology* (1992) 184, 161–70.
7. Perlman SE, Leach EE, Dominguez L, Ruszkowski AM, Rudy SJ. "Be smart, be safe, be sure". The revised pregnancy prevention program for women on isotretinoin. *J Reprod Med* (2001), 46 (Suppl), 179–85.
8. Holmes SC, Bankowska U, Mackie RM. The prescription of isotretinoin to women: is every precaution taken? *Br J Dermatol* (1998) 138, 450–5.

9. Accutane (Isotretinoin). Roche Laboratories Inc. US Prescribing information, August 2005.
10. Roaccutane (Isotretinoin). Roche Products Ltd. UK Summary of product characteristics, October 2006.

Hormonal contraceptives + Rifamycins

Hormonal contraceptives are less reliable during treatment with rifampicin. Breakthrough bleeding and spotting commonly occur, and pregnancy may not be prevented. Rifabutin also reduces the reliability of hormonal contraceptives, although it interacts to a lesser extent, and no contraceptive failures appear to have been reported.

Clinical evidence

(a) Rifabutin

In two studies rifabutin 300 mg daily for 10 or 14 days reduced the plasma levels of **ethinylestradiol** and **norethisterone** in women taking a combined oral contraceptive, but to a lesser extent than rifampicin. The AUC for **ethinylestradiol** decreased by about 35% in both studies, and the AUC of **norethisterone** decreased by 17%. In one study, spotting occurred in 21.7% of women when they took rifabutin (compared with 3.7% in the control cycle and 36% with rifampicin).[1] Ovulation did not occur with rifabutin or rifampicin in either study.[1,2] There appear to be no reports of contraceptive failure attributed to rifabutin.

(b) Rifampicin (Rifampin)

A report in 1971 noted a marked increase in the frequency of intermenstrual breakthrough bleeding (regarded as loss of reliability of the contraceptive) in women taking a **combined oral contraceptive** and rifampicin.[3] In a later report by the same researchers, 62 out of 88 women taking a combined oral contraceptive had menstrual cycle disorders of various kinds (spotting, bleeding, failure to menstruate) while taking a rifampicin-based regimen for tuberculosis, compared with only 1 of 26 treated with a streptomycin-based regimen. In addition, 5 pregnancies occurred in women taking the rifampicin-based regimen.[4,5] Other case reports have confirmed this interaction, and there have been a total of at least 11 other pregnancies reported.[6-13] Combined oral contraceptives commonly mentioned in these reports include **ethinylestradiol** with **norgestrel** or **norethisterone**.[7,9-13] There has also been a report of a pregnancy occurring in a women who was using a **progestogen-only implant**: a 29-year-old woman who had been fitted with an **etonogestrel** implant *(Implanon)* for approximately 2 years was prescribed rifampicin 300 mg twice daily for hidradenitis suppurativa and was found to be 5 weeks pregnant about 6 months later.[14]

One pharmacodynamic study found that 11 out of 21 women taking a triphasic oral contraceptive (**ethinylestradiol/levonorgestrel** 30 to 40 micrograms/50 to 125 micrograms) ovulated (assessed by increased progesterone levels) while taking rifampicin 300 mg daily.[15] In another study, 2 out of 7 women taking a combined oral contraceptive (**ethinylestradiol/norethisterone** 30 micrograms/1 mg) ovulated while taking rifampicin. In addition, rifampicin reduced the AUC of **norethisterone** by 30%.[16] Conversely, two other studies did not detect ovulation in 34 women taking a combined oral contraceptive (**ethinylestradiol/norethisterone** 35 micrograms/1 mg) and rifampicin.[1,2] However, an increased incidence of spotting was noted in one of these studies (36% versus 3.7% in the control cycle).[1] Furthermore, both of these studies found that rifampicin 300 mg daily for 10 days or 600 mg daily for 14 days reduced the AUC of **ethinylestradiol** by about 63% and **norethisterone** by about 55%. These pharmacokinetic results confirm the findings of earlier studies.[17,18] Rifampicin plasma levels[19] and efficacy[3] are reported to be unchanged by oral contraceptives.

Mechanism

Rifampicin is a potent non-specific enzyme inducer, which has been shown to increase the hydroxylation of ethinylestradiol fourfold in an *in vitro* study,[20,21] and twofold in an *in vivo* study.[22] Another study showed that the metabolism of ethinylestradiol derived from mestranol was similarly affected.[23] As a result, the reduced steroid levels may be insufficient to prevent the re-establishment of a normal menstrual cycle with ovulation, which would explain the breakthrough bleeding and pregnancies that have occurred. Rifabutin similarly acts as an enzyme inducer, but it is less potent than rifampicin (said to be half as potent in reducing contraceptive steroid levels).[2]

Importance and management

The interaction between the combined oral contraceptives and rifampicin is well documented, well established and clinically important. Menstrual cycle disturbances of 36 to 70%,[1,3,4] and an ovulation rate of up to 52%[15,16] show very clearly that women receiving **combined oral contraceptives** should use an alternative or additional form of contraception while taking rifampicin, and for 4 to 8 weeks after its withdrawal.[24,25] Direct information about the interaction between combined oral contraceptives and rifabutin seems to be limited to the pharmacodynamic studies cited, but it is supported by the well-recognised enzyme-inducing properties of rifabutin. It would clearly be prudent for women receiving rifabutin to take the same precautions as with rifampicin, although the risks are lower because rifabutin is a less potent enzyme inducer. No cases of contraceptive failure appear to have been attributed to the use of rifabutin. Nevertheless, to be on the safe side, the Faculty of Family Planning and Reproductive Health Care (FFPRHC) Clinical Effectiveness Unit, the manufacturers and the CSM in the UK say that patients using these contraceptives and rifabutin should be advised to use other methods of contraception.[25-27] Note that the combined hormonal contraceptive patch is also affected by liver enzyme-inducers such as rifamycins.

No contraceptive failures due to rifampicin or rifabutin have been reported with the **progestogen-only oral contraceptives**, but their reliability in the presence of either drug is doubtful because both rifampicin and rifabutin are known to increase the metabolism of the progestogen component of combined oral contraceptives.[1,2,16,17] The FFPRHC recommends that alternative methods of contraception to the progestogen-only oral pill should be used when receiving liver-enzyme inducing antibacterials.[25]

There has been a report of a pregnancy in a women who was using a **progestogen-only implant** about 6 months after starting rifampicin.[14] The FFPRHC recommends that patients with a progestogen-only implant should use additional methods of contraception during and for 4 weeks after stopping a short course of a liver enzyme-inducing antibacterial. Alternative forms of contraception should be considered in patients requiring long-term treatment with these antibacterials.[25]

The **progestogen-only injection** and **levonorgestrel-releasing IUD** do not appear to be affected, so no additional protection is required.[25]

The effectiveness of the **emergency progestogen-containing oral contraceptive** will also be reduced in women taking liver enzyme inducers. In the UK it is possible to purchase this type of emergency hormonal contraceptive without a prescription; however, it is recommended that patients taking liver enzyme inducing antibacterials should not be supplied with the emergency contraceptive but should be referred to a doctor or family planning service.[25]

The FFPRHC has issued guidance on the use of liver enzyme inducers, such as rifampicin and rifabutin, with all forms of hormonal contraceptives, including the emergency hormonal contraceptive, and these are given in detail elsewhere, see 'Hormonal contraceptives + Antiepileptics; Barbiturates or Phenytoin', p.985.

1. LeBel M, Masson E, Guilbert E, Colborn D, Paquet F, Allard S, Vallée F, Narang PK. Effects of rifabutin and rifampicin on the pharmacokinetics of ethinylestradiol and norethindrone. *J Clin Pharmacol* (1998) 38, 1042–50.
2. Barditch-Crovo P, Braun Trapnell C, Ette E, Zacur HA, Coresh J, Rocco LE, Hendrix CW, Flexner C. The effects of rifampin and rifabutin on the pharmacokinetics and pharmacodynamics of a combination oral contraceptive. *Clin Pharmacol Ther* (1999) 65, 428–38.
3. Reimers D, Ježek A. Rifampicin und andere Antituberkulotika bei gleichzeitiger oraler Kontrazeption. *Prax Pneumol* (1971) 25, 255–62.
4. Nocke-Finck L, Breuer H, Reimers D. Wirkung von Rifampicin auf den Menstruationszyklus und die Östrogenausscheidung bei Einnahme oraler Kontrazeptiva. *Dtsch Med Wochenschr* (1973) 98, 1521–3.
5. Reimers D, Nocke-Finck L, Breuer H. Rifampicin causes a lowering in efficacy of oral contraceptives by influencing oestrogen excretion. Reports on Rifampicin: XXII International Tuberculosis Conference, Tokyo, September 1973, 87–9.
6. Kropp R. Rifampicin und Ovulationshemmer. *Prax Pneumol* (1974) 28, 270–2.
7. Bessot J-C, Vandevenne A, Petitjean R, Burghard G. Effets opposés de la rifampicine et de l'isoniazide sur le métabolisme des contraceptifs oraux? *Nouv Presse Med* (1977) 6, 1568.
8. Hirsch A. Pilules endormies. *Nouv Presse Med* (1973) 2, 2957.
9. Piguet B, Muglioni JF, Chaline G. Contraception orale et rifampicine. *Nouv Presse Med* (1975) 4, 115–16.
10. Skolnick JL, Stoler BS, Katz DB, Anderson WH. Rifampicin, oral contraceptives and pregnancy. *JAMA* (1976) 236, 1382.
11. Gupta KC, Ali MY. Failure of oral contraceptive with rifampicin. *Med J Zambia* (1980/81) 15, 23.
12. Hirsch A, Tillement JP, Chrétein J. Effects contrariants de la rifampicine sur les contraceptifs oraux: a propos de trois grossesses non désirées observées chez deux malades. *Rev Fr Mal Respir* (1975) 3, 174–82.
13. Lafaix Ch, Cadoz M, Richard A, Patouillard P. L'effect "antipilule" de la rifampicine. *Med Hyg (Geneve)* (1976) 1181, 181–2.
14. Bacon L, Mina M. Unintended pregnancies with Implanon. *Contraception* (2006) 73, 111.

15. Meyer B, Müller F, Wessels P, Maree J. A model to detect interactions between roxithromycin and oral contraceptives. *Clin Pharmacol Ther* (1990) 47, 671–4.
16. Joshi JV, Joshi UM, Sankolli GM, Gupta K, Rao AP, Hazari K, Sheth UK, Saxena BN. A study of interaction of low-dose combination oral contraceptive with anti-tubercular drugs. *Contraception* (1980) 21, 617–29.
17. Back DJ, Breckenridge AM, Crawford F, MacIver M, Orme ML'E, Park BK, Rowe PH, Smith E. The effect of rifampicin on norethisterone pharmacokinetics. *Eur J Clin Pharmacol* (1979) 15, 193–7.
18. Back DJ, Breckenridge AM, Crawford FE, Hall JM, MacIver M, Orme ML'E, Rowe PH, Smith E, Watts MJ. The effect of rifampicin on the pharmacokinetics of ethynylestradiol in women. *Contraception* (1980) 21, 135–43.
19. Gupta KC, Joshi JV, Anklesaria PS, Shah RS, Satoskar RS. Plasma rifampicin levels during oral contraception. *J Assoc Physicians India* (1988) 36, 365–6.
20. Bolt HM, Kappus H, Bolt M. Rifampicin and oral contraception. *Lancet* (1974) i, 1280–1.
21. Bolt HM, Kappus H, Bolt M. Effect of rifampicin treatment on the metabolism of oestradiol and 17α-ethinyloestradiol by human liver microsomes. *Eur J Clin Pharmacol* (1975) 8, 301–7.
22. Bolt HM, Bolt M, Kappus H. Interaction of rifampicin treatment with pharmacokinetics and metabolism of ethinyloestradiol in man. *Acta Endocrinol (Copenh)* (1977) 85, 189–97.
23. Gelbke HP, Gethmann U, Knuppen R. Influence of rifampicin treatment on the metabolic fate of [4-^{14}C] mestranol in women. *Horm Metab Res* (1977) 9, 415–19.
24. Orme M, Back DJ. Oral contraceptive steroids – pharmacological issues of interest to the prescribing physician. *Adv Contracept* (1991) 7, 325–31.
25. Faculty of Family Planning and Reproductive Health Care Clinical Effectiveness Unit. FFPRHC Guidance: Drug interactions with hormonal contraception. April 2005. Available at: http://www.ffprhc.org.uk/admin/uploads/DrugInteractionsFinal.pdf (accessed 23/08/07).
26. Committee on Safety of Medicines (CSM)/Medicines Control Agency (MCA). Revised indication and drug interactions of rifabutin. Current Problems 1997, 23, 14.
27. Mycobutin (Rifabutin). Pharmacia Ltd. UK Summary of product characteristics, October 2006.

Hormonal contraceptives + St John's wort (*Hypericum perforatum*)

St John's wort may affect the pharmacokinetics of desogestrel, ethinylestradiol, and norethisterone. Both breakthrough bleeding and, more rarely, combined oral contraceptive failure have been reported in women taking St John's wort. Two cases describe the failure of emergency hormonal contraception, which was attributed to the use of St John's wort.

Clinical evidence

(a) Combined hormonal contraceptives

A study in 17 healthy women taking **ethinylestradiol/desogestrel** 20/150 micrograms daily found that St John's wort (300 mg twice or three times daily) did not affect the AUC or maximum levels of **ethinylestradiol**. However, the AUC and maximum levels of the active metabolite of **desogestrel** were significantly decreased by about 40% and 20%, respectively. There was no evidence that ovulation occurred. However, the frequency of breakthrough bleeding increased significantly from 35% to around 80%, which may affect compliance.[1] Another study in 12 healthy women taking **ethinylestradiol/norethisterone** 35 micrograms/1 mg (*Ortho-Novum*) found that St John's wort 300 mg three times daily for 8 weeks increased the oral clearance of **norethisterone** and reduced the half-life of **ethinylestradiol,** but the serum levels of LH, FSH and progesterone were unaffected. However, of more importance, was the increase in breakthrough bleeding, which the authors state as a major cause of patients stopping hormonal contraceptives.[2] A further study in 16 subjects also found reductions in the levels of low-dose **ethinylestradiol/norethisterone** 20 micrograms/1 mg. Furthermore, they found increased progesterone levels of more than 3 nanograms/mL (an indication that ovulation occurred) in 3 patients who also took St John's wort compared with one subject who took placebo. Breakthrough bleeding occurred in was also increased.[3]

The Adverse Drug Reactions Database of the Swedish Medical Products Agency has on record 2 cases of pregnancy due to the failure of a combined oral contraceptive, which was attributed to the use of products containing St John's wort (*Esbericum* and *Kira*). One woman was taking **ethinylestradiol** and **norethisterone** and the other was taking **ethinylestradiol** and **levonorgestrel.**[4] This follows an earlier report from the Swedish Medical Products Agency of 8 cases of breakthrough bleeding in women aged 23 to 31 taking long-term oral contraceptives and St John's wort. Breakthrough bleeding occurred within about a week of starting St John's wort in 5 of the cases, and was known to have resolved in 3 cases when the St John's wort was stopped.[5] The CSM in the UK has on record a further 7 cases of pregnancy in women taking St John's wort and oral contraceptives in the two-year period from February 2000 to February 2002.[6] Another earlier brief report describes 3 women taking a combined oral contraceptive (**ethinylestradiol/desogestrel** 30/150 micrograms) who developed breakthrough bleeding one week (2 cases) and 3 months (1 case) after starting to take St John's wort.[7] A single case of pregnancy has also been reported in a patient taking St John's wort with **ethinylestradiol/dienogest** (*Valette*).[8] The German Federal Institute for Drugs and Medical Devices has received a total of 8 case reports of ineffective contraception with St John's wort.[9]

(b) Emergency hormonal contraceptives

The CSM in the UK has received reports of 2 women taking St John's wort who became pregnant despite taking **emergency hormonal contraception**. One of them was also taking an oral contraceptive.[6]

Mechanism

It is believed that St John's wort can induce the cytochrome P450-mediated metabolism of the contraceptive steroids, thereby reducing their serum levels and their effects.[5,7,10] This can lead to breakthrough bleeding and, in some cases, contraceptive failure. This is consistent with the way St John's wort appears to lower the serum levels of some other drugs. Note that St John's wort is a herbal preparation, and the specific constituents responsible for enzyme induction are currently unknown. Also, the levels of individual constituents can vary between different preparations of the herb.

Importance and management

Information appears to be limited to these reports but the interaction between hormonal contraceptives and St John's wort appears to be established. Its incidence is not known but the evidence so far suggests that breakthrough bleeding may be a problem, although pregnancy resulting from this interaction appears to be uncommon. However, since it is not known who is particularly likely to be at risk, women taking oral contraceptives should either avoid St John's wort (the recommendation of the CSM/MCA and the FFPRHC in the UK[10,11]) or they should use an additional form of contraception. Only two cases of emergency hormonal contraceptive failure attributed to an interaction with St John's wort have so far been reported, but the effects of any interaction here would be very difficult to assess. The Faculty of Family Planning and Reproductive Health Care (FFPRHC) Clinical Effectiveness Unit is in agreement with the CSM advice but recommends that, if St John's wort must be continued, the guidelines for the use of liver enzyme inducers with hormonal contraceptives should be followed, see 'Hormonal contraceptives + Antiepileptics; Barbiturates or Phenytoin', p.985, for details of this guidance. Note that combined hormonal contraceptive patch, progestogen-only pills and implants may also be affected.

See also 'Emergency hormonal contraceptives + Enzyme inducers', p.977 for information on how to manage the interaction with emergency hormonal contraception.

Although the considerable worldwide popularity of St John's wort is fairly recent, it is currently the most widely used antidepressant in Germany and has been used for very many years in both Germany and Austria. Yet, there seems to be no published evidence that oral contraceptive failure in those countries is more frequent than anywhere else. This would seem to confirm that contraceptive failure leading to pregnancy occurring as a result of this interaction is very uncommon, or perhaps that it has failed to be identified as a possible cause.

1. Pfrunder A, Schiesser M, Gerber S, Haschke M, Bitzer J, Drewe J. Interaction of St John's wort with low-dose oral contraceptive therapy: a randomized controlled trial. *Br J Clin Pharmacol* (2003) 56, 683–90.
2. Hall SD, Wang Z, Huang S-M, Hamman MA, Vasavada N, Adigun AQ, Hilligoss JK, Miller M, Gorski JC. The interaction between St John's wort and an oral contraceptive. *Clin Pharmacol Ther* (2003) 74, 525–35.
3. Murphy PA, Kern SE, Stanczyk FZ, Westhoff CL. Interaction of St John's wort with oral contraceptives: effects on the pharmacokinetics of norethindrone and ethinyl estradiol, ovarian activity and breakthrough bleeding. *Contraception* (2005) 71, 402–8.
4. Swedish Medical Products Agency. St John's wort may influence other medication. Data on file, 2002.
5. Yue Q-Y, Bergquist C, Gerdén B. Safety of St John's wort (Hypericum perforatum). *Lancet* (2000) 355, 576–7.
6. Committee on Safety of Medicines. Personal communication, February 15th, 2002.
7. Bon S, Hartmann K, Kuhn M. Johanniskraut: Ein Enzyminduktor? *Schweiz Apothekerzeitung* (1999) 16, 535–6.
8. Schwarz UI, Büschel B, Kirch W. Unwanted pregnancy on self-medication with St John's wort despite hormonal contraception. *Br J Clin Pharmacol* (2003) 55, 112–13.
9. Bundesinstitut für Arzneimittel und Medizinprodukte. Personal communication, March 2007.

10. Committee on Safety of Medicines. Message from Professor A Breckenridge (Chairman of CSM) and Fact Sheet for Health Care Professionals. Important interactions between St John's wort (*Hypericum perforatum*) preparations and prescribed medicines, 29th February 2000. Available at: http://www.mhra.gov.uk/home/idcplg?IdcService=SS_GET_PAGE&useSecondary=true&ssDocName=CON2015756&ssTargetNodeId=221 (accessed 23/08/2007).
11. Faculty of Family Planning and Reproductive Health Care Clinical Effectiveness Unit. FFPRHC Guidance: Drug interactions with hormonal contraception. April 2005. Available at: http://www.ffprhc.org.uk/admin/uploads/DrugInteractionsFinal.pdf (accessed 23/08/07).

Hormonal contraceptives or HRT + Statins

Atorvastatin and rosuvastatin may modestly increase the plasma levels of combined oral contraceptives. Rosuvastatin pharmacokinetics and lipid-lowering effects were unaffected by an oral contraceptive containing ethinylestradiol and norgestimate. The pharmacokinetics of a single dose of pravastatin were also unaffected by combined oral contraceptives. However, norethisterone abolished the beneficial effects of atorvastatin and/or estradiol on the lipid profile.

Clinical evidence, mechanism, importance and management

(a) Atorvastatin

A study in 12 healthy women taking a combined oral contraceptive (**ethinylestradiol/norethisterone** 35 micrograms/1 mg) found that atorvastatin 40 mg daily increased the AUC of **norethisterone** and **ethinylestradiol** by about 28% and 19%, respectively, and increased their maximum plasma levels by 24% and 30%, respectively.[1] These increases are only moderate and unlikely to be clinically important, but the manufacturers say that they should be considered when selecting an appropriate oral contraceptive dosage for women given atorvastatin.[2,3]

A double-blind, randomised, placebo-controlled study in postmenopausal women with hypercholesterolaemia and arterial hypertension found that whilst atorvastatin alone, **estradiol** alone, or the combination of both had beneficial effects on the lipid profile and endothelium-dependent vasodilatation, these effects were abolished by the addition of **norethisterone**. It was suggested that progesterone derivatives with high androgenic activity, such as norethisterone, have a negative effect on lipid profile.[4]

(b) Pravastatin

The pharmacokinetics of a single 20-mg dose of pravastatin were found to be unaffected in 15 young women taking combined oral contraceptives (**ethinylestradiol** with **norethisterone**, **norgestrel** or **levonorgestrel**), when compared with similar women not taking contraceptives. No adverse effects attributable to concurrent use were seen.[5]

(c) Rosuvastatin

A non-randomised study in 18 healthy women taking a combined oral contraceptive (*Ortho Tri-Cyclen;* **ethinylestradiol** 35 micrograms for 21 days with **norgestimate** 180/215/250 micrograms, 7 days of each) found that the addition of rosuvastatin 40 mg daily increased the AUC and maximum concentration of ethinylestradiol by 26% and 25%, respectively, and increased the AUC and maximum concentration of norgestrel, an active metabolite of norgestimate, by 34% and 23%, respectively. The contraceptive efficacy was unchanged as measured by FSH, LH and progesterone levels.[6] These increases in hormonal steroid levels are unlikely to be clinically significant in patients taking low-dose oral contraceptives,[6] although the manufacturer notes that these changes should be considered when choosing a hormonal contraceptive preparation.[7] The pharmacokinetics and lipid-lowering effects of rosuvastatin were unaffected.[6]

1. Yang B-B, Siedlik PH, Smithers JA, Sedman AJ, Stern RH. Atorvastatin pharmacokinetic interactions with other CYP3A4 substrates: erythromycin and ethinyl estradiol. *Pharm Res* (1996) 13 (9 Suppl), S-437.
2. Lipitor (Atorvastatin). Pfizer Ltd. UK Summary of product characteristics, September 2006.
3. Lipitor (Atorvastatin calcium). Pfizer Inc. US Prescribing information, March 2007.
4. Faludi AA, Aldrighi JM, Bertolami MC, Saleh MH, Silva RA, Nakamura Y, Pereira IRO, Abdalla DSP, Ramires JAF, Sousa JEMR. Progesterone abolishes estrogen and/or atorvastatin endothelium dependent vasodilatory effects. *Atherosclerosis* (2004) 177, 89–96.
5. Pan HY, Waclawski AP, Funke PT, Whigan D. Pharmacokinetics of pravastatin in elderly versus young men and women. *Ann Pharmacother* (1993) 27, 1029–33.
6. Simonson SG, Martin PD, Warwick MJ, Mitchell PD, Schneck DW. The effect of rosuvastatin on oestrogen & progestin pharmacokinetics in healthy women taking an oral contraceptive. *Br J Clin Pharmacol* (2004) 57, 279–86.
7. Crestor (Rosuvastatin calcium). AstraZeneca UK Ltd. UK Summary of product characteristics, June 2007.

Hormonal contraceptives + Sucrose polyesters

Sucrose polyesters do not interact with oral contraceptives.

Clinical evidence, mechanism, importance and management

When 28 healthy women took 18 g of sucrose polyester (*Olestra*) daily for 28 days, the pharmacokinetics of the components of a combined oral contraceptive (**ethinylestradiol/norgestrel** 30/300 micrograms) were unchanged. Serum progesterone levels also remained unaltered, suggesting no ovulation occurred.[1] This agrees with the findings of earlier single-dose studies, which found that sucrose polyester had no effect on the bioavailability of single doses of **ethinylestradiol** or **norethisterone**.[2] No special contraceptive precautions appear to be necessary.

1. Miller KW, Williams DS, Carter SB, Jones MB, Mishell DR. The effect of olestra on systemic levels of oral contraceptives. *Clin Pharmacol Ther* (1990) 48, 34–40.
2. Roberts RJ, Leff RD. Influence of absorbable and nonabsorbable lipids and lipidlike substances on drug availability. *Clin Pharmacol Ther* (1989) 45, 299–304.

Hormonal contraceptives + Terbinafine

Terbinafine does not have a clinically significant interaction with oral contraceptives.

Clinical evidence, mechanism, importance and management

An *in vitro* study in human livers found that terbinafine did not alter the pharmacokinetics of **ethinylestradiol**.[1] However, the manufacturer of terbinafine notes that menstrual disturbances have occurred in patients taking both oral contraceptives and terbinafine.[2] In a post-marketing survey, which included 314 patients taking both oral contraceptives and terbinafine, the rate of menstrual disorders was within the rate reported for patients taking oral contraceptives alone.[3]

1. Back DJ, Stevenson P, Tjia JF. Comparative effects of two antimycotic agents, ketoconazole and terbinafine, on the metabolism of tolbutamide, ethinyloestradiol, cyclosporin and ethoxycoumarin by human liver microsomes *in vitro*. *Br J Clin Pharmacol* (1989) 28, 166–70.
2. Lamisil Tablets (Terbinafine hydrochloride). Novartis Pharmaceuticals UK Ltd. UK Summary of product characteristics, February 2007.
3. O'Sullivan DP, Needham CA, Bangs A, Atkin K, Kendall FD. Postmarketing surveillance of oral terbinafine in the UK: report of a large cohort study. *Br J Clin Pharmacol* (1996) 42, 559–65.

Hormonal contraceptives + Tobacco

There is some evidence that smoking increases the risk of breakthrough bleeding with combined oral contraceptives, although smoking appears not to alter contraceptive steroid levels. The risk of cardiovascular disease in women taking combined oral contraceptives is greatly increased if they smoke, particularly in the older age group. Progestogen-only oral contraceptives are an alternative.

Clinical evidence

(a) Cardiovascular effects

Early after the introduction of combined oral contraceptives it was realised that they increase the risk of cardiovascular effects such as thromboembolism, myocardial infarction, and stroke, and that the risks were markedly increased in women who also smoked.[1-5] For example, one of these studies found a relative risk of non-fatal myocardial infarction in women taking an oral contraceptive of 4.5 in non-smokers and 39 in heavy smokers.[4] Another study found a relative risk of subarachnoid haemorrhage in women taking oral contraceptives of 6.5 for non-smokers and 22 for smokers.[5] Heavy smokers (who smoke more than 15 cigarettes daily) have a threefold increased risk of myocardial infarction and a twofold increase in the risk of stroke compared with non-smokers, and these risks are further increased by the use of combined oral contraceptives.[6] A study involving 17,032 women aged 25 to 39 years at entry, who had used oral contraceptives (mainly containing 50 micrograms of oestrogen), a diaphragm, or an intrauterine device, found that the risk of death from ischaemic heart disease was slightly, but not statistically significantly, raised in all oral contraceptive users. However, smoking had a substantial effect on mortality from ischaemic heart disease; in heavy smokers (more that 15 cigarettes daily) the mortality rate ratios for oral contraceptive use for 48 months or less, for 49 to 96 months, and for 97 months or more compared with non-use were 2.4, 4.8, and 2.8, respectively.[7]

(b) Contraceptive efficacy

An analysis of data from three large clinical studies in a total of 2956 women found that smoking was associated with an increased incidence of spotting and bleeding in users of combined oral contraceptives. The relative risk was 1.3 during the first cycle of use and increased to 1.9 by the sixth cycle.[8] Similarly, in a study of women who became pregnant while taking oral contraceptives, smokers were more likely to have menstrual disturbances, and smokers taking the combined oral contraceptive had a 20% greater pill failure rate than expected,.[9] This association was not noted for **progestogen-only oral contraceptive** failure.[9] Conversely, in a large cohort study in the UK, the failure rate of oral contraceptives was not increased in smokers.[10] In one study in 311 women taking oral contraceptives, plasma levels of ethinylestradiol and norgestrel were similar in smokers and non-smokers,[11] and another study found only a small increase in ethinylestradiol clearance in smokers.[12]

Mechanism

The cardiovascular effects reported do not appear to be attributable to any effect of smoking on the metabolism of contraceptives steroids (see below). Rather, the adverse effects of combined oral contraceptives on cardiovascular risk factors, such as plasma lipids and coagulation parameters, appear to be accentuated by smoking.

Smoking increased the metabolism (2-hydroxylation) of *endogenous* estradiol in one study in premenopausal women.[13] Smoking does not appear to alter the levels of contraceptive steroids to a clinically relevant extent.

Importance and management

The cardiovascular interaction between smoking and **combined hormonal contraceptives** is well established. The Faculty of Family Planning and Reproductive Health Care (FFPRHC) Clinical Effectiveness Unit and Royal College of Obstetricians and Gynaecologists guidelines on criteria for the use of contraceptives recommend that the combined hormonal contraceptive should not be used in women aged over 35 who are current smokers or who stopped smoking less than one year ago as the risks, particularly of cardiovascular disease, outweigh the benefits.[6,14] Women over the age of 35 years with no additional risk factors (such as diabetes, hypertension etc) and who stopped smoking more than one year ago may consider using a combined hormonal contraceptive. This is because the risk of cardiovascular disease reduces by as much as 50% one year after stopping smoking, although it may not become comparable to that of a non-smoker for up to 4 to 10 years.[6,14] Women aged under 35 years who smoke and have no other associated risk factors may use a combined hormonal contraceptive, but should be informed about the increased risk of cardiovascular disease. Any woman with multiple risk factors for cardiovascular disease (older age, smoking, diabetes, hypertension, obesity, family history of arterial disease, migraine) should not take the combined hormonal contraceptive.[14,15] The BNF recommends that women who smoke 40 or more cigarettes a day should not receive combined oral contraceptives.[15] In women who smoke, for whom a combined oral contraceptive is not contraindicated, ones with the lowest doses of ethinylestradiol may be safer.[16] All smokers should be encouraged to stop.[16] In the UK, **progestogen-only oral contraceptives** are considered suitable for women who are heavy smokers,[14] although it should be remembered that they have a higher failure rate than the combined oral contraceptives.

Smoking may increase the incidence of breakthrough bleeding. This may decrease the acceptability of the oral contraceptive, and lead to the use of less effective contraceptive methods.[8] However, it also raises the question of whether smoking increases the failure rate of oral contraceptives. The only evidence that this may occur is anecdotal. Further study is needed.

1. Arntzenius AC, van Gent CM, van der Voort H, Stegerhoek CI, Styblo K. Reduced high-density lipoprotein in women aged 40–41 using oral contraceptives. *Lancet* (1978) i, 1221–3.
2. Frederiksen H, Ravenholt RT. Thromboembolism, oral contraceptives and cigarettes. *Public Health Rep* (1970) 85, 197–205.
3. Collaborative Group for the study of stroke in young women. Oral contraceptives and stroke in young women: associated risk factors. *JAMA* (1975) 231, 718–22.
4. Shapiro S, Slone D, Rosenberg L, Kaufman DW, Stolley PD, Miettinen OS. Oral-contraceptive use in relation to myocardial infarction. *Lancet* (1979) i, 743–7.
5. Petitti DB, Wingerd J. Use of oral contraceptives, cigarette smoking, and risk of subarachnoid haemorrhage. *Lancet* (1978) ii, 234–6.
6. Faculty of Family Planning and Reproductive Health Care Clinical Effectiveness Unit. FFPRHC Guidance: Contraception for women aged over 40 years, January 2005. Available at: http://www.ffprhc.org.uk/admin/uploads/ContraceptionOver40.pdf (accessed 23/08/07).
7. Vessey M, Painter R, Yeates D. Mortality in relation to oral contraceptive use and cigarette smoking. *Lancet* (2003) 362, 185–91.
8. Rosenberg MJ, Waugh MS, Stevens CM. Smoking and cycle control among oral contraceptive users. *Am J Obstet Gynecol* (1996) 174, 628–32.
9. Sparrow MJ. Pregnancies in reliable pill takers. *N Z Med J* (1989) 102, 575–7.
10. Vessey MP, Villard-Mackintosh L, Jacobs HS. Anti-estrogenic effect of cigarette smoking. *N Engl J Med* (1987) 317, 769–70.
11. Crawford FE, Back DJ, Orme ML'E, Breckenridge AM. Oral contraceptive steroid plasma concentrations in smokers and non-smokers. *BMJ* (1981) 282, 1829–30.
12. Kanarkowski R, Tornatore KM, D'Ambrosio R, Gardner MJ, Jusko WJ. Pharmacokinetics of single and multiple doses of ethinyl estradiol and levonorgestrel in relation to smoking. *Clin Pharmacol Ther* (1988) 43, 23–31.
13. Michnovicz JJ, Hershcopf RJ, Naganuma H, Bradlow HL, Fishman J. Increased 2-hydroxylation of estradiol as a possible mechanism for the anti-estrogenic effect of cigarette smoking. *N Engl J Med* (1986) 315, 1305–9.
14. Faculty of Family Planning and Reproductive Health Care and Royal College of Obstetricians and Gynaecologists. UK Medical eligibility criteria for contraceptive use (UKMEC 2005/2006), July 2006. Available at: http://www.ffprhc.org.uk/admin/uploads/298_UKMEC_200506.pdf (accessed 23/08/07).
15. British National Formulary. 53rd ed. London: The British Medical Association and The Pharmaceutical Press; 2007. p. 422.
16. Schiff I, Bell WR, Davis V, Kessler CM, Meyers C, Nakajima S, Sexton BJ. Oral contraceptives and smoking, current considerations: recommendations of a consensus panel. *Am J Obstet Gynecol* (1999) 180 (Part 2) S383–S384.

Hormonal contraceptives + Tolterodine

Tolterodine does not appear to interact with combined oral contraceptives.

Clinical evidence, mechanism, importance and management

A randomised, crossover study in 24 women found that tolterodine 2 mg twice daily on days 1 to 14 of two 28-day contraceptive cycles had no effect on the pharmacokinetics of the steroids in a combined oral contraceptive (**ethinylestradiol/levonorgestrel** 30/150 micrograms). The pharmacokinetics of the tolterodine were also not significantly altered, and the serum levels of estradiol and progesterone indicated that suppression of ovulation continued during both periods of treatment.[1] No special precautions would therefore seem to be needed if these drugs are used concurrently.

1. Olsson B, Landgren B-M. The effect of tolterodine on the pharmacokinetics and pharmacodynamics of a combination oral contraceptive containing ethinyl estradiol and levonorgestrel. *Clin Ther* (2001) 23, 1876–88.

Hormonal contraceptives or HRT + Triptans

Oral contraceptives appear to modestly raise the levels of frovatriptan, naratriptan and zolmitriptan, and slightly increase those of sumatriptan. These changes are not considered clinically significant. HRT did not appear to affect the pharmacokinetics of naratriptan.

Almotriptan, rizatriptan and sumatriptan appear not to alter the levels of oral contraceptives.

Clinical evidence

(a) Almotriptan

A study in 21 women found that a single 12.5-mg dose of almotriptan had no clinically significant effect on the pharmacokinetics of a combined oral contraceptive containing **ethinylestradiol** 30 micrograms and **desogestrel** 150 micrograms, taken for two cycles.[1]

(b) Frovatriptan

In a retrospective analysis of pharmacokinetic data from phase I studies, the mean maximum concentration and AUC of frovatriptan were 25% and 30% higher, respectively, in women taking oral contraceptives than in women not taking oral contraceptives.[2]

(c) Naratriptan

The clearance of naratriptan was reduced by 32% by oral contraceptives leading to a slightly higher level of naratriptan. HRT had no effect on the pharmacokinetics of naratriptan.[3] A case of ischaemic colitis has been reported in a patient taking an oral contraceptive containing ethinylestradiol 30 micrograms and drospirenone 3 mg long-term with naratriptan 2.5 mg, taken to relieve migraine attacks.[4]

(d) Rizatriptan

A placebo-controlled study in 20 healthy young women taking a combined oral contraceptive (**ethinylestradiol/norethisterone** 35 micrograms/1 mg) found that the concurrent use of rizatriptan (6 days of 10 mg daily followed by 2 days of 10 mg every 4 hours to a total of 3 doses daily) did not affect the pharmacokinetics of either contraceptive steroid. Blood pressure, heart rate and temperature were unaffected and adverse effects were similar to those seen with placebo.[5]

(e) Sumatriptan

A study to investigate the effects of a combined oral contraceptive (**ethinylestradiol/norethisterone** 35 micrograms/1 mg) on the pharmacokinetics of sumatriptan was done in 26 women who had been taking this contraceptive for at least 3 months. A single 50-mg oral dose of sumatriptan was given once after 21 days of active treatment with the oral contraceptive, and again after 7 days of placebo (day 28). A 16% higher AUC and a 17% higher maximum concentration of sumatriptan was noted on day 21, compared with day 29. There was an 18% reduction in the maximum concentration of **norethisterone** when it was given with sumatriptan, but no change in its AUC. Similarly, there was no change in the AUC or maximum concentration of **ethinylestradiol** when it was given with sumatriptan.[6]

(f) Zolmitriptan

In a retrospective analysis of pharmacokinetic data from several studies, the mean maximum concentration and AUC of zolmitriptan were 30 to 50% higher, respectively, in women taking oral contraceptives than in women not taking oral contraceptives.[7] The effects of zolmitriptan on oral contraceptive steroids have not been studied.[7]

Mechanism

Not known.

Importance and management

Although data are limited, the minor to modest possible increases in frovatriptan, naratriptan, sumatriptan and zolmitriptan pharmacokinetics described are not likely to produce clinically relevant adverse effects. Almotriptan, rizatriptan and sumatriptan do not appear to have any clinically important effect on levels of contraceptive steroids. The significance of the single case report of ischaemic colitis associated with concurrent use of naratriptan and a combined oral contraceptive is unclear. Note that ischaemic colitis has, rarely, been reported with naratriptan itself.[8] The manufacturers have found no cases of ischaemic colitis in approximately 450 women on oral contraceptives and taking naratriptan for prophylaxis for 5 to 6 days.[8] However, caution may be needed with concurrent use in those patients with risk factors for ischaemic colitis, such as those with a history of abdominal surgery, low blood pressure, diabetes, cardiovascular disease or stroke.

More importantly, women who suffer from migraine and take a combined oral contraceptive are at increased risk of a stroke compared with those using combined oral contraceptives who do not suffer from migraine.[9-11] The Faculty of Family Planning and Reproductive Health Care(FFPRHC) guidance states that women of all ages who currently have migraines *with* aura should not use a combined hormonal contraceptive. Women over the age of 35 who have migraine attacks *without* aura and those of any age with a past history of migraine *with* aura should also not use combined hormonal contraceptives.[11] Women taking any hormonal contraceptive who develop migraine with aura as a new symptom should have their contraceptive choices reviewed. The FFPRHC guidance gives advice on alternative choices of contraceptive method for women with migraine or a history of migraine.[11]

1. Cabarrocas X, Macher J-P. Lack of a pharmacokinetic interaction between almotriptan and oral contraceptives: a double-blind, placebo-controlled, crossover study in healthy female volunteers. *Cephalalgia* (2003) 23, 716.
2. Buchan P. Effects of alcohol, smoking and oral contraceptives on the pharmacokinetics of frovatriptan. *Eur J Neurol* (2000) 7 (Suppl 3), 86–7.
3. Amerge (Naratriptan hydrochloride). GlaxoSmithKline. US Prescribing information, April 2007.
4. Charles JA, Pullicino PM, Stoopack PM, Shroff Y. Ischemic colitis associated with naratriptan and oral contraceptive use. *Headache* (2005) 45, 386–9.
5. Shadle CR, Liu G, Goldberg MR. A double-blind, placebo-controlled evaluation of the effect of oral doses of rizatriptan 10 mg on oral contraceptive pharmacokinetics in healthy female volunteers. *J Clin Pharmacol* (2000) 40, 309–15.
6. Moore KHP, McNeal S, Britto MR, Bye C, Sale M, Richardson MS. The pharmacokinetics of sumatriptan when administered with norethindrone 1 mg/ethinyl estradiol 0.035 mg in healthy volunteers. *Clin Ther* (2002) 24, 1887–1901.
7. Zomig (Zolmitriptan). AstraZeneca Pharmaceuticals LP. US Prescribing information, January 2007.
8. Malone TD, Kori SH. Ischemic colitis associated with naratriptan and oral contraceptive use: A response. *Headache* (2005) 45, 1419–20.
9. Faculty of Family Planning and Reproductive Health (FFPRHC) Clinical Effectiveness Unit. Contraception for women aged over 40 years, January 2005. Available at: http://www.ffprhc.org.uk/admin/uploads/ContraceptionOver40.pdf (accessed 23/08/07).
10. Faculty of Family Planning and Reproductive Health Care Clinical Guidance: First prescription of combined oral contraception, July 2006 (updated January 2007). Available at: http://www.ffprhc.org.uk/admin/uploads/FirstPrescCombOralContJan06.pdf (accessed 23/08/07).
11. Faculty of Family Planning and Reproductive Health Care (FFPRHC) & Royal College of Obstetricians & Gynaecologists. UK Medical eligibility criteria for contraceptive use (UK-MEC 2005/2006), July 2006. Available at: http://www.ffprhc.org.uk/admin/uploads/298_UKMEC_200506.pdf (accessed 23/08/07).

Hormonal contraceptives + Ziprasidone

Ziprasidone appears not to interact to a clinically relevant extent with combined oral contraceptives.

Clinical evidence, mechanism, importance and management

In a placebo-controlled, crossover study, 18 women taking an oral contraceptive (**ethinylestradiol/levonorgestrel** 30/150 micrograms) for at least 3 months were also given ziprasidone 20 mg twice daily for 8 days. The only change in the pharmacokinetics of the two steroids was an approximately 30-minute increase in the time to maximum plasma concentration of the **levonorgestrel**, but this was not considered to be clinically significant. No adverse effects occurred. It was concluded that combined use is safe and that ziprasidone does not affect the efficacy of this oral contraceptive[1] and is also unlikely to affect the metabolism and therefore efficacy of other similar contraceptives.

1. Muirhead GJ, Harness J, Holt PR, Oliver S, Anziano RJ. Ziprasidone and the pharmacokinetics of a combined oral contraceptive. *Br J Clin Pharmacol* (2000) 49 (Suppl 1), 49S–56S.

HRT + Enzyme inducers

Enzyme inducers that increase the metabolism of contraceptive steroids might also be expected to reduce the efficacy of menopausal HRT. An isolated case describes reduced efficacy of oral conjugated oestrogens in a patient taking phenytoin.

Clinical evidence, mechanism, importance and management

A report describes a 28-year-old woman taking oral **conjugated oestrogens** (*Premarin*) 1.25 mg daily after ovidectomy, who had a dramatic increase in the incidence of hot flushes when she began to take **phenytoin** 300 mg daily. Her estrone and estradiol levels were found to be very low, and they subsequently increased by four to sixfold after the **phenytoin** was stopped, at which point the incidence of hot flushes decreased.[1] This seems to be the only report of this interaction.

However, it is not unreasonable to assume that enzyme inducers that increase the metabolism of contraceptive steroids (see 'Table 28.1', (p.975)) would also increase the metabolism of oestrogens used for HRT. Some manufacturers state that these drugs may reduce the efficacy of HRT preparations. This would be most likely to be noticed where HRT is prescribed for menopausal vasomotor symptoms, but might be difficult to detect where the indication is osteoporosis. The interaction is not relevant to HRT applied locally for menopausal vaginitis. It has also been suggested that any interaction is less likely with transdermal HRT, which bypasses hepatic first-pass metabolism. Further study is needed to confirm the importance of this possible interaction.

1. Notelovitz M, Tjapkes J, Ware M. Interaction between estrogen and Dilantin in a menopausal woman. *N Engl J Med* (1981) 304, 788–9.

HRT + Moexipril

Moexipril is reported not to interact adversely with HRT.

Clinical evidence, mechanism, importance and management

A placebo-controlled study involving 95 hypertensive postmenopausal women taking HRT found that moexipril, given for 12 weeks, did not affect metabolic parameters associated with cardiovascular disease and concurrent use was considered to be safe and effective.[1] HRT had no effect on the blood pressure-lowering ability of moexipril.[1] Consider also 'Drospirenone + Potassium-sparing drugs', p.977, for a possible interaction between ACE inhibitors and drospirenone.

1. Koch B, Oparil S, Stimpel M. Co-administration of an ACE-inhibitor (moexipril) and hormonal replacement therapy in postmenopausal women. *J Hum Hypertens* (1999) 13, 337–42.

IUDs; Copper + Anti-inflammatory drugs

There are a few early reports suggesting that the very occasional contraceptive failure of a copper IUD may have been due to an interaction with a corticosteroid, aspirin or NSAID.

Clinical evidence, mechanism, importance and management

The cases of 4 women who, despite being fitted with copper IUDs, each had two successive pregnancies have been reported. Two were taking **corticosteroids** regularly and the other two often took **aspirin** for migraine.[1,2] Unwanted pregnancies have also been reported in 3 women with copper IUDs who were taking **corticosteroids,**[3-5] and in 2 women taking **NSAIDs** (**indometacin** and **naproxen**).[5] A later case-control study found that **aspirin** and **NSAIDs** were used more frequently in 717 women who became pregnant while using IUDs than in 717 non-pregnant IUD users (the majority of IUDs were copper). The difference was significant only for **aspirin** (102 IUD failures, 59 control failures). It is possible that this finding could have resulted from bias in recall or reporting.[2] The postulated mechanism for any interaction was that part of the efficacy of copper IUDs may be based on local inflammatory effects, and that anti-inflammatory drugs might reduce this.

The evidence for this possible interaction is very slim and inconclusive, and there appear to be no further reports of any problems. Modern copper-containing IUDs are one of the most effective methods of contraception. Also, intermittent use of anti-inflammatory drugs such as NSAIDs is widespread. A recent Cochrane Database Systematic Review of studies on the use of NSAIDs to reduce pain and/or bleeding with IUDs recommends the use of NSAIDs as first-line drugs to reduce these adverse effects.[6] One manufacturer of copper IUDs states that the evidence does not justify general precautions.[7] No special precautions therefore appear to be necessary.

1. Buhler M, Papiernik E. Successive pregnancies in women fitted with intrauterine devices who take anti-inflammatory drugs. *Lancet* (1983) 1, 483.
2. Papiernik R, Rozenbaum H, Amblard P, Dephot N, de Mouzon J. Intra-uterine device failure: relation with drug use. *Eur J Obstet Gynecol Reprod Biol* (1989) 32, 205–12.
3. Inkeles DM, Hansen RI. Unexpected pregnancy in a woman using an intrauterine device and receiving steroid therapy. *Ann Ophthalmol* (1982) 14, 975.
4. Zerner J, Miller AB, Festino MJ. Failure of an intrauterine device concurrent with administration of corticosteroids. *Fertil Steril* (1976) 27, 1467–8.
5. Thomas P-R, Stérilet et anti-inflammatoires: à propos de quatre observations. *Concours Med* (1977) 45, 7095–6.
6. Grimes DA, Hubacher D, Lopez LM, Schulz KF. Non-steroidal anti-inflammatory drugs for heavy bleeding or pain associated with intrauterine-device use. Available in The Cochrane Database of Systematic Reviews; Issue 2. Chichester: John Wiley; 2007 (accessed 04/01/07).
7. NOVA T 380 (copper containing intrauterine contraceptive device). Schering Health Care Limited. Technical data sheet, May 2003.

Medroxyprogesterone acetate or Megestrol + Aminoglutethimide

Aminoglutethimide markedly reduces the plasma levels of medroxyprogesterone and megestrol.

Clinical evidence

(a) Medroxyprogesterone acetate

In 6 postmenopausal women with breast cancer aminoglutethimide 250 mg two to four times daily approximately halved the plasma levels of medroxyprogesterone acetate 500 mg three times daily.[1] Another study in 6 postmenopausal women found that aminoglutethimide 250 mg four times daily reduced medroxyprogesterone levels by 63% after oral, but not intravenous, medroxyprogesterone.[2] In another study in 6 women with advanced breast cancer, it was found that as the dosage of aminoglutethimide was gradually reduced from 250 mg twice daily and finally withdrawn, the plasma levels of medroxyprogesterone steadily climbed to three times their initial level, although the dose remained constant at a total of 800 mg daily.[3]

(b) Megestrol

Aminoglutethimide 250 mg four times daily reduced the serum levels of megestrol 160 mg daily by 78% in 6 postmenopausal women.[2]

Mechanism

The most likely reason for this interaction is that aminoglutethimide acts as an enzyme inducer, increasing the metabolism of the progestogens, thereby decreasing their levels. When the aminoglutethimide is withdrawn, the enzyme induction ceases, and the progestogen level rises.

Importance and management

Both interactions appear to be established and are possibly clinically important. A 50% reduction in the plasma levels of medroxyprogesterone and megestrol should be expected during concurrent use, and this may reduce the adrenal suppressive effect.[1] The authors of one report[3] say that to achieve adequate plasma medroxyprogesterone acetate levels in breast cancer (above 100 nanograms/mL) a daily dose of 800 mg of *Provera* is probably necessary in the presence of aminoglutethimide 125 or 250 mg twice daily. This is double the usual recommended dose for this condition.

1. Van Deijk WA, Blijham GH, Mellink WAM, Meulenberg PMM. Influence of aminoglutethimide on plasma levels of medroxyprogesterone acetate: its correlation with serum cortisol. *Cancer Treat Rep* (1985) 69, 85–90.
2. Lundgren S, Lønning PE, Aakvaag A, Kvinnsland S. Influence of aminoglutethimide on the metabolism of medroxyprogesterone acetate and megestrol acetate in postmenopausal patients with advanced breast cancer. *Cancer Chemother Pharmacol* (1990) 27, 101–5.
3. Halpenny O, Bye A, Cranny A, Feely J, Daly PA. Influence of aminoglutethimide on plasma levels of medroxyprogesterone acetate. *Med Oncol Tumor Pharmacother* (1990) 7, 241–7.

Oestrogens + Diltiazem

Diltiazem may slightly raise estradiol levels but the clinical significance of this is unclear.

Clinical evidence, mechanism, importance and management

A study in 5 healthy postmenopausal women given diltiazem 30 mg twice daily for 4 days with a single 2-mg oral dose of estradiol on day 2, found that there was a slight but non-significant increase in the maximum levels of estrone. Diltiazem is a moderate inhibitor of the cytochrome P450 isoenzyme CYP3A4 and would be expected to decrease the metabolism of estradiol. This single-dose study appears to suggest that the increase in oestrogen levels caused by diltiazem is small and unlikely to cause any clinically significant adverse effects. However, the dose of diltiazem given was much lower than commonly prescribed doses, the number of patients involved in the study was small, and therefore these results may not accurately reflect the effect of concurrent use.[1] More study is needed.

1. Annas A, Carlström K, Alván G, AL-Shurbaji A. The effect of ketoconazole and diltiazem on oestrogen metabolism in postmenopausal women after single dose oestradiol treatment. *Br J Clin Pharmacol* (2003) 56, 334–6.

Oestrogens + Grapefruit juice

No clinically significant interaction appears to occur between grapefruit juice and a single dose of either estradiol or ethinylestradiol, although their levels are modestly increased by grapefruit juice.

Clinical evidence, mechanism, importance and management

(a) Estradiol

In women given a single 2-mg dose of estradiol, grapefruit juice produced a small 16% increase in the AUC of estrone, a metabolite of estradiol, but did not affect the AUC of estradiol.[1]

(b) Ethinylestradiol

In 13 healthy young women given a single 50-microgram dose of ethinylestradiol, grapefruit juice increased the mean maximum plasma level and AUC_{0-8} of ethinylestradiol by 37% and 30%, respectively, when compared with a control drink (herb tea). There was wide intersubject variation in the increase, but the mean 28% rise in the AUC_{0-12} was not significant. The subjects drank grapefruit juice 100 mL or herb tea

30 minutes before the ethinylestradiol, a further 100 mL with the ethinylestradiol, and then 200 mL every 3 hours for 12 hours after taking the ethinylestradiol. It is thought that this increase in bioavailability probably occurs because grapefruit juice inhibits intestinal cytochrome P450 isoenzyme CYP3A4, which metabolises ethinylestradiol.[2] Grapefruit juice may be taken at the same time of day as the combined oral contraceptive (which usually contains ethinylestradiol) but it seems unlikely that this interaction is of practical importance because the increased bioavailability is still less than the extent of known variability between individuals. However, this requires confirmation in a longer-term study. The authors suggest that diet may be a factor in the known inter-individual variability of contraceptive steroid levels.[2]

1. Schubert W, Cullberg G, Edgar B, Hedner T. Inhibition of 17 beta-estradiol metabolism by grapefruit juice in ovariectomized women. *Maturitas* (1994) 20, 155–63.
2. Weber A, Jäger R, Börner A, Klinger G, Vollanth R, Matthey K, Balogh A. Can grapefruit juice influence ethinylestradiol bioavailability? *Contraception* (1996) 53, 41–7.

Progestogen-only contraceptives + Antibacterials

The reliability of progestogen-only methods of hormonal contraception are not affected by antibacterials that do not induce liver enzymes, such as the penicillins and tetracyclines.

Clinical evidence, mechanism, importance and management

Four of the 63 contraceptive failures attributed to antibacterials in the records of the CSM in the UK for 1968 to 1984 occurred with a progestogen-only contraceptive (unspecified).[1] In another study, 2 of 37 cases of contraceptive failure attributed to antibacterials occurred with a progestogen-only contraceptive (unspecified).[2]

Note that the mechanism behind the rare cases of failure of *combined* oral contraceptives seen with various broad-spectrum antibacterials is postulated to be reduced enterohepatic recycling of ethinylestradiol (see 'Hormonal contraceptives + Antibacterials; Penicillins', p.981). Since progestogens are largely metabolised to inactive substances before they are conjugated, they do not undergo enterohepatic recycling of the active substance.

Pharmacokinetic data show that the progestogen component (**levonorgestrel, norethisterone**) of *combined* oral contraceptives is not affected by **ampicillin**,[3,4] **clarithromycin**,[5] **doxycycline**,[6] **metronidazole**,[4] **moxifloxacin**,[7] or **tetracycline**.[8] There is no reason to expect that the contraceptive efficacy of the various progestogen-only methods (tablets, implants, injections, IUDs) would be affected by antibacterials that alter gut flora and do not induce liver enzymes.

It is generally accepted that no interaction occurs,[9] and it is likely that the few cases seen with progestogen-only contraceptives are chance associations.[1] The Faculty of Family Planning and Reproductive Health Care (FFPRHC) Clinical Effectiveness Unit does not recommend any additional contraceptive precautions when antibacterials that do not induce liver enzymes are taken with any method of progestogen-only hormonal contraception, including the emergency contraceptive pill.[10] However, note that **rifampicin** and **rifabutin** are likely to reduce the efficacy of most forms of hormonal contraceptives, as they induce the metabolism of both oestrogens and progestogens, see 'Hormonal contraceptives + Rifamycins', p.1001.

1. Back DJ, Grimmer SFM, Orme ML'E, Proudlove C, Mann RD, Breckenridge AM. Evaluation of Committee on Safety of Medicines yellow card reports on oral contraceptive-drug interactions with anticonvulsants and antibiotics. *Br J Clin Pharmacol* (1988) 25, 527–32.
2. Sparrow MJ. Pill method failures. *N Z Med J* (1987) 100, 102–5.
3. Back DJ, Breckenridge AM, MacIver M, Orme M, Rowe PH, Staiger Ch, Thomas E, Tjia J. The effects of ampicillin on oral contraceptive steroids in women. *Br J Clin Pharmacol* (1982) 14, 43–8.
4. Joshi JV, Joshi UM, Sankholi GM, Krishna U, Mandlekar A, Chowdhury V, Hazari K, Gupta K, Sheth UK, Saxena BN. A study of interaction of low-dose combination oral contraceptive with ampicillin and metronidazole. *Contraception* (1980) 22, 643–52.
5. Back DJ, Tjia J, Martin C, Millar E, Salmon P, Orme M. The interaction between clarithromycin and combined oral-contraceptive steroids. *J Pharm Med* (1991) 2, 81–7.
6. Neely JL, Abate M, Swinker M, D'Angio R. The effect of doxycycline on serum levels of ethinyl estradiol, norethindrone, and endogenous progesterone. *Obstet Gynecol* (1991) 77, 416–20.
7. Staß H, Sachse R, Heinig R, Zühlsdorf M, Horstmann R. Pharmacokinetics (PK) of steroid hormones in oral contraceptives (OC) are not altered by oral moxifloxacin (MOX). *J Antimicrob Chemother* (1999) 44 (Suppl A) 138–9.
8. Murphy AA, Zacur HA, Charache P, Burkman RT. The effect of tetracycline on levels of oral contraceptives. *Am J Obstet Gynecol* (1991) 164, 28–33.
9. McCann MF, Potter LS. Progestin-only contraception: a comprehensive review. *Contraception* (1994) 50, S1–S198.
10. Faculty of Family Planning and Reproductive Health Care Clinical Effectiveness Unit. FFPRHC Guidance: Drug interactions with hormonal contraception. April 2005. Available at: http://www.ffprhc.org.uk/admin/uploads/DrugInteractionsFinal.pdf (accessed 23/08/07).

Progestogen-only contraceptives + Enzyme inducers

Enzyme inducers appear to reduce the contraceptive reliability of the levonorgestrel implant, and pregnancies have been reported following the use of carbamazepine, phenytoin, and phenobarbital. Pregnancies have also been reported when the etonogestrel implant was used in women taking enzyme-inducing antiepileptics, particularly carbamazepine. The efficacy of medroxyprogesterone depot injection does not appear to be affected by enzyme inducers. Similarly, norethisterone depot injection is thought unlikely to be affected. The contraceptive reliability of the progestogen-releasing intrauterine system is also not thought to be affected.

Clinical evidence, mechanism, importance and management

(a) Implants

A woman taking **phenytoin** 300 mg daily became pregnant 9 months after the insertion of a **levonorgestrel**-releasing subdermal contraceptive implant (*Norplant*). **Levonorgestrel** levels increased by 50% after discontinuation of the **phenytoin**, and progesterone levels fell, suggesting greater suppression of ovulation.[1] In another report plasma **levonorgestrel** levels (from an implant) were 38% lower in 6 women taking **phenytoin** alone or in combination with **carbamazepine** or valproate than in 10 subjects taking no medication. Two of the 6 women became pregnant (one taking **phenytoin** and one taking **phenytoin** with **carbamazepine**).[2] Similarly, one woman taking **phenobarbital** 210 mg daily became pregnant about 17 months after the insertion of a **levonorgestrel** implant.[3] Another report[4] briefly mentions that one woman taking enzyme-inducing antiepileptics became pregnant while using a **levonorgestrel** implant, and mentions that the manufacturer had 30 other similar cases on file as of 1995.

Pregnancy has been reported in a patient taking **carbamazepine** 600 mg daily and using the **etonogestrel** implant (*Implanon*).[5] A report describes 8 other cases of contraceptive failure with this implant in Australian patients who were taking liver enzyme-inducing antiepileptics (7 of the 8 were taking carbamazepine).[6] The Faculty of Family Planning and Reproductive Health Care (FFPRHC) Clinical Effectiveness Unit recommends that the progestogen-only implant may be continued with short courses of enzyme inducers but only if combined with additional contraceptive methods, see 'Hormonal contraceptives + Antiepileptics; Barbiturates or Phenytoin', p.985, for more detailed guidance. The progestogen-only implant should be reviewed to an alternative form of contraceptive with long-term use of liver enzyme inducers.[7] A list of enzyme inducers can be found in 'Table 28.1', (p.975)).

(b) Injectable preparations

The manufacturer states that the clearance of **medroxyprogesterone acetate** is approximately equal to hepatic blood flow, and as such, would not be expected to be affected by drugs that alter hepatic enzyme activity. Therefore, they say that no dosage adjustment is needed.[8] This is in line with the FFPRHC guidance.[7]

There are data showing that **rifamycins** can reduce the plasma levels of **norethisterone** when it is used as a component of combined oral contraceptives (see 'Hormonal contraceptives + Rifamycins', p.1001). The manufacturer of *Noristerat* notes that enzyme inducers may reduce the efficacy of the norethisterone enantate injection .[9] However, guidance from the FFPRHC Clinical Effectiveness Unit is to continue with the normal injection schedule for norethisterone.[7].

(c) Progestogen-releasing intrauterine system (IUS)

Some enzyme inducers increase the metabolism and reduce the efficacy of combined oral contraceptives (see 'Table 28.1', (p.975), for a list). The manufacturer has not studied the influence of these drugs on the efficacy of the **levonorgestrel**-releasing IUS (*Mirena*),[10] and has said that they cannot be sure that the foreign body effect (i.e. the effect whereby the presence of the IUS prevents implantation) and/or locally acting hormone will provide reliable contraception when systemic hormone levels and suppression of ovaries are reduced by drug interactions.[11] However, this appears to be overly cautious. The systemic absorption of **levonorgestrel** from the IUS leads to lower blood levels than are seen with standard progestogen-only oral contraceptives, and women using a **levonorgestrel** IUS usually continue to ovulate. Thus, the contraceptive effects of the **levonorgestrel** IUS are mainly local.[10] Also, a pilot study in 56 women (49 epileptics) using a **levonorgestrel** IUS, most of them also taking enzyme inducers, who accumulated 1075 months of use, found only one apparent contraceptive failure.[12]

The FFPRHC Clinical Effectiveness Unit considers that the levonorgestrel-releasing IUS is unlikely to be affected by enzyme inducers and recommends that no additional contraceptive protection is required.[7] It is therefore a suitable contraceptive for women taking these drugs.[13]

1. Odlind V, Olsson S-E. Enhanced metabolism of levonorgestrel during phenytoin treatment in a woman with Norplant® implants. *Contraception* (1986) 33, 257–61.
2. Haukkamaa M. Contraception by Norplant® subdermal capsules is not reliable in epileptic patients on anticonvulsant treatment. *Contraception* (1986) 33, 559–65.
3. Shane-McWhorter L, Cerveny JD, MacFarlane LL, Osborn C. Enhanced metabolism of levonorgestrel during phenobarbital treatment and resultant pregnancy. *Pharmacotherapy* (1998) 18, 1360–4.
4. Krauss GL, Brandt J, Campbell M, Plate C, Summerfield M. Antiepileptic medication and oral contraceptive interactions: a national survey of neurologists and obstetricians. *Neurology* (1996) 46, 1534–9.
5. Schindlbeck C, Janni W, Friese K. Failure of implanon contraception in a patient taking carbamazepin for epilepsia. *Arch Gynecol Obstet* (2006) 273, 255–6.
6. Harrison-Woolrych M, Hill R. Unintended pregnancies with the etonogestrel implant (Implanon): a case series from postmarketing experience in Australia. *Contraception* (2005) 71, 306–8.
7. Faculty of Family Planning and Reproductive Health Care Clinical Effectiveness Unit. FFPRHC Guidance: Drug interactions with hormonal contraception. April 2005. Available at: http://www.ffprhc.org.uk/admin/uploads/DrugInteractionsFinal.pdf (accessed 23/08/07).
8. Depo-Provera (Medroxyprogesterone acetate). Pharmacia Ltd. UK Summary of product characteristics, November 2004.
9. Noristerat (Norethisterone enantate). Schering Health Care Ltd. UK Summary of product characteristics, April 2004.
10. Mirena (Levonorgestrel Intrauterine System). Schering Health Care Ltd. UK Summary of product characteristics, July 2004.
11. Personal communication. Schering Health Care Limited. April 2001.
12. Bounds W, Guillebaud J. Observational series on women using the contraceptive Mirena concurrently with anti-epileptic and other enzyme-inducing drugs. *J Fam Plann Reprod Health Care* (2002) 28, 78–80.
13. Crawford P. Interactions between antiepileptic drugs and hormonal contraception. *CNS Drugs* (2002) 16, 263–72.

Tibolone + Enzyme inducers

On theoretical grounds the manufacturer of tibolone says that the effects of tibolone may be reduced by enzyme-inducing antiepileptics and rifampicin.

Clinical evidence, mechanism, importance and management

The manufacturer says that on a theoretical basis enzyme inducers such as the **barbiturates**, **carbamazepine**, **phenytoin** and **rifampicin** may accelerate the metabolism of tibolone and thus decrease its efficacy.[1] However, they note that no examples of these interactions have been reported in clinical practice, and pharmacokinetic studies are required to demonstrate this interaction. Nevertheless it would be prudent to monitor concurrent use.

1. Livial (Tibolone). Organon Laboratories Ltd. UK Summary of product characteristics, May 2006.

29

Immunosuppressants

The immunosuppressants dealt with in this section are the corticosteroids, basiliximab, daclizumab, etanercept, infliximab, ciclosporin, everolimus, leflunomide, muromonab-CD3, mycophenolate, sirolimus, and tacrolimus. A classification is given in 'Table 29.1', (see below). When any of these drugs acts as the interacting agent the relevant monograph is categorised in the section dealing with the drug whose effects are changed. Other drugs that are also used for immunosuppression (e.g. azathioprine and methotrexate) are found in the section on antineoplastic drugs.

Table 29.1 Immunosuppressant drugs

Group	*Drugs*
Corticosteroids	Beclometasone, Budesonide, Ciclesonide, Deflazacort, Dexamethasone, Fludrocortisone, Fluticasone, Hydrocortisone, Methylprednisolone, Prednisolone, Predisone, Triamcinolone
Monoclonal antibodies	
Causing lysis of B-lymphocytes	Alemtuzumab, Rituximab
Preventing T-lymphocyte proliferation	Basiliximab, Daclizumab
Blocking T-cell generation and function	Muromonab-CD3
Inhibitors of tumour necrosis factor	Adalimumab, Infliximab
Others	
Calcineurin inhibitors	Ciclosporin (Cyclosporine), Tacrolimus
Inhibitors of tumour necrosis factor	Etanercept
Miscellaneous	Everolimus, Leflunomide (DMARD), Mycophenolate, Sirolimus

Basiliximab + Miscellaneous

The concurrent use of basiliximab with azathioprine, muromonab-CD3 or mycophenolate is not associated with an increase in adverse effects or infections. The dose requirements of ciclosporin or tacrolimus may be altered by basiliximab. Basiliximab is reported not to interact with analgesics, anti-infective drugs, diuretics, beta blockers or calcium-channel blockers.

Clinical evidence, mechanism, importance and management

(a) Azathioprine

Azathioprine, added to regimens including basiliximab, ciclosporin microemulsion and corticosteroids reduced the clearance of basiliximab by 22%. However, the use of basiliximab in triple regimens with azathioprine did not increase adverse effects or infections.[1]

(b) Ciclosporin

A study in 39 paediatric renal transplant patients taking ciclosporin found that in 24 patients, who were also given basiliximab 10 or 20 mg on days 0 and 4 after transplantation, lower doses of ciclosporin resulted in significantly higher trough levels and some evidence of early ciclosporin toxicity within the first 10 days. At days 28 to 50 ciclosporin levels declined and 20% higher doses were required to maintain adequate trough levels in the basiliximab group.[2] Another study in 54 paediatric liver transplant patients found that the addition of basiliximab to ciclosporin and corticosteroids did not significantly alter the overall ciclosporin dose requirements. However, 9 basiliximab-treated patients experienced acute rejection at 21 to 28 days after transplantation, and this was associated with low ciclosporin trough levels, requiring an increased ciclosporin dosage in 6 of the 9 patients.[3] It was considered that the effect on ciclosporin was due to an interleukin-2 receptor mediated alteration of the cytochrome P450 enzyme system.[2] This was considered to only play a minor role in the liver-transplant patients because of significantly lower target trough levels in these patients.[3] However, a further study found no increase in rejection episodes between days 28 to 50 in kidney-transplant patients treated with basiliximab and ciclosporin.[4]

The authors of the first study[2] recommend that the initial dose of ciclosporin should be limited to 400 mg/m^2 in children receiving renal transplants who are also given with basiliximab. Dose reductions were not considered necessary by other authors, but close monitoring was recommended.[3,4]

A retrospective analysis of renal transplant patients compared the rates of acute rejection within 6 months in patients given ciclosporin, mycophenolate mofetil and prednisone, with or without basiliximab. Overall the rates of acute rejection were 11% and 23% in the basiliximab and no-basiliximab groups, respectively. In 74 patients not given basiliximab, low therapeutic ciclosporin exposure on day 3 was associated with increased acute rejection within the first 6 months post-transplantation (45% with ciclosporin AUC less than 4400 nanogram.h/mL compared with 15% with a ciclosporin AUC of greater than 4400 nanogram.h/mL). In 93 patients given basiliximab, rates of acute rejection were similar (about 10%) in patients with low or therapeutic ciclosporin exposure at day 3. It was suggested that achieving early ciclosporin therapeutic targets may not be required if basiliximab is also used.[5]

(c) Muromonab-CD3

The manufacturers of basiliximab say that patients in phase 3 studies received basiliximab with muromonab-CD3 for episodes of rejection, with no increase in adverse events or infections. Human antimurine antibody responses were reported in 2 of 138 patients receiving basiliximab and 4 of 34 patients receiving both basiliximab and muromonab-CD3. Therefore, the manufacturers say that if basiliximab has been given, muromonab-CD3 or other murine antilymphocytic antibody preparations can still subsequently be given.[1]

(d) Mycophenolate

Azathioprine, added to regimens including basiliximab, ciclosporin microemulsion and corticosteroids, reduced the clearance of basiliximab by 51%. However, the use of basiliximab in triple regimens with mycophenolate did not increase adverse effects or infections.[1]

(e) Tacrolimus

A study in 12 adult renal-transplant patients found that trough tacrolimus levels on day 3 were increased by 63% in patients also given basiliximab and in 50% of these patients this was associated with the development of acute tubular necrosis. By day 30, tacrolimus trough levels showed a downward trend in the basiliximab treated group, despite similar dose requirements to those on day 10. Tacrolimus dose requirements were lower in the basiliximab group compared to the control group throughout the 60-day study period.[6] Dose reductions were not considered necessary by the authors, but close monitoring was recommended.[6]

(f) Other drugs

The manufacturers report that basiliximab has been used with **analgesics, antibacterials, antifungals, antivirals, diuretics, beta blockers** and **calcium-channel blockers** without any increase in adverse reactions. None of the drugs was individually named.[1]

1. Simulect (Basiliximab). Novartis Pharmaceuticals UK Ltd. UK Summary of product characteristics, January 2006.
2. Strehlau J, Pape L, Offner G, Bjoern N, Ehrich JHH. Interleukin-2 receptor antibody-induced alterations of ciclosporin dose requirements in paediatric transplant patients. *Lancet* (2000) 356, 1327–8.
3. Ganschow R, Grabhorn E, Burdelski M. Basiliximab in paediatric liver-transplant recipients. *Lancet* (2001) 357, 388.
4. Vester U, Kranz B, Treichel U, Hoyer PF. Basiliximab in paediatric liver-transplant recipients. *Lancet* (2001) 357, 388–9.
5. Balbontin FG, Kiberd B, Singh D, Fraser A, Belitsky P, Lawen J. Basiliximab lowers the therapeutic threshold for cyclosporine exposure in the early post kidney transplant period. *J Am Soc Nephrol* (2003) 14, 650A.
6. Sifontis NM, Benedetti E, Vasquez EM. Clinically significant drug interaction between basiliximab and tacrolimus in renal transplant recipients. *Transplant Proc* (2002) 34, 1730–2.

Ciclosporin + ACE inhibitors and Angiotensin II receptor antagonists

Acute renal failure developed in four kidney transplant patients taking ciclosporin when they were given enalapril. Oliguria was seen in another patient taking ciclosporin with captopril. Other studies have found no significant changes in renal function with candesartan and losartan or with enalapril. Hyperkalaemia may develop in patients taking ACE inhibitors or angiotensin II receptor antagonists with ciclosporin.

Clinical evidence

(a) ACE Inhibitors

Two kidney transplant patients on ciclosporin developed acute renal failure 10 to 42 days after starting to take **enalapril** 5 to 10 mg twice daily. Recovery was complete when the **enalapril** was stopped in one of the patients, and when both **enalapril** and ciclosporin were stopped in the other. The latter patient had no problems when the ciclosporin was restarted. Both recovered renal function after 10 to 30 days. Neither had any previous evidence of renal artery stenosis or chronic rejection, which are conditions known to predispose to renal failure during ACE inhibitor treatment. Two other patients appeared to tolerate concurrent use well.[1] Two further kidney transplant patients developed acute renal failure when given **enalapril**. Neither had renal arterial stenosis or acute rejection.[2] The manufacturer briefly mentions that transient oliguria was seen in a kidney transplant patient given ciclosporin and **captopril**.[3]

A study in 13 kidney transplant patients taking ciclosporin found that concurrent treatment with **enalapril** 5 or 10 mg daily for 3 weeks caused a larger increase in potassium levels (mean increase of 0.5 mmol/L) than in those patients given **losartan** 50 mg daily (mean increase of 0.2 mmol/L). Potassium levels were not increased above 5.5 mmol/L in any of the patients studied. Uric acid levels were also increased by **enalapril** but decreased by **losartan**, although this was not statistically significant. No changes in ciclosporin trough levels were seen during the study and the serum creatinine remained stable.[4] Another study in kidney transplant patients taking ciclosporin with either **enalapril** (33 patients) or **enalapril** plus amlodipine (32 patients) found that the potassium and serum creatinine levels did not increase in the **enalapril**/amlodipine group whereas they increased by 0.2 mmol/L and 9 micromol/L, respectively, in the group who received **enalapril** alone. Ciclosporin levels remained stable in all patients.[5]

(b) Angiotensin II receptor antagonists

A study in kidney transplant patients taking ciclosporin with **losartan** found that the serum creatinine was only slightly and non-significantly increased in 5 patients. Losartan was stopped in 3 patients because of a rise in creatinine levels. Transient hyperkalaemia (potassium above 5.5 mmol/L) developed in 4 patients but the potassium had fallen to below 5.5 mmol/L by week 12 in all patients. Ciclosporin levels were remained stable during the study and no significant dose changes were made, although one patient was withdrawn from the study due to ciclosporin toxicity which the authors state was not related to the use of losartan.[6] Another study in 14 kidney transplant patients taking ciclosporin with **losartan** 50 to 100 mg daily for 8 weeks found serum creatinine, potassium and ciclosporin levels were unaffected.[7] Another study in 41 kidney transplant patients with proteinuria taking ciclosporin found that the addition of **candesartan** 4 to 12 mg daily had no significant effects on the creatinine clearance or ciclosporin levels.[8]

Mechanism

Not understood. One suggestion is that ciclosporin reduces renal blood flow and reduces perfusion through the glomerulus, which is worsened when angiotensin II is inhibited by the ACE inhibitor.[1] One study suggested that the larger increase in potassium levels may be related to changes in aldosterone levels seen with enalapril.[4]

Importance and management

There have been few specific case reports of renal failure and hyperkalaemia with ciclosporin and ACE inhibitors or angiotensin II receptor antagonists. Data from the efficacy studies above suggest that the incidence of renal failure and hyperkalaemia is low, nevertheless care and good monitoring are needed if ACE inhibitors or angiotensin II receptor antagonists and ciclosporin are used concurrently. Also note that the manufacturers of ciclosporin warn about the possible risk of hyperkalaemia with ACE inhibitors and angiotensin II receptor antagonists with ciclosporin as these drugs may raise potassium levels.[9] Monitor potassium levels more closely in the initial weeks of concurrent use, bearing in mind that an increase in potassium levels may be due to worsening renal function as well as these drugs.

1. Murray BM, Venuto RC, Kohli R, Cunningham EE. Enalapril-associated renal failure in renal transplants: possible role of cyclosporine. *Am J Kidney Dis* (1990) 16, 66–9.
2. Garcia TM, da Costa JA, Costa RS, Ferraz AS. Acute tubular renal necrosis in kidney transplant patients treated with enalapril. *Ren Fail* (1994) 16, 419–23.
3. Cockburn I. Cyclosporine A: a clinical evaluation of drug interactions. *Transplant Proc* (1986) 18 (Suppl 5), 50–5.
4. Schmidt A, Gruber U, Böhmig G, Köller E, Mayer G. The effect of ACE inhibitor and angiotensin II receptor antagonist therapy on serum uric acid levels and potassium homeostasis in hypertensive renal transplant recipients treated with CsA. *Nephrol Dial Transplant* (2001) 16, 1034–7.
5. Halimi JM, Giraudeau B, Buchler M, Al-Najjar A, Etienne I, Laouad I, Bruyere F, Lebranchu Y. Enalapril/amlodipine combination in cyclosporine-treated renal transplant recipients: a prospective randomized trial. *Clin Transplant* (2007) 21, 277–84.
6. del Castillo D, Campistol JM, Guirado L, Capdevilla L, Martínez JG, Pereira P, Bravo J, Pérez R. Efficacy and safety of losartan in the treatment of hypertension in renal transplant patients. *Kidney Int* (1998) 54, (Suppl 68) S135–S139.
7. Tylicki L, Biedunkiewicz B, Chamienia A, Wojnarowski K, Zdrojewski Z, Rutkowski B. Randomized placebo-controlled study on the effects of losartan and carvedilol on albuminuria in renal transplant recipients. *Transplantation* (2006) 81, 52–6.
8. Omoto K, Tanabe K, Tokumoto T, Shimmura H, Ishida H, Toma H. Use of candesartan cilexetil decreases proteinuria in renal transplant patients with chronic allograft dysfunction. *Transplantation* (2003) 76, 1170–4.
9. Neoral (Ciclosporin). Novartis Pharmaceuticals UK Ltd. UK Summary of product characteristics, December 2004.

Ciclosporin + Acetazolamide

There is some limited evidence to suggest that acetazolamide can cause a marked and rapid rise in ciclosporin serum levels, possibly accompanied by renal toxicity.

Clinical evidence, mechanism, importance and management

A study in 3 men found that 72 hours after they started taking acetazolamide (dose not stated) their trough serum ciclosporin levels rose by more than sixfold, from a range of 54 to 270 nanograms/mL up to 517 to 1827 nanograms/mL.[1] Another man with a heart transplant had a fivefold increase in his serum ciclosporin levels, marked renal impairment, and neurotoxicity when he was given oral acetazolamide for raised intra-ocular pressure secondary to panuveitis.[2] The increase in ciclosporin serum levels has also been seen in *animal* studies.[3]

Information seems to be limited to these reports but it seems that the concurrent use of ciclosporin and acetazolamide should be closely monitored, being alert of the need to reduce the ciclosporin dosage. The interaction can apparently develop very rapidly.

1. Tabbara KF, Al-Faisal Z, Al-Rashed W. Interaction between acetazolamide and cyclosporine. *Arch Ophthalmol* (1998) 116, 832–3.
2. Keogh A, Esmore D, Spratt P, Savdie E, McClusky P, Chang V. Acetazolamide and cyclosporine. *Transplantation* (1988) 46, 478–9.
3. El-Sayed YM, Tabbara KF, Gouda MW. Effect of acetazolamide on the pharmacokinetics of cyclosporine in rabbits. *Int J Pharmaceutics* (1995) 121, 181–6.

Ciclosporin + Aciclovir and related drugs

Aciclovir does not normally seem to affect ciclosporin serum levels nor worsen renal function, but a very small number of cases of nephrotoxicity and increased serum ciclosporin levels have been seen following concurrent use. Valaciclovir, a prodrug of aciclovir, is expected to interact similarly.

Clinical evidence

A retrospective study in kidney transplant patients taking ciclosporin (serum levels in the range 100 to 250 nanograms/mL) found that in 12 patients oral aciclovir 800 mg four times daily for 3 months had no significant effect on their ciclosporin serum levels or on nephrotoxicity when compared with 9 control subjects.[1] No significant changes in renal function were seen in 11 patients taking ciclosporin when they were given intravenous aciclovir 750 to 1500 mg/m^2 daily for at least 7 days to treat herpes infections.[2] No significant changes in serum creatinine or ciclosporin levels were seen during the 14 days following kidney transplant in 17 patients given aciclovir 800 mg daily.[3] Fifty-three kidney transplant patients were given ciclosporin and aciclovir 800 mg to 3.2 g daily for 12 weeks. The aciclovir was withdrawn from 2 patients because of unexplained and temporary increases in serum creatinine levels. The serum ciclosporin levels were not reported.[4] Five patients (2 adults and 3 children) taking ciclosporin, prednisone and azathioprine were given aciclovir 200 mg five times daily for 6 days for herpes zoster or chicken pox. Ciclosporin serum levels remained unchanged and renal function improved.[5]

In contrast to the cases cited above, 3 of 7 bone marrow transplant patients given ciclosporin and intravenous aciclovir 500 mg/m^2 every 8 or 12 hours (depending on renal function) developed nephrotoxicity, which was fatal in one case. Histological evidence suggested ciclosporin nephrotoxicity.[6] The manufacturer briefly notes that an increase in serum creatinine was seen in ciclosporin recipients in one report, and increased aciclovir levels accompanied by reversible acute tubular necrosis in another.[7] Yet another report describes a threefold increase in ciclosporin serum levels, which occurred when a child with a heart transplant was given intravenous aciclovir.[8]

Mechanism

Not understood; although both drugs are known to be nephrotoxic, all be it rarely in the case of aciclovir.

Importance and management

Well documented. The evidence available indicates that ciclosporin levels and renal function are usually unaltered by the concurrent use of aciclovir, but the handful of cases where problems have arisen clearly indicate that renal function should be well monitored. One group of workers suggest that aciclovir, in doses of 250 mg/m^2 by slow infusion, does not adversely affect renal function in well-hydrated patients taking ciclosporin if their ciclosporin levels are carefully monitored.[2] **Valaciclovir**, a prodrug of aciclovir, is rapidly converted to the active drug, aciclovir. Therefore the advice given for aciclovir equally applies to valaciclovir. The manufacturers recommend that renal function is closely monitored if high doses of valaciclovir (more than 4 g daily) are given with drugs that affect renal function, such as ciclosporin.[9]

1. Dugandzic RM, Sketris IS, Belitsky P, Schlech WF, Givner ML. Effect of coadministration of acyclovir and cyclosporine on kidney function and cyclosporine concentrations in renal transplant patients. *DICP Ann Pharmacother* (1991) 25, 316–7.

2. Johnson PC, Kumor K, Welsh MS, Woo J, Kahan BD. Effects of coadministration of cyclosporine and acyclovir on renal function of renal allograft recipients. *Transplantation* (1987) 44, 329–31.
3. Stoffel M, Squifflet JP, Pirson Y, Lamy M, Alexandre GPJ. Effectiveness of oral acyclovir prophylaxis in renal transplant recipients. *Transplant Proc* (1987) 19, 2190–3.
4. Balfour HH, Chace BA, Stapleton JT, Simmons RL, Fryd DS. A randomized, placebo-controlled trial of oral acyclovir for the prevention of cytomegalovirus disease in recipients of renal allografts. *N Engl J Med* (1989) 320, 1381–7.
5. Hayes K, Shakuntala V, Pingle A, Dhawan IK, Masri MA. Safe use of acyclovir (Zovirax) in renal transplant patients on cyclosporine A therapy: case reports. *Transplant Proc* (1992) 24, 1926.
6. Shepp DH, Dandliker PS, Meyers JD. Treatment of varicella-zoster virus infection in severely immunocompromised patients: a randomized comparison of acyclovir and vidarabine. *N Engl J Med* (1986) 314, 208–12.
7. Cockburn I. Cyclosporine A: a clinical evaluation of drug interactions. *Transplant Proc* (1986) 18 (Suppl 5), 50–5.
8. Boardman M, Yodur Purdy C. Cyclosporine and aciclovir; report of a drug interaction. Am Soc Hosp Pharmacists Midyear Clinical Meeting, Dallas, Texas. December 1988, Abstract SP-16.
9. Valtrex (Valaciclovir). GlaxoSmithKline UK. UK Summary of product characteristics, September 2005.

Ciclosporin + Alcohol

An isolated report describes a marked increase in serum ciclosporin levels in a patient after an episode of binge drinking, but a subsequent study found that moderate, single doses of alcohol in other patients had no such effect. Red wine decreases ciclosporin bioavailability.

Clinical evidence

The serum ciclosporin levels of a kidney transplant patient doubled, from 101 to 205 nanograms/mL, and remained high for about 4 days after he went on a 2-day alcohol binge. A subsequent study in 8 other patients with kidney transplants found no changes in serum ciclosporin or creatinine levels when they drank 50 mL of 100% alcohol in orange juice (about equivalent to 4 oz of whisky).[1]

A crossover study in 12 healthy subjects given a single 8 mg/kg dose of ciclosporin with water or 350 mL (12 oz) of Californian red wine found that red wine caused a 50% increase in the oral clearance of ciclosporin. The ciclosporin AUC was reduced by 30% and the maximum blood levels were reduced by 38%, from 1258 to 779 micrograms/L. There was a high degree of variability, with increases in oral clearance ranging from 1.5 to 129%, with Caucasians experiencing a greater degree of change than Asians.[2]

Mechanism

A study in *animals* found that pretreatment with oral ciclosporin had no effect on the pharmacokinetics of alcohol or acetaldehyde. This suggests that any difference in the alcohol consumption of patients taking ciclosporin is unlikely to have a pharmacokinetic basis.[3] The mechanism by which red wine exerts its effect is not known. White wine does not appear to affect ciclosporin pharmacokinetics,[4] so the interaction is not believed to be an effect of alcohol. Antioxidants in red wine such as resveratrol may inactivate the cytochrome P450 isoenzyme CYP3A4 and this would also be expected to increase ciclosporin levels. The solubility of ciclosporin is decreased in red wine and it is possible that substances in red wine bind ciclosporin in the gastrointestinal tract and reduce its bioavailability.[2] Another study by the same authors suggested that ciclosporin absorption is possibly impaired by P-glycoprotein induction.[5]

Importance and management

The authors of the first study[1] say that they currently advise their renal transplant patients to avoid heavy drinking, but that an occasional drink probably does not affect ciclosporin levels. Patients may be advised to avoid alcohol after transplantation, but those who do drink alcohol should exercise caution if drinking red wine while taking ciclosporin.

1. Paul MD, Parfrey PS, Smart M, Gault H. The effect of ethanol on serum cyclosporine A levels in renal transplant patients. *Am J Kidney Dis* (1987) 10, 133–5.
2. Tsunoda SM, Harris RZ, Christians U, Velez RL, Freeman RB, Benet LZ, Warshaw A. Red wine decreases cyclosporine bioavailability. *Clin Pharmacol Ther* (2001) 70, 462–7.
3. Giles HG, Orrego H, Sandrin S, Saldivia V. The influence of cyclosporine on abstinence from alcohol in transplant patients. *Transplantation* (1990) 49, 1201–2.
4. Tsunoda SM, Harris RZ, Freeman RB, Warshaw A. Acute and chronic wine effects on cyclosporine disposition. *Br J Clin Pharmacol* (2000) 42.
5. Tsunoda SM, Christians U, Velez RL, Benet LZ, Harris RZ. Red wine (RW) effects on cyclosporine (CyA) metabolites. *Clin Pharmacol Ther* (2000) 67, 150.

Ciclosporin + Allopurinol

Isolated cases of markedly raised ciclosporin levels have been reported in patients given allopurinol. However, in two clinical studies, a trend towards lower ciclosporin levels with low-dose allopurinol has been seen.

Clinical evidence, mechanism, importance and management

The ciclosporin levels of a kidney transplant patient rose by about threefold, accompanied by an increase in serum creatinine from 124 to 194 micromol/L, after allopurinol 100 mg daily was taken for 12 days.[1] Another previously stable kidney transplant patient had a two- to threefold rise in her ciclosporin level when allopurinol 200 mg daily was given. Her serum creatinine remained unchanged throughout.[2] The general importance of these two reports of increased ciclosporin levels is unknown, although increases in ciclosporin levels are associated with increased risk of nephrotoxicity.

Two clinical studies in renal transplant patients taking ciclosporin, azathioprine and prednisolone with low-dose allopurinol 25 mg daily or on alternate days found a reduction in ciclosporin levels (significant in one group), as well as a beneficial reduction in the acute rejection rate.[3] Note that azathioprine levels can be raised significantly by allopurinol usually requiring a dose reduction, see 'Thiopurines + Allopurinol', p.664. The case reports above and the clinical studies are probably insufficient to recommend increased monitoring of ciclosporin levels in all patients given allopurinol, but bear them in mind in the event of an unexpected response to treatment.

1. Stevens SL, Goldman MH. Cyclosporine toxicity associated with allopurinol. *South Med J* (1992) 85, 1265–6.
2. Gorrie M, Beaman M, Nicholls A, Backwell P. Allopurinol interaction with cyclosporine. *BMJ* (1994) 308, 113.
3. Chocair PR, Duley JA, Cameron JS, Arap S, Ianhez L, Sabbaga E, Simmonds HA. Does low-dose allopurinol, with azathioprine, cyclosporin and prednisolone, improve renal transplant immunosuppression? *Adv Exp Med Biol* (1994) 370, 205–8.

Ciclosporin + Amiodarone

Ciclosporin serum levels can be increased or decreased by amiodarone, and nephrotoxicity has occurred as a result of increased levels. Increased amiodarone levels and pulmonary toxicity have been reported in patients also given ciclosporin.

Clinical evidence

(a) Ciclosporin affected

Eight patients with heart transplants and 3 patients with heart-lung transplants taking ciclosporin were also given amiodarone for atrial flutter or fibrillation. Their serum ciclosporin levels rose by 9% despite a 13 to 14% reduction in the ciclosporin dosage, serum creatinine levels rose by 38% (from 157 to 216 micromol/L), and blood urea nitrogen rose by 30%.[1] In another report by some of the same authors, one patient is said to have shown a 50% decrease in the clearance of ciclosporin when given amiodarone.[2] Eight other patients with heart or heart-lung transplants were effectively treated with amiodarone for atrial flutter and/or atrial fibrillation, but they had a 31% rise in serum ciclosporin levels, from 248 to 325 nanograms/mL despite a 44% reduction in the ciclosporin dosage (from 6.2 to 3.5 mg/kg daily). Serum creatinine levels rose by 39%.[3] The serum ciclosporin levels of a kidney transplant patient doubled when amiodarone was given.[4]

In contrast, in 5 heart transplant patients amiodarone was discontinued and ciclosporin initiated, but the metabolism of ciclosporin was increased for 4 to 5 weeks (total plasma metabolites increased from 720 to 1437 nanograms/mL). The mean maintenance ciclosporin level was *reduced* by 15 nanograms/mL.[5]

(b) Amiodarone affected

In two heart transplant patients who had stopped amiodarone and started ciclosporin an increase in the plasma levels of amiodarone and its main metabolite, desethylamiodarone, was seen for 4 to 5 weeks. During this period increased adverse effects, including pulmonary toxicity, were seen.[5]

Mechanism

Uncertain. A reduction[2] or an increase[5] in the metabolism of the ciclosporin by the amiodarone has been suggested. An interaction between amiodarone and phospholipids in the plasma membrane may inhibit transport processes. Blocking of P-glycoprotein in the intestinal mucosa and liver by both amiodarone and ciclosporin may result in decreased excretion and increased toxicity of amiodarone as well as accumulation of ciclosporin metabolites.[5]

Importance and management

An established and clinically important interaction. Concurrent use need not be avoided but close monitoring and ciclosporin dosage reductions are needed to minimise the potential nephrotoxicity. Remember to re-adjust the ciclosporin dosage if the amiodarone is stopped, bearing in mind that it may take weeks before the amiodarone is totally cleared from the body.

The significance of the increase in amiodarone levels in two patients and the occurrence of pulmonary toxicity in another, all of whom had stopped amiodarone and started ciclosporin, is unclear but bear these reports in mind.

1. Egami J, Mullins PA, Mamprin F, Chauhan A, Large SR, Wallwork J, Schofield PM. Increase in cyclosporine levels due to amiodarone therapy after heart and heart-lung transplantation. *J Am Coll Cardiol* (1993) 21, 141A.
2. Nicolau DP, Uber WE, Crumbley AJ, Strange C. Amiodarone-cyclosporine interaction in a heart transplant patient. *J Heart Lung Transplant* (1992) 11, 564–8.
3. Mamprin F, Mullins P, Graham T, Kendall S, Biocine B, Large S, Wallwork J, Schofield P. Amiodarone-cyclosporine interaction in cardiac transplantation. *Am Heart J* (1992) 123, 1725–6.
4. Chitwood KK, Abdul-Haqq AJ, Heim-Duthoy KL. Cyclosporine-amiodarone interaction. *Ann Pharmacother* (1993) 27, 569–71.
5. Preuner JG, Lehle K, Keyser A, Merk J, Rupprecht L, Goebels R. Development of severe adverse effects after discontinuing amiodarone therapy in human heart transplant recipients. *Transplant Proc* (1998) 30, 3943–4.

Ciclosporin + Amphotericin B

There is some good evidence to suggest that the risk of nephrotoxicity is increased if ciclosporin and amphotericin B are used concurrently. However, other evidence suggests that a liposomal form of amphotericin B (*AmBisome*) does not increase nephrotoxicity or hepatotoxicity when given to infants taking ciclosporin. Ciclosporin blood levels may be increased or decreased by amphotericin B.

Clinical evidence

(a) Toxic effects

1. Nephrotoxicity. The concurrent use of ciclosporin and amphotericin B increased the incidence of nephrotoxicity in 47 patients with bone marrow transplants. Out of 10 patients who had received both drugs, 5 doubled and 3 tripled their serum creatinine levels within 5 days. In contrast only 8 out of 21 (38%) taking ciclosporin alone and 3 out of 16 (19%) taking methotrexate and amphotericin B doubled their serum creatinine within 14 to 30 days and 5 days, respectively.[1] Two studies of the risk factors associated with amphotericin B identified the concurrent use of ciclosporin as posing a particularly significant risk for the development of the moderate to severe nephrotoxicity in 8 to 12% of patients given amphotericin.[2,3] Two other studies in bone marrow transplant patients taking ciclosporin found that amphotericin B contributed significantly to nephrotoxicity and renal failure.[4,5] It can apparently develop even after amphotericin B has been withdrawn.[4] Marked nephrotoxicity is described in one patient in another report.[6] However, a retrospective study of patients taking ciclosporin also found an increase in creatinine levels during the concurrent use of a continuous infusion of amphotericin B (sodium deoxycholate complex; *Fungizone*) in 22 patients (compared with 62 patients taking ciclosporin alone), but severe reductions in renal function (creatinine clearance less than 30 mL/minute) were not found.[7] In contrast, a study including 8 severely ill infants undergoing bone marrow transplantation for severe immunodeficiency, found no evidence of significant nephrotoxicity or hepatotoxicity when liposomal amphotericin B (*AmBisome*) was given with ciclosporin. The average course of treatment lasted for 29 days.[8]

2. Neurotoxicity. An isolated case report described severe tremors, later becoming myoclonic, attributed to the concurrent use of liposomal amphotericin B (*AmBisome*) and ciclosporin. Serum ciclosporin levels were unaltered and creatinine levels only rose slightly.[9] This alleged neurotoxicity was challenged in a letter citing 187 transplant patients who had received ciclosporin and *AmBisome*, none of whom developed neurotoxicity attributable to an interaction.[10]

3. Other adverse effects. Renal tubular acidosis and hypomagnesaemia were noted to be the most common adverse effects of concurrent low-dose amphotericin B 5 to 10 mg daily with ciclosporin in a retrospective analysis in bone marrow transplant patients.[11]

(b) Ciclosporin levels

A retrospective analysis in allogeneic bone marrow transplant patients found that those patients taking high-dose prednisone with continuous infusion ciclosporin and also given prophylactic amphotericin B 5 to 10 mg daily had 13 to 23% lower plasma levels of ciclosporin in the first four weeks post-transplant when compared with those on the same GVHD (graft-versus-host-disease) prophylaxis regimen who did not receive amphotericin B. No obvious dose reductions or changes in renal function were noted in these patients. It was also noted in this study that patients with ciclosporin plasma levels of 500 nanograms/mL had a 2.2-fold increased risk of developing GVHD when compared with patients with levels of 1000 nanograms/mL.[11]

In contrast, a study in 187 transplant patients given an average dose of ciclosporin 10 mg/kg daily found that ciclosporin blood levels increased significantly from 275 nanograms/mL to 328 nanograms/mL during treatment with liposomal amphotericin B (*AmBisome)* and decreased to 242 nanograms/mL one week after amphotericin B was stopped.[12] A retrospective study found a non-significant increase in mean ciclosporin blood levels (from 259 to 296 nanograms/mL) with the concurrent use of amphotericin B (0.6 to 2 mg/kg daily for 3 to 112 days) in 22 patients who had undergone allogeneic stem cell transplants. However, a lower maximum mean ciclosporin blood level of 775 nanograms/mL was seen in those patients who received amphotericin B compared with 1240 nanograms/mL in 62 patients receiving ciclosporin without amphotericin B, although again this was not significant.[7]

Mechanism

The precise mechanism of the effects of amphotericin B on ciclosporin blood levels and the nephrotoxicity is not understood, although simple additive nephrotoxicity is a likely explanation for the latter.

Importance and management

The increased nephrotoxicity associated with ciclosporin and amphotericin B appears to be established and clinically important. The authors of one report[1] say that "if amphotericin must be given, withholding ciclosporin until the serum level is less than about 150 nanograms/mL may be a means of decreasing renal toxicity without losing the immunosuppressive effect."

The reports supporting a lack of significant nephrotoxicity all used liposomal amphotericin B, a formulation that is recommended when amphotericin toxicity (particularly nephrotoxicity) is considered to be a significant risk. This would seem to suggest that in patients taking ciclosporin, the less nephrotoxic forms of amphotericin B are advisable. Renal function should be closely monitored during concurrent use.

The changes in ciclosporin blood levels reported with amphotericin B are inconsistent. However, these studies should be borne in mind when using both drugs, and ciclosporin levels as well as renal function should be closely monitored.

1. Kennedy MS, Deeg HJ, Siegel M, Crowley JJ, Storb R, Thomas ED. Acute renal toxicity with combined use of amphotericin B and cyclosporine after bone marrow transplantation. *Transplantation* (1983) 35, 211–15.
2. Luber AD, Maa L, Lam M, Guglielmo BJ. Risk factors for amphotericin B- induced nephrotoxicity. *J Antimicrob Chemother* (1999) 43, 267–71.
3. Harbarth S, Pestotnik SL, Lloyd JF, Burke JP, Samore MH. The epidemiology of nephrotoxicity associated with conventional amphotericin B therapy. *Am J Med* (2001) 111, 528–34.
4. Tutschka PJ, Beschorner WE, Hess AD, Santos GW. Cyclosporin-A to prevent graft-versus-host-disease: a pilot study in 22 patients receiving allogeneic marrow transplants. *Blood* (1983) 61, 318–25.
5. Miller KB, Schenkein DP, Comenzo R, Erban JK, Fogaren T, Hirsch CA, Berkman E, Rabson A. Adjusted-dose continuous-infusion cyclosporin A to prevent graft-versus-host disease following allogeneic bone marrow transplantation. *Ann Hematol* (1994) 68, 15–20.
6. Conti DJ, Tolkoff-Rubin NE, Baker GP, Doran M, Cosimi AB, Delmonico F, Auchincloss H, Russell PS, Rubin RH. Successful treatment of invasive fungal infection with fluconazole in organ transplant recipients. *Transplantation* (1989) 48, 692–5.
7. Furrer K, Schaffner A, Vavricka SR, Halter J, Imhof A, Schanz U. Nephrotoxicity of cyclosporine A and amphotericin B-deoxycholate as continuous infusion in allogeneic stem cell transplantation. *Swiss Med Wkly* (2002) 132, 316–20.
8. Pasic S, Flannagan L, Cant AJ. Liposomal amphotericin (AmBisome) is safe in bone marrow transplantation for primary immunodeficiency. *Bone Marrow Transplant* (1997) 19, 1229–32.

9. Ellis ME, Spence D, Ernst P, Meunier F. Is cyclosporin neurotoxicity enhanced in the presence of liposomal amphotericin B? *J Infect* (1994) 29, 106–7.
10. Ringdén O, Andström EE, Remberger M, Svahn B-M, Tollemar J. No increase in cyclosporin neurotoxicity in transplant recipients treated with liposomal amphotericin B. *Infection* (1996) 24, 269.
11. O'Donnell MR, Schmidt GM, Tegtmeier BR, Faucett C, Fahey JL, Ito J, Nademanee A, Niland J, Parker P, Smith EP, Snyder DS, Stein AS, Blume KG, Forman SJ. Prediction of systemic fungal infection in allogeneic marrow recipients: impact of amphotericin prophylaxis in high-risk patients. *J Clin Oncol* (1994) 12, 827–34.
12. Ringdén O, Andström E, Remberger M, Svahn B-M, Tollemar J. Safety of liposomal amphotericin B (AmBisome) in 187 transplant recipients treated with ciclosporin. *Bone Marrow Transplant* (1994) 14, (Suppl 5) S10–S14.

Ciclosporin + Anabolic steroids and Androgens

Raised ciclosporin levels occurred in two patients given methyltestosterone. Hepatotoxicity has been seen in three patients given ciclosporin and norethandrolone.

Clinical evidence

(a) Methyltestosterone

A man with a kidney transplant who had been stable taking ciclosporin, prednisolone and azathioprine for 23 months was given methyltestosterone 5 mg three times daily for impotence. After 4 weeks he developed anorexia and pruritus. He was found to have a raised bilirubin level and his ciclosporin level had risen from 70 to 252 nanograms/mL, with an accompanying decrease in his renal function. The methyltestosterone was withdrawn and he was later restabilised.[1] Another case describes abnormally high ciclosporin levels (in excess of 2000 nanograms/mL) when a patient taking methyltestosterone was given ciclosporin 15 mg/kg daily.[2]

(b) Norethandrolone

Three out of four patients with bone marrow aplasia taking ciclosporin and prednisone developed liver toxicity. The adverse effects developed in 2 of them when norethandrolone was added. No toxicity occurred when they were given either of the drugs alone.[3] Jaundice associated with toxic hepatitis that occurred in a 14-year-old girl during the post-transplant period was attributed to the concurrent use of ciclosporin and norethandrolone.[4]

Mechanism

Uncertain. In the first case, the increase in ciclosporin levels were attributed to cholestatic jaundice brought on by the methyltestosterone.[2] Both norethandrolone and ciclosporin are known to be hepatotoxic, so additive hepatotoxicity may occur.

Importance and management

Information is limited. However, it would seem prudent to avoid the use of androgens or anabolic steroids in patients taking ciclosporin wherever possible. If no alternative is available it may be prudent to increase the frequency of liver function monitoring.

1. Møller BB, Ekelund B. Toxicity of cyclosporine during treatment with androgens. *N Engl J Med* (1985) 313, 1416.
2. Goffin E, Pirson Y, Geubel A, van Ypersele de Strihou C. Cyclosporine-methyltestosterone interaction. *Nephron* (1991) 59, 174–5.
3. Sahnoun Z, Frikha M, Zeghal KM, Souissi T. Toxicité hépatique de la ciclosporine et interaction médicamenteuse avec les androgènes. *Sem Hop Paris* (1993) 69, 26–8.
4. Vinot O, Cochat P, Dubourg-Derain L, Bouvier R, Vial T, Philippe N. Jaundice associated with concomitant use of norethandrolone and cyclosporine. *Transplantation* (1993) 56, 470–1.

Ciclosporin + Antibacterials; Aminoglycosides

Both *animal* and human studies indicate that nephrotoxicity may be increased by the concurrent use of ciclosporin and gentamicin. This has also been shown for tobramycin. Cases of renal impairment have been reported for amikacin and gentamicin.

Clinical evidence

A comparative study in patients given **gentamicin** 30 mg with lincomycin just before renal transplantation found that the concurrent use of ciclosporin increased the incidence of nephrotoxicity from 5% to 67%.[1] When **gentamicin** and lincomycin were replaced with ampicillin, ceftazidime and lincomycin the incidence of nephrotoxicity was 10%.[1] Another study describes increased nephrotoxicity associated with the concurrent use of ciclosporin and **tobramycin** in bone marrow transplant recipients.[2,3] The interaction between ciclosporin and **gentamicin** has also been well demonstrated in *animals*.[4,5] One case report describes reversible acute worsening of renal function in a renal transplant patient receiving ciclosporin with **gentamicin**,[6] and another case report describes impaired renal function in a heart transplant patient taking ciclosporin and given **amikacin**.[7]

In contrast, a retrospective analysis of the medical records of bone marrow transplant patients suggested that aminoglycosides can be safely given with a continuous infusion of ciclosporin without excessive nephrotoxicity, if the patient is carefully monitored.[8]

Mechanism

Uncertain. Since both ciclosporin and the aminoglycosides can individually be nephrotoxic, it seems that their toxicities can be additive.

Importance and management

Established and clinically important interactions. The concurrent use of ciclosporin and aminoglycosides should be avoided where possible, and only undertaken with care and very close monitoring of renal function.

1. Termeer A, Hoitsma AJ, Koene RAP. Severe nephrotoxicity caused by the combined use of gentamicin and cyclosporine in renal allograft recipients. *Transplantation* (1986) 42, 220–1.
2. Hows JM, Chipping PM, Fairhead S, Smith J, Baughan A, Gordon-Smith EC. Nephrotoxicity in bone marrow transplant recipients treated with cyclosporin A. *Br J Haematol* (1983) 54, 69–78.
3. Hows JM, Palmer S, Want S, Dearden C, Gordon-Smith EC. Serum levels of cyclosporin A and nephrotoxicity in bone marrow transplant patients. *Lancet* (1981) ii, 145–6.
4. Whiting PH, Simpson JG. The enhancement of cyclosporin A-induced nephrotoxicity by gentamicin. *Biochem Pharmacol* (1983) 32, 2025–8.
5. Ryffel B, Müller AM, Mihatsch MJ. Experimental cyclosporine nephrotoxicity: risk of concomitant chemotherapy. *Clin Nephrol* (1986) 25 (Suppl 1), S121–S125.
6. Morales JM, Andres A, Prieto C, Diaz Rolòn JA, Rodicio JL. Reversible acute renal toxicity by toxic sinergic effect between gentamicin and cyclosporine. *Clin Nephrol* (1988) 29, 272.
7. Thaler F, Gotainer B, Teodori G, Dubois C, Loirat Ph. Mediastinitis due to *Nocardia asteroides* after cardiac transplantation. *Intensive Care Med* (1992) 18, 127–8.
8. Chandrasekar PH, Cronin SM. Nephrotoxicity in bone marrow transplant recipients receiving aminoglycoside plus cyclosporine or aminoglycoside alone. *J Antimicrob Chemother* (1991) 27, 845–9.

Ciclosporin + Antibacterials; Aztreonam

Aztreonam does not appear to alter ciclosporin levels.

Clinical evidence, mechanism, importance and management

A study in 20 kidney transplant patients taking ciclosporin found that when aztreonam was added for the treatment of various infections the ciclosporin serum levels were not significantly changed. The ciclosporin blood levels before, during, and after aztreonam treatment were 517, 534, and 592 nanograms/mL, respectively.[1] On the basis of this study there would seem to be no need to take special precautions if ciclosporin and aztreonam are used concurrently.

1. Alonso Hernandez A. Effects of aztreonam on cyclosporine levels in kidney transplant patients. *Transplantology J Cell Organ Transplant* (1993) 4, 85–6.

Ciclosporin + Antibacterials; Cephalosporins

Isolated case reports suggest that ceftazidime, ceftriaxone, and latamoxef may increase ciclosporin levels, whereas one report suggested ceftazidime, ceftriaxone, and cefuroxime did not, although ceftazidime caused deterioration in some measures of renal function.

Clinical evidence, mechanism, importance and management

Two kidney transplant patients had two- to fourfold rises in ciclosporin blood levels within 2 to 3 days of starting **ceftriaxone** 1 g twice daily. Levels fell when the antibacterial was stopped. The reason is uncertain but it was suggested that **ceftriaxone** possibly inhibits the metabolism of ciclosporin by the liver.[1] However, a report of 51 kidney transplant patients stated that **ceftriaxone** and **cefuroxime** had no effect on ciclosporin blood levels and also that they were not nephrotoxic. This report also stated that **ceftazidime** did not affect serum ciclosporin levels, but it increased blood urea nitrogen and creatinine levels, indicating that it was nephrotoxic.[2] A report briefly mentions that **ceftazidime** and **latamoxef** have also been implicated in an increase in ciclosporin plasma levels.[3] However, the manufacturers of **ceftazidime** state that there is no evidence to suggest that **ceftazidime** itself is nephrotoxic when used in the recommended doses, although dose adjustment is required in renal failure.[4] A study in 28 bone marrow transplant patients taking ciclosporin found no evidence that **ceftazidime** 2 g three times daily worsened renal function.[5]

Information about these cephalosporins is very limited indeed. The general relevance of these reports is uncertain, but bear them in mind in the event of unexpected response to treatment.

1. Alvarez JS, Del Castillo JAS, Ortiz MJA. Interaction between ciclosporin and ceftriaxone. *Nephron* (1991) 59, 681–2.
2. Xu F, Wu Z, Zou H. Effects on renal function and cyclosporine blood concentration by combination with three cephalosporins in renal transplant patients. *Zhongguo Kang Sheng Su Za Zhi* (1997) 22, 223–5.
3. Cockburn I. Cyclosporin A: a clinical evaluation of drug interactions. *Transplant Proc* (1986) 18 (Suppl 5), 50–5.
4. Fortum Injection (Ceftazidime pentahydrate). GlaxoSmithKline UK. UK Summary of product characteristics, May 2007.
5. Verhagen C, de Pauw BE, de Witte T, Holdrinet RSG, Janssen JTP, Williams KJ. Ceftazidime does not enhance cyclosporin-A nephrotoxicity in febrile bone marrow transplantation patients. *Blut* (1986) 53, 333–9.

Ciclosporin + Antibacterials; Chloramphenicol

Four patients had a marked rise in serum ciclosporin levels when they were given chloramphenicol. A small study supports these findings.

Clinical evidence

A retrospective study identified 3 transplant patients taking ciclosporin who had received a total of 6 courses of intravenous chloramphenicol, each lasting for at least 12 days. By day 4 of concurrent use ciclosporin blood levels had increased on average by 41.3%. Ciclosporin doses tended to be slightly reduced over the course of treatment, and by day 10, ciclosporin levels were about 31% below baseline.[1]

A woman with a heart-lung transplant and with a trough ciclosporin level of 84 nanograms/mL started taking oral chloramphenicol (dosage not stated) to treat an infection with *Xanthomonas maltophilia*. On the next day the ciclosporin levels had risen to 240 micrograms/L. The chloramphenicol was continued but the ciclosporin dosage was reduced from 300 to 225 mg daily. By day 8 the ciclosporin levels were back within the therapeutic range.[2]

Two kidney transplant patients had marked increases in ciclosporin blood levels (almost doubled in one case) when they were given chloramphenicol for urinary tract infections.[3]

There is another report of this interaction, but the case is greatly complicated by the presence of ciprofloxacin, vancomycin, ceftazidime, and a recent course of rifampicin taken by the patient.[4]

Mechanism

Uncertain. Chloramphenicol is a recognised enzyme inhibitor and it seems possible that it may reduce the metabolism of the ciclosporin by the liver.[4]

Importance and management

Information seems to be limited to these reports, so although the interaction appears to be established, its incidence is obviously uncertain. It would now be prudent to monitor ciclosporin levels if systemic chloramphenicol is added, being alert for the need to reduce the ciclosporin dosage. The study[1] highlights the need to monitor levels closely throughout the whole chloramphenicol course.

It seems doubtful if there will be enough chloramphenicol absorbed from eye drops to interact with ciclosporin, but this needs confirmation.

1. Mathis AS, Shah N, Knipp GT, Friedman GS. Interaction of chloramphenicol and the calcineurin inhibitors in renal transplant recipients. *Transpl Infect Dis* (2002) 4, 169–74.
2. Steinfort CL, McConachy KA. Cyclosporin-chloramphenicol drug interaction in a heart-lung transplant recipient. *Med J Aust* (1994) 161, 455.
3. Zawadzki J, Prokurat S, Smirska E, Jelonek A. Interaction between cyclosporine A and chloramphenicol after kidney transplantation. *Pediatr Nephrol* (1991) 5, C49.
4. Bui LL, Huang DD. Possible interaction between cyclosporine and chloramphenicol. *Ann Pharmacother* (1999) 33, 252–3.

Ciclosporin + Antibacterials; Clindamycin

Two patients had a marked reduction in their serum ciclosporin levels when they took clindamycin.

Clinical evidence, mechanism, importance and management

A lung transplant patient receiving ciclosporin in a dose to maintain levels of 100 to 150 nanograms/mL required dose increases to achieve this level when clindamycin 600 mg three times daily was given. Initially the levels were almost halved by the addition of clindamycin. Ciclosporin was reduced to the original dose when the clindamycin was stopped.[1]

In a second lung transplant patient, the use of clindamycin 600 mg three times daily necessitated ciclosporin dose increases from 325 mg daily to 1.1 g daily over 4 weeks to maintain serum levels of about 200 nanograms/mL. The reasons for the interaction are not understood, but the authors suggest close monitoring of ciclosporin levels to prevent underdosing if clindamycin is given;[1] however, this seems exceptionally cautious as these two cases appear to be all that have been reported.

1. Thurnheer R, Laube I, Speich R. Possible interaction between clindamycin and cyclosporin. *BMJ* (1999) 319, 163.

Ciclosporin + Antibacterials; Imipenem/Cilastatin

Several transplant patients with impaired renal function have experienced adverse CNS effects (including convulsions and tremors) while taking imipenem/cilastatin and ciclosporin. Imipenem/cilastatin may affect ciclosporin levels.

Clinical evidence, mechanism, importance and management

A woman taking ciclosporin following a kidney transplant developed a urinary-tract infection for which she was given imipenem/cilastatin 500 mg intravenously every 12 hours (dose adjusted for renal function). About 20 minutes after the second dose she became confused, disorientated, agitated, and developed motor aphasia and intense tremor. This was interpreted as being a combination of the adverse CNS effects of both drugs. The imipenem/cilastatin was not given again and the effects subsided over the next few days. However, it was noted that the ciclosporin blood levels rose over the next 4 days from about 400 to 1000 nanograms/mL.[1]

Four transplant patients who were taking ciclosporin developed seizures when they were given imipenem/cilastatin 1 g daily, and a fifth patient developed myoclonia. These patients all had chronic renal impairment.[2] In contrast, imipenem/cilastatin 2 g daily for 4 weeks, given with ciprofloxacin, was effectively and successfully used in another patient taking ciclosporin after a heart transplant. This patient was switched to imipenem/cilastatin and ciprofloxacin after developing acute renal failure while receiving amikacin.[3] Reduced serum ciclosporin levels following the use of imipenem/cilastatin have been seen in *rats*.[4]

It should be noted that focal tremors, myoclonus and convulsions are a known adverse effects of imipenem/cilastatin and are most likely to occur in patients with reduced renal function. However, the patients cited above received imipenem/cilastatin in doses adjusted for their renal function. The manufacturers of imipenem/cilastatin recommend that patients who develop focal tremors, myoclonus and convulsions while receiving the antibacterial should be started on an antiepileptic drug. If symptoms persist the dose should be reduced, or the drug withdrawn.[5]

1. Zazgornik J, Schein W, Heimberger K, Shaheen FAM, Stockenhuber F. Potentiation of neurotoxic side effects by coadministration of imipenem to cyclosporine therapy in a kidney transplant recipient--synergism of side effects or drug interaction? *Clin Nephrol* (1986) 26, 265–6.
2. Bösmüller C, Steurer W, Königsrainer A, Willeit J, Margreiter R. Increased risk of central nervous system toxicity inpatients treated with ciclosporin and imipenem/cilastatin. *Nephron* (1991) 58, 362–4.
3. Thaler F, Gotainer B, Teodori G, Dubois C, Loirat Ph. Mediastinitis due to *Nocardia asteroides* after cardiac transplantation. *Intensive Care Med* (1992) 18, 127–8.

4. Mraz W, Sido B, Knedel M, Hammer C. Concomitant immunosuppressive and antibiotic therapy-reduction of cyclosporine A blood levels due to treatment with imipenem/cilastatin. *Transplant Proc* (1987) 19, 4017–20.
5. Primaxin IV Injection (Imipenem monohydrate/Cilastatin sodium). Merck Sharp & Dohme Ltd. UK Summary of product characteristics, October 2005.

Ciclosporin + Antibacterials; Macrolides

Ciclosporin levels can be markedly raised by clarithromycin, erythromycin, josamycin, pristinamycin and possibly midecamycin. Rokitamycin and troleandomycin are predicted to interact similarly. Roxithromycin appears to interact minimally, while no interaction is normally seen with azithromycin, dirithromycin or spiramycin, although there are isolated reports of an interaction with azithromycin.

Clinical evidence

(a) Azithromycin

Eight healthy subjects were given ciclosporin 3.75 to 7.5 mg/kg alone and then after taking azithromycin 500 mg initially then 250 mg daily for 4 days. Azithromycin did not alter ciclosporin levels.[1] Other studies have also found no evidence of a clinically significant interaction between ciclosporin and azithromycin in a total of 62 kidney transplant patients,[2-4] but there are case reports describing a marked increase in ciclosporin levels in 2 patients attributed to azithromycin.[5,6]

(b) Clarithromycin

In a study in 8 healthy subjects, ciclosporin 3.75 to 7.5 mg/kg was given alone and after they took clarithromycin 250 mg every 12 hours for 7 days. The maximum ciclosporin levels were raised by 50% by the clarithromycin. In another study a mean 30% reduction in the dosage of ciclosporin was needed in 6 transplant patients also given clarithromycin.[7] Clarithromycin 500 mg twice daily as part of a *Helicobacter pylori* eradication regimen caused a two- to threefold increase in ciclosporin levels in 27 kidney transplant patients.[8,9] The ciclosporin levels in 4 renal transplant patients with stable renal function increased by approximately 72% when clarithromycin 250 mg twice daily for 6 days was added to treat gingival hyperplasia. Ciclosporin levels returned to baseline levels within 7 days of stopping clarithromycin. Only two patients required a ciclosporin dose reduction.[10]

Numerous case reports also describe this interaction: ciclosporin levels or AUC have been increased by two- to threefold,[11-14] with changes being seen within 3 to 6 days of clarithromycin 250 or 500 mg twice daily being started.[11,14] Another patient had a seven- to twelvefold rise in serum ciclosporin levels and acute renal failure within 3 weeks of starting to take clarithromycin 1 g daily.[15] Another case report in a heart transplant patient taking ciclosporin found that the addition of rifampicin to clarithromycin negated the increase in ciclosporin levels seen with clarithromycin alone, and the ciclosporin dose requirement with concurrent clarithromycin plus rifampicin was similar to that before clarithromycin or rifampicin were started.[16]

(c) Dirithromycin

Dirithromycin 500 mg daily for 14 days did not significantly affect the pharmacokinetics of a single 15-mg/kg oral dose of ciclosporin in 8 healthy subjects.[17]

(d) Erythromycin

A study in 9 transplant patients taking ciclosporin found that erythromycin increased the mean trough serum levels of 3 kidney transplant patients sevenfold, from 147 to 1125 nanograms/mL, and of 6 heart transplant patients four- to fivefold, from 185 to 815 nanograms/mL. Acute nephrotoxicity occurred in all 9 patients, and 7 showed mild to severe hepatotoxicity caused by the increased ciclosporin levels.[18]

Markedly raised ciclosporin blood levels and/or toxicity have been described in a number of other studies and case reports with erythromycin given orally or intravenously to about 50 other patients.[19-34] The interaction has also been demonstrated in healthy subjects.[1,35] Oral erythromycin may possibly have a greater effect than intravenous erythromycin.[30,36] Erythromycin-related ototoxicity, possibly associated with the use of ciclosporin, has been reported in liver transplant patients.[37]

(e) Josamycin

A man with a renal transplant who was taking azathioprine, prednisone and ciclosporin 330 mg daily had a marked rise in his plasma ciclosporin levels from about 90 to 600 nanograms/mL when he took josamycin 2 g daily for 5 days. He responded in the same way when later rechallenged with josamycin. Another patient also reacted in the same way.[38] Two- to fourfold rises in ciclosporin levels have been seen in 9 other patients given josamycin 2 to 3 g (50 mg/kg) daily.[39-41] Another patient had a 40% rise in ciclosporin levels when given josamycin 500 mg twice daily.[42]

(f) Midecamycin

The steady-state ciclosporin blood levels of 10 kidney transplant patients were roughly doubled when they took midecamycin 800 mg twice daily.[43] A 43-year-old kidney transplant patient taking ciclosporin, azathioprine and prednisone, began further treatment on day 27 after the transplant with midecamycin diacetate 600 mg twice daily and co-trimoxazole three times daily for pneumonia. By day 33 the concentration/dose ratio of the ciclosporin had doubled, and ciclosporin levels had reached 700 nanograms/mL, accompanied by a rise in serum creatinine levels. When the midecamycin was replaced by cefuroxime, the concentrations of both ciclosporin and creatinine fell to their former levels within 3 days.[44] Ciclosporin levels in another kidney transplant patient taking ciclosporin 120 mg twice daily increased from 95 to 380 nanograms/mL 3 days after starting midecamycin 800 mg twice daily.[45] Blood levels of ciclosporin in a kidney transplant patient also increased from 97 to 203 nanograms/mL 4 days after starting midecamycin diacetate 600 mg twice daily.[46]

(g) Pristinamycin

A kidney transplant patient had a tenfold increase in plasma ciclosporin levels from 30 to 290 nanograms/mL after taking pristinamycin 2 g daily for 8 days. Blood creatinine levels rose from 75 to 120 micromol/L. Another patient given pristinamycin 1.25 g had a rise in ciclosporin levels from 78 to 855 nanograms/mL after 6 days. Ciclosporin and creatinine levels fell to normal levels within 2 days of stopping both drugs.[47]

Pristinamycin 50 mg/kg daily raised the ciclosporin blood levels of 10 patients by 65% from 560 to 925 nanograms/mL. Ciclosporin levels fell when the pristinamycin was stopped.[48] Within 5 days of starting to take pristinamycin 4 g daily the ciclosporin levels of another patient more than doubled. His serum creatinine levels also rose. Both fell back to baseline levels within 3 days of stopping the antibacterial.[49]

(h) Roxithromycin

Eight patients with heart transplants taking ciclosporin 8 mg/kg daily, prednisolone and azathioprine for at least one month, were given roxithromycin 150 mg twice daily for 11 days. A 37.5% rise in plasma ciclosporin levels occurred at the time the roxithromycin was given, and a 60% rise occurred 4 hours later. Ciclosporin levels fell again when the roxithromycin was stopped. A small (10%) increase in serum creatinine levels occurred. There was no evidence of a deterioration in renal function.[50] The half-life of roxithromycin was found in one study to be doubled, from 17 to 34.4 hours, in patients with kidney transplants who were taking ciclosporin.[51]

(i) Spiramycin

The ciclosporin plasma levels of 6 heart transplant patients taking corticosteroids, azathioprine and ciclosporin remained unchanged when they were given spiramycin 3 MIU twice daily for 10 days.[52] Similarly, no interaction was found between ciclosporin and spiramycin in other studies in patients with renal transplants.[53-56]

(j) Telithromycin

There appears to be no clinical reports of an interaction between ciclosporin and telithromycin. However, the manufacturers of telithromycin note that it is an inhibitor of the cytochrome P450 isoenzyme CYP3A4 and it may therefore increase ciclosporin levels, requiring dose adjustment.[57]

(k) Other macrolides

In vitro studies (see 'Mechanism' below) suggest that **rokitamycin** and **troleandomycin** interact with ciclosporin in the same way as erythromycin,[58] but as yet there seems to be no direct clinical evidence of an interaction.

Mechanism

In vitro studies with human liver microsomes have found that clarithromycin, erythromycin, josamycin, rokitamycin, roxithromycin and troleandomycin

domycin (but not spiramycin) inhibit ciclosporin metabolism in the liver, which is catalysed by the cytochrome P450 isoenzyme CYP3A.[15,58] This would be expected to result in raised ciclosporin levels. Telithromycin is also an inhibitor of CYP3A4 and may increase ciclosporin levels.[57] Erythromycin[30,34] and clarithromycin[13] also possibly increase the absorption of ciclosporin from the gut by inhibiting intestinal wall metabolism.

Azithromycin is believed to be metabolised by routes independent of the cytochrome P450 enzyme system. Intravenous azithromycin was thought to have increased ciclosporin levels through P-glycoprotein inhibition and/or competition for biliary excretion in one case report.[6]

Importance and management

The interaction between ciclosporin and erythromycin is well documented, well established and potentially serious. If concurrent use is thought appropriate, monitor the ciclosporin blood levels closely and reduce the dosage appropriately. A reduction of about 35% has been calculated to be necessary.[32] The dosage should be increased again when the erythromycin is stopped. The effect of intravenous erythromycin is less than oral erythromycin so if the route of administration is changed, be alert for the need to change the ciclosporin dosage.[30,36]

Information about the interactions with clarithromycin, josamycin, midecamycin, and pristinamycin is much more limited, but they appear to behave like erythromycin. The same precautions should be taken. There seems to be no direct clinical information about telithromycin, troleandomycin and rokitamycin but they would be expected to interact like erythromycin. Note that troleandomycin is usually a more potent inhibitor of CYP3A4 than erythromycin, so it may be expected to have a larger effect on ciclosporin levels.

Dirithromycin and spiramycin normally appear not to interact and roxithromycin appears only to interact very minimally. Also bear in mind that roxithromycin serum levels may be increased.

Although most reports suggest that azithromycin does not interact, increased monitoring is recommended by some, because of the isolated reports of increased ciclosporin levels.[6]

1. Bottorff MB, Marien ML, Clendening C. Macrolide antibiotics and inhibition of CYP3A isozymes: differences in cyclosporin pharmacokinetics. *Clin Pharmacol Ther* (1997) 56, 224.
2. Gómez E, Sánchez JE, Aguado S, Alvarez Grande J. Interaction between azithromycin and cyclosporin? *Nephron* (1996) 73, 724.
3. Bubic-Filipi Lj, Puretic Z, Thune S, Glavas-Boras S, Pasini J, Marekovic Z. Influence of azithromycin on cyclosporin levels in patients with a kidney transplant. *Nephrol Dial Transplant* (1998) 13, A276.
4. Bachmann K, Jauregui L, Chandra R, Thakker K. Influence of a 3-day regimen of azithromycin on the disposition kinetics of cyclosporine A in stable renal transplant patients. *Pharmacol Res* (2003) 47, 549–54.
5. Ljutic D, Rumboldt Z. Possible interaction between azithromycin and cyclosporine: a case report. *Nephron* (1995) 70, 130.
6. Page RL, Ruscin JM, Fish D, LaPointe M. Possible interaction between intravenous azithromycin and oral cyclosporine. *Pharmacotherapy* (2001) 21, 1436–43.
7. Sádaba B, López De Ocáriz A, Azanza JR, Quiroga J, Cienfuegos JA. Concurrent clarithromycin and cyclosporin A treatment. *J Antimicrob Chemother* (1998) 42, 393–5.
8. Skálová P, Marečková O, Skála I, Lácha J, Teplan V, Vítko Š, Petrásek R. Eradication of *Helicobacter pylori* with clarithromycin: danger of toxic levels of cyclosporin A. *Gut* (1998) 43 (Suppl 2), A109.
9. Skalova P, Mareckova O, Skala I, Lacha J, Teplan V, Vitko S, Petrasek R. Toxic levels of cyclosporin A after renal transplantation on clarithromycin therapy. *Nephrol Dial Transplant* (1998) 13, A256.
10. Sánchez-Nuñez ML, Gómez E, Sánchez JE, Portal C, Alvarez-Grande J. Clarithromycin in the treatment of cyclosporin-associated gingival hyperplasia. *Nephrol Dial Transplant* (1997) 12, 2040–1.
11. Gersema LM, Porter CB, Russell EH. Suspected drug interaction between cyclosporine and clarithromycin. *J Heart Lung Transplant* (1994) 13, 343–5.
12. Ferrari SL, Goffin E, Mourad M, Wallemacq P, Squifflet J-P, Pirson Y. The interaction between clarithromycin and cyclosporine in kidney transplant recipients. *Transplantation* (1994) 58, 725–7.
13. Sketris IS, Wright MR, West ML. Possible role of intestinal P-450 enzyme system in a cyclosporine-clarithromycin interaction. *Pharmacotherapy* (1996) 16, 301–5.
14. Treille S, Quoidbach A, Demol H, Vereerstraeten P, Abramowicz D. Kidney graft dysfunction after drug interaction between clarithromycin and cyclosporin. *Nephrol Dial Transplant* (1996) 11, 1192–3.
15. Spicer ST, Liddle C, Chapman JR, Barclay P, Nankivell BJ, Thomas P, O'Connell PJ. The mechanism of cyclosporine toxicity induced by clarithromycin. *Br J Clin Pharmacol* (1997) 43, 194–6.
16. Plemmons RM, McAllister CK, Garces MC, Ward RL. Osteomyelitis due to *Mycobacterium haemophilum* in a cardiac transplant patient: case report and analysis of interactions among clarithromycin, rifampin, and cyclosporine. *Clin Infect Dis* (1997) 24, 995–7.
17. Bachmann K, Sullivan TJ, Resse JH, Miller K, Scott M, Jauregui L, Sides G. The pharmacokinetics of oral cyclosporine A are not affected by dirithromycin. *Intersci Conf Antimicrob Agents Chemother* (1994) 34, 4.
18. Jensen CWB, Flechner SM, Van Buren CT, Frazier OH, Cooley DA, Lorber MI, Kahan BD. Exacerbation of cyclosporine toxicity by concomitant administration of erythromycin. *Transplantation* (1987) 43, 263–70.
19. Kohan DE. Possible interaction between cyclosporine and erythromycin. *N Engl J Med* (1986), 314, 448.
20. Hourmant M, Le Bigot JF, Vernillet L, Sagniez G, Remi JP, Soulillou JP. Coadministration of erythromycin results in an increase of blood cyclosporine to toxic levels. *Transplant Proc* (1985) 17, 2723–7.
21. Wadhwa NK, Schroeder TJ, O'Flaherty E, Pesce AJ, Myre SA, Munda R, First MR. Interaction between erythromycin and cyclosporine in a kidney and pancreas allograft recipient. *Ther Drug Monit* (1987) 9, 123–5.
22. Murray BM, Edwards L, Morse GD, Kohli RR, Venuto RC. Clinically important interaction of cyclosporine and erythromycin. *Transplantation* (1987) 43, 602–4.
23. Griño JM, Sabate I, Castelao AM, Guardia M, Seron D, Alsina J. Erythromycin and cyclosporine. *Ann Intern Med* (1986) 105, 467–8.
24. Gonwa TA, Nghiem DD, Schulak JA, Corry RJ. Erythromycin and cyclosporine. *Transplantation* (1986) 41, 797–9.
25. Harnett JD, Parfrey PS, Paul MD, Gault MH. Erythromycin-cyclosporine interaction in renal transplant patients. *Transplantation* (1987) 43, 316–18.
26. Kessler M, Louis J, Renoult E, Vigneron B, Netter P. Interaction between cyclosporin and erythromycin in a kidney transplant patient. *Eur J Clin Pharmacol* (1986) 30, 633–4.
27. Godin JRP, Sketris IS, Belitsky P. Erythromycin-cyclosporine interaction. *Drug Intell Clin Pharm* (1986) 20, 504–5.
28. Martell R, Heinrichs D, Stiller CR, Jenner M, Keown PA, Dupre J. The effects of erythromycin in patients treated with cyclosporine. *Ann Intern Med* (1986) 104, 660–1.
29. Ptachcinski PJ, Carpenter BJ, Burckart GJ, Venkataramanan R, Rosenthal JT. Effect of erythromycin on cyclosporine levels. *N Engl J Med* (1985) 313, 1416–17.
30. Gupta SK, Bakran A, Johnson RWG, Rowland M. Erythromycin enhances the absorption of cyclosporin. *Br J Clin Pharmacol* (1988) 25, 401–2.
31. Morales JM, Andres A, Prieto C, Arenas J, Ortuño B, Praga M, Ruilope LM, Rodicio JL. Severe reversible cyclosporine-induced acute renal failure. A role for urinary PGE_2 deficiency? *Transplantation* (1988) 46, 163–5.
32. Vereerstraeten P, Thiry P, Kinnaert P, Toussaint C. Influence of erythromycin on cyclosporine pharmacokinetics. *Transplantation* (1987) 44, 155–6.
33. Ben-Ari J, Eisenstein B, Davidovits M, Shmueli D, Shapira Z, Stark H. Effect of erythromycin on blood cyclosporine concentrations in kidney transplant patients. *J Pediatr* (1988) 112, 992–3.
34. Gupta SK, Bakran A, Johnson RWG, Rowland M. Cyclosporin-erythromycin interaction in renal transplant patients. *Br J Clin Pharmacol* (1989) 27, 475–81.
35. Freeman DJ, Martell R, Carruthers SG, Heinrichs D, Keown PA, Stiller CR. Cyclosporin-erythromycin interaction in normal subjects. *Br J Clin Pharmacol* (1987) 23, 776–8.
36. Zylber-Katz E. Multiple drug interactions with cyclosporine in a heart transplant patient. *Ann Pharmacother* (1995) 29, 127–31. Correction. ibid. 790.
37. Moral A, Navasa M, Rimola A, García-Valdecasas JC, Grande L, Visa J, Rodés J. Erythromycin ototoxicity in liver transplant patients. *Transpl Int* (1994) 7, 62–4.
38. Kreft-Jais C, Billaud EM, Gaudry C, Bedrossian J. Effect of josamycin on plasma cyclosporine levels. *Eur J Clin Pharmacol* (1987) 32, 327–8.
39. Azanza JR, Catalán M, Alvarez MP, Sádaba B, Honorato J, Llorens R, Harreros J. Possible interaction between cyclosporine and josamycin: a description of three cases. *Clin Pharmacol Ther* (1992) 51, 572–5.
40. Torregrosa JV, Campistol JM, Franco A, Andreu J. Interaction of josamycin with cyclosporin A. *Nephron* (1993) 65, 476–7.
41. Azanza J, Catalán M, Alvarez P, Honorato J, Herreros J, Llorens R. Possible interaction between cyclosporine and josamycin. *J Heart Transplant* (1990) 9, 265–6.
42. Capone D, Gentile A, Stanziale P, Imperatore P, D'Alessandro R, D'Alto V, Basile V. Drug interaction between cyclosporine and josamycin in a kidney transplanted patient. *Fundam Clin Pharmacol* (1996) 10, 172.
43. Couet W, Istin B, Seniuta P, Morel D, Potaux L, Fourtillan JB. Effect of ponsinomycin on cyclosporin pharmacokinetics. *Eur J Clin Pharmacol* (1990) 39, 165–7.
44. Alfonso I, Alcalde G, Garcia-Sáiz M, de Cos MA, Mediavilla A. Interaction between cyclosporine a and midecamycin. *Eur J Clin Pharmacol* (1997) 52, 79–80.
45. Finielz P, Mondon J-M, Chuet C, Guiserix J. Drug interaction between midecamycin and cyclosporin. *Nephron* (1995) 70, 136.
46. Treille S, Quoidbach A, Demol H, Juvenois A, Dehout F, Abramowicz D. Kidney graft dysfunction after drug interaction between miocamycin and cyclosporin. *Transpl Int* (1999) 12, 157.
47. Gagnadoux MF, Loirat C, Pillion G, Bertheleme JP, Pouliquen M, Guest G, Broyer M. Néphrotoxicité due à l'interaction pristinamycine-cyclosporine chez le transplanté rénal. *Presse Med* (1987) 16, 1761.
48. Herbrecht R, Garcia J-J, Bergerat J-P, Oberling F. Effect of pristinamycin on cyclosporin levels in bone marrow transplant recipients. *Bone Marrow Transplant* (1989) 4, 457–8.
49. Garraffo R, Monnier B, Lapalus P, Duplay H. Pristinamycin increases cyclosporin blood levels. *Med Sci Res* (1987) 15, 461.
50. Billaud E M, Guillemain R, Fortineau N, Kitzis M-D, Dreyfus G, Amrein C, Kreft-Jaïs C, Husson J-M, Chrétien P. Interaction between roxithromycin and cyclosporin in heart transplant patients. *Clin Pharmacokinet* (1990) 19, 499–502.
51. Morávek J, Matoušovic K, Prát V, Šedivý J. Pharmacokinetics of roxithromycin in kidney grafted patients under cyclosporin A or azathioprine immunosuppression and in healthy volunteers. *Int J Clin Pharmacol Ther Toxicol* (1990) 28, 262–7.
52. Guillemain R, Billaud E, Dreyfus G, Amrein C, Kitzis M, Jebara VA and Kreft-Jais C. The effects of spiramycin on plasma cyclosporin A concentrations in heart transplant patients. *Eur J Clin Pharmacol* (1989) 36, 97–8.
53. Kessler M, Netter P, Zerrouki M, Renoult E, Trechot P, Dousset B, Jonon B, Mur JM. Spiramycin does not increase plasma cyclosporin concentrations in renal transplant patients. *Eur J Clin Pharmacol* (1988) 35, 331–2.
54. Vernillet L, Bertault-Peres P, Berland Y, Barradas J, Durand A, Olmer M. Lack of effect of spiramycin on cyclosporin pharmacokinetics. *Br J Clin Pharmacol* (1989) 27, 789–94.
55. Birmele B, Lebranchu Y, Beliveau F, Rateau H, Furet Y, Nivet H, Bagros PH. Absence of interaction between cyclosporine and spiramycin. *Transplantation* (1989) 47, 927–8.
56. Kessler M, Netter P, Renoult E, Trechot P, Dousset B, Bannwarth B. Lack of effect of spiramycin on cyclosporin pharmacokinetics. *Br J Clin Pharmacol* (1990) 29, 370–1.
57. Ketek (Telithromycin). Sanofi-Aventis. UK Summary of product characteristics, May 2007.
58. Marre R, de Sousa G, Orloff AM, Rahmani R. *In vitro* interaction between cyclosporin A and macrolide antibiotics. *Br J Clin Pharmacol* (1993) 35, 447–8.

Ciclosporin + Antibacterials; Metronidazole

Three reports describe an increase in ciclosporin levels in patients given metronidazole.

Clinical evidence, mechanism, importance and management

The ciclosporin blood levels of a kidney transplant patient rose from 850 to 1930 nanograms/mL when metronidazole 2.25 g daily and cimetidine 800 mg daily were started. The levels fell to about 1500 nanograms/mL when the metronidazole dosage was halved and the cimetidine stopped. Because the levels of ciclosporin were still so high, the dose of ciclosporin was reduced from 7.1 to 5.7 mg/kg daily, which resulted in a further decrease in the ciclosporin level to about 1200 to 1380 nanograms/mL. Finally the metronidazole was stopped and the ciclosporin levels fell to a range of 501 to 885 nanograms/mL.[1]

Another kidney transplant patient developed a raised serum creatinine (increased from 223 to 304 micromol/L) with virtually doubled ciclosporin blood levels when metronidazole 1.5 g daily was given.[2]

Ciclosporin levels in yet another kidney transplant patient doubled (from 134 to 264 micrograms/L) accompanied by a modest elevation in serum creatinine when metronidazole 400 mg three times daily was also given. The levels fell again when metronidazole was stopped.[3]

These three cases appear to be the only reports of an interaction, one of which is confused by the presence of cimetidine (see also 'Ciclosporin + H_2-receptor antagonists', p.1035). There is insufficient evidence to advocate monitoring every patient given the combination, but it would be prudent to at least bear this interaction in mind if using metronidazole in patients taking ciclosporin.

1. Zylber-Katz E, Rubinger D and Berlatzky Y. Cyclosporine interactions with metronidazole and cimetidine. *Drug Intell Clin Pharm* (1988) 22, 504–5.
2. Vincent F, Glotz D, Kreft-Jais C, Boudjeltia S, Duboust A, Bariety J. Insuffisance rénale aiguë chez un transplanté rénal traité par cyclosporine A et métronidazole. *Therapie* (1994) 49, 155.
3. Herzig K, Johnson DW. Marked elevation of blood cyclosporin and tacrolimus levels due to concurrent metronidazole therapy. *Nephrol Dial Transplant* (1999) 14, 521–3.

Ciclosporin + Antibacterials; Penicillins

Ampicillin does not interact adversely with ciclosporin. Increased nephrotoxicity has been seen in lung transplant patients given nafcillin prophylactically, whereas an isolated report describes a fall in ciclosporin levels in a patient treated with nafcillin. A case of raised ciclosporin levels in a patient taking ticarcillin has been described.

Clinical evidence

(a) Ampicillin

Seventy-one kidney transplant patients taking ciclosporin had no changes in serum urea, creatinine or ciclosporin levels when ampicillin was given.[1]

(b) Nafcillin

A retrospective study of 19 lung transplant patients taking ciclosporin found that those given nafcillin for one week as prophylaxis against staphylococci had a greater degree of renal impairment than those not taking nafcillin. Serum creatinine levels rose steadily over 6 days until the nafcillin was stopped, whereas the patients not taking nafcillin had no changes in creatinine levels. Three of the nafcillin group temporarily needed haemodialysis. Ciclosporin doses in the nafcillin group were higher but the blood levels in both groups were not significantly different. The incidence of viral infections was also greater in the nafcillin group.[2]

A kidney transplant patient taking ciclosporin and prednisone experienced a marked fall in her serum ciclosporin levels on two occasions when given nafcillin 2 g every 6 hours. Trough blood levels fell from 229 to 119 nanograms/mL and then to 68 nanograms/mL after 3 and 7 days of nafcillin, respectively, and rose when the nafcillin was stopped. On the second occasion ciclosporin levels fell from 272 to 42 nanograms/mL after 9 days of treatment with nafcillin.[3]

(c) Ticarcillin

Rises in plasma ciclosporin levels from 90 to 230 nanograms/mL, and from 120 to 300 nanograms/mL occurred in a man within 5 to 10 days of starting ticarcillin 10 g daily.[4]

Mechanism

The authors of the study using nafcillin[2] postulate that it may have interfered with the ciclosporin assay, resulting in an underestimate of the actual levels, so that the nephrotoxicity was simply due to higher ciclosporin levels.[2] The fall in ciclosporin levels in the individual patient taking nafcillin[3] is not understood, nor is the rise in levels seen in the patient taking ticarcillin.[4]

Importance and management

Information seems to be limited to the studies and cases cited. No special precautions would seem necessary with ampicillin, but an alternative to nafcillin would seem prudent for anti-staphylococcal prophylaxis. The isolated report with ticarcillin is of unknown general significance. More study is needed.

1. Xu F, Shi XH. Interaction between ampicillin, norfloxacin and cyclosporine in renal transplant recipients. *Zhongguo Kang Sheng Su Za Zhi* (1992) 17, 290–2.
2. Jahansouz F, Kriett JM, Smith CM, Jamieson SW. Potentiation of cyclosporin nephrotoxicity by nafcillin in lung transplant recipients. *Transplantation* (1993) 55, 1045–8.
3. Veremis SA, Maddux MS, Pollak R, Mozes MF. Subtherapeutic cyclosporine concentrations during nafcillin therapy. *Transplantation* (1987) 43, 913–5.
4. Lambert C, Pointet P, Ducret F. Interaction ciclosporine-ticarcilline chez un transplanté rénal. *Presse Med* (1989) 18, 230.

Ciclosporin + Antibacterials; Quinolones

Ciclosporin serum levels are normally unchanged by the use of ciprofloxacin, but increased serum levels and nephrotoxicity may occur in a small number of patients. There is also some evidence that the immunosuppressant effects of ciclosporin are reduced by ciprofloxacin. One study, and two case reports describe rises in ciclosporin levels in patients given norfloxacin, but another study found no change. Similar results have been found with levofloxacin. No significant interaction appears to occur between ciclosporin and enoxacin, ofloxacin, pefloxacin and trovafloxacin.

Clinical evidence

(a) Ciprofloxacin

A single-dose study in 10 healthy subjects found that after taking ciprofloxacin 500 mg twice daily for 7 days the pharmacokinetics of oral ciclosporin 5 mg/kg were unchanged.[1] Five other studies confirm the lack of a pharmacokinetic interaction in:

- kidney transplant patients taking ciprofloxacin 750 mg twice daily for 13 days;[2]
- kidney transplant patients taking ciprofloxacin 500 mg twice daily for 7 days;[3]
- bone marrow transplant patients given ciprofloxacin 500 mg twice daily for 4 days;[4]
- heart transplant patients given ciprofloxacin 250 to 500 mg for 7 to 140 days;[5]
- heart transplant patients given ciprofloxacin 800 mg to 1.5 g daily.[6]

There were no changes in serum ciclosporin levels or evidence of nephrotoxicity.

In contrast, a handful of cases of nephrotoxicity have been reported, with three cases of increased ciclosporin levels.[7,8] A heart transplant patient developed acute renal failure within 4 days of being given ciprofloxacin 750 mg every 8 hours.[9] Another patient who had undergone a kidney transplant developed reversible nephrotoxicity.[10] Decreased renal function in a heart-lung transplant patient has been described in another report.[7] This patient and another also had increased ciclosporin blood levels when given ciprofloxacin 500 mg three times daily.[7] Acute interstitial nephritis in a cardiac transplant patient has also been reported.[11-13] A patient taking ciclosporin for red cell aplasia had an increase in ciclosporin levels from 120 nanograms/mL to 297 nanograms/mL, requiring a dose reduction from 250 mg to 200 mg daily, when intravenous ciprofloxacin 200 mg two or three times daily [exact dose unclear] was started. A ciclosporin dose increase back to 250 mg daily was required when the ciprofloxacin course was finished.[8]

A case-control study in 42 kidney transplant patients suggested that the proportion of cases experiencing at least one episode of biopsy-proved rejection within 1 to 3 months of receiving a transplant were significantly greater in those who had taken ciprofloxacin (45%) than in those who had not (19%). There was also a marked increase in the incidence of rejection associated with ciprofloxacin use (29%) compared with the controls (2%).[14]

(b) Enoxacin

Enoxacin 400 mg twice daily for 5 days had little effect on either blood or plasma levels of single doses of ciclosporin in 10 healthy subjects.[15]

(c) Levofloxacin

A single-dose study in 12 healthy subjects found that levofloxacin 500 mg had no effect on the pharmacokinetics of ciclosporin oral solution (*Sandimmune*).[16] A case report in a patient taking oral ciclosporin 250 mg daily (as the emulsion formulation) found no change in ciclosporin levels when he was given intravenous levofloxacin 500 mg daily for 9 days.[8]

In contrast, in a study in 5 kidney transplant patients taking ciclosporin (microemulsion formulation) the maximum ciclosporin blood concentration was increased by 23% when levofloxacin 500 mg twice daily for 5 days was taken for a urinary-tract infection. The authors concluded that this interaction may be clinically significant, and warned about extrapolating the results from single-dose studies in healthy subjects (as above) to patients with transplants.[17]

(d) Norfloxacin

Six renal transplant patients given norfloxacin 400 mg twice daily for 3 to 23 days for urinary tract infections,[18] and 4 heart transplant patients given norfloxacin 400 mg for 7 to 140 days had no changes in their serum ciclosporin levels.[5] However, two reports describe rises, one marked, in serum ciclosporin levels in a heart transplant patient and a kidney transplant patient given norfloxacin.[19] A comparative study in 5 children (mean age, 8 years) found that while receiving norfloxacin 5 to 10 mg/kg daily their daily dose of ciclosporin was 4.5 mg/kg daily compared with a control group of 6 children not taking norfloxacin who needed 7.4 mg/kg daily.[20]

(e) Ofloxacin

Thirty-nine patients with kidney transplants taking ciclosporin and prednisolone had no evidence of nephrotoxicity nor of any other interaction when they were given ofloxacin 100 to 400 mg daily for periods of 3 to 500 days.[21]

(f) Pefloxacin

A study in kidney transplant patients taking corticosteroids, azathioprine and ciclosporin found that the pharmacokinetics of the ciclosporin were not significantly changed by pefloxacin 400 mg twice daily for 4 days.[22]

(g) Trovafloxacin

A placebo-controlled crossover study in 7 stable kidney transplant patients treated with ciclosporin (*Sandimmune*) found that the pharmacokinetics of the ciclosporin were not significantly altered by trovafloxacin 200 mg daily for 7 days.[23]

Mechanism

The interaction between ciclosporin and norfloxacin probably occurs because norfloxacin inhibits the cytochrome P450 isoenzyme CYP3A4, resulting in a reduction in ciclosporin metabolism.[20] The interaction between ciclosporin and ciprofloxacin may possibly be due to some antagonism by ciprofloxacin of the ciclosporin-dependent inhibition of interleukin-2, which thereby opposes its immunosuppressant action.[14]

Importance and management

Information seems to be limited to these reports. They indicate that in children and adults the dosage of ciclosporin will probably need to be reduced in the presence of norfloxacin. Information with levofloxacin is currently limited, but a modest increase in ciclosporin levels may occur, and increased monitoring seems advisable.

No pharmacokinetic interaction usually occurs between ciclosporin and ciprofloxacin but very occasionally and unpredictably an increase in serum ciclosporin levels and/or kidney toxicity occurs. There is also some evidence that the immunosuppressant effects of ciclosporin may be reduced.[14] Bear these interactions in mind if both drugs are given.

There seem to be no reports of problems with enoxacin, ofloxacin, pefloxacin or trovafloxacin.

1. Tan KKC, Trull AK, Shawket S. Co-administration of ciprofloxacin and cyclosporin: lack of evidence for a pharmacokinetic interaction. *Br J Clin Pharmacol* (1989) 28, 185–7.
2. Lang J, Finaz de Villaine J, Garraffo R, Touraine J-L. Cyclosporine (cyclosporin A) pharmacokinetics in renal transplant patients receiving ciprofloxacin. *Am J Med* (1989) 87 (Suppl 5A), 82S–85S.
3. Van Buren DH, Koestner J, Adedoyin A, McCune T, MacDonell R, Johnson HK, Carroll J, Nylander W, Richie RE. Effect of ciprofloxacin on cyclosporine pharmacokinetics. *Transplantation* (1990) 50, 888–9.
4. Krüger HU, Schuler U, Proksch B, Göbel M, Ehninger G. Investigation of potential interaction of ciprofloxacin with cyclosporine in bone marrow transplant recipients. *Antimicrob Agents Chemother* (1990) 34, 1048–52.
5. Robinson JA, Venezio FR, Costanzo-Nordin MR, Pifarre R, O'Keefe PJ. Patients receiving quinolones and cyclosporine after heart transplantation. *J Heart Transplant* (1990) 9, 30–1.
6. Hooper TL, Gould FK, Swinburn CR, Featherstone G, Odom NJ, Corris PA, Freeman R, McGregor CGA. Ciprofloxacin: a preferred treatment for legionella infections in patients receiving cyclosporin A. *J Antimicrob Chemother* (1988) 22, 952–3.
7. Nasir M, Rotellar C, Hand M, Kulczycki L, Alijani MR, Winchester JF. Interaction between ciclosporin and ciprofloxacin. *Nephron* (1991) 57, 245–6.
8. Borrás-Blasco J, Conesa-García V, Navarro-Ruiz A, Marín-Jiménez F, González-Delgado M, Gomez-Corrons A. Ciprofloxacin, but not levofloxacin, affects cyclosporine blood levels in a patient with pure red blood cell aplasia. *Am J Med Sci* (2005) 330, 144–6.
9. Avent CK, Krinsky JK, Kirklin JK, Bourge RC, Figg WD. Synergistic nephrotoxicity due to ciprofloxacin and cyclosporine. *Am J Med* (1988) 85, 452–3.
10. Elston RA, Taylor J. Possible interaction of ciprofloxacin with cyclosporin A. *J Antimicrob Chemother* (1988) 21, 679–80.
11. Rosado LJ, Siskind MS, Copeland JG. Acute interstitial nephritis in a cardiac transplant patient receiving ciprofloxacin. *J Thorac Cardiovasc Surg* (1994) 107, 1364.
12. Bourge RC. Invited letter concerning: acute interstitial nephritis in a cardiac transplant recipients receiving ciprofloxacin. *J Thorac Cardiovasc Surg* (1994) 107, 1364–5.
13. Rosado LJ, Siskind MS, Nolan PE, Copeland JG. Invited letter concerning: acute interstitial nephritis in a cardiac transplant recipients receiving ciprofloxacin. *J Thorac Cardiovasc Surg* (1994) 107, 1365–6.
14. Wrishko RE, Levine M, Primmett DRN, Kim S, Partovi N, Lewis S, Landsberg D, Keown PA. Investigation of a possible interaction between ciprofloxacin and cyclosporine in renal transplant patients. *Transplantation* (1997) 64, 996–999.
15. Ryerson BA, Toothaker RD, Posvar EL, Sedman AJ, Koup JR. Effect of enoxacin on cyclosporine pharmacokinetics in healthy subjects. *Intersci Conf Antimicrob Agents Chemother* (1991) 31, 198.
16. Doose DR, Walker SA, Chien SC, Williams RR, Nayak RK. Levofloxacin does not alter cyclosporine disposition. *J Clin Pharmacol* (1998) 38, 90–3.
17. Federico S, Carrano R, Capone D, Gentile A, Palmiero G, Basile V. Pharmacokinetic interaction between levofloxacin and ciclosporin or tacrolimus in kidney transplant recipients. *Clin Pharmacokinet* (2006) 45, 169–75.
18. Jadoul M, Pirson Y, van Ypersele de Strihou C. Norfloxacin and cyclosporine-a safe combination. *Transplantation* (1989) 47, 747–8.
19. Thomson DJ, Menkis AH, McKenzie FN. Norfloxacin-cyclosporine interaction. *Transplantation* (1988) 46, 312–13.
20. McLellan RA, Drobitch RK, McLellan DH, Acott PD, Crocker JFS, Renton KW. Norfloxacin interferes with cyclosporine disposition in pediatric patients undergoing renal transplantation. *Clin Pharmacol Ther* (1995) 58, 322–7.
21. Vogt P, Schorn T, Frei U. Ofloxacin in the treatment of urinary tract infection in renal transplant recipients. *Infection* (1988) 16, 175–8.
22. Lang J, Finaz de Villaine J, Guemei A, Touraine JL, Faucon C. Absence of pharmacokinetic interaction between pefloxacin and cyclosporin A in patients with renal transplants. *Rev Infect Dis* (1989) 11 (Suppl 5), S1094.
23. Johnson HJ, Swan SK, Heim-Duthoy KL, Pelletier SM, Teng R, Vincent J. The effect of trovafloxacin on steady-state pharmacokinetics of cyclosporine (CSA) in stable renal transplant patients. *Pharm Res* (1997) 14 (11 Suppl), S-509.

Ciclosporin + Antibacterials; Quinupristin/Dalfopristin

A study found that quinupristin/dalfopristin increased the AUC and maximum blood levels of ciclosporin. In an isolated case quinupristin/dalfopristin was found to increase ciclosporin levels by about threefold.

Clinical evidence, mechanism, importance and management

In a study in 24 subjects given a single 300-mg dose of ciclosporin, taken 1.5 hours before the fourth of 9 infusions of quinupristin/dalfopristin (7.5 mg/kg given at intervals of 8 hours) the AUC and maximum blood levels of ciclosporin were increased by 63% and 30%, respectively, and ciclosporin clearance was decreased by 34%.[1]

A kidney transplant patient taking ciclosporin with trough blood levels of between 80 and 105 nanograms/mL developed a vancomycin-resistant enterococcal infection. After a series of antibacterials had failed to clear the infection she was given intravenous quinupristin/dalfopristin 300 mg every 8 hours. After 3 days of treatment her ciclosporin trough level rose to almost 300 nanograms/mL. A ciclosporin dose reduction from 75 to 50 mg twice daily returned her levels to baseline. However, 2 days after the antibacterials were discontinued she was found to have a trough ciclosporin level of only 34 nanograms/mL. She was subsequently restabilised on her original dose of ciclosporin.[2]

Information is limited. However, the manufacturers state that quinupristin/dalfopristin has been shown *in vitro* to inhibit the cytochrome P450 isoenzyme CYP3A4 and advise that ciclosporin levels are closely monitored during concurrent use;[3,4] ciclosporin dose reductions may be necessary.

1. Ballow C, Chevalier P, Geary W, Pasquier O, Forrest A, Montay G, Rey J. Randomized, crossover, phase I study of the interaction between quinupristin/dalfopristin (RP 59500) at steady state and cyclosporine in healthy volunteers. Nordic Pharma UK, data on file (Ref-Syn-0188).
2. Stamatakis MK, Richards JG. Interaction between quinupristin/dalfopristin and cyclosporine. *Ann Pharmacother* (1997) 31, 576–8.
3. Synercid (Quinupristin/Dalfopristin). DSM Pharmaceuticals, Inc. US Prescribing information, July 2003.
4. Synercid (Quinupristin/Dalfopristin). Monarch Pharmaceuticals. UK Summary of product characteristics, March 2005.

Ciclosporin + Antibacterials; Sulfonamides and/or Trimethoprim

In isolated cases, sulfadiazine given orally or sulfadimidine given intravenously with trimethoprim have caused a reduction in se-

rum ciclosporin levels. Sulfametoxydiazine possibly caused a minor reduction in ciclosporin levels in one case. Although co-trimoxazole increases serum creatinine levels in kidney transplant patients taking ciclosporin, it normally appears to be safe and effective.

Clinical evidence

(a) Co-trimoxazole

A large-scale study in 132 kidney transplant patients taking ciclosporin encompassing 33 876 patient days found that co-trimoxazole was effective and well tolerated. Ciclosporin pharmacokinetics remained unchanged. A 15% rise in serum creatinine levels occurred, which reversed when the co-trimoxazole was stopped. This rise was not interpreted as a sign of nephrotoxicity but appeared to be due to inhibition of the tubular excretion of creatinine by the co-trimoxazole.[1]

Other reports describe a few patients given ciclosporin with co-trimoxazole who developed rises in creatinine levels (interpreted as evidence of nephrotoxicity),[2-5] interstitial nephritis,[6] granulocytopenia and thrombocytopenia.[7,8] Apparent nephrotoxicity has also been seen with **trimethoprim** and ciclosporin.[9]

(b) Sulfadiazine or Sulfametoxydiazine

Three heart transplant patients treated for toxoplasmosis had a reduction in their ciclosporin levels when they were given sulfadiazine 4 to 6 g daily. Their dosage-to-level ciclosporin ratios rose by 58%, 82%, and 29%, respectively. Two had previously been given sulfametoxydiazine and this had caused a minor reduction in ciclosporin levels in one of these patients.[10]

(c) Sulfadimidine with trimethoprim

A heart transplant patient taking ciclosporin and prednisolone developed undetectable serum ciclosporin levels 7 days after starting intravenous sulfadimidine 2 g four times daily and **trimethoprim** 300 to 500 mg twice daily. Doubling the ciclosporin dosage had little effect and evidence of transplant rejection was seen. Within 10 days of starting to take the antibacterials orally instead of intravenously the serum ciclosporin levels returned to roughly their former levels and the rejection problems disappeared.[11]

Another report by some of the same authors describes a similar marked fall in serum ciclosporin levels in 5 heart transplant patients (one of them the same as the report already cited[11]) when given sulfadimidine and **trimethoprim** intravenously.[12]

Mechanism

Uncertain. Co-trimoxazole and trimethoprim can raise serum creatinine levels, possibly due to inhibition of creatinine secretion by the kidney tubules.[13] The reduction in serum ciclosporin levels apparently caused by the sulfonamides is not understood.

Importance and management

The documentation is only moderate, and these interactions are not firmly established. Be aware that intravenous sulfadimidine with trimethoprim may cause a marked reduction in serum ciclosporin levels with accompanying inadequate immunosuppression. Sulfadiazine may also reduce ciclosporin levels. The evidence suggests that oral sulfadimidine with trimethoprim, sulfametoxydiazine, and co-trimoxazole do not interact adversely and are normally safe and effective, although toxicity can apparently occur in a small number of patients. Until more information is available it would be prudent to keep a close check on ciclosporin levels if any sulphonamide is added to established treatment with ciclosporin. The manufacturer recommends close monitoring of renal function when ciclosporin is used with co-trimoxazole.[14]

1. Maki DG, Fox BC, Kuntz J, Sollinger HW, Belzer FO. A prospective, randomized, double-blind study of trimethoprim-sulfamethoxazole for prophylaxis of infection in renal transplantation. Side effects of trimethoprim-sulfamethoxazole interaction with cyclosporine. *J Lab Clin Med* (1992) 119, 11–24.
2. Thompson JF, Chalmers DHK, Hunnisett AGW, Wood RFM, Morris PJ. Nephrotoxicity of trimethoprim and cotrimoxazole in renal allograft recipients treated with cyclosporine. *Transplantation* (1983) 36, 204–6.
3. Ringdén O, Myrenfors P, Klintmalm G, Tydén G, Öst L. Nephrotoxicity by co-trimoxazole and cyclosporin in transplanted patients. *Lancet* (1984) i, 1016–17.
4. Klintmalm G, Säwe J, Ringdén O, von Bahr C, Magnusson A. Cyclosporine plasma levels in renal transplant patients. Association with renal toxicity and allograft rejection. *Transplantation* (1985) 39, 132–7.
5. Klintmalm G, Ringdén O, Groth CG. Clinical and laboratory signs in nephrotoxicity and rejection in cyclosporine treated renal allograft recipients. *Transplant Proc* (1983) 15 (Suppl 1), 2815–20.
6. Smith EJ, Light JA, Filo RS, Yum MN. Interstitial nephritis caused by trimethoprim-sulfamethoxazole in renal transplant recipients. *JAMA* (1980) 244, 360–1.
7. Bradley PP, Warden GD, Maxwell JG, Rothstein G. Neutropenia and thrombocytopenia in renal allograft recipients treated with trimethoprim-sulfamethoxazole. *Ann Intern Med* (1980) 93, 560–2.
8. Hulme B, Reeves DS. Leucopenia associated with trimethoprim-sulfamethoxazole after renal transplantation. *BMJ* (1971) 3, 610–2.
9. Nyberg G, Gäbel H, Althoff P, Bjoörk S, Herlitz H, Brynger H. Adverse effect of trimethoprim on kidney function in renal transplant patients. *Lancet* (1984) i, 394–5.
10. Spes CH, Angermann CE, Stempfle HU, Wenke K, Theisen K. Sulfadiazine therapy for toxoplasmosis in heart transplant recipients decreases cyclosporine concentration. *Clin Investig* (1992) 70, 752–4.
11. Wallwork J, McGregor CGA, Wells FC, Cory-Pearce R, English TAH. Cyclosporin and intravenous sulphadimidine and trimethoprim therapy. *Lancet* (1983) i, 336–7.
12. Jones DK, Hakim M, Wallwork J, Higenbottam TW, White DJG. Serious interaction between cyclosporin A and sulphadimidine. *BMJ* (1986) 292, 728–9.
13. Berg KJ, Gjellestad A, Norby G, Rootwelt K, Djøseland O, Fauchald P, Mehl A, Narverud J, Talseth T. Renal effects of trimethoprim in ciclosporin- and azathioprine-treated kidney-allografted patients. *Nephron* (1989) 53, 218–22.
14. Neoral (Ciclosporin). Novartis Pharmaceuticals UK Ltd. Summary of UK product characteristics, December 2004.

Ciclosporin + Antidiabetics

Some preliminary evidence suggests that glibenclamide (glyburide) can raise serum ciclosporin levels to a moderate extent. Glipizide caused about a twofold increase in ciclosporin levels in 2 patients, but no change was noted in a study in 11 patients. A single-dose study found ciclosporin significantly increased repaglinide bioavailability. However a study in kidney transplant patients found no consistent increase in blood glucose-lowering effects in patients taking both drugs. Pioglitazone and rosiglitazone are predicted to not interact with ciclosporin.

Clinical evidence, mechanism, importance and management

(a) Pioglitazone

In vitro and human studies have shown that pioglitazone does not affect cytochrome P450 isoenzymes, including CYP3A4. Therefore no interaction would be expected with ciclosporin, which is mainly metabolised by CYP3A4.[1]

(b) Repaglinide

A placebo-controlled study in 12 healthy subjects given ciclosporin 100 mg twice daily for two doses, with a single 250-microgram dose of repaglinide on day 2, found that ciclosporin significantly increased the maximum plasma level and AUC of repaglinide by 175% and 244%, respectively. It was suggested that ciclosporin inhibited the cytochrome P450 isoenzyme CYP3A4-mediated metabolism of repaglinide, as well as affecting OAT-mediated liver uptake of repaglinide.[2,3]

No significant changes were seen in ciclosporin, sirolimus or tacrolimus blood levels and no dosage changes were required in a study in kidney transplant patients taking repaglinide (18 as monotherapy and 5 combined with either metformin or rosiglitazone). The effects of ciclosporin on repaglinide metabolism were not investigated in this study, although concurrent use was found to be effective.[4] Commenting further, the authors noted that they were unable to demonstrate a consistent, increased blood glucose-lowering effect with concurrent use of repaglinide and ciclosporin,[5] although other authors, citing the study above,[2] noted that ciclosporin may markedly increase plasma repaglinide levels and enhance its blood glucose-lowering effects.[3]

Although the clinical study found no serious adverse effects with concurrent ciclosporin and repaglinide, the situation is not clear. The large increases in repaglinide levels seen were significant, although they were found in a single-dose study in healthy subjects taking no other potentially interacting medication. The possibility of increased hypoglycaemia should be borne in mind if ciclosporin and repaglinide are used concurrently. Patients should be advised to report any adverse effects, particularly an increase in the number of hypoglycaemic events.

(c) Sulphonylureas

A review of 6 post-transplant diabetic patients taking ciclosporin found that their steady-state plasma ciclosporin levels rose by 57% when they were given **glibenclamide (glyburide)**. Hepatic and renal function were unchanged. The reason for this reaction is not known, but it is suggested that **glibenclamide** possibly inhibits the cytochrome P450 isoenzyme CYP3A4, the major isoenzyme involved in the metabolism of ciclosporin, resulting in a reduction in its clearance.[6]

Ciclosporin blood levels in 2 patients were more than doubled, and they needed reductions of 20 to 30% in their ciclosporin dosage when they were also given **glipizide** 10 mg daily.[7] In contrast, a study in 11 post-transplant diabetic patients found no significant alterations in ciclosporin pharmacokinetics when **glipizide** was given.[8] This interaction is unconfirmed and of uncertain clinical significance. However, note that one of the rare adverse effects of ciclosporin is hyperglycaemia. There is insufficient evidence to recommend increased monitoring, but be aware of the potential for an interaction in the case of an unexpected response to treatment. Information about other sulphonylureas appears not to be available.

1. Actos (Pioglitazone hydrochloride). Takeda UK Ltd. UK Summary of product characteristics, January 2007.
2. Kajosaari LI, Niemi M, Neuvonen M, Laitila J, Neuvonen PJ, Backman JT. Cyclosporine markedly raises the plasma concentrations of repaglinide. *Clin Pharmacol Ther* (2005) 78, 388–99.
3. Backman JT, Kajosaari LI, Niemi M, Neuvonen PJ. Cyclosporine A increases plasma concentrations and effects of repaglinide. *Am J Transplant* (2006) 6, 2221–2.
4. Türk T, Peitruck F, Dolff S, Kribben A, Janssen OE, Mann K, Philipp T, Heemann U, Witzke O. Repaglinide in the management of new-onset diabetes mellitus after renal transplantation. *Am J Transplant* (2006) 6, 842–6.
5. Türk T, Witzke O. Pharmacological interaction between cyclosporine A and repaglinide. Is it clinically relevant? *Am J Transplant* (2006) 6, 2223.
6. Islam SI, Masuda QN, Bolaji OO, Shaheen FM, Sheikh IA. Possible interaction between cyclosporine and glibenclamide in posttransplant diabetic patients. *Ther Drug Monit* (1996) 18, 624–6.
7. Chidester PD, Connito DJ. Interaction between glipizide and cyclosporine: report of two cases. *Transplant Proc* (1993) 25, 2136–7.
8. Sagedal S, Åsberg A, Hartmann A, Bergan S, Berg KJ. Glipizide treatment of post-transplant diabetes does not interfere with cyclosporine pharmacokinetics in renal allograft recipients. *Clin Transplant* (1998) 12, 553–6.

Ciclosporin + Antiepileptics

Serum ciclosporin levels are markedly reduced by carbamazepine, phenobarbital, or phenytoin. The dosage of ciclosporin may need to be increased two- to fourfold to maintain adequate immunosuppression. Oxcarbazepine may cause a small decrease in ciclosporin levels. Valproate appears not to affect ciclosporin levels but two case reports suggest that it may damage renal grafts and cause hepatotoxicity in patients taking ciclosporin.

Clinical evidence

(a) Carbamazepine

The ciclosporin serum levels of a kidney transplant patient fell from 346 to 64 nanograms/mL within 3 days of starting to take carbamazepine 200 mg three times daily. A week later serum levels were down to 37 nanograms/mL. They rose again when the carbamazepine was stopped but fell once more when it was restarted. The ciclosporin dosage was increased to keep the levels within the therapeutic range.[1]

The mean average steady-state blood levels of ciclosporin (adjusted for dose) in a group of 3 children with kidney transplants taking carbamazepine were 50% lower than in 3 other matched patients not taking carbamazepine.[2] Four other individual patients have also shown this interaction.[3-5] One needed her ciclosporin dosage to be doubled in order to maintain adequate blood levels while taking carbamazepine 800 mg daily.[3] When the carbamazepine was replaced by sodium valproate in 3 patients, the ciclosporin dosages could be reduced to their previous level.[3,4]

(b) Oxcarbazepine

A kidney transplant patient taking ciclosporin 270 mg daily and valproate, gabapentin, prednisone, doxepin, allopurinol, levothyroxine and pravastatin was also given oxcarbazepine. Fourteen days later, with the dose of oxcarbazepine at 750 mg daily, the ciclosporin trough level fell below 100 nanograms/mL and after a further 2 days was 87 nanograms/mL. The ciclosporin dose was increased to 290 mg daily and the oxcarbazepine dose reduced to 600 mg daily. Ciclosporin levels then remained stable above 100 nanograms/mL and seizure frequency was reduced by 95%.[6]

(c) Phenobarbital

A 4-year-old child with a bone marrow transplant who was receiving phenobarbital 50 mg twice daily had serum ciclosporin levels of less than 60 nanograms/mL even after raising the ciclosporin dosage to 18 mg/kg daily. When the phenobarbital dosage was reduced to 25% of the original dose the trough serum ciclosporin levels rose to 205 nanograms/mL.[7] Another report describes an increase in ciclosporin levels from 512 to 810 nanograms/mL after phenytoin and phenobarbital were replaced by sodium valproate in one patient.[8]

A threefold increase in ciclosporin clearance was seen in another child with a kidney transplant while taking phenobarbital.[9] Reductions in ciclosporin levels due to phenobarbital have been described in other patients.[10-13]

(d) Phenytoin

The observation that 5 patients taking ciclosporin needed dosage increases while taking phenytoin prompted a further study in 6 healthy subjects. Phenytoin 300 or 400 mg daily reduced the maximum ciclosporin blood levels and AUC by 37% (from 1325 to 831 micrograms/L) and 47%, respectively.[14]

Other reports describe patients who needed two- to fourfold increases in their ciclosporin dosages when they were given phenytoin.[15-19]

Another report describes an increase in ciclosporin levels from 512 to 810 nanograms/mL after phenytoin and phenobarbital were replaced by sodium valproate.[8]

A report of severe gingival overgrowth in a kidney transplant patient was attributed to the additive adverse effects of ciclosporin and phenytoin. Ciclosporin was replaced by tacrolimus, which may have fewer oral adverse effects, and almost complete reversal of gingival overgrowth was achieved within 6 months.[20]

(e) Sodium valproate

In 5 cases an interacting antiepileptic was successfully replaced by sodium valproate,[3,4,8,21] see *Carbamazepine*, *Phenobarbital* and *Phenytoin*, above.[13,21] However, sodium valproate may not always be without problems because interstitial nephritis was suspected in one patient with a renal graft taking ciclosporin and valproate,[10] and fatal valproate-induced hepatotoxicity occurred in another patient taking ciclosporin.[22]

Mechanism

It is thought that phenytoin,[14,15] carbamazepine[1,2] and phenobarbital[7,11] increase the metabolism of the ciclosporin by the liver (hepatic cytochrome P450 oxygenase system) thereby decreasing the serum levels. Oxcarbazepine produced only small reductions in ciclosporin levels, and the effect is probably due to weak induction of the cytochrome P450 isoenzyme CYP3A.[6] Phenytoin also possibly reduces the absorption of the ciclosporin.[23]

Importance and management

None of these interactions is extensively documented but all appear to be established and of clinical importance. Serum ciclosporin levels should be well monitored if carbamazepine, phenobarbital or phenytoin are added and the ciclosporin dosage increased appropriately. **Primidone** is metabolised to phenobarbital by the liver, and therefore would be expected to reduce ciclosporin levels. Information about oxcarbazepine is very limited but small reductions in its dose, together with an increase in ciclosporin dose, may be adequate to control any interaction. However, more study is required before oxcarbazepine can be recommended as a suitable alternative.[6] The effects of the interaction may persist for a week or more after the anticonvulsant is withdrawn. Sodium valproate seems not to alter ciclosporin levels, but the case reports of nephritis and hepatotoxicity suggest some caution is warranted.

1. Lele P, Peterson P, Yang S, Jarell B, Burke JF. Cyclosporine and tegretol — another drug interaction. *Kidney Int* (1985) 27, 344.
2. Cooney GF, Mochon M, Kaiser B, Dunn SP, Goldsmith B. Effects of carbamazepine on cyclosporine metabolism in pediatric renal transplant recipients. *Pharmacotherapy* (1995) 15, 353–6.
3. Hillebrand G, Castro LA, van Scheidt W, Beukelmann D, Land W, Schmidt D. Valproate for epilepsy in renal transplant recipients receiving cyclosporine. *Transplantation* (1987) 43, 915–16.
4. Schofield OMV, Camp RDR, Levene GM. Cyclosporin A in psoriasis: interaction with carbamazepine. *Br J Dermatol* (1990) 122, 425–6.
5. Alvarez JS, Del Castillo JAC, Ortiz MJA. Effect of carbamazepine on ciclosporin blood level. *Nephron* (1991) 58, 235–6.
6. Rösche J, Fröscher W, Abendroth D, Liebel J. Possible oxcarbazepine interaction with cyclosporine serum levels: a single case study. *Clin Neuropharmacol* (2001) 24, 113–16.
7. Carstensen H, Jacobsen N, Dieperink H. Interaction between cyclosporin A and phenobarbitone. *Br J Clin Pharmacol* (1986) 21, 550–1.
8. Noguchi M, Kiuchi C, Akiyama H, Sakamaki H, Onozawa Y. Interaction between cyclosporin A and anticonvulsants. *Bone Marrow Transplant* (1992) 9, 391.
9. Burckart GJ, Venkataramanan R, Starzl T, Ptachcinski JR, Gartner JC, Rosenthal T. Cyclosporine clearance in children following organ transplantation. *J Clin Pharmacol* (1984) 24, 412.
10. Kramer G, Dillmann U, Tettenborn B. Cyclosporine-phenobarbital interaction. *Epilepsia* (1989) 30, 701.
11. Beierle FA, Bailey L. Cyclosporine metabolism impeded/blocked by co-administration of phenobarbital. *Clin Chem* (1989) 35, 1160.

12. Wideman CA. Pharmacokinetic monitoring of cyclosporine. *Transplant Proc* (1983) 15 (Suppl 1), 3168–75.
13. Matsuura T, Akiyama T, Kurita T. Interaction between phenobarbital and ciclosporin following renal transplantation: a case report. *Hinyokika Kiyo* (1990) 36, 447–50.
14. Freeman DJ, Laupacis A, Keown PA, Stiller CR, Carruthers SG. Evaluation of cyclosporin-phenytoin interaction with observations on cyclosporin metabolites. *Br J Clin Pharmacol* (1984) 18, 887–93.
15. Keown PA, Laupacis A, Carruthers G, Stawecki M, Koegler J, McKenzie FN, Wall W, Stiller CR. Interaction between phenytoin and cyclosporine following organ transplantation. *Transplantation* (1984) 38, 304–6.
16. Grigg-Damberger MM, Costanzo-Nordin R, Kelly MA, Bahamon-Dussan JE, Silver M, Zucker MJ, Celesia GG. Phenytoin may compromise efficacy of cyclosporine immunosuppression in cardiac transplant patients. *Epilepsia* (1988) 29, 693.
17. Schmidt H, Naumann R, Jaschonek K, Einsele H, Dopfer R, Ehninger G. Drug interaction between cyclosporin and phenytoin in allogeneic bone marrow transplantation. *Bone Marrow Transplant* (1989) 4, 212–13.
18. Schweitzer EJ, Canafax DM, Gillingham KJ, Najarian JS, Matas AJ. Phenytoin administration in kidney recipients on CSA immunosuppression. *J Am Soc Nephrol* (1991) 2, 816.
19. Castelao AM. Cyclosporine A – drug interactions. 2nd Int Conf Therapeutic Drug Monitoring Toxicology, Barcelona, Spain 1992. 203–9.
20. Hernandez G, Arriba L, Lucas M, de Andres A. Reduction of severe gingival overgrowth in a kidney transplant patient by replacing cyclosporin A with tacrolimus. *J Periodontol* (2000) 71, 1630–6.
21. Nishioka T, Ikegami M, Imanishi M, Ishii T, Uemura T, Kunikata S, Kanda H, Matsuura T, Akiyama T, Kurita T. Interaction between phenobarbital and ciclosporin following renal transplantation: a case report. *Hinyokika Kiyo* (1990) 36, 447–50.
22. Fischman MA, Hull D, Bartus SA, Schweizer RT. Valproate for epilepsy in renal transplant recipients receiving cyclosporine. *Transplantation* (1989) 48, 542.
23. Rowland M, Gupta SK. Cyclosporin-phenytoin interaction: re-evaluation using metabolite data. *Br J Clin Pharmacol* (1987) 24, 329–34.

Ciclosporin + Antimycobacterials

Ciclosporin serum levels are markedly reduced by rifampicin and transplant rejection can rapidly develop. Rifamycin seems to interact similarly, but limited evidence suggests that rifabutin interacts to a lesser extent. Ethambutol and isoniazid do not generally appear to interact with ciclosporin although case reports have described alterations in ciclosporin levels.

Clinical evidence

(a) Rifabutin

The clearance of ciclosporin in a patient with a kidney transplant doubled when isoniazid, ethambutol, pyridoxine and rifampicin 600 mg daily were given. When these drugs were replaced by rifabutin 150 mg and clofazimine 100 mg daily the ciclosporin clearance fell to about its former levels, but after about 3 weeks the clearance was about 20% greater than before the antimycobacterial drugs were given.[1]

(b) Rifampicin (Rifampin)

A study in 39 kidney transplant patients taking ciclosporin at a mean dose of 158 mg daily found that the ciclosporin dose needed to be increased by between 150 to 525 mg daily (an average dose of 469 mg daily) when rifampicin 450 to 600 mg daily was taken as part of a regimen for tuberculosis. An increased incidence of acute rejection occurred during treatment with ciclosporin and rifampicin and 16 patients had kidney graft failure and needed to go back on haemodialysis because of this interaction.[2]

A heart transplant patient taking ciclosporin started taking rifampicin 600 mg daily with amphotericin B for the treatment of an *Aspergillus fumigatus* infection. Within 11 days her serum ciclosporin levels had fallen from 473 to less than 31 nanograms/mL and severe acute graft rejection occurred. The dosage of ciclosporin was increased stepwise and the levels climbed to a plateau before suddenly falling again. The dosage had to be increased to more than 30 mg/kg daily to achieve serum levels in the range 100 to 300 nanograms/mL.[3]

A considerable number of other reports about individual patients, both adult and paediatric, confirm that a very marked fall in serum ciclosporin levels occurs, often to undetectable levels, accompanied by transplantation rejection in many instances, if rifampicin is given either intravenously or orally without raising the ciclosporin dosage.[1,4-28] Ciclosporin levels become toxic within 2 weeks of stopping the rifampicin unless the previously adjusted ciclosporin dosage is reduced.[4,6]

Three patients needed increases in the dosage of ciclosporin when given rifampicin and erythromycin, although the latter normally reduces ciclosporin requirements.[19,29,30] Another patient whose ciclosporin levels had been raised by 'clarithromycin', (p.1016), had a fall in their levels when rifampicin was added.[31]

(c) Rifamycin sodium

Rifamycin sodium used to irrigate a wound has been reported to reduce the serum levels of ciclosporin in a kidney transplant patient.[32]

(d) Other antituberculars

Isoniazid[12,22,23] and **ethambutol**[22,23] do not normally interact with ciclosporin. However, there is one case report describing a patient who had a gradual rise in serum ciclosporin levels when isoniazid and ethambutol were stopped,[14] and another which attributed a marked rise in ciclosporin levels to the use of isoniazid.[33] There have been several other case reports of successful treatment of tuberculosis in heart and kidney transplant patients using **isoniazid**, **ethambutol**, pyrazinamide with ofloxacin, or **streptomycin**.[34,35] Consider also 'pyrazinamide', (p.1044), and 'quinolones', (p.1018).

Mechanism

Rifampicin stimulates the metabolism of the ciclosporin by the cytochrome P450 isoenzyme CYP3A[36] resulting in a marked increase in ciclosporin clearance. In addition, rifampicin decreases ciclosporin absorption by inducing its metabolism by the gut wall,[37] thus producing a significant fall in ciclosporin levels. If rifampicin is given with erythromycin or clarithromycin, the enzyme inhibitory effects of the macrolides are swamped by the more potent enzyme-inducing effects of rifampicin. Rifabutin has some enzyme-inducing properties but the extent is quite small compared with rifampicin, and the onset may be delayed.[38]

Importance and management

The interaction between ciclosporin and rifampicin is very well documented, well established and clinically important, as transplant rejection may occur unless the ciclosporin dosage is markedly increased. In one study 27% of patients taking rifampicin lost grafts due to rejection, and this was directly attributed to the interaction.[22] The interaction develops within a few days (within a single day in one case[20]). Monitor the effects of concurrent use and increase the ciclosporin dosage appropriately. Three- to fivefold dosage increases (sometimes frequency-increases from two to three times daily) have proved to be effective, with daily monitoring. Remember also to reduce the ciclosporin dosage when rifampicin is stopped to reduce the risk of ciclosporin toxicity.

The authors of one large study concluded that it is better to avoid rifampicin in patients taking ciclosporin and to use other antimycobacterials instead.[22] They found that the use of three antitubercular drugs (not including rifampicin) for at least 9 months reduced mortality. Other reports similarly found that regimens without rifampicin were suitable for the treatment of tuberculosis in transplant patients.[23,34,35]

Another suggested alternative is to replace the ciclosporin with another non-interacting immunosuppressant, such as azathioprine and low-dose prednisolone for immunosuppression, if rifampicin is needed.[13]

Other rifamycins may also be an option; limited evidence suggests that rifabutin interacts minimally. However, the manufacturer[39] and the CSM in the UK[40] caution about the possibility of an interaction, and close monitoring of ciclosporin levels would still be advisable. Topical rifamycin interacted like rifampicin in one patient when it was applied to a wound.[32]

1. Vandevelde C, Chang A, Andrews D, Riggs W, Jewesson P. Rifampin and ansamycin interactions with cyclosporine after renal transplantation. *Pharmacotherapy* (1991) 11, 88–9.
2. El-Agroudy AE, Refaie AF, Moussa OM, Ghoneim MA. Tuberculosis in Egyptian kidney transplant recipients: study of clinical course and outcome. *J Nephrol* (2003) 16, 404–11.
3. Modry DL, Stinson EB, Oyer PE, Jamieson SW, Baldwin JC, Shumway NE. Acute rejection and massive cyclosporine requirements in heart transplant recipients treated with rifampin. *Transplantation* (1985) 39, 313–14.
4. Langhoff E, Madsen S. Rapid metabolism of cyclosporin and prednisone in kidney transplant patients on tuberculostatic treatment. *Lancet* (1983) ii, 1303.
5. Cassidy MJD, Van Zyl-Smit R, Pascoe MD, Swanepoel CR, Jacobson JE. Effect of rifampicin on cyclosporin A blood levels in a renal transplant recipient. *Nephron* (1985) 41, 207–8.
6. Coward RA, Raferty AT, Brown CB. Cyclosporin and antituberculous therapy. *Lancet* (1985) i, 1342–3.
7. Howard P, Bixler TJ, Gill B. Cyclosporine-rifampin drug interaction. *Drug Intell Clin Pharm* (1985) 19, 763–4.
8. Van Buren D, Wideman CA, Ried M, Gibbons S, Van Buren CT, Jarowenko M, Flechner SM, Frazier OH, Cooley DA, Kahan BD. The antagonistic effect of rifampin upon cyclosporine bioavailability. *Transplant Proc* (1984) 16, 1642–5.
9. Allen RDM, Hunnisett AG, Morris PJ. Cyclosporin and rifampicin in renal transplantation. *Lancet* (1985) i, 980.
10. Langhoff E, Madsen S. Rapid metabolism of cyclosporin and prednisone in kidney transplant patient receiving tuberculostatic treatment. *Lancet* (1983) ii, 1031.
11. Offermann G, Keller F, Molzahn M. Low cyclosporin A blood levels and acute graft rejection in a renal transplant recipient during rifampin treatment. *Am J Nephrol* (1985) 5, 385–7.
12. Jurewicz WA, Gunson BK, Ismail T, Angrisani L, McMaster P. Cyclosporin and antituberculous therapy. *Lancet* (1985) i, 1343.
13. Daniels NJ, Dover JS, Schachter RK. Interaction between cyclosporin and rifampicin. *Lancet* (1984) ii, 639.

14. Leimenstoll G, Schlegelberger T, Fulde R, Niedermayer W. Interaktion von Ciclosporin und Ethambutol-Isoniazid. *Dtsch Med Wochenschr* (1988) 113, 514–15.
15. Prado A, Ramirez M, Aguirre EC, Martin RS, Zucchini A. Interaccion entre ciclosporina y rifampicina en un caso de transplante renal. *Medicina (B Aires)* (1987) 47, 521–4.
16. Al-Sulaiman MH, Dhar JM, Al-Khader AA. Successful use of rifampicin in the treatment of tuberculosis in renal transplant patients immunosuppressed with cyclosporine. *Transplantation* (1990) 50, 597–8.
17. Sánchez DM, Rincón LC, Asensio JM, Serna AB. Interacción entre ciclosporina y rifampicina. *Rev Clin Esp* (1988) 183, 217.
18. Peschke B, Ernst W, Gossmann J, Kachel HG, Schoeppe W, Scheuermann EH. Antituberculous drugs in kidney transplant recipients treated with cyclosporine. *Transplantation* (1993) 56, 236–8.
19. Zylber-Katz E. Multiple drug interactions with cyclosporine in a heart transplant patient. *Ann Pharmacother* (1995) 29, 127–31. Correction. ibid. 790.
20. Wandel C, Böhrer H, Böcker R. Rifampicin and cyclosporine dosing in heart transplant patients. *J Cardiothorac Vasc Anesth* (1995) 9, 621–2.
21. Capone D, Aiello C, Santoro GA, Gentile A, Stanziale P, D'Alessandro R, Imperatore P, Basile V. Drug interaction between cyclosporine and two antimicrobial agents, josamycin and rifampicin, in organ-transplanted patients. *Int J Clin Pharmacol Res* (1996) 16, 73–6.
22. Aguado JM, Herrero JA, Gavaldá J, Torre-Cisneros J, Blanes M, Rufí G, Moreno A, Gurguí A, Hayek M, Lumbreras C and the Spanish Transplantation Infection Study Group, GESITRA. Clinical presentation and outcome of tuberculosis in kidney, liver, and heart transplant recipients in Spain. *Transplantation* (1997) 63, 1276–86.
23. Muñoz P, Palomo J, Muños R, Rodriguez-Creixéms M, Pelaez T, Bouza E. Tuberculosis in heart transplant recipients. *Clin Infect Dis* (1995) 21, 398–402.
24. Freitag VL, Skifton RD, Lake KD. Effect of short-term rifampin on stable cyclosporine concentration. *Ann Pharmacother* (1999) 33, 871–2.
25. Almeida RV, Carvalho JGR, Mulinari A, Hauck P. Tuberculosis in renal transplant recipients. *J Am Soc Nephrol* (1997) 8, 709A.
26. Kim YH, Yoon YR, Kim YW, Shin JG, Cha IJ. Effects of rifampin on cyclosporine disposition in kidney recipients with tuberculosis. *Transplant Proc* (1998) 30, 3570–2.
27. Zelunka EJ. Intravenous cyclosporine-rifampin interaction in a pediatric bone marrow transplant recipient. *Pharmacotherapy* (2002) 22, 387–90.
28. Koselj M, Bren A, Kandus A, Kovac D. Drug interactions between cyclosporine and rifampicin, erythromycin, and azoles in kidney recipients with opportunistic infections. *Transplant Proc* (1994) 26, 2823–4.
29. Hooper TL, Gould FK, Swinburne CR, Featherstone G, Odom NJ, Corris PA, Freeman R, McGregor CGA. Ciprofloxacin: a preferred treatment for legionella infections in patients receiving cyclosporin A. *J Antimicrob Chemother* (1988) 22, 952–3.
30. Soto J, Sacristan JA, Alsar MJ. Effect of the simultaneous administration of rifampicin and erythromycin on the metabolism of cyclosporine. *Clin Transplant* (1992) 6, 312–14.
31. Plemmons RM, McAllister CK, Garces MC, Ward RL. Osteomyelitis due to *Mycobacterium haemophilum* in a cardiac transplant patient: case report and analysis of interactions among clarithromycin, rifampin and cyclosporine. *Clin Infect Dis* (1997) 24, 995–7.
32. Renoult E, Hubert J, Trechot Ph, Hestin D, Kessler M, L'Hermite J. Effect of topical rifamycin SV treatment on cyclosporin A blood levels in a renal transplant patient. *Eur J Clin Pharmacol* (1991) 40, 433–4.
33. Diaz Couselo FA, Porato F, Turin M, Etchegoyen FP, Diez RA. Interacciones de la ciclosporina en transplantados renales. *Medicina (B Aires)* (1992) 52, 296–302.
34. Jastrzębski D, Zaklicyński M, Kozielski J, Siola M, Dworniczak S, Wojdyla A, Zembala M. Possibility to treat lung tuberculosis without using rifampicin in heart transplant recipients-two case reports. *Ann Transplant* (2003) 8, 42–4.
35. Vachharajani TJ, Oza UG, Phadke AG, Kirpalani AL. Tuberculosis in renal transplant recipients: rifampicin sparing treatment protocol. *Int Urol Nephrol* (2002) 34, 551–3.
36. Pichard L, Fabre JM, Domergue J, Fabre G, Saint-Aubert B, Mourad G, Maurel P. Molecular mechanism of cyclosporine A drug interactions: inducers and inhibitors of cytochrome P450 screening in primary cultures of human hepatocytes. *Transplant Proc* (1991) 23, 978–9.
37. Hebert MF, Roberts JP, Prueksaritanont T, Benet LZ. Bioavailability of cyclosporine with concomitant rifampin administration is markedly less than predicted by hepatic enzyme induction. *Clin Pharmacol Ther* (1992) 52, 453–7.
38. Perucca E, Grimaldi R, Frigo GM, Sardi A, Möning H, Ohnhaus EE. Comparative effects of rifabutin and rifampicin on hepatic microsomal enzyme activity in normal subjects. *Eur J Clin Pharmacol* (1988) 34, 595–9.
39. Mycobutin (Rifabutin). Pharmacia Ltd. UK Summary of product characteristics, October 2006.
40. Committee on the Safety of Medicines/Medicines Control Agency. Revised indication and drug interactions of rifabutin. *Current Problems* (1997) 23, 14.

Ciclosporin + Azoles

The evidence suggests that all the azole antifungals can raise ciclosporin levels to a greater or lesser degree. Ketoconazole may cause five- to tenfold rises, while itraconazole, fluconazole and voriconazole may cause two- to threefold rises. A case report suggests that intravenous miconazole interacts similarly and in theory, miconazole oral gel may also interact. Posaconazole may also modestly raise ciclosporin levels. Rhabdomyolysis has been reported with the combination of ciclosporin and itraconazole, but four of these cases were complicated by the presence of statins.

Clinical evidence

(a) Fluconazole

Fluconazole 200 mg daily for 14 days roughly doubled the ciclosporin trough blood levels of 8 kidney transplant patients, from 27 to 58 nanograms/mL. The AUC increased 1.8-fold but serum creatinine levels were unchanged.[1,2]

Other reports describe two- to threefold rises in ciclosporin blood levels in kidney transplant patients within 6 to 11 days of starting treatment with fluconazole 100 to 200 mg daily.[3-8] One patient developed nephrotoxicity, which resolved when the dosages of both drugs were reduced.[9]

In contrast, some patients have had little or no changes in serum ciclosporin or creatinine levels when fluconazole was given.[8,10-15] This may have been because the interaction is dose-dependent.[14,16] One study found a lack of interaction in females and African-American patients, suggesting that gender and ethnicity may also be factors.[17] Another study found that there was only a 20% increase in ciclosporin levels when intravenous ciclosporin was given with high-dose intravenous fluconazole, which was not considered clinically relevant.[18]

An *in vitro* study suggests that the activity of fluconazole against *Candida albicans* may be enhanced by ciclosporin.[19]

(b) Itraconazole

In 4 heart-lung, 2 heart and one lung transplant patient an average 56% reduction (range 33 to 84%) in the ciclosporin dosages were needed when itraconazole (dosage not stated) was given. Serum creatinine levels rose temporarily until the ciclosporin dosage had been readjusted.[20] Two- to threefold rises in ciclosporin levels were seen in another 2 patients given itraconazole 200 mg daily,[21,22] and in one case the raised levels persisted for more than 4 weeks after the itraconazole was stopped.[22] Intravenous itraconazole 200 mg twice daily for 2 days then 200 mg daily caused a twofold increase in the levels of intravenous ciclosporin in 2 patients.[23]

Other case reports and studies suggest that dosage reductions of about 50 to 80% (where stated) were needed when patients taking ciclosporin were given itraconazole.[24,25,26] Enhanced itraconazole absorption in the presence of a carbonated drink that increased stomach acidity was found to allow decreases in ciclosporin dose and increases in its dose interval.[27]

These reports contrast with another describing 14 bone marrow transplant patients taking ciclosporin. Those given itraconazole 100 mg twice daily had no significant changes in ciclosporin or creatinine serum levels.[28] Another patient required only a 10% reduction in ciclosporin dose when given itraconazole 400 mg daily for 40 days.[8]

Rhabdomyolysis has been reported in 3 lung transplant patients[24,29] and 2 heart transplant patients[30,31] when itraconazole was used in combination with ciclosporin. However, in three of these cases the concurrent use of simvastatin and in one case concurrent simvastatin and gemfibrozil would also have been factors,[24,29-31] as both ciclosporin and itraconazole can increase simvastatin levels (see 'Statins + Ciclosporin', p.1097, and also 'Statins + Azoles', p.1093).

(c) Ketoconazole

Ketoconazole 200 mg daily caused a marked and rapid rise in the ciclosporin blood levels of 36 renal transplant patients. On the basis of experience with previous patients, the ciclosporin dosage was reduced by 70% when ketoconazole was started, and after a year the dosage reduction was 85% (from 420 mg to 66 mg daily). Minimal nephrotoxicity was seen.[32-34] A study in children with nephrotic syndrome found the addition of ketoconazole allowed a ciclosporin dose reduction of approximately 37%. They also found that those in the ketoconazole treated group (153 patients) had a lower frequency of renal impairment, were more likely to be able to stop taking steroids and had a better chance of staying in remission than those not given ketoconazole (54 patients).[35]

Other reports[8,36-50] describe essentially similar rises in ciclosporin levels during the use of ketoconazole. The effects of ketoconazole on ciclosporin were found to be slightly increased (from 80 to 85%) when diltiazem was also given.[51] Ketoconazole 2% cream has been found not interact with ciclosporin 1 mg/kg daily in the treatment of contact allergic dermatitis and the ciclosporin dosage does not need to be reduced.[52] Impaired glucose tolerance has been attributed to the use of ketoconazole and ciclosporin in one patient.[53]

(d) Miconazole

A single case report describes a rise of about 65% in ciclosporin serum levels within 3 days of intravenous miconazole 1 g every 8 hours being started. Ciclosporin levels rose again during subsequent treatment with miconazole.[54]

(e) Posaconazole

Posaconazole 200 mg daily was given to 4 heart transplant patients receiving stable doses of ciclosporin. Three of the 4 required dose reductions of between about 15 and 27% to maintain ciclosporin levels.[55] Although these dosage adjustments were considered low, they do indicate that posaconazole interacts in a similar manner to the other azoles. The manufacturers also report cases of ciclosporin toxicity which resulted in significant adverse effects, including nephrotoxicity and one fatal case of leukoencephalopathy.[56]

(f) Voriconazole

In a placebo-controlled, crossover study, 14 kidney transplant patients receiving stable doses of ciclosporin were given voriconazole 200 mg every 12 hours for 15 doses. Of the 14 patients, 7 discontinued treatment during the voriconazole phase due to adverse effects, 4 due to raised ciclosporin levels (mean 2.48-fold), one due to raised liver function, one due to asthenia, dyspnoea and oedema, and one due to an underlying condition unrelated to the voriconazole. In the remaining 7 patients voriconazole caused 1.7-fold increases in the ciclosporin AUC.[57] Ciclosporin levels were significantly *reduced* in a bone marrow transplant patient, from a range of 150 to 184 nanograms/mL to 56 to 111 nanograms/mL, when prophylactic voriconazole was *stopped* due to abnormal liver function tests. The levels returned to range when the voriconazole was restarted.[58]

Mechanism

In vitro studies show that these azole antifungals inhibit the metabolism of ciclosporin by human liver microsomal enzymes, ketoconazole being the most potent.[59,60] As a result ciclosporin blood levels rise. Fluconazole and ketoconazole also appear to inhibit the metabolism of ciclosporin by the gut wall.[18,46]

Importance and management

The interaction between ciclosporin and ketoconazole is very well established and clinically important. Ciclosporin blood levels rise rapidly and sharply, but they can be controlled by reducing the ciclosporin dosage by about 70 to 80%[8,25,32,38,50] thereby preventing kidney damage. A ciclosporin dosage reduction of 68 to 89% was required over a 13-month period in one study, with no adverse changes in immunosuppressive activity, resulting in a total cost saving of about 65%, partially offset because of the need for more frequent patient follow-up and the cost of the ketoconazole.[32,33] Other studies have suggested that this interaction can be exploited to make cost savings.[47,48,50] Reviews of the pros and cons of concurrent use have been published.[34,61] Ketoconazole may possibly have a kidney-protective effect.[32,33] A study in renal transplant patients suggested that variability in absorption and in the response to metabolic inhibition by ketoconazole made the ciclosporin blood level response difficult to predict and monitor.[62] There are also other confounding factors. For example, a patient who was given ketoconazole to increase ciclosporin levels was subsequently given famotidine. The famotidine raised gastric pH, which resulted in a reduction in the ketoconazole absorption, and the ciclosporin levels consequently fell.[63]

Information about ciclosporin with fluconazole or itraconazole is less extensive, but concurrent use should be closely monitored, being alert for the need to reduce the ciclosporin dosage, in some cases by up to 50% or more, although some patients may demonstrate no significant changes at all. There is also some evidence that in the case of fluconazole, the interaction may possibly depend on its dosage,[14] gender and ethnicity,[17] and the route of ciclosporin administration.[18]

The interaction between *intravenous* miconazole and ciclosporin may be potentially serious and of clinical importance. There is no evidence of an interaction with other forms of miconazole. However, a large proportion of miconazole *oral* gel (both prescription and non-prescription doses) may be swallowed and therefore adequate systemic absorption may occur for interactions with other medications. The manufacturers of miconazole oral gel recommend close monitoring and possible dose reduction of ciclosporin if given concurrently.[64] An interaction with *intravaginal* miconazole would not normally be expected because its systemic absorption is usually very low (less than 2%) in healthy women of child-bearing age.[65]

The manufacturers of voriconazole suggest that the dose of ciclosporin should be halved when initiating voriconazole, and that ciclosporin levels should be carefully monitored during voriconazole treatment. It is important that the ciclosporin dose is increased again as necessary if voriconazole is withdrawn.[58,66,67]

The dose of ciclosporin should be reduced by about 25% when posaconazole is started, with careful monitoring of ciclosporin levels and dose adjustment as needed.[55,56]

Additional caution is required where ciclosporin and azoles are used in patients taking statins, and either ciclosporin dose reduction,[24] replacement of ciclosporin with tacrolimus,[29] reducing the statin dose or stopping the statin[30] have been recommended.

1. Canafax DM, Graves NM, Hilligoss DM, Carleton BC, Gardner MJ, Matas AJ. Interaction between cyclosporine and fluconazole in renal allograft recipients. *Transplantation* (1991) 51, 1014–8.
2. Canafax DM, Graves NM, Hilligoss DM, Carleton BC, Gardner MJ, Matas AJ. Increased cyclosporine levels as a result of simultaneous fluconazole and cyclosporine therapy in renal transplant recipients: a double-blind, randomized pharmacokinetic and safety study. *Transplant Proc* (1991) 23, 1041–2.
3. Torregrosa V, De la Torre M, Campistol JM, Oppenheimer F, Ricart MJ, Vilardell J, Andreu J. Interaction of fluconazole with ciclosporin A. *Nephron* (1992) 60, 125–6.
4. Sugar AM, Saunders C, Idelson BA, Bernard DB. Interaction of fluconazole and cyclosporine. *Ann Intern Med* (1989) 110, 844.
5. Barbara JAJ, Clarkson AR, LaBrooy J, McNeil JD, Woodroffe AJ. Candida albicans arthritis in a renal allograft recipient with an interaction between cyclosporin and fluconazole. *Nephrol Dial Transplant* (1993) 8, 263–6.
6. Tett S, Carey D, Lee H-S. Drug interactions with fluconazole. *Med J Aust* (1992) 156, 365.
7. Foradori A, Mezzano S, Videla C, Pefaur J, Elberg A. Modification of the pharmacokinetics of cyclosporine A and metabolites by the concomitant use of Neoral and diltiazem or ketoconazol in stable adult kidney transplants. *Transplant Proc* (1998) 30, 1685–7.
8. Koselj M, Bren A, Kandus A, Kovac D. Drug interactions between cyclosporine and rifampicin, erythromycin, and azoles in kidney recipients with opportunistic infections. *Transplant Proc* (1994) 26, 2823–4.
9. Collignon P, Hurley B, Mitchell D. Interaction of fluconazole with cyclosporin. *Lancet* (1989) i, 1262.
10. Ehninger G, Jaschonek K, Schuler U, Krüger HU. Interaction of fluconazole with cyclosporin. *Lancet* (1989) ii, 104–5.
11. Krüger HU, Schuler U, Zimmermann R, Ehninger G. Absence of significant interaction of fluconazole with cyclosporin. *J Antimicrob Chemother* (1989) 24, 781–6.
12. Conti DJ, Tolkoff-Rubin NE, Baker GP, Doran M, Cosimi AB, Delmonico F, Auchincloss H, Russell PS, Rubin RH. Successful treatment of invasive fungal infection with fluconazole in organ transplant recipients. *Transplantation* (1989) 48, 692–5.
13. Rubin RH, Debruin MF, Knirsch AK. Fluconazole therapy for patients with serious *Candida* infections who have failed standard therapies. *Intersci Conf Antimicrob Agents Chemother* (1989), 112.
14. López-Gil JA. Fluconazole-cyclosporine interaction: a dose-dependent effect? *Ann Pharmacother* (1993) 27, 427–30.
15. Lumbreras C, Cuervas-Mons V, Jara P, del Palacio A, Turrión VS, Barrios C, Moreno E, Noriega AR, Paya CV. Randomized trial of fluconazole versus nystatin for the prophylaxis of *Candida* infection following liver transplantation. *J Infect Dis* (1996) 174, 583–8.
16. Sud K, Singh B, Krishna VS, Thennarasu K, Kohli HS, Jha V, Gupta KL, Sakhuja V. Unpredictable cyclosporin-fluconazole interaction in renal transplant recipients. *Nephrol Dial Transplant* (1999) 14, 1698–1703.
17. Mathis AS, DiRenzo T, Friedman GS, Kaplan B, Adamson R. Sex and ethnicity may chiefly influence the interaction of fluconazole with calcineurin inhibitors. *Transplantation* (2001) 71, 1069–75.
18. Osowski CL, Dix SP, Lin LS, Mullins RE, Geller RB, Wingard JR. Evaluation of the drug interaction between intravenous high-dose fluconazole and cyclosporine or tacrolimus in bone marrow transplant patients. *Transplantation* (1996) 61, 1268–72.
19. Marchetti O, Moreillon P, Glauser MP, Bille J, Sanglard D. Potent synergism of the combination of fluconazole and cyclosporine in *Candida albicans*. *Antimicrob Agents Chemother* (2000) 44, 2373–81.
20. Kramer MR, Marshall SE, Denning DW, Keogh AM, Tucker RM, Galgiani JN, Lewiston NJ, Stevens DA, Theodore J. Cyclosporine and itraconazole interaction in heart and lung transplant recipients. *Ann Intern Med* (1990) 113, 327–9.
21. Kwan JT C, Foxall PJD, Davidson DGC, Bending MR, Eisinger AJ. Interaction of cyclosporin and itraconazole. *Lancet* (1987) ii, 282.
22. Trenk D, Brett W, Jähnchen E, Birnbaum D. Time course of cyclosporin/itraconazole interaction. *Lancet* (1987) ii, 1335–6.
23. Leather HL, Boyette R, Wingard JR. Evaluation of the pharmacokinetic drug interaction between intravenous itraconazole and IV tacrolimus or IV cyclosporin in allogeneic bone marrow transplant patients. *Blood* (2000) 96, 390a.
24. Malouf MA, Bicknell M, Glanville AR. Rhabdomyolysis after lung transplantation. *Aust N Z J Med* (1997) 27, 186.
25. Faggian G, Livi U, Bortolotti U, Mazzucco A, Stellin G, Chiominto B, Viviani MA, Gallucci V. Itraconazole therapy for acute invasive pulmonary aspergillosis in heart transplantation. *Transplant Proc* (1989) 21, 2506–7.
26. Florea NR, Capitano B, Nightingale CH, Hull D, Leitz GJ, Nicolau DP. Beneficial pharmacokinetic interaction between cyclosporine and itraconazole in renal transplant recipients. *Transplant Proc* (2003) 35, 2873–7.
27. Wimberley SL, Haug MT, Shermock K, Maurer J, Mehta A, Schilz R, Gordon S. Enhanced cyclosporine (CSA)-itraconazole (ICZ) interaction with cola in lung transplant recipients (LTR). *Intersci Conf Antimicrob Agents Chemother* (1999) 39, 4.
28. Novakova I, Donnelly P, de Witte T, de Pauw B, Boezeman J, Veltman G. Itraconazole and cyclosporin nephrotoxicity. *Lancet* (1987) ii, 920–1.
29. Cohen E, Kramer MR, Maoz C, Ben-Dayan D, Garty M. Cyclosporin drug-interaction-induced rhabdomyolysis. A report of two cases in lung transplant recipients. *Transplantation* (2000) 70, 119–22.
30. Vlahakos DV, Manginas A, Childou D, Zamanika C, Alivizatos PA. Itraconazole-induced rhabdomyolysis and acute renal failure in a heart transplant recipient treated with simvastatin and cyclosporine. *Transplantation* (2002) 73, 1962–4.
31. Maxa JL, Melton LB, Ogu CC, Sills MN, Limanni A. Rhabdomyolysis after concomitant use of cyclosporine, simvastatin, gemfibrozil, and itraconazole. *Ann Pharmacother* (2002) 36, 820–2.
32. First MR, Schroeder TJ, Weiskittel P, Myre SA, Alexander JW, Pesce AJ. Concomitant administration of cyclosporin and ketoconazole in renal transplant patients. *Lancet* (1989) ii, 1198–1201.
33. First MR, Schroeder TJ, Alexander JW, Stephens GW, Weiskittel P, Myre SA, Pesce AJ. Cyclosporine dose reduction by ketoconazole administration in renal transplant recipients. *Transplantation* (1991) 51, 365–70.
34. First MR, Schroeder TJ, Michael A, Hariharan S, Weiskittel P, Alexander JW. Cyclosporin-ketoconazole interaction. Long-term follow-up and preliminary results of a randomized trial. *Transplantation* (1993) 55, 1000–4.
35. El-Husseini A, El-Basuony F, Donia A, Mahmoud I, Hassan N, Sayed-Ahmad N, Sobh M. Concomitant administration of cyclosporine and ketoconazole in idiopathic nephrotic syndrome. *Nephrol Dial Transplant* (2004) 19, 2266–71.
36. Ferguson RM, Sutherland DER, Simmons RL, Najarian JS. Ketoconazole, cyclosporin metabolism and renal transplantation. *Lancet* (1982) ii, 882–3.
37. Morgenstern GR, Powles R, Robinson B, McElwain TJ. Cyclosporin interaction with ketoconazole and melphalan. *Lancet* (1982) ii, 1342.
38. Dieperink H, Møller J. Ketoconazole and cyclosporin. *Lancet* (1982) ii, 1217.

39. Gluckman E, Devergie A, Lokiec F, Poirier O, Baumelou A. Nephrotoxicity of cyclosporin in bone-marrow transplantation. *Lancet* (1981) ii, 144–5.
40. Shepard JH, Canafax DM, Simmons RL, Najarian JS. Cyclosporine-ketoconazole: a potentially dangerous drug-drug interaction. *Clin Pharm* (1986) 5, 468.
41. Schroeder TJ, Melvin DB, Clardy CW, Wadhwa NK, Myre SA, Reising JM, Wolf RK, Collins JA, Pesce AJ, First MR. Use of cyclosporine and ketoconazole without nephrotoxicity in two heart transplant recipients. *J Heart Transplant* (1987) 6, 84–9.
42. Girardet RE, Melo JC, Fox MS, Whalen C, Lusk R, Masri ZH, Lansing AM. Concomitant administration of cyclosporine and ketoconazole for three and a half years in one heart transplant recipient. *Transplantation* (1989) 48, 887–90.
43. Schroeder TJ, Weiskittel P, Pesce AJ, Myre SA, Alexander JW, First MR. Cyclosporine pharmacokinetics with concomitant ketoconazole therapy. *Clin Chem* (1989) 35, 1176–7.
44. Charles BG, Ravenscroft PJ, Rigby RJ. The ketoconazole-cyclosporin interaction in an elderly renal transplant patient. *Aust N Z J Med* (1989) 19, 292–3.
45. Veraldi S, Menni S. Severe gingival hyperplasia following cyclosporin and ketoconazole therapy. *Int J Dermatol* (1988) 27, 730.
46. Gomez DY, Wacher VJ, Tomlanovich SJ, Hebert MF, Benet LZ. The effects of ketoconazole on the intestinal metabolism and bioavailability of cyclosporine. *Clin Pharmacol Ther* (1995) 58, 15–9.
47. Kriett JM, Jahansouz F, Smith CM, Hayden AM, Fox KJ, Kapelanski DP, Jamieson SW. The cyclosporine-ketoconazole interaction:safety and economic impact in lung transplantation. *J Heart Lung Transplant* (1994) 13, S43.
48. Keogh A, Spratt P, McCosker C, Macdonald P, Mundy J, Kaan A. Ketoconazole to reduce the need for cyclosporine after cardiac transplantation. *N Engl J Med* (1995) 333, 628–33.
49. McLachlan AJ, Tett SE. Effect of metabolic inhibitors on cyclosporine pharmacokinetics using a population approach. *Ther Drug Monit* (1998) 20, 390–5.
50. Butman SM, Wild JC, Nolan PE, Fagan TC, Finley PR, Hicks MJ, Mackie MJ, Copeland JG. Prospective study of the safety and financial benefit of ketoconazole as adjunctive therapy to cyclosporine after heart transplantation. *J Heart Lung Transplant* (1991) 10, 351–8.
51. Hariharan S, Schroeder T, First MR. The effect of diltiazem on cyclosporin A (CYA) bioavailability in patients treated with CYA and ketoconazole. *J Am Soc Nephrol* (1992) 3, 861.
52. McLelland J, Shuster S. Topical ketoconazole does not potentiate oral cyclosporin A in allergic contact dermatitis. *Acta Derm Venereol (Stockh)* (1992) 72, 285.
53. Kiss D, Thiel G. Glucose-intolerance and prolonged renal-transplant insufficiency due to ketoconazole-cyclosporin A interaction. *Clin Nephrol* (1990) 33, 207–8.
54. Horton CM, Freeman CD, Nolan PE, Copeland JG. Cyclosporine interactions with miconazole and other azole-antimycotics: a case report and review of the literature. *J Heart Lung Transplant* (1992) 11, 1127–32.
55. Courtney RD, Statkevich P, Laughlin M, Lim J, Clement RP, Batra VK. Effect of posaconazole on the pharmacokinetics of cyclosporine. *Intersci Conf Antimicrob Agents Chemother* (2001) 41, 4.
56. Noxafil (Posaconazole). Schering-Plough Ltd. UK Summary of product characteristics, October 2006.
57. Romero AJ, Le Pogamp P, Nilsson L-G, Wood N. Effect of voriconazole on the pharmacokinetics of cyclosporine in renal transplant patients. *Clin Pharmacol Ther* (2002) 71, 226–34.
58. Groll AH, Kolve H, Ehlert K, Paulussen M, Vormoor J. Pharmacokinetic interaction between voriconazole and ciclosporin following allogeneic bone marrow transplantation. *J Antimicrob Chemother* (2004) 53, 113–4.
59. Back DJ, Tjia JF. Comparative effects of the antimycotic drugs ketoconazole, fluconazole, itraconazole and terbinafine on the metabolism of cyclosporin by human liver microsomes. *Br J Clin Pharmacol* (1991) 32, 624–6.
60. Omar G, Whiting PH, Hawksworth GM, Humphrey MJ, Burke MD. Ketoconazole and fluconazole inhibition of the metabolism of cyclosporin A by human liver in vitro. *Ther Drug Monit* (1997) 19, 436–45.
61. Albengres E, Tillement JP. Cyclosporin and ketoconazole, drug interaction or therapeutic association? *Int J Clin Pharmacol Ther Toxicol* (1992) 30, 555–70.
62. Sorenson AL, Lovdahl M, Hewitt JM, Granger DK, Almond PS, Russlie HQ, Barber D, Matas AJ, Canafax DM. Effects of ketoconazole on cyclosporine metabolism in renal allograft recipients. *Transplant Proc* (1994) 26, 2822.
63. Karlix JL, Cheng MA, Brunson ME, Ramos EL, Howard RJ, Peterson JC, Patton PR, Pfaff WW. Decreased cyclosporine concentrations with the addition of an H_2-receptor antagonist in a patient on ketoconazole. *Transplantation* (1993) 56, 1554–5.
64. Daktarin Oral Gel (Miconazole). Janssen-Cilag Ltd. UK Summary of product characteristics, May 2006.
65. Daneshmend TK. Systemic absorption of miconazole from the vagina. *J Antimicrob Chemother* (1986) 18, 507–11.
66. VFEND (Voriconazole). Pfizer Ltd. UK Summary of product characteristics, July 2007.
67. VFEND (Voriconazole). Pfizer Inc. US Prescribing information, November 2006.

Ciclosporin + Benzbromarone

Benzbromarone does not interact adversely with ciclosporin.

Clinical evidence, mechanism, importance and management

Twenty-five kidney transplant patients taking ciclosporin were given benzbromarone 100 mg daily to treat hyperuricaemia. The plasma uric acid levels decreased from 579 to 313 micromol/L and the 24-hour urinary uric acid secretion rose from 2082 to 3233 micromol after 4 weeks of treatment. The plasma uric acid levels normalised in 21 of the patients who had creatinine clearances of over 25 mL/minute. No significant adverse effects developed and the ciclosporin serum levels remained unchanged. The authors of the report emphasise the advantages of benzbromarone over allopurinol because of its efficacy, lack of significant adverse effects and because, unlike allopurinol, it does not interact with azathioprine, which often accompanies ciclosporin treatment.[1]

1. Zürcher RM, Bock HA, Thiel G. Excellent uricosuric efficacy of benzbromarone in cyclosporin-A-treated renal transplant patients. A prospective study. *Nephrol Dial Transplant* (1994) 9, 548–51.

Ciclosporin + Beta blockers

Carvedilol may increase ciclosporin levels in some patients. Atenolol and metoprolol do not appear to interact with ciclosporin.

Clinical evidence, mechanism, importance and management

A study in 21 kidney transplant patients found that when **atenolol** was gradually replaced by **carvedilol** in a stepwise manner, starting with **carvedilol** 6.25 mg daily, gradually increasing to 50 mg daily, the ciclosporin dosage had to be gradually reduced. At 90 days the daily ciclosporin dosage had been reduced by 20% (from 3.7 to 3 mg/kg) to maintain levels within the therapeutic range but considerable inter-individual variations were seen.[1] A retrospective study in 12 heart transplant patients found that **carvedilol** increased the ciclosporin level in 10 patients from a mean of 257 nanograms/mL to 380 nanograms/mL. This required a mean dose reduction of 31 mg daily (10%). In the same study, 20 patients taking **metoprolol** did require any significant ciclosporin dosage alterations.[2] A study in 30 renal transplant patients found no change in the ciclosporin levels of those taking **atenolol** 25 to 100 mg daily.[3]

The reason for the interaction with **carvedilol** is not understood. The manufacturers of carvedilol recommend close monitoring of ciclosporin levels with appropriate dose adjustment when carvedilol is added.[4] Information about other beta blockers seems to be lacking, although metoprolol and atenolol do not appear to interact.

1. Kaijser M, Johnsson C, Zezina L, Backman U, Dimeny E, Fellstrom B. Elevation of cyclosporin A blood levels during carvedilol treatment in renal transplant patients. *Clin Transplant* (1997) 11, 577–81.
2. Bader FM, Hagan ME, Crompton JA, Gilbert EM. The effect of β-blocker use on cyclosporine level in cardiac transplant recipients. *J Heart Lung Transplant* (2005) 24, 2144–7.
3. Hausberg M, Barenbrock M, Hohage H, Müller S, Heidenreich S, Rahn K-H. ACE inhibitor versus β-blocker for the treatment of hypertension in renal allograft recipients. *Hypertension* (1999) 33, 862–8.
4. Eucardic (Carvedilol). Roche Products Ltd. UK Summary of product characteristics, September 2005.

Ciclosporin + Bifendate

Two case reports show that bifendate can cause a gradual fall in the serum levels of ciclosporin.

Clinical evidence, mechanism, importance and management

Two kidney transplant patients were successfully treated with ciclosporin and prednisolone for 30 and 36 months, respectively. When they were given bifendate 75 mg daily for the treatment of chronic hepatitis, both of them had a gradual fall in their trough serum ciclosporin levels. The ciclosporin levels of the first patient fell from 97.7 to 78 nanograms/mL at 4 weeks and to 49 nanograms/mL at 6 weeks. The other patient had a fall from 127.5 to 70.5 nanograms/mL at 8 weeks and to 45 nanograms/mL at 16 weeks. The reasons are not understood. The ciclosporin dosages remained unchanged throughout, and despite the low serum levels that occurred, no graft rejection was seen. When the bifendate was stopped, the ciclosporin levels gradually climbed again, at about the same rate as their decline, to about their former levels.[1] There would seem to be no clear reason for avoiding concurrent use but it would be prudent to monitor the outcome, being alert for the need to increase the ciclosporin dosage. Bifendate is derived from *Schisandra* and is a 'hepatonic' preparation with actions that are not understood.

1. Kim YS, Kim DH, Kim DO, Lee BK, Kim KW, Park JN, Lee JC, Choi YS, Rim H. The effect of diphenyl-dimethyl-dicarboxylate on cyclosporine-A blood level in kidney transplants with chronic hepatitis. *Korean J Intern Med* (1997) 12, 67–9.

Ciclosporin + Bile acids or Ursodeoxycholic acid (Ursodiol)

Ursodeoxycholic acid unpredictably increases the absorption and raises the serum levels of ciclosporin in some but not all patients. Bile acids (cholic/dehydrocholic acids) appear not to interact with ciclosporin.

Clinical evidence

(a) Bile acids (Cholic/dehydrocholic acids)

Eleven healthy subjects were given a single oral dose of ciclosporin on three occasions: while fasting, with breakfast, and with breakfast plus bile acid tablets (**cholic acid** 400 mg, **dehydrocholic acid** 100 mg). The mean ciclosporin AUCs were 7283, 7453 and 9078 nanograms/mL, respectively, indicating that the bile acids increased the absorption of the ciclosporin by 22%. However, a related study in 19 transplant patients found that their 12-hour trough ciclosporin serum levels were unchanged by the concurrent use of this dosage of bile acids over an 8-day period.[1]

(b) Ursodeoxycholic acid

A patient who had previously had his entire ileum removed and about 1 metre of the residual jejunum anastomosed to the transverse colon, had a heart transplant. It was possible to reduce his ciclosporin dosage from 1.6 to 1.2 g daily when he started taking ursodeoxycholic acid 1 to 2 g daily. However, when the ursodeoxycholic acid was stopped, his ciclosporin serum levels became subtherapeutic and severe acute rejection developed. The ciclosporin levels rose once again when ursodeoxycholic acid was restarted, and the ciclosporin AUC was increased by more than threefold.[2] The trough serum ciclosporin levels of a patient with chronic active hepatitis C increased from 150 to 500 nanograms/mL when he was given ursodeoxycholic acid, and it was necessary to halve his daily ciclosporin dosage to keep the ciclosporin levels at 150 nanograms/mL.[3]

In contrast, a study in 7 liver transplant patients found no statistically significant changes in mean ciclosporin levels when a single 600-mg dose of ursodeoxycholic acid was given at the same time as the ciclosporin.[4] Yet another study in 12 liver transplant patients, 6 of whom were cholestatic, found that ciclosporin was absorbed more rapidly after a single dose of ursodeoxycholic acid in 8 patients, but, although 7 patients had some rise in their AUC, the mean 24-hour AUC was not significantly changed. There was no consistent improvement in ciclosporin pharmacokinetics in the cholestatic patients.[5]

Mechanism

When an interaction occurs it is thought to do so because the ursodeoxycholic acid improves micellation of the oil-containing oral ciclosporin formulation so that its absorption is increased.[2]

Importance and management

Information is limited but bile acids do not apparently interact with ciclosporin, while the interaction with ursodeoxycholic acid appears to be uncertain and unpredictable. It would therefore be prudent to monitor the effects of adding or stopping ursodeoxycholic acid in any patient taking ciclosporin, being alert for the need to adjust the ciclosporin dosage. More study is needed.

1. Lindholm A, Henricsson S, Dahlqvist R. The effect of food and bile acid administration on the relative bioavailability of cyclosporin. *Br J Clin Pharmacol* (1990) 29, 541–8.
2. Gutzler F, Zimmermann R, Ring GH, Sauer P, Stiehl A. Ursodeoxycholic acid enhances the absorption of cyclosporine in a heart transplant patient with short bowel syndrome. *Transplant Proc* (1992) 24, 2620–1.
3. Sharobeem R, Bacq Y, Furet Y, Grezard O, Nivet H, Breteau M, Bagros P, Lebranchu Y. Cyclosporine A and ursodeoxycholic acid interaction. *Clin Transplant* (1993) 7, 223–6.
4. Maboundou CW, Paintaud G, Vanlemmens C, Magnette J, Bresson-Hadni S, Mantion G, Miguet JP, Bechtel PR. A single dose of ursodiol does not affect cyclosporine absorption in liver transplant patients. *Eur J Clin Pharmacol* (1996) 50, 335–7.
5. al-Quaiz MN, O'Grady JG, Tredger JM, Williams R. Variable effect of ursodeoxycholic acid on cyclosporin absorption after orthotopic liver transplantation. *Transpl Int* (1994) 7, 190–4.

Ciclosporin + Bosentan

Bosentan modestly decreases ciclosporin levels, and ciclosporin increases bosentan levels. The manufacturer of bosentan contraindicates the combination, because of the possible increased risk of liver toxicity.

Clinical evidence, mechanism, importance and management

In a study designed to assess the effects of bosentan on ciclosporin renal toxicity, 7 healthy subjects were given bosentan 500 mg and ciclosporin 300 mg, both twice daily, for 7 days. Bosentan did maintain renal plasma flow, which is markedly decreased by ciclosporin. However, bosentan was calculated to have reduced the AUC of ciclosporin by about 50%. In addition, bosentan had no effect on the ciclosporin-induced rise in blood pressure, and headache, nausea, and vomiting were a problem with the combination. Moreover, the steady-state AUC of bosentan was raised 1.7-fold when compared with the AUC of a single dose of bosentan.[1] It should be noted that bosentan induces its own metabolism, and after 7 days, plasma levels are about 50 to 65% of those seen after a single dose.[2] Therefore, the effect of ciclosporin on the bosentan AUC may be twice those described in this study (i.e. up to a fourfold increase in the AUC of bosentan). The manufacturers of bosentan say that when bosentan is given with ciclosporin its plasma levels were markedly raised (30-fold after a single dose and three- to fourfold at steady state). They also list ciclosporin as an example of a drug, like bosentan, that inhibits the bile salt export pump, and is therefore expected to increase the risk of liver toxicity when used with bosentan. They therefore contraindicate the combination.[2] Further study is needed, as some consider the combination to have clinical potential.

The combination of **tacrolimus** or **sirolimus** with bosentan has not been studied but based on the information available for ciclosporin, the manufacturers of bosentan advise against concurrent use, but if it is required, close monitoring is recommended.[2]

1. Binet I, Wallnöfer A, Weber C, Jones R, Thiel G. Renal hemodynamics and pharmacokinetics of bosentan with and without cyclosporine A. *Kidney Int* (2000) 57, 224–31.
2. Tracleer (Bosentan monohydrate). Actelion Pharmaceuticals UK. UK Summary of product characteristics, October 2006.

Ciclosporin + Bupropion

An isolated case describes a large fall in ciclosporin levels in a 10-year-old boy given bupropion.

Clinical evidence, mechanism, importance and management

A 10-year-old boy, who had received a heart transplant 6 years previously started taking bupropion 75 mg twice daily in addition to his usual transplant medication, which included ciclosporin. After taking bupropion for 22 days, his ciclosporin level was found to be only 39 nanograms/mL. The last level taken before bupropion treatment had been 197 nanograms/mL. Despite an increase in his ciclosporin dose from 420 to 500 mg daily, the ciclosporin levels fell further, to 27 nanograms/mL. The ciclosporin dosage was then increased to 550 mg daily and bupropion was stopped.[1]

The reason for this probable interaction is unclear, although an interaction via the cytochrome P450 isoenzyme CYP3A4 is a possibility. This appears to be the only reported case of an interaction between ciclosporin and bupropion, and its general importance is unknown.

1. Lewis BR, Aoun SL, Bernstein GA, Crow SJ. Pharmacokinetic interactions between cyclosporin and bupropion or methylphenidate. *J Child Adolesc Psychopharmacol* (2001) 11, 193–8.

Ciclosporin + Busulfan and Cyclophosphamide

The development of seizures in patients taking ciclosporin after bone marrow transplants has been attributed to previous treatment with busulfan and cyclophosphamide. Cyclophosphamide was found to reduce ciclosporin levels.

Clinical evidence, mechanism, importance and management

A study in stem cell transplant patients found that the ciclosporin levels in 47 patients whose pre-transplant conditioning regimens contained cyclophosphamide were reduced to a mean of 149.7 nanograms/mL, compared with a mean of 217.3 nanograms/mL in 56 patients whose regimens did not contain cyclophosphamide.[1] Five of 182 patients receiving allogenic bone marrow transplants developed seizures within 22 to 61 days of starting ciclosporin and methylprednisolone. All of them had received busulfan 16 mg/kg and cyclophosphamide 120 mg/kg as preparative therapy without radiation. Magnetic resonance imaging found brain abnormalities, which resolved a few days after the ciclosporin was withdrawn.[2] The reasons for the effects on ciclosporin levels and the increase in adverse effects seen are not understood, nor is the association between the use of the preparative drugs, the ciclosporin, and the development of the seizure clearly established. The authors of the report[2] recommend that if seizures develop the ciclosporin should be stopped and antiepileptics started.

1. Nagamura F, Takahashi T, Takeuchi M, Iseki T, Ooi J, Tomonari A, Uchimaru K, Takahashi S, Tojo A, Tani K, Asano S. Effect of cyclophosphamide on serum cyclosporine levels at the conditioning of hematopoietic stem cell transplantation. *Bone Marrow Transplant* (2003) 32, 1051–8.
2. Ghany AM, Tutschka PJ, McGhee RB, Avalos BR, Cunningham I, Kapoor N, Copelan EA. Cyclosporine-associated seizures in bone marrow transplant recipients given busulfan and cyclophosphamide preparative therapy. *Transplantation* (1991) 52, 310–15.

Ciclosporin + Calcium-channel blockers

Diltiazem, nicardipine and verapamil markedly raise serum ciclosporin levels but also appear to possess kidney protective effects. A single case describes elevated ciclosporin levels caused by nisoldipine. Nifedipine normally appears not to interact, but rises and falls in ciclosporin levels have been seen in a few patients. Felodipine, isradipine, lacidipine and nitrendipine normally appear not to raise serum ciclosporin levels. Amlodipine has modestly increased ciclosporin levels in some studies, but not in others, and it may also have kidney-protective properties.

Clinical evidence

(a) Amlodipine

Ten hypertensive patients with kidney transplants taking ciclosporin (3 of them also taking azathioprine) were also given amlodipine 5 to 10 mg daily for 4 weeks. The hypertension was well controlled, the drug well tolerated, and the pharmacokinetics of the ciclosporin remained unaltered.[1] However, another study in 11 hypertensive kidney transplant patients found that amlodipine, given for 7 weeks, raised the ciclosporin levels by an average of 40%, without affecting creatinine levels.[2] A review identified two other studies that have found increases in ciclosporin levels of 23% and 43% with amlodipine, whereas four studies have found no change.[3] Amlodipine is reported to reduce ciclosporin-associated nephrotoxicity in a study in patients with psoriasis,[4] and in a review of kidney-transplant recipients.[3]

(b) Diltiazem

A pharmacokinetic study in 9 patients taking ciclosporin found that the addition of diltiazem 180 mg daily increased the trough blood level, maximum blood level and half-life of ciclosporin by 112%, 37%, and 43%, respectively.[5] Sixty-five kidney transplant patients taking ciclosporin and diltiazem were found to need less ciclosporin when compared with 63 control patients not given diltiazem (7.3 mg/kg daily compared with 9 mg/kg daily). There were considerable individual differences in dose requirements.[6] Other studies clearly confirm that diltiazem can raise ciclosporin blood levels.[7-32] In some cases the ciclosporin blood levels were not only controlled by reducing the ciclosporin dosage by 30 to 60%, but it appeared that diltiazem had a kidney protective role (reduced nephrotoxicity, fewer rejection episodes and haemodialysis sessions).[11,22,33-37] Another study found that a reduction in ciclosporin dose of about 21% was required for both men and women during chronic administration of diltiazem 90 mg twice daily, despite reports of higher activity of the cytochrome P450 isoenzyme CYP3A4 in women than in men.[38]

(c) Felodipine

Thirteen kidney transplant patients had no significant changes in their serum ciclosporin levels when they took felodipine 2.5 to 10 mg daily and serum creatinine levels were also unchanged. Mean blood pressures fell from 161/100 to 152/90 mmHg.[39] Another study found no significant changes in ciclosporin levels in patients also given felodipine.[40] A single 10-mg dose of felodipine was found to have beneficial effects on blood pressure, renal haemodynamics, renal tubular sodium and water handling in ciclosporin-treated kidney transplant patients. The effects of long-term use were not studied.[41] A single-dose study in 12 healthy subjects found that the maximum serum levels of ciclosporin 5 mg/kg were slightly raised by 16% by felodipine 10 mg, while the AUC and maximum plasma level of the felodipine were raised by 58% and 151%, respectively, but blood pressures were unchanged.[42] The same group of workers also briefly described acute and short-term studies in groups of kidney transplant and dermatological patients, which found that felodipine 5 to 10 mg reduced blood pressure and opposed ciclosporin nephrotoxicity.[43] A study in heart transplant patients taking ciclosporin found that felodipine attenuated the hypertrophic effects of ciclosporin on transplanted hearts.[44]

(d) Isradipine

Twelve kidney transplant patient had no changes in their ciclosporin levels over 4 weeks while taking up to 2.5 mg of isradipine twice daily.[45] Similar findings are noted in another study.[40] Three other studies in 31 kidney transplant patients confirmed that ciclosporin blood levels are unchanged by isradipine and blood pressures are reduced.[46-48]

(e) Lacidipine

Ten kidney transplant patients taking ciclosporin, prednisone and azathioprine started taking lacidipine 4 mg daily. A very small increase in the trough blood levels (6%) and AUC (14%) of the ciclosporin occurred. The blood pressures fell from 142/93 to 125/79 mmHg, and the 14-hour urinary output rose from 1401 to 2050 mL.[49]

(f) Lercanidipine

The manufacturers of lercanidipine contraindicate the concurrent use of ciclosporin as the plasma levels of lercanidipine were raised threefold by ciclosporin, and the ciclosporin AUC was raised by 21% by lercanidipine.[50]

(g) Nicardipine

Nicardipine 20 mg three times daily raised the ciclosporin blood levels in 9 patients by 110% (from 226 to 430 nanograms/mL, range 24 to 341%). Their serum creatinine concentrations rose from 136 to 147 micromol/L.[51]

Other studies have found increases in serum ciclosporin levels, in some cases as much as two to threefold, when nicardipine was given.[52-58]

(h) Nifedipine

Five of 9 patients who had an interaction with nicardipine (see above) had no interaction when they were given nifedipine.[51] No changes in ciclosporin levels were seen in other studies,[36,59-63] but raised[17,20] and reduced levels[64] have been reported in others. Two studies found that nifedipine appeared to protect patients against the nephrotoxicity of ciclosporin.[65,66] However, there is some evidence that the adverse effects of nifedipine such as flushing, rash[67] and gingival overgrowth may be increased.[68-71] However, another study in 121 renal transplant patients found the prevalence of gingival overgrowth in patients taking ciclosporin was increased (but not to a statistically significant extent) by the concurrent use of calcium-channel blockers (not specified).[72]

(i) Nisoldipine

A 46-year-old man taking azathioprine, prednisolone and ciclosporin after a kidney transplant 18 months previously was given nisoldipine 5 mg twice daily. During the following month his ciclosporin levels rose from a range of 100 to 150 micrograms/L up to 200 micrograms/L and an increase in serum creatinine levels occurred. His ciclosporin dose was gradually reduced from 325 to 250 mg daily, and his ciclosporin and creatinine levels returned to the acceptable range.[73]

(j) Nitrendipine

Nitrendipine 20 mg daily for 3 weeks had no significant effect on the ciclosporin blood levels in 16 kidney transplant patients.[74]

(k) Verapamil

Twenty-two kidney transplant patients given ciclosporin and verapamil had ciclosporin blood levels that were 50 to 70% higher than in 18 other patients not given verapamil, despite similar ciclosporin doses in both groups. Serum creatinine levels were lower in those taking verapamil. Moreover, only 3 of the 22 had rejection episodes within 4 weeks compared with 10 out of 18 not given verapamil.[75]

Other studies have found that verapamil 120 to 320 mg daily can increase, double or even triple ciclosporin blood levels in individual patients with kidney or heart transplants.[24,40,62,64,76-80] Combined use does not apparently increase the severity or prevalence of gingival overgrowth caused by ciclosporin.[81]

Mechanism

The increased ciclosporin levels are largely due to the calcium-channel blockers inhibiting ciclosporin metabolism by the cytochrome P450 isoenzyme CYP3A4 in the liver. Note that, of the calcium-channel blockers, diltiazem and verapamil are the strongest CYP3A4 inhibitors (see 'Calcium-channel blockers', (p.860)). Diltiazem also appears to reduce ischaemia-induced renal tubular necrosis.[82] Other calcium-channel blockers also seem to have a kidney-protective effect. The raised felodipine levels are possibly due to competitive inhibition by ciclosporin of intestinal and liver metabolism, or changes in P-glycoprotein activity.

Importance and management

The interactions of ciclosporin with diltiazem, nicardipine and verapamil are established and relatively well documented. Concurrent use need not be avoided, but ciclosporin levels should be well monitored and dosage reductions made as necessary. Even though ciclosporin blood levels are increased, these calcium-channel blockers appear to have a kidney-protective effect. One study[83] noted that, although calcium-channel blockers increase ciclosporin blood levels, this is of no harm to the patient, since no changes in renal function were observed. With diltiazem and verapamil the ciclosporin dosage can apparently be reduced by about 25 to 50% and possibly more with nicardipine. One case suggests that this is also true with nisoldipine. Several studies suggest that substantial cost savings can be made by combining either diltiazem[13,84,85] or verapamil[24] with ciclosporin. Take care not to substitute one diltiazem product for another after the patient has been stabilised because there is evidence that their bioequivalence differences may alter the extent of the interaction.[27,86] Concurrent use with lercanidipine is contraindicated by the manufacturers.[50]

The situation with nifedipine is not totally clear (no effect or decreases or increases) but it appears to have a kidney-protective effect[63] as does felodipine. The manufacturers of ciclosporin recommend avoiding nifedipine in patients who develop gingival overgrowth.[87]

The situation with amlodipine is also uncertain, but isradipine, lacidipine and nitrendipine appear to be non-interacting alternatives. Many of the calcium channel blockers have a kidney-protective effect.

1. Toupance O, Lavaud S, Canivet E, Bernaud C, Hotton J-M, Chanard J. Antihypertensive effect of amlodipine and lack of interference with cyclosporine metabolism in renal transplant recipients. *Hypertension* (1994) 24, 297–300.
2. Pesavento TE, Jones PA, Julian BA, Curtis JJ. Amlodipine increases cyclosporine levels in hypertensive renal transplant patients: results of a prospective study. *J Am Soc Nephrol* (1996) 7, 831–5.
3. Schrama YC, Koomans HA. Interactions of cyclosporin A and amlodipine: blood cyclosporin A levels, hypertension and kidney function. *J Hypertens* (1998) 16 (Suppl 4), S33–S38.
4. Raman GV, Campbell SK, Farrer A, Albano JDM, Cook J. Modifying effects of amlodipine on cyclosporin A-induced changes in renal function in patients with psoriasis. *J Hypertens* (1998) 16 (Suppl 4), S39–S41.
5. Foradori A, Mezzano S, Videla C, Pefaur J, Elberg A. Modification of the pharmacokinetics of cyclosporine A and metabolites by the concomitant use of Neoral and diltiazem or ketoconazole in stable adult kidney transplants. *Transplant Proc* (1998) 30, 1685–7.
6. Kohlhaw K, Wonigeit K, Frei U, Oldhafer K, Neumann K, Pichlmayr R. Effect of calcium channel blocker diltiazem on cyclosporine A blood levels and dose requirements. *Transplant Proc* (1988) 20 (Suppl 2), 572–4.
7. Pochet JM, Pirson Y. Cyclosporin-diltiazem interaction. *Lancet* (1986) i, 979.
8. Griño JM, Sabate I, Castelao AM, Alsina J. Influence of diltiazem on cyclosporin clearance. *Lancet* (1986) i, 1387.
9. Kunzendorf U, Walz G, Neumayer H-H, Wagner K, Keller F, Offermann G. Einfluss von Diltiazem auf die Ciclosporin-Blutspiegel. *Klin Wochenschr* (1987) 65, 1101–3.
10. Sabaté I, Griñó JM, Castelao AM, Huguet J, Serón D, Blanco A. Cyclosporin-diltiazem interaction: comparison of cyclosporin levels measured with two monoclonal antibodies. *Transplant Proc* (1989) 21, 1460–1.
11. Choi KC, Kang YJ, Kim SK, Ryu SB. Effects of the calcium channel blocker diltiazem on the blood and serum levels of cyclosporin A. *Chonnam J Med Sci* (1989) 2, 131–6.
12. Campistol JM, Oppenheimer F, Vilardell J, Ricart MJ, Alcaraz A, Ponz E, Andreu J. Interaction between ciclosporin and diltiazem in renal transplant patients. *Nephron* (1991) 57, 241–2.
13. Valantine H, Keogh A, McIntosh N, Hunt S, Oyer P, Schroeder J. Cost containment-Coadministration of diltiazem with cyclosporine following cardiac transplant. *J Heart Transplant* (1990) 9, 68.
14. Bourge RC, Kirklin JK, Naftel DC, Figg WD, White-Williams C, Ketchum C. Diltiazem-cyclosporine interaction in cardiac transplant recipients: impact on cyclosporine dose and medication costs. *Am J Med* (1991) 90, 402–4.
15. Maddux MS, Veremis SA, Bauma WD, Pollak R. Significant drug interactions with cyclosporine. *Hosp Ther* (1987) 12, 56–70.
16. Brockmöller J, Neumayer H-H, Wagner K, Weber W, Heinemeyer G, Kewitz H, Roots I. Pharmacokinetic interaction between cyclosporin and diltiazem. *Eur J Clin Pharmacol* (1990) 38, 237–42.
17. Diaz C, Gillum DM. Interaction of diltiazem and nifedipine with cyclosporine in renal transplant recipients. *Kidney Int* (1989) 35, 513.
18. Wagner K, Albrecht S, Neumayer H-H. Prevention of posttransplant acute tubular necrosis by the calcium antagonist diltiazem: a prospective randomized study. *Am J Nephrol* (1987) 7, 287–91.
19. McCauley J, Ptachcinski RJ, Shapiro R. The cyclosporine-sparing effects of diltiazem in renal transplantation. *Transplant Proc* (1989) 21, 3955–7.
20. Castelao AM. Cyclosporine A - drug interactions. 2nd Int Conf Therapeutic Drug Monitoring Toxicology, Barcelona, Spain, 1992. 203–9.
21. Shennib H, Auger J-L. Diltiazem improves cyclosporine dosage in cystic fibrosis lung transplant recipients. *J Heart Lung Transplant* (1994) 13, 292–6.
22. Macdonald P, Keogh A, Connell J, Harvison A, Richens D, Spratt P. Diltiazem co-administration reduces cylosporine toxicity after heart transplantation: a prospective randomised study. *Transplant Proc* (1992) 24, 2259–62.
23. Masri MA, Shakuntala V, Shanwaz M, Zaher M, Dhawan I, Yasin I, Pingle A. Pharmacokinetics of cyclosporine in renal transplant patients on diltiazem. *Transplant Proc* (1994) 26, 1921.
24. Sketris IS, Methot ME, Nicol D, Belitsky P, Knox MG. Effect of calcium-channel blockers on cyclosporine clearance and use in renal transplant patients. *Ann Pharmacother* (1994) 28, 1227–31.
25. Bleck JS, Thiesemann C, Kliem V, Christians U, Hecker H, Repp H, Frei U, Westhoff-Bleck M, Manns M, Sewing KF. Diltiazem increases blood concentrations of cyclized cyclosporine metabolites resulting in different cyclosporine metabolite patterns in stable male and female renal allograft recipients. *Br J Clin Pharmacol* (1996) 41, 551–6.
26. Morris RG, Jones TE. Diltiazem disposition and metabolism in recipients of renal transplants. *Ther Drug Monit* (1998) 20, 365–70.
27. Jones TE, Morris RG, Mathew TH. Formulation of diltiazem affects cyclosporin-sparing activity. *Eur J Clin Pharmacol* (1997) 52, 55–8.
28. Jones TE, Morris RG, Mathew TH. Diltiazem-cyclosporin pharmacokinetic interaction — dose-response relationship. *Br J Clin Pharmacol* (1997) 44, 499–504.
29. Sharma A, Bell L, Drolet D, Drouin E, Gaul M, Girardin P, Goodyer P, Schreiber R. Cyclosporine (CSA) Neoral kinetics in children treated with diltiazem. *J Am Soc Nephrol* (1996) 7, 1923.
30. Wagner C, Sperschneider H, Korn A, Christians U. Influence of diltiazem on cyclosporine metabolites in renal graft recipients treated with Sandimmun® and Neoral®. *J Am Soc Nephrol* (1997) 8, 707A.
31. Åsberg A, Christensen H, Hartmann A, Carlson E, Molden E, Berg KJ. Pharmacokinetic interactions between microemulsion formulated cyclosporine A and diltiazem in renal transplant recipients. *Eur J Clin Pharmacol* (1999) 55, 383–7.
32. Kumana CR, Tong MKL, Li C-S, Lauder IJ, Lee JSK, Kou M, Walley T, Haycox A, Chan TM. Diltiazem co-treatment in renal transplant patients receiving microemulsion cyclosporin. *Br J Clin Pharmacol* (2003) 56, 670–8.
33. Neumayer H-H, Wagner K. Diltiazem and economic use of cyclosporin. *Lancet* (1986) ii, 523.
34. Wagner K, Albrecht S, Neumayer H-H. Prevention of delayed graft function in cadaveric kidney transplantation by a calcium antagonist. Preliminary results of two prospective randomized trials. *Transplant Proc* (1986) 18, 510–15.
35. Wagner K, Albrecht S, Neumayer H-H. Prevention of delayed graft function by a calcium antagonist- a randomized trial in renal graft recipients on cyclosporine A. *Transplant Proc* (1986) 18, 1269–71.
36. Wagner K, Philipp T, Heinemeyer G, Brockmüller F, Roots I, Neumayer HH. Interaction of cyclosporin and calcium antagonists. *Transplant Proc* (1989) 21, 1453–6.
37. Neumayer H-H, Kunzendorf U, Schreiber M. Protective effects of calcium antagonists in human renal transplantation. *Kidney Int* (1992) 41 (Suppl 36), S87–S93.
38. Aros CA, Ardiles LG, Schneider HO, Flores CA, Alruiz PA, Jerez VR, Mezzano SA. No gender-associated differences of cyclosporine pharmacokinetics in stable renal transplant patients treated with diltiazem. *Transplant Proc* (2005) 37, 3364–6.
39. Cohen DJ, Teng S-N, Valeri A, Appel GB. Influence of oral felodipine on serum cyclosporine concentrations in renal transplant patients. *J Am Soc Nephrol* (1993) 4, 929.
40. Yildiz A, Sever MŞ, Türkmen A, Ecder T, Türk S, Akkaya V, Ark E. Interaction between cyclosporin A and verapamil, felodipine, and isradipine. *Nephron* (1999) 81, 117–18.
41. Pedersen EB, Sørensen SS, Eiskjær H, Skovbon H, Thomsen K. Interaction between cyclosporine and felodipine in renal transplant recipients. *Kidney Int* (1992) 41 (Suppl 36), S82–S86.
42. Madsen JK, Jensen JD, Jensen LW, Pedersen EB. Pharmacokinetic interaction between cyclosporine and the dihydropyridine calcium antagonist felodipine. *Eur J Clin Pharmacol* (1996) 50, 203–8.
43. Madsen JK, Kornerup HJ, Sørensen SS, Zachariae H, Pedersen EB. Ciclosporine nephrotoxicity can be counteracted by a calcium antagonist (felodipine) in acute and short-term studies. *J Am Soc Nephrol* (1995) 6, 1102.
44. Schwitter J, DeMarco T, Globits S, Sakuma H, Klinski C, Chatterjee K, Parmley WW, Higgins CB. Influence of felodipine on left ventricular hypertrophy and systolic function in orthoptic heart transplant recipients: possible interaction with cyclosporine medication. *J Heart Lung Transplant* (1999) 18, 1003–13.
45. Endresen L, Bergan S, Holdaas H, Pran T, Sinding-Larsen B, Berg KJ. Lack of effect of the calcium antagonist isradipine on cyclosporine pharmacokinetics in renal transplant patients. *Ther Drug Monit* (1991) 13, 490–5.
46. Martinez F, Pirson Y, Wallemacq P, van Ypersele de Strihou C. No clinically significant interaction between ciclosporin and isradipine. *Nephron* (1991) 59, 658–9.
47. Vernillet L, Bourbigot B, Codet JP, Le Saux L, Moal MC, Morin JF. Lack of effect of isradipine on cyclosporin pharmacokinetics. *Fundam Clin Pharmacol* (1992) 6, 367–74.
48. Ahmed K, Michael B, Burke JF. Effects of isradipine on renal hemodynamics in renal transplant patients treated with cyclosporine. *Clin Nephrol* (1997) 48, 307–10.
49. Ruggenenti P, Perico N, Mosconi L, Gaspari F, Benigni A, Amuchastegui CS, Bruzzi I, Remuzzi G. Calcium channel blockers protect transplant patients from cyclosporine-induced daily renal hypoperfusion. *Kidney Int* (1993) 43, 706–11.
50. Zanidip (Lercanidipine hydrochloride). Recordati Pharmaceuticals Ltd. UK Summary of product characteristics, October 2004.
51. Bourbigot B, Guiserix J, Airiau J, Bressollette L, Morin JF, Cledes J. Nicardipine increases cyclosporin blood levels. *Lancet* (1986) i, 1447.
52. Cantarovich M, Hiesse C, Lockiec F, Charpentier B, Fries D. Confirmation of the interaction between cyclosporine and the calcium channel blocker nicardipine in renal transplant patients. *Clin Nephrol* (1987) 28, 190–3.
53. Kessler M, Renoult E, Jonon B, Vigneron B, Huu TC, Netter P. Interaction ciclosporine-nicardipine chez le transplanté rénal. *Therapie* (1987) 42, 273–5.
54. Deray G, Aupetit B, Martinez F, Baumelou A, Worcel A, Benhmida M, Legrand JC, Jacobs C. Cyclosporin-nicardipine interaction. *Am J Nephrol* (1989) 9, 349.
55. Kessler M, Netter P, Renoult E, Jonon B, Mur JM, Trechot P, Dousset B. Influence of nicardipine on renal function and plasma cyclosporin in renal transplant patients. *Eur J Clin Pharmacol* (1989) 36, 637–8.
56. Todd P, Garioch JJ, Rademaker M, Thomson J. Nicardipine interacts with cyclosporin. *Br J Dermatol* (1989) 121, 820.
57. Bouquet S, Chapelle G, Barrier L, Boutaud P, Menu P, Courtois P Interactions ciclosporine-nicardipine chez un transplanté cardiaque, adaptation posologique. *J Pharm Clin* (1992) 11, 59.
58. Mabin D, Fourquet I, Richard P, Esnault S, Islam MS, Bourbigot B. Leucoencéphalopathie régressive au cours d'un surdosage en cyclosporine A. *Rev Neurol (Paris)* (1993) 149, 576–8.
59. McNally P, Mistry N, Idle J, Walls J, Feehally J. Calcium channel blockers and cyclosporine metabolism. *Transplantation* (1989) 48, 1071.
60. Rossi SJ, Hariharan S, Schroeder TJ, First MR. Cyclosporine dosing and blood levels in renal transplants receiving Procardia XL. *Clin Pharmacol Ther* (1993) 53, 238.
61. Rossi SJ, Hariharan S, Schroeder TJ, First MR. Cyclosporine dosing and blood levels in renal transplant recipients receiving Procardia XL. *J Am Soc Nephrol* (1992) 3, 877.
62. Ogborn MR, Crocker JFS, Grimm PC. Nifedipine, verapamil and cyclosporin A pharmacokinetics in children. *Pediatr Nephrol* (1989) 3, 314–16.
63. Propper DJ, Whiting PH, Power DA, Edward N, Catto GRD. The effect of nifedipine on graft function in renal allograft recipients treated with cyclosporin A. *Clin Nephrol* (1989) 32, 62–7.
64. Howard RL, Shapiro JI, Babcock S, Chan L. The effect of calcium channel blockers on the cyclosporine dose requirement in renal transplant recipients. *Ren Fail* (1990) 12, 89–92.
65. Feehally J, Walls J, Mistry N, Horsburgh T, Taylor J, Veitch PS, Bell PRF. Does nifedipine ameliorate cyclosporin A nephrotoxicity? *BMJ* (1987) 295, 310.
66. Morales JM, Andrés A, Alvarez C, Prieto C, Ortuño B, Ortuño T, Paternina ER, Hernandez Poblete G, Praga M, Ruilope LM, Rodicio JL. Calcium channel blockers and early cyclosporine nephrotoxicity after renal transplantation: a prospective randomized study. *Transplant Proc* (1990) 22, 1733–5.
67. McFadden JP, Pontin JE, Powles AV, Fry L, Idle JR. Cyclosporin decreases nifedipine metabolism. *BMJ* (1989) 299, 1224.
68. Thomason JM, Seymour RA, Rice N. The prevalence and severity of cyclosporin and nifedipine-induced gingival overgrowth. *J Clin Periodontol* (1993) 20, 37–40.

69. Jackson C, Babich S. Gingival hyperplasia: interaction between cyclosporin A and nifedipine? A case report. *N Y State Dent J* (1997) 63, 46–8.
70. Thomason JM, Ellis JS, Kelly PJ, Seymour RA. Nifedipine pharmacological variables as risk factors for gingival overgrowth in organ-transplant patients. *Clin Oral Investig* (1997) 1, 35–9.
71. Morgan JDT, Swarbrick MJ, Edwards CM, Donnelly PK. Cyclosporin, nifedipine and gingival hyperplasia: a randomized controlled study. *Transpl Int* (1994) 7 (Suppl 1), S320–S321.
72. Vescovi P, Meleti M, Manfredi M, Merigo E, Pedrazzi G. Cyclosporin-induced gingival overgrowth: a clinical-epidemiological evaluation of 121 Italian renal transplant recipients. *J Periodontol* (2005) 76, 1259–63.
73. Fourtounas C, Kopelias I, Kiriaki D, Agroyannis B. Increased cyclosporine blood levels after nisoldipine administration in a renal transplant recipient. *Transpl Int* (2002) 15, 586–8.
74. Çopur MS, Tasdemir I, Turgan Ç, Yasavul Ü, Çaglar S. Effects of nitrendipine on blood pressure and blood ciclosporin A level in patients with posttransplant hypertension. *Nephron* (1989) 52, 227–30.
75. Dawidson I, Rooth P, Fry WR, Sandor Z, Willms C, Coorpender L, Alway C, Reisch J. Prevention of acute cyclosporine-induced renal blood flow inhibition and improved immunosuppression with verapamil. *Transplantation* (1989) 48, 575–80.
76. Lindholm A, Henricsson S. Verapamil inhibits cyclosporin metabolism. *Lancet* (1987) i, 1262–3.
77. Hampton EM, Stewart CF, Herrod HG, Valenski WR. Augmentation of in- vitro immunosuppressive effects of cyclosporin by verapamil. *Clin Pharmacol Ther* (1987) 41, 169.
78. Robson RA, Fraenkel M, Barratt LJ, Birkett DJ. Cyclosporin-verapamil interaction. *Br J Clin Pharmacol* (1988) 25, 402–3.
79. Angermann CE, Spes CH, Anthuber M, Kemkes BM, Theisen K. Verapamil increases cyclosporin-A blood trough levels in cardiac recipients. *J Am Coll Cardiol* (1988) 11, 206A.
80. Sabaté I, Griñó JM, Castelao AM, Ortolá J. Evaluation of cyclosporin-verapamil interaction, with observations on parent cyclosporin and metabolites. *Clin Chem* (1988) 34, 2151.
81. Cebeci I, Kantarci A, Firatli E, Çarin M, Tuncer Ö. The effect of verapamil on the prevalence and severity of cyclosporine-induced gingival overgrowth in renal allograft recipients. *J Periodontol* (1996) 67, 1201–5.
82. Oppenheimer F, Alcaraz A, Mañalich M, Ricart MJ, Vilardell J, Campistol JM, Andreu J, Talbot-Wright R, Fernandez-Cruz L. Influence of the calcium blocker diltiazem on the prevention of acute renal failure after renal transplantation. *Transplant Proc* (1992) 24, 50–1.
83. Wagner K, Henkel M, Heinemeyer G, Neumayer H-H. Interaction of calcium blockers and cyclosporine. *Transplant Proc* (1988) 20 (Suppl 2), 561–8.
84. Smith CL, Hampton EM, Pederson JA, Pennington LR, Bourne DWA. Clinical and medicoeconomic impact of the cyclosporine-diltiazem interaction in renal transplant recipients. *Pharmacotherapy* (1994) 14, 471–81.
85. Iqbal S, Holland D, Toffelmire EB. Diltiazem inhibition of cyclosporin metabolism provides cost effective therapy. *Clin Pharmacol Ther* (1995) 57, 219.
86. Cooke CE. Nontherapeutic cyclosporine levels. Sustained-release diltiazem products are not the same. *Transplantation* (1994) 57, 1687.
87. Neoral (Ciclosporin). Novartis Pharmaceuticals UK Ltd. UK Summary of product characteristics, December 2004.

Ciclosporin + Chlorambucil

An isolated report describes a reduction in ciclosporin levels in a patient given chlorambucil.

Clinical evidence, mechanism, importance and management

A woman with B-chronic lymphocytic leukaemia and autoimmune haemolytic anaemia controlled with ciclosporin started taking chlorambucil 5 mg daily because of disease progression. When she reached a total cumulative dose of chlorambucil of 200 mg she suddenly relapsed, and her serum ciclosporin levels were found to have dropped to 60 nanograms/mL from a range of 200 to 400 nanograms/mL. The ciclosporin levels remained low despite a doubling of the ciclosporin dosage and withdrawal of the chlorambucil. Only after one month did the anaemia respond and the ciclosporin levels rise again.[1]

This appears to be an isolated report so the general significance of this interaction is unclear.

1. Emilia G, Messora C. Interaction between cyclosporin and chlorambucil. *Eur J Haematol* (1993) 51, 179.

Ciclosporin + Chloroquine or Hydroxychloroquine

Three patients had rapid rises in serum ciclosporin levels, with evidence of nephrotoxicity in two of them, when they were given chloroquine. Some loss of renal function has even been seen with low doses of ciclosporin used with chloroquine for rheumatoid arthritis. Hydroxychloroquine is expected to interact similarly

Clinical evidence

A kidney transplant patient taking ciclosporin, azathioprine and prednisolone had a threefold rise in ciclosporin blood levels, from 148 to 420 nanograms/mL, accompanied by a rise in serum creatinine levels within 48 hours of starting chloroquine 900 mg daily for suspected malarial fever. On days 2 and 3 the chloroquine dosage was reduced to 300 mg daily. The ciclosporin and creatinine returned to their former levels 7 days after the chloroquine was stopped.[1]

When another kidney transplant patient taking ciclosporin, azathioprine and prednisolone was given chloroquine 100 mg daily for 6 days, his ciclosporin serum levels rose from 105 to 470 nanograms/mL and his serum creatinine levels rose from 200 to 234 micromol/L, accompanied by a rise in blood pressure from 130/80 to 160/100 mmHg. These changes reversed when the chloroquine was stopped, and occurred again when chloroquine was restarted.[2] The ciclosporin serum levels of another patient were doubled by chloroquine 100 mg daily.[3]

A randomised, controlled study in 88 patients with recent onset rheumatoid arthritis found that the addition of ciclosporin (1.25 or 2.5 mg/kg daily) to chloroquine 100 mg daily was moderately effective, but changes in serum creatinine levels occurred. In the presence of chloroquine the creatinine was not significantly altered by placebo or ciclosporin 1.25 mg/kg, but was raised by 10 micromol/L by ciclosporin 2.5 mg/kg, indicating that some renal effects can occur.[4]

Mechanism

Not understood. Both chloroquine and ciclosporin can impair renal function.[4]

Importance and management

Information is limited but it would be prudent to monitor the effects of giving chloroquine to any patient taking ciclosporin, being alert for any changes in renal function, even with low doses of both drugs, and additionally looking for increases in serum ciclosporin levels when using high ciclosporin doses. The authors of the study do not recommend further studies of the combination in rheumatoid arthritis.[4] There do not appear to be any published case reports or studies of an interaction with **hydroxychloroquine**, but the manufacturers note that it has a similar metabolic profile to chloroquine,[5] and would therefore be expected to interact similarly. The same precautions would therefore seem appropriate if hydroxychloroquine is given with ciclosporin.

1. Nampoory MRN, Nessim J, Gupta RK, Johny KV. Drug interaction of chloroquine and ciclosporin. *Nephron* (1992) 62, 108–9.
2. Finielz P, Gendoo Z, Chuet C, Guiserix J. Interaction between cyclosporin and chloroquine. *Nephron* (1993) 65, 333.
3. Guiserix J, Aizel A. Interactions ciclosporine-chloroquine. *Presse Med* (1996) 25, 1214.
4. van den Borne BEEM, Landewé RBM, Goei The HS, Rietveld JH, Zwinderman AH, Bruyn GAW, Breedveld FC, Dijkmans BAC. Combination therapy in recent onset rheumatoid arthritis: a randomized double blind trial of the addition of low dose cyclosporine to patients treated with low dose chloroquine. *J Rheumatol* (1998) 25, 1493–8.
5. Plaquenil (Hydroxychloroquine sulfate). Sanofi-Aventis. UK Summary of product characteristics, March 2003.

Ciclosporin + Clodronate

Clodronate does not appear to alter ciclosporin blood levels.

Clinical evidence, mechanism, importance and management

Ten heart transplant patients taking ciclosporin, azathioprine and diltiazem were also given clodronate 800 mg daily for one week. No statistically significant differences were seen in their ciclosporin blood levels or AUCs while they were taking clodronate. Three of them were also taking simvastatin, two were taking ranitidine and one was taking propafenone, furosemide and cyclophosphamide. There would seem to be no reason for avoiding concurrent use, but the authors of the report suggest that longer-term use of clodronate should be well monitored.[1] There seems to be no information about other bisphosphonates.

1. Baraldo M, Furlanut M, Puricelli C. No effect of clodronate on cyclosporin A blood levels in heart transplant patients simultaneously treated with diltiazem and azathioprine. *Ther Drug Monit* (1994) 16, 435.

Ciclosporin + Clonidine

A child taking ciclosporin had a marked rise in his ciclosporin blood levels when clonidine was also given.

Clinical evidence, mechanism, importance and management

A 3-year-old kidney transplant patient taking ciclosporin, azathioprine and prednisone was given a combination of propranolol, hydralazine, furosemide and nifedipine postoperatively in an attempt to control his blood pressure. Minoxidil was added, but was considered unacceptable because of adverse cosmetic effects. When it was replaced with clonidine, the ciclosporin levels increased about threefold to 927 nanograms/mL, despite a dose reduction. Ciclosporin levels returned to the patient's normal range of 150 to 300 nanograms/mL when the clonidine was withdrawn, and blood pressure was controlled by the addition of an ACE inhibitor. It is possible that clonidine inhibited the metabolism of ciclosporin by cytochrome P450.[1]

As this appears to be the only report of an interaction, there is insufficient evidence to recommend routinely increasing the monitoring of ciclosporin levels in every patient taking these drugs. However, the possibility of an interaction should still be considered if both drugs are given.

1. Gilbert RD, Kahn D, Cassidy M. Interaction between clonidine and cyclosporine A. *Nephron* (1995) 71, 105.

Ciclosporin + Colchicine

A number of cases of ciclosporin toxicity, multiple organ failure and serious muscle disorders (myopathy, rhabdomyolysis) have been seen when colchicine and ciclosporin were given concurrently.

Clinical evidence and mechanism

A patient with a kidney transplant had a transient rise (lasting 2 to 3 days) in serum creatinine and ciclosporin blood levels, from 100 to 200 nanograms/mL up to 1519 nanograms/mL one day after receiving a total of 4 mg of colchicine.[1] Another kidney transplant patient taking ciclosporin, azathioprine and prednisone developed colchicine neuromyopathy (possibly rhabdomyolysis), ciclosporin nephrotoxicity and liver function abnormalities when given colchicine.[2] Acute myopathy (muscle weakness, myalgia) or rhabdomyolysis occurred in a further 11 patients who took ciclosporin and colchicine.[3-9] There is also a report of colchicine-induced myopathy and hepatonephropathy in a heart transplant patient who took both ciclosporin and colchicine.[10] A syndrome of myopathy, gastrointestinal disturbances and mild hepatic and renal impairment has been described in 6 patients and was attributed to the use of colchicine with ciclosporin.[10-12] This may be due to inhibition of P-glycoprotein by ciclosporin and subsequent impairment of colchicine excretion in to the bile and urine, resulting in elevated, toxic colchicine levels.[10]

Importance and management

The overall picture presented by these reports is unclear. It is not known whether the colchicine toxicity is made worse by ciclosporin, or the ciclosporin toxicity is made worse by colchicine, or the reaction is a result of both effects. If concurrent use is thought to be appropriate, it should be very carefully monitored because the outcome can be serious. Rhabdomyolysis appears to be a rare complication and the manufacturer of ciclosporin advises a change of treatment if any signs and symptoms develop.[5] Patients should be reminded to report any unexplained muscle pain, tenderness or weakness. More study is needed.

1. Menta R, Rossi E, Guariglia A, David S, Cambi V. Reversible acute cyclosporin nephrotoxicity induced by colchicine administration. *Nephrol Dial Transplant* (1987) 2, 380–1.
2. Rieger EH, Halasz NA, Wahlstrom HE. Colchicine neuromyopathy after renal transplantation. *Transplantation* (1990) 49, 1196–8.
3. Lee BI, Shin SJ, Yoon SN, Choi YJ, Yang CW, Bang BK. Acute myopathy induced by colchicine in a cyclosporine-treated renal recipient. A case report and review of the literature. *J Korean Med Sci* (1997) 12, 160–1.
4. Noppen M, Velkeniers B, Dierckx R, Bruyland M, Vanhaelst L. Cyclosporine and myopathy. *Ann Intern Med* (1987) 107, 945–6.
5. Arellano F, Krupp P. Muscular disorders associated with cyclosporin. *Lancet* (1991), 337, 915.
6. Rumpf KW, Henning HV. Is myopathy in renal transplant patients induced by cyclosporin or colchicine? *Lancet* (1990) 335, 800–1.
7. Jagose JT, Bailey RR. Muscle weakness due to colchicine in a renal transplant recipient. *N Z Med J* (1997) 110, 343.
8. Çağlar K, Safali M, Yavuz I, OdabaŞi Z, Yenicesu M, Vural A. Colchicine-induced myopathy with normal creatinine phosphokinase level in a renal transplant patient. *Nephron* (2002) 92, 922–4.
9. Ducloux D, Schuller V, Bresson-Vautrin C, Chalopin J-M. Colchicine myopathy in renal transplant recipients on cyclosporin. *Nephrol Dial Transplant* (1997) 12, 2389–92.
10. Gruberg L, Har-Zahav Y, Agranat O, Freimark D. Acute myopathy induced by colchicine in a cyclosporine treated heart transplant recipient: possible role of the multidrug resistance transporter. *Transplant Proc* (1999) 31, 2157–8.
11. Yussim A, Bar-Nathan N, Lustig S, Shaharabani E, Geier E, Shmuely D, Nakache R, Shapira Z. Gastrointestinal, hepatorenal, and neuromuscular toxicity caused by cyclosporine-colchicine interaction in renal transplantation. *Transplant Proc* (1994) 26, 2825–6.
12. Minetti EE, Minetti L. Multiple organ failure in a kidney transplant patient receiving both colchicine and cyclosporine. *J Nephrol* (2003) 16, 421–5.

Ciclosporin + Colestyramine

Colestyramine can interact with ciclosporin in some patients but the outcome appears to be unpredictable.

Clinical evidence, mechanism, importance and management

Four transplant patients taking ciclosporin and prednisolone, given colestyramine for one week, then simultaneously with ciclosporin on the day of testing, had only a very small average increase (6%) in the AUC of ciclosporin, but one patient had a 55% increase and another a 23% decrease.[1] Another study[2] in 6 kidney transplant patients found that colestyramine 4 g daily caused no significant changes in ciclosporin pharmacokinetics. The ciclosporin was given at 8 am and 8 pm, with the colestyramine at noon.

It would seem prudent to separate administration of colestyramine and ciclosporin. It is usually advised that colestyramine is given 1 hour before or 4 to 6 hours after other drugs.

1. Keogh A, Day R, Critchley L, Duggin G, Baron D. The effect of food and cholestyramine on the absorption of cyclosporine in cardiac transplant patients. *Transplant Proc* (1988) 20, 27–30.
2. Jensen RA, Lal SM, Diaz-Arias A, James-Kracke M, Van Stone JC, Ross G. Does cholestyramine interfere with cyclosporine absorption? A prospective study in renal transplant patients. *ASAIO J* (1995) 41, M704–M706.

Ciclosporin + Corticosteroids

The concurrent use of ciclosporin and corticosteroids is very common, but some evidence suggests that ciclosporin serum levels are raised by corticosteroids. Ciclosporin can reduce the clearance of corticosteroids. Convulsions have also been described during concurrent use, and the incidence of diabetes mellitus may be increased following the use of ciclosporin with methylprednisolone. One case of osteonecrosis has been reported with topical betamethasone and ciclosporin.

Clinical evidence

(b) Betamethasone

A patient with psoriasis taking ciclosporin and applying an average of betamethasone 30 mg daily (as 15 g to 150 g of topical betamethasone 0.05% cream or ointment) developed avascular osteonecrosis of the femoral heads of both hip joints.[1]

(b) Methylprednisolone

A study found that the pharmacokinetics of methylprednisolone in patients taking ciclosporin and azathioprine varied widely between individual kidney transplant patients, but the mean values were similar to those found in normal subjects.[2]

The plasma ciclosporin levels of 22 out of 33 patients were reported to be more than doubled by intravenous methylprednisolone and the ciclosporin dosage needed to be reduced in 6 patients.[3,4] Other studies have found that high doses of methylprednisolone increased or more than doubled ciclosporin levels.[5-7] However, another study found that the clearance of ciclosporin was increased by high-dose methylprednisolone, although trough ciclosporin levels were unchanged.[8]

A report describes 4 young patients (aged 10, 12, 13 and 18 years) who had undergone bone marrow transplants for severe aplastic anaemia and who developed convulsions when given high-dose methylprednisolone (5 to 20 mg/kg daily) and ciclosporin.[9] Convulsions also occurred in a 25-year-old woman given ciclosporin with high-dose methylprednisolone.[10]

A study of 314 kidney transplant patients during the period 1979 to 1987 found that the incidence of diabetes mellitus in those given ciclosporin and methylprednisolone was twice that of other patients given azathioprine and methylprednisolone. The diabetes developed within less than 2 months.[11]

(c) Prednisolone or Prednisone

A pharmacokinetic study in 40 patients found that the clearance of prednisolone was reduced by about 30% in those taking ciclosporin when compared with those taking azathioprine.[12]

Another study in patients with kidney transplants by the same group of workers reported a 25% reduction in the clearance of prednisolone in the presence of ciclosporin.[13] Other studies[3,14,15] confirm that ciclosporin reduces the clearance of prednisolone by about one-third, and as a result some patients develop signs of steroid toxicity (cushingoid symptoms such as steroid-induced diabetes, osteonecrosis of the hip joints).[3] These studies have all been questioned by the authors of another study, which found that the metabolism of prednisolone was not affected by ciclosporin.[16]

A comparative study over a year, in two groups of kidney transplant patients taking ciclosporin and azathioprine, one group with and the other without prednisone, found that those taking prednisone had lower trough ciclosporin levels (about 10 to 20%) despite using the same or higher doses of ciclosporin.[17]

There is other evidence that low-dose prednisolone does not increase the immunosuppression of ciclosporin, but it can reduce ciclosporin nephrotoxicity.[18]

Mechanism

The evidence suggests that ciclosporin reduces the metabolism of the corticosteroids by the liver thereby raising their levels.[14,19] Corticosteroids are known to cause osteonecrosis and ciclosporin may depress bone resorption as well as bone remodelling.[1]

Importance and management

None of these adverse interactions is well established, and the picture is confusing. Concurrent use is common and advantageous but be alert for any evidence of increased ciclosporin and corticosteroid effects. It is not clear whether high-dose corticosteroids cause a rise in serum ciclosporin levels or not. Ciclosporin levels measured by RIA (radioimmunoassay) should be interpreted with caution in patients taking high-dose corticosteroids as the levels of ciclosporin metabolites, which can interfere with the test, may be altered.[20] The authors of one report point out that this interaction could possibly lead to a misinterpretation of clinical data as a rise in serum creatinine levels in patients with kidney transplants is assumed to be due to rejection, unless proven otherwise. If a corticosteroid is then given, this could lead to increased ciclosporin levels, which might be interpreted as ciclosporin nephrotoxicity.[4] The contribution of ciclosporin and *topical* corticosteroid to the development of osteonecrosis in the isolated case report is not known. More study is needed.

1. Reichert-Pénétrat S, Tréchot P, Barbaud A, Gillet P, Schmutz J-L. Bilateral femoral avascular necrosis in a man with psoriasis: responsibility of topical corticosteroids and role of cyclosporine. *Dermatology* (2001) 203, 356–7.
2. Tornatore KM, Morse GD, Jusko WJ, Walshe JJ. Methylprednisolone disposition in renal transplant recipients receiving triple-drug immunosuppression. *Transplantation* (1989) 48, 962–5.
3. Öst L, Klintmalm G, Ringdén O. Mutual interaction between prednisolone and cyclosporine in renal transplant patients. *Transplant Proc* (1985) 17, 1252–5.
4. Klintmalm G, Säwe J. High dose methylprednisolone increases plasma cyclosporin levels in renal transplant recipients. *Lancet* (1984) i, 731.
5. Klintmalm G, Säwe J, Ringdéen O, von Bahr C, Magnusson A. Cyclosporine plasma levels in renal transplant patients. Association with renal toxicity and allograft rejection. *Transplantation* (1985) 39, 132–7.
6. Hall TG. Effect of methylprednisolone on cyclosporine blood levels. *Pharmacotherapy* (1990) 10, 248.
7. Rogerson ME, Marsden JT, Reid KE, Bewick M, Holt DW. Cyclosporine blood concentrations in the management of renal transplant recipients. *Transplantation* (1986) 41, 276–8.
8. Ptachcinski RJ, Venkataramanan R, Burckart GJ, Hakala TR, Rosenthal JT, Carpenter BJ, Taylor RJ. Cyclosporine–high-dose steroid interaction in renal transplant recipients: assessment by HPLC. *Transplant Proc* (1987) 19, 1728–9.
9. Durrant S, Chipping PM, Palmer S, Gordon-Smith EC. Cyclosporin A, methylprednisolone and convulsions. *Lancet* (1982) ii, 829–30.
10. Boogaerts MA, Zachee P, Verwilghen RL. Cyclosporin, methylprednisolone and convulsions. *Lancet* (1982) ii, 1216–17.
11. Roth D, Milgrom M, Esquenazi V, Fuller L, Burke G, Miller J. Posttransplant hyperglycaemia. Increased incidence in cyclosporine-treated renal allograft recipients. *Transplantation* (1989) 47, 278–81.
12. Langhoff E, Madsen S, Olgaard K, Ladefoged J. Clinical results and cyclosporine effect on prednisolone metabolism. *Kidney Int* (1984) 26, 642.
13. Langhoff E, Madsen S, Flachs H, Olgaard K, Ladefoged J, Hvidberg EF. Inhibition of prednisolone metabolism by cyclosporine in kidney-transplanted patients. *Transplantation* (1985) 39, 107–9.
14. Öst L. Effects of cyclosporin on prednisolone metabolism. *Lancet* (1984) i, 451.
15. Öst L. Impairment of prednisolone metabolism by cyclosporine treatment in renal graft recipients. *Transplantation* (1987) 44, 533–35.
16. Frey FJ, Schnetzer A, Horber FF, Frey BM. Evidence that cyclosporine does not affect the metabolism of prednisolone after renal transplantation. *Transplantation* (1987) 43, 494–8.
17. Hricik DE, Moritz C, Mayes JT, Schulak JA. Association of the absence of steroid therapy with increased cyclosporine blood levels in renal transplant recipients. *Transplantation* (1990) 49, 221–3.
18. Nott D, Griffin PJA, Salaman JR. Low-dose steroids do not augment cyclosporine immunosuppression but do diminish cyclosporine nephrotoxicity. *Transplant Proc* (1985) 17, 1289–90.
19. Henricsson S, Lindholm A, Aravoglou M. Cyclosporin metabolism in human liver microsomes and its inhibition by other drugs. *Pharmacol Toxicol* (1990) 66, 49–52.
20. Ptachcinski RJ, Burckart GJ, Venkataramanan R, Rosenthal JT, Carpenter BJ, Hakala TR. Effect of high-dose steroids on cyclosporine blood concentrations using RIA and HPLC analysis. *Drug Intell Clin Pharm* (1987) 21, 20A.

Ciclosporin + Coumarins

The ciclosporin levels of a patient were reduced when warfarin was given. When the ciclosporin dosage was raised an increase in the warfarin dosage was needed. The INR of another patient taking warfarin was reduced when she was given ciclosporin. A further report describes a rise in serum ciclosporin levels when an unnamed anticoagulant was given. Other reports describe increased or decreased acenocoumarol effects and decreased ciclosporin levels in two patients.

Clinical evidence

(a) Acenocoumarol

The anticoagulant dosage of a patient taking acenocoumarol needed to be reduced by about half to maintain a therapeutic INR when he was given ciclosporin after a kidney transplant. The required dose of ciclosporin slightly decreased.[1] Conversely, a patient taking acenocoumarol 32 mg per week was given ciclosporin for nephrotic syndrome. After 10 days his acenocoumarol dose needed to be increased to maintain a therapeutic INR, and the ciclosporin level was considered too low and so the dose was increased from 100 to 150 mg daily. However, a further 10 days later (after the increase in acenocoumarol dose) the ciclosporin level was even lower. Eventually the patient achieved therapeutic levels in the presence of acenocoumarol with a ciclosporin dose of 200 mg daily.[2]

(b) Warfarin

A man with erythrocyte aplasia effectively treated with ciclosporin for 18 months, relapsed within a week of starting warfarin. His ciclosporin levels had fallen from a range of 300 to 350 nanograms/mL down to 170 nanograms/mL. He responded well when the ciclosporin dosage was increased from 3 to 7 mg/kg daily, but his prothrombin activity rose from 17% of control to 64% and he needed an increase in the warfarin dosage to achieve satisfactory anticoagulation.[3] The patient was also taking 'phenobarbital', (p.1021). A woman with angioimmunoblastic T-cell lymphoma receiving chemotherapy developed a deep vein thrombosis and was therefore treated firstly with heparin and later warfarin. When ciclosporin 300 mg daily was added, her INR decreased by about 40% and she needed a progressive warfarin dosage increase from 18.75 to 27.5 mg per week.[4] Another report briefly says that serum ciclosporin levels rose in a patient given a warfarin derivative.[5]

Mechanism

Acenocoumarol, warfarin and ciclosporin are all metabolised, at least in part, by the cytochrome P450 isoenzyme CYP3A4. It is possible that some competition occurs for metabolism, leading to increased or decreased effects of the anticoagulants and decreased ciclosporin levels.

Importance and management

Information about the interactions of the oral anticoagulants and ciclosporin seems to be limited to these reports. They simply serve to emphasise the need to monitor concurrent use because the outcome is clearly uncertain.

1. Campistol JM, Maragall D, Andreu J. Interaction between cyclosporin A and sintrom. *Nephron* (1989) 53, 291–2.
2. Borrás-Blasco J, Enriquez R, Navarro-Ruiz A, Martinez-Ramirez M, Cabezuelo JB, Gonzalez-Delgado M. Interaction between cyclosporine and acenocoumarol in a patient with nephrotic syndrome. *Clin Nephrol* (2001) 55, 338–40.
3. Snyder DS. Interaction between cyclosporine and warfarin. *Ann Intern Med* (1988) 108, 311.

4. Turri D, Lannitto E, Caracciolo C, Mariani G. Oral anticoagulants and cyclosporin A. *Haematologica* (2000) 85, 893–4.
5. Cockburn I. Cyclosporin A: a clinical evaluation of drug interactions. *Transplant Proc* (1986) 18 (Suppl 5), 50–5.

Ciclosporin + Danazol

Marked increases in serum ciclosporin levels have been seen in seven patients taking danazol.

Clinical evidence

A 15-year-old girl, one-year post kidney transplant, taking ciclosporin and prednisone, had a marked rise in serum ciclosporin levels over about 2 weeks (from a range of 250 to 325 nanomol/mL up to 700 to 850 nanomol/mL) when she was given danazol 200 mg twice daily, even though the ciclosporin dosage was reduced from 350 to 250 mg daily.[1]

Similar rises in ciclosporin levels, from about 400 to 600 nanograms/mL, and from 150 to about 450 nanograms/mL, were seen in another patient on two occasions over about a 6-week period when danazol 400 mg daily and later 600 mg daily was given.[2] A 12-year-old boy needed a reduction in his ciclosporin dosage from 10 to 2 mg/kg daily when danazol 400 mg twice daily was added.[3] A marked rise in ciclosporin blood levels has been described in 2 other patients when given danazol 200 mg three or four times daily.[4,5]

A pharmacokinetic study in one kidney transplant patient found that danazol 200 mg three times daily for 16 days reduced the ciclosporin clearance by 50%, prolonged its half-life by 66%, and raised its AUC by 65%.[6]

A patient with aplastic anaemia taking ciclosporin was given danazol 200 mg daily for pancytopenia and endometriosis. Within 4 days the patient had epigastric pain and elevated serum ciclosporin and creatinine levels. Danazol was stopped and the ciclosporin dose was halved. Two weeks later abrupt severe hepatic injury occurred and the patient died of hepatic failure, although this was thought to be due to danazol toxicity rather than the interaction.[7]

Mechanism

Danazol is a known inhibitor of the cytochrome P450 isoenzyme system.[3,7] Ciclosporin is predominantly metabolised by the cytochrome P450 isoenzyme CYP3A4. It therefore seems likely that danazol raises ciclosporin levels by inhibiting its metabolism.

Importance and management

Although the information seems to be limited to these few reports the interaction is established. The ciclosporin levels of any patient who is given danazol should be carefully monitored, and dosage adjustments made as necessary.

1. Ross WB, Roberts D, Griffin PJA and Salaman JR. Cyclosporin interaction with danazol and norethisterone. *Lancet* (1986) i, 330.
2. Schröder O, Schmitz N, Kayser W, Euler HH, Löffler H. Erhöhte Ciclosporin-A-spiegel bei gleichzeitiger Therapie mit Danazol. *Dtsch Med Wochenschr* (1986) 111, 602–3.
3. Blatt J, Howrie D, Orlando S. Burckart G. Interaction between cyclosporine and danazol in a pediatric patient. *J Pediatr Hematol Oncol* (1996) 18, 95.
4. Borrás-Blasco J, Rosique-Robles JD, Peris-Marti J, Navarro-Ruiz J, Gonzalez-Delgado M, Conesa-Garcia V. Possible cyclosporin-danazol interaction in a patient with aplastic anaemia. *Am J Hematol* (1999) 62, 63–4.
5. Koneru B, Hartner C, Iwatsuki S, Starzl TE. Effect of danazol on cyclosporine pharmacokinetics. *Transplantation* (1988) 45, 1001.
6. Passfall J, Keller F. Pharmacokinetics of danazol-cyclosporin interaction. *Nephrol Dial Transplant* (1994) 9, 1055.
7. Hayashi T, Takahashi T, Minami T, Akaike J, Kasahara K, Adachi M, Hinoda Y, Takahashi S, Hirayama T, Imai K. Fatal acute hepatic failure induced by danazol in a patient with endometriosis and aplastic anemia. *J Gastroenterol* (2001) 36, 783–6.

Ciclosporin + Disopyramide

An isolated report describes the development of nephrotoxicity, which was attributed to an interaction between ciclosporin and disopyramide.

Clinical evidence, mechanism, importance and management

Ten months after receiving a kidney transplant a 40-year-old woman developed premature ventricular beats and was therefore given oxprenolol in addition to her usual ciclosporin and methylprednisolone. After 2 months she had shown no improvement so she started taking disopyramide 100 mg three times daily. Over the next week her serum creatinine rose from 88 to 159 micromol/L, at which point the disopyramide was stopped. Her renal function returned to normal over the next week. As she had previously been stable taking ciclosporin, and, as nephrotoxicity had not been reported with disopyramide, an interaction was suspected.[1]

This interaction is unconfirmed and of uncertain clinical significance. There is insufficient evidence to recommend increased monitoring, but be aware of the potential for an interaction in the case of an unexpected response to treatment.

1. Nanni G, Magalini SC, Serino F, Castagneto M. Effect of disopyramide in a cyclosporine-treated patient. *Transplantation* (1988) 45, 257.

Ciclosporin + Diuretics

Isolated cases of nephrotoxicity have been described when patients taking ciclosporin were given either amiloride with hydrochlorothiazide, metolazone, or mannitol. Furosemide can possibly protect the kidney against ciclosporin damage. The concurrent use of ciclosporin with thiazides, but not loop diuretics, may increase serum magnesium levels. The concurrent use of ciclosporin with potassium-sparing diuretics may cause hyperkalaemia.

Clinical evidence, mechanism, importance and management

A 39-year-old man taking ciclosporin, whose second kidney transplant functioned subnormally, and who required treatment for hypertension with atenolol and minoxidil, developed ankle oedema, which was resistant to **furosemide**, despite doses of up to 750 mg daily. When **metolazone** 2.5 mg daily was added for 2 weeks his serum creatinine levels more than doubled, from 193 to 449 micromol/L. When **metolazone** was stopped the creatinine levels fell again. Ciclosporin serum levels were unchanged and neither graft rejection nor hypovolaemia occurred.[1]

The kidney transplant of another patient taking ciclosporin almost ceased to function when **mannitol** was given, and a biopsy indicated severe ciclosporin nephrotoxicity. Transplant function recovered when the **mannitol** was stopped.[2] The same reaction was demonstrated in *rats*.[2]

A woman taking ciclosporin had a rise in serum creatinine levels from 121 to 171 micromol/L three weeks after she started to take *Moduretic* (**amiloride** with [**hydro**]**chlorothiazide**). Trough serum ciclosporin levels were unchanged.[3]

Although *animal* studies suggested that **furosemide** might increase the nephrotoxicity of ciclosporin,[4] more recent human studies suggest that it may have a protective effect.[5]

Although ciclosporin and **loop diuretics** are both known to cause magnesium wasting, a review of magnesium serum levels, magnesium replacement doses and diuretic use in 50 heart transplant recipients indicated that magnesium requirements were not altered by the use of ciclosporin with **loop diuretics**. However, the use of **thiazides** with ciclosporin resulted in increases in serum magnesium and decreases in magnesium replacement.[6]

Ciclosporin alone can cause hyperkalaemia, especially if renal function is impaired. Because of this, the US manufacturers suggest that ciclosporin should not be used with **potassium-sparing diuretics**,[7] whereas the UK manufacturers suggest that caution is required with combined use, with close control of potassium levels.[8]

The general importance of all these adverse interactions is not clear, but good monitoring is obviously needed if diuretics are given with ciclosporin.

1. Christensen P, Leski M. Nephrotoxic drug interaction between metolazone and cyclosporin. *BMJ* (1987) 294, 578.
2. Brunner FP, Hermle M, Mihatsch MJ, Thiel G. Mannitol potentiates cyclosporine nephrotoxicity. *Clin Nephrol* (1986) 25 (Suppl 1), S130–S136.
3. Deray G, Baumelou B, Le Hoang P, Aupetit B, Girard B, Baumelou A, Legrand JC, Jacobs C. Enhancement of cyclosporin nephrotoxicity by diuretic therapy. *Clin Nephrol* (1989) 32, 47.
4. Whiting PH, Cunningham C, Thomson AW, Simpson JG. Enhancement of high dose cyclosporin A toxicity by frusemide. *Biochem Pharmacol* (1984) 33, 1075–9.
5. Driscoll DF, Pinson CW, Jenkins RL, Bistrian BR. Potential protective effects of furosemide against early cyclosporine-induced renal injury in hepatic transplant recipients. *Transplant Proc* (1989) 21, 3549–50.
6. Arthur JM, Shamin S. Interaction of cyclosporine and FK506 with diuretics in transplant patients. *Kidney Int* (2000) 58, 325–30.

7. Neoral (Ciclosporin). Novartis. US Prescribing information, August 2005.
8. Neoral (Ciclosporin). Novartis Pharmaceuticals UK Ltd. UK Summary of product characteristics, December 2004.

Ciclosporin + Fibrates

The use of bezafibrate with ciclosporin has resulted in significantly increased serum creatinine and reductions, no change, or increased serum ciclosporin levels. The use of fenofibrate has also been associated with reduced renal function and possibly reduced serum ciclosporin levels. Two studies found no pharmacokinetic interaction between ciclosporin and gemfibrozil while a third found gemfibrozil caused a significant reduction in ciclosporin levels.

Clinical evidence, mechanism, importance and management

(a) Bezafibrate

A kidney transplant patient had a rise in his previously stable ciclosporin blood levels from a range of 150 to 200 nanograms/mL to about 340 nanograms/mL over a 6-week period after bezafibrate 200 mg twice daily was given. The rise was accompanied by increases in blood urea nitrogen and creatinine levels. Renal biopsy found evidence of possible ciclosporin toxicity, and rejection. The patient recovered when the bezafibrate was stopped.[1]

Two other transplant patients (one kidney and the other heart) had a reversible deterioration in renal function when they were given bezafibrate. This was severe in one, and the other had the effect on two occasions. Neither had any changes in ciclosporin blood levels.[2,3] Two other similar cases have been reported, one of whom was subsequently given gemfibrozil without problems.[4]

Another study over 3 months in 40 heart transplant patients taking ciclosporin found that bezafibrate was associated with a rise in serum creatinine levels, although none of the patients had to be withdrawn from the study because of this. The ciclosporin level tended to be lower (198 nanograms/mL at baseline, compared with 144 nanograms/mL after 3 months).[5]

Neither the incidence nor the reasons for these reactions are known, but because the outcome is uncertain and potentially serious, keep a close check on the effects of adding bezafibrate to ciclosporin in any patient. The manufacturers of bezafibrate suggest close monitoring of renal function.[6]

(b) Fenofibrate

Fenofibrate 200 mg once daily effectively reduced the blood cholesterol levels of 10 heart transplant patients from 7.7 to 6.5 mmol/L without significantly altering ciclosporin blood levels over a 2-week period. The only possible adverse effect was an increase in creatinine levels from 145 to 157 mmol/L, suggesting some possible nephrotoxicity. No other clinically adverse effects were seen. However, the authors of this study suggested that longer follow-up studies were needed to confirm the safety of using these drugs together.[7] They followed this up with a 1-year study[8] in 43 heart transplant patients, only 14 of whom completed the study (67% withdrew for various reasons). Fourteen patients had a rise in blood creatinine levels and a decrease in renal function, which improved when the fenofibrate was stopped. There was also some evidence of a reduction in ciclosporin levels in 5 patients, who developed rejection, and 14 patients, who had to stop fenofibrate because ciclosporin levels could not be maintained without adversely affecting renal function.

The evidence from these reports emphasises the importance of monitoring the long-term concurrent use of these two drugs because there are clearly some potential hazards.

(c) Gemfibrozil

Forty kidney transplant patients taking ciclosporin had a reduction in their hypertriglyceridaemia when gemfibrozil was added, and their ciclosporin blood levels and serum creatinine remained unaltered.[9] Another study in 12 patients similarly found that gemfibrozil did not affect ciclosporin blood levels.[10]

However, in contrast to these findings, another study in 7 kidney transplant patients with hyperlipidaemia found that gemfibrozil 450 mg once or twice daily was associated with a decline in trough ciclosporin levels. Levels declined from 93 to 76 nanograms/mL after 6 weeks of treatment and after dose increases in 3 patients the level at 3 months was 88 nanograms/mL. In 8 similar patients not given gemfibrozil, and with the same ciclosporin dose throughout, trough levels changed from 99 to 98 nanograms/mL at 6 weeks and to 123 nanograms/mL at 3 months. In 2 patients there was a significant increase in serum creatinine, and biopsy revealed chronic rejection in one and ciclosporin toxicity in the other. The study was stopped at 6 months because a drug interaction was suspected. The mechanism is not known, but changes in distribution of lipoproteins during gemfibrozil treatment may cause changes in the free fraction of ciclosporin. Ciclosporin absorption may also be reduced. Close monitoring is recommended during concomitant use.[11]

1. Hirai M, Tatuso E, Sakurai M, Ichikawa M, Matsuya F, Saito Y. Elevated blood concentrations of cyclosporine and kidney failure after bezafibrate in renal graft recipient. *Ann Pharmacother* (1996) 30, 883–4.
2. Lipkin GW, Tomson CRV. Severe reversible renal failure with bezafibrate. *Lancet* (1993) 341, 371.
3. Jespersen B, Tvedegaard E. Bezafibrate induced reduction of renal function in a renal transplant recipient. *Nephrol Dial Transplant* (1995) 10, 702–3.
4. Devuyst O, Goffin E, Pirson Y, van Ypersele de Strihou C. Creatinine rise after fibrate therapy in renal graft recipients. *Lancet* (1993) 341, 840.
5. Barbir M, Hunt B, Kushwaha S, Kehely A, Prescot R, Thompson GR, Mitchell A, Yacoub M. Maxepa versus bezafibrate in hyperlipidemic cardiac transplant recipients. *Am J Cardiol* (1992) 70, 1596–1601.
6. Bezalip (Bezafibrate). Roche Products Ltd. UK Summary of product characteristics, November 2005.
7. deLorgeril M, Boissonnat P, Bizollon CA, Guidollet J, Faucon G, Guichard JP, Levy-Prades-Sauron R, Renaud S, Dureau G. Pharmacokinetics of cyclosporine in hyperlipidaemic long-term survivors of heart transplantation. Lack of interaction with the lipid-lowering agent, fenofibrate. *Eur J Clin Pharmacol* (1992) 43, 161–5.
8. Boissonnat P, Salen P, Guidollet J, Ferrara R, Dureau G, Ninet J, Renaud S, de Lorgeril M. The long-term effects of the lipid-lowering agent fenofibrate in hyperlipidemic heart transplant recipients. *Transplantation* (1994) 58, 245–7.
9. Pisanti N, Stanziale P, Imperatore P, D'Alessandro R, De Marino V, Capone D, De Marino V. Lack of effect of gemfibrozil on cyclosporine blood concentrations in kidney-transplanted patients. *Am J Nephrol* (1998) 18, 199–203.
10. Valino RN, Reiss WG, Hanes D, White M, Hoehn-Saric E, Klassen D, Bartlett S, Weir MR. Examination of the potential interaction between HMG-CoA reductase inhibitors and cyclosporine in transplant patients. *Pharmacotherapy* (1996) 16, 511.
11. Fehrman-Ekholm I, Jogestrand T, Angelin B. Decreased cyclosporine levels during gemfibrozil treatment of hyperlipidemia after kidney transplantation. *Nephron* (1996) 72, 483.

Ciclosporin + Food or Drinks

Food and milk can increase the bioavailability of ciclosporin. Lipid admixtures for parenteral nutrition appear not to affect ciclosporin pharmacokinetics.

Clinical evidence

(a) Food or Milk

Patients taking ciclosporin with milk had a 39% higher AUC after food and 23% higher AUC when fasting, compared with other patients taking ciclosporin with orange juice (which is not known to interact).[1] Food more than doubled the AUC of ciclosporin (bioavailability increased from about 21% to 53%) and almost tripled its maximum serum levels, from 783 to 2062 nanograms/mL.[2] When 18 patients with kidney transplants were given ciclosporin mixed with 240 mL of chocolate milk and taken with a standard hospital breakfast, their peak ciclosporin levels rose by 31%, from 1120 to 1465 nanograms/mL, trough blood levels rose by 17%, from 228 to 267 nanograms/mL, and the AUC rose by 45%. Very considerable individual variations occurred.[3]

A study in 10 patients undergoing bone-marrow transplantation and given isocaloric and isonitrogenous parenteral nutrition with or without lipids found that ciclosporin pharmacokinetics are not affected by **lipid-enriched admixtures**.[4]

(b) Soft drinks

A lung transplant patient taking ciclosporin had large variations in his ciclosporin levels, which ranged between 319 and 761 nanograms/mL, on discharge from hospital, which were unexplained by changes in his current medication or ciclosporin dose changes. It was found that on the days when the ciclosporin levels were increased, the patient had drunk a citrus soft drink (*Sun Drop*) at breakfast. These fluctuations resolved when he stopped drinking the soft drink.[5] However, a subsequent pharmacokinetic study in 12 healthy subjects found that neither *Sun Drop* nor another citrus soft drink, *Fresca*, had any significant effects on the pharmacokinetics of a single 2.5-mg/kg dose of ciclosporin. Both *Sun Drop* and *Fresca* were tested, and found to contain bergamottin 0.078 and 6.5 mg/L, respectively (note that 'grapefruit', (p.1034), contains about 5.6 mg/L). The authors note that factors that such as genetic and disease-related variability in ciclosporin metabolism as well as changes in the bergamottin content between batches of the drinks may account for the contrasting results.[6]

Mechanism

The authors of the report of an interaction with a citrus soda drink confirmed with the manufacturers that it contained furanocoumarins such as bergamottin which are thought to inhibit CYP3A4,[5,6] the major isoenzyme involved in the metabolism of ciclosporin.

Importance and management

The food and milk interactions are established, clinically important, and result in an increase in the bioavailability of ciclosporin. The situation should therefore be monitored if any changes are made to the diet of patients taking ciclosporin. Patients should be warned because increased ciclosporin levels are associated with increased nephrotoxicity. Lipid admixtures in parenteral nutrition do not appear to affect ciclosporin pharmacokinetics and it is speculated that they may protect against ciclosporin-induced nephrotoxicity. Close supervision and monitoring is required. There is insufficient evidence to allow extrapolation of the results to bone-marrow transplant recipients with risk factors such as dyslipidaemia, liver, or renal impairment.[4]

The isolated report[5] of an interaction between a citrus soft drink (containing furanocoumarins) and ciclosporin was not confirmed by a subsequent single-dose pharmacokinetic study in healthy subjects[6] and therefore its significance is unclear. The case does highlight the influence diet can have on ciclosporin and it should be borne in mind should any unexpected changes in ciclosporin levels occur.

1. Keogh A, Day R, Critchley L, Duggin G, Baron D. The effect of food and cholestyramine on the absorption of cyclosporine in cardiac transplant recipients. *Transplant Proc* (1988) 20, 27–30.
2. Gupta SK, Benet LZ. Food increases the bioavailability of cyclosporin in healthy volunteers. *Clin Pharmacol Ther* (1989) 45,148.
3. Ptachcinski RJ, Venkataramanan R, Rosenthal JT, Burckart GJ, Taylor RJ, Hakala TR. The effect of food on cyclosporine absorption. *Transplantation* (1985) 40, 174–6.
4. Santos P, Lourenço R, Camilo ME, Oliveira AG, Figueira I, Pereira ME, Ferreira B, Carmo JA, Lacerda JMF. Parenteral nutrition and cyclosporine: do lipids make a difference? A prospective randomized crossover trial. *Clin Nutr* (2001) 20, 31–6.
5. Johnston PE, Milstone A. Probable interaction of bergamottin and cyclosporine in a lung transplant recipient. *Transplantation* (2005) 79, 746.
6. Schwarz UI, Johnston PE, Bailey DG, Kim RB, Mayo G, Milstone A. Impact of citrus soft drinks relative to grapefruit juice on ciclosporin disposition. *Br J Clin Pharmacol* (2005) 62, 485–91.

Ciclosporin + Foscarnet

Acute but reversible renal failure occurred in two transplant patients when foscarnet was given with ciclosporin.

Clinical evidence

A man with a kidney transplant taking corticosteroids and ciclosporin developed a cytomegalovirus infection that was treated with foscarnet 85 mg/kg daily. Despite efforts to minimise the nephrotoxic effects of the foscarnet (hydration with 2.5 litres of isotonic saline daily and nifedipine 80 mg the day before and during treatment) the patient developed non-oliguric worsening of his renal function after 8 days. Nine days after stopping the foscarnet, the former renal function was restored.[1]

A liver transplant patient taking steroids, azathioprine and ciclosporin was given foscarnet 180 mg/kg daily for a hepatitis B infection. Acute renal failure occurred 5 days after the foscarnet was started, and renal function was restored 10 days after the foscarnet was stopped. The ciclosporin blood levels were therapeutic and not significantly altered at any time in either patient.[1]

Mechanism

Not understood. It seems that the nephrotoxic effects of the ciclosporin and foscarnet may be additive.

Importance and management

Direct information appears to be limited to this report, but it is consistent with the known potential toxicity of both drugs. Acute renal failure can clearly occur despite the preventative measures taken. The authors of this report[1] say that monitoring of renal function is mandatory when both drugs are given.

1. Morales JM, Muñoz MA, Fernández Zataraín G, Garcia Cantón C, García Rubiales MA, Andrés A, Aguado JM, Pinto IG. Reversible acute renal failure caused by the combined use of foscarnet and cyclosporin in organ transplanted patients. *Nephrol Dial Transplant* (1995) 10, 882–3.

Ciclosporin + Ganciclovir

Four patients given ciclosporin and ganciclovir developed an acute but reversible eye movement disorder.

Clinical evidence, mechanism, importance and management

In a USA hospital, 582 allogeneic bone marrow transplants were carried out between 1988 and 1994. All the patients were given ciclosporin and about 45% also had ganciclovir at some time during the first 3 months after the transplant. Four patients (0.7%) developed an acute eye movement disorder (unilateral or bilateral sixth nerve palsies) within 4 to 34 days of starting ganciclovir. Three of the 4 patients also had bilateral ptosis. The problem cleared 24 to 48 hours after withdrawal of both drugs from 3 patients, and the withdrawal of just ciclosporin from the other patient. Objective eye movement abnormality with diplopia recurred in one patient when both drugs were restarted, but not when ciclosporin alone was given.[1]

The reason for this toxic reaction is not known but the authors of the report postulate a transient brain stem or neuromuscular dysfunction caused by both drugs.[1] It is an uncommon reaction and reversible, so that concurrent use need not be avoided but both drugs should be stopped if it happens. The report cited here seems to be the only report of this interaction.

1. Openshaw H, Slatkin NE, Smith E. Eye movement disorders in bone marrow transplant patients on cyclosporin and ganciclovir. *Bone Marrow Transplant* (1997) 19, 503–5.

Ciclosporin + Grapefruit and other fruit juices

Grapefruit juice and pomelo juice, but not cranberry or orange juice, can increase the bioavailability of ciclosporin.

Clinical evidence

A considerable number of single and multiple dose studies in healthy subjects, transplant recipients, and other patients with haematological diseases have shown that if oral ciclosporin is taken with 150 to 250 mL (5 to 8 ozs) of **grapefruit juice**, the trough and peak blood levels and the bioavailability of the ciclosporin may be significantly increased. The increases reported vary considerably. Increases in trough blood levels range from 23 to 85%,[1-8] increases in peak blood levels range from 0 to 69%,[4-6,9-13] and increases in AUCs range from 0 to 72%.[2-6,9,10,14,15]

In one study the AUC of the microemulsion formulation of ciclosporin was increased by 38% (range 12 to 194%) by **grapefruit juice** but the maximum levels were unchanged.[16] A further study with the microemulsion formulation found that both the peak levels and AUC were increased by **grapefruit juice**, but while increases of 39% and 60%, respectively, were observed in African-American patients, smaller increases of 8% and 44% were observed in Caucasian patients.[17]

A study in 6 paediatric kidney transplant patients found that giving ciclosporin oral solution with **grapefruit juice** produced a significant increase (109%) in the 12-hour trough level although the AUC was not significantly changed. When ciclosporin was given as a microemulsion, **grapefruit juice** did not significantly affect the pharmacokinetics of ciclosporin.[18] **Grapefruit juice** has no effect on ciclosporin levels when the ciclosporin is given intravenously.[19]

Ciclosporin levels are unaffected by **orange juice**.[2,8]

A study in 12 healthy subjects given a single 200-mg dose of ciclosporin found that **pomelo juice** significantly increased the AUC and maximum level of ciclosporin by about 19% and 12%, respectively, whereas **cranberry juice** did not have any significant effects on ciclosporin pharmacokinetics.[20]

Mechanism

It is suggested that grapefruit juice inhibits the activity of the cytochrome P450 isoenzyme CYP3A in the gut wall and liver. Ciclosporin is primarily metabolised by CYP3A4 and so its levels rise. Pomelo is related to grapefruit and therefore potentially interacts by the same mechanism.

Importance and management

The interaction between grapefruit juice and ciclosporin is established and clinically important, and results in increases in the bioavailability of ciclosporin. Patients taking ciclosporin should be warned about drinking grapefruit juice because increased ciclosporin levels are associated with increased nephrotoxicity. In general, grapefruit juice should be avoided.

It has been suggested[2] that the interaction between grapefruit juice and ciclosporin could be exploited to save money. One group of authors has suggested that grapefruit juice is roughly as effective as diltiazem in raising ciclosporin blood levels, and has the advantage of being inexpensive, nutritious and lacking the systemic effects of diltiazem and ketoconazole which have been used in this way, see 'Ciclosporin + Calcium-channel blockers', p.1027 and 'Ciclosporin + Azoles', p.1023. However, it has also been pointed out that it may be risky to try to exploit this interaction in this way because the increases appear to be so variable and difficult, if not impossible, to control. This is because batches of grapefruit juice vary so much, and also considerable patient variation occurs with this interaction.[21-23] The US manufacturers suggest that patients taking ciclosporin should avoid whole grapefruit, as well as the juice.[24]

The significance of the single report of the small increases in ciclosporin bioavailability and blood levels seen with pomelo juice in healthy subjects is unclear.[20] However, a similar interaction has been seen in a kidney transplant patient taking tacrolimus, see 'Tacrolimus + Grapefruit and other fruit juices', p.1079. There is insufficient evidence to recommend avoiding pomelo juice or pomelo fruit when taking ciclosporin but bear this potential interaction in mind. More study is needed.

1. Ducharme MP, Provenzano R, Dehoorne-Smith M, Edwards DJ. Trough concentrations of cyclosporine in blood following administration with grapefruit juice. *Br J Clin Pharmacol* (1993) 36, 457–9.
2. Yee GC, Stanley DL, Pessa LJ, Costa TD, Beltz SE, Ruiz J, Lowenthal DT. Effect of grapefruit juice on blood cyclosporine concentration. *Lancet* (1995) 345, 955–6.
3. Proppe DG, Hoch OD, McLean AJ, Visser KE. Influence of chronic ingestion of grapefruit juice on steady-state blood concentrations of cyclosporine A in renal transplant patients with stable graft function. *Br J Clin Pharmacol* (1995) 39, 337–8.
4. Min DI, Ku Y-M, Perry PJ, Ukah FO, Ashton K, Martin MF, Hunsicker LG. Effect of grapefruit juice on cyclosporine pharmacokinetics in renal transplant patients. *Transplantation* (1996) 62, 123–5.
5. Herlitz H, Edgar B, Hedner T, Lidman K, Karlberg I. Grapefruit juice: a possible source of variability in blood concentration of cyclosporin A. *Nephrol Dial Transplant* (1993) 8, 375.
6. Brunner L, Munar MY, Vallian J, Wolfson M, Stennett DJ, Meyer MM, Bennett WM. Interaction between cyclosporine and grapefruit juice requires long-term ingestion in stable renal transplant recipients. *Pharmacotherapy* (1998) 18, 23–9.
7. Emilia G, Longo G, Bertesi M, Gandini G, Ferrara L, Valenti C. Clinical interaction between grapefruit juice and cyclosporine: is there any interest for the hematologists? *Blood* (1998) 91, 362–3.
8. Edwards DJ, Fitzsimmons ME, Schuetz EG, Yasuda K, Ducharme MP, Warbasse LH, Woster PM, Schuetz JD, Watkins P. 6',7'-dihydroxybergamottin in grapefruit juice and Seville orange juice: effects on cyclosporine disposition, enterocyte CYP3A4, and P-glycoprotein. *Clin Pharmacol Ther* (1999) 65, 237–44.
9. Ku Y-M, Min DI, Flanigan M. Effect of grapefruit juice on the pharmacokinetics of microemulsion cyclosporine and its metabolite in healthy volunteers: does the formulation difference matter? *J Clin Pharmacol* (1998) 38, 959–65.
10. Proppe D, Visser K, Hoch O, Bartels R, Meier H, McLean AJ. Differential influence on cyclosporin A metabolism by chronic grapefruit juice exposure. *Eur J Clin Invest* (1996) 26 (Suppl 1), A20.
11. Ioannides-Demos LL, Christophidis N, Ryan P, Angelis P, Liolios L, McLean AJ. Dosing implications of a clinical interaction between grapefruit juice and cyclosporine and metabolite concentrations in patients with autoimmune diseases. *J Rheumatol* (1997) 24, 49–54.
12. Hollander AAMJ, van Rooij J, Lentjes EGWM, Arbouw F, van Bree JB, Schoemaker RC, van Es LA, van der Woude FJ, Cohen AF. The effect of grapefruit juice on cyclosporine and prednisone metabolism in transplant patients. *Clin Pharmacol Ther* (1995) 57, 318–24.
13. Mehrsai AR, Pourmand G, Mansour D, Zand S, Rezaali A. Effect of grapefruit juice on serum concentration of cyclosporine in Iranian renal transplant patients. *Transplant Proc* (2003) 35, 2739–41.
14. Yee GC, Adams VR, Pessa L, Braddock RJ, Ruiz J, Lowenthal DT. Comparison of one versus two doses of grapefruit juice on oral cyclosporine pharmacokinetics. *Pharmacotherapy* (1997) 17, 1112.
15. Proppe D, Visser K, Bartels R, Hoch O, Meyer H, McLean AJ. Grapefruit juice selectively modifies cyclosporin A metabolite patterns in renal transplant patients. *Clin Pharmacol Ther* (1996) 59, 138.
16. Bistrup C, Nielsen FT, Jeppesen UE, Dieperink H. Effect of grapefruit juice on Sandimmun Neoral® absorption among stable renal allograft recipients. *Nephrol Dial Transplant* (2001) 16, 373–7.
17. Lee M, Min DI, Ku Y-M, Flanigan M. Effect of grapefruit juice on pharmacokinetics of microemulsion cyclosporine in African American subjects compared with Caucasian subjects: does ethnic difference matter? *J Clin Pharmacol* (2001) 41, 317–23.
18. Brunner LJ, Pai K-S, Munar MY, Lande MB, Olyaei AJ, Mowry JA. Effect of grapefruit juice on cyclosporin A pharmacokinetics in pediatric renal transplant patients. *Pediatr Transplant* (2000) 4, 313–21.
19. Ducharme MP, Warbasse LH, Edwards DJ. Disposition of intravenous and oral cyclosporine after administration with grapefruit juice. *Clin Pharmacol Ther* (1995) 57, 485–91.
20. Grenier J, Fradette C, Morelli G, Merritt GJ, Vranderick M, Ducharme MP. Pomelo juice, but not cranberry juice, affects the pharmacokinetics of cyclosporine in humans. *Clin Pharmacol Ther* (2006) 79, 255–62.
21. Johnston A, Holt DW. Effect of grapefruit juice on blood cyclosporin concentration. *Lancet* (1995) 346, 122–3.
22. Hollander AAMJ, van der Woude FJ, Cohen AF. Effect of grapefruit juice on blood cyclosporin concentration. *Lancet* (1995) 346, 123.
23. Yee GC, Lowenthal DT. Effect of grapefruit juice on blood cyclosporin concentration. *Lancet* (1995) 346, 123–4.
24. Neoral (Ciclosporin). Novartis. US Prescribing information, August 2005.

Ciclosporin + Griseofulvin

An isolated report describes decreased ciclosporin levels in a patient given griseofulvin.

Clinical evidence, mechanism, importance and management

A 57-year-old-man, who had been stable for almost one year taking ciclosporin, azathioprine and prednisolone following a kidney transplant, was given griseofulvin 500 mg daily for onychomycosis. Two weeks later his trough ciclosporin levels had dropped from 90 to 50 nanograms/mL and remained low, despite an increase in his ciclosporin dose from 2.8 to 4.8 mg/kg. When the griseofulvin was later stopped, his ciclosporin levels rose to over 200 nanograms/mL and his dose of ciclosporin was readjusted.[1]

This appears to be the only report of an interaction with griseofulvin, and its general significance is unclear.

1. Abu-Romeh SH, Rashed A. Ciclosporin A and griseofulvin: another drug interaction. *Nephron* (1991) 58, 237.

Ciclosporin + H_2-receptor antagonists

Reports are inconsistent. Cimetidine and famotidine have been reported to increase ciclosporin levels, whereas in other studies cimetidine, famotidine and ranitidine have been reported to not affect ciclosporin levels. Both cimetidine and ranitidine have been reported to cause an increase in serum creatinine levels, in some but not all studies, but this may possibly not be a reliable indicator of increased nephrotoxicity. Isolated cases of thrombocytopenia and hepatotoxicity have been reported with ranitidine and ciclosporin.

Clinical evidence

(a) Cimetidine

A study in 5 liver transplant patients taking ciclosporin found that cimetidine 800 mg given every 12 hours for 3 doses raised peak ciclosporin levels, but no changes in trough levels were seen after 4 hours. Similarly, no change in trough ciclosporin levels was seen in 2 patients who received cimetidine 400 mg four times daily for 4 weeks, and the conclusion was reached that it was safe to use cimetidine over at least a 4-week period.[1] In a retrospective study it was reported that heart transplant patients taking cimetidine had a lower dosage/level quotient leading to higher ciclosporin blood levels for the same dosage.[2] Similarly, a study in 6 healthy subjects found a 30% rise in the AUC of ciclosporin 300 mg given after a 3-day course of cimetidine 400 mg daily.[3] Raised ciclosporin blood levels have also been seen in a patient given cimetidine and metronidazole[4] (see 'Ciclosporin + Antibacterials; Metronidazole', p.1017).

Cimetidine or **ranitidine** increased the mean serum creatinine levels in 7 kidney transplant patients taking ciclosporin by 41%, from 202 to 285 micromol/L. All of the patients had a rise, whereas only 2 out of 5 other patients with heart transplants had a rise in their serum creatinine levels when given either cimetidine or **ranitidine**, nevertheless the mean rise was 37%, from 152 to 209 micromol/L. Ciclosporin levels were not altered.[5] A transient increase in creatinine serum levels at days 2 and 5 was seen in another study of 7 kidney transplant patients given cimetidine 400 mg daily for 7 days. Again ciclosporin levels were not altered.[6] Similarly, cimetidine did not alter ciclosporin blood levels in 2 studies in healthy subjects.[7,8]

(b) Famotidine

Famotidine is reported not to affect ciclosporin blood levels.[9-11] However, higher ciclosporin blood levels were found in a study of heart transplant patients given famotidine.[2] No significant changes in the pharmacokinetics of ciclosporin was seen in a single-dose study in 8 healthy subjects[8] and no changes in serum creatinine or BUN levels were seen in 7 kidney transplant patients.[11]

(c) Ranitidine

One report (see *Cimetidine* above), where the effects of cimetidine and ranitidine were examined together, suggests that ranitidine raises creatinine levels in patients taking ciclosporin, without affecting ciclosporin levels.[5] Similarly, several other reports say that ranitidine does not alter ciclosporin blood levels.[12-15] One also notes that ranitidine does not alter creatinine levels and inulin clearance.[13]

A report describes thrombocytopenia in a man taking ciclosporin after a kidney transplant who was given ranitidine.[16] Another patient experienced hepatotoxicity while taking ciclosporin with ranitidine.[17]

Mechanism

It is not clear why these reports are inconsistent, nor how the H_2-receptor antagonists might raise ciclosporin blood levels. It has also been suggested that any rise in serum creatinine levels could simply be because these H_2-receptor antagonists compete with creatinine for secretion by the kidney tubules, and therefore rises are not an indicator of nephrotoxicity[18,19]

Importance and management

Information about the possible interactions of ciclosporin and cimetidine, famotidine or ranitidine is inconsistent, but there appear to be very few reports of confirmed toxicity. Moreover the reported increases in serum creatinine levels seen with the H_2-receptor antagonists may not be a reflection of increased nephrotoxicity (see 'Mechanism'). Thus there is little to suggest that concurrent use should be avoided, but good initial monitoring is advisable.

1. Puff MR, Carey WD. The effect of cimetidine on cyclosporine A levels in liver transplant recipients: a preliminary report. *Am J Gastroenterol* (1992) 87, 287–91.
2. Reichenspurner H, Meiser BM, Muschiol F, Nolltert G, Überfuhr P, Markewitz A, Wagner F, Pfeiffer M, Reichart B. The influence of gastrointestinal agents on resorption and metabolism of cyclosporine after heart transplantation: experimental and clinical results. *J Heart Lung Transplant* (1993) 12, 987–92.
3. Choi J-S, Choi I, Min DI. Effect of cimetidine on pharmacokinetics of cyclosporine in healthy volunteers. *Pharmacotherapy* (1997) 17, 1120.
4. Zylber-Katz E, Rubinger D, Berlatzky Y. Cyclosporine interactions with metronidazole and cimetidine. *Drug Intell Clin Pharm* (1988) 22, 504–5.
5. Jarowenko MV, Van Buren CT, Kramer WG, Lorber MI, Flechner SM, Kahan BD. Ranitidine, cimetidine, and the cyclosporine-treated recipient. *Transplantation* (1986) 42, 311–12.
6. Barn YM, Ramos EL, Balagtas RS, Peterson JC, Karlix JL. Cimetidine or ranitidine in prophylactic doses do not affect renal function or cyclosporine levels in renal transplant patients (RTP). *J Am Soc Nephrol* (1993) 4, 925.
7. Freeman DJ, Laupacis A, Keown P, Stiller C, Carruthers G. The effect of agents that alter drug metabolizing enzyme activity on the pharmacokinetics of cyclosporine. *Ann R Coll Physicians Surg Can* (1984) 17, 301.
8. Shaefer MS, Rossi SJ, McGuire TR, Schaaf LJ, Collier DS, Stratta RJ. Evaluation of the pharmacokinetic interaction between cimetidine or famotidine and cyclosporine in healthy men. *Ann Pharmacother* (1995) 29, 1088–91.
9. Schütz A, Kemkes BM. Ciclosporinspiegel unter Gabe von Famotidin. *Fortschr Med* (1990) 23, 457–8.
10. Morel D, Bannwarth B, Vinçon G, Penouil F, Elouaer-Blanc L, Aparicio M, Potaux L. Effect of famotidine on renal transplant patients treated with ciclosporine A. *Fundam Clin Pharmacol* (1993) 7, 167–70.
11. Inoue S, Sugimoto H, Nagao T, Akiyama N. Does H_2-receptor antagonist alter the renal function of cyclosporine-treated kidney grafts? *Jpn J Surg* (1990) 20, 553–8.
12. Zazgornik J, Schindler J, Gremmel F, Balcke P, Kopsa H, Derfler K, Minar E. Ranitidine does not influence the blood ciclosporin levels in renal transplant patients (RTP). *Kidney Int* (1985) 28, 401.
13. Jadoul M, Hené RJ. Ranitidine and the cyclosporine-treated recipient. *Transplantation* (1989) 48, 359.
14. Popovic J, Cameron JS. Effects of ranitidine on renal function in transplant recipients. *Nephrol Dial Transplant* (1990) 5, 980–1.
15. Tsang VT, Johnston A, Heritier F, Leaver N, Hodson ME, Yacoub M. Cyclosporin pharmacokinetics in heart-lung transplant recipients with cystic fibrosis. *Eur J Clin Pharmacol* (1994) 46, 261–5.
16. Bailey RR, Walker RJ, Swainson CP. Some new problems with cyclosporin A? *N Z Med J* (1985) 98, 915–6.
17. Hiesse C, Cantarovich M, Santelli C, Francais P, Charpentier B, Fries D, Buffet C. Ranitidine hepatotoxicity in a renal transplant patient. *Lancet* (1985) i, 1280.
18. Pachon J, Lorber MI, Bia MJ. Effects of H_2-receptor antagonists on renal function in cyclosporine-treated renal transplant patients. *Transplantation* (1989) 47, 254–9.
19. Lewis SM, McClosky WW. Potentiation of nephrotoxicity by H_2-antagonists in patients receiving cyclosporine. *Ann Pharmacother* (1997) 31, 363–5.

Ciclosporin + Herbal medicines; Alfalfa and Black cohosh

An isolated report describes acute rejection and vasculitis with black cohosh and/or alfalfa in a renal transplant patient taking ciclosporin.

Clinical evidence, mechanism, importance and management

A stable kidney transplant patient taking ciclosporin 75 mg twice daily began to take alfalfa (*Medicago sativa*) and black cohosh (*Cimicifuga racemosa*) supplements on medical advice. Her serum creatinine rose from between about 97 to 124 micromol/L up to 168 micromol/L in 4 weeks and, to 256 micromol/L at 6 weeks with no associated change in her ciclosporin levels. Severe acute rejection with vasculitis was diagnosed and treated with corticosteroids and anti-T lymphocyte immunoglobulin. Alfalfa has been reported to cause worsening of lupus and immunostimulation and it was suggested that immunostimulation may have contributed to the acute rejection in this patient.[1] The evidence of for this interaction is limited, but as the effects were so severe in this case it would seem prudent to avoid concurrent use.

1. Light TD, Light JA. Acute renal transplant rejection possibly related to herbal medications. *Am J Transplant* (2003) 3, 1608–9.

Ciclosporin + Herbal medicines; Berberine

Berberine appears to increase the bioavailability and trough blood levels of ciclosporin.

Clinical evidence, mechanism, importance and management

A study in 6 kidney transplant patients looked at the effects of the Chinese herbal medicine berberine on the pharmacokinetics of ciclosporin. The patients were taking ciclosporin 3 mg/kg twice daily for an average of 12 days before berberine 200 mg three times daily for 12 days was added. The AUC and trough blood levels of ciclosporin were increased by 34.5% and 88.3%, respectively. The peak ciclosporin level was decreased but this was not statistically significant.[1] A clinical study by the same authors in 52 kidney transplant patients stable taking ciclosporin and given berberine 200 mg three times daily for 3 months found that the ciclosporin trough levels were increased by 24.4% in the berberine-treated group, when compared with 52 similar patients taking ciclosporin without berberine. The ciclosporin levels in 8 patients fell after berberine was stopped.[1]

A single-dose study in healthy subjects found conflicting results. Six subjects given a single 6-mg/kg dose of ciclosporin daily found that berberine 300 mg twice daily, taken for 10 days before the dose of ciclosporin, had no significant effects on the pharmacokinetics of ciclosporin. However, a separate study in another 6 subjects given a single 3-mg/kg dose of ciclosporin found that a single 300 mg dose of berberine increased the AUC of ciclosporin by 19.2%.[2]

The mechanism for the increase in ciclosporin levels is unclear. Although the increase is not sufficiently severe to suggest that concurrent use should be avoided, it may make ciclosporin levels less stable and therefore be undesirable (see 'drug-herb interactions', (p.10)). If concurrent use is undertaken it should be well monitored.

1. Wu X, Li Q, Xin H, Yu A, Zhong M. Effects of berberine on the blood concentration of cyclosporin A in renal transplanted recipients: clinical and pharmacokinetic study. *Eur J Clin Pharmacol* (2005) 61, 567–72.
2. Xin HW, Wu XC, Li Q, Yu AR, Zhong MY, Liu YY. The effects of berberine on the pharmacokinetics of cyclosporin A in healthy volunteers. *Methods Find Exp Clin Pharmacol* (2006) 28, 25–9.

Ciclosporin + Herbal medicines; *Geum chiloense*

A single case report describes a marked and rapid increase in the serum ciclosporin levels of a man after he drank an infusion of *Geum chiloense.*

Clinical evidence, mechanism, importance and management

A 54-year-old kidney transplant patient taking ciclosporin, prednisone, azathioprine, diltiazem and nifedipine had a sudden and very marked rise in his ciclosporin levels from his usual range of 60 to 90 [mg/dL] up to a range of 469 to 600 [mg/dL]. He had been taking ciclosporin 2 to 3 mg/kg daily for 15 months since the transplant. His serum creatinine levels were found to be 115 micromol/L. It eventually turned out that about 2 weeks earlier he had started to drink an infusion of *Geum chiloense* (or *Geum quellyon),* a herbal remedy claimed to increase virility and to treat prostatism. When the herbal remedy was stopped, his serum ciclosporin levels rapidly returned to their normal values. The reasons for this apparent interaction are not known.[1]

This appears to be the only case on record but it serves, along with reports about other herbs, to emphasise that herbal remedies may not be safe just because they are 'natural'. In this instance the herbal remedy markedly increased the potential nephrotoxicity of the ciclosporin. Patients should be warned.

1. Duclos J, Goecke H. "Hierba del clavo" *(Geum chiloense)* interfiere niveles de ciclosporin: potencial riesgo para trasplantados. *Rev Med Chil* (2001) 129, 789–90.

Ciclosporin + Herbal medicines; Quercetin

A study found that quercetin increased the bioavailability of ciclosporin.

Clinical evidence, mechanism, importance and management

In a study in 8 healthy subjects a single 300-mg dose of ciclosporin was given four times: alone, with oral quercetin 5 mg/kg, 30 minutes after oral quercetin 5 mg/kg, or after a 3-day course of quercetin 5 mg/kg twice daily. It was found that the AUC of ciclosporin was increased by 16% by the concurrent use of a single dose of quercetin, by 36% when given after single-dose quercetin, and by 46% when given after multiple-dose quercetin. These correlate with results from previous *animal* studies.[1] Quercetin is a flavonoid, found in many foods and drinks as well as supplements such as ginkgo, and it has also been found to affect the cytochrome P450 isoenzyme CYP3A4, the main isoenzyme involved in ciclosporin metabolism. Quercetin is also found in citrus fruits. Although the increase in ciclosporin levels is modest, and the interaction is not sufficiently severe to suggest that concurrent use should be avoided, it may make ciclosporin levels less stable as the quercetin content of different herbs and preparations is likely to vary. Concurrent use may therefore be undesirable. If concurrent use of ciclosporin and a quercetin-containing product is undertaken it should be well monitored.

1. Choi JS, Choi BC, Choi KE. Effect of quercetin on the pharmacokinetics of oral cyclosporine. *Am J Health-Syst Pharm* (2004) 61, 2406–9.

Ciclosporin + Herbal medicines; Red yeast rice (*Monascus purpureus*)

Red yeast rice has been reported to cause rhabdomyolysis in a kidney transplant patient taking ciclosporin.

Clinical evidence, mechanism, importance and management

A kidney transplant patient taking ciclosporin 300 mg daily developed asymptomatic rhabdomyolysis when she started to take a herbal preparation of red yeast rice (*Monascus purpureus*) containing rice fermented with red yeast, beta-sitosterol, danshen root (*Salvia mitorriza*) and garlic bulb (*Allium sativum*). Two months later, her creatine phosphokinase rose to 1050 units/L but reduced to 600 units/L 2 weeks after stopping the herbal preparation. It is thought that a component of the red yeast rice called monacolin K (identical to lovastatin) probably caused the muscle toxicity.[1] Although this appears to be an isolated case it would be expected to be generally significant as ciclosporin is well known to interact with the statins, and this interaction appeared to be mediated by a statin-like component. Concurrent use need not be avoided, but it would seem prudent to discuss the potential effects with patients and describe the symptoms of myopathy. Patients should report any unexplained muscle pain, tenderness or weakness.

1. Prasad GVR, Wong T, Meliton G, Bhaloo S. Rhabdomyolysis due to red yeast rice (*Monascus purpureus*) in a renal transplant recipient. *Transplantation* (2002) 74, 1200–1.

Ciclosporin + Herbal medicines; St John's wort (*Hypericum perforatum*)

Marked reductions in ciclosporin blood levels and transplant rejection can occur within a few weeks of starting St John's wort.

Clinical evidence

A marked drop in ciclosporin blood levels was identified in one kidney transplant patient as being due to the addition of St John's wort extract 300 mg three times daily. When the St John's wort was stopped the ciclosporin levels rose. The authors of this report identified another 35 kidney and 10 liver transplant patients whose ciclosporin levels had dropped by an average of 49% (range 30 to 64%) after starting St John's wort. Two of them had rejection episodes.[1,2] In addition, subtherapeutic ciclosporin levels in 7 kidney transplant patients,[3-7] one liver transplant patient,[8] and 6 heart transplant patients[9-11] have been attributed to self-medication with St John's wort. Acute graft rejection episodes occurred in 7 cases,[3,5,7-9,11] and one patient subsequently developed chronic rejection, requiring a return to dialysis.[5] Another case of subtherapeutic ciclosporin levels occurred in a kidney transplant patient during the concurrent use of a herbal tea containing St John's wort. The patient's levels remained subtherapeutic despite a ciclosporin dose increase from 150 to 250 mg daily. The levels recovered within 5 days of stopping the herbal tea and the ciclosporin dose was reduced to 175 mg daily.[12]

These case reports are supported by a small study in which 11 renal transplant patients, with stable dose requirements for ciclosporin, were given St John's wort extract (*Jarsin 300*) 600 mg daily for 14 days. Pharmacokinetic changes were noted 3 days after the St John's wort was added. By day 10 the ciclosporin dose had to be increased from an average of 2.7 to 4.2 mg/kg daily in an attempt to keep ciclosporin levels within the therapeutic range. Two weeks after the St John's wort was stopped, only 3 patients had been successfully re-stabilised on their baseline ciclosporin dose. Additionally, the pharmacokinetics of various ciclosporin metabolites were substantially altered.[13]

Another study in 10 kidney transplant patients stable taking ciclosporin found that the content of hyperforin in the St John's wort affected the extent of the interaction with ciclosporin. In patients taking St John's wort with a high hyperforin content (hyperforin 7 mg; hypericin 0.45 mg) the reduction in the AUC_{0-12} of ciclosporin was 45% greater than that in patients taking St John's wort with a low hyperforin content (hyperforin 0.1 mg; hypericin 0.45 mg). The maximum blood ciclosporin level and the trough ciclosporin level were also reduced by 36% and 45%, respectively, in the patients taking the higher hyperforin-containing St John's wort preparation, when compared with the patients taking the preparation with a lower hyperforin content. The patients taking the high-hyperforin preparation required a mean ciclosporin dose increase of 65% whereas the patients taking the low-hyperforin preparation did not require any ciclosporin dose alterations.[14]

Mechanism

St John's wort is a known inducer of the cytochrome P450 isoenzyme CYP3A4 by which ciclosporin is metabolised. Concurrent use therefore reduces ciclosporin levels. It has also been suggested that St John's wort affects ciclosporin reabsorption by inducing the drug transporter protein, P-glycoprotein, in the intestine.[9,13]

Importance and management

An established and clinically important interaction. The incidence is not known, but all patients taking ciclosporin should avoid St John's wort because of the potential severity of this interaction. Transplant rejection can develop within 3 to 4 weeks. It is possible to accommodate this interaction by increasing the ciclosporin dosage[11] (possibly about doubled) but this raises the costs of an already expensive drug. Also, the varying content of natural products would make this hard to monitor. The advice of the CSM in the UK is that patients receiving ciclosporin should avoid or stop taking St John's wort. In the latter situation, the ciclosporin blood levels should be well monitored and the dosage adjusted as necessary.[15] The study described above suggests that increased monitoring will be needed for at least 2 weeks after the St John's wort is stopped.[13]

1. Breidenbach Th, Hoffmann MW, Becker Th, Schlitt H, Klempnauer J. Drug interaction of St John's wort with ciclosporin. *Lancet* (2000) 355, 1912.
2. Breidenbach T, Kliem V, Burg M, Radermacher J, Hoffmann MW, Klempnauer J. Profound drop of cyclosporin A whole blood trough levels caused by St John's wort (Hypericum perforatum). *Transplantation* (2000) 69, 2229–30.
3. Barone GW, Gurley BJ, Ketel BL, Abul-Ezz SR. Herbal supplements: a potential for drug interactions in transplant recipients. *Transplantation* (2001) 71, 239–41.
4. Mai I, Kreuger H, Budde K, Johne A, Brockmoeller J, Neumayer H-H, Roots I. Hazardous pharmacokinetic interaction of Saint John's wort (Hypericum perforatum) with the immunosuppressant cyclosporin. *Int J Clin Pharmacol Ther* (2000) 38, 500–2.
5. Barone GW, Gurley BJ, Ketel BL, Lightfoot ML, Abul-Ezz SR. Drug interaction between St John's wort and cyclosporine. *Ann Pharmacother* (2000) 34, 1013–16.

6. Moschella PA-C, Jaber BL. Interaction between cyclosporine and Hypericum perforatum (St John's wort) after organ transplantation. *Am J Kidney Dis* (2001) 38, 1105–7.
7. Turton-Weeks SM, Barone GW, Gurley BJ, Ketel BL, Lightfoot ML, Abul-Ezz SR. St John's wort: a hidden risk for transplant patients. *Prog Transplant* (2001) 11, 116–20.
8. Karliova M, Treichel U, Malagò M, Frilling A, Gerken G, Broelsch CE. Interaction of *hypericum perforatum* (St John's wort) with cyclosporin A metabolism in a patient after liver transplantation. *J Hepatol* (2000) 33, 853–5.
9. Ruschitzka F, Meier PJ, Turina M, Lüscher TF, Noll G. Acute heart transplant rejection due to Saint John's wort. *Lancet* (2000) 355, 548–9.
10. Ahmed SM, Banner NR, Dubrey SW. Low cyclosporin-A level due to Saint-John's-wort in heart-transplant patients. *J Heart Lung Transplant* (2001) 20, 795.
11. Bon S, Hartmann K, Kuhn M. Johanniskraut: ein enzyminducktor? *Schweiz Apothekerzeitung* (1999) 16, 535–6.
12. Alscher DM, Klotz U. Drug interaction of herbal tea containing St. John's wort with cyclosporine. *Transpl Int* (2003) 16, 543–4.
13. Bauer S, Störmer E, Johne A, Krüger H, Budde K, Neumayer H-H, Roots I, Mai I. Alterations in cyclosporin A pharmacokinetics and metabolism during treatment with St John's wort in renal transplant patients. *Br J Clin Pharmacol* (2003) 55, 203–11.
14. Mai I, Bauer S, Perloff ES, Johne A, Uehleke B, Frank B, Budde K, Roots I. Hyperforin content determines the magnitude of the St John's wort–cyclosporine drug interaction. *Clin Pharmacol Ther* (2004) 76, 330–40.
15. Committee on Safety of Medicines (UK). Message from Professor A Breckenridge (Chairman of CSM) and Fact Sheet for Health Care Professionals, 29th February 2000.

Ciclosporin + Hormonal contraceptives and Progestogens

Hepatotoxicity has been described in two patients given ciclosporin and combined oral contraceptives. Rises in serum ciclosporin levels may also occur. Some increase in ciclosporin levels has been seen with norethisterone.

Clinical evidence

(a) Contraceptives

A woman with uveitis taking ciclosporin 5 mg/kg daily had an increase in her trough plasma ciclosporin levels (roughly doubled) on two occasions within 8 to 10 days of starting an oral contraceptive (**levonorgestrel/ethinylestradiol** 150/30 micrograms). She also experienced nausea, vomiting and hepatic pain, and had evidence of severe hepatotoxicity (very marked increases in AST and ALT, and rises in serum bilirubin and alkaline phosphatase).The woman had previously taken this oral contraceptive for 5 years without problems.[1]

Another report describes hepatotoxicity in a patient taking ciclosporin 2 weeks after she started an oral contraceptive (**desogestrel/ethinylestradiol** 150/30 micrograms). The contraceptive was stopped, and liver enzyme levels promptly started to fall, but ciclosporin levels continued to rise, and peaked about 10 days later, at a level about threefold higher than they had been.[2]

(b) Norethisterone

A 15-year-old girl taking ciclosporin who had a marked increase in serum ciclosporin levels when she was given 'danazol', (p.1032), continued to have elevated levels, but not as high, when the danazol was replaced by norethisterone 5 mg three times daily. The levels returned to her previous normal range when the norethisterone was stopped.[3] No changes in ciclosporin levels were seen in another patient who was intermittently given norethisterone.[4] Two women had a mild rise in ciclosporin levels with no changes in creatinine levels when they were given norethisterone 10 mg daily for 10 days.[5]

Mechanism

Uncertain. It seems possible that some of these compounds inhibit the metabolism of the ciclosporin by the liver, thereby leading to an increase in its serum levels. The mechanism of the hepatotoxicity is not understood, but in some cases it seems that it occurs simply as a rare adverse effect of the sex hormone.

Importance and management

This interaction with oral contraceptives and norethisterone is unconfirmed and of uncertain clinical significance. There is insufficient evidence to recommend increased monitoring but be aware of the potential for an interaction in the case of an unexpected response to treatment.

1. Deray G, le Hoang P, Cacoub P, Assogba U, Grippon P, Baumelou A. Oral contraceptive interaction with cyclosporin. *Lancet* (1987) i, 158–9.
2. Leimenstoll G, Jessen P, Zabel P, Niedermayer W. Arzneimittelschaädigung der leber bei kombination von cyclosporin A und einem antikonzeptivum. *Dtsch Med Wochenschr* (1984) 109, 1989–90.
3. Ross WB, Roberts D, Griffin PJA and Salaman JR. Cyclosporin interaction with danazol and norethisterone. *Lancet* (1986) i, 330.
4. Koneru B, Hartner C, Iwatsuki S, Starzl TE. Effect of danazol on cyclosporine pharmacokinetics. *Transplantation* (1988) 45, 1001.
5. Castelao AM. Cyclosporine A — drug interactions. 2nd Int Conf Therapeutic Drug Monitoring Toxicology, Barcelona, Spain, 1992. 203–9.

Ciclosporin + Melphalan

Melphalan appears to increase the nephrotoxic effects of ciclosporin.

Clinical evidence, mechanism, importance and management

A comparative study found that 13 out of 17 patients receiving bone marrow transplants and given ciclosporin 12.5 mg/kg daily with high-dose melphalan (single injection of 140 to 250 mg/m^2) developed renal failure, compared with no cases of renal failure in 7 other patients given melphalan but no ciclosporin.[1] In another study, one out of 4 patients given both drugs developed nephrotoxicity.[2] The reasons are not understood. Renal function should be monitored closely on concurrent use.

1. Morgenstern GR, Powles R, Robinson B, McElwain TJ. Cyclosporin interaction with ketoconazole and melphalan. *Lancet* (1982) ii, 1342.
2. Dale BM, Sage RE, Norman JE, Barber S, Kotasek D. Bone marrow transplantation following treatment with high-dose melphalan. *Transplant Proc* (1985) 17, 1711–13.

Ciclosporin + Methotrexate

Previous or concurrent treatment with methotrexate may possibly increase the risk of liver and other toxicity in those given ciclosporin, but effective and valuable concurrent use has also been reported. Ciclosporin causes a moderate rise in serum methotrexate levels, but methotrexate does not appear to affect the pharmacokinetics of ciclosporin.

Clinical evidence

(a) Evidence of an interaction

A limited comparative study in patients with chronic plaque psoriasis suggested that the previous use of methotrexate, which can cause liver damage, possibly increases the risk of ciclosporin toxicity (higher ciclosporin blood levels and serum creatinine levels, hypertension).[1] This was confirmed by another study in 4 patients with resistant psoriasis in whom ciclosporin 5 mg/kg daily given with methotrexate 2.5 mg every 12 hours for three doses at weekly intervals increased the blood levels of both drugs, and increased the adverse effects (nausea, vomiting, mouth ulcers). Rises in creatinine levels and liver enzymes (AST, ALT) also occurred.[2]

An open-label pharmacokinetic study in 26 patients with rheumatoid arthritis taking methotrexate 7.5 to 22.5 mg weekly with ciclosporin 1.5 mg/kg every 12 hours for 14 days, found that the AUC of the weekly dose of methotrexate increased by 26%, whereas the plasma levels of its major metabolite (7-hydroxymethotrexate), which is much less active and may be associated with toxicity, were reduced by 80%.[3] Another study in patients with rheumatoid arthritis found that the pharmacokinetics of ciclosporin after the first dose did not differ between those who had been receiving intramuscular methotrexate 10 mg each week for 6 months and those not receiving methotrexate.[4]

(b) Evidence of concurrent use without toxicity

A pilot study described the effective use of ciclosporin and methotrexate for the control of acute graft-versus-host disease in bone marrow transplant patients, with the ciclosporin dosage reduced by 50% to 1.5 mg/kg/day during the first 2 weeks. The methotrexate dosages were 10 to 15 mg/m^2 on days 1, 3, 6, and 11 after grafting. Hepatotoxicity appeared to be reduced.[5] Another study in three bone marrow transplant patients found that low-dose methotrexate (15 mg/m^2 on day 1, and 10 mg/m^2 on days 3, 6 and 11) given with ciclosporin did not significantly affect clinical care and no interaction of clinical significance was seen.[6]

Mechanism

Not understood.

Importance and management

The reports cited here give an inconsistent picture. On the one hand there is the strong recommendation by the authors of the second study[2] that combined use should be avoided, even in patients with severe unresponsive psoriasis, whereas it seems from the other studies in patients with rheumatoid arthritis, or those undergoing bone marrow transplant[5,6] that concurrent use can be valuable, effective and apparently safe. Patients receiving ciclosporin should routinely be monitored for renal effects, and those receiving methotrexate routinely monitored for hepatotoxicity. If both drugs are used concurrently it may be worth increasing the frequency of this monitoring to aid rapid detection of any adverse effects.

1. Powles AV, Baker BS, Fry L, Valdimarsson H. Cyclosporin toxicity. *Lancet* (1990) 335, 610.
2. Korstanje MJ, van Breda Vriesman CJP, van de Staak WJBM. Cyclosporine and methotrexate: a dangerous combination. *J Am Acad Dermatol* (1990) 23, 320–1.
3. Fox RI, Morgan SL, Smith HT, Robbins BA, Choc MG, Baggott JE. Combined oral cyclosporin and methotrexate therapy in patients with rheumatoid arthritis elevates methotrexate levels and reduces 7-hydroxymethotrexate levels when compared with methotrexate alone. *Rheumatology (Oxford)* (2003) 42, 989–94.
4. Baraldo M, Ferraccioli G, Pea F, Gremese E, Furlanut M. Cyclosporine A pharmacokinetics in rheumatoid arthritis patients after 6 months of methotrexate therapy. *Pharm Res* (1999) 40, 483–6.
5. Stockschlaeder M, Storb R, Pepe M, Longton G, McDonald G, Anasetti C, Appelbaum F, Doney K, Martin P, Sullivan K, Witherspoon R. A pilot study of low-dose cyclosporin for graft-versus-host prophylaxis in marrow transplantation. *Br J Haematol* (1991) 80, 49–54.
6. Dix S, Devine SM, Geller RB, Wingard JR. Re: severe interaction between methotrexate and a macrolide antibiotic. *J Natl Cancer Inst* (1995) 87, 1641–2.

Ciclosporin + Methoxsalen

In a single-dose study, methoxsalen increased the bioavailability of ciclosporin .

Clinical evidence, mechanism, importance and management

A study in 12 healthy subjects found that a single 40-mg dose of methoxsalen significantly increased the AUC and peak plasma level of a single 200-mg dose of ciclosporin by about 14% and 8%, respectively. In two patients the AUCs increased by 1.8-fold and 2.7-fold, respectively. The half-life and time to peak levels were not affected. As methoxsalen absorption is subject to high interindividual variation, this particular study was unable to detect a significant difference in methoxsalen pharmacokinetics although the AUC and peak levels tended to be reduced by concurrent ciclosporin.[1]

Methoxsalen may act by reducing the absorption of ciclosporin. Further study is required to see if this interaction is clinically significant. However, bear this interaction in mind in patients taking ciclosporin if levels are increased.

1. Rheeders M, Bouwer M, Goosen TC. Drug-drug interaction after single oral doses of the furanocoumarin methoxsalen and cyclosporine. *J Clin Pharmacol* (2006) 46, 768–75.

Ciclosporin + Methylphenidate

In an isolated case, the ciclosporin levels of a 10-year-old-boy were raised by 50% after he started to take methylphenidate.

Clinical evidence, mechanism, importance and management

A 10-year-old boy, who had received a heart transplant 6 years previously, started taking methylphenidate 5 mg twice daily in addition to his transplant medication, which included ciclosporin. After 4 days his ciclosporin level was found to have risen from 195 to 302 nanograms/mL. His ciclosporin dosage was therefore reduced from 550 to 500 mg daily, and at the same time the methylphenidate was increased to 7.5 mg twice daily. As the next ciclosporin level was still elevated at 251 nanograms/mL, the ciclosporin dose was further reduced to 450 mg daily. The boy then remained on this dose of ciclosporin with acceptable levels, despite further dose increases in the methylphenidate to an eventual dose of 20 mg daily.[1]

The reason for this probable interaction is unclear. This appears to be the only reported case of an interaction between ciclosporin and methylphenidate, and its general importance is unknown.

1. Lewis BR, Aoun SL, Bernstein GA, Crow SJ. Pharmacokinetic interactions between cyclosporin and bupropion or methylphenidate. *J Child Adolesc Psychopharmacol* (2001) 11, 193–8.

Ciclosporin + Metoclopramide

Metoclopramide moderately increases the absorption of ciclosporin and raises its blood levels.

Clinical evidence, mechanism, importance and management

When 14 kidney transplant patients were given metoclopramide their peak ciclosporin blood levels were increased by 46%, from 388 to 567 nanograms/mL and the ciclosporin AUC was increased by 22%. The dosage of metoclopramide was 10 mg by mouth 30 minutes before, 5 mg with, and 5 mg 30 minutes after the morning dose of ciclosporin.[1] Ciclosporin is largely absorbed by the small intestine so the likely mechanism for this interaction is increased absorption of ciclosporin because metoclopramide hastens gastric emptying. The clinical importance of this interaction is uncertain. Concurrent use should be well monitored to ensure that any increase in ciclosporin peak levels does not increase adverse effects. Note that the increase in the AUC of ciclosporin is only modest.

1. Wadhwa NK, Schroeder TJ, O'Flaherty E, Pesce AJ, Myre SA, First MR. The effect of oral metoclopramide on the absorption of cyclosporine. *Transplant Proc* (1987) 19, 1730–3.

Ciclosporin + Midazolam

On the basis of an experimental study in 9 patients it was concluded that the dosage of midazolam needs no adjustment in those taking ciclosporin. Midazolam also appears to have no effect on ciclosporin pharmacokinetics.[1]

1. Li G, Treiber G, Meinshausen J, Wolf J, Werringloer J, Klotz U. Is cyclosporin A an inhibitor of drug metabolism? *Br J Clin Pharmacol* (1990) 30, 71–7.

Ciclosporin + Minoxidil

The concurrent use of ciclosporin and minoxidil can cause excessive hairiness (hypertrichosis).

Clinical evidence, mechanism, importance and management

Six male kidney transplant patients taking ciclosporin (blood levels of 100 to 200 nanograms/mL) were given methyldopa, a diuretic and minoxidil 15 to 40 mg daily for intractable hypertension. After 4 weeks of treatment all of them complained of severe and unpleasant hypertrichosis (excessive hairiness). Two months after stopping the minoxidil the hypertrichosis had significantly improved.[1] Both ciclosporin and minoxidil cause hypertrichosis and it would seem that their effects may be additive. The authors of the report point out that this is not a life-threatening problem, but it limits the concurrent use of these drugs in both men and women.[1]

1. Sever MS, Sonmez YE, Kocak N. Limited use of minoxidil in renal transplant recipients because of the additive side-effects of cyclosporine on hypertrichosis. *Transplantation* (1990) 50, 536.

Ciclosporin + Modafinil

Ciclosporin serum levels were reported to be reduced by modafinil in one patient.

Clinical evidence, mechanism, importance and management

A kidney transplant patient, stabilised for 9 years taking ciclosporin 200 mg daily, developed Gélineau's syndrome (narcoleptic syndrome) and was given modafinil 200 mg daily. Within a few weeks her ciclosporin blood levels were noted to have fallen, and it was necessary to raise her ciclosporin dosage stepwise to 300 mg daily before her blood levels were back to their former values.[1] This is the first reported case of an interaction between ciclosporin and modafinil, and its general importance is unknown. However, the manufacturers state that in interaction studies modafinil induced the cytochrome P450 isoenzyme CYP3A4, the major enzyme involved in the metabolism of ciclosporin,[2] which would suggest that the interaction may be of general importance.

1. LeCacheux Ph, Charasse C, Mourtada R, Muh Ph, Boulahrouz R, Simon P. Syndrome de Gélineau chez une transplantée rénale. Mise en évidence d'une interaction cyclosporine-modafinil. *Presse Med* (1997) 26, 466.
2. Provigil (Modafinil). Cephalon Ltd. UK Summary of product characteristics, July 2007.

Ciclosporin + Muromonab-CD3

Muromonab-CD3 increases ciclosporin blood levels.

Clinical evidence, mechanism, importance and management

When muromonab-CD3 5 mg daily for 10 days was given to 10 kidney transplant patients to treat acute rejection, their mean trough ciclosporin levels on day 8 were higher than before the muromonab-CD3 was started, despite a 50% reduction in the ciclosporin dosage. When the muromonab-CD3 was withdrawn, the ciclosporin dosage needed to be increased again.[1] The reasons are not understood. It is clearly necessary to titrate the dosage of ciclosporin downwards if muromonab-CD3 is given to prevent an excessive rise in ciclosporin levels with the attendant risks of renal toxicity.

1. Vrahnos D, Sanchez J, Vasquez EM, Pollak R, Maddux MS. Cyclosporine levels during OKT3 treatment of acute renal allograft rejection. *Pharmacotherapy* (1991) 11, 278.

Ciclosporin + NNRTIs

The ciclosporin levels of one patient dramatically decreased following the addition of efavirenz.

Clinical evidence

A patient was diagnosed as HIV-positive 3 years after a kidney transplant, for which he was taking ciclosporin. He was started on efavirenz 600 mg daily, lamivudine and zidovudine, and 7 days later, after an initial rise, his ciclosporin level dropped from about 203 to 80 nanograms/mL. A nadir of 50 nanograms/mL was reached one month later.[1]

Mechanism

Efavirenz induces the cytochrome P450 isoenzyme CYP3A4. Ciclosporin is extensively metabolised by CYP3A4, so concurrent use decreases ciclosporin levels.

Importance and management

There appears to be only one report of a reduction in ciclosporin levels with efavirenz. However, as subtherapeutic levels of ciclosporin may have significant consequences, including transplant rejection, it would be prudent to monitor ciclosporin levels closely in patients given efavirenz.

1. Tseng A, Nguyen ME, Cardella C, Humar A, Conly J. Probable interaction between efavirenz and cyclosporine. *AIDS* (2002) 16, 505–6.

Ciclosporin + NRTIs

No change in ciclosporin levels was seen in a study in 6 kidney transplant patients taking ciclosporin when lamivudine 100 to 150 mg daily was added to treat chronic hepatitis B.[1] Another study in 15 kidney transplant patients also found that lamivudine 50 to 100 mg daily did not affect ciclosporin levels.[2]

1. Jung YO, Lee YS, Yang WS, Han DJ, Park JS, Park S-K. Treatment of chronic hepatitis B with lamivudine in renal transplant recipients. *Transplantation* (1998) 66, 733–7.
2. Mouquet C, Bernard B, Poynard T, Thibault V, Opolon P, Coriat P, Bitker MO. Chronic hepatitis B treatment with lamivudine in kidney transplant patients. *Transplant Proc* (2000) 32, 2762.

Ciclosporin + NSAIDs, Aspirin or Paracetamol (Acetaminophen)

NSAIDs sometimes reduce renal function in individual patients, which is reflected in serum creatinine level rises and possibly in changes in ciclosporin levels, but concurrent use can also be uneventful. Diclofenac serum levels can be doubled by ciclosporin. There is an isolated report of colitis in a child treated with ciclosporin and diclofenac or indometacin.

Clinical evidence

(a) Aspirin

No pharmacokinetic interaction was found when ciclosporin was given with aspirin 960 mg three times daily in healthy subjects.[1]

(b) Diclofenac

A study in 20 patients with rheumatoid arthritis given ciclosporin and diclofenac found that 7 of them had a high probability of an interaction (rises in serum creatinine levels and blood pressures), and 9 possibly had an interaction.[2] A kidney transplant patient taking ciclosporin, digoxin, furosemide, prednisolone, and spironolactone had a marked rise in serum creatinine levels immediately after starting to take diclofenac 25 mg three times daily. A fall in serum ciclosporin levels from 409 to 285 nanograms/mL also occurred.[3] Increased nephrotoxicity was seen in another patient taking ciclosporin for idiopathic uveitis when given diclofenac 150 mg daily.[4]

A 6-month study in 20 patients with severe rheumatoid arthritis given diclofenac 100 to 200 mg with ciclosporin 3 mg/kg daily found that the AUC of diclofenac was doubled and serum creatinine levels raised from 71 to 88.4 micromol/L. The overall pattern of adverse events and laboratory abnormalities were similar to those in patients with rheumatoid arthritis treated with ciclosporin and other NSAIDs. It was suggested that it would be prudent to start with low doses of diclofenac and to monitor well.[5] A study in 24 healthy subjects found that diclofenac 50 mg every 8 hours for 8 days caused no changes in the pharmacokinetics of ciclosporin, but there was some inconclusive evidence that diclofenac serum levels were increased.[6]

A child with rheumatoid arthritis taking ciclosporin 10 mg/kg daily developed colitis when diclofenac was given. The NSAID was stopped and her symptoms resolved while the ciclosporin was continued.[7]

(c) Dipyrone (Metamizole sodium)

A placebo-controlled, crossover study in 6 kidney and 2 heart transplant patients taking ciclosporin found that while they were taking dipyrone 500 mg three times daily for 4 days the pharmacokinetics of the ciclosporin (AUC, trough and peak blood levels, elimination half-life) were unchanged, but the time to reach maximum blood levels was slightly prolonged, from 2.1 to 3.8 hours. It is not known what the effects of more prolonged use might be.[8]

(d) Indometacin

A study in 16 healthy subjects found that indometacin 100 mg twice daily for 9 days reduced the maximum blood levels of a single 300-mg dose of ciclosporin by 18% and slowed its absorption (time to maximum concentration increased by 30 minutes) but the extent of absorption was not changed, indicating the absence of a clinically relevant pharmacokinetic interaction. Further, the pharmacokinetics of indometacin were not affected by ciclosporin.[9] A study in rheumatoid arthritis patients taking ciclosporin 2.5 mg/kg daily, found that creatinine clearances were reduced by 6% in those taking indometacin 50 mg four times daily, but this was not considered to be clinically important.[10] An experimental study in healthy subjects found that ciclosporin 10 mg/kg twice daily for 4 days had no effect on effective renal plasma flow (ERPF) or the glomerular filtration rate (GFR), but when indometacin 50 mg twice daily was added the ERPF fell by 32% and the GFR by 37%.[11]

A child with rheumatoid arthritis on ciclosporin 10 mg/kg daily developed colitis when indometacin was given. The NSAID was stopped and her symptoms resolved the ciclosporin was continued.[7]

(e) Ketoprofen

A study in rheumatoid arthritis patients taking ciclosporin 2.5 mg/kg daily, found that creatinine clearances were reduced by 2.3% in those taking ketoprofen 50 mg four times daily, but this was not considered to be clinically important.[10] Another report describes increased serum creatinine levels in a patient with rheumatoid arthritis who took ciclosporin and ketoprofen.[12]

(f) Mefenamic acid

The ciclosporin blood levels in a renal transplant patient doubled, accompanied by rise in creatinine levels from 113 to 168 micromol/L within a day of starting to take mefenamic acid. Levels fell to normal within a week of stopping the mefenamic acid.[13]

(g) Naproxen

In 11 patients with rheumatoid arthritis taking ciclosporin, naproxen and sulindac increased serum creatinine levels by 24% and reduced renal function (glomerular filtration rate reduced from 98 mL/minute at baseline to 67 mL/minute while taking an NSAID and ciclosporin). All patients had a clinical improvement in their rheumatoid arthritis.[14]

(h) Paracetamol (Acetaminophen)

A study in rheumatoid arthritis patients taking ciclosporin 2.5 mg/kg daily, found that creatinine clearances were reduced by 3.5% in those taking paracetamol 650 mg four times daily, but this was not considered to be clinically important.[10]

(i) Piroxicam

Piroxicam is reported to have increased the serum creatinine levels of a patient with rheumatoid arthritis by an unknown amount (but classed as a significant adverse event). This resolved when the piroxicam was withdrawn.[12] A study in healthy subjects given piroxicam 20 mg daily for 11 days and a single 300-mg dose of ciclosporin on day 10 found no clinically relevant pharmacokinetic interaction.[9]

(j) Sulindac

A study in rheumatoid arthritis patients taking ciclosporin 2.5 mg/kg daily, found that creatinine clearances were reduced by 2.6% in those taking sulindac 100 mg four times daily, but this was not considered to be clinically important.[10]

A patient with a kidney transplant had a rise in serum creatinine levels when sulindac was used. Ciclosporin blood levels fell and rose again when the sulindac was stopped.[3] Another report states that the ciclosporin levels of a woman with a kidney transplant were more than doubled within 3 days of her starting to take sulindac 150 mg twice daily.[15] In 11 patients with rheumatoid arthritis taking ciclosporin, both sulindac and naproxen increased serum creatinine levels by 24% and reduced renal function (glomerular filtration rate reduced from 98 mL/minute at baseline to 67 mL/minute while taking an NSAID and ciclosporin). All patients had a clinical improvement in their rheumatoid arthritis.[14]

Another report describes a patient with rheumatoid arthritis taking ciclosporin who developed increased serum creatinine levels when given ketoprofen, but not when given sulindac.[12]

Mechanism

Uncertain. One idea is that intact kidney prostacyclin synthesis is needed to maintain the glomerular filtration rate and renal blood flow in patients given ciclosporin, which may possibly protect the kidney from the development of ciclosporin-induced nephrotoxicity. If NSAIDs that inhibit prostaglandin production in the kidney are given, the nephrotoxic effects of the ciclosporin manifest themselves, possibly independently of changes in serum ciclosporin levels.[3] A study in *rats* found that indometacin and ciclosporin together can cause rises in serum creatinine levels that are much greater than with either drug alone.[16]

The occurrence of colitis in a child receiving ciclosporin and either diclofenac or indometacin appeared to be independent of changes in ciclosporin levels and may be a result of additive effects of both drugs.[7]

Importance and management

Information about the NSAIDs listed here is sparse and limited, but the overall picture appears to be that concurrent use in rheumatoid arthritis need not be avoided but renal function should be very well monitored. The manufacturers of ciclosporin also specifically recommend that patients with rheumatoid arthritis taking ciclosporin and an NSAID should have their hepatic function measured as well as renal function, because hepatotoxicity is a potential adverse effect of both drugs.[17] It has been suggested that gastrointestinal symptoms should also be carefully evaluated.[7] It is clearly difficult to generalise about what will or will not happen if any particular NSAID is given but in the case of diclofenac it has been recommended that doses at the lower end of the range should be used at the start because its serum levels can be doubled by ciclosporin.

1. Kovarik JM, Mueller EA, Gaber M, Johnston A, Jähnchen E. Pharmacokinetics of cyclosporine and steady-state aspirin during coadministration. *J Clin Pharmacol* (1993) 33, 513–21.
2. Branthwaite JP, Nicholls A. Cyclosporin and diclofenac interaction in rheumatoid arthritis. *Lancet* (1991) 337, 252.
3. Harris KP, Jenkins D, Walls J. Nonsteroidal antiinflammatory drugs and cyclosporine. A potentially serious adverse interaction. *Transplantation* (1988) 46, 598–9.
4. Deray G, Le Hoang P, Aupetit B, Achour A, Rottembourg J, Baumelou A. Enhancement of cyclosporine A nephrotoxicity by diclofenac. *Clin Nephrol* (1987) 27, 213–14.
5. Kovarik JM, Kurki P, Mueller E, Guerret M, Markert E, Alten R, Zeidler H, Genth-Stolzenburg S. Diclofenac combined with cyclosporine in treatment of refractory rheumatoid arthritis: longitudinal safety assessment and evidence of a pharmacokinetic/dynamic interaction. *J Rheumatol* (1996) 23, 2033–8.
6. Mueller EA, Kovarik JM, Koelle EU, Merdjan H, Johnston A, Hitzenberger G. Pharmacokinetics of cyclosporine and multiple-dose diclofenac during coadministration. *J Clin Pharmacol* (1993) 33, 936–43.
7. Constantopoulos A. Colitis induced by interaction of cyclosporine A and non-steroidal anti-inflammatory drugs. *Pediatr Int* (1999) 41, 184–6.
8. Caraco Y, Zylber-Katz E, Fridlander M, Admon D, Levy M. The effect of short-term dipyrone administration on cyclosporin pharmacokinetics. *Eur J Clin Pharmacol* (1999) 55, 475–8.
9. Kovarik JM, Mueller EA, Gerbeau C, Tarral A, Francheteau P, Guerret M. Cyclosporine and nonsteroidal antiinflammatory drugs: exploring potential drug interactions and their implications for the treatment of rheumatoid arthritis. *J Clin Pharmacol* (1997) 37, 336–43.
10. Tugwell P, Ludwin D, Gent M, Roberts R, Bensen W, Grace E, Baker P. Interaction between cyclosporin A and nonsteroidal antiinflammatory drugs. *J Rheumatol* (1997) 24, 1122–5.
11. Sturrock NDC, Lang CC, Struthers AD. Indomethacin and cyclosporin together produce marked renal vasoconstriction in humans. *J Hypertens* (1994) 12, 919–24.
12. Ludwin D, Bennett KJ, Grace EM, Buchanan WA, Bensen W, Bombardier C, Tugwell PX. Nephrotoxicity in patients with rheumatoid arthritis treated with cyclosporine. *Transplant Proc* (1988) 20 (Suppl 4), 367–70.
13. Agar JWMacD. Cyclosporin A and mefenamic acid in a renal transplant patient. *Aust N Z J Med* (1991) 21, 784–5.
14. Altman RD, Perez GO, Sfakianakis GN. Interaction of cyclosporine A and nonsteroidal anti-inflammatory drugs on renal function in patients with rheumatoid arthritis. *Am J Med* (1992) 93, 396–402.
15. Sesin GP, O'Keefe E, Roberto P. Sulindac-induced elevation of serum cyclosporine concentration. *Clin Pharm* (1989) 8, 445–6.
16. Whiting PH, Burke MD, Thomson AW. Drug interactions with cyclosporine. Implications from animal studies. *Transplant Proc* (1986) 18 (Suppl 5), 56–70.
17. Neoral (Ciclosporin). Novartis Pharmaceuticals UK Ltd. UK Summary of product characteristics, December 2004.

Ciclosporin + Opioids

An isolated report describes neuropsychosis in a patient who was given intravenous ciclosporin and morphine. A single case report describes a patient taking ciclosporin who developed opioid withdrawal on stopping low-dose, transdermal fentanyl.

Clinical evidence, mechanism, importance and management

A patient who underwent renal transplantation was given ciclosporin 6 mg/kg daily by intravenous infusion over 2 hours and intravenous methylprednisolone postoperatively. He also received patient-controlled analgesia (PCA) as bolus doses of **morphine** 0.5 mg to a total dose of 13 mg on the first day and 11 mg on the second day. On the third day he developed insomnia, anxiety, amnesia, aphasia and severe confusion. The morphine was discontinued and the symptoms subsided after treatment with propofol, diazepam and haloperidol. It was suggested that ciclosporin may have decreased the excitation threshold of neuronal cells, which potentiated the dysphoric effects of **morphine**.[1]

A patient taking ciclosporin following a stem cell transplant developed opioid withdrawal symptoms when transdermal **fentanyl** 25 micrograms/hour was discontinued. The authors suggested that elevation of **fentanyl** levels due to inhibition of the cytochrome P450 isoenzyme CYP3A4 by ciclosporin during concurrent use may have been a possible cause, as withdrawal symptoms are not usual with this dose of **fentanyl**. However, they also note that other factors may have played a role, such as the physical and mental status of the patient after the stem cell transplant.[2] Further, ciclosporin does not usually appear to interact with other drugs by inhibiting CYP3A4.

These appear to be isolated cases and almost certainly not of general importance.

1. Lee P-C, Hung C-J, Lei H-Y, Tsai Y-C. Suspected acute post-transplant neuropsychosis due to interaction of morphine and cyclosporin after a renal transplant. *Anaesthesia* (2000) 55, 827–8.
2. Tsutsumi Y, Kanamori H, Tanaka J, Asaka M, Imamura M, Masauzi N. Withdrawal symptoms from transdermal fentanyl (TDF) after an allogeneic blood stem cell transplant. *Pain Med* (2006) 7, 164–5.

Ciclosporin + Orlistat

The absorption of ciclosporin is significantly reduced by orlistat. In one case, orlistat appeared to have less effect on the microemulsion formulation of ciclosporin (*Neoral*) than the oil formulation (*Sandimmun*). Nevertheless, an episode of acute graft rejection (said to be non-significant) has been reported with the microemulsion formulation.

Clinical evidence

In a heart transplant patient taking ciclosporin (*Sandimmun*), orlistat 120 mg three times daily reduced the trough blood levels of ciclosporin by 47%, to 52 nanograms/mL. The peak levels and the AUC of ciclosporin were increased by 86% and 75%, respectively.[1] Another heart transplant patient taking ciclosporin (*Neoral*) had a nonsignificant acute rejection episode on routine endocardial biopsy, with trough ciclosporin levels of 38 nanograms/mL, 24 days after starting to take orlistat. Ciclosporin trough levels increased to about 90 to 110 nanograms/mL when the orlistat was stopped.[2] In a further patient taking ciclosporin (*Sandimmun*) 250 mg daily, orlistat 360 mg daily reduced the ciclosporin levels from 150 to 50 nanograms/mL. Increasing the dose of ciclosporin did not result in an increased level, so the patient was given *Neoral* instead. Adequate levels of 160 nanograms/mL were finally achieved with ciclosporin (*Neoral*) 375 mg daily.[3] Details of this patient are also briefly given elsewhere.[4] Another report describes 6 transplant recipients who developed subtherapeutic ciclosporin trough levels after also taking orlistat.[5] Another heart transplant patient had a progressive reduction in her ciclosporin (*Sandimmune*) level when she started to take orlistat. Note that this patient was also reported to have severe diarrhoea secondary to poor adherence to a low-fat diet when taking orlistat, which may have contributed to the low levels seen.[6]

Mechanism

Orlistat inhibits pancreatic lipase and prevents the absorption of dietary fat and lipophilic molecules such as ciclosporin. Absorption of ciclosporin from the oil suspension formulation (*Sandimmun*) is more dependent on the lipid absorption stage and thus may be more affected by orlistat than the microemulsion form (*Neoral*).[3]

Importance and management

Information appears to be limited to these reports, but the interaction seems to be established. It has been suggested that the effects of the interaction may be reduced by using the microemulsion formulation of ciclosporin (*Neoral*)[3] (which has generally replaced the corn oil suspension). Monitoring is required if the two drugs are used together, either in the standard or microemulsion form because there is a risk of subtherapeutic levels even with the microemulsion preparation.[2] Some authors recommend avoidance of the combination.[1] The UK manufacturers of orlistat do not recommend concurrent use, but if such use is unavoidable more frequent ciclosporin monitoring is recommended.[7] The US manufacturers recommend taking ciclosporin at least 2 hours before or 2 hours after orlistat, and that ciclosporin levels should be monitored more frequently in these patients.[8]

1. Nägele H, Petersen B, Bonacker U, Rödiger W. Effect of orlistat on blood cyclosporin concentration in an obese heart transplant patient. *Eur J Clin Pharmacol* (1999) 55, 667–9.
2. Schnetzler B, Kondo-Oestreicher M, Vala D, Khatchatourian G, Faidutti B. Orlistat decreases the plasma level of cyclosporine and may be responsible for the development of acute rejection episodes. *Transplantation* (2000) 70, 1540–1.
3. Le Beller C, Bezie Y, Chabatte C, Guillemain R, Amrein C, Billaud EM. Co-administration of orlistat and cyclosporine in a heart transplant recipient. *Transplantation* (2000) 70, 1541–2.
4. Chavatte C, Le Beller C, Guillemain R, Amrein C, Billaud EM. Cyclosporine/orlistat drug interaction in heart transplant recipient. *Fundam Clin Pharmacol* (2000) 14, 246.
5. Colman E, Fossler M. Reduction in blood cyclosporine concentrations by orlistat. *N Engl J Med* (2000) 342, 1141–2.
6. Barbaro D, Orsini P, Pallini S, Piazza F, Pasquini C. Obesity in transplant patients: case report showing interference of orlistat with absorption of cyclosporine and review of literature. *Endocr Pract* (2002) 8, 124–6.
7. Xenical (Orlistat). Roche Products Ltd. UK Summary of product characteristics, May 2006.
8. Xenical (Orlistat). Roche Pharmaceuticals. US Prescribing information, January 2007.

Ciclosporin + Oxybutynin

Oxybutynin did not appear to affect ciclosporin levels in two children.

Clinical evidence, mechanism, importance and management

In a retrospective analysis, one child with a kidney transplant taking ciclosporin had no change in his ciclosporin level and dosage over the 2 months before and the 2 months after he started oxybutynin 2 mg twice daily. Another patient had no change in ciclosporin levels and dosage over the 3 months before and 3 months after stopping oxybutynin 5 mg twice daily.[1] This analysis was prompted by evidence suggesting oxybutynin may induce the cytochrome P450 isoenzyme CYP3A4, which is involved in the metabolism of ciclosporin. Although the evidence is limited, it suggests that oxybutynin is unlikely to have an important effect on ciclosporin levels.

1. Springate JE. Oxybutynin does not affect cyclosporin blood levels. *Ther Drug Monit* (2001) 23, 155–6.

Ciclosporin + Pancreatic enzymes

Pancreatic enzyme extracts do not increase the bioavailability of ciclosporin in cystic fibrosis patients.

Clinical evidence, mechanism, importance and management

A study in heart-lung transplant patients with cystic fibrosis found that they needed almost five times the oral dose of ciclosporin of other patients, confirming other studies in these patients that had shown a very much reduced bioavailability of oral ciclosporin. This is probably a reflection of the generally poor digestion and absorption in cystic fibrosis patients. The addition of pancreatic enzymes (*Creon*) was not found to improve this poor ciclosporin bioavailability. No adverse effects were reported.[1]

1. Tsang VT, Johnston A, Heritier F, Leaver N, Hodson ME, Yacoub M. Cyclosporin pharmacokinetics in heart-lung transplant recipients with cystic fibrosis. *Eur J Clin Pharmacol* (1994) 46, 261–5.

Ciclosporin + Prazosin

Preliminary studies show that prazosin causes a small reduction in the glomerular filtration rate in kidney transplant patients taking ciclosporin.

Clinical evidence, mechanism, importance and management

A study in 8 patients with kidney transplants found that prazosin 1 mg twice daily for one week did not alter their ciclosporin blood levels, and arterial blood pressures and renal vascular resistance were reduced. However, the glomerular filtration rate (GFR) was reduced by about 10% (from 47 to 42 mL/minute).[1] Previous studies in kidney transplant patients taking azathioprine, prednisone and prazosin found no reduction in GFR.[2] There would seem to be no strong reasons for totally avoiding prazosin in patients taking ciclosporin, but the authors of the report point out that the fall in GFR makes prazosin a less attractive antihypertensive than a calcium-channel blocker.

1. Kiberd BA. Effects of prazosin therapy in renal allograft recipients receiving cyclosporine. *Transplantation* (1990) 49, 1200–1.
2. Curtis JR, Bateman FJA. Use of prazosin in management of hypertension in patients with chronic renal failure and in renal transplant recipients. *BMJ* (1975) 4, 432.

Ciclosporin + Probucol

Probucol reduces blood ciclosporin levels by about 40%.

Clinical evidence

A study in 6 heart transplant patients taking ciclosporin found that the concurrent use of probucol 500 mg every 12 hours decreased trough whole blood ciclosporin levels from 139 to 81 nanograms/mL and the AUC_{0-9} by 28%. The clearance was increased by 60% and volume of distribution also increased.[1]

Another group of workers similarly found that 9 out 10 kidney transplant patients had a reduction in their trough blood ciclosporin levels while taking probucol.[2]

Mechanism

Not understood. Evidence from *in vitro* and *animal* studies suggest that probucol may form complexes with ciclosporin in the gut, preventing absorption. The studies also found that probucol does not affect ciclosporin absorption via P-glycoprotein-mediated transport.[3]

Importance and management

Information appears to be limited to these studies, but the interaction appears to be well established. The ciclosporin dosage may need to be increased if probucol is added. Monitor the effects and adjust the dosage appropriately.

1. Sundararajan V, Cooper DKC, Muchmore J, Manion CV, Liguori C, Zuhdi N, Novitzky D, Chen P-N, Bourne DWA, Corder CN. Interaction of cyclosporine and probucol in heart transplant patients. *Transplant Proc* (1991) 23, 2028–32.
2. Gallego C, Sánchez P, Planells C, Sánchez S, Monte E, Romá E, Sánchez J, Pallardó LM. Interaction between probucol and cyclosporine in renal transplant patients. *Ann Pharmacother* (1994) 28, 940–2.
3. Sugimoto K-I, Sudoh T, Tsuruoka S, Yamamoto Y, Maezono S, Watanabe Y, Fujimura A. Effect of probucol on oral bioavailability of cyclosporine A. *Eur J Pharm Sci* (2004) 22, 71–7.

Ciclosporin + Propafenone

In an isolated report, propafenone caused a 60% increase in the ciclosporin levels of a patient.

Clinical evidence

A heart transplant patient taking ciclosporin, azathioprine and prednisolone developed ventricular tachycardia 9 months after transplantation, for which he was given propafenone 600 or 750 mg daily. After the first day, his ciclosporin level had risen from about 160 to 190 nanograms/mL, and after 5 days the levels had reached around 260 nanograms/mL. Over the same time period his serum creatinine rose from 168 to 212 micromol/L. His ciclosporin dose was reduced from 240 mg daily to a final dose of 200 mg daily after which his renal function and ciclosporin levels were re-established at about the level before propafenone was started.[1]

Mechanism

The authors suggest that propafenone interferes with the metabolism of ciclosporin by affecting hepatic cytochrome P450, or that propafenone may enhance the absorption of ciclosporin.

Importance and management

Information appears to be limited to this one report, the general importance of which is unknown.

1. Spes CH, Angermann CE, Horn K, Strasser T, Mudra H, Landgraf R, Theisen K. Ciclosporin-propafenone interaction. *Klin Wochenschr* (1990) 68, 872.

Ciclosporin or Tacrolimus + Potassium compounds

Ciclosporin and tacrolimus can cause or worsen pre-existing hyperkalaemia. The concurrent use of potassium compounds should be closely monitored.

Clinical evidence, mechanism, importance and management

Both ciclosporin and tacrolimus can cause hyperkalaemia.[1,2] Tacrolimus has been reported in one study in 34 liver transplant patients to cause hyperkalaemia (defined in this study as potassium greater than 4.5 mmol/L) in 21% of patients, even when the trough level was within therapeutic range.[3] Another study in kidney transplant patients found that the incidence of hyperkalaemia was higher in tacrolimus treated patients, when compared with ciclosporin treated patients.[4]

Hyperkalaemia can in itself be a sign of worsening renal function but may be exacerbated by ciclosporin or tacrolimus. This can be worsened further by the use of potassium supplements.

The manufacturers of tacrolimus recommend that patients should avoid a high potassium intake, such as in supplements.[1] The manufacturers of ciclosporin however recommend potassium level monitoring with concurrent use of any potassium supplement or a potassium-rich diet.[2]

1. Prograf (Tacrolimus monohydrate). Astellas Pharma Ltd. UK Summary of product characteristics, May 2007.
2. Neoral (Ciclosporin). Novartis Pharmaceuticals UK Ltd. UK Summary of product characteristics, December 2004.
3. Dansirikul C, Staatz CE, Duffull SB, Taylor PJ, Lynch SV, Tett SE. Relationships of tacrolimus pharmacokinetic measures and adverse outcomes in stable adult liver transplant recipients. *J Clin Pharm Ther* (2006) 31, 17–25.
4. Higgins R, Ramaiyan K, Dasgupta T, Kanji H, Fletcher S, Lam F, Kashi H. Hyponatraemia and hyperkalaemia are more frequent in renal transplant recipients treated with tacrolimus than with cyclosporin. Further evidence for differences between cyclosporin and tacrolimus nephrotoxicities. *Nephrol Dial Transplant* (2004) 444–50.

Ciclosporin + Protease inhibitors

Protease inhibitors significantly increase the levels of ciclosporin. Ciclosporin may increase the time to maximum nelfinavir levels.

Clinical evidence

(a) Fosamprenavir

A HIV-positive patient taking ciclosporin 250 to 350 mg twice daily (to maintain a therapeutic ciclosporin trough level of 300 to 400 nanograms/mL) was restarted on his usual HAART regimen of tenofovir, lamivudine and fosamprenavir 1.4 g twice daily on day 12 post-liver transplantation. Within 2 days, the ciclosporin level had increased to 600 nanograms/mL, requiring a ciclosporin dose reduction to 100 mg twice daily.[1]

(b) Nelfinavir

A pilot study in 7 HIV-positive subjects taking nelfinavir 1.25 g twice daily found that a single 4-mg/kg oral dose of ciclosporin increased the time to maximum serum level for nelfinavir from 2.6 to 3.2 hours. The AUC of nelfinavir was also increased but this was not significant. In the same study, a single 2-mg/kg intravenous dose of ciclosporin given over 2.5 hours had little effect on the pharmacokinetics of oral nelfinavir. Nelfinavir did not significantly affect the pharmacokinetics of either oral or intravenous ciclosporin.[2]

(c) Ritonavir-boosted regimens

Three HIV-positive patients who had undergone liver transplantation required reductions in their ciclosporin doses when they started taking ritonavir-boosted HAART. One patient taking ciclosporin 150 mg twice daily had an increase in his ciclosporin levels to 900 nanograms/mL when ritonavir-boosted HAART was started, and needed a dose reduction of 95% to maintain a usual ciclosporin trough level of 75 to 150 nanograms/mL. A second patient also required a similar reduction. The third patient needed a dose reduction of 80% when taking ritonavir-boosted **lopinavir**, but no further ciclosporin dose alteration was needed when his treatment was changed to ritonavir-boosted indinavir.[3]

(d) Saquinavir

An HIV-positive patient taking lamivudine and zidovudine, and ciclosporin for a kidney transplant, started taking saquinavir 1.2 g three times daily. Within 2 days he started to complain of fatigue, headache and gastrointestinal discomfort. On investigation his ciclosporin level was found to have risen from a range of 150 to 200 nanograms/mL up to 580 nanograms/mL, and his saquinavir AUC was increased 4.3-fold (by comparison with subjects not taking ciclosporin). His ciclosporin dose was reduced from 150 mg twice daily to 75 mg twice daily, and his saquinavir dose was reduced to 600 mg three times daily, which resulted in ciclosporin levels similar to those achieved previously.[4]

Mechanism

All protease inhibitors can inhibit the cytochrome P450 isoenzyme CYP3A4 to varying degrees, see 'Antivirals', (p.772). Ciclosporin is extensively metabolised by CYP3A4, so any inhibition of this isoenzyme is likely to increase ciclosporin levels. Ciclosporin and the protease inhibitors are substrates for P-glycoprotein, which may explain the raised nelfinavir and saquinavir levels.

Importance and management

The increase in ciclosporin levels seen with ritonavir may occur irrespective of whether it is used as an antiretroviral in its own right or as a pharmacokinetic enhancer with other antiretrovirals[5] (usually in a lower dose of 100 mg twice daily). The inhibition of ciclosporin metabolism by other protease inhibitors, either alone or in combination with ritonavir, may lead to significant increases in ciclosporin levels. Therefore, ciclosporin levels should be carefully monitored and the dose adjusted accordingly during concurrent use, bearing in mind that large dose reductions may be required in some patients, as seen with ritonavir. It is also important to reduce or alter the ciclosporin dose should the protease inhibitor be stopped or changed to avoid ciclosporin toxicity. The clinical significance of the effects of ciclosporin on nelfinavir pharmacokinetics are unclear, and further study is needed.

1. Guaraldi G, Cocchi S, Codeluppi M, Di Benedetto F, Bonora S, Motta A, Luzi K, Pecorari M, Gennari W, Masetti M, Gerunda GE, Esposito R. Pharmacokinetic interaction between amprenavir/ritonavir and fosamprenavir on cyclosporine in two patients with human immunodeficiency virus infection undergoing orthotopic liver transplantation. *Transplant Proc* (2006) 38, 1138–40.
2. Frassetto L, Tahi T, Aggarwal AM, Bucher P, Jacobsen W, Christians U, Benet LZ, Floren LC. Pharmacokinetic interactions between cyclosporine and protease inhibitors in HIV+ subjects. *Drug Metab Pharmacokinet* (2003) 18, 114–20.
3. Vogel M, Voight E, Michaelis H-C, Sudhop T, Wolff M, Türler A, Sauerbruch T, Rockstroh JK, Spengler U. Management of drug-to-drug interactions between cyclosporine A and the protease-inhibitor lopinavir/ritonavir in liver-transplanted HIV-infected patients. *Liver Transpl* (2004) 10, 939–44.
4. Brinkman K, Huysmans F, Burger DM. Pharmacokinetic interaction between saquinavir and cyclosporine. *Ann Intern Med* (1998) 129, 914–15.
5. Norvir (Ritonavir). Abbott Laboratories Ltd. UK Summary of product characteristics, May 2007.

Ciclosporin + Proton pump inhibitors

Omeprazole does not normally appear to affect serum ciclosporin levels, but two isolated reports describe doubled serum ciclosporin levels in one patient, and more than halved serum ciclosporin levels in another. Pantoprazole does not affect serum ciclosporin levels.

Clinical evidence

(a) Omeprazole

Ten kidney transplant patients had no significant changes in ciclosporin levels when given omeprazole 20 mg daily for 2 weeks.[1] Eight kidney transplant patients similarly had no significant changes in ciclosporin levels when given omeprazole 20 mg daily for 6 days.[2] No significant changes in ciclosporin levels were seen in another kidney transplant patient when omeprazole 20 mg daily was given for 8 weeks.[3]

In contrast, the ciclosporin blood levels of a liver transplant patient roughly doubled (from a range of 187 to 261 up to 510 nanograms/mL) about 2 weeks after omeprazole 40 mg daily was started. His ciclosporin levels were readjusted by reducing the dose from 130 to 80 mg twice daily. The levels then remained steady at about 171 nanograms/mL for the following 4 months.[4] In contrast, the serum ciclosporin levels of a bone marrow transplant patient fell from 254 to about 100 nanograms/mL over 14 days in the presence of omeprazole 40 mg daily. The ciclosporin levels climbed again rapidly when the omeprazole was stopped.[5]

(b) Pantoprazole

Studies in kidney transplant patients have found that pantoprazole 40 mg once daily does not affect ciclosporin blood levels when given in the evening,[6] or when both drugs are given together in the morning.[7]

Mechanism

Not understood.

Importance and management

Information is limited but what is known suggests that no interaction normally occurs. However, bear the case reports in mind in the case of an unexpected response to treatment. Note that, in the studies cited in which no interaction occurred, the dose of omeprazole was 20 mg daily, whereas the two cases of interaction involved 40 mg daily so some caution would be appropriate if initiating omeprazole at this higher dose. There would seem to be no reason for avoiding concurrent use of ciclosporin and pantoprazole.[8]

1. Blohmé I, Idström J-P, Andersson T. A study of the interaction between omeprazole and cyclosporine in renal transplant patients. *Br J Clin Pharmacol* (1993) 35, 156–60.
2. Kahn D, Manas D, Hamilton H, Pascoe MD, Pontin AR. The effect of omeprazole on cyclosporine metabolism in renal transplant recipients. *S Afr Med J* (1993) 83, 785.
3. Castellote E, Bonet J, Lauzurica R, Pastor C, Cofan F, Caralps A. Does interaction between omeprazole and cyclosporin exist? *Nephron* (1993) 65, 478.
4. Schouler L, Dumas F, Couzigou P, Janvier G, Winnock S, Saric J. Omeprazole-cyclosporin interaction. *Am J Gastroenterol* (1991) 86, 1097.
5. Arranz R, Yañez E, Franceschi JL, Fernandez-Rañada JM. More about omeprazole-cyclosporine interaction. *Am J Gastroenterol* (1993) 88, 154–5.
6. Lorf T, Ramadori G, Ringe B, Schwörer H. Pantoprazole does not affect cyclosporin A blood concentration in kidney-transplant patients. *Eur J Clin Pharmacol* (2000) 55, 733–5.
7. Lorf T, Ramadori G, Ringe B, Schwörer H. The effect of pantoprazole on tacrolimus and cyclosporin A blood concentration in transplant patients. *Eur J Clin Pharmacol* (2000) 56, 439–40.
8. Schwrer H, Lorf T, Ringe B, Ramadori G. Pantoprazole and cyclosporine or tacrolimus. *Aliment Pharmacol Ther* (2001) 15, 561–2.

Ciclosporin + Pyrazinamide

Pyrazinamide does not normally appear to interact with ciclosporin but one isolated report suggests that it may possibly have contributed to the effects of rifampicin in one patient, which resulted in lowered ciclosporin levels. Another patient developed toxic myopathy attributed to the use of pyrazinamide with ciclosporin.

Clinical evidence, mechanism, importance and management

A 12-year-old girl with a kidney transplant taking ciclosporin and prednisolone had a rejection episode while taking rifampicin and isoniazid, apparently due to the fall in serum ciclosporin levels caused by the rifampicin. The rejection settled when the rifampicin was replaced by pyrazinamide.[1] Other patients taking ciclosporin have been given pyrazinamide combined with ethambutol and/or streptomycin without any apparent interaction problems.[2] However, an anecdotal report suggested that when pyrazinamide was given with rifampicin and isoniazid it appeared to add to the effects of the rifampicin causing an additional reduction in ciclosporin blood levels.[3] Another report attributed the development of toxic myopathy in a kidney transplant patient to the concurrent use of pyrazinamide and ciclosporin.[4]

There would therefore seem to be no reason for avoiding pyrazinamide in patients taking ciclosporin, but be aware of these rare complications.

1. Coward RA, Raftery AT, Brown CB. Cyclosporin and antituberculous therapy. *Lancet* (1985) i, 1342–3.
2. Aguado JM, Herrero JA, Gavaldá J, Torre-Cisneros J, Blanes M, Rufí G, Moreno A, Gurguí A, Hayek M, Lumbreras C and the Spanish Transplantation Infection Study Group, GESITRA. Clinical presentation and outcome of tuberculosis in kidney, liver, and heart transplant recipients in Spain. *Transplantation* (1997) 63, 1276–86.
3. Jiménez del Cerro LA, Hernández FR. Effect of pyrazinamide on ciclosporin levels. *Nephron* (1992) 62, 113.
4. Fernández-Solà J, Campistol JM, Miró Ó, Garcés N, Soy D, Grau JM. Acute toxic myopathy due to pyrazinamide in a patient with renal transplantation and cyclosporine therapy. *Nephrol Dial Transplant* (1996) 11, 1850–2.

Ciclosporin + Quinine

An isolated case suggests that quinine reduces ciclosporin levels.

Clinical evidence, mechanism, importance and management

A man with a kidney transplant and mild cerebral falciparum malaria had a gradual decrease in his ciclosporin blood levels, from 328 to 107 nanograms/mL, over 7 days when he was given quinine 600 mg every 8 hours, and a gradual rise when the quinine was stopped.[1]

The reason for this apparently isolated report is unclear and its general importance is unknown. There is insufficient evidence to recommend increased monitoring, but be aware of the potential for an interaction in the case of an unexpected response to treatment. The effects of lower quinine doses used for cramps are unclear.

1. Tan HW, Ch'ng SL. Drug interaction between cyclosporine A and quinine in a renal transplant patient with malaria. *Singapore Med J* (1991) 32, 189–90.

Ciclosporin + Retinoids

An increase in ciclosporin blood levels occurred in one patient given etretinate, but studies have not found this effect. In two patients taking isotretinoin and ciclosporin, rises in ciclosporin levels occurred, although another patient taking both drugs had no alteration in ciclosporin levels.

Clinical evidence

(a) Etretinate

In one case, a woman with generalised pustular psoriasis who had been taking ciclosporin 200 mg daily had a considerable rise in her ciclosporin blood levels to 540 micrograms/L when the dosage was raised to 300 mg daily and etretinate 50 mg daily was added. An interaction was suspected as contributing to this effect because it was found possible to reduce the ciclosporin dosage gradually to 150 mg daily (accompanied by a fall in the trough ciclosporin blood levels to 168 micrograms/L), without any loss in the control of the disease.[1] However, only a modest ciclosporin dosage reduction was needed in another study when etretinate was given.[2]

Other reports suggest successful and uncomplicated concurrent use. There was no improvement when a patient with erythrodermic psoriasis was given ciclosporin 5 to 10 mg/kg daily, but ciclosporin 5 mg/kg daily with etretinate 700 micrograms/kg daily cleared the psoriasis by 90%. Reducing the dose of either drug resulted in exacerbation of symptoms.[3] Another 5 patients with plaque-type psoriasis had a relapse when the ciclosporin dosage was reduced in the presence of etretinate, but no additive therapeutic effect was seen. All of them had elevated serum creatinine levels.[4] No obvious advantages but no increase in adverse effects were found in another study that gave ciclosporin with etretinate.[5]

(b) Isotretinoin

A 27-year old man with a heart transplant taking ciclosporin was given isotretinoin 40 mg daily for 2 months, then 80 mg daily up to 20 weeks. His ciclosporin trough levels remained within the recommended range, and there was no evidence of graft rejection.[6] Another man with a heart transplant taking ciclosporin received isotretinoin 1 mg/kg daily for 4 months. His daily ciclosporin dose was reduced from 7 mg/kg to 6 mg/kg one month after starting isotretinoin because of a rise in ciclosporin level to 587 nanograms/mL. However, it was noted that this may have had nothing to do with the isotretinoin, since the patient required alterations in ciclosporin dose in 3 instances before isotretinoin was started. No laboratory abnormalities were noted, nor was ciclosporin toxicity seen, and the heart transplant function remained satisfactory.[7] A 13-year-old girl with aplastic anaemia and taking ciclosporin was given isotretinoin 40 mg daily for 20 weeks. She had a threefold increase in trough ciclosporin level at week 17, which was considered probably unrelated to isotretinoin, and was managed by reducing her ciclosporin dose. Serum lipids did not change during concurrent use.[8]

Mechanism

Uncertain. An *in vitro* study using human liver microsomes found that concentrations of 100 micromol of acitretin, etretinate and isotretinoin inhibited the total ciclosporin metabolism and total primary ciclosporin metabolite production to the same extent (32 to 45%).[1] These figures suggest that the retinoids may inhibit ciclosporin metabolism. However, another *in vitro* study using human liver microsomes did not find that etretinate inhibits the metabolism of ciclosporin.[9]

Importance and management

The overall picture seems to be that etretinate has only a modest effect, or no effect at all, on ciclosporin blood levels in most patients. Nevertheless, this possible interaction is worth bearing in mind because of the possibility of isolated cases of raised ciclosporin levels. There seems to be no marked therapeutic advantage in using both drugs together for psoriasis. From the cases presented, it is unclear if isotretinoin alters ciclosporin levels. In addition, it has been suggested that serum lipids should be monitored because both drugs can cause an increase.[6] **Acitretin** (the major metabolite of etretinate) probably behaves like etretinate, although this needs confirmation.

1. Shah IA, Whiting PH, Omar G, Ormerod AD, Burke MD. The effects of retinoids and terbinafine on the human hepatic microsomal metabolism of cyclosporin. *Br J Dermatol* (1993) 129, 395–8.
2. Meinardi MMHM, Bos JD. Cyclosporine maintenance therapy in psoriasis. *Transplant Proc* (1988) 20 (Suppl 4), 42–9.
3. Korstanje MJ, Bessems PJMJ, van de Staak WJBM. Combination therapy cyclosporin-etretinate effective in erythrodermic psoriasis. *Dermatologica* (1989) 179, 94.
4. Korstanje MJ, van de Staak WJBM. Combination-therapy cyclosporin-A-etretinate for psoriasis. *Clin Exp Dermatol* (1990) 15, 172–3.
5. Brechtel B, Wellenreuther U, Toppe E, Czarnetzki BM. Combination of etretinate with cyclosporine in the treatment of severe recalcitrant psoriasis. *J Am Acad Dermatol* (1994) 30, 1023–4.
6. Abel EA. Isotretinoin treatment of severe cystic acne in a heart transplant patient receiving cyclosporine: consideration of drug interactions. *J Am Acad Dermatol* (1991) 24, 511.
7. Bunker CB, Rustin MHA, Dowd PM. Isotretinoin treatment of severe acne in posttransplant patients taking cyclosporine. *J Am Acad Dermatol* (1990) 22, 693–4.
8. Hazen PE, Walker AE, Stewart JJ, Carney JF, Engstrom CW, Turgeon KL, Shurin S. Successful use of isotretinoin in a patient on cyclosporine: apparent lack of toxicity. *Int J Dermatol* (1993) 32, 466–7.
9. Webber IR, Back DJ. Effect of etretinate on cyclosporin metabolism *in vitro*. *Br J Dermatol* (1993) 128, 42–4.

Ciclosporin + Sevelamer

One study suggests sevelamer does not appear to alter ciclosporin levels, but a report describes markedly reduced ciclosporin levels in a patient who took sevelamer.

Clinical evidence, mechanism, importance and management

The pharmacokinetics of ciclosporin were unchanged in a study in 18 kidney transplant patients taking ciclosporin, (with 9 patients also taking mycophenolate) after they took sevelamer as a single 1.6- or 1.2-g dose and when sevelamer was given in the same dose, three times daily for 4 days.[1] Eight of the patients were children (average age 12 years).[1] However, the findings in this study have been criticised by other authors,[2] who, in contrast, report a case of reduced ciclosporin levels in a liver transplant patient. The patient had been stable taking ciclosporin 60 mg daily, but when she was given sevelamer 806 mg three times daily a dose increase to 85 mg daily was needed to maintain ciclosporin levels.[3] This may be due to binding of sevelamer with ciclosporin in the gut preventing ciclosporin absorption.[3,4] The manufacturers of sevelamer recommend close monitoring of ciclosporin levels with concurrent use or when sevelamer is stopped, and they also recommend that ciclosporin is taken at least 1 hour before or 3 hours after sevelamer.[5]

1. Pieper A-K, Buhle F, Bauer S, Mai I, Budde K, Haffner D, Neumayer H-H, Querfeld U. The effect of sevelamer on the pharmacokinetics of cyclosporin A and mycophenolate mofetil in patients following renal transplantation. *Nephrol Dial Transplant* (2004) 19, 2630–3.
2. Uehlinger D, Marti H-P, Jadoul M, Wauters J-P. Sevelamer and pharmacokinetics of cyclosporin A after kidney transplantation. *Nephrol Dial Transplant* (2005) 20, 661.
3. Guillen-Ananya M-A, Jadoul M. Drug interaction between sevelamer and cyclosporin. *Nephrol Dial Transplant* (2004) 19, 515.
4. Wauters J-P, Uelinger D, Marti H-P. Drug interaction between sevelamer and cyclosporin. *Nephrol Dial Transplant* (2005) 20, 660–1.
5. Renagel (Sevelamer). Genzyme Therapeutics. UK Summary of product characteristics, June 2007.

Ciclosporin + Sibutramine

Ciclosporin is predicted to raise sibutramine levels. One case report describes an increase in ciclosporin levels when a patient was changed from orlistat to sibutramine.

Clinical evidence, mechanism, importance and management

A kidney transplant patient taking ciclosporin 100 mg twice daily took orlistat for 27 months with no problems or changes in her ciclosporin levels or dosage reported. As orlistat was unsuccessful for weight reduction in this patient, sibutramine 10 mg daily was given instead. One week later her trough ciclosporin level had increased from 79 to 152 nanograms/mL and her ciclosporin daily dose was reduced by 25 mg. Her ciclosporin level was still raised one week later at 162 nanograms/mL and her ciclosporin daily dose was again reduced by 25 mg. No increase in blood pressure or serum creatinine occurred.[1]

Sibutramine is metabolised by the cytochrome P450 isoenzyme CYP3A4 although it is not known to have any effects on this isoenzyme. Ciclosporin is also metabolised by CYP3A4 and the changes in levels seen may therefore have been due to competition for metabolism. In contrast to what was seen in this case, the manufacturers predict that inhibitors of CYP3A4 (they name ciclosporin, but note that this drug does not usually interact by inhibiting this isoenzyme) may lead to an increase in levels of the active metabolite of sibutramine, but no effects on ciclosporin levels are expected.[2]

This appears to be the only case report of an increase in ciclosporin levels with sibutramine.[1] However, orlistat has been reported to reduce ciclosporin absorption, and therefore levels, see ' orlistat', (p.1042), so there is a possibility that the increase in ciclosporin levels was due to stopping orlistat rather than starting sibutramine, but this was not investigated.

1. Clerbaux G, Goffin E, Pirson Y. Interaction between sibutramine and cyclosporine. *Am J Transplant* (2003) 3, 906.
2. Reductil (Sibutramine hydrochloride monohydrate). Abbott Laboratories Ltd. UK Summary of product characteristics, November 2005.

Ciclosporin + Somatostatin analogues

Octreotide causes a marked reduction in the blood levels of ciclosporin and inadequate immunosuppression may result. Lanreotide is predicted to interact similarly.

Clinical evidence

A diabetic man with kidney and pancreatic segment transplants was successfully immunosuppressed with azathioprine, methylprednisolone and ciclosporin. When he was also given subcutaneous **octreotide** 100 micrograms twice daily to reduce fluid collection around the pancreatic graft, his trough ciclosporin blood levels fell below the assay detection limit of 50 nanograms/mL. Serum creatinine increased dramatically, which was interpreted as a selective rejection episode of the kidney transplant. Nine other diabetics similarly treated with **octreotide** for peripancreatic fluid collection and fistulas after pancreatic transplantation also had significant falls in their ciclosporin blood levels within 24 to 48 hours, in 3 of them to undetectable levels.[1] A similar interaction was seen in another patient.[2]

Mechanism

Uncertain. A suggestion is that the octreotide reduces the intestinal absorption of the ciclosporin.[1,2]

Importance and management

The interaction between octreotide and ciclosporin is established and clinically important, although the documentation is limited. The authors of one report recommend that before giving octreotide the oral dosage of ciclosporin should be increased on average by 50% and the serum levels monitored daily.[1] The manufacturers of **lanreotide** say that, as with other somatostatin analogues, it may reduce the absorption of ciclosporin from the gut.[3] As yet there appear to be no reports of this interaction in practice; however, it would be prudent to monitor the outcome of the use of lanreotide with ciclosporin.

1. Landgraf R, Landgraf-Leurs MMC, Nusser J, Hillebrand G, Illner W-D, Abendroth D, Land W. Effect of somatostatin analogue (SMS 201–995) on cyclosporine levels. *Transplantation* (1987) 44, 724–5.
2. Rosenberg L, Dafoe DC, Schwartz R, Campbell DA, Turcotte JG, Tsai S-T, Vinik A. Administration of somatostatin analog (SMS 201–995) in the treatment of a fistula occurring after pancreas transplantation. Interference with cyclosporine suppression. *Transplantation* (1987) 43, 764–6.
3. Somatuline LA (Lanreotide acetate). Ipsen Ltd. UK Summary of product characteristics, August 2003.

Ciclosporin + SSRIs and related antidepressants

Four cases of raised ciclosporin levels have been seen in patients taking nefazodone and ciclosporin, one with raised creatinine levels and tremor, and one with raised liver enzymes. A small study found no evidence of an interaction between fluoxetine and ciclosporin although one case of increased ciclosporin levels has been seen with fluoxetine. Fluvoxamine may inhibit the metabolism of ciclosporin and one case of increased ciclosporin levels has been reported with fluvoxamine. The serotonin syndrome has been seen in a patient taking ciclosporin and sertraline. Limited evidence suggests that citalopram and sertraline do not alter ciclosporin levels.

Clinical evidence

(a) Citalopram

In 5 transplant patients the pharmacokinetics of ciclosporin were not significantly affected by citalopram 10 to 20 mg daily.[1]

(b) Fluoxetine

A small, retrospective study in 9 liver transplant and 4 heart transplant patients found no evidence that fluoxetine 5 to 20 mg daily increased ciclosporin blood levels.[2] However, the ciclosporin blood levels of a heart transplant patient were doubled by fluoxetine 20 mg daily for 10 days. They fell when the ciclosporin dosage was reduced and needed to be increased again when the fluoxetine was stopped.[3]

(c) Fluvoxamine

A patient had increased ciclosporin blood levels and serum creatinine levels and fine tremor 2 weeks after starting fluvoxamine 100 mg daily, and the ciclosporin dosage was subsequently reduced by 33%.[4]

(d) Sertraline

A 53-year-old man taking ciclosporin following a renal transplant developed the serotonin syndrome 5 days after starting to take sertraline 50 mg daily. Ciclosporin is known to increase serotonin turnover within the brain, and so the reaction was attributed to an interaction between sertraline and ciclosporin.[5] One report briefly mentions that a patient taking ciclosporin had her antidepressant medication switched from nefazodone to sertraline, because sertraline did not affect ciclosporin levels.[6]

(e) Nefazodone

A kidney transplant patient had a 70% rise in trough serum ciclosporin levels within 3 days of starting to take nefazodone 25 mg twice daily.[7] Another kidney transplant patient had a two- to threefold rise in ciclosporin levels associated with raised creatinine levels and marked generalised tremors after starting nefazodone 100 mg twice daily. The patient was eventually stabilised on a 50% lower dose of ciclosporin.[4] Similarly, a cardiac transplant patient taking ciclosporin had a tenfold increase in ciclosporin levels shortly after the addition of nefazodone 150 mg twice daily. Levels returned to baseline over 6 days after nefazodone was stopped.[6] A patient taking nefazodone developed significantly raised liver enzymes AST and ALT one month after kidney transplantation. His ciclosporin level was high, at 614 nanograms/mL, and both ciclosporin and nefazodone were stopped. He had previously taken nefazodone uneventfully, and subsequently took ciclosporin uneventfully, so the raised liver enzymes were attributed to a pharmacokinetic interaction between the two drugs.[8] However, note that nefazodone has generally been withdrawn due to its adverse effects on the liver.

Mechanism

Fluvoxamine and nefazodone are inhibitors of the cytochrome P450 isoenzyme CYP3A4, the main isoenzyme by which ciclosporin is metabolised. Concurrent use can therefore lead to increased ciclosporin levels. Fluoxetine may interact similarly. Citalopram and sertraline do not usually significantly inhibit CYP3A4 and would therefore not be expected to interact.

Importance and management

Although the evidence is limited, it appears that nefazodone can cause a marked rise in ciclosporin levels, with an increase in adverse effects. Alternative antidepressants should probably be used, or concurrent therapy very well monitored. Similar caution would seem prudent with fluvoxamine, and possibly fluoxetine. Citalopram, and sertraline do not appear to alter ciclosporin levels and may therefore be suitable alternatives. Serotonin syndrome is a rare adverse effect, usually associated with the use of more than one serotonergic drug (see 'The serotonin syndrome', (p.9)).

1. Liston HL, Markowitz JS, Hunt N, DeVane CL, Boulton DW, Ashcraft E. Lack of citalopram effect on the pharmacokinetics of cyclosporine. *Psychosomatics* (2001) 42, 370–2.
2. Strouse TB, Fairbanks LA, Skotzko CE, Fawzy FI. Fluoxetine and cyclosporine in organ transplantation: failure to detect significant drug interactions or adverse clinical events in depressed organ recipients. *Psychosomatics* (1996) 37, 23–30.
3. Horton RC, Bonser RS. Interaction between cyclosporin and fluoxetine. *BMJ* (1995) 311, 422.
4. Vella JP, Sayegh MH. Interactions between cyclosporine and newer antidepressant medications. *Am J Kidney Dis* (1998) 31, 320–3.

5. Wong EH, Chan NN, Sze KH, Or KH. Serotonin syndrome in a renal transplant patient. *J R Soc Med* (2002) 95, 304–5.
6. Wright DH, Lake KD, Bruhn PS, Emery RW. Nefazodone and cyclosporine drug-drug interaction. *J Heart Lung Transplant* (1999) 18, 913–15.
7. Helms-Smith KM, Curtis SL, Hatton RC. Apparent interaction between nefazodone and cyclosporine. *Ann Intern Med* (1996) 125, 424.
8. Garton T, Nefazodone and CYP450 3A4 interactions with cyclosporine and tacrolimus. *Transplantation* (2002) 74, 745.

Ciclosporin + Sucrose polyesters

Sucrose polyesters (e.g. *Olestra*) may reduce the bioavailability and peak levels of ciclosporin.

Clinical evidence, mechanism, importance and management

A study in 7 kidney transplant patients aged 9 to 18 years, found that the addition of sucrose polyesters (*Olestra)*, in a single 0.35-g/kg dose (maximum of 16 g) reduced the ciclosporin AUC and peak levels by almost 19% and 27%, respectively. Ciclosporin trough levels and elimination rate were not affected by *Olestra*. The reduced bioavailability was thought to be due to *Olestra* reducing the absorption of ciclosporin. *Olestra* is marketed as a non-absorbable, non-calorific fat ingredient in snack foods. The authors note that *Olestra* is mainly consumed by children and adolescents, with the age group of 13 to 17-year-olds being reported to eat 16.2 g of *Olestra* per snack, and therefore this interaction could be of particular significance for young transplant patients taking ciclosporin.[1] However, note that changes in the AUC of ciclosporin of this size are very modest.

1. Terrill CJ, Lill J, Somerville KT, Sherbotie JR. Modifications in cyclosporine (CsA) microemulsion blood concentrations by Olestra. *J Ren Nutr* (2003) 13, 26–30.

Ciclosporin + Sulfasalazine

An isolated report describes elevated ciclosporin levels in a kidney transplant patient that developed when sulfasalazine was stopped.

Clinical evidence

A patient with a kidney transplant was taking azathioprine, ciclosporin, prednisone and sulfasalazine 1.5 g daily. After initial adjustments the dose of ciclosporin remained at 480 mg daily for 8 months. The dose of prednisone was reduced and treatment stopped at 8 months, and azathioprine was stopped at 12 months without any need to adjust the ciclosporin dosage. Sulfasalazine was stopped 13.5 months after transplantation and the mean ciclosporin level increased from 205 nanograms/mL to 360 nanograms/mL within 5 days, and to 389 nanograms/mL after 10 days. The ciclosporin dosage was reduced over the following 2 months from 9.6 mg/kg to 5.6 mg/kg to maintain blood levels at about 200 nanograms/mL.[1]

Mechanism

Not understood. The time course of the interaction, noted after 5 days probably excludes decreased absorption. It is possible that the interaction is due to induction of the cytochrome P450 enzymes.

Importance and management

Information appears to be limited to this isolated case report. There is insufficient evidence to recommend increased monitoring, but be aware of the potential for an interaction in the case of an unexpected response to treatment.

1. Du Cheyron D, Debruyne D, Lobbedez T, Richer C, Ryckelynck J-P, Hurault de Ligny B. Effect of sulfasalazine on cyclosporin blood concentration. *Eur J Clin Pharmacol* (1999) 55, 227–8.

Ciclosporin + Sulfinpyrazone

Sulfinpyrazone can reduce ciclosporin levels and episodes of transplant rejection have resulted.

Clinical evidence

A study in 120 heart transplant patients found that sulfinpyrazone 200 mg daily was effective in the treatment of hyperuricaemia. The mean uricaemia over 4 to 8 months fell by 22%, from 0.51 to 0.4 mmol/L, but unexpectedly the mean trough ciclosporin levels fell by 39%, from 183 to 121 micrograms/L, despite a 7.7% increase in the ciclosporin daily dosage. Two of the patients developed rejection: one after 4 months of taking sulphinpyrazone when the ciclosporin levels fell to 50 micrograms/L, and the other after 7 months of taking sulfinpyrazone, when the ciclosporin levels fell to 20 micrograms/L.[1]

Another report describes a patient who needed unusually high doses of ciclosporin while taking sulfinpyrazone,[2] while yet another report describes *increased* ciclosporin levels in a patient taking sulfinpyrazone. In this latter case there is the possibility that it may have been an artefact due to interference with the assay method.[3]

Mechanism

Not understood.

Importance and management

Information appears to be limited to these reports but the interaction would seem to be established and clinically important. If sulfinpyrazone is added to established treatment with ciclosporin, be alert for the need to raise the ciclosporin dosage. The mean fall in trough ciclosporin levels seen in the major study cited was 39%.[1] This study does comment on how quickly this interaction develops but the two cases of transplant rejection occurred after 4 months and 7 months, which implies that it can possibly be slow. Long-term monitoring would therefore be a prudent precaution. The authors of this report say that sulfinpyrazone is an effective alternative to allopurinol and no additional adverse effects occur including myelotoxicity when it is used with azathioprine.

1. Caforio ALP, Gambino A, Tona F, Feltrin G, Marchini F, Pompei E, Testolin L, Angelini A, Dalla Volta S, Casarotto D. Sulfinpyrazone reduces cyclosporine levels: a new drug interaction in heart transplant recipients. *J Heart Lung Transplant* (2000) 19, 1205–8.
2. Dossetor JB, Kovithavongs T, Salkie M, Preiksaitis J. Cyclosporine-associated lymphoproliferation, despite controlled cyclosporine blood concentrations, in a renal allograft recipient. *Proc Eur Dial Transplant Assoc Eur Ren Assoc* (1985) 21, 1021–6.
3. Cockburn I. Cyclosporin A: a clinical evaluation of drug interactions. *Transplant Proc* (1986) 18 (Suppl 5), 50–5.

Ciclosporin + Terbinafine

Terbinafine causes a small but usually clinically unimportant reduction in ciclosporin serum levels.

Clinical evidence, mechanism, importance and management

After taking terbinafine 250 mg daily for 6 to 7 days the mean AUC of a single 300-mg dose of ciclosporin was decreased by 13% and the maximum blood level was reduced by 14% in a study in 20 healthy subjects. It was suggested that as *Sandimmun* was used in the study, inter- and intra-individual variations in ciclosporin absorption caused these differences, rather than any drug interaction.[1,2] Another study in 11 patients with kidney, heart or lung transplants found that terbinafine 250 mg daily for 12 weeks caused a small but clinically irrelevant decrease in serum ciclosporin levels.[3] Another study in 30 kidney transplant patients taking ciclosporin and given terbinafine 250 mg daily for 6 to 12 weeks found no significant interaction and none of the patients required ciclosporin dose changes.[4]

Four kidney transplant patients taking ciclosporin were given terbinafine 250 mg daily for fungal skin and nail infections. Ciclosporin levels were reduced during concurrent treatment in all patients. However, in 3 of the patients ciclosporin levels remained within the therapeutic range and therefore no dose adjustment was made. One patient required an increase in the ciclosporin dose to maintain levels within the therapeutic range, and then a reduction in dose on stopping terbinafine.[5] These studies broadly confirm previous *in vitro* work with human liver microsomal enzymes, which found that terbinafine either does not inhibit ciclosporin metabolism or only causes modest inhibition.[6-8] In general, the changes in the pharmacokinetics of ciclosporin appear to be clinically unimportant. However, patients whose ciclosporin levels are at the lower end of the therapeutic range should be closely monitored if they are given terbinafine.[5]

1. Long CC, Hill SA, Thomas RC, Holt DW, Finlay AY. The effect of terbinafine on the pharmacokinetics of cyclosporin in vivo. *Skin Pharmacol* (1992) 5, 200–1.

2. Long CC, Hill SA, Thomas RC, Johnston A, Smith SG, Kendall F, Finlay AY. Effect of terbinafine on the pharmacokinetics of cyclosporin in humans. *J Invest Dermatol* (1994) 102, 740–3.

3. Jensen P, Lehne G, Fauchald P, Simonsen S. Effect of oral terbinafine treatment on cyclosporin pharmacokinetics in organ transplant recipients with dermatophyte nail infection. *Acta Derm Venereol (Stockh)* (1996) 76, 280–1.

4. Lee KH, Kim YS, Kim MS, Chung HS, Park K. Study of the efficacy and tolerability of oral terbinafine in the treatment of oncychomycosis in renal transplant patients. *Transplant Proc* (1996) 28, 1488–9.

5. Lo ACY, Lui S-L, Lo W-K, Chan DTM, Cheng IKP. The interaction of terbinafine and cyclosporine A in renal transplant patients. *Br J Clin Pharmacol* (1997) 43, 340–1.

6. Back DJ, Stevenson P, Tjia JF. Comparative effects of two antimycotic agents, ketoconazole and terbinafine, on the metabolism of tolbutamide, ethinyloestradiol, cyclosporin and ethoxycoumarin by human liver microsomes *in vitro*. *Br J Clin Pharmacol* (1989) 28, 166–70.

7. Shah IA, Whiting PH, Omar G, Ormerod AD, Burke MD. The effects of retinoids and terbinafine on the human hepatic microsomal metabolism of cyclosporin. *Br J Dermatol* (1993) 129, 395–8.

8. Back DJ, Tjia JF, Abel SM. Azoles, allylamines and drug metabolism. *Br J Dermatol* (1992) 126 (Suppl 39), 14–18.

Ciclosporin + Ticlopidine

Three case reports describe marked falls in ciclosporin blood levels, and one study noted that trough ciclosporin levels were halved by ticlopidine. However, another study reported that ticlopidine did not affect ciclosporin bioavailability.

Clinical evidence

The ciclosporin blood levels of a patient with nephrotic syndrome were roughly halved on two occasions when he was given ticlopidine 500 mg daily.[1] Another two patients with kidney transplants had similar falls (one patient on two occasions) when ticlopidine 250 mg daily was given.[2,3]

Twelve heart transplant patients were given ticlopidine 250 mg twice daily. The mean whole blood trough ciclosporin levels were noted to be halved but the mean ciclosporin dosage was not altered over a 3-month period. The neutrophil, platelet and whole blood leucocyte counts and haemoglobin levels were not significantly altered, but adverse effects included epistaxis (1 patient), haematuria (1 patient), which both necessitated a 50% dosage reduction, and neutropenia (1 patient), which resolved when the ticlopidine was withdrawn.[4]

A later study by the same group in 20 heart transplant patients given ticlopidine 250 mg daily found that the bioavailability of the ciclosporin was not clearly altered by ticlopidine, although one patient was withdrawn from the study after 3 days because of a 60% fall in ciclosporin levels, attributed to poor compliance rather than an interaction. No clinically significant adverse haematological, biochemical or ECG or echocardiography changes occurred.[5]

Mechanism

Not understood.

Importance and management

Information appears to be limited to the reports cited. It appears that the occasional patient may unpredictably have marked reductions in ciclosporin blood levels. For this reason close monitoring of ciclosporin levels is needed, particularly when ticlopidine is first added, so that any problems can be quickly identified and any dosage alterations made as needed.

1. Birmelé B, Lebranchu Y, Bagros Ph, Nivet H, Furet Y, Pengloan J. Interaction of cyclosporin and ticlopidine. *Nephrol Dial Transplant* (1991) 6, 150–1.

2. Verdejo A, de Cos MA, Zubimendi JA. Probable interaction between cyclosporin A and low dose ticlopidine. *BMJ* (2000) 320, 1037.

3. Feriozzi S, Massimetti C, Anacarani E. Treatment with ticlopidine is associated with reduction of cyclosporin A blood levels. *Nephron* (2002) 92, 249–50.

4. de Lorgeril M, Boissonnat P, Dureau G, Guidollet J, Renaud S. Evaluation of ticlopidine, a novel inhibitor of platelet aggregation, in heart transplant recipients. *Transplantation* (1993) 55, 1195–6.

5. Boissonat P, de Lorgeril M, Perroux V, Salen P, Batt AM, Barthelemy JC, Brouard R, Serres E, Delaye J. A drug interaction study between ticlopidine and cyclosporin in heart transplant recipients. *Eur J Clin Pharmacol* (1997) 53, 39–45.

Ciclosporin + Trimetazidine

Trimetazidine appears not to alter the pharmacokinetics or immunosuppressive effects of ciclosporin.

Clinical evidence, mechanism, importance and management

To find out if the concurrent use of trimetazidine and ciclosporin was associated with any adverse effects, 12 kidney transplant patients taking ciclosporin were given trimetazidine 40 mg twice daily for 5 days. No changes in the pharmacokinetics of the ciclosporin were seen, and there were no alterations in interleukin-2 concentrations or soluble interleukin-2 receptors.[1] An associated study by the same group of workers using two models (the lymphoproliferative response of normal human lymphocytes to phytohaemagglutinin and a delayed *mouse* hypersensitivity model) similarly found that trimetazidine did not interfere with the effects of ciclosporin.[2] It was concluded on the basis of these two studies that the concurrent use of ciclosporin and trimetazidine need not be avoided.

1. Simon N, Brunet P, Roumenov D, Dussol B, Barre J, Duche JC, Albengres E, D'Athis Ph, Crevat A, Berland Y, Tillement JP. The effects of trimetazidine-cyclosporin A coadministration on interleukin 2 and cyclosporin A blood levels in renal transplant patients. *Therapie* (1995) 50 (Suppl), 498.

2. Albengres E, Tillement JP, d'Athis P, Salducci D, Chauvet-Monges AM, Crevat A. Lack of pharmacodynamic interaction between trimetazidine and cyclosporin A in human lymphoproliferative and mouse delayed hypersensitivity response models. *Fundam Clin Pharmacol* (1996) 10, 264–8.

Ciclosporin + Vitamins

In a single-dose study, the ciclosporin AUC was increased by vitamin E, while in another study vitamin E decreased the ciclosporin AUC. Ciclosporin levels were also reduced by vitamin C and vitamin E with or without betacarotene.

Clinical evidence and mechanism

Ten healthy subjects were given a single 10-mg/kg oral dose of ciclosporin with and without a 0.1-mL/kg oral dose of vitamin E (d-alpha tocopheryl polyethylene glucose 1000 succinate; *Liqui-E*). The AUC of the ciclosporin increased by 60%, and it was suggested that absorption was increased due to improved solubilisation and micelle formation within the gut, or that decreased intestinal metabolism occurred.[1] In contrast, another study in 12 healthy subjects found that vitamin E 800 units daily for 6 weeks reduced the AUC of a single 5-mg/kg dose of ciclosporin by 21%.[2]

A study in 10 kidney transplant patients taking ciclosporin found that the addition of an antoxidant vitamin supplement for 6 months containing vitamin C 500 mg, vitamin E 400 units and betacarotene (vitamin A precursor) 6 mg daily reduced the ciclosporin blood level by 24%. An associated improvement in renal function, indicated by an increase in glomerular filtration rate (GFR) of 17%, was also seen and may have been associated with reduced ciclosporin levels. The reason for the reduction is unclear.[3] A study in 56 kidney transplant patients taking ciclosporin with vitamin C 1000 mg daily and vitamin E 300 mg daily found that ciclosporin levels were significantly lower in the vitamin-treated group when compared with a placebo group. A reduction in serum creatinine was also seen.[4]

Importance and management

The clinical significance of these studies is unclear as there appear to be no published case reports of any adverse effects due to this interaction. However, in some patients, changes in ciclosporin levels may significantly affect ciclosporin immunosuppression, and dose modification may be required. Patients should be questioned about their intake of vitamin supplements before starting or when taking ciclosporin, particularly if a sudden or unexplained reduction in stable ciclosporin levels occurs. More study is needed, particularly with regard to the concurrent use of standard, commercially available multivitamin preparations.

1. Chang T, Benet LZ, Hebert MF. The effect of water-soluble vitamin E on cyclosporine pharmacokinetics in healthy volunteers. *Clin Pharmacol Ther* (1996) 59, 297–303.
2. Bárány P, Stenvinkel P, Ottosson-Seeberger A, Alvestrand A, Morrow J, Roberts JJ, Salahudeen AK. Effect of 6 weeks of vitamin E administration on renal haemodynamic alterations following a single dose of neoral in healthy volunteers. *Nephrol Dial Transplant* (2001) 16, 580–4.
3. Blackhall ML, Fassett RG, Sharman JE, Geraghty DP, Coombes JS. Effects of antioxidant supplementation on blood cyclosporin A and glomerular filtration rate in renal transplant recipients. *Nephrol Dial Transplant* (2005) 20, 1970–75.
4. de Vries APJ, Oterdoom LH, Gans ROB, Bakker SJL. Supplementation with anti-oxidants vitamin C and E decreases cyclosporine A trough-levels in renal transplant recipients. *Nephrol Dial Transplant* (2006) 21, 231–2.

Corticosteroids + Aminoglutethimide

The effects of dexamethasone, but not hydrocortisone, can be reduced or abolished by aminoglutethimide.

Clinical evidence

(a) Dexamethasone

Aminoglutethimide 500 to 750 mg daily reduced the half-life of dexamethasone 1 mg from 264 to 120 minutes in 6 patients.[1] In another 22 patients it was found that larger doses of dexamethasone (1.5 to 3 mg daily) compensated for the increased dexamethasone metabolism caused by aminoglutethimide and complete adrenal suppression was achieved over a prolonged period.[1] Another study found a fourfold increase in dexamethasone clearance in 10 patients taking aminoglutethimide 1 g daily.[2]

A patient, dependent on dexamethasone due to brain oedema caused by a tumour, deteriorated rapidly, with headache and lethargy, when aminoglutethimide was also given. The problem was solved by withdrawing the aminoglutethimide and temporarily increasing the dexamethasone dosage from 6 to 16 mg daily.[3]

(b) Hydrocortisone

One study found that aminoglutethimide did not affect the response to hydrocortisone, and that hydrocortisone 40 mg was adequate replacement therapy in patients taking aminoglutethimide 1 g daily. In this study, aminoglutethimide did not affect the half-life of ^{3}H-cortisol, which suggests that it does not affect hydrocortisone metabolism.[2] Hydrocortisone 30 mg daily is normally adequate replacement in patients taking aminoglutethimide.[4]

Mechanism

Aminoglutethimide is an enzyme inducer and it seems likely that it interacts by increasing the metabolism and clearance of dexamethasone by the liver, thereby reducing its effects.[5]

Importance and management

Information is limited but the interaction between dexamethasone and aminoglutethimide is established. The reduction in the serum corticosteroid levels can be enough to reduce or even abolish the effects of corticosteroid replacement therapy[1] or to cause loss of control of a disease condition.[3] This has been successfully accommodated by increasing the dosage of the dexamethasone. Hydrocortisone is routinely used with aminoglutethimide as replacement therapy, and would seem to be a suitable alternative to dexamethasone, where clinically appropriate. Other synthetic corticosteroids are predicted to interact in the same way as dexamethasone, but this needs confirmation.

1. Santen RJ, Lipton A, Kendall J. Successful medical adrenalectomy with amino-glutethimide. Role of altered drug metabolism. *JAMA* (1974) 230, 1661–5.
2. Santen RJ, Wells SA, Runić S, Gupta C, Kendall J, Rudy EB, Samojlik E. Adrenal suppression with aminoglutethimide. I. Differential effects of aminoglutethimide on glucocorticoid metabolism as a rationale for the use of hydrocortisone. *J Clin Endocrinol Metab* (1977) 45, 469–79.
3. Halpern J, Catane R, Baerwald H. A call for caution in the use of aminoglutethimide: negative interactions with dexamethasone and beta blocker treatment. *J Med* (1984) 15, 59–63.
4. Cytadren (Aminoglutethimide). Novartis Pharmaceuticals Corporation. US Prescribing information, March 2002.
5. Santen RJ, Brodie AMH. Suppression of oestrogen production as treatment of breast carcinoma: pharmacological and clinical studies with aromatase inhibitors. *Clin Oncol* (1982) 1, 77–130.

Corticosteroids + Antacids

The absorption of prednisone, and probably prednisolone, can be reduced by large but not small doses of aluminium/magnesium hydroxide antacids. Dexamethasone absorption is reduced by magnesium trisilicate.

Clinical evidence

(a) Dexamethasone

In 6 healthy subjects **magnesium trisilicate** 5 g in 100 mL of water considerably reduced the bioavailability of a single 1-mg oral dose of dexamethasone. Using the urinary excretion of 11-hydroxycorticosteroids as a measure, the reduction in bioavailability was about 75%.[1]

(b) Prednisolone or Prednisone

Gastrogel (**aluminium/magnesium hydroxide** and **magnesium trisilicate**) 20 mL had no significant effect on the serum levels, half-life or AUC of 10- or 20-mg doses of prednisone in 5 patients and 2 healthy subjects.[2]

Another study in 8 healthy subjects given a 20-mg dose of prednisolone found that 30 mL of **Magnesium Trisilicate Mixture BP** or *Aludrox* (**aluminium hydroxide gel**) caused small changes in peak prednisolone levels and absorption, but these did not reach statistical significance. However, one subject given **magnesium trisilicate** had considerably reduced prednisolone levels.[3] **Aluminium phosphate** has also been found not to affect prednisolone absorption.[4,5] In contrast, another study in healthy subjects and patients given 60 mL of *Aldrox* or *Melox* (both containing **aluminium/magnesium hydroxide**) found that the bioavailability of prednisone 10 mg was reduced by 30% on average, and even by 40% in some individuals.[6]

Mechanism

The reduction in dexamethasone absorption is attributed to adsorption onto the surface of the magnesium trisilicate.[1,7]

Importance and management

Information seems to be limited to these studies. The indication is that large doses of some antacids can reduce the bioavailability of corticosteroids, but small doses do not, although this needs confirmation. One manufacturer of dexamethasone suggests that the doses of antacid should be spaced as far as possible from the dexamethasone,[8] while another suggests an interval of at least 2 hours.[9] In other similar antacid interactions 2 to 3 hours is usually sufficient. The manufacturers of **deflazacort** also suggest an interval of at least 2 hours between administration of deflazacort and antacids.[10] Concurrent use should be monitored to confirm that the therapeutic response is adequate. Information about the interaction of other corticosteroids and antacids is lacking.

1. Naggar VF, Khalil SA, Gouda MW. Effect of concomitant administration of magnesium trisilicate on GI absorption of dexamethasone in humans. *J Pharm Sci* (1978) 67, 1029–30.
2. Tanner AR, Caffin JA, Halliday JW, Powell LW. Concurrent administration of antacids and prednisone: effect on serum levels of prednisolone. *Br J Clin Pharmacol* (1979) 7, 397–400.
3. Lee DAH, Taylor GM, Walker JG, James VHT. The effect of concurrent administration of antacids on prednisolone absorption. *Br J Clin Pharmacol* (1979) 8, 92–4.
4. Albin H, Vinçon G, Demotes-Mainard F, Begaud B, Bedjaoui A. Effects of aluminium phosphate on the bioavailability of cimetidine and prednisolone. *Eur J Clin Pharmacol* (1984) 26, 271–3.
5. Albin H, Vinçon G, Pehourcq F, Lecorre C, Fleury B, Conri C. Influence d'un anti-acide sur la biodisponibilité de la prednisolone. *Therapie* (1983) 38, 61–5.
6. Uribe M, Casian C, Rojas S, Sierra JG, Go VLW, Muñoz RM, Gil S. Decreased bioavailability of prednisone due to antacids in patients with chronic active liver disease and in healthy volunteers. *Gastroenterology* (1981) 80, 661–5.
7. Prakash A, Verma RK. *In vitro* adsorption of dexamethasone and betamethasone on antacids. *Indian J Pharm Sci* (1984) Jan-Feb, 55–6.
8. Dexamethasone Tablets. Organon Laboratories Ltd. UK Summary of product characteristics, March 2007.
9. Dexsol Oral Solution (Dexamethasone sodium phosphate). Rosemont Pharmaceuticals Ltd. UK Summary of product characteristics, October 2005.
10. Calcort (Deflazacort). Shire Pharmaceuticals Ltd. UK Summary of product characteristics, January 2005.

Corticosteroids + Antithyroid drugs

Prednisolone clearance is increased by the use of carbimazole or thiamazole.

Clinical evidence

A comparative study was conducted in:

A. 8 women taking levothyroxine with thiamazole 2.5 mg daily or carbimazole 5 mg daily for Graves' ophthalmology,

B. 6 women taking levothyroxine who had undergone subtotal thyroidectomy, and

C. 6 other healthy women.

All were euthyroid. It was found that the clearance of a 540 microgram/kg dose of intravenous **prednisolone** in those in group A was much greater than in groups B and C (0.37, 0.24 and 0.2 L/h.kg respectively). After 6 hours the plasma **prednisolone** levels in group A were only about 10% of those in the healthy women (group C) and was undetectable after 8 hours, whereas total and unbound **prednisolone** levels were much higher and measurable over the 10 hour study period in groups B and C.[1]

In another group of previously hyperthyroid patients, now euthyroid because of carbimazole treatment, the total **prednisolone** clearance was 0.4 L/hour.[1]

Mechanism

Not established. It seems possible that the thiamazole and carbimazole increase the metabolism of the prednisolone by the liver microsomal enzymes, thereby increasing its clearance.

Importance and management

Direct information seems to be limited to this study, although the authors point out that there is a clinical impression that higher doses of prednisolone are needed in patients with Graves' disease. Be alert for the need to use higher doses of prednisolone in patients taking either thiamazole or carbimazole. Also note that a hypothyroid state may increase corticosteroid effects, and thus corticosteroids are cautioned in hypothyroid patients.

1. Legler UF. Impairment of prednisolone disposition in patients with Graves' disease taking methimazole. *J Clin Endocrinol Metab* (1988) 66, 221–3.

Corticosteroids + Aprepitant

In the short-term, aprepitant increases the plasma levels of dexamethasone and methylprednisolone.

Clinical evidence

(a) Dexamethasone

In a crossover study in 20 subjects, aprepitant 125 mg on day one, and 80 mg on days 2 to 5 given with a standard dexamethasone regimen (20 mg on day one, and 8 mg on days 2 to 5) increased the dexamethasone AUC by 2.2-fold. When the same dose of aprepitant was given with a reduced-dose dexamethasone regimen (12 mg on day one, and 4 mg on days 2 to 5), the AUC of dexamethasone was similar to that seen with the standard dexamethasone regimen given alone. All regimens in this study also included intravenous ondansetron 32 mg on day one.[1]

(b) Methylprednisolone

In a crossover study in 10 subjects, aprepitant 125 mg on day one, and 80 mg on days 2 and 3, given with a methylprednisolone regimen (125 mg intravenously on day one, and 40 mg orally on days 2 and 3), increased the AUC of methylprednisolone by 1.3-fold on day one and 2.5-fold on day 3.[1]

Mechanism

Aprepitant is a moderate inhibitor of the cytochrome P450 isoenzyme CYP3A4, and probably raises levels of these corticosteroids in the short-term by inhibiting their metabolism via CYP3A4. However, if the corticosteroids were given longer term, at later time points within 2 weeks after starting aprepitant, an inductive effect on CYP3A4 may occur; see 'Benzodiazepines + Aprepitant', p.721 for a more detailed explanation.

Importance and management

An established interaction of clinical importance. The manufacturer[2,3] recommends that the usual dose of dexamethasone should be reduced by about 50% when given with aprepitant (although note that the dose given in the manufacturers dexamethasone/aprepitant antiemetic regimen accounts for the interaction). In clinical studies a dexamethasone regimen of 12 mg on day one and 8 mg on days 2 to 4 was used, and this is the recommended regimen. The manufacturer recommends that the usual dose of intravenous methylprednisolone should be reduced by 25%, and the usual oral dose by 50%, when given with aprepitant. However, the manufacturer also notes that during continuous treatment with methylprednisolone, corticosteroid levels would be expected to *decrease* at later time points within 2 weeks of starting aprepitant and the effect is expected to be greater if methylprednisolone is given orally rather than intravenously.

1. McCrea JB, Majumdar AK, Goldberg MR, Iwamoto M, Gargano C, Panebianco DL, Hesney M, Lines CR, Petty KJ, Deutsch PJ, Murphy MG, Gottesdiener KM, Goldwater DR, Blum RA. Effects of the neurokinin1 receptor antagonist aprepitant on the pharmacokinetics of dexamethasone and methylprednisolone. *Clin Pharmacol Ther* (2003) 74, 17–24.
2. Emend (Aprepitant). Merck Sharp & Dohme Ltd. UK Summary of product characteristics, February 2007.
3. Emend (Aprepitant). Merck & Co., Inc. US Prescribing information, June 2006.

Corticosteroids + Azoles; Itraconazole

There is some evidence to suggest that itraconazole can increase the levels and/or effects of inhaled budesonide, the active metabolite of ciclesonide, deflazacort, dexamethasone and methylprednisolone, and, to a lesser extent, prednisolone and prednisone. A few case reports describe the development of secondary Cushing's syndrome in patients taking itraconazole and budesonide, fluticasone and deflazacort.

Clinical evidence

(a) Budesonide

A 70-year-old patient receiving long-term treatment for asthma, which included inhaled budesonide 1.2 to 1.6 mg daily and diltiazem, developed Cushing's syndrome after taking itraconazole 200 mg twice daily for 8 weeks for a fungal infection of the skin and subcutaneous tissues. Corticosteroid levels may already have been increased by the use of 'diltiazem', (p.1054), with the effects becoming more pronounced after starting itraconazole. Budesonide and itraconazole were discontinued but she subsequently required long-term oral hydrocortisone for secondary adrenal insufficiency. A recurrence of the fungal infection was treated with voriconazole 200 mg twice daily, which appeared not to interact with the oral hydrocortisone.[1]

Two other reports describe the development of Cushing's syndrome in patients with cystic fibrosis given inhaled budesonide, and then itraconazole for bronchopulmonary aspergillosis.[2] One patient was also taking clarithromycin. which may have contributed to the increased budesonide effects (see also 'Corticosteroids + Macrolides', p.1056). The other patient was a 4-year-old boy who developed Cushing's syndrome 2 weeks after starting treatment with itraconazole 200 mg daily and inhaled budesonide 400 micrograms daily.[3]

In a double-blind, randomised, crossover study, 10 healthy subjects were given 1 mg of inhaled budesonide over a period of 2 minutes after taking itraconazole 200 mg daily for 5 days. The AUC of budesonide was increased 4.2-fold by the itraconazole, and the plasma cortisol levels of the patients were suppressed, indicating an increased budesonide effect.[4] Another study compared the results of the ACTH (tetracosactide) test in 25 patients taking itraconazole 400 to 600 mg daily and high-dose inhaled budesonide 800 micrograms to 1.6 mg daily with patients receiving either drug alone. Adrenal insufficiency was detected in 44% of those treated with both drugs, but in none of the patients taking itraconazole or budesonide alone.[5]

(b) Ciclesonide

The manufacturer notes that giving itraconazole with ciclesonide may increase serum levels of the active metabolite of ciclesonide (seen with ketoconazole) and that the risk of adverse effects such as Cushing's syndrome may be increased.[6]

(c) Deflazacort

A patient with cystic fibrosis taking deflazacort developed Cushing's syndrome soon after starting itraconazole 200 mg twice daily. The effects gradually disappeared when the itraconazole was stopped.[7]

(d) Dexamethasone

A study in 8 healthy subjects found that itraconazole 200 mg daily for 4 days increased the AUC, peak plasma level, and elimination half-life of a single 4.5-mg dose of dexamethasone by 3.7-, 1.7-, and 2.8-fold, respectively. In another phase of the study itraconazole decreased the systemic clearance of intravenous dexamethasone 5 mg by 68% and increased the AUC and elimination half-life 3.3- and 3.2-fold, respectively. The adrenal-suppressant effects of dexamethasone were enhanced by itraconazole.[8]

(e) Fluticasone

A case report describes profound adrenal suppression with secondary Cushing's syndrome in a patient with cystic fibrosis given itraconazole 200 mg twice daily and low-dose inhaled fluticasone 250 micrograms daily.[9] Another report describes a patient with asthma who had been taking inhaled fluticasone 1 to 1.5 mg twice daily for 2 years who developed secondary Cushing's syndrome and adrenal suppression 6 weeks after starting itraconazole (initially 100 mg daily then 200 mg daily).[10]

(f) Methylprednisolone

A study in 14 healthy subjects found that itraconazole 400 mg for one day and then 200 mg daily for the next 3 days, increased the AUC of a single 48-mg dose of methylprednisolone by more than 2.5-fold.[11] Other studies in healthy subjects have found that itraconazole decreases the clearance, and increases the elimination half-life and AUC of both oral and intravenous methylprednisolone. Enhanced adrenal suppression also occurred.[12,13]

A man with a lung transplant taking methylprednisolone, ciclosporin and azathioprine was given itraconazole 200 mg twice daily to treat a suspected *Aspergillus fumigatus* infection. Three weeks later signs of corticosteroid toxicity developed, namely myopathy (confirmed by electromyography) and diabetes mellitus. Ten days after stopping the itraconazole the muscle force had improved and the daily dose of insulin had decreased from 120 to 20 units.[14]

(g) Prednisolone or Prednisone

Six patients with allergic bronchopulmonary aspergillosis (3 with underlying cystic fibrosis and 3 with severe asthma) were given itraconazole 200 mg twice daily for 1 to 6 months. Four of the patients also taking systemic prednisone were able to reduce the corticosteroid dosage by 44% (from 43 to 24 mg daily) without any clinical deterioration.[15] Another study found no clinically significant pharmacokinetic interaction between itraconazole (400 mg on day one then 200 mg daily for 3 days) and a single 60-mg dose of prednisone in healthy subjects.[11]

A study in 10 healthy subjects found that itraconazole 200 mg daily for 4 days increased the AUC of a single 20-mg oral dose of prednisolone by 24%, but this was considered to be of limited clinical significance.[16]

Mechanism

It seems probable that the itraconazole inhibits the metabolism of these corticosteroids by the cytochrome P450 isoenzyme CYP3A4 in the liver leading to higher levels and therefore increased effects. The active metabolite of ciclesonide is also metabolised by CYP3A4.[6] Prednisolone is less likely than methylprednisolone to interact with CYP3A4 inhibitors.[16]

Importance and management

These interactions appear to be established. There is currently too little data to assess the incidence, but it would be prudent to monitor the outcome of adding itraconazole to any patient taking deflazacort, dexamethasone or methylprednisolone, being alert for the need to reduce the steroid dosage. The manufacturers of ciclesonide suggest that the concurrent use of itraconazole should be avoided unless the benefits outweigh the risks.[6] Adrenal function should also be monitored in patients receiving inhaled budesonide or fluticasone given itraconazole, as Cushing's syndrome has been reported in a few patients during concurrent use. Itraconazole appears to interact with prednisone and prednisolone to a lesser extent, but the effects may still be clinically important in some patients. Information about other corticosteroids is lacking but good monitoring seems advisable with all of them.

1. Bolland MJ, Bagg W, Thomas MG, Lucas JA, Ticehurst R, Black PN. Cushing's syndrome due to interaction between inhaled corticosteroids and itraconazole. *Ann Pharmacother* (2004) 38, 46–9.
2. Main KM, Skov M, Sillesen IB, Dige-Petersen H, Müller J, Koch C, Lanng S. Cushing's syndrome due to pharmacological interaction in a cystic fibrosis patient. *Acta Paediatr* (2002) 91, 1008–11.
3. De Wachter E, Malfroot A, De Schutter I, Vanbesien J, De Schepper J. Inhaled budesonide induced Cushing's syndrome in cystic fibrosis patients, due to drug inhibition of cytochrome P450. *J Cyst Fibros* (2003) 2, 72–5.
4. Raaska K, Niemi M, Neuvonen M, Neuvonen PJ, Kivistö KT. Plasma concentrations of inhaled budesonide and its effects on plasma cortisol are increased by the cytochrome P4503A4 inhibitor itraconazole. *Clin Pharmacol Ther* (2002) 72, 362–9.
5. Skov M, Main KM, Sillesen IB, Müller J, Koch C, Lanng S. Iatrogenic adrenal insufficiency as a side-effect of combined treatment of itraconazole and budesonide. *Eur Respir J* (2002) 20,127–33.
6. Alvesco (Ciclesonide). Altana Pharma Ltd. UK Summary of product characteristics, January 2007.
7. Sauty A, Leuenberger PH, Fitting JW. Cushing's syndrome in a patient with cystic fibrosis treated with itraconazole and deflazacort for allergic bronchopulmonary aspergillosis. *Eur Respir J* (1995) 8 (Suppl 19), 441S.
8. Varis T, Kivistö KT, Backman JT, Neuvonen PJ. The cytochrome P450 3A4 inhibitor itraconazole markedly increases the plasma concentrations of dexamethasone and enhances its adrenal-suppressant effect. *Clin Pharmacol Ther* (2000) 68, 487–94.
9. Parmar JS, Howell T, Kelly J, Bilton D. Profound adrenal suppression secondary to treatment with low dose inhaled steroids and itraconazole in allergic bronchopulmonary aspergillosis in cystic fibrosis. *Thorax* (2002) 57, 749–50.
10. Woods DR, Arun CS, Corris PA, Perros P. Cushing's syndrome without excess cortisol. *BMJ* (2006) 332, 469–70.
11. Lebrun-Vignes B, Corbrion Archer V, Diquet B, Levron JC, Chosidow O, Puech AJ, Warot D. Effect of itraconazole on the pharmacokinetics of prednisolone and methylprednisolone and cortisol secretion in healthy subjects. *Br J Clin Pharmacol* (2001) 51, 443–50.
12. Varis T, Kaukonen K-M, Kivistö KT, Neuvonen PJ. Plasma concentrations and effects of oral methylprednisolone are considerably increased by itraconazole. *Clin Pharmacol Ther* (1998) 64, 363–8.
13. Varis T, Kivistö KT, Backman JT, Neuvonen PJ. Itraconazole decreases the clearance and enhances the effects of intravenously administered methylprednisolone in healthy volunteers. *Pharmacol Toxicol* (1999) 85, 29–32.
14. Linthoudt H, Van Raemdonck D, Lerut T, Demedts M, Verleden G. The association of itraconazole and methylprednisolone may give rise to important steroid-related side effects. *J Heart Lung Transplant* (1996) 15, 1165.
15. Denning DW, Van Wye JE, Lewiston NJ, Stevens DA. Adjunctive therapy of allergic bronchopulmonary aspergillosis with itraconazole. *Chest* (1991) 100, 813–9.
16. Varis T, Kivistö KT, Neuvonen PJ. The effect of itraconazole on the pharmacokinetics and pharmacodynamics of oral prednisolone. *Eur J Clin Pharmacol* (2000) 56, 57–60.

Corticosteroids + Azoles; Ketoconazole

Ketoconazole reduces the metabolism and clearance of methylprednisolone. Ketoconazole may increase levels of the active metabolite of ciclesonide. Ketoconazole modestly increases the systemic effect of inhaled budesonide and possibly fluticasone, and markedly increases the AUC of oral budesonide. The situation with prednisone and prednisolone is uncertain: studies have shown some moderate pharmacokinetic effects, but this does not appear to alter the action of either drug.

Clinical evidence

(a) Budesonide

Sixteen healthy subjects were given a single 1-mg inhaled dose of budesonide after taking ketoconazole 200 mg daily for 2 days. Plasma cortisol levels and urinary cortisol excretion were used as a measure of how much budesonide was absorbed systemically, and ketoconazole was found to cause a 37% decrease in the AUC_{0-24} of cortisol.[1]

Another study in 8 healthy subjects found that the AUC of a single 3-mg oral dose of budesonide was increased 6.5-fold when it was given with the last dose of ketoconazole 200 mg daily for 4 days. When budesonide was given 12 hours before the last dose of ketoconazole, the AUC was increased 3.8-fold.[2]

(b) Ciclesonide

The manufacturer notes that the use of ketoconazole with ciclesonide increase the serum levels of the active metabolite of ciclesonide 3.5-fold and that an increased risk of adverse effects such as cushingoid syndrome cannot be excluded.[3]

(c) Fluticasone

Sixteen healthy subjects were given a single 500-microgram inhaled dose of fluticasone after taking ketoconazole 200 mg daily for 2 days. Plasma cortisol levels and urinary cortisol excretion were used as a measure of how much fluticasone was absorbed systemically, and it was found that ketoconazole had no effect on fluticasone absorption.[1] However, the manufacturers of fluticasone cite a study in which the exposure to fluticasone was increased by 150% by ketoconazole, which resulted in reductions in plasma cortisol levels.[4]

(d) Methylprednisolone

In 6 healthy subjects ketoconazole 200 mg daily for 6 days increased the mean AUC of a single 20-mg intravenous dose of methylprednisolone by 135% and decreased the clearance by 60%. The 24-hour cortisol AUC was reduced by 44%.[5] These findings were confirmed in another study by the same group of workers.[6]

(e) Prednisolone or Prednisone

In 10 healthy subjects ketoconazole 200 mg daily for 6 to 7 days caused a 50% rise in the levels of both total and unbound prednisolone, following a dose of either oral prednisone or intravenous prednisolone.[7] In contrast, two other studies found that ketoconazole 200 mg daily for 6 days did not affect either the pharmacokinetics or the pharmacodynamics of prednisolone, as measured by the suppressive effects on serum cortisol, blood basophil and helper T-lymphocyte values of prednisolone.[8,9]

Mechanism

Ketoconazole inhibits the cytochrome P450 isoenzyme CYP3A4 in the intestinal wall and liver so that the metabolism of some corticosteroids is reduced and therefore their levels increase. The active metabolite of ciclesonide is also metabolised by CYP3A4,[3] and it may therefore be similarly affected.

Importance and management

The interaction between methylprednisolone and ketoconazole appears to be established and clinically important. A 50% reduction in the dose of methylprednisolone was recommended by the authors of one study.[6] It has been pointed out that increased corticosteroid serum levels have an increased immunosuppressive effect, which may be undesirable in those with a fungal infection needing treatment with ketoconazole.[7] The situation with prednisone and prednisolone is as yet uncertain,[10,11] and more study is needed. The study using inhaled budesonide indicates that ketoconazole increases the systemic effect of inhaled budesonide. Some manufacturers[12,13] recommend that if the combination cannot be avoided the interval between giving the two drugs should be as great as possible; a reduction in the dose of budesonide should also be considered. In addition, a significant interaction may occur with oral budesonide; the effects of ketoconazole on budesonide may be reduced by about half by separating the administration of the two drugs by 12 hours.[2] The manufacturers suggest reducing the oral budesonide dose if adverse effects occur.[14]

The situation with inhaled fluticasone is less clear, with one study finding an effect and another finding no effect. The manufacturers of fluticasone suggest that caution is warranted and where possible long-term concurrent use should be avoided.[4] Similarly, the manufacturer of ciclesonide suggests that it should not be used with ketoconazole unless the benefits outweigh the risks.[3] It would seem prudent to bear this possible interaction in mind if any corticosteroid is given with ketoconazole. Patients should be warned to be alert for any evidence of increased corticosteroid effects (such as moon face, weight gain, hyperglycaemia) and to seek medical advice if these occur.

1. Falcoz C, Lawlor C, Hefting NR, Borgstein NG, Smeets FWM, Wemer J, Jonkman JHG, House F. Effects of CYP3A4 inhibition by ketoconazole on systemic activity of inhaled fluticasone propionate and budesonide. *Eur Respir J* (1997) 10 (Suppl 25), 175S–176S.
2. Seidegård J. Reduction of the inhibitory effect of ketoconazole on budesonide pharmacokinetics by separation of their time of administration. *Clin Pharmacol Ther* (2000) 68, 13–17.
3. Alvesco (Ciclesonide). Altana Pharma Ltd. UK Summary of product characteristics, January 2007.
4. Flixotide Evohaler (Fluticasone propionate). Allen & Hanburys. UK Summary of product characteristics, March 2006.
5. Glynn AM, Slaughter RL, Brass C, D'Ambrosio R, Jusko WJ. Effects of ketoconazole on methylprednisolone pharmacokinetics and cortisol secretion. *Clin Pharmacol Ther* (1986) 39, 654–9.
6. Kandrotas RJ, Slaughter RL, Brass C, Jusko WJ. Ketoconazole effects on methylprednisolone disposition and their joint suppression of endogenous cortisol. *Clin Pharmacol Ther* (1987) 42, 465–70.
7. Zürcher RM, Frey BM, Frey FJ. Impact of ketoconazole on the metabolism of prednisolone. *Clin Pharmacol Ther* (1989) 45, 366–72.
8. Yamashita SK, Ludwig EA, Middleton E, Jusko WJ. Lack of pharmacokinetic and pharmacodynamic interactions between ketoconazole and prednisolone. *Clin Pharmacol Ther* (1991) 49, 558–70.
9. Ludwig EA, Slaughter RL, Savliwala M, Brass C, Jusko WJ. Steroid-specific effects of ketoconazole disposition: unaltered prednisolone elimination. *Drug Intell Clin Pharm* (1989) 23, 858–61.
10. Jusko WJ. Ketoconazole effects on corticosteroid disposition. *Clin Pharmacol Ther* (1990) 47, 418–9.
11. Zürcher RM, Frey BM, Frey FJ. Ketoconazole effects on corticosteroid disposition. *Clin Pharmacol Ther* (1990) 47, 419–21.
12. Pulmicort Inhaler (Budesonide). AstraZeneca UK Ltd. UK Summary of product characteristics, April 2005.
13. Novolizer (Budesonide). Meda Pharmaceuticals. UK Summary of product characteristics, June 2006.
14. Entocort CR (Budesonide) AstraZeneca UK Ltd. UK Summary of product characteristics, April 2006.

Corticosteroids + Azoles; Voriconazole

Voriconazole increases plasma levels of prednisolone but not to a clinically significant extent. A case report notes that voriconazole appears not to interact with oral hydrocortisone.

Clinical evidence

In healthy subjects, voriconazole 200 mg twice daily for 30 days increased the maximum plasma levels and AUC of a single 60-mg dose of **prednisolone** by 11% and 34%, respectively.[1,2]

A patient who developed Cushing's syndrome and secondary adrenal insufficiency during treatment with itraconazole and inhaled budesonide was given oral **hydrocortisone** replacement. The patient was then also given voriconazole 200 mg twice daily for 3 months without any apparent effects on the **hydrocortisone**.[3]

Mechanism

Voriconazole is an inhibitor of the cytochrome P450 isoenzyme CYP3A4, but its inhibitory effects are much less than those of itraconazole.[3] Therefore voriconazole is less likely than 'itraconazole', (p.1050), or 'ketoconazole', (p.1051) to affect the pharmacokinetics of the corticosteroids.

Importance and management

No dosage adjustment of the corticosteroid is said to be necessary if voriconazole is given with prednisolone,[1,2] and this also appears to be the case if voriconazole is given with hydrocortisone.[3]

1. VFEND (Voriconazole). Pfizer Ltd. UK Summary of product characteristics, July 2007.
2. VFEND (Voriconazole). Pfizer Inc. US Prescribing information, November 2006.
3. Bolland MJ, Bagg W, Thomas MG, Lucas JA, Ticehurst R, Black PN. Cushing's syndrome due to interaction between inhaled corticosteroids and itraconazole. *Ann Pharmacother* (2004) 38, 46–9.

Corticosteroids + Barbiturates

The therapeutic effects of systemic dexamethasone, methylprednisolone, prednisone and prednisolone are decreased by phenobarbital. Other barbiturates, including primidone, probably interact similarly.

Clinical evidence

(a) Dexamethasone

A 14-year-old girl with congenital adrenal hyperplasia taking dexamethasone rapidly became over-treated (weight gain, signs of hypercortisolism) when treatment with **primidone** 250 mg twice daily was withdrawn over a month. Satisfactory control was only achieved when the dexamethasone dosage was reduced threefold.[1] A reduction in the effects of dexamethasone has also been described when another patient with congenital adrenal hyperplasia was given **primidone** for petit mal seizures.[2]

(b) Methylprednisolone

Phenobarbital increased the clearance of methylprednisolone in asthmatic children by 209%.[3]

(c) Prednisolone or Prednisone

Three prednisone-dependent patients with bronchial asthma taking prednisone 10 to 40 mg daily had a marked worsening of their symptoms within a few days of starting to take **phenobarbital** 120 mg daily. There was a deterioration in their pulmonary function tests (FEV_1, degree of bronchospasm) and a rise in eosinophil counts, all of which improved when the **phenobarbital** was stopped. The prednisone clearance was increased by the **phenobarbital**.[4] In a group of 75 children with kidney transplants taking azathioprine and prednisone, the incidence of graft failure was increased in those taking **phenobarbital** 60 to 120 mg daily. Two of the 11 epileptic children were also taking phenytoin 100 mg daily.[5] Another study in renal transplant patients found that prednisolone elimination is increased by **phenobarbital**.[6]

Nine patients with rheumatoid arthritis taking prednisolone 8 to 15 mg daily had strong evidence of clinical deterioration (worsening joint tenderness, pain, morning stiffness, fall in grip strength) when they took **phenobarbital** for 2 weeks (plasma levels 0 to 86.2 micromol/L). The prednisolone half-life fell by 25%.[7]

In contrast, the prednisone requirements of children were unaltered when they took a compound preparation containing **phenobarbital** 24 mg daily.[8]

Mechanism

Phenobarbital is a recognised potent liver enzyme inducer that increases the metabolism of corticosteroids, thereby reducing their effects. Pharmacokinetic studies have shown that phenobarbital reduces the half-lives of these corticosteroids and increases their clearances by 40 to 209%.[3,4,9] Primidone interacts in a similar way because it is metabolised in the body to phenobarbital.[1]

Importance and management

The interaction between the corticosteroids and phenobarbital is well documented, well established and of clinical importance. Concurrent use need not be avoided but the outcome should be monitored. Increase the corticosteroid dosage as necessary. The extent of the increase is variable. Dexamethasone,[4] **hydrocortisone**,[10] methylprednisolone,[3,9] prednisone[4,5] and prednisolone[3,7] are all known to be affected. Prednisone and prednisolone appear to be less affected than methylprednisolone and may be preferred.[3] Be alert for the same interaction with other corticosteroids and other barbiturates, which also are enzyme-inducers, although direct evidence seems to be lacking. The dexamethasone adrenal suppression test may be expected to be unreliable in those taking phenobarbital, just as it is with phenytoin, another potent enzyme-inducer. See 'Corticosteroids + Phenytoin', p.1059.

1. Young MC, Hughes IA. Loss of therapeutic control in congenital adrenal hyperplasia due to interaction between dexamethasone and primidone. *Acta Paediatr Scand* (1991) 80, 120–4.
2. Hancock KW, Levell A. Primidone/dexamethasone interaction. *Lancet* (1978) ii, 97–8.
3. Bartoszek M, Brenner AM, Szefler SJ. Prednisolone and methylprednisolone kinetics in children receiving anticonvulsant therapy. *Clin Pharmacol Ther* (1987) 42, 424–32.
4. Brooks SM, Werk EE, Ackerman SJ, Sullivan I, Thrasher K. Adverse effects of phenobarbital on corticosteroid metabolism in patients with bronchial asthma. *N Engl J Med* (1972) 286, 1125–8.
5. Wassner SJ, Pennisi AJ, Malekzadeh MH, Fine RN. The adverse effect of anticonvulsant therapy on renal allograft survival. *J Pediatr* (1976) 88, 134–7.
6. Gambertoglio JG, Holford NHG, Kapusnik JE, Nishikawa R, Saltiel M, Stanik-Lizak P, Birnbaum JL, Hau T, Amend WJC. Disposition of total and unbound prednisolone in renal transplant patients receiving anticonvulsants. *Kidney Int* (1984) 25, 119–23.
7. Brooks PM, Buchanan WW, Grove M, Downie WW. Effects of enzyme induction on metabolism of prednisolone. Clinical and laboratory study. *Ann Rheum Dis* (1976) 35, 339–43.
8. Falliers CJ. Corticosteroids and phenobarbital in asthma. *N Engl J Med* (1972) 287, 201.
9. Stjernholm MR, Katz FH. Effects of diphenylhydantoin, phenobarbital, and diazepam on the metabolism of methylprednisolone and its sodium succinate. *J Clin Endocrinol Metab* (1975) 41, 887–93.
10. Burstein S, Klaiber EL. Phenobarbital-induced increase in 6-β-hydroxycortisol excretion: clue to its significance in human urine. *J Clin Endocrinol Metab* (1965) 25, 293–6.

Corticosteroids + Bile-acid binding resins

Colestyramine and possibly colestipol reduce the absorption of oral hydrocortisone. Colestyramine does not appear to affect prednisolone absorption.

Clinical evidence

(a) Colestyramine

In 10 healthy subjects, colestyramine 4 g reduced the AUC of a 50-mg oral dose of **hydrocortisone** by 43%. Peak levels were reduced and delayed (by about 50 minutes).[1] Two of the subjects were given both 4 g and 8 g of colestyramine, and their AUCs were reduced by 47% and 59% by the 4-g dose and by 97% and 86% by the 8-g dose.[1]

In contrast, an 8-g dose of colestyramine did not affect the bioavailability of **prednisolone** in 2 patients receiving long-term **prednisolone**.[2]

(b) Colestipol

A man with hypopituitarism taking **hydrocortisone** 20 mg each morning and 10 mg each evening became lethargic, ataxic, and developed headaches (all signs of **hydrocortisone** insufficiency) within 4 days of starting to take colestipol 15 g three times daily for hypercholesterolaemia. He responded rapidly when given intravenous **hydrocortisone** 100 mg, and was discharged with the colestipol replaced by a statin.[3]

Mechanism

It seems that hydrocortisone can become bound to colestyramine or colestipol in the gut, thereby reducing its absorption.[1,4]

Importance and management

Information is limited, but these interactions with hydrocortisone appear to be established (they are consistent with the interactions of both of these bile-acid resins with other drugs). Separate the administration of the drugs as much as possible to minimise admixture in the gut, although the authors of one report warn that this may not necessarily avoid this interaction because their data show that the colestyramine may remain in the gut for a considerable time.[1] The usual recommendation is to give other drugs one hour before or 4 to 6 hours after taking colestyramine, and one hour before or 4 hours after taking colestipol. Monitor the effects and increase the hydrocortisone dosage, or use an alternative to colestyramine, if necessary. Prednisolone may be a non-interacting alternative, but the evidence for this is extremely limited.

1. Johansson C, Adamsson U, Stierner U, Lindsten T. Interaction of cholestyramine on the uptake of hydrocortisone in the gastrointestinal tract. *Acta Med Scand* (1978) 204, 509–12.
2. Audétat V, Paumgartner G, Bircher J. Beeinträchtigt Cholestyramin die biologische Verfügbarkeit von Prednisolon? *Schweiz Med Wochenschr* (1977) 107, 527–8.
3. Nekl KE, Aron DC. Hydrocortisone-colestipol interaction. *Ann Pharmacother* (1993) 27, 980–1.
4. Ware AJ, Combes B. Influence of sodium taurocholate, cholestyramine and Mylanta on the intestinal absorption of glucocorticoids in the rat. *Gastroenterology* (1973) 64, 1150–5.

Corticosteroids + Caffeine

The results of the dexamethasone suppression test can be falsified by the acute ingestion of caffeine but chronic caffeine use does not appear to have an effect.

Clinical evidence, mechanism, importance and management

In one study, 22 healthy subjects and 6 depressed patients were given a single 480-mg dose of caffeine or placebo at 2 pm following a single 1-mg dose of **dexamethasone** given at 11 pm the previous evening. Caffeine significantly increased the cortisol levels following the **dexamethasone** dose; cortisol levels taken at 4 pm were about 146 nanomol/L with caffeine, compared with about 64 nanomol/L with placebo.[1] Thus the equivalent of about 4 to 5 cups of coffee may effectively falsify the results of the **dexamethasone** suppression test. However, in a study in 121 patients with depression, there was no correlation between chronic low to high intake of caffeine (6 mg to 2.3 g daily) and cortisol levels at 8 am, 4 pm or 11 pm on the day after a 1-mg dose of **dexamethasone** given at 11 pm the previous evening. It was suggested that chronic caffeine intake produces tolerance to the effects of acute caffeine on the hypothalamic-pituitary adrenal (HPA) axis.[2]

1. Uhde TW, Bierer LM, Post RM. Caffeine-induced escape from dexamethasone suppression. *Arch Gen Psychiatry* (1985) 42, 737–8.
2. Lee MA, Flegel P, Cameron OG, Greden JF. Chronic caffeine consumption and the dexamethasone suppression test in depression. *Psychiatry Res* (1988) 24, 61–5.

Corticosteroids + Carbamazepine

The clearance of dexamethasone, methylprednisolone and prednisolone is increased in patients taking carbamazepine, and the results of the dexamethasone suppression test may be invalid in those taking carbamazepine.

Clinical evidence

A study in 8 patients receiving long-term treatment with carbamazepine found that the elimination half-life of **prednisolone** was about 45 minutes shorter, and the clearance was 42% higher, than in 9 healthy subjects not taking carbamazepine.[1]

A study in asthmatic children found that carbamazepine increased the clearance of **prednisolone** by 79% and increased the clearance of **methylprednisolone** by 342%.[2] A patient taking carbamazepine and valproate required high-dose **prednisolone** (20 to 60 mg daily) for polymyalgia rheumatica. It was noted that when carbamazepine was discontinued her response to **prednisolone** improve, allowing the dose to be reduced to 20 mg then 10 mg daily.[3]

A report describes two patients suspected of having Cushing's syndrome because the overnight suppression test with **dexamethasone** 1 mg had not suppressed their cortisol levels. Further investigation found no clinical evidence of Cushing's syndrome and the false-positive test results were attributed to the fact that both patients were taking carbamazepine 400 mg three times daily at the time of the test. The test was repeated in one patient 3 weeks after carbamazepine was stopped and it indicated normal cortisol suppression.[4] A study in 8 healthy subjects found that, in the presence of carbamazepine 800 mg daily, the dosage of **dexamethasone** needed to suppress cortisol secretion (as part of the **dexamethasone** adrenal suppression test) was increased two to fourfold.[5] A further study found that it took 2 to 13 days for false-positive results to occur after carbamazepine was started, and 3 to 12 days to recover when the carbamazepine was stopped.[6]

Mechanism

Carbamazepine induces liver enzymes, which results in the increased metabolism of the steroids.

Importance and management

Information is limited but the interaction appears to be established. Patients taking carbamazepine are likely to need increased doses of dexamethasone, methylprednisolone or prednisolone. Prednisolone is less affected than methylprednisolone and is probably preferred. The same interaction seems likely with other corticosteroids but more study is needed to confirm this. Note that **hydrocortisone** and **prednisone** are affected by another potent enzyme inducer, 'phenobarbital', (p.1052), and would therefore also be expected to interact with carbamazepine.

1. Olivesi A. Modified elimination of prednisolone in epileptic patients on carbamazepine monotherapy, and in women using low-dose oral contraceptives. *Biomed Pharmacother* (1986) 40, 301–8.
2. Bartoszek M, Brenner AM, Szefler SJ. Prednisolone and methylprednisolone kinetics in children receiving anticonvulsant therapy. *Clin Pharmacol Ther* (1987) 42, 424–32.
3. Sato A, Katada S, Sato M, Kobayashi H. A case of polymyalgia rheumatica with improved steroid-responsibility after discontinuing carbamazepine. *No To Shinkei* (2004) 56, 61–3.
4. Ma RCW, Chan WB, So WY, Tong PCY, Chan JCN, Chow CC. Carbamazepine and false positive dexamethasone suppression tests for Cushing's syndrome. *BMJ* (2005) 330, 299–300.
5. Köbberling J, v zur Mühlen A. The influence of diphenylhydantoin and carbamazepine on the circadian rhythm of free urinary corticoids and on the suppressibility of the basal and the 'impulsive' activity by dexamethasone. *Acta Endocrinol (Copenh)* (1973) 72, 308–18.
6. Privitera MR, Greden JF, Gardner RW, Ritchie JC, Carroll BJ. Interference by carbamazepine with the dexamethasone suppression test. *Biol Psychiatry* (1982) 17, 611–20.

Corticosteroids + Diltiazem

Diltiazem increases the AUC of intravenous and oral methylprednisolone, but the clinical significance of this is unclear.

Clinical evidence

In a study, 5 healthy subjects were given diltiazem 180 mg daily for 4 days, with and without *intravenous* **methylprednisolone** 300 micrograms/kg (based on ideal body-weight) on day 5. Diltiazem increased the AUC of **methylprednisolone** by 50%, prolonged its half-life by 37% and reduced the **methylprednisolone** clearance by 33%. Although the morning cortisol concentration was only 12% of that during the placebo phase, overall the suppressive effects of **methylprednisolone** on cortisol excretion were unchanged.[1] Another similar study in which patients were given diltiazem and a single 16-mg oral dose of **methylprednisolone** found much larger effects: the AUC of **methylprednisolone** was increased 2.6-fold, and the morning cortisol excretion was only 12% of that in the absence of diltiazem,[2] suggesting an enhanced effect.

Mechanism

Diltiazem is an inhibitor of the cytochrome P450 isoenzyme CYP3A4. As methylprednisolone is metabolised by CYP3A4 any inhibition of its activity would be expected to raise methylprednisolone levels.[1,2] It has been suggested that P-glycoprotein may also play a role.[1,2] Inhibition of intestinal/hepatic CYP3A4 may increase the oral bioavailability of methylprednisolone, which could contribute to the pharmacokinetic differences seen in the interaction when methylprednisolone is given orally rather than intravenously.

Importance and management

Information about the interaction between diltiazem and methylprednisolone seems limited to these two studies, but the effect of concurrent use is clear. However, the clinical significance of the raised methylprednisolone levels has not been established. Monitoring for an increase in the adverse effects of methylprednisolone, as suggested by one of the authors, seems a prudent measure.[1]

1. Booker BM, Magee MH, Blum RA, Lates CD, Jusko WJ. Pharmacokinetic and pharmacodynamic interactions between diltiazem and methylprednisone in healthy volunteers. *Clin Pharmacol Ther* (2002) 72, 370–82.
2. Varis T, Backman JT, Kivistö KT, Neuvonen PJ. Diltiazem and mibefradil increase the plasma concentrations and greatly enhance the adrenal-suppressant effect of oral methylprednisolone. *Clin Pharmacol Ther* (2000) 67, 215–21.

Corticosteroids + Diuretics; Potassium-depleting

Since both corticosteroids and the loop or thiazide diuretics can cause potassium loss, severe depletion is possible if they are used together.

Clinical evidence, mechanism, importance and management

There seem to be no formal clinical studies about the extent of the additive potassium depletion that can occur when potassium-depleting diuretics and corticosteroids are given together but an exaggeration of the potassium loss undoubtedly occurs (e.g. seen with **hydrocortisone** and **furosemide**[1]). One study looking at hypokalaemia with potassium-depleting diuretics found that corticosteroids were a significant risk factor for hypokalaemic events; 19.9% of patients taking a potassium-depleting diuretic developed hypokalaemia, whereas 31.1% of patients taking a potassium-depleting diuretic and a corticosteroid developed hypokalaemia.[2] Hypokalaemia in patients taking potassium-depleting diuretics should be corrected before a corticosteroid is started. Concurrent use should be well monitored and the potassium intake increased as appropriate to balance this loss.

The greatest potassium loss occurs with the naturally occurring corticosteroids such as **cortisone** and **hydrocortisone**. **Corticotropin (ACTH)**, which is a pituitary hormone, and **tetracosactrin** (a synthetic polypeptide) stimulate corticosteroid secretion by the adrenal cortex and can thereby indirectly cause potassium loss. **Fludrocortisone** also causes potassium loss. The synthetic corticosteroids (**glucocorticoids**) have a less marked potassium-depleting effect and are therefore less likely to cause problems. These include **betamethasone**, **dexamethasone**, **prednisolone**, **prednisone** and **triamcinolone**.

The potassium-depleting diuretics (i.e. **loop diuretics** or **thiazide** and related diuretics) are listed in 'Table 26.1', (p.944). **Acetazolamide**, a weak diuretic, has also been predicted to cause hypokalaemia in the presence of corticosteroids. However, hypokalaemia seen with **acetazolamide** is rarely clinically significant, and therefore the risks are lower

1. Manchon ND, Bercoff E, Lemarchand P, Chassagne P, Senant J, Bourreille J. Fréquence et gravité des interactions médicamenteuses dans une population âgée: étude prospective concernant 639 malades. *Rev Med Interne* (1989) 10, 521–5.
2. Widmer P, Maibach R, Künzi UP, Capaul R, Mueller U, Galeazzi R, Hoigné R. Diuretic-related hypokalaemia: the role of diuretics, potassium supplements, glucocorticoids and β_2-adrenoceptor agonists. *Eur J Clin Pharmacol* (1995) 49, 31–6.

Corticosteroids + Ephedrine

Ephedrine increases the clearance of dexamethasone.

Clinical evidence, mechanism, importance and management

Nine asthmatic patients had a 40% increase in the clearance and a similar reduction in the half-life of **dexamethasone** when they were given ephedrine 100 mg daily for 3 weeks.[1] This would be expected to reduce the overall effects of **dexamethasone**, but this requires confirmation. Be alert for any evidence that the **dexamethasone** effects are reduced if both drugs are given. It is not clear whether other corticosteroids behave similarly.

1. Brooks SM, Sholiton LJ, Werk EE, Altenau P. The effects of ephedrine and theophylline on dexamethasone metabolism in bronchial asthma. *J Clin Pharmacol* (1977) 17, 308–18.

Corticosteroids + Fluoxetine

Fluoxetine does not affect the pharmacokinetics of prednisolone or its effects on cortisol suppression.

Clinical evidence, mechanism, importance and management

In healthy subjects, fluoxetine 20 mg daily for 5 days then 60 mg daily for 9 days did not significantly affect the pharmacokinetics of a single 40-mg dose of **prednisolone succinate**, given as an intravenous bolus, or the duration of cortisol suppression.[1] Fluoxetine is a potent inhibitor of the cytochrome P450 isoenzyme CYP2D6 but it also inhibits other isoenzymes including CYP3A4 and thus may inhibit the metabolism of corticosteroids that are CYP3A4 substrates. However, **prednisolone** is less likely than other corticosteroids, such as **methylprednisolone**, to interact with CYP3A4 inhibitors.[2] No clinically important interaction is likely if **prednisolone** and fluoxetine are given concurrently. The situation with other corticosteroids that may be more likely to interact is not known. More study is needed.

1. Carson SW, Letrent KJ, Kotlyar M, Foose G, Tancer ME. Lack of fluoxetine effect on prednisolone disposition and cortisol suppression. *Pharmacotherapy* (2004) 24, 482–7.
2. Varis T, Kivistö KT, Neuvonen PJ. The effect of itraconazole on the pharmacokinetics and pharmacodynamics of oral prednisolone. *Eur J Clin Pharmacol* (2000) 56, 57–60.

Corticosteroids + Glycyrrhizin (Liquorice)

Glycyrrhizin can reduce the clearance of prednisolone.

Clinical evidence, mechanism, importance and management

A study in 6 healthy subjects found that after taking 50-mg oral doses of glycyrrhizin every 8 hours for 4 doses, followed by a bolus injection of **prednisolone hemisuccinate** 96 micrograms/kg, the AUC of total **prednisolone** was increased by 50% and the AUC of free **prednisolone** was increased by 55%.[1] This confirms the findings of two previous studies in which the glycyrrhizin was given orally,[1] or by intravenous infusion,[2] and one study where the route of administration is not clear.[3]

A study that included 4 patients taking **hydrocortisone** found glycyrrhizin also increased the corticosteroid AUC and half-life.[3]

The probable reason for this reaction is that glycyrrhizin inhibits the metabolism of **prednisolone** by the liver. In one of the studies it was also found that glycyrrhizin increased the effects of **prednisolone** in some patients with rheumatoid arthritis and polyarteritis nodosa.[2]

The clinical importance of these observations is uncertain, but some increase in effects may be beneficial whereas excess effects may be toxic. Concurrent use should be well monitored.

1. Chen M-F, Shimada F, Kato H, Yano S, Kanaoka M. Effect of oral administration of glycyrrhizin on the pharmacokinetics of prednisolone. *Endocrinol Jpn* (1991) 38, 167–74.
2. Chen M-F, Shimada F, Kato H, Yano S, Kanaoka M. Effect of glycyrrhizin on the pharmacokinetics of prednisolone following low dosage of prednisolone hemisuccinate. *Endocrinol Jpn* (1990) 37, 331–41.
3. Ojima M, Satoh K, Gomibuchi T, Itoh N, Kin S, Fukuchi S, Miyachi Y. The inhibitory effects of glycyrrhizin and glycyrrhetinic acid on the metabolism of cortisol and prednisolone—*in vivo* and *in vitro* studies. *Nippon Naibunpi Gakkai Zasshi* (1990) 66, 584–96.

Corticosteroids + Grapefruit juice

Grapefruit juice increases plasma levels of methylprednisolone and is predicted to increase plasma levels of rectal budesonide. Grapefruit juice does not affect the pharmacokinetics of prednisone or prednisolone.

Clinical evidence, mechanism, importance and management

(a) Budesonide

One of the manufacturers of rectal budesonide predict that grapefruit juice will increase budesonide levels and therefore advise that concurrent use should be avoided. Even though budesonide plasma levels are higher after rectal use than after oral or inhaled use, this seems a very cautious approach.[1]

(b) Methylprednisolone

In a crossover study, 10 healthy subjects were given either double-strength grapefruit juice 200 mL, or water, three times daily for 2 days. On day 3, grapefruit juice 200 mL or water was given with, and 30 and 90 minutes after, a single 16-mg dose of methylprednisolone. Grapefruit juice increased the AUC and peak plasma level of methylprednisolone by 75% and 27%, respectively. The time to reach peak levels was increased from 2 to 3 hours and the elimination half-life was increased by 35%. Plasma cortisol levels after methylprednisolone was given with grapefruit juice or water were not significantly different, although grapefruit juice slightly decreased plasma cortisol levels before the morning dose of methylprednisolone. As the effects on plasma cortisol levels were slight this interaction is unlikely to be of clinical significance in most patients' although the authors note that in some sensitive subjects large amounts of grapefruit juice might enhance the effects of oral methylprednisolone.[2]

(c) Prednisolone or Prednisone

A study in 12 kidney transplant patients taking ciclosporin and corticosteroids found that grapefruit juice, given every 3 hours for 30 hours, increased ciclosporin levels, but had no significant effect on the AUC of prednisone or prednisolone. It was concluded that grapefruit juice does not affect the metabolism of prednisone or prednisolone.[3] No special precautions are therefore needed if patients drink grapefruit juice while taking these corticosteroids.

1. Budenofalk Rectal Foam (Budesonide). Dr. Falk Pharma UK Ltd. UK Summary of product characteristics, June 2006.
2. Varis T, Kivistö KT, Neuvonen PJ. Grapefruit juice can increase the plasma concentrations of oral methylprednisolone. *Eur J Clin Pharmacol* (2000) 56, 489–93.
3. Hollander AA, van Rooij J, Lentjes EGWM, Arbouw F, van Bree JB, Schoemaker RC, van Es LA, van der Woude FJ, Cohen AF. The effect of grapefruit juice on cyclosporine and prednisone metabolism in transplant patients. *Clin Pharmacol Ther* (1995) 57, 318–24.

Corticosteroids + H_2-receptor antagonists

Cimetidine does not interact with prednisolone, prednisone or dexamethasone, and ranitidine does not interact with prednisone.

Clinical evidence, mechanism, importance and management

Prednisone is a pro-drug, which must be converted to prednisolone within the body to become active. A double-blind crossover study in 9 healthy subjects found that **cimetidine** 300 mg every 6 hours or **ranitidine** 150 mg twice daily for 4 days did not significantly alter the pharmacokinetics of prednisolone after a single 40-mg oral dose of **prednisone**.[1] Another double-blind, crossover study found that **cimetidine** 1 g daily only caused minor changes in plasma **prednisolone** levels following a 10-mg dose of enteric-coated **prednisolone**.[2] Similarly, another study found that **cimetidine** 600 mg twice daily for 7 days had no effect on the pharmacokinetics of a single 8-mg intravenous dose of **dexamethasone sodium phosphate**.[3]

There would therefore seem to be no reason for avoiding concurrent use. Information about other corticosteroids appears to be lacking, but no interaction is anticipated.

1. Sirgo MA, Rocci ML, Ferguson RK, Eshelman FN Vlasses PH. Effects of cimetidine and ranitidine on the conversion of prednisone to prednisolone. *Clin Pharmacol Ther* (1985) 37, 534–8.
2. Morrison PJ, Rogers HJ, Bradbrook ID, Parsons C. Concurrent administration of cimetidine and enteric-coated prednisolone: effect on plasma levels of prednisolone. *Br J Clin Pharmacol* (1980) 10, 87–9.
3. Peden NR, Rewhorn I, Champion MC, Mussani R, Ooi TC. Cortisol and dexamethasone elimination during treatment with cimetidine. *Br J Clin Pharmacol* (1984) 18, 101–3.

Corticosteroids + Hormonal contraceptives and Sex hormones

The serum levels of prednisone, prednisolone, cloprednol, methylprednisolone and possibly other corticosteroids are increased by oral contraceptives. In theory, both the therapeutic and toxic effects would be expected to be increased, but in practice it is uncertain whether these changes are important. Fluocortolone and oral budesonide levels were not affected by oral contracep-

tives. Prasterone did not affect the pharmacokinetics of prednisone or the effects of prednisolone on cortisol secretion. Progesterone appears not to affect the metabolism of prednisolone.

Clinical evidence

(a) Oral contraceptives

1. Budesonide. In 20 women taking an oral contraceptive (**ethinylestradiol/desogestrel**) the plasma levels of an oral budesonide 4.5 mg daily for 7 days, and cortisol suppression were no different, when compared with 20 women not taking an oral contraceptive.[1]

2. Cloprednol. The clearance of cloprednol 20 mg was decreased by about one-third in 7 women taking an oral contraceptive (**ethinylestradiol/norethisterone**), when compared with women not taking an oral contraceptive.[2]

3. Fluocortolone. A study in 7 women found that the pharmacokinetics of fluocortolone 20 mg were unaffected by an oral contraceptive (**ethinylestradiol/norethisterone**).[3]

4. Methylprednisolone. A study in two groups of 6 patients found that the clearance of methylprednisolone was decreased to about half in the group taking oral contraceptives, when compared with the group not taking oral contraceptives. The oral contraceptive group were less sensitive to the suppressive effects of methylprednisolone on the secretion of cortisol, and had more suppression of basophils, but no changes in the T-helper cell response patterns.[4]

5. Prednisolone or prednisone. In a placebo-controlled study, 20 healthy women took an oral contraceptive (**ethinylestradiol/desogestrel** 30/150 micrograms) for at least 4 months before being given prednisolone 20 mg daily for 7 days. The prednisolone AUC and steady-state levels were 2.3-fold higher, when compared with those in 20 women not taking oral contraceptives.[1] Several other studies have found similar results, with the prednisolone AUC increasing 1.6- to 6-fold,[5,6] and the clearance reducing by about 35 to 85%[5-10] in the presence of oral contraceptives containing **ethinylestradiol** or **mestranol** and various progestogens such as **levonorgestrel**, **norgestrel** and **norethisterone**. Similarly, a 2.3-fold increase in the AUC of prednisolone and a 45% decrease in its clearance was seen when prednisone was given to women taking an oral contraceptive.[11]

(b) Prasterone

In a study in 14 healthy women, prasterone 200 mg daily for one menstrual cycle (approximately 28 days) did not affect the pharmacokinetics of a single 20-mg dose of **prednisone** or its inhibition of cortisol secretion.[12]

(c) Progesterone

Intravenous and oral **prednisolone** was given to 6 post-menopausal women before and after they took progesterone 5 mg for 2 months. The pharmacokinetics of the **prednisolone** were not significantly altered.[13]

Mechanism

Not understood. The possibilities include a change in the metabolism of the corticosteroids, or in their binding to serum proteins.[11] The absence of an interaction with progesterone suggests that the oestrogenic component of the oral contraceptives is possibly responsible for any interaction.[13]

Importance and management

It is established that the pharmacokinetics of some corticosteroids are affected by oral contraceptives, but the clinical importance of any such changes is not known. The therapeutic and adverse effects would be expected to be increased but there appear to be no clinical reports of adverse reactions arising from concurrent use. In fact the authors of one study[4] concluded that women can be dosed similarly with methylprednisolone irrespective of oral contraceptive use.

However, until more is known it would be prudent to bear this interaction in mind when using any corticosteroid and oral contraceptive together. Only prednisone, prednisolone, cloprednol and methylprednisolone have been reported to interact and other corticosteroids possibly behave similarly, the exception apparently being fluocortolone and oral budesonide. Progesterone appears not to interact with prednisolone.

1. Seidegård J, Simonsson M, Edsbäcker S. Effect of an oral contraceptive on the plasma levels of budesonide and prednisolone and the influence on plasma cortisol. *Clin Pharmacol Ther* (2000) 67, 373–81.
2. Legler UF. Altered cloprednol disposition in oral contraceptive users. *Clin Pharmacol Ther* (1987) 41, 237.
3. Legler UF. Lack of impairment of fluocortolone disposition in oral contraceptive users. *Eur J Clin Pharmacol* (1988) 35, 101–3.
4. Slayter KL, Ludwig EA, Lew KH, Middleton E, Ferry JJ, Jusko WJ. Oral contraceptive effects on methylprednisolone pharmacokinetics and pharmacodynamics. *Clin Pharmacol Ther* (1996) 59, 312–21.
5. Legler UF, Benet LZ. Marked alterations in prednisolone elimination for women taking oral contraceptives. *Clin Pharmacol Ther* (1982) 31, 243.
6. Olivesi A. Modified elimination of prednisolone in epileptic patients on carbamazepine monotherapy, and in women using low-dose oral contraceptives. *Biomed Pharmacother* (1986) 40, 301–8.
7. Boekenoogen SJ, Szefler SJ, Jusko WJ. Prednisolone disposition and protein binding in oral contraceptive users. *J Clin Endocrinol Metab* (1983) 56, 702–9.
8. Kozower M, Veatch L, Kaplan MM. Decreased clearance of prednisolone, a factor in the development of corticosteroid side effects. *J Clin Endocrinol Metab* (1974) 38, 407–12.
9. Legler UF, Benet LZ. Marked alterations in dose-dependent prednisolone kinetics in women taking oral contraceptives. *Clin Pharmacol Ther* (1986) 39, 425–9.
10. Meffin PJ, Wing LMH, Sallustio BC, Brooks PM. Alterations in prednisolone disposition as a result of oral contraceptive use and dose. *Br J Clin Pharmacol* (1984) 17, 655–64.
11. Frey BM, Schaad HJ, Frey FJ. Pharmacokinetic interaction of contraceptive steroids with prednisone and prednisolone. *Eur J Clin Pharmacol* (1984) 26, 505–11.
12. Meno-Tetang GML, Blum RA, Schwartz KE, Jusko WJ. Effects of oral prasterone (dehydroepiandrosterone) on single-dose pharmacokinetics of oral prednisone and cortisol suppression in normal women. *J Clin Pharmacol* (2001) 41, 1195–1205.
13. Tsunoda SM, Harris RZ, Mroczkowski PJ, Hebert MF, Benet LZ. Oral progesterone therapy does not affect the pharmacokinetics of prednisolone and erythromycin in post-menopausal women. *Clin Pharmacol Ther* (1995) 57, 182.

Corticosteroids + Macrolides

Troleandomycin and, to a lesser extent, clarithromycin and erythromycin can reduce the clearance of methylprednisolone, thereby increasing both its therapeutic and adverse effects. A patient receiving long-term clarithromycin developed Cushing's syndrome after starting treatment with inhaled budesonide. There appears to be no pharmacokinetic interaction between erythromycin and inhaled ciclesonide. Similarly, prednisolone appears not to be affected by macrolides, except possibly in those also taking enzyme-inducers such as phenobarbital. Isolated case reports describe the development of acute mania and psychosis in two patients, apparently due to an interaction between prednisone and clarithromycin.

Clinical evidence

(a) Budesonide

A 40-year-old woman with cystic fibrosis given **clarithromycin** 500 mg twice daily for 4 years for a *Mycobacterium abscessus* infection developed Cushing's syndrome with adrenal suppression 6 weeks after starting to use inhaled budesonide 400 micrograms daily. A slow rise in morning free cortisol levels was found 4 weeks after stopping budesonide, but she died 8 weeks later of severe respiratory failure.[1]

(b) Ciclesonide

In a crossover study, healthy subjects were given a single 500-mg dose of **erythromycin** and inhaled ciclesonide 640 micrograms, alone or together. Concurrent use did not alter the pharmacokinetics of either drug.[2]

(c) Methylprednisolone

1. Azithromycin. A review by the manufacturers briefly mentions that azithromycin did not alter the pharmacokinetics of methylprednisolone.[3]

2. Clarithromycin. A study in 6 asthmatic patients found that clarithromycin 500 mg twice daily for 9 days reduced the clearance of a single dose of methylprednisolone by 65% and resulted in significantly higher plasma methylprednisolone levels.[4]

3. Erythromycin. A study in 9 asthmatic patients aged 9 to 18 found that after taking erythromycin 250 mg four times daily for a week, the clearance of methylprednisolone was decreased by 46% (range 28 to 61%) and the half-life was increased by 47%, from 2.34 to 3.45 hours.[5]

4. Troleandomycin. A pharmacokinetic study in 4 children and 6 adult corticosteroid-dependent asthmatics found that troleandomycin 14 mg/kg daily for one week increased the half-life of methylprednisolone by 88%, from 2.46 to 4.63 hours, and reduced the total body clearance by 64%. All 10 had cushingoid symptoms (cushingoid facies and weight gain), which resolved when the methylprednisolone dosage was reduced, without any loss in the control of the asthma.[6] Another study found that the dose of methylprednisolone could be reduced by 50% in the presence of troleandomycin, without loss of disease control.[7] Other studies have found similar effects.[8-13] However, a randomised, placebo-controlled 2-year study found that although troleandomycin modestly reduced the required dose of methylprednisolone, this did not reduce corticosteroid-related adverse effects.[13] A case report describes a fatal varicella infection attributed to the potentiation of steroid effects by troleandomycin.[14]

(d) Prednisolone or Prednisone

1. Clarithromycin. A 30-year-old woman with no history of mental illness was treated for acute sinusitis with prednisone 20 mg daily for 2 days, followed by 40 mg for a further 2 days and clarithromycin 1 g daily. After 5 days she stopped taking both drugs (for unknown reasons), but a further 5 days later she was hospitalised with acute mania (disorganised thoughts and behaviour, pressured speech, increased energy, reduced need for sleep and labile effect). She spontaneously recovered after a further 5 days and had no evidence of psychiatric illness 4 months later.[15] A 50-year-old man with emphysema was given prednisone 20 mg daily to improve dyspnoea. After about 2 weeks he was also given clarithromycin 500 mg twice daily for purulent bronchitis. Shortly afterwards his family noticed psychiatric symptoms characterised by paranoia, delusions and what was described as dangerous behaviour. He recovered following treatment with low-dose olanzapine, a gradual reduction of the prednisone dosage and discontinuation of the clarithromycin. An interaction was suspected as the patient had previously received prednisone on a number of occasions without the development of psychosis.[16]
A study in 6 asthmatic patients found that clarithromycin 500 mg twice daily for 9 days had no significant effect on prednisone pharmacokinetics.[4]

2. Troleandomycin. A study found that prednisolone clearance was not affected by troleandomycin in 3 patients, but was reduced by about 50% by troleandomycin in one patient who was also taking **phenobarbital**, which is an enzyme inducer.[8]

Mechanism

What is known suggests that clarithromycin, erythromycin and troleandomycin can inhibit the metabolism of methylprednisolone. The volume of distribution is also decreased.[5,6,8,17] Clarithromycin may inhibit the metabolism of budesonide.[1]

Importance and management

Information about the clarithromycin or erythromycin interactions with methylprednisolone is much more limited than with the interaction between troleandomycin and methylprednisolone, but they all appear to be established and of clinical importance. The effect should be taken into account during concurrent use and appropriate dosage reductions made to avoid the development of corticosteroid adverse effects. The authors of one study[6] suggest that this reduction should be empirical, based primarily on clinical symptomatology. Another group found that a 68% reduction in methylprednisolone dosage was possible within 2 weeks.[10] Troleandomycin appears to have a greater effect than erythromycin or clarithromycin.

Prednisolone seems not to interact with troleandomycin and may be a non-interacting alternative, except possibly in those taking enzyme-inducers (e.g. phenobarbital).

The evidence for the interaction leading to psychosis between prednisone and clarithromycin is limited and its general importance is uncertain, but prescribers should be aware of the reports of psychosis if both drugs are used together. Note that psychosis is a rare adverse effect of high-dose corticosteroids given alone.

One case report indicates that clarithromycin may enhance the effects of inhaled budesonide and although the authors suggest that prolonged use of clarithromycin and the terminal condition of the patient may have been factors, they advise close monitoring if the combination is used.[1] Note that rectal budesonide produces higher plasma levels than the oral or inhaled use. The manufacturers of one UK rectal preparation advise that potent inhibitors of CYP3A4 (they name clarithromycin) should be avoided.[18] However, given the evidence available, this seems a very cautious approach.

In general the concurrent use of corticosteroids and macrolides need not be avoided, but it would seem prudent to monitor for corticosteroid adverse effects and suspect an interaction if symptoms occur.

1. De Wachter E, Malfroot A, De Schutter I, Vanbesien J, De Schepper J. Inhaled budesonide induced Cushing's syndrome in cystic fibrosis patients, due to drug inhibition of cytochrome P450. *J Cyst Fibros* (2003) 2, 72–5.
2. Nave R, Drollmann A, Steinijans VW, Zech K, Bethke TD. Lack of pharmacokinetic drug-drug interaction between ciclesonide and erythromycin. *Int J Clin Pharmacol Ther* (2005) 43, 264–70.
3. Hopkins S. Clinical toleration and safety of azithromycin. *Am J Med* (1991) 91 (Suppl 3A), 40S–45S.
4. Fost DA, Leung DY, Martin RJ, Brown EE, Szefler SJ, Spahn JD. Inhibition of methylprednisolone elimination in the presence of clarithromycin therapy. *J Allergy Clin Immunol* (1999) 103, 1031–5.
5. LaForce CF, Szefler SJ, Miller MF, Ebling W, Brenner M. Inhibition of methylprednisolone elimination in the presence of erythromycin therapy. *J Allergy Clin Immunol* (1983) 72, 34–9.
6. Szefler SJ, Rose JQ, Ellis EF, Spector SL, Green AW, Jusko WJ. The effect of troleandomycin on methylprednisolone elimination. *J Allergy Clin Immunol* (1980) 66, 447–51.
7. Ball BD, Hill M, Brenner M, Sanks R, Szefler SJ. Critical assessment of troleandomycin in severe steroid-requiring asthmatic children. *Ann Allergy* (1988) 60, 155.
8. Szefler SJ, Ellis EF, Brenner M, Rose JQ, Spector SL, Yurchak A, Andrews F, Jusko WJ. Steroid-specific and anticonvulsant interaction aspects of triacetyloleandomycin-steroid therapy. *J Allergy Clin Immunol* (1982) 69, 455–60.
9. Itkin IH, Menzel M. The use of macrolide antibiotic substances in the treatment of asthma. *J Allergy* (1970) 45, 146–62.
10. Wald JA, Friedman BF, Farr RS. An improved protocol for the use of troleandomycin (TAO) in the treatment of steroid-requiring asthma. *J Allergy Clin Immunol* (1986) 78, 36–43.
11. Zeiger RS, Schatz M, Sperling W, Simon RA, Stevenson DD. Efficacy of troleandomycin in outpatients with severe, corticosteroid-dependent asthma. *J Allergy Clin Immunol* (1980) 66, 438–46.
12. Kamada AK, Hill MR, Brenner AM, Szefler SJ. Glucocorticoid reduction with troleandomycin in chronic, severe asthmatic children: implications for future trials and clinical application. *J Allergy Clin Immunol* (1992) 89, 285.
13. Nelson HS, Hamilos DL, Corsello PR, Levesque NV, Buchmeier AD, Bucher BL. A double-blind study of troleandomycin and methylprednisolone in asthmatic subjects who require daily corticosteroids. *Am Rev Respir Dis* (1993) 147, 398–404.
14. Lantner R, Rockoff JB, DeMasi J, Boran-Ragotzy R, Middleton E. Fatal varicella in a corticosteroid-dependent asthmatic receiving troleandomycin. *Allergy Proc* (1990) 11, 83–7.
15. Finkenbine R, Gill HS. Case of mania due to prednisone-clarithromycin interaction. *Can J Psychiatry* (1997) 42, 778.
16. Finkenbine RD, Frye MD. Case of psychosis due to prednisone-clarithromycin interaction. *Gen Hosp Psychiatry* (1998) 20, 325–6.
17. Szefler SJ, Brenner M, Jusko WJ, Spector SL, Flesher KA, Ellis EF. Dose- and time-related effect of troleandomycin on methylprednisolone elimination. *Clin Pharmacol Ther* (1982) 32, 166–171.
18. Budenofalk Rectal Foam (Budesonide). Dr. Falk Pharma UK Ltd. UK Summary of product characteristics, June 2006.

Corticosteroids + Mifepristone

The UK manufacturers of mifepristone say that the efficacy of corticosteroids (included inhaled corticosteroids) is expected to be reduced in the 3 to 4 days following the use of mifepristone, because of the antiglucocorticoid activity of mifepristone.[1] Patients taking corticosteroids should be monitored during this time, and consideration given to increasing the corticosteroid dose. However, the US manufacturers contraindicate the use of mifepristone in those receiving long-term corticosteroid therapy.[2]

1. Mifegyne (Mifepristone). Exelgyn Laboratories. UK Summary of product characteristics, February 2006.
2. Mifeprex (Mifepristone). Danco Laboratories, LLC. US Prescribing information, July 2005.

Corticosteroids + Nefazodone

Nefazodone inhibits the metabolism of methylprednisolone and prolongs its effects on cortisol suppression.

Clinical evidence

In healthy subjects, nefazodone for 9 days (initial dose of 100 mg, increased to 150 mg, then 200 mg, twice daily) increased the AUC of a single 0.6-mg/kg intravenous dose of **methylprednisolone** by twofold and increased its half-life from 2.28 to 3.32 hours. **Methylprednisolone** clearance was decreased from 28.7 to 14.6 L/hour. The duration of cortisol suppression after **methylprednisolone** alone was 23.3 hours, which increased to more than 32 hours when nefazodone was also given.[1]

Mechanism

Nefazodone probably inhibits methylprednisolone metabolism by cytochrome P450 isoenzyme CYP3A4.[1]

Importance and management

At clinically relevant doses nefazodone decreases methylprednisolone clearance and significantly prolongs methylprednisolone induced cortisol suppression. Care is recommended during concurrent use.[1] Note that nefazodone has been generally withdrawn from the market.

1. Kotlyar M, Brewer ER, Golding M, Carson SW. Nefazodone inhibits methylprednisolone disposition and enhances its adrenal-suppressant effect. *J Clin Psychopharmacol* (2003) 23, 652–6.

Corticosteroids + NSAIDs

Corticosteroids or NSAIDs alone may be risk factors for gastrointestinal bleeding and ulceration. The concurrent use of NSAIDs and corticosteroids increases the risk of gastrointestinal bleeding and probably ulceration.
Ibuprofen, indometacin and naproxen may increase the levels of free prednisolone, and plasma levels of diclofenac are modestly increased by triamcinolone.

Clinical evidence, mechanism, importance and management

(a) Gastrointestinal bleeding and ulceration

A retrospective study of more than 20 000 patients who had received corticosteroids found that the incidence of upper gastrointestinal bleeding was no greater than in the control group who had not received corticosteroids (bleeds occurred in 95 patients compared with 91 patients). However, the risk of bleeding was increased if the patients were also taking aspirin or other NSAIDs.[1] This is consistent with the results of another study in patients taking **prednisone** and **indometacin**.[2]

A case control study reviewed 1415 patients aged 65 years or older, hospitalised between 1984 and 1986 for peptic ulcer or upper gastrointestinal haemorrhage of unknown cause, and 7063 control patients. The relative risk for the development of peptic ulcer disease was estimated to be 2 in those taking oral corticosteroids, and 4.4 in those taking corticosteroids with NSAIDs. It was estimated that patients taking corticosteroids with NSAIDs have a 15-fold greater risk for peptic ulcer disease than patients taking neither drug.[3] Another study compared 1121 patients aged 60 or over who were admitted to hospital with bleeding peptic ulcers, with 989 control patients, to investigate factors other than NSAIDs that may have contributed to the risk of bleeding.[4] The risk was threefold greater for the use of corticosteroids alone, but when corticosteroids were used with NSAIDs, the risk was tenfold greater.[4]

NSAIDs alone increase the risk of gastrointestinal adverse effects.[5-8] Most patients with NSAID-associated ulcers are elderly: this is because there is a greater prevalence of ulcer disease in the elderly, and they are more likely to be taking NSAIDs and be sensitive to them.[7] A history of ulcer disease is a further risk factor.[7] Corticosteroids alone are reported not to be a risk factor in some studies,[1,2,9] while other studies found they were a risk factor for gastrointestinal adverse effects.[4,10] However, several studies have found that the risk of gastrointestinal adverse effects is increased by the combined use of corticosteroids and NSAIDs[3-5,10] and caution with concurrent use has been suggested.[3] It may be prudent to consider the use of gastroprotection in patients taking NSAIDs and corticosteroids, especially if they are elderly.

Consider also 'Aspirin or other Salicylates + Corticosteroids or Corticotropin', p.136.

(b) Pharmacokinetic interactions

A patient with rheumatoid arthritis taking **prednisolone** 5 to 10 mg daily with an NSAID (aspirin 700 mg to 2.8 g daily, **ibuprofen** 400 mg to 1.2 g daily, or **naproxen** 250 to 500 mg daily) intermittently, developed osteonecrosis of the upper third of the femoral head that was attributed to increased free levels of **prednisolone** due to displacement by the NSAID.[11] A study in 11 patients with stable rheumatoid disease regularly taking a corticosteroid found that **indometacin** 75 mg or **naproxen** 250 mg twice daily for 2 weeks did not alter the total plasma levels of a single 7.5-mg dose of **prednisolone** but the amount of unbound (free) **prednisolone** increased by 30 to 60%.[12] The probable reason is that these NSAIDs displace both administered and endogenous corticosteroids from their plasma protein binding sites, although the clinical relevance of this change is unclear. In a double-blind, crossover study 12 healthy subjects were given **rofecoxib** 250 mg daily or placebo for 14 days, with a single 30-mg dose of either intravenous **prednisolone** or oral **prednisone** on days 10 and 14. **Rofecoxib** did not affect the pharmacokinetics of the corticosteroids, even in a dose 10 times greater than that used clinically.[13]

In a double-blind, crossover study in healthy subjects given a single intramuscular dose of **diclofenac sodium** 75 mg alone and with **triamcinolone diacetate** 40 mg, the maximum plasma levels of **diclofenac** were increased by 24% by **triamcinolone**. This was possibly due to an increased rate of absorption but this is unlikely to be of clinical relevance. Other pharmacokinetic parameters of **diclofenac** were not significantly changed.[14] The majority of these pharmacokinetic interactions seem unlikely to be of clinical significance, but they may well contribute to the adverse effects of both drugs, particularly the corticosteroids. No particular action appears to be necessary to account for these pharmacokinetic effects.

1. Carson JL, Strom BL, Schinnar R, Sim E, Maislin G, Morse ML. Do corticosteroids really cause upper GI bleeding? *Clin Res* (1987) 35, 340A.
2. Emmanuel JH, Montgomery RD. Gastric ulcer and anti-arthritic drugs. *Postgrad Med J* (1971) 47, 227–32.
3. Piper JM, Ray WA, Daugherty JR, Griffin MR. Corticosteroid use and peptic ulcer disease: role of nonsteroidal anti-inflammatory drugs. *Ann Intern Med* (1991) 114, 735–40.
4. Weil J, Langman MJS, Wainwright P, Lawson DH, Rawlins M, Logan RFA, Brown TP, Vessey MP, Murphy M, Colin-Jones DG. Peptic ulcer bleeding: accessory risk factors and interactions with non-steroidal anti-inflammatory drugs. *Gut* (2000) 46, 27–31.
5. Langman MJ, Weil J, Wainwright P, Lawson DH, Rawlins MD, Logan RF, Murphy M, Vessey MP, Colin-Jones DG. Risks of bleeding peptic ulcer associated with individual non-steroidal anti-inflammatory drugs. *Lancet* (1994) 343, 1075–9.
6. Weil J, Colin-Jones D, Langman M, Lawson D, Logan R, Murphy M, Rawlins M, Vessey M, Wainwright P. Prophylactic aspirin and risk of peptic ulcer bleeding. *BMJ* (1995) 310, 827–30.
7. Seager JM, Hawkey CJ. ABC of the upper gastrointestinal tract: indigestion and non-steroidal anti-inflammatory drugs. *BMJ* (2001) 323, 1236–9.
8. CSM/MCA. Non-steroidal anti-inflammatory drugs (NSAIDs) and gastrointestinal (GI) safety. *Current Problems* (2002) 28, 5.
9. Conn HO, Blitzer BL. Nonassociation of adrenocorticosteroid therapy and peptic ulcer. *N Engl J Med* (1976) 294, 473–9.
10. Messer J, Reitman D, Sacks HS, Smith H, Chalmers TC. Association of adrenocorticosteroid therapy and peptic-ulcer disease. *N Engl J Med* (1983) 309, 21–4.
11. Patial RK, Bansal SK, Kashyap S, Negi A. Drug interaction–induced osteonecrosis of femoral head. *J Assoc Physicians India* (1990) 38, 446–7.
12. Rae SA, Williams IA, English J, Baylis EM. Alteration of plasma prednisolone levels by indomethacin and naproxen. *Br J Clin Pharmacol* (1982) 14, 459–61.
13. Schwartz JI, Mukhopadhyay S, Porras AG, Viswanathan-Aiyer K-J, Adcock S, Ebel DL, Gertz BJ. Effect of rofecoxib on prednisolone and prednisone pharmacokinetics in healthy subjects. *J Clin Pharmacol* (2003) 43, 187–92.
14. Derendorf H, Mullersman G, Barth J, Grüner A, Möllmann H. Pharmacokinetics of diclofenac sodium after intramuscular administration in combination with triamcinolone acetate. *Eur J Clin Pharmacol* (1986) 31, 363–5.

Corticosteroids + Omeprazole

Omeprazole had no effect on oral budesonide or prednisone pharmacokinetics in healthy subjects, but an isolated and unexplained report describes a reduction in the effects of prednisone in a patient taking omeprazole.

Clinical evidence, mechanism, importance and management

A placebo-controlled, randomised study in 18 healthy subjects found that omeprazole 40 mg daily had no effect on the pharmacokinetics of a single 40-mg dose of **prednisone**.[1] This contrasts with an isolated and unexplained report of a patient suffering from pemphigus who was given **prednisone** 1 mg/kg daily with, a week later, ranitidine 200 mg daily for a gastric ulcer. Four weeks later, when the skin lesions were well controlled, it was decided to replace the ranitidine with omeprazole 40 mg daily. Within 4 days the skin lesions began to worsen progressively, although the **prednisone** dosage remained unchanged. After 3 weeks it was decided to stop the omeprazole and restart the ranitidine because an adverse interaction between the **prednisone** and the omeprazole was suspected. Within about a week, the skin condition had begun to improve.[2] The suggested explanation for the interaction is that the omeprazole inhibited the liver enzyme (11β-hydroxylase) that normally converts **prednisone** into its active form (prednisolone) resulting in inadequate treatment of the pemphigus.[2]

A placebo-controlled, randomised study in 11 healthy subjects found that omeprazole 20 mg daily for 5 days had no effect on the pharmacokinetics of a single 9-mg dose of **budesonide** (*Entocort CR* capsules).[3]

It would seem that adverse interactions between oral **budesonide** or **prednisone** and omeprazole are unlikely, but the isolated case should be borne in mind in the event of an unexpected response to treatment.

1. Cavanaugh JH, Karol M. Lack of pharmacokinetic interaction after administration of lansoprazole or omeprazole with prednisone. *J Clin Pharmacol* (1996) 36, 1064–71.
2. Joly P, Chosidow O, Laurent-Puig P, Delchier J-C, Roujeau J-C, Revuz J. Possible interaction prednisone-oméprazole dans la pemphigoïde bulleuse. *Gastroenterol Clin Biol* (1990) 14, 682–3.
3. Edsbäcker S, Larsson P, Bergstrand M. Pharmacokinetics of budesonide controlled-release capsules when taken with omeprazole. *Aliment Pharmacol Ther* (2003) 17, 403–8.

Table 29.2 A comparison of the effects of phenytoin on the pharmacokinetics of different glucocorticoids (after Petereit and colleagues[1])

Corticosteroid	*Daily dosage of phenytoin (mg)*	*Half-life without phenytoin (minutes)*	*Decreased half-life with phenytoin (%)*	*Increased mean clearance rate with phenytoin (%)*	*Refs*
Hydrocortisone	300 to 400	60 to 90	15	25	2
Methylprednisolone	300				3
Prednisone	Prednisolone is the biologically active metabolite of prednisone so that the values for prednisone and prednisolone should be similar				4
Prednisolone	300	190 to 240	45	77	2
Dexamethasone	300	250	51	140	5, 6

1. Petereit LB, Meikle AW. Effectiveness of prednisolone during phenytoin therapy. *Clin Pharmacol Ther* (1977) 22, 912–16.
2. Choi Y, Thrasher K, Werk EE, Sholiton LJ, Olinger C. Effect of diphenylhydantoin on cortisol kinetics in humans. *J Pharmacol Exp Ther* (1971) 176, 27–34.
3. Stjernholm MR, Katz FH. Effects of diphenylhydantoin, phenobarbital, and diazepam on the metabolism of methylprednisolone and its sodium succinate. *J Clin Endocrinol Metab* (1975) 41, 887–93.
4. Meikle AW, Weed JA, Tyler FH. Kinetics and interconversion of prednisolone and prednisone studies with new radio-immunoassays. *J Clin Endocrinol Metab* (1975) 41, 717.
5. Brooks SM, Werk EE, Ackerman SJ, Sullivan I, Thrasher K. Adverse effects of phenobarbital on corticosteroid metabolism in patients with bronchial asthma. *N Engl J Med* (1972) 286, 1125–8.
6. Haque N, Thrasher K, Werk EE, Knowles HC, Sholiton LJ. Studies of dexamethasone metabolism in man. Effect of diphenylhydantoin. *J Clin Endocrinol Metab* (1972) 34, 44–50.

Corticosteroids + Phenytoin

The therapeutic effects of dexamethasone, methylprednisolone, prednisolone, prednisone (and probably other glucocorticoids) and fludrocortisone can be markedly reduced by phenytoin. One study suggested that dexamethasone may modestly increase serum phenytoin levels, but another study and two case reports of patients with brain metastases suggest that an important *decrease* can occur. The results of the dexamethasone adrenal suppression test may prove to be unreliable in those taking phenytoin.

Clinical evidence

(a) Reduced corticosteroid levels

A comparative pharmacokinetic study in 6 neurological or neurosurgical patients taking oral **dexamethasone** and phenytoin found that the average amount of **dexamethasone** that reached the general circulation was a quarter of that observed in 9 other patients taking **dexamethasone** alone(mean oral bioavailability fractions of 0.21 and 0.84, respectively).[1] Another report describes patients who needed increased doses of **dexamethasone** while taking phenytoin.[2]

The **fludrocortisone** dosages of two patients required 4-fold and 10- to 20-fold increases, respectively, in the presence of phenytoin.[3]

Renal allograft survival is decreased in patients taking **prednisone** and phenytoin, due (it is believed) to a reduction in the immunosuppressant effects of the corticosteroid.[4]

Several studies suggest that phenytoin may affect the half-life and clearance of a number of corticosteroids. These are shown in 'Table 29.2', (see above).

(b) Interference with the dexamethasone adrenal suppression test

A study in 7 patients found that phenytoin 300 to 400 mg daily reduced the plasma cortisol levels in response to **dexamethasone** from 22 to 19 microgram%, compared with a reduction from 18 to 4 microgram% in the absence of phenytoin.[5] Other studies confirm that plasma cortisol and urinary 17-hydroxycorticosteroid levels are suppressed far less than might be expected with small doses of **dexamethasone** (500 micrograms every 6 hours for 8 doses), but with larger doses (2 mg every 6 hours for 8 doses) suppression was normal.[6] However, one case describes a patient in whom even 16 mg of **dexamethasone** failed to cause cortisol depression while she was taking phenytoin, but when she was re-tested in the absence of phenytoin only 1 mg of **dexamethasone** was needed to elicit a response.[7]

(c) Serum phenytoin levels increased or decreased

A study into epilepsy prophylaxis post-trauma found that the serum phenytoin levels in those taking **dexamethasone** 16 to 150 mg (mean 63.6 mg) was 40% higher than those taking phenytoin alone (17.3 micrograms/mL compared with 12.5 micrograms/mL). The phenytoin was given as a loading dose of 11 mg/kg intravenously and then 13 mg/kg intramuscularly.[8]

Conversely, a retrospective study of 40 patient records (diagnosis unspecified) indicated that **dexamethasone** reduced serum phenytoin levels: the serum phenytoin levels of 6 patients receiving fixed doses of phenytoin were halved by **dexamethasone**.[9] Another report describes a patient with brain metastases who required over 8 mg/kg of phenytoin (600 mg) to achieve therapeutic phenytoin levels in the presence of **dexamethasone** 16 mg. When the **dexamethasone** was increased to 28 mg daily he experienced seizures, and an increase in his phenytoin dose from 600 mg to 1 g only resulted in an increase in his levels from 13.9 to 16.4 micrograms/mL.[10] Another patient, also with a brain metastasis, needed a large dose of phenytoin (greater than 10 mg/kg) while taking **dexamethasone**. He had an almost fourfold rise in serum phenytoin levels when **dexamethasone** was stopped.[11]

Mechanism

Phenytoin is a potent liver enzyme inducer that increases the metabolism of the corticosteroids so that they are cleared from the body more quickly, reducing both their therapeutic and adrenal suppressant effects.

Importance and management

The fall in serum corticosteroid levels is established and of clinical importance in systemic treatment, but it seems unlikely to affect the response to steroids given topically or by inhalation, intra-articular injection or enema.[12] The interaction can be accommodated in several ways:

- Increase the corticosteroid dosage proportionately to the increase in clearance (see 'Table 29.2', (see above)). With prednisolone an average increase of 100% (range 58 to 260% in 5 subjects) proved effective.[12] A fourfold increase may be necessary with dexamethasone,[1] and much greater increases have been required with fludrocortisone.[3]
- Exchange the corticosteroid for another that is less affected (see 'Table 29.2', (see above)). A switch from dexamethasone to equivalent doses of methylprednisolone has been reported to be effective[13] but another report found that methylprednisolone was more affected than prednisolone.[14] In another case the exchange of dexamethasone 16 mg daily for prednisone 100 mg daily was successful.[15]
- Exchange the phenytoin for another antiepileptic: barbiturates (including primidone[16]) and carbamazepine, are also enzyme-inducers, but valproate is a possible non-interacting alternative[2] where clinically appropriate. However, remember that corticosteroids should only be given to epileptics with care and good monitoring because of the risk that they will exacerbate the disease condition.

The effects of phenytoin on the dexamethasone adrenal suppression test can apparently be accommodated by using larger than usual doses of dexamethasone (2 mg every 6 hours for 8 doses)[6] or by an overnight test using 50 mg of hydrocortisone.[13]

The reports on the changes in serum phenytoin levels are inconsistent (both increases and decreases have been seen). The effects of concurrent use should be closely monitored.

1. Chalk JB, Ridgeway K, Brophy TRO'R, Yelland JDN, Eadie MJ. Phenytoin impairs the bioavailability of dexamethasone in neurological and neurosurgical patients. *J Neurol Neurosurg Psychiatry* (1984) 47, 1087–90.
2. McLelland J, Jack W. Phenytoin/dexamethasone interaction: a clinical problem. *Lancet* (1978) i, 1096–7.
3. Keilholz U, Guthrie GP. Case report: adverse effect of phenytoin on mineralocorticoid replacement with fludrocortisone in adrenal insufficiency. *Am J Med Sci* (1986) 291, 280–3.
4. Wassner SJ, Pennisi AJ, Malekzadeh MH, Fine RN. The adverse effect of anticonvulsant therapy on renal allograft survival. *J Pediatr* (1976) 88, 134–7.
5. Werk EE, Choi Y, Sholiton L, Olinger C, Haque N. Interference in the effect of dexamethasone by diphenylhydantoin. *N Engl J Med* (1969) 281, 32–4.
6. Jubiz W, Meikle AW, Levinson RA, Mizutani S, West CD, Tyler FH. Effect of diphenylhydantoin on the metabolism of dexamethasone. *N Engl J Med* (1970) 283, 11–14.
7. Debrunner J, Schmid C, Schneeman M. Falsely positive dexamethasone suppression test in a patient treated with phenytoin to prevent seizures due to nocardia brain abscesses. *Swiss Med Wkly* (2002) 132, 267.
8. Lawson LA, Blouin RA, Smith RB, Rapp RP, Young AB. Phenytoin-dexamethasone interaction: a previously unreported observation. *Surg Neurol* (1981) 16, 23–4.
9. Wong DD, Longenecker RG, Liepman M, Baker S, LaVergne M. Phenytoin-dexamethasone: a possible drug-drug interaction. *JAMA* (1985) 254, 2062–3.
10. Recuenco I, Espinosa E, García B, Carcas A. Effect of dexamethasone on the decrease of serum phenytoin concentrations. *Ann Pharmacother* (1995) 29, 935.
11. Lackner TE. Interaction of dexamethasone with phenytoin. *Pharmacotherapy* (1991) 11, 344–7.
12. Petereit LB, Meikle AW. Effectiveness of prednisolone during phenytoin therapy. *Clin Pharmacol Ther* (1977) 22, 912–6.
13. Meikle AW, Stanchfield JB, West CD, Tyler FH. Hydrocortisone suppression test for Cushing syndrome: therapy with anticonvulsants. *Arch Intern Med* (1974) 134, 1068–71.
14. Bartoszek M, Brenner AM, Szefler SJ. Prednisolone and methylprednisolone kinetics in children receiving anticonvulsant therapy. *Clin Pharmacol Ther* (1987) 42, 424–32.
15. Boylan JJ, Owen DS, Chin JB. Phenytoin interference with dexamethasone. *JAMA* (1976) 235, 803–4.
16. Hancock KW, Levell MJ. Primidone/dexamethasone interaction. *Lancet* (1978) ii, 97–8.

Corticosteroids + Protease inhibitors

Several cases of Cushing's syndrome have been seen in patients using inhaled or intranasal fluticasone when ritonavir was also given. Ritonavir may reduce the clearance of prednisone, and ritonavir or nelfinavir may increase levels of the active metabolite of ciclesonide. Dexamethasone may reduce the levels of indinavir and saquinavir.

Clinical evidence

An HIV-positive 32-year-old man who had been using intranasal **fluticasone** 200 micrograms twice daily for 3 years for allergic rhinitis, developed a cushingoid face and gained 6.5 kg in weight within 5 months of starting to take **ritonavir**, zidovudine and lamivudine.[1] Another HIV-positive man receiving inhaled **beclometasone** 400 to 800 micrograms daily for asthma and intranasal **fluticasone** 800 micrograms daily for allergic rhinitis was also given **ritonavir**, **saquinavir**, stavudine and nevirapine, after which he developed mild cushingoid facial changes. Both patients had high plasma levels of **fluticasone**. The problems resolved when the **fluticasone** was withdrawn. A third HIV-positive patient receiving inhaled **beclometasone**, intranasal **fluticasone**, **ritonavir**, zidovudine and lamivudine had increased **fluticasone** levels but no signs of Cushing's syndrome.[1]

There are reports of at least 9 other patients, including 2 children,[2] who have developed Cushing's syndrome within 2 to 5 months of using regimens of inhaled[2-7] or intranasal[8] **fluticasone**, with **ritonavir**,[8] **ritonavir/amprenavir**,[3,7] **ritonavir/lopinavir**,[2,5] **ritonavir/saquinavir**,[4] **ritonavir/indinavir**[7] or **ritonavir/lopinavir/saquinavir**.[6] The interaction was confirmed in one patient by replacing the **ritonavir** with nevirapine for 3 weeks and then restarting the **ritonavir**.[8] Another six HIV-positive patients taking protease inhibitors including low doses of **ritonavir** and with HIV-lipodystrophy developed symptomatic Cushing's syndrome when also given inhaled **fluticasone**. All had adrenal suppression, and after withdrawal of **fluticasone**, 3 patients required oral corticosteroids for several months. Exacerbation of pre-existing diabetes mellitus occurred in one patient and 4 patients had osteoporosis (1 with fractures).[9] The manufacturer of ciclesonide notes that giving **ritonavir** or **nelfinavir** with ciclesonide may increase the serum levels of the active metabolite of ciclesonide and that an increased risk of adverse effects such as cushingoid syndrome cannot be excluded.[10]

A study in healthy subjects found that the AUC of a single 20-mg dose of **prednisone**, given before and on days 4 and 14 of a 14.5 day course of **ritonavir** 200 mg twice daily, were increased by about 30% by the **ritonavir**. The apparent oral clearance of **prednisolone** was reduced from 8.84 L/hour to 6.45 and 6.88 L/hour on days 4 and 14, respectively.[11]

Mechanism

Ritonavir, and all protease inhibitors, inhibit the cytochrome P450 isoenzyme CYP3A4 to varying degrees. Fluticasone is metabolised by this isoenzyme and therefore the protease inhibitors cause its plasma levels to rise. The active metabolite of ciclesonide is also metabolised by CYP3A4,[10] and is therefore similarly affected.

Importance and management

Information is limited but the interaction between ritonavir and fluticasone appears to be an established and clinically important. The incidence is not known. Patients using these two drugs should be very well monitored for any signs of corticosteroid overdose. The problem may take months to manifest itself. It has been suggested that if an inhaled corticosteroid is required by a patient taking ritonavir, a corticosteroid with less systemic availability should be given at the lowest effective dose.[12] The manufacturers of the fluticasone inhaler[13,14] and nasal spray[15,16] advise against their concurrent use with ritonavir unless the potential benefit is considered to outweigh the risk of systemic corticosteroid adverse effects.

Ritonavir may increase the levels of prednisone and some manufacturers of **betamethasone**,[17] **budesonide**,[18] ciclesonide,[10] or **dexamethasone**[19,20] predict a similar interaction with ritonavir or nelfinavir.[10].

The manufacturers of **dexamethasone** note that it is a modest inducer of CYP3A4 and state that it may reduce the plasma levels of **indinavir**,[20,21] and saquinavir,[20] or other drugs metabolised by CYP3A4.[21] The clinical outcome of this predicted effect is unknown, but until more is known, it would seem prudent to monitor antiviral efficacy if these combinations are used.

1. Chen F, Kearney T, Robinson S, Daley-Yates PT, Waldron S, Churchill DR. Cushing's syndrome and severe adrenal suppression in patients treated with ritonavir and inhaled nasal fluticasone. *Sex Transm Infect* (1999) 75, 274.
2. Johnson SR, Marion AA, Vrchotichy T, Emmanuel PJ, Lujan-Zilbermann J. Cushing syndrome with secondary adrenal insufficiency from concomitant therapy with ritonavir and fluticasone. *J Pediatr* (2006) 148, 386–8.
3. Clevenbergh P, Corcostegui M, Gérard D, Hieronimus S, Mondain V, Chichmanian RM, Sadoul JL, Dellamonica P. Iatrogenic Cushing's syndrome in an HIV-infected patient treated with inhaled corticosteroids (fluticasone propionate) and low dose ritonavir enhanced PI containing regimen. *J Infect* (2002) 44, 194–5.
4. Gupta SK, Dubé MP. Exogenous Cushing syndrome mimicking human immunodeficiency virus lipodystrophy. *Clin Infect Dis* (2002) 35, e69–e71.
5. Rouanet I, Peyrière H, Mauboussin JM, Vincent D. Cushing's syndrome in a patient treated by ritonavir/lopinavir and inhaled fluticasone. *HIV Med* (2003) 4, 149–50.
6. Gillett MJ, Cameron PU, Nguyen HV, Hurley DM, Mallal SA. Iatrogenic Cushing's syndrome in an HIV-infected patient treated with ritonavir and inhaled fluticasone. *AIDS* (2005) 19, 740–1.
7. Soldatos G, Sztal-Mazer S, Woolley I, Stockigt J. Exogenous glucocorticoid excess as a result of ritonavir-fluticasone interaction. *Intern Med J* (2005) 35, 67–8.
8. Hillebrand-Haverkort ME, Prummel MF, ten Veen JH. Ritonavir-induced Cushing's syndrome in a patient treated with nasal fluticasone. *AIDS* (1999) 13, 1803.
9. Samaras K, Pett S, Gowers A, McMurchie M, Cooper DA. Iatrogenic Cushing's syndrome with osteoporosis and secondary adrenal failure in human immunodeficiency virus-infected patients receiving corticosteroids and ritonavir-boosted protease inhibitors: six cases. *J Clin Endocrinol Metab* (2005) 90, 4394–8.
10. Alvesco (Ciclesonide). Altana Pharma Ltd. UK Summary of product characteristics, January 2007.
11. Penzak SR, Formentini E, Alfaro RM, Long M, Natarajan V, Kovacs J. Prednisolone pharmacokinetics in the presence and absence of ritonavir after oral prednisone administration to healthy volunteers. *J Acquir Immune Defic Syndr* (2005) 40, 573–80.
12. Li AM. Ritonavir and fluticasone: beware of this potentially fatal combination. *J Pediatr* (2006) 148, 294–5.
13. Flixotide Evohaler (Fluticasone propionate). Allen & Hanburys. UK Summary of product characteristics, March 2006.
14. Flovent (Fluticasone propionate) GlaxoSmithKline. US Prescribing information, January 2007.
15. Flixonase Aqueous Nasal Spray (Fluticasone propionate) Allen & Hanburys. UK Summary of product characteristics, April 2007.
16. Flonase (Fluticasone propionate) GlaxoSmithKline. US Prescribing information, March 2004.
17. Betnesol Tablets (Betamethasone sodium phosphate). UCB Pharma Ltd. UK Summary of product characteristics, June 2005.
18. Budenofalk Rectal Foam (Budesonide). Dr. Falk Pharma UK Ltd. UK Summary of product characteristics, June 2006.
19. Dexsol Oral Solution (Dexamethasone sodium phosphate). Rosemont Pharmaceuticals Ltd. UK Summary of product characteristics, October 2005.
20. Dexamethasone Tablets. Organon Laboratories Ltd. UK Summary of product characteristics, March 2007.
21. Decadron Tablets (Dexamethasone). Merck & Co.,Inc. US Prescribing information, May 2004.

Corticosteroids + Rifampicin (Rifampin)

The effects of systemic cortisone, dexamethasone, fludrocortisone, hydrocortisone, methylprednisolone, prednisone and prednisolone can be markedly reduced by rifampicin, but aldosterone appears not to be affected. Rifabutin and rifapentine are predicted to interact similarly, all be it to a lesser extent.

Clinical evidence

(a) Aldosterone

Seven patients with Addison's disease due to tuberculosis had no changes in the pharmacokinetics of intravenous aldosterone after being given rifampicin 600 mg daily for 6 days.[1]

(b) Cortisone and fludrocortisone

A patient with Addison's disease taking cortisone and fludrocortisone had typical signs of corticosteroid overdosage when the rifampicin he was taking was replaced by ethambutol,[2] suggesting that the rifampicin reduces the levels of these corticosteroids. Another Addisonian patient needed an increase in her dosage of cortisone from 37.5 to 50 mg daily, plus fludrocortisone 100 micrograms daily, when rifampicin 450 mg daily was started.[3] When rifampicin was added to **prednisolone** or **dexamethasone** and fludrocortisone it caused an Addisonian crisis in two patients.[4]

(c) Dexamethasone

Rifampicin markedly increases the clearance of dexamethasone.[5,6] See also under (b) above.

(d) Hydrocortisone

A metabolic study in an Addisonian patient taking hydrocortisone found that rifampicin shortened its half-life and reduced its AUC.[7]

(e) Methylprednisolone, Prednisone or Prednisolone

A child with nephrotic syndrome taking prednisolone, and accidentally given a BCG vaccine, was given rifampicin and isoniazid to prevent possible dissemination of the vaccine. When the nephrotic condition did not respond, the prednisolone dosage was raised from 2 to 3 mg/kg daily without any evidence of corticosteroid overdosage. Later when the rifampicin and isoniazid were withdrawn, remission of the nephrotic condition was achieved with the original dosage of prednisolone.[8] A number of other reports describe a reduction in the response to prednisone, prednisolone or methylprednisolone in patients given rifampicin.[4,9-17] Pharmacokinetic studies in patients have shown that the AUC of prednisolone is reduced by about 60% by rifampicin, and its half-life is decreased by 40 to 60%.[11,15,18]

Mechanism

Rifampicin is a potent liver enzyme inducer, which increases the metabolism of the corticosteroids by the liver,[10,19] thereby decreasing their levels and reducing their effects.

Importance and management

The interactions between the corticosteroids and rifampicin are established, well documented and clinically important. The need to increase the dosages of cortisone, dexamethasone, fludrocortisone, hydrocortisone, methylprednisolone, prednisolone and prednisone should be expected if rifampicin is given. It has been suggested that as an initial adjustment the dosage of prednisolone should be increased two to threefold, and reduced proportionately if the rifampicin is withdrawn.[10,11,18,20] The dosage increases needed for other corticosteroids await assessment. In the case of prednisolone the interaction develops maximally by 14 days and disappears about 14 days after withdrawal of the rifampicin.[21] There seems to be no direct information about other glucocorticoids but be alert for them to be similarly affected. It is not clear whether any of the topically applied corticosteroids will interact with rifampicin but any clinically significant interaction would be expected to be very rare. The systemic corticosteroids are usually considered as contraindicated, or only to be used with great care, in patients with active or quiescent tuberculosis. There does not seem to be any information regarding the other rifamycins, **rifabutin** (a weak enzyme inducer) and **rifapentine** (a moderate enzyme inducer). However, the UK manufacturers and the CSM in the UK warn that rifabutin may possibly reduce the effects of a number of drugs, including corticosteroids,[22,23] and therefore some caution is probably prudent.

1. Schulte HM, Monig H, Benker G, Pagel H, Reinwein D, Ohnhaus EE. Pharmacokinetics of aldosterone in patients with Addison's disease: effect of rifampicin treatment on glucocorticoid and mineralocorticoid metabolism. *Clin Endocrinol (Oxf)* (1987) 27, 655–62.
2. Edwards OM, Courtenay-Evans RJ, Galley JM, Hunter J, Tait AD. Changes in cortisol metabolism following rifampicin therapy. *Lancet* (1974) ii, 549–51.
3. Maisey DN, Brown RC, Day JL. Rifampicin and cortisone replacement therapy. *Lancet* (1974) ii, 896–7.
4. Kyriazopoulou V, Parparousi O, Vagenakis AG. Rifampicin-induced adrenal crisis in Addisonian patients receiving corticosteroid replacement therapy. *J Clin Endocrinol Metab* (1984) 59, 1204–6.
5. Ediger SK, Isley WL. Rifampicin-induced adrenal insufficiency in the acquired immunodeficiency syndrome: difficulties in diagnosis and treatment. *Postgrad Med J* (1988) 64, 405–6.
6. Kawai SA. A comparative study of the accelerated metabolism of cortisol, prednisolone and dexamethasone in patients under rifampicin therapy. *Nippon Naibunpi Gakkai Zasshi* (1985) 61, 145–61.
7. Wang YH, Shi YF, Xiang HD. Effect of rifampin on the metabolism of glucocorticoids in Addison's disease. *Zhonghua Nei Ke Za Zhi* (1990) 29, 108–11,127.
8. Hendrickse W, McKiernan J, Pickup M, Lowe J. Rifampicin-induced non-responsiveness to corticosteroid treatment in nephrotic syndrome. *BMJ* (1979) i, 306.
9. van Marle W, Woods KL, Beeley L. Concurrent steroid and rifampicin therapy. *BMJ* (1979) i, 1020.
10. Buffington GA, Dominguez JH, Piering WF, Hebert LA, Kauffman HM, Lemann J. Interaction of rifampin and glucocorticoids. Adverse effect on renal allograft function. *JAMA* (1976) 236, 1958–60.
11. McAllister WAC, Thompson PJ, Al-Habet SM, Rogers HJ. Rifampicin reduces effectiveness and bioavailability of prednisolone. *BMJ* (1983) 286, 923–5.
12. Powell-Jackson PR, Gray BJ, Heaton RW, Costello JF, Williams R, English J. Adverse effect of rifampicin administration on steroid-dependent asthma. *Am Rev Respir Dis* (1983) 128, 307–10.
13. Bitaudeau Ph, Clément S, Chartier JPh, Papapietro PM, Bonnafoux A, Arnaud M, Trèves R, Desproges-Gotteron R. Interaction rifampicine-prednisolone. A propos de deux cas au cours d'une maladie de Horton. *Rev Rhum Mal Osteoartic* (1989) 56, 87–8.
14. Kawai S, Ichikawa Y. Drug interactions between glucocorticoids and other drugs. *Nippon Rinsho* (1994) 52, 773–8.
15. Carrie F, Roblot P, Bouquet S, Delon A, Roblot F, Becq-Giraudon B. Rifampin-induced nonresponsiveness of giant cell arteritis to prednisone treatment. *Arch Intern Med* (1994) 154, 1521–4.
16. Verma M, Singh T, Chhatwal J, Saini V, Pawar B. Rifampicin induced steroid unresponsiveness in nephrotic syndrome. *Indian Pediatr* (1994) 31, 1437.
17. Lin FL. Rifampin-induced deterioration in steroid-dependent asthma. *J Allergy Clin Immunol* (1996) 98, 1125.
18. Bergrem H, Refvem OK. Altered prednisolone pharmacokinetics in patients treated with rifampicin. *Acta Med Scand* (1983) 213, 339–43.
19. Sotaniemi EA, Medzihradsky F, Eliasson G. Glutaric acid as an indicator of use of enzyme-inducing drugs. *Clin Pharmacol Ther* (1974) 15, 417–23.
20. Löfdahl C-G, Mellstrand T, Svedmyr N, Wåhlén P. Increased metabolism of prednisolone and rifampicin after rifampicin treatment. *Am Rev Respir Dis* (1984) 129, A201.
21. Lee KH, Shin JG, Chong WS, Kim S, Lee JS, Jang IJ, Shin SG. Time course of the changes in prednisolone pharmacokinetics after co-administration or discontinuation of rifampicin. *Eur J Clin Pharmacol* (1993) 45, 287–89.
22. Mycobutin (Rifabutin). Pharmacia Ltd. UK Summary of product characteristics, October 2006.
23. Committee on the Safety of Medicines/Medicines Control Agency. Revised indication and drug interactions of rifabutin. *Current Problems* (1997) 23, 14.

Corticosteroids + Sucralfate

Sucralfate appears not to interact with prednisone.

Clinical evidence, mechanism, importance and management

In 12 healthy subjects sucralfate 1 g every 6 hours had no significant effect on the pharmacokinetics of a single 20-mg dose of **prednisone**; however, the peak plasma levels were delayed by about 45 minutes when the drugs were given at the same time, but not when the sucralfate was given 2 hours after the **prednisone**.[1] No particular precautions are likely to be needed in patients given both drugs. Information about other corticosteroids is lacking.

1. Gambertoglio JG, Romac DR, Yong C-L, Birnbaum J, Lizak P, Amend WJC. Lack of effect of sucralfate on prednisone bioavailability. *Am J Gastroenterol* (1987) 82, 42–5.

Corticosteroids + Vaccines; Live

Patients who are immunised with live vaccines while receiving immunosuppressive doses of corticosteroids may develop generalised, possibly life-threatening, infections.

Clinical evidence, mechanism, importance and management

The use of corticosteroids can reduce the number of circulating lymphocytes and suppress the normal immune response, so that concurrent immunisation with live vaccines can lead to generalised infection. It is suggested that **prednisone** in doses of greater than 10 to 15 mg daily will suppress the immune response, whereas 40 to 60-mg doses on alternate days probably does not,[1] although this is debated.

A patient with lymphosarcoma and hypogammaglobulinaemia, taking **prednisone** 15 mg daily, developed a generalised vaccinial infection when she was given **smallpox vaccine**.[2] A fatal vaccinial infection developed following **smallpox vaccination** in another patient taking **cortisone**.[3] This type of problem can be controlled with immunoglobulin to give cover against a general infection while immunity develops, and this has been successfully used in steroid-dependent patients needing **smallpox vaccination**.[4]

The principles applied to **smallpox** may be generally applicable to other live attenuated vaccines (e.g. **measles, mumps, rubella, poliomyelitis, BCG**), but no studies seem to have been done to establish what is safe.[1] It is generally accepted that patients taking immunosuppressants should not be given live vaccines. Problems with topical or inhaled steroids in normal dosages seem unlikely because the amounts absorbed are relatively small.[1] However, this needs confirmation. The British National Formulary states that live vaccination should be postponed for at least 3 months after stopping high-dose corticosteroids.[5]

Consider also 'Immunosuppressants + Vaccines', p.1064.

1. Shapiro L. Questions and Answers. Live virus vaccine and corticosteroid therapy: answered by Fauci AS, Bellanti JA, Polk IJ, Cherry JD. *JAMA* (1981) 246, 2075–6.
2. Rosenbaum EH, Cohen RA, Glatstein HR. Vaccination of a patient receiving immunosuppressive therapy for lymphosarcoma. *JAMA* (1966) 198, 737–40.
3. Olansky S, Smith JG, Hansen-Pruss OCE. Fatal vaccinia associated with cortisone therapy. *JAMA* (1956) 162, 887–8.
4. Joseph MR. Vaccination of patients on steroid therapy. *Med J Aust* (1974) 2, 181.
5. British National Formulary. 53rd ed. London: The British Medical Association and The Pharmaceutical Press; 2007. p. 630.

Corticosteroids + Valspodar

Dexamethasone does not affect the pharmacokinetics of valspodar. Valspodar modestly increases the AUC of dexamethasone.

Clinical evidence, mechanism, importance and management

In a crossover study healthy fasting subjects were given single doses of **dexamethasone** 8 mg and valspodar 400 mg either alone or together. **Dexamethasone** had no effect on the pharmacokinetics of valspodar. The AUC of **dexamethasone** was increased by 24% by valspodar. This change is modest and therefore dosage alterations are probably not required if concurrent use is of a short duration.[1]

1. Kovarik JM, Purba HS, Pongowski M, Gerbeau C, Humbert H, Mueller EA. Pharmacokinetics of dexamethasone and valspodar, a P-glycoprotein (*mdr1*) modulator: implications for coadministration. *Pharmacotherapy* (1998) 18, 1230–6.

Corticosteroids + Zileuton

No clinically relevant pharmacokinetic interaction occurs between prednisone and zileuton.

Clinical evidence, mechanism, importance and management

In a randomised, double-blind, crossover study, 16 healthy subjects were given zileuton 600 mg every 6 hours for a week, with either a 40-mg dose of **prednisone** or placebo on day 6. The pharmacokinetics of both drugs were slightly altered but this was not considered to be clinically relevant. The **prednisone** half-life increased from 2.8 to 2.9 hours, while the zileuton AUC and the time to achieve maximum serum levels were decreased by 13% and 26%, respectively. It was concluded that concurrent use carries a minimal risk of a clinically important pharmacokinetic interaction.[1] No special precautions would appear to be needed.

1. Awni WM, Cavanaugh JH, Tzeng T-B, Witt G, Granneman GR, Dube LM. Pharmacokinetic interactions between zileuton and prednisone. *Clin Pharmacokinet* (1995) 29 (Suppl 2), 105–111.

Daclizumab + Miscellaneous

No adverse drug interactions appear to have been reported with daclizumab, although its use with another antilymphocyte antibody in transplant patients receiving intensive immunosuppression may be a factor in fatal infection.

Clinical evidence, mechanism, importance and management

The manufacturers of daclizumab say that because it is an immunoglobulin, no metabolic drug interactions (i.e. those mediated by inhibitory or inducing effects on cytochrome P450 enzymes) would be expected,[1,2] and none seems to have been reported. The manufacturers say that daclizumab has been given in clinical studies with the following drugs without any adverse interactions: **aciclovir, azathioprine, antithymocyte immune globulin, ciclosporin, corticosteroids, ganciclovir, muromonab-CD3, mycophenolate mofetil** and **tacrolimus**.[1]

However, in one clinical study in heart transplant patients taking ciclosporin, **mycophenolate**, and corticosteroids, use of daclizumab with another antilymphocyte (such as **muromonab-CD3** or **antithymocyte immunoglobulin**) appeared to be associated with a higher incidence of fatal infection: 8 of 40 patients died, compared with 2 of 37 who received an antilymphocyte and placebo. The manufacturer suggests that concurrent use of daclizumab with another antilymphocyte antibody in patients receiving intensive immunosuppression may be a factor leading to fatal infection.[1,2] Caution may be warranted, and more study is needed.

1. Zenapax (Daclizumab). Roche Products Ltd. UK Summary of product characteristics, August 2006.
2. Zenapax (Daclizumab). Roche Pharmaceuticals. US Prescribing information, September 2005.

Etanercept + Miscellaneous

An increased risk of serious infection and neutropenia is reported if etanercept is given with anakinra. A higher incidence of malignancies has been reported in patients with Wegener's granulomatosis when given both cyclophosphamide and etanercept. No clinically significant pharmacokinetic interactions occur between etanercept and methotrexate. Etanercept did not affect the pharmacodynamics of warfarin. A reduced neutrophil count may occur in patients treated with etanercept and sulfasalazine. No interactions have been found when etanercept was given with salicylates (other than sulfasalazine), corticosteroids, or NSAIDs. Live vaccines should not been given to patients taking etanercept.

Clinical evidence, mechanism, importance and management

(a) Anakinra

In a study in patients with active rheumatoid arthritis taking etanercept and anakinra for up to 24 weeks, serious infections occurred in 7% of patients, compared with none in patients taking etanercept alone. Neutropenia occurred in 2% of patients taking both drugs.[1] Infections are very common adverse effects of treatment with etanercept but serious infections are reported to be uncommon (occurring in about 1% of etanercept- and placebo-treated groups in clinical studies).[1,2] Further, the combination of etanercept with anakinra has not increased clinical benefit and the manufacturers say that concurrent use is not recommended.[1,2]

(b) Cyclophosphamide

The US manufacturers say that etanercept is not recommended in patients receiving cyclophosphamide. They state that in a study in patients with Wegener's granulomatosis, the addition of etanercept to standard treatment, including cyclophosphamide, was associated with a higher incidence of non-cutaneous solid malignancies.[1]

(c) Methotrexate

A double-blind study in 98 patients with rheumatoid arthritis receiving subcutaneous etanercept 25 mg twice weekly, or etanercept with oral methotrexate (median weekly dose of 20 mg) were randomly selected for a pharmacokinetic study from 682 patients in a clinical study. The pharmacokinetics of etanercept were not altered by concurrent methotrexate and no dosage adjustment is required during concurrent use.[3]

(d) Sulfasalazine

A study in patients taking sulfasalazine found that when etanercept was also given, patients had a decrease in neutrophil counts, when compared to other groups of patients receiving either drug alone. The clinical significance is not known.[1,2]

(e) Vaccines, live

As no data are available on the secondary transmission of infection by live vaccines in patients receiving etanercept, the manufacturers recommend that live vaccines should not be given.[1,2]

(f) Other drugs

The UK manufacturers note that no interactions have been found when etanercept was given with **corticosteroids**, **salicylates** (except sulfasalazine, see under (e) above), **NSAIDs** or other analgesics.[2]

1. Enbrel (Etanercept) Amgen & Wyeth Pharmaceuticals. US Prescribing information, February 2007.
2. Enbrel (Etanercept). Wyeth Pharmaceuticals. UK Summary of product characteristics, April 2007.
3. Zhou H, Mayer PR, Wajdula J, Fatenejad S. Unaltered etanercept pharmacokinetics with concurrent methotrexate in patients with rheumatoid arthritis. *J Clin Pharmacol* (2004) 44, 1235–43.

Everolimus + Azoles

Ketoconazole significantly increases everolimus levels. A case report describes reduced everolimus clearance in a patient also given itraconazole. Pharmacokinetic modelling suggests that fluconazole will not interact to a clinically relevant extent.

Clinical evidence, mechanism, importance and management

In a study, 12 healthy subjects were given a single 1-mg dose of everolimus on day 4 of an 8-day course of **ketoconazole** 200 mg twice daily. Ketoconazole increased the AUC, peak blood level and half-life of everolimus by 15-fold, 3.9-fold, and 1.9 fold, respectively.[1] Similarly, a patient taking everolimus with ciclosporin and prednisone had a 74% decrease in everolimus clearance when **itraconazole** was given. However, in 16 patients, pharmacokinetic modelling suggested that everolimus clearance was reduced by a non-significant 7% when fluconazole was given.[2] More study is needed to confirm this finding.

Patients who are given **ketoconazole**, and possibly any azole that is also a potent inhibitor of the cytochrome P450 isoenzyme CYP3A4, such as **itraconazole**, should have their everolimus levels monitored closely and dose adjustments made as required.[1]

1. Kovarik JM, Beyer D, Bizot MN, Jiang Q, Shenouda M, Schmouder RL. Blood concentrations of everolimus are markedly increased by ketoconazole. *J Clin Pharmacol* (2005) 45, 514–8.
2. Kovarik JM, Hsu C-H, McMahon L, Berthier S, Rordorf C. Population pharmacokinetics of everolimus in de novo renal transplant patients: impact of ethnicity and comedications. *Clin Pharmacol Ther* (2001) 70, 247–54.

Everolimus + Ciclosporin

Ciclosporin increases the AUC of everolimus. Everolimus appears to have no significant effects on ciclosporin levels.

Clinical evidence

(a) Effects on ciclosporin

In a placebo-controlled study in 54 kidney transplant patients taking ciclosporin (93% also taking prednisone), everolimus 0.75 mg to 10 mg daily in single or divided doses in 44 patients had no consistent, clinically significant effect on ciclosporin levels, when compared with the 10 patients given placebo, although because of wide interpatient variability, there is a possibility that a significant interaction could occur in some patients.[1] Another study in 101 kidney transplant patients taking ciclosporin and prednisone with everolimus 0.5 to 2 mg twice daily for 1 year also found no evidence that everolimus affected ciclosporin pharmacokinetics.[2]

(b) Effects on everolimus

The possibility of a drug interaction was assessed in a crossover study in 24 healthy subjects who were given a single 2-mg dose of everolimus, alone and with single doses of ciclosporin, either *Neoral* (microemulsion) 175 mg or *Sandimmune* (corn oil suspension) 300 mg. *Neoral* increased the peak levels and AUC of everolimus by 82% and 168% respectively. *Sandimmune* did not affect the peak levels of everolimus but increased its AUC by 74%.[3]

Mechanism

Not fully understood. Both everolimus and ciclosporin are metabolised by the cytochrome P450 isoenzyme CYP3A4 and both are substrates of P-glycoprotein. Competition via one or both of these pathways in the liver or gut wall may contribute to the interaction.[3]

Importance and management

Information on the effects on everolimus levels when it is used with ciclosporin appear to be limited to the single-dose study.[3] However, it has been suggested if ciclosporin (either *Neoral* or *Sandimmune*) is removed from an everolimus/ciclosporin regimen, a two- to threefold decrease in everolimus exposure could be expected. Monitoring is recommended.[3] Note that sirolimus (of which everolimus is a derivative) interacts similarly, see 'Sirolimus + Ciclosporin', p.1072.

It would appear that, in general, everolimus has no clinically significant effects on the pharmacokinetics of ciclosporin.

1. Budde K, Lehne G, Winkler M, Renders L, Lison A, Fritsche L, Soulillou J-P, Fauchald P, Neumayer H-H, Dantal J and RADW 102 Renal Transplant Study Group. Influence of everolimus on steady-state pharmacokinetics of cyclosporine in maintenance renal transplant patients. *J Clin Pharmacol* (2005) 45, 781–91.
2. Kovarik JM, Kahan BD, Kaplan B, Lorber M, Winkler M, Rouilly M, Gerbeau C, Cambon N, Boger R, Rordorf C on behalf of the Everolimus Phase II Study Group. Longitudinal assessment of everolimus in de novo renal transplant recipients over the first post-transplant year: pharmacokinetics, exposure-response relationships, and influence of cyclosporine. *Clin Pharmacol Ther* (2001). 69, 48–56.
3. Kovarik JM, Kalbag J, Figueiredo J, Rouilly M, O'Bannon LF, Rordorf C. Differential influence of two cyclosporine formulations on everolimus pharmacokinetics: a clinically relevant pharmacokinetic interaction. *J Clin Pharmacol* (2002) 42, 95–9.

Everolimus + Macrolides

Erythromycin increases everolimus levels. Other macrolides probably interact similarly.

Clinical evidence, mechanism, importance and management

Sixteen healthy subjects were given a single 4-mg dose of everolimus before and on day 5 of a 9-day course of erythromycin 500 mg three times daily. The peak blood levels and AUC of everolimus were increased twofold and 4.4-fold, respectively, and its half-life was prolonged by 39%. Erythromycin probably inhibited the metabolism of everolimus by the cytochrome P450 isoenzyme CYP3A4. There was wide inter-subject variability in the levels of erythromycin and therefore they could not be correlated with the extent of the interaction with everolimus. The authors recommend that appropriate everolimus dose reductions based on frequently monitored blood levels should be made when patients are given erythromycin.[1] Other macrolides that inhibit CYP3A4 (such as **clarithromycin** and **telithromycin**, but not **azithromycin**) would be expected to interact similarly, and therefore concurrent use of these drugs with everolimus should also be monitored.

1. Kovarik JM, Beyer D, Bizot MN, Jiang Q, Shenouda M, Schmouder R. Effect of multiple-dose erythromycin on everolimus pharmacokinetics. *Eur J Clin Pharmacol* (2005) 61, 35–8.

Everolimus + Rifampicin (Rifampin)

Rifampicin reduces the bioavailability and increases the clearance of everolimus.

Clinical evidence, mechanism, importance and management

Twelve healthy subjects were given a single 4-mg dose of everolimus before and after taking rifampicin 600 mg daily for 7 days. Rifampicin increased the clearance of everolimus by 172%, and increased its AUC and peak blood levels by 63% and 58%, respectively, although there was a large inter-individual variation in the AUC. Induction of both cytochrome P450 isoenzyme CYP3A4 and P-glycoprotein (everolimus is metabolised by CYP3A4 and is a substrate for P-glycoprotein) by rifampicin may have increased metabolism and reduced the bioavailability of everolimus.[1]

There appear to be no other published clinical studies or case reports of this interaction but what happened is in line with the way both drugs are known to interact. Monitor concurrent use for everolimus efficacy, anticipating the need to increase the dose of everolimus.

1. Kovarik JM, Hartmann S, Figueiredo J, Rouilly M, Port A, Rordorf C. Effect of rifampicin on apparent clearance of everolimus. *Ann Pharmacother* (2002) 36, 981–5.

Everolimus + Verapamil

Increased levels of both everolimus and verapamil can occur on concurrent use.

Clinical evidence, mechanism, importance and management

A study in 16 healthy subjects given a single 2 mg dose of everolimus before and on day 2 of a 6-day course of verapamil 80 mg three times daily found that verapamil increased the AUC and peak blood level of everolimus by 3.5-fold and 2.3-fold, respectively. Everolimus also increased the plasma levels of verapamil by 2.3-fold.[1]

Verapamil is an inhibitor of the cytochrome P450 isoenzyme CYP3A4, the isoenzyme primarily involved in the metabolism of everolimus, and inhibits P-glycoprotein, a transporter for which everolimus is a substrate. Therefore concurrent use raises everolimus levels. It is not known exactly why verapamil levels are raised. This appears to be the only evidence for an interaction, but it is in line with the way these drugs are known to interact. If both drugs are given it would seem prudent to monitor everolimus blood levels as well as monitor for adverse effects due to verapamil, such as hypotension, flushing and oedema, and adjust the dose of both drugs as needed.

1. Kovarik JM, Beyer D, Bizot MN, Jiang Q, Allison MJ, Schmouder RL. Pharmacokinetic interaction between verapamil and everolimus. *Br J Clin Pharmacol* (2005) 60, 434–7.

Immunosuppressants + Vaccines

The body's immune response is suppressed by immunosuppressants such as ciclosporin, mycophenolate, sirolimus, and tacrolimus. The antibody response to vaccines may be reduced, although even partial protection may be of benefit. In general, the use of live attenuated vaccines is considered contraindicated because of the possible risk of generalised infection. Inactivated vaccines may be used.

Clinical evidence

(a) Diphtheria, tetanus, and inactivated polio vaccines

In organ transplant recipients taking immunosuppressants, tetanus vaccines[1,2] and inactivated polio vaccines[1] produced protective antibody titres. The response to diphtheria vaccine was lower than in healthy controls[1] and the antibody titre had fallen below the protective level by 12 months in 38% of patients in one study,[1] and 24% in another.[2] Note that live polio vaccines are not recommended in immunosuppressed patients (see *Live vaccines*, below).

(b) Hepatitis vaccines

The antibody response to **hepatitis B vaccine** is generally poor in patients taking immunosuppressants after organ transplantation,[3,4] although one research group reported a sustained antibody response in half of their patients,[5] and an overall 85% seroconversion rate was seen in one study in children (aged between 4 and 16 years).[6] In this latter study,[6] children receiving **ciclosporin** monotherapy had a higher seroconversion rate (100%) than those receiving **ciclosporin** and **corticosteroids** (84%) and those receiving **ciclosporin**, **azathioprine**, and **corticosteroids** (66%).

The antibody response to **hepatitis A vaccine** in patients taking immunosuppressants after organ transplantation is variable,[7-9] and declines quicker than in healthy controls.[9] In renal transplant recipients, there is some evidence that the response is inversely related to the number of immunosuppressant drugs.[8]

(c) Influenza vaccine

A number of studies have been published on the efficacy of influenza vaccination in organ transplant recipients taking immunosuppressants. Many have found a reduction in the proportion of patients developing a protective antibody titre compared with healthy control subjects,[10,11] whereas some have found no reduction.[12] A few studies have looked at the effects of individual drugs in the immunosuppressive regimen. In one comparative study in 59 kidney transplant patients, 21 patients taking **ciclosporin** and **prednisone** had a significantly lower immune response to influenza vaccine (inactivated trivalent) than 38 patients taking **azathioprine** and **prednisone** or 29 healthy subjects taking no drugs. All of the immune response measurements were reduced by 20 to 30% in those taking **ciclosporin**.[13] In another study, 13 patients taking **mycophenolate**, **ciclosporin**, and **prednisolone** had a marked reduction in antibody response to influenza vaccine, when compared with 25 patients taking **ciclosporin**, **azathioprine** and **prednisolone**.[14] In yet another study, patients receiving **ciclosporin** had lower antibody responses when compared with patients receiving **tacrolimus**.[15] Patients given a higher dose of **prednisolone** per kg had a reduced antibody response to influenza vaccine in one study, and those given a daily dose had a reduced response, when compared with those given an alternate day schedule.[16]

Confirmation of the practical importance of the reduced antibody titre in some patients is described in a case report of a heart transplant patient taking **ciclosporin** who did not respond to influenza vaccination while taking **ciclosporin** and **prednisone**. He had two episodes of influenza, one serologically confirmed, and it was later shown that vaccination had not resulted in seroconversion.[17] Similarly, a patient taking **tacrolimus** after a liver transplant developed influenza A myocarditis despite prophylactic vaccination.[18]

(d) Live vaccines

The use of live vaccines in patients receiving corticosteroids has caused generalised infection, see 'Corticosteroids + Vaccines; Live', p.1061. Similarly, the use of live vaccines in patients taking other immunosuppressants is not recommended: probably as a consequence of this there are few published reports about the use of live vaccines with immunosuppressants. One study found that measles vaccine was effective in 7 of 18 children under 3 years old after liver transplantation, and that there were no complications directly attributable to the vaccine.[19]

(e) Pneumococcal vaccines

Good responses to pneumococcal vaccines in patients taking immunosuppressant drugs after organ transplantation have been seen,[10,20] but protective antibody titres may not persist as long as in healthy subjects.[21]

Mechanism

Immunosuppression by these drugs diminishes the ability of the body to respond immunologically both to transplants and to vaccination.

Importance and management

These are established and clinically important interactions. The UK Department of Health[22] recommends the following:

- Live vaccines: patients taking immunosuppressive drugs such as ciclosporin, methotrexate, cyclophosphamide, leflunomide, and cytokine inhibitors should not be given live vaccines during or for up to 6 months after treatment has stopped, as they can cause severe or fatal infections.
- Inactivated vaccines: ideally should be given at least 2 weeks before immunosuppressive therapy is started.
- Bone marrow transplant patients may lose their antibodies against most diseases and should be considered for re-immunisation under specialist supervision.

The proportion of patients developing protective antibody titres to vaccines is often reduced in patients taking immunosuppressants. Nevertheless, for many vaccines, the reduced response seen is still considered clinically useful, and, for example, in the case of kidney transplant patients,[23] and in patients who are immunosuppressed (either by drugs or disease), influenza vaccination is actively recommended.[22,23] Pneumococcal vaccine should also be given to these patients. If a vaccine is given, it may be prudent to monitor the response, so that alternative prophylactic measures can be considered where it is considered inadequate. For influenza vaccine, one suggestion is that if patients remain unprotected after a single vaccination and a booster dose, amantadine 200 mg daily should be given during an influenza epidemic. It will protect against influenza A but not B infection.[17] Note that, even where effective antibody titres are produced, these may not persist as long as in healthy subjects, and more frequent booster doses may be required.

There appears to be little published experience of the use of live vaccines in patients receiving immunosuppressants (apart from 'corticosteroids', (p.1061)), and live vaccines should generally not be used in these patients. The manufacturers of **leflunomide** say that no clinical data are available on the efficacy of vaccines given to patients taking leflunomide, and live vaccines are not recommended.[24,25]

1. Huzly D, Neifer S, Reinke P, Schröder K, Schönfeld C, Hofmann T, Bienzle U. Routine immunizations in adult renal transplant recipients. *Transplantation* (1997) 63, 839–45.
2. Enke BU, Bökenkamp A, Offner G, Bartmann P, Brodehl J. Response to diphtheria and tetanus booster vaccination in pediatric renal transplant recipients. *Transplantation* (1997) 64, 237–41.
3. Angelico M, Di Paolo D, Trinito MO, Petrolati A, Araco A, Zazza S, Lionetti R, Casciani CU, Tisone G. Failure of a reinforced triple course of hepatitis B vaccination in patients transplanted for HBV-related cirrhosis. *Hepatology* (2002) 35, 176–81.
4. Loinaz C, Ramón de Juanes J, Moreno Gonzalez E, López A, Lumbreras C, Gómez R, Gonzalez-Pinto I, Jiménez C, Garcia I, Fuertes A. Hepatitis B vaccination results in 140 liver transplant recipients. *Hepatogastroenterology* (1997) 44, 235–8.
5. Bienzle U, Günther M, Neuhaus R, Neuhaus P. Successful hepatitis B vaccination in patients who underwent transplantation for hepatitis B virus-related cirrhosis: preliminary results. *Liver Transpl* (2002) 8, 562–4.
6. Duca P, Del Pont JM, D'Agostino D. Successful immune response to a recombinant hepatitis B vaccine in children after liver transplantation. *J Pediatr Gastroenterol Nutr* (2001) 32, 168–70.
7. Arslan M, Wiesner RH, Poterucha JJ, Zein NN. Safety and efficacy of hepatitis A vaccination in liver transplantation recipients. *Transplantation* (2001) 72, 272–6.
8. Stark K, Günther M, Neuhaus R, Reinke P, Schröder K, Linnig S, Bienzle U. Immunogenicity and safety of hepatitis A vaccine in liver and renal transplant recipients. *J Infect Dis* (1999) 180, 2014–17.
9. Günther M, Stark K, Neuhaus R, Reinke P, Schröder K, Bienzle U. Rapid decline of antibodies after hepatitis A immunization in liver and renal transplant recipients. *Transplantation* (2001) 71, 477–90.
10. Dengler TJ, Strnad N, Buhring I, Zimmermann R, Girgsdies O, Kubler WE, Zielen S. Differential immune response to influenza and pneumococcal vaccination in immunosuppressed patients after heart transplantation. *Transplantation* (1998) 66, 1340–47.
11. Soesman NMR, Rimmelzwaan GF, Nieuwkoop NJ, Beyer WEP, Tilanus HW, Kemmeren MH, Metselaar HJ, de Man RA, Osterhaus ADME. Efficacy of influenza vaccination in adult liver transplant recipients. *J Med Virol* (2000) 61, 85–93.
12. Edvardsson VO, Flynn JT, Deforest A, Kaiser BA, Schulman SL, Bradley A, Palmer J, Polinsky MS, Baluarte HJ. Effective immunization against influenza in pediatric renal transplant recipients. *Clin Transplant* (1996) 10, 556–60.
13. Versluis DJ, Beyer WEP, Masurel N, Wenting GJ, Weimar W. Impairment of the immune response to influenza vaccination in renal transplant recipients by cyclosporine, but not azathioprine. *Transplantation* (1986) 42, 376–9.
14. Smith KGC, Isbel NM, Catton MG, Leydon JA, Becker GJ, Walker RG. Suppression of the humoral immune response by mycophenolate mofetil. *Nephrol Dial Transplant* (1998) 13, 160–4.
15. Mazzone PJ, Mossad SB, Mawhorter SD, Mehta AC, Schilz RJ, Maurer JR. The humoral immune response to influenza vaccination in lung transplant patients. *Eur Respir J* (2001) 18, 971–6.
16. Mack DR, Chartrand SA, Ruby EI, Antonson DL, Shaw BW, Heffron TG. Influenza vaccination following liver transplantation in children. *Liver Transpl Surg* (1996) 2, 431–7.
17. Beyer WEP, Diepersloot RJA, Masurel N, Simoons ML, Weimar W. Double failure of influenza vaccination in a heart transplant patient. *Transplantation* (1987) 43, 319.
18. Vilchez RA, Fung JJ, Kusne S, Influenza A myocarditis developing in an adult liver transplant recipient despite vaccination: a case report and review of the literature. *Transplantation* (2000) 70, 543–5.
19. Rand EB, McCarthy CA, Whitington PF. Measles vaccination after orthotopic liver transplantation. *J Pediatr* (1993) 123, 87–9.
20. Kazancioğlu R, Sever MŞ, Yüksel-Önel D, Eraksoy H, Yildiz A, Çelik AV, Kauacan SM, Badur S. Immunization of renal transplant recipients with pneumococcal polysaccharide vaccine. *Clin Transplant* (2000) 14, 61–5.
21. Linnemann CC, First MR, Schiffman G. Revaccination of renal transplant and hemodialysis recipients with pneumococcal vaccine. *Arch Intern Med* (1986) 146, 1554–6.
22. Department of Health. *Immunisation Against Infectious Disease* 2006: "The Green Book". Available at: http://www.dh.gov.uk/en/Policyandguidance/Healthandsocialcaretopics/Greenbook/DH_4097254 (accessed 23/08/07).
23. UK Department of Health. Adult Immunisation Update, 8 August 2003. Available at http://www.dh.gov.uk/assetRoot/04/02/99/70/04029970.pdf (accessed 23/08/07).
24. Arava (Leflunomide). Sanofi-Aventis. UK Summary of product characteristics, January 2006.
25. Arava (Leflunomide). Sanofi-Aventis US LLC. US Prescribing information, July 2007.

Infliximab + Miscellaneous

Live vaccines should not be given to patients undergoing treatment with infliximab. Serious infection and neutropenia is predicted to occur if infliximab is given with anakinra. Infliximab may increase serum levels of azathioprine metabolites, and a rare T-cell lymphoma has been reported in adolescents and young adults treated with infliximab and also given azathioprine or mercaptopurine. Serum levels of infliximab appear to be unaffected by aminosalicylates, corticosteroids, ciprofloxacin or metronidazole.

Clinical evidence, mechanism, importance and management

(a) Anakinra

Infliximab inhibits the activity of tumour necrosis factor (TNFα). In clinical studies the use of anakinra with another TNFα inhibitor, 'etanercept', (p.1062) has been associated with an increased risk of serious infection and neutropenia and no additional benefit, when compared to the use of these drugs alone.[1,2] As a result of this the manufacturers of infliximab note that similar toxicity may occur if anakinra is given with infliximab and therefore advise against concurrent use.[1,2]

(b) Azathioprine or Mercaptopurine

In 32 patients with Crohn's disease taking azathioprine (mean dose 2.81 mg/kg) and with stable levels of 6-tioguanine nucleotides (the active metabolites of azathioprine), infusions of infliximab 5 mg/kg over 2 hours resulted in a significant increase in 6-tioguanine nucleotide levels in 21 patients after 1 to 3 weeks, when compared to pre-infusion levels. The leucocyte count was significantly decreased and mean corpuscular volume increased. Significant increases in 6-tioguanine nucleotides were associated with good tolerance and favourable response to infliximab. These changes were transient: levels returned to normal 3 months later.[3] Although this study suggests that concurrent use did not result in adverse effects the manufacturers report that rare post-marketing cases of an aggressive and usually fatal hepatosplenic T-cell lymphoma have been reported in adolescent and young adult patients with Crohn's disease treated with infliximab. All cases occurred in patients also receiving azathioprine or mercaptopurine. A causal relationship is unclear.[1,2]

(c) Vaccines (live)

As no data are available on the response to vaccination with live vaccines or on the secondary transmission of infection by live vaccines in patients receiving anti-TNF therapy, the manufacturers recommend that live vaccines should not be given concurrently with infliximab.[1,2]

(d) Miscellaneous

The manufacturers note that serum levels of infliximab appear to be unaffected by baseline use of medications to treat Crohn's disease including aminosalicylates, ciprofloxacin, corticosteroids and metronidazole.[2]

1. Remicade (Infliximab). Schering-Plough Ltd. UK Summary of product characteristics, May 2007.
2. Remicade (Infliximab). Centocor, Inc. US Prescribing information, April 2007.
3. Roblin X, Serre-Debeauvais F, Phelip J-M, Bessard G, Bonaz B. Drug interaction between infliximab and azathioprine in patients with Crohn's disease. *Aliment Pharmacol Ther* (2003) 18, 917–25.

Leflunomide + Miscellaneous

The serum levels of the active metabolite of leflunomide are reduced by activated charcoal, and colestyramine. The manufacturers advise against the concurrent use of alcohol because of the potential for hepatotoxicity. Methotrexate may also increase leflunomide hepatotoxicity, so in general the combination is not recommended. A case of fatal fulminant hepatic failure has been reported in a patient taking leflunomide and itraconazole. A case of peripheral neuropathy has been reported in a patient taking leflunomide and tegafur/uracil. The manufacturers predict interactions between leflunomide and phenytoin or tolbutamide, and advise caution with rifampicin as it may increase leflunomide metabolite levels. No clinically relevant interaction occurs with cimetidine, corticosteroids or NSAIDs.

Clinical evidence, mechanism, importance and management

(a) Alcohol

The UK manufacturers say that because of the potential for additive hepatotoxic effects, it is recommended that alcohol should be avoided by patients taking leflunomide.[1]

(b) Charcoal or Colestyramine

Studies in healthy subjects found that colestyramine 8 g three times daily reduced the serum levels of the active metabolite of leflunomide (A771726) by 48% after 24 hours and by 49 to 65% after 48 hours.[1,2]

Treatment with activated charcoal 50 g every 6 hours for 24 hours, either orally or by nasogastric tube, reduced A771726 levels by 37% after 24 hours and by 48% after 48 hours.[1,2]

These drugs are thought to bind with the A771726 in the gut, thereby interrupting the enterohepatic cycle or possibly its gastrointestinal dialysis.[1] Patients should therefore not be given either colestyramine or activated charcoal with leflunomide, unless the intention is to remove the leflunomide, for example following overdosage or when switching from leflunomide to another DMARD (see (e) and (f), below), or where there is any other good reason to clear leflunomide from the body more quickly.[1,2]

(c) Cimetidine

The manufacturers say that no clinically significant interaction occurs between leflunomide and cimetidine.[1,2]

(d) Corticosteroids

The manufacturers say that corticosteroids may continue to be used if leflunomide is given.[1,2]

(e) CYP2C9 substrates

The manufacturers advise caution if leflunomide is given with **phenytoin** or **tolbutamide**.[1] The reason is that the active metabolite of leflunomide (A771726) has been shown by *in vitro* studies to be an inhibitor of the cytochrome P450 isoenzyme CYP2C9, which is concerned with the metabolism of these two drugs. If this inhibition were to occur *in vivo* it could possibly lead to a decrease in their metabolism and an increase in their toxicity. Although so far there appear to be no clinical reports of an interaction, the manufacturers made a similar prediction with warfarin, another CYP2C9 substrate, which has, in isolated cases, been borne out in practice. See 'Coumarins + Leflunomide', p.423.

(f) DMARDs other than methotrexate

The manufacturers say that the concurrent use of leflunomide and other DMARDs (they list **azathioprine**, **chloroquine**, **hydroxychloroquine**, intramuscular or oral **gold** and **penicillamine**) has not yet been studied but they say that combined use is not advisable because of the increased risk of serious adverse reactions (haemo- or hepatotoxicity). As the active metabolite of leflunomide has a long half life of 1 to 4 weeks the manufacturers say that a washout of colestyramine or activated charcoal should be given if patients are to be started on other DMARDs.[1,2] See also *Methotrexate*, below.

(g) Itraconazole

A 68-year-old woman who had been taking leflunomide 10 mg daily for about 4 months was started on itraconazole 300 mg daily for a fungal infection. About one month later her leflunomide dose was increased to 20 mg daily, and liver function tests were normal. The following month, she developed abdominal pain, vomiting, and weakness. Despite symptomatic treatment and washout with colestyramine, fatal fulminant hepatic failure occurred. The authors of the report attribute the reaction to additive hepatotoxicity between the leflunomide and itraconazole.[3] This interaction serves to highlight the cautions about the use of other hepatotoxic drugs, see (a) and (h).

(h) Methotrexate

No pharmacokinetic interaction was seen in patients taking methotrexate (mean dose 17.2 mg per week) with leflunomide 100 mg daily for 2 days as a loading dose followed by 10 to 20 mg daily.[4] However, elevated liver enzyme levels have been seen following concurrent use.[1] By March 2001, the European Agency for the Evaluation of Medicinal Products was aware of 129 cases of serious hepatic reactions in patients taking leflunomide, and 78% of these were in patients concurrently treated with hepatotoxic medications. In patients with elevated liver function tests, 58% were also being treated with methotrexate and/or NSAIDs.[5] Because of the possible risks of additive or synergistic liver toxicity or haematotoxicity, particularly when used long-term, the UK manufacturers say that the concurrent use of methotrexate is not advisable.[1] The US manufacturers say that if concurrent use is undertaken, chronic monitoring should be increased to monthly intervals.[2] Close liver enzyme monitoring is also recommended if switching between these drugs, and colestyramine or activated charcoal washout should be performed when switching from leflunomide to methotrexate.[1,2]

(i) NSAIDs

Leflunomide inhibits the activity of the cytochrome P450 isoenzyme CYP2C9 *in vitro* and might therefore be expected to increase the serum levels of NSAIDs that are metabolised by this isoenzyme (e.g. **diclofenac**, **ibuprofen**) but the manufacturers say that no safety problems were seem in clinical studies with leflunomide and NSAIDs. No special precautions would seem to be needed if any of these or any other NSAID drugs are given concurrently.[1]

(j) Rifampicin (Rifampin)

When a single dose of leflunomide was given to subjects after taking multiple dose rifampicin, the peak levels of the active metabolite of leflunomide (A771726) were increased by 40% but the AUC was unchanged.[1,2] The reasons are not understood. There would seem to be no reason for avoiding concurrent use, but the manufacturers advise caution as A771721 levels may build up over time.[2] It may be prudent to increase the frequency of leflunomide monitoring if these two drugs are used together.

(k) Tegafur with Uracil

A 75-year-old man with rectal cancer was given a 28-day course of tegafur/uracil 200 mg three times daily and calcium folinate 30 mg daily. Treatment was withheld because of an episode of minor duodenal bleeding and 3 months later he was given leflunomide 100 mg daily for 3 days followed by 20 mg daily to treat rheumatoid arthritis. A further two courses of tegafur/uracil (separated by 7 days) was given because of tumour progression, after which the patient had increasing numbness of the lower extremities, diagnosed as polyneuropathy. He also had severe diarrhoea and hand-foot syndrome. Tegafur is a prodrug of fluorouracil. Uracil prevents fluorouracil degradation by inhibiting dihydropyrimidine dehydrogenase. Both tegafur/uracil and leflunomide may cause neurotoxicity. As these symptoms had not occurred when tegafur/uracil had been given without leflunomide, it was suggested that leflunomide may increase fluorouracil toxicity by increasing its conversion to fluorouracil monophosphate, or by enhancing the effect of uracil by additional inhibition of dihydropyrimidine dehydrogenase.[6] This is an isolated case and its general importance is unclear.

1. Arava (Leflunomide). Sanofi-Aventis. UK Summary of product characteristics, January 2006.
2. Arava (Leflunomide). Sanofi-Aventis US LLC. US Prescribing information, July 2007.
3. Legras A, Bergemer-Fouquet A-M, Jonville-Bera A-P. Fatal hepatitis with leflunomide and itraconazole. *Am J Med* (2002) 113, 352–3.
4. Weinblatt ME, Kremer JM, Coblyn JS, Maier AL, Helfgott SM, Morrell M, Byrne VM, Kaymakcian MV, Strand V. Pharmacokinetics, safety, and efficacy of combination treatment with methotrexate and leflunomide in patients with active rheumatoid arthritis. *Arthritis Rheum* (1999) 42, 1322–8.
5. EMEA. EMEA public statement on leflunomide (Arava) - severe and serious hepatic reactions. London, 12 March 2001. Available at: http://www.emea.eu.int/pdfs/human/press/pus/561101en.pdf (accessed 23/08/07).
6. Kopp H-G, Kanz L, Hartmann JT, Moerike K. Leflunomide and peripheral neuropathy: a potential interaction between uracil/tegafur and leflunomide. *Clin Pharmacol Ther* (2005) 78, 89–90.

Muromonab-CD3 + Indometacin

One report suggested that indometacin may possibly increase the incidence of encephalopathy and psychosis in patients given muromonab-CD3.

Clinical evidence, mechanism, importance and management

A study of patient records found that 4 out of a total of 55 kidney transplant patients (7.3%) given muromonab-CD3 and indometacin 50 mg orally or rectally every 6 to 8 hours for 48 to 72 hours developed serious encephalopathy and psychosis compared with only two out of 173 patients (1.2%) who had received muromonab-CD3 without indometacin.[1] This appears to be an isolated report, and its general significance is unknown. Indometacin has been used to reduce the adverse effects of muromonab-CD3, and in one analysis concurrent use was associated with reduced fever, headache, and gastrointestinal disturbances.[2] Muromonab-CD3 alone is associated with encephalopathy and other CNS adverse effects, and the manufacturer warns that patients should be closely monitored for these effects.[3]

1. Chan GL, Weinstein SS, Wright CE, Bowers VD, Alveranga DY, Shires DL, Ackermann JR, LeFor WW, Kahana L. Encephalopathy associated with OKT3 administration. Possible interaction with indomethacin. *Transplantation* (1991) 52, 148–50.
2. Gaughan WJ, Francos BB, Dunn SR, Francos GC, Burke JF. A retrospective analysis of indomethacin on adverse reactions to orthoclone OKT3 in the therapy of acute renal allograft rejection. *Am J Kidney Dis* (1994) 24, 486–90.
3. Orthoclone OKT3 (Muromonab-CD3). Ortho Biotech Products, LP. US Prescribing information, November 2004.

Mycophenolate + Allopurinol

No clinically relevant interactions have been seen between mycophenolate mofetil and allopurinol.

Clinical evidence, mechanism, importance and management

A study in 5 kidney transplant patients with gouty arthritis, who were switched from azathioprine to mycophenolate mofetil 2 g daily (to avoid the risk of an azathioprine/allopurinol interaction), found that no adverse effects occurred when they were given allopurinol 100 or 200 mg daily. On average, 10 weeks after the switch had taken place, uricaemia had fallen by 21%, mean serum creatinine levels were only slightly raised, by 12%, and white cell counts were unchanged.[1] Another study in 19 kidney transplant patients taking mycophenolate 2 g daily, ciclosporin and prednisolone also found a significant reduction in uricaemia without any adverse effects on white cell count, after allopurinol 100 mg daily was also taken, for 60 days.[2]

No special precautions would therefore seem necessary if allopurinol is used with mycophenolate, although the authors of both studies suggest that long-term randomised studies are needed to confirm safety.

1. Jacobs F, Mamzer-Bruneel MF, Skhiri H, Thervet E, Legendre Ch, Kreis H. Safety of the mycophenolate mofetil-allopurinol combination in kidney transplant recipients with gout. *Transplantation* (1997) 64, 1087–8.
2. Navascués RA, Gómez E, Rodriguez M, Laures AS, Baltar J, Grande JA. Safety of the allopurinol-mycophenolate mofetil combination in the treatment of hyperuricemia of kidney transplant patients. *Nephron* (2002) 91, 173–4.

Mycophenolate + Antacids

An aluminium/magnesium hydroxide antacid reduced the absorption of mycophenolate in one study, but the clinical relevance of this is uncertain.

Clinical evidence, mechanism, importance and management

When 10 mL of an **aluminium/magnesium hydroxide** antacid (*Maalox TC*) was given four times daily to 10 patients with a single 2-g dose of mycophenolate mofetil, the AUC of mycophenolic acid (the active form of the drug) was reduced by 17% and the maximum plasma concentration of mycophenolic acid was reduced by 38%.[1] The clinical importance of this reduction has not been assessed, but the authors of the report suggest that since 80% of transplant patients receive antacids, in practice, this interaction is of no great significance. The US manufacturers say that **aluminium/magnesium** antacids can be used in patients taking mycophenolate, but that they should not be given simultaneously.[2] With many other (but not all) antacid interactions, a 2-hour separation is usually sufficient to avoid an interaction. It would seem prudent to check that the immunosuppressant effects of mycophenolate remain adequate in the presence of this or any other antacid.

1. Bullingham R, Shah J, Goldblum R, Schiff M. Effects of food and antacid on the pharmacokinetics of single doses of mycophenolate mofetil in rheumatoid arthritis patients. *Br J Clin Pharmacol* (1996) 41, 513–16.
2. CellCept (Mycophenolate mofetil). Roche Laboratories Inc. US Prescribing information, October 2005.

Mycophenolate + Azathioprine

The manufacturers have recommended that mycophenolate mofetil should not be given with azathioprine because they say that concurrent use has not been studied,[1,2] and both drugs have the potential to cause bone marrow suppression.[1]

1. CellCept (Mycophenolate mofetil). Roche Laboratories Inc. US Prescribing information, October 2005.
2. CellCept (Mycophenolate mofetil). Roche Products Ltd. UK Summary of product characteristics, March 2006.

Mycophenolate + Ciclosporin or Tacrolimus

Ciclosporin reduces the levels of mycophenolic acid. Tacrolimus may increase mycophenolic acid levels in some patient groups, but the clinical significance of this is unclear.

Clinical evidence

(a) Mycophenolate with Ciclosporin or Tacrolimus

A study in 78 kidney transplant patients taking corticosteroids with mycophenolate 1 g two or three times daily, and also taking either ciclosporin (68 patients) or tacrolimus (10 patients), found lower trough levels of the active metabolite, mycophenolic acid, and higher levels of the glucuronide metabolite in patients taking ciclosporin during the first 3 months post-transplant, when compared with those taking tacrolimus. Of interest is that of the 11 patients changed from ciclosporin to tacrolimus during the study, 5 patients subsequently required mycophenolate dose reductions because of adverse effects.[1] Another study found that despite a higher dose of mycophenolate, patients also taking ciclosporin had a 50% lower trough mycophenolic acid level when compared with those taking mycophenolate with tacrolimus.[2] Other studies have found similar results.[3-5] In another study, 12 stable kidney transplant patients taking ciclosporin (*Neoral)* were given enteric-coated mycophenolate sodium (*Mycofortic)* 720 mg twice daily for 14 days. After pharmacokinetic assessment, they were then changed over to tacrolimus with the same dose and formulation of mycophenolate sodium. This study found that when tacrolimus was given the mycophenolic acid AUC was 20% greater than when ciclosporin was taken, but maximum concentration of mycophenolic acid was 24% greater with ciclosporin than with tacrolimus.[6] However, a recent study in 22 kidney transplant patients taking mycophenolate found that neither ciclosporin (13 patients) nor tacrolimus (9 patients) affected the plasma levels of mycophenolic acid. Levels of the glucuronide metabolite were increased by ciclosporin but not tacrolimus.[7] The manufacturers report that in one study in renal transplant patients receiving ciclosporin and mycophenolate mofetil, the AUC of mycophenolic acid was increased by about 30% when ciclosporin was replaced by tacrolimus.[8]

(b) Mycophenolate with Ciclosporin

There are reports that the trough levels of the active metabolite of mycophenolate, mycophenolic acid, may be reduced in the presence of ciclosporin.[9] In a study, 52 kidney transplant patients were given mycophenolate mofetil 1 g twice daily with ciclosporin and prednisone. Six months after transplantation 19 patients continued triple therapy, 19 discontinued ciclosporin and 14 discontinued prednisone. Three months later, patients in whom ciclosporin had been discontinued had higher trough mycophenolic acid levels compared with the other groups of patients. Discontinuing ciclosporin resulted in almost a doubling of mycophenolic acid trough levels.[10] Other studies note similar effects on mycophenolic acid levels in adult[11] and paediatric patients.[12]

A study in 33 children taking ciclosporin with prednisolone and 15 children additionally taking mycophenolate mofetil found that the ciclosporin levels 2 hours after the ciclosporin dose, was significantly reduced in those patients taking mycophenolate.[13] Another study in children found similar results.[14]

(c) Mycophenolate with Tacrolimus

A study in stable kidney transplant patients taking tacrolimus long-term found that the addition of mycophenolate mofetil resulted in a increase in the tacrolimus AUC, but this was not considered significant.[15] Another study in renal transplant patients found no change in tacrolimus levels when mycophenolate was given.[8] However a 20% increase in tacrolimus levels has been reported in a study in liver transplant patients given mycophenolate 1.5 g twice daily.[8]

Mechanism

Mycophenolate is hydrolysed to its active drug, mycophenolic acid. This then undergoes glucuronidation by uridine diphosphate glucuronosyltransferase (UGT) to form an inactive glucuronide metabolite. This metabolite is then either excreted in urine or undergoes enterohepatic recirculation, where it is converted back into the active form, mycophenolic acid. Ciclosporin is thought to inhibit the enterohepatic conversion of the glucuronide metabolite back to the active metabolite, mycophenolic acid, leading to lower levels of the mycophenolic acid.[8]

Tacrolimus may inhibit uridine diphosphate glucuronosyltransferase (UGT) which metabolises mycophenolic acid to the glucuronide metabolite,[1,7] and may also interfere with the enterohepatic recycling of the glucuronide metabolite.[8]

Importance and management

The addition of mycophenolate mofetil to ciclosporin has been found to reduce the incidence of rejection episodes in kidney transplant patients[16] and it is licensed for combined use.[8] From the studies above, ciclosporin appears to reduce the levels of the active metabolite, mycophenolic acid, and increase the levels of the glucuronide metabolite (which is associated with mycophenolate adverse effects). The UK manufacturers point out that as efficacy studies were conducted in patients using ciclosporin, mycophenolate and corticosteroids, the finding that ciclosporin reduces the mycophenolic acid AUC by 19% to 38% does not affect the recommended dose requirements.[8] They also state that ciclosporin pharmacokinetics are not affected by mycophenolate.[8] However, this is in contrast to the studies in children reported above.[13,14] It has also been observed that the use of triple therapy with corticosteroids, ciclosporin and mycophenolate mofetil rather than with azathioprine makes it possible to use a lower dose of ciclosporin.[17] However, other studies have noted that adjusting ciclosporin doses affects mycophenolic acid levels, and therefore the overall effect on immunosuppression needs careful monitoring.[12]

The significance of the reported increases in mycophenolic acid levels with concurrent tacrolimus is not clear, and the manufacturers note that the benefit of concurrent use with tacrolimus has not been established.[8] There are also inherent problems in interpretation of the results of studies comparing ciclosporin or tacrolimus with mycophenolate.[2,4,18,19] It has been suggested that the changes in mycophenolic acid trough levels are because tacrolimus increases mycophenolic acid levels;[4] however, another interpretation may be that the differences in mycophenolic acid trough levels and AUCs seen are because ciclosporin decreases mycophenolic acid exposure.[18]

Patients taking either ciclosporin or tacrolimus with mycophenolate should have their immunosuppressive response closely monitored, particularly if changing from ciclosporin to tacrolimus or *vice versa*, and dose adjustment of mycophenolate should be considered if patients develop mycophenolate-related adverse effects on switching from ciclosporin to tacrolimus.

1. Mandla R, Midtvedt K, Line P-D, Hartmann A, Bergan S. Mycophenolic acid clinical pharmacokinetics influenced by a cyclosporine C2 based immunosuppressive regimen in renal allograft recipients. *Transpl Int* (2006) 19, 44–53.
2. Gerbase MW, Fathi M, Spiliopoulos A, Rochat T, Nicod LP. Pharmacokinetics of mycophenolic acid associated with calcineurin inhibitors: long-term monitoring in stable lung recipients with and without cystic fibrosis. *J Heart Lung Transplant* (2003) 22, 587–90.
3. Pou L, Brunet M, Cantarell C, Vidal E, Oppenheimer F, Monforte V, Vilardell J, Roman A, Martorell J, Capdevila L. Mycophenolic acid plasma concentrations: influence of co-medication. *Ther Drug Monit* (2001) 23, 35–8.
4. Hübner GI, Eismann R, Sziegoleit W. Drug interaction between mycophenolate mofetil and tacrolimus detectable within therapeutic mycophenolic acid monitoring in renal transplant patients. *Ther Drug Monit* (1999) 21, 536–9.
5. Vidal E, Cantarell C, Capdevila L, Monforte V, Roman A, Pou L. Mycophenolate mofetil pharmacokinetics in transplant patients receiving cyclosporine or tacrolimus in combination therapy. *Pharmacol Toxicol* (2000) 87, 182–4.
6. Kaplan B, Meier-Kriesche H-U, Minnick P, Bastien M-C, Sechaud R, Yeh C-M, Balez S, Picard F, Schmouder R. Pharmacokinetics (PK) of enteric-coated mycophenolate sodium (EC-MPS, *Myfortic*) in stable renal transplant patients with Neoral or tacrolimus. *J Am Soc Nephrol* (2003) 14, 910A.
7. Naito T, Shinno K, Maeda T, Kagawa Y, Hashimoto H, Otsuka A, Takayama T, Ushiyama T, Suzuki K, Ozono S. Effects of calcineurin inhibitors on pharmacokinetics of mycophenolic acid and its glucuronide metabolite during the maintenance period following renal transplantation. *Biol Pharm Bull* (2006) 29, 275–80.
8. CellCept (Mycophenolate mofetil). Roche Products Ltd. UK Summary of product characteristics, March 2006.
9. Weber SW, Keller F. Low mycophenolate predose levels with cyclosporine co-medication. *Kidney Blood Press Res* (1999) 22, 390.
10. Gregoor PJ, de Sevaux RG, Hene RJ, Hesse CJ, Hilbrands LB, Vos P, van Gelder T, Hoitsma AJ, Weimar W. Effect of cyclosporine on mycophenolic acid trough levels in kidney transplant recipients. *Transplantation* (1999) 68, 1603–6.
11. Smak Gregoor PJ, Van Gelder T, Hesse CJ, van der Mast BJ, van Be NM, Weimar W. Mycophenolic acid plasma concentrations in kidney allograft recipients with or without cyclosporin: a cross-sectional study. *Nephrol Dial Transplant* (1999) 14, 706–8.
12. Filler G, Lepage N, Delisle B, Mai I. Effect of cyclosporine on mycophenolic acid area under the concentration-time curve in pediatric kidney transplant recipients. *Ther Drug Monit* (2001) 23, 514–19.
13. Pape L, Froede K, Strehlau J, Ehrich JHH, Offner G. Alterations of cyclosporin A metabolism induced by mycophenolate mofetil. *Pediatr Transplant* (2003) 7, 302–4.
14. Filler G, Drug interactions between mycophenolate and cyclosporine. *Pediatr Transplant* (2004) 8, 201–4.
15. Pirsch J, Bekersky I, Vincenti F, Boswell G, Woodle ES, Alak A, Kruelle M, Fass N, Facklam D, Mekki Q. Coadministration of tacrolimus and mycophenolate mofetil in stable kidney transplant patients: pharmacokinetics and tolerability. *J Clin Pharmacol* (2000) 40, 527–32.
16. Sollinger HW. Mycophenolate mofetil for the prevention of acute rejection in primary care cadaveric renal allograft recipients. *Transplantation* (1995) 60, 225–32.
17. Sanz Moreno C, Gomez Sanchez M, Fdez Fdez J, Botella J. Cyclosporine A (CsA) needs are reduced with substitution of azathioprine (Aza) by mycophenolate mofetil (MMF). *Nephrol Dial Transplant* (1998) 13, A260.
18. van Gelder T, Smak Gregoor PJH, Weimar W. Letter to the editor. *Ther Drug Monit* (2000) 22, 639.
19. Hübner GI, Sziegoleit W. Response to letter from van Gelder. *Ther Drug Monit* (2000) 22, 498–9.

Mycophenolate + Colestyramine

Colestyramine reduces the absorption of mycophenolate but the clinical relevance of this is uncertain.

Clinical evidence, mechanism, importance and management

Colestyramine 4 g three times daily for 4 days reduced the AUC of mycophenolic acid by 40% in a group of healthy subjects after they took a single 1.5-g oral dose of mycophenolate mofetil.[1] The UK manufacturers advise caution with concurrent use,[1] while the US manufacturers say that this combination is not recommended.[2] Separating the administration of colestyramine and mycophenolate is not likely to eliminate this interaction, as colestyramine affects the enterohepatic recirculation of mycophenolate.[2]

The clinical importance of the reduction in mycophenolic acid levels has not been assessed but, if colestyramine is also given, it would seem prudent to confirm that the immunosuppressant effects of mycophenolate remain adequate.

1. CellCept (Mycophenolate mofetil). Roche Products Ltd. UK Summary of product characteristics, March 2006.
2. CellCept (Mycophenolate mofetil). Roche Laboratories Inc. US Prescribing information, October 2005.

Mycophenolate + Iron compounds

One study found that oral iron preparations significantly reduced the absorption of mycophenolate. However, other studies found that oral iron had no significant effect on the absorption of mycophenolate mofetil.

Clinical evidence, mechanism, importance and management

A study in 10 kidney transplant patients taking mycophenolate mofetil 1 g daily found that a single 105-mg dose of **ferrous sulfate** had no significant effect on the absorption of mycophenolate.[1] Another study in 40 kidney transplant patients found that two sustained-release tablets of **ferrous sulfate** (*Ferrogradumet*) daily, given either at the same time or 4 hours after the morning dose of mycophenolate (for 5 days after kidney transplantation), had no significant effect on the absorption of mycophenolate 1 g twice daily, when compared with patients not given an iron supplement. Mycophenolate toxicity occurred in 29% of the patients receiving concurrent iron, in 23% of the patients taking iron 4 hours after mycophenolate, and in 15% of patients not taking iron, Rejection occurred in 29%, 15%, and 8%, respectively, and anaemia in 0%, 21% and 15%, respectively, although the differences were not statistically significant (although this may have been due to the small study size).[2] A study in 16 healthy subjects given a single 1-g dose of mycophenolate mofetil with two sustained-release **ferrous sulfate** tablets (105 mg elemental iron per tablet) found no evidence of reduced mycophenolate absorption.[3]

These studies are in contrast with an earlier study in 7 healthy subjects, which found that a single 1050-mg dose of **ferrous sulfate** (210 mg of elemental iron) reduced the AUC and maximum levels of mycophenolic acid by more than 90%.[4] In general, it would appear that no significant interaction usually occurs and concurrent use has no significant effect on the immunosuppressive effects of mycophenolate.

1. Lorenz M, Wolzt M, Wiegel G, Puttinger H, Horl WH, Fodinger M, Speiser W, Sunder-Plassmann G. Ferrous sulfate does not affect mycophenolic acid pharmacokinetics in kidney transplant patients. *Am J Kidney Dis* (2004) 43, 1098–103.
2. Mudge DW, Atcheson B, Taylor PJ, Sturtevant JM, Hawley CM, Campbell SB, Isbel NM, Nicol DL, Pillans PI, Johnson DW. The effect of oral iron administration on mycophenolate mofetil absorption in renal transplant recipients: a randomized, controlled trial. *Transplantation* (2004) 77, 206–9.
3. Ducray PS, Banken L, Gerber M, Boutouyrie B, Zandt H. Absence of an interaction between iron and mycophenolate mofetil absorption. *Br J Clin Pharmacol* (2006) 62, 492–5.
4. Morii M, Ueno K, Ogawa A, Kato R, Yoshimura H, Wada K, Hashimoto H, Takeda M, Tanaka K, Nakatani T, Shibakawa M. Impairment of mycophenolate mofetil absorption by iron ion. *Clin Pharmacol Ther* (2000) 68, 613–16.

Mycophenolate + Methotrexate

A study in patients with rheumatoid arthritis found that the combination of methotrexate and mycophenolate mofetil was well tolerated and there were no pharmacokinetic interactions.[1] There would appear to be no need for dose adjustments if both drugs are given for rheumatoid arthritis.

1. Yocum D, Kremer J, Blackburn W, Caldwell J, Furst D, Nunez M, Zuzga J, Zeig S, Gutierrez M, Merrill J, Dumont E, B Leishman. Cellcept® (mycophenolate mofetil - MMF) and methotrexate (MTX) safety and pharmacokinetic (PK) interaction study in rheumatoid arthritis patients. *Arthritis Rheum* (1999) 42 (9 Suppl), S83.

Mycophenolate + Metronidazole

Metronidazole may reduce the bioavailability of mycophenolate mofetil.

Clinical evidence, mechanism, importance and management

A study in 9 healthy subjects found that metronidazole 500 mg three times daily for 5 days reduced the AUC of a single 1-g oral dose of mycophenolate mofetil given two hours after the antibacterial on day 4 by 19% The AUC of the glucuronide metabolite was also reduced, by 27%. When norfloxacin 400 mg twice daily was also given, the AUC of mycophenolate and its glucuronide metabolite were reduced by 33% and 41%, respectively. This interaction was thought to be due to interference of the enterohepatic recirculation of mycophenolate by the antibacterials.[1] There appear to be no further clinical reports of an interaction between metronidazole and mycophenolate. The changes with metronidazole alone were modest, and possibly of minor clinical significance, but the larger reductions seen when norfloxacin was also given suggest that some caution may be prudent. Monitor the outcome of concurrent use to ensure that mycophenolate remains effective.

1. Naderer OJ, Dupuis RE, Heinzen EL, Wiwattanawongsa MS, Johnson MW, Smith PC. The influence of norfloxacin and metronidazole on the disposition of mycophenolate mofetil. *J Clin Pharmacol* (2005) 45, 219–26.

Mycophenolate + Miscellaneous

Co-trimoxazole appears to have no effect on the bioavailability of mycophenolic acid. Probenecid increased the AUC of the glucuronide metabolite of mycophenolic acid threefold in *animals*. However, as there appear to be no clinical reports of this interaction, the clinical significance of this is unclear. Further study is needed.[1]

1. CellCept (Mycophenolate mofetil). Roche Products Ltd. UK Summary of product characteristics, March 2006.

Mycophenolate + Polycarbophil calcium

Polycarbophil calcium reduces the bioavailability of mycophenolate.

Clinical evidence, mechanism, importance and management

A study in 5 healthy subjects given a single 1-g dose of mycophenolate alone or with polycarbophil calcium 2.4 g found that the AUC and peak serum levels of mycophenolic acid were reduced by about 51% and 69%, respectively. The authors suggest that this interaction was probably the result of reduced absorption due to chelate-complex formation between mycophenolate and the calcium ions, which they demonstrated in an *in vitro* study. It was concluded that mycophenolate and polycarbophil calcium should not be taken at the same time.[1] A suitable interval was not specified, but a separation of 2 hours has been suggested with 'antacids', (p.1067), which interact by a similar mechanism. Further study is needed.

1. Kato R, Ooi K, Ikura-Morii M, Tsuchishita Y, Hashimoto H, Yoshimura H, Uenishi K, Kawai M, Tanaka K, Ueno K. Impairment of mycophenolate mofetil absorption by calcium polycarbophil. *J Clin Pharmacol* (2002) 42, 1275–80.

Mycophenolate + Quinolones

Norfloxacin may reduce the bioavailability of mycophenolate mofetil.

Clinical evidence, mechanism, importance and management

A study in 11 healthy subjects found that norfloxacin 400 mg twice daily reduced the AUC of a single 1-g oral dose of mycophenolate mofetil given two hours after the antibacterial on day 4 by 10%. The AUC of the glucuronide metabolite was also reduced by 10%. When norfloxacin 400 mg twice daily was also given, the AUC of mycophenolate and its glucuronide metabolite were reduced by 33% and 41%, respectively. This interaction was thought to be due to interference of the enterohepatic recirculation of mycophenolate by the antibacterials.[1] There appear to be no further clinical reports of an interaction between these antibacterials and mycophenolate. The changes with norfloxacin alone were modest, and unlikely to be of clinical significance, but the larger reductions seen when metronidazole was also given suggest that some caution may be prudent. Monitor the outcome of concurrent use to ensure that mycophenolate remains effective. There is no information about the use of other quinolones and metronidazole given with mycophenolate, but, if the mechanism is correct, until more information is available, it would be prudent to assume that they will interact similarly.

1. Naderer OJ, Dupuis RE, Heinzen EL, Wiwattanawongsa MS, Johnson MW, Smith PC. The influence of norfloxacin and metronidazole on the disposition of mycophenolate mofetil. *J Clin Pharmacol* (2005) 45, 219–26.

Mycophenolate + Rifampicin (Rifampin)

Rifampicin reduces the levels of mycophenolic acid (the active metabolite of mycophenolate) and increases the levels of the metabolite associated with mycophenolate adverse effects.

Clinical evidence

A heart-lung transplant patient taking tacrolimus 7 mg twice daily and mycophenolate mofetil 1 g twice daily was given rifampicin 600 mg daily, pyrazinamide 1 g daily, isoniazid 300 mg daily and pyridoxine 250 mg weekly for suspected mycobacterial infection. As expected, the tacrolimus dose needed to be substantially increased when rifampicin was started, and the rifampicin dose was reduced to 450 mg daily to try to minimise the interaction. However, the mycophenolate mofetil dose also needed to be increased to 6 g daily without achieving an adequate level (target trough plasma level of 2.5 micrograms/mL). Rifampicin was then stopped and the patient continued taking isoniazid and pyrazinamide. Pharmacokinetic analysis of mycophenolate, before and 13 days after rifampicin was stopped, found that the dose-corrected trough level of mycophenolic acid increased 18-fold and the AUC_{0-12} increased by 221%.

A subsequent study by the same authors in 8 kidney transplant patients taking mycophenolate 750 mg to 1 g twice daily found that rifampicin 600 mg daily for 8 days decreased the AUC_{0-12} and peak levels of mycophenolic acid by 17.5% and 18.5%, respectively. Glucuronide levels were increased and the AUC_{0-12} and peak levels of the acyl glucuronide metabolite, which has been associated with an increase in mycophenolate adverse effects, was significantly increased by 193% and 121%, respectively.[1]

Mechanism

The exact mechanism of this interaction is unknown. Mycophenolate is a pro-drug and is metabolised to its active form, mycophenolic acid, which undergoes glucuronidation by uridine diphosphate-glucuronosyltransferases (UGTs) in the liver, kidney and intestine to its inactive 7-*O*-glucuronide metabolite. The authors of these reports suggest that rifampicin induces intestinal, kidney and liver glucuronidation of mycophenolic acid by UGT and reduces its enterohepatic recirculation and absorption.[1,2]

Importance and management

These appear to be the only reports of an interaction between rifampicin and mycophenolate. However, the effects of reduced mycophenolic acid levels could be significant in terms of acute graft rejection. Also the increases in the levels of the acyl glucuronide metabolite could put the patient at greater risk of adverse effects, although this was not seen in these studies. Mycophenolate should be monitored closely during concurrent use with rifampicin and the dose adjusted as required, both on starting or stopping rifampicin. .

1. Naesens M, Kupyers DRJ, Streit F, Armstrong VW, Oellerich M, Verbeke K, Vanrenterghem Y. Rifampin induces alterations in mycophenolic acid glucuronidation and elimination: implications for drug exposure in renal allograft recipients. *Clin Pharmacol Ther* (2006) 80, 509–21.
2. Kupyers DRJ, Verleden G, Naesens M, Vanrenterghem Y. Drug interaction between mycophenolate mofetil and rifampin: possible induction of uridine diphosphate-glucuronosyltransferase. *Clin Pharmacol Ther* (2005) 78, 81–8.

Mycophenolate + Sevelamer

Sevelamer moderately reduces mycophenolate levels.

Clinical evidence, mechanism, importance and management

In a pharmacokinetic study, 3 adult and 6 paediatric kidney transplant patients taking mycophenolate and ciclosporin were given sevelamer, either as a single 1.6-g dose (adults), or 1.2-g dose (children), or for 4 days (same dose given three times daily). The average age of the children was 12 years. The single dose of sevelamer reduced the AUC of mycophenolate by 25%, and multiple-dosing with sevelamer reduced the AUC of mycophenolate by 30%. The interaction was thought to be due to sevelamer reducing the absorption of mycophenolate.[1]

The clinical significance of this interaction is unclear although the manufacturers note that graft rejection has not been reported.[2] However, it would seem prudent to monitor mycophenolate levels in any patient given sevelamer. The manufacturers of sevelamer recommend that mycophenolate is given at least one hour before or three hours after taking sevelamer.[3]

1. Pieper A-K, Buhle F, Bauer S, Mai I, Budde K, Haffner D, Neumayer H-H, Querfeld U. The effect of sevelamer on pharmacokinetics of cyclosporin A and mycophenolate-mofetil after renal transplantation. *Nephrol Dial Transplant* (2004) 19, 2630–3.
2. CellCept (Mycophenolate mofetil). Roche Products Ltd. UK Summary of product characteristics, March 2006.
3. Renagel (Sevelamer). Genzyme Therapeutics. UK Summary of product characteristics, June 2007.

Mycophenolate + Sirolimus

Higher levels of mycophenolic acid have been seen in kidney transplant patients taking mycophenolate with sirolimus when compared with similar patients taking mycophenolate with ciclosporin.

Clinical evidence and mechanism

A study in 12 kidney transplant patients taking mycophenolate 1 g twice daily at the same time as sirolimus (dose adjusted to attain therapeutic trough blood levels of 10 to 15 nanograms/mL), for 30 days found that the AUC_{0-9} of the active metabolite of mycophenolate, mycophenolic acid, was 1.5-fold higher in the sirolimus-treated group when compared to a similar group of 19 patients taking ciclosporin instead of sirolimus.[1] A study in 13 kidney transplant patients taking mycophenolate 1 g twice daily with sirolimus (trough blood levels of 10 to 20 nanograms/mL), found that the mycophenolic acid trough levels and AUC were significantly higher in patients taking sirolimus, compared with a similar group of 17 patients given ciclosporin, although peak mycophenolic acid levels were similar. Mycophenolate dose reductions were required in 2 patients in the first month, another 3 patients in the second month and 6 patients in the third month (total of 11 patients), compared with the ciclosporin group where 5 patients needed mycophenolate dose reductions. A higher incidence of leucopenia at months 1 and 2 after transplantation was reported in patients taking sirolimus, rather than ciclosporin, with mycophenolate.[2]

Another study in 11 kidney transplant patients taking low-dose mycophenolate 500 mg twice daily with low-dose sirolimus (mean dose of between 3.6 to 4.3 mg daily adjusted to achieve a trough blood level of 5 to 10 nanograms/mL) found that the sirolimus-based regimen had a 4.4-fold higher dose-adjusted mycophenolic acid trough level than those found in another similar group of 10 patients taking a ciclosporin-based regimen.[3]

Yet another study in 15 kidney transplant patients taking mycophenolate with sirolimus looked at the effects of sirolimus on mycophenolate dose regimens of 500 mg, 750 mg, and 1 g twice daily and compared them with the effects of ciclosporin on mycophenolate 1 g twice daily in 12 similar patients. They found that mycophenolate 750 mg twice daily with sirolimus produced a comparable AUC_{0-12} and trough mycophenolic acid levels to mycophenolate 1 g twice daily with ciclosporin.

Importance and management

Ciclosporin is known to inhibit the metabolism of mycophenolate, producing lower levels of mycophenolic acid, see 'Mycophenolate + Ciclosporin or Tacrolimus', p.1067. Whether sirolimus specifically raises mycophenolate levels compared with mycophenolate taken on its own is unclear, however raised mycophenolic acid levels have been associated with an increased risk of adverse effects.[1-3] The authors of one of the studies[4] suggest that the mycophenolate dose should be reduced from 1 g to 750 mg twice daily in patients taking sirolimus, as this produced comparable mycophenolic acid levels values with the recommended dose of mycophenolate 1 g twice daily with ciclosporin.

However, until further information is available, patients taking mycophenolate and changed from ciclosporin to sirolimus should be closely monitored for signs of adverse effects, and the dose of mycophenolate reduced accordingly.

1. Picard, N, Prémaud, Rousseau A, Le Meur Y, Marquet P. A comparison of the effect of ciclosporin and sirolimus on the pharmacokinetics of mycophenolate in renal transplant patients. *Br J Clin Pharmacol* (2006) 62, 477–84.
2. Büchler M, Lebranchu Y, Bénéton M, Le Meur Y, Heng AE, Westeel PF, le Guellec C, Libert F, Hary L, Marquet P, Paintaud G. Higher exposure to mycophenolic acid with sirolimus than with cyclosporine cotreatment. *Clin Pharmacol Ther* (2005) 78, 34–42.
3. Cattaneo D, Merlini S, Zenoni S, Baldelli S, Gotti E, Remuzzi G, Perico N. Influence of comedication with sirolimus or cyclosporine on mycophenolic acid pharmacokinetics in kidney transplantation. *Am J Transplant* (2005) 5, 2937–44.
4. El Haggan W, Ficheux M, Debruyne D, Rognant N, Lobbedez T, Allard C, Coquerel A, Ryckelynck JP, Hurault de Ligny B, Pharmacokinetics of mycophenolic acid in kidney transplant patients receiving sirolimus versus cyclosporine. *Transplant Proc* (2005) 37, 864–6.

Mycophenolate + St John's wort (*Hypericum perforatum*)

St John's wort does not appear to alter the pharmacokinetics of mycophenolate.

Clinical evidence, mechanism, importance and management

In a pharmacokinetic study, 8 stable kidney transplant patients taking mycophenolate and tacrolimus were given 600 mg of St John's wort extract (*Jarsin 300*) daily for 14 days. The study intended to make dose adjustments to keep the trough mycophenolic acid levels within the desired range, but dosage adjustment was not found to be necessary in any of the 8 patients.[1]

1. Mai I, Störmer E, Bauer S, Krüger H, Budde K, Roots I. Impact of St John's wort treatment on the pharmacokinetics of tacrolimus and mycophenolic acid in renal transplant patients. *Nephrol Dial Transplant* (2003) 18, 819–22.

Mycophenolate + Voriconazole

Voriconazole had no effect on the pharmacokinetics of a single 1-g dose of mycophenolate.[1]

1. Wood N, Abel, Fielding A, Nichols DJ, Bygrave E. Voriconazole does not affect the pharmacokinetics of mycophenolic acid. *Intersci Conf Antimicrob Agents Chemother* (2001) 41, 3.

Sirolimus + ACE inhibitors

Oedema of the tongue, face, lips, neck and chest has been reported in patients taking sirolimus with enalapril or ramipril.

Clinical evidence

A study in 52 kidney transplant patients taking sirolimus 2 to 5 mg daily with **ramipril** 2.5 to 5 mg daily found that 5 of these patients developed non-life threatening tongue oedema within one month of starting **ramipril**. All of these patients had taken **ramipril** before their transplant without any adverse effects or signs of angioedema. The tongue oedema resolved within 2 weeks of stopping ramipril. The authors noted that at that time all 5 patients were taking sirolimus 5 mg daily and ramipril 5 mg daily, with their sirolimus levels in the higher end of the range between 16 to 20 nanograms/mL. Three months after their transplant, when sirolimus had been stabilised at a lower dose of 2 to 4 mg daily, resulting in blood levels of 8 to 12 nanograms/mL, ramipril was restarted at a 2.5 mg daily with no adverse effects.[1]

A kidney transplant patient taking sirolimus 9 mg daily developed non-pitting oedema of the eyelid, cheek and lips when he started to take **ramipril** (dose not specified).[2] Another kidney transplant patient who had taken **enalapril** 2.5 mg daily for two months developed erythematous skin lesions with non-pitting oedema of the neck, face and chest 9 days after she was switched from tacrolimus to sirolimus 2 mg daily. Symptoms resolved in both patients when the ACE inhibitor was stopped and corticosteroid therapy was increased.[2]

Mechanism, importance and management

ACE inhibitors alone can cause angioedema but in the study above, all 5 patients had previously taken an ACE inhibitor without any allergic reaction or adverse effects.[1] Although not life-threatening, these reports of oedema suggest that caution should be used when either starting an ACE inhibitor in a patient already taking sirolimus or when starting sirolimus in a patient taking an ACE inhibitor. The effect may be dose-related, with higher doses of both drugs potentially posing a greater risk.

1. Stallone G, Infante B, Di Paolo S, Schena A, Grandaliano G, Gesualdo L, Schena FP. Sirolimus and angiotensin-converting enzyme inhibitors together induce tongue oedema in renal transplant recipients. *Nephrol Dial Transplant* (2004) 19, 2906–8.
2. Burdese M, Rossetti M, Guarena C, Consiglio V, Mezza E, Soragna G, Gai M, Segoloni GP, Piccoli GB. Sirolimus and ACE-inhibitors: a note of caution. *Transplantation* (2005) 79, 251–2.

Sirolimus or Tacrolimus + Amiodarone

There is an isolated case report of increased sirolimus and tacrolimus levels associated with the concurrent use of amiodarone in a paediatric patient.

Clinical evidence, mechanism, importance and management

A 2-year-old heart transplant patient given tacrolimus 0.02 mg/kg daily was given amiodarone to control ventricular arrhythmias. Her tacrolimus trough levels were reported as within target range of 8 to 10 micrograms/L on both day 1 and day 3 after starting the amiodarone. She was then switched from tacrolimus to sirolimus 0.06 mg/kg daily, increased to 0.12 mg/kg after 2 days, with tacrolimus continued until therapeutic sirolimus levels were achieved. The sirolimus levels and tacrolimus levels 9 days after starting amiodarone were found to be 53 micrograms/L and 13 micrograms/L, respectively. Subsequent sirolimus doses were put on hold and tacrolimus was stopped. The sirolimus levels were raised for a further 14 days. Sirolimus was restarted at a lower dose (0.03 mg/kg daily) but the levels remained above 10 micrograms/L and the sirolimus dose was reduced further to 0.02 mg/kg daily.[1] The elevated levels of both drugs were attributed to an interaction with amiodarone, which can inhibit the cytochrome P450 isoenzyme CYP3A4, and affect P-glycoprotein, which have effects on sirolimus and tacrolimus metabolism and clearance.[1]

The authors of this report advise that, because of the long half-life of sirolimus, and the difficulty in reducing elevated levels quickly, prescribers should consider reducing the sirolimus and tacrolimus doses before starting amiodarone[1] rather than waiting for the interaction to occur. They also advise more frequent monitoring of sirolimus and tacrolimus levels if amiodarone is also given. This appears to be the only published report of this interaction at present.

1. Nalli N, Stewart-Texeira L, Dipchand AI. Amiodarone-sirolimus/tacrolimus interaction in a pediatric heart transplant patient. *Pediatr Transplant* (2006) 10, 736–739.

Sirolimus + Azoles

Sirolimus levels are markedly raised by ketoconazole, and itraconazole, posaconazole and voriconazole appear to interact similarly. Clotrimazole is are also predicted to interact with sirolimus. A case report suggests that fluconazole also raises sirolimus levels. In theory it is possible that miconazole oral gel may also interact with sirolimus.

Clinical evidence

(a) Fluconazole

A patient taking sirolimus after a kidney transplant was given fluconazole 200 mg daily for oesophageal candidiasis. Because an interaction was anticipated, the sirolimus dosage was reduced from 4 to 3 mg daily. After 4 days the sirolimus level had risen from about 10 micrograms/L to 22.8 micrograms/L. The dose of sirolimus was then reduced to 2 mg daily, but by the seventh day of fluconazole treatment the sirolimus level had reached 35 micrograms/L, after which they began to fall. The patient then had a hyperkalaemic arrest and died.[1] The sirolimus levels of another kidney transplant patient were raised almost fivefold about 3 weeks after she started to take fluconazole.[2]

(b) Itraconazole

A heart transplant patient needed only half of his normal sirolimus dose to maintain about the same trough levels when he took itraconazole 400 mg daily for a year.[2] A kidney transplant patient taking sirolimus 5 mg daily was given an initial dose of itraconazole 600 mg daily on post-transplant day 10 followed by 400 mg daily. The sirolimus trough level was subtherapeutic at 6.8 nanograms/mL one day after starting itraconazole so the sirolimus dose was increased to 10 mg daily. The sirolimus level then increased rapidly and reached a level of 82.5 nanograms/mL 6 days after itraconazole was started.[3] A haematopoietic stem cell transplant patient taking itraconazole 200 mg twice daily was changed from tacrolimus to sirolimus 7 mg daily. The sirolimus dose was reduced to 5 mg daily 6 days later because the sirolimus level was 17.5 nanograms/mL (therapeutic range 5 to 15 nanograms/mL). The sirolimus level was found to be 35.6 nanograms/mL two days later and sirolimus was stopped until the level had fallen back to the normal range. It was subsequently restarted and the dose adjusted between 0.5 mg and 2 mg daily according to levels.[4]

(c) Ketoconazole

A clinical study in 23 healthy subjects found that while taking ketoconazole 200 mg daily for 10 days, the maximum serum levels and AUC of a single 5-mg dose of sirolimus were increased 4.3-fold and 10.9-fold, respectively.[5] In a study in 6 kidney transplant patients, ciclosporin was stopped because of toxicity or rejection episodes and sirolimus was started. They were given a lower than recommended dose of sirolimus (250 to 500 micrograms daily) but were also given ketoconazole 100 to 200 mg daily, adjusted to maintain sirolimus levels within the therapeutic range. The serum creatinine of the patients improved and reduced from 230 micromol/L to 194 micromol/L.[6]

(d) Voriconazole

Voriconazole 400 mg twice daily for one day, then 200 mg twice daily for 8 days markedly raised the maximum serum levels and AUC of a single 2-mg dose of sirolimus by about 7-fold and 11-fold, respectively.[7] In a retrospective study of allogeneic haematopoietic stem cell transplant patients, 11 patients were found to have received both sirolimus and voriconazole for a median of 33 days (range, 3 to 100 days). Three patients had increased trough sirolimus levels of between 10 and 19 nanograms/mL and serious toxicity occurred in 2 of them. The other eight patients had their sirolimus dose reduced by 90% when voriconazole was started, in anticipation of the interaction Trough sirolimus levels were similar to those before voriconazole administration and no significant toxicity from either drug was found.[8] A patient taking sirolimus, who had markedly raised sirolimus levels with itraconazole, was given voriconazole, and the sirolimus dose was decreased to 0.5 mg daily in anticipation of a similar interaction. The sirolimus trough level was 6.4 nanograms/mL, about the patients' usual range, two days after starting voriconazole.[4]

A case report describes a patient with a heart transplant who was given two doses of voriconazole 400 mg then 200 mg twice daily for 16 days. When sirolimus was started a dose of 1 mg gave a sirolimus trough level of 12.8 nanograms/mL, but after the voriconazole was stopped a dose of 3 mg only gave trough sirolimus levels of 7.4 nanograms/mL.[2] Voriconazole has been seen to markedly raise sirolimus levels in a number of other patients.[2,9]

Mechanism

Ketoconazole, itraconazole, posaconazole and voriconazole are potent inhibitors of the cytochrome P450 isoenzyme CYP3A4, the isoenzyme that is at least partly responsible for the metabolism of sirolimus.[10] Therefore these azoles probably cause raised sirolimus levels by inhibiting its metabolism. Fluconazole and miconazole also inhibit CYP3A4, but are less potent than ketoconazole. Hence sirolimus levels rise when fluconazole is given, but the rise is not as great as that seen with ketoconazole. Sirolimus is also a substrate for P-glycoprotein and, as azole antifungals may inhibit intestinal P-glycoprotein, this may also contribute to the interaction by increasing the oral bioavailability of sirolimus.[3]

Importance and management

The concurrent use of sirolimus is contraindicated by the manufacturers of **voriconazole**.[7,11] The rises in sirolimus levels caused by voriconazole are probably too large to be easily accommodated by reducing the dosage of the sirolimus. One study found that an initial empiric reduction in sirolimus dose by 90% at the start of treatment with voriconazole was adequate. However, more study is required to confirm the safety of such regimens.[8]

The manufacturers of sirolimus say that concurrent use of strong inhibitors of CYP3A4, including **ketoconazole**, voriconazole and **itraconazole** is not recommended,[10,12] but note that any patient given these drugs should have their trough sirolimus levels closely monitored both during use and after they are stopped. **Clotrimazole**[10,12] and **posaconazole**[13] are predicted to interact similarly. **Fluconazole**, although a weaker inhibitor of CYP3A4 than ketoconazole, voriconazole or itraconazole, has been reported to interact in two cases. Sirolimus plasma levels should be monitored during treatment with and following the withdrawal of any of these antifungals.

There appear to be no reports of an interaction between **miconazole** and sirolimus. However, a large proportion of miconazole oral gel (both prescription and non-prescription doses) may be swallowed and therefore adequate systemic absorption may occur to produce an interaction. The manufacturers of miconazole oral gel recommend close monitoring and possible dose reduction of sirolimus if both drugs are given.[14] An interaction with intravaginal miconazole would not normally be expected because its systemic absorption is usually very low (less than 2%).[15]

1. Cervelli MJ. Fluconazole-sirolimus drug interaction. *Transplantation* (2002) 74, 1477–8.
2. Sádaba B, Campanero MA, Quetglas EG, Azanza JR. Clinical relevance of sirolimus drug interactions in transplant patients. *Transplant Proc* (2004) 36, 3226–8.
3. Kupyers DR, Claes K, Evenepoel P, Maes B, Vandecasteele S, Vanrenterghem Y, Van Damme B, Desmet K. Drug interaction between itraconazole and sirolimus in a primary renal allograft recipient. *Transplantation* (2005) 79, 737.
4. Said A, Garnick JJ, Dieterle N, Peres E, Abidi MH, Ibrahim RB. Sirolimus-itraconazole interaction in a hematopoietic stem cell transplant recipient. *Pharmacotherapy* (2006) 26, 289–95.
5. Floren LC, Christians U, Zimmerman JJ, Neefe L, Schorer R, Rushowrth D, Harper D, Renz J, Benet LZ. Sirolimus oral bioavailability increases ten-fold with concomitant ketoconazole. *Clin Pharmacol Ther* (1999) 65, 159.
6. Thomas PP, Manivannan J, John GT, Jacob CK. Sirolimus and ketoconazole co-prescription in renal transplant recipients. *Transplantation* (2004) 77, 474–5.
7. VFEND (Voriconazole). Pfizer Inc. US Prescribing information, November 2006.
8. Marty FM, Lowry CM, Cutler CS, Campbell BJ, Fiumara K, Baden LR, Antin JH. Voriconazole and sirolimus coadministration after allogeneic hematopoietic stem cell transplantation. *Biol Blood Marrow Transplant* (2006) 12, 552–9.
9. Mathis AS, Shah NK, Friedman GS. Combined use of sirolimus and voriconazole in renal transplantation: a report of two cases. *Transplant Proc* (2004) 36, 2708–9.
10. Rapamune (Sirolimus). Wyeth Pharmaceuticals. UK Summary of product characteristics, March 2007.
11. VFEND (Voriconazole). Pfizer Ltd. UK Summary of product characteristics, July 2007.
12. Rapamune (Sirolimus). Wyeth Pharmaceuticals Inc. US Prescribing information, May 2007.
13. Noxafil (Posaconazole). Schering-Plough Ltd. UK Summary of product characteristics, October 2006.
14. Daktarin Oral Gel (Miconazole). Janssen-Cilag Ltd. UK Summary of product characteristics, May 2006.
15. Daneshmend TK. Systemic absorption of miconazole from the vagina. *J Antimicrob Chemother* (1986) 18, 507–11.

Sirolimus + Calcium-channel blockers

Diltiazem and verapamil raise sirolimus levels, and dosage adjustments may be necessary. Nicardipine is predicted to interact similarly. Nifedipine appears not to interact with sirolimus.

Clinical evidence, mechanism, importance and management

A randomised, crossover study in 18 healthy subjects found that a single 120-mg oral dose of **diltiazem** increased the AUC and the maximum serum levels of a single 10-mg oral dose of sirolimus by 60% and 43%, respectively. The pharmacokinetics of **diltiazem** and its metabolites were unchanged. The likely reason for this interaction is that **diltiazem** inhibits the cytochrome P450 isoenzyme CYP3A4 in the intestinal wall and liver, which is the primary route of sirolimus metabolism. **Diltiazem** may also inhibit P-glycoprotein activity, which leads to increased sirolimus absorption.[1] This was a single-dose study, but the evidence suggests that this interaction will also occur with multiple doses of both drugs, for which reason the manufacturers recommend whole blood monitoring and a possible sirolimus dosage reduction (based on sirolimus levels) if **diltiazem** is used concurrently.[2,3]

In 26 healthy subjects the concurrent use of sirolimus oral solution 2 g daily and **verapamil** 180 mg every 12 hours resulted in an increase in the sirolimus maximum levels and AUC, of 2.3-fold and 2.2-fold, respectively, and an increase in the maximum levels and AUC of ***S*-verapamil** of 1.5-fold.[2,3] The manufacturer notes that other calcium-channel blockers that inhibit CYP3A4 might interact similarly, and they specifically name **nicardipine**.[2,3]

Nifedipine [which does not inhibit CYP3A4] is said not to interact,[2,3] and a study comparing 16 patients taking **nifedipine** and sirolimus with 10 patients taking sirolimus alone found no significant differences in sirolimus pharmacokinetics between the two groups.[4]

1. Böttinger Y, Säwe J, Brattström C, Tollemar J, Burke JT, Häss G, Zimmerman JJ. Pharmacokinetic interaction between single oral doses of diltiazem and sirolimus in healthy volunteers. *Clin Pharmacol Ther* (2001) 69, 32–40.
2. Rapamune (Sirolimus). Wyeth Pharmaceuticals Inc. US Prescribing information, May 2007.
3. Rapamune (Sirolimus). Wyeth Pharmaceuticals. UK Summary of product characteristics, March 2007.
4. Zimmerman JJ, Kahan BD. Pharmacokinetics of sirolimus in stable renal transplant patients after multiple oral dose administration. *J Clin Pharmacol* (1997) 37, 405–15.

Sirolimus + Ciclosporin

Ciclosporin raises sirolimus serum levels, and this can be reduced by giving the drugs at least 4 hours apart. Concurrent use for longer than 3 to 4 months possibly increases renal toxicity, and should be used with caution only when the benefits outweigh the risks. Sirolimus has been reported to increase ciclosporin levels.

Clinical evidence

(a) Effects on ciclosporin

A randomised study found that when sirolimus was added to a ciclosporin/corticosteroid regimen in kidney transplant patients, the steady-state ciclosporin levels remained unchanged. Blood pressure, glomerular filtration rate, creatinine levels, triglyceride levels and liver enzymes (ALT, AST) were unchanged.[1] A 2-week pharmacokinetic study in 40 kidney transplant patients found that sirolimus 0.5 to 6.5 mg/m^2 given twice daily did not affect the pharmacokinetics of ciclosporin 75 to 400 mg twice daily. The patients were also taking prednisone.[2] Two related studies in kidney transplant patients confirmed the absence of an effect of sirolimus on ciclosporin pharmacokinetics.[3] Similarly, in another study in healthy subjects, single doses of sirolimus did not affect the pharmacokinetics of a single dose of ciclosporin (microemulsion formulation, *Neoral*) when given either at the same time or 4 hours apart.[4]

However, another study in kidney transplant patients taking ciclosporin (*Neoral*) and sirolimus (taken 4 hours after ciclosporin) over a 6 month period found that the oral clearance of ciclosporin was decreased, and lower doses of ciclosporin were needed to maintain therapeutic levels.[5] A kidney transplant patient taking ciclosporin 400 mg daily with prednisone started taking sirolimus 2 mg daily. Within 2 weeks, she was readmitted to hospital with signs of ciclosporin toxicity, including raised creatinine, urea, and high blood pressure, and her ciclosporin level was found to have increased to 536 nanograms/mL. The ciclosporin dose was reduced to 300 mg daily, sirolimus continued, and her ciclosporin level reduced to 276 nanograms/mL. The sirolimus levels remained at 5.2 to 10.6 nanograms/mL, within the therapeutic range.[6]

(b) Effects on sirolimus

In a single-dose study in healthy subjects, ciclosporin (microemulsion formulation, *Neoral*) given 4 hours before sirolimus increased the maximum serum levels of sirolimus 1.4-fold and increased its AUC 1.8-fold. When the drugs were given at the same time, the effect was even greater, with a 2.2-fold increase in maximum sirolimus level and 3.3-fold increase in the AUC.[4] This study confirmed the findings of a previous multiple-dose study in kidney transplant recipients,[7] and similar results have been seen in other studies.[8] Ciclosporin 300 mg taken at the same time, 2 hours after, or 4 hours after sirolimus 5 mg increased the AUC of sirolimus by 183%, 141%, and 80%, respectively, but when sirolimus was taken 2 hours before ciclosporin, there was no increase in the AUC or peak levels of sirolimus.[9] The US manufacturer of sirolimus also presents data showing that ciclosporin oral solution (*Sandimmune*) given at the same time as sirolimus, increased sirolimus trough levels by 67% to 86% in 150 patients with psoriasis.[5]

Mechanism

It appears that ciclosporin inhibits the metabolism of sirolimus by the cytochrome P450 isoenzyme CYP3A4 in the gut and liver leading to increased sirolimus levels.[4,5,9] P-glycoprotein inhibition may also contribute to the interaction.

Importance and management

An established interaction. The manufacturers recommend that sirolimus should be given 4 hours after microemulsion ciclosporin, and consistently, either with or without food.[5,9] Despite this, it may still be necessary to reduce the sirolimus dose.[4] Renal function should be closely monitored, and if serum creatinine levels increase, discontinuation of sirolimus or ciclosporin should be considered.[5] If ciclosporin is withdrawn, the sirolimus dosage will need to be raised fourfold to take into account the absence of the interaction (twofold increase needed) and the need for increased immunosuppression (twofold increase needed). A target trough sirolimus level of 12 to 20 nanograms/mL (chromatographic assay) is recommended when ciclosporin has been withdrawn.[9]

Until further clinical data are available, the manufacturer does not recommend continued usage of the combination beyond 3 months[9] to 4 months.[5] In patients taking sirolimus and ciclosporin for more than 3 months, higher serum creatinine levels and lower glomerular filtration rates have been seen. Patients who were successfully withdrawn from ciclosporin had improved creatinine levels, higher glomerular filtration rates and a lower risk of malignancy.[9]

The UK manufacturers do not recommend the use of sirolimus in high-risk patients (e.g. those with renal impairment, markers of rejection of multi-organ transplants) as insufficient numbers of this type of patient were studied.[9] However, the US manufacturers state that it may be used in combination with ciclosporin in high-risk patients for up to 1 year.[5]

The concurrent use of both drugs increases the risk of developing calcineurin inhibitor-induced haemolytic uraemic syndrome/thrombotic thrombocytopenic purpura/thrombotic microangiopathy.[5,9] An increased risk of hepatic artery thrombosis, leading to graft loss and/or death in most cases, has also been seen in clinical studies in *de novo* liver transplant patients taking sirolimus with ciclosporin, and the manufacturers do not recommend using sirolimus in liver or lung transplant patients as safety and effectiveness have not been proven.[5,9]

1. Murgia MG, Jordan S, Kahan BD. The side effect profile of sirolimus: a phase I study in quiescent cyclosporine-prednisone-treated renal transplant patients. *Kidney Int* (1996) 49, 209–16.
2. Zimmerman JJ, Kahan BD. Pharmacokinetics of sirolimus in stable renal transplant patients after multiple oral dose administration. *J Clin Pharmacol* (1997) 37, 405–15.
3. Ferron GM, Mishina EV, Zimmerman JJ, Jusko WJ. Population pharmacokinetics of sirolimus in kidney transplant patients. *Clin Pharmacol Ther* (1997) 61, 416–28.
4. Zimmerman JJ, Harper D, Getsy J, Jusko WJ. Pharmacokinetic interactions between sirolimus and microemulsion cyclosporine when orally administered jointly and 4 hours apart in healthy volunteers. *J Clin Pharmacol* (2003) 42, 1168–76.
5. Rapamune (Sirolimus). Wyeth Pharmaceuticals Inc. US Prescribing information, May 2007.
6. Dąbrowska-Zamojcin E, Pawlik A, Domański L, Różański J, Droździk M. Cyclosporine and sirolimus interaction in a kidney transplant patient. *Transplant Proc* (2005) 37, 2317–19.
7. Kaplan B, Meier-Kriesche H-U, Napoli KL, Kahan BD. The effects of relative timing of sirolimus and cyclosporine microemulsion formulation coadministration on the pharmacokinetics of each agent. *Clin Pharmacol Ther* (1998) 63, 48–53.
8. Wu FLL, Tsai M-K, Chen RR-L, Sun S-W, Huang J-D, Hu R-H, Chen K-H, Lee P-H. Effects of calcineurin inhibitors on sirolimus pharmacokinetics during staggered administration in renal transplant recipients. *Pharmacotherapy* (2005) 25, 646–53.
9. Rapamune (Sirolimus). Wyeth Pharmaceuticals. UK Summary of product characteristics, March 2007.

Sirolimus + Corticosteroids

Intravenous methylprednisolone had no effect on trough sirolimus levels. Sirolimus slightly increased prednisolone levels (derived from prednisone), but this is probably not clinically relevant.

Clinical evidence, mechanism, importance and management

(a) Methylprednisolone

When 14 patients taking sirolimus (and also taking either azathioprine or mycophenolate) were given methylprednisolone as a daily intravenous bolus for 1 to 5 days (total dose of between 500 mg and 3 g) the sirolimus trough concentrations were not significantly altered.[1] No additional precautions seem necessary on concurrent use.[1]

(b) Prednisolone or Prednisone

In a study in kidney transplant patients taking ciclosporin and prednisone 5 to 20 mg daily, only minor to moderate changes occurred in the pharmacokinetics of prednisolone when sirolimus 6 to 13 mg/m^2 daily was given for 2 weeks.[2] The maximum plasma prednisolone levels were raised by 14%, and the AUC was raised by 18%. The clinical relevance of these findings is uncertain, but they are likely to be minor.

1. Bäckman L, Kreis H, Morales JM, Wilczek H, Taylor R, Burke JT. Sirolimus steady-state trough concentrations are not affected by bolus methylprednisolone therapy in renal allograft recipients. *Br J Clin Pharmacol* (2002) 54, 65–8.
2. Jusko WJ, Ferron GM, SM Mis, Kahan BD, Zimmerman JJ. Pharmacokinetics of prednisolone during administration of sirolimus in patients with renal transplants. *J Clin Pharmacol* (1996) 36, 1100–6.

Sirolimus + CYP3A4 inducers

Drugs that induce the cytochrome P450 isoenzyme CYP3A4 are predicted to lower sirolimus levels. Close monitoring is recommended.

Clinical evidence, mechanism, importance and management

Sirolimus is extensively metabolised by the cytochrome P450 isoenzyme CYP3A4 in the intestinal wall and by the drug transporter protein P-glycoprotein: drugs that induce their activity are predicted to lower sirolimus levels.[1,2]

'Rifampicin', (p.1074), and 'phenytoin', (p.1074), are known potent enzyme inducers, and have been seen to lower sirolimus levels, and the manufacturers predict that **carbamazepine**, **phenobarbital** (and thus, primidone), and **St John's wort** will interact similarly.[1,2] These predictions are as yet unconfirmed, but it would certainly be prudent to monitor sirolimus levels closely if any of these drugs are used concurrently. In the case of **St John's wort**, it may be best to avoid the combination all together (see 'drug-herb interactions', (p.10)). What should be remembered is that the extent of the inducing effects of these drugs is not identical, so that very marked effects like those observed with rifampicin may not occur; nevertheless the interaction may still be clinically important.

1. Rapamune (Sirolimus). Wyeth Pharmaceuticals Inc. US Prescribing information, May 2007.
2. Rapamune (Sirolimus). Wyeth Pharmaceuticals. UK Summary of product characteristics, March 2007.

Sirolimus + CYP3A4 inhibitors

Drugs that inhibit the cytochrome P450 isoenzyme CYP3A4 are predicted to raise sirolimus levels. Monitoring is recommended.

Clinical evidence, mechanism, importance and management

Sirolimus is extensively metabolised by cytochrome P450 isoenzyme CYP3A4 in the intestinal wall and by the drug transporter protein, P-glycoprotein: drugs that inhibit their activity may raise sirolimus levels.[1,2]

'Ketoconazole and voriconazole', (p.1071), 'diltiazem and verapamil', (p.1072), 'erythromycin', (below) and 'nelfinavir', (p.1074) have been shown to raise sirolimus levels, and the manufacturers name a number of others that also inhibit CYP3A4, which they predict will interact similarly. They list **bromocriptine** (although there appear to be no reported interactions with bromocriptine due to CYP3A4 inhibition), **cimetidine**, and **danazol**.[1,2]

These predictions are as yet unconfirmed, but it would certainly be prudent to monitor sirolimus levels closely if these drugs are used concurrently. What should be remembered is that the extent of the inhibitory effects of these drugs is not identical, so that very marked effects like those observed with ketoconazole may not occur, nevertheless the interaction may still be clinically important. **Grapefruit juice** also inhibits CYP3A4 (potentially raising sirolimus levels), and in this case the manufacturers recommend that concurrent use should be avoided.[1,2]

1. Rapamune (Sirolimus). Wyeth Pharmaceuticals Inc. US Prescribing information, May 2007.
2. Rapamune (Sirolimus). Wyeth Pharmaceuticals. UK Summary of product characteristics, March 2007.

Sirolimus + Macrolides

Two patients had large elevations in their sirolimus levels when they were given erythromycin. Other macrolides are expected to interact similarly.

Clinical evidence, mechanism, importance and management

A case report describes 2 patients taking sirolimus who were also given **erythromycin** 1 g three times daily for suspected Legionella pneumonia. Despite reductions in the sirolimus dosage, the sirolimus levels of both patients rose fivefold.[1]

In 24 healthy subjects the concurrent use of **erythromycin** 800 mg three times daily with sirolimus oral solution 2 mg daily resulted in a significant increase in the peak blood levels and AUC of sirolimus, by 4.2- and 4.4-fold, respectively. The peak plasma levels and AUC of erythromycin were also increased, by 1.6- and 1.7-fold, respectively.[2,3]

Erythromycin is an inhibitor of the cytochrome P450 isoenzyme CYP3A4, which is the main enzyme responsible for the metabolism of sirolimus. Therefore **erythromycin** probably inhibited the metabolism of sirolimus, causing the levels to rise.

The manufacturers predict that other inhibitors of CYP3A4 (they name **clarithromycin** and **telithromycin**) will interact similarly, and should be avoided.[2,3] The manufacturers of **telithromycin** specifically advise that if concurrent use is needed, sirolimus levels should be closely monitored and the dose altered as required, both when starting treatment and also when telithromycin is stopped.[4]

The manufacturers of sirolimus also name **troleandomycin** as a moderate inhibitor of CYP3A4, which may possibly interact.[2,3] However, **troleandomycin** tends to be a more potent inhibitor of CYP3A4 than **clarithromycin**, so it would seem prudent to at least monitor concurrent use closely, or even consider avoiding the combination, as recommended with **clarithromycin**.

1. Claesson K, Brattström C, Burke JT. Sirolimus and erythromycin interaction: two cases. *Transplant Proc* (2001) 33, 2136.
2. Rapamune (Sirolimus). Wyeth Pharmaceuticals. UK Summary of product characteristics, March 2007.
3. Rapamune (Sirolimus). Wyeth Pharmaceuticals Inc. US Prescribing information, May 2007.
4. Ketek (Telithromycin). Sanofi-Aventis. UK Summary of product characteristics, May 2007.

Sirolimus + Miscellaneous

The manufacturers of sirolimus note that cisapride and metoclopramide may increase sirolimus levels, although there do not appear to be any published reports of this interaction.[1,2] No significant pharmacokinetic interaction has been found with aciclovir, digoxin, glibenclamide or co-trimoxazole.[13,4] There is an isolated case report of atorvastatin increasing sirolimus trough serum levels twofold in one patient, and a reduction in the sirolimus dose was required.[5]

1. Rapamune (Sirolimus). Wyeth Pharmaceuticals. UK Summary of product characteristics, March 2007.
2. Rapamune (Sirolimus). Wyeth Pharmaceuticals Inc. US Prescribing information, May 2007.
3. 4. Zimmerman JJ. Exposure-response relationships and drug interactions of sirolimus. *AAPS J* (2004) 6, 1–12.
5. Barshes, NR, Goodpastor SE, Goss JA, DeBakey ME. Sirolimus-atorvastatin drug interaction in the pancreatic islet transplant recipient. *Transplantation* (2003) 76, 1649–50.

Sirolimus + Phenytoin

Two case reports describe increased sirolimus dose requirements in the presence of phenytoin.

Clinical evidence, mechanism, importance and management

An 11-year-old girl with a kidney transplant taking phenytoin started taking sirolimus 30 micrograms/kg twice daily following an episode of acute rejection. The dose of sirolimus was increased tenfold over the next few weeks in an attempt to achieve the target trough level of 10 to 20 nanograms/mL, and two further episodes of acute rejection occurred. About one month after the sirolimus had been started, tacrolimus was added, and her phenytoin was stopped. Over the next few weeks her sirolimus level rose to about 40 nanograms/mL. The patient subsequently recovered.[1]

A 62-year-old woman started taking phenytoin 100 mg twice daily because she developed a seizure disorder following a liver transplant. At this time she was taking ciclosporin, but it was decided to start sirolimus because of neurological complications. The initial sirolimus dose of 5 mg daily produced subtherapeutic sirolimus levels. She was subsequently stabilised taking sirolimus 15 mg daily, with trough levels of less than 5 nanograms/mL. Phenytoin was stopped, and about 5 days later her trough sirolimus level was found to be around 15 to 20 nanograms/mL. After a further 5 days, the sirolimus dose was reduced to 10 mg daily. The authors of this report suggest that the initial high sirolimus dose was necessary as phenytoin, a potent inducer of the cytochrome P450 isoenzyme CYP3A4, increased the metabolism of sirolimus, which is mainly metabolised by this isoenzyme. When the phenytoin was withdrawn, sirolimus metabolism returned to normal, resulting in high sirolimus levels.[2]

These appear to be the only reports of this interaction, but they are consistent with the way both drugs are known to interact. It would therefore seem prudent to monitor sirolimus levels in any patient in whom phenytoin is started or withdrawn, and to adjust the dose as necessary.

1. Hodges CB, Maxwell H, Beattie TJ, Murphy AV, Jindal RM. Use of rapamycin in a transplant patient who developed ciclosporin neurotoxicity. *Pediatr Nephrol* (2001) 16, 777–8.
2. Fridell JA, Jain AKB, Patel K, Virji M, Rao KN, Fung JJ, Venkataramanan R. Phenytoin decreases the blood concentrations of sirolimus in a liver transplant recipient: a case report. *Ther Drug Monit* (2003) 25, 117–19.

Sirolimus + Protease inhibitors

Nelfinavir increased the levels of sirolimus in one patient. Other protease inhibitors are predicted to also raise sirolimus levels.

Clinical evidence, mechanism, importance and management

An HIV-positive, liver transplant patient taking sirolimus 5 mg daily was given **nelfinavir** 250 mg twice daily (one-fifth of normal dose), lamivudine and zidovudine. Three weeks later, because of a reduced full blood count,her sirolimus blood levels were checked, and found to be 24.7 nanograms/mL. Her sirolimus dose was reduced to 3 mg daily and then 2 mg daily and her levels rechecked 5 days later. The trough sirolimus level was found to be 4.6 nanograms/mL, which was almost fivefold higher than the trough levels of 3 control patients taking sirolimus 5 to 7 mg daily but not taking nelfinavir. The peak level and AUC were also much higher in the patient taking nelfinavir.[1]

The manufacturers point out that sirolimus is extensively metabolised by cytochrome P450 isoenzyme CYP3A4 and cleared by P-glycoprotein, so drugs such as the protease inhibitors, which inhibit their activity may raise sirolimus levels.[2,3] Close monitoring with dose adjustments are recommended during the concurrent use of sirolimus and nelfinavir, or any other protease inhibitor.

1. Jain AKB, Venkataramanan R, Fridell JA, Gadomski M, Shaw LM, Ragni M, Korecka M, Fung J. Nelfinavir, a protease inhibitor, increases sirolimus levels in a liver transplantation patient: a case report. *Liver Transpl* (2002) 8, 838–40.
2. Rapamune (Sirolimus). Wyeth Pharmaceuticals Inc. US Prescribing information, May 2007.
3. Rapamune (Sirolimus). Wyeth Pharmaceuticals. UK Summary of product characteristics, March 2007.

Sirolimus + Rifamycins

Rifampicin (rifampin) significantly decreases sirolimus levels. Rifabutin and rifapentine are predicted to interact similarly, although to a lesser extent.

Clinical evidence, mechanism, importance and management

A clinical study in 14 healthy subjects found that **rifampicin (rifampin)** 600 mg daily for 6 days increased the clearance of a single 10-mg oral dose of sirolimus 5.5-fold, and reduced the AUC and maximum serum levels of sirolimus by 82% and 71%, respectively. **Rifampicin** is a potent inducer of the cytochrome P450 isoenzyme CYP3A4, the isoenzyme by which sirolimus is metabolised.[1,2] Therefore concurrent use increases sirolimus metabolism and reduces its levels. The manufacturers say that concurrent use is not recommended.[1] **Rifabutin** [a weak CYP3A4 inhibitor] and **rifapentine** [a moderate CYP3A4 inhibitor] are predicted to also lower sirolimus levels,[1,2] but not to the same extent as **rifampicin**. Nevertheless, the concurrent use of **rifabutin** is not recommended.[1]

1. Rapamune (Sirolimus). Wyeth Pharmaceuticals. UK Summary of product characteristics, March 2007.
2. Rapamune (Sirolimus). Wyeth Pharmaceuticals Inc. US Prescribing information, May 2007.

Tacrolimus + ACE inhibitors and Angiotensin II receptor antagonists

Candesartan and losartan do not appear to affect the pharmacokinetics of tacrolimus, although concurrent use may increase the risk of developing hyperkalaemia.

Clinical evidence, mechanism, importance and management

A study in 12 kidney transplant patients taking tacrolimus twice daily for 12 days with **candesartan cilexetil** (2 mg daily for 3 days, then 4 mg daily for 3 days, and then 16 mg daily for 3 days) found that the pharmacokinetics of tacrolimus were unchanged. Renal function remained stable and unchanged, and no adverse effects were reported.[1] Another study in a group of 21 kidney transplant patients taking tacrolimus found no significant change in the serum creatinine or the levels of tacrolimus when they also took **candesartan cilexetil** 4 to 12 mg daily for one year. Serum potassium levels were reported to have increased by an average of 0.34 mmol/L, although it is unclear from the study if this was specifically in the tacrolimus group or also included another group taking candesartan and ciclosporin.[2] A study in kidney transplant patients taking tacrolimus and given losartan 50 mg daily for 12 weeks (some receiving 100 mg daily from week 8) for hypertension found no significant changes in the tacrolimus levels. Transient hyperkalaemia occurred in 4 of the 67 patients.[3]

Tacrolimus may cause nephrotoxicity and hyperkalaemia, and thus both renal function and potassium levels should be monitored when ACE inhibitors or angiotensin II receptor antagonists are also given.

1. Pietruck F, Kiel G, Birkel M, Stahlheber-Dilg B, Philipp T. Evaluation of the effect of candesartan cilexetil on the steady-state pharmacokinetics of tacrolimus in renal transplant patients. *Biopharm Drug Dispos* (2005) 26, 135–41.
2. Omoto K, Tanabe K, Tokumoto T, Shimmura H, Ishida H, Toma H. Use of candesartan cilexetil decreases proteinuria in renal transplant patients with chronic allograft dysfunction. *Transplantation* (2003) 76, 117–4.
3. del Castillo D, Campistol JM, Guirado L, Capdevilla L, Martínez JG, Pereira P, Bravo J, Pérez R. Efficacy and safety of losartan in the treatment of hypertension in renal transplant patients. *Kidney Int* (1998) (Suppl 68) 54, S-135–S-139.

Tacrolimus + Antacids

There is some evidence to suggest that some antacids may possibly reduce the blood levels of tacrolimus, but the clinical importance of this awaits confirmation.

Clinical evidence, mechanism, importance and management

A very brief report states that widely variable trough plasma tacrolimus levels have been seen in patients taking **sodium bicarbonate** close to the time when the tacrolimus was given, and that the use of **sodium bicarbonate** results in lower blood levels of tacrolimus. No details were given.[1] It was suggested that their administration should be separated by at least 2 hours, or the **sodium bicarbonate** replaced by **sodium citrate** and **citric acid**, to ensure stable trough tacrolimus levels are achieved.[1]

A crossover study in healthy subjects found that a single dose of **aluminium/magnesium hydroxide** increased the mean AUC of tacrolimus by 21% and decreased the mean peak level of tacrolimus by 10%.[2]

In vitro studies also found that **aluminium hydroxide** gel and **magnesium oxide** can cause a significant reduction in tacrolimus concentrations due to pH-mediated degradation and as a result it was suggested that the administration of antacids and tacrolimus should be separated.[3]

However, a study in 18 renal transplant patients found that the concurrent use of *Maalox* (**aluminium/magnesium hydroxide**) or **sodium bicarbonate** did not reduce tacrolimus blood levels and no patients required a tacrolimus dose increase.[4]

More study is needed to confirm and assess the extent and clinical importance of these interactions, but good monitoring would be appropriate if tacrolimus is given with any antacids, being alert for the need to separate the dosages by at least 2 hours.

1. Venkataramanan R, Swaminathan A, Prasad T, Jain A, Zuckerman S, Warty V, McMichael J, Lever J, Burckart G, Starzl T. Clinical pharmacokinetics of tacrolimus. *Clin Pharmacokinet* (1995) 29, 404–30.
2. Prograf (Tacrolimus). Astellas Pharma US Inc. US Prescribing information, April 2006.
3. Steeves M, Abdallah HY, Venkataramanan R, Burckart GT, Ptachcinski RJ, Abu-Elmagd K, Jain AK, Fung F, Todo S, Starzl TE. In-vitro interaction of a novel immunosuppressant, FK506, and antacids. *J Pharm Pharmacol* (1991) 43, 574–7.
4. Chisholm MA, Mulloy LL, Jagadeesan M, DiPiro JT. Coadministration of tacrolimus with anti-acid drugs. *Transplantation* (2003) 76, 665–6.

Tacrolimus + Azoles

When tacrolimus is given orally, its serum levels are considerably increased by oral fluconazole, and tacrolimus dose reductions may be needed. Itraconazole, ketoconazole, posaconazole, voriconazole, and oral clotrimazole, also raise tacrolimus levels. There is some evidence that the levels of intravenous tacrolimus are minimally affected by fluconazole and ketoconazole. In theory it is possible that miconazole oral gel may also interact with tacrolimus.

Clinical evidence

(a) Clotrimazole

A study in 35 kidney transplant patients taking tacrolimus 150 micrograms/kg twice daily and clotrimazole 10 mg three times daily (17 patients) or nystatin (control group, 18 patients) found that clotrimazole significantly increased tacrolimus trough blood levels from 15 to 20 nanograms/mL up to 53 nanograms/mL at day 5. Tacrolimus levels were not affected by nystatin and by day 7 patients in the clotrimazole group were found to require significantly lower tacrolimus doses than those in the nystatin group.[1] In a liver transplant patient the trough plasma levels of tacrolimus 6 mg daily rose from 3.5 to 5.6 nanograms/mL within a day of clotrimazole 10 mg four times daily being started, and reached more than 9 nanograms/mL within 8 days. Later studies and rechallenge confirmed that the clotrimazole was responsible for the rise in tacrolimus levels. The tacrolimus AUC was nearly doubled.[2]

(b) Fluconazole

Twenty organ transplant patients (11 livers, 6 kidneys, 2 hearts and one bone marrow) taking tacrolimus were also given fluconazole 100 or 200 mg daily for various fungal infections. On day 1 the median plasma trough levels of those given fluconazole 100 mg rose 1.4-fold, and in those taking 200 mg it rose 3.1-fold. The dosage of tacrolimus was reduced to accommodate this rise: the median dosage reduction was 56% (range 0 to 88%). The highest tacrolimus level was seen within 3 days. A pharmacokinetic study in one patient found that when fluconazole 100 mg daily was stopped, the tacrolimus AUC fell by about 60%.[3]

Other studies in adult[4] and paediatric patients[5] and individual case reports[6,7] have confirmed that tacrolimus levels are increased by oral fluconazole, increasing the risk of nephrotoxicity.[5] In a retrospective study, patients given fluconazole required a 40% reduction in tacrolimus dose to achieve similar trough levels.[8] A bone-marrow transplant patient taking tacrolimus and given fluconazole for oral candidiasis experienced headache and was found to have glycosuria, increased serum creatinine and Pelger-Huet anomaly of granulocytes, which disappeared after tacrolimus was discontinued. The effects were thought to be due to tacrolimus toxicity due to an interaction with fluconazole.[9] However, one study found that if intravenous tacrolimus is given with intravenous fluconazole 400 mg, the steady-state levels of tacrolimus are only slightly increased (by about 16%), which was considered to be clinically unimportant.[10]

(c) Itraconazole

A study in 40 lung transplant patients taking tacrolimus with prophylactic itraconazole 200 mg twice daily for 6 months found that when itraconazole was stopped the mean tacrolimus dose to maintain therapeutic levels increased by 76% (to 5.74 mg daily). The adverse effects and rejection rate were not affected by itraconazole.[11] Similar findings are reported in another study in heart and lung transplant patients.[12] Trough blood levels of tacrolimus in a heart-lung transplant patient increased threefold from 16 to 57 nanograms/mL and serum creatinine levels also rose after she was given itraconazole 200 mg daily.[13] A kidney transplant recipient taking tacrolimus 6 mg daily was given itraconazole 100 mg twice daily for a urinary candida infection. Within a day, the tacrolimus trough levels increased from 12.6 to 21 nanograms/mL and the tacrolimus dose was progressively reduced to 3 mg daily. Four days after the itraconazole was discontinued tacrolimus had to be progressively increased back to its initial dose.[14] The interaction has been reported in three other renal transplant recipients.[15-17]

(d) Ketoconazole

In a kidney transplant patient taking tacrolimus and prednisone, the addition of ketoconazole 200 mg daily resulted in an increase in tacrolimus blood levels from 11.1 to 27.9 nanograms/mL, despite a 45% decrease in the dose of tacrolimus. Eventually the dose of tacrolimus had to be reduced by 80% to keep the levels within the therapeutic range. Tacrolimus levels decreased to 5.8 nanograms/mL within a week of discontinuing ketoconazole and so the dose was raised.[18] A pharmacokinetic study in 6 healthy subjects found that ketoconazole 200 mg orally at bedtime for 12 days increased the bioavailability of a single 100 microgram/kg dose of oral tacrolimus from 14% to 30%.[19] The manufacturer notes that the clearance of intravenous tacrolimus was not significantly changed by ketoconazole, although it was highly variable between patients.[20]

(e) Posaconazole

The peak blood level and AUC of a single 50 microgram/kg dose of tacrolimus was reported to be increased by 121% and 358%, respectively, by the addition of posaconazole.[21]

(f) Voriconazole

A small study comparing the tacrolimus levels of two patients, one taking voriconazole 200 mg twice daily, the other placebo, found that the tacrolimus levels were nearly tenfold higher in the patient taking voriconazole. This was originally designed as a larger study, but the study was stopped after the finding in these initial two subjects.[22] Another study in 14 healthy subjects found that voriconazole 400 mg twice daily on day one, then 200 mg twice daily for 6 days increased the AUC and maximum plasma levels of a single 100 microgram/kg dose of tacrolimus by 3.2-fold and 2.3-fold, respectively.[23] A liver transplant patient taking tacrolimus was hospitalised with multiple complaints, and was found to have a high tacrolimus level. Tacrolimus was withheld and later restarted at 3 mg daily and then gradually reduced to 1.5 mg daily. When voriconazole 400 mg twice daily was started, the tacrolimus dose was reduced by one-third to 0.5 mg daily, but eventually needed to be reduced to 0.15 mg daily (90% overall dose reduction) as a result of rising tacrolimus levels.[24] A kidney transplant patient taking tacrolimus 2 mg daily had an increase in tacrolimus levels from less than 12 nanograms/mL to 25 nanograms/mL when voriconazole 4 mg/kg twice daily was added. His renal function also worsened. The tacrolimus dose was eventually reduced to 0.5 mg on alternate days, with an improvement in his renal function.[25]

Mechanism

Fluconazole, itraconazole, ketoconazole, posaconazole and voriconazole inhibit the metabolism of the tacrolimus by the gut wall and/or liver by the cytochrome P450 isoenzyme CYP3A4, and/or inhibit the activity of P-glycoprotein so that more tacrolimus is absorbed.[10,14,19,22] Therefore, intravenous tacrolimus is little affected.[10]

Importance and management

The interaction between tacrolimus and **fluconazole** is established, clinically important and can develop rapidly (within 3 days). The authors of one of the reports say that up to 200 mg of oral fluconazole daily can be used safely and effectively provided that the tacrolimus dosage is reduced by half.[3] One study specifically examining dose adjustments suggests that fluconazole can be safely used if 60% of the original tacrolimus dose is given.[8] If tacrolimus is given intravenously, no clinically important interaction appears to occur.[10]

The interactions of tacrolimus with **itraconazole** and **ketoconazole** also appear to be established, and the manufacturer states that nearly all patients will require tacrolimus dose reductions when given these drugs.[20,26]

Information about **clotrimazole** is limited, but on the basis of the case report and study it would be prudent to monitor tacrolimus levels, and adjust the dose as necessary.

The manufacturers of **posaconazole** recommend that the tacrolimus dose is reduced by about two-thirds in patients given posaconazole.[21] Tacrolimus levels should be closely monitored and further dose adjustments made if needed.

The manufacturers of **voriconazole** advise reducing the tacrolimus dose to one-third when starting voriconazole, closely monitoring tacrolimus levels throughout, and increasing the tacrolimus dose in response to levels obtained when voriconazole is stopped.[27,28] However, greater reductions in tacrolimus dose may be needed in some patients,[22,24] and raised tacrolimus levels requiring a total 90% tacrolimus dose reduction were reported in one patient.[24]

In vitro studies with human liver microsomes have shown that **miconazole**[29] also inhibits liver and small intestine microsomes that metabolise tacrolimus and it seems possible that it may interact like fluconazole but this needs confirmation. There appear to be no clinical reports of an interaction between miconazole and tacrolimus. However, a large proportion of miconazole oral gel (both prescription and non-prescription doses) may be swallowed and therefore adequate systemic absorption may occur to produce an interaction. The manufacturers of miconazole oral gel recommend close monitoring and possible dose reduction of tacrolimus if both drugs are given concurrently.[30] An interaction with intravaginal miconazole would not normally be expected because its systemic absorption is usually very low (less than 2%) in healthy women of child-bearing age.[31] No interaction would be expected if miconazole is applied to the skin.

1. Vasquez EM, Pollak R, Benedetti E. Clotrimazole increases tacrolimus blood levels: a drug interaction in kidney transplant patients. *Clin Transplant* (2001) 15, 95–9.
2. Mieles L, Venkataramanan R, Yokoyama I, Warty VJ, Starzl TE. Interaction between FK506 and clotrimazole in a liver transplant recipient. *Transplantation* (1991) 52, 1086–7.
3. Mañez R, Martin M, Raman V, Silverman D, Jain A, Warty V, Gonzalez-Pinto I, Kusne S, Starzl TE. Fluconazole therapy in transplant recipients receiving FK506. *Transplantation* (1994) 57, 1521–23.
4. Toy S, Tata P, Jain A, Patsy K, Lever J, Burckart G, Warty V, Kusne S, Abu-Elmagd K, Fung J, Starzl T, Venkataramanan R. A pharmacokinetic interaction between tacrolimus and fluconazole. *Pharm Res* (1996) 13 (9 Suppl), S435.
5. Vincent I, Furlan V, Debray D, Jacquemin E, Taburet AM. Effects of antifungal agents on the pharmacokinetics and nephrotoxicity of FK506 in paediatric liver transplant recipients. *Intersci Conf Antimicrob Agents Chemother* (1995) 35, 5.
6. Assan R, Fredj G, Larger E, Feutren G, Bismuth H. FK 506/fluconazole interaction enhances FK506 nephrotoxicity. *Diabete Metab* (1994) 20, 49–52.
7. Chamorey E, Nouveau B, Viard L, Garcia-Credoz F, Durand A, Pisano P. Interaction tacrolimus-fluconazole chez un enfant transplanté coeur-poumons. A propos d'un cas clinique. *J Pharm Clin* (1998) 17, 51–3.
8. Toda F, Tanabe K, Ito S, Shinmura H, Tokumoto T, Ishida H, Toma H. Tacrolimus trough level adjustment after administration of fluconazole to kidney recipients. *Transplant Proc* (2002) 34, 1733–5.
9. Gondo H, Okamura C, Osaki K, Shimoda K, Asano Y, Okamura T. Acquired Pelger-Huet anomaly in association with concomitant tacrolimus and fluconazole therapy following allogenic bone marrow transplantation. *Bone Marrow Transplant* (2000) 26, 1255–7.
10. Osowski CL, Dix SP, Lin LS, Mullins RE, Geller RB, Wingard JR. Evaluation of the drug interaction between intravenous high-dose fluconazole and cyclosporine or tacrolimus in bone marrow transplant patients. *Transplantation* (1996) 61, 1268–72.
11. Shitrit D, Ollech JE, Ollech A, Bakal I, Saute M, Sahar G, Kramer MR. Itraconazole prophylaxis in lung transplant recipients receiving tacrolimus (FK506): efficacy and drug interaction. *J Heart Lung Transplant* (2005) 24, 2148–52.
12. Banerjee R, Leaver N, Lyster H, Banner NR. Coadministration of itraconazole and tacrolimus after thoracic organ transplantation. *Transplant Proc* (2001) 33, 1600–2.
13. Furlan V, Parquin F, Penaud JF, Cerrina J, Le Roy Ladurie F, Dartevelle P, Taburet AM. Interaction between tacrolimus and itraconazole in a heart-lung transplant recipient. *Transplant Proc* (1998) 30, 187–8.
14. Capone D, Gentile A, Imperatore P, Palmiero G, Basile V. Effects of itraconazole on tacrolimus blood concentrations in a renal transplant recipient. *Ann Pharmacother* (1999) 33, 1124–5.
15. Katari SR, Magnone M, Shapiro R, Jordan M, Scantlebury V, Vivas C, Gritsch A, McCauley J, Demetris AJ, Randhawa PS. Clinical features of acute reversible tacrolimus (FK506) nephrotoxicity in kidney transplant recipients. *Clin Transplant* (1997) 11, 237–42.
16. Macías MO, Salvador P, Hurtado JL, Martín I. Tacrolimus-itraconazole interaction in a kidney transplant patient. *Ann Pharmacother* (2000) 34, 536.
17. Ideura T, Muramatsu T, Higuchi M, Tachibana N, Hora K, Kiyosawa K. Tacrolimus/itraconazole interactions: a case report of ABO-incompatible living-related renal transplantation. *Nephrol Dial Transplant* (2000) 15, 1721–3.
18. Moreno M, Latorre C, Manzanares C, Morales E, Herrero JC, Dominguez-Gil B, Carreño A, Cubas A, Delgado M, Andres A, Morales JM. Clinical management of tacrolimus drug interactions in renal transplant patients. *Transplant Proc* (1999) 31, 2252–3.
19. Floren LC, Bekersky I, Benet LZ, Mekki Q, Dressler D, Lee JW, Roberts JP, Hebert MF. Tacrolimus oral bioavailability doubles with coadministration of ketoconazole. *Clin Pharmacol Ther* (1997) 62, 41–9.
20. Prograf (Tacrolimus). Astellas Pharma US Inc. US Prescribing information, April 2006.
21. Noxafil (Posaconazole). Schering Plough Ltd. UK Summary of product characteristics, October 2006.
22. Venkataramanan R, Zang S, Gayowski T, Singh N. Voriconazole inhibition of the metabolism of tacrolimus in a liver transplant recipient and in human liver microsomes. *Antimicrob Agents Chemother* (2002) 46, 3091–3.
23. Wood N, Tan K, Allan R, Fielding A, Nichols DJ. Effect of voriconazole on the pharmacokinetics of tacrolimus. *Intersci Conf Antimicrob Agents Chemother* (2001) 41, 2.
24. Pai MP, Allen S. Voriconazole inhibition of tacrolimus metabolism. *Clin Infect Dis* (2003) 36, 1089–91.
25. Tintillier M, Kirch L, Goffin E, Cuvelier C, Pochet J-M. Interaction between voriconazole and tacrolimus in a kidney-transplanted patient. *Nephrol Dial Transplant* (2005) 20, 664–5.
26. Prograf (Tacrolimus monohydrate). Astellas Pharma Ltd. UK Summary of product characteristics, May 2007.
27. VFEND (Voriconazole). Pfizer Ltd. UK Summary of product characteristics, July 2007.
28. VFEND (Voriconazole). Pfizer Inc. US Prescribing information, November 2006.
29. Christians U, Schmidt G, Bader A, Lampen A, Schottmann R, Linck A, Sewing K-F. Identification of drugs inhibiting the *in vitro* metabolism of tacrolimus by human liver microsomes. *Br J Clin Pharmacol* (1996) 41, 187–90.

30. Daktarin Oral Gel (Miconazole). Janssen-Cilag Ltd. UK Summary of product characteristics, May 2006.
31. Daneshmend TK. Systemic absorption of miconazole from the vagina. *J Antimicrob Chemother* (1986) 18, 507–11.

Tacrolimus + Calcium-channel blockers

Nifedipine causes a moderate rise in tacrolimus blood levels and also appears to be kidney protective. Case reports suggest that diltiazem and felodipine also elevate tacrolimus levels; nicardipine, nilvadipine and verapamil are predicted to interact similarly.

Clinical evidence

(a) Diltiazem

The trough blood levels of tacrolimus 8 mg twice daily increased from 12.9 to 55 nanograms/mL in a liver transplant patient within 3 days of him starting diltiazem (initially 5 to 10 mg/hour intravenously for one day, then 30 mg orally every 8 hours). The patient became delirious, confused and agitated. Both drugs were stopped, and over the next 3 days his mental state improved and his tacrolimus levels fell to 6.7 nanograms/mL. Tacrolimus was then restarted, gradually increasing to a dose of 5 mg twice daily, which produced levels of 9 to 10 nanograms/mL.[1]

A study in 2 liver and 2 kidney transplant patients found that diltiazem increased the AUC of tacrolimus. In the kidney transplant patients the increase appeared to be dose related; a 20-mg dose of diltiazem caused a 26% and 67% rise, while a 180-mg dose caused a 48% and 177% rise in each patient, respectively. The liver transplant patients did not have any alteration in the AUC of tacrolimus until they were given higher doses of diltiazem; one patient had an 18% rise following a 120-mg dose, the other a 22% rise following a 180-mg dose.[2]

A study in 7 liver transplant patients given tacrolimus 100 micrograms/kg twice daily found that modified-release diltiazem 90 mg daily did not significantly alter the absorption or metabolism of tacrolimus when compared to 7 similar patients not given diltiazem.[3] The authors of the other study[2] suggest that this lack of effect may have been because only 90 mg of diltiazem was used.

(b) Felodipine

A 13-year-old boy taking tacrolimus 4 mg twice daily was given felodipine 2.5 mg daily 15 days after receiving a kidney transplant. Two weeks later his tacrolimus level was reported as greater than 30 nanograms/mL (previous levels ranged from 10.6 to 20 nanograms/mL), and despite a reduction in the dose of tacrolimus to 3 mg twice daily a subsequent tacrolimus level was 53.9 nanograms/mL. He was eventually stabilised at the original tacrolimus levels with tacrolimus 500 micrograms twice daily. When the felodipine was stopped several months later, his tacrolimus dose needed to be raised to maintain therapeutic levels.[4]

(c) Nifedipine

A 1-year retrospective study of two groups of liver transplant patients found that in the 22 patients taking nifedipine 30 or 60 mg daily there was a 55% increase in the tacrolimus blood levels after 1 month. By 6 months the tacrolimus dosage had been reduced by a total of 25.5% in the nifedipine group and by 12 months by 31.4% when compared with the group not taking nifedipine. The nifedipine group also had improved renal function (lowered serum creatinine).[5]

Mechanism

Uncertain, but it seems likely that some calcium-channel blockers inhibit the cytochrome P450 isoenzyme CYP3A4 and/or P-glycoprotein, thereby reducing the metabolism of tacrolimus leading to increased blood levels.[1,5] This is consistent with the findings of an *in vitro* study using human liver microsomes.[6]

Importance and management

In the case of nifedipine, this seems to be an established and clinically important interaction. However, the increase seems slow, and it seems likely that any decrease in the dose requirements of tacrolimus will be detected by routine monitoring. Although the information about diltiazem is less conclusive it would seem wise to follow the same precautions, as the effect of diltiazem on tacrolimus seems to vary greatly between the few patients studied. The manufacturers of felodipine advise monitoring tacrolimus levels if felodipine is given.[7,8] Direct information about other calcium-channel blockers appears to be lacking, but the US and UK manufacturers of tacrolimus[9,10] predict that **nicardipine** and **verapamil** may raise tacrolimus levels by inhibiting CYP3A4 (see Mechanism), and the UK manufacturers additionally suggest that **nilvadipine** may interact similarly.[10]

1. Hebert MF, Lam AY. Diltiazem increases tacrolimus concentrations. *Ann Pharmacother* (1999) 33, 680–2.
2. Jones TE, Morris RG. Pharmacokinetic interaction between tacrolimus and diltiazem: dose-response relationship in kidney and liver transplant recipients. *Clin Pharmacokinet* (2002) 41, 381–8.
3. Teperman L, Turgut S, Negron C, John D, Diflo T, Morgan G, Tobias H. Diltiazem is a safe drug in transplant patients on Prograf and does not affect Prograf levels. *Hepatology* (1996) 24, 180A.
4. Butani L, Berg G, Makker SP. Effect of felodipine on tacrolimus pharmacokinetics in a renal transplant recipient. *Transplantation* (2002) 73, 159.
5. Seifeldin RA, Marcos-Alvarez A, Gordon FD, Lewis WD, Jenkins RL. Nifedipine interaction with tacrolimus in liver transplant recipients. *Ann Pharmacother* (1997) 31, 571–5.
6. Iwasaki K, Matsuda H, Nagase K, Shiraga T, Tokuma Y, Uchida K. Effects of twenty-three drugs on the metabolism of FK506 by human liver microsomes. *Res Commun Chem Pathol Pharmacol* (1993) 82, 209–16.
7. Plendil (Felodipine). AstraZeneca UK Ltd. UK Summary of product characteristics, March 2006.
8. Plendil (Felodipine). AstraZeneca. US Prescribing information, November 2003.
9. Prograf (Tacrolimus). Astellas Pharma US Inc. US Prescribing information, April 2006.
10. Prograf (Tacrolimus monohydrate). Astellas Pharma Ltd. UK Summary of product characteristics, May 2007.

Tacrolimus + Chloramphenicol

A marked rise in tacrolimus trough blood levels has been reported in several patients who were given systemic chloramphenicol.

Clinical evidence

A retrospective study identified 3 patients taking tacrolimus who had received a total of 5 courses of intravenous chloramphenicol, each lasting for at least 12 days. Tacrolimus trough blood levels were doubled by day 2, and had risen by 207% at their peak, on day 6. The tacrolimus dose had been decreased by about one-third by day 12, and the tacrolimus levels returned to around the baseline value.[1]

An adolescent patient with a kidney transplant developed toxic tacrolimus levels on the second day of starting chloramphenicol for a vancomycin-resistant enterococcal infection. The tacrolimus dosage had to be reduced by 83% to achieve safe serum levels, and it was found that the dose-adjusted tacrolimus AUC was 7.5-fold greater in the presence of chloramphenicol.[2] Another report describes a similar interaction in a liver transplant patient taking tacrolimus 4 mg twice daily. The patient was given intravenous chloramphenicol, but at the unintentionally high dose of 1850 mg every 6 hours. After about 3 days the patient complained of lethargy, fatigue, headaches and tremors so both drugs were stopped. His tacrolimus trough level had increased from a range of 9 to 11 nanograms/mL to more than 60 nanograms/mL. Seven days after chloramphenicol had been stopped his tacrolimus level was 8.2 nanograms/mL and his symptoms had resolved.[3] Another case report in a kidney-pancreas transplant patient taking tacrolimus 4 mg twice daily found that the addition of oral chloramphenicol 750 mg four times daily increased the tacrolimus trough blood level to more than 30 micrograms/L within 3 days. After 10 days, the dose of tacrolimus was reduced to 1.5 mg twice daily and the tacrolimus level fell to between 18 to 25 micrograms/L. Chloramphenicol was stopped 5 days later and the tacrolimus dose was increased to 3 mg twice daily. However the tacrolimus level fell to below 5 micrograms/L for several days leading to an episode of acute organ rejection. The tacrolimus level then returned to within the therapeutic range and the patient stabilised.[4]

Mechanism

Chloramphenicol (a known enzyme inhibitor) is thought to raise tacrolimus levels by rapidly reducing its metabolism.[2]

Importance and management

These appear to be the only reports of this interaction, but it is consistent with the known metabolic characteristics of both drugs and therefore it is expected to be an interaction of general importance. Monitor the outcome closely if systemic chloramphenicol is given to any patient taking tacrolimus, being alert for the need to reduce the tacrolimus dosage. It seems doubtful if a clinically relevant interaction will occur with topical chloramphenicol because the dosage and the systemic absorption is small, but this needs confirmation.

1. Mathis AS, Shah N, Knipp GT, Friedman GS. Interaction of chloramphenicol and the calcineurin inhibitors in renal transplant recipients. *Transpl Infect Dis* (2002) 4, 169–74.
2. Schulman SL, Shaw LM, Jabs K, Leonard MB, Brayman KL. Interaction between tacrolimus and chloramphenicol in a renal transplant recipient. *Transplantation* (1998) 65, 1397–8.
3. Taber DJ, Dupuis RE, Hollar KD, Strzalka AL, Johnson MW. Drug-drug interaction between chloramphenicol and tacrolimus in a liver transplant recipient. *Transplant Proc* (2000) 32, 660–62.
4. Bakri R, Breen C, Maclean D, Taylor J, Goldsmith D. Serious interaction between tacrolimus FK506 and chloramphenicol in a kidney-pancreas transplant recipient. *Transpl Int* (2003) 16, 441–3.

Tacrolimus + Ciclosporin

The manufacturers say that tacrolimus and ciclosporin should not be used concurrently because of the increased risk of nephrotoxicity.

Clinical evidence, mechanism, importance and management

One study found that, in patients with normal bilirubin levels, the half-life of ciclosporin was prolonged from a range of 6 to 15 hours up to 26 to 74 hours, and the ciclosporin serum levels, measured by a fluorescent polarisation immunoassay, were raised by tacrolimus.[1] On the other hand another study found no changes in the pharmacokinetics of ciclosporin, as measured by HPLC, in patients given tacrolimus, but creatinine levels were almost doubled (suggesting kidney damage),[2] which confirmed a previous report suggesting that severe renal impairment may develop when both drugs are given.[3] Tacrolimus levels may also be raised by ciclosporin.[4] The manufacturers of tacrolimus say that it should not be given with ciclosporin because of the risk of additive/synergistic nephrotoxicity, and, if ciclosporin is being replaced by tacrolimus, 12 to 24 hours should elapse between stopping one drug and starting the other. If ciclosporin levels are raised, the introduction of tacrolimus should be further delayed.[4,5]

1. Venkataramanan R, Jain A, Cadoff E, Warty V, Iwasaki K, Nagase K, Krajack A, Imventarza O, Todo S, Fung JJ, Starzl TE. Pharmacokinetics of FK 506: preclinical and clinical studies. *Transplant Proc* (1990) 22 (Suppl 1), 52–6.
2. Jain AB, Venkataramanan R, Fung J, Burckart G, Emeigh J, Diven W, Warty V, Abu-Elmagd K, Todo S, Alessiani M, Starzl TE. Pharmacokinetics of cyclosporine and nephrotoxicity in orthoptic liver transplant patients rescued with FK 506. *Transplant Proc* (1991) 23, 2777–9.
3. McCauley J, Fung J, Jain A, Todo S, Starzl TE. The effects of FK506 on renal function after liver transplantation. *Transplant Proc* (1990) 22 (Suppl 1), 17–20.
4. Prograf (Tacrolimus). Astellas Pharma US Inc. US Prescribing information, April 2006.
5. Prograf (Tacrolimus monohydrate). Astellas Pharma Ltd. UK Summary of product characteristics, May 2007.

Tacrolimus + Corticosteroids

The effects of methylprednisolone on tacrolimus pharmacokinetics are uncertain. Prednisone appears to reduce the levels of tacrolimus.

Clinical evidence, mechanism, importance and management

A review of early studies of tacrolimus stated that serum levels were said to have been increased on 10 occasions, decreased on 5 occasions, and unaltered on 2 occasions by **methylprednisolone**.[1]

In a randomised study conducted over 3 months, 31 patients receiving tacrolimus, mycophenolate and daclizumab were compared with 34 patients receiving tacrolimus, mycophenolate and **prednisone**. Higher tacrolimus doses were required to maintain therapeutic tacrolimus levels in the **prednisone** group. This reached a maximum after one month, when a 30% larger tacrolimus dose was necessary.[2] A further study found that patients taking higher doses of **prednisone** (more than 0.25 mg/kg daily) also needed larger doses of tacrolimus to maintain therapeutic trough blood levels. The authors considered that this was possibly due to induction of the cytochrome P450 isoenzyme CYP3A4 by **prednisone** and recommended that tacrolimus levels be closely monitored and adjusted according to any changes in corticosteroid dose.[3]

1. Venkataramanan R, Jain A, Cadoff E, Warty V, Iwasaki K, Nagase K, Krajack A, Imventarza O, Todo S, Fung JJ, Starzl TE. Pharmacokinetics of FK 506: preclinical and clinical studies. *Transplant Proc* (1990) 22 (Suppl 1), 52–6.
2. Hesselink DA, Ngyuen H, Wabbijn M, Smak Gregoor PJH, Steyerberg EW, van Riemsdijk IC, Weimar W, van Gelder T. Tacrolimus dose requirement in renal transplant recipients is significantly higher when used in combination with corticosteroids. *Br J Clin Pharmacol* (2003) 56, 327–30.
3. Anglicheau D, Flamant M, Schlageter MH, Martinez F, Cassinat B, Beaune P, Legendre C, Thervet E. Pharmacokinetic interaction between corticosteroids and tacrolimus after renal transplantation. *Nephrol Dial Transplant* (2003) 18, 2409–14.

Tacrolimus + Danazol

An isolated report describes an increase in tacrolimus levels in a patient given danazol.

Clinical evidence, mechanism, importance and management

The trough serum levels of tacrolimus 10 mg daily rose from 0.7 to 2.7 nanograms/mL in a kidney transplant patient within 4 days of danazol 400 mg to 1.2 g daily being started. Despite a reduction in the danazol dosage to 600 mg and then 400 mg daily, her tacrolimus and creatinine serum levels remained high for one month until the danazol was withdrawn. The reason is not known, but the authors suggest that danazol possibly inhibits the metabolism (demethylation and hydroxylation) of tacrolimus by the liver so that it is cleared from the body more slowly.[1] Tacrolimus is metabolised by the cytochrome P450 isoenzyme CYP3A4, and danazol has been shown to inhibit this pathway (consider 'Statins + Danazol', p.1099). Therefore although this is an isolated case it seems possible that it will be of general significance. Monitor the effects of concurrent use in any patient, reducing the tacrolimus dosage as necessary.

1. Shapiro R, Venkataramanan R, Warty VS, Scantlebury VP, Rybka W, McCauley J, Fung JJ, Starzl TE. FK 506 interaction with danazol. *Lancet* (1993) 341, 1344–5.

Tacrolimus + Echinocandins

Caspofungin moderately decreases tacrolimus levels. Anidulafungin and micafungin do not appear to affect tacrolimus pharmacokinetics, and tacrolimus does not affect the pharmacokinetics of anidulafungin, caspofungin, or micafungin.

Clinical evidence, mechanism, importance and management

(a) Anidulafungin

Thirty-five healthy subjects were given a single 5-mg oral dose of tacrolimus 3 days before and on day 10 of a course of intravenous anidulafungin (200 mg loading dose and then 100 mg daily). Anidulafungin did not have any significant effects on the pharmacokinetics of tacrolimus and no serious adverse effects were reported. The pharmacokinetics of anidulafungin were not affected by tacrolimus.[1] No additional monitoring would seem to be required with this combination; however, bear in mind that the study above was a single-dose study in healthy subjects. More study is required in patients taking long-term tacrolimus.

(b) Caspofungin

The preliminary results of one study suggest that caspofungin reduces the AUC of tacrolimus by 20% in healthy subjects,[2] and reduces the trough tacrolimus levels by 26%.[3] Tacrolimus did not alter the pharmacokinetics of caspofungin.[2] The manufacturers of caspofungin advise that tacrolimus levels should be monitored if caspofungin is given, and tacrolimus doses adjusted as appropriate.[3,4] Note that this change is relatively modest.

(c) Micafungin

Twenty-six healthy subjects were given single 5-mg doses of tacrolimus alone, after intravenous micafungin 100 mg, and one day after intravenous micafungin 100 mg daily for 5 days. The pharmacokinetics of tacrolimus were not affected by micafungin, and single-dose tacrolimus had no effects on the pharmacokinetics of micafungin.[5] No additional monitoring would seem to be required with this combination.

1. Dowell JA, Stogniew M, Krause D, Henkel T, Damle B. Lack of pharmacokinetic interaction between anidulafungin and tacrolimus. *J Clin Pharmacol* (2007) 47, 305–14.
2. Stone J, Holland S, Wickersham P, Deutsch P, Winchell G, Hesney M, Miller R, Freeman A, Dilzer S, Lasseter K. Drug interactions between caspofungin and tacrolimus. *Intersci Conf Antimicrob Agents Chemother* (2001) 41, 1.
3. Cancidas (Caspofungin acetate). Merck Sharp & Dohme Ltd. UK Summary of product characteristics, January 2007.

4. Cancidas (Caspofungin acetate). Merck & Co., Inc. US Prescribing information, February 2005.
5. Hebert MF, Blough DK, Townsend RW, Allison M, Buell D, Keirns J, Bekersky I. Concomitant tacrolimus and micafungin pharmacokinetics in healthy volunteers. *J Clin Pharmacol* (2005) 45, 1018–23.

Tacrolimus + Grapefruit and other fruit juices

Grapefruit juice can markedly increase the serum levels of tacrolimus. Pomelo may interact similarly.

Clinical evidence and mechanism

(a) Grapefruit juice

Eight liver transplant patients were given 12 oz (about 360 mL) of grapefruit juice twice daily, which they drank within 45 minutes of taking their dose of tacrolimus. After one week it was found that their 12-hour trough, and 1-hour and 4-hour tacrolimus levels were raised by 300%, 195%, and 400%, respectively. Two patients had headaches, one had diarrhoea and one had an increased creatinine level, that reversed, but none of the 12 developed rejection or irreversible toxicity. Two of the patients continued to drink the grapefruit juice and it was possible to halve their tacrolimus dosage.[1] Similarly, 6 kidney transplant patients had their dose of tacrolimus reduced by an average of 40% after drinking 100 mL of grapefruit juice daily for 5 days.[2] A liver transplant patient was advised to drink grapefruit juice in an effort to increase her tacrolimus trough blood levels, which were subtherapeutic (below 5 nanograms/mL) despite a dose of tacrolimus 10 mg daily. She drank 250 mL of grapefruit juice four times daily for 3 days during which time the tacrolimus level did not increase. However, one week after she stopped the grapefruit juice the tacrolimus level was found to have increased to 37 nanograms/mL.[3]

(b) Pomelo

A case report describes a kidney transplant patient taking tacrolimus whose tacrolimus level rose from a range of 8 to 10 nanograms/mL up to 25.2 nanograms/mL after he ate about 100 g of pomelo (*Citrus grandis,* a fruit related to grapefruit).[4] The same authors subsequently found that pomelo juice extract inhibited the cytochrome P450 isoenzyme CYP3A4 *in vitro* but had no effect on P-glycoprotein.[5]

Importance and management

The reason for the rise in tacrolimus levels is not known, but it seems likely that it is due to inhibition of the metabolism of tacrolimus by some component of grapefruit juice and pomelo fruit. In practical terms the authors of the first report suggest that this interaction means that the dosage of tacrolimus can possibly be reduced (to save money) although there is a clear need to monitor the effects closely not only because of the inter-individual factors affecting tacrolimus dosing but also because of the difficulties of standardising grapefruit juice.[1] However, the manufacturers of tacrolimus suggest that the combination should be avoided.[6,7] Patients should be informed of the potential risk of this interaction.

1. Westveer MK, Farquhar ML, George P, Mayes JT. Co-administration of grapefruit juice increases tacrolimus levels in liver transplant patients. Proceedings of the 15th Annual Meeting of the American Society of Transplant Physicians 1996. Abstract P-115.
2. Michelangelo V, Piero D, Elisa C, Enrico S, Mauro B, Pietro B. Grapefruit juice and kinetics of tacrolimus. *J Am Soc Nephrol* (2001) 12, 862A.
3. Fukatsu S, Fukudo M, Masuda S, Yano I, Katsura T, Ogura Y, Oike F, Takada Y, Inui K-I. Delayed effect of grapefruit juice on pharmacokinetics and pharmacodynamics of tacrolimus in a living-donor liver transplant recipient. *Drug Metab Pharmacokinet* (2006) 21, 122–5.
4. Egashira K, Fukuda E, Onga T, Yogi Y, Matsuya F, Koyabu N, Ohtani H, Sawada Y. Pomelo-induced increase in the blood level of tacrolimus in a renal transplant patient. *Transplantation* (2003) 75, 1057.
5. Egashira K, Ohtani H, Itoh S, Koyabu N, Tsujimoto M, Murakami H, Sawada Y. Inhibitory effects of pomelo on the metabolism of tacrolimus and the activities of CYP3A4 and P-glycoprotein. *Drug Metab Dispos* (2004) 32, 828–33.
6. Prograf (Tacrolimus). Astellas Pharma US Inc. US Prescribing information, April 2006.
7. Prograf (Tacrolimus monohydrate). Astellas Pharma Ltd. UK Summary of product characteristics, May 2007.

Tacrolimus + Macrolides

Patients have had marked increases in serum tacrolimus levels accompanied by evidence of renal toxicity when they were given erythromycin. The same interaction has been seen in patients given clarithromycin, and is predicted with josamycin and troleandomycin. Although azithromycin would not be expected to interact, an isolated case reports an increase in tacrolimus levels on concurrent use.

Clinical evidence

(a) Azithromycin

One report briefly describes a patient taking tacrolimus following a bone marrow transplant who took a 10-day course of azithromycin (dose not stated) without any significant alteration in his serum creatinine or trough tacrolimus levels.[1] However, a isolated case report describes an increase in tacrolimus levels from a range of 15.8 to 17.5 nanograms/mL to greater than 30 nanograms/mL in a patient who had been receiving intravenous tacrolimus 20 micrograms/kg daily 3 days after azithromycin 500 mg daily was started.[2]

(b) Clarithromycin

A woman with a kidney transplant taking tacrolimus, prednisone and azathioprine was given clarithromycin 500 mg twice daily for 4 days, then 250 mg daily to treat a severe *Mycoplasma pneumoniae* infection. Despite a 64% reduction in the dosage of the tacrolimus, the trough tacrolimus concentrations rose sharply, from 2.8 to 36.1 nanograms/mL by day 6 and creatinine levels increased from 309 to 442 micromol/L. The tacrolimus dosage was further reduced and then stopped, and not restarted until the clarithromycin treatment was completed.[3] In another 2 kidney transplant patients, tacrolimus levels increased by 146% and 131%, respectively, following 9 doses of clarithromycin 250 mg. Creatinine levels increased by 91% and 30%, respectively.[4] Similarly the tacrolimus levels of a bone marrow transplant patient rose from below 1.1 to 10.1 nanograms/mL after he took clarithromycin 500 mg twice daily for about 4 days.[1] A similar increase in tacrolimus levels has been reported in a heart transplant patient, despite an initial reduction in tacrolimus dose in anticipation of the interaction,[5] and in another kidney transplant patient.[6]

(c) Erythromycin

A liver transplant patient taking tacrolimus 6 mg twice daily for one year had a marked rise in serum tacrolimus levels from about 1.4 to 6.5 nanomol/L when intravenous ampicillin/sulbactam 3 g every 6 hours and oral erythromycin 250 mg every 6 hours were given for 4 days to treat pneumonia. Renal toxicity, demonstrated by increased blood urea and creatinine levels also occurred. The erythromycin was stopped, and the next day the tacrolimus was also stopped. Over the next week the plasma levels of the tacrolimus, blood urea nitrogen and creatinine fell.[7] A kidney transplant patient had an increase in his plasma tacrolimus levels from 1.3 to 8.5 nanograms/mL 4 days after starting erythromycin 400 mg four times daily. His serum creatinine levels almost doubled.[8] A man with a kidney transplant had a sixfold rise in tacrolimus blood levels when he took erythromycin.[9] Another similar case has been described.[10] Two children aged 3 and 7 years also had rises in tacrolimus blood levels, which were accompanied by renal toxicity when erythromycin was added.[11]

Mechanism

The macrolides inhibit tacrolimus metabolism by the cytochrome P450 isoenzyme CYP3A. Azithromycin is less likely to interact with tacrolimus because it does not inhibit CYP3A.[12]

Importance and management

Direct information seems to be limited to these case reports. However, it would be prudent to closely monitor the effects of adding clarithromycin or erythromycin in any patient, being alert for the need to reduce the tacrolimus dosage to avoid nephrotoxicity. The manufacturers predict that **josamycin**[13] and **troleandomycin**[14] will interact similarly and so the same precautions would also be appropriate. The manufacturers of **telithromycin** also recommend close monitoring of tacrolimus levels and reducing the tacrolimus dose as required.[15] Most other macrolides would also be expected to interact although they do not all behave identically.

The significance of the single case report of azithromycin increasing tacrolimus levels is unclear as azithromycin does not affect CYP3A4, and therefore has been predicted not to interact, as suggested by the other case.

1. Ibrahim RB, Abella EM, Chandrasekar PH. Tacrolimus-clarithromycin interaction in a patient receiving bone marrow transplantation. *Ann Pharmacother* (2002) 36, 1971–2.
2. Mori T, Aisa Y, Nakazato T, Yamazaki R, Ikeda Y, Okamoto S. Tacrolimus-azithromycin interaction in a recipient of allogeneic bone marrow transplantation. *Transpl Int* (2005) 18, 757–8.

3. Wolter K, Wagner K, Philipp T, Fritschka E. Interaction between FK 506 and clarithromycin in a renal transplant patient. *Eur J Clin Pharmacol* (1994) 47, 207–8.
4. Gómez G, Álvarez ML, Errasti P, Lavilla FJ, García N, Ballester B, García I, Purroy A. Acute tacrolimus nephrotoxicity in renal transplant patients treated with clarithromycin. *Transplant Proc* (1999) 31, 2250–1.
5. Kunicki PW, Sobieszczańska-Malek M. Pharmacokinetic interaction between tacrolimus and clarithromycin in a heart transplant patient. *Ther Drug Monit* (2005) 27, 107–8.
6. Katari SR, Magnone M, Shapiro R, Jordan M, Scantlebury V, Vivas C, Gritsch A, McCauley J, Starzl T, Demetris J, Randhawa PS. Clinical features of acute reversible tacrolimus (FK 506) nephrotoxicity in kidney transplant recipients. *Clin Transplant* (1997) 11, 237–42.
7. Shaeffer MS, Collier D, Sorrell MF. Interaction between FK506 and erythromycin. *Ann Pharmacother* (1994) 28, 280–1.
8. Jensen C, Jordan M, Shapiro R, Scantelbury V, Hakala T, Fung J, Stasrzl T, Venkataramanan R. Interaction between tacrolimus and erythromycin. *Lancet* (1994) 344, 825.
9. Padhi ID, Long P, Basha M, Anandan JV. Interaction between tacrolimus and erythromycin. *Ther Drug Monit* (1997) 19, 120–2.
10. Moreno M, Latorre C, Manzanares C, Morales E, Herrero JC, Dominguez-Gil B, Carreño A, Cubas A, Delgado M, Andres A, Morales JM. Clinical management of tacrolimus drug interactions in renal transplant patients. *Transplant Proc* (1999) 31, 2252–3.
11. Furlan V, Perello L, Jacquemin E, Debray D, Taburet A-M. Interactions between FK506 and rifampicin or erythromycin in pediatric liver recipients. *Transplantation* (1995) 59, 1217–18.
12. Paterson DL, Singh N. Interactions between tacrolimus and antimicrobial agents. *Clin Infect Dis* (1997) 25, 1430–40.
13. Prograf (Tacrolimus monohydrate). Astellas Pharma Ltd. UK Summary of product characteristics, May 2007.
14. Prograf (Tacrolimus). Astellas Pharma US Inc. US Prescribing information, April 2006.
15. Ketek (Telithromycin). Sanofi-Aventis. UK Summary of product characteristics, May 2007.

Tacrolimus + Metoclopramide

In an isolated case, metoclopramide may have increased tacrolimus levels, resulting in tacrolimus toxicity and acute renal failure.

Clinical evidence, mechanism, importance and management

A case report describes a liver transplant patient taking several drugs, including tacrolimus up to 28 mg twice daily, who had subtherapeutic tacrolimus levels, which were increased when she took metoclopramide, initially 10 mg four times daily, then 20 mg four times daily, for gastric dysmotility. Her tacrolimus trough levels increased from less than 2 nanograms/mL to greater than 30 nanograms/mL within 5 to 6 days, and she developed tremor, weakness, nausea, vomiting, diarrhoea and acute renal failure. The authors considered that the increase in tacrolimus levels was due to metoclopramide, possibly due to its effects in increasing gut motility and hence, tacrolimus absorption. However several other factors may have contributed, such as diarrhoea and the use of cimetidine and ketoconazole.[1]

This appears to be the only reported case of tacrolimus toxicity, with metoclopramide, and, because of the number of complicating factors, it is by no means established. Its general significance is unclear.

1. Prescott WA, Callahan BL, Park JM. Tacrolimus toxicity associated with concomitant metoclopramide therapy. *Pharmacotherapy* (2004) 24, 532–7.

Tacrolimus + Metronidazole

Two reports describe increases in tacrolimus levels in patients also given metronidazole.

Clinical evidence

A kidney transplant patient taking tacrolimus 3 mg twice daily had a threefold increase in his tacrolimus levels when he was given metronidazole 500 mg four times daily for 14 days. His trough level increased from 9.2 nanograms/mL to 26.3 nanograms/mL within 4 days of starting the metronidazole, requiring a tacrolimus dose reduction to 1 mg twice daily. Five days after stopping the metronidazole his trough level had returned to 9.2 nanograms/mL and his dose was increased back up to 2 mg twice daily.[1] A similar increase in tacrolimus trough levels was seen in a kidney transplant patient taking tacrolimus 3 mg in the morning and 2 mg at night. His tacrolimus level rose from 9 nanograms/mL to nearly 18 nanograms/mL when he started taking metronidazole 400 mg three times daily for a *C. difficile* infection. The tacrolimus dose was reduced to 1 mg twice daily and the tacrolimus level fell to 8.1 nanograms/mL. When the metronidazole was stopped, his tacrolimus level decreased further to 5.2 nanograms/mL and his tacrolimus dosage needed to be increased to 2 mg twice daily.[2]

Mechanism

Metronidazole is a weak inhibitor of cytochrome P450 isoenzyme CYP3A4[1] and it has also been suggested that metronidazole is also an inhibitor or substrate for P-glycoprotein.[1] As tacrolimus is a metabolised by CYP3A4 and is also a substrate for P-glycoprotein, one or both of these mechanisms may be involved in this interaction.

Importance and management

These two cases appear to be the only reports of a possible interaction between tacrolimus and metronidazole. There is insufficient evidence to advocate monitoring in every patient given the combination, but it would be prudent to at least bear this interaction in mind if using metronidazole in patients taking tacrolimus.

1. Page RL, Klem PM, Rogers C. Potential elevation of tacrolimus trough concentrations with concomitant metronidazole therapy. *Ann Pharmacother* (2005) 39, 1109–13.
2. Herzig K, Johnson DW. Marked elevation of blood cyclosporin and tacrolimus levels due to concurrent metronidazole therapy. *Nephrol Dial Transplant* (1999) 14, 521–3.

Tacrolimus + Miscellaneous

Tacrolimus is metabolised by CYP3A4, the induction and inhibition of which may affect the serum levels of tacrolimus. The manufacturers also issue cautions about the concurrent use of tacrolimus and anticoagulants, antidiabetics, nephrotoxic and neurotoxic drugs.

Clinical evidence, mechanism, importance and management

(a) CYP3A4 inducers

In vitro studies with *rat* and human liver microsomes[1,2] have found that tacrolimus is extensively metabolised by the cytochrome P450 isoenzyme CYP3A4. This means that drugs that induce CYP3A4 may potentially reduce the serum levels of tacrolimus.

Rifampicin (rifampin) and possibly **phenytoin**, known potent enzyme inducers, have been seen to lower tacrolimus levels (see 'Tacrolimus + Rifamycins', p.1083, and 'Tacrolimus + Phenytoin', p.1081), and the manufacturers suggest that **carbamazepine**, **isoniazid** and **phenobarbital** will interact similarly.[3,4] However, note that there is little to suggest that **isoniazid** has a clinically significant effect on this isoenzyme.

These predictions are as yet unconfirmed, but it would certainly be prudent to monitor tacrolimus levels closely if any of these drugs (with the possible exception of isoniazid) are used concurrently. The manufacturers also note that in *animal* studies, tacrolimus has been shown to decrease the clearance and increase the half-life of **pentobarbital**,[3] and a report also describes the use of a **phenobarbital** infusion to treat a tacrolimus overdose.[5]

(b) CYP3A4 inhibitors

In vitro studies with *rat* and human liver microsomes[1,2] have found that tacrolimus is extensively metabolised by the cytochrome P450 isoenzyme CYP3A4. This means that drugs that inhibit CYP3A4 may potentially increase the serum levels of tacrolimus. Most of the known inhibitors of CYP3A4 (such as the 'azoles', (p.1075), 'protease inhibitors', (p.1082) and 'macrolides', (p.1079)) have clearly been shown to interact with tacrolimus. The manufacturers of tacrolimus suggest that other enzyme-inhibiting drugs may also inhibit tacrolimus metabolism and therefore suggest that its levels are monitored if they are given. They name **bromocriptine**, **cimetidine**, **dapsone**, **ergotamine**, **lidocaine**, **midazolam**, **quinidine** and **tamoxifen**.[3,4] These predictions are as yet unconfirmed, and note that, with exception of **cimetidine**, these drugs are not commonly associated with clinically significant interactions by this mechanism.

(c) Neurotoxicity or nephrotoxicity

Other predicted interactions of tacrolimus include additive neuro- or nephrotoxicity with **aciclovir**, **aminoglycosides**, **co-trimoxazole**, **ganciclovir**, **gyrase inhibitors**, **NSAIDs** (see 'NSAIDs', (p.1081)) or **vancomycin** (nephrotoxicity has been seen with **amphotericin B** and tacrolimus).[3]

(d) Protein-binding interactions

Because tacrolimus is extensively bound to plasma proteins, the UK manufacturers mention the possibility of protein-binding interactions with oral

anticoagulants or **antidiabetics,**[3] (but this has largely been discredited as a mechanism, see 'Protein-binding interactions', (p.3)).

1. Shah IA, Whiting PH, Omar G, Thomson AW, Burke MD. Effects of FK 506 on human microsomal cytochrome P–450–dependent drug metabolism in vitro. *Transplant Proc* (1991) 23, 2783–5.
2. Pichard L, Fabre I, Domergue J, Joyeux H, Maurel P. Effect of FK 506 on human hepatic cytochromes P–450: interaction with CyA. *Transplant Proc* (1991) 23, 2791–3.
3. Prograf (Tacrolimus monohydrate). Astellas Pharma Ltd. UK Summary of product characteristics, May 2007.
4. Prograf (Tacrolimus). Astellas Pharma US Inc. US Prescribing information, April 2006.
5. McLaughlin GE, Rossique-Gonzalez M, Gelman B, Kato T. Use of phenobarbital in the management of acute tacrolimus toxicity: a case report. *Transplant Proc* (2000) 32, 665–8.

Tacrolimus + NNRTIs

Efavirenz appears to decrease the metabolism of tacrolimus.

Clinical evidence, mechanism, importance and management

An HIV-positive liver transplant patient who had taken **efavirenz**, lamivudine and zidovudine pre-transplantation and then again post-transplantation with concurrent tacrolimus and corticosteroids, had therapeutic tacrolimus levels for 6 days despite tacrolimus and the antiretrovirals being stopped because of zidovudine-induced rhabdomyolysis.[1] **Efavirenz** is a known inducer of the cytochrome P450 isoenzyme CYP3A4 by which tacrolimus is metabolised. It seems likely that the effect of **efavirenz** was sufficient to dramatically reduce tacrolimus clearance. Although this is only an isolated case it is in line with the way both drugs are known to interact. It would seem prudent to closely monitor tacrolimus levels in any patient given **efavirenz**.

1. Antonini M, Ettorre GM, Vennarecci G, D'Offizi G, Narciso P, Del Nonno F, Perracchio L, Visco G, Santoro E. Anti-retrovirals and immunosuppressive drug interactions in a HIV-positive patient after liver transplantation. *Hepatogastroenterology* (2004) 51, 646–8.

Tacrolimus + NSAIDs

Two liver transplant patients taking tacrolimus developed acute renal failure after also taking ibuprofen.

Clinical evidence, mechanism, importance and management

Two patients with liver transplants taking tacrolimus developed acute but reversible renal failure, one after taking four *Motrin* (**ibuprofen**) tablets (strength not stated) and the other after three 400-mg tablets of **ibuprofen** taken over 24 hours. Both had stable renal function before taking the **ibuprofen.**[1]

NSAIDs are known to inhibit prostaglandin synthesis and as a result may decrease renal blood flow, which in certain circumstances can lead to renal failure. Renal impairment is more likely to occur in the presence of renal vasoconstrictors. Tacrolimus is known to cause renal vasoconstriction and thus the combined effects of **ibuprofen** and tacrolimus may have led to acute renal failure. Both patients also had a degree of liver impairment, which the authors suggest may have potentiated the toxicity of tacrolimus with **ibuprofen**.

The authors of the report say that if renal toxicity develops, tacrolimus should be withdrawn. They used intravenous prostaglandin-E1 effectively in one patient. They also suggest that NSAIDs should not be given to patients taking tacrolimus, especially if it is being used as rescue therapy for abnormal graft function.[1] There seems to be nothing documented about adverse interactions with other NSAIDs but if the suggested mechanism is true, they may possibly behave like **ibuprofen**. The UK manufacturers of tacrolimus suggest that all NSAIDs may have additive nephrotoxic effects with tacrolimus.[2]

1. Sheiner PA, Mor E, Chodoff L, Glabman S, Emre S, Schwartz ME, Miller CM. Acute renal failure associated with the use of ibuprofen in two liver transplant recipients on FK506. *Transplantation* (1994) 57, 1132–3.
2. Prograf (Tacrolimus monohydrate). Astellas Pharma Ltd. UK Summary of product characteristics, May 2007.

Tacrolimus + Orlistat

Orlistat does not appear to significantly affect the pharmacokinetics of tacrolimus, although small dosage adjustments may be needed in some patients.

Clinical evidence, mechanism, importance and management

A study in 12 liver transplant patients taking tacrolimus with orlistat 120 mg three times daily for 6 months found that concurrent use was well tolerated. However, 4 patients required a reduction and 2 required an increase in their tacrolimus dose, although these adjustments were only minor dose changes. No diarrhoea was reported by the patients in this study, concurrent use was well tolerated and no episodes of rejection occurred. The authors concluded that orlistat could be safely used in patients taking tacrolimus provided that tacrolimus levels are carefully monitored.[1]

1. Cassiman D, Roelants M, Vandenplas G, Van der Merwe SW, Mertens A, Libbrecht L, Verslype C, Fevery J, Aerts R, Pirenne J, Muls E, Nevens F. Orlistat treatment is safe in overweight and obese liver transplant recipients: a prospective, open label trial. *Transpl Int* (2006) 19, 1000–5.

Tacrolimus + Phenytoin

An isolated report describes an increase in serum phenytoin levels attributed to the use of tacrolimus. Phenytoin decreased tacrolimus levels in one case, and has been used to reduce tacrolimus levels after an overdose.

Clinical evidence

(a) Phenytoin levels

A kidney transplant patient taking phenytoin 500 and 600 mg on alternate days (and also taking azathioprine, bumetanide, digoxin, diltiazem, heparin, insulin and prednisone) had his immunosuppressant treatment changed from ciclosporin, to tacrolimus 14 to 16 mg daily. About 7 weeks later he presented to hospital because of a fainting episode and his phenytoin levels were found to have risen from 18.4 to 36.2 micrograms/mL. The phenytoin was temporarily stopped until his serum levels had fallen, and he was then discharged on a reduced phenytoin dosage of 400 and 500 mg on alternate days with no further problems.[1] The presumption is that the fainting episode was due to the raised serum phenytoin levels.

(b) Tacrolimus levels

In one kidney transplant patient taking phenytoin, tacrolimus 250 micrograms/kg daily was needed to give a blood level of 9 nanograms/mL. Three months later phenytoin was gradually stopped, with gradual tapering of the tacrolimus dose. The patient was eventually stabilised with a tacrolimus dose of 160 micrograms/kg daily giving a blood level of 11 nanograms/mL.[2]

Another report describes the use of an intravenous phenytoin infusion to treat acute tacrolimus overdoses in 2 patients, with the aim of enhancing tacrolimus metabolism.[3]

Mechanism

Tacrolimus is extensively metabolised by the cytochrome P450 isoenzyme CYP3A4, and phenytoin is a known inducer of this system. Phenytoin is therefore predicted to decrease tacrolimus levels. In the first case, it was suggested that tacrolimus might have inhibited the metabolism of phenytoin, although other factors may have had some part to play in the raised phenytoin levels.[1]

Importance and management

No interaction is established, but based on the known metabolism of these drugs it would be prudent to monitor tacrolimus levels in a patient given phenytoin. Similarly, based on the single case of phenytoin toxicity, it may also be advisable to monitor phenytoin levels.

1. Thompson PA, Mosley CA. Tacrolimus-phenytoin interaction. *Ann Pharmacother* (1996) 30, 544.

2. Moreno M, Latorre C, Manzanares C, Morales E, Herrero JC, Dominguez-Gil B, Carreño A, Cubas A, Delgado M, Andres A, Morales JM. Clinical management of tacrolimus drug interactions in renal transplant patients. *Transplant Proc* (1999) 31, 2252–3.
3. Karasu Z, Gurakar A, Carlson J, Pennington S, Kerwin B, Wright H, Nour B, Sebastian A. Acute tacrolimus overdose and treatment with phenytoin in liver transplant recipients. *J Okla State Med Assoc* (2001) 94, 121–3.

Tacrolimus + Protease inhibitors

Protease inhibitors including lopinavir, nelfinavir, ritonavir and saquinavir significantly inhibit the metabolism of tacrolimus and increase its blood levels.

Clinical evidence

A retrospective study in 10 HIV-positive kidney transplant patients found that all of the patients taking a **protease inhibitor** (not specified) required a tacrolimus dose reduction, and 3 of them needed to be changed from a protease inhibitor to an alternative antiretroviral.[1]

(a) Lopinavir

A liver transplant patient taking tacrolimus 5 mg twice daily to give a tacrolimus trough blood level of 10.6 nanograms/mL had a large increase in tacrolimus levels to 78.5 nanograms/mL when lopinavir/ritonavir was started, despite a tacrolimus dose reduction to 6 mg daily. Tacrolimus neurotoxicity developed, but no nephrotoxicity was seen. The patient was eventually stabilised taking tacrolimus 500 micrograms weekly while taking lopinavir/ritonavir. Other patients have developed raised tacrolimus levels and been eventually restabilised on tacrolimus dosages of 500 micrograms to 1 mg weekly, while taking lopinavir/ritonavir: tacrolimus levels have continued to increase despite tacrolimus doses being withheld.[2,3]

(b) Nelfinavir

An HIV-positive patient, with hepatitis C following a liver transplant was given stavudine, lamivudine, and nelfinavir 500 mg three times daily. Tacrolimus 6 mg daily was started postoperatively but high blood levels were observed and the dose was reduced over the next 3 months to a maintenance dose of 500 micrograms weekly, which achieved levels of between 7 and 25.9 nanograms/mL.[4] A patient had a tacrolimus level of 10.9 nanograms/mL while taking tacrolimus 4 mg twice daily without antiretrovirals. When he was given a combination of didanosine, nelfinavir and stavudine, he had a tacrolimus level of 23.7 nanograms/mL, despite a dosage reduction to tacrolimus 500 micrograms daily.[5] A brief report describes petit mal seizures brought on by high tacrolimus levels, which were thought to be as a result of an interaction with nelfinavir. The patient was stabilised on once weekly tacrolimus.[6] In a study HIV-positive patients who underwent liver transplantation were given tacrolimus and a HAART regimen, which included a protease inhibitor. Tacrolimus dosing was reduced in all patients on HAART to between 1 and 3 mg daily. A patient developed acute organ rejection due to low tacrolimus levels when nelfinavir was stopped without an increase in the tacrolimus dose.[7]

(c) Ritonavir

A case report describes an HIV-positive, kidney transplant patient who developed an increase in tacrolimus levels requiring a large dose reduction to tacrolimus 500 micrograms weekly when ritonavir and **saquinavir** were also given.[8] A patient had a tacrolimus level of 10.9 nanograms/mL while taking tacrolimus 4 mg twice daily without antiretrovirals. When he was given a combination of didanosine, nelfinavir and stavudine, he had a tacrolimus level of 23.7 nanograms/mL, despite a reduction in the dose of tacrolimus to 500 micrograms daily. When nelfinavir was replaced by, ritonavir and **saquinavir**, tacrolimus 1 mg twice daily resulted in tacrolimus levels in excess of 120 nanograms/mL with severe, prolonged toxicity.[5] In a study HIV-positive patients who underwent liver transplantation were given tacrolimus with a HAART regimen, which included a protease inhibitor. Tacrolimus dosing was reduced in all patients on HAART to between 1 to 3 mg daily. One patient taking ritonavir had a tacrolimus level of 50 nanograms/mL despite the initial dose of tacrolimus being reduced to 3 mg daily. Another patient developed tacrolimus toxicity due to ritonavir and her tacrolimus dose needed to be reduced to 250 micrograms every 4 days to keep the tacrolimus levels within range.[7]

Mechanism

All protease inhibitors are, to varying degrees, inhibitors of the cytochrome P450 isoenzyme CYP3A4, by which tacrolimus is metabolised. It therefore seems likely that the protease inhibitors reduced tacrolimus metabolism resulting in the extremely high levels seen. The protease inhibitors also inhibit P-glycoprotein, of which tacrolimus is a substrate. See also 'Antiretrovirals', (p.772). It has been suggested that this could lead to increased levels of unmetabolised tacrolimus in the bile which may be reabsorbed through the enterohepatic circulation system, thus further increasing tacrolimus levels.[2]

Importance and management

An established and clinically important interaction. It is advised that when protease inhibitors are given to patients taking tacrolimus, a significant reduction in the dose of tacrolimus is required, with close and frequent monitoring of tacrolimus blood levels. One centre said that they routinely decreased the tacrolimus dose to 1 mg to 3 mg daily in patients requiring a protease inhibitor-based HAART regimen, although some patients still developed toxicity despite this initial reduction.[7]

1. Mazuecos A, Pascual J, Gómez E, Sola E, Cofán F, López F, Puig-Hooper CE, Baltar JM, González-Molina M, Oppenheimer F, Marcén R, Rivero M. Renal transplantation in HIV-infected patients in Spain. *Nefrologia* (2006) 26, 113–20.
2. Jain AB, Venkataramanan R, Eghtesad B, Marcos A, Ragni M, Shapiro R, Rafail AB, Fung JJ. Effect of coadministered lopinavir and ritonavir (Kaletra) on tacrolimus blood concentration in liver transplanted patients. *Liver Transpl* (2003) 9, 954–60.
3. Schonder KS, Shullo MA, Okusanya O. Tacrolimus and lopinavir/ritonavir interaction in liver transplantation. *Ann Pharmacother* (2003) 37, 1793–6.
4. Schvarcz R, Rudbeck G, Söderdahl G, Ståhle L. Interaction between nelfinavir and tacrolimus after orthoptic liver transplantation in a patient coinfected with HIV and hepatitis C virus (HCV). *Transplantation* (2000) 69, 2194–5.
5. Sheikh AM, Wolf DC, Lebovics E, Goldberg R, Horowitz HW. Concomitant human immunodeficiency virus protease inhibitor therapy markedly reduces tacrolimus metabolism and increases blood levels. *Transplantation* (1999) 68, 307–9.
6. Ragni M, Dodson SF, Hunt SC, Bontempo FA, Fung JJ. Liver transplantation in a hemophilia patient with acquired immunodeficiency syndrome. *Blood* (1999) 93, 1113–14.
7. Neff GW, Bonham A, Tzakis AG, Ragni M, Jayaweera D, Schiff ER, Shakil O, Fung JJ. Orthoptic liver transplantation in patients with human immunodeficiency virus and end-stage liver disease. *Liver Transpl* (2003) 9, 239–47.
8. Hardy G, Stanke-Labesque F, Contamin C, Serre-Debeauvais F, Bayle F, Zaoui P, Bessard G. Protease inhibitors and diltiazem increase tacrolimus blood concentration in a patient with renal transplantation: a case report. *Eur J Clin Pharmacol* (2004) 60, 603–5.

Tacrolimus + Proton pump inhibitors

Lansoprazole may increase tacrolimus levels in patients with low levels of the cytochrome P450 isoenzyme CYP2C19. Pantoprazole and omeprazole are predicted to interact similarly. Rabeprazole appears not to interact with tacrolimus.

Clinical evidence

A 57-year-old woman taking tacrolimus following a kidney transplant started taking **lansoprazole** 30 mg daily 19 days after her transplant because of a peptic ulcer. After 3 days her tacrolimus trough level rose from a range of 16.3 to 17.6 nanograms/mL up to 26.7 nanograms/mL. The tacrolimus dose was reduced, and levels of 12 to 15.4 nanograms/mL were achieved. When **lansoprazole** was replaced by famotidine the tacrolimus levels reduced to 8 nanograms/mL. The patient was later switched from famotidine to **rabeprazole** 10 mg daily without any further alteration in tacrolimus levels.[1,2]

Another report describes a patient who had no significant alteration in tacrolimus levels when **rabeprazole** 10 mg daily was started and stopped.[2]

A study in 6 transplant patients taking tacrolimus found that **pantoprazole** 40 mg once daily for 5 days did not significantly affect the trough levels of tacrolimus.[3]

A study in 51 kidney transplant patients taking tacrolimus and **omeprazole** 20 mg daily found no significant interaction.[4] A retrospective study in 48 kidney transplant patients found that when patients switched from cimetidine 400 mg daily to **omeprazole** 20 mg daily resulted in a 15% decrease in the dose/weight normalised tacrolimus trough levels.[5]

Mechanism

Two of the patients reported above[1,2] had decreased activity of the cytochrome P450 isoenzyme CYP2C19, by which lansoprazole is mainly metabolised. When levels of this enzyme are low, CYP3A4 (which normally only metabolises a fraction of lansoprazole) becomes more important in the metabolism of lansoprazole, and interactions with drugs that affect CYP3A4 become more likely. Tacrolimus is metabolised by CYP3A4, and therefore competition with lansoprazole for metabolism may have led to raised tacrolimus levels in these patients. Pantoprazole may interact similarly in poor metabolisers.[3] The decreased tacrolimus levels in one study with omeprazole[5] may have been more to do with stopping the cimetidine (a known enzyme inhibitor) than an effect of omeprazole. Rabeprazole is metabolised non-enzymatically and therefore does not seem to interact.[1,2]

Importance and management

The incidence of the interaction between tacrolimus and lansoprazole is unknown. It would seem to most frequently occur in those with decreased CYP2C19 activity,[6] and therefore it is not easy to predict which patients would be affected. The manufacturers of tacrolimus say that this interaction may also occur with omeprazole, which is metabolised in the same way as lansoprazole. It would seem prudent to monitor tacrolimus levels if either of these proton pump inhibitors is started or stopped. Although no interaction was noted in the study with pantoprazole[3] the authors do note that it may interact like lansoprazole in patients with CYP2C19 deficiency. Rabeprazole may be a suitable alternative proton pump inhibitor as limited evidence suggests that it does not interact, and nor would it be expected to do so.

1. Homma M, Itagaki F, Yuzawa K, Fukao K, Kohda Y. Effects of lansoprazole and rabeprazole on tacrolimus blood concentration: case of a renal transplant recipient with CYP2C19 gene mutation. *Transplantation* (2002) 73, 303–4.
2. Itagaki F, Homma M, Yuzawa K, Fukao K, Kohda Y. Drug interaction of tacrolimus and proton pump inhibitors in renal transplant recipients with CYP2C19 gene mutation. *Transplant Proc* (2002) 34, 2777–8.
3. Lorf T, Ramadori G, Ringe B, Schwörer H. The effect of pantoprazole on tacrolimus and cyclosporin A blood concentration in transplant recipients. *Eur J Clin Pharmacol* (2000) 56, 439–40.
4. Pascual J, Marcén R, Orea OE, Navarro M, Alarcón MC, Ocaña J, Villafruela JJ, Burgos FJ, Ortuño J. Interaction between omeprazole and tacrolimus in renal allograft recipients: a clinical-analytical study. *Transplant Proc* (2005) 37, 3752–3.
5. Lemahieu WPD, Maes BD, Verbeke K, Vanrenterghem Y. Impact of gastric acid suppressants on cytochrome P450 3A4 and P-glycoprotein: consequences for FK506 assimilation. *Kidney Int* (2005) 67, 1152–60.
6. Prograf (Tacrolimus). Astellas Pharma US Inc. US Prescribing information, April 2006.

Tacrolimus + Quinolones

Levofloxacin modestly increased the bioavailability of tacrolimus in one study. *In vitro*, enoxacin had no effect on tacrolimus metabolism.

Clinical evidence, mechanism, importance and management

A study in 5 kidney transplant patients found that **levofloxacin** 500 mg twice daily for 5 days increased the AUC_{0-12} of tacrolimus by about 27%.[1]

On the basis of the study above[1] and of some quite unexpected rises in drug levels and subsequent nephrotoxicity in a handful of patients taking the similarly metabolised immunosuppressant, ciclosporin, with a quinolone antibacterial (see 'Ciclosporin + Antibacterials; Quinolones', p.1018), one review suggested that close monitoring would be appropriate if tacrolimus is given with any quinolone.[2] However, *in vitro* studies have suggested that enoxacin does not affect the metabolism of tacrolimus, and ciprofloxacin does not affect the immunosuppressant activity of tacrolimus. Further study is needed.

1. Federico S, Carrano R, Capone D, Gentile A, Palmiero G, Basile V. Pharmacokinetic interaction between levofloxacin and ciclosporin or tacrolimus in kidney transplant recipients: ciclosporin, tacrolimus and levofloxacin in renal transplantation. *Clin Pharmacokinet* (2006) 45, 169–75.
2. Petersen DL, Singh N. Interactions between tacrolimus and antimicrobial agents. *Clin Infect Dis* (1997) 25, 1430–40.

Tacrolimus + Quinupristin/Dalfopristin

Tacrolimus levels have been reported to increase by 15% during the concurrent use of quinupristin/dalfopristin. The manufacturers state that quinupristin/dalfopristin has been shown *in vitro* to inhibit the cytochrome P450 isoenzyme CYP3A4, the main isoenzyme involved in the metabolism of tacrolimus. Tacrolimus levels should therefore be closely monitored during concurrent use.[1]

1. Synercid (Quinupristin/Dalfopristin). Monarch Pharmaceuticals. UK Summary of product characteristics, March 2005.

Tacrolimus + Rifamycins

A number of liver transplant patients have needed markedly increased tacrolimus dosages when rifampicin (rifampin) was added. A pharmacokinetic study has shown that rifampicin increases the clearance and decreases the bioavailability of intravenous and oral tacrolimus. Rifabutin is unlikely to interact to the same extent, but given the magnitude of the interaction with rifampicin, caution is still warranted.

Clinical evidence

The trough tacrolimus blood levels of a 10-year-old boy with a liver transplant fell from 10 nanograms/mL to unmeasurable levels within 2 days of **rifampicin** (**rifampin**) 150 mg twice daily being started. His tacrolimus dosage was therefore doubled from 4 to 8 mg twice daily. When the **rifampicin** was later stopped, the tacrolimus dosage had to be reduced to 3 mg twice daily to keep the blood levels in the region of 10 nanograms/mL.[1]

An extremely marked reduction in tacrolimus trough levels occurred in a 10-month-old child with a liver transplant when **rifampicin** was given with tacrolimus. Tacrolimus levels fell to about one-tenth of baseline levels.[2] This case has also been reported elsewhere.[3] In another case, this time in an adult, a tenfold increase was needed in the tacrolimus dosage to keep trough blood levels within the target range when **rifampicin** was started. However, despite levels within the acceptable range, a biopsy showed suspected tacrolimus nephrotoxicity, which was considered to be possibly due to the cumulative tacrolimus dose, or to high levels of tacrolimus metabolites (which were not measured).[4] Another patient with a kidney transplant had a decrease in tacrolimus levels from 9.2 to 1.4 nanograms/mL 2 days after starting **rifampicin**. **Rifampicin** was stopped and replaced by pyrazinamide, with a gradual return to the baseline tacrolimus level.[5] A study in 6 healthy subjects supports the findings of these case reports. In the study, **rifampicin** 600 mg daily significantly increased the clearance and decreased the bioavailability of both oral and intravenous tacrolimus.[6]

Mechanism

This interaction is thought to occur because rifampicin, a known enzyme inducer, increases the metabolism of the tacrolimus by the cytochrome P450 isoenzyme CYP3A4 in the liver and small bowel, and by inducing P-glycoprotein, so that the tacrolimus is cleared more rapidly.

Importance and management

These reports are consistent with the way rifampicin interacts with many other drugs and therefore this interaction would seem to be of general clinical importance. It would be prudent to be alert for the need to raise the dosage of tacrolimus if rifampicin is added in any patient.

Direct information about **rifabutin** seems to be lacking, but any interaction with tacrolimus is likely to be much less marked than with rifampicin because its enzyme-inducing effects are considerably less. Nevertheless until the situation is clear it would be prudent to closely monitor concurrent use with any rifamycin, being alert for the need to raise the tacrolimus dosage.

1. Furlan V, Perello L, Jacquemin E, Debray D, Taburet A-M. Interactions between FK506 and rifampicin or erythromycin in pediatric liver recipients. *Transplantation* (1995) 59, 1217–18.
2. Kiuchi T, Inomata Y, Uemoto S, Satomura K, Egawa H, Okajima H, Yamaoka Y, Tanaka K. A hepatic graft tuberculosis transmitted from a living-related donor. *Transplantation* (1997) 63, 905–7.
3. Kiuchi T, Tanaka K, Inomata Y, Uemoto S, Satomura K, Egawa H, Uyama S, Sano K, Okajima H, Yamaoka Y. Experience of tacrolimus-based immunosuppression in a living-related liver transplantation complicated with graft tuberculosis: interaction with rifampicin and side effects. *Transplant Proc* (1996) 28, 3171–2.
4. Chenhsu R-Y, Loong C-C, Chou M-H, Lin M-F, Yang W-C. Renal allograft dysfunction associated with rifampin-tacrolimus interaction. *Ann Pharmacother* (2000) 34, 27–31.
5. Moreno M, Latorre C, Manzanares C, Morales E, Herrero JC, Dominguez-Gil B, Carreño A, Cubas A, Delgado M, Andres A, Morales JM. Clinical management of tacrolimus drug interactions in renal transplant patients. *Transplant Proc* (1999) 31, 2252–3.
6. Hebert MF, Fisher RM, Marsh CL, Dressler D, Bekersky I. Effects of rifampin on tacrolimus pharmacokinetics in healthy volunteers. *J Clin Pharmacol* (1999) 39, 91–6.

Tacrolimus + Sevelamer

Sevelamer may reduce the absorption of tacrolimus.

Clinical evidence, mechanism, importance and management

A kidney transplant patient had a progressive reduction in tacrolimus levels requiring an increase in his tacrolimus dose after he started to take sevelamer 800 mg three times daily. A small pharmacokinetic study in the same patient found that the peak level was increased from 9.9 to 13.1 nanograms/mL and the AUC_{0-7} was increased 2.4-fold, 3 days after sevelamer was stopped.[1] Sevelamer can affect the absorption of drugs and the reduction in tacrolimus levels may be due to binding with sevelamer in the gut preventing its absorption.

This appears to be the only case report of an interaction between these two drugs, but sevelamer has been seen to have similar effects on a number of other drugs. It is recommended that any drug for which a reduction in the bioavailability may be clinically significant should be taken at least one hour before or three hours after sevelamer.[2] Tacrolimus levels should be closely monitored and the dose adjusted as needed if concurrent use is required.

1. Merkle M, Wornle M, Rupprecht HD. The effect of sevelamer on tacrolimus target levels. *Transplantation* (2005) 80, 707.
2. Renagel (Sevelamer). Genzyme Therapeutics. UK Summary of product characteristics, June 2007.

Tacrolimus + Sildenafil

Sildenafil does not appear to affect the pharmacokinetics of tacrolimus. The levels of sildenafil were higher in patients taking tacrolimus than in healthy subjects, but it is not clear whether this was due to tacrolimus alone. A marked blood pressure drop occurred when both drugs were given in one study.

Clinical evidence, mechanism, importance and management

In 10 men with erectile dysfunction, taking tacrolimus after a kidney transplant, a single 50-mg dose of sildenafil did not affect the pharmacokinetics of tacrolimus. When the pharmacokinetics of sildenafil were compared with those quoted by the manufacturer it was found that the maximum plasma concentration and AUC of tacrolimus were increased by 55% and 90%, respectively in patients taking tacrolimus. The AUC of the sildenafil metabolite was also raised. There are several possible reasons for these differences. The pharmacokinetics quoted by the manufacturers are from healthy subjects, not patients, and the patients in the study were taking a multitude of other drugs, some of which could have affected sildenafil. Apart from the pharmacokinetic effects, it was noted that the mean blood pressure dropped by 27/20 mmHg after sildenafil was given, which could be of significance in patients with cardiovascular disease.[1] A subsequent study by the same authors, in 9 men with erectile dysfunction taking tacrolimus after a kidney transplant, found that sildenafil 25 mg daily for 9 days had no significant effects on the pharmacokinetics of tacrolimus.[2] Another study in 4 patients taking tacrolimus found that sildenafil 50 or 100 mg produced no change in tacrolimus levels.[3]

It would appear that sildenafil does not affect tacrolimus levels, however, given the reduction in blood pressure seen in one study,[1] it may be prudent to initially prescribe sildenafil at the 25 mg dose, as the authors of this study advise, and increase it as required and tolerated.

1. Christ B, Brockmeier D, Hauck EW, Friemann S. Interactions of sildenafil and tacrolimus in men with erectile dysfunction after kidney transplantation. *Urology* (2001) 58, 589–93.
2. Christ B, Brockmeier D, Hauck EW, Kamali-Ernst S. Investigation on interaction between tacrolimus and sildenafil in kidney-transplanted patients with erectile dysfunction. *Int J Clin Pharmacol Ther* (2004) 42, 149–56.
3. Cofán F, Gutiérrez R, Beardo P, Campistol JM, Oppenheimer F, Alcover J. Interacción entre sildenafilo y los inhibidores de la calcineurina en trasplantados renales con disfunción eréctile. *Nefrologia* (2002) 22, 470–6.

Tacrolimus + Sirolimus

Sirolimus may reduce tacrolimus blood levels. There is some evidence to suggest that tacrolimus may increase the clearance of sirolimus.

Clinical evidence, mechanism, importance and management

A study in 18 liver transplant and 7 kidney-pancreas transplant patients taking tacrolimus and sirolimus found no difference in the pharmacokinetics of either drug and no nephrotoxicity when the drugs were taken either simultaneously or 4 hours apart.[1] A single-dose study in 28 healthy subjects found no pharmacokinetic interaction between sirolimus and tacrolimus when they were given either at the same time or 4 hours apart.[2]

However subsequent studies have found decreases in tacrolimus levels due to the concurrent use of sirolimus. A study in 7 children with kidney transplants taking tacrolimus and prednisone found that the addition of sirolimus to treat chronic allograft nephropathy resulted in a decrease in dose-normalised tacrolimus trough blood levels from 0.14 kg/L to 0.1 kg/L on day 3 and 0.08 kg/L on day 28. All patients required a tacrolimus dose increase, with a mean increase of about 70% (range 21.9 to 245.4%) in order to keep the tacrolimus blood levels above 3 nanograms/mL. This was thought to be due to a reduction in the bioavailability of tacrolimus rather than increased excretion.[3] Another study in 28 kidney transplant patients taking tacrolimus and given sirolimus 0.5, 1, or 2 mg daily also found an initial reduction in the tacrolimus level with the first dose. The tacrolimus levels recovered, but a trend towards reduced tacrolimus levels was seen with continued dosing. Tacrolimus did not appear to alter sirolimus levels, when compared with previous data in studies with sirolimus alone.[4]

A study in 16 adult kidney transplant patients taking tacrolimus and fixed-dose sirolimus 500 micrograms or 2 mg daily found a significant, dose-dependent increase in the AUC of tacrolimus of 16% and 31%, respectively, and an increase in the peak levels of tacrolimus of 19% and 33%, respectively, when sirolimus was stopped.[5]

A study in paediatric kidney transplant patients found the clearance of sirolimus in patients was increased in those taking tacrolimus, when compared with those not taking a calcineurin inhibitor.[6] A retrospective study in adult kidney transplant patients taking tacrolimus and sirolimus found that concurrent use may be associated with extensive tubular cell injury and a unique form of cast nephropathy.[7]

The manufacturers of sirolimus note that clinical studies in *de novo* liver transplant patients have found an increased risk of hepatic artery thrombosis when tacrolimus is also given: concurrent use is not recommended in this patient group.[8]

Patients taking sirolimus with tacrolimus should have their tacrolimus and probably sirolimus levels closely monitored and the dose adjusted if needed.

1. McAlister VC, Mahalati K, Peltekian KM, Fraser A, MacDonald AS. A clinical pharmacokinetic study of tacrolimus and sirolimus combination immunosuppression comparing simultaneous to separated administration. *Ther Drug Monit* (2002) 24, 346–50.
2. Patat A, Zimmerman JJ, Parks V, Souan M. Lack of pharmacokinetic interaction co-administered of sirolimus and tacrolimus. *Clin Pharmacol Ther* (2003) 73, P43.
3. Filler G, Womiloju T, Feber J, Lepage N, Christians U. Adding sirolimus to tacrolimus-based immunosuppression in pediatric renal transplant recipients reduces tacrolimus exposure. *Am J Transplant* (2005) 5, 2005–10.
4. Undre NA. Pharmacokinetics of tacrolimus-based combination therapies. *Nephrol Dial Transplant* (2003) 18 (Suppl 1), i12–i15.
5. Baldan N, Rigotti P, Furian L, Margani G, Ekser B, Frison L, De Martin S, Palatini P. Co-administration of sirolimus alters tacrolimus pharmacokinetics in a dose-dependent manner in adult renal transplant recipients. *Pharmacol Res* (2006) 54, 181–5.
6. Schacter AD, Benfield MR, Wyatt RJ, Grimm PC, Fennell RS, Herrin JT, Lirenman DS, McDonald RA, Munoz-Arizpe R, Harmon WE. Sirolimus pharmacokinetics in pediatric renal transplant recipients receiving calcineurin inhibitor co-therapy. *Pediatr Transplant* (2006) 10, 914–9.
7. Smith KD, Wrenshall LE, Nicosia RF, Pichler R, Marsh CL, Alpers CE, Polissar N, Davis CL. Delayed graft function and cast nephropathy associated with tacrolimus plus rapamycin use. *J Am Soc Nephrol* (2003) 14, 1037–45.
8. Rapamune (Sirolimus). Wyeth Pharmaceuticals. UK Summary of product characteristics, March 2007.

Tacrolimus + SSRIs and related antidepressants

Marked increases in tacrolimus levels and toxicity were observed when three patients were also given nefazodone. In theory, fluvoxamine may increase tacrolimus levels. Paroxetine and sertraline may not interact, but the situation is not clear.

Clinical evidence

A kidney transplant patient taking tacrolimus 5 mg daily developed delirium and renal failure 4 weeks after starting to take **nefazodone** 150 mg daily. The tacrolimus levels had been 9.4 nanograms/mL some 3 months earlier when he was taking a dose of 6 mg daily, but in the presence of **nefazodone** the tacrolimus level increased to 46.4 nanograms/mL with a tacrolimus dose of 5 mg daily. His serum creatinine had doubled. The tacrolimus level fell to 29.6 nanograms/mL within 2 days of the dose being reduced to 3 mg daily. **Nefazodone** was then replaced by **paroxetine** 20 mg daily. After 3 days the tacrolimus dose was increased to 5 mg daily and satisfactory levels of 12.4 nanograms/mL were observed.[1]

A kidney transplant patient taking prednisone, azathioprine and tacrolimus 5 mg daily for 2 years experienced headache, confusion and 'grey areas' in her vision within one week of starting **nefazodone** 50 mg twice daily in place of **sertraline**, for depression. Her serum creatinine had risen from 132 to 195 micromol/Land her trough tacrolimus level was greater than 30 nanograms/mL. **Nefazodone** was replaced by **sertraline**, and tacrolimus was withheld for 4 days. Signs of tacrolimus-induced neurotoxicity disappeared within 36 hours and serum creatinine and tacrolimus levels returned to pretreatment levels within 2 weeks.[2]

Another patient developed raised liver enzymes and raised tacrolimus levels after taking **nefazodone** and tacrolimus for 2 weeks. When the **nefazodone** was stopped his liver enzymes normalised over the next 5 days, and his tacrolimus levels fell from 23 to 9.5 nanograms/mL over 10 days.[3]

Mechanism

Tacrolimus is metabolised by the cytochrome P450 isoenzyme CYP3A4, which is inhibited by nefazodone, concurrent use therefore results in increased levels of tacrolimus. Paroxetine and sertraline do not have significant effects on CYP3A4 and are therefore not expected to interact with tacrolimus.

Importance and management

Information appears to be limited but what is known indicates that tacrolimus levels or at least signs of toxicity should be well monitored if nefazodone is also given. In view of the narrow therapeutic index of tacrolimus, it may be advisable to avoid concurrent nefazodone.

Fluvoxamine is an inhibitor of CYP3A4[4] and so theoretically could affect the metabolism of tacrolimus. Close monitoring of tacrolimus levels is therefore advised. Paroxetine and sertraline and possibly other SSRIs may be suitable alternative antidepressants, but the evidence is slim, so additional monitoring may still be warranted.[1] Further study on the use of antidepressants with tacrolimus is needed.

1. Campo JV, Smith C, Perel JM. Tacrolimus toxic reaction associated with the use of nefazodone: paroxetine as an alternative agent. *Arch Gen Psychiatry* (1998) 55, 1050–2.
2. Olyaei AJ, deMattos AM, Norman DJ, Bennett WM. Interaction between tacrolimus and nefazodone in a stable renal transplant recipient. *Pharmacotherapy* (1998) 18, 1356–9.
3. Garton T, Nefazodone and CYP450 3A4 interactions with cyclosporine and tacrolimus. *Transplantation* (2002) 74, 745.
4. Faverin (Fluvoxamine). Solvay Healthcare Ltd. UK Summary of product characteristics, June 2006.

Tacrolimus + St John's wort (*Hypericum perforatum*)

St John's wort decreases tacrolimus levels.

Clinical evidence

In a clinical study, 10 healthy subjects were given a single 100-microgram/kg dose of tacrolimus alone, or after they took St John's wort 300 mg three times daily for 14 days. On average St John's wort decreased the maximum blood level of tacrolimus by 65% and its AUC by 32%. However, the decrease in AUC ranged from 15% to 64%, with one patient having a 31% *increase* in AUC.[1] Similar results have been found in a study in 10 kidney transplant patients given St John's wort (*Jarsin300*) 600 mg daily for 2 weeks. In order to achieve target levels, the tacrolimus dose was increased in all patients, from a median of 4.5 mg daily to 8 mg daily. Two weeks after stopping St John's wort, tacrolimus doses were reduced to a median of 6.5 mg daily, and then to the original dose of 4.5 mg daily after about 4 weeks.[2]

A case report describes a 65-year-old patient taking tacrolimus following a kidney transplant. The patient started to take St John's wort (*Neuroplant*) 600 mg daily, and after one month the tacrolimus trough blood levels had dropped from a range of 6 to 10 nanograms/mL down to 1.6 nanograms/mL, with an unexpected improvement in creatinine levels. When the St John's wort was stopped, tacrolimus levels and creatinine returned to the previous range. Subsequently a lower target range of tacrolimus was set.[3]

Mechanism

St John's wort induces the cytochrome P450 isoenzyme CYP3A4 and affects the transporter protein P-glycoprotein. CYP3A4 and P-glycoprotein are involved in the metabolism and clearance of tacrolimus, so an increase in their effects would be expected to result in a decrease in tacrolimus levels.[1,3]

Importance and management

Although the evidence currently seems limited to these reports the interaction between tacrolimus and St John's wort has been predicted from the pharmacokinetics of these two drugs. Given the unpredictability of the interaction (and the variability in content of St John's wort products) it would seem prudent to avoid St John's wort in transplant patients, and possibly other types of patient taking tacrolimus. If St John's wort is started or stopped, monitor tacrolimus levels and adjust the dose accordingly.

1. Hebert MF, Park JM, Chen Y-L, Akhtar S, Larson AM. Effects of St John's wort (Hypericum perforatum) on tacrolimus pharmacokinetics in healthy volunteers. *J Clin Pharmacol* (2004) 44, 89–94.
2. Mai I, Störmer E, Bauer S, Krüger H, Budde K, Roots I. Impact of St John's wort treatment on the pharmacokinetics of tacrolimus and mycophenolic acid in renal transplant patients. *Nephrol Dial Transplant* (2003) 18, 819–22.
3. Bolley R, Zülke C, Kammerl M, Fischereder M, Krämer BK. Tacrolimus-induced nephrotoxicity unmasked by induction of the CYP3A4 system with St John's wort. *Transplantation* (2002) 73, 1009.

Tacrolimus + Theophylline

An isolated report suggests that theophylline may increase tacrolimus blood levels.

Clinical evidence

A kidney transplant patient taking tacrolimus 7 mg daily was given theophylline 600 mg daily to treat post-transplant erythrocytosis. After 1 month serum creatinine increased from 110 to 145 micromol/L and the tacrolimus trough blood level increased to 16 nanograms/mL, from a range of 5 to 15 nanograms/mL. The theophylline dosage was reduced to 300 mg daily on 4 days of each week and one month later the serum creatinine was 175 micromol/L and the trough tacrolimus level was 48.5 nanograms/mL. Theophylline was discontinued and the renal function and trough tacrolimus levels rapidly returned to normal. The pharmacokinetics of tacrolimus were later assessed in the same patient. Theophylline 125 mg daily for 4 days was associated with an almost five-fold increase in the AUC of tacrolimus and an increase in the peak tacrolimus blood levels from 19.3 to 37.4 nanograms/mL, without significant alterations in renal function on this occasion.[1]

Mechanism

Unclear. An *in vitro* study found that tacrolimus and theophylline each exhibited a negligible effect on the metabolism of the other drug.[2] However, the authors of the case report suggest that theophylline levels in their patient could have been sufficient to inhibit the cytochrome P450 isoenzyme-mediated metabolism of tacrolimus.[1]

Importance and management

Direct information seems to be limited to this single case report. The authors conclude that low-dose theophylline may be given to transplant patients with erythrocytosis provided that tacrolimus levels are closely monitored.[1] However, this interaction is unconfirmed and of uncertain clinical significance. There is insufficient evidence to recommend increased monitoring in every patient, but be aware of the potential for an interaction in the case of an unexpected response to treatment.

1. Boubenider S, Vincent I, Lambotte O, Roy S, Hiesse C, Taburet A-M, Charpentier B. Interaction between theophylline and tacrolimus in a renal transplant patient. *Nephrol Dial Transplant* (2000) 15, 1066–8.
2. Matsuda H, Iwasaki K, Shiraga T, Tozuka Z, Hata T, Guengerich FP. Interactions of FK506 (tacrolimus) with clinically important drugs. *Res Commun Mol Pathol Pharmacol* (1996) 91, 57–64.

30

Lipid regulating drugs

This section is concerned with the drugs that are used for dyslipidaemias (i.e. disturbed levels of lipids in the blood). In the very broadest of terms (and ideally) they lower the blood levels of cholesterol and low-density lipoprotein (LDL), and raise those of high-density lipoprotein (HDL). Such drugs include the statins (more properly known as HMG-CoA (hydroxymethylglutaryl-coenzyme A) reductase inhibitors), fibrates, ezetimibe, bile-acid binding resins (e.g. colestipol, colestyramine) and nicotinic acid (niacin) and related drugs. These are listed in 'Table 30.1', (below). Where lipid regulating drugs affect other drugs the interactions are covered elsewhere.

Table 30.1 Lipid-regulating drugs

Group	*Drugs*
Bile-acid binding resins	Colesevelam, Colestilan, Colestipol, Colestyramine
Fibrates	Bezafibrate, Ciprofibrate, Clofibrate, Fenofibrate, Gemfibrozil
Statins	Atorvastatin, Fluvastatin, Lovastatin, Pravastatin, Rosuvastatin, Simvastatin
Miscellaneous	Acipimox, Ezetimibe, Nicotinic acid, Omega-3 marine triglycerides

(a) Statins

1. Muscle toxicity. Statins are generally well-tolerated, but have two major but relatively uncommon adverse effects. They raise liver enzymes and can cause skeletal muscle disorders (e.g. myalgia, myopathy and rhabdomyolysis). Rhabdomyolysis is a syndrome resulting from skeletal muscle injury, which results in the release of the enzyme creatine kinase (among other things) into the circulation. Creatine kinase (CK) is also known as creatine phosphokinase (CPK). Both terms are used throughout the text, the choice being dependent on the term used in the source quoted. Rhabdomyolysis can range from asymptomatic elevations in creatine kinase to acute renal failure, and in its severest form may be life-threatening. As well as elevated creatinine kinase levels, signs and symptoms of rhabdomyolysis include muscle pain and weakness, reddish-brown urine (myoglobinuria).[1]

Just how statins cause muscle disorders is as yet unclear, although it is thought to be connected to elevated statin levels.[2] Any pharmacokinetic interaction that results in a marked rise in statin levels is therefore to be regarded seriously.

One of the ways blood statin levels can become elevated is if the interacting drug inhibits the metabolism of the statin, with the result that it is cleared from the body more slowly and it begins to accumulate (see pharmacokinetics below). The overall risk of myopathy with the statins is quite low and commonly quoted as 0.5%, although one report[3] puts the incidence of mild myopathies with a statin alone as up to 7%. The incidence seems to rise markedly if other drugs are being taken concurrently. Thus a literature review of published reports for the period 1985 to 2000 found 15 cases of rhabdomyolysis with statins alone, but 54 cases when combined with other drugs.[2] Other patient-related risk factors for myopathy include:[4]

- age greater than 80 years,
- frailty,
- multisystem disease (e.g. chronic renal impairment),
- perioperative periods,
- hypothyroidism,
- alcohol abuse,
- female sex.

In order to reduce the risk of myopathy the CSM in the UK have advised that statins should be used with care in patients who are at increased risk of this adverse effect. Among other risk factors, they mention concomitant use with fibrates, such as 'gemfibrozil', (p.1100), and with inhibitors of CYP3A4 such as 'ciclosporin', (p.1097), 'macrolides', (p.1104), 'azoles', (p.1093), and 'protease inhibitors', (p.1108). They also recommend that patients should be made aware of the risks of myopathy and rhabdomyolysis, and asked to promptly report muscle pain, tenderness, or weakness, especially if accompanied by malaise, fever, or dark urine.[5] A 2002 advisory[4] on the use of statins gives some important safety recommendations, which are useful in the context of interactions:

- Routine monitoring of creatinine kinase is of little value in the absence of clinical symptoms.
- If a patient has a creatinine kinase value 10 times the upper limit of normal, and is symptomatic, statin treatment should be immediately discontinued (if also taking a fibrate or nicotinic acid these too should be discontinued).
- If a patient has symptoms of muscle pain with a creatinine kinase of up to 10 times the upper limit of normal they should be monitored closely until either symptoms resolve of the creatinine kinase becomes greater than 10 times the upper limit of normal.
- If progressive creatinine kinase elevations occur consider a dose reduction or temporary discontinuation of the statin.
- Liver enzyme values of up to 3 times the upper limit of normal do not represent a contraindication to treatment but patients should be carefully monitored.

2. Pharmacokinetics. Lovastatin and simvastatin are extensively metabolised by the cytochrome P450 isoenzyme CYP3A4 so that drugs that can inhibit this enzyme can cause marked rises in blood statin levels. Atorvastatin is also metabolised by CYP3A4, but to a lesser extent than lovastatin or simvastatin. Some of the statins are not metabolised by this enzyme so they interact differently. Fluvastatin is metabolised primarily by CYP2C9 (with a minor contribution from CYP3A4), 10% of rosuvastatin is metabolised, and the isoenzymes involved appear to be CYP2C9 and CYP2C19, while the cytochrome P450 system does not appear to be involved in the metabolism of pravastatin.[6]

The statins are also P-glycoprotein substrates, and may therefore interact due to competition for this carrier, generally resulting in altered oral bioavailability.[6] However, *in vitro* study has suggested that, due to the low affinity of atorvastatin and simvastatin for P-glycoprotein this is unlikely to be a clinically significant cause of statin drug interactions.[7] Some metabolites of atorvastatin, lovastatin and simvastatin have been shown to inhibit P-glycoprotein, while fluvastatin and pravastatin seem to have little effect.[8] There appears to be no data on the effect of rosuvastatin on P-glycoprotein.[9]

(b) Bile-acid binding resins

Bile-acid binding resins lower cholesterol by binding with bile acids in the gastrointestinal tract to form an insoluble complex that is excreted in the faeces. This predisposes them to interactions by binding with other drugs in the same way as they do with bile acids, which prevents absorption or local action of the affected drug. These binding interactions are not covered here, but are covered under the affected drugs. A new bile-acid binding resin, colesevelam, is supposed to be devoid of clinically significant drug-binding interactions.[10]

(c) Ezetimibe

Ezetimibe is a cholesterol absorption inhibitor, and, as the name suggests, it and the major metabolite, ezetimibe glucuronide, impair the intestinal absorption of cholesterol, both from the diet and biliary cholesterol.[11] The absorption of other fats is not affected. Ezetimibe has not been found to have significant effects on cytochrome P450, suggesting it is unlikely to interact by this mechanism.

(d) Fibrates

Fibrates are protein-bound drugs that are metabolised via the cytochrome P450 isoenzyme CYP3A4. They are not generally recognised as inhibitors of this enzyme. Although protein binding contributes to their interactions, this mechanism alone does not usually lead to serious interactions. This leaves their mechanism of interaction largely unexplained, although it has been suggested that they may act as inhibitors of glucuronidation.[12] As with the statins (see above), fibrates are also recognised as causing myopathies, and the risk of this appears to be greatly increased when they are given with statins, see 'Statins + Fibrates', p.1100.

(e) Nicotinic acid

Nicotinic acid has little effect on the cytochrome P450 isoenzyme system and is therefore unlikely to result in significant pharmacokinetic interactions. It also appears to increase the risk of myopathies when given with statins, see 'Statins + Nicotinic acid (Niacin)', p.1106. Also note that although no interaction has been generally shown with **acipimox** the manufacturers recommend caution with drugs that interact with nicotinic acid.[13] This is because nicotinic acid is an analog of **acipimox**, and so may share its interactions.

1. Allison RC, Bedsole DL. The other medical causes of rhabdomyolysis. *Am J Med Sci* (2003) 326, 79–88.
2. Omar MA, Wilson JP, Cox TS. Rhabdomyolysis and HMG-CoA reductase inhibitors. *Ann Pharmacother* (2001) 35, 1096–1107.
3. Ucar M, Mjorndal T, Dahlqvist R, HMG CoA reductase inhibitors and myotoxicity. *Drug Safety* (2000) 22, 441–57.
4. Pasternak RC, Smith SC, Bairey-Merz CN, Grundy SM, Cleeman JI, Lenfant C. ACC/AHA/NHLBI clinical advisory on the use and safety of statins. *J Am Coll Cardiol* (2002) 40, 567–72.
5. Committee on Safety of Medicines/Medicines Control Agency. HMG CoA reductase inhibitors (statins) and myopathy. *Current Problems* (2002) 28, 8–9.
6. Williams D, Feely J. Pharmacokinetic-pharmacodynamic drug interactions with HMG-CoA reductase inhibitors. *Clin Pharmacokinet* (2002) 41, 343–70.
7. Hochman JH, Pudvah N, Qiu J, Yamazaki M, Tang C, Lin JH, Prueksaritanont T. Interactions of human P-glycoprotein with simvastatin, simvastatin acid, and atorvastatin. *Pharm Res* (2004) 21, 1686–91.
8. Bogman K, Peyer AK, Torok M, Kusters E, Drewe J. HMG-CoA reductase inhibitors and P-glycoprotein modulation. *Br J Pharmacol* (2001) 132, 1183–92.
9. Roach AE, Tsikouris JP, Haase KK. Rosuvastatin. A new HMG-CoA reductase inhibitor for hypercholesterolemia. *Formulary* (2002) 37, 179–85.
10. Donovan JM, Stypinski D, Stiles MR, Olson TA, Burke SK. Drug interactions with colesevelam hydrochloride, a novel, potent lipid-lowering agent. *Cardiovasc Drugs Ther* (2000) 14, 681–90.
11. Simard C, Turgeon J. The pharmacokinetics of ezetimibe. *Can J Clin Pharmacol* (2003) 10 (Suppl A), 13A–20A.
12. Prueksaritanont T, Zhao JJ, Ma B, Roadcap BA, Tang C, Qui Y, Liu L, Lin JH, Pearson PG, Baillie TA. Mechanistic studies on metabolic interactions between gemfibrozil and statins. *J Pharmacol Exp Ther* (2002) 301, 1042–51.
13. Olbetam (Acipimox). Pharmacia Ltd. UK Summary of product characteristics, March 2007.

Acipimox + Colestyramine

Colestyramine does not appear to significantly affect the pharmacokinetics of acipimox.

Clinical evidence, mechanism, importance and management

A randomised crossover study in 7 healthy subjects given acipimox 150 mg with three 4-g doses of colestyramine (taken concurrently, and then 8 and 16 hours later) found that the pharmacokinetics of acipimox were slightly but not significantly altered by the colestyramine.[1] There would seem to be no good reason for avoiding concurrent use.

1. de Paolis C, Farina R, Pianezzola E, Valzelli G, Celotti F, Pontiroli AE. Lack of pharmacokinetic interaction between cholestyramine and acipimox, a new lipid lowering agent. *Br J Clin Pharmacol* (1986) 22, 496–7.

Colestyramine + Food

A study in 10 patients with type IIA hyperlipoproteinaemia found that the efficacy of colestyramine in controlling total cholesterol and low density lipoprotein levels was unaltered whether the colestyramine was taken with or before meals.[1]

1. Sirtori M, Pazzucconi F, Gianfranceschi G, Sirtori CR. Efficacy of cholestyramine does not vary when taken before or during meals. *Atherosclerosis* (1991) 88, 249–52.

Ezetimibe + Ciclosporin

The levels of ezetimibe and possibly ciclosporin may be elevated by their concurrent use, and so the combination should be used with caution.

Clinical evidence, mechanism, importance and management

A randomised, crossover study in 12 healthy subjects found that ezetimibe 20 mg daily for 8 days increased the AUC of a single 100-mg dose of ciclosporin by 15%. The authors noted that it would be difficult to determine the outcome of long-term concurrent use, but the modest effect seen suggested that caution was necessary if the combination was given.[1] However, an efficacy study noted that in 16 renal transplant patients the addition of ezetimibe 10 mg daily had no effect on ciclosporin levels.[2]

In one study, 8 stable renal transplant patients taking ciclosporin were given a single 10-mg dose of ezetimibe. When compared with other data from healthy control subjects, the AUC of ezetimibe was found to be 3.4-fold higher in the patients taking ciclosporin.[3] A further patient with severe renal impairment taking multiple drugs, including ciclosporin, had a 12-fold increase in the AUC of ezetimibe.[3] A case report describes a heart transplant patient taking ciclosporin 100 mg twice daily with atorvastatin 40 mg daily. As his LDL-cholesterol was inadequately lowered by the atorvastatin, and greater doses had not been tolerated due to elevated creatine kinase levels, ezetimibe 10 mg daily was added. His LDL-cholesterol then decreased from 126 mg/dL to 51 mg/dL (target less than 100 mg/dL), and so his dose of ezetimibe was decreased to 5 mg daily.[4] The authors of this case report note that only about 50% of heart transplant patients are able to achieve LDL-cholesterol of less than 100 mg/dL and attribute the effects seen in their patient to an interaction. However, the validity of any interaction has been debated,[5,6] and an efficacy study in which renal transplant patients taking ciclosporin and a statin were given ezetimibe 10 mg daily noted an enhanced but not excessive effect on lipids.[2]

Therefore it seems that ciclosporin can greatly raise ezetimibe levels, possibly resulting in an increased effect on lipid reduction, and that ciclosporin levels can be raised, possibly significantly in some patients, by ezetimibe. If concurrent use is necessary, until the effects of concurrent treatment are better established, it would seem prudent to monitor both ciclosporin levels and the effects on lipid levels, anticipating the need to reduce the dosage of either drug. The authors of the case report cited suggest that, in patients taking ciclosporin, ezetimibe should be started at a dose of 5 mg daily or less and slowly titrated upwards.[6]

1. Bergman AJ, Burke J, Larson P, Johnson-Levonas AO, Reyderman L, Statkevich P, Kosoglou T, Greenberg HE, Kraft WK, Frick G, Murphy G, Gottesdiener K, Paolini JF. Effects of ezetimibe on cyclosporine pharmacokinetics in healthy subjects. *J Clin Pharmacol* (2006) 46, 321–7.
2. Kohnle M, Pietruck F, Kribben A, Philipp T, Heemann U, Witzke O. Ezetimibe for the treatment of uncontrolled hypercholesterolemia in patients with high-dose statin therapy after renal transplantation. *Am J Transplant* (2006) 205–8.
3. Bergman AJ, Burke J, Larson P, Johnson-Levonas AO, Reyderman L, Statkevich P, Maxwell SE, Kosoglou T, Murphy G, Gottesdiener K, Robson R, Paolini JF. Interaction of single-dose ezetimibe and steady-state cyclosporine in renal transplant patients. *J Clin Pharmacol* (2006) 46, 328–36.
4. Koshman SL, Lalonde LD, Burton I, Tymchak WJ, Pearson GJ. Supratherapeutic response to ezetimibe administered with cyclosporine. *Ann Pharmacother* (2005) 39, 1561–5.
5. Ito MK. Comment: supratherapeutic response to ezetimibe administered with cyclosporine. *Ann Pharmacother* (2005) 39, 2141.
6. Pearson GJ, Koshman SL, Lalonde LD, Burton I, Tymchak WJ. Comment: supratherapeutic response to ezetimibe administered with cyclosporine. Author's reply. *Ann Pharmacother* (2005) 39, 2142.

Ezetimibe + Colestyramine

In a study of 40 healthy hypercholesterolaemic subjects, colestyramine 4 g twice daily decreased the mean AUC of ezetimibe by about 80% and decreased the mean AUC of total ezetimibe (ezetimibe plus metabolites) by about 55%.[1] Colestyramine may therefore be expected to decrease the lipid-lowering effects of ezetimibe. Note that ezetimibe undergoes enterohepatic recirculation, so separating administration may not fully resolve this interaction.

1. Zetia (Ezetimibe). Merck/Schering-Plough Pharmaceuticals. US Prescribing information, June 2007.

Ezetimibe + Rifampicin (Rifampin)

Single-dose rifampicin increases ezetimibe levels without altering its effects on sterols, whereas multiple doses of rifampicin decrease ezetimibe levels and almost totally abolish its effects.

Clinical evidence

In a single-dose study investigating the disposition of ezetimibe 8 healthy subjects were given ezetimibe 20 mg with rifampicin 600 mg. Rifampicin increased the ezetimibe maximum serum levels by about 2.5-fold, without affecting the AUC. The maximum serum levels of ezetimibe glucuronide (the major active metabolite of ezetimibe) were similarly increased, and its AUC was also increased, by about twofold. The sterol-lowering effects of ezetimibe were also more rapid in the presence of rifampicin, but the overall effect was unchanged, possibly because ezetimibe and its glucuronide were excreted more rapidly.[1] In another study by the same researchers ezetimibe 20 mg was given 12 hours after the last dose of an 8-day course of rifampicin 600 mg daily. This time both the AUC and maximum serum levels of ezetimibe and its glucuronide were *decreased* (AUC decreased by more than 50%) and the effect of ezetimibe on sterols was almost completely abolished.[2]

Mechanism

The raised ezetimibe levels seen in the single-dose study are thought to occur because rifampicin enhances the absorption of ezetimibe, probably by inhibiting intestinal P-glycoprotein, and another transporter protein, MRP2. However, inhibition of MRP2 appears to reduce enterohepatic circulation, which is needed for the long duration of ezetimibe effects, and therefore shortens the sterol-lowering effects of ezetimibe.[1] It seems likely that the balance of these factors is altered when rifampicin is given in multiple doses, which leads to a reduction in the effects of ezetimibe. Other factors are possibly also involved.[2]

Importance and management

Information about the interaction between ezetimibe and rifampicin appears to be limited to these studies, which were primarily designed to investigate ezetimibe disposition. However, it seems likely that the effects of ezetimibe will be reduced in patients who are also given multiple doses of rifampicin. If both drugs are given it would be prudent to closely monitor the effects on lipid levels.

1. Oswald S, Giessmann T, Luetjohann D, Wegner D, Rosskopf D, Weitschies W, Siegmund W. Disposition and sterol-lowering effect of ezetimibe are influenced by single-dose coadministration of rifampin, an inhibitor of multidrug transport proteins. *Clin Pharmacol Ther* (2006) 80, 477–85.
2. Oswald S, Haenisch S, Fricke C, Sudhop T, Remmler C, Giessmann T, Jedlitschky G, Adam U, Dazert E, Warzok R, Wacke W, Cascorbi I, Kroemer HK, Weitschies W, von Bergmann K, Siegmund W. Intestinal expression of P-glycoprotein (*ABCB1*), multidrug resistance associated protein 2 (*ABCC2*), and uridine diphosphate–glucuronosyltransferase 1A1 predicts the disposition and modulates the effects of the cholesterol absorption inhibitor ezetimibe in humans. *Clin Pharmacol Ther* (2006) 79, 206–17.

Fibrates + Bile-acid binding resins

Colestyramine does not alter the pharmacokinetics of clofibrate when both drugs are given at the same time. Similarly colestipol does not alter the pharmacokinetics of clofibrate or fenofibrate, and colesevelam does not alter the pharmacokinetics of fenofibrate. Colestipol can reduce the absorption of gemfibrozil if given at the same time, but not if administration is separated by 2 hours. A similar interaction occurs between bezafibrate and colestyramine

Clinical evidence, mechanism, importance and management

(a) Bezafibrate

The manufacturers of bezafibrate recommend that there should be a 2-hour interval between administration of [drugs such as **colestyramine**] and bezafibrate, as the absorption of bezafibrate may otherwise be impaired.[1]

(b) Clofibrate

Over a 6-day period no clinically relevant changes in the pharmacokinetics of clofibrate occurred in 24 healthy subjects, who were given daily doses of **colestipol** 10 g at the same time as clofibrate 500 mg.[2] **Colestyramine** 4 g four times daily had no effect on the fasting plasma levels, urinary and faecal excretion, or the half-life of clofibrate in 6 patients taking 1 g of clofibrate twice daily. In this study, the morning and evening doses of **colestyramine** were taken at the same time as the clofibrate.[3]

(c) Fenofibrate

Over a 6-day period no clinically relevant changes in the pharmacokinetics of fenofibrate occurred in 18 healthy subjects, who were given daily doses of **colestipol** 10 g at the same time as fenofibrate 200 mg in the morning, and **colestipol** 5 g at the same time as fenofibrate 100 mg in the evening.[4] In a randomised, crossover study 27 healthy subjects took fenofibrate 160 mg with **colesevelam** 3.75 g, four hours before **colesevelam**, or alone. **Colesevelam** caused some slight changes in the pharmacokinetics of fenofibrate when both drugs were given simultaneously but this was not considered to be clinically significant.[5]

(d) Gemfibrozil

A study in 10 patients with raised serum cholesterol and triglyceride levels found that if gemfibrozil 600 mg was given alone, 2 hours before or 2 hours after **colestipol** 5 g, the serum gemfibrozil concentration curves were similar. However, when both drugs were given at the same time, the AUC of gemfibrozil was reduced by about a third.[6] Another study found that combined use of gemfibrozil and **colestipol** (doses not separated) enhanced the LDL-lowering effects of both drugs, but tended to mitigate the HDL-raising effects of the gemfibrozil.[7] Combined use is effective, but information is very limited about the clinical importance of the reduction in gemfibrozil bioavailability. However, the interaction can be avoided by separating the administration of the two drugs by at least 2 hours.

1. Bezalip (Bezafibrate). Roche Products Ltd. UK Summary of product characteristics, November 2005.
2. DeSante KA, DiSante AR, Albert KS, Weber DJ, Welch RD, Vecchio TJ. The effect of colestipol hydrochloride on the bioavailability and pharmacokinetics of clofibrate. *J Clin Pharmacol* (1979) 19, 721–25.
3. Sedaghat A, Ahrens EH. Lack of effect of cholestyramine on the pharmacokinetics of clofibrate in man. *Eur J Clin Invest* (1975) 5, 177–85.
4. Harvengt C, Desager JP. Lack of pharmacokinetic interaction of colestipol and fenofibrate in volunteers. *Eur J Clin Pharmacol* (1980) 17, 459–63.
5. Jones MR, Baker BA, Mathew P. Effect of colesevelam HCl on single-dose fenofibrate pharmacokinetics. *Clin Pharmacokinet* (2004) 43, 943–50.
6. Forland SC, Feng Y, Cutler RE. Apparent reduced absorption of gemfibrozil when given with colestipol. *J Clin Pharmacol* (1990) 30, 29–32.
7. East C, Bilheimer DW, Grundy SM. Combination drug therapy for familial combined hyperlipidemia. *Ann Intern Med* (1988) 109, 25–32.

Fibrates + Colchicine

Case reports suggest that the current use of fibrates and colchicine can result in rhabdomyolysis or neuromyopathy.

Clinical evidence

A 40-year-old man with chronic hepatitis and nephritic syndrome, who had been taking colchicine 500 micrograms three times daily uneventfully for 2 to 3 years, started taking **gemfibrozil** 600 mg twice daily. About one month later he presented with muscle pain and dark brown urine, and had a creatinine kinase of 3 559 units/L, and he was diagnosed as having rhabdomyolysis. Both drugs were stopped, and he recovered over the following 9 days.[1] Another case report describes neuromyopathy (creatinine kinase level 15 084 units/L), in a patient who had been taking **bezafibrate** 400 mg daily with colchicine 3 mg daily for 14 days.[2] This patient was known to have renal impairment.

Mechanism

Colchicine alone can, rarely, cause myopathy. However, it is more common in those given colchicine long term (as in the case with gemfibrozil), in high dose, or in the presence or renal impairment (as in the case with bezafibrate).[2] As the fibrates can also, rarely, cause myopathy, an additive or synergistic effect seems possible.

Importance and management

Although information seems limited to these two cases, the effects seen are known to be associated with both colchicine and the fibrates, so an interaction, all be it rare, seems to be established. It would be prudent to suspect this interaction in any patient presenting with muscle pain or a raised creatinine kinase level. The section on 'muscle toxicity', (p.1086), discusses risk factors for myopathy and it would seem prudent to be aware of these, as both patients in the cases above had other risk factors for rhabdomyolysis.

1. Atmacca H, Sayarlioğu, Külah E, Demircan N, Akpolat T. Rhabdomyolysis associated with gemfibrozil-colchicine therapy. *Ann Pharmacother* (2002) 36, 1719–21.
2. Sugie M, Kuriki A, Arai D, Ichikawa H, Kawamura M. A case report of acute neuromyopathy induced by concomitant use of colchicine and bezafibrate. *No To Shinkei* (2005) 57, 785–90.

Fibrates + Diuretics

Treatment with clofibrate in patients with nephrotic syndrome receiving furosemide has sometimes led to marked diuresis and severe and disabling adverse muscular effects. An isolated report describes rhabdomyolysis in a patient taking bezafibrate and furosemide.

Clinical evidence

(a) Bezafibrate

An isolated report attributed a case of acute renal failure and rhabdomyolysis to treatment with bezafibrate 400 mg daily and **furosemide** 25 mg on alternate days.[1]

(b) Clofibrate

Three patients with hyperlipoproteinaemia secondary to nephrotic syndrome, taking **furosemide** 80 to 500 mg daily, developed severe muscle pain, low lumbar backache, stiffness, and general malaise with pronounced diuresis within 3 days of starting to take clofibrate 1 to 2 g daily. Similarly, a patient taking **bendroflumethiazide** 10 mg daily developed adverse muscle effects within 3 days of starting clofibrate. Of these 4 patients, 3 had documented raised serum transaminases or creatine phosphokinase.

Two other patients had raised levels of serum transaminases or creatine phosphokinase while taking clofibrate with **furosemide**.

A further study in 4 of the 6 patients discussed above and 4 healthy controls, free serum clofibrate was markedly higher in the patients, and this correlated with low serum albumin. Urinary clofibrate excretion was markedly delayed.[2]

Mechanism

Not understood. The marked diuresis may have been due to competition and displacement of the furosemide by the clofibrate from its plasma protein binding sites. Clofibrate occasionally causes a muscle toxicity, which could have been exacerbated by the urinary loss of Na^+ and K^+ and the increase in the half-life of clofibrate. The reason for the bezafibrate/furosemide-induced rhabdomyolysis is unknown.

Importance and management

The clinical documentation seems to be limited to these reports. It appears to be a combination of a drug-drug interaction (clofibrate with furosemide) with or without a drug-disease interaction (clofibrate with nephrotic syndrome). The authors of one report[2] suggest that serum proteins and renal function should be checked before giving clofibrate to any patient. If serum albumin is low, the total daily dosage of clofibrate should not exceed 500 mg for each 1 g per 100 mL of the albumin concentration. However, note that this guidance is old.

1. Venzano C, Cordì GC, Corsi L, Dapelo M, De Micheli A, Grimaldi GP. Un caso di rabdomiolisi acuta con insufficienza renale acuta da assunzione contemporanea di furosemide e bezafibrato. *Minerva Med* (1990) 81, 909–11.
2. Bridgman JF, Rosen SM, Thorp JM. Complications during clofibrate treatment of nephrotic-syndrome hyperlipoproteinaemia. *Lancet* (1972) ii, 506–9.

Fibrates + Ezetimibe

Ezetimibe does not alter fenofibrate or gemfibrozil pharmacokinetics. Fenofibrate and gemfibrozil may modestly increase ezetimibe levels, although this is unlikely to be clinically relevant. The manufacturers currently advise caution if ezetimibe is given with a fibrate, because of the theoretical increased risk of gallstone formation.

Clinical evidence

(a) Fenofibrate

In a randomised, crossover study 18 healthy subjects were given ezetimibe 10 mg daily with fenofibrate 145 mg daily for 10 days, or either drug alone. Ezetimibe did not affect the AUC of fenofibrate, and, although fenofibrate increased the total AUC of ezetimibe and ezetimibe-glucuronide by 1.5-fold this was not considered to be clinically significant.[1] This expectation appears to have largely been borne out by safety studies. In a randomised, placebo-controlled study, 32 otherwise healthy patients with hypercholesterolaemia were given fenofibrate 200 mg daily, ezetimibe 10 mg daily, both drugs in combination, or placebo daily for 14 days. The combination was well-tolerated, and resulted in an increased reduction in LDL-cholesterol than that achieved by either active drug alone. Concurrent use did not affect the pharmacokinetics of either drug.[2] A further efficacy and safety study in 172 patients taking ezetimibe 10 mg daily with fenofibrate 160 mg daily, found that there was a trend towards increased treatment-related adverse effects, when compared with patients taking either drug alone. However, the incidence of musculoskeletal disorders was similar.[3]

(b) Gemfibrozil

In a randomised, crossover study 12 healthy subjects were given ezetimibe 10 mg daily with gemfibrozil 600 mg twice daily for 7 days, or either drug alone. Ezetimibe did not affect the AUC of gemfibrozil, and, although gemfibrozil increased the total AUC of ezetimibe and ezetimibe glucuronide by about 1.7-fold this was not considered to be clinically significant.[4].

Mechanism, importance and management

Despite these seemingly favourable results, the UK manufacturers of ezetimibe state that the safety of combined use with fibrates is not yet established. This is because both fibrates and ezetimibe increase cholesterol excretion into the bile, which could promote the production of gallstones.[5] They say that if gallstones or gall bladder disease is suspected then the combination should be discontinued.

1. Gustavson LE, Schweitzer SM, Burt DA, Achari R, Rieser MJ, Edeki T, Chira T, Yannicelli HD, Kelly MT. Evaluation of the potential for pharmacokinetic interaction between fenofibrate and ezetimibe: a phase I, open-label, multiple-dose, three-period crossover study in healthy subjects. *Clin Ther* (2006) 28, 373–87.
2. Kosoglou T, Guillaume M, Sun S, Pember LJC, Reyderman L, Statkevich P, Cutler DL, Veltri EP, Affrime MB. Pharmacodynamic interaction between fenofibrate and the cholesterol absorption inhibitor ezetimibe. *Atherosclerosis* (2001) 2 (Suppl 2), 38.
3. Farnier M, Freeman MW, Macdonell G, Perevozskaya I, Davies MJ, Mitchel YB, Gumbiner B for the Ezetimibe Study Group. Efficacy and safety of the coadministration of ezetimibe with fenofibrate in patients with mixed hyperlipidaemia. *Eur Heart J* (2005) 26, 897–905.
4. Reyderman L, Kosoglou T, Statkevich P, Pember L, Boutros T, Maxwell SE, Affrime M, Batra V. Assessment of a multiple-dose drug interaction between ezetimibe, a novel selective cholesterol absorption inhibitor and gemfibrozil. *Int J Clin Pharmacol Ther* (2004) 42, 512–18.
5. Ezetrol (Ezetimibe). MSD-SP Ltd. UK Summary of product characteristics, December 2006.

Fibrates + Nifedipine

It has been suggested that three cases of rhabdomyolysis occurred because of an interaction between bezafibrate and nifedipine, but it seems more likely that the dose of bezafibrate was too high.

Clinical evidence, mechanism, importance and management

Rhabdomyolysis developed in 4 of 5 patients undergoing CAPD, who were given **bezafibrate** 200 to 400 mg daily for raised cholesterol and triglyceride levels. Of these, 3 patients were also taking nifedipine, and one of these 3 was also taking lovastatin. Raised creatinine kinase levels developed within 8 to 16 days of concurrent use, and resolved within 48 hours of stopping the **bezafibrate**. The authors suggest that nifedipine may have competed with **bezafibrate** for metabolism by the cytochrome P450 isoenzyme CYP3A4. They therefore say that patients with renal failure needing a fibrate should avoid taking CYP3A4 substrates.[1] However, as the recommended dose for **bezafibrate** in CAPD patients is 200 mg every 72 hours[2] it appears likely that the high dose, and not an interaction, was responsible for the rhabdomyolysis. No precautions therefore seem necessary.

1. Weissgarten J, Zaidenstein R, Fishman S, Dishi V, Michovitz-Koren M, Averbukh Z, Golik A. *Perit Dial Int* (1999) 19, 180–2.
2. Ashley C, Currie A, ed. The Renal Drug Handbook. 2nd ed. Oxford: Radcliffe Medical Press; 2004. p62.

Fibrates + Rifampicin (Rifampin)

Preliminary evidence suggests that rifampicin can reduce the plasma levels of the active metabolite of clofibrate, but rifampicin apparently has no effect on gemfibrozil pharmacokinetics.

Clinical evidence, mechanism, importance and management

(a) Clofibrate

A 35% reduction in the steady-state plasma levels of the active metabolite of clofibrate, chlorophenoxyisobutyric acid (CIPB), was seen in 5 healthy subjects after they took rifampicin 600 mg daily for 7 days.[1] This appears to occur because the metabolism of CIPB by the liver and/or the kidneys is increased.[1] On the basis of this study it would now be prudent to monitor serum lipid levels of patients taking clofibrate if rifampicin is added, and to increase the clofibrate dosage if necessary. More study is needed to establish this interaction.

(b) Gemfibrozil

Rifampicin 600 mg daily for 6 days did not significantly affect the pharmacokinetics of gemfibrozil 600 mg in a study in 10 healthy subjects.[2] No special precautions seem necessary.

1. Houin G, Tillement J-P. Clofibrate and enzymatic induction in man. *Int J Clin Pharmacol Ther Toxicol* (1978) 16, 150–4.
2. Forland SC, Feng Y, Cutler RE. The effect of rifampin on the pharmacokinetics of gemfibrozil. *J Clin Pharmacol* (1988) 28, 930.

Fibrates; Ciprofibrate + Ibuprofen

An isolated report describes a patient taking ciprofibrate who developed acute renal failure and rhabdomyolysis after taking ibuprofen.

Clinical evidence, mechanism, importance and management

A 29-year-old man with type M hyperlipidaemia[1] who had been taking ciprofibrate 100 mg daily for 6 months began to take ibuprofen 200 mg and then 400 mg daily for a painful heel. The pain became general, his urine turned 'muddy', he complained of having a 'stiff body', and he rapidly developed acute renal failure. His serum creatinine concentration was found to be 647 micromol/L and his creatine kinase was 13 740 units/L.

The reasons for this reaction are not known, but the authors of the report postulate that the ibuprofen displaced the ciprofibrate from its binding sites, thereby turning a safe dose into a toxic one.[1] However, it should be said that this mechanism of interaction is rarely important on its own, so it seems likely that some other factors may have contributed to what happened.

This is an isolated case so that its general importance is unknown, but it is probably very small.

1. Ramachandran S, Giles PD, Hartland A. Acute renal failure due to rhabdomyolysis in presence of concurrent ciprofibrate and ibuprofen treatment. *BMJ* (1997) 314, 1593.

Fibrates; Clofibrate + Hormonal contraceptives

Oral contraceptives increase the clearance of clofibrate but the significance of this is unclear.

Clinical evidence, mechanism, importance and management

A comparative study in men, women, and women taking combined oral contraceptives found that the clearance of clofibrate was increased by 48% in those taking combined oral contraceptives, apparently due to an increase in clofibrate glucuronidation.[1] Another study found that combined oral contraceptives increased the excretion of clofibric acid glucuronide (the pharmacologically active form of clofibrate) by 25%.[2] None of these studies addressed the question of whether concurrent use significantly reduces clofibrate efficacy, but it would seem prudent to monitor for increases in blood lipid levels. It should be noted that combined oral contraceptives themselves can have various adverse effects on lipid levels, and these may impair the effects of treatment.

1. Miners JO, Robson RA, Birkett DJ. Gender and oral contraceptive steroids as determinants of drug glucuronidation: effects on clofibric acid elimination. *Br J Clin Pharmacol* (1984) 18, 240–43.
2. Liu H-F, Magdalou J, Nicolas A, Lafaurie C, Siest G. Oral contraceptives stimulate the excretion of clofibric acid glucuronide in women and female rats. *Gen Pharmacol* (1991) 22, 393–7.

Fibrates; Clofibrate + Probenecid

Plasma clofibrate levels can be approximately doubled by probenecid, but the clinical significance of this is unclear.

Clinical evidence, mechanism, importance and management

A pharmacokinetic study in 4 healthy subjects taking clofibrate 500 mg every 12 hours found that probenecid 500 mg every 6 hours for 7 days almost doubled the steady-state clofibric acid levels, from 72 to 129 mg/L, and raised the free clofibric acid levels from 2.5 to 9.1 mg/L. The suggested reason is that the probenecid reduces the renal and metabolic clearance of the clofibrate by inhibiting its conjugation with glucuronic acid.[1] The clinical importance of this interaction is uncertain. It appears not to have been assessed.

1. Veenendaal JR, Brooks PM, Meffin PJ. Probenecid-clofibrate interaction. *Clin Pharmacol Ther* (1981) 29, 351–8.

Fibrates; Gemfibrozil + Antacids

Antacids can reduce the absorption of gemfibrozil.

Clinical evidence, mechanism, importance and management

A study in patients with kidney and liver disease found that the concurrent use of antacids (**aluminium hydroxide**, **aluminium magnesium silica hydrate**) reduced the maximum plasma gemfibrozil levels by about 50 to 70%, and the AUC by about 30 to 60%. The precise values are not given in the text. The reasons for these reductions are not known, but it was suggested that the gemfibrozil is adsorbed onto the antacids in the gut. The authors recommend that gemfibrozil is given 1 to 2 hours before antacids.[1] More study is needed to confirm these findings.

1. Knauf H, Kölle EU, Mutschler E. Gemfibrozil absorption and elimination in kidney and liver disease. *Klin Wochenschr* (1990) 68, 692–8.

Fibrates; Gemfibrozil + Psyllium

When 10 healthy subjects took gemfibrozil 600 mg with, or 2 hours after, 3 g of psyllium in 240 mL water, the AUC of gemfibrozil was reduced by about 10%.[1] This change in bioavailability is almost certainly too small to be clinically significant.

1. Forland SC, Cutler RE. The effect of psyllium on the pharmacokinetics of gemfibrozil. *Clin Res* (1990) 38, 94A.

Nicotinic acid (Niacin) + Aspirin

Aspirin reduces the flushing reaction that often occurs with nicotinic acid, but there is some evidence that it can also increase nicotinic acid plasma levels.

Clinical evidence, mechanism, importance and management

Nicotinic acid (70 to 100 micrograms/kg per minute as an infusion over 6 hours) was given to 6 healthy subjects. When the subjects were also given aspirin 1 g orally 2 hours after the infusion was started, the plasma nicotinic acid levels rose markedly, and its clearance was reduced by 30 to 54%.[1] The probable reason is that the salicylate competes with the nicotinic acid for metabolism by glycine conjugation in the liver so that the clearance of nicotinic acid is reduced, resulting in a rise in its levels. The clinical importance of this effect when aspirin is given to reduce the annoying nicotinic acid flushing reaction[2] is not known. However, as nicotinic acid is titrated upwards, according to efficacy and tolerability, any increase in its levels caused by aspirin is probably naturally accounted for.

1. Ding RW, Kolbe K, Merz B, de Vries J, Weber E, Benet LZ. Pharmacokinetics of nicotinic acid-salicylic acid interaction. *Clin Pharmacol Ther* (1989) 46, 642–7.
2. Jungnickel PW, Maloley PA, Vander Tuin EL, Peddicord TE, Campbell JR. Effect of two aspirin pretreatment regimens on niacin-induced cutaneous reactions. *J Gen Intern Med* (1997) 12, 591–6.

Nicotinic acid (Niacin) + Nicotine

An isolated report describes an unpleasant flushing reaction that developed in a woman taking nicotinic acid when she started to use nicotine transdermal patches.

Clinical evidence, mechanism, importance and management

A case report describes a woman who had taken nicotinic acid 250 mg twice daily for 3 years without problems, as well as nifedipine, ranitidine, colestyramine and ferrous sulfate. Following laryngectomy for cancer of the larynx, she restarted all of the drugs except the colestyramine and began to use nicotine transdermal patches 21 mg daily to try to give up smoking. On several occasions, shortly after taking the nicotinic acid, she developed unpleasant flushing episodes lasting about 30 minutes. No further episodes developed when the nicotinic acid was stopped.[1] The reasons are not understood, but flushing is a very common adverse effect of nicotinic acid, and it would seem that in this case the nicotine patch may have been responsible for its emergence. A comment on this report suggests that this reaction may possibly have an immunological basis.[2] Either way, this reaction is more unpleasant than serious.

1. Rockwell KA. Potential interaction between niacin and transdermal nicotine. *Ann Pharmacother* (1993) 27, 1283–4.
2. Sudan BJL. Comment: niacin, nicotine, and flushing. *Ann Pharmacother* (1994) 28, 1113.

Statins + ACE inhibitors

In general the statins do not appear to interact with the ACE inhibitors. An isolated report describes severe hyperkalaemia in a diabetic given lisinopril with lovastatin, and acute pancreatitis has been attributed to the use of lisinopril with atorvastatin.

Clinical evidence, mechanism, importance and management

Retrospective analysis of clinical study data found no evidence that the safety of **lovastatin** was altered by the use of unspecified ACE inhibitors in 142 patients.[1] Another retrospective analysis of clinical study data found no evidence that the safety or efficacy of **fluvastatin** was altered by the use of unspecified ACE inhibitors.[2] Likewise, the UK manufacturer of **atorvastatin**[3] says that in clinical studies it was given with ACE inhibitors without evidence of significant adverse interactions. A study in healthy subjects found that **simvastatin** had no effect on the pharmacokinetics or ACE-inhibitory effects of **ramipril** or its metabolites.[4] Similarly, no evidence of clinically important adverse interactions was found when **moexipril** was used with **cholesterol-lowering drugs** [not specifically named].[5] An isolated report describes a type I diabetic (receiving insulin) with hypertension and hyperlipidaemia who developed myositis and severe hyperkalaemia (serum potassium 8.4 mmol/L) when given **lovastatin** 20 to 40 mg daily with **lisinopril** 50 mg daily. His serum potassium returned to about 5.5 mmol/L after the **lovastatin** was stopped and the dosage of **lisinopril** lowered (to 20 mg daily). About 3 months later, the patient resumed taking the **lovastatin**, but after only 2 doses he again had severe myositis and hyperkalaemia, which resolved after the **lovastatin** was discontinued. The reason seemed to be a combination of the hyperkalaemic effects of the **lisinopril**, the release of intracellular potassium into the blood stream associated with the myositis caused by the **lovastatin**, and a predisposition to hyperkalaemia due to the diabetes and mild renal impairment.[6] Another case report describes the development of acute pancreatitis in a patient who had been taking **lisinopril** 10 mg daily with **atorvastatin** 20 mg daily for 9 months. No other cause for the pancreatitis was identified, and both drugs alone have, rarely, been associated with the development of pancreatitis.[7] These are unusual cases and, given the widespread use of drugs from these classes they seem unlikely to be of general importance. No special precautions would seem to be necessary if ACE inhibitors are given with statins.

1. Pool JL, Shear CL, Downton M, Schnaper H, Stinnett S, Dujovne C, Bradford RH, Chremos AN. Lovastatin and coadministered antihypertensive/cardiovascular agents. *Hypertension* (1992) 19, 242–8.
2. Peters TK, Jewitt-Harris J, Mehra M, Muratti EN. Safety and tolerability of fluvastatin with concomitant use of antihypertensive agents. An analysis of a clinical trial database. *Am J Hypertens* (1993) 6, 346S–352S.
3. Lipitor (Atorvastatin). Pfizer Ltd. UK Summary of product characteristics, September 2006.
4. Meyer BH, Scholtz HE, Müller FO, Luus HG, de la Rey N, Seibert-Grafe M, Eckert HG, Metzger H. Lack of interaction between ramipril and simvastatin. *Eur J Clin Pharmacol* (1994) 47, 373–5.
5. Moexipril and Hydrochlorothiazide Tablets. Teva Pharmaceuticals USA. US Prescribing information, June 2004.
6. Edelman S, Witztum JL. Hyperkalemia during treatment with HMG-CoA reductase inhibitor. *N Engl J Med* (1989) 320, 1219–20.
7. Kanbay M, Sekuk H, Yilmaz U, Gur G, Boyacioglu S. Acute pancreatitis associated with combined lisinopril and atorvastatin therapy. *Dig Dis* (2005) 23, 92–4.

Statins + Amiodarone

There is some evidence of a high incidence of myopathy when amiodarone is given with high doses of simvastatin. Cases of myopathy and rhabdomyolysis have been reported in patients taking the combination.

Clinical evidence, mechanism, importance and management

The manufacturers of **simvastatin** note that in an ongoing unpublished clinical study, myopathy (clinically significant muscle pain with a creatinine kinase at least 10 times the upper limit of normal[1]) has been reported in 6% of patients receiving **simvastatin** 80 mg daily with amiodarone.[2-4] There is some evidence from reports to the US FDA that the concurrent use of **simvastatin** with amiodarone is associated with a higher incidence of muscle toxicity than **pravastatin** with amiodarone. They reported that the percentage of reports of muscle, liver, pancreas, and bone marrow toxicity associated with statins and involving concurrent amiodarone was 1% for **simvastatin** and 0.4% for **pravastatin**.[5]

A 63-year-old man developed diffuse muscle pain with generalised muscular weakness 4 weeks after starting to take **simvastatin** 40 mg daily, and about 2 weeks after starting to take amiodarone (1 g daily for 10 days, then 200 mg daily thereafter). There was a marked increase in creatinine kinase, which normalised after stopping both drugs.[6] A 77-year-old man taking multiple medications including amiodarone 100 mg daily and **simvastatin** 20 mg daily, developed increasing lower-extremity pain and darkening of his urine 3 weeks after his **simvastatin** dose was increased to 40 mg daily. He was diagnosed with rhabdomyolysis secondary to **simvastatin** use,[7] although a later comment suggested that amiodarone could have contributed.[8] Two other cases of rhabdomyolysis in patients taking amiodarone with **simvastatin**[9,10] (one involving clarithromycin),[10] have also been reported. One of these patients had pneumonia,[10] and the other diabetes,[9] both of which have been suggested as risk factors for rhabdomyolysis.

Amiodarone is an inhibitor of various cytochrome P450 isoenzymes. Whether it inhibits the metabolism of **simvastatin** and other extensively-metabolised statins, and thereby increases the risk of muscle toxicity, is not known. Amiodarone alone may sometimes cause myopathy.

The interaction is not established. However, one manufacturer in the UK recommends that the dose of **simvastatin** should not exceed 20 mg daily in patients also taking amiodarone unless the clinical benefit is likely to outweigh the increased risk of myopathy and rhabdomyolysis.[2] Another contraindicates the combination.[3] The US manufacturer advises only using doses of **simvastatin** above 20 mg if the benefits outweigh the risks.[4]

Until more is known, caution is certainly warranted. See also 'muscle toxicity', (p.1086), for further guidance on monitoring and risk factors for muscle toxicity. **Lovastatin** is metabolised in the same way as **simvastatin**, and shares many of its interactions: the manufacturers of **lovastatin** suggest a maximum dose of 40 mg daily in the presence of amiodarone.[11] **Pravastatin** appears less likely to interact.

1. Ponte CD, Wratchford P. Amiodarone's role in simvastatin-associated rhabdomyolysis. *Am J Health-Syst Pharm* (2003) 60, 1791–2.
2. Zocor (Simvastatin). Merck Sharp & Dohme Ltd. UK Summary of product characteristics, December 2005.
3. Simvador (Simvastatin). Discovery Pharmaceuticals Ltd. UK Summary of product characteristics, July 2003.
4. Zocor (Simvastatin). Merck & Co., Inc. US Prescribing information, May 2007.
5. Alsheikh-Ali AA, Karas RH. Adverse events with concomitant amiodarone and statin therapy. *Prev Cardiol* (2005) 8, 95–7.
6. Roten L, Schoenenberger RA, Krähenbühl S, Schlienger RG. Rhabdomyolysis in association with simvastatin and amiodarone. *Ann Pharmacother* (2004) 38, 978–81.
7. Wratchford P, Ponte CD. High-dose simvastatin and rhabdomyolysis. *Am J Health-Syst Pharm* (2003) 60, 698–700.
8. de Denus S, Spinler SA. Amiodarone's role in simvastatin-associated rhabdomyolysis. *Am J Health-Syst Pharm* (2003) 60, 1791.
9. Ricuarte B, Guirguis A, Taylor HC, Zabriskie D. Simvastatin–amiodarone interaction resulting in rhabdomyolysis, azotemia, and possible hepatotoxicity. *Ann Pharmacother* (2006) 40, 753–7.
10. Chouhan UM, Chakrabarti S, Millward LJ. Simvastatin interaction with clarithromycin and amiodarone causing myositis. *Ann Pharmacother* (2005) 39, 1760–1.
11. Mevacor (Lovastatin). Merck & Co., Inc. US Prescribing information, May 2007.

Statins + Angiotensin II receptor antagonists

Irbesartan and telmisartan appear not to alter the pharmacokinetics of simvastatin, fluvastatin does not alter the pharmacokinetics of losartan or its active metabolite, and olmesartan appears not to interact with pravastatin.

Clinical evidence, mechanism, importance and management

(a) Fluvastatin

In a crossover study 12 healthy subjects were given **losartan** 50 mg in the morning for 7 days, followed by fluvastatin 40 mg at bedtime for 7 days, and then both drugs together for another 7 days. It was found that the steady-state pharmacokinetics of **losartan** and its active metabolite, E-3174, were not significantly altered by fluvastatin.[1] It was anticipated that fluvastatin might inhibit the conversion of losartan to E-3174 by inhibiting the cytochrome P450 isoenzyme CYP2C9 (compare 'Angiotensin II receptor antagonists + Azoles', p.35). The findings of this study indicate that a clinically relevant pharmacokinetic interaction is unlikely, and no **losartan** dose adjustment is required on combined use.

(b) Pravastatin

The manufacturer of **olmesartan** states that it has no clinically relevant interaction with pravastatin in healthy subjects.[2]

(c) Simvastatin

A study in 12 healthy subjects found that **irbesartan** 300 mg had no significant effect on the pharmacokinetics of a single 50-mg dose of simvastatin, or its metabolite simvastatin acid, and the combination was well-tolerated.[3] No clinically relevant interaction was noted when **telmisartan** was given with simvastatin.[4]

1. Meadowcroft AM, Williamson KM, Patterson JH, Hinderliter AL, Pieper JA. The effects of fluvastatin, a CYP2C9 inhibitor, on losartan pharmacokinetics in healthy volunteers. *J Clin Pharmacol* (1999) 39, 418–24.
2. Olmetec (Olmesartan medoxomil). Daiichi Sankyo UK Ltd. UK Summary of product characteristics, August 2006.

3. Marino MR, Vachharajani NN, Hadjilambris OW. Irbesartan does not affect the pharmacokinetics of simvastatin in healthy subjects. *J Clin Pharmacol* (2000) 40, 875–9.
4. Micardis (Telmisartan). Boehringer Ingelheim Pharmaceuticals Inc. US Prescribing information, May 2006.

Statins + Antacids

An aluminium/magnesium hydroxide antacid (*Maalox*) causes a moderate reduction in the bioavailability of atorvastatin, pravastatin, and rosuvastatin, but the lipid-lowering efficacy of atorvastatin and pravastatin is not affected.

Clinical evidence, mechanism, importance and management

In a multiple-dose study, 18 patients were given **atorvastatin** 10 mg daily for 15 days with 30 mL of an **aluminium/magnesium hydroxide** antacid (*Maalox TC*) four times daily for a further 17 days. The maximum serum levels and AUC of **atorvastatin** were reduced by 34%, and the absorption rate was also reduced by the antacid. However, the LDL-cholesterol reduction remained the same.[1] The concurrent use of the same antacid (*Maalox TC*) 15 mL four times daily, given one hour before **pravastatin**, reduced the bioavailability of a single 20-mg dose of **pravastatin** by 28%. This change was less than that seen with food, which did not alter **pravastatin** efficacy.[2] There is therefore no need to avoid the concurrent use of **aluminium/magnesium hydroxide** antacids such as *Maalox,* nor does the dosage of **atorvastatin** or **pravastatin** need to be raised.

The US manufacturers of **rosuvastatin** quote a study in which an **aluminium/magnesium hydroxide** antacid reduced the levels of a 40-mg dose of **rosuvastatin** by 54%. No clinically significant interaction was seen when the doses were given 2 hours apart, and a 2-hour separation is therefore recommended on concurrent use.[3]

1. Yang B-B, Smithers JA, Abel RB, Stern RH, Sedman AJ, Olson SC. Effects of Maalox TC® on pharmacokinetics and pharmacodynamics of atorvastatin. *Pharm Res* (1996) 13 (9 Suppl), S437.
2. ER Squibb . A report on the comparative pharmacokinetics of pravastatin in the presence and absence of cimetidine or antacids in healthy male subjects. Data on file. (Protocol No 27, 201-43), 1988.
3. Crestor (Rosuvastatin calcium). AstraZeneca. US Prescribing information, July 2007.

Statins + Azoles

Fluconazole modestly increases the levels of fluvastatin and rosuvastatin, but not pravastatin. Miconazole would be expected to interact similarly. Itraconazole causes a marked rise in the serum levels of atorvastatin, lovastatin, pravastatin and simvastatin, but no change in fluvastatin or rosuvastatin levels. Ketoconazole would be expected to interact similarly. Rhabdomyolysis has been reported in some cases. Due to the risk of myopathy, the manufacturers of voriconazole caution, and the manufacturers of posaconazole contraindicate, concurrent use with atorvastatin, lovastatin and simvastatin.

Clinical evidence

(a) Atorvastatin

A case report describes a 76-year-old man taking multiple medications, including pravastatin 80 mg daily with **fluconazole** 150 mg daily, uneventfully for about 18 months. Due to an inadequate response to the pravastatin he was changed to atorvastatin 40 mg daily. Within one week he developed dyspnoea, myopathy, rhabdomyolysis and renal failure. Although both drugs were stopped he later died of multi-organ failure. The authors considered an interaction between atorvastatin and **fluconazole** as the most likely explanation for the rhabdomyolysis.[1]

Ten healthy subjects were given **itraconazole** 200 mg daily for 5 days with a single 40-mg dose of atorvastatin on day 4. The **itraconazole** increased the AUC of atorvastatin acid and atorvastatin lactone fourfold and threefold, respectively, and increased their half-lives threefold and twofold, respectively. The AUC values of active and total HMG-CoA reductase inhibitors were increased 1.6- and 1.7-fold, respectively.[2] In a similar study,[3] the same dose of **itraconazole** increased the AUC of atorvastatin by 2.5-fold and of atorvastatin lactone by about threefold. Another study has also shown that **itraconazole** raises atorvastatin levels.[4]

In a review of the FDA spontaneous reports of statin-associated rhabdomyolysis covering the period November 1997 to March 2000, an azole antifungal was potentially implicated in 2 cases of rhabdomyolysis involving atorvastatin.[5]

(b) Fluvastatin

A randomised, double-blind study in 12 healthy subjects found that **fluconazole** (400 mg on day 1 followed by 200 mg daily for 3 days) increased the AUC of a single 40-mg dose of fluvastatin by 84% and increased its maximum plasma level by 44%. The pharmacokinetics of the **fluconazole** were unaffected.[6] In a similar study, **itraconazole** 100 mg daily for 4 days did not significantly affect the pharmacokinetics of fluvastatin, apart from a small increase in its half-life.[7]

(c) Lovastatin

In a double-blind, crossover study in 12 healthy subjects **itraconazole** 200 mg daily or a placebo was given for 4 days with a single 40-mg oral dose of lovastatin on day 4. On average the peak plasma concentration and the 24-hour AUC of the lovastatin were increased more than 20-fold. The peak plasma concentration of the active metabolite of lovastatin, lovastatin acid, was increased 13-fold (range 10 to 23-fold) and its AUC was increased 20-fold. The creatine kinase activity of one subject increased 10-fold, but in the other 11 subjects it remained unchanged.[8] Another study also found similar pharmacokinetic changes.[7] Brief mention is also made of severe rhabdomyolysis in one patient given lovastatin and **itraconazole**.[8]

A 63-year-old woman who had been taking lovastatin 80 mg, nicotinic acid 3 g daily, timolol and aspirin for almost 10 years without problems, developed weakness and tenderness in her arms, back and legs within 2 weeks of starting to take **itraconazole** 100 mg twice daily. A few days later her urine became brown, and positive for haem. She was diagnosed as having acute rhabdomyolysis and hepatotoxicity. The lovastatin, nicotinic acid and **itraconazole** were stopped, and she was treated with ubidecarenone. Over the next 18 days her elevated serum enzymes returned to normal, although her plasma cholesterol levels almost doubled. She was restarted on nicotinic acid 11 weeks later without problems.[9]

In a review of the FDA spontaneous reports of statin-associated rhabdomyolysis covering the period November 1997 to March 2000, an azole antifungal was potentially implicated in 6 cases of rhabdomyolysis involving lovastatin.[5]

(d) Pravastatin

A randomised, double-blind study in 12 healthy subjects found that **fluconazole** (400 mg on day 1 followed by 200 mg daily for 3 days) had no significant effect on the pharmacokinetics of a single 40-mg dose of pravastatin.[6]

The AUC of a single 40-mg dose of pravastatin was increased by 71% in 10 healthy subjects who took **itraconazole** 200 mg daily for 4 days, although this did not reach statistical significance.[10] In a similar study, the same dosage of **itraconazole** caused a modest 51% increase in the AUC of pravastatin.[3] In contrast, one study in 104 subjects found that **itraconazole** had no effect on pravastatin pharmacokinetics.[4]

(e) Rosuvastatin

Fluconazole 200 mg once daily for 11 days increased the AUC and maximum plasma concentration of rosuvastatin (given on day 8) by 14% and 9%, respectively, in 14 healthy subjects. The proportion of circulating active HMG-CoA reductase inhibitors was not affected by **fluconazole**.[11] In similar studies by the same workers, **itraconazole**[12] and **ketoconazole**[13] also had no clinically significant effect on the levels of rosuvastatin.

(f) Simvastatin

An 83-year-old man who had been taking multiple medications including simvastatin 40 mg daily for 2 years was given **fluconazole** 400 mg daily as part of a prophylactic regimen against chemotherapy-induced neutropenic sepsis. After one week he developed generalised muscle weakness and was found to have brown urine and an elevated serum creatine kinase. His medication was stopped, and he was treated with hydration and diuretics, after which his symptoms resolved.[14]

In a two-phase crossover study, 10 healthy subjects were given **itraconazole** 200 mg daily or a placebo for 4 days, with a single 40-mg dose of simvastatin on day 4. The peak serum levels of total simvastatin acid (simvastatin acid plus simvastatin lactone) were increased 17-fold and the AUC was increased 19-fold. The maximum serum levels and the AUC of total HMG-CoA reductase inhibitors increased about 3-fold and 5-fold, respectively.[10]

A 74-year-old who had been taking simvastatin 40 mg daily, lisinopril and aspirin for about a year without problems developed pain in his feet, and then in his arms and neck, within 3 weeks of starting **itraconazole** 200 mg daily. His urine turned brown, his muscles were tender, and abnormal serum creatine kinase and other enzyme levels were found. A diagnosis of rhabdomyolysis was made.[15] A 70-year-old with a kidney transplant was taking, among many other drugs, ciclosporin and simvastatin 40 mg daily. Despite the high dose of simvastatin, even in conjunction with ciclosporin (see also 'Statins + Ciclosporin', p.1097), he had experienced no problems. Within 2 weeks of starting **itraconazole** 100 mg twice daily he developed malaise and general muscle weakness with elevated creatine kinase levels, which was diagnosed as rhabdomyolysis. His serum simvastatin levels were found to be raised. A later subject also had an increase in simvastatin serum levels, from 0.5 to 6.5 nanogram/mL within a day of starting **itraconazole** 200 mg daily.[16] Three further similar cases have also been reported with the combination of simvastatin, ciclosporin and **itraconazole**.[17-19] Gemfibrozil was also taken in one of these cases.[19] In addition, three similar cases have been reported in patients taking simvastatin, which developed between 10 days and 4 weeks after starting **ketoconazole** 200 or 400 mg daily.[20-22] In a review of the FDA spontaneous reports of statin-associated rhabdomyolysis covering the period November 1997 to March 2000, an azole antifungal was potentially implicated in 4 cases of rhabdomyolysis involving simvastatin.[5]

Mechanism

Fluconazole and **miconazole** inhibit the cytochrome P450 isoenzymes CYP2C9 and CYP3A4, whereas itraconazole and ketoconazole are potent inhibitors of CYP3A4. Consequently their interaction profiles differ amongst the various statins depending on which isoenzymes are involved in the metabolism of the statins in question: this has been shown in several studies.[3,6,7] From these studies it appears that the effect of itraconazole is greatest on lovastatin and simvastatin, with a marked effect on atorvastatin, a modest effect on pravastatin or rosuvastatin, and no effect on fluvastatin. Fluconazole has a marked effect on fluvastatin, but no effect on pravastatin. See 'Lipid regulating drugs', (p.1086) for further discussion on the metabolism of the statins.

Importance and management

An established interaction of clinical importance, which differs depending on the drug pair used. The differing risks and management of the various drug pairs are discussed below. See also 'muscle toxicity', (p.1086), for further guidance on monitoring, and risk factors for muscle toxicity.

1. Lovastatin or simvastatin. The very marked increases in levels of lovastatin and simvastatin that can occur considerably increase the risk of severe muscle damage and therefore the use of these statins with **itraconazole** or **ketoconazole** should be avoided. If a short course of an azole antifungal is considered essential, the manufacturers suggest temporary withdrawal of the statin.[23-25] The manufacturers of **voriconazole** predict that it will interact with statins metabolised by the cytochrome P450 isoenzyme CYP3A4, resulting in elevated statin levels, and possibly rhabdomyolysis. They suggest that a dosage reduction of the statin should be considered during concurrent use.[26,27] The manufacturer of **posaconazole** (also a CYP3A4 inhibitor) contraindicates its use with simvastatin or lovastatin.[28]

2. Atorvastatin. Although the increase in the levels of atorvastatin are not as great as those with lovastatin or simvastatin, they are still marked, and unless the benefits outweigh the risks the combination of an azole antifungal with atorvastatin should, where possible, be avoided. As a general rule, any patient given atorvastatin with an azole should be told to report any signs of myopathy and possible rhabdomyolysis (i.e. otherwise unexplained muscle pain, tenderness or weakness or dark coloured urine). If myopathy does occur, the statin should be stopped immediately. Note that the manufacturer of **posaconazole** contraindicates its use with atorvastatin,[28] and the manufacturers of **voriconazole** suggest considering a dosage reduction of the statin.[26,27]

3. Fluvastatin. The clinical relevance of the modest changes in fluvastatin levels with different azole antifungals is unclear. Note that in a review of the FDA spontaneous reports of statin-associated rhabdomyolysis for the period November 1997 to March 2000, azole antifungals were not identified as a potentially interacting drug in any of the reports for fluvastatin.[5] However, fluconazole and miconazole are inhibitors of CYP2C9 by which fluvastatin is metabolised and so a degree of caution seems warranted. Therefore any patient given fluconazole (or **miconazole** in preparations such as the oral gel, which is absorbed) with fluvastatin should be told to report any signs of myopathy and possible rhabdomyolysis (i.e. otherwise unexplained muscle pain, tenderness or weakness or dark coloured urine). If myopathy does occur, the statin should be stopped immediately.

4. Pravastatin. The clinical relevance of the modest changes in pravastatin levels with different azole antifungals seems likely to be small, and a clinically significant interaction would not be expected. Note that in a review of the FDA spontaneous reports of statin-associated rhabdomyolysis for the period November 1997 to March 2000, azole antifungals were not identified as a potentially interacting drug in any of the reports for pravastatin.[5]

1. Kahri J, Valkonen M, Bäcklund T, Vuoristo M, Kivistö KT. Rhabdomyolysis in a patient receiving atorvastatin and fluconazole. *Eur J Clin Pharmacol* (2005) 60, 905–7.
2. Kantola T, Kivistö KT, Neuvonen PJ. Effect of itraconazole on the pharmacokinetics of atorvastatin. *Clin Pharmacol Ther* (1998) 64, 58–65.
3. Mazzu AL, Lasseter KC, Shamblen E, Cooper BS, Agarwal V, Lettieri J, Sundaresen P. Itraconazole alters the pharmacokinetics of atorvastatin to a greater extent than either cerivastatin or pravastatin. *Clin Pharmacol Ther* (2000) 68, 391–400.
4. Jacobson TA. Comparative pharmacokinetic interaction profiles of pravastatin, simvastatin, and atorvastatin when coadministered with cytochrome P450 inhibitors. *Am J Cardiol* (2004) 94, 1140–6.
5. Omar MA, Wilson JP. FDA adverse event reports on statin-associated rhabdomyolysis. *Ann Pharmacother* (2002) 36, 288–95.
6. Kantola T, Backman JT, Niemi M, Kivistö KT, Neuvonen PJ. Effect of fluconazole on plasma fluvastatin and pravastatin concentrations. *Eur J Clin Pharmacol* (2000) 56, 225–9.
7. Kivistö KT, Kantola T, Neuvonen PJ. Different effects of itraconazole on the pharmacokinetics of fluvastatin and lovastatin. *Br J Clin Pharmacol* (1998) 46, 49–53.
8. Neuvonen PJ, Jalava K-M. Itraconazole drastically increases plasma concentrations of lovastatin and lovastatin acid. *Clin Pharmacol Ther* (1996) 60, 54–61.
9. Lees RS, Lees AM. Rhabdomyolysis from the coadministration of lovastatin and the antifungal agent itraconazole. *N Engl J Med* (1995) 333, 664–5.
10. Neuvonen PJ, Kantola T, Kivistö KT. Simvastatin but not pravastatin is very susceptible to interaction with CYP3A4 inhibitor itraconazole. *Clin Pharmacol Ther* (1998) 332–41.
11. Cooper KJ, Martin PD, Dane AL, Warwick MJ, Schneck DW, Cantarini MV. The effect of fluconazole on the pharmacokinetics of rosuvastatin. *Eur J Clin Pharmacol* (2002) 58, 527–31.
12. Cooper KJ, Martin PD, Dane AL, Warwick MJ, Schneck DW, Cantarini MV. Effect of itraconazole on the pharmacokinetics of rosuvastatin. *Clin Pharmacol Ther* (2003) 73, 322–9.
13. Cooper KJ, Martin PD, Dane AL, Warwick MJ, Raza A, Schneck DW. Lack of effect of ketoconazole on the pharmacokinetics of rosuvastatin in healthy subjects. *Br J Clin Pharmacol* (2003) 55, 94–9.
14. Shaukat A, Benekli M, Vladutiu GD, Slack JL, Wetzler M, Baer MR. Simvastatin–fluconazole causing rhabdomyolysis. *Ann Pharmacother* (2003) 37, 1032–5.
15. Horn M. Coadministration of itraconazole with hypolipidemic agents may induce rhabdomyolysis in healthy individuals. *Arch Dermatol* (1996) 132, 1254.
16. Segaert MF, De Soete C, Vandewiele I, Verbanck J. Drug-interaction-induced rhabdomyolysis. *Nephrol Dial Transplant* (1996) 11, 1846–7.
17. Malouf MA, Bicknell M, Glanville AR. Rhabdomyolysis after lung transplantation. *Aust N Z J Med* (1997) 27, 186.
18. Vlahakos DV, Manginas A, Chilidou D, Zamanika C, Alivizatos PA. Itraconazole-induced rhabdomyolysis and acute renal failure in a heart transplant recipient treated with simvastatin and cyclosporine. *Transplantation* (2002) 73, 1962–4.
19. Maxa JL, Melton LB, Ogu CC, Sills MN, Limanni A. Rhabdomyolysis after concomitant use of cyclosporine, simvastatin, gemfibrozil, and itraconazole. *Ann Pharmacother* (2002) 36, 820–23.
20. Gilad R, Lampl Y. Rhabdomyolysis induced by simvastatin and ketoconazole treatment. *Clin Neuropharmacol* (1999) 22, 295–7.
21. Itakura H, Vaughn D, Haller DG, O'Dwyer PJ. Rhabdomyolysis from cytochrome P-450 interaction of ketoconazole and simvastatin in prostate cancer. *J Urol (Baltimore)* (2003) 169, 613.
22. McKelvie PA, Dennett X. Myopathy associated with HMG-CoA reductase inhibitors (statins): a series of 10 patients and review of the literature. *J Clin Neuromusc Dis* (2002) 3,143–8.
23. Mevacor (Lovastatin). Merck & Co., Inc. US Prescribing information, May 2007.
24. Zocor (Simvastatin). Merck Sharp & Dohme Ltd. UK Summary of product characteristics, December 2005.
25. Zocor (Simvastatin). Merck & Co., Inc. US Prescribing information, May 2007.
26. VFEND (Voriconazole). Pfizer Ltd. UK Summary of product characteristics, July 2007.
27. VFEND (Voriconazole). Pfizer Inc. US Prescribing information, November 2006.
28. Noxafil (Posaconazole). Schering-Plough Ltd. UK Summary of product characteristics, October 2006.

Statins + Beta blockers

Propranolol does not cause any clinically relevant changes to the pharmacokinetics of fluvastatin, lovastatin or pravastatin. In clinical studies, the safety and efficacy of statins were not altered by the concurrent use of beta blockers as a class.

Clinical evidence, mechanism, importance and management

In a study in 24 healthy subjects the pharmacokinetics of a single 40-mg dose of **fluvastatin** was not affected by the concurrent use of **propranolol** 40 mg every 12 hours for 3 days.[1] Similarly, the same dose of **propranolol** caused less than an 18% reduction in the AUC of **lovastatin** 20 mg and its metabolites, and modestly reduced the AUC of **pravastatin** 20 mg and its metabolites by 16 to 23%.[2] These changes are small and unlikely to be clinically relevant.

Retrospective analysis of clinical study data found no evidence that the safety or efficacy of **fluvastatin** was altered by the use of beta blockers (unspecified).[3] Similarly, in another analysis, there was no evidence that the safety or efficacy of **lovastatin** was altered by selective beta blockers (primarily **atenolol**, **metoprolol** and **labetalol**) or non-selective beta blockers (primarily **propranolol**, **nadolol** and **timolol**).[4] Likewise, the manufacturer of **atorvastatin**[5] says that in clinical studies it was used concurrently with beta blockers without evidence of significant adverse interactions.

No special precautions would seem to be necessary if beta blockers are given concurrently with statins.

1. Smith HT, Jokubaitis LA, Troendle AJ, Hwang DS, Robinson WT. Pharmacokinetics of fluvastatin and specific drug interactions. *Am J Hypertens* (1993) 6, 375S–382S.
2. Pan HY, Triscari J, DeVault AR, Smith SA, Wang-Iverson D, Swanson BN, Willard DA. Pharmacokinetic interaction between propranolol and the HMG-CoA reductase inhibitors pravastatin and lovastatin. *Br J Clin Pharmacol* (1991) 31, 665–70.
3. Peters TK, Jewitt-Harris J, Mehra M, Muratti EN. Safety and tolerability of fluvastatin with concomitant use of antihypertensive agents. An analysis of a clinical trial database. *Am J Hypertens* (1993) 6, 346S–352S.
4. Pool JL, Shear CL, Downton M, Schnaper H, Stinnett S, Dujovne C, Bradford RH, Chremos AN. Lovastatin and coadministered antihypertensive/cardiovascular agents. *Hypertension* (1992) 19, 242–8.
5. Lipitor (Atorvastatin). Pfizer Ltd. UK Summary of product characteristics, September 2006.

Statins + Bile-acid binding resins

Although colestyramine and colestipol reduce plasma fluvastatin and pravastatin levels, the overall total lipid-lowering effect is increased by concurrent use. Separating their administration minimises this interaction. Colestipol appears to interact with atorvastatin similarly. Colesevelam appears not to interact with lovastatin.

Clinical evidence

(a) Atorvastatin

A study in which atorvastatin and **colestipol** were given concurrently found that although the serum levels of atorvastatin were reduced by about 25%, the total reduction in the LDL-cholesterol levels was greater than when each drug was given alone.[1]

(b) Fluvastatin

Colestyramine 8 g given at the same time as fluvastatin 20 mg decreased the AUC and the maximum plasma levels of fluvastatin by 89 and 96%, respectively, in 19 healthy subjects. When the fluvastatin was given 2 hours after the **colestyramine**, the AUC and the maximum plasma levels of fluvastatin were reduced by just over 50%.[2] In another study in 20 healthy subjects, the AUC and maximum plasma levels of fluvastatin were reduced by 51 and 82%, respectively, when fluvastatin was taken 4 hours after **colestyramine** 8 g and a meal.[2]

Despite these marked reductions in fluvastatin bioavailability, other studies in large numbers of hypercholesterolaemic patients have shown that concurrent use actually has additive lipid-lowering effects.[2,3] In the first of these studies, fluvastatin was given 4 hours after **colestyramine**,[2] but the other study did not indicate whether or not doses were separated.[3]

(c) Lovastatin

An open-label crossover study in 22 healthy subjects found that the pharmacokinetics of lovastatin 20 mg given with a meal were not significantly affected when **colesevelam** 2.25 g was given at the same time.[4]

(d) Pravastatin

In a randomised study 33 patients with primary hypercholesterolaemia were given pravastatin 5, 10, or 20 mg twice daily before their morning and evening meals for 4 weeks and then for a further 4 weeks they also took **colestyramine** 24 g daily. The **colestyramine** was taken at least an hour after the pravastatin. Despite the fact that the **colestyramine** reduced the bioavailability of the pravastatin by 18 to 49%, the reduction in blood lipid levels was enhanced by concurrent use.[5] A related study in 18 subjects found that **colestyramine** reduced the bioavailability of pravastatin by about 40% when given at the same time, but only small and clinically insignificant pharmacokinetic changes occurred when the pravastatin was given one hour before, or 4 hours after the **colestyramine**.[6] Similarly, a multicentre study involving 311 patients found that the combined use of pravastatin 40 mg daily and **colestyramine** 12 g daily was highly effective in the treatment of hypercholesterolaemia. The **colestyramine** was taken at least one hour after the pravastatin.[7]

Colestipol reduced the bioavailability of pravastatin in 18 subjects by about 50%, but no reduction in bioavailability was seen when pravastatin was given 1 hour before **colestipol** and a meal.[6]

Mechanism

It seems probable that these bile-acid binding resins bind with statins in the gut and thereby reduce the amount of statin available for absorption.

Importance and management

Established interactions but of only relatively minor importance. Despite the reduction in the bioavailability of pravastatin caused by colestyramine or colestipol, the overall lipid-lowering effect is increased by concurrent use.[5,7] The effects of the interaction can be minimised by separating their administration as described above. This can be easily achieved by taking the colestyramine or colestipol with meals, and the pravastatin at bedtime. Similarly, any interaction between fluvastatin and colestyramine can be minimised by taking fluvastatin at least 4 hours after colestyramine. There would appear to be no reason for avoiding concurrent use of atorvastatin and colestipol, nor lovastatin and colesevelam.

1. Lipitor (Atorvastatin). Pfizer Ltd. UK Summary of product characteristics, September 2006.
2. Smith HT, Jokubaitis LA, Troendle AJ, Hwang DS, Robinson WT. Pharmacokinetics of fluvastatin and specific drug interactions. *Am J Hypertens* (1993) 6, 375S–382S.
3. Hagen E, Istad H, Ose L, Bodd E, Eriksen H-M, Selvig V, Bard JM, Fruchart JC, Borge M, Wolf M-C, Pfister P. Fluvastatin efficacy and tolerability in comparison and in combination with cholestyramine. *Eur J Clin Pharmacol* (1994) 46, 445–9.
4. Donovan JM, Kisicki JC, Stiles MR, Tracewell WG, Burke SK. Effect of colesevelam on lovastatin pharmacokinetics. *Ann Pharmacother* (2002) 36, 392–7.
5. Pan HY, DeVault AR, Swites BJ, Whigan D, Ivashkiv E, Willard DA, Brescia D. Pharmacokinetics and pharmacodynamics of pravastatin alone and with cholestyramine in hypercholesterolemia. *Clin Pharmacol Ther* (1990) 48, 201–7.
6. Pan HY, DeVault AR, Ivashkiv E, Whigan D, Brennan JJ, Willard DA. Pharmacokinetic interaction studies of pravastatin with bile-acid-binding resins. 8th International Symposium on Atherosclerosis, Rome, October 9-13, 1988. 711.
7. Pravastatin Multicenter Study Group II. Comparative efficacy and safety of pravastatin and cholestyramine alone and combined in patients with hypercholesterolemia. *Arch Intern Med* (1993) 153, 1321–9.

Statins + Calcium-channel blockers

Marked rises in statin plasma levels have been seen when lovastatin or simvastatin were given with diltiazem, and when simvastatin was given with verapamil. Isolated cases of rhabdomyolysis have occurred as a result of these interactions. However, overall, it seems that problems with combinations of statins and calcium-channel blockers (particularly the dihydropyridine-type) are rare.

Clinical evidence

(a) Atorvastatin

The manufacturers of **amlodipine** state that it does not affect the pharmacokinetics of atorvastatin.[1] They also note that no clinically significant interactions were seen in clinical studies in which atorvastatin was used with antihypertensives, including unspecified calcium-channel blockers.[1] However, they do warn that drugs that are metabolised by the cytochrome P450 isoenzyme CYP3A4 (e.g. calcium-channel blockers) do have the potential to interact.[1]

A 60-year-old man taking atorvastatin 20 mg daily, developed rhabdomyolysis 3 weeks after **diltiazem** (an *inhibitor* of CYP3A4) was started.[2] Another similar case has also been reported.[3]

(b) Fluvastatin

A retrospective study of the effects of antihypertensives on the efficacy of fluvastatin found that the concurrent use of unspecified calcium-channel blockers did not significantly affect the safety or lipid-lowering effects of fluvastatin, although there was a trend towards enhanced lowering of triglycerides.[4]

(c) Lovastatin

A retrospective study of the effects of lovastatin and antihypertensive medication found that when calcium-channel blockers (**diltiazem**, **nifedipine** or **verapamil**) were used in combination with lovastatin there was an additional 3 to 5% lowering in the LDL-cholesterol, which was of marginal significance.[5] Pharmacokinetic studies have shown that oral **diltiazem** increases the AUC and maximum serum levels of lovastatin by about fourfold.[6,7] In another study, lovastatin 20 mg and **isradipine** 5 mg was given to 12 healthy subjects either alone or together for 5 days. **Isradipine** reduced the AUC of lovastatin by 40%, in males but not females.[8]

(d) Pravastatin

A study in 10 healthy subjects found that sustained-release **diltiazem** 120 mg twice daily had no effect on the pharmacokinetics of a single 20-mg dose of pravastatin.[6] Similarly, a study in 15 healthy subjects found that extended-release **verapamil** 480 mg daily for 3 days did not affect the pharmacokinetics of pravastatin 40 mg daily.[9]

(e) Simvastatin

1. Amlodipine. In a study in 8 patients taking simvastatin 5 mg daily the addition of amlodipine 5 mg daily for 4 weeks increased the maximum levels and AUC of simvastatin by a modest 1.4- and 1.3-fold, respectively, without affecting the lipid profiles of the patients.[10]

2. Diltiazem. A single 20-mg dose of simvastatin was given to 10 healthy subjects after they had taken sustained-release diltiazem 120 mg twice daily for 2 weeks. Diltiazem caused about a fivefold increase in the simvastatin AUC, a fourfold increase in the maximum serum levels, and a 2.5-fold increase in the half-life.[11]
The clinical relevance of the diltiazem interaction was demonstrated in a 53-year-old man, who developed rhabdomyolysis 3 months after diltiazem 30 mg four times daily was added to established treatment with simvastatin 40 mg daily. Both drugs were discontinued and he recovered over the following 10 days.[12] Other similar cases have also been reported.[3,13]
An *in vitro* study using human liver microsomes also found that diltiazem moderately inhibits simvastatin metabolism.[14]

3. Lacidipine. In a randomised, crossover study simvastatin 40 mg daily was given for 8 days, with or without lacidipine 4 mg daily. Lacidipine raised the AUC of simvastatin by 35%, which was considered to be modest and unlikely to be of clinical significance.[15]

4. Verapamil. A study in which 12 subjects were given verapamil 80 mg three times daily, found a 4.6-fold increase in the AUC of simvastatin, a 2.6-fold increase in its maximum serum levels, and about a twofold increase in its half-life.[16] Similarly, a study in 12 healthy subjects found that extended-release verapamil 480 mg daily for 3 days caused a fivefold increase in the maximum serum levels of simvastatin 40 mg, and about a fourfold increase in its AUC.[9]
The clinical relevance of the verapamil interaction was demonstrated in a 63-year-old man, who developed rhabdomyolysis about 1 month after extended-release verapamil 240 mg daily was added to established treatment with simvastatin 40 mg daily and ciclosporin. Verapamil and simvastatin were discontinued and he recovered over the following 14 days.[17] An *in vitro* study using human liver microsomes also found that verapamil moderately inhibits simvastatin metabolism.[14]

Mechanism

Diltiazem and verapamil inhibit the cytochrome P450 isoenzyme CYP3A4, which is responsible for the metabolism of lovastatin, simvastatin and to an extent, atorvastatin. Therefore concurrent use of these drugs results in an increase in the levels of the statin. One study found that oral, but not intravenous diltiazem interacts, suggesting that it is CYP3A4 in the gut wall that is the site of the interaction.[18] Isradipine and lovastatin are both metabolised by CYP3A4, and therefore the modest interaction may have occurred as a result of competition for metabolism. A similar mechanism probably accounts for the modest interaction between simvastatin and lacidipine or amlodipine. See 'Lipid regulating drugs', (p.1086), and 'Calcium-channel blockers', (p.860), for more information about the way these groups of drugs are metabolised.

Importance and management

Information is limited, but what is known suggests that the concurrent use of these drugs is normally uneventful. Even with those pairs of drugs where the increases in plasma levels are quite large (such as when simvastatin was given with diltiazem or verapamil) problems seem to be very rare. Indeed an analysis of the 4S study and the Heart Protection Study (which used maximum simvastatin doses of 40 mg) found no evidence that the concurrent use of a calcium-channel blocker increases the risk of myopathy.[19] Therefore concurrent use need not be avoided, but it has been suggested that treatment with a statin in a patient taking diltiazem (and probably verapamil) should be started with the lowest possible dose and titrated upwards, or, if diltiazem (or verapamil) is started, the dose of the statin should be considerably reduced.[16] The manufacturers of lovastatin recommend restricting the dose to 40 mg daily if verapamil is given,[20] and the manufacturers of simvastatin suggest restricting the dose to 20 mg daily.[21,22] Note that one UK manufacturer[23] recommends that the combination should be avoided, which seems somewhat over-cautious. In the UK it has been suggested that the dose of simvastatin should be restricted to 40 mg daily in the presence of diltiazem.[22]. See also 'muscle toxicity', (p.1086), for further guidance on monitoring and risk factors for muscle toxicity.

1. Lipitor (Atorvastatin). Pfizer Ltd. UK Summary of product characteristics, September 2006.
2. Lewin JJ, Nappi JM, Taylor MH. Rhabdomyolysis with concurrent atorvastatin and diltiazem. *Ann Pharmacother* (2002) 36, 1546–9.
3. Gladding P, Pilmore H, Edwards C. Potentially fatal interaction between diltiazem and statins. *Ann Intern Med* (2004) 140, W31.
4. Peters TK, Jewitt-Harris J, Mehra M, Muratti EN. Safety and tolerability of fluvastatin with concomitant use of antihypertensive agents. An analysis of a clinical trial database. *Am J Hypertens* (1993) 6, 346S–352S.
5. Pool JI, Shear CL, Downton M, Schnaper H, Stinnett S, Dujovne C, Bradford RH, Chremos AN. Lovastatin and coadministered antihypertensive/cardiovascular agents. *Hypertension* (1992) 19, 242–8.
6. Azie NE, Brater DC, Becker PA, Jones DR, Hall SD. The interaction of diltiazem with lovastatin and pravastatin. *Clin Pharmacol Ther* (1998) 64, 369–77.
7. Jones DR, Azie NE, Masica BA, Brater DC, Hall SD. Oral but not intravenous (IV) diltiazem impairs lovastatin clearance. *Clin Pharmacol Ther* (1999) 65, 149.
8. Zhou LX, Finley DK, Hassell AE, Holtzman JL. Pharmacokinetic interaction between isradipine and lovastatin in normal, female and male volunteers. *J Pharmacol Exp Ther* (1995) 273, 121–7.
9. Jacobson TA. Comparative pharmacokinetic interaction profiles of pravastatin, simvastatin, and atorvastatin when coadministered with cytochrome P450 inhibitors. *Am J Cardiol* (2004) 94, 1140–6.
10. Nishio S, Watanabe H, Kosuge K, Uchida S, Hayashi H, Ohashi K. Interaction between amlodipine and simvastatin in patients with hypercholesterolemia and hypertension. *Hypertens Res* (2005) 28, 223–7.
11. Mousa O, Brater DC, Sunblad KJ, Hall SD. The interaction of diltiazem with simvastatin. *Clin Pharmacol Ther* (2000) 67, 267–74.
12. Kanathur N, Mathai MG, Byrd RP, Fields CL, Roy TM. Simvastatin-diltiazem drug interaction resulting in rhabdomyolysis and hepatitis. *Tenn Med* (2001) 94, 339–41.
13. Peces R, Pobes A. Rhabdomyolysis associated with concurrent use of simvastatin and diltiazem. *Nephron* (2001) 89, 117–18.
14. Yeo KR, Yeo WW. Inhibitory effects of verapamil and diltiazem on simvastatin metabolism in human liver microsomes. *Br J Clin Pharmacol* (2001) 51, 461–70.
15. Ziviani L, Da Ros L, Squassante L, Milleri S, Cugola M, Iavarone LE. The effects of lacidipine on the steady/state plasma concentrations of simvastatin in healthy subjects. *Br J Clin Pharmacol* (2001) 51, 147–52.
16. Kantola T, Kivistö KT, Neuvonen PJ. Erythromycin and verapamil considerably increase serum simvastatin and simvastatin acid concentrations. *Clin Pharmacol Ther* (1998) 64, 177–82.
17. Chiffoleau A, Tochu J-N, Veyrac G, Petit T, Abadie P, Bourin M, Jolliet P. Rhabdomyolyse liée à l'ajout du vérapamil à un traitement par simvastatine et cyclosporine chez un patient transplanté cardiaque. *Therapie* (2003) 58, 168–70.
18. Masica AL, Azie NE, Brater C, Hall SD, Jones DR. Intravenous diltiazem and CYP3A-mediated metabolism. *Br J Clin Pharmacol* (2000) 50, 273–6.
19. Gruer PJK, Vega JM, Mercuri MF, Dobrinska MR, Tobert JA. Concomitant use of cytochrome P450 3A4 inhibitors and simvastatin. *Am J Cardiol* (1999) 84, 811–15.
20. Mevacor (Lovastatin). Merck & Co., Inc. US Prescribing information, May 2007.
21. Zocor (Simvastatin). Merck & Co., Inc. US Prescribing information, May 2007.
22. Zocor (Simvastatin). Merck Sharp & Dohme Ltd. UK Summary of product characteristics, December 2005.
23. Simvador (Simvastatin). Discovery Pharmaceuticals Ltd. UK Summary of product characteristics, July 2003.

Statins + Carbamazepine

Carbamazepine dramatically reduces simvastatin levels.

Clinical evidence

In a randomised, crossover study 12 healthy subjects were given carbamazepine 200 mg daily for 2 days, then 300 mg twice daily for 12 days, with a single 80-mg dose of **simvastatin** 12 hours after the last dose of carbamazepine. The AUC and maximum serum levels of **simvastatin** were reduced by 75% and 68%, respectively, and the AUC and maximum serum levels of simvastatin acid (the active metabolite of **simvastatin**) were reduced by 82% and 69%, respectively.[1]

Mechanism

Carbamazepine is a known potent inducer of the cytochrome P450 isoenzyme CYP3A4 by which simvastatin is metabolised. Carbamazepine therefore increases simvastatin metabolism, leading to reduced levels. **Lovastatin**, and to a lesser extent, **atorvastatin** are also metabolised by CYP3A4.

Importance and management

Although this appears to be the only study, the effects of concurrent use are consistent with both the way carbamazepine interacts with many other CYP3A4 substrates and the way simvastatin interacts with other CYP3A4 inducers. The effects of simvastatin are likely to be greatly reduced on concurrent use and a dose increase seems likely to be necessary. Monitor concurrent use to check simvastatin is effective. It seems unlikely that other statins, such as fluvastatin or pravastatin, which are not metabolised by CYP3A4, will interact, and they may therefore be preferable. However, this needs confirmation.

1. Ucar M, Neuvonen M, Luurila H, Dahlqvist R, Neuvonen PJ, Mjörndal T. Carbamazepine markedly reduces serum concentrations of simvastatin and simvastatin acid. *Eur J Clin Pharmacol* (2004) 59, 879–82.

Statins + Ciclosporin

Ciclosporin can cause marked rises in the plasma levels of atorvastatin, fluvastatin, lovastatin, pravastatin, rosuvastatin, and simvastatin, and for some of the statins this has led to the development of serious myopathy (rhabdomyolysis) accompanied by renal failure. The plasma levels of ciclosporin appear not to be affected by fluvastatin, lovastatin, pravastatin, or rosuvastatin, but some moderate changes in ciclosporin levels have been seen when atorvastatin or simvastatin were given.

Clinical evidence

(a) Atorvastatin

1. Effect on ciclosporin. In a study of 10 patients taking ciclosporin following a kidney transplant, 4 showed increases in their trough ciclosporin levels of between 26 and 54% when atorvastatin 10 mg was added, necessitating a dosage reduction of ciclosporin. No changes were seen in 6 other patients, and the incidence of adverse effects was no greater than in a control transplant group not given atorvastatin.[1] When atorvastatin 10 mg daily was given to 21 renal transplant patients taking ciclosporin, the maximum serum levels of ciclosporin generally decreased (by a mean of 13.5%). However, 4 patients needed a *decrease* in their ciclosporin dose and one patient needed an increase.[2] Another study suggests that ciclosporin causes a negligible increase in ciclosporin levels in liver transplant patients.[3]

2. Effect on atorvastatin. In an open study the concurrent use of atorvastatin 10 mg daily with ciclosporin resulted in a sixfold increase in atorvastatin levels, when compared with historical controls not taking ciclosporin.[2] A further analysis of this study has been reported elsewhere.[4] A case of rhabdomyolysis has been described in a woman who took both drugs for 2 months. She had also been taking diltiazem.[5] In a review of the FDA spontaneous reports of statin-associated rhabdomyolysis covering the period November 1997 to March 2000, ciclosporin was potentially implicated in 5 cases of rhabdomyolysis involving atorvastatin.[6]

(b) Fluvastatin

1. Effect on ciclosporin. When fluvastatin 20 mg daily was given to 16 patients taking ciclosporin 21 to 103 months after renal transplantation, no significant changes were seen in their ciclosporin levels.[7,8] Similar results were seen in other studies, one using fluvastatin 20 mg twice daily,[9] and one in 17 renal transplant recipients taking extended-release fluvastatin.[10]

2. Effect on fluvastatin. In a double-blind study 52 heart transplant patients taking ciclosporin were randomised to receive fluvastatin 40 mg daily for 1 year. Fluvastatin had a positive effect on lipid profiles, and, although creatine phosphokinase levels rose, the maximum reached was 4.5 times normal, which did not require cessation of the fluvastatin and normalised without intervention. There was no increase in the reported rate of myalgia, and no patients developed rhabdomyolysis.[11] The AUC and maximum serum concentration of fluvastatin were found to be about 94% and 30% higher, respectively, in transplant patients taking ciclosporin than in historical control patients not taking ciclosporin.[12] Similarly, the AUC and maximum serum concentration of fluvastatin were threefold and sixfold greater in transplant patients taking ciclosporin than in healthy subjects not given ciclosporin.[13] A further study in 20 renal transplant patients receiving fluvastatin 20 mg daily reported 2 patients with mild myalgia without creatine phosphokinase rises, and a patient with elevated creatine phosphokinase without myalgia, when ciclosporin was also given.[14] Further studies suggest that concurrent use does not affect creatine phosphokinase or result in additional adverse effects.[7-9]

(c) Lovastatin

1. Effect on ciclosporin. Ciclosporin and creatine phosphokinase levels were not significantly changed in 6 renal transplant patients taking ciclosporin and lovastatin (10 mg for 8 weeks, then 20 mg for 12 weeks).[15] Similar results were found in another study.[16]

2. Effect on lovastatin. The plasma levels of lovastatin 10 to 20 mg daily in 6 patients also taking ciclosporin were about the same as those seen in healthy subjects taking lovastatin 40 mg alone (i.e. the levels were increased by up to fourfold by ciclosporin).[15] In another study in 21 renal transplant patients taking ciclosporin, the maximum serum levels and AUC of lovastatin 20 mg daily were 40 and 47% higher, respectively, 28 days after beginning therapy than on day 1 (suggesting accumulation) and were estimated to be 20-fold higher than values reported in healthy subjects not taking ciclosporin.[17] A further study found that the AUC of lovastatin was five times greater in patients taking ciclosporin than in patients not taking ciclosporin, irrespective of whether the patients had received transplants or were receiving other immunosuppressants.[18]

There are at least 9 documented cases of rhabdomyolysis, often resulting in acute renal failure, in patients taking ciclosporin and lovastatin.[19-23] In each of these cases the patient was taking lovastatin 40 to 80 mg daily. Several other studies suggest that this interaction may be dose-related. In one study, 15 patients taking ciclosporin were given lovastatin 20 mg daily without problem, but 4 of 5 other patients, who were given lovastatin 40 to 80 mg daily developed rhabdomyolysis, which was associated with renal failure in two of them.[24] In a further study 24 patients were given lovastatin 10 or 20 mg daily in addition to ciclosporin. Of the 12 receiving the 20-mg dose, 7 developed either myalgia and muscle weakness or raised creatine phosphokinase levels, but only one patient from the 10-mg group did.[25] A report describes a case of rhabdomyolysis when clopidogrel was added to treatment with ciclosporin and lovastatin.[26] The incidence of myopathies with lovastatin is about 0.1 to 0.2%,[17] but in the presence of ciclosporin the incidence is said to be as high as 30%.[27]

(d) Pravastatin

1. Effect on ciclosporin. Several studies have shown no significant change in ciclosporin levels in patients also taking pravastatin.[17,28]

2. Effect on pravastatin. A study in 19 paediatric and adolescent cardiac transplant patients (mean age 12.1 years) found that triple immunosuppressant therapy (17 patients taking ciclosporin) raised the maximum levels and AUC of pravastatin 10 mg daily for 8 weeks by about eightfold and tenfold, respectively, when compared with control subjects not receiving immunosuppressants. There was extremely large intersubject variation in the pravastatin AUC and maximum levels.[29] Similar results have been found in other studies in adults.[30,31] Although a study in patients taking ciclosporin found that the AUC of pravastatin 20 mg daily did not differ between day 1 and day 28 of therapy (suggesting no accumulation), the AUC values were estimated to be five to sevenfold higher than in patients not taking ciclosporin.[17] In a review of the FDA spontaneous reports of statin-associated rhabdomyolysis covering the period November 1997 to March 2000, ciclosporin was potentially implicated in 2 cases of rhabdomyolysis involving pravastatin.[6]

Several studies have shown no rises in creatine phosphokinase levels,[28,32,33] and no increase in adverse effects[17,32,34] when pravastatin in doses of 10 to 40 mg daily was given with ciclosporin.

(e) Rosuvastatin

In an open-label study 10 stable heart transplant patients taking ciclosporin were given rosuvastatin 10 mg daily for 10 days. When compared to healthy historical controls, the rosuvastatin maximum levels and AUC_{0-24} were found to have been increased by 10.6-fold and 7.1-fold, respectively. Rosuvastatin had little effect on ciclosporin levels.[35]

(f) Simvastatin

1. Effect on ciclosporin. A study found that the ciclosporin levels of 12 renal transplant patients fell from 334 to 235 micrograms/L after simvastatin 5 to 15 mg daily was added.[36] A retrospective study by the same authors confirmed these results in 12 patients.[36] In contrast, a single-dose pharmacokinetic study suggested that simvastatin increases the maximum levels and AUC of ciclosporin by a modest 8% and 13%, respectively.[37]

2. Effect on simvastatin. A group of 20 heart transplant patients were given simvastatin 10 mg daily and ciclosporin over a period of 4 months. The plasma levels of simvastatin acid were at least 6 times higher in 7 patients taking ciclosporin than in 7 control patients not taking ciclosporin.[38] Similarly, a study comparing 5 renal transplant patients taking ciclosporin and simvastatin 20 mg daily with 5 renal transplant patients not given ciclosporin found that the AUC and maximum serum levels of simvastatin were 2.5-fold and 2-fold greater, respectively, in the patients taking ciclosporin.[39]

There are at least 5 documented cases of rhabdomyolysis,[40-43] one of which was fatal,[41] in patients given ciclosporin and simvastatin. Another report describes a case of rhabdomyolysis when clopidogrel was added to treatment with ciclosporin and simvastatin.[26] In a review of the FDA spontaneous reports of statin-associated rhabdomyolysis covering the period November 1997 to March 2000, ciclosporin was potentially implicated in 31 cases of rhabdomyolysis involving simvastatin.[6]

In the first study cited above,[38] significant changes in ciclosporin levels and creatine kinase were seen and the combination was well tolerated. Similar results were found in another study over 8 months.[44]

Mechanism

The marked rises in statin levels and/or toxicity (rhabdomyolysis) probably occur because both the statin and ciclosporin compete for the same metabolising enzyme, the cytochrome P450 isoenzyme CYP3A4. The extent of the interaction seems to depend on the relative affinities of the different statins for this isoenzyme, and also on whether they can be metabolised by alternative pathways. P-glycoprotein and other transporter proteins may also have a part to play, especially in the raised ciclosporin levels seen with pravastatin. See 'Lipid regulating drugs', (p.1086) for more information about the metabolism of the statins.

In the cases where rhabdomyolysis developed when clopidogrel was added to treatment with ciclosporin and a statin it was thought that the addition of clopidogrel (which may also inhibit the cytochrome P450 enzyme system) may have destabilised the delicate metabolic equilibrium between the statins and ciclosporin precipitating the development of rhabdomyolysis.[26]

Importance and management

The interacting effect of ciclosporin on the statins is well documented, well established and clinically important. Concurrent use need not be avoided (except in the case of rosuvastatin, where concurrent use is contraindicated in the UK[45]) but it should be very well monitored, a precautionary recommendation being to start (or reduce) the statin to the lowest daily dose appropriate to the patient's condition.[46,47] The manufacturers of simvastatin suggest that the dose should not exceed 10 mg daily,[48-50] and the manufacturer of lovastatin suggests its dose should not exceed 20 mg daily.[46] The manufacturer of pravastatin suggests a starting dose of 20 mg.[47] Note that, unlike the UK manufacturers, the US manufacturers do not contraindicate rosuvastatin. However, they do warn that the risk of myopathy is increased, and advise that this should be taken into consideration when deciding on a dose. Therefore, as with other statins, it would seem that the lowest daily dose of rosuvastatin should be used.[51] Any patient given ciclosporin with a statin should be told to report any signs of myopathy and possible rhabdomyolysis (i.e. otherwise unexplained muscle pain, tenderness or weakness or dark coloured urine). If myopathy does occur, withdrawing the statin has been shown to resolve the symptoms.

Alterations in ciclosporin levels with the statins are generally small and seem likely to be identified by routine ciclosporin monitoring. However, note that of the statins, simvastatin, and possibly atorvastatin had somewhat larger effects, and an increase in the frequency of ciclosporin monitoring may be desirable if these statins are used. See also 'muscle toxicity', (p.1086), for further guidance on monitoring and risk factors for muscle toxicity.

1. Renders L, Mayer-Kadner I, Koch C, Schärffe S, Burkhardt K, Veelken R, Schmieder RE, Hauser IA. Efficacy and drug interactions of the new HMG-CoA reductase inhibitors cerivastatin and atorvastatin in CsA-treated renal transplant recipients. *Nephrol Dial Transplant* (2001) 16, 141–6.
2. Åsberg A, Hartmann A, Fjeldså E, Bergan S, Holdaas H. Bilateral pharmacokinetic interaction between cyclosporine A and atorvastatin in renal transplant recipients. *Am J Transplant* (2001) 1, 382–6.
3. Taylor PJ, Kubler PA, Lynch SV, Allen J, Butler M, Pillans PI. Effect of atorvastatin on cyclosporine pharmacokinetics in liver transplant recipients. *Ann Pharmacother* (2004) 38, 205–8.
4. Hermann M, Åsberg A, Christensen H, Holdaas H, Hartmann A, Reubsaet JLE. Substantially elevated levels of atorvastatin and metabolites in cyclosporine-treated renal transplant recipients. *Clin Pharmacol Ther* (2004) 76, 388–91.
5. Maltz HC, Balog DL, Cheigh JS. Rhabdomyolysis associated with concomitant use of atorvastatin and cyclosporine. *Ann Pharmacother* (1999) 33, 1176–9.
6. Omar MA, Wilson JP. FDA adverse event reports on statin-associated rhabdomyolysis. *Ann Pharmacother* (2002) 36, 288–95.
7. Li PKT, Mak TWL, Wang AYM, Lee YT, Leung CB, Lui SF, Lam CWK, Lai KN. The interaction of fluvastatin and cyclosporin A in renal-transplant patients. *Int J Clin Pharmacol Ther* (1995) 33, 246–8.
8. Li PKT, Mak TWL, Chan TH, Wang A, Lam CWK, Lai KN. Effect of fluvastatin on lipoprotein profiles in treating renal transplant recipients with dyslipoproteinemia. *Transplantation* (1995) 60, 652–6.
9. Holdaas H, Hartmann A, Stenstrøm J, Dahl KJ, Borge M, Pfister P. Effect of fluvastatin for safely lowering atherogenic lipids in renal transplant patients receiving cyclosporine. *Am J Cardiol* (1995) 76, 102A–106A.
10. Holdaas H, Hagen E, Åsberg A, Lund K, Hartman A, Vaidyanathan, Prasad P, He Y-L, Yeh C-M, Bigler H, Rouilly M, Denouel J. Evaluation of the pharmacokinetic interaction between fluvastatin XL and cyclosporine in renal transplant recipients. *Int J Clin Pharmacol Ther* (2006) 44, 163–71.
11. O'Rourke B, Barbir M, Mitchell AG, Yacoub MH, Banner NR. Efficacy and safety of fluvastatin therapy for hypercholesterolemia after heart transplantation. Results of a randomised double blind placebo controlled study. *Int J Cardiol* (2004) 94, 235–40.
12. Goldberg R, Roth D. Evaluation of fluvastatin in the treatment of hypercholesterolemia in renal transplant recipients taking cyclosporine. *Transplantation* (1996) 62, 1559–64.
13. Park J-W, Siekmeier R, Lattke P, Merz M, Mix C, Schüler S, Jaross W. Pharmacokinetics and pharmacodynamics of fluvastatin in heart transplant recipients taking cyclosporine A. *J Cardiovasc Pharmacol Ther* (2001) 6, 351–61.
14. Goldberg RB, Roth D. A preliminary report of the safety and efficacy of fluvastatin for hypercholesterolemia in renal transplant patients receiving cyclosporine. *Am J Cardiol* (1995) 76, 107A–109A.
15. Cheung AK, DeVault GA, Gregory MC. A prospective study on treatment of hypercholesterolemia with lovastatin in renal transplant patients receiving cyclosporine. *J Am Soc Nephrol* (1993) 3, 1884–91.
16. Castelao AM, Griñó JM, Andrés E, Gilvernet S, Serón D, Castiñeiras MJ, Roca M, Galcerán JM, González MT, Alsina J. HMGCoA reductase inhibitors lovastatin and simvastatin in the treatment of hypercholesterolemia after renal transplantation. *Transplant Proc* (1993) 25, 1043–6.
17. Olbricht C, Wanner C, Eisenhauer T, Kliem V, Doll R, Boddaert M, O'Grady P, Krekler M, Mangold B, Christians U. Accumulation of lovastatin, but not pravastatin, in the blood of cyclosporine-treated kidney graft patients after multiple doses. *Clin Pharmacol Ther* (1997) 62, 311–21.
18. Gullestad L, Nordal KP, Berg KJ, Cheng H, Schwartz MS, Simonsen S. Interaction between lovastatin and cyclosporine A after heart and kidney transplantation. *Transplant Proc* (1999) 31, 2163–5.
19. Alejandro DSJ, Petersen J. Myoglobinuric acute renal failure in a cardiac transplant patient taking lovastatin and cyclosporine. *J Am Soc Nephrol* (1994) 5, 153–160.
20. Corpier CL, Jones PH, Suki WN, Lederer ED, Quinones MA, Schmidt SW, Young JB. Rhabdomyolysis and renal injury with lovastatin use. Report of two cases in cardiac transplant recipients. *JAMA* (1988) 260, 239–41.
21. East C, Alivizatos PA, Grundy SM, Jones PH, Farmer JA. Rhabdomyolysis in patients receiving lovastatin after cardiac transplantation. *N Engl J Med* (1988) 318, 47–8.
22. Norman DJ, Illingworth DR, Munson J, Hosenpud J. Myolysis and acute renal failure in a heart-transplant recipient receiving lovastatin. *N Engl J Med* (1988) 318, 46–7.
23. Kobashigawa JA, Murphy F, Stevenson LW, Moriguchi JD, Kawata N, Chuck C, Wilmarth J, Leonard L, Drinkwater D, Laks H. Low dose of lovastatin safely lowers cholesterol after cardiac transplantation. *Circulation* (1989) 80 (Suppl II), II-641.
24. Ballantyne CM, Radovancevic B, Farmer JA, Frazier OH, Chandler L, Payton-Ross C, Cocanougher B, Jones PH, Young JB, Gotto AM. Hyperlipidemia after heart transplantation: report of a 6-year experience, with treatment recommendations. *J Am Coll Cardiol* (1992) 19, 1315–21.
25. Heroux AL, Thompson JA, Katz S, Hastillo AK, Katz M, Quigg RJ, Hess ML. Elimination of the lovastatin-cyclosporine adverse interaction in heart transplant patients. *Circulation* (1989) 80, II-641.
26. Uber PA, Mehra MR, Park MH, Scott RL. Clopidogrel and rhabdomyolysis after heart transplantation. *J Heart Lung Transplant* (2003) 22, 107–8.
27. Tobert JA. Rhabdomyolysis in patients receiving lovastatin after cardiac transplantation. *N Engl J Med* (1988) 318, 48.
28. Cassem JD, Hamilton MA, Albanese E, Sabad A, Kobashigawa JA. Does pravastatin affect cyclosporine pharmacokinetics in cardiac transplant recipients. *J Investig Med* (1997) 45, 139A.
29. Hedman M, Neuvonen PJ, Neuvonen M, Holmberg C, Antikainen M. Pharmacokinetics and pharmacodynamics of pravastatin in pediatric and adolescent cardiac transplant recipients on a regimen of triple immunosuppression. *Clin Pharmacol Ther* (2004) 75, 101–109.
30. Park J-W, Siekmeier R, Merz M, Krell B, Harder S, März W, Seidel D, Schüler S, Groß W. Pharmacokinetics of pravastatin in heart-transplant patients taking cyclosporin A. *Int J Clin Pharmacol Ther* (2002) 40, 439–50.
31. Regazzi MB, Iacona I, Campana C, Raddato V, Lesi C, Perani G, Gavazzi A, Viganò M. Altered disposition of pravastatin following concomitant drug therapy with cyclosporin A in transplant recipients. *Transplant Proc* (1993) 25, 2732–4.
32. Yoshimura N, Oka T, Okamoto M, Ohmori Y. The effects of pravastatin on hyperlipidemia in renal transplant recipients. *Transplantation* (1992) 53, 94–9.
33. Muhlmeister HF, Hamilton MA, Cogert GA, Cassem JD, Sabad A, Kobashigawa JA. Long-term HMG-CoA reductase inhibition appears safe and effective after cardiac transplantation. *J Investig Med* (1997) 45, 139A.
34. Kobashigawa JA, Brownfield ED, Stevenson LW, Gleeson MP, Moriguchi JD, Kawata N, Hamilton MA, Hage AS, Minkley R, Salamandra J, Ruzevich S, Drinkwater DC, Laks H. Effects of pravastatin for hypercholesterolemia in cardiac transplant recipients. *J Am Coll Cardiol* (1993) 21, 141A.
35. Simonson SG, Raza A, Martin PD, Mitchell PD, Jarcho JA, Brown CDA, Windass AS, Schneck DW. Rosuvastatin pharmacokinetics in heart transplant recipients administered an antirejection regimen including cyclosporine. *Clin Pharmacol Ther* (2004) 76, 167–77.
36. Akhlaghi F, McLachlan AJ, Keogh AM, Brown KF. Effect of simvastatin on cyclosporine unbound fraction and apparent blood clearance in heart transplant recipients. *Br J Clin Pharmacol* (1997) 44, 537–42.
37. Xu F, Wu Z-H, Zhang Z-Y, Zou H-Q. Delay of metabolism rate of ciclosporin by simvastatin in 7 Chinese healthy men. *Acta Pharmacol Sin* (1998) 19, 443–4.
38. Campana C, Iacona I, Regazzi MB, Gavazzi A, Perani G, Raddato V, Montemartini C, Viganò M. Efficacy and pharmacokinetics of simvastatin in heart transplant recipients. *Ann Pharmacother* (1995) 29, 235–9.
39. Arnadottir M, Eriksson L-O, Thysell H, Karkas JD. Plasma concentration profiles of simvastatin 3-hydroxy-3-methyl-glutaryl-coenzyme A reductase inhibitory activity in kidney transplant recipients with and without ciclosporin. *Nephron* (1993) 65, 410–13.
40. Blaison G, Weber JC, Sachs D, Korganow AS, Martin T, Kretz JG, Pasquali JL. Rhabdomyolyse causée par la simvastatine chez un transplanté cardiaque sous ciclosporine. *Rev Med Interne* (1992) 13, 61–3.
41. Weise WJ, Possidente CJ. Fatal rhabdomyolysis associated with simvastatin in a renal transplant patient. *Am J Med* (2000) 108, 351–2.
42. Meier C, Stey C, Brack T, Maggiorini M, Risti B, Krahenbuhl S. Rhabdomyolyse bei mit Simvastatin und Ciclosporin behandelten Patienten: Rolle der aktivitat des Cytochrom-P450-Enzymsystems der Leber. *Schweiz Med Wochenschr* (1995) 125, 1342–6.

43. Gumprecht J, Zychma M, Grzeszczak W, Kuźniewicz R, Burak W, Żywiec J, Karasek D, Otulski I, Mosur M. Simvastatin-induced rhabdomyolysis in a CsA-treated renal transplant recipient. *Med Sci Monit* (2003) 9, CS89–CS91.
44. Barbir M, Rose M, Kushwaha S, Akl S, Mitchell A, Yacoub M. Low-dose simvastatin for the treatment of hypercholesterolaemia in recipients of cardiac transplantation. *Int J Cardiol* (1991) 33, 241–6.
45. Crestor (Rosuvastatin calcium). AstraZeneca UK Ltd. UK Summary of product characteristics, June 2007.
46. Mevacor (Lovastatin). Merck & Co., Inc. US Prescribing information, May 2007.
47. Lipostat (Pravastatin). Bristol-Myers Squibb Pharmaceuticals Ltd. UK Summary of product characteristics, December 2005.
48. Zocor (Simvastatin). Merck Sharp & Dohme Ltd. UK Summary of product characteristics, December 2005.
49. Zocor (Simvastatin). Merck & Co., Inc. US Prescribing information, May 2007.
50. Simvador (Simvastatin). Discovery Pharmaceuticals Ltd. UK Summary of product characteristics, July 2003.
51. Crestor (Rosuvastatin calcium). AstraZeneca. US Prescribing information, July 2007.

Statins + Colchicine

Three case reports describe myopathy or rhabdomyolysis in patients given colchicine with fluvastatin, pravastatin or simvastatin. It seems possible that this interaction could occur with colchicine and any statin.

Clinical evidence

(a) Fluvastatin

A 70-year-old man who had been taking fluvastatin 80 mg daily for 2 years started taking colchicine 1.5 mg daily for an attack of gouty arthritis. Within 3 days he felt nauseous and began to develop muscle pains and weakness. On admission to hospital he was found to have acute renal failure and a raised creatine kinase, and was diagnosed with rhabdomyolysis. Both drugs were stopped and he made a full recovery over 2 months. He was eventually restabilised on fluvastatin without incident.[1]

(b) Pravastatin

A 65-year-old woman who had been taking pravastatin 20 mg daily for 6 years was given colchicine 1.5 mg daily for an episode of gout. Within 20 days she had developed muscle weakness in the legs and had a slightly raised creatine kinase. A diagnosis of myopathy was made and so both the colchicine and pravastatin were stopped. The weakness resolved over the following week. The colchicine was subsequently given alone, and myopathy did not occur.[2]

(c) Simvastatin

A patient with chronic renal failure who had been taking simvastatin for 2 years was given colchicine for gout. Within 2 weeks he developed muscle weakness, which was diagnosed as myopathy. Both drugs were stopped and the symptoms resolved.[3]

Mechanism

It has been suggested that the interaction between simvastatin occurs because both drugs are metabolised by the cytochrome P450 isoenzyme CYP3A4.[3] However, as the interaction has subsequently been seen with fluvastatin and pravastatin this seems unlikely to be the full explanation. P-glycoprotein has also been implicated.[2] Colchicine alone can, rarely, cause myopathy. However, it is more common in those given colchicine long term, in high dose, or in the presence of renal impairment.[2] As the statins can also cause myopathy, an additive or synergistic effect seems possible.[1]

Importance and management

Although this interaction is rare it is serious. Given the evidence available it seems likely to occur with all statins, although this has not been clearly demonstrated. All patients taking statins should be warned about the symptoms of myopathy and told to report muscle pain or weakness. It would be prudent to reinforce this advice if they are given colchicine. See also 'muscle toxicity', (p.1086), for further guidance on monitoring and risk factors for muscle toxicity.

1. Atasoyu EM, Evrenkaya TR, Solmazgul E. Possible colchicine rhabdomyolysis in a fluvastatin-treated patient. *Ann Pharmacother* (2005) 39, 1368–9.
2. Alayli G, Cengiz K, Cantürk F, Durmuş D, Akyol Y, Menekşe EB. Acute myopathy in a patient with concomitant use of pravastatin and colchicine. *Ann Pharmacother* (2005) 39, 1358–61.
3. Hsu W-C, Chen W-H, Chang M-T, Chiu H-C. Colchicine-induced acute myopathy in a patient with concomitant use of simvastatin. *Clin Neuropharmacol* (2002) 25, 266–8.

Statins + Danazol

Severe rhabdomyolysis and myoglobinuria developed in a man taking lovastatin about two months after danazol was added. Another report describes a similar interaction with simvastatin.

Clinical evidence

(a) Lovastatin

A 72-year-old man taking atenolol, aspirin, dipyridamole and lovastatin 20 mg twice daily was admitted to hospital after complaining of myalgia over the last 12 days, and brown urine over the last 5 days. His condition was diagnosed as severe rhabdomyolysis and myoglobinuria. About 2 months previously he had started taking danazol 200 mg three times daily and prednisone, and one month previously he had received a 10-day course of doxycycline 100 mg twice daily. The aspirin and lovastatin were stopped (danazol was stopped 4 days before admission and the doxycycline was stopped 5 days before the onset of symptoms), and all the symptoms resolved. Laboratory tests were normal within 2 weeks.[1]

(b) Simvastatin

A 68-year-old man who had been taking simvastatin 40 mg daily long-term without problem developed rhabdomyolysis (progressive muscle pain and weakness, tea-coloured urine, renal impairment, and a raised creatine phosphokinase) within 3 weeks of starting to take danazol 200 mg three times daily. He was given haemodialysis and subsequently recovered.

Mechanism

It has been suggested that danazol (and the doxycycline) were possibly hepatotoxic, which led to decreased lovastatin metabolism, or that the danazol had a direct toxic effect on the muscles.[1] Danazol inhibits the cytochrome P450 isoenzyme CYP3A4 by which simvastatin and lovastatin are metabolised, which would result in raised statin levels, and therefore myopathy and rhabdomyolysis.[1,2] This seems a more likely explanation for the effects seen.

Importance and management

These appear to be the only reports of this apparent interaction, but the pharmacokinetic basis of the interaction seems to be established. The US manufacturers of lovastatin[3] suggest that the dose should not exceed 20 mg daily in the presence of danazol. Similarly the manufacturers of simvastatin suggest that the dose should not exceed 10 mg daily in the presence of danazol.[4,5] It would seem prudent to reinforce the symptoms of myopathy and tell patients to report any unexplained muscle pain, tenderness or weakness. The authors of the lovastatin report[1] point out that, as in this case, severe lovastatin muscle toxicity may be very slow to develop. See also 'muscle toxicity', (p.1086), for further guidance on monitoring, and risk factors for muscle toxicity.

The statins that are not significantly metabolised by CYP3A4 (**fluvastatin**, **pravastatin**, **rosuvastatin**) are not expected to interact.

1. Dallaire M, Chamberland M, Rhabdomyolyse sévère chez un patient recevant lovastatine, danazol et doxycycline. *Can Med Assoc J* (1994) 150, 1991–4.
2. Andreou ER, Ledger S. Potential drug interaction between simvastatin and danazol causing rhabdomyolysis. *Can J Clin Pharmacol* (2003) 10, 172–4.
3. Mevacor (Lovastatin). Merck & Co., Inc. US Prescribing information, May 2007.
4. Zocor (Simvastatin). Merck Sharp & Dohme Ltd. UK Summary of product characteristics, December 2005.
5. Zocor (Simvastatin). Merck & Co., Inc. US Prescribing information, May 2007.

Statins + Diuretics

In clinical studies, the safety and efficacy of statins were not altered by concurrent use of diuretics.

Clinical evidence, mechanism, importance and management

Retrospective analysis of clinical study data[1] found no evidence that the safety or efficacy of **lovastatin** was altered by the use of **potassium-sparing diuretics** (hydrochlorothiazide with **triamterene** or **amiloride**), or **thiazide diuretics** (mostly **hydrochlorothiazide**). Another retrospective study of 19 patients found that the addition of **lovastatin** to diuretic treatment caused an initial 30% fall in total serum cholesterol levels for one month, followed by a rise of about 20%. In a further 13 patients, the addition of diuretic treatment to **lovastatin** caused a 20% fall in total serum cholesterol for one month and then a 20% rise back to baseline values. The diuretics used were **furosemide** (16 patients), **triamterene/hydrochlorothiazide** (7), **hydrochlorothiazide** (8), **indapamide** (1). The fall and subsequent rise in serum cholesterol levels occurred in all of the patients except just the one taking **indapamide**.[2] The reason for this initial fall in cholesterol, particularly when the diuretic was added to the statin, is unknown, and the findings of this study are difficult to interpret.

Retrospective analysis of clinical trial data found no evidence that the safety or efficacy of **fluvastatin** was altered by the use of unspecified **diuretics**.[3] Likewise, the manufacturer of **atorvastatin**[4] says that in clinical studies it was used concurrently with unnamed **diuretics** without evidence of significant adverse interactions.

The bulk of the evidence suggests no special precautions are necessary if diuretics are given concurrently with statins.

1. Pool JL, Shear CL, Downton M, Schnaper H, Stinnett S, Dujovne C, Bradford RH, Chremos AN. Lovastatin and coadministered antihypertensive/cardiovascular agents. *Hypertension* (1992) 19, 242–8.
2. Aruna AS, Akula SK, Sarpong DF. Interaction between potassium-depleting diuretics and lovastatin in hypercholesterolemic ambulatory care patients. *J Pharm Technol* (1997) 13, 21–6.
3. Peters TK, Jewitt-Harris J, Mehra M, Muratti EN. Safety and tolerability of fluvastatin with concomitant use of antihypertensive agents. An analysis of a clinical trial database. *Am J Hypertens* (1993) 6, 346S–352S.
4. Lipitor (Atorvastatin). Pfizer Ltd. UK Summary of product characteristics, September 2006.

Statins + Everolimus

In a single-dose study in healthy subjects everolimus did not alter the pharmacokinetics or HMG-CoA reductase activity of atorvastatin or pravastatin to a clinically relevant extent. Everolimus pharmacokinetics were unaltered by the statins.[1]

1. Kovarik JM, Hartmann S, Hubert M, Berthier S, Schneider W, Rosenkranz B, Rordorf C. Pharmacokinetic and pharmacodynamic assessments of HMG-CoA reductase inhibitors when coadministered with everolimus. *J Clin Pharmacol* (2002) 42, 222–8.

Statins + Ezetimibe

Ezetimibe does not appear to have adverse pharmacokinetic interactions with atorvastatin, fluvastatin, lovastatin, rosuvastatin or simvastatin. However, some evidence suggests that concurrent use may increase the risk of myopathy.

Clinical evidence

(a) Atorvastatin

In a three-arm study patients were given atorvastatin 80 mg daily, atorvastatin 80 mg daily with ezetimibe 10 mg daily, or atorvastatin 40 mg daily with ezetimibe 10 mg daily. No difference in adverse events was noted between each of the 3 groups and there were no significant elevations in creatine kinase. No cases of myopathy or rhabdomyolysis occurred, and the combination was well-tolerated.[1] Similarly, an efficacy study found that ezetimibe did not worsen statin intolerance or toxicity in 628 patients with hypercholesterolaemia who were taking atorvastatin.[2] However, a case report describes a 43-year-old man taking atorvastatin 80 mg daily who developed severe muscle pain with elevated creatinine kinase levels 3 weeks after he started taking ezetimibe 10 mg daily. Symptoms resolved when both drugs were withdrawn and he later restarted the atorvastatin without problems.[3] A further similar case has also been reported.[4]

(b) Fluvastatin

In a randomised, crossover study 32 otherwise healthy subjects with hypercholesterolaemia were given either ezetimibe 10 mg daily, fluvastatin 20 mg daily or both drugs in combination for 14 days. The combination was well tolerated, no significant pharmacokinetic interaction occurred, and an enhanced lowering of LDL-cholesterol was noted, which was considered to be clinically favourable.[5] However, a case report describes a 52-year-old man taking fluvastatin 80 mg daily who developed elevated creatinine kinase levels 8 weeks after ezetimibe 10 mg daily was added. His creatinine kinase levels returned to normal 4 weeks after the ezetimibe was withdrawn.[3]

(c) Lovastatin

In a randomised, crossover study 18 healthy subjects were given either ezetimibe 10 mg daily, lovastatin 20 mg daily or both drugs in combination for 7 days. The combination was well tolerated, and no significant pharmacokinetic interaction was noted.[6]

(d) Rosuvastatin

In a placebo-controlled study 12 otherwise healthy subjects with hypercholesterolaemia were given ezetimibe 10 mg daily with rosuvastatin 10 mg daily for 14 days. The combination was well tolerated (no significant changes in liver enzymes or creatinine phosphokinase noted), the pharmacokinetics of both drugs were not significantly changed, and an enhanced lowering of LDL-cholesterol was noted, which was considered to be clinically favourable.[7]

(e) Simvastatin

In a three-arm study, patients were given simvastatin 80 mg daily, simvastatin 80 mg daily with ezetimibe 10 mg daily, or simvastatin 40 mg daily with ezetimibe 10 mg daily. No difference in adverse events was noted between each of the 3 groups and there were no significant elevations in creatine kinase. No cases of myopathy or rhabdomyolysis occurred, and the combination was well-tolerated.[1] In another study, ezetimibe 0.25 mg, 1 mg or 10 mg daily had no effect on the pharmacokinetics of simvastatin 10 mg daily, when both were given for 14 days. In addition, 10 and 20-mg doses of simvastatin were well-tolerated in combination with ezetimibe.[8]

Mechanism, importance and management

The available evidence suggests that on the whole the concurrent use of a statin with ezetimibe does not result in a change in the pharmacokinetics of either drug. However, there is some evidence to suggest that concurrent use may increase the risk of myopathy. Therefore any patient taking a statin who is also given ezetimibe should be told to report any signs of myopathy and possible rhabdomyolysis (i.e. otherwise unexplained muscle pain, tenderness or weakness or dark coloured urine). See also 'muscle toxicity', (p.1086), for further guidance on monitoring, and risk factors for muscle toxicity.

Note that a combination preparation containing simvastatin and ezetimibe is widely available.

1. Gagné C, Gaudet D, Bruckert E for the Ezetimibe Study Group. Efficacy and safety of ezetimibe coadministered with atorvastatin or simvastatin in patients with homozygous familial hypercholesterolemia. *Circulation* (2002) 105, 2469–75.
2. Ballantyne CM, Houri J, Notarbartolo A, Melani L, Lipka LJ, Suresh R, Sun S, LeBeaut AP, Sager PT, Veltri EP for the Ezetimibe Study Group. Effect of ezetimibe coadministered with atorvastatin in 628 patients with primary hypercholesterolemia: A prospective, randomised, double-blind trial. *Circulation* (2003) 107, 2409–15.
3. Fux R, Mörike K, Gundel U-F, Hartmann R, Gleiter CH. Ezetimibe and statin-associated myopathy. *Ann Intern Med* (2004) 140, 671–2.
4. Simard C, Poirier P. Ezetimibe-associated myopathy in monotherapy and in combination with a 3-hydroxy-3-methylglutaryl coenzyme A reductase inhibitor. *Can J Cardiol* (2006) 22, 141–44.
5. Reyderman L, Kosoglou T, Cutler DL, Maxwell S, Statkevich P. The effect of fluvastatin on the pharmacokinetics and pharmacodynamics of ezetimibe. *Curr Med Res Opin* (2005) 21, 1171–9.
6. Reyderman L, Kosoglou T, Boutros T, Sieberling M, Statkevich P. Pharmacokinetic interaction between ezetimibe and lovastatin in healthy volunteers. *Curr Med Res Opin* (2004) 20, 1493–1500.
7. Kosoglou T, Statkevich P, Yang B, Suresh R, Zhu Y, Boutros T, Maxwell SE, Tiessen R, Cutler DL. Pharmacodynamic interaction between ezetimibe and rosuvastatin. *Curr Med Res Opin* (2004) 20, 1185–95.
8. Kosoglou T, Meyer I, Veltri EP, Statkevich P, Yang B, Zhu Y, Mellars L, Maxwell SE, Patrick JE, Cutler DL, Batra VK, Affrime MB. Pharmacodynamic interaction between the new selective cholesterol absorption inhibitor ezetimibe and simvastatin. *Br J Clin Pharmacol* (2002) 54, 309–19.

Statins + Fibrates

The plasma levels of lovastatin, simvastatin, atorvastatin and pravastatin are increased by gemfibrozil, the levels of fluvastatin are increased by bezafibrate, and the levels of pravastatin are increased by fenofibrate. No pharmacokinetic interactions occur with the combinations of fluvastatin with gemfibrozil, lovastatin with bezafibrate, and pravastatin, rosuvastatin or simvastatin with fenofibrate. Both statins and fibrates are known to cause rhabdomyolysis, and their concurrent use increases the risk of this reaction.

Clinical evidence

A. Bezafibrate

(a) Fluvastatin

In one study bezafibrate 200 mg three times daily increased the AUC and maximum levels of fluvastatin 20 mg daily by about 50 to 60%. Bezafibrate pharmacokinetics were not affected.[1]

(b) Lovastatin

In a study in 11 healthy subjects the pharmacokinetics of a single 40-mg dose of lovastatin were not altered by bezafibrate 400 mg daily for 3 days.[2]

B. Fenofibrate

(a) Pravastatin

A single-dose study in 23 healthy subjects found that the concurrent use of pravastatin 40 mg and fenofibrate 201 mg had no effect on the pharmacokinetics of either drug, but a moderate increase in the formation of a non-toxic pravastatin metabolite was seen. This was not thought to be clinically important.[3] In a multiple-dose study pravastatin 40 mg daily was given to 23 healthy subjects with fenofibrate 160 mg daily. Fenofibrate increased the maximum levels and AUC of pravastatin by about 40% and 30%, respectively. Similar increases were seen for the main pravastatin metabolite. The combination was well tolerated, and the increases were considered to be modest.[4] However, a case report describes a patient taking fenofibrate 300 mg daily, who developed rhabdomyolysis after starting pravastatin 10 mg daily.[5]

(b) Rosuvastatin

A 7-day course of fenofibrate 67 mg three times daily and rosuvastatin 10 mg daily resulted in only minor changes in fenofibric acid and rosuvastatin exposure in 14 healthy subjects, when compared with either drug given alone.[6]

(c) Simvastatin

In a randomised, crossover study 25 healthy subjects were given simvastatin 80 mg daily with fenofibrate 160 mg daily for 7 days. The pharmacokinetics of both drugs and their main metabolites (as assessed in 12 subjects) were unchanged by concurrent use. All 25 subjects were assessed for safety, and the combination was found to be well tolerated.[7]

C. Gemfibrozil

(a) Atorvastatin

A pharmacokinetic study in 10 healthy subjects found that gemfibrozil 600 mg twice daily increased the AUC of atorvastatin and its metabolites by 24% and 30 to 80%, respectively, which was considered a moderate increase.[8] A 43-year-old woman with multiple medical problems was taking gemfibrozil 600 mg twice daily. After a recurrent attack of pancreatitis, atorvastatin 10 mg and glibenclamide (glyburide) 2.5 mg, both twice daily, were added to her treatment. About 3 weeks later she developed brown and turbid urine (suggesting urinary myoglobin), creatine kinase levels of 4633 units/L and had myalgia. She was diagnosed as having rhabdomyolysis. Her serum creatine kinase levels rapidly fell when the atorvastatin and gemfibrozil were withdrawn.[9]

In a case series of 10 patients taking a statin who presented for muscle biopsy, one patient taking gemfibrozil developed myopathy 3 months after his dose of atorvastatin was increased from 10 to 20 mg.[10]

(b) Fluvastatin

In a randomised, crossover study 15 patients were given fluvastatin 20 mg and gemfibrozil 600 mg twice daily. The pharmacokinetics of both gemfibrozil and fluvastatin were unchanged by concurrent use and no significant adverse effects were noted.[11]

(c) Lovastatin

In a pharmacokinetic study, 11 healthy subjects were given gemfibrozil 1.2 g daily for 3 days, with a single 40-mg dose of lovastatin on day 3. The AUC and maximum plasma level of lovastatin acid (a metabolite) were nearly threefold greater in the presence of gemfibrozil.[2]

By 1990 the FDA had documented 12 case reports of severe myopathy or rhabdomyolysis associated with the concurrent use of lovastatin and gemfibrozil. The mean serum creatine kinase levels of the patients reached 15 250 units/L. Four of those tested showed myoglobinuria and five had acute renal failure.[12] Details of cases of rhabdomyolysis associated with the concurrent use of these drugs,[13-18] three involving renal failure,[14,15,17] have been given elsewhere. Other cases of rhabdomyolysis have been seen in patients taking lovastatin and gemfibrozil, with ciclosporin,[19] or niacin.[20] Aside from these cases, a review of combined statin/fibrate use identified a further 4 cases of rhabdomyolysis involving gemfibrozil and lovastatin, all involving lovastatin doses of 40 mg and above.[21]

However, in contrast, other reports[22-25] describe apparently safe and effective concurrent use under very well controlled conditions, although elevated creatine phosphokinase levels, without rhabdomyolysis, were seen in up to 8% of cases.

(d) Pravastatin

In a study in 18 healthy subjects gemfibrozil 600 mg caused no clinically significant changes in the bioavailability of a single 20-mg dose of pravastatin.[26] However, another study using pravastatin 40 mg found that the AUC and maximum levels of pravastatin were increased roughly threefold and twofold, respectively.[27] A 12-week study with pravastatin 40 mg daily and gemfibrozil 600 mg twice daily found that marked abnormalities in creatine kinase concentrations (four times the pretreatment values) occurred in 1 of 71 patients taking pravastatin alone, 1 of 73 patients taking placebo, 2 of 72 patients taking gemfibrozil alone, and 4 of 75 patients taking gemfibrozil with pravastatin. The differences between treatments were not statistically significant. Two patients taking combination therapy had this withdrawn because of asymptomatic creatine kinase elevations. Severe myopathy or rhabdomyolysis was not seen in any patient, although 14 patients had musculoskeletal pain, but in most cases this was not considered to be related to treatment.[28]

(e) Rosuvastatin

In a randomised, crossover study 20 healthy subjects were given gemfibrozil 600 mg twice daily for 7 days, with a single 80-mg dose of rosuvastatin on day 4. The AUC of rosuvastatin was increased 1.88-fold (11 subjects assessed) and the maximum levels of rosuvastatin were increased 2.21-fold. Three subjects had asymptomatic increases in ALT levels (less than 2.5 times upper limit of normal).[29]

(f) Simvastatin

A 62-year-old man with diabetes taking simvastatin 20 mg daily and gemfibrozil 600 mg daily (as well as acenocoumarol, glibenclamide (glyburide) and diclofenac) was hospitalised because of melaena, generalised myalgia, malaise and brown urine. Laboratory tests confirmed the diagnosis of rhabdomyolysis. He recovered when the simvastatin and gemfibrozil were stopped.[30] Another diabetic patient had been taking simvastatin and gemfibrozil 600 mg daily for 2½ years (as well as felodipine, indapamide, calcium carbonate, bumetanide, psyllium, acenocoumarol and insulin). She complained of tiredness, generalised myalgia and anuria 3 months after her dosage of simvastatin had been increased to 80 mg daily. Rhabdomyolysis with exaggerated renal impairment were diagnosed and confirmed. She recovered when the simvastatin and gemfibrozil were stopped.[30] Three further cases of rhabdomyolysis have been reported in patients taking simvastatin, 3 weeks to 3 months after starting gemfibrozil.[31-33] One of these cases was fatal.[31]

A pharmacokinetic study found that when gemfibrozil was given with simvastatin the AUC of simvastatin acid (an active metabolite of simvastatin) was increased nearly twofold and the peak concentration was doubled.[34]

In a case series of 10 patients taking a statin who presented for muscle biopsy, two patient taking gemfibrozil developed myopathy while also taking simvastatin.[10]

D. Unspecified Fibrates

In a review[35] of the FDA spontaneous reports of statin-associated rhabdomyolysis covering the period November 1997 to March 2000, fibrates (unspecified) were potentially implicated in 10 of 73 cases of rhabdomyolysis seen with **atorvastatin**, 4 of 10 with **fluvastatin**, 5 of 40 with **lovastatin**, 6 of 71 with **pravastatin**, and 33 of 215 with **simvastatin**.

Mechanism

Not understood. Myopathy can occur with statins and fibrates alone and their effects may therefore be additive or synergistic. There is also some evidence that the fibrates may inhibit the metabolism of the statins, but *not* because they inhibit the cytochrome P450 isoenzyme CYP3A4.[2,34] More recent study has shown that gemfibrozil may inhibit the glucuronidation of some of the statin metabolites, and that gemfibrozil is an inhibitor of some of the CYP2C isoenzymes.[36] Other evidence suggests that drug transporter proteins (such as OATP2) may also be involved.[27,29]

Importance and management

There are many studies showing efficacious use of many pairs of statins and fibrates, and the overall incidence of myopathy with a statin and a fibrate has been put at 0.12%.[21] Nevertheless, the risks of these combinations are evident, at least for individual patients, and generally the combinations should only be used if the benefits of use outweigh the risks.

The manufacturer of bezafibrate contraindicates the use of a statin if a number of conditions considered to be risk factors for myopathy (such as renal impairment and hypothyroidism) are present.[37] Monitoring of creatine kinase has been suggested in patients taking a statin with a fibrate, but this will not necessarily identify all cases of developing rhabdomyolysis. As a general rule, any patient given a statin and a fibrate should be told to report any signs of myopathy and possible rhabdomyolysis (i.e. otherwise unexplained muscle pain, tenderness or weakness or dark coloured urine). If myopathy does occur, the statin should be stopped immediately. See also 'muscle toxicity', (p.1086), for further guidance on monitoring and risk factors for muscle toxicity.

Individual combinations of statins and fibrates are associated with different levels of risk. The interactions of lovastatin and simvastatin with fibrates, particularly gemfibrozil, are established and clinically important. The FDA discourage the concurrent use of lovastatin with gemfibrozil in any patient, but suggest that it should be completely avoided in patients with compromised liver or renal function.[12] The manufacturers of lovastatin and simvastatin recommend that combined use with fibrates should generally be avoided, but if the benefits are considered to outweigh the risks, a low dose of the statin should be used. In the presence of a fibrate, the maximum generally recommended dose for lovastatin is 20 mg and for simvastatin is 10 mg. Fenofibrate is excluded from this recommendation for simvastatin, and gemfibrozil is particularly cautioned.[38-40] The UK manufacturer of rosuvastatin recommends starting with a 5 mg dose of rosuvastatin, and contraindicates the 40-mg dose, in any patient taking a fibrate.[41] Further, the US manufacturer recommends a maximum dose of 10 mg of rosuvastatin in patients taking gemfibrozil.[42]

1. Lescol (Fluvastatin sodium). Novartis Pharmaceuticals UK Ltd. UK Summary of product characteristics, October 2006.
2. Kyrklund C, Backman JT, Kivistö KT, Neuvonen M, Laitila J, Neuvonen PJ. Plasma concentrations of active lovastatin acid are markedly increased by gemfibrozil but not bezafibrate. *Clin Pharmacol Ther* (2001) 69, 340–5.
3. Pan W-J, Gustavson LE, Achari R, Rieser MJ, Ye X, Gutterman C, Wallin BA. Lack of a clinically significant pharmacokinetic interaction between fenofibrate and pravastatin in healthy volunteers. *J Clin Pharmacol* (2000) 40, 316–23.
4. Gustavson LE, Schweitzer SM, Koehne-Voss S, Achari R, Chira TO, Esslinger H-U, Yannicelli HD. The effects of multiple doses of fenofibrate on the pharmacokinetics of pravastatin and its 3α-hydroxy isomeric metabolite. *J Clin Pharmacol* (2005) 45, 947–53.
5. Raimondeau J, Le Marec H, Chevallier JC, Bouhour JB. Myolyse biologique survenue à l'occasion d'un relais thérapeutique fénofibrate-pravastatine. *Presse Med* (1992) 21, 663–4.
6. Martin PD, Dane AL, Schneck DW, Warwick MJ. An open-label, randomized, three-way crossover trial of the effect of coadministration of rosuvastatin and fenofibrate on the pharmacokinetic properties of rosuvastatin and fenofibric acid in healthy male volunteers. *Clin Ther* (2003) 25, 459–71.
7. Bergman AJ, Murphy G, Burke J, Zhao JJ, Valesky R, Liu L, Lasseter KC, He W, Prueksaritanont T, Qiu Y, Hartford A, Vega JM, Paolini JF. Simvastatin does not have a clinically significant pharmacokinetic interaction with fenofibrate in humans. *J Clin Pharmacol* (2004) 44, 1054–62.
8. Backman JT, Luurila H, Neuvonen M, Neuvonen PJ. Rifampin markedly decreases and gemfibrozil increases the plasma concentrations of atorvastatin and its metabolites. *Clin Pharmacol Ther* (2005) 78, 154–67.
9. Duell PB, Connor WE, Illingworth DR. Rhabdomyolysis after taking atorvastatin with gemfibrozil. *Am J Cardiol* (1998) 81, 368–9.
10. McKelvie PA, Dennett X. Myopathy associated with HMG-CoA reductase inhibitors (statins): a series of 10 patients and review of the literature. *J Clin Neuromusc Dis* (2002) 3,143–8.
11. Spence JD, Munoz CE, Hendricks L, Latchinian L, Khouri HE. Pharmacokinetics of the combination of fluvastatin and gemfibrozil. *Am J Cardiol* (1995) 76, 80A–83A.
12. Pierce LR, Wysowski DK, Gross TP. Myopathy and rhabdomyolysis associated with lovastatin-gemfibrozil combination therapy. *JAMA* (1990) 264, 71–75.
13. Tobert JA. Myolysis and acute renal failure in a heart-transplant recipient receiving lovastatin. *N Engl J Med* (1988) 318, 48.
14. Marais GE, Larson KK. Rhabdomyolysis and acute renal failure induced by combination lovastatin and gemfibrozil therapy. *Ann Intern Med* (1990) 112, 228–30.
15. Manoukian AA, Bhagavan NV, Hayashi T, Nestor TA, Rios C, Scottolini AG. Rhabdomyolysis secondary to lovastatin therapy. *Clin Chem* (1990) 36, 2145–7.
16. Kogan AD, Orenstein S. Lovastatin-induced acute rhabdomyolysis. *Postgrad Med J* (1990) 66, 294–6.
17. Goldman JA, Fisherman AB, Lee JE, Johnson RJ. The role of cholesterol-lowering agents in drug-induced rhabdomyolysis and polymyositis. *Arthritis Rheum* (1989) 32, 358–9.
18. Abdul-Ghaffar NUAMA, El-Sonbaty MR. Pancreatitis and rhabdomyolysis associated with lovastatin-gemfibrozil therapy. *J Clin Gastroenterol* (1995) 21, 340–1.
19. East C, Alivizatos PA, Grundy SM, Jones PH, Farmer JA. Rhabdomyolysis in patients receiving lovastatin after cardiac transplantation. *N Engl J Med* (1988) 318, 47–8.
20. Knoll RW, Ciafone R, Galen M. Rhabdomyolysis and renal failure secondary to combination therapy of hyperlipidemia with lovastatin and gemfibrozil. *Conn Med* (1993) 593–4.
21. Shek A, Ferrill J. Statin-fibrate combination therapy. *Ann Pharmacother* (2001) 35, 908–17.
22. Illingworth DR, Bacon S. Influence of lovastatin plus gemfibrozil on plasma lipids and lipoproteins in patients with heterozygous familial hypercholesterolemia. *Circulation* (1989) 79, 590–6.
23. Glueck CJ, Oakes N, Speirs J, Tracy T, Lang J. Gemfibrozil-lovastatin therapy for primary hyperlipoproteinemias. *Am J Cardiol* (1992) 70, 1–9.
24. East C, Bilheimer DW, Grundy SM. Combination drug therapy for familial combined hyperlipidemia. *Ann Intern Med* (1988) 109, 25–32.
25. Wirebaugh SR, Shapiro ML, McIntyre TH, Whitney EJ. A retrospective review of the use of lipid-lowering agents in combination, specifically, gemfibrozil and lovastatin. *Pharmacotherapy* (1992) 12, 445–50.
26. ER Squibb. A report on the bioavailability of pravastatin in the presence and absence of gemfibrozil or probucol in healthy male subjects. Data on file (Protocol No 27, 201-18), 1988.
27. Kyrklund C, Backman JT, Neuvonen M, Neuvonen PJ. Gemfibrozil increases plasma pravastatin concentrations and reduces pravastatin renal clearance. *Clin Pharmacol Ther* (2003) 73, 538–44.
28. Wiklund O, Angelin B, Bergman M, Berglund L, Bondjers G, Carlsson A, Lindén T, Miettinen T, Ödman B, Olofsson S-O, Saarinen I, Sipilä R, Sjöström P, Kron B, Vanhanen H, Wright I. Pravastatin and gemfibrozil alone and in combination for the treatment of hypercholesterolemia. *Am J Med* (1993) 94, 13–20.
29. Schneck DW, Birmingham BK, Zalikowski JA, Mitchell PD, Wang Y, Martin PD, Lasseter KC, Brown CDA, Windass AS, Raza A. The effect of gemfibrozil on the pharmacokinetics of rosuvastatin. *Clin Pharmacol Ther* (2004) 75, 455–63.
30. Van Puijenbroek EP, Du Buf-Vereijken PWG, Spooren PFMJ, Van Doormaal JJ. Possible increased risk of rhabdomyolysis during concomitant use of simvastatin and gemfibrozil. *J Intern Med* (1996) 240, 403–4.
31. Federman DG, Hussain F, Walters JB. Fatal rhabdomyolysis caused by lipid-lowering therapy. *South Med J* (2001) 94, 1023–6.
32. Tal A, Rajeshawari M, Isley W. Rhabdomyolysis associated with simvastatin-gemfibrozil therapy. *South Med J* (1997) 90, 546–7.
33. Berland Y, Vacher Coponat H, Durand C, Baz M, Laugier R, Musso JL. Rhabdomyolysis with simvastatin use. *Nephron* (1991) 57, 365–6.
34. Backman JT, Kyrklund C, Kivistö KT, Wang J-S, Neuvonen PJ. Plasma concentrations of active simvastatin acid are increased by gemfibrozil. *Clin Pharmacol Ther* (2001) 68, 122–9.
35. Omar MA, Wilson JP. FDA adverse event reports on statin-associated rhabdomyolysis. *Ann Pharmacother* (2002) 36, 288–95.
36. Prueksaritanont T, Zhao JJ, Ma B, Roadcap BA, Tang C, Qui Y, Liu L, Lin JH, Pearson PG, Baillie TA. Mechanistic studies on metabolic interactions between gemfibrozil and statins. *J Pharmacol Exp Ther* (2002) 301, 1042–51.
37. Bezalip Mono (Bezafibrate). Roche Products Ltd. UK Summary of product characteristics, November 2005.
38. Zocor (Simvastatin). Merck Sharp & Dohme Ltd. UK Summary of product characteristics, December 2005.
39. Mevacor (Lovastatin). Merck & Co., Inc. US Prescribing information, May 2007.
40. Zocor (Simvastatin). Merck & Co., Inc. US Prescribing information, May 2007.
41. Crestor (Rosuvastatin calcium). AstraZeneca UK Ltd. UK Summary of product characteristics, June 2007.
42. Crestor (Rosuvastatin calcium). AstraZeneca. US Prescribing information, July 2007.

Statins + Fusidic acid

Rhabdomyolysis has been described in patients given atorvastatin or simvastatin with fusidic acid.

Clinical evidence, mechanism, importance and management

A patient with a renal transplant and diabetes taking various drugs was given **atorvastatin** 10 mg daily for hyperlipidaemia. Six weeks later, because of a resistant infection, clindamycin and ciprofloxacin were discontinued and fusidic acid 1.5 g daily was started. At this time serum creatine kinase was 54 units/L. Two weeks later the patient was admitted with progressive muscle weakness and pain in both legs. His serum creatinine kinase was 3550 units/L, and he also had raised myoglobin levels. Both continued to rise for 5 days after the **atorvastatin** and fusidic acid were stopped, then gradually returned to normal over one week. Serum levels of both fusidic acid and **atorvastatin** were higher than expected, and it was considered that an interaction was likely.[1] Another patient who had been taking **simvastatin** 10 mg daily for 10 months, developed rhabdomyolysis 15 days after starting to take fusidic acid. She recovered after stopping both drugs.[2] Another case involving **simvastatin** and fusidic acid, which was initially mistaken for drug induced hepatitis, has also been reported.[3] Furthermore, fusidic acid was a possible contributing factor to another case of rhabdomyolysis seen in a patient given 'simvastatin and tacrolimus', (p.1109).

The clinical significance of this possible interaction is unclear, but it would seem wise to remind patients taking either **atorvastatin** or **simvastatin** with fusidic acid to be on the look out for the symptoms of myopathy and rhabdomyolysis (i.e. otherwise unexplained muscle pain, tenderness or weakness or dark coloured urine). If myopathy does occur, the statin should be stopped immediately. See also 'muscle toxicity', (p.1086), for further guidance on monitoring, and risk factors for muscle toxicity.

1. Wenisch C, Krause R, Fladerer P, El Menjawi I, Pohanka E. Acute rhabdomyolysis after atorvastatin and fusidic acid therapy. *Am J Med* (2000) 109, 78.
2. Dromer C, Vedrenne C, Billey T, Pages M, Fournié B, Fournié A. Rhabdomyolyse à la simvastatine: a propos d'un cas avec revue de la littérature. *Rev Rhum Mal Osteoartic* (1992) 59, 281–3.
3. Yuen SLS, McGarity B. Rhabdomyolysis secondary to interaction of fusidic acid and simvastatin. *Med J Aust* (2003) 179, 172.

Statins + Grapefruit and other fruit juices

Large amounts of grapefruit juice markedly increase the plasma levels of lovastatin and simvastatin, but only modestly affect the plasma levels of atorvastatin. Pravastatin seems not to interact. The clinical significance of the possible effects of pomegranate juice on rosuvastatin, and orange juice on pravastatin are unclear.

Clinical evidence

(a) Atorvastatin

Twelve healthy subjects were given 200 mL of double-strength grapefruit juice three times daily for 5 days. On day 3 they were given a single 40-mg dose of atorvastatin with the grapefruit juice then two more 200-mL doses of grapefruit juice, one after 30 minutes and the other after 90 minutes. The AUC_{0-72} of atorvastatin acid and total HMG-CoA reductase inhibitors were increased 2.5-fold and 1.5-fold, respectively.[1] Other studies, using 250 mL of single-strength grapefruit three times a day, have found broadly similar increases in atorvastatin levels.[2,3]

(b) Lovastatin

Ten healthy subjects were given 200 mL of double-strength grapefruit juice three times daily for 3 days. On day 3 they took lovastatin 80 mg with 200 mL of grapefruit juice, then two more 200-mL doses of grapefruit juice, one after 30 minutes and the other after 90 minutes. The mean peak serum levels of the lovastatin and its active metabolite, lovastatin acid, were increased 12-fold and 4-fold, respectively, and the mean AUCs were increased 15-fold and 5-fold, respectively.[4] However, another study in which lovastatin 40 mg was given the evening after single-strength grapefruit juice was taken with breakfast found that the AUC and maximum serum level of lovastatin were approximately doubled, and the AUC and maximum serum level of lovastatin acid were only increased 1.6-fold.[5] It has been suggested that if the grapefruit juice had been given at the same time as the lovastatin in the latter study[5] then much greater increases in the AUC and maximum serum levels would have been found.[6]

(c) Pravastatin

Grapefruit juice did not significantly affect the pharmacokinetics of a single 40-mg dose of pravastatin. In this study, 200-mL of double-strength grapefruit juice was given three times daily for 2 days, and then on the third day 200 mL was given with the pravastatin and again after 30 and 90 minutes.[1] A further study using 10 mg of pravastatin similarly found that grapefruit juice did not significantly affect pravastatin pharmacokinetics.[3]

In a study in 14 healthy subjects a total of 800 mL of **orange juice**, was given over about 3 hours, starting 15 minutes before a 10-mg dose of pravastatin. **Orange juice** increased the AUC of pravastatin by a modest 1.5-fold, without affecting the maximum pravastatin levels.[7]

(d) Rosuvastatin

A case report describes a 48-year-old man taking ezetimibe 10 mg daily, and rosuvastatin 5 mg on alternate days, who developed rhabdomyolysis within 3 weeks of starting to drink 200 mL of **pomegranate juice** twice weekly. Although the patient had been stable taking ezetimibe with rosuvastatin for 15 months he had a history of myopathy with statins and had an elevated creatine kinase before statin treatment had started.[8]

(e) Simvastatin

Ten healthy subjects were given 200 mL of double-strength grapefruit juice three times daily for 2 days. On day 3 they took 60 mg of simvastatin with 200 mL of grapefruit juice, then two more 200-mL doses of grapefruit juice, one after 30 minutes and the other after 90 minutes. The mean peak serum levels of the simvastatin and simvastatin acid, were increased 9-fold and 7-fold, respectively, and the mean AUCs were increased 16-fold and 7-fold, respectively.[9] In a further study by the same research group, when simvastatin was given 24 hours after the last dose of grapefruit juice (same dosage regimen as the previous study) the effect was only 10% of that observed during concurrent use, and had disappeared within 3 to 7 days.[10] The manufacturer notes that the effect of 240 mL of standard grapefruit juice on simvastatin was minimal (13% increase in AUC of active plasma HMG-CoA reductase inhibitors).[11] However, another study found as little as 200 mL of grapefruit juice taken daily for 3 days could increase the maximum levels of simvastatin and simvastatin acid by up to about fourfold.[12]

A case report describes rhabdomyolysis in a patient taking simvastatin 80 mg daily (dose increased 6 months prior to presentation), which occurred 4 days after she started to eat one fresh grapefruit a day.[13]

Mechanism

It seems almost certain that some components of the grapefruit juice (not yet positively identified but possibly naringenin), inhibit the activity of the cytochrome P450 isoenzyme CYP3A4 in the gut wall, thereby reducing the metabolism of the statins as they are absorbed, and allowing more to pass into the body. See 'Lipid regulating drugs', (p.1086) for more information about the metabolism of the statins.

Importance and management

Information about the interaction of statins and grapefruit juice seems to be mainly limited to pharmacokinetic reports (i.e. few adverse case reports) but they are consistent with the way other CYP3A4 inhibitors interact with the statins.

Large increases in the serum levels of lovastatin and simvastatin are potentially hazardous because elevated statin levels carry the risk of toxicity (muscle damage and the possible development of rhabdomyolysis). As even small quantities of grapefruit juice taken in the morning can significantly affect simvastatin levels the UK manufacturers say that concurrent use should generally be avoided.[11,14] In the US the manufacturers suggest that intake of grapefruit juice should be restricted to less than 1 quart [roughly 1 litre] daily.[15,16] See also 'muscle toxicity', (p.1086), for further guidance on monitoring and risk factors for muscle toxicity.

The modest increase in atorvastatin levels when taken with high doses of grapefruit juice seems less likely to be clinically relevant, but the UK manufacturer suggests that large quantities should be avoided.[17] In general, the occasional glass of grapefruit juice would not appear to be a problem. Pravastatin seems not to interact. Information about other statins appears to be lacking, but no interaction would be expected with **fluvastatin** or **rosuvastatin**.

The interaction of **pomegranate juice** with rosuvastatin and ezetimibe seems to be limited to one case report, which is clouded by other possible contributory factors. Furthermore, although pomegranate juice has been shown to inhibit CYP3A4,[8] rosuvastatin is not metabolised by this route. Although it is possible that other mechanisms may be responsible, no firm conclusions can be drawn from this case.

The interaction of pravastatin with **orange juice** would be expected to be of little clinical significance in most patients, but this needs confirmation.

1. Lilja JJ, Kivistö KT, Neuvonen PJ. Grapefruit juice increases serum concentrations of atorvastatin and has no effect on pravastatin. *Clin Pharmacol Ther* (1999) 66, 118–27.
2. Ando H, Tsuruoka S, Yanagihara H, Sugimoto K, Miyata M, Yamazoe Y, Takamura T, Kaneko S, Fujimura A. Effects of grapefruit juice on the pharmacokinetics of pitavastatin and atorvastatin. *Br J Clin Pharmacol* (2005) 60, 494–7.
3. Fukazawa I, Uchida N, Uchida E, Yasuhara H. Effects of grapefruit juice on pharmacokinetics of atorvastatin and pravastatin in Japanese. *Br J Clin Pharmacol* (2004) 57, 448–55.
4. Kantola T, Kivistö KT, Neuvonen PJ. Grapefruit juice greatly increases serum concentrations of lovastatin and lovastatin acid. *Clin Pharmacol Ther* (1998) 63, 397–402.
5. Rogers JD, Zhao J, Liu L, Amin RD, Gagliano KD, Porras AG, Blum RA, Wilson MF, Stepanavage M, Vega JM. Grapefruit juice has minimal effects on plasma concentrations of lovastatin-derived 3-hydroxy-3-methylglutaryl coenzyme A reductase inhibitors. *Clin Pharmacol Ther* (1999) 66, 358–66.
6. Bailey DG, Dresser GK. Grapefruit juice-lovastatin interaction. *Clin Pharmacol Ther* (2000) 67, 690.
7. Koitabashi Y, Kumai T, Matsumoto N, Watanabe M, Sekine S, Yanagida Y, Kobayashi S. Orange juice increased the bioavailability of pravastatin, 3-hydroxy-3-methylglutaryl CoA reductase inhibitor, in rats and healthy human subjects. *Life Sci* (2006) 78, 2852–9.
8. Sorokin AV, Duncan B, Panetta R, Thompson PD. Rhabdomyolysis with pomegranate juice consumption. *Am J Cardiol* (2006) 98, 705–6.
9. Lilja JJ, Kivistö KT, Neuvonen PJ. Grapefruit juice-simvastatin interaction: effect on serum concentrations of simvastatin, simvastatin acid, and HMG-CoA reductase inhibitors. *Clin Pharmacol Ther* (1998) 64, 477–83.
10. Lilja JJ, Kivistö KT, Neuvonen PJ. Duration of effect of grapefruit juice on the pharmacokinetics of the CYP3A4 substrate simvastatin. *Clin Pharmacol Ther* (2000) 68, 384–90.
11. Zocor (Simvastatin). Merck Sharp & Dohme Ltd. UK Summary of product characteristics, December 2005.
12. Lilja JJ, Neuvonen M, Neuvonen PJ. Effects of regular consumption of grapefruit juice on the pharmacokinetics of simvastatin. *Br J Clin Pharmacol* (2004) 58, 56–60.
13. Dreier JP, Endres M. Statin-associated rhabdomyolysis triggered by grapefruit consumption. *Neurology* (2004) 62, 670.
14. Simvador (Simvastatin). Discovery Pharmaceuticals Ltd. UK Summary of product characteristics, July 2003.
15. Mevacor (Lovastatin). Merck & Co., Inc. US Prescribing information, May 2007.
16. Zocor (Simvastatin). Merck & Co., Inc. US Prescribing information, May 2007.
17. Lipitor (Atorvastatin). Pfizer Ltd. UK Summary of product characteristics, September 2006.

Statins + H_2-receptor antagonists or Proton pump inhibitors

No clinically significant interaction appears to occur between cimetidine and atorvastatin, fluvastatin, or pravastatin, between ranitidine and fluvastatin, or between fluvastatin and omeprazole.

Clinical evidence, mechanism, importance and management

(a) Atorvastatin

In a crossover study, 12 healthy subjects were given atorvastatin for 15 days with and without **cimetidine** 300 mg four times daily. **Cimetidine** had no effect on the maximum serum levels or AUC of atorvastatin. **Cimetidine** had little effect on the lipid-lowering ability of atorvastatin, except that the reduction in triglycerides was slightly less, but this difference was considered to be of little clinical significance.[1] There would appear to be no reason for avoiding concurrent use. **Esomeprazole** has been implicated in a case of rhabdomyolysis involving atorvastatin and clarithromycin. See 'Statins + Macrolides', below.

(b) Fluvastatin

The manufacturers of fluvastatin say that its bioavailability is increased by **cimetidine**, **omeprazole**, and **ranitidine** (AUC increased by 24 to 33%[2]), but they say that this is of no clinical relevance.[3] No special precautions would seem to be necessary.

(c) Pravastatin

Cimetidine 300 mg four times daily for 3 days increased the bioavailability of a single 20-mg dose of pravastatin by 58%. The dose of pravastatin was given on day 3, one hour after the first dose of **cimetidine**.[4] However, the manufacturers say that it is unlikely that the changes caused by **cimetidine** will affect the clinical efficacy of pravastatin.[4]

1. Stern RH, Gibson DM, Whitfield LR. Cimetidine does not alter atorvastatin pharmacokinetics or LDL-cholesterol reduction. *Eur J Clin Pharmacol* (1998) 53, 475–8.
2. Lescol (Fluvastatin sodium). Novartis Pharmaceuticals Corp. US Prescribing information, October 2006.
3. Lescol (Fluvastatin sodium). Novartis Pharmaceuticals UK Ltd. UK Summary of product characteristics, October 2006.
4. ER Squibb. A report on the comparative pharmacokinetics of pravastatin in the presence and absence of cimetidine or antacids in healthy male subjects. Data on file (Protocol No 27, 201-43), 1988.

Statins + Imatinib

Imatinib raises simvastatin serum levels, increasing the risk of toxicity. It seems likely that lovastatin and possibly atorvastatin may also be similarly affected.

Clinical evidence, mechanism, importance and management

In a single-dose study, 20 patients with chronic myeloid leukaemia were given **simvastatin** 40 mg prior to and on the last day of a 7-day course of imatinib 400 mg daily. Imatinib increased the maximum serum levels of **simvastatin** twofold and the AUC threefold. The authors conclude that caution is warranted if **simvastatin** and imatinib are taken concurrently.[1]

Imatinib inhibits the cytochrome P450 isoenzyme CYP3A4,[1] by which **simvastatin** is metabolised. It therefore seems likely that **lovastatin** will be similarly affected, and **atorvastatin** may be affected to some extent (see 'Lipid regulating drugs', (p.1086)). These rises increase the risk of **simvastatin** toxicity (myopathy and rhabdomyolysis), for which reason a dosage reduction should be considered.

As a general rule, any patient given imatinib with **atorvastatin, lovastatin** or **simvastatin** should be told to report any signs of myopathy and possible rhabdomyolysis (i.e. otherwise unexplained muscle pain, tenderness or weakness or dark coloured urine). If myopathy does occur, the statin should be stopped immediately. See also 'muscle toxicity', (p.1086), for further guidance on monitoring, and risk factors for muscle toxicity.

1. O'Brien SG, Meinhardt P, Bond E, Beck J, Peng B, Dutreix C, Mehring G, Milosavljev S, Huber C, Capdeville R, Fischer T. Effects of imatinib mesylate (STI571, Glivec) on the pharmacokinetics of simvastatin, a cytochrome P450 3A4 substrate, in patients with chronic myeloid leukaemia. *Br J Cancer* (2003) 89, 1855–9.

Statins + Macrolides

Cases of acute rhabdomyolysis have been reported between lovastatin and azithromycin, clarithromycin, or erythromycin and between simvastatin and clarithromycin or roxithromycin. Macrolide antibacterials have also been potentially implicated in cases of rhabdomyolysis with atorvastatin and pravastatin. Pharmacokinetic studies suggest that the macrolides increase the levels of the statins metabolised by CYP3A4 (namely atorvastatin, lovastatin and simvastatin).

Clinical evidence

(a) Azithromycin

A 51-year-old man who had been taking **lovastatin** 40 mg daily for 5 years developed muscle aches and fever one day after finishing a 5-day course of azithromycin 250 mg daily. His creatine phosphokinase levels were elevated and he was diagnosed as having rhabdomyolysis. This patient was also taking colestyramine, diltiazem, doxazosin, glibenclamide (glyburide), 'thyroid', allopurinol, naproxen, prednisone, loratadine and inhaled beclometasone.[1]

In a randomised study, two groups of 12 healthy subjects were given **atorvastatin** 10 mg daily for 8 days with azithromycin 500 mg daily or placebo for the final 3 days. When the azithromycin group were compared with the placebo group no change in **atorvastatin** pharmacokinetics were noted.[2]

(b) Clarithromycin

A 76-year-old woman who had been taking **lovastatin** 40 mg daily for 5 years developed muscle pain and weakness 2 days after completing a 10-day course of clarithromycin 500 mg twice daily. Later, when hospitalised, she was found to have elevated creatine phosphokinase levels and was diagnosed as having acute rhabdomyolysis.[1] In a similar case, a 64-year-old man with multiple pathologies, including renal impairment, developed rhabdomyolysis 3 weeks after clarithromycin was added to his treatment, which included **simvastatin** 80 mg daily.[3] Other reports describe 7 further cases of rhabdomyolysis in patients taking **simvastatin**,[4-7] **atorvastatin**,[8,9] or **lovastatin**,[10] which in some cases occurred within days of the clarithromycin being started. In 5 of these cases the patients were also taking amiodarone,[6] ciclosporin,[5,7] efavirenz/lopinavir/ritonavir,[9] **esomeprazole**,[8] or gemfibrozil,[10] which may also have had some part to play in the reaction.

A preliminary report of a pharmacokinetic study suggests that clarithromycin 500 mg twice daily for 7 days can increase the AUC and maximum levels of a single 40-mg dose of **simvastatin** eightfold.[11]

In a randomised study, two groups of 12 healthy subjects were given **atorvastatin** 10 mg daily for 8 days with clarithromycin 500 mg twice daily or placebo for the final 3 days. When the clarithromycin group were compared with the placebo group the **atorvastatin** AUC was 82% higher and the maximum serum levels 50% higher.[2]

In a randomised study 3 groups of 15 healthy subjects were given **atorvastatin** 80 mg daily, **pravastatin** 40 mg daily or **simvastatin** 40 mg daily with clarithromycin 500 mg twice daily for 8 days. Clarithromycin increased the AUC of **atorvastatin** by fourfold, **pravastatin** by twofold and **simvastatin** by tenfold.[12]

(c) Erythromycin

Twelve healthy subjects were given a single 10-mg dose of **atorvastatin** on day 7 of an 11-day course of erythromycin 500 mg four times daily. The maximum serum **atorvastatin** levels were raised by 38% and the AUC was raised by 33% by the erythromycin.[13] Either **lovastatin** or **pravastatin** 40 mg daily was given to 12 healthy subjects for 14 days, with erythromycin 500 mg three times daily for the last 7 days. The erythromycin caused the maximum serum levels and AUC of **lovastatin** to rise more than fivefold. The pharmacokinetics of the **pravastatin** remained unchanged.[14] Similarly, **fluvastatin** levels are not significantly altered by erythromycin.[15]

A man taking **lovastatin** 20 mg three times daily, diltiazem, allopurinol and aspirin developed progressive weakness and diffuse myalgia after taking erythromycin 500 mg every 6 hours for 13 days. When admitted to hospital his creatine kinase level was high (35 200 units/L) and his urine was reddish-brown. The rhabdomyolysis was treated by stopping the **lovastatin**, and by giving furosemide with vigorous intravenous hydration.[16]

A woman who had been taking **lovastatin** for 7 years developed multiple organ toxicity (rhabdomyolysis, acute renal failure, pancreatitis, livedo reticularis and raised aminotransferase levels) when erythromycin was added.[17] Four other cases of rhabdomyolysis attributed to an interaction between **lovastatin** and erythromycin have been reported,[17-19] although it should be noted that one of these patients[18] was also taking ciclosporin, which may have contributed to the effects seen.

A study in which 12 subjects were given erythromycin 500 mg three times daily, found a 6.2-fold increase in the AUC of a single 40-mg dose of **simvastatin**, and a 3.4-fold increase in its maximum serum levels. The major active metabolite, simvastatin acid, was similarly affected.[20]

Erythromycin 500 mg four times daily for 7 days did not raise the levels of a single 80-mg dose of **rosuvastatin** in 11 healthy subjects. In fact, **rosuvastatin** levels were slightly lowered, although this was not considered to be of clinical relevance if short-term courses of erythromycin are used.[21]

(d) Roxithromycin

A 73-year-old woman, who had been stable for 6 months while taking a combination of gemfibrozil 600 mg twice daily, **simvastatin** 80 mg daily and diltiazem, developed muscular weakness and myalgia 7 days after starting roxithromycin. All drugs were stopped, and initially she developed myoglobinuria and had a further elevation in her creatine kinase level, but this normalised over the following 18 days. She was discharged after 6 weeks, by which time she had regained full strength.[22] In a randomised, crossover study, 12 healthy subjects were given **lovastatin** 80 mg either alone or following 5 days of pre-treatment with roxithromycin 300 mg four times daily. Roxithromycin increased the maximum level and AUC of lovastatin acid by 38% and 42%, respectively, and decreased the maximum level and AUC of lovastatin lactone by a similar amount.[23]

(e) Telithromycin

In a randomised, crossover study, 14 healthy subjects were given telithromycin 800 mg daily for 5 days, with a single 40-mg dose of **simvastatin** either with, or 12 hours after, the last dose of telithromycin. Although separating administration decreased the effect of telithromycin on **simvastatin** levels by over 50%, the AUC and maximum serum levels of **simvastatin** were still raised by 4-fold and 3.4-fold, respectively.[24]

(f) Unspecified macrolides

In a review of the FDA spontaneous reports of statin-associated rhabdomyolysis covering the period November 1997 to March 2000, macrolide antibacterials (unspecified) were potentially implicated in 13 of 73 cases of rhabdomyolysis seen with **atorvastatin**, 11 of 40 with **lovastatin**, 6 of 71 with **pravastatin**, and 10 of 215 with **simvastatin**.[25]

Mechanism

Most macrolides inhibit the cytochrome P450 isoenzyme CYP3A4, by which lovastatin, simvastatin and, to some extent, atorvastatin are metabolised. Hence the concurrent use of a macrolide raises the levels of these statins, leading in some instances to toxicity (myopathy and rhabdomyolysis). No interaction would be expected with pravastatin because it is not metabolised by CYP3A4, (although a moderate effect has been found with clarithromycin) and no interaction would be expected with **azithromycin** as it does not appear to inhibit CYP3A4. See 'Lipid regulating drugs', (p.1086) for a more detailed discussion of statin metabolism.

Importance and management

Information about the interactions between statins and macrolide antibacterials seems to be limited to the reports cited here. In general it appears that the macrolides raise the levels of statins metabolised by CYP3A4 (i.e. atorvastatin, lovastatin and simvastatin), but not all patients are affected. One study found a large interpatient variation in results,[20] which may account for this. It should be noted that the manufacturers of lovastatin and simvastatin specifically recommend that these drugs are not used with clarithromycin, erythromycin or telithromycin, and suggest that the statin be temporarily withdrawn if these antibacterials are required.[26-28] The risk is smaller with atorvastatin, but as the cases illustrate adverse interactions are possible. The US manufacturers therefore recommend that concurrent use should only be undertaken if the benefits outweigh the risks.[29] Pravastatin and fluvastatin are not metabolised by CYP3A4, and so would not be expected to interact with macrolides via this mechanism, but potential cases have been identified. This is worth noting when considering rosuvastatin, which is also said to have a low propensity for interactions with CYP3A4.

To be on the safe side, any patient taking any statin who is given a macrolide (except probably azithromycin) should be warned to be alert for any signs of myopathy (i.e. otherwise unexplained muscle pain, tenderness or weakness or dark coloured urine). If myopathy does occur, the statin should be stopped immediately. See also 'muscle toxicity', (p.1086), for further guidance on monitoring, and risk factors for muscle toxicity.

1. Grunden JW, Fisher KA. Lovastatin-induced rhabdomyolysis possibly associated with clarithromycin and azithromycin. *Ann Pharmacother* (1997) 31, 859–63.
2. Amsden GW, Kuye O, Wei GCG. A study of the interaction potential of azithromycin and clarithromycin with atorvastatin in healthy volunteers. *J Clin Pharmacol* (2002) 42, 442–7.
3. Lee AJ, Maddix DS. Rhabdomyolysis secondary to a drug interaction between simvastatin and clarithromycin. *Ann Pharmacother* (2001) 35, 26–31.
4. Kahri AJ, Valkonen MM, Vuoristo MKE, Pentikäinen PJ. Rhabdomyolysis associated with concomitant use of simvastatin and clarithromycin. *Ann Pharmacother* (2004) 38, 719.
5. Valero R, Rodrigo E, Zubimendi JA, Arias M. Rabdomiolisis secundaria a interacción de estatinas con macrólidos en un paciente con trasplante renal. *Nefrologia* (2004) 24, 382–3.
6. Chouhan UM, Chakrabarti S, Millward LJ. Simvastatin interaction with clarithromycin and amiodarone causing myositis. *Ann Pharmacother* (2005) 39, 1760–1.
7. Meier C, Stey C, Brack T, Maggiorini M, Risti B, Krähenbühl S. Rhabdomyolyse bei mit simvastatin und ciclosporin behandelten patienten: Rolle der aktivität des cytochrom-P450-enzymsystems der leber. *Schweiz Med Wochenschr* (1995) 125, 1342–6.
8. Sipe BE, Jones RJ, Bokhart GH. Rhabdomyolysis causing AV blockade due to possible atorvastatin, esomeprazole, and clarithromycin interaction. *Ann Pharmacother* (2003) 37, 808–11.
9. Mah Ming JB, Gill MJ. Drug-induced rhabdomyolysis after concomitant use of clarithromycin, atorvastatin, and lopinavir/ritonavir in a patient with HIV. *AIDS Patient Care STDS* (2003) 17, 207–10.
10. Landesman KA, Stozek M, Freeman NJ. Rhabdomyolysis associated with the combined use of hydroxymethylglutaryl-coenzyme A reductase inhibitors with gemfibrozil and macrolide antibiotics. *Conn Med* (1999) 63, 455–7.
11. Montay G, Chevalier P, Guimart C, Guillaume M, Shi J, Bhargava V. Effects of clarithromycin on the pharmacokinetics of simvastatin. *Intersci Conf Antimicrob Agents Chemother* (2003) 43, 38.
12. Jacobson TA. Comparative pharmacokinetic interaction profiles of pravastatin, simvastatin, and atorvastatin when coadministered with cytochrome P450 inhibitors. *Am J Cardiol* (2004) 94, 1140–6.
13. Siedlik PH, Olson SC, Yang B-B, Stern RH. Erythromycin coadministration increases plasma atorvastatin concentrations. *J Clin Pharmacol* (1999) 39, 501–4.
14. Bottorff MB, Behrens DH, Gross A, Markel M. Differences in metabolism of lovastatin and pravastatin as assessed by CYP3A inhibition with erythromycin. *Pharmacotherapy* (1997) 17, 184.
15. Lescol (Fluvastatin sodium). Novartis Pharmaceuticals Corp. US Prescribing information, October 2006.
16. Ayanian JZ, Fuchs CS, Stone RM. Lovastatin and rhabdomyolysis. *Ann Intern Med* (1988) 109, 682–3.
17. Wong PWK, Dillard TA, Kroenke K. Multiple organ toxicity from addition of erythromycin to long-term lovastatin therapy. *South Med J* (1998) 91, 202–5.
18. Corpier CL, Jones PH, Suki WN, Lederer ED, Quinones MA, Schmidt SW, Young JB. Rhabdomyolysis and renal injury with lovastatin use. Report of two cases in cardiac transplant recipients. *JAMA* (1988) 260, 239–41.
19. Spach DH, Bauwens JE, Clark CD, Burke WG. Rhabdomyolysis associated with lovastatin and erythromycin use. *West J Med* (1991) 154, 213–15.
20. Kantola T, Kivistö KT, Neuvonen PJ. Erythromycin and verapamil considerably increase serum simvastatin and simvastatin acid concentrations. *Clin Pharmacol Ther* (1998) 64, 177–82.
21. Cooper KJ, Martin PD, Dane AL, Warwick MJ, Raza A, Schneck DW. The effect of erythromycin on the pharmacokinetics of rosuvastatin. *Eur J Clin Pharmacol* (2003), 59, 51–6.
22. Huynh T, Cordato D, Yang F, Choy T, Johnstone K, Bagnall F, Hitchens N, Dunn R. HMG CoA reductase-inhibitor-related myopathy and the influence of drug interactions. *Intern Med J* (2002) 32, 486–90.
23. Bucher M, Mair G, Kees F. Effect of roxithromycin on the pharmacokinetics of lovastatin in volunteers. *Eur J Clin Pharmacol* (2002) 57, 787–91.
24. Montay G, Chevalier P, Guimart C, Boudraa Y, Guillaume M, Shi J, Bhargava V. A 12-hour dosing interval reduces pharmacokinetic interaction between telithromycin and simvastatin. *Intersci Conf Antimicrob Agents Chemother* (2003) 43, 38.
25. Omar MA, Wilson JP. FDA adverse event reports on statin-associated rhabdomyolysis. *Ann Pharmacother* (2002) 36, 288–95.
26. Mevacor (Lovastatin). Merck & Co., Inc. US Prescribing information, May 2007.
27. Zocor (Simvastatin). Merck Sharp & Dohme Ltd. UK Summary of product characteristics, December 2005.
28. Zocor (Simvastatin). Merck & Co., Inc. US Prescribing information, May 2007.
29. Lipitor (Atorvastatin calcium). Pfizer Inc. US Prescribing information, March 2007.

Statins + Nefazodone

Nefazodone has been implicated in cases of muscle toxicity and rhabdomyolysis in patients taking simvastatin, lovastatin, and possibly pravastatin.

Clinical evidence

(a) Lovastatin

In a review of the FDA spontaneous reports of statin-associated rhabdomyolysis covering the period November 1997 to March 2000, nefazodone was potentially implicated in 2 cases of rhabdomyolysis involving lovastatin.[1]

(b) Pravastatin

A 74-year-old man taking atenolol, aspirin and pravastatin had his treatment with citalopram replaced by nefazodone 50 mg twice daily. Because the possibility of an interaction was suspected, his plasma creatine kinase levels were monitored and were found to be 877 units/L (range 0 to 190 units/L) at 36 hours. Lactate dehydrogenase, aspartate aminotransferase and alanine aminotransferase were all slightly elevated and this was interpreted as indicating muscle toxicity. The nefazodone was withdrawn and although creatine kinase levels were falling they were still above the normal range when the pravastatin was withdrawn 14 days later. Pravastatin was subsequently re-introduced and then venlafaxine 75 mg twice daily was added without problems.[2] However, the diagnosis of muscle toxicity has been questioned, and, because pravastatin levels were not measured, the possibility of an interaction has also been questioned.[3]

(c) Simvastatin

A 44-year-old man who had uneventfully taken simvastatin 40 mg daily for 19 weeks developed 'tea-coloured' urine, initially misdiagnosed as a urinary tract infection, a month after starting to take nefazodone 100 mg twice daily. A month later he was also complaining of severe myalgias of the thighs and calves, and was found to have muscle weakness and tenderness. Laboratory tests confirmed a diagnosis of rhabdomyolysis and myositis. He was asymptomatic within 3 weeks of stopping both drugs, and remained problem-free 5 weeks after restarting simvastatin 40 mg daily.[4] A further case of rhabdomyolysis has been reported in a 72-year-old man taking simvastatin. Symptoms developed 6 weeks after nefazodone was initiated (2 weeks after a dose increment). He recovered with rehydration after the nefazodone was stopped.[5] Similarly, another case report describes rhabdomyolysis in a 56-year-old man taking simvastatin, which developed about 5 weeks after nefazodone was initiated (4 weeks after a dose increment).[6] In a review of the FDA spontaneous reports of statin-associated rhabdomyolysis covering the period November 1997 to March 2000, nefazodone was potentially implicated in 2 cases of rhabdomyolysis involving simvastatin.[1]

Mechanism

Uncertain. The suggestion is that nefazodone (an inhibitor of the cytochrome P450 isoenzyme CYP3A4, an enzyme involved in the metabolism of simvastatin) caused a marked increase in the serum levels of the simvastatin with accompanying toxicity.[4] The same mechanism might also account for the interaction with lovastatin, but the explanation for the case with pravastatin is less clear. See, 'Lipid regulating drugs', (p.1086) for a more detailed discussion of statin metabolism.

Importance and management

Information about interactions between nefazodone and the statins seems to be limited to these reports so that the risks associated with using nefazodone are uncertain. The manufacturers of lovastatin and simvastatin advise avoiding the combination.[7-9] Some caution is probably prudent with atorvastatin as it is also metabolised by CYP3A4. Patients given atorvastatin with nefazodone should be told to report any signs of myopathy and possible rhabdomyolysis (i.e. otherwise unexplained muscle pain, tenderness or weakness or dark coloured urine). If myopathy does occur, the statin should be stopped immediately. See also 'muscle toxicity', (p.1086), for further guidance on monitoring, and risk factors for muscle toxicity.

Other statins seem unlikely to interact. Note that in 2003 nefazodone was withdrawn in many countries due to cases of liver toxicity.

1. Omar MA, Wilson JP. FDA adverse event reports on statin-associated rhabdomyolysis. *Ann Pharmacother* (2002) 36, 288–95.
2. Alderman CP. Possible interaction between nefazodone and pravastatin. *Ann Pharmacother* (1999) 33, 871.
3. Bottorf MB. Comment: possible interaction between nefazodone and pravastatin. *Ann Pharmacother* (2000) 34, 538.
4. Jacobsen RH, Wang P, Glueck CJ. Myositis and rhabdomyolysis associated with concurrent use of simvastatin and nefazodone. *JAMA* (1997) 277, 296.
5. Thompson M, Samuels S. Rhabdomyolysis with simvastatin and nefazodone. *Am J Psychiatry* (2002) 159, 1067.
6. Skrabal MZ, Stading JA, Monaghan MS. Rhabdomyolysis associated with simvastatin-nefazodone therapy. *South Med J* (2003) 96, 1034–5.
7. Mevacor (Lovastatin). Merck & Co., Inc. US Prescribing information, May 2007.
8. Zocor (Simvastatin). Merck Sharp & Dohme Ltd. UK Summary of product characteristics, December 2005.
9. Zocor (Simvastatin). Merck & Co., Inc. US Prescribing information, May 2007.

Statins + Nicotinic acid (Niacin)

The risk of muscle toxicity, such as rhabdomyolysis, may be increased in patients taking a statin with nicotinic acid.

Clinical evidence, mechanism, importance and management

A patient taking **lovastatin** developed rhabdomyolysis, which was attributed to the addition of nicotinic acid 2.5 g daily.[1] A similar reaction occurred in another patient taking the same combination[2] as well as in a further patient taking ciclosporin, nicotinic acid and **lovastatin**[3] (see also 'Statins + Ciclosporin', p.1097). Myositis has also been briefly reported in a patient taking **lovastatin** and nicotinic acid.[1] These adverse reports are isolated and it is by no means certain that nicotinic acid contributed to what happened. Myopathy does occur with **lovastatin** alone,[4] with a reported incidence of 0.1%. A combined preparation of **lovastatin**/nicotinic acid is marketed (*Advicor,* USA), and in a 52-week study investigating efficacy and tolerability, none of the 814 patients experienced drug-induced myopathy, although 7 patients were withdrawn from the study due to elevated creatine kinase levels.[5] Similarly, a review of the use of extended-release niacin with **lovastatin** found that myopathy, which was reported in 3% of patients, tended to be associated with higher initial doses of statins.[6] There do not appear to be any published reports of myopathy occurring with nicotinic acid and any other statins. However, in a review of the FDA spontaneous reports of statin-associated rhabdomyolysis covering the period November 1997 to March 2000, nicotinic acid was identified as a potentially interacting drug in 2 of 215 cases for **simvastatin**, 1 of 71 cases for **pravastatin**, and 1 of 40 cases for **lovastatin**. Nicotinic acid was not identified as an interacting drug in any reports for **atorvastatin** or **fluvastatin**.[7]

Nicotinic acid does not alter the bioavailability of **fluvastatin**[8] or **pravastatin**.[9]

Although these cases are isolated, some caution is certainly warranted. The US manufacturers of **lovastatin** recommend a maximum dose of 20 mg in patients taking nicotinic acid in doses of 1 g or more daily.[10] Similarly the UK manufacturers of **simvastatin** recommend a maximum dose of 10 mg in patients taking nicotinic acid in doses of 1 g or more daily.[11] To be on the safe side, if the decision is made to use nicotinic acid with any statin the outcome should be very well monitored. Patients should be told to report otherwise unexplained muscle pain, tenderness or weakness or dark coloured urine). See also 'muscle toxicity', (p.1086), for further guidance on monitoring, and risk factors for muscle toxicity.

1. Reaven P, Witztum JL. Lovastatin, nicotinic acid and rhabdomyolysis. *Ann Intern Med* (1988) 109, 597–8.
2. Hill MD, Bilbao JM. Case of the month: February 1999 – 54 year old man with severe muscle weakness. *Brain Pathol* (1999) 9, 607–8.
3. Norman DJ, Illingworth DR, Munson J, Hosenpud J. Myolysis and acute renal failure in a heart-transplant recipient receiving lovastatin. *N Engl J Med* (1988) 318, 46–7.
4. Bilheimer DW. Long term clinical tolerance of lovastatin (Mevinolin) and Simvastatin (Epistatin). An overview. *Drug Invest* (1990) 2 (Suppl 2), 58–67.
5. Kashyap ML, McGovern ME, Berra K, Guyton JR, Kwiterovich PO, Harper WL, Toth PD, Favrot LK, Kerzner B, Nash SD, Bays HE, Simmons PD. Long-term safety and efficacy of a once-daily niacin/lovastatin formulation for patients with dyslipidaemia. *Am J Cardiol* (2002) 89, 672–8.
6. Yim BT, Chong PH. Niacin-ER and lovastatin treatment of hypercholesterolemia and mixed dyslipidemia. *Ann Pharmacother* (2003) 37, 106–15.
7. Omar MA, Wilson JP. FDA adverse event reports on statin-associated rhabdomyolysis. *Ann Pharmacother* (2002) 36, 288–95.
8. Smith HT, Jokubaitis LA, Troendle AJ, Hwang DS, Robinson WT. Pharmacokinetics of fluvastatin and specific drug interactions. *Am J Hypertens* (1993) 6, 375S–382S.
9. ER Squibb. A report on the effect of nicotinic acid alone and in the presence of aspirin on the bioavailability of SQ 31,000 in healthy male subjects. Data on file (Protocol No 27, 201-6), 1987.
10. Mevacor (Lovastatin). Merck & Co., Inc. US Prescribing information, May 2007.
11. Zocor (Simvastatin). Merck Sharp & Dohme Ltd. UK Summary of product characteristics, December 2005.

Statins + NNRTIs

Delavirdine is expected to raise the levels of atorvastatin, simvastatin and lovastatin. This expectation is supported by a case of rhabdomyolysis, which developed in a patient taking atorvastatin and delavirdine. Efavirenz (and possibly nevirapine) *lower* the levels of atorvastatin, simvastatin, and pravastatin.

Clinical evidence, mechanism, importance and management

(a) Delavirdine

An isolated case report describes a 63-year-old HIV-positive man, who had been taking **atorvastatin** 20 mg daily with indinavir, lamivudine and stavudine, and who was admitted to hospital 2 months after indinavir was replaced with delavirdine. He had a one-month history of malaise, muscle pain, vomiting, and dark urine. Laboratory tests confirmed a diagnosis of rhabdomyolysis, and he was found to have acute renal failure. All drugs were withheld, and he gradually recovered over the following month. It was suggested that delavirdine inhibited the metabolism of **atorvastatin**.[1] Although the possible interaction between **simvastatin** or **lovastatin** and delavirdine does not appear to have been studied it would be expected to be similar, if not greater in magnitude, to that seen with **atorvastatin**. One of the manufacturers of **simvastatin** contraindicates concurrent use,[2] and the US manufacturer of delavirdine advises against the use of either **simvastatin** or **lovastatin**. They also advise caution with **atorvastatin**, due to the risk of rhabdomyolysis.[3] See also 'muscle toxicity', (p.1086), for further guidance on monitoring, and risk factors for muscle toxicity.

(b) Efavirenz

In an open-label study 42 healthy subjects were given efavirenz 600 mg daily for 11 days, with **atorvastatin** 10 mg daily, **simvastatin** 40 mg daily, or **pravastatin** 40 mg daily for the last 2 days. Efavirenz reduced the AUC of **simvastatin** and its active metabolites by about 45 to 55%, reduced the AUC of **atorvastatin** and its active metabolites by 35 to 45% and reduced the AUC of **pravastatin** by about 40%. The pharmacokinetics of efavirenz were not changed. Decreases in LDL-cholesterol were attenuated when efavirenz was given with **simvastatin**.[4] The changes with **atorvastatin** and **simvastatin** were expected, as efavirenz induces the cytochrome P450 isoenzyme CYP3A4, by which **simvastatin**, and to an extent **atorvastatin** are metabolised. The authors note that similar results would be expected with **nevirapine**, which also induces CYP3A4. The reasons for the reduction in the **pravastatin** AUC are less clear, as it is not metabolised by CYP3A4.[4] It would seem prudent to monitor the lipid-profile of patients taking efavirenz and any of these statins, although bear in mind that NNRTIs are often used with 'protease inhibitors', (p.1108), which dramatically raise the levels of some statins.

1. Castro JG, Gutierrez L. Rhabdomyolysis with acute renal failure probably related to the interaction of atorvastatin and delavirdine. *Am J Med* (2002) 112, 505.
2. Simvador (Simvastatin). Discovery Pharmaceuticals Ltd. UK Summary of product characteristics, July 2003.
3. Rescriptor (Delavirdine mesylate). Pfizer Inc. US Prescribing information, June 2006.
4. Gerber JG, Rosenkranz SL, Fichtenbaum CJ, Vega JM, Yang A, Alston BL, Brobst SW, Segal Y, Aberg JA. Effect of efavirenz on the pharmacokinetics of simvastatin, atorvastatin, and pravastatin: results of AIDS Clinical Trials Group 5108 study. *J Acquir Immune Defic Syndr* (2005) 39, 307–12.

Statins + Orlistat

No clinically relevant interaction has been seen between orlistat and atorvastatin, pravastatin or simvastatin.

Clinical evidence, mechanism, importance and management

(a) Atorvastatin

In a randomised study, 32 healthy subjects were given atorvastatin 20 mg daily for 6 days, with or without orlistat 120 mg three times daily for 6 days. Orlistat had no significant effect on the pharmacokinetics of atorvastatin.[1]

(b) Pravastatin

In a placebo-controlled, crossover study in 24 subjects with mild hypercholesterolaemia, orlistat 120 mg three times daily was reported to have no effect on the pharmacokinetics, or lipid-lowering effects, of pravastatin 40 mg daily, when both drugs were given for 6 days.[2]

A review includes brief details of a comparative study in two groups of healthy subjects given pravastatin, either with orlistat or placebo. After 10 days there was no significant difference in the pravastatin AUC between the groups, but the maximum serum concentration did show a tendency to be higher in the orlistat group.[3]

(c) Simvastatin

In a placebo-controlled, randomised study in 29 healthy subjects orlistat 120 mg three times daily had no effect on the pharmacokinetics of simvastatin 40 mg daily.[4]

1. Zhi J, Moore R, Kanitra L, Mulligan TE. Pharmacokinetic evaluation of the possible interaction between selected concomitant medications and orlistat at steady state in healthy subjects. *J Clin Pharmacol* (2002) 42, 1011–19.
2. Oo CY, Akbari B, Lee S, Nichols G, Hellmann CR. Effect of orlistat, a novel anti-obesity agent, on the pharmacokinetics and pharmacodynamics of pravastatin in patients with mild hypercholesterolaemia. *Clin Drug Invest* (1999) 17, 217–23.
3. Guerciolini R. Mode of action of orlistat. *Int J Obes* (1997) 21 (Suppl 3), S12–S23.
4. Zhi J, Moore R, Kanitra L, Mulligan TE. Effects of orlistat, a lipase inhibitor, on the pharmacokinetics of three highly lipophilic drugs (amiodarone, fluoxetine, and simvastatin) in healthy volunteers. *J Clin Pharmacol* (2003) 43, 428–34.

Statins + Phenytoin

In an isolated case, phenytoin reduced the cholesterol-lowering effect of simvastatin, fluvastatin and atorvastatin. The concurrent use of phenytoin and fluvastatin modestly raises the levels of both drugs.

Clinical evidence, mechanism, importance and management

A 50-year-old woman taking **simvastatin** 10 mg daily had her antiepileptic medication changed from sodium valproate to phenytoin 325 mg daily. Over the following 3 months her total cholesterol rose from 9.4 to 15.99 mmol/L. The dose of **simvastatin** was gradually increased to 40 mg daily without significant effect on her cholesterol levels. Despite further changes (to **fluvastatin** 40 mg daily, then to **atorvastatin** 80 mg daily) her cholesterol level remained above 10 mmol/L. Finally phenytoin was discontinued and her cholesterol dropped to 6.24 mmol/L with **atorvastatin** 80 mg daily.[1] The reasons are not known, but it is possible that phenytoin induced the metabolism of the statins, so that they were cleared from the body more quickly and were therefore less effective. The concurrent use of phenytoin 300 mg and **fluvastatin** 40 mg increased the maximum levels and AUC of **fluvastatin** by 27% and 40%, respectively, and increased the maximum levels and AUC of phenytoin by 5% and 20%, respectively.[2] These changes are relatively modest and probably occur because both drugs are metabolised by the cytochrome P450 isoenzyme CYP2C9.

Evidence of an interaction currently appears to be limited to these two reports and the clinical significance remains unclear. The change in phenytoin levels seems unlikely to be clinically significant. There is a small risk that the concurrent use of **fluvastatin** and phenytoin could result in myopathy. Patients should be told to report any signs of myopathy and possible rhabdomyolysis (i.e. otherwise unexplained muscle pain, tenderness or weakness or dark coloured urine). If myopathy does occur, the statin should be stopped immediately. See also 'muscle toxicity', (p.1086), for further guidance on monitoring, and risk factors for muscle toxicity.

1. Murphy MJ, Dominiczak MH. Efficacy of statin therapy: possible effect of phenytoin. *Postgrad Med J* (1999) 75, 359–60.
2. Lescol (Fluvastatin sodium). Novartis Pharmaceuticals Corp. US Prescribing information, October 2006.

Statins + Phosphodiesterase type-5 inhibitors

A man taking simvastatin developed symptoms of rhabdomyolysis after taking a single dose of sildenafil. The pharmacokinetics of atorvastatin and sildenafil do not appear to be altered by concurrent use, and tadalafil does not alter lovastatin pharmacokinetics.

Clinical evidence

(a) Sildenafil

A 76-year-old man who had been taking **simvastatin** 10 mg daily for 3 years, presented at a clinic with a 3-day history of severe and unexplained muscle aches, particularly in the lower part of his legs and feet. The problem had started within 10 hours of taking a single 50-mg dose of sildenafil. When examined he showed no muscle tenderness or swelling but his creatine phosphokinase level was slightly raised (406 units/L). There was also a mild elevation of blood urea nitrogen and an increase in creatinine and potassium levels. A tentative diagnosis of rhabdomyolysis was made, there being no other obvious identifiable cause for the myalgia. Both **simvastatin** and sildenafil were stopped, and he made a full recovery.[1] A study in 24 healthy subjects found that the pharmacokinetics of sildenafil (single 100-mg dose) and **atorvastatin** (10 mg daily for 7 days) were unchanged by concurrent use.[2]

(b) Tadalafil

In a study in 16 healthy subjects, tadalafil 20 mg daily for 14 days did not affect the pharmacokinetics of a 40-mg dose of **lovastatin**.[3]

Mechanism, importance and management

The reasons for this possible interaction are not known. This is as yet an isolated case, and no broad generalisations can be based on such slim evidence. Based on the current evidence no further precautions currently seem necessary.

1. Gutierrez CA. Sildenafil-simvastatin interaction: possible cause of rhabdomyolysis? *Am Fam Physician* (2001) 63, 636–7.
2. Chung M, DiRico A, Calcagni A, Messig M, Scott R. Lack of a drug interaction between sildenafil and atorvastatin. *J Clin Pharmacol* (2000) 40, 1057.
3. Ring BJ, Patterson BE, Mitchell MI, Vandenbranden M, Gillespie J, Bedding AW, Jewell H, Payne CD, Forgue ST, Eckstein J, Wrighton SA, Phillips DL. Effect of tadalafil on cytochrome P450 3A4-mediated clearance: studies in vitro and in vivo. *Clin Pharmacol Ther* (2005) 77, 63–75.

Statins + Protease inhibitors

The levels of atorvastatin and simvastatin are markedly increased by lopinavir and saquinavir (with ritonavir), nelfinavir, and ritonavir alone. Pravastatin seems only moderately affected. Several cases of rhabdomyolysis have been attributed to this interaction.

Clinical evidence

(a) Indinavir

In a non-randomised study patients receiving HAART were given **pravastatin** or **fluvastatin**. Neither of the statins altered the pharmacokinetics of indinavir, the combination was well tolerated, and no increase in adverse events was seen.[1]

(b) Lopinavir/Ritonavir

Either **atorvastatin** 20 mg daily or **pravastatin** 20 mg daily were given to 24 healthy subjects for 4 days during a 14-day course of lopinavir/ritonavir 400/100 mg twice daily. The maximum serum levels and AUC of **atorvastatin** were increased by between 4.7- and 5.9-fold and the maximum serum levels and AUC of **pravastatin** were only increased by about 30%. **Atorvastatin** and **pravastatin** had no effect on the pharmacokinetics of lopinavir or ritonavir.[2]

(c) Nelfinavir

In an open label study, 31 healthy subjects were given either **atorvastatin** 10 mg daily or **simvastatin** 20 mg daily for 28 days, with nelfinavir 1.25 g twice daily for the last 14 days. Nelfinavir increased the maximum serum levels and AUC of **atorvastatin** approximately twofold and the maximum serum levels and AUC of **simvastatin** approximately sixfold. No significant adverse effects, or any signs of rhabdomyolysis were noted throughout the study.[3]

One study found that nelfinavir 750 mg three times daily increased the maximum serum levels and AUC of **pravastatin** 40 mg daily by 29% and 35%, respectively, and increased the maximum serum levels and AUC of **atorvastatin** 40 mg daily by 32% and 209%, respectively.[4] A further study, in which 14 healthy subjects took nelfinavir 1.25 g twice daily for 12 days, with **pravastatin** 40 mg daily for the final 4 days, found that the AUC of **pravastatin** ranged from a decrease of 65% to an increase of 11%, and the maximum serum levels ranged from a decrease of 77% to an increase of 154%.[5]

In another study, 14 healthy subjects were given nelfinavir 1.25 g twice daily for 18 days, with **pravastatin** 40 mg daily for the last 4 days. No significant change was noted in the pharmacokinetics of nelfinavir, nor of its major metabolite.[6]

A case report describes a 70-year-old HIV-positive man taking nelfinavir who developed rhabdomyolysis and died, about 3 weeks after being given **simvastatin** 80 mg daily. He had previously tolerated both **pravastatin** 40 mg daily and **simvastatin** 10 mg daily.[7]

(d) Ritonavir

A 51-year-old woman was admitted to hospital with a 4-day history of muscular aches and weakness. Among other drugs, she had been taking zidovudine, lamivudine, indinavir, and **simvastatin** for 2 years. Ritonavir 100 mg twice daily had been added to her usual regimen 2 weeks previously. The rhabdomyolysis was therefore attributed to an interaction between ritonavir and **simvastatin**.[8] Another similar case has also been reported.[9] See also (b) above and (e) below for interactions of ritonavir combined with other protease inhibitors.

(e) Saquinavir/Ritonavir

Ritonavir 300 mg twice daily and saquinavir 400 mg twice daily were given to healthy subjects for 3 days, after which the dose was increased to ritonavir 400 mg twice daily and saquinavir 400 mg twice daily for a further 11 days. On the last 4 days **atorvastatin, pravastatin**, or **simvastatin** (all 40 mg daily) were also given. The mean **pravastatin** AUC was approximately halved (13 subjects), the mean **atorvastatin** AUC was increased approximately fourfold (14 subjects) and the mean **simvastatin** acid AUC was increased approximately 32-fold (14 subjects). No cases of rhabdomyolysis were noted.[6]

Mechanism

The protease inhibitors, especially ritonavir, are known to be strong inhibitors of the cytochrome P450 isoenzyme CYP3A4. The levels of statins metabolised by this isoenzyme (notably simvastatin, and to some extent atorvastatin) are therefore increased. See 'Lipid regulating drugs', (p.1086) for information on the metabolism of the individual statins.

Importance and management

The interactions of the protease inhibitors and atorvastatin or simvastatin appear to be established by the pharmacokinetic studies cited here, and supported by a few case reports. It is generally recommended that simvastatin and lovastatin, which is similarly metabolised, should be avoided in patients taking protease inhibitors, and several manufacturers of simvastatin contraindicate concurrent use.[10,11] Atorvastatin should be used in low doses (i.e.10 mg) with care. See also 'muscle toxicity', (p.1086), for further guidance on monitoring, and risk factors for muscle toxicity.

Pravastatin and fluvastatin can probably be used without dose adjustments, but monitoring is needed to confirm this as one study with nelfinavir and pravastatin[5] suggested a trend towards *reduced* pravastatin efficacy.

1. Benesic A, Zilly M, Kluge F, Weißbrich B, Winzer R, Klinker H, Langmann P. Lipid lowering therapy with fluvastatin and pravastatin in patients with HIV infection and antiretroviral therapy: comparison of efficacy and interaction with indinavir. *Infection* (2004) 32, 229–33.
2. Carr RA, Andre AK, Bertz RJ, Hsu A, Lam W, Chang M, Chen P, Williams L, Bernstein B, Sun E. Concomitant administration of ABT-378/ritonavir (ABT-378/r) results in a clinically important pharmacokinetic (PK) interaction with atorvastatin (ATO) but not pravastatin (PRA). *Intersci Conf Antimicrob Agents Chemother* (2000) 40, 334.
3. Hsyu P-H, Schultz-Smith MD, Lillibridge JH, Lewis RH, Kerr BM. Pharmacokinetic interactions between nelfinavir and 3-hydroxy-methylglutaryl coenzyme A reductase inhibitors atorvastatin and simvastatin. *Antimicrob Agents Chemother* (2001) 45, 3445–50.
4. Barry M, Belz G, Roll S, O'Grady P, Swaminathan A, Geraldes M, Mangold B. Interaction of nelfinavir with atorvastatin and pravastatin in normal healthy volunteers. *AIDS* (2000) 14 (Suppl 4), S90.
5. Aberg JA, Rosenkranz SL, Fichtenbaum CJ, Alston BL, Brobst SW, Segal Y, Gerber JG for the ACTG A5108 team. Pharmacokinetic interaction between nelfinavir and pravastatin in HIV-seronegative volunteers: ATCG study A5108. *AIDS* (2006) 20, 725–9.
6. Fichtenbaum CJ, Gerber JG, Rosenkranz SL, Segal Y, Aberg JA, Blaschke T, Alston B, Fang F, Kosel B, Aweeka F and the NIAID AIDS Clinical Trials Group. Pharmacokinetic interactions between protease inhibitors and statins in HIV seronegative volunteers: ACTG study A5047. *AIDS* (2002) 16, 569–77.
7. Hare CB, Vu MP, Grunfeld C, Lampiris HW. Simvastatin-nelfinavir interaction implicated in rhabdomyolysis and death. *Clin Infect Dis* (2002) 35, e111–e112.
8. Cheng CH, Miller C, Lowe C, Pearson VE. Rhabdomyolysis due to probable interaction between simvastatin and ritonavir. *Am J Health-Syst Pharm* (2002) 59, 728–30.
9. Martin CM, Hoffman V, Berggren RE. Rhabdomyolysis in a patient receiving simvastatin concurrently with highly active antiretroviral therapy. *Intersci Conf Antimicrob Agents Chemother* (2000) 40, 316.
10. Zocor (Simvastatin). Merck Sharp & Dohme Ltd. UK Summary of product characteristics, December 2005.
11. Simvador (Simvastatin). Discovery Pharmaceuticals Ltd. UK Summary of product characteristics, July 2003.

Statins + Rifampicin (Rifampin)

Rifampicin lowers the serum levels of atorvastatin, fluvastatin, pravastatin, and simvastatin.

Clinical evidence, mechanism, importance and management

It was briefly mentioned in a review by the manufacturer of **fluvastatin** that rifampicin reduced the AUC and the maximum serum levels of **fluvastatin** by 51% and 59%, respectively. No further study details were given.[1] In a randomised, crossover study in 10 healthy subjects, 5 days pretreatment with rifampicin 600 mg daily reduced the AUCs of **simvastatin** and simvastatin acid by 87% and 93%, respectively.[2] A study of the same design with a 40-mg dose of **atorvastatin** found that rifampicin decreased the AUC of **atorvastatin** by 80% and decreased the AUCs of its two active metabolites by 43% and 81%, respectively. There was considerable intersubject variation in these values.[3] In a further study by the same authors, this time with **pravastatin** 40 mg, it was found that rifampicin reduced the AUC of **pravastatin** by 31%, but again there were large interindividual differences in the results, with some subjects having an *increase* in AUC.[4] It might therefore be necessary to increase the dosage of **atorvastatin**, **fluvastatin**, **simvastatin**, and possibly **pravastatin** in some subjects, if rifampicin is given concurrently, but this needs confirmation.

1. Jokubaitis LA. Updated clinical safety experience with fluvastatin. *Am J Cardiol* (1994) 73, 18D–24D.
2. Kyrklund C, Backman JT, Kivistö KT, Neuvonen M, Laitila J, Neuvonen PJ. Rifampin greatly reduces plasma simvastatin and simvastatin acid concentrations. *Clin Pharmacol Ther* (2000) 68, 592–7.
3. Backman JT, Luurila H, Neuvonen M, Neuvonen PJ. Rifampin markedly decreases and gemfibrozil increases the plasma concentrations of atorvastatin and its metabolites. *Clin Pharmacol Ther* (2005) 78, 154–67.
4. Kyrklund C, Backman JT, Neuvonen M, Neuvonen PJ. Effect of rifampicin on pravastatin pharmacokinetics in healthy subjects. *Br J Clin Pharmacol* (2004) 57, 181–7.

Statins + St John's wort (*Hypericum perforatum*)

St John's wort modestly decreases the plasma level of simvastatin, but not pravastatin.

Clinical evidence, mechanism, importance and management

In a placebo-controlled, crossover study, 16 healthy subjects took St John's wort 300 mg three times daily for 14 days. On day 14 **simvastatin** 10 mg was given to 8 subjects and **pravastatin** 20 mg was given to the other 8 subjects. St John's wort did not affect the plasma concentration of **pravastatin**, but it tended to reduce the **simvastatin** AUC and significantly reduced the AUC of its active metabolite, **simvastatin** hydroxy acid, by 62%.[1] The reason for this interaction is unknown, but St John's wort may reduce the levels of **simvastatin** and its metabolite by inhibiting the cytochrome P450 isoenzyme CYP3A4 or by having some effect on P-glycoprotein. The clinical significance of these reductions is unclear, but it may be prudent to consider an interaction if lipid-lowering targets are not met.

1. Sugimoto K, Ohmori M, Tsuruoka S, Nishiki K, Kawaguchi A, Harada K, Arakawa M, Sakomoto K, Masada M, Miyamori I, Fujimura A. Different effects of St John's wort on the pharmacokinetics of simvastatin and pravastatin. *Clin Pharmacol Ther* (2001) 70, 518–24.

Statins + Tacrolimus

An isolated case of rhabdomyolysis occurred in a patient taking tacrolimus with simvastatin. Tacrolimus does not appear to affect atorvastatin pharmacokinetics.

Clinical evidence, mechanism, importance and management

A 51-year-old woman, who was taking tacrolimus after a kidney transplant, started taking **simvastatin** 10 mg daily following a stroke. After 5 months, the dose was increased to 20 mg daily, and fusidic acid was started for osteomyelitis. Muscle pain developed 2 weeks later, and after a further 3 weeks she was admitted to hospital, when her creatinine kinase level was found to be 24 000 units/mL (reported range 10 to 70 units/mL) and she had renal impairment. The **simvastatin** and fusidic acid were immediately stopped and the patient recovered over the following 2 weeks. She was later treated with a combination of **fluvastatin**, tacrolimus and fusidic acid without incident, leading the authors to suspect that the rhabdomyolysis was caused by an interaction between **simvastatin** and tacrolimus.[1] However, note that 'fusidic acid', (p.1102), has been implicated in cases of rhabdomyolysis with **simvastatin**. The clinical significance of this case report is therefore unclear.

A pharmacokinetic study in 13 healthy subjects found that the short-term use of tacrolimus (2 doses 12 hours apart) did not affect the pharmacokinetics of **atorvastatin**.[2]

1. Kotanko P, Kiristis W, Skrabal F. Rhabdomyolysis and acute renal graft impairment in a patient treated with simvastatin, tacrolimus, and fusidic acid. *Nephron* (2002) 90, 234–5.
2. Lemahieu WPD, Hermann M, Asberg A, Verbeke K, Holdaas H, Vanrenterghem Y, Maes BD. Combined therapy with atorvastatin and calcineurin inhibitors: no interactions with tacrolimus. *Am J Transplant* (2005) 5, 2236–43.

Statins; Atorvastatin + Sirolimus

A case report describes elevated sirolimus levels in a patient, which occurred after atorvastatin was started.

Clinical evidence, mechanism, importance and management

A case report describes a patient who had undergone a pancreatic islet transplant and who had been stable taking sirolimus 8 to 11 mg daily for 5 months. A routine lipid evaluation at 6 months found raised cholesterol and triglyceride levels, and so atorvastatin was started. Six weeks later the trough sirolimus level was 20.5 nanograms/mL (target 7 to 10 nanograms/mL) and so the sirolimus dose was reduced. Further reductions were subsequently needed, and 3 months after the atorvastatin was started the sirolimus dose had been halved.[1] The authors suggested that the atorvastatin competed with sirolimus for metabolism by the cytochrome P40 isoenzyme CYP3A4, which resulted in reduced sirolimus metabolism and the elevated levels seen.[1] This case report seems to be the only evidence of an interaction and so its general significance is unknown. However, it may be prudent to be aware of the possibility of an interaction if both drugs are given.

1. Barshes NR, Goodpastor SE, Goss JA, DeBakey ME. Sirolimus-atorvastatin drug interaction in the pancreatic islet transplant recipient. *Transplantation* (2003) 76, 1649–50.

Statins; Lovastatin + Fibre or Pectin

Pectin and oat bran can reduce the cholesterol-lowering effects of lovastatin.

Clinical evidence, mechanism, importance and management

The serum LDL-cholesterol levels of 3 patients taking lovastatin 80 mg daily showed a marked rise from 4.48 to 6.36 mmol/L when they were also given pectin 15 g daily. One patient had a 59% rise in LDL-cholesterol.[1] Two other patients taking lovastatin had a rise in LDL-cholesterol from 5.03 to 6.54 mmol/L when they were also given 50 to 100 g of **oat bran** daily. One patient had a 41% rise in LDL-cholesterol.[1] When the pectin and **oat bran** were stopped, the serum levels of the LDL-cholesterol fell. It is presumed that both pectin and **oat bran** reduced the absorption of lovastatin from the gut.[1] Evidence is still very limited but if patients are adding these fibres to their diets it would seem prudent to separate the ingestion of lovastatin by as much as possible.

1. Richter WO, Jacob BG, Schwandt P. Interaction between fibre and lovastatin. *Lancet* (1991) 338, 706.

Statins; Pravastatin + Aspirin

Aspirin 324 mg did not significantly affect the pharmacokinetics of a single 20-mg dose of pravastatin.[1]

1. ER Squibb. A report on the effect of nicotinic acid alone and in the presence of aspirin on the bioavailability of SQ 31,000 in healthy male subjects. Data on file (Protocol No 27, 201-6), 1987.

Statins; Pravastatin + Mianserin

An isolated report describes rhabdomyolysis attributed to the long-term concurrent use of pravastatin and mianserin, triggered by a cold.

Clinical evidence, mechanism, importance and management

An isolated report describes a 72-year-old woman taking pravastatin 20 mg daily and mianserin 10 mg daily for 2 years, who was hospitalised because of weakness in her legs that began 2 days previously, shortly after she developed a cold. She could stand, but was unable to walk unaided. Laboratory data revealed evidence of increased serum enzymes, all of which suggested rhabdomyolysis. Within a week of stopping the pravastatin the leg weakness had disappeared and all of the laboratory results had returned to normal. The authors of the report attributed the toxicity to the long-term use of both drugs, ageing and the development of a cold.[1] However, what part these factors and/or the presence of mianserin actually played in the development of this toxicity is not known. It seems unlikely that this case is of general significance.

1. Takei A, Chiba S. Rhabdomyolysis associated with pravastatin treatment for major depression. *Psychiatry Clin Neurosci* (1999) 53, 539.

Statins; Pravastatin + Probucol

Probucol 500 mg did not cause any clinically significant changes in the bioavailability of a single 20-mg dose of pravastatin in a study in 20 healthy subjects.[1]

1. ER Squibb. A report on the bioavailability of pravastatin in the presence and absence of gemfibrozil or probucol in healthy male subjects. Data on file (Protocol No 27, 201-18), 1988.

Statins; Simvastatin + Bosentan

Bosentan modestly reduces the AUC of simvastatin and its active metabolite, which could lead to a reduction in simvastatin efficacy.

Clinical evidence

In a three-way, crossover study, 9 healthy subjects were given either bosentan 125 mg twice daily for 5.5 days, simvastatin 40 mg daily for 6 days, or both treatments together. Simvastatin had no effect on the pharmacokinetics of bosentan, but bosentan reduced the AUC of simvastatin and its β-hydroxyacid metabolite by 34% and 46%, respectively.[1]

Mechanism

Bosentan is known to be a mild inducer of the cytochrome P450 isoenzyme CYP3A4, which is involved in the metabolism of simvastatin. Induction of simvastatin metabolism may have led to the reduced levels seen. See 'Lipid regulating drugs', (p.1086) for more information on the metabolism of all the statins.

Importance and management

A 40% reduction in the AUC of simvastatin is potentially clinically significant. If bosentan and simvastatin are used concurrently it would seem prudent to monitor the outcome to ensure that simvastatin is effective.

1. Dingemanse J, Schaarschmidt D, van Giersbergen PLM. Investigation of the mutual pharmacokinetic interactions between bosentan, a dual endothelin receptor antagonist, and simvastatin. *Clin Pharmacokinet* (2003) 42, 293–301.

Statins; Simvastatin + Fish oils

In a randomised, crossover study in 23 subjects, omega-3-acid ethyl esters (*Omacor*) 4 g daily did not significantly affect the pharmacokinetics of simvastatin 80 mg daily when both drugs were given together for 14 days. The combination was also well tolerated.[1] No additional precautions would appear to be necessary on concurrent use.

1. McKenney JM, Swearingen D, Di Spirito M, Doyle R, Pantaleon C, Kling D, Shalwitz RA. Study of the pharmacokinetic interaction between simvastatin and prescription omega-3-acid ethyl esters. *J Clin Pharmacol* (2006) 46, 785–91.

31

Lithium

Lithium is used in the management of mania, bipolar disorder (formerly manic depression) and recurrent depressive illnesses. The dosage of lithium is adjusted to give therapeutic serum concentrations of 0.4 to 1 mmol/L, although it should be noted that this is the range used in the UK, and other ranges have been quoted.

Lithium is given under close supervision with regular monitoring of serum concentrations because there is a narrow margin between therapeutic concentrations and those that are toxic. Initially weekly monitoring is advised, dropping to every 3 months for those on stable regimens. It is usual to take serum-lithium samples about 10 to 12 hours after the last oral dose.

Adverse effects that are not usually considered serious include nausea, weakness, fine tremor, mild polydipsia and polyuria. If serum concentrations rise into the 1.5 to 2 mmol/L range, toxicity usually occurs, and may present as lethargy, drowsiness, coarse hand tremor, lack of coordination, muscular weakness, increased nausea and vomiting, or diarrhoea. Higher levels result in neurotoxicity, which manifests as ataxia, giddiness, tinnitus, confusion, dysarthria, muscle twitching, nystagmus, and even coma or seizures. Cardiovascular symptoms may also develop and include ECG changes and circulatory problems, and there may be a worsening of polyuria.[1-3] Lithium levels of over 2 mmol/L can be extremely dangerous and therefore require urgent attention. Chronic lithium toxicity has been reported to have a 9% mortality, whilst acute toxicity has a 25% mortality.[4] However, patients with chronic lithium toxicity are more likely to experience severe symptoms at lower serum-lithium levels. Concurrent medications, older age and prior neurological illness may increase the susceptibility to lithium toxicity.[5]

In addition to the effects described above, lithium can induce diabetes insipidus and hypothyroidism in some patients, and is contraindicated in those with renal or cardiac insufficiency.

Just how lithium exerts its beneficial effects is not known, but it may compete with sodium ions in various parts of the body, and it alters the electrolyte composition of body fluids.

Many of the interactions involving lithium occur because of altered serum-lithium concentrations. Lithium is mainly excreted by the kidney; it undergoes glomerular filtration and then tubular reabsorption competitively with sodium. Therefore, drugs that affect renal excretion (e.g. 'thiazide diuretics', (p.1123)) or electrolyte balance (e.g. 'sodium compounds', (p.1128)) are likely to interact. Drug interactions may be an important cause of lithium neurotoxicity occurring when serum-lithium levels are within the therapeutic range.[6] This tends to occur with centrally active drugs e.g. 'antipsychotics', (p.710), 'carbamazepine', (p.1118), 'SSRIs', (p.1115), and 'tricyclic antidepressants', (p.1117). Most of the interactions involving lithium are discussed in this section but a few are found elsewhere in this publication. Virtually all of the reports are concerned with the carbonate, but sometimes lithium is given as the acetate, aspartate, chloride, citrate, gluconate, orotate or sulphate instead. There is no reason to believe that these lithium compounds will interact any differently to lithium carbonate.

1. Finley PR, Warner MD, Peabody CA. Clinical relevance of drug interactions with lithium. *Clin Pharmacokinet* (1995) 29, 172–91.
2. Camcolit (Lithium carbonate). Norgine Ltd. UK Summary of product characteristics, September 2006.
3. Eskalith (Lithium carbonate). GlaxoSmithKline. US Prescribing Information, September 2003.
4. Vipond AJ, Bakewell S, Telford R, Nicholls AJ. Lithium toxicity. *Anaesthesia* (1996) 51, 1156–8.
5. Chen K-P, Shen WW, Lu M-L. Implication of serum concentration monitoring in patients with lithium intoxication. *Psychiatry Clin Neurosci* (2004) 58, 25–9.
6. Emilien G, Maloteaux JM. Lithium neurotoxicity at low therapeutic doses. Hypotheses for causes and mechanism of action following a retrospective analysis of published case reports. *Acta Neurol Belg* (1996) 96, 281–93.

Lithium + ACE inhibitors

ACE inhibitors can raise lithium levels, and in some individuals two to fourfold increases have been recorded. Cases of lithium toxicity have been reported in patients when given captopril, enalapril or lisinopril (and possibly perindopril). One analysis found an increased relative risk of 7.6 for lithium toxicity requiring hospitalisation in elderly patients newly started on an ACE inhibitor. Risk factors for this interaction seem to be poor renal function, heart failure, volume depletion, and increased age.

Clinical evidence

An analysis of 10,615 elderly patients receiving lithium found that 413 (3.9%) were admitted to hospital at least once for lithium toxicity during a 10-year study period. The prescriptions for any ACE inhibitor (not specifically named) were compared between these 413 hospitalised patients and 1651 control patients. For any use of ACE inhibitor (63 cases and 110 controls) there was an increased relative risk of hospitalisation for lithium toxicity of 1.6. When patients who had started taking an ACE inhibitor within the last month were evaluated (14 cases and 5 controls), a dramatically increased risk of lithium toxicity was found (relative risk 7.6).[1]

Studies and case reports of the interaction between lithium and specific named ACE inhibitors are outlined in the subsections below.

(a) Captopril

A patient taking lithium carbonate developed a serum-lithium level of 2.35 mmol/L and toxicity (tremor, dysarthria, digestive problems) within 10 days of starting to take captopril 50 mg daily. He was restabilised on half his previous dose of lithium.[2] A retrospective study also reports a case of increased lithium levels with captopril (see under *(c) Lisinopril*, below).

(b) Enalapril

A woman taking lithium carbonate developed signs of lithium toxicity (ataxia, dysarthria, tremor, confusion) within 2 to 3 weeks of starting to take enalapril 20 mg daily. After 5 weeks her plasma-lithium levels had risen from 0.88 to 3.3 mmol/L, and moderate renal impairment was noted.[3] No toxicity occurred when the enalapril was later replaced by nifedipine.[3] Lithium toxicity following the use of enalapril, and associated in some cases with a decrease in renal function, has been seen in another 5 patients,[4-8] and a reduced lithium dosage was found adequate in another patient.[9] Enalapril 5 mg daily for 9 days had no effect on the mean serum-lithium levels of 9 healthy male subjects. However, one subject had a 31% increase in lithium levels.[10]

A retrospective study also reports several cases of increased lithium levels with enalapril (see under *(c) Lisinopril*, below).

(c) Lisinopril

A retrospective study of patient records identified 20 patients who were stabilised on lithium and then started on an ACE inhibitor (13 given lisinopril, 6 enalapril and one captopril). Their serum-lithium levels rose by an average of 35% (from 0.64 to 0.86 mmol/L) and there was a 26% decrease in lithium clearance. Signs and symptoms suggestive of toxicity (increased tremor, confusion, ataxia), necessitating a dosage reduction or lithium withdrawal, developed in four (20%) of these patients. In three patients the development of the interaction was delayed for several weeks.[11] A woman taking lithium developed lithium toxicity and a trough-serum level of 3 mmol/L within 3 weeks of stopping clonidine and starting lisinopril 20 mg daily.[12] Other reports similarly describe acute lithium toxicity in 4 patients when they were given lisinopril.[8,13-15] One of them was also taking verapamil,[15] which has also been shown to interact with lithium, but not usually to raise lithium levels (see 'Lithium + Calcium-channel blockers', p.1121).

(d) Perindopril

A patient taking lithium developed toxicity 3 months after starting to take perindopril and bendroflumethiazide,[16] which may also interact, see 'Lithium + Diuretics; Thiazide and related', p.1123.

(e) Ramipril

Ramipril has been shown to decrease renal lithium excretion in *rats*.[17]

Mechanism

Not fully understood. It has been suggested that as both ACE inhibitors and lithium cause sodium to be lost in the urine, and also ACE inhibitors reduce thirst stimulation, fluid depletion can occur. The normal compensatory reaction for fluid depletion is constriction of the efferent renal arterioles to maintain the glomerular filtration rate, but this mechanism is blocked by the ACE inhibitor. In addition, lithium and sodium ions are competitively reabsorbed, mainly in the proximal tubule, and with less sodium available, more lithium is retained. Consequently the renal excretion of lithium falls and toxicity develops.

Importance and management

The interaction between lithium and the ACE inhibitors is established and of clinical importance, although its incidence is probably small. One manufacturer has suggested that the concurrent use of ACE inhibitors and lithium carbonate should generally be avoided.[18] However, although lithium levels can rise, this is not always of clinical importance. The risk of lithium toxicity increases when other risk factors are also present (see below).

If any ACE inhibitor is added to established lithium treatment, monitor well for symptoms of lithium toxicity (see 'Lithium', (p.1111)) and consider measuring lithium levels more frequently. Be alert for the need to reduce the lithium dosage (possibly by between one-third to one-half).[12,14] The development of the interaction may be delayed, so monitoring lithium levels every week[12] or every two weeks[11] for several weeks has been advised.

Risk factors for increased lithium toxicity include: advanced age,[1,11] congestive heart failure,[10,12] renal insufficiency[7,12] and volume depletion.[6,12] Some consider these to be contraindications to the use of lithium.[7,12,18] Only captopril, enalapril, lisinopril (and possibly perindopril) have been reported to interact, but it seems likely, given the proposed mechanism, that this interaction will occur with any other ACE inhibitor.

1. Juurlink DN, Mamdani MM, Kopp A, Rochon PA, Shulman KI, Redelmeier DA. Drug-induced lithium toxicity in the elderly: a population-based study. *J Am Geriatr Soc* (2004) 52, 794–8.
2. Pulik M, Lida H. Interaction lithium-inhibiteurs de l'enzyme de conversion. *Presse Med* (1988) 17, 755.
3. Douste-Blazy P, Rostin M, Livarek B, Tordjman E, Montastruc JL, Galinier F. Angiotensin converting enzyme inhibitors and lithium treatment. *Lancet* (1986) i, 1448.
4. Mahieu M, Houvenagel E, Leduc JJ, Choteau P. Lithium-inhibiteurs de l'enzyme conversion: une association á éviter? *Presse Med* (1988) 17, 281.
5. Drouet A, Bouvet O. Lithium et inhibiteurs de l'enzyme de conversion. *Encephale* (1990) 16, 51–2.
6. Navis GJ, de Jong PE, de Zeeuw D. Volume homeostasis, angiotensin converting enzyme inhibition, and lithium therapy. *Am J Med* (1989) 86, 621.
7. Simon G. Combination angiotensin converting enzyme inhibitor/lithium therapy contraindicated in renal disease. *Am J Med* (1988) 85, 893–4.
8. Correa FJ, Eiser AR. Angiotensin-converting enzyme inhibitors and lithium toxicity. *Am J Med* (1992) 93, 108–9.
9. Ahmad S. Sudden hypothyroidism and amiodarone-lithium combination: an interaction. *Cardiovasc Drugs Ther* (1995) 9, 827–8.
10. DasGupta K, Jefferson JW, Kobak KA, Greist JH. The effect of enalapril on serum lithium levels in healthy men. *J Clin Psychiatry* (1992) 53, 398–400.
11. Finley PR, O'Brien JG, Coleman RW. Lithium and angiotensin-converting enzyme inhibitors: evaluation of a potential interaction. *J Clin Psychopharmacol* (1996) 16, 68–71.
12. Baldwin CM, Safferman AZ. A case of lisinopril-induced lithium toxicity. *DICP Ann Pharmacother* (1990) 24, 946–7.
13. Griffin JH, Hahn SM. Lisinopril-induced lithium toxicity. *DICP Ann Pharmacother* (1991) 25, 101.
14. Anon. ACE inhibitors and lithium toxicity. *Biol Ther Psychiatry* (1988) 11, 43.
15. Chandragiri SS, Pasol E, Gallagher RM. Lithium, ACE inhibitors, NSAIDs, and verapamil. A possible fatal combination. *Psychosomatics* (1998) 39, 281–2.
16. Vipond AJ, Bakewell S, Telford R, Nicholls AJ. Lithium toxicity. *Anaesthesia* (1996) 51, 1156–8.
17. Barthelmebs M, Grima M, Imbs J-L. Ramipril-induced decrease in renal lithium excretion in the rat. *Br J Pharmacol* (1995) 116, 2161–5.
18. Eskalith (Lithium carbonate). GlaxoSmithKline. US Prescribing Information, September 2003.

Lithium + Acetazolamide

There is some evidence that the excretion of lithium can be increased by the short-term use of acetazolamide. However, lithium toxicity has been seen in one patient given the combination for a month.

Clinical evidence, mechanism, importance and management

A single-dose study in 6 subjects given lithium 600 mg ten hours before acetazolamide 500 or 750 mg found a 31% increase in the urinary excretion of lithium.[1] A woman was successfully treated for a lithium overdose with acetazolamide, intravenous fluids, sodium bicarbonate, potassium chloride and mannitol.[2]

Paradoxically, lithium toxicity occurred in another patient after a month of treatment with acetazolamide. Lithium levels rose from 0.8 to 5 mmol/L, although it should be noted that the later measurement was taken 8 hours post-dose.[3] See 'Lithium', (p.1111) for details of lithium monitoring.

1. Thomsen K, Schou M. Renal lithium excretion in man. *Am J Physiol* (1968) 215, 823–7.
2. Horowitz LC, Fisher GU. Acute lithium toxicity. *N Engl J Med* (1969) 281, 1369.
3. Gay C, Plas J, Granger B, Olie JP, Loo H. Intoxication au lithium. Deux interactions inédites: l'acétazolamide et l'acide niflumique. *Encephale* (1985) 11, 261–2.

Lithium + Aciclovir

An isolated case report describes lithium toxicity caused by high-dose intravenous aciclovir.

Clinical evidence, mechanism, importance and management

A 42-year-old woman, taking lithium carbonate 450 mg twice daily, developed signs of lithium toxicity 6 days after starting treatment with intravenous aciclovir 10 mg/kg, which was given every 8 hours for a severe herpes zoster infection following chemotherapy. Her serum-lithium levels had risen over fourfold to 3.4 mmol/L. The reasons for this interaction are unknown but the authors of the report postulate that aciclovir may have inhibited the renal excretion of lithium.[1]

This appears to be the first and only report of this interaction, but it would now be prudent to monitor for symptoms of lithium toxicity (see 'Lithium', (p.1111)) and consider monitoring lithium levels if high-dose intravenous aciclovir is given to any patient. The report recommends measuring lithium levels every second or third day.[1] Oral aciclovir is predicted not to interact because of its low bioavailability, and no interaction would be expected with topical aciclovir as the plasma levels achieved by this route are minimal.

1. Sylvester RK, Leitch J, Granum C. Does acyclovir increase serum lithium levels? *Pharmacotherapy* (1996) 16, 466–8.

Lithium + Angiotensin II receptor antagonists

Case reports describe lithium toxicity in patients given candesartan, losartan, valsartan, and possibly irbesartan. Other angiotensin II receptor antagonists would be expected to interact similarly.

Clinical evidence

(a) Candesartan

A 58-year-old woman taking long-term lithium for depression (stable serum-lithium levels between 0.6 and 0.7 mmol/L), and unnamed calcium antagonists for hypertension, was additionally given candesartan 16 mg daily. She was hospitalised 8 weeks later with a 10-day history of ataxia, increasing confusion, disorientation and agitation, and was found to have a serum-lithium level of 3.25 mmol/L. She recovered completely when all the drugs were stopped. She was later restabilised on her original lithium dosage with a change to urapidil for her hypertension.[1]

(b) Irbesartan

A report describes a 74-year-old woman with increased lithium levels of 2.3 mmol/L and symptoms of lithium toxicity, which were associated with several drugs including irbesartan, lisinopril, escitalopram, levomepromazine, furosemide and spironolactone. It was suggested that these drugs could have delayed lithium excretion or worsened neurotoxic effects. An increase in the lisinopril dose and the addition of irbesartan several weeks before admission may have contributed to the lithium toxicity.[2]

(c) Losartan

An elderly woman taking lithium carbonate developed lithium toxicity (ataxia, dysarthria, and confusion) after starting to take losartan 50 mg daily. Her serum-lithium levels rose from 0.63 to 2 mmol/L over 5 weeks. The lithium and losartan were stopped and her symptoms had disappeared 2 days later. When lithium therapy was restarted and the losartan was replaced by nicardipine, her lithium levels were restabilised at 0.77 mmol/L within 2 weeks.[3]

(d) Valsartan

A woman with a long history of bipolar disorder was treated with lithium carbonate (serum levels consistently at 0.9 mmol/L) and a number of other drugs (L-tryptophan, lorazepam, glibenclamide, conjugated oestrogens and ciprofloxacin). Two weeks before being hospitalised for a manic relapse she was additionally started on valsartan 80 mg daily. While in hospital the ciprofloxacin was stopped, lorazepam was replaced by zopiclone, and quetiapine was added. On day 3 of her hospitalisation her serum-lithium levels were 1.1 mmol/L and she became increasingly delirious, confused and ataxic over the next week. By day 11 her serum-lithium levels had risen to 1.4 mmol/L. When an interaction was suspected, the valsartan was replaced by diltiazem. She later recovered and was stabilised on her original lithium carbonate dosage with lithium levels of 0.8 mmol/L.[4]

Mechanism

Not fully understood. It could be that, as with the ACE inhibitors, angiotensin II receptor antagonists inhibit aldosterone secretion, resulting in increased sodium loss by the kidney tubules. This causes lithium retention and thus an increase in lithium levels. However, angiotensin II receptor antagonists have less effect on aldosterone than the ACE inhibitors, making a clinically significant interaction less likely. *Animal* studies show that ramipril,[5] but not losartan,[6] decreases the excretion of lithium by the kidney, which would support this idea.

Importance and management

Direct information about interactions between lithium and angiotensin II receptor antagonists seems to be limited to these reports, although the interaction has been predicted to occur with all drugs of this class. Such sparse evidence is not enough to recommend contraindicating the concurrent use of angiotensin II receptor antagonists with lithium, although the UK manufacturers of irbesartan[7] and **olmesartan**[8] do not recommend the combination. Several manufacturers (including the UK manufacturers of **eprosartan** and **telmisartan**)[9,10] advise careful monitoring of serum-lithium levels, and this seems a sensible precaution, even though the risk of an interaction is probably fairly low. One report suggests weekly monitoring for the first month of concurrent use,[4] but any rise in serum-lithium levels may be gradual so that toxicity might take as long as 3 to 7 weeks to develop fully. Be mindful that the lithium dosage may need to be decreased.[11]

Patients on lithium should be aware of the symptoms of lithium toxicity and told to report them immediately should they occur. This should be reinforced when they are given angiotensin II receptor antagonists. As with 'ACE inhibitors', (p.1112), the risk of lithium toxicity would be expected to increase when risk factors such as advanced age, renal insufficiency, heart failure and volume depletion are also present.

1. Zwanzger P, Marcuse A, Boerner RJ, Walther A, Rupprecht R. Lithium intoxication after administration of AT_1 blockers. *J Clin Psychiatry* (2001) 62, 208–9.
2. Spinewine A, Schoevaerdts D, Mwenge GB, Swine C, Dive A. Drug-induced lithium intoxication: a case report. *J Am Geriatr Soc* (2005) 53, 360–1.
3. Blanche P, Raynaud E, Kerob D, Galezowski N. Lithium intoxication in an elderly patient after combined treatment with losartan. *Eur J Clin Pharmacol* (1997) 52, 501.
4. Leung M, Remick RA. Potential drug interaction between lithium and valsartan. *J Clin Psychopharmacol* (2000) 20, 392–3.
5. Barthelmebs M, Grima M, Imbs J-L. Ramipril-induced decrease in renal lithium excretion in the rat. *Br J Pharmacol* (1995) 116, 2161–5.
6. Barthelmebs M, Alt-Tebacher M, Madonna O, Grima M, Imbs J-L. Absence of a losartan interaction with renal lithium excretion in the rat. *Br J Pharmacol* (1995) 116, 2166–9.
7. Aprovel (Irbesartan). Sanofi-Aventis. UK Summary of product characteristics, May 2006.
8. Olmetec (Olmesartan medoxomil). Daiichi Sankyo UK Ltd. UK Summary of product characteristics, August 2006.
9. Teveten (Eprosartan mesilate). Solvay Healthcare Ltd. UK Summary of product characteristics, June 2006.
10. Micardis (Telmisartan). Boehringer Ingelheim Ltd. UK Summary of product characteristics, March 2007.
11. Eskalith (Lithium carbonate). GlaxoSmithKline. US Prescribing information, September 2003.

Lithium + Antibacterials

A retrospective study of patients receiving long-term lithium therapy found that concurrent medication, especially antibiotics, tended to be associated with a higher risk of elevated serum-lithium levels. However, the underlying infection and poor fluid intake might have contributed.

Clinical evidence, mechanism, importance and management

A multicentre, retrospective study of patients receiving long-term lithium therapy found 51 patients with elevated serum-lithium levels (greater than or equal to 1.3 mmol/L) which was at least 50% greater than the previous serum level. Fifteen patients had used potentially interacting medication and, of these, 7 patients had used antibacterials (6 different unnamed antibacterials). It was suggested that the underlying infection, associated fever and poor fluid intake might have contributed to the elevated lithium levels in these patients rather than the use of the antibacterial *per se*.[1] See under 'co-trimoxazole or trimethoprim', (below), 'quinolones', (below), 'metronidazole', (below), 'spectinomycin', (below), and 'tetracyclines', (below) for case reports of lithium toxicity with specific antibacterials.

1. Wilting I, Movig KLL, Moolenaar M, Hekster YA, Brouwers JRBJ, Heerdink ER, Nolen WA, Egberts ACG. Drug-drug interactions as a determinant of elevated lithium serum levels in daily clinical practice. *Bipolar Disord* (2005) 7, 274–80.

Lithium + Antibacterials; Co-trimoxazole or Trimethoprim

Two reports describe lithium toxicity in three patients given co-trimoxazole; in two of these patients toxicity was paradoxically accompanied by a fall in serum-lithium levels. A further report describes lithium toxicity accompanied by an increase in serum-lithium levels in a patient given trimethoprim.

Clinical evidence, mechanism, importance and management

Two patients stabilised on lithium carbonate (serum level 0.75 mmol/L) showed signs of lithium toxicity (tremor, fasciculations, muscular weakness, dysarthria, apathy) within a few days of being given co-trimoxazole [dose not stated], yet their serum-lithium levels were found to have fallen to about 0.4 mmol/L. Within 48 hours of withdrawing the co-trimoxazole, the signs of toxicity had gone, and their serum-lithium concentrations had returned to their former levels.[1] Another report very briefly states that ataxia, tremor and diarrhoea developed in a patient on lithium and timolol when co-trimoxazole was given.[2]

A 40-year-old woman taking lithium 1.2 g daily, experienced nausea, diarrhoea, malaise, difficulty concentrating, trembling, an uncertain gait and muscle spasms after trimethoprim 300 mg daily was started; her serum-lithium levels appeared to be elevated. She made a good recovery following rehydration.[3]

The reasons for this interaction are not understood, although trimethoprim may affect the renal excretion of lithium.[3] The general importance of this interaction is uncertain. If concurrent use is undertaken it would clearly be prudent to monitor the clinical response, as it would appear that in this situation serum level monitoring might not always be a reliable guide to toxicity. Consider also 'Lithium + Antibacterials', p.1113.

1. Desvilles M, Sevestre P. Effet paradoxal de l'association lithium et sulfaméthoxazol-triméthoprime. *Nouv Presse Med* (1982) 11, 3267–8.
2. Edwards IR. Medicines Adverse Reactions Committee: eighteenth annual report, 1983. *N Z Med J* (1984) 97, 729–32.
3. de Vries PL. Lithiumintoxicatie bij gelijktijdig gebruik van trimethoprim. *Ned Tijdschr Geneeskd* (2001) 145, 539–40.

Lithium + Antibacterials; Metronidazole

The lithium levels of three patients rose, to toxic levels in two cases, after they took metronidazole. Renal impairment was also reported in two of these patients.

Clinical evidence, mechanism, importance and management

A 40-year-old woman taking lithium carbonate 1.8 g daily, levothyroxine 150 micrograms daily and propranolol 60 mg daily developed signs of lithium toxicity (ataxia, rigidity, poor cognitive function, impaired co-ordination) after completing a one-week course of metronidazole 500 mg twice daily. Her serum-lithium levels had risen by 46% (from 1.3 to 1.9 mmol/L).[1] Another report describes 2 patients whose serum-lithium levels rose by about 20 and 125%, 5 to 12 days, respectively, after they finished a one-week course of metronidazole (750 mg or 1 g daily in divided doses).[2] A degree of renal impairment occurred during concurrent treatment and was still present 5 and 6 months later.[2] In contrast, one other patient is said to have taken both drugs together uneventfully.[1]

There seems to be no reason for avoiding concurrent use, but the outcome should be well monitored. Some have recommended that a reduction in the lithium dose should be considered, especially in patients maintained at relatively high serum-lithium levels.[1,2] Patients taking lithium should be aware of the symptoms of lithium toxicity and told to report them immediately should they occur. This should be reinforced when they are given metronidazole. The authors of one of the reports also recommend frequent analysis of creatinine and electrolyte levels and urine osmolality in order to detect any renal problems in patients on this combination.[2]

Consider also 'Lithium + Antibacterials', p.1113.

1. Ayd FJ. Metronidazole-induced lithium intoxication. *Int Drug Ther Newslett* (1982) 17, 15–16.
2. Teicher MH, Altesman RI, Cole JO, Schatzberg AF. Possible nephrotoxic interaction of lithium and metronidazole. *JAMA* (1987) 257, 3365–6.

Lithium + Antibacterials; Quinolones

An isolated case of lithium toxicity has been reported in a patient taking lithium and levofloxacin. Another possible case has been reported with ciprofloxacin.

Clinical evidence, mechanism, importance and management

A 56-year-old man taking lithium carbonate 400 mg three times daily for a bipolar disorder was admitted to hospital with bronchitis. He was started on **levofloxacin** 300 mg daily, and within 2 days was noted to have developed gait ataxia, dysarthria, coarse tremor, dizziness, vomiting, and confusion. Lithium toxicity was suspected, and because of the time course of the symptoms, an interaction with **levofloxacin** was considered responsible. Serum-lithium levels were found to have risen from 0.89 mmol/L (measured 2 weeks previously) to 2.53 mmol/L, and a reduction in his renal function was noted. Both drugs were stopped and the patient recovered over the following 4 days. His lithium level was found to be 1.12 mmol/L at that time.[1]

The mechanism of this interaction between lithium and **levofloxacin** is unclear, and this appears to be the only report. However, it would seem prudent to bear this interaction in mind if a patient on lithium is prescribed **levofloxacin**. Patients on lithium should be aware of the symptoms of lithium toxicity and told to report them immediately should they occur. This should be reinforced when they are given **levofloxacin**. For a report of lithium toxicity with raised lithium levels in a patient started on **ciprofloxacin** and nimesulide, which was attributed to the NSAID, see *Nimesulide*, under 'Lithium + NSAIDs', p.1125, and consider also 'Lithium + Antibacterials', p.1113.

1. Takahashi H, Higuchi H, Shimizu T. Severe lithium toxicity induced by combined levofloxacin administration. *J Clin Psychiatry* (2000) 61, 949–50.

Lithium + Antibacterials; Spectinomycin

An isolated case report describes a patient who developed lithium toxicity when given spectinomycin.

Clinical evidence, mechanism, importance and management

A woman developed lithium toxicity (tremor, nausea, vomiting, ataxia and dysarthria) when given spectinomycin injections [dose not stated] in addition to her long-term treatment with lithium.[1] Her serum-lithium levels had risen from a range of 0.8 to 1.1 mmol/L up to 3.2 mmol/L. Spectinomycin reduces urinary output, and so it was suggested that a reduced renal clearance of lithium led to these elevated levels. Information seems to be limited to this report, but it would seem prudent to bear this interaction in mind in any patient given both drugs.

Consider also 'Lithium + Antibacterials', p.1113.

1. Conroy RW. Quoted as a personal communication by Ayd FJ. Possible adverse drug-drug interaction report. *Int Drug Ther Newslett* (1978) 13, 15.

Lithium + Antibacterials; Tetracyclines

The concurrent use of lithium and the tetracyclines is normally uneventful, but two isolated reports describe increased serum-lithium levels and lithium toxicity, one in a woman taking tetracy-

cline, and the other in a man taking doxycycline. An isolated case of pseudotumor cerebri occurred in one patient taking lithium and minocycline.

Clinical evidence

(a) Doxycycline

A man on long-term treatment with lithium carbonate became confused within a day of starting to take doxycycline 100 mg twice daily. By the end of a week he had developed symptoms of lithium toxicity (ataxia, dysarthria, worsened tremor, fatigue, etc.). His serum-lithium levels had risen from a range of 0.8 to 1.1 mmol/L up to 1.8 mmol/L; his renal function remained normal. He recovered when the doxycycline was withdrawn.[1]

(b) Minocycline

A case report describes pseudotumor cerebri in an obese 15-year-old girl taking lithium, 4 months after she started taking minocycline 75 mg twice daily for acne.[2]

(c) Tetracycline

An isolated report describes a woman, who had been taking lithium for 3 years, with serum levels within the range of 0.5 to 0.84 mmol/L. Within 2 days of starting to take a sustained-release form of tetracycline *(Tetrabid)* her serum-lithium levels had risen to 1.7 mmol/L, and 2 days later they had further risen to 2.74 mmol/L. By then she showed clear symptoms of lithium toxicity (slight drowsiness, slurring of the speech, fine tremor and thirst).[3]

In contrast, 13 healthy subjects taking lithium carbonate 450 mg twice daily or 900 mg once daily had a small reduction in serum-lithium levels (from 0.51 to 0.47 mmol/L) when they were given tetracycline 500 mg twice daily for 7 days.[4] The incidence of adverse reactions remained largely unchanged, except for a slight increase in CNS and gastrointestinal adverse effects.

Mechanism

Not understood. One suggested reason for increased serum-lithium levels is that tetracycline (known to have nephrotoxic potential) may have adversely affected the renal clearance of lithium.[3]

Importance and management

These adverse interaction reports are isolated and unexplained. Two reports make the point that these drugs are commonly used for acne caused by lithium,[1,5] so any common interaction resulting in raised lithium levels would be expected to have come to light by now. The case of pseudotumor cerebri also appears rare, but note that the female gender and obesity are risk factors for its development and so greater caution may be warranted in this type of patient.[2] The authors advise frequent enquiry about headaches and visual changes.

There would seem to be no reason for avoiding the concurrent use of lithium and tetracycline, doxycycline or minocycline, but be aware of the potential for a rare interaction. Consider also 'Lithium + Antibacterials', p.1113.

1. Miller SC. Doxycycline-induced lithium toxicity. *J Clin Psychopharmacol* (1997) 17, 54–5.
2. Jonnalagadda J, Saito E, Kafantaris V. Lithium, minocycline, and pseudotumor cerebri. *J Am Acad Child Adolesc Psychiatry* (2005) 44, 209.
3. McGennis AJ. Lithium carbonate and tetracycline interaction. *BMJ* (1978) 2, 1183.
4. Fankhauser MP, Lindon JL, Connolly B, Healey WJ. Evaluation of lithium–tetracycline interaction. *Clin Pharm* (1988) 7, 314–17.
5. Jefferson JW. Lithium and tetracycline. *Br J Dermatol* (1982) 107, 370.

Lithium + Antidepressants; Mirtazapine

No pharmacokinetic or pharmacodynamic interactions appeared to occur between lithium and mirtazapine in one study in healthy subjects.

Clinical evidence, mechanism, importance and management

In a randomised, double-blind, crossover study, 12 healthy subjects were given lithium carbonate 600 mg daily or placebo for 10 days, with a single 30-mg dose of mirtazapine on day 10. The pharmacokinetics of both mirtazapine and lithium were unaltered by concurrent use. In addition, no pharmacodynamic changes, as studied by psychometric testing, were identified.[1]

1. Sitsen JMA, Voortman G, Timmer CJ. Pharmacokinetics of mirtazapine and lithium in healthy male subjects. *J Psychopharmacol* (2000) 14, 172–6.

Lithium + Antidepressants; Nefazodone

No pharmacokinetic interaction occurs between lithium and nefazodone.

Clinical evidence, mechanism, importance and management

In a study in 12 healthy subjects, nefazodone 200 mg twice daily was given alone for 5 days. After a washout period, lithium was given for 11 days, in escalating doses from 250 mg twice daily to 500 mg twice daily. When therapeutic steady-state lithium levels were achieved nefazodone 200 mg twice daily was added for 5 days. The pharmacokinetics of both nefazodone and lithium were unaltered by concurrent use, although there were some small changes in the pharmacokinetics of the nefazodone metabolites. However, since the combination was well tolerated, no dosage adjustments were considered necessary on concurrent use.[1]

1. Laroudie C, Salazar DE, Cosson J-P, Cheuvart B, Istin B, Girault J, Ingrand I, Decourt J-P. *Eur J Clin Pharmacol* (1999) 54, 923–8.

Lithium + Antidepressants; SSRIs

The concurrent use of lithium and SSRIs can be advantageous and uneventful, but various kinds of neurotoxicities have occurred in some patients. Isolated reports describe the development of symptoms similar to those of the serotonin syndrome in patients taking lithium and fluoxetine, fluvoxamine, paroxetine and possibly citalopram. In addition, increases and decreases in serum-lithium levels have been seen with fluoxetine.

Clinical evidence

(a) Citalopram

No pharmacokinetic changes were seen in one study in 8 healthy subjects when lithium 30 mmol/day (as lithium sulfate 1.98 g daily) was added to citalopram 40 mg daily.[1] Another study, in 24 patients who had previously not responded to citalopram alone, found that the concurrent use of citalopram 40 or 60 mg and lithium carbonate 800 mg daily was effective and did not increase adverse effects.[2] Even so, the manufacturers of citalopram suggest that concurrent use should be undertaken with caution, as they are aware of reports of enhanced serotonergic effects when lithium and SSRIs are used together.[3,4]

For a report of the serotonin syndrome in a patient with bipolar affective disorder treated with lithium, citalopram and olanzapine, see 'Olanzapine + Lithium', p.756.

(b) Fluoxetine

A woman with bipolar affective disorder, successfully maintained for 20 years on lithium carbonate 1.2 g daily, developed stiffness of her arms and legs, dizziness, unsteadiness in walking and speech difficulties within a few days of starting fluoxetine 20 mg daily. Her serum-lithium levels had risen from a range of 0.75 to 1.15 mmol/L up to 1.7 mmol/L. The lithium dosage was reduced to 900 mg daily and the fluoxetine withdrawn. Within 7 days, the toxic symptoms had disappeared and the lithium levels had fallen to 0.9 mmol/L.[5] Two other patients had increases in serum-lithium levels of about 45 and 70% (but no lithium toxicity) about a month after starting fluoxetine 20 or 40 mg daily, respectively. The problem resolved when the lithium dosage was reduced by 40 and 30%, respectively, and in the second case, the fluoxetine was withdrawn. Both patients also developed mania, either after readjustment of the lithium dose or during the combined treatment.[6] The US manufacturer of fluoxetine[7] says that concurrent use of these two drugs has resulted in both increased and decreased serum-lithium concentrations.

Toxicity (confusion, ataxia, coarse tremor, incoordination, movement disorders, fever) was seen in a patient when lithium was added to fluoxetine treatment, although the serum-lithium levels remained within the therapeutic range.[8] A woman maintained on clonazepam and then started on fluoxetine 20 mg then 40 mg daily, developed tremor and ataxia 6 days after lithium carbonate 100 mg increased to 400 mg daily was added. The problems resolved when the lithium and fluoxetine were withdrawn.[9] Extrapyramidal effects and ataxia were seen in one patient on lithium and fluoxetine, and dystonia in another patient who was also taking carbamazepine, captopril and trimipramine.[10] The development of the serotonin syndrome is also reported to have occurred in 2 patients on lithium and fluoxetine.[11,12] Heat stroke developed in a man on lithium and fluoxetine, attributed to synergistic impairment of his temperature regulatory system by the two drugs.[13] Absence seizures occurred in another patient given both drugs.[14]

(c) Fluvoxamine

A woman taking fluvoxamine became somnolent within a day of starting lithium. The lithium level 20 hours after the last dose was 0.2 mmol/L. She recovered when both drugs were stopped and she was discharged on lithium alone. The excessive somnolence was considered to have been possibly caused by increased serotonin levels caused by this drug combination.[15] A woman on long-term lithium treatment was started on fluvoxamine 50 mg daily, increased to 200 mg daily over 10 days. She gradually developed tremor, difficulties in making fine hand movements, impaired motor co-ordination and hyperreflexia. Serum lithium-levels remained therapeutic throughout. The reaction was interpreted as a mild form of the serotonin syndrome.[16]

The Committee on Safety of Medicines in the UK had received 19 reports of adverse reactions when fluvoxamine was given with lithium (5 reports of convulsions and one of hyperpyrexia) by 1989.[17]

In contrast to these reports, a study in 6 patients found that lithium (dosed to achieve plasma levels of 0.3 to 0.65 mmol/L) and fluvoxamine 100 to 150 mg daily (for between 3 and 23 weeks) was safe and effective, and no adverse interaction of any kind occurred.[18] Another study in 6 depressed patients found that lithium did not affect the pharmacokinetics of fluvoxamine 100 mg daily and combined use was more effective than fluvoxamine alone.[19] It would seem therefore that concurrent use can be valuable, but there is a clear need to monitor the outcome so that any problems can be quickly identified.

(d) Paroxetine

A study in 14 patients taking lithium found that tremor increased significantly when paroxetine 20 to 40 mg daily was added. The greatest increments occurred approximately 3 weeks after combined treatment was started, but tremor activity was still significantly greater than baseline after 6 weeks. No patient discontinued treatment because of the increase in tremor.[20]

A 59-year-old woman with a long-standing bipolar disorder who had taken paroxetine 10 mg increased to 30 mg daily for 3 weeks, developed symptoms suggestive of the serotonin syndrome (shivering, tremor of her arms and legs, flushed face, agitation, and some impairment of mental focussing) after lithium 400 mg daily was added.[21] Her serum lithium and paroxetine levels were found to be 0.63 mmol/L and 690 nanograms/mL respectively (the latter being sixfold higher than the upper levels seen in other patients). The paroxetine dosage was reduced to 10 mg daily, which decreased the serum levels to 390 nanograms/mL, whereupon she became symptom-free and her depression was relieved. It is not clear whether this reaction was due to an interaction or not as she never took the higher dose of paroxetine in the absence of lithium.

There is a report of seizures, unsteady gait and blurred speech in a patient with bipolar disorder and cystic fibrosis taking lithium and paroxetine; both drugs were discontinued. However, this patient was abusing oxycodone and clonazepam and was also on a variety of anti-asthma medications (salbutamol, salmeterol, budesonide, montelukast and cromoglicate), so the exact cause of the seizures is unclear.[22]

(e) Sertraline

In a randomised, placebo-controlled study, 16 healthy subjects were given lithium 600 mg twice daily for 9 days. On day 8, half of the subjects received two 100-mg doses of sertraline 8 hours apart, while the other half received placebo. Sertraline caused a statistically insignificant fall of 1.4% in steady-state lithium levels, and a statistically insignificant rise in renal lithium excretion. However, there was a high incidence of adverse effects (mainly tremor and nausea) with the combined treatment: tremor occurred in 7 out of the 8 taking sertraline, whereas no adverse effects were reported in the placebo group.[23]

Severe priapism occurred in a patient taking lithium carbonate 600 mg daily within 2 weeks of having the dosage of sertraline increased from 50 to 100 mg daily. It was not clear whether this was purely a reaction to the increased sertraline dosage, although it was suggested that the effect may have been due to the serotonergic effects of both drugs.[24]

The UK manufacturer of sertraline suggests that reports of increased tremor indicate a possible pharmacodynamic interaction, and therefore they advise caution if both drugs are used.[25]

Mechanism

Not fully understood although it seems likely that many of the symptoms could be due to the effects of both lithium and SSRIs on serotonin.

Importance and management

Concurrent use can be uneventful. A review of the safety of the combined use of lithium and the SSRIs identified 503 subjects who had received the combination without any evidence of serious adverse events.[26] However, occasionally and unpredictably adverse reactions develop, but the precise incidence is not known. Most manufacturers of the SSRIs, and the US manufacturers of lithium,[27] suggest that the combination of lithium and the SSRIs should be used with caution, and patients should be monitored closely. The UK manufacturers of lithium say that the combination may precipitate a serotonergic syndrome,[28,29] which justifies immediate discontinuation of treatment.[28]

If lithium is used in conjunction with an SSRI be alert for any evidence of toxicity. The symptoms may include tremor, dysarthria, ataxia, confusion, and many other symptoms of the serotonin syndrome. Heat stroke has also been seen and the serum-lithium levels may rise. It would clearly be prudent to monitor concurrent use carefully. For more information on the serotonin syndrome, see 'Additive or synergistic interactions', (p.9).

1. Gram LF, Hansen MGJ, Sindrup SH, Brøsen K, Poulsen JH, Aaes-Jørgensen T, Overø KF. Citalopram: interaction studies with levomepromazine, imipramine, and lithium. *Ther Drug Monit* (1993) 15, 18–24.
2. Baumann P, Souche A, Montaldi S, Baettig D, Lambert S, Uehlinger C, Kasas A, Amey M, Jonzier-Perey M. A double-blind, placebo-controlled study of citalopram with and without lithium in the treatment of therapy-resistant depressive patients: a clinical, pharmacokinetic, and pharmacogenetic investigation. *J Clin Psychopharmacol* (1996) 16, 307–14.
3. Cipramil (Citalopram hydrobromide). Lundbeck Ltd. UK Summary of product characteristics, January 2007.
4. Celexa (Citalopram hydrobromide). Forest Pharmaceuticals, Inc. US Prescribing information, May 2007.
5. Salama AA, Shafey M. A case of severe lithium toxicity induced by combined fluoxetine and lithium carbonate. *Am J Psychiatry* (1989) 146, 278.
6. Hadley A, Cason MP. Mania resulting from lithium-fluoxetine combination. *Am J Psychiatry* (1989) 146, 1637–8.
7. Prozac (Fluoxetine hydrochloride). Eli Lilly and Company. US Prescribing information, May 2007.
8. Noveske FG, Hahn KR, Flynn RJ. Possible toxicity of combined fluoxetine and lithium. *Am J Psychiatry* (1989) 146, 1515.
9. Austin LS, Arana GW, Melvin JA. Toxicity resulting from lithium augmentation of antidepressant treatment in elderly patients. *J Clin Psychiatry* (1990) 51, 344–5.
10. Coulter DM, Pillans PI. Fluoxetine and extrapyramidal side effects. *Am J Psychiatry* (1995) 152, 122–5.
11. Karle J, Bjørndal F. Serotonergt syndrom - ved kombineret behandling med litium og fluoxetin. *Ugeskr Laeger* (1995) 157, 1204–5.
12. Muly EC, McDonald W, Steffens D, Book S. Serotonin syndrome produced by a combination of fluoxetine and lithium. *Am J Psychiatry* (1993) 150, 1565.
13. Albukrek D, Moran DS, Epstein Y. A depressed workman with heatstroke. *Lancet* (1996) 347, 1016.
14. Sacristan JA, Iglesias C, Arellano F, Lequerica J. Absence seizures induced by lithium: possible interaction with fluoxetine. *Am J Psychiatry* (1991) 148, 146–7.
15. Evans M, Marwick P. Fluvoxamine and lithium: an unusual interaction. *Br J Psychiatry* (1990) 156, 286.
16. Öhman R, Spigset O. Serotonin syndrome induced by fluvoxamine-lithium interaction. *Pharmacopsychiatry* (1993) 26, 263–4.
17. Committee on the Safety of Medicines. *Current Problems* (1989) 26, 3. Correction. Ibid. 1989, 27, 3.
18. Hendrickx B, Floris M. A controlled pilot study of the combination of fluvoxamine and lithium. *Curr Ther Res* (1991) 49, 106–10.
19. Miljković BR, Pokrajac M, Timotijević I, Varagić V. The influence of lithium on fluvoxamine therapeutic efficacy and pharmacokinetics in depressed patients on combined fluvoxamine-lithium therapy. *Int Clin Psychopharmacol* (1997) 12, 207–12.
20. Zanninelli R, Bauer M, Jobert M, Müller-Oerlinghausen B. Changes in quantitatively assessed tremor during treatment of major depression with lithium augmented by paroxetine or amitriptyline. *J Clin Psychopharmacol* (2001) 21, 190–8.
21. Sobanski T, Bagli M, Laux G, Rao ML. Serotonin syndrome after lithium add-on medication to paroxetine. *Pharmacopsychiatry* (1997) 30, 106–7.
22. Munera PA, Perel JM, Asato M. Medication interaction causing seizures in a patient with bipolar disorder and cystic fibrosis. *J Child Adolesc Psychopharmacol* (2002) 12, 275–6.
23. Apseloff G, Wilner KD, von Deutsch DA, Henry EB, Tremaine LM, Gerber N, Lazar JD. Sertraline does not alter steady-state concentrations or renal clearance of lithium in healthy volunteers. *J Clin Pharmacol* (1992) 32, 643–6.
24. Mendelson WB, Franko T. Priapism with sertraline and lithium. *J Clin Psychopharmacol* (1994) 14, 434–5.
25. Lustral (Sertraline hydrochloride). Pfizer Ltd. UK Summary of product characteristics, October 2005.
26. Hawley CJ, Loughlin PJ, Quick SJ, Gale TM, Sivakumaran T, Hayes J, McPhee S, for the Hertfordshire Neuroscience Research Group. Efficacy, safety and tolerability of combined administration of lithium and selective serotonin reuptake inhibitors: a review of the current evidence. *Int Clin Psychopharmacol* (2000) 15, 197–206.
27. Eskalith (Lithium carbonate). GlaxoSmithKline. US Prescribing information, September 2003.

28. Priadel (Lithium carbonate). Sanofi-Aventis. UK Summary of product characteristics, August 2006.
29. Li-Liquid (Lithium citrate). Rosemont Pharmaceuticals Ltd. UK Summary of product characteristics, July 2007.

Lithium + Antidepressants; Tricyclic and related

The concurrent use of a tricyclic antidepressant and lithium can be successful in some patients, but others may develop adverse effects, a few of them severe. Cases of neurotoxicity, the serotonin syndrome and the neuroleptic malignant syndrome have been reported.

Clinical evidence

A study in 14 treatment-resistant depressed patients aged between 61 and 82 found that 7 showed complete improvement and 3 showed partial improvement, 3 to 21 days after lithium was added to treatment with the tricyclic or related antidepressants. Lithium adverse effects occurred in 6 patients; 4 of whom stopped lithium as a result. One of them was successfully restarted at a lower dose. Tremor was the most frequent adverse effect, and reversible neurotoxicity with a stroke-like syndrome was the most severe. The antidepressants used were **amitriptyline**, **doxepin**, **maprotiline** and **trazodone**.[1] A meta-analysis of 9 studies on the acute treatment of unipolar or bipolar depression indicated that the combined use of a mood stabiliser (lithium in 6 studies) and a tricyclic antidepressant was associated with an increased risk of switches into (hypo)mania, when compared with a mood stabiliser alone. It was suggested that monotherapy with a mood stabiliser should be tried to see if it is effective, before adding an antidepressant. Tricyclics were considered to be second-line antidepressants, with SSRIs the preferred choice.[2]

Reports relating to specific tricyclics are outlined below.

(a) Amitriptyline

A study in 17 lithium-maintained patients found that tremor increased significantly when amitriptyline 75 to 150 mg daily was added. The greatest increments occurred within approximately 3 weeks of starting the combined treatment, but tremor activity was still significantly greater than baseline after 6 weeks. No patient discontinued treatment because of the increase in tremor.[3] Seizures occurred in a patient on amitriptyline 300 mg daily, 13 days after lithium carbonate 300 mg three times daily was started. After recovery, combined therapy was resumed, but further seizures occurred 10 days later. Her lithium levels were 0.9 mmol/L three days before this second episode. She later took amitriptyline 500 mg daily without adverse effect.[4] Another patient developed neuroleptic malignant syndrome after one week of treatment with lithium carbonate 300 mg and amitriptyline 25 mg, both three times daily. The patient had also received chlorpromazine for one week, just before the lithium-antidepressant therapy was started.[5] No pharmacokinetic interaction was found in 10 therapy-resistant patients with major depression who were given amitriptyline and lithium for 4 weeks.[6]

(b) Clomipramine

A depressed man taking clomipramine 175 mg, levomepromazine 25 mg and flunitrazepam 2 mg daily, was started on lithium 600 mg daily. About one week later, after his dosage of lithium was raised to 1 g daily and he developed the serotonin syndrome (myoclonus, shivering, tremors, incoordination). Due to this reaction, and because his serum-lithium levels were 1.6 mmol/L, the lithium was stopped. The serotonin syndrome then abated. The clomipramine dosage was reduced, but some mild symptoms remained until the clomipramine was stopped. He responded well to lithium 600 mg daily alone, without developing the serotonin syndrome.[7]

(c) Doxepin

A 64-year-old man developed periods of confusion and disorientation within 2 weeks of starting to take lithium 300 mg twice daily with doxepin 100 mg at bedtime. He was admitted to hospital because of urinary retention, and he was also lethargic and became confused, but despite the withdrawal of both drugs he developed a condition similar to the neuroleptic malignant syndrome (fever, muscle rigidity, changes in consciousness, autonomic dysfunction), which was successfully treated with dantrolene.[8]

(d) Nortriptyline

A 65-year-old woman developed tremor, memory difficulties, disorganised thinking and auditory hallucinations when given lithium carbonate 300 mg twice daily (lithium level 0.82 mmol/L) and nortriptyline 50 mg daily. However, because she only ever received lithium with nortriptyline, the possibility that this was an effect of lithium alone cannot be excluded.[9]

Mechanism

Not fully understood. Tremor is a relatively frequent adverse effect of both lithium and antidepressants with serotonergic properties. It might be expected that combinations of lithium (which is itself serotonergic) with such antidepressants will enhance not only efficacy, but also increase the incidence of adverse effects.[3] For more information about the serotonin syndrome, see 'Additive or synergistic interactions', (p.9).

Importance and management

The concurrent use of lithium and tricyclics can be valuable, but the reports cited here clearly show the need to monitor the outcome closely so that any problems can be dealt with quickly. The incidence of these serious reactions is not known.

1. Lafferman J, Solomon K, Ruskin P. Lithium augmentation for treatment-resistant depression in the elderly. *J Geriatr Psychiatry Neurol* (1988) 1, 49–52.
2. Nolen WA, Bloemkolk D. Treatment of bipolar depression, a review of the literature and a suggestion for an algorithm. *Neuropsychobiology* (2000) 42 (Suppl 1), 11–17.
3. Zaninelli R, Bauer M, Jobert M, Müller-Oerlinghausen B. Changes in quantitatively assessed tremor during treatment of major depression with lithium augmented by paroxetine or amitriptyline. *J Clin Psychopharmacol* (2001) 21, 190–8.
4. Solomon JG. Seizures during lithium-amitriptyline therapy. *Postgrad Med* (1979) 66, 145–8.
5. Fava S, Galizia AC. Neuroleptic malignant syndrome and lithium carbonate. *J Psychiatry Neurosci* (1995) 20, 305–6.
6. Jaspert A, Ebert D, Loew T, Martus P. Lithium increases the response to tricyclic antidepressant medication – no evidence of influences of pharmacokinetic interactions. *Pharmacopsychiatry* (1993) 26, 165.
7. Kojima H, Terao T, Yoshimura R. Serotonin syndrome during clomipramine and lithium treatment. *Am J Psychiatry* (1993) 150, 1897.
8. Rosenberg PB, Pearlman CA. NMS-like syndrome with a lithium/doxepin combination. *J Clin Psychopharmacol* (1991) 11, 75–6.
9. Austin LS, Arana GW, Melvin JA. Toxicity resulting from lithium augmentation of antidepressant treatment in elderly patients. *J Clin Psychiatry* (1990) 51, 344–5.

Lithium + Antidepressants; Venlafaxine

Symptoms similar to those of the serotonin syndrome have developed in a few patients taking lithium with venlafaxine. No clinically significant pharmacokinetic interaction appears to occur between these two drugs.

Clinical evidence, mechanism, importance and management

In an open study of 13 major depressive patients who did not respond to a 4-week course of venlafaxine 300 mg daily, lithium was added and continued for 4 weeks. After 12 days of combined treatment, 2 patients experienced symptoms of hypomania, marked nausea and trembling (considered to be a moderate form of the serotonin syndrome), and had to stop lithium treatment. Their lithium-plasma levels were within the therapeutic range (0.83 and 0.77 mmol/L on day 7). Lithium was well tolerated by most of the other patients, with trembling being the most frequent adverse effect (4 out of 11).[1]

A case report describes a 50-year-old woman who developed the serotonin syndrome 45 days after starting to take lithium and venlafaxine (and within 10 days of the most recent dose increase of venlafaxine). Both drugs were immediately stopped and she recovered over the next 4 to 5 days. Plasma levels of venlafaxine, its metabolite *O*-desmethylvenlafaxine (ODV), and lithium had remained within the normal therapeutic range throughout. As she had previously experienced profound adverse effects with two different SSRIs, the authors concluded that the patient was unusually sensitive to serotonergic medication.[2]

In a pharmacokinetic study, 12 healthy subjects were given a single 600-mg dose of lithium carbonate on day 1 and day 8, with venlafaxine 50 mg every 8 hours for 7 days from day 4. The renal clearance of venlafaxine was reduced by about 50% and that of its active metabolite ODV was reduced by 15%. Neither of these changes was considered clinically relevant, as the total clearance was not affected. The maximum serum levels of the lithium were increased by about 10%, and the time to reach this was reduced by about 30 minutes, but these changes met the criteria for bioequivalence, and the other pharmacokinetic parameters of lithium were unchanged.[3] The general picture that emerged was that no clinically important pharmacokinetic interaction normally occurs if these two drugs are used together.

There seems to be no good reason for avoiding concurrent use, but be aware that an interaction is possible and monitor the outcome carefully. For more information about the serotonin syndrome, see 'Additive or synergistic interactions', (p.9).

1. Bertschy G, Ragama-Pardos E, Aït-Ameur A, Muscionico M, Favre S, Roth L. Lithium augmentation in venlafaxine non-responders: an open study. *Eur Psychiatry* (2003) 18, 314–17.
2. Mekler G, Woggon B. A case of serotonin syndrome caused by venlafaxine and lithium. *Pharmacopsychiatry* (1997) 30, 272–3.
3. Troy SM, Parker VD, Hicks DR, Boudino FD, Chiang ST. Pharmacokinetic interaction between multiple-dose venlafaxine and single-dose lithium. *J Clin Pharmacol* (1996) 36, 175–81.

Lithium + Antiepileptics; Carbamazepine

Although the combined use of lithium and carbamazepine is beneficial in many patients, it may increase the risk of neurotoxicity. Sinus node dysfunction has also occurred in a few patients. An isolated report describes a patient who had a marked rise in lithium levels and lithium toxicity, which was apparently caused by carbamazepine-induced renal impairment.

Clinical evidence

(a) Neurotoxicity with normal drug levels

A patient taking lithium 1.8 g daily developed severe neurotoxicity (ataxia, truncal tremors, nystagmus, limb hyperreflexia, muscle fasciculation) within 3 days of starting to take carbamazepine 600 mg daily. Blood levels of both drugs remained within the therapeutic range. The symptoms resolved when each drug was withdrawn in turn, and re-occurred within 3 days of restarting concurrent treatment.[1] Five patients with rapid-cycling bipolar disorder developed similar neurotoxic symptoms (confusion, drowsiness, generalised weakness, lethargy, coarse tremor, hyperreflexia, cerebellar signs) when they were given lithium carbonate with carbamazepine [doses not stated]. Plasma levels of both drugs remained within the accepted range.[2] Other reports describe adverse neurological effects during the concurrent use of lithium and carbamazepine, which were also not accompanied by significant changes in lithium levels,[3-7] although in one patient raised serum levels of both drugs were seen.[8] A systematic search through the Medline database, for reports of neurotoxic adverse effects in patients taking lithium at low therapeutic concentrations, found a total of 41 cases over approximately 30 years from 1966. Carbamazepine had been taken concurrently in 22% of these cases, in some instances with other potentially interacting drugs.[9] Another retrospective study of 46 type I bipolar patients found significant benefits of long-term combined lithium and carbamazepine therapy compared with monotherapy with lithium (31 patients) or carbamazepine (15). However, rates of adverse effects increased 2.5-fold compared with monotherapy, and there were particular excesses of tremor and drowsiness.[10]

In other patients the combined use of lithium and carbamazepine was said to be well tolerated and beneficial,[11,12] but one report suggests that the dosages may need to be carefully titrated to avoid adverse effects.[13]

(b) Sinus node dysfunction

A 9-year study in a psychiatric hospital found that, of 5 patients on lithium who developed sinus node dysfunction, 4 were also on carbamazepine.[14]

(c) Toxic lithium levels

An isolated case report describes carbamazepine-induced acute renal failure, which resulted in a 3.5-fold rise in lithium levels and lithium toxicity 3 weeks after carbamazepine was started.[15]

Mechanism

Not understood. A paper that plotted the serum levels of lithium and carbamazepine on a two-dimensional graph failed to find any evidence of synergistic toxicity.[16] Sinus node dysfunction can be caused by either lithium or carbamazepine, but this is rare. However, the effects may possibly be additive.

Importance and management

The neurotoxic interaction is established, but its incidence is not known. The incidence of severe neurotoxicity may be quite small, but increased mild adverse events such as tremor and drowsiness seem to be fairly common.[10] The authors of one paper suggest that the risk factors appear to be a history of neurotoxicity with lithium, and compromised medical or neurological function.[2] If concurrent use is undertaken, the outcome should be closely monitored. This is particularly important because neurotoxicity can develop even though the levels remain within the accepted therapeutic range. If severe neurotoxicity develops the lithium treatment should be discontinued promptly, whatever the lithium level.[9]

1. Chaudhry RP, Waters BGH. Lithium and carbamazepine interaction: possible neurotoxicity. *J Clin Psychiatry* (1983) 44, 30–1.
2. Shukla S, Godwin CD, Long LEB, Miller MG. Lithium-carbamazepine neurotoxicity and risk factors. *Am J Psychiatry* (1984) 141, 1604–6.
3. Andrus PF. Lithium and carbamazepine. *J Clin Psychiatry* (1984) 45, 525.
4. Marcoux AW. Carbamazepine-lithium drug interaction. *Ann Pharmacother* (1996) 30, 547.
5. Manto M-U, Jacquy J, Hildebrand J. Cerebellar ataxia in upper limbs triggered by addition of carbamazepine to lithium treatment. *Acta Neurol Belg* (1996) 96, 316–17.
6. Ghose K. Effect of carbamazepine in polyuria associated with lithium therapy. *Pharmakopsychiatr Neuropsychopharmakol* (1978) 11, 241–5.
7. Price WA, Zimmer B. Lithium-carbamazepine neurotoxicity in the elderly. *J Am Geriatr Soc* (1985) 33, 876–7.
8. Hassan MN, Thakar J, Weinberg AL, Grimes JD. Lithium-carbamazepine interaction: clinical and laboratory observations. *Neurology* (1987) 37 (Suppl 1), 172.
9. Emilien G, Maloteaux JM. Lithium neurotoxicity at low therapeutic doses. Hypotheses for causes and mechanism of action following a retrospective analysis of published case reports. *Acta Neurol Belg* (1996) 96, 281–93.
10. Baethge C, Baldessarini RJ, Mathiske-Schmidt K, Hennen J, Berghöfer A, Müller-Oerlinghausen B, Bschor T, Adli M, Bauer M. Long-term combination therapy versus monotherapy with lithium and carbamazepine in 46 bipolar I patients. *J Clin Psychiatry* (2005) 66, 174–82.
11. Laird LK, Knox EP. The use of carbamazepine and lithium in controlling a case of chronic rapid cycling. *Pharmacotherapy* (1987) 7, 130–2.
12. Pies R. Combining lithium and anticonvulsants in bipolar disorder: a review. *Ann Clin Psychiatry* (2002) 14, 223–32.
13. Kramlinger KG, Post RM. The addition of lithium to carbamazepine. Antidepressant efficacy in treatment-resistant depression. *Arch Gen Psychiatry* (1989) 46, 794–800.
14. Steckler TL. Lithium- and carbamazepine-associated sinus node dysfunction: nine-year experience in a psychiatric hospital. *J Clin Psychopharmacol* (1994) 14, 336–9.
15. Mayan H, Golubev N, Dinour D, Farfel Z. Lithium intoxication due to carbamazepine-induced renal failure. *Ann Pharmacother* (2001) 35, 560–2.
16. McGinness J, Kishimoto A, Hollister LE. Avoiding neurotoxicity with lithium-carbamazepine combinations. *Psychopharmacol Bull* (1990) 26, 181–4.

Lithium + Antiepileptics; Gabapentin

Gabapentin did not alter the pharmacokinetics of single-dose lithium in patients with normal renal function.

Clinical evidence, mechanism, importance and management

In a double-blind study, 13 patients with normal renal function were given a single 600-mg dose of lithium either with or without gabapentin at steady state. Gabapentin did not significantly alter the pharmacokinetics of the lithium, and no increase in adverse effects was noted. More long-term studies will be needed to confirm this lack of interaction, especially in patients with impaired renal function as both drugs are eliminated by renal excretion.[1]

1. Frye MA, Kimbrell TA, Dunn RT, Piscitelli S, Grothe D, Vanderham E, Corá-Locatelli G, Post RM, Ketter TA. Gabapentin does not alter single-dose lithium pharmacokinetics. *J Clin Psychopharmacol* (1998) 18, 461–4.

Lithium + Antiepileptics; Lamotrigine

Lamotrigine does not appear to cause a clinically significant alteration in lithium levels. Cognitive adverse effects have been reported in one patient taking the combination.

Clinical evidence, mechanism, importance and management

In an open, randomised, two-period, crossover study, 20 healthy men were given 2 g of anhydrous lithium gluconate (9.8 mmol of lithium) every 12 hours for 11 doses, either with or without lamotrigine 100 mg daily. It was found that the serum-lithium levels were decreased by about 8% by lamotrigine, but these small changes were not considered to be clinically relevant.[1]

A 2002 review of the few published reports on the use of lithium with lamotrigine suggested that the combination appears to be well tolerated.[2] However, one woman taking lithium who had been treated with lamotrigine 50 mg for 4 weeks, experienced delirium when the dose of lamotrigine was increased to 150 mg daily. The symptoms disappeared when the lamotrigine dose was reduced to 100 mg daily.[3] It is not clear whether these effects were directly caused by the combination of lithium and lamotrigine. However; the author of the review considered that if cognitive adverse effects occur, it might be worth considering a reduction in the dose of either or both drugs.[2] More study is needed.

1. Chen C, Veronese L, Yin Y. The effects of lamotrigine on the pharmacokinetics of lithium. *Br J Clin Pharmacol* (2000) 50, 193–5.
2. Pies R. Combining lithium and anticonvulsants in bipolar disorder: a review. *Ann Clin Psychiatry* (2002) 14, 223–32.
3. Sporn J, Sachs G. The anticonvulsant lamotrigine in treatment-resistant manic-depressive illness. *J Clin Psychopharmacol* (1997) 17, 185–9.

Lithium + Antiepileptics; Phenytoin

Symptoms of lithium toxicity (sometimes with unchanged lithium levels) have been seen in a few patients concurrently treated with phenytoin, although the interaction has not been clearly demonstrated.

Clinical evidence, mechanism, importance and management

A patient with a history of depression and convulsions was treated with increasing doses of lithium carbonate and phenytoin over a period of about 4 years. Although the serum levels of both drugs remained within the therapeutic range, he eventually began to develop symptoms of lithium toxicity (thirst, polyuria, polydipsia and tremor) that disappeared when the lithium was stopped. Later, when lithium was restarted, the symptoms returned, this time abating when the phenytoin was replaced by carbamazepine. The patient then claimed that he felt normal for the first time in years.[1] Another report describes symptoms of lithium toxicity in a patient with lithium levels within the normal range. This patient was also taking phenytoin.[2]

In a further case[3] a man taking phenytoin became ataxic within 3 days of starting to take lithium. He had no other toxic symptoms and his serum-lithium level was 2 mmol/L. However, as he only ever took lithium in the presence of phenytoin, it is not possible to say whether the effects were as a result of an interaction, or whether toxic levels would have occurred with the lithium alone. Another similar case has also been reported.[4]

Information seems to be limited to these reports and none of them presents a clear picture of the role of phenytoin in the reactions described.[1-4] The interaction is not well established. Patients taking lithium should be aware of the symptoms of lithium toxicity and told to report them immediately should they occur. This should be reinforced when they are given phenytoin. Increased serum lithium monitoring does not appear to be of value in this situation as the interaction occurred in patients with lithium levels within the normally accepted range.

1. MacCallum WAG. Interaction of lithium and phenytoin. *BMJ* (1980) 280, 610–11.
2. Speirs J, Hirsch SR. Severe lithium toxicity with "normal" serum concentrations. *BMJ* (1978) 1, 815–16.
3. Salem RB, Director K, Muniz CE. Ataxia as the primary symptom of lithium toxicity. *Drug Intell Clin Pharm* (1980) 14, 622–3.
4. Raskin DE. Lithium and phenytoin interaction. *J Clin Psychopharmacol* (1984) 4, 120.

Lithium + Antiepileptics; Topiramate

Two isolated reports describe elevated serum-lithium levels and evidence of toxicity in patients also taking topiramate. No important pharmacokinetic interaction has been seen in healthy subjects.

Clinical evidence, mechanism, importance and management

A 42-year-old woman with type II bipolar disorder was started on lithium carbonate 1.5 g and topiramate 500 mg daily, resulting in a steady-state trough serum-lithium level of 0.5 mmol/L after 10 days. She was also started on citalopram 10 mg daily. The patient raised the topiramate dose to 800 mg daily in an attempt to lose weight, and 5 weeks later began to complain of severe anorexia, nausea, fatigue and impaired concentration. She had managed to lose 35 lb (almost 16 kg) of weight she had gained whilst on a previous drug combination. When examined she was lethargic, with tremors, nystagmus, bradycardia and memory loss. Her trough serum-lithium level had risen by 180% to 1.4 mmol/L. The symptoms disappeared over 4 days when the lithium was stopped. Two months later she was stabilised once again on lithium carbonate 1.2 g and topiramate 500 mg daily, with a steady-state serum-lithium level of 0.5 mmol/L.[1] Another report describes a case of increased lithium levels and toxicity (worsening concentration, confusion, lethargy) after topiramate was added to lithium therapy. The lithium was stopped and then restarted at half the original dose, which produced therapeutic lithium levels of 0.67 mmol/L. In addition, while maintaining the dose of lithium at 450 mg daily, further increases in the topiramate dose from 75 to 125 mg daily over 4 weeks resulted in parallel elevations of lithium levels (from 0.67 to 0.92 mmol/L).[2]

However, a review of the pharmacokinetic interactions of topiramate reported a study that had found that there was little pharmacokinetic interaction with lithium when topiramate (50 mg twice daily titrated to 100 mg twice daily) was given to 12 healthy subjects receiving lithium carbonate 300 mg three times daily. The AUC of lithium was about 18% lower and the clearance 21.7% higher. When compared with historical data, the clearance of topiramate appeared to be lower.[3]

The reasons for these reactions are not known, but topiramate is mainly eliminated by renal excretion and high doses of topiramate may competitively interfere with lithium excretion.[1] Similarly, lithium may affect topiramate clearance.[3] Some of the toxicity could have been due to the adverse effects of either drug, with the weight loss in the first case possibly disturbing the sodium excretion, which could have affected the loss of lithium in the urine.

These cases highlight the possible risk of elevated serum-lithium levels especially if high doses of topiramate are used. Patients on lithium should be aware of the symptoms of lithium toxicity and told to report them immediately should they occur. This should be reinforced when they are given topiramate. Consider monitoring lithium levels in patients newly started on this combination and carefully adjusting the dose of topiramate and/or lithium to minimise adverse effects.[4,5]

1. Pinninti NR, Zelinski G. Does topiramate elevate serum lithium levels? *J Clin Psychopharmacol* (2002) 22, 340.
2. Abraham G, Owen J. Topiramate can cause lithium toxicity. *J Clin Psychopharmacol* (2004) 24, 565–7.
3. Bialer M, Doose DR, Murthy B, Curtin C, Wang S-S, Twyman RE, Schwabe S. Pharmacokinetic interactions of topiramate. *Clin Pharmacokinet* (2004) 43, 763–80.
4. Chengappa KNR, Gershon S, Levine J. The evolving role of topiramate among other mood stabilizers in the management of bipolar disorder. *Bipolar Disord* (2001) 3, 215–32.
5. Pies R. Combining lithium and anticonvulsants in bipolar disorder: a review. *Ann Clin Psychiatry* (2002) 14, 223–32.

Lithium + Antiepileptics; Valproate

No clinically relevant adverse interaction appears to occur between lithium carbonate and valproate.

Clinical evidence, mechanism, importance and management

In a crossover study, 16 healthy subjects were given valproate (as valproate semisodium) or a placebo twice daily for 12 days, to which lithium carbonate 300 mg three times daily was added on days 6 to 10. The valproate-serum levels and AUC rose slightly, while the serum-lithium levels were unaltered. Adverse events did not change significantly. It was concluded that the concurrent use of these drugs is safe.[1] A review on the efficacy of lithium/anticonvulsant combinations in bipolar disorder lists several studies in which the combination of valproate (as valproate semisodium) and lithium was used. On the whole the combination was considered safe and well tolerated, although a few patients discontinued treatment due to adverse effects, which included gastrointestinal symptoms and raised liver transaminases. It was, however, difficult to know if these adverse effects were due to the individual drugs or the result of an interaction. Other adverse effects that have been reported with the combined treatment include tremor, cognitive impairment and alopecia.[2]

1. Granneman GR, Schneck DW, Cavanaugh JH, Witt GF. Pharmacokinetic interactions and side effects resulting from concomitant administration of lithium and divalproex sodium. *J Clin Psychiatry* (1996) 57, 204–6.
2. Pies R. Combining lithium and anticonvulsants in bipolar disorder: a review. *Ann Clin Psychiatry* (2002) 14, 223–32.

Lithium + Aspirin or other Salicylates

No clinically significant pharmacokinetic interaction appears to occur between aspirin, lysine aspirin and sodium salicylate and lithium.

Clinical evidence, mechanism, importance and management

In a steady-state study 10 healthy women with average plasma-lithium levels of 0.63 mmol/L had a slight 6% rise in their renal excretion of lithium when they were given aspirin 1 g four times daily for 7 days. However, no statistically significant alteration in lithium levels was found.[1]

No change in serum lithium levels was seen in 7 patients taking lithium when they were given aspirin 975 mg four times daily for 6 days.[2] Another report states that aspirin 600 mg four times daily had no effect on the absorption or renal excretion of single doses of lithium carbonate given to 6 healthy subjects.[3] Further reports describe no change in serum lithium levels with **lysine aspirin**,[4] intravenous aspirin,[5] or intravenous **sodium salicylate**.[5] However, lithium clearance was slightly reduced by 22% by intravenous **sodium salicylate**,[5] and a study in one healthy subject found a 32% increase in mean serum-lithium levels from 0.41 to 0.54 mmol/L after 5 days of oral aspirin treatment (975 mg four times daily for 2 days, then 650 mg four times daily for 3 days).[6]

1. Reimann IW, Diener U, Frölich JC. Indomethacin but not aspirin increases plasma lithium ion levels. *Arch Gen Psychiatry* (1983) 40, 283–6.
2. Ragheb MA. Aspirin does not significantly affect patients' serum lithium levels. *J Clin Psychiatry* (1987) 48, 425.
3. Bikin D, Conrad KA, Mayersohn M. Lack of influence of caffeine and aspirin on lithium elimination. *Clin Res* (1982) 30, 249A.
4. Singer L, Imbs JL, Danion JM, Singer P, Krieger-Finance F, Schmidt M, Schwartz J. Risque d'intoxication par le lithium en cas de traitement associé par les anti-inflammatoires non stéroïdiens. *Therapie* (1981) 36, 323–6.
5. Reimann IW, Golbs E, Fischer C, Frölich JC. Influence of intravenous acetylsalicylic acid and sodium salicylate on human renal function and lithium clearance. *Eur J Clin Pharmacol* (1985) 29, 435–41.
6. Bendz H, Feinberg M. Aspirin increases serum lithium ion levels. *Arch Gen Psychiatry* (1984) 41, 310–11.

Lithium + Baclofen

The hyperkinetic symptoms of two patients with Huntington's chorea were aggravated within a few days of starting concurrent lithium and baclofen. One patient took lithium first, the other baclofen.

Clinical evidence, mechanism, importance and management

A patient with Huntington's chorea, treated with lithium and haloperidol, was additionally given baclofen, and another patient being treated with imipramine, clopenthixol, chlorpromazine and baclofen was additionally given lithium. Within a few days both patients showed a severe aggravation of their hyperkinetic symptoms, which disappeared within 3 days of withdrawing the baclofen.[1] Other patients with Huntington's chorea showed no major changes in their mental state or movement disorders when given up to 90 mg of baclofen daily,[2,3] which suggests that an interaction with lithium may have been the cause of the hyperkinesis in these two patients. On the basis of this very limited evidence it would seem prudent to monitor the effects of concurrent use and consider stopping one of the drugs if hyperkinesis develops.

1. Andén N-E, Dalén P, Johansson B. Baclofen and lithium in Huntington's chorea. *Lancet* (1973) ii, 93.
2. Barbeau A. G.A.B.A. and Huntington's chorea. *Lancet* (1973) ii, 1499–1500.
3. Paulson GW. Lioresal in Huntington's disease. *Dis Nerv Syst* (1976) 37, 465–7.

Lithium + Benzodiazepines

Neurotoxicity and increased serum-lithium levels were reported in five patients when clonazepam was added to treatment with lithium. An isolated case of serious hypothermia has been reported during the concurrent use of lithium and diazepam. Alprazolam seems unlikely to cause a clinically important rise in serum-lithium levels.

Clinical evidence, mechanism, importance and management

(a) Alprazolam

Alprazolam 2 mg daily for 4 days slightly increased the steady-state AUC of lithium by about 8% and reduced its urinary recovery from 93.6 to 78.2% in 10 healthy subjects taking lithium 900 mg to 1.5 g daily. It was suggested that these changes were unlikely to be clinically significant, but confirmation of this is needed.[1]

(b) Clonazepam

A retrospective study of patient records revealed 5 patients with bipolar affective disorder, treated with lithium carbonate 900 mg to 2.4 g daily, who had developed a reversible neurotoxic syndrome with ataxia, dysarthria, drowsiness and confusion when they were given clonazepam 2 to 16 mg daily. In one case the clonazepam was added to their antipsychotics (chlorpromazine, perphenazine, haloperidol) and in 4 cases the clonazepam replaced the antipsychotic treatment. In all cases the lithium levels rose, and in two of these cases they reached toxic levels. The authors of the report suggest that the neurotoxicity was caused either by the increase in lithium levels, or by synergistic toxicity, however, the use of antipsychotics may also have increased CNS sensitivity. It was recommended that lithium levels should be measured more frequently if clonazepam is added, and the effects of concurrent use well monitored.[2]

(c) Diazepam

A mentally retarded patient had occasional hypothermic episodes (below 35°C) while taking lithium and diazepam, but not while taking either drug alone. After taking lithium 1 g and diazepam 30 mg daily for 17 days, the patient's temperature fell from 35.4 to 32°C over 2 hours, and he became comatose with reduced reflexes, dilated pupils, a systolic blood pressure of 40 to 60 mmHg, a pulse rate of 40 and no piloerector response.[3] The reasons for this reaction are not known. This is an isolated case and therefore concurrent use need not be avoided, but be alert for any evidence of hypothermia. There seems to be no evidence of this adverse interaction with any of the other benzodiazepines.

1. Evans RL, Nelson MV, Melethil S, Townsend R, Hornstra RK, Smith RB. Evaluation of the interaction of lithium and alprazolam. *J Clin Psychopharmacol* (1990) 10, 355–9.
2. Koczerginski D, Kennedy SH, Swinson RP. Clonazepam and lithium—a toxic combination in the treatment of mania? *Int Clin Psychopharmacol* (1989) 4, 195–9.
3. Naylor GJ, McHarg A. Profound hypothermia on combined lithium carbonate and diazepam treatment. *BMJ* (1977) 3, 22.

Lithium + Caffeine

The heavy consumption of caffeine-containing drinks may cause a small to moderate reduction in serum-lithium levels.

Clinical evidence, mechanism, importance and management

A study in 11 psychiatric patients taking lithium 600 mg to 1.2 g daily who were also regular **coffee** drinkers (4 to 8 cups daily containing 70 to 120 mg of caffeine per cup) found that when the **coffee** was withdrawn, their serum-lithium levels rose by an average of 24%, although the levels of 3 patients did not change.[1] These findings are consistent with another report of 2 patients with lithium-induced tremors that were aggravated when they stopped drinking large amounts of **coffee**. One of the patients had a 50% rise in lithium levels, and required a reduction in lithium dose from 1.5 g daily to 1.2 g daily.[2] An early single-dose study found that the intake of xanthines such as caffeine caused an increase in lithium excretion.[3] However, another single-dose study did not find any significant changes in urinary clearance of lithium in 6 subjects given caffeine 200 mg four times daily compared with a caffeine-free control period.[4]

It is not clear exactly how caffeine affects the excretion of lithium by the renal tubules, but other xanthines have a similar effect (see 'Lithium + Theophylline', p.1129). The weight of evidence cited here suggests that although there is no need for those on lithium to avoid caffeine (**coffee**, **tea**, **cola drinks** etc.), in cases where a reduction in caffeine intake is desirable, it should be withdrawn cautiously. This is particularly important in those whose serum-lithium levels are already high, because of the risk of toxicity. When caffeine is withdrawn it may be necessary to reduce the dose of lithium. In addition, remember that there is a caffeine-withdrawal syndrome (headache and fatigue being the major symptoms) that might worsen some of the major psychiatric disorders (such as affective and schizophrenic disorders).[1]

1. Mester R, Toren P, Mizrachi I, Wolmer L, Karni N, Weizman A. Caffeine withdrawal increases lithium blood levels. *Biol Psychiatry* (1995) 37, 348–50.
2. Jefferson JW. Lithium tremor and caffeine intake: two cases of drinking less and shaking more. *J Clin Psychiatry* (1988) 49, 72–3.
3. Thomsen K, Schou M. Renal lithium excretion in man. *Am J Physiol* (1968) 215, 823–7.
4. Bikin D, Conrad KA, Mayersohn M. Lack of influence of caffeine and aspirin on lithium elimination. *Clin Res* (1982) 30, 249A.

Lithium + Calcitonin (Salcatonin)

A study in 4 depressed women found that calcitonin (salcatonin) caused a small reduction in serum-lithium levels, the clinical importance of which is not known.

Clinical evidence

Prompted by the occasional observation of decreased serum-lithium levels in outpatients receiving calcitonin, a study was undertaken in 4 bipolar depressive women. The patients, who had been stable on lithium for 10 years, were additionally given salmon calcitonin (salcatonin) 100 units subcutaneously for 3 consecutive days for postmenopausal osteoporosis. It was found that their serum-lithium levels fell, on average, from 0.73 to 0.59 mmol/L. The clearance of lithium in the urine was tested in 2 of the patients, and both showed increases (9.8 and 16.2%).[1]

Mechanism

Not known. Increased renal excretion and possibly some reduced intestinal absorption of the lithium have been suggested by the authors of the report.[1]

Importance and management

Information seems to be limited to this study, which only lasted for 3 days. The study found only a small fall in serum-lithium levels, and did not assess the effect on the control of depression. It seems unlikely that this interaction will be clinically important in most patients, but as some patients may be affected, monitor the outcome of concurrent use, and consider monitoring lithium levels.

1. Passiu G, Bocchetta A, Martinelli V, Garau P, Del Zompo M, Mathieu A. Calcitonin decreases lithium plasma levels in man. Preliminary report. *Int J Clin Pharmacol Res* (1998) 18, 179–81.

Lithium + Calcium-channel blockers

The concurrent use of lithium and verapamil can be uneventful, but neurotoxicity (ataxia, movement disorders, tremors) with unchanged lithium levels has been reported in a few patients. Reduced and increased lithium levels have also occurred with verapamil. An acute parkinsonian syndrome and marked psychosis has been seen in at least one patient taking lithium and diltiazem. Reduced lithium clearance, and one possible case of increased lithium levels have been reported with nifedipine.

Clinical evidence

(a) Diltiazem

A woman stable on lithium for several years developed marked psychosis and parkinsonism within a week of starting to take diltiazem 30 mg three times daily.[1] An acute parkinsonism syndrome developed in a 58-year-old man within 4 days of adding 30 mg of diltiazem three times daily to his treatment with lithium and tiotixene.[2] However, this report has been questioned as the symptoms may have been attributable to an adverse effect of the tiotixene, and, even if the lithium toxicity was genuine, it is thought to have been more likely due to recent increases in the lithium dose, or the patient's diuretic therapy than diltiazem.[3]

(b) Nifedipine

In a study of patients with essential hypertension, two doses of nifedipine 20 mg did not affect single-dose lithium clearance, but nifedipine 40 to 80 mg daily for 6 and 12 weeks was found to decrease single-dose lithium clearance by 30%.[4] A man, on lithium carbonate 1.5 g daily with a level of 0.8 mmol/L, developed ataxia and dysarthria 7 days after starting nifedipine 30 mg daily for 48 hours, then 60 mg daily. His lithium dose was reduced by 40%, but his serum-lithium level first increased to 1.1 mmol/L (about 2 weeks after starting the nifedipine), before restabilising at 0.9 mmol/L.[5] In contrast, a patient taking lithium, who developed dysarthria and ataxia after verapamil was added to her treatment (see *(c)* below), was subsequently well controlled on lithium and nifedipine 40 mg daily.[6]

(c) Verapamil

A 42-year-old woman taking lithium carbonate 900 mg daily developed toxicity (nausea, vomiting, muscular weakness, ataxia and tinnitus) within 9 days of starting to take verapamil 80 mg three times daily. Her bipolar depressive disorder improved even though her serum-lithium levels remained unchanged at 1.1 mmol/L. The toxicity disappeared within 48 hours of stopping the verapamil, but her disorder worsened. The same pattern was repeated when verapamil was re-started and then withdrawn.[7] Another 3 cases of movement disorders (including ataxia, tremors and choreoathetosis) resulting from the concurrent use of lithium and verapamil have also been reported,[6,8,9] two of which had documented unchanged serum-lithium levels.[6,8] In one case the patient was restabilised by halving the dose of lithium.[8]

Conversely, a patient stable on lithium 900 mg to 1.2 g daily for over 8 years had a marked fall in his serum-lithium levels from about 1.04 to 0.5 mmol/L when he was given verapamil 80 mg four times daily. He was restabilised on approximately double the dose of lithium.[10] Another patient had an increased lithium clearance when given verapamil for 3 days, and a fall in serum-lithium levels from 0.61 to 0.53 mmol/L.[10]

In addition to unchanged or decreased lithium levels with verapamil, one manufacturer notes that increased lithium levels have occurred.[11]

Mechanism

Not understood. However, it has been suggested that calcium-channel blockers and lithium affect neurotransmitter production[1,2,9] (several pathways have been described), which results in CNS sensitivity. This produces movement disorders, which are said to mimic lithium toxicity. In most of the cases mentioned above, symptoms of toxicity were present at therapeutic lithium levels, which would support this suggested mechanism.

Importance and management

The neurotoxic adverse reactions cited above for lithium and verapamil contrast with two other case reports describing uneventful concurrent use.[12,13] Variable reports of altered serum-lithium levels have also occurred. This unpredictability emphasises the need to monitor the effects closely where it is thought appropriate to give lithium and verapamil. Only a couple of isolated reports of neurotoxicity have been reported with lithium and diltiazem, and their general relevance is uncertain, but bear them in mind in the event of an unexpected response to treatment. Some limited data suggest that nifedipine may slightly reduce lithium clearance, and the clinical relevance of this is again uncertain.

1. Binder EF, Cayabyab L, Ritchie DJ, Birge SJ. Diltiazem-induced psychosis and a possible diltiazem-lithium interaction. *Arch Intern Med* (1991) 151, 373–4.
2. Valdiserri EV. A possible interaction between lithium and diltiazem: case report. *J Clin Psychiatry* (1985) 46, 540–1.
3. Flicker MR, Quigley MA, Caldwell EG. Diltiazem-lithium interaction: an opposing viewpoint. *J Clin Psychiatry* (1988) 49, 325–6.
4. Bruun NE, Ibsen H, Skøtt P, Toftdahl D, Giese J, Holstein-Rathlou NH. Lithium clearance and renal tubular sodium handling during acute and long-term nifedipine treatment in essential hypertension. *Clin Sci* (1988) 75, 609–13.
5. Pinkofsky HB, Sabu R, Reeves RR. A nifedipine-induced inhibition of lithium clearance. *Psychosomatics* (1997) 38, 400–1.
6. Wright BA, Jarrett DB. Lithium and calcium channel blockers: possible neurotoxicity. *Biol Psychiatry* (1991) 30, 635–6.
7. Price WA, Giannini AJ. Neurotoxicity caused by lithium-verapamil synergism. *J Clin Pharmacol* (1986) 26, 717–19.
8. Price WA, Shalley JE. Lithium-verapamil toxicity in the elderly. *J Am Geriatr Soc* (1987) 35, 177–8.
9. Helmuth D, Ljaljevic Z, Ramirez L, Meltzer HY. Choreoathetosis induced by verapamil and lithium treatment. *J Clin Psychopharmacol* (1989) 9, 454–5.
10. Weinrauch LA, Belok S, D'Elia JA. Decreased serum lithium during verapamil therapy. *Am Heart J* (1984) 108, 1378–80.
11. Covera-HS (Verapamil). Pfizer Inc. US Prescribing Information, May 2004.
12. Brotman AW, Farhadi AM, Gelenberg AJ. Verapamil treatment of acute mania. *J Clin Psychiatry* (1986) 47, 136–8.
13. Gitlin MJ, Weiss J. Verapamil as maintenance treatment in bipolar illness: a case report. *J Clin Psychopharmacol* (1984) 4, 341–3.

Lithium + Cisplatin

Isolated case reports describe either a fall or no alteration in serum-lithium levels in patients given cisplatin. However, note that cisplatin-induced renal impairment may cause an increase in lithium levels.

Clinical evidence, mechanism, importance and management

The serum-lithium levels of a woman taking lithium carbonate 300 mg four times daily fell, over a period of 2 days, from 1 to 0.3 mmol/L, and from 0.8 to 0.5 mmol/L, on two occasions when given cisplatin (100 mg/m^2 intravenously over 2 hours). To prevent cisplatin-induced renal toxicity, she was also given a fluid load over a total of 24 hours, which included one litre of sodium chloride 0.9% over 4 hours, one litre of mannitol 20% over 4 hours, and one litre of dextrose 5% in sodium chloride 0.9%. Serum-lithium levels returned to normal at the end of 2 days. No change in the control of the psychotic symptoms was seen.[1]

A man had a transient 64% decrease in serum-lithium levels, without perceptible clinical consequences, during the first of four courses of cisplatin, bleomycin, and etoposide. The effect became less pronounced during the subsequent courses.[2] It is not clear whether the fall in serum-lithium levels in these cases was due to increased renal clearance caused by the cisplatin or the sodium load, dilution from the fluid load, or a combination of all three factors.

In contrast, one patient had no clinically significant changes in her serum-lithium levels when treated with cisplatin, but 2 months later her deteriorating renal function resulted in a rise in her serum-lithium levels.[3]

None of these interactions was of great clinical importance, but the authors of the first report pointed out that some regimens of cisplatin involve the use of higher doses (40 mg/m^2 daily) with a sodium chloride 0.9% fluid load over 5 days, and under these circumstances it would be prudent to monitor the serum-lithium levels carefully. Concurrent use should be monitored in all patients.

1. Pietruszka LJ, Biermann WA, Vlasses PH. Evaluation of cisplatin-lithium interaction. *Drug Intell Clin Pharm* (1985) 19, 31–2.
2. Beijnen JH, Bais EM, ten Bokkel Huinink WW. Lithium pharmacokinetics during cisplatin-based chemotherapy: a case report. *Cancer Chemother Pharmacol* (1994) 33, 523–6.
3. Beijnen JH, Vlasveld LT, Wanders J, ten Bokkel Huinink WW, Rodenhuis S. Effect of cisplatin-containing chemotherapy on lithium serum concentrations. *Ann Pharmacother* (1992) 26, 488–90.

Lithium + Corticosteroids

Corticosteroids may disturb electrolyte balance, which in theory could affect serum-lithium levels, but there do not appear to be any reports of significant interactions.

Clinical evidence, mechanism, importance and management

A patient with systemic lupus erythematosus suffering from steroid-induced depression and moderate renal impairment was given lithium 600 mg daily and her depression improved. However, serum-lithium levels increased from 0.4 to 0.8 mmol/L within one week and the lithium treatment caused an exacerbation of a finger tremor. The lithium was discontinued and then restarted at 400 mg daily, resulting in serum levels of 0.4 mmol/L, which improved her depression and was associated with only a fine finger tremor. Three other patients with steroid-induced depression were also successfully treated with lithium.[1]

One UK manufacturer warns that drugs affecting electrolyte balance, such as corticosteroids, may alter lithium excretion and should therefore be avoided,[2] but other manufacturers do not appear to mention this potential interaction. An early study in *rats* reported increased lithium clearance with methylprednisolone.[3] The available evidence is insufficient to recommend routine monitoring. However, it may be prudent to consider monitoring lithium effects in patients with renal impairment, or other conditions pre-disposing to lithium toxicity, taking levels if early symptoms suggest a potential problem.

1. Terao T. Lithium therapy for corticosteroid-induced mood disorder. *J Clin Psychiatry* (2001) 62, 57.
2. Priadel (Lithium carbonate). Sanofi-Aventis. UK Summary of product characteristics, August 2006.
3. Imbs JL, Singer L, Danion JM, Schmidt M, Zawilslak R. Effects of indomethacin and methylprednisolone on renal elimination of lithium in the rat. *Int Pharmacopsychiatry* (1980) 15, 143–9.

Lithium + Diuretics; Loop

The concurrent use of lithium carbonate and furosemide can be safe and uneventful, but serious lithium toxicity has been described. Bumetanide interacts similarly. The risk of lithium toxicity with a loop diuretic is greatly increased during the first month of concurrent use.

Clinical evidence

An analysis of 10,615 elderly patients receiving lithium found that 413 (3.9%) were admitted to hospital at least once for lithium toxicity during a 10-year study period. The prescriptions for any loop diuretic (not specifically named) were compared between these 413 hospitalised patients and 1651 control patients. For any use of a loop diuretic (54 cases and 71 controls) there was an increased relative risk of hospitalisation for lithium toxicity of 1.7. When patients who were newly started on a loop diuretic were analysed (12 cases and 6 controls), a dramatically increased risk of lithium toxicity within a month of initiating treatment was found (relative risk 5.5).[1] Reports relating to specific named loop diuretics are discussed below.

(a) Bumetanide

Bumetanide has been responsible for the development of lithium toxicity in 2 patients[2,3] one of whom was on a salt-restricted diet.[3]

(b) Furosemide

Six healthy subjects stabilised on lithium carbonate 300 mg three times daily (mean serum levels 0.43 mmol/L) were given furosemide 40 mg daily for 14 days. Five experienced some minor adverse effects, probably attributable to the furosemide, without significant changes in serum-lithium levels, but one subject experienced such a marked increase in the toxic effects of lithium that she withdrew from the study after taking both drugs for only 5 days. Her serum-lithium levels were found to have risen from 0.44 to 0.71 mmol/L.[4]

There are another 4 case reports of individual patients who experienced serious lithium toxicity or other adverse reactions when given lithium and furosemide.[5-8] One of the patients was also on a salt-restricted diet,[5] which has also been implicated in episodes of lithium toxicity, see 'Lithium + Sodium compounds', p.1128. In contrast, 6 patients who had been stabilised on lithium for over 6 years had no significant changes in their serum-lithium levels over a 12-week period while taking furosemide 20 to 80 mg daily.[9] Other studies in healthy subjects also found no significant changes in lithium levels when furosemide 40 or 80 mg daily was given.[10,11]

Mechanism

Not fully understood. If and when a rise in serum-lithium levels occurs, it may be related to the salt depletion that can accompany the use of furosemide (for a more detailed explanation see 'Lithium + Sodium compounds', p.1128). As with the 'thiazide diuretics', (p.1123) such an interaction would take a few days to develop. This may explain why one study in subjects given a single dose of lithium failed to demonstrate that furosemide had any effect on the urinary excretion of lithium.[12]

Importance and management

Information seems to be limited to the reports cited. The incidence of this interaction is uncertain and its development unpredictable. It would be imprudent to give furosemide or bumetanide to patients stabilised on lithium unless the effects can be well monitored because some patients may develop serious toxicity. Patients on lithium should be aware of the symptoms of lithium toxicity (see 'Lithium', (p.1111)) and told to report them immediately should they occur. Consider increased monitoring of lithium levels in patients newly started on this combination.

1. Juurlink DN, Mamdani MM, Kopp A, Rochon PA, Shulman KI, Redelmeier DA. Drug-induced lithium toxicity in the elderly: a population-based study. *J Am Geriatr Soc* (2004) 52, 794–8.
2. Kerry RJ, Ludlow JM, Owen G. Diuretics are dangerous with lithium. *BMJ* (1980) 281, 371.
3. Huang LG. Lithium intoxication with coadministration of a loop-diuretic. *J Clin Psychopharmacol* (1990) 10, 228.
4. Jefferson JW, Kalin NH. Serum lithium levels and long-term diuretic use. *JAMA* (1979) 241, 1134–6.
5. Hurtig HI, Dyson WL. Lithium toxicity enhanced by diuresis. *N Engl J Med* (1974) 290, 748–9.
6. Oh TE. Frusemide and lithium toxicity. *Anaesth Intensive Care* (1977) 5, 60–2.
7. Grau Segura E, Pinet Ogue MC, Franco Peral M. Intoxicación por sales de litio. Presentación de un caso. *Med Clin (Barc)* (1984) 83, 294–6.
8. Thornton WE, Pray BJ. Lithium intoxication: a report of two cases. *Can Psychiatr Assoc J* (1975) 20, 281–2.
9. Saffer D, Coppen A. Frusemide: a safe diuretic during lithium therapy? *J Affect Disord* (1983) 5, 289–92.
10. Crabtree BL, Mack JE, Johnson CD, Amyx BC. Comparison of the effects of hydrochlorothiazide and furosemide on lithium disposition. *Am J Psychiatry* (1991) 148, 1060–3.
11. Shalmi M, Rasmusen H, Amtorp O, Christensen S. Effect of chronic oral furosemide administration on the 24-hour cycle of lithium clearance and electrolyte excretion in humans. *Eur J Clin Pharmacol* (1990) 38, 275–80.
12. Thomsen K, Schou M. Renal lithium excretion in man. *Am J Physiol* (1968) 215, 823–7.

Lithium + Diuretics; Potassium-sparing

There is evidence that the excretion of lithium can be increased by triamterene. In contrast, serum-lithium levels may rise if spironolactone is used. Amiloride appears not to interact. See also 'Lithium + Diuretics; Loop', above, and 'Lithium + Diuretics; Thiazide and related', p. 1123.

Clinical evidence and mechanism

(a) Amiloride

Amiloride has been found to have no significant effect on serum-lithium levels when used in the treatment of lithium-induced polyuria.[1,2] One review briefly mentions a case report in which amiloride was successfully used as a replacement for bendroflumethiazide, which had caused lithium toxicity.[3] However, some manufacturers[4,5] suggest that, as a diuretic, amiloride reduces the renal clearance of lithium, thereby increasing the risk of lithium toxicity. There appears to be no evidence to confirm this alleged interaction.

(b) Spironolactone

One study found that spironolactone had no statistically significant effect on the excretion of lithium.[6] Whereas, in another report, the use of spironolactone 100 mg daily was accompanied by a rise in serum-lithium levels from 0.63 to 0.9 mmol/L. The levels continued to rise for several days after the spironolactone was stopped.[7]

(c) Triamterene

Triamterene, given to a patient taking lithium while on a salt-restricted diet, is said to have led to a strong lithium diuresis.[8] Similarly, triamterene increased lithium excretion in 8 healthy subjects.[9]

Importance and management

These diuretics have been available for a very considerable time and it might have been expected that by now any serious adverse interactions with lithium would have emerged, but information is very sparse. None of the reports available gives a clear indication of the outcome of concurrent use, but some monitoring would be a prudent precaution. Patients on lithium should be aware of the symptoms of lithium toxicity (see 'Lithium', (p.1111)) and told to report them immediately should they occur.

1. Batlle DC, von Riotte AB, Gaviria M, Grupp M. Amelioration of polyuria by amiloride in patients receiving long-term lithium therapy. *N Engl J Med* (1985) 312, 408–14.
2. Kosten TR, Forrest JN. Treatment of severe lithium-induced polyuria with amiloride. *Am J Psychiatry* (1986) 143, 1563–8.
3. Aronson JK, Reynolds DJM. ABC of monitoring drug therapy. Lithium. *BMJ* (1992) 305, 1273–6.
4. Midamor (Amiloride hydrochloride). Merck & Co., Inc. US Prescribing information, November 2002.
5. Amilamont (Amiloride). Rosemont Pharmaceuticals Ltd. UK Summary of product characteristics, December 2000.
6. Thomsen K, Schou M. Renal lithium excretion in man. *Am J Physiol* (1968) 215, 823–7.
7. Baer L, Platman SR, Kassir S, Fieve RR. Mechanisms of renal lithium handling and their relationship to mineralocorticoids: a dissociation between sodium and lithium ions. *J Psychiatr Res* (1971) 8, 91–105.
8. Williams, Katz, Shield eds. Recent Advances in the Psychobiology of the Depressive Illnesses. Washington DC: DHEW Publications, 1972 p 49–58.
9. Wetzels JFM, van Bergeijk JD, Hoitsma AJ, Huysmans FTM, Koene RAP. Triamterene increases lithium excretion in healthy subjects: evidence for lithium transport in the cortical collecting tubule. *Nephrol Dial Transplant* (1989) 4, 939–42.

Lithium + Diuretics; Thiazide and related

Thiazide and related diuretics can cause a rapid rise in serum-lithium levels, leading to toxicity unless the lithium dosage is reduced appropriately. This interaction has been seen with bendroflumethiazide, chlorothiazide, chlortalidone, hydrochlorothiazide and indapamide, and potentially occurs with hydroflumethiazide. Other thiazides and related diuretics are expected to behave similarly.

Clinical evidence

A retrospective analysis of 10 615 elderly patients receiving lithium found that 413 (3.9%) were admitted to hospital at least once for lithium toxicity during a 10-year study period. The prescriptions for a thiazide-type diuretic were compared between these 413 hospitalised patients and 1651 control patients. For any use of a thiazide diuretic (16 cases and 37 controls) there was a non-significant increased relative risk of 1.3 for hospitalisation due to lithium toxicity. When treatment for patients who were newly started on a thiazide diuretic was analysed (5 cases and 6 controls), the increased relative risk of toxicity was also non-significant (1.3). The authors considered that these findings suggest that the use of thiazide diuretics and lithium may not be as hazardous as previously thought. However, the authors also suggest that another explanation is that clinicians were aware of the potential interaction and so adjusted doses or observed patients more closely in the outpatient setting, thereby avoiding any hospitalisations for toxicity.[1]

Case reports and studies for named thiazide diuretics are outlined below.

(a) Bendroflumethiazide

A study in 22 patients, who had been treated with either bendroflumethiazide 2.5 mg or hydroflumethiazide 25 mg daily for at least 2 months, found that these diuretics caused a 24% reduction in the urinary clearance of a single 600-mg dose of lithium carbonate.[2] There is also a case report of a roughly twofold increase in serum-lithium levels,[3] and a case of lithium toxicity with a roughly threefold increase in serum-lithium levels mentioned in a review article,[4] both following the addition of bendroflumethiazide to treatment with lithium. In a further case, lithium toxicity, with serum-lithium levels of 4.28 mmol/L was detected 3 months after the addition of bendroflumethiazide.[5] However, this case was complicated by the presence of perindopril, which might also raise lithium levels, as has occurred with other 'ACE inhibitors', (p.1112).

In contrast to these reports, one single-dose study found that bendroflumethiazide 7.5 mg given 10 hours after lithium carbonate 600 mg had no effect on lithium clearance.[6] However, it seems unlikely that single-dose studies will detect an interaction (see Mechanism below).

(b) Chlorothiazide

A single 300-mg dose of lithium carbonate was given to 4 healthy subjects alone and following 7 days of treatment with chlorothiazide 500 mg daily. Lithium-plasma levels were increased and lithium clearance was decreased by about 26% following chlorothiazide treatment.[7]

Lithium toxicity developed in a patient taking lithium after she was given chlorothiazide, spironolactone and amiloride.[8] The lithium levels rose from 0.6 to 2.2 mmol/L.

A 54-year-old patient developed nephrogenic diabetes insipidus when she was treated with lithium carbonate. The addition of chlorothiazide reduced her polyuria, but resulted in an elevation in her lithium level from 1.3 to more than 2 mmol/L, with accompanying signs of toxicity. The patient was later successfully treated with chlorothiazide and a reduced dose of lithium.[9]

(c) Chlortalidone

A 58-year-old woman developed lithium toxicity within 10 days of starting chlortalidone [dose unknown].[10] Her lithium levels rose from 0.8 to 3.7 mmol/L.

(d) Hydrochlorothiazide

In a placebo-controlled study, the serum-lithium levels of 13 healthy subjects taking lithium 300 mg twice daily rose by 23% (from 0.3 to 0.37 mmol/L), when they were given hydrochlorothiazide 25 mg twice daily for 5 days.[11] Similar results were found in another small study.[12]

In addition to these studies at least 6 cases of lithium toxicity have been seen when hydrochlorothiazide was given to patients taking lithium.[13-17] Hydrochlorothiazide was either given with amiloride,[13-15] spironolactone[16] or triamterene.[17] See also 'Lithium + Diuretics; Potassium-sparing', p.1122.

(e) Hydroflumethiazide

A study in 22 patients who had been treated with either bendroflumethiazide 2.5 mg or hydroflumethiazide 25 mg daily for at least 2 months found that these diuretics caused a 24% reduction in the urinary clearance of a single 600-mg dose of lithium carbonate.[2]

(f) Indapamide

A 64-year-old man developed lithium toxicity one week after starting to take indapamide 5 mg daily.[18] His serum-lithium level was 3.93 mmol/L.

Mechanism

Not fully understood. The interaction occurs even though the thiazides and related diuretics exert their major actions in the distal part of the kidney tubule whereas lithium is mainly reabsorbed in the proximal part. However, thiazide diuresis is accompanied by sodium loss which, within a few days, is compensated by retention of sodium, this time in the proximal part of the tubule. Since both sodium and lithium ions are treated similarly, the increased reabsorption of sodium would include lithium as well, hence a significant and measurable reduction in its excretion.[5,19]

Importance and management

Established, well-documented and potentially serious interactions. The rise in serum-lithium levels and the accompanying toxicity develops most commonly within about a week to 10 days,[4,7,9-11,13,17] although it has apparently been seen after 19 days[16] and even 3 months.[5] Not every patient necessarily develops a clinically important interaction, but it is not possible to predict which patients will be affected. The lack of serious cases of toxicity in the case-control study either suggests the interaction is rare, or that appropriate precautions are used when the combination is prescribed.[1]

Although only the diuretics named above have been implicated in this interaction, it seems likely that all thiazides and related diuretics will interact similarly. None of the thiazide or related diuretics should be given to patients on lithium unless the serum-lithium levels can be closely monitored and appropriate downward dosage adjustments made. The US manufacturers also say that caution should be used and serum-lithium levels monitored closely with adjustment of the lithium dosage.[20] One UK manufacturer says that if a thiazide diuretic has to be prescribed for a patient treated with lithium, then the lithium dosage should first be reduced, and the patient then stabilised by frequent monitoring of lithium levels. Similar precautions should be exercised on diuretic withdrawal.[21] However, this does not seem to be in line with most other recommendations. Patients on lithium should be aware of the symptoms of lithium toxicity (see 'Lithium', (p.1111)) and told to report them immediately should they occur.

Concurrent use under controlled conditions has been advocated for certain psychiatric conditions and for the control of lithium-induced nephrogenic diabetes insipidus. A successful case is described above.[9] It has been suggested that a 40 to 70% reduction in the lithium dose would be needed with doses of 0.5 to 1 g of chlorothiazide,[22,23] but it would seem sensible to base any dose adjustments on individual lithium levels.

1. Juurlink DN, Mamdani MM, Kopp A, Rochon PA, Shulman KI, Redelmeier DA. Drug-induced lithium toxicity in the elderly: a population-based study. *J Am Geriatr Soc* (2004) 52, 794–8.
2. Petersen V, Hvidt S, Thomsen K, Schou M. Effect of prolonged thiazide treatment on renal lithium clearance. *BMJ* (1974) 3, 143–5.
3. Kerry RJ, Ludlow JM, Owen G. Diuretics are dangerous with lithium. *BMJ* (1980) 281, 371.
4. Aronson JK, Reynolds DJM. ABC of monitoring drug therapy. Lithium. *BMJ* (1992) 305, 1273–6.
5. Vipond AJ, Bakewell S, Telford R, Nicholls AJ. Lithium toxicity. *Anaesthesia* (1996) 51, 1156–8.
6. Thomsen K, Schou M. Renal lithium excretion in man. *Am J Physiol* (1968) 215, 823–7.
7. Poust RI, Mallinger AG, Mallinger J, Himmelhoch JM, Neil JF, Hanin I. Effect of chlorothiazide on the pharmacokinetics of lithium in plasma and erythrocytes. *Psychopharmacol Comm* (1976) 2, 273–84.
8. Basdevant A, Beaufils M, Corvol P. Influence des diurétiques sur l'élimination rénale du lithium. *Nouv Presse Med* (1976) 5, 2085–6.
9. Levy ST, Forrest JN, Heninger GR. Lithium-induced diabetes insipidus: manic symptoms, brain and electrolyte correlates, and chlorothiazide treatment. *Am J Psychiatry* (1973) 130, 1014–18.
10. Solomon JG. Lithium toxicity precipitated by a diuretic. *Psychosomatics* (1980) 21, 425, 429.
11. Crabtree BL, Mack JE, Johnson CD, Amyx BC. Comparison of the effects of hydrochlorothiazide and furosemide on lithium disposition. *Am J Psychiatry* (1991) 148, 1060–3.
12. Jefferson JW, Kalin NH. Serum lithium levels and long-term diuretic use. *JAMA* (1979) 241, 1134–6.
13. Macfie AC. Lithium poisoning precipitated by diuretics. *BMJ* (1975) 1, 516.
14. König P, Küfferle B, Lenz G. Ein fall von Lithiumtoxikation bei therapeutischen Lithiumdosen infolge zusätzlicher Gabe eines Diuretikums. *Wien Klin Wochenschr* (1978) 90, 380–2.
15. Dorevitch A, Baruch E. Lithium toxicity induced by combined amiloride HCl-hydrochlorothiazide administration. *Am J Psychiatry* (1986) 143, 257–8.
16. Lutz EG. Lithium toxicity precipitated by diuretics. *J Med Soc New Jers* (1975) 72, 439–40.
17. Mehta BR, Robinson BHB. Lithium toxicity induced by triamterene-hydrochlorothiazide. *Postgrad Med J* (1980) 56, 783–4.
18. Hanna ME, Lobao CB, Stewart JT. Severe lithium toxicity associated with indapamide therapy. *J Clin Psychopharmacol* (1990) 10, 379–80.
19. Schwarcz G. The problem of antihypertensive treatment in lithium patients. *Compr Psychiatry* (1982) 23, 50–54.
20. Eskalith (Lithium carbonate). GlaxoSmithKline. US Prescribing information, September 2003.
21. Priadel (Lithium carbonate). Sanofi-Aventis. UK Summary of product characteristics, August 2006.
22. Himmelhoch JM, Poust RI, Mallinger AG, Hanin I, Neil JF. Adjustment of lithium dose during lithium-chlorothiazide therapy. *Clin Pharmacol Ther* (1977) 22, 225–7.
23. Himmelhoch JM, Forrest J, Neil JF, Detre TP. Thiazide-lithium synergy in refractory mood swings. *Am J Psychiatry* (1977) 134, 149–52.

Lithium + Herbal medicines

A woman developed lithium toxicity after taking a herbal diuretic remedy. A brief report describes mania in a patient taking lithium who also took St John's wort.

Clinical evidence, mechanism, importance and management

(a) Herbal diuretics

A 26-year-old woman who had been taking lithium 900 mg twice daily for 5 months, with hydroxyzine, lorazepam, propranolol, risperidone and sertraline, came to an emergency clinic complaining of nausea, diarrhoea, unsteady gait, tremor, nystagmus and drowsiness, (all symptoms of lithium toxicity). Her lithium level, which had previously been stable at 1.1 mmol/L was found to be 4.5 mmol/L. For the past 2 to 3 weeks she had been taking a non-prescription **herbal diuretic** containing **corn silk**, ***Equisetum hyemale***, **juniper**, **ovate buchu**, **parsley** and **uva ursi**, all of which are believed to have diuretic actions. The other ingredients were bromelain, paprika, potassium and vitamin B_6.[1]

The most likely explanation for what happened is that the **herbal diuretic** caused the lithium toxicity. It is impossible to know which herb or combination of herbs actually caused the toxicity, or how, but this case once again emphasises that herbal remedies are not risk-free just because they are natural. It also underscores the need for patients to avoid self-medication without first seeking informed advice and supervision if they are taking potentially hazardous drugs like lithium.

(b) St John's wort (Hypericum perforatum)

A search of Health Canada's database of spontaneous adverse reactions identified one case in which St John's wort was suspected of inducing mania in a patient also taking lithium.[2] No further details were given of this case.

1. Pyevich D, Bogenschutz MP. Herbal diuretics and lithium toxicity. *Am J Psychiatry* (2001) 158, 1329.
2. Natural health products and adverse reactions. *Can Adverse React News* (2004) 14 , 2–3. Available at: http://www.hc-sc.gc.ca/dhp-mps/alt_formats/hpfb-dgpsa/pdf/medeff/carn-bcei_v14n1_e.pdf (accessed 23/08/07).

Lithium + Iodides

The hypothyroid and goitrogenic effects of lithium carbonate and iodides may be additive if given concurrently. Other factors such as geographical location, age and gender may also be important.

Clinical evidence

A man with normal thyroid function showed evidence of hypothyroidism after 3 weeks of treatment with lithium carbonate 750 mg to 1.5 g daily. After 2 further weeks, during which he was also treated with **potassium iodide**, the hypothyroidism became even more marked, but resolved completely within 2 weeks of the withdrawal of both drugs. This patient was studied before the potential risk of hypothyroidism with iodine was well-recognised.[1]

In another study of the possible effects of iodide intake on thyroid function in 10 patients on lithium therapy, 3 to 5 weeks of **potassium iodide** caused hypothyroidism in 2 patients and hyperthyroidism in one. Little effect on thyroid function was seen in 5 control patients given **potassium iodide** without lithium.[2] A case of hypothyroidism involving lithium and a product containing **isopropamide iodide** plus haloperidol (*Vesalium*) has also been reported.[3,4]

Mechanism

Lithium accumulates in the thyroid gland and blocks the release of the thyroid hormones by thyroid-stimulating hormone, and can therefore cause clinical hypothyroidism.[1,5-12] The prevalence of hypothyroidism may be higher in women, in middle-age,[12] and in countries with a higher level of nutritional iodine.[13] Potassium iodide temporarily prevents the production of thyroid hormones but, as time goes on, synthesis recommences. Thus, both lithium and iodide ions can depress the production or release of the hormones and therefore have additive hypothyroid effects.

Importance and management

The pharmacological interaction of altered thyroid function with lithium and iodides would appear to be established. However, the clinical use of iodides is now very limited (mostly to the pre-operative treatment of thyrotoxicosis). It is therefore unlikely that iodides will be used in patients on lithium. Where countries are adopting iodization programmes to prevent iodine deficiency, there may be an increased risk of clinical hypothyroidism in patients taking lithium.[13] Lithium-induced hypothyroidism can be treated with thyroxine replacement.

1. Shopsin B, Shenkman L, Blum M, Hollander CS. Iodine and lithium-induced hypothyroidism. Documentation of synergism. *Am J Med* (1973) 55, 695–9.
2. Spaulding SW, Burrow GN, Ramey JN, Donabedian RK. Effect of increased iodide intake on thyroid function in subjects on chronic lithium therapy. *Acta Endocrinol (Copenh)* (1977) 84, 290–6.
3. Luby ED, Schwartz D, Rosenbaum H. Lithium-carbonate-induced myxedema. *JAMA* (1971) 218, 1298–9.
4. Wiener JD. Lithium carbonate-induced myxedema. *JAMA* (1972) 220, 587.
5. Schou M, Amdisen A, Jensen SE, Olsen T. Occurrence of goitre during lithium treatment. *BMJ* (1968) 3, 710–13.
6. Shopsin B, Blum M, Gershon S. Lithium-induced thyroid disturbance: case report and review. *Compr Psychiatry* (1969) 10, 215–23.
7. Emerson CH, Dyson WL, Utiger RD. Serum thyrotropin and thyroxine concentrations in patients receiving lithium carbonate. *J Clin Endocrinol Metab* (1973) 36, 338–46.
8. Candy J. Severe hypothyroidism — an early complication of lithium therapy. *BMJ* (1972) 3, 277.
9. Villeneuve A, Gautier J, Jus A, Perron D. Effect of lithium on thyroid in man. *Lancet* (1973) ii, 502.
10. Lloyd GG, Rosser RM, Crowe MJ. Effect of lithium on thyroid in man. *Lancet* (1973) ii, 619.
11. Bocchetta A, Bernardi F, Pedditzi M, Loviselli A, Velluzzi F, Martino E, Del Zompo M. Thyroid abnormalities during lithium treatment. *Acta Psychiatr Scand* (1991) 83, 193–8.
12. Johnston AM, Eagles JM. Lithium-associated clinical hypothyroidism: prevalence and risk factors. *Br J Psychiatry* (1999) 175, 336–9.
13. Leutgeb U. Ambient iodine and lithium-associated clinical hypothyroidism. *Br J Psychiatry* (2000) 176, 495–6.

Lithium + Ispaghula (Psyllium)

In an isolated case, the withdrawal of ispaghula husk resulted in an increase in lithium levels. Psyllium slightly reduced the absorption of lithium in a study in healthy subjects.

Clinical evidence

A 47-year-old woman recently started on lithium was found to have blood-lithium levels of 0.4 mmol/L five days after an increment in her lithium dose and whilst also taking one teaspoonful of ispaghula husk twice daily. The ispaghula husk was stopped 3 days later and lithium levels measured 4 days later were found to be 0.76 mmol/L.[1]

A study in 6 healthy subjects similarly showed that the absorption of lithium (as measured by the urinary excretion) was reduced by about 14% by psyllium.[2]

Mechanism

Not understood. One idea is that the absorption of the lithium from the gut is reduced.[1,2]

Importance and management

Information is very limited and the general importance of this interaction is uncertain, but it would now seem prudent to bear this interaction in mind in patients given ispaghula or psyllium preparations. If an interaction is suspected consider monitoring lithium levels and separating the administration of the two drugs by at least an hour, or use an alternative laxative.

1. Perlman BB. Interaction between lithium salts and ispaghula husk. *Lancet* (1990) 335, 416.
2. Toutoungi M, Schulz P, Widmer J, Tissot R. Probable interaction entre le psyllium et le lithium. *Therapie* (1990) 45, 358–60.

Lithium + Mazindol

An isolated report describes a case of lithium toxicity, which was attributed to the concurrent use of mazindol.

Clinical evidence, mechanism, importance and management

A bipolar depressive woman, stabilised on lithium carbonate, showed signs of lithium toxicity (sluggishness, ataxia) within 3 days of starting to take mazindol 2 mg daily. After 9 days she developed twitching, limb rigidity and muscle fasciculation, and was both dehydrated and stuporose. Her serum-lithium levels were found to have risen from a range of 0.4 to 1.3 mmol/L up to 3.2 mmol/L. The mazindol was stopped, and she recovered over the next 48 hours whilst being rehydrated.[1] It is not known whether this was a direct interaction between the two drugs, but the authors suggest that the anorectic effect of mazindol led to this toxicity [i.e. the reduced intake of sodium and water caused a reduction in the renal excretion of lithium]. There seem to be no other reports of interactions between lithium and other anorectic drugs confirming this possibility.

This is an isolated case and its general importance is uncertain, but bear it in mind in the case of an unexpected response to treatment. Note that stimulants such as mazindol are no longer generally recommended as appetite suppressants.[2]

1. Hendy MS, Dove AF, Arblaster PG. Mazindol-induced lithium toxicity. *BMJ* (1980) 280, 684–5.
2. Sweetman SC, ed. Martindale: The complete drug reference. 35th ed. London: Pharmaceutical Press; 2007. p. 1959.

Lithium + Methyldopa

Symptoms of lithium toxicity, not always associated with raised lithium levels, have been described in four patients and four healthy subjects when they were also given methyldopa.

Clinical evidence

A manic-depressive woman, taking lithium carbonate 900 mg daily was hospitalised for signs of manic decompensation and her lithium dose was increased to 1.8 g daily. When she was also given methyldopa 1 g daily for hypertension, she developed signs of lithium toxicity (blurred vision, hand tremors, mild diarrhoea, confusion, and slurred speech), even though her serum-lithium levels were within the range of 0.5 to 0.7 mmol/L. The methyldopa was then stopped and the lithium carbonate dose reduced to 1.5 g daily. Ten days later the lithium level was 1.4 mmol/L, and the lithium dose was decreased to 900 mg daily.[1] Later the author of this report demonstrated this interaction on himself.[2] He took lithium carbonate 150 mg four times daily for a week (lithium level 0.5 mmol/L), and then added methyldopa 250 mg every 8 hours. Within 2 days, signs of lithium toxicity had clearly developed, and the following day his lithium level had increased to 0.8 mmol/L. He then stopped the methyldopa, and about 36 hours later his lithium level was 0.7 mmol/L.

There are 3 other cases of patients who took methyldopa with lithium, and developed symptoms of lithium toxicity. In one of these cases the patient had lithium levels within the normal therapeutic range,[3] but in the other two the lithium levels increased to 1.5 and 1.87 mmol/l.[4,5] A small study in 3 healthy subjects also found that the combination of lithium and methyldopa resulted in increased confusion, sedation and dysphoria.[6]

Mechanism

Not understood. Both a central effect and an effect on renal excretion have been proposed.[3-5]

Importance and management

Information appears to be limited to the reports cited, but the interaction would seem to be established. Avoid concurrent use whenever possible, but if this is not workable then the effects should be closely monitored. Serum-lithium measurements may be unreliable because symptoms of toxicity can occur even though the levels remain within the normally accepted therapeutic range.

1. Byrd GJ. Methyldopa and lithium carbonate: suspected interaction. *JAMA* (1975) 233, 320.
2. Byrd GJ. Lithium carbonate and methyldopa: apparent interaction in man. *Clin Toxicol* (1977) 11, 1–4.
3. Osanloo E, Deglin JH. Interaction of lithium and methyldopa. *Ann Intern Med* (1980) 92, 433–4.
4. O'Regan JB. Adverse interaction of lithium carbonate and methyldopa. *Can Med Assoc J* (1976) 115, 385–6.
5. Yassa R. Lithium-methyldopa interaction. *Can Med Assoc J* (1986) 134, 141–2.
6. Walker N, White K, Tornatore F, Boyd JL, Cohen JL. Lithium-methyldopa interactions in normal subjects. *Drug Intell Clin Pharm* (1980) 14, 638–9.

Lithium + NSAIDs

NSAIDs may increase serum-lithium levels leading to toxicity, but there is great variability between different NSAIDs and also between individuals taking the same NSAID. For example, studies have found that celecoxib causes a modest 17% increase in lithium levels, yet case reports describe increases of up to 344%. Similar effects occur with other NSAIDs, and it seems likely that all NSAIDs will interact similarly. However, note that sulindac seems unique in that it is the only NSAID that has also been reported to cause a decrease in lithium levels.

Clinical evidence

A retrospective analysis of 10 615 elderly patients receiving lithium found that 413 (3.9%) were admitted to hospital at least once for lithium toxicity during a 10-year study period. The prescriptions for any NSAID were compared between these 413 hospitalised patients and 1651 control patients. For any use of an NSAID (63 cases and 187 controls) there was no increased relative risk of hospitalisation for lithium toxicity (relative risk 1.1). Similarly, when patients who were newly started on an NSAID were analysed (4 cases and 17 controls), there was still no increased risk (relative risk 0.6). The authors considered that these findings suggest that the use of NSAIDs and lithium may not be as hazardous as previously thought, although they do suggest that another explanation could be that clinicians were aware of the potential interaction, and so adjusted doses or observed patients more closely in the outpatient setting, thereby avoiding any hospitalisations for toxicity.[1]

Case reports and studies about individual, named NSAIDs are outlined in the following subsections, and 'Table 31.1', (p.1127) summarises the effects of NSAIDs on lithium concentrations.

(a) Celecoxib

A 58-year-old woman, with a stable serum-lithium level of between 0.5 and 0.9 mmol/L, developed renal impairment associated with severe lithium toxicity, within 5 days of starting to take celecoxib 400 mg twice daily. Her lithium level was 4 mmol/L. Of note, and a possible contributory factor, was the presence of ibuprofen, which she had taken with her lithium for several years without incident.[2]

In addition to 3 of the cases in 'Table 31.1', (p.1127), a review of the FDA's Adverse Event Reporting System database in January 2003 found 2 cases of increased lithium levels and symptoms of lithium toxicity in patients who also took celecoxib.[3]

(b) Ibuprofen

Three patients stabilised on lithium, with plasma levels of 0.7 to 0.9 mmol/L, were given ibuprofen 1.2 or 2.4 g daily for 7 days. The serum-lithium levels of one patient rose from 0.8 to 1 mmol/L and he experienced nausea and drowsiness. The 2 other patients, including the one on the 1.2-g ibuprofen dose, did not show this interaction.[4]

Three other case reports describe patients with symptoms of lithium toxicity that occurred within 1 to 7 days of them starting to take ibuprofen 1.2 g daily.[5-7] In another case, episodes of unsteadiness and tremor associated with raised lithium levels were attributed to varying use of prescribed ibuprofen 400 mg three times daily.[8]

(c) Indometacin

A case report describes lithium toxicity in a man given indometacin 50 mg every 6 hours. Three days after he started the indometacin his serum creatinine was raised, and 9 days later he had symptoms of lithium toxicity and was found to have a lithium levels of 3.5 mmol/L. It was suggested that the indometacin caused renal impairment, which led to lithium retention and toxicity.[9]

(d) Ketorolac

An 80-year-old man taking haloperidol, procyclidine, clonazepam, aspirin, digoxin and lithium (serum levels between 0.5 and 0.7 mmol/L) was additionally given indometacin 100 mg daily for arthritis, which was replaced, after 13 days, by ketorolac 30 mg daily. The next day his serum-lithium level was 0.9 mmol/L and 6 days later 1.1 mmol/L. Subsequently the patient developed severe nausea and vomiting, and both drugs were stopped.[10]

(e) Mefenamic acid

Acute lithium toxicity, accompanied by a sharp deterioration in renal function, was seen in a patient taking lithium carbonate with mefenamic acid 500 mg three times daily for 2 weeks. Withdrawal of the drugs and subsequent rechallenge confirmed this interaction.[11] Another case of toxicity was seen in a patient on lithium given mefenamic acid. Her renal function was impaired when the lithium was started, but it had been stable for about 6 months before the NSAID was added.[12] A brief report also mentions another case of this interaction.[13]

(f) Niflumic acid

An isolated report describes lithium toxicity in a woman who took niflumic acid (said to be three capsules daily) for 7 days with the addition of aspirin 1.5 g daily after 5 days. Her serum-lithium levels rose from 0.8 to 1.6 mmol/L.[14]

(g) Nimesulide

A 42-year old woman taking lithium was given nimesulide 100 mg and ciprofloxacin 250 mg, both twice daily, for flank pain and dysuria. After 72 hours, she developed symptoms of lithium toxicity and the dose of lithium was reduced. After 98 hours she had vomiting, ataxia, and oliguria, and lithium levels were found to be 3.23 mmol/L (previous level 1.08 mmol/L) and her serum creatinine was raised.[15]

(h) Oxyphenbutazone

In an apparently isolated case, a 49-year-old woman is reported to have developed nausea and vomiting associated with a rise in lithium levels following the addition of oxyphenbutazone suppositories 500 mg daily. She responded well to a reduction in the lithium dosage.[16]

(i) Parecoxib

The manufacturers of parecoxib say that valdecoxib, the main active metabolite of parecoxib, has been shown to cause decreases in the clearance of lithium (serum clearance reduced by 25%, renal clearance reduced by 30%), resulting in a 34% increase in its serum levels. Valdecoxib pharmacokinetics were unchanged by lithium.[17]

(j) Piroxicam

A 56-year-old woman, stabilised for over 9 years on lithium, with levels usually between 0.8 and 1 mmol/L, experienced lithium toxicity (unsteadiness, trembling, confusion) and was admitted to hospital on three occasions after taking piroxicam. Her serum levels on two occasions had risen to 2.7 and 1.6 mmol/L, although in the latter instance the lithium had been withdrawn the day before the levels were taken. In a subsequent study her serum-lithium levels rose from 1 to 1.5 mmol/L after she took piroxicam 20 mg daily.[18] Two other case reports describe lithium toxicity, which occurred 4 weeks and 4 months after piroxicam was started.[19,20]

(k) Rofecoxib

A 73-year-old man, with lithium levels of between 0.6 and 0.9 mmol/L for the past 13 years, developed symptoms of lithium toxicity (serum-lithium level 1.5 mmol/L) within 9 days of starting to take rofecoxib 12.5 mg daily. An interaction was strongly suspected. However, it should be noted that the patient had required his lithium dose to be successively decreased over the 13 years to maintain his lithium levels within the desired range. Captopril 6.25 mg daily had also been started during this time,[21] although it is unclear whether it had a part to play either in the lithium dose reduction or the development of an interaction.

In addition to 6 of the cases in 'Table 31.1', (p.1127), a review of the FDA's Adverse Event Reporting System database in January 2003 found 7 cases of increased serum-lithium concentrations after the addition of rofecoxib.[3]

(l) Sulindac

1. Lithium levels reduced. A patient stabilised on lithium had a marked fall in serum-lithium levels from 0.65 to 0.39 mmol/L after 2 weeks of concurrent treatment with sulindac 100 mg twice daily. Her serum-lithium levels gradually climbed over the next 6 weeks to 0.71 mmol/L and restabilised without any change in the dosage of either lithium or sulindac. She needed amitriptyline for depression while the lithium levels were low, but bouts of depression had not been uncommon, even when lithium levels were stable.[22] The serum-lithium levels of another patient were approximately halved a week after his dosage of sulindac was doubled to 200 mg twice daily. He remained on both drugs, but a higher dose of lithium was needed.[22]

2. Lithium levels unaffected. Two small studies (in a total of 10 patients)[23,24] and a case report[25] found that serum-lithium levels were unaffected by the use of sulindac.

3. Lithium levels increased. Two patients developed increased serum-lithium levels apparently due to the use of sulindac.[26] In one case the lithium levels rose from 1 to 2 mmol/L after 19 days of treatment with sulindac 150 mg twice daily, and symptoms of toxicity were seen. The levels fell to 0.8 mmol/L within 5 days of stopping the sulindac. The other patient had a rise from 0.9 to 1.7 mmol/L within a week of adding sulindac 150 mg twice daily. The sulindac was continued and the lithium dosage was reduced from 1.8 to 1.5 g daily. The serum-lithium levels fell and were 1.2 mmol/L at 37 days and 1 mmol/L at 70 days. No symptoms of lithium toxicity occurred.[26]

(m) Tiaprofenic acid

A 79-year-old woman on lithium (as well as fosinopril, nifedipine, oxazepam and haloperidol) had a rise in her trough serum-lithium levels

Table 31.1 Summary of the effects of NSAIDs on lithium levels

NSAID	*Dose*	*Subjects*	*Increase in lithium levels*	*Time to symptoms or increase in levels*	*Refs*
Celecoxib	200 to 800 mg daily	4 cases	56 to 248%	10 days to 10 weeks	1, 2
	200 mg twice daily	Study in healthy subjects	17%		3, 4
Diclofenac	75 mg daily	Case	86%	25 days	5
	50 mg three times daily	Study in 5 healthy subjects	26%	7 to 10 days	6
Flurbiprofen	100 mg twice daily	Placebo-controlled study in 11 otherwise healthy subjects with bipolar disorder	19%	7 days	7
Ibuprofen	1.6 to 1.8 g daily in divided doses	Studies in 11 healthy subjects and 9 subjects with bipolar disorder	12 to 67%	6 to 9 days	8, 9
Indometacin	150 mg daily	Studies in 9 healthy subjects and 6 subjects with bipolar disorder	30 to 61%	6 to 10 days	10-12
Ketoprofen	400 mg daily	Case	About 90%	3 weeks	13
Ketorolac	60 mg daily	Case	50%	3 weeks	14
	40 mg daily	Study in 5 healthy subjects	29%	5 days	15
Lornoxicam	4 mg twice daily	Study in 12 healthy subjects	20% (61% in one subject)	7 days	16
Meloxicam	15 mg daily	Study in 16 healthy subjects	21%	14 days	17
Naproxen	220 or 250 mg three times daily	Study in 9 healthy subjects and 7 bipolar or schizoaffective disorder	0 to 42%	5 to 6 days	18, 19
Phenylbutazone	750 mg daily (suppositories)	Case	106%	36 hours	20
	100 mg three times daily	Study in 5 subjects with bipolar disorder	0 to 15%	6 days	21
Piroxicam	20 mg daily	2 cases	130 to 235%	1 to 2 months	22, 23
Rofecoxib	Not stated or 25 mg once or twice daily	7 cases	58 to 448%	6 days to about 3 months	2, 24
	50 mg [daily]	Study in 10 healthy subjects	Unstated rise in 9 subjects, of these 3 were withdrawn early with levels of 1.26 mmol/L or more	Up to 5 days	25

1. Gunja N, Graudins A, Dowsett R. Lithium toxicity: a potential interaction with celecoxib. *Intern Med J* (2002) 32, 494-5.
2. Phelan KM, Mosholder AD, Lu S. Lithium interaction with the cyclooxygenase 2 inhibitors rofecoxib and celecoxib and other non-steroidal anti-inflammatory drugs. *J Clin Psychiatry* (2003) 64, 1328-34.
3. Celebrex (Celecoxib). Pharmacia Ltd. UK Summary of product characteristics, November 2005.
4. Celebrex (Celecoxib). Searle Ltd. US Prescribing Information, July 2005.
5. Monji A, Maekawa T, Miura T, Nishi D, Horikawa H, Nakagawa Y, Tashiro N. Interactions between lithium and non-steroidal antiinflammatory drugs. *Clin Neuropharmacol* (2002) 25, 241-2.
6. Reimann IW, Frölich JC. Effects of diclofenac on lithium kinetics. *Clin Pharmacol Ther* (1981) 30, 348-52.
7. Hughes BM, Small RE, Brink D, McKenzie ND. The effect of flurbiprofen on steady-state plasma lithium levels. *Pharmacotherapy* (1997) 17, 113-20.
8. Kristoff CA, Hayes PE, Barr WH, Small RE, Townsend RJ, Ettigi PG. Effect of ibuprofen on lithium plasma and red blood cell concentrations. *Clin Pharm* (1986) 5, 51-5.
9. Ragheb M. Ibuprofen can increase serum lithium level in lithium-treated patients. *J Clin Psychiatry* (1987) 48, 161-3.
10. Ragheb M, Ban TA, Buchanan D, Frolich JC. Interaction of indomethacin and ibuprofen with lithium in manic patients under a steady-state lithium level. *J Clin Psychiatry* (1980) 41, 397-8.
11. Frölich JC, Leftwich R, Ragheb M, Oates JA, Reimann I, Buchanan D. Indomethacin increases plasma lithium. *BMJ* (1979) 1, 1115-16.
12. Reimann IW, Diener U, Frölich JC. Indomethacin but not aspirin increases plasma lithium ion levels. *Arch Gen Psychiatry* (1983) 40, 283-6.
13. Singer L, Imbs JL, Danion JM, Singer P, Krieger-Finance F, Schmidt M, Schwartz J. Risque d'intoxication par le lithium en cas de traitement associé par les anti-inflammatories non stéroïdiens. *Therapie* (1981) 36, 323-6.
14. Iyer V, Ketorolac (Toradol®) induced lithium toxicity. *Headache* (1994) 34, 442-4.
15. Cold JA, ZumBrunnen TL, Simpson MA, Augustin BG, Awad E, Jann MW. Increased lithium serum and red blood cell concentrations during ketorolac coadministration. *J Clin Psychopharmacol* (1998) 18, 33-7.
16. Ravic M, Salas-Herrera I, Johnston A, Turner P, Foley K, Rosenow D. Influence of lornoxicam a new non-steroidal anti-inflammatory drug on lithium pharmacokinetics. *Hum Psychopharmacol* (1993) 8, 289-92.
17. Türck D, Heinzel G, Luik G. Steady-state pharmacokinetics of lithium in healthy volunteers receiving concomitant meloxicam. *Br J Clin Pharmacol* (2000) 50, 197-204.
18. Ragheb M, Powell AL. Lithium interaction with sulindac and naproxen. *J Clin Psychopharmacol* (1986) 6, 150-4.
19. Levin GM, Grum C, Eisele G. Effect of over-the-counter dosages of naproxen sodium and acetaminophen on plasma lithium concentrations in normal volunteers. *J Clin Psychopharmacol* (1998) 18, 237-40.
20. Singer L, Imbs JL, Schmidt M, Mack G, Sebban M, Danion JM. Baisse de la clearance rénale du lithium sous l'effet de la phénylbutazone. *Encephale* (1978) 4, 33-40.
21. Ragheb M. The interaction of lithium with phenylbutazone in bipolar affective patients. *J Clin Psychopharmacol* (1990) 10, 149-150.
22. Kelly CB, Cooper SJ. Toxic elevation of serum lithium concentration by non-steroidal anti-inflammatory drugs. *Ulster Med J* (1991) 60, 240-2.
23. Harrison TM, Wynne Davies D, Norris CM. Lithium carbonate and piroxicam. *Br J Psychiatry* (1986) 149, 124-5.
24. Rätz Bravo AE, Egger SS, Crespo S, Probst WL, Krähenbühl S. Lithium intoxication as a result of an interaction with rofecoxib. *Ann Pharmacother* (2004) 38, 1189-93.
25. Sajbel TA, Carter GW, Wiley RB. Pharmacokinetic effects of rofecoxib therapy on lithium. *Pharmacotherapy* (2001) 21, 380.

from 0.36 to 0.57 mmol/L within 3 days of starting to take tiaprofenic acid 200 mg three times daily. The serum-lithium levels had risen to 0.65 mmol/L by the next day and, despite halving the lithium dosage, were found to be 0.69 mmol/L five days later. These rises were attributed to an interaction with the tiaprofenic acid exacerbated by the fosinopril,[27] see 'Lithium + ACE inhibitors', p.1112.

Mechanism

Not understood. It has been suggested that the interacting NSAIDs inhibit the synthesis of the renal prostaglandins (PGE_2) so that the renal blood flow is reduced, thereby reducing the renal excretion of the lithium. In addition, reduced renal PGE_2 levels may be associated with increased reabsorption of sodium and lithium. However, this fails to explain why aspirin, which blocks renal prostaglandin synthesis by 65 to 70%, does not usually affect serum-lithium levels, see 'Lithium + Aspirin or other Salicylates', p.1119.

Importance and management

The interaction between NSAIDs and lithium is well established, although the incidence is unknown. The increase in serum-lithium levels appears to vary between the different NSAIDs and also between individuals taking the same NSAID (see 'Table 31.1', (p.1127)). Factors such as advanced age, impaired renal function, decreased sodium intake, volume depletion, renal artery stenosis, and heart failure increase the risk.

The documentation of these interactions is variable and limited, and although only some NSAIDs have been shown to interact, it seems likely that they will all interact to a greater or lesser extent. What is known indicates that most NSAIDs should be avoided, especially if other risk factors are present, unless serum-lithium levels can be very well monitored (initially every few days) and the dosage reduced appropriately. The effects of sulindac appear to be unpredictable (serum levels raised, lowered or unchanged) so that good monitoring is still necessary.

Patients on lithium should be aware of the symptoms of lithium toxicity and told to report them immediately should they occur. This should be reinforced when they are given an NSAID.

1. Juurlink DN, Mamdani MM, Kopp A, Rochon PA, Shulman KI, Redelmeier DA. Drug-induced lithium toxicity in the elderly: a population-based study. *J Am Geriatr Soc* (2004) 52, 794–8.
2. Slørdal L, Samstad S, Bathen J, Spigset O. A life-threatening interaction between lithium and celecoxib. *Br J Clin Pharmacol* (2003) 55, 413–14.
3. Phelan KM, Mosholder AD, Lu S. Lithium interaction with the cyclooxygenase 2 inhibitors rofecoxib and celecoxib and other nonsteroidal anti-inflammatory drugs. *J Clin Psychiatry* (2003) 64, 1328–34.
4. Ragheb M, Ban TA, Buchanan D, Frolich JC. Interaction of indomethacin and ibuprofen with lithium in manic patients under a steady-state lithium level. *J Clin Psychiatry* (1980) 41, 397–8.
5. Bailey CE, Stewart JT, McElroy RA. Ibuprofen-induced lithium toxicity. *South Med J* (1989) 82, 1197.
6. Ayd FJ. Ibuprofen-induced lithium intoxication. *Int Drug Ther Newslett* (1985) 20, 16.
7. Khan IH. Lithium and non-steroidal anti-inflammatory drugs. *BMJ* (1991) 302, 1537–8.
8. Kelly CB, Cooper SJ. Toxic elevation of serum lithium concentration by non-steroidal anti-inflammatory drugs. *Ulster Med J* (1991) 60, 240–2.
9. Herschberg SN, Sierles FS. Indomethacin-induced lithium toxicity. *Am Fam Physician* (1983) 28, 155–7.
10. Langlois R, Paquette D. Increased serum lithium levels due to ketorolac therapy. *Can Med Assoc J* (1994) 150, 1455–6.
11. MacDonald J, Neale TJ. Toxic interaction of lithium carbonate and mefenamic acid. *BMJ* (1988) 297, 1339.
12. Shelley RK. Lithium toxicity and mefenamic acid: a possible interaction and the role of prostaglandin inhibition. *Br J Psychiatry* (1987) 151, 847–8.
13. Honey J. Lithium-mefenamic acid interaction: Quoted by Ayd FJ. *Int Drug Ther Newslett* (1982) 17, 16.
14. Gay C, Plas J, Granger B, Olie JP, Loo H. Intoxication au lithium. Deux interactions inédites: l'acétazolamide et l'acide niflumique. *Encephale* (1985) 11, 261–2.
15. Bocchia M, Bertola G, Morganti D, Toscano M, Colombo E. Intossicazione da litio e uso di nimesulide. *Recenti Prog Med* (2001) 92, 462.
16. Singer L, Imbs JL, Danion JM, Singer P, Krieger-Finance F, Schmidt M, Schwartz J. Risque d'intoxication par le lithium en cas de traitement associé par les anti-inflammatoires non stéroïdiens. *Therapie* (1981) 36, 323–6.
17. Dynastat Injection (Parecoxib sodium). Pfizer Ltd. UK Summary of product characteristics, April 2007.
18. Kerry RJ, Owen G, Michaelson S. Possible toxic interaction between lithium and piroxicam. *Lancet* (1983) i, 418–19.
19. Nadarajah J, Stein GS. Piroxicam induced lithium toxicity. *Ann Rheum Dis* (1985) 44, 502.
20. Walbridge DG, Bazire SR. An interaction between lithium carbonate and piroxicam presenting as lithium toxicity. *Br J Psychiatry* (1985) 147, 206–7.
21. Lundmark J, Gunnarsson T, Bengtsson F. A possible interaction between lithium and rofecoxib. *Br J Clin Pharmacol* (2002) 53, 403–4.
22. Furnell MM, Davies J. The effect of sulindac on lithium therapy. *Drug Intell Clin Pharm* (1985) 19, 374–6.
23. Ragheb M, Powell AL. Lithium interaction with sulindac and naproxen. *J Clin Psychopharmacol* (1986) 6, 150–4.
24. Ragheb MA, Powell AL. Failure of sulindac to increase serum lithium levels. *J Clin Psychiatry* (1986) 47, 33–4.
25. Miller LG, Bowman RC, Bakht F. Sparing effect of sulindac on lithium levels. *J Fam Pract* (1989) 28, 592–3.
26. Jones MT, Stoner SC. Increased lithium concentrations reported in patients treated with sulindac. *J Clin Psychiatry* (2000) 61, 527–8.
27. Alderman CP, Lindsay KSW. Increased serum lithium concentration secondary to treatment with tiaprofenic acid and fosinopril. *Ann Pharmacother* (1996) 30, 1411–13.

Lithium + Paracetamol (Acetaminophen)

Paracetamol appears not to alter lithium levels.

Clinical evidence, mechanism, importance and management

A study in 9 healthy subjects given lithium carbonate 300 mg every 12 hours to achieve steady state, followed by the addition of 650 mg of paracetamol every 6 hours for 5 days, found no evidence that paracetamol increased serum-lithium levels. Six subjects had no change in lithium levels, one subject had a 0.1 mmol/L decrease, and two had a 0.1 mmol/L increase.[1] One patient whose serum lithium level doubled while taking rofecoxib was later given paracetamol without any problems.[2] No precautions seem necessary on concurrent use.

1. Levin GM, Grum C, Eisele G. Effect of over-the-counter dosages of naproxen sodium and acetaminophen on plasma lithium concentrations in normal volunteers. *J Clin Psychopharmacol* (1998) 18, 237–40.
2. Rätz Bravo AE, Egger SS, Crespo S, Probst WL, Krähenbühl S. Lithium intoxication as a result of an interaction with rofecoxib. *Ann Pharmacother* (2004) 38, 1189–93.

Lithium + Propranolol

One study suggests that propranolol may decrease the clearance of lithium, but the significance of this is unclear. An isolated report describes a patient taking lithium who developed marked bradycardia after he took propranolol 30 mg daily.

Clinical evidence, mechanism, importance and management

A study in lithium-treated manic-depressive patients found that the clearance of lithium was about 20% lower in 23 patients also taking propranolol than in 292 similar patients on lithium alone.[1] However, the clinical effects of this difference were not evaluated, so the significance of this finding is unclear. A 70-year-old man who had been stable on lithium for 16 years was additionally started on propranolol 30 mg daily for lithium-induced tremor. Six weeks later he was hospitalised because of vomiting, dizziness, headache and a fainting episode. His pulse rate was 35 to 40 bpm and his serum-lithium level was 0.3 mmol/L. When later discharged on lithium without propranolol his pulse rate had risen to a range of 64 to 80 bpm.[2]

The authors attribute the bradycardia to an interaction with lithium as the low dose of propranolol was considered unlikely to cause bradycardia alone. They also point out that both drugs affect the movement of calcium across cell membranes, which could account for the decreased contraction rate of the heart muscle, and thus bradycardia in this patient. They suggest careful monitoring in elderly patients with atherosclerotic cardiovascular problems.[2]

The general importance of this interaction, if it is such, is uncertain, but it seems possible with all beta blockers because they can all cause bradycardia. However, as beta blockers are used to treat lithium-induced tremor, any serious problem would be expected to have come to light by now.

1. Schou M, Vestergaard P. Use of propranolol during lithium treatment: an enquiry and a suggestion. *Pharmacopsychiatry* (1987) 20, 131.
2. Becker D. Lithium and propranolol: possible synergism? *J Clin Psychiatry* (1989) 50, 473.

Lithium + Sodium compounds

The ingestion of marked amounts of sodium can prevent the establishment or maintenance of adequate serum-lithium levels. Conversely, dietary salt restriction can cause serum-lithium levels to rise to toxic concentrations if the lithium dosage is not reduced appropriately.

Clinical evidence

(a) Lithium response reduced by the ingestion of sodium

A 35-year-old man, started on lithium carbonate 250 mg four times a day, had a serum-lithium level of 0.5 mmol/L by the following morning. When the dosage frequency was progressively increased to five, and later six times a day, his serum-lithium levels did not exceed 0.6 mmol/L because, unknown to his doctor, he was also taking **sodium bicarbonate**.

The patient's wife said he had been taking **"Soda Bic"** for years but since he started on lithium he had been "shovelling it in." When the **sodium bicarbonate** was stopped, relatively stable serum-lithium levels of 0.8 mmol/L were achieved on the initial dosage of lithium carbonate.[1]

An investigation to find out why a number of inpatients failed either to reach or maintain adequate therapeutic serum-lithium levels over a period of 2 months, revealed that a clinic nurse had been giving the patients *Efferdex*, a product containing about 50% **sodium bicarbonate**, because the patients complained of nausea. The reduction in the expected serum-lithium levels was as much as 40% in some cases.[2]

Other studies confirm that the serum-lithium levels can fall, and the effectiveness of treatment can lessen, if the intake of sodium is increased.[3-5]

(b) Lithium response increased by sodium restriction

The serum-lithium levels of 4 patients rose more rapidly and achieved a higher peak when salt was restricted to less than 10 mmol of sodium per day compared with the situation when the patients took a **dietary salt supplement**.[6]

Mechanism

The situation is complex and not fully established, but the mechanism can be broadly described in simplistic terms.

Sodium balance is controlled by the kidney; if the serum sodium is low the kidney can reabsorb more sodium to maintain the balance. The kidney excretes and reabsorbs both lithium and sodium, but it does not appear to clearly distinguish between lithium and sodium ions. Therefore, if a patient taking lithium restricts sodium intake, the kidney may reabsorb both sodium and lithium, causing a rise in serum-lithium levels. A corresponding decrease in lithium levels can occur when sodium intake is supplemented.[7,8]

Importance and management

Well established and clinically important interactions. The establishment and maintenance of therapeutic serum-lithium levels can be jeopardised if the intake of sodium is altered. Warn patients not to take non-prescription antacids or urinary alkalinisers without first seeking informed advice. Sodium bicarbonate comes in various guises and disguises e.g. *Alka-Seltzer* (55.8%), *Andrews Salts* (22.6%), *Eno* (46.4%), *Jaap's Health Salts* (21.3%), *Peptac* (28.8%). Substantial amounts of sodium also occur in some **urinary alkalinising agents** (e.g. *Citralka*, *Citravescent*).[9] There are many similar preparations available throughout the world. An antacid containing **aluminium/magnesium hydroxide** with simeticone has been found to have no effect on the bioavailability of lithium carbonate,[10] so that antacids of this type would appear to be safer alternatives.

Patients already stabilised on lithium should not begin to limit their intake of salt unless their serum-lithium levels can be monitored and suitable dosage adjustments made, because their lithium levels can rise quite rapidly.

1. Arthur RK. Lithium levels and "Soda Bic". *Med J Aust* (1975) 2, 918.
2. McSwiggan C. Interaction of lithium and bicarbonate. *Med J Aust* (1978) 1, 38–9.
3. Bleiweiss H. Salt supplements with lithium. *Lancet* (1970) i, 416.
4. Demers RG, Heninger GR. Sodium intake and lithium treatment in mania. *Am J Psychiatry* (1971) 128, 100–104.
5. Baer L, Platman SR, Kassir S, Fieve RR. Mechanisms of renal lithium handling and their relationship to mineralocorticoids: a dissociation between sodium and lithium ions. *J Psychiatr Res* (1971) 8, 91–105.
6. Platman SR, Fieve RR. Lithium retention and excretion: The effect of sodium and fluid intake. *Arch Gen Psychiatry* (1969) 20, 285–9.
7. Thomsen K, Schou M. Renal lithium excretion in man. *Am J Physiol* (1968) 215, 823–7.
8. Singer I, Rotenberg D. Mechanisms of lithium action. *N Engl J Med* (1973) 289, 254–60.
9. Beard TC, Wilkinson SJ, Vial JH. Hazards of urinary alkalizing agents. *Med J Aust* (1988) 149, 723.
10. Goode DL, Newton DW, Ueda CT, Wilson JE, Wulf BG, Kafonek D. Effect of antacid on the bioavailability of lithium carbonate. *Clin Pharm* (1984) 3, 284–7.

Lithium + Theophylline

Serum-lithium levels are moderately reduced by 20 to 30% by the concurrent use of theophylline, which may cause patients to relapse.

Clinical evidence

The serum-lithium levels of 10 healthy subjects taking lithium carbonate 900 mg daily fell by 20 to 30%, and the urinary clearance increased by 30%, when they were given theophylline *(Theo-dur)*. Steady-state theophylline levels of 5.4 to 12.7 micrograms/mL were achieved, and it was noted that higher theophylline levels were strongly correlated with increased lithium clearance.[1] This study has been reported in brief elsewhere.[2]

A man taking theophylline was diagnosed with a bipolar disorder and started on lithium while in hospital for an exacerbation of COPD. When the dose of theophylline was raised, because of a worsening in his condition, his lithium dose also had to be increased to control the emergence of manic symptoms. He received a maximum theophylline dose of 1.5 g daily, during which time he needed 2.7 g of lithium daily. When the theophylline was stopped, he only needed around 1.5 g of lithium daily to control his manic symptoms.[3] Two studies support the evidence from these cases with the finding that lithium excretion is increased by about 50% by **aminophylline** or theophylline.[4,5]

Mechanism

Uncertain. Theophylline has an effect on the renal clearance of lithium.

Importance and management

Information is very limited but the interaction appears to be established. Depressive and manic relapses may occur if the dosage of lithium is not raised appropriately when theophylline is given. Serum-lithium levels should be monitored if theophylline or aminophylline is stopped, started, or if the dosage is altered.

Other xanthines e.g. caffeine appear to have a similar effect, see 'Lithium + Caffeine', p.1120.

1. Perry PJ, Calloway RA, Cook BL, Smith RE. Theophylline precipitated alterations of lithium clearance. *Acta Psychiatr Scand* (1984) 69, 528–37.
2. Cook BL, Smith RE, Perry PJ, Calloway RA. Theophylline-lithium interaction. *J Clin Psychiatry* (1985) 46, 278–9.
3. Sierles FS, Ossowski MG. Concurrent use of theophylline and lithium in a patient with chronic obstructive lung disease and bipolar disorder. *Am J Psychiatry* (1982) 139, 117–18.
4. Thomsen K, Schou M. Renal lithium excretion in man. *Am J Physiol* (1968) 215, 823–7.
5. Holstad SG, Perry PJ, Kathol RG, Carson RW, Krummel SJ. The effects of intravenous theophylline infusion versus intravenous sodium bicarbonate infusion on lithium clearance in normal subjects. *Psychiatry Res* (1988) 25, 203–11.

Lithium + Triptans

In two cases patients on lithium developed symptoms suggestive of the serotonin syndrome after taking sumatriptan.

Clinical evidence, mechanism, importance and management

A comprehensive literature search published in 1998 identified several cases of adverse events reported with **sumatriptan** and lithium, although in most cases other medications were also being taken. Two patients taking **sumatriptan** and lithium concurrently were identified with symptoms suggestive of the serotonin syndrome, but these were mild to moderate and self-limiting. The number of patients taking lithium and **sumatriptan** was not stated, so the incidence is unknown.[1] The conclusion was reached that **sumatriptan** can be used cautiously in patients receiving lithium.[1] The manufacturers of **sumatriptan** and other triptans (e.g. **almotriptan**)[2] do not appear to have studied the effects of these drugs on lithium and there seem to be no other reports of problems with lithium and triptans. More study is needed.

1. Gardner DM, Lynd LD. Sumatriptan contraindications and the serotonin syndrome. *Ann Pharmacother* (1998) 32, 33–8.
2. Lundbeck Ltd. Personal communication, March 2001.

32

MAOIs

The intended target of the MAOIs (monoamine oxidase inhibitors) is MAO within the brain, but MAO is also found in other parts of the body. Particularly high concentrations occur in the gut and liver, where it acts as a protective detoxifying enzyme against tyramine and possibly other potentially hazardous amines, which exist in foods that have undergone bacterial degradation. There are at least two forms of MAO: MAO-A metabolises (deaminates) noradrenaline (norepinephrine) and serotonin (5-HT), while MAO-B metabolises phenylethylamine. Substances like tyramine and dopamine are metabolised by both forms of MAO.

The older MAOIs (see 'Table 32.1', (below)) are non-selective or non-specific, and inhibit both isoenzymes A and B. They are irreversible and long-acting, because the return of MAO activity depends upon the regeneration of new enzymes. As a result their effects (both beneficial and adverse) can last for 2 to 3 weeks after they have been withdrawn. Tranylcypromine differs in being a more reversible inhibitor of MAO, so the onset and disappearance of its actions are quicker than the other non-selective MAOIs. However, its effects still last for a number of weeks after withdrawal (e.g. see 'MAOIs or RIMAs + Tyramine-rich foods', p.1153), so it is still effectively an irreversible inhibitor, and is usually classified as such. These non-selective MAOIs cause serious and potentially life-threatening hypertensive interactions with the sympathomimetics found in some proprietary 'cough and cold remedies', (p.1147), and with 'tyramine-rich foods', (p.1153), and 'drinks', (p.1151).

Some of the newer and more recently developed drugs with MAO inhibitory activity (see 'Table 32.1', (below)) interact to a lesser extent than the older MAOIs. This is because they are largely selective. One group of these selective inhibitors targets MAO-A, and are relatively rapidly reversible; inhibition of this enzyme is responsible for the antidepressant effect. These selective MAO-A inhibitors (moclobemide, toloxatone) have been given the acronym RIMAs (Reversible Inhibitors of Monoamine oxidase A). They leave MAO-B largely uninhibited so that there is still a metabolic pathway available for the breakdown of amines, such as tyramine, that can cause a rise in blood pressure. In practical terms this means that the amount of tyramine needed to cause a hypertensive crisis is about tenfold greater than with the non-selective MAOIs (see 'tyramine-rich foods', (p.1153)).

The other newer selective MAOIs that specifically inhibit MAO-B are ineffective for the treatment of depression and are mainly used for Parkinson's disease, and so are covered elsewhere, see 'Antiparkinsonian and related drugs', (p.672). In low doses they inhibit MAO-B, leaving MAO-A largely uninhibited. However, selegiline loses some of its selectivity at doses of more than 10 mg daily and will therefore be subject to the same interactions as the non-selective MAOIs. Rasagiline is another irreversible selective inhibitor of MAO-B used for Parkinson's disease.

Some other drugs covered elsewhere also have MAOI activity. Furazolidone is an antiprotozoal with MAOI activity. Linezolid is an oxazolidinone antibacterial with reversible nonselective MAOI activity. Interactions typical of MAOI inhibitors might therefore occur with furazolidone and linezolid.

If you look at the product information issued by manufacturers, you will frequently see warnings about real and alleged interactions with MAOIs. Blackwell,[1] who has done much work on the interactions of the MAOIs, has rightly pointed out that the MAOIs are among the drugs that accumulate much myth and misinformation. He notes that the MAOIs have developed such a sinister reputation that manufacturers often issue a reflexive admonition to avoid co-administration with new drugs.

This means that many of the warnings about potential interactions with the MAOIs may lack a sound scientific basis. However, equally this does not mean that the proven serious life-threatening interactions that are associated with the MAOIs should be dismissed, and it should be noted that any drug with indirectly-acting sympathomimetic activity is likely to interact.

1. Blackwell B. Monoamine oxidase inhibitor interactions with other drugs. *J Clin Psychopharmacol* (1991) 11, 55–59.

Table 32.1 Monoamine oxidase inhibitors (MAOIs)

Irreversible non-selective MAO-inhibitors (MAO-A and MAO-B)	*Reversible Inhibitors of MAO-A (RIMAs)*	*Irreversible inhibitors of MAO-B**
Iproniazid	Brofaromine	Rasagiline
Isocarboxazid	Moclobemide	Selegiline
Mebanazine	Toloxatone	
Nialamide		
Phenelzine		
Tranylcypromine		
Tranylcypromine with trifluoperazine		

*MAO-B inhibitors are used in Parkinson's disease, so are covered elsewhere

MAOIs + Antihistamines

The alleged interaction between the MAOIs and antihistamines appears to be based on a single *animal* study, and is probably more theoretical than real. The exception seems to be cyproheptadine, which can reduce the effect of MAOIs because of its serotonin antagonist effect, see 'MAOIs or RIMAs + Antihistamines; Cyproheptadine', below.

Clinical evidence, mechanism, importance and management

A number of lists, charts and books about adverse interactions suggest that potentially serious interactions can occur between the MAOIs and the antihistamines. This appears to be based on a study in *rabbits* from 1972, which showed that some antihistamines (notably alkylamine antihistamines such as **chlorphenamine**, **brompheniramine**, and also **diphenhydramine**) produced a fatal hyperpyrexia, thought to be due to serotonin potentiation, when given intravenously to **phenelzine** pretreated *rabbits*.[1] This reaction was considered to be similar to that seen with 'pethidine', (p.1140), or the 'tricyclics', (p.1149). However, in over 20 years since the publication of this data, the manufacturers of various antihistamines did not identify any clinical reports of adverse interactions attributed to the use of any antihistamine with an MAOI.[2-6] Nevertheless, the UK manufacturers of most of the sedating antihistamines (**alimemazine**, **brompheniramine**, **chlorphenamine**, **diphenhydramine**, **promethazine**) state that MAOIs may intensify the antimuscarinic effect of antihistamines, and many contraindicate or caution concurrent use[7-11] (see also 'MAOIs + Antimuscarinics', p.1132). No such warning is given for non-sedating antihistamines. There would appear to be no good reason to avoid the concurrent use of sedating or non-sedating antihistamines and MAOIs. Note that cyproheptadine is an exception, because of its specific serotonin antagonist properties, see 'MAOIs or RIMAs + Antihistamines; Cyproheptadine', below.

1. Sinclair JG. Antihistamine-monoamine oxidase inhibitor interaction in rabbits. *J Pharm Pharmacol* (1972) 24, 955–61.
2. Intercare Products (Sandoz). Personal communication, May 1995.
3. Rhône-Poulenc Rorer, Personal communication, December 1997.
4. Glaxo Wellcome. Personal communication, December 1995.
5. Stafford Miller. Personal communication, November 1995.
6. Hoechst Roussel. Personal communication, November 1995.
7. Nytol (Diphenydramine hydrochloride). GlaxoSmithKline Consumer Healthcare. UK Summary of product characteristics, February 2002.
8. Piriton (Chlorphenamine maleate). GlaxoSmithKline Consumer Healthcare. UK Summary of product characteristics, October 2004.
9. Dimotane Plus Paediatric (Brompheniramine maleate). Wyeth Pharmaceuticals. UK Summary of product characteristics, June 2003.
10. Phenergan (Promethazine). Sanofi-Aventis. UK Summary of product characteristics, July 2006.
11. Vallergan Tablets (Alimemazine). Sanofi-Aventis. UK Summary of product characteristics, January 2007.

MAOIs or RIMAs + Antihistamines; Cyproheptadine

Isolated reports describe delayed hallucinations in a patient on phenelzine and cyproheptadine, and the rapid re-emergence of depression in two other patients on brofaromine or phenelzine when given cyproheptadine.

Clinical evidence

A woman who had responded well to **brofaromine** rapidly became depressed again when she took cyproheptadine. She had to be hospitalised due to suicidal ideation, but eventually she responded to treatment and she then took **brofaromine** and cyproheptadine for 6 months.[1] A man whose depression responded well to **phenelzine** 75 mg daily was given cyproheptadine 4 mg to treat associated sexual dysfunction and anorgasmia. Within 3 days of adding the cyproheptadine his depression returned, but the anorgasmia did not improve. When the cyproheptadine was stopped his depression was relieved.[2] Hallucinations developed in a woman taking **phenelzine** 2 months after cyproheptadine was started.[3]

Mechanism

Cyproheptadine is a serotonin antagonist. The reversal of the effects of the brofaromine was therefore attributed by the authors of one report[1] to the blockage of 5-HT (serotonin) receptors by cyproheptadine (brofaromine has both MAO-A inhibitory and 5-HT uptake inhibitory properties).

Cyproheptadine has also been observed to block the activity of serotonin reuptake inhibitors (see 'SSRIs + Cyproheptadine', p.1216).

Importance and management

Information seems to be limited to these reports but it would now be prudent to be alert for a reduction in efficacy or an adverse response if cyproheptadine is given with any MAOI or RIMA. The manufacturer of cyproheptadine actually contraindicates concurrent used with MAOIs.[4] However, there appears to be no reason why cyproheptadine cannot be used to treat the serotonin syndrome occurring in a patient on an MAOI.

As with other sedative antihistamines (see 'MAOIs + Antihistamines', above), the UK manufacturers of cyproheptadine also say that MAOIs prolong and intensify the antimuscarinic effects of antihistamines,[4] but there seems to be no clinical data to support this.

1. Katz RJ, Rosenthal M. Adverse interaction of cyproheptadine with serotonergic antidepressants. *J Clin Psychiatry* (1994) 55, 314–15.
2. Zubieta JK, Demitrack MA. Depression after cyproheptadine: MAO treatment. *Biol Psychiatry* (1992) 31, 1177–8.
3. Kahn DA. Possible toxic interaction between cyproheptadine and phenelzine. *Am J Psychiatry* (1987) 144, 1242–3.
4. Periactin (Cyproheptadine hydrochloride). Merck Sharp & Dohme Ltd. UK Summary of product characteristics, January 2004.

MAOIs or RIMAs + Antihypertensives

Bradycardia has been reported in two patients taking nadolol or metoprolol with phenelzine. MAOIs commonly cause hypotension, and might reasonably be expected to have additive hypotensive effects with antihypertensive drugs, although this was not seen with phenelzine and atenolol in a study in normotensive patients. In one small study, the RIMA, moclobemide increased the hypotensive effect of metoprolol, but did not alter the effect of nifedipine or hydrochlorothiazide on blood pressure.

Clinical evidence, mechanism, importance and management

(a) MAOIs

It had been claimed[1] that MAOIs should be discontinued at least 2 weeks before starting **propranolol**, but studies in *animals*[2] using **mebanazine** as a representative MAOI failed to show any undesirable property of **propranolol** following the use of an MAOI. Bradycardia of 46 to 53 bpm has been described in two patients taking **nadolol** 40 mg or **metoprolol** 150 mg daily for hypertension within 8 to 11 days of starting **phenelzine** 60 mg daily. No noticeable adverse effects were seen, but the authors recommend careful monitoring, particularly in the elderly, who may tolerate bradycardia poorly.[3] MAOIs can cause symptomatic hypotension, and therefore additive blood pressure lowering effects with antihypertensive drugs might occur. However, in one small study in normotensive patients with migraine, 11 (33%) of patients had orthostatic hypotension when they were given **phenelzine** alone, but none of these had orthostatic hypotension when they were also given **atenolol**.[4] Nevertheless, it would be prudent to monitor blood pressure more closely in patients taking antihypertensives with MAOIs.

(b) RIMAs

A study in 5 hypertensive subjects taking **metoprolol** found that **moclobemide** 200 mg three times daily for 2 weeks increased the hypotensive effect of **metoprolol** (systolic 10 to 15 mmHg lower, diastolic 5 to 10 mmHg lower). However, no comparable effects were seen when **moclobemide** was given to 7 subjects taking **hydrochlorothiazide** or 6 subjects taking **nifedipine**. No orthostatic hypotension occurred with any of the drug combinations.[5] The reason for the differing effect with **metoprolol** is unknown, and further study is needed. Be aware that **moclobemide** may add to the effect of **metoprolol**, and consider increased monitoring if either drug is started or stopped.

1. Frieden J. Propranolol as an antiarrhythmic agent. *Am Heart J* (1967) 74, 283–5.
2. Barrett AM, Cullum VA. Lack of inter-action between propranolol and mebanazine. *J Pharm Pharmacol* (1968) 20, 911–15.
3. Reggev A, Vollhardt BR. Bradycardia induced by an interaction between phenelzine and beta blockers. *Psychosomatics* (1989) 30, 106–8.

4. Merikangas KR, Merikangas JR. Combination monoamine oxidase inhibitor and β-blocker treatment of migraine, with anxiety and depression. *Biol Psychiatry* (1995) 38, 603–10.
5. Amrein R, Güntert TW, Dingemanse J, Lorscheid T, Stabl M, Schmid-Burgk W. Interactions of moclobemide with concomitantly administered medication: evidence from pharmacological and clinical studies. *Psychopharmacology (Berl)* (1992) 106, S24–S31.

MAOIs + Antimuscarinics

No adverse interactions between the MAOIs and antimuscarinics have been reported, although the possibility has been suggested.

Clinical evidence, mechanism, importance and management

A hyperthermic reaction has been reported in some *animals* given **tranylcypromine** or **nialamide** with **procyclidine** or **benzatropine**. It was considered that this might be due to an exaggerated dopamine response.[1] However, there do not appear to be any reports of such an interaction occurring clinically. Nevertheless, some manufacturers of irreversible non-selective MAOIs[2,3] and antimuscarinics[4] issue cautions about the possibility of increased effects of antimuscarinics when given with MAOIs. This is presumably because, in theory, inhibition of drug-metabolising enzymes by MAOIs may possibly enhance the effects of antimuscarinics.

1. Pedersen V, Nielsen IM. Hyperthermia in rabbits caused by interaction between M.A.O.I.s, antiparkinson drugs, and neuroleptics. *Lancet* (1975) i, 409–10.
2. Isocarboxazid. Cambridge Laboratories. UK Summary of product characteristics, March 2000.
3. Nardil (Phenelzine sulfate). Link Pharmaceuticals Ltd. UK Summary of product characteristics, July 2003.
4. Kemadrin (Procyclidine). GlaxoSmithKline UK. UK Summary of product characteristics, September 2006.

MAOIs + Barbiturates

Although the MAOIs can enhance and prolong the activity of barbiturates in *animals*, only a few isolated cases of adverse responses attributed to an interaction have been described.

Clinical evidence

One reviewer[1] briefly mentions that on three or four occasions patients taking an MAOI continued, without the prescriber's knowledge, to take their usual barbiturate hypnotic and thereby "... unknowingly raised their dose of barbiturate by five to ten times, and as a consequence barely managed to stagger through the day." No details are given, so it is not known whether the serum barbiturate levels of these patients were measured, or whether the raised levels are only a surmise.

A patient taking **tranylcypromine** 10 mg three times daily was inadvertently given intramuscular **amobarbital sodium** 250 mg for sedation. Within an hour she became ataxic, and fell to the floor, repeatedly hitting her head. After complaining of nausea and dizziness the patient became semicomatose and remained in that state for a further 36 hours. To what extent the head trauma played a part is uncertain.[2]

A man taking **amobarbital sodium** 195 mg at night suffered severe headache, and became confused after also taking **phenelzine** 15 mg three times daily for 4 weeks. On admission to hospital he was comatose, and he had a temperature of 40°C, blood pressure of 150/90 mmHg, tachycardia, stertorous respiration, fixed dilated pupils, exaggerated tendon reflexes and extensor plantar responses. His condition deteriorated and he died 2 hours after admission.[3] Pathology suggested a rise in intracranial pressure was responsible. The authors attribute this response to the drugs, but do not rule out a possible contribution of alcohol.[3]

Mechanism

Not known. *Animal* studies[2,4] show that MAOIs prolong the activity of barbiturates, and that this is possibly because they inhibit the metabolism of barbiturates by a mechanism independent of MAO inhibition. Whether this occurs in man as well is uncertain.

Importance and management

The evidence for these interactions seem to be confined to a few unconfirmed anecdotal reports. There is no well-documented evidence showing that concurrent use should be avoided, although some caution is clearly appropriate. For mention of successful anaesthesia including the use of **thiopental** in patients on MAOIs, see 'Anaesthetics, general + MAOIs', p.100.

1. Kline NS. Psychopharmaceuticals: effects and side effects. *Bull WHO* (1959) 21, 397–410.
2. Domino EF, Sullivan TS, Luby ED. Barbiturate intoxication in a patient treated with a MAO inhibitor. *Am J Psychiatry* (1962) 118, 941–3.
3. MacLeod I. Fatal reaction to phenelzine. *BMJ* (1965) 1, 1554.
4. Buchel L, Lévy J. Mécanisme des phénomènes de synergie du sommeil expérimental. II. Étude des associations iproniazide-hypnotiques, chez le rat et la souris. *Arch Sci Physiol (Paris)* (1965) 19, 161–79.

MAOIs or RIMAs + Benzodiazepines

Isolated cases of adverse reactions (chorea, severe headache, facial flushing, massive oedema, and prolonged coma) attributed to interactions between phenelzine and chlordiazepoxide, clonazepam or nitrazepam, and between isocarboxazid and chlordiazepoxide have been described. Evidence from clinical trials suggests that there is no interaction between moclobemide and benzodiazepines, although one study found a slight progressive worsening in driving performance.

Clinical evidence and mechanism

(a) MAOIs (non-selective, irreversible)

A patient who had been taking **phenelzine** 45 mg daily for 9 years developed a severe occipital headache after taking 500 micrograms of clonazepam. A similar but milder headache occurred the next night when she took the same dose. No blood pressure measurements were taken.[1] Another report describes facial flushing in a patient taking clonazepam, which occurred after **phenelzine** was started, and which responded to a reduction in the clonazepam dose.[2]

A patient with depression responded well when given **phenelzine** 15 mg and chlordiazepoxide 10 mg three times a day, but 4 to 5 months later developed choreiform movements of moderate severity, and slight dysarthria. These symptoms subsided when both drugs were withdrawn.[3]

Two patients taking chlordiazepoxide and either **phenelzine** or **isocarboxazid** developed severe oedema, which was attributed to the use of the combination.[4,5]

A patient became unconscious and hyperreflexic, with a low blood pressure (100/60 mmHg), increased heart rate (100 bpm), and increased temperature (38.4şC) about 29 hours after taking an overdose of **phenelzine** and chlordiazepoxide.[6] Another report briefly mentions a case of prolonged coma lasting 3 days in a patient who overdosed with **phenelzine** and chlordiazepoxide.[7]

A patient taking **phenelzine** 30 mg twice daily was started on nitrazepam 5 mg at night and the dose was gradually increased to 15 mg at night over 2 months. He developed MAOI toxicity (excessive sweating, postural hypotension) within 10 days of increasing his dose of nitrazepam to 15 mg daily. Both drugs were stopped and he recovered after 3 days. The **phenelzine** was restarted 2 weeks later without problems. It was suggested that since the patient was a slow acetylator, metabolism of nitrazepam by *N*-acetyl transferase would have been decreased, which may have affected the metabolism of **phenelzine**, thereby increasing its levels.[8]

(b) RIMAs

A meta-analysis of 879 patients taking **moclobemide** is reported to have found that insomnia, restlessness, agitation and anxiety occurred twice as often in the 467 patients taking one or more benzodiazepines than in those not taking concurrent benzodiazepines. However, these adverse events were often already present when **moclobemide** was started, so it is suggested that the patient groups were probably different. Apart from this difference between the patient groups, there was no evidence of any relevant pharmacokinetic or pharmacodynamic interaction.[9] Another review briefly reported that no clinically relevant interaction was noted between **moclobemide** and benzodiazepines in clinical studies.[10]

Driving performance gradually worsened over 6 weeks in a double-blind study in depressed patients given **moclobemide** (22 subjects) or fluoxetine (19 subjects). Thirty-one patients were taking long-term benzodiazepines, and at the start of the study their driving was no different to the patients not taking benzodiazepines. In an attempt to suggest a possible reason for the worsening performance, various variables were assessed in a regression analysis. It was found that patients taking **moclobemide** who were also taking a benzodiazepine with nordiazepam among its metabolites (**clorazepate**, **prazepam**, **diazepam**, **cloxazolam**, **clotiazepam**) experienced a progressive worsening in their driving, whereas patients on other benzodiazepines (**bromazepam**, **alprazolam**, **oxazepam**, **lorazepam**) tended to have no change in driving ability. It was tentatively suggested that **moclobemide** may have inhibited the metabolism of nordiazepam by the cytochrome P450 isoenzyme CYP2C19, so increasing the effect of the benzodiazepine, and worsening driving performance.[11]

Importance and management

The case reports of adverse interactions cited here appear to be isolated, and it is by no means certain that all the responses were in fact due to drug interactions. However, bear them in mind in the event of unexpected responses to treatment. No special precautions would normally be required during concurrent use, although a reminder that benzodiazepines may affect the performance of skilled tasks, such as driving, may be appropriate when a patient's medication is changed. Note that the manufacturer of moclobemide says that if depressed patients with excitation or agitation are first treated with moclobemide, a sedative such as a benzodiazepine should also be given for up to 2 to 3 weeks.[12] Further study is required to find out if there are any clinically important pharmacokinetic interactions between moclobemide and any of the benzodiazepines.

1. Eppel AB. Interaction between clonazepam and phenelzine. *Can J Psychiatry* (1990) 35, 647.
2. Karagianis JL, March H. Flushing reaction associated with the interaction of phenelzine and clonazepam. *Can J Psychiatry* (1991) 36, 389.
3. Macleod DM. Chorea induced by tranquillisers. *Lancet* (1964) i, 388–9.
4. Goonewardene A, Toghill PJ. Gross oedema occurring during treatment for depression. *BMJ* (1977) 1, 879–80.
5. Pathak SK. Gross oedema during treatment for depression. *BMJ* (1977) 1, 1220.
6. Young S, Walpole BG. Tranylcypromine and chlordiazepoxide intoxication. *Med J Aust* (1986) 144, 166–7.
7. Denton PH, Borrelli VM, Edwards NV. Dangers of monoamine oxidase inhibitors. *BMJ* (1962) 2, 1752–3.
8. Harris AL, McIntyre N. Interaction of phenelzine and nitrazepam in a slow acetylator. *Br J Clin Pharmacol* (1981) 12, 254–5.
9. Amrein R, Güntert TW, Dingesmanse J, Lorscheid T, Stabl M, Schmid-Burgk W. Interactions of moclobemide with concomitantly administered medication: evidence from pharmacological and clinical studies. *Psychopharmacology (Berl)* (1992) 106, S24–S31.
10. Zimmer R, Gieschke R, Fischbach R, Gasic S. Interaction studies with moclobemide. *Acta Psychiatr Scand* (1990) 82 (Suppl 360), 84–6.
11. Ramaekers JG, Ansseau M, Muntjewerff ND, Sweens JP, O'Hanlon JF. Considering the P450 cytochrome system as determining combined effects of antidepressants and benzodiazepines on actual driving performance of depressed outpatients. *Int Clin Psychopharmacol* (1997) 12, 159–69.
12. Manerix (Moclobemide). Roche Products Ltd. UK Summary of product characteristics, September 2005.

MAOIs or RIMAs + Buspirone

Elevated blood pressure has been reported in four patients taking buspirone and either phenelzine or tranylcypromine. Buspirone may have contributed to a case of the serotonin syndrome in a patient who overdosed on moclobemide and clomipramine.

Clinical evidence, mechanism, importance and management

(a) MAOIs

Four cases of significant blood pressure elevation, which occurred during the use of buspirone and either **phenelzine** or **tranylcypromine**, have been reported to the FDA's Spontaneous Reporting System. One patient was a 75-year-old woman and the other 3 patients were men aged between 30 and 42 years. The report does not say how much the blood pressure rose, or how quickly, and no other details are given.[1] On the basis of this rather sparse information the manufacturers of buspirone[2,3] recommend that it should not be used concurrently with an MAOI.

(b) RIMAs

A severe case[4] of the serotonin syndrome (including hyperthermia and muscle rigidity requiring mechanical ventilation) has been reported in a patient who took an overdose of '**moclobemide**, clomipramine and buspirone', (p.1149). Concurrent use of more than one serotonergic drug is thought to be a risk factor for the development of 'the serotonin syndrome', (p.9).

1. Anon. BuSpar Update. *Psychiatry Drug Alert* (1987) 1, 43.
2. Buspar (Buspirone hydrochloride). Bristol-Myers Pharmaceuticals. UK Summary of product characteristics, March 2007.
3. BuSpar (Buspirone hydrochloride). Bristol-Myers Squibb Company. US Prescribing information, March 2007.
4. Höjer J, Personne M, Skagius A-S, Hansson O. Serotoninergt syndrom: flera allvarliga fall med denna ofta förbisedda diagnos. *Lakartidningen* (2002) 99, 2054–5, 2058–60.

MAOIs + Caffeine or Choline theophyllinate

Isolated reports suggest that the CNS stimulant effects of caffeine may possibly be increased by the MAOIs. Another isolated report describes the development of tachycardia and apprehension in a patient taking phenelzine after she also took a cough syrup, containing choline theophyllinate.

Clinical evidence

(a) Caffeine

One reviewer briefly mentions that a patient who normally drank 10 or 12 cups of **coffee** daily, without adverse effects, experienced extreme jitteriness during treatment with an MAOI, which subsided when the **coffee** consumption was reduced to 2 or 3 cups a day. The same reaction was also said to have occurred in other patients taking MAOIs who drank **tea** or some of the **'Cola' drinks**, which contain caffeine.[1] This reviewer also mentions another patient taking an MAOI who claimed that a single cup of **coffee** taken in the morning kept him jittery all day and up the entire night as well, a reaction that occurred on three separate occasions.[1] In another report, a woman taking **phenelzine** experienced a severe headache with a slight blood pressure rise on two occasions after drinking **cola** containing 35 to 55 mg of caffeine.[2] Similarly, a brief mention is made of 2 patients taking **phenelzine** who experienced extreme restlessness, agitation, tremor, and insomnia after starting to drink large quantities of **diet cola**. This was attributed to an interaction between **phenelzine** and **aspartame**,[3] but could equally well be attributed to an interaction with caffeine, or indeed a reaction to caffeine alone. Caffeine and **theophylline** may have contributed to the serious reaction that occurred in a woman the day after discontinuing **phenelzine**, who took a *Do-Do* tablet (containing ephedrine, caffeine, theophylline),[4] see also 'MAOIs or RIMAs + Sympathomimetics; Indirectly-acting', p.1147.

(b) Choline theophyllinate

A woman with agoraphobia, being treated with **phenelzine** 45 mg daily, developed tachycardia, palpitations and apprehension lasting for about 4 hours after she had taken a cough syrup containing choline theophyllinate and guaifenesin. The symptoms recurred when she was again given the cough syrup, and yet again when given choline theophyllinate alone, but not when given guaifenesin alone.[5]

Mechanism

Unknown. Caffeine alone can cause headache, tachycardia, and jitteriness, and individuals vary in their susceptibility to these effects. The effects of caffeine, theophylline, and theobromine in *rats* were enhanced by MAOIs.[6]

Importance and management

Apart from these few reports, the literature appears to be otherwise silent about an interaction between the MAOIs and xanthines. Whether this reflects their mildness and unimportance, or their rarity, is not clear. There would seem to be no need for any special precautions in patients taking MAOIs who are given xanthine bronchodilators or consuming caffeine-containing beverages or pharmaceuticals, but bear these adverse reports in mind in the event of any unexpected response. Nevertheless, some manufacturers of MAOIs recommend the avoidance of excessive amounts of tea and coffee,[7] or caffeine in any form.[8-10]

1. Kline NS. Psychopharmaceuticals: effects and side-effects. *Bull WHO* (1959) 21, 397–410.
2. Pakes GE. Phenelzine-cola headache. *Am J Hosp Pharm* (1979) 36, 736.
3. Shader RI, Greenblatt DJ. Phenelzine and the dream machine—ramblings and reflections. *J Clin Psychopharmacol* (1985) 5, 65.
4. Dawson JK, Earnshaw SM, Graham CS. Dangerous monoamine oxidase inhibitor interactions are still occurring in the 1990s. *J Accid Emerg Med* (1995) 12, 49–51.
5. Shader RI, Greenblatt DJ. MAOIs and drug interactions—a proposal for a clearinghouse. *J Clin Psychopharmacol* (1985) 5, A17.
6. Berkowitz BA, Spector S, Pool W. The interaction of caffeine, theophylline and theobromine with monoamine oxidase inhibitors. *Eur J Pharmacol* (1971) 16, 315–21.
7. Nardil (Phenelzine sulfate). Link Pharmaceuticals Ltd. UK Summary of product characteristics, July 2003.
8. Marplan (Isocarboxazid). Oxford Pharmaceutical Services Inc. US Prescribing information, January 2000.
9. Nardil (Phenelzine sulfate). Pfizer Inc. US Prescribing information, June 2007.
10. Parnate (Tranylcypromine sulfate). GlaxoSmithKline. US Prescribing information, June 2007.

MAOIs + Cloral hydrate

A case of fatal hyperpyrexia and another case of serious hypertension have been linked to interactions between cloral hydrate and phenelzine, but in both cases there are other plausible explanations for the reactions seen.

Clinical evidence, mechanism, importance and management

A woman taking **phenelzine** 15 mg three times daily was found in bed deeply comatose with marked muscular rigidity, twitching down one side and a temperature of 41°C. She died without regaining consciousness. A postmortem failed to establish the cause of death, but it subsequently came to light that she had started drinking whisky, and she had access to cloral hydrate, of which she may have taken a fatal dose.[1] Another patient, also taking **phenelzine** 15 mg three times daily and cloral hydrate to aid sleep, developed an excruciating headache followed by nausea, photophobia and a substantial rise in blood pressure.[2] This latter reaction is similar to the 'cheese reaction', see 'tyramine-rich foods', (p.1153), but at the time the authors of the report were unaware of this type of reaction so that they failed to find out if any tyramine-rich foods had been eaten on the day of the attack.[2]

There is no clear evidence that either of these adverse reactions was due to an interaction between **phenelzine** and cloral hydrate, and there do not seem to be any other reports to suggest that an interaction between these drugs is likely.

1. Howarth E. Possible synergistic effects of the new thymoleptics in connection with poisoning. *J Ment Sci* (1961) 107, 100–103.
2. Dillon H, Leopold RL. Acute cerebro-vascular symptoms produced by an antidepressant. *Am J Psychiatry* (1965) 121, 1012–14.

MAOIs + Cocaine

Some reports suggest that patients on MAOIs may experience a severe headache if they abuse cocaine. Two isolated reports describe the delayed development of hyperpyrexia, and other symptoms including coma, agitation, muscle tremors and rigidity after patients taking phenelzine or iproniazid were given a cocaine spray during surgery.

Clinical evidence, mechanism, importance and management

The use of cocaine is generally contraindicated in patients taking MAOIs[1-3] because it is expected to interact like 'indirectly-acting sympathomimetics', (p.1147). This is supported by a report of hypertensive reactions in 2 patients taking **phenelzine** who became drunk and used cocaine. Both experienced frightening reactions including headache, a rise in blood pressure, palpitations, and chest tightness. One required no treatment, and the other was treated with propranolol and diazepam.[4] Because this reaction was not considered as dangerous as expected, **phenelzine** has been tried as a deterrent to the abuse of cocaine: one uncontrolled study reports its use in 26 patients without mentioning any adverse reactions.[4] Another report mentions a man given **phenelzine** for cocaine abuse who experienced no reaction to the use of cocaine. He was then given **tranylcypromine**, and after 10 weeks risked sniffing cocaine, which did produce a severe occipital headache and nausea. However, after abstaining for another 10 weeks he again used cocaine, this time without any reaction.[5]

A man taking **phenelzine** 15 mg twice daily underwent vocal chord surgery. He was anaesthetised with thiopental, and later nitrous oxide and isoflurane 0.5% in oxygen. Muscle paralysis was produced with suxamethonium and gallamine. During the operation his vocal chords were sprayed with 1 mL of a 10% cocaine spray. He regained consciousness 30 minutes after the surgery and was returned to the ward, but a further 30 minutes later he was found unconscious, with generalised coarse tremors and marked muscle rigidity. His rectal temperature was 41.5°C. He was initially thought to have malignant hyperpyrexia and was treated accordingly with wet blankets, as well as with intravenous fluids and oxygen, and he largely recovered within 7 hours. However, later it seemed more likely that the reaction had been due to an adverse interaction between the **phenelzine** and cocaine, because he had been similarly and uneventfully treated with cocaine in the absence of **phenelzine** on two previous occasions.[6] A similar case was described in a woman taking **iproniazid** who had her trachea sprayed with 1 mL of 10% cocaine before intubation during surgery. She was also given pethidine 20 mg, and shortly after surgery became pyrexial, flushed, agitated and sweated profusely. She was treated with intravenous chlorpromazine.[7] In this case, the reaction could have been due to the pethidine alone (see 'MAOIs or RIMAs + Opioids; Pethidine (Meperidine)', p.1140), or both the cocaine and the pethidine. The reasons for these adverse reactions are not understood, but a delayed excitatory reaction due to increased 5-HT (serotonin) concentrations has been suggested.[6] The general importance of these cases is not known, but bear them in mind if cocaine is used in a patient on an MAOI.

1. Nardil (Phenelzine sulfate). Link Pharmaceuticals Ltd. UK Summary of product characteristics, July 2003.
2. Nardil (Phenelzine sulfate). Pfizer Inc. US Prescribing information, June 2007.
3. Parnate (Tranylcypromine sulfate). GlaxoSmithKline. US Prescribing information, June 2007.
4. Golwyn DH. Cocaine abuse treated with phenelzine. *Int J Addict* (1988) 23, 897–905.
5. Brewer C. Treatment of cocaine abuse with monoamine oxidase inhibitors. *Br J Psychiatry* (1993) 163, 815–16.
6. Tordoff SG, Stubbing JF, Linter SPK. Delayed excitatory reaction following interaction of cocaine and monoamine oxidase inhibitor (phenelzine). *Br J Anaesth* (1991) 66, 516–18.
7. Clement AJ, Benazon D. Reactions to other drugs in patients taking monoamine-oxidase inhibitors. *Lancet* (1962) 2, 197–8.

MAOIs or RIMAs + Dextromethorphan

Two fatal cases of hyperpyrexia and coma (symptoms similar to the serotonin syndrome) have occurred in patients taking phenelzine with dextromethorphan (in overdosage in one case). Three other serious but non-fatal reactions occurred in patients taking dextromethorphan with isocarboxazid or phenelzine. MAOIs should not be used with dextromethorphan. Moclobemide inhibits the metabolism of dextromethorphan, and isolated cases of severe CNS reactions have occurred with the combination, which is also contraindicated.

Clinical evidence

(a) MAOIs

A woman taking **phenelzine** 15 mg four times daily complained of nausea and dizziness before collapsing, 30 minutes after drinking about 55 mL of a cough mixture containing dextromethorphan. She remained hyperpyrexic (42°C), hypotensive (systolic blood pressure below 70 mmHg) and unconscious for 4 hours, before dying after a cardiac arrest.[1]

A 15-year-old girl taking **phenelzine** 15 mg three times daily (as well as thioridazine, procyclidine and metronidazole) took 13 capsules of *Romilar CF* (containing dextromethorphan hydrobromide 15 mg, phenindamine tartrate 6.25 mg, phenylephrine hydrochloride 5 mg and paracetamol (acetaminophen) 120 mg in each capsule). She became comatose, hyperpyrexic (103°F), had a blood pressure of 100/60 mmHg, a pulse of 160 bpm and later died of a cardiac arrest.[2] This case is complicated by the overdosage and multiplicity of drugs present, particularly the phenylephrine. See 'MAOIs or RIMAs + Sympathomimetics; Phenylephrine', p.1148.

A 28-year-old woman developed severe myoclonus and rigidity, and became largely unresponsive after taking **phenelzine** and *Robitussin DM* (dextromethorphan hydrobromide 15 mg with guaifenesin 100 mg).[3] Yet another patient taking **phenelzine** developed muscular rigidity, uncontrollable shaking, generalised hyperreflexia and sweating when given *Robitussin DM*. Within 2 hours he had responded to 10 mg of intravenous diazepam and oral activated charcoal.[4]

A woman taking **isocarboxazid** 30 mg daily took diazepam 1 mg and 10 mL of *Robitussin DM*. Within 20 minutes she was nauseated and dizzy, and within 45 minutes she began to have fine bilateral leg tremor and muscle spasms of the abdomen and lower back. These were followed by bilateral and persistent myoclonic jerks of legs, occasional choreoathetoid movements and marked urinary retention. These adverse effects persisted for about 19 hours, gradually becoming less severe.[5]

The US manufacturer of **tranylcypromine** notes that the concurrent use of MAOIs and dextromethorphan has resulted in brief episodes of psychosis or bizarre behaviour.[6] Similarly, the US manufacturer of **phenelzine** mentions one case of drowsiness and bizarre behaviour when dextromethorphan lozenges were used by a patient taking phenelzine. They also note that concurrent use of dextromethorphan may cause a reaction similar to that seen with pethidine (meperidine),[7] as described in some of the cases above.

(b) RIMAs

Moclobemide 300 mg twice daily for 9 days markedly reduced the *O*-demethylation of dextromethorphan (seven 20-mg doses given every 4 hours over 2 days), in 4 healthy subjects.[8] The manufacturer notes that isolated cases of severe CNS adverse reactions have been seen with the combination.[9] Concurrent use of dextromethorphan may have contributed to a fatality involving the illicit use of **moclobemide** and 'ecstasy', (p.1144).

Mechanism

(a) The authors of three of the reports[3-5] suggest that these effects may have been due to an increase in serotonin activity in the CNS 'the serotonin syndrome', (p.9). Symptoms similar to the serotonin syndrome (hyperpyrexia, dilated pupils, hyperexcitability and motor restlessness) have been seen in *rabbits* treated with dextromethorphan and **nialamide**, phenelzine or **pargyline**,[10] and also with MAOIs and 'pethidine', (p.1140).

(b) Moclobemide appears to inhibit the metabolism of dextromethorphan by the cytochrome P450 isoenzyme CYP2D6, and the combination may also cause adverse CNS effects.

Importance and management

Despite the very limited information available, the severity of the reactions indicates that patients taking MAOIs should avoid taking dextromethorphan. The manufacturer of moclobemide also contraindicates the concurrent use of dextromethorphan.[9] Patients should be warned that many cough preparations contain dextromethorphan.

1. Rivers N, Horner B. Possible lethal reaction between Nardil and dextromethorphan. *Can Med Assoc J* (1970) 103, 85.
2. Shamsie JC, Barriga C. The hazards of use of monoamine oxidase inhibitors in disturbed adolescents. *Can Med Assoc J* (1971) 104, 715.
3. Nierenberg DW, Semprebon M. The central nervous system serotonin syndrome. *Clin Pharmacol Ther* (1993) 53, 84–8.
4. Sauter D, Macneil P, Weinstein E, Azar A. Phenelzine sulfate-dextromethorphan interaction: a case report. *Vet Hum Toxicol* (1991) 33, 365.
5. Sovner R, Wolfe J. Interaction between dextromethorphan and monoamine oxidase inhibitor therapy with isocarboxazid. *N Engl J Med* (1988) 319, 1671.
6. Parnate (Tranylcypromine sulfate). GlaxoSmithKline. US Prescribing information, June 2007.
7. Nardil (Phenelzine sulfate). Pfizer Inc. US Prescribing information, June 2007.
8. Härtter S, Dingemanse J, Baier D, Ziegler G, Hiemke C. Inhibition of dextromethorphan metabolism by moclobemide. *Psychopharmacology (Berl)* (1998) 135, 22–6.
9. Manerix (Moclobemide). Roche Products Ltd. UK Summary of product characteristics, September 2005.
10. Sinclair JG. Dextromethorphan-monoamine oxidase inhibitor interaction in rabbits. *J Pharm Pharmacol* (1973) 25, 803–8.

MAOIs + Disulfiram

An isolated report describes delirium in a man taking lithium and disulfiram when the moclobemide he was also taking was replaced by tranylcypromine.

Clinical evidence, mechanism, importance and management

A man with disulfiram implants taking long-term lithium had his MAOI changed from **moclobemide** [dosage not stated] to **tranylcypromine** 10 mg twice daily. Within 2 days he became acutely delirious (agitated, disoriented, incoherent, visual hallucinations) and later subcomatose, with nystagmus and a downward gaze. He was successfully treated with haloperidol and promethazine, and recovered within 24 hours. No alcohol was detected in his blood, and serum **tranylcypromine** levels were below 50 micrograms/L, which was considered normal.[1]

The authors of this report attribute the reaction to an interaction between **tranylcypromine** and disulfiram. However, there would seem to be other possible explanations for this reaction. MAOIs have rarely been seen to interact adversely with 'lithium', (p.1136), and there also seems potential for an interaction between the two 'MAOIs', (p.1137).

This seems to be the only report of an adverse reaction between disulfiram and an MAOI, so it is possible that this is just an idiosyncratic reaction. However, warnings about this drug combination, based on theoretical considerations and studies in *animals*, have previously been given, and **tranylcypromine** was considered to be the MAOI that presented the greatest risk.[2] Consequently, the US manufacturers of **tranylcypromine**[3] and **isocarboxazid**[4] recommend caution with the concurrent use of disulfiram. It seems that this particular patient had no problems while taking **moclobemide**, which is a RIMA.

1. Blansjaar BA, Egberts TCG. Delirium in a patient treated with disulfiram and tranylcypromine. *Am J Psychiatry* (1995) 152, 296.
2. Ciraulo DA. Can disulfiram (Antabuse) be safely co-administered with the monoamine oxidase inhibitor (MAOI) antidepressants? . *J Clin Psychopharmacol* (1989) 9, 315–16.
3. Parnate (Tranylcypromine sulfate). GlaxoSmithKline. US Prescribing information, June 2007.
4. Marplan (Isocarboxazid). Oxford Pharmaceutical Services Inc. US Prescribing information, January 2000.

MAOIs + Dopa-rich foods

A few reports describe a rapid, serious and potentially life-threatening hypertensive reaction in patients taking MAOIs if they eat young broad bean pods, which contain dopa. No serious hypertensive reaction is likely to occur with moclobemide.

Clinical evidence

A 65-year-old hypertensive man taking **pargyline** had a severe headache and palpitations on two occasions after eating "whole, cooked, broad beans" (young broad bean pods). A controlled study in this man found that he had a rise in systolic blood pressure from 165 to 262 mmHg about 20 minutes after eating whole broad bean pods. The pods alone had the same effect, but the beans on their own had little effect. This rise in blood pressure was also seen in two other patients on **pargyline**, and was reversed by intravenous phentolamine. Two normotensive subjects taking pargyline 50 mg daily also had an increase in blood pressure (over 70 mmHg systolic in one subject) following the ingestion of bean pods.[1] Another case report describes a man taking **phenelzine** 15 mg three times daily who had a very severe headache after eating a meal including fresh, young, sliced, broad bean pods from his garden.[2] One other case has been briefly mentioned, although it was not known whether the broad beans were eaten with or without the pods.[3]

Mechanism

Broad bean (*Vicia faba*) pods contain dopa,[1] which is enzymatically converted in the body, firstly to dopamine and then to noradrenaline, both of which are normally broken down by monoamine oxidase. In the presence of an MAOI this breakdown is suppressed, which means that the total levels of dopamine and noradrenaline are increased. Precisely how this then leads to a sharp rise in blood pressure is not clear, but either dopamine or noradrenaline, or both, directly or indirectly stimulate the alpha-receptors of the cardiovascular system.

Importance and management

Although there are only a few cases of the interaction between the non-selective MAOIs (listed in 'Table 32.1', (p.1130)) and broad bean pods, the interaction would appear to be established and is serious and potentially life-threatening. Patients should not eat young broad bean *pods* during treatment with any of these MAOIs, nor for a period of 2 to 3 weeks after their withdrawal. It should be noted that this prohibition does not apply to 'mature' broad beans (the seeds) removed from their pods, which is the more common way of eating broad beans.

1. Hodge JV, Nye ER, Emerson GW. Monoamine-oxidase inhibitors, broad beans, and hypertension. *Lancet* (1964) i, 1108.
2. Blomley DJ. Monoamine-oxidase inhibitors. *Lancet* (1964) ii, 1181–2.
3. McQueen EG. Interactions with monoamine oxidase inhibitors. *BMJ* (1975) 4, 101.

MAOIs + Doxapram

No adverse interactions have been reported between the MAOIs and doxapram, although *animal* studies suggest that an increased pressor effect is theoretically possible.

Clinical evidence, mechanism, importance and management

The manufacturers note that *animal* studies have shown that the actions of doxapram may be potentiated by pretreatment with an MAOI,[1] and that the pressor effects of MAOIs and doxapram may be additive.[2] Based on this, they advise that concurrent use should be undertaken with great care.[1,2] To date, there appear to be no clinical reports of this interaction.

1. Dopram Infusion (Doxapram). Anpharm Ltd. UK Summary of product characteristics, February 2001.
2. Dopram (Doxapram hydrochloride). Baxter Healthcare Corporation. US Prescribing information, March 2004.

MAOIs + Erythromycin

An isolated case report describes severe hypotension and fainting in a woman taking phenelzine, which occurred shortly after she started a course of erythromycin.

Clinical evidence, mechanism, importance and management

A woman taking **phenelzine** 15 mg daily experienced three syncopal episodes 4 days after starting to take erythromycin 250 mg four times daily for pneumonia. When admitted to hospital her supine systolic blood pressure was only 70 mmHg. When she sat up, it was unrecordable. Although she was not dehydrated, she was given 4 litres of sodium chloride 0.9%, without any effect on her blood pressure. Within 24 hours of stopping the **phenelzine** her blood pressure had returned to normal.[1] The reasons for this severe hypotensive reaction are not known, but it was suggested that the erythromycin may have caused rapid gastric emptying, which resulted in a very rapid absorption of the **phenelzine** (described by the author as rapid dumping into the blood stream), which resulted in the adverse effect of hypotension.[1] This seems to be the first and only report of this interaction, and so its general importance is uncertain.

1. Bernstein AE. Drug interaction. *Hosp Community Psychiatry* (1990) 41, 806–7.

MAOIs + Ginseng

Isolated reports describe two patients taking phenelzine who developed adverse effects (including headache and insomnia) after taking ginseng.

Clinical evidence, mechanism, importance and management

A 64-year-old woman taking **phenelzine** developed headache, insomnia, and tremulousness on two occasions after taking ginseng.[1] Three years later, she experienced the same symptoms and an increase in depression 72 hours after starting to take ginseng capsules.[2] Another depressed woman taking ginseng and bee pollen experienced a relief of her depression and became active and extremely optimistic when she was started on **phenelzine** 45 mg daily, but this was accompanied by insomnia, irritability, headaches and vague visual hallucinations. When the **phenelzine** was stopped and then re-started in the absence of the ginseng and bee pollen, her depression was not relieved.[3] It seems unlikely that the bee pollen had any part to play in these reactions and suspicion therefore falls on the ginseng. It would seem that the psychoactive effects of the ginsenosides from the ginseng and the MAOI were somehow additive. Ginseng has stimulant effects, but its adverse effects include insomnia, nervousness, hypertension and euphoria. These two cases once again illustrate that herbal medicines are not necessarily problem-free if combined with orthodox drugs.

1. Shader RI, Greenblatt DJ. Phenelzine and the dream machine—ramblings and reflections. *J Clin Psychopharmacol* (1985) 5, 65.
2. Shader RI, Greenblatt DJ. Bees, ginseng and MAOIs revisited. *J Clin Psychopharmacol* (1988) 8, 235.
3. Jones BD, Runikis AM. Interaction of ginseng with phenelzine. *J Clin Psychopharmacol* (1987) 7, 201–2.

MAOIs or RIMAs + Levodopa

A rapid, serious and potentially life-threatening hypertensive reaction can occur in patients taking MAOIs if they are also given levodopa. An interaction with levodopa given with carbidopa or benserazide is unlikely. No serious hypertensive reaction has been reported to occur with moclobemide. See also 'MAOIs + Dopa-rich foods', p.1135.

Clinical evidence

(a) MAOIs

A patient who had been taking **phenelzine** daily for 10 days was given 50 mg of oral levodopa. In just over an hour his blood pressure had risen from 135/90 mmHg to about 190/130 mmHg, and despite a 5 mg intravenous injection of phentolamine it continued to rise over the next 10 minutes to 200/135 mmHg, before falling after a further 4 mg injection of phentolamine. The following day the experiment was repeated with levodopa 25 mg, but no blood pressure changes were seen. Three weeks after withdrawal of the **phenelzine** even 500 mg of levodopa had no hypertensive effect.[1]

Similar cases of severe, acute hypertension, accompanied in most instances by flushing, throbbing and pounding in the head, neck and chest, and light-headedness have been described in other case reports and studies involving the concurrent use of levodopa with **pargyline**,[2] **nialamide**,[3] **tranylcypromine**,[4,5] **phenelzine**[6] and **isocarboxazid**.[1]

(b) RIMAs

A study in 12 healthy subjects given a single dose of levodopa/benserazide with **moclobemide** 200 mg twice daily found that nausea, vomiting and dizziness were increased, but no significant hypertensive reaction was seen.[7]

Mechanism

Not fully understood. Levodopa is enzymatically converted in the body, firstly to dopamine and then to noradrenaline, both of which are normally broken down by monoamine oxidase. But in the presence of an MAOI this breakdown is suppressed, which means that the total levels of dopamine and noradrenaline are increased. Precisely how this then leads to a sharp rise in blood pressure is not clear, but either dopamine or noradrenaline, or both, directly or indirectly stimulate the alpha-receptors of the cardiovascular system.

Importance and management

The interaction between the non-selective MAOIs (listed in 'Table 32.1', (p.1130)) and levodopa on its own is well documented, serious and potentially life-threatening. Patients should not be given levodopa on its own during treatment with any of these MAOIs, nor for a period of 2 to 3 weeks after their withdrawal. Note that this interaction is inhibited by the presence of dopa-decarboxylase inhibitors[4] such as carbidopa and benserazide (as in *Sinemet* and *Madopar*) so that a serious interaction is unlikely to occur with these preparations. Even so, the manufacturers continue to list the MAOIs among their contraindications.

No important acute adverse interaction appears to occur between levodopa/benserazide and moclobemide, but some adverse effects can apparently occur.

1. Hunter KR, Boakes AJ, Laurence DR, Stern GM. Monoamine oxidase inhibitors and L-dopa. *BMJ* (1970) 3, 388.
2. Hodge JV. Use of monoamine-oxidase inhibitors. *Lancet* (1965) i, 764–5.
3. Friend DG, Bell WR, Kline NS. The action of L-dihydroxyphenylalanine in patients receiving nialamide. *Clin Pharmacol Ther* (1965) 6, 362–6.
4. Teychenne PF, Calne DB, Lewis PJ, Findley LJ. Interactions of levodopa with inhibitors of monoamine oxidase and L-aromatic amino acid decarboxylase. *Clin Pharmacol Ther* (1975) 18, 273–7.
5. Sharpe J, Marquez-Julio A, Ashby P. Idiopathic orthostatic hypotension treated with levodopa and MAO inhibitor: a preliminary report. *Can Med Assoc J* (1972) 107, 296–300.
6. Kassirer JP, Kopelman RI. A modern medical Descartes. *Hosp Pract* (1987) 22, 17–25.
7. Dingemanse J. An update of recent moclobemide interaction data. *Int Clin Psychopharmacol* (1993) 7, 167–80.

MAOIs or RIMAs + Lithium

Two cases of tardive dyskinesia have been described following the long-term use of tranylcypromine and lithium, which did not resolve when the MAOI was stopped. Limited evidence suggests that no problems occur when moclobemide is given with lithium.

Clinical evidence, mechanism, importance and management

(a) MAOIs

One report describes 2 patients with bipolar affective disorder who developed a buccolingual-masticatory syndrome after taking **tranylcypromine** 30 or 40 mg daily and lithium carbonate 900 or 1200 mg daily for 1.5 or 3 years. These symptoms did not resolve when the **tranylcypromine** was stopped. This reaction was attributed to dopamine receptor hypersensitivity.[1]

There appear to be no other reports suggesting that the combination of MAOIs and lithium is unsafe. However, there are a few reports of patients taking MAOIs and lithium who developed hyperpyrexia when given 'tryptophan', (p.1151). The role (if any) of lithium in these cases is unknown. Note that lithium has been used to augment antidepressants although most of the data relate to tricyclics or SSRIs.[2] Bear these cases in mind in the event of any unexpected response to treatment with MAOIs and lithium.

(b) RIMAs

There was no evidence of any adverse interaction when **moclobemide** 150 to 675 mg daily was given for 3 to 52 weeks to 50 patients taking lithium.[3] Similarly, lithium augmentation was used in a small uncontrolled study in patients on high-dose **moclobemide** without any evidence of important adverse effects.[4]

1. Stancer HC. Tardive dyskinesia not associated with neuroleptics. *Am J Psychiatry* (1979) 136, 727.
2. Nelson JC. Augmentation strategies in depression 2000. *J Clin Psychiatry* (2000) 61 (Suppl 2), 13–19.
3. Amrein R, Güntert TW, Dingemanse J, Lorscheid T, Stabl M, Schmid-Burgk W. Interactions of moclobemide with concomitantly administered medication: evidence from pharmacological and clinical studies. *Psychopharmacology (Berl)* (1992) 106, S24–S31.
4. Magder DM, Aleksic I, Kennedy SH. Tolerability and efficacy of high-dose moclobemide alone and in combination with lithium and trazodone. *J Clin Psychopharmacol* (2000) 20, 394–5.

MAOIs + MAOIs or RIMAs

Strokes, fatal reactions (possibly including the serotonin syndrome), hypertensive reactions and CNS disturbances have been seen, either when one MAOI was abruptly replaced by another, when the two MAOIs were given together, or when there was an insufficient MAOI-free interval. A case of serotonin syndrome occurred in a patient who overdosed on moclobemide and tranylcypromine.

Clinical evidence, mechanism, importance and management

(a) MAOIs + MAOIs

A patient who had been taking **isocarboxazid** for 3.5 weeks (starting at 10 mg daily and gradually increased to 30 mg daily) was switched to **tranylcypromine** 10 mg, starting the same day, followed by 10 mg three times daily on the following day. Later that night she complained of feeling 'funny', had difficulty in talking, developed a headache, was restless, flushed, sweating, had an elevated temperature of 39.5°C, and a pulse rate of 130 bpm. She died the following day.[1] Another patient, switched without a drug-free period, from **phenelzine** 75 mg daily (by tapering the dose by 15 mg daily until discontinued) to **tranylcypromine** (starting at 10 mg daily, increasing by 10 mg daily, until a dose of 20 mg twice daily was reached), suffered a subcortical cerebral haemorrhage on the fourth day following the morning 20-mg dose of **tranylcypromine**, which resulted in total right-sided hemiplegia.[2,3] The patient remained significantly disabled from the sequelae of her stroke.[4] A third patient experienced a mild cerebral haemorrhage, without residual problems, when she took **phenelzine** 45 mg and **tranylcypromine** 20 mg at bedtime; the MAOIs were being switched by reducing the dose of phenelzine and gradually increasing the dose of **tranylcypromine**. Consumption of 'soy sauce', (p.1153), may have contributed to this reaction.[5] In a fourth case, **phenelzine** 45 mg daily was stopped, and then after a two-day drug-free period **tranylcypromine** 20 mg was given, with a further 30-mg dose the next day. The patient experienced a rise in blood pressure to 240/130 mmHg, but recovered uneventfully, and a year later was successfully switched from **phenelzine** to **tranylcypromine** with a 2-week drug-free interval.[2] In another case, hypertension with severe headache, inability to walk and slurred speech, but without permanent sequelae, resulted from starting **tranylcypromine** 30 mg seven days after discontinuing **phenelzine**. **Tranylcypromine** 10 mg daily was restarted 3 days later (10 days after discontinuing the **phenelzine**) with no adverse effects, but when the dose was increased to 20 mg daily (14 days after discontinuing **phenelzine**) the patient experienced a milder version of the same symptoms.[6]

Acute CNS toxicity, hypertension, tachycardia, tremor and urinary retention occurred in a woman 48 hours after **phenelzine** was abruptly stopped and **isocarboxazid** started. In this patient, **phenelzine** was poorly tolerated causing hypertension and headache.[7]

Switching from **iproniazid** to **tranylcypromine**/trifluoperazine may have been the cause of a fatal reaction (fever, shivering, sweating, cyanosis) in a patient also given ephedrine[8,9] (see also 'MAOIs or RIMAs + Sympathomimetics; Indirectly-acting', p.1147).

In contrast, one woman was switched directly from **phenelzine** 60 mg daily to **tranylcypromine** 20 mg daily without any obvious problems (blood pressure was on the high side, but within the usual range for this patient). She was abruptly switched directly back to **phenelzine**, again without any adverse effect.[10,11] Similarly, a review of 8 cases of patients who were switched rapidly from **tranylcypromine** to **phenelzine** (3 cases) or *vice versa* (5 cases) found that 7 patients tolerated the switch well with minimal or no adverse effects. However the eighth patient experienced anxiety, nausea, hyperventilation, flushing, sense of doom, and increased insomnia, which may have been a mild form of the serotonin syndrome.[12]

The reasons for these reactions are not understood, but one idea is that the amphetamine-like properties of **tranylcypromine** may have had some part to play. Certainly there are cases of spontaneous rises in blood pressure and intracranial bleeding in patients given **tranylcypromine**.[13] Not all patients experience adverse reactions when switched from one MAOI to another,[10,12] but because of the sometimes severe reactions, it would seem prudent to have a drug-free wash-out interval when doing so, and to start dosing in a conservative and step-wise manner.

(b) RIMAs + MAOIs

The serotonin syndrome occurred in a patient who took an overdose of **moclobemide** and **tranylcypromine**. In this analysis of moclobemide overdoses, the risk of developing serotonin toxicity was increased 35-fold in patients who also took another serotonergic drug, of which this case with **tranylcypromine** was one of 11 mentioned.[14]

1. Bazire SR. Sudden death associated with switching monoamine oxidase inhibitors. *Drug Intell Clin Pharm* (1986) 20, 954–6.
2. Gelenberg AJ. Switching MAOI. *Biol Ther Psychiatry* (1984) 7, 33 and 36.
3. Gelenberg AJ. Switching MAOI. The sequel. *Biol Ther Psychiatry* (1985) 8, 41.
4. Mattes JA. Stroke resulting from a rapid switch from phenelzine to tranylcypromine. *J Clin Psychiatry* (1998) 59, 382.
5. Anon. Switching MAOIs: part three. *Biol Ther Psychiatry* (1987) 10, 7.
6. Chandler JD. Switching MAOIs. *J Clin Psychopharmacol* (1987) 7, 438.
7. Safferman AZ, Masiar SJ. Central nervous system toxicity after abrupt monoamine oxidase inhibitor switch: a case report. *Ann Pharmacother* (1992) 26, 337–8.
8. Low-Beer GA, Tidmarsh D. Collapse after "Parstelin". *BMJ* (1963) 2, 683–4.
9. Schrire I. Collapse after "Parstelin". *BMJ* (1963) 2, 748.
10. True BL, Alexander B, Carter B. Switching monoamine oxidase inhibitors. *Drug Intell Clin Pharm* (1985) 19, 825–7.
11. True BL, Alexander B, Carter BL. Comment: switching MAO inhibitors. *Drug Intell Clin Pharm* (1986) 20, 384–5.
12. Szuba MP, Hornig-Rohan M, Amsterdam JD. Rapid converson from one monoamine oxidase inhibitor to another. *J Clin Psychiatry* (1997) 58, 307–10.
13. Cooper AJ, Magnus RV, Rose MJ. A hypertensive syndrome with tranylcypromine medication. *Lancet* (1964) 1, 527–9.
14. Isbister GK, Hackett LP, Dawson AH, Whyte IM, Smith AJ. Moclobemide poisoning: toxicokinetics and occurrence of serotonin toxicity. *Br J Clin Pharmacol* (2003) 56, 441–50.

MAOIs + Mazindol

An isolated report describes a patient taking phenelzine who had a marked rise in blood pressure when given a single dose of mazindol.

Clinical evidence, mechanism, importance and management

A woman taking **phenelzine** 30 mg three times daily had a rise in blood pressure from 110/60 to 200/100 mmHg within 2 hours of receiving a 10-mg test dose of mazindol. The blood pressure remained elevated for another hour, but had fallen again after another 3 hours. The patient experienced no subjective symptoms.[1] It is uncertain whether this hypertensive reaction was the result of an interaction, or simply a direct response to the mazindol alone (the dose was large compared with the manufacturer's recommended dosage of 2 to 3 mg daily). The general importance is uncertain. The manufacturer advises avoiding the combination, and say that mazindol should not be used until 14 days after MAOIs have been stopped.[2]

1. Oliver RM. Interaction between phenelzine and mazindol: Personal communication, 1981.
2. Sanorex (Mazindol). Novartis Pharmaceuticals. Canadian prescribing information. Compendium of Pharmaceuticals and Specialities, 2004.

MAOIs + Methyldopa

Theoretically hypertension may occur when non-selective MAOIs are taken with methyldopa, although additive blood-pressure lowering effects are also a possibility. The concurrent use of antidepressant MAOIs and methyldopa may not be desirable because methyldopa can sometimes cause depression.

Clinical evidence, mechanism, importance and management

Theoretically, methyldopa might cause hypertension in patients treated with non-selective MAOIs, by releasing catecholamines into the circulation[1,2] On the basis of this the manufacturers of some MAOIs[3,4] and methyldopa[5] contraindicate concurrent use. Nevertheless, there do not appear to be any reports of hypertension occurring as a result of concurrent use. Conversely, the UK manufacturer of **isocarboxazid**[6] mentions that it may potentiate the hypotensive effect of methyldopa. MAOIs alone have hypotensive effects and additional blood pressure lowering effects have been reported in a few patients given **pargyline** (an MAOI formerly used in the treatment of hypertension) with methyldopa.[7,8] Note that the potential depressant adverse effects of methyldopa may make it an unsuitable drug for patients with depression.

1. van Rossum JM. Potential danger of monoamineoxidase inhibitors and α-methyldopa. *Lancet* (1963) i, 950–1.
2. Natarajan S. Potential danger of monoamineoxidase inhibitors and α-methyldopa. *Lancet* (1964) i, 1330.
3. Nardil (Phenelzine sulfate). Pfizer Inc. US Prescribing information, June 2007.
4. Parnate (Tranylcypromine sulfate). GlaxoSmithKline. US Prescribing information, June 2007.
5. Aldomet (Methyldopa). Merck Sharp & Dohme Ltd. UK Summary of product characteristics, August 2001.
6. Isocarboxazid. Cambridge Laboratories. UK Summary of product characteristics, March 2000.
7. Herting RL. Monoamine oxidase inhibitors. *Lancet* (1963) i, 1324.
8. Gillespsie L, Oates JA, Crout JR, Sjoerdsma A. Clinical and chemical studies with α-methyldopa in patients with hypertension. *Circulation* (1962) 25, 281–91.

MAOIs + Monosodium glutamate

Hypertension in patients taking MAOIs who had eaten certain foods (soy sauce, chicken nuggets) has been attributed, in anecdotal reports, to an interaction with monosodium glutamate. However, a small controlled study found no evidence to support this idea, and the reaction was probably related to 'tyramine', (p.1153).

Clinical evidence

Five healthy subjects were given monosodium glutamate 400 to 1600 mg or a placebo with or without **tranylcypromine** for at least 2 weeks. Episodes of hypertension were seen in 2 subjects taking **tranylcypromine** with both placebo and monosodium glutamate, but no changes in blood pressure or heart rate occurred that could be attributed to an interaction while taking monosodium glutamate. The largest dose of monosodium glutamate used was about twice the amount usually found in meals containing large amounts of monosodium glutamate.[1]

There have been anecdotal reports of hypertensive reactions in patients taking MAOIs that were attributed to interactions with the monosodium glutamate contained in **soy sauce**[2] and **chicken nuggets**.[3]

Mechanism

Monosodium glutamate alone can cause a small rise in blood pressure, and MAOIs alone very occasionally cause hypertensive episodes. However, the reactions reported with soy sauce and chicken nuggets were probably due to a high tyramine content, as a high tyramine content has subsequently been detected in some soy sauces,[4] (see also 'MAOIs or RIMAs + Tyramine-rich foods', p.1153).

Importance and management

No interaction between monosodium glutamate *per se* and MAOIs has been established, although it should be pointed out that the number of subjects studied was very small. It is quite possible that the anecdotal reports were due to the tyramine content of the foods, and not to monosodium glutamate. In Hong Kong, patients on MAOIs are not advised to avoid monosodium glutamate, but are instructed to avoid excessive soy sauce because of its possible high tyramine content.[4]

1. Balon R, Pohl R, Yeragani VK, Berchou R, Gershon S. Monosodium glutamate and tranylcypromine administration in healthy subjects. *J Clin Psychiatry* (1990) 51, 303–6.
2. McCabe B, Tsuang MT. Dietary consideration in MAO inhibitor regimens. *J Clin Psychiatry* (1982) 43, 178–81.
3. Pohl R, Balon R, Berchou R. Reaction to chicken nuggets in a patient taking an MAOI. *Am J Psychiatry* (1988) 145, 651.
4. Lee S, Wing YK. MAOI and monosodium glutamate interaction. *J Clin Psychiatry* (1991) 52, 43.

MAOIs + Opioids; Fentanyl and related drugs

Fentanyl has been used without problems in a few reports, but one fatal case of hyperthermia has occurred, and also a case of hypertension and tachycardia. Case reports describe the uneventful use of alfentanil, remifentanil and sufentanil in patients taking MAOIs.

Clinical evidence

(a) Alfentanil

A 54-year-old woman taking **tranylcypromine** with trifluoperazine underwent general anaesthesia with no problems. She received temazepam as premedication, and propofol induction. Supplementary alfentanil was given in increments of 250 micrograms to a total of 2.5 mg. Atracurium was given for neuromuscular block with 100% oxygen for ventilation.[1] Similarly, another report describes successful anaesthesia using propofol, alfentanil 25 micrograms/kg, and succinylcholine during ECT therapy in two patients taking a variety of drugs including **phenelzine**.[2]

(b) Fentanyl

A 71-year-old woman taking ***Parstelin*** (**tranylcypromine** with trifluoperazine) was given an intravenous test dose of fentanyl 20 micrograms and diazepam before surgery, without problems. She was then given another 20-microgram intravenous dose of fentanyl during surgery, followed by an epidural bolus infusion of fentanyl 50 micrograms 15 minutes before the end of the surgery. After surgery she was given a continuous epidural infusion of fentanyl 50 to 70 micrograms/hour for 4 days to control postoperative pain, also without problems.[3] Similarly, another report describes 2 patients who had stopped taking **phenelzine** 36 hours and 10 days before undergoing uneventful cardiac surgery using fentanyl, pancuronium and 100% oxygen.[4] Four further patients taking **tranylcypromine**, **isocarboxazid**, or **pargyline** had no adverse reactions to fentanyl given during surgery (3 cases) or for postoperative pain relief (3 cases).[5]

In contrast, a man taking **tranylcypromine** who received fentanyl during and after surgery developed postoperative hypertension, hyperthermia, and severe shivering followed by resistant hypotension, and finally died.[6] Another patient taking **phenelzine** who underwent cardiac surgery, with anaesthesia maintained by fentanyl and midazolam, developed hypertension and supraventricular tachycardia, which did not respond to digoxin and esmolol. About 15 minutes after stopping the fentanyl/midazolam and starting enflurane, the haemodynamics gradually improved, and analgesia was subsequently managed with ketorolac without problems.[7]

(c) Remifentanil

A patient taking **phenelzine** was given remifentanil for the maintenance of anaesthesia without adverse effect. An adverse interaction was considered unlikely with this combination.[8]

(d) Sufentanil

A 43-year-old woman taking **tranylcypromine** 60 mg daily underwent general anaesthesia with sufentanil, isoflurane, and nitrous oxide without problem.[9]

Mechanism, importance and management

Fentanyl has been used safely in a number of patients receiving MAOIs. However, a fatality due to a serotonin-like syndrome has occurred in a patient taking an MAOI given fentanyl, and another case of hypertension and tachycardia has occurred. The authors of one of these reports, considered that there was insufficient evidence to conclude that patients on MAOIs can be given fentanyl safely, and call for all cases of combined use to be reported.[6] Case reports also describe the safe use of alfentanil, remifentanil, and sufentanil. However, one UK manufacturer of fentanyl *patches* recommends that they should not be used during the use of, or within 14 days of stopping, an MAOI.[10]

Note that fentanyl and related drugs are frequently used during surgery, and it is generally considered that MAOIs should be discontinued 2 weeks before surgery, see 'Anaesthetics, general + MAOIs', p.100.

1. Powell H. Use of alfentanil in a patient receiving monoamine oxidase inhibitor therapy. *Br J Anaesth* (1990) 64, 528.
2. Beresford BJ, Glick D, Dinwiddie SH. Combination propofol-alfentanil anesthesia for electroconvulsive therapy in patients receiving monoamine oxidase inhibitors. *J ECT* (2004) 20, 120–2.
3. Youssef MS, Wilkinson PA. Epidural fentanyl and monoamine oxidase inhibitors. *Anaesthesia* (1988) 43, 210–12.
4. Michaels I, Serrins M, Shier NQ, Barash PG. Anesthesia for cardiac surgery in patients receiving monoamine oxidase inhibitors. *Anesth Analg* (1984) 63, 1041–4.
5. El-Ganzouri AR, Ivankovich AD, Braverman B, McCarthy R. Monoamine oxidase inhibitors: should they be discontinued preoperatively? *Anesth Analg* (1985) 64, 592–6.
6. Noble WH, Baker A. MAO inhibitors and coronary artery surgery: a patient death. *Can J Anaesth* (1992) 39, 1061–6.
7. Insler SR, Kraenzler EJ, Licina MG, Savage RM, Starr NJ. Cardiac surgery in a patient taking monoamine oxidase inhibitors: an adverse fentanyl reaction. *Anesth Analg* (1994) 78, 593–7.
8. Ure DS, Gillies MA, James KS. Safe use of remifentanil in a patient treated with the monoamine oxidase inhibitor phenelzine. *Br J Anaesth* (2000) 84, 414–16.
9. O'Hara JF, Maurer WG, Smith MP. Sufentanil-isoflurane-nitrous oxide anesthesia for a patient treated with monoamine oxidase inhibitor and tricyclic antidepressant. *J Clin Anesth* (1995) 7, 148–50.
10. Matrifen (Fentanyl). Nycomed UK Ltd. UK Summary of product characteristics, June 2007.

MAOIs or RIMAs + Opioids; Dextropropoxyphene (Propoxyphene)

An isolated report describes 'leg shakes', diaphoresis and severe hypotension in a woman taking phenelzine when she was given dextropropoxyphene. Another isolated report describes a marked increase in sedation when a woman was given phenelzine and dextropropoxyphene. *Animal* data show moclobemide potentiates dextropropoxyphene.

Clinical evidence, mechanism, importance and management

(a) MAOIs

A woman taking **phenelzine** 15 mg three times daily, sodium valproate, lithium and trazodone, was given dextropropoxyphene 100 mg and paracetamol (acetaminophen) 650 mg for back pain and headache. Some 12 hours later she was admitted to hospital for leg shakes, discomfort and weakness. She was confused and anxious, and intensely diaphoretic. The next day she became severely hypotensive (systolic BP 55 to 60 mmHg) and needed large fluid volume resuscitation in intensive care. She later recovered fully.[1] Another woman taking propranolol, oestrogen-replacement therapy and **phenelzine** became very sedated and groggy, causing her to have to lie down on two occasions, both within 2 hours of taking dextropropoxyphene 100 mg and paracetamol 650 mg. She had experienced no problems with either paracetamol or dextropropoxyphene/paracetamol before starting the **phenelzine**, and subsequently had no problems with paracetamol alone while continuing the **phenelzine**.[2] The mechanisms of these interactions are not understood but some of the symptoms in the first case were not unlike those seen in the serotonin syndrome.

Apart from these two isolated reports, there seems to be no other clinical evidence of adverse interactions between MAOIs and dextropropoxyphene. For reports of the serotonin syndrome seen with pethidine (meperidine) and MAOIs, see 'MAOIs or RIMAs + Opioids; Pethidine (Meperidine)', p.1140.

(b) RIMAs

In *animals,* the effects of dextropropoxyphene were increased by **moclobemide**.[3] A brief mention is made of 3 patients, taking **moclobemide** and codeine (2 patients) or dextropropoxyphene (1 patient): one of these patients developed moderate agitation.[3]

1. Zornberg GL, Hegarty JD. Adverse interaction between propoxyphene and phenelzine. *Am J Psychiatry* (1993) 150, 1270–1.
2. Garbutt JC. Potentiation of propoxyphene by phenelzine. *Am J Psychiatry* (1987) 144, 251–2.
3. Amrein R, Güntert TW, Dingemanse J, Lorscheid T, Stabl M, Schmid-Burgk W. Interactions of moclobemide with concomitantly administered medication: evidence from pharmacological and clinical studies. *Psychopharmacology (Berl)* (1992) 106, S24–S31.

MAOIs + Opioids; Miscellaneous

Hypotension (profound in one case) has been seen in a few patients given morphine and an MAOI. One case of hypotension and stupor has occurred with papaveretum. Single cases of the safe use of methadone and hydromorphone have also been described.

Clinical evidence

(a) Hydromorphone

No problems were encountered when a patient taking **tranylcypromine** was given hydromorphone via a patient-controlled device for postoperative pain.[1] This patient also received sufentanil during surgery without problem.

(b) Methadone

A patient receiving methadone maintenance therapy (30 mg daily) was successfully and uneventfully treated for depression with **tranylcypromine**, initially 10 mg daily gradually increased to 30 mg daily.[2]

(c) Morphine

A study in 15 patients who had been taking either **phenelzine**, **isocarboxazid**, **iproniazid** or *Parstelin* (**tranylcypromine** with trifluoperazine) for 3 to 8 weeks, had no changes in blood pressure, pulse rate or state of awareness when given test doses of up to 4 mg of intramuscular morphine. However, note that none of these patients showed an interaction with test doses of up to 40 mg of **pethidine** (meperidine).[3] One other study reported no adverse interaction in 3 patients taking **isocarboxazid** when they were given morphine premedication,[4] and a further study revealed no problems in 9 patients taking **tranylcypromine** who were given morphine for postoperative pain relief.[5] Another patient taking **phenelzine** was uneventfully treated with morphine postoperatively.[6] Two further patients taking MAOIs, who reacted adversely to **pethidine** (meperidine),[7,8] had not previously done so when given morphine. In an early report, intramuscular morphine was given without apparent problem to 5 patients who had developed severe headache while taking **tranylcypromine**.[9] Another author briefly noted that he knew of about 10 cases where morphine had been used in patients taking MAOIs with no adverse effects except a more prolonged morphine action.[10]

However, a patient taking **tranylcypromine** 40 mg and trifluoperazine 20 mg daily and undergoing a preoperative test with morphine, developed pin point pupils, became unconscious and unresponsive to stimuli, and had a systolic blood pressure fall from 160 to 40 mmHg after receiving a total of 6 mg of morphine intravenously. Within 2 minutes of being given naloxone 4 mg intravenously, the patient was awake and rational with a systolic blood pressure fully restored.[11] A moderate fall in blood pressure (from 140/90 to 90/60 mmHg) was seen in another patient taking an MAOI given morphine,[12] and a brief episode of hypotension treated with phenylephrine occurred in a patient taking **phenelzine** receiving continuous epidural morphine during surgery.[5]

(d) Papaveretum

A 54-year-old woman taking **phenelzine** was given papaveretum 10 mg as premedication, and 50 minutes later she was found to be unrousable, sweating and hypotensive.[13]

Mechanism, importance and management

This serious MAOI/pethidine interaction also casts a shadow over morphine, which probably accounts for its inclusion in a number of lists and charts of drugs said to interact with the MAOIs. However, there is some limited evidence that patients on MAOIs who had reacted adversely with pethidine did not do so when given morphine,[7,8] and quite a number of reports of its safe use. The few hypotensive reactions cited here[5,11,12] are of a different character and appear to be rare. There would therefore seem to be no good reason for avoiding morphine in patients taking MAOIs, but be alert for the rare adverse response. However, several manufacturers have contraindicated concurrent use of morphine in patients taking MAOIs or within 2 weeks of stopping an MAOI,[14-16] because they can cause CNS adverse effects with hyper- or hypotension.[14,15] A similar situation exists with codeine: one UK manufacturer of a codeine/paracetamol product states that concurrent use of codeine with an MAOI may increase the effects of both drugs;[17] however another contraindicates the use of codeine, both with and within 14 days of stopping an MAOI.[18] Some recommend lower initial dosages of morphine or oxycodone, frequent monitoring, and gradual upward dose titration.[19] One case report suggests that MAOIs can be given to patients on methadone, but the evidence is clearly limited.

1. O'Hara JF, Maurer WG, Smith MP. Sufentanil-isoflurane-nitrous oxide anesthesia for a patient treated with monoamine oxidase inhibitor and tricyclic antidepressant. *J Clin Anesth* (1995) 7, 148–50.
2. Mendelson G. Narcotics and monoamine oxidase-inhibitors. *Med J Aust* (1979) 1, 400.
3. Evans-Prosser CDG. The use of pethidine and morphine in the presence of monoamine oxidase inhibitors. *Br J Anaesth* (1968) 40, 279–82.
4. Ebrahim ZY, O'Hara J, Borden L, Tetzlaff J. Monoamine oxidase inhibitors and elective surgery. *Cleve Clin J Med* (1993) 60, 129–130.
5. El-Ganzouri AR, Ivankovich AD, Braverman B, McCarthy R. Monoamine oxidase inhibitors: should they be discontinued preoperatively? *Anesth Analg* (1985) 64, 592–6.
6. Ure DS, Gillies MA, James KS. Safe use of remifentanil in a patient treated with the monoamine oxidase inhibitor phenelzine. *Br J Anaesth* (2000) 84, 414–16.
7. Shee JC. Dangerous potentiation of pethidine by iproniazid, and its treatment. *BMJ* (1960) 2, 507–9.
8. Palmer H. Potentiation of pethidine. *BMJ* (1960) 2, 944.
9. Brown DD, Waldron DH. An unusual reaction to tranylcypromine. *Practitioner* (1962) 189, 83–6.
10. Sargant W. Interactions with monoamine oxidase inhibitors. *BMJ* (1975) 4, 101.
11. Barry BJ. Adverse effects of MAO inhibitors with narcotics reversed with naloxone. *Anaesth Intensive Care* (1979) 7, 194.
12. Jenkins LC, Graves HB. Potential hazards of psychoactive drugs in association with anaesthesia. *Can Anaesth Soc J* (1965) 12, 121–8.
13. Spencer GT, Smith SE. Dangers of monoamine oxidase inhibitors. *BMJ* (1963) 1,750.
14. MST Continus (Morphine sulfate). Napp Pharmaceuticals Ltd. UK summary of product characteristics, June 2001.
15. Oramorph (Morphine sulfate). Boehringer Ingelheim. UK Summary of product characteristics, July 2006.
16. Morphgesic SR (Morphine sulfate). Amdipharm. UK Summary of product characteristics, January 2003
17. Tylex (Codeine/Paracetamol). Schwartz Pharma Ltd. UK Summary of product characteristics, October 2006.
18. Solpadol (Codeine/Paracetamol). Sanofi-Aventis. UK Summary of product characteristics, July 2006.
19. Gratz SS, Simpson GM. MAOI-Narcotic interactions. *J Clin Psychiatry* (1993) 54, 439.

MAOIs or RIMAs + Opioids; Pethidine (Meperidine)

The concurrent use of pethidine and MAOIs has resulted in a serious and potentially life-threatening reaction in several patients, and one possible case has been reported with moclobemide. Excitement, muscle rigidity, hyperpyrexia, flushing, sweating and unconsciousness can occur very rapidly. Respiratory depression and hypertension or hypotension have also been seen. Pethidine should not be given to patients taking any MAOI or RIMA.

Clinical evidence

(a) MAOIs

Severe, rapid and potentially fatal toxic reactions, both excitatory and depressant can occur:

A woman stopped taking **iproniazid** 50 mg twice daily and about a day and a half later became restless and incoherent almost immediately after being given pethidine 100 mg for chest pain. She was comatose within 20 minutes. An hour after receiving the injection she was flushed, sweating and showed Cheyne-Stokes respiration. Her pupils were dilated and unreactive. Deep reflexes could not be initiated and plantar reflexes were extensor. Her pulse rate was 82 bpm and blood pressure 156/110 mmHg. She was rousable within 10 minutes of receiving an intravenous injection of prednisolone hemisuccinate 25 mg. A very similar reaction was described in another patient.[1]

A woman who, unknown to her doctor, was taking **tranylcypromine**, was given pethidine 100 mg. Within minutes she became unconscious, noisy and restless, having to be held down by 3 people. Her breathing was stertorous and the pulse impalpable. Generalised tonic spasm developed, with ankle clonus, extensor plantar reflexes, shallow respiration and cyanosis. On admission to hospital she had a pulse rate of 160 bpm, a blood pressure of 90/60 mmHg and was sweating profusely (temperature 38.3°C). Her condition gradually improved and 4 hours after admission she was conscious but drowsy. Recovery was complete the next day.[2]

Other cases of this interaction have been reported in patients treated with **iproniazid**,[3-5] **pargyline**,[6,7] **phenelzine**,[8-13] and **mebanazine**.[14] Fatalities have occurred. One of 8 patients taking an MAOI and given test doses of pethidine experienced a drop in systolic blood pressure of 30 mmHg and a rise in pulse rate of 20 bpm after the first 5-mg dose of pethidine.[15] However, a study in 15 patients who had been taking either **phenelzine**, **isocarboxazid**, **iproniazid** or *Parstelin* (**tranylcypromine** with trifluoperazine) for 3 to 8 weeks, found no changes in blood pressure, pulse rate or state of awareness with test doses of up to 40 mg of pethidine.[16] Similarly, no major problems were noted in a retrospective review of 45 episodes of anaesthesia in patients taking **isocarboxazid** who were given pethidine as part of premedication.[17]

(b) RIMAs

One report suggests that on the basis of *animal* studies the combination of **moclobemide** and pethidine should be avoided or used with caution.[18] A report of suspected serotonin syndrome in a 73-year-old woman, given pethidine in addition to her usual treatment with **moclobemide** 750 mg daily, nortriptyline 100 mg daily and lithium 750 mg daily, adds some weight to this suggestion.[19]

Mechanism

Not understood, despite the extensive studies undertaken.[20-22] The reaction has proved difficult to study in *animals*, since mice appear to be more sensitive to the reaction than humans. There is some evidence that the reactions may be due to an increase in levels of 5-HT within the brain, causing 'the serotonin syndrome', (p.9). Tramadol, an opioid with additional noradrenergic and serotonergic properties, has clearly caused the serotonin syndrome when used with MAOIs, see 'tramadol', (p.1141).

Importance and management

The interaction between pethidine and the MAOIs, which was first observed in the mid-1950s, is based on case reports. One case has been reported with RIMA moclobemide. It is serious and potentially fatal. Its incidence is unknown, but it is probably quite low, because one study that attempted to produce the interaction by giving increasing test doses of pethidine to 15 patients taking various MAOIs did not show the interaction.[16] It may therefore be an idiosyncratic reaction. Nevertheless, it would be imprudent to give pethidine to any patients on an MAOI or RIMA. Bear in mind that the older MAOIs are all essentially irreversible so that an interaction is possible for many days after their withdrawal (at least 2 weeks is the official advice), whereas the newer RIMAs (e.g. moclobemide) are reversible and unlikely still to interact 48 hours after they have been stopped.

Sensitivity test

A sensitivity test has been suggested,[15] but given the fact that there are many alternatives to pethidine and MAOIs readily available, and given that a drop in systolic blood pressure of 30 mmHg has been reported even with the first step of the test dose (5 mg of pethidine)[15] it would seem prudent to avoid the combination. Also, the test dose procedure is unlikely to be suitable when opioids are required in an emergency situation.

1. Shee JC. Dangerous potentiation of pethidine by iproniazid, and its treatment. *BMJ* (1960) 2, 507–9.
2. Denton PH, Borrelli VM, Edwards NV. Dangers of monoamine oxidase inhibitors. *BMJ* (1962) 2, 1752–3.
3. Clement AJ, Benazon D. Reactions to other drugs in patients taking monoamine-oxidase inhibitors. *Lancet* (1962) ii, 197–8.
4. Papp C, Benaim S. Toxic effects of iproniazid in a patient with angina. *BMJ* (1958) 2, 1070–2.
5. Mitchell RS. Fatal toxic encephalitis occurring during iproniazid therapy in pulmonary tuberculosis. *Ann Intern Med* (1955) 42, 417–24.
6. Vigran IM. Dangerous potentiation of meperidine hydrochloride by pargyline hydrochloride. *JAMA* (1964) 187, 953–4.
7. Jenkins LC, Graves HB. Potential hazards of psychoactive drugs in association with anaesthesia. *Can Anaesth Soc J* (1965) 12, 121–8.
8. Palmer H. Potentiation of pethidine. *BMJ* (1960) 2, 944.
9. Taylor DC. Alarming reaction to pethidine in patients on phenelzine. *Lancet* (1962) ii, 401–2.
10. Cocks DP, Passmore-Rowe A. Dangers of monoamine oxidase inhibitors. *BMJ* (1962) 2, 1545–6.
11. Reid NCRW, Jones D. Pethidine and phenelzine. *BMJ* (1962) 1, 408.
12. Meyer D, Halfin V. Toxicity secondary to meperidine in patients on monoamine oxidase inhibitors: a case report and critical review. *J Clin Psychopharmacol* (1981) 1, 319–21.
13. Asch DA, Parker RM. Sounding board. The Libby Zion case. One step forward or two steps backward? *N Engl J Med* (1988) 318, 771–5.
14. Anon. Death from drugs combination. *Pharm J* (1965) 195, 341.
15. Churchill-Davidson HC. Anaesthesia and monoamine oxidase inhibitors. *BMJ* (1965) 1, 520.
16. Evans-Prosser CDG. The use of pethidine and morphine in the presence of monoamine oxidase inhibitors. *Br J Anaesth* (1968) 40, 279–82.
17. Ebrahim ZY, O'Hara J, Borden L, Tetzlaff J. Monoamine oxidase inhibitors and elective surgery. *Cleve Clin J Med* (1993) 60, 129–130.
18. Amrein R, Güntert TW, Dingemanse J, Lorscheid T, Stabl M, Schmid-Burgk W. Interactions of moclobemide with concomitantly administered medication: evidence from pharmacological and clinical studies. *Psychopharmacology (Berl)* (1992) 106, S24–S31.
19. Gillman PK. Possible serotonin syndrome with moclobemide and pethidine. *Med J Aust* (1995) 162, 554.

20. Leander JD, Batten J, Hargis GW. Pethidine interaction with clorgyline, pargyline or 5-hydroxytryptophan: lack of enhanced pethidine lethality or hyperpyrexia in mice. *J Pharm Pharmacol* (1978) 30, 396–8.
21. Rogers KJ, Thornton JA. The interaction between monoamine oxidase inhibitors and narcotic analgesics in mice. *Br J Pharmacol* (1969) 36, 470–80.
22. Gessner PK, Soble AG. A study of the tranylcypromine-meperidine interaction: effects of *p*-chlorophenylalanine and *l*-5-hydroxytryptophan. *J Pharmacol Exp Ther* (1973) 186, 276–87.

MAOIs + Opioids; Tramadol

The serotonin syndrome developed in one patient on iproniazid and tramadol, and delirium in another given tramadol shortly after stopping phenelzine. A fatal case of possible serotonin syndrome has been seen with tramadol, moclobemide and clomipramine.

Clinical evidence, mechanism, importance and management

The manufacturers of tramadol contraindicated its use with the MAOIs[1,2] on the basis that it is an opioid agonist, like pethidine (meperidine). This may mean the serotonin syndrome could develop (see 'MAOIs or RIMAs + Opioids; Pethidine (Meperidine)', p.1140). This prediction was confirmed by a report[3] of the development of the serotonin syndrome (myoclonus, tremor, sweating, hyperreflexia, tachycardia) in a patient on **iproniazid** when tramadol was added to his drug regimen. When the tramadol was stopped the patient recovered within 48 hours. Another single case report describes the development of severe delirium in a patient within 3 days of stopping long term treatment with **phenelzine** 45 mg daily and starting intramuscular tramadol 100 mg three times daily. The patient became anxious and confused, and developed visual hallucinations and persecutory ideation. The symptoms disappeared within 48 hours of stopping the tramadol.[4] Another report suggests that tramadol may have contributed to the development of a fatal serotonin syndrome in a patient abusing tramadol, **moclobemide** and clomipramine.[5]

This demonstrates that there are sound practical and theoretical reasons for patients on MAOIs to avoid tramadol. Note that the serotonin syndrome has also occurred with 'tramadol and SSRIs', (p.1222).

1. Zydol SR (Tramadol hydrochloride). Grünenthal Ltd. UK Summary of product characteristics, February 2005.
2. Ultram (Tramadol hydrochloride). Ortho-McNeil Pharmaceutical, Inc. US Prescribing information, May 2004.
3. de Larquier A, Vial T, Bréjoux G, Descotes J. Syndrome sérotoninergique lors de l'association tramadol et iproniazide. *Therapie* (1999) 54, 767–8.
4. Calvisi V, Ansseau M. Confusion mentale liée à l'administration de tramadol chez une patiente sous IMAO. *Rev Med Liege* (1999) 54, 912–3.
5. Hernandez AF, Montero MN, Pla A, Villanueva E. Fatal moclobemide overdose or death caused by serotonin syndrome? *J Forensic Sci* (1995) 40, 128–30.

MAOIs or RIMAs + Phenothiazines

The concurrent use of MAOIs and phenothiazines is usually safe and effective. However, rarely, cases of possible neuroleptic malignant syndrome or hyperpyrexia have been reported with MAOIs and chlorpromazine, levomepromazine or trifluoperazine. Some of these cases were fatal. Chlorpromazine has been successfully used for treatment of the serotonin syndrome occurring with MAOIs and other drugs. Moclobemide has been used with various phenothiazines without problem, but one case of fatal overdose is attributed to an interaction between moclobemide and perazine.

Clinical evidence

(a) MAOIs

MAOIs and phenothiazines have been safe and effective when used together in the treatment of psychiatric conditions, particularly in the form of a preparation containing both **tranylcypromine** and **trifluoperazine**,[1-3] which is still marketed in some countries. There is also a report of the beneficial use of **tranylcypromine** with **chlorpromazine**.[4]

However, rarely, cases suggestive of the neuroleptic malignant syndrome or similar have been reported. In one case, a 70-year-old woman taking **isocarboxazid** 10 mg daily and **chlorpromazine** 25 mg three times daily, suddenly developed dyspnoea, tachycardia, pyrexia, muscular rigidity, hypotension, and became comatose. Her condition initially improved over 24 hours, but she later died from acute renal failure as a result of rhabdomyolysis. Throughout the previous 2 years of inpatient care, the patient had received neuroleptics intermittently and had developed an unexplained toxic confusional state on 6 occasions, which suggested that the neuroleptic malignant syndrome had a milder chronic course in this patient before the full acute syndrome developed.[5] In another case, a woman presented with symptoms of the neuroleptic malignant syndrome one week after starting **tranylcypromine/trifluoperazine** 10/1 mg and immediately after doubling the dose. She was intubated and treated with dantrolene and intravenous sodium bicarbonate, and made a full recovery.[6] Interpretation of her case is complicated by the fact she had been previously taking imipramine, and was switched to tranylcypromine/trifluoperazine without a break (see also 'MAOIs or RIMAs + Tricyclic and related antidepressants', p.1149). One study mentions an unexplained fatality in a woman who suddenly developed hyperthermia and coma while taking **levomepromazine** and **pargyline**.[7] Another report briefly mentions a woman who developed fatal hyperthermia while taking **levomepromazine** and **tranylcypromine**,[8] and a fatality following the use of an unnamed MAOI/phenothiazine combination.[8] Note that **chlorpromazine**[9] has 5-HT antagonist activity, and has been successfully used in the treatment of severe serotonin syndrome occurring with 'MAOIs and tricyclic antidepressants', (p.1149).

One early reviewer stated that MAOIs increase the potency of phenothiazine derivatives such that their initial dose should be reduced by three-quarters. He briefly mentions a case of a patient taking long-term **perphenazine** who developed a Parkinson-like syndrome with extrapyramidal symptoms a few hours after starting an MAOI.[10] The US manufacturers note that, based on the increased incidence of extrapyramidal effects reported with concurrent use of some MAOIs and phenothiazines, this possibility should be considered with **promethazine**.[11]

A report attributes 2 cases of fatal fulminant hepatitis to an interaction between **iproniazid** and **prochlorperazine**.[12]

A single report[13] describes a woman taking an MAOI who developed a severe occipital headache after taking 30 mL of a paediatric cough linctus. Initially this interaction was attributed to **promethazine**, but it is now known that the linctus in question contained phenylpropanolamine, which is much more likely to have been the cause.[14] See 'MAOIs or RIMAs + Sympathomimetics; Indirectly-acting', p.1147 for the interaction with phenylpropanolamine.

(b) RIMAs

Clinically relevant interactions were not noted when **moclobemide** was given with one or more neuroleptics (including phenothiazines such as **chlorpromazine**, **levomepromazine**, **thioridazine**). Adverse effects such as hypotension, tachycardia, drowsiness, tremor, and constipation were somewhat more frequent, probably due to additive effects.[15] A fatal case of overdose with **moclobemide** and **perazine** was attributed to synergistic effects resulting in functional cardiovascular disorder.[16]

Mechanism

Neuroleptic malignant syndrome (NMS) is a rare condition associated with a reduction in dopamine activity in the brain, which has occurred with a wide variety of dopamine antagonists including the phenothiazines. It is unclear what role, if any, is played by the MAOIs in the few possible cases cited here. Note that MAOIs can cause the similar serotonin syndrome, and it is important to differentiate between the two conditions, especially since phenothiazines would aggravate NMS, but can successfully treat the serotonin syndrome.

Importance and management

No special precautions would normally seem to be necessary during the concurrent use of MAOIs and phenothiazines. However, bear in mind that serious, sometimes fatal, cases of the neuroleptic malignant syndrome or hyperpyrexia have rarely occurred with combinations of MAOIs and **chlorpromazine**, **levomepromazine** and **trifluoperazine**. The role of the MAOI in these cases is unclear. Chlorpromazine has been used successfully to treat the serotonin syndrome occurring with MAOIs and other serotonergic drugs, but note that it should be avoided if neuroleptic malignant syndrome is a possible diagnosis, or if the patient is hypotensive, see 'MAOIs or RIMAs + Tricyclic and related antidepressants', p.1149.

1. Winkelman NW. Three evaluations of a monoamine oxidase inhibitor and phenothiazine combination (a methodological and clinical study). *Dis Nerv Syst* (1965) 26, 160–4.
2. Chesrow EJ, Kaplitz SE. Anxiety and depression in the geriatric and chronically ill patient. *Clin Med* (1965) 72, 1281–4.

3. Janecek J, Schiele BC, Bellville T, Anderson R. The effects of withdrawal of trifluoperazine on patients maintained on the combination of tranylcypromine and trifluoperazine. A double blind study. *Curr Ther Res* (1963) 5, 608–15.
4. Bucci L. The negative symptoms of schizophrenia and the monoamine oxidase inhibitors. *Psychopharmacology (Berl)* (1987) 91, 104–8.
5. Jones EM, Dawson A. Neuroleptic malignant syndrome: a case report with post-mortem brain and muscle pathology. *J Neurol Neurosurg Psychiatry* (1989) 52, 1006–9.
6. Lappa A, Podestà M. Capelli O, Castagna A, Di Placido G, Alampi D, Semeraro F. Successful treatment of a complicated case of neuroleptic malignant syndrome. *Intensive Care Med* (2002) 28, 976–7.
7. Barsa JA, Saunders JC. A comparative study of tranylcypromine and pargyline. *Psychopharmacologia* (1964) 6, 295–8.
8. McQueen EG. New Zealand Committee on Adverse Drug Reactions: fourteenth annual report 1979. *N Z Med J* (1980) 91, 226–9.
9. Graham PM. Successful treatment of the toxic serotonin syndrome with chlorpromazine. *Med J Aust* (1997) 166, 166–7.
10. Kline NS. Psychopharmaceuticals: effects and side effects. *Bull WHO* (1959) 21, 397–410.
11. Phenergan (Promethazine). Wyeth Pharmaceuticals Inc. US Prescribing information. July 2005.
12. Capron J-P, Gineston J-L, Opolon P, Dupas J-L, Denis J, Quénum C, Lorriaux A. Hépatite fulminante mortelle due a l'association iproniazide-prochlorpérazine: deux cas. *Gastroenterol Clin Biol* (1980) 4, 123–7.
13. Mitchell L. Psychotropic drugs. *BMJ* (1968) 1, 381.
14. Griffin JP, D'Arcy PF eds. A Manual of Adverse Drug Interactions. 2nd ed Bristol: Wright; 1979. p. 174.
15. Amrein R, Güntert TW, Dingemanse J, Lorscheid T, Stabl M, Schmid-Burgk W. Interactions of moclobemide with concomitantly administered medication: evidence from pharmacological and clinical studies. *Psychopharmacology (Berl)* (1992) 106, S24–S31.
16. Musshoff F, Varchmin-Schultheiss K, Madea B. Suicide with moclobemide and perazine. *Int J Legal Med* (1998) 111, 196–8.

MAOIs + Rauwolfia alkaloids or Tetrabenazine

Central excitation and possibly hypertension can occur if rauwolfia alkaloids are given to patients already taking an MAOI, but is less likely if the rauwolfia alkaloid is given first. Theoretically additive blood-pressure lowering effects are also a possibility. The use of drugs that have the potential to cause depression, such as the rauwolfia alkaloids or tetrabenazine, is generally contraindicated in patients needing treatment for depression.

Clinical evidence

A woman with a history of manic depression who had been in a depressed phase for 5 years was given **nialamide** 100 mg three times daily. Two days later, **reserpine** 500 micrograms three times daily was also started. The following day she became frankly hypomanic and almost immediately went into mania.[1]

In another report,[2] a patient, who was started on **tetrabenazine** 10 mg three times daily, 2 days after stopping a week of treatment with **nialamide** 25 mg daily, collapsed 6 hours after the first dose, and demonstrated epileptiform convulsions, partial unconsciousness, rapid respiration and tachycardia. He recovered within 15 minutes, but 3 days later he had a similar attack and the **tetrabenazine** was stopped.

Another author states that the use of **reserpine** or **tetrabenazine** after pretreatment with **iproniazid** can lead to a temporary disturbance of affect and memory, associated with autonomic excitation, delirious agitation, disorientation and illusions of experience and recognition, which lasts for up to 3 days.[3,4]

A prolonged period of increased motor activity after starting **reserpine** ('reserpine-reversal') possibly occurred in 3 patients with schizophrenia treated firstly with **phenelzine** for 12 weeks, then a placebo for 16 to 33 weeks, and lastly **reserpine** for 12 weeks, when compared with patients receiving **reserpine** who had not received an MAOI. Their blood pressures rose slightly and persistently, and their psychomotor activity was considerably increased, lasting in two cases throughout the 12-week period of treatment.[5]

Theoretically, **reserpine** might cause hypertension in patients treated with non-selective MAOIs (see Mechanism). On the basis of this the US manufacturer of **tranylcypromine**[6] contraindicates concurrent use. Conversely, the UK manufacturer of **isocarboxazid**[7] mentions that it may potentiate the hypotensive effect of **reserpine** (MAOIs alone can have hypotensive effects).

Mechanism

Rauwolfia alkaloids such as reserpine cause adrenergic neurones to become depleted of their normal stores of noradrenaline (norepinephrine). In this way they prevent or reduce the normal transmission of impulses at the adrenergic nerve endings of the sympathetic nervous system and thereby act as antihypertensives. Since the brain also possesses adrenergic neurones, failure of transmission in the CNS could account for the sedation and depression observed with these drugs. If rauwolfia alkaloids are given to patients already taking an MAOI, large amounts of accumulated noradrenaline can be released throughout the body. In the brain, 5-HT is also released. The release of these substances results in marked central excitation and hypertension. This would account for the case reports cited and the effects seen in *animals*.[8-10] These stimulant effects are sometimes called 'reserpine-reversal' because instead of the expected sedation or depression, excitation or delayed depression is seen. It depends upon the order in which the drugs are given.

Importance and management

The use of drugs that have the potential to cause depression is generally contraindicated in patients needing treatment for depression. However, one report suggests that if concurrent use is considered desirable, the MAOIs should be given after, and not before the rauwolfia alkaloid, so that sedation rather than excitation will occur.[11] Bear in mind the possibility of hypo- or hypertension.

1. Gradwell BG. Psychotic reactions and phenelzine. *BMJ* (1960) 2, 1018.
2. Davies TS. Monoamine oxidase inhibitors and rauwolfia compounds. *BMJ* (1960) 2, 739–40.
3. Voelkel A. Klinische Wirkung von Pharmaka mit Einfluss auf den Monoaminestoffwechsel de Gehirns. *Confin Neurol* (1958) 18, 144–9.
4. Voelkel A. Clinical experiences with amine oxidase inhibitors in psychiatry. *Ann N Y Acad Sci* (1959) 80, 680–6.
5. Esser AH. Clinical observations on reserpine reversal after prolonged MAO inhibition. *Psychiatr Neurol Neurochir* (1967) 70, 59–63.
6. Parnate (Tranylcypromine sulfate). GlaxoSmithKline. US Prescribing information, June 2007.
7. Isocarboxazid. Cambridge Laboratories. UK Summary of product characteristics, March 2000.
8. Shore PA, Brodie BB. LSD-like effects elicited by reserpine in rabbits pretreated with isoniazid. *Proc Soc Exp Biol Med* (1957) 94, 433–5.
9. Chessin M, Kramer ER, Scott CC. Modification of the pharmacology of reserpine and serotonin by iproniazid. *J Pharmacol Exp Ther* (1957) 119, 453–60.
10. von Euler US, Bygdeman S, Persson N-Å. Interaction of reserpine and monoamine oxidase inhibitors on adrenergic transmitter release. *Biochim Biol Sper* (1970) 9, 215–20.
11. Natarajan S. Potential danger of monoamineoxidase inhibitors and α-methyldopa. *Lancet* (1964) i, 1330.

MAOIs or RIMAs + SSRIs

A number of case reports describe the serotonin syndrome in patients given SSRIs with MAOIs: some have been fatal. Concurrent use is contraindicated. Some studies suggest that moclobemide may not interact with the SSRIs, but there have also been case reports of the serotonin syndrome and concurrent use is contraindicated. A suitable washout interval is needed when switching between MAOIs or RIMAs and SSRIs.

Clinical evidence, mechanism, importance and management

A. MAOIs

(a) Fluoxetine

A very high incidence (25 to 50%) of adverse effects occurred in 12 patients taking fluoxetine 10 to 100 mg daily with either **phenelzine** 30 to 60 mg daily or **tranylcypromine** 10 to 140 mg daily, and in 6 other patients started on either of these MAOIs 10 days or more after stopping fluoxetine. There were mental changes such as hypomania, racing thoughts, agitation, restlessness and confusion. The physical symptoms included myoclonus, hypertension, tremor, teeth chattering and diarrhoea.[1]

A detailed review of cases reported to the manufacturers described 8 acute cases, 7 of them fatal, in patients given fluoxetine with either **tranylcypromine** or **phenelzine**.[2] Uncontrollable shivering, teeth chattering, double vision, nausea, confusion, and anxiety developed in a woman given **tranylcypromine** after stopping fluoxetine. The problem resolved within a day of stopping the **tranylcypromine**, and did not recur when fluoxetine was tried again 6 weeks later.[3]

A number of other reports describe similar reactions in patients given fluoxetine and **tranylcypromine**,[3-8] some occurring up to 6 weeks after the SSRI was stopped,[6] and several resulting in fatalities.[3,7]

(b) Sertraline

A man taking **tranylcypromine** and clonazepam was additionally given sertraline 25 to 50 mg daily. Within 4 days he began to experience chills, increasing confusion, sedation, exhaustion, unsteadiness and incoordination. Other symptoms included impotence, urinary hesitancy and constipation. These problems rapidly resolved when the sertraline was stopped and the **tranylcypromine** dosage reduced from 30 to 20 mg daily.[9]

A woman with a major depressive disorder taking lithium, thioridazine, doxepin and **phenelzine** was also given sertraline 100 mg daily for worsening depression. Within 3 hours she became semi-comatose, with a temperature of 41°C, a heart rate of 154 bpm and symptoms of rigidity and shivering. She was treated with diazepam, midazolam, ice-packs and dantrolene.[10] Two other similar cases, involving the use of sertraline with **isocarboxazid**[11] and **phenelzine**[12] have been reported. The latter case was fatal.[12] Another case of mild serotonin syndrome (managed with cyproheptadine) occurred in a woman who took a single dose of sertraline 11 days after stopping **isocarboxazid**.[13]

B. RIMAs

(a) Citalopram

A 34-year-old man who had been taking **moclobemide** 100 mg every 8 hours for several months was switched to citalopram 20 mg daily without a break. An hour later he started getting agitated and had involuntary movements of the legs, which progressed to generalised rigidity. Apart from a heart rate of 100 bpm all other vital signs were normal. He was treated with benzodiazepines and recovered uneventfully.[14] Three patients developed the serotonin syndrome (tremor, convulsions, hyperthermia, unconsciousness) and died 3 to 16 hours after taking overdoses of **moclobemide** and citalopram.[15] Other cases of the serotonin syndrome after overdose of **moclobemide** and citalopram have been reported:[16,17] one also included **sertraline** and sumatriptan.[16]

(b) Fluoxetine

A placebo-controlled trial in 18 healthy subjects found that the use of fluoxetine 20 mg with **moclobemide** 100 to 600 mg daily for 9 days gave no evidence of an adverse interaction.[18] Other studies in healthy subjects and patients similarly found no evidence of the serotonin syndrome.[19,20]

A post-marketing analysis found that at least 30 patients switched from fluoxetine to **moclobemide** within a week had experienced no adverse effects.[18,21]

However, 3 patients have developed the serotonin syndrome[22-24] and one developed agitation and confusion[25] following the use of **moclobemide** and fluoxetine. A fatal case of the serotonin syndrome occurred in a patient who took an overdose of **moclobemide**, fluoxetine, and clomipramine,[26] and another patient taking **moclobemide** developed the serotonin syndrome after taking an overdose of fluoxetine.[27] A study suggests that the combination may cause a high rate of adverse effects (insomnia, dizziness, nausea and headache).[22]

A double-blind study in 41 healthy subjects found that when they were given fluoxetine 40 mg daily for 7 days, then 20 mg for 9 days, immediately followed by **befloxatone** (2.5, 5, 10 or 20 mg daily) for 5 days, no unusual adverse reactions occurred and no changes in body temperature, haemodynamics or ECGs were seen.[28]

(c) Fluvoxamine

When 13 of 22 healthy subjects given fluvoxamine 100 mg daily for 9 days were also given **moclobemide** in increasing doses of 50 to 400 mg daily for 4 days from day 7, no serious adverse reactions occurred. Any adverse events were mild to moderate (some increase in headaches, fatigue, dizziness, all of which may occur with both drugs alone) and there was no evidence of the serious serotonin syndrome.[18,29] An open study in 6 depressed patients given **moclobemide** 225 to 800 mg daily and fluvoxamine 50 to 200 mg daily found a marked improvement in depression. Insomnia was the commonest adverse effect (treated with trazodone) but none of the patients showed any evidence of the serotonin syndrome.[30] Similar results were found in other studies.[20,31] However, a fatal case of the serotonin syndrome occurred in a woman who took an overdose of **moclobemide** and fluvoxamine, and another fatal overdose was attributed to the same combination.[32]

(d) Paroxetine

An open 6-week study in 19 patients with major depression taking paroxetine (or fluoxetine) 20 mg daily to which **moclobemide** up to 600 mg daily was added, indicated that these combinations were possibly effective.[33] An extension of this study with 50 patients is reported elsewhere.[22] However, a range of adverse effects occurred in some patients, the clearest one being insomnia, and the serotonin syndrome was seen in one patient.[22,33] Conversely, the serotonin syndrome was not seen in another study, where low initial doses and gradual up-titration of both paroxetine and **moclobemide** was used.[20] Two possible cases of mild serotonin syndrome occurred in women on **moclobemide** within 2 to 24 hours of starting additional paroxetine.[34] Similarly, cases of severe serotonin syndrome have been reported with overdoses of **moclobemide** and paroxetine.[35,36]

(e) Sertraline

In one study, 31 severely ill patients were given **moclobemide** 35 to 800 mg daily with SSRIs including sertraline 25 to 100 mg daily, initially using lower than usual starting doses of both drugs and then gradually titrating them slowly upwards. The other SSRIs used were fluoxetine, fluvoxamine and paroxetine. There was no evidence of the serotonin syndrome.[20] An open study in 5 depressed patients given **moclobemide** 150 to 600 mg daily and sertraline 25 to 200 mg daily found improvements ranging from minimal to complete remission. Insomnia was the commonest adverse effect (treated with trazodone) but none of the patients showed any evidence of the serotonin syndrome.[30] However, one case of possible serotonin syndrome occurred in a woman who took an overdose of **moclobemide** and sertraline,[34] and another after an overdose of **moclobemide**, **citalopram**, sertraline and sumatriptan.[16] Similarly, a fatality has been reported with an overdose of **moclobemide**, sertraline and pimozide, with blood levels suggesting that none of the drugs individually would have been fatal.[37]

(f) Unspecified SSRIs

Serotonin toxicity (the serotonin syndrome) occurred in 5 patients who took an overdose of **moclobemide** with an SSRI [specific drugs not mentioned]. In this analysis of **moclobemide** overdoses, the risk of developing serotonin toxicity was increased 35 times in patients who also took another serotonergic drug. Of the 11 cases mentioned 5 patients were taking SSRIs.[38]

Mechanism

MAO-A is involved in the metabolism of serotonin, so combined use of MAOIs or RIMAs with SSRIs may lead to excessive serotonin levels, which can result in the serotonin syndrome. For more information see 'the serotonin syndrome', (p.9).

Importance and management

Direct information about the interaction between MAOIs and SSRIs is limited. However, it is clear that severe, sometimes fatal interactions (the serotonin syndrome or similar) have occurred with MAOIs and fluoxetine or sertraline, so these reports should certainly be taken seriously. The incidence appears to be low, possibly as the combined use of any MAOI and any SSRI is contraindicated. In addition, at least 2 weeks should elapse between stopping any MAOI and starting any SSRI to allow for the effects of the MAOI to diminish. Moreover, the manufacturers of each SSRI give guidance on the appropriate intervals that should be left between stopping the SSRI and starting an MAOI, that is, 14 days for sertraline,[39,40] seven days for citalopram,[41] **escitalopram**,[42] fluvoxamine[43] or paroxetine[44] (14 days in the US),[45-47] and at least 5 weeks for fluoxetine, with an even longer interval if long-term or high-dose fluoxetine has been used.[48,49]

The RIMAs (e.g. moclobemide) also have serotonergic effects, and so they are unlikely to be any safer than the non-selective MAOIs in regard to interactions with SSRIs. The few cases of serotonin syndrome cited with therapeutic doses of this combination confirm that it is not necessarily safe. The combination may be particularly problematic in overdose, and negates the generally benign course of moclobemide overdose alone. It should be noted that the manufacturer of moclobemide contraindicates its use with SSRIs.[50] Because the effects of moclobemide are readily reversible, only one day need elapse between stopping moclobemide and starting an SSRI. However, if stopping an SSRI and starting moclobemide, the same intervals are required as for the irreversible MAOIs.

For the management of serotonin syndrome, see Importance and management under 'MAOIs or RIMAs + Tricyclic and related antidepressants', p.1149.

1. Feighner JP, Boyer WF, Tyler DL, Neborsky RJ. Adverse consequences of fluoxetine-MAOI combination therapy. *J Clin Psychiatry* (1990) 51, 222–5.
2. Beasley CM, Masica DN, Heiligenstein JH, Wheadon DE, Zerbe RL. Possible monoamine oxidase inhibitor — serotonin uptake inhibitor interaction: fluoxetine clinical data and preclinical findings. *J Clin Psychopharmacol* (1993) 13, 312–20.
3. Sternbach H. Danger of MAOI therapy after fluoxetine withdrawal. *Lancet* (1988) ii, 850–1.
4. Ooi, TK. The serotonin syndrome. *Anaesthesia* (1991) 46, 507–8.
5. Spiller HA, Morse S, Muir C. Fluoxetine ingestion: A one year retrospective study. *Vet Hum Toxicol* (1990) 32, 153–5.
6. Coplan JD, Gorman JM. Detectable levels of fluoxetine metabolites after discontinuation: an unexpected serotonin syndrome. *Am J Psychiatry* (1993) 150, 837.
7. Kline SS, Mauro LS, Scala-Barnett DM, Zick D. Serotonin syndrome versus neuroleptic malignant syndrome as a cause of death. *Clin Pharm* (1989) 8, 510–14.

8. Miller F, Friedman R, Tanenbaum J, Griffin A. Disseminated intravascular coagulation and acute myoglobinuric renal failure: a consequence of the serotonergic syndrome. *J Clin Psychopharmacol* (1991) 11, 277–9.
9. Bhatara VS, Bandettini FC. Possible interaction between sertraline and tranylcypromine. *Clin Pharm* (1993) 12, 222–5.
10. Graber MA, Hoehns TB, Perry PJ. Sertraline-phenelzine drug interaction: a serotonin syndrome reaction. *Ann Pharmacother* (1994) 28, 732–5.
11. Brannan SK, Talley BJ, Bowden CL. Sertraline and isocarboxazid cause a serotonin syndrome. *J Clin Psychopharmacol* (1994) 14, 144–5.
12. Keltner N. Serotonin syndrome: a case of fatal SSRI/MAOI interaction. *Perspect Psychiatr Care* (1994) 30, 26–31.
13. Lappin RI, Auchincloss EL. Treatment of the serotonin syndrome with cyproheptadine. *N Engl J Med* (1994) 331, 1021–2.
14. Gumà M, Clemente F, Segura A, Costa J. Síndrome serotoninérgico: moclobemida y citalopram. *Med Clin (Barc)* (1999) 113, 677–8.
15. Neuvonen PJ, Pohjola-Sintonen S, Tacke U, Vuori E. Five fatal cases of serotonin syndrome after moclobemide-citalopram or moclobemide-clomipramine overdoses. *Lancet* (1993) 342, 1419.
16. Höjer J, Personne M, Skagius A-S, Hansson O. Serotoninergt syndrom: flera allvarliga fall med denna ofta förbisedda diagnos. *Lakartidningen* (2002) 99, 2054–5, 2058–60.
17. Dams R, Benijts THP, Lambert WE, Van Bocxlaer JF, Van Varenbergh D, Van Peteghem C, De Leenheer AP. A fatal case of serotonin syndrome after combined moclobemide–citalopram intoxication. *J Anal Toxicol* (2001) 25, 147–51.
18. Dingemanse J. An update of recent moclobemide interaction data. *Int Clin Psychopharmacol* (1993) 7, 167–80.
19. Dingemanse J, Wallnöfer A, Gieschke R, Guentert T, Amrein R. Pharmacokinetic and pharmacodynamic interactions between fluoxetine and moclobemide in the investigation of development of the "serotonin syndrome". *Clin Pharmacol Ther* (1998) 63, 403–13.
20. Bakish D, Hooper CL, West DL, Miller C, Blanchard A, Bashir F. Moclobemide and specific serotonin re-uptake inhibitor combination treatment of resistant anxiety and depressive disorders. *Hum Psychopharmacol* (1995) 10, 105–9.
21. Dingemanse J, Guentert TW, Moritz E, Eckernas S-A. Pharmacodynamic and pharmacokinetic interactions between fluoxetine and moclobemide. *Clin Pharmacol Ther* (1993) 53, 178.
22. Hawley CJ, Quick SJ, Ratnam S, Pattinson HA, McPhee S. Safety and tolerability of combined treatment with moclobemide and SSRIs: a systematic study of 50 patients. *Int Clin Psychopharmacol* (1996) 11, 187–91.
23. Benazzi F. Serotonin syndrome with moclobemide-fluoxetine combination. *Pharmacopsychiatry* (1996) 29, 162.
24. Liebenberg R, Berk M, Winkler G. Serotonergic syndrome after concomitant use of moclobemide and fluoxetine. *Hum Psychopharmacol* (1996) 11, 146–7.
25. Chan BSH, Graudins A, Whyte IM, Dawson AH, Braitberg G, Duggin GG. Serotonin syndrome resulting from drug interactions. *Med J Aust* (1998) 169, 523–5.
26. Power BM, Pinder M, Hackett LP, Ilett KF. Fatal serotonin syndrome following a combined overdose of moclobemide, clomipramine and fluoxetine. *Anaesth Intensive Care* (1995) 23, 499–502.
27. Chambost M, Liron L, Peillon D, Combe C. Syndrome serotoninergique lors d'une intoxication par la fluoxetine chez une patiente prenant du moclobemide. *Can J Anesth* (2000) 47, 246–50.
28. Pinquier JL, Caplain H, Durrieu G, Zieleniuk I, Rosenzweig P. Safety and pharmacodynamic study of befloxatone after fluoxetine withdrawal. *Clin Pharmacol Ther* (1998) 63, 187.
29. Wallnöfer A, Guentert TW, Eckernäs SA, Dingemanse J. Moclobemide and fluvoxamine co-administration: a prospective study in healthy volunteers to investigate the potential development of the 'serotonin syndrome'. *Hum Psychopharmacol* (1995) 10, 25–31.
30. Joffe RT, Bakish D. Combined SSRI-moclobemide treatment of psychiatric illness. *J Clin Psychiatry* (1994) 55, 24–5.
31. Ebert D, Albert R, May A, Stosiek I, Kaschka W. Combined SSRI-RIMA treatment in refractory depression. Safety data and efficacy. *Psychopharmacology (Berl)* (1995) 119, 342–4.
32. Rogde S, Hilberg T, Teige B. Fatal combined intoxication with new antidepressants. Human cases and an experimental study of postmortem moclobemide redistribution. *Forensic Sci Int* (1999) 100, 109–16.
33. Hawley CJ, Ratnam S, Pattinson HA, Quick SJ, Echlin D. Safety and tolerability of combined treatment with moclobemide and SSRIs: a preliminary study of 19 patients. *J Psychopharmacol* (1996) 10, 241–5.
34. Graudins A, Stearman A, Chan B. Treatment of the serotonin syndrome with cyproheptadine. *J Emerg Med* (1998) 16, 615–19.
35. Robert P, Senard JM, Fabre M, Cabot C, Cathala B. Syndrome sérotoninergique lors d'une intoxication aiguë aux antidépresseurs. *Ann Fr Anesth Reanim* (1996) 15, 663–5.
36. FitzSimmons CR, Metha S. Serotonin syndrome caused by overdose with paroxetine and moclobemide. *J Accid Emerg Med* (1999) 16, 293–5.
37. McIntyre IM, King CV, Staikos V, Gall J, Drummer OH. A fatality involving moclobemide, sertraline, and pimozide. *J Forensic Sci* (1997) 42, 951–3.
38. Isbister GK, Hackett LP, Dawson AH, Whyte IM, Smith AJ. Moclobemide poisoning: toxicokinetics and occurrence of serotonin toxicity. *Br J Clin Pharmacol* (2003) 56, 441–50.
39. Lustral (Sertraline hydrochloride). Pfizer Ltd. UK Summary of product characteristics, October 2005.
40. Zoloft (Sertraline). Pfizer Inc. US Product information, December 2005.
41. Cipramil (Citalopram hydrobromide). Lundbeck Ltd. UK Summary of product characteristics, January 2007.
42. Cipralex (Escitalopram oxalate). Lundbeck Ltd. UK Summary of product characteristics, December 2005.
43. Faverin (Fluvoxamine). Solvay Healthcare Ltd. UK Summary of product characteristics, June 2006.
44. Seroxat (Paroxetine hydrochloride hemihydrate). GlaxoSmithKline UK. UK Summary of product characteristics, April 2007.
45. Celexa (Citalopram hydrobromide). Forest Pharmaceuticals, Inc. US Prescribing information, May 2007.
46. Lexapro (Escitalopram oxalate). Forest Pharmaceuticals Inc. US Prescribing information, May 2007.
47. Paxil (Paroxetine hydrochloride). GlaxoSmithKline. US Prescribing information, July 2006.
48. Prozac (Fluoxetine hydrochloride). Eli Lilly and Company Ltd. UK Summary of product characteristics, March 2007.
49. Prozac (Fluoxetine hydrochloride). Eli Lilly and Company. US Prescribing information, May 2007.
50. Manerix (Moclobemide). Roche Products Ltd. UK Summary of product characteristics, September 2005.

MAOIs + Sulfafurazole (Sulfisoxazole)

An isolated report describes a patient taking phenelzine who developed weakness and ataxia after also taking sulfafurazole.

Clinical evidence, mechanism, importance and management

A woman who had been taking **phenelzine** 15 mg three times daily for about 3 weeks complained of weakness, ataxia, vertigo, tinnitus, muscle pains and paraesthesias within 7 days of starting to take sulfafurazole 1 g four times daily. These adverse effects continued until the 10-day sulfonamide course was completed, and did not occur again in the following 8 weeks.[1] The reasons are not understood, but as these adverse effects are a combination of the adverse effects of both drugs, it seems possible that a mutual interaction (perhaps saturation of the acetylating mechanisms in the liver) was responsible. This appears to be an isolated report, but bear it in mind in the event of an unexpected response to treatment.

1. Boyer WF, Lake CR. Interaction of phenelzine and sulfisoxazole. *Am J Psychiatry* (1983) 140, 264–5.

MAOIs or RIMAs + Sympathomimetics; Amfetamines and related drugs

The concurrent use of non-selective MAOIs and amfetamines and related drugs can result in a potentially fatal hypertensive crisis and/or serotonin syndrome. Interactions have been reported for amfetamine, dexamfetamine, metamfetamine, and methylphenidate. Interactions have also been reported with the illicit drug ecstasy (MDMA, methylenedioxymethamfetamine) when taken with phenelzine or moclobemide. The manufacturers of fenfluramine and dexfenfluramine contraindicated their use with MAOIs.

Clinical evidence

A. MAOIs

(a) Amfetamines

A 30-year-old depressed woman who was taking **phenelzine** 15 mg three times daily and trifluoperazine 2 mg at night, acquired some **dexamfetamine sulfate** tablets from a friend and took 20 mg. Within 15 minutes she complained of severe headache, which she described as if "her head was bursting". An hour later her blood pressure was 150/100 mmHg. Later she became comatose with a blood pressure of 170/100 mmHg and died. A postmortem examination revealed a haemorrhage in the left cerebral hemisphere, disrupting the internal capsule and adjacent areas of the corpus striatum.[1]

This interaction has been reported with single oral doses of **amfetamine**,[2,3] single intravenous doses of **amfetamine**,[4] single doses of illicit **amfetamine/dexamfetamine**,[5,6] or single doses of intravenous **metamfetamine**,[7-10] in patients taking **tranylcypromine**,[2,7,8] **phenelzine**,[3,5,6,8,9] and **isocarboxazid**.[8,10] A woman who had been addicted to high-dose **dexamfetamine**/amobarbital was hospitalised and had the **dexamfetamine**/amobarbital withdrawn. Five days later she was given a single dose of **tranylcypromine** and within an hour had a 20 minute episode of hypertension, tachycardia, headache, sweating, lacrimation and altered consciousness, which abated without treatment. She had similar attacks at 2-hourly intervals over about 5 days when they gradually became milder and shorter.[11]

Extreme hyperpyrexia, apparently without hypertension, has been described in a woman who took **tranylcypromine** with **dexamfetamine**/amobarbital. She developed progressive agitation, diaphoresis, hyperkinesis, opisthotonus, coma and convulsions, but recovered following the use of an ice bath and other supportive measures.[12,13]

(b) Dexfenfluramine or fenfluramine

The manufacturer recommended that fenfluramine should not be used in patients with a history of depression, or during treatment with antidepressants (especially the MAOIs), and there should be an interval of 3 weeks between stopping the MAOIs and starting fenfluramine.[14] A woman taking **phenelzine** developed severe headache, neck stiffness and nausea within an hour of taking fenfluramine 20 mg, and then collapsed and remained stuporous for about 4 hours. This reaction was considered similar to that seen with MAOIs and amfetamines.[15]

The manufacturer of dexfenfluramine similarly contraindicated its use with or within 2 weeks of stopping an MAOI,[16] and advised waiting 3 weeks between stopping dexfenfluramine and starting an MAOI. This is due to the potential risk of the serotonin syndrome,[17,18] which has rarely occurred with the concurrent use of two or more serotonergic drugs (see 'the serotonin syndrome', (p.9)). The manufacturer of dexfenfluramine and fenfluramine had found no clinical evidence of serious problems with either of these drugs when taken with MAOIs,[19] so that the published warnings about possible interactions would appear to be based on theoretical considerations.

Note that dexfenfluramine and fenfluramine have generally been withdrawn because their use was found to be associated with a high incidence of abnormal echocardiograms indicating abnormal functioning of heart valves.

(c) Ecstasy (MDMA, methylenedioxymethamfetamine)

Marked hypertension, diaphoresis, altered mental status and hypertonicity (slow forceful twisting and arching movements) occurred in one patient taking **phenelzine** with ecstasy.[20] Increased muscle tension, decorticate-like posturing, fever, tachycardia and coma occurred in another patient taking **phenelzine**, 15 minutes after drinking juice containing ecstasy.[21] Both patients recovered.[20,21]

(d) Methylphenidate

A patient started treatment with **tranylcypromine**, then 4 days later methylphenidate was added. After 15 days of concurrent use he had a hypertensive crisis and both drugs were stopped.[22] In a study of the use of **phenelzine** as an antagonist to stimulants, 3 patients took oral or intravenous methylphenidate and all three experienced moderate to severe headache.[6] An episode of symptoms consistent with the serotonin syndrome occurred in a man taking **isocarboxazid** and trazodone, 2 months after the dose of these drugs was increased and methylphenidate was added. He had experienced two similar episodes 4 and 8 weeks previously, which had each resolved spontaneously over 12 hours. All three drugs have serotonergic properties and where thought to have contributed to the reaction.[23] Conversely, a man taking **tranylcypromine** for depression was successfully treated with methylphenidate for attention deficit/hyperactivity disorder (ADHD). He was given methylphenidate 2.5 mg daily, which was very gradually increased over a number of months to 45 mg daily. He was successfully treated with the combination for 6 months and periodic blood pressure measurements did not change significantly from baseline.[24] Another similar case has been described with **phenelzine** and methylphenidate.[25] No cases of hypertensive crisis were seen in 4 patients taking **tranylcypromine** or **phenelzine** when treated concurrently with methylphenidate for periods of 6 to 30 months.[26]

B. RIMAs

Four patients died after taking **moclobemide** and **ecstasy** (MDMA, methylenedioxymethamfetamine). The clinical evidence is limited, but in each case the forensic pathologist concluded that the cause of death was the combined use of these drugs. It was suggested that what happened is consistent with the serotonin syndrome, although the evidence is fairly slim. Two patients had taken maximum therapeutic doses and two moderate overdoses of **moclobemide**. Note that **moclobemide** had not been prescribed to any of them. Post-mortem analysis also found the presence of **dextromethorphan** in one patient, which was thought to have contributed,[27] see also 'MAOIs or RIMAs + Dextromethorphan', p.1134.

Mechanism

The hypertensive reaction can be attributed to overstimulation of the adrenergic receptors of the cardiovascular system.[28] During treatment with non-selective MAOIs, large amounts of noradrenaline (norepinephrine) accumulate at adrenergic nerve endings not only in the brain, but also within the sympathetic nerve endings, which innervate arterial blood vessels. Stimulation of these latter nerve endings by sympathomimetic amines with indirect actions causes the release of the accumulated noradrenaline and results in the massive stimulation of the receptors. An exaggerated blood vessel constriction occurs and the blood pressure rise is proportionately excessive. Intracranial haemorrhage can occur if the pressure is so high that a blood vessel ruptures.[1]

Some of the reactions may also possibly be related to the serotonin syndrome. Amfetamines act by releasing serotonin (and possibly also dopamine) from neurones in the brain, so that increased stimulation of the serotonin receptors occurs. This possibly explains their mood-modifying effects. MAOIs prevent the breakdown of serotonin within neurones so that more serotonin is available for release, and in excess this can apparently result in the toxic and even fatal serotonin syndrome. The RIMAs (such as moclobemide) appear to behave like the older non-selective MAOIs in this context.

Importance and management

The hypertensive reaction is a very well-documented, serious, and potentially fatal interaction, whereas the serotonin syndrome appears to be rarer. Patients taking any of the non-selective MAOIs should not normally take amfetamines, or related drugs such as methylphenidate. A possible exception to this prohibition is that under very well controlled conditions dexamfetamine and methylphenidate may sometimes be effectively (and apparently safely) used with MAOIs for refractory depression,[25,26,29] or ADHD.[24] Direct evidence implicating central stimulants such as **diethylpropion**, **mazindol**, **pemoline**, **phendimetrazine**, and **phenmetrazine** seems not to have been documented, but on the basis of their known pharmacology their concurrent use with the MAOIs should be avoided. Patients on MAOIs should also be warned to avoid the illicit use of amfetamines and ecstasy. It would also be prudent to avoid moclobemide with amfetamines and related drugs, although the incidence of the interactions with moclobemide is unlikely to be as great as that seen with the non-selective MAOIs. In the cases with ecstasy, it seems likely that high doses of moclobemide were used to try to enhance the actions of the ecstasy, but these cases, nevertheless, show that combined use is potentially life threatening.

Treatment

For a brief mention of the treatment of hypertensive crisis, see Importance and Management under 'MAOIs or RIMAs + Sympathomimetics; Indirectly-acting', p.1147. For the management of fever and other symptoms of the serotonin syndrome, see Importance and management under 'MAOIs or RIMAs + Tricyclic and related antidepressants', p.1149.

1. Lloyd JTA, Walker DRH. Death after combined dexamphetamine and phenelzine. *BMJ* (1965) 2, 168–9.
2. Zeck P. The dangers of some antidepressant drugs. *Med J Aust* (1961) 2, 607–8.
3. Tonks CM, Livingston D. Monoamineoxidase inhibitors. *Lancet* (1963) i, 1323–4.
4. Feinberg M, de Vigne J-P, Kronfol Z, Young E. Duration of action of phenelzine in two patients. *Am J Psychiatry* (1981) 138, 379–80.
5. Devabhaktuni RV, Jampala VC. Using street drugs while on MAOI therapy. *J Clin Psychopharmacol* (1987) 7, 60–1.
6. Maletzky BM. Phenelzine as a stimulant drug antagonist: a preliminary report. *Int J Addict* (1977) 12, 651–5.
7. Macdonald R. Tranylcypromine. *Lancet* (1963) i, 269.
8. Mason A. Fatal reaction associated with tranylcypromine and methylamphetamine. *Lancet* (1962) i, 1073.
9. Dally PJ. Fatal reaction associated with tranylcypromine and methylamphetamine. *Lancet* (1962) i, 1235–6.
10. Bethune HC, Burrell RH, Culpan RH. Headache associated with monoamine oxidase inhibitors. *Lancet* (1963) ii, 1233–4.
11. Hay G. Severe reaction to monoamine-oxidase inhibitor in a dexamphetamine addict. *Lancet* (1962) ii, 665.
12. Lewis E. Hyperpyrexia with antidepressant drugs. *BMJ* (1965) 1, 1671–2.
13. Kriskó I, Lewis E, Johnson JE. Severe hyperpyrexia due to tranylcypromine–amphetamine toxicity. *Ann Intern Med* (1969) 70, 559–64.
14. Ponderax Pacaps (Fenfluramine). Servier Laboratories Ltd. ABPI Compendium of Data Sheets and Summaries of Product Characteristics 1998–9, p. 1307.
15. Brandon S. Unusual effect of fenfluramine. *BMJ* (1969) 4, 557–8.
16. Adifax (Dexfenfluramine). Servier Laboratories Ltd. ABPI Compendium of Data Sheets and Summaries of Product Characteristics 1998–9, p. 1302.
17. Dolan JA, Amchin J, Albano D. Potential hazard of serotonin syndrome associated with dexfenfluramine hydrochloride (Redux): Reply. *JAMA* (1996) 276, 1220–1.
18. Schenck CH, Mahowald MW. Potential hazard of serotonin syndrome associated with dexfenfluramine hydrochloride (Redux). *JAMA* (1996) 276, 1220.
19. Servier Laboratories Ltd. Personal communication, July 1997.
20. Smilkstein MJ, Smolinske SC, Rumack BH. A case of MAO inhibitor/MDMA interaction: agony after ecstasy. *Clin Toxicol* (1987) 25, 149–59.
21. Kaskey GB. Possible interaction between an MAOI and "Ecstasy". *Am J Psychiatry* (1992) 149, 411–2.
22. Sherman M, Hauser GC, Glover BH. Toxic reactions to tranylcypromine. *Am J Psychiatry* (1964) 120, 1019–21.
23. Bodner RA, Lynch T, Lewis L, Kahn D. Serotonin syndrome. *Neurology* (1995) 45, 219–23.
24. Feinberg SS. Combining stimulants with monoamine oxidase inhibitors: a review of uses and one possible additional indication. *J Clin Psychiatry* (2004) 65, 1520–4.
25. Shelton Clauson A, Elliott ES, Watson BD, Treacy J. Coadministration of phenelzine and methylphenidate for treatment-resistant depression. *Ann Pharmacother* (2004) 38, 508.
26. Feighner JP, Herbstein J, Damlouji N. Combined MAOI, TCA, and direct stimulant therapy of treatment-resistant depression. *J Clin Psychiatry* (1985) 46, 206–9.
27. Vuori E, Henry JA, Ojanoperä I, Nieminen R, Savolainen T, Wahlsten P, Jäntti M. Death following ingestion of MDMA (ecstasy) and moclobemide. *Addiction* (2003) 98, 365–8.
28. Simpson LL. Mechanism of the adverse interaction between monoamine oxidase inhibitors and amphetamine. *J Pharmacol Exp Ther* (1978) 205, 392–9.
29. Fawcett J, Kravitz HM, Zajecka JM, Schaff MR. CNS stimulant potentiation of monoamine oxidase inhibitors in treatment-refractory depression. *J Clin Psychopharmacol* (1991) 11, 127–32.

MAOIs or RIMAs + Sympathomimetics; Beta-agonist bronchodilators

An isolated case of tachycardia and apprehension has been described in an asthmatic taking phenelzine after salbutamol (albuterol) was added. Hypomania was seen in another asthmatic taking phenelzine when inhaled isoetarine was added. Hypertensive crisis occurred in a woman taking toloxatone and phenylephrine when given [oral] terbutaline.

Clinical evidence

(a) MAOIs

A report briefly describes a case of tachycardia and apprehension in a patient taking **phenelzine** when **salbutamol** (**albuterol**) was started [route of administration not stated].[1] Hypomania has been described in a patient taking **phenelzine** in the few weeks after starting inhaled **isoetarine** 680 micrograms up to every 4 hours.[2]

(b) RIMAs

A 72-year old woman taking long-term levothyroxine, **toloxatone** 400 mg daily (for 2 months), and phenylephrine (for 3 weeks) developed episodes of hypertension, sweating, tachycardia, and headache within 3 days after starting [oral] **terbutaline** 10 mg daily. She had extremely high plasma catecholamine levels. All drugs were stopped on admission to hospital and she recovered over 2 to 3 days.[3]

Mechanism

Note that drugs with directly-acting sympathomimetic effects (of which beta agonists are an example) do not normally interact to cause hypertension with MAOIs, see 'sympathomimetics; directly-acting', (below). However, phenylephrine (which has some indirect actions, see 'sympathomimetics; phenylephrine', (p.1148)) may have contributed to the reaction between toloxatone and terbutaline, and the fact that terbutaline seems to have been given orally would also have contributed. The hypomania reaction is not understood.

Importance and management

These appear to be isolated cases, and are possibly not of general importance. Bear them in mind in the event of an unexpected response to treatment.

1. Shader RI, Greenblatt DJ. MAOIs and drug interactions—a proposal for a clearinghouse. *J Clin Psychopharmacol* (1985) 5, A17.
2. Goldman LS, Tiller JA. Hypomania related to phenelzine and isoetharine interaction in one patient. *J Clin Psychiatry* (1987) 48, 170.
3. Lefebvre H, Richard R, Noblet C, Moore N, Wolf L-M. Life-threatening pseudo-phaeochromocytoma after toloxatone, terbutaline, and phenylephrine. *Lancet* (1993) 341, 555–6.

MAOIs or RIMAs + Sympathomimetics; Directly-acting

The pressor effects of adrenaline (epinephrine), isoprenaline (isoproterenol), noradrenaline (norepinephrine) and methoxamine may be unchanged or only moderately increased in patients taking MAOIs. There is limited evidence that the increase may be somewhat greater in those who show a significant hypotensive response to the MAOI. Moclobemide does not appear to interact.

Clinical evidence

(a) MAOIs

In a randomised, double-blind, placebo-controlled study in 12 healthy subjects, **phenelzine** 15 mg three times daily for 7 days had no effect on the dose of intravenous **noradrenaline** (**norepinephrine**) required to raise the systolic blood pressure by 25 mmHg. In addition, **phenelzine** had no effect on the diastolic blood pressure rises and heart rate reductions seen with **noradrenaline**. In this study, **phenelzine** itself had no effect on blood pressure or heart rate.[1] Similarly, in an earlier study in two healthy subjects given **phenelzine** 15 mg three times daily and two given **tranylcypromine** 10 mg three times daily for 7 days, there was no significant change in pressor response to intravenous **adrenaline** (**epinephrine**) or **isoprenaline** (**isoproterenol**) after treatment with the MAOI. However, the tachycardia caused by **isoprenaline** was antagonised by the MAOIs (109 bpm with the MAOI versus 127 bpm without). No clinically significant potentiation of the pressor effect of **noradrenaline** was seen, although one of the subjects taking **tranylcypromine** had a twofold increase in the pressor response in the mid-range of **noradrenaline** concentrations infused, but not in the upper or lower ranges. None of these 4 subjects had a change in blood pressure or heart rate caused by the MAOI alone.[2] In yet another study in 3 healthy subjects given **tranylcypromine** for 8 to 14 days, the effects of intravenous **noradrenaline** were slightly increased, while with intravenous **adrenaline** a moderate two to fourfold increase in the effects on heart rate and diastolic pressure took place, but a less marked increase in systolic pressure. Intravenous **isoprenaline** behaved very much like **adrenaline**, but there was no enhancement of systolic pressure. This study did not state the effect of the MAOI alone on blood pressure.[3]

A patient using 1% **adrenaline** eye drops twice daily had no increase in blood pressure or heart rate when treated with **tranylcypromine** 20 mg, rising to 50 mg daily.[4] Another patient taking **phenelzine** presented with severe anaphylaxis after taking two doses of flucloxacillin, and was initially treated unsuccessfully with hydrocortisone, chlorphenamine and ranitidine because of concerns about using **adrenaline** with MAOIs. However, as her condition worsened she was given two 100-microgram boluses of intravenous **adrenaline**, with rapid improvement. No adverse reaction was noted.[5] In another study, one healthy subject given **phenelzine** for 8 days experienced a marked reduction in blood pressure, but showed no significant changes in pressor response to **noradrenaline**.[6]

In contrast, in a study in hypertensive patients who had postural hypotension after being given either **pheniprazine** (a formerly investigational older MAOI) (6 patients) or **tranylcypromine** (one patient), the dose of **noradrenaline** required to produce a 25 mmHg rise in systolic pressure was reduced by 62 to 87%. In three of these patients on **pheniprazine** the dose of **methoxamine** was reduced by 61 to 70% compared with that required in the absence of an MAOI. Three patients were later given **nialamide**: augmentation of the pressor response of **noradrenaline** or **methoxamine** only occurred in the one patient who had developed postural hypotension.[7]

(b) RIMAs

In a randomised, double-blind, placebo-controlled study in 12 healthy subjects, **moclobemide** 100 mg three times daily for 7 days had no effect on the dose of intravenous **noradrenaline** required to raise the systolic blood pressure by 25 mmHg. In addition, **moclobemide** had no effect on the diastolic blood pressure rises and heart rate reductions seen with **noradrenaline**. In this study, **moclobemide** itself had no effect on blood pressure or heart rate.[1] A review paper also briefly mentions that **moclobemide** 600 mg daily for 3 weeks had no relevant effect on the heart rate response to intravenous **isoprenaline**.[8]

Mechanism

These sympathomimetic amines act directly on the receptors at the nerve endings, which innervate arterial blood vessels, so that the presence of the MAOI-induced accumulation of noradrenaline within these nerve endings would not be expected to alter the extent of direct stimulation (contrast 'Sympathomimetics; Indirectly-acting', (p.1147)). The enhancement seen in those patients whose blood pressure was lowered by the MAOI might possibly be due to an increased sensitivity of the receptors, which is seen if the nerves are cut, and is also seen during temporary 'pharmacological severance'.

Importance and management

The overall picture is that no clinically relevant enhancement of the effects of noradrenaline or adrenaline occurs in patients taking MAOIs, although some uncertainty remains about those who show MAOI-induced hypotension. The authors of three of the reports cited[2-4] are in broad agreement that problems are unlikely to occur, and others consider that intravenous adrenaline may be used in life-threatening situations in patients on MAOIs, albeit with caution.[5] Others also consider that the use of adrenaline in eye drops or as a component of local anaesthesia in dental and other procedures may be used in patients receiving MAOIs,[4,9] and that there is no justification for the continued listing of an interaction between MAOIs and local anaesthetics with vasoconstrictors in US prescribing information.[9] It is worth noting that there are no case reports of interactions with these drugs.

Direct evidence about methoxamine is even more limited, but it seems to behave similarly. None of the studies demonstrated any marked changes in the effects of isoprenaline.

The situation in patients who show a reduced blood pressure due to the use of an MAOI is less clear. One early study[7] found an increase in the pressor effects of noradrenaline and methoxamine in hypertensive patients who had developed orthostatic hypotension on pheniprazine or tranylcypromine. Bear this possibility in mind.

Moclobemide does not appear to alter the pressor response to noradrenaline.

The interaction between phenylephrine and the MAOIs is dealt with elsewhere (see 'MAOIs or RIMAs + Sympathomimetics; Phenylephrine', p.1148). Consider also 'MAOIs or RIMAs + Sympathomimetics; Beta-agonist bronchodilators', p.1146 and 'Inotropes and Vasopressors; Dopamine + Selegiline', p.893, for dosing advice with when dopamine is given to patients taking MAOIs.

1. Cusson JR, Goldenberg E, Larochelle P. Effect of a novel monoamine-oxidase inhibitor, moclobemide on the sensitivity to intravenous tyramine and norepinephrine in humans. *J Clin Pharmacol* (1991) 31, 462–7.
2. Boakes AJ, Laurence DR, Teoh PC, Barar FSK, Benedikter LT, Prichard BNC. Interactions between sympathomimetic amines and antidepressant agents in man. *BMJ* (1973) 1, 311–15.
3. Cuthbert MF, Vere DW. Potentiation of the cardiovascular effects of some catecholamines by a monoamine oxidase inhibitor. *Br J Pharmacol* (1971) 43, 471P–472P.
4. Thompson DS, Sweet RA, Marzula K, Peredes JC. Lack of interaction of monoamine oxidase inhibitors and epinephrine in an older patient. *J Clin Psychopharmacol* (1997) 17, 322–3.
5. Fenwick MJ, Muwanga CL. Anaphylaxis and monoamine oxidase inhibitors–the use of adrenaline. *J Accid Emerg Med* (2000) 17, 143–4.
6. Elis J, Laurence DR, Mattie H, Prichard BNC. Modification by monoamine oxidase inhibitors of the effect of some sympathomimetics on blood pressure. *BMJ* (1967) 2, 75–8.
7. Horwitz D, Goldberg LI, Sjoerdsma A. Increased blood pressure responses to dopamine and norepinephrine produced by monoamine oxidase inhibitors in man. *J Lab Clin Med* (1960) 56, 747–53.
8. Zimmer R, Gieschke R, Fischbach R, Gasic S. Interaction studies with moclobemide. *Acta Psychiatr Scand* (1990) 82 (Suppl 360), 84–6.
9. Yagiela JA. Adverse drug interactions in dental practice: interactions associated with vasoconstrictors. Part V of a series. *J Am Dent Assoc* (1999) 130, 701–9.

MAOIs or RIMAs + Sympathomimetics; Indirectly-acting

The use of indirectly-acting sympathomimetic amines concurrently with, and for 2 weeks after stopping, non-selective MAOIs can result in a potentially fatal hypertensive crisis and should be avoided. Note that these amines are commonly used as vasoconstrictor decongestants (e.g. ephedrine, phenylpropanolamine and pseudoephedrine) in many proprietary cough, cold and influenza preparations, or for their vasoconstrictor effects in migraine (e.g. isometheptene). Indirectly-acting amines are also used parenterally for treating hypotension occurring during spinal anaesthesia (e.g. ephedrine, mephentermine, metaraminol). Potentially serious interactions have also been seen with moclobemide and indirectly-acting sympathomimetics.

Clinical evidence

(a) MAOIs

A study in 3 healthy subjects, given **phenelzine** 45 mg or **tranylcypromine** 30 mg daily for 5 to 14 days, found that the blood pressure rise following oral **ephedrine** 30 mg was enhanced. The maximal increase in mean arterial pressure was 22 mmHg (compared with 4 to 6 mmHg without the MAOI). A similar increase was seen up to 10 days after discontinuation of the MAOI. A similar increase in blood pressure was also seen in one of the subjects given intravenous **ephedrine** 2 mg per minute for 6 minutes.[1] In another subject given **tranylcypromine** 30 mg daily for 20 to 30 days, **phenylpropanolamine** in capsules or a linctus preparation caused a rapid and marked rise in blood pressure to 210/140 mmHg within 2 hours, necessitating the use of phentolamine to reverse the effect.[2] Slow-release **phenylpropanolamine** caused a smaller and more gradual rise to 160/100 mmHg over 2 hours.[2] Similarly, the pressor effect of intravenous **phenylpropanolamine** was potentiated about four to fivefold (systolic) and three to tenfold (diastolic) in 3 subjects given **tranylcypromine** 30 mg daily for 8 to 14 days, and the reflex bradycardia was potentiated about 2.5- to 6-fold.[3]

Numerous case reports describe similar rapid and serious rises in blood pressure, accompanied by tachycardia, chest pains and severe occipital headache with concurrent use of MAOIs and indirectly-acting sympathomimetics. Other symptoms that have occurred include neck stiffness, flushing, sweating, nausea, vomiting, hypertonicity of the limbs, and sometimes epileptiform convulsions, and fatal intracranial haemorrhage, cardiac arrhythmias and cardiac arrest have resulted.

This interaction has been reported with oral **ephedrine**,[4] oral **isometheptene mucate**,[5] intravenous **mephentermine**,[6] intramuscular **metaraminol**,[7] oral **phenylpropanolamine**,[8-13] and oral **pseudoephedrine**,[12,14,15] in patients taking **nialamide**,[4] **phenelzine**,[5,6,9-13] **iproniazid**,[15] **mebanazine**,[9] and **pargyline**.[7,8]

Tachycardia and *hypotension*, then pyrexia has been described in a woman who took a single *Do-Do* tablet (**ephedrine,** caffeine, theophylline) the day after stopping **phenelzine**.[16] Similarly, fatal hyperpyrexia without hypertension occurred in a man taking **tranylcypromine**/trifluoperazine given oral **ephedrine**,[17] although switching his MAOI without a full washout period may have caused, or contributed to, this reaction[18] (see 'MAOIs + MAOIs or RIMAs', p.1137). A woman taking **phenelzine** developed bradycardia (40 bpm) after taking one tablet of *Sinutab* (without codeine),[19] which probably contained **pseudoephedrine**.

(b) RIMAs

No interaction was seen in subjects taking **brofaromine** 75 mg twice daily for 10 days when given 75 mg of slow-release **phenylpropanolamine** (*Acutrim Late Day*), but immediate-release **phenylpropanolamine** in gelatin capsules caused a 3.3-fold increase in pressor sensitivity.[20] The pressor effects of high-dose oral **ephedrine** (two doses of 50 mg with a 4-hour interval) in 11 healthy subjects taking **moclobemide** 300 mg twice daily were increased about three to fourfold, and this resulted in an increase in palpitations and headache.[21,22]

Mechanism

The reaction can be attributed to overstimulation of the adrenergic receptors of the cardiovascular system. During treatment with non-selective MAOIs, large amounts of noradrenaline (norepinephrine) accumulate at adrenergic nerve endings not only in the brain, but also within the sympathetic nerve endings, which innervate arterial blood vessels. Stimulation of these latter nerve endings by sympathomimetic amines with indirect actions causes the release of the accumulated noradrenaline and results in the massive stimulation of the receptors. An exaggerated blood vessel constriction occurs and the blood pressure rise is proportionately excessive. Intracranial haemorrhage can occur if the pressure is so high that a blood vessel ruptures. Directly-acting sympathomimetics do not cause this effect, see 'MAOIs or RIMAs + Sympathomimetics; Directly-acting', p.1146.

Importance and management

(a) MAOIs

A very well-documented, serious, and potentially fatal interaction. Patients taking any of the MAOIs should not normally take any sympathomimetic amine with indirect activity. These include ephedrine, isometheptene mucate, mephentermine, metaraminol, phenylpropanolamine and pseudoephedrine. Direct evidence implicating **methylephedrine** and **pholedrine** seems not to have been documented, but on the basis of their known pharmacology their concurrent use with the MAOIs should be avoided.

Note that some of the indirectly-acting amines, including ephedrine, phenylpropanolamine and pseudoephedrine, are used as vasoconstrictor decongestants in numerous oral non-prescription cough, cold and influenza preparations. Isometheptene is used in non-prescription analgesic preparations for migraine. Patients on MAOIs should be strongly warned not to take any of these drugs concurrently or for 2 weeks after stopping their MAOI. Also, note that serious interactions have occurred because of confusion between non-prescription products with very similar names that contain different active ingredients.[12]

Physicians should also avoid the use of indirectly-acting vasoconstrictor amines such as ephedrine, mephentermine and metaraminol for reversing hypotension during spinal anaesthesia in patients taking MAOIs or who have recently stopped these (within the previous 2 weeks).

(b) RIMAs

The data with high-dose ephedrine show that moclobemide is not free of this interaction, and the manufacturers of moclobemide[23] advise avoiding sympathomimetics such as ephedrine, pseudoephedrine and phenylpropanolamine. It would also be prudent to avoid moclobemide with any of the other indirectly-acting sympathomimetics cited here, although the severity of the interactions with moclobemide is unlikely to be as great as that seen with the MAOIs. For example, ephedrine and phenylephrine have been successfully and uneventfully used in the presence of moclobemide (omitted on the day of surgery) during anaesthesia to control hypotension.[24]

(c) Treatment

Hypertensive reactions have been controlled by intravenous phentolamine, phenoxybenzamine, intramuscular chlorpromazine, labetalol or sublingual nifedipine. The manufacturers of phenelzine state that on the basis of present evidence, slow intravenous injection of phentolamine is recommended.[25,26] However, it is advisable to refer to current guidelines on the management of hypertensive crises for up-to-date advice. See also Importance and Management under 'MAOIs or RIMAs + Tyramine-rich foods', p.1153.

1. Elis J, Laurence DR, Mattie H, Prichard BNC. Modification by monoamine oxidase inhibitors of the effect of some sympathomimetics on blood pressure. *BMJ* (1967) 2, 75–8.
2. Cuthbert MF, Greenberg MP, Morley SW. Cough and cold remedies: a potential danger to patients on monoamine oxidase inhibitors. *BMJ* (1969) 1, 404–6.
3. Cuthbert MF, Vere DW. Potentiation of the cardiovascular effects of some catecholamines by a monoamine oxidase inhibitor. *Br J Pharmacol* (1971) 43, 471P–472P.
4. Hirsch MS, Walter RM, Hasterlik RJ. Subarachnoid hemorrhage following ephedrine and MAO inhibitor. *JAMA* (1965) 194, 1259.
5. Kraft KE, Dore FH. Computerized drug interaction programs: how reliable ? *JAMA* (1996) 275, 1087.
6. Stark DCC. Effects of giving vasopressors to patients on monoamine-oxidase inhibitors. *Lancet* (1962) i, 1405–6.
7. Horler AR, Wynne NA. Hypertensive crisis due to pargyline and metaraminol. *BMJ* (1965) 2, 460–1.
8. Jenkins LC, Graves HB. Potential hazards of psychoactive drugs in association with anaesthesia. *Can Anaesth Soc J* (1965) 12, 121–8.
9. Tonks CM, Lloyd AT. Hazards with monoamine-oxidase inhibitors. *BMJ* (1965) 1, 589.
10. Mason AMS, Buckle RM. "Cold" cures and monoamine-oxidase inhibitors. *BMJ* (1969) 1, 845–6.
11. Humberstone PM. Hypertension from cold remedies. *BMJ* (1969) 1, 846.
12. Harrison WM, McGrath PJ, Stewart JW, Quitkin F. MAOIs and hypertensive crises: the role of OTC drugs. *J Clin Psychiatry* (1989) 50, 64–5. Correction. Magurno JAJ, Board AW. ibid. (1990) 51, 212–3. [drug].
13. Smookler S, Bermudez AJ. Hypertensive crisis resulting from an MAO inhibitor and an over-the-counter appetite suppressant. *Ann Emerg Med* (1982) 11, 482–4.
14. Wright SP. Hazards with monoamine-oxidase inhibitors: a persistent problem. *Lancet* (1978) i, 284–5.
15. Davies R. Patient medication records. *Pharm J* (1982) 228, 652.
16. Dawson JK, Earnshaw SM, Graham CS. Dangerous monoamine oxidase inhibitor interactions are still occurring in the 1990s. *J Accid Emerg Med* (1995) 12, 49–51.
17. Low-Beer GA, Tidmarsh D. Collapse after "Parstelin". *BMJ* (1963) 2, 683–4.
18. Schrire I. Collapse after "Parstelin". *BMJ* (1963) 2, 748.
19. Terry R, Kaye AH, McDonald M. Sinutab. *Med J Aust* (1975) 1, 763.
20. Gleiter CH, Mühlbauer B, Gradin-Frimmer G, Antonin KH, Bieck PR. Administration of sympathomimetic drugs with the selective MAO-A inhibitor brofaromine. Effect on blood pressure. *Drug Invest* (1992) 4, 149–54.
21. Dingemanse J. An update of recent moclobemide interaction data. *Int Clin Psychopharmacol* (1993) 7, 167–80.
22. Dingemanse J, Guentert T, Gieschke R, Stabl M. Modification of the cardiovascular effects of ephedrine by the reversible monoamine oxidase A-inhibitor moclobemide. *J Cardiovasc Pharmacol* (1996) 28, 856–61.
23. Manerix (Moclobemide). Roche Products Ltd. UK Summary of product characteristics, September 2005.
24. Martyr JW, Orlikowski CEP. Epidural anaesthesia, ephedrine and phenylephrine in a patient taking moclobemide, a new monoamine oxidase inhibitor. *Anaesthesia* (1996) 51, 1150–2.
25. Nardil (Phenelzine sulfate). Link Pharmaceuticals Ltd. UK Summary of product characteristics, July 2003.
26. Nardil (Phenelzine sulfate). Pfizer inc. US Prescribing information, June 2007.

MAOIs or RIMAs + Sympathomimetics; Phenylephrine

The concurrent use of oral phenylephrine and the non-selective MAOIs can result in a potentially life-threatening hypertensive crisis. Phenylephrine is commonly found in proprietary cough, cold and influenza preparations. The effects of parenteral phenylephrine may be approximately doubled by MAOIs. Some interaction occurs between phenylephrine and the RIMAs moclobemide or brofaromine, but the blood pressure response appears to be much smaller than that seen with the non-selective MAOIs.

Clinical evidence

(a) MAOIs

A study in 3 healthy subjects, given **phenelzine** 45 mg or **tranylcypromine** 30 mg daily for 7 days, found that the blood pressure rise following oral phenylephrine was markedly enhanced. On 2 of 3 occasions when 45 mg of phenylephrine was given orally, the rise in blood pressure became potentially disastrous and had to be reversed with phentolamine. On these two occasions the maximal increase in mean arterial pressure was 67 mmHg (compared with 1 or 11 mmHg without the MAOI). On the other occasion, the maximal increase in mean arterial pressure was 48 mmHg. The rise in blood pressure was accompanied by a severe headache. With 3 and 10 mg of phenylephrine, the maximal increase was 7 and 20 mmHg, respectively. After intravenous phenylephrine 3 mg was given over 20 minutes, the maximal increase in mean arterial pressure was 45 mmHg, compared with 23 mmHg without an MAOI.[1]

Another study describes a similar 2- to 2.5-fold increase in the pressor effects of *intravenous* phenylephrine following the use of **phenelzine** or **tranylcypromine**.[2] A patient taking **tranylcypromine** who developed hypotension (40/0 mmHg) during surgery had an exaggerated pressor response (250/140 mmHg) when an intravenous infusion of phenylephrine 4 mg/500 mL was started.[3] However, in another report repeated 100-microgram doses of intravenous phenylephrine were successfully used to treat hypotension in a patient on an MAOI, without any hypertensive reaction.[4]

A case report of hypertension that was initially attributed to phenylephrine was later corrected to pseudoephedrine.[5]

(b) RIMAs

No clinically important interaction occurred in healthy subjects taking **brofaromine** 75 mg twice daily when they were given a single 2.5-mg dose of phenylephrine as nasal drops.[6] However, higher doses [exact amount not stated] did produce a blood pressure response,[6] with a maximum recorded diastolic blood pressure of 100 mmHg.

A study in 7 healthy subjects found that **moclobemide** 100 mg three times daily for one week had no effect on the increase in blood pressure induced by intravenous phenylephrine.[7] Another study reported similar results.[8] However, when **moclobemide** was given in a dose of 200 mg three times daily for up to 3 weeks the blood pressure response to infusions of phenylephrine was increased by up to 1.8-fold.[7] In one patient taking **moclobemide** (dose withheld on the morning of surgery), ephedrine and phenylephrine were used successfully and uneventfully to control hypotension during anaesthesia.[9]

A case of life-threatening hypertension[10] occurred in a patient taking **toloxatone**, non-prescription phenylephrine and **'terbutaline'**, (p.1146).

Mechanism

If given by mouth phenylephrine is used in large doses because much of it is destroyed by MAO in the gut and liver, and only a small amount gets into the general circulation. If MAO is inhibited, most of the oral dose escapes destruction and passes freely into circulation, hence the gross enhancement of the pressor effects. Phenylephrine has mainly direct sympathomimetic activity, but it may also have some minor indirect activity as well, which would be expected to result in the release of some of the MAOI-accumulated noradrenaline (norepinephrine) at adrenergic nerve endings (see also 'MAOIs or RIMAs + Sympathomimetics; Indirectly-acting', p.1147). This might account for the increased response to phenylephrine given parenterally.

Importance and management

The interaction between the MAOIs and oral phenylephrine is established, serious and potentially life-threatening. Phenylephrine commonly occurs in oral non-prescription cough, cold and influenza preparations, so patients should be strongly warned about them. Whether the effects of nasal drops and sprays and eye drops are also enhanced is uncertain, but it would be prudent to avoid them until they have been shown to be safe. The response to parenteral administration is also approximately doubled, so that a dosage reduction is necessary.

The few studies that are available suggest that any interaction with RIMAs is less severe than that with MAOIs, but this needs confirmation.

Treatment

These hypertensive reactions have been controlled by intravenous phentolamine,[1] chlorpromazine, or nifedipine.[11] However, it is advisable to refer to current guidelines on the management of hypertensive crises for up-to-date advice. In the US, the manufacturers of phenelzine advise intravenous **phentolamine** 5 mg, given slowly to avoid excessive hypotension.[12] See also Importance and management under 'MAOIs or RIMAs + Tyramine-rich foods', p.1153.

1. Elis J, Laurence DR, Mattie H, Prichard BNC. Modification by monoamine oxidase inhibitors of the effect of some sympathomimetics on blood pressure. *BMJ* (1967) 2, 75–8.

2. Boakes AJ, Laurence DR, Teoh PC, Barar FSK, Benedikter L, Prichard BNC. Interactions between sympathomimetic amines and antidepressant agents in man. *BMJ* (1973) 1, 311–15.
3. Jenkins LC, Graves HB. Potential hazards of psychoactive drugs in association with anaesthesia. *Can Anaesth Soc J* (1965) 12, 121–8.
4. El-Ganzouri A, Ivankovich AD, Braverman B, Land PC. Should MAOI be discontinued preoperatively? *Anesthesiology* (1983) 59, A384.
5. Harrison WM, McGrath PJ, Stewart JW, Quitkin F. MAOIs and hypertensive crises: the role of OTC drugs. *J Clin Psychiatry* (1989) 50, 64–5. Correction. Magurno JAJ, Board AW. ibid. (1990) 51, 212–3. [drug].
6. Gleiter CH, Mühlbauer B, Gradin-Frimmer G, Antonin KH, Bieck PR. Administration of sympathomimetic drugs with the selective MAO-A inhibitor brofaromine. Effect on blood pressure. *Drug Invest* (1992) 4, 149–54.
7. Amrein R, Güntert TW, Dingemanse J, Lorscheid T, Stabl M, Schmid-Burgk W. Interactions of moclobemide with concomitantly administered medication: evidence from pharmacological and clinical studies. *Psychopharmacology (Berl)* (1992) 106, S24–S31.
8. Korn A, Eichler HG, Gasić S. Moclobemide, a new specific MAO-inhibitor does not interact with direct adrenergic agonists. The Second Amine Oxidase Workshop, Uppsala. August 1986. *Pharmacol Toxicol* (1987) 60 (Suppl I), 31.
9. Martyr JW, Orlikowski CEP. Epidural anaesthesia, ephedrine and phenylephrine in a patient taking moclobemide, a new monoamine oxidase inhibitor. *Anaesthesia* (1996) 51, 1150–2.
10. Lefebvre H, Richard R, Noblet C, Moore N, Wolf L-M. Life-threatening pseudo-phaeochromocytoma after toloxatone, terbutaline, and phenylephrine. *Lancet* (1993) 341, 555–6.
11. Golwyn DH, Weinstock RC. MAOIs, OTC drugs, and hypertensive crisis. *J Clin Psychiatry* (1990) 51, 213.
12. Nardil (Phenelzine sulfate). Pfizer Inc. US Prescribing information, June 2007.

MAOIs or RIMAs + Tricyclic and related antidepressants

Because of the very toxic and sometimes fatal reactions (the serotonin syndrome or similar) that have occurred in patients taking either MAOIs or RIMAs with tricyclic antidepressants, concurrent use is regarded as contraindicated in all but rare circumstances, and a suitable washout interval is needed when switching between MAOIs or RIMAs and tricyclics. Of the tricyclics, clomipramine and imipramine have been most frequently implicated in adverse reactions with the MAOIs.

Clinical evidence

A. MAOIs

The toxic reactions that occur when the tricyclics are given with MAOIs have included (with variations) sweating, flushing, hyperpyrexia, restlessness, excitement, tremor, muscle twitching and rigidity, convulsions and coma. Two illustrative examples:

A woman who had been taking **tranylcypromine** 10 mg twice daily for about 3 weeks, stopped taking it 3 days before she took a single tablet of **imipramine**. Within a few hours she complained of an excruciating headache, and soon afterwards lost consciousness and started to convulse. The toxic reactions manifested were a temperature of 40.6°C, pulse rate of 120 bpm, severe extensor rigidity, carpal spasm, opisthotonos and cyanosis. She was treated with amobarbital and phenytoin, and her temperature was reduced with alcohol-ice-soaked towels. The treatment was effective and she recovered.[1]

In a recent case, a patient was treated with **imipramine** 75 mg daily for 7 weeks with lithium as well for the last 3 weeks. These drugs were discontinued and after one week of washout he started **tranylcypromine**, which was gradually increased to 50 mg twice daily. After 2 weeks at this dose, he received a single 225-mg dose of **imipramine** in error. Four hours later his condition deteriorated rapidly. He was agitated, confused, with severe rigidity, myoclonic jerks, hyperthermia, hypertension and tachycardia, and 2 hours later had a cardiac and respiratory arrest. He was resuscitated and treated with midazolam, pancuronium, dantrolene sodium, and a cooling mattress. The following day he had a sudden fall in blood pressure, and was eventually pronounced brain dead, and artificial respiration was terminated.[2]

Similar reactions have been recorded with oral therapeutic doses of:

- **amitriptyline** with **phenelzine**[3,4]
- **clomipramine** with **phenelzine**[5-7] or **tranylcypromine** (with or without trifluoperazine)[8-10]
- **desipramine** with **phenelzine**[11]
- **imipramine** with **iproniazid**,[12] **isocarboxazid**,[12] **pargyline**,[13] **phenelzine**[14-16] or **tranylcypromine**.[12,17]

There have been a number of fatalities.[8,9,11,18] Reactions have also occurred when intramuscular **imipramine** was given with **phenelzine**.[19-21] In some instances the drugs were not taken together, but were substituted without a washout period in between.[6,17] In some other reports there was an overdose of one or both drugs,[22-25] and/or the presence of other potentially interacting drugs.[23,24] There are many more reports of these interactions than are listed here: those published prior to 1977 have been extensively reviewed elsewhere.[16,26,27]

Three patients with bipolar disorder developed mania when treated with **isocarboxazid** and **amitriptyline**.[28]

In contrast, there are a number of other uncontrolled studies[29-31] and reviews[26,27] describing the beneficial use of an MAOI with a tricyclic antidepressant. In addition, one study has reported switching 178 patients from tricyclics to MAOIs within 4 days or less. Of these patients, 63 were given the MAOI while still being tapered from the tricyclic, all without any apparent problems.[32] Nevertheless, in a 6-week randomised double-blind trial, the combinations of **phenelzine** or **isocarboxazid** plus **trimipramine** were less effective than **trimipramine** alone in patients with mild to moderate depression.[33] Similarly, in a smaller randomised open study, the combination of **amitriptyline** and **tranylcypromine** was no more effective than either drug alone.[34]

B. RIMAs

(a) Amitriptyline

Two small studies in healthy subjects and patients found no problems when **moclobemide** was given with, or 24 hours after, amitriptyline,[35,36] or when amitriptyline was given immediately after **moclobemide**.[35] However, a patient taking amitriptyline and **clomipramine** developed the serotonin syndrome after taking a dose of **moclobemide** and died[37] (see also **clomipramine** below).

Only a minor and clinically unimportant change in the pharmacokinetics of amitriptyline occurs in patients given **toloxatone**.[38]

(b) Clomipramine

A small study in healthy subjects found no problems when **moclobemide** was given 24 hours after clomipramine.[36] However, the serotonin syndrome occurred in 3 patients when clomipramine was replaced by **moclobemide** without a washout period[39,40] or with only a 24-hour washout period,[41] and in another patient when **moclobemide** was replaced by clomipramine after only 12 hours.[42] A fatal case of the serotonin syndrome occurred in a patient taking clomipramine and **amitriptyline**, with symptoms manifesting within 30 minutes of a 300-mg dose of **moclobemide**.[37] Two other patients developed fatal serotonin syndrome after taking moderate overdoses of **moclobemide** and clomipramine.[43] The serotonin syndrome has been reported in at least 8 other cases of **moclobemide** and clomipramine overdose,[44-50] one of which also involved tramadol[45] (see also 'MAOIs + Opioids; Tramadol', p.1141), another fluoxetine[46] (see also 'MAOIs or RIMAs + SSRIs', p.1142), and yet another buspirone[50] (see also 'MAOIs or RIMAs + Buspirone', p.1133). Conversely, a case of an overdose of moclobemide and clomipramine resulted in no adverse effects except sinus tachycardia.[51]

(c) Desipramine

A small single dose study in healthy subjects found no problems when **moclobemide** was given with desipramine.[35]

(d) Doxepin

Serotonin toxicity (the serotonin syndrome) occurred in a patient who took an overdose of **moclobemide** and doxepin. In this analysis of **moclobemide** overdoses, the risk of developing serotonin toxicity was increased 35 times in patients who also took another serotonergic drug, of which this case with doxepin was one of 11 mentioned.[52]

(e) Imipramine

The serotonin syndrome occurred in a patient who had been taking **moclobemide** for about a month and imipramine (50 mg at night increased to 200 mg at night) for about 17 days.[53]

(f) Maprotiline

One study found a nonsignificant 25% rise in serum levels of maprotiline (a tetracyclic antidepressant) in 6 patients also taking **moclobemide**. No serious toxic reactions were reported.[54]

(g) Trimipramine

One study found a 39% rise in serum trimipramine levels in 15 patients also taking **moclobemide**. No serious toxic reactions were reported.[54]

Mechanism

Not understood. One idea is that both drugs cause grossly elevated monoamine levels (5-HT, noradrenaline (norepinephrine)) in the brain, which 'spill-over' into areas not concerned with mood elevation. It may be related to, or the same as 'the serotonin syndrome', (p.9). Of the tricyclics, clomipramine in particular is a potent inhibitor of serotonin uptake. Less likely suggestions are that the MAOIs inhibit the metabolism of the tricyclic antidepressants, or that active and unusual metabolites of the tricyclic antidepressants are produced.[26]

Importance and management

An established and fairly common interaction, but serious and life-threatening occurrences seem rare. If concurrent use is to be avoided, the following guidelines[55] are recommended:

- Tricyclic antidepressants should *not* be started for 2 weeks after treatment with MAOIs has been stopped (3 weeks if starting clomipramine or imipramine).
- An MAOI should *not* be started until at least 7 to 14 days after a tricyclic or related antidepressant has been stopped (3 weeks in the case of clomipramine or imipramine).
- Moclobemide has a short duration of action so no treatment-free period is required after it has been stopped before starting a tricyclic antidepressant. [Note however that some recommend waiting 24 hours.[42]]
- Moclobemide should *not* be started until at least a week after a tricyclic antidepressant has been stopped.

No detailed clinical work has been done to find out precisely what sets the scene when the interaction does occur, but some general empirical guidelines have been suggested so that it can, as far as possible, be avoided when concurrent treatment is thought appropriate:[15,16,26,27,56]

- Treatment with both types of drug should only be undertaken by those well aware of the problems and who can undertake adequate supervision.
- Only patients refractory to all other types of treatment should be considered.
- Tranylcypromine, phenelzine, clomipramine and imipramine appear to be high on the list of drugs that have interacted adversely. Combination of clomipramine with tranylcypromine is particularly dangerous. Amitriptyline, trimipramine and isocarboxazid are possibly safer.
- Absence of information documenting unsuitability or hazard does not necessarily imply that the two drugs may be used safely together, but may merely reflect an untried combination.[56]
- Drugs should be given orally, not parenterally.
- It seems safer to give the tricyclic antidepressants first, or together with the MAOI, than to give the MAOI first. If the patient is already taking an MAOI, it may not be safe to start the tricyclic antidepressant until recovery from MAO-inhibition is complete.
- Small doses should be given initially, increasing the levels of each drug, one at a time, over a period of 2 to 3 weeks to levels generally about half[56] those used for each one individually.

Treatment of the serotonin syndrome

In the management of serotonin syndrome, it is important to recognise the possibility of the syndrome early, as the patient's condition can rapidly deteriorate. Potentially precipitating drugs should be stopped and agitation should be managed with benzodiazepines. The intensity of therapy depends on the severity of the condition. Moderately ill patients may benefit from the administration of 5-HT antagonists such as cyproheptadine. The 5-HT antagonist, chlorpromazine has also been used and can be beneficial, but should not be given if the patient is hypotensive or if the neuroleptic malignant syndrome is a possible diagnosis. Hyperthermic patients should be immediately sedated, given neuromuscular blockers and intubated, since the rise in temperature is due to muscular activity. MAOI-induced hypotension should be managed with low doses of direct-acting sympathomimetics. Propranolol, bromocriptine, and dantrolene have been used, but these are no longer recommended. Because of the potential severity of the condition, a poison-control centre, clinical pharmacology service or medical toxicologist should be consulted for up-to-date advice.[57]

1. Brachfeld J, Wirtshafter A, Wolfe S. Imipramine-tranylcypromine incompatibility. Near-fatal toxic reaction. *JAMA* (1963) 186, 1172–3.
2. Otte W, Birkenhager TK, van den Broek WW. Fatal interaction between tranylcypromine and imipramine. *Eur Psychiatry* (2003) 18, 264–5.
3. Heyland D, Sauvé M. Neuroleptic malignant syndrome without the use of neuroleptics. *Can Med Assoc J* (1991) 145, 817–19.
4. Teas GA. Toxic delirium resulting from combination antidepressant therapy. *Am J Psychiatry* (1981) 138, 1127.
5. Beeley L, Daly M. *Bulletin of West Midlands Centre for Adverse Drug Reaction Reporting* (1986) 23, 16.
6. Stern TA, Schwartz JH, Shuster JL. Catastrophic illness associated with the combination of clomipramine, phenelzine, and chlorpromazine. *Ann Clin Psychiatry* (1992) 4, 81–5.
7. Pascual J, Combarros O, Berciano J. Partial status epilepticus following single low dose of clorimipramine in a patient on MAO-inhibitor treatment. *Clin Neuropharmacol* (1987) 10, 565–7.
8. Beaumont G. Drug interactions with clomipramine (Anafranil). *J Int Med Res* (1973) 1, 480–4.
9. Tackley RM, Tregaskis B. Fatal disseminated intravascular coagulation following a monoamine oxidase inhibitor/tricyclic interaction. *Anaesthesia* (1987) 42, 760–3.
10. Gillman PK. Successful treatment of serotonin syndrome with chlorpromazine. *Med J Aust* (1996) 165, 345–6.
11. Bowen LW. Fatal hyperpyrexia with antidepressant drugs. *BMJ* (1964) 2, 1465–6.
12. Ayd FJ. Toxic somatic and psychopathological reactions to antidepressant drugs. *J Neuropsychiatr* (1961) 2 (Suppl 1), S119–S122.
13. McCurdy RL, Kane FJ. Transient brain syndrome as a non-fatal reaction to combined pargyline imipramine treatment. *Am J Psychiatry* (1964), 121, 397–8.
14. Howarth E. Possible synergistic effects of the new thymoleptics in connection with poisoning. *J Ment Sci* (1961) 107, 100–103.
15. Graham PM, Potter JM, Paterson JW. Combination monoamine oxidase inhibitor/tricyclic antidepressant interaction. *Lancet* (1982) ii, 440.
16. Schuckit M, Robins E, Feighner J. Tricyclic antidepressants and monoamine oxidase inhibitors. Combination therapy in the treatment of depression. *Arch Gen Psychiatry* (1971) 24, 509–14.
17. Grantham J, Neel W, Brown RW. Toxicity reversed. Reversal of imipramine-monoamine oxidase inhibitor induced toxicity by chlorpromazine. *J Kans Med Soc* (1964) 65, 279–80.
18. Wright SP. Hazards with monoamine-oxidase inhibitors: a persistent problem. *Lancet* (1978) i, 284–5.
19. Hills NF. Combining the antidepressant drugs. *BMJ* (1965) 1, 859.
20. Lockett MF, Milner G. Combining the antidepressant drugs. *BMJ* (1965) 1, 921.
21. Singh H. Atropine-like poisoning due to tranquillizing agents. *Am J Psychiatry* (1960) 117, 360–1.
22. Davies G. Side-effects of phenelzine. *BMJ* (1960) 2, 1019.
23. Nierenberg DW, Semprebon M. The central nervous system serotonin syndrome. *Clin Pharmacol Ther* (1993) 53, 84–8.
24. Richards GA, Fritz VU, Pincus P, Reyneke J. Unusual drug interactions between monoamine oxidase inhibitors and tricyclic antidepressants. *J Neurol Neurosurg Psychiatry* (1987) 50, 1240–1.
25. Stanley B, Pal NR. Fatal hyperpyrexia with phenelzine and imipramine. *BMJ* (1964) 2, 1011.
26. Ponto LB, Perry PJ, Liskow BI, Seaba HH. Drug therapy reviews: tricyclic antidepressant and monoamine oxidase inhibitor combination therapy. *Am J Hosp Pharm* (1977) 34, 954–61.
27. Ananth J, Luchins D. A review of combined tricyclic and MAOI therapy. *Compr Psychiatry* (1977) 18, 221–30.
28. de la Fuente JR, Berlanga C, León-Andrade C. Mania induced by tricyclic-MAOI combination therapy in bipolar treatment-resistant disorder: case reports. *J Clin Psychiatry* (1986) 47, 40–1.
29. Gander GA. The clinical value of monoamine oxidase inhibitors and tricyclic antidepressants in combination. *Int Congr Ser* (1966) 122, 336–43.
30. Gander DR. Treatment of depressive illnesses with combined antidepressants. *Lancet* (1965) ii, 107–9.
31. Berlanga C. Ortego-Soto HA. A 3-year follow-up of a group of treatment-resistant depressed patients with a MAOI/tricyclic combination. *J Affect Disord* (1995) 34, 187–92.
32. Kahn D, Silver JM, Opler LA. The safety of switching rapidly from tricyclic antidepressants to monoamine oxidase inhibitors. *J Clin Psychopharmacol* (1989) 9, 198–202.
33. Young JPR, Lader MH, Hughes WC. Controlled trial of trimipramine, monoamine oxidase inhibitors, and combined treatment in depressed outpatients. *BMJ* (1979) 2, 1315–17.
34. White K, Pistole T, Boyd JL. Combined monoamine oxidase inhibitor-tricyclic antidepressant treatment: a pilot study. *Am J Psychiatry* (1980) 137, 1422–5.
35. Korn A, Eichler HG, Fischbach R, Gasic S. Moclobemide, a new reversible MAO inhibitor – interaction with tyramine and tricyclic antidepressants in healthy volunteers and depressive patients. *Psychopharmacology (Berl)* (1986) 88, 153–7.
36. Dingemanse J, Kneer J, Fotteler B, Groen H, Peeters PAM, Jonkman JHG. Switch in treatment from tricyclic antidepressants to moclobemide: a new generation monoamine oxidase inhibitor. *J Clin Psychopharmacol* (1995) 15, 41–8.
37. Kuisma MJ. Fatal serotonin syndrome with trismus. *Ann Emerg Med* (1995) 26, 108.
38. Vandel S, Bertschy G, Perault MC, Sandoz M, Bouquet S, Chakroun R, Guibert S, Vandel B. Minor and clinically non-significant interaction between toloxatone and amitriptyline. *Eur J Clin Pharmacol* (1993) 44, 97–9.
39. Spigset O, Mjorndal T, Lovheim O. Serotonin syndrome caused by a moclobemide-clomipramine interaction. *BMJ* (1993) 306, 248.
40. Chan BSH, Graudins A, Whyte IM, Dawson AH, Braitberg G, Duggin GG. Serotonin syndrome resulting from drug interactions. *Med J Aust* (1998) 169, 523–5.
41. Dardennes RM, Even C, Ballon N, Bange F. Serotonin syndrome caused by a clomipramine–moclobemide interaction. *J Clin Psychiatry* (1998) 59, 382–3.
42. Gillman PK. Serotonin syndrome – clomipramine too soon after moclobemide? *Int Clin Psychopharmacol* (1997) 12, 339–42.
43. Neuvonen PJ, Pohjola-Sintonen S, Tacke U, Vuori E. Five fatal cases of serotonin syndrome after moclobemide-citalopram or moclobemide-clomipramine overdoses. *Lancet* (1993) 342, 1419.
44. Myrenfors PG, Eriksson T, Sandstedt CS, Sjöberg G. Moclobemide overdose. *J Intern Med* (1993) 233, 113–15.
45. Hernandez AF, Montero MN, Pla A, Villaneuva E. Fatal moclobemide overdose or death caused by serotonin syndrome? *J Forensic Sci* (1995) 40, 128–30.
46. Power BM, Pinder M, Hackett LP, Ilett KF. Fatal serotonin syndrome following a combined overdose of moclobemide, clomipramine and fluoxetine. *Anaesth Intensive Care* (1995) 23, 499–502.
47. François B, Marquet P, Desachy A, Roustan J, Lachatre G, Gastinne H. Serotonin syndrome due to an overdose of moclobemide and clomipramine: a potentially life-threatening association. *Intensive Care Med* (1997) 23, 122–4.
48. Finge T, Malavialle C, Lambert J. Forme mortelle de syndrome sérotoninergique. *Ann Fr Anesth Reanim* (1997), 16, 80–1.
49. Ferrer-Dufol A, Perez-Aradros C, Murillo EC. Fatal serotonin syndrome caused by moclobemide-clomipramine overdose. *Clin Toxicol* (1998) 36, 31–2.
50. Höjer J, Personne M, Skagius A-S, Hansson O. Serotoninergt syndrom: flera allvarliga fall med denna ofta förbisedda diagnos. *Lakartidningen* (2002) 99, 2054–5, 2058–60.
51. Iwersen S, Schmoldt A. Three suicide attempts with moclobemide. *J Toxicol Clin Toxicol* (1996) 34, 223–5.
52. Isbister GK, Hackett LP, Dawson AH, Whyte IM, Smith AJ. Moclobemide poisoning: toxicokinetics and occurrence of serotonin toxicity. *Br J Clin Pharmacol* (2003) 56, 441–50.

53. Brodribb TR, Downey M, Gilbar PJ. Efficacy and adverse effects of moclobemide. *Lancet* (1994) 343, 475–6.
54. König F, Wolfersdorf M, Löble M, Wößner S, Hauger B. Trimipramine and maprotiline plasma levels during combined treatment with moclobemide in therapy-resistant depression. *Pharmacopsychiatry* (1997) 30, 125–7.
55. British National Formulary. 53rd ed. London: The British Medical Association and The Pharmaceutical Press; 2007, p. 205–6.
56. Sweetman SC, ed. Martindale: The complete drug reference. 35th ed. London: Pharmaceutical Press; 2007, p. 378.
57. Boyer EW, Shannon M. The serotonin syndrome. *N Engl J Med* (2005) 352, 1112–20.

MAOIs + Tryptophan

A number of patients have developed severe behavioural and neurological signs of toxicity (some similar to the serotonin syndrome) after taking MAOIs with tryptophan, and fatalities have occurred.

Clinical evidence

A man taking **phenelzine** 90 mg daily developed behavioural and neurological toxicity within 2 hours of being given 6 g of tryptophan.[1] He had shivering and diaphoresis, his psychomotor retardation disappeared and he became jocular, fearful, and moderately labile. His neurological signs included bilateral Babinski signs, hyperreflexia, rapid horizontal ocular oscillations, shivering of the jaw, trunk and limbs, mild dysmetria and ataxia. The situation resolved on withdrawal of the drugs.[1]

Similar symptoms have been reported in other studies and cases. In an early study, giving tryptophan 20 to 50 mg/kg to 7 patients with hypertension taking an unknown MAOI produced neurological effects including alcohol-like intoxication, drowsiness, hyperreflexia and clonus.[2] Similar symptoms with the addition of sweating, flushing and paraesthesias were described in 5 patients in an experimental study of tryptophan 30 mg/kg orally combined with **pargyline** or **isocarboxazid**.[3] In another study in 14 depressed patients taking various MAOIs, 4 patients had muscular jactitation and hyperreflexia when also given tryptophan 2.5 to 5 g three times daily, and in 2 patients this was severe enough to discontinue the tryptophan.[4] Other reports describe similar symptoms in patients taking **phenelzine**[5,6] or **tranylcypromine**[7] when they were given tryptophan.

One patient taking **tranylcypromine** and lithium had transient episodes of toxicity with hyperthermia (and other symptoms of neurological toxicity) when the dose of tryptophan was increased to 2 g at night. He had a total of about 12 of these episodes over several weeks before tryptophan was stopped and the episodes ceased.[8] Malignant hyperpyrexia occurred in a patient taking **phenelzine** and tryptophan,[9] and fatal cases have occurred in two patients on **phenelzine**, tryptophan and lithium.[10,11] Another patient who had been taking **tranylcypromine** for 2 weeks developed serious hyperpyrexia and muscular rigidity 2 days after starting tryptophan 6 g daily: she had discontinued levodopa-carbidopa one month previously.[12] Tryptophan may have contributed to a fatal case of the serotonin syndrome in a patient switched from fluoxetine to **tranylcypromine**.[13]

Hypomania without neurological symptoms has occurred in 2 patients when tryptophan was added to **phenelzine** or **tranylcypromine**,[14] and delirium or disorientation, (sometimes with neurological symptoms) has occurred in 8 patients on **tranylcypromine** within 2 to 4 days of starting tryptophan, or within 1 day of increasing the dose of tryptophan.[15] A further patient also experienced delirium within hours of tryptophan being added to her **phenelzine** treatment.[16]

In contrast, concurrent use has been reported as both safe and effective.[17]

Mechanism

Not understood. The reactions appear to be related to the serotonin syndrome, which can occur with two or more serotonergic drugs (see 'The serotonin syndrome', (p.9)). MAOIs may inhibit the metabolism of 5-hydroxytryptamine (serotonin), formed from tryptophan, so resulting in its accumulation.[3,9]

Importance and management

Information seems to be confined to the reports listed. Concurrent use can be effective in the treatment of depression,[17] but occasionally and unpredictably severe and even life-threatening toxicity occurs. The authors of one of the reports detailed above[1] recommend that patients on MAOIs should be started on a low dose of tryptophan (0.5 g). This should be gradually increased while monitoring the mental status of the patient for changes suggesting hypomania, and neurological changes, including ocular oscillations and upper motor neurone signs.

Note that products containing tryptophan for the treatment of depression were withdrawn in the USA, UK, and many other countries because of a possible association with the development of an eosinophilia-myalgia syndrome. However, since the syndrome appeared to have been associated with tryptophan from one manufacturer, tryptophan preparations were reintroduced in the UK in 1994 for restricted use.[18,19]

1. Thomas JN, Rubin EH. Case report of a toxic reaction from a combination of tryptophan and phenelzine. *Am J Psychiatry* (1984) 141, 281–3.
2. Oates JA, Sjoerdsma A. Neurological effects of tryptophan in patients receiving a monoamine oxidase inhibitor. *Neurology* (1960) 10, 1076–8.
3. Hodge JV, Oates JA, Sjoerdsma A. Reduction of the central effects of tryptophan by a decarboxylase inhibitor. *Clin Pharmacol Ther* (1964) 5, 149–55.
4. Pare CMB. Potentiation of monoamine-oxidase inhibitors by tryptophan. *Lancet* (1963) 2, 527–8.
5. Glassman AH, Platman SR. Potentiation of monoamine oxidase inhibitor by tryptophan. *J Psychiatr Res* (1969) 7, 83–8.
6. Levy AB, Bucher P, Votolato N. Myoclonus, hyperreflexia and diaphoresis in patients on phenelzine-tryptophan combination treatment. *Can J Psychiatry* (1985) 30, 434–6.
7. Baloh RW, Dietz J, Spooner JW. Myoclonus and ocular oscillations induced by l-tryptophan. *Ann Neurol* (1982) 11, 95–7.
8. Price WA, Zimmer B, Kucas P. Serotonin syndrome: a case report. *J Clin Pharmacol* (1986) 26, 77–8.
9. Kim SY, Mueller PD. Life-threatening interaction between phenelzine and L-tryptophan. *Vet Hum Toxicol* (1989) 31, 370.
10. Staufenberg EF, Tantam D. Malignant hyperpyrexia syndrome in combined treatment. *Br J Psychiatry* (1989) 154, 577–8.
11. Brennan D, MacManus M, Howe J, McLoughlin J. 'Neuroleptic malignant syndrome' without neuroleptics. *Br J Psychiatry* (1988) 152, 578–9.
12. Parsa MA, Rohr T, Ramirez LF, Meltzer HY. Neuroleptic malignant syndrome without neuroleptics. *J Clin Psychopharmacol* (1990) 10, 437–8.
13. Kline SS, Mauro LS, Scala-Barnett DM, Zick D. Serotonin syndrome versus neuroleptic malignant syndrome as a cause of death. *Clin Pharm* (1989) 8, 510–14.
14. Goff DC. Two cases of hypomania following the addition of l-tryptophan to a monoamine oxidase inhibitor. *Am J Psychiatry* (1985) 142, 1487–8.
15. Pope HG, Jonas JM, Hudson JI, Kafka MP. Toxic reactions to the combination of monoamine oxidase inhibitors and tryptophan. *Am J Psychiatry* (1985) 142, 491–2.
16. Alvine G, Black DW, Tsuang D. Case of delirium secondary to phenelzine/l-tryptophan combination. *J Clin Psychiatry* (1990) 51, 311.
17. Nelson JC. Augmentation strategies in depression 2000. *J Clin Psychiatry* (2000) 61 (Suppl 2), 13–19.
18. Committee on Safety of Medicines/Medicines Control Agency. L-Tryptophan (Optimax): limited availability for resistant depression. *Current Problems* (1994) 20, 2.
19. Optimax (Tryptophan). Merck Pharmaceuticals. UK Summary of product characteristics, November 2004.

MAOIs or RIMAs + Tyramine-rich drinks

Patients taking the non-selective MAOIs (e.g. tranylcypromine, phenelzine) can suffer a serious hypertensive reaction if they drink tyramine-rich drinks (some beers or lagers, including low-alcohol brands, or wines), but no serious interaction is likely with the RIMAs (e.g. moclobemide). The hypotensive adverse effects of the MAOIs may be exaggerated in a few patients by alcohol, and they may experience dizziness and faintness after drinking relatively modest amounts. Moclobemide does not appear to alter the psychomotor effects of alcohol to a clinically relevant extent.

Clinical evidence, mechanism, importance and management

A. Hypertensive reactions

A severe and potentially life-threatening hypertensive reaction can occur in patients taking MAOIs if they consume alcoholic drinks containing significant amounts of tyramine. The details of the tyramine/MAOI reaction, its mechanism, the names of the non-selective MAOIs that interact, and the RIMAs that are unlikely to do so are described in the monograph 'MAOIs or RIMAs + Tyramine-rich foods', p.1153. The specific case reports for various tyramine-containing drinks are outlined in the sub-sections below. Note that an 8 to 20-mg dose of tyramine is required before an important rise in blood pressure takes place in a patient taking **tranylcypromine**, and this dose may be higher for other MAOIs (see under 'tyramine-rich foods', (p.1153)). 'Table 32.2', (p.1152) summarises the reported tyramine-content of some drinks,[1-7] and more extensive lists have been published elsewhere.[6-8] These can be used as a broad general guide when advising patients, but they cannot be an absolute guide because alcoholic drinks are the end-product of a biological fermentation process and no two batches are ever absolutely identical. For example there may be a 50-fold difference even between wines from the same grape stock.[5] There is no way of knowing for certain the tyramine-content of a particular drink without a detailed analysis.

Table 32.2 The tyramine-content of some drinks

	Tyramine content (mg/L)	*Refs*
Ales, beers and lagers		
Beer (Canada)	0 to 11.2, 27.1, 29.5, 112.9	1,2
Beer (Former Czechoslovakia)	10.4, 47 to 60	3
Beer (Germany)	1	3
Beer (Ireland)	0.5 to 4, 54	2,3
Beer (Netherlands)	1	3
Beer (UK)	0.3 to 1.34	2-4
Beer (USA)	0.7 to 4.4	2,3,5
Low-alcohol beers	0 to 10	2,6
Wines		
Chianti (Italy)		
Governo process	1.8 to 10.4, 25.4	1, 5
Newer process	0.0 to 4.7	3,4,7,8
Champagne	1, 13.7 to 18	3,9
Wine, red (Canada, France, Italy, Spain, USA)	0 to 8.6 (mean 5.2)	9
Wine, white (France, Germany, Italy, Portugal, Spain, Former Yugoslavia)	0.4 to 6.5	4,5,9
Fortified wines and spirits		
Gin	0	8
Port	Less than 0.2 (undetectable)	5
Sherry	0.2 to 3.6	1,3,5,8
Vodka	0	8
Whiskey	0	8

1. Sen NP. Analysis and significance of tyramine in foods. *J Food Sci* (1969) 34, 22-6.
2. Tailor SAN, Shulman KI, Walker SE, Moss J, Gardner D. Hypertensive episode associated with phenelzine and tap beer - a reanalysis of the role of pressor amines in beer. *J Clin Psychopharmacol* (1994) 14, 5-14.
3. Da Prada M, Zürcher G, Wüthrich I, Haefely WE. On tyramine, food, beverages and the reversible MAO inhibitor moclobemide. *J Neural Transm* (1988) (Suppl 26), 31.
4. Hannah P, Glover V, Sandler M. Tyramine in wine and beer. *Lancet* (1988) i, 879.
5. Horwitz D, Lovenberg W, Engelman K, Sjoerdsma A. Monoamine oxidase inhibitors, tyramine and cheese. *JAMA* (1964) 188, 1108-10.
6. Draper R, Sandler M, Walker PL. Clinical curio: monoamine oxidase inhibitors and non-alcoholic beer. BMJ (1984) 289, 308.
7. Korn A, Eichler HG, Fischbach R, Gasic S. Moclobemide, a new reversible MAO inhibitor - interaction with tyramine and tricyclic antidepressants in healthy volunteers and depressive patients. *Psychopharmacology (Berl)* (1986) 88, 153-7.
8. Shulman KI, Walker SE, MacKenzie S, Knowles S. Dietary restriction, tyramine, and use of monoamine oxidase inhibitors. *J Clin Psychopharmacol* (1989) 9, 397-402.
9. Zee JA, Simard RE, L'Heureux L, Tremblay J. Biogenic amines in wines. *Am J Enol Vitic* (1983) 34, 6-9.

(a) Ales, Beers and Lagers

Some ales, beers and lagers in 'social' amounts contain enough tyramine to reach the 8 to 20 mg dose needed to provoke a reaction; for example a litre (a little under two pints) of some samples of **Canadian ale or beer** (see 'Table 32.3', (p.1154)). Case reports of reactions have been published. A man taking **phenelzine** 60 mg daily developed a typical hypertensive reaction after drinking only 14 oz. (about 400 mL) of **Upper Canada lager beer on tap** (containing about 113 mg of tyramine/litre).[8] In addition, **alcohol-free beer** and **lager** may have a tyramine-content that is equal to ordinary beer and lager.[9,10] One patient taking **tranylcypromine** suffered an acute cerebral haemorrhage after drinking a **de-alcoholised Irish beer**,[9] hypertensive reactions occurred in three other patients taking **tranylcypromine** or **phenelzine** after drinking no more than about 375 mL of **alcohol-free beer or lager**[10] and a further patient taking **tranylcypromine** developed a vascular headache after drinking 3 bottles of non-alcoholic beer.[11] A very extensive study of 79 different brands of beer (from Canada, England, France, Germany, Holland, Ireland, Scotland, USA) found that the tyramine content of the **bottled** and **canned beers** examined was generally too low to matter (less than 10 mg/L), but four of 37 **beers on tap** (all 4 were lagers) contained more than enough tyramine (27 to 113 mg/L) to cause a hypertensive reaction.[8] It was concluded in this report that the consumption of **canned** or **bottled beer**, including **de-alcoholised beer**, in moderation (fewer than four bottles, 1.5 litres in a 4-hour period) was safe in patients on MAOIs, but, to be on the cautious side, all **beers on tap**, including **lagers** should be avoided.[8] The RIMAs are less likely to interact, see 'MAOIs or RIMAs + Tyramine-rich foods', p.1153.

(b) Spirits

Gin, whisky, vodka and **other spirits** do not contain significant amounts of tyramine because they are distilled, and the volumes drunk are relatively small.[7] There seem to be no reports of hypertensive reactions in patients taking MAOIs after drinking spirits and none would be expected. One author[12] anecdotally noted that "bottles of whisky have been drunk by some patients on the MAOIs, the only result being that they got drunk more easily and cheaply." However, a 38-year-old man collapsed with tachycardia the morning after taking an overdose of **moclobemide** and drinking half a bottle of **whisky** (more than 350 mL). He then suffered a cardiac arrest, and resuscitation was unsuccessful. Blood pressure was not recorded. The authors attributed this case to an interaction between moclobemide and tyramine,[13] although the tyramine content of the whisky was not assessed, so any interaction is not established, especially since whisky does not usually contain tyramine.

(c) Wines

In the context of adverse interactions with MAOIs, **Chianti** has developed a sinister reputation, because 400 mL of one early sample of **Italian Chianti** wine (see 'Table 32.2', (above)) contained enough tyramine to reach the 8 to 20 mg threshold for causing important hypertensive reactions. However, it is claimed by the **Chianti** producers[14] and others[15] that the newer methods that have replaced the ancient 'governo alla toscana' process result in negligible amounts of tyramine in today's **Chianti**. This seems to be borne out by the results of analyses,[3,5-7] two of which failed to find any tyramine at all in some samples.[3,7] Some of the other wines listed in 'Table 32.2', (above) also contain tyramine, but patients would have to drink as much as 2 litres or more before reaching what is believed to be the threshold dosage. This suggests that small or moderate amounts (1 or 2 glasses) are unlikely to be hazardous in patients taking MAOIs.

B. Hypotensive reactions

Some degree of hypotension can occur in patients taking MAOIs and this may be exaggerated by the vasodilation and reduced cardiac output caused by alcohol. In one report, a patient on an MAOI describes having a **gin** and orange and then becoming unsteady when standing up and hitting her head on the wall.[16] Patients should therefore be warned of the possibility of orthostatic hypotension and syncope if they drink. They should be advised not to stand up too quickly, and to remain sitting or lying if they feel faint or begin to 'black out'.

C. Psychomotor performance

The possibility that **alcohol**-induced deterioration in psychomotor skills (i.e. those associated with safe driving) might be increased by the RIMAs has been studied. Moclobemide appears to have only a minor and clinically unimportant effect.[17,18]

1. Horwitz D, Lovenberg W, Engelman K, Sjoerdsma A. Monoamine oxidase inhibitors, tyramine and cheese. *JAMA* (1964) 188, 1108–10.
2. Sen NP. Analysis and significance of tyramine in foods. *J Food Sci* (1969) 34, 22–6.
3. Korn A, Eichler HG, Fischbach R, Gasic S. Moclobemide, a new reversible MAO inhibitor – interaction with tyramine and tricyclic antidepressants in healthy volunteers and depressive patients. *Psychopharmacology (Berl)* (1986) 88, 153–7.
4. Zee JA, Simard RE, L'Heureux L, Tremblay J. Biogenic amines in wines. *Am J Enol Vitic* (1983) 34, 6–9.
5. Hannah P, Glover V, Sandler M. Tyramine in wine and beer. *Lancet* (1988) i, 879.
6. Da Prada M, Zürcher G, Wüthrich I, Haefely WE. On tyramine, food, beverages and the reversible MAO inhibitor moclobemide. *J Neural Transm* (1988) (Suppl 26), 31–56.

7. Shulman KI, Walker SE, MacKenzie S, Knowles S. Dietary restriction, tyramine, and use of monoamine oxidase inhibitors. *J Clin Psychopharmacol* (1989) 9, 397–402.
8. Tailor SAN, Shulman KI, Walker SE, Moss J, Gardner D. Hypertensive episode associated with phenelzine and tap beer—a reanalysis of the role of pressor amines in beer. *J Clin Psychopharmacol* (1994) 14, 5–14.
9. Murray JA, Walker JF, Doyle JS. Tyramine in alcohol-free beer. *Lancet* (1988) i, 1167–8.
10. Thakore J, Dinan TG, Kelleher M. Alcohol-free beer and the irreversible monoamine oxidase inhibitors. *Int Clin Psychopharmacol* (1992) 7, 59–60.
11. Draper R, Sandler M, Walker PL. Clinical curio: monoamine oxidase inhibitors and non-alcoholic beer. *BMJ* (1984) 289, 308.
12. Sargant W. Interactions with monoamine oxidase inhibitors. *BMJ* (1975) 4, 101.
13. Bleumink GS, van Vliet ACM, van der Tholen A, Stricker BHC. Fatal combination of moclobemide overdose and whisky. *Neth J Med* (2003) 61, 88–90.
14. Anon. Statement from the Consorzio Vino Chianti Classico, London. Undated (circa 1984).
15. Kalish G. Chianti myth. *The Wine Spectator* (1981) July 31st.
16. Anon. MAOIs — a patient's tale. *Pulse* (1981) December 5th, p 69.
17. Berlin I, Cournot A, Zimmer R, Pedarriosse A-M, Manfredi R, Molinier P, Puech AJ. Evaluation and comparison of the interaction between alcohol and moclobemide or clomipramine in healthy subjects. *Psychopharmacology (Berl)* (1990) 100, 40–5.
18. Tiller JWG. Antidepressants, alcohol and psychomotor performance. *Acta Psychiatr Scand* (1990) (Suppl 360), 13–17.

MAOIs or RIMAs + Tyramine-rich foods

A potentially life-threatening hypertensive reaction can develop in patients on the non-selective MAOIs (tranylcypromine, phenelzine etc.) who eat tyramine-rich foods. Deaths from intracranial haemorrhage have occurred. Significant amounts of tyramine occur in some aged cheeses, yeast extracts (e.g. *Marmite*) and some types of salami. Caviar, pickled herrings, soy sauce, avocados and other foods have been implicated in this interaction. Note that any food high in aromatic amino acids can become high in tyramine if spoilage occurs or after storage. The RIMAs (moclobemide, toloxatone) interact with tyramine to a lesser extent, such that dietary restrictions are generally unnecessary.

Clinical evidence

A. Reactions to foods

(a) MAOIs

A rapid, serious, and potentially fatal rise in blood pressure can occur in patients taking MAOIs who ingest tyramine-rich foods or drinks. A violent occipital headache, pounding heart, neck stiffness, flushing, sweating, nausea and vomiting may be experienced. One of the earliest recorded observations specifically linking this reaction to **cheese** was in 1963 by a pharmacist called Rowe, who wrote to Blackwell[1] after seeing the reaction in his wife who was taking ***Parstelin*** (**tranylcypromine** with trifluoperazine).

"After **cheese on toast**; within a few minutes face flushed, felt very ill; head and heart pounded most violently, and perspiration was running down her neck. She vomited several times, and her condition looked so severe that I dashed over the road to consult her GP. He diagnosed 'palpitations' and agreed to call if the symptoms had not subsided in an hour. In fact the severity diminished and after about 3 hours she was normal, other than a severe headache — but 'not of the throbbing kind'. She described the early part of the attack 'as though her head must burst'."

Blackwell and his colleagues[1] discuss a series of 25 early cases, and the information that led to this interaction becoming established. **Tranylcypromine** was the most frequently implicated MAOI: of 25 cases, 17 were with **tranylcypromine**, 6 with **phenelzine** and one each with **pargyline** and **mebanazine**. In addition, **cheese** was the most frequently implicated food, in 18 of 25 cases, with ***Marmite*** (**yeast** extract) in 3 and **pickled herrings** in one. Four patients had intracranial haemorrhages and one died.[1] From 1961 up to February 1964 the US FDA found about 500 cases of induced hypertension with **tranylcypromine** and 38 cases of cerebral vascular accidents with 21 deaths. As a result, **tranylcypromine** was withdrawn in the US, although it was later reintroduced with many restrictions, including the need to avoid **cheese** while taking the drug.[2]

In addition to reactions to **cheese**, cases of hypertensive reactions have been reported with **avocados**,[3] **beef livers**[4] and **chicken livers**,[5] **caviar**,[6] **pickled herrings**,[7] **soused herrings**,[8] **tinned fish**,[8] **tinned milk**,[1] **peanuts**,[8] **soy sauce**,[9] **miso**,[10] **a powdered protein diet supplement** (***Ever-so-slim***[11] or ***Complan***[1]) **packet soup** (containing hydrolysed **yeast**),[12] **sour cream** in coffee,[8] and **New Zealand prickly spinach**[13] (*Tetragonia tetragonoides*). [Note this is not a true spinach as found in the USA or Europe.] These reactions occurred with **tranylcypromine**,[3,5-9] **phenelzine**[4,10,11,13] or unspecified MAOIs.[8,12]

(b) Moclobemide

There do not appear to be any published reports of the '**cheese** reaction' with moclobemide. The combination of ***Bovril*** (**yeast** extract) 12 g and moclobemide 150 mg, both three times daily, was used to normalise blood pressure in a patient with severe postural hypotension as a result of central autonomic failure.[14]

B. Tyramine studies

Pharmacodynamic studies comparing RIMAs with MAOIs using oral tyramine sensitivity tests have revealed that only 20 to 50 mg of oral tyramine (given with a meal) is required to raise the systolic BP by 30 mmHg in subjects taking **tranylcypromine** 10 mg twice daily.[15] In another study, the pressor tyramine dose was only 8 mg in those given **tranylcypromine**, but higher (33 mg) in those taking **phenelzine**.[16] These pharmacodynamic studies confirm the clinical evidence that the **cheese** reaction is more likely with **tranylcypromine**.

The mean dose of oral tyramine (added to a meal) required to raise systolic BP by 30 mmHg (the tyramine 30 dose) was decreased fivefold (from 1450 mg to 306 mg, range 150 to 500 mg) by moclobemide 200 mg three times daily, in a double-blind, parallel group, placebo-controlled study in healthy subjects. In comparison, **tranylcypromine** 10 mg twice daily decreased the tyramine 30 dose by about 38-fold.[15] In another study, the reduction in the tyramine 30 dose for **moclobemide** 150 mg three times daily was sevenfold; for **phenelzine** 60 mg daily, 13-fold; and for **tranylcypromine** 20 mg daily, 55-fold. After stopping the drugs, the pressor effect to tyramine normalised within 3 days for **moclobemide**, and 30 days for **tranylcypromine**. However, the pressor response had normalised in only 2 subjects 2 to 4 weeks after they stopped **phenelzine**, and had not normalised during the 11-week study period in the other 4 subjects.[16] In a further study the tyramine 30 dose was reduced by about 4-fold by **moclobemide** 100 mg three times daily and 10.3-fold by **phenelzine** 15 mg three times daily.[17] Numerous other pharmacological studies have confirmed the low increase in pressor response to tyramine with **moclobemide**.[18-21]

The pressor response to oral tyramine 200 mg was not altered by pretreatment with **toloxatone** 200 mg or 400 mg three times daily in healthy subjects, although the effect of higher doses of tyramine was increased.[22] Similar results were reported in an earlier study.[23]

Mechanism

Tyramine is formed in foods such as cheese by the bacterial degradation of milk and other proteins, firstly to tyrosine and other amino acids, and the subsequent decarboxylation of the tyrosine to tyramine. This interaction is therefore not associated with fresh foods, but with those which have been allowed to over-ripen or 'mature' in some way,[3] or if spoilage occurs. Tyramine is an indirectly-acting sympathomimetic amine, one of its actions being to release noradrenaline (norepinephrine) from the adrenergic neurones associated with blood vessels, which causes a rise in blood pressure by stimulating their constriction.[3]

Normally any ingested tyramine is rapidly metabolised by the enzyme monoamine oxidase in the gut wall and liver before it reaches the general circulation. However, if the activity of the enzyme at these sites is inhibited (by the presence of an MAOI), any tyramine passes freely into the circulation, causing not just a rise in blood pressure, but a highly exaggerated rise due to the release from the adrenergic neurones of the large amounts of noradrenaline that accumulate there during inhibition of MAO.[3] This final step in the interaction is identical to that which occurs with any other indirectly-acting sympathomimetic amine in the presence of an MAOI (see 'MAOIs or RIMAs + Sympathomimetics; Indirectly-acting', p.1147).

RIMAs such as moclobemide and toloxatone selectively inhibit MAO-A, which leaves MAO-B still available to metabolise tyramine. This means that they have less effect on the tyramine pressor response than non-selective MAOIs.

Importance and management

An extremely well-documented, well-established, serious interaction. A potentially fatal hypertensive reaction can occur between the irreversible, non-selective MAOIs (see 'Table 32.1', (p.1130)) and tyramine-rich foods. Tranylcypromine is more likely to cause the reaction than phenelzine. The incidence is uncertain, but early estimates of hypertensive reactions to tranylcypromine (before restrictions in its use with indirectly-acting sympathomimetics and foods) range from 0.03% to 20%.[2,24,25] Patients taking any of the non-selective MAOIs (**isocarboxazid**, **nialamide**,

Table 32.3 The tyramine-content of some foods

Food	*Tyramine content (mg/kg or mg/L)*	*Refs*
Avocado	Higher in ripe fruit, 23, 0	1-3
Banana peel	52, 65	2,4
Banana pulp	7, 0	2-4
Caviar (Iranian)	680	5
Cheese - see Table 32.4, p.1155, and Pizza toppings, below		
Country cured ham	not detectable	6
Farmer salami sausage	314	6
Genoa salami sausage	0 to 1237 (average 534)	6
Hard salami	0 to 392 (average 210)	6
Herring (pickled)	3030	7
Lebanon bologna	0 to 333 (average 224)	6
Liver-chicken	94 to 113	8
Liver-beef	0 to 274	9
Orange pulp	10	2
Pepperoni sausage	0 to 195 (average 39)	6
Pizza toppings (cheese and pepperoni)	0 to 3.6 (0 to 0.38 mg on half a medium pizza)	10
Plum, red	6	2
Sauerkraut	55	4
Soy sauce	0 to 878	4,10-12
Soya bean curd (tofu)	0.6 to 16	10
Soya beans, fermented	713	12
Soya bean paste, fermented	206	12
Smoked landjaeger sausage	396	6
Summer sausage	184	6
Tomato	4, 0	2,3
Thuringer cervelat	0 to 162	6
Yeast extracts		
Bovril	200 to 500	13
Bovril beef cubes	200 to 500	13
Bovril chicken cubes	50 to 200	13
Marmite (UK product)	500 to 3000	3,4,13
Oxo chicken cubes	130	14
Red Oxo cubes	250	14
Yoghurt	0 to 4	3,4,15

1. Generali JA, Hogan LC, McFarlane M, Schwab S, Hartman CR. Hypertensive crisis resulting from avocados and a MAO inhibitor. *Drug Intell Clin Pharm* (1981) 15, 904-6.
2. Udenfriend S, Lovenberg W, Sjoerdsma A. Physiologically active amines in common fruits and vegetables. *Arch Biochem* (1959) 85, 487.
3. Da Prada M, Zürcher G, Wüthrich I, Haefely WE. On tyramine, food, beverages and the reversible MAO inhibitor moclobemide. *J Neural Transm* (1988) (Suppl 26), 31-56.
4. Shulman KI, Walker SE, MacKenzie S, Knowles S. Dietary restriction, tyramine, and the use of monoamine oxidase inhibitors. *J Clin Psychopharmacol* (1989) 9, 397-402.
5. Isaac P, Mitchell B, Grahame-Smith DG. Monoamine-oxidase inhibitors and caviar. *Lancet* (1977) ii, 816.

Continued

Table 32.3 The tyramine-content of some foods (continued)

6. Rice S, Eitenmiller RR, Koehler PE. Histamine and tyramine content of meat products. *J Milk Food Technol* (1975) 38, 256-8.
7. Nuessle WF, Norman FC, Miller HE. Pickled herring and tranylcypromine reaction. *JAMA* (1965) 192, 726.
8. Heberg DL, Gordon MW, Glueck BC. Six cases of hypertensive crisis in patients on tranylcypromine after eating chicken livers. *Am J Psychiatry* (1966) 122, 933-5.
9. Boulton AA, Cookson B, Paulton R. Hypertensive crisis in a patient on MAOI antidepressants following a meal of beef liver. *Can Med Assoc J* (1970) 102, 1394-5.
10. Shulman KI, Walker SE. Refining the MAOI diet: tyramine content of pizzas and soy products. *J Clin Psychiatry* (1999) 60, 191-3.
11. Lee S, Wing YK. MAOI and monosodium glutamate interaction. *J Clin Psychiatry* (1991) 52, 43.
12. Da Prada M, Zürcher G. Tyramine content of preserved and fermented foods or condiments of Far Eastern cuisine. *Psychopharmacology (Berl)* (1992) 106, S32-S34.
13. Clarke A. (Bovril Ltd). Personal communication (1987).
14. Oxo Ltd. Personal communication (1987).
15. Horwitz D, Lovenberg W, Engelman K, Sjoerdsma A. Monoamine oxidase inhibitors, tyramine, and cheese. *JAMA* (1964) 188, 1108-10.

phenelzine, pargyline, tranylcypromine, and **iproniazid**) should not eat foods reported to contain substantial amounts of tyramine (see 'Table 32.3', (above) and 'Table 32.4', (p.1155)). As little as 8 to 20 mg of tyramine can raise the blood pressure in patients taking tranylcypromine, and this may be present in usual portions of hard cheeses.[16] In addition, avoidance of the prohibited foods should be continued for 2 to 3 weeks after stopping the MAOI to allow full recovery of the enzymes. However, note that in one study some patients took over 11 weeks to recover from the effects of phenelzine.[16]

Because tyramine levels vary so much it is impossible to guess the amount present in any food or drink. Old, over-ripe strong smelling cheeses with a salty, biting taste or those with characteristic holes due to fermentation should be avoided as they generally contain high levels of tyramine. Fresh cheeses made from pasteurised milk tend to have lower levels of tyramine.[26] The tyramine-content can even differ significantly within a single cheese: the centre having the lowest levels of tyramine, and the rind, containing the most.[26,27] There is no guarantee that patients who have uneventfully eaten these hazardous foodstuffs on many occasions may not eventually experience a full-scale hypertensive crisis, if all the many variables conspire together.[28]

The need to plan a sensible and safe diet for those taking MAOIs is clear, and over the years attempts have been made to produce simplified, practical diets for those taking MAOIs.[29-35] A total prohibition should be imposed on the following: **aged cheese** and **yeast extracts** such as ***Marmite,*** and possibly also ***Bovril*** and **pickled herrings** (see 'Table 32.3', (above)). A number of other foods should also be viewed with suspicion such as **sauerkraut**, **fermented bologna** and **salami**, **pepperoni**, and **summer sausage** because some of them may contain significant amounts of tyramine (see 'Table 32.3', (above)). Some preserved and fermented Far Eastern foods such as **fermented soya beans**, **soya bean paste** and **soya bean curd (Tofu)** can also contain relatively high tyramine levels.[33,36] However, **yoghurt**, **fresh cream** and possibly **chocolate** are often viewed with unjustifiable suspicion. It also seems very doubtful if either **cream cheese** or **cottage cheese** represent a hazard, or **processed cheese** slices.[32] **Whole green bananas** contain up to 65 micrograms of tyramine per gram, but this is mostly in the skin as the **pulp** contains relatively small amounts. Although case reports have occurred with a variety of other foods, it is generally acknowledged that widespread restrictions should not be imposed on a food based solely on an unsubstantiated isolated report,[29,30,32] and that some reports could equally be attributed to spoilage.[30,37] Therefore, of perhaps more importance is the advice to only eat protein-based foods (particularly meat, fish and liver) when fresh (within their sell-by date and after correct storage).[30,32] Note that cooking does not inactivate tyramine. For the need to avoid broad-bean pods because of their dopamine content, see 'MAOIs + Dopa-rich foods', p.1135. The RIMAs are safer (in the context of interactions with tyramine-rich foods and drinks) than the older MAOIs, because they are more readily reversible and selective. Therefore the risk of a serious hypertensive reaction with moclobemide is very much reduced. The authors of one study calculate

Table 32.4 The tyramine content of some cheeses
This table is principally intended to show the extent and the variation that can occur

Variety of cheese	*Tyramine content (mg/kg)*	*Approximate mg/60g portion*	*Refs*
American processed	50	3	1
Argenti	188	11	2
Blue	31 to 997	2 to 60	2-4
Boursault	1116	67	3
Brick	194	12	2
Brie	3 to 473	0.2 to 28	1,4,5
Cambozola Blue Vein	18	1	4
Camembert	3 to 519	0.2 to 31	1–3,5
Cheddar	8 to 1530	0.5 to 92	2-6
Cheshire	24 to 418	1.4 to 25	5
Cream cheese	undetectable (less than 0.2), 9	0 to 0.5	1,4
Cottage cheese	undetectable (less than 0.2), 5	0 to 0.3	1,5
Danish Blue	31 to 743	2 to 45	3-5
d'Oka	158, 310	9.5, 19	2
Double Gloucester	43	2.6	5
Edam	100, 214	6, 13	2
Emmental	11 to 958	0.7 to 57	1,4,5
Feta	5.8, 20, 76	0.3 to 4.6	4-6
Gorgonzola	56 to 768	3.4 to 46	4,5
Gouda	54, 95	3.2, 5.7	2
Gouda type (Canadian)	20	1.2	3
Gourmandise	216	13	3
Gruyere	64 to 516	3.8 to 31	1,4,5,7
Kashar	44 (mean of seven samples)	2.6	7
Liederkrantz	1226, 1683	74, 101	2
Limburger	44 to 416	2.6, 25	2,5
Mozzarella	17 to 410	1 to 25	3-6
Munster	87 to 110	5.2 to 6.6	2,4,5
Mycella	1340	80	3
Parmesan	4 to 290	0.2 to 17	3-5
Provolone	38	2.3	3
Red Leicester	41	2.5	5
Ricotta	0	0	4
Romano	4, 197, 238	0.2 to 14	2,3,6
Roquefort	13 to 520	0.8 to 31	2,3,5
Stilton	359 to 2170	28 to 130	1,3-5
Tulum	208 (mean of seven samples)	12.5	7
White (Turkish)	17.5 (mean of seven samples)	1	7

1. Horwitz D, Lovenberg W, Engelman K, Sjoerdsma A. Monoamine oxidase inhibitors, tyramine and cheese. *JAMA* (1964) 188, 1108-10.

Continued

Table 32.4 The tyramine content of some cheeses (continued)
This table is principally intended to show the extent and the variation that can occur

2. Kosikowsky FV, Dahlberg AC. The tyramine content of cheese. *J Dairy Sci* (1948) 31, 293-303.
3. Sen NP. Analysis and significance of tyramine in foods. *J Food Sci* (1969) 34, 22-6.
4. Shulman KI, Walker SE, MacKenzie S, Knowles S. Dietary restriction, tyramine, and the use of monoamine oxidase inhibitors. *J Clin Psychopharmacol* (1989) 9, 397-402.
5. Da Prada M, Zürcher G, Wüthrich I, Haefely WE. On tyramine, food, beverages and the reversible MAO inhibitor moclobemide. *J Neural Transm* (1988) (Suppl 26), 31-56.
6. Shulman KI, Walker SE. Refining the MAOI diet: tyramine content of pizzas and soy products. *J Clin Psychiatry* (1999) 60, 191-3.
7. Kayaalp SO, Renda N, Kaymakcalan S, Özer A. Tyramine content of some cheeses. *Toxicol Appl Pharmacol* (1970) 16, 459-60.

that the lowest amount of tyramine (150 mg) found to cause a 30 mmHg rise in systolic BP with moclobemide is equivalent to that found in about 200 g of Stilton cheese or 300 g of Gorgonzola cheese, which are really excessive amounts of cheese to be eaten in a few minutes.[15] Moreover, no 'cheese reactions' appear to have been published for moclobemide. Most patients therefore do not need to follow the special dietary restrictions required with the older MAOIs, but, to be on the safe side, the manufacturers of moclobemide advise all patients to avoid large amounts of tyramine-rich foods, because a few individuals may be particularly sensitive to tyramine.[38] This warning would also seem appropriate for all of the other RIMAs. Note that if moclobemide were given with an MAO-B inhibitor such as selegiline, it would essentially be the same as giving a non-selective MAOI, and dietary tyramine restrictions would then be required, see 'MAO-B inhibitors + Tyramine-rich foods', p.693.

Treatment

Severe hypertensive reactions require urgent immediate treatment. The drug most commonly used to control hypertensive reactions with MAOIs is phentolamine, given as a slow intravenous injection. However, the need for the patient to get to an emergency treatment centre delays treatment, and as a consequence, providing the patient with a drug they could self administer has been suggested. Sublingual nifedipine has been advocated,[39] but does not appear to have been widely adopted, perhaps because the possibility of a sudden dramatic drop in blood pressure is just as dangerous. Another similar option is a small dose of chlorpromazine.[40]

It is advisable to refer to current guidelines on the management of hypertensive crises for up-to-date advice.

1. Blackwell B, Marley E, Price J, Taylor D. Hypertensive interactions between monoamine oxidase inhibitors and foodstuffs. *Br J Psychiatry* (1967) 113, 349–65.
2. Sadusk JF. The physician and the Food and Drug Administration. *JAMA* (1964) 190, 907–9.
3. Generali JA, Hogan LC, McFarlane M, Schwab S, Hartman CR. Hypertensive crisis resulting from avocados and a MAO inhibitor. *Drug Intell Clin Pharm* (1981) 15, 904–6.
4. Boulton AA, Cookson B, Paulton R. Hypertensive crisis in a patient on MAOI antidepressants following a meal of beef liver. *Can Med Assoc J* (1970) 102, 1394–5.
5. Hedberg DL, Gordon MW, Glueck BC. Six cases of hypertensive crisis in patients on tranylcypromine after eating chicken livers. *Am J Psychiatry* (1966) 122, 933–7.
6. Isaac P, Mitchell B, Grahame-Smith DG. Monoamine-oxidase inhibitors and caviar. *Lancet* (1977) ii, 816.
7. Nuessle WF, Norman FC, Miller HE. Pickled herring and tranylcypromine reaction. *JAMA* (1965) 192, 726–7.
8. Kelly D, Guirguis W, Frommer E, Mitchell-Heggs N, Sargant W. Treatment of phobic states with antidepressants. A retrospective study of 246 patients. *Br J Psychiatry* (1970) 116, 387–98.
9. Abrams JH, Schulman P, White WB. Successful treatment of a monoamine oxidase inhibitor-tyramine hypertensive emergency with intravenous labetalol. *N Engl J Med* (1985) 313, 52.
10. Mesmer RE. Don't mix miso with MAOIs. *JAMA* (1987) 258, 3515.
11. Zetin M, Plon L, DeAntonio M. MAOI reaction with powdered protein dietary supplement. *J Clin Psychiatry* (1987) 48, 499.
12. McQueen EG. Interactions with monoamine oxidase inhibitors. *BMJ* (1975) 4, 101.
13. Comfort A. Hypertensive reaction to New Zealand prickly spinach in a woman taking phenelzine. *Lancet* (1981) ii, 472.
14. Karet FE, Dickerson JEC, Brown J, Brown MJ. Bovril and moclobemide: a novel therapeutic strategy for central autonomic failure. *Lancet* (1994) 344, 1263–5.
15. Berlin I, Zimmer R, Cournot A, Payan C, Pedarriosse AM, Puech AJ. Determination and comparison of the pressor effect of tyramine during long-term moclobemide and tranylcypromine treatment in healthy volunteers. *Clin Pharmacol Ther* (1989) 46, 344–51.

16. Bieck PR, Antonin KH. Tyramine potentiation during treatment with MAO inhibitors: brofaromine and moclobemide vs irreversible inhibitors. *J Neural Transm* (1989) (Suppl 28), 21–31.
17. Warrington SJ, Turner P, Mant TGK, Morrison P, Haywood G, Glover V, Goodwin BL, Sandler M, St John-Smith P, McClelland GR. Clinical pharmacology of moclobemide, a new reversible monoamine oxidase inhibitor. *J Psychopharmacol* (1991) 5, 82–91.
18. Korn A, Eichler HG, Fischbach R, Gasic S. Moclobemide, a new reversible MAO inhibitor – interaction with tyramine and tricyclic antidepressants in healthy volunteers and depressive patients. *Psychopharmacology (Berl)* (1986) 88, 153–7.
19. Korn A, Da Prada M, Raffesberg W, Gasic S, Eichler HG. Effect of moclobemide, a new reversible monoamine oxidase inhibitor, on absorption and pressor effect of tyramine. *J Cardiovasc Pharmacol* (1988) 11, 17–23.
20. Burgess CD, Mellsop GW. Interaction between moclobemide and oral tyramine in depressed patients. *Fundam Clin Pharmacol* (1989) 3, 47–52.
21. Audebert C, Blin O, Monjanel-Mouterde S, Auquier P, Pedarriosse AM, Dingemanse J, Durand A, Cano JP. Influence of food on the tyramine pressor effect during chronic moclobemide treatment of healthy volunteers. *Eur J Clin Pharmacol* (1992) 43, 507–12.
22. Provost J-C, Funck-Brentano C, Rovei V, D'Estanque J, Ego D, Jaillon P. Pharmacokinetic and pharmacodynamic interaction between toloxatone, a new reversible monoamine oxidase-A inhibitor, and oral tyramine in healthy subjects. *Clin Pharmacol Ther* (1992) 52, 384–93.
23. Tipton KF, Dostert P, Strolin Benedetti M, eds. Monoamine Oxidase and Disease: Pressor amines and monoamine oxidase inhibitors. London: Academic Press; 1984. p. 429–41.
24. Cooper AJ, Magnus RV, Rose MJ. A hypertensive syndrome with tranylcypromine medication. *Lancet* (1964) i, 527–9.
25. Anon. Hypertensive reactions to monoamine oxidase inhibitors. *BMJ* (1964) i, 578–9.
26. Da Prada M, Zürcher G, Wüthrich I, Haefely WE. On tyramine, food, beverages and the reversible MAO inhibitor moclobemide. *J Neural Transm* (1988) (Suppl 26), 31–56.
27. Price K, Smith SE. Cheese reaction and tyramine. *Lancet* (1971) i, 130–1.
28. Hutchison JC. Toxic effects of monoamine-oxidase inhibitors. *Lancet* (1964) ii, 151.
29. Sullivan EA, Shulman KI. Diet and monoamine oxidase inhibitors: a re-examination. *Can J Psychiatry* (1984) 29, 707–11.
30. McCabe BJ. Dietary tyramine and other pressor amines in MAOI regimens: a review. *J Am Diet Assoc* (1986) 86, 1059–64.
31. Brown C, Taniguchi G, Yip K. The monoamine oxidase inhibitor-tyramine interaction. *J Clin Pharmacol* (1989) 29, 529–32.
32. Gardner DM, Shulman KI, Walker SE, Tailor SAN. The making of a user friendly MAOI diet. *J Clin Psychiatry* (1996) 57, 99–104.
33. Shulman KI, Walker SE. Refining the MAOI diet: tyramine content of pizzas and soy products. *J Clin Psychiatry* (1999) 60, 191–3.
34. Shulman KI, Walker SE. Clarifying the safety of the MAOI diet and pizza: reply. *J Clin Psychiatry* (2000) 61, 145–6.
35. Marcason W. What is the bottom line for dietary guidelines when taking monoamine oxidase inhibitors? *J Am Diet Assoc* (2005) 105, 163.
36. Da Prada M, Zürcher G. Tyramine content of preserved and fermented foods or condiments of Far Eastern cuisine. *Psychopharmacology (Berl)* (1992) 106, S32–S34.
37. Sen NP. Analysis and significance of tyramine in foods. *J Food Sci* (1969) 34, 22–26.
38. Manerix (Moclobemide). Roche Products Ltd. UK Summary of product characteristics, September 2005.
39. Fier M. Safer use of MAOIs. *Am J Psychiatry* (1991) 148, 391–2.
40. Lippman SB, Nash K. Monoamine oxidase inhibitor update. Potential adverse food and drug interactions. *Drug Safety* (1990) 5, 195–204.

MAOIs or RIMAs + Venlafaxine

Serious and potentially life-threatening reactions (the serotonin syndrome) can develop if venlafaxine and non-selective MAOIs (isocarboxazid, phenelzine, tranylcypromine) are given concurrently, or even sequentially if insufficient time is left in between. The situation with moclobemide, in therapeutic doses, is uncertain.

Clinical evidence

(a) MAOIs

1. Isocarboxazid. A man with recurrent depression taking isocarboxazid 30 mg daily was additionally given venlafaxine 75 mg. After the second dose he developed agitation, hypomania, diaphoresis, shivering and dilated pupils. These symptoms subsided when the venlafaxine was stopped. He subsequently developed myoclonic jerks and diaphoresis when given both drugs.[1]

2. Phenelzine. A woman who had stopped taking phenelzine 45 mg daily 7 days previously, developed sweating, lightheadedness and dizziness within 45 minutes of taking a single 37.5-mg dose of venlafaxine. In the emergency department she was found to be lethargic, agitated and extremely diaphoretic. The agitation was treated with lorazepam. A week later, after she had recovered, she was again started on the same regimen of venlafaxine without problems.[2] A man similarly developed the serotonin syndrome when he started venlafaxine the day after he stopped taking phenelzine.[3] A woman developed the serotonin syndrome within less than an hour of taking phenelzine and venlafaxine together,[4] and 4 other patients similarly developed the reaction when phenelzine was replaced by venlafaxine.[5]

Twelve days after an overdose of phenelzine (53 tablets of 15 mg), benztropine, haloperidol and lorazepam, a 31-year-old man was given venlafaxine 75 mg every 12 hours in addition to existing treatment with olanzapine and diazepam. About an hour after the first dose, he developed leg shakiness and stiffness, diaphoresis, blurred vision, difficulty breathing, chills, nausea and palpitations. Venlafaxine and olanzapine were discontinued and the man recovered within 24 hours, after treatment with intravenous fluids, propranolol and paracetamol.[6]

3. Tranylcypromine. A woman who had been taking tranylcypromine for 3 weeks developed a serious case of the serotonin syndrome within 4 hours of inadvertently taking a single tablet of venlafaxine. She recovered within 24 hours, when treated with ice packs, a cooling blanket, diazepam and dantrolene.[7] The serotonin syndrome developed in a man taking tranylcypromine within 2 hours of taking half a venlafaxine tablet.[8] Another case of the serotonin syndrome has been described in a man taking tranylcypromine 60 mg daily who accidentally took venlafaxine 300 mg.[9]

(b) RIMAs

A 32-year-old man taking **moclobemide** 20 mg twice daily and diazepam developed the serotonin syndrome 40 minutes after taking a single 150-mg dose of venlafaxine.[10] Serotonin toxicity (the serotonin syndrome) occurred in 4 patients who took an overdose of **moclobemide** with venlafaxine (just 150 mg in one case and 750 mg in another). In this analysis of **moclobemide** overdoses, the risk of developing serotonin toxicity was increased 35 times in patients who also took another serotonergic drug. Venlafaxine was taken in 4 of the 11 cases mentioned.[11] Another man very rapidly developed the serotonin syndrome after taking considerable overdoses of **moclobemide** (3 g) and venlafaxine (2.625 g).[12]

Mechanism

The serotonin syndrome is thought to occur because venlafaxine can inhibit serotonin re-uptake (its antidepressant effect is related to this activity), and MAOIs and RIMAs inhibit the metabolism of serotonin. The result is an increase in the concentrations of serotonin apparently causing overstimulation of the 5-HT_{1A} receptors in the brain and spinal cord. See also 'the serotonin syndrome', (p.9).

Importance and management

An established, serious and potentially life-threatening interaction. The manufacturers of venlafaxine say that adverse reactions, some serious, have been seen in patients who had recently stopped taking an MAOI and started venlafaxine, or who had stopped venlafaxine and then started an MAOI. Some have been fatal.[13,14] They recommend that venlafaxine should not be used in combination with an MAOI or within 14 days of stopping treatment with the MAOI.[13,14] Based on the half-life of venlafaxine they say that at least 7 days should elapse between stopping venlafaxine and starting an MAOI. The manufacturers do not distinguish in this recommendation between the irreversible older non-selective MAOIs and the RIMAs such as moclobemide. In one of the studies it was suggested that a wash-out period of several weeks is required between stopping MAOIs such as phenelzine and initiating a second serotonergic drug such as venlafaxine.[6]

1. Klysner R, Larsen JK, Sørensen P, Hyllested M, Pedersen BD. Toxic interaction of venlafaxine and isocarboxazide. *Lancet* (1995) 346, 1298–9.
2. Phillips SD, Ringo P. Phenelzine and venlafaxine interaction. *Am J Psychiatry* (1995) 152, 1400–1401.
3. Heisler MA, Guidry JR, Arnecke B. Serotonin syndrome induced by administration of venlafaxine and phenelzine. *Ann Pharmacother* (1996) 30, 84.
4. Weiner LA, Smythe M, Cisek J. Serotonin syndrome secondary to phenelzine-venlafaxine interaction. *Pharmacotherapy* (1998) 18, 399–403.
5. Diamond S, Pepper BJ, Diamond ML, Freitag FG, Urban GJ, Erdemoglu AK. Serotonin syndrome induced by transitioning from phenelzine to venlafaxine: four patient reports. *Neurology* (1998) 51, 274–6.
6. Mason PJ, Morris VA, Balcezak TJ. Serotonin syndrome. Presentation of 2 cases and review of the literature. *Medicine* (2000) 79, 201–9.
7. Hodgman M, Martin T, Dean B, Krenzelok E. Severe serotonin syndrome secondary to venlafaxine and maintenance tranylcypromine therapy. *J Toxicol Clin Toxicol* (1995) 33, 554.
8. Brubacher JR, Hoffman RS, Lurin MJ. Serotonin syndrome from venlafaxine-tranylcypromine interaction. *Vet Hum Toxicol* (1996) 38, 358–61.
9. Claassen JAHR, Gelissen HPMM. The serotonin syndrome. *N Engl J Med* (2005) 352, 2455.
10. Chan BSH, Graudins A, Whyte IM, Dawson AH, Braitberg G, Duggin GG. Serotonin syndrome resulting from drug interactions. *Med J Aust* (1998) 169, 523–5.
11. Isbister GK, Hackett LP, Dawson AH, Whyte IM, Smith AJ. Moclobemide poisoning: toxicokinetics and occurrence of serotonin toxicity. *Br J Clin Pharmacol* (2003) 56, 441–50.
12. Roxanas MG, Machado JFD. Serotonin syndrome in combined moclobemide and venlafaxine ingestion. *Med J Aust* (1998) 168, 523–4.
13. Efexor (Venlafaxine hydrochloride). Wyeth Pharmaceuticals. UK Summary of product characteristics, May 2006.
14. Effexor XR (Venlafaxine hydrochloride). Wyeth Pharmaceuticals Inc. US Prescribing information, June 2007.

RIMAs; Moclobemide + Antipsychotics

The manufacturer of moclobemide noted that in 1992 there were data available from 110 patients given moclobemide 150 to 400 mg daily with various antipsychotics, namely acepromazine, aceprometazine, alimemazine, bromperidol, chlorpromazine, chlorprothixene, clothiapine, clozapine, cyamemazine, flupenthixol, fluphenazine, fluspirilene, haloperidol, levomepromazine, penfluridol, pipamperone, prothipendyl, sulpiride, thioridazine, or zuclopenthixol. There was no evidence of any clinically relevant interactions. There was, however, some evidence that hypotension, tachycardia, sleepiness, tremor and constipation were more common, suggesting synergistic adverse effects.[1]

1. Amrein R, Güntert TW, Dingemanse J, Lorscheid T, Stabl M, Schmid-Burgk W. Interactions of moclobemide with concomitantly administered medication: evidence from pharmacological and clinical studies. *Psychopharmacology (Berl)* (1992) 106, S24–S31.

RIMAs; Moclobemide + Cimetidine

Cimetidine increases the plasma levels of moclobemide. Moclobemide dosage reductions are recommended.

Clinical evidence, mechanism, importance and management

After taking cimetidine 200 mg five times daily for 2 weeks the maximum plasma levels of a single 100-mg dose of moclobemide in 8 healthy subjects was increased by 39% and the clearance was reduced by 52%.[1] The probable reason is that the cimetidine (a well-recognised enzyme inhibitor) reduces the first-pass metabolism of the moclobemide.

It has been recommended that if moclobemide is added to treatment with cimetidine it should be started at the lowest therapeutic dose, and titrated as required. If cimetidine is added to treatment with moclobemide, the dosage of the moclobemide should initially be reduced by 50% and later adjusted as necessary.[2,3]

1. Schoerlin M-P, Mayersohn M, Hoevels B, Eggers H, Dellenbach M, Pfefen J-P. Cimetidine alters the disposition kinetics of the monoamine oxidase-A inhibitor moclobemide. *Clin Pharmacol Ther* (1991) 49, 32–8.
2. Amrein R, Güntert TW, Dingemanse J, Lorscheid T, Stabl M, Schmid-Burgk W. Interactions of moclobemide with concomitantly administered medication: evidence from pharmacological and clinical studies. *Psychopharmacology (Berl)* (1992) 106, S24–S31.
3. Manerix (Moclobemide). Roche Products Ltd. UK Summary of product characteristics, September 2005.

RIMAs; Moclobemide + Omeprazole

Omeprazole doubled the AUC of moclobemide in extensive metabolisers of CYP2C19, effectively making them poor metabolisers. The clinical relevance of this is uncertain.

Clinical evidence

Omeprazole 40 mg daily for 7 days increased the AUC of a single 300-mg dose of moclobemide by about twofold in 8 healthy subjects who were extensive metabolisers of CYP2C19.[1] After this increase, the AUC of moclobemide in these subjects was still lower than that seen in 8 healthy subjects who were poor metabolisers of CYP2C19 (without omeprazole). Omeprazole had no appreciable effect on the pharmacokinetics of moclobemide in the 8 subjects who were poor metabolisers of CYP2C19.

Mechanism

Omeprazole is an inhibitor of cytochrome P450 isoenzyme CYP2C19, by which moclobemide is extensively metabolised. Activity of this enzyme is genetically determined with about 5% of Caucasians and up to 20% of Asians being poor metabolisers. Consider also 'Genetic factors', (p.4).

Importance and management

The pharmacokinetic interaction is established, but its clinical relevance is unclear. Omeprazole effectively makes extensive metabolisers of moclobemide into poor metabolisers. Moclobemide is a fairly safe drug, and metaboliser status is usually unknown. Bear in mind the possibility of an interaction if adverse effects are seen in a patient on moclobemide given omeprazole.

1. Yu K-S, Yim D-S, Cho J-Y, Soon S, Park JY, Lee K-H, Jang I-J, Yi S-Y, Bae K-S, Shin S-g. Effect of omeprazole on the pharmacokinetics of moclobemide according to the genetic polymorphism of CYP2C19. *Clin Pharmacol Ther* (2001) 69, 266–73.

33

Respiratory drugs

This section includes the diverse drugs that are principally used in the management of asthma and chronic obstructive pulmonary disease (COPD), with the exception of corticosteroids, which are covered elsewhere.

(a) Antimuscarinic bronchodilators

The parasympathetic nervous system is involved in the regulation of bronchomotor tone and antimuscarinic drugs have bronchodilator properties. Ipratropium bromide and other antimuscarinic bronchodilators used in COPD are listed in 'Table 33.1', (p.1159). A wide range of drugs have antimuscarinic (anticholinergic) adverse effects. Enhanced antimuscarinic effects occur when drugs with these properties are given concurrently, see 'Antimuscarinics + Antimuscarinics', p.674. However, these interactions do not usually occur with drugs such as ipratropium, given by inhalation.

(b) Beta$_2$-agonist bronchodilators

Salbutamol and terbutaline are examples of short-acting beta agonists that selectively stimulate the beta$_2$ receptors in the bronchi causing bronchodilation. They are used in the treatment of asthma and the management of COPD. Long-acting beta$_2$ agonists such as salmeterol are used in patients with asthma who also require anti-inflammatory therapy. 'Table 33.1', (p.1159) lists the beta$_2$ agonists available. The beta$_2$ agonists represent a significant improvement on isoprenaline (isoproterenol), which also stimulates beta$_1$ receptors in the heart, and on ephedrine, which also stimulates alpha receptors. The beta$_2$ agonists can cause hypokalaemia, which can be increased by the concurrent use of other 'potassium-depleting drugs', (p.1162).

(c) Leukotriene antagonists

Montelukast and zafirlukast block the effects of cysteinyl leukotrienes, which cause effects such as airways oedema, bronchoconstriction and inflammation. The leukotriene antagonists are used in the treatment of asthma, either alone, or with inhaled corticosteroids. They should not be used to relieve an acute asthma attack. Both drugs are metabolised in the liver by the cytochrome P450 isoenzymes such as CYP3A4 and CYP2C9 (montelukast) and CYP2C9 (zafirlukast). Zafirlukast is thought to inhibit CYP2C9 and CYP3A4, and this is thought to be the mechanism for its interaction with 'warfarin', (p.423). There is therefore a possibility that interactions could occur with other drugs that undergo metabolism by these isoenzymes but clinical evidence of this varies.

(d) Xanthines

The main xanthines used in medicine are theophylline and aminophylline, the latter generally being preferred when greater water solubility is needed (e.g. in the formulation of injections). Xanthines are given in the treatment of asthma because they relax the bronchial smooth muscle. In an attempt to improve upon theophylline, various different derivatives have been made, such as diprophylline and enprofylline. 'Table 33.1', (p.1159) lists these xanthines. Theophylline is metabolised by the cytochrome P450 isoenzymes in the liver, principally CYP1A2, to demethylated and hydroxylated products. Many drugs interact with theophylline by inhibition or potentiation of its metabolism. Theophylline has a narrow therapeutic range, and small increases in serum levels can result in toxicity. Moreover, symptoms of serious toxicity such as convulsions and arrhythmias can occur before minor symptoms suggestive of toxicity. Within the context of interactions, aminophylline generally behaves like theophylline, because it is a complex of theophylline with ethylenediamine.

Caffeine is also a xanthine and it is principally used as a central nervous system stimulant, increasing wakefulness, and mental and physical activity. It is most commonly taken in the form of tea, coffee, cola drinks ('*Coke*') and cocoa. 'Table 33.2', (p.1159) lists the usual caffeine content of these drinks. Caffeine is also included in hundreds of non-prescription analgesic preparations with aspirin, codeine and/or paracetamol, but whether it enhances the analgesic effect is debatable. Caffeine is also used to assess the activity of hepatic enzyme systems (particularly the cytochrome P450 isoenzyme CYP1A2) and can usefully demonstrate altered liver function, notably from drugs, as well as disease states.

Caffeine, like theophylline, also undergoes extensive hepatic metabolism, principally by CYP1A2, and interacts with many drugs, but it has a wider therapeutic range. However, other xanthines may act differently (e.g. diprophylline does not undergo hepatic metabolism), so it should not be assumed that they all share common interactions.

Note though, that all xanthines can potentiate hypokalaemia caused by other drugs and that the toxic effects of different xanthines are additive.

Table 33.1 Respiratory drugs

Group	*Route*	*Drugs*
Antimuscarinics (Anticholinergics)	Inhaled	Ipratropium bromide, Oxitropium, Tiotropium
Beta-2 adrenoceptor agonists	Oral	Bambuterol, Clenbuterol, Reproterol, Salbutamol (Albuterol), Terbutaline
	Inhaled	Short-acting: Bitolterol, Clenbuterol, Fenoterol, Levosalbutamol, Pirbuterol, Procaterol, Reproterol, Salbutamol (Albuterol), Terbutaline, Tolubuterol Long-acting: Arformoterol, Formoterol, Salmeterol
	Intravenous	Reproterol, Salbutamol (Albuterol), Terbutaline
Leukotriene antagonists and inhibitors	Oral	Amlexanox, Ibudilast, Montelukast, Pemirolast, Pranlukast, Zafirlukast
Lipoxygenase inhibitors	Oral	Zileuton
Mast cell stabilisers	Inhaled	Nedocromil sodium, Sodium cromoglicate
	Oral	Amlexanox, Ketotifen, Pemirolast, Tranilast
Sympathomimetics	Oral	Ephedrine, Hexoprenaline, Orciprenaline
Xanthine derivatives	Oral	Aminophylline, Bamifylline, Bufylline, Choline theophyllinate, Diprophylline, Doxofylline, Etofylline, Etamiphylline camsilate, Heptaminol acefyllinate, Proxyphylline, Theophylline
	Intravenous	Aminophylline, Bamifylline

Table 33.2 Caffeine-containing herbs and caffeine-containing drinks

Source	*Caffeine-content*	*Caffeine-content of drink*
Cocoa[1]		about 5 mg/100 mL
Coffee beans[2]	1 to 2%	up to 100 mg/100 mL, decaffeinated up to about 3 mg/100 mL
Guarana[3*]	2.5 to 7%	
Kola (Cola)[2]	1.5 to 2.5%	up to 20 mg/100 mL in 'cola' drinks
Maté (Paraguay tea)[2]	0.2 to 2%	
Tea[2]	1 to 5%	up to 60 mg/100 mL

*Note that guarana contains guaranine (which is known to be identical to caffeine) as well as small quantities of other xanthines.

1. Information taken from research conducted by the US Department of Nutritional Services. Available at http://www.holymtn.com/tea/caffeine_content.htm (accessed 22/08/07).
2. Sweetman SC, editor. Martindale: The complete drug reference. 35th ed. London: Pharmaceutical Press; 2007 p. 2188.
3. Houghton P. Herbal products 7. Guarana. *Pharm J* (1995) 254, 435-6.

Anti-asthma drugs + Areca (Betel nuts)

The chewing of betel nuts may worsen the symptoms of asthma.

Clinical evidence

A study of a possible interaction with betel nuts was prompted by the observation of two Bangladeshi patients with severe asthma that appeared to have been considerably worsened by chewing betel nuts. One out of 4 other asthmatic patients who regularly chewed betel nuts developed severe bronchoconstriction (a 30% fall in FEV_1) on two occasions when given betel nuts to chew, and all 4 patients said that prolonged betel nut chewing induced coughing and wheezing. A double-blind study found that the inhalation of **arecoline** (the major constituent of the nut) caused bronchoconstriction in 6 of 7 asthmatics, and 1 of 6 healthy control subjects.[1] A study in asthmatic patients who regularly chewed betel nuts found that 4 patients had a mean increase in their FEV_1 of 10 to 25%, whereas 11 patients had significant falls in their FEV_1 of 11 to 25%. Interestingly, 5 of the patients who did not think chewing betel nut affected their asthma experienced a reduction in their FEV_1.[2]

A survey in 61 asthmatic patients found that 22 of the 34 patients who still chewed betel nut, either for occasional use or regularly, reported that it worsened their asthma.[3]

Mechanism

Betel nut 'quids' consist of areca nut (*Areca catechu*) wrapped in betel vine leaf (*Piper betle*) and smeared with a paste of burnt (slaked) lime. It is chewed for the euphoric effects of the major constituent, arecoline, a cholinergic alkaloid, which appears to be absorbed through the mucous membrane of the mouth. Arecoline has identical properties to pilocarpine and normally has only mild systemic cholinergic properties; however asthmatic subjects seem to be particularly sensitive to the bronchoconstrictor effects of this alkaloid and possibly other substances contained in the nut.

Importance and management

Direct evidence appears to be limited to the above reports, but the interaction seems to be established. It would not normally appear to be a serious interaction, but asthmatics should be encouraged to avoid betel nuts. This is a drug-disease interaction rather than a drug-drug interaction.

1. Taylor RFH, Al-Jarad N, John LME, Conroy DM, Barnes NC. Betel-nut chewing and asthma. *Lancet* (1992) 339, 1134–6.
2. Sekkadde Kiyingi K, Saweri A. Betel nut chewing causes bronchoconstriction in some asthma patients. *P N G Med J* (1994) 37, 90–9.
3. Kiyingi KS. Betel-nut chewing may aggravate asthma. *P N G Med J* (1991) 34, 117–21.

Anti-asthma drugs + Beta blockers

Non-cardioselective beta blockers (e.g. propranolol, timolol) should not be used in asthmatic subjects because they may cause serious bronchoconstriction, even if given as eye drops. Non-cardioselective beta blockers oppose the bronchodilator effects of beta-agonist bronchodilators, and higher doses may be required to reverse bronchospasm. Even cardioselective blockers (e.g. atenolol) can sometimes cause acute bronchospasm in asthmatics. However, cardioselective beta blockers do not generally inhibit the bronchodilator effect of beta-agonist bronchodilators.

Clinical evidence

(a) Cardioselective beta blockers

A review of 29 studies (including 19 single-dose studies) on the use of cardioselective beta blockers in patients with reversible airway disease indicated that in patients with mild to moderate disease, the short-term use of cardioselective beta blockers does not cause significant adverse respiratory effects. Information on the effects in patients with more severe or less reversible disease, or on the frequency or severity of acute exacerbations was not available.[1] Another review indicated that when low doses of cardioselective beta blockers are given to patients with mild, intermittent or persistent asthma, or moderate persistent asthma, and heart failure or myocardial infarction, the benefits of treatment outweigh the risks. However, it was considered that further study is required to establish long-term safety, and also that beta blockers should be avoided in severe persistent asthma.[2]

The cardioselective beta blockers would not be expected to affect the beta receptors in the bronchi, but bronchospasm can sometimes occur following their use by asthmatics and others with obstructive airways diseases, particularly if high doses are used. Deterioration of asthma was reported in a patient taking oral **betaxolol** with **theophylline** and **pranlukast**, although **betaxolol** is considered to be highly cardioselective and less likely to cause pulmonary adverse effects than other cardioselective beta blockers.[3]

No adverse pharmacodynamic interaction normally occurs between beta-agonist bronchodilators and cardioselective beta blockers. This has been demonstrated in studies with:

- **Atenolol** with **salbutamol** (**albuterol**) inhalation.[4,5]
- **Celiprolol** in asthmatic patients with **isoprenaline** (**isoproterenol**), or **salbutamol**,[4,6,7] or **terbutaline** infusion or inhalation[8]
- **Metoprolol** in asthmatic patients at rest with **isoprenaline** infusion[9,10]

In contrast, another study found that the increase in forced expiratory volume (FEV) with a **terbutaline** inhalation and infusion was reduced by about 300 mL by **atenolol** and **metoprolol**. The authors considered that this would be clinically relevant in severe asthma.[11] Another study in 12 patients with mild asthma found that single doses of **celiprolol** 200 mg or **nebivolol** 5 mg reduced the FEV_1 by 272 mL and 193 mL, respectively, when compared with placebo. Increasing inhalation of **salbutamol** to a total dose of 800 micrograms reversed these reductions but did not restore the FEV_1 back to its initial value. None of these changes was considered to be clinically significant by the authors.[12]

Fifteen patients with mild to moderate COPD and airways hyperresponsiveness were given **celiprolol** 200 mg daily, **metoprolol** 100 mg daily or **propranolol** 80 mg daily for 4 days. Propranolol significantly reduced the FEV_1 and increased airways hyper-responsiveness compared with placebo whereas metoprolol only increased airways hyper-responsiveness. Celiprolol had no significant effects on pulmonary function. The bronchodilating effects of a single 12-microgram dose of **formoterol** were significantly reduced by propranolol, but not by metoprolol or celiprolol.[7]

(b) Non-selective beta blockers

Non-selective beta blockers (e.g. **propranolol**) are contraindicated in asthmatic subjects because they can cause bronchospasm, reduce lung ventilation and may possibly precipitate a severe asthmatic attack in some subjects. An example of the danger is illustrated by an asthmatic patient who developed fatal status asthmaticus after taking just one dose of **propranolol**.[13] Another case report describes a patient with bronchial asthma receiving **salbutamol** who collapsed and died after taking three 20-mg **propranolol** tablets, which had been supplied in error instead of 20-mg prednisone tablets.[14] The manufacturers of **propranolol** note that from 1965 to 1996, the CSM in the UK had received 51 reports of bronchospasm due to **propranolol**, 13 of them fatal, and 5 of them in patients who had a history of asthma, bronchospasm or wheeze.[15] The non-cardioselective beta blockers **oxprenolol**[5] and **propranolol**[4,5,8-10] oppose the effects of bronchodilators such as **isoprenaline** (**isoproterenol**),[4,9,10] **salbutamol** (**albuterol**),[4,5] and **terbutaline**.[8] Even eye drops containing the non-selective beta blockers **timolol**[16,17] and **metipranolol**[18] have been reported to precipitate acute bronchospasm. In patients with heart failure treated with **carvedilol**, 3 of 12 with concurrent asthma had wheezing requiring **carvedilol** withdrawal. In contrast, only 1 of 31 patients with COPD had wheezing.[19]

Mechanism

Non-selective beta blockers such as propranolol also block the $beta_2$ receptors in the bronchi so that the normal bronchodilation, which is under the control of the sympathetic nervous system, is reduced or abolished. As a result the bronchoconstriction of asthma can be made worse. Cardioselective beta blockers on the other hand, preferentially block $beta_1$ receptors in the heart, with less effect on the $beta_2$ receptors, so that $beta_2$ stimulating bronchodilators, such as isoprenaline, salbutamol and terbutaline, continue to have bronchodilator effects.

Importance and management

A well established drug-disease interaction. In 1996, the CSM in the UK[20] re-issued the following advice: "Beta blockers, including those considered to be cardioselective, should not be given to patients with a history of asthma/bronchospasm." Non-cardioselective beta blockers (indicated in 'Table 22.1', (p.833)) should certainly be avoided in asthmatics and those with chronic obstructive pulmonary disease, whether given systemically or in eye drops, because serious and life-threatening bronchospasm may occur. The cardioselective beta blockers are generally safer but not entirely free from risk in some patients, particularly in high dosage. In contrast to the 1996 recommendations of the CSM on cardioselective beta blockers, one recent review from 2002/3[1,21] recommends that "cardioselective beta blockers should not be withheld from patients with mild to moderate reversible airway disease". However, some concern has been expressed that this conclusion was based on results from short-term studies and state that the question of safety in asthmatics over the long term has not been answered.[22] Further, there are no studies to suggest the safety of cardioselective beta blockers in patients with exacerbations of asthma,[23] and even a highly cardioselective drug such as betaxolol may cause bronchospasm.[3] In 2004, the American College of Cardiology and American Heart Association guidelines for management of ST-elevation myocardial infarction stated that the benefits of using beta blockers strongly outweigh the risk of adverse events in patients with COPD or mild asthma (non-active), and noted that most patients with asthma are able to tolerate cardioselective beta blockers. Therefore if a beta blocker is required a cardioselective beta blocker should be used, and the patient's pulmonary function monitored.[24] A recent Cochrane review concluded that cardioselective beta blockers did not produce any significant adverse respiratory effects or reduction in the response to beta_2 agonists, and it recommended that cardioselective beta blockers should not be withheld from patients with COPD.[25]

Celiprolol (a cardioselective beta blocker) appears to be exceptional in causing mild bronchodilatation in asthmatics and not bronchoconstriction, although it may still produce a reduction in expiratory volume, as seen in the study above,[12] but some caution is still necessary as this requires confirmation.[6]

The bronchoconstrictive effects of the beta blockers can be opposed by beta_2 agonist bronchodilators such a salbutamol, but as the manufacturers point out, large doses may be needed and they suggest that ipratropium and intravenous aminophylline may also be needed.[15]

1. Salpeter S, Ormiston T, Salpeter EE. Cardioselective β-blockers in patients with reversible airway disease: a meta-analysis. *Ann Intern Med* (2002) 137, 715–25.
2. Self T, Soberman JE, Bubla JM, Chafin CC. Cardioselective beta-blockers in patients with asthma and concomitant heart failure or history of myocardial infarction: when do benefits outweigh risks? *J Asthma* (2003) 40, 839–45.
3. Miki A, Tanaka Y, Ohtani H, Sawada Y. Betaxolol-induced deterioration of asthma and a pharmacodynamic analysis based on β-receptor occupancy. *Int J Clin Pharmacol Ther* (2003) 41, 358–64.
4. Doshan HD, Rosenthal RR, Brown R, Slutsky A, Applin WJ, Caruso FS. Celiprolol, atenolol and propranolol: a comparison of pulmonary effects in asthmatic patients. *J Cardiovasc Pharmacol* (1986) 8 (Suppl 4), S105–S108.
5. Fogari R, Zoppi A, Tettamanti F, Poletti L, Rizzardi G, Fiocchi G. Comparative effects of celiprolol, propranolol, oxprenolol, and atenolol on respiratory function in hypertensive patients with chronic obstructive lung disease. *Cardiovasc Drugs Ther* (1990) 4, 1145–50.
6. Pujet JC, Dubreuil C, Fleury B, Provendier O, Abella ML. Effects of celiprolol, a cardioselective beta-blocker, on respiratory function in asthmatic patients. *Eur Respir J* (1992) 5, 196–200.
7. Van der Woude HJ, Zaagsma J, Postma DS, Winter TH, Van Hulst M, Aalbers R. Detrimental effects of β-blockers in COPD: A concern for nonselective β-blockers. *Chest* (2005) 127, 818–24.
8. Matthys H, Doshan HD, Rühle K-H, Applin WJ, Braig H, Pohl M. Bronchosparing properties of celiprolol, a new β_1, α_2 blocker, in propranolol-sensitive asthmatic patients. *J Cardiovasc Pharmacol* (1986) 8 (Suppl 4), S40–S42.
9. Thiringer G, Svedmyr N. Interaction of orally administered metoprolol, practolol and propranolol with isoprenaline in asthmatics. *Eur J Clin Pharmacol* (1976) 10, 163–70.
10. Johnsson G, Svedmyr N, Thiringer G. Effects of intravenous propranolol and metoprolol and their interaction with isoprenaline on pulmonary function, heart rate and blood pressure in asthmatics. *Eur J Clin Pharmacol* (1975) 8, 175–80.
11. Löfdahl C-G, Svedmyr N. Cardioselectivity of atenolol and metoprolol. A study in asthmatic patients. *Eur J Respir Dis* (1981) 62, 396–404.
12. Cazzola M, Noschese P, D'Amato M, D'Amato G. Comparison of the effects of single oral doses of nebivolol and celiprolol on airways in patients with mild asthma. *Chest* (2000) 118, 1322–6.
13. Anon. Beta-blocker caused death of asthmatic. *Pharm J* (1991) 247, 185.
14. Spitz DJ. An unusual death in an asthmatic patient. *Am J Forensic Med Pathol* (2003) 24, 271–2.
15. Fallowfield JM, Marlow HF. Propranolol is contraindicated in asthma. *BMJ* (1996) 313, 1486.
16. Charan NB, Lakshminarayan S. Pulmonary effects of topical timolol. *Arch Intern Med* (1980) 140, 843–4.
17. Jones FL, Ekberg NL. Exacerbation of obstructive airway disease by timolol. *JAMA* (1980) 244, 2730.
18. Vinti H, Chichmanian RM, Fournier JP, Pesce A, Taillan B, Fuzibet JG, Cassuto JP, Dujardin P. Accidents systémiques des bêta-bloquants en collyres. A propos de six observations. *Rev Med Interne* (1989) 10, 41–4.
19. Kotlyar E, Keogh AM, Macdonald PS, Arnold RH, McCaffrey DJ, Glanville AR. Tolerability of carvedilol in patients with heart failure and concomitant chronic obstructive pulmonary disease or asthma. *J Heart Lung Transplant* (2002), 21, 1290–5.
20. Committee on Safety of Medicines/Medicines Control Agency. Reminder: Beta-blockers contraindicated in asthma. *Current Problems* (1996) 22, 2.
21. Salpeter SR, Ormiston TM. Use of β-blockers in patients with reactive airway disease. *Ann Intern Med* (2003) 139, 304.
22. Shulan DJ, Katlan M, Lavsky-Shulan M. Use of β-blockers in patients with reactive airway disease. *Ann Intern Med* (2003) 139, 304.
23. Epstein PE. Fresh air and β-blockade. *Ann Intern Med* (2002) 137, 766–7.
24. Antman EM, Anbe DT, Armstrong PW, Bates ER, Green LA, Hand M, Hochman JS, Krumholz HM, Kushner FG, Lamas GA, Mullany CJ, Ornato JP, Pearle DL, Sloan MA, Smith SC, Alpert JS, Anderson JL, Faxon DP, Fuster V, Gibbons RJ, Gregoratos G, Halperin JL, Hiratzka LF, Hunt SA, Jacobs AK.. ACC/AHA guidelines for the management of patients with ST-elevation myocardial infarction. A report of the American College of Cardiology/American Heart Association Task Force on Practice Guidelines (Committee to revise the 1999 guidelines for the management of patients with acute myocardial infarction). *J Am Coll Cardiol* (2004) 44, E1–E212. Available at: http://www.acc.org/qualityandscience/clinical/guidelines/stemi/Guideline1/index.pdf (accessed 22/08/2007).
25. Salpeter S, Ormiston T, Salpeter E. Cardioselective beta-blockers for chronic obstructive pulmonary disease (review). Available in The Cochrane Database of Systematic Reviews; Issue 4. Chichester: John Wiley; 2005 (accessed 22/08/2007).

Anti-asthma drugs + NSAIDs

Aspirin and many other NSAIDs can cause bronchoconstriction in some asthmatic patients. Celecoxib, etoricoxib and meloxicam do not usually cause bronchospasm in aspirin or NSAID-sensitive patients. Aspirin, nimesulide and piroxicam appear not to alter theophylline pharmacokinetics.

Clinical evidence, mechanism, importance and management

(a) NSAIDs in asthma

About 10% of asthmatics are hypersensitive to **aspirin**, and in some individuals life-threatening bronchoconstriction can occur. This is not a drug-drug interaction but an adverse response of asthmatic patients to **aspirin**, whether taking an anti-asthmatic drug or not. The reasons are not fully understood. Those known to be sensitive to **aspirin** may also possibly react to other NSAIDs, in particular the **acetylated salicylates**, the **indole** and **indene acetic acids**, and the **propionic acid derivatives** (see 'Table 6.1', (p.134)). The **fenamates**, **oxicams**, **pyrazolones** and **pyrazolidinediones** are better tolerated.[1] The nonacetylated salicylates (**sodium salicylate**, **salicylamide**, **choline magnesium trisalicylate**) are normally well tolerated. Aspirin-sensitive individuals are also less likely to react to **nimesulide**.[1,2]

In 60 patients with proven **aspirin**-sensitivity, **celecoxib** 100 mg on day one and 200 mg on day two caused no decline in forced expiratory volume.[3] Two more studies found similar results.[4,5] **Celecoxib** is a selective inhibitor of cyclo-oxygenase-2 and this supports the suggestion that inhibition of cyclo-oxygenase-1 may be critical factor in the precipitation of respiratory reactions in **aspirin**-exacerbated respiratory disease.[3] This suggests that **celecoxib** may be an alternative in patients who are known to be aspirin sensitive. Nevertheless, the manufacturer of **celecoxib** contraindicates its use in patients who are sensitive to aspirin or NSAIDs.[6] In a study in 21 patients with either asthma, nasal polyps, allergic rhinitis or a combination of these, challenged with **meloxicam** 7.5 mg, only one patient with a history of aspirin allergy developed bronchospasm and erythema with meloxicam.[7] Another study found no reaction in 24 patients with a history of NSAID-induced respiratory hypersensitivity given meloxicam 7.5 to 15 mg daily.[4]

However, the manufacturer of **meloxicam** contraindicates its use in patients who are sensitive to aspirin or NSAIDs.[8] Seventy-seven rheumatology patients with a history of asthma caused by aspirin or a NSAID and given ascending doses of **etoricoxib** 60 to 120 mg daily for 3 days had no respiratory or cutaneous reaction to etoricoxib even after rechallenge 5 days later.[9]

(b) NSAIDs with theophylline

Piroxicam 20 mg daily for 7 days had no effect on the pharmacokinetics of theophylline (given as a single 6-mg/kg intravenous dose of aminophylline) in 6 healthy subjects.[10] **Enteric-coated aspirin** 650 mg daily for 4 weeks had no effect on the steady-state serum levels of theophylline in 8 elderly patients (aged 60 to 81) with chronic obstructive pulmonary disease.[11] **Nimesulide** 100 mg twice daily for 7 days did not affect lung function in 10 patients with chronic obstructive airways disease taking slow-release theophylline 200 mg twice daily, although there was a slight, clinically insignificant fall in theophylline levels, possibly due to enzyme induction. The pharmacokinetics of the nimesulide were unchanged.[12]

Apart from checking that the patient is not sensitive to **aspirin** or any other NSAID (see (*a*) above), there would seem to be no reason for avoiding **aspirin** or **piroxicam** in patients taking theophylline.

1. Bianco S, Robuschi M, Petrigni G, Scuri M, Pieroni MG, Refini RM, Vaghi A, Sestini PS. Efficacy and tolerability of nimesulide in asthmatic patients intolerant to aspirin. *Drugs* (1993) 46 (Suppl 1), 115–120.
2. Senna GE, Passalacqua G, Dama A, Crivellaro M, Schiappoli M, Bonadonna P, Canonica GW. Nimesulide and meloxicam are a safe alternative drugs for patients intolerant to nonsteroidal anti-inflammatory drugs. *Allerg Immunol (Paris)* (2003) 35, 393–6.

3. Woessner KM, Simon RA, Stevenson DD. The safety of celecoxib in patients with aspirin-sensitive asthma. *Arthritis Rheum* (2002) 46, 2201–6.
4. Senna G, Bilò M-B, Antonicelli L, Schiappoli M, Crivellaro M-A, Bonadonna P, Dama A-R. Tolerability of three selective cyclo-oxygenase-2 inhibitors, meloxicam, celecoxib and rofecoxib in NSAID-sensitive patients. *Allerg Immunol (Paris)* (2004) 36, 215–8.
5. Martín-Garcia C, Hinojosa M, Berges P, Camacho E, García-Rodriguez R, Alfaya T. Celecoxib, a highly selective COX-2 inhibitor, is safe in aspirin-induced asthma patients. *J Investig Allergol Clin Immunol* (2003) 13, 20–5.
6. Celebrex (Celecoxib). Pharmacia Ltd. UK Summary of product characteristics, February 2007.
7. Bavbek S, Dursun AB, Dursun E, Eryilmaz A, Misirligil Z. Safety of meloxicam in aspirin-hypersensitive patients with asthma and/or nasal polyps. *Int Arch Allergy Immunol* (2007) 142, 64–9.
8. Mobic (Meloxicam). Boehringer Ingelheim Ltd. UK Summary of product characteristics, April 2006.
9. El Miedany Y, Youssef S, Ahmed I, El Gaafary M. Safety of etoricoxib, a specific cyclooxygenase-2 inhibitor, in asthmatic patients with aspirin-exacerbated respiratory disease. *Ann Allergy Asthma Immunol* (2006) 97, 105–9.
10. Maponga C, Barlow JC, Schentag JJ. Lack of effect of piroxicam on theophylline clearance in healthy volunteers. *DICP Ann Pharmacother* (1990) 24, 123–6.
11. Daigneault EA, Hamdy RC, Ferslew KE, Rice PJ, Singh J, Harvill LM, Kalbfleisch JH. Investigation of the influence of acetylsalicylic acid on the steady state of long-term therapy with theophylline in elderly male patients with normal renal function. *J Clin Pharmacol* (1994) 34, 86–90.
12. Auteri A, Blardi P, Bruni F, Domini L, Pasqui AL, Saletti M, Verzuri MS, Scicabarozzi I, Vargui G, Di Perri T. Pharmacokinetics and pharmacodynamics of slow-release theophylline during treatment with nimesulide. *Int J Clin Pharmacol Res* (1991) 11, 211–7.

Beta-agonist bronchodilators + Potassium-depleting drugs

Beta agonists (e.g. fenoterol, salbutamol (albuterol), terbutaline) can cause hypokalaemia. This can be increased by other potassium-depleting drugs such as the corticosteroids, diuretics (e.g. bendroflumethiazide, furosemide) and theophylline. The risk of serious cardiac arrhythmias in asthmatic patients may be increased.

Clinical evidence

(a) Corticosteroids

1. Hypokalaemia. The hypokalaemic effects of beta$_2$ agonists may be increased by corticosteroids. Twenty-four healthy subjects had a fall in their serum potassium levels when they were given either **salbutamol (albuterol)** 5 mg or **fenoterol** 5 mg by nebuliser over 30 minutes. The fall in potassium levels was increased after they took **prednisone** 30 mg daily for a week. The greatest fall (from 3.75 to 2.78 mmol/L) was found 90 minutes after **fenoterol** and **prednisone** were taken. The ECG effects observed included ectopic beats and transient T wave inversion, but no significant ECG disturbances were noted in these healthy subjects.[1]

2. Anti-inflammatory/bronchodilator effects. A marked rise in asthma deaths was noted in New Zealand in the 1980s. A case-control study found that the risk of death was increased in oral corticosteroid-dependent asthmatics (severe asthma) who were also taking inhaled **fenoterol**.[2] This, and other data, suggested the possibility that combined use of short-acting beta$_2$ agonists and corticosteroids might be deleterious in some situations, prompting numerous studies, which were reviewed in 2000.[3] The overall findings were, that although inhaled corticosteroids do not prevent the pro-inflammatory effects of short-acting beta$_2$ agonists, the combination is beneficial in the treatment of asthma at usual therapeutic doses of both drugs. The authors caution that this might not apply with excessive use of short-acting beta$_2$ agonists.[3]

The addition of a long-acting beta$_2$ agonist (e.g. **salmeterol**) to treatment in patients with chronic asthma inadequately controlled by inhaled corticosteroids and 'as required' short-acting beta$_2$ agonists is beneficial.[3,4]

(b) Diuretics

The serum potassium level of 15 healthy subjects was measured after they were given inhaled **terbutaline** 5 mg with either a placebo, **furosemide** 40 mg daily, or **furosemide** 40 mg with **triamterene** 50 mg daily for 4 days. With **terbutaline** alone the potassium levels fell by 0.53 mmol/L; after taking **furosemide** as well they fell by 0.75 mmol/L; and after **furosemide** and **triamterene** they fell by 0.59 mmol/L. These falls were reflected in some ECG (T wave) changes.[5]

After 7 days of treatment with **bendroflumethiazide** 5 mg daily the serum potassium levels of 10 healthy subjects had fallen by 0.71 mmol/L. After taking 100 micrograms to 2 mg of inhaled **salbutamol (albuterol)** as well, the levels fell by 1.06 mmol/L, to 2.72 mmol/L. ECG changes consistent with hypokalaemia and hypomagnesaemia were seen.[6] In another study the same authors found that the addition of **bendroflumethiazide** 5 mg daily to inhaled **salbutamol** 2 mg further reduced serum potassium levels by 0.4 mmol/L, to 2.92 mmol/L. This reduction was abolished by the addition of **triamterene** 200 mg (serum potassium increased to 3.43 mmol/L) or **spironolactone** 100 mg (serum potassium increased to 3.53 mmol/L) but **triamterene** 50 mg only attenuated the effect of **bendroflumethiazide** (serum potassium 3.1 mmol/L). ECG effects with this combination were also reduced by the addition of triamterene or spironolactone.[7]

Other diuretics that can cause potassium loss include **bumetanide, furosemide, etacrynic acid**, the **thiazides**, and many other related diuretics, see 'Table 26.1', (p.944).

(c) Theophylline

The concurrent use of **salbutamol (albuterol)** or **terbutaline** and theophylline can cause an additional fall in serum potassium levels, and other beta$_2$ agonists will interact similarly. See 'Theophylline + Beta-agonist bronchodilators', p.1174.

Mechanism

Additive potassium-depleting effects.

Importance and management

Established interactions. The CSM in the UK[8] advises that, as potentially serious hypokalaemia may result from beta$_2$ agonist therapy, particular caution is required in severe asthma, as this effect may be potentiated by theophylline and its derivatives, corticosteroids, diuretics, and by hypoxia. Hypokalaemia with concurrent use of thiazide and loop diuretics may be reduced or even abolished by the addition of spironolactone or high-dose triamterene. Plasma potassium levels should therefore be monitored in patients with severe asthma. Hypokalaemia may result in cardiac arrhythmias in patients with ischaemic heart disease and may also affect the response of patients to drugs such as the digitalis glycosides and antiarrhythmics.

Note that the combined use of beta$_2$ agonists and corticosteroids in asthma is usually beneficial.

1. Taylor DR, Wilkins GT, Herbison GP, Flannery EM. Interaction between corticosteroid and β-agonist drugs. Biochemical and cardiovascular effects in normal subjects. *Chest* (1992) 102, 519–24.
2. Crane J, Pearce N, Flatt A, Burgess C, Jackson R, Kwong T, Ball M, Beasley R. Prescribed fenoterol and death from asthma in New Zealand, 1981–1983: case-control study. *Lancet* (1989) i, 917–22.
3. Taylor DR, Hancox RJ. Interactions between corticosteroids and β agonists. *Thorax* (2000) 55, 595–602.
4. Shrewsbury S, Pyke S, Britton M. Meta-analysis of increased dose of inhaled steroid or addition of salmeterol in symptomatic asthma (MIASMA). *BMJ* (2000) 320, 1368–73.
5. Newnham DM, McDevitt DG, Lipworth BJ. The effects of frusemide and triamterene on the hypokalaemic and electrocardiographic responses to inhaled terbutaline. *Br J Clin Pharmacol* (1991) 32, 630–2.
6. Lipworth BJ, McDevitt DG, Struthers AD. Prior treatment with diuretic augments the hypokalemic and electrocardiographic effects of inhaled albuterol. *Am J Med* (1989) 86, 653–7.
7. Lipworth BJ, McDevitt DG, Struthers AD. Hypokalemic and ECG sequelae of combined beta-agonist/diuretic therapy. Protection by conventional doses of spironolactone but not triamterene. *Chest* (1990) 98, 811–15.
8. Committee on Safety of Medicines. β_2 agonists, xanthines and hypokalaemia. *Current Problems* (1990) 28.

Caffeine + Allopurinol

Allopurinol may invalidate the results of studies using caffeine as a probe drug for determining acetylator status or activity of CYP1A2.

Clinical evidence, mechanism, importance and management

In 21 healthy subjects, allopurinol 300 mg daily for 8 days altered the levels of urinary caffeine metabolites of a single 200-mg dose of caffeine. In particular, the metabolic ratio used to determine whether people are fast or slow acetylators was substantially changed. Thus, allopurinol may invalidate the results of phenotyping with the urinary caffeine test. In addition, the caffeine metabolite ratio used to express the activity of the cytochrome P450 isoenzyme CYP1A2 was not stable when allopurinol was used.[1] This interaction is of relevance to research rather than clinical practice.

1. Fuchs P, Haefeli WE, Ledermann HR, Wenk M. Xanthine oxidase inhibition by allopurinol affects the reliability of urinary caffeine metabolic ratios as markers for *N*-acetyltransferase 2 and CYP1A2 activities. *Eur J Clin Pharmacol* (1999) 54, 869–76.

Caffeine + Antiepileptics

Phenytoin can increase the clearance of caffeine, and possibly invalidates the caffeine breath test. Whether carbamazepine increases caffeine metabolism is unclear. Valproate appears not to have any effect on caffeine.

Clinical evidence

The clearance of caffeine was about twofold higher and its half-life was reduced by about 50% in patients with epilepsy taking **phenytoin**, when compared with healthy subjects not taking any medications. In the same study, there were no significant differences in caffeine pharmacokinetics between healthy subjects and patients receiving **carbamazepine** or **sodium valproate**.[1] Conversely, **carbamazepine** was considered to have induced the metabolism of caffeine in 5 children with epilepsy, as assessed by the caffeine breath test.[2] In another study in healthy subjects, there was a reduction in the AUC of **carbamazepine** when it was given with caffeine, but caffeine had no effect on the pharmacokinetics of **sodium valproate**.[3]

Mechanism

Phenytoin acts as an enzyme inducer, thereby increasing the metabolism of caffeine, lowering its levels. Carbamazepine possibly has the same effect.

Importance and management

Phenytoin may possibly invalidate the caffeine breath test, but normally no special precautions are needed if both drugs are taken. The interaction between carbamazepine and caffeine requires further study.

1. Wietholtz H, Zysset T, Kreiten K, Kohl D, Büchsel R, Matern S. Effect of phenytoin, carbamazepine, and valproic acid on caffeine metabolism. *Eur J Clin Pharmacol* (1989) 36, 401–6.
2. Parker AC, Pritchard P, Preston T, Choonara I. Induction of CYP1A2 activity by carbamazepine in children using the caffeine breath test. *Br J Clin Pharmacol* (1998) 45, 176–8.
3. Vaz J, Kulkarni C, Joy D, Joseph T. Influence of caffeine on pharmacokinetic profile of sodium valproate and carbamazepine in normal healthy volunteers. *Indian J Exp Biol* (1998) 36, 112–14.

Caffeine + Antifungals

Fluconazole and terbinafine cause a modest rise in serum caffeine levels. Ketoconazole appears to have less effect.

Clinical evidence, mechanism, importance and management

A study in 6 young subjects (average age 24) given **fluconazole** 400 mg daily and 5 elderly subjects (average age 69) given **fluconazole** 200 mg daily for 10 days found that fluconazole reduced the plasma clearance of caffeine by an average of 25% (32% in the young and 17% in the old).[1] In a single-dose study in 8 healthy subjects, **terbinafine** 500 mg and **ketoconazole** 400 mg decreased caffeine clearance by 21% and 10%, respectively, and increased its half-life by 31% and 16%, respectively.[2]

It seems unlikely that these moderately increased serum caffeine levels will have a clinically important effect, but this needs confirmation.

1. Nix DE, Zelenitsky SA, Symonds WT, Spivey JM, Norman A. The effect of fluconazole on the pharmacokinetics of caffeine in young and elderly subjects. *Clin Pharmacol Ther* (1992) 51, 183.
2. Wahlländer A, Paumgartner G. Effect of ketoconazole and terbinafine on the pharmacokinetics of caffeine in healthy volunteers. *Eur J Clin Pharmacol* (1989) 37, 279–83.

Caffeine + Artemisinin

Artemisinin reduces the metabolism of caffeine.

Clinical evidence, mechanism, importance and management

A study in 7 healthy subjects found that a single 500-mg dose of artemisinin reduced clearance of a single 136.5-mg dose of caffeine by 35%. The metabolism of caffeine to one of its major metabolites, paraxanthine, was reduced by 66%.[1] It was suggested that artemisinin inhibits the metabolism of caffeine by the cytochrome P450 isoenzyme CYP1A2 in the liver.[1]

There is too little information to advise patients taking artemisinin to completely avoid caffeine-containing beverages, foods or medication, but bear this interaction in mind if the adverse effects of caffeine (insomnia, jitteriness etc) become troublesome.

1. Bapiro TE, Sayi J, Hasler JA, Jande M, Rimoy G, Masselle A, Masimirembwa CM. Artemisinin and thiabendazole are potent inhibitors of cytochrome P450 1A2 (CYP1A2) activity in humans. *Eur J Clin Pharmacol* (2005) 61, 755–61.

Caffeine + Cimetidine

The clearance of caffeine is decreased by cimetidine but this seems unlikely to be clinically significant.

Clinical evidence, mechanism, importance and management

In 5 subjects cimetidine 1 g daily for 6 days increased the half-life of a single 300-mg dose of caffeine by about 70% and reduced caffeine clearance.[1] In another study, cimetidine 1.2 g daily for 4 days increased the caffeine half-life by 45% in 6 smokers and by 96% in 6 non-smokers. The caffeine clearance was reduced by 31% in the smokers and by 42% in the non-smokers.[2] A further study found that the caffeine half-life was increased by 59% and the clearance decreased by 40% by cimetidine.[3] Conversely, in a further study in children, cimetidine was not found to affect caffeine metabolism as assessed by the caffeine breath test.[4]

The changes seen in some studies probably occurred because cimetidine, a well-known non-specific enzyme inhibitor reduced the metabolism of caffeine by the liver, resulting in its accumulation in the body.

Any increased caffeine effects are normally unlikely to be of much importance in most people, but they might have a small part to play in exaggerating the undesirable effects of caffeine from food, drinks (e.g. tea, coffee, cola drinks, chocolate) and analgesics, which are sometimes formulated with caffeine.

1. Broughton LJ, Rogers HJ. Decreased systemic clearance of caffeine due to cimetidine. *Br J Clin Pharmacol* (1981) 12, 155–9.
2. May DC, Jarboe CH, VanBakel AB, Williams WM. Effects of cimetidine on caffeine disposition in smokers and nonsmokers. *Clin Pharmacol Ther* (1982) 31, 656–61.
3. Beach CA, Gerber N, Ross J, Bianchine JR. Inhibition of elimination of caffeine by cimetidine in man. *Clin Res* (1982) 30, 248A.
4. Parker AC, Pritchard P, Preston T, Dalzell AM, Choonara I. Lack of inhibitory effect of cimetidine on caffeine metabolism in children using the caffeine breath test. *Br J Clin Pharmacol* (1997) 43, 467–70.

Caffeine + Class I antiarrhythmics

Caffeine clearance is reduced by 30 to 60% by mexiletine, resulting in raised serum caffeine levels. Whether this might result in caffeine toxicity is uncertain. Lidocaine, flecainide and tocainide do not appear to affect caffeine clearance. Caffeine does not significantly alter mexiletine levels.

Clinical evidence

(a) Mexiletine

In a study in 7 patients with cardiac arrhythmias taking long-term mexiletine 600 mg daily the clearance of caffeine was found to be reduced by 48%.[1] In 5 healthy subjects given a single 200-mg dose of mexiletine, the clearance of a single 366-mg dose of caffeine was reduced by 57%, from 126 to 54 mL/minute, and the elimination half-life rose from approximately 4 to 7 hours.[1] The clearance of mexiletine was not affected by caffeine. A preliminary report of this study also noted that fasting caffeine levels were almost sixfold higher during the mexiletine treatment period (1.99 compared with 0.35 micrograms/mL).[2]

Another study in 14 healthy subjects found that caffeine 100 mg four times daily, for 2 days before and 2 days after mexiletine, did not cause any significant changes in the plasma levels of a single 200-mg dose of mexiletine. Caffeine levels tended to be increased 24 hours after taking mexiletine.[3]

(b) Other antiarrhythmics

Single doses of **lidocaine** 200 mg, **flecainide** 100 mg and **tocainide** 500 mg had no effect on caffeine clearance in 7 healthy subjects given a single 366-mg dose of caffeine.[2]

Mechanism

It is likely that, as with theophylline (see 'Theophylline + Mexiletine or Tocainide', p.1188), mexiletine inhibits the hepatic metabolism of caffeine by the cytochrome P450 isoenzyme CYP1A2.

Importance and management

The interaction between caffeine and mexiletine appears to be established, but its clinical importance is uncertain. Some of the adverse effects of mexiletine might be partially due to caffeine-retention (from drinking tea, coffee, cola drinks, etc.).[1] In excess, caffeine can cause jitteriness, tremor and insomnia. It has also been suggested that the caffeine test for liver function might be impaired by mexiletine.[1] Be alert for these possible effects.

1. Joeres R, Klinker H, Heusler H, Epping J, Richter E. Influence of mexiletine on caffeine elimination. *Pharmacol Ther* (1987) 33, 163–9.
2. Joeres R, Richter E. Mexiletine and caffeine elimination. *N Engl J Med* (1987) 317, 117.
3. Labbé L, Abolfathi Z, Robitaille NM, St-Maurice F, Gilbert M, Turegon J. Stereoselective disposition of the antiarrhythmic agent mexiletine during the concomitant administration of caffeine. *Ther Drug Monit* (1999) 21, 191–9.

Caffeine + Disulfiram

Disulfiram reduces the clearance of caffeine, which might complicate the withdrawal from alcohol.

Clinical evidence, mechanism, importance and management

A study in healthy subjects and recovering alcoholics found that disulfiram 250 or 500 mg daily reduced the clearance of caffeine by about 30%, but a few of the alcoholics had a more than 50% reduction.[1] As a result the levels of caffeine in the body increased. Raised levels of caffeine can cause irritability, insomnia and anxiety, similar to the symptoms of alcohol withdrawal. As coffee consumption is often particularly high among recovering alcoholics, there is the risk that they may turn to alcohol to calm themselves down. To avoid this possible complication it might be wise for recovering alcoholics not to drink too much tea or coffee. Decaffeinated coffee and tea are widely available.

1. Beach CA, Mays DC, Guiler RC, Jacober CH, Gerber N. Inhibition of elimination of caffeine by disulfiram in normal subjects and recovering alcoholics. *Clin Pharmacol Ther* (1986) 39, 265–70.

Caffeine + Echinacea

Echinacea appears to have a variable effect on the pharmacokinetics of caffeine.

Clinical evidence, mechanism, importance and management

In a pharmacokinetic study, 12 healthy subjects were given an 8-day course of *Echinacea purpurea* root 400 mg four times daily, with a single 200-mg oral dose of caffeine on day 6. The maximum serum concentration and AUC of caffeine were increased by about 30%. There was a large variation between subjects, with some having a 50% increase in caffeine clearance, and some a 90% decrease. The paraxanthine-to-caffeine ratio (a measure of CYP1A2 activity) was reduced by just 10%.[1] In another study in 12 healthy subjects given *Echinacea purpurea* 800 mg twice daily for 28 days, the paraxanthine-to-caffeine ratio was not significantly affected when a single 100-mg dose of caffeine was given at the end of the treatment with *Echinacea purpurea*.[2]

It is possible that drugs that are metabolised by the cytochrome P450 isoenzyme CYP1A2 and have a narrow therapeutic index may be adversely affected by the concurrent use of Echinacea-containing products. For a list of drugs that are substrates of this enzyme, see 'Table 1.2', (p.4). Further study is required.

1. Gorski JC, Huang S-M, Pinto A, Hamman MA, Hilligoss JK, Zaheer NA, Desai M, Miller M, Hall SD. The effect of echinacea (*Echinacea purpurea* root) on cytochrome P450 activity in vivo. *Clin Pharmacol Ther* (2004) 75, 89–100.
2. Gurley BJ, Gardner SF, Hubbard MA, Williams DK, Gentry WB, Carrier J, Khan IA, Edwards DJ, Shah A. In vivo assessment of botanical supplementation on human cytochrome P450 phenotypes: *Citrus aurantium*, *Echinacea purpurea*, milk thistle, and saw palmetto. *Clin Pharmacol Ther* (2004) 76, 428–40.

Caffeine + Fluvoxamine

The clearance of caffeine is considerably reduced by fluvoxamine. An increase in the stimulant and adverse effects of caffeine would be expected, however this was not demonstrated in one study. Caffeine may cause a reduction in the bioavailability of fluvoxamine.

Clinical evidence

In a randomised, crossover study, fluvoxamine 50 mg daily for 4 days and then 100 mg daily for a further 8 days was given to 8 healthy subjects, with a single 200-mg oral dose of caffeine before and on day 8 of fluvoxamine use. Fluvoxamine reduced the total clearance of caffeine by about 80% (from 107 to 21 mL/minute) and increased its half-life from 5 to 31 hours. Specifically, the clearance of caffeine by *N*3-, *N*1- and *N*7-demethylation was decreased.[1] Another study in 30 patients found a positive correlation between plasma fluvoxamine and plasma caffeine levels, suggesting that the interaction is dose-related.[2] A further study found that low, sub-therapeutic doses of fluvoxamine 10 or 20 mg daily were sufficient to markedly inhibit caffeine metabolism.[3] A study in 7 subjects found that fluvoxamine 100 mg twice daily for 4 doses significantly increased the maximum levels of a single 250-mg dose of caffeine by 40%, and increased the AUC and half-life of caffeine by 12.7-fold and 10-fold, respectively. However, this did not result in an increase in caffeine-related adverse effects, and none of the subjects felt they were more alert with the combination than with either drug alone.[4]

A study in 12 healthy subjects (6 smokers and 6 non-smokers, none were poor metabolisers of CYP2D6) found that caffeine 150 mg twice daily for 11 days reduced the AUC of a single 50-mg dose of fluvoxamine taken on day 8, by approximately 24%. The plasma concentration of fluvoxamine was also decreased by 12% but this was not significant.[5]

Mechanism

Fluvoxamine is a potent inhibitor of the cytochrome P450 isoenzyme CYP1A2, which is the principal enzyme concerned with the metabolism of caffeine. As a result the caffeine is cleared from the body much more slowly and accumulates.[1-3]

Importance and management

The increase in caffeine levels with concurrent use would seem to be established. There are no reports of caffeine toxicity arising from this interaction and one study[4] found no increase in the pharmacodynamic or adverse effects of caffeine despite a large increase in the levels. However, an increase in the stimulant and adverse effects of caffeine (headache, jitteriness, restlessness, insomnia) may be possible in susceptible patients if they continue to consume large amounts of caffeine-containing food or drinks (tea, coffee, cola drinks, chocolate, etc.) or take caffeine-containing medications. They should be warned to reduce their caffeine intake if problems develop. It has been suggested that some of the adverse effects of fluvoxamine (i.e. nervousness, restlessness and insomnia) could in fact be caused by caffeine toxicity. However, a preliminary study, as well as the study reported above,[4] found that caffeine intake had a limited effect on the frequency of adverse effects of fluvoxamine.[6]

The clinical significance of the change in the AUC of fluvoxamine with caffeine intake is unclear. This slight decrease is unlikely to be important in most patients.

1. Jeppesen U, Loft S, Poulsen HE, Brøsen K. A fluvoxamine-caffeine interaction study. *Pharmacogenetics* (1996) 6, 213–222.
2. Yoshimura R, Ueda N, Nakamura J, Eto S, Matsushita M. Interaction between fluvoxamine and cotinine or caffeine. *Neuropsychobiology* (2002) 45, 32–5.
3. Christensen M, Tybring G, Mihara K, Yasui-Furokori N, Carrillo JA, Ramos SI, Andersson K, Dahl M-L, Bertilsson L. Low daily 10-mg and 20-mg doses of fluvoxamine inhibit the metabolism of both caffeine (cytochrome P4501A2) and omeprazole (cytochrome P4502C19). *Clin Pharmacol Ther* (2002) 71, 141–52.
4. Culm-Merdek KE, von Moltke LL, Harmatz JS, Greenblatt DJ. Fluvoxamine impairs single-dose caffeine clearance without altering caffeine pharmacodynamics. *Br J Clin Pharmacol* (2005) 60, 486–93.
5. Fukasawa T, Yasui-Furukori N, Suzuki A, Ishii G, Inoue Y, Tateishi T, Otani K. Effects of caffeine on the kinetics of fluvoxamine and its major metabolite in plasma after a single oral dose of the drug. *Ther Drug Monit* (2006) 28, 308–11.
6. Spigset O. Are adverse drug reactions attributed to fluvoxamine caused by concomitant intake of caffeine? *Eur J Clin Pharmacol* (1998) 54, 665–6.

Caffeine + Grapefruit juice

Grapefruit juice does not interact with caffeine to a clinically relevant extent.

Clinical evidence, mechanism, importance and management

In 12 healthy subjects grapefruit juice, at a dose of 1.2 litres, decreased the clearance of caffeine from coffee by 23% and prolonged its half-life by 31%, but these changes were not considered clinically relevant.[1] A crossover study in 6 healthy subjects given caffeine 3.3 mg/kg found that multiple doses of grapefruit juice (equivalent to 6 glasses) caused a non-significant increase in the AUC of caffeine. No changes in ambulatory systolic or diastolic blood pressure or heart rate were seen.[2]

1. Fuhr U, Klittich K, Staib AH. Inhibitory effect of grapefruit juice and the active component, naringenin on CYP1A2 dependent metabolism of caffeine in man. *Br J Clin Pharmacol* (1993) 35, 431–6. [Title corrected by erratum].
2. Maish WA, Hampton EM, Whitsett TL, Shepard JD, Lovallo WR. Influence of grapefruit juice on caffeine pharmacokinetics and pharmacodynamics. *Pharmacotherapy* (1996) 16, 1046–52.

Caffeine + Hormonal contraceptives or HRT

The half-life of caffeine is prolonged to some extent in women taking combined oral contraceptives or HRT.

Clinical evidence

(a) Contraceptives

The clearance of a single 162-mg dose of caffeine was reduced, the half-life prolonged (7.9 compared with 5.4 hours), and the plasma levels were raised in 9 women taking low-dose combined oral contraceptives for at least 3 months, when compared with 9 other women not taking an oral contraceptive.[1] This finding was confirmed in three other studies,[2-4] which found that caffeine elimination was prolonged, from 4 to 6 hours before the use of combined oral contraceptives, to about 9 hours by the end of the first cycle, and to about 11 hours by the end of the third cycle.[3,4] A further study found that there was little difference between the effects of two oral contraceptives (**ethinylestradiol** 30 micrograms with gestodene 75 micrograms or levonorgestrel 125 micrograms) on caffeine: both increased the half-life of caffeine by a little over 50%, but the maximum serum levels were unchanged.[5]

(b) HRT

In one study, 12 healthy postmenopausal women were given a single 200-mg dose of caffeine after taking **estradiol** (*Estrace*) for 8 weeks, titrated to give **estradiol** plasma concentrations of 50 to 150 picograms/mL. The metabolism of caffeine was reduced by 29% overall. If the data for 2 subjects who were found to have taken extra caffeine during the study period are excluded, the caffeine metabolism showed an even greater average reduction of 38%.[6]

Mechanism

Uncertain. Estrogens can inhibit the cytochrome P450 isoenzyme CYP1A2, by which caffeine is metabolised, which may explain its accumulation in the body.

Importance and management

An established interaction that is probably of limited clinical importance. Women taking oral contraceptives containing estrogens or HRT who take caffeine-containing analgesics or drink caffeine-containing drinks (tea, coffee, cola drinks, etc.) may find the effects of caffeine, such as jitteriness and insomnia, increased and prolonged.

1. Abernethy DR, Todd EL. Impairment of caffeine clearance by chronic use of low-dose oestrogen-containing oral contraceptives. *Eur J Clin Pharmacol* (1985) 28, 425–8.
2. Patwardhan RV, Desmond PV, Johnson RF, Schenker S. Impaired elimination of caffeine by oral contraceptive steroids. *J Lab Clin Med* (1980) 95, 603–8.
3. Meyer FP, Canzler E, Giers H, Walther H. Langzeituntersuchung zum Einfluß von Non-Ovlon auf die Pharmakokinetik von Coffein im intraindividuellen Vergleich. *Zentralbl Gynakol* (1988) 110, 1449–54.
4. Rietveld EC, Broekman MMM, Houben JJG, Eskes TKAB, van Rossum JM. Rapid onset of an increase in caffeine residence time in young women due to oral contraceptive steroids. *Eur J Clin Pharmacol* (1984) 26, 371–3.
5. Balogh A, Klinger G, Henschel L, Börner A, Vollanth R, Kuhnz W. Influence of ethinylestradiol-containing combination oral contraceptives with gestodene or levonorgestrel on caffeine elimination. *Eur J Clin Pharmacol* (1995) 48, 161–6.
6. Pollock BG, Wylie M, Stack JA, Sorisio DA, Thompson DS, Kirshner MA, Folan MM, Condifer KA. Inhibition of caffeine metabolism by estrogen replacement therapy in postmenopausal women. *J Clin Pharmacol* (1999) 39, 936–40.

Caffeine + Idrocilamide

Oral idrocilamide reduces the clearance of caffeine, which can lead to caffeine toxicity.

Clinical evidence, mechanism, importance and management

The possibility that caffeine ingestion might have had some part to play in the development of psychiatric disorders seen in patients taking idrocilamide, prompted a pharmacokinetic study in 4 healthy subjects. While taking oral idrocilamide 400 mg three times a day the half-life of caffeine (150 to 200 mg of caffeine from one cup of coffee) was prolonged from about 7 to 59 hours. The overall clearance of caffeine was decreased by about 90%.[1,2]

Idrocilamide can inhibit the cytochrome P450 isoenzyme CYP1A2 by which caffeine is metabolised, leading to its accumulation.

Evidence is limited but the interaction appears to be established. Patients taking oral idrocilamide should probably avoid or minimise their intake of caffeine, including caffeine-containing drinks (tea, coffee, cola drinks, etc.), otherwise caffeine toxicity may develop. Decaffeinated teas and coffee are widely available. Some medicines may contain caffeine, so these should also be used with care.

1. Brazier JL, Descotes J, Lery N, Ollagnier M, Evreux J-C. Inhibition by idrocilamide of the disposition of caffeine. *Eur J Clin Pharmacol* (1980) 17, 37–43.
2. Evreux JC, Bayere JJ, Descotes J, Lery N, Ollagnier M, Brazier JL. Les accidents neuro-psychiques de l'idrocilamide: conséquence d'une inhibition due métabolisme de la caféine? *Lyon Med* (1979) 241, 89–91.

Caffeine + Kava

There are conflicting results from studies of the interaction of kava and caffeine. It appears that kava is unlikely to affect the pharmacokinetics of caffeine, although further study is required to confirm this.

Clinical evidence, mechanism, importance and management

In a study in 6 subjects (3 of whom smoked tobacco) who regularly took 7 to 27 g of kavalactones weekly as an aqueous kava extract, the metabolic ratio of caffeine was increased twofold when kava was withheld for 30 days, which suggested that kava inhibits the cytochrome P450 isoenzyme CYP1A2, which is involved in the metabolism of caffeine.[1]

However, in a study in 12 non-smoking healthy subjects given kava kava root extract 1 g twice daily for 28 days before receiving a single 100-mg dose of oral caffeine, no significant change in the metabolic ratio of caffeine was noted.[2] It is possible that the inhibitory effect of tobacco smoke on CYP1A2, and the lack of standardisation of kava intake may have influenced the results.

1. Russman S, Lauterburg BH, Barguil Y, Choblet E, Cabalion P, Rentsch K, Wenk M. Traditional aqueous kava extracts inhibit cytochrome P450 1A2 in humans: protective effect against environmental carcinogens? *Clin Pharmacol Ther* (2005) 77, 451–4.
2. Gurley BJ, Gardner SF, Hubbard MA, Williams DK, Gentry WB, Khan IA, Shah A. In vivo effects of goldenseal, kava kava, black cohosh, and valerian on human cytochrome P450 1A2, 2D6, 2E1, and 3A4/5 phenotypes. *Clin Pharmacol Ther* (2005) 77, 415–26.

Caffeine + Menthol

A crossover study in 11 healthy subjects found that a single 100-mg dose of menthol taken with coffee containing 200 mg caffeine increased the time to maximum caffeine concentration by about 30 minutes. The increase in the actual maximum concentration was not significant, and there were no significant effects on caffeine half-life. It was thought that menthol reduced the rate of caf-

feine absorption.[1] The clinical importance of this is not clear but it is seems likely to be small.

1. Gelal A, Guven H, Balkan D, Artok L, Benowitz NL. Influence of menthol on caffeine disposition and pharmacodynamics in healthy female volunteers. *Eur J Clin Pharmacol* (2003) 59, 417–22.

Caffeine + Psoralens

Oral methoxsalen and 5-methoxypsoralen markedly reduce caffeine clearance but the clinical significance of this is uncertain. Topical methoxsalen does not interact with caffeine.

Clinical evidence

A single 1.2-mg/kg oral dose of **methoxsalen** (8-methoxypsoralen), given to 5 subjects with psoriasis 1 hour before a single 200-mg oral dose of caffeine, reduced the clearance of caffeine by 69%. The elimination half-life of caffeine over the period from 2 to 16 hours after taking the **methoxsalen** increased tenfold (from 5.6 to 57 hours).[1] In a similar study, 8 patients with psoriasis were given caffeine 200 mg with or without **5-methoxypsoralen** 1.2 mg/kg. The AUC of caffeine increased by about threefold and there was a threefold decrease in its clearance.[2]

A study in patients receiving PUVA therapy (**methoxsalen** either orally, in 4 patients, or topically as a bath in 7 patients, plus UVA) found that the clearance of a single 150-mg dose of caffeine was markedly reduced in the patients given oral **methoxsalen** but not altered in those given topical **methoxsalen**.[3]

Mechanism

Both methoxsalen and 5-methoxypsoralen inhibit the hepatic metabolism of caffeine by the cytochrome P450 isoenzyme CYP1A2, thereby markedly increasing caffeine levels.[2,3]

Importance and management

The practical consequences of this interaction are as yet uncertain, but it seems possible that the toxic effects of caffeine will be increased. In excess, caffeine (including that from tea, coffee and cola drinks) can cause jitteriness, headache and insomnia. The interaction does not appear to occur with topical methoxsalen.

1. Mays DC, Camisa C, Cheney P, Pacula CM, Nawoot S, Gerber N. Methoxsalen is a potent inhibitor of the metabolism of caffeine in humans. *Clin Pharmacol Ther* (1987) 42, 621–6.
2. Bendriss EK, Bechtel Y, Bendriss A, Humbert P, Paintaud G, Megnette J, Agache P, Bechtel PR. Inhibition of caffeine metabolism by 5-methoxypsoralen in patients with psoriasis. *Br J Clin Pharmacol* (1996) 41, 421–4.
3. Tantcheva-Poór I, Servera-Llaneras M, Scharffetter-Kochanek K, Fuhr U. Liver cytochrome P450 CYP1A2 is markedly inhibited by systemic but not by bath PUVA in dermatological patients. *Br J Dermatol* (2001) 144, 1127–32.

Caffeine + Quinolones

Enoxacin markedly increases caffeine levels. The effects of caffeine derived from drinks such as tea, coffee or cola, would be expected to be increased. Pipemidic acid interacts to a lesser extent, and ciprofloxacin, norfloxacin and pefloxacin interact less still. Fleroxacin, lomefloxacin, ofloxacin, rufloxacin, and trovafloxacin appear not to interact.

Clinical evidence

The effects of various quinolones on the pharmacokinetics of caffeine[1-13] are summarised in 'Table 33.3', (p.1167). In one study ciprofloxacin and fleroxacin increased caffeine levels more in women than men, but this difference in effect was not significant when the results were normalised for body weight.[13]

Mechanism

It would seem that the metabolism (*N*-demethylation) of caffeine is markedly reduced by some quinolones (notably pipemidic acid and enoxacin) resulting in greater levels and possibly greater effects. Other quinolones have either a much smaller effect or no effect at all. The quinolones that interact appear to inhibit the cytochrome P450 isoenzyme CYP1A2[14] by which caffeine is metabolised.

Importance and management

Established interactions. Based on the results of two studies, on a scale of 100 to 0, the relative potencies of these quinolones as inhibitors of caffeine elimination have been determined as follows: enoxacin 100, pipemidic acid 29, ciprofloxacin 11, norfloxacin 9 and ofloxacin 0.[15] From further studies, clinafloxacin appears to be similar to enoxacin (profound effect), pefloxacin to norfloxacin (to which it is metabolised; modest effect), and fleroxacin, lomefloxacin, rufloxacin, and trovafloxacin appear to behave like ofloxacin (no effect). Patients taking enoxacin might be expected to experience an increase in the effects of caffeine (such as headache, jitteriness, restlessness, insomnia) if, for example, they continue to drink their usual amounts of caffeine-containing drinks (tea, coffee, cola drinks, etc.). They should be warned to cut out or reduce their intake of caffeine if this occurs. The authors of one report[1] suggest that patients with hepatic disorders, cardiac arrhythmias or latent epilepsy should avoid caffeine if they take enoxacin for one week or more. The effects of pipemidic acid are less, and those of ciprofloxacin, norfloxacin and pefloxacin are probably of little or no clinical importance. Fleroxacin, lomefloxacin, ofloxacin, rufloxacin, and trovafloxacin do not interact.

1. Staib AH, Stille W, Dietlein G, Shah PM, Harder S, Mieke S, Beer C. Interaction between quinolones and caffeine. *Drugs* (1987) 34 (Suppl 1), 170–4.
2. Carbó M, Segura J, De la Torre R, Badenas JM, Camí J. Effect of quinolones on caffeine disposition. *Clin Pharmacol Ther* (1989) 45, 234–40.
3. Harder S, Staib AH, Beer C, Papenburg A, Stille W, Shah PM. 4-Quinolones inhibit biotransformation of caffeine. *Eur J Clin Pharmacol* (1988) 35, 651–6.
4. Stille W, Harder S, Mieke S, Beer C, Shah PM, Frech K, Staib AH. Decrease of caffeine elimination in man during co-administration of 4-quinolones. *J Antimicrob Chemother* (1987) 20, 729–34.
5. Healy DP, Schoenle JR, Stotka J, Polk RE. Lack of interaction between lomefloxacin and caffeine in normal volunteers. *Antimicrob Agents Chemother* (1991) 35, 660–4.
6. Peloquin CA, Nix DE, Sedman AJ, Wilton JH, Toothaker RD, Harrison NJ, Schentag JJ. Pharmacokinetics and clinical effects of caffeine alone and in combination with oral enoxacin. *Rev Infect Dis* (1989) II (Suppl 5), S1095.
7. Healy DP, Polk RE, Kanawati L, Rock DT, Mooney ML. Interaction between oral ciprofloxacin and caffeine in normal volunteers. *Antimicrob Agents Chemother* (1989) 33, 474–8.
8. Nicolau DP, Nightingale CH, Tessier PR, Fu Q, Xuan D-w, Esguerra EM, Quintiliani R. The effect of fleroxacin and ciprofloxacin on the pharmacokinetics of multiple dose caffeine. *Drugs* (1995) 49 (Suppl 2), 357–9.
9. LeBel M, Teng R, Dogolo LC, Willavize S, Friedman HL, Vincent J. The influence of steady-state trovafloxacin on the steady-state pharmacokinetics of caffeine in healthy subjects. *Pharm Res* (1996) 13 (Suppl 9), S434.
10. Randinitis EJ, Koup JR, Rausch G, Vassos AB. Effect of (CLX) administration on the single-dose pharmacokinetics of theophylline and caffeine. *Intersci Conf Antimicrob Agents Chemother* (1998) 38, 6.
11. Cesana M, Broccali G, Imbimbo BP, Crema A. Effect of single doses of rufloxacin on the disposition of theophylline and caffeine after single administration. *Int J Clin Pharmacol Ther Toxicol* (1991) 29, 133–8.
12. Kinzig-Schippers M, Fuhr U, Zaigler M, Dammeyer J, Rüsing G, Labedzki A, Bulitta J, Sörgel F. Interaction of pefloxacin and enoxacin with the human cytochrome P450 enzyme CYP1A2. *Clin Pharmacol Ther* (1999) 65, 262–74.
13. Kim M-Y, Nightingale CH, Nicolau DP. Influence of sex on the pharmacokinetic interaction of fleroxacin and ciprofloxacin with caffeine. *Clin Pharmacokinet* (2003), 42, 985–96.
14. Fuhr U, Wolff T, Harder S, Schymanski P, Staib AH. Quinolone inhibition of cytochrome P450-dependent caffeine metabolism in human liver microsomes. *Drug Metab Dispos* (1990) 18, 1005–10.
15. Barnett G, Segura J, de la Torre R, Carbó M. Pharmacokinetic determination of relative potency of quinolone inhibition of caffeine disposition. *Eur J Clin Pharmacol* (1990) 39, 63–9.

Caffeine + Saw palmetto

Saw palmetto does not appear to affect the pharmacokinetics of caffeine.

Clinical evidence, mechanism, importance and management

Saw palmetto 160 mg twice daily was given to 12 healthy subjects for 28 days with a single 100-mg dose of caffeine at the end of treatment with saw palmetto. The metabolism of caffeine was not affected by the concurrent use of saw palmetto, which suggests that saw palmetto does not significantly affect the cytochrome P450 isoenzyme CYP1A2. Therefore the metabolism of other drugs that are substrates of CYP1A2 would not be expected to be affected by saw palmetto.[1] For a list of drugs that are substrates of this isoenzyme, see 'Table 1.2', (p.4).

1. Gurley BJ, Gardner SF, Hubbard MA, Williams DK, Gentry WB, Carrier J, Khan IA, Edwards DJ, Shah A. In vivo assessment of botanical supplementation on human cytochrome P450 phenotypes: *Citrus aurantium*, *Echinacea purpurea*, milk thistle, and saw palmetto. *Clin Pharmacol Ther* (2004) 76, 428–40.

Table 33.3 Effect of quinolones on caffeine pharmacokinetics in healthy subjects

Quinolone[*]	*Daily caffeine intake*[†]	*Change in AUC*	*Change in clearance*	*Refs*
Ciprofloxacin				
100 mg twice daily	220 to 230 mg	+17%		1
250 mg twice daily	220 to 230 mg	+57%	-33%	1-3
500 mg twice daily	230 mg	+58%		1
500 mg twice daily	100 mg three times daily	+127%	-49%	4
500 mg twice daily	100 mg three times daily	+101% women +80% men	-53% women -47% men	5
750 mg (3 x 12-hourly doses)	100 mg	+59%	-45%	6
Clinafloxacin				
400 mg twice daily	200 mg		-84%	7
Enoxacin				
100 mg twice daily	230 mg	+138%		1
200 mg twice daily	230 mg	+176%		1
400 mg twice daily	220 to 230 mg	+346%	-78%	1-3
400 mg twice daily	200 mg daily	+370%	-79%	8
400 mg twice daily	183 mg daily		-83%	9
Fleroxacin				
400 mg daily	100 mg three times daily	+18% women No change in men	No change in women No change in men	4
Lomefloxacin				
400 mg daily	200 mg daily	No change	No change	10
Norfloxacin				
200 mg twice daily	230 mg	+16%		1
800 mg twice daily	350 mg	+52%	-35%	11
Ofloxacin				
200 mg twice daily	220 to 230 mg	No change	No change	1-3
Pefloxacin				
400 mg twice daily	183 mg daily		-47%	9
Pipemidic acid				
400 mg twice daily	230 mg	+179%		1
800 mg twice daily	350 mg	+119%	-63%	11
Rufloxacin				
400 mg (single dose)	200 mg	-18%	No change	12
Trovafloxacin				
200 mg daily	183 mg daily	+17%		13

*Unless otherwise stated quinolones were given for 3 to 5 days.
†Unless otherwise stated caffeine was given as a single dose.

1. Harder S, Staib AH, Beer C, Papenburg A, Stille W, Shah PM. 4-Quinolones inhibit biotransformation of caffeine. *Eur J Clin Pharmacol* (1988) 35, 651-6.
2. Staib AH, Stille W, Dietlein G, Shah PM, Harder S, Mieke S, Beer C. Interaction between quinolones and caffeine. *Drugs* (1987) 34 (Suppl 1), 170-4.
3. Stille W, Harder S, Mieke S, Beer C, Shah PM, Frech K, Staib AH. Decrease of caffeine elimination in man during co-administration of 4-quinolones. *J Antimicrob Chemother* (1987) 20, 729-34.
4. Nicolau DP, Nightingale CH, Tessier PR, Fu Q, Xuan D-W, Esguerra EM, Quintiliani R. The effect of fleroxacin and ciprofloxacin on the pharmacokinetics of multiple dose caffeine. *Drugs* (1995) 49 (Suppl 2), 357-9.
5. Kim M-Y, Nightingale CH, Nicolau DP. Influence of sex on the pharmacokinetic interaction of fleroxacin and ciprofloxacin with caffeine. *Clin Pharmacokinet* (2003), 42, 985–96.
6. Healy DP, Polk RE, Kanawati L, Rock DT, Mooney ML. Interaction between oral ciprofloxacin and caffeine in normal volunteers. *Antimicrob Agents Chemother* (1989) 33, 474-8.
7. Randinitis EJ, Koup JR, Rausch G, Vassos AB. Effect of (CLX) administration on the single-dose pharmacokinetics of theophylline and caffeine. *Intersci Conf Antimicrob Agents Chemother* (1998) 38, 6.

Continued

Table 33.3 Effect of quinolones on caffeine pharmacokinetics in healthy subjects (continued)

8. Peloquin CA, Nix DE, Sedman AJ, Wilton JH, Toothaker RD, Harrison NJ, Schentag JJ. Pharmacokinetics and clinical effects of caffeine alone and in combination with oral enoxacin. *Rev Infect Dis* (1989) II (Suppl 5), S1095.
9. Kinzig-Schippers M, Fuhr U, Zaigler M, Dammeyer J, Rüsing G, Labedzki A, Bulitta J, Sörgel F. Interaction of pefloxacin and enoxacin with the human cytochrome P450 enzyme CYP1A2. *Clin Pharmacol Ther* (1999) 65, 262-74.
10. Healy DP, Schoenle JR, Stotka J, Polk RE. Lack of interaction between lomefloxacin and caffeine in normal volunteers. *Antimicrob Agents Chemother* (1991) 35, 660-4.
11. Carbó M, Segura J, De la Torre R, Badenas JM, Camí J. Effect of quinolones on caffeine disposition. *Clin Pharmacol Ther* (1989) 45, 234-40.
12. Cesana M, Broccali G, Imbimbo BP, Crema A. Effect of single doses of rufloxacin on the disposition of theophylline and caffeine after single administration. *Int J Clin Pharmacol Ther Toxicol* (1991) 29, 133-8.
13. LeBel M, Teng R, Dogolo LC, Willavize S, Friedman HL, Vincent J. The influence of steady-state trovafloxacin on the steady-state pharmacokinetics of caffeine in healthy subjects. *Pharm Res* (1996) 13 (Suppl 9), S434.

Caffeine + Sho-saiko-to

Sho-saiko-to slightly reduces the metabolism of caffeine, but this is not expected to be clinically important.

Clinical evidence, mechanism, importance and management

In a study, 26 healthy subjects were given sho-saiko-to 2.5 g twice daily for 5 days, with a single 150-mg dose of caffeine on days 1 and 5. By assessing the metabolites of caffeine, it was estimated that sho-saiko-to caused a 16% inhibition of the cytochrome P450 isoenzyme CYP1A2. The clinical significance of this finding is unclear, but is likely to be small, although further studies will help clarify this.[1]

1. Saruwatari J, Nakagawa K, Shindo J, Nachi S, Echizen H, Ishizaki T. The in-vivo effects of sho-saiko-to, a traditional Chinese herbal medicine, on two cytochrome P450 enzymes (1A2 and 3A) and xanthine oxidase in man. *J Pharm Pharmacol* (2003) 55, 1553–9.

Caffeine + St John's wort (*Hypericum perforatum*)

St John's wort appears to increase the metabolism of caffeine in women, but not men.

Clinical evidence, mechanism, importance and management

A study in 16 healthy subjects given a single 200-mg dose of caffeine before and after St John's wort 300 mg (containing 900 micrograms of hypericin) three times daily for 14 days, found no overall change in the pharmacokinetics of caffeine. However, when the subset of 8 female patients was considered, it was found that there was an induction of CYP1A2 in this group of patients resulting in an increase in the production of caffeine metabolites.[1] More study is needed, as this may have important implications for other CYP1A2 substrates.

1. Wenk M, Todesco L, Krähenbühl S. Effect of St John's wort on the activities of CYP1A2, CYP3A4, CYP2D6, N-acetyltransferase 2, and xanthine oxidase in healthy males and females. *Br J Clin Pharmacol* (2004) 57, 494–9.

Caffeine + Tiabendazole

Tiabendazole reduces the metabolism of caffeine.

Clinical evidence, mechanism, importance and management

A study in 7 healthy subjects found that a single 500-mg dose of tiabendazole reduced the clearance of caffeine by 66% and increased the half-life and AUC by 140% and 57%, respectively. The metabolism of caffeine to one of its major metabolites, paraxanthine, was reduced by 92%.[1] It was suggested that tiabendazole inhibits the metabolism of caffeine by the cytochrome P450 isoenzyme CYP1A2 in the liver.

Tiabendazole is known to have clinically significant inhibitory effects on the metabolism of 'theophylline', (p.1171), and therefore would also be expected to affect caffeine metabolism. There is too little information to suggest that patients taking tiabendazole should avoid caffeine-containing beverages, foods or medication, but bear this interaction in mind if the adverse effects of caffeine (e.g. insomnia, jitteriness) become troublesome.

1. Bapiro TE, Sayi J, Hasler JA, Jande M, Rimoy G, Masselle A, Masimirembwa CM. Artemisinin and thiabendazole are potent inhibitors of cytochrome P450 1A2 (CYP1A2) activity in humans. *Eur J Clin Pharmacol* (2005) 61, 755–61.

Caffeine + Venlafaxine

Venlafaxine does not affect the pharmacokinetics of caffeine.

Clinical evidence, mechanism, importance and management

In 15 healthy subjects venlafaxine 37.5 mg twice daily for 3 days then 75 mg twice daily for 4 days did not affect the AUC or clearance of caffeine 200 mg daily (equivalent to about 3 cups of coffee). A slight but significant decrease in the half-life from 6.1 to 5.5 hours was noted.[1] On the basis of this study, no special precautions are needed if both drugs are taken together.

1. Amchin J, Zarycranski W, Taylor KP, Albano D, Klockowski PM. Effect of venlafaxine on CYP1A2-dependent pharmacokinetics and metabolism of caffeine. *J Clin Pharmacol* (1999) 39, 252–9.

Caffeine + Verapamil

A small and relatively unimportant decrease in the clearance of caffeine may occur in patients given verapamil.

Clinical evidence, mechanism, importance and management

In 6 healthy subjects verapamil 80 mg three times daily for 2 days decreased the total clearance of a single 200-mg dose of caffeine by 25%, and increased its half-life by 25% (from 4.6 to 5.8 hours).[1] These changes are small, and unlikely to be of much importance in most patients.

1. Nawoot S, Wong D, Mays DC, Gerber N. Inhibition of caffeine elimination by verapamil. *Clin Pharmacol Ther* (1988) 43, 148.

Doxofylline + Miscellaneous

There is some limited evidence to suggest that erythromycin may increase the effects of doxofylline, but the clinical importance of this is uncertain. Digoxin initially raises, then lowers serum doxofylline levels, but the bronchodilator effects do not appear to be significantly affected. Allopurinol and lithium carbonate appear to have no significant effects on doxofylline.

Clinical evidence, mechanism, importance and management

Healthy subjects were given doxofylline 400 mg three times daily, either alone, or with **allopurinol** 100 mg once daily, **erythromycin** 400 mg three times daily or **lithium carbonate** 300 mg three times daily. None of the pharmacokinetic parameters measured, including the maximum serum levels, were significantly altered by any of these drugs apart from the AUC of doxofylline, which was raised by about 40% by **allopurinol**, 70% by **erythromycin**, and 35% by **lithium carbonate**. Only the **erythromycin** result was statistically significant.[1] The clinical significance of these changes is uncertain, and their mechanism is not understood. Until the situation is much clearer it would be prudent to check the outcome of adding **erythromycin** to established treatment with doxofylline, being alert for evidence of increased effects.

In a comparative study in 9 patients taking doxofylline 800 mg daily, **digoxin** 500 micrograms daily was given to 5 patients. It was found that **digoxin** *increased* the serum levels of doxofylline by 50% on the first day of treatment, 3 hours after administration but then *reduced* doxofylline levels by about 30% at steady-state (day 30). Nevertheless, the bronchodilating effects of the doxofylline were little different between the two groups. It was concluded that concurrent use is normally safe and effective, but the initial doxofylline dose should be chosen to avoid too high a serum level on the first day, and pulmonary function should be well monitored.[2]

1. Harning R, Sekora D, O'Connell K, Wilson J. A crossover study of the effect of erythromycin, lithium carbonate, and allopurinol on doxofylline pharmacokinetics. *Clin Pharmacol Ther* (1994) 55, 158.
2. Provvedi D, Rubegni M, Biffignandi P. Pharmacokinetic interaction between doxofylline and digitalis in elderly patients with chronic obstructive bronchitis. *Acta Ther* (1990) 16, 239–46.

Ipratropium bromide + Salbutamol (Albuterol)

Acute angle-closure glaucoma developed rapidly in eight patients given nebulised ipratropium and salbutamol. Increased intra-ocular pressure has been reported in others, including one patient using an ipratropium metered-dose inhaler with nebulised salbutamol.

Clinical evidence

Five patients with an acute exacerbation of chronic obstructive airways disease given nebulised ipratropium and salbutamol, developed acute angle-closure glaucoma, four of them within 1 to 36 hours of starting treatment. Two of the patients had a history of angle-closure glaucoma.[1] Three other similar cases of acute angle-closure glaucoma due to the concurrent use of salbutamol and ipratropium are reported elsewhere.[2,3] An increase in intra-ocular pressure has also been reported in other patients given both drugs by nebuliser.[4] One case of acute angle-closure glaucoma has been reported in a patient treated with inhaled ipratropium, via a metered-dose inhaler, and nebulised salbutamol.[5]

Mechanism

This reaction appears to occur because the antimuscarinic action of the ipratropium causes semi-dilatation of the pupil, partially blocking the flow of aqueous humour from the posterior to the anterior chamber, thereby bowing the iris anteriorly and obstructing the drainage angle. The salbutamol increases the production of aqueous humour and makes things worse. Additional factors are that higher levels of both drugs are achieved by using a nebuliser, and that some drug may escape round the edge of the mask and have a direct action on the eye.[1]

Importance and management

An established but uncommon interaction, which appears to occur mainly in patients receiving these drugs by nebuliser and those already predisposed to angle-closure glaucoma. The authors of the first report[1] advise care in the placing of the mask to avoid the escape of droplets (the use of goggles and continuing the application of any glaucoma treatment is also effective[4]) and, if possible, the avoidance of their concurrent use by nebuliser in patients predisposed to angle-closure glaucoma.

1. Shah P, Dhurjon L, Metcalfe T, Gibson JM. Acute angle closure glaucoma associated with nebulised ipratropium bromide and salbutamol. *BMJ* (1992) 304, 40–1.
2. Packe GE, Cayton RM, Mashoudi N. Nebulised ipratropium bromide and salbutamol causing closed-angle glaucoma. *Lancet* (1984) ii, 691.
3. Reuser T, Flanagan DW, Borland C, Bannerjee DK. Acute angle closure glaucoma occurring after nebulized bronchodilator treatment with ipratropium bromide and salbutamol. *J R Soc Med* (1992) 85, 499–500.
4. Kalra L, Bone M. The effect of nebulized bronchodilator therapy on intraocular pressures in patients with glaucoma. *Chest* (1988) 93, 739–41.
5. Hall SK. Acute angle-closure glaucoma as a complication of combined β-agonist and ipratropium bromide therapy in the emergency department. *Ann Emerg Med* (1994) 23, 884–7.

Montelukast + Anti-asthma drugs

There is an isolated report of severe oedema in a patient taking oral prednisone and montelukast, but studies suggest that the concurrent use of montelukast and prednisolone or prednisone are useful and well-tolerated. Montelukast in normal doses does not interact to a clinically relevant extent with salbutamol (albuterol)

Clinical evidence, mechanism, importance and management

(a) Beta agonists

A study in patients with moderately severe asthma found no adverse interactions when **salbutamol (albuterol)** was given with montelukast 100 mg or 250 mg, with or without inhaled corticosteroids.[1] The British Thoracic Society guidelines recommend that a leukotriene antagonist is used as an add-on therapy in patients using short-acting inhaled $beta_2$ agonists.[2]

(b) Corticosteroids

A study in healthy subjects (55 taking montelukast and 36 taking a placebo) found that the plasma profiles of oral **prednisone** 20 mg and of intravenous **prednisolone** 250 mg were unaffected by montelukast 200 mg daily for 6 weeks.[3] The manufacturers also report that licensed doses of montelukast do not have any clinically significant effect on the pharmacokinetics of prednisone and prednisolone.[4] Other studies in patients using inhaled and/or oral corticosteroids have found that concurrent use is beneficial and well tolerated.[5-7]

However, an isolated report describes a case of marked peripheral oedema possibly linked to the use of **prednisone** and montelukast. A 23-year-old patient with severe allergic and exercise-induced asthma and rhinoconjunctivitis treated with salmeterol and fluticasone by inhalation and oral cetirizine was given **prednisone** 40 mg daily for one week then 20 mg daily for a further week. When **prednisone** was stopped, severe asthma reoccurred and he was given **prednisone** 60 mg daily for one week then 40 mg daily for a further week with montelukast 10 mg daily. After 10 days of treatment he developed severe peripheral oedema, gaining 13 kg in weight. Renal and cardiovascular function were normal. **Prednisone** was stopped and the asthma was controlled by continued montelukast and the excess weight was lost as the oedema resolved. The patient had good tolerance of both **prednisone** and montelukast alone. Corticosteroid-induced renal tubular sodium and fluid retention may have occurred when montelukast was also given.[8]

This isolated report is of uncertain general relevance. Usually, no special precautions appear to be needed if these drugs are used concurrently, and the British Thoracic Society guidelines recommend that a leukotriene antagonist is used as an add-on therapy to inhaled steroids in adults and children over five years of age.[2]

1. Botto A, Kundu S, Reiss T. A double-blind, placebo-controlled, 3-period, crossover study to investigate the bronchodilating ability of oral doses of MK-0476 and to investigate the interaction with inhaled albuterol in moderately severe asthmatic patients. Merck Sharp & Dohme. Data on file (Protocol 066) 1996.
2. British Thoracic Society & Scottish Intercollegiate Guidelines Network. British guideline on the management of asthma, November 2005. Available at: http://www.enterpriseportal2.co.uk/filestore/bts/asthmaupdatenov05.pdf (accessed 22/08/07).
3. Noonan T, Shingo S, Kundu S, Reiss TF. A double-blind, placebo-controlled, parallel-group study in healthy male volunteers to investigate the safety and tolerability of 6 weeks of administration of MK-0476, and in subgroups, the effect of 6 weeks of administration of MK-0476 on the single dose pharmacokinetics of po and iv theophylline and corticosteroids. Merck Sharp & Dohme. Data on file.
4. Singulair (Montelukast sodium). Merck Sharp & Dohme Ltd. UK Summary of product characteristics, November 2006.
5. Dahlén S-E, Malmström K, Nizankowska E, Dahlén B, Kuna P, Kowalski M, Lumry WR, Picado C, Stevenson DD, Bousquet J, Pauwels R, Holgate ST, Shahane A, Zhang J, Reiss TF, Szczeklik A. Improvement of aspirin-intolerant asthma by montelukast, a leukotriene antagonist. *Am J Respir Crit Care Med* (2002) 165, 9–14.
6. Knorr B, Matz J, Bernstein JA, Nguyen H, Seidenberg BC, Reiss TF, Becker A, for the Pediatric Montelukast Study Group. Montelukast for chronic asthma in 6- to 14-year-old children. A randomized, double-blind trial. *JAMA* (1998) 279, 1181–6.
7. Phipatanakul W, Greene C, Downes SJ, Cronin B, Eller TJ, Schneider LC, Irani A-M. Montelukast improves asthma control in asthmatic children maintained on inhaled corticosteroids. *Ann Allergy Asthma Immunol* (2003) 91, 49–54.
8. Geller M. Marked peripheral edema associated with montelukast and prednisone. *Ann Intern Med* (2000) 132, 924.

Montelukast + Antiepileptics

Phenobarbital modestly reduces montelukast levels, but this is not thought to be clinically significant. Phenytoin is predicted to interact similarly.

Clinical evidence, mechanism, importance and management

Montelukast 10 mg was given to 14 healthy subjects before and after they took **phenobarbital** 100 mg daily for 14 days. It was found that the geometric mean AUC and the maximum serum levels of the montelukast were reduced by 38% and 20%, respectively, but it was concluded that no montelukast dosage adjustment is needed.[1] The reason for these reductions is almost certainly because phenobarbital induces the cytochrome P450 isoenzyme CYP3A4 so that montelukast metabolism is increased. The manufacturers therefore caution the use of montelukast with inducers of CYP3A4, such as **phenytoin** and **phenobarbital**, especially in children.[2] However, there is so far no clinical evidence that the montelukast dosage needs adjustment in the presence of any of these drugs.

1. Holland S, Shahane A, Rogers JD, Porras A, Grasing K, Lasseter K, Pinto M, Freeman A, Gertz B, Amin R. Metabolism of montelukast (M) is increased by multiple doses of phenobarbital (P). *Clin Pharmacol Ther* (1998) 63, 231.
2. Singulair (Montelukast sodium). Merck Sharp & Dohme Ltd. UK Summary of product characteristics, November 2006.

Montelukast + Antihistamines

Montelukast does not interact to a clinically relevant extent with loratadine or terfenadine.

Clinical evidence, mechanism, importance and management

Healthy subjects were given terfenadine 60 mg every 12 hours for 14 days, with montelukast 10 mg daily from day 8 to day 14. It was found that the **terfenadine** pharmacokinetics and the QTc interval were unaltered by concurrent use.[1] No adverse interactions were seen in large numbers of patients given montelukast 10 or 20 mg and **loratadine** 10 mg, and the combination was found to be beneficial in the treatment of allergic rhinitis and conjunctivitis.[2] No special precautions are therefore needed if these drugs are given concurrently.

1. Holland S, Gertz B, DeSmet M, Michiels N, Larson P, Freeman A, Keymeulen B. Montelukast (MON) has no effect on terfenadine (T) pharmacokinetics (PK) or QTc. *Clin Pharmacol Ther* (1998) 63, 232.
2. Malstrom K, Meltzer E, Prenner B, Lu S, Weinstein S, Wolfe J, Wei LX, Reiss TF. Effects of montelukast (a leukotriene receptor antagonist), loratadine, montelukast + loratadine and placebo in seasonal allergic rhinitis and conjunctivitis. *J Allergy Clin Immunol* (1998) 101, S97.

Montelukast + Rifampicin (Rifampin)

The manufacturers of montelukast caution its use with inducers of the cytochrome P450 isoenzyme CYP3A4, such as rifampicin, especially in children.[1] This is because phenobarbital (an inducer of CYP3A4) has been found to reduce the AUC and serum levels of montelukast.[1] However, there is currently no clinical evidence that the montelukast dosage needs adjustment in patients taking rifampicin.

1. Singulair (Montelukast sodium). Merck Sharp & Dohme Ltd. UK Summary of product characteristics, November 2006.

Terbutaline + Magnesium sulfate

Subcutaneous terbutaline and intravenous magnesium sulfate appear not to interact adversely.

Clinical evidence, mechanism, importance and management

Eight healthy adults were given two subcutaneous doses of terbutaline 250 micrograms 30 minutes apart, with and without intravenous magnesium sulfate 4 g in 250 mL of sodium chloride 0.9%, given over the same 30-minute period.[1] Most of the effects of terbutaline, such as those on respiratory rate, blood pressure, glucose and calcium levels, were found to be moderately increased by magnesium sulfate at 60 minutes but these changes were all considered to be small. It was concluded that there appear to be no good reasons for avoiding their concurrent use, for example in the emergency treatment of asthma and other conditions.

1. Skorodin MS, Freebeck PC, Yetter B, Nelson JE, Van de Graaff WB, Walsh JM. Magnesium sulfate potentiates several cardiovascular and metabolic actions of terbutaline. *Chest* (1994) 105, 701–5.

Theophylline + Aciclovir

Preliminary evidence suggests that aciclovir can increase the serum levels of theophylline.

Clinical evidence

Prompted by a case of increased theophylline adverse effects in a patient given aciclovir, a study was carried out in 5 healthy subjects who were given single 320-mg doses of theophylline (as 400 mg of aminophylline) before and with the sixth dose of aciclovir 800 mg five times daily for 2 days. The AUC of the theophylline was increased by 45% and its total body clearance was reduced by 30% by the aciclovir.[1]

Mechanism

Uncertain, but the evidence suggests that aciclovir inhibits the oxidative metabolism of theophylline, resulting in accumulation.[1]

Importance and management

Evidence appears to be limited to this report. However, be alert for an increase in adverse effects of theophylline (nausea, headache, tremor) if aciclovir is added to established treatment, and consider monitoring levels. More study is needed.

1. Maeda Y, Konishi T, Omoda K, Takeda Y, Fukuhara S, Fukuzawa M, Ohune T, Tsuya T, Tsukiai S. Inhibition of theophylline metabolism by aciclovir. *Biol Pharm Bull* (1996) 19, 1591–5.

Theophylline + Allopurinol

Evidence from clinical studies and a single case report indicate that the effects of theophylline may be increased by allopurinol.

Clinical evidence

The peak plasma levels of theophylline 450 mg daily rose by 38% in a patient who took allopurinol for 3 days.[1] In a study in 12 healthy subjects, allopurinol 300 mg twice daily for 14 days increased the half-life of a single 5-mg/kg oral dose of theophylline by 25%, and increased its AUC by 27%.[2] Similar increases were seen when a second dose of theophylline was given 28 days after starting the allopurinol.[2]

However, in two other studies allopurinol 300 mg daily for 7 days did not have any effect on the pharmacokinetics of theophylline, following a single 5-mg/kg intravenous dose of aminophylline.[3,4] Similarly, steady-state theophylline levels were not affected by allopurinol 100 mg three times daily in 4 subjects. However, there was an alteration in the proportion of different urinary theophylline metabolites: methyluric acid decreased and methylxanthine increased.[4]

Mechanism

Uncertain. Allopurinol, a xanthine oxidase inhibitor, can block the conversion of methylxanthine to methyluric acid, but this had no effect on theophylline levels in two studies. One suggestion is that allopurinol inhibits the oxidative metabolism of theophylline by the liver.[1]

Importance and management

Evidence appears to be limited to a single case report and the studies in healthy subjects. The interaction only appears to be of moderate importance. Nevertheless, it would seem prudent to check for any signs of theophylline adverse effects (headache, nausea, tremor) during concurrent use, particularly in situations where the metabolism of the theophylline may already be reduced (other drugs or diseases), or where high doses of allopurinol are used. For mention that allopurinol may invalidate the results of phenotyping tests using caffeine, see 'Caffeine + Allopurinol', p.1162.

1. Barry M, Feeley J. Allopurinol influences aminophenazone elimination. *Clin Pharmacokinet* (1990) 19, 167–9.
2. Manfredi RL, Vesell ES. Inhibition of theophylline metabolism by long-term allopurinol administration. *Clin Pharmacol Ther* (1981) 29, 224–9.
3. Vozeh S, Powell JR, Cupit GC, Riegelman S, Sheiner LB. Influence of allopurinol on theophylline disposition in adults. *Clin Pharmacol Ther* (1980) 27, 194–7.
4. Grygiel JJ, Wing LMH, Farkas J, Birkett DJ. Effects of allopurinol on theophylline metabolism and clearance. *Clin Pharmacol Ther* (1979) 26, 660–7.498708

Theophylline + Alosetron

Alosetron does not alter theophylline pharmacokinetics.

Clinical evidence, mechanism, importance and management

In a placebo-controlled study, 10 healthy women were given alosetron 1 mg twice daily for 16 days with oral theophylline 200 mg twice daily from day 8 to day 16. No clinically relevant changes in the pharmacokinetics of theophylline were seen, and concurrent use was well tolerated. The effect of theophylline on alosetron pharmacokinetics was not measured but the authors of the report say that no metabolic interaction seems likely.[1] No special precautions would therefore appear to be needed if these drugs are used together.

1. Koch KM, Ricci BM, Hedayetullah NS, Jewell D, Kersey KE. Effect of alosetron on theophylline pharmacokinetics. *Br J Clin Pharmacol* (2001) 52, 596–600.

Theophylline + Aminoglutethimide

Theophylline clearance is increased by aminoglutethimide, which may result in a moderate reduction in the serum levels and therapeutic effects of theophylline.

Clinical evidence, mechanism, importance and management

Aminoglutethimide 250 mg four times a day increased the clearance of sustained-release theophylline 200 mg twice daily by 18 to 43% in 3 patients.[1] Theophylline clearance was assessed before starting aminoglutethimide as well as during weeks 2 to 12 of concurrent use.

It seems probable that aminoglutethimide, a known enzyme inducer, increases the metabolism of theophylline by the liver, thereby decreasing its levels. The clinical importance is uncertain, but it seems likely that the effects of theophylline would be reduced to some extent. Monitor the effects and if necessary take theophylline levels. Increase the theophylline dosage accordingly.

1. Lønning PE, Kvinnsland S, Bakke OM. Effect of aminoglutethimide on antipyrine, theophylline and digitoxin disposition in breast cancer. *Clin Pharmacol Ther* (1984) 36, 796–802.

Theophylline + Amiodarone

An isolated case report describes an elderly man who developed raised theophylline levels and toxicity when he was given amiodarone.

Clinical evidence, mechanism, importance and management

An 86-year-old man taking furosemide, digoxin, domperidone and sustained-release theophylline developed signs of theophylline toxicity when amiodarone 600 mg daily was given. After 9 days his serum theophylline levels had doubled, from about 16.8 to 35 mg/L. The toxicity disappeared when the theophylline was stopped.[1] The reason for this adverse reaction is not understood but it has been suggested that amiodarone may reduce the metabolism of the theophylline by the liver.[1] This is an isolated case and its general importance is uncertain. More study is needed.

Amiodarone may cause thyroid dysfunction, which may affect theophylline requirements, see also 'Theophylline + Thyroid and Antithyroid compounds', p.1200.

1. Soto J, Sacristán JA, Arellano F, Hazas J. Possible theophylline-amiodarone interaction. *DICP Ann Pharmacother* (1990) 24, 1115.

Theophylline + Antacids

The extent of absorption of theophylline from the gut does not appear to be significantly affected by aluminium or magnesium hydroxide antacids. However, an increase in the rate of absorption of some sustained-release theophylline preparations may occur.

Clinical evidence, mechanism, importance and management

In a study in 12 healthy subjects, there was no difference in the steady-state maximum serum concentrations or AUC of theophylline given as *Nuelin-Depot* or *Theodur* when an antacid (*Novalucid*, containing **aluminium/magnesium hydroxide** and **magnesium carbonate**) was given. However, the antacid caused a faster absorption of theophylline from *Nuelin-Depot*, which resulted in greater fluctuations in the serum levels. It was considered that the adverse effects of theophylline might be increased in those patients with serum levels at the top of the range.[1] Similar results have been found in single-dose studies when aminophylline,[2] *Slo-Phyllin Gyrocaps,*[3] *Somophyllin CRT,*[4] and *Theo-Dur*[5] were given with **aluminium/magnesium hydroxide** antacids, and in multiple dose studies in patients when *Armophylline*,[6] *Aminophyllin*[7] or *Theodur*[7] were given with **aluminium/magnesium hydroxide** antacids. Administration of 30 mL of an **aluminium/magnesium hydroxide** antacid (*Maalox)* four times daily did not affect the trough levels of theophylline in a patient taking *Theo-Dur* 400 mg three times daily.[8] Care should be taken extrapolating this information to other sustained-release preparations of theophylline, but generally speaking no special precautions seem to be necessary if antacids are given with theophylline.

1. Myhre KI, Walstad RA. The influence of antacid on the absorption of two different sustained-release formulations of theophylline. *Br J Clin Pharmacol* (1983) 15, 683–7.
2. Arnold LA, Spurbeck GH, Shelver WH, Henderson WM. Effect of an antacid on gastrointestinal absorption of theophylline. *Am J Hosp Pharm* (1979) 36, 1059–62.
3. Shargel L, Stevens JA, Fuchs JE, Yu ABC. Effect of antacid on bioavailability of theophylline from rapid and timed-release drug products. *J Pharm Sci* (1981) 70, 599–602.
4. Ferrari M, Olivieri M, Romito D, Biasin C, Barozzi E, Bassetti S. Influence of gastric pH changes on pharmacokinetic of a sustained-release formulation of theophylline. *Riv Eur Sci Med Farmacol* (1991) 13, 269–74.
5. Darzentas LJ, Stewart RB, Curry SH, Yost RL. Effect of antacid on bioavailability of a sustained-release theophylline preparation. *Drug Intell Clin Pharm* (1983) 17, 555–7.
6. Muir JF, Peiffer G, Richard MO, Benhamou D, Andrejak M, Hary L, Moore N. Lack of effect of magnesium-aluminium hydroxide on the absorption of theophylline given as a pH-dependent sustained release preparation. *Eur J Clin Pharmacol* (1993) 44, 85–8.
7. Reed RC, Schwartz HJ. Lack of influence of an intensive antacid regimen on theophylline bioavailability. *J Pharmacokinet Biopharm* (1984) 12, 315–331.
8. Fernandes E, Melewicz FM. Antacids and theophylline-ranitidine interaction. *Ann Intern Med* (1984) 101, 279.

Theophylline + Anthelmintics; Benzimidazoles

Theophylline serum levels can be markedly increased by tiabendazole and toxicity may develop. Neither albendazole nor mebendazole appear to interact with theophylline.

Clinical evidence

(a) Albendazole

A study in 6 healthy subjects found that the pharmacokinetics of a single dose of theophylline were unaffected by a single 400-mg dose of albendazole.[1]

(b) Mebendazole

A study in 6 healthy subjects found that the pharmacokinetics of a single dose of intravenous aminophylline were unaffected by mebendazole 100 mg twice daily for 3 days.[1] The absence of a significant interaction was reported in another similar study using the same mebendazole dosage.[2]

(c) Tiabendazole

An elderly man taking prednisone, furosemide, terbutaline and orciprenaline was switched from oral to intravenous aminophylline, giving a stable serum level of 21 mg/L after 48 hours. When he was also given tiabendazole 4 g daily for 5 days, for persistence of a *Strongyloides stercoralis* infestation, he developed theophylline toxicity (severe nausea) and his serum levels were found to be 46 mg/L. Three months previously, he had been treated with tiabendazole 3 g daily for 3 days without any symptoms of toxicity (no theophylline levels were measured).[3] The theophylline levels of another patient rose from 15 to 22 mg/L when he was given tiabendazole 1.8 g twice daily for 3 days, despite a theophylline dosage reduction of one-third, made in anticipation of the interaction. Theophylline levels were still elevated 2 days after the tiabendazole was stopped, and the theophylline dose was further reduced. Levels returned to normal after 5 days, and the theophylline dose was eventually increased again.[4]

A retrospective study of patients given theophylline and tiabendazole found that 9 out of 40 (23%) had developed elevated serum theophylline levels and of those 9 patients, 5 experienced significant toxicity, with 3 requiring hospitalisation. The other 31 patients did not have theophylline levels taken.[5] A further report describes a patient receiving intravenous aminophylline who had an increase in theophylline levels from 18 to 26 mg/L within 2 days of starting tiabendazole 1.5 g twice daily.[2] The authors of this report then studied 6 healthy subjects who received a single dose of aminophylline before and while taking tiabendazole 1.5 g twice daily for 3 days. Three of the subjects had to discontinue the study because of severe nausea, vomiting or dizziness. In the remaining three, tiabendazole markedly affected the pharmacokinetics of aminophylline; the half-life increased from 6.7 to 18.6 hours, the clearance fell by 66% and the elimination rate constant decreased by 65%.[2]

Mechanism

Uncertain. It is suggested that tiabendazole inhibits the metabolism of theophylline, probably by the cytochrome P450 isoenzyme CYP1A2 in the liver, thereby prolonging its stay in the body and raising its serum levels. The nausea and vomiting may have been due to the adverse effects of both theophylline and tiabendazole.

Importance and management

The interaction between theophylline and tiabendazole is established and of clinical importance. Monitor theophylline levels and reduce the theophylline dosage accordingly. A 50% reduction in the theophylline dosage has been suggested,[4] or, where practical, stopping theophylline for 2 to 3 days while giving the tiabendazole.[5] Albendazole and mebendazole do not appear to interact with theophylline, and therefore may be suitable alternative anthelmintics depending on the condition being treated.

1. Adebayo GI, Mabadeje AFB. Theophylline disposition — effects of cimetidine, mebendazole and albendazole. *Aliment Pharmacol Ther* (1988) 2, 341–6.
2. Schneider D, Gannon R, Sweeney K, Shore E. Theophylline and antiparasitic drug interactions. A case report and a study of the influence of thiabendazole and mebendazole on theophylline pharmacokinetics in adults. *Chest* (1990) 97, 84–7.
3. Sugar AM, Kearns PJ, Haulk AA, Rushing JL. Possible thiabendazole-induced theophylline toxicity. *Am Rev Respir Dis* (1980) 122, 501–3.
4. Lew G, Murray WE, Lane JR, Haeger E. Theophylline—thiabendazole drug interaction. *Clin Pharm* (1989) 8, 225–7.
5. German T, Berger R. Interaction of theophylline and thiabendazole in patients with chronic obstructive lung disease. *Am Rev Respir Dis* (1992) 145, A807.

Theophylline + Anticholinesterases; Centrally acting

The serum levels of theophylline are increased by tacrine. Donepezil has no effect on theophylline levels.

Clinical evidence, mechanism, importance and management

(a) Donepezil

An open-label, crossover study in 12 healthy subjects found that donepezil 5 mg daily for 10 days had no significant effects on the pharmacokinetics of theophylline. Dose modification or additional monitoring is not required during concurrent use.[1]

(b) Tacrine

Healthy subjects were given theophylline 158 mg alone or while taking tacrine 20 mg every 6 hours. The clearance of the theophylline was reduced by 50%, probably because the tacrine inhibits its metabolism by the cytochrome P450 isoenzyme CYP1A2 in the liver.[2] Be alert for the need to reduce the theophylline dosage to avoid toxicity if tacrine is added. More study of this interaction is needed in patients given multiple doses of both drugs.

1. Tiseo PJ, Foley K, Friedhoff LT. Concurrent administration of donepezil HCl and theophylline; assessment of pharmacokinetic changes following multiple-dose administration in healthy volunteers. *Br J Clin Pharmacol* (1998) 46 (Suppl 1), 35–9.
2. deVries TM, Siedlik P, Smithers JA, Brown RR, Reece PA, Posvar EL, Sedman AJ, Koup JR, Forgue ST. Effect of multiple-dose tacrine administration on single-dose pharmacokinetics of digoxin, diazepam, and theophylline. *Pharm Res* (1993) 10 (10 Suppl), S-333.

Theophylline + Antihistamines and related drugs

Azelastine, cetirizine, ketotifen, mequitazine, mizolastine, pemirolast, repirinast, and terfenadine do not appear to alter the pharmacokinetics of theophylline.

Clinical evidence, mechanism, importance and management

Azelastine 2 mg twice daily had no significant effect on the clearance of theophylline 300 mg twice daily in 10 subjects with bronchial asthma. However, one patient had a 20.8% increase and another a 25.3% decrease in clearance.[1]

A single 240-mg dose of *intravenous* theophylline was given to 6 healthy subjects after they had taken **cetirizine** 10 mg twice daily for 3.5 days. There was no change in theophylline pharmacokinetics, but the half-life of cetirizine was decreased by 19%. This change in cetirizine pharmacokinetics was not considered to be clinically relevant.[2]

Two studies, one in healthy adults[3] and one in asthmatic children,[4] showed that **ketotifen** did not affect the pharmacokinetics of a single oral dose of either theophylline[3] or aminophylline.[4] It was suggested that concurrent use might actually decrease the CNS adverse effects of each drug.[3]

In 7 asthmatic patients the steady-state pharmacokinetics of theophylline were not significantly affected when **mequitazine** 6 mg daily was given for 3 weeks.[5]

Mizolastine 10 mg daily had virtually no effect on the steady-state pharmacokinetics of theophylline in 17 healthy subjects, although a 13% increase in mean trough level and an 8% increase in the AUC was seen. These changes were not considered clinically relevant.[6]

Pemirolast 10 mg daily for 4 days was found to have no significant effect on the steady-state serum levels or clearance of theophylline in 7 healthy subjects.[7]

Repirinast 300 mg daily had no effect on the pharmacokinetics of theophylline in 10 asthmatics given a single dose of aminophylline.[8] Another study in 7 asthmatics found that **repirinast** (dosage unclear) for 3 weeks had no effect on the pharmacokinetics of theophylline 400 to 800 mg, given in two divided doses.[9]

In 10 healthy subjects the pharmacokinetics of a single 250-mg dose of theophylline were unchanged by **terfenadine** 120 mg twice daily for 16 days.[10] Similarly, **terfenadine** 60 mg twice daily did not affect the steady-state pharmacokinetics of theophylline 4 mg/kg daily.[11] Another study in 17 healthy, male subjects found no change in the pharmacokinetics of a single 4-mg/kg oral dose of theophylline (rounded to nearest 50 mg) when taken with a single 60-mg dose of **terfenadine**.[12]

No special precautions seem to be necessary if any of these drugs is given with theophylline.

1. Asamoto H, Kokura M, Kawakami A, Sasaki Y, Fujii H, Sawano T, Iso S, Ooishi T, Horiuchi Y, Ohara N, Kitamura Y, Morishita H. Effect of azelastine on theophylline clearance in asthma patients. *Arerugi* (1988) 37, 1033–7.
2. Hulhoven R, Desager JP, Harvengt C. Lack of clinically relevant interaction of cetirizine on theophylline disposition in healthy subjects: a placebo-controlled study. *Am J Ther* (1995) 2, 71–4.
3. Matejcek M, Irwin P, Neff G, Abt K, Wehrli W. Determination of the central effects of the asthma prophylactic ketotifen, the bronchodilator theophylline, and both in combination: an application of quantitative electroencephalography to the study of drug interactions. *Int J Clin Pharmacol Ther Toxicol* (1985) 23, 258–66.
4. Garty M, Scolnik D, Danziger Y, Volovitz B, Ilfeld DN, Varsano I. Non-interaction of ketotifen and theophylline in children with asthma an acute study. *Eur J Clin Pharmacol* (1987) 32, 187–9.
5. Hasegawa T, Takagi K, Kuzuya T, Nadai M, Apichartpichean R, Muraoka I. Effect of mequitazine on the pharmacokinetics of theophylline in asthmatic patients. *Eur J Clin Pharmacol* (1990) 38, 255–8.
6. Pinquier JL, Salva P, Deschamps C, Ascalone V, Costa J. Effect of mizolastine, a new non sedative H1 antagonist on the pharmacokinetics of theophylline. *Therapie* (1995) 50 (Suppl), 148.
7. Hasegawa T, Takagi K, Nadai M, Ogura Y, Nabeshima T. Kinetic interaction between theophylline and a newly developed anti-allergic drug, pemirolast potassium. *Eur J Clin Pharmacol* (1994) 46, 55–8.
8. Nagata M, Tabe K, Houya I, Kiuchi H, Sakamoto Y, Yamamoto K, Dohi Y. The influence of repirinast, an anti-allergic drug, on theophylline pharmacokinetics in patients with bronchial asthma. *Nihon Kyobu Shikkan Gakkai Zasshi* (1991) 29, 413–19.
9. Takagi K, Kuzuya T, Horiuchi T, Nadai M, Apichartpichean R, Ogura Y, Hasegawa T. Lack of effect of repirinast on the pharmacokinetics of theophylline in asthmatic patients. *Eur J Clin Pharmacol* (1989) 37, 301–3.
10. Brion N, Naline E, Beaumont D, Pays M, Advenier C. Lack of effect of terfenadine on theophylline pharmacokinetics and metabolism in normal subjects. *Br J Clin Pharmacol* (1989) 27, 391–5.
11. Luskin SS, Fitzsimmons WE, MacLeod CM, Luskin AT. Pharmacokinetic evaluation of the terfenadine-theophylline interaction. *J Allergy Clin Immunol* (1989) 83, 406–11.
12. Fitzsimmons WE, Luskin SS, MacLeod CM, Luskin AT. Single-dose study of the effect of terfenadine on theophylline absorption and disposition. *Ann Allergy* (1989) 62, 213–14.

Theophylline + Azoles

Theophylline levels are normally unaffected or only minimally affected by fluconazole and ketoconazole. An isolated report describes a rise in serum theophylline levels due to fluconazole, and another describes falls in theophylline levels in three patients taking ketoconazole.

Clinical evidence

(a) Fluconazole

A crossover study in 5 healthy subjects found that fluconazole 100 mg given every 12 hours for 7 doses caused only a non-significant 16% decrease in the clearance of a single 300-mg oral dose of aminophylline.[1] Another study in 10 healthy subjects found that fluconazole 100 mg daily for one week had no significant effect on the serum levels of theophylline 150 mg twice daily.[2] The clearance of a single 6-mg/kg oral dose of theophylline was reduced by 13.4% in 9 subjects who took fluconazole 400 mg daily for 10 days.[3] In contrast, an isolated and brief report says that one of 2 patients given theophylline and fluconazole had a rise (amount not specified) in serum theophylline levels.[4]

(b) Ketoconazole

No significant changes in the pharmacokinetics of a single 3-mg/kg intravenous dose of theophylline (given as aminophylline) were seen in 12 healthy subjects who took a single 400-mg dose of ketoconazole, or in 4 subjects who took ketoconazole 400 mg daily for 5 days.[5] Similar results were found in another study in 10 healthy subjects who took ketoconazole 200 mg daily for 7 days.[6] Ketoconazole 400 mg daily for 6 days increased the half-life of a single 250-mg oral dose of theophylline by 21.7% in 6 healthy subjects, but had no effect on its clearance.[7] In contrast, a case report describes a man whose serum theophylline levels fell sharply from about 16.5 to 9 mg/L (reference range 10 to 20 mg/L) over the 2 hours immediately after taking 200 mg of ketoconazole. A less striking fall was seen in 2 other patients.[8]

Mechanism

These antifungals appear to have minimal effects on the cytochrome P450 isoenzyme CYP1A2, which is concerned with the oxidative metabolism of theophylline.[1,7] It is not clear why a few individuals show some changes in theophylline levels.

Importance and management

Information seems to be limited to these reports. Neither fluconazole nor ketoconazole normally appears to interact to a relevant extent in most patients. However, it seems that very occasionally some changes occur so bear this interaction in mind in the case of unexpected changes in theophylline levels, adverse effects or uncontrolled symptoms. Other azole antifungals such as itraconazole, posaconazole and voriconazole, which are substrates for and inhibitors of CYP2C19, CYP2C9, and/or CYP3A4, are also unlikely to interact with theophylline.

1. Konishi H, Morita K, Yamaji A. Effect of fluconazole on theophylline disposition in humans. *Eur J Clin Pharmacol* (1994) 46, 309–12.
2. Feil RA, Rindone JP, Morrill GB, Habib MP. Effect of low-dose fluconazole on theophylline serum concentrations in healthy volunteers. *J Pharm Technol* (1995) 11, 267–9.
3. Foisy MM, Nix D, Middleton E, Kotas T, Symonds WT. The effects of single dose fluconazole (SD FLU) versus multiple dose fluconazole (MD FLU) on the pharmacokinetics (PK) of theophylline (THL) in young healthy volunteers. *Intersci Conf Antimicrob Agents Chemother* (1995) 39, 7.
4. Tett S, Carey D, Lee H-S. Drug interactions with fluconazole. *Med J Aust* (1992) 156, 365.
5. Brown MW, Maldonado AL, Meredith CG, Speeg KV. Effect of ketoconazole on hepatic oxidative drug metabolism. *Clin Pharmacol Ther* (1985) 37, 290–7.
6. Heusner JJ, Dukes GE, Rollins DE, Tolman KG, Galinsky RE. Effect of chronically administered ketoconazole on the elimination of theophylline in man. *Drug Intell Clin Pharm* (1987) 21, 514–17.
7. Naline E, Sanceaume M, Pays M, Advenier C. Application of theophylline metabolite assays to the exploration of liver microsome oxidative function in man. *Fundam Clin Pharmacol* (1988) 2, 341–51.
8. Murphy E, Hannon D, Callaghan B. Ketoconazole—theophylline interaction. *Ir Med J* (1987) 80, 123–4.

Theophylline + Barbiturates

Theophylline serum levels can be reduced by phenobarbital or pentobarbital. A single report describes a similar interaction with secobarbital and it would be expected to occur with other barbiturates.

Clinical evidence

(a) Pentobarbital

A single case report describes a man receiving intravenous aminophylline who had a 95% rise in the clearance of theophylline after he was given high-dose intravenous pentobarbital.[1] In healthy subjects pentobarbital 100 mg daily for 10 days increased the clearance of oral theophylline by a mean of 40% and reduced the AUC by 26%, although there were marked intersubject differences.[2]

(b) Phenobarbital

After taking phenobarbital (2 mg/kg daily to a maximum of 60 mg) for 19 days the mean steady-state serum theophylline levels in 7 asthmatic children aged 6 to 12 years were reduced by 30%, and the clearance was increased by 35% (range 12 to 71%).[3] In contrast, two earlier studies (one by the same group of authors) found no significant change in the pharmacokinetics of theophylline, in asthmatic children given phenobarbital 2 mg/kg daily, or 16 or 32 mg three times daily.[4,5]

The mean theophylline clearance, from a single intravenous dose of aminophylline, was increased by 34% in healthy adult subjects given phenobarbital.[6] In another study the clearance of theophylline was increased by 17% when phenobarbital was given for 2 weeks, although this was not significant.[7] The effects of phenobarbital can be additive with the effects of phenytoin and smoking; one patient required 4 g of theophylline daily to maintain therapeutic serum levels and to control her asthma.[8]

One retrospective study found that premature infants needed a higher dose of intravenous aminophylline for neonatal apnoea when they were given phenobarbital,[9] but a later prospective study failed to confirm this.[10] A study in one set of newborn twins given intravenous aminophylline found that the serum theophylline levels of the twin given phenobarbital were about half those of the twin not given phenobarbital.[11]

(c) Secobarbital

The clearance of theophylline increased by 337% over a 4-week period in a child treated with periodic doses of secobarbital and regular doses of **phenobarbital**.[12]

Mechanism

The barbiturates are potent liver enzyme inducers, which possibly increase the metabolism of theophylline by the liver, thereby hastening its removal from the body. This has been shown in *animal* studies, although *N*-demethylation (the main metabolic route for theophylline) was not affected.[13]

Importance and management

A moderately well documented, established and clinically important interaction. Patients given phenobarbital or pentobarbital may need above-average doses of theophylline to achieve and maintain adequate serum levels. Concurrent use should be monitored and appropriate theophylline dosage increases made. All of the barbiturates can cause enzyme induction and may, to a greater or lesser extent, be expected to behave similarly. This is illustrated by the single report involving secobarbital. However, direct information about other barbiturates seems to be lacking. Note that theophylline itself can cause seizures, although mostly in overdose, and should be used with caution in patients with epilepsy.

1. Gibson GA, Blouin RA, Bauer LA, Rapp RP, Tibbs PA. Influence of high-dose pentobarbital on theophylline pharmacokinetics: A case report. *Ther Drug Monit* (1985) 7, 181–4.
2. Dahlqvist R, Steiner E, Koike Y, von Bahr C, Lind M, Billing B. Induction of theophylline metabolism by pentobarbital. *Ther Drug Monit* (1989) 11, 408–10.
3. Saccar CL, Danish M, Ragni MC, Rocci ML, Greene J, Yaffe SJ, Mansmann HC. The effect of phenobarbital on theophylline disposition in children with asthma. *J Allergy Clin Immunol* (1985) 75, 716–9.
4. Goldstein EO, Eney RD, Mellits ED, Solomon H, Johnson G. Effect of phenobarbital on theophylline metabolism in asthmatic children. *Ann Allergy* (1977) 39, 69.
5. Greene J, Danish M, Ragni M, Lecks H, Yaffe S. The effect of phenobarbital upon theophylline elimination kinetics in asthmatic children. *Ann Allergy* (1977) 39, 69.
6. Landay RA, Gonzalez MA, Taylor JC. Effect of phenobarbital on theophylline disposition. *J Allergy Clin Immunol* (1978) 62, 27–9.
7. Piafsky KM, Sitar DS, Ogilvie RI. Effect of phenobarbital on the disposition of intravenous theophylline. *Clin Pharmacol Ther* (1977) 22, 336–9.
8. Nicholson JP, Basile SA, Cury JD. Massive theophylline dosing in a heavy smoker receiving both phenytoin and phenobarbital. *Ann Pharmacother* (1992) 26, 334–6.
9. Yazdani M, Kissling GE, Tran TH, Gottschalk SK, Schuth CR. Phenobarbital increases the theophylline requirement of premature infants being treated for apnea. *Am J Dis Child* (1987) 141, 97–9.

10. Kandrotas RJ, Cranfield TL, Gal P, Ransom J, Weaver RL. Effect of phenobarbital administration on theophylline clearance in premature neonates. *Ther Drug Monit* (1990) 12, 139–43.
11. Delgado E, Carrasco JM, García B, Pérez E, García Lacalle C, Bermejo T, De Juana P. Interacción teofilina-fenobarbital en un neonato. *Farm Clin* (1996) 13, 142–5.
12. Paladino JA, Blumer NA, Maddox RR. Effect of secobarbital on theophylline clearance. *Ther Drug Monit* (1983) 5, 135–9.
13. Williams JF, Szentivanyi A. Implications of hepatic drug-metabolizing activity in the therapy of bronchial asthma. *J Allergy Clin Immunol* (1975) 55, 125.

Theophylline + BCG vaccine

BCG vaccine can increase the half-life of theophylline, but the clinical importance of this is uncertain.

Clinical evidence, mechanism, importance and management

Two weeks after 12 healthy subjects were vaccinated with 0.1 mL of BCG vaccine, the clearance of a single 128-mg dose of theophylline (as choline theophyllinate) was reduced by 21% and the theophylline half-life was prolonged by 14% (range: 10% reduction to 47% increase).[1] It therefore seems possible that the occasional patient may develop some signs of theophylline toxicity if their serum levels are already towards the top end of the therapeutic range but theophylline levels are unlikely to be affected in most patients given BCG vaccine.

1. Gray JD, Renton KW, Hung OR. Depression of theophylline elimination following BCG vaccination. *Br J Clin Pharmacol* (1983) 16, 735–7.

Theophylline + Beta-agonist bronchodilators

The concurrent use of xanthines such as theophylline and beta-agonist bronchodilators is a useful option in the management of asthma and chronic obstructive pulmonary disease, but potentiation of some adverse reactions can occur, the most serious being hypokalaemia and tachycardia, particularly with high-dose theophylline. Some patients may have a significant fall in serum theophylline levels if given oral or intravenous salbutamol (albuterol) or intravenous isoprenaline (isoproterenol).

Clinical evidence

(a) Fenoterol

A study in 12 patients with chronic airways disease found that oral fenoterol 2.5 mg three times daily did not affect the steady-state level of sustained-release theophylline 10.1 mg/kg twice daily.[1]

Another study in 8 healthy subjects found that the addition of sustained-release theophylline to inhaled fenoterol 600 and 800 micrograms increased the heart rate and systolic blood pressure. Theophylline levels were not affected.[2]

(b) Formoterol

In a single-dose study, 8 healthy subjects were given oral doses of theophylline 375 mg and formoterol 144 micrograms. Combined use caused no significant pharmacokinetic interaction, but a significantly greater drop in the potassium level was seen, when compared with either drug given alone.[3]

(c) Isoprenaline (Isoproterenol)

An infusion of isoprenaline increased the clearance of theophylline (given as intravenous aminophylline) by a mean of 19% in 6 children with status asthmaticus and respiratory failure. Two of them had increases in clearance of greater than 30%.[4] Another study in 12 patients with status asthmaticus found that an isoprenaline infusion (mean maximum rate 0.77 micrograms/kg per minute) caused a mean fall in serum theophylline levels of almost 6 micrograms/mL.[5] The levels rose again when isoprenaline was stopped.[5] A critically ill patient receiving intravenous aminophylline, phenytoin and nebulised terbutaline had a marked 4.5-fold increase in theophylline clearance when an isoprenaline infusion and intravenous methylprednisolone were added to the regimen.[6]

(d) Orciprenaline (Metaproterenol)

In 6 healthy subjects orciprenaline 20 mg given every 8 hours by mouth or 1.95 mg given every 6 hours by inhalation for 3 days had no effect on the pharmacokinetics of theophylline (given as a single intravenous dose of aminophylline).[7] This confirms a previous finding in asthmatic children, in whom it was shown that oral orciprenaline did not alter steady-state serum theophylline levels.[8]

(e) Salbutamol (Albuterol)

1. Effects on heart rate or potassium levels. Pretreatment with oral theophylline for 9 days significantly increased the hypokalaemia and tachycardia caused by an infusion of salbutamol (4 micrograms/kg loading dose then 8 micrograms/kg for an hour) in healthy subjects.[9] A potentially dangerous additive increase in heart rate of about 35 to 40% was seen in one study in 9 patients with COPD given infusions of aminophylline and salbutamol.[10] Similarly, heart rate was significantly higher in 15 asthmatic children given single doses of oral theophylline and salbutamol (109 bpm) when compared with a control group given oral theophylline alone (91 bpm).[11] However, another study in 18 patients with COPD and heart disease found that neither the occurrence nor the severity of arrhythmias seemed to be changed when oral theophylline was given with inhaled salbutamol.[12] A 10-year-old girl given theophylline and salbutamol had a respiratory arrest, possibly related to hypokalaemia.[13]

2. Effects on theophylline levels. Theophylline clearance was increased by a mean of 14%, and in 3 cases by greater than 30%, when salbutamol was given orally to 10 healthy subjects, but no changes in clearance were seen when salbutamol was given by inhalation.[14] Another study reported a 25% reduction in serum theophylline levels in 10 patients who took oral salbutamol 16 mg.[15] A child of 19 months given intravenous theophylline was also given an infusion of salbutamol: theophylline clearance was increased and the theophylline dose needed to be increased threefold to compensate.[16] Peak flow readings were decreased in 15 children (aged 5 to 13 years) given single doses of oral salbutamol and theophylline, but theophylline levels were not significantly decreased.[11] These reports contrast with another study in 8 healthy subjects, which found no change in the steady-state pharmacokinetics of oral theophylline given with oral salbutamol.[17]

(f) Terbutaline

In 7 healthy subjects pretreatment with oral theophylline for at least 4 days significantly increased the fall in serum potassium levels and rises in blood glucose, pulse rate, and systolic blood pressure caused by an infusion of terbutaline.[18] A study in children given slow-release formulations of both theophylline and terbutaline found no increases in reported adverse effects and simple additive effects on the control of their asthma.[19]

Oral terbutaline decreased serum theophylline levels by about 10% in 6 asthmatics, but the control of asthma was improved.[20] Another study in asthmatic children, found that terbutaline elixir 75 micrograms/kg three times daily reduced steady-state serum levels of theophylline by 22%, but the symptoms of cough and wheeze improved.[21] Yet another study found no changes in the pharmacokinetics of aminophylline in asthmatic children given terbutaline.[22]

(g) Unspecified beta$_2$ agonists

In 1990, the CSM in the UK noted that, of 26 reports they had on record of hypokalaemia with unnamed **xanthines** or beta$_2$ agonists, 9 occurred in patients receiving both groups of drugs. In 5 of these 9 cases, the hypokalaemia had no clinical consequence. However, in 2 cases it resulted in cardiorespiratory arrest, in another case confusion, and in a further case intestinal pseudo-obstruction.[23]

Mechanism

Beta$_2$ agonists can cause hypokalaemia, particularly when they are given parenterally or by nebulisation. Xanthines such as theophylline can also cause hypokalaemia, and this is a common feature of theophylline toxicity. The potassium-lowering effects of both these groups of drugs are additive. Why some beta agonists lower serum theophylline levels is not known.

Importance and management

Concurrent use is beneficial, but the reports outlined above illustrate some of the disadvantages and adverse effects that have been identified. In particular, it has been suggested that the use of intravenous beta agonists in acutely ill patients receiving theophylline may be hazardous because of the risk of profound hypokalaemia and cardiac arrhythmias.[9,18] Monitoring of serum potassium in these situations was suggested.[18] Moreover, the CSM in the UK particularly recommends monitoring potassium levels in those with severe asthma as the hypokalaemic effects of beta$_2$ agonists can be potentiated by theophylline and its derivatives, corticosteroids, diuretics and hypoxia.[23]

1. Lucena MI, Almagro J, Rius F, Sanchez de la Cuesta F. Bronchodilator effect and serum theophylline level after combined treatment with fenoterol and theophylline in reversible chronic airflow obstruction. *Eur J Clin Pharmacol* (1988) 35, 669–71.
2. Flatt A, Burgess C, Windom H, Beasley R, Purdie G, Crane J. The cardiovascular effects of inhaled fenoterol alone and during treatment with oral theophylline. *Chest* (1989) 96, 1317–20.
3. van den Berg BTJ, Derks MGM, Koolen MGJ, Braat MCP, Butter JJ, van Boxtel CJ. Pharmacokinetic/pharmacodynamic modelling of the eosinopenic and hypokalemic effects of formoterol and theophylline combination in healthy men. *Pulm Pharmacol Ther* (1999) 12, 185–92.
4. Hemstreet MP, Miles MV, Rutland RO. Effect of intravenous isoproterenol on theophylline kinetics. *J Allergy Clin Immunol* (1982) 69, 360–4.
5. O'Rourke PP, Crone RK. Effect of isoproterenol on measured theophylline levels. *Crit Care Med* (1984) 12, 373–5.
6. Griffith JA, Kozloski GD. Isoproterenol-theophylline interaction: possible potentiation by other drugs. *Clin Pharm* (1990) 9, 54–7.
7. Conrad KA, Woodworth JR. Orciprenaline does not alter theophylline elimination. *Br J Clin Pharmacol* (1981) 12, 756–7.
8. Rachelefsky GS, Katz RM, Mickey MR, Siegel SC. Metaproterenol and theophylline in asthmatic children. *Ann Allergy* (1980) 45, 207–12.
9. Whyte KF, Reid C, Addis GJ, Whitesmith R, Reid JL. Salbutamol induced hypokalaemia: the effect of theophylline alone and in combination with adrenaline. *Br J Clin Pharmacol* (1988) 25, 571–8.
10. Georgopoulos D, Wong D, Anthonisen NR. Interactive effects of systemically administered salbutamol and aminophylline in patients with chronic obstructive pulmonary disease. *Am Rev Respir Dis* (1988) 138, 1499–1503.
11. Dawson KP, Fergusson DM. Effects of oral theophylline and oral salbutamol in the treatment of asthma. *Arch Dis Child* (1982) 57, 674–6.
12. Poukkula A, Korhonen UR, Huikuri H, Linnaluoto M. Theophylline and salbutamol in combination in patients with obstructive pulmonary disease and concurrent heart disease: effect on cardiac arrhythmias. *J Intern Med* (1989) 226, 229–34.
13. Epelbaum S, Benhamou PH, Pautard JC, Devoldere C, Kremp O, Piussan C. Arrêt respiratoire chez une enfant asthmatique traitée par bêta-2-mimétiques et théophylline. Rôle possible de l'hypokaliémie dans les décès subits des asthmatiques. *Ann Pediatr (Paris)* (1989) 36, 473–5.
14. Amitai Y, Glustein J, Godfrey S. Enhancement of theophylline clearance by oral albuterol. *Chest* (1992) 102, 786–9.
15. Terra Filho M, Santos SRCJ, Cukier A, Verrastro C, Carvalho-Pinto RM, Fiss E, Vargas FS.Efeitos dos agonistas beta-2-adrenérgicos por via oral, sobre os níveis séricos de teofilina. *Rev Hosp Clin Fac Med Sao Paulo* (1991) 46, 170–2.
16. Amirav I, Amitai Y, Avital A, Godfrey S. Enhancement of theophylline clearance by intravenous albuterol. *Chest* (1988) 94, 444–5.
17. McCann JP, McElnay JC, Nicholls DP, Scott MG, Stanford CF. Oral salbutamol does not affect theophylline kinetics. *Br J Pharmacol* (1986) 89 (Proc Suppl), 715P.
18. Smith SR, Kendall MJ. Potentiation of the adverse effects of intravenous terbutaline by oral theophylline. *Br J Clin Pharmacol* (1986) 21, 451–3.
19. Chow OKW, Fung KP. Slow-release terbutaline and theophylline for the long-term therapy of children with asthma: A latin square and factorial study of drug effects and interactions. *Pediatrics* (1989) 84, 119–25.
20. Garty MS, Keslin LS, Ilfeld DN, Mazar A, Spitzer S, Rosenfeld JB. Increased theophylline clearance by terbutaline in asthmatic adults. *Clin Pharmacol Ther* (1988) 43, 150.
21. Danziger Y, Garty M, Volwitz B, Ilfeld D, Varsano I, Rosenfeld JB. Reduction of serum theophylline levels by terbutaline in children with asthma. *Clin Pharmacol Ther* (1985) 37, 469–71.
22. Wang Y, Yin A, Yu Z. Effects of bricanyl on the pharmacokinetics of aminophylline in asthmatic patients [In Chinese]. *Zhongguo Yiyuan Yaoxue Zazhi* (1992) 12, 389–90.
23. Committee on Safety of Medicines. β_2-Agonists, xanthines and hypokalaemia. *Current Problems* (1990) 28.

Theophylline + Beta blockers

Propranolol reduces the clearance of theophylline. More importantly, non-cardioselective beta blockers such as nadolol and propranolol, should not be given to asthmatic patients because they can cause bronchospasm. The concurrent use of theophylline and cardioselective beta blockers such as atenolol, bisoprolol or metoprolol is not contraindicated, but some caution is still appropriate. Atenolol and bisoprolol do not affect the pharmacokinetics of theophylline.

Clinical evidence

(a) Pharmacokinetics

A study in 8 healthy subjects (5 of whom smoked 10 to 30 cigarettes daily) found that the clearance of a single 5.7 to 6.4 mg/kg dose of theophylline (as intravenous aminophylline) was reduced by 37% by **propranolol** 40 mg every 6 hours, when compared with theophylline alone. **Metoprolol** 50 mg every 6 hours did not alter the clearance in the group as a whole, but the smokers had an 11% reduction in clearance.[1] Another study, in 7 healthy subjects, found that the steady-state plasma clearance of theophylline was reduced by 30% by **propranolol** 40 mg every 8 hours, and by 52% by **propranolol** 240 mg every 8 hours.[2] However, a further study found no significant pharmacokinetic interaction between theophylline and **propranolol**.[3] Three other studies found that the cardioselective beta blockers **atenolol** 50 to 150 mg,[4,5] and **bisoprolol** 10 mg,[6] and the non-selective beta blocker **nadolol** 80 mg[4] did not affect the pharmacokinetics of theophylline.

(b) Pharmacodynamics

Beta blockers, particularly those that are not cardioselective, can cause bronchoconstriction, which opposes the bronchodilatory effects of theophylline. See 'betaxolol with theophylline and pranlukast', (p.1160), for mention of a patient who had a deterioration of asthma with this combination.

In a study in 8 healthy subjects both **propranolol** 40 mg every 6 hours and **metoprolol** 50 mg every 6 hours prevented the mild inotropic effect seen with theophylline alone.[7]

An infusion of **propranolol** reduced the hypokalaemia and tachycardia that occurred after a theophylline overdose.[8,9] **Esmolol** has been used similarly.[10]

Mechanism

Propranolol possibly affects the clearance of theophylline by inhibiting its metabolism (demethylation and hydroxylation).[2,11]

Importance and management

The risk of severe, possibly even fatal bronchospasm when beta blockers are taken by asthmatics would seem to be far more important than any pharmacokinetic interaction with theophylline. See the warning in 'Anti-asthma drugs + Beta blockers', p.1160. Therefore the non-cardioselective beta blockers, such as propranolol, are contraindicated in patients with asthma or chronic obstructive pulmonary disease (COPD). Bronchospasm can occur with beta blockers given by any route of administration, even topically as eye drops. Cardioselective beta blockers have less effect on the airways, but can still cause bronchoconstriction. See 'Table 22.1', (p.833), for details of the selectivity of beta blockers.

1. Conrad KA, Nyman DW. Effects of metoprolol and propranolol on theophylline elimination. *Clin Pharmacol Ther* (1980) 28, 463–7.
2. Miners JO, Wing LMH, Lillywhite KJ, Robson RA. Selectivity and dose-dependency of the inhibitory effect of propranolol on theophylline metabolism in man. *Br J Clin Pharmacol* (1985) 20, 219–23.
3. Minton NA, Turner J, Henry JA. Pharmacodynamic and pharmacokinetic interactions between theophylline and propranolol during dynamic exercise. *Br J Clin Pharmacol* (1995) 40, 521P.
4. Corsi CM, Nafziger AN, Pieper JA, Bertino JS. Lack of effect of atenolol and nadolol on the metabolism of theophylline. *Br J Clin Pharmacol* (1990) 29, 265–8.
5. Cerasa LA, Bertino JS, Ludwig EA, Savliwala M, Middleton E, Slaughter RL. Lack of effect of atenolol on the pharmacokinetics of theophylline. *Br J Clin Pharmacol* (1988) 26, 800–802.
6. Warrington SJ, Johnston A, Lewis Y, Murphy M. Bisoprolol: Studies of potential interactions with theophylline and warfarin in healthy volunteers. *J Cardiovasc Pharmacol* (1990) 16 (Suppl 5), S164–S168.
7. Conrad KA, Prosnitz EH. Cardiovascular effects of theophylline. Partial attenuation by beta-blockade. *Eur J Clin Pharmacol* (1981) 21, 109–114.
8. Kearney TE, Manoguerra AS, Curtis GP, Ziegler MG. Theophylline toxicity and the beta-adrenergic system. *Ann Intern Med* (1985) 102, 766–9.
9. Amin DN, Henry JA. Propranolol administration in theophylline overdose. *Lancet* (1985) i, 520–1.
10. Seneff M, Scott J, Freidman B, Smith M. Acute theophylline toxicity and the use of esmolol to reverse cardiovascular instability. *Ann Emerg Med* (1990) 19, 671–3.
11. Greenblatt DJ, Franke K, Huffman DH. Impairment of antipyrine clearance in humans by propranolol. *Circulation* (1978) 57, 1161–4.

Theophylline + Caffeine

Consumption of caffeine-containing beverages can raise serum theophylline levels, but the clinical relevance of this is unclear.

Clinical evidence, mechanism, importance and management

Caffeine can decrease the clearance of theophylline by 18 to 29%, prolong its half-life by up to 44% and increase its average serum levels by as much as 23%.[1-3] In addition, caffeine plasma levels were increased about twofold when theophylline was given.[2] In these studies, caffeine was given in the form of tablets[1,2] or as 2 to 7 cups of instant coffee.[3] In one study, 2 of the subjects who did not normally drink coffee experienced headaches and nausea.[2] The probable mechanism of the interaction is that the two drugs compete for the same metabolic pathway resulting in a reduction in their metabolism and accumulation. In addition, when caffeine levels are high, a small percentage of it is converted to theophylline. There would, however, seem to be no good reason for patients taking theophylline to avoid caffeine (in **coffee**, **tea**, **cola drinks**, medications, etc.), but if otherwise unexplained adverse effects occur it might be worth checking if caffeine is responsible. In addition, caffeine intake could have an impact on the interaction of theophylline with other drugs.

1. Loi CM, Jue SG, Bush ED, Crowley JJ, Vestal RE. Effect of caffeine dose on theophylline metabolism. *Clin Res* (1987) 35, 377A.
2. Jonkman JHG, Sollie FAE, Sauter R, Steinijans VW. The influence of caffeine on the steady-state pharmacokinetics of theophylline. *Clin Pharmacol Ther* (1991) 49, 248–55.
3. Sato J, Nakata H, Owada E, Kikuta T, Umetsu M, Ito K. Influence of usual intake of dietary caffeine on single-dose kinetics of theophylline in healthy human subjects. *Eur J Clin Pharmacol* (1993) 44, 295–8.

Theophylline + Calcium-channel blockers

Giving calcium-channel blockers to patients taking theophylline normally has no adverse effect on the control of asthma, despite the small or modest alteration that may occur in serum theophylline levels with diltiazem, felodipine, nifedipine and verapamil. However, there are isolated case reports of unexplained theophylline toxicity in two patients given nifedipine and two patients given verapamil. Isradipine appears not to interact.

Clinical evidence

(a) Diltiazem

In 9 healthy subjects diltiazem 90 mg twice daily for 10 days reduced the clearance of theophylline (given as a single 6-mg/kg dose of aminophylline) by 21%, and increased its half-life from 6.1 to 7.5 hours.[1] A 12% fall in the clearance of a single 5-mg/kg oral dose of theophylline was found when healthy subjects were given diltiazem 90 mg three times daily.[2] In 8 patients with asthma or chronic obstructive pulmonary disease (COPD), diltiazem 60 mg three times daily for 5 days reduced the clearance of steady-state theophylline (given as a continuous infusion of aminophylline 12 mg/kg/day) by 22% and increased its half-life from 5.7 to 7.5 hours.[3]

Conversely, other studies found no significant changes in peak steady-state theophylline levels in 18 patients with asthma given diltiazem 240 to 480 mg daily for 7 days,[4] or in 7 healthy subjects given diltiazem 120 mg twice daily for 7 days.[5] Similarly, there was no significant change in the half-life or clearance of theophylline (given as a single 250-mg intravenous dose of aminophylline) in healthy subjects given diltiazem 120 mg three times daily for 6 days.[6]

(b) Felodipine

In 10 healthy subjects felodipine 5 mg every 8 hours for 4 days reduced the plasma AUC of theophylline (given as theophylline aminopropanol; *Oxyphylline*) by 18.3%, but had no effect on metabolic or renal clearance.[7]

(c) Isradipine

A three-way, crossover study in 11 healthy subjects found that isradipine 2.5 or 5 mg every 12 hours for 6 days had no significant effect on the pharmacokinetics of a single 5-mg/kg dose of aminophylline oral solution.[8]

(d) Nifedipine

In one study, slow-release nifedipine 20 mg twice daily reduced the mean steady-state theophylline levels of 8 asthmatics by 30%, from 9.7 to 6.8 mg/L. Levels fell by 50%, 56%, and 64% in three of the patients, but no changes in the control of the asthma (as measured by peak flow determinations and symptom scores) were seen.[9] However, many other studies have found no changes, or only small to modest changes, in the pharmacokinetics of theophylline (given as oral theophylline or as intravenous lysine theophylline[10] or aminophylline[11]) in healthy subjects[5,10-12] or asthmatic patients[4,13,14] given nifedipine. The control of the asthma was unchanged by nifedipine.[13,14] Yet another study found that the combined use of slow-release theophylline and nifedipine improved pulmonary function and blood pressure control.[15]

In contrast, there are 2 case reports of patients who developed theophylline toxicity (theophylline levels raised to 30 mg/L and 41 mg/L), apparently due to the addition of nifedipine.[16,17] In one case, the toxicity recurred on rechallenge, and resolved when the theophylline dosage was reduced by 60%.[17] During a Swan Ganz catheter study of patient response to nifedipine for pulmonary hypertension, 2 patients developed serious nifedipine adverse effects, which responded to intravenous aminophylline.[18]

(e) Verapamil

In one study, verapamil 80 mg every 6 hours for 2 days had no effect on the pharmacokinetics of theophylline (200 mg aminophylline every 6 hours) given to 5 asthmatics, and no effect on their spirometry (FVC, FEV_1, FEF_{25-75}).[19] Similarly, another study found that verapamil 80 mg every 8 hours had no effect on the steady-state levels of sustained-release theophylline 3 mg/kg per day in healthy subjects.[20] In contrast, numerous other studies in healthy subjects (given intravenous or oral aminophylline or theophylline) have found modest reductions in theophylline clearance of between 8 and 23% with verapamil 40 to 120 mg taken every 6 to 8 hours.[2,6,12,21-23] One study showed that the extent of reduction in clearance depended on the verapamil dosage.[23] An isolated report describes a woman taking digoxin and sustained-release theophylline who developed signs of toxicity (tachycardia, nausea, vomiting) after starting to take verapamil 80 mg, increased to 120 mg every 8 hours. Her theophylline serum levels doubled over a 6-day period. Theophylline was later successfully reintroduced at one-third of the original dosage.[24] Another isolated report describes a patient who needed a 50% reduction in their theophylline dose while taking verapamil 120 mg daily.[25]

Mechanism

It is believed that diltiazem and verapamil can, to a limited extent, decrease the metabolism of theophylline by the liver, possibly by inhibiting the cytochrome P450 isoenzyme CYP1A2.[26] Similarly, nifedipine may alter hepatic theophylline metabolism,[12] or it may increase the volume of distribution of theophylline.[10,11] Felodipine possibly reduces theophylline absorption.[7]

Importance and management

The evidence for this interaction is adequately documented but the results are not entirely consistent. However, the overall picture is that the concurrent use of theophylline and these calcium-channel blockers is normally safe. Despite the small or modest decreases in the clearance or absorption of theophylline seen with diltiazem, felodipine and verapamil, and the quite large reductions in serum levels seen in one study with nifedipine, no adverse changes in the control of the asthma were seen in any of the studies. However, very occasionally and unpredictably theophylline levels have risen enough to cause toxicity in patients given nifedipine (2 case reports) or verapamil (2 case reports), so that it would be prudent to be aware of the possibility of an interaction when these drugs are given.

1. Nafziger AN, May JJ, Bertino JS. Inhibition of theophylline elimination by diltiazem therapy. *J Clin Pharmacol* (1987) 27, 862–5.
2. Sirmans SM, Pieper JA, Lalonde RL, Smith DG, Self TH. Effect of calcium channel blockers on theophylline disposition. *Clin Pharmacol Ther* (1988) 44, 29–34.
3. Soto J, Sacristan JA, Alsar MJ. Diltiazem treatment impairs theophylline elimination in patients with bronchospastic airway disease. *Ther Drug Monit* (1994) 16, 49–52.
4. Christopher MA, Harman E, Hendeles L. Clinical relevance of the interaction of theophylline with diltiazem or nifedipine. *Chest* (1989) 95, 309–13.
5. Smith SR, Haffner CA, Kendall MJ. The influence of nifedipine and diltiazem on serum theophylline concentration-time profiles. *J Clin Pharm Ther* (1989) 14, 403–8.
6. Abernethy DR, Egan JM, Dickinson TH, Carrum G. Substrate-selective inhibition by verapamil and diltiazem: differential disposition of antipyrine and theophylline in humans. *J Pharmacol Exp Ther* (1988) 244, 994–9.
7. Bratel T, Billing B, Dahlqvist R. Felodipine reduces the absorption of theophylline in man. *Eur J Clin Pharmacol* (1989) 36, 481–5.
8. Perreault MM, Kazierad DJ, Wilton JH, Izzo JL. The effect of isradipine on theophylline pharmacokinetics in healthy volunteers. *Pharmacotherapy* (1993) 13, 149–53.
9. Smith SR, Wiggins J, Stableforth DE, Skinner C, Kendall MJ. Effect of nifedipine on serum theophylline concentrations and asthma control. *Thorax* (1987) 42, 794–6.
10. Jackson SHD, Shah K, Debbas NMG, Johnston A, Peverel-Cooper CA, Turner P. The interaction between i.v. theophylline and chronic oral dosing with slow release nifedipine in volunteers. *Br J Clin Pharmacol* (1986) 21, 389–92.
11. Adebayo GI, Mabadeje AFB. Effect of nifedipine on antipyrine and theophylline disposition. *Biopharm Drug Dispos* (1990) 11, 157–64.
12. Robson RA, Miners JO, Birkett DJ. Selective inhibitory effects of nifedipine and verapamil on oxidative metabolism: effects on theophylline. *Br J Clin Pharmacol* (1988) 25, 397–400.
13. Garty M, Cohen E, Mazar A, Ilfeld DN, Spitzer S, Rosenfeld JB. Effect of nifedipine and theophylline in asthma. *Clin Pharmacol Ther* (1986) 40, 195–8.
14. Yilmaz E, Canberk A, Eroğlu L. Nifedipine alters serum theophylline levels in asthmatic patients with hypertension. *Fundam Clin Pharmacol* (1991) 5, 341–5.
15. Spedini C, Lombardi C. Long-term treatment with oral nifedipine plus theophylline in the management of chronic bronchial asthma. *Eur J Clin Pharmacol* (1986) 31, 105–6.
16. Parrillo SJ, Venditto M. Elevated theophylline blood levels from institution of nifedipine therapy. *Ann Emerg Med* (1984) 13, 216–17.
17. Harrod CS. Theophylline toxicity and nifedipine. *Ann Intern Med* (1987) 106, 480.
18. Kalra L, Bone MF, Ariaraj SJP. Nifedipine-aminophylline interaction. *J Clin Pharmacol* (1988) 28, 1056–7.
19. Gotz VP, Russell WL. Effect of verapamil on theophylline disposition. *Chest* (1987) 92, 75S.
20. Rindone JP, Zuniga R, Sock JA. The influence of verapamil on theophylline serum concentrations. *Drug Metabol Drug Interact* (1989) 7, 143–7.
21. Nielsen-Kudsk JE, Buhl JS, Johannessen AC. Verapamil-induced inhibition of theophylline elimination in healthy humans. *Pharmacol Toxicol* (1990) 66, 101–3.
22. Gin AS, Stringer KA, Welage LS, Wilton JH, Matthews GE. The effect of verapamil on the pharmacokinetic disposition of theophylline in cigarette smokers. *J Clin Pharmacol* (1989) 29, 728–32.
23. Stringer KA, Mallet J, Clarke M, Lindenfeld JA. The effect of three different oral doses of verapamil on the disposition of theophylline. *Eur J Clin Pharmacol* (1992) 43, 35–8.
24. Burnakis TG, Seldon M, Czaplicki AD. Increased serum theophylline concentrations secondary to oral verapamil. *Clin Pharm* (1983) 2, 458–61.

25. Bangura L, Malesker MA, Dewan NA. Theophylline and verapamil: Clinically significant drug interaction. *J Pharm Technol* (1997) 13, 241–3.
26. Fuhr U, Woodcock BG, Siewert M. Verapamil and drug metabolism by the cytochrome P450 isoform CYP1A2. *Eur J Clin Pharmacol* (1992) 42, 463–4.

Theophylline + Cannabis

Cannabis smokers may need more theophylline than non-smokers to achieve the same therapeutic benefits, because the theophylline is cleared from the body more quickly.

Clinical evidence, mechanism, importance and management

One study found that tobacco or cannabis smoking similarly caused higher total clearances of theophylline (given as oral aminophylline) than in non-smokers (about 74 mL/kg per hour compared with 52 mL/kg per hour), and that clearance was even higher (93 mL/kg per hour) in those who smoked both.[1] A later analysis by the same authors, of factors affecting theophylline clearance, found that smoking 2 or more joints of cannabis weekly was associated with a higher total clearance of theophylline than non-use (82.9 mL/kg per hour versus 56.1 mL/kg per hour).[2]

Tobacco and cannabis smoke contain polycyclic hydrocarbons, which act as inducers of the cytochrome P450 isoenzyme CYP1A2, and this results in a more rapid clearance of theophylline from the body.

Little is known about the effects of smoking cannabis on theophylline levels, but be alert for the need to increase the theophylline dosage in regular users.

Consider also 'Theophylline + Tobacco', p.1201.

1. Jusko WJ, Schentag JJ, Clark JH, Gardner M, Yurchak AM. Enhanced biotransformation of theophylline in marihuana and tobacco smokers. *Clin Pharmacol Ther* (1978) 24, 406–10.
2. Jusko WJ, Gardner MJ, Mangione A, Schentag JJ, Koup JR, Vance JW. Factors affecting theophylline clearances: age, tobacco, marijuana, cirrhosis, congestive heart failure, obesity, oral contraceptives, benzodiazepines, barbiturates, and ethanol. *J Pharm Sci* (1979) 68, 1358–66.

Theophylline + Carbamazepine

Two case reports describe a marked fall in serum theophylline levels when carbamazepine was given. Another single case report and a pharmacokinetic study describe a fall in serum carbamazepine levels when theophylline was given.

Clinical evidence

(a) Theophylline serum levels reduced

An 11-year-old girl with asthma was stable for 2 months taking theophylline, and phenobarbital until the phenobarbital was replaced by carbamazepine. The asthma worsened, her theophylline serum levels became subtherapeutic and the half-life of the theophylline was reduced from 5.25 to 2.75 hours. Asthmatic control was restored, and the half-life returned to pre-treatment levels 3 weeks after the carbamazepine was replaced by ethotoin.[1] The clearance of theophylline in an adult patient was doubled by carbamazepine 600 mg daily.[2]

(b) Carbamazepine serum levels reduced

The trough carbamazepine levels of a 10-year-old girl were roughly halved when she was given theophylline for 2 days, and she experienced a grand mal seizure. Her serum theophylline levels were also unusually high at 26 mg/L for the 5 mg/kg dosage she was taking, so it may be that the convulsions were as much due to this as to the fall in carbamazepine levels.[3]

A single-dose pharmacokinetic study in healthy subjects found that the AUC and maximum serum levels of carbamazepine were reduced by 31% and 45%, respectively, by oral aminophylline.[4]

Mechanism

Not established, but it seems probable that each drug increases the liver metabolism and clearance of the other drug, resulting in a reduction in their effects.[1,3] It is also possible that aminophylline interferes with the absorption of carbamazepine.[4]

Importance and management

Information seems to be limited to the reports cited so that the general importance is uncertain. Concurrent use need not be avoided, but it would be prudent to check that the serum concentrations of each drug (and their effects) do not become subtherapeutic. Note that theophylline should be used with caution in patients with epilepsy as it can cause seizures, although this is usually a sign of toxicity.

1. Rosenberry KR, Defusco CJ, Mansmann HC, McGeady SJ. Reduced theophylline half-life induced by carbamazepine therapy. *J Pediatr* (1983) 102, 472–4.
2. Reed RC, Schwartz HJ. Phenytoin-theophylline-quinidine interaction. *N Engl J Med* (1983) 308, 724–5.
3. Mitchell EA, Dower JC, Green RJ. Interaction between carbamazepine and theophylline. *N Z Med J* (1986) 99, 69–70.
4. Kulkarni C, Vaz J, David J, Joseph T. Aminophylline alters pharmacokinetics of carbamazepine but not that of sodium valproate — a single dose pharmacokinetic study in human volunteers. *Indian J Physiol Pharmacol* (1995) 39, 122–6.

Theophylline + Cephalosporins

Ceftibuten and cefalexin appear not to interact with theophylline. Cefaclor has been implicated in two cases of theophylline toxicity in children, but studies in adult subjects found no pharmacokinetic interaction.

Clinical evidence, mechanism, importance and management

Ceftibuten 200 mg twice daily for 7 days was found to have no significant effect on the pharmacokinetics of a single intravenous dose of theophylline given to 12 healthy subjects.[1] A study in 9 healthy adults given a single 5-mg/kg intravenous dose of aminophylline found that **cefalexin** 500 mg, then 250 mg every 6 hours for 48 hours, had no significant effect on the pharmacokinetics of theophylline.[2]

A case report[3] suggested that **cefaclor** might have been responsible for the development of theophylline toxicity in 2 children. However, a single-dose study[4] and a steady-state study[5] in healthy adults found that **cefaclor** 250 mg three times daily for 8 and 9 days, respectively, had no effect on the pharmacokinetics of oral or intravenous theophylline. Although the pharmacokinetics of theophylline differ in adults and children a significant interaction with **cefaclor** seems unlikely.

No special precautions seem to be necessary with any of these antibacterials. Note that acute infections *per se* can alter theophylline pharmacokinetics.

1. Bachmann K, Schwartz J, Jauregui L, Martin M, Nunlee M. Failure of ceftibuten to alter single dose theophylline clearance. *J Clin Pharmacol* (1990) 30, 444–8.
2. Pfeifer HJ, Greenblatt DJ, Friedman P. Effects of three antibiotics on theophylline kinetics. *Clin Pharmacol Ther* (1979) 26, 36–40.
3. Hammond D, Abate MA. Theophylline toxicity, acute illness, and cefaclor administration. *DICP Ann Pharmacother* (1989) 23, 339–40.
4. Bachmann K, Schwartz J, Forney RB, Jauregui L. Impact of cefaclor on the pharmacokinetics of theophylline. *Ther Drug Monit* (1986) 8, 151–4.
5. Jonkman JHG, van der Boon WJV, Schoenmaker R, Holtkamp A, Hempenius J. Clinical pharmacokinetics of theophylline during co-treatment with cefaclor. *Int J Clin Pharmacol Ther Toxicol* (1986) 24, 88–92.

Theophylline + Clopidogrel or Ticlopidine

Ticlopidine reduces the clearance of theophylline and is expected to raise its serum levels. Clopidogrel, an analogue of ticlopidine, appears not to interact.

Clinical evidence, mechanism, importance and management

(a) Clopidogrel

Clopidogrel 75 mg daily for 10 days did not alter the steady-state pharmacokinetics of theophylline given to 12 healthy subjects.[1] No problems are therefore anticipated with the concurrent use of these two drugs.

(b) Ticlopidine

In 10 healthy subjects ticlopidine 250 mg twice daily for 10 days reduced the clearance of a single 5-mg/kg oral dose of theophylline by 37% and increased the half-life by 44%, from about 8.5 hours to 12 hours.[2] The reason for these effects is not known but it seems possible that ticlopidine inhibits the metabolism of theophylline by the liver. Information is limited, but it would seem prudent to monitor the effects of concurrent use: it may be necessary to reduce the dosage of theophylline, particularly when serum levels are already at the top end of the range.

1. Caplain H, Thebault J-J, Necciari J. Clopidogrel does not affect the pharmacokinetics of theophylline. *Semin Thromb Hemost* (1999) 24, 65–8.
2. Colli A, Buccino G, Cocciolo M, Parravicini R, Elli GM, Scaltrini G. Ticlopidine-theophylline interaction. *Clin Pharmacol Ther* (1987) 41, 358–62.

Theophylline + Codeine

A study in 6 healthy subjects found that codeine 30 mg prolonged the oral to caecal transit time of a single 500-mg dose of sustained-release theophylline (*Theo-Dur*). The mean amount left to be absorbed from the colon was reduced from 58% to 33%, but the time to 90% absorption of theophylline was not significantly affected (7.1 hours compared with 8.5 hours). Therefore codeine does not appear to significantly affect the rate or extent of absorption of theophylline, and concurrent use need not be avoided.[1]

1. Sommers DK, Meyer EC, Van Wyk M, Moncrieff J, Snyman JR, Grimbeek RJ. The influence of codeine, propantheline and metoclopramide on small bowel transit and theophylline absorption from a sustained-release formulation. *Br J Clin Pharmacol* (1992) 33, 305–8.

Theophylline + Corticosteroids

Theophylline and corticosteroids have established roles in the management of asthma and their concurrent use is not uncommon. There are isolated reports of increases in serum theophylline levels (sometimes associated with toxicity) when oral or parenteral corticosteroids are given, but other reports show no changes. The general clinical importance of these findings is uncertain. Both theophylline and corticosteroids can cause hypokalaemia, which may be additive.

Clinical evidence

(a) Betamethasone

The elimination half-life of theophylline (given as intravenous aminophylline) was no different in premature infants who had been exposed to betamethasone *in utero* than in those who had not, although the exposed neonates had a wider range of theophylline metabolites indicating greater hepatic metabolism.[1,2]

(b) Dexamethasone

In one study it was briefly mentioned that theophylline did not appear to affect dexamethasone metabolism.[3]

(c) Hydrocortisone

Three patients in status asthmaticus with relatively stable serum concentrations of theophylline were given a 500-mg intravenous bolus of hydrocortisone followed 6 hours later by 200 mg of hydrocortisone given every 2 hours for 3 doses. In each case the serum theophylline levels rose from about 20 mg/L to between 30 and 50 mg/L. At least 2 of the patients complained of nausea and headache.[4] In contrast, 7 healthy subjects given sustained-release theophylline had no significant change in steady-state theophylline clearance when they were given a single 33-mg/kg dose of intravenous hydrocortisone, although there was a trend towards increased clearance.[5] Intravenous bolus doses of hydrocortisone 500 mg or 1 g did not affect theophylline levels in patients taking choline theophyllinate 400 mg every 12 hours for 8 days.[6]

(d) Methylprednisolone

An 88% increase in the clearance of a single dose of intravenous aminophylline was seen in one of 3 healthy subjects pretreated with oral methylprednisolone.[7] There was no significant change in clearance in the other 2 subjects. Another study in 10 children (aged 2 to 6) with status asthmaticus found that intramuscular methylprednisolone tended to increase the half-life of theophylline (given as oral aminophylline or theophylline).[8] A further study also reported that when intravenous aminophylline was given to 16 children taking corticosteroids (route and type not specified) the theophylline half-life was prolonged from 5 to 6.2 hours, and the clearance was reduced by about one-third, when compared with 10 children not taking corticosteroids.[9] Similarly, 7 healthy subjects given sustained-release theophylline had no significant change in steady-state theophylline clearance when they were given a single 1.6-mg/kg dose of intravenous methylprednisolone, although there was a trend towards increased clearance.[5]

(e) Prednisone or Prednisolone

A study in 6 healthy subjects showed that a single 20-mg oral dose of prednisone had no significant effect on the pharmacokinetics of a single 200-mg oral dose of aminophylline.[10] The pharmacokinetics of a single 5.6-mg/kg intravenous dose of aminophylline was unchanged in 9 patients with chronic airflow obstruction when they were given prednisolone 20 mg daily for 3 weeks.[11]

Mechanism

Not understood.

Importance and management

The concurrent use of theophylline and corticosteroids is common and therapeutically valuable, whereas the few reported interactions of theophylline with oral or parenteral corticosteroids are poorly documented and their clinical importance is difficult to assess because both increases, small decreases and no changes in the serum levels of theophylline have been seen. It is also questionable whether the results of studies in healthy subjects can validly be extrapolated to patients with status asthmaticus. There do not appear to be any data on the effect of *inhaled* corticosteroids on the clearance of theophylline. Both theophylline and corticosteroids can cause hypokalaemia, and the possibility that this may be potentiated by concurrent use should be considered.

1. Jager-Roman E, Doyle PE, Thomas D, Baird-Lambert J, Cvejic M, Buchanan N. Increased theophylline metabolism in premature infants after prenatal betamethasone administration. *Dev Pharmacol Ther* (1982) 5, 127–35.
2. Baird-Lambert J, Doyle PE, Thomas D, Jager-Roman E, Cvejic M, Buchanan N. Theophylline metabolism in preterm neonates during the first weeks of life. *Dev Pharmacol Ther* (1984) 7, 239–44.
3. Brooks SM, Sholiton LJ, Werk EE, Altenau P. The effects of ephedrine and theophylline on dexamethasone metabolism in bronchial asthma. *J Clin Pharmacol* (1977) 17, 308.
4. Buchanan N, Hurwitz S, Butler P. Asthma—a possible interaction between hydrocortisone and theophylline. *S Afr Med J* (1979) 56, 1147–8.
5. Leavengood DC, Bunker-Soler AL, Nelson HS. The effect of corticosteroids on theophylline metabolism. *Ann Allergy* (1983) 50, 249–51.
6. Tatsis G, Orphanidou D, Douratsos D, Mellissinos C, Pantelakis D, Pipini E, Jordanoglou J. The effect of steroids on theophylline absorption. *J Int Med Res* (1991) 19, 326–9.
7. Squire EN, Nelson HS. Corticosteroids and theophylline clearance. *N Engl Reg Allergy Proc* (1987) 8, 113–15.
8. De La Morena E, Borges MT, Garcia Rebollar C, Escorihuela R. Efecto de la metil-prednisolona sobre los niveles séricos de teofilina. *Rev Clin Esp* (1982) 167, 297–300.
9. Elvey SM, Saccar CL, Rocci ML, Mansmann HC, Martynec DM, Kester MB. The effect of corticosteroids on theophylline metabolism in asthmatic children. *Ann Allergy* (1986) 56, 520.
10. Anderson JL, Ayres JW, Hall CA. Potential pharmacokinetic interaction between theophylline and prednisone. *Clin Pharm* (1984) 3, 187–9.
11. Fergusson RJ, Scott CM, Rafferty P, Gaddie J. Effect of prednisolone on theophylline pharmacokinetics in patients with chronic airflow obstruction. *Thorax* (1987) 42, 195–8.

Theophylline + Co-trimoxazole

Co-trimoxazole (trimethoprim/sulfamethoxazole) does not alter the pharmacokinetics of theophylline.

Clinical evidence, mechanism, importance and management

In 6 healthy subjects co-trimoxazole 960 mg twice daily for 8 days had no effect on the pharmacokinetics of theophylline, given as a single 341-mg intravenous dose of aminophylline.[1] Another study, in 8 healthy subjects, found that co-trimoxazole 960 mg twice daily for 5 days had no effect on the pharmacokinetics of a single 267-mg oral dose of theophylline.[2] No special precautions would seem necessary if these drugs are given concurrently. However, note that acute infections *per se* can alter theophylline pharmacokinetics.

1. Jonkman JHG, Van Der Boon WJV, Schoenmaker R, Holtkamp AH, Hempenius J. Lack of influence of co-trimoxazole on theophylline pharmacokinetics. *J Pharm Sci* (1985) 74, 1103–4.
2. Lo KF, Nation RL, Sansom LN. Lack of effect of co-trimoxazole on the pharmacokinetics of orally administered theophylline. *Biopharm Drug Dispos* (1989) 10, 573–80.

Theophylline + Dextropropoxyphene (Propoxyphene)

Dextropropoxyphene does not significantly alter steady-state theophylline levels.

Clinical evidence, mechanism, importance and management

In 6 healthy subjects pre-treatment with dextropropoxyphene 65 mg every 8 hours for 5 days did not significantly change the total plasma clearance of steady-state theophylline 125 mg every 8 hours.[1] There was a small reduction in the formation of the hydroxylated metabolite of theophylline. There would seem to be no need to avoid concurrent use or to take particular precautions.

1. Robson RA, Miners JO, Whitehead AG, Birkett DJ. Specificity of the inhibitory effect of dextropropoxyphene on oxidative drug metabolism in man: effects on theophylline and tolbutamide disposition. *Br J Clin Pharmacol* (1987) 23, 772–5.

Theophylline + Disulfiram

Theophylline clearance is decreased by disulfiram.

Clinical evidence

After taking disulfiram 250 mg daily for one week, the clearance of a 5-mg/kg intravenous dose of theophylline was decreased by a mean of about 21% (range 14.6 to 29.6%) in 20 recovering alcoholics. Those taking disulfiram 500 mg daily had a mean decrease of 32.5% (range 21.6 to 49.6%).[1] Smoking appeared to have no important effects on the extent of this interaction. None of the patients were reported to have any significant liver disease, such as cirrhosis, which may also affect theophylline metabolism.

Mechanism

Disulfiram inhibits the liver enzymes concerned with the both the hydroxylation and demethylation of theophylline, thereby reducing its clearance from the body.

Importance and management

Information appears to be limited to this study but it would seem to be a clinically important interaction. Monitor the serum levels of theophylline and its effects if disulfiram is added, anticipating the need to reduce the theophylline dosage. Note that the extent of this interaction appears to depend upon the dosage of disulfiram used.

1. Loi C-M, Day JD, Jue SG, Bush ED, Costello P, Dewey LV, Vestal RE. Dose-dependent inhibition of theophylline metabolism by disulfiram in recovering alcoholics. *Clin Pharmacol Ther* (1989) 45, 476–86.

Theophylline + Dobutamine

A man taking theophylline developed marked tachycardia when he was given dobutamine.

Clinical evidence, mechanism, importance and management

An asthmatic patient taking sustained-release theophylline 150 mg twice daily, digoxin and spironolactone was anaesthetised for an aortic valve replacement with fentanyl, midazolam and pipecuronium. Following induction, intubation, and ventilation with 100% oxygen, his systolic blood pressure fell from 120 to 80 mmHg, and his heart rate slowed from 70 to 50 bpm. Dobutamine was given at a dose of 5 micrograms/kg per minute, and after 2 to 3 minutes his heart rate rose to 150 bpm and his systolic pressure rose to 190 mmHg. The authors of the report[1] attribute the tachycardia to an interaction between dobutamine and theophylline. They suggested that the interaction was possibly as a result of a synergistic increase in cyclic AMP levels in cardiac muscle and/or theophylline-induced potentiation of catecholamine action. They advise the careful titration of dobutamine in any asthmatic taking theophylline, particularly if a slow-release preparation is being used. However, more study of this apparent interaction is needed as this appears to be the only report, and so it's general importance is unknown.

1. Baraka A, Darwish R, Rizkallah P. Excessive dobutamine-induced tachycardia in the asthmatic cardiac patient: possible potentiation by theophylline therapy. *J Cardiothorac Vasc Anesth* (1993) 7, 641–2.

Theophylline + Doxapram

Doxapram pharmacokinetics are unchanged by theophylline in premature infants, but agitation and increased muscle activity may occur in adults.

Clinical evidence, mechanism, importance and management

Intravenous theophylline does not affect the pharmacokinetics of doxapram given to treat apnoea in premature infants. No adjustment of the dosage of doxapram is needed in the presence of theophylline.[1] However, the manufacturers of doxapram say that there may be an interaction between doxapram and aminophylline or theophylline, which is manifested by agitation and increased skeletal muscle activity. Care should therefore be taken if these drugs are used together.[2]

1. Jamali F, Coutts RT, Malek F, Finer NN, Peliowski A. Lack of a pharmacokinetic interaction between doxapram and theophylline in apnea of prematurity. *Dev Pharmacol Ther* (1991) 16, 78–82.
2. Dopram (Doxapram hydrochloride). Baxter Healthcare Corporation. US Prescribing information, March 2004.

Theophylline + Enoximone

Aminophylline possibly reduces the beneficial cardiovascular effects of enoximone. Theoretically, milrinone would be expected to interact similarly.

Clinical evidence, mechanism, importance and management

An experimental study into the mechanism of action of enoximone in 14 patients with ischaemic or idiopathic dilative cardiomyopathy found that pretreatment with intravenous aminophylline 7 mg/kg given over 15 minutes reduced the beneficial haemodynamic effects of intravenous enoximone 1 mg/kg given over 15 minutes.[1] This appears to occur because each drug competes for inhibition of cAMP specific phosphodiesterases in cardiac and vascular smooth muscle. **Milrinone**, another phosphodiesterase inhibitor similar to enoximone, would be expected to interact in the same way. However, there are, at present, no published reports of a possible interaction with milrinone, and no case reports of a problem occurring with the concurrent use of either drug with theophylline. The clinical importance of this study therefore awaits evaluation.

1. Morgagni GL, Bugiardini R, Borghi A, Pozzati A, Ottani F, Puddu P. Aminophylline counteracts the hemodynamic effects of enoximone. *Clin Pharmacol Ther* (1990) 47, 140.

Theophylline + Ephedrine

Some data suggest that an increased frequency of adverse effects occurs when ephedrine is used with theophylline.

Clinical evidence, mechanism, importance and management

A double-blind, randomised study in 23 children aged 4 to 14 found that when ephedrine was given with theophylline (in a ratio of 25 mg ephedrine to 130 mg theophylline), the number of adverse reactions increased significantly, when compared with each drug taken separately. Moreover, the combination was no more effective than theophylline alone. The combination was associated with insomnia (14 patients), nervousness (13) and gastrointestinal complaints (18), including vomiting (12). The serum theophylline levels were unchanged by ephedrine.[1] A previous study by the same authors in 12 asthmatic children given ephedrine and aminophylline found similar results.[2] In contrast, a later study suggested that ephedrine 25 mg every 8 hours given with aminophylline did produce improvements in spirometry and no adverse effects were seen. However, it was calculated that the theophylline dosage used was about half that used in the previous study.[3]

In the treatment of asthma, ephedrine has been largely superseded by more selective sympathomimetics, which have fewer adverse effects. Ephedrine is still an ingredient of a number of non-prescription cough and cold remedies, when it may be combined with theophylline (e.g. *Franol*).

Patients taking theophylline requiring ephedrine should be advised report any adverse effects.

1. Weinberger M, Bronsky E, Bensch GW, Bock GN, Yecies JJ. Interaction of ephedrine and theophylline. *Clin Pharmacol Ther* (1975) 17, 585–92.
2. Weinberger MM, Bronsky EA. Evaluation of oral bronchodilator therapy in asthmatic children. *J Pediatr* (1974) 84, 421–7.
3. Tinkelman DG, Avner SE. Ephedrine therapy in asthmatic children. Clinical tolerance and absence of side effects. *JAMA* (1977) 237, 553–7.

Theophylline + Food

The effect of food on theophylline bioavailability is unclear. In general it appears that fat or fibre in food has no effect, whereas high-protein and high-carbohydrate diets decrease and increase the theophylline half-life, respectively. Significant changes in theophylline bioavailability have been seen in patients given both enteral feeds and total parenteral nutrition.

Clinical evidence

(a) Food

The bioavailability of theophylline from sustained-release preparations has been shown to be reduced,[1,2] increased,[1,3] or unaffected[4-8] when the theophylline was given immediately after **breakfast**. Dose dumping, leading to signs of theophylline toxicity, was seen in 3 children with asthma who were given a dose of *Uniphyllin* immediately after **breakfast**.[6] The **fat** content[9,10] or **fibre** content[11] of meals does not seem to significantly affect theophylline absorption. **High-protein** meals appear to decrease theophylline half-life,[12,13] whereas **high-carbohydrate** meals seem to increase it.[13] There was no difference in theophylline metabolism in one study when patients were changed from a **high-carbohydrate/low-protein** diet to a **high-protein/low-carbohydrate** diet.[14] One study found that changing from a **high-protein** to a **high-carbohydrate** meal had an effect on the metabolism of theophylline similar to that of cimetidine, and that the effects of the meal change and cimetidine were additive.[15] The effects of **spicy food** have been studied, but the clinical significance of the changes are uncertain.[16]

(b) Enteral feeds

A patient with chronic obstructive pulmonary disease had a 53% reduction in his serum theophylline levels accompanied by bronchospasm when he was fed continuously through a nasogastric tube with ***Osmolite***. The interaction occurred with both theophylline tablets (*Theo-Dur*) and liquid theophylline, but not when the theophylline was given intravenously as aminophylline. It was also found that the interaction could be avoided by interrupting feeding 1 hour either side of the oral liquid theophylline dose.[17] Conversely, hourly administration of 100 mL of ***Osmolite*** did not affect the extent of theophylline absorption from a slow-release preparation (*Slo-bid Gyrocaps*) in healthy subjects, although the rate of absorption was slowed.[18] Similarly, in healthy subjects, hourly administration of 100 mL of ***Ensure*** for 10 hours did not affect the rate or extent of absorption of theophylline from *Theo-24* tablets.[19]

(c) Parenteral nutrition

An isolated report describes an elderly woman treated with aminophylline by intravenous infusion who had a marked fall in her serum theophylline levels (from 16.3 to 6.3 mg/L) when the amino acid concentration of her parenteral nutrition regimen was increased from 4.25 to 7%.[20] A study in 7 patients with malnutrition (marasmus-kwashiorkor) found only a small, probably clinically irrelevant increase in the elimination of a single intravenous dose of theophylline when they were fed intravenously.[21]

Mechanism

Not fully understood. As with any sustained-release formulation, the presence of food in the gut may alter the rate or extent of drug absorption by altering gastrointestinal transit time. It has been suggested that high-protein diets stimulate liver enzymes thereby increasing the metabolism of the theophylline and hastening its clearance from the body. High carbohydrate diets have the opposite effect. The cytochrome P450 isoenzyme CYP1A2 (the principal enzyme involved in the metabolism of theophylline) is known to be induced by chemicals contained in cruciferous vegetables[22] or formed by the action of high temperatures or smoke on meat.[23] This suggestion is supported by a study in which charcoal-grilled (broiled) beef decreased the half-life of theophylline by an average of 22%.[24] Further, high doses of daidzein, the principal isoflavone in soybeans, may inhibit CYP1A2 resulting in an increase in theophylline levels and half-life of about 33% and 41%, respectively.[25]

Importance and management

Interactions between theophylline and food have been thoroughly studied but there seems to be no consistent pattern in the way the absorption of different theophylline preparations is affected. Be alert for any evidence of an inadequate response that can be related to food intake. Avoid switching between different preparations, and monitor the effects if this is necessary. Consult the product literature for any specific information on food and encourage patients to take their theophylline consistently in relation to meals where this is considered necessary. Advise patients not make major changes in their diet without consultation. Monitor the effects of both enteral and parenteral nutrition, since theophylline dosage adjustments may be required.

1. Karim A, Burns T, Wearley L, Streicher J, Palmer M. Food-induced changes in theophylline absorption from controlled-release formulations. Part I. Substantial increased and decreased absorption with Uniphyl tablets and Theo-Dur Sprinkle. *Clin Pharmacol Ther* (1985) 38, 77–83.
2. Lohmann A, Dingler E, Sommer W. Influence of food on the bioavailability of theophylline from a sustained-release theophylline preparation. *Arzneimittelforschung* (1991) 41, 732–4.
3. Vaughan L, Milavetz G, Hill M, Weinberger M, Hendeles L. Food-induced dose-dumping of Theo-24, a 'once-daily' slow-release theophylline product. *Drug Intell Clin Pharm* (1984) 18, 510.
4. Johansson Ö, Lindberg T, Melander A, Wåhlin-Boll E. Different effects of different nutrients on theophylline absorption in man. *Drug Nutr Interact* (1985) 3, 205–11.
5. Sips AP, Edelbroek PM, Kulstad S, de Wolff FA, Dijkman JH. Food does not effect bioavailability of theophylline from Theolin Retard. *Eur J Clin Pharmacol* (1984) 26, 405–7.
6. Steffensen G, Pedersen S. Food induced changes in theophylline absorption from a once-a-day theophylline product. *Br J Clin Pharmacol* (1986) 22, 571–7.
7. Ürmös I, Grézal G, Balogh Nemes K, Szállási T, Drabant S, Csörgo M, Klebovich I. Food interaction study of a new theophylline (Egifilin) 200 and 400 mg retard tablet in healthy volunteers. *Int J Clin Pharmacol Ther* (1997) 35, 65–70.
8. González MA, Straughn AB. Effect of meals and dosage-form modification on theophylline bioavailability from a 24-hour sustained-release delivery system. *Clin Ther* (1994) 16, 804–14.
9. Thebault JJ, Aiache JM, Mazoyer F, Cardot JM. The influence of food on the bioavailability of a slow release theophylline preparation. *Clin Pharmacokinet* (1987) 13, 267–72.
10. Lefebvre RA, Belpaire FM, Bogaert MG. Influence of food on steady state serum concentrations of theophylline from two controlled-release preparations. *Int J Clin Pharmacol Ther Toxicol* (1988) 26, 375–9.
11. Fassihi AR, Dowse R, Robertson SSD. Effect of dietary cellulose on the absorption and bioavailability of theophylline. *Int J Pharmaceutics* (1989) 50, 79–82.
12. Kappas A, Anderson KE, Conney AH, Alvares AP. Influence of dietary protein and carbohydrate on antipyrine and theophylline metabolism in man. *Clin Pharmacol Ther* (1976) 20, 643–53.
13. Feldman CH, Hutchinson VE, Pippenger CE, Blumenfeld TA, Feldman BR, Davis WJ. Effect of dietary protein and carbohydrate on theophylline metabolism in children. *Pediatrics* (1980) 66, 956–62.
14. Thompson PJ, Skypala I, Dawson S, McAllister WAC, Turner Warwick M. The effect of diet upon serum concentrations of theophylline. *Br J Clin Pharmacol* (1983) 16, 267–70.
15. Anderson KE, McCleery RB, Vesell ES, Vickers FF, Kappas A. Diet and cimetidine induce comparable changes in theophylline metabolism in normal subjects. *Hepatology* (1991) 13, 941–6.
16. Bouraoui A, Toumi A, Bouchahcha S, Boukef K, Brazier JL. Influence de l'alimentation épicée et piquante sur l'absorption de la théophylline. *Therapie* (1986) 41, 467–71.
17. Gal P, Layson R. Interference with oral theophylline absorption by continuous nasogastric feedings. *Ther Drug Monit* (1986) 8, 421–3.
18. Bhargava VO, Schaaf LJ, Berlinger WG, Jungnickel PW. Effect of an enteral nutrient formula on sustained-release theophylline absorption. *Ther Drug Monit* (1989) 11, 515–19.
19. Plezia PM, Thornley SM, Kramer TH, Armstrong EP. The influence of enteral feedings on sustained-release theophylline absorption. *Pharmacotherapy* (1990) 10, 356–61.
20. Ziegenbein RC. Theophylline clearance increase from increased amino acid in a CPN regimen. *Drug Intell Clin Pharm* (1987) 21, 220–1.
21. Cuddy PG, Bealer JF, Lyman EL, Pemberton LB. Theophylline disposition following parenteral feeding of malnourished patients. *Ann Pharmacother* (1993) 27, 846–51.
22. Pantuck EJ, Pantuck CB, Garland WA, Min BH, Wattenberg LW, Anderson KE, Kappas A, Conney AH. Stimulatory effect of Brussels sprouts and cabbage on human drug metabolism. *Clin Pharmacol Ther* (1979) 25, 88–95.
23. Kleman MI, Overvik E, Poellinger L, Gustafsson JA. Induction of cytochrome P4501A isoenzymes by heterocyclic amines and other food-derived compounds. *Princess Takamatsu Symp* (1995) 23, 163–71.
24. Kappas A, Alvares AP, Anderson KE, Pantuck EJ, Pantuck CB, Chang R, Conney AH. Effect of charcoal-broiled beef on antipyrine and theophylline metabolism. *Clin Pharmacol Ther* (1979) 23, 445–50.
25. Peng W-X, Li H-D, Zhou H-H. Effect of daidzein on CYP1A2 activity and pharmacokinetics of theophylline in healthy volunteers. *Eur J Clin Pharmacol* (2002) 59, 237–41.

Theophylline + Furosemide

Furosemide is reported to increase, decrease or to have no effect on serum theophylline levels. Both theophylline and diuretics can cause hypokalaemia, which may be additive.

Clinical evidence

In 8 asthmatics the mean peak serum level of a 300-mg dose of sustained-release theophylline was reduced by 41%, from 12.14 to 7.16 mg/L by a single 25-mg oral dose of furosemide.[1] Conversely, 10 patients with asthma, chronic bronchitis or emphysema, receiving a continuous maintenance infusion of aminophylline, had a 21% rise in their serum theophylline levels, from 13.7 to 16.6 mg/L, 4 hours after being given a 40-mg intravenous dose of furosemide over 2 minutes.[2] A crossover study in 12 healthy subjects failed to find any change in steady-state plasma theophylline levels when two 20-mg doses of oral furosemide were given 4 hours apart, although the overall renal clearance of theophylline was reduced.[3]

Four premature neonates, two given oral and two given intravenous theophylline with furosemide had a fall in steady-state serum theophylline levels from 8 mg/L down to 2 to 3 mg/L when furosemide was given within 30 minutes of the theophylline.[4]

A randomised, placebo-controlled study in 24 infants receiving ECMO (extracorporeal membrane oxygenation) found that theophylline 2 mg/kg enhanced the response to diuresis with furosemide 1 mg/kg. If the response were maintained over a 24-hour period an extra 110 mL/kg of fluid would have been lost.[5]

Mechanism

Not understood, although in theory furosemide may cause increased renal excretion of theophylline, which could explain the reduced levels.

Importance and management

Information is limited and the outcome of concurrent use is inconsistent and uncertain. If both drugs are used be aware of the potential for changes in serum theophylline levels. Consider measuring levels, and make appropriate dosage adjustments as necessary. Both theophylline and diuretics can cause hypokalaemia, and the possibility that this may additive on concurrent use should be considered. More study is needed to assess the clinical significance of the effects of theophylline and furosemide on diuresis.

1. Carpentiere G, Marino S, Castello F. Furosemide and theophylline. *Ann Intern Med* (1985) 103, 957.
2. Conlon PF, Grambau GR, Johnson CE, Weg JG. Effect of intravenous furosemide on serum theophylline concentration. *Am J Hosp Pharm* (1981) 38, 1345–7.
3. Jänicke U-A, Krüdewagen B, Schulz A, Gundert-Remy U. Absence of a clinically significant interaction between theophylline and furosemide. *Eur J Clin Pharmacol* (1987) 33, 487–91.
4. Toback JW, Gilman ME. Theophylline-furosemide inactivation? *Pediatrics* (1983) 71, 140–1.
5. Lochan SR, Adeniyi-Jones S, Assadi FK, Frey BM, Marcus S, Baumgart S. Coadministration of theophylline enhances diuretic response to furosemide in infants during extracorporeal membrane oxygenation: a randomized controlled pilot study. *J Pediatr* (1998) 133, 86–9.

Theophylline + Grapefruit juice

Grapefruit juice does not significantly alter theophylline pharmacokinetics.

Clinical evidence, mechanism, importance and management

In one study, 12 healthy subjects were given a single 200-mg oral dose of theophylline solution (*Euphyllin*) diluted in either 100 mL of grapefruit juice or water, followed by another 900 mL of juice or water over the next 16 hours. The pharmacokinetics of the theophylline were found to be unchanged by the grapefruit juice.[1]

The authors of this study had previously shown that grapefruit juice had a small effect on the pharmacokinetics of 'caffeine', (p.1165), and that one of the constituents of grapefruit juice (naringenin) inhibited the cytochrome P450 isoenzyme CYP1A2 (the principal enzyme in theophylline metabolism) *in vitro*. However, most clinically relevant interactions between drugs and grapefruit juice are considered to occur because grapefruit juice inhibits intestinal CYP3A4.

There would seem to be no reason why patients taking theophylline should avoid grapefruit juice.

1. Fuhr U, Maier A, Keller A, Steinijans VW, Sauter R, Staib AH. Lacking effect of grapefruit juice on theophylline pharmacokinetics. *Int J Clin Pharmacol Ther* (1995) 33, 311–14.

Theophylline + Griseofulvin

Griseofulvin does not appear to alter the pharmacokinetics of theophylline to a clinically relevant extent.

Clinical evidence, mechanism, importance and management

A study was initiated because it was suspected that griseofulvin might possibly interact with theophylline. In 12 healthy subjects griseofulvin 500 mg daily for 8 days reduced the half-life of theophylline from 6.6 to 5.7 hours, and increased the clearance of two of its metabolites, after a single oral dose of aminophylline (*Teofylamin*). However, these changes are far too small to usually have any clinical relevance.[1] There would appear to be no reason for avoiding concurrent use.

1. Rasmussen BB, Jeppesen U, Gaist D, Brøsen K. Griseofulvin and fluvoxamine interactions with the metabolism of theophylline. *Ther Drug Monit* (1997) 19, 56–62.

Theophylline + H_2-receptor antagonists

Cimetidine raises theophylline serum levels and toxicity may develop. However, the extent of the interaction is unlikely to be clinically relevant in most patients with low-dose cimetidine. Famotidine, nizatidine, ranitidine and roxatidine appear not to interact.

Clinical evidence

(a) Cimetidine

A number of case reports describe significantly increased theophylline levels, including many that were toxic, in patients (adults and children) given oral or intravenous aminophylline or theophylline with cimetidine.[1-6] A few cases describe serious adverse effects such as seizures.[3,4]

In a large number of pharmacokinetic studies healthy subjects were given oral or intravenous aminophylline or theophylline[7-15] and patients were given oral or intravenous theophylline[16-20] with oral cimetidine 800 mg to 1.2 g daily in divided doses for 4 to 10 days. It was clearly shown that cimetidine prolonged the theophylline half-life by about 30 to 65% and reduced theophylline clearance by about 20 to 40%. Steady-state serum theophylline levels were raised about one-third.[16,17,20] The effect of cimetidine was maximal in 3 days in the one study assessing this.[16] The extent of the interaction did not differ between cimetidine 1.2 g daily and 2.4 g daily in one study,[10] although two further studies found that cimetidine 800 mg daily had less effect than cimetidine 1.2 g daily.[12,21] A study investigating low-dose cimetidine (200 mg twice daily; UK non-prescription dosage) found only a 12% decrease in theophylline clearance.[22]

Two studies found that the effect of cimetidine did not differ between young and elderly subjects,[12,23] whereas another found it was more pronounced in the elderly.[21] The effects of cimetidine did not differ between smokers and non-smokers in one study,[24] but were more pronounced in smokers in another.[25] In a further study the effects of cimetidine were not affected by gender.[21] Three studies found that the inhibitory effects of cimetidine and 'ciprofloxacin', (p.1192), were additive.[23,26,27]

Three studies found that intravenous cimetidine also inhibited the clearance of theophylline (given as intravenous aminophylline or sustained-release theophylline).[28-30] In one of these, oral and intravenous cimetidine reduced theophylline clearance to the same extent, but when clearance was corrected for the lower bioavailability of the oral cimetidine, oral cimetidine resulted in a greater inhibition than intravenous cimetidine.[28] Another study found that the effects of a continuous 50-mg/hour infusion of cimetidine were similar to those of an intermittent infusion of 300 mg every 6 hours.[29]

In contrast, a further study[31] in healthy subjects found no clinically important interaction between intravenous aminophylline and an intravenous cimetidine infusion, but the aminophylline was given only 12 hours after starting the cimetidine, which may be insufficient for cimetidine to have had an effect. Similarly, a more recent study in 18 critically ill patients given a continuous 50-mg/hour intravenous infusion of cimetidine and low-dose aminophylline 10.8 mg/hour for just 48 hours found no clinically important interaction.[32]

(b) Famotidine

Famotidine 40 mg twice daily for 5 days had no effect on the pharmacokinetics of theophylline (given as intravenous aminophylline) in 10 healthy subjects.[14] In another study, 16 patients with bronchial asthma or chronic obstructive pulmonary disease (COPD) found that famotidine 20 mg twice daily for at least 3 days did not affect the clearance of theophylline.[33] Two further studies also found no interaction between intravenous theophylline and famotidine 20 or 40 mg twice daily for 4 or 9 days in COPD patients.[19,34] In a post-marketing surveillance study it was noted that 4 asthmatics taking theophylline had also taken famotidine 40 mg daily for 4 to 8 weeks without any problems.[35] In contrast, in a patient with COPD and liver impairment, the AUC and serum levels of an intravenous dose of theophylline were raised by 78% and the clearance was halved by famotidine 40 mg daily for 8 days.[36] A later study by the same authors in 7 patients with COPD similarly treated, but with normal liver function, found that the AUC of theophylline was increased by 56% and its clearance was reduced by 35% by famotidine.[37]

(c) Nizatidine

A study in 17 patients with chronic obstructive pulmonary disease found that nizatidine 150 mg twice daily for a month had no effect on the steady-state pharmacokinetics of theophylline.[20] However, there were 6 reports of apparent interactions in the Spontaneous Adverse Drug Reaction Database of the FDA in the US up to the end of August 1989. Four patients taking theophylline developed elevated serum theophylline levels, with symptoms of toxicity in at least one case, when given nizatidine. The problems resolved when either both drugs, or just nizatidine were stopped.[38]

(d) Ranitidine

Many studies in healthy subjects (given intravenous aminophylline or oral theophylline)[10,11,15,39-41] and patients (given sustained-release theophylline)[17,20,42-45] have failed to find that ranitidine affects the pharmacokinetics of theophylline, even in daily doses far in excess of those used clinically (up to 4.2 g of ranitidine daily).[39] However, there are 7 reports describing a total of 10 patients, who developed theophylline toxicity when given ranitidine with sustained-release theophylline[46-51] or intravenous aminophylline.[52] The validity of a number of these reports has been questioned,[53-56] with the authors subsequently modifying some.[57,58]

(e) Roxatidine

Roxatidine 150 mg daily did not affect the clearance of theophylline.[59] Similarly, in 9 healthy subjects, roxatidine 150 mg twice daily did not significantly change the pharmacokinetics of a single 250-mg intravenous dose of aminophylline.[60]

Mechanism

Cimetidine is an enzyme inhibitor that reduces the metabolism (predominantly *N*-demethylation)[61] of theophylline by the cytochrome P450 isoenzyme CYP1A2 in the liver, thereby raising its serum levels. Famotidine, nizatidine and ranitidine do not have enzyme-inhibiting effects so that it is not clear why they sometimes appear to behave like cimetidine.

Importance and management

The interaction between theophylline and cimetidine is very well documented (not all the references being listed here), very well established and clinically important. Theophylline serum levels normally rise by about one-third, but much greater increases have been seen in individual patients. Monitor theophylline levels closely. Note that in one study the peak effect was reached in 3 days. Initial theophylline dose reductions of 30 to 50% have been suggested to avoid toxicity.[4] Alternatively, use one of the other H_2-receptor antagonists, or consider changing to a proton pump inhibitor, see 'Theophylline + Proton pump inhibitors', p.1191. The effect of low-dose (e.g. UK non-prescription dose) cimetidine is unlikely to be clinically relevant unless theophylline levels are at the higher end of the therapeutic range. The situation with famotidine, nizatidine and ranitidine is not totally clear. They would not be expected to interact because they are not enzyme inhibitors like cimetidine, but very occasionally and unpredictably they appear to do so. Nevertheless, current opinion is that normally no special precautions are needed with these H_2-receptor antagonists,[54] or roxatidine.

Note that some of the symptoms of theophylline toxicity, such as nausea, vomiting and abdominal pain, are similar to those of gastrointestinal ulceration. It is important to check the theophylline level should patients present with these symptoms, to prevent a misdiagnosis.

1. Weinberger MM, Smith G, Milavetz G, Hendeles L. Decreased theophylline clearance due to cimetidine. *N Engl J Med* (1981) 304, 672.
2. Campbell MA, Plachetka JR, Jackson JE, Moon JF, Finley PR. Cimetidine decreases theophylline clearance. *Ann Intern Med* (1981) 95, 68–9.
3. Lofgren RP, Gilbertson RA. Cimetidine and theophylline. *Ann Intern Med* (1982) 96, 378.
4. Bauman JH, Kimelblatt BJ, Carracio TR, Silverman HM, Simon GI, Beck GJ. Cimetidine-theophylline interaction. Report of four patients. *Ann Allergy* (1982) 48, 100–102.
5. Fenje PC, Isles AF, Baltodano A, MacLeod SM, Soldin S. Interaction of cimetidine and theophylline in two infants. *Can Med Assoc J* (1982) 126, 1178.
6. Uzzan D, Uzzan B, Bernard N, Caubarrere I. Interaction médicamenteuse de la cimétidine et de la théophylline. *Nouv Presse Med* (1982) 11, 1950.
7. Jackson JE, Powell JR, Wandell M, Bentley J, Dorr R. Cimetidine decreases theophylline clearance. *Am Rev Respir Dis* (1981) 123, 615–17.
8. Roberts RK, Grice J, Wood L, Petroff V, McGuffie C. Cimetidine impairs the elimination of theophylline and antipyrine. *Gastroenterology* (1981) 81, 19–21.
9. Reitberg DP, Bernhard H, Schentag JJ. Alteration of theophylline clearance and half-life by cimetidine in normal volunteers. *Ann Intern Med* (1981) 95, 582–5.
10. Powell JR, Rogers JF, Wargin WA, Cross RE, Eshelman FN. Inhibition of theophylline clearance by cimetidine but not ranitidine. *Arch Intern Med* (1984) 144, 484–6.
11. Ferrari M, Angelini GP, Barozzi E, Olivieri M, Penna S, Accardi R. A comparative study of ranitidine and cimetidine effects on theophylline metabolism. *G Ital Mal Torace* (1984) 38, 31–4.
12. Cohen IA, Johnson CE, Berardi RR, Hyneck ML, Achem SR. Cimetidine-theophylline interaction: effects of age and cimetidine dose. *Ther Drug Monit* (1985) 7, 426–34.
13. Mulkey PM, Murphy JE, Shleifer NH. Steady-state theophylline pharmacokinetics during and after short-term cimetidine administration. *Clin Pharm* (1983) 2, 439–41.
14. Lin JH, Chremos AN, Chiou R, Yeh KC, Williams R. Comparative effect of famotidine and cimetidine on the pharmacokinetics of theophylline in normal volunteers. *Br J Clin Pharmacol* (1987) 24, 669–72.
15. Adebayo GI. Effects of equimolar doses of cimetidine and ranitidine on theophylline elimination. *Biopharm Drug Dispos* (1989) 10, 77–85.
16. Vestal RE, Thummel KE, Musser B, Mercer GD. Cimetidine inhibits theophylline clearance in patients with chronic obstructive pulmonary disease: A study using stable isotope methodology during multiple oral dose administration. *Br J Clin Pharmacol* (1983) 15, 411–18.
17. Boehning W. Effect of cimetidine and ranitidine on plasma theophylline in patients with chronic obstructive airways disease treated with theophylline and corticosteroids. *Eur J Clin Pharmacol* (1990) 38, 43–5.
18. Roberts RK, Grice J, McGuffie C. Cimetidine-theophylline interaction in patients with chronic obstructive airways disease. *Med J Aust* (1984) 140, 279–80.
19. Bachmann K, Sullivan TJ, Reese JH, Jauregui L, Miller K, Scott M, Yeh KC, Stepanavage M, King JD, Schwartz J. Controlled study of the putative interaction between famotidine and theophylline in patients with chronic obstructive pulmonary disease. *J Clin Pharmacol* (1995) 35, 529–35.
20. Bachmann K, Sullivan TJ, Mauro LS, Martin M, Jauregui L, Levine L. Comparative investigation of the influence of nizatidine, ranitidine, and cimetidine on the steady-state pharmacokinetics of theophylline in COPD patients. *J Clin Pharmacol* (1992) 32, 476–82.
21. Seaman JJ, Randolph WC, Peace KE, Frank WO, Dickson B, Putterman K, Young MD. Effects of two cimetidine dosage regimens on serum theophylline levels. *Postgrad Med: Custom Comm* (1985) 78, 47–53.
22. Nix DE, Di Cicco RA, Miller AK, Boyle DA, Boike SC, Zariffa N, Jorkasky DK, Schentag JJ. The effect of low-dose cimetidine (200 mg twice daily) on the pharmacokinetics of theophylline. *J Clin Pharmacol* (1999) 39, 855–65.
23. Loi C-M, Parker BM, Cusack BJ, Vestal RE. Aging and drug interactions.III. Individual and combined effects of cimetidine and ciprofloxacin on theophylline metabolism in healthy male and female nonsmokers. *J Pharmacol Exp Ther* (1997) 280, 627–37.
24. Cusack BJ, Dawson GW, Mercer GD, Vestal RE. Cigarette smoking and theophylline metabolism: effects of cimetidine. *Clin Pharmacol Ther* (1985) 37, 330–6.
25. Grygiel JJ, Miners JO, Drew R, Birkett DJ. Differential effects of cimetidine on theophylline metabolic pathways. *Eur J Clin Pharmacol* (1984) 26, 335–40.
26. Davis RL, Quenzer RW, Kelly HW, Powell JR. Effect of the addition of ciprofloxacin on theophylline pharmacokinetics in subjects inhibited by cimetidine. *Ann Pharmacother* (1992) 26, 11–13.
27. Loi C-M, Parker BM, Cusack BJ, Vestal RE. Individual and combined effects of cimetidine and ciprofloxacin on theophylline metabolism in male nonsmokers. *Br J Clin Pharmacol* (1993) 36, 195–200.
28. Cremer KF, Secor J, Speeg KV. Effect of route of administration on the cimetidine-theophylline drug interaction. *J Clin Pharmacol* (1989) 29, 451–6.
29. Gutfeld MB, Welage LS, Walawander CA, Wilton JH, Harrison NJ. The influence of intravenous cimetidine dosing regimens on the disposition of theophylline. *J Clin Pharmacol* (1989) 29, 665–9.
30. Krstenansky PM, Javaheri S, Thomas JP, Thomas RL. Effect of continuous cimetidine infusion on steady-state theophylline concentration. *Clin Pharm* (1989) 8, 206–9.
31. Gaska JA, Tietze KJ, Rocci ML, Vlasses PH. Theophylline pharmacokinetics: effect of continuous versus intermittent cimetidine IV infusion. *J Clin Pharmacol* (1991) 31, 668–72.
32. Mojtahedzadeh M, Sadray S, Hadjibabaie M, Fasihi M, Rezaee S. Determination of theophylline clearance after cimetidine infusion in critically ill patients. *J Infus Nurs* (2003) 26, 234–8.
33. Asamoto H, Kokura M, Kawakami A, Sawano T, Sasaki Y, Kohara N, Kitamura Y, Oishi T, Morishita H. Effect of famotidine on theophylline clearance in asthma and COPD patients. *Arerugi* (1987) 36, 1012–17.
34. Verdiani P, DiCarlo S, Baronti A. Famotidine effects on theophylline pharmacokinetics in subjects affected by COPD. Comparison with cimetidine and placebo. *Chest* (1988) 94, 807–10.
35. Chichmanian RM, Mignot G, Spreux A, Jean-Girard C, Hofliger P. Tolérance de la famotidine. Étude due réseau médecins sentinelles en pharmacovigilance. *Therapie* (1992) 47, 239–43.
36. Dal Negro R, Turco P, Pomari C, Trevisan F. Famotidina e teofillina: interferenza farmacocinetica cimetidino-simile? *G Ital Mal Torace* (1988) 42, 185–6.
37. Dal Negro R, Pomari C, Turco P. Famotidine and theophylline pharmacokinetics. An unexpected cimetidine-like interaction in patients with chronic obstructive pulmonary disease. *Clin Pharmacokinet* (1993) 24, 255–8.
38. Shinn AF. Unrecognized drug interactions with famotidine and nizatidine. *Arch Intern Med* (1991) 151, 810–14.
39. Kelly HW, Powell JR, Donohue JF. Ranitidine at very large doses does not inhibit theophylline elimination. *Clin Pharmacol Ther* (1986) 39, 577–81.
40. McEwen J, McMurdo MET, Moreland TA. The effects of once-daily dosing with ranitidine and cimetidine on theophylline pharmacokinetics. *Eur J Drug Metab Pharmacokinet* (1988) 13, 201–5.
41. Kehoe WA, Sands CD, Feng Long L, Hui Lan H, Harralson AF. The effect of ranitidine on theophylline metabolism in healthy ethnic Koreans. *Pharmacotherapy* (1994) 14, 373.
42. Seggev JS, Barzilay M, Schey G. No evidence for interaction between ranitidine and theophylline. *Arch Intern Med* (1987) 147, 179–80.
43. Zarogoulidis K, Economidis D, Paparoglou A, Pneumaticos I, Sevastou P, Tsopouridis A, Papaioanou A. Effect of ranitidine on theophylline plasma levels in patients with COPD. *Eur Respir J* (1988) 1 (Suppl 2), 195S.
44. Pérez-Blanco FJ, Huertas González JM, Morata Garcia de la Puerta IJ, Saucedo Sánchez R. Interacción de ranitidina con teofilina. *Rev Clin Esp* (1995) 195, 359–60.
45. Cukier A, Vargas FS, Santos SRCJ, Donzella H, Terra-Filho M, Teixeira LR, Light RW. Theophylline-ranitidine interaction in elderly COPD patients. *Braz J Med Biol Res* (1995) 28, 875–9.
46. Fernandes E, Melewicz FM. Ranitidine and theophylline. *Ann Intern Med* (1984) 100, 459.
47. Gardner ME, Sikorski GW. Ranitidine and theophylline. *Ann Intern Med* (1985) 102, 559.
48. Roy AK, Cuda MP, Levine RA. Induction of theophylline toxicity and inhibition of clearance rates by ranitidine. *Am J Med* (1988) 85, 525–7.

49. Dietemann-Molard A, Popin E, Oswald-Mammosser M, Colas des Francs V, Pauli G. Intoxication à la théophylline par interaction avec la ranitidine à dose élevée. *Presse Med* (1988) 17, 280.
50. Skinner MH, Lenert L, Blaschke TF. Theophylline toxicity subsequent to ranitidine administration: a possible drug-drug interaction. *Am J Med* (1989) 86, 129–32.
51. Hegman GW, Gilbert RP. Ranitidine-theophylline interaction — fact or fiction? *DICP Ann Pharmacother* (1991) 25, 21–5.
52. Murialdo G, Piovano PL, Costelli P, Fonzi S, Barberis A, Ghia M. Seizures during concomitant treatment with theophylline and ranitidine: a case report. *Ann Ital Med Int* (1990) 5, 413–17.
53. Muir JG, Powell JR, Baumann JH. Induction of theophylline toxicity and inhibition of clearance rates by ranitidine. *Am J Med* (1989) 86, 513–14.
54. Kelly HW. Comment: ranitidine does not inhibit theophylline metabolism. *Ann Pharmacother* (1991) 25, 1139.
55. Williams DM, Figg WD, Pleasants RA. Comment: ranitidine does not inhibit theophylline metabolism. *Ann Pharmacother* (1991) 25, 1140.
56. Dobbs JH, Smith RN. Ranitidine and theophylline. *Ann Intern Med* (1984) 100, 769.
57. Roy AK. Induction of theophylline toxicity and inhibition of clearance rates by ranitidine. *Am J Med* (1989) 86, 513.
58. Hegman GW. Comment: ranitidine does not inhibit theophylline metabolism. *Ann Pharmacother* (1991) 25, 1140–41.
59. Labs RA. Interaction of roxatidine acetate with antacids, food and other drugs. *Drugs* (1988) 35 (Suppl 3), 82–9.
60. Yoshimura N, Takeuchi H, Ogata H, Ishioka T, Aoi R. Effects of roxatidine acetate hydrochloride and cimetidine on the pharmacokinetics of theophylline in healthy subjects. *Int J Clin Pharmacol Ther Toxicol* (1989) 27, 308–12.
61. Naline E, Sanceaume M, Pays M, Advenier C. Application of theophylline metabolite assays to the exploration of liver microsome oxidative function in man. *Fundam Clin Pharmacol* (1988) 2, 341–51.

Theophylline + Hormonal contraceptives

Theophylline clearance is reduced to some extent in women taking a combined oral contraceptive, but no toxicity has been reported.

Clinical evidence

The total plasma clearance of a single 4-mg/kg oral dose of aminophylline was about 30% lower in 8 women taking a combined oral contraceptive (**ethinylestradiol/norgestrel**, *Ovral*) than in 8 other women not taking oral contraceptives.[1] The theophylline half-life was also prolonged by about 30%, from 7.34 to 9.79 hours. Similar results were found in other studies in subjects given intravenous or oral aminophylline and combined oral contraceptives (**ethinylestradiol/norgestrel**, *Ovral* and **mestranol/etynodiol diacetate**, *Ovulen* or unnamed products).[2,3] In contrast, no significant differences were seen in the pharmacokinetics of theophylline (given as intravenous aminophylline) in 10 adolescent women (15 to 18 years) taking low-dose combined or sequential oral contraceptives (**ethinylestradiol/norethisterone**), when compared with age matched controls.[4] However, in the same women the clearance of oral theophylline was found to be reduced by 33% after they took a triphasic combined oral contraceptive for 3 to 4 months.[5] In a retrospective analysis of factors affecting theophylline clearance, the use of oral contraceptives was associated with a reduced theophylline clearance in women who smoked.[6]

Mechanism

Uncertain, but it seems possible that the oestrogenic component may inhibit the metabolism of the theophylline by the liver microsomal enzymes, thereby reducing its clearance.

Importance and management

An established interaction, but there seem to be no reports of theophylline toxicity resulting from concurrent use. Women taking combined oral contraceptives may need less theophylline than those not taking oral contraceptives. There is a small risk that patients with serum theophylline levels at the top end of the range may show some toxicity when oral contraceptives are added. It has been proposed that the effects may be more apparent with long-term, high-dose contraceptive use.[1,4]

1. Tornatore KM, Kanarkowski R, McCarthy TL, Gardner MJ, Yurchak AM, Jusko WJ. Effect of chronic oral contraceptive steroids on theophylline disposition. *Eur J Clin Pharmacol* (1982) 23, 129–34.
2. Roberts RK, Grice J, McGuffie C, Heilbronn L. Oral contraceptive steroids impair the elimination of theophylline. *J Lab Clin Med* (1983) 101, 821–5.
3. Gardner MJ, Tornatore KM, Jusko WJ, Kanarkowski R. Effects of tobacco smoking and oral contraceptive use on theophylline disposition. *Br J Clin Pharmacol* (1983) 16, 271–80.
4. Koren G, Chin TF, Correia J, Tesoro A, MacLeod S. Theophylline pharmacokinetics in adolescent females following coadministration of oral contraceptives. *Clin Invest Med* (1985) 8, 222–6.
5. Long DR, Roberts EA, Brill-Edwards M, Quaggin S, Correia J, Koren G, MacLeod SM. The effect of the oral contraceptive Ortho 7/7/7® on theophylline (T) clearance in non-smoking women aged 18–22. *Clin Invest Med* (1987) 10 (4 Suppl B), B59.
6. Jusko WJ, Gardner MJ, Mangione A, Schentag JJ, Koup JR, Vance JW. Factors affecting theophylline clearances: age, tobacco, marijuana, cirrhosis, congestive heart failure, obesity, oral contraceptives, benzodiazepines, barbiturates, and ethanol. *J Pharm Sci* (1979) 68, 1358–66.

Theophylline + Idrocilamide

Idrocilamide given orally can increase serum theophylline levels.

Clinical evidence, mechanism, importance and management

In 6 healthy subjects oral idrocilamide 600 mg daily for 3 days then 1.2 g for 4 days increased the half-life of a single dose of theophylline 2.5-fold, from 8.5 to 21.6 hours, and reduced the clearance by 67%.[1] This is due to a reduction in the liver metabolism caused by the idrocilamide (see also 'Caffeine + Idrocilamide', p.1165). Information is very limited but it indicates that concurrent use should be closely monitored. Anticipate the need to reduce the theophylline dosage with *oral* idrocilamide.

1. Lacroix C, Nouveau J, Hubscher Ph, Tardif D, Ray M, Goulle JP. Influence de l'idrocilamide sur le metabolisme de la theophylline. *Rev Pneumol Clin* (1986) 42, 164–6.

Theophylline + Imipenem

Seizures developed in three patients taking aminophylline or theophylline when they were given imipenem.

Clinical evidence, mechanism, importance and management

Two patients receiving intravenous aminophylline developed seizures within 11 to 56 hours of starting treatment with intravenous imipenem 500 mg every 6 to 8 hours. Seizures developed in a third patient taking theophylline after imipenem had been given for 6 days. In all 3, seizures occurred 2 to 3 hours after a dose of imipenem.[1] The reasons for this effect are not known. Theophylline serum levels appeared to be unchanged.[1] In an analysis of data from 1754 patients who had received imipenem in dose-ranging studies, 3% had seizures, and imipenem was judged to be associated with a third of these cases. However, the concurrent use of theophylline or aminophylline was not found to be a significant risk factor for the development of seizures with imipenem.[2] The general importance of these cases is therefore uncertain.

1. Semel JD, Allen N. Seizures in patients simultaneously receiving theophylline and imipenem or ciprofloxacin or metronidazole. *South Med J* (1991) 84, 465–8.
2. Calandra G, Lydick E, Carrigan J, Weiss L, Guess H. Factors predisposing to seizures in seriously ill infected patients receiving antibiotics: experience with imipenem/cilastatin. *Am J Med* (1988) 84, 911–18.

Theophylline + Influenza vaccines

Normally none of the influenza vaccines (whole-virion, split-virion and surface antigen) interact with theophylline, but there are three reports describing rises in serum theophylline levels in a few patients (some to toxic levels), which was attributed to the use of an influenza vaccine.

Clinical evidence

(a) Evidence of no interaction

Mean steady-state serum theophylline levels were not altered by a trivalent split-virion influenza vaccine (*Fluzone*) in 12 patients with asthma, although one patient had an increase in levels (see (*b*), below). Levels were measured before vaccination and 1, 3, 7 and 14 days after vaccination.[1] Theophylline levels were unchanged in 5 patients with COPD when they were given 0.5 mL of influenza vaccine (*Fluogen*).[2] Similarly, no evidence of a rise in theophylline levels was found in a number of other studies in healthy subjects, both adults and children, receiving maintenance theophylline or aminophylline, and given various trivalent split-virion vaccines[3-6] including *Fluzone*,[7] *Fluogen*,[8-10] *Influvac*,[11] Mutagrip.[12] In addition, no change in the pharmacokinetics of theophylline (given as oral aminophylline) was found after use of a whole-virion vaccine in healthy adults.[13] No evidence of serious theophylline toxicity was seen in 119 elderly people taking maintenance theophylline and given an unspecified influenza vaccine.[14]

(b) Evidence of an interaction

Three patients who had been taking oral choline theophyllinate (oxtriphylline) 200 mg (equivalent to 128 mg of theophylline) every 6 hours for at least 7 days had a rise in their serum theophylline levels of 219%, 89%, and 85%, respectively, within 12 to 24 hours of receiving 0.5 mL of trivalent split-virion influenza vaccine (*Fluogen*, Parke Davis). In some cases effects persisted for up to 72 hours, and two patients showed signs of theophylline toxicity. A subsequent study in 4 healthy subjects found that the same dose of vaccine more than doubled the half-life of theophylline, from 3.3 to 7.3 hours, and halved its clearance.[15]

A girl had a rise in theophylline levels from 20 to 34 mg/L (with no sign of toxicity) within 5 hours of being given a trivalent split-virion vaccine.[16] In a study where 11 of 12 patients had no increase in theophylline levels after vaccination with *Fluzone*, one woman showed a rise in levels (from 10 to 24.5 mg/L) accompanied by headaches and palpitations.[1]

The clearance of theophylline (given as choline theophyllinate) was reduced by 25% one day after influenza vaccination (trivalent influenza vaccine, *Fluogen*, Parke Davis) in 8 healthy subjects, but this was of borderline significance. Theophylline metabolism had returned to pre-vaccination levels after 7 days.[17]

A patient with COPD treated with sustained-release theophylline 300 mg twice daily (theophylline levels between 7 and 12 mg/L) developed nausea and palpitations the day after he received a trivalent influenza vaccination (*Fluogen*). His theophylline level was increased to 26 [mg/L]. His dose was reduced to 200 mg twice daily and the adverse effects resolved. However, a few days later his COPD had become symptomatic and the theophylline level was found to be subtherapeutic, so the dose was raised to 300 mg twice daily, as before.[18]

Mechanism

Uncertain. If an interaction occurs, it has been suggested it is probably due to inhibition of the liver enzymes concerned with the metabolism of theophylline, possibly secondary to interferon production, resulting in theophylline accumulation in the body.[15,17] One suggestion is that vaccine contaminants, which are potent interferon-inducing agents, may be responsible (rather than the vaccine itself), so that an interaction would seem to be less likely with modern highly-purified subunit vaccines.[19] In one study where an interaction occurred, an increase in serum interferon levels was detected,[17] whereas, in two of the studies showing no interaction, no interferon production was detected.[10,13] Influenza infection *per se* can result in decreased theophylline clearance and theophylline toxicity.[20]

Importance and management

A very thoroughly investigated interaction, the weight of evidence being that no adverse interaction normally occurs with any type of influenza vaccine in children, adults or the elderly. Even so, bearing in mind the occasional and unexplained reports of an interaction[1,15,16,18] it would seem prudent to monitor the effects of concurrent use (for nausea headaches, palpitations), although problems are very unlikely to arise now that purer vaccines are available (see 'Mechanism'). Note that any rise in theophylline levels is likely to be transient.

1. Fischer RG, Booth BH, Mitchell DQ, Kibbe AH. Influence of trivalent influenza vaccine on serum theophylline levels. *Can Med Assoc J* (1982) 126, 1312–13.
2. Britton L, Ruben FL. Serum theophylline levels after influenza vaccine. *Can Med Assoc J* (1982) 126, 1375.
3. Stults BM, Hashisaki PA. Influenza vaccination and theophylline pharmacokinetics in patients with chronic obstructive lung disease. *West J Med* (1983) 139, 651–4.
4. Gomolin IH, Chapron DJ, Luhan PA. Lack of effect of influenza vaccine on theophylline levels and warfarin anticoagulation in the elderly. *J Am Geriatr Soc* (1985) 33, 269–72.
5. Feldman CH, Rabinowitz A, Levison M, Klein R, Feldman BR, Davis WJ. Effects of influenza vaccine on theophylline metabolism in children with asthma. *Am Rev Respir Dis* (1985) 131 (4 Suppl), A9.
6. Bryett KA, Levy J, Pariente R, Gobert P, Falquet JCV. Influenza vaccine and theophylline metabolism. Is there an interaction? *Acta Ther* (1989) 15, 49–58.
7. Goldstein RS, Cheung OT, Seguin R, Lobley G, Johnson AC. Decreased elimination of theophylline after influenza vaccination. *Can Med Assoc J* (1982) 126, 470.
8. San Joaquin VH, Reyes S, Marks MI. Influenza vaccination in asthmatic children on maintenance theophylline therapy. *Clin Pediatr (Phila)* (1982) 21, 724–6.
9. Bukowskyj M, Munt PW, Wigle R, Nakatsu K. Theophylline clearance. Lack of effect of influenza vaccination and ascorbic acid. *Am Rev Respir Dis* (1984) 129, 672–5.
10. Grabowski N, May JJ, Pratt DS, Richtsmeier WJ, Bertino JS, Sorge KF. The effect of split virus influenza vaccination on theophylline pharmacokinetics. *Am Rev Respir Dis* (1985) 131, 934–8.
11. Winstanley PA, Tjia J, Back DJ, Hobson D, Breckenridge AM. Lack of effect of highly purified subunit influenza vaccination on theophylline metabolism. *Br J Clin Pharmacol* (1985) 20, 47–53.
12. Jonkman JHG, Wymenga ASC, de Zeeuw RA, van der Boon WVJ, Beugelink JK, Oosterhuis B, Jedema JN. No effect of influenza vaccination on the theophylline pharmacokinetics as studied by ultraviolet spectrophotometry, HPLC, and EMIT assay methods. *Ther Drug Monit* (1988) 10, 345–8.
13. Hannan SE, May JJ, Pratt DS, Richtsmeier WJ, Bertino JS. The effect of whole virus influenza vaccination on theophylline pharmacokinetics. *Am Rev Respir Dis* (1988) 137, 903–6.
14. Patriarca PA, Kendal AP, Stricof RL, Weber JA, Meissner MK, Dateno B. Influenza vaccination and warfarin or theophylline toxicity in nursing-home residents. *N Engl J Med* (1983) 308, 1601–2.
15. Renton KW, Gray JD, Hall RI. Decreased elimination of theophylline after influenza vaccination. *Can Med Assoc J* (1980) 123, 288–90.
16. Walker S, Schreiber L, Middelkamp JN. Serum theophylline levels after influenza vaccination. *Can Med Assoc J* (1981) 125, 243–4.
17. Meredith CG, Christian CD, Johnson RF, Troxell R, Davis GL, Schenker S. Effects of influenza virus vaccine on hepatic drug metabolism. *Clin Pharmacol Ther* (1985) 37, 396–401.
18. Hamdy RC, Micklewright M, Beecham VF, Moore SW. Influenza vaccine may enhance theophylline toxicity. A case report and review of the literature. *J Tenn Med Assoc* (1995) 88, 463–4.
19. Winstanley PA, Back DJ, Breckenridge AM. Inhibition of theophylline metabolism by interferon. *Lancet* (1987) ii, 1340.
20. Kraemer MJ, Furukawa CT, Koup JR, Shapiro GG, Pierson WE, Bierman CW. Altered theophylline clearance during an influenza B outbreak. *Pediatrics* (1982) 69, 476–80.

Theophylline + Interferons

Theophylline clearance is reduced by up to 50% by interferon alfa and by about 25% by interferon beta.

Clinical evidence

A study in 5 patients with stable chronic active hepatitis B and 4 healthy subjects found that 20 hours after being given a single 9- or 18-million unit intramuscular injection of interferon (recombinant human interferon alfa A), the clearance of theophylline (given as intravenous aminophylline) was approximately halved (range 33 to 81%) in 8 of the 9 subjects. The mean theophylline elimination half-life was increased from 6.3 to 10.7 hours (1.5 to sixfold increases). In the healthy subjects the theophylline clearances were noted to have returned to their former values 4 weeks after the study.[1]

Another study, in 11 healthy subjects given interferon alfa (*Roferon-A*) 3 million units daily for 3 days, found that the terminal half-life and AUC of theophylline (given as aminophylline) were only increased by 10 to 15%, with a similar decrease in clearance.[2] In 7 patients with cancer interferon alfa (*Intron-A*) 3 million units given 3 times a week for 2 weeks decreased the clearance of a single 150-mg oral dose of theophylline by 33%.[3]

Seven patients with chronic hepatitis C receiving interferon beta 3 to 9 million units daily for 8 weeks were given a single 250-mg dose of intravenous aminophylline. Interferon beta reduced the total body clearance of theophylline by 26% (range 5.8 to 57%) and increased the elimination half-life by 39% (range 27 to 139%), but had no significant effect on the volume of distribution, although there was wide inter-patient variability.[4]

Mechanism

Interferon alfa inhibits the liver enzymes[5] concerned with the metabolism of some drugs, such as theophylline. Therefore the metabolism of theophylline is reduced, and it accumulates. Interferon beta also appears to inhibit liver enzymes.[4]

Importance and management

Direct information appears to be limited to these reports, only one of which found clear evidence of a clinically important interaction. So far there appear to be no reports of toxicity but it would seem prudent to monitor concurrent use closely (nausea, headaches, palpitations), taking theophylline levels if necessary. Patients with enhanced metabolism (e.g. smokers) are predicted to be most at risk.[1]

1. Williams SJ, Baird-Lambert JA, Farrell GC. Inhibition of theophylline metabolism by interferon. *Lancet* (1987) ii, 939–41.
2. Jonkman JHG, Nicholson KG, Farrow PR, Eckert M, Grasmeijer G, Oosterhuis B, De Noorde OE, Guentert TW. Effects of α-interferon on theophylline pharmacokinetics and metabolism. *Br J Clin Pharmacol* (1989) 27, 795–802.
3. Israel BC, Blouin RA, McIntyre W, Shedlofsky SI. Effects of interferon-α monotherapy on hepatic drug metabolism in cancer patients. *Br J Clin Pharmacol* (1993) 36, 229–35.
4. Okuno H, Takasu M, Kano H, Seki T, Shiozaki Y, Inoue K. Depression of drug-metabolising activity in the human liver by interferon-β. *Hepatology* (1993) 17, 65–9.
5. Williams SJ, Farrell GC. Inhibition of antipyrine metabolism by interferon. *Br J Clin Pharmacol* (1986) 22, 610–12.

Theophylline + Ipriflavone

An isolated report describes increased theophylline levels in a patient given ipriflavone.

Clinical evidence, mechanism, importance and management

The theophylline serum levels of a patient with chronic obstructive pulmonary disease, taking sustained-release theophylline 300 mg twice daily, rose from 9.5 to 17.3 mg/L when ipriflavone 600 mg daily for about 4 weeks was taken. No symptoms of toxicity occurred. The serum theophylline levels returned to roughly the initial level when the ipriflavone was stopped, and rose again when it was restarted.[1] *In vitro* studies with human liver microsomes suggest that ipriflavone can inhibit the cytochrome P450 isoenzyme CYP1A2 and the demethylation of theophylline,[2,3] which would reduce the metabolism of theophylline and increase its levels.

Although so far only one case of this interaction has been reported, the *in vitro* studies suggest that it would be prudent to monitor the theophylline levels of any patient given ipriflavone, making any dosage reductions as necessary.

1. Takahashi J, Kawakatsu K, Wakayama T, Sawaoka H. Elevation of serum theophylline levels by ipriflavone in a patient with chronic obstructive pulmonary disease. *Eur J Clin Pharmacol* (1992) 43, 207–8.
2. Monostory K, Vereczkey L. The effect of ipriflavone and its main metabolites on theophylline biotransformation. *Eur J Drug Metab Pharmacokinet* (1996) 21, 61–6.
3. Monostory K, Vereczkey L, Lévai F, Szatmári I. Ipriflavone as an inhibitor of human cytochrome P450 enzymes. *Br J Pharmacol* (1998) 123, 605–10.

Theophylline + Leukotriene antagonists

Montelukast does not appear to alter theophylline levels. A single case report describes a rapid rise in theophylline levels in a patient given zafirlukast. Zafirlukast levels are modestly reduced by theophylline, but this does not appear to be clinically important.

Clinical evidence

(a) Montelukast

In a study in 16 healthy subjects, the pharmacokinetics of a single intravenous dose of theophylline were not significantly changed by montelukast 10 mg daily for 10 days, but when they were given montelukast 200 mg and 600 mg daily, the AUC of theophylline was reduced by 43% and 66%, respectively. These doses are 20 and 60-fold higher than the usual 10 mg daily dose,[1] and therefore the clinical relevance of these effects is unclear.

(b) Zafirlukast

When zafirlukast was given with theophylline, the mean serum levels of zafirlukast were reduced by 30%, but the serum theophylline levels remained unchanged.[2] In contrast, an isolated report describes a 15-year-old asthmatic taking sustained-release theophylline 300 mg twice daily (as well as inhaled fluticasone, salbutamol (albuterol) and salmeterol, and oral prednisolone) who became nauseous shortly after zafirlukast (dose not stated) was added to her treatment. An increase in her theophylline level from 11 to 24 mg/L was noted. The theophylline was stopped, and later attempts to reintroduce theophylline at lower doses resulted in the same dramatic increases in serum theophylline levels.[3]

Mechanism

Not understood.

Importance and management

Information about interactions between theophylline and montelukast seems to be limited. The study above indicates that when using normal clinical doses of montelukast no special precautions or dosage alterations are needed. Similarly, no adverse interaction would normally seem to occur with zafirlukast and theophylline; the isolated case is of doubtful general significance.

1. Malmstrom K, Schwartz J, Reiss TF, Sullivan TJ, Reese JH, Jauregui L, Miller K, Scott M, Shingo S, Peszek I, Larson P, Ebel D, Hunt TL, Huhn RD, Bachmann K. Effect of montelukast on single-dose theophylline pharmacokinetics. *Am J Ther* (1998) 5, 189–95.
2. Accolate (Zafirlukast). AstraZeneca UK Ltd. UK Summary of product characteristics, December 2004.
3. Katial RK, Stelzle RC, Bonner MW, Marino M, Cantilena LR, Smith LJ. A drug interaction between zafirlukast and theophylline. *Arch Intern Med* (1998) 158, 1713–5.

Theophylline + Loperamide

Loperamide delays the absorption of theophylline from a sustained-release preparation.

Clinical evidence, mechanism, importance and management

A study of the effects of altering the transit time of drugs through the small intestine found that when 12 healthy subjects were given high-dose loperamide (8 mg every 6 hours for a total of 8 doses), the rate, but not extent, of absorption of a single 600-mg dose of sustained-release theophylline (*Theo-24*) was decreased. The maximum serum theophylline levels were reduced from 4.6 to 3.2 micrograms/mL, and this peak level occurred at 20 hours instead of 11 hours. One suggested reason for these effects is that loperamide inhibits the movement of the gut, thereby decreasing the dissolution rate of the *Theo-24* pellets.[1] More study is needed to establish the clinical significance of the interaction in patients receiving long-term theophylline.

1. Bryson JC, Dukes GE, Kirby MG, Heizer WD, Powell JR. Effect of altering small bowel transit time on sustained release theophylline absorption. *J Clin Pharmacol* (1989) 29, 733–8.

Theophylline + Macrolides

Troleandomycin can increase serum theophylline levels, causing toxicity if the dosage is not reduced. Azithromycin, clarithromycin, dirithromycin, josamycin, midecamycin, rokitamycin, spiramycin, and telithromycin normally only cause modest changes in theophylline levels or do not interact at all. There are unexplained and isolated case reports of theophylline toxicity with josamycin and clarithromycin. Roxithromycin usually has no relevant interaction but a significant increase in theophylline levels was seen in one study. See also 'Theophylline + Macrolides; Erythromycin', p.1187.

Clinical evidence

(a) Azithromycin

In an analysis of the safety data from clinical studies of azithromycin, there was no evidence that the plasma levels of theophylline were affected in patients given both drugs.[1] Similarly, no adverse effects were reported in another clinical study of patients taking azithromycin and theophylline.[2] Azithromycin 250 mg twice daily did not affect the clearance or serum levels of theophylline in patients with asthma.[3] However, a 68-year-old man had a marked but transient fall in his serum theophylline level when azithromycin was withdrawn, and this was confirmed on rechallenge.[4] The same authors conducted a study in 4 healthy subjects given azithromycin 500 mg on day 1 then 250 mg daily for 4 days and sustained-release theophylline 200 mg twice daily. Theophylline levels were slightly elevated during the use of azithromycin, and a transient drop occurred 5 days after azithromycin was stopped.[5]

(b) Clarithromycin

Clarithromycin 250 mg twice daily for 7 days had no effect on the steady-state serum theophylline levels of 10 elderly patients with COPD.[6] Similarly, two other studies found that clarithromycin had little or no effect on theophylline pharmacokinetics.[3,7] Another study in healthy subjects given clarithromycin 500 mg twice daily for 4 days found a 17% increase in the AUC and an 18% increase in the maximum plasma levels of theophylline, but this was considered clinically unimportant.[8] In two clinical studies in patients with an acute bacterial exacerbation of chronic bronchitis the number of patients requiring an adjustment in theophylline dosage was similar when those who took clarithromycin were compared with those who took ampicillin.[9,10] However, there are isolated reports of possible theophylline toxicity, including a case that resulted in rhabdomyolysis with renal failure requiring haemodialysis.[11,12] For a report of theophylline toxicity in a patient also taking clarithromycin and levofloxacin, see 'Theophylline + Quinolones', p.1192.

(c) Dirithromycin

In one study, 13 healthy subjects had a fall in their steady-state trough theophylline level of 18%, and a fall in their peak serum level of 26% while taking dirithromycin 500 mg daily for 10 days, although this was not considered clinically relevant.[13] No significant changes in theophylline pharmacokinetics were seen in 14 patients with COPD who were given dirithromycin 500 mg daily for 10 days.[14] This is supported by a similar single-dose study in 12 healthy subjects.[15]

(d) Josamycin

No clinically significant changes in serum theophylline levels were seen in 5 studies in patients (both adults and children)[16-18] or healthy subjects[19] given josamycin, but a modest rise in theophylline levels was described in one study in children.[20] Another study reported a 23% reduction in the levels of theophylline (given as intravenous aminophylline) in 5 patients with particularly severe respiratory impairment, but no significant effect in 5 other patients with less severe disease.[21] However, an isolated report describes theophylline toxicity in a 80-year-old man who was given josamycin.[22]

(e) Midecamycin/Midecamycin diacetate

In one study, 18 asthmatic children had a slight decrease in serum theophylline levels when they were given midecamycin 40 mg/kg daily for 10 days for a bronchopulmonary infection, but no changes were seen in 5 healthy adult subjects.[23]

Similarly, no significant changes in serum theophylline levels were seen in 20 patients taking slow-release theophylline (*Theo-dur*) 300 mg twice daily, or intravenous theophylline 4 mg/kg three times daily, when they were given midecamycin diacetate (miocamycin; ponsinomycin) 1.2 g daily for 10 days.[24] A number of other studies confirm the absence of a clinically important interaction between oral or intravenous theophylline or intravenous aminophylline and midecamycin diacetate in children and adults.[25-28]

(f) Rokitamycin

Two studies in 12 adults with COPD and 11 elderly patients taking theophylline found no significant changes in serum theophylline levels when they were given rokitamycin 600 to 800 mg daily for a week.[29,30]

(g) Roxithromycin

One study in 12 healthy subjects and another in 16 patients with chronic obstructive pulmonary disease found only minor increases in steady-state theophylline levels, which were not considered clinically relevant, when they were given roxithromycin 150 mg twice daily.[31,32] Another study in 5 healthy subjects similarly showed that roxithromycin 300 mg twice daily did not affect the pharmacokinetics of theophylline.[33] However, further study reported a significant increase in serum theophylline levels in 14 patients with asthma who were given roxithromycin 150 mg twice daily, but since the rise was not quantified it is difficult to assess the clinical relevance of this finding.[3]

(h) Spiramycin

A study in 15 asthmatic patients taking theophylline found that spiramycin 1 g twice daily for at least 5 days had no significant effect on their steady-state serum theophylline levels.[34]

(i) Telithromycin

A study in 24 healthy subjects given theophylline found that telithromycin 800 mg daily for 4 days did not have a clinically relevant effect on theophylline exposure.[35]

(j) Troleandomycin

A series of 8 patients with severe chronic asthma found that troleandomycin 250 mg four times daily caused an average reduction in the clearance of theophylline (given as intravenous aminophylline) of 50%. One patient had a theophylline-induced seizure after 10 days, with a serum theophylline level of 43 mg/mL (reference range 10 to 20 mg/L). The theophylline half-life in this patient had increased from 4.6 to 11.3 hours.[36] Other studies in healthy subjects[23,37] and patients[18] given oral theophylline with troleandomycin have also found reductions in theophylline clearance and marked rises in serum theophylline levels and half-life, even at low troleandomycin doses.[38]

Mechanism

It is believed that troleandomycin forms inactive cytochrome P450-metabolite complexes within the liver, the effect of which is to reduce the metabolism (*N*-demethylation and 8-hydroxylation)[37] of theophylline, thereby reducing its clearance and increasing its levels. Clarithromycin, josamycin, midecamycin, and roxithromycin are thought to rarely form complexes, and azithromycin, dirithromycin, rokitamycin and spiramycin are not thought to inactivate cytochrome P450.[39]

Importance and management

The interaction between theophylline and troleandomycin is established and well documented. If troleandomycin is given, monitor the levels of theophylline closely and adjust the dose as necessary. Reductions of 25 to 50% may be needed.[38,40] The situation with roxithromycin is uncertain since only 1 of 4 studies suggested an interaction, but it would be prudent to be alert for the need to reduce the theophylline dosage. Alternative macrolides that usually interact only moderately, or not at all are azithromycin, clarithromycin, dirithromycin, josamycin, midecamycin, rokitamycin and spiramycin. Telithromycin may also be a suitable alternative. However, even with these macrolides it would still be prudent to monitor the outcome because a few patients, especially those with theophylline levels at the high end of the range, may need some small theophylline dosage adjustments. In the case of azithromycin, care should be taken in adjusting the dose based on theophylline levels taken after about 5 days of concurrent use, as they may only be a reflection of a transient drop. In addition, acute infection *per se* may alter theophylline pharmacokinetics.

1. Hopkins S. Clinical toleration and safety of azithromycin. *Am J Med* (1991) 91 (Suppl 3A), 40S–45S.
2. Davies BI, Maesen FPV, Gubbelmans R. Azithromycin (CP-62,993) in acute exacerbations of chronic bronchitis: an open, clinical, microbiological and pharmacokinetic study. *J Antimicrob Chemother* (1989) 23, 743–51.
3. Rhee YK, Lee HB, Lee YC. Effects of erythromycin and new macrolides on the serum theophylline level and clearance. *Allergy* (1998) 53 (Suppl 43), 142.
4. Pollak PT, Slayter KL. Reduced serum theophylline concentrations after discontinuation of azithromycin: evidence for an usual interaction. *Pharmacotherapy* (1997) 17, 827–9.
5. Pollack PT, MacNeil DM. Azithromycin-theophylline inhibition-induction interaction. *Clin Pharmacol Ther* (1999) 65, 144.
6. Gaffuri-Riva V, Crippa F, Guffanti EE. Theophylline interaction with new quinolones and macrolides in COPD patients. *Am Rev Respir Dis* (1991) 143, A498.
7. Gillum JG, Israel DS, Scott RB, Climo MW, Polk RE. Effect of combination therapy with ciprofloxacin and clarithromycin on theophylline pharmacokinetics in healthy volunteers. *Antimicrob Agents Chemother* (1996) 40, 1715–16.
8. Ruff F, Chu S-Y, Sonders RC, Sennello LT. Effect of multiple doses of clarithromycin (C) on the pharmacokinetics (Pks) of theophylline (T). *Intersci Conf Antimicrob Agents Chemother* (1990) 30, 213.
9. Bachand RT. Comparative study of clarithromycin and ampicillin in the treatment of patients with acute bacterial exacerbations of chronic bronchitis. *J Antimicrob Chemother* (1991) 27 (Suppl A), 91–100.
10. Aldons PM. A comparison of clarithromycin with ampicillin in the treatment of outpatients with acute bacterial exacerbation of chronic bronchitis. *J Antimicrob Chemother* (1991) 27 (Suppl A), 101–8.
11. Abbott Labs. Personal communication, February 1995.
12. Shimada N, Omuro H, Saka S, Ebihara I, Koide H. A case of acute renal failure with rhabdomyolysis caused by the interaction of theophylline and clarithromycin. *Nippon Jinzo Gakkai Shi* (1999) 41, 460–3.
13. Bachmann K, Nunlee M, Martin M, Sullivan T, Jauregui L, DeSante K, Sides GD. Changes in the steady-state pharmacokinetics of theophylline during treatment with dirithromycin. *J Clin Pharmacol* (1990) 30, 1001–5.
14. Bachmann K, Jauregui L, Sides G, Sullivan TJ. Steady-state pharmacokinetics of theophylline in COPD patients treated with dirithromycin. *J Clin Pharmacol* (1993) 33, 861–5.
15. McConnell SA, Nafziger AN, Amsden GW. Lack of effect of dirithromycin on theophylline pharmacokinetics in healthy volunteers. *J Antimicrob Chemother* (1999) 43, 733–6.
16. Ruff F, Prosper M, Pujet JC. Théophylline et antibiotiques. Absence d'interaction avec la josamycine. *Therapie* (1984) 39, 1–6.
17. Jiménez Baos R, Casado de Frías E, Cadórniga R, Moreno M. Estudio de posibles interacciones entre josamicina y teofilina en niños. *Rev Farmacol Clin Exp* (1985) 2, 345–8.
18. Brazier JL, Kofman J, Faucon G, Perrin-Fayolle M, Lepape A, Lanoue R. Retard d'élimination de la théophylline dû á la troléandomycine. Absence d'effet de la josamycine. *Therapie* (1980) 35, 545–9.
19. Selles JP, Panis G, Jaber H, Bres J, Armando P. Influence of josamycine on theophylline kinetics. 13th International Congress on Chemotherapy, Vienna, Aug 28–Sept 2 1983. 15–20.
20. Vallarino G, Merlini M, Vallarino R. Josamicina e teofillinici nella patologia respiratoria pediatrica. *G Ital Chemioter* (1982) 29 (Suppl 1), 129–33.
21. Bartolucci L, Gradoli C, Vincenzi V, Iapadre M, Valori C. Macrolide antibiotics and serum theophylline levels in relation to the severity of the respiratory impairment: a comparison between the effects of erythromycin and josamycin. *Chemioterapia* (1984) 3, 286–90.
22. Barbare JC, Martin F, Biour M. Surdosage en théophylline at anomalies des tests hépatiques associés à la prise de josamycine. *Therapie* (1990) 45, 357–58.
23. Lavarenne J, Paire M, Talon O. Influence d'un nouveau macrolide, la midécamycine, sur les taux sanguins de théophylline. *Therapie* (1981) 36, 451–6.
24. Rimoldi R, Bandera M, Fioretti M, Giorcelli R. Miocamycin and theophylline blood levels. *Chemioterapia* (1986) 5, 213–16.
25. Principi N, Onorato J, Giuliani MG, Vigano A. Effect of miocamycin on theophylline kinetics in children. *Eur J Clin Pharmacol* (1987) 31, 701–4.
26. Couet W, Ingrand I, Reigner B, Girault J, Bizouard J, Fourtillan JB. Lack of effect of ponsinomycin on the plasma pharmacokinetics of theophylline. *Eur J Clin Pharmacol* (1989) 37, 101–4.
27. Dal Negro R, Turco P, Pomari C, de Conti F. Miocamycin doesn't affect theophylline serum levels in COPD patients. *Int J Clin Pharmacol Ther Toxicol* (1988) 26, 27–9.
28. Principi N, Onorato J, Giuliani M, Viganó A. Effect of miocamycin on theophylline kinetics in asthmatic children. *Chemioterapia* (1987) 6 (Suppl 2), 339–40.

29. Ishioka T. Effect of a new macrolide antibiotic, 3'-O-propionyl-leucomycin A5 (Rokitamycin), on serum concentrations of theophylline and digoxin in the elderly. *Acta Ther* (1987) 13, 17–23.
30. Cazzola M, Matera MG, Paternò E, Scaglione F, Santangelo G, Rossi F. Impact of rokitamycin, a new 16-membered macrolide, on serum theophylline. *J Chemother* (1991) 3, 240–4.
31. Saint-Salvi B, Tremblay D, Surjus A, Lefebvre MA. A study of the interaction of roxithromycin with theophylline and carbamazepine. *J Antimicrob Chemother* (1987) 20 (Suppl B), 121–9.
32. Bandera M, Fioretti M, Rimoldi R, Lazzarini A, Anelli M. Roxithromycin and controlled release theophylline, an interaction study. *Chemioterapia* (1988) 7, 313–16.
33. Hashiguchi K, Niki Y, Soejima R. Roxithromycin does not raise serum theophylline levels. *Chest* (1992) 102, 653–4.
34. Debruyne D, Jehan A, Bigot M-C, Lechevalier B, Prevost J-N, Moulin M. Spiramycin has no effect on serum theophylline in asthmatic patients. *Eur J Clin Pharmacol* (1986) 30, 505–7.
35. Bhargava V, Leroy B, Shi J, Montay G. Effect of telithromycin on the pharmacokinetics of theophylline in healthy volunteers. *Intersci Conf Antimicrob Agents Chemother* (2002) 42, 28.
36. Weinberger M, Hudgel D, Spector S, Chidsey C. Inhibition of theophylline clearance by troleandomycin. *J Allergy Clin Immunol* (1977) 59, 228–31.
37. Naline E, Sanceaume M, Pays M, Advenier C. Application of theophylline metabolite assays to the exploration of liver microsome oxidative function in man. *Fundam Clin Pharmacol* (1988) 2, 341–51.
38. Kamada AK, Hill MR, Brenner AM, Szefler SJ. Effect of low-dose troleandomycin on theophylline clearance: implications for therapeutic drug monitoring. *Pharmacotherapy* (1992) 12, 98–102.
39. Periti P, Mazzei T, Mini E, Novelli A. Pharmacokinetic drug interactions of macrolides. *Clin Pharmacokinet* (1992) 23, 106–31. Correction. ibid. (1993) 24, 70.
40. Eitches RW, Rachelefsky GS, Katz RM, Mendoza GR, Siegel SC. Methylprednisolone and troleandomycin in treatment of steroid-dependent asthmatic children. *Am J Dis Child* (1985) 139, 264–8.

Theophylline + Macrolides; Erythromycin

Theophylline serum levels can be increased by erythromycin. Toxicity may develop in those patients whose serum levels are at the higher end of the therapeutic range unless the dosage is reduced. The onset may be delayed for several days, and not all patients demonstrate this interaction. Erythromycin levels may possibly fall to subtherapeutic concentrations.

Clinical evidence

(a) Effect on theophylline

The peak serum theophylline levels of 12 patients with COPD given aminophylline 4 mg/kg orally every 6 hours were raised by 28% by erythromycin stearate 500 mg every 6 hours for 2 days. The clearance was reduced by 22%. Only one patient developed clinical signs of toxicity, although the authors suggest this may be because the other patients had low theophylline levels (11 mg/L) to start with and they may not have been studied for long enough to detect the full effect of the erythromycin.[1] Several single-dose studies in healthy or asthmatic adults given aminophylline or theophylline have demonstrated this interaction[2-6] and multiple-dose studies with aminophylline have also shown that erythromycin alters theophylline pharmacokinetics.[7,8] A multiple-dose study in asthmatic children showed a 40% rise in the levels of theophylline (given as intravenous aminophylline).[9] There was often wide inter-subject variability, and not all patients demonstrated the interaction.[1,4,6-9] In addition to the studies, there are several case reports where erythromycin was thought to have caused previously therapeutic theophylline levels to rise to become toxic. In 3 cases the level rose twofold, with accompanying symptoms of toxicity,[10-12] and in one case the patient developed a fatal cardiac arrhythmia.[13] Toxic theophylline levels of 41 mg/L have also been reported in one patient 3 days after a 6-day course of erythromycin was finished, although this patient did not have any clinical signs or symptoms or theophylline toxicity.[14]

Several studies in both healthy adults,[15-18] and adults with COPD[5,19] did not demonstrate any clinically significant interaction, although two of these studies did find a reduction in the clearance of theophylline in some subjects.[15,19]

(b) Effect on erythromycin

The peak serum levels of erythromycin 500 mg every 8 hours were almost halved and the AUC_{0-8h} was reduced by 38% when 6 healthy subjects were given a single 250-mg intravenous dose of theophylline.[6] Another pharmacokinetic study found that serum erythromycin levels fell by more than 30% when intravenous theophylline was given with oral erythromycin.[8] Other studies using intravenous erythromycin found no significant pharmacokinetic changes. The renal clearance was increased, but this did not affect the overall clearance.[18,20]

Mechanism

The mechanism for the effects of erythromycin on theophylline levels is not fully understood. It seems most likely that erythromycin inhibits the metabolism of theophylline by the liver resulting in a reduction in its clearance and a rise in its serum levels. The human organic anion transporter 2 (hOat2) found in the liver may also be involved in this interaction.[21] The reduction in erythromycin levels may be caused by theophylline affecting the absorption of oral erythromycin.[18]

Importance and management

The effects of erythromycin on theophylline are established (but still debated) and well documented. Not all the reports are referenced here. It does not seem to matter which erythromycin salt is used. Monitor theophylline levels and anticipate the need to reduce the theophylline dosage to avoid toxicity. Not all patients will show this interaction but remember it may take several days (most commonly 2 to 7 days) to manifest itself. Some patients may have a high theophylline level but no clinical signs or symptoms, therefore do not rely on symptoms alone to monitor for toxicity.[14] Limited evidence suggests that levels may return to normal 2 to 7 days after stopping erythromycin.[10-12,14] There are many factors, such as smoking,[3,19] which also affect theophylline kinetics, and which may play a role in altering the significance of the interaction in different patients. Those particularly at risk are patients with already high serum theophylline levels and/or taking high dosages (20 mg/kg or more). Ideally, use a non-interacting antibacterial if possible. However, where concurrent treatment cannot be avoided, a 25% reduction in theophylline dose has been recommended for patients with levels in the 15 to 20 mg/L range,[1,2,22] but little dosage adjustment is probably needed for those at the lower end of the range, (below 15 mg/L) unless toxic symptoms appear.[1,4] In practice erythromycin can probably be safely started with theophylline, with the levels monitored after 48 hours and appropriate dosage adjustments then made.

The fall in erythromycin levels caused by theophylline is not well documented, but what is known suggests that it may be clinically important. Be alert for any evidence of an inadequate response to the erythromycin and increase the dosage or change the antibacterial if necessary. Intravenous erythromycin appears not to be affected.

1. Reisz G, Pingleton SK, Melethil S, Ryan PB. The effect of erythromycin on theophylline pharmacokinetics in chronic bronchitis. *Am Rev Respir Dis* (1983) 127, 581–4.
2. Prince RA, Wing DS, Weinberger MM, Hendeles LS, Riegelman S. Effect of erythromycin on theophylline kinetics. *J Allergy Clin Immunol* (1981) 68, 427–31.
3. May DC, Jarboe CH, Ellenburg DT, Roe EJ, Karibo J. The effects of erythromycin on theophylline elimination in normal males. *J Clin Pharmacol* (1982) 22, 125–30.
4. Zarowitz BJM, Szefler SJ, Lasezkay GM. Effect of erythromycin base on theophylline kinetics. *Clin Pharmacol Ther* (1981) 29, 601–5.
5. Richer C, Mathieu M, Bah H, Thuillez C, Duroux P, Giudicelli J-F. Theophylline kinetics and ventilatory flow in bronchial asthma and chronic airflow obstruction: Influence of erythromycin. *Clin Pharmacol Ther* (1982) 31, 579–86.
6. Iliopoulou A, Aldhous ME, Johnston A, Turner P. Pharmacokinetic interaction between theophylline and erythromycin. *Br J Clin Pharmacol* (1982) 14, 495–9.
7. Branigan TA, Robbins RA, Cady WJ, Nickols JG, Ueda CT. The effects of erythromycin on the absorption and disposition kinetics of theophylline. *Eur J Clin Pharmacol* (1981) 21, 115–20.
8. Paulsen O, Höglund P, Nilsson L-G, Bengtsson H-I. The interaction of erythromycin with theophylline. *Eur J Clin Pharmacol* (1987) 32, 493–8.
9. LaForce CF, Miller MF, Chai H. Effect of erythromycin on theophylline clearance in asthmatic children. *J Pediatr* (1981) 99, 153–6.
10. Cummins LH, Kozak PP, Gillman SA. Erythromycin's effect on theophylline blood level. *Pediatrics* (1977) 59, 144–5.
11. Cummins LH, Kozak PP, Gillman SA. Theophylline determinations. *Ann Allergy* (1976) 37, 450–51.
12. Green JA, Clementi WA. Decrease in theophylline clearance after the administration of erythromycin to a patient with obstructive lung disease. *Drug Intell Clin Pharm* (1983) 17, 370–2.
13. Andrews PA. Interactions with ciprofloxacin and erythromycin leading to aminophylline toxicity. *Nephrol Dial Transplant* (1998) 13, 1006–8.
14. Wiggins J, Arbab O, Ayres JG, Skinner C. Elevated serum theophylline concentration following cessation of erythromycin treatment. *Eur J Respir Dis* (1986) 68, 298–300.
15. Pfeifer HJ, Greenblatt DJ, Friedman P. Effects of three antibiotics on theophylline kinetics. *Clin Pharmacol Ther* (1979) 26, 36–40.
16. Kelly SJ, Pingleton SK, Ryan PB, Melethil S. The lack of influence of erythromycin on plasma theophylline levels. *Chest* (1980) 78, 523.
17. Maddux MS, Leeds NH, Organek HW, Hasegawa GR, Bauman JL. The effect of erythromycin on theophylline pharmacokinetics at steady state. *Chest* (1982) 81, 563–5.
18. Pasic J, Jackson SHD, Johnston A, Peverel-Cooper CA, Turner P, Downey K, Chaput de Saintonge DM. The interaction between chronic oral slow-release theophylline and single-dose intravenous erythromycin. *Xenobiotica* (1987) 17, 493–7.
19. Stults BM, Felice-Johnson J, Higbee MD, Hardigan K. Effect of erythromycin stearate on serum theophylline concentration in patients with chronic obstructive lung disease. *South Med J* (1983) 76, 714–18.
20. Hildebrandt R, Möller H, Gundert-Remy U. Influence of theophylline on the renal clearance of erythromycin. *Int J Clin Pharmacol Ther Toxicol* (1987) 25, 601–4.
21. Kobayashi Y, Sakai R, Ohshiro N, Ohbayashi M, Kohyama N, Yamamoto T. Possible involvement of organic anion transporter 2 on the interaction of theophylline with erythromycin in the human liver. *Drug Metab Dispos* (2005) 33, 619–22.
22. Aronson JK, Hardman M, Reynolds DJM. ABC of monitoring drug therapy. Theophylline. *BMJ* (1992) 305, 1355–8.

Theophylline + Methoxsalen

Oral methoxsalen markedly increases theophylline levels. Topical methoxsalen would not be expected to interact.

Clinical evidence, mechanism, importance and management

In a single-dose study in 3 healthy subjects a 1.2-mg/kg oral dose of methoxsalen increased the AUC of a single 600-mg dose of theophylline (given 1 hour later) 1.7-fold, 2.1-fold and 2.7-fold, in the 3 subjects, respectively.[1] Methoxsalen probably inhibits the metabolism of theophylline[2] by the cytochrome P450 isoenzyme CYP1A2. Although information is limited, the findings support what is known about caffeine and 'psoralens', (p.1166). Theophylline dose reductions are likely to be required during concurrent use with systemic methoxsalen but seem unlikely to be necessary with topical treatment such as PUVA therapy.

1. Apseloff G, Shepard DR, Chambers MA, Nawoot S, Mays DC, Gerber N. Inhibition and induction of theophylline metabolism by 8-methoxypsoralen. In vitro study in rats and humans. *Drug Metab Dispos* (1990) 18, 298–303.
2. Tantcheva-Poór I, Servera-Llaneras M, Scharffetter-Kochanek K, Fuhr U. Liver cytochrome P450 CYP1A2 is markedly inhibited by systemic but not by bath PUVA in dermatological patients. *Br J Dermatol* (2001) 144, 1127–32.

Theophylline + Metoclopramide

Metoclopramide does not appear to interact with slow-release theophylline.

Clinical evidence, mechanism, importance and management

In 8 healthy subjects a single 10-mg dose of metoclopramide taken 20 minutes before a 600-mg dose of slow-release theophylline (*Theo-Dur*), caused a small but insignificant 14.5% reduction in the bioavailability of theophylline. However, adverse effects (nausea, headache, tremors, CNS stimulation) were seen more often in those taking metoclopramide than in those taking placebo, possibly because metoclopramide caused an earlier rise in theophylline levels, and because some of the adverse effects of these two drugs may be additive.[1] A later study in 12 healthy subjects found that metoclopramide 15 mg every 6 hours had no effect on the rate or extent of absorption of a 600–mg dose of sustained-release theophylline (*Theo-24*).[2] A similar lack of interaction was found in another study using *Theo-Dur*.[3] There would seem to be no reason for avoiding concurrent use.

1. Steeves RA, Robinson JD, McKenzie MW, Justus PG. Effects of metoclopramide on the pharmacokinetics of a slow-release theophylline product. *Clin Pharm* (1982) 1, 356–60.
2. Bryson JC, Dukes GE, Kirby MG, Heizer WD, Powell JR. Effect of altering small bowel transit time on sustained release theophylline absorption. *J Clin Pharmacol* (1989) 29, 733–8.
3. Sommers DK, Meyer EC, Van Wyk M, Moncrieff J, Snyman JR, Grimbeek RJ. The influence of codeine, propantheline and metoclopramide on small bowel transit and theophylline absorption from a sustained-release formulation. *Br J Clin Pharmacol* (1992) 33, 305–8.

Theophylline + Metronidazole

No interaction of clinical importance normally takes place if metronidazole is given to patients taking theophylline, but an isolated report describes seizures in one patient also taking ciprofloxacin.

Clinical evidence, mechanism, importance and management

There were no significant changes in the pharmacokinetics of theophylline given as a single intravenous dose of aminophylline to 5 women taking metronidazole 250 mg three times a day for trichomoniasis.[1] Another study in 10 healthy subjects confirmed this finding.[2] However, an acutely ill elderly woman taking theophylline had a generalised seizure while being treated with metronidazole and ciprofloxacin, despite her theophylline level being within the therapeutic range (10 to 20 mg/L).[3] Both ciprofloxacin and, more rarely, metronidazole are associated with seizures.[3] Although the evidence is limited, no special precautions would seem to be necessary during concurrent use.

1. Reitberg DP, Klarnet JP, Carlson JK, Schentag JJ. Effect of metronidazole on theophylline pharmacokinetics. *Clin Pharm* (1983) 2, 441–4.
2. Adebayo GI, Mabadeje AFB. Lack of inhibitory effect of metronidazole on theophylline disposition in healthy subjects. *Br J Clin Pharmacol* (1987) 24, 110–13.
3. Semel JD, Allen N. Seizures in patients simultaneously receiving theophylline and imipenem or ciprofloxacin or metronidazole. *South Med J* (1991) 84, 465–8.

Theophylline + Mexiletine or Tocainide

Serum theophylline levels are increased by mexiletine and toxicity may occur. Tocainide has only a small and probably clinically unimportant effect on theophylline pharmacokinetics.

Clinical evidence

(a) Mexiletine

A man developed theophylline toxicity within a few days of starting to take mexiletine 200 mg three times daily. His serum theophylline level rose from 15.3 to 25 mg/L, but fell to 14.2 mg/L, and the symptoms of toxicity resolved, when the theophylline dosage was reduced by two-thirds.[1]

Other case reports describe 1.5 to threefold increases in theophylline serum levels (accompanied by clear signs of toxicity in some instances) in a total of 10 patients who were given mexiletine.[2-7] Theophylline dose reductions of 50% were required in 3 cases,[2,6] although 2 of the patients that did not require dose reductions had initial theophylline levels below the therapeutic range.[3] The arrhythmia of one patient was aggravated even at therapeutic serum theophylline levels, and mexiletine was discontinued.[4]

In 15 healthy subjects, mexiletine 200 mg three times a day for 5 days reduced the clearance of a single 5-mg/kg intravenous dose of theophylline by 46% in women and 40% in men. The theophylline half-life was prolonged by 96% (from 7.4 to 14.5 hours) in women and 71% (from 8.7 to 14.9 hours) in men.[8] Two further studies in healthy subjects given theophylline with mexiletine for 5 days found a reduction in steady-state theophylline clearance of about 45%, and an increase in the AUC of about 60%.[9,10]

(b) Tocainide

After taking tocainide 400 mg every 8 hours for 5 days, the pharmacokinetics of a single 5-mg/kg intravenous dose of theophylline was measured in 8 healthy subjects. The clearance was decreased by about 10% and the half-life slightly prolonged (from 9.7 to 10.4 hours), but these changes were not thought to be large enough to warrant altering theophylline doses.[11]

Mechanism

Mexiletine inhibits the metabolism (demethylation) of theophylline by the liver, thereby increasing its effects.[8,10,12] It is possible that the interaction is due to competitive inhibition of the cytochrome P450 isoenzyme CYP1A2.[13]

Importance and management

The interaction between theophylline and mexiletine is established and of clinical importance. Monitor concurrent use and reduce the theophylline dosage as necessary to prevent the development of theophylline toxicity. It has been suggested that 50% dose reductions may be necessary.[8] It seems doubtful if the interaction between theophylline and tocainide is clinically important but this needs confirmation.

1. Katz A, Buskila D, Sukenik S. Oral mexiletine-theophylline interaction. *Int J Cardiol* (1987) 17, 227–8.
2. Stanley R, Comer T, Taylor JL, Saliba D. Mexiletine-theophylline interaction. *Am J Med* (1989) 86, 733–4.
3. Ueno K, Miyai K, Seki T, Kawaguchi Y. Interaction between theophylline and mexiletine. *DICP Ann Pharmacother* (1990) 24, 471–2.
4. Kessler KM, Interian A, Cox M, Topaz O, De Marchena EJ, Myerburg RJ. Proarrhythmia related to a kinetic and dynamic interaction of mexiletine and theophylline. *Am Heart J* (1989) 117, 964–6.292
5. Kendall JD, Chrymko MM, Cooper BE. Theophylline-mexiletine interaction: a case report. *Pharmacotherapy* (1992) 12, 416–18.
6. Inafuku M, Suzuki T, Ohtsu F, Hariya Y, Nagasawa K, Yoshioka Y, Nakahara Y, Hayakawa H. The effect of mexiletine on theophylline pharmacokinetics in patients with bronchial asthma. *J Cardiol* (1992) 22, 227–33.
7. Ellison MJ, Lyman DJ, San Miguel E. Threefold increase in theophylline serum concentration after addition of mexiletine. *Am J Emerg Med* (1992) 10, 506–8.
8. Loi C-M, Wei X, Vestal RE. Inhibition of theophylline metabolism by mexiletine in young male and female nonsmokers. *Clin Pharmacol Ther* (1991) 49, 571–80.
9. Stoysich AM, Mohiuddin SM, Destache CJ, Nipper HC, Hilleman DE. Influence of mexiletine on the pharmacokinetics of theophylline in healthy volunteers. *J Clin Pharmacol* (1991) 31, 354–7.
10. Hurwitz A, Vacek JL, Botteron GW, Sztern MI, Hughes EM, Jayaraj A. Mexiletine effects on theophylline disposition. *Clin Pharmacol Ther* (1991) 50, 299–307.
11. Loi C-M, Wei X, Parker BM, Korrapati MR, Vestal RE. The effect of tocainide on theophylline metabolism. *Br J Clin Pharmacol* (1993) 35, 437–40.
12. Ueno K, Miyai K, Kato M, Kawaguchi Y, Suzuki T. Mechanism of interaction between theophylline and mexiletine. *DICP Ann Pharmacother* (1991) 25, 727–30.
13. Nakajima M, Kobayashi K, Shimada N, Tokudome S, Yamamoto T, Kuroiwa Y. Involvement of CYP1A2 in mexiletine metabolism. *Br J Clin Pharmacol* (1998) 46, 55–62.

Theophylline + Moracizine

Moracizine modestly increases theophylline clearance, although conversely *animal* data suggest that moracizine inhibits theophylline metabolism.

Clinical evidence

Single oral doses of aminophylline and a sustained-release theophylline preparation (*TheoDur*) were given to 12 healthy subjects. After they took moracizine 250 mg three times daily for 2 weeks, the AUC of theophylline was reduced by 32% and 36%, its clearance was increased by 44% and 66%, and the elimination half-life decreased by 33% and 20%, for aminophylline and theophylline respectively.[1]

Mechanism

Uncertain. Moracizine is an enzyme inducer and appears to increase the metabolism of theophylline.[1] In contrast, *in vitro* and *animal* data show moracizine to be an inhibitor of the cytochrome P450 isoenzyme CYP1A2, which is the main isoenzyme involved in the metabolism of theophylline.[2] This would, in theory, be expected to lead to raised theophylline levels.

Importance and management

Information seems to be limited to this study. The clinical importance of this interaction has not been assessed, but monitor the effects of concurrent use and be alert for the need to adjust the theophylline dose. More study is needed.

1. Pieniaszek HJ, Davidson AF, Benedek IH. Effect of moricizine on the pharmacokinetics of single-dose theophylline in healthy subjects. *Ther Drug Monit* (1993) 15, 199–203.
2. Konishi H, Morita K, Minouchi T, Yamaji A. Moricizine, an antiarrhythmic agent, as a potent inhibitor of hepatic microsomal CYP1A. *Pharmacology* (2002) 66, 190–8.

Theophylline + Nefazodone

Nefazodone does not appear to interact adversely with theophylline.

Clinical evidence, mechanism, importance and management

Nefazodone 200 mg twice daily for 7 days had no effect on the pharmacokinetics or pharmacodynamics of theophylline 600 mg to 1.2 g daily in patients with chronic obstructive airways disease, nor was there any effect on their FEV_1 values.[1] No special precautions would seem necessary if both drugs are used.

1. Dockens RC, Rapoport D, Roberts D, Greene DS, Barbhaiya RH. Lack of an effect of nefazodone on the pharmacokinetics and pharmacodynamics of theophylline during concurrent administration in patients with chronic obstructive airways disease. *Br J Clin Pharmacol* (1995) 40, 598–601.

Theophylline + Non-prescription theophylline products

Patients taking theophylline should not take other medications containing theophylline (some of which are non-prescription products) unless the total dosage of theophylline can be adjusted appropriately.

Clinical evidence, mechanism, importance and management

A patient taking theophylline developed elevated serum theophylline levels of 35.7 micrograms/mL while taking *Quinamm* for leg cramps (old formulation containing quinine 260 mg and aminophylline 195 mg). This case report highlights the need to avoid the inadvertent intake of additional doses of theophylline if toxicity is to be avoided. The newer formulation of *Quinamm* does not contain theophylline.[1] Note that non-prescription preparations containing theophylline are available in many countries. For example, some cough and cold preparations in the UK contain theophylline (e.g. *Do-Do Chesteze, Franol Plus*). Patients should be warned.

1. Shane R. Potential toxicity of theophylline in combination with *Quinamm*. *Am J Hosp Pharm* (1982) 39, 40.

Theophylline + Olanzapine

There appears to be no significant pharmacokinetic interaction between theophylline and olanzapine.

Clinical evidence, mechanism, importance and management

A study in 18 healthy subjects given olanzapine 5 mg on day one, 7.5 mg on day 2 and then 10 mg daily for 7 days found no significant changes in the pharmacokinetics of theophylline (given as a single 350-mg intravenous dose of aminophylline). The pharmacokinetics of olanzapine also appeared to be unchanged when both drugs were given.[1] No special precautions would appear to be necessary on concurrent use. The authors also conclude that olanzapine would not be expected to affect the pharmacokinetics of other drugs that are (like theophylline) substrates for the cytochrome P450 isoenzyme CYP1A2, see 'Table 1.2', (p.4).

1. Macias WL, Bergstrom RF, Cerimele BJ, Kassahun K, Tatum DE, Callaghan JT. Lack of effect of olanzapine on the pharmacokinetics of a single aminophylline dose in healthy men. *Pharmacotherapy* (1998) 18, 1237–48.

Theophylline + Ozagrel

Ozagrel does not appear to alter theophylline pharmacokinetics.

Clinical evidence, mechanism, importance and management

Ozagrel 200 mg twice daily was given to 4 patients with asthma taking sustained-release theophylline. After 24 weeks the ozagrel was stopped without any significant effect on the pharmacokinetics of theophylline. Similarly, in another 8 patients with bronchial asthma, there were no significant differences in the pharmacokinetics of theophylline (given as a single infusion of aminophylline) before and after taking ozagrel 200 mg twice daily for 7 days.[1] No special precautions would seem to be needed during concurrent use.

1. Kawakatsu K, Kino T, Yasuba H, Kawaguchi H, Tsubata R, Satake N, Oshima S. Effect of ozagrel (OKY-046), a thromboxane synthetase inhibitor, on theophylline pharmacokinetics in asthmatic patients. *Int J Clin Pharmacol Ther Toxicol* (1990) 28, 158–63.

Theophylline + Penicillins

Ampicillin, with or without sulbactam, and amoxicillin do not alter the pharmacokinetics of theophylline.

Clinical evidence, mechanism, importance and management

A retrospective study in asthmatic children aged 3 months to 6 years found that the mean half-life of theophylline did not differ between those treated with ampicillin and those not.[1] The pharmacokinetics of theophylline 8.5 mg/kg daily were not altered in 12 adult patients with chronic obstructive pulmonary disease when they were given ampicillin 1 g plus sulbactam 500 mg every 12 hours for 7 days.[2]

A study in 9 healthy adult subjects showed that amoxicillin 750 mg daily for 9 days did not affect the pharmacokinetics of theophylline 540 mg twice daily.[3,4]

No special precautions would seem to be necessary during concurrent use of these antibacterials and theophylline. However, note that acute infections *per se* can alter theophylline pharmacokinetics.

1. Kadlec GJ, Ha LT, Jarboe CH, Richards D, Karibo JM. Effect of ampicillin on theophylline half-life in infants and young children. *South Med J* (1978) 71, 1584.
2. Cazzola M, Santangelo G, Guidetti E, Mattina R, Caputi M, Girbino G. Influence of sulbactam plus ampicillin on theophylline clearance. *Int J Clin Pharmacol Res* (1991) 11, 11–15.
3. Jonkman JHG, van der Boon WJV, Schoenmaker R, Holtkamp A, Hempenius J. Lack of effect of amoxicillin on theophylline pharmacokinetics. *Br J Clin Pharmacol* (1985) 19, 99–101.
4. Jonkman JHG, van der Boon WJV, Schoenmaker R, Holtkamp AH, Hempenius J. Clinical pharmacokinetics of amoxycillin and theophylline during cotreatment with both medicaments. *Chemotherapy* (1985) 31, 329–35.

Theophylline + Pentoxifylline

Pentoxifylline can raise serum theophylline serum levels.

Clinical evidence, mechanism, importance and management

The mean trough steady-state theophylline serum levels of 9 healthy subjects given sustained-release theophylline *(TheoDur)* 200 or 300 mg twice daily for 7 days were increased by 30% by pentoxifylline 400 mg three times daily. However, the change in levels ranged from a 12.8% decrease to a 94.8% increase. The subjects complained of insomnia, nausea, diarrhoea and tachycardia more frequently while taking both drugs, but this did not reach statistical significance.[1] The mechanism of this interaction is not understood, although note, pentoxifylline is also a xanthine derivative. Patients should be well monitored for theophylline adverse effects (headache, nausea, palpitations) while taking both drugs. More study is needed to clarify this highly variable interaction.

1. Ellison MJ, Horner RD, Willis SE, Cummings DM. Influence of pentoxifylline on steady-state theophylline serum concentrations from sustained-release formulations. *Pharmacotherapy* (1990) 10, 383–6.

Theophylline + Phenylpropanolamine

Phenylpropanolamine reduces the clearance of theophylline.

Clinical evidence, mechanism, importance and management

In 8 healthy subjects a single 150-mg oral dose of phenylpropanolamine decreased the clearance of theophylline (given as a single 4-mg/kg intravenous dose of aminophylline 1 hour after the phenylpropanolamine) by 50%.[1] Such a large reduction in clearance would be expected to result in some increase in serum theophylline levels, but so far no studies of this potentially clinically important interaction seem to have been carried out in patients. Be alert for evidence of toxicity if both drugs are used. More study is needed. See also 'Pseudoephedrine and related drugs + Caffeine', p.1276.

1. Wilson HA, Chin R, Adair NE, Zaloga GP. Phenylpropanolamine significantly reduces the clearance of theophylline. *Am Rev Respir Dis* (1991) 143, A629.

Theophylline + Phenytoin

The serum levels of theophylline can be markedly reduced by phenytoin. Some limited evidence suggests that theophylline may also reduce phenytoin levels.

Clinical evidence

(a) Reduced phenytoin serum levels

A preliminary report noted that the seizure frequency of an epileptic woman taking phenytoin 100 mg four times daily increased when she was given intravenous, and then later oral, theophylline. Her serum phenytoin levels had more than halved, from 15.7 mg/L to around 5 to 8 mg/L. An increase in the phenytoin dosage to 200 mg three times daily raised her serum phenytoin levels to only 7 to 11 mg/L until the drugs were given 1 to 2 hours apart. The patient then developed phenytoin toxicity with a serum level of 33 mg/L. A subsequent single-dose study in 4 healthy subjects confirmed that higher serum levels of both drugs were achieved when the theophylline and phenytoin were given 2 hours apart rather than simultaneously.[1] Another study in 7 healthy subjects found that the AUC of a single 400-mg dose of phenytoin was reduced by 21% when it was given at the same time as a single 7.5-mg/kg dose of theophylline compared with a reduction of 7% when the same doses were given 2 hours apart.[2]

A later preliminary study in 14 subjects (by some of the same authors) found that after 2 weeks of concurrent use, the mean serum phenytoin levels of 5 of the subjects rose by 40% and the mean levels of the group as a whole rose by about 27% when the theophylline was stopped. Urinary concentrations of a phenytoin metabolite were raised.[3]

(b) Reduced theophylline serum levels

The observation that a patient taking phenytoin had lower than expected theophylline levels prompted a study in 10 healthy subjects. After taking phenytoin for 10 days the clearance of theophylline (after a single intravenous dose of aminophylline) was increased by 73%, and both its AUC and half-life were reduced by about 50%.[4] Another study in 6 healthy subjects showed that after taking phenytoin 300 mg daily for 3 weeks the mean clearance of theophylline (after a single intravenous dose of aminophylline) was increased by 45% (range 31 to 65%).[5] Similar results were found in a further study.[6] Other reports on individual asthmatic patients have shown that phenytoin can increase the clearance of theophylline by about 1.3- to 3.5-fold.[7-9] Another study[10] and a case report[11] show that the reduction in theophylline levels caused by phenytoin can be additive with the effects of smoking. A subsequent study found that the extent of phenytoin-induced metabolism of theophylline was not affected by age, despite an age-related reduction in theophylline metabolism.[12] Consider also 'Theophylline + Tobacco', p.1201.

Mechanism

Uncertain. It has been suggested that theophylline either impairs phenytoin absorption or induces phenytoin metabolism, but neither suggestion seem likely.

It seems probable that phenytoin, a known enzyme inducer, increases the metabolism of theophylline by the cytochrome P450 isoenzyme CYP1A2 in the liver, thereby increasing its clearance .

Importance and management

The effect of phenytoin on theophylline is established and of clinical importance. Patients given both drugs should be monitored to confirm that theophylline remains effective. Ideally the serum levels should be measured to confirm that they remain within the therapeutic range. Theophylline dosage increases of up to 50% or more may be required.[13] Conversely, patients should be monitored for signs of toxicity and theophylline levels should be checked in patients who stop phenytoin. The effect of theophylline on phenytoin is not established and the documentation is limited. It may be prudent to monitor phenytoin levels as well. Separating the doses appears to minimise any interaction. Note that theophylline itself can cause seizures, although mostly in overdose, and should be used with caution in patients with epilepsy.

1. Wada JA, Perry JK, eds. Advances in Epileptology: Phenytoin-theophylline interaction; a case report. New York: Raven Press; 1980 p. 505.
2. Hendeles L, Wyatt R, Weinberger M, Schottelius D, Fincham R. Decreased oral phenytoin absorption following concurrent theophylline administration. *J Allergy Clin Immunol* (1979) 63, 156.
3. Taylor JW, Hendeles L, Weinberger M, Lyon LW, Wyatt R, Riegelman S. The interaction of phenytoin and theophylline. *Drug Intell Clin Pharm* (1980) 14, 638.
4. Marquis J-F, Carruthers SG, Spence JD, Brownstone YS, Toogood JH. Phenytoin-theophylline interaction. *N Engl J Med* (1982) 307, 1189–90.
5. Miller M, Cosgriff J, Kwong T, Morken DA. Influence of phenytoin on theophylline clearance. *Clin Pharmacol Ther* (1984) 35, 666–9.
6. Adebayo GI. Interaction between phenytoin and theophylline in healthy volunteers. *Clin Exp Pharmacol Physiol* (1988) 15, 883–7.
7. Sklar SJ, Wagner JC. Enhanced theophylline clearance secondary to phenytoin therapy. *Drug Intell Clin Pharm* (1985) 19, 34–6.
8. Reed RC, Schwartz HJ. Phenytoin-theophylline-quinidine interaction. *N Engl J Med* (1983) 308, 724–5.
9. Landsberg K, Shalansky S. Interaction between phenytoin and theophylline. *Can J Hosp Pharm* (1988) 41, 31–2.
10. Crowley JJ, Cusack BJ, Jue SG, Koup JR, Vestal RE. Cigarette smoking and theophylline metabolism: effects of phenytoin. *Clin Pharmacol Ther* (1987) 42, 334–40.
11. Nicholson JP, Basile SA, Cury JD. Massive theophylline dosing in a heavy smoker receiving both phenytoin and phenobarbital. *Ann Pharmacother* (1992) 26, 334–6.
12. Crowley JJ, Cusack BJ, Jue SG, Koup JR, Park BK, Vestal RE. Aging and drug interactions. II. Effect of phenytoin and smoking on the oxidation of theophylline and cortisol in healthy men. *J Pharmacol Exp Ther* (1988) 245, 513–23.
13. Slugg PH, Pippenger CE. Theophylline and its interactions. *Cleve Clin Q* (1985) 52, 417–24.

Theophylline + Pirenzepine

Pirenzepine does not appear to alter the pharmacokinetics of theophylline.

Clinical evidence, mechanism, importance and management

Pirenzepine 50 mg twice daily for 5 days had no effect on the pharmacokinetics of theophylline (given as aminophylline 6.5 mg/kg, intravenously) in 5 healthy subjects.[1] This would suggest that no special precautions are needed on concurrent use.

1. Sertl K, Rameis H, Meryn S. Pirenzepin does not alter the pharmacokinetics of theophylline. *Int J Clin Pharmacol Ther Toxicol* (1987) 25, 15–17.

Theophylline + Pneumococcal vaccine

Pneumococcal vaccination does not appear to affect theophylline pharmacokinetics.

Clinical evidence, mechanism, importance and management

The pharmacokinetics of oral theophylline 250 mg three times daily for 10 days were unaltered in 6 healthy subjects both the day after and one week after they received 0.5 mL of a pneumococcal vaccine.[1] These findings need confirmation in patients, but what is known suggests that no special precautions are needed during concurrent use.

1. Cupit GC, Self TH, Bekemeyer WB. The effect of pneumococcal vaccine on the disposition of theophylline. *Eur J Clin Pharmacol* (1988) 34, 505–7.

Theophylline or Diprophylline + Probenecid

Theophylline levels are unaffected by probenecid, but diprophylline levels can be raised.

Clinical evidence

(a) Diprophylline

A study in 12 healthy subjects showed that the half-life of a single 20-mg/kg oral dose of diprophylline was doubled (from 2.6 to 4.9 hours) and the clearance approximately halved by probenecid 1 g, which resulted in raised serum diprophylline levels.[1]

(b) Theophylline

A study in 7 healthy subjects found that probenecid 1 g given 30 minutes before a 5.6-mg/kg oral dose of aminophylline had no significant effect on the pharmacokinetics of theophylline.[2]

Mechanism

Diprophylline is largely excreted unchanged by the kidneys, and probenecid inhibits its renal tubular secretion.[3] Theophylline is largely cleared from the body by hepatic metabolism, and would therefore not be expected to be affected by probenecid.

Importance and management

Based on the findings of this single-dose study, it would seem to be prudent to monitor serum diprophylline levels if probenecid is started or stopped. No special precautions are needed if theophylline and probenecid are given concurrently.

1. May DC, Jarboe CH. Effect of probenecid on dyphylline elimination. *Clin Pharmacol Ther* (1983) 33, 822–5.
2. Chen TWD, Patton TF. Effect of probenecid on the pharmacokinetics of aminophylline. *Drug Intell Clin Pharm* (1983) 17, 465–6.
3. Nadai M, Apichartpichean R, Hasegawa T, Nabeshima T. Pharmacokinetics and the effect of probenecid on the renal excretion mechanism of diprophylline. *J Pharm Sci* (1992) 81, 1024–7.

Theophylline + Propafenone

Two isolated reports describe raised serum theophylline levels, with symptoms of toxicity, when two patients were given propafenone.

Clinical evidence

In a 71-year-old man, propafenone 150 mg daily raised the levels of sustained-release theophylline 300 mg twice daily from a range of 10.2 to 12.8 mg/L to 19 mg/L, and signs of theophylline toxicity developed. The day after propafenone was withdrawn the level fell to 10.8 mg/L. When the propafenone was later restarted the theophylline levels rose again to 17.7 mg/L within one week, but fell when the theophylline dosage was reduced by one-third.[1]

In another report, a 63-year-old man had a marked reduction in the clearance of sustained-release theophylline and a rise in theophylline levels from 10.8 mg/L to a maximum of 20.3 mg/L over 7 days when he took propafenone 150 mg every 8 hours, increasing to 300 mg every 8 hours.[2] Theophylline was discontinued.

Mechanism

Uncertain. It has been suggested that propafenone may reduce the metabolism of theophylline by the liver, thereby increasing its levels.

Importance and management

Information is limited to these two reports, but it would seem prudent to monitor the effect of adding propafenone to established treatment with theophylline in any patient. Be alert for increased theophylline levels and signs of toxicity. Controlled studies are needed to further investigate this potential interaction.

1. Lee BL, Dohrmann ML. Theophylline toxicity after propafenone treatment: evidence for drug interaction. *Clin Pharmacol Ther* (1992) 51, 353–5.
2. Spinler SA, Gammaitoni A, Charland SL, Hurwitz J. Propafenone-theophylline interaction. *Pharmacotherapy* (1993) 13, 68–71.

Theophylline + Propantheline

A study in 6 healthy subjects found that propantheline 30 mg did not affect the rate or extent of absorption of a single 500-mg dose of theophylline (*Theo-Dur*). No special precautions would seem necessary on concurrent use.[1]

1. Sommers DK, Meyer EC, Van Wyk M, Moncrieff J, Snyman JR, Grimbeek RJ. The influence of codeine, propantheline and metoclopramide on small bowel transit and theophylline absorption from a sustained-release formulation. *Br J Clin Pharmacol* (1992) 33, 305–8.

Theophylline + Protease inhibitors

Ritonavir can reduce the serum levels of theophylline. Indinavir appears not to interact.

Clinical evidence, mechanism, importance and management

(a) Indinavir

A study in 12 healthy subjects given a single 250-mg oral dose of theophylline before and after 5 days of treatment with indinavir 800 mg three times daily found an 18% increase in the AUC of theophylline, which was not considered clinically significant.[1] There have been no further published studies or cases to date to confirm this result, and as indinavir does not inhibit CYP1A2 (see 'Table 21.2', (p.773)), the main isoenzyme that metabolises theophylline, it would seem unlikely that special precautions are necessary during concurrent use.

(b) Ritonavir

In a placebo-controlled study, 27 subjects taking theophylline 3 mg/kg every 8 hours were given ritonavir 300 mg increased to 500 mg twice daily for 10 days. Ritonavir reduced the AUC of theophylline by 43% and reduced the maximum and minimum steady-state theophylline levels by 32% and 57%, respectively. The interaction achieved its maximal effect 6 days after starting ritonavir.[2] Ritonavir induces the metabolism of theophylline by CYP1A2. Information is very limited but the interaction appears to be established. Consider monitoring theophylline levels if ritonavir is started and be alert for the need to increase the theophylline dose.

1. Mistry GC, Laurent A, Sterrett AT, Deutsch PJ. Effect of indinavir on the single-dose pharmacokinetics of theophylline in healthy subjects. *J Clin Pharmacol* (1999) 39, 636–42.
2. Hsu A, Granneman GR, Witt G, Cavanaugh JH, Leonard J. Assessment of multiple doses of ritonavir on the pharmacokinetics of theophylline. 11th Int Conf AIDS, Vancouver, 1996. Mo.B.1200.

Theophylline + Proton pump inhibitors

Omeprazole may cause a small increase in theophylline clearance, and lansoprazole may cause a small decrease in theophylline levels, neither of which are likely to be clinically relevant. Pantoprazole and rabeprazole do not appear to interact with theophylline.

Clinical evidence

(a) Lansoprazole

Lansoprazole 60 mg daily for 9 days caused only a very slight reduction in the steady-state theophylline levels of 14 healthy subjects.[1] Other studies have also shown little or no change in theophylline pharmacokinetics on concurrent use.[2-6]

(b) Omeprazole

The changes in the half-life and clearance of theophylline caused by omeprazole were found to be small and clinically unimportant in two studies.[7,8] No changes in the steady-state pharmacokinetics of theophylline were found in other studies.[5,9,10] However, one study found that omeprazole produced an 11% increase in the clearance of theophylline in poor metabolisers of omeprazole (i.e. those with low levels of the cytochrome P450 isoenzyme CYP2C19 and therefore higher levels of omeprazole),[11] but this seems unlikely to be clinically significant.

(c) Pantoprazole

A crossover study in 8 healthy subjects showed that intravenous pantoprazole 30 mg daily had no clinically important effect on the pharmacokinetics of theophylline given by infusion. No clinically relevant changes in blood pressure, heart rate, ECG and routine clinical laboratory parameters were seen.[12] Other studies have also found no significant change in theophylline pharmacokinetics when pantoprazole was given.[4,5]

(d) Rabeprazole

A single 250-mg oral dose of theophylline was given to 25 patients before and after taking rabeprazole 20 mg or a placebo daily for 7 days. No significant changes in the pharmacokinetics of theophylline were seen.[13,14]

Mechanism, importance and management

Lansoprazole possibly induces cytochrome P450 isoenzyme CYP1A2 (the enzyme by which theophylline is metabolised) to a small extent, but this is unlikely to be significant unless an individual is particularly sensitive to this effect.[1] Other proton pump inhibitors are unlikely to interact with theophylline, and so no special precautions would seem necessary on concurrent use.

1. Granneman GR, Karol MD, Locke CS, Cavanaugh JH. Pharmacokinetic interaction between lansoprazole and theophylline. *Ther Drug Monit* (1995) 17, 460–4.
2. Kokufu T, Ihara N, Sugioka N, Koyama H, Ohta T, Mori S, Nakajima K. Effects of lansoprazole on pharmacokinetics and metabolism of theophylline. *Eur J Clin Pharmacol* (1995) 48, 391–5.
3. Ko J-W, Jang I-J, Shin S-G, Flockhart DA. Effect of lansoprazole on theophylline clearance in extensive and poor metabolizers of cytochrome P450 2C19. *Clin Pharmacol Ther* (1998) 63, 217.
4. Pan WJ, Goldwater DR, Zhang Y, Pilmer BL, Hunt RH. Lack of a pharmacokinetic interaction between lansoprazole or pantoprazole and theophylline. *Aliment Pharmacol Ther* (2000) 14, 345–52.
5. Dilger K, Zheng Z, Klotz U. Lack of drug interaction between omeprazole, lansoprazole, pantoprazole and theophylline. *Br J Clin Pharmacol* (1999) 48, 438–44.
6. Ko J-W, Jang I-J, Shin J-G, Nam S-K, Shin S-G, Flockhart DA. Theophylline pharmacokinetics are not altered by lansoprazole in CYP2C19 poor metabolizers. *Clin Pharmacol Ther* (1999) 65, 606–14.
7. Oosterhuis B, Jonkman JHG, Andersson T, Zuiderwijk PBM. No influence of single intravenous doses of omeprazole on theophylline elimination kinetics. *J Clin Pharmacol* (1992) 32, 470–5.
8. Sommers De K, van Wyk M, Snyman JR, Moncrieff J. The effects of omeprazole-induced hypochlorhydria on absorption of theophylline from a sustained-release formulation. *Eur J Clin Pharmacol* (1992) 43, 141–3.
9. Taburet AM, Geneve J, Bocquentin M, Simoneau G, Caulin C, Singlas E. Theophylline steady state pharmacokinetics is not altered by omeprazole. *Eur J Clin Pharmacol* (1992) 42, 343–5.
10. Pilotto A, Franceschi M, Lagni M, Fabrello R, Fortunato A, Meggiato T, Soffiati G, Oliani G, Di Mario F. The effect of omeprazole on serum concentrations of theophylline, pepsinogens A and C, and gastrin in elderly duodenal ulcer patients. *Am J Ther* (1995) 2, 43–6.
11. Cavuto NJ, Sukhova N, Hewett J, Balian JD, Woosley RL, Flockhart MD. Effect of omeprazole on theophylline clearance in poor metabolizers of omeprazole. *Clin Pharmacol Ther* (1995) 57, 215.
12. Schulz H-U, Hartmann M, Steinijans VW, Huber R, Lührmann B, Bliessath H, Wurst W. Lack of influence of pantoprazole on the disposition kinetics of theophylline in man. *Int J Clin Pharmacol Ther Toxicol* (1991) 29, 369–75.
13. Humphries TJ, Nardi RV, Spera AC, Lazar JD, Laurent AL, Spanyers SA. Coadministration of rabeprazole sodium (E3810) does not effect the pharmacokinetics of anhydrous theophylline or warfarin. *Gastroenterology* (1996) 110 (Suppl), A138.
14. Humphries TJ, Nardi RV, Lazar JD, Spanyers SA. Drug-drug interaction evaluation of rabeprazole sodium: a clean/expected slate? *Gut* (1996) 39 (Suppl 3), A47.

Theophylline + Pyrantel

A single case report describes increased serum theophylline levels when a child was also given pyrantel.

Clinical evidence

An 8-year-old boy with status asthmaticus was treated firstly with intravenous aminophylline and then switched to sustained-release oral theophylline on day 3, at which point his serum theophylline level was 15 mg/L. On day 4 he was given a single 160-mg dose of pyrantel (for an *Ascaris lumbricoides* infection) at the same time as his second theophylline dose. About 2.5 hours later his serum theophylline level was 24 mg/L, and a further 1.5 hours later it had risen to 30 mg/L. No further theophylline was given and no symptoms of theophylline toxicity occurred. The patient was discharged later in the day without theophylline.[1]

Mechanism

Not understood. One suggestion is that the pyrantel inhibited the liver enzymes concerned with the metabolism of the theophylline, thereby increasing its levels. However, this is unlikely as the interaction occurred so rapidly. Another suggestion was that pyrantel may have increased drug release from the sustained-release theophylline preparation.

Importance and management

Information is limited to this single case report. No general conclusions can be based on such slim evidence, but concurrent use should be well monitored because, in this case, the serum theophylline concentration increase was very rapid. More study is needed.

1. Hecht L, Murray WE, Rubenstein S. Theophylline-pyrantel pamoate interaction. *DICP Ann Pharmacother* (1989) 23, 258.

Theophylline + Pyridoxal

There is no evidence of an adverse interaction if pyridoxal (a vitamin B_6 substance) and theophylline are taken concurrently. There may be some reduction in theophylline-induced hand tremor.

Clinical evidence, mechanism, importance and management

In a crossover study, 15 young healthy adults were given theophylline (*Theo-Dur*) for 4 weeks, with the dose adjusted to give plasma levels of 10 mg/L, combined with daily doses of either a placebo or a vitamin B_6 supplement containing pyridoxal hydrochloride 15 mg. A variety of psychomotor and electrophysiological tests and self-report questionnaires failed to distinguish between the effects of the placebo or the vitamin B_6 supplement, except that the hand tremor induced by the theophylline tended to be reduced.[1] In another study by the same research group, 15 healthy subjects (smoking status not indicated) took pyridoxal 15 mg daily for 2 weeks prior to starting, and when also taking, sustained-release theophylline (*Theo-Dur*), 5 mg/kg daily for one week increased to 8 mg/kg daily for the next 3 weeks. Theophylline levels were subtherapeutic and ranged from 7.6 to 9.9 [mg/L]. Supplementation with pyridoxal did not prevent theophylline-induced reductions in pyridoxine 5-phosphate levels, as an indicator of vitamin B_6 status, although these did not drop below the normal reference range.[2]

There would seem to be no reason for avoiding concurrent use and it may even have some advantage.

1. Bartel PR, Ubbink JB, Delport R, Lotz BP, Becker PJ. Vitamin B-6 supplementation and theophylline-related effects in humans. *Am J Clin Nutr* (1994) 60, 93–9.
2. Delport R, Ubbink JB, Vermaak WJH, Becker PJ. Theophylline increases pyridoxal kinase activity independently from vitamin B6 nutritional status. *Res Commun Chem Pathol Pharmacol* (1993) 79, 325–33.

Theophylline + Quinolones

Theophylline serum levels can be markedly increased in most patients by enoxacin. Pipemidic acid and clinafloxacin probably interact similarly. Theophylline levels can also be markedly increased in some patients by ciprofloxacin, and possibly pefloxacin. Norfloxacin, ofloxacin, pazufloxacin, or prulifloxacin normally cause a much smaller rise in theophylline levels. However, serious toxicity has been seen in few patients given norfloxacin. Fleroxacin, flumequine, gatifloxacin, gemifloxacin, levofloxacin, lomefloxacin, moxifloxacin, nalidixic acid, rufloxacin, sparfloxacin and trovafloxacin appear not to interact.

Table 33.4 Effect of quinolones on theophylline pharmacokinetics in order of magnitude of the potential interaction

Quinolone (daily dose)	*Increase in theophylline level*	*Increase in AUC*	*Decrease in clearance*	*Refs*
Enoxacin 600 to 1200 mg	72 to 243%	84 to 248%	42 to 74%	1–8
Pipemidic acid 800 to 1500 mg	71%	76 to 79%	49%	3, 9
Clinafloxacin 400 to 800 mg			46 to 69%	10
Grepafloxacin 200 to 600 mg	28 to 82%	93 to 113%	33 to 54%	11, 12
Ciprofloxacin 600 to 1500 mg	17 to 50%	22 to 52%	18 to 31%	2, 3, 13–18
Pazufloxacin 500 mg	up to 27%	up to 33%	25%	19
Pefloxacin 400 to 800 mg	17 to 20%	19 to 53%	29%	2, 3
Norfloxacin 600 to 800 mg	up to 22%	up to 17%	up to 15%	7, 16, 20–23
Prulifloxacin 600 mg		16%	15%	24
Ofloxacin 400 to 600 mg	up to 10%	up to 10%	up to 12%	2, 3, 7, 22, 25–27
Trovafloxacin 200 to 300 mg		up to 8%		28, 29
Fleroxacin 400 mg	No significant change	up to 8%	up to 6%	30–33
Flumequine 1200 mg	No significant change	No significant change	No significant change	34
Gatifloxacin 400 mg	No significant change	No significant change		35
Gemifloxacin 400 to 600 mg	No significant change	No significant change		36
Levofloxacin 300 to 1000 mg	No significant change	No significant change	No significant change	11, 37, 38
Lomefloxacin 400 to 800 mg	No significant change	No significant change	No significant change	9, 15, 39–42
Moxifloxacin 200 mg to 400 mg	No significant change	No significant change	No significant change	43
Nalidixic acid 400 to 600 mg		No significant change	No significant change	2, 16
Rufloxacin 200 to 400 mg	No significant change	No significant change	No significant change	44, 45
Sparfloxacin 200 to 400 mg	No significant change	No significant change	No significant change	46–49

1. Wijnands WJA, Vree TB, van Herwaarden CLA. Enoxacin decreases the clearance of theophylline in man. *Br J Clin Pharmacol* (1985) 20, 583-8.
2. Wijnands WJA, Vree TB, van Herwaarden CLA. The influence of quinolone derivatives on theophylline clearance. *Br J Clin Pharmacol* (1986) 22, 677-83.
3. Niki Y, Soejima R, Kawane H, Sumi M, Umeki S. New synthetic quinolone antibacterial agents and serum concentration of theophylline. *Chest* (1987) 92, 663-9.
4. Beckmann J, Elsäßer W, Gundert-Remy U, Hertrampf R. Enoxacin - a potent inhibitor of theophylline metabolism. *Eur J Clin Pharmacol* (1987) 33, 227-30.
5. Takagi K, Hasegawa T, Yamaki K, Suzuki R, Watanabe T, Satake T. Interaction between theophylline and enoxacin. *Int J Clin Pharmacol Ther Toxicol* (1988) 26, 288-92.
6. Rogge MC, Solomon WR, Sedman AJ, Welling PG, Koup JR, Wagner JG. The theophylline-enoxacin interaction: II. Changes in the disposition of theophylline and its metabolites during intermittent administration of enoxacin. *Clin Pharmacol Ther* (1989) 46, 420-8.
7. Sano M, Kawakatsu K, Ohkita C, Yamamoto I, Takeyama M, Yamashina H, Goto M. Effects of enoxacin, ofloxacin and norfloxacin on theophylline disposition in humans. *Eur J Clin Pharmacol* (1988) 35, 161-5.
8. Sörgel F, Mahr G, Granneman GR, Stephan U, Nickel P, Muth P. Effects of 2 quinolone antibacterials, temafloxacin and enoxacin, on theophylline pharmacokinetics. *Clin Pharmacokinet* (1992) 22 (Suppl 1), 65-74.
9. Staib AH, Harder S, Fuhr U, Wack C. Interaction of quinolones with the theophylline metabolism in man: investigations with lomefloxacin and pipemidic acid. *Int J Clin Pharmacol Ther Toxicol* (1989) 27, 289-93.

Continued

Table 33.4 Effect of quinolones on theophylline pharmacokinetics in order of magnitude of the potential interaction (continued)

10. Randinitis EJ, Alvey CW, Koup JR, Rausch G, Abel R, Bron NJ, Hounslow NJ, Vassos AB, Sedman AJ. Drug interactions with clinafloxacin. *Antimicrob Agents Chemother* (2001) 45, 2543-52.
11. Niki Y, Hashiguchi K, Okimoto N, Soejima R. Quinolone antimicrobial agents and theophylline. *Chest* (1992) 101, 881.
12. Efthymiopoulos C, Bramer SL, Maroli A, Blum B. Theophylline and warfarin interaction studies with grepafloxacin. *Clin Pharmacokinet* (1997) 33 (Suppl 1), 39-46.
13. Nix DE, DeVito JM, Whitbread MA, Schentag JJ. Effect of multiple dose oral ciprofloxacin on the pharmacokinetics of theophylline and indocyanine green. *J Antimicrob Chemother* (1987) 19, 263-9.
14. Schwartz J, Jauregui L, Lettieri J, Bachmann K. Impact of ciprofloxacin on theophylline clearance and steady-state concentrations in serum. *Antimicrob Agents Chemother* (1988) 32, 75-7.
15. Robson RA, Begg EJ, Atkinson HC, Saunders DA, Frampton CM. Comparative effects of ciprofloxacin and lomefloxacin on the oxidative metabolism of theophylline. *Br J Clin Pharmacol* (1990) 29, 491-3.
16. Prince RA, Casabar E, Adair CG, Wexler DB, Lettieri J, Kasik JE. Effect of quinolone antimicrobials on theophylline pharmacokinetics. *J Clin Pharmacol* (1989) 29, 650-4.
17. Batty KT, Davis TME, Ilett KF, Dusci LJ, Langton SR. The effect of ciprofloxacin on theophylline pharmacokinetics in healthy subjects. *Br J Clin Pharmacol* (1995) 39, 305-11.
18. Gillum JG, Israel DS, Scott RB, Climo MW, Polk RE. Effect of combination therapy with ciprofloxacin and clarithromycin on theophylline pharmacokinetics in healthy volunteers. *Antimicrob Agents Chemother* (1996) 40, 1715-16.
19. Niki Y, Watanabe S, Yoshida K, Miyashita N, Nakajima M, Matsushima T. Effect of pazufloxacin mesilate on the serum concentration of theophylline. *J Infect Chemother* (2002) 8, 33–6.
20. Bowles SK, Popovski Z, Rybak MJ, Beckman HB, Edwards DJ. Effect of norfloxacin on theophylline pharmacokinetics at steady state. *Antimicrob Agents Chemother* (1988) 32, 510-12.
21. Sano M, Yamamoto I, Ueda J, Yoshikawa E, Yamashina H, Goto M. Comparative pharmacokinetics of theophylline following two fluoroquinolones co-administration. *Eur J Clin Pharmacol* (1987) 32, 431-2.
22. Ho G, Tierney MG, Dales RE. Evaluation of the effect of norfloxacin on the pharmacokinetics of theophylline. *Clin Pharmacol Ther* (1988) 44, 35–8.
23. Davis RL, Kelly HW, Quenzer RW, Standefer J, Steinberg B, Gallegos J. Effect of norfloxacin on theophylline metabolism. *Antimicrob Agents Chemother* (1989) 33, 212-4.
24. Fattore C, Cipolla G, Gatti G, Bartoli A, Orticelli G, Picollo R, Millerioux L, Ciotolli GB, Perucca E. Pharmacokinetic interactions between theophylline and prulifloxacin in healthy volunteers. *Clin Drug Invest* (1998) 16, 387-92.
25. Gregoire SL, Grasela TH, Freer JP, Tack KJ, Schentag JJ. Inhibition of theophylline clearance by coadministered ofloxacin without alteration of theophylline effects. *Antimicrob Agents Chemother* (1987) 31, 375-8.
26. Al-Turk WA, Shaheen OM, Othman S, Khalaf RM, Awidi AS. Effect of ofloxacin on the pharmacokinetics of a single intravenous theophylline dose. *Ther Drug Monit* (1988) 10, 160-3.
27. Fourtillan JB, Granier J, Saint-Salvi B, Salmon J, Surjus A, Tremblay D, Vincent du Laurier M, Beck S. Pharmacokinetics of ofloxacin and theophylline alone and in combination. *Infection* (1986) 14 (Suppl 1), S67-S69.
28. Dickens GR, Wermeling D, Vincent J. Phase I pilot study of the effects of trovafloxacin (CP-99,219) on the pharmacokinetics of theophylline in healthy men. *J Clin Pharmacol* (1997) 37, 248-52.
29. Vincent J, Teng R, Dogolo LC, Willavize SA, Friedman HL. Effect of trovafloxacin, a new fluoroquinolone antibiotic, on the steady-state pharmacokinetics of theophylline in healthy volunteers. *J Antimicrob Chemother* (1997) 39 (Suppl B), 81-6.
30. Niki Y, Tasaka Y, Kishimoto T, Nakajima M, Tsukiyama K, Nakagawa Y, Umeki S, Hino J, Okimoto N, Yagi S, Kawane H, Soejima R. Effect of fleroxacin on serum concentration of theophylline. *Chemotherapy* (1990) 38, 364-71.
31. Seelmann R, Mahr G, Gottschalk B, Stephan U, Sörgel F. Influence of fleroxacin on the pharmacokinetics of theophylline. *Rev Infect Dis* (1989) 11 (Suppl 5), S1100.
32. Soejima R, Niki Y, Sumi M. Effect of fleroxacin on serum concentrations of theophylline. *Rev Infect Dis* (1989) 11 (Suppl 5), S1099.
33. Parent M, St-Laurent M, LeBel M. Safety of fleroxacin coadministered with theophylline to young and elderly volunteers. *Antimicrob Agents Chemother* (1990) 34, 1249-53.
34. Lacarelle B, Blin O, Auderbert C, Auquier P, Karsenty H, Horriere F, Durand A. The quinolone, flumequine, has no effect on theophylline pharmacokinetics. *Eur J Clin Pharmacol* (1994) 46, 477-8.
35. Stahlberg HJ, Göhler K, Guillaume M, Mignot A. Effects of gatifloxacin (GTX) on the pharmacokinetics of theophylline in healthy young volunteers. *J Antimicrob Chemother* (1999) 44 (Suppl A), 136.
36. Davy M, Allen A, Bird N, Rost KL, Fuder H. Lack of effect of gemifloxacin on the steady-state pharmacokinetics of theophylline in healthy volunteers. *Chemotherapy* (1999) 45, 478-84.
37. Okimoto N, Niki Y, Soejima R. Effect of levofloxacin on serum concentration of theophylline. *Chemotherapy* (1992) 40, 68-74.
38. Gisclon LG, Curtin CR, Fowler CL, Williams RR, Hafkin B, Natarajan J. Absence of a pharmacokinetic interaction between intravenous theophylline and orally administered levofloxacin. *J Clin Pharmacol* (1997) 37, 744-50.
39. Nix DE, Norman A, Schentag JJ. Effect of lomefloxacin on theophylline pharmacokinetics. *Antimicrob Agents Chemother* (1989) 33, 1006-8.
40. Wijnands GJA, Cornel JH, Martea M, Vree TB. The effect of multiple-dose oral lomefloxacin on theophylline metabolism in man. *Chest* (1990) 98, 1440-4.
41. LeBel M, Vallé F, St-Laurent M. Influence of lomefloxacin on the pharmacokinetics of theophylline. *Antimicrob Agents Chemother* (1990) 34, 1254-6.
42. Kuzuya T, Takagi K, Apichartpichean R, Muraoka I, Nadai M, Hasegawa T. Kinetic interaction between theophylline and a newly developed quinolone, NY-198. *J Pharmacobiodyn* (1989) 12, 405-9.
43. Stass H, Kubitza D. Lack of pharmacokinetic interaction between moxifloxacin, a novel 8-methoxyfluoroquinolone, and theophylline. *Clin Pharmacokinet* (2001) 40 (Suppl 1) 63–70.
44. Cesana M, Broccali G, Imbimbo BP, Crema A. Effect of single doses of rufloxacin on the disposition of theophylline and caffeine after single administration. *Int J Clin Pharmacol Ther Toxicol* (1991) 29, 133-8.
45. Kinzig-Schippers M, Fuhr U, Cesana M, Müller C, Staib AH, Rietbrock S. Sörgel F. Absence of effect of rufloxacin on theophylline pharmacokinetics in steady state. *Antimicrob Agents Chemother* (1998) 42, 2359-64.
46. Takagi K, Yamaki K, Nadai M, Kuzuya T, Hasegawa T. Effect of a new quinolone, sparfloxacin, on the pharmacokinetics of theophylline in asthmatic patients. *Antimicrob Agents Chemother* (1991) 35, 1137-41.
47. Okimoto N, Niki Y, Sumi M, Nakagawa Y, Soejima R. Effect of sparfloxacin on plasma concentration of theophylline. *Chemotherapy (Tokyo)* (1991) 39 (Suppl 4), 158-60.
48. Mahr G, Seelmann R, Gottschalk B, Stephan U, Sörgel F. No effect of sparfloxacin (SPFX) on the metabolism of theophylline (THE) in man. *Intersci Conf Antimicrob Agents Chemother* (1990) 30, 296.
49. Yamaki K, Miyatake H, Taki F, Suzuki R, Takagi K, Satake T. Studies on sparfloxacin (SPFX) against respiratory tract infections and its effect on theophylline pharmacokinetics. *Chemotherapy* (1991) 39 (Suppl 4), 280-5.

Clinical evidence

A. Pharmacokinetic studies

The effects of the quinolones on the pharmacokinetics of theophylline in clinical studies in healthy subjects or patients are listed in 'Table 33.4', (p.1193).

B. Case reports

(a) Ciprofloxacin

There are numerous cases that describe the interaction between ciprofloxacin and theophylline or aminophylline, which commonly report large increases in serum theophylline levels (32 to 478% or 1.3 to 5.6-fold increases), often associated with toxicity.[1-11] From 1987 to 1988, the CSM in the UK had received 8 reports of clinically important adverse interactions between these two drugs, with one fatal case.[1] By 1991, the FDA in the US had received 39 reports of the interaction, with three deaths.[9]

An elderly woman taking theophylline developed toxic serum levels and died shortly after starting to take ciprofloxacin.[7] Seizures, associated with toxic levels of theophylline, were described in a number of the case reports.[5,9-11] Seizures have also occurred when ciprofloxacin was used with theophylline or aminophylline, even when theophylline levels were within the therapeutic range (10 to 20 mg/L).[9,12,13] Ciprofloxacin and toxic levels of theophylline are both known to cause seizures independently. It was suggested that, in the case of seizures, there may be a pharmacodynamic interaction between theophylline and the fluoroquinolones as well as a pharmacokinetic interaction.[9] In each case seizures began within 1 to 7 days of starting the combination and were reported as being either partial or grand mal. The addition of clarithromycin does not appear to increase the effects of ciprofloxacin on theophylline.[14]

(b) Clinafloxacin

The apparently stable serum theophylline levels of a 78-year-old man with steroid-dependent chronic obstructive pulmonary disease were approximately doubled after he received intravenous clinafloxacin 200 mg every 12 hours for 5 days. Two theophylline doses were withheld, and then the dosage was reduced from 300 mg every 8 hours to 200 mg every 8 hours. Within another 5 days his serum theophylline levels had returned to his previous steady-state level.[15]

(c) Enoxacin

Some patients in early studies of enoxacin experienced adverse effects (serious nausea and vomiting, tachycardia, seizures)[16,17] and this was found to be associated with unexpectedly high plasma theophylline levels.[16,18]

(d) Levofloxacin

Levofloxacin has not significantly altered the pharmacokinetics of theophylline in studies, see 'Table 33.4', (p.1193). However, a 59-year-old man developed theophylline toxicity 7 and 5 days after starting clarithromycin and levofloxacin, respectively. His theophylline clearance decreased by about 40% when compared to the value before starting these drugs and so the theophylline dosage was reduced. After stopping the levofloxacin, the theophylline level fell, and the theophylline clearance returned to the initial value, even though clarithromycin was continued.[19]

(e) Norfloxacin

No clinically significant changes in theophylline levels occurred in a patient given norfloxacin who subsequently had marked changes when given ciprofloxacin.[3] This report and the studies in 'Table 33.4', (p.1193) contrast with the records of the FDA in the US, which describe 3 patients (up to 1989)[20] and 9 patients (up to 1991)[9] who experienced marked increases in theophylline levels ranging from 64 to 171% (mean 103%). Three patients developed seizures, and one died.[9]

(f) Pefloxacin

An isolated report describes convulsions in a patient, which were attributed to the use of theophylline with pefloxacin.[21]

Mechanism

The interacting quinolones appear to inhibit the metabolism (*N*-demethylation) of theophylline to different extents (some hardly at all), so that it is cleared from the body more slowly and its serum levels rise. The quinolones are known to inhibit the cytochrome P450 isoenzyme CYP1A2 by which theophylline is metabolised. Although neither levofloxacin and clarithromycin alone usually interact, the case report suggests that together they may.[19] There is some evidence that combined use of theophyllines and quinolones may amplify the epileptogenic activity of the quinolones.[9,22]

Importance and management

The interactions of enoxacin and ciprofloxacin with theophylline are well documented, well established and of clinical importance. The effect of enoxacin is marked and occurs in most patients, whereas the incidence with ciprofloxacin is uncertain and problems do not develop in all patients. The risk seems greatest in the elderly[23] and those with theophylline levels already towards the top end of the therapeutic range. Toxicity may develop rapidly (within 2 to 3 days) unless the theophylline dosage is reduced.

With enoxacin, it has been suggested that the dose of theophylline should be reduced by 50%,[18,24-26] although reductions of 75% may possibly be necessary for those with high theophylline clearances.[26] Alterations in the theophylline dose should be based on careful monitoring of theophylline levels. New steady-state serum theophylline levels are achieved within about 2 to 3 days of starting and stopping enoxacin.[26,27]

Although problems do not develop in all patients taking theophylline and ciprofloxacin it would be prudent to be alert for this interaction in any patient. Some recommend an initial reduction in theophylline dose, in the order of 30 to 50% when ciprofloxacin is started.[9,28,29] However, since a proportion of patients will not require a dose reduction, others suggest that the dose should be modified based on the theophylline level on day 2 of ciprofloxacin use.[11,24,30-32]

Direct information about clinafloxacin and pipemidic acid is more limited, but they also appear to cause a considerable rise in serum theophylline levels, similar to enoxacin, and therefore it would seem prudent to anticipate the need for a dosage reduction and monitor theophylline levels closely.

Keep a check on the effects if norfloxacin, ofloxacin, pazufloxacin, or pefloxacin are used because theophylline serum levels may possibly rise to a small extent (10 to 22%), but these antibacterials normally appear to be much safer. However, be aware that norfloxacin has caused a much larger rise on occasions.[9,20] Fleroxacin, flumequine, gatifloxacin, gemifloxacin, levofloxacin, lomefloxacin, moxifloxacin, nalidixic acid, rufloxacin, sparfloxacin and trovafloxacin appear not to interact significantly, and no special precautions seem necessary with these drugs. However, note that acute infection *per se* can alter theophylline pharmacokinetics. The manufacturers of some quinolones include a warning in their product literature about the risk of combining theophylline with quinolones because of their potential additive effects on reducing the seizure threshold. Convulsions have been reported with theophylline and ciprofloxacin, norfloxacin, or pefloxacin. With some of these cases it is difficult to know whether what happened was due to increased theophylline levels, to patient pre-disposition, to potential additive effects on the seizure threshold, or to all three factors combined. However, the literature suggests that seizures attributed to concurrent use are relatively rare, so that the general warning about the risks with all quinolones may possibly be an overstatement.

1. Bem JL, Mann RD. Danger of interaction between ciprofloxacin and theophylline. *BMJ* (1988) 296, 1131.
2. Thomson AH, Thomson GD, Hepburn M, Whiting B. A clinically significant interaction between ciprofloxacin and theophylline. *Eur J Clin Pharmacol* (1987) 33, 435–6.
3. Richardson JP. Theophylline toxicity associated with the administration of ciprofloxacin in a nursing home patient. *J Am Geriatr Soc* (1990) 38, 236–8.
4. Duraski RM. Ciprofloxacin-induced theophylline toxicity. *South Med J* (1988) 81,1206.
5. Holden R. Probable fatal interaction between ciprofloxacin and theophylline. *BMJ* (1988) 297, 1339.
6. Rybak MJ, Bowles SK, Chandraseker PH, Edwards DJ. Increased theophylline concentrations secondary to ciprofloxacin. *Drug Intell Clin Pharm* (1987) 21, 879–81.
7. Paidipaty B, Erickson S. Ciprofloxacin-theophylline drug interaction. *Crit Care Med* (1990) 18, 685–6.
8. Spivey JM, Laughlin PH, Goss TF, Nix DE. Theophylline toxicity secondary to ciprofloxacin administration. *Ann Emerg Med* (1991) 20, 1131–4.
9. Grasela TH, Dreis MW. An evaluation of the quinolone-theophylline interaction using the Food and Drug Administration spontaneous reporting system. *Arch Intern Med* (1992) 152, 617–621.
10. Schlienger RG, Wyser C, Ritz R, Haefeli WE. Der klinisch-pharmakologische fall (4). Epileptischer Anfall als unerwünschte Arzneimittelwirkung bei Theophyllinintoxikation. *Schweiz Rundsch Med Prax* (1996) 85, 1407–12.
11. Andrews PA. Interactions with ciprofloxacin and erythromycin leading to aminophylline toxicity. *Nephrol Dial Transplant* (1998) 13, 1006–8.
12. Semel JD, Allen N. Seizures in patients simultaneously receiving theophylline and imipenem or ciprofloxacin or metronidazole. *South Med J* (1991) 84, 465–8.
13. Bader MB. Role of ciprofloxacin in fatal seizures. *Chest* (1992) 101, 883–4.
14. Gillum JG, Israel DS, Scott RB, Climo MW, Polk RE. Effect of combination therapy with ciprofloxacin and clarithromycin on theophylline pharmacokinetics in healthy volunteers. *Antimicrob Agents Chemother* (1996) 40, 1715–16.
15. Matuschka PR, Vissing RS. Clinafloxacin-theophylline drug interaction. *Ann Pharmacother* (1995) 29, 378–80.

16. Wijnands WJA, van Herwaarden CLA, Vree TB. Enoxacin raises plasma theophylline concentrations. *Lancet* (1984) ii, 108–9.
17. Davies BI, Maesen FPV, Teengs JP. Serum and sputum concentrations of enoxacin after single oral dosing in a clinical and bacteriological study. *J Antimicrob Chemother* (1984) 14 (Suppl C), 83–9.
18. Wijnands WJA, Vree TB, van Herwaarden CLA. Enoxacin decreases the clearance of theophylline in man. *Br J Clin Pharmacol* (1985) 20, 583–8.
19. Nakamura H, Ohtsuka T, Enomoto H, Hasegawa A, Kawana H, Kuriyama T, Ohmori S, Kitada M. Effect of levofloxacin on theophylline clearance during theophylline and clarithromycin combination therapy. *Ann Pharmacother* (2001) 35, 691–3.
20. Green L, Clark J. Fluoroquinolones and theophylline toxicity: norfloxacin. *JAMA* (1989) 262, 2383.
21. Conri C, Lartigue MC, Abs L, Mestre MC, Vincent MP, Haramburu F, Constans J. Convulsions chez une malade traitée par péfloxacine et théophylline. *Therapie* (1990) 45, 358.
22. Segev S, Rehavi M, Rubinstein E. Quinolones, theophylline, and diclofenac interactions with the γ-aminobutyric acid receptor. *Antimicrob Agents Chemother* (1988) 32, 1624–6.
23. Raoof S, Wollschlager C, Khan FA. Ciprofloxacin increases serum levels of theophylline. *Am J Med* (1987) 82 (Suppl 4A), 115–18.
24. Wijnands WJA, Vree TB, van Herwaarden CLA. The influence of quinolone derivatives on theophylline clearance. *Br J Clin Pharmacol* (1986) 22, 677–83.
25. Takagi K, Hasegawa T, Yamaki K, Suzuki R, Watanabe T, Satake T. Interaction between theophylline and enoxacin. *Int J Clin Pharmacol Ther Toxicol* (1988) 26, 288–92.
26. Koup JR, Toothaker RD, Posvar E, Sedman AJ, Colburn WA. Theophylline dosage adjustment during enoxacin coadministration. *Antimicrob Agents Chemother* (1990) 34, 803–7.
27. Rogge MC, Solomon WR, Sedman AJ, Welling PG, Koup JR, Wagner JG. The theophylline-enoxacin interaction: II. Changes in the disposition of theophylline and its metabolites during intermittent administration of enoxacin. *Clin Pharmacol Ther* (1989) 46, 420–8.
28. Robson RA, Begg EJ, Atkinson HC, Saunders DA, Frampton CM. Comparative effects of ciprofloxacin and lomefloxacin on the oxidative metabolism of theophylline. *Br J Clin Pharmacol* (1990) 29, 491–3.
29. Prince RA, Casabar E, Adair CG, Wexler DB, Lettieri J, Kasik JE. Effect of quinolone antimicrobials on theophylline pharmacokinetics. *J Clin Pharmacol* (1989) 29, 650–4.
30. Nix DE, DeVito JM, Whitbread MA, Schentag JJ. Effect of multiple dose oral ciprofloxacin on the pharmacokinetics of theophylline and indocyanine green. *J Antimicrob Chemother* (1987) 19, 263–9.
31. Schwartz J, Jauregui L, Lettieri J, Bachmann K. Impact of ciprofloxacin on theophylline clearance and steady-state concentrations in serum. *Antimicrob Agents Chemother* (1988) 32, 75–7.
32. Batty KT, Davis TME, Ilett KF, Dusci LJ, Langton SR. The effect of ciprofloxacin on theophylline pharmacokinetics in healthy subjects. *Br J Clin Pharmacol* (1995) 39, 305–11.

Theophylline + Repaglinide

Repaglinide 2 mg three times a day for 4 days did not significantly affect the steady-state pharmacokinetics of theophylline in 14 healthy subjects, although the peak plasma concentration was slightly reduced.[1] No special precautions would appear to be necessary during concurrent use.

1. Hartop V, Thomsen MS. Drug interaction studies with repaglinide: repaglinide on digoxin or theophylline pharmacokinetics and cimetidine on repaglinide pharmacokinetics. *J Clin Pharmacol* (2000) 40, 184–92.

Theophylline + Ribavirin

Ribavirin does not alter theophylline levels.

Clinical evidence, mechanism, importance and management

Oral ribavirin 200 mg every 6 hours had no effect on the plasma theophylline levels of 13 healthy subjects given immediate or sustained-release aminophylline. Similarly, ribavirin 10 mg/kg daily did not affect the plasma theophylline levels in 6 children with influenza and asthma.[1] No special precautions seem necessary on concurrent use.

1. Fraschini F, Scaglione F, Maierna G, Cogo R, Furcolo F, Gattei R, Borghi C, Palazzini E. Ribavirin influence on theophylline plasma levels in adult and children. *Int J Clin Pharmacol Ther Toxicol* (1988) 26, 30–2.

Theophylline + Rifamycins and/or Isoniazid

Rifampicin (rifampin) lowers the serum levels of theophylline, but rifabutin appears to have little effect. Isoniazid may decrease or increase theophylline clearance and may increase theophylline levels. An isolated report describes theophylline toxicity one month after a patient started to take theophylline with isoniazid. Isoniazid and rifampicin increased theophylline clearance during the initial few days of tuberculosis treatment in one study, but there is some evidence that it decreases it within 4 weeks in another.

Clinical evidence

A. Effects of the individual antimycobacterial drugs on theophylline

(a) Isoniazid alone

Theophylline toxicity has been described in one patient receiving isoniazid 5 mg/kg daily and theophylline, and this subsequently recurred on rechallenge.[1] In 7 healthy subjects, high-dose isoniazid (10 mg/kg daily) for 10 days increased the AUC_{0-6} of theophylline by only 8%. The theophylline was given as an intravenous infusion of aminophylline and the plasma levels after 6 hours were 22% higher (about 10.5 mg/L compared with 8.7 mg/L). Five subjects also had an increase in the half-life and AUC of isoniazid, but these changes were not statistically significant.[2] Another study, in 13 healthy subjects, found that isoniazid 400 mg daily for 2 weeks reduced the mean clearance of theophylline (given as intravenous aminophylline) by 21%.[3]

However, another study in 4 healthy subjects given isoniazid 300 mg daily for 6 days found that the clearance of oral theophylline was increased by 16%, but no consistent changes were seen in any of the other pharmacokinetic parameters measured.[4]

(b) Rifabutin

The AUC of a single 5-mg/kg dose of theophylline was reduced by 6% in 11 healthy subjects who took rifabutin 300 mg daily for 12 days. The half-life and clearance of theophylline were not affected.[5]

(c) Rifampicin (Rifampin)

The AUC of theophylline (given as sustained-release aminophylline 450 mg) was reduced by 18% in 7 healthy subjects who took rifampicin 600 mg daily for one week. A parallel study in another 8 healthy subjects given the same dosage of rifampicin showed that the metabolic clearance of theophylline (given as intravenous aminophylline 5 mg/kg) was increased by 45%.[6]

Similarly, other studies in healthy subjects given oral or intravenous theophylline or intravenous aminophylline and rifampicin 300 to 600 mg daily for 6 to 14 days found 25 to 82% rises in theophylline clearance, and 19 to 31% decreases in its half-life.[5,7-12] A 61% fall in the 5-hour post-dose serum levels of theophylline (given as choline theophyllinate) occurred in a 15-month-old boy when he was given a 4-day course of rifampicin 20 mg/kg daily as meningitis prophylaxis.[13]

B. Effects of combined antimycobacterial drugs on theophylline

A study in patients taking a combination of **isoniazid**, **rifampicin**, **ethambutol** and **pyrazinamide** for pulmonary tuberculosis with intravenous aminophylline 7.35 mg/kg daily for 7 days found that the clearance of theophylline progressively increased, and was 53% faster on day seven.[14] In contrast, in an earlier study by the same authors, after 4 weeks of the same antimycobacterials (isoniazid, rifampicin, ethambutol with or without pyrazinamide) the theophylline clearance in patients receiving long-term theophylline was about 35% slower than in a control group of similar patients not taking antimycobacterials.[15] A single report describes unexpectedly *high* serum theophylline levels 4 days after theophylline 300 mg twice daily was started in an alcoholic patient with hepatic impairment who had started to take **rifampicin** and **isoniazid** 2 weeks previously.[16]

Mechanism

Rifampicin is a potent liver enzyme inducer, which increases the metabolism of the theophylline, thereby increasing its clearance and reducing its serum levels.[8] It has been suggested that isoniazid inhibits the metabolism of theophylline by the liver, thereby reducing its clearance and increasing its plasma levels. Rifabutin is a much less potent liver enzyme inducer than rifampicin, and consequently has less of an effect on theophylline metabolism.

With combined therapy, it was suggested that the effects of rifampicin might be more apparent during the initial 7 days, but that by week 4 the effect of isoniazid might predominate, because of its reduced inactivation by rifampicin combined with a reduction in the effect of rifampicin by auto-induction of its own metabolism.[15] High theophylline levels in the isolated case above may have been due to liver impairment brought about by the combined use of rifampicin and isoniazid, or alcoholism.[13]

Importance and management

The interaction between theophylline and **rifampicin** is established. The levels and therapeutic effects of theophylline are likely to be reduced during concurrent treatment, and this effect can usually be detected within

36 hours.[13] The wide range of increases in clearance that have been reported (25 to 82%) and the large inter-subject variation make it difficult to predict the increase in theophylline dosage required, but in some instances a twofold increase may be needed.[8] Monitor theophylline levels if rifampicin is started or stopped and adjust the theophylline dose accordingly.

The effects of **rifabutin** are considerably less than those of rifampicin, with the one available study showing no significant interaction. On the basis of this, no special precautions appear to be necessary, but it may be prudent to monitor the efficacy of theophylline on concurrent use.

The reason for the inconsistent results with **isoniazid** alone is not understood, nor is this interaction well established. It has been suggested that it may take 3 to 4 weeks for any significant increase in theophylline levels to occur.[1] However, if enzyme inhibition was the cause, the effects would be expected more rapidly than this. All of the studies cited covered a period of only 6 to 14 days, whereas the case report describes the effects over a period up to 55 days.[1] It has also been suggested that the dose of isoniazid may be important, with the clearance of theophylline being unaffected by 'usual doses' of isoniazid, but reduced by larger doses.[17] The outcome of concurrent isoniazid and theophylline use is uncertain and may be affected by other antimycobacterials, but it would clearly be prudent to be alert for any evidence of changes in theophylline levels and toxicity if isoniazid is given.

Isoniazid and rifampicin are usually taken as part of a combination chemotherapy regimen in the treatment of tuberculosis. There is some evidence that, in the short-term, combined use of these drugs will decrease theophylline levels, but that theophylline levels may increase during long-term therapy. However this requires confirmation. Patients taking theophylline with a combined anti-tubercular regimen including isoniazid and rifampicin should have their theophylline levels closely monitored and the dose adjusted according to the response, bearing in mind that these changes may occur over a longer period of time as reported in the case with isoniazid.

1. Torrent J, Izquierdo I, Cabezas R, Jané F. Theophylline-isoniazid interaction. *DICP Ann Pharmacother* (1989) 23, 143–5.
2. Höglund P, Nilsson L-G, Paulsen O. Interaction between isoniazid and theophylline. *Eur J Respir Dis* (1987) 70, 110–16.
3. Samigun, Mulyono, Santoso B. Lowering of theophylline clearance by isoniazid in slow and rapid acetylators. *Br J Clin Pharmacol* (1990) 29, 570–3.
4. Thompson JR, Burckart GJ, Self TH, Brown RE, Straughn AB. Isoniazid-induced alterations in theophylline pharmacokinetics. *Curr Ther Res* (1982) 32, 921–5.
5. Gillum JG, Sesler JM, Bruzzese VL, Israel DS, Polk RE. Induction of theophylline clearance by rifampin and rifabutin in healthy male volunteers. *Antimicrob Agents Chemother* (1996) 40, 1866–9.
6. Powell-Jackson PR, Jamieson AP, Gray BJ, Moxham J, Williams R. Effect of rifampicin administration on theophylline pharmacokinetics in humans. *Am Rev Respir Dis* (1985) 131, 939–40.
7. Straughn AB, Henderson RP, Lieberman PL, Self TH. Effect of rifampin on theophylline disposition. *Ther Drug Monit* (1984) 6, 153–6.
8. Robson RA, Miners JO, Wing LMH, Birkett DJ. Theophylline-rifampicin interaction: non-selective induction of theophylline metabolic pathways. *Br J Clin Pharmacol* (1984) 18, 445–8.
9. Löfdahl CG, Mellstrand T, Svedmyr N. Increased metabolism of theophylline by rifampicin. *Respiration* (1984) 46 (Suppl 1), 104.
10. Hauser AR, Lee C, Teague RB, Mullins C. The effect of rifampin on theophylline disposition. *Clin Pharmacol Ther* (1983) 33, 254.
11. Boyce EG, Dukes GE, Rollins DE, Sudds TW. The effect of rifampin on theophylline kinetics. *J Clin Pharmacol* (1986) 26, 696–9.
12. Rao S, Singh SK, Narang RK, Rajagopalan PT. Effect of rifampicin on theophylline pharmacokinetics in human beings. *J Assoc Physicians India* (1994) 42, 881–2.
13. Brocks DR, Lee KC, Weppler CP, Tam YK. Theophylline-rifampin interaction in a pediatric patient. *Clin Pharm* (1986) 5, 602–4.
14. Ahn HC, Lee YC. The clearance of theophylline is increased during the initial period of tuberculosis treatment. *Int J Tuberc Lung Dis* (2003) 7, 587–91.
15. Ahn HC, Yang JH, Lee HB, Rhee YK, Lee YC. Effect of combined therapy of oral anti-tubercular agents on theophylline pharmacokinetics. *Int J Tuberc Lung Dis* (2000) 4, 784–7.
16. Dal Negro R, Turco P, Trevisan F, De Conti F. Rifampicin-isoniazid and delayed elimination of theophylline: a case report. *Int J Clin Pharmacol Res* (1988) 8, 275–7.
17. Thompson JR, Self TH. Theophylline and isoniazid. *Br J Clin Pharmacol* (1990) 30, 909.

Theophylline + Ropinirole

Theophylline and ropinirole do not appear to interact.

Clinical evidence, mechanism, importance and management

In one study, 12 patients with parkinsonism were given ropinirole, increased from 0.5 mg to 2 mg three times daily over 28 days, then continued for a further 19 days. The pharmacokinetics of theophylline, given as a single intravenous dose of aminophylline, were assessed before ropinirole was started and on day 27. The pharmacokinetics of ropinirole were then assessed before, during and after, the use of oral controlled-release theophylline twice daily for 13 days (dose titrated to achieve plasma levels in the range 8 to 15 micrograms/mL). In both cases it was found that concurrent use did not alter the pharmacokinetics of either drug, and concurrent use was well tolerated.[1] There would therefore appear to be no reason to take special precautions if both drugs are used, and no need to adjust the dosage of either drug. An interaction had originally been suspected because both drugs are metabolised by the cytochrome P450 isoenzyme CYP1A2.

1. Thalamas C, Taylor A, Brefel-Courbon C, Eagle S, Fitzpatrick K, Rascol O. Lack of pharmacokinetic interaction between ropinirole and theophylline in patients with Parkinson's disease. *Eur J Clin Pharmacol* (1999) 55, 299–303.

Theophylline + SSRIs

Theophylline serum levels can be markedly and rapidly increased by fluvoxamine. Toxicity will develop if the theophylline dosage is not suitably reduced. Some preliminary clinical evidence suggests that fluoxetine and citalopram may not interact, and *in vitro* evidence suggests that paroxetine and sertraline are also unlikely to interact.

Clinical evidence

(a) Citalopram

In a study in 13 healthy subjects citalopram 40 mg daily for 21 days (to achieve steady-state) did not affect the pharmacokinetics of a single 300-mg oral dose of theophylline.[1]

(b) Fluoxetine

The pharmacokinetics of theophylline were unchanged in 8 healthy subjects when they were given a 6-mg/kg infusion of aminophylline over 30 minutes, 8 hours after a single 40-mg dose of fluoxetine.[2]

(c) Fluvoxamine

The effect of fluvoxamine on theophylline pharmacokinetics has been characterised in two studies in healthy subjects. In the first study the AUC of theophylline (given as a single 442-mg oral dose of aminophylline) was increased almost threefold, the clearance was reduced by 62% and the half-life was prolonged from 7.4 to 32.1 hours by fluvoxamine 50 mg daily for 3 days then 100 mg daily for 13 days.[3] In the second study, the clearance of theophylline (given as a single 300-mg oral dose of aminophylline) was reduced by about 70% and the half-life was increased from 6.6 to 22 hours by fluvoxamine 50 to 100 mg daily for 7 days.[4] This interaction was shown to be reduced in patients with mild and severe liver cirrhosis (Child class A and C, respectively), whereas the clearance of a single 4-mg/kg dose of theophylline elixir was reduced by 62%, 52%, and 10.5% in healthy subjects, patients with mild cirrhosis, and patients with severe cirrhosis, respectively. The half-life of theophylline was increased by 13.6 hours in healthy subjects compared with 10.5 hours in patients with mild cirrhosis and 1 hour in patients with severe cirrhosis, demonstrating the reduced metabolic capabilities of the cirrhotic liver.[5]

A number of case reports have described fluvoxamine-induced theophylline toxicity. Agitation and tachycardia (120 bpm) developed in an 83-year-old man taking theophylline 600 mg daily (*Theostat*) about a week after he started to take fluvoxamine 100 mg daily. His serum theophylline levels were found to have risen from under 15 mg/L to 40 mg/L.[6] A 70-year-old man similarly developed theophylline toxicity, with theophylline levels of about 32 mg/L (reference range 10 to 20 mg/L), when fluvoxamine was added. Subsequently the theophylline concentrations were found to parallel a number of changes in the fluvoxamine dosage.[7] The clearance of theophylline in an 84-year-old man was approximately halved while he was taking fluvoxamine.[8] An 11-year-old boy complained of headaches, tiredness and vomiting within a week of starting to take fluvoxamine. His serum theophylline levels were found to have doubled, from 14.2 to 27.4 mg/L.[9] A 78-year-old woman became nauseous within 2 days of starting to take fluvoxamine 50 mg daily, and by day 6, when the fluvoxamine was stopped, her serum theophylline levels were found to have increased about threefold. She experienced a seizure, became comatose, and had supraventricular tachycardia (200 bpm) requiring intravenous digoxin and verapamil. She recovered uneventfully.[10] A patient taking fluvoxamine 100 mg daily developed nausea, vomiting, confusion, reduced sleep and a poor appetite 5 days after she began to take theophylline 300 mg twice daily for COPD. Her theophylline level was found to be 25.9 mg/L.[11]

Mechanism

In vitro studies with human liver microsomes have shown that fluvoxamine inhibits the cytochrome P450 isoenzyme CYP1A2, the principal enzyme responsible for the metabolism of theophylline.[12,13] This results in raised theophylline levels and toxicity. This metabolic function, and hence interaction, appears to be severely reduced in patients with severe cirrhosis, probably due to reduced hepatic expression of CYP1A2 and reduced uptake of fluvoxamine.[5] The other SSRIs, citalopram, fluoxetine, **paroxetine** and **sertraline** only weakly inhibited CYP1A2 *in vitro*, and consequently would not be expected to interact.[12,13]

Importance and management

The interaction between fluvoxamine and theophylline is established and clinically important. The CSM in the UK advise that concurrent use should usually be avoided, but that if this is not possible, reduce the theophylline dosage by half when fluvoxamine is added and monitor theophylline levels.[14]. There is evidence to suggest that the extent of this interaction is markedly reduced in patients with liver cirrhosis, particularly severe Child class C, despite higher levels of fluvoxamine,[5] although caution should still be applied with concurrent use in this patient group as they are more likely to have high levels of theophylline due to reduced metabolism. There is good *in vitro* evidence to suggest that fluvoxamine is the only SSRI likely to interact (because it is the only one that significantly affects CYP1A2). This would seem to be borne out by the lack of studies and case reports in the literature describing problems with any of the other SSRIs.

1. Møller SE, Larsen F, Pitsiu M, Rolan PE. Effect of citalopram on plasma levels of oral theophylline. *Clin Ther* (2000) 22, 1494–1501.
2. Mauro VF, Mauro LS, Klions HA. Effect of single dose fluoxetine on aminophylline pharmacokinetics. *Pharmacotherapy* (1994) 14, 367.
3. Donaldson KM, Wright DM, Mathlener IS, Harry JD. The effect of fluvoxamine at steady state on the pharmacokinetics of theophylline after a single dose in healthy male volunteers. *Br J Clin Pharmacol* (1994) 37, 492P.
4. Rasmussen BB, Jeppesen U, Gaist D, Brøsen K. Griseofulvin and fluvoxamine interactions with the metabolism of theophylline. *Ther Drug Monit* (1997) 19, 56–62.
5. Orlando R, Padrini R, Perazzi M, De Martin S, Piccoli P, Palatini P. Liver dysfunction markedly decreases the inhibition of cytochrome P450 1A2-mediated theophylline metabolism by fluvoxamine. *Clin Pharmacol Ther* (2006) 79, 489–99.
6. Diot P, Jonville AP, Gerard F, Bonnelle M, Autret E, Breteau M, Lemarie E, Lavandier M. Possible interaction entre théophylline et fluvoxamine. *Therapie* (1991) 46, 170–71.
7. Thomson AH, McGovern EM, Bennie P, Caldwell G, Smith M. Interaction between fluvoxamine and theophylline. Pharm J (1992) 249, 137. Correction. ibid. (1992) 249, 214.
8. Puranik A, Fitzpatrick R, Ananthanarayanan TS. Monitor serum theophylline. *Care Elder* (1993) 5, 237.
9. Sperber AD. Toxic interaction between fluvoxamine and sustained release theophylline in an 11-year-old boy. *Drug Safety* (1991) 6, 460–2.
10. van den Brekel AM, Harrington L. Toxic effects of theophylline caused by fluvoxamine. *Can Med Assoc J* (1994) 151, 1289–90.
11. DeVane CL, Markowitz JS, Hardesty SJ, Mundy S, Gill HS. Fluvoxamine-induced theophylline toxicity. *Am J Psychiatry* (1997) 154, 1317–18.
12. Brøsen K, Skjelbo E, Rasmussen BB, Poulsen HE, Loft S. Fluvoxamine is a potent inhibitor of cytochrome P4501A2. *Biochem Pharmacol* (1993) 45, 1211–14.
13. Rasmussen BB, Mäenpää J, Pelkonen O, Loft S, Poulsen HE, Lykkesfeldt J, Brøsen K. Selective serotonin reuptake inhibitors and theophylline metabolism in human liver microsomes: potent inhibition by fluvoxamine. *Br J Clin Pharmacol* (1995) 39, 151–9.
14. Committee on Safety of Medicines/Medicines Control Agency. Fluvoxamine increases plasma theophylline levels. *Current Problems* (1994) 20, 12.

Theophylline + St John's wort (*Hypericum perforatum*)

A patient needed a marked increase in the dosage of theophylline while taking St John's wort, but no pharmacokinetic interaction was found in a 2-week study in healthy subjects.

Clinical evidence

A woman, who had previously been stable for several months taking theophylline 300 mg twice daily, was found to need a markedly increased theophylline dosage of 800 mg twice daily to achieve serum levels of 9.2 mg/L. It turned out that 2 months previously she had started to take 300 mg of a St John's wort supplement (hypericin 0.3%) each day. When she stopped taking the St John's wort, her serum theophylline levels doubled within a week to 19.6 mg/L and her theophylline dosage was consequently reduced. This patient was also taking a whole spectrum of other drugs (amitriptyline, furosemide, ibuprofen, inhaled triamcinolone, morphine, potassium, prednisone, salbutamol (albuterol), valproic acid, zolpidem and zafirlukast) and was also a smoker. No changes in the use of these drugs or altered compliance were identified that might have offered an alternative explanation for the changed theophylline requirements.[1]

However, a study in 12 healthy subjects found that a standardised preparation of St John's wort 300 mg (hypericin 0.27%) three times daily for 15 days had no significant effects on the plasma level of a single 400-mg oral dose of theophylline.[2]

Mechanism

Uncertain. *In vitro* data suggest one component of St John's wort (hypericin) can act as an inducer of the cytochrome P450 isoenzyme CYP1A2.[1] It has also been suggested that treatment with St John's wort for 15 days was unlikely to induce the isoenzymes sufficiently to cause changes in plasma theophylline.[2] The patient in the case report had been taking St John's wort for 2 months, although at a lower dose, therefore differences in duration of treatment may account for the discrepancy. This is supported by studies in which 4-week[3] but not 2-week treatment[4] with St John's wort modestly increased the paraxanthine/caffeine ratio, used as a measure of CYP1A2 activity.

Importance and management

Direct information about this apparent interaction between theophylline and St John's wort appears to be limited. No pharmacokinetic interaction was noted in healthy subjects, but the case report describes a marked decrease in theophylline levels. Mechanistic studies suggest a modest interaction at most. Furthermore most clinically significant interactions with St John's wort are mediated by the cytochrome P450 isoenzyme CYP3A4. However, it would be prudent to monitor the effects and serum levels of theophylline if St John's wort is started or stopped, and patients should be warned of the possible effects of concurrent use. In 2000, the CSM in the UK recommended that patients taking theophylline should not take St John's wort. In those patients already taking the combination, the St John's wort should be stopped and the theophylline dosage monitored and adjusted if necessary.[5,6] More study is needed, as this interaction is potentially of little clinical significance.

1. Nebel A, Schneider BJ, Baker RK, Kroll DJ. Potential metabolic interaction between St John's wort and theophylline. *Ann Pharmacother* (1999) 33, 502.
2. Morimoto T, Kotegawa T, Tsutsumi K, Ohtani Y, Imai H, Nakano S. Effect of St John's wort on the pharmacokinetics of theophylline in healthy volunteers. *J Clin Pharmacol* (2004) 44, 95–101
3. Gurley BJ, Gardner SF, Hubbard MA, Williams DK, Gentry WB, Cui Y, Ang CYW. Cytochrome P450 phenotypic ratios for predicting herb-drug interactions in humans. *Clin Pharmacol Ther* (2002) 72, 276–287.
4. Wang Z, Gorski JC, Hamman MA, Huang S-M, Lesko LJ, Hall SD. The effects of St John's wort (*Hypericum perforatum*) on human cytochrome P450 activity. *Clin Pharmacol Ther* (2001) 70, 317–326.
5. Committee on Safety of Medicines (UK). Message from Professor A Breckenridge (Chairman of CSM) and Fact Sheet for Health Care Professionals, 29th February 2000.
6. Committee on Safety of Medicines/Medicines Control Agency. Reminder: St John's wort *(Hypericum perforatum)* interactions. *Current Problems* (2000) 26, 6–7.

Theophylline + Succimer

A single case report describes a 36% reduction in the serum theophylline levels of a man treated with succimer.

Clinical evidence, mechanism, importance and management

A 65-year old man with chronic obstructive airways disease and chronic lead intoxication was given a 19-day course of lead chelation with succimer. His theophylline level was found to be reduced from about 11 mg/L to 7 mg/L on day 6 and remained at this level until about 9 days after the course of succimer was completed, when it returned to pretreatment levels. His clinical status did not alter despite these changes; possibly because he was also taking prednisone.[1] The reason for these alterations is not understood.

The general importance of this interaction is not known, but it would now be prudent to monitor the situation closely if succimer is added to established treatment with theophylline.

1. Harchelroad R. Pharmacokinetic interaction between dimercaptosuccinic acid (DMSA) and theophylline (THEO). *Vet Hum Toxicol* (1994) 36, 376.

Theophylline + Sucralfate

Two studies found that sucralfate caused only minor changes in theophylline pharmacokinetics, but another suggests that the ab-

sorption of sustained-release theophylline is significantly reduced by sucralfate.

Clinical evidence, mechanism, importance and management

In 8 healthy subjects no clinically important changes occurred in the absorption of a single 5-mg/kg dose of an oral non-sustained release theophylline preparation given at the same time as sucralfate 1 g four times daily. A slight 5% decrease in the AUC was detected.[1] Another study found that sucralfate 1 g four times daily reduced the AUC of a single dose of a sustained-release theophylline preparation (*Theodur*) by 9% (timing of the theophylline dose in relation to the sucralfate dose not noted).[2] In contrast, another group of workers found that when sucralfate 1 g was given 30 minutes before a 350 mg dose of sustained-release theophylline (*PEG capsules*), the theophylline AUC was reduced by 40%.[3] Many patients are given sustained-release theophylline preparations, but neither of these studies clearly shows what is likely to happen in clinical practice, so be alert for any evidence of a reduced response to theophylline. Usually, separating the administration of sucralfate from other drugs by 2 hours is considered sufficient to avoid interactions that occur by reduced absorption.[4] However, the study showing decreased theophylline absorption did not examine the effect of separating the doses. Further study is needed.

1. Cantral KA, Schaaf LJ, Jungnickel PW, Monsour HP. Effect of sucralfate on theophylline absorption in healthy volunteers. *Clin Pharm* (1988) 7, 58–61.
2. Kisor DF, Livengood B, Vieira-Fattahi S, Sterchele JA. Effect of sucralfate administration on the absorption of sustained released theophylline. *Pharmacotherapy* (1990) 10, 253.
3. Fleischmann R, Bozler G, Boekstegers P. Bioverfügbarkeit von Theophylline unter Ulkustherapeutika. *Verh Dtsch Ges Inn Med* (1984) 90, 1876–9.
4. Antepsin (Sucralfate). Chugai Pharma UK Ltd. UK Summary of product characteristics, November 2006.

Theophylline + Sulfinpyrazone

Sulfinpyrazone can cause a small increase in theophylline clearance.

Clinical evidence, mechanism, importance and management

In 6 healthy subjects the total clearance of theophylline 125 mg every 8 hours for 4 days was increased by 22% (range 8.5 to 42%) when they were given sulfinpyrazone 200 mg every 6 hours.[1] This appeared to be the sum of an increase in the metabolism of theophylline by the liver and a decrease in its renal clearance.

Information seems to be limited to this study. The resulting fall in serum theophylline levels is unlikely to be clinically relevant.

1. Birkett DJ, Miners JO, Attwood J. Evidence for a dual action of sulphinpyrazone on drug metabolism in man: theophylline-sulphinpyrazone interaction. *Br J Clin Pharmacol* (1983) 15, 567–9.

Theophylline + Tadalafil

Tadalafil does not alter the pharmacokinetics of theophylline.

Clinical evidence, mechanism, importance and management

A double-blind, placebo-controlled, randomised, crossover study in 17 healthy subjects given enough oral theophylline (a non-selective phosphodiesterase inhibitor) to achieve steady-state levels of about 12 mg/L found that the concurrent use of tadalafil 10 mg daily for 7 days did not affect the pharmacokinetics of either drug. There was a small increase of 3.5 bpm in the heart rate, which was not considered to be clinically relevant in the healthy subjects,[1] but the UK manufacturers advise that this should be considered when both drugs are used concurrently.[2]

1. Eli Lilly and Company. Personal communication, March 2003.
2. Cialis (Tadalafil). Eli Lilly and Company Ltd. UK Summary of product characteristics, July 2006.

Theophylline + Tamsulosin

No clinically relevant pharmacokinetic interaction occurs between theophylline and tamsulosin.

Clinical evidence, mechanism, importance and management

In a double-blind study 10 healthy subjects were given tamsulosin 400 micrograms 30 minutes after breakfast for 2 days then 800 micrograms on the following 5 days with a single 5-mg/kg dose of intravenous theophylline one hour after the last dose of tamsulosin. The pharmacokinetics of theophylline and tamsulosin were not affected by concurrent use. Theophylline is mainly metabolised by the cytochrome isoenzyme CYP1A2, while tamsulosin is metabolised by CYP3A4 and CYP2D6, and therefore a pharmacokinetic interaction would not be expected.[1] The safety of combined use was considered acceptable and dose adjustments were not considered necessary during concurrent use.[1]

1. Miyazawa Y, Starkey LP, Forrest A, Schentag JJ, Kamimura H, Swarz H, Ito Y. Effects of the concomitant administration of tamsulosin (0.8 mg/day) on the pharmacokinetics and safety profile of theophylline (5 mg/kg): a placebo-controlled evaluation. *J Int Med Res* (2002) 30, 34–43.

Theophylline + Tegaserod

Tegaserod does not appear to alter the pharmacokinetics of theophylline.

Clinical evidence, mechanism, importance and management

In 18 healthy subjects, the pharmacokinetics of a single 600-mg dose of controlled-release theophylline were unchanged when it was given with three doses of tegaserod 6 mg (the first was given about 24 hours before the theophylline, the second simultaneously, and the third 12 hours later).[1] It was suggested that tegaserod would not be expected to affect the pharmacokinetics of other drugs that are (like theophylline) substrates for the cytochrome P450 isoenzyme CYP1A2, see 'Table 1.2', (p.4).

1. Zhou H, Khalilieh S, Svendsen K, Pommier F, Osborne S, Appel-Dingemanse S, Lasseter K, McLeod JF. Tegaserod coadministration does not alter the pharmacokinetics of theophylline in healthy subjects. *J Clin Pharmacol* (2001) 41, 987–93.

Theophylline + Teicoplanin

Clinical studies in 20 patients with chronic obstructive pulmonary disease found that teicoplanin 200 mg twice daily and aminophylline 240 mg twice daily (both given as intravenous infusions) had no significant effect on the steady-state pharmacokinetics of either drug.[1] No special precautions would seem necessary during concurrent use.

1. Angrisani M, Cazzola M, Loffreda A, Losasso C, Lucarelli C, Rossi F. Clinical pharmacokinetics of teicoplanin and aminophylline during cotreatment with both medicaments. *Int J Clin Pharmacol Res* (1992) 12, 165–71.

Theophylline + Terbinafine

Preliminary evidence indicates that terbinafine can increase the serum levels of theophylline to some extent, but the clinical importance of this is uncertain.

Clinical evidence, mechanism, importance and management

In an open-label, randomised, crossover study 12 healthy subjects were given a single 5-mg/kg oral dose of aminophylline before and after taking terbinafine 250 mg daily for 3 days. The AUC and half-life of theophylline were increased by 16% and 23%, respectively, and the theophylline clearance was reduced by 14%. It was suggested[1] that this is due to the inhibitory effect of terbinafine on the activity of the cytochrome P450 isoenzyme CYP1A2, which is the main isoenzyme involved in the metabolism of theophylline. The changes seen were only relatively small, but the study periods only lasted 3 days so that the effects of longer concurrent use are uncertain, but a clinically significant interaction seems unlikely. More study is needed.

1. Trépanier EF, Nafziger AN, Amsden GW. Effect of terbinafine on theophylline pharmacokinetics in healthy volunteers. *Antimicrob Agents Chemother* (1998) 42, 695–7.

Theophylline + Tetracyclines

Serum theophylline levels increased in two patients who were also given minocycline or tetracycline. Some controlled studies have shown both increases and decreases in theophylline clearance with doxycycline and tetracycline, with no significant changes overall.

Clinical evidence

(a) Doxycycline

A study in 10 asthmatic subjects given doxycycline 100 mg twice daily on day 1 and then 100 mg daily for 4 days found that the mean serum theophylline level was not significantly altered. However, there was large inter-individual variation, with 4 subjects showing rises of more than 20% (range 24 to 31%) and 2 having decreases of 22% and 33%.[1] Fluctuations of this size are not unusual with theophylline. Another study in 8 healthy subjects given doxycycline 100 mg daily for 7 days with theophylline 350 mg twice daily failed to find any significant changes in theophylline pharmacokinetics.[2]

(b) Minocycline

The serum theophylline levels of a 70-year-old woman with normal liver function increased from 9.8 to 15.5 mg/L after she was given minocycline 100 mg twice daily by infusion for 6 days. Her serum theophylline level was 10.9 mg/L 14 days after the minocycline was stopped.[3]

(c) Tetracycline

After taking tetracycline hydrochloride 250 mg four times daily for 8 days a patient with chronic obstructive pulmonary disease (COPD) showed evidence of theophylline toxicity. After 10 days of tetracycline her serum theophylline levels had risen from about 13 mg/L to 30.8 mg/L. Both drugs were stopped, and after 24 hours her theophylline level was 12.4 mg/L. A later rechallenge in this patient confirmed that the tetracycline was responsible for the raised theophylline levels.[4]

In an earlier study in 8 healthy subjects tetracycline 250 mg four times daily for 7 days did not affect the mean pharmacokinetics of theophylline (given as a single intravenous dose of aminophylline), although there was large inter-individual variation. Four subjects had a decrease in clearance of over 15%, (32% in one subject), and conversely, one subject had a 21% increase in clearance.[5] Other studies in subjects and patients given tetracycline for shorter periods have not found evidence of an important interaction. A study in 9 healthy adults given single 5-mg/kg intravenous doses of aminophylline found that tetracycline 250 mg every 6 hours for 48 hours had no significant effect on theophylline pharmacokinetics.[6] Five non-smoking patients with COPD or asthma had an average rise in serum theophylline levels of 14% after 5 days of treatment with tetracycline 250 mg four times daily, and an 11% decrease in clearance. However, when a sixth patient was included (a smoker) the results were no longer statistically significant.[7]

Mechanism

Not understood. Inhibition of theophylline metabolism and clearance by the tetracyclines has been suggested.[4]

Importance and management

Information seems to be limited. There are two isolated cases of increased theophylline levels with minocycline and tetracycline, but controlled studies have not shown any significant changes in overall theophylline pharmacokinetics. It has been suggested that a clinically important interaction may possibly only occur in a few patients.[1,4] Further study is needed. There seems to be no evidence of adverse interactions with any of the other tetracyclines. However, note that acute infections *per se* can alter theophylline pharmacokinetics.

1. Seggev JS, Shefi M, Schey G, Farfel Z. Serum theophylline concentrations are not affected by coadministration of doxycycline. *Ann Allergy* (1986) 56, 156–7.
2. Jonkman JHG, van der Boon WJV, Schoenmaker R, Holtkamp A, Hempenius J. No influence of doxycycline on theophylline pharmacokinetics. *Ther Drug Monit* (1985) 7, 92–4.
3. Kawai M, Honda A, Yoshida H, Goto M, Shimokata T. Possible theophylline-minocycline interaction. *Ann Pharmacother* (1992) 26, 1300–1.
4. McCormack JP, Reid SE, Lawson LM. Theophylline toxicity induced by tetracycline. *Clin Pharm* (1990) 9, 546–9.
5. Mathis JW, Prince RA, Weinberger MM, McElnay JC. Effect of tetracycline hydrochloride on theophylline kinetics. *Clin Pharm* (1982) 1, 446–8.
6. Pfeifer HJ, Greenblatt DJ, Friedman P. Effects of three antibiotics on theophylline kinetics. *Clin Pharmacol Ther* (1979) 26, 36–40.
7. Gotz VP, Ryerson GG. Evaluation of tetracycline on theophylline disposition in patients with chronic obstructive airways disease. *Drug Intell Clin Pharm* (1986) 20, 694–7.

Theophylline + Thyroid and Antithyroid compounds

Thyroid dysfunction may modestly affect theophylline requirements. There are two isolated cases of theophylline toxicity in patients being treated for hypothyroidism.

Clinical evidence

The theophylline elimination rate constant after a single intravenous dose of aminophylline was found to be greater in hyperthyroid patients (0.155 h^{-1}) than in euthyroid (0.107 h^{-1}) or hypothyroid patients (0.060 h^{-1}); some other pharmacokinetic parameters were also changed.[1] The authors concluded that thyroid dysfunction may modestly alter theophylline requirements. It is therefore also likely that drug-induced changes in the thyroid status, such as those caused by amiodarone, may also alter the amount of theophylline needed to maintain therapeutic levels.

(a) Antithyroid compounds

The serum theophylline level of an asthmatic patient was found to have doubled, from 15.2 to 30.9 mg/L, accompanied by toxicity, 3 months after treatment for hyperthyroidism with **radioactive iodine** (^{131}I). At this point the patient was hypothyroid, and after treatment with levothyroxine was started, his serum theophylline returned to approximately the same level as before radioactive iodine treatment (13.9 mg/L).[2] Another patient with Graves' disease treated with a combination of **thiamazole** (**methimazole**) 10 mg three times daily and Lugol's solution (**iodine** and **potassium iodide**) and taking theophylline 500 mg twice daily (*TheoDur*), had a theophylline level of 4.7 mg/L before radioactive iodine therapy. His level increased to 13.6 mg/L 7 months after thyroid ablation.[3] Five hyperthyroid patients had a 20% reduction in theophylline clearance and an increase in their theophylline half-life, from 4.6 to 5.9 hours, when they were given **carbimazole** 45 mg and propranolol 60 mg daily. In this study, a single intravenous dose of aminophylline was given before the treatment of thyrotoxicosis and after the euthyroid state had been achieved.[4] Note that propranolol can reduce the clearance of theophylline but should be avoided in patients with respiratory disease, see 'beta blockers', (p.1175), for more information.

(b) Thyroid hormones

One week after starting to take theophylline 1 g daily, a patient who was hypothyroid (serum thyroxine 1.4 micrograms/dL, reference range 4 to 11 micrograms/dL) developed severe theophylline toxicity, with serum theophylline levels of 34.7 mg/L, manifested by ventricular fibrillation (from which he was successfully resuscitated) and repeated seizures over 24 hours. After 2 months treatment with **thyroid hormones**, which increased his serum thyroxine levels to 4.3 micrograms/dL, his serum theophylline level was 13.2 mg/L, 10 days after reinstitution of the same theophylline dosage.[5]

Mechanism

Thyroid status may affect the rate at which theophylline is metabolised. In hyperthyroidism it is increased, whereas in hypothyroidism it is decreased.

Importance and management

It is established that changes in thyroid status may affect how the body handles theophylline. Monitor the effects and anticipate the possible need to begin to reduce the theophylline dosage if treatment for hyperthyroidism is started (e.g. with radioactive iodine, carbimazole, **thiamazole**, **propylthiouracil**, etc.). Similarly, anticipate the possible need to increase the theophylline dosage if treatment is started for hypothyroidism (e.g. with levothyroxine). Stabilisation of the thyroid status may take weeks or even months to achieve so that if monitoring of the theophylline dosage is considered necessary, it will need to extend over the whole of this period.

This monitoring would also apply to drugs that may cause thyroid dysfunction such as amiodarone.

1. Pokrajac M, Simić D, Varagić VM. Pharmacokinetics of theophylline in hyperthyroid and hypothyroid patients with chronic obstructive pulmonary disease. *Eur J Clin Pharmacol* (1987) 33, 483–6.
2. Johnson CE, Cohen IA. Theophylline toxicity after iodine 131 treatment for hyperthyroidism. *Clin Pharm* (1988) 7, 620–2.
3. Bauman JH, Teichman S, Wible DA. Increased theophylline clearance in a patient with hyperthyroidism. *Ann Allergy* (1984) 52, 94–6.
4. Vozeh S, Otten M, Staub J-J, Follath F. Influence of thyroid function on theophylline kinetics. *Clin Pharmacol Ther* (1984) 36, 634–40.
5. Aderka D, Shavit G, Garfinkel D, Santo M, Gitter S, Pinkhas J. Life-threatening theophylline intoxication in a hypothyroidic patient. *Respiration* (1983) 44, 77–80.

Theophylline + Tobacco

Tobacco smokers, and non-smokers heavily exposed to tobacco smoke, may need more theophylline than non-smokers to achieve the same therapeutic benefits, because the theophylline is cleared from the body more quickly. This may also occur in those who chew tobacco or take snuff but not if they chew nicotine gum.

Clinical evidence

A study found that the mean half-life of theophylline (given as a single oral dose of aminophylline) was 4.3 hours in a group of tobacco smokers (20 to 40 cigarettes a day) compared with 7 hours in a group of non-smokers, and that theophylline clearance was higher (mean 126%) and more variable in the smokers.[1] Almost identical results were found in an earlier study,[2] and a number of later studies in subjects given oral or intravenous theophylline or aminophylline confirm these findings.[3-7] The ability of smoking to increase theophylline clearance occurs irrespective of gender,[3,6] and in the presence of congestive heart failure or liver impairment.[7] The effects of ageing on the induction of theophylline metabolism by tobacco smoking is less clear. One study has found that in both young subjects (less than 30-years-old) and elderly subjects (more than 67-years-old) smoking decreased the half-life and increased the clearance of theophylline, when compared with non-smokers. The effect was greater in the young subjects.[4] However, another study found no difference in the pharmacokinetics of theophylline between asthmatic and healthy smokers and non-smokers aged over 65 years.[8] A similar high clearance of theophylline (given as intravenous aminophylline) has been seen in a patient who chewed tobacco (1.11 mL/kg per minute compared with the more usual 0.59 mL/kg per minute).[9] The half-life of theophylline (given as intravenous aminophylline) in passive smokers (non-smokers regularly exposed to tobacco smoke in the air they breathe, for 4 hours a day in this study) is reported to be shorter than in non-smokers (6.93 hours compared with 8.69 hours).[10] The clearance of theophylline (given as intravenous aminophylline) in asthmatic children exposed to passive tobacco smoke was also found to be greater (1.36 mL/kg per minute compared with 0.09 mL/kg per minute) and their steady-state serum theophylline levels were lower than in similar children not exposed to passive smoking.[11]

In one study, 3 of 4 patients who stopped smoking for 3 months (confirmed by serum thiocyanate levels) had a longer theophylline half-life, but only 2 had a slight decrease in theophylline clearance.[1] In another study, ex-smokers who had stopped heavy smoking 2 years previously had values for theophylline clearance and half-life that were intermediate between non-smokers and current heavy smokers.[3] In another study, 7 hospitalised smokers who abstained from smoking for 7 days had a 35.8% increase in theophylline half-life and a 37.6% decrease in clearance (although clearance after abstinence was still higher than values usually found in non-smokers).[12]

Mechanism

Tobacco smoke contains polycyclic hydrocarbons, which act as inducers of the cytochrome P450 isoenzyme CYP1A2, and this results in a more rapid clearance of theophylline from the body. Both the *N*-demethylation and 8-hydroxylation of theophylline is induced.[13] Ageing appears to offset the effects of smoking on theophylline metabolism.[8]

Importance and management

An established interaction of clinical importance. Heavy smokers (20 to 40 cigarettes daily) may need much greater theophylline dosage than non-smokers,[1] and increased doses are likely for those who chew tobacco or take snuff,[9] but not for those who chew nicotine gum.[12,14] In patients who stop smoking, a reduction in the theophylline dosage of up to 25 to 33% may be needed after one week,[12] but full normalisation of hepatic function appears to take many months or even years.[1,3] Investigators of the possible interactions of theophylline with other drugs should take smoking habits into account when selecting their subjects.[6,10,11] Note that the effects of 'cannabis', (p.1177), may be additive with those of tobacco smoking.

1. Hunt SN, Jusko WJ, Yurchak AM. Effect of smoking on theophylline disposition. *Clin Pharmacol Ther* (1976) 19, 546–51.
2. Jenne J, Nagasawa H, McHugh R, MacDonald F, Wyse E. Decreased theophylline half-life in cigarette smokers. *Life Sci* (1975) 17, 195–8.
3. Powell JR, Thiercelin J-F, Vozeh S, Sansom L, Riegelman S. The influence of cigarette smoking and sex on theophylline disposition. *Am Rev Respir Dis* (1977) 116, 17–23.
4. Cusack B, Kelly JG, Lavan J, Noel J, O'Malley K. Theophylline kinetics in relation to age: the importance of smoking. *Br J Clin Pharmacol* (1980) 10, 109–14.
5. Jusko WJ, Schentag JJ, Clark JH, Gardner M, Yurchak AM. Enhanced biotransformation of theophylline in marihuana and tobacco smokers. *Clin Pharmacol Ther* (1978) 24, 406–10.
6. Jennings TS, Nafziger AN, Davidson L, Bertino JS. Gender differences in hepatic induction and inhibition of theophylline pharmacokinetics and metabolism. *J Lab Clin Med* (1993) 122, 208–16.
7. Harralson AF, Kehoe WA, Chen J-D. The effect of smoking on theophylline disposition in patients with hepatic disease and congestive heart failure. *J Clin Pharmacol* (1996) 36, 862.
8. Samaan S, Fox R. The effect of smoking on theophylline kinetics in healthy and asthmatic elderly males. *J Clin Pharmacol* (1989) 29, 448–50.
9. Rockwood R, Henann N. Smokeless tobacco and theophylline clearance. *Drug Intell Clin Pharm* (1986) 20, 624–5.
10. Matsunga SK, Plezia PM, Karol MD, Katz MD, Camilli AE, Benowitz NL. Effects of passive smoking on theophylline clearance. *Clin Pharmacol Ther* (1989) 46, 399–407.
11. Mayo PR. Effect of passive smoking on theophylline clearance in children. *Ther Drug Monit* (2001) 23, 503–5.
12. Lee BL, Benowitz NL, Jacob P. Cigarette abstinence, nicotine gum, and theophylline disposition. *Ann Intern Med* (1987) 106, 553–5.
13. Grygiel J, Birkett DJ. Cigarette smoking and theophylline clearance and metabolism. *Clin Pharmacol Ther* (1981) 30, 491–6.
14. Benowitz NL, Lee BL, Jacob P. Nicotine gum and theophylline metabolism. *Biomed Pharmacother* (1989) 43, 1–3.

Theophylline + Trimetazidine

Trimetazidine does not appear to alter the pharmacokinetics of theophylline.

Clinical evidence, mechanism, importance and management

In a study in 13 healthy subjects trimetazidine 20 mg twice daily for at least 14 days did not alter the pharmacokinetics of a single 375-mg dose of theophylline.[1] These results suggest that treatment with theophylline is unlikely to be altered in patients concurrently treated with trimetazidine, but this needs confirmation in multiple-dose studies.

1. Edeki TI, Johnston A, Campbell DB, Ings RMJ, Brownsill R, Genissel P, Turner P. An examination of the possible pharmacokinetic interaction of trimetazidine with theophylline, digoxin and antipyrine. *Br J Clin Pharmacol* (1989) 26, 657P.

Theophylline + Vidarabine

A single case report describes a woman who had a rise in serum theophylline levels when she took aminophylline oral liquid with vidarabine.

Clinical evidence, mechanism, importance and management

A woman taking aminophylline oral liquid developed elevated serum theophylline levels (an increase from 14 mg/L to 24 mg/L) four days after starting to take vidarabine 400 mg daily for herpes zoster.[1] She was also being treated with ampicillin, gentamicin, clindamycin and digoxin, for congestive heart failure, chronic pulmonary disease and suspected sepsis. It was suggested that the vidarabine inhibited the metabolism of the theophylline resulting in the raised levels seen. The general significance of this case is uncertain, but it would now seem prudent to bear this interaction in mind if vidarabine is given with aminophylline or theophylline.

1. Gannon R, Sullman S, Levy RM, Grober J. Possible interaction between vidarabine and theophylline. *Ann Intern Med* (1984) 101, 148–9.

Theophylline + Viloxazine

Viloxazine increases serum theophylline levels and toxicity may occur.

Clinical evidence

A study in 8 healthy subjects given a single 200-mg dose of theophylline suggested that pretreatment with viloxazine 100 mg three times daily for 3 days increased the AUC_{0-24} of theophylline by 47%, increased its maximum serum concentration, and reduced its clearance.[1] An elderly woman hospitalised for respiratory failure and treated with a variety of drugs including theophylline, developed acute theophylline toxicity (a grand mal seizure) 2 days after starting to take viloxazine 200 mg daily. Her serum theophylline levels had increased threefold, from about 10 to 28 mg/L, but the levels were reduced when the viloxazine was withdrawn.[2] Nausea and vomiting, associated with raised serum theophylline levels, occurred in another patient treated with viloxazine. Theophylline was stopped, and then reintroduced at one quarter of the original dose. The theophylline level subsequently became subtherapeutic when the viloxazine was stopped.[3] A further case report in an elderly man describes a marked rise in serum theophylline levels to toxic concentrations (55.3 mg/L) when viloxazine, 100 mg then 300 mg daily, was started.[4]

Mechanism

It is suggested that the viloxazine competitively antagonises the metabolism of the theophylline by the liver, thereby reducing its clearance and resulting in an increase in its serum levels.

Importance and management

Information seems to be limited to these reports but it would appear to be a clinically important interaction. Theophylline serum levels should be well monitored if viloxazine is added, anticipating the need to reduce the dosage.

1. Perault MC, Griesemann E, Bouquet S, Lavoisy J, Vandel B. A study of the interaction of viloxazine with theophylline. *Ther Drug Monit* (1989) 11, 520–2.
2. Laaban JP, Dupeyron JP, Lafay M, Sofeir M, Rochemaure J, Fabiani P. Theophylline intoxication following viloxazine induced decrease in clearance. *Eur J Clin Pharmacol* (1986) 30, 351–3.
3. Thomson AH, Addis GJ, McGovern EM, McDonald NJ. Theophylline toxicity following coadministration of viloxazine. *Ther Drug Monit* (1988) 10, 359–60.
4. Vial T, Bertholon P, Lafond P, Pionchon C, Grangeon C, Bruel M, Antoine JC, Ollagnier M, Evreux JC. Surdosage en théophylline secondaire à un traitement par viloxazine. *Rev Med Interne* (1994) 15, 696–8.

Theophylline + Zileuton

Zileuton raises theophylline levels and increases the incidence of adverse effects.

Clinical evidence

In a double-blind, crossover study, 13 healthy subjects were given 200 mg of theophylline (*Slo-Phyllin*) four times daily for 5 days and either zileuton 800 mg twice daily or a placebo. Zileuton caused a 73% rise in the mean steady-state peak serum levels of theophylline (from 12 to 21 mg/L), a 92% increase in its AUC, and halved its apparent plasma clearance. During the use of zileuton the incidence of adverse effects increased (headache, gastrointestinal effects), which was attributed to theophylline toxicity, and this caused 3 of the original 16 subjects to withdraw from the study.[1]

Mechanism

Not fully established but it seems highly likely that zileuton inhibits the metabolism of the theophylline by the cytochrome P450 enzymes (probably the isoenzymes CYP1A2 and CYP3A) so that its serum levels rise.

Importance and management

Information is limited but the interaction appears to be established and of clinical importance. Concurrent use need not be avoided but monitor theophylline levels and reduce the dosage of theophylline as necessary. The report quoted above suggests that a typical asthma patient may initially need the theophylline dosage to be halved, and this dose reduction is recommended by the US manufacturers.[2] Similarly, the dose of theophylline should be reduced if it is given to a patient already taking zileuton, and adjusted according to theophylline levels.[2] This is based on the results of a study in over 1000 patients taking zileuton 600 mg four times daily without apparent problems when this course of action was followed.[1]

1. Granneman GR, Braeckman RA, Locke CS, Cavanaugh JH, Dubé LM, Awni WM. Effect of zileuton on theophylline pharmacokinetics. *Clin Pharmacokinet* (1995) 29 (Suppl 2), 77–83.
2. Zyflo (Zileuton). Critical Therapeutics Inc. US Prescribing information, November 2005.

Zafirlukast + Aspirin

Aspirin 650 mg four times daily is reported to have resulted in a mean increase in the plasma levels of zafirlukast 40 mg daily of 45%. No further details are available.[1,2] The clinical importance of this interaction awaits assessment but the manufacturers do not suggest any alteration in the zafirlukast dosage.[3]

1. Accolate (Zafirlukast). AstraZeneca Pharmaceuticals LP. US Prescribing information, July 2004.
2. Accolate (Zafirlukast). AstraZeneca UK Ltd. UK Summary of product characteristics, December 2004.
3. Zeneca Pharmaceuticals, Personal communication, July 1997.

Zafirlukast + Macrolides

Zafirlukast plasma levels are decreased by erythromycin, but this does not appear to be clinically important. No interaction has been found between zafirlukast and azithromycin or clarithromycin.

Clinical evidence, mechanism, importance and management

A study in 11 asthmatic patients found that **erythromycin** 500 mg three times daily for 5 days reduced the mean plasma level of zafirlukast 40 mg by about 40%.[1,2] This reduction in levels would be expected to reduce its antiasthmatic effects. If these drugs are given concurrently, be alert for a reduced response. However, note that the manufacturers do not suggest any alteration in the zafirlukast dosage.[3]

Zafirlukast is an inhibitor of the cytochrome P450 isoenzyme CYP3A4 *in vitro*. However, a study in 12 healthy subjects found that zafirlukast 20 mg twice daily for 12 days did not significantly affect the pharmacokinetics of a single 500-mg dose of **azithromycin** or **clarithromycin**.[4] No precaution would seem necessary if zafirlukast is given with azithromycin or clarithromycin.

1. Accolate (Zafirlukast). AstraZeneca Pharmaceuticals LP. US Prescribing information, July 2004.
2. Accolate (Zafirlukast). AstraZeneca UK Ltd. UK Summary of product characteristics, December 2004.
3. Zeneca Pharmaceuticals, Personal communication, July 1997.
4. Garey KW, Peloquin CA, Godo PG, Nafziger AN, Amsden GW. Lack of effect of zafirlukast on the pharmacokinetics of azithromycin, clarithromycin and 14-hydroxyclarithromycin in healthy volunteers. *Antimicrob Agents Chemother* (1999) 43, 1152–5.

Zafirlukast + Terfenadine

Zafirlukast plasma levels are decreased by terfenadine but the clinical significance of this is unclear. Zafirlukast does not increase the levels of terfenadine, and concurrent use does not prolong the QTc interval.

Clinical evidence, mechanism, importance and management

A study in 16 healthy men given zafirlukast 160 mg twice daily for 16 days with terfenadine 60 mg twice daily on days 8 to 16 found that the mean maximum serum levels and AUC of zafirlukast were reduced by 70% and 60%, respectively. There was a small, non-significant reduction in the terfenadine AUC and serum levels.[1] A study in 8 healthy subjects given zafirlukast 160 mg twice daily with terfenadine 60 mg twice daily for 8 days found that the AUC of terfenadine and the QTc interval were not significantly increased with concurrent use, despite the fact that zafirlukast appears to inhibit CYP3A4 *in vitro*, the major enzyme involved in terfenadine metabolism.[2] The reduction in zafirlukast serum levels would be expected to reduce its antiasthmatic effects, but this needs assessment. If both drugs are given be alert for a reduced response to zafirlukast.

1. Suttle AB, Birmingham BK, Vargo DL, Wilkinson LA, Morganroth J. Pharmacokinetics of zafirlukast and terfenadine after coadministration to healthy men. *J Clin Pharmacol* (1997) 37, 870.
2. Vargo DL, Suttle AB, Wilkinson LA, Thyrum PT, Tschan JH, Morganroth J. Effect of zafirlukast on QTc and area under the curve of terfenadine in healthy men. *J Clin Pharmacol* (1997) 37, 870.

34

SSRIs, Tricyclics and related antidepressants

The development of the tricyclic antidepressants arose out of work carried out on phenothiazine compounds related to chlorpromazine. The earlier molecules possessed two benzene rings joined by a third ring of carbon atoms, with sometimes a nitrogen, and had antidepressant activity, hence their name. Some of the later antidepressants have one, two or even four rings. 'Table 34.1', (see below) lists the common tricyclic antidepressants, the selective serotonin reuptake inhibitors (SSRIs) and a number of other drugs that are also used for depression.

SSRIs

These antidepressants act on neurones in a similar way to the tricyclics (see below) but they selectively inhibit the reuptake of serotonin (5-hydroxytryptamine or 5-HT). They have fewer antimuscarinic effects and are also less sedative and cardiotoxic.

Tricyclic antidepressants

The tricyclic antidepressants inhibit the activity of the 'uptake' mechanism by which some chemical transmitters (serotonin (5-HT) or noradrenaline (norepinephrine)) re-enter nerve endings in the CNS. In this way they raise the concentrations of the chemical transmitter in the receptor area. If depression represents some inadequacy in transmission between the nerves in the brain, increasing the amount of transmitter may go some way towards reversing this by improving transmission.

The tricyclics also have antimuscarinic (sometimes referred to as anticholinergic or atropine-like) activity and can cause dry mouth, blurred vision, constipation, urinary retention and an increase in ocular pressure. Postural hypotension and cardiotoxic effects may also occur, but they are less frequent. CNS adverse effects include sedation, the precipitation of seizures in certain individuals, and extrapyramidal reactions.

Other antidepressant drugs

(a) Nefazodone and Trazodone

Nefazodone is a phenylpiperazine structurally related to trazodone. Both nefazodone and trazodone block the reuptake of serotonin at presynaptic neurones and block α_1-adrenoceptors, but have no apparent effect on dopamine. Unlike trazodone, nefazodone blocks the reuptake of noradrenaline. Compared to the tricyclics, neither drug has very significant antimuscarinic effects, but trazodone also has marked sedative properties. Nefazodone is an inhibitor of the cytochrome P450 isoenzyme CYP3A4 and therefore it will inhibit the metabolism of drugs by this route. For a list of CYP3A4 substrates see 'Table 1.4', (p.6). Note that, nefazodone has largely been withdrawn due to adverse hepatic effects.

(b) Reboxetine

Reboxetine is a potent inhibitor of noradrenaline reuptake. It has a weak effect on serotonin reuptake and no significant affinity for muscarinic receptors.

(c) Serotonin and noradrenaline reuptake inhibitors (SNRIs)

Antidepressants in this group include duloxetine, milnacipran and venlafaxine. They inhibit both serotonin and noradrenaline reuptake but with differing selectivity. Milnacipran blocks serotonin and noradrenaline reuptake approximately equally, but duloxetine and to a greater extent venlafaxine have selectivity for serotonin. Duloxetine and venlafaxine are reported to weakly inhibit dopamine reuptake. They are also reported to have no significant affinity for histaminergic, muscarinic or adrenergic receptors, and, compared with the tricyclics, appear to lack significant sedative and antimuscarinic effects.

(d) Tetracyclic antidepressants and related drugs

Mianserin and maprotiline are tetracyclic antidepressants, which have actions similar to those of the tricyclic antidepressants. However, while the tetracyclics are more sedating, their antimuscarinic effects are less marked. Maprotiline inhibits the reuptake of noradrenaline (norepinephrine) and has weak affinity for central adrenergic (α_1) receptors. Mianserin does not prevent the peripheral reuptake of noradrenaline; it blocks presynaptic adrenergic (α_2) receptors and increases the turnover of brain noradrenaline. It is also an antagonist of serotonin receptors in some parts of the brain.

Mirtazapine is a piperazinoazepine and an analogue of mianserin. It is a presynaptic adrenergic α_2-antagonist that increases central noradrenergic and serotonergic transmission. It is a potent inhibitor of histamine (H_1) receptors and this accounts for its sedative properties. It has little antimuscarinic activity.

Table 34.1 SSRIs, Tricyclics and related antidepressants

Group	*Drugs*
SSRIs (Selective serotonin reuptake inhibitors)	Citalopram, Escitalopram, Femoxetine, Fluoxetine, Fluvoxamine, Paroxetine, Sertraline
Tetracyclic antidepressants	Maprotiline, Mianserin
Tricyclic antidepressants	Amineptine, Amitriptyline, Amoxapine, Butriptyline, Clomipramine, Desipramine, Dibenzepin, Dosulepin, Doxepin, Imipramine, Lofepramine, Melitracen, Nortriptyline, Opipramol, Protriptyline, Trimipramine
Other antidepressants	Duloxetine, Iprindole, Mirtazapine, Milnacipran, Nefazodone, Reboxetine, Trazodone, Venlafaxine, Viloxazine

Bupropion + Antiepileptics

Carbamazepine decreases bupropion levels and increases the levels of its active metabolite hydroxybupropion. Phenobarbital and phenytoin are predicted to interact similarly. The concurrent use of bupropion and valproate has led to increased levels of valproate and hydroxybupropion, and hallucinations have been reported in patients taking both drugs. Hypomania has been reported in a patient taking bupropion and lamotrigine.

Clinical evidence, mechanism, importance and management

(a) Carbamazepine, Phenobarbital, Phenytoin

One study found that carbamazepine at steady-state decreased the maximum plasma levels and AUC of bupropion and two of its metabolites (threohydrobupropion and erythrohydrobupropion) by about 81 to 96%. These two metabolites have only weak potential antidepressant activities. However, the AUC of another metabolite, hydroxybupropion (which has similar potency to the parent compound) was increased by 50% and its maximum plasma levels by 71%.[1] Two patients with bipolar illness have been described who were initially given bupropion 450 mg daily, later increased up to 600 mg daily. They had undetectable bupropion plasma levels while taking carbamazepine but their plasma levels of hydroxybupropion were markedly increased.[2]

What the sum of all these changes is likely to mean is uncertain, but good monitoring for any evidence of reduced efficacy and/or increased toxicity (due to the raised hydroxybupropion) is clearly needed. The same good monitoring would also be appropriate with phenytoin and phenobarbital, which would be expected to interact similarly, but clinical studies appear to be lacking.

(b) Lamotrigine

A study in 12 healthy subjects found that bupropion 150 mg twice daily did not affect the pharmacokinetics of a single 100-mg dose of lamotrigine.[3] A 23-year-old patient with a DSM-IV diagnosis of major depression taking bupropion 400 mg daily had an improvement in mood when she was also given lamotrigine 25 mg at night, and there was further improvement in mood, decreased anxiety and increased energy when lamotrigine was increased to 50 mg daily for 3 weeks. However, when the dose of lamotrigine was increased to 75 mg daily she reported decreased sleep, increased energy, mood lability and increased spending, which was diagnosed as hypomania. The symptoms resolved over about 2 weeks when the lamotrigine dose was reduced to 50 mg at bedtime. Antidepressants in high doses or in combination can induce hypomania and in this case the effect was attributed to a potentiation of the effects of bupropion, caused by lamotrigine.[4]

(c) Sodium valproate

A study found that the AUC of hydroxybupropion, an active metabolite of bupropion, almost doubled when bupropion was given with valproate at steady-state, but the pharmacokinetics of the parent compound and the two other less active metabolites were unaffected.[1] An increase in valproate levels of almost 30% was seen in another report in one patient.[2] Visual and auditory hallucinations were reported in a patient given bupropion and valproate.[5] The UK manufacturer recommends caution when using drugs which may inhibit bupropion metabolism, such as valproate.[6] As valproate levels may also be increased by bupropion, good monitoring for evidence of increased adverse effects of both drugs would seem appropriate.

1. Ketter TA, Jenkins JB, Schroeder DH, Pazzaglia PJ, Marangell LB, George MS, Callahan AM, Hinton ML, Chao J, Post RM. Carbamazepine but not valproate induces bupropion metabolism. *J Clin Psychopharmacol* (1995) 15, 327–33.
2. Popli AP, Tanquary J, Lamparella V, Masand PS. Bupropion and anticonvulsant drug interactions. *Ann Clin Psychiatry* (1995) 7, 99–101.
3. Odishaw J, Chen C. Effects of steady-state bupropion on the pharmacokinetics of lamotrigine in healthy subjects. *Pharmacotherapy* (2000) 20, 1448–53.
4. Margolese HC, Beauclair L, Szkrumelak N, Chouinard G. Hypomania induced by adjunctive lamotrigine. *Am J Psychiatry* (2003) 160, 183–4.
5. Filteau M-J, Leblanc J, Lefrançoise S, Demers M-F. Visual and auditory hallucinations with the association of bupropion and valproate. *Can J Psychiatry* (2000) 45, 198–9.
6. Zyban (Bupropion hydrochloride). GlaxoSmithKline UK. UK Summary of product characteristics, October 2006.

Bupropion + Antiretrovirals

Ritonavir, efavirenz and nelfinavir inhibit the cytochrome P450 isoenzyme CYP2B6 *in vitro* and may, theoretically, increase bupropion levels. However, an *in vivo* study suggests that ritonavir may *decrease* bupropion levels.

Clinical evidence, mechanism, importance and management

In vitro data[1] indicate that the antiretroviral drugs **efavirenz**, **nelfinavir** and **ritonavir** are capable of inhibiting the cytochrome P450 isoenzyme CYP2B6, which is the isoenzyme primarily involved in bupropion metabolism. The potential therefore exists for a drug interaction causing an *increase* in bupropion concentrations, which may lead to an increased risk of seizures. The US manufacturer of **ritonavir** predicts that the metabolism of bupropion might possibly be inhibited, leading to increased plasma levels and toxicity,[2] and they recommend caution with a possible decrease in bupropion dose.[2] However, a retrospective study identified 10 HIV-positive patients who had taken bupropion 150 mg once or twice daily together with **nelfinavir**, **ritonavir** or **efavirenz** for 3 weeks to 2 years (median 8 months) without having seizures, but note that the number of patients was small and the 2 patients who received **ritonavir** were only given 100 mg twice daily.[3]

In contrast, the manufacturers of bupropion report a study in healthy subjects, in which **ritonavir** 600 mg twice daily for 20 days *decreased* the AUC and maximum serum levels of bupropion by about 65% and 60%, respectively. The plasma levels of the active metabolites of bupropion were also decreased.[4] This contrasting information suggests that further study is needed. In the meantime, patients given bupropion with **ritonavir** should be monitored for increased bupropion effects and decreased bupropion effects. It would seem prudent to start bupropion at the lowest recommended dose and titrate to effect.

1. Hesse LM, von Moltke LL, Shader RI, Greenblatt DJ. Ritonavir, efavirenz, and nelfinavir inhibit CYP2B6 activity in vitro: potential drug interactions with bupropion. *Drug Metab Dispos* (2001) 29, 100–102.
2. Norvir (Ritonavir). Abbott Laboratories. US Prescribing information, January 2006.
3. Park-Wyllie LY, Antoniou T. Concurrent use of bupropion with CYP2B6 inhibitors, nelfinavir, ritonavir and efavirenz: a case series. *AIDS* (2003) 17, 638–40.
4. Zyban (Bupropion hydrochloride). GlaxoSmithKline UK. UK Summary of product characteristics, October 2006.

Bupropion + Benzodiazepines and related drugs

Visual hallucinations have been seen in one patient given zolpidem with bupropion. Bupropion is contraindicated during the abrupt withdrawal from any drug known to be associated with seizures on withdrawal, particularly benzodiazepines and related drugs.

Clinical evidence, mechanism, importance and management

Visual hallucinations lasting 3 to 4 hours occurred in a 17-year-old boy who had been taking bupropion 450 mg daily for one month and **zolpidem** 5 to 10 mg daily for about 6 months, when he increased the **zolpidem** dose to 60 mg.[1] Note that the recommended dose of **zolpidem** is 10 mg daily and that **zolpidem** itself can cause psychiatric adverse effects such as hallucinations. Therefore an interaction is not established. Bupropion is contraindicated during abrupt withdrawal from any drug known to be associated with seizures on withdrawal, particularly benzodiazepines and benzodiazepine-like drugs.[2,3]

1. Elko CJ, Burgess JL, Robertson WO. Zolpidem-associated hallucinations and serotonin reuptake inhibition: a possible interaction. *Clin Toxicol* (1998), 36, 195–203.
2. Zyban (Bupropion hydrochloride). GlaxoSmithKline UK. UK Summary of product characteristics, October 2006.
3. Zyban (Bupropion hydrochloride). GlaxoSmithKline. US Prescribing information, August 2007.

Bupropion + Carbimazole

An isolated report describes acute liver failure in a patient taking bupropion and carbimazole.

Clinical evidence, mechanism, importance and management

A 41-year-old man treated for hyperthyroidism with carbimazole 15 mg daily and propranolol 10 mg daily for 5 years received a 10-day course of bupropion 150 mg daily to aid smoking cessation. Ten weeks after completing the course of bupropion he was admitted to hospital with severe jaundice, nausea, dyspepsia, lethargy, and epigastric discomfort persisting for 5 days. The only other medication he had taken was paracetamol (acetaminophen) 500 mg to 1 g daily for up to 2 days, about 2 weeks before admission. Both carbimazole and propranolol were discontinued. He developed acute liver failure and a rapid deterioration of renal function, complicated by sepsis and coagulopathy. Liver biopsy showed evidence of non-specific drug-induced acute liver injury. The patient died 19 days after the onset of symptoms. Both bupropion and carbimazole may cause liver damage. In this case the hepatotoxicity was attributed to bupropion or a combined toxic effect of bupropion and carbimazole. The potential for serious hepatotoxicity should be borne in mind if bupropion is given with other hepatotoxic drugs.[1]

1. Khoo A-L, Tham L-S, Lee K-H, Lim G-K. Acute liver failure with concurrent bupropion and carbimazole therapy. *Ann Pharmacother* (2003) 37, 220–3.

Bupropion + Cimetidine

A randomised, open-label, crossover study in 24 healthy subjects found no evidence of any significant pharmacokinetic interaction between a single 300-mg dose of bupropion (sustained release preparation) and a single 800-mg dose of cimetidine.[1] No special precautions would seem to be necessary on concurrent use.

1. Kustra R, Corrigan B, Dunn J, Duncan B, Hsyu P-H. Lack of effect of cimetidine on the pharmacokinetics of sustained-release bupropion. *J Clin Pharmacol* (1999) 39, 1184–8.

Bupropion + Corticosteroids

A patient taking bupropion had a seizure after being given an intra-articular injection of methylprednisolone.

Clinical evidence, mechanism, importance and management

A case report describes a patient taking bupropion, who experienced a severe, prolonged seizure 24 hours after receiving **methylprednisolone** 30 mg for subacromial bursitis.[1] The author notes that there could be a risk of seizures in patients taking bupropion who are given prophylactic oral steroids.[1] This is in line with the manufacturers' suggestion that systemic steroids could increase the risk of seizures, see 'Bupropion + Miscellaneous', p.1206.

1. White P. Interaction of intra-articular steroids and bupropion. *Clin Radiol* (2002) 57, 235.

Bupropion + Guanfacine

A grand mal seizure in a child, which was attributed to an interaction between bupropion and guanfacine, was later identified as being more probably due to a bupropion overdose.

Clinical evidence, mechanism, importance and management

A 10-year-old girl, being treated for attention deficit hyperactivity disorder, was prescribed increasing doses of bupropion up to 100 mg three times daily, to which guanfacine, initially 500 micrograms twice daily then 500 micrograms three times daily, was added. Ten days later she had a grand mal seizure, which the author of the report attributed to an interaction between the two drugs.[1,2] This was challenged in subsequent correspondence.[3] Furthermore, 2 years later the author of the original report wrote to say that he had now discovered that the girl had in fact taken 500 mg of bupropion and 5 mg of guanfacine before the seizure took place, so that what happened was much more likely to have been due to an overdose of the bupropion than to an interaction with guanfacine.[4] Bupropion is associated with seizures at high doses (see 'Bupropion + Miscellaneous', p.1206). There is insufficient evidence to suggest that the concurrent use of these two drugs should be avoided.

1. Tilton P. Bupropion and guanfacine. *J Am Acad Child Adolesc Psychiatry* (1998) 37, 682–3.
2. Tilton P. Seizure associated with bupropion and guanfacine. *J Am Acad Child Adolesc Psychiatry* (1999) 38, 3.
3. Namerow LB. Seizure associated with bupropion and guanfacine. *J Am Acad Child Adolesc Psychiatry* (1999) 38, 2.
4. Tilton P. Seizure after guanfacine plus bupropion: correction. *J Am Acad Child Adolesc Psychiatry* (2000) 39, 1341.

Bupropion + MAOIs and related drugs

Bupropion is contraindicated with MAOIs, although there is little clinical evidence of serious problems. Orthostatic hypotension occurred in a patient given bupropion and selegiline, and an isolated report describes hypertension in a patient receiving bupropion and the antibacterial linezolid, which has weak MAO inhibitory activity.

Clinical evidence, mechanism, importance and management

In an uncontrolled study, 10 patients were treated for major affective disorder (8 unipolar, 2 bipolar) with bupropion in daily doses of 225 to 450 mg and an MAOI: **isocarboxazid** (1 patient), **phenelzine** (5), **tranylcypromine** (2), and the MAO-B inhibitor **selegiline** (2). Four were transferred from the MAOI to bupropion without any washout period, and the other 6 were given both drugs concurrently. No untoward cardiovascular events occurred, except for one patient taking bupropion and **selegiline**, who experienced orthostatic hypotension. Notable weight loss occurred in two others when transferred from the MAOI to bupropion.[1] A Medline search (1962 to 2003) and review of published literature found no documented reports of hypertensive crises or fatalities when a stimulant drug (including bupropion) was cautiously added to an MAOI, although orthostatic hypotension and elevated blood pressure were reported.[2]

Despite very limited clinical evidence, the manufacturers of bupropion are apparently wary of a possible interaction with MAOIs because of the toxicity seen in studies in *animals* when **phenelzine** and bupropion were given concurrently.[3] They contraindicate bupropion with MAOIs and recommend that at least 14 days should elapse between stopping irreversible MAOIs and starting bupropion.[3,4] This precaution would therefore apply particularly to the older MAOIs (**phenelzine**, **tranylcypromine**, **isocarboxazid** etc). For reversible MAOIs such as **moclobemide**, the manufacturers advise that a 24-hour period is sufficient.[4] Note also, that an isolated report describes severe intermittent intraoperative hypertension possibly due to an interaction between maintenance bupropion and **linezolid,** which had been started 24 hours previously for treatment of a resistant gram-positive infection.[5] Linezolid is known to have weak MAOI properties, and, although concurrent use need not be avoided, this report therefore introduces a note of caution if both drugs are given together.

1. Abuzzahab Sr, FS. Combination therapy: monoamino oxidase inhibitors and bupropion HCl. *Neuropsychopharmacology* (1994) 10, 74S.
2. Feinberg SS. Combining stimulants with monoamine oxidase inhibitors: a review of uses and one possible additional indication. *J Clin Psychiatry* (2004) 65, 1520–4.
3. Zyban (Bupropion hydrochloride). GlaxoSmithKline. US Prescribing information, August 2007.
4. Zyban (Bupropion hydrochloride). GlaxoSmithKline UK. UK Summary of product characteristics, October 2006.
5. Marcucci C, Sandson NB, Dunlap JA. Linezolid-bupropion interaction as possible etiology of severe intermittent intraoperative hypertension? *Anesthesiology* (2004) 101, 1487–8.

Bupropion + Methylphenidate

Isolated reports describe grand mal seizures in one patient and myocardial infarction in another, associated with bupropion and methylphenidate.

Clinical evidence, mechanism, importance and management

A 14-year-old boy taking methylphenidate 60 mg daily was additionally given bupropion 200 mg increased to 300 mg daily. The patient experienced grand mal seizures 4 weeks after the dosage increase, but remained seizure-free once the bupropion was discontinued.[1] Another report describes acute myocardial infarction in a 16-year-old boy associated with methylphenidate, bupropion and erythromycin. It was proposed that the erythromycin might have caused elevated levels of bupropion leading to a hyperadrenergic state and this, together with the sympathetic effects of the methylphenidate, resulted in excessive vasospasm, leading to myocardial damage.[2]

The report of the myocardial infarction is isolated and of uncertain general significance. Note that the manufacturers of bupropion list stimulants as drugs that increase the risk of seizures with bupropion (see 'Bupropion + Miscellaneous', below) and this case adds weight to that warning.

1. Ickowicz A. Bupropion-methylphenidate combination and grand mal seizures. *Can J Psychiatry* (2002) 47, 790–1.
2. George AK, Kunwar AR, Awasthi A. Acute myocardial infarction in a young male on methylphenidate, bupropion, and erythromycin. *J Child Adolesc Psychopharmacol* (2005) 15, 693–5.

Bupropion + Miscellaneous

The manufacturers issue warnings about the concurrent use of bupropion with alcohol, amantadine, levodopa, drugs that can lower the convulsive threshold, drugs metabolised by the cytochrome P450 isoenzyme CYP2D6, drugs which affect CYP2B6, and also the use of nicotine.

Clinical evidence, mechanism, importance and management

(a) Alcohol

The manufacturers report rare adverse neuropsychiatric events or reduced alcohol tolerance in patients drinking alcohol during bupropion treatment. They recommend that the consumption of alcohol should be minimised or avoided.[1,2] For comment on the increased risk of seizures with alcohol see *(d)*, below.

(b) Antiparkinsonian drugs

The manufacturers say that the concurrent use of bupropion and **levodopa** or **amantadine** should be undertaken with caution because limited clinical data suggest a higher incidence of undesirable effects (nausea, vomiting, excitement, restlessness, postural tremor) in patients given bupropion with either drug. Good monitoring is therefore appropriate and patients should be given small initial bupropion doses, which are increased gradually.[1,2]

(c) CYP2B6 substrates

The manufacturers advise caution if bupropion is used with drugs such as **clopidogrel**, **cyclophosphamide**, **ifosfamide**, **orphenadrine**, and **ticlopidine** as bupropion is metabolised to its major metabolite hydroxybupropion by CYP2B6 and these drugs are also metabolised by this isoenzyme.[1,2] However, there is no evidence to suggest that this is a problem in practice.

(d) CYP2D6 substrates

The manufacturers of bupropion predict that it may inhibit the metabolism of drugs by the cytochrome P450 isoenzyme CYP2D6, which might result in a rise in their plasma levels. They name **haloperidol**, **risperidone**, **thioridazine**, **flecainide**, **propafenone**. The recommendation is that if any of these drugs is added to treatment with bupropion, doses at the lower end of the range should be used. If bupropion is added to existing treatment, decreased dosages should be considered.[1,2] This seems a prudent precaution as bupropion raises the levels of 'desipramine', (p.1232), 'dextromethorphan', (p.1255), 'metoprolol', (p.838), all of which are metabolised by this isoenzyme.

(e) Drugs and circumstances that can lower the convulsive threshold

There is a small dose-related risk of seizures with bupropion. At a daily dose of 300 mg of the sustained-release formulation the risk is 0.1%, which increases to 0.4% at a dose of 450 mg of the immediate-release formulation, and increases tenfold between doses of 450 and 600 mg daily.[2] The manufacturers caution the use of other drugs that lower the convulsive threshold, the concern being that these drugs might further increase the risk of seizures. The UK[1] and US[2] manufacturers list **antipsychotics**, antidepressants (see 'SSRIs', (p.1215) and 'tricyclics', (p.1232)), 'systemic steroids', (p.1205), and **theophylline**. The UK manufacturers additionally list **antimalarials**, **tramadol**, **quinolones** and **sedating antihistamines**. A maximum dose of 150 mg of bupropion should be considered for patients prescribed such drugs.[1] Caution is also urged with regard to circumstances that may lower the convulsive threshold, including the use of **anorectics** or '**stimulants**', (p.1205), excessive use of **alcohol** or **sedatives**, addiction to **cocaine** or **opiates**. Bupropion is contraindicated during abrupt withdrawal from **alcohol** or any drug known to be associated with seizures on withdrawal.[1,2]

(f) Nicotine

Nicotine transdermal patches are reported not to affect the pharmacokinetics of bupropion or its metabolites.[1] The manufacturers of bupropion say that limited data suggest that giving up smoking is more easily achieved if bupropion is taken while using a nicotine transdermal system, but a higher rate of treatment-emergent hypertension has been noted with the combined treatment.[1,2] They recommend weekly monitoring to check for any evidence of a blood pressure increase.[1] The same warning would also seem to be applicable to the use of nicotine in any other form (oral or nasal).

For a report of acute myocardial ischaemia attributed to combined use of bupropion, nicotine (from smoking) and pseudoephedrine, see 'Bupropion + Pseudoephedrine', below.

1. Zyban (Bupropion hydrochloride). GlaxoSmithKline UK. UK Summary of product characteristics, October 2006.
2. Zyban (Bupropion hydrochloride). GlaxoSmithKline. US Prescribing information, August 2007.

Bupropion + Pseudoephedrine

An isolated report describes acute myocardial ischaemia associated with bupropion, nicotine and pseudoephedrine.

Clinical evidence, mechanism, importance and management

A 21-year-old man presented in a hospital emergency department with severe chest pain, radiating pain into both arms and between the shoulder blades, diaphoresis and shortness of breath. Initially this was diagnosed as an acute myocardial infarction, but a later angiogram showed normal coronary arteries and it was concluded that these symptoms were due to acute myocardial ischaemia apparently brought on by the combined use of pseudoephedrine (9 tablets of 30 mg taken over the previous 3 days), bupropion for smoking cessation and **nicotine** (he smoked 25 cigarettes daily). The authors of the report postulate that all these drugs acted on the alpha receptors of the coronary arteries to cause vasospasm and acute ischaemia. He had been taking both drugs and erythromycin for 3 days, and had taken pseudoephedrine on numerous previous occasions without problems. He recovered fully.[1]

This is an isolated case from which no general conclusions can be drawn, but some warning might be appropriate for patients who are at risk of coronary ischaemia. For comment on the use of **nicotine** with bupropion, see 'Bupropion + Miscellaneous', above.

1. Pederson KJ, Kuntz DH, Garbe GJ. Acute myocardial ischemia associated with ingestion of bupropion and pseudoephedrine in a 21-year-old man. *Can J Cardiol* (2001) 17, 599–601.

Bupropion + St John's wort (*Hypericum perforatum*)

A brief report describes the development of mania in one patient, which was associated with the concurrent use of St John's wort and bupropion.[1] No general conclusions can be drawn from this isolated report.

1. Griffiths J, Jordan S, Pilan K. Natural health products and adverse reactions. *Can Adverse React News* (2004) 14 (1), 2–3.

Maprotiline + Hormonal contraceptives or Tobacco

Neither tobacco smoking nor the use of oral contraceptives affect the levels of maprotiline.

Clinical evidence, mechanism, importance and management

A study in women showed that, over a 28-day period, the use of oral contraceptives did not significantly affect the steady-state blood levels of maprotiline 75 mg given at night, nor was its therapeutic effectiveness changed.[1] Smoking also has no effect on maprotiline efficacy and blood levels.[1,2]

1. Luscombe DK. Interaction studies: the influence of age, cigarette smoking and the oral contraceptive on blood concentrations of maprotiline. In 'Depressive Illness — Far Horizons?' McIntyre JNM (ed), Cambridge Med Publ, Northampton 1982, p 61–2.
2. Holman RM. Maprotiline and cigarette smoking: an interaction study: clinical findings. In 'Depressive Illness — Far Horizons?' McIntyre JNM (ed), Cambridge Med Publ, Northampton 1982, p 66–7.

Maprotiline + Propranolol

Maprotiline toxicity, attributed to the concurrent use of propranolol, has been described in three patients.

Clinical evidence

A patient experienced maprotiline toxicity (dizziness, hypotension, dry mouth, blurred vision, etc.) after taking propranolol 120 mg daily for 2 weeks. His trough maprotiline levels had risen by 40%. The levels fell and the adverse effects disappeared when the propranolol was withdrawn.[1] Another patient taking propranolol 120 mg daily began to experience visual hallucinations and psychomotor agitation within a few days of starting to take maprotiline 200 mg daily.[2] Another man taking haloperidol, benzatropine, triamterene, hydrochlorothiazide and propranolol became disorientated, agitated and uncooperative, with visual hallucinations and incoherent speech, within a week of starting to take maprotiline 150 mg daily. These symptoms disappeared when all the drugs were withdrawn. Reintroduction of the antihypertensive drugs with haloperidol and desipramine proved effective and uneventful.[3]

Mechanism

Not understood. A suggested reason is that the propranolol reduces the blood flow to the liver so that the metabolism of the maprotiline is reduced, leading to its accumulation in the body.

Importance and management

Information seems to be limited to the cases cited. The general importance of this interaction is uncertain. The authors of one of the reports[2] say that simultaneous use is inadvisable, but on the basis of just three cases, and with no further information, this seems over-cautious.

1. Tollefson G, Lesar T. Effect of propranolol on maprotiline clearance. *Am J Psychiatry* (1984) 141, 148–9.
2. Saiz-Ruiz J, Moral L. Delirium induced by association of propranolol and maprotiline. *J Clin Psychopharmacol* (1988) 8, 77–8.
3. Malek-Ahmadi P, Tran T. Propranolol and maprotiline toxic interaction. *Neurobehav Toxicol Teratol* (1985) 7, 203.

Maprotiline + Risperidone

Risperidone appears to increase the plasma levels of maprotiline.

Clinical evidence, mechanism, importance and management

A 39-year-old patient with a schizodepressive disorder taking pipamperone and lorazepam, and taking maprotiline 175 mg daily for a severe depressive episode had plasma levels of maprotiline of 145 and 166 nanograms/mL after 4 and 6 weeks, respectively. After 8 weeks, she was given risperidone to treat acute psychotic symptoms. The dose of risperidone was titrated over 5 days up to 5 mg daily and the dose of pipamperone was increased from 40 to 80 mg at night. She had a rapid remission of the psychotic symptoms and almost complete remission of the depression, but gradually developed antimuscarinic adverse effects. Ten days after starting risperidone and with maprotiline at a dose of 150 mg daily, maprotiline plasma levels had increased to 266 nanograms/mL. The doses of maprotiline and risperidone were reduced to 100 mg and 3 mg daily, respectively, and this reduced the severity of the adverse effects.[1]

Gradual increases in maprotiline levels over 6 to 7 weeks during concurrent risperidone therapy have been found in 2 other patients. One of the patients was also taking **nortriptyline**, but its levels were unaltered.[1]

Maprotiline is mainly metabolised by the cytochrome P450 isoenzyme CYP2D6. The increased levels of maprotiline may be due to an inhibition of CYP2D6-mediated metabolism by risperidone.[1] This interaction is unconfirmed but be aware of the possibility of an interaction if maprotiline adverse effects are troublesome.

1. Normann C, Lieb K, Walden J. Increased plasma concentration of maprotiline by coadministration of risperidone. *J Clin Psychopharmacol* (2002) 22, 92–4.

Maprotiline or Mianserin + Sympathomimetics

No adverse interaction would usually be expected in patients taking maprotiline or mianserin who are also given sympathomimetics (commonly used as vasopressors or in cough and cold remedies).

Clinical evidence, mechanism, importance and management

The pressor (increased blood pressure) responses to **tyramine** and **noradrenaline** (**norepinephrine**) in depressed patients remained virtually unchanged after 14 days of treatment with mianserin 60 mg daily.[1-4] In 5 healthy subjects taking maprotiline the pressor response to **tyramine** was reduced threefold while the **noradrenaline** response remained unchanged.[5]

The practical importance of these observations is that, unlike the tricyclic antidepressants, no special precautions normally seem necessary if patients taking maprotiline or mianserin are given **noradrenaline** or other directly-acting sympathomimetics. Similarly, none of the dietary precautions against eating **tyramine**-rich foods or drinks, or any precautions against the administration of indirectly-acting sympathomimetics such as **phenylpropanolamine** in cough and cold remedies, would appear to be necessary.

1. Ghose K, Coppen A, Turner P. Autonomic actions and interactions of mianserin hydrochloride (Org GB94) and amitriptyline in patients with depressive illness. *Psychopharmacology (Berl)* (1976) 49, 201–4.
2. Coppen A, Ghose K, Swade C, Wood K. Effect of mianserin hydrochloride on peripheral uptake mechanisms for noradrenaline and 5-hydroxytryptamine in man. *Br J Clin Pharmacol* (1978) 5, 13S–17S.
3. Ghose K. Studies on the interaction between mianserin and noradrenaline in patients suffering from depressive illness. *Br J Clin Pharmacol* (1977) 4, 712–14.
4. Coppen AJ, Ghose K. Clinical and pharmacological effects of treatment with a new antidepressant. *Arzneimittelforschung* (1976) 26, 1166–7.
5. Briant RH, George CF. The assessment of potential drug interactions with a new tricyclic antidepressant drug. *Br J Clin Pharmacol* (1974) 1, 113–18.

Mianserin + Antiepileptics

Plasma levels of mianserin can be markedly reduced by the concurrent use of carbamazepine, phenobarbital or phenytoin.

Clinical evidence

A comparative study in 6 epileptics and 6 healthy subjects showed that **phenytoin** with either **phenobarbital** or **carbamazepine** markedly reduced the plasma levels of a single dose of mianserin.[1,2] The mean half-life of mianserin was reduced by 75% (from 16.9 to 4.8 hours) and the AUC was reduced by 86%. Another study in 4 patients found that **carbamazepine** reduced serum mianserin levels by 70%.[3] In another study 12 patients taking mianserin 60 mg daily were also given **carbamazepine** 400 mg daily for 4 weeks. Average plasma levels of total *S*-mianserin (the more potent enantiomer) and total *R*-mianserin were reduced by about 45% in the presence of **carbamazepine**.[4]

Mechanism

It seems probable that these antiepileptics increase the metabolism of mianserin by the liver, thereby increasing its loss from the body. Carbamazepine may increase the metabolism of mianserin by cytochrome P450 isoenzyme CYP3A4.[4]

Importance and management

Information seems to be limited to these studies, but the interaction appears to be established and of clinical importance. Monitor concurrent use and increase the dosage of mianserin as necessary. One study suggests that the dose of mianserin may need to be approximately doubled if carbamazepine 400 mg daily is added.[4]

1. Nawishy S, Hathway N, Turner P. Interactions of anticonvulsant drugs with mianserin and nomifensine. *Lancet* (1981) ii, 871–2.

2. Richens A, Nawishy S, Trimble M. Antidepressant drugs, convulsions and epilepsy. *Br J Clin Pharmacol* (1983) 15, 295S–298S.
3. Leinonen E, Lillsunde P, Laukkanen V, Ylitalo P. Effects of carbamazepine on serum antidepressant concentrations in psychiatric patients. *J Clin Psychopharmacol* (1991) 11, 313–18.
4. Eap CB, Yasui N, Kaneko S, Baumann P, Powell K, Otani K. Effects of carbamazepine coadministration on plasma concentrations of the enantiomers of mianserin and of its metabolites. *Ther Drug Monit* (1999) 21, 166–70.

Mirtazapine + Antidepressants

The manufacturers say that two weeks should elapse between taking an MAOI and mirtazapine. Mirtazapine combined with other serotonergic antidepressants may possibly increase the risk of bleeding and/or the serotonin syndrome. SSRIs may increase plasma levels of mirtazapine and there is a report of hypomania associated with combined use. The concurrent use of mirtazapine with amitriptyline may have a minor effect on the levels of both drugs.

Clinical evidence

(a) MAOIs

No adverse interactions have been reported between mirtazapine and the MAOIs[1,2] but, to be on the safe side, the manufacturers say that the concurrent use of mirtazapine and MAOIs should be avoided both during and within two weeks of stopping treatment.[2,3]

(b) SNRIs

For mention of the serotonin syndrome and an increased risk of bleeding in patients given mirtazapine and **venlafaxine,** see 'SNRIs; Venlafaxine + Antidepressants', p.1212.

(c) SSRIs

1. Escitalopram. For a report of bleeding associated with the combined use of escitalopram, mirtazapine and venlafaxine, see 'SNRIs; Venlafaxine + Antidepressants', p.1212.

2. Fluoxetine. There is an isolated report[4] of the serotonin syndrome in a 75-year-old woman when fluoxetine 20 mg daily was discontinued and mirtazapine 30 mg daily started soon afterwards (exact interval not stated). Symptoms including dizziness, headache, nausea, dry mouth, anxiety, agitation, suicidal ideas and difficulty in walking occurred within hours of the first dose of mirtazapine. Symptoms worsened until mirtazapine was discontinued on day 5, after which an improvement was noticed. Fluoxetine was restarted on day 7.

3. Fluvoxamine. A 26-year-old woman with a 12-year history of anorexia nervosa, taking fluvoxamine 200 mg daily, developed symptoms consistent with the serotonin syndrome (tremors, restlessness, twitching, flushing, diaphoresis, nausea) about 4 days after starting mirtazapine 30 mg daily.[5] A 17-year-old boy taking mirtazapine 30 mg daily experienced increased anxiety when fluvoxamine 100 mg daily was also given. Mirtazapine serum levels were increased threefold. In a second patient taking mirtazapine 15 mg daily, the addition of fluvoxamine 50 mg daily resulted in a fourfold increase in serum mirtazapine concentrations, accompanied by mood improvements.[6]

4. Paroxetine. A study in 21 healthy subjects given mirtazapine 30 mg, paroxetine 40 mg or a combination of both, daily for 9 days, found that paroxetine inhibited the metabolism of mirtazapine (AUC of mirtazapine increased by about 17%). Mirtazapine did not alter the pharmacokinetics of paroxetine. The results of psychometric assessments suggested that concurrent use of mirtazapine and paroxetine did not alter cognitive function, or cause major changes in mood or sleep, compared with the use of either drug alone.[7]

5. Sertraline. A woman taking sertraline 250 mg daily was also given mirtazapine 15 mg daily because of inadequately controlled depression. Within 4 days she developed hypomanic symptoms and she stopped taking the mirtazapine. The hypomania resolved within 3 days but her depression then recurred.[8]

(d) Tricyclic antidepressants

In a single-blind, crossover study involving 24 healthy subjects, mirtazapine 15 to 30 mg daily, **amitriptyline** 25 to 75 mg daily or both drugs were given for periods of 9 days and in addition, 8 subjects received placebo. **Amitriptyline** increased the maximum plasma levels of mirtazapine, in male subjects only, by 36%. Mirtazapine increased the maximum plasma levels of **amitriptyline** in male subjects by 23% but in female subjects the maximum plasma levels were *decreased* by 23%. Other pharmacokinetic parameters and tolerability were not affected by concurrent use.[9]

Mechanism

The cytochrome P450 isoenzyme CYP2D6 is inhibited by fluoxetine and paroxetine and CYP1A2 is inhibited by fluvoxamine. Both of these isoenzymes are involved in the metabolism of mirtazapine, which may explain the raised mirtazapine levels reported.

SNRIs, SSRIs and mirtazapine affect serotonin transmission, which may lead to increased serotonin levels[4,5] and therefore cause the symptoms described as the serotonin syndrome. For more about the serotonin syndrome see 'Additive or synergistic interactions', (p.9).

Importance and management

These isolated reports would seem to suggest that the combined use of mirtazapine and the SSRIs can lead to the serotonin syndrome. However, whether these are cases of the serotonin syndrome has been disputed.[10] Low body weight and a decrease in total body fat may also have contributed in one case.[5] This and other reports of anxiety and hypomania highlight the need for some caution during concurrent use. One manufacturer reported that, from postmarketing experience, it appears that the serotonin syndrome occurs very rarely in patients taking mirtazapine alone or in combination with SSRIs. They recommend that if the combination is required, dosage alterations should be made with caution and patients closely monitored for any signs of excessive serotonin stimulation.[11] Similar caution would also seem appropriate with SNRIs.

1. Akzo Nobel, Organon Laboratories Ltd. Personal communication, January 1999.
2. Remeron (Mirtazapine). Organon USA Inc. US Prescribing information, June 2005.
3. Zispin (Mirtazapine). Organon Laboratories Ltd. UK Summary of product characteristics, September 2005.
4. Benazzi F. Serotonin syndrome with mirtazapine-fluoxetine combination. *Int J Geriatr Psychiatry* (1998) 13, 495–6.
5. Demers JC, Malone M. Serotonin syndrome induced by fluvoxamine and mirtazapine. *Ann Pharmacother* (2001) 35, 1217–20.
6. Anttila SAK, Rasanen I, Leinonen EVJ. Fluvoxamine augmentation increases serum mirtazapine concentrations three- to fourfold. *Ann Pharmacother* (2001) 35, 1221–3.
7. Ruwe FJL, Smulders RA, Kleijn HJ, Hartmans HLA, Sitsen JMA. Mirtazapine and paroxetine: a drug-drug interaction study in healthy subjects. *Hum Psychopharmacol* (2001) 16, 449–59.
8. Soutullo CA, McElroy SL, Keck PE. Hypomania associated with mirtazapine augmentation of sertraline. *J Clin Psychiatry* (1998) 59, 320.
9. Sennef C, Timmer CJ, Sitsen JMA. Mirtazapine in combination with amitriptyline: a drug-drug interaction study in healthy subjects. *Hum Psychopharmacol* (2003) 18, 91–101.
10. Isbister GK, Dawson AH, Whyte IM. Comment: serotonin syndrome induced by fluvoxamine and mirtazapine. *Ann Pharmacother* (2001) 35, 1674–5.
11. Mirtazapine. Genus Pharmaceuticals. UK Summary of product characteristics, May 2005.

Mirtazapine + Antiepileptics

Carbamazepine and phenytoin can decrease the plasma levels of mirtazapine.

Clinical evidence, mechanism, importance and management

In a placebo-controlled study, healthy subjects were given **carbamazepine** (at steady state) with mirtazapine for 7 days. It was found that **carbamazepine** (an inducer of cytochrome P450 isoenzyme CYP3A4) decreased the AUC and maximum plasma levels of mirtazapine, by 63% and 44%, respectively, and increased the peak levels of demethylmirtazapine. Another related study found that mirtazapine did not affect the pharmacokinetics of **carbamazepine** (also a CYP3A4 substrate).[1]

A study in 9 healthy subjects given **phenytoin** 200 mg daily for 17 days, and from day 11, mirtazapine 15 mg daily for 2 days then 30 mg daily for 5 days, found that mirtazapine had no effect on the steady-state pharmacokinetics of **phenytoin**.[2] In a second associated study, 8 healthy subjects were given mirtazapine 15 mg daily for 2 days then 30 mg daily for 15 days with **phenytoin** 200 mg daily on days 8 to 17. It was found that **phenytoin** (an inducer of CYP3A4) decreased the AUC and maximum plasma levels of mirtazapine by 47% and 33%, respectively.[2]

The manufacturers advise that if **carbamazepine** or other drugs that induce drug metabolism (such as **phenytoin**) are given with mirtazapine, the mirtazapine dose may have to be increased. Further, if treatment with an inducer is stopped, the mirtazapine dosage may have to be reduced.[3,4] Although not specifically named, **phenobarbital** and **primidone** can also induce CYP3A4, and they therefore may interact similarly. Note that, mirtazapine can lower the seizure threshold, and therefore its use should be carefully considered in patients taking these drugs for epilepsy.

1. Sitsen JMA, Maris FA, Timmer CJ. Drug-drug interaction studies with mirtazapine and carbamazepine in healthy male subjects. *Eur J Drug Metab Pharmacokinet* (2001) 26, 109–21.
2. Spaans E, van den Heuvel MW, Schnabel PG, Peeters PAM, Chin-Kon-Sung UG, Colbers EPH, Sitsen JMA. Concomitant use of mirtazapine and phenytoin: a drug-drug interaction study in healthy male subjects. *Eur J Clin Pharmacol* (2002) 58, 423–9.
3. Zispin (Mirtazapine). Organon Laboratories Ltd. UK Summary of product characteristics, September 2005.
4. Mirtazapine. Genus Pharmaceuticals. UK Summary of product characteristics, May 2005.

Mirtazapine + Antipsychotics

Limited evidence suggests that risperidone does not appear to affect mirtazapine pharmacokinetics. Mirtazapine does not appear to interact to a clinically relevant extent with clozapine, olanzapine or risperidone.

Clinical evidence, mechanism, importance and management

A pilot study in 6 psychiatric patients taking **risperidone** 1 to 3 mg twice a day for 1 to 4 weeks followed by 2 to 4 weeks of combined treatment with mirtazapine 15 to 30 mg at night, found that mirtazapine did not affect the plasma levels of **risperidone** or its 9-hydroxy metabolite. Data from another patient suggest that giving **risperidone** with mirtazapine does not result in clinically relevant changes in the plasma levels of mirtazapine. Concurrent use did not appear to increase the incidence of adverse effects, but the number of patients was limited.[1]

Another study in 24 schizophrenic patients investigated the effect of adding mirtazapine 30 mg at bedtime, for 6 weeks, to treatment with **clozapine** (9 patients), **risperidone** (8), or **olanzapine** (7). Mirtazapine had a negligible effect on the metabolism of all three drugs and the combination was well tolerated.[2]

1. Loonen AJM, Doorschot CH, Oostelbos MCJM, Sitsen JMA. Lack of drug interactions between mirtazapine and risperidone in psychiatric patients: a pilot study. *Eur Neuropsychopharmacol* (1999) 10, 51–7.
2. Zoccali R, Muscatello MR, La Torre D, Malara G, Canale A, Crucitti D, D'Arrigo C, Spina E. Lack of a pharmacokinetic interaction between mirtazapine and the newer antipsychotics clozapine, risperidone and olanzapine in patients with chronic schizophrenia. *Pharmacol Res* (2003) 48, 411–14.

Mirtazapine + Benzodiazepines

The sedative effects of mirtazapine may be increased by the benzodiazepines.

Clinical evidence, mechanism, importance and management

A single-dose study in 12 healthy subjects found that the pharmacokinetics of mirtazapine and **diazepam** were not affected by concurrent use, but **diazepam** further impaired the action of mirtazapine on objectively measured skill performance; the combined actions were mostly additive.[1] The impairment of psychomotor performance and learning caused by **diazepam** is increased by mirtazapine and therefore the manufacturers warn that the sedative effects of benzodiazepines in general may be potentiated by concurrent use with mirtazapine.[2,3]

1. Mattila M, Mattila MJ, Vrijmoed-de Vries M, Kuitunen T. Actions and interactions of psychotropic drugs on human performance and mood: single doses of ORG 3770, amitriptyline and diazepam. *Pharmacol Toxicol* (1989) 65, 81–8.
2. Zispin (Mirtazapine). Organon Laboratories Ltd. UK Summary of product characteristics, September 2005.
3. Remeron (Mirtazapine). Organon USA Inc. US Prescribing information, June 2005.

Mirtazapine + Cimetidine

Cimetidine increases the bioavailability of mirtazapine.

Clinical evidence, mechanism, importance and management

In a double-blind, crossover study in 12 healthy subjects, placebo or cimetidine 800 mg twice daily were given for 14 days. Mirtazapine 30 mg was given at night on days 6 to 12. Concurrent administration of cimetidine with mirtazapine increased the AUC and peak plasma levels of mirtazapine by 54% and 22%, respectively. Trough and average mirtazapine plasma levels, at steady state, were increased by 61% and 54%, respectively, by cimetidine. Mirtazapine did not affect the pharmacokinetics of cimetidine.[1] The manufacturers advise that mirtazapine dosage may need to be reduced during concurrent treatment and increased when cimetidine treatment is stopped.[2,3]

1. Sitsen JMA, Maris FA, Timmer CJ. Concomitant use of mirtazapine and cimetidine: a drug-drug interaction study in healthy male subjects. *Eur J Clin Pharmacol* (2000) 56, 389–94.
2. Zispin (Mirtazapine). Organon Laboratories Ltd. UK Summary of product characteristics, September 2005.
3. Mirtazapine. Genus Pharmaceuticals. UK Summary of product characteristics, May 2005.

Mirtazapine + Miscellaneous

Pharmacokinetic interactions may occur between mirtazapine and inhibitors or inducers of the cytochrome P450 isoenzyme CYP3A4.

Clinical evidence, mechanism, importance and management

(a) CYP3A4 inhibitors

Ketoconazole is reported to increase the peak plasma levels and AUC of mirtazapine by about 30% and 45%, respectively.[1] Mirtazapine is extensively metabolised and the cytochrome P450 isoenzyme CYP3A4 is thought to be responsible for the formation of the N-demethyl and N-oxide metabolites.[2] The manufacturers advise caution when potent inhibitors of CYP3A4 such as **azole antifungals**, **protease inhibitors**, **erythromycin**, or **nefazodone** are given with mirtazapine.[1,2]

(b) Rifampicin (Rifampin)

The manufacturers advise that if drugs such as rifampicin, that induce drug metabolism, are given with mirtazapine, the mirtazapine dose may have to be increased. Further, if treatment with an inducer is stopped, mirtazapine dosage may have to be reduced.[1,2]

1. Zispin (Mirtazapine). Organon Laboratories Ltd. UK Summary of product characteristics, September 2005.
2. Mirtazapine. Genus Pharmaceuticals. UK Summary of product characteristics, May 2005.

Nefazodone + Antidepressants

An isolated report describes a woman who developed marked and acute hypotension and weakness when desipramine, fluoxetine and venlafaxine were replaced by nefazodone. Isolated cases describe the serotonin syndrome in patients given nefazodone together, or sequentially, with another serotonergic drug (amitriptyline, paroxetine, St John's wort, or trazodone). The manufacturer recommended that nefazodone should not be used with an MAOI or within 14 days of discontinuing an MAOI. Note that, due to adverse hepatic effects nefazodone was widely withdrawn from the market.

Clinical evidence, mechanism, importance and management

(a) MAOIs

The manufacturer stated that nefazodone should not be used with an MAOI or within 2 weeks of discontinuing treatment with an MAOI. Conversely at least one week should be allowed after stopping nefazodone before starting an MAOI.[1] There appears to be no direct clinical evidence that an adverse interaction occurs.

(b) Reboxetine

Nefazodone may increase the plasma concentrations of reboxetine, see 'Reboxetine + Antidepressants', p.1210.

(c) SSRIs

Anecdotal evidence has suggested that patients who are switched from an SSRI to nefazodone may tolerate nefazodone poorly. Nevertheless, in a 12-week, open study involving 26 depressed patients, nefazodone 100 to 600 mg daily was equally well tolerated in the 13 patients who had discontinued an SSRI within 1 to 4 weeks compared with the other 13 patients who had received no antidepressant treatment for the previous 6 months. However, the patients who had recent exposure to an SSRI (within the previous 4 weeks) were given a washout period of 4 to 5 days for short half-life SSRIs or a full week washout period for **fluoxetine** prior to initiating nefazodone.[2] Cases with specific SSRIs are discussed in the subsections below.

1. Fluoxetine. A woman with a one-year history of DSM-IV major depressive disorder and panic disorder was given daily doses of **desipramine** 75 mg, fluoxetine 20 mg, **venlafaxine** 37.5 mg, **clonazepam** 3 mg and **valproate** 400 mg with no adverse effects, except a dry mouth and sexual difficulties.[3] The first three drugs were stopped and replaced by nefazodone 100 mg twice daily, started about 12 hours later. Within an hour of the first dose she felt very weak and her blood pressure was found to have fallen to only 90/60 mmHg (normally 120/90 mmHg). On waking the next day she had severe weakness, unsteady gait, pale, cool and sweaty skin, and paraesthesia. During the day she took two further 100-mg doses of nefazodone and her condition persisted and worsened with continuing hypotension. The nefazodone was discontinued and by the following day the weakness had improved, disappearing over the next few days. Within a week nefazodone 200 mg daily was reintroduced without problems.
The US manufacturer of nefazodone noted that nefazodone did not alter the pharmacokinetics of fluoxetine, but fluoxetine increased the AUC of the metabolites of nefazodone by up to 6-fold.[1] When nefazodone 200 mg twice was given to patients who had been taking fluoxetine for 7 days adverse effects (including headache and nausea) were increased. The manufacturers advised allowing a washout period of at least one week (more may be needed depending on dose and individual patient characteristics) to minimise these effects.[1] It therefore seems likely that fluoxetine was the interacting drug, but it is impossible to rule out a contribution from the other drugs.

2. Paroxetine. A woman was withdrawn from nefazodone after about 6 months of treatment, tapering over the last fortnight to 75 mg every 12 hours. Within a day she started taking paroxetine 20 mg daily and valproic acid, and was admitted the next day with muscle rigidity, uncoordinated muscle tremors, flailing arms and twitching legs, diaphoresis and agitation. This was identified as the serotonin syndrome. Rechallenge with paroxetine 7 days later was uneventful.[4]

(d) St John's wort

An elderly patient taking nefazodone 100 mg twice daily, developed symptoms similar to the serotonin syndrome within 3 days of starting to take St John's wort 300 mg three times daily. The symptoms included nausea, vomiting, and restlessness. She was asked to stop both medications, but continued the St John's wort and her symptoms gradually improved over a 1-week period.[5]

(e) Trazodone

A woman taking irbesartan for hypertension was also given nefazodone at an initial dosage of 200 mg daily, followed by 400 mg daily for about 5 weeks. Four days after the dose was increased to 500 mg daily, and trazodone 25 to 50 mg daily was also added as a hypnotic, she was admitted to hospital with a blood pressure of 240/120 mmHg. She was confused, had difficulty concentrating and had numbness on the right side of her lips, nose and right-hand fingers, flushed pruritic skin, nausea, and loose stools. On examination she was restless, hyperreflexic, and diaphoretic. Nefazodone and trazodone were discontinued. She recovered after treatment with labetalol, clonidine, amlodipine and increased irbesartan dosage.[6] Although trazodone is used with other serotonergic drugs, it is important to be aware that this may lead to the potentially fatal 'serotonin syndrome', (p.9).

The manufacturers of trazodone say that *in vitro* drug metabolism studies suggest that there is a potential for drug interactions when trazodone is given with a potent CYP3A4 inhibitor such as nefazodone. There may be substantial increases in trazodone levels, with the potential for adverse effects, and a lower dose of trazodone should be considered.[7,8] The UK manufacturer suggests avoidance of the combination where possible.[7]

(f) Tricyclic antidepressants

1. Amitriptyline. A woman who had been taking amitriptyline 10 mg at night and thioridazine developed the serotonin syndrome after taking half a tablet of nefazodone (dosage unspecified).[9]

2. Desipramine. The manufacturer of nefazodone reported that desipramine 75 mg daily did not change the pharmacokinetics of nefazodone 150 mg twice daily, but levels of the nefazodone metabolite, meta-chlorophenylpiperazine, were increased by up to 50%. There was no change in the pharmacokinetics of desipramine or its metabolite. No specific dosage adjustments were said to be required on concurrent use.[1]

1. Nefazodone hydrochloride. Watson Laboratories Inc. US Prescribing information, June 2004.
2. Mischoulon D, Opitz G, Kelly K, Fava M, Rosenbaum JF. A preliminary open study of the tolerability and effectiveness of nefazodone in major depressive disorder: comparing patients who recently discontinued an SSRI with those on no recent antidepressant treatment. *Depress Anxiety* (2004) 19, 43–50.
3. Benazzi F. Dangerous interaction with nefazodone added to fluoxetine, desipramine, venlafaxine, valproate and clonazepam combination therapy. *J Psychopharmacol* (1997) 11, 190–1.
4. John L, Perreault MM, Tao T, Blew PG. Serotonin syndrome associated with nefazodone and paroxetine. *Ann Emerg Med* (1997) 29, 287–9.
5. Lantz MS, Buchalter E, Giambanco V. St. John's wort and antidepressant drug interactions in the elderly. *J Geriatr Psychiatry Neurol* (1999) 12, 7–10.
6. Margolese HC, Chouinard G. Serotonin syndrome from addition of low-dose trazodone to nefazodone. *Am J Psychiatry* (2000) 157, 1022.
7. Molipaxin (Trazodone hydrochloride). Sanofi-Aventis. UK Summary of product characteristics, July 2005.
8. Desyrel (Trazodone hydrochloride). Bristol-Myers Squibb Company. US Prescribing information, January 2005.
9. Chan BSH, Graudins A, Whyte IM, Dawson AH, Braitberg G, Duggin GG. Serotonin syndrome resulting from drug interactions. *Med J Aust* (1998) 169, 523–5.

Nefazodone + Cimetidine

No changes in the steady-state pharmacokinetics of either cimetidine or nefazodone were seen in a week long study in 18 healthy subjects given cimetidine 300 mg four times daily and nefazodone 200 mg every 12 hours. No special precautions would seem to be necessary if both drugs are used concurrently.[1]

1. Barbhaiya RH, Shukla UA, Greene DS. Lack of interaction between nefazodone and cimetidine: a steady state pharmacokinetic study in humans. *Br J Clin Pharmacol* (1995) 40, 161–5.

Reboxetine + Antidepressants

The manufacturer of reboxetine recommends avoiding the concurrent use of potent CYP3A4 inhibitors as reboxetine levels may be increased. They also recommend avoiding the concurrent use of MAOIs, because of the possible risk of hypertensive crises. The concurrent use of fluoxetine and reboxetine does not appear to alter the pharmacokinetics of either drug.

Clinical evidence, mechanism, importance and management

A study in 30 healthy subjects given reboxetine 4 mg twice daily and **fluoxetine** 20 mg daily found no significant changes in the pharmacokinetics of either drug.[1]

The manufacturer of reboxetine suggests that because **fluvoxamine** is a potent inhibitor of CYP3A4 it may increase plasma concentrations of reboxetine, and, because of the narrow therapeutic margin of reboxetine, concurrent use should be avoided.[2] However, note that **fluvoxamine** is more usually considered a potent inhibitor of CYP1A2 and is generally considered a weak inhibitor of CYP3A4.

No data seem to be available about the concurrent use of reboxetine with **MAOIs** and the manufacturer currently advises the avoidance of **MAOIs** because of the potential risk of a tyramine-like effect [hypertensive crisis].[2]

1. Fleishaker JC, Herman BD, Pearson LK, Ionita A, Mucci M. Evaluation of the potential pharmacokinetic/pharmacodynamic interaction between fluoxetine and reboxetine in healthy volunteers. *Clin Drug Invest* (1999) 18, 141–50.
2. Edronax (Reboxetine methanesulphonate). Pharmacia Ltd. UK Summary of product characteristics, May 2006.

Reboxetine + CYP3A4 inhibitors

Ketoconazole may inhibit the metabolism of reboxetine. The manufacturer therefore advises avoiding the concurrent use of azoles, macrolides and nefazodone.

Clinical evidence, mechanism, importance and management

A study in 11 healthy subjects found that **ketoconazole** 200 mg daily for 5 days increased the plasma concentrations of a single 4-mg dose of reboxetine, taken on the second day, by about 50%. Although the adverse effect profile of reboxetine was not altered, because reboxetine has a narrow therapeutic index it was concluded that caution should be used and a reduction in reboxetine dosage considered if it is given with **ketoconazole**.[1] The manufacturer recommends that potent inhibitors of CYP3A4, including **azoles**, **macrolides** (**erythromycin**) and **nefazodone** should not be given with reboxetine.[2] For a list of clinically significant CYP3A4 inhibitors see 'Table 1.4', (p.6).

1. Herman BD, Fleishaker JC, Brown MT. Ketoconazole inhibits the clearance of the enantiomers of the antidepressant reboxetine in humans. *Clin Pharmacol Ther* (1999) 66, 374–9.
2. Edronax (Reboxetine methanesulphonate). Pharmacia Ltd. UK Summary of product characteristics, May 2006.

Reboxetine + Dextromethorphan

A study in 10 healthy subjects who were of the CYP2D6 extensive metaboliser phenotype (the most commonly found phenotype) found that the pharmacokinetics of reboxetine 8 mg daily were not affected by a single 30-mg dose of dextromethorphan.[1]

1. Avenoso A, Facciolà G, Scordo MG, Spina E. No effect of the new antidepressant reboxetine on CYP2D6 activity in healthy volunteers. *Ther Drug Monit* (1999) 21, 577–9.

Reboxetine + Miscellaneous

The manufacturer points out the possibility of hypokalaemia if reboxetine is used with potassium-depleting diuretics. Experience with reboxetine in elderly patients suggests it reduces potassium by up to 0.8 mmol/L, starting after 14 weeks of use. They also suggest that the concurrent use of reboxetine and ergot derivatives might result in increased blood pressure although no clinical data are quoted, and the concurrent use of lorazepam results in mild to moderate drowsiness and an orthostatic increase in heart rate, but no pharmacokinetic interaction occurs.[1]

1. Edronax (Reboxetine methanesulphonate). Pharmacia Ltd. UK Summary of product characteristics, May 2006.

SNRIs + H_2-receptor antagonists

Cimetidine may increase duloxetine and venlafaxine plasma levels, which may lead to an increase in their adverse effects. Famotidine does not appear to interact with duloxetine.

Clinical evidence, mechanism, importance and management

(a) Duloxetine

The metabolism of duloxetine is reduced by cytochrome P450 isoenzyme CYP1A2 inhibitors and it has been suggested that drugs with this effect should be avoided (see 'fluvoxamine', (p.1212)). The US manufacturer of duloxetine specifically mentions **cimetidine** as an inhibitor of this enzyme[1] and therefore if duloxetine is given with **cimetidine** it would seem prudent to monitor duloxetine plasma levels and adverse effects. **Famotidine** has no effect on the rate or extent of absorption of a single 40-mg dose of duloxetine,[1] and it may therefore be a suitable alternative to **cimetidine** in patients taking duloxetine.

(b) Venlafaxine

Cimetidine 800 mg daily for 5 days was found to reduce the oral clearance of venlafaxine 50 mg every 8 hours by 40%, and to increase the AUC by 62% in 18 healthy subjects. It had no effect on the formation or elimination of the major active metabolite of venlafaxine, *O*-desmethylvenlafaxine (ODV). The total level of venlafaxine with ODV was found to be increased by only 13%. Thus the overall pharmacological activity of the two was only slightly increased by **cimetidine**[2] and no special precautions would seem to be necessary on concurrent use. However, the manufacturers of venlafaxine suggest that the elderly and those with hepatic impairment may possibly show a more pronounced effect, and such patients should be monitored more closely,[3,4] for venlafaxine adverse effects.

1. Cymbalta (Duloxetine hydrochloride). Eli Lilly and Company. US Prescribing information, May 2007.
2. Troy SM, Rudolph R, Mayersohn M, Chiang ST. The influence of cimetidine on the disposition kinetics of the antidepressant venlafaxine. *J Clin Pharmacol* (1998) 38, 467–74.
3. Efexor (Venlafaxine hydrochloride). Wyeth Pharmaceuticals. UK Summary of product characteristics, May 2006.
4. Effexor XR (Venlafaxine hydrochloride). Wyeth Pharmaceuticals Inc. US Prescribing information, June 2007.

SNRIs + Propafenone

An isolated report describes psychosis, which occurred when a patient took venlafaxine with propafenone. Duloxetine may increase propafenone levels.

Clinical evidence, mechanism, importance and management

(a) Duloxetine

Duloxetine is a moderate inhibitor of the cytochrome P450 isoenzyme CYP2D6 and may increase the levels of drugs metabolised by CYP2D6 such as propafenone. The US manufacturer recommends that the concurrent use of duloxetine and propafenone should be approached with caution.[1]

(b) Venlafaxine

A 67-year-old woman with bipolar disorder taking venlafaxine 300 mg daily experienced symptoms of paranoia, visual hallucinations and marked confusion, about 2 weeks after starting propafenone 600 mg daily for intermittent atrial fibrillation. Serum levels of venlafaxine had increased from 85 nanograms/mL to 520 nanograms/mL (upper level of normal range 150 nanograms/mL) and levels of the metabolite *O*-desmethylvenlafaxine had increased but were still within normal ranges. Venlafaxine was stopped for a few days then restarted at the lower dose of 75 mg daily and her mental condition (diagnosed as organic psychosis) improved. However, as she also had orthostatic hypotension her propafenone dosage was subsequently reduced to 300 mg daily, which necessitated dosage adjustments of venlafaxine because of a marked drop in serum level. When propafenone was again increased to 600 mg daily the venlafaxine had to be reduced to 50 mg daily.[2] The reasons for the interaction are not known, but venlafaxine is partly metabolised by CYP2D6 and propafenone may compete for this metabolic pathway. Information is limited to this single case report, and therefore its general significance is unclear..

1. Cymbalta (Duloxetine hydrochloride). Eli Lilly and Company. US Prescribing information, May 2007
2. Pfeffer F, Grube M. An organic psychosis due to a venlafaxine-propafenone interaction. *Int J Psychiatry Med* (2001) 31, 427–32.

SNRIs + St John's wort (*Hypericum perforatum*)

The serotonin syndrome has been reported in one patient taking venlafaxine and St John's wort.

Clinical evidence, mechanism, importance and management

An interaction between **venlafaxine** and St John's wort *(Hypericum perforatum)* was reported to the Centre Régional de Pharmacovigilance de Marseille involving a 32-year-old man who had been taking **venlafaxine** 250 mg daily for several months. He started taking St John's wort at a dose of 200 drops 3 times daily (usual dose up to 160 drops daily) and on the third day felt faint and anxious, and had symptoms of diaphoresis, shivering and tachycardia. The St John's wort was stopped and his symptoms resolved in 3 days without altering the dose of **venlafaxine**.[1] A search of Health Canada's database of spontaneous adverse reactions for the period 1998 to 2003 also found one case of suspected serotonin syndrome as a result of an interaction between **venlafaxine** and St John's wort.[2] **Duloxetine** would be expected to interact similarly. The manufacturers of both **duloxetine** and **venlafaxine** generally advise caution if they are given with drugs that affect the serotonergic neurotransmitter systems,[3-5]

1. Prost N, Tichadou L, Rodor F, Nguyen N, David JM, Jean-Pastor MJ. Interaction millepertuis-venlafaxine. *Presse Med* (2000) 29, 1285–6.
2. Griffiths J, Jordan S, Pilan K. Natural health products and adverse reactions. *Can Adverse React News* (2004) 14 (1), 2–3.
3. Efexor (Venlafaxine hydrochloride). Wyeth Pharmaceuticals. UK Summary of product characteristics, May 2006.

4. Effexor XR (Venlafaxine hydrochloride). Wyeth Pharmaceuticals Inc. US Prescribing information, June 2007.
5. Cymbalta (Duloxetine hydrochloride). Eli Lilly and Company Ltd. UK Summary of product characteristics, November 2006.

SNRIs; Duloxetine + Antidepressants

The manufacturers of duloxetine contraindicate the concurrent use of MAOIs because of the theoretical risk of the serotonin syndrome. Similarly they recommend caution with other serotonergic drugs, including the SSRIs, venlafaxine, and tryptophan. Fluvoxamine should not be used with duloxetine, because it markedly increases duloxetine levels. Low-dose paroxetine caused a modest increase in the duloxetine AUC, and fluoxetine is predicted to interact similarly.

Clinical evidence, mechanism, importance and management

The manufacturer advises caution if duloxetine is used with **SSRIs** (see below), 'tricyclic antidepressants', (p.1240), 'St John's wort', (p.1224), **venlafaxine**, or **tryptophan**, because the concurrent use of more than one serotonergic drug has rarely resulted in 'the serotonin syndrome', (p.9).[1,2]

(a) SSRIs

1. Fluvoxamine. Fluvoxamine 100 mg daily increased the AUC of duloxetine five- to sixfold, and decreased its clearance by about 77% in 14 healthy subjects.[1-3] Similar increases in duloxetine plasma levels were found in 15 healthy subjects who were given fluvoxamine 50 to 100 mg daily and duloxetine 40 mg twice daily.[4]
Fluvoxamine is a potent inhibitor of the cytochrome P450 isoenzyme CYP1A2, by which duloxetine is, in part, metabolised.[3] Therefore concurrent use raises duloxetine levels. Although the clinical relevance of the increases in duloxetine levels have not been assessed, the manufacturer considers that the rise with fluvoxamine is so marked that the combination should be avoided.[1-3] The UK manufacturers specifically contraindicate concurrent use.[1,2] Other SSRIs have minimal effects on this isoenzyme, and would therefore not be expected to interact by *this* route, but see also paroxetine, below.

2. Paroxetine. The concurrent use of paroxetine 20 mg daily and duloxetine 40 mg daily increased the AUC of duloxetine at steady state by about 60% in healthy subjects.[5] Paroxetine is an inhibitor of CYP2D6, which has a role in duloxetine metabolism. Therefore concurrent use raises duloxetine levels. The rise in duloxetine levels with paroxetine 20 mg daily is probably not clinically relevant, but the manufacturer notes that greater increases would be expected with higher doses.[3] Caution is warranted. Other SSRIs (notably **fluoxetine**) also inhibit this isoenzyme, and would therefore be expected to interact similarly.

(b) MAOIs

The manufacturers contraindicate the use of duloxetine with non-selective irreversible MAOIs, and for 14 days after discontinuing an MAOI, and at least 5 days should be allowed after stopping duloxetine before starting an MAOI. This is because of the possible risk of serotonin syndrome.[1-3] Although the risk would be lower with selective, reversible MAOIs such as **moclobemide**, the manufacturer still says concurrent use is not recommended.[1,2]

1. Cymbalta (Duloxetine hydrochloride). Eli Lilly and Company Ltd. UK Summary of product characteristics, November 2006.
2. Yentreve (Duloxetine hydrochloride). Eli Lilly and Company Ltd. UK Summary of product characteristics, November 2006.
3. Cymbalta (Duloxetine hydrochloride). Eli Lilly and Company. US Prescribing information, May 2007.
4. Small D, Loghin C, Lucas R, Knadler MP, Zhang L, Chappell J, Bergstrom R, Callaghan JT. Pharmacokinetic evaluation of combined duloxetine and fluvoxamine dosing in CYP2D6 poor metabolizers. *Clin Pharmacol Ther* (2005) 77, P37.
5. Skinner MH, Kuan H-Y, Pan A, Sathirakul K, Knadler MP, Gonzales CR, Yeo KP, Reddy S, Lim M, Ayan-Oshodi M, Wise SD. Duloxetine is both an inhibitor and a substrate of cytochrome P4502D6 in healthy volunteers. *Clin Pharmacol Ther* (2003) 73, 170–7.

SNRIs; Duloxetine + Miscellaneous

Ciprofloxacin, enoxacin and quinidine are predicted to raise duloxetine levels. Duloxetine is predicted to raise the levels of flecainide and thioridazine. Due to the theoretical risk of serotonin syndrome, the manufacturers of duloxetine recommend caution with other serotonergic drugs or other CNS depressants. The pharmacokinetics of duloxetine were not affected by antacids.

Clinical evidence, mechanism, importance and management

(a) Antacids

Aluminium/magnesium-containing antacids had no effect on the rate or extent of absorption of a single 40-mg dose of duloxetine.[1-3] No special precautions appear to be necessary on concurrent use.

(b) CYP1A2

1. Inducers. Population pharmacokinetic studies have shown that **smokers** have almost 50% lower plasma concentrations of duloxetine, when compared with **non-smokers**.[1] The clinical significance of this finding is unclear.

2. Inhibitors. 'Fluvoxamine', (above), a potent inhibitor of the cytochrome P450 isoenzyme CYP1A2, markedly increases duloxetine levels. The manufacturers predict that some **quinolones** (they name **ciprofloxacin** and **enoxacin**) will have the same effect and suggest that their concurrent use with duloxetine should be avoided.[1-3] For a list of clinically significant CYP1A2 inhibitors, see 'Table 1.2', (p.4).

(c) CYP2D6

1. Inhibitors. Paroxetine, an inhibitor of the cytochrome P450 isoenzyme CYP2D6, increases duloxetine levels. The manufacturer suggests that other CYP2D6 inhibitors will interact similarly, and specifically names **quinidine**.[3] For a list of clinically significant CYP2D6 inhibitors, see 'Table 1.3', (p.6).

2. Substrates. Duloxetine is a moderate inhibitor of the cytochrome P450 isoenzyme CYP2D6. The manufacturers advise caution if duloxetine is given with drugs that are predominantly metabolised by CYP2D6 and have a narrow therapeutic index,[1-3] including **flecainide**, and **thioridazine** which is contraindicated in the US because of the risk of arrhythmias with elevated levels of this drug.[3] This seems prudent as the CYP2D6 inhibitory effects of duloxetine have been shown to be modest (see 'tolterodine', (p.1289) and 'desipramine', (p.1240)), and changes of this size may be clinically significant with narrow therapeutic index drugs.

(d) Serotonergic drugs

Because the concurrent use of more than one serotonergic drug has rarely resulted in 'the serotonin syndrome', (p.9), the manufacturer advises caution if duloxetine is used with 'tricyclic antidepressants', (p.1240), or other 'antidepressants', (above), **triptans**, **tramadol**, and **pethidine**.[1,2]

1. Cymbalta (Duloxetine hydrochloride). Eli Lilly and Company Ltd. UK Summary of product characteristics, November 2006.
2. Yentreve (Duloxetine hydrochloride). Eli Lilly and Company Ltd. UK Summary of product characteristics, November 2006.
3. Cymbalta (Duloxetine hydrochloride). Eli Lilly and Company. US Prescribing information, May 2007.

SNRIs; Venlafaxine + Antidepressants

Bupropion may increase venlafaxine plasma levels. Antimuscarinic adverse effects can develop in patients taking fluoxetine and venlafaxine. Venlafaxine combined with other serotonergic antidepressants may increase the risk of bleeding and/or the serotonin syndrome. The serotonin syndrome has also been reported in patients taking venlafaxine with mirtazapine or trazodone; some of these patients were also taking other serotonergic drugs.

Clinical evidence and mechanism

(a) Bupropion

Bupropion was found to increase venlafaxine plasma levels and decrease the levels of the metabolite, O-desmethylvenlafaxine, in 7 patients who had been given venlafaxine alone for a minimum of 6 weeks and then with bupropion SR 150 mg daily for a further 8 weeks.[1]

For a report of worsening symptoms of the serotonin syndrome when venlafaxine was given with bupropion and sertraline, see 'SSRIs + Bupropion', p.1215.

(b) MAOIs

For reports of the serotonin syndrome with venlafaxine and MAOIs, see 'MAOIs or RIMAs + Venlafaxine', p.1156.

(c) Mirtazapine

The serotonin syndrome occurred in a patient given extended-release venlafaxine 75 mg daily and mirtazapine 30 mg daily, during cross-tapering of the two drugs (reducing mirtazapine dose and starting venlafaxine).[2] Another case occurred when tramadol was given to a patient taking venlafaxine and mirtazapine.[3]

For a report of haemorrhages associated with the use of mirtazapine, venlafaxine and escitalopram, see *(d)* below.

(d) SSRIs

1. Antimuscarinic adverse effects. A woman taking **fluoxetine** 20 mg and clonazepam 1 mg daily developed blurred vision, dry mouth, constipation, dizziness, insomnia and a hand tremor within a week of starting to take venlafaxine 37.5 mg daily. These symptoms worsened by the second week and persisted until the venlafaxine was stopped.[4,5] Four patients (aged 21, 24, 51 and 70) taking **fluoxetine** developed antimuscarinic adverse effects (constipation, blurred vision, urinary retention and dry mouth) within a week of starting venlafaxine, which persisted until the venlafaxine was stopped.[6] A 61-year-old man taking **fluoxetine** 20 mg daily had extreme difficulty in urinating within 2 days of starting to take venlafaxine 37.5 mg daily. The effect became intolerable after 10 days but no other obvious antimuscarinic adverse effects (blurred vision, constipation, dry mouth, tachycardia) were seen. This patient had some prostate enlargement and had previously had some moderate urinary problems while taking **fluoxetine** and nortriptyline.[5,7]

One possible explanation is that **fluoxetine** inhibits the cytochrome P450 isoenzyme CYP2D6, which is concerned with the metabolism of venlafaxine, leading to an increase in its serum levels and in its usually minimal antimuscarinic adverse effects.[4-7] An alternative explanation is that these adverse effects are due to an adrenergic mechanism.[7]

2. Haemorrhages. A 60-year-old man experienced haemorrhages from his nose and rectum one week after venlafaxine 150 mg daily and **mirtazapine** 15 mg daily were added to treatment with **escitalopram** 20 mg daily. The bleeding progressively worsened during the following 3 weeks and then the patient reduced the dosages to **escitalopram** 15 mg, **mirtazapine** 7.5 mg and venlafaxine 100 mg daily, and the bleeding decreased over the following week. He continued weekly tapering of the medications and the bleeding progressively decreased until it stopped when the doses were **escitalopram** 5 mg, **mirtazapine** 7.5 mg and venlafaxine 37.5 mg daily. Previous treatments with these three drugs used alone had not caused haemorrhages and it was suggested that the bleeding was due to the combined drugs causing high levels of serotonin.[8]

3. Serotonin syndrome. A 39-year-old woman with depression and panic attacks was taking cimetidine, trazodone, clonazepam and **fluoxetine**. Within 24 hours of abruptly stopping clonazepam and **fluoxetine** and starting lorazepam and venlafaxine, she developed the serotonin syndrome (diaphoresis, tremors, slurred speech, myoclonus, restlessness and diarrhoea).[9]

A 21-year-old woman whose long-term treatment with **paroxetine** was stopped a week before starting venlafaxine (37.5 mg daily for 5 days then 75 mg daily for 2 days) developed vomiting, dizziness, incoordination, anxiety and electric shock sensations in her arms and legs within 3 days of starting venlafaxine. She stopped venlafaxine after 7 days of treatment, but symptoms persisted for 5 days until she was treated with cyproheptadine.[10]

A 75-year-old man developed the serotonin syndrome after discontinuing **sertraline** and starting venlafaxine 48 hours later, although the onset of symptoms did not develop until after 14 days of therapy with venlafaxine. The venlafaxine was discontinued and the symptoms subsided over a 6-day period. However, 2 weeks later **amitriptyline** was introduced and a recurrence of symptoms was seen over the following 48 hours. The author commented that any drug with serotonergic activity might potentially cause a serotonin syndrome when serotonin transmission has been enhanced by concomitant or recently withdrawn serotonergic drugs.[11] Other reports of the serotonin syndrome have been described with venlafaxine and 'amitriptyline', (p.1240), and 'sertraline and bupropion', (p.1215).

(e) Trazodone

A 50-year-old HIV-positive man, who was receiving methadone for opioid dependence, developed signs of the serotonin syndrome 18 days after starting to take extended-release venlafaxine (dose increased to 225 mg daily over 7 days) and trazodone 100 mg at bedtime. His clinical status improved rapidly over 24 hours when all medications were discontinued. The serotonin syndrome was thought to have been precipitated by the combination of venlafaxine and trazodone, both of which inhibit the reuptake of serotonin, but methadone may have also been a contributing factor. He was not taking any concurrent medication for his HIV infection.[12]

(f) Tricyclic antidepressants

For reports of increased antimuscarinic effects and the serotonin syndrome, see 'Tricyclic antidepressants + SNRIs; Venlafaxine', p.1240.

Importance and management

Information about the adverse antimuscarinic adverse effects due to an interaction between fluoxetine and venlafaxine seems to be limited to the reports cited, all by the same author. The incidence is not known, but if venlafaxine and fluoxetine are given concurrently, be alert for any evidence of increased antimuscarinic adverse effects (such as dry mouth, blurred vision and urinary retention). It may be necessary to withdraw one or other of the two drugs.

Also note that the development of the serotonin syndrome has been attributed to the sequential use of an SSRI (fluoxetine, paroxetine, or sertraline) and venlafaxine. It has also occurred with concurrent use of venlafaxine and mirtazapine or trazodone. The manufacturers of venlafaxine caution its use with other drugs that affect serotonergic transmission, such as the SSRIs[13,14] because of the potential risks of the serotonin syndrome. For more about the serotonin syndrome see 'Additive or synergistic interactions', (p.9).

1. Kennedy SH, McCann SM, Masellis M, McIntyre RS, Raskin J, McKay G, Baker GB. Combining bupropion SR with venlafaxine, paroxetine, or fluoxetine: a preliminary report on pharmacokinetic, therapeutic, and sexual dysfunction effects. *J Clin Psychiatry* (2002) 63, 181–6.
2. Dimellis D. Serotonin syndrome produced by a combination of venlafaxine and mirtazapine. *World J Biol Psychiatry* (2002) 3, 167.
3. Houlihan DJ. Serotonin syndrome resulting from coadministration of tramadol, venlafaxine, and mirtazapine. *Ann Pharmacother* (2004) 38, 411–13.
4. Benazzi F. Severe anticholinergic side effects with venlafaxine-fluoxetine combination. *Can J Psychiatry* (1997) 42, 980–1.
5. Benazzi F. Venlafaxine-fluoxetine interaction. *J Clin Psychopharmacol* (1999) 19, 96–8.
6. Benazzi F. Venlafaxine drug-drug interactions in clinical practice. *J Psychiatry Neurosci* (1998) 23, 181–2.
7. Benazzi F. Urinary retention with venlafaxine-fluoxetine combination. *Hum Psychopharmacol* (1998) 13, 139–40.
8. Benazzi F. Hemorrhages during escitalopram–venlafaxine–mirtazapine combination treatment of depression. *Can J Psychiatry* (2005) 50, 184.
9. Bhatara VS, Magnus RD, Paul KL, Preskorn SH. Serotonin syndrome induced by venlafaxine and fluoxetine: a case study in polypharmacy and potential pharmacodynamic and pharmacokinetic mechanisms. *Ann Pharmacother* (1998) 32, 432–6.
10. Chan BSH, Graudins A, Whyte IM, Dawson AH, Braitberg G, Duggin GG. Serotonin syndrome resulting from drug interactions. *Med J Aust* (1998) 169, 523–5.
11. Perry NK. Venlafaxine-induced serotonin syndrome with relapse following amitriptyline. *Postgrad Med J* (2000) 76, 254–6.
12. McCue RE, Joseph M. Venlafaxine- and trazodone-induced serotonin syndrome. *Am J Psychiatry* (2001) 158, 2088–9.
13. Effexor XR (Venlafaxine hydrochloride). Wyeth Pharmaceuticals Inc. US Prescribing information, June 2007.
14. Efexor (Venlafaxine hydrochloride). Wyeth Pharmaceuticals. UK Summary of product characteristics, May 2006.

SNRIs; Venlafaxine + Antihypertensives

No important interactions normally appear to occur with venlafaxine and ACE inhibitors, beta blockers or diuretics, but an isolated report suggests that propranolol, particularly if it is given with other CYP2D6 substrates, may affect the metabolism of venlafaxine.

Clinical evidence, mechanism, importance and management

During the phase II and III clinical studies of venlafaxine, 267 patients were also taking antihypertensive medications, including **beta blockers**, **diuretics**, **ACE inhibitors** (specific drugs were not named in the report) without any reported adverse interactions, but note that no specific pharmacokinetic studies were undertaken.[1] A case study reports high trough plasma levels of venlafaxine and low levels of O-desmethylvenlafaxine in a patient also taking **propranolol** and mianserin.[2] It was thought that these drugs competitively inhibited the metabolism of venlafaxine by the cytochrome P450 isoenzyme CYP2D6. The general significance of this report is unclear.

1. Wyeth Laboratories. Data on file (Study S).
2. Eap CB, Bertel-Laubscher R, Zullino D, Amey M, Baumann P. Marked increase of venlafaxine enantiomer concentrations as a consequence of metabolic interactions: A case report. *Pharmacopsychiatry* (2000) 33, 112–15.

SNRIs; Venlafaxine + Co-amoxiclav

An isolated case of the serotonin syndrome has been attributed to the concurrent use of venlafaxine and co-amoxiclav.

Clinical evidence, mechanism, importance and management

A 56-year-old man taking venlafaxine 37.5 mg twice daily for 10 months was given a course of co-amoxiclav (**amoxicillin** with **clavulanate**) 375 mg three times daily to treat gingivitis and a dental abscess. Within 3 hours of a dose of co-amoxiclav he developed tingling in the tip of his tongue, intense paraesthesia in the fingers, severe abdominal cramps, profuse diarrhoea, cold sweats, tremor and uncontrollable shivering. He was also agitated and frightened, but not confused. The symptoms lasted for 6 hours and were initially assumed to be due to gastroenteritis. However, 2 months later while still taking venlafaxine, he developed identical symptoms after a single dose of co-amoxiclav, which was then diagnosed as the serotonin syndrome. The patient had taken co-amoxiclav without problem when not taking venlafaxine and after the second episode continued venlafaxine without further episodes of the serotonin syndrome. Venlafaxine is metabolised mainly by the cytochrome P450 isoenzyme CYP2D6, but co-amoxiclav is not a substrate for this isoenzyme and its ability to inhibit CYP2D6 is not known. It is probable that many patients have received both venlafaxine and co-amoxiclav without adverse effects, so the general importance of this isolated report is unknown, but it seems likely to be small.[1]

1. Connor H. Serotonin syndrome after single doses of co-amoxiclav during treatment with venlafaxine. *J R Soc Med* (2003) 96, 233–4.

SNRIs; Venlafaxine + Dexamfetamine

An isolated case of the serotonin syndrome has been attributed to the concurrent use of dexamfetamine and venlafaxine.

Clinical evidence, mechanism, importance and management

A 32-year-old patient taking dexamfetamine 5 mg three times daily for adult attention deficit hyperactivity disorder (ADHD) presented with marked agitation, anxiety, shivering and tremor 2 weeks after also starting to take venlafaxine 75 mg to 150 mg daily. Other symptoms included generalised hypertonia, hyperreflexia, frequent myoclonic jerking, tonic spasm of the orbicularis oris muscle, and sinus tachycardia. His symptoms resolved completely when both drugs were withdrawn and cyproheptadine, to a total dose of 32 mg over 3 hours, was given. Dexamfetamine was restarted after 3 days. It was suggested that the combination of serotonin re-uptake blockade and either presynaptic release of serotonin or monoamine oxidase inhibition by dexamfetamine could cause increased serotonin in the CNS. Caution is advised when dexamfetamine is given with venlafaxine.[1] For more information about the serotonin syndrome, see 'Additive or synergistic interactions', (p.9).

1. Prior FH, Isbister GK, Dawson AH, Whyte IM. Serotonin toxicity with therapeutic doses of dexamphetamine and venlafaxine. *Med J Aust* (2002) 176, 240–1.

SNRIs; Venlafaxine + Jujube (*Ziziphus jujuba*)

An isolated report describes an acute serotonin reaction when venlafaxine was given with a Chinese herbal remedy, jujube (sour date nut).

Clinical evidence, mechanism, importance and management

A 40-year-old woman with intermittent depression took jujube 500 mg daily (**sour date nut; suanzaoren**; *Ziziphus jujuba*), prescribed by a traditional Chinese healer, for several weeks, with minor improvement. She was then prescribed venlafaxine 37.5 mg daily by a psychiatrist, but approximately one hour after taking the first dose of venlafaxine together with the jujube she became agitated, restless, nauseated, dizzy and ataxic, and subsequently collapsed. She showed symptoms of a severe acute serotonin reaction with some anaphylactic features, which improved over the following 8 hours. She stopped taking the jujube and subsequently took venlafaxine 150 mg daily for 1 month without adverse effects.[1] This highlights the need for physicians to ask patients about the use of herbal remedies and to advise their discontinuation before prescribing antidepressant drugs if there is any possibility of an interaction.

1. Stewart DE. Venlafaxine and sour date nut. *Am J Psychiatry* (2004) 161, 1129–30.

SNRIs; Venlafaxine + Metoclopramide

An isolated case of the serotonin syndrome has been attributed to the concurrent use of metoclopramide and venlafaxine.

Clinical evidence, mechanism, importance and management

A 32-year-old woman with depression who had been taking venlafaxine 225 mg daily in divided doses for 3 years was admitted to hospital after a fall. She developed a movement disorder and a period of unresponsiveness after being given a 10-mg intravenous dose of metoclopramide. After a second dose of metoclopramide the symptoms recurred and were associated with confusion, agitation, fever, diaphoresis, tachypnoea, tachycardia, and hypertension. The symptoms were consistent with the serotonin syndrome, with a serious extrapyramidal movement disorder. The venlafaxine was withheld and she was given diazepam. The symptoms resolved over the next two days, after which she continued to take venlafaxine.[1] Information seems to be limited to this report, and the general significance of this interaction is unclear.

1. Fisher AA, Davis MW. Serotonin syndrome caused by selective serotonin reuptake-inhibitors–metoclopramide interaction. *Ann Pharmacother* (2002) 36, 67–71.

SNRIs; Venlafaxine + Miscellaneous

Theoretically the metabolism of venlafaxine may be inhibited by CYP2D6 inhibitors or substrates such as diphenhydramine, melperone, quinidine or thioridazine. CYP3A4 inhibitors such as ketoconazole may also have some effect. An isolated case describes a hypertensive crisis associated with venlafaxine and disulfiram. The manufacturers predict that the use of triptans with venlafaxine may have additive effects on serotonin, which could lead to the serotonin syndrome.

Clinical evidence, mechanism, importance and management

(a) CYP2D6 inhibitors or substrates

Venlafaxine is primarily metabolised to its active metabolite *O*-desmethylvenlafaxine by CYP2D6.[1,2] Some studies suggest that the metabolism of venlafaxine may be inhibited by inhibitors or substrates of CYP2D6 such as **diphenhydramine**,[3] **melperone**,[4] **quinidine**,[5] or **thioridazine**,[6] especially in patients who are extensive metabolisers (i.e. have normal levels) of this isoenzyme.[3,6] However, the US manufacturer says that the concurrent use of these drugs would produce plasma levels of venlafaxine similar to those seen in patients who are genetically CYP2D6 poor metabolisers (about 5 to 10% of general population) and therefore no dosage adjustment is necessary.[2] However, the UK manufacturer suggests caution particularly if venlafaxine, another drug that inhibits CYP3A4, is also given to patients who are poor metabolisers of CYP2D6, see below under CYP3A4 inhibitors.[1]

(b) CYP3A4 inhibitors

CYP3A4 plays a minor role in the metabolism of venlafaxine to the inactive metabolite *N*-desmethylvenlafaxine[7]. However, the manufacturers suggest than in poor CYP2D6 metabolisers, CYP3A4 could become more important, and clinically significant drug interactions with CYP3A4 inhibitors may then occur.[1] In one study involving CYP2D6 extensive and poor metabolisers, **ketoconazole** (a potent CYP3A4 inhibitor) increased the plasma levels of venlafaxine and *O*-desmethylvenlafaxine (AUCs increased 36% and 26%, respectively). However, the response in poor metabolisers was erratic with 3 out of 6 displaying marked increases in AUC (81%,126% and 206%, respectively) whilst the other 3 showed little or no change.[7]

(c) Disulfiram

An isolated report describes a hypertensive crisis associated with a low dose of venlafaxine (75 mg daily). It was thought that the concurrent use of disulfiram might have increased the toxicity of venlafaxine by interfering with its metabolism via CYP3A4. However disulfiram predominantly inhibits CYP2E1 and has not been reported to significantly affect CYP3A4. Note that disulfiram may provoke hypertension through its interaction with alcohol; however the authors state they found no evidence of a reaction with alcohol in this patient.[8] This is an isolated and unexplained case, which is of unknown general significance.

(d) Triptans

The manufacturers caution the use of drugs that affect serotonergic transmission, such as the triptans.[1,2] This is because of the possible risks of the serotonin syndrome. For more about the serotonin syndrome see 'Additive or synergistic interactions', (p.9). This interaction has been seen, rarely, to occur with a number of other serotonergic drugs and venlafaxine, which gives weight to this prediction.

1. Efexor (Venlafaxine hydrochloride). Wyeth Pharmaceuticals. UK Summary of product characteristics, May 2006.
2. Effexor XR (Venlafaxine hydrochloride). Wyeth Pharmaceuticals Inc. US Prescribing information, June 2007.
3. Lessard E, Yessine MA, Hamelin BA, Gauvin C, Labbe L, O'Hara G, LeBlanc J, Turgeon J. Diphenhydramine alters the disposition of venlafaxine through inhibition of CYP2D6 activity in humans. *J Clin Psychopharmacol* (2001) 21, 175–84.
4. Grözinger M, Dragicevic A, Hiemke C, Shams M, Müller MJ, Härtter S. Melperone is an inhibitor of the CYP2D6 catalyzed O-demethylation of venlafaxine. *Pharmacopsychiatry* (2003) 36, 3–6.
5. Fogelman SM, Schmider J, Venkatakrishnan K, von Moltke LL, Harmatz JS, Shader RI, Greenblatt DJ. *O*- and *N*-demethylation of venlafaxine *in vitro* by human liver microsomes and by microsomes from cDNA-transfected cells: effect of metabolic inhibitors and SSRI antidepressants. *Neuropsychopharmacology* (1999) 20, 480–90.
6. Eap CB, Bertel-Laubscher R, Zullino D, Amey M, Baumann P. Marked increase of venlafaxine enantiomer concentrations as a consequence of metabolic interactions: A case report. *Pharmacopsychiatry* (2000) 33, 112–15.
7. Lindh JD, Annas A, Meurling L, Dahl M-L, AL-Shurbaji A. Effect of ketoconazole on venlafaxine plasma concentrations in extensive and poor metabolisers of debrisoquine. *Eur J Clin Pharmacol* (2003) 59, 401–6.
8. Khurana RN, Baudendistel TE. Hypertensive crisis associated with venlafaxine. *Am J Med* (2003) 115, 676–7.

SNRIs; Venlafaxine + Tramadol

Two cases of the serotonin syndrome have been reported when tramadol was given with venlafaxine; one patient was also receiving mirtazapine. Fatal seizures occurred in an alcoholic man receiving tramadol, venlafaxine, quetiapine and trazodone.

Clinical evidence, mechanism, importance and management

A 47-year-old man who had been stable taking venlafaxine 300 mg daily and mirtazapine 30 mg daily for 4 months was given tramadol, titrated to 300 mg daily over 4 weeks, without adverse effects. However, approximately 7 weeks after increasing the dose of tramadol to 400 mg daily he experienced agitation, confusion, severe shivering, diaphoresis, myoclonus, hyperreflexia, mydriasis, and tachycardia. His symptoms resolved over 36 hours after all medications were discontinued and did not recur when venlafaxine and mirtazapine were restarted without tramadol.[1] A 65-year-old woman who had been taking venlafaxine 100 mg daily for 3 weeks, developed symptoms of the serotonin syndrome 3 days after tramadol 300 mg daily was added. The symptoms resolved completely 3 days after venlafaxine withdrawal, when tramadol was also withdrawn. No symptoms occurred on rechallenge with venlafaxine alone, 2 weeks later.[2] A 36-year-old alcoholic died after developing seizures while taking tramadol several drugs, including venlafaxine, trazodone and quetiapine, all of which interact with the neurotransmitter serotonin. It was thought that the combination of these drugs and alcohol withdrawal lowered the seizure threshold.[3]

1. Houlihan DJ. Serotonin syndrome resulting from coadministration of tramadol, venlafaxine, and mirtazapine. *Ann Pharmacother* (2004) 38, 411–13.
2. Anon. Venlafaxine + tramadol: serotonin syndrome. *Prescrire Int* (2004) 13, 57.
3. Ripple MG, Pestaner JP, Levine BS, Smialek JE. Lethal combination of tramadol and multiple drugs affecting serotonin. *Am J Forensic Med Pathol* (2000) 21, 370–4.

SSRIs + Azoles

Anorexia developed in a patient taking fluoxetine when itraconazole was started, and it disappeared when the itraconazole was stopped. The pharmacokinetics of citalopram in healthy subjects were not affected by ketoconazole. The clearance of escitalopram was not affected by ketoconazole in an *in vitro* study.

Clinical evidence, mechanism, importance and management

(a) Citalopram or Escitalopram

In a double-blind, placebo-controlled, crossover study in 18 healthy subjects, a single 200-mg dose of **ketoconazole** did not affect the pharmacokinetics of citalopram 40 mg.[1] **Ketoconazole** is a potent inhibitor of cytochrome P450 isoenzyme CYP3A4, which, in part, metabolises citalopram, but as several other cytochrome P450 isoenzymes are also involved in citalopram metabolism it would seem that inhibition of only one pathway does not result in clinically significant effects. Similarly, escitalopram is metabolised by CYP3A4, CYP2C19, and CYP2D6, and it has been suggested that its clearance is also unlikely to be affected by impaired activity of only one CYP isoform.[2]

(b) Fluoxetine

A man taking fluoxetine 20 mg daily, diazepam and several anti-asthma drugs (salbutamol (albuterol), salmeterol, budesonide, theophylline) was given **itraconazole** 200 mg daily for allergic bronchopulmonary aspergillosis. Within 1 to 2 days he developed anorexia without nausea. He stopped the **itraconazole** after a week, and the anorexia resolved 1 to 2 days later. The author of the report suggested that **itraconazole,** a potent enzyme inhibitor, increased the levels of the fluoxetine metabolite, norfluoxetine, which resulted in the anorexia.[3] Anorexia is a recognised adverse effect of fluoxetine. However, drug levels were not taken, so this suggestion has not been confirmed.

This report and the conclusions reached are uncertain, but they draw attention to the possibility of an interaction between fluoxetine and **itraconazole**. Consider this interaction if fluoxetine adverse effects are troublesome.

1. Gutierrez M, Abramowitz W. Lack of effect of a single dose of ketoconazole on the pharmacokinetics of citalopram. *Pharmacotherapy* (2001) 21, 163–8.
2. Von Moltke LL, Greenblatt DJ, Giancarlo GM, Granda BW, Harmatz JS, Shader RI. Escitalopram (*S*-citalopram) and its metabolites in vitro: cytochromes mediating biotransformation, inhibitory effects, and comparison to *R*-citalopram. *Drug Metab Dispos* (2001) 29, 1102–9.
3. Black PN. Probable interaction between fluoxetine and itraconazole. *Ann Pharmacother* (1995) 29, 1048–9.

SSRIs + Bupropion

There are isolated reports of psychosis, mania and seizures associated with the use of bupropion and fluoxetine and an isolated report of the serotonin syndrome with bupropion and sertraline. Hypersexuality has also been reported with bupropion and fluoxetine or sertraline.

Clinical evidence

(a) Fluoxetine

The day after stopping fluoxetine 60 mg daily, a 41-year-old man was started taking 75 mg and later 100 mg of bupropion three times daily. After 10 days he became edgy and anxious and after 12 days he developed myoclonus. After 14 days he became severely agitated and psychotic, with delirium and hallucinations. His behaviour returned to normal 6 days after the bupropion was stopped.[1] Another patient taking lithium carbonate for bipolar disorder developed anxiety, panic and eventually mania a little over a week after stopping fluoxetine and starting bupropion.[2]

A further patient developed a grand mal seizure after being given fluoxetine and bupropion 300 mg daily.[3]

A 35-year old woman taking fluoxetine 40 mg daily was given low-dose bupropion (100 mg daily) to treat fluoxetine-induced sexual dysfunction. Despite a good initial response, hypersexuality developed leading to discontinuation of bupropion.[4]

(b) Sertraline

A 62-year-old woman treated with therapeutic doses of bupropion and sertraline experienced upper extremity tremor, clumsiness and gait difficulties, with fluctuating symptoms of confusion, forgetfulness, and alternating agitation and lethargy, which started after a few days on this regimen. **Venlafaxine** was then added and the clinical picture worsened with deterioration of mental status, hallucinations, insomnia, myoclonic jerks, postural and balance difficulties, incoordination and incontinence. The medications were discontinued and the symptoms, which were indicative of the serotonin syndrome, gradually resolved.[5]

An isolated case describes spontaneous orgasm with the combined use of bupropion and sertraline. Bupropion had been successfully used to treat SSRI-induced impaired sexual function, but after 6 weeks of combined therapy she experienced a sudden-onset, spontaneous orgasm; this occurred again on rechallenge with bupropion.[6]

Mechanism

Several mechanisms have been proposed. Bupropion inhibits the cytochrome P450 isoenzyme CYP2D6, which may interfere with the metabolism of some SSRIs, causing an increase in plasma levels and increased toxicity. However, a small study found no statistically significant changes in plasma levels of fluoxetine or **paroxetine** when combined with bupropion.[7] An *in vitro* study demonstrated that several SSRIs (paroxetine, sertraline, norfluoxetine, and **fluvoxamine**) could inhibit CYP2B6, the isoenzyme involved in bupropion hydroxylation,[8] and in one of the cases described above it was suggested that residual fluoxetine may have inhibited the metabolism of bupropion, leading to toxic levels.[1] A pharmacodynamic mechanism has also been proposed. Bupropion can cause seizures and antidepressants may further lower the seizure threshold, see 'Bupropion + Miscellaneous', p.1206.

Importance and management

Information is very limited but these reports suggest that if concurrent or sequential use is thought appropriate, the outcome should be well monitored and reduced doses should be considered. The UK and US manufacturers recommend that drugs that are metabolised by CYP2D6 should be given with bupropion with caution and initiated at the lower end of the dose range. If bupropion is added to the treatment of a patient already taking a drug metabolised by CYP2D6, the need to decrease the dose of this drug should be considered.[9,10] The UK manufacturers specifically name paroxetine and the US manufacturers additionally name fluoxetine and sertraline. In addition, the manufacturers advise extreme caution if bupropion is given with antidepressants that lower seizure threshold[10] and recommend reducing the dose of bupropion to a maximum of 150 mg daily.[9]

1. van Putten T, Shaffer I. Delirium associated with bupropion. *J Clin Psychopharmacol* (1990) 10, 234.
2. Zubieta JK, Demitrack MA. Possible bupropion precipitation of mania and a mixed affective state. *J Clin Psychopharmacol* (1991) 11, 327–8.
3. Ciraulo DA, Shader RI. Fluoxetine drug-drug interactions.II. *J Clin Psychopharmacol* (1990) 10, 213–17.
4. Chollet CAS, Andreatini R. Effect of bupropion on sexual dysfunction induced by fluoxetine: a case report of hypersexuality. *J Clin Psychiatry* (2003) 64, 1268–9.
5. Munhoz RP. Serotonin syndrome induced by a combination of bupropion and SSRIs. *Clin Neuropharmacol* (2004) 27, 219–22.
6. Grimes JB, Labbate LA. Spontaneous orgasm with the combined use of bupropion and sertraline. *Biol Psychiatry* (1996) 40, 1184–5.
7. Kennedy SH, McCann SM, Masellis M, McIntyre RS, Raskin J, McKay G, Baker GB. Combining bupropion SR with venlafaxine, paroxetine, or fluoxetine: a preliminary report on pharmacokinetic, therapeutic, and sexual dysfunction effects. *J Clin Psychiatry* (2002) 63, 181–6.
8. Hesse LM, Venkatakrishnan K, Court MH, von Moltke LL, Duan SX, Shader RI, Greenblatt DJ. CYP2B6 mediates the in vitro hydroxylation of bupropion: potential drug interactions with other antidepressants. *Drug Metab Dispos* (2000) 28, 1176–83.
9. Zyban (Bupropion hydrochloride). GlaxoSmithKline UK. UK Summary of product characteristics, October 2006.
10. Zyban (Bupropion hydrochloride). GlaxoSmithKline. US Prescribing information, August 2007.

SSRIs + Cocaine

An isolated report describes a fatal multiple drug intoxication involving citalopram and cocaine. *Animal* studies have suggested that SSRIs may potentiate the pro-convulsive effects of cocaine.

Clinical evidence, mechanism, importance and management

An isolated report describes a fatal multiple drug intoxication involving **citalopram** and cocaine. It was suggested that SSRIs and cocaine bind to the same receptor site and their concurrent use may have an additive effect through inhibition of serotonin reuptake. The patient also took other drugs including omeprazole, which may have further potentiated the effects of **citalopram**.[1]

A study in *animals* suggested that most SSRIs potentiate cocaine-induced convulsions, although **sertraline** appeared to have no effect on convulsions or lethality.[2]

1. Fu K, Konrad RJ, Hardy RW, Brissie RM, Robinson CA. An unusual multiple drug intoxication case involving citalopram. *J Anal Toxicol* (2000) 24, 648–50.
2. O'Dell LE, George FR, Ritz MC. Antidepressant drugs appear to enhance cocaine-induced toxicity. *Exp Clin Psychopharmacol* (2000) 8, 133–41.

SSRIs + Cyproheptadine

Several reports suggest that cyproheptadine can oppose the antidepressant effects of fluoxetine, and another describes the same effect with paroxetine.

Clinical evidence

(a) Fluoxetine

Three depressed men complained of anorgasmia when taking fluoxetine. When this was treated with cyproheptadine their depressive symptoms returned, decreasing again when cyproheptadine was stopped.[1] Two women also complained of anorgasmia within 1 to 3 months of starting to take fluoxetine 40 to 60 mg daily for bulimia nervosa. When cyproheptadine was added to treat this sexual dysfunction, the urge to binge on food returned in both of them and one experienced increased depression. These symptoms resolved 4 to 7 days after stopping cyproheptadine.[2] A woman successfully treated with fluoxetine 40 mg daily showed a re-emergence of her depressive symptoms on two occasions within 36 hours of starting to take cyproheptadine.[3] In a further case, a woman who responded well to fluoxetine 20 mg daily for depression had a recurrence of her depression after she began to take cyproheptadine for migraine. Increasing the dose of fluoxetine to 40 mg daily controlled the depressive symptoms while cyproheptadine was continued for migraine.[4] In contrast, no exacerbation of depression was seen in a study in which both cyproheptadine and fluoxetine were used in 2 patients.[5]

(b) Paroxetine

A woman taking paroxetine 20 mg daily for depression relapsed and worsened, and developed confusion and psychotic symptoms, within 2 days of starting to take cyproheptadine 2 mg twice daily for the treatment of anorgasmia.[6] Psychotic symptoms resolved 2 days after stopping cyproheptadine. However, cyproheptadine (8 mg followed by 12 mg in 3 divided doses over 24 hours) seemed to have little effect on the course of the serotonin syndrome caused by a massive overdose of paroxetine (3.6 g) taken with alcohol. It was thought that the dosing of cyproheptadine might have been insufficient for such a large overdose. The patient recovered over the next 6 days with supportive measures.[7]

Mechanism

Although the mechanism is not fully understood, it has been suggested that because cyproheptadine is a serotonin antagonist it blocks or opposes the serotonergic effects of these SSRIs.[1-3,6,7]

Importance and management

Direct information about this interaction appears to be limited to these studies although cyproheptadine has also been found to oppose the antidepressant effects of MAOIs (see 'MAOIs or RIMAs + Antihistamines; Cyproheptadine', p.1131). One study suggests that not every patient is affected.[5] If concurrent use is thought appropriate, the outcome should be very well monitored for evidence of a reduced antidepressant response.

1. Feder R. Reversal of antidepressant activity of fluoxetine by cyproheptadine in three patients. *J Clin Psychiatry* (1991) 52, 163–4.
2. Goldbloom DS, Kennedy SH. Adverse interaction of fluoxetine and cyproheptadine in two patients with bulimia nervosa. *J Clin Psychiatry* (1991) 52, 261–2.
3. Katz RJ, Rosenthal M. Adverse interaction of cyproheptadine with serotonergic antidepressants. *J Clin Psychiatry* (1994) 55, 314–15.
4. Boon F. Cyproheptadine and SSRIs. *J Am Acad Child Adolesc Psychiatry* (1999) 38, 112.

5. McCormick S, Olin J, Brotman AW. Reversal of fluoxetine-induced anorgasmia by cyproheptadine in two patients. *J Clin Psychiatry* (1990) 51, 383–4.
6. Christensen RC. Adverse interaction of paroxetine and cyproheptadine. *J Clin Psychiatry* (1995) 56, 433–4.
7. Velez LI, Shepherd G, Roth BA, Benitez FL. Serotonin syndrome with elevated paroxetine concentrations. *Ann Pharmacother* (2004) 38, 269–72.

SSRIs and related antidepressants + Dextromethorphan

Three reports describe the development of a serotonin-like syndrome in two patients taking paroxetine and one taking citalopram and nefazodone, when they were given dextromethorphan. Another report describes hallucinations in a woman taking fluoxetine and dextromethorphan.

Clinical evidence

(a) Citalopram

A man who had been taking citalopram 30 mg, nefazodone 600 mg and long-acting oxycodone 10 mg at bedtime without problems, started taking a cough syrup containing dextromethorphan and within a day he began to experience fatigue, lethargy, jitteriness and headache. He stopped taking the dextromethorphan and his symptoms gradually disappeared over several hours.[1]

(b) Fluoxetine

A woman who had been taking fluoxetine 20 mg daily for 17 days took about 10 mL of a cough syrup containing dextromethorphan, and a further dose the next morning, with the next dose of fluoxetine. Within 2 hours vivid hallucinations developed (bright colours, distortions of shapes and sizes), which lasted 6 to 8 hours. The patient said they were similar to her past experience with LSD 12 years earlier.[2] However, in a report of an extensive metabolic study[3] in which depressed patients taking fluoxetine were given a single 30-mg dose of dextromethorphan, no mention was made of adverse effects.[3]

(c) Paroxetine

A man with multiple medical problems was admitted to hospital as an emergency, mainly because he was vomiting blood. He was taking diazepam, diltiazem, glyceryl trinitrate, paroxetine, piroxicam, ranitidine and ticlopidine. Four days previously he had begun to take ***Nyquil***, a non-prescription remedy for colds, containing dextromethorphan, pseudoephedrine, paracetamol (acetaminophen) and doxylamine. After two days he developed shortness of breath, nausea, headache and confusion, and on admission he was also diaphoretic, tremulous, tachycardic and hypertensive. Later he became rigid. The eventual diagnosis was that he was suffering from the serotonin syndrome, attributed to an interaction between paroxetine and dextromethorphan in the presence of vascular disease. He was successfully treated with lorazepam 16 mg intravenously over 1 hour. The bleeding was thought to be from a small prepyloric ulcer.[4]

The authors of this report very briefly describe another patient taking paroxetine who developed symptoms consistent with the serotonin syndrome within a few hours of taking a non-prescription cough remedy containing dextromethorphan and guaifenesin. She needed intensive care treatment.[5]

Mechanism

Not understood. The symptoms that developed with citalopram or paroxetine and dextromethorphan were attributed by the authors of the reports to the serotonin syndrome, caused by the additive effects of the SSRIs and dextromethorphan on serotonin transmission. It has also been suggested that paroxetine inhibited the cytochrome P450 isoenzyme CYP2D6, by which dextromethorphan is metabolised, resulting in increased dextromethorphan levels.[5,6] Fluoxetine also inhibits CYP2D6.[3]

Importance and management

These seem to be, so far, the only reports of the serotonin syndrome being attributed to an interaction between an SSRI and dextromethorphan. However, it has been suggested that the incidence of mild serotonin excess (as seen in with citalopram) may be more common than is known.[1] The general importance of this apparent interaction is therefore very uncertain. The SSRIs are now very widely prescribed and dextromethorphan is a relatively common ingredient of non-prescription medicines. More study is therefore needed to establish this apparent interaction, but in the meantime it would seem prudent for patients taking citalopram, fluoxetine, or paroxetine to be cautious using dextromethorphan-containing products because the risks of the serotonin syndrome, which, if it occurs, can be serious. Concurrent use should be well monitored. It is not clear whether other SSRIs would interact with dextromethorphan similarly, but it has been predicted that **sertraline** and **fluvoxamine** are less likely to do so.[6] This prediction has been challenged.[5] The outcome will largely depend on the mechanism of this interaction, as **sertraline** and **fluvoxamine** do not usually have clinically significant effects on CYP2D6. For more information about the serotonin syndrome, see 'Additive or synergistic interactions', (p.9).

1. Ener RA, Meglathery SB, Van Decker WA, Gallagher RM. Serotonin syndrome and other serotonergic disorders. *Pain Med* (2003) 4, 63–74.
2. Achamallah NS. Visual hallucinations after combining fluoxetine and dextromethorphan. *Am J Psychiatry* (1992) 149, 1406.
3. Otton SV, Wu D, Joffe RT, Cheung SW, Sellers EM. Inhibition by fluoxetine of cytochrome P450 2D6 activity. *Clin Pharmacol Ther* (1993) 53, 401–9.
4. Skop BP, Finkelstein JA, Mareth TR, Magoon MR, Brown TM. The serotonin syndrome associated with paroxetine, an over-the-counter cold remedy, and vascular disease. *Am J Emerg Med* (1994) 12, 642–4.
5. Skop BP, Brown TM, Mareth TR. The serotonin syndrome associated with paroxetine. *Am J Emerg Med* (1995) 13, 606–7.
6. Harvey AT, Burke M. Comment on: The serotonin syndrome associated with paroxetine, an over-the-counter-cold remedy, and vascular disease. *Am J Emerg Med* (1995) 13, 605–6.

SSRIs + Grapefruit juice

Excessive consumption of grapefruit caused symptoms similar to the serotonin syndrome in a patient taking fluoxetine and trazodone.
Grapefruit juice appears to raise fluvoxamine levels, which resulted in adverse effects in one patient. Sertraline plasma levels are also increased by grapefruit juice.

Clinical evidence

A 57-year-old HIV-positive man had been receiving indinavir, stavudine and lamivudine, as well as other medications including **fluoxetine** 20 mg daily and trazodone 200 mg daily. He complained of dizziness, mild confusion, diarrhoea, visual changes, and a general feeling of being "out of sorts" for approximately one month. On further questioning it was found that the patient had been having one grapefruit each morning but had increased his consumption to 3 per day. His symptoms resolved when he stopped eating grapefruit.[1]

A randomised, placebo-controlled, crossover study in 10 healthy subjects found that 250 mL of grapefruit juice three times daily for 6 days increased the AUC of a single 75-mg dose of **fluvoxamine** by 60% and increased the maximum plasma levels by 33%.[2] A 75-year-old woman taking **fluvoxamine** 150 mg at night experienced palpitations when on holiday in Florida, which stopped when she returned home. The only change identified was that she drank grapefruit juice daily while in Florida. She had previously experienced palpitations when taking a higher dose of **fluvoxamine** (200 mg at night).[3]

A study in 5 patients taking **sertraline** 50 to 75 mg daily found that the concurrent use of grapefruit juice for one week increased serum trough levels by almost 50%.[4]

Mechanism

Grapefruit juice is an inhibitor of the cytochrome P450 isoenzyme CYP3A4 and sertraline is partially metabolised by this enzyme. Therefore grapefruit juice would be expected to reduce the metabolism of sertraline. This has been demonstrated *in vitro*; grapefruit juice inhibited the formation of desmethylsertraline in a dose-dependent manner.[4] The other SSRIs mentioned above are not significantly affected by CYP3A4, but grapefruit juice also inhibits other isoenzymes that could affect the metabolism of SSRIs especially if the patient is also a poor metaboliser of CYP2D6.[2,3]

Importance and management

There are very few reports of clinically significant interaction between grapefruit and SSRIs, but the possibility of an interaction should be borne in mind especially if unusual amounts of grapefruit have been consumed.

1. DeSilva KE, Le Flore DB, Marston BJ, Rimland D. Serotonin syndrome in HIV-infected individuals receiving antiretroviral therapy and fluoxetine. *AIDS* (2001) 15, 1281–5.

2. Hori H, Yoshimura R, Ueda N, Eto S, Shinkai K, Sakata S, Ohmori O, Terao T, Nakamura J. Grapefruit juice-fluvoxamine interaction. Is it risky or not? *J Clin Psychopharmacol* (2003) 23, 422–4.
3. Wiens A. How does grapefruit juice affect psychotropic medications? *J Psychiatry Neurosci* (2000) 25, 198.
4. Lee AJ, Chan WK, Harralson AF, Buffum J, Bui B-CC. The effects of grapefruit juice on sertraline metabolism: an in vitro and in vivo study. *Clin Ther* (1999) 21, 1890–9.

SSRIs + H_2-receptor antagonists

Citalopram, escitalopram, paroxetine and sertraline levels are moderately increased by cimetidine but the only clinically relevant effect appears to be a slight increase in adverse effects with sertraline.

Clinical evidence

(a) Citalopram

Twelve healthy subjects were given citalopram 40 mg daily for 21 days and then for the next 8 days they were also given **cimetidine** 400 mg twice daily. The **cimetidine** caused a 29% decrease in the oral clearance of the citalopram, a 39% rise in its maximum serum levels and a 43% increase in its AUC. Some changes in the renal clearance of the citalopram metabolites were also seen.[1]

(b) Escitalopram

Cimetidine 400 mg twice daily increased the mean plasma level of escitalopram by about 70%. There was also a 22% increase in the maximum plasma level of citalopram, but this was not considered to be clinically significant.[2]

(c) Paroxetine

Cimetidine 200 mg four times daily for 8 days did not affect the mean pharmacokinetic values or bioavailability of a single 30-mg dose of paroxetine in 10 healthy subjects. However, 2 subjects had AUC increases of 55% and 81%, respectively, while taking **cimetidine** and 4 others also had some minor increases.[3] Another study in 11 healthy subjects found that **cimetidine** 300 mg three times a day increased the AUC of paroxetine 30 mg daily by 50% after 1 week of concurrent use.[4]

(d) Sertraline

In a randomised, two-way, crossover study, 12 healthy subjects were given a single 100-mg oral dose of sertraline after taking either **cimetidine** 800 mg or a placebo at bedtime for 7 days. **Cimetidine** increased the AUC of sertraline by 50%, the maximum serum levels of sertraline by 24%, and the half-life by 26%.[5,6] There was a small increase in sertraline adverse effects (not specified) while taking the **cimetidine**.[5]

Mechanism

The apparent reason for all these changes is that cimetidine inhibits the activity of cytochrome P450 so that the metabolism of the SSRIs is reduced, and as a result their serum levels rise.

Importance and management

The authors of the citalopram study say that while cimetidine certainly causes an increase in the serum levels of citalopram, the extent is only moderate and because the drug is well tolerated and there are very considerable pharmacokinetic variations between individual subjects, they consider that there is no need to reduce the citalopram dosage.[1] This advice is most likely applicable to escitalopram, the *S*-isomer of citalopram. However, the manufacturer of escitalopram suggests caution, and advises that a reduction in the dose of escitalopram may be necessary (based on monitoring of adverse effects) during concurrent treatment.[7]

Information on the concurrent use of cimetidine and paroxetine or sertraline seems to be limited and the clinical significance of the changes in clearance is not known. However, it would be prudent to monitor the outcome for excessive adverse effects (dry mouth, nausea, diarrhoea, dyspepsia, tremor, ejaculatory delay, sweating) if cimetidine is used with either of these SSRIs and reduce the sertraline or paroxetine dosage if necessary.

If the suggested mechanism of interaction is true, one of the other H_2-receptor antagonists that lack enzyme inhibitory activity, such as **ranitidine** or **famotidine**, might be a non-interacting alternative for cimetidine. This needs confirmation.

1. Priskorn M, Larsen F, Segonzac A, Moulin M. Pharmacokinetic interaction study of citalopram and cimetidine in healthy subjects. *Eur J Clin Pharmacol* (1997) 52, 241–2.
2. Malling D, Poulsen MN, Søgaard B. The effect of cimetidine or omeprazole on the pharmacokinetics of escitalopram in healthy subjects. *Br J Clin Pharmacol* (2005) 60, 287–90.
3. Greb WH, Buscher G, Dierdorf H-D, Köster FE, Wolf D, Mellows G. The effect of liver enzyme inhibition by cimetidine and enzyme induction by phenobarbitone on the pharmacokinetics of paroxetine. *Acta Psychiatr Scand* (1989) 80 (Suppl 350), 95–8.
4. Bannister SJ, Houser VP, Hulse JD, Kisicki JC, Rasmussen JGC. Evaluation of the potential for interactions of paroxetine with diazepam, cimetidine, warfarin, and digoxin. *Acta Psychiatr Scand* (1989) 80 (Suppl 350), 102–6.
5. Invicta Pharmaceuticals. Phase 1 study to assess the potential of cimetidine to alter the disposition of sertraline in normal, healthy male volunteers. Data on file (Study 050-019), 1991.
6. Zoloft (Sertraline hydrochloride). Pfizer Inc. US Prescribing information, June 2007.
7. Cipralex (Escitalopram oxalate). Lundbeck Ltd. UK Summary of product characteristics, December 2005.

SSRIs + Herbal medicines

A man taking fluoxetine experienced symptoms of the serotonin syndrome after ingesting the psychoactive beverage ayahuasca, which contains monoamine oxidase-inhibiting harmala alkaloids. The Japanese herbal medicine *Gorei-san* does not appear to interact with fluvoxamine or paroxetine.

Clinical evidence, mechanism, importance and management

A 36-year-old man who was receiving **fluoxetine** 20 mg daily for mild depression participated in a religious ceremony using **ayahuasca** (also known as **caapi, daime, hoasca, natema, yage**) which is a psychoactive beverage characteristically containing harmala alkaloids (primarily **harmine** and **harmaline**) derived from the vine *Banisteriopsis caapi*. One hour after ingesting 100 mL of **ayahuasca** he experienced tremors, sweating, shivering and confusion. His condition deteriorated over the next few hours with gross motor tremors and severe nausea and vomiting, but he rapidly recovered four hours after ingestion of the **ayahuasca**, with no treatment. The harmala alkaloids are capable of blocking the enzymatic activity of MAO for several hours, and consequently inhibit the metabolic breakdown of neurotransmitters. There is, therefore, the potential for the serotonin syndrome with SSRIs and **ayahuasca**.[1]

For reports of the serotonin syndrome and other adverse effects when St John's wort was taken together with SSRIs, see 'SSRIs + St John's wort (*Hypericum perforatum*)', p.1224.

An efficacy study in 20 patients taking **fluvoxamine** (19 patients) or **paroxetine** (1 patient) reported that the addition of the Japanese herbal medicine ***Gorei-san*** (TJ-17), which is composed of 5 herbs *(Alismatis rhizoma, Atractylodis lanceae rhizoma, Polyporus, Hoelen,* and *Cinnamomi cortex)*, caused no additional adverse events.[2] However, note that this study was not specifically looking at drug interactions and therefore only gives a broad indication that concurrent use is safe and effective.

1. Callaway JC, Grob CS. Ayahuasca preparations and serotonin reuptake inhibitors: a potential combination for severe adverse interactions. *J Psychoactive Drugs* (1998) 30, 367–9.
2. Yamada K, Yagi G, Kanba S. Effectiveness of *Gorei-san* (TJ-17) for treatment of SSRI-induced nausea and dyspepsia: preliminary observations. *Clin Neuropharmacol* (2003) 26, 112–14.

SSRIs + 5-HT_3-receptor antagonists

Symptoms similar to the serotonin syndrome have been reported in two patients receiving paroxetine and ondansetron or sertraline and dolasetron.

Clinical evidence, mechanism, importance and management

A possible case of the serotonin syndrome (or possibly neuroleptic malignant syndrome) was reported in a 49-year-old woman who developed postoperative delirium. She had been taking **paroxetine** 30 mg daily up to 2 days before surgery and was given **ondansetron** 4 mg during surgery and morphine during and after surgery. Approximately one hour after leaving theatre she became agitated and confused. She also displayed uncontrolled limb movements, brisk reflexes, ankle clonus, abnormal ocular function, hypertension, pyrexia, and raised creatinine kinase levels. The delirium did not respond to naloxone, diazepam or flumazenil and lasted for nearly 2 days. Several explanations involving the disruption of serotonergic and/or dopaminergic transmission were suggested.[1] There has been some debate about whether inhibition of CYP2D6 was another possible mechanism, but this seems unlikely.[1,2]

Similarly, a 49-year-old woman, who had been receiving **sertraline** for some time without incident was premedicated with **dolasetron** 100 mg before receiving her first cycle of adjuvant chemotherapy for breast cancer. Shortly afterwards she developed symptoms of profound agitation and elation, but with an overwhelming desire to commit suicide and was disoriented. The symptoms resolved within hours without pharmacological intervention. Three weeks later she received the same medications except **ondansetron** was substituted for **dolasetron** and she experienced no adverse effects. The author concluded that a variant of the serotonin syndrome may rarely be seen when 5-HT_3-receptor antagonists and SSRIs are given together, and clinicians should consider this possibility if these adverse effects occur.[3]

1. Stanford BJ, Stanford SC. Postoperative delirium indicating an adverse drug interaction involving the selective serotonin reuptake inhibitor, paroxetine? *J Psychopharmacol* (1999) 13, 313–17.
2. Palmer JL. Postoperative delirium indicating an adverse drug interaction involving the selective serotonin reuptake inhibitor, paroxetine? *J Psychopharmacol* (2000) 14, 186–8.
3. Sorscher SM. Probable serotonin syndrome variant in a patient receiving a selective serotonin reuptake inhibitor and a 5-HT_3 receptor antagonist. *J Psychopharmacol* (2002) 16, 191.

SSRIs + Interferons

The antidepressant effects of paroxetine and trazodone may be reversed by interferon.

Clinical evidence, mechanism, importance and management

A 31-year-old woman, whose mood and other depressive symptoms improved during treatment with **paroxetine** 50 mg daily and trazodone 50 mg at night, was later found to have essential thrombocythaemia. After unsuccessful treatment with dipyridamole, she was given **interferon alfa**, stabilised at 3 million units 3 times weekly. After 3 months her depressive symptoms returned, and worsened over a period of 6 months, despite increased doses of trazodone and cognitive therapy. **Interferon alfa** was discontinued and replaced by hydroxycarbamide, and then anagrelide. After a good response to a course of ECT, her depressive symptoms were controlled by **paroxetine** 50 mg daily and trazodone 150 mg at night.[1]

Interferon is associated with a risk of depression, but in this case it appeared to reverse the antidepressant response. It was suggested that this might have been due to the capacity of interferon to impair serotonin synthesis, by inducing enzymes that degrade the serotonin precursor tryptophan. If this mechanism is true then all SSRIs have the potential to interact. Bear the possibility of an interaction in mind if the response to an SSRIs is poor in a patient given interferon.

1. McAllister-Williams RH, Young AH, Menkes DB. Antidepressant response reversed by interferon. *Br J Psychiatry* (2000) 176, 93.

SSRIs + Lysergide (LSD)

Three patients with a history of lysergide (LSD) abuse experienced the new onset or worsening of the LSD flashback syndrome when given fluoxetine, paroxetine or sertraline. Grand mal convulsions occurred when one patient taking LSD was given fluoxetine. In contrast, one study found that SSRIs reduced or eliminated the subjective responses to LSD.

Clinical evidence

An 18-year-old girl with depression, panic and anxiety disorders, and with a long history of illicit drug abuse experienced a 15-hour LSD flashback within 2 days of starting to take **sertraline** 50 mg daily. Another flashback lasting a day occurred when the **sertraline** was replaced by **paroxetine**. No further flashbacks occurred when the SSRIs were stopped. A 17-year-old boy with depression, also with a long history of illicit drug abuse (including LSD), began to experience LSD flashbacks 2 weeks after starting to take **paroxetine**. His father, a chronic drug abuser, had taken both **fluoxetine** and **paroxetine** for depression and had also reported new onset of a flashback syndrome.[1] An isolated report describes grand mal convulsions in a patient while taking **fluoxetine**, tentatively attributed to the concurrent abuse of LSD.[2] In contrast, a retrospective study found that 28 of 32 subjects (88%) who took LSD and who had taken an SSRI (**fluoxetine**, **paroxetine** or **sertraline**) or trazodone for more than 3 weeks had a subjective decrease or virtual elimination of their responses to LSD. However, another subject who had taken **fluoxetine** for only one week had an increased response to LSD.[3]

Mechanism

Not understood. Lysergide increases serotonin in the brain, and one suggestion is that when the serotonin re-uptake is blocked in the brain, there is an increased stimulation of 5-HT_1 and 5-HT_2 receptors.[1] Changes in brain catecholamine systems may also be involved.[3]

Importance and management

Information is very limited and conflicting. The authors of the first report suggest that patients who are given SSRIs should be warned about the possibility of flashback or hallucinations if they have a known history of LSD abuse.

1. Markel H, Lee A, Holmes RD, Domino EF. Clinical and laboratory observations. LSD flashback syndrome exacerbated by selective serotonin reuptake inhibitor antidepressants in adolescents. *J Pediatr* (1994) 125, 817–9.
2. Picker W, Lerman A, Hajal F. Potential interaction of LSD and fluoxetine. *Am J Psychiatry* (1992) 149, 843–4.
3. Bonson KR, Buckholtz JW, Murphy DL. Chronic administration of serotonergic antidepressants attenuates the subjective effects of LSD in humans. *Neuropsychopharmacology* (1996) 14, 425–36.

SSRIs + Macrolides

An isolated case report describes apparent acute fluoxetine toxicity in a man brought about by the use of clarithromycin. Another isolated report describes the development of what is thought to be the serotonin syndrome in a 12-year-old boy taking sertraline and erythromycin.

Clinical evidence

(a) Fluoxetine

A 53-year-old-man taking fluoxetine 80 mg and nitrazepam 10 mg at bedtime for depression and insomnia, was given **clarithromycin** 250 mg twice daily for a respiratory infection. Within a day he started to become increasingly confused and after 3 days was admitted to hospital with a diagnosis of psychosis and delirium. When no organic cause for the delirium could be found, all his medications were stopped, and **erythromycin** was started. His mental state returned to normal after 36 hours. Once the antibacterial course had finished, the fluoxetine and nitrazepam were restarted and no further problems occurred.[1]

(b) Sertraline

A 12-year-old boy with severe obsessive-compulsive disorder and simple phobia, responded to sertraline 12.5 mg daily, titrated over 12 weeks to 37.5 mg daily. He began to feel mildly nervous within 4 days of starting to take **erythromycin** 400 mg daily for an infection. Over the next 10 days his nervousness grew, culminating in panic, restlessness, irritability, agitation, paraesthesias, tremulousness, decreased concentration and confusion. The symptoms abated within 72 hours of stopping both drugs.[2]

Mechanism

The authors attribute what was seen to fluoxetine toxicity in the first case, and to the serotonin syndrome in the second case. They postulated that erythromycin (a known and potent inhibitor of cytochrome P450 isoenzyme CYP3A4) and the related macrolide clarithromycin, reduced the metabolism of the SSRIs, thereby raising their serum levels and precipitating the observed toxicity.[1,2]

Importance and management

These are isolated reports and their general importance is unknown. Nor is it unequivocally established that the second case was the serotonin syndrome and not an idiosyncratic reaction. Nevertheless, be aware of these cases when using macrolides with fluoxetine or sertraline.

1. Pollak PT, Sketris IS, MacKenzie SL, Hewlett TJ. Delirium probably induced by clarithromycin in a patient receiving fluoxetine. *Ann Pharmacother* (1995) 29, 486–8.
2. Lee DO, Lee CD. Serotonin syndrome in a child associated with erythromycin and sertraline. *Pharmacotherapy* (1999) 19, 894–6.

SSRIs + Metoclopramide

There are two reports of the serotonin syndrome in patients taking sertraline when metoclopramide was added. Extrapyramidal symptoms have occurred in patients given fluoxetine, fluvoxamine or sertraline with metoclopramide.

Clinical evidence

(a) Extrapyramidal symptoms

Two patients developed extrapyramidal symptoms while taking **fluoxetine** and metoclopramide.[1,2]

A 14-year-old boy receiving **fluvoxamine** 50 mg daily for anorexia nervosa was, after day 7, given metoclopramide 10 mg three times daily. On the third day of concurrent use he developed acute movement disorders including acute dystonia, jaw rigidity, horizontal nystagmus, uncontrolled tongue movements and dysarthria. The boy had taken the same dose of metoclopramide alone on other occasions without experiencing extrapyramidal reactions. A pharmacokinetic interaction was considered unlikely since both drugs use different metabolic pathways.[3]

In another report a woman with gastro-oesophageal reflux, controlled with metoclopramide 15 mg four times daily, developed symptoms consistent with a mandibular dystonia (periauricular pain, jaw tightness, the sensation of her teeth clenching and grinding) 2 days after starting **sertraline** 50 mg daily. A 50-mg dose of diphenhydramine resolved the problem within 30 minutes, but the same symptoms recurred the next day, 8 hours after taking **sertraline**. The symptoms were relieved by 2 mg of oral benzatropine.[4]

A regional pharmacovigilance centre in France reported 37 cases of extrapyramidal adverse effects linked to concurrent use of an SSRI and a neuroleptic (said to be metoclopramide in 4 cases).[5]

(b) Serotonin syndrome

A patient who had been taking **sertraline** 100 mg daily started taking metoclopramide 10 mg four times daily for nausea. After 24 hours his symptoms had worsened and he developed malaise, cardiac arrhythmia, visual hallucinations, diaphoresis, sialosis, hyperreflexia, and tremor. The serotonin syndrome was diagnosed and his symptoms improved with cyproheptadine.[6] Another patient taking **sertraline** 100 mg daily for depression over an 18-month period developed agitation, dysarthria, diaphoresis, and a movement disorder within 2 hours of receiving a single 10-mg intravenous dose of metoclopramide. The symptoms, diagnosed as the serotonin syndrome with serious extrapyramidal movement disorder, resolved within 6 hours of treatment with diazepam.[7]

Mechanism

Both SSRIs and metoclopramide can cause extrapyramidal reactions; metoclopramide by blocking dopamine D_2 receptors in the basal ganglia, and SSRIs by inhibition of dopamine neurotransmission.[3,4] Metoclopramide has also been reported to have intermediate affinity to certain serotonin receptors.[7]

Importance and management

Information seems to be limited to these reports, but they highlight the fact that care should be taken if two drugs with the potential to cause the same adverse effects are used together.

1. Coulter DM, Pillans PI. Fluoxetine and extrapyramidal side effects. *Am J Psychiatry* (1995) 152, 122–5.
2. Fallon BA, Liebowitz MR. Fluoxetine and extrapyramidal symptoms in CNS lupus. *J Clin Psychopharmacol* (1991) 11, 147–8.
3. Palop V, Jimenez MJ, Catalán C, Martínez-Mir I. Acute dystonia associated with fluvoxamine-metoclopramide. *Ann Pharmacother* (1999) 33, 382.
4. Christensen RC, Byerly MJ. Mandibular dystonia associated with the combination of sertraline and metoclopramide. *J Clin Psychiatry* (1996) 57, 596.
5. Anon. Extrapyramidal reactions to SSRI antidepressant + neuroleptic combinations. *Prescrire Int* (2004) 13, 57.
6. Vandemergel X, Beukinga I, Nève P. Syndrome sérotoninergique secondaire à la prise de sertraline et de metoclopramide. *Rev Med Brux* (2000) 3, 161–3.
7. Fisher AA, Davis MW. Serotonin syndrome caused by selective serotonin reuptake-inhibitors–metoclopramide interaction. *Ann Pharmacother* (2002) 36, 67–71.

SSRIs + NNRTIs

A case of the serotonin syndrome occurred in a woman taking fluoxetine when efavirenz was added. Nevirapine decreased fluoxetine plasma levels, but fluvoxamine increased nevirapine levels.

Clinical evidence, mechanism, importance and management

(a) Efavirenz

A case of serotonin syndrome in a woman taking **fluoxetine** coincided with the start of a new antiretroviral regimen including efavirenz. Symptoms resolved when the **fluoxetine** dose was halved. It was suggested that efavirenz inhibited the metabolism of **fluoxetine**.[1] Until further information is available, caution may be warranted if both drugs are given.

(b) Nevirapine

A study involving 60 HIV-positive patients taking a nevirapine-containing regimen found that **fluoxetine** had no influence on the pharmacokinetics of nevirapine, but nevirapine significantly lowered the combined plasma levels of **fluoxetine** and norfluoxetine.[2] If nevirapine is given with **fluoxetine**, the clinical response to **fluoxetine** should be monitored and the dosage increased if necessary. In the same study the concurrent use of **fluvoxamine** resulted in a significant 34% reduction in the apparent clearance of nevirapine, and this appeared to be dependent on the dose of **fluvoxamine**. The pharmacokinetics of **fluvoxamine** were not affected.[2] If both drugs are given be aware that **fluvoxamine** could be a cause of increased nevirapine adverse effects.

1. DeSilva KE, Le Flore DB, Marston BJ, Rimland D. Serotonin syndrome in HIV-infected individuals receiving antiretroviral therapy and fluoxetine. *AIDS* (2001) 15, 1281–5.
2. De Maat MMR, Huitema ADR, Mulder JW, Meenhorst PL, van Gorp ECM, Mairuhu ATA, Beijnen JH. Drug interaction of fluvoxamine and fluoxetine with nevirapine in HIV-1-infected individuals. *Clin Drug Invest* (2003) 23, 629–37.

SSRIs + Opioids

Symptoms of the serotonin syndrome have been reported with opioids including hydromorphone, oxycodone, pentazocine, pethidine and tramadol and possibly morphine when given with various SSRIs. Seizures have been seen when dextropropoxyphene was given with an SSRI.

Fluoxetine has slightly reduced the analgesic effects of morphine and oxycodone. Buprenorphine metabolism is inhibited by fluvoxamine *in vitro*, but this is probably not clinically relevant.

Clinical evidence

(a) Buprenorphine

Fluvoxamine inhibited the metabolism of buprenorphine *in vitro*, but the inhibition was not thought sufficient to be clinically significant.[1]

Fluoxetine did not inhibit buprenorphine dealkylation *in vitro*, although norfluoxetine did so, but this was also thought unlikely to be significant *in vivo*.[1]

(b) Dextropropoxyphene

Ten of 32 cases of seizures or myoclonus associated with antidepressant treatment reported to the Swedish Adverse Drug Reactions Advisory Committee involved SSRIs (**fluvoxamine** 6, **citalopram** 2, **paroxetine** 2). An important risk factor appeared to be concurrent treatment with other drugs, such as dextropropoxyphene (2 cases), that decrease the seizure threshold.[2]

(c) Hydrocodone

Visual hallucinations occurred in a 90-year-old woman taking hydrocodone when her antidepressant was changed from **citalopram** 10 mg daily to **escitalopram** 10 mg daily. The hallucinations stopped after her hydrocodone was discontinued because of improvement in pain control. The patient had previously taken **paroxetine** and the same dose of hydrocodone, without experiencing hallucinations or other serotonin-related symptoms.[3]

(d) Hydromorphone

An 81-year-old woman who had been taking **fluoxetine** 20 mg daily along with other medication for several years, developed abnormal movements, confusion, incoherent speech, sweating, facial redness, tremor, hyperreflexia and muscle spasm 2 days after starting to take hydromorphone 12 mg daily. The symptoms resolved within 2 weeks of stopping the **fluoxetine** (the hydromorphone was continued).[4]

(e) Methadone

The SSRIs, particularly fluvoxamine, can raise methadone levels. See 'SSRIs + Opioids; Methadone', below.

(f) Morphine

A double-blind, placebo-controlled study in 35 patients found that the preoperative use of **fluoxetine** 10 mg daily for 7 days reduced the analgesic effect of intravenous morphine given for postoperative dental pain.[5] In contrast, a double-blind, crossover study in 15 healthy subjects found that a single 60-mg dose of **fluoxetine** slightly improved (by 3 to 8%) the analgesic effect (as assessed by dental electrical stimulation) of morphine sulfate in doses tailored to produce and maintain steady-state plasma levels of 15, 30 and 60 nanograms/mL for 60 minutes. Plasma levels of morphine were not affected by **fluoxetine**, and morphine was found not to affect plasma levels of **fluoxetine** or norfluoxetine. The subjects experienced less nausea and drowsiness, but the psychomotor and respiratory depressant effects of morphine were not altered.[6]

A patient experienced postoperative delirium which lasted for nearly 2 days and included agitation, confusion, uncontrolled limb movements, abnormal ocular function, hypertension, pyrexia, brisk reflexes, ankle clonus and raised creatinine kinase. She had been taking **paroxetine** before surgery and during surgery she was given morphine and ondansetron.[7]

(g) Oxycodone

A man with advanced multiple sclerosis found that when he began to take **fluoxetine** 20 mg daily for depression he needed to increase his analgesic dosage of oxycodone (for painful muscle spasms) about fourfold, from 65 to 75 mg daily to about 250 to 275 mg daily.[8]

A bone-marrow transplant recipient taking, amongst other drugs, **sertraline** 50 mg daily, ciclosporin 75 mg daily, and oxycodone 10 mg as needed, developed severe tremors and visual hallucinations. This coincided with him taking oxycodone 200 mg over 48 hours for severe pain. An adverse reaction to ciclosporin was initially suspected (although serum levels were not high), and this was temporarily discontinued along with the oxycodone. The visual hallucinations decreased but the tremors continued, and did not lessen until **sertraline** was discontinued and cyproheptadine given. It was concluded that the patient was experiencing a form of the serotonin syndrome as a result of markedly increased opioid use while taking an SSRI.[9] Two other cases describe probable serotonin syndrome in elderly patients receiving either **sertraline** or **escitalopram** together with extended-release oxycodone. In both cases symptoms of the serotonin syndrome (agitation, increased muscle tone, ataxia, tremor and/or myoclonic jerks) occurred after increasing the opioid dose.[3] Another case of severe serotonergic symptoms including confusion, nausea, fever, shivering, agitation, clonus, hyperreflexia, hypertonia, and tachycardia occurred in a 70-year-old woman taking **fluvoxamine** 200 mg daily when she started taking oxycodone 40 mg twice daily. Discontinuation of these two drugs resulted in resolution of her symptoms over 48 hours.[10]

(h) Pentazocine

A double-blind, placebo-controlled study in 35 patients has shown that oral **fluoxetine** 10 mg daily for 7 days preoperatively did not to reduce the analgesic effects of pentazocine 45 mg given intravenously for postoperative dental pain.[5]

A man who had been taking **fluoxetine** 20 mg daily, later increased to 40 mg daily, was given a single 100-mg oral dose of pentazocine (*Talwin Nx* containing pentazocine 50 mg and naloxone 500 micrograms) for a severe headache. Within 30 minutes he complained of lightheadedness, anxiety, nausea and paraesthesias of the hands. He was diaphoretic, flushed, and ataxic, and had a mild tremor of his arms. His blood pressure was 178/114 mmHg, pulse 62 bpm and respiration 16 breaths per minute. He was given intramuscular diphenhydramine 50 mg and recovered over the following 4 hours.[11]

(i) Pethidine (Meperidine)

A 43-year-old man who had been taking **fluoxetine** approximately every other day experienced symptoms of the serotonin syndrome immediately after receiving pethidine 50 mg intravenously for an endoscopic procedure.[12]

(j) Tramadol

The serotonin syndrome has occurred in a number of patients taking SSRIs with tramadol. See 'SSRIs + Opioids; Tramadol', p.1222.

Mechanism

Fluoxetine inhibits the activity of the cytochrome P450 isoenzyme CYP2D6 within the liver so that the metabolism of oxycodone to an active metabolite oxymorphone is reduced. The metabolism of hydrocodone and similar opioids may also be affected by CYP2D6 inhibitors, see 'Opioids; Codeine and related drugs + Quinidine', p.184. Buprenorphine and morphine are not metabolised by CYP2D6, so their metabolism would not be expected to be affected by fluoxetine. Buprenorphine is metabolised by CYP3A4 and so fluvoxamine might be expected to inhibit its metabolism to some extent.

Dextropropoxyphene may have inhibited the metabolism of the SSRIs leading to an increase in seizures.

It has been suggested that the reason for the reduced morphine analgesia may have something to do with the initial effects of SSRIs on serotonergic neurotransmission.[6] The serotonin syndrome seems to develop unpredictably in some patients given two or more serotonergic drugs, in this case, opioids and SSRIs.

Importance and management

Adverse interactions between SSRIs and opioids seem rare (although see 'methadone', (below)) and there is little to suggest that they cannot be used together safely and effectively. The evidence suggesting that fluoxetine may decrease morphine or oxycodone analgesia is limited and insufficient to suggest any change in practice. However, if a patient does not seem to respond well to either of these opioids consider an interaction as a possible cause. Buprenorphine metabolism might be slightly reduced by fluvoxamine, but this does not appear to be clinically relevant.

The incidence of serotonin syndrome-like reactions with opioids and SSRIs is fairly rare (although see 'tramadol', (p.1222)); however, the possibility of 'the serotonin syndrome', (p.9), should be considered in patients experiencing altered mental status, autonomic dysfunction and neuromuscular adverse effects while receiving these drugs.

1. Iribarne C, Picart D, Dréano Y, Berthou F. In vitro interactions between fluoxetine or fluvoxamine and methadone or buprenorphine. *Fundam Clin Pharmacol* (1998) 12, 194–9.
2. Spigset O, Hedenmalm K, Dahl M-L, Wiholm B-E, Dahlqvist R. Seizures and myoclonus associated with antidepressant treatment: assessment of potential risk factors, including CYP2D6 and CYP2C19 polymorphisms, and treatment with CYP2D6 inhibitors. *Acta Psychiatr Scand* (1997) 96, 379–84.
3. Gnanadesigan N, Espinoza RT, Smith R, Israel M, Reuben DB. Interaction of serotonergic antidepressants and opioid analgesics: is serotonin syndrome going undetected? *J Am Med Dir Assoc* (2005) 6, 265–9.
4. Anon. Fluoxetine + hydromorphone: serotonin syndrome? *Prescrire Int* (2004) 13, 57.
5. Gordon NC, Heller PH, Gear RW, Levine JD. Interactions between fluoxetine and opiate analgesia for postoperative dental pain. *Pain* (1994) 58, 85–8.
6. Erjavec MK, Coda BA, Nguyen Q, Donaldson G, Risler L, Shen DD. Morphine-fluoxetine interactions in healthy volunteers: analgesia and side effects. *J Clin Pharmacol* (2000) 40, 1286–95.
7. Stanford BJ, Stanford SC. Postoperative delirium indicating an adverse drug interaction involving the selective serotonin reuptake inhibitor, paroxetine? *J Psychopharmacol* (1999) 13, 313–17.
8. Otton SV, Wu D, Joffe RT, Cheung SW, Sellers EM. Inhibition by fluoxetine of cytochrome P450 2D6 activity. *Clin Pharmacol Ther* (1993) 53, 401–9.
9. Rosebraugh CJ, Flockhart DA, Yasuda SU, Woosley RL. Visual hallucination and tremor induced by sertraline and oxycodone in a bone marrow transplant patient. *J Clin Pharmacol* (2001) 41, 224–7.
10. Karunatilake H, Buckley NA. Serotonin syndrome induced by fluvoxamine and oxycodone. *Ann Pharmacother* (2006) 40, 155–7.
11. Hansen TE, Dieter K, Keepers GA. Interaction of fluoxetine and pentazocine. *Am J Psychiatry* (1990) 147, 949–50.
12. Tissot TA. Probable meperidine-induced serotonin syndrome in a patient with a history of fluoxetine use. *Anesthesiology* (2003) 98, 1511–12.

SSRIs + Opioids; Methadone

Methadone serum levels may rise if fluvoxamine is added, sometimes resulting in increased adverse effects. Sertraline, paroxetine, and possibly fluoxetine, may also modestly increase methadone levels.

Clinical evidence

(a) Fluoxetine

Methadone 30 to 100 mg daily, and fluoxetine 20 mg daily were given to 9 patients (two of them were also taking fluvoxamine). Although there were possible compliance problems with some of the patients, the methadone plasma/dose ratio of the group as a whole was not altered by the addition of the fluoxetine.[1] This is consistent with the results of two other studies, which found that fluoxetine did not appear to alter the plasma methadone levels of patients treated for cocaine dependence.[2,3] However, the plasma samples for 7 of the 9 patients in the first study[1] were subsequently analysed again to measure the *S*- and *R*-enantiomers of methadone separately. This analysis revealed that fluoxetine 20 mg daily modestly increased the levels-to-dose ratio of the active *R*-methadone (by 33%) without significantly changing either the total or inactive *S*-methadone level-to-dose ratios.[4] Moreover, a patient taking methadone developed opioid toxicity when given ciprofloxacin and fluoxetine, see 'Opioids; Methadone + Ciprofloxacin', p.189.

(b) Fluvoxamine

Five patients taking maintenance doses of methadone were given fluvoxamine. Two of them had an increase of about 20% in the methadone plasma/dose ratio, while the other 3 showed 40 to 100% rises (suggesting increased methadone levels). One of them developed asthenia, marked drowsiness and nausea, which disappeared when both drug dosages were reduced.[5] A subsequent analysis of the enantiomers of methadone revealed that fluvoxamine increased the levels of both *R*- and *S*-methadone.[4] A report describes one patient who was unable to maintain adequate methadone levels, despite a daily dosage of 200 mg, and experienced withdrawal symptoms until fluvoxamine was added.[6] Another patient taking methadone 70 mg daily and diazepam 2 mg twice daily was admitted to hospital with an acute exacerbation of asthma and intractable cough 3 weeks after starting fluvoxamine 100 mg daily. Blood gas measurements indicated severe hypoxaemia and hypercapnia. The symptoms resolved when the methadone dose was reduced to 50 mg daily and diazepam was gradually withdrawn, at which point methadone levels fell by about 23% (from 262 to 202 nanograms/mL).[7]

(c) Paroxetine

Paroxetine 20 mg daily increased steady-state methadone levels by 35% in 10 patients taking maintenance doses of methadone. Both *R*- and *S*-methadone levels were increased in the 8 patients who were extensive metabolisers of the cytochrome P450 isoenzyme CYP2D6 (see 'Genetic factors', (p.4)), but in the 2 patients who were poor metabolisers, only the *S*-methadone levels were increased. Apart from one patient who reported feeling high during the first night after starting paroxetine, no symptoms of over-medication or toxicity were noted.[8]

(d) Sertraline

A placebo-controlled study in 31 depressed methadone-maintained patients found that sertraline significantly increased the methadone plasma level/dose ratio by 26% while patients on placebo had a 16% decrease after 6 weeks treatment, but by 12 weeks ratios had shifted towards baseline values. Adverse effects were similar in both groups.[9] A 31-year-old woman taking methadone 230 mg daily was found to have a prolonged QT interval after taking sertraline 50 mg daily was added to her medications, although she was asymptomatic. The QT interval returned to normal when the methadone and sertraline were stopped and her methadone was replaced with morphine.[10]

Mechanism

Fluvoxamine, and to a lesser extent fluoxetine, paroxetine, and sertraline, can inhibit the liver metabolism of the methadone (possibly by the cytochrome P450 isoenzymes CYP3A4,[11] CYP2D6,[11,12] and/or CYP1A2[4]) thereby allowing it to accumulate in the body.

Importance and management

Information is limited, but it indicates that the effects of starting or stopping fluvoxamine should be monitored in patients taking methadone, being alert for the need to adjust the methadone dosage. Although the increase in methadone levels with sertraline and paroxetine, and possibly also fluoxetine, is unlikely to have clinical effects in most patients, the possibility should be borne in mind, especially if high doses of methadone are being used. Note that methadone can prolong the QT-interval in high doses, see 'drugs that prolong the QT-interval', (p.257).

1. Bertschy G, Eap CB, Powell K, Baumann P. Fluoxetine addition to methadone in addicts: pharmacokinetic aspects. *Ther Drug Monit* (1996) 18, 570–2.
2. Batki SL, Manfredi LB, Jacob P, Jones RT. Fluoxetine for cocaine dependence in methadone maintenance: quantitative plasma and urine cocaine-benzoylecgonine concentrations. *J Clin Psychopharmacol* (1993) 13, 243–50.
3. Baño MD, Agujetas M, M, López ML, Tena T, Rodríguez A, Lora-Tamayo C, Guillén JL. Eficacia de la fluoxetina (FX) en el tratamiento de la adicción a cocaína en pacientes en mantenimiento con metadona y su interacción en los niveles plasmáticos. *Actas Esp Psiquiatr* (1999) 27, 321–4.
4. Eap CB, Bertschy G, Powell K, Baumann P. Fluvoxamine and fluoxetine do not interact in the same way with the metabolism of the enantiomers of methadone. *J Clin Psychopharmacol* (1997) 17, 113–17.
5. Bertschy G, Baumann P, Eap CB, Baettig D. Probable metabolic interaction between methadone and fluvoxamine in addict patients. *Ther Drug Monit* (1994) 16, 42–5.
6. DeMaria PA, Serota RD. A therapeutic use of the methadone fluvoxamine drug interaction. *J Addict Dis* (1999) 18, 5–12.
7. Alderman CP, Frith PA. Fluvoxamine-methadone interaction. *Aust N Z J Psychiatry* (1999) 33, 99–101.
8. Begré S, von Bardeleben U, Ladewig D, Jaquet-Rochat S, Cosendai-Savary L, Golay KP, Kosel M, Baumann P, Eap CB. Paroxetine increases steady-state concentrations of (R)-methadone in CYP2D6 extensive but not poor metabolizers. *J Clin Psychopharmacol* (2002) 22, 211–15.
9. Hamilton SP, Nunes EV, Janal M, Weber L. The effect of sertraline on methadone plasma levels in methadone-maintenance patients. *Am J Addict* (2000) 9, 63–9.
10. Piguet V, Desmeules J, Ehret G, Stoller R, Dayer P. QT interval prolongation in patients on methadone with concomitant drugs. *J Clin Psychopharmacol* (2004) 24, 446–8.
11. Iribarne C, Picart D, Dréano Y, Berthou F. In vitro interactions between fluoxetine or fluvoxamine and methadone or buprenorphine. *Fundam Clin Pharmacol* (1998) 12, 194–9.
12. Wang J-S, DeVane CL. Involvement of CYP3A4, CYP2C8, and CYP2D6 in the metabolism of (*R*)- and (*S*)-methadone in vitro. *Drug Metab Dispos* (2003) 31, 742–7.

SSRIs + Opioids; Tramadol

Tramadol should be used with caution with SSRIs because of the increased risk of seizures. Several reports describe the development of the serotonin syndrome in patients taking SSRIs with tramadol. Another patient developed hallucinations with tramadol and paroxetine.

Clinical evidence

(a) Seizures

The CSM in the UK has publicised 27 reports of convulsions and one of worsening epilepsy with tramadol, a reporting rate of 1 in 7000 patients. Some of the patients were given doses well in excess of those recommended, and some were taking SSRIs (5 patients) or 'tricyclic antidepressants', (p.187), both of which are known to reduce the convulsive threshold.[1] Similarly, of 124 seizure cases associated with tramadol reported to the FDA in the US, 20 included the concurrent use of SSRIs.[2]

(b) Serotonin syndrome

The Australian Adverse Drug Reaction Advisory Committee has stated that tramadol may cause the serotonin syndrome, particularly when it is used at high doses or in combination with other drugs increasing serotonin levels; of 20 reported cases of the serotonin syndrome associated with tramadol, 16 were taking potentially interacting medicines including SSRIs.[3] Cases of the serotonin syndrome with specific SSRIs are discussed below.

1. Citalopram. A 70-year-old woman who had been taking citalopram 10 mg daily for 3 years developed tremors, restlessness, fever, confusion, and visual hallucinations after starting to take tramadol 50 mg daily for pain relief following an operation. Her symptoms stopped after tramadol was stopped. However, she continued to take citalopram and one year later she developed identical symptoms after taking tramadol 20 mg daily. Citalopram is metabolised by the cytochrome P450 enzyme CYP2C19 and tramadol is *O*-demethylated by CYP2D6 and the patient was found to be deficient in both CYP2C19 and CYP2D6, suggesting that her metabolising capacity of both pathways was reduced.[4]

2. Fluoxetine. A woman who had been taking fluoxetine 20 mg daily for 3 years developed what was eventually diagnosed as the serotonin syndrome. A month previously she had started to take tramadol 50 mg four times daily, increased after a fortnight to 100 mg four times daily. Ten days before hospitalisation she had developed a tremor of the right hand and face, and in hospital she showed agitation, marked facial blepharospasm, some sweating and pyrexia, and stuttering. The symptoms began to subside 7 days after both drugs were stopped, and after 2 months she had recovered fully.[5]

3. Paroxetine. A man who had been taking paroxetine 20 mg daily for 4 months without problems developed shivering, diaphoresis and myoclonus and became subcomatose within 12 hours of taking tramadol 100 mg. This was diagnosed as the serotonin syndrome. Tramadol was stopped, the paroxetine dosage halved and he became conscious within a day. The other symptoms gradually disappeared over the next week.[6] A 78-year-old woman taking paroxetine 20 mg daily developed nausea, diaphoresis and irritability 3 days after starting tramadol 50 mg three times a day. The next day she developed muscular weakness and confusion, and was found to have a temperature of about 38.2°C and a pulse rate of 110 bpm. She recovered when the drugs were withdrawn. Similar symptoms occurred in another elderly woman taking paroxetine 10 mg daily within 2 days of starting tramadol 50 mg four times daily. Both women were later able to continue taking paroxetine alone without problems.[7]
A tetraparetic patient with chronic pain developed nightmares and hallucinations 56 days after starting to take tramadol, paroxetine and dosulepin, which only stopped when the drugs were withdrawn.[8]

4. Sertraline. A 42-year-old woman was admitted to intensive care with atypical chest pain, sinus tachycardia, confusion, psychosis, sundowning [increased agitation, activity and negative behaviours, which happen late in the day or evening], agitation, diaphoresis and tremor. She was taking a large number of drugs, including sertraline and tramadol. She was diagnosed as having the serotonin syndrome, attributed to an increase in the dosage of tramadol (from 150 mg daily to 300 mg daily in increments of 50 mg every 2 to 3 days), and an increased sertraline dosage [original amounts not stated but 100 mg daily when the adverse events developed]. The tramadol had been started 3 weeks previously and she had been taking the sertraline for a year.[9]
An 88-year-old woman taking sertraline 50 mg daily (later increased to 100 mg daily), as well as several other medications was given dextropropoxyphene with paracetamol and tramadol 200 mg daily increased to 400 mg daily for pain relief after a fracture. Ten days after starting tramadol she became confused, with alterations in cognitive function, tremor, problems with co-ordination and muscle weakness. The serotonin syndrome was suspected and therefore sertraline was withdrawn over a period of 2 days, the dose of tramadol was reduced from 400 to 200 mg daily, and the patient recovered over a period of about 2 weeks.[10]
In another report, the serotonin syndrome occurred after the first dose of sertraline 50 mg in a 75-year-old woman who had been taking tramadol 50 mg daily for 3 days. The concentration of serotonin (5-hydroxytryptamine) in her CSF was found to be elevated to 38.5 nanograms/mL (normal value less than 10 picograms/mL).[11]

(c) Pharmacokinetic effect

A double-blind, placebo-controlled, crossover study in 16 healthy extensive metabolisers found that pretreatment with paroxetine 20 mg daily for 3 days increased the AUC of (+)- and (–)-tramadol by 37% and 32%, respectively and decreased the AUCs of the *O*-demethylated metabolites of tramadol by 67% and 40%, respectively. The analgesic effect of tramadol was reduced, but not abolished.[12]

Mechanism

Tramadol may cause seizures and SSRIs can reduce the seizure threshold, thus if both are taken together the risk is increased. 'The serotonin syndrome', (p.9), seems to develop unpredictably in some patients given two or more serotonergic drugs (in this case, tramadol and SSRIs).

Paroxetine is a potent inhibitor of the cytochrome P450 isoenzyme CYP2D6 and inhibits the CYP2D6 mediated formation of the *O*-demethylated metabolites of tramadol. The reduction in these metabolites may result in reduced analgesia as the opioid effect of tramadol is thought to be mediated mainly by (+)-*O*-desmethyltramadol.[12]

Importance and management

Because of the possible increased risk of seizures, tramadol should be used with caution in patients taking drugs such as the SSRIs, which can lower the seizure threshold. The concurrent use of tramadol and SSRIs may also lead to an increase in serotonin-associated effects, which can include the serotonin syndrome. However, the relatively few reported cases of the serotonin syndrome or other reactions due to an interaction between an SSRI and tramadol need to be set in the wider context of apparently uneventful and advantageous use in other patients,[12-14] although some workers have suggested that the incidence of serotonin syndrome may be underreported.[15] There would seem to be little reason for totally avoiding the concurrent use of the SSRIs and tramadol but it would clearly be prudent to monitor the outcome closely.

Tramadol analgesia may possibly be altered by paroxetine and potentially by other drugs that inhibit CYP2D6, such as fluoxetine.[12]

1. Committee on Safety of Medicines/Medicines Control Agency. In focus–tramadol. *Current Problems* (1996) 22, 11.
2. Kahn LH, Alderfer RJ, Graham DJ. Seizures reported with tramadol. *JAMA* (1997) 278, 1661.
3. Adverse Drug Reactions Advisory Committee (ADRAC). Tramadol – four years' experience. *Aust Adverse Drug React Bull* (2003) 22, 2.
4. Mahlberg R, Kunz D, Sasse J, Kirchheiner J. Serotonin syndrome with tramadol and citalopram. *Am J Psychiatry* (2004) 161, 1129.
5. Kesavan S, Sobala GM. Serotonin syndrome with fluoxetine plus tramadol. *J R Soc Med* (1999) 92, 474–5.
6. Egberts ACG, ter Borgh J, Brodie-Meijer CCE. Serotonin syndrome attributed to tramadol addition to paroxetine therapy. *Int Clin Psychopharmacol* (1997) 12, 181–182.
7. Lantz MS, Buchalter EN, Giambanco V. Serotonin syndrome following the administration of tramadol with paroxetine. *Int J Geriatr Psychiatry* (1998) 13, 343–5.
8. Devulder J, De Laat M, Dumoulin K, Renson A, Rolly G. Nightmares and hallucinations after long term intake of tramadol combined with antidepressants. *Acta Clin Belg* (1996) 51, 184–6.
9. Mason BJ, Blackburn KH. Possible serotonin syndrome associated with tramadol and sertraline coadministration. *Ann Pharmacother* (1997) 31, 175–7.
10. Sauget D, Franco PS, Amaniou M, Mazere J, Dantoine T. Possible syndrome sérotoninergique induit par l'association de tramadol à de la sertraline chez une femme âgée. *Therapie* (2002) 57, 309–10.
11. Mittino D, Mula M, Monaco F. Serotonin syndrome associated with tramadol-sertraline coadministration. *Clin Neuropharmacol* (2004) 27, 150–1.
12. Laugesen S, Enggaard TP, Pedersen RS, Sindrup SH, Brøsen K. Paroxetine, a cytochrome P450 2D6 inhibitor, diminishes the stereoselective *O*-demethylation and reduces the hypoalgesic effect of tramadol. *Clin Pharmacol Ther* (2005) 77, 312–23.
13. Fanelli J, Montgomery C. Use of the analgesic tramadol in antidepressant potentiation. *Psychopharmacol Bull* (1996) 32, 442.
14. Barkin RL. Alternative dosing for tramadol aids effectiveness. *Formulary* (1995) 30, 542–3.
15. Freeman WD, Chabolla DR. 36-Year-old woman with loss of consciousness, fever, and tachycardia. *Mayo Clin Proc* (2005) 80, 667–70.

SSRIs + Protease inhibitors

Fluoxetine modestly raised the levels of ritonavir, and ritonavir is predicted to raise levels of fluoxetine, paroxetine and sertraline. A few cases of the serotonin syndrome have been attributed to the use of fluoxetine and ritonavir. The concurrent use of escitalopram and ritonavir do not appear to affect the pharmacokinetics of either drug.

Clinical evidence, mechanism, importance and management

In a single-dose study involving 18 healthy subjects, no significant pharmacokinetic interaction was seen when **ritonavir** was given with **escitalopram**.[1]

Ritonavir 600 mg was given to 16 healthy subjects before and after 8 days of treatment with **fluoxetine** 30 mg twice daily. The maximum plasma levels of **ritonavir** were unaffected, but its AUC rose by 19%. These changes were not considered large enough to warrant changing the dose of **ritonavir**.[2] The study was criticised for not achieving steady state before assessing the pharmacokinetics and thus possibly underestimating the interaction.[3] However, the authors point out that **fluoxetine** levels were equivalent to those seen at steady state, and multiple dosing of **ritonavir** is likely to induce its own metabolism, so if anything, the interaction would be lessened at steady state.[4]

The UK manufacturers of **ritonavir** predict that it may raise the levels of SSRIs (**fluoxetine**, **paroxetine**, **sertraline**) due to the inhibitory effect of **ritonavir** on the cytochrome P450 isoenzymes CYP2D6.[5] The US manufacturers do not mention any specific SSRIs.[6] Both manufacturers suggest careful monitoring of adverse effects when these drugs are used with **ritonavir**; a dose reduction of the SSRI may be required.[5,6]

Two cases of serotonin syndrome were attributed to adding **ritonavir** to established **fluoxetine** treatment. In one patient this was managed by halving the **fluoxetine** dose, and in the other **ritonavir** was withdrawn. Other cases of the serotonin syndrome have been seen in patients taking **ritonavir** or **indinavir** with fluoxetine. One involved the additional use of 'trazodone', (p.1229), and the other involved large quantities of 'grapefruit', (p.1217).

1. Gutierrez, MM, Rosenberg J, Abramowitz W. An evaluation of the potential for pharmacokinetic interaction between escitalopram and the cytochrome P450 3A4 inhibitor ritonavir. *Clin Ther* (2003) 25, 1200–10.
2. Ouellet D, Hsu A, Qian J, Lamm JE, Cavanaugh JH, Leonard JM, Granneman GR. Effect of fluoxetine on the pharmacokinetics of ritonavir. *Antimicrob Agents Chemother* (1998) 42, 3107–12.
3. Bellibas SE. Ritonavir-fluoxetine interaction. *Antimicrob Agents Chemother* (1999) 43, 1815.
4. Ouellet D, Hsu A. Ritonavir-fluoxetine interaction. *Antimicrob Agents Chemother* (1999) 43, 1815.

5. Norvir (Ritonavir). Abbott Laboratories Ltd. UK Summary of product characteristics, May 2007.
6. Norvir (Ritonavir). Abbott Laboratories. US Prescribing information, January 2006.

SSRIs + Rifampicin (Rifampin)

In two isolated cases rifampicin decreased the efficacy of citalopram and sertraline.

Clinical evidence

A 34-year-old man, with a long-standing history of anxiety disorder being treated with **sertraline** 200 mg at bedtime, reported that the medication was no longer working well. He was experiencing a significant amount of anxiety, excessive worry, and poor energy. He additionally reported feeling "spaced out," and having dizziness exacerbated by movement, lethargy, and insomnia. He had started taking rifampicin 300 mg twice daily and co-trimoxazole 7 days earlier and it was found that his **sertraline** and *N*-desmethylsertraline levels were only 39% and 46%, respectively, of the levels achieved when he was not taking rifampicin and co-trimoxazole. He later experienced similar symptoms when the **sertraline** dose was tapered so that paroxetine could be substituted.[1] Similarly, a 55-year-old man taking **citalopram** 40 to 60 mg daily reported a decrease in therapeutic efficacy (increased crying and panic attacks) after starting rifampicin 600 mg twice daily. His condition improved when the rifampicin was stopped.[2]

Mechanism

Both sertraline and citalopram are metabolised by cytochrome P450 isoenzymes including CYP3A4 and rifampicin is a potent inducer of the hepatic CYP450 system, particularly CYP3A4. It would therefore appear that rifampicin induced the metabolism of these two drugs resulting in decreased plasma levels.

Importance and management

There seem to be very few reports of this interaction, but rifampicin is a potent enzyme inducer and so clinicians should be aware that rifampicin may reduce citalopram or sertraline plasma levels leading to decreased efficacy or symptoms of SSRI withdrawal. In theory, rifampicin could affect other SSRIs metabolised via other cytochrome P450 isoenzymes, but there appear to be no reports of this. The UK manufacturer of **paroxetine** suggests that no initial dosage adjustment is considered necessary when **paroxetine** is given with enzyme inducing drugs such as rifampicin. Any subsequent dosage adjustment should be guided by clinical effect (tolerability and efficacy).[3] Until more is known this would seem to be a sensible approach with rifampicin and any SSRI.

1. Markowitz JS, DeVane CL. Rifampin-induced selective serotonin reuptake inhibitor withdrawal syndrome in a patient treated with sertraline. *J Clin Psychopharmacol* (2000) 20, 109–10.
2. Kukoyi O, Argo TR, Carnaham RM. Exacerbation of panic disorder with rifampin therapy in a patient receiving citalopram. *Pharmacotherapy* (2005) 25, 435–7.
3. Seroxat (Paroxetine hydrochloride hemihydrate). GlaxoSmithKline UK. UK Summary of product characteristics, April 2007.

SSRIs + SSRIs

An isolated report describes an adverse reaction (hypertension, tachycardia, fever, auditory hallucinations and confusion) in a man when he started sertraline within a day of stopping fluoxetine. A small study found that the concurrent use of citalopram and fluvoxamine increased citalopram plasma levels with beneficial effects and the manufacturers of escitalopram predict that it may be similarly affected.

Clinical evidence, mechanism, importance and management

(a) Citalopram or Escitalopram with Fluvoxamine

A study in 7 depressed patients who had not responded to treatment with citalopram 40 mg daily for 3 weeks, found that the addition of fluvoxamine 50 to 100 mg daily for another 3 weeks improved the control of the depression. Plasma *S*-and *R*-citalopram levels rose two- to threefold. None of the patients developed the serotonin syndrome, and no changes in vital signs or ECGs were seen.[1] The manufacturers of escitalopram, the *S*-isomer of citalopram therefore suggest that its levels may similarly be raised by fluvoxamine.[2]

(b) Fluoxetine with Sertraline

One of 16 healthy subjects who began to take sertraline 50 mg daily on the day after stopping a 2-week trial of fluoxetine 20 mg daily, rapidly developed hypertension, tachycardia, fever, auditory hallucinations and confusion. Most of these symptoms disappeared 48 hours after stopping the sertraline, but the confusion took a week to subside.[3] The other 15 subjects had no clinically significant adverse effects. This subject was later found to have a history of psychosis so that the picture is a little confused, but the rapid abatement of the symptoms when the sertraline was stopped suggests that they were due either to the sertraline alone, or to an interaction with the residual fluoxetine.

It is therefore not clear whether a washout period is needed between these two drugs, but a decision on this will depend on the severity of the depression in the particular patient being treated. The manufacturers of sertraline imply caution when they say that the duration of a washout period when switching from one SSRI to another has not yet been established.[4,5]

1. Bondolfi G, Chautems C, Rochat B, Bertschy G, Baumann P. Non-response to citalopram in depressive patients: pharmacokinetic and clinical consequences of a fluvoxamine augmentation. *Psychopharmacology (Berl)* (1996) 128, 421–5.
2. Cipralex (Escitalopram oxalate). Lundbeck Ltd. UK Summary of product characteristics, December 2005.
3. Rosenblatt JE, Rosenblatt NC. How long a hiatus between discontinuing fluoxetine and beginning sertraline? *Curr Affect Illn* (1992) 11, 2.
4. Lustral (Sertraline hydrochloride). Pfizer Ltd. UK Summary of product characteristics, October 2005.
5. Zoloft (Sertraline hydrochloride). Pfizer Inc. US Prescribing information, June 2007.

SSRIs + St John's wort (*Hypericum perforatum*)

Several patients taking sertraline developed symptoms diagnosed as the serotonin syndrome after also taking St John's wort. Another patient taking St John's wort developed severe sedation after taking a single dose of paroxetine. Isolated cases of mania have also been reported when SSRIs were taken with St John's wort.

Clinical evidence

(a) Fluoxetine

For a report of hypomania when St John's wort and Ginkgo biloba were added to treatment with fluoxetine and buspirone, see 'Buspirone + Herbal medicines', p.741.

(b) Paroxetine

In one report, a woman stopped taking paroxetine 40 mg daily after 8 months, and 10 days later started to take 600 mg of St John's wort powder daily. No problems occurred until the next night when she took a single 20-mg dose of paroxetine because she thought it might help her sleep. The following day at noon she was found still to be in bed, rousable but incoherent, groggy and slow moving and almost unable to get out of bed. Two hours later she still complained of nausea, weakness and fatigue, but her vital signs and mental status were normal. Within 24 hours all symptoms had resolved.[1]

(c) Sertraline

Four elderly patients taking sertraline developed symptoms characteristic of the serotonin syndrome within 2 to 4 days of also taking St John's wort 300 mg, either two or three times daily. The symptoms included dizziness, nausea, vomiting, headache, anxiety, confusion, restlessness, and irritability. Two of them were treated with oral cyproheptadine 4 mg either two or three times daily, and the symptoms of all of them resolved within a week. They later resumed treatment with sertraline without problems.[2] A search of Health Canada's database of spontaneous adverse reactions from 1998 to 2003 found 2 cases of suspected serotonin syndrome as a result of an interaction between sertraline and St John's wort.[3]

Mania developed in a 28-year-old man, who continued to take St John's wort against medical advice whilst also receiving sertraline 50 mg daily for depression; he was also receiving testosterone replacement post-orchidectomy.[4]

Mechanism

A pharmacodynamic interaction may occur between St John's wort and SSRIs because they can both inhibit the reuptake of 5-hydroxytryptamine (serotonin).[5] The serotonin syndrome has been seen with St John's wort alone,[6] and so additive serotonergic effects appear to be the explanation for what occurred in the cases described here.

Importance and management

Information appears to be limited to these reports, but interactions between SSRIs and St John's wort would seem to be established. The incidence is not known but it is probably small, nevertheless because of the potential severity of the reaction it would seem prudent to avoid concurrent use. The advice of the CSM in the UK is that St John's wort should be stopped if patients are taking any SSRI because of the risk of increased serotonergic effects and an increased incidence of adverse reactions.[7]

1. Gordon JB. SSRIs and St. John's wort: possible toxicity? *Am Fam Physician* (1998) 57, 950–3.
2. Lantz MS, Buchalter E, Giambanco V. St. John's wort and antidepressant drug interactions in the elderly. *J Geriatr Psychiatry Neurol* (1999) 12, 7–10.
3. Griffiths J, Jordan S, Pilon K. Natural health products and adverse reactions. *Can Adverse React News* (2004) 14 (1), 2–3.
4. Barbenel DM, Yusufi B, O'Shea D, Bench CJ. Mania in a patient receiving testosterone replacement post-orchidectomy taking St John's wort and sertraline. *J Psychopharmacol* (2000) 14, 84–6.
5. Izzo AA. Drug interactions with St. John's wort (Hypericum perforatum): a review of the clinical evidence. *Int J Clin Pharmacol Ther* (2004) 42, 139–48.
6. Demott K. St. John's wort tied to serotonin syndrome. *Clin Psychiatry News* (1998) 26, 28.
7. Committee on Safety of Medicines (UK). Message from Professor A Breckenridge (Chairman of CSM) and Fact Sheet for Health Care Professionals, 29th February 2000.

SSRIs + Sympathomimetics

Isolated reports describe delirium in one patient and a seizure in another when methylphenidate was taken with sertraline. Schizophrenia and symptoms of amfetamine toxicity have also been reported in two patients taking amfetamine and fluoxetine. There is an isolated report of the serotonin syndrome associated with concurrent citalopram and dexamfetamine and another associated with sertraline and etilefrine. There is also a report of adverse effects associated with fluoxetine and phenylpropanolamine.

Clinical evidence, mechanism, importance and management

(a) Amfetamines

1. Amfetamine. A man who had taken a small, unspecified, but previously tolerated dose of amfetamine developed signs of amfetamine overdosage (restlessness, agitation, hyperventilation, etc.) while taking **fluoxetine** 60 mg daily. Another man taking **fluoxetine** 20 mg daily developed symptoms of schizophrenia after taking two unspecified doses of amfetamine.[1] It was suggested that this occurred because **fluoxetine** inhibits the cytochrome P450 isoenzyme CYP2D6, which is involved in the metabolism of amfetamine, thereby increasing amfetamine levels.[2] The general importance of these apparent interactions is uncertain.

2. Dexamfetamine. A patient who experienced the serotonin syndrome with concurrent 'venlafaxine', (p.1214) and dexamfetamine had a second episode when **citalopram** was given with the dexamfetamine.[3]

3. Ecstasy (MDMA, methylenedioxymethamfetamine). For comments on the effects of SSRIs on the metabolism of ecstasy and the possibility of increased serotonin effects, see 'Amfetamines and related drugs + SSRIs', p.201.

(b) Etilefrine

A case of the serotonin syndrome was reported due to an interaction between **sertraline** and etilefrine.[4]

(c) Methylphenidate

A 61-year-old man with major depression was prescribed **sertraline** 50 mg daily without response. Three months later the dose was increased to 100 mg daily and methylphenidate 2.5 mg daily was started. His symptoms improved and the dose of methylphenidate was increased to 2.5 mg twice daily and then 5 mg twice daily. After several days at the higher dose, the patient experienced visual hallucinations and confusion. The methylphenidate was discontinued and a day later the psychosis resolved. He was maintained on **sertraline** 100 mg daily and his mood and motivation remained good.[5]

An isolated report describes a tonic-clonic seizure in a 13-year-old boy after he had been taking **sertraline** 25 to 50 mg daily and methylphenidate 80 mg daily for about 2 weeks. He had been receiving methylphenidate without significant adverse effects for about 10 months before the seizure and following discontinuation of the **sertraline** experienced no further seizures.[6]

In contrast, beneficial augmentation of effects has been reported with methylphenidate and SSRIs (**fluoxetine**, **paroxetine**, **sertraline**) without significant adverse effects.[7,8]

(d) Phenylpropanolamine

A 16-year-old girl with an eating disorder, taking **fluoxetine** 20 mg daily, developed vague medical complaints of dizziness, 'hyper' feelings, diarrhoea, palpitations and a reported weight loss of 14 lbs within 2 weeks. The author of the report suggested that these effects might have been the result of an interaction with phenylpropanolamine (1 to 2 capsules of *Dexatrim* once daily), which the patient was surreptitiously taking, associated with a restricted food and fluid intake.[9]

1. Barrett J, Meehan O, Fahy T. SSRI and sympathomimetic interaction. *Br J Psychiatry* (1996) 168, 253.
2. Glue P. SSRI and sympathomimetic interaction. *Br J Psychiatry* (1996) 168, 653.
3. Prior FH, Isbister GK, Dawson AH, Whyte IM. Serotonin toxicity with therapeutic doses of dexamphetamine and venlafaxine. *Med J Aust* (2002) 176, 240–1.
4. Martínez Hernanz A, Pérez Sales P. Síndrome serotoninérgico por sertralina y etilefrina: una interacción no descrita. *Psiquis* (2001) 2, 222–4.
5. McGlohn SE, Bostwick JM. Sertraline with methylphenidate in an ICU patient. *Psychosomatics* (1995) 36, 584–5.
6. Feeney DJ, Klykylo WM. Medication-induced seizures. *J Am Acad Child Adolesc Psychiatry* (1997) 36, 1018–19.
7. Gammon GD, Brown TE. Fluoxetine and methylphenidate in combination for treatment of attention deficit disorder and comorbid depressive disorder. *J Child Adolesc Psychopharmacol* (1993) 3, 1–10.
8. Stoll AL, Pillay SS, Diamond L, Workum SB, Cole JO. Methylphenidate augmentation of serotonin selective reuptake inhibitors: a case series. *J Clin Psychiatry* (1996) 57, 72–6.
9. Walters AM. Sympathomimetic-fluoxetine interaction. *J Am Acad Child Adolesc Psychiatry* (1992) 31, 565–6.

SSRIs + Tobacco

Smoking does not appear to alter citalopram pharmacokinetics, and has only modest effects on fluvoxamine pharmacokinetics.

Clinical evidence, mechanism, importance and management

(a) Citalopram

In a pharmacokinetic study involving 44 adolescent patients (under 21 years of age), there was considerable inter-individual variation in serum levels of citalopram and its metabolites at all doses studied. However, smoking did appear to influence the disposition of citalopram.[1] The clinical significance of this is unknown and more study is required.

(b) Fluvoxamine

A comparative study in 12 smokers and 12 non-smokers given single 50-mg oral doses of fluvoxamine found that smoking reduced the fluvoxamine AUC and the maximum serum levels by about 30%.[2] However, a study in Japanese patients found no significant difference in steady-state plasma levels of fluvoxamine and its metabolite (fluvoxamino acid) between 34 non-smokers and 15 smokers.[3] This suggests that the overall pharmacokinetic effect of smoking is probably minimal, although the effects of a sudden withdrawal from heavy smoking has not been investigated.

1. Reis M, Olsson G, Carlsson B, Lundmark J, Dahl ML, Walinder J, Ahlner J, Bengtsson F. Serum levels of citalopram and its main metabolites in adolescent patients treated in a naturalistic clinical setting. *J Clin Psychopharmacol* (2002) 22, 406–13.
2. Spigset O, Carleborg L, Hedenmalm K, Dahlqvist R. Effect of cigarette smoking on fluvoxamine pharmacokinetics in humans. *Clin Pharmacol Ther* (1995) 58, 399–403.
3. Gerstenberg G, Aoshima T, Fukasawa T, Yoshida K, Takahashi H, Higuchi H, Murata Y, Shimoyama R, Ohkubo T, Shimizu T, Otani K. Effects of the CYP 2D6 genotype and cigarette smoking on the steady-state plasma concentrations of fluvoxamine and its major metabolite fluvoxamino acid in Japanese depressed patients. *Ther Drug Monit* (2003) 25, 463–8.

SSRIs + Tryptophan

Central and peripheral toxicity developed in five patients taking fluoxetine when they were given tryptophan. On theoretical grounds an adverse reaction seems possible between fluvoxamine (and probably other SSRIs) and tryptophan or oxitriptan.

Clinical evidence

(a) Fluoxetine

The concurrent use of tryptophan with fluoxetine 20 mg daily has been reported to be tolerated.[1] A more recent placebo-controlled, double-blind study involving 30 patients with depression found that the use of tryptophan 2 g daily during the initial phase of treatment with fluoxetine 20 mg daily was beneficial and well-tolerated,[2] but problems have been seen when higher doses of both drugs have been given together. Five patients taking fluoxetine 50 to 100 mg daily for at least 3 months developed a number of reactions including central toxicity (agitation, restlessness, aggressive behaviour, worsening of obsessive-compulsive disorders) and peripheral toxicity (abdominal cramps, nausea, diarrhoea) within a few days of starting tryptophan 1 to 4 g daily. These symptoms disappeared when the tryptophan was stopped. Some of the patients had taken tryptophan in the absence of fluoxetine without problems.[3]

(b) Fluvoxamine

A warning by the CSM in the UK about the risks of giving fluvoxamine with tryptophan appears to be an extrapolation from the serious reaction (the serotonin syndrome) which has been seen with fluoxetine[4] (see above).

Mechanism, importance and management

Tryptophan is a precursor of serotonin (5-hydroxytryptamine) and the authors point out that the symptoms resemble the serotonin syndrome, which occurs when serotonin levels are increased. They warn against the concurrent use of tryptophan with fluoxetine or other serotonin reuptake inhibitors.[3] This caution is echoed by most of the manufacturers of the SSRIs; the UK manufacturer of paroxetine additionally mentions **oxitriptan** [L-5-hydroxytryptophan].[5]

1. Ciraulo DA, Shader RI. Fluoxetine drug-drug interactions II. *J Clin Psychopharmacol* (1990) 10, 213–17.
2. Levitan RD, Shen J-H, Jindal R, Driver HS, Kennedy SH, Shapiro CM. Preliminary randomized double-blind placebo-controlled trial of tryptophan combined with fluoxetine to treat major depressive disorder: antidepressant and hypnotic effects. *J Psychiatry Neurosci* (2000) 25, 337–46.
3. Steiner W, Fontaine R. Toxic reaction following the combined administration of fluoxetine and L-tryptophan: five case reports. *Biol Psychiatry* (1986) 21, 1067–71.
4. Committee on Safety of Medicines. Current Problems, May 1989, 26, 3. Correction. ibid. December 1989, 27, 3.
5. Seroxat (Paroxetine hydrochloride hemihydrate). GlaxoSmithKline UK. UK Summary of product characteristics, April 2007.

SSRIs; Citalopram + Irinotecan

An isolated report describes rhabdomyolysis in a patient receiving citalopram and irinotecan. However, an interaction is by no means established.

Clinical evidence, mechanism, importance and management

A 74-year-old man who had been taking citalopram for 2 months developed rhabdomyolysis after undergoing initial treatment for gastrointestinal cancer with irinotecan. All medications were discontinued, but the rhabdomyolysis was exacerbated upon restarting the citalopram for depression. The citalopram was discontinued and he improved over the next 5 days. It was thought that levels of citalopram might have increased because citalopram and irinotecan share at least one metabolic pathway (CYP3A4), and the cytochrome system may also have been compromised in the cancer patient.[1] However, the patient was also taking **simvastatin**, which is known to be associated with rhabdomyolysis and which is also metabolised by CYP3A4; however the authors make no mention of this. An interaction between citalopram and irinotecan is therefore by no means established, and speculatively, this could perhaps be an interaction between irinotecan and simvastatin, which was exacerbated by citalopram.

1. Richards S, Umbreit JN, Fanucchi MP, Giblin J, Khuri F. Selective serotonin reuptake inhibitor-induced rhabdomyolysis associated with irinotecan. South Med J 92003) 96, 1031–33.

SSRIs; Fluoxetine + Alosetron

Alosetron had no clinically significant effect on fluoxetine pharmacokinetics in healthy subjects.

Clinical evidence, mechanism, importance and management

An open study in 12 healthy subjects found that alosetron 1 mg twice daily for 15 days had no clinically significant effect on the pharmacokinetics of a single 20-mg dose of fluoxetine. There was a median 3-hour delay in time to reach peak levels of both *S*- and *R*-fluoxetine, but this was thought unlikely to be clinically relevant for a drug that requires several weeks to achieve its full therapeutic effect.[1]

1. D'Souza DL, Dimmitt DC, Robbins DK, Nezamis J, Simms L, Koch KM. Effect of alosetron on the pharmacokinetics of fluoxetine. *J Clin Pharmacol* (2001) 41, 455–8.

SSRIs; Fluoxetine + Aminoglutethimide

Limited evidence suggests that the effects of fluoxetine are increased by aminoglutethimide.

Clinical evidence, mechanism, importance and management

A patient with severe obsessive-compulsive disorder, resistant to clomipramine combined with SSRIs, improved when given fluoxetine 40 mg daily and aminoglutethimide 250 mg four times daily. Over a four-and-a-half year period, whenever attempts were made to reduce the dosage of either drug, the patient started to relapse.[1] Thus at least one patient has taken both drugs together without problems, and the evidence suggests that the aminoglutethimide has a potentiating effect on the fluoxetine. However, more study is needed to confirm the efficacy and safety of this drug combination in other patients.

1. Chouinard G, Bélanger M-C, Beauclair L, Sultan S, Murphy BEP. Potentiation of fluoxetine by aminoglutethimide, an adrenal steroid suppressant, in obsessive-compulsive disorder resistant to SSRIs: a case report. *Prog Neuropsychopharmacol Biol Psychiatry* (1996) 20, 1067–79.

SSRIs; Fluoxetine + Cannabis

An isolated report describes mania when a patient taking fluoxetine smoked cannabis.

Clinical evidence, mechanism, importance and management

A 21-year-old woman with a 9-year history of bulimia and depression was taking fluoxetine 20 mg daily. A month later, about 2 days after smoking two 'joints' of cannabis (**marijuana**), she experienced a persistent sense of well-being, increased energy, hypersexuality and pressured speech. These symptoms progressed into grandiose delusions, for which she was hospitalised. Her mania and excitement were controlled with lorazepam and perphenazine, and she largely recovered after about 8 days. The reasons for this reaction are not understood but the authors of the report point out that one of the active components of cannabis, **dronabinol** (**Δ^9-tetrahydrocannabinol**) is, like fluoxetine, a potent inhibitor of serotonin uptake. Thus a synergistic effect on central serotonergic neurones might have occurred.[1] This seems to be the first and only report of an apparent adverse interaction between cannabis and fluoxetine, but it emphasises the risks of concurrent use.

1. Stoll AL, Cole JO, Lukas SE. A case of mania as a result of fluoxetine-marijuana interaction. *J Clin Psychiatry* (1991) 52, 280–1.

SSRIs; Fluoxetine + Chlorothiazide

Fluoxetine is reported not to affect the pharmacokinetics of chlorothiazide.[1] No special precautions would seem necessary on concurrent use.

1. Lemberger L, Bergstrom RF, Wolen RL, Farid NA, Enas GG, Aronoff GR. Fluoxetine: clinical pharmacology and physiologic disposition. *J Clin Psychiatry* (1985) 46, 14–19.

SSRIs; Fluoxetine + CYP2D6 substrates

There is *in vitro* evidence that the effects of flecainide and mexiletine may possibly be increased by fluoxetine. The plasma levels of other drugs predominantly metabolised by CYP2D6 (such as encainide and thioridazine) may also be increased by fluoxetine. The

US manufacturer of fluoxetine contraindicates its use with thioridazine due to the risk of ventricular arrhythmias.

Clinical evidence, mechanism, importance and management

Studies in patients and *in vitro* investigations using human liver microsomes have shown that fluoxetine and its metabolite, norfluoxetine have a strong inhibitory effect on the activity of the cytochrome P450 isoenzyme CYP2D6 in the liver.[1,2] This means that in practice, fluoxetine may increase and prolong the effects of drugs metabolised by this isoenzyme.

Flecainide and **mexiletine** are predominantly or partly metabolised by CYP2D6 but there appear to be no clinical cases of interactions between these drugs and fluoxetine. However, fluoxetine does interact with 'propafenone', (p.275), which is also metabolised by CYP2D6 so it would seem prudent to be alert for increased and prolonged effects of these drugs if fluoxetine is added.

The manufacturers of fluoxetine warn that drugs predominantly metabolised by CYP2D6, and which have a narrow therapeutic index, should be initiated at or adjusted to the low end of their dose range in patients taking fluoxetine. This will also apply if fluoxetine has been taken in the previous 5 weeks because of its long elimination half-life.[3,4] The UK manufacturer[3] specifically mentions **flecainide**, **encainide**, and 'tricyclic antidepressants', (p.1241)). For a list of CYP2D6 substrates, see 'Table 1.3', (p.6). Of interest, the US manufacturer also lists vinblastine as a CYP2D6 substrate, and therefore cautions its use, but note that vinblastine is more usually considered to be a CYP3A4 substrate.

1. Otton SV, Wu D, Joffe RT, Cheung SW, Sellers EM. Inhibition by fluoxetine of cytochrome P450 2D6 activity. *Clin Pharmacol Ther* (1993) 53, 401–9.
2. Brøsen K, Skjelbo E. Fluoxetine and norfluoxetine are potent inhibitors of P450IID6 — the source of the sparteine/debrisoquine oxidation polymorphism. *Br J Clin Pharmacol* (1991) 32, 136–7.
3. Prozac (Fluoxetine hydrochloride). Eli Lilly and Company Ltd. UK Summary of product characteristics, March 2007.
4. Prozac (Fluoxetine). Eli Lilly and Company. US Prescribing information, May 2007.

SSRIs; Fluoxetine + Orlistat

The pharmacokinetics of a single 40-mg oral dose of fluoxetine (a lipophilic drug) were not affected by orlistat 120 mg three times daily in healthy subjects.[1]

1. Zhi J, Moore R, Kanitra L, Mulligan TE. Effects of orlistat, a lipase inhibitor, on the pharmacokinetics of three highly lipophilic drugs (amiodarone, fluoxetine, and simvastatin) in healthy volunteers. *J Clin Pharmacol* (2003) 43, 428–35.

SSRIs; Fluvoxamine + Enoxacin

A study in healthy subjects suggested that enoxacin slightly inhibits the metabolism of fluvoxamine.

Clinical evidence, mechanism, importance and management

A placebo-controlled study in 10 healthy subjects given enoxacin 200 mg daily for 11 days and a single 50-mg dose of fluvoxamine on the eighth day, found that enoxacin increased the plasma levels of fluvoxamine at 2 and 3 hours and the maximum plasma level was increased from 10.2 to 11.6 nanograms/mL. The scores of the Stanford sleepiness scale were also increased. Enoxacin appears to slightly inhibit the metabolism of fluvoxamine, presumably by interfering with cytochrome P450 isoenzyme CYP1A2-mediated pathways, although the exact pathway was not clear.[1]

1. Kunii T, Fukasawa T, Yasui-Furukori N, Aoshima T, Suzuki A, Tateishi T, Inoue Y, Otani K. Interaction study between enoxacin and fluvoxamine. *Ther Drug Monit* (2005) 27, 349–53.

SSRIs; Paroxetine + Barbiturates

Paroxetine appears not to interact to a clinically important extent with amobarbital, but phenobarbital may reduce the AUC of paroxetine. Two cases of hepatotoxicity have been reported when paroxetine was given with a barbiturate.

Clinical evidence, mechanism, importance and management

Phenobarbital 100 mg once daily given to 10 healthy subjects for 14 days caused reductions of 10 to 86% in the AUC of paroxetine in 6 subjects, but the mean AUC values were unaltered. One subject showed a 56% *increase* in AUC.[1] The sedative effects and impairment of psychomotor performance caused by **amobarbital** 100 mg were not increased by paroxetine 30 mg.[2] Two cases of hepatitis in young women were considered to be caused by the concurrent use of ***Atrium*** (a barbiturate complex) and paroxetine, which are both hepatotoxic.[3]

For an isolated report of a tonic clonic seizure in a woman taking paroxetine who was anaesthetised with methohexital, see 'Anaesthetics, general + SSRIs', p.105.

1. Greb WH, Buscher G, Dierdorf H-D, Köster FE, Wolf D, Mellows G. The effect of liver enzyme inhibition by cimetidine and enzyme induction by phenobarbitone on the pharmacokinetics of paroxetine. *Acta Psychiatr Scand* (1989) 80 (Suppl 350), 95–8.
2. Cooper SM, Jackson D, Loudon JM, McClelland GR, Raptopoulos P. The psychomotor effects of paroxetine alone and in combination with haloperidol, amylobarbitone, oxazepam, or alcohol. *Acta Psychiatr Scand* (1989) 80 (Suppl 350), 53–55.
3. Cadranel J-F, Di Martino V, Cazier A, Pras V, Bachmeyer C, Olympio P, Gonzenbach A, Mofredj A, Coutarel P, Devergie B, Biour M. *Atrium* and paroxetine-related severe hepatitis. *J Clin Gastroenterol* (1999) 28, 52–5.

SSRIs; Paroxetine + Miscellaneous

Paroxetine appears not to interact to a clinically important extent with aluminium hydroxide or food, although absorption may be reduced by large quantities of milk. Concurrent use of paroxetine and aprepitant may slightly reduce the plasma levels of both drugs, but this is probably not clinically significant.

Clinical evidence, mechanism, importance and management

(a) Aluminium hydroxide

Aludrox (aluminium hydroxide) 15 mL twice daily increased the absorption of a single 30-mg dose of paroxetine in healthy subjects by about 12%, and increased the maximum plasma concentration by 14%.[1] This is unlikely to be clinically important. No particular precautions would seem to be necessary on concurrent use.

(b) Aprepitant

The US manufacturer of aprepitant notes that the concurrent use of paroxetine 20 mg daily and aprepitant 85 or 170 mg daily reduced the AUC of both drugs by about 25%, and reduced the maximum serum levels by about 20%.[2] These changes are unlikely to be clinically important.

(c) Food or drink

A study in healthy subjects found that the absorption of paroxetine was not markedly changed by food. A 40% reduction in absorption was seen when paroxetine was taken with one litre of **milk**,[1] but few people are likely to drink such a large amount regularly, and so this interaction is unlikely to be clinically significant.

1. Greb WH, Brett MA, Buscher G, Dierdorf H-D, von Schrader HW, Wolf D, Mellows G, Zussman BD. Absorption of paroxetine under various dietary conditions and following antacid intake. *Acta Psychiatr Scand* (1989) 80 (Suppl 350), 99–101.
2. Emend (Aprepitant). Merck & Co., Inc. US Prescribing information, June 2006.

Tianeptine + Oxazepam

A study in healthy subjects given tianeptine 12.5 mg and oxazepam 10 mg both three times daily found no significant changes in the pharmacokinetics of either drug.[1]

1. Toon S, Holt BL, Langley SJ, Mullins FGP, Rowland M, Halliday MS, Salvadori C, Delalleau B. Pharmacokinetic and pharmacodynamic interaction between the antidepressant tianeptine and oxazepam at steady-state. *Psychopharmacology (Berl)* (1990) 101, 226–32.

Trazodone + Antidepressants

Trazodone and fluoxetine have been used concurrently with advantage, but some patients develop increased adverse effects. There have been isolated reports of the serotonin syndrome in patients receiving trazodone and MAOIs, usually in association with

other serotonergic drugs. A single case report describes the development of anorexia, psychosis and hypomania in a patient receiving trazodone and tryptophan.

Clinical evidence, mechanism, importance and management

(a) MAOIs

A case report describes a patient treated with trazodone, **isocarboxazid** and methylphenidate who developed symptoms of the serotonin syndrome.[1] The US manufacturer says due to the absence of clinical experience, if MAOIs are discontinued shortly before or are to be given concurrently with trazodone, therapy should be initiated cautiously with a gradual increase in dosage until optimum response is achieved.[2] However, the UK manufacturer of trazodone says possible interactions with MAOIs have occasionally been reported; they do not recommend concurrent use, nor should trazodone be given within 2 weeks of stopping an MAOI. MAOIs should not be taken within one week of stopping trazodone.[3]

(b) SSRIs

A patient taking trazodone showed a 31% increase in the antidepressant/dose ratio (suggesting increased trazodone levels) when **fluoxetine** 40 mg daily was added. She became sedated and developed an unstable gait.[4] A study involving 27 patients also found that **fluoxetine** increases plasma trazodone levels.[5] However, another study reported **citalopram** and **fluoxetine** had no significant impact on trazodone serum levels, even though the mean concentration/dose ratios were nearly 30% higher with the combined therapy than with trazodone monotherapy.[6]

A man with traumatic brain injury showed new-onset dysarthria and speech blocking when **fluoxetine** was added to trazodone. His speech returned to normal when the **fluoxetine** was stopped.[7] A 39-year-old HIV-positive man taking multiple antiviral and antibacterial drugs experienced bilateral hand tremor while receiving trazodone 50 mg at bedtime, which worsened when the dose of trazodone was increased to 100 mg and **fluoxetine** 20 mg daily was added. The trazodone and **fluoxetine** were discontinued and the tremor completely disappeared after 7 days without specific treatment for myoclonus.[8]

Five out of 16 patients receiving **fluoxetine** stopped taking trazodone 25 to 75 mg, which was given for insomnia, because of excessive sedation the next day.[9] Three out of 8 patients had improvement in sleep and depression when given both drugs but the other 5 were either unaffected or had intolerable adverse effects (headaches, dizziness, daytime sedation, fatigue).[10] However, another report described advantageous concurrent use in 6 patients without an increase in adverse effects.[11]

It appears that the plasma levels of trazodone may be increased by **fluoxetine** due to inhibition of cytochrome P450 isoenzymes by **fluoxetine** and/or norfluoxetine.[5] Trazodone is a substrate for CYP3A4 and, although **fluoxetine** is a weak inhibitor, its metabolite norfluoxetine is a moderate inhibitor of this enzyme.[8] *In vitro* data suggest **citalopram** has little inhibitory effect on CYP3A4.[6,12]

These cases and studies suggest that the concurrent use of trazodone and **fluoxetine** can be useful and uneventful but it would seem prudent to monitor the outcome for any evidence of increased adverse effects. **Citalopram** would not be expected to have a pharmacokinetic interaction. However, the cases with **fluoxetine** suggest that a pharmacodynamic interaction may be possible, and therefore a degree of caution would be prudent if trazodone is given with any SSRI.

(c) Tryptophan

A single report describes the effective use of trazodone 100 mg and tryptophan 500 mg, both three times weekly with clonazepam in a patient with schizophrenia and congenital defects. However, the patient stopped eating, lost 4.5 kg in weight over 3 weeks, developed signs of psychosis or hypomania, and soon afterwards she became drowsy and withdrawn. When the drugs were withdrawn the aggressive behaviour restarted, but she responded again to lower doses of trazodone and tryptophan although the signs of psychosis re-emerged.[13]

(d) Venlafaxine

For a report of the serotonin syndrome in a patient taking trazodone and venlafaxine, see 'SNRIs; Venlafaxine + Antidepressants', p.1212.

1. Bodner RA, Lynch T, Lewis L, Kahn D. Serotonin syndrome. *Neurology* (1995) 45, 219–23.
2. Desyrel (Trazodone hydrochloride). Bristol-Myers Squibb Company. US Prescribing information, January 2005.
3. Molipaxin (Trazodone hydrochloride). Sanofi-Aventis. UK Summary of product characteristics, July 2005.
4. Aranow RB, Hudson JI, Pope HG, Grady TA, Laage TA, Bell IR, Cole JO. Elevated antidepressant plasma levels after addition of fluoxetine. *Am J Psychiatry* (1989) 146, 911–13.
5. Maes M, Westenberg H, Vandoolaeghe E, Demedts P, Wauters A, Neels H, Meltzer HY. Effects of trazodone and fluoxetine in the treatment of major depression: therapeutic pharmacokinetic and pharmacodynamic interactions through formation of meta-chlorophenylpiperazine. *J Clin Psychopharmacol* (1997) 17, 358–64.
6. Prapotnik M, Waschgler R, König P, Moll W, Conca A. Therapeutic drug monitoring of trazodone: are there pharmacokinetic interactions involving citalopram and fluoxetine? *Int J Clin Pharmacol Ther* (2004) 42, 120–4.
7. Patterson DE, Braverman SE, Belandres PV. Speech dysfunction due to trazodone-fluoxetine combination in traumatic brain injury. *Brain Inj* (1997) 11, 287–91.
8. Darko W, Guharoy R, Rose F, Lehman D, Pappas V. Myoclonus secondary to the concurrent use of trazodone and fluoxetine. *Vet Hum Toxicol* (2001) 43, 214–5.
9. Metz A, Shader RI. Adverse interactions encountered when using trazodone to treat insomnia associated with fluoxetine. *Int Clin Psychopharmacol* (1990) 5, 191–4.
10. Nierenberg AA, Cole JO, Glass L. Possible trazodone potentiation of fluoxetine: a case series. *J Clin Psychiatry* (1992) 53, 83–5.
11. Swerdlow NR, Andia AM. Trazodone-fluoxetine combination for treatment of obsessive-compulsive disorder. *Am J Psychiatry* (1989) 146, 1637.
12. Celexa (Citalopram hydrobromide). Forest Pharmaceuticals, Inc. US Prescribing information, May 2007.
13. Patterson BD, Srisopark MM. Severe anorexia and possible psychosis or hypomania after trazodone-tryptophan treatment of aggression. *Lancet* (1989) i, 1017.

Trazodone + Azoles

Ketoconazole or itraconazole may inhibit the metabolism of trazodone.

Clinical evidence, mechanism, importance and management

An *in vitro* study demonstrated that **ketoconazole** inhibited the metabolism of trazodone to its principal metabolite, meta-chlorophenylpiperazine.[1] Trazodone is a substrate for the cytochrome P450 isoenzyme CYP3A4 and inhibitors of this enzyme such as **ketoconazole** or **itraconazole** may inhibit its metabolism, leading to substantial increases in trazodone plasma concentrations with the potential for adverse effects.[2-4] The FDA in the US and the manufacturers of trazodone recommend that a lower dose of trazodone should be considered if it is given with a potent CYP3A4 inhibitor such as **ketoconazole** or **itraconazole**.[2-4] However, the UK manufacturer also suggests that the combination should be avoided where possible.[4]

1. Zalma A, von Moltke LL, Granda BW, Harmatz JS, Shader RI, Greenblatt DJ. In vitro metabolism of trazodone by CYP3A: inhibition by ketoconazole and human immunodeficiency viral protease inhibitors. *Biol Psychiatry* (2000) 47, 655–61.
2. Desyrel (Trazodone hydrochloride). Bristol-Myers Squibb Company. US Prescribing information, January 2005.
3. Lewis-Hall FC. Bristol-Myers Squibb Company. Letter to healthcare professionals, April 2004.
4. Molipaxin (Trazodone hydrochloride). Sanofi-Aventis. UK Summary of product characteristics, July 2005.

Trazodone + *Ginkgo biloba*

Coma developed in an elderly patient with Alzheimer's disease after she took trazodone with ginkgo biloba.

Clinical evidence, mechanism, importance and management

An 80-year-old woman with Alzheimer's disease developed coma a few days after starting low-dose trazodone 20 mg twice daily and ginkgo biloba. The patient woke immediately after being given flumazenil 1 mg intravenously. It was suggested that the flavonoids in the ginkgo had a subclinical direct effect on the benzodiazepine receptor. In addition, increased CYP3A4 metabolism of trazodone to its active metabolite, 1-(m-chlorophenyl)piperazine (mCPP), was thought to have enhanced the release of GABA (gamma-amino butyric acid). Flumazenil may have blocked the direct effect of the flavonoids, thus causing the GABA activity to fall below the level required to have a clinical effect.[1] This appears to be an isolated case, from which no general conclusions can be drawn.

1. Galluzzi S, Zanetti O, Binetti G, Trabucchi M, Frisoni GB. Coma in a patient with Alzheimer's disease taking low dose trazodone and ginkgo biloba. *J Neurol Neurosurg Psychiatry* (2000) 68, 679–80.

Trazodone + Haloperidol

Low-dose haloperidol is reported not to interact to a clinically relevant extent with trazodone.

Clinical evidence, mechanism, importance and management

Nine depressed patients who had been taking trazodone 150 to 300 mg at bedtime for 2 to 19 weeks were given haloperidol 4 mg daily for a week. Plasma trazodone levels were not significantly changed but levels of its metabolite (*m*-chlorophenylpiperazine) were slightly raised (from 78 to 92 nanograms/mL). This study[1] was carried out to investigate the way trazodone is metabolised, but it also demonstrated that no clinically relevant pharmacokinetic interaction occurs between these two drugs at these dosages.

1. Mihara K, Otani K, Ishida M, Yasui N, Suzuki A, Ohkubo T, Osanai T, Kaneko S, Sugawara K. Increases in plasma concentration of m-chlorophenylpiperazine, but not trazodone, with low-dose haloperidol. *Ther Drug Monit* (1997) 19, 43–5.

Trazodone + Lysergide (LSD)

A retrospective study found that 28 of 32 subjects (88%) who took LSD and who had taken an SSRI or trazodone for more than 3 weeks had a subjective decrease or virtual elimination of their responses to LSD.[1]

1. Bonson KR, Buckholtz JW, Murphy DL. Chronic administration of serotonergic antidepressants attenuates the subjective effects of LSD in humans. *Neuropsychopharmacology* (1996) 14, 425–36.

Trazodone + Macrolides

Clarithromycin impaired the clearance of trazodone and enhanced its sedative effects in healthy subjects. Erythromycin is also likely to increase trazodone plasma levels.

Clinical evidence, mechanism, importance and management

In a placebo-controlled study in healthy subjects, **clarithromycin** impaired the clearance and enhanced the sedative effects of a 50-mg dose of trazodone.[1] The manufacturers comment that trazodone is a substrate for the cytochrome P450 isoenzyme CYP3A4 and inhibitors of this enzyme may inhibit its metabolism leading to substantial increases in trazodone plasma levels, with the potential for adverse effects.[2,3] The UK manufacturer of trazodone recommends that a lower dose of trazodone should be considered if it is given with a CYP3A4 inhibitor such as **erythromycin**, but that concurrent use should be avoided where possible.[3] It seems likely that all macrolides that inhibit CYP3A4 will interact to some extent. As **azithromycin** does not significantly affect CYP3A4 it would not be expected to interact.

1. Greenblatt DJ, von Moltke LL, Harmatz JS. Clarithromycin impairs clearance and potentiates clinical effects of trazodone but not of zolpidem. *Clin Pharmacol Ther* (2005) 77, P28.
2. Desyrel (Trazodone hydrochloride). Bristol-Myers Squibb Company. US Prescribing information, January 2005.
3. Molipaxin (Trazodone hydrochloride). Sanofi-Aventis. UK Summary of product characteristics, July 2005.

Trazodone + Protease inhibitors

Ritonavir impairs the clearance of trazodone with an increased potential for adverse effects. Other protease inhibitors may interact similarly.

Clinical evidence

A randomised, placebo-controlled, crossover study in 10 healthy subjects found that short-term exposure to low-dose **ritonavir** (200 mg twice daily for 2 days) impaired the clearance of a single 50-mg dose of trazodone by 52%. Mean peak plasma levels of trazodone were increased by 34%, and the AUC increased more than twofold. In addition, **ritonavir** enhanced the adverse effects of trazodone with increased sedation, fatigue and performance impairment.[1] Symptoms of the serotonin syndrome occurred in an HIV-positive patient taking antiretrovirals and other drugs, including fluoxetine and trazodone, when **ritonavir** was added. The symptoms resolved on discontinuing the trazodone and halving the **ritonavir** dose.[2] The serotonin syndrome has also been seen in a patient taking trazodone, **indinavir** and excessive amounts of 'grapefruit', (p.1217).

An *in vitro* study demonstrated that the metabolism of trazodone to its principal metabolite, meta-chlorophenylpiperazine (mCPP), was inhibited by **ritonavir**, which is a potent inhibitor of the cytochrome P450 isoenzyme CYP3A4. **Indinavir** was also a strong inhibitor of mCPP formation, whereas **saquinavir** and **nelfinavir** were considerably less potent inhibitors.[3]

Mechanism

Trazodone is a substrate for CYP3A4 and inhibitors of this enzyme such as ritonavir and indinavir may inhibit its metabolism, leading to substantial increases in trazodone plasma concentrations with the potential for adverse effects.[4-6]

Importance and management

The FDA in the US and the manufacturers of trazodone recommend that a lower dose of trazodone should be considered if it is given with potent CYP3A4 inhibitors such as the protease inhibitors ritonavir and indinavir.[4-6] However, the UK manufacturer also suggests that the combination should be avoided where possible.[5]

1. Greenblatt DJ, von Moltke LL, Harmatz JS, Fogelman SM, Chen G, Graf JA, Mertzanis P, Byron S, Culm KE, Granda BW, Daily JP, Shader RI. Short-term exposure to low-dose ritonavir impairs clearance and enhances adverse effects of trazodone. *J Clin Pharmacol* (2003) 43, 414–22.
2. DeSilva KE, Le Flore DB, Marston BJ, Rimland D. Serotonin syndrome in HIV-infected individuals receiving antiretroviral therapy and fluoxetine. *AIDS* (2001) 15, 1281–5.
3. Zalma A, von Moltke LL, Granda BW, Harmatz JS, Shader RI, Greenblatt DJ. In vitro metabolism of trazodone by CYP3A: inhibition by ketoconazole and human immunodeficiency viral protease inhibitors. *Biol Psychiatry* (2000) 47, 655–61.
4. Lewis-Hall FC. Bristol-Myers Squibb Company. Letter to healthcare professionals, April 2004.
5. Molipaxin (Trazodone hydrochloride). Sanofi-Aventis. UK Summary of product characteristics, July 2005.
6. Desyrel (Trazodone hydrochloride). Bristol-Myers Squibb Company. US Prescribing information, January 2005.

Trazodone + Pseudoephedrine

A single report describes toxicity in a woman treated with trazodone when she took pseudoephedrine.

Clinical evidence, mechanism, importance and management

An isolated report describes a woman who had been taking trazodone 250 mg daily for 2 years who took two doses of a non-prescription medicine containing pseudoephedrine. Within 6 hours she experienced dread, anxiety, panic, confusion, depersonalisation and the sensation that parts of her body were separating. None of these symptoms had been experienced in the past when she was taking either preparation alone.[1] The reasons for this reaction are not understood. This appears to be an isolated case, and therefore no general conclusions can be drawn.

1. Weddige RL. Possible trazodone-pseudoephedrine toxicity: a case report. *Neurobehav Toxicol Teratol* (1985) 7, 204.

Tricyclic antidepressants + ACE inhibitors

Preliminary evidence from two patients suggests that enalapril may increase the effects of clomipramine, resulting in toxicity.

Clinical evidence

Two patients taking **enalapril** (one taking 20 mg daily and the other taking 20 mg five times weekly) were given **clomipramine** for depression. The **clomipramine** dosage of one of them was increased from 25 to 50 mg, and 10 days later he became euphoric and exalted. The problem resolved when the **clomipramine** dosage was reduced to 25 mg again. The other patient had been stable taking **enalapril** for over a year when **clomipramine** and disulfiram 400 mg daily were added. Within 2 weeks he developed confusion, irritability and insomnia. These adverse effects diminished when the **clomipramine** dosage was reduced to 50 mg daily.[1]

Mechanism

The ratio of clomipramine to its metabolite (desmethylclomipramine) is normally less than 1, but both of these patients demonstrated a ratio of more than 1. This suggests that the normal metabolism (demethylation) of the clomipramine was inhibited, thus allowing the clomipramine to accumulate and its toxic effects to manifest themselves. In the second patient the disulfiram may also have had a minor additional enzyme inhibitory effect.[1]

Importance and management

Information is limited to these two cases and the interaction is not firmly established. More study is needed. There seems to be nothing documented about adverse effects from the concurrent use of the other ACE inhibitors and tricyclic antidepressants, although postural hypotension is a possibility.

1. Toutoungi M. Potential effect of enalapril on clomipramine metabolism. *Hum Psychopharmacol* (1992) 7, 347–9.

Tricyclic antidepressants + Amfetamines and related drugs

Methylphenidate can increase the levels and rate of response to tricyclic antidepressants. This has led to both increased beneficial and adverse effects. No significant pharmacokinetic interaction has been reported between desipramine and dexamfetamine or methylphenidate. An isolated report describes a blood dyscrasia in a child given methylphenidate and imipramine.

Clinical evidence

A study in 'several patients' demonstrated a dramatic increase in the plasma levels of **imipramine** and its active metabolite desipramine when they took **methylphenidate**. In one patient taking **imipramine** 150 mg daily, methylphenidate 20 mg daily increased the plasma levels of **imipramine** from 100 to 700 micrograms/L and of the metabolite desipramine from 200 to 850 micrograms/L over a period of 16 days. Clinical improvement occurred in several of the patients.[1] Similar effects have been described in other reports.[2-5] It seems that elevation of drug levels takes several days to occur, and several days to wear off.[3]

A study of the combined use of tricyclic antidepressants (**desipramine**, **imipramine**, **nortriptyline**, **doxepin**) with **methylphenidate** 5 to 15 mg twice daily was undertaken in 20 of 41 patients with depression who responded to a test dose of **methylphenidate**. Combined use accelerated the antidepressant response to tricyclics with 6 of 20 patients responding after 1 week and 10 of 16 patients responding after 2 weeks. Adverse effects included insomnia, dizziness, hypotension and dry mouth. **Methylphenidate** was discontinued after less than 2 weeks concurrent use in 3 patients because of increased anxiety, irritability and hypomania.[6] There is also a report of a 9-year-old boy and a 15-year-old boy who exhibited severe behavioural problems until the **imipramine** and **methylphenidate** they were taking were stopped.[7] Another report describes more frequent adverse effects in 10 paediatric patients taking **methylphenidate** with **desipramine** than with **methylphenidate** alone.[8] Three patients taking tricyclic antidepressants and with labile blood pressure experienced hypertensive episodes when **methylphenidate** was also given. They responded to withdrawal of **methylphenidate** and two patients had further hypertensive episodes when rechallenged with **methylphenidate**.[9] An isolated report describes leucopenia, anaemia, eosinophilia and thrombocytosis in a child of 10 when given **imipramine** and **methylphenidate**.[10] In one patient taking **desipramine** 250 mg daily, concurrent **methylphenidate** 40 mg daily resulted in a small decrease in serum **desipramine** levels, but a marked improvement in mood.[11]

In contrast, a retrospective review in 142 children and adolescents taking either **desipramine** alone, or **desipramine** with **dexamfetamine** or **methylphenidate**, indicated the absence of a clinically significant interaction between **desipramine** and either stimulant. Pharmacokinetic parameters were similar in each group.[12]

Mechanism

In vitro experiments with human liver slices indicate that methylphenidate inhibits the metabolism of imipramine, resulting in raised blood levels.[3] The accelerated response to tricyclic antidepressants may also be partly due to increased serum levels in the presence of methylphenidate, although the adverse effects observed were not entirely consistent with elevated levels of tricyclics.[6] There are also reports suggesting that methylphenidate does not significantly affect desipramine levels.[8,11] The blood dyscrasia may have been due to the rare additive effects of both drugs.[10]

Importance and management

Information is limited. Some therapeutic improvement including accelerated response is seen in some patients. This may be partially because of the very marked rise in the blood levels of the antidepressant due to methylphenidate, but may also be due to an additional effect on mood attributable to methylphenidate. Concurrent use may cause adverse effects sufficiently severe to necessitate withdrawal of methylphenidate, but it is not certain whether this can solely be attributed to increases in serum levels of tricyclic antidepressants. Information about other tricyclic antidepressants is lacking. However, it has been suggested that concurrent use in children and adolescents may be undesirable, due to case reports of adverse behavioural effects.[7] If concurrent use is deemed necessary it would seem prudent to monitor concurrent use for adverse tricyclic effects (e.g. dry mouth, blurred vision, urinary retention) and adjust the dose as necessary.

1. Sellers EM. Ed. Clinical Pharmacology of Psychoactive Drugs.Toronto: Alcoholism and Drug Addiction Research Foundation; 1975 p 183–202.
2. Cooper TB, Simpson GM. Concomitant imipramine and methylphenidate administration: a case report. *Am J Psychiatry* (1973) 130, 721.
3. Wharton RN, Perel JM, Dayton PG, Malitz S. A potential clinical use for methylphenidate with tricyclic antidepressants. *Am J Psychiatry* (1971) 127, 1619–25.
4. Zeidenberg P, Perel JM, Kanzler M, Wharton RN, Malitz S. Clinical and metabolic studies with imipramine in man. *Am J Psychiatry* (1971) 127, 1321–6.
5. Cooper TB, Simpson GM. Concomitant imipramine and methylphenidate administration: a case report. *Am J Psychiatry* (1973) 130, 721.
6. Gwirtsman HE, Szuba MP, Toren L, Feist M. The antidepressant response to tricyclics in major depressives is accelerated with adjunctive use of methylphenidate. *Psychopharmacol Bull* (1994) 30, 157–64.
7. Grob CS, Coyle JT. Suspected adverse methylphenidate-imipramine interactions in children. *J Dev Behav Pediatr* (1986) 7, 265–7.
8. Pataki CS, Carlson GA, Kelly KL, Rapport MD, Biancaniello TM. Side effects of methylphenidate and desipramine alone and in combination in children. *J Am Acad Child Adolesc Psychiatry* (1993) 32, 1065–72.
9. Flemenbaum A. Hypertensive episodes after adding methylphenidate (Ritalin) to tricyclic antidepressants. *Psychosomatics* (1972) 13, 265–8.
10. Burke MS, Josephson A, Lightsey A. Combined methylphenidate and imipramine complication. *J Am Acad Child Adolesc Psychiatry* (1995) 34, 403–4.
11. Drimmer EJ, Gitlin MJ, Gwirtsman HE. Desipramine and methylphenidate combination treatment for depression: case report. *Am J Psychiatry* (1983) 140, 241–2.
12. Cohen LG, Prince J, Biederman J, Wilens T, Faraone SV, Whitt S, Mick E, Spencer T, Meyer MC, Polisner D, Flood JG. Absence of effect of stimulants on the pharmacokinetics of desipramine in children. *Pharmacotherapy* (1999) 19, 746–52.

Tricyclic antidepressants + Azoles; Fluconazole

Markedly increased serum amitriptyline levels developed in five patients and increased serum nortriptyline levels in another patient when they took fluconazole. Mental changes, syncope, and prolonged QTc interval occurred in some of these patients and there is also a report of prolonged QT interval and torsades de pointes associated with the concurrent use of amitriptyline and fluconazole in a further patient.

Clinical evidence

(a) Amitriptyline

A man with AIDS given fluconazole 200 mg daily and amitriptyline 25 mg then 50 mg three times a day developed mental changes and visual hallucinations within 3 days. His serum amitriptyline levels were found to be 724 nanograms/mL (therapeutic levels 150 to 250 nanograms/mL). The confusion resolved within 4 days of stopping the amitriptyline when the levels had fallen to 270 nanograms/mL. Two similar cases were described in this report, in one case in a patient with renal impairment.[1] A woman taking amitriptyline 100 mg twice daily, isosorbide mononitrate and metoprolol became lethargic, drowsy and confused 4 days after starting fluconazole 100 mg daily. She was found to have elevated serum levels of amitriptyline plus nortriptyline of 956 nanograms/mL (patient's usual range 150 to 250 nanograms/mL) and a prolonged QTc interval. At first, amitriptyline overdose was suspected. The patient was intubated but became delirious, agitated and disorientated. She recovered over the next 24 hours and the amitriptyline level had fallen to 190 nanograms/mL after 4 days. It was concluded that the amitriptyline toxicity was due to an interaction with fluconazole.[2]

Other reports similarly describe increased amitriptyline levels when fluconazole was given; in a child who developed syncope as a result[3] and in a 57-year-old woman who developed QT-interval prolongation (although hypokalaemia and the use of sertraline, which can increase serum tricyclic levels, may have contributed to this effect).[4]

(b) Nortriptyline

An elderly woman taking nortriptyline 75 mg daily and other drugs (ciclosporin, morphine, metoclopramide, bumetanide as well as an unnamed antibacterial) was given fluconazole (loading dose of 200 mg, followed by 100 mg daily). After concurrent use for 13 days her trough serum nortriptyline levels had risen by 70% (from 149 to 252 nanograms/mL).[5]

Mechanism

Not understood, but it has been suggested that the fluconazole inhibits the cytochrome P450 isoenzymes CYP2C9, CYP2C19, CYP3A4 and possibly CYP2D6, which are concerned with the metabolism of these tricyclics, and as a result their serum levels rise.[1,3]

Importance and management

Information about an interaction between tricyclics and fluconazole seems to be limited to these reports, which, bearing in mind the widespread use of these drugs, would suggest that these interactions are uncommon. The evidence suggests that other factors (such as renal impairment and other potentially interacting medications) may be necessary before this interaction occurs. Bear this possible interaction in mind if tricyclic adverse effects become troublesome.

1. Newberry DL, Bass SN, Mbanefo CO. A fluconazole/amitriptyline drug interaction in three male adults. *Clin Infect Dis* (1997) 24, 270–1.
2. Duggal HS. Delirium associated with amitriptyline/fluconazole drug. *Gen Hosp Psychiatry* (2003) 25, 297–8.
3. Robinson RF, Nahata MC, Olshefski RS. Syncope associated with concurrent amitriptyline and fluconazole therapy. *Ann Pharmacother* (2000) 34, 1406–9.
4. Dorsey ST, Biblo LA. Prolonged QT interval and torsades de pointes caused by the combination of fluconazole and amitriptyline. *Am J Emerg Med* (2000) 18, 227–9.
5. Gannon RH, Anderson ML. Fluconazole-nortriptyline drug interaction. *Ann Pharmacother* (1992) 26, 1456–7.

Tricyclic antidepressants + Azoles; Ketoconazole

Ketoconazole appears not to interact with desipramine, and only interacts to a small and clinically irrelevant extent with imipramine.

Clinical evidence, mechanism, importance and management

Two groups of 6 healthy subjects were given a single 100-mg dose of either **imipramine** or **desipramine** alone, and then again on day 10 of a 14-day course of ketoconazole 200 mg once daily. It was found that the ketoconazole caused the oral clearance of the **imipramine** to fall by 17%, its half-life to rise by 15% and the AUC of **desipramine**, derived from the **imipramine**, to fall by 9%. No significant changes in the pharmacokinetics of the **desipramine** were seen.[1]

These findings show that ketoconazole inhibits the demethylation of **imipramine** without affecting the 2-hydroxylation of **imipramine** and **desipramine**, and confirms that cytochrome P450 isoenzyme CYP3A4 has a role in the metabolism of these tricyclic antidepressants.[1] However, in practical terms it would seem that any changes are small and unlikely to be of any clinical significance. No special precautions would appear necessary if ketoconazole is used with either of these two drugs. Information about other tricyclics seems to be lacking.

1. Spina E, Avenoso A, Campo GM, Scordo MG, Caputi AP, Perucca E. Effect of ketoconazole on the pharmacokinetics of imipramine and desipramine in healthy subjects. *Br J Clin Pharmacol* (1997) 43, 315–8.

Tricyclic antidepressants + Baclofen

An isolated report describes a patient with multiple sclerosis taking baclofen who was unable to stand within a few days of starting to take nortriptyline, and later imipramine.

Clinical evidence, mechanism, importance and management

A man with multiple sclerosis, who was taking baclofen 10 mg four times a day to relieve spasticity, complained of leg weakness and was unable to stand within 6 days of starting to take **nortriptyline** 50 mg at bedtime. His muscle tone returned 48 hours after stopping the **nortriptyline**. Two weeks later he was given **imipramine** 75 mg daily and once again his muscle tone was lost.[1] The reason is not understood. There seems to be nothing documented about any other tricyclic antidepressant and baclofen. Prescribers should be aware of this report if considering the use of both drugs, but its general importance is not known. It is probably small.

1. Silverglat MJ. Baclofen and tricyclic antidepressants: possible interaction. *JAMA* (1981) 246, 1659.

Tricyclic antidepressants + Barbiturates

The plasma levels of amitriptyline, imipramine and nortriptyline can be reduced by the barbiturates. A reduced therapeutic response would be expected. The tricyclics also lower the convulsive threshold and may be inappropriate for patients with convulsive disorders.

Clinical evidence

A comparative study in 5 pairs of twins given **nortriptyline** found that the twins also taking unnamed barbiturates had considerably lower steady-state plasma **nortriptyline** levels.[1]

Similar observations have been made in patients and healthy subjects taking **nortriptyline** with **amobarbital**[2,3] or **pentobarbital**,[4] and **protriptyline** with **amobarbital sodium**.[5] Another patient had a reduction in blood **imipramine** levels of about 50% (and loss of antidepressant control) within 2 weeks of starting to take about 400 mg of **butalbital** daily.[6]

Mechanism

The barbiturates are potent liver enzyme inducers and may therefore increase the metabolism and clearance of the tricyclic antidepressants from the body.

Importance and management

The interaction between tricyclic antidepressants and barbiturates is established. By no means every drug pair has been studied but since the barbiturates as a whole are potent liver enzyme inducers one should be alert for this interaction with any of them. Some reduction in the effects of the tricyclic would be expected, but the general clinical importance is uncertain.

Note that the tricyclics lower the convulsive threshold and may therefore be inappropriate for patients with convulsive disorders.

1. Alexanderson B, Price Evans DA, Sjöqvist F. Steady-state plasma levels of nortriptyline in twins: influence of genetic factors and drug therapy. *BMJ* (1969) 4, 764–8.
2. Burrows GD, Davies B. Antidepressants and barbiturates. *BMJ* (1971) 4, 113.
3. Silverman G, Braithwaite R. Interaction of benzodiazepines and tricyclic antidepressants. *BMJ* (1972) 4, 111.
4. Steiner E, Koike Y, Lind M, von Bahr C. Increased nortriptyline metabolism after treatment with pentobarbital in man. *Acta Pharmacol Toxicol (Copenh)* (1986) 59 (Suppl 4), 91.
5. Moody JP, Whyte SF, MacDonald AJ and Naylor GJ. Pharmacokinetic aspects of protriptyline plasma levels. *Eur J Clin Pharmacol* (1977) 11, 51–6.
6. Garey KW, Amsden GW, Johns CA. Possible interaction between imipramine and butalbital. *Pharmacotherapy* (1997) 17, 1041–2.

Tricyclic antidepressants + Benzodiazepines and related drugs

Concurrent use is not uncommon and normally appears to be uneventful. However, three patients became drowsy, forgetful and appeared uncoordinated and drunk while taking amitriptyline and chlordiazepoxide. A combined preparation of amitriptyline and chlordiazepoxide (*Limbitrol*) is available but its advantages have been questioned: adverse effects have been seen in four patients. Diazepam may increase the risks of carrying out complex tasks (e.g. driving) if added to amitriptyline, as may other combinations of benzodiazepines and tricyclics.

Clinical evidence

(a) Amitriptyline

1. Chlordiazepoxide. Clinical studies in large numbers of patients have shown that the incidence of adverse reactions while taking amitriptyline and chlordiazepoxide was no greater than might have been expected with either of the drugs used alone,[1-3] but a few adverse reports have been documented. A depressed patient taking amitriptyline 150 mg and chlordiazepoxide 40 mg daily became confused, forgetful and uncoordinated. He acted as though he was drunk.[4] Two other patients taking amitriptyline and chlordiazepoxide experienced drowsiness, memory impairment, slurring of the speech and an inability to concentrate. Both were unable to work and one described himself as feeling drunk.[5] Four patients taking *Limbitrol* are reported to have experienced some manifestations of toxicity (delusions, confusion, agitation, disorientation, dry mouth, blurred vision).[6] Some of these effects seem to arise from increased CNS depression (possibly additive) and/or an increase in the antimuscarinic adverse effects of the tricyclic.

2. Diazepam. A study demonstrated an increase in amitriptyline levels when diazepam was given,[7] and two others found that the addition of diazepam to amitriptyline 50 to 75 mg further reduced attention and the performance of a number of psychomotor tests.[8,9] In contrast, two studies suggested that diazepam did not affect amitriptyline levels.[3,10]

3. Nitrazepam or Oxazepam. Studies on the effects of nitrazepam and oxazepam on the steady-state plasma levels of amitriptyline;[3] did not find any interactions.

(b) Clomipramine

One study suggested that alprazolam does not affect clomipramine levels.[11]

(c) Desipramine

1. Alprazolam. An *in vitro* study in human liver microsomes found that alprazolam does not affect the metabolism (hydroxylation) of desipramine.[12]

2. Clonazepam. An isolated report describes a patient taking desipramine 300 mg daily whose serum desipramine levels were halved when he was given clonazepam 3 mg daily and rose again when it was withdrawn.[13]

3. Zolpidem. Visual hallucinations have been seen in one patient given zolpidem and desipramine.[14]

(d) Imipramine

1. Alprazolam. Alprazolam seems to raise imipramine levels by about 20 to 30%.[15]

2. Triazolam. Triazolam is effective in treating insomnia in depressed patients taking imipramine, and does not reduce the effects of the antidepressant.[16,17]

3. Zaleplon. A single 75-mg dose of imipramine had no effect on the pharmacokinetics of zaleplon 20 mg, and psychomotor tests showed only short term additive effects lasting 1 to 2 hours.[18]

4. Zolpidem. A single-dose study using zolpidem 20 mg and imipramine 75 mg found no effect on the pharmacokinetics of either drug. However, imipramine increased the sedative effects of zolpidem, and anterograde amnesia was seen.[19]

(e) Nortriptyline

Lorazepam may be useful for anxiety or insomnia in elderly depressed patients without impairing the response to treatment with nortriptyline.[20]

Studies on the effects of alprazolam, chlordiazepoxide, diazepam, nitrazepam and oxazepam on the steady-state plasma levels of nortriptyline[3,12,21] found no interactions.

(f) Trimipramine

In a study in 10 healthy subjects, when zopiclone and trimipramine were given concurrently for a week, the bioavailability of zopiclone was reduced by almost 14% and the bioavailability of the trimipramine by almost 27%, but neither of these changes were statistically significant.[22]

Mechanism

Uncertain. Additive CNS depression and increased antimuscarinic effects are a possibility with some combinations.

Importance and management

There seems to be no reason for avoiding the concurrent use of benzodiazepines and tricyclics although the advantages and disadvantages remain the subject of debate. Other combinations of tricyclic antidepressants and benzodiazepines would not be expected to behave differently from those described here. Some patients will possibly experience increased drowsiness and inattention with the more sedative antidepressants such as amitriptyline, particularly during the first few days, and this may be exaggerated by benzodiazepines such as diazepam. Driving risks may therefore be increased.

1. Haider I. A comparative trial of Ro4–6270 and amitriptyline in depressive illness. *Br J Psychiatry* (1967) 113, 993–8.
2. General Practitioner Clinical Trials. Chlordiazepoxide with amitriptyline in neurotic depression. *Practitioner* (1969) 202, 437–40.
3. Silverman G, Braithwaite RA. Benzodiazepines and tricyclic antidepressant plasma levels. *BMJ* (1973) 3, 18–20.
4. Kane FJ, Taylor TW. A toxic reaction to combined Elavil-Librium therapy. *Am J Psychiatry* (1963) 119, 1179–80.
5. Abdou FA. Elavil-Librium combination. *Am J Psychiatry* (1964) 120, 1204.
6. Beresford TP, Feinsilver DL, Hall RCW. Adverse reactions to a benzodiazepine-tricyclic antidepressant compound. *J Clin Psychopharmacol* (1981) 1, 392–4.
7. Dugal R, Caille G, Albert J-M, Cooper SF. Apparent pharmacokinetic interaction of diazepam and amitriptyline in psychiatric patients: a pilot study. *Curr Ther Res* (1975) 18, 679–87.
8. Patat A, Klein MJ, Hucher M, Granier J. Acute effects of amitriptyline on human performance and interactions with diazepam. *Eur J Clin Pharmacol* (1988) 35, 585–92.
9. Moskowitz H, Burns M. The effects on performance of two antidepressants, alone and in combination with diazepam. *Prog Neuropsychopharmacol Biol Psychiatry* (1988) 12, 783–92.
10. Otani K, Nordin C, Bertilsson L. No interaction of diazepam on amitriptyline disposition in depressed patients. *Ther Drug Monit* (1987) 9, 120–2.
11. Carson SW, Wright CE, Millikin SP, Lyon J, Chambers JH. Pharmacokinetic evaluation of the combined administration of alprazolam and clomipramine. *Clin Pharmacol Ther* (1992) 51, 154.
12. Bertilsson L, Åberg-Wistedt A, Lidén A, Otani K, Spina E. Alprazolam does not inhibit the metabolism of nortriptyline in depressed patients or inhibit the metabolism of desipramine in human liver microsomes. *Ther Drug Monit* (1988) 10, 231–3.
13. Deicken RF. Clonazepam-induced reduction in serum desipramine concentration. *J Clin Psychopharmacol* (1988) 8, 71–3.
14. Elko CJ, Burgess JL, Robertson WO. Zolpidem-associated hallucinations and serotonin reuptake inhibition: a possible interaction. *Clin Toxicol* (1998) 36, 195–203.
15. Grasela TH, Antal EJ, Ereshefsky L, Wells BG, Evans RL, Smith RB. An evaluation of population pharmacokinetics in therapeutic trials. Part II. Detection of a drug-drug interaction. *Clin Pharmacol Ther* (1987) 42, 433–41.
16. Cohn JB. Triazolam treatment of insomnia in depressed patients taking tricyclics. *J Clin Psychiatry* (1983) 44, 401–6.
17. Dominguez RA, Jacobson AF, Goldstein BJ, Steinbook RM. Comparison of triazolam and placebo in the treatment of insomnia in depressed patients. *Curr Ther Res* (1984) 36, 856–65.
18. Darwish M. Overview of drug interaction studies with zaleplon. Poster presented at 13th Annual Meeting of Associated Professional Sleep Studies (APSS), Orlando, Florida, June 23rd, 1999.
19. Sauvanet JP, Langer SZ, Morselli PL, eds. Imidazopyridines in Sleep Disorders. New York: Raven Press; 1988 p. 165–73.
20. Buysse DJ, Reynolds CF, Houck PR, Perel JM, Frank E, Begley AE, Mazumdar S, Kupfer DJ. Does lorazepam impair the antidepressant response to nortriptyline and psychotherapy? *J Clin Psychiatry* (1997) 58, 426–432.
21. Gram LF, Overo KF and Kirk L. Influence of neuroleptics and benzodiazepines on metabolism of tricyclic antidepressants in man. *Am J Psychiatry* (1974) 131, 863.
22. Caille G, Du Souich P, Spenard J, Lacasse Y, Vezina M. Pharmacokinetic and clinical parameters of zopiclone and trimipramine when administered simultaneously to volunteers. *Biopharm Drug Dispos* (1984) 5, 117–25.

Tricyclic antidepressants + Bupropion

Bupropion may increase the levels of tricyclic antidepressants that are metabolised by CYP2D6, including desipramine, imipramine, and nortriptyline. Adverse effects including confusion, lethargy and unsteadiness have been reported with nortriptyline and bupropion. A seizure occurred in a patient given trimipramine and bupropion.

Clinical evidence

A pharmacokinetic study in healthy subjects known to be extensive metabolisers of CYP2D6 found that bupropion doubled the maximum plasma levels of **desipramine** and increased its AUC fivefold.[1,2] Another study in a 64-year-old woman taking **imipramine** 150 to 200 mg daily found that when bupropion 225 mg daily was added, there was a fourfold rise in the plasma levels of **imipramine** and its metabolite desipramine, but no problems were reported. A comparison of the estimated clearances were: without bupropion, **imipramine** 1.7 mL/minute and **desipramine** 1.7 mL/minute; with bupropion, **imipramine** 0.73 mL/minute and **desipramine** 0.31 mL/minute.[3]

Nortriptyline toxicity occurred in an 83-year-old woman when sustained-release bupropion was also given. **Nortriptyline** 75 mg at night produced a plasma level of 96 nanograms/mL, but when bupropion

150 mg twice daily was added she became unsteady, confused and lethargic and her plasma **nortriptyline** level increased by about 200% (to 274 nanograms/mL). The increased plasma **nortriptyline** level and toxicity occurred again when she was rechallenged with bupropion.[4] An isolated report describes a seizure when **trimipramine** 100 mg daily was taken with bupropion 150 mg twice daily. The addition of bupropion resulted in a substantial increase in her plasma levels of **trimipramine** into the 'toxic' range. She was later successfully treated with lower doses of both drugs (**trimipramine** 50 mg at night and bupropion 150 mg daily).[5]

Mechanism

In vitro studies[1,2] have shown that both bupropion and its active metabolite, hydroxybupropion, are inhibitors of CYP2D6, the isoenzyme involved with the metabolism of these tricyclics, which would explain why their levels rose.

Importance and management

Although clinical evidence is limited it is supported by *in vitro* data, and so an interaction would seem to be established. It would seem prudent to be alert for increased tricyclic adverse effects if any of these drugs listed here is given with bupropion, and reduce the tricyclic dose as necessary. Note that bupropion is predicted to increase the risk of seizures with tricyclics, and this effect is dose-related. See 'Bupropion + Miscellaneous', p.1206.

1. Zyban (Bupropion hydrochloride). GlaxoSmithKline UK. UK Summary of product characteristics, October 2006.
2. Zyban (Bupropion hydrochloride). GlaxoSmithKline. US Prescribing information, August 2007.
3. Shad MU, Preskorn SH. A possible bupropion and imipramine interaction. *J Clin Psychopharmacol* (1997) 17, 118–19.
4. Weintraub D. Nortriptyline toxicity secondary to interaction with bupropion sustained-release. *Depress Anxiety* (2001) 13, 50–2.
5. Enns MW. Seizure during combination of trimipramine and bupropion. *J Clin Psychiatry* (2001) 62, 476–7.

Tricyclic antidepressants + Butyrophenones

Serum desipramine levels can be considerably increased in a few patients by haloperidol. This may have caused a grand mal seizure in one case but toxic reactions appear to be uncommon. Desipramine and bromperidol appear not to interact.

Clinical evidence

(a) Bromperidol

When 13 schizophrenics taking bromperidol 12 to 24 mg daily for 1 to 20 weeks were additionally given **desipramine** 50 mg daily for a week, bromperidol plasma levels remained unchanged and no adverse clinical events were seen.[1]

(b) Haloperidol

1. Desipramine. A comparative study in patients taking similar doses of desipramine (2.5 to 2.55 mg/kg) showed that the two patients also taking haloperidol had steady-state plasma desipramine levels that were more than double those of 15 others not taking haloperidol (255 nanograms/mL compared with 110 nanograms/mL).[2]
A case report describes a patient who had a grand mal seizure when taking desipramine with haloperidol. Her serum desipramine levels were unusually high at 610 nanograms/mL.[3]

2. Imipramine. The urinary excretion of a test dose of ^{14}C-imipramine given to two schizophrenic patients was reduced by about 35 to 40% when they took haloperidol 12 to 20 mg daily.[4] The plasma metabolite levels of ^{14}C-nortriptyline of another schizophrenic fell while taking haloperidol 16 mg daily, whereas plasma levels of unchanged nortriptyline rose.[5]

Mechanism

Haloperidol reduces the metabolism of the tricyclic antidepressants, thereby reducing their clearance, which results in a rise in their plasma levels.

Importance and management

The interaction between the tricyclic antidepressants and haloperidol is established though its documentation is sparse. Concurrent use is common whereas adverse reactions are not, but be aware that serum desipramine levels may be elevated. This may have been the cause of the grand mal seizure in the case cited.[3] Imipramine appears to interact similarly. Monitor the outcome if haloperidol is added to established treatment with tricyclic antidepressants.

Note that bromperidol and haloperidol prolong the QT-interval, and this effect has been seen with tricyclics, usually in overdose, see also 'Drugs that prolong the QT interval + Other drugs that prolong the QT interval', p.257.

1. Suzuki A, Otani K, Ishida M, Yasui N, Kondo T, Mihara K, Kaneko S, Inoue Y. No interaction between desipramine and bromperidol. *Prog Neuropsychopharmacol Biol Psychiatry* (1996) 20, 1265–71.
2. Nelson JC, Jatlow PI. Neuroleptic effect on desipramine steady-state plasma concentrations. *Am J Psychiatry* (1980) 137, 1232–4.
3. Mahr GC, Berchou R, Balon R. A grand mal seizure associated with desipramine and haloperidol. *Can J Psychiatry* (1987) 32, 463–4.
4. Gram LF, Overø KF. Drug interaction: inhibitory effect of neuroleptics on metabolism of tricyclic antidepressants in man. *BMJ* (1972) 1, 463–5.
5. Gram LF, Overø KF, Kirk L. Influence of neuroleptics and benzodiazepines on metabolism of tricyclic antidepressants in man. *Am J Psychiatry* (1974) 131, 863–6.

Tricyclic antidepressants + Calcium-channel blockers

Diltiazem and verapamil can increase plasma imipramine levels, possibly accompanied by undesirable ECG changes. Two isolated reports describe increased nortriptyline and trimipramine levels in two patients given diltiazem.

Clinical evidence

(a) Imipramine

Twelve healthy subjects were given a 7-day course of **verapamil** 120 mg every 8 hours and 13 healthy subjects were given a 7-day course of **diltiazem** 90 mg every 8 hours. The AUCs of a single 100-mg dose of imipramine given on day 4 were increased by 15% by **verapamil**, and 30% by **diltiazem**. One hour after taking imipramine (2 hours after taking the calcium-channel blockers), the average PR interval was greater than 200 milliseconds, which represented first-degree heart block. Two subjects developed second-degree heart block after taking imipramine with **verapamil**.[1]

(b) Nortriptyline

A diabetic patient taking glipizide and aspirin started taking nortriptyline, and, at the same time, his treatment with **nifedipine** was replaced by **diltiazem** 180 mg daily initially, raised to 240 mg daily after a week. Several changes in the nortriptyline dosage were made over a 4-week period because its plasma levels became unexpectedly high (the ratio of plasma nortriptyline to its dosage were approximately doubled).[2]

(c) Trimipramine

A depressed woman taking trimipramine 125 mg daily developed high plasma levels of 546 micrograms/L while taking **diltiazem** 60 mg three times daily. Two weeks later they reached 708 micrograms/L, despite a reduction in the trimipramine dosage to 75 mg daily. She showed no toxicity and her ECG was normal.[3]

Mechanism

It has been suggested that diltiazem and verapamil increase the bioavailability of imipramine by decreasing its clearance. The ECG changes appear to result from the increased imipramine levels and the additive effects of both drugs on the atrioventricular conduction time. Diltiazem may similarly affect nortriptyline and trimipramine.

Importance and management

Information appears to be limited to these reports so that the general clinical importance of each of these interactions is uncertain. However it would now seem prudent to be alert for evidence of increases in the levels of tricyclic antidepressants if diltiazem or verapamil is added. The evidence of heart block with imipramine and diltiazem is of particular concern.

1. Hermann DJ, Krol TF, Dukes GE, Hussey EK, Danis M, Han Y-H, Powell JR, Hak LJ. Comparison of verapamil, diltiazem, and labetalol on the bioavailability and metabolism of imipramine. *J Clin Pharmacol* (1992) 32, 176–83.

2. Krähenbühl S, Smith-Gamble V, Hoppel CL. Pharmacokinetic interaction between diltiazem and nortriptyline. *Eur J Clin Pharmacol* (1996) 49, 417–19.
3. Cotter PA, Raven PW, Hudson M. Asymptomatic tricyclic toxicity associated with diltiazem. *Ir J Psychol Med* (1996) 13, 168–9.

Tricyclic antidepressants + Cannabis

Tachycardia has been described when patients taking tricyclic antidepressants smoked cannabis.

Clinical evidence, mechanism, importance and management

A 21-year-old woman taking **nortriptyline** 30 mg daily experienced marked tachycardia (an increase from 90 to 160 bpm) after smoking a cannabis cigarette. It was controlled with propranolol.[1] A 26-year-old complained of restlessness, dizziness and tachycardia (120 bpm) after smoking cannabis while taking **imipramine** 50 mg daily.[2] Four adolescents aged 15 to 18 taking tricyclic antidepressants for attention-deficit hyperactivity disorder had transient cognitive changes, delirium and tachycardia after smoking cannabis.[3]

Increased heart rates are well-documented adverse effects of both the tricyclic antidepressants and cannabis, and what occurred was probably due to the additive beta-adrenergic and antimuscarinic effects of the tricyclics, with the beta-adrenergic effect of the cannabis. Direct information is limited but it has been suggested that concurrent use should be avoided.[1]

1. Hillard JR, Vieweg WVR. Marked sinus tachycardia resulting from the synergistic effects of marijuana and nortriptyline. *Am J Psychiatry* (1983) 140, 626–7.
2. Kizer KW. Possible interaction of TCA and marijuana. *Ann Emerg Med* (1980) 9, 444.
3. Wilens TE, Biederman J, Spencer TJ. Case study: adverse effects of smoking marijuana while receiving tricyclic antidepressants. *J Am Acad Child Adolesc Psychiatry* (1997) 36, 45–8.

Tricyclic antidepressants + Carbamazepine

The serum levels of amitriptyline, desipramine, doxepin, imipramine and nortriptyline can be reduced (halved or more) by carbamazepine but there is evidence that this is not necessarily clinically important. In contrast raised clomipramine levels have been seen in patients taking carbamazepine. An isolated report describes carbamazepine toxicity in a patient shortly after she started to take desipramine.

Clinical evidence

(a) Carbamazepine levels increased

A woman receiving long-term treatment with carbamazepine developed toxicity (nausea, vomiting, blurred vision with visual hallucinations, slurred speech, ataxia) within 6 days of starting to take **desipramine** daily (3 days at 150 mg daily). Her carbamazepine levels were found to have doubled from 7.7 to 15 micrograms/mL.[1]

(b) Tricyclic levels increased

A study confirming the value of carbamazepine and **clomipramine** in the treatment of post-herpetic neuralgia found that carbamazepine appeared to raise both **clomipramine** plasma levels and those of its major metabolite (desmethylclomipramine).[2]

(c) Tricyclic levels reduced

A study found that carbamazepine reduced the serum levels of **nortriptyline** by 58% and of **amitriptyline** plus its metabolite, **nortriptyline**, by 60% in 8 psychiatric patients. In 17 other patients carbamazepine reduced serum **doxepin** levels by 54% and **doxepin** plus its metabolite, **nordoxepin**, by 55%.[3] A retrospective study of very large numbers of patients confirmed that carbamazepine approximately halves the serum levels of **amitriptyline** and **nortriptyline**.[4] An elderly woman needed her **nortriptyline** dosage to be increased from 75 to 150 mg daily to achieve effective antidepressant serum levels when carbamazepine 500 to 600 mg daily was added.[5]

In a study in 36 children (aged 5 to 16 years) with attention-deficit disorder taking **imipramine**, or **imipramine** and carbamazepine for 1 to 6 months, found that even though the **imipramine** dosage was significantly higher in the combined treatment group, the plasma levels were significantly lower; and the total plasma antidepressant levels were approximately half of those found in the children not taking carbamazepine.[6] A study[7] in 6 healthy subjects found that carbamazepine 200 mg twice daily for a month increased the apparent oral clearance of a single 100-mg dose of **desipramine** (given on day 24) by 31% and shortened its half-life from 22.1 to 17.8 hours. A patient given **desipramine** and carbamazepine is reported to have had exceptionally low serum **desipramine** levels and cardiac complaints, which may have been due to the presence of increased levels of the hydroxy metabolite of **desipramine**.[8]

A study in 13 patients with endogenous depression (DSM-III-R) taking **imipramine**, which confirmed that carbamazepine reduced the total serum levels of **imipramine** and desipramine, found that levels of the pharmacologically active free drugs remained unchanged.[9,10] Moreover 10 of the patients demonstrated a positive therapeutic response (greater than a 50% decrease in the Hamilton Depression Rating Scale) and a reduction in adverse drug reactions.[9]

Mechanism

It seems likely that the carbamazepine (a recognised enzyme-inducing drug) increases the metabolism and loss of these tricyclics from the body, thereby reducing their serum levels. The reason for the increased serum carbamazepine and clomipramine levels is not understood.

Importance and management

The reduction in the serum levels of amitriptyline, desipramine, doxepin, imipramine and nortriptyline caused by the interaction with carbamazepine appears to be established but the clinical importance is very much less certain. Evidence from one study,[9] that achieved a beneficial response in patients taking tricyclics and carbamazepine suggests that it is possibly not necessary to increase the tricyclic dosage to accommodate this interaction. The fact that a retrospective study found that increased imipramine doses were being given to those taking carbamazepine suggests that this interaction will be naturally accounted for. If carbamazepine is added to treatment with any of these tricyclics, be aware that the dose of the tricyclic may need to be titrated up to achieve the desired therapeutic response. Remember too that the tricyclics can lower the convulsive threshold and should therefore be used with caution in patients with epilepsy.

1. Lesser I. Carbamazepine and desipramine: a toxic reaction. *J Clin Psychiatry* (1984) 45, 360.
2. Gerson GR, Jones RB, Luscombe DK. Studies on the concomitant use of carbamazepine and clomipramine for the relief of post-herpetic neuralgia. *Postgrad Med J* (1977) 53 (Suppl 4), 104–9.
3. Leinonen E, Lillsunde P, Laukkanen V, Ylitalo P. Effects of carbamazepine on serum antidepressant concentrations in psychiatric patients. *J Clin Psychopharmacol* (1991) 11, 313–18.
4. Jerling M, Bertilsson L, Sjöqvist F. The use of therapeutic drug monitoring data to document kinetic drug interactions: an example with amitriptyline and nortriptyline. *Ther Drug Monit* (1994) 16, 1–12.
5. Brøsen K, Kragh-Sørensen P. Concomitant intake of nortriptyline and carbamazepine. *Ther Drug Monit* (1993) 15, 258–60.
6. Brown CS, Wells BG, Cold JA, Froemming JH, Self TH, Jabbour JT. Possible influence of carbamazepine on plasma imipramine concentrations in children with attention deficit hyperactivity disorder. *J Clin Psychopharmacol* (1990) 10, 359–62.
7. Spina E, Avenoso A, Campo GM, Caputi AP, Perucca E. The effect of carbamazepine on the 2-hydroxylation of desipramine. *Psychopharmacology (Berl)* (1995) 117, 413–16.
8. Baldessarini RJ, Teicher MH, Cassidy JW, Stein MH. Anticonvulsant cotreatment may increase toxic metabolites of antidepressants and other psychotropic drugs. *J Clin Psychopharmacol* (1988) 8, 381–2.
9. Szymura-Oleksiak J, Wyska E, Wasieczko A. Effects of carbamazepine coadministration on free and total serum concentrations of imipramine and its metabolites. *Eur J Clin Pharmacol* (1997) 52 (Suppl) A141.
10. Szymura-Oleksiak J, Wyska E, Wasieczko A. Pharmacokinetic interaction between imipramine and carbamazepine in patients with major depression. *Psychopharmacology (Berl)* (2001) 154, 38–42.

Tricyclic antidepressants + Colestyramine

Colestyramine causes a moderate fall in the plasma levels of imipramine. *In vitro* evidence suggests that amitriptyline, desipramine and nortriptyline are likely to be similarly affected. One patient who had an unusual gut pathology and depression controlled by doxepin became depressed again when colestyramine was added.

Clinical evidence

Six depressed patients taking **imipramine** 75 to 150 mg, usually twice daily, were given colestyramine 4 g three times daily for 5 days. The plasma levels of **imipramine** fell by an average of 23% (range 11 to 30%) and the plasma levels of desipramine (the major metabolite) fell, although this was less consistent and said not to be statistically significant.

The effect of these reduced levels on the control of the depression was not assessed.[1]

A man whose depression was controlled with **doxepin** relapsed within a week of starting to take colestyramine 6 g twice daily. Within 3 weeks of increasing the dosage separation of the two drugs from 4 to 6 hours his combined serum antidepressant levels (i.e. **doxepin** plus *n*-desmethyldoxepin) had risen from 39 to 81 nanograms/mL and his depression had improved. Reducing the colestyramine dosage to a single 6-g dose daily, separated from the **doxepin** by 15 hours, resulted in a further rise in his serum antidepressant levels to 117 nanograms/mL accompanied by relief of his depression.[2]

Mechanism

It seems almost certain that these tricyclics become bound to the colestyramine (an anion-exchange resin) within the gut, thereby reducing their absorption. An *in vitro* study[3] with simulated gastric fluid found that, at pH 1, **amitriptyline**, **desipramine**, doxepin, imipramine and **nortriptyline** were approximately 79 to 90% bound by colestyramine: at pH 4 they were 36 to 48% bound and at pH 6.5 they were 62 to 76% bound. In an earlier study,[4] binding of these tricyclics at pH 1 had ranged from 76 to 100%.

Importance and management

The interaction between imipramine and colestyramine is established but of uncertain clinical importance because the fall in the plasma imipramine levels quoted above was only moderate (23%) and the effects were not measured. The single case involving doxepin[2] was unusual because the patient had an abnormal gastrointestinal tract (hemigastrectomy with pyloroplasty and chronic diarrhoea). Nevertheless it would now be prudent to be alert for any evidence of a reduced antidepressant response if colestyramine is given concurrently. A simple way of minimising the admixture of the drugs in the gut is to separate their administration. It is usually suggested that these drugs should be given 1 hour before or 4 to 6 hours after colestyramine. There seems to be no direct clinical information about other tricyclics but *in vitro* studies suggest that amitriptyline, desipramine and nortriptyline probably interact like imipramine.

1. Spina E, Avenoso A, Campo GM, Caputi AP, Perucca E. Decreased plasma concentrations of imipramine and desipramine following cholestyramine intake in depressed patients. *Ther Drug Monit* (1994) 16, 432–4.

2. Geeze DS, Wise MG, Stigelman WH. Doxepin-cholestyramine interaction. *Psychosomatics* (1988) 29, 233–6.

3. Bailey DN. Effect of pH changes and ethanol on the binding of tricyclic antidepressants to cholestyramine in simulated gastric fluid. *Ther Drug Monit* (1992) 14, 343–6.

4. Bailey DN, Coffee JJ, Anderson B, Manoguerra AS. Interactions of tricyclic antidepressants with cholestyramine in vitro. *Ther Drug Monit* (1992) 14, 339–42.

Tricyclic and related antidepressants + Co-trimoxazole

Four patients taking tricyclic antidepressants and one taking viloxazine relapsed when they took co-trimoxazole. Recurrence of panic attacks occurred in another patient taking imipramine when she also took co-trimoxazole.

Clinical evidence, mechanism, importance and management

Four patients taking tricyclic antidepressants (**imipramine**, **clomipramine**, **dibenzepin**) and one taking **viloxazine** relapsed into depression when they took co-trimoxazole (trimethoprim with sulfamethoxazole) for 2 to 9 days.[1] The reasons are not known. Another patient treated for 5 years with alprazolam and **imipramine** for panic disorder and who had not had panic attacks for several months developed insomnia, anxiety and panic attacks within 6 days of starting to take co-trimoxazole. The panic attacks stopped when she stopped taking co-trimoxazole. It is not known whether co-trimoxazole interacted with alprazolam and **imipramine** to reduce their effects or whether co-trimoxazole, which may cause nervousness, had exacerbated the panic disorder.[2] These seem to be the only reports of a possible interaction between these drugs so that the general importance is very uncertain.

1. Brion S, Orssaud E, Chevalier JF, Plas J, Waroquaux O. Interaction entre le cotrimoxazole et les antidépresseurs. *Encephale* (1987) 13, 123–6.

2. Zealberg JJ, Lydiard RB, Christie S. Exacerbation of panic disorder in a woman treated with trimethoprim-sulfamethoxazole. *J Clin Psychopharmacol* (1991) 11, 144–5.

Tricyclic antidepressants + Disulfiram

Disulfiram reduces the clearance of imipramine and desipramine. The concurrent use of amitriptyline and disulfiram has been reported to cause a therapeutically useful increase in the effects of disulfiram but 'organic brain syndrome' has been seen in two patients.

Clinical evidence, mechanism, importance and management

It has been noted that **amitriptyline** increases the effects of both disulfiram and citrated **calcium carbimide** without any increase in adverse effects.[1] However, there is also some evidence that an adverse interaction can occur. A study in two men found that disulfiram 500 mg daily increased the AUC of **imipramine** (12.5 mg given intravenously after an overnight fast) by about 30%, and of **desipramine** 12.5 mg given intravenously in one subject by a similar amount.[2] Peak plasma levels were also increased. The suggested reason is that the disulfiram inhibits the metabolism of the antidepressants by the liver. There is also a report of a man taking disulfiram who, when given **amitriptyline**, complained of dizziness, visual and auditory hallucinations, and who became disorientated to person, place and time. A similar reaction was seen in another patient.[3] Concurrent use should therefore be well monitored for any evidence of toxicity.

1. MacCallum WAG. Drug interactions in alcoholism treatment. *Lancet* (1969) i, 313.

2. Ciraulo DA, Barnhill J, Boxenbaum H. Pharmacokinetic interaction of disulfiram and antidepressants. *Am J Psychiatry* (1985) 142, 1373–4.

3. Maany I, Hayashida M, Pfeffer SL, Kron RE. Possible toxic interaction between disulfiram and amitriptyline. *Arch Gen Psychiatry* (1982) 39, 743–4.

Tricyclic antidepressants + Fenfluramine

It has been said that the concurrent use of tricyclics and fenfluramine is safe and effective; however, others have suggested that as fenfluramine can cause depression, concurrent use should be avoided if the tricyclic is given for depression.

Clinical evidence, mechanism, importance and management

Exacerbation of depression has been seen in some patients given fenfluramine[1] and several cases of withdrawal depression have been observed in patients taking amitriptyline and fenfluramine, following episodes of severe depression.[2] The manufacturers have advised that fenfluramine should not be used in patients with a history of depression or in those being treated with antidepressants.[3] On the other hand it has also been claimed that fenfluramine can be used safely and effectively with tricyclic antidepressants.[4,5] One report describes a rise in the plasma levels of amitriptyline when fenfluramine 60 mg daily was given to patients taking amitriptyline 150 mg daily.[6]

Note that fenfluramine was widely withdrawn in 1997 because its use was found to be associated with a high incidence of abnormal echocardiograms indicating abnormal functioning of heart valves.

1. Gaind R. Fenfluramine (Ponderax) in the treatment of obese psychiatric out-patients. *Br J Psychiatry* (1969) 115, 963–4.

2. Harding T. Fenfluramine dependence. *BMJ* (1971) 3, 305.

3. ABPI Data Sheet Compendium, 1998–99 p 1307. Datapharm publications, London.

4. Pinder RM, Brogden RN, Sawyer PR, Speight TM, Avery GS. Fenfluramine: a review of its pharmacological properties and therapeutic efficacy in obesity. *Drugs* (1975) 10, 241–323.

5. Mason EC. Servier Laboratories Ltd. Personal Communication, February 1976.
6. Gunne L-M, Antonijevic S, Jonsson J. Effect of fenfluramine on steady state plasma levels of amitriptyline. *Postgrad Med J* (1975) 51 (Suppl 1), 117.

Tricyclic antidepressants + Flupentixol

Flupentixol did not inhibit the metabolism of imipramine in two patients but high levels of imipramine and its metabolite, desipramine, were found in another patient.

Clinical evidence, mechanism, importance and management

A study using ^{14}C-**imipramine** showed that, unlike the situation with the 'phenothiazines', (p.760), flupentixol 3 to 6 mg daily did not inhibit the metabolism of **imipramine** in 2 patients.[1] However, there is an isolated report of very high plasma levels of **imipramine** and its metabolite desipramine in a patient with schizophrenia who was given flupentixol decanoate 40 mg intramuscularly once every 2 weeks and **imipramine** 150 mg daily. It was suggested that this may have resulted from competitive inhibition of liver enzymes.[2] This is an isolated case and its general significance is unknown.

1. Gram LF, Overø KF. Drug interaction: inhibitory effect of neuroleptics on metabolism of tricyclic antidepressants in man. *BMJ* (1972) 1, 463–5.
2. Cook PE, Dermer SW, Cardamone J. Imipramine-flupenthixol decanoate interaction. *Can J Psychiatry* (1986) 31, 235–7.

Tricyclic antidepressants + Food

Limited evidence suggests that very high fibre diets can reduce the serum levels of doxepin and desipramine, and therefore decrease their effects. The bioavailability of amitriptyline may be affected by food.

Clinical evidence, mechanism, importance and management

Three patients showed no response to **doxepin** or **desipramine** and had reduced serum tricyclic antidepressant levels while taking very high **fibre diets** (**wheat bran**, **wheat germ**, **oat bran**, **rolled oats**, **sunflower seeds**, **coconut shreds**, **raisins**, **bran muffins**). When the diet was changed or stopped, the serum tricyclic antidepressant levels rose and the depression was relieved.[1] The reasons for this effect are not known. This interaction may possibly provide an explanation for otherwise unaccountable relapses or inadequate responses to tricyclic antidepressant treatment. Another study in 12 healthy subjects found that **breakfast** had no effect on the bioavailability of a 50-mg dose of **imipramine**, or on its peak levels or the time to peak levels.[2] A study in 9 healthy subjects given a single 25-mg dose of **amitriptyline** in the fasting state and with a standardised **breakfast** found that there were no consistent significant changes in the bioavailability of **amitriptyline** or its main metabolite nortriptyline. Similar results were found in a parallel study in which the same subjects were given a single 25-mg dose of **nortriptyline**. However, there were large inter-individual changes in the AUC of **amitriptyline** after food, ranging from an increase of 94% to a decrease of about 40%. The largest food-related **amitriptyline** AUC *increases* occurred among the subjects with the lowest fasting AUC values and the only major food-related *decrease* occurred in the subject with the largest fasting AUC. It was concluded that for an individual patient, the timing of **amitriptyline** administration in relation to food intake should be standardised to avoid large variations in drug levels.[3]

1. Stewart DE. High-fiber diet and serum tricyclic antidepressant levels. *J Clin Psychopharmacol* (1992) 12, 438–40.
2. Abernethy DR, Divoll M, Greenblatt DJ, Shader RI. Imipramine pharmacokinetics and absolute bioavailability: effect of food. *Clin Res* (1983) 31, 626A.
3. Liedholm H, Lidén A. Food intake and the presystemic metabolism of single doses of amitriptyline and nortriptyline. *Fundam Clin Pharmacol* (1998) 12, 636–42.

Tricyclic antidepressants + Grapefruit juice

Grapefruit juice does not appear to have a clinically significant affect on amitriptyline or clomipramine levels or imipramine absorption.

Clinical evidence, mechanism, importance and management

A study in 6 patients given **clomipramine** 112.5 to 225 mg daily found that grapefruit juice 250 mL increased the mean plasma levels of **clomipramine** and desmethylclomipramine by 4.5% and 10.5%, respectively. In another 7 patients taking **amitriptyline** 100 to 150 mg daily grapefruit juice did not affect tricyclic plasma levels.[1]

1. Vandel P, Regina W, Reix I, Vandel S, Sechter D, Bizouard P. Faut-il contre-indiquer le jus de pamplemousse? Une approche en psychiatrie. [Grapefruit juice as a contraindication? An approach in psychiatry]. *Encephale* (1999) 25, 67–71.

Tricyclic antidepressants + H_2-receptor antagonists

Cimetidine can raise the plasma levels of amitriptyline, desipramine, doxepin, imipramine and nortriptyline. Other tricyclic antidepressants are expected to interact similarly. Ranitidine does not appear to interact with the tricyclics.

Clinical evidence

(a) Amitriptyline

After a group of healthy subjects took **cimetidine** 300 mg every 6 hours for two days, the peak plasma levels and the AUC of a single 25-mg dose of amitriptyline were raised by 37% and 80%, respectively.[1]

Another study by the same authors found that **ranitidine** does not interact with amitriptyline.[2]

(b) Desipramine

In a study in 8 patients **cimetidine** 1 g daily for 4 days raised the plasma levels of desipramine 100 to 250 mg daily by 51%, and its hydroxylated metabolite (2-hydroxydesipramine) was raised by 46%.[3] Another study showed that this interaction only occurs in those individuals who are [CYP2D6 extensive metabolisers].[4]

(c) Doxepin

A study in 10 healthy subjects given a single 100-mg oral dose of doxepin 12 hours after starting to take **cimetidine** 300 mg every 6 hours found that the peak plasma level and AUC of doxepin were raised by 28% and 31%, respectively.[5]

In another study **cimetidine** 600 mg twice daily was found to double the steady-state plasma levels of doxepin 50 mg daily, whereas **ranitidine** 300 mg daily had no effect.[6] A patient taking doxepin complained that the normally mild adverse effects (urinary hesitancy, dry mouth and decreased visual acuity) became incapacitating when he also took **cimetidine**. His serum doxepin levels were found to be elevated.[7]

(d) Imipramine

In 12 healthy subjects **cimetidine** 300 mg every 6 hours for 3 days raised the peak plasma levels and the AUC of a single 100-mg dose of imipramine by 65% and 172%, respectively. After taking **ranitidine** 150 mg twice daily for 3 days the pharmacokinetics of imipramine were unaltered.[8] These findings with **cimetidine** confirm those of previous studies.[9,10]

There are case reports of patients taking imipramine who developed severe antimuscarinic adverse effects (dry mouth, urine retention, blurred vision) associated with very marked rises in serum imipramine levels when they also took **cimetidine**.[11,12]

(e) Nortriptyline

After taking **cimetidine** 300 mg four times daily for 2 days, the peak plasma nortriptyline levels of 6 healthy subjects were not significantly raised, but the AUC was increased by 20%.[9]

A case report describes a patient whose serum nortriptyline levels were raised about one-third while taking **cimetidine**.[13] Another patient complained of abdominal pain and distention (but no other antimuscarinic adverse effects) when treated with nortriptyline and **cimetidine**.[14]

Mechanism

Cimetidine is a potent liver enzyme inhibitor, which reduces the metabolism of the tricyclic antidepressants, and may also reduce the hepatic clearance of these drugs. This results in a rise in their serum levels. Ranitidine does not interact because it is not an enzyme inhibitor.

Importance and management

The interactions with cimetidine are well established, well documented and of clinical importance. The incidence is uncertain but most patients could be affected. Those taking amitriptyline, desipramine, doxepin, imipramine or nortriptyline who are given cimetidine should be warned that adverse effects such as mouth dryness, urine retention, blurred vision, constipation, tachycardia, postural hypotension may be more likely to occur. Other tricyclic antidepressants would be expected to be similarly affected. If symptoms are troublesome reduce the dosage of the antidepressant (33 to 50% has been suggested) or replace the cimetidine with ranitidine, which does not appear to interact. Other H_2-receptor antagonists that do not cause enzyme inhibition (e.g. **famotidine** and **nizatidine**) would also not be expected to interact.

1. Curry SH, DeVane CL, Wolfe MM. Cimetidine interaction with amitriptyline. *Eur J Clin Pharmacol* (1985) 29, 429–33.
2. Curry SH, DeVane CL, Wolfe MM. Lack of interaction of ranitidine with amitriptyline. *Eur J Clin Pharmacol* (1987) 32, 317–20.
3. Amsterdam JD, Brunswick DJ, Potter L, Kaplan MJ. Cimetidine-induced alterations in desipramine plasma concentrations. *Psychopharmacology (Berl)* (1984) 83, 373–5.
4. Steiner E, Spina E. Differences in the inhibitory effect of cimetidine on desipramine metabolism between rapid and slow debrisoquin hydroxylators. *Clin Pharmacol Ther* (1987) 42, 278–82.
5. Abernethy DR, Todd EL. Doxepin-cimetidine interaction: increased doxepin bioavailability during cimetidine treatment. *J Clin Psychopharmacol* (1986) 6, 8–12.
6. Sutherland DL, Remillard AJ, Haight KR, Brown MA, Old L. The influence of cimetidine versus ranitidine on doxepin pharmacokinetics. *Eur J Clin Pharmacol* (1987) 32, 159–64.
7. Brown MA, Haight KR, McKay G. Cimetidine-doxepin interaction. *J Clin Psychopharmacol* (1985) 5, 245–7.
8. Wells BG, Pieper JA, Self TH, Stewart CF, Waldon SL, Bobo L, Warner C. The effect of ranitidine and cimetidine on imipramine disposition. *Eur J Clin Pharmacol* (1986) 31, 285–90.
9. Henauer SA, Hollister LE. Cimetidine interaction with imipramine and nortriptyline. *Clin Pharmacol Ther* (1984) 35, 183–7.
10. Abernethy DR, Greenblatt DJ, Shader RI. Imipramine-cimetidine interaction: impairment of clearance and enhanced absolute bioavailability. *J Pharmacol Exp Ther* (1984) 229, 702–705.
11. Shapiro PA. Cimetidine-imipramine interaction: case report and comments. *Am J Psychiatry* (1984) 141, 152.
12. Miller DD, Macklin M. Cimetidine-imipramine interaction: a case report. *Am J Psychiatry* (1983) 140, 351–2.
13. Miller DD, Sawyer JB, Duffy JP. Cimetidine's effect on steady-state serum nortriptyline concentrations. *Drug Intell Clin Pharm* (1983) 17, 904–5.
14. Lerro FA. Abdominal distention syndrome in a patient receiving cimetidine-nortriptyline therapy. *J Med Soc New Jers* (1983) 80, 631–2.

Tricyclic antidepressants + Inotropes and Vasopressors

Patients taking tricyclic antidepressants show a grossly exaggerated response (hypertension, cardiac arrhythmias, etc.) to parenteral noradrenaline (norepinephrine), adrenaline (epinephrine) and to a lesser extent to phenylephrine. Case reports suggest that this interaction only occurs rarely with local anaesthetics containing these vasoconstrictors.

Clinical evidence

The effects of intravenous infusions of **noradrenaline (norepinephrine)** were increased approximately ninefold, and of **adrenaline (epinephrine)** approximately threefold, in 6 healthy subjects who had been taking **protriptyline** 60 mg daily for 4 days.[1,2]

The pressor effects of intravenous infusions of **noradrenaline** were increased four to eightfold, of **adrenaline** two to fourfold, and of **phenylephrine** two to threefold in 4 healthy subjects who had been taking **imipramine** 75 mg daily for 5 days. There were no noticeable or consistent changes in their response to **isoprenaline (isoproterenol)**.[3] However, in a study of possible adverse interactions between **imipramine** and **isoprenaline**, although no abnormalities of heart rhythm were seen, one out of the 4 healthy subjects studied showed potentiation of **isoprenaline**- induced tachycardia.[4]

Five patients taking **nortriptyline**, **desipramine** or other unnamed tricyclic antidepressants experienced adverse reactions, some of them severe (throbbing headache, chest pain) following the injection of ***Xylestesin*** (lidocaine with 1:25 000 **noradrenaline**) during dental treatment.[5] Several episodes of marked increases in blood pressure, dilated pupils, intense malaise, violent but transitory tremor, and palpitations have been reported in patients taking unnamed tricyclic antidepressants when they were given local anaesthetics containing **adrenaline** or **noradrenaline** for dental treatment.[6]

There are other reports describing this interaction of:

- **noradrenaline** with **imipramine**,[7-9] **clomipramine**,[9] **desipramine**,[8,10] **nortriptyline**,[11] **protriptyline**[10] and **amitriptyline**;[8,10]
- **adrenaline** with **amitriptyline**,[12]
- **corbadrine** with **desipramine** (in *dogs*).[13]

Mechanism

The tricyclics and some related antidepressants block or inhibit the uptake of noradrenaline (norepinephrine) into adrenergic neurones. Thus the most important means by which noradrenaline is removed from the adrenoceptor area is inactivated and the concentration of noradrenaline outside the neurone can rise. If more noradrenaline (or one of the other directly acting alpha or alpha/beta agonists) is then given, the adrenoceptors of the cardiovascular system concerned with raising blood pressure become grossly stimulated by this superabundance of amines, and the normal response becomes exaggerated.

Importance and management

A well documented, well established and potentially serious interaction. The parenteral use of noradrenaline (norepinephrine), adrenaline (epinephrine), phenylephrine or any other sympathomimetic amines with predominantly direct activity should be avoided in patients taking tricyclic antidepressants. If these inotropes must be used, the rate and amount injected must be very much reduced to accommodate the exaggerated responses that will occur. However, the situation where adrenaline or noradrenaline are used with a local anaesthetic for surface or infiltration anaesthesia, or nerve block is less clear. The cases cited are all from the 1960s or 1970s, and the preparations concerned contained concentrations of adrenaline or noradrenaline several times greater than those used currently. However, it should be noted that preparations such as *Xylocaine* with adrenaline still carry a caution about their use with tricyclic antidepressants.[14] Anecdotal evidence suggests that local anaesthetics containing sympathomimetics are, in practice, commonly used in patients receiving tricyclic antidepressants,[15] so the sparsity of reports, especially recent ones, would add weight to the argument that the interaction is only rarely significant. However, it would still seem advisable to be aware of the potential for interaction. Aspiration has been recommended to avoid inadvertent intravenous administration. **Felypressin** has been shown to be a safe alternative.[16-18] If an adverse interaction occurs it can be controlled by the use of an alpha-receptor blocker, such as phentolamine.

Doxepin in doses of less than 150 to 200 mg daily blocks neuronal uptake much less than other tricyclic antidepressants and so is unlikely to show this interaction to the same degree, but in larger doses it will interact like other tricyclics.[19,20] It does not seem to have been established whether the response to oral doses or nasal drops containing phenylephrine is enhanced by the presence of a tricyclic, but there seem to be no reports of problems.

1. Svedmyr N. The influence of a tricyclic antidepressive agent (protriptyline) on some of the circulatory effects of noradrenaline and adrenaline in man. *Life Sci* (1968) 7, 77–84.
2. Svedmyr N. Potentieringsrisker vid tillförsel av katekolaminer till patienter som behandlas med tricykliska antidepressiva medel. *Lakartidningen* (1968) 65 (Suppl 1), 72–6.
3. Boakes AJ, Laurence DR, Teoh PC, Barar FSK, Benedikter LT, Prichard BNC. Interactions between sympathomimetic amines and antidepressant agents in man. *BMJ* (1973) 1, 311–15.
4. Boakes AJ, Laurence DR, Teoh PC, Barar FSK, Benedikter LT, Prichard BNC. Interactions between sympathomimetic amines and antidepressant agents in man. *BMJ* (1973) 1, 311–15.
5. Boakes AJ, Laurence DR, Lovel KW, O'Neil R, Verrill PJ. Adverse reactions to local anaesthetic/vasoconstrictor preparations. A study of the cardiovascular responses to Xylestesin and Hostacain-with-Noradrenaline. *Br Dent J* (1972) 133, 137–40.
6. Dam WH. Personal communication cited by Kristoffersen MB. Antidepressivas potensering af katekolaminvirkning. *Ugeskr Laeger* (1969) 131, 1013–14.
7. Gershon S, Holmberg G, Mattsson E, Mattsson N, Marshall A. Imipramine hydrochloride. Its effects on clinical, autonomic and psychological functions. *Arch Gen Psychiatry* (1962) 6, 96–101.
8. Fischbach R, Harrer G, Harrer H. Verstärkung der noradrenalin-wirkung durch psychopharmaka beim menschen. *Arzneimittelforschung* (1966) 16, 263–5.
9. Borg K-O, Johnsson G, Jordö L, Lundborg P, Rönn O, Welin-Fogelberg I. Interaction studies between three antidepressant drugs (zimelidine, imipramine and chlorimipramine) and noradrenaline in healthy volunteers and some pharmacokinetics of the drugs studied. *Acta Pharmacol Toxicol (Copenh)* (1979) 45, 198–205.
10. Mitchell JR, Cavanaugh JH, Arias L, Oates JA. Guanethidine and related agents. III. Antagonism by drugs which inhibit the norepinephrine pump in man. *J Clin Invest* (1970) 49, 1596–1604.
11. Persson G, Siwers B. The risk of potentiating effect of local anaesthesia with adrenalin in patients treated with tricyclic antidepressants. *Swed Dent J* (1975) 68, 9–18.
12. Siemkowicz E. Hjertestop efter amitriptylin og adrenalin. *Ugeskr Laeger* (1975) 137, 1403–4.
13. Dreyer AC, Offermeier J. The influence of desipramine on the blood pressure elevation and heart rate stimulation of levonordefrin and felypressin alone and in the presence of local anaesthetics. *J Dent Assoc S Afr* (1986) 41, 615–18.

14. Xylocaine 1% and 2% with Adrenaline (Lidocaine with Adrenaline). AstraZeneca UK Ltd. UK Summary of product characteristics, September 2006.
15. Brown RS, Lewis VA. More on the contraindications to vasoconstrictors in dentistry. *Oral Surg Oral Med Oral Pathol* (1993) 76, 2–3.
16. Aellig WH, Laurence DR, O'Neil R, Verrill PJ. Cardiac effects of adrenaline and felypressin as vasoconstrictors in local anaesthesia for oral surgery under diazepam sedation. *Br J Anaesth* (1970) 42, 174–6.
17. Goldman V, Astrom A, Evers H. The effect of a tricyclic antidepressant on the cardiovascular effects of local anaesthetic solutions containing different vasoconstrictors. *Anaesthesia* (1971) 26, 91.
18. Perovic J, Terzic M, Todorovic L. Safety of local anaesthesia induced by prilocaine with felypressin in patients on tricyclic antidepressants. *Bull Group Int Rech Sci Stomatol Odontol* (1979) 22, 57–62.
19. Fann WE, Cavanaugh JH, Kaufmann JS, Griffith JD, Davis JM, Janowsky DS, Oates JA. Doxepin: effects on transport of biogenic amines in man. *Psychopharmacologia* (1971) 22, 111–25.
20. Oates JA, Fann WE, Cavanaugh JH. Effect of doxepin on the norepinephrine pump. *Psychosomatics* (1969) 10, 12–13.

Tricyclic antidepressants + Macrolides

Troleandomycin increases the plasma levels of imipramine, and an isolated report suggests that josamycin may possibly increase amitriptyline serum levels. Erythromycin may possibly raise clomipramine levels, but was not found to interact with other tricyclic antidepressants in one study.

Clinical evidence, mechanism, importance and management

(a) Erythromycin

Erythromycin 250 mg four times daily for 6 days was found not to affect the tricyclic antidepressant levels of 8 patients taking **desipramine**, **imipramine**, **doxepin**, or **nortriptyline**.[1] Behavioural changes have been reported in a 15-year-old patient when erythromycin was added to a regimen of **clomipramine** and risperidone,[2] resulting in symptoms compatible with the serotonin syndrome, although mental confusion and autonomic instability were absent.[3] It was suggested that erythromycin increased **clomipramine** levels by inhibiting its metabolism by the cytochrome P450 isoenzyme CYP3A4.[4] **Clomipramine** levels may also have been raised by competition with risperidone for metabolism by CYP2D6.

(b) Josamycin

A patient taking **amitriptyline** had a marked increase in the total serum levels of **amitriptyline** and its metabolite, nortriptyline, after taking josamycin but no toxicity was reported. It was suggested that josamycin had inhibited **amitriptyline** metabolism.[5] This is only an isolated case and its general significance is unknown.

(c) Troleandomycin

A study in 9 healthy Chinese men found that when they were given troleandomycin 250 mg daily for 2 days before a single 100-mg oral dose of **imipramine**, the AUC of the **imipramine** was increased by 59% and its oral clearance was reduced by 30%. It is thought that troleandomycin inhibits the *N*-demethylation of **imipramine** by inhibiting the cytochrome P450 isoenzyme subfamily CYP3A.[6] The clinical importance of this interaction is uncertain, but it may be prudent to be alert for increased antimuscarinic adverse effects (e.g. dry mouth, blurred vision, urinary retention).

1. Amsterdam JD, Maislin G. Effect of erythromycin on tricyclic antidepressant metabolism. *J Clin Psychopharmacol* (1991) 11, 203–6.
2. Fisman S, Reniers D, Diaz P. Erythromycin interaction with risperidone or clomipramine in an adolescent. *J Child Adolesc Psychopharmacol* (1996) 6, 133–8.
3. Fisman S, Diaz P. Erythromycin and clomipramine: Noncompetitive inhibition of demethylation. Reply. *J Child Adolesc Psychopharmacol* (1996) 6, 213.
4. Oesterheld JR. Erythromycin and clomipramine: Noncompetitive inhibition of demethylation. *J Child Adolesc Psychopharmacol* (1996) 6, 211–12.
5. Sánchez Romero A, Calzado Solaz C. Posible interacción entre josamicina y amitriptilina. *Med Clin (Barc)* (1992) 98, 279.
6. Wang J-S, Wang W, Xie H-G, Huang S-L, Zhou H-H. Effect of troleandomycin on the pharmacokinetics of imipramine in Chinese: the role of CYP3A. *Br J Clin Pharmacol* (1997) 44, 195–8.

Tricyclic antidepressants + Modafinil

Clomipramine serum levels were reported to be increased by modafinil in one patient. However, a study found no pharmacokinetic interaction.

Clinical evidence, mechanism, importance and management

In a placebo-controlled, crossover study, 18 patients were given a single 50-mg dose of **clomipramine** on day 1 and modafinil 200 mg daily on days 1 to 3. No pharmacokinetic changes were found to have occurred with either of the two drugs.[1] However, a single case report describes a patient taking **clomipramine** 75 mg daily who had a rise in serum **clomipramine** and desmethylclomipramine levels when modafinil 200 mg was added.[2] It was suggested that she had low levels of the cytochrome P450 isoenzyme CYP2D6 (a 'poor metaboliser') so that the additional inhibition of CYP2C19 by modafinil resulted in elevated serum levels.

Information about other tricyclic antidepressants is lacking, but the manufacturers of modafinil point out that other poor metabolisers (about 7 to 10% of the Caucasian population) may possibly also show increased serum tricyclic antidepressant levels in the presence of modafinil.[3,4] Therefore monitoring concurrent use would seem to be a prudent precaution.

1. Wong YN, Gorman S, Simcoe D, McCormick GC, Grebow P. A double-blind placebo-controlled crossover study to investigate the kinetics and acute tolerability of modafinil and clomipramine alone and in combination in healthy male volunteers. Association of Professional Sleep Societies meeting, San Francisco, June 1997, Abstract 117.
2. Grözinger M, Härtter S, Hiemke C, Griese E-U, Röschke J. Interaction of modafinil and clomipramine as comedication in a narcoleptic patient. *Clin Neuropharmacol* (1998) 21, 127–9.
3. Provigil (Modafinil). Cephalon, Inc. US Prescribing information, December 2004.
4. Provigil (Modafinil). Cephalon Ltd. UK Summary of product characteristics, July 2007.

Tricyclic antidepressants + Nasal decongestants

The effects of phenylpropanolamine, pseudoephedrine and other related drugs would be expected to be reduced by the tricyclic antidepressants, but so far only one case, involving ephedrine and amitriptyline, seems to have been reported.

Clinical evidence, mechanism, importance and management

Drugs such as **phenylpropanolamine** and **pseudoephedrine** exert their effects by causing the release of noradrenaline (norepinephrine) from adrenergic neurones. In the presence of a tricyclic antidepressant, the uptake of these amines into adrenergic neurones is partially or totally prevented and the noradrenaline-releasing effects are therefore blocked. Consequently the effects of drugs such as **phenylpropanolamine** would be expected to be reduced by tricyclic antidepressants. This predicted interaction has been listed by the manufacturers in some data sheets. However, the almost total lack of evidence in the literature suggests that this is no more than a theoretical interaction. The only report found describes an elderly woman taking **amitriptyline** 75 mg daily, who developed hypotension (70 mmHg systolic) during subarachnoid anaesthesia. Her blood pressure rose only minimally when she was given intravenous boluses of **ephedrine** totalling 90 mg.[1]

Bearing in mind how long and how widely both groups of drugs have been in use, the absence of any other reports would suggest that any interaction between them is rarely of practical importance.

1. Serle DG. Amitriptyline and ephedrine in subarachnoid anesthesia. *Anaesth Intensive Care* (1985) 13, 214.

Tricyclic antidepressants + Oestrogens

There is evidence that oestrogens can sometimes reduce the effects of imipramine, yet at the same time paradoxically cause imipramine toxicity. The general clinical importance of this interaction has yet to be evaluated.

Clinical evidence

A study in women taking **imipramine** 150 mg daily for primary depression found that those given **ethinylestradiol** 25 or 50 micrograms [daily] for one week showed greater improvement than those given **imipramine** alone. However, after 2 weeks, those given **ethinylestradiol** 50 micrograms daily showed less improvement than other women given only 25 micrograms of **ethinylestradiol** [daily] or a placebo.[1] In an earlier associated study 5 patients taking **imipramine** 150 mg and **ethinylestradiol** 50 micrograms daily developed signs of **imipramine** toxicity (severe lethargy (4 patients), hypotension (4), coarse tremor (2), mild depersonalisation (2)) that was dealt with by halving the **imipramine** dose.[1] Another study found that oral contraceptives increased the absolute bioavailability of **imipramine** by 60%.[2]

Long-standing **imipramine** toxicity was relieved in a woman taking **imipramine** 100 mg daily when her dosage of conjugated oestrogen was reduced to 25%.[3] However, although several studies have shown that serum **clomipramine** levels were raised or remained unaffected by the concurrent use of oestrogen-containing contraceptives, they failed to confirm that tricyclic antidepressant toxicity occurs more often in those taking oral contraceptives than those who are not.[4-7] Akathisia in 3 patients has been attributed to an interaction between conjugated oestrogens and **amitriptyline** or **clomipramine**.[8]

Mechanism

Among the possible reasons for these effects are that the oestrogens increase the bioavailability of imipramine,[2] or inhibit its metabolism.[9]

Importance and management

These interactions are inadequately established. There is no obvious reason for avoiding concurrent use, but it would seem reasonable to be alert for any evidence of toxicity and/or lack of response to tricyclic antidepressant treatment in those taking oestrogens in any form. One study suggested that the imipramine dosage should be reduced by about one-third.[2] More study is needed.

1. Prange AJ, Wilson IC, Alltop LB. Estrogen may well affect response to antidepressant. *JAMA* (1972) 219, 143–4.
2. Abernethy DR, Greenblatt DJ, Shader RI. Imipramine disposition in users of oral contraceptive steroids. *Clin Pharmacol Ther* (1984) 35, 792–7.
3. Khurana RC. Estrogen-imipramine interaction. *JAMA* (1972) 222, 702–3.
4. Beaumont G. Drug interactions with clomipramine (Anafranil). *J Int Med Res* (1973) 1, 480–84.
5. Gringras M, Beaumont G, Grieve A. Clomipramine and oral contraceptives: an interaction study — clinical findings. *J Int Med Res* (1980) 8 (Suppl 3), 76–80.
6. Luscombe DK, Jones RB. Effects of concomitantly administered drugs on plasma levels of clomipramine and desmethylclomipramine in depressive patients receiving clomipramine therapy. *Postgrad Med J* (1977) 53 (Suppl 4), 77.
7. John VA, Luscombe DK, Kemp H. Effects of age, cigarette smoking and the oral contraceptive on the pharmacokinetics of clomipramine and its desmethyl metabolite during chronic dosing. *J Int Med Res* (1980) 8 (Suppl 3), 88–95.
8. Krishnan KRR, France RD, Ellinwood EH Jr. Tricyclic-induced akathisia in patients taking conjugated estrogens. *Am J Psychiatry* (1984) 141, 696–7.
9. Somani SM, Khurana RC. Mechanism of estrogen-imipramine interaction. *JAMA* (1973) 223, 560.

Tricyclic antidepressants + Orlistat

Orlistat appears not to affect the plasma levels of clomipramine or desipramine in patients, or the pharmacokinetics of amitriptyline in healthy subjects.

Clinical evidence, mechanism, importance and management

A preliminary study in patients who had been taking psychotropic drugs long-term found no clinically relevant changes in plasma levels of **clomipramine** (3 patients) or **desipramine** (1 patient) when they were given orlistat over an 8-week period.[1] A study in 20 healthy subjects found that orlistat 120 mg three times daily for 6 days did not affect the pharmacokinetics of **amitriptyline** 25 mg three times daily.[2]

Although evidence is limited no particular precautions seem likely to be necessary on concurrent use.

1. Hilger E, Quiner S, Ginzel I, Walter H, Saria L, Barnas C. The effect of orlistat on plasma levels of psychotropic drugs in patients with long-term psychopharmacotherapy. *J Clin Psychopharmacol* (2002) 22, 68–70.
2. Zhi J, Moore R, Kanitra L, Mulligan TE. Pharmacokinetic evaluation of the possible interaction between selected concomitant medications and orlistat at steady state in healthy subjects. *J Clin Pharmacol* (2002) 42, 1011–19.

Tricyclic antidepressants + Protease inhibitors

Ritonavir raises desipramine levels and is predicted to also raise the levels of other tricyclic antidepressants.

Clinical evidence, mechanism, importance and management

A single 100-mg dose of **desipramine** was given to 14 healthy subjects before and after they took **ritonavir** 500 mg twice daily for 10 days. The AUC and half-life of **desipramine** increased nearly 2.5-fold and 2-fold, respectively. The maximum plasma levels were also increased by about 22%. These changes are considered to be clinically significant, so the authors suggest that a lower initial dose of **desipramine** should be used if it is to be started in patients taking **ritonavir**, and careful monitoring should be carried out in the first few weeks of treatment.[1] These effects are likely to be due to the inhibitory effects of **ritonavir** on the cytochrome P450 isoenzyme CYP2D6.[2] Because of this, the manufacturers of **ritonavir** also predict that the levels of other tricyclic antidepressants (e.g. **amitriptyline**, **imipramine**, **nortriptyline**) will also be raised, and they suggest careful monitoring of adverse effects if any tricyclic is used with **ritonavir**. A dose reduction of the tricyclic may be required.[3,4] *In vitro* data show that other protease inhibitors also inhibit **desipramine** hydroxylation (in order of potency; **indinavir**, **saquinavir**, and then **nelfinavir**), but all of these drugs have less of an effect than **ritonavir**.[2]

1. Bertz RI, Cao G, Cavanaugh JH, Hsu A, Granneman GR, Leonard JM. Effect of ritonavir on the pharmacokinetics of desipramine. 11th International Conference on AIDS, Vancouver, 1996. Abstract Mo.B.1201.
2. Von Moltke LL, Greenblatt DJ, Duan SX, Daily JP, Harmatz JS, Shader RI. Inhibition of desipramine hydroxylation (cytochrome P450-2D6) in vitro by quinidine and by viral protease inhibitors: relation to drug interactions in vivo. *J Pharm Sci* (1998) 87, 1184–9.
3. Norvir (Ritonavir). Abbott Laboratories. US Prescribing information, January 2006.
4. Norvir (Ritonavir). Abbott Laboratories Ltd. UK Summary of product characteristics, May 2007.

Tricyclic antidepressants + Quinidine or Quinine

Quinidine can reduce the clearance of desipramine, imipramine, nortriptyline and trimipramine, and quinine can reduce the clearance of desipramine, thereby increasing their serum levels.

Clinical evidence

(a) Quinidine

In a study in 5 healthy subjects quinidine 50 mg given 1 hour before a single 50-mg dose of **nortriptyline** increased the **nortriptyline** AUC fourfold, and the half-life threefold (from 14.2 to 44.7 hours).[1] The clearance fell from 5.4 to 1.9 mL/minute.

A single-dose study in healthy subjects found that quinidine 200 mg daily reduced the clearance of **imipramine** 100 mg by 30% and **desipramine** 100 mg by 85%.[2] A further study in 2 healthy subjects similarly found that quinidine 50 mg almost doubled the half-life of a single 75-mg dose of **trimipramine**, which was reflected in some waking EEG changes.[3]

In healthy subjects given quinidine 800 mg daily for 2 days, the urinary excretion of 2-hydroxydesipramine from a single 25-mg dose of **desipramine** was reduced by 97% and 68% in rapid and slow hydroxylators, respectively.[4]

(b) Quinine

Quinine 750 mg daily for 2 days reduced the urinary excretion of 2-hydroxydesipramine from a single 25-mg dose of **desipramine** in rapid hydroxylators by 56% but had no significant effect on the clearance in slow hydroxylators.[4]

Mechanism

Quinidine reduces the metabolism (hydroxylation) of these tricyclic antidepressants, by inhibiting the cytochrome P450 isoenzyme CYP2D6, and thereby reduces their loss from the body.[5,6] Quinine inhibits the metabolism of desipramine to a lesser extent than quinidine.

Importance and management

The clinical importance of these interactions awaits assessment, but be alert for evidence of increased tricyclic antidepressant effects and possibly toxicity if quinidine is added. One report suggested steady-state increases of 30% with imipramine and more than 500% with desipramine in extensive metabolisers.[2] More study is needed. There seems to be no information about the effect of quinidine on other tricyclics. Information about the effect of quinine on tricyclics is very limited, but the effects are smaller than those of quinidine and therefore less likely to result in clinically significant adverse effects. Note that quinidine, possibly quinine, and the tricyclics (notably in overdose) may prolong the QT interval, see also 'Drugs that prolong the QT interval + Other drugs that prolong the QT interval', p.257.

1. Ayesh R, Dawling S, Widdop B, Idle JR, Smith RL. Influence of quinidine on the pharmacokinetics of nortriptyline and desipramine. *Br J Clin Pharmacol* (1988) 25, 140P–141P.
2. Brøsen K, Gram LF. Quinidine inhibits the 2-hydroxylation of imipramine and desipramine, but not the demethylation of imipramine. *Eur J Clin Pharmacol* (1989) 37, 155–60.

3. Eap CB, Laurian S, Souche A, Koeb L, Reymond P, Buclin T, Baumann P. Influence of quinidine on the pharmacokinetics of trimipramine and on its effect on the waking EEG of healthy volunteers. A pilot study on two subjects. *Neuropsychobiology* (1992) 25, 214–20.
4. Steiner E, Dumont E, Spina E, Dahlqvist R. Inhibition of desipramine 2-hydroxylation by quinidine and quinine. *Clin Pharmacol Ther* (1988) 43, 577–81.
5. Pfandl B, Mörike K, Winne D, Schareck W, Breyer-Pfaff U. Stereoselective inhibition of nortriptyline hydroxylation in man by quinidine. *Xenobiotica* (1992) 22, 721–30.
6. Von Moltke LL, Greenblatt DJ, Cotreau-Bibbo MM, Duan SX, Harmatz JS, Shader RI. Inhibition of desipramine hydroxylation *in vitro* by serotonin-reuptake-inhibitor antidepressants, and by quinidine and ketoconazole: a model system to predict drug interactions *in vivo*. *J Pharmacol Exp Ther* (1994) 268, 1278–83.

Tricyclic antidepressants + Rifampicin (Rifampin)

In three patients a marked reduction in nortriptyline or amitriptyline levels occurred when rifampicin was given.

Clinical evidence

A man with tuberculosis needed to take 175-mg doses of **nortriptyline** to achieve therapeutic serum levels while taking isoniazid 300 mg, rifampicin 600 mg, pyrazinamide 1.5 g and pyridoxine 25 mg daily. Three weeks after stopping the antitubercular drugs, the patient suddenly became drowsy and his **nortriptyline** serum levels were found to have risen from 193 nanomol/L to 562 nanomol/L, and later to 671 nanomol/L. It was then found possible to maintain his **nortriptyline** serum levels in the range of 150 to 500 nanomol/L with only 75 mg of **nortriptyline** daily.[1] A woman taking **amitriptyline** and fluoxetine had a marked fall in her plasma **amitriptyline** levels when she took rifampicin 600 mg, isoniazid 200 mg and ethambutol 1.2 g daily. When these antitubercular drugs were stopped, her **amitriptyline** plasma levels rose once again.[2] In a further case in a 43-year-old woman taking **nortriptyline** 50 mg daily, serum levels were not detectable when rifampicin 600 mg daily was given. Increasing the dose of **nortriptyline** to 75 mg daily failed to produce detectable serum levels. Two weeks after discontinuation of rifampicin, **nortriptyline** levels increased significantly.[3]

Mechanism

It seems highly probable that rifampicin (a well recognised and potent enzyme inducer) increased the metabolism of nortriptyline and amitriptyline by the liver thereby reducing their levels.

Importance and management

Information about the interaction between tricyclic antidepressants and rifampicin seems to be limited to just these three reports, which is a little surprising since both have been widely used for a considerable time. This suggests that generally this interaction may have limited clinical importance. However, bear this interaction in mind if patients taking rifampicin seem unresponsive to treatment with tricyclics. Increase the tricyclic dosage if necessary, and remember to readjust the dose if rifampicin is stopped.

1. Bebchuk JM, Stewart DE. Drug interaction between rifampin and nortriptyline: a case report. *Int J Psychiatry Med* (1991) 21, 183–7.
2. Bertschy G, Vandel S, Perault MC. Un cas d'interaction métabolique: amitriptyline, fluoxétine, antituberculeux. *Therapie* (1994) 49, 509–12.
3. Self T, Corley CR, Nabhan S, Abell T. Case report: interaction of rifampin and nortriptyline. *Am J Med Sci* (1996) 311, 80–1.

Tricyclic antidepressants + SNRIs; Duloxetine

Duloxetine markedly increased the AUC of desipramine; other tricyclics metabolised by CYP2D6 are expected to interact similarly. Note that the use of duloxetine with other serotonergic drugs such as the tricyclics should be undertaken with caution or avoided because of the theoretical increased risk of serotonin syndrome.

Clinical evidence

Duloxetine 60 mg twice daily increased the AUC of a single 50-mg dose of **desipramine** by 2.9-fold in subjects who were extensive metabolisers of the cytochrome P450 isoenzyme CYP2D6.[1]

Mechanism

Desipramine is extensively metabolised by the cytochrome P450 isoenzyme CYP2D6, and can be used as a probe drug for assessment of the effect of drugs on this isoenzyme in extensive metabolisers (see 'Genetic factors', (p.4)).

Importance and management

The pharmacokinetic interaction with desipramine is established. Although the clinical relevance of the increased levels has not been assessed, the manufacturer recommends caution if duloxetine is given to patients taking desipramine and other similarly metabolised tricyclics, such as **nortriptyline**, **amitriptyline** and **imipramine**.[2,3]

The manufacturers note that tricyclics like **clomipramine** or **amitriptyline** should be used with caution[3] or avoided[4] with duloxetine, because of the possible risks of 'the serotonin syndrome', (p.9).

1. Skinner MH, Kuan H-Y, Pan A, Sathirakul K, Knadler MP, Gonzales CR, Yeo KP, Reddy S, Lim M, Ayan-Oshodi M, Wise SD. Duloxetine is both an inhibitor and a substrate of cytochrome P4502D6 in healthy volunteers. *Clin Pharmacol Ther* (2003) 73, 170–7.
2. Cymbalta (Duloxetine hydrochloride). Eli Lilly and Company. US Prescribing information, May 2007.
3. Cymbalta (Duloxetine hydrochloride). Eli Lilly and Company Ltd. UK Summary of product characteristics, November 2006.
4. Yentreve (Duloxetine hydrochloride). Eli Lilly and Company Ltd. UK Summary of product characteristics, November 2006.

Tricyclic antidepressants + SNRIs; Venlafaxine

Venlafaxine can cause a marked increase in the antimuscarinic adverse effects of clomipramine, desipramine and nortriptyline. There are isolated reports of seizures in a patient taking venlafaxine and trimipramine and the serotonin syndrome has been seen in patients taking venlafaxine with, or shortly before, the use of tricyclics.

Clinical evidence

A 74-year-old man taking venlafaxine 150 mg daily and thioridazine had his treatment changed to daily doses of venlafaxine 75 mg, **desipramine** 50 mg, haloperidol 500 micrograms and alprazolam 250 micrograms. Within 5 days he exhibited severe antimuscarinic adverse effects (acute confusion, delirium, stupor, urinary retention and paralytic ileus). This was attributed to an interaction between the venlafaxine and amitriptyline.[1] Similarly, a 75-year-old man taking haloperidol, alprazolam and venlafaxine developed urinary retention and became delirious when he also took **desipramine**.[2] A woman taking **nortriptyline** 20 mg and fluoxetine 20 mg daily with only mild antimuscarinic adverse effects developed much more severe effects (dry mouth, worsened constipation, blurred vision) over 4 weeks following the replacement of the fluoxetine by venlafaxine 75 mg daily.[3] Similar effects were seen in a 73-year-old man taking venlafaxine with and **nortriptyline** 20 mg daily and a 61-year-old man taking venlafaxine with **clomipramine** 150 mg daily.[2]

A 69-year-old man with bipolar disorder, who had been taking venlafaxine up to 337.5 mg daily, thioridazine 25 mg at night, and sodium valproate 1.2 g daily for several months with no adverse motor symptoms, experienced extrapyramidal effects 3 to 4 days after the venlafaxine had been gradually replaced by **nortriptyline** 50 mg daily. Symptoms persisted despite withdrawal of thioridazine, but improved on reduction of the **nortriptyline** dosage to 20 mg daily.[4] The cause of the reaction was not known, but it was suggested that there may have been an interaction between venlafaxine and **nortriptyline** possibly modulated by thioridazine or sodium valproate.

A 25-year-old woman taking venlafaxine 150 mg daily and **trimipramine** 50 mg daily for depression developed seizures within 11 days of the **trimipramine** dose being increased to 100 mg daily. Both drugs were stopped and the patient had no further seizures.[5]

There is also a report of the serotonin syndrome occurring in a 21-year-old patient when **amitriptyline** 10 mg at night was added to the range of medications she was receiving, which included venlafaxine 37.5 mg daily, pethidine (meperidine) 400 mg daily and fluconazole 200 mg daily.[6] There are two other reports of the serotonin syndrome in patients who had discontinued venlafaxine 3 days and 2 weeks, respectively, before starting **amitriptyline**.[7,8]

Mechanism

Not fully established but it is suggested that venlafaxine can inhibit the metabolism of these tricyclics by the cytochrome P450 isoenzyme CYP2D6, leading to an increase in their serum levels and a marked increase in their antimuscarinic adverse effects.[2]

Both venlafaxine and trimipramine can cause seizures, although usually after overdose. Either a pharmacokinetic interaction involving inhibition of drug metabolism by the isoenzyme CYP2D6, or a pharmacodynamic interaction may have resulted in seizures.[5]

'The serotonin syndrome', (p.9), has been reported in patients taking venlafaxine and amitriptyline alone or with other serotonergic drugs. Both can increase serotonergic activity by inhibition of serotonin re-uptake at presynaptic neurones. In addition, one of the cases described above[6] is complicated by the fact that pethidine also has serotonergic activity and the metabolism of amitriptyline can be inhibited by 'fluconazole', (p.1230).

Importance and management

Information appears to be limited to these reports, three of which are by the same author. The incidence is not known but if venlafaxine and any tricyclic antidepressant are given concurrently, be alert for any evidence of increased antimuscarinic adverse effects. Although there appears to be only one report, the possibility of an increased risk of seizures with concurrent use should be borne in mind. It may be necessary to withdraw one or other of the two drugs. The reports of the serotonin syndrome highlight the need for caution when one or more serotonergic drugs are given either concurrently or within a short period of each other.

1. Benazzi F. Anticholinergic toxic syndrome with venlafaxine-desipramine combination. *Pharmacopsychiatry* (1998) 31, 36–7.
2. Benazzi F. Venlafaxine drug-drug interactions in clinical practice. *J Psychiatry Neurosci* (1998) 23, 181–2.
3. Benazzi F. Venlafaxine-fluoxetine-nortriptyline interaction. *J Psychiatry Neurosci* (1997) 22, 278–9.
4. Conforti D, Borgherini G, Fiorellini Bernardis LA, Magni G. Extrapyramidal symptoms associated with the adjunct of nortriptyline to a venlafaxine-valproic acid combination. *Int Clin Psychopharmacol* (1999) 14, 197–8.
5. Schlienger RG, Klink MH, Eggenberger C, Drewe J. Seizures associated with therapeutic doses of venlafaxine and trimipramine. *Ann Pharmacother* (2000) 34, 1402–5.
6. Dougherty JA, Young H, Shafi T. Serotonin syndrome induced by amitriptyline, meperidine, and venlafaxine. *Ann Pharmacother* (2002) 36, 1647–8.
7. McDaniel WW. Serotonin syndrome: early management with cyproheptadine. *Ann Pharmacother* (2001) 35, 870–3.
8. Perry NK. Venlafaxine-induced serotonin syndrome with relapse following amitriptyline. *Postgrad Med J* (2000) 76, 254–6.

Tricyclic and related antidepressants + SSRIs

The levels of the tricyclic antidepressants can be raised by the SSRIs, but the extent varies greatly, from 20% to tenfold: fluvoxamine, fluoxetine and paroxetine appear to have the greatest effects. Tricyclic toxicity has been seen in a number of cases. Tricyclics may increase the levels of citalopram and possibly fluvoxamine, but the significance of this is unclear. There are several case reports of the serotonin syndrome following concurrent and even sequential use of the SSRIs and tricyclics.

Clinical evidence

(a) Citalopram

In one study[1] citalopram caused an increase of about 50% in the AUC of desipramine (the primary metabolite of **imipramine**), and a reduction in the levels of the subsequently formed metabolite of desipramine (2-hydroxydesipramine) after a single 100-mg oral dose of **imipramine**. In contrast, 5 patients taking **amitriptyline**, **clomipramine** or **maprotiline** had no changes in their plasma tricyclic antidepressant levels when citalopram 20 to 60 mg daily was also given.[2] In another general study, in which 18 patients were given citalopram and tricyclic antidepressants, serum levels of citalopram were doubled in those receiving the tricyclic **clomipramine**; pooled results for all the tricyclics showed a 44% rise in serum citalopram levels.[3] An increase of this size is of doubtful clinical importance with citalopram. In 2 patients the plasma levels of **clomipramine** 100 mg daily remained stable when the dose was reduced to 75 mg daily and citalopram 40 mg daily was started.[4,5] One had elevated levels of desmethylclomipramine[4] and the other had elevated levels of the active metabolite, 8-hydroxydesmethylclomipramine.[5]

A case report describes elevated **desipramine** levels in a patient taking paroxetine that resolved when the patient was switched to citalopram.[6]

(b) Escitalopram

Escitalopram 20 mg daily for 21 days increased the maximum serum levels and AUC of a single 50-mg dose of **desipramine** by 40% and 100%, respectively.[7] The UK manufacturers predict that **clomipramine** and **nortriptyline** will be similarly affected.[8]

(c) Fluoxetine

Four patients given daily doses of **desipramine** 300 mg, **imipramine** 150 mg or **nortriptyline** 100 mg had two to fourfold increases in plasma tricyclic antidepressant levels within 1 to 2 weeks of starting fluoxetine 10 to 60 mg daily. Two of them developed antimuscarinic adverse effects (constipation, urinary hesitancy).[9]

A number of other reports and studies clearly confirm that marked increases occur in the levels of **amitriptyline**,[10-13] **clomipramine**,[11,14] **desipramine**,[15-24] **imipramine**[11,19-21,25,26] and **nortriptyline**,[17,18,27-29] accompanied by toxicity, if fluoxetine is added without reducing the dosage of the tricyclic antidepressant. Delirium and seizures have also been described,[20,30] and a death has been attributed to chronic **amitriptyline** toxicity caused by fluoxetine.[31] The pharmacokinetics of fluoxetine appear not to be affected by **amitriptyline**.[13]

A migraine-like stroke developed in a woman 48 hours after her long-standing treatment with fluoxetine 100 mg daily was abruptly changed to **clomipramine** 200 mg daily.[32]

(d) Fluvoxamine

The **amitriptyline** plasma levels of 8 patients rose (range 15 to 233%) when they were also given fluvoxamine 100 to 300 mg daily. Even larger rises in plasma **clomipramine** levels occurred (up to eightfold) in four other patients given fluvoxamine 100 to 300 mg daily. The tricyclic dosages remained the same or were slightly lower. No toxicity was seen.[33-35]

A number of other reports and studies confirm that increases occur in the levels of **amitriptyline**,[36-39] **clomipramine**,[36-41] **desipramine**,[42-45] **imipramine**,[36,37,42-46] **maprotiline**[36] and **trimipramine**[47] in the presence of fluvoxamine. This interaction seems severe with **clomipramine** (a 10-fold rise in one case)[41] and mild with **desipramine**.[44,45] One study also suggested that fluvoxamine levels may be raised.[36] An isolated report describes worsening depression in a patient taking **dosulepin** 75 mg daily and mianserin within 24 hours of replacing the **dosulepin** with fluvoxamine 75 mg daily. The symptoms continued during the next day but were reversed within a day of fluvoxamine being replaced with **dosulepin**.[48]

(e) Paroxetine

A study in 17 healthy subjects who were extensive metabolisers and taking **desipramine** 50 mg daily found that when they were also given paroxetine 20 mg daily for 10 days the maximum plasma levels of the **desipramine** rose by 358%, the trough plasma levels rose by 511% and the AUC rose by 421%. An approximately tenfold increase in the maximum plasma levels and the AUC of the paroxetine also occurred.[49] Another study found a fivefold decrease in **desipramine** clearance in extensive metabolisers given paroxetine 20 mg daily.[50] Paroxetine has also been shown to increase the levels of **clomipramine**,[51] **desipramine**,[6] **imipramine**,[52,53] and **trimipramine**.[54] This resulted in a variety of adverse effects including dizziness,[51] confusion,[6] sedation[54] and memory impairment.[54]

A 21-year-old man developed the serotonin syndrome when he took one tablet of paroxetine only one day after stopping **desipramine**, which he had taken for 5 days. He recovered after treatment with cyproheptadine.[55] A woman taking paroxetine 30 mg daily developed the serotonin syndrome (tachycardia, delirium, bizarre movements, myoclonus) within 2 hours of taking a single 50-mg dose of **imipramine**. She recovered when treated with intravenous fluids, sedation and cyproheptadine.[56]

(f) Sertraline

In 9 healthy subjects, sertraline 50 mg daily increased the maximum plasma levels of **desipramine** 50 mg daily by 31% at steady-state, and increased the AUC by 23%.[24] A later related study in 17 healthy subjects by the same group of workers found that, using the same drug dosages, sertraline increased the **desipramine** maximum plasma levels by 44%, the minimum levels by 19% and the AUC by 37%. The maximum plasma levels and AUC of the sertraline were increased about twofold.[49] Other studies have found that sertraline increases **desipramine**,[57-60] **imipramine**,[57] and **nortriptyline**[61] levels, but it has also been suggested that sertraline has no effect on **imipramine** levels.[62,63]

A woman who had been taking sertraline 50 mg daily (as well as morphine sulfate and periciazine) developed the serotonin syndrome within 3 days of starting to take **amitriptyline** 75 mg daily. She recovered when all of the psychotropic drugs were withdrawn.[64]

Mechanism

Fluoxetine, paroxetine, and to a lesser extent sertraline and citalopram, inhibit the cytochrome P450 isoenzyme CYP2D6, which is involved in the metabolism of the tricyclic antidepressants. Hence these SSRIs cause tricyclic levels to rise. Fluvoxamine causes a similar effect, possibly by inhibiting the latter stages of metabolism through CYP1A2 and CYP3A4. The elevated levels of 8-hydroxydesmethylclomipramine during concurrent clomipramine and citalopram administration in one patient may have been due to the inhibition of glucuronidation by citalopram.[5]

The serotonin syndrome possibly develops because both the tricyclics and SSRIs affect serotonin transmission, which may result in increased serotonin levels. For more on the serotonin syndrome, see 'Additive or synergistic interactions', (p.9).

Importance and management

The interactions of the SSRIs and tricyclic antidepressants are established and of clinical significance. The SSRIs increase tricyclic levels, with fluvoxamine, fluoxetine and paroxetine apparently having the greatest effects. The increased tricyclic levels can be beneficial.[36,39,65] However, it has been suggested that patients given fluoxetine should have their tricyclic dose reduced to one-quarter.[19] Similar recommendations have been made with fluvoxamine (reduction in tricyclic dose to one-third)[42] and sertraline.[66] It would also seem prudent to consider a dosage reduction of the tricyclic if paroxetine is added. Some suggest that a small initial dose of the SSRI should also be used.[66]

Patients taking any combination of tricyclic and SSRI should be monitored for adverse effects (e.g. dry mouth, sedation, confusion) with tricyclic levels monitored where possible. Remember that the active metabolite of fluoxetine has a half-life of 7 to 15 days, and so any interaction may persist for some time after the fluoxetine is withdrawn,[67-69] and may occur on sequential use.

The serotonin syndrome seems to occur rarely but patients and prescribers should be aware of the symptoms so that prompt action can be taken if problems occur. For more about the serotonin syndrome see, 'Additive or synergistic interactions', (p.9).

1. Gram LF, Hansen MG, Sindrup SH, Brøsen K, Poulsen JH, Aaes-Jørgensen T, Overø KF. Citalopram: interaction studies with levomepromazine, imipramine and lithium. *Ther Drug Monit* (1993) 15, 18–24.
2. Baettig D, Bondolfi G, Montaldi S, Amey M, Baumann P. Tricyclic antidepressant plasma levels after augmentation with citalopram: a case study. *Eur J Clin Pharmacol* (1993) 44, 403–5.
3. Leinonen E, Lepola U, Koponen H, Kinnunen I. The effect of age and concomitant treatment with other psychoactive drugs on serum concentrations of citalopram measured with a nonenantioselective method. *Ther Drug Monit* (1996) 18, 111–17.
4. Haffen E, Vandel P, Broly F, Vandel S, Sechter D, Bizouard P, Bechtel PR. Citalopram: an interaction study with clomipramine in a patient heterozygous for CYP2D6 genotype. *Pharmacopsychiatry* (1999) 32, 232–4.
5. Haffen E, Vandel P, Bonin B, Vandel S. Citalopram pharmacokinetic interaction with clomipramine. UDP-glucuronosyltransferase inhibition? A case report. *Therapie* (1999) 54, 768–70.
6. Ashton AK. Lack of desipramine toxicity with citalopram. *J Clin Psychiatry* (2000) 61, 144.
7. Lexapro (Escitalopram oxalate). Forest Pharmaceuticals Inc. US Prescribing information, May 2007.
8. Cipralex (Escitalopram oxalate). Lundbeck Ltd. UK Summary of product characteristics, December 2005.
9. Aranow RB, Hudson JI, Pope HG, Grady TA, Laage TA, Bell IR, Cole JO. Elevated antidepressant plasma levels after addition of fluoxetine. *Am J Psychiatry* (1989) 146, 911–13.
10. March JS, Moon RL, Johnston H. Fluoxetine-TCA interaction. *J Am Acad Child Adolesc Psychiatry* (1990) 29, 985–6.
11. Vandel S, Bertschy G, Bonin B, Nezelof S, François TH, Vandel B, Sechter D, Bizouard P. Tricyclic antidepressant plasma levels after fluoxetine addition. *Neuropsychobiology* (1992) 25, 202–7.
12. Bertschy G, Vandel S, Perault MC. Un cas d'interaction métabolique: amitriptyline, fluoxétine, antituberculeux. *Therapie* (1994) 49, 509–12.
13. El-Yazigi A, Chaleby K, Gad A, Raines DA. Steady-state kinetics of fluoxetine and amitriptyline in patients treated with a combination of these drugs as compared with those treated with amitriptyline alone. *J Clin Pharmacol* (1995) 35, 17–21.
14. Balant-Gorgia AE, Ries C, Balant LP. Metabolic interaction between fluoxetine and clomipramine: A case report. *Pharmacopsychiatry* (1996) 29, 38–41.
15. Bell IR, Cole JO. Fluoxetine induces elevation of desipramine level and exacerbation of geriatric nonpsychotic depression. *J Clin Psychopharmacol* (1988) 8, 447–8.
16. Goodnick PJ. Influence of fluoxetine on plasma levels of desipramine. *Am J Psychiatry* (1989) 146, 552.
17. Vaughan DA. Interaction of fluoxetine with tricyclic antidepressants. *Am J Psychiatry* (1988) 145, 1478.
18. von Ammon Cavanaugh S. Drug-drug interactions of fluoxetine with tricyclics. *Psychosomatics* (1990) 31, 273–6.
19. Westermeyer J. Fluoxetine-induced tricyclic toxicity: extent and duration. *J Clin Pharmacol* (1991) 31, 388–92.
20. Preskorn SH, Beber JH, Faul JC, Hirschfeld RMA. Serious adverse effects of combining fluoxetine and tricyclic antidepressants. *Am J Psychiatry* (1990) 147, 532.
21. Bergstrom RF, Peyton AL, Lemberger L. Quantification and mechanism of the fluoxetine and tricyclic antidepressant interaction. *Clin Pharmacol Ther* (1992) 51, 239–48.
22. Nelson JC, Mazure CM, Bowers MB, Jatlow PI. A preliminary, open study of the combination of fluoxetine and desipramine for rapid treatment of major depression. *Arch Gen Psychiatry* (1991) 48, 303–7.
23. Wilens TE, Biederman J, Baldessarini RJ, McDermott SP, Puopolo PR, Flood JG. Fluoxetine inhibits desipramine metabolism. *Arch Gen Psychiatry* (1992) 49, 752.
24. Preskorn SH, Alderman J, Chung M, Harrison W, Messig M, Harris S. Pharmacokinetics of desipramine coadministered with sertraline or fluoxetine. *J Clin Psychopharmacol* (1994) 14, 90–8.
25. Faynor SM, Espina V. Fluoxetine inhibition of imipramine metabolism. *Clin Chem* (1989) 35, 1180.
26. Hahn SM, Griffin JH. Comment: fluoxetine adverse effects and drug interactions. *DICP Ann Pharmacother* (1991) 25, 1273–4.
27. Kahn DG. Increased plasma nortriptyline concentration in a patient cotreated with fluoxetine. *J Clin Psychiatry* (1990) 51, 36.
28. Schraml F, Benedetti G, Hoyle K, Clayton A. Fluoxetine and nortriptyline combination therapy. *Am J Psychiatry* (1989) 146, 1636–7.
29. Downs JM, Downs AD, Rosenthal TL, Deal N, Akiskal HS. Increased plasma tricyclic antidepressant concentrations in two patients concurrently treated with fluoxetine. *J Clin Psychiatry* (1989) 50, 226–7.
30. Sternbach H. Fluoxetine-clomipramine interaction. *J Clin Psychiatry* (1995) 56, 171–2.
31. Preskorn SH, Baker B. Fatality associated with combined fluoxetine-amitriptyline therapy. *JAMA* (1997) 277, 1682.
32. Molaie M. Serotonin syndrome presenting with migraine like stroke. *Headache* (1997) 37, 519–21.
33. Vandel S, Bertschy G, Allers G. Fluvoxamine tricyclic antidepressant interaction. *Therapie* (1990) 45, 21.
34. Bertschy G, Vandel S, Vandel B, Allers G, Vomat R. Fluvoxamine-tricyclic antidepressant interaction. An accidental finding. *Eur J Clin Pharmacol* (1991) 40, 119–120.
35. Bertschy G, Vandel S, Nezelof S, Bizouard P, Bechtel P. L'interaction fluvoxamine-antidépresseurs tricycliques. *Therapie* (1993) 48, 63–4.
36. Härtter S, Wetzel H, Hammes E, Hiemke C. Inhibition of antidepressant demethylation and hydroxylation by fluvoxamine in depressed patients. *Psychopharmacology (Berl)* (1993) 110, 302–8.
37. Szegedi A, Wetzel H, Leal M, Härtter S, Hiemke C. Combination treatment with clomipramine and fluvoxamine: drug monitoring, safety, and tolerability data. *J Clin Psychiatry* (1996) 57, 257–64.
38. Vandel S, Bertschy G, Baumann P, Bouquet S, Bonin B, Francois T, Sechter D, Bizouard P. Fluvoxamine and fluoxetine: Interaction studies with amitriptyline, clomipramine and neuroleptics in phenotyped patients. *Pharmacol Res* (1995) 31, 347–53.
39. Vandel P, Bonin B, Bertschy G, Baumann P, Bouquet S, Vandel S, Sechter D, Bizouard P. Observations of the interaction between tricyclic antidepressants and fluvoxamine in poor metabolisers of dextromethorphan and mephenytoin. *Therapie* (1997) 52, 74–6.
40. Conus P, Bondolfi G, Eap CB, Macciardi F, Baumann P. Pharmacokinetic fluvoxamine-clomipramine interaction with favorable therapeutic consequences in therapy-resistant depressive patient. *Pharmacopsychiatry* (1996) 29, 108–110.
41. Roberge C, Lecordier-Maret F, Beljean-Leymarie M, Heriault F, Starace J. Major drug interaction between fluvoxamine and clomipramine: about a case report. *J Pharm Clin* (1998) 17, 117–19.
42. Spina E, Campo GM, Avenoso A, Pollicino MA, Caputi AP. Interaction between fluvoxamine and imipramine/desipramine in four patients. *Ther Drug Monit* (1992) 14, 194–6.
43. Maskall DD, Lam RW. Increased plasma concentration of imipramine following augmentation with fluvoxamine. *Am J Psychiatry* (1993) 150, 1566.
44. Spina E, Pollicino AM, Avenso A, Campo GM, Caputi AP. Fluvoxamine-induced alterations in plasma concentrations of imipramine and desipramine in depressed patients. *Int J Clin Pharmacol Res* (1993) 13, 167–71.
45. Spina E, Pollicino AM, Avenoso A, Campo GM, Perucca E, Caputi AP. Effect of fluvoxamine on the pharmacokinetics of imipramine and desipramine in healthy subjects. *Ther Drug Monit* (1993) 15, 243–6.
46. Xu ZH, Huang S-L, Zhou H-H. Inhibition of imipramine *N*-demethylation by fluvoxamine in Chinese young men. *Acta Pharmacol Sin* (1996) 17, 399–402.
47. Seifritz E, Holsboer-Trachsler E, Hemmeter U, Eap CB, Baumann P. Increased trimipramine plasma levels during fluvoxamine comedication. *Eur Neuropsychopharmacol* (1994) 4, 15–20.
48. Sato K, Yoshida K, Higuchi H, Shimizu T. Rapid worsening of depressive symptoms in a patient with depression after switching from a TCA to an SSRI. *J Neuropsychiatr Clin Neurosci* (2002) 14, 357.
49. Alderman J, Preskorn SH, Greenblatt DJ, Harrison W, Penenberg D, Allison J, Chung M. Desipramine pharmacokinetics when coadministered with paroxetine or sertraline in extensive metabolizers. *J Clin Psychopharmacol* (1997) 17, 284–91.
50. Brøsen K, Hansen JG, Nielsen KK, Sindrup SH, Gram LF. Inhibition by paroxetine of desipramine metabolism in extensive but not in poor metabolizers of sparteine. *Eur J Clin Pharmacol* (1993) 44, 349–55.
51. Skjelbo EF, Brøsen K. Interaktion imellem paroxetin og clomipramin som mulig årsag til indlæggelse på medicinsk afdeling. *Ugeskr Laeger* (1998) 160, 5665–6.
52. Albers LJ, Reist C, Helmeste D, Vu R, Tang SW. Paroxetine shifts imipramine metabolism. *Psychiatry Res* (1996) 59, 189–96.
53. Yoon YR, Shim JC, Shin JG, Shon JH, Kim YH, Cha IJ. Drug interaction between paroxetine and imipramine. Kor Soc Pharmacol Meeting, Seoul, S Korea, October 1997, p168.
54. Leinonen E, Koponen HJ, Lepola U. Paroxetine increases serum trimipramine concentration. A report of two cases. *Hum Psychopharmacol* (1995) 10, 345–7.
55. Chan BSH, Graudins A, Whyte IM, Dawson AH, Braitberg G, Duggin GG. Serotonin syndrome resulting from drug interactions. *Med J Aust* (1998) 169, 523–5.
56. Weiner AL, Tilden FF, McKay CA. Serotonin syndrome: case report and review of the literature. *Conn Med* (1997) 61, 717–21.
57. Kurtz DL, Bergstrom RF, Goldberg MJ, Cerimele BJ. The effect of sertraline on the pharmacokinetics of desipramine and imipramine. *Clin Pharmacol Ther* (1997) 62, 145–56.
58. Zussman BD, Davie CC, Fowles SE, Kumar R, Lang U, Wargenau M, Sourgens H. Sertraline, like other SSRIs, is a significant inhibitor of desipramine metabolism in vivo. *Br J Clin Pharmacol* (1995) 39, 550P–551P.
59. Lydiard RB, Anton RF, Cunningham T. Interactions between sertraline and tricyclic antidepressants. *Am J Psychiatry* (1993) 150, 1125–6.
60. Barros J, Asnis G. An interaction of sertraline and desipramine. *Am J Psychiatry* (1993) 150, 1751.
61. Solai LK, Mulsant BH, Pollock BG, Sweet RA, Rosen J, Yu K, Reynolds CF. Effect of sertraline on plasma nortriptyline levels in depressed elderly. *J Clin Psychiatry* (1997) 58, 440–3.
62. Erikson SM, Carson SW, Grimsley S, Carter JG, Kumar A, Jann MW. Effect of sertraline on steady-state serum concentrations of imipramine and its metabolites. *Pharmacotherapy* (1994) 14, 368.
63. Jann MW, Carson SW, Grimsley SR, Erikson S, Kumar A, Carter JG. Effects of sertraline upon imipramine pharmacodynamics. *Clin Pharmacol Ther* (1995) 57, 207.

64. Alderman CP, Lee PC. Comment: serotonin syndrome associated with combined sertraline-amitriptyline treatment. *Ann Pharmacother* (1996) 30, 1499–1500.
65. Wetzel H, Härtter A, Szegedi A, Hammes E, Leal M, Hiemke C. Fluvoxamine co-medication to tricyclic antidepressants: metabolic interactions, clinical efficiency and side-effects. *Pharmacopsychiatry* (1993) 26, 211.
66. Eiber R, Escande M. Associations et interactions: les antidépresseurs tricycliques et les inhibiteurs spécifiques de la recapture de la sérotonine. *Encephale* (1999) 25, 584–9.
67. Downs JM, Dahmer SK. Fluoxetine and elevated plasma levels of tricyclic antidepressants. *Am J Psychiatry* (1990) 147, 1251.
68. Skowron DM, Gutierrez MA, Epstein S. Precaution with titrating nortriptyline after the use of fluoxetine. *DICP Ann Pharmacother* (1990) 24, 1008.
69. Müller N, Brockmöller J, Roots I. Extremely long plasma half-life of amitriptyline in a woman with the cytochrome P450IID6 29/29-kilobase wild-type allele — a slowly reversible interaction with fluoxetine. *Ther Drug Monit* (1991) 13, 533–6.

Tricyclic antidepressants + St John's wort (*Hypericum perforatum*)

The plasma levels of amitriptyline can be reduced by St John's wort, but the clinical importance of this interaction is unknown.

Clinical evidence

Twelve depressed patients were given 75 mg of **amitriptyline** twice daily and 900 mg of St John's wort extract (*Lichtwer Pharma, Berlin*) daily for at least 14 days. The AUC_{0-12} of the **amitriptyline** was reduced by about 22% and the AUC of nortriptyline (its metabolite) was reduced by about 41%.[1]

Mechanism

Not fully understood, but there is evidence that St John's wort is an enzyme inducer, which can increase liver metabolism by cytochrome P450 isoenzymes, thereby reducing the plasma levels of both amitriptyline and its metabolite (nortriptyline). Induction of P-glycoprotein by St John's wort may also contribute.

Importance and management

The interaction appears to be established, but its clinical importance is uncertain. Both the tricyclics and St John's wort are antidepressants, but whether the final sum of this interaction is more or less antidepressant activity is not known. It was not assessed in this study.[1] Other tricyclics probably interact similarly because they too can be affected by enzyme-inducing drugs. Monitor for antidepressant efficacy and increased adverse effects if St John's wort is given with any tricyclic. More study is needed.

1. Johne A, Schmider J, Brockmöller J, Stadelmann AM, Störmer E, Bauer S, Scholler G, Langheinrich M, Roots I. Decreased plasma levels of amitriptyline and its metabolites on comedication with an extract from St. John's wort (*Hypericum perforatum*). *J Clin Psychopharmacol* (2002) 22, 46–54.

Tricyclic antidepressants + Terbinafine

Terbinafine markedly increased the AUC of desipramine in a pharmacokinetic study. Case reports describe increases in the serum levels of amitriptyline, desipramine, imipramine and nortriptyline, with associated toxicity, in patients additionally given oral terbinafine.

Clinical evidence

(a) Amitriptyline

A 37-year-old woman who had been taking amitriptyline 75 mg daily, valproate and olanzapine for 3 years, developed extreme dryness of the mouth, nausea and dizziness shortly after starting to take terbinafine 250 mg daily. Serum levels of amitriptyline and its metabolite nortriptyline rose from just under 400 nanomol/L to over 1800 nanomol/L. Terbinafine was stopped, and the amitriptyline dose reduced to 25 mg daily, but the amitriptyline and nortriptyline levels did not return to baseline for several months. The patient had normal CYP2D6 metaboliser status.[1]

(b) Desipramine

In a pharmacokinetic study terbinafine 250 mg daily for 21 days markedly increased the AUC of a single 50-mg dose of desipramine by fivefold, and increased the maximum levels twofold. The AUC of desipramine was still more than double the baseline levels 4 weeks after stopping desipramine. In this study, healthy subjects were extensive CYP2D6 metabolisers, which is the usual phenotype.[2]

A case report describes a 3.5-fold increase in desipramine levels, with associated toxicity (dizziness, ataxia, incoordination, and difficulty swallowing), in a 52-year-old man taking desipramine 350 mg daily, which occurred within 2 to 3 weeks of him starting terbinafine. The desipramine was stopped for a few days and restarted at a dose of just 50 mg daily, which gave similar serum levels to those seen before terbinafine was started. When the terbinafine was stopped, the dose of desipramine needed to be gradually titrated up to the initial amount.[3]

(c) Imipramine

A 51-year-old man who had been taking lithium carbonate and varying doses of imipramine 150 to 200 mg daily for 10 years was also given oral terbinafine 250 mg daily for onychomycosis. About a week later he complained of dizziness, muscle twitching and excessive mouth dryness. His serum imipramine levels, measured 5 days later, had risen from his usual range of 100 to 200 nanograms/mL up to 530 nanograms/mL. Within 10 days of reducing his daily imipramine dose from 200 to 75 mg daily, his serum levels had fallen to 229 nanograms/mL. His liver function was normal.[4]

(d) Nortriptyline

A report describes a marked increase in the serum levels of nortriptyline (about doubled) accompanied by evidence of toxicity (fatigue, vertigo, loss of energy and appetite, and falls) in a 74-year-old man taking nortriptyline 125 mg daily, roughly 14 days after he started to take terbinafine 250 mg daily. His symptoms responded to a dose reduction to 75 mg daily. His serum levels were similarly elevated when he was later re-challenged with terbinafine. His liver function was normal.[5] The same authors reported a similar case in a woman who had been taking nortriptyline and terbinafine for one month before she showed signs of an interaction. A later re-challenge with terbinafine confirmed the interaction.[6]

Mechanism

Terbinafine is an inhibitor of the cytochrome P450 isoenzyme CYP2D6, which is the principal enzyme involved in the metabolism of many tricyclics. Terbinafine can have a very prolonged half-life, so an interaction may occur/continue for a number of weeks after stopping the drug.

Importance and management

Although there are only a few case reports, the increase in levels of tricyclic antidepressant in the presence of terbinafine appears to be clinically important. Caution is recommended if terbinafine is given to patients taking drugs metabolised by CYP2D6 such as tricyclic antidepressants.[2] It would seem prudent to monitor for tricyclic adverse effects (such as dry mouth, blurred vision and urinary retention). Tricyclic levels may return to normal only slowly after discontinuation of terbinafine.[1,2,6] It is also suggested that there may be a risk of clinically significant interactions if these drugs are given within 3 months of stopping terbinafine.[1]

1. Castberg I, Helle J, Aamo TO. Prolonged pharmacokinetic drug interaction between terbinafine and amitriptyline. *Ther Drug Monit* (2005) 27, 680–2.
2. Madani S, Barilla D, Cramer J, Wang Y, Paul C. Effect of terbinafine on the pharmacokinetics and pharmacodynamics of desipramine in healthy volunteers identified as cytochrome P450 2D6 (CYP2D6) extensive metabolizers. *J Clin Pharmacol* (2002) 42, 1211–18.
3. O'Reardon JP, Hetznecker JM, Rynn MA, Baldassano CF, Szuba MP. Desipramine toxicity with terbinafine. *Am J Psychiatry* (2002) 159, 492. Erratum ibid. 1076.
4. Teitelbaum ML, Pearson VE. Imipramine toxicity and terbinafine. *Am J Psychiatry* (2001) 158, 2086.
5. van der Kuy P-HM, Hooymans PM, Verkaaik AJB. Nortriptyline intoxication induced by terbinafine. *BMJ* (1998) 316, 441.
6. van der Kuy P-HM, van den Heuvel HA, Kempen RW, Vanmolkot LML. Pharmacokinetic interaction between nortriptyline and terfenadine. *Ann Pharmacother* (2002) 36, 1712–14.

Tricyclic antidepressants + Thyroid hormones

The antidepressant response to imipramine, amitriptyline and possibly other tricyclics can be accelerated by the use of thyroid hormones. However, isolated cases of paroxysmal atrial tachycardia, thyrotoxicosis and hypothyroidism have occurred on concurrent use.

Clinical evidence, mechanism, importance and management

The addition of **liothyronine** 25 micrograms daily was found to increase the speed and efficacy of **imipramine** in relieving depression.[1] Similar results have been described in other studies with **desipramine**[2] or **amitriptyline**[3] but the reasons are not understood. One possible explanation is that the patients had overt or subclinical hypothyroidism, which after correction with **liothyronine** allowed them to overcome an impaired response to tricyclic antidepressants.[4] However, adverse reactions have also been seen. A patient being treated for both hypothyroidism and depression with **thyroid** 60 mg and **imipramine** 150 mg daily complained of dizziness and nausea. She was found to have developed paroxysmal atrial tachycardia.[5] A 10-year-old girl with congenital hypothyroidism, well controlled on desiccated **thyroid** 150 mg daily, developed severe thyrotoxicosis after taking **imipramine** 25 mg daily for 5 months for enuresis. The problem disappeared when the **imipramine** was withdrawn.[6] In another patient the effect of **levothyroxine** was lost and hypothyroidism developed when **dosulepin** was started.[7]

This is normally an advantageous interaction,[8] in which **liothyronine** appears to have a significantly greater antidepressant-potentiating effect than **levothyroxine**.[9] These apparent interactions remain unexplained. There would seem to be no good reason, generally speaking, for avoiding concurrent use unless problems arise.

1. Wilson IC, Prange AJ, McClane TK, Rabon AM, Lipton MA. Thyroid-hormone enhancement of imipramine in nonretarded depressions. *N Engl J Med* (1970) 282, 1063–7.
2. Extein I. Case reports of l-triiodothyronine potentiation. *Am J Psychiatry* (1982) 139, 966–7.
3. Wheatley D. Potentiation of amitriptyline by thyroid hormone. *Arch Gen Psychiatry* (1972) 26, 229–33.
4. Berlin I, Corruble E. Thyroid hormones and antidepressant response. *Am J Psychiatry* (2002) 159, 1441.
5. Prange AJ. Paroxysmal auricular tachycardia apparently resulting from combined thyroid-imipramine treatment. *Am J Psychiatry* (1963) 119, 994–5.
6. Colantonio LA, Orson JM. Triiodothyronine thyrotoxicosis. Induction by desiccated thyroid and imipramine. *Am J Dis Child* (1974) 128, 396–7.
7. Beeley L, Beadle F, Lawrence R. *Bulletin of the West Midlands Centre for Adverse Drug Reaction Reporting* (1984) 19, 11.
8. Altshuler LL, Bauer M, Frye MA, Gitlin MJ, Mintz J, Szuba MP, Leight KL, Whybrow PC. Does thyroid supplementation accelerate tricyclic antidepressant response? A review and meta-analysis of the literature. *Am J Psychiatry* (2001) 158, 1617–22.
9. Joffe RT, Singer W. A comparison of triiodothyronine and thyroxine in the potentiation of tricyclic antidepressants. *Psychiatry Res* (1990) 32, 241–51.

Tricyclic antidepressants + Tobacco

Smoking tobacco reduces the plasma levels of amitriptyline, clomipramine, desipramine, imipramine and nortriptyline, but this does not appear to result in a clinically significant interaction.

Clinical evidence

Two studies found no difference between the steady-state **nortriptyline** plasma levels of tobacco smokers and non-smokers,[1,2] but others have found that smoking tobacco lowers the plasma levels of **amitriptyline**, **clomipramine**,[3] **desipramine**, **imipramine**[4] and **nortriptyline**.[5] For example a 25% reduction in plasma **nortriptyline** levels was found in one study,[5] and a 45% reduction in total levels of **imipramine** and its metabolite, desipramine, was found in another.[4]

Mechanism

The probable reason for the reduced tricyclic levels is that some of the components of tobacco smoke are enzyme inducers, which increase the metabolism of these antidepressants by the liver.

Importance and management

These interactions are established but it might wrongly be concluded from the figures quoted that smokers need larger doses to control their depression. Some evidence suggests that the plasma levels of free (and pharmacologically active) nortriptyline are greater in smokers than non-smokers (10.2% compared with 7.4%), which probably offsets the fall in total plasma levels.[5] Thus the lower plasma levels in smokers may be as therapeutically effective as the higher levels in non-smokers, so that there is probably no need to raise the dosage to accommodate this interaction.

1. Norman TR, Burrows GD, Maguire KP, Rubinstein G, Scoggins BA, Davies B. Cigarette smoking and plasma nortriptyline levels. *Clin Pharmacol Ther* (1977) 21, 453–6.
2. Alexanderson B, Price Evans DA, Sjöqvist F. Steady-state plasma levels of nortriptyline in twins: influence of genetic factors and drug therapy. *BMJ* (1969) 4, 764–8.
3. John VA, Luscombe DK, Kemp H. Effects of age, cigarette smoking and the oral contraceptive on the pharmacokinetics of clomipramine and its desmethyl metabolite during chronic dosing. *J Int Med Res* (1980) 8 (Suppl 3), 88–95.
4. Perel JM, Hurwic MJ, Kanzler MB. Pharmacodynamics of imipramine in depressed patients. *Psychopharmacol Bull* (1975) 11, 16–18.
5. Perry PJ, Browne JL, Prince RA, Alexander B, Tsuang MT. Effects of smoking on nortriptyline plasma concentrations in depressed patients. *Ther Drug Monit* (1986) 8, 279–84.

Tricyclic antidepressants + Urinary acidifiers or alkalinisers

The urinary excretion of desipramine, nortriptyline and other tricyclic antidepressants are not significantly affected by drugs that alter urinary pH.

Clinical evidence, mechanism, importance and management

Because the tricyclics are bases it might be expected that changes in the urinary pH would have an effect on their excretion, but in fact the excretion of unchanged drug is small (less than 5% with **nortriptyline** and **desipramine**) compared with the amounts metabolised by the liver.[1] Only in the case of hepatic impairment is simple urinary clearance likely to take on a more important role.

1. Sjöqvist F, Berglund F, Borgå O, Hammer W, Andersson S, Thorstrand C. The pH-dependent excretion of monomethylated tricyclic antidepressants. *Clin Pharmacol Ther* (1969) 10, 826–33.

Tricyclic antidepressants + Valproate

Amitriptyline and nortriptyline plasma levels can be increased by sodium valproate and valpromide, but in contrast, an isolated report attributes a paradoxical rise in serum desipramine levels to the withdrawal of valproic acid. Valproate pharmacokinetics may be moderately affected by amitriptyline. Status epilepticus has been attributed to elevated clomipramine levels in a patient taking valproic acid.

Clinical evidence

(a) Sodium or Semisodium valproate

In one study, 15 healthy subjects were given a single 50-mg dose of **amitriptyline** 2 hours after taking the ninth dose of semisodium valproate 500 mg every 12 hours. The maximum plasma levels and AUC of **amitriptyline** were raised by 19% and 30%, respectively. The corresponding values for the nortriptyline metabolite were 28% and 55%, respectively.[1] A study in 6 patients with depression found that **amitriptyline** 100 mg daily for 3 weeks produced a 43% increase in the volume of distribution and a 16% increase in the plasma half-life of a single 400-mg intravenous dose of sodium valproate. The AUC and total body clearance of valproate were not significantly changed.[2]

One patient developed delirium within 3 days, and another developed grossly elevated **nortriptyline** plasma levels (393 nanograms/mL, about threefold higher than the therapeutic range) and evidence of toxicity (tremulousness of hands and fingers) about one week after starting valproate 750 mg to 1 g daily. The toxicity rapidly disappeared when both drugs were stopped. Another patient also developed elevated **nortriptyline** plasma levels, attributed to the addition of valproate.[3] A patient taking **clomipramine** 150 mg daily suffered feelings of numbness and sleep disturbances attributed to elevated serum levels of **clomipramine** and desmethylclomipramine, caused by valproate 1 to 1.4 g daily. Halving the dose of **clomipramine** restored serum concentrations to therapeutic levels.[4]

(b) Valproic acid

An epileptic patient who had been seizure-free for 3 years while taking valproic acid developed a prolonged episode of status epilepticus 12 days after starting to taking **clomipramine** 75 mg daily. The **clomipramine** serum level 7 hours after the last dose was 341.6 nanograms/mL (usual levels 68 to 272 nanograms/mL). The seizure was attributed to the elevated **clomipramine** levels.[5] In contrast, a woman taking valproic acid, tiotixene and **desipramine** developed elevated and potentially toxic serum **desipramine** levels (a rise from 259 to 324 nanograms/mL) at the end of a 3-month period during which valproic acid was gradually withdrawn and replaced by clorazepate. The authors of the report attributed this reaction to the valproic acid withdrawal.[6]

(c) Valpromide

In 10 patients valpromide 600 mg daily for 10 days caused a 65% rise in the plasma levels of **nortriptyline** (from 61 to 100.5 nanograms/mL) and a 50% rise in the levels of **amitriptyline** (from 70.5 to 105.5 nanograms/mL).[7,8]

Mechanism

Uncertain. Inhibition of the metabolism of these tricyclics by valproate has been suggested.[3-5]

Importance and management

Information seems to be limited to these reports. It would seem prudent to monitor for tricyclic adverse effects (such as dry mouth, blurred vision and urinary retention) in patients given valproate and amitriptyline, clomipramine, or nortriptyline and to reduce the dosage of the tricyclic if necessary. Where possible consider monitoring tricyclic levels. Information about other tricyclic antidepressants seems to be lacking. The occurrence of status epilepticus in another patient reinforces the fact that the tricyclics can lower the convulsive threshold and should therefore be used with caution in patients with epilepsy.

1. Wong SL, Cavanaugh J, Shi H, Awni WM, Granneman GR. Effects of divalproex sodium on amitriptyline and nortriptyline pharmacokinetics. *Clin Pharmacol Ther* (1996) 60, 48–53.
2. Pisani F, Primerano G, D'Agostino AA, Spina E, Fazio A. Valproic acid-amitriptyline interaction in man. *Ther Drug Monit* (1986) 8, 382–3.
3. Fu C, Katzman M, Goldbloom DS. Valproate/nortriptyline interaction. *J Clin Psychopharmacol* (1994) 14, 205–6.
4. Fehr C, Gründer G, Hiemke C, Dahmen N. Increase in serum clomipramine concentrations caused by valproate. *J Clin Psychopharmacol* (2000) 20, 493–4.
5. DeToledo JC, Haddad H, Ramsay RE. Status epilepticus associated with the combination of valproic acid and clomipramine. *Ther Drug Monit* (1997) 19, 71–3.
6. Joseph AB, Wroblewski BA. Potentially toxic serum concentrations of desipramine after discontinuation of valproic acid. *Brain Inj* (1993) 7, 463–5.
7. Bertschy G, Vandel S, Jounet JM, Allers G. Interaction valpromide-amitriptyline. Augmentation de la biodisponibilité de l'amitriptyline et de la nortriptyline par le valpromide. *Encephale* (1990) 16, 43–5.
8. Vandel S, Bertschy G, Jounet JM, Allers G. Valpromide increases the plasma concentrations of amitriptyline and its metabolite nortriptyline in depressive patients. *Ther Drug Monit* (1988) 10, 386–9.

Tricyclic antidepressants; Amitriptyline + Ethchlorvynol

Transient delirium has been attributed to the concurrent use of amitriptyline and ethchlorvynol,[1] but no details were given and there appear to be no other reports confirming this alleged interaction.

1. Hussar DA. Tabular compilation of drug interactions. *Am J Pharm* (1969) 141, 109–156.

Tricyclic antidepressants; Amitriptyline + Furazolidone

A report describes the development of toxic psychosis, hyperactivity, sweating and hot and cold flushes in a woman taking amitriptyline with furazolidone, and diphenoxylate with atropine.

Clinical evidence, mechanism, importance and management

A depressed woman taking daily doses of conjugated oestrogens 1.25 mg and amitriptyline 75 mg, was also given furazolidone 300 mg daily and diphenoxylate with atropine sulfate. Two days later she began to experience blurred vision, profuse perspiration followed by alternate chills and hot flushes, restlessness, motor activity, persecutory delusions, auditory hallucinations and visual illusions. The symptoms cleared within a day of stopping the furazolidone.[1] The reasons are not understood but the authors point out that furazolidone has MAO-inhibitory properties and that the symptoms were similar to those seen when the tricyclic antidepressants and MAOIs interact. However the MAO-inhibitory activity of furazolidone normally develops over several days. Whether the concurrent use of atropine and amitriptyline (both of which have antimuscarinic activity) had some part to play in the reaction is uncertain. No firm conclusions can be drawn from this slim evidence, but clinicians should be aware of this case when considering the concurrent use of tricyclic antidepressants and furazolidone.

1. Aderhold RM and Muniz CE. Acute psychosis with amitriptyline and furazolidone. *JAMA* (1970) 213, 2080.

Tricyclic antidepressants; Amitriptyline + Sucralfate

Sucralfate causes a marked reduction in the absorption of amitriptyline.

Clinical evidence, mechanism, importance and management

When 6 healthy subjects took a single 75-mg dose of amitriptyline with a single 1-g dose of sucralfate, the AUC of the amitriptyline was reduced by 50%.[1] Concurrent use should be monitored to confirm that the therapeutic effects of the antidepressant are not lost. An increase in the dosage may be needed. There seems to be nothing documented about other tricyclics.

1. Ryan R, Carlson J, Farris F. Effect of sucralfate on the absorption and disposition of amitriptyline in humans. *Fedn Proc* (1986) 45, 205.

Tricyclic antidepressants; Clomipramine + Ademetionine

A severe reaction, diagnosed as the serotonin syndrome, developed in a woman taking ademetionine shortly after her clomipramine dosage was raised.

Clinical evidence, mechanism, importance and management

An elderly woman with a major affective disorder was treated with intramuscular ademetionine 100 mg daily and clomipramine 25 mg daily for 10 days. About 2 to 3 days after the clomipramine dosage was raised to 75 mg daily, she became progressively agitated, anxious and confused. On admission to hospital she was stuporous, with a pulse rate of 130 bpm, a respiratory rate of 30 breaths per minute, and she had diarrhoea, myoclonus, generalised tremors, rigidity, hyperreflexia, shivering, profound diaphoresis and dehydration. Her temperature rose from 40.5 to 43°C. She had no infection, and the diagnosis was of 'the serotonin syndrome', (p.9). The drugs were withdrawn and she was given dantrolene 50 mg intravenously every 6 hours for 48 hours. She made a complete recovery.[1] The reason for this severe adverse reaction is not understood.

1. Iruela LM, Minguez L, Merino J, Monedero G. Toxic interaction of *S*-adenosylmethionine and clomipramine. *Am J Psychiatry* (1993) 150, 522.

Tricyclic antidepressants; Clomipramine + Oxybutynin

Oxybutynin reduced the blood levels of clomipramine in one patient.

Clinical evidence, mechanism, importance and management

An elderly woman had clomipramine and desmethylclomipramine blood levels of 405 and 50 nanograms/mL, respectively, after taking clomipramine 25 mg daily and fluvoxamine 100 mg daily for 18 days. Within one week of starting oxybutynin 5 mg daily, the levels of clomipramine and desmethylclomipramine had fallen to 133 and less than 25 nanograms/mL, respectively, and remained low during a further week of concurrent treatment.[1]

Clomipramine levels may be reduced because oxybutynin is an inducer of cytochrome P450 isoenzymes, which could increase the metabolism of clomipramine, and therefore reduce it levels.[1] This appears to be the only report of an interaction, the mechanism of which is not fully clear. It is therefore of unknown general significance. However, note that both tricyclic antidepressants and oxybutynin have antimuscarinic effects, which may be additive on concurrent use. Consider 'Antimuscarinics + Antimuscarinics', p.674, for more on this potential interaction.

1. Grozinger M, Hartter S, Hiemke C, Roschke J. Oxybutynin enhances the metabolism of clomipramine and dextrorphan possibly by induction of a cytochrome P450 isoenzyme. *J Clin Psychopharmacol* (1999) 19, 287–9.

Tricyclic antidepressants; Desipramine + Propafenone

An isolated report describes markedly raised serum desipramine levels in a patient who also took propafenone.

Clinical evidence, mechanism, importance and management

A man with major depression responded well to desipramine 175 mg daily with serum desipramine levels in the range of 500 to 1000 nanomol/L. When he was treated for paroxysmal atrial fibrillation with digoxin 250 micrograms daily and propafenone 150 mg twice daily and 300 mg at night he developed markedly elevated serum desipramine levels (2092 nanomol/L) and toxicity (dry mouth, sedation, shakiness) while taking desipramine 150 mg daily. The adverse effects resolved when the desipramine was stopped for 5 days, but when it was restarted at 75 mg daily his serum desipramine levels were still raised (1130 nanomol/L).

The raised desipramine levels are thought to result from decreased metabolism and clearance, caused by propafenone.[1] The general importance of this case is uncertain, but be alert for signs of desipramine toxicity in any patient given propafenone concurrently. Adjust the desipramine dosage appropriately.

1. Katz MR. Raised serum levels of desipramine with the antiarrhythmic propafenone. *J Clin Psychiatry* (1991) 52, 432–3.

Tricyclic antidepressants; Doxepin + Tamoxifen

An isolated report describes a reduction in doxepin serum levels attributed to the use of tamoxifen.

Clinical evidence, mechanism, importance and management

A 79-year-old woman with a long history of bipolar disorder, stabilised on lithium carbonate and doxepin 200 mg at bedtime and also taking propranolol, was given tamoxifen 20 mg daily after a mastectomy for breast cancer. It was noted that her total blood levels of doxepin and its major metabolite were reduced by about 25% over the next 11 months. The control of her depression remained unchanged. The reasons for this apparent interaction are not known.[1] The manufacturer of tamoxifen has another undetailed and isolated report of a possible interaction.[2]

This appears to be the first and only clear report of an interaction between a tricyclic antidepressant and tamoxifen so that its general importance is not known. It seems likely to be small.

1. Jefferson JW. Tamoxifen-associated reduction in tricyclic antidepressant levels in blood. *J Clin Psychopharmacol* (1995) 15, 223–4.
2. Zeneca, Personal communication. November 1995.

Tricyclic antidepressants; Imipramine + Beta blockers

Propranolol increased the imipramine levels in two children. Labetalol has been found to increase imipramine levels in adults. The clinical importance of these interactions is uncertain.

Clinical evidence

(a) Labetalol

In 13 healthy subjects labetalol 200 mg every 12 hours for 4 days, increased the AUC of a single 100-mg dose of imipramine by 53%, when compared with a placebo.[1] The maximum plasma level increased by 28%.

(b) Propranolol

A 9-year-old boy was given propranolol for the control of anger and aggression, and imipramine for stress and depression. When his imipramine dosage was raised from 60 to 80 mg daily and his propranolol dose was also raised, from 360 to 400 mg daily, his levels of imipramine plus metabolite (desipramine) rose sharply from a total of 139 nanograms/mL to 469 nanograms/mL. Reducing the imipramine to 60 mg and raising the propranolol to 440 mg daily only reduced the total imipramine/desipramine levels to 426 nanograms/mL. Another imipramine reduction to 40 mg and an increase in the propranolol dose to 480 mg daily resulted in a final total imipramine/desipramine level of 207 nanograms/mL. No significant adverse effects or heart block occurred.[2]

A 9-year-old girl taking imipramine 75 mg daily with a total imipramine/desipramine level of 260 nanograms/mL, had a marked rise to 408 nanograms/mL within 3 days of starting to take propranolol 10 mg three times daily. Two days after stopping the imipramine, her desipramine level (imipramine not measured) had fallen from 382 to 222 nanograms/mL.[2]

Mechanism

Uncertain. The suggestion is that these drugs compete for metabolism (hydroxylation) by the same cytochrome P450 isoenzymes (CYP2D6 and CYP2C8) in the liver, with imipramine being the 'loser', resulting in its accumulation in the body.[2]

Importance and management

Information seems to be limited to these two studies. The clinical importance of this interaction is uncertain, but it would now be prudent to monitor the outcome if propranolol or labetalol is added to treatment with imipramine. Tricyclic adverse effects include dry mouth, blurred vision and urinary retention. Where possible consider monitoring the plasma imipramine levels. There seems to be no information as yet about other beta blockers or tricyclic antidepressants.

1. Hermann DJ, Krol TF, Dukes GE, Hussey EK, Danis M, Han Y-H, Powell JR, Hak LJ. Comparison of verapamil, diltiazem, and labetalol on the bioavailability and metabolism of imipramine. *J Clin Pharmacol* (1992) 32, 176–83.
2. Gillette DW, Tannery LP. Beta blocker inhibits tricyclic metabolism. *J Am Acad Child Adolesc Psychiatry* (1994) 33, 223–4.

Tricyclic antidepressants; Imipramine + Vinpocetine

Vinpocetine does not appear to affect plasma imipramine levels.

Clinical evidence, mechanism, importance and management

In 18 healthy subjects the steady-state plasma levels of imipramine 25 mg three times daily were unaffected by vinpocetine 10 mg three times daily, taken concurrently for 10 days.[1] No special precautions would seem to be necessary. There seems to be nothing documented about any of the other tricyclic antidepressants.

1. Hitzenberger G, Schmid R, Braun W, Grandt R. Vinpocetine therapy does not change imipramine pharmacokinetics in man. *Int J Clin Pharmacol Ther Toxicol* (1990) 28, 99–104.

35

Miscellaneous drugs

Acamprosate + Miscellaneous

Naltrexone modestly increases the rate and extent of acamprosate absorption. There is no pharmacokinetic interaction between acamprosate and alcohol or diazepam. Disulfiram does not alter the pharmacokinetics of acamprosate, and acamprosate does not alter the pharmacokinetics of imipramine. The combination of acamprosate and barbiturates, meprobamate, or oxazepam does not appear to increase the risk of adverse effects.

Clinical evidence, mechanism, importance and management

(a) Alcohol

In studies in healthy subjects, the pharmacokinetics of both alcohol and acamprosate were unchanged by concurrent use.[1]

(b) Antidepressants, anxiolytics and hypnotics

A 15-day study in 591 patients, to assess the effects of the concurrent use of acamprosate with other drugs commonly used in the management of alcohol withdrawal, found no evidence of additional adverse effects with **meprobamate**, **oxazepam**, or the barbiturate complex **tetrabamate** (that includes **phenobarbital**).[2] Other studies found that acamprosate caused no clinically relevant changes in **imipramine** pharmacokinetics, and the pharmacokinetics of both **diazepam** and acamprosate were unchanged by concurrent use.[1]

No special precautions would therefore appear to be needed with any of these drugs.

(c) Disulfiram

In a study in 12 healthy subjects, disulfiram 500 mg once daily for 7 days did not alter the plasma levels of acamprosate 666 mg three times daily.[1]

(d) Naltrexone

In a study in 24 healthy subjects, the concurrent use of naltrexone 50 mg daily and acamprosate 2 g daily for 7 days modestly increased the rate and extent of absorption of acamprosate, as indicated by a 33% increase in maximum level, a 33% reduction in time to maximum level, and a 25% increase in AUC. There was no change in naltrexone pharmacokinetics.[3] Similarly, an increase in acamprosate levels was seen in a study of the use of acamprosate and naltrexone in alcohol-dependent subjects.[4] No particular adverse events were identified on concurrent use,[3,4] suggesting that the drugs may be used together.

1. Saivin S, Hulot T, Chabac S, Potgieter A, Durbin P, Houin G. Clinical pharmacokinetics of acamprosate. *Clin Pharmacokinet* (1998) 35, 331–45.
2. Aubin HJ, Lehert P, Beaupère B, Parot P, Barrucand D. Tolerability of the combination of acamprosate with drugs used to prevent alcohol withdrawal syndrome. *Alcoholism* (1995) 31, 25–38.
3. Mason BJ, Goodman AM, Dixon RM, Hameed MHA, Hulot T, Wesnes K, Hunter JA, Boyeson MG. A pharmacokinetic and pharmacodynamic drug interaction study of acamprosate and naltrexone. Neuropsychopharmacology. (2002) 27, 596–606.
4. Johnson BA, O'Malley SS, Ciraulo DA, Roache JD, Chambers RA, Sarid-Segal O, Couper D. Dose-ranging kinetics and behavioral pharmacology of naltrexone and acamprosate, both alone and combined, in alcohol-dependent subjects. *J Clin Psychopharmacol* (2003) 23, 281–93.

Agalsidase + Miscellaneous

Agalsidase alfa and agalsidase beta should not be given with amiodarone, chloroquine, gentamicin, monobenzone due to a theoretical risk of inhibition of intra-cellular alpha-galactosidase activity.[1,2] These enzymes are unlikely to interact via cytochrome p450-mediated mechanisms.[1]

1. Replagal (Agalsidase alfa). Shire Human Genetic Therapies. UK Summary of product characteristics, February 2007.
2. Fabrazyme (Agalsidase beta). Genzyme Therapeutics. UK Summary of product characteristics, February 2007.

Allopurinol + Aluminium hydroxide

Three haemodialysis patients had a marked reduction in the effects of allopurinol while taking aluminium hydroxide. Separating the doses by 3 hours reduced the effects of this interaction.

Clinical evidence

Three patients receiving haemodialysis, taking 5.7 g of aluminium hydroxide daily and allopurinol 300 mg daily for high phosphate and uric acid levels, had no reduction in their hyperuricaemia until the aluminium hydroxide was given 3 hours before the allopurinol, whereupon their uric acid levels fell by 40 to 65%. When one patient returned to taking both preparations together, her uric acid levels began to rise.[1]

Mechanism

Not understood, but it seems likely that aluminium and allopurinol may bind in the gut, resulting in impaired allopurinol absorption.

Importance and management

Information seems to be limited to this report. Renal patients taking large doses of aluminium should be advised to separate the administration of these two drugs by 3 hours or more to avoid admixture in the gut. The effects of lower doses of aluminium and the effects in patients with normal renal function do not appear to have been studied.

1. Weissman I, Krivoy N. Interaction of aluminum hydroxide and allopurinol in patients on chronic hemodialysis. *Ann Intern Med* (1987) 107, 787.

Allopurinol + Iron compounds

No adverse interaction occurs if iron and allopurinol are given concurrently.

Clinical evidence, mechanism, importance and management

Some early *animal* studies, where allopurinol was given in very large doses, suggested that allopurinol might have an inhibitory effect on the release of iron from hepatic stores. It was feared that this might result in hepatic iron overload. This led the manufacturers of allopurinol in some countries to issue a warning about their concurrent use.[1] However, subsequent research suggests that no special precautions are needed.[1-3]

1. Ascione FJ. Allopurinol and iron. *JAMA* (1975) 232, 1010.

2. Emmerson BT. Effects of allopurinol on iron metabolism in man. *Ann Rheum Dis* (1966) 25, 700–703.
3. Davis PS, Deller DJ. Effect of a xanthine-oxidase inhibitor (allopurinol) on radioiron absorption in man. *Lancet* (1966) ii, 470–2.

Allopurinol + Tamoxifen

A single case report describes allopurinol hepatotoxicity in a man given tamoxifen.

Clinical evidence, mechanism, importance and management

An elderly man who had been taking allopurinol 300 mg daily for 12 years developed fever and marked increases in his serum levels of lactic dehydrogenase and alkaline phosphatase within a day of starting to take tamoxifen 10 mg twice daily.[1] He rapidly recovered when the allopurinol was stopped. The reasons for the reaction are not understood, but the authors suggested that the increased hepatotoxic effect may have resulted from tamoxifen inhibiting allopurinol metabolism, thereby increasing the serum levels of allopurinol and its metabolite. The general importance of this isolated report is not known.

1. Shah KA, Levin J, Rosen N, Greenwald E, Zumoff B. Allopurinol hepatotoxicity potentiated by tamoxifen. *N Y State J Med* (1982) 82, 1745–6.

Allopurinol + Thiazide diuretics

Severe allergic reactions to allopurinol have been seen in a few patients with renal impairment who were also taking thiazide diuretics.

Clinical evidence, mechanism, importance and management

Most patients tolerate allopurinol very well, but life-threatening hypersensitivity reactions (e.g. rash, vasculitis, hepatitis, eosinophilia, progressive renal impairment) develop very occasionally with doses of 200 to 400 mg of allopurinol daily.[1] A report of six such hypersensitivity reactions found that all of the reported cases were associated with pre-existing renal impairment, and in half of these, the patients were also taking thiazide diuretics.[1] Another report describes two patients who developed a hypersensitivity vasculitis while taking allopurinol and **hydrochlorothiazide**.[2] The excretion of oxipurinol (the major metabolite of allopurinol) is reduced in renal impairment, but studies indicate that in healthy subjects with normal renal function thiazide diuretics, such as **hydrochlorothiazide**, do not appear to affect either the plasma levels of oxipurinol or its excretion.[3,4] However, other studies have shown that the effects of allopurinol on pyrimidine metabolism are enhanced by the use of thiazides (i.e. they potentially increase hyperuricaemia, which may lead to renal damage).[5] Some caution is therefore appropriate if both drugs are used, particularly if renal function is impaired, but more study is needed to confirm this possible interaction.

1. Hande KR, Noone RM, Stone WJ. Severe allopurinol toxicity. Description and guidelines for prevention in patients with renal insufficiency. *Am J Med* (1984) 76, 47–56.
2. Young JL, Boswell RB, Nies AS. Severe allopurinol hypersensitivity. Association with thiazides and prior renal compromise. *Arch Intern Med* (1974) 134, 553–8.
3. Hande KR. Evaluation of a thiazide-allopurinol drug interaction. *Am J Med Sci* (1986) 292, 213–16.
4. Löffler W, Landthaler R, de Vries JX, Walter-Sack I, Ittensohn A, Voss A, Zöllner N. Interaction of allopurinol and hydrochlorothiazide during prolonged oral administration of both drugs in normal subjects. I. Uric acid kinetics. *Clin Investig* (1994) 72, 1071–5.
5. Wood MH, O'Sullivan WJ, Wilson M, Tiller DJ. Potentiation of an effect of allopurinol on pyrimidine metabolism by chlorothiazide in man. *Clin Exp Pharmacol Physiol* (1974) 1, 53–8.

Allopurinol + Uricosuric drugs

Probenecid and benzbromarone increase the renal excretion of oxipurinol, the active metabolite of allopurinol, but this probably does not alter clinical efficacy. Theoretically, the use of uricosuric drugs with allopurinol could lead to uric acid precipitation in the kidneys and therefore maintenance of a high urine output is recommended when allopurinol is given by injection. Probenecid markedly increases the serum levels of allopurinol riboside, which may be advantageous in some circumstances.

Clinical evidence, mechanism, importance and management

(a) Allopurinol

Probenecid appears to increase the renal excretion of the active metabolite of allopurinol, oxipurinol,[1] while allopurinol is thought to inhibit the metabolism of **probenecid**.[2] Allopurinol can increase the half-life and raise the serum levels of **probenecid** by about 50% and 20%, respectively.[2] In another study, **benzbromarone** lowered the AUC of oxipurinol by about 40%, but did not affect allopurinol levels.[3]

It has been suggested that the use of allopurinol and **probenecid** might lead to an increase in the excretion of uric acid, which could result in the precipitation of uric acid in the kidneys. Conversely, increased renal excretion of oxipurinol might decrease the efficacy of allopurinol. However, the clinical importance of these mutual interactions seems to be minimal. No problems were reported in two studies in patients given 100 to 600 mg of allopurinol and 500 mg to 2.5 g of **probenecid** daily for between 8 and 16 weeks.[4] Similarly, combined use of allopurinol and **benzbromarone** was more effective in lowering serum uric acid than allopurinol alone.[3] Nevertheless, the UK manufacturer recommends that the significance of any reduction in efficacy, which may occur when uricosuric drugs are given with allopurinol, should be assessed in each case.[5] For allopurinol injection, the US manufacturer recommends that to help prevent renal precipitation of urates in patients receiving concurrent uricosuric drugs, a fluid intake sufficient to give a urinary output of at least 2 litres daily, and the maintenance of neutral or slightly alkaline urine, are desirable.[6]

(b) Allopurinol riboside

A study in 3 healthy subjects found that **probenecid** halved the clearance, increased the peak plasma levels and AUC, and extended the half life of allopurinol riboside.[7] In some circumstances such an interaction may be advantageous as there is some evidence that the cure rate of American trypanosomiasis (Chagas' disease) and cutaneous leishmaniasis is better when the two drugs are used together.[7,8]

1. Elion GB, Yü T-F, Gutman AB, Hitchings GH. Renal clearance of oxipurinol, the chief metabolite of allopurinol. *Am J Med* (1968) 45, 69–77.
2. Horwitz D, Thorgeirsson SS, Mitchell JR. The influence of allopurinol and size of dose on the metabolism of phenylbutazone in patients with gout. *Eur J Clin Pharmacol* (1977) 12, 133–6.
3. Müller FO, Schall R, Groenewoud G, Hundt HKL, van der Merwe JC, van Dyk M. The effect of benzbromarone on allopurinol/oxypurinol kinetics in patients with gout. *Eur J Clin Pharmacol* (1993) 44, 69–72.
4. Yü T-F, Gutman AB. Effect of allopurinol (4-hydroxypyrazolo(3,4-d)pyrimidine) on serum and urinary uric acid in primary and secondary gout. *Am J Med* (1964) 37, 885–98.
5. Zyloric (Allopurinol). GlaxoSmithKline UK. UK Summary of product characteristics, September 2006.
6. Aloprim (Allopurinol sodium). Bedford Laboratories. US Prescribing information, June 2004.
7. Were JBO, Shapiro TA. Effects of probenecid on the pharmacokinetics of allopurinol riboside. *Antimicrob Agents Chemother* (1993) 37, 1193–6.
8. Saenz RE, Paz HM, Johnson CM, Marr JJ, Nelson DJ, Pattishall KH, Rogers MD. Treatment of American cutaneous leishmaniasis with orally administered allopurinol riboside. *J Infect Dis* (1989) 160, 153–8.

Alprostadil + Miscellaneous

Some manufacturers advise that intracavernosal alprostadil and other drugs used for erectile dysfunction should not be given concurrently.

Clinical evidence, mechanism, importance and management

There appear to be no published reports of adverse interactions between intracavernous alprostadil (prostaglandin E_1) and other drugs used for erectile dysfunction, but some manufacturers say that smooth muscle relaxants such as **papaverine** and other drugs used to induce erections such as **alpha-blocking drugs** [e.g. intracavernosal **phentolamine**] should not be used concurrently because of the risks of priapism (painful prolonged abnormal erection).[1]

1. Viridal DUO (Alprostadil). Schwarz Pharma Ltd. UK Summary of product characteristics, July 2006.

Aluminium hydroxide + Ascorbic acid (Vitamin C) or Citrates

Patients with renal failure, given aluminium and oral citrate, can develop a potentially fatal encephalopathy due to a very marked rise in blood aluminium levels. There is evidence that aluminium and vitamin C may interact similarly. Some also suggest that

those with normal renal function should not take aluminium antacids within 2 to 3 hours of foods and drinks that contain citrates. It is worth noting that formulations of a wide range of drugs (including many non-prescription preparations) contain citrates as the effervescing or dispersing agent.

Clinical evidence

(a) Ascorbic acid

A study in 13 healthy subjects given aluminium hydroxide 900 mg three times daily found that ascorbic acid (vitamin C) 2 g daily increased the urinary excretion of aluminium threefold.[1] Ascorbic acid significantly increases the concentration of aluminium in the liver, brain, and bones of *rats* given aluminium hydroxide.[2]

(b) Citrates

Four patients with advanced chronic renal impairment taking aluminium hydroxide and citrate (**Shohl's**) solution died due to hyperaluminaemia.[3] Comparison of these 4 patients with another 34 renal patients revealed that they had taken more aluminium hydroxide, more citrate, and were older. In the group as a whole, increased serum aluminium levels were correlated with increased citrate intake.[4] Five healthy subjects were then given aluminium hydroxide with or without citrate solution: aluminium levels were 11 micrograms/L at baseline, rising to 44 micrograms/L when aluminium hydroxide was given, and rising to 98 micrograms/L when citrate was added. Aluminium clearance also dramatically increased in the presence of citrate.[4] Another report describes this interaction in 2 patients with renal impairment, and in a possible further 6 patients, all of whom died.[5] In a further single-dose study in 6 patients with end-stage renal disease, sodium citrate/citric acid 30 mL markedly increased the AUC of aluminium, from a 30-mL dose of aluminium hydroxide gel, by 4.6-fold.[6] A number of other studies in healthy subjects have confirmed that citrate markedly increases aluminium absorption, see mechanism, below.

A tenfold rise in serum aluminium levels that occurred in a haemodialysis patient given **effervescent co-codamol**, was attributed to the presence of sodium citrate in the formulation, which is used to produce the effervescence.[7]

Mechanism

Studies in healthy subjects clearly demonstrate that citrate markedly increases the absorption of aluminium from the gut.[4,8,9] The absorption is increased threefold if taken with **lemon juice**,[10] eight to tenfold if taken with **orange juice**,[11,12] and five to 50-fold if taken with citrate,[4,8,9,11] but the reason is not understood. It could be that a highly soluble aluminium citrate complex is formed.[5,8]

Importance and management

(a) Patients with renal impairment

The interaction between aluminium and citrates in patients with renal impairment is established and clinically important: it is potentially fatal. Concurrent use should be strictly avoided. The authors of one report emphasise the risks associated with any of the commonly used citrates (sodium, calcium or potassium citrates, citric acid, Shohl's solution (citric acid/sodium citrate), etc).[8] Remember too that some effervescent and dispersible tablets (including many proprietary non-prescription analgesics, indigestion and hangover remedies such as *Alka-Seltzer*) contain citric acid or citrates,[7,13] and they may also occur in soft drinks.[13] Haemodialysis patients should be strongly warned about these. The interaction between aluminium and ascorbic acid is not yet well established, but the information available so far suggests that this combination should also be avoided. It is not clear whether orange juice is also unsafe but the available evidence suggests that concurrent administration is probably best avoided.

(b) Patients with normal renal function

The importance of the interaction between aluminium and citrates in subjects with normal renal function is by no means clear, because it is still not known whether increased aluminium absorption results in aluminium accumulation over the long term, in those with normal renal function.[12] However, some authors have recommended that food or drinks containing citric acid (citrus fruits and fruit juices) should not be taken at the same time as aluminium-containing medicines, but that their ingestion should be separated by 2 to 3 hours.[12]

1. Domingo JL, Gomez M, Llobet JM, Richart C. Effect of ascorbic acid on gastrointestinal aluminium absorption. *Lancet* (1991) 338, 1467.
2. Domingo JL, Gomez M, Llobet JM, Corbella J. Influence of some dietary constituents on aluminum absorption and retention in rats. *Kidney Int* (1991) 39, 598–601.
3. Bakir AA, Hryhorczuk DO, Berman E, Dunea G. Acute fatal hyperaluminemic encephalopathy in undialyzed and recently dialyzed uremic patients. *Trans Am Soc Artif Intern Organs* (1986) 32, 171–6.
4. Bakir AA, Hryhorczuk DO, Ahmed S, Hessl SM, Levy PS, Spengler R, Dunea G. Hyperaluminemia in renal failure: the influence of age and citrate intake. *Clin Nephrol* (1989) 31, 40–4.
5. Kirschbaum HB, Schoolwerth AC. Acute aluminum toxicity associated with oral citrate and aluminum-containing antacids. *Am J Med Sci* (1989) 297, 9–11.
6. Rudy D, Sica DA, Comstock T, Davis J, Savory J, Schoolwerth AC. Aluminum-citrate interaction in end-stage renal disease. *Int J Artif Organs* (1991) 14, 625–9.
7. Main J, Ward MK. Potentiation of aluminium absorption by effervescent analgesic tablets in a haemodialysis patient. *BMJ* (1992) 304, 1686.
8. Coburn JW, Mischel MG, Goodman WG, Salusky IB. Calcium citrate markedly enhances aluminum absorption from aluminium hydroxide. *Am J Kidney Dis* (1991) 17, 708–11.
9. Walker JA, Sherman RA, Cody RP. The effect of oral bases on enteral aluminum absorption. *Arch Intern Med* (1990) 150, 2037–9.
10. Slanina P, Frech W, Ekström L-G, Lööf L, Slorach S, Cedergren A. Dietary citric acid enhances absorption of aluminum in antacids. *Clin Chem* (1986) 32, 539–41.
11. Weberg R, Berstad A. Gastrointestinal absorption of aluminium from single doses of aluminium containing antacids in man. *Eur J Clin Invest* (1986) 16, 428–32.
12. Fairweather-Tait S, Hickson K, McGaw B, Reid M. Orange juice enhances aluminium absorption from antacid preparation. *Eur J Clin Nutr* (1994) 48, 71–3.
13. Dorhout Mees EJ, Basçi A. Citric acid in calcium effervescent tablets may favour aluminium intoxication. *Nephron* (1991) 59, 322.

Aprepitant + CYP2C9 substrates

Aprepitant slightly reduces the plasma levels of 'warfarin', (p.385) and 'tolbutamide' (p.515), because it is an inducer of the cytochrome P450 isoenzyme CYP2C9. The manufacturers therefore recommend caution when aprepitant is given with other drugs that are known to be metabolised by CYP2C9, because of the possibility that their plasma levels may be reduced.[1,2] They specifically mention phenytoin. They also note that, because phenytoin is a 'CYP3A4 inducer', (below), it is predicted to decrease levels of aprepitant and might reduce its efficacy.[1,2] Consequently, the UK manufacturer advises avoiding the concurrent use of phenytoin.[1] Other CYP2C9 substrates are listed in 'Table 1.3', (p.6).

1. Emend (Aprepitant). Merck Sharp & Dohme Ltd. UK Summary of product characteristics, February 2007.
2. Emend (Aprepitant). Merck & Co., Inc. US Prescribing information, June 2006.

Aprepitant + CYP3A4 inducers

Rifampicin markedly reduced the AUC of aprepitant, and reduced efficacy would be expected. In the UK, the manufacturer recommends that concurrent use of aprepitant and other strong inducers of CYP3A4 should be avoided.

Clinical evidence, mechanism, importance and management

The manufacturers note that when a single 375-mg dose of aprepitant was given on day 9 of a 14-day regimen of **rifampicin** 600 mg daily, the AUC of aprepitant was decreased about 11-fold (91%), and the half-life about threefold (68%).[1,2]

Rifampicin is an inducer of the cytochrome P450 isoenzyme CYP3A4, by which aprepitant is metabolised. Concurrent use therefore decreases aprepitant levels

Although not assessed, this marked reduction in aprepitant levels could result in reduced efficacy. In the UK, the manufacturer recommends that concurrent use of aprepitant and strong inducers of CYP3A4, such as **rifampicin**, be avoided.[1] They also name **phenytoin** (see also 'Aprepitant + CYP2C9 substrates', above), **carbamazepine**, and **phenobarbital**, and also recommend that concurrent use of **St John's wort** is avoided.[1] Other inducers of CYP3A4 are listed in 'Table 1.4', (p.6).

1. Emend (Aprepitant). Merck Sharp & Dohme Ltd. UK Summary of product characteristics, February 2007.
2. Emend (Aprepitant). Merck & Co., Inc. US Prescribing information, June 2006.

Aprepitant + CYP3A4 inhibitors

Ketoconazole markedly increases aprepitant levels. The manufacturer recommends caution when aprepitant is used with ketoconazole or other strong inhibitors of CYP3A4.

Clinical evidence, mechanism, importance and management

The manufacturers note that when a single 125-mg dose of aprepitant was given on day 5 of a 10-day course of **ketoconazole** 400 mg daily, the AUC of aprepitant was increased by about fivefold, and the half-life by about threefold.[1,2]

Ketoconazole is an inhibitor of the cytochrome P450 isoenzyme CYP3A4, by which aprepitant is metabolised. Concurrent use therefore raises aprepitant levels.

Although the effect of these increases has not been assessed, such marked increases in levels could increase adverse effects. The manufacturers recommend caution when aprepitant is given with **ketoconazole** and other drugs that are strong inhibitors of CYP3A4. They specifically name **ritonavir**, **clarithromycin**,[1,2] **telithromycin**,[1] **itraconazole**, **nefazodone**, **troleandomycin**, and **nelfinavir**.[2] For the effect of **diltiazem** (a moderate CYP3A4 inhibitor), see 'Calcium-channel blockers + Aprepitant', p.861. Other inhibitors of CYP3A4 are listed in 'Table 1.4', (p.6).

1. Emend (Aprepitant). Merck Sharp & Dohme Ltd. UK Summary of product characteristics, February 2007.
2. Emend (Aprepitant). Merck & Co., Inc. US Prescribing information, June 2006.

Aprepitant + CYP3A4 substrates

Aprepitant can increase the levels of CYP3A4 substrates in the short-term, then reduce them within 2 weeks. Caution is advised. Note that the manufacturers of aprepitant specifically contraindicate its concurrent use with pimozide, terfenadine, astemizole or cisapride.

Clinical evidence, mechanism, importance and management

In the first few days of use, aprepitant 125/80 mg markedly increased levels of midazolam, a probe drug substrate for the cytochrome P450 isoenzyme CYP3A4. Then, within 2 weeks, a reduction in levels was seen, see 'Benzodiazepines + Aprepitant', p.721. This effect was not seen with the 40/25 mg dose regimen. Aprepitant is therefore both a dose-dependent inhibitor and an inducer of CYP3A4.

Because of this, aprepitant is expected to increase drug levels of other CYP3A4 substrates during treatment by up to about threefold, and the manufacturer recommends caution.[1,2] They specifically recommend caution with **ergot derivatives**. Moreover, because of the risk of life-threatening torsade de pointes arrhythmias with increased levels of **pimozide**, **terfenadine**, **astemizole** or **cisapride**, they specifically contraindicate the concurrent use of aprepitant with these CYP3A4 substrates. For a list of CYP3A4 substrates, see 'Table 1.4', (p.6). Within 2 weeks of aprepitant therapy, a reduced level of CYP3A4 substrates might occur, and caution is also advised during this time.

1. Emend (Aprepitant). Merck Sharp & Dohme Ltd. UK Summary of product characteristics, February 2007.
2. Emend (Aprepitant). Merck & Co., Inc. US Prescribing information, June 2006.

Ascorbic acid (Vitamin C) + Salicylates

Aspirin reduces the absorption of ascorbic acid by about one-third. Serum salicylate levels do not appear to be affected by ascorbic acid.

Clinical evidence, mechanism, importance and management

A study in healthy subjects found that the absorption of a single 500-mg dose of ascorbic acid was about one-third lower in those given **aspirin** 900 mg concurrently, and the urinary excretion was about 50% lower.[1] The clinical importance of this is uncertain. It has been suggested that the normal physiological requirement of 30 to 60 mg of ascorbic acid daily may need to be increased to 100 to 200 mg daily in the presence of **aspirin**.[1] Another study in 9 healthy subjects found that ascorbic acid 1 g three times daily did not significantly affect serum salicylate levels of **choline salicylate**.[2]

1. Basu TK. Vitamin C-aspirin interactions. *Int J Vitam Nutr Res* (1982) 23 (Suppl), 83–90.
2. Hansten PD, Hayton WL. Effect of antacid and ascorbic acid on serum salicylate concentration. *J Clin Pharmacol* (1980) 24, 326–31.

Baclofen + Ibuprofen

A man developed baclofen toxicity when given ibuprofen.

Clinical evidence, mechanism, importance and management

An isolated report describes a man taking baclofen 20 mg three times a day, who developed baclofen toxicity (confusion, disorientation, bradycardia, blurred vision, hypotension and hypothermia) after taking 8 doses of ibuprofen 600 mg three times daily. It appeared that the toxicity was caused by ibuprofen-induced acute renal impairment leading to baclofen accumulation.[1] Renal impairment is a relatively rare adverse effect of ibuprofen. The general importance of this interaction is likely to be very small. There appears to be no information about baclofen and other NSAIDs, and little reason for avoiding concurrent use.

1. Dahlin PA, George J. Baclofen toxicity associated with declining renal clearance after ibuprofen. *Drug Intell Clin Pharm* (1984) 18, 805–8.

Baclofen + Tizanidine

No clinically significant pharmacokinetic interaction appears to occur between baclofen and tizanidine.

Clinical evidence, mechanism, importance and management

In a randomised, three-period study, 15 healthy subjects were given baclofen 10 mg three times daily and tizanidine 4 mg three times daily, together and alone, for 7 consecutive doses. None of the pharmacokinetic parameters of either drug were changed by more than 30%, a figure calculated to indicate the presence of an interaction.[1] No changes in the dosages of either drug are therefore likely to be needed if they are taken concurrently.

1. Shellenberger MK, Groves L, Shah J, Novak GD. A controlled pharmacokinetic evaluation of tizanidine and baclofen at steady state. *Drug Metab Dispos* (1999) 27, 201–204.

Benzbromarone + Aspirin

Aspirin antagonises the uricosuric effects of benzbromarone.

Clinical evidence, mechanism, importance and management

A single 160-mg dose of benzbromarone increased the percent ratio of urate to creatinine clearance by 371% at its peak in 6 subjects with gout (i.e. benzbromarone increases urate clearance). However, when the same dose of benzbromarone was given with a single 600-mg dose of aspirin, the peak ratio of urate to creatinine clearance with benzbromarone 160 mg was reduced by about 75%[1] (i.e. aspirin reduces the effect of benzbromarone on urate clearance). In another study aspirin, in divided doses of 650 mg, up to a total of 5.2 g daily, was given to 29 healthy subjects taking benzbromarone 40 to 80 mg daily. The urate lowering effects of benzbromarone were most affected by aspirin 2.7 g; benzbromarone reduced the urate levels by 60%, but in the presence of aspirin 2.7 g the levels were only reduced by 48%.[2] Aspirin and other **salicylates** antagonise the effects of uricosuric drugs such as benzbromarone, and should generally be avoided in those with hyperuricaemia or gout (see also 'Aspirin or other Salicylates + Probenecid', p.138).

1. Sinclair DS, Fox IH. The pharmacology of hypouricemic effect of benzbromarone. *J Rheumatol* (1975) 2, 437–45.
2. Sorensen LB, Levinson DJ. Clinical evaluation of benzbromarone. *Arthritis Rheum* (1976) 19, 183–90.

Benzbromarone + Chlorothiazide

Benzbromarone lowers uric acid levels in patients taking chlorothiazide, without affecting diuretic activity.[1,2]

1. Heel RC, Brogden RN, Speight TM, Avery GS. Benzbromarone: a review of its pharmacological properties and therapeutic use in gout and hyperuricaemia. *Drugs* (1977) 14, 349–66.
2. Gross A, Giraud V. Über die Wirkung von Benzbromaron auf Urikämie und Urikosurie. *Med Welt* (1972) 23, 133–6.

Betahistine + Terfenadine

A single report describes the re-emergence of labyrinthine symptoms when a patient taking betahistine was given terfenadine.

Clinical evidence, mechanism, importance and management

An isolated and very brief report describes a patient whose labyrinthine symptoms (vertigo, dizziness, nausea and vomiting), controlled by betahistine, returned during the concurrent use of terfenadine and other unspecified drugs.[1] This interaction had been predicted on theoretical grounds because betahistine, is an analogue of histamine, and would therefore be expected to interact like this with any antihistamine.[2] The use of antihistamines should be carefully considered in patients taking betahistine.

1. Beeley L, Cunningham H, Brennan A. *Bulletin of the West Midlands Centre for Adverse Drug Reaction Reporting* (1993) 36, 28.
2. Serc (Betahistine). Solvay Healthcare Ltd. UK Summary of product characteristics, October 2006.

Bisphosphonates + Aminoglycosides

Severe hypocalcaemia occurred in two patients taking sodium clodronate when they were given netilmicin or amikacin. Theoretically, additive calcium lowering effects could occur with any bisphosphonate aminoglycoside combination.

Clinical evidence

A 62-year-old woman with multiple myeloma was given **sodium clodronate** 2.4 g daily for osteolysis and bone pain. After 7 days she developed grand mal seizures, and her serum calcium was found to be 1.72 mmol/L (normal range 2.25 to 2.6 mmol/L). Despite daily calcium infusions her calcium remained low. The authors state that symptomatic hypocalcaemia with clodronate is rare, and attributed the dramatic response in this patient to an interaction with a course of **netilmicin** given 5 days earlier for septicaemia.[1]

A 69-year-old man with prostate cancer had been taking **sodium clodronate** 2.4 g daily for bone pain for 13 months, and serum calcium levels had always remained within normal limits. After being admitted with febrile neutropenia following a course of chemotherapy, the clodronate was withdrawn and he was given intravenous **amikacin** and ceftazidime. After 7 days he became unconscious, and developed spontaneous twitching movements in his arms and legs. His calcium was found to be 1.39 mmol/L and he was diagnosed with hypocalcaemic tetany. He was given calcium infusions, and his serum calcium returned to normal over the next 12 hours.[2]

Mechanism

Not fully understood, but one suggestion is that any fall in blood calcium levels brought about by the use of clodronate is normally balanced to some extent by the excretion of parathyroid hormone, which raises blood calcium levels. However, the aminoglycoside antibacterials can damage the kidneys, not only causing the loss of calcium, but of magnesium as well. Any hypomagnesaemia inhibits the activity of the parathyroid gland, so that the normal homoeostatic response to hypocalcaemia is reduced or even abolished.[1,2] Clodronate itself can sometimes be nephrotoxic.

Importance and management

Direct information seems to be limited to these two reports. Biochemical hypocalcaemia is believed to occur in about 10% of patients taking bisphosphonates,[3] but symptomatic hypocalcaemia is said to be rare.[2] It seems therefore that the addition of the aminoglycoside in these two cases precipitated severe clinical hypocalcaemia. The authors of both reports therefore advise care if bisphosphonates are given with aminoglycosides, and recommend close monitoring of calcium and magnesium levels. They also point out that the renal loss of calcium and magnesium can continue for weeks after aminoglycosides are stopped, and that bisphosphonates can also persist in bone for weeks.[1,2] This means that the interaction is potentially possible whether the drugs are given concurrently or sequentially.

1. Pedersen-Bjergaard U, Myhre J. Severe hypoglycaemia (sic) after treatment with diphosphonate and aminoglycoside. *BMJ* (1991) 302, 295.
2. Mayordomo JI, Rivera F. Severe hypocalcaemia after treatment with oral clodronate and aminoglycoside. *Ann Oncol* (1993) 4, 432–5.
3. Jodrell DI, Iveson TJ, Smith IE. Symptomatic hypocalcaemia after treatment with high-dose aminohydroxypropylidene diphosphonate. *Lancet* (1987) i, 622.

Bisphosphonates + Aspirin or NSAIDs

The concurrent use of alendronate and naproxen increased the incidence of gastric mucosal damage in a small pharmacological study, and increased the risk of upper gastrointestinal disorders in a case-control study. However, two analyses of placebo-controlled studies found no increased risk of gastrointestinal damage with the combination. There was no increased risk of gastrointestinal adverse effects in NSAID users given risedronate.
Indometacin raises tiludronate bioavailability, whereas aspirin and diclofenac do not appear to affect the pharmacokinetics of tiludronate. NSAIDs may exacerbate the renal dysfunction sometimes seen with clodronate.

Clinical evidence, mechanism, importance and management

(a) Alendronate

In a short-term endoscopy study in 26 healthy subjects, gastric mucosal damage developed in 8% of those given alendronate alone, in 12% of those given **naproxen** alone, and 38% of those given both drugs.[1] In a case-control study,[2] the risk of having an acid-related upper gastrointestinal disorder with alendronate was increased by the concurrent use of NSAIDs (relative risk 1.7). However, retrospective analysis of data from a very large long-term placebo-controlled study found no evidence that the risk of upper gastrointestinal adverse effects with concurrent use of NSAIDs and alendronate was any greater than with NSAIDs and placebo.[3] Note that this finding has been questioned,[4] and some of the issues responded to.[5] Similarly, in a retrospective analysis of a 12-week placebo-controlled study, in those taking regular NSAIDs (about half of the patients) there was no difference in incidence of upper gastrointestinal adverse events between those given alendronate and those given placebo. The most commonly used NSAIDs in this study were **aspirin**, **celecoxib**, **rofecoxib**, **ibuprofen** and **naproxen**.[6]

Alendronate is commonly known to be associated with oesophageal adverse effects, and there are strict dosing instructions to minimise this risk.[7] It may also cause local irritation of the stomach, although its potential to cause gastric ulcers is not considered established.[3,7]

The status of this interaction is currently controversial. Some consider that alendronate should not be given to patients receiving NSAIDs,[4] while others urge caution in their use together.[1,2] However, some consider that there is no evidence that alendronate adds to the known gastrointestinal toxicity of NSAIDs,[5] and the manufacturer issues no caution about the concurrent use of NSAIDs.[7] Until further evidence is available, it would seem sensible to monitor the concurrent use of alendronate and NSAIDs carefully.

(b) Clodronate

The manufacturer notes that patients receiving NSAIDs in addition to clodronate have developed renal impairment, although a synergistic action has not been established.[8] Clodronate alone may cause renal impairment, and the manufacturers suggest that renal function should be assessed before giving clodronate.[8] This would seem particularly important in those taking NSAIDs.

(c) Risedronate

The manufacturer notes that in phase III osteoporosis studies of risedronate, no clinically relevant interactions were noted, even though aspirin and NSAIDs being used by 33% and 45% of patients, respectively.[9] Similarly, in a retrospective analysis of a 2-year placebo-controlled study, in those using regular NSAIDs (about two-thirds of patients) there was no difference in incidence of upper gastrointestinal adverse events between those given risedronate and those given placebo.[10]

(d) Tiludronate

Single-dose studies in 12 healthy subjects found that **diclofenac** 25 mg and aspirin 600 mg had no significant effect on the pharmacokinetics of tiludronate. On the other hand, **indometacin** 50 mg increased the maximum serum concentration and the AUC of tiludronate about twofold when these drugs were taken together, but not when they were given 2 hours apart.[11] For this reason the manufacturers advise that **indometacin** and tiludronate should be given 2 hours apart.[12]

1. Graham DY, Malaty HM. Alendronate and naproxen are synergistic for development of gastric ulcers. *Arch Intern Med* (2001) 161, 107–110.
2. Ettinger B, Pressman A, Schein J. Clinic visits and hospital admissions for care of acid-related upper gastrointestinal disorders in women using alendronate for osteoporosis. *Am J Manag Care* (1998) 4, 1377–82.
3. Bauer DC, Black D, Ensrud K, Thompson D, Hochberg M, Nevitt M, Musliner T, Freedholm D, for the Fracture Intervention Trial Research Group. Upper gastrointestinal tract safety profile of alendronate. *Arch Intern Med* (2000) 160, 517–25.
4. Rothschild BM. Alendronate and nonsteroidal anti-inflammatory drug interaction safety is not established. *Arch Intern Med* (2000) 160, 1702.
5. Bauer DC, for the Fracture Intervention Trial Research Group. Alendronate and nonsteroidal anti-inflammatory drug interaction safety is not established: a reply. *Arch Intern Med* (2000) 160, 2686.
6. Cryer B, Miller P, Petruschke RA, Chen E, Geba GP, de Papp AE. Upper gastrointestinal tolerability of once weekly alendronate 70 mg with concomitant non-steroidal anti-inflammatory drug use. *Aliment Pharmacol Ther* (2005) 21, 599–607.
7. Fosamax Once Weekly (Alendronate sodium). Merck Sharp & Dohme Ltd. UK Summary of product characteristics, November 2006.
8. Bonefos Capsules (Sodium clodronate). Schering Health Care Ltd. UK Summary of product characteristics, November 2006.
9. Actonel (Risedronate sodium). Procter & Gamble Pharmaceuticals UK Limited. UK Summary of product characteristics, October 2006.
10. Adami S, Pavelka K, Cline GA, Hosterman MA, Barton IP, Cohen SB, Bensen WG. Upper gastrointestinal tract safety of daily oral risedronate in patients taking NSAIDs: a randomized, double-blind, placebo-controlled trial. *Mayo Clin Proc* (2005) 80, 1278–85.
11. Sanofi Winthrop. Data on file, June 1996.
12. Skelid (Disodium tiludronate). Sanofi-Aventis. UK Summary of product characteristics, January 2006.

Bisphosphonates + Polyvalent cations

The oral absorption of bisphosphonates is reduced by *Maalox* and by other antacids, calcium-rich foods, calcium supplements, iron preparations, magnesium-containing laxatives or milk.

Clinical evidence

(a) Clodronate

In a randomised study in 31 healthy subjects the AUC of clodronate was reduced to 10% of the optimum level when it was taken with breakfast. Delaying administration until 2 hours after breakfast only slightly improved the AUC (34% of optimum). The best AUC was achieved when clodronate was given 2 hours before breakfast, although the AUC one hour before was similar (91% of optimum).[1]

(b) Tiludronate

The maximum serum levels and AUC of tiludronate in 12 healthy subjects were halved when *Maalox* (**aluminium/magnesium hydroxide**) was taken one hour before tiludronate, but the bioavailability was only slightly affected when *Maalox* was taken 2 hours after the tiludronate.[2]

Mechanism

The bisphosphonates can form complexes with a number of polyvalent metallic ions (e.g. Al^{3+}, Ca^{2+}, Fe, Mg^{2+}), which can impair their absorption.

Importance and management

Established and important interactions, although the documentation is limited. Bisphosphonates should be prevented from coming into contact with a range of preparations such as **antacids** (containing **aluminium, bismuth, calcium, magnesium**), **laxatives** (containing magnesium), **iron preparations** and **calcium** or other **mineral supplements**. **Food**, **milk** and **dairy products** in particular, contain calcium, and may also impair absorption.

Recommendations on the timing of administration of bisphosphonates in relation to food and other drugs varies.

- The manufacturers of **alendronate**[3] suggest that, in order to avoid absorption interactions, patients should wait at least 30 minutes after taking alendronate before taking any other drug or food, and that alendronate should be taken with plain water only.
- The manufacturers of **tiludronate**[4] recommend that it is taken with water on an empty stomach (at least two hours before or after meals). In addition, they recommend administration of tiludronate and antacids or calcium compounds should be separated by 2 hours.
- The manufacturers of **clodronate**[5] suggest leaving 1 hour between the administration of food and clodronate.
- The manufacturers of **risedronate**[6] recommend it is taken with water at least 30 minutes before the first food or drink of the day. Alternatively, they say it should be given at least 2 hours from any food or drink at any other time of the day, at least 30 minutes before going to bed.
- Similarly, the manufacturers of **etidronate**[7] recommend it is given on an empty stomach at least 2 hours from any food or medicines containing polyvalent cations (as listed above).

1. Laitinen K, Patronen A, Harju P, Löyttyniemi E, Pylkkänen L, Kleimola T, Perttunen K. Timing of food intake has a marked effect on the bioavailability of clodronate. *Bone* (2000) 27, 293–6.
2. Sanofi Winthrop. Data on file, June 1996.
3. Fosamax Once Weekly (Alendronate sodium). Merck Sharp & Dohme Ltd. UK Summary of product characteristics, November 2006.
4. Skelid (Disodium tiluronate). Sanofi-Aventis. UK Summary of product characteristics, January 2006.
5. Bonefos Capsules (Sodium clodronate). Schering Health Care Ltd. UK Summary of product characteristics, November 2006.
6. Actonel 30 mg Film Coated Tablets (Risedronate sodium). Procter & Gamble Pharmaceuticals UK Limited. UK Summary of product characteristics, October 2006.
7. Didronel (Etidronate disodium). Procter & Gamble Pharmaceuticals UK Ltd. UK Summary of product characteristics, October 2006.

Bitter orange + Cytochrome P450 isoenzyme substrates

Bitter orange does not alter the metabolism of caffeine, chlorzoxazone, debrisoquine, or midazolam, and is therefore unlikely to interact with drugs that are metabolised by CYP1A2, CYP2E1, CYP2D6 or CYP3A4.

Clinical evidence, mechanism, importance and management

Bitter orange (*Citrus aurantium*) 350 mg, standardised to 4% synephrine, was given to 12 healthy subjects twice daily for 28 days. Single doses of **caffeine** 100 mg, **chlorzoxazone** 250 mg, **debrisoquine** 5 mg, and **midazolam** 8 mg were given before and at the end of the treatment with bitter orange. The metabolism of these drugs was not affected by the concurrent use of bitter orange, which suggests that bitter orange is unlikely to affect the metabolism of other drugs that are substrates of the cytochrome P450 isoenzymes CYP1A2, CYP2E1, CYP2D6 or CYP3A4.[1] For a list of drugs that are substrates of these enzymes, see 'Table 1.2',(p.4), 'Table 1.3',(p.6), and 'Table 1.4',(p.6).

1. Gurley BJ, Gardner SF, Hubbard MA, Williams DK, Gentry WB, Carrier J, Khan IA, Edwards DJ, Shah A. In vivo assessment of botanical supplementation on human cytochrome P450 phenotypes: *Citrus aurantium*, *Echinacea purpurea*, milk thistle, and saw palmetto. *Clin Pharmacol Ther* (2004) 76, 428–40.

Black cohosh + Cytochrome P450 isoenzyme substrates

Black cohosh does not affect the metabolism of caffeine, chlorzoxazone and debrisoquine, and is therefore unlikely to affect the metabolism of drugs that are substrates for CYP1A2, CYP2E1 and CYP2D6.

Clinical evidence, mechanism, importance and management

In a study in 12 non-smoking healthy subjects given black cohosh root extract 1090 mg twice daily for 28 days before receiving single doses of **caffeine**, **chlorzoxazone** and **debrisoquine**, no clinically significant changes in the metabolism of these drugs were noted. It is therefore unlikely that other drugs metabolised by CYP1A2, CYP2E1, or CYP2D6 (see 'Table 1.2', (p.4), and 'Table 1.3', (p.6)) will be affected by the use of black cohosh (cimicifuga).[1] For the lack of effect of black cohosh on midazolam, see 'benzodiazepines', (p.724).

1. Gurley BJ, Gardner SF, Hubbard MA, Williams DK, Gentry WB, Khan IA, Shah A. In vivo effects of goldenseal, kava kava, black cohosh, and valerian on human cytochrome P450 1A2, 2D6, 2E1, and 3A4/5 phenotypes. *Clin Pharmacol Ther* (2005) 77, 415–26.

Charcoal, activated + Miscellaneous

Small doses of activated charcoal appear to have little effect on the absorption of ciprofloxacin and oral contraceptives (administration separated), and only modestly reduces nizatidine absorption. Case reports describe the lack of efficacy of mitobronitol and reduced serum phenobarbital levels in the presence of small doses of activated charcoal.

Clinical evidence, mechanism, importance and management

The use of activated charcoal, in a usual dose of 50 g, to reduce the absorption of drugs and poisons after acute overdose is well established, as is repeated doses of activated charcoal to enhance the elimination of some drugs taken in overdose after they have been absorbed (e.g. **carbamazepine**, **theophylline**). Studies and references supporting these therapeutic uses of activated charcoal are not reviewed here.

Activated charcoal is also included in various remedies used for gastrointestinal disorders such as flatulence or diarrhoea. Doses in these instances are very much lower (1 to 2 g daily) than those used in the treatment of poisoning, and there seems to be little reported about the effects of these doses on the absorption of other drugs. In one single-dose study in healthy subjects, **nizatidine** absorption was reduced by about 30% when it was taken one hour before activated charcoal 2 g.[1] In another single-dose study in 6 subjects, taking activated charcoal 1 g soon after ciprofloxacin 500 mg, had little effect on the pharmacokinetics of **ciprofloxacin** 500 mg (AUC reduced by 10%).[2]

In one case report, an antiemetic complementary remedy containing activated charcoal was thought to be the cause of a lack of effect of **mitobronitol** 125 mg used to treat primary thrombocythaemia in one patient.[3] In another case report,[4] activated charcoal 2 g three times daily was given with **phenobarbital** and enteral nutrition via a gastric fistula tube. The charcoal appeared to reduce the absorption of **phenobarbital** (serum level 4.3 mg/L compared with a previous level of 24.8 mg/L). Giving the activated charcoal at least one hour apart from the **phenobarbital** resulted in an increase in serum levels to about 16 to 18 mg/L.

Activated charcoal 5 g four times daily was taken for 3 days, mid-cycle, with the first daily dose taken 3 hours after the morning dose of a **combined oral contraceptive** (ethinylestradiol/norethisterone or ethinylestradiol/gestodene), had no effect on the pharmacokinetics of the contraceptive steroids in 9 healthy subjects,[5] and ovulation (assessed by hormone measurements and ultrasonography) did not occur.[6] The authors concluded that repeated charcoal treatment, given 3 hours after and at least 12 hours before a **combined oral contraceptive**, can be used to treat diarrhoea in women taking **combined oral contraceptives**.[5,6]

1. Knadler MP, Bergstrom RF, Callaghan JT, Obermeyer BD, Rubin A. Absorption studies of the H_2-blocker nizatidine. *Clin Pharmacol Ther* (1987) 42, 514–20.

2. Torre D, Sampietro C, Rossi S, Bianchi W, Maggiolo F. Ciprofloxacin and activated charcoal: pharmacokinetic data. *Rev Infect Dis* (1989) 11 (Suppl 5), S1015–S1016.

3. Windrum P, Hull DR, Morris TCM. Herb-drug interactions. *Lancet* (2000) 355, 1019–20.

4. Tanaka C, Yagi H, Sakamoto M, Koyama Y, Ohmura T, Ohtani H, Sawada Y. Decreased phenobarbital absorption with charcoal administration for chronic renal failure. *Ann Pharmacother* (2004) 38, 73–6.

5. Elomaa K, Ranta S, Tuominen J, Lähteenmäki P. The possible role of enterohepatic cycling on bioavailability of norethisterone and gestodene in women using combined oral contraceptives. *Contraception* (2001) 63, 13–8.

6. Elomaa K, Ranta S, Tuominen J, Lähteenmäki P. Charcoal treatment and risk of escape ovulation in oral contraceptive users. *Hum Reprod* (2001) 16, 76–81.

Chlorzoxazone + Disulfiram

Disulfiram markedly increases the plasma levels of chlorzoxazone.

Clinical evidence, mechanism, importance and management

A study in 6 healthy subjects to identify the activity of cytochrome P450 isoenzyme CYP2E1 found that a single 500-mg dose of disulfiram markedly inhibited the metabolism of a single 750-mg dose of chlorzoxazone (clearance reduced by 85%, half-life increased from 0.92 to 5.1 hours, and a two-fold increase in peak plasma levels).[1]

No increased adverse effects were seen while using these single doses, but an increase in toxicity would be expected (sedation, headache, nausea) with multiple doses. Be alert for the need to reduce the chlorzoxazone dosage if disulfiram is given concurrently.

1. Kharasch ED, Thummel KE, Mhyre J, Lillibridge JH. Single-dose disulfiram inhibition of chlorzoxazone metabolism: a clinical probe for P450 2E1. *Clin Pharmacol Ther* (1993) 53, 643–50.

Chlorzoxazone + Isoniazid

The adverse effects of chlorzoxazone may be increased in some patients (particularly slow-acetylators of isoniazid) if they also take isoniazid.

Clinical evidence

Five out of 10 healthy slow acetylators of isoniazid experienced an increase in the adverse effects of a 750-mg dose of chlorzoxazone (sedation, headache, nausea) after taking isoniazid 300 mg daily for 7 days. These symptoms disappeared within 2 days of withdrawing the isoniazid.[1] Pharmacokinetic analysis showed that the clearance of chlorzoxazone was reduced by 56% when given on the last day of isoniazid administration, then increased by 56% when given 2 days after stopping isoniazid.[1] Similar findings were reported in another study in slow acetylators of isoniazid: chlorzoxazone clearance was reduced by 78% when subjects had taken isoniazid 300 mg daily for 14 days, at which point the isoniazid was stopped. Two days later chlorzoxazone clearance was increased by 58%, and it had returned to normal 2 weeks later.[2] Rapid acetylators of isoniazid also had a 60% reduction in chlorzoxazone clearance on the last day of isoniazid administration, but did not have any increase 2 days later.[2]

Mechanism

Isoniazid appears to cause a dual interaction. During administration, it inhibits the activity of cytochrome P450 isoenzyme CYP2E1, the enzyme involved in the metabolism of chlorzoxazone. Shortly after stopping isoniazid, the metabolism of chlorzoxazone is increased, possibly because of induction of CYP2E1, although this effect was only evident in the slow acetylators.[1,2]

Importance and management

The increase in chlorzoxazone levels is established, and occurs in both slow and fast acetylators of isoniazid, although the increase in levels is slightly greater in slow acetylators. In practical terms this means that it may be necessary to reduce the chlorzoxazone dosage in some patients if they take isoniazid. Monitor concurrent use carefully. The rebound increase in chlorzoxazone clearance in slow acetylators on stopping isoniazid was short-lived and is probably of little clinical importance.

1. Zand R, Nelson SD, Slattery JT, Thummel KE, Kalhorn TF, Adams SP, Wright JM. Inhibition and induction of cytochrome P4502E1-catalyzed oxidation by isoniazid in humans. *Clin Pharmacol Ther* (1993) 54, 142–9.
2. O'Shea D, Kim RB, Wilkinson GR. Modulation of CYP2E1 activity by isoniazid in rapid and slow *N*-acetylators. *Br J Clin Pharmacol* (1997) 43, 99–103.

CNS depressants + CNS depressants

The concurrent use of two or more drugs that depress the CNS may be expected to result in increased CNS depression. This may have undesirable and even life-threatening consequences.

Clinical evidence, mechanism, importance and management

Many drugs have the propensity to cause depression of the central nervous system, resulting in drowsiness, sedation, respiratory depression and at the extreme, death. If more than one CNS depressant is taken, their effects may be additive. It is not uncommon for patients, particularly the elderly, to be taking numerous drugs (and possibly alcohol as well). Such patients are therefore at risk of cumulative CNS depression ranging from mild drowsiness through to a befuddled stupor, which can make the performance of the simplest everyday task more difficult or even impossible. The importance of this will depend on the context: it may considerably increase the risk of accident in the kitchen, at work, in a busy street, driving a car, or handling other potentially dangerous machinery where alertness is at a premium. It has been estimated that as many as 600 traffic accident fatalities each year in the UK can be attributed to the sedative effects of psychoactive drugs.[1] In a Spanish study of fatal road traffic accidents, blood samples were analysed from 9.7% of drivers killed in road accidents over a 10-year period. Of these drivers, medicines were detected in 4.7% (269 cases), and of these benzodiazepines were the most common (73%). Other drugs present in 6% to 12% of cases included antidepressants, analgesics, antiepileptics, barbiturates and antihistamines. Of the benzodiazepine cases, almost three quarters had another substance detected, mainly illicit drugs (cocaine, opiates, or cannabis) or alcohol. Only 7.7% had taken benzodiazepines or another medicinal drug alone.[2] **Alcohol** almost certainly makes things worse.

An example of the lethal effects of combining an **antihistamine**, a **benzodiazepine** and **alcohol** is briefly mentioned in the monograph 'Alcohol + Antihistamines', p.47. A less spectacular but socially distressing example is that of a woman accused of shop-lifting while in a confused state arising from the combined sedative effects of *Actifed*, a *Beechams Powder* and *Dolobid* (containing **triprolidine**, **salicylamide** and **diflunisal**, respectively).[3]

Few if any well-controlled studies have investigated the cumulative or additive detrimental effects of CNS depressants (except with **alcohol**), but the following is a list of some of the groups of drugs that to a greater or lesser extent possess CNS depressant activity and which might be expected to interact in this way: **alcohol**, **opioid analgesics**, **anticonvulsants**, **antidepressants**, **antihistamines**, **antiemetics**, **antipsychotics**, **anxiolytics** and **hypnotics**. Some of the interactions of **alcohol** with these drugs are dealt with in individual monographs.

1. Anon. Sedative effects of drugs linked to accidents. *Pharm J* (1994) 253, 564.
2. Carmen del Río M, Gómez J, Sancho M, Alvarez FJ. Alcohol, illicit drugs and medicinal drugs in fatally injured drivers in Spain between 1991 and 2000. *Forensic Sci Int* (2002) 127, 63–70.
3. Herxheimer A, Haffner BD. Prosecution for alleged shoplifting: successful pharmacological defence. *Lancet* (1982) i, 634.

Colchicine + Macrolides

Several case reports describe acute life-threatening colchicine toxicity caused by the addition of erythromycin or clarithromycin, and one retrospective study found that 9 of 88 patients who had received the combination of colchicine and clarithromycin died.

Clinical evidence

A 29-year-old woman with familial Mediterranean fever and amyloidosis, who was taking long-term colchicine 1 mg daily, developed acute and life-threatening colchicine toxicity (fever, diarrhoea, myalgia, pancytopenia and later alopecia) 16 days after starting to take **erythromycin** 2 g daily. This patient had both cholestasis and renal impairment, factors that would be expected to reduce colchicine clearance and therefore predispose her to colchicine toxicity.[1] Colchicine levels rose from below 12.6 nanograms/mL to 22 nanograms/mL after the addition of **erythromycin**.[1] In another patient, who had been taking colchicine 1.5 mg daily for 6 years, similar signs of acute colchicine toxicity developed 4 days after starting a 7-day course of **clarithromycin** 1 g daily, amoxicillin and omeprazole for *H. pylori* associated gastritis. The colchicine dose was reduced to 500 micrograms daily and then, after recovery, gradually increased slowly back to 1.5 mg daily.[2]

In another case, a 67-year-old man on CAPD taking colchicine 500 micrograms twice daily was admitted with symptoms of colchicine toxicity (including pancytopenia) 4 days after starting a course of **clarithromycin** 500 mg twice daily for an upper respiratory tract infection. All drugs were stopped and supportive treatment given, but he later died from multi-organ failure.[3]

These case reports led to a retrospective study of patients who had received the combination of colchicine and **clarithromycin** as inpatients. Of 116 patients given the drugs, 88 had received them concurrently and 28 received them sequentially. Nine of the concurrent group died (compared with only 1 of the sequential group), and of the nine, five had pancytopenia, and six had renal impairment. In the 88 patients receiving the drugs concurrently, longer overlapping therapy increased the relative risk of death 2.16-fold, the presence of renal impairment increased the risk 9.1-fold, and the development of pancytopenia increased the risk 23.4-fold.[4]

Two further cases of fatal agranulocytosis, presumed to result from use of colchicine with **clarithromycin**, have been reported,[5] and 2 other cases describe colchicine toxicity during **clarithromycin** use in patients with renal impairment.[6]

Mechanism

Erythromycin and clarithromycin may inhibit the hepatic metabolism of colchicine via the cytochrome P450 isoenzyme CYP3A4, and/or might increase its bioavailability via effects on P-glycoprotein.[2,4] These effects would be more marked in patients with renal impairment.

Importance and management

Information on this interaction is limited, but it appears that macrolide antibacterials can provoke acute colchicine toxicity, at the very least in predisposed individuals. If any patient is given colchicine and a macrolide (except probably azithromycin, which is not a notable CYP3A4 inhibitor), be aware of the potential for toxicity, especially in patients with pre-existing renal impairment.

1. Caraco Y, Putterman C, Rahamimov R, Ben-Chetrit E. Acute colchicine intoxication - possible role of erythromycin administration. *J Rheumatol* (1992) 19, 494–6.
2. Rollot F, Pajot O, Chauvelot-Moachon L, Nazal EM, Kélaïdi C, Blanche P. Acute colchicine intoxication during clarithromycin administration. *Ann Pharmacother* (2004) 38, 2074–7.
3. Dogukan A, Oymak FS, Taskapan H, Güven M, Tokgoz B, Utas C. Acute fatal colchicine intoxication in a patient on continuous ambulatory peritoneal dialysis (CAPD). Possible role of clarithromycin administration. *Clin Nephrol* (2001) 55, 181–2.
4. Hung IFN, Wu AKL, Cheng VCC, Tang BSF, To KW, Yeung CK, Woo PCY, Lau SKP, Cheung BMY, Yuen KY. Fatal interaction between clarithromycin and colchicine in patients with renal insufficiency: a retrospective study. *Clin Infect Dis* (2005) 41, 291–300.
5. Cheng VCC, Ho PL, Yuen KY. Two probable cases of serious drug interaction between clarithromycin and colchicine. *South Med J* (2005) 98, 811–13.
6. Akdag I, Ersoy A, Kahvecioglu S, Gullulu M, Dilek K. Acute colchicine intoxication during clarithromycin administration in patients with chronic renal failure. *J Nephrol* (2006) 19, 515–17.

Contrast media + Phenothiazines

Two isolated case reports describe epileptiform reactions in two patients when metrizamide was used for lumbar myelography in the presence of chlorpromazine or dixyrazine. No such cases appear to have been reported for intrathecal iohexol: nevertheless, the manufacturer of iohexol advises the avoidance of phenothiazines and other drugs that lower seizure threshold when iohexol is used intrathecally.

Clinical evidence

A patient receiving long-term treatment with **chlorpromazine** 75 mg daily had a grand mal seizure three-and-a-half hours after being given **metrizamide** (16 mL of 170 mg iodine per mL by the lumbar route). He had another seizure 5 hours later.[1] One out of 34 other patients demonstrated epileptogenic activity on an EEG when given **metrizamide** for lumbar myelography. The patient was taking **dixyrazine** 10 mg three times daily.[2] However, a clinical study in 26 patients given **levomepromazine** for the relief of lumbago-sciatic pain found no evidence of an increased risk of seizures after receiving **metrizamide** for myelography.[3]

Mechanism

Intrathecal metrizamide or iohexol alone are rarely associated with seizures. Theoretically, this risk might be increased in patients taking other drugs that lower the seizure threshold, such as the phenothiazines.

Importance and management

The case report with intrathecal metrizamide led to the advice to stop phenothiazines prior to giving this contrast agent.[4] Intrathecal iohexol has also rarely been associated with seizures, and consequently, the US manufacturer recommends that drugs that lower seizure threshold, especially phenothiazines are not recommended for use with iohexol by this route.[5] They should be stopped 48 hours before the procedure and not restarted until at least 24 hours after the procedure. This advice specifically includes phenothiazines used for their antiemetic properties. Although this risk is theoretical this would seem to be a prudent precaution. This advice does not apply to other routes of iohexol administration.[5]

1. Hindmarsh T, Grepe A and Widen L. Metrizamide-phenothiazine interaction. Report of a case with seizures following myelography. *Acta Radiol Diagnosis* (1975) 16, 129–34.
2. Hindmarsh T. Lumbar myelography with meglumine iocarmate and metrizamide. *Acta Radiol Diagnosis* (1975) 16, 209–22.
3. Standnes B, Oftedal S-I, Weber H. Effect of levomepromazine on EEG and on clinical side effects after lumbar myelography with metrizamide. *Acta Radiol Diagnosis* (1982) 23, 111–14.
4. Fedutes BA, Ansani NT. Seizure potential of concomitant medications and radiographic contrast media agents. *Ann Pharmacother* (2003) 37, 1506–10.
5. Omnipaque (Iohexol). GE Healthcare Inc. US Prescribing information, May 2006.

Contrast media; Iopanoic acid + Colestyramine

A single report describes poor radiographic visualisation of the gall bladder in a man due to an interaction between iopanoic acid and colestyramine within the gut.

Clinical evidence, mechanism, importance and management

The cholecystogram of a man with post-gastrectomy syndrome taking colestyramine who was given oral iopanoic acid as an x-ray contrast medium, suggested that he had an abnormal and apparently collapsed gall bladder. A week after stopping the colestyramine a repeat cholecystogram gave excellent visualisation of a gall bladder of normal appearance.[1] The same effects have been observed experimentally in *dogs*.[1] The reason seems to be that the colestyramine binds with the iopanoic acid in the gut so that little is absorbed and little is available for secretion in the bile, hence the poor visualisation of the gall bladder.

On the basis of reports about other drugs that similarly bind to colestyramine, it seems probable that this interaction could be avoided if the administration of the iopanoic acid and the colestyramine were to be separated as much as possible (note that it is usually recommended that other drugs are given 1 hour before or 4 to 6 hours after colestyramine). Whether other oral acidic x-ray contrast media bind in a similar way to colestyramine is uncertain, but this possibility should be considered.

1. Nelson JA. Effect of cholestyramine on telepaque oral cholecystography. *Am J Roentgenol Radium Ther Nucl Med* (1974) 122, 333–4.

Cyclobenzaprine + Fluoxetine and Droperidol

A patient taking cyclobenzaprine and fluoxetine developed torsade de pointes arrhythmia and ventricular fibrillation when droperidol was added.

Clinical evidence, mechanism, importance and management

A 59-year-old woman receiving long-term treatment with fluoxetine and cyclobenzaprine, who had a prolonged baseline QTc interval of 497 milliseconds, was given droperidol before surgery on her Achilles tendon. During the surgery she developed torsade de pointes arrhythmia, which progressed to ventricular fibrillation. On the first postoperative day after the cyclobenzaprine had been withdrawn, her QTc interval had decreased towards normal (440 milliseconds).[1]

A likely explanation is that her cyclobenzaprine serum levels were already raised by fluoxetine (a known inhibitor of cytochrome P450 isoenzyme CYP2D6, an enzyme involved in the metabolism of cyclobenzaprine) and as a result her QTc interval was prolonged. Cyclobenzaprine is structurally like the tricyclic antidepressants and shares their ability to cause arrhythmias, particularly in high doses. Therefore the addition of the droperidol, also known to prolong the QT interval, simply further extended the QTc interval and precipitated the torsade de pointes. This case not only illustrates the existence of an interaction between cyclobenzaprine and fluoxetine, but also the life-threatening risks of taking multiple 'drugs that can further prolong the QT interval', (p.257).

1. Michalets EL, Smith LK, Van Tassel ED. Torsade de pointes resulting from the addition of droperidol to an existing cytochrome P450 drug interaction. *Ann Pharmacother* (1998) 32, 761–5.

Dantrolene + Metoclopramide

Metoclopramide increases the bioavailability of dantrolene.

Clinical evidence, mechanism, importance and management

A study in 7 paraplegics and 6 quadriplegics with spinal cord injuries found that a single 10-mg intravenous dose of metoclopramide increased the bioavailability of a single 100-mg oral dose of dantrolene by 57%. The reasons are not known, although it was suggested that absorption may have been affected. The clinical relevance of this interaction is uncertain but the authors of the study suggest that patients should be well monitored if metoclopramide is added or withdrawn from patients who are taking dantrolene.[1]

1. Gilman TM, Segal JL, Brunnemann SR. Metoclopramide increases the bioavailability of dantrolene in spinal cord injury. *J Clin Pharmacol* (1996) 36, 64–71.

Dextromethorphan + Amiodarone

Amiodarone can reduce the clearance of dextromethorphan.

Clinical evidence

A study in 8 patients with cardiac arrhythmias found that amiodarone (1 g daily for 10 days followed by 200 to 400 mg daily for a mean duration of 76 days) changed their excretion of dextromethorphan 40 mg and its metabolite. The amount of unchanged dextromethorphan in the urine rose by nearly 150%, whereas the amount of its metabolite (dextrorphan) fell by about 25%.[1]

Mechanism

In vitro studies using liver microsomes have shown that amiodarone inhibits the metabolism (*O*-demethylation) of dextromethorphan by inhibiting the cytochrome P450 isoenzyme CYP2D6 within the liver.[1] Thus the dextromethorphan is cleared more slowly.

Importance and management

Information seems to be limited to this study. The clinical implications are that amiodarone may interfere with the results of phenotyping if dextromethorphan is used to determine CYP2D6 activity, and that dextromethorphan toxicity (excitation, confusion) may possibly develop in patients taking amiodarone. Be alert for any signs of toxicity if both are used. As yet, too little is known about this interaction to say by how much the dextromethorphan dosage should be reduced. Remember that dextromethorphan occurs in a considerable number of proprietary cough preparations.

1. Funck-Brentano C, Jacqz-Aigrain E, Leenhardt A, Roux A, Poirier J-M, Jaillon P. Influence of amiodarone on genetically determined drug metabolism in humans. *Clin Pharmacol Ther* (1991) 50, 259–66.

Dextromethorphan + Bupropion

Bupropion may reduce the metabolism of dextromethorphan in some patients.

Clinical evidence, mechanism, importance and management

A study in 21 subjects who were quitting smoking and were CYP2D6 extensive metabolisers, found that 6 of 13 subjects who received bupropion 150 mg once daily for 3 days and then twice daily for 14 days had metabolic ratios of dextromethorphan 30 mg similar to those seen in poor metabolisers: the metabolism of dextromethorphan to dextrorphan was substantially reduced. No such change was seen in the 8 subjects who received placebo. It has been suggested that care should be taken when initiating or discontinuing bupropion in patients taking dextromethorphan, due to the possibility of raised dextromethorphan levels.[1] Patients should be warned that they may experience increased adverse effects to dextromethorphan and advised that this is found in non-prescription preparations such as cough suppressants.

1. Kotlyar M, Brauer LH, Tracy TS, Hatsukami DK, Harris J, Bronars CA, Adson DE. Inhibition of CYP2D6 activity by bupropion. *J Clin Psychopharmacol* (2005) 25, 226–9.

Dextromethorphan + Echinacea

Echinacea does not appear to have a clinically relevant effect on the pharmacokinetics of dextromethorphan.

Clinical evidence, mechanism, importance and management

In a study, 12 healthy subjects were given *Echinacea purpurea* root 400 mg four times daily for 8 days with a single 30-mg dose of **dextromethorphan** on day 6. In the 11 subjects who were of the cytochrome P450 isoenzyme CYP2D6 extensive metaboliser phenotype (see 'Genetic factors in drug metabolism', (p.4)), there were no changes in the pharmacokinetics of **dextromethorphan**. In contrast, the one subject who was a poor metaboliser had a 42% increase in the AUC of **dextromethorphan** and a 31% increase in its half-life.[1] In another study, in 12 healthy subjects given *Echinacea purpurea* 800 mg twice daily for 28 days, there was no change in the debrisoquine urinary ratio after a single dose of debrisoquine 5 mg, suggesting that *Echinacea purpurea* does not alter the activity of the cytochrome P450 isoenzyme CYP2D6.[2]

The findings of these studies suggest that echinacea is unlikely to have a clinically relevant effect on CYP2D6 substrates (see 'Table 1.3', (p.6), for a list).

1. Gorski JC, Huang S-M, Pinto A, Hamman MA, Hilligoss JK, Zaheer NA, Desai M, Miller M, Hall SD. The effect of echinacea (*Echinacea purpurea* root) on cytochrome P450 activity in vivo. *Clin Pharmacol Ther* (2004) 75, 89–100.

2. Gurley BJ, Gardner SF, Hubbard MA, Williams DK, Gentry WB, Carrier J, Khan IA, Edwards DJ, Shah A. In vivo assessment of botanical supplementation on human cytochrome P450 phenotypes: *Citrus aurantium*, *Echinacea purpurea*, milk thistle, and saw palmetto. *Clin Pharmacol Ther* (2004) 76, 428–40.

Dextromethorphan + *Ginkgo biloba*

***Ginkgo biloba* does not affect the metabolism of dextromethorphan.**

Clinical evidence, mechanism, importance and management

Ginkgo biloba leaf extract 120 mg twice daily for 16 days was given to 12 healthy subjects with a single 30-mg dose of dextromethorphan on day 14 day. The *Ginkgo biloba* preparation (*Ginkgold*) contained ginkgo flavonol glycosides 24% and terpene lactones 6%. There was no change in the metabolism of dextromethorphan when it was taken after the *Ginkgo biloba*.[1] Dextromethorphan is a probe substrate for the cytochrome P450 isoenzyme CYP2D6, and the findings suggest that *Ginkgo biloba* is unlikely to interact with other drugs that are substrates of CYP2D6, see 'Table 1.3', (p.6).

1. Markowitz JS, Donovan JL, DeVane CL, Sipkes L, Chavin KD. Multiple-dose administration of *Ginkgo biloba* did not affect cytochrome P-450 2D6 or 3A4 activity in normal volunteers. *J Clin Psychopharmacol* (2003) 23, 576–81.

Dextromethorphan + Quinidine

Quinidine markedly increases the plasma levels of dextromethorphan in those who are of the extensive CYP2D6 metaboliser phenotype (the most common phenotype). This effect is maximal at low doses of quinidine (25 to 30 mg).

Clinical evidence

In a study in 6 extensive CYP2D6 metabolisers given dextromethorphan 60 mg twice daily, steady-state plasma dextromethorphan levels averaged only 12 nanograms/mL. However, after being given quinidine 75 mg twice daily for a week, then a single 60-mg dose of dextromethorphan, their plasma dextromethorphan levels were over threefold higher, at 38 nanograms/mL.[1] Some of the patients given the combination had an increase in dextromethorphan adverse effects (nervousness, tremors, restlessness, dizziness, shortness of breath, confusion etc).[1] Similarly, other pharmacokinetic studies have found increases in dextromethorphan levels in extensive CYP2D6 metabolisers, but not in poor CYP2D6 metabolisers.[2-4] In a dose-ranging study, quinidine 25 to 30 mg daily produced maximal increases in dextromethorphan levels, with higher doses producing no further increases, and lower doses producing smaller increases.[5] In one experimental study of citric acid-induced cough, quinidine increased the cough-suppressant effect of dextromethorphan.[6,7]

Mechanism

Quinidine inhibits the oxidative metabolism of dextromethorphan by the cytochrome P450 isoenzyme CYP2D6 to dextrorphan, effectively making extensive metabolisers of CYP2D6 into the poor metaboliser phenotype, see 'Genetic factors in drug metabolism', (p.4), for further discussion of metaboliser phenotypes.

Importance and management

An established interaction. Extensive metabolisers of CYP2D6 are likely to become more sensitive to dextromethorphan if they are taking quinidine.

Low-dose quinidine has been combined with dextromethorphan to sustain therapeutic levels of dextromethorphan and thereby try and improve its efficacy in various neurological disorders (dextromethorphan is a *N*-methyl-D-aspartate antagonist, which means it can affect pain transmission). A fixed dose combination is being investigated.[8]

1. Zhang Y, Britto MR, Valderhaug KL, Wedlund PJ, Smith RA. Dextromethorphan: enhancing its systemic availability by way of low-dose quinidine-mediated inhibition of cytochrome P4502D6. *Clin Pharmacol Ther* (1992) 51, 647–55.

2. Schadel M, Wu D, Otton SV, Kalow W, Sellers EM. Pharmacokinetics of dextromethorphan and metabolites in humans: influence of CYP2D6 phenotype and quinidine inhibition. *J Clin Psychopharmacol* (1995) 15, 263–9.

3. Desmeules JA, Oestreicher MK, Piguet V, Allaz A-F, Dayer P. Contribution of cytochrome P-4502D6 phenotype to the neuromodulatory effects of dextromethorphan. *J Pharmacol Exp Ther* (1999) 288, 607–12.

4. Capon DA, Bochner F, Kerry N, Mikus G, Danz C, Somogyi AA. The influence of CYP2D6 polymorphism and quinidine on the disposition and antitussive effect of dextromethorphan in humans. *Clin Pharmacol Ther* (1996) 60, 295–307.

5. Pope LE, Khalil MH, Berg JE, Stiles M, Yakatan GJ, Sellers EM. Pharmacokinetics of dextromethorphan after single or multiple dosing in combination with quinidine in extensive and poor metabolizers. *J Clin Pharmacol* (2004) 44, 1132–42.

6. Abdul Manap R, Wright CE, Gregory A, Rostami-Hodjegan A, Meller ST, Kelm GR, Lennard MS, Tucker GT, Morice AH. The antitussive effect of dextromethorphan in relation to CYP2D6 activity. *Br J Clin Pharmacol* (1999) 48, 382–7.

7. Moghadamnia AA, Rostami-Hodjegan A, Abdul-Manap R, Wright CE, Morice AH, Tucker GT. Physiologically based modelling of inhibition of metabolism and assessment of relative potency of drug and metabolite: dextromethorphan vs. dextrorphan using quinidine inhibition. *Br J Clin Pharmacol* (2003) 56, 57–67.

8. Anon. Dextromethorphan/quinidine: AVP 923, dextromethorphan/cytochrome P450-2D6 inhibitor, quinidine/dextromethorphan. *Drugs R D* (2005) 6, 174–7.

Dextromethorphan + Saw palmetto

Saw palmetto does not alter the metabolism of dextromethorphan.

Clinical evidence, mechanism, importance and management

Saw palmetto 320 mg daily, given to 12 subjects for 16 days, did not affect the metabolism of a single 30-mg dose of dextromethorphan given on day 14. No change was seen in the dextromethorphan metabolic ratio.[1] This suggests that saw palmetto is unlikely to alter the pharmacokinetics of drugs that are metabolised by the cytochrome P450 isoenzyme CYP2D6, of which dextromethorphan is a probe substrate.[1] This finding was confirmed by a further study in 12 healthy subjects who were given saw palmetto and debrisoquine, another substrate of CYP2D6.[2]

For a list of drugs that are substrates of this enzyme, see 'Table 1.3',(p.6).

1. Markowitz JS, Donovan JL, DeVane L, Taylor RM, Ruan Y, Wang J-S, Chavin KD. Multiple doses of saw palmetto (*Serenoa repens*) did not alter cytochrome P450 2D6 and 3A4 activity in normal volunteers. *Clin Pharmacol Ther* (2003) 74, 536–42.
2. Gurley BJ, Gardner SF, Hubbard MA, Williams DK, Gentry WB, Carrier J, Khan IA, Edwards DJ, Shah A. In vivo assessment of botanical supplementation on human cytochrome P450 phenotypes: *Citrus aurantium, Echinacea purpurea*, milk thistle, and saw palmetto. *Clin Pharmacol Ther* (2004) 76, 428–40.

Dextromethorphan + St John's wort (*Hypericum perforatum*)

St John's wort does not affect the pharmacokinetics of dextromethorphan.

Clinical evidence, mechanism, importance and management

St John's wort (*LI160, Lichtwer Pharma*, 0.12 to 0.3% hypericin) 300 mg three times daily was given to 12 healthy subjects for 16 days with a single 30-mg dose of dextromethorphan on day 14. There was no consistent change in the urinary dextromethorphan to dextrorphan metabolic ratio: 6 subjects had an increase in the production of dextrorphan while the other 6 subjects had a reduction in dextrorphan production. This finding was within the normal inter-patient variation in dextromethorphan metabolism,[1] and suggests that St John's wort does not significantly affect the cytochrome P450 isoenzyme CYP2D6. Similar findings were reported in another study in 16 healthy subjects given a single 25-mg dose of dextromethorphan on the last day of a 14-day course of St John's wort (*Jarsin*; 900 micrograms of hypericin*)* 300 mg three times daily.[2]

St John's wort would not therefore be expected to alter the pharmacokinetics of other substrates of CYP2D6, for a list see 'Table 1.3', (p.6).

1. Markowitz JS, Donovan JL, DeVane CL, Taylor RM, Ruan Y, Wang J-S, Chavin KD. Effect of St John's wort on drug metabolism by induction of cytochrome P450 3A4 enzyme. *JAMA* (2003) 290, 1500–4.
2. Wenk M, Todesco L, Krähenbühl S. Effect of St John's wort on the activities of CYP1A2, CYP3A4, CYP2D6, N-acetyltransferase 2, and xanthine oxidase in healthy males and females. *Br J Clin Pharmacol* (2004) 57, 494–9.

Disulfiram + Cannabis

An isolated case report describes a hypomanic-like reaction when a man taking disulfiram used cannabis.

Clinical evidence, mechanism, importance and management

A man with a 10-year history of drug abuse (alcohol, amfetamines, cocaine, cannabis) taking disulfiram 250 mg daily, experienced a hypomanic-like reaction (euphoria, hyperactivity, insomnia, irritability) on two occasions, associated with the concurrent use of cannabis. The patient said that he felt as though he had been taking amfetamine.[1] The reason for this reaction is not understood. In a randomised study in alcohol dependent subjects who had previously used cannabis, no unusual interaction effects were found in a group of 11 subjects receiving disulfiram and smoking cannabis twice weekly for 4 weeks.[2] Therefore the interaction described in the case report would not appear to be of general significance.

1. Lacoursiere RB, Swatek R. Adverse interaction between disulfiram and marijuana: a case report. *Am J Psychiatry* (1983) 140, 243–4.
2. Rosenberg CM, Gerrein JR, Schnell C. Cannabis in the treatment of alcoholism. *J Stud Alcohol* (1978) 39, 1955–8.

Dutasteride + Miscellaneous

Preliminary evidence suggests that diltiazem and verapamil, inhibitors of cytochrome P450 isoenzyme CYP3A4, cause moderate increases in dutasteride levels but this is probably not clinically significant. In the UK, the manufacturer says that dutasteride dosage adjustments may be needed with potent inhibitors of CYP3A4 such as indinavir, itraconazole, ketoconazole, nefazodone and ritonavir. No clinically significant interaction appears to occur between dutasteride and amlodipine, digoxin, or warfarin. There is no interaction when dutasteride is given one hour before colestyramine.

Clinical evidence, mechanism, importance and management

(a) Colestyramine

In a study in 12 healthy subjects the absorption of dutasteride 5 mg was not affected when it was given one hour before a single 12-g dose of colestyramine.[1,2] No precautions seem necessary if this dosing interval is observed.

(b) CYP3A4 inhibitors and substrates

When dutasteride was given with **amlodipine** (4 subjects), **diltiazem** (5 subjects) or **verapamil** (6 subjects) during dose-ranging studies, **amlodipine** did not significantly affect the clearance of dutasteride but **diltiazem** and **verapamil** were associated with a decrease of 44% and 37%, respectively.[2] This was thought to be due to the inhibitory effect of **diltiazem** and **verapamil** on P-glycoprotein and the cytochrome P450 isoenzyme CYP3A4. Dutasteride has a wide safety margin, so these changes were not thought to be clinically significant.[2] However, in the UK, the manufacturers warn that potent CYP3A4 inhibitors (they name **indinavir**, **itraconazole**, **ketoconazole**, **nefazodone** and **ritonavir**) may cause a clinically significant increase in dutasteride levels, and so they suggest reducing the dosing frequency if increased dutasteride adverse effects occur in the presence of these drugs.[1]

(c) Digoxin

A placebo-controlled study in 20 healthy subjects taking digoxin found that its pharmacokinetics were unchanged by dutasteride 500 micrograms daily for 3 weeks.[2] No digoxin dose adjustment would be expected to be necessary on concurrent use.

(d) Warfarin

Dutasteride 500 micrograms daily, given to 23 healthy subjects with warfarin for 35 days had no effect on the pharmacokinetics of *S*- or *R*-warfarin, and the prothrombin time was unaffected by the presence of dutasteride.[2] No warfarin dose adjustment would be expected to be necessary on concurrent use.

1. Avodart (Dutasteride). GlaxoSmithKline UK. UK Summary of product characteristics, January 2006.
2. Avodart (Dutasteride). GlaxoSmithKline. US Prescribing information, May 2005.

Enteric-coated, delayed-release preparations + Drugs that affect gastric pH

Theoretically, enteric-coated, delayed-release preparations may possibly dissolve prematurely if they are taken at the same time as antacids. This has been seen with some preparations, but not others. Release characteristics are likely to depend on the specific coating, and the manufacturers advice should be followed.

Clinical evidence

(a) Antacid

A placebo-controlled, crossover study in 21 healthy subjects, found that when extended-release **oxybutynin** 10 mg (*Ditropan XL*) was given at the same time as *Maalox* 20 mL (**aluminium/magnesium hydroxide** and **simethicone**) there was no change in the pharmacokinetics of **oxybutynin** or its metabolite.[1]

In an identical study in 23 healthy subjects, *Maalox* increased the maximum plasma level of a single 4-mg dose of extended-release **tolterodine** (*Detrol LA*) by 50%, but did not change any other pharmacokinetic parameter (time to maximum level, elimination half-life, AUC).[1]

(b) Omeprazole

In a placebo-controlled, crossover study in 39 healthy subjects, pre-treatment with omeprazole 20 mg daily for 4 days did not alter the pharmacokinetics of extended-release oxybutynin 10 mg [*Ditropan XL*]. The metabolites of oxybutynin were similarly unaffected. Pretreatment with omeprazole increased the maximum plasma level a single 4-mg dose of extended release tolterodine [*Detrol LA*] by 38%, but did not change any other pharmacokinetic parameter (time to maximum level, elimination half-life, AUC).[2]

The bioavailability of enteric-coated preparations of aspirin, diclofenac, and ketoprofen are unaffected by omeprazole, see 'NSAIDs or Aspirin + Proton pump inhibitors', p.155.

Mechanism

A marked rise in pH caused by antacids might cause premature dissolution of the coating of preparations formulated to prevent release of the contents until they reach the more alkaline conditions within the small intestine. Other types of delayed release preparations that have release characteristics independent of pH, such as those based on the osmotic principle, would not be expected to be affected.

Importance and management

Traditionally, it has been considered that drugs formulated with enteric coatings to resist gastric acid, or formulated as delayed release preparations, should not be given with antacids. Accelerated drug release from a delayed release product (dose dumping) might lead to increased adverse effects and lack of efficacy for the duration of the dose interval. The evidence above for extended-release tolterodine suggest that an antacid did cause a faster release of tolterodine from this product, but whether the 50% increase in maximum level is sufficient to cause an increase in adverse effects is not known. Pre-treatment with omeprazole caused a smaller 38% increase in maximum tolterodine levels. The extended-release oxybutynin product was not affected by antacid or omeprazole, which was not unexpected since release from this product is osmotically driven and pH independent.

Release characteristics are likely to depend on the specific coating, and therefore no general advice can be given. The manufacturers advice should be followed.

1. Sathyan G, Dmochowski RR, Appell RA, Guo C, Gupta SK. Effect of antacid on the pharmacokinetics of extended-release formulations of tolterodine and oxybutynin. *Clin Pharmacokinet* (2004) 43, 1059–68.
2. Dmochowski R, Chen A, Sathyan G, MacDiarmid S, Gidwani S, Gupta S. Effect of the proton pump inhibitor omeprazole on the pharmacokinetics of extended-release formulations of oxybutynin and tolterodine. *J Clin Pharmacol* (2005) 45, 961–8.

Ethylene dibromide + Disulfiram

The very high incidence of malignant tumours in *rats* exposed to both ethylene dibromide and disulfiram is the basis of the recommendation that concurrent exposure to these compounds should be avoided.

Clinical evidence, mechanism, importance and management

Research conducted to establish the occupational safety of exposure to ethylene dibromide found that the incidence of malignant tumours in *rats* exposed to 20 ppm ethylene dibromide (7 hours daily, 5 days weekly), while receiving a diet containing 0.05% disulfiram by weight, is very high indeed.[1,2] The reasons are not understood. In addition to the precautions needed to protect workers from the toxic effects of ethylene dibromide, it has been strongly recommended that disulfiram should not be given to those who may be exposed to this compound.[2] This information is also summarised in another report.[3]

1. Plotnick HB. Carcinogenesis in rats of combined ethylene dibromide and disulfiram. *JAMA* (1978) 239, 1609.
2. Anon. Ethylene dibromide and disulfiram toxic interaction. *NIOSH Current Intelligence Bulletin: US Department of Health, Education and Welfare Publication* (1978) No 78–145.
3. Stein HP, Bahlman LJ, Leidel NA, Parker JC, Thomas AW, Millar JD. Ethylene dibromide and disulfiram toxic interaction. *Am Ind Hyg Assoc J* (1978) 39, A35–A37.

Evening primrose oil + Phenothiazines

Although seizures have occurred in a few schizophrenics taking phenothiazines and evening primrose oil, no adverse effects were seen in others, and there appears to be no firm evidence that evening primrose oil should be avoided by epileptic patients.

Clinical evidence

Twenty-three patients were enrolled in a placebo-controlled study of evening primrose oil in schizophrenia. During the treatment phase, patients were given 8 capsules of *Efamol* in addition to their normal medication. Seizures developed in 3 patients, one during treatment with placebo. The other two patients were taking evening primrose oil, one was receiving **fluphenazine decanoate** 50 mg once every 2 weeks and the other **fluphenazine decanoate** 25 mg once every 2 weeks with **thioridazine**, which was later changed to **chlorpromazine**.[1] In another study, 3 long-stay hospitalised schizophrenics were taking evening primrose oil. Their schizophrenia became much worse and all 3 patients showed EEG evidence of temporal lobe epilepsy.[2]

In contrast, no seizures or epileptiform events were reported in a crossover study of 48 patients (most of them schizophrenics) taking **phenothiazines** when they were given evening primrose oil for 4 months.[3] Concurrent use was also apparently uneventful in another study in schizophrenic patients.[4]

Mechanism

Not understood. One suggestion is that evening primrose oil possibly increases the well-recognised epileptogenic effects of the phenothiazines, rather than having an epileptogenic action of its own.[1] Another idea is that it might unmask temporal lobe epilepsy.[1,2]

Importance and management

The interaction between phenothiazines and evening primrose oil is not well established, nor is its incidence known, but clearly some caution is appropriate during concurrent use, because seizures may develop in a few individuals. There seems to be no way of identifying the patients at particular risk. The extent to which the underlying disease condition might affect what happens is also unclear.

No interaction between anticonvulsants and evening primrose oil has been established and the reports cited above[1,2] appear to be the sole basis for the suggestion that evening primrose oil should be avoided by epileptics. No seizures appear to have been reported in patients taking evening primrose oil in the absence of phenothiazines. The manufacturers of *Epogam*, an evening primrose oil preparation, claim that it is known to have improved the control of epilepsy in patients previously uncontrolled with conventional antiepileptic drugs, and other patients are said to have had no problems during concurrent treatment.[5] Even so, until the situation is formally examined it would seem prudent to monitor concurrent use.

1. Holman CP, Bell AFJ. A trial of evening primrose oil in the treatment of chronic schizophrenia. *J Orthomol Psychiatry* (1983) 12, 302–4.
2. Vaddadi KS. The use of gamma-linolenic acid and linoleic acid to differentiate between temporal lobe epilepsy and schizophrenia. *Prostaglandins Med* (1981) 6, 375–9.
3. Vaddadi KS, Courtney P, Gilleard CJ, Manku MS, Horrobin DF. A double-blind trial of essential fatty acid supplementation in patients with tardive dyskinesia. *Psychiatry Res* (1989) 27, 313–23.
4. Vaddadi KS, Horrobin DF. Weight loss produced by evening primrose oil administration in normal and schizophrenic individuals. *IRCS Med Sci* (1979) 7, 52.
5. Scotia Pharmaceuticals Ltd. Personal Communication, January 1991.

Folic acid + Adsorbents

***In vitro* studies show that folic acid is markedly adsorbed by magnesium trisilicate and edible clay.[1] This would be expected to reduce its absorption from the gut, but the clinical importance of this awaits assessment.**

1. Iwuagwu MA, Jideonwo A. Preliminary investigations into the in-vitro interaction of folic acid with magnesium trisilicate and edible clay. *Int J Pharmaceutics* (1990) 65, 63–7.

Folic acid + Sulfasalazine

Sulfasalazine can reduce the absorption of folic acid.

Clinical evidence, mechanism, importance and management

The absorption of folic acid was reduced by about one-third (from 65 to 44.5%) in patients with ulcerative and granulomatous colitis, when compared with healthy subjects, and even further reduced (down to 32%) when sulfasalazine was taken.[1] Another study confirmed that serum folate levels are lower in patients with ulcerative colitis taking sulfasalazine, and that the impairment of the absorption of folates by sulfasalazine was a mechanism in this.[2] Sulfasalazine is also known to interfere with folate metabolism.

It is well established that sulfasalazine is, rarely, associated with blood dyscrasias due to folate deficiency and also other haematological toxicities, and consequently regular blood counts are recommended to detect this. The effects of folate deficiency (e.g. macrocytosis, pancytopenia) can be normalised by the administration of folic acid or folinic acid.

1. Franklin JL, Rosenberg IH. Impaired folic acid absorption in inflammatory bowel disease: effects of salicylazosulfapyridine (Azulfidine). *Gastroenterology* (1973) 64, 517–25.

2. Halsted CH, Gandhi G, Tamura T. Sulfasalazine inhibits the absorption of folates in ulcerative colitis. *N Engl J Med* (1981) 305, 1513–17.

Garlic + Cytochrome P450 isoenzyme substrates

Garlic dose not affect the pharmacokinetics of alprazolam or dextromethorphan, and is therefore not expected to interact with drugs metabolised by CYP3A4 or CYP2D6.

Clinical evidence, mechanism, importance and management

A study in 14 healthy subjects found that garlic (*Allium sativum*), 600 mg twice daily for 14 days, did not affect the pharmacokinetics of a single 2-mg dose of **alprazolam** or the metabolism of a single 30-mg dose of **dextromethorphan**. This suggests that garlic is unlikely to affect the metabolism of other drugs that are substrates of the cytochrome P450 isoenzymes CYP3A4 or CYP2D6.[1] For a list of drugs that are substrates of these enzymes, see 'Table 1.3',(p.6), and 'Table 1.4',(p.6).

1. Markowitz JS, DeVane CL, Chavin KD, Taylor RM, Ruan Y, Donovan JL. Effects of garlic (*Allium* sativum L.) supplementation on cytochrome P450 2D6 and 3A4 activity in healthy volunteers. *Clin Pharmacol Ther* (2003) 74, 170–7.

Ginseng + Cytochrome P450 isoenzyme substrates

Ginseng does not appear to affect the metabolism of alprazolam or dextromethorphan.

Clinical evidence, mechanism, importance and management

A study in 12 healthy subjects found that Siberian ginseng, 485 mg twice daily for 14 days, did not affect the pharmacokinetics of a single 2-mg dose of **alprazolam** or the metabolism of a single 30-mg dose of **dextromethorphan**. This suggests that Siberian ginseng is unlikely to affect the metabolism of other drugs that are substrates of the cytochrome P450 isoenzymes CYP2D6 or CYP3A4.[1] For a list of drugs that are substrates of these enzymes, see 'Table 1.3', (p.6), and 'Table 1.4', (p.6), respectively.

1. Donovan JL, DeVane CL, Chavin KD, Taylor RM, Markowitz JS. Siberian ginseng (*Eleutheroccus* [sic] *senticosus*) effects on CYP2D6 and CYP3A4 activity in normal volunteers. *Drug Metab Dispos* (2003) 31, 519–22.

Glucagon + Beta blockers

The blood glucose-elevating effects of glucagon may be reduced by propranolol.

Clinical evidence, mechanism, importance and management

The blood glucose-elevating effects of glucagon was reduced in the presence of **propranolol** in 5 healthy subjects.[1] Blood glucose levels increased by about 45% in the presence of glucagon, but when **propranolol** was also given the increase was only about 15%. The reason is uncertain, but one suggestion is that the **propranolol** inhibits the effects of the catecholamines that are released by glucagon. The clinical importance of this interaction is uncertain.

1. Messerli FH, Kuchel O, Tolis G, Hamet P, Frayasse J, Genest J. Effects of β-adrenergic blockage on plasma cyclic AMP and blood sugar responses to glucagon and isoproterenol in man. *Int J Clin Pharmacol Biopharm* (1976) 14, 189–94.

Goldenseal (*Hydrastis*) + Cytochrome P450 isoenzyme substrates

Goldenseal modestly decreased the metabolism of midazolam and debrisoquine but had no effect on the metabolism of caffeine or chlorzoxazone.

Clinical evidence, mechanism, importance and management

In a study 12 non-smoking healthy subjects were given goldenseal root extract 900 mg three times daily for 28 days before receiving single doses of **caffeine**, **chlorzoxazone**, **debrisoquine** and **midazolam**. No significant changes in the metabolism of **caffeine** or **chlorzoxazone** were noted. Goldenseal (hydrastis) appeared to reduce the activity of the cytochrome P450 isoenzymes CYP2D6 and CYP3A4/5 by 40%, measured by the effect on the urinary recovery of **debrisoquine**, and the reduced production of the 1-hydroxy metabolite of **midazolam**.[1]

On the basis of this pharmacokinetic probe study it was suggested that goldenseal may have a clinically relevant effect on midazolam (and other substrates of CYP3A4/5, see 'Table 1.4', (p.6)), and debrisoquine (and other substrates of CYP2D6, see 'Table 1.3', (p.6)). Some caution might be required as raised levels of these drugs are possible.

1. Gurley BJ, Gardner SF, Hubbard MA, Williams DK, Gentry WB, Khan IA, Shah A. In vivo effects of goldenseal, kava kava, black cohosh, and valerian on human cytochrome P450 1A2, 2D6, 2E1, and 3A4/5 phenotypes. *Clin Pharmacol Ther* (2005) 77, 415–26.

5-HT$_3$-receptor antagonists + Aprepitant

Aprepitant had no clinically relevant effect on the pharmacokinetics of dolasetron, granisetron, ondansetron or palonosetron.

Clinical evidence

(a) Dolasetron

In a study in 12 healthy subjects, aprepitant 125 mg on day one, then 80 mg on days 2 and 3 had no effect on the pharmacokinetics of a single 100-mg oral dose of dolasetron given on day one, regardless of CYP2D6 metaboliser type.[1]

(b) Granisetron

Aprepitant 125 mg on day one, then 80 mg on days 2 and 3 had no effect on the pharmacokinetics of oral granisetron 2 mg given to healthy subjects on day one.[2]

(c) Ondansetron

In a study in healthy subjects, aprepitant 375 mg on day one, then 250 mg on days 2 to 5 caused a minor 15% increase in the AUC of intravenous ondansetron 32 mg given on day one.[2]

(d) Palonosetron

Aprepitant 125 mg on day one, then 80 mg on days 2 and 3 had no effect on the pharmacokinetics of a single 250-microgram intravenous dose of palonosetron given to healthy subjects on day one.[3]

Mechanism

None.

Importance and management

No important pharmacokinetic interactions occur, therefore no dosage adjustment is required when aprepitant is given with dolasetron, ondansetron, granisetron or palonosetron.

1. Li SX, Pequignot E, Panebianco D, Lupinacci P, Majumdar A, Rosen L, Ahmed T, Royalty JE, Rushmore TH, Murphy MG, Petty KJ. Lack of effect of aprepitant on hydrodolasetron pharmacokinetics in CYP2D6 extensive and poor metabolizers. *J Clin Pharmacol* (2006) 46, 792–801.

2. Blum RA, Majumdar A, McCrea J, Busillo J, Orlowski LH, Panebianco D, Hesney M, Petty KJ, Goldberg MR, Murphy MG, Gottesdiener KM, Hustad CM, Lates C, Kraft WK, Van Buren S, Waldman SA, Greenberg HE. Effects of aprepitant on the pharmacokinetics of ondansetron and granisetron in healthy subjects. *Clin Ther* (2003) 25, 1407–19.
3. Shah AK, Hunt TL, Gallagher SC, Cullen MT. Pharmacokinetics of palonosetron in combination with aprepitant in healthy volunteers. *Curr Med Res Opin* (2005) 21, 595–601.

5-HT$_3$-receptor antagonists + Cimetidine

Cimetidine had no important effect on dolasetron or granisetron pharmacokinetics.

Clinical evidence, mechanism, importance and management

(a) Dolasetron

A study in 18 healthy subjects given dolasetron 200 mg daily found that cimetidine 300 mg four times daily for 7 days increased the AUC and maximum plasma level of the active metabolite of dolasetron, hydrodolasetron, by 24% and 15%, respectively, probably due to the inhibitory effect of cimetidine on the cytochrome P450-mediated metabolism of dolasetron. As 400-mg oral doses of dolasetron have been shown to be well tolerated (the usual oral dose is up to 200 mg) these changes were not considered to be clinically significant.[1] Therefore no special precautions appear necessary if cimetidine and dolasetron are used concurrently.

(b) Granisetron

Pretreatment with cimetidine 200 mg four times daily for 8 days had no effect on the pharmacokinetics of a single 40-microgram/kg intravenous dose of granisetron given on day 8 in a study in 12 healthy subjects.[2] No granisetron dose adjustments are likely to be necessary if cimetidine is given.

1. Dimmitt DC, Cramer MB, Keung A, Arumugham T, Weir SJ. Pharmacokinetics of dolasetron with coadministration of cimetidine or rifampin in healthy subjects. *Cancer Chemother Pharmacol* (1999) 43, 126–32.
2. Youlten L. The effect of repeat dosing with cimetidine on the pharmacokinetics of intravenous granisetron in healthy volunteers. *J Pharm Pharmacol* (2004) 56, 169–75.

5-HT$_3$-receptor antagonists + Drugs that prolong the QT interval

All available 5-HT$_3$-receptor antagonists (dolasetron, granisetron, ondansetron, palonosetron, tropisetron) have caused small increases (generally not exceeding 15 milliseconds) in the QTc interval. Some consider that these changes are not clinically relevant. Nevertheless, many of the manufacturers give various cautions about using 5-HT$_3$-receptor antagonists together with other drugs known to prolong the QT interval.

Clinical evidence, mechanism, importance and management

The 5-HT$_3$-receptor antagonists are now known to cause small increases (generally not exceeding 15 milliseconds) in the QTc interval.[1] It has been concluded that this class effect is too small to be of clinical relevance,[1,2] and that there is insufficient evidence to differentiate the 5-HT$_3$-receptor antagonists by this effect.[3] Nevertheless, manufacturers issue differing guidance about concurrent use with other QT prolonging drugs as follows:

- **Dolasetron**: the UK manufacturer contraindicates[4] the concurrent use of dolasetron and **class I** or **class III antiarrhythmics**, and recommends caution with other drugs that prolong ECG intervals in patients at risk. The US manufacturer advises caution with all drugs that may prolong the QT interval. They include **diuretics**, with potential for inducing electrolyte abnormalities.[5]
- **Granisetron**: Neither the UK nor the UK manufacturers mention QT prolongation.[6,7]
- **Ondansetron**: the UK manufacturer recommends caution in patients treated with **antiarrhythmics** or **beta blockers**,[8] whereas the US manufacturer does not issue any cautions regarding QT-prolongation.[9]
- **Palonosetron**: the UK and US manufacturers recommend caution with other drugs that increase the QT interval.[10,11] The US manufacturer specifically mentions **antiarrhythmics** and **diuretics** with potential for inducing electrolyte abnormalities.[11]
- **Tropisetron**: the UK manufacturer recommends care when it is used with other drugs that are likely to prolong the QT interval, and specifically mentions **antiarrhythmics** and **beta blockers**.[12]

For further information about drug interactions involving the QT interval see 'Drugs that prolong the QT interval + Other drugs that prolong the QT interval', p.257.

1. Navari RM, Koeller JM. Electrocardiographic and cardiovascular effects of the 5-hydroxytryptamine$_3$ receptor antagonists. *Ann Pharmacother* (2003) 37,1276–86.
2. Kovac AL. Benefits and risks of newer treatments for chemotherapy-induced and postoperative nausea and vomiting. *Drug Safety* (2003) 26, 227–59.
3. Navari RM, Koeller JM. Comment: electrocardiographic and cardiovascular effects of the 5-hydroxytryptamine-3 receptor antagonists. Authors' reply. *Ann Pharmacother* (2003) 37, 1918–19.
4. Anzemet Tablets (Dolasetron mesilate). Amdipharm. UK Summary of product characteristics, May 2006.
5. Anzemet (Dolasetron mesylate). Sanofi Aventis US LLC. US Prescribing information, June 2006.
6. Kytril Tablets (Granisetron hydrochloride). Roche Products Ltd. UK Summary of product characteristics, July 2007.
7. Kytril (Granisetron hydrochloride). Roche Laboratories Inc. US Prescribing information, November 2005.
8. Zofran Tablets (Ondansetron). GlaxoSmithKline UK. UK summary of product characteristics, October 2006.
9. Zofran (Ondansetron hydrochloride). GlaxoSmithKline. US Prescribing information, February 2006.
10. Aloxi (Palonosetron hydrochloride). Cambridge Laboratories. UK Summary of product characteristics, March 2005.
11. Aloxi (Palonosetron hydrochloride). MGI Pharma Inc. US Prescribing information, January 2006.
12. Navoban (Tropisetron hydrochloride). Novartis Pharmaceuticals UK Ltd. UK Summary of product characteristics, August 2006.

5-HT$_3$-receptor antagonists + Enzyme inducers

Rifampicin causes a minor reduction in dolasetron levels and a modest reduction in ondansetron levels, and may affect granisetron and tropisetron similarly, but does not appear to alter palonosetron levels. However, with the possible exception of ondansetron, none of the changes are thought to be clinically relevant.

Clinical evidence, mechanism, importance and management

(a) Dolasetron

In a study in 17 healthy subjects given dolasetron 200 mg daily, **rifampicin** (rifampin) 600 mg daily for 7 days decreased the AUC and maximum plasma level of the active metabolite of dolasetron, hydrodolasetron, by 28% and 17%, respectively, probably due to induction of hydrodolasetron metabolism by **rifampicin**.[1] These changes were not considered to be clinically significant and therefore no special precautions appear necessary if **rifampicin** and dolasetron are used concurrently.

(b) Granisetron

The US manufacturer notes that, in a pharmacokinetic study, the enzyme inducer **phenobarbital** increased the clearance of granisetron by 25%. They say that the clinical relevance of this change is unknown,[2] but such a modest change is not likely to be important.

(c) Ondansetron

Pretreatment with **rifampicin** 600 mg once daily for 5 days markedly decreased the AUC of a single 8-mg dose of oral ondansetron by 65% and intravenous ondansetron by 48% in a study in 10 healthy subjects. This is most likely due to the induction of CYP3A4-mediated metabolism of ondansetron by **rifampicin**. The authors concluded that ondansetron may not be as effective if given to patients taking **rifampicin**.[3] Nevertheless, the US manufacturer says that, although the potent inducers CYP3A4, **phenytoin**, **carbamazepine**, and rifampicin increased ondansetron clearance, on the basis of available data, no ondansetron dose adjustment is recommended for patients taking these drugs.[4]

(d) Palonosetron

The UK manufacturer notes that, in a population pharmacokinetic analysis, enzyme inducers (**dexamethasone** and **rifampicin**) had no effect on palonosetron clearance.[5] No palonosetron dose adjustment is likely to be necessary when given with these drugs.

(e) Tropisetron

The manufacturer states that drugs known to induce hepatic enzymes might lower tropisetron plasma concentrations. However, they say that such changes are unlikely to be of practical importance with the recommended dosage regimen.[6]

1. Dimmitt DC, Cramer MB, Keung A, Arumugham T, Weir SJ. Pharmacokinetics of dolasetron with coadministration of cimetidine or rifampin in healthy subjects. *Cancer Chemother Pharmacol* (1999) 43, 126–32.
2. Kytril (Granisetron hydrochloride). Roche Laboratories Inc. US Prescribing information. November 2005.
3. Villikka K, Kivistö KT, Neuvonen PJ. The effect of rifampin on the pharmacokinetics of oral and intravenous ondansetron. *Clin Pharmacol Ther* (1999) 65, 377–81.
4. Zofran Tablets (Ondansetron hydrochloride). GlaxoSmithKline. US Prescribing information, February 2006.
5. Aloxi (Palonosetron hydrochloride). Cambridge Laboratories. UK Summary of product characteristics, March 2005.
6. Navoban (Tropisetron hydrochloride). Novartis Pharmaceuticals UK Ltd. UK Summary of product characteristics, August 2006.

5-HT$_3$-receptor antagonists; Dolasetron + Miscellaneous

Food does not affect dolasetron absorption. Atenolol modestly reduced the clearance of the active metabolite of dolasetron. One patient taking verapamil and given dolasetron experienced heart block.

Clinical evidence, mechanism, importance and management

(a) Atenolol

The US manufacturer[1] notes that atenolol reduced the clearance of the active metabolite of dolasetron, hydrodolasetron, by 27%. This change is not likely to be clinically significant.

(b) Food

In a single-dose study, 23 healthy subjects were given 200 mg of dolasetron orally either alone, or following a **high-fat breakfast** (containing fat 55 g, protein 33 g and carbohydrate 58 g). Although there was a slight delay in absorption, dosing with a meal and dosing without a meal were considered to be bioequivalent. Therefore dolasetron may be given without regard to meals.[2]

(c) Verapamil

The US manufacturer notes that, in one case, a 61-year-old woman taking verapamil developed complete heart block following the use of dolasetron,[1] although this was not proven to be as a result of an interaction. In other patients taking verapamil, the clearance of hydrodolasetron (the active metabolite of dolasetron) was unchanged.[1]

1. Anzemet (Dolasetron mesylate). Sanofi-Aventis US LCC. US Prescribing information, June 2006.
2. Lippert C, Keung A, Arumugham T, Eller M, Hahne W, Weir S. The effect of food on the bioavailability of dolasetron mesylate tablets. *Biopharm Drug Dispos* (1998) 19, 17–19.

5-HT$_3$-receptor antagonists; Ondansetron + Food or Antacids

Food slightly increases the bioavailability of ondansetron, but an antacid was found to have no effect.

Clinical evidence, mechanism, importance and management

When 12 healthy subjects were given an 8 mg ondansetron tablet 5 minutes after a **meal**, its bioavailability was slightly increased (AUC raised by 17%) but the concurrent use of an **aluminium/magnesium hydroxide** antacid (*Maalox*) had no effect on ondansetron.[1]

1. Bozigian HP, Pritchard JF, Gooding AE, Pakes GE. Ondansetron absorption in adults: effect of dosage form, food, and antacids. *J Pharm Sci* (1994) 83, 1011–13.

5-HT$_3$-receptor antagonists; Palonosetron + Metoclopramide

Metoclopramide 10 mg four times daily did not alter the pharmacokinetics of a single 750-microgram intravenous dose of palonosetron in healthy subjects.[1]

1. Aloxi (Palonosetron hydrochloride). MGI Pharma, Inc. US Prescribing information, January 2006.

Iron chelators + Ascorbic acid (Vitamin C)

High-dose vitamin C may cause cardiac disorders in some patients treated with desferrioxamine. Doses of up to 200 mg daily appear to be without adverse effect.

Clinical evidence, mechanism, importance and management

Vitamin C is given with iron chelators to patients with iron overload because it mobilises iron stores and thus promotes the excretion of iron. One study in 11 patients with thalassaemia noted that a striking deterioration in left ventricular function occurred when the patients were given 500 mg of vitamin C with intramuscular **desferrioxamine**. In most patients left ventricular function returned to normal when the vitamin C was stopped.[1] For this reason it has been suggested that vitamin C should be used with **desferrioxamine** with caution,[2] only where there is a demonstrated need,[3] and in the lowest possible dose.[1] The manufacturers of **desferrioxamine** recommend that a maximum daily dose of 200 mg of vitamin C should be used in adults, that vitamin C should not be given within the first month of **desferrioxamine** treatment, and that it should not be given to those with cardiac failure.[4,5]

The manufacturers of the oral iron chelator **deferasirox** note that, although concurrent use with vitamin C has not been formally studied, doses of vitamin C up to 200 mg daily were allowed in clinical studies of **deferasirox** without adverse consequences.[6,7]

1. Henry W. Echocardiographic evaluation of the heart in thalassemia major. *Ann Intern Med* (1979) 91, 892–4.
2. Cohen A, Cohen IJ, Schwartz E. Scurvy and altered iron stores in thalassemia major. *N Engl J Med* (1981) 304, 158–60.
3. Nienhuis AW. Vitamin C and iron. *N Engl J Med* (1981) 304, 170–1.
4. Desferal Vials (Desferrioxamine mesilate). Novartis Pharmaceuticals UK Ltd. UK Summary of product characteristics, August 2006.
5. Desferal Vials (Desferoxamine mesylate). Novartis. US Prescribing information, February 2006.
6. Exjade (Deferasirox). Novartis Pharmaceuticals UK Ltd. UK Summary of product characteristics, August 2006.
7. Exjade (Deferasirox). Novartis. US Prescribing information, April 2007.

Iron chelators; Deferasirox + Miscellaneous

Deferasirox did not alter the pharmacokinetics of digoxin. Food increases the bioavailability of deferasirox, and it should be taken on an empty stomach. The use of deferasirox with aluminium antacids is not recommended. Rifampicin, phenobarbital and phenytoin are predicted to increase the metabolism of deferasirox, and, until more is known, concurrent use should be monitored. Based on *in vitro* data, deferasirox might inhibit the metabolism of CYP2C8 substrates like paclitaxel and repaglinide. Hydroxycarbamide does not alter deferasirox metabolism.

Clinical evidence, mechanism, importance and management

(a) Aluminium-containing antacids

Although concurrent use has not been formally studied, the manufacturer recommends that deferasirox is not taken with aluminium-containing antacids.[1,2] Deferasirox has a lower affinity for aluminium than for iron, but theoretically aluminium might reduce the efficacy of deferasirox.

(b) CYP2C8 substrates

In vitro studies suggested that the only cytochrome P450 isoenzyme that was inhibited by deferasirox at concentrations similar to those that might be achieved clinically was CYP2C8. For this reason, the EMEA have requested that a clinical drug-drug interaction study be conducted to exclude a potential interaction with CYP2C8 substrates.[3] Pending the findings of this, the UK manufacturers warn that an interaction between deferasirox and CYP2C8 substrates, such as **paclitaxel** and **repaglinide** cannot be excluded.[1] Therefore, bear the possibility of an interaction in mind. See 'Table 1.3', (p.6), for a list of clinically relevant CYP2C8 substrates.

(c) Digoxin

In healthy subjects, deferasirox had no effect on the pharmacokinetics of digoxin.[1,2] No digoxin dose adjustment would be expected to be necessary on concurrent use.

(d) Food

Food increased the bioavailability of deferasirox to a variable extent, and the manufacturer recommends that it is taken on an empty stomach at least 30 minutes before food.[1,2] The tablets for oral suspension can be dispersed in water, orange juice, or apple juice.[2]

(e) Hydroxycarbamide

In vitro, hydroxycarbamide did not inhibit the metabolism of deferasirox.[2,3] Although an interaction has not been formally studied, the manufacturer considers it unlikely that concurrent use in patients with sickle cell anaemia will result in an interaction.[2,3]

(f) UGT enzyme inducers

Deferasirox metabolism is predicted to be increased if it is given with UGT enzyme inducers such as **rifampicin (rifampin)**, **phenobarbital** or **phenytoin** because deferasirox is metabolised principally by glucuronidation. Pending the results of a drug-interaction study,[3] the UK manufacturer recommends that the efficacy of deferasirox (serum ferritin levels) should be monitored if these drugs are used together with deferasirox, and when they are stopped, and the dose of deferasirox adjusted if necessary.[1]

1. Exjade (Deferasirox). Novartis Pharmaceuticals UK Ltd. UK Summary of product characteristics, August 2006.
2. Exjade (Deferasirox). Novartis. US Prescribing information, April 2007.
3. European Medicines Agency. Exjade. European Public Assessment Report. Scientific discussion, 2006. Available at: http://www.emea.europa.eu/humandocs/PDFs/EPAR/exjade/H-670-en6.pdf (accessed 23/08/2007).

Iron chelators; Desferrioxamine (Deferoxamine) + Prochlorperazine

Prochlorperazine caused unconsciousness in two patients being treated with desferrioxamine.

Clinical evidence, mechanism, importance and management

Administration of prochlorperazine to 2 patients receiving desferrioxamine resulted in unconsciousness for 48 to 72 hours. It was suggested that the drug combination resulted in increased removal of iron from the central nervous system, thereby impairing noradrenergic and serotonergic systems.[1] It has also been suggested that desferrioxamine-induced damage of the retina may be more likely in the presence of phenothiazines.[2] It would seem wise to avoid the concurrent use of desferrioxamine and prochlorperazine, but there seems to be no direct evidence of adverse interactions with any of the other phenothiazines.

1. Blake DR, Winyard P, Lunec J, Williams A, Good PA, Crewes SJ, Gutteridge JMC, Rowley D, Halliwell B, Cornish A, Hider RC. Cerebral and ocular toxicity induced by desferrioxamine. *Q J Med* (1985) 56, 345–55.
2. Pall H, Blake DR, Good PA, Wynyard P, Williams AC. Copper chelation and the neuro-ophthalmic toxicity of desferrioxamine. *Lancet* (1986) ii, 1279.

Iron compounds + Antacids

The absorption of iron and the expected haematological response can be reduced by the concurrent use of antacids.

Clinical evidence

A study in healthy subjects who were mildly iron-deficient (due to blood donation or menstruation) found that about 5 mL of *Mylanta II* (**aluminium/magnesium hydroxide** with simeticone) had little effect on the absorption of 10 or 20 mg of **ferrous sulfate** at 2 hours. However, **sodium bicarbonate** 1 g almost halved the absorption of **ferrous sulfate**, and **calcium carbonate** 500 mg reduced it by two-thirds. Conversely, iron absorption from a **multivitamin** and **mineral** preparation was little affected by whether or not the tablet contained 200 mg of calcium (as **calcium carbonate**).[1] Another study found that an antacid containing **aluminium/magnesium hydroxides** and **magnesium carbonate** reduced the absorption of **ferrous sulfate** and **ferrous fumarate** (both containing 100 mg of ferrous iron) in healthy iron-replete subjects by 37% and 31%, respectively.[2] Poor absorption of iron during treatment with **sodium bicarbonate** and **aluminium hydroxide** has been described elsewhere.[3,4] One study did not find that the absorption of **ferrous sulfate** (iron 10 mg/kg) was affected by doses of **magnesium hydroxide** (5 mg for every 1 mg of iron) when given 30 minutes apart.[5] However, it has been suggested that iron absorption was not measured for a sufficient period to fully rule out a reduction in absorption.[6]

When oral iron failed to cause an expected rise in haemoglobin levels in patients taking non-absorbable alkalis such as **magnesium trisilicate**, a study was undertaken in 9 patients. Each patient was given 5 mg of isotopically labelled **ferrous sulfate** after a 35-g dose of **magnesium trisilicate**. The **magnesium** reduced the absorption of iron by an average of 70 to 88%, the reduction being small in some patients, but one individual had a fall from 67% to 5%.[7]

Mechanism

Uncertain. One suggestion is that magnesium sulfate changes ferrous sulfate into less easily absorbed salts, or increases its polymerisation.[7] Carbonates possibly cause the formation of poorly soluble iron complexes.[3] Aluminium hydroxide is believed to precipitate iron as the hydroxide and ferric ions can become intercalated into the aluminium hydroxide crystal lattice,[8] leaving less available for absorption.

Importance and management

Information is limited and difficult to assess because of the many variables (e.g. different dosages ranging from very small to those mimicking overdose, and a mix of subjects and patients). However, a reasonable 'blanket precaution' to achieve maximal absorption would be to separate the administration of iron preparations and antacids as much as possible to avoid admixture in the gut. This may not prove to be necessary with some preparations.

1. O'Neil-Cutting MA, Crosby WH. The effect of antacids on the absorption of simultaneously ingested iron. *JAMA* (1986) 255, 1468–70.
2. Ekenved G, Halvorsen L, Sölvell L. Influence of a liquid antacid on the absorption of different iron salts. *Scand J Haematol* (1976) 28 (Suppl), 65–77.
3. Benjamin BI, Cortell S, Conrad ME. Bicarbonate-induced iron complexes and iron absorption: one effect of pancreatic secretions. *Gastroenterology* (1967) 35, 389–96.
4. Rastogi SP, Padilla F, Boyd CM. Effect of aluminum hydroxide on iron absorption. *J Arkansas Med Soc* (1976) 73, 133–4.
5. Snyder BK, Clark RF. Effect of magnesium hydroxide administration on iron absorption after a supratherapeutic dose of ferrous sulfate in human volunteers: a randomized controlled trial. *Ann Emerg Med* (1999) 33, 400–405.
6. Wallace KL, Curry SC, LoVecchio F, Raschke RA. Effect of magnesium hydroxide on iron absorption after ferrous sulfate. *Ann Emerg Med* (1999) 34, 685–6.
7. Hall GJL, Davis AE. Inhibition of iron absorption by magnesium trisilicate. *Med J Aust* (1969) 2, 95–6.
8. Coste JF, De Bari VA, Keil LB, Needle MA. *In-vitro* interactions of oral hematinics and antacid suspensions. *Curr Ther Res* (1977) 22, 205–15.

Iron compounds or Vitamin B_{12} + Chloramphenicol

In addition to the serious and potentially fatal bone marrow depression that can occur with chloramphenicol, it may also cause a milder, reversible bone marrow depression, which can oppose the treatment of anaemias with iron or vitamin B_{12}.

Clinical evidence

Ten out of 22 patients receiving **iron dextran** for iron-deficiency anaemia and also given chloramphenicol, failed to show the expected haematological response to the iron.[1] Four patients receiving vitamin B_{12} for pernicious anaemia were all similarly refractory to treatment until the chloramphenicol was withdrawn.[1]

Mechanism

Chloramphenicol can cause two forms of bone marrow depression. One is serious and irreversible, and can result in fatal aplastic anaemia, whereas the other is probably unrelated, milder and reversible, and appears to occur at chloramphenicol serum levels of 25 micrograms/mL or more. This occurs because chloramphenicol can inhibit protein synthesis, the first sign of which is a fall in the reticulocyte count, which reflects inadequate red cell maturation. This response to chloramphenicol has been seen in *animals*,[2] healthy individuals,[3] a series of patients with liver disease,[4] and in anaemic patients[1] being treated with iron dextran or vitamin B_{12}.

Importance and management

An established interaction of clinical importance. The authors of one study recommend that chloramphenicol dosages of 25 to 30 mg/kg are usually adequate for treating infections without running the risk of elevating serum levels to 25 micrograms/mL or more, which is when this type of marrow depression can occur.[5] Monitor the effects of using iron or vitamin B_{12} together with chloramphenicol. A preferable alternative would be to use a different antibacterial. Note that chloramphenicol should not be used in patients with pre-existing bone-marrow depression or blood dyscrasias.

1. Saidi P, Wallerstein RO, Aggeler PM. Effect of chloramphenicol on erythropoiesis. *J Lab Clin Med* (1961) 57, 247–56.
2. Rigdon RH, Crass G, Martin N. Anemia produced by chloramphenicol (Chloromycetin) in the duck. *AMA Arch Pathol* (1954) 58, 85–93.
3. Jiji RM, Gangarosa EJ, de la Macorra F. Chloramphenicol and its sulfamoyl analogue. Report of reversible erythropoietic toxicity in healthy volunteers. *Arch Intern Med* (1963) 111, 116–28.
4. McCurdy PR. Chloramphenicol bone marrow toxicity. *JAMA* (1961) 176, 588–93.
5. Scott JL, Finegold SM, Belkin GA, Lawrence JS. A controlled double-blind study of the hematologic toxicity of chloramphenicol. *N Engl J Med* (1965) 272, 1137–42.

Iron compounds + Coffee or Tea

Coffee may possibly contribute towards the development of iron-deficiency anaemia in pregnant women, and reduce the levels of iron in breast milk. As a result their babies may also be iron deficient. Tea may also possibly be associated with microcytic anaemia in children.

Clinical evidence

(a) Coffee

A controlled study among pregnant women in Costa Rica found that coffee consumption was associated with reductions in the haemoglobin levels and haematocrits of the mothers during pregnancy, and of their babies shortly after birth, despite the fact that the women were taking **ferric sulfate** 200 mg and 500 micrograms of folate daily. The babies also had a slightly lower birth weight (3189 g versus 3310 g). Almost a quarter of the mothers were considered to have iron-deficiency anaemia (haemoglobin levels of less than 11 g/dL), compared with none among the control group of non-coffee drinkers. Levels of iron in breast milk were reduced by about one-third. The coffee drinkers drank more than 450 mL of coffee daily, equivalent to more than 10 g of ground coffee.[1]

(b) Tea

A much higher incidence of microcytic anaemia has been described in tea-drinking infants in Israel. The tea-drinkers consumed a median of 250 mL of tea each day, and the incidence of anaemia was 64%, which was about twice that of the non-tea drinking control group (31%).[2] A case report describes an impaired response to iron, given to correct an iron-deficiency anaemia, in the presence of 2 litres of black tea taken daily. The patient recovered when the black tea was stopped.[3] Another report describes no change in the absorption of **iron supplements** in daily doses of 2 to 15.8 mg/kg in 10 iron-deficient tea-drinking children, although note that the children were only given 150 mL of tea.[4]

Mechanism

Tannins are thought to form insoluble complexes with iron and thus reduce its absorption.[2,4]

Importance and management

The general importance of these findings is uncertain, but be aware that coffee or tea consumption may contribute to iron-deficiency anaemia. Note that tea and coffee are not generally considered to be suitable drinks for babies and children, because of their effects on iron absorption. More study is needed.

1. Muñoz LM, Lönnerdal B, Keen CL, Dewey KG. Coffee consumption as a factor in iron deficiency anemia among pregnant women and their infants in Costa Rica. *Am J Clin Nutr* (1988) 48, 645–51.
2. Merhav H, Amitai Y, Palti H, Godfrey S. Tea drinking and microcytic anemia in infants. *Am J Clin Nutr* (1985) 41, 1210–13.
3. Mahlknecht U, Weidmann E, Seipelt G. Black tea delays recovery from iron-deficiency anaemia. *Haematologica* (2001) 86, 559.
4. Koren G, Boichis H, Keren G. Effects of tea on the absorption of pharmacological doses of an oral iron preparation. *Isr J Med Sci* (1982) 18, 547.

Iron compounds + Colestyramine

Colestyramine binds with ferrous sulfate in the gut and reduces its absorption, but the clinical importance of this is uncertain.

Clinical evidence, mechanism, importance and management

Studies have shown that colestyramine binds with iron, and in *rats* this was found to halve the absorption of a single 100-microgram dose of **ferrous sulfate**.[1] Nobody seems to have checked on the general clinical importance of this in patients. Until more is known it would seem prudent to separate the dosages of the iron and colestyramine to avoid mixing in the gut, thereby minimising the effects of this possible interaction. The standard recommendation is to avoid other drugs one hour before or 4 to 6 hours after colestyramine.

1. Thomas FB, McCullough F, Greenberger NJ. Inhibition of the intestinal absorption of inorganic and hemoglobin iron by cholestyramine. *J Lab Clin Med* (1971) 78, 70–80.

Iron compounds + H_2-receptor antagonists

Apart from a brief and unconfirmed report alleging that cimetidine reduced the response to ferrous sulfate in three patients, there appears to be no other evidence that H_2-receptor antagonists reduce the absorption of iron to a clinically relevant extent. Iron causes only a small and clinically irrelevant reduction in the serum levels of cimetidine and famotidine.

Clinical evidence, mechanism, importance and management

(a) Effect on iron

A brief report describes 3 patients taking **cimetidine** 1 g and **ferrous sulfate** 600 mg daily whose ulcers healed after 2 months, but their anaemia and altered iron metabolism persisted. When the **cimetidine** was reduced to 400 mg daily, but with the same dose of iron, the blood picture resolved satisfactorily within a month.[1] The author of the report attributed this response to the **cimetidine**-induced rise in gastric pH, which reduced the absorption of the iron. However, this suggested mechanism was subsequently disputed, as medicinal iron is already in the most absorbable form, Fe^{2+}, and so does not need an acidic environment to aid absorption.[2] A study in patients with iron deficiency, or iron-deficiency anaemia, found that the concurrent use of **famotidine**, **nizatidine**, or **ranitidine**, did not affect their response to 2.4 g of **iron succinyl-protein complex** (equivalent to 60 mg of iron twice daily).[3] No special precautions would seem necessary on concurrent use.

(b) Effect on H_2-receptor antagonists

In a series of 3 studies, healthy subjects were given a 300-mg tablet of **cimetidine** with either a 300-mg tablet of **ferrous sulfate** or 300 mg of **ferrous sulfate** in solution. The reductions in the AUC and the maximum serum levels of the **cimetidine** were small (less than 16%). In the third experiment they were given **famotidine** 40 mg with a 300-mg tablet of **ferrous sulfate**. Again, the AUC and maximum serum level reductions were also very small (10% or less). These small reductions are almost certainly due to the formation of a weak complex between the iron and these H_2-receptor antagonists.[4] An *in vitro* study with **ranitidine** found that, while it also binds with iron, it forms a very weak complex, and is less likely to bind than **cimetidine** or **famotidine**.[4] It was concluded that no clinically relevant interaction occurs between **ferrous sulfate** and any of these H_2-receptor antagonists.[4]

1. Esposito R. Cimetidine and iron-deficiency anaemia. *Lancet* (1977) ii, 1132.
2. Rosner F. Cimetidine and iron absorption. *Lancet* (1978) i, 95.

3. Bianchi FM, Cavassini GB, Leo P. Iron protein succinylate in the treatment of iron deficiency: Potential interaction with H_2-receptor antagonists. *Int J Clin Pharmacol Ther Toxicol* (1993) 31, 209–17.

4. Partlow ES, Campbell NRC, Chan SC, Pap KM, Granberg K, Hasinoff BB. Ferrous sulfate does not reduce serum levels of famotidine or cimetidine after concurrent ingestion. *Clin Pharmacol Ther* (1996) 59, 389–93.

Iron compounds + Neomycin

Neomycin may alter the absorption of iron.

Clinical evidence, mechanism, importance and management

A study in 6 patients found that neomycin markedly reduced the absorption of iron (iron^{59} as **ferrous citrate**) in 4 patients, but increased the absorption in the other 2 patients who initially had low serum iron levels. None of the patients were anaemic at any time.[1] The importance of this is uncertain, but consider this possible interaction if the response to iron is poor.

1. Jacobson ED, Chodos RB, Faloon WW. An experimental malabsorption syndrome induced by neomycin. *Am J Med* (1960) 28, 524–33.

Iron compounds + Phosphate binders

Calcium carbonate and calcium acetate (in phosphate-binding doses) caused a modest reduction in the absorption of iron from ferrous sulfate, whereas sevelamer had only a minor effect.

Clinical evidence, mechanism, importance and management

In a single-dose study in 23 fasting healthy subjects,[1] the bioavailability of iron from **ferrous sulfate** 200 mg was reduced by 27% by **calcium acetate** 2.7 g, 19% by **calcium carbonate** 3 g, and 10% by **sevelamer** 2.8 g.

It was suggested that calcium may form insoluble complexes with iron, so reducing its absorption.

This study suggests that these calcium phosphate-binders may have a clinically relevant effect on iron absorption, whereas **sevelamer** probably does not. However, the findings need replicating in an appropriate patient group taking the phosphate binders long-term with meals. See also 'antacids', (p.1262) for data suggesting that lower doses of **calcium carbonate** may or may not reduce iron absorption.

1. Pruchnicki MC, Coyle JD, Hoshaw-Woodard S, Bay WH. Effect of phosphate binders on supplemental iron absorption in healthy subjects. *J Clin Pharmacol* (2002) 42, 1171–6.

Iron compounds + Vitamin E substances

Vitamin E impaired the response to iron in a group of anaemic children.

Clinical evidence, mechanism, importance and management

A group of 26 anaemic children aged 7 to 40 months were given **iron dextran** 5 mg/kg daily for 3 days. Vitamin E 200 units daily was also given to 9 of the children, starting 24 hours before the **iron dextran** and continued for a total of 4 days. It was noted that after 6 days, those taking vitamin E had a reticulocyte response of only 4.4% compared with 14.4% in the patients not given vitamin E. The vitamin E group also had reduced haemoglobin levels and a lower haematocrit. The reasons are not understood. Check for any evidence of a reduced haematological response in anaemic patients given iron and vitamin E. The authors of the report point out that this dosage of vitamin E was well above the recommended daily dietary intake.[1]

1. Melhorn DK, Gross S. Relationships between iron-dextran and vitamin E in iron deficiency anemia in children. *J Lab Clin Med* (1969) 74, 789–802.

Kava + Cytochrome P450 isoenzyme substrates

Kava does not appear to affect the metabolism of debrisoquine and mephenytoin. Kava may inhibit the metabolism of chlorzoxazone but not all studies have found this effect.

Clinical evidence, mechanism, importance and management

In a study in 6 subjects (3 of whom smoked tobacco), who usually took 7 to 27 g of kavalactones weekly as an aqueous kava extract, the metabolism of **chlorzoxazone**, **debrisoquine**, and **mephenytoin** (which are substrates of CYP2E1, CYP2D6, and CYP2C19, respectively), was not affected when the subjects stopped taking kava for 30 days.[1] Similar results were found in a study in 12 healthy subjects given kava kava root extract 1 g twice daily for 28 days before receiving a single dose of **debrisoquine**, but when the interaction between kava kava root extract and **chlorzoxazone** was also studied in these subjects a 40% inhibitory effect of kava on CYP2E1 was seen, which is in contrast to the previous study.[2] For a list of drugs which are substrates of CYP2E1, CYP2D6, and CYP2C19, see 'Table 1.3', (p.6).

Consider also 'midazolam', (p.730), 'caffeine', (p.1165), which are substrates for CYP3A4 and CYP1A2, respectively.

1. Russman S, Lauterburg BH, Barguil Y, Choblet E, Cabalion P, Rentsch K, Wenk M. Traditional aqueous kava extracts inhibit cytochrome P450 1A2 in humans: protective effect against environmental carcinogens? *Clin Pharmacol Ther* (2005) 77, 451–4.

2. Gurley BJ, Gardner SF, Hubbard MA, Williams DK, Gentry WB, Khan IA, Shah A. In vivo effects of goldenseal, kava kava, black cohosh, and valerian on human cytochrome P450 1A2, 2D6, 2E1, and 3A4/5 phenotypes. *Clin Pharmacol Ther* (2005) 77, 415–26.

Melatonin + Caffeine

Caffeine increases the levels of both endogenous and orally administered melatonin.

Clinical evidence

A crossover study in 12 healthy subjects found that a single 200-mg dose of caffeine (equivalent to one large or two small cups of coffee), taken 1 hour before and 1 and 3 hours after a single 6-mg oral dose of melatonin, increased the average AUC and maximum levels of melatonin by 120% and 137%, respectively, although the half-life of melatonin was not significantly affected. The interaction was less pronounced in smokers (6 subjects) than in non-smokers (6 subjects).[1]

Another crossover study in 12 healthy subjects (by the same authors) found that a single 200-mg dose of caffeine, taken 12 or 24 hours before a single 6-mg dose of melatonin, did not affect the melatonin levels, although 2 subjects had raised melatonin levels when caffeine was taken 12 hours, but not 24 hours, before melatonin.[2]

In 12 healthy subjects given a single 200-mg dose of caffeine, taken in the evening, endogenous, nocturnal melatonin levels were found to be increased, and the AUC of melatonin was increased by 32%.[3]

Mechanism

Caffeine is thought to reduce the metabolism of melatonin by competing for metabolism by the cytochrome P450 isoenzyme CYP1A2.[1-3]

Importance and management

Melatonin is produced by the pineal gland in the body and is also available as a supplement in some parts of the world. However, the effects of long-term use of this supplement are unknown. From the above studies, it appears that caffeine significantly increases the levels of single doses of supplementary melatonin, however the long-term effects of caffeine and concurrent multiple dosing of melatonin do not appear to have been studied. Melatonin can cause drowsiness when taken on its own, so patients who take melatonin should be advised that this effect may be increased if they also take caffeine. This increased drowsiness may oppose the stimulating effect of caffeine.

1. Härtter S, Nordmark A, Rose D-M, Bertilsson L, Tybring G, Laine K. Effects of caffeine intake on the pharmacokinetics of melatonin, a probe drug for CYP1A2 activity. *Br J Clin Pharmacol* (2003) 56, 679–682.

2. Härtter S, Korhonen T, Lundgren S, Rane A, Tolonen A, Turpeinen M, Laine K. Effect of caffeine intake 12 or 24 hours prior to melatonin intake and *CYP1A2*1F* polymorphism on CYP1A2 phenotyping by melatonin. *Basic Clin Pharmacol Toxicol* (2006) 99, 300–4.
3. Ursing C, Wikner J, Brismar K, Röjdmark S. Caffeine raises the serum melatonin level in healthy subjects: an indication of melatonin metabolism by cytochrome P450 (CYP)1A2. *J Endocrinol Invest* (2003) 26, 403–6.

Methoxsalen + Phenytoin

The serum levels of methoxsalen can be markedly reduced by the concurrent use of phenytoin. This resulted in failure of treatment for psoriasis in one patient.

Clinical evidence, mechanism, importance and management

A patient with epilepsy failed to respond to treatment for psoriasis with PUVA (12 treatments of methoxsalen 30 mg given orally and ultraviolet A irradiation) while taking phenytoin 250 mg daily. Methoxsalen serum levels were normal in the absence of phenytoin, but abnormally low while taking phenytoin,[1] due, it is suggested, to the enzyme inducing effects of the phenytoin. This interaction could lead to serious erythema and blistering if the phenytoin dose is reduced during therapy, as methoxsalen levels rise and therefore photosensitivity caused by the methoxsalen may be increased. Concurrent use should be avoided or very closely monitored.

1. Staberg B, Hueg B. Interaction between 8-methoxypsoralen and phenytoin. Consequence for PUVA therapy. *Acta Derm Venereol* (1985) 65, 553–5.

Metyrapone + Miscellaneous

The results of the metyrapone test for Cushing's syndrome are unreliable in patients taking cyproheptadine or phenytoin. The manufacturer also states that barbiturates, antidepressants, some hormones, and antipsychotics may influence the results of the test.

Clinical evidence

(a) Cyproheptadine

Pretreatment with cyproheptadine 4 mg every 6 hours, 2 days before and throughout a standard metyrapone test (750 mg every 4 hours for 6 doses), reduced the metyrapone-induced urinary 17-hydroxycorticosteroid response in 9 healthy subjects by 32%, and also reduced the serum 11-deoxycortisol response.[1]

(b) Phenytoin

A study in 5 healthy subjects and 3 patients taking phenytoin 300 mg showed that their serum metyrapone levels 4 hours after taking a regular 750-mg dose were very low, when compared with a control group (6.5 versus 48.2 micrograms/100 mL). The response to metyrapone (i.e. the fall in circulating glucocorticoids) is related to serum levels and was therefore proportionately lower.[2] Other reports confirm that the urinary steroid response to metyrapone is subnormal in patients taking phenytoin.[3,4]

Doubling the dose of metyrapone from 750 mg every 4 hours to every 2 hours has been shown to give results similar to those in subjects not taking phenytoin.[2]

Mechanism

Phenytoin is a potent liver enzyme inducer that increases the metabolism of metyrapone, thereby reducing its effects.[2,5]

Importance and management

The results of metyrapone tests for Cushing's syndrome will be unreliable in patients taking cyproheptadine and phenytoin, and therefore these should be withdrawn prior to the test. The manufacturer also states that **barbiturates**, antidepressants (they name **amitriptyline**) and antipsychotics (they name **chlorpromazine**), hormones that affect the hypothalamo-pituitary axis, and **antithyroid drugs** may influence the results of the test. They recommend that, if any of these drugs cannot be withdrawn prior to the test, the necessity of carrying out the metyrapone test should be reviewed.[6]

1. Plonk J, Feldman JM, Keagle D. Modification of adrenal function by the anti-serotonin agent cyproheptadine. *J Clin Endocrinol Metab* (1976) 42, 291–5.
2. Meikle AW, Jubiz W, Matsukura S, West CD, Tyler FH. Effect of diphenylhydantoin on the metabolism of metyrapone and release of ACTH in man. *J Clin Endocrinol Metab* (1969) 29, 1553–8.
3. Krieger DT. Effect of diphenylhydantoin on pituitary-adrenal interrelations. *J Clin Endocrinol Metab* (1962) 22, 490–3.
4. Werk EE, Thrasher K, Choi Y, Sholiton LJ. Failure of metyrapone to inhibit 11-hydroxylation of 11-deoxycortisol during drug therapy. *J Clin Endocrinol Metab* (1967) 27, 1358–60.
5. Jubiz W, Levinson RA, Meikle AW, West CD, Tyler FH. Absorption and conjugation of metyrapone during diphenylhydantoin therapy: mechanism of the abnormal response to oral metyrapone. *Endocrinology* (1970) 86, 328–31.
6. Metopirone (Metyrapone). Alliance Pharmaceuticals. UK Summary of product characteristics, February 2005.

Mifepristone + Aspirin or NSAIDs

The manufacturers of mifepristone say that the antiprostaglandin effects of NSAIDs including aspirin could theoretically decrease the efficacy of mifepristone. They recommend using non-NSAID analgesics.[1]

1. Mifegyne (Mifepristone). Exelgyn Laboratories. UK Summary of product characteristics, February 2006.

Milk thistle + Cytochrome P450 isoenzyme substrates

Milk thistle does not alter the metabolism of caffeine, chlorzoxazone, or debrisoquine.

Clinical evidence, mechanism, importance and management

Milk thistle 175 mg, standardised to 80% silymarins, was given to 12 healthy subjects twice daily for 28 days. Subjects also received single doses of **caffeine** 100 mg, **chlorzoxazone** 250 mg, and **debrisoquine** 5 mg, before and at the end of the treatment with milk thistle. The metabolism of these drugs was not affected by the concurrent use of milk thistle, which suggests that milk thistle is unlikely to affect the metabolism of drugs that are substrates of the cytochrome P450 isoenzymes CYP1A2, CYP2E1, or CYP2D6.[1] For a list of drugs that are substrates of these isoenzymes, see 'Table 1.2', (p.4), and 'Table 1.3', (p.6).

For the lack of effect of milk thistle on CYP3A4, see 'Benzodiazepines + Milk thistle', p.732.

1. Gurley BJ, Gardner SF, Hubbard MA, Williams DK, Gentry WB, Carrier J, Khan IA, Edwards DJ, Shah A. In vivo assessment of botanical supplementation on human cytochrome P450 phenotypes: *Citrus aurantium*, *Echinacea purpurea*, milk thistle, and saw palmetto. *Clin Pharmacol Ther* (2004) 76, 428–40.

Moxisylyte + Miscellaneous

There is a theoretical possibility of increased blood pressure lowering effects if moxisylyte is used with antihypertensives or tricyclic antidepressants.

Clinical evidence, mechanism, importance and management

Moxisylyte is an alpha-1, and to a lesser extent, an alpha-2 blocker, which may be used orally as a peripheral vasodilator in Raynaud's syndrome. The manufacturers suggest that if moxisylyte is used by patients taking antihypertensives, it may theoretically potentiate the antihypertensive effect, although at the recommended doses this has not been reported.[1]

They also say that tricyclic antidepressants might increase any hypotensive effect of moxisylyte.[1]

1. Opilon (Moxisylyte hydrochloride). Concord Pharmaceuticals Ltd. UK Summary of product characteristics, April 2004.

Nicotine + Vasopressin

A case report described marked hypotension and bradycardia in a young woman during surgery, attributed to the combined effects of vasopressin and nicotine from a transdermal patch.

Clinical evidence

A 22-year-old woman in good health was anaesthetised for surgery with nitrous oxide/oxygen and isoflurane. Twenty minutes after induction she was given an injection of 0.2 units of vasopressin into the cervix. Within seconds she developed severe hypotension and bradycardia, and over the next 30 minutes blood pressures as low as 70/35 mmHg and heart rates as low as 38 bpm were recorded. She was treated with atropine and adrenaline (epinephrine), and eventually made a full recovery. This patient was wearing a transdermal nicotine patch.[1]

Mechanism

The circulatory collapse was attributed by the authors to the combined effects of the injected vasopressin and the nicotine from the transdermal patch. Both of these drugs can increase afterload and cause coronary artery vasoconstriction, which the authors suggest may have decreased the blood supply to the heart and resulted in cardiac depression.[1]

Importance and management

This is an isolated report and any interaction is therefore not well established. Nevertheless the recommendation of the authors seems sensible, namely that nicotine patches should be removed the night before or 24 hours before surgery, and that patients should be asked to avoid smoking before surgery to make sure that nicotine levels are minimal. More study is needed.

1. Groudine SB, Morley JN. Recent problems with paracervical vasopressin: a possible synergistic reaction with nicotine. *Med Hypotheses* (1996) 47, 19–21.

Oxiracetam + Antiepileptics

The half-life of oxiracetam was shorter in patients taking carbamazepine and valproate or clobazam, but oxiracetam did not affect the serum levels of sodium valproate, carbamazepine or clobazam.

Clinical evidence, mechanism, importance and management

Oxiracetam 800 mg twice daily for 14 days did not affect the serum levels of **sodium valproate**, **carbamazepine**, or **clobazam** and their metabolites in 3 epileptics taking **carbamazepine** and **valproate** and one taking **carbamazepine** and **clobazam**.[1] However, it was noted that the oxiracetam half-life was 2.8 to 7.56 hours,[1] which tended to be shorter than that seen in a previous study in healthy subjects who had been given oxiracetam 2 g (half-life 5.6 to 11.7 hours).[2] The clinical relevance of this is uncertain, but the authors suggest that it may be necessary to raise the oxiracetam dosage or give it more frequently in the presence of these drugs.[1]

1. van Wieringen A, Meijer JWA, van Emde Boas W, Vermeij TAC. Pilot study to determine the interaction of oxiracetam with antiepileptic drugs. *Clin Pharmacokinet* (1990) 18, 332–8.

2. Perucca E, Albrici A, Gatti G, Spalluto R, Visconti M, Crema A. Pharmacokinetics of oxiracetam following intravenous and oral administration in healthy volunteers. *Eur J Drug Metab Pharmacokinet* (1984) 9, 267–74.

Oxygen; hyperbaric + Miscellaneous

It has been suggested, but not confirmed, that because increased levels of carbon dioxide in the tissues can increase the 'sensitivity' to oxygen-induced convulsions, carbonic anhydrase inhibitors, such as acetazolamide, are contraindicated in those given hyperbaric oxygen, because they cause carbon dioxide to persist in the tissues. Nor should hyperbaric oxygen be given during opioid or barbiturate withdrawal because the convulsive threshold of such patients is already low.[1]

1. Gunby P. HBO can interact with preexisting patient conditions. *JAMA* (1981) 246, 1177–8.

Papaverine + Diazepam

Two men given normal test doses of papaverine for the investigation of impotence had prolonged erections attributed to the concurrent use of diazepam.

Clinical evidence, mechanism, importance and management

Undesirably prolonged erections (duration of 5 and 6 hours) occurred in 2 patients who had been given 5 or 10 mg of diazepam intravenously for anxiety before a 60-mg intracavernosal injection of papaverine.[1] Papaverine acts by relaxing the arterioles that supply the corpora so that the pressure rises. The increased pressure in the corpora compresses the trabecular venules so that the pressure continues to maintain the erection. Diazepam also relaxes smooth muscle and it would seem that this can be additive with the effects of papaverine. The authors of the report say that caution should be exercised in the choice of papaverine dosage in patients taking anxiolytics (i.e. use less) although these two cases involving diazepam seem to be the only ones recorded.[1]

1. Vale JA, Kirby RS, Lees W. Papaverine, benzodiazepines, and prolonged erections. *Lancet* (1991) 337, 1552.

Penicillamine + Antacids

The absorption of penicillamine from the gut can be reduced by 30 to 40% if antacids containing aluminium/magnesium hydroxide are taken.

Clinical evidence

Maalox-plus (**aluminium/magnesium hydroxide, simeticone**) 30 mL reduced the absorption of a single 500-mg dose of penicillamine in 6 healthy subjects by one-third.[1] Another study found that 30 mL of *Aludrox* (**aluminium/magnesium hydroxide**) reduced the absorption of penicillamine by about 40%.[2]

Mechanism

The most likely explanation is that the penicillamine forms less soluble chelates with magnesium and aluminium ions in the gut, which reduces its absorption.[2] Another idea is that the penicillamine is possibly less stable at the higher pH values caused by the antacid.[1]

Importance and management

An established interaction of clinical importance. If maximal absorption is needed the administration of the two drugs should be separated to avoid mixing in the gut. Two hours or so has been found enough for most other drugs which interact similarly. There seems to be nothing documented about other antacids.

1. Osman MA, Patel RB, Schuna A, Sundstrom WR, Welling PG. Reduction in oral penicillamine absorption by food, antacid and ferrous sulphate. *Clin Pharmacol Ther* (1983) 33, 465–70.
2. Ifan A, Welling PG. Pharmacokinetics of oral 500-mg penicillamine: effect of antacids on absorption. *Biopharm Drug Dispos* (1986) 7, 401–5.

Penicillamine + Food

Food can reduce the absorption of penicillamine by as much as a half.

Clinical evidence

The presence of food reduced the plasma levels of penicillamine 500 mg by about 50% in healthy subjects. The total amount absorbed was similarly reduced.[1,2] These figures are in good agreement with previous findings.[3]

Mechanism

Uncertain. One suggestion is that food delays gastric emptying so that the penicillamine is exposed to more prolonged degradation in the stomach.[2] Another idea is that the protein in food reduces penicillamine absorption.

Importance and management

An established interaction. If maximal effects are required the penicillamine should be taken at least 30 minutes before food.

1. Schuna A, Osman MA, Patel RB, Welling PG, Sundstrom WR. Influence of food on the bioavailability of penicillamine. *J Rheumatol* (1983) 10, 95–7.
2. Osman MA, Patel RB, Schuna A, Sundstrom WR, Welling PG. Reduction in oral penicillamine absorption by food, antacid and ferrous sulphate. *Clin Pharmacol Ther* (1983) 33, 465–70.
3. Bergstrom RF, Kay DR, Harkcom TM, Wagner JG. Penicillamine kinetics in normal subjects. *Clin Pharmacol Ther* (1981) 30, 404–13.

Penicillamine + Iron compounds

The absorption of penicillamine can be reduced as much as two-thirds by oral iron compounds.

Clinical evidence

Ferrous iron 90 mg (as *Fersamal*) reduced the absorption of penicillamine 250 mg in 5 healthy subjects by about two-thirds (using the cupruretic effects of penicillamine as a measure).[1]

A two-thirds reduction in absorption has been described in 6 other subjects given penicillamine 500 mg and **ferrous sulfate** 300 mg.[2] Other studies confirm this interaction.[3,4] There is also evidence that the withdrawal of iron from patients stabilised on penicillamine can lead to the development of toxicity (nephropathy) unless the penicillamine dosage is reduced.[5]

Mechanism

It is believed that the iron and penicillamine form a chemical complex or chelate within the gut, which is less easily absorbed.

Importance and management

An established and clinically important interaction. For maximal absorption give the iron at least 2 hours after the penicillamine. This should reduce their admixture in the gut.[1] Do not withdraw iron suddenly from patients stabilised on penicillamine because the marked increase in absorption that follows may precipitate penicillamine toxicity. The toxic effects of penicillamine seem to be dependent on the size of the dose and possibly also related to the rate at which the dosage is increased.[5] Only ferrous sulfate and fumarate have been studied but other iron compounds would be expected to interact similarly.

1. Lyle WH. Penicillamine and iron. *Lancet* (1976) ii, 420.
2. Osman MA, Patel RB, Schuna A, Sundstrom WR, Welling PG. Reduction in oral penicillamine absorption by food, antacid, and ferrous sulphate. *Clin Pharmacol Ther* (1983) 33, 465–70.
3. Lyle WH, Pearcey DF, Hui M. Inhibition of penicillamine-induced cupruresis by oral iron. *Proc R Soc Med* (1977) 70 (Suppl 3), 48–9.
4. Hall ND, Blake DR, Alexander GJM, Vaisey C, Bacon PA. Serum SH reactivity: a simple assessment of D-penicillamine absorption? *Rheumatol Int* (1981) 1, 39–41.
5. Harkness JAL, Blake DR. Penicillamine nephropathy and iron. *Lancet* (1982) ii, 1368–9.

Penicillamine + Miscellaneous

Penicillamine plasma levels are increased by chloroquine and an increase in penicillamine toxicity is possible. Penicillamine should not be used with gold. Indometacin slightly increases penicillamine levels, and its use with any NSAID might increase the risk of renal damage. An isolated report describes penicillamine-induced breast enlargement in a woman taking a combined oral contraceptive.

Clinical evidence, mechanism, importance and management

(a) Disease-modifying antirheumatic drugs

Studies in which **chloroquine** was given to patients taking penicillamine found that it was more effective, less effective, or indistinguishable from penicillamine alone. However in some instances penicillamine toxicity was reported to be increased.[1] A pharmacokinetic study in patients with rheumatoid arthritis taking penicillamine 250 mg daily found that a single 250-mg dose of **chloroquine phosphate** increased the AUC by 34%, and raised the peak plasma levels by about 55%.[1] It therefore seems possible that any increased toxicity is simply a reflection of increased plasma penicillamine levels. Be alert for evidence of toxicity if both drugs are used. Note that the US manufacturer states that penicillamine should not be used in patients who are receiving antimalarials (which would include **chloroquine** and **hydroxychloroquine**) because these drugs are also associated with serious haematological effects.[2]

There is some evidence that using **gold** with penicillamine may increase the risk of adverse effects, and the manufacturer says that they should not be used together.[2,3] In addition, patients who have had an adverse reaction to **gold** may be at a greater risk of serious adverse reactions to penicillamine,[2,3] and caution is recommended.[3]

(b) NSAIDs

Indometacin has been found to increase the AUC of penicillamine by 26% and the peak plasma levels by about 22%.[1] The UK manufacturer notes that use of NSAIDs may increase the risk of renal damage with penicillamine.[3] The US manufacturer specifically recommends avoiding **oxyphenbutazone** or **phenylbutazone** because these drugs are also associated with serious haematological and renal effects.[2] Urinalysis for detection of haematuria or proteinuria should be regularly carried out in patients taking penicillamine.[2,3] Be alert for evidence of toxicity if NSAIDs and penicillamine are used together.

(c) Oral contraceptives

A woman with Wilson's disease began to develop dark facial hair about 10 months after starting to take penicillamine 1.25 to 1.5 g daily. After 20 months her testosterone levels were found to be slightly raised, and so she was given a combined oral contraceptive, but within a month her breasts began to enlarge and become more tender. After a further 6 months the penicillamine was replaced by trientine hydrochloride.[4] The reasons are not understood, but the authors of the report suggest that the penicillamine was the prime cause of the macromastia, but it possibly needed the presence of a 'second trigger' (i.e. the oral contraceptive) to set things in motion.[4]

There are 12 other cases of macromastia and gynaecomastia on record associated with the use of penicillamine, in some of which the second trigger may possibly have been a **corticosteroid** or **cimetidine**.[4] Macromastia appears to be an unusual adverse effect of penicillamine and there would seem to be no general reason for patients taking penicillamine to avoid oral contraceptives.

1. Seideman P, Lindström B. Pharmacokinetic interactions of penicillamine in rheumatoid arthritis. *J Rheumatol* (1989) 16, 473–4.
2. Cuprimine (Penicillamine). Merck & Co., Inc. US Prescribing information, October 2004.
3. Distamine (Penicillamine). Alliance Pharmaceuticals. UK Summary of product characteristics, October 2005.
4. Rose BI, LeMaire WJ, Jeffers LJ. Macromastia in a woman treated with penicillamine and oral contraceptives. *J Reprod Med* (1990) 35, 43–5.

Phenylpropanolamine + Indinavir

A report describes a hypertensive crisis when a patient taking indinavir was also given phenylpropanolamine.

Clinical evidence, mechanism, importance and management

A 28-year-old woman was prescribed HIV-prophylaxis following a needle stick injury. She was initially given zidovudine, indinavir and lamivudine, but after one week stavudine was substituted for zidovudine as she was experiencing nausea and vomiting. Six hours after taking *Tavist-D* (clemastine with phenylpropanolamine) for a sinus complaint she had a feeling of chest tightness associated with difficulty in breathing, and shortly afterwards she experienced left-sided upper extremity weakness, followed by a severe right-sided temporal headache. Her blood pressure was 220/120 mmHg, but returned to normal within 4 hours, and the neurological deficit resolved over the next 8 hours. However, 12 hours later, the same neurological deficit recurred, although no increase in blood pressure was noted. The neurological deficit was thought to be due to reversible cerebral vasoconstriction, secondary to phenylpropanolamine toxicity. She was treated with nimodipine 60 mg every 4 hours and aspirin 325 mg daily, and her symptoms did not recur.[1]

The patient had been taking phenylpropanolamine intermittently for several years without any adverse reaction and it was thought that the recent addition of the anti-HIV regimen potentiated the effect of the phenylpropanolamine.[1] It seems likely that the indinavir was responsible for the interaction as it is a potent enzyme inhibitor. This is an isolated report and its general significance is not known, but it would be prudent to be alert for this interaction in patients given both drugs.

1. Khurana V, de la Fuente M, Bradley TP. Hypertensive crisis secondary to phenylpropanolamine interacting with triple-drug therapy for HIV prophylaxis. *Am J Med* (1999) 106, 118–19.

Phenylpropanolamine + Indometacin

An isolated report describes a patient taking phenylpropanolamine who developed serious hypertension after taking a single dose of indometacin, but a controlled study in other subjects failed to find any evidence of an adverse interaction.

Clinical evidence

A woman who had been taking phenylpropanolamine 85 mg daily for several months as an appetite suppressant, developed a severe bifrontal headache within 15 minutes of taking indometacin 25 mg. Thirty minutes later her systolic blood pressure was 210 mmHg and her diastolic blood pressure was unrecordable. A later study in this patient confirmed that neither drug on its own caused this response, but when they were taken together the blood pressure rose to a maximum of 200/150 mmHg within about 30 minutes of taking the indometacin, and was associated with bradycardia. The blood pressure was rapidly reduced by phentolamine.[1]

In contrast, a controlled study in 14 healthy young women found no evidence that sustained-release indometacin 75 mg twice daily given with sustained-release phenylpropanolamine 75 mg daily caused a rise in blood pressure.[2]

Mechanism

Not understood.

Importance and management

Direct information seems to be limited to these reports. They suggest that an adverse hypertensive response is unlikely in most individuals given these drugs. However, note that phenylpropanolamine alone has been associated with severe hypertension and has been implicated in causing stroke.[3] It is therefore no longer available in the US and UK and its use has been restricted in many other countries.

1. Lee KY, Beilin LJ, Vandongen R. Severe hypertension after ingestion of an appetite suppressant (phenylpropanolamine) with indomethacin. *Lancet* (1979) i, 1110–11.
2. McKenney JM, Wright JT, Katz GM, Goodman RP. The effect of phenylpropanolamine on 24-hour blood pressure in normotensive subjects administered indomethacin. *DICP Ann Pharmacother* (1991) 25, 234–9.
3. Brust JCM. Editorial comment: over-the-counter cold remedies and stroke. *Stroke* (2003) 34, 1673.

Phosphodiesterase type-5 inhibitors + Alpha blockers

Postural hypotension may occur with higher doses of sildenafil, tadalafil or vardenafil given at the same time as doxazosin or terazosin. The effect may be less marked with tamsulosin.

Clinical evidence, mechanism, importance and management

(a) Sildenafil

Retrospective analysis of pooled data from various clinical studies including patients taking non-nitrate antihypertensives such as the alpha blockers suggests that the adverse effect profile, blood pressure, or heart rate were not significantly different when they also took sildenafil or placebo.[1] However, the manufacturer notes that when sildenafil 100 mg was given simultaneously with **doxazosin** 4 mg after at least 14 consecutive daily doses of **doxazosin**, severe postural hypotension occurred in one of 4 subjects with benign prostatic hypertrophy, and 2 others had mild dizziness. Two of the subjects had a standing systolic BP of less than 85 mmHg. This did not occur in a further 17 subjects who, as a result of these effects, were given a lower dose of sildenafil 25 mg. In two other studies, 2 of 19 and 3 of 20 patients had a standing systolic BP of less than 85 mmHg after receiving 14 days of **doxazosin** then a single simultaneous dose of sildenafil 50 mg or 100 mg with **doxazosin**.[2]

The manufacturers recommend that patients should be stable on an alpha blocker before sildenafil is started and that consideration should be given to starting sildenafil at the lowest dose (25 mg).[2,3] The UK manufacturer notes that a hypotensive effect is most likely within 4 hours of taking an alpha blocker. When starting an alpha blocker in a patient taking sildenafil, the US manufacturer states that the alpha blocker should be started at the lowest dose.[2]

(b) Tadalafil

A placebo-controlled, randomised, two-period, crossover study in 18 healthy subjects found that a single 20-mg dose of tadalafil increased the blood pressure-reducing effects of **doxazosin** following 7 days of treatment with **doxazosin** 8 mg daily. The mean maximum systolic falls for the combination were 3.6 mmHg when lying and 9.8 mmHg when standing. Some of the subjects felt dizzy, but none of them fainted.[4] Conversely, a small and clinically irrelevant effect was seen when tadalafil 10 or 20 mg was given with **tamsulosin**.[4,5] A further study in which a single 20-mg oral dose of tadalafil or placebo was given to 17 healthy subjects on the seventh day of taking extended-release **alfuzosin** 10 mg daily found that none of the subjects had a decrease in standing systolic BP of more than 30 mmHg. No syncope or severe adverse events were reported. However, note that the doses were separated by 4 hours.[4]

The UK manufacturer of tadalafil says that the concurrent use of alpha blockers and tadalafil is not recommended as it may lead to symptomatic hypotension in some patients.[5] Conversely, the US manufacturer recommends that patients should be stable on their alpha blocker before tadalafil is used, and that tadalafil should be initiated at the lowest recommended dose. When starting an alpha blocker in a patient taking the optimum dose of tadalafil, the alpha blocker should be initiated at the lowest possible dose.[4]

(c) Vardenafil

The manufacturers of vardenafil have conducted several placebo-controlled, randomised, crossover studies, in patients with BPH and in healthy subjects taking alpha blockers, to assess the effects of concurrent vardenafil on blood pressure.

Vardenafil 5 mg was given to 21 patients taking **terazosin** 5 or 10 mg daily. Vardenafil given simultaneously caused significant hypotension in one patient (BP 80/60 mmHg) and 5 patients experienced postural hypotension of greater than 30 mmHg (compared with only 2 patients in the placebo group). When vardenafil was given 6 hours after the alpha blocker no adverse effects were reported.[6] Vardenafil 10 or 20 mg was also given to healthy subjects taking **terazosin** 10 mg daily. Due to significant hypotension in a large number of the subjects the study was halted.[6]

Vardenafil 5 mg was given to 21 patients taking **tamsulosin** 400 micrograms daily. Vardenafil given simultaneously caused significant hypotension in 2 patients (systolic BP less than 85 mmHg) and 2 patients experienced postural hypotension of greater then 30 mmHg (compared with only one patient in the placebo group). When vardenafil was given 6 hours after the alpha blocker significant hypotension still occurred in 2 patients and one experienced postural hypotension of greater than 30 mmHg.[6] Larger doses of vardenafil (10 or 20 mg) given to 23 patients taking **tamsulosin** 400 or 800 micrograms resulted in postural hypotension of greater then 30 mmHg in one patient, and 3 patients became dizzy. When vardenafil was given to 20 healthy subjects with **tamsulosin** 400 micrograms daily 7 subjects became dizzy.[6]

The manufacturer recommends that patients should be stable on their alpha blocker before using vardenafil, and that vardenafil should be initiated at a dose of 5 mg[6,7] (or less in the presence of potent inhibitors of CYP3A4 such as the 'azoles', (p.1270) or the 'protease inhibitors', (p.1273)).[6] The UK manufacturer also says that the doses should be separated if vardenafil is to be given with an alpha blocker (with the exception of **tamsulosin**, where they consider this precaution unnecessary).[7] From the data above, 6 hours would seem adequate. When starting an alpha blocker in a patient taking vardenafil, the US manufacturer states that the alpha blocker should be started at the lowest dose.[6]

1. Zusman RM, Prisant LM, Brown MJ. Effect of sildenafil citrate on blood pressure and heart rate in men with erectile dysfunction taking concomitant antihypertensive medication. *J Hypertens* (2000) 18, 1865–9.
2. Viagra (Sildenafil citrate). Pfizer Inc. US Prescribing information, October 2006.
3. Viagra (Sildenafil citrate). Pfizer Ltd. UK Summary of product characteristics, June 2006.
4. Cialis (Tadalafil). Eli Lilly and Company Ltd. US Prescribing information, January 2007.
5. Cialis (Tadalafil). Eli Lilly and Company Ltd. UK Summary of product characteristics, July 2006.

6. Levitra (Vardenafil hydrochloride). Bayer pharmaceuticals Corporation. US prescribing information, March 2007.
7. Levitra (Vardenafil hydrochloride trihydrate). Bayer plc. UK Summary of product characteristics, November 2006.

Phosphodiesterase type-5 inhibitors + Antacids

No clinically significant interaction appears to occur between sildenafil, tadalafil or vardenafil and aluminium/magnesium hydroxide antacids.

Clinical evidence, mechanism, importance and management

(a) Sildenafil

In a single dose study in 12 healthy subjects the bioavailability of sildenafil was not affected by single 30-mL doses of an **aluminium/magnesium hydroxide** antacid.[1]

(b) Tadalafil

An open-label, randomised, crossover study in 12 healthy subjects found that 20 mL of *Maalox* (**aluminium/magnesium hydroxide**) reduced the mean maximum serum level of a single 10-mg dose of tadalafil by 30%. Although peak tadalafil levels were delayed by 2.5 hours, the total amount of tadalafil absorbed was unchanged. None of the changes caused were considered to be clinically relevant, and there would appear to be no reason for avoiding concurrent use.[2]

(c) Vardenafil

In a two-way crossover study a single 20-mg dose of vardenafil was given to 12 healthy subjects with 10 mL of an **aluminium/magnesium hydroxide** antacid (*Maalox 70*). The bioavailability of vardenafil was not significantly altered by the antacid, therefore no additional precautions are needed if these drugs are used together.[3]

1. Wilner K, Laboy L, LeBel M. The effects of cimetidine and antacid on the pharmacokinetic profile of sildenafil citrate in healthy male volunteers. *Br J Clin Pharmacol* (2002) 53, 31S–36S.
2. Eli Lilly and Company. Personal communication, March 2003.
3. Rohde G, Wensing G, Sachse R. The pharmacokinetics of vardenafil, a new selective PDE5 inhibitor, are not affected by the antacid, Maalox 70. *Pharmacotherapy* (2001) 21, 1254.

Phosphodiesterase type-5 inhibitors + Antihypertensives

No clinically relevant interactions appear to occur between sildenafil, tadalafil or vardenafil and most antihypertensive drugs. The exceptions may be diltiazem and verapamil. The potentially serious interactions of sildenafil, tadalafil and vardenafil with the alpha blockers and nitrates are discussed elsewhere. See 'Phosphodiesterase type-5 inhibitors + Alpha blockers', p.1268 and 'Phosphodiesterase type-5 inhibitors + Nitrates', p.1272.

Clinical evidence, mechanism, importance and management

(a) Sildenafil

In a study in 8 hypertensive men taking one to five antihypertensives (**amlodipine** (5 patients), a **diuretic** (4), an **ACE inhibitor** (3), an **angiotensin II receptor antagonist** (2), **diltiazem** (1)), a single 50-mg dose of sildenafil reduced the systolic BP by a mean maximum of 24 mmHg, compared with only 6 mmHg for placebo. One patient had a blood pressure fall of 48/23 mmHg, but none complained of hypotensive symptoms.[1] Two retrospective analyses of pooled data from various clinical trials suggests that patients on non-nitrate antihypertensives (**ACE inhibitors**, alpha blockers, **beta blockers**, **calcium-channel blockers**, **diuretics**) and sildenafil showed no significant difference blood pressure, or heart rate compared with those taking antihypertensives and placebo,[2] and that the incidence of dizziness did not differ between sildenafil recipients on antihypertensives and those not.[2,3] In a placebo-controlled study in patients with hypertension receiving stable therapy with 2 or more antihypertensives (including **diuretics**, **calcium-channel blockers**, **ACE inhibitors**, **beta blockers**, alpha blockers, **angiotensin II receptor antagonists**), the occurrence of adverse events potentially related to hypotensive effects (dizziness, hypotension, labile BP, vertigo) was less than 4% in sildenafil recipients.[4] Note that combined use with alpha blockers may be especially likely to induce hypotensive events, see 'Phosphodiesterase type-5 inhibitors + Alpha blockers', p.1268.

The manufacturers report that in population pharmacokinetic analysis, there was no effect on sildenafil pharmacokinetics in those taking **ACE inhibitors**, **calcium-channel blockers** and **thiazide** and **related diuretics**[5,6] whereas the AUC of the less potent active metabolite of sildenafil is increased by 62% by **loop** and **potassium-sparing diuretics** and by 102% by **non-selective beta blockers**, although these changes were not considered clinically relevant.[6]

When sildenafil 100 mg was given to hypertensive patients taking **amlodipine** the mean additional fall in blood pressure (8/7 mmHg) was of the same magnitude as that seen when sildenafil was given alone to healthy subjects.[5,6]

It should be noted that some calcium-channel blockers (e.g. **diltiazem**, **verapamil**) are known to inhibit the cytochrome P450 isoenzyme CYP3A4, by which sildenafil is metabolised, and so these calcium-channel blockers have the potential to raise sildenafil levels. Although the manufacturers do not specifically mention these drugs, they do recommend a lower starting dose of sildenafil in patients taking potent inhibitors of CYP3A4,[5,6] and this would seem a sensible precaution in patients taking **diltiazem** or **verapamil** (usually considered to be moderate CYP3A4 inhibitors). There is a case of a patient taking **diltiazem** 30 mg three times daily who underwent coronary angiography 48 hours after taking sildenafil 50 mg, and who developed profound and persistent hypotension (BP 90/60 mmHg) after receiving sublingual nitrate for pain related to angina during the procedure.[7] It was suggested that **diltiazem** may have inhibited the metabolism of sildenafil so that it interacted with the nitrate,[7,8] although the time scale for this interaction has been disputed.[9]

The manufacturer notes that in population pharmacokinetic analysis of patients with pulmonary hypertension, there appeared to be an increase in sildenafil exposure when it was taken with beta blockers (none named) in combination with CYP3A4 substrates (none named).[10,11] The clinical relevance of this is uncertain, and further study is needed.

(b) Tadalafil

Placebo-controlled studies in patients taking **enalapril**, **metoprolol** or **bendroflumethiazide**, found that a 10-mg dose of tadalafil did not affect blood pressure or heart rate.[12] Similar results were seen in a study in patients taking **amlodipine** and given tadalafil 20 mg.[12] In another study in patients taking unnamed **angiotensin II receptor antagonists** (alone or in combination with thiazides, **calcium-channel blockers** or **beta blockers**[13]), tadalafil 20 mg lowered the mean BP by 8/4 mmHg more than placebo, and about twice as many patients had a potentially clinically relevant decrease in blood pressure, although no potential hypotensive symptoms (e.g. dizziness) occurred.[12] In phase III studies, there was no difference in blood pressure changes in patients taking antihypertensives (**ACE inhibitors**, **calcium-channel blockers**, **thiazide diuretics**, **beta blockers**, **angiotensin II receptor antagonists**, alpha blockers and **loop diuretics**) between those given tadalafil and those given placebo, and there was no difference in the number of patients with a potentially clinically relevant reduction in systolic BP (greater than 30 mmHg). Similarly, in patients taking tadalafil, there was a similar incidence of dizziness between those taking antihypertensives and those not.[12] The manufacturers say that tadalafil 20 mg may induce a small fall in blood pressure in patients taking antihypertensives, but this is unlikely to be clinically relevant, with the exception of 'alpha blockers', (p.1268). Nevertheless, they still advise caution on concurrent use as some patients with underlying cardiovascular disease may possibly be affected.[13,14]

There would therefore appear to be no reason for avoiding the concurrent use of any of these drugs nor (the implication is) with other drugs that fall into these drug classes. However, it should be noted that some **calcium-channel blockers** (e.g. **diltiazem**, **verapamil**) are known to have a moderate inhibitory effect on the cytochrome P450 isoenzyme CYP3A4, an enzyme involved in the metabolism of tadalafil, and so may have the potential to raise tadalafil levels.[13] Although the manufacturers do not specifically mention these **calcium-channel blockers**, they do recommend caution[13] or a lower dose of tadalafil[14] in patients taking *potent* inhibitors of CYP3A4. Some caution is therefore appropriate.

(c) Vardenafil

In a randomised, double-blind, crossover study, 22 patients with hypertension, stabilised on slow-release **nifedipine** 30 or 60 mg daily were given a single 20-mg dose of vardenafil, or placebo. Vardenafil slightly decreased the maximum plasma levels and relative bioavailability of **nifedipine**, as well as causing a further decrease in supine blood pressure of about 6/5 mmHg. Heart rate was increased by 4 bpm.[15] **Nifedipine** did not alter vardenafil levels.[16]

Vardenafil alone may decrease blood pressure, and the US manufacturer cautions that vardenafil may add to the blood pressure lowering effects of antihypertensive drugs.[16]

The UK manufacturers say that, although not specifically studied, population pharmacokinetic analysis has suggested that **ACE inhibitors, beta blockers**, and **diuretics** have no effect on vardenafil pharmacokinetics.[17]

1. Mahmud A, Hennessy M, Feely J. Effect of sildenafil on blood pressure and arterial wave reflection in treated hypertensive men. *J Hum Hypertens* (2001) 15, 707–13.
2. Zusman RM, Prisant LM, Brown MJ. Effect of sildenafil citrate on blood pressure and heart rate in men with erectile dysfunction taking concomitant antihypertensive medication. *J Hypertens* (2000) 18, 1865–9.
3. Kloner RA, Brown M, Prisant LM, Collins M, for the Sildenafil Study Group. Effect of sildenafil in patients with erectile dysfunction taking antihypertensive therapy. *Am J Hypertens* (2001) 14, 70–3.
4. Pickering TG, Shepherd AMM, Puddey I, Glasser DB, Orazem J, Sherman N, Mancia G. Sildenafil citrate for erectile dysfunction in men receiving multiple antihypertensive agents: a randomized controlled trial. *Am J Hypertens* (2004) 17, 1135–42.
5. Viagra (Sildenafil citrate). Pfizer Ltd. UK Summary of product characteristics, June 2006.
6. Viagra (Sildenafil citrate). Pfizer Inc. US Prescribing information, October 2006.
7. Khoury V, Kritharides L. Diltiazem-mediated inhibition of sildenafil metabolism may promote nitrate-induced hypotension. *Aust N Z J Med* (2000) 30, 641–2.
8. Kiritharides L. Diltiazem-mediated inhibition of sildenafil metabolism may promote nitrate-induced hypotension. Reply. *Intern Med J* (2001) 31, 374–5.
9. Howes L. Diltiazem-mediated inhibition of sildenafil metabolism may promote nitrate-induced hypotension. *Intern Med J* (2001) 31, 373.
10. Revatio (Sildenafil citrate). Pfizer Ltd. UK Summary of product characteristics, March 2007.
11. Revatio (Sildenafil citrate). Pfizer Inc. US Prescribing information, July 2006.
12. Kloner RA, Mitchell M, Emmick JT. Cardiovascular effects of tadalafil in patients on common antihypertensive therapies. *Am J Cardiol* (2003) 92 (Suppl), 47M–57M.
13. Cialis (Tadalafil). Eli Lilly and Company Ltd. UK Summary of product characteristics, July 2006.
14. Cialis (Tadalafil). Eli Lilly and Company Ltd. US Prescribing information, January 2007.
15. Rohde G, Jordaan PJ. Influence of vardenafil on blood pressure and pharmacokinetics in hypertensive patients on nifedipine therapy. 31th Annual Meeting of the American College of Clinical Pharmacology, San Francisco, California, 2002.
16. Levitra (Vardenafil hydrochloride). Bayer Pharmaceuticals Corporation. US Prescribing information, March 2007.
17. Levitra (Vardenafil hydrochloride trihydrate). Bayer plc. UK Summary of product characteristics, November 2006.

Phosphodiesterase type-5 inhibitors + Aspirin

Sildenafil, tadalafil and vardenafil do not potentiate the increased bleeding time seen with aspirin.

Clinical evidence, mechanism, importance and management

(a) Sildenafil

In a pharmacological study, sildenafil 50 mg did not potentiate the increase in bleeding time seen with aspirin 150 mg.[1] No additional precautions therefore seem necessary on concurrent use.

(b) Tadalafil

A randomised, double-blind, parallel-group study in a total of 28 subjects found that a single 10-mg dose of tadalafil did not increase the bleeding time after aspirin 300 mg daily was taken for 5 days.[2] There would seem to be no reason for taking special precautions if both drugs are used.

(c) Vardenafil

The manufacturers say that population pharmacokinetic analysis suggests that aspirin had no effect on vardenafil pharmacokinetics.[3] In addition, vardenafil 10 mg and 20 mg did not potentiate the bleeding time caused by aspirin 162 mg.[3,4] No additional precautions therefore seem necessary on concurrent use.

1. Viagra (Sildenafil citrate). Pfizer Inc. US Prescribing information, October 2006.
2. Eli Lilly and Company. Personal communication, March 2003.
3. Levitra (Vardenafil hydrochloride trihydrate). Bayer plc. UK Summary of product characteristics, November 2006.
4. Levitra (Vardenafil hydrochloride). Bayer Pharmaceuticals Corporation. US Prescribing information, March 2007.

Phosphodiesterase type-5 inhibitors + Azoles

Ketoconazole and itraconazole markedly raise the levels of sildenafil, tadalafil and vardenafil.

Clinical evidence

(a) Sildenafil

'Erythromycin', (p.1272), increases sildenafil levels threefold. The manufacturers therefore predict that other more potent CYP3A4 inhibitors such as **itraconazole** and **ketoconazole** will have even greater effects.[1,2] They say that population data from clinical studies suggests that CYP3A4 inhibitors such as **ketoconazole** reduced sildenafil clearance without increasing the incidence of adverse effects.[1,2] In a study in *dogs*, the concurrent use of **itraconazole** enhanced and prolonged the adverse effects of sildenafil.[3] However, a case report describes the apparently uneventful concurrent use of sildenafil 100 mg with **itraconazole** 400 mg daily for 7 days each month in a 56-year-old man.[4]

(b) Tadalafil

In an open label, randomised study in 12 healthy subjects, **ketoconazole** 200 mg daily increased the AUC of a single 10-mg dose of tadalafil by twofold,[5,6] and **ketoconazole** 400 mg daily increased the AUC fourfold.[5,6] The manufacturers predict that **itraconazole** will interact similarly.[5,6] This prediction has been borne out by a case report of a 56-year-old man who was taking **itraconazole** 400 mg daily for 7 days each month. Within a few hours of his first 10-mg dose of tadalafil he developed priapism, which lasted for more than 4 hours. The same reaction occurred when he took tadalafil during the following month. He had seemingly previously taken sildenafil with **itraconazole** without adverse effect.[4]

(c) Vardenafil

Ketoconazole 200 mg daily increased the AUC of a 5-mg dose of vardenafil tenfold, and increased the maximum plasma levels fourfold. Although not specifically studied, **itraconazole** is expected to cause similar rises in vardenafil levels.[7,8]

Mechanism

Sildenafil, tadalafil and vardenafil are all metabolised by the cytochrome P450 isoenzyme CYP3A4. Ketoconazole and itraconazole are potent inhibitors of CYP3A4, and therefore inhibit sildenafil, tadalafil and vardenafil metabolism, which leads to an increase in their levels.

Importance and management

Information about the interaction between phosphodiesterase type-5 inhibitors and azoles is sparse, but what is known is in line with the predicted effects.

For **sildenafil**, when used for erectile dysfunction, the manufacturers recommend that a low starting dose of sildenafil (25 mg) should be considered if ketoconazole or itraconazole are used concurrently.[1,2] When used for pulmonary hypertension, the manufacturers say that concurrent use of sildenafil with ketoconazole and itraconazole is contraindicated in the UK,[9] or not recommended in the US.[10]

For **tadalafil**, the UK manufacturer advises caution[5] and the US manufacturer advises that the dose of tadalafil should not exceed 10 mg in a 72-hour period for patients taking potent CYP3A4 inhibitors such as ketoconazole.[6] However, note that this dose has caused priapism in one patient taking itraconazole.

Vardenafil levels are greatly increased by ketoconazole and probably itraconazole so the UK manufacturer advises avoiding concurrent use in all patients. The use of ketoconazole or itraconazole in patients over 75 years is specifically contraindicated with vardenafil.[7] In contrast, the US prescribing information recommends that the dose of vardenafil should not exceed 5 mg in 24 hours when used with ketoconazole or itraconazole 200 mg daily, or 2.5-mg in 24 hours with ketoconazole or itraconazole 400 mg daily.[8]

1. Viagra (Sildenafil citrate). Pfizer Ltd. UK Summary of product characteristics, June 2006.
2. Viagra (Sildenafil citrate). Pfizer Inc. US Prescribing information, October 2006.
3. Kim EJ, Seo JW, Hwang JY, Han SS. Effects of combined treatment with sildenafil and itraconazole on the cardiovascular system in telemetered conscious dogs. *Drug Chem Toxicol* (2005) 28, 177–86.
4. Galatti L, Fioravanti A, Salvo F, Polimeni G, Giustini SE. Interaction between tadalafil and itraconazole. *Ann Pharmacother* (2005) 39, 200.
5. Cialis (Tadalafil). Eli Lilly and Company Ltd. UK Summary of product characteristics, July 2006.
6. Cialis (Tadalafil). Eli Lilly and Company Ltd. US Prescribing information, January 2007.
7. Levitra (Vardenafil hydrochloride trihydrate). Bayer plc. UK Summary of product characteristics, November 2006.
8. Levitra (Vardenafil hydrochloride). Bayer Pharmaceuticals Corporation. US prescribing information, March 2007.

9. Revatio (Sildenafil citrate). Pfizer Ltd. UK Summary of product characteristics, March 2007.
10. Revatio (Sildenafil citrate). Pfizer Inc. US Prescribing information, July 2006.

Phosphodiesterase type-5 inhibitors + CYP3A4 inducers

Rifampicin markedly reduced tadalafil levels, and is predicted to interact similarly with sildenafil and vardenafil. Other CYP3A4 inducers are likely to have the same effect with these phosphodiesterase type-5 inhibitors.

Clinical evidence

(a) Sildenafil

On the basis of the 63% reduction in AUC seen with the moderate CYP3A4 inducer 'bosentan', (p.1274), the US manufacturer of sildenafil says that concurrent use with potent inducers of CYP3A4 such as **rifampicin** is predicted to cause a greater reduction in sildenafil levels.[1,2]

(b) Tadalafil

A study[3,4] in 12 healthy subjects found that **rifampicin** 600 mg daily given for 13 days decreased the AUC of a single 10-mg dose of tadalafil by 88%.

Mechanism

Rifampicin induces the activity of the cytochrome P450 isoenzyme CYP3A4, the principal enzyme concerned with the metabolism of sildenafil, tadalafil and vardenafil.

Importance and management

The pharmacokinetic interaction between rifampicin and tadalafil is established, and will almost certainly occur with sildenafil. It is unlikely that standard doses of these phosphodiesterase type-5 inhibitors would be as effective as usual in patients taking rifampicin. Other CYP3A4 inducers such as **barbiturates**,[2] **carbamazepine**,[2-5] **efavirenz**,[2] **nevirapine**,[2] **phenobarbital**,[3-5] **phenytoin**,[2-5] **rifabutin**,[2] and **St John's wort**[5] are predicted by the manufacturers to do the same (for a list of CYP3A4 inducers see 'Table 1.4', (p.6)). Despite the marked interaction, the US manufacturer of tadalafil states that no dosage adjustment is warranted.[4] Conversely, the manufacturers of sildenafil state that efficacy should be closely monitored in patients taking CYP3A4 inducers,[5] or that dose adjustment may be necessary.[2] If these phosphodiesterase type-5 inhibitors are not effective in a patients taking a CYP3A4 inducer, it would seem sensible to try a higher dose with close monitoring.

Although the manufacturer of **vardenafil** does not mention CYP3A4 inducers,[6,7] like tadalafil and sildenafil, vardenafil is principally metabolised by CYP3A4, and its levels are markedly raised by CYP3A4 inhibitors such as 'ketoconazole', (p.1270). It is therefore very likely that vardenafil levels will be reduced by rifampicin and similar drugs, and concurrent use should be monitored.

1. Viagra (Sildenafil citrate). Pfizer Inc. US Prescribing information, October 2006.
2. Revatio (Sildenafil citrate). Pfizer Inc. US Prescribing information, July 2006.
3. Cialis (Tadalafil). Eli Lilly and Company Ltd. UK Summary of product characteristics, July 2006.
4. Cialis (Tadalafil). Eli Lilly and Company Ltd. US Prescribing information, January 2007.
5. Revatio (Sildenafil citrate). Pfizer Ltd. UK Summary of product characteristics, March 2007.
6. Levitra (Vardenafil hydrochloride trihydrate). Bayer plc. UK Summary of product characteristics, November 2006.
7. Levitra (Vardenafil hydrochloride). Bayer Pharmaceuticals Corporation. US prescribing information, March 2007.

Phosphodiesterase type-5 inhibitors + Grapefruit juice

Grapefruit juice modestly increases the absorption of sildenafil. Tadalafil and vardenafil are predicted to interact similarly.

Clinical evidence, mechanism, importance and management

Grapefruit juice 250 mL was given to 24 healthy subjects both one hour before and with a 50-mg dose of **sildenafil**. The AUC of **sildenafil** was increased by 23% by grapefruit juice, but the maximum plasma level was not significantly changed. Inter-individual variation in **sildenafil** pharmacokinetics was also increased by grapefruit juice. The authors suggest that although the slight rise in AUC is unlikely to be clinically significant, the combination is best avoided due to the increased variability in **sildenafil** pharmacokinetics.[1] However, this seems overcautious, since the manufacture permits reduced doses of **sildenafil** with much more potent inhibitors of CYP3A4, such as 'itraconazole', (p.1270).

The manufacturers of **tadalafil** predict that grapefruit juice will increase its levels[2,3] and the UK manufacturer advises caution with concurrent use.[2]

The manufacturers of **vardenafil** also predict that grapefruit juice will increase its levels[4,5] and recommend avoiding this combination.[4]

1. Jetter A, Kinzig-Schippers M, Walchner-Bonjean M, Hering U, Bulitta J, Schreiner P, Sörgel F, Fuhr U. Effects of grapefruit juice on the pharmacokinetics of sildenafil. *Clin Pharmacol Ther* (2002) 71, 21–9.
2. Cialis (Tadalafil). Eli Lilly and Company Ltd. UK Summary of product characteristics, July 2006.
3. Cialis (Tadalafil). Eli Lilly and Company Ltd. US Prescribing information, January 2007.
4. Levitra (Vardenafil hydrochloride trihydrate). Bayer plc. UK Summary of product characteristics, November 2006.
5. Levitra (Vardenafil hydrochloride). Bayer Pharmaceuticals Corporation. US prescribing information, March 2007.

Phosphodiesterase type-5 inhibitors + H_2-receptor antagonists

Sildenafil levels are modestly raised by cimetidine. No interaction appears to occur when nizatidine is given with tadalafil and when cimetidine or ranitidine is given with vardenafil.

Clinical evidence, mechanism, importance and management

(a) Sildenafil

In a study in 10 healthy subjects, **cimetidine** 800 mg daily for 4 days increased the AUC of a single 50-mg dose of sildenafil given on day 3 by 56%, when compared with 10 healthy subjects given sildenafil and placebo.[1] It has been suggested that these changes occur because **cimetidine** is a non-specific cytochrome P450 inhibitor.[2] The manufacturers say that population pharmacokinetic analysis revealed a reduced clearance of sildenafil in patients taking CYP3A4 inhibitors, such as ketoconazole, erythromycin and **cimetidine**.[2,3] The UK manufacturers say that, although no increase in adverse effects was seen, a starting dose of 25 mg of sildenafil should be considered.[3] For **cimetidine**, studies suggest the increase is modest, compared to 'erythromycin', (p.1272), and this therefore seems overcautious. Furthermore, no recommendation is made about the sildenafil dose with **cimetidine** by the US manufacturer.[2]

(b) Tadalafil

An open-label, randomised, three-period, crossover study in 12 healthy subjects found that **nizatidine** 300 mg reduced the mean maximum serum levels of tadalafil by 14% following a single 10-mg dose, but other pharmacokinetic parameters, including the extent of absorption, were largely unchanged. None of the changes caused were considered to be clinically relevant and there would appear to be no reason for avoiding concurrent use.[4]

Any alterations in the absorption of tadalafil are therefore unlikely to be caused by changes in gastric pH.[4]

(c) Vardenafil

In a three-way crossover study, a single 20-mg dose of vardenafil was given to 10 healthy subjects following a 3-day course of **cimetidine** 400 mg twice daily, **ranitidine** 150 mg twice daily or with no pre-treatment. **Cimetidine** slightly increased the relative bioavailability of vardenafil (by about 12%, not considered clinically relevant), while **ranitidine** had no effect. It was concluded that any alterations in the absorption of vardenafil are not caused by changes in gastric pH.[5] No special precautions appear to be necessary during concurrent use.

1. Wilner K, Laboy L, LeBel M. The effects of cimetidine and antacid on the pharmacokinetic profile of sildenafil citrate in healthy male volunteers. *Br J Clin Pharmacol* (2002) 53, 31S–36S.
2. Viagra (Sildenafil citrate). Pfizer Inc. US Prescribing information, October 2006.
3. Viagra (Sildenafil citrate). Pfizer Ltd. UK Summary of product characteristics, June 2006.

4. Eli Lilly and Company. Personal communication, March 2003.
5. Rohde G, Wensing G, Unger S, Sachse R. The pharmacokinetics of vardenafil, a new selective PDE5 inhibitor, is minimally affected by coadministration with cimetidine or ranitidine. *Pharmacotherapy* (2001) 21, 1254.

Phosphodiesterase type-5 inhibitors + Macrolides

Erythromycin raises sildenafil levels almost threefold and raises vardenafil levels fourfold. Clarithromycin raises sildenafil levels about twofold. Erythromycin is predicted to similarly raise tadalafil levels. Azithromycin does not interact with sildenafil.

Clinical evidence

(a) Sildenafil

In a study in 24 healthy subjects, **erythromycin** 500 mg twice daily for 5 days was found to increase the AUC of single 100-mg doses of sildenafil almost threefold.[1] In the same study, **azithromycin** 500 mg once daily for 3 days had no effect on the pharmacokinetics of sildenafil.[1] In another study, in 12 healthy subjects, **clarithromycin** 500 mg increased the AUC of sildenafil 50 mg 2.3-fold, and the maximum level 2.4-fold.[2]

(b) Tadalafil

'Ketoconazole', (p.1270), doubles tadalafil levels. The manufacturers therefore predict that other CYP3A4 inhibitors such as **erythromycin**[3,4] will interact similarly.

(c) Vardenafil

Erythromycin 500 mg three times daily increased the AUC of a 5-mg dose of vardenafil fourfold, and increased the maximum plasma levels threefold in healthy subjects.[5,6]

Mechanism

Sildenafil, tadalafil and vardenafil are all metabolised by the cytochrome P450 isoenzyme CYP3A4. Many macrolides are moderate inhibitors of this isoenzyme and therefore inhibit sildenafil, tadalafil and vardenafil metabolism, which leads to increased levels of the phosphodiesterase inhibitors. Azithromycin does not usually act as a CYP3A4 inhibitor and therefore does not interact.

Importance and management

The interaction of the macrolides with the phosphodiesterase type-5 inhibitors is established, although most of the studies concern the use of erythromycin. These interactions are expected to result in both increased efficacy and increased incidence of adverse effects.

For **sildenafil**, the manufacturers recommend that a low starting dose of sildenafil 25 mg should be considered in patients with erectile dysfunction taking inhibitors of CYP3A4 such as erythromycin.[7,8] For pulmonary hypertension, the UK manufacturer says that a downward reduction of the sildenafil dose to 20 mg twice daily should be considered with erythromycin, and 20 mg once daily with clarithromycin or **telithromycin**,[9] (however, note that erythromycin had a greater effect than clarithromycin in the studies above) whereas the US manufacturer says that no dose adjustment is needed with erythromycin.[10]

For **tadalafil**, caution is advised by the UK manufacturers as adverse effects may be increased in some patients. They specifically mention erythromycin and clarithromycin.[3]

For **vardenafil,** the UK manufacturer says that dosage adjustment might be necessary in patients taking erythromycin, and recommend that the dose of vardenafil should not exceed 5 mg.[5] The US prescribing information similarly recommends that the dose of vardenafil should not exceed 5 mg in 24 hours for erythromycin, but further restricts the dose in the presence of clarithromycin to 2.5 mg in 24 hours.[6]

Dosing guidance is not given for the other macrolides, but it would seem prudent to follow the advice given for erythromycin in patients taking any macrolide known to inhibit CYP3A4 (e.g. clarithromycin, **telithromycin**). Azithromycin seems unlikely to interact.

1. Muirhead GJ, Faulkner S, Harness JA, Taubel J. The effects of steady-state erythromycin and azithromycin on the pharmacokinetics of sildenafil citrate in healthy volunteers. *Br J Clin Pharmacol* (2002) 53, 37S–43S.
2. Hedaya MA, El-Afify DR, El-Maghraby GM. The effect of ciprofloxacin and clarithromycin on sildenafil oral bioavailability in human volunteers. *Biopharm Drug Dispos* (2006) 27, 103–10.
3. Cialis (Tadalafil). Eli Lilly and Company Ltd. UK Summary of product characteristics, July 2006.
4. Cialis (Tadalafil). Eli Lilly and Company Ltd. US Prescribing information, January 2007.
5. Levitra (Vardenafil hydrochloride trihydrate). Bayer plc. UK Summary of product characteristics, November 2006.
6. Levitra (Vardenafil hydrochloride). Bayer pharmaceuticals Corporation. US prescribing information, March 2007.
7. Viagra (Sildenafil citrate). Pfizer Ltd. UK Summary of product characteristics, June 2006.
8. Viagra (Sildenafil citrate). Pfizer Inc. US Prescribing information, October 2006.
9. Revatio (Sildenafil citrate). Pfizer Ltd. UK Summary of product characteristics, March 2007.
10. Revatio (Sildenafil citrate). Pfizer Inc. US Prescribing information, July 2006.

Phosphodiesterase type-5 inhibitors + Nitrates

The phosphodiesterase type-5 inhibitors potentiate the hypotensive effects of nitrates in a proportion of patients, which might result in potentially serious hypotension or even precipitate myocardial infarction. Therefore, the concurrent use of sildenafil, tadalafil or vardenafil with organic nitrates (glyceryl trinitrate (nitroglycerin), isosorbide dinitrate, isosorbide mononitrate, etc.) is contraindicated. The concurrent use of nicorandil and all phosphodiesterase type-5 inhibitors is also contraindicated.

Clinical evidence

(a) Sildenafil

1. Erectile dysfunction. Two double-blind, placebo-controlled studies in groups of 15 or 16 men with angina found that the fall in blood pressure seen when taking nitrates and a single 50-mg dose of sildenafil was about doubled. Those given sildenafil and **isosorbide dinitrate** 20 mg twice daily had a mean blood pressure fall of 44/26 mmHg compared with 22/13 mmHg with placebo. Those who used 500 micrograms of sublingual **glyceryl trinitrate** one hour before the sildenafil had a mean blood pressure fall of 36/21 mmHg compared with 26/11 mmHg with **glyceryl trinitrate** and placebo. Individual blood pressure falls as great as 84/52 mmHg were seen.[1]

A postmarketing report from the FDA in the US for the period late March to July 1998 briefly lists 69 fatalities after taking sildenafil. These were mostly in middle-aged and elderly men (average age 64), 12 of whom had also taken **glyceryl trinitrate** (**nitroglycerin**) or a nitrate medication, but it is not clear what part (if any) the nitrates played in the deaths.[2]

In a limited and preliminary study it was reported that no blood pressure alteration was seen when a small dose of **glyceryl trinitrate** (amount not specified) was given as a dermal patch while subjects were taking 50 mg of sildenafil. In addition, the beneficial effects of the **glyceryl trinitrate** on the radial artery pressure waveform were approximately doubled, and persisted for up to 8 hours.[3]

2. Pulmonary hypertension. In a study of the combined use of intravenous sildenafil and **inhaled nitric oxide** in the management of pulmonary hypertension in 15 infants, significant hypotension occurred, which, along with a decrease in oxygenation, was considered sufficiently detrimental for the study to be stopped early.[4] Conversely, beneficial combined use has been described in one adult patient with severe hypoxemia caused by pulmonary hypotension.[5] Note that **nitric oxide** is not to be confused with the anaesthetic **nitrous oxide**, which is not a nitric oxide donor and therefore poses no risk,[6] see Mechanism below.

(b) Tadalafil

In a double-blind, randomised, placebo-controlled study, 51 patients with chronic stable angina were given tadalafil 5 mg, 10 mg or a placebo, followed 2 hours later by a single 400-microgram dose of sublingual **glyceryl trinitrate**. Although tadalafil caused little additional decrease in blood pressure to that seen with **glyceryl trinitrate**, a potentially clinically significant blood pressure reduction (standing systolic BP less than 85 mmHg) was seen in 13 and 11 of the patients when given tadalafil 5 and 10 mg, respectively, compared with one patient in the placebo group.[7,8] In a similar study in 45 patients taking long-term oral **isosorbide mononitrate**, tadalafil 5 or 10 mg had minimal effects on the decrease in blood pressure caused by this nitrate, but again, more patients had a standing systolic BP of less than 85 mmHg when receiving tadalafil 10 mg than placebo (6 versus 0).[7,8] Another similar study in 48 healthy subjects compared the effects of tadalafil 10 mg, sildenafil 50 mg, and placebo, in combination with sublingual **glyceryl trinitrate** 400 micrograms. Again, it was found that the presence of the tadalafil had minimal effects on the mean maximum decreases in blood pressure, but it was noted that 23 patients given tadalafil and 23 given sildenafil had a standing systolic blood pressure of 85 mmHg or less following the use of the nitrate, compared with 12 in the placebo group.[8,9] In a further study, a haemodynamic interaction between tadalafil 20 mg and sublingual **glyceryl trinitrate** was seen when the **glyceryl trinitrate** was given 4, 8 and 24 hours after the tadalafil, and was not seen at 48 hours and beyond. Note that no time points between 24 and 48 hours were examined.[10]

An analysis of the rates of serious cardiovascular adverse events (mortality, myocardial infarction, thrombotic strokes) in clinical studies involving tadalafil indicated that adverse events were no more frequent than in the general population of men with erectile dysfunction.[8]

(c) Vardenafil

A single 400-microgram dose of sublingual **glyceryl trinitrate** (nitroglycerin) given to 18 healthy subjects 1 to 24 hours after a single 10-mg dose of vardenafil was found to be no different to placebo in causing changes in seated heart rate and blood pressure.[11,12] However, a single 20-mg dose of vardenafil did potentiate the blood pressure-lowering effects and increases in heart rate (about an 8 mmHg additional drop in systolic BP compared with placebo) seen with **sublingual nitrates** (400 micrograms) taken 1 and 4 hours after the vardenafil. These effects were not seen when the nitrate was taken 24 hours after the vardenafil dose.[11,13]

Mechanism

Sexual stimulation causes the endothelium of the penis to release nitric oxide (NO), which in turn activates guanylate cyclase to increase the production of cyclic guanosine monophosphate (cGMP). This relaxes the blood vessel musculature of the corpus cavernosum thus allowing it to fill with blood and cause an erection. The erection ends when the guanosine monophosphate is removed by an enzyme (type 5 cGMP phosphodiesterase, or PDE5). Sildenafil, tadalafil and vardenafil inhibit this enzyme thereby increasing and prolonging the effects of the guanosine monophosphate. Because this vasodilation is usually fairly localised (these drugs are highly selective for PDE5) it normally only causes mild to moderate falls in blood pressure (on average about 10 mmHg) with mild headache or flushing. However, if other nitrates (e.g. glyceryl trinitrate) are taken concurrently, high levels of nitric oxide enter the circulation, and this markedly increases systemic vasodilation and hence the hypotensive effect.

Importance and management

The interaction between phosphodiesterase type-5 inhibitors and nitrates is established, clinically important, potentially serious and even possibly fatal. Sildenafil and organic nitrates of any form are contraindicated both for erectile dysfunction[14,15] (within 24 hours of each other[6]) and for pulmonary hypertension[16,17] because of the risk of precipitating serious hypotension, or even myocardial infarction.[18] The ACC/AHA Expert consensus document provides a useful list of many of the organic nitrates available, which include glyceryl trinitrate (nitroglycerin), isosorbide mononitrate, **isosorbide dinitrate** and illicit substances such as **amyl nitrite**.[6]

Similarly, the manufacturers of vardenafil[11,13] and tadalafil[19,20] say that their combination with nitrates (taken either regularly and/or intermittently) is contraindicated. Nitrates should not be given for at least 48 hours after the last dose of tadalafil.[19,20]

It is not yet known whether **nicorandil** interacts with the phosphodiesterase inhibitors to a clinically relevant extent or not,[21] but because part of its vasodilatory actions are mediated by the release of nitric oxide (like conventional nitrates), the manufacturers of **nicorandil** contraindicate its use with all phosphodiesterase inhibitors.[22]

1. Webb DJ, Muirhead G, Wulff M, Sutton A, Levi R, Dinsmore WW. Sildenafil citrate potentiates the hypotensive effects of nitric oxide donor drugs in male patients with stable angina. *J Am Coll Cardiol* (2000) 36, 25–31.
2. FDA (US Food and Drug Administration) postmarketing information sildenafil citrate (Viagra): Postmarketing safety of sildenafil citrate (Viagra). Reports of death in Viagra users received from marketing (late March) through July 1998. August 27th 1998.
3. O'Rourke M, Jiang X-J. Sildenafil/nitrate interaction. *Circulation* (2000) 101, e90.
4. Stocker C, Penny DJ, Brizard CP, Cochrane AD, Soto R, Shekerdemian LS. Intravenous sildenafil and inhaled nitric oxide: a randomised trial in infants after cardiac surgery. *Intensive Care Med* (2003) 29, 1996–2003.
5. Bigatello LM, Hess D, Dennehy KC, Medoff BD, Hurford WE. Sildenafil can increase the response to inhaled nitric oxide. *Anesthesiology* (2000) 92, 1827–9.
6. ACC/AHA Expert consensus document. Use of sildenafil (Viagra) in patients with cardiovascular disease. *J Am Coll Cardiol* (1999) 33, 273–82.
7. Kloner RA, Emmick J, Bedding A, Humen D. Pharmacodynamic interactions between tadalafil and nitrates. *Int J Impot Res* (2002) 14 (Suppl 3) S29.
8. Kloner RA, Mitchell M, Emmick J. Cardiovascular effect of tadalafil. *Am J Cardiol* (2003) 92 (Suppl) 37M–46M.
9. Kloner RA, Mitchell MI, Bedding A, Emmick J. Pharmacodynamic interactions between tadalafil and nitrates compared with sildenafil. *J Urol (Baltimore)* (2002) 167 (Suppl) 176–7.
10. Kloner RA, Hutter AM, Emmick JT, Mitchell MI, Denne J, Jackson G. Time course of the interaction between tadalafil and nitrates. *J Am Coll Cardiol* (2003) 42, 1855–60.
11. Levitra (Vardenafil hydrochloride trihydrate). Bayer plc. UK Summary of product characteristics, November 2006.
12. Mazzu AL, Nicholls AJ, Zinny M. Vardenafil, a new selective PDE-5 inhibitor, interacts minimally with nitroglycerin in healthy middle-aged male subjects. *Int J Impot Res* (2001) 13 (Suppl 5) S64.
13. Levitra (Vardenafil hydrochloride). Bayer Pharmaceuticals Corporation. US prescribing information, March 2007.
14. Viagra (Sildenafil citrate). Pfizer Ltd. UK Summary of product characteristics, June 2006.
15. Viagra (Sildenafil citrate). Pfizer Inc. US Prescribing information, October 2006.
16. Revatio (Sildenafil citrate). Pfizer Ltd. UK Summary of product characteristics, March 2007.
17. Revatio (Sildenafil citrate). Pfizer Inc. US Prescribing information, July 2006.
18. Viagra (Sildenafil). Pfizer Inc. Dear Doctor letter, May 1998.
19. Cialis (Tadalafil). Eli Lilly and Company Ltd. UK Summary of product characteristics, July 2006.
20. Cialis (Tadalafil). Eli Lilly and Company Ltd. US Prescribing information, January 2007.
21. Aventis Pharma, Personnal communication, February 2000.
22. Ikorel (Nicorandil). Sanofi-Aventis. UK Summary of product characteristics, June 2004.

Phosphodiesterase type-5 inhibitors + Protease inhibitors

Indinavir, saquinavir and ritonavir can cause marked rises in serum sildenafil levels. A fatal heart attack occurred in a man taking ritonavir and saquinavir when he also took sildenafil. Similar marked interactions occur between vardenafil and indinavir or ritonavir, and are predicted to occur between vardenafil and the other protease inhibitors. Ritonavir caused less marked increases in tadalafil levels.

Clinical evidence

A. Sildenafil

(a) Indinavir

A study in 6 HIV-positive patients found that sildenafil 25 mg did not significantly alter the plasma levels of indinavir. However, the sildenafil AUC was about 4.4-fold higher than the AUC in historical control patients taking sildenafil (data normalised to a 25 mg dose) without indinavir.[1] A study in 2 HIV-positive patients found that sildenafil 25 mg did not affect the pharmacokinetics of indinavir.[2]

(b) Nelfinavir

A study in 5 HIV-positive patients found that sildenafil 25 mg did not affect the pharmacokinetics of nelfinavir.[2]

(c) Ritonavir

In a randomised, placebo-controlled, double-blind, crossover study, 28 healthy subjects were given sildenafil 100 mg before and after taking ritonavir for 7 days (300, 400 and 500 mg twice daily on days 1, 2 and 3 to 7, respectively). It was found that the sildenafil AUC was increased 11-fold and the maximum serum levels 3.9-fold by ritonavir, but the incidence and severity of the sildenafil adverse effects and the steady-state levels of ritonavir remained unchanged.[3] However, the clinical significance of this interaction is highlighted by a case report of a 47-year-old man, with no cardiovascular risk factors apart from smoking, who had a fatal heart attack when he took sildenafil 25 mg while he was also taking ritonavir and **saquinavir**. One hour after the ninth dose, he had an onset of severe chest pain, and died soon after.[4]

A study in 2 HIV-positive patients found that sildenafil 25 mg did not affect the pharmacokinetics of ritonavir (given with **saquinavir**).[2]

(d) Saquinavir

In a randomised, placebo-controlled, double-blind crossover study, 28 healthy subjects were given sildenafil 100 mg before and after taking saquinavir 1.2 g three times daily for 7 days. It was found that the sildenafil AUC was increased 3.1-fold and the maximum serum levels 2.4-fold, but the incidence and severity of the sildenafil adverse effects and the steady-state levels of saquinavir remained unchanged.[3] Also see (c) above for a case report of a fatal interaction involving sildenafil, **ritonavir** and saquinavir.

A study in 2 HIV-positive patients found that sildenafil 25 mg did not affect the pharmacokinetics of **ritonavir**-boosted saquinavir.[2]

B. Tadalafil

Ritonavir 200 mg twice daily increased the AUC of a single 20-mg dose of tadalafil twofold (124%), without affecting the maximum serum levels.[5,6]

C. Vardenafil

When a single 10-mg dose of vardenafil was given with **indinavir** 800 mg three times daily, the AUC of vardenafil was increased 16-fold, and the maximum plasma level was increased sevenfold.[7,8] Moreover, **ritonavir** 600 mg twice daily produced a 49-fold increase in the AUC of vardenafil, and prolonged the half-life to 26 hours.[8]

Mechanism

Protease inhibitors inhibit the activity of the cytochrome P450 isoenzyme CYP3A4, the enzyme that metabolises sildenafil, tadalafil and vardenafil. This results in an increase in their serum levels. Ritonavir is the most potent CYP3A4 inhibitor, followed by indinavir, nelfinavir, amprenavir, and then saquinavir, see 'Antivirals', (p.772)).

Importance and management

Information about interactions between phosphodiesterase type-5 inhibitors and protease inhibitors appears to be limited to the studies and case cited, but the interactions would seem to be established and of clinical importance.

For **sildenafil**, because of the very marked rises in levels, concurrent use of ritonavir and sildenafil for pulmonary hypertension is not advised,[9] or in the UK, contraindicated.[10] When single doses of sildenafil are used for erectile dysfunction, the UK manufacturer also says concurrent use with ritonavir is not advised.[11] In this situation, if the decision is taken to use sildenafil in a patient taking ritonavir, the dose of sildenafil should not exceed a single 25-mg dose in a 48-hour period,[3,11,12] but note that the fatality described above[4] occurred despite the use of this dose. For other CYP3A4 inhibitors such as saquinavir, the recommendation for erectile dysfunction is that a low starting dose (25 mg) should be considered.[3,11,12] For pulmonary hypertension, the UK manufacturer says that a downward reduction of the sildenafil dose to 20 mg twice daily should be considered with saquinavir,[10] whereas the US manufacturer says that no dose adjustment is needed with saquinavir.[9] The authors of the indinavir study suggest that a starting dose of 12.5 mg may be more appropriate for erectile dysfunction in those taking indinavir, and that the maximum dosage frequency should be reduced to once or twice weekly.[1] Direct evidence for other protease inhibitors is lacking but they would be expected to interact similarly (see Mechanism above) and it would seem consistent to follow the broad principle of starting with a low sildenafil dosage.

For **tadalafil**, the US manufacturer advises that the dose should not exceed 10 mg every 72 hours in patients taking ritonavir,[5] whereas the UK manufacturer advises caution on concurrent use.[6] It is probably prudent to apply this advice to patients taking any protease inhibitor.

For **vardenafil**, due to the very large rises in levels, the UK manufacturer contraindicates its use with protease inhibitors that are potent CYP3A4 inhibitors (they name ritonavir and indinavir).[7] In contrast, the US prescribing information recommends dose restrictions as follows: the dose of vardenafil should not exceed 2.5 mg in 24 hours when used with atazanavir, indinavir, or saquinavir, and should not exceed 2.5 mg in 72 hours when used with ritonavir.[8]

1. Merry C, Barry MG, Ryan M, Tjia JF, Hennessy M, Eagling V, Mulcahy F, Back DJ. Interaction of sildenafil and indinavir when co-administered to HIV positive patients. AIDS (Hagerstown) 1999, 13, F101–F107.
2. Bratt G, Ståhle L. Sildenafil does not alter nelfinavir pharmacokinetics. *Ther Drug Monit* (2003) 25, 240–42.
3. Muirhead GJ, Wulff MB, Fielding A, Kleinermans D, Buss N. Pharmacokinetic interactions between sildenafil and saquinavir/ritonavir. *Br J Clin Pharmacol* (2000) 50, 99–107.
4. Hall MCS, Ahmad S. Interaction between sildenafil and HIV-1 combination therapy. *Lancet* (1999) 353, 2071–2.
5. Cialis (Tadalafil). Eli Lilly and Company Ltd. US Prescribing information, January 2007.
6. Cialis (Tadalafil). Eli Lilly and Company Ltd. UK Summary of product characteristics, July 2006.
7. Levitra (Vardenafil hydrochloride trihydrate). Bayer plc. UK Summary of product characteristics, November 2006.
8. Levitra (Vardenafil hydrochloride). Bayer Pharmaceuticals Corporation. US prescribing information, March 2007.
9. Revatio (Sildenafil citrate). Pfizer Inc. US Prescribing information, July 2006.
10. Revatio (Sildenafil citrate). Pfizer Ltd. UK Summary of product characteristics, March 2007.
11. Viagra (Sildenafil citrate). Pfizer Ltd. UK Summary of product characteristics, June 2006.
12. Viagra (Sildenafil citrate). Pfizer Inc. US Prescribing information, October 2006.

Phosphodiesterase type-5 inhibitors; Sildenafil + Antidepressants

Retrospective analysis of clinical study data suggested that SSRIs and tricyclic antidepressants did not alter sildenafil pharmacokinetics. However, in one study fluvoxamine was found to modestly increase the levels and vascular effects of sildenafil.

Clinical evidence

The manufacturer notes that population pharmacokinetic analysis of clinical study data indicate that inhibitors of cytochrome P450 isoenzyme CYP2D6 such as **SSRIs** and **tricyclic antidepressants** do not have any effect on the pharmacokinetics of sildenafil.[1,2] However, in a double-blind, placebo-controlled study in healthy subjects, pre-treatment with **fluvoxamine** 50 mg daily for 3 days then 100 mg daily for 6 days increased the AUC of sildenafil 50 mg by 40%. This resulted in an increase in the vascular effects of sildenafil.[3]

Mechanism

Sildenafil is principally metabolised by cytochrome P450 isoenzyme CYP3A4, and to a lesser extent by CYP2C9. Fluvoxamine probably raises sildenafil by inhibition of both of these isoenzymes. Grouping all SSRIs and tricyclics together in a retrospective analysis would not be a sensitive enough technique to have picked up this modest effect of fluvoxamine.

Importance and management

The increases in sildenafil levels with fluvoxamine are modest, and the authors concluded that they do not suggest a large clinically relevant interaction. Nevertheless, they suggest it may be prudent to consider a 25-mg starting dose of sildenafil in patients taking fluvoxamine.[3] This may be sensible. Although retrospective analyses of clinical study data are useful to identify potentially important drug interactions, they are not sensitive enough to rule out interactions, and should not replace prospective pharmacokinetic studies.

1. Viagra (Sildenafil citrate). Pfizer Ltd. UK Summary of product characteristics, June 2006.
2. Viagra (Sildenafil citrate). Pfizer Inc. US Prescribing information, October 2006.
3. Hesse C, Siedler H, Burhenne J, Riedel K-D, Haefeli WE. Fluvoxamine affects sildenafil kinetics and dynamics. *J Clin Psychopharmacol* (2005) 25, 589–92.

Phosphodiesterase type-5 inhibitors; Sildenafil + Bosentan

Bosentan markedly reduces sildenafil levels.

Clinical evidence

In 10 patients with pulmonary hypertension, bosentan 62.5 mg twice daily for one month decreased the AUC of a single 100-mg dose of sildenafil by 53% and increased its clearance 2.3-fold. After a second month of bosentan at an increased dose of 125 mg twice daily, the AUC of a single 100-mg dose of sildenafil was reduced by 69%, and the clearance increased 3.4-fold. The AUC of the primary metabolite, desmethylsildenafil, was also decreased in a dose-dependent manner by bosentan.[1] In a further study in healthy subjects, the concurrent use of bosentan 125 mg twice daily and sildenafil 80 mg three times daily for 6 days decreased the AUC of sildenafil by 63%.[2]

Mechanism

Bosentan induces the cytochrome P450 isoenzyme CYP3A4 and CYP2C9, by which sildenafil is metabolised.

Importance and management

This pharmacokinetic interaction is established and potentially clinically important. The efficacy of sildenafil is likely to be reduced in patients taking bosentan, and should be closely monitored.

1. Paul GA, Gibbs JSR, Boobis AR, Abbas A, Wilkins MR. Bosentan decreases the plasma concentration of sildenafil when coprescribed in pulmonary hypertension. *Br J Clin Pharmacol* (2005) 60, 107–12.
2. Revatio (Sildenafil citrate). Pfizer Ltd. UK Summary of product characteristics, March 2007.

Phosphodiesterase type-5 inhibitors; Sildenafil + Dihydrocodeine

Two men using sildenafil had prolonged erections following orgasm while also taking dihydrocodeine.

Clinical evidence, mechanism, importance and management

Two men, successfully treated with 100-mg doses of sildenafil for erectile dysfunction, experienced prolonged erections after orgasm while also taking dihydrocodeine 30 to 60 mg every 6 hours for soft tissue injuries. One of them had two erections lasting 4 and 5 hours, and this did not occur on subsequent occasions when the dihydrocodeine was stopped. The other had 2 to 3 hour erections on three occasions during the first week of dihydrocodeine use, but no problems over the next 2 weeks while continuing to take the dihydrocodeine.[1] The reasons are not understood.

According to the manufacturers of sildenafil, priapism (painful prolonged abnormal erection) associated with its use is rare, and there appear to be no other reports about an interaction between sildenafil and dihydrocodeine. Excessively prolonged erections can have serious consequences and may need urgent treatment. Therefore, the authors suggest it would now be prudent to warn patients about this possible (though remote) problem if opioids are being used, and advise them to contact the prescriber if priapism occurs.[1]

1. Goldmeier D, Lamba H. Prolonged erections produced by dihydrocodeine and sildenafil. *BMJ* (2002) 324, 1555.

Phosphodiesterase type-5 inhibitors; Sildenafil + Ecstasy

The abuse of sildenafil and ecstasy (MDMA, methylenedioxymethamfetamine) has been reported to result in serious headache and priapism requiring emergency treatment.

Clinical evidence, mechanism, importance and management

A journalist's account, based purely on anecdotal reports, claims that the illicit use of sildenafil with ecstasy (MDMA, methylenedioxymethamfetamine) causes "hammerheading" because of the pounding headache and the prolonged and painful penile erections that require emergency medical treatment.[1] The report does not say how much of each of these drugs is taken to produce these adverse effects. The outcome can clearly be unpleasant, painful and, the priapism, potentially serious.

1. Breslau K, Peraino K, Fantz A. The 'sextasy' craze. Newsweek, June 3, 2002, 30.

Phosphodiesterase type-5 inhibitors; Sildenafil + Miscellaneous

No pharmacokinetic interaction appears to occur between sildenafil and a combined oral contraceptive or tolbutamide.

Clinical evidence, mechanism, importance and management

(a) Oral contraceptives

The pharmacokinetics of sildenafil were not altered by concurrent use of a combined oral contraceptive (**ethinylestradiol/levonorgestrel**), and the plasma levels of these contraceptive steroids were not altered by sildenafil.[1,2]

(b) Tolbutamide

Sildenafil 50 mg did not alter the pharmacokinetics of tolbutamide 250 mg,[3,4] probably because sildenafil is only a weak inhibitor of the cytochrome P450 isoenzyme CYP2C9 (consider also 'warfarin', (p.441)).

1. Revatio (Sildenafil citrate). Pfizer Ltd. UK Summary of product characteristics, March 2007.
2. Revatio (Sildenafil citrate). Pfizer Inc. US Prescribing information, July 2006.
3. Viagra (Sildenafil citrate). Pfizer Ltd. UK Summary of product characteristics, June 2006.
4. Viagra (Sildenafil citrate). Pfizer Inc. US Prescribing information, October 2006.

Phosphodiesterase type-5 inhibitors; Vardenafil + Miscellaneous

The manufacturers of vardenafil suggest the avoidance of class Ia and III antiarrhythmics because of fears of possible QT interval prolongation. No clinically significant interaction has been seen between vardenafil and food, glibenclamide (glyburide), metformin or sulphonylureas.

Clinical evidence, mechanism, importance and management

(a) Antiarrhythmics (class Ia and III)

Vardenafil 10 mg and 80 mg caused very small (8 and 10 millisecond) increases in the corrected QT interval in healthy subjects.[1,2] This increase was similar to that seen with a single 400-mg dose of moxifloxacin,[2] a drug known to cause moderate QT-prolongation. Because of this, the manufacturers recommend that vardenafil is not used in those taking class Ia antiarrhythmics (e.g. **quinidine**, **procainamide**) or class III antiarrhythmics (e.g. **amiodarone**, **sotalol**), which are also known to prolong the QT interval.[1,2] Note that prolongation of the QT interval is associated with an increased risk of the potentially fatal torsade de pointes arrhythmia (see also 'Drugs that prolong the QT interval + Other drugs that prolong the QT interval', p.257).

(b) Antidiabetics

The manufacturers say that the pharmacokinetics of **glibenclamide** (**glyburide**) were not affected by a single 20-mg dose of vardenafil,[1] and that vardenafil had no effect on **glibenclamide** pharmacodynamics (glucose and insulin levels).[2] Also, although no specific pharmacokinetic study has been conducted, the manufacturers say that population pharmacokinetic analysis suggests that **sulphonylureas** (not named) and **metformin** have no effect on vardenafil pharmacokinetics. No additional precautions therefore seem necessary on concurrent use.[1]

(c) Food

In a single-dose study, healthy subjects were given a single 20-mg dose of vardenafil on four occasions; after an overnight fast, on an empty stomach, following a **high-fat breakfast** (fat 58 g), or following a **moderate-fat evening meal** (fat 23 g). No pharmacokinetic changes were noted in the fasting or moderate-fat periods. Although the **high-fat breakfast** caused a slight decrease and a slight delay in the absorption of vardenafil this was not considered to be sufficient to warrant changing the dosing time or making dosage adjustments. Therefore vardenafil may be given without regard to meals.[3]

1. Levitra (Vardenafil hydrochloride trihydrate). Bayer plc. UK Summary of product characteristics, November 2006.
2. Levitra (Vardenafil hydrochloride). Bayer Pharmaceuticals Corporation. US Prescribing information, March 2007.
3. Rajagopalan P, Mazzu A, Xia C, Dawkins R, Sundaresan P. Effect of high-fat breakfast and moderate-fat evening meal on the pharmacokinetics of vardenafil, an oral phosphodiesterase-5 inhibitor for the treatment of erectile dysfunction. *J Clin Pharmacol* (2003) 43, 1–8.

Pseudoephedrine + Antacids or Antidiarrhoeals

Kaolin does not appear to interact significantly with pseudoephedrine, but aluminium hydroxide may possibly cause a more rapid onset of action.

Clinical evidence

In a single-dose crossover study in 6 healthy subjects, 30 mL of **aluminium hydroxide gel** did not affect the total amount of pseudoephedrine absorbed from a single 60-mg dose over 24 hours, but the rate of absorption was significantly increased during the first 3 hours.[1] Conversely, 30 mL of a 30% suspension of **kaolin** reduced the amount of pseudoephedrine absorbed from a single 60-mg dose by just 10%. The rate of absorption was also decreased.[1]

Mechanism

The increased rate of absorption of pseudoephedrine seen with aluminium hydroxide is probably also due to pH rises, which favour the formation of the lipid-soluble absorbable form of pseudoephedrine. The reduced absorption with kaolin is probably due to adsorption of the pseudoephedrine onto the surface of the kaolin.

Importance and management

Aluminium hydroxide may possibly cause a more rapid onset of pseudoephedrine activity (but this needs confirmation). Any interaction seems unlikely to be clinically significant. Similarly, the effects of kaolin on absorption are small and unlikely to be clinically important. For the effect of sodium bicarbonate on pseudoephedrine and ephedrine, see 'urinary alkalinisers', (p.1277).

1. Lucarotti RL, Colaizzi JL, Barry H, Poust RI. Enhanced pseudoephedrine absorption by concurrent administration of aluminium hydroxide gel in humans. *J Pharm Sci* (1972) 61, 903–5.

Pseudoephedrine and related drugs + Caffeine

Phenylpropanolamine can raise blood pressure and in some cases this may be further increased by caffeine. Combined use has resulted in hypertensive crises in a few individuals. Ephedrine may interact similarly. Phenylpropanolamine can markedly raise plasma caffeine levels, and isolated reports describe the development of acute psychosis when caffeine was given with phenylpropanolamine or ephedrine.

Clinical evidence

(a) Ephedrine

In a single-dose, randomised study, 15 healthy subjects were given ephedrine 25 mg, caffeine 200 mg, both drugs together, or placebo. An assessment of systolic blood pressure found that ephedrine had no significant effect, caffeine caused a 9.1 mmHg increase, and the use of both drugs resulted in an 11.7 mmHg increase. Caffeine alone did not increase heart rate, but both ephedrine and ephedrine plus caffeine caused increases of roughly 11%. Subjective tests suggested that there was no significant difference in feelings of headache, chest pain, heart pounding or shortness of breath between the treatments There was no significant pharmacokinetic interaction between the drugs.[1] In another randomised study, investigating the combination of ephedrine 20 mg and caffeine 200 mg, both three times daily, for weight loss, did not find any significant hypertensive effects with the combination, although the authors suggested that this may have been due to the favourable effects of weight loss on blood pressure. However, one patient was withdrawn due to a rise in blood pressure, to 185/125 mmHg.[2]

A review of reports from the FDA in the US revealed that several patients have experienced severe adverse effects (subarachnoid haemorrhage, cardiac arrest, hypertension, tachycardia and neurosis) after taking dietary supplements containing ephedrine or **ephedra** alkaloids with caffeine.[3] However, it is not possible to definitively say that these effects were the result of an interaction because none of the patients took either drug separately. Similarly, a meta-analysis assessing the safety of ephedra or ephedrine and caffeine found a two- to threefold increase in the risk of adverse events (including psychiatric symptoms and palpitations) with ephedra or ephedrine, but concluded that it was not possible to assess the contribution of caffeine to these events.[4]

Two episodes of acute psychosis occurred in a 32-year-old man after he took *vigueur fit* tablets (containing **ephedra** alkaloids and caffeine), *Red Bull* (containing caffeine) and alcohol. He had no previous record of aberrant behaviour despite regularly taking 6 to 9 tablets of *vigueur fit* daily (about twice the recommended dose). However, on this occasion, over a 10-hour period, he consumed 3 or 4 bottles of *Red Bull* (containing about 95 mg of caffeine per 250-mg bottle) and enough alcohol to reach a blood-alcohol level of about 335 mg%. No more episodes occurred after he stopped taking the *vigueur fit* tablets. **Ephedra** alkaloids (ephedrine and **pseudoephedrine**) may cause psychosis and it appears that their effects may be exaggerated by an interaction with caffeine and alcohol.[5]

(b) Phenylpropanolamine

In a placebo-controlled study, the mean blood pressure of 16 healthy subjects rose by 11/12 mmHg after they took caffeine 400 mg, by 12/13 mmHg after they took phenylpropanolamine 75 mg, and by 12/11 mmHg when both drugs were taken. Phenylpropanolamine 150 mg caused a greater rise of 36/18 mmHg. One of the subjects had a hypertensive crisis after taking phenylpropanolamine 150 mg and again 2 hours after taking caffeine 400 mg. This needed antihypertensive treatment.[6] The same group of workers describe a similar study in which the AUC of caffeine 400 mg increased by more than threefold, and the mean peak caffeine concentration increased almost fourfold (from 2.1 to 8 micrograms/mL) after phenylpropanolamine 75 mg was given.[7] Additive increases in blood pressure are described in another report.[8]

Mania with psychotic delusions occurred in a healthy woman (who normally drank 7 to 8 cups of **coffee** daily) within 3 days of her starting to take a phenylpropanolamine-containing decongestant. She recovered within a week of stopping both the **coffee** and the phenylpropanolamine.[9]

Mechanism

Uncertain. Simple additive hypertensive effects would seem to be part of the explanation. The effects of caffeine may compound the effects of these sympathomimetic drugs on the cardiovascular and central nervous systems by blocking adenosine receptors (causing vasoconstriction) and also augmenting the release of catecholamines.[3,5]

Importance and management

Fairly well established interactions. These studies illustrate the potential hazards of these drugs, even in normal healthy individuals. However, it has to be said that there seem to be no other reports of adverse interactions, which is perhaps surprising bearing in mind that coffee/caffeine is very widely used and ephedrine and phenylpropanolamine have also been widely available over the counter. One possible explanation for this could be that these interactions may go unrecognised or be attributed to one drug only e.g. phenylpropanolamine, whereas caffeine has also been taken either as part of the preparation[3,10] or in beverages (often not reported).Nevertheless, serious adverse events have been reported with caffeine and phenylpropanolamine or dietary supplements containing ephedra alkaloids (sometimes called ma huang) and therefore these preparations may pose a serious health risk to some users.[3] The risk may be affected by individual susceptibility, the additive stimulant effects of caffeine, the variability in the contents of alkaloids in non-prescription dietary supplements, or pre-existing medical conditions.[3] One study in healthy subjects that found no adverse clinical response to the enhanced cardiac effects of the combination concluded that the cardiac effects could be clinically significant in patients with compromised cardiac function.[1] The authors of one report[6] advised that likely users of phenylpropanolamine (those with allergies or the overweight) and those particularly vulnerable (elderly or hypertensive patients) should be warned about taking more than the recommended dose of phenylpropanolamine, and also about taking caffeine at the same time, because of the possible risk of intracranial haemorrhage.

Note that, phenylpropanolamine is no longer available in the US and UK and its use has been restricted in many other countries. In addition, because of the associated health risks, the FDA bans combinations of caffeine with ephedrine or pseudoephedrine, and also bans herbal products containing ephedra.

1. Haller CA, Jacob P, Benowitz NL. Enhanced stimulant and metabolic effects of combined ephedrine and caffeine. *Clin Pharmacol Ther* (2004) 75, 259–73.
2. Astrup A, Breum L, Toubro S, Hein P, Quaade F. The effect and safety of an ephedrine/caffeine compound compared to ephedrine, caffeine and placebo in obese subjects on an energy restricted diet. A double blind trial. *Int J Obes Relat Metab Disord* (1992) 16, 269–77.
3. Haller CA, Benowitz NL. Adverse cardiovascular and central nervous system events associated with dietary supplements containing ephedra alkaloids. *N Engl J Med* (2000) 343, 1833–8.
4. Shekelle PG, Hardy ML, Morton SC, Maglione M, Mojica WA, Suttorp MJ, Rhodes SL, Jungvig L, Gagné J. Efficacy and safety of ephedra and ephedrine for weight loss and athletic performance: a meta-analysis. *JAMA* (2003) 280, 1537–45.
5. Tormey WP, Bruzzi A. Acute psychosis due to the interaction of legal compounds – ephedra alkaloids in 'Vigueur Fit' tablets, caffeine in 'Red Bull' and alcohol. *Med Sci Law* (2001) 41, 331–6.
6. Lake CR, Zaloga G, Bray J, Rosenberg D, Chernow B. Transient hypertension after two phenylpropanolamine diet aids and the effects of caffeine: a placebo-controlled follow-up study. *Am J Med* (1989) 86, 427–32.
7. Lake CR, Rosenberg DB, Gallant S, Zaloga G, Chernow B. Phenylpropanolamine increases plasma caffeine levels. *Clin Pharmacol Ther* (1990) 47, 675–85.
8. Brown NJ, Ryder D, Branch RA. A pharmacodynamic interaction between caffeine and phenylpropanolamine. *Clin Pharmacol Ther* (1991) 50, 363–71.

9. Lake CR. Manic psychosis after coffee and phenylpropanolamine. *Biol Psychiatry* (1991) 30, 401–4.
10. Lake CR, Gallant S, Masson E, Miller P. Adverse drug effects attributed to phenylpropanolamine: a review of 142 case reports. *Am J Med* (1990) 89, 195–208.

Pseudoephedrine and related drugs + Urinary acidifiers or alkalinisers

Alkalinisation of the urine (e.g. by sodium bicarbonate) causes retention of ephedrine and pseudoephedrine by the kidneys, leading to the possible development of toxicity (tremors, anxiety, insomnia, tachycardia). Acidification of the urine (e.g. with ammonium chloride) has the opposite effect.

Clinical evidence

(a) Ephedrine

When the urine was made acidic (pH of about 5) with **ammonium chloride**, the excretion of ephedrine in the urine of three healthy subjects was two to fourfold higher than when the urine was made alkaline (pH of about 8) with **sodium bicarbonate**.[1]

(b) Pseudoephedrine

A patient with renal tubular acidosis and persistently alkaline urine developed unexpected toxicity (cachexia and personality changes) when given therapeutic doses (not stated) of pseudoephedrine for 2.5 months. She was found to have a very prolonged pseudoephedrine half-life of 50 hours (10 times normal). Therefore 8 subjects (adults and children) were studied, to establish the possible effects of changing the urinary pH on pseudoephedrine elimination. When the urinary pH was adjusted using **ammonium chloride** or **sodium bicarbonate**, within the approximate range of 5.7 to 7.8, the half-life of a single dose of pseudoephedrine (about 5 mg/kg) was found to increase from 1.9 hours at the lowest pH to 21 hours at the highest pH.[2]

This confirms an earlier study, in which it was found that at a urinary pH of 8, the half-life of pseudoephedrine was 16, 9.2, and 15 hours in 3 subjects, respectively. At a urinary pH of about 5, the half-life was 4.8, 3, and 6.4 hours, respectively.[3] **Sodium bicarbonate** was given to raise urinary pH and **ammonium chloride** to lower urinary pH.

Another study in 6 healthy subjects found that **sodium bicarbonate** 5 g initially increased the excretion rate of a single 60-mg dose of pseudoephedrine, but as the urinary pH increased the excretion of pseudoephedrine was reduced.[4]

Mechanism

Ephedrine and pseudoephedrine are basic drugs, which are mainly excreted unchanged in the urine. In acidic urine, most of the drug is ionised in the tubular filtrate and unable to diffuse passively back into the circulation, and is therefore lost in the urine. In alkaline urine, these drugs mostly exist in the lipid-soluble form, which are reabsorbed.

The increased rate of absorption of pseudoephedrine seen with sodium bicarbonate is probably also due to pH rises, which favour the formation of the lipid-soluble absorbable form of pseudoephedrine.

Importance and management

The interaction between ephedrine or pseudoephedrine and urinary alkalinisers are established but reports of adverse reactions in patients appear to be rare. Be aware that any increase in the adverse effects of these drugs (tremor, anxiety, insomnia, tachycardia, etc.) could be due to drug retention brought about by this interaction. **Acetazolamide** makes the urine alkaline and would be expected to interact with ephedrine and pseudoephedrine in the same way as sodium bicarbonate.

Acidification of the urine with ammonium chloride increases the loss of ephedrine and pseudoephedrine in the urine and could be exploited in cases of drug overdosage.

1. Wilkinson GR, Beckett AH. Absorption, metabolism and excretion of the ephedrines in man. I. The influence of urinary pH and urine volume output. *J Pharmacol Exp Ther* (1968) 162, 139–47.
2. Brater DC, Kaojarern S, Benet LZ, Lin ET, Lockwood T, Morris RC, McSherry EJ, Melmon KL. Renal excretion of pseudoephedrine. *Clin Pharmacol Ther* (1980) 28, 690–4.
3. Kuntzman RG, Tsai I, Brand L, Mark LC. The influence of urinary pH on the plasma half-life of pseudoephedrine in man and dog and a sensitive assay for its determination in human plasma. *Clin Pharmacol Ther* (1971) 12, 62–7.
4. Lucarotti RL, Colaizzi JL, Barry H, Poust RI. Enhanced pseudoephedrine absorption by concurrent administration of aluminium hydroxide gel in humans. *J Pharm Sci* (1972) 61, 903–5.

PUVA therapy + Herbal medicines or Foods

Two case reports describe photosensitivity, one in a patient taking rue (*Ruta graveolens*) and another in a patient who ate large amounts of celery soup.

Clinical evidence, mechanism, importance and management

A 35-year-old woman taking methoxsalen and undergoing PUVA for psoriasis unexpectedly developed increased photosensitivity. Over the previous weekend and on the morning of therapy she had been drinking a concoction of **rue *(Ruta graveolens)***.[1] This plant naturally contains 5-methoxypsoralen so it would appear that a pharmacodynamic interaction occurred, which resulted in the photosensitivity.

The authors note that other herbal products contain photosensitising substances (e.g. those containing members of the **Umbelliferae** family; such as **celery**, or ***Chlorella*** species), and so suggest that patients undergoing PUVA should be warned about the potential interactions.[1] This warning appears justified by the case of a woman taking methoxsalen and undergoing PUVA, who developed photosensitivity after eating a large quantity of soup containing **celery**, parsnip and parsley.[2]

1. Puig L. Pharmacodynamic interaction with phototoxic plants during PUVA therapy. *Br J Dermatol* (1997) 136, 973–4.
2. Boffa MJ, Gilmour E, Ead RD. Celery soup causing severe phototoxicity during PUVA therapy. *Br J Dermatol* (1996) 135, 330–45.

Raloxifene + Miscellaneous

The absorption of raloxifene is reduced by colestyramine, and their concurrent use is not recommended. No clinically relevant changes in raloxifene pharmacokinetics occur with aluminium/magnesium hydroxide, amoxicillin, ampicillin or calcium carbonate. Raloxifene does not alter digoxin or methylprednisolone levels. Oral antibacterials, antihistamines, aspirin, benzodiazepines, H_2-receptor antagonists, ibuprofen or paracetamol (acetaminophen) were used in clinical studies without any obvious effect on raloxifene levels. Smoking does not appear to alter the efficacy of raloxifene.

Clinical evidence, mechanism, importance and management

(a) Ampicillin and Amoxicillin

Ampicillin is reported to reduce the maximum serum levels of raloxifene by 28% and the extent of the absorption by 14% without affecting the elimination rate.[1] This is thought to be because ampicillin reduces the number of enteric bacteria and so reduces enterohepatic recycling of raloxifene. These small changes are unlikely to be clinically relevant. In another clinical efficacy study, there was no discernible difference in plasma raloxifene levels when taken with amoxicillin.[1]

(b) Antacids

The manufacturers of raloxifene report that in studies, an antacid containing **aluminium/magnesium hydroxide** given 1 hour before and 2 hours after raloxifene had no effect on its absorption. Also, no interaction was seen with **calcium carbonate**.[2] There would therefore appear to be no reason for avoiding concurrent use.

(c) Colestyramine

The manufacturers report that colestyramine reduced the absorption of raloxifene by about 60% due to an interruption in enterohepatic cycling.[1] It is recommended that these two drugs should not be used concurrently.[1,3]

(d) Digoxin

Raloxifene is reported not to affect the steady-state AUC of digoxin, while the maximum serum levels of digoxin were increased by less than 5%.[3]

(e) Methylprednisolone

Steady state raloxifene had no effect on the pharmacokinetics of a single oral dose of methylprednisolone.[1,3]

(f) Tobacco

Retrospective analysis of data from a placebo-controlled study of raloxifene found that raloxifene was equally effective in current tobacco smokers as non-smokers, although smokers had a lower baseline bone mineral density.[4]

(g) Miscellaneous

Data from clinical efficacy studies revealed no clinically relevant differences in the plasma levels of raloxifene when stratified according to concurrent drug use. These drugs included **oral antibacterials** (not named), **antihistamines** (not named), **aspirin**, **benzodiazepines** (not named), **H_2-receptor antagonists** (not named), NSAIDs (**ibuprofen**, **naproxen**), and **paracetamol** (**acetaminophen**).[3] There would therefore appear to be no reason for avoiding the concurrent use of any of these drugs with raloxifene.

1. Evista (Raloxifene hydrochloride). Eli Lilly and Company. US Prescribing information, July 2007.
2. Eli Lilly and Company Limited. Personal communication, September 1998.
3. Evista (Raloxifene hydrochloride). Eli Lilly and Company Ltd. UK Summary of product characteristics, May 2007.
4. Chapurlat RD, Ewing SK, Bauer DC, Cummings SR. Influence of smoking on the antiosteoporotic efficacy of raloxifene. *J Clin Endocrinol Metab* (2001) 86, 4178–82.

Retinoids + Food

Fatty foods increase the absorption of acitretin, etretinate and isotretinoin.

Clinical evidence

(a) Acitretin

The absorption of acitretin was increased by 90% and the peak plasma concentrations were increased by 70% when acitretin 50 mg was taken by 18 healthy subjects with a **standard breakfast**. The **breakfast** consisted of two poached eggs, two slices of toast, two pats of margarine and 8 oz (about 240 mL) of skimmed milk.[1]

(b) Etretinate

Studies have found that **high-fat meals** and **milk** cause about a two to fivefold increase in the absorption of **etretinate**, when compared with **high-carbohydrate meals** or when fasting.[2,3]

(c) Isotretinoin

In a study in 20 healthy subjects the AUC of a single 80-mg dose of isotretinoin was increased 1.4-fold, 1.7-fold, and 1.9-fold when taken one hour before a **standard breakfast**, during **breakfast**, and one hour after **breakfast**, respectively, when compared with the same dose of isotretinoin taken 4 hours before breakfast.[4]

Mechanism

It is thought that because these retinoids are lipid soluble they become absorbed into the lymphatic system by becoming incorporated into the bile-acid micelles of the fats in the food. In this way losses due to first-pass liver metabolism and gut wall metabolism are minimised, and bioavailability increased.

Importance and management

Established interactions of clinical importance. The manufacturers of acitretin recommend taking it with meals[5,6] or with milk,[5] and the manufacturers of isotretinoin recommend taking it with food.[7,8] Similar recommendations were made with etretinate.[9]

1. McNamara PJ, Jewell RC, Jensen BK, Brindley CJ. Food increases the bioavailability of acitretin. *J Clin Pharmacol* (1988) 28, 1051–5.
2. DiGiovanna JJ, Cross EG, McClean SW, Ruddel ME, Gantt G, Peck GL. Etretinate: effect of milk intake on absorption. *J Invest Dermatol* (1984) 82, 636–40.
3. Colburn WA, Gibson DM, Rodriguez LC, Buggé CJL, Blumenthal HP. Effect of meals on the kinetics of etretinate. *J Clin Pharmacol* (1985) 25, 583–9.
4. Colburn WA, Gibson DM, Wiens RE, Hanigan JJ. Food increases the bioavailability of isotretinoin. *J Clin Pharmacol* (1983) 23, 534–9.
5. Neotigason (Acitretin). Roche Products Ltd. UK Summary of product characteristics, April 2007.
6. Soriatane (Acitretin). Connectics. US Prescribing information, July 2004.
7. Isotretinoin. Beacon Pharmaceuticals. UK Summary of product characteristics, November 2006.
8. Accutane (Isotretinoin). Roche Laboratories Inc. US Prescribing information, August 2005.
9. Tigason (Etretinate). Roche Products Ltd. ABPI Datasheet Compendium, 1993–1994, p.1347–9.

Retinoids + Tetracyclines

The development of 'pseudotumour cerebri' (benign intracranial hypertension) has been associated with the concurrent use of acitretin or isotretinoin and tetracyclines.

Clinical evidence, mechanism, importance and management

The concurrent use of **isotretinoin** and a tetracycline has resulted in the development of 'pseudotumour cerebri' (i.e. a clinical picture of cranial hypertension with headache, dizziness and visual disturbances). By 1983, the FDA in the US had received reports of 10 patients with 'pseudotumour cerebri' and/or papilloedema associated with the use of **isotretinoin**. Four had retinal haemorrhages, and 5 of the 10 were also taking a tetracycline.[1] The manufacturers also have similar reports on file of 3 patients given **isotretinoin** and either **minocycline** or **tetracycline**.[2] The same reaction has been seen in a patient given **etretinate** with **minocycline**.[3] It seems that the tetracyclines and retinoids have an additive effect in increasing intracranial pressure. The manufacturers of **acitretin**[4,5] and **isotretinoin**[6,7] contraindicate their use with tetracyclines.

1. Anon. Adverse effects with isotretinoin. *FDA Drug Bull* (1983) 13, 21–3.
2. Shalita AR, Cunningham WJ, Leyden JJ, Pochi PE, Strauss JS. Isotretinoin treatment of acne and related disorders: an update. *J Am Acad Dermatol* (1983) 9, 629–38.
3. Viraben R, Mathieu C, Fonton B. Benign intracranial hypertension during etretinate therapy for mycosis fungoides. *J Am Acad Dermatol* (1985) 13, 515–17.
4. Neotigason (Acitretin). Roche Products Ltd. UK Summary of product characteristics, April 2007.
5. Soriatane (Acitretin). Connectics. US Prescribing information, July 2004.
6. Isotretinoin. Beacon Pharmaceuticals. UK Summary of product characteristics, November 2006.
7. Accutane (Isotretinoin). Roche Laboratories Inc. US Prescribing information, August 2005.

Retinoids + Vitamin A (Retinol)

A condition similar to vitamin A (retinol) overdosage may occur if acitretin or isotretinoin are given with vitamin A.

Clinical evidence, mechanism, importance and management

Combined treatment with **isotretinoin** and vitamin A may result in a condition similar to overdosage with vitamin A. Concurrent use should therefore be avoided or very closely monitored because changes in bone structure can occur, including premature fusion of the epiphyseal discs in children.[1]

The manufacturers of **acitretin**[2] say that the concurrent use of vitamin A should be avoided. In the UK[2] they advise no more than 4000 to 5000 units daily, which is the recommended daily allowance, and in the US[3] they advise doses of no more than the minimum recommended daily allowance. Similarly, the manufacturers of **isotretinoin** say that vitamin A should be avoided.[4,5]

1. Milstone LM, McGuire J, Ablow RC. Premature epiphyseal closure in a child receiving oral 13-*cis*-retinoic acid. *J Am Acad Dermatol* (1982) 7, 663–6.
2. Neotigason (Acitretin). Roche Products Ltd. UK Summary of product characteristics, April 2007.
3. Soriatane (Acitretin). Connectics. US Prescribing information, July 2004.
4. Isotretinoin. Beacon Pharmaceuticals. UK Summary of product characteristics, November 2006.
5. Accutane (Isotretinoin). Roche Laboratories Inc. US Prescribing information, August 2005.

Ritodrine + Miscellaneous

Supraventricular tachycardia developed in a woman given ritodrine when she was also given glycopyrronium (glycopyrrolate). Tachycardia has also been reported in two patients when atropine was used with ritodrine. Hypertension has been reported when cyclopropane was given to patients who had recently received ritodrine. The abuse of cocaine does not appear to increase the incidence of adverse effects in patients given ritodrine.

Clinical evidence, mechanism, importance and management

(a) Anaesthetics

In an analysis of 43 women who had a caesarean section under **cyclopropane** anaesthesia, all of the 6 who had previously been given ritodrine developed unacceptably high blood pressure (185/103 mmHg) after **cyclopropane** was started. Arrhythmias were reported in 2 of these patients.[1]

(b) Antimuscarinics

Premature labour in a 39-year-old woman who was 28 weeks pregnant was arrested with an intravenous infusion of ritodrine hydrochloride. Two weeks later, while she was on the maximum dose of ritodrine (300 micrograms/minute), her uterine contractions began again and she was scheduled for emergency caesarean section. The ritodrine was discontinued 40 minutes before the operation. It was noted in the operating room that she had copious oral secretions so she was given 100% oxygen by mask and 200 micrograms of intravenous **glycopyrronium (glycopyrrolate)**. Shortly afterwards she developed a supraventricular tachycardia (a rise in heart rate from 80 up to 180 bpm), which was converted to sinus tachycardia of 130 bpm when she was given intravenous propranolol 500 micrograms, in divided doses over several minutes.[2]

The reason for this reaction is not understood. Ritodrine alone has been responsible for tachyarrhythmias and one possible explanation for this interaction is that the effects of these two drugs were additive. Two other patients given intravenous ritodrine 6 mg over 3 minutes developed tachyarrhythmias when they were premedicated with **atropine**.[3] Information is very limited and the interaction is not well established but some caution is clearly appropriate if both drugs are used. The authors of the first report advise avoidance.

Other sympathomimetics have also been seen to interact with antimuscarinics, see 'Inotropes and Vasopressors + Antimuscarinics', p.889.

(c) Cocaine

A study in 51 pregnant patients given ritodrine for premature labour found no evidence of an increase in adverse effects in 17 of the patients who had been abusing cocaine.[4]

1. Johannsen G. Ritodrine and cyclopropane interaction. *Anaesthesia* (1980) 35, 84–85.
2. Simpson JI, Giffin JP. A glycopyrrolate-ritodrine drug-drug interaction. *Can J Anaesth* (1988) 35, 187–9.
3. Sheybany S, Murphy JF, Evans D, Newcombe RG, Pearson JF. Ritodrine in the management of fetal distress. *Br J Obstet Gynaecol* (1982) 89, 723–6.
4. Darby MJ, Mazdisnian F. Does recent cocaine use increase the risk of side effects with β-adrenergic tocolysis? *Am J Obstet Gynecol* (1991) 164, 377.

Sodium oxybate + Miscellaneous

Patients taking sodium oxybate should not drink alcoholic beverages with sodium oxybate. Additive CNS depressant effects are predicted with other CNS depressant drugs, and concurrent use of sedative hypnotics should be avoided. No pharmacokinetic interaction occurs with omeprazole, protriptyline, zolpidem or modafinil, but a pharmacodynamic interaction cannot be ruled out. Food markedly delays and modestly reduces the absorption of sodium oxybate.

Clinical evidence, mechanism, importance and management

(a) Alcohol and other CNS depressants

Sodium oxybate is the sodium salt of **gamma hydroxybutyrate** (GHB) a CNS depressant substance with well known abuse potential. When used clinically it is predicted to have additive effects with alcohol and other CNS depressants and the manufacturers specifically say it should not be used with these.[1,2] Patients should be warned not to drink alcoholic beverages while taking sodium oxybate.[1,2]

1. Antidepressants. The manufacturer notes that there was no pharmacokinetic interaction between sodium oxybate and **protriptyline**, but that the possibility of a pharmacodynamic interaction was not assessed.[1,2] The UK manufacturer states that the rate of adverse effects was increased when sodium oxybate was given with **tricyclic antidepressants**.[1]

2. Barbiturates. The UK manufacturer specifically contraindicates the use of sodium oxybate in patients taking barbiturates.[1]

3. Benzodiazepines and related hypnotics. The manufacturer states that sodium oxybate should not be given in combination with sedative hypnotics,[1,2] and the UK manufacturer specifically cautions against the concurrent use of benzodiazepines because of the possibility of increased risk of respiratory depression.[1]

The manufacturer notes that there was no pharmacokinetic interaction between sodium oxybate and **zolpidem**, but that the possibility of a pharmacodynamic interaction was not assessed,[1] and cannot be ruled out.[2]

4. Opioids. The UK manufacturer specifically contraindicates the use of sodium oxybate in patients taking opioids.[1]

(b) Food

In a study in 34 healthy subjects 4.5 g of sodium oxybate solution was given after a high-fat meal. It was found that food delayed the time to maximum level from 0.75 to 2 hours, reduced the maximum level by 58% and reduced the AUC by 35%, when compared with the fasted state.[3] The first dose of sodium oxybate should be taken at least 2 to 3 hours after the evening meal, and patients should always try to keep the same timing of dosing in relation to meals.[1,2]

(c) Modafinil and other CNS stimulants

The manufacturer notes that there was no pharmacokinetic interaction between sodium oxybate and **modafinil**, but that the possibility of a pharmacodynamic interaction was not assessed.[1,2] About 80% of patients in clinical studies were also taking CNS stimulants.[1]

(d) Proton pump inhibitors

In a crossover study in 44 healthy subjects pretreatment with **omeprazole** 40 mg daily for 5 days did not alter the pharmacokinetics of a single 3-g dose of sodium oxybate. There was no difference in the frequency and severity of adverse events.[4] No sodium oxybate dose adjustment is therefore expected to be needed in patients taking proton pump inhibitors.[1]

1. Xyrem (Sodium oxybate). UCB Pharma Ltd. UK Summary of product characteristics, March 2007.
2. Xyrem (Sodium oxybate). Jazz Pharmaceuticals, Inc. US Prescribing information, November 2005.
3. Borgen LA, Okerholm R, Morrison D, Lai A. The influence of gender and food on the pharmacokinetics of sodium oxybate oral solution in healthy subjects. *J Clin Pharmacol* (2003) 43, 59–65.
4. Borgen LA, Morrison D, Lai A. The effect of omeprazole on the bioavailability of sodium oxybate. *Clin Pharmacol Ther* (2004) 75, P21.

Sodium polystyrene sulfonate + Antacids

The concurrent use of antacids with sodium polystyrene sulfonate can result in metabolic alkalosis. Use with aluminium hydroxide has resulted in intestinal obstruction.

Clinical evidence, mechanism, importance and management

A man with hyperkalaemia developed metabolic alkalosis when given 30 g of sodium polystyrene sulfonate with 30 mL of **magnesium hydroxide** mixture three times daily.[1] Alkalosis has also been described in a study in a number of patients given this cation exchange resin with *Maalox* (**magnesium/aluminium hydroxide**) and **calcium carbonate**.[2] The suggested reason is that the breakdown of the **magnesium hydroxide** usually requires equal amounts of bicarbonate and hydrogen ions, and so does not cause any acid-base disturbance. However, when sodium polystyrene sulfonate is given, it binds the **magnesium**, while the hydroxide is neutralised by the hydrogen ions. This results in a relative excess of bicarbonate ions, which are absorbed, leading to metabolic alkalosis. This interaction appears to be established. Concurrent use should be undertaken with caution and serum electrolytes should be closely monitored. Administration of the resin rectally as an enema can avoid the problem.

In addition to alkalosis, the manufacturer also notes that concurrent use of **aluminium hydroxide** and the resin has resulted in intestinal obstruction due to 'concretions' of **aluminium hydroxide**.[3] Caution is advised.

1. Fernandez PC, Kovnat PJ. Metabolic acidosis reversed by the combination of magnesium and a cation-exchange resin. *N Engl J Med* (1972) 286, 23–4.

2. Schroeder ET. Alkalosis resulting from combined administration of a 'nonsystemic' antacid and a cation-exchange resin. *Gastroenterology* (1969) 56, 868–74.

3. Resonium A (Sodium polystyrene sulfonate). Sanofi-Aventis. UK Summary of product characteristics, February 2005.

Sodium polystyrene sulfonate + Sorbitol

Potentially fatal colonic necrosis may occur if sodium polystyrene sulfonate is given as an enema with sorbitol.

Clinical evidence

Five patients with uraemia developed severe colonic necrosis after being given enemas containing sodium polystyrene sulfonate and sorbitol for the treatment of hyperkalaemia. Four of the 5 died as a result. Associated studies in uraemic *rats* found that all of them died over a 2-day period after being given enemas of sodium polystyrene sulfonate with sorbitol. Extensive haemorrhage and transmural necrosis developed. No deaths occurred when enemas without sorbitol were given.[1]

Mechanism

Not understood.

Importance and management

Information is very limited and the interaction is not firmly established, nevertheless its seriousness indicates that sodium polystyrene sulfonate should not be given as an enema in aqueous vehicles containing sorbitol. More study is needed. Note that the manufacturer advises against the concurrent use of both *oral* and rectal sorbitol with sodium polystyrene sulfonate, because of the risk of colonic necrosis.[2]

1. Lillemoe KD, Romolo JL, Hamilton SR, Pennington LR, Burdick JF, Williams GM. Intestinal necrosis due to sodium polystyrene (Kayexalate) in sorbitol enemas: clinical and experimental support for the hypothesis. *Surgery* (1987) 101, 267–72.

2. Resonium A (Sodium polystyrene sulfonate). Sanofi-Aventis. UK Summary of product characteristics, February 2005.

St John's wort (*Hypericum perforatum*) + Cimetidine

Cimetidine does not significantly alter the metabolism of the constituents of St John's wort, hypericin and pseudohypericin.

Clinical evidence, mechanism, importance and management

A placebo-controlled study in healthy subjects taking St John's wort (*LI160, Lichtwer Pharma*) 300 mg three times daily found that, apart from a modest 25% increase in the AUC of pseudohypericin, cimetidine 1 g daily (in divided doses) did not significantly affect the pharmacokinetics of either the hypericin or pseudohypericin constituents of St John's wort. The available evidence therefore suggests that cimetidine is unlikely to affect the dose requirements of St John's wort.[1]

1. Johne A, Perloff ES, Bauer S, Schmider J, Mai I, Brockmöller J, Roots I. Impact of cytochrome P-450 inhibition by cimetidine and induction by carbamazepine on the kinetics of hypericin and pseudohypericin in healthy volunteers. *Eur J Clin Pharmacol* (2004) 60, 617–22.

Strontium ranelate + Miscellaneous

Food, dairy products and calcium compounds markedly reduce the absorption of strontium ranelate, and administration should be separated by at least 2 hours. Aluminium and magnesium antacids only slightly reduce strontium ranelate absorption. Strontium ranelate is predicted to reduce the absorption of the quinolones and the tetracyclines, and strontium should be stopped during courses of these antibacterials. Vitamin D does not affect strontium ranelate bioavailability.

Clinical evidence, mechanism, importance and management

(a) Antacids

The manufacturer notes that **aluminium/magnesium hydroxide** slightly reduced the absorption of strontium ranelate (AUC decreased by 20 to 25%) when given either at the same time or 2 hours before the strontium. However, when the antacid was given 2 hours *after* strontium, absorption was barely affected.[1] Therefore, the manufacturers recommend that antacids should be taken 2 hours after strontium ranelate. However, because it is also recommended that strontium ranelate is taken at bedtime, they say that, if this is impractical, concurrent intake is acceptable.[1] Note that **calcium**-containing antacids would have a greater effect, see (b) below, and concurrent intake would not be recommended.

(b) Food, Dairy products, and Calcium compounds

The manufacturers note that food, milk, dairy products, and calcium supplements reduce the bioavailability of strontium ranelate by about 60 to 70%, when compared with administration 3 hours after a meal.[1] This is because divalent cations such as calcium form complexes with strontium ranelate so preventing its absorption. Therefore, strontium ranelate should not be taken within 2 hours of eating, or presumably within 2 hours of any calcium compound. The manufacturer recommends that strontium ranelate should be taken at bedtime, at least 2 hours after eating.[1]

(c) Quinolones and Tetracyclines

The manufacturer predicts that strontium will complex with quinolones and tetracyclines, so preventing their absorption. Because of this, they recommend that when treatment with quinolones or tetracyclines is required, strontium ranelate therapy should be temporarily suspended.[1]

(d) Vitamin D

The manufacturer notes that vitamin D supplements had no effect on strontium ranelate bioavailability.[1]

1. Protelos (Strontium ranelate). Servier Laboratories Ltd. UK Summary of product characteristics, February 2007.

Sulfinpyrazone + NSAIDs

The uricosuric effects of sulfinpyrazone are not opposed by the concurrent use of flufenamic acid, meclofenamic acid or mefenamic acid.[1,2] Consider also 'Aspirin or other Salicylates + Sulfinpyrazone', p.138.

1. Latham BA, Radcliff F, Robinson RG. The effect of mefenamic acid and flufenamic acid on plasma uric acid levels. *Ann Phys Med* (1966) 8, 242–3.

2. Robinson RG, Radcliff FJ. The effect of meclofenamic acid on plasma uric acid levels. *Med J Aust* (1972) 1, 1079–80.

Sulfinpyrazone + Probenecid

Probenecid reduces the urinary excretion of sulfinpyrazone, but the overall uric acid clearance remains unaltered.

Clinical evidence, mechanism, importance and management

A study in 8 patients with gout showed that while probenecid was able to inhibit the renal tubular excretion of sulfinpyrazone, reducing it by about 75%, the maximal uric acid clearance was about the same as when either drug was given alone.[1] There would therefore seem to be no advantage in using these drugs together. The possibility of an increase in the adverse effects of sulfinpyrazone does not seem to have been studied.

1. Perel JM, Dayton PG, Snell MM, Yü TF, Gutman AB. Studies of interactions among drugs in man at the renal level: probenecid and sulphinpyrazone. *Clin Pharmacol Ther* (1969) 10, 834–40.

Thyroid hormones + Antacids

A few reports describe reduced levothyroxine effects in patients given aluminium or magnesium-containing antacids.

Clinical evidence, mechanism, importance and management

A man with hypothyroidism corrected with **levothyroxine** 150 micrograms daily developed high serum TSH levels (a rise from 1.1 up to 36 mU/L) while taking an **aluminium/magnesium hydroxide** antacid (*Silain-Gel*), and on two subsequent occasions when rechallenged. The reasons are not understood. Although he remained asymptomatic throughout,[1] the rise in the levels of TSH indicated that the dosage of the **levothyroxine** had become insufficient in the presence of the antacid. Two similar cases have also been reported, where the presence of an **aluminium/magnesium** antacid or **magnesium oxide** reduced the response to **levothyroxine**. One patient required four times her normal dose of **levothyroxine**.[2]

The general importance of this interaction is not known, but be alert for the need to increase the **levothyroxine** dosage in any patient given antacids. More study is needed. See also 'calcium carbonate', (below), which can reduce levothyroxine effects.

1. Sperber AD, Liel Y. Evidence for interference with the intestinal absorption of levothyroxine sodium by aluminum hydroxide. *Arch Intern Med* (1991) 152, 183–4.
2. Mersebach H, Rasmussen ÅK, Kirkegaard L, Feldt-Rasmussen U. Intestinal adsorption of levothyroxine by antacids and laxatives: case stories and *in vitro* experiments. *Pharmacol Toxicol* (1999) 84, 107–9.

Thyroid hormones + Antiepileptics

An isolated report describes a patient, previously stable taking levothyroxine, who developed clinical hypothyroidism when phenytoin was given. Both carbamazepine and phenytoin can reduce endogenous serum thyroid hormone levels, but clinical hypothyroidism caused by an interaction seems to be rare.

Clinical evidence

A patient with hypothyroidism had been successfully managed with 150 micrograms of **levothyroxine** daily for 4 years, developed hypothyroidism when given 300 mg of **phenytoin** daily. Doubling the **levothyroxine** dosage proved to be effective. Later this interaction was confirmed when stopping and restarting the **phenytoin** produced the same effect.[1]

A number of other reports describe very significant reductions in endogenous markers of thyroid function in subjects and patients taking **phenytoin**[2-5] or **carbamazepine**,[4-6] but not **sodium valproate**.[5] However, there seems to be only two cases in which reversible hypothyroidism was seen, one with **carbamazepine** and **phenytoin**, and the other with **carbamazepine** alone.[7] There is also a report of an arrhythmia in a patient with hypothyroidism and rheumatic heart disease given **phenytoin**; this was attributed to the displacement of protein bound **levothyroxine** by **phenytoin** leading to an increase in free **levothyroxine** in the plasma.[8] This report was later criticised by others, who suggested that the arrhythmia, if indeed there was one, was caused directly by the cardiac actions of **phenytoin**.[9,10]

Mechanism

Both phenytoin and carbamazepine can increase the metabolism of endogenous thyroid hormones, thereby reducing their plasma levels. Phenytoin can also displace levothyroxine and triiodothyronine from thyroxine binding globulin.[11]

Importance and management

Despite very clear evidence that both carbamazepine and phenytoin can cause a marked reduction in endogenous serum thyroid hormone levels, the development of clinical hypothyroidism seems to be very rare, and there seems to be only one case on record of an interaction between levothyroxine and phenytoin. There seems to be little reason for avoiding concurrent use, but the outcome should be monitored. Increase the levothyroxine dosage if necessary. Consider also 'Thyroid hormones + Barbiturates', below.

1. Blackshear JL, Schultz AL, Napier JS, Stuart DD. Thyroxine replacement requirements in hypothyroid patients receiving phenytoin. *Ann Intern Med* (1983) 99, 341–2.
2. Hansen JM, Skovsted L, Lauridsen UB, Kirkegaard C, Siersbæk-Nielsen K. The effect of diphenylhydantoin on thyroid function. *J Clin Endocrinol Metab* (1974) 39, 785–9.
3. Oppenheimer JH, Fisher LV, Nelson KM, Jailer JW. Depression of the serum protein-bound iodine level by diphenylhydantoin. *J Clin Endocrinol Metab* (1961) 21, 252–62.
4. Rootwelt K, Ganes T, Johannessen SI. Effect of carbamazepine, phenytoin and phenobarbitone on serum levels of thyroid hormones and thyrotropin in humans. *Scand J Clin Lab Invest* (1978) 38, 731–6.
5. Larkin JG, Macphee GJA, Beastall GH, Brodie MJ. Thyroid hormone concentrations in epileptic patients. *Eur J Clin Pharmacol* (1989) 36, 213–16.
6. Connell JMC, Rapeport WG, Gordon S, Brodie MJ. Changes in circulating thyroid hormones during short-term hepatic enzyme induction with carbamazepine. *Eur J Clin Pharmacol* (1984) 26, 453–6.
7. Aanderud S, Strandjord RE. Hypothyroidism induced by anti-epileptic therapy. *Acta Neurol Scand* (1980) 61, 330–2.
8. Fulop M, Widrow DR, Colmers RA, Epstein EJ. Possible diphenylhydantoin-induced arrhythmia in hypothyroidism. *JAMA* (1966) 196, 454–6.
9. Farzan S. Diphenylhydantoin and arrhythmia. *JAMA* (1966) 197, 133.
10. Gaspar HL. Diphenylhydantoin and arrhythmia. *JAMA* (1966) 197, 133.
11. Franklyn JA, Sheppard MC, Ramsden DB. Measurement of free thyroid hormones in patients on long-term phenytoin therapy. *Eur J Clin Pharmacol* (1984) 26, 633–4.

Thyroid hormones + Barbiturates

An isolated report describes a reduction in the response to levothyroxine when a woman also took a barbiturate. See also 'Thyroid hormones + Antiepileptics', p.1281.

Clinical evidence, mechanism, importance and management

An elderly woman taking 300 micrograms of **levothyroxine** daily for hypothyroidism complained of severe breathlessness within a week of reducing her nightly dose of *Tuinal* (**secobarbital** 100 mg with **amobarbital** 100 mg) from two capsules to one capsule. She was subsequently found to be thyrotoxic. She became symptom-free again when the dosage of the **levothyroxine** was halved.[1] The reason for this effect is not known, but **phenobarbital** has been shown to reduce the serum levels of endogenous thyroid hormones in some studies,[2] and it seems possible that in this case these other two barbiturates acted in the same way, probably by enzyme induction. The general importance of this interaction is almost certainly small, but be alert for any evidence of changes in thyroid status if barbiturates are added or withdrawn from patients taking **levothyroxine**. Consider also 'Thyroid hormones + Antiepileptics', above.

1. Hoffbrand BI. Barbiturate/thyroid-hormone interaction. *Lancet* (1979) ii, 903–4.
2. Ohnhaus EE, Studer H. A link between liver microsomal enzyme activity and thyroid hormone metabolism in man. *Br J Clin Pharmacol* (1983) 15, 71–6.

Thyroid hormones + Calcium carbonate

The efficacy of levothyroxine can be reduced by calcium carbonate.

Clinical evidence

Twenty patients with hypothyroidism were given **levothyroxine**, to which calcium carbonate 1.2 g daily was then added for 3 months. While taking the calcium carbonate their mean free thyroxine levels fell from 16.7 to 15.4 picomol/L and rose again to 18 picomol/L when it was stopped. The mean total thyroxine levels over the same period were about 118, 111 and 120 nanomol/L, respectively, and the mean TSH levels were 1.6, 2.7 and 1.4 mU/L, respectively.[1]

A woman with thyroid cancer taking **levothyroxine** 125 micrograms daily to suppress serum TSH levels had a reduced response (fatigue, weight gain) when she took *Tums* containing calcium carbonate, for the prevention of osteoporosis. She often took the two together. Over a 5-month period her serum TSH levels rose from 0.08 mU/L to 13.3 mU/L. Within 3 weeks of stopping the calcium carbonate, her serum TSH levels had fallen to 0.68 mU/L.[2] Other reports have described 4 patients who had elevations in their TSH levels while taking calcium carbonate concurrently with **levothyroxine**. All levels returned to normal when administration was separated by about 4 hours.[2-4]

Mechanism

In vitro studies indicate that levothyroxine is adsorbed onto calcium carbonate when the pH is low (as in the stomach), which would reduce the amount available for absorption.[1]

Importance and management

An established interaction, which seems to be of limited clinical significance. The study cited[1] shows that the mean reduction in the absorption of levothyroxine is quite small, but the case reports[2,3] show that some individuals can experience a reduction in the absorption that is clinically important. Since it is impossible to predict which patients are likely to be affected significantly, the cautious approach would be to advise all patients to separate the dosages of the two preparations by at least 4 hours to avoid admixture in the gut. This interaction would be expected to occur with calcium carbonate in any form but it is not known whether other thyroid hormone preparations interact in the same way as levothyroxine.

1. Singh N, Singh PN, Hershmann JM. Effect of calcium carbonate on the absorption of levothyroxine. *JAMA* (2000) 283, 2822–25.
2. Schneyer CR. Calcium carbonate and reduction of levothyroxine efficacy. *JAMA* (1998) 279, 750.
3. Butner LE, Fulco PP, Feldman G. Calcium carbonate-induced hypothyroidism. *Ann Intern Med* (2000) 132, 595.
4. Csako G, McGriff NJ, Rotman-Pikielny P, Sarlis NJ, Pucino F. Exaggerated levothyroxine malabsorption due to calcium carbonate supplementation in gastrointestinal disorders. *Ann Pharmacother* (2001) 35, 1578–83.

Thyroid hormones + Ciprofloxacin

There is a report of unexplained hypothyroidism in two patients taking levothyroxine who had also been taking oral ciprofloxacin for 3 to 4 weeks.

Clinical evidence, mechanism, importance and management

An 80-year-old patient with advanced thyroid cancer taking **levothyroxine** 125 micrograms daily required treatment with oral ciprofloxacin 750 mg twice daily and intravenous dicloxacillin for osteomyelitis complicating a fracture. After 4 weeks of treatment she complained of increasing tiredness, and was found to have a markedly raised TSH level (10 times of the upper limit of normal). Increasing the **levothyroxine** dose to 200 micrograms daily did not have any effect on TSH, so the dose was returned to 125 micrograms. The ciprofloxacin was then stopped, and the thyroid function tests rapidly normalised.[1]

Another women stable taking **levothyroxine** 150 micrograms daily had a more than 10-fold increase in TSH levels after taking ciprofloxacin 500 mg twice daily for 3 weeks.[1] When administration of **levothyroxine** and ciprofloxacin was separated by 6 hours, thyroid function tests normalised, which suggests that concurrent administration somehow reduces the absorption of **levothyroxine**.

This interaction is not established, but the two cases suggest that long-term ciprofloxacin should be considered as a possible cause of hypothyroidism in patients taking **levothyroxine**. Further study is needed.

1. Cooper JG, Harboe K, Frost SK, Skadberg Ø. Ciprofloxacin interacts with thyroid replacement therapy. *BMJ* (2005) 330, 1002.

Thyroid hormones + Colestyramine

The absorption of thyroid extract, levothyroxine, and tri-iodothyronine from the gut is reduced by the concurrent use of colestyramine.

Clinical evidence

A patient with hypothyroidism, taking **levothyroxine**, had a fall in his basal metabolic rate when given colestyramine: this prompted a further study in two similar patients taking **thyroid extract** 60 mg daily or **levothyroxine sodium** 100 micrograms daily, and 5 healthy subjects. Colestyramine 4 g four times daily reduced their absorption of **levothyroxine**[131], the amount recovered in the faeces being roughly doubled. One of the patients had a worsening of her hypothyroidism. Giving the **levothyroxine** 4 to 5 hours after the colestyramine reduced but did not completely prevent the interaction.[1]

Another report describes a patient taking **levothyroxine** whose TSH levels rose when colestyramine was taken, and fell again when it was stopped, indicating an impairment of **levothyroxine** absorption.[2]

Mechanism

Colestyramine binds to levothyroxine in the gut, thereby reducing its absorption. Since levothyroxine probably also undergoes enterohepatic recirculation, continued contact with the colestyramine is possible and separating administration may not entirely eliminate the interaction.

Importance and management

An established interaction (although the documentation is very limited) and of clinical importance. *In vitro* tests show that **liothyronine** interacts similarly.[1] The interaction can be minimised by separating the dosages by 4 to 6 hours (but see 'Mechanism'). Even so, the outcome should be monitored so that any necessary thyroid hormone dosage adjustments can be made.

1. Northcutt RC, Stiel JN, Hollifield JW, Stant EG. The influence of cholestyramine on thyroxine absorption. *JAMA* (1969) 208, 1857–61.
2. Harmon SM, Seifert CF. Levothyroxine-cholestyramine interaction reemphasized. *Ann Intern Med* (1991) 115, 658–9.

Thyroid hormones + Grapefruit juice

In a pharmacokinetic study, grapefruit juice had little effect on the absorption of levothyroxine, suggesting a clinically relevant interaction is unlikely. However, there is one case of unexplained hypothyroidism in a patient taking levothyroxine, which resolved when grapefruit juice consumption was reduced.

Clinical evidence, mechanism, importance and management

A 36-year-old woman previously stable taking **levothyroxine** 100 micrograms daily and with a marked consumption of grapefruit juice (specific volumes not stated) had a very high TSH level even after an increase in her **levothyroxine** dose to 150 micrograms daily. When she was advised to drink less grapefruit juice, her TSH fell to within the normal range.[1]

This case prompted a crossover study in 10 healthy subjects; however, grapefruit juice caused only a slight 11% reduction in the maximal increase in thyroxine after a single 600-microgram dose of **levothyroxine**. In this study, normal-strength grapefruit juice 200 mL was taken 3 times a day for 2 days, then on the third day, grapefruit juice 200 mL was taken one hour before, simultaneously with, and one hour after, **levothyroxine**.[1]

The pharmacokinetic study established that grapefruit juice appears to have only small effects on **levothyroxine** levels, which suggests that a clinically relevant interaction is unlikely. However, consider this case in the event of an unexpected decreased response to **levothyroxine**.

1. Lilja JJ, Laitinen K, Neuvonen PJ. Effects of grapefruit juice on the absorption of levothyroxine. *Br J Clin Pharmacol* (2005) 60, 337–41.

Thyroid hormones + H_2-receptor antagonists

Cimetidine, but not ranitidine, causes a small reduction in the absorption of levothyroxine.

Clinical evidence, mechanism, importance and management

When 10 women with simple goitre were given 400 mg of **cimetidine** 90 minutes before a single capsule of **levothyroxine**, the absorption of **levothyroxine** was reduced over the first 4 hours by about 21%. The reasons are not understood. A single 300-mg dose of **ranitidine** was found not to affect the **levothyroxine** absorption in a matched group of 10 women.[1]

The clinical importance of this interaction with **cimetidine** awaits assessment, but it seems unlikely to be generally significant.

1. Jonderko G, Jonderko K, Marcisz CZ, Kotulska A. Effect of cimetidine and ranitidine on absorption of [^{125}I] levothyroxine administered orally. *Acta Pharmacol Sin* (1992) 13, 391–4.

Thyroid hormones + HRT

HRT appears to increase the requirement for levothyroxine in some patients.

Clinical evidence

In 25 postmenopausal women taking stable doses of **levothyroxine** (for hypothyroidism or TSH suppression), the addition of hormone replacement therapy (**conjugated estrogens** 0.625 mg daily with or without **medroxyprogesterone acetate** 5 mg daily for 12 days each month) decreased serum free thyroxine levels and increased TSH levels. The changes in TSH were clinically important in 10 of the 25 women, requiring increased doses of **levothyroxine**, although only one woman had symptoms of hypothyroidism.[1]

Mechanism

Estrogens increase thyroxine binding-globulin. In women with normal thyroid function this does not alter free thyroxine levels or TSH levels,[1] as the thyroxine secretion can increase to accommodate the changes. However, in women with hypothyroidism who cannot compensate for the increased thyroxine binding, decreased free thyroxine and therefore increased TSH can result.

Importance and management

Although this study appears to be the only evidence of an interaction, it would now be prudent to monitor thyroid function several months after starting or stopping HRT to check levothyroxine requirements.

1. Arafah BM. Increased need for thyroxine in women with hypothyroidism during estrogen therapy. *N Engl J Med* (2001) 344, 1743–9.

Thyroid hormones + Imatinib

Imatinib appears to cause hypothyroidism in thyroidectomy patients taking levothyroxine.

Clinical evidence, mechanism, importance and management

Retrospective analysis of 11 patients taking **levothyroxine** and with thyroid cancer found that 8 patients who had previously undergone a total thyroidectomy developed markedly elevated TSH levels and were clinically hypothyroid after receiving treatment with imatinib. Despite a mean increase in the dose of **levothyroxine** of about 200%, hypothyroidism was reversed in only 3 patients. Thyroid function tests normalised on discontinuing imatinib. Conversely, no effect on thyroid status was seen in the 3 patients who had not had their thyroid gland removed.[1]

The authors postulated that imatinib might increase the clearance of the thyroid hormones thyroxine and tri-iodothyronine by induction of glucuronosyltransferases (UGTs).[1] Patients who have undergone a thyroidectomy cannot respond to these changes and therefore become hypothyroid.

The findings from this study appear to be established. TSH levels should be closely monitored in thyroidectomy patients taking **levothyroxine** if they are given imatinib, anticipate the need to increase the **levothyroxine** dose. The authors suggest that in thyroidectomy patients the dose of **levothyroxine** should be doubled before starting imatinib.[1]

1. de Groot JWB, Zonnenberg BA, Plukker JTM, van Der Graaf WTA, Links TP. Imatinib induces hypothyroidism in patients receiving levothyroxine. *Clin Pharmacol Ther* (2005) 78, 433–8.

Thyroid hormones + Iron compounds

Ferrous sulfate causes a reduction in the effects of levothyroxine in patients with hypothyroidism.

Clinical evidence

Fourteen patients with primary hypothyroidism had an increase in TSH levels from 1.6 to 5.4 mU/L when given **ferrous sulfate** 300 mg daily for 12 weeks along with their usual **levothyroxine** dose. The symptoms of hypothyroidism in 9 patients worsened.[1] In another report a woman with hypothyroidism, taking **levothyroxine**, had a very marked rise in TSH levels when she took **ferrous sulfate**. Her **levothyroxine** dosage needed to be raised from 175 to 200 micrograms daily.[2]

Mechanism

The addition of iron to levothyroxine *in vitro* was found to produce a poorly soluble purple iron-levothyroxine complex suggesting that this might also occur in the gut.[1]

Importance and management

Information is limited to these reports but it appears to be a clinically important interaction. Monitor the effects of concurrent use and separate the doses of ferrous sulfate and levothyroxine by 2 hours or more on the assumption that reduced absorption accounts for this interaction. Monitor well. The same precautions would seem appropriate with any other iron compound.

1. Campbell NRC, Hasinoff BB, Stalts H, Rao B, Wong NCW. Ferrous sulfate reduces thyroxine efficacy in patients with hypothyroidism. *Ann Intern Med* (1992) 117, 1010–3.
2. Schlienger JL. Accroissement des besoins en thyroxine par le sulfate de fer. *Presse Med* (1994) 23, 492.

Thyroid hormones + Protease inhibitors

A man needed to have his levothyroxine dosage doubled when he took ritonavir/saquinavir, and another woman possibly had a similar reaction when given indinavir then nelfinavir. Conversely, another woman needed a markedly reduced dose of levothyroxine when given indinavir.

Clinical evidence, mechanism, importance and management

An HIV-positive man, taking **levothyroxine** for autoimmune thyroiditis, developed an enlarged thyroid gland and marked lethargy about a month after his HIV treatment was changed to include stavudine, lamivudine, **saquinavir** and **ritonavir**. It became necessary to double his maintenance dose of levothyroxine to re-stabilise him. When the **ritonavir** and **saquinavir** were withdrawn and replaced by **indinavir**, the patient was able to go back to the original dose of **levothyroxine**. It is thought that this interaction occurred because **ritonavir** *increases* the activity of the glucuronosyl transferases, which are concerned with the metabolism (conjugation) of **levothyroxine**.[1]

Although this case suggested that **indinavir** did not interact with **levothyroxine**, a further case suggests the opposite. A 36-year-old HIV-positive woman taking **levothyroxine** 750 micrograms daily (following partial thyroid gland destruction for Grave's disease) was started on stavudine, lamivudine and **indinavir**. After about 7 weeks she presented with symptoms of hyperthyroidism (including nervousness, palpitations and weight loss). Her serum TSH was low and thyroxine was high. After stepped dose decreases she was finally restabilised on **levothyroxine** 120 micrograms daily, with normal thyroid indices. The authors postulated that **indinavir** *reduces* the activity of glucuronosyl transferases (in contrast to **ritonavir**).[2]

Conversely, in another woman a 4-week course of antiretroviral prophylaxis, including 2 weeks of **indinavir** then 2 weeks of **nelfinavir**, tended to reduce the efficacy of **levothyroxine** 125 micrograms daily. She was fatigued and had elevated TSH and hypercholesterolaemia, which resolved after the antiretroviral therapy was stopped.[3]

Direct information of the interactions of protease inhibitors and thyroid hormones seems limited. Whether or not an interaction occurs seems to depend on the individual protease inhibitor, how it affects glucuronidation, and how much remaining thyroid function a patient has.[3] Until more is known about this interaction it would seem prudent to monitor thyroid function more closely if a protease inhibitor is given to a patient with pre-existing hypothyroidism.

1. Tseng A, Fletcher D. Interaction between ritonavir and levothyroxine. *AIDS* (1998) 12, 2235–6.
2. Lanzafame M, Trevenzoli M, Faggian F, Marcati P, Gatti F, Carolo G, Concia E. Interaction between levothyroxine and indinavir in a patient with HIV infection. *Infection* (2002) 30, 54–5.
3. Nerad JL, Kessler HA. Hypercholesterolemia in a health care worker receiving thyroxine after postexposure prophylaxis for human immunodeficiency virus infection. *Clin Infect Dis* (2001) 32, 1635–6.

Thyroid hormones + Proton pump inhibitors

In one study, patients who had been taking levothyroxine and omeprazole for a least 6 months required a modest 37% increase in the median levothyroxine dose required to suppress TSH levels to those seen before starting omeprazole. Conversely, in a pharmacokinetic study, pantoprazole did not alter the absorption of a single dose of levothyroxine.

Clinical evidence

In a randomised, crossover study in 20 healthy subjects, pre-treatment with **pantoprazole** 40 mg daily for one week had no effect on the AUCs of TSH or thyroxine after a single 4-micrograms/kg dose of **levothyroxine**.[1]

In contrast, in a non-randomised study in 10 women with multinodular goitre and gastroesophageal reflux disease taking a stable dose of **levothyroxine** to suppress thyroid growth, the use of **omeprazole** 40 mg daily for at least 6 months caused a variable increase in TSH levels (median 1.7 mU/L versus 0.1 mU/L before treatment). At that time, the dose of **levothyroxine** was increased to suppress TSH levels: this required a median dose of **levothyroxine** of 2.16 micrograms/kg compared with 1.58 micrograms/kg before starting **omeprazole** (a 37% increase).[2]

Mechanism

A decrease in gastric acidity might decrease levothyroxine absorption. Supporting this is the finding that in patients with impaired gastric acid secretion the required dose of levothyroxine was 22 to 34% higher than in patients free of gastric disease.[2] However, this effect could be due to the disease rather than gastric acid *per se*.[3]

Importance and management

An interaction between levothyroxine and proton pump inhibitors is not established. The pharmacokinetic study with pantoprazole did not reveal a change in levothyroxine absorption, whereas the study in patients who had been taking omeprazole for 6 months suggested that patients may need a modest increase in levothyroxine dose. Bear in mind the possibility of an interaction if a patient starting a proton pump inhibitor shows signs of reduced levothyroxine efficacy. Any interaction may take several months to develop. Further study is needed.

1. Dietrich JW, Gieselbrecht K, Holl RW, Boehm BO. Absorption kinetics of levothyroxine is not altered by proton-pump inhibitor therapy. *Horm Metab Res* (2006) 38, 57–9.
2. Centanni M, Gargano L, Canettieri G, Viceconti N, Franchi A, Delle Fave G, Annibale B. Thyroxine in goiter, Helicobacter pylori infection, and chronic gastritis. *N Engl J Med* (2006) 354, 1787–95.
3. Dietrich JW, Boehm BO. Thyroxine in goiter, H. pylori infection, and gastritis. *N Engl J Med* (2006) 355, 1177.

Thyroid hormones + Raloxifene

There are two reports of patients who developed increased levothyroxine requirements after taking raloxifene for a number of months.

Clinical evidence

A 79-year-old woman taking **levothyroxine** 150 micrograms daily developed elevated TSH levels and symptoms of hypothyroidism within 2 to 3 months of starting to take raloxifene 60 mg daily. Over the next 6 months the **levothyroxine** dose was progressively increased to 300 micrograms daily without normalising TSH levels. This patient took the raloxifene early in the morning at the same time as the **levothyroxine**. Subsequently, separating the dose of raloxifene and **levothyroxine** by 12 hours led to a drop in TSH levels. In a single-dose study in this patient, serum thyroxine levels were reduced when **levothyroxine** 1 mg was given with raloxifene 60 mg, and separating the doses of raloxifene and **levothyroxine** by 12 hours was found to reduce TSH levels.[1] Another very similar case has been reported in a 47-year-old woman, which also, resolved on separating administration by 12 hours.[2]

Mechanism

Raloxifene is known to increase levels of thyroxine binding globulin, which results in increased levels of total thyroxine, without altering free thyroxine.[3] However, this is not likely to be the mechanism in the cases described, since separating the doses would not reduce any effect by this mechanism. It appears that raloxifene reduced the absorption of levothyroxine, but the mechanism for this is not known.

Importance and management

The interaction is not established, but the similar outcomes in both case reports suggest that an interaction may occur. Further study is needed, but until then it would be prudent to monitor TSH levels in patients taking levothyroxine and starting raloxifene, especially if they complain of tiredness. If TSH levels are raised, try separating administration by 12 hours before increasing the levothyroxine dose.

1. Siraj ES, Gupta MK, Reddy SSK. Raloxifene causing malabsorption of levothyroxine. *Arch Intern Med* (2003) 163, 1367–70.
2. Garwood CL, Van Schepen KA, McDonough RP, Sullivan AL. Increased thyroid-stimulating hormone levels associated with concomitant administration of levothyroxine and raloxifene. *Pharmacotherapy* (2006) 26, 881–5.
3. Evista (Raloxifene hydrochloride). Eli Lilly and Company Ltd. UK Summary of product characteristics, May 2007.

Thyroid hormones + Rifampicin (Rifampin)

Two case reports suggest that rifampicin might possibly reduce the effects of thyroid hormones.

Clinical evidence, mechanism, importance and management

A woman with Turner's syndrome, who had undergone a total thyroidectomy and who was being treated with **levothyroxine** 100 micrograms daily, had a marked fall in serum **levothyroxine** levels and free **levothyroxine** index with a dramatic rise in TSH levels when given rifampicin. However, no symptoms of clinical hypothyroidism developed, and the drop in serum **levothyroxine** occurred prior to starting rifampicin, which may reflect the clinical picture of an acute infection.[1] Another case describes a *fall* in TSH levels when rifampicin was discontinued.[2]

A possible reason for the changes is that rifampicin, a potent enzyme inducer, can markedly increase the metabolism of many drugs and thereby reduce their effects. Rifampicin has been found to reduce endogenous serum thyroxine levels in healthy subjects[3] and possibly in patients.[2]

There seem to be no reports of adverse effects in other patients given both drugs and the evidence for this interaction is by no means conclusive. Although rifampicin can affect thyroid hormones, it appears that healthy individuals can compensate for this. Since hypothyroid patients may not be able to compensate in the same way, bear this interaction in mind if rifampicin is given to a patient taking **levothyroxine**.

1. Isley WL. Effect of rifampin therapy on thyroid function tests in a hypothyroid patient on replacement L-thyroxine. *Ann Intern Med* (1987) 107, 517–18.
2. Nolan SR, Self TH, Norwood JM. Interaction between rifampin and levothyroxine. *South Med J* (1999) 92, 529–31.
3. Ohnhaus EE, Studer H. A link between liver microsomal enzyme activity and thyroid hormone metabolism in man. *Br J Clin Pharmacol* (1983) 15, 71–6.

Thyroid hormones + Sertraline

Limited evidence suggests that the effects of levothyroxine can be opposed in some patients by sertraline.

Clinical evidence, mechanism, importance and management

Nine patients with hypothyroidism were noted to have elevated TSH levels (indicating a decrease in the efficacy of their treatment with **levothyroxine**, when they also received sertraline. Two other patients with thyroid cancer, whose TSH levels had been deliberately depressed, developed TSH levels in the normal range while taking sertraline. None of the patients showed any signs of hypothyroidism at the time, and all of them had been taking the same dose of **levothyroxine** for at least 6 months. TSH levels of up to almost 17 mU/L (normal range 0.3 to 5 mU/L) were seen in some patients. The **levothyroxine** dosages were increased by 11 to 50%, until the TSH levels were back to normal. The authors of this report say that they know of 3 patients whose TSH levels were unaltered by sertraline.[1]

The manufacturers of sertraline say that their early-alert safety database to the end of July 1997 had identified 14 cases of hypothyroidism where a possible relation to sertraline could not be excluded. Seven of the patients were taking **levothyroxine**.[2]

The mechanism of this interaction (if such it is) is not known, but these cases draw attention to the need to monitor the effects of adding sertraline in patients taking **levothyroxine**, the dosage of which may need to be increased. More study is needed.

1. McCowen KC, Spark R. Elevated serum thyrotropin in thyroxine-treated patients with hypothyroidism given sertraline. *N Engl J Med* (1997) 337, 1010–11.

2. Clary CM, Harrison WM. Elevated serum thyrotropin in thyroxine-treated patients with hypothyroidism given sertraline. *N Engl J Med* (1997) 337, 1011.

Thyroid hormones + Sodium polystyrene sulfonate

A woman with hypothyroidism taking levothyroxine relapsed when she took sodium polystyrene sulfonate.

Clinical evidence

A woman taking **levothyroxine** 150 micrograms daily for hypothyroidism, following total thyroidectomy, later developed renal impairment and required dialysis. She was also taking digoxin, clofibrate, calcium carbonate, ferrous sulfate, nicotinic acid, folic acid, and magnesium sulfate. Because of persistent hyperkalaemia she started taking sodium polystyrene sulfonate 15 g daily. After 6 months, she developed lethargy, a hoarse voice, facial fullness and weight gain (all symptoms of hypothyroidism). These symptoms resolved within 6 weeks of raising the **levothyroxine** dosage to 200 micrograms daily and separating its administration from the sodium polystyrene sulfonate by 10 hours (previously taken at the same time as the **levothyroxine**).[1]

Mechanism

Sodium polystyrene sulfonate is a cation-exchange resin that is used to bind potassium ions in exchange for sodium. An *in vitro* study found that when levothyroxine 200 micrograms was dispersed in 100 mL water with 15 g sodium polystyrene sulfonate, the concentration of the levothyroxine at pH 2 fell by 93% and at pH 7 by 98%.[1] This drop in concentration would almost certainly occur in the gut as well, thereby markedly reducing the amount of levothyroxine available for absorption.

Importance and management

Information seems to be limited to this study, but the interaction would appear to be of general importance. Separate the dosages of levothyroxine and sodium polystyrene sulfonate as much as possible (10 hours seems to be effective) and monitor the thyroid function to confirm that this is effective.

1. McLean M, Kirkwood I, Epstein M, Jones B, Hall C. Cation-exchange resin and inhibition of intestinal absorption of thyroxine. *Lancet* (1993) 341, 1286.

Thyroid hormones + Statins

An isolated report describes raised serum thyroid hormone levels and evidence of thyrotoxicosis in a man taking levothyroxine with lovastatin. In contrast another isolated case report describes hypothyroidism in a woman taking levothyroxine with lovastatin. Another report describes reduced efficacy of levothyroxine in two patients taking simvastatin, one of whom was successfully treated with pravastatin.

Clinical evidence, mechanism, importance and management

(a) Lovastatin

A 54-year-old diabetic man taking 150 micrograms of **levothyroxine** daily for Hashimoto's thyroiditis, and a number of other drugs (gemfibrozil, clofibrate, propranolol, diltiazem, quinidine, aspirin, dipyridamole, insulin) started taking lovastatin 20 mg daily. Weakness and muscle aches (with a normal creatinine phosphokinase) developed within 2 to 3 days and over a 27-day period he lost 10% of his body weight. His serum **levothyroxine** levels rose from 11.3 to 27.2 micrograms/dL. The author of the report postulated that the lovastatin may have displaced the thyroid hormones from their binding sites, thereby increasing their effects and causing this acute thyrotoxic state. It was suggested that the patient did not have any cardiac symptoms because of his pre-existing drug regimen.[1]

In contrast, a woman with goitrous hypothyroidism due to Hashimoto's thyroiditis, which was being treated with 125 micrograms of **levothyroxine sodium** daily, developed evidence of hypothyroidism (elevated TSH) on two occasions while taking lovastatin 20 or 60 mg daily. No clinical signs of hypothyroidism developed, apart from some increased fatigue, and possibly an increased sensitivity to insulin. The author suggested that lovastatin may have influenced the absorption or clearance of **levothyroxine**.[2]

When the second report was published, the manufacturers of lovastatin reported that at that time (August 1989) more than 1 million patients had taken lovastatin, and hypothyroidism had only been reported in 3 patients.[3] It seems that any interaction is a very rare event and consequently unlikely to happen in most patients. No special precautions would therefore seem to be necessary.

(b) Simvastatin

A 75-year-old woman who had been stable taking **levothyroxine** 800 micrograms weekly for many years had a gradual increase in TSH levels and increasing tiredness after starting to take simvastatin 10 mg daily. After 4 months the **levothyroxine** dose was increased to 900 micrograms daily, but the patient's symptoms had not improved in 2 weeks and the simvastatin was stopped. The patient's symptoms gradually resolved, and the dose of levothyroxine was reduced back to the previous level.[4]

Another patient, who had recently started taking **levothyroxine** 50 micrograms daily, because of rising TSH levels, was also given simvastatin 10 mg daily. TSH levels continued to increase, so the simvastatin was stopped, and the TSH levels decreased to the normal range within 4 weeks without the need for an alteration in the **levothyroxine** dose. This patient was subsequently treated with **pravastatin** without a change in thyroid status.[4]

The authors conclude that any interaction must be extremely rare given the frequent use of simvastatin and **levothyroxine**.[4] No special precautions would appear to be required on concurrent use, but bear the possibility of this interaction in mind in the event of an unexpected response to treatment.

1. Lustgarten BP. Catabolic response to lovastatin therapy. *Ann Intern Med* (1988) 109, 171–2.

2. Demke DM. Drug interaction between thyroxine and lovastatin. *N Engl J Med* (1989) 321, 1341–2.

3. Gormley GJ, Tobert JA. Drug interaction between thyroxine and lovastatin. *N Engl J Med* (1989) 321, 1342.

4. Kisch E, Segall HS. Interaction between simvastatin and L-thyroxine. *Ann Intern Med* (2005) 143, 547.

Thyroid hormones + Sucralfate

An isolated report describes a marked reduction in the effects of levothyroxine in a patient taking sucralfate, whereas a subsequent study in patients did not find any interaction.

Clinical evidence, mechanism, importance and management

A woman with hypothyroidism did not respond to **levothyroxine** despite taking 4.8 micrograms/kg daily while taking sucralfate (dose not stated). Her response remained inadequate (TSH levels high, thyroxine levels low) even when the **levothyroxine** was taken 2.5 hours after the sucralfate, but when **levothyroxine** was taken 4.5 hours before the sucralfate, the thyroxine and TSH levels gradually became normal. A later *in vitro* study demonstrated that sucralfate binds strongly to **levothyroxine**, and it is presumed that this can also occur in the gut, thereby reducing its absorption.[1] However, sucralfate 1 g daily taken with **levothyroxine** in the morning for 6 weeks did not alter levels of thyroxine or TSH in 10 patients with hypothyroidism taking stable doses of levothyroxine.[2]

This seems to be the first and only report of this interaction, and its findings were not backed up by the subsequent study. Nevertheless, it might be prudent not to take sucralfate until a few hours after the **levothyroxine**. Patients should be advised accordingly and the response well monitored.

1. Havrankova J, Lahaie R. Levothyroxine binding by sucralfate. *Ann Intern Med* (1992) 117, 445–6.
2. Khan F, Jeanniton E, Renedo M. Does sucralfate impede levothyroxine therapy? *Ann Intern Med* (1993) 118, 317.

Tizanidine + Antihypertensives

Tizanidine may increase the effects of antihypertensive drugs. There are two case reports of severe hypotension with lisinopril. The manufacturer of tizanidine contraindicates the concurrent use of α_2-adrenergic agonists (e.g. clonidine).

Clinical evidence

A 10-year-old child taking **lisinopril** developed severe hypotension within a week of starting to take tizanidine.[1] Similarly, a 48-year-old stroke patient taking **amlodipine**, **nimodipine**, **lisinopril**, and **labetalol**, which had been added sequentially to control hypertension, had a dramatic reduction in blood pressure (from 130/85 to 66/42 mmHg) within 2 hours of her first dose of tizanidine 2 mg. She was given dopamine to maintain her blood pressure, and tizanidine and all the antihypertensives were withdrawn. Later **labetalol**, **amlodipine**, **nimodipine** and tizanidine were successfully resumed without producing similar problems.[2]

Mechanism

Tizanidine is a centrally acting α_2-adrenergic agonist structurally related to clonidine and can cause dose related hypotension (66% of patients given a single 8-mg dose of tizanidine had a 20% reduction in blood pressure). This can result in bradycardia, dizziness or light-headedness, and rarely syncope. The antihypertensive effects of tizanidine are said to be less than one-tenth of those of clonidine.[3] These effects are expected to be additive with other antihypertensive drugs. However, in the cases with lisinopril, it was suggested that ACE inhibition, combined with the alpha-agonist effects of tizanidine prevented the usual sympathetic response to hypotension (that is, it was not thought to be due to simple additive hypotensive effects).[1,2]

Importance and management

Tizanidine alone can cause hypotension, an effect which is usually minimised by titration of the dose. Patients should be warned about this effect. Because of this, the manufacturers caution that tizanidine might increase the effects of antihypertensive drugs, including **diuretics**, and recommend caution on concurrent use. This is a prudent precaution. The US manufacturer specifically states that tizanidine (an α_2-adrenergic agonist that is structurally related to clonidine) should not be used with other α_2-adrenergic agonists [e.g. **clonidine**, **methyldopa**].[3]

The UK manufacturers also say that the concurrent use of **beta blockers** may potentiate bradycardia and hypotension.[4]

1. Johnson TR, Tobias JD. Hypotension following the initiation of tizanidine in a patient treated with an angiotensin converting enzyme inhibitor for chronic hypertension. *J Child Neurol* (2000) 15, 818–19.
2. Kao C-D, Chang J-B, Chen J-T, Wu Z-A, Shan D-E, Liao K-K. Hypotension due to interaction between lisinopril and tizanidine. *Ann Pharmacother* (2004) 38, 1840–43.
3. Zanaflex (Tizanidine hydrochloride). Acorda Therapeutics, Inc. US Prescribing information, July 2006.
4. Zanaflex (Tizanidine hydrochloride). Cephalon Ltd. UK Summary of product characteristics, December 2006.

Tizanidine + CYP1A2 inhibitors

Fluvoxamine causes a very marked 33-fold increase in tizanidine levels with a consequent increase in hypotensive and sedative effects. The combination is potentially hazardous and should be avoided. Ciprofloxacin markedly increases tizanidine levels and adverse effects, and particular caution is required if this combination is considered essential. Combined oral contraceptives increase tizanidine levels fourfold and might increase adverse effects. Other inhibitors of CYP1A2 are predicted to interact similarly.

Clinical evidence

(a) Ciprofloxacin

In a placebo-controlled, crossover study in 10 healthy subjects ciprofloxacin 500 mg twice daily for 3 days markedly increased the AUC of a single 4-mg dose of tizanidine by tenfold and the maximum level by sevenfold, without significantly affecting the half-life. The hypotensive and sedative effects of tizanidine were also markedly increased by ciprofloxacin.[1]

A 45-year-old Japanese woman with multiple sclerosis taking tizanidine 3 mg daily had a reduction in blood pressure (from 124/88 to 102/74 mmHg) and heart rate (from 86 to 58 bpm) shortly after starting to take ciprofloxacin 400 mg daily. After 2 days she complained of drowsiness and her blood pressure was 92/54 mmHg.[2] Retrospective analysis revealed 8 patients who had received tizanidine and ciprofloxacin concurrently. In these patients, the mean reduction in blood pressure on starting ciprofloxacin was 21.3/15.4 mmHg, and the heart rate reduction was 14.9 bpm. Adverse effects attributable to tizanidine occurred in three of the patients.[2]

(b) Fluvoxamine

In a placebo-controlled, crossover study in 10 healthy subjects fluvoxamine 100 mg once daily for 4 days very markedly increased the AUC of a single 4-mg dose of tizanidine by 33-fold and the maximum level by 12-fold. The elimination half-life was prolonged from 1.5 to 4.3 hours. The hypotensive and sedative effects of tizanidine were also markedly increased by fluvoxamine, with all of the 10 subjects somnolent and dizzy for 3 to 6 hours.[3]

A 70-year-old Japanese woman started taking tizanidine 3 mg daily 15 days after starting fluvoxamine 100 mg increased to 150 mg daily. Her heart rate dropped from about 85 bpm to a range of 56 to 60 bpm. After tizanidine was stopped, the symptoms improved immediately.[4] Retrospective analysis revealed 23 patient who had received tizanidine with fluvoxamine. Of these patients, 6 had adverse effects including low heart rate, dizziness, drowsiness and hypotension. The patients with adverse effects were, on average, taking higher doses of fluvoxamine and tizanidine than those without adverse effects.[4]

(c) Oral contraceptives

In a study in 15 healthy women taking a combined oral contraceptive (**ethinylestradiol/gestodene**), the AUC of a single 4-mg dose of tizanidine was 3.9-fold higher than in 15 healthy women not taking an oral contraceptive, without any difference in the elimination half-life. In addition, the blood pressure-lowering effect of tizanidine was increased by 12/8 mmHg in the oral contraceptive users.[5] The manufacturer also notes that retrospective analysis of population pharmacokinetic data showed that the clearance of tizanidine is about 50% lower in women taking oral contraceptives.[6,7]

(d) Rofecoxib

In a placebo-controlled, crossover study in 9 healthy subjects rofecoxib 25 mg daily for 4 days markedly increased the AUC of a single 4-mg dose of tizanidine by 13.6-fold and the maximum level by 6.1-fold. The hypotensive and sedative effects of tizanidine were also markedly increased by rofecoxib. There was no evidence of QT prolongation in this study.[8]

An otherwise healthy 59-year-old woman developed extreme sinus bradycardia (30 bpm) with chest pain and acute right heart failure while taking tizanidine, diclofenac and rofecoxib. This resolved promptly after stopping the medication.[9] Note that rofecoxib was generally withdrawn worldwide in 2004 because of its cardiovascular adverse effects, but these data are included here for completeness.

Mechanism

Tizanidine is a substrate of the cytochrome P450 isoenzyme CYP1A2, which undergoes substantial presystemic metabolism by this isoenzyme. Ciprofloxacin appears to inhibit mainly the presystemic metabolism leading to increased absorption, as reflected by the increase in maximum level without a change in elimination half-life. Rofecoxib and fluvoxamine inhibited both presystemic metabolism and the elimination phase. Fluvoxamine, which is a known potent inhibitor of CYP1A2, had the most marked effect. The contraceptive steroids were modest inhibitors of CYP1A2 by comparison.

Importance and management

These pharmacokinetic interactions are well established, and clinically important. The common adverse effects of tizanidine, such as hypotension and sedation, are dose related, and consequently the manufacturers recommend starting with a low dose of tizanidine (2 or 4 mg) and carefully titrating to the usual maximum of 24 mg daily, and not exceeding 36 mg daily.[6,7] This represents a maximum 18-fold variation in dosage. **Fluvoxamine** increases the exposure to tizanidine by a mean of 33-fold, which, broadly speaking, changes a 2 mg dose into a 66 mg dose, which is far higher than the maximum recommended dose. For this reason, the authors of one of the studies conclude that the combination is potentially hazardous and should be avoided.[3] The US manufacturer also contraindicates the combination.[7] Given the available data this is sensible advice. Note that other **SSRIs** are generally not considered to inhibit CYP1A2, see 'Theophylline + SSRIs', p.1197, and may therefore be suitable alternatives to fluvoxamine.

For **ciprofloxacin,** there is a marked tenfold increase in exposure to tizanidine, with a consequent increase in adverse effects. Some authors recommend that this combination be avoided,[2] whereas others recommend caution.[1] The US manufacturer contraindicates the combination,[7] whereas the UK manufacturers do not mention this potential interaction.[6] If ciprofloxacin is considered the most appropriate antibacterial to use in a patient already taking tizanidine, anticipate the need to reduce the tizanidine dose before starting the ciprofloxacin, and closely monitor adverse effects: starting ciprofloxacin may cause marked hypotension, bradycardia, and sedation. Other quinolones also inhibit CYP1A2, but to varying degrees, see 'Table 33.4', (p.1193).

For **combined oral contraceptives**, the increase in exposure to tizanidine is a more moderate fourfold. The manufacturer states that clinical response or adverse effects might occur at lower doses of tizanidine in patients taking oral contraceptives,[6] and that during dose titration, individual doses should be reduced.[7] Care is needed.[7]

In addition, the US manufacturer also recommends caution if tizanidine is given with other inhibitors of CYP1A2, of which they mention **amiodarone**, **mexiletine**, **propafenone**, **cimetidine** and **ticlopidine**.[7] For a list of clinically important CYP1A2 inhibitors, see 'Table 1.2', (p.4).

1. Granfors MT, Backman JT, Neuvonen M, Neuvonen PJ. Ciprofloxacin greatly increases concentrations and hypotensive effect of tizanidine by inhibiting its cytochrome P450 1A2-mediated presystemic metabolism. *Clin Pharmacol Ther* (2004) 76, 598–606.
2. Momo K, Homma M, Kohda Y, Ohkoshi N, Yoshizawa T, Tamaoka A. Drug interaction of tizanidine and ciprofloxacin: case report. *Clin Pharmacol Ther* (2006) 80, 717–9.
3. Granfors MT, Backman JT, Neuvonen M, Ahonen J, Neuvonen PJ. Fluvoxamine drastically increases concentrations and effects of tizanidine: a potentially hazardous interaction. *Clin Pharmacol Ther* (2004) 75, 331–41.
4. Momo K, Doki K, Hosono H, Homma M, Kohda Y. Drug interaction of tizanidine and fluvoxamine. *Clin Pharmacol Ther* (2004) 76, 509–10.
5. Granfors MT, Backman JT, Laitila J, Neuvonen PJ. Oral contraceptives containing ethinyl estradiol and gestodene markedly increase plasma concentrations and effects of tizanidine by inhibiting cytochrome P450 1A2. *Clin Pharmacol Ther* (2005) 78, 400–11.
6. Zanaflex (Tizanidine hydrochloride). Cephalon Ltd. UK Summary of product characteristics, December 2006.
7. Zanaflex (Tizanidine hydrochloride). Acorda Therapeutics, Inc. US Prescribing information, July 2006.
8. Backman JT, Karjalainen MJ, Neuvonen M, Laitila J, Neuvonen PJ. Rofecoxib is a potent inhibitor of cytochrome P450 1A2: studies with tizanidine and caffeine in healthy subjects. *Br J Clin Pharmacol* (2006) 62, 345–57.
9. Kick R, Bertoli R, Moschovitis G, Caduff Janosa P, Cerny A. [Extreme sinus bradycardia (30/min) with acute right heart failure under tizanidine (Sirdalud). Possible pharmacological interaction with rofecoxib (Vioxx)]. *Med Klin* (2005) 100, 213–16.

Tizanidine + Miscellaneous

The sedative effects of tizanidine and other sedative drugs and alcohol are additive. Increased bradycardia might occur with digoxin. It is unclear whether tizanidine prolongs the QT interval in humans. No interaction occurs with paracetamol (acetaminophen).

Clinical evidence, mechanism, importance and management

(a) CNS depressants

One of the most common adverse effects of tizanidine is somnolence or drowsiness (occurring in up to 50% of patients[1]) for which reason the manufacturers warn about the possibility of increased sedation with other **sedative drugs**, and **alcohol**.[2,3] In addition to additive sedative effects, **alcohol** increased the AUC of tizanidine by about 20% and its maximum level by 15%, which was associated with an increase in adverse effects of tizanidine.[3] Patients should be warned.

(b) Digoxin

Tizanidine alone can cause bradycardia.[2,3] The UK manufacturers say that the concurrent use of digoxin may potentiate bradycardia.[2]

(c) Drugs that prolong the QT interval

The US manufacturer information states that prolongation of the QT interval and bradycardia were noted in chronic toxicity studies in *dogs* at doses equal to the maximum dose.[3] The UK information states that caution should be exercised when tizanidine is prescribed with drugs known to increase the QT interval.[2] In one pharmacological interaction study in healthy subjects, there was no evidence of QT prolongation either with tizanidine 4 mg, or almost 14-fold increased tizanidine levels caused by 'rofecoxib', (p.1286), despite increased bradycardia and hypotension.[4] This suggests that a clinically significant interaction resulting in QT-prolongation is unlikely.

(d) Paracetamol

In 20 healthy subjects, no clinically significant interaction occurred between 325 mg of paracetamol (acetaminophen) and 4 mg of tizanidine.[1]

1. Wagstaff AJ, Bryson HM. Tizanidine. A review of its pharmacology, clinical efficacy and tolerability in the management of spasticity associated with cerebral and spinal disorders. *Drugs* (1997) 53, 435–52.
2. Zanaflex (Tizanidine hydrochloride). Cephalon Ltd. UK Summary of product characteristics, December 2006.
3. Zanaflex (Tizanidine hydrochloride). Acorda Therapeutics, Inc. US Prescribing information, July 2006.
4. Backman JT, Karjalainen MJ, Neuvonen M, Laitila J, Neuvonen PJ. Rofecoxib is a potent inhibitor of cytochrome P450 1A2: studies with tizanidine and caffeine in healthy subjects. *Br J Clin Pharmacol* (2006) 62, 345–57.

Tizanidine + Rifampicin

Rifampicin moderately decreases the plasma concentrations of tizanidine.

Clinical evidence, mechanism, importance and management

In a placebo-controlled, crossover study in 10 healthy subjects, pre-treatment with rifampicin 600 mg daily for 5 days moderately reduced the AUC and peak level of a single 4-mg dose of tizanidine given on day 6 by about 50%, without altering the half-life.[1]

Rifampicin appears to be only a weak inducer of the cytochrome P450 isoenzyme CYP1A2, by which tizanidine is metabolised.[1]

Rifampicin moderately reduces the levels and effects of tizanidine. Because tizanidine dose is titrated to effect, this is probably not that clinically important. A small increase in dose might be required.

1. Backman JT, Granfors MT, Neuvonen PJ. Rifampicin is only a weak inducer of CYP1A2-mediated presystemic and systemic metabolism: studies with tizanidine and caffeine. *Eur J Clin Pharmacol* (2006) 62, 451–61.

Trientine + Miscellaneous

Trientine can possibly chelate with iron thereby reducing its absorption. On theoretical grounds a similar chelation interaction may occur with calcium and magnesium antacids and mineral supplements.

Clinical evidence, mechanism, importance and management

(a) Iron compounds

Trientine is a copper chelating agent used for Wilson's disease. One of the adverse effects of trientine is that it can cause iron deficiency, probably because it chelates with iron in the gut and thereby reduces its absorption. It is usual to make good this iron deficiency where necessary by giving an iron supplement. The manufacturers suggest that the iron supplement should be given at a different time of the day from trientine to minimise their admixture in the gut.[1,2] A separation of at least 2 hours is recommended.[2]

(b) Other mineral supplements and antacids

Trientine may be inactivated by metal binding in the gastrointestinal tract. The UK manufacturers say that there is no evidence that **calcium** or **magnesium antacids** alter the efficacy of trientine, but it is good practice to separate their administration.[1] The US manufactures say that, in general, mineral supplements should not be given with trientine. They say that it is important that trientine is taken at least one hour apart from any other drug or **milk**.[2]

1. Trientine dihydrochloride. Univar Ltd. UK Summary of product characteristics, July 2003.
2. Syprine (Trientine hydrochloride). Merck & Co., Inc. US Prescribing information, January 2001.

Tyramine + Cimetidine

A woman taking cimetidine experienced a severe headache and hypertension when she drank *Bovril* and ate some cheese.

Clinical evidence, mechanism, importance and management

A 77-year-old woman with hiatus hernia, who had been taking cimetidine 400 mg four times daily for 3 years, experienced a severe frontal headache and hypertension, which appeared to be related to the ingestion of a cup of ***Bovril*** and some **English cheddar cheese**, both of which can contain substantial amounts of tyramine.[1] Although the authors point out the similarity between this reaction and that seen in patients on MAOIs who eat tyramine-rich foods (see 'MAOIs or RIMAs + Tyramine-rich foods', p.1153), there is no satisfactory explanation for what occurred. They note that she was also taking salbutamol (another sympathomimetic) but rule out any contribution from this drug.

This is an isolated report and there is no reason why in general patients taking cimetidine should avoid tyramine-rich foods.

1. Griffin MJJ, Morris JS. MAOI-like reaction associated with cimetidine. *Drug Intell Clin Pharm* (1987) 21, 219.

Urinary antimuscarinics; Darifenacin + CYP3A4 inhibitors

Ketoconazole markedly increases darifenacin levels, whereas erythromycin and fluconazole have only a modest effect on darifenacin levels.

Clinical evidence

(a) Azoles

The manufacturers note that, in a study in 16 healthy subjects, **ketoconazole** 400 mg daily for 6 days markedly increased the steady-state AUC of darifenacin 30 mg once daily by about tenfold.[1,2] The UK manufacturers also note that **ketoconazole** 400 mg caused a fivefold increase in the AUC of a 7.5-mg dose of darifenacin.[3]

Fluconazole 200 mg then 100 mg daily had much less effect, causing an 84% increase in the steady-state AUC of darifenacin 30 mg once daily.[1,2]

(b) Erythromycin

The manufacturers note that erythromycin 500 mg daily increased the steady-state AUC of darifenacin 30 mg once daily by 95% in a study in healthy subjects.[1,2]

Mechanism

Darifenacin is principally metabolised by the cytochrome P450 isoenzyme CYP3A4, of which ketoconazole is a potent inhibitor, and erythromycin and fluconazole are moderate inhibitors.

Importance and management

Although the clinical relevance of these pharmacokinetic interactions have not been assessed, the manufacturers recommend that the daily dose of darifenacin is limited to 7.5 mg if it is given with ketoconazole or other potent inhibitors of CYP3A4.[1] They specifically name **clarithromycin**, **itraconazole**, (**miconazole**[2]), **nefazodone**, **nelfinavir** and **ritonavir**.[1] They say that dose adjustments are not required for moderate CYP3A4 inhibitors of which they list **erythromycin**, **fluconazole**, **diltiazem** and **verapamil**.[1] The UK manufacturers of darifenacin say that the concurrent use of potent CYP3A4 inhibitors is contraindicated. They specifically name **ritonavir**, **ketoconazole** and **itraconazole**. They then recommend a 7.5 mg dose of darifenacin in those taking moderate CYP3A4 inhibitors (they specifically name **grapefruit juice**, **clarithromycin**, **erythromycin**, **telithromycin** and **fluconazole**). For a list of CYP3A4 inhibitors, see 'Table 1.4', (p.6).

1. Enablex (Darifenacin hydrobromide). Novartis. US Prescribing information, February 2007.
2. Skerjanec A. The clinical pharmacokinetics of darifenacin. *Clin Pharmacokinet* (2006) 45, 325–50.
3. Emselex (Darifenacin hydrobromide). Novartis Pharmaceuticals UK Ltd. UK Summary of product characteristics, March 2007.

Urinary antimuscarinics; Darifenacin + Miscellaneous

Paroxetine and cimetidine cause small, clinically irrelevant, increases in darifenacin levels. Darifenacin increases imipramine levels, and caution is required with this and other tricyclics. Darifenacin does not significantly affect the pharmacokinetics of midazolam or combined oral contraceptives.

Clinical evidence, mechanism, importance and management

(a) Cimetidine

The manufacturers note that, in a study in healthy subjects, cimetidine 800 mg twice daily increased the steady-state AUC of darifenacin 30 mg once daily by 34%.[1,2] This change is unlikely to be clinically relevant. However, the UK manufacturers recommend that the dose of darifenacin should be started at 7.5 mg daily and, if well tolerated, titrated to 15 mg daily in the presence of cimetidine.[3] This seems a cautious approach.

(b) CYP2D6 inhibitors

The manufacturers note that, in a study in healthy subjects, **paroxetine** 20 mg daily increased the steady-state AUC of darifenacin 30 mg once daily by 33%.[1,2] This change is unlikely to be clinically relevant, and no dosage adjustments are recommended by the US manufacturers in the presence of CYP2D6 inhibitors.[1] However, the UK manufacturers recommend that the dose of darifenacin should be started at 7.5 mg daily and, if well tolerated, titrated to 15 mg daily in the presence of CYP2D6 inhibitors (they name **paroxetine**, **terbinafine** and **quinidine**).[3] This seems a cautious approach. For a list of CYP2D6 inhibitors, see 'Table 1.3', (p.6).

(c) CYP2D6 substrates

The manufacturers note that steady-state darifenacin 30 mg once daily increased the AUC of **imipramine** by 70% and increased the AUC of its active metabolite, desipramine, 2.6-fold in a study in healthy subjects.[2] Because of these changes, the manufacturer recommends caution with tricyclic antidepressants and other CYP2D6 substrates that have a narrow therapeutic window.[1,3] They name **flecainide** and **thioridazine** (see 'Table 1.3', (p.6), for a list).

(d) Midazolam

The manufacturers note that darifenacin 30 mg daily increased the AUC of a single 7.5-mg dose of midazolam by just 17% in a study in healthy subjects.[1-3] This change is not clinically important.[3]

(e) Oral contraceptives

The manufacturers note that steady-state darifenacin 10 mg three times daily had no effect on the pharmacokinetics of a combined oral contraceptive (**ethinylestradiol/levonorgestrel**) in a study in 22 healthy women.[1,2]

1. Enablex (Darifenacin hydrobromide). Novartis. US Prescribing information, February 2007.
2. Skerjanec A. The clinical pharmacokinetics of darifenacin. *Clin Pharmacokinet* (2006) 45, 325–50.
3. Emselex (Darifenacin hydrobromide). Novartis Pharmaceuticals UK Ltd. UK Summary of product characteristics, March 2007.

Urinary antimuscarinics; Oxybutynin + CYP3A4 inhibitors

Itraconazole and ketoconazole double the serum levels of oxybutynin. The clinical relevance of this is uncertain.

Clinical evidence

A single 5-mg dose of oxybutynin was given to 10 healthy subjects after they had taken **itraconazole** 200 mg daily or placebo for 4 days. The peak serum levels and the AUC of the oxybutynin were approximately doubled, while the pharmacokinetics of the active metabolite of oxybutynin were unchanged. The sum of the oxybutynin and its metabolite concentrations were on average about 13% higher than with the placebo. No increase in adverse effects was seen. Similarly, some manufacturers note that **ketoconazole** increases oxybutynin levels about twofold.[1,2]

Mechanism

This interaction is almost certainly due to itraconazole and ketoconazole inhibiting the metabolism of oxybutynin by the cytochrome P450 isoenzyme CYP3A4, in the intestinal wall and liver.

Importance and management

The authors of this report consider that this interaction is only of minor importance, but note that this was only a single-dose study and may not necessarily reflect the full picture in practice. Nevertheless, because itraconazole is a known and potent enzyme inhibitor, they predict that other CYP3A4 inhibitors that are less potent (they name **erythromycin**, **diltiazem**, and **verapamil**) are unlikely to interact with oxybutynin significantly.[3] Nevertheless, some manufacturers recommend caution with concurrent use,[1,2] and until more is known this seem prudent. Bear in mind the possibility of an interaction if antimuscarinic effects (dry mouth, constipation, drowsiness) are increased.

1. Ditropan XL (Oxybutynin chloride). Ortho-McNeil Pharmaceutical, Inc. US Prescribing information, June 2004.
2. Lyrinel XL (Oxybutynin hydrochloride). Janssen-Cilag Ltd. UK Summary of product characteristics, June 2006.
3. Lukkari E, Juhakoski A, Aranko K, Neuvonen PJ. Itraconazole moderately increases serum concentrations of oxybutynin but does not affect those of the active metabolite. *Eur J Clin Pharmacol* (1997) 52, 403–6.

Urinary antimuscarinics; Solifenacin + CYP3A4 inhibitors

Ketoconazole markedly increases solifenacin levels, and the solifenacin dose should be limited if ketoconazole or other potent inhibitors of CYP3A4 are used.

Clinical evidence

In a crossover study in healthy subjects, **ketoconazole** 200 mg daily for 20 days increased the AUC of a single 10-mg dose of solifenacin given on day 7 twofold.[1] Moreover, the manufacturer notes that a higher dose of **ketoconazole** 400 mg daily increased the AUC threefold.[2,3]

Mechanism

Solifenacin is principally metabolised by the cytochrome P450 isoenzyme CYP3A4, of which ketoconazole is a known, potent inhibitor.

Importance and management

Although the clinical relevance of this interaction has not been assessed, the manufacturers recommend that the daily dose of solifenacin succinate is limited to 5 mg if it is given with ketoconazole or other potent inhibitors of CYP3A4.[2,3] The UK manufacturer specifically names **itraconazole**, **nelfinavir** and **ritonavir**.[2] In addition, in patients with severe renal impairment or moderate hepatic impairment, the combined use of solifenacin and potent CYP3A4 inhibitors is contraindicated.[2] For a list of clinically significant CYP3A4 inhibitors, see 'Table 1.4', (p.6).

1. Swart PJ, Krauwinkel WJJ, Smulders RA, Smith NN. Pharmacokinetic effect of ketoconazole on solifenacin in healthy volunteers. *Basic Clin Pharmacol Toxicol* (2006) 99, 33–6.
2. Vesicare (Solifenacin succinate). Astellas Pharma Ltd. UK Summary of product characteristics, September 2005.
3. VESIcare (Solifenacin succinate). GlaxoSmithKline. US Prescribing information, November 2004.

Urinary antimuscarinics; Solifenacin + Miscellaneous

The manufacturer notes that solifenacin had no significant effect on the pharmacokinetics of an oral contraceptive containing ethinylestradiol and levonorgestrel.[1,2] They predict that inducers of the cytochrome P450 isoenzyme CYP3A4 such as carbamazepine, phenytoin, and rifampicin will interact with solifenacin;[1] reduced efficacy is possible. Note that, as significant interactions have occurred with potent CYP3A4 inhibitors (such as 'ketoconazole', (p.1289), this prediction seems reasonable. Food did not affect solifenacin pharmacokinetics.[3]

1. Vesicare (Solifenacin succinate). Astellas Pharma Ltd, UK Summary of product characteristics, September 2005.
2. VESIcare (Solifenacin succinate). GlaxoSmithKline. US Prescribing information, November 2004.
3. Uchida T, Krauwinkel WJ, Mulder H, Smulders RA. Food does not affect the pharmacokinetics of solifenacin, a new muscarinic receptor antagonist: results of a randomized crossover trial. *Br J Clin Pharmacol* (2004) 58, 4–7.

Urinary antimuscarinics; Tolterodine + CYP3A4 inhibitors

Ketoconazole can increase tolterodine levels in those who are deficient in the cytochrome P450 isoenzyme CYP2D6 (poor metabolisers). The manufacturers of tolterodine currently say that potent CYP3A4 inhibitors such as clarithromycin, erythromycin, itraconazole and ketoconazole, and protease inhibitors should be used with caution or avoided because of a risk of increased tolterodine effects.

Clinical evidence

A study[1] in 8 healthy subjects who were deficient in the cytochrome P450 isoenzyme CYP2D6 (poor metabolisers) found that after taking **ketoconazole** 200 mg daily for 4 days the clearance of a single 2-mg dose of tolterodine was reduced by 61% and its AUC was increased 2.5-fold. A subsequent multiple-dose study in 6 of the original subjects given tolterodine 1 mg twice daily (half the usual dose) found similar increased levels: **ketoconazole** 200 mg once daily caused a 2.1-fold increase in tolterodine AUC, and a 2.2-fold increase in the AUC of the active moiety (unbound tolterodine plus metabolite).[1]

Mechanism

Although tolterodine is normally metabolised to its active metabolite by CYP2D6, in those with low levels of this isoenzyme (about 5 to 10% of the population), metabolism by CYP3A4, becomes more important. It should be noted that tolterodine levels are already higher in poor CYP2D6 metabolisers than extensive metabolisers[2] but are likely to rise even further when a potent CYP3A4 inhibitor such as ketoconazole blocks this other route of metabolism.

Importance and management

The UK manufacturers[3] consider that this increase in levels represents a risk of overdose in poor CYP2D6 metabolisers. Consequently, they do not recommend the use of potent CYP3A4 inhibitors (they name **clarithromycin**, **erythromycin**, **ketoconazole**, and **itraconazole**, and **protease inhibitors**) with tolterodine in any patient (note that metaboliser status is rarely known). However, the US manufacturers[2] recommend only that the dose of tolterodine be reduced to 1 mg twice daily in patients currently taking drugs that are potent inhibitors of CYP3A4, and this seems the more sensible advice. It may be prudent to assess experience of adverse effects in these patients, and to reduce the dose further or withdraw the drug if it is not tolerated.

1. Brynne N, Forslund C, Hallén B, Gustafsson LL, Bertilsson L. Ketoconazole inhibits the metabolism of tolterodine in subjects with deficient CYP2D6 activity. *Br J Clin Pharmacol* (1999) 48, 564–72.
2. Detrol (Tolterodine tartrate). Pharmacia & Upjohn Company. US prescribing information, December 2006.
3. Detrusitol (Tolterodine tartrate). Pharmacia Ltd. UK Summary of product characteristics, May 2007.

Urinary antimuscarinics; Tolterodine + Duloxetine

Duloxetine increased the maximum levels of tolterodine by 64%, but this was not considered to be clinically significant.

Clinical evidence, mechanism, importance and management

In a placebo-controlled, crossover study, 14 healthy subjects received duloxetine 40 mg twice daily and tolterodine 2 mg twice daily for 5 days. Duloxetine increased the steady-state AUC of tolterodine by 71% and its maximum level by 64%. However, duloxetine had no effect on the pharmacokinetics of 5-hydroxymethyl-tolterodine the active metabolite of tolterodine.[1]

Duloxetine is an inhibitor of the cytochrome P450 isoenzyme CYP2D6, by which tolterodine is metabolised.

The increases in tolterodine levels were not considered to be clinically relevant, and no routine dosage adjustment of tolterodine dosage was considered necessary when given with duloxetine.[1] Consider also 'Urinary antimuscarinics; Tolterodine + Fluoxetine', p.1290.

1. Hua TC, Pan A, Chan C, Poo YK, Skinner MH, Knadler MP, Gonzales CR, Wise SD. Effect of duloxetine on tolterodine pharmacokinetics in healthy volunteers. *Br J Clin Pharmacol* (2004) 57, 652–6.

Urinary antimuscarinics; Tolterodine + Fluoxetine

Although fluoxetine can markedly inhibit the metabolism of tolterodine in some patients this is unlikely to cause a clinically important increase in the effects of tolterodine.

Clinical evidence, mechanism, importance and management

Thirteen psychiatric patients with symptoms of urinary incontinence were given tolterodine 2 mg twice daily for 5 doses, followed by fluoxetine 20 mg daily for 3 weeks, and then both drugs for a further 3 days. Nine of the 13 completed the study, the other 4 withdrew because of fluoxetine-related adverse effects. Fluoxetine is an inhibitor of the cytochrome P450 isoenzyme CYP2D6, the main enzyme involved in the metabolism of tolterodine. However, levels of this enzyme can vary between individuals and in the 7 patients with high CYP2D6 levels (extensive metabolisers) there was a 4.8-fold increase in the AUC of tolterodine and a minor reduction in its active and equipotent metabolite. In contrast the AUC of tolterodine increased by about 25% in 2 patients with low levels of CYP2D6 (poor metabolisers). These changes in AUC represent an increase of about 25% in active moiety (unbound tolterodine plus metabolite) for both poor and extensive metabolisers, a figure within normal variation.[1]

In practical terms this means that the antimuscarinic (anticholinergic) effects of the tolterodine are only moderately increased, and it seems unlikely that any tolterodine dosage changes are likely to be needed. Consider also 'Antimuscarinics + Antimuscarinics', p.674.

1. Brynne N, Svanström C, Åberg-Wistedt A, Hallén B, Bertlisson L. Fluoxetine inhibits the metabolism of tolterodine—pharmacokinetic implications and proposed clinical relevance. *Br J Clin Pharmacol* (1999) 48, 553–63.

Ursodeoxycholic acid (Ursodiol) + Bile-acid binding resins

The absorption of ursodeoxycholic acid can be more than halved by colestilan or colestyramine given simultaneously, and efficacy might be reduced.

Clinical evidence

(a) Colestilan

Following a test meal with an overnight fast, 5 healthy subjects were given 200 mg of ursodeoxycholic acid alone or with 1.5 g of colestilan granules. It was found that the ursodeoxycholic acid serum levels at 30 minutes were reduced by the colestilan by more than 50% in 4 out of the 5 subjects, and the mean level was decreased from 9.2 to 3.4 micromol/L.[1]

(b) Colestyramine

Simultaneous administration of colestyramine 4 g daily with ursodeoxycholic acid reduced the fasting serum levels of ursodeoxycholic acid by about 60% in a study in 5 healthy subjects. Separation of administration by 5 hours tended to diminish the reduction (serum levels reduced by less than 40%).[2]

Mechanism

The mechanism of this interaction would appear to be that the bile-acid binding resins bind with ursodeoxycholic acid (a bile acid) in the intestine and thereby reduce its absorption.

Importance and management

These interactions would appear to be established, and are probably clinically important. One UK manufacturer actually advises that **colestipol** and colestyramine should be avoided when ursodeoxycholic acid is given, as they may limit the effectiveness of therapy.[3] The authors of the reports recommend that in order to reduce the effects of this interaction, these two drugs should be separated,[1,2] by at least 2 hours.[1]

1. Takikawa H, Ogasawara T, Sato A, Ohashi M, Hasegawa Y, Hojo M. Effect of colestimide on intestinal absorption of ursodeoxycholic acid in men. *Int J Clin Pharmacol Ther* (2001) 39, 558–60.
2. Rust C, Sauter GH, Oswald M, Büttner J, Kullak-Ublick GA, Paumgartner G, Beuers U. Effect of cholestyramine on bile acid pattern and synthesis during administration of ursodeoxycholic acid in man. *Eur J Clin Invest* (2000) 30, 135–9.
3. Urdox (Urosodeoxycholic acid). Wockhardt UK Ltd. UK Summary of product characteristics, January 2002.

Valerian + Cytochrome P450 isoenzyme substrates

Valerian root extract does not affect the metabolism of caffeine, chlorzoxazone, debrisoquine and metabolism.

Clinical evidence, mechanism, importance and management

In a study 12 non-smoking healthy subjects were given valerian root extract 125 mg three daily for 28 days before receiving single doses of caffeine, chlorzoxazone, debrisoquine and midazolam. Valerian root extract caused no significant changes in the metabolism of these drugs, and it is therefore unlikely that other drugs metabolised by the cytochrome P450 isoenzymes CYP1A2, CYP2E1, CYP2D6 or CYP3A4 will be affected by the use of valerian.[1] See tables 'Table 1.2', (p.4), 'Table 1.3', (p.6), and 'Table 1.4', (p.6), for a list of substrates for these isoenzymes.

1. Gurley BJ, Gardner SF, Hubbard MA, Williams DK, Gentry WB, Khan IA, Shah A. In vivo effects of goldenseal, kava kava, black cohosh, and valerian on human cytochrome P450 1A2, 2D6, 2E1, and 3A4/5 phenotypes. *Clin Pharmacol Ther* (2005) 77, 415–26.

Vinpocetine + Antacids

Aluminium/magnesium hydroxide gel (1 sachet four times daily) had no significant effects on the serum levels of vinpocetine (20 mg three times daily) in 18 healthy subjects.[1] No special precautions seem necessary if they are taken together.

1. Lohmann A, Grobara P, Dingler E. Investigation of the possible influence of the absorption of vinpocetine with concomitant application of magnesium-aluminium-hydroxide gel. *Arzneimittelforschung* (1991) 41, 1164–7.

Vitamin A (Retinol) + Neomycin

Neomycin can markedly reduce the absorption of vitamin A (retinol) from the gut.

Clinical evidence, mechanism, importance and management

Neomycin 2 g markedly reduced the absorption of a test dose of vitamin A in 5 healthy subjects. It is suggested that this was due to a direct chemical interference between the neomycin and bile in the gut, which disrupted the absorption of fats and fat-soluble vitamins.[1] The extent to which long-term treatment with neomycin (or other aminoglycosides) would impair the treatment of vitamin A deficiency has not been determined.

1. Barrowman JA, D'Mello A, Herxheimer A. A single dose of neomycin impairs absorption of vitamin A (Retinol) in man. *Eur J Clin Pharmacol* (1973) 5, 199–201.

Vitamin B_{12} + Miscellaneous

Neomycin, aminosalicylic acid and the H_2-receptor antagonists can reduce the absorption of vitamin B_{12} from the gut, but no interaction is likely when B_{12} is given by injection.

Clinical evidence, mechanism, importance and management

Neomycin causes a generalised malabsorption syndrome, which has been shown[1] to reduce the absorption of vitamin B_{12}. **Colchicine** has also been shown to decrease B_{12} absorption.[1] **Aminosalicylic acid** reduces vitamin B_{12} absorption for reasons that are not understood, but which are possibly related to a mild generalised malabsorption syndrome.[2] Review of the literature[3] suggests that H_2-receptor antagonists (such as **cimetidine** and **ranitidine**) can also reduce vitamin B_{12} absorption, primarily because they reduce gastric acid production. The acid is needed to aid the release of B_{12} from dietary protein sources. There is therefore a possibility that on long-term use patients could become vitamin B_{12} deficient.

Within the context of adverse drug interactions, none of these drugs is normally likely to be clinically important, because for anaemia, vitamin B_{12} should be given parenterally for convenience and to avoid well-established problems with absorption.

1. Faloon WW, Chodos RB. Vitamin B_{12} absorption studies using colchicine, neomycin and continuous 57Co B_{12} administration. *Gastroenterology* (1969) 56, 1251.
2. Palva IP, Rytkönen U, Alatulkkila M, Palva HLA. Drug-induced malabsorption of vitamin B_{12}. V. Intestinal pH and absorption of vitamin B_{12} during treatment with para-aminosalicylic acid. *Scand J Haematol* (1972) 9, 5–7.
3. Force RW, Nahata MC. Effect of histamine H_2-receptor antagonists on vitamin B_{12} absorption. *Ann Pharmacother* (1992) 26, 1283–6.

Vitamin D substances; Alfacalcidol + Danazol

An isolated report describes hypercalcaemia when a woman taking alfacalcidol also took danazol.

Clinical evidence, mechanism, importance and management

A woman with idiopathic hypoparathyroidism, treated with alfacalcidol, developed hypercalcaemia when she was given danazol 400 mg daily for endometriosis. She needed a reduction in the dosage of alfacalcidol from 4 to 0.75 micrograms daily. When the danazol was stopped 6 months later, the alfacalcidol dosage was raised to 4 micrograms daily and she remained normocalcaemic.[1] The reasons for this interaction are not understood and the general importance is limited as this appears to be an isolated case.

1. Hepburn NC, Abdul-Aziz LAS, Whiteoak R. Danazol-induced hypercalcaemia in alphacalcidol-treated hypoparathyroidism. *Postgrad Med J* (1989) 65, 849–50.

Vitamin D substances + Phenytoin and Barbiturates

The long-term use of phenytoin, phenobarbital, or primidone can disturb vitamin D and calcium metabolism and may result in osteomalacia. There are a few reports of patients taking vitamin D supplements who responded poorly to vitamin replacement while taking phenytoin or barbiturates. Serum phenytoin levels are not altered by vitamin D.

Clinical evidence

(a) Effect on vitamin D

A 16-year-old with grand mal epilepsy and idiopathic hypoparathyroidism did not adequately respond to daily doses of **alfacalcidol** 10 micrograms and 6 to 12 g of calcium, apparently because phenytoin 200 mg and **primidone** 500 mg daily were also being taken. However, when **dihydrotachysterol** 0.6 to 2.4 mg daily was given normal calcium levels were achieved.[1]

Other reports describe patients whose response to usual doses of vitamin D was poor, because of concurrent anticonvulsant treatment with phenytoin and **phenobarbital** or **primidone**.[2-4] Other reports clearly show low serum calcium levels,[5,6] low serum vitamin D levels,[7] osteomalacia,[6] and bone structure alterations[5,7] in the presence of phenytoin.

(b) Effect on phenytoin

A controlled study in 151 epileptic patients taking phenytoin and calcium showed that the addition of 2000 units of vitamin D_2 daily over a 3-month period had no significant effect on serum phenytoin levels.[8]

Mechanism

The enzyme-inducing effects of phenytoin and other anticonvulsants increase the metabolism of the vitamin D, thereby reducing its effects and disturbing calcium metabolism.[3] In addition, phenytoin may possibly reduce the absorption of calcium from the gut.[1]

Importance and management

The disturbance of calcium metabolism by phenytoin and other anticonvulsants is very well established, but there are only a few reports describing a poor response to vitamin D. The effects of concurrent treatment should be well monitored. Those who need vitamin D supplements may possibly need greater than usual doses.

1. Rubinger D, Korn-Lubetzki I, Feldman S, Popovtzer MM. Delayed response to 1 α-hydroxycholecalciferol therapy in a case of hypoparathyroidism during anticonvulsant therapy. *Isr J Med Sci* (1980) 16, 772–4.
2. Asherov J, Weinberger A, Pinkhas J. Lack of response to vitamin D therapy in a patient with hypoparathyroidism under anticonvulsant drugs. *Helv Paediatr Acta* (1977) 32, 369–73.
3. Chan JCM, Oldham SB, Holick MF, DeLuca HF. 1-α-Hydroxyvitamin D_3 in chronic renal failure. A potent analogue of the kidney hormone, 1,25-dihydroxycholecalciferol. *JAMA* (1975) 234, 47–52.
4. Maclaren N, Lifshitz F. Vitamin D-dependency rickets in institutionalized, mentally retarded children on long term anticonvulsant therapy. II. The response to 25-hydroxycholecalciferol and to vitamin D_2. *Pediatr Res* (1973) 7, 914–22.
5. Mosekilde L, Melsen F. Anticonvulsant osteomalacia determined by quantitative analyses of bone changes. Population study and possible risk factors. *Acta Med Scand* (1976) 199, 349–55.
6. Hunter J, Maxwell JD, Stewart DA, Parson V, Williams R. Altered calcium metabolism in epileptic children on anticonvulsants. *BMJ* (1971) 4, 202–4.
7. Hahn TJ, Avioli LV. Anticonvulsant osteomalacia. *Arch Intern Med* (1975) 135, 997–1000.
8. Christiansen C, Rødbro P. Effect of vitamin D_2 on serum phenytoin. A controlled therapeutical trial. *Acta Neurol Scand* (1974) 50, 661–4.

Vitamin K substances + Antibacterials

Seven patients in intensive care did not respond to intravenous vitamin K for hypoprothrombinaemia while receiving gentamicin and clindamycin.

Clinical evidence, mechanism, importance and management

Some patients, particularly those in intensive care who are not eating, can quite rapidly develop acute vitamin K deficiency, which leads to prolonged prothrombin times and possibly bleeding.[1,2] This can normally be controlled by giving vitamin K parenterally. However, one report describes 7 such patients, all with normal liver function, who unexpectedly did not respond to intravenous **phytomenadione**. Examination of their records showed that all were receiving **gentamicin** and **clindamycin**.[2] Just why, or if, these two antibacterials might have opposed the effects of intravenous vitamin K is not understood. More study is needed.

1. Ham JM. Hypoprothrombinaemia in patients undergoing prolonged intensive care. *Med J Aust* (1971) 2, 716–18.
2. Rodriguez-Erdmann F, Hoff JV, Carmody G. Interaction of antibiotics with vitamin K. *JAMA* (1981) 246, 937.

Vitamins + Orlistat

Orlistat decreases the absorption of supplemental beta-carotene and vitamin E. There is some evidence to suggest that some patients may have low vitamin D levels while taking orlistat, even if they are also taking multivitamins.

Clinical evidence

Studies in healthy subjects have found that about two-thirds of a supplemental dose of **beta-carotene**[1] and roughly half the dose of **vitamin E** (**α-tocopherol**)[2] was absorbed in the presence of orlistat, while the absorption of **vitamin A** was not affected.[2] In the first study, beta-carotene was given within about 30 minutes of the orlistat,[1] whereas in the second, the vitamin supplement was given at the same time as orlistat.[2] In another study, 17 obese adolescents were given orlistat 120 mg three times daily with meals and a daily multivitamin (containing **vitamins A, D, E,** and **K**) to be taken at night. Levels of **vitamins A, E** and **K** were not significantly altered over 6 months of orlistat use, but **vitamin D** concentrations dropped after the first month, but had returned to baseline by 3 months. Three subjects (all African-Americans) required additional **vitamin D** supplementation, but all had a low dietary intake of **vitamin D**.[3,4]

Mechanism

Orlistat reduces dietary fat absorption by inhibiting gastrointestinal lipase. Consequently, it reduces the absorption of fat soluble vitamins.

Importance and management

To maximise vitamin absorption, the manufacturers recommend that any multivitamin preparations should be taken at least 2 hours before or after orlistat, such as at bedtime.[5,6] The US manufacturers suggest that patients taking orlistat should be advised to take multivitamins, because of the possibility of reduced vitamin levels.[6] Note that the authors of the study in adolescents suggest that monitoring of vitamin D may be required, even if multivitamins are given.[3]

1. Zhi J, Melia AT, Koss-Twardy SG, Arora S, Patel IH. The effect of orlistat, an inhibitor of dietary fat absorption, on the pharmacokinetics of β-carotene in healthy volunteers. *J Clin Pharmacol* (1996) 36, 152–9.
2. Melia AT, Koss-Twardy SG, Zhi J. The effect of orlistat, an inhibitor of dietary fat absorption, on the absorption of vitamins A and E in healthy volunteers. *J Clin Pharmacol* (1996) 36, 647–53.
3. McDuffie JR, Calis KA, Booth SL, Uwaifo GI, Yanovski JA. Effects of orlistat on fat-soluble vitamins in obese adolescents. *Pharmacotherapy* (2002) 22, 814–22.
4. McDuffie JR, Calis KA, Uwaifo GI, Sebring NG, Fallon EM, Hubbard VS, Yanovski JA. Three-month tolerability of orlistat in adolescents with obesity-related comorbid conditions. *Obes Res* (2002) 10, 642–50.
5. Xenical (Orlistat). Roche Products Ltd. UK Summary of product characteristics, May 2006.
6. Xenical (Orlistat). Roche Pharmaceuticals. US Prescribing information, January 2007.

Zinc sulphate + Calcium compounds

Calcium compounds reduce the absorption of zinc.

Clinical evidence, mechanism, importance and management

Elemental calcium in doses of 600 mg (either as **calcium carbonate** or **calcium citrate**) was given to 9 healthy women with a single 20-mg oral dose of zinc sulphate.[1] The AUC of zinc was reduced by 72% by **calcium carbonate** and by 80% by **calcium citrate**. The reason for this interaction is not understood, nor is the clinical importance of this interaction known, but it would seem prudent to separate the administration of zinc from the administration of any calcium compound. Two to three hours separation is often sufficient to achieve maximal absorption with interactions like this. More study of this interaction is needed to confirm the extent and to determine if separation of the doses is an adequate precaution.

1. Argiratos V, Samman S. The effect of calcium carbonate and calcium citrate on the absorption of zinc in healthy female subjects. *Eur J Clin Nutr* (1994) 48, 198–204.

Index

All of the pairs of drugs included in this book, whether interacting or not, are listed in this index. They may also be listed under the group names if the interaction is thought to apply to the group as a whole, or if several members of the group have been shown to interact. Note that in some circumstances, broad terms (e.g. analgesics) have been used, where the information is insufficient to allow more specific indexing. It is therefore advisable to look up both the individual drug and its group to ensure all the relevant information is obtained. It may also be advisable to look up both drugs of interest if you don't initally find what you are looking for as drug name synonyms are also included as lead-ins. You can possibly get a lead on the way unlisted drugs behave if you look up those which are related, but bear in mind that none of them are identical and any conclusions reached should only be tentative.